Rothman-Simeone and Herkowitz's

The Spine

Rothman-Simeone and Herkowitz's

The Spine

SEVENTH EDITION

Steven R. Garfin, MD
Distinguished Professor and Chair
Department of Orthopaedic Surgery
University of California, San Diego
San Diego, California

Frank J. Eismont, MD
Leonard M. Miller Professor and Chairman
Department of Orthopaedic Surgery
University of Miami Miller School of Medicine
Miami, Florida

Gordon R. Bell, MD
Emeritus Staff
Former Director, Center for Spine Health
Cleveland Clinic
Cleveland, Ohio

Jeffrey S. Fischgrund, MD
Harry N. Herkowitz Professor and Chairman
Department of Orthopaedic Surgery
Beaumont Health
Royal Oak, Michigan

Christopher M. Bono, MD
Chief, Orthopaedic Spine Service
Department of Orthopaedic Surgery
Associate Professor of Orthopaedic Surgery
Harvard Medical School
Brigham and Women's Hospital
Boston, Massachusetts

ELSEVIER

ELSEVIER

1600 John F. Kennedy Blvd.
Ste 1800
Philadelphia, PA 19103-2899

ROTHMAN-SIMEONE AND HERKOWITZ'S THE SPINE, SEVENTH EDITION

ISBN: 978-0-323-39397-3

Notices

Knowledge and best practice in this field are constantly changing. As new research and experience broaden our understanding, changes in research methods, professional practices, or medical treatment may become necessary.

Practitioners and researchers must always rely on their own experience and knowledge in evaluating and using any information, methods, compounds, or experiments described herein. In using such information or methods they should be mindful of their own safety and the safety of others, including parties for whom they have a professional responsibility.

With respect to any drug or pharmaceutical products identified, readers are advised to check the most current information provided (i) on procedures featured or (ii) by the manufacturer of each product to be administered, to verify the recommended dose or formula, the method and duration of administration, and contraindications. It is the responsibility of practitioners, relying on their own experience and knowledge of their patients, to make diagnoses, to determine dosages and the best treatment for each individual patient, and to take all appropriate safety precautions.

To the fullest extent of the law, neither the Publisher nor the authors, contributors, or editors, assume any liability for any injury and/or damage to persons or property as a matter of products liability, negligence or otherwise, or from any use or operation of any methods, products, instructions, or ideas contained in the material herein.

Senior Content Strategist: Kristine Jones
Senior Content Development Specialist: Joanie Milnes
Publishing Services Manager: Patricia Tannian
Senior Project Manager: Carrie Stetz
Design Direction: Maggie Reid

Printed in China

Last digit is the print number: 9 8 7 6 5 4 3 2 1

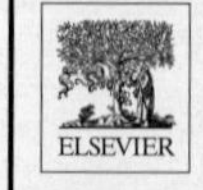

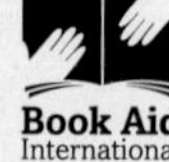

This edition is dedicated to our esteemed colleague and close friend, Harry N. Herkowitz, MD, who passed away, too early, in June 2013. In a humble attempt to honor him and his legacy, we list Harry's name along with our mentors, thus changing the title of this book to *Rothman-Simeone and Herkowitz's The Spine.* Harry abruptly and unintentionally left the editorship of this great work, of which he truly was the lead and driving force for the first six editions. We present this seventh edition proudly and with the hope that our departed friend would approve. To fill the void left by this one man, we have added two new editors whom Harry respected immensely.

Harry was a luminary in spine. Orthopedic surgeons and neurosurgeons worldwide have benefited from his extensive and significant contributions to the field. Harry worked incredibly hard and accomplished much during his career, rising to the presidency of multiple organizations. He was an excellent and exceptionally active surgeon. He was a surgeon's surgeon, as we say, who was respected as a superb educator, a leader among leaders, and a shining example of a clinical researcher. Harry emphasized and fostered patient-oriented care long before it was in vogue. His manner of practice and teaching epitomized evidence-based medicine, once again before it became a defined process. With an intrinsic drive, he continued to search for excellence. His accomplishments, for a single person, were extraordinary.

Unlike most of us, Harry did not begin his career in a university setting with its attendant peer pressure to publish and produce; his was an internal force. Ultimately he surpassed his original goals. "Don't worry, I will get it done," was a consoling and affirming phrase he used often. And after he uttered those words, we didn't worry, and he would always get it done. Today, it would be unusual to get through a round of fellowship candidate interviews without hearing the word "privademics," and it is to this type of practice that many of our young colleagues aspire. Harry, under the guidance of our mentor Richard Rothman, MD, PhD, blazed a trail into this heretofore unknown hybrid world brilliantly and selflessly, setting aside his and his group's personal finances and time.

In so many ways and in so many settings, Harry changed the lives of patients, colleagues, and trainees. He rewarded those who lived up to his expectations with a lifetime of honor and friendship. He changed the course of contemporary spine surgery through his research and his leadership of numerous professional organizations, not the least of which was the American Board of Orthopaedic Surgery.

Harry was cordial to everyone, tough when needed, and extremely loyal to his friends. His professional and personal life was about giving and sharing with others what he had learned along the way (much of which was from Richard Rothman). Those of us who knew him well saw his softer side. Besides being a great, loyal, and true friend, he was, most importantly, a devoted family man. He adored his wife, Jan, and children, Seth (and wife Lauren) and Rachel (and husband Michael). Sadly, he never met his granddaughter.

We all strive to move forward, improving on the past when possible and appropriate. But the spine world, and the friends Harry left behind, are not the same without him. He bound contemporary orthopedic and spine communities together.

Thank you to Harry's mentors, and family, who shared this giant with us.

Contributors

Muhammad M. Abd-El-Barr, MD, PhD
Resident Neurosurgeon
Harvard Medical School
Brigham and Women's Hospital
Boston Children's Hospital
Boston, Massachusetts

Steven S. Agabegi, MD
Assistant Professor
Department of Orthopaedic Surgery and Sports Medicine
Division of Spine Surgery
University of Cincinnati College of Medicine
Cincinnati, Ohio

Todd J. Albert, MD
Surgeon in Chief and Medical Director
Korein-Wilson Professor of Orthopaedic Surgery
Hospital for Special Surgery
Weill Cornell Medical College
New York, New York

Ilyas S. Aleem, MD, MSc, FRCSC
Assistant Professor, Spine Surgery
Departments of Orthopaedic Surgery and Neurosurgery
University of Michigan
Ann Arbor, Michigan

R. Todd Allen, MD, PhD
Assistant Clinical Professor
Spine Fellowship Program Director
Department of Orthopaedic Surgery
University of California, San Diego
San Diego, California

Howard S. An, MD
The Morton International Endowed Chair
Professor of Orthopaedic Surgery
Director of Spine Surgery and Spine Fellowship Program
Department of Orthopaedic Surgery
Rush University Medical Center
Chicago, Illinois

Dheera Ananthakrishnan, MD, MSE
Assistant Professor
Department of Orthopaedic Surgery
Emory University
Atlanta, Georgia

D. Greg Anderson, MD
Professor
Departments of Orthopaedic and Neurological Surgery
Rothman Institute, Thomas Jefferson University
Philadelphia, Pennsylvania

Paul A. Anderson, MD
Professor
Orthopedic Surgery and Rehabilitation
University of Wisconsin
Madison, Wisconsin

Gunnar B.J. Andersson, MD, PhD
Professor and Chairman Emeritus
Department of Orthopedic Surgery
Rush University Medical Center
Chicago, Illinois

M. Saeid Asadollahi
Graduate Research Assistant
Engineering Center for Orthopaedic Research Excellence (E-CORE)
Department of Bioengineering
College of Engineering
University of Toledo
Toledo, Ohio

John Attenello, MD
Orthopaedic Surgery Resident
Division of Orthopaedic Surgery
University of Hawaii
Honolulu, Hawaii

Raghav Badrinath, MD
Resident
Department of Orthopedic Surgery
University of California, San Diego
San Diego, California

Michele C. Battié, PhD
Professor
Faculty of Rehabilitation Medicine
University of Alberta
Edmonton, Alberta, Canada

Jennifer J. Beck, MD
Assistant Professor
Orthopedic Surgery
Orthopedic Institute for Children/UCLA
Los Angeles, California

Gordon R. Bell, MD
Emeritus Staff
Former Director, Center for Spine Health
Cleveland Clinic
Cleveland, Ohio

Carlo Bellabarba, MD
Professor
Orthopaedic and Neurological Surgery
University of Washington;
Chief, Orthopaedics and Sports Medicine
Harborview Medical Center
Seattle, Washington

David M. Benglis Jr, MD
Atlanta Brain and Spine Care
Atlanta, Georgia

Amandeep Bhalla, MD
Spine Surgery Fellow
Department of Orthopaedic Surgery
Harvard Medical School
Boston, Massachusetts

Mohit Bhandari, MD, PhD, FRCSC
Professor and Academic Head
Canada Research Chair in Evidence-Based Orthopaedics
Division of Orthopaedic Surgery
McMaster University
Hamilton, Ontario, Canada

Nitin N. Bhatia, MD
Vice Chairman
Chief, Spine Service
Residency Program Director
Department of Orthopaedic Surgery
University of California, Irvine
Orange, California

Jesse E. Bible, MD, MHS
Assistant Professor
Department of Orthopaedics
Penn State Milton S. Hershey Medical Center
Hershey, Pennsylvania

Christopher M. Bono, MD
Chief, Orthopaedic Spine Service
Department of Orthopaedic Surgery
Brigham and Women's Hospital;
Associate Professor of Orthopaedic Surgery
Harvard Medical School
Boston, Massachusetts

Barrett S. Boody, MD
Resident Physician
Department of Orthopaedic Surgery
Northwestern University
Chicago, Illinois

David G. Borenstein, MD
Clinical Professor of Medicine
Division of Rheumatology
Department of Medicine
George Washington University Medical Center;
Partner, Arthritis and Rheumatism Associates
Washington, DC

Richard J. Bransford, MD
Professor
Orthopaedic and Neurological Surgery
University of Washington
Harborview Medical Center
Seattle, Washington

Zorica Buser, PhD
Senior Research Associate
Department of Orthopaedic Surgery
Keck School of Medicine
University of Southern California
Hoffman Medical Research Center
Los Angeles, California

Eugene Carragee, MD
Professor
Department of Orthopedics
Stanford University School of Medicine
Stanford, California

Jose Manuel Casamitjana, MD
Senior Consultant
Orthopaedic Surgeon
Cervical Spine Pathology
Orthopaedic and Trauma Hospital
Barcelona, Spain

Samuel H. Cass, BS
MD Candidate
University of Miami Miller School of Medicine
Miami, Florida

Saad B. Chaudhary, MD, MBA
Assistant Professor
Minimally Invasive and Complex Spine Surgery
Department of Orthopaedic Surgery
Icahn School of Medicine at Mount Sinai
New York, New York

Jeffrey L. Chen, MD, MHS
Assistant Clinical Professor
Department of Anesthesiology
Center for Pain Medicine
University of California San Diego
La Jolla, California

Boyle C. Cheng, PhD
Director of Research
Neuroscience Institute
Allegheny Health Network
Pittsburgh, Pennsylvania

Daniel Cher, MD
Vice President of Clinical Affairs
SI-BONE, Inc.
San Jose, California

Jason Pui Yin Cheung, MBBS, MMedSc
Clinical Assistant Professor
Department of Orthopaedics and Traumatology
University of Hong Kong
Pokfulam, Hong Kong

Kenneth M.C. Cheung, MBBS(UK), MD(HK)
Jessie Ho Professor in Spine Surgery
Chair Professor and Head
Department of Orthopaedics and Traumatology
University of Hong Kong
Pokfulam, Hong Kong

Matthew R. Cohn, MD
Department of Orthopedic Surgery
Rush University Medical Center
Chicago, Illinois

Daniel Cook, BS
Laboratory Manager, Spine and Biomechanics Laboratory
Neuroscience Institute
Allegheny Health Network
Pittsburgh, Pennsylvania

Edward C. Covington, MD
Medical Consulting and Education
Emeritus Staff
Neurologic Institute
Cleveland Clinic
Cleveland, Ohio

Alvin H. Crawford, MD
Professor Emeritus
Orthopaedic Surgery
University of Cincinnati, College of Medicine;
Founding Director, Crawford Spine Center
Cincinnati Children's Hospital;
Orthopaedic Surgery
Christ Hospital
Westchester Community Hospital
Cincinnati, Ohio

Shari Cui, MD
Assistant Professor, Spine Surgery
Department of Orthopaedic Surgery
West Virginia University
Morgantown, West Virginia

Bradford L. Currier, MD
Professor of Orthopedics
Mayo Clinic College of Medicine;
Director, Spinal Fellowship Program
Mayo Clinic College of Medicine
Rochester, Minnesota

Scott D. Daffner, MD
Associate Professor
Department of Orthopaedics
West Virginia University School of Medicine
Morgantown, West Virginia

Kevin L. Dalal, MD
Assistant Professor
Department of Physical Medicine and Rehabilitation
University of Miami Miller School of Medicine
Miami, Florida

Bruce V. Darden II, MD
Fellowship Director
Orthocarolina Spine Center
Charlotte, North Carolina

Sara Davin, PsyD, MPH
Staff Psychologist
Chronic Pain Rehabilitation Section
Center for Neurological Restoration
Cleveland Clinic
Cleveland, Ohio

Scott Delp, PhD
James H. Clark Professor
Departments of Bioengineering, Mechanical Engineering, and Orthopaedic Surgery
Schools of Engineering and Medicine
Stanford University
Stanford, California

Richard Derby, MD
Medical Director
Spinal Diagnostics and Treatment Center
Daly City, California

Peter B. Derman, MD
Orthopedic Surgery Resident
Hospital for Special Surgery
New York, New York

Clinton J. Devin, MD
Associate Professor of Orthopaedic Surgery and Neurosurgery
Vanderbilt University Medical Center
Nashville, Tennessee

Elizabeth A. Dugan, PhD
Postdoctoral Associate
Miami Project to Cure Paralysis
University of Miami Miller School of Medicine
Miami, Florida

Alexandra Miller Dunham, MD
Resident
Orthopaedic Surgery
Johns Hopkins University School of Medicine
Baltimore, Maryland

Richard W. Easton, MD
Assistant Professor
Department of Orthopaedic Surgery
Oakland University William Beaumont School of Medicine
Rochester Hills, Michigan;
Section Head
Orthopaedic and Spine Surgery
Beaumont Hospital
Troy, Michigan

Jason C. Eck, DO, MS
Spine Surgeon
Center for Sports Medicine and Orthopaedics
Chattanooga, Tennessee

Frank J. Eismont
Leonard M. Miller Professor and Chairman
Department of Orthopaedic Surgery
University of Miami Miller School of Medicine
Miami, Florida

Todd M. Emch, MD
Staff
Division of Neuroradiology
Imaging Institute
Cleveland Clinic
Cleveland, Ohio

Sanford E. Emery, MD, MBA
Professor and Chairman
Department of Orthopaedics
West Virginia University
Morgantown, West Virginia

Yashar Eshraghi, MD
Assistant Clinical Professor
Department of Anesthesiology and Perioperative Care
School of Medicine
University of California, Irvine
Irvine, California

Saif Aldeen Farhan, MD
Research Spine Fellow
Department of Orthopaedic Surgery
University of California, Irvine
Irivine, California

Timothy J. Furnish, MD
Associate Clinical Professor of Anesthesiology
Center for Pain Medicine
Pain Fellowship Program Director
University of California, San Diego Medical Center
San Diego, California

Shyam Gajavelli, PhD
Associate Scientist
Department of Neurosurgery
Miami Project to Cure Paralysis
University of Miami Miller School of Medicine
Miami, Florida

Steven R. Garfin, MD
Distinguished Professor and Chair
Department of Orthopaedic Surgery
University of California, San Diego
San Diego, California

Bhavuk Garg, MD
Associate Professor
Department of Orthopaedics
All India Institute of Medical Sciences
New Delhi, India

Matthew F. Gary, MD
Assistant Professor of Neurosurgery and Orthopaedic Surgery
Emory Spine Center
Emory University School of Medicine
Atlanta, Georgia

Joseph P. Gjolaj, MD
Assistant Professor
Orthopaedic Surgery
University of Miami Miller School of Medicine;
Orthopaedic Spine Surgeon
Orthopaedic Surgery
Jackson Memorial Hospital
Miami, Florida

Paul Glazer, MD
Spine Specialists of Boston
Chestnut Hill, Massachusetts

Michael P. Glotzbecker, MD
Assistant Professor
Department of Orthopaedic Surgery
Boston Children's Hospital
Boston, Massachusetts

Vijay K. Goel, PhD
Distinguished University Professor
Endowed Chair and McMaster-Gardner Professor of Orthopaedic Bioengineering
Co-Director, Engineering Center for Orthopaedic Research Excellence (E-CORE)
Departments of Bioengineering and Orthopaedic Surgery
Colleges of Engineering and Medicine
University of Toledo
Toledo, Ohio

Jonathan N. Grauer, MD
Associate Professor
Department of Orthopaedics and Rehabilitation
Yale University School of Medicine
New Haven, Connecticut

Barth A. Green, MD
Professor of Neurological Surgery
University of Miami Miller School of Medicine
Miami, Florida

Ajay Gupta, MD
Head, Pediatric Epilepsy
Director, Tuberous Sclerosis Program
Associate Professor, Cleveland Clinic Lerner College of Medicine
Cleveland Clinic Foundation
Cleveland, Ohio

Richard D. Guyer, MD
Past President
Director, Spine Fellowship
Texas Back Institute
Plano, Texas;
Clinical Associate Professor
Department of Orthopaedic Surgery
University of Texas Southwestern School of Medicine
Dallas, Texas

Aldric Hama, PhD
Study Director
Hamamatsu Pharma Research
Hamamatsu, Japan

Hamid Hassanzadeh, MD
Assistant Professor
Department of Orthopaedic Surgery
University of Virginia
Charlottesville, Virginia

Spencer Hauser, MD
Fellow, Orthopaedic Surgery
Duke University School of Medicine
Durham, North Carolina

Robert F. Heary, MD
Professor of Neurosurgery
Rutgers New Jersey Medical School
Director, Spine Center of New Jersey
Newark, New Jersey

Daniel J. Hedequist, MD
Associate Professor
Department of Orthopaedic Surgery
Boston Children's Hospital
Boston, Massachusetts

Stanley A. Herring, MD
Clinical Professor
Rehabilitation Medicine, Orthopaedics and Sports Medicine and Neurological Surgery
University of Washington;
Director, UW Medicine Sports Health and Safety System
Co-Medical Director, UW Medicine Sports Concussion Program
Harborview Medical Center and Seattle Children's Hospital
Seattle, Washington

Kenneth A. Hood, DO
Assistant Clinical Professor, Spine Surgery
Department of Orthopaedic Surgery
University of Arizona
Tucson, Arizona

Wellington K. Hsu, MD
Clifford C. Raisbeck Distinguished Professor of Orthopaedic Surgery
Director of Research
Department of Orthopaedic Surgery
Northwestern University Feinberg School of Medicine
Chicago, Illinois

Serena S. Hu, MD
Professor and Vice Chair
Chief, Spine Service
Department of Orthopedic Surgery
Stanford University
Stanford, California

Xiaobang Hu, PhD
Research Director
Scoliosis and Spine Tumor Center
Texas Back Institute
Texas Health Presbyterian Hospital
Plano, Texas

Kevin T. Huang, MD
Department of Neurosurgery
Boston Children's Hospital
Harvard Medical School
Boston, Massachusetts

Andre M. Jakoi, MD
Department of Orthopedic Surgery
Spine Division
University of Southern California
Los Angeles, California

Pawel P. Jankowski, MD
Chief Resident
Department of Neurosurgery
University of California, San Diego
San Diego, California

Andrew Jea, MHA, FACS, FAAP
Pediatric Neurosurgeon
Goodman Campbell Brain and Spine;
Professor and Chief
Section of Pediatric Neurosurgery
Department of Neurological Surgery
Indiana University School of Medicine
Indianapolis, Indiana

Walter J. Jermakowicz, MD, PhD
Resident
Department of Neurological Surgery
University of Miami Miller School of Medicine
Miami, Florida

Xavier F. Jimenez, MD
Medical Director
Chronic Pain Rehabilitation Program
Chronic Pain Rehabilitation Section
Cleveland Clinic
Cleveland, Ohio

Jeremiah N. Johnson, MD
Assistant Professor
Department of Neurosurgery
Baylor College of Medicine
Houston, Texas

Robert Johnson, DO
Orthopaedic Spine Surgeon
Idaho Back Institute
Blackfoot, Idaho

James D. Kang, MD
Thornhill Family Professor of Orthopaedic Surgery
Harvard Medical School;
Chairman, Department of Orthopaedic Surgery
Brigham and Women's Hospital
Boston, Massachusetts

Abhishek Kannan, MD
Resident Physician
Department of Orthopaedic Surgery
Northwestern University Feinberg School of Medicine
Chicago, Illinois

Jaakko Kaprio, MD, PhD
Academy Professor
Director, Institute for Molecular Medicine Finland (FIMM)
Nordic EMBL Partnership for Molecular Medicine
University of Helsinki
Helsinki, Finland

Lori A. Karol, MD
Assistant Chief of Staff
Orthopaedic Surgery
Texas Scottish Rite Hospital for Children;
Professor
Orthopaedic Surgery
University of Texas-Southwestern
Dallas, Texas

Jad G. Khalil, MD
Attending Spine Surgeon
William Beaumont Hospital
Royal Oak, Michigan

Safdar N. Khan, MD
Benjamin R. and Helen Slack Wiltberger Endowed Chair in Orthopaedic Spine Surgery
Associate Professor and Chief, Division of Spine Surgery
Department of Orthopaedic Surgery
Associate Professor, Department of Integrated Systems Engineering
Clinical Co-Director, Spine Research Institute
Ohio State University Wexner Medical Center
Columbus, Ohio;
Director, The Spine Program at Wooster Hospital
Wooster, Ohio

A. Jay Khanna, MD, MBA
Vice Chair and Professor
Department of Orthopaedic Surgery
Johns Hopkins University
Baltimore, Maryland

Shinichi Kikuchi, MD, PhD
Orthopedic Department
Fukushima Medical University
Fukushima, Japan

Choll W. Kim, MD, PhD
Director, Advanced Spine and Joint Institute
University of California, San Diego;
Spine Institute of San Diego
Center for Minimally Invasive Spine Surgery at Alvarado Hospital
San Diego, California

David H. Kim, MD
Associate Clinical Professor
Orthopaedic Surgery
Tufts University School of Medicine;
Director of Medical Education
Department of Orthopaedic Surgery
New England Baptist Hospital
Boston, Massachusetts

Theodore D. Koreckij, MD
Dickson-Diveley Midwest Orthopaedic Clinic;
Clinical Assistant Professor
Orthopaedic Surgery
University of Missouri-Kansas City;
Kansas City Orthopaedic Institute
Leawood, Kansas

Tyler Kreitz, MD
Department of Orthopaedic Surgery
Thomas Jefferson University
Philadelphia, Pennsylvania

Jonathan D. Krystal, MD
Clinical Instructor
Orthopedic Surgery
Thomas Jefferson University Hospital;
Spine Fellow
Spine Surgery
Rothman Institute
Philadelphia, Pennsylvania

Mark F. Kurd, MD
Assistant Professor
Department of Orthopaedic Surgery
Thomas Jefferson University
Rothman Institute
Philadelphia, Pennsylvania

Swamy Kurra, MBBS
Research Fellow
SUNY Upstate Medical University
Syracuse, New York

Kenny Kwan, BMBCh(Oxon)
Clinical Assistant Professor
Department of Orthopaedics and Traumatology
Li Ka Shing Faculty of Medicine
University of Hong Kong
Pokfulam, Hong Kong

Brian Kwon, MD
Assistant Clinical Professor
Orthopedic Surgery
Tufts University School of Medicine;
Department of Orthopaedic Surgery
New England Baptist Hospital
Boston, Massachusetts

Lauren LaMont, MD
Orthopedic Surgeon
Department of Pediatric Orthopedics
Cook Children's Hospital
Fort Worth, Texas

Joseph M. Lane, MD
Professor of Orthopaedic Surgery
Orthopaedic Surgery
Chief, Metabolic Bone Disease Service
Hospital for Special Surgery
New York, New York

William F. Lavelle, MD
Associate Professor
Departments of Orthopaedic Surgery and Pediatrics
SUNY Upstate Medical University
Syracuse, New York

Darren R. Lebl, MD
Spine and Scoliosis Surgery
Hospital for Special Surgery
New York, New York

Nathan H. Lebwohl, MD
Chief of Spinal Deformity Surgery
Department of Orthopaedics
University of Miami Miller School of Medicine
Miami, Florida

Joon Yung Lee, MD
Associate Professor, Department of Orthopedic Surgery
Medical Director, Ferguson Laboratory
Associate Program Director, Orthopedic Residency
University of Pittsburgh Medical Center
Pittsburgh, Pennsylvania

Scott I. Lee, MD
Orthopedic Spine Surgeon
Adventist Health
White Memorial Medical Center
Los Angeles, California;
Glendale Adventist Medical Center
Glendale, California

Yu-Po Lee, MD
Clinical Professor
Department of Orthopaedic Surgery
University of California, Irvine
Irvine, California

Ronald A. Lehman Jr, MD
Professor of Orthopaedic Surgery
Chief, Degenerative, MIS, and Robotic Spine Surgery
Director, Athletics Spine Center
Director, Spine Research
Co-Director, Adult and Pediatric Spine Fellowship
Advanced Pediatric and Adult Deformity Service
The Spine Hospital
New York–Presbyterian/The Allen Hospital
New York, New York

Lawrence G. Lenke, MD
Professor and Chief of Spinal Surgery
Chief of Spinal Deformity Surgery
Department of Orthopedic Surgery
Columbia University College of Physicians and Surgeons;
Surgeon-in-Chief
The Spine Hospital
New York–Presbyterian/The Allen Hospital
New York, New York

Dante Leven, MD
Total Orthopedics and Sports Medicine
Associate Professor
Nassau University Medical Center
East Meadow, New York

Allan D. Levi, MD, PhD
Chair, Department of Neurological Surgery
Professor of Neurological Surgery, Orthopedics, and Rehabilitation Medicine
University of Miami Miller School of Medicine
Chief of Neurosurgery
Jackson Memorial Hospital
Miami, Florida

Richard L. Lieber, PhD
Senior Vice President and Chief Scientific Officer
Rehabilitation Institute of Chicago;
Professor of Physiology and Biomedical Engineering
Northwestern University
Chicago, Illinois

Isador H. Lieberman, MD
Director
Scoliosis and Spine Tumor Center
Texas Back Institute
Texas Health Presbyterian Hospital
Plano, Texas

Richard A. Lindtner, MD, PhD
Trauma Surgeon
Department of Trauma Surgery and Sports Medicine
Medical University of Innsbruck
Innsbruck, Austria

Gregory Lopez, MD
Assistant Professor of Spine Surgery
Rush University
Chicago, Illinois

J. Diego Lozano, MD
Interventional Neuroradiologist
Providence Little Company of Mary Medical Center
Mechanical Thrombectomy-Ready Advanced Primary Stroke Center
Torrance, California

Prasath Mageswaran, PhD
Research Associate
Spine Research Institute
Ohio State University
Columbus, Ohio

Kamran Majid, MD
Physician
Orthopedic Spine Surgery
Kaiser Permanente
Oakland, California

Antonios Mammis, MD
Assistant Professor, Neurological Surgery and Anesthesiology
Director, Center for Neuromodulation
Director, Functional and Restorative Neurosurgery
Senator, Rutgers University
Rutgers New Jersey Medical School
Newark, New Jersey

Satyajit Marawar, MD
Orthopedic Spine Surgeon
Veterans Affairs Medical Center
Syracuse, New York

William S. Marras, PhD, CPE
Honda Chair Professor
Integrated Systems Engineering/Spine Research Institute
Ohio State University
Columbus, Ohio

Eric A.K. Mayer, MD
Associate Director, Clinical Transformation
Cleveland Clinic Center for Spine Health
Cleveland, Ohio

Tom G. Mayer, MD
Harvard College
Columbia College of Physicians and Surgeons
New York, New York

Daniel Mazanec, MD
Physician Emeritus
Cleveland Clinic
Cleveland, Ohio;
Chief Medical Officer
Dorsata
Arlington, Virginia

Steven J. McAnany, MD
Spine Surgery
Assistant Professor of Orthopaedic Surgery
Washington University Orthopaedics
St. Louis, Missouri

Paul C. McCormick, MD, MPH
Herbert and Linda Gallen Professor of Neurological Surgery
Director
Spine Hospital at the Neurological Institute of New York;
Attending Physician
New York–Presbyterian/Columbia University Medical Center
New York, New York

Zachary McCormick, MD
Assistant Professor of Physical Medicine and Rehabilitation
Department of Orthopaedics
University of California, San Francisco
San Francisco, California

Nagy A. Mekhail, MD, PhD
Carl Wasmuth Professor and Chair
Director, Evidence-Based Pain Management and Research
Cleveland Clinic
Cleveland, Ohio

Ehud Mendel, MD
President Elect, Ohio State Neurosurgical Society
Justine Skestos Endowed Chair
Professor of Neurosurgery, Oncology, Orthopedics, and Systems Engineering
Vice Chair Clinical/Academic Affairs
Clinical Director, OSU Spine Research Institute
Director, Spine Program, Complex/Oncological Fellowship Program
Ohio State University Wexner Medical Center
James Cancer Hospital
Columbus, Ohio

Addisu Mesfin, MD
Associate Professor
Orthopaedic Surgery
University of Rochester
Rochester, New York

Umesh Metkar, MD
Orthopaedic Spine Surgeon
Spine Center at Beth Israel Deaconess Medical Center
Boston, Massachusetts

Lyle J. Micheli, MD
Director
Division of Sports Medicine
O'Donnell Family Professor of Orthopaedics and Sports Medicine
Boston Children's Hospital
Boston, Massachusetts

Megan Mignemi, MD
Assistant Professor of Orthopedics and Rehabilitation
Division of Pediatric Orthopedics
Monroe Carell Jr. Children's Hospital at Vanderbilt
Nashville, Tennessee

Andrew Z. Mo, MD
Orthopaedic Surgery
Lenox Hill Hospital
New York, New York

William J. Molinari III, MD
Orthopedic Surgeon
Residency Program Site Director
Department of Orthopedics
Malcolm Randall VA Medical Center;
Spine Surgeon
Assistant Residency Program Director
Department of Orthopedics
University of Florida
Gainesville, Florida

David M. Montgomery, MD
Associate Professor
Department of Orthopaedic Surgery
Oakland University/William Beaumont School of Medicine
Royal Oak, Michigan

Thomas Mroz, MD
Director, Center for Spine Health
Director, Clinical Research
Center for Spine Health
Departments of Orthopaedic and Neurological Surgery
Cleveland Clinic
Cleveland, Ohio

Scott J. Mubarak, MD
Surgeon in Chief
Emeritus Chair, Division of Pediatric Orthopedics
Rady Children's Hospital;
Clinical Professor
Department of Orthopedics
University of California, San Diego Medical Center
San Diego, California

Charles N. Munyon, MD
Director of Functional and Restorative Neurosurgery
Assistant Professor of Neurosurgery
Lewis Katz School of Medicine at Temple University
Philadelphia, Pennsylvania

Robert F. Murphy, MD
Assistant Professor
Department of Orthopaedics
Medical University of South Carolina
Charleston, South Carolina

George F. Muschler, MD
Vice Chair, Orthopaedic and Rheumatologic Institute
Cleveland Clinic Foundation
Cleveland, Ohio

Robert R. Myers, PhD
Professor of Anesthesiology and Pathology
University of California, San Diego School of Medicine
San Diego, California

Dileep R. Nair, MD
Section Head of Adult Epilepsy
Epilepsy Center
Cleveland Clinic
Cleveland, Ohio

Sreeharsha V. Nandyala, MD
Orthopaedic Surgery Resident
Massachusetts General Hospital
Harvard Medical School
Boston, Massachusetts

Raj Nangunoori, MD
Department of Neurosurgery
Allegheny Health Network
Pittsburgh, Pennsylvania

Randy Neblett, MA, LPC, BCB
Psychology Department Coordinator and Biofeedback Coordinator
Productive Rehabilitation Institute of Dallas for Ergonomics (PRIDE);
Research Coordinator
PRIDE Research Foundation
Dallas, Texas

David Nelles, MD
Orthopedic Spine Surgery
Muir Orthopedic Surgeons
Walnut Creek, California

Peter O. Newton, MD
Chief
Department of Pediatric Orthopedics
Rady Children's Hospital;
Clinical Professor
Orthopaedic Surgery
University of California, San Diego
San Diego, California

Christopher O'Boynick, MD
Physician
Premier Care Orthopedics and Sports Medicine
St. Louis, Missouri

Joseph R. O'Brien, MD, MPH
Washington Spine and Scoliosis Clinic
Medical Director, Minimally Invasive Spine Surgery
Virginia Hospital Center
Mayo Clinic Care Network
Arlington, Virginia

Kjell Olmarker, MD, PhD
Musculoskeletal Research
Department of Medical Chemistry and Cell Biology
Institute of Biomedicine
Sahlgrenska Academy
University of Gothenburg
Gothenburg, Sweden

Adam S. Olsen, MD
Resident Physician
Department of Orthopaedic Surgery
University of Pittsburgh Medical Center
Pittsburgh, Pennsylvania

John E. O'Toole, MD
Professor
Department of Neurosurgery
Rush University Medical Center
Chicago, Illinois

Sohrab Pahlavan, MD
Spine Surgery Fellow
Department of Orthopaedic Surgery
University of Miami/Jackson Memorial Hospital
Miami, Florida

Daniel Park, MD
Assistant Professor
Department of Orthopedics
William Beaumont Hospital
Royal Oak, Michigan

Alpesh A. Patel, MD
Professor of Orthopaedic Surgery
Director, Orthopaedic Spine Surgery
Co-director, Northwest Spine Center
Northwestern University Feinberg School of Medicine
Chicago, Illinois

Chetan K. Patel, MD
Medical Director
Spine Health Institute
Florida Hospital Medical Group
Altemonte Springs, Florida

Neil N. Patel, MD
Orthopedic Spine Surgeon
Spine Team Texas
Southlake, Texas

Adam M. Pearson, MD
Assistant Professor
Orthopaedic Surgery
Geisel School of Medicine at Dartmouth
Hanover, New Hampshire

Martin H. Pham, MD
Resident Physician
Department of Neurosurgery
University of Southern California
Los Angeles, California

Frank M. Phillips, MD
Professor
Department of Orthopaedic Surgery
Rush University Medical Center;
Co-Director, Spine Fellowship
Rush University Medical Center
Chicago, Illinois

Christine Piper, MD
Resident Physician
Department of Orthopaedic Surgery
George Washington University
Washington, DC

Nicolas S. Piuzzi, MD
Orthopaedic Regenerative Medicine and Cellular Therapy Clinical Scholar
Department of Orthopaedic Surgery and Biomedical Engineering
Cleveland Clinic
Cleveland, Ohio

Michael P. Planalp, MD
Orthopaedic Surgery Resident
William Beaumont Hospital
Royal Oak, Michigan

Peter B. Polatin, MD, MPH
Consultant Physician
Production Rehabilitation Institute of Dallas for Ergonomics;
Senior Faculty
Harvard Program in Refugee Trauma
Boston, Massachusetts

Sina Pourtaheri, MD
Assistant Professor
Department of Orthopaedic Surgery
University of California, San Diego
San Diego, California;
Assistant Professor
Department of Orthopaedic Surgery
University of California, Los Angeles
Los Angeles, California

Mark R. Proctor, MD
Associate Professor of Neurosurgery
Harvard Medical School
Boston Children's Hospital
Boston, Massachusetts

Andrew J. Pugely, MD
Assistant Professor of Spine Surgery
Department of Orthopaedic Surgery
University of Iowa
Iowa City, Iowa

Ajit S. Puri, MD
Associate Professor of Radiology, Neurology, and Neurosurgery
Division of Neuroimaging and Intervention
University of Massachusetts Medical School
Worcester, Massachusetts

Varun Puvanesarajah, MD
Department of Orthopaedic Surgery
Johns Hopkins University
Baltimore, Maryland

Sheeraz A. Qureshi, MD, MBA
Associate Professor, Orthopaedic Surgery
Minimally Invasive Spine Surgery
Hospital for Special Surgery
Weill Cornell Medical College
New York, New York

Dipak B. Ramkumar, MD
Resident in Orthopaedic Surgery
Instructor in Anatomy
Department of Orthopaedic Surgery
Dartmouth-Hitchcock Medical Center
Geisel School of Medicine at Dartmouth
Lebanon, New Hampshire

Raj Rao, MD
Professor of Orthopaedic Surgery and Neurosurgery
Chairman, Department of Orthopaedic Surgery
George Washington University
Washington, DC

Alexandre Rasouli, MD
Spinal Surgeon
Center of Excellence
Cedars-Sinai Medical Center
Los Angeles, California

Brandon L. Raudenbush, MD
Fellow
Orthopaedic Surgery
University of Rochester
Rochester, New York

W. Carlton Reckling, MD, MBA
Chief Medical Officer and Vice President of Medical Affairs
SI-BONE, Inc.
San Jose, California

K. Daniel Riew, MD
Professor of Orthopaedic Surgery
Columbia University;
Chief, Cervical Spine Surgery and Co-Director, Spine Division
Co-Director, Columbia University Spine Fellowship
Department of Orthopaedic Surgery
The Spine Hospital
New York–Presbyterian/The Allen Hospital
New York, New York

Jeffrey Rihn, MD
Associate Professor
Department of Orthopedic Surgery
Rothman Institute
Thomas Jefferson University Hospital
Philadelphia, Pennsylvania

Makarand V. Risbud, PhD
James J. Maguire Jr. Professor of Spine Research
Director of Spine Research Program
Department of Orthopaedic Surgery
Professor and Co-Director, Cell Biology and Regenerative Medicine PhD Program
Thomas Jefferson University
Philadelphia, Pennsylvania

Brett D. Rosenthal, MD
Senior Housestaff Physician
Department of Orthopaedic Surgery
Northwestern University
Chicago, Illinois

Jeffrey S. Ross, MD
Neuroradiology Division
Department of Radiology
Senior Associate Consultant
Mayo Clinic Arizona;
Professor of Radiology
Mayo Clinic College of Medicine
Phoenix, Arizona

Glenn Russo, MD, MS
Department of Orthopaedics and Rehabilitation
Yale University School of Medicine
New Haven, Connecticut

Björn Rydevik, MD, PhD
Department of Orthopaedics
University of Gothenburg
Gothenburg, Sweden

Jacqueline Sagen, PhD
Professor of Neurosurgery
Miami Project to Cure Paralysis
University of Miami Miller School of Medicine
Miami, Florida

Comron Saifi, MD
Assistant Professor of Orthopaedic Surgery and Neurosurgery
Director of Clinical Spine Research
University of Pennsylvania
Philadelphia, Pennsylvania

Rajiv Saigal, MD, PhD
Assistant Professor of Surgery
Department of Surgery
University of Washington
Seattle, Washington

Lawrence Samkoff, MD
Associate Professor of Neurology
Attending Neurologist
Neuroimmunology Unit
Department of Neurology
University of Rochester Medical Center
Rochester, New York

Rick C. Sasso, MD
Professor
Chief of Spine Surgery
Department of Orthopaedic Surgery
Indiana University School of Medicine
Carmel, Indiana

Michael Saulino, MD, PhD
Physiatrist
MossRehab
Elkins Park, Pennsylvania;
Assistant Professor
Rehabilitation Medicine
Jefferson Medical College
Philadelphia, Pennsylvania

Judith Scheman, PhD
Director, Behavioral Medicine
Digestive Disease and Surgery Institute
Cleveland Clinic
Cleveland, Ohio

Andrew J. Schoenfeld, MD, MSc
Assistant Professor
Department of Orthopaedic Surgery
Brigham and Women's Hospital
Harvard Medical School
Boston, Massachusetts

Gregory D. Schroeder, MD
Rothman Institute
Thomas Jefferson University
Philadelphia, Pennsylvania

Alexandra Schwartz, MD
Clinical Professor
Orthopaedic Surgery
University of California, San Diego
San Diego, California

James D. Schwender, MD
Staff Surgeon
Twin Cities Spine Center
Minneapolis, Minnesota

R. Michael Scott, MD
Fellows Family Chair in Pediatric Neurosurgery
Neurosurgeon-in-Chief, Emeritus
Boston Children's Hospital;
Professor of Neurosurgery
Harvard Medical School
Boston, Massachusetts

Olga Selioutski, DO
Assistant Professor
Strong Epilepsy Center
Department of Neurosurgery
University of Rochester
Rochester, New York

Dilip K. Sengupta, MD, DrMed
Director
Center for Scoliosis and Advanced Spine Surgery
Dallas, Texas

Eiman Shafa, MD
Fellow in Spine Surgery
Twin Cities Spine Center
Minneapolis, Minnesota

Ashish H. Shah, MD
Jackson Memorial Hospital
University of Miami
Miami, Florida

Neel Shah, MD
Department of Orthopedic Surgery
New England Baptist Hospital
Boston, Massachusetts

Suken A. Shah, MD
Division Chief, Spine and Scoliosis Center
Department of Orthopaedics
Nemours/Alfred I. duPont Hospital for Children
Wilmington, Delaware;
Associate Professor of Orthopaedic Surgery and Pediatrics
Department of Orthopaedic Surgery
Sidney Kimmel Medical College of Thomas Jefferson University
Philadelphia, Pennsylvania

Alok Sharan, MD, MHCDS
Co-Director, WESTMED Spine Center
Yonkers, New York;
Assistant Professor
Albert Einstein College of Medicine
New York, New York;
Distinguished Visiting Research Fellow
Center for Complex Systems and Enterprises
Stevens Institute of Technology
Hoboken, New Jersey

Andrew L. Sherman, MD, MS
Professor and Vice Chair
Department of Physical Medicine and Rehabilitation
University of Miami Miller School of Medicine
Miami, Florida

Adam L. Shimer, MD
Associate Professor
Orthopedic Surgery
University of Virginia
Charlottesville, Virginia

Shyam Shridharani, MD
Section Chief, Spine Surgery
Department of Orthopaedic Surgery
University of Arizona
Tucson, Arizona

J. Alex Sielatycki
Department of Orthopaedics
Vanderbilt University
Nashville, Tennessee

Krzysztof B. Siemionow, MD, PhD
Chief of Spine Surgery
Department of Orthopedic Surgery
University of Illinois
Chicago, Illinois

Fernando E. Silva, MD
Southeast Texas Spine Center
CHRISTUS Southeast Texas St. Elizabeth Hospital
Beaumont, Texas

Andrew K. Simpson, MD
Spine Surgeon
Texas Back Institute
Dallas, Texas

J. David Sinclair, MD
Medical Director, Paradigm Outcomes
Walnut Creek, California;
Independent Consultant for the Management of Chronic Pain
Seattle, Washington

Evan J. Smith, MD
Resident Physician
Department of Orthopaedic Surgery
George Washington University
Washington, DC

Gwendolyn Sowa, MD, PhD
Professor and Chair, Department of Physical Medicine and Rehabilitation
Co-Director, Ferguson Laboratory for Orthopaedic and Spine Research
Pittsburgh, Pennsylvania

Paul D. Sponseller, MD, MBA
Professor and Head
Pediatric Orthopaedics
Johns Hopkins Bloomberg Children's Center
Baltimore, Maryland

Kevin Spratt, MD
Dartmouth-Hitchcock Medical Center
Lebanon, New Hampshire;
Geisel School of Medicine at Dartmouth
Hanover, New Hampshire

Christopher J. Standaert, MD
Clinical Professor
Department of Rehabilitation Medicine
University of Washington
Seattle, Washington

Michael Stauff, MD
Assistant Professor
Department of Orthopedics and Physical Rehabilitation
University of Massachusetts Medical School
Worcester, Massachusetts

T. Barrett Sullivan, MD
Resident Physician
Department of Orthopedic Surgery
University of California, San Diego
San Diego, California

Ryan A. Tauzell, PT, MA, CMDT
Physical Therapist
Choice Physical Therapy and Wellness
Christiansburg, Virginia

Jinny Tavee, MD
Neuromuscular Fellowship Program Director
Associate Professor
Cleveland Clinic Lerner College of Medicine
Cleveland, Ohio

Bobby K.-B. Tay, MD
Professor
Orthopaedic Surgery
UCSF Medical Center
San Francisco, California

Dinesh P. Thawrani, MD
Assistant Professor
Department of Orthopedic Surgery
University of Cincinnati College of Medicine;
Attending Physician
Orthopaedic Surgery
Cincinnati VA Medical Center
Cincinnati, Ohio

Clifford B. Tribus, MD
Professor
Department of Orthopedic Surgery and Rehabilitative Medicine
University of Wisconsin-Madison
Madison, Wisconsin

Eeric Truumees, MD
Professor of Surgery and Perioperative Care
Dell Medical School
University of Texas;
Chief Executive Officer
Seton Brain and Spine Institute
Austin, Texas

Alexander R. Vaccaro, MD, PhD, MBA
Richard H. Rothman Professor and Chairman
Department of Orthopaedic Surgery
Professor of Neurosurgery
Co-Director, Delaware Valley Spinal Cord Injury Center
Co-Chief of Spine Surgery
Sidney Kimmel Medical Center at Thomas Jefferson University
President, Rothman Institute
Philadelphia, Pennsylvania

Steve Vanni, DO
University of Miami
Miami, Florida

Arya G. Varthi, MD
Spine Surgery Fellow
Rush University Medical Center
Chicago, Illinois

Anita Vasavada, PhD
Associate Professor
Voiland School of Chemical Engineering and Bioengineering
Department of Integrative Physiology and Neuroscience
Washington State University
Pullman, Washington

Michael J. Vives, MD
Associate Professor and Chief of Spine Surgery
Department of Orthopedics
Rutgers University–New Jersey Medical School
Newark, New Jersey

Nam Vo, PhD
Associate Professor
Co-Director, Ferguson Laboratory for Spine Research
Department of Orthopaedic Surgery
Department of Pathology
McGowan Institute for Regenerative Medicine
Stimulating Pittsburgh in Geroscience (SPRIG)
Pittsburgh, Pennsylvania

Ajay K. Wakhloo, MD, PhD, FAHA
Professor of Radiology, Neurology, and Neurosurgery
Division of Neuroimaging and Intervention
University of Massachusetts Medical School
Worcester, Massachusetts

Mark S. Wallace, MD
Professor of Clinical Anesthesiology
Department of Anesthesiology
Division of Pain Medicine
University of California, San Diego
San Diego, California

Emily Walsh, BA
Research Intern
Neuroscience Institute
Allegheny Health Network
Pittsburgh, Pennsylvania

Jeffrey C. Wang, MD
Chief, Orthopaedic Spine Service
Professor of Orthopaedic Surgery and Neurosurgery
Co-Director, USC Spine Center
Los Angeles, California

Samuel R. Ward, PT, PhD
Professor of Radiology, Orthopaedic Surgery, and Bioengineering
University of California, San Diego
San Diego, California

Matthew L. Webb, MD
Resident Physician
Department of Orthopaedic Surgery
Hospital of the University of Pennsylvania
Philadelphia, Pennsylvania

James N. Weinstein, MD
Dartmouth-Hitchcock Health
Dartmouth Institute for Health Policy and Clinical Practice
Lebanon, New Hampshire;
Geisel School of Medicine at Dartmouth
Hanover, New Hampshire

Dennis R. Wenger, MD
Director of Orthopedic Training Program
Rady Children's Hospital
Clinical Professor of Orthopedic Surgery (volunteer)
University of California, San Diego
San Diego, California

F. Todd Wetzel, AB, MD
Professor and Vice Chair
Department of Orthopaedic Surgery and Sports Medicine
Professor
Department of Neurosurgery
Temple University School of Medicine
Philadelphia, Pennsylvania

Peter G. Whang, MD, FACS
Associate Professor
Orthopaedics and Rehabilitation
Yale University School of Medicine
New Haven, Connecticut

Seth K. Williams, MD
Assistant Professor
Department of Orthopedics and Rehabilitation
University of Wisconsin School of Medicine and Public Health
Madison, Wisconsin

Lee Wolfer, MD
Medical Director
Bay Area Integrative Orthopedics
San Francisco, California

Kuan Wen Wu, MD
Department of Orthopaedic Surgery
National Taiwan University Hospital
Taipan, Taiwan

Burt Yaszay, MD
Associate Clinical Professor
Rady Children's Hospital
University of California, San Diego
San Diego, California

Anthony T. Yeung, MD
Associate, Desert Institute for Spine Care
Voluntary Professor, University of New Mexico School of Medicine
Albuquerque, New Mexico

Christopher A. Yeung, MD
President
Desert Institute for Spine Care
Phoenix, Arizona

Terri A. Zachos, MD, PhD, DVM
Diplomate, American College of Veterinary Surgeons
Clinical Research Fellow in Orthopaedic Traumatology
Department of Orthopaedic Surgery
Geisinger Health Systems
Geisinger Commonwealth School of Medicine
Danville, Pennsylvania

Jie Zheng, MD
Department of Neurosurgery
Allegheny Health Network
Pittsburgh, Pennsylvania

Jack E. Zigler, MD
Medical Director
Texas Back Institute
Plano, Texas

Vinko Zlomislic, MD
Assistant Clinical Professor
Department of Orthopaedic Surgery
University of California, San Diego
San Diego, California

Preface

As can be seen from the Dedication and Acknowledgment pages, the Editorial Board for this seventh edition of *The Spine* has undergone some changes. With the passing of Harry N. Herkowitz, MD, and the fact this may be the last edition for some of the remaining long-term editors, two new editors—Christopher N. Bono, MD, and Jeffrey S. Fischgrund, MD—have stepped in, and up, to help us create this new edition of *Rothman-Simeone and Herkowitz's The Spine*. We hope readers will find this edition—as well as future editions—as important and useful as previous ones.

This edition of *The Spine* comes 7 years after the sixth edition. We have strived to continue the original concepts of Richard H. Rothman, MD, PhD, and Frederick A. Simeone, MD, which was to correlate basic science, knowledge of the natural history, and clinical course of spinal disorders with current treatments based on established scientific principles and evidence-based literature. This edition, as in those of the past, provides a comprehensive look at spinal disorders affecting adults and children. It is directed at clinicians of all levels and specialties who treat spinal conditions and who need and appreciate our underlying principles, which ultimately lead to enhanced quality of care for patients.

Since this may be the last edition for some of the editors, we feel it is important to briefly describe the background for this seventh edition of *The Spine*. In our Preface to the sixth edition, we highlighted each of the previous editions by choosing important wording from the Prefaces. We have followed the same pattern here so that new readers, as well as long-term ones, can put this edition in historical perspective.

The forerunner to *The Spine* was *The Intervertebral Disc* by Drs. Rothman and DePalma. In their preface written in 1970, the authors wrote: "The role of the intervertebral disc in the production of neck and back pain, with or without radiation into one of the extremities, has been the subject of much investigation for many decades…The disc has been attacked from every conceivable angle, the most important of which is its biochemical nature and its response to physiologic aging and trauma. In spite of the exhaustive studies recorded in the literature, it is alarming to find how little of this knowledge has been acquired by those concerned with neck and back disorders…We are sure that much that is recorded in this book is still very controversial. Yet, we believe that our approach to this complex problem will be helpful and rewarding to others." This comprehensive monograph on the disc totaled 373 pages. It crystallized concepts of the disc for spine physicians of the day and served as the forerunner of many books to follow.

In the Preface to the first edition, Rothman and Simeone stated, "*The Spine* had as its genesis a strong feeling on the part of its editors that a need existed for a comprehensive textbook to include all aspects of diagnosis and treatment of spinal disease. Our goals were to lower the traditional disciplinary barriers and biases and to present a uniform guideline to problem solving in this area…This book has been designed to include all facets of disease related to the spine, whether orthopedic, neurosurgical, or medical in nature… An attempt has been made to achieve completeness without exhaustive and burdensome details. The contributing authors have not merely recorded the possibilities in diagnosis and treatment of spinal disorders, but have relied on their personal experience to offer concrete recommendations." The first edition of *The Spine,* following the dictates of the editors, covered the full range of knowledge of spinal disorders known at the time and became an essential component of the libraries of all medical personnel who dealt with spinal disorders. The authors, one a neurosurgeon (F.A.S.) and one an orthopedic surgeon (R.H.R.), combined their efforts to teach the world not only diseases of the spine, but also the importance of working together in an attempt to understand and treat the disease processes. Their spinal fellowship, as well as personal fellowship, was based on this multidisciplinary yet regimented approach to the spine and has been the model that we have sought to achieve in our own clinical and teaching environments.

The Preface to the second edition of *The Spine* stated, "Advancements in medicine generally follow broader scientific and even social trends. The treatment of spine diseases is no exception. Consequently, increments of new information have been added to the general body of knowledge in spotty, but predictable, areas. These new developments constitute the raison d'être for this second edition. The dramatic progress in radiologic imaging stands out as the most useful innovation [at that time, computed tomography]. Each contributor has demonstrated his commitment to summarizing the most recent information in a manner useful to students and clinicians alike, and for this the editors are proud and appreciative."

The Preface to the third edition included the following: "The current edition has new editorial leadership. Those of us involved in the direction of this project have tried to follow the model previously established by Drs. Rothman and Simeone in finding the best authors for each chapter. We, hopefully, have emphasized, as in the past editions, the importance of understanding the basic science in a concise manner, which leads to the ability to make appropriate decisions and manage patients with simple or complex spinal problems. We have attempted to update each section, have eliminated those areas that are not current, and have separated some components of the basic science from the clinical to aid readers in locating pertinent information in the ever-increasing body of knowledge related to the spine."

The Editorial Board for the fourth edition of *Rothman-Simeone The Spine* carried over from the third edition. "It provided expanded information on magnetic resonance imaging and laparoscopic and endoscopic surgery. It contained a comprehensive discussion of disc degeneration and its treatment. This edition also introduces a chapter on outcomes research and its importance to our assessment of functional outcome in addition to the more traditional measurements of success, including radiographic parameters."

The fifth edition of *The Spine* added much new information, along with significant updates in content and references. This edition introduced Key Points, which were four or five important concepts and facts contained at the end of many of the clinical chapters. A Key References section was added for each chapter that highlighted the most significant references. Chapters new to the fifth edition included surgical management of osteopenic fractures, disc and nuclear replacement, management of flat back deformity, use of transforaminal lumbar interbody fusion, and use of bone graft extenders and bone morphogenetic protein in the lumbar spine. Other new chapters included thoracoscopic surgery and its clinical applications and intraoperative monitoring, including motor-evoked potentials. A new chapter on genetic application and its exciting role for future treatments of degenerative disease was included in the basic science section. Minimally invasive posterior approaches to the lumbar spine were also introduced in that edition.

The sixth continued under the same Editorial Board as the fifth edition. The editors were charged with ensuring that the chapters within their sections contained the latest evidence-based information whenever available. New chapters included those devoted to arthroplasty for cervical and lumbar degenerative disorders. In addition, revision strategies for failed disc replacements highlighted the potential difficulties in dealing with this complex surgical problem. The sixth edition also significantly expanded the discussion of minimally invasive techniques with six chapters devoted to the rationale for minimally invasive surgery and the surgical techniques, results, and complications. A chapter devoted to soft stabilization for lumbar fixation was also added. Also new to that edition were a chapter devoted to anulus repair and a chapter devoted to the basic science of spinal cord injury. As had been done in previous editions, chapter updates were incorporated throughout the book whenever appropriate.

This, the seventh edition of *The Spine*, includes many of the chapters and authors from the sixth edition. However, all have been updated to include what is new in the basic and clinical sciences related to the topic, with relevant references and updates on clinical outcomes where warranted. In essence, as in all other editions, these chapters epitomize the newer academic catchphrase of "clinical translational research."

We have also expanded international authorship, including adding new contributors. The genetics chapters have been enhanced with both basic and clinically relevant information. Even more content on minimally invasive surgery has been added, with updates on outcomes, approaches, and techniques. We have eliminated some topics (e.g., facet replacement) that have fallen out of favor and/or use. We have added discussion on the sacroiliac joint, since that is one of the newest areas in spine care. We have updated the current status on motion-sparing techniques, including disc replacement with now longer-term follow-up and experiential updates in complications and their treatment. Although this is specifically important to disc replacement, it is the crux of change in most preexisting chapters.

The current Editorial Board remains committed to the broad-based appeal of this book. The authors include basic scientists, neuroradiologists, neurologists, physiatrists, and rheumatologists, along with orthopedic surgeons and neurosurgeons. In addition, this book remains unique in providing comprehensive sections on pediatric disorders and adult disease. Its comprehensive content ranges from degenerative disease to deformity to trauma and tumor. Afflictions of the spinal cord, along with detailed discussions of complications and their management, contribute to this book's broad appeal.

We feel this edition of *The Spine* continues to be the primary reference resource for all physicians and other clinicians with an interest in spinal disorders and treatments.

Steven R. Garfin
Frank J. Eismont
Gordon R. Bell
Jeffrey S. Fischgrund
Christopher M. Bono

Acknowledgment

In the past six editions, the editors have always dedicated this book to our mentors Drs. Rothman and Simeone, our families, and our associates, who have given us the time, support, love, and energy to pursue our careers as well as to coordinate, write, and edit this tome, which in fact was a dedication of love toward Drs. Rothman and Simeone. All of this is still true today. This edition, however, represents our feelings toward Harry N. Herkowitz, MD, our deceased lead editor and organizer, colleague, and close, close friend (see Dedication). The senior editors would like to thank and acknowledge our new "junior" editors, Christopher M. Bono, MD, and Jeffrey S. Fischgrund, MD, who have accepted this responsibility for now and the future—carrying on the spine care educational lineage provided by Drs. Rothman, Simeone, and Herkowitz. They stepped in as if they had been with us since the first edition. In addition, the full editorial team would like to thank all of the authors and contributors, some who have done this many times before and accepted our request to submit an updated chapter because it was dedicated to Harry, as well as the new contributors, who did the same thing. It is a monumental effort on everyone's part. We truly appreciate all of them and their hard work. We also thank the readers and the publishers, who have made this one of, if not the, longest-lasting and most-read complete texts on spine care in the world.

Contents

VOLUME 1

SECTION I
BASIC SCIENCE

SECTION I

1 CHAPTER Development of the Spine

Christopher M. Bono
Amandeep Bhalla
Steven R. Garfin

The embryologic development of the human spine is an enormously complex process that is only partially understood. Differentiation of the pluripotent tissues of the embryo leads to early formation of a repetitive segmented vertebral structure. Because the embryo is exquisitely susceptible to malformation and developmental error, each step of formation is critical.[1-4] Familiarity with these various steps can be helpful in understanding not only congenital syndromes, but also the possible developmental role concerning predisposition to some degenerative spinal processes, typically considered "wear and tear" conditions.[5,6] The continuously expanding understanding of the genetic basis of life, with the genetics of spinal development no exception, has aided the understanding of these syndromes.[7-13]

Fundamental to understanding spinal embryology is the concept of metamerism. In principle, *metamerism* is the development of a highly specialized organism, with multifunctional organ systems, from many anatomically similar segments arranged in a linear fashion. This is particularly easy to conceptualize in the spine because the fully developed spine comprises numerous units with similar shape, arrangement, and function. Metamerism also pertains to the development of the appendages from the metameres, however, which do not have such repetitive arrangement of consecutive units.

In embryonic development, the metameric segments are called *somites*. Primitively, all somites have the same developmental potential. Genetic signaling, specific to the species, determines the degree of regional specialization, such as limbs in mammals versus fins in fish or the lack thereof in snakes. Using these comparative examples, one can also understand the concepts of isomerism and anisomerism. *Isomerism* is characteristic of more primitive animals, in which the number of somites is greater but more uniform and not so highly specialized. This is akin to the snake, which has a great number of vertebral units sustaining its long body, but no limbs. In contrast, *anisomerism* is present in more developed species, such as mammals, in which many of the somites have been deleted (resulting in a lesser number of vertebrae), whereas the remaining somites are more highly specialized so that complex, specialized appendages can be developed.

Although the mature vertebral column is composed of numerous similar units, the tissues within each of those units are highly specialized. The vertebrae, discs, nerves, and blood vessels have embryologic precursors that form according to rapidly dynamic interstructural relationships. This chapter provides the essentials of human spinal development as they relate to the fully developed structure to understand its form, function, and various pathologic possibilities better.

Early Embryologic Spine Precursors: Day 17 to Week 4

The development of the human spine begins on the seventeenth day of gestation. This is within the triploblastic stage of the embryo, during which it is shaped as a disc (Figs. 1.1 and 1.2). On one side of the disc is the amnion cavity, and on the other is the yolk sac. On the dorsal layer (which is in contact with the amnion) of the disc, there are epiblastic cells that converge and invaginate into the disc to form the primitive pit or node. When embedded within the tissue, it forms a tubelike structure that extends craniad, "burrowing" deep to the embryonic disc along its ventral surface. The tube cavity is in continuity with the amniotic fluid. This extension is known as the *notochordal tube*.

At this point, the ventral wall of the notochordal tube is in contact with the yolk sac, which causes disintegration of these cells. A flat remnant of dorsal wall cells from the notochordal tube forms the notochordal plate on the nineteenth day. This plate matures and thickens to form a solid round structure known as the *notochord*. The yolk sac reforms, which obliterates the temporary communication between the amnion and the yolk sac (persistence of this yolk sac/amnion communication is lethal). The presence of the notochord induces a thickening in the overlying ectodermal cells, which are fated to become neuroectodermal cells. The thickening forms the neural plate. At this time, the neural plate is in continuity with the amniotic cavity. On the eighteenth day, the sides of the plate begin to curl up to form a tube. When the edges have

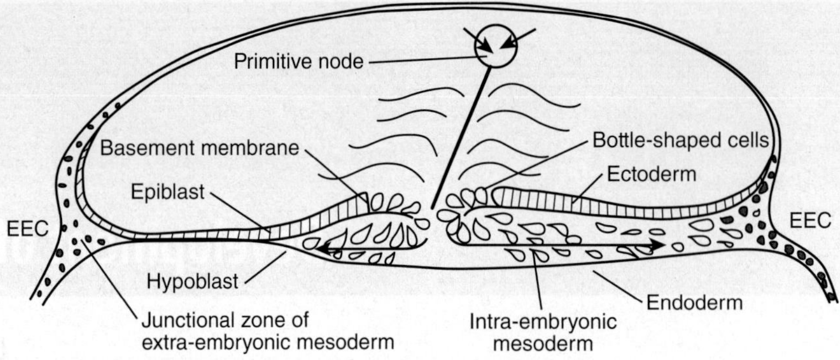

FIG. 1.1 During triploblastic stage (seventeenth day of gestation), the embryo is shaped as a disc. *EEC*, extraembryonic coelom. (From Brooks M, Zietman AL. *Clinical Embryology: A Color Atlas and Text*. Boca Raton, FL: CRC Press; 1998:57.)

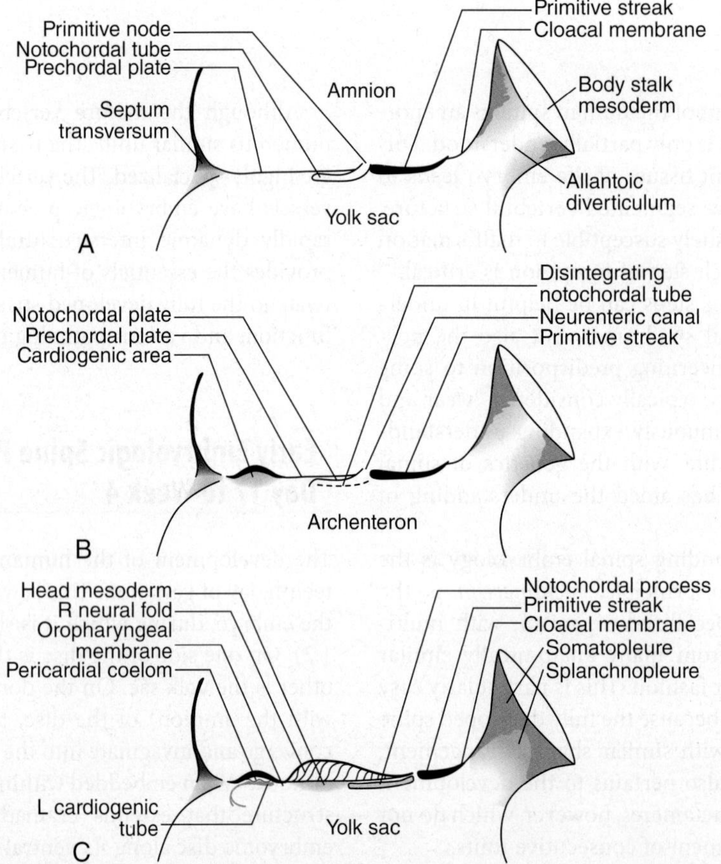

FIG. 1.2 (A) On one side of the disc is the amniotic cavity, and on the other is the yolk sac. The notochordal tube "burrows" deep into the embryonic disc. (B) When the ventral wall of the notochordal tube contacts the yolk sac, it disintegrates. (C) Remaining dorsal wall cells thicken to form the notochordal plate; this matures and thickens to become the notochord. *L*, left; *R*, right. (From Brooks M, Zietman AL. *Clinical Embryology: A Color Atlas and Text*. Boca Raton, FL: CRC Press; 1998:57.)

fused together, it is known as the *neural tube*. The amniotic fluid trapped inside is the precursor to spinal fluid.

The notochord lies ventral to the neural tube in the midline. Mesodermal tissues on either side of these structures condense to form longitudinal columns. By the nineteenth day, there are three distinct columns on either side of the midline: (1) medial paraxial columns, which give rise to the somites; (2) intermediate mesodermal columns, which form the urogenital organs; and (3) lateral mesodermal plates, which form the gut cavities. In considering the development of the spine, attention is focused on the medial paraxial columns. The juxtaposition to the intermediate columns may help explain, however, why abnormalities of the urogenital tract are frequently associated with vertebral anomalies.[1]

The somites are arranged in consecutive fashion along the dorsal aspect of the embryo. They are first formed in the rostral (or cranial) aspect of the embryo, continuing caudad to form 42 to 44 individual segments over a period of days where the medial paraxial columns previously existed. Because they are close to the dorsal surface, they are visibly apparent as a series of beaded elevations (Fig. 1.3).

Within the somite different regions have specialized fates (Figs. 1.4 and 1.5). The dorsolateral cells become the dermomyotomes. These eventually give rise to the skin (lateral) and muscle (medial) overlying the spine. The ventromedial cells within the somite become the sclerotomes. These are the precursors of the skeletal components (vertebrae) of the spine. The neural tube is fated to become the spinal cord.

From Somites to Spinal Column

The sclerotomes, myotomes, notochord, and neural tube eventually develop into the discoligamentous vertebral complex, paraspinal musculature, nucleus pulposus, and neural elements. This development is achieved through numerous sequential steps and stages.

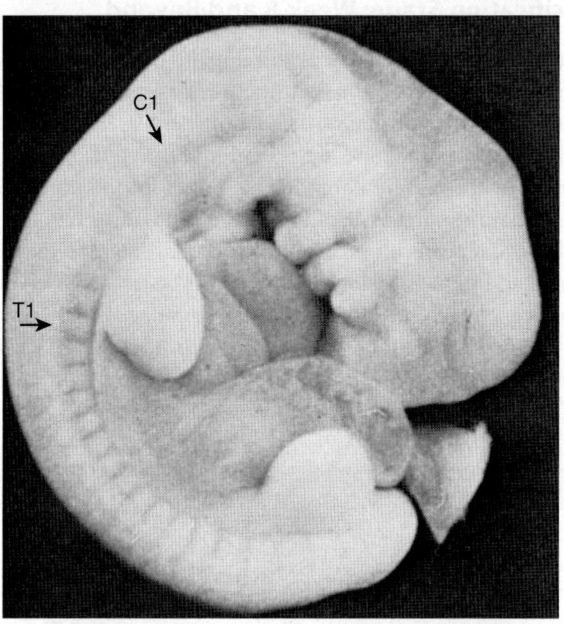

FIG. 1.3 Somites of the human embryo are externally represented as a series of dorsolateral swellings.

Precartilaginous (Mesenchymal) Stage: Weeks 4 and 5

The mesenchymal cells within the sclerotome divide into three main regions. One immediately surrounds the notochord. This region is the precursor for the vertebral bodies and the anulus fibrosus portion of the intervertebral discs. A second region surrounds the neural tube; this is destined to develop into the posterior arch of the vertebra. The third region of cells is within the body wall and is related to extraspinal tissue.

In metameric fashion, the sclerotomes are organized into a consecutively stacked arrangement. The next step in spinal development has been explained by the "resegmentation" theory.[14-18] *Resegmentation* describes the division of each sclerotome into a cranial and caudal half. The cranial half is loosely arranged, whereas the caudal half is composed of densely packed cells. A small portion of the densely packed

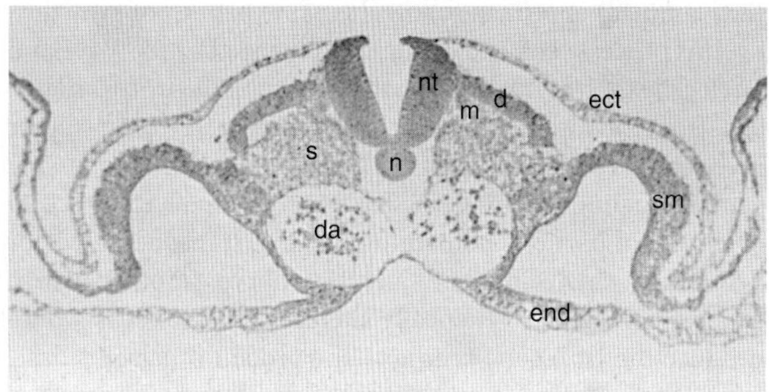

FIG. 1.4 Cross section of thoracic somite in a chick embryo. The notochord (n) underlies the neural tube (nt). The somite is divided into dermatome (d), myotome (m), and sclerotome (s). Lateral to this, the somatic mesoderm (sm), endoderm (end), and ectoderm (ect) are shown. Ventral to the sclerotomes lie the paired dorsal aortae (da).

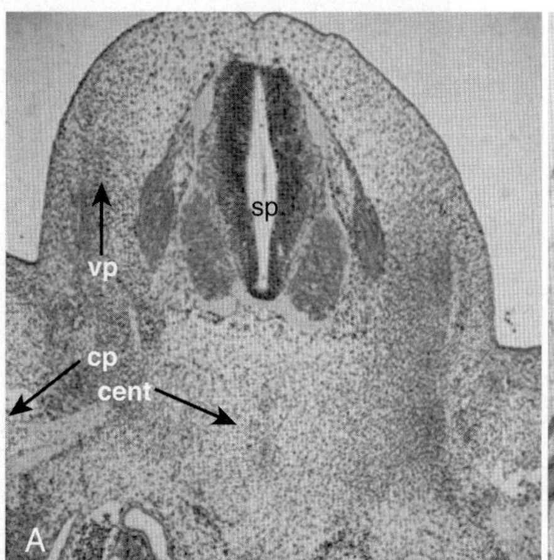

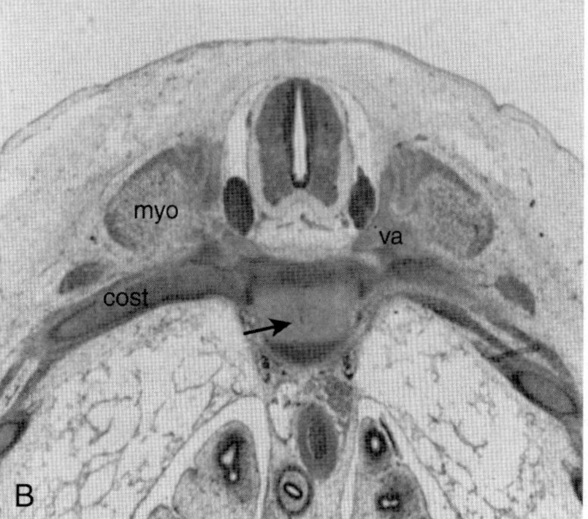

FIG. 1.5 (A) Cross section of pig embryo. *Arrows* indicate the direction of somite cell migration to form the vertebral process (vp), costal process (cp), and centrum (cent). The neural tube shows the anterior horn masses and the dorsal root ganglia. (B) Cartilaginous vertebral arch (va) and costal process (cost) are evident, as is the myotomic precursor to the spinal muscles (myo). *Arrow* indicates the intracentral vestige of the notochord, called the mucoid streak.

cells migrate superiorly to form the annular portion of the intervertebral disc, surrounding the notochord. Most of the densely packed cells fuse with the loosely packed cells of the adjacent caudal sclerotome. This fusion creates the centrum, the precursor of the vertebral body. The centrum develops from portions of two neighboring sclerotomes. This has significance on the anatomy of the fully developed spinal column. Initially, the segmental nerve precursors are located at the midportion of each sclerotome, whereas the segmental artery lies at the junction between two adjacent levels. After resegmentation, the nerve lies at the level of the disc and the artery lies at the mid-centrum, where one would expect to find them in the fully developed specimen.

Experimental data support the resegmentation theory.[8,19-22] The crux of these experiments includes implanting a quail somite (from a quail embryo) within a chick embryo's native somites. The quail somite is juxtaposed to a chick somite, and they develop together as the embryo grows. The quail tissue can be differentiated from the chick tissue using special staining techniques. Eventually, the somites give rise to sclerotomes that develop into centra. With the use of this model, it has been shown that the centrum does arise from the caudal and cranial halves of adjacent sclerotomes. The posterior arches (i.e., laminae) appear to follow this same pattern of growth.

This process seems to be highly influenced by the *Pax1* and *Pax9* genes.[22] It is unclear whether the spinous process develops from one sclerotome or two adjacent levels.[8,22] Other investigators have produced evidence of resegmentation using genetic labeling techniques.[20] These studies involved injection of retroviral particles containing the lacZ transducing vector BAG into a single somite of a chick embryo. In other words, a single somite was genetically altered so that its cells would produce the lacZ gene product—the protein β-galactosidase. When the investigators evaluated the developed embryo, they detected β-galactosidase in the caudal and cranial halves of two adjacent vertebrae, suggesting that cells from the labeled somite were incorporated into two neighboring vertebrae.

Cartilaginous Stage: Weeks 6 and 7

Before the sixth week, the embryonic spinal precursor is composed of mesenchymal cells. Starting in the sixth week, cartilage-producing centers, or chondrification centers, form within each developing vertebra. Although type II collagen production within the extracellular matrix has been detected in the fifth week, it is most active during the cartilaginous stage; it tapers off during the ossification stage, but its production persists within the notochordal remnants of the nucleus pulposus.[12] Two chondrification centers form in each half of the centrum, which eventually fuse into a solid block of cartilage. A hemivertebra is formed because of a failure of chondrification in one half of the vertebral body. The segmental arteries from either side of the centrum fuse at its middle aspect. Chondrification centers also form within each half of the vertebral arch and eventually fuse with each other in the midline and to the posterior aspect of the centrum.

Next, primitive cartilaginous transverse processes and spinous processes develop from the vertebral arch. More recent evidence has shown that the cartilaginous spinous process is formed from Msx1 and Msx2 (two embryologic proteins), producing mesenchymal cells, which require BMP4 to differentiate.[23] These relationships highlight the important interactions of primordial proteins in governing further development of the spine.

The developing centrum and vertebra have the notochord as a central axis. Intervening segments of loosely packed cells are present between the regions of densely packed cells. The outer disc is formed by these loosely packed cells of the sclerotome, which are fated to become the anulus fibrosus. The notochord disintegrates within the centrum during resegmentation and chondrification except in the region of the intervertebral disc, where some of its cells remain. The nucleus fibrosus is the replacement of the embryologic notochord.

Ossification Stage: Week 8 and Beyond

Primary ossification centers develop in utero. In the spine, ossification centers form within the cartilaginous template. There are three primary ossification centers in the typical embryonic vertebra: one in the center of the centrum and one in each of the vertebra arch halves. At about the ninth week, the preparation for ossification of the centrum is heralded by anterior and posterior excavations of the cartilaginous centrum produced by the invasion of pericostal vessels.[24] These vessels produce ventral and dorsal vascular lacunae, which support the initial ossification (Fig. 1.6). Ossification of the centra starts first at the lower thoracic spine working craniad and caudad from that point.[25]

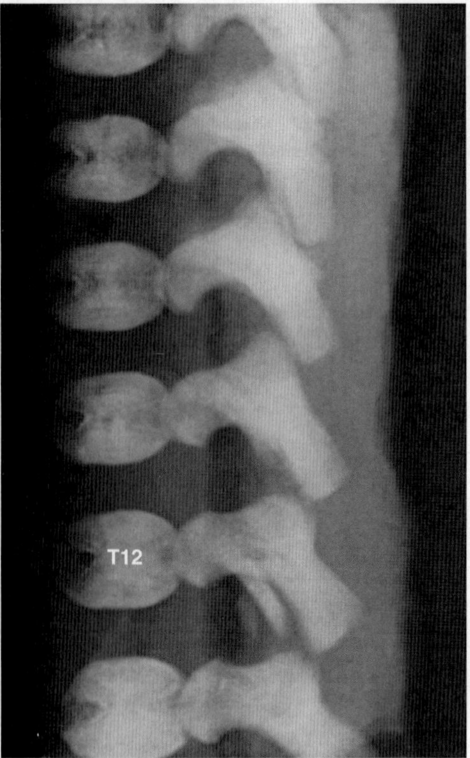

FIG. 1.6 Lateral radiograph of a 34-week spine. Ossification of the centra starts first at the lower thoracic spine, working craniad and caudad from that point.

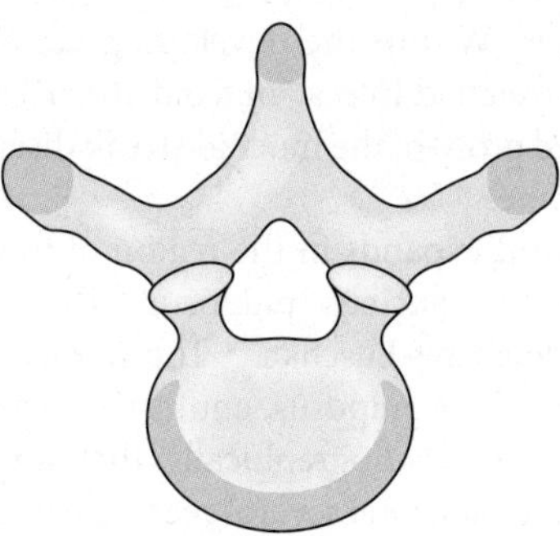

FIG. 1.7 Secondary centers of ossification of a thoracic vertebra. The centers at the tips of the spinous and transverse processes appear at 16 years and fuse at approximately 25 years. The ring apophysis of the centrum ossifies at around 14 years and fuses at about 25 years.

Secondary ossification centers develop after birth. In the spine, these appear after puberty. There are five centers: one in the tip of the spinous process, one in each transverse process tip, and one ring epiphysis in the superior and inferior endplates of the vertebral bodies. This development occurs at about 15 or 16 years of age, but eventually these ossification centers fuse in the middle of the third decade (Fig. 1.7).[26] The transverse processes of the lower cervical vertebrae, particularly C7, may show an additional costal center of ossification that produces the troublesome cervical rib; this reinforces the concept that all vertebrae primitively had the potential of forming ribs.

A pair of embryologic joints, known as *neurocentral joints,* is not present in the fully developed spine. These are located at the junction of the vertebral arches and the centrum but are anterior to the site of the future pedicle. Although not true "joints," they allow expansion of the vertebral arch and spinal canal along with growth of the vertebral body. This expansion is most rapid between 18 and 36 weeks of gestation.[2] At birth, the spinal canal diameter at L1 through L4 is approximately 70% of adult size, whereas at L5 it is only 50%.[2] This indicates differential growth within regions of the vertebral column during fetal development. Full adult dimensions are reached by 1 year of life at L3 and L4 levels. The neurocentral joints persist until 3 to 6 years of age. The fusion of the fetal vertebral arches to the centra occurs well anterior to the pedicles, at the site of the neurocentral joints. The definitive vertebral body includes more than just the bone derived from the ossification center of the centrum, so the terms *body* and *centrum* are not accurately interchangeable (Figs. 1.8 and 1.9).

It is commonly thought that isthmic spondylolysis occurs because of a stress-type fracture within the pars interarticularis of the lower lumbar vertebrae, most commonly L5. Specific anatomic features of the adult lumbar spine, such as variation of the dimensions of the "lateral buttress" within the lumbar spine, have been described. Prenatal factors have been sought, but with limited success. Sagi and colleagues[5] analyzed histomorphologically the lumbar spines of fetal spines aged 8 to 20 weeks to determine the sequence and location of ossification of the pars interarticularis of the various levels. They reported several findings. First, the pars begins to ossify in the twelfth to thirteenth week of gestation. In the upper lumbar levels,

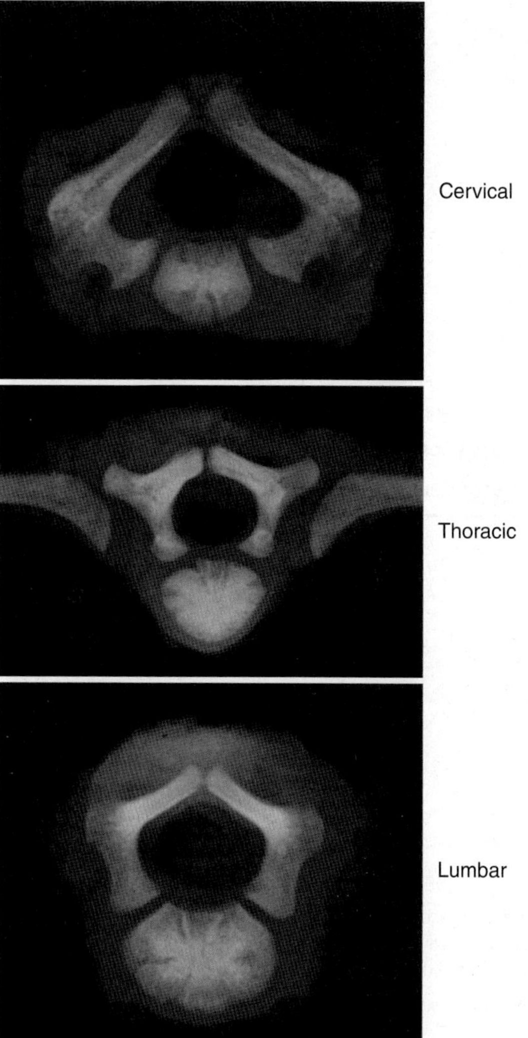

FIG. 1.8 Fusion of the fetal vertebral arches to the centra occurs well anterior to the pedicles, at the site of the neurocentral joints. The contributions of the vertebral arches to the dorsolateral parts of the bodies are apparent. The definitive vertebral body includes more than just the bone derived from the ossification center of the centrum, so that the terms *body* and *centrum* are not accurately interchangeable.

ossification begins at the posterior portion of the pedicle and continues caudad, creating uniform ossification and trabeculation of the pars interarticularis. In contrast, the pars of the lower lumbar levels begins within the center of the pars itself, extending from this point to connect to the neighboring structures. Sagi and colleagues[5] found that this resulted in uneven ossification. This finding may help explain areas of weakness within the pars interarticularis of the lower lumbar levels and may suggest that there is a prenatal predilection for a stress fracture in most individuals.

Fate of the Notochord

In the early embryo, the notochord serves as a rigid template around which the future vertebral column develops. It is a uniform structure that is present throughout the entire length

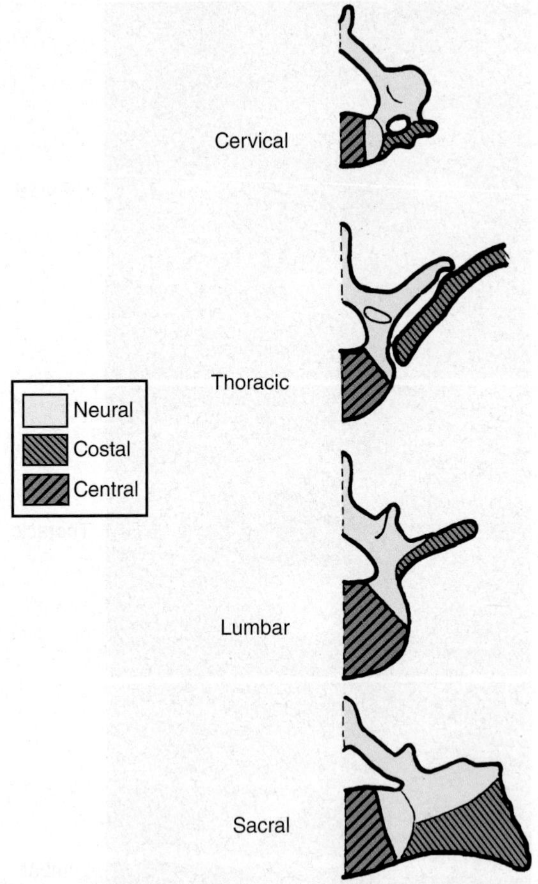

FIG. 1.9 Neurocentral synchondroses lie well within the vertebral body in all cases. Normally, costovertebral synchondroses develop a true diarthrodial joint only in the thoracic region.

of the primordial spinal column. A sheath exists around the notochord in its early stages. Immunohistochemical staining studies of 4- and 5-week embryos identified that a complex of extracellular matrix molecules is already present within this sheath, including sulfated glycosaminoglycans, hyaluronic acid, fibronectin, laminin, tenascin, and collagen II.[27] Aggrecan, keratan sulfate, and other large aggregating proteoglycans (present in the mature spine) were not detected at this stage, suggesting that these appear later in development. The notochordal cells themselves showed reactivity to transforming growth factor-β (TGF-β), suggesting an early influence of this growth factor on the developing extracellular matrix, and the formation of vasculature, cartilage, and bones.[27,28] Disruptions in the TGF-β signaling pathways have been implicated in the abnormal bone morphology and ligamentous laxity found in Loeys-Dietz syndrome, an autosomal dominant mutation of TGF-BR1 or TGF-BR2. Patients with this syndrome, first described in 2005, may have cervical osseous deformity and instability.[29]

In the 20-mm embryo, the notochord becomes an intrinsically segmented structure in the thoracic and lumbar region; in the 30-mm embryo, this structure is evident in the cervical region as well. Segmentation leads to areas of fusiform enlargements in the region of the intervertebral disc, while the notochord is slowly obliterated in the region of the developing vertebral bodies. Within the developing vertebral body, the notochord is stretched into a "mucoid streak" (see Fig. 1.5B). With continued growth, the mucoid streak disappears, leaving behind only bone.

The notochord expands in the region of the intervertebral disc to form the nucleus pulposus. This was originally described in detail by Luschka.[30] The notochord is a major source of the nucleus pulposus, and it has been shown histochemically and autoradiographically that notochordal cells proliferate and remain vital several years after birth.[31] Although notochordal cells generally do not seem to be demonstrable in the human nucleus pulposus of individuals older than 5 years of age, Schwabe[32] reported their survival in the incarcerated discs of the sacrum in a series of specimens ranging from 22 to 45 years in age. A chordoma is abnormal neoplastic growth of notochord cells that remain within the spine in adult life. This suggests that notochordal rest cells can persist well into middle age in some individuals. These neoplasms may develop at any point along the original notochordal track but are usually in the rostral (basisphenoid or basiocciput) and caudal (sacral) regions.

As a theme of development of the spine, the region of the previous notochord lies anterior to the center of the fully developed vertebral body. This has been verified by Nolting and colleagues,[25] who detected remnants of notochordal tissue anterior to the cartilaginous body center in 13 fetal spines aged 10 to 24 weeks. This finding further reinforces that using the terms *centrum* and *vertebral body* interchangeably is inaccurate.

From Neural Tube to Spinal Cord

On the twentieth day, ectodermal tissues on either side of the neural plate become thick and "pucker up." This area is known as the *neural crest,* which contains cells that eventually compose the neural elements. The mesenchymal tissue beneath the neural crest is the neural fold. As the folds grow toward the midline, the two neural crests meet and fuse on day 22. The underlying neural plate forms a tube, known as the *neural tube,* whose walls are composed of the previous neural plate. The neural tube invaginates itself within the dorsum of the embryo. On the twenty-sixth day, the fused neural crest cells invaginate into the embryo and divide into right and left globules. They are termed the *dorsal root ganglia*. They are oval and appear before ossification of the spine.[33]

By the fifth week, the neural tube has changed into a diamond shape and is termed the *neural canal.* A sulcus limitans forms between its anterior (basal) and posterior (alar) halves, which are destined to become motor and sensory tracts. The dorsal root ganglion is composed of sensory cells alone. It develops two "arms." One arm is an extension toward the posterior aspect of the neural canal, which eventually joins the future site of the posterior column of the spinal cord. The other arm is a lateral extension that projects from the dorsal ganglion to reach peripheral tissues.

During the sixth week, the sulcus limitans disappears, and the basal and alar halves join together, while keeping their respective motor and sensory functions. Ventral horns form in the basal portion, which appear as gray matter because they are composed of motor cell bodies. Axons grow out from the ventral horns to peripheral structures. These axons join with the dorsal root ganglion to form the spinal nerves, which exit the vertebral column as a single unit.

In the seventh to eighth week, white matter finally develops within the spinal cord, representing myelin formation along axon sheaths; this occurs in ascending and descending tracts. The central part of the spinal cord retains a small cavity lined with ependymal cells that allows the transfer of fluid. This cavity was previously filled with amnion, the early embryologic analogue of cerebrospinal fluid.

Development of the Costal Elements

The costal elements persist only in the thoracic spine of the fully developed normal spinal column. During the fifth week, costal processes are formed and project from either side of the centrum. By the seventh week, they become sequestrated, or separated, from the centrum, by forming costovertebral and costotransverse joints. The cartilaginous structures begin to ossify in the eighth week, recognizable as ribs. In the cervical spine, the primordial costal processes fuse with transverse processes to form the costotransverse bar. Eventually, the unique cervical transverse processes form, which contain the transverse foramen for the vertebral artery. In the lumbar spine, the costal processes do not fully form. They persist only partially as the transverse processes of the fully developed spine. The embryonic transverse process forms the mammillary process (not the transverse process). The transverse and mammillary processes eventually fuse. In the sacrum, the costal processes fuse with the embryonic transverse processes and merge to become the anlage of bone of the lateral sacral mass.

Development of the Intervertebral Disc

The intervertebral disc warrants special attention because it is the pathologic focus of many spinal conditions. In the early stages of embryonic development, there are an increasing number of cells in the peripheral portion of the disc and a decreasing number adjacent to the notochord. As the embryo grows beyond a crown-rump length of 10 mm, the cells in the peripheral zone become elongated and are arranged in a lamellar pattern. When it reaches a length of 20 to 40 mm, collagen fibers begin to be synthesized and are exported from the cells, forming a collagen-rich extracellular matrix. The collagen fibers follow the pattern of the cells and are arranged in a lamellar pattern as well, giving the peripheral disc (or anulus fibrosus) its characteristic composition of circumferential bands of tissue. No fully continuous fibers span the entire periphery of the disc; rather, multiple strands interdigitate to create a highly tensile structure. These lamellar bundles appear to be more densely arranged in the anterior anulus and less dense in the posterior anulus of the developing spine, which may explain the propensity for posterior disc rupture in young patients.[6] As the embryo passes into the fetal stage at 2 months, the cells begin to decrease in number, and the production of extracellular matrix is increased.

By the start of the fetal period, the disc has three distinct regions: (1) an external fibrous zone, (2) an internal hyaline zone surrounding the notochord, and (3) a fibrocartilaginous zone. The disc grows by interstitial and appositional growth.[34] *Interstitial growth* refers to growth that occurs at the outer attachment of the anulus to the cartilaginous endplates. *Appositional growth* refers to growth that occurs longitudinally between the vertebra and the disc. Lamellar fibers form attachments to the cartilaginous endplates in the region of the nucleus pulposus, which completely encases the gel-like structure. The outer layers of the anulus become deeply embedded into the peripheral portion of the endplate cartilage.

As the endplate ossifies, forming the ring apophysis, the inserted annular fibers become tightly fixed. The "weak link" in this complex is between the ring apophysis and its corresponding vertebral body, so that apophyseal separation fractures are more common than rupture of the intervertebral disc in the immature spine. The interval between the apophysis and the vertebral ossification center provides an entrance for vessels to supply nutrition to the endplate and to the intervertebral disc by diffusion. This supply is obliterated after union of the ring apophysis to the vertebral body.

There is a lack of agreement regarding the extent of the vascularity of the fetal intervertebral disc. In the fetal disc, the anulus pulposus seems to be vascularized. Taylor and Twomney[35] found that a plexus of vessels around the circumference of the disc sent branches deep within the anulus. In contrast, Whalen and colleagues[36] reported that these vessels entered only the outermost lamellae of the anulus fibrosus. In addition to vessels within the anulus, regularly spaced vascular channels within the cartilage have been shown within the interface between the cartilaginous endplate and the disc (Fig. 1.10). These channels most likely do not act as blood vessels but rather as a sinusoidal "cul-de-sac" system that delivers nutritional factors by diffusion. The deep regions of the disc

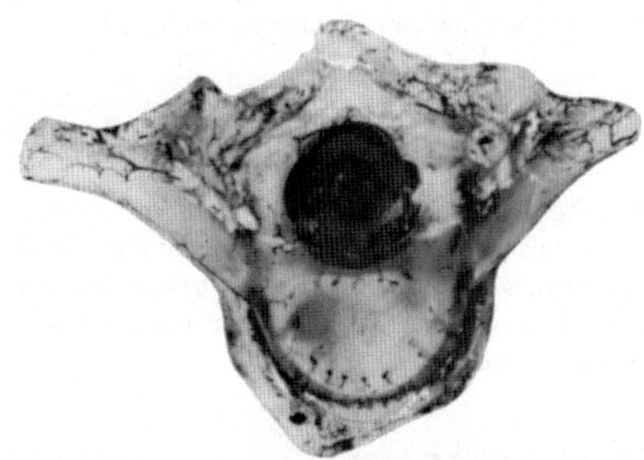

FIG. 1.10 Section through cartilaginous vertebra of 30 weeks after vascular injection. Note the coronal vascular pattern. Each tuft consists of a central artery entwined by recurrent veins that end in a chondrous lacuna as a terminal arteriovenous anastomotic sinusoid (cul-de-sac). Nutrients diffuse from the sinusoid into the surrounding tissues.

are probably not vascularized at any point in development. The adult intervertebral disc is avascular, receiving nutrition only through diffusion through the endplates aided by the flux of fluid to and from the nucleus pulposus. This avascularity may be present at 17 to 24 weeks.[24]

Spinal Ligament Development

There is a paucity of literature concerning the development of the spinal ligaments in the human fetus. Misawa and colleagues[37] dissected 25 human fetuses 6 to 24 weeks of age. They found that, at 6 to 7 weeks, "light zones" represented areas of low cell density that correlated with vertebral bodies, whereas "dark zones" were areas of high cell density and corresponded to the intervertebral regions. The posterior longitudinal ligament was first recognized at 10 weeks, whereas the appearance of the ligamentum flavum was concomitant with that of the lamina at 12 weeks. The fibers of the ligamentum flavum became discernible only at 15 weeks.

Influence of Fetal Movement

Development of the human skeleton seems to be strongly influenced by the interaction of its immature moving parts. In the appendicular skeleton, the opposing surfaces of the femoral head and acetabulum are codependent on each other for normal development into a highly mobile, but stable, weight-bearing joint. In the spine, the development of facet joints is thought to be influenced by torsional loading. It is commonly thought, however, that these demands are placed on the spine only postnatally during upright posture.

The importance of fetal spinal movement has been recognized only more recently. Boszczyk and colleagues[38] used ultrasonography to study the movements of 52 normal fetal spines in utero. They found that rotational movements of 4 to 10 degrees were measurable in fetuses at 9 to 36 weeks. These investigators concluded that this amount of rotation influenced the ultimate morphology of the joint and that torsional stresses are present prenatally and postnatally. Functional demands on the spine may begin even before birth.

Development of Specialized Vertebral Regions

Most of the spine develops in a very uniform manner. The more particular mechanical requirements of the cranial and caudal extremes of the spine have led to unique development processes, however, enabling functional transition between the head and lower limbs.

Occipitocervical Complex

Four occipital myotomes can be readily identified in the human embryo of 4-mm crown-rump length.[39] The first is small, the second is of intermediate size, and the third and fourth are equivalent to the succeeding cervical segments. The first cervical nerve and the hypoglossal artery clearly delimit the most caudal occipital segment. Eight rootlets of the hypoglossal nerve can be discerned rostral to the hypoglossal artery, and these usually unite into four, but no less than three, main roots. This confirms the involvement of at least three precervical segments in the formation of the occiput. DeBeer[40] claimed that a total of nine segments might be involved in skull formation. The first four appear very primitive but contribute to the preotic cranium, whereas the fifth is rudimentary, without a myotome. The last four segments are definite precursors of the occipital complex.

The definitive hypoglossal nerve shows some retention of its multisegmental origins. Its rootlets usually coalesce into two distinct fascicles that exit through separate openings in the dura, and occasionally these do not unite until they have left the skull. The formation of the hypoglossal canal may also indicate a multisegmental relationship. The usual single aperture has been regarded in some texts as homologous to the intervertebral foramen between the neural arch equivalents of two occipital somites, but during chondrification a membranous strut that separates the two main fascicles of the nerve may be observed. By further chondrification and ossification, a double hypoglossal canal accommodating both strands of the nerve may result. Most likely, this mesenchymal strut is a representative of the membranous neural arch process of an intervening segment and is a good indicator that at least three somitic levels were involved in forming the part of the occipital bone surrounding the hypoglossal canal.

Atlantoaxial Complex

The axis and atlas, although considered two vertebral levels in the fully developed spine, actually arise from three different centra. Sensenig[41] first described this in detail in 1937, and later O'Rahilly and Meyer[42] provided a description. These three centra have been named the *X, Y,* and *Z* components. The apical *X component* at first projects into the early foramen magnum and forms an occipitoaxial joint. It has come to be known as the *proatlas* and constitutes the main portion of the odontoid process. Although it is commonly written that the odontoid process develops from the centrum of C1, this is probably not entirely true.[43] Remains of the occipitocervical syndesmosis are apparent by the formation of the alar ligaments. The *Y component* becomes the centrum of the atlas, and the *Z component* becomes the centrum of the axis (C2). The X, Y, and Z components are related to the first, second, and third cervical nerves, which explains the redundancy of the numbering of the upper cervical nerves. Muller and O'Rahilly[44] determined that these three components actually develop from only two and a half sclerotomes in the chick embryo.

Considering the segmental complexities involved in the development of the normal human craniocervical articulations, the occasional occurrence of anomalous separations, fusions, and intercalated ossicles should not be surprising. The odontoid process has origins from the axial portion of the

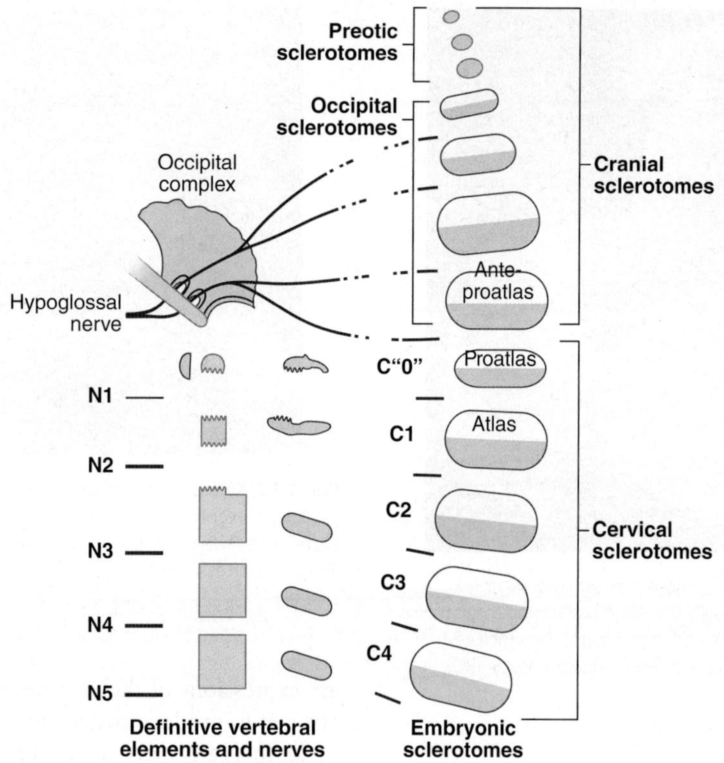

FIG. 1.11 Schematic representation of craniocervical sclerotomes and their segmentally related definitive cranial and vertebral elements and nerves. The cranial and cervical sclerotomes originally formed a continuum. The axis incorporates three sclerotomic elements. The caudal four cranial sclerotomes contribute to the occiput, and their nerves coalesce to form the hypoglossal nerve.

occipital and upper two cervical sclerotomes and is formed from two separate ossification centers that fuse by the seventh month of gestation.[45] A second ossification center, forming the tip of the odontoid, appears by age 3 to 6 and fuses by puberty. Because the odontoid process develops from its own centrum, it can be better understood how an os odontoideum may arise. This anomaly is manifested as a spherule of bone suspended between the two alar ligaments without any apparent bony connection to the C2 body. Os odontoideum has been theorized to be related to prior injury to the odontoid process, but its etiology may also be developmental. Os odontoideum can manifest clinically as neck pain, myelopathy, or even sudden death.[45] Its embryologic development also helps explain the region at the base of the odontoid process that predisposes to nonunion after displaced fractures.

Morphologic anomalies of the odontoid have been described and are attributable to early development. With absence of the midline integration of the primary ossification centers, bifid odontoid process may result, which may lead to craniocervical instability. Furthermore, inclination of the odontoid process may be influenced by traction of the apical ligament on the tip of the odontoid process during development of the craniocervical junction.[46] Retroflexion of the odontoid has been described in patients with Chiari I malformations.[47]

The most frequent manifestation of variant segmentation is the appearance of a third (midline) occipital condyle, also known as a *basilar tubercle*. This structure occurs as a projection on the basion (anterior central point) of the foramen magnum. Sometimes it is expressed as a simple rounded tubercle, but in better developed cases there is actually an articular facet that receives the tip of the odontoid process forming a true diarthrosis (joint). Occasionally, accessory facets lateral to the central projection are present. In a series of 600 skulls, some suggestion of a third condyle was present in 14% of specimens.[48]

Toro and Szepe[49] observed that the third condyle often occurs with occipitalization of the atlas. They also thought that it may be the expression of the hypochordal arch of the "ante-proatlas." As they used this term, it seems to designate the most caudal occipital somite (Fig. 1.11). A more complete separation of this ante-proatlas may form a true occipital vertebra. First described by Meckel in 1815, this malformation forms a more or less complete ring inferior to the foramen magnum, and its anterior arch is often fused to the skull, bearing a third condyle. This condition is distinguished from occipitalization of the atlas by the radiologic identification of the true atlas beneath it. Transverse processes of variable relative size may be present in occipital vertebrae, but these do not show a transverse foramen.[50] Because bony eminences on either side of the third condyle are common to these structures, they may encroach on the foramen magnum, causing neurologic sequelae.

Occipitalization of the atlas occurs in 0.1% to 0.8% of the population according to the series of skulls examined. If the occipitalization is complete, there is no movable atlanto-occipital articulation, and the atlas ring is more constricted. Also, the level of the odontoid tip shows a higher relative

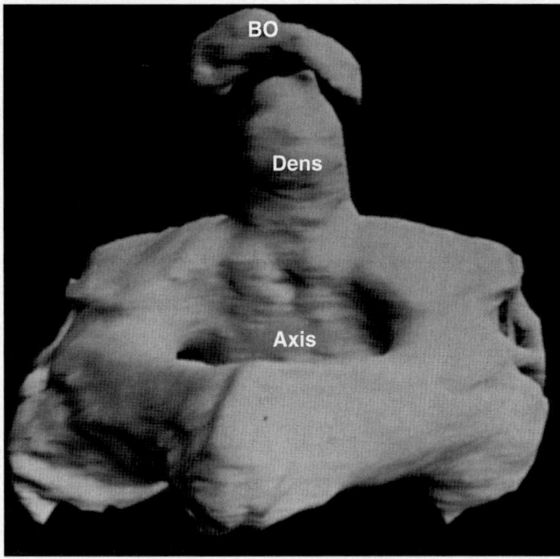

FIG. 1.12 Nonfused "floating" ossicles may occur within craniocervical syndesmoses. A variably shaped, usually pea-sized ossification that occurs between the basion and the tip of the odontoid (in the presence of a complete odontoid process) has been labeled Bergmann ossicle (BO).

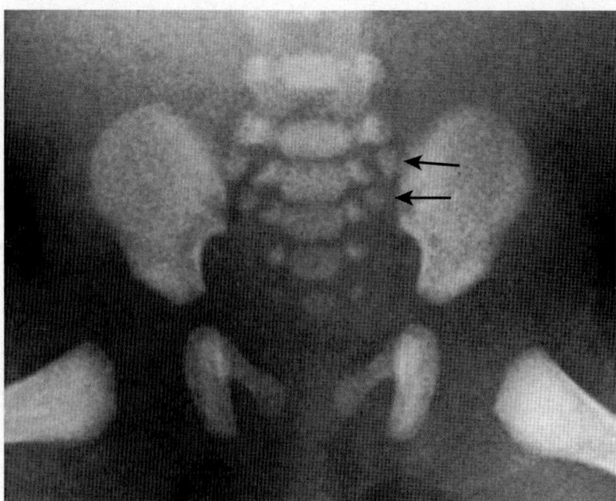

FIG. 1.13 Anteroposterior radiograph of a 34-week fetal pelvis showing two of the eventual three ossific centers (*arrows*) of the costal contributions to the alae. These form in the cartilage that anchors the fetal sacrum to the auricular processes of the iliac wings.

position, and the fusion is often asymmetrical. Inglemark's series of skulls showed that in 78% of the true congenital cases the posterior arch was fused to the posterior rim of the foramen magnum; the anterior arch was fused in 54%, and lateral fusions occurred in 23%.[51] Toro and Szepe[49] suggested that the variable expressions of fragments of the proatlas arch, which normally form parts of the atlas, may enhance the predilection of this segment to fuse to the skull.

Nonfused "floating" ossicles may occur within the craniocervical syndesmoses. A variably shaped, usually pea-sized ossification that occurs between the basion and the tip of the odontoid (in the presence of a complete odontoid process) has been labeled Bergmann ossicle (Fig. 1.12)[52] and is most likely a variant derivative of the ante-proatlas mesenchyme. Putz[53] also recorded the incidence of a small ossicle between the anterior lip of the foramen magnum and the anterior arch of the atlas and within the anterior atlanto-occipital membrane. He was convinced that this was a manifestation of the hypochordal potential of the last occipital (ante-proatlas) somite.

Sacrum

Ossification of the bodies of the sacral vertebrae is unique in that, in addition to the single central ossific zone, two true epiphyseal plates later provide accessory ossification to the superior and inferior surfaces of each segment. The central centers for the superior three sacral vertebrae are evident at week 9, whereas these centers for the fourth and fifth segments do not appear until after week 24. Each vertebral arch of the sacrum shows the conventional bilateral centers, but in addition six centers produce the sacral alae. Between weeks 24 and 32, these centers appear anterolateral to the anterior sacral foramina of the upper three sacral vertebrae. They are expressions of the ever-present potential of the vertebral anlagen to produce costal equivalents (Fig. 1.13).

In the early part of the first year after birth, the sacral vertebrae are still separated by intervertebral discs, and the lower two are the first to fuse in late adolescence. Before this, the ossific centers for the superior and inferior epiphyseal plates of the bodies appear, and between 18 and 20 years of age, lateral epiphyseal plates form on the auricular surfaces of the sacral alae. By the middle of the third decade, the entire sacrum should be fused, although internal remnants of the intervertebral plates remain throughout life. These may be visualized in a sagittal section or in radiographs taken at the appropriate anteroposterior angle.

The coccygeal segments lack neural arch equivalents and form a single ossific center for their bodies. The first usually appears before 5 years of age, and the succeeding three ossify during consecutive 5-year intervals.

Genetic Control of Spinal Segmentation

In the previous edition, an extensive discussion of the genetic control of segmentation was presented. This discussion focused on the wealth of information provided by studies performed on the fruit fly, *Drosophila*. The most essential concept provided by these studies is the fact that the individual aspects of the advanced stages of development are the result of a sequential action of numerous genes, and the mutation of single-effect genes, whose phenotypic expressions have provided the classic mendelian patterns of heredity, usually show errors in only a single step in this concatenation of events. *Drosophila* development shows that a set of maternal effect genes (so labeled because they are exclusively derived from the maternal genome) initially establishes the axial symmetry of the body within the ovum. A group of approximately 20 segmentation genes guides cellular construction of the defined segments. Mutations of these genes are manifest as deletions affecting the normal segment number. Most mutations of the segmentation genes are lethal, and knowledge of them has been obtained from the doomed larval forms. Because they are commonly recessive, however, the mutant strain can be propagated for continuous study. The equivalent genetic effects would not be so readily observable in vertebrates, but comparative evidence strongly indicates that similar genetic mechanisms are operable.

Only after the segmental boundaries have been established can the structures characteristic of each segment be determined. These designations are effected by the homeotic selector genes. The term *homeotic* (from the Greek *homoeos,* meaning "similar") was originally used by Bateson[54] to label the mutant substitution of segment appendages because he surmised that they indicated a similarity (genetic homology) in their underlying developmental mechanisms. In contrast to the segmentation genes whose mutations affect the whole segment, mutations of the homeotic genes are expressed as homologous structures (e.g., legs and wings) grotesquely appearing on inappropriate segments. It is now known that these homeotic genes are closely grouped in two locations on the third chromosome of *Drosophila*'s four chromosomes.

Another significant outcome of *Drosophila* genetic research has been the identification of a sequence of nucleotide base pairs that is common to the homeotic selector genes.[10] Intergenetic cross homologies of certain gene regions are not unusual, but the relatively small sequence common to these homeotic genes contained only a 180–base pair unit that could easily be used as a probe to identify the locations of its homologues. This compact genetic fragment was called the *homeobox* by McGinnis and associates,[55] and the protein it encodes is known as the *homeodomain.*[10]

Links Between Fly and Human

Evolution recognized a fundamental advantage in deriving a body plan from the regional diversification of a series of basically similar modules because virtually all higher organisms develop from some type of segmental organization. Although vertebrate segmentation is not externally obvious in the postembryonic stages, the sclerotomic contributions to the axial skeleton retain the original metameric organization; the common neurologic examination based on a knowledge of the myotomic and dermatomic distribution of the cranial and spinal nerves pays perpetual homage to the truth that humans and the other vertebrates are segmentally constructed animals.

As would be expected, the homeobox-containing genes discovered in humans[9] do not act in exactly the same manner as they do in *Drosophila* because the types of segmental organization are quite different. Nevertheless, the nucleotide sequence cognates of the *Drosophila* homeobox genes found in mammals seem to have considerable influence in the early establishment of brainstem and spinal cord formation.[13] As in the more primitive forms, malfunctions of the genes controlling the more fundamental aspects of segmentation most likely produce early lethal mutations. Because higher vertebrates do not have an autonomous larval stage, the occurrence of such mutations would be lost to general observation. Nevertheless, some gross errors of segmentation that may reach parturition do show genetic implication.

Congenital Syndromes: Genetic Evidence of Segmentation in Humans

Klippel-Feil Syndrome

In humans, congenital vertebral fusions, most commonly manifested in the various types of Klippel-Feil syndrome, serve as a prime example of segmentation. Many instances of this syndrome seem to result from spontaneous mutations or individual teratogenic accidents in the early developmental sequences because most reports present single case histories without examination of the extended family and the family's pedigree. Gunderson and colleagues[11] provided substantial evidence, however, that many cases of Klippel-Feil syndrome are probands of a familial history of the condition. These authors provided the pedigrees of 11 probands. Of particular interest is their type II of the syndrome, which exhibits fusions limited to the cervical regions at C2–C3 and C5–C6. Gunderson and colleagues[11] concluded that this disorder, which produced segmentation errors at consistent spine levels through several successive generations, strongly indicated a dominant mutant defect of a gene that controls these specific levels of segmentation.

Caudal Dysplasias

Another class of segmental spinal malformations that indicates genetic import is grouped under the generic term of *caudal dysplasias.*[4] This malformation complex has proved to be heritable and has a marked association with maternal diabetes. From this complex, certain insights into genetic mechanisms of mammalian spinal development may be derived. That some degree of caudal segment regression is a natural phenomenon is shown by the reduction of the original postsacral somites from eight (±2) to four (±1) in normal human development. In more severe forms of lumbosacral agenesis, all vertebral elements as far cephalad as the upper lumbar region may fail to develop. The association with maternal diabetes has been attributed to a teratogenic effect of hyperglycemia because experimental elevations of blood glucose have produced varying degrees of caudal deficiencies in animals.[53] Similar effects have been induced by various toxic insults during embryogenesis of the spine.

Because caudal agenesis is not a consistent occurrence in the offspring of diabetic mothers, a more complex genetic association has been suspected, particularly as diabetes mellitus and spine defects have been associated with human leukocyte antigen (HLA)-type histocompatibility genes.[4] This inference has been supported by studies of the T-locus genes in the mouse. This locus apparently is a segment of the mouse chromosomes with a collection of genes that have a profound effect on spine development and other aspects of embryogenesis.[56] There is evidence that a gene complex, functionally similar to the mouse T locus, may be operable in humans because an association between histocompatibility antigens of the HLA type and the inheritance of human spina bifida has been reported.[57]

The HLAs are controlled by a cluster of contiguous genes located on the human chromosome 6. As in the mouse T locus, each gene in this group has several alleles, and numerous serologically discrete forms of cell surface antigens may be coded by the gene complex. The total ensemble of the HLAs produced within an individual determines its HLA "personality."[57] The comparative evidence suggests that the HLA complex, because of its defined chromosomal localization, its coding for the antigen complex, and its effect on spine development, is a reasonable candidate for the human analogue of the mouse T locus.

In vertebrates, as in other forms of segmented animals, a definite sequence of genetically controlled events establishes the basic aspects of segment formation. When this has been accomplished, some analogue of the homeotic system of genes most likely determines the regional specializations of the individual segments. This system provides an early determination within the vertebrate sclerotome because these embryonic cell masses exhibit a marked "position effect" before any regional differentiation of the somite is visibly evident. This effect has been shown in the chick embryo, in which the transplantation of an early thoracic sclerotome into the cervical region results in a rib-bearing thoracic vertebra whose specific character development was not modified by its heterotopic location.[58] This early position identity may be because vertebrate embryonic patterns are mostly established through early cell-to-cell interactions subsequent to cell cleavages, and these involve the antigen-mediated cell surface recognitions and adhesions as shown by the HLAs. Nevertheless, some analogues of the homeotic mechanisms in *Drosophila,* although differing in their modes of expression, must determine whether a given vertebra exhibits cervical, thoracic, or sacral characteristics.

The range of anomalies observed in the human spine well support the concept that regional vertebral specification may be the result of a homeotic type of selective repression. In addition to the obvious articulated ribs of the thoracic region, each human vertebral level shows some expression of the costal element potential, but it is usually incorporated as an immovable projection. Anomalous free or articulated rib components have been observed at virtually every vertebral level, including the sacrum and coccyx.[59] The hypochordal potential may best indicate the existence of early segmental totipotency in the vertebrates, however. This component is normally expressed at only the C1 level in humans and in the caudal region in other mammals. If there is some interference in the normal control mechanisms, it may also arise at other levels because hypochordal elements have been observed to occur below the last normal vertebra in some cases of lumbosacral agenesis.

Acknowledgment

We acknowledge Wesley W. Parke, PhD (deceased), an original author of this chapter in previous editions who was responsible for much of the critical information included in this work.

KEY REFERENCES

1. Akobo S, Rizk E, Loukas M, et al. The odontoid process: a comprehensive review of its anatomy, embryology, and variations. *Childs Nerv Syst.* 2015;31(11):2025-2034.
2. Cesmebasi A, Loukas M, Hogan E, et al. The Chiari malformations: a review with emphasis on anatomical traits. *Clin Anat.* 2015;28(2):184-194.
3. Cohen MM Jr. TGF beta/Smad signaling system and its pathologic correlates. *Am J Med Genet A.* 2003;116A(1):1-10.
4. Fuhrhop SK, McElroy MJ, Dietz HC 3rd, MacCarrick GL, Sponseller PD. High prevalence of cervical deformity and instability requires surveillance in Loeys-Dietz syndrome. *J Bone Joint Surg Am.* 2015;97(5):411-419.
5. Vijayasaradhi M, Phaniraj GL, Kumar BL. Anteverted odontoid: a rare congenital bony anomaly of craniovertebral junction. *Neurol India.* 2010;58(3):490-492.

REFERENCES

1. Rai AS, Taylor TK, Smith GH, et al. Congenital abnormalities of the urogenital tract in association with congenital vertebral malformations. *J Bone Joint Surg Br.* 2002;84:891-895.
2. Ursu TR, Porter RW, Navaratnam V. Development of the lumbar and sacral vertebral canal in utero. *Spine.* 1996;21:2705-2708.
3. Wakimoto BT, Turner FR, Kaufman TC. Defects in embryogenesis in mutants associated with the antennapedia gene complex of *Drosophila melanogaster. Dev Biol.* 1984;102:147-172.
4. Welch JP, Alterman K. The syndrome of caudal dysplasia. *Pediatr Pathol.* 1984;2:313-327.
5. Sagi HC, Jarvis JG, Uhtoff HK. Histomorphic analysis of the development of the pars interarticularis and its association with isthmic spondylosis. *Spine.* 1998;23:1635-1639.
6. Tsuji H, Hirano N, Ohshima H, et al. Structural variation of the anterior and posterior annulus fibrosus in the development of human lumbar intervertebral disc: a risk factor for intervertebral disc rupture. *Spine.* 1993;18:204-210.
7. Akam ME. The molecular basis for metameric pattern in the *Drosophila* embryo. *Development.* 1987;101:1-22.
8. Aoyama H, Asamoto K. The development fate of the rostral/caudal half of a somite for vertebra and rib formation: experimental confirmation of the resegmentation theory using chick-quail chimeras. *Mech Dev.* 2000;99:71-82.
9. Cannizzaro LA, Croce CM, Griffin CA, et al. Human homeobox containing genes located at chromosome regions 2q31-2q37 and 12q12-12q13. *Am J Hum Genet.* 1987;41:1-15.
10. Genring WJ, Hiromi Y. Homeotic genes and the homeobox. *Annu Rev Genet.* 1986;20:147-173.
11. Gunderson CH, Greenspan RH, Glasner GH, et al. The Klippel-Feil syndrome: genetic and clinical reevaluation of cervical fusion. *Medicine (Baltimore).* 1967;46:491-511.
12. Krengel S, Gotz W, Herken R. Expression pattern of type II collagen mRNA during early vertebral development in the human embryo. *Anat Embryol (Berl).* 1996;193:43-51.
13. Tribioli C, Lufkin T. The murine Bapx1 homeobox gene plays a critical role in embryonic development of the axial skeleton and spleen. *Development.* 1999;126:699-711.
14. Baur R. Zum Problem der neugliederung der Wirbelsaule. *Acta Anat (Basel).* 1969;72:321-356.
15. Dalgleish AE. A study of the development of the thoracic vertebrae in the mouse assisted by autoradiography. *Acta Anat (Basel).* 1985;122:91-98.

16. Remak R. *Untersuchungen uber die entwicklung der Wirbeltiere.* Berlin: Riemer; 1855.
17. Verbout AJ. A critical review of the "Neugliederung" concept in relation to the development of the vertebral columns. *Acta Biotheor.* 1976;25:219-258.
18. VonEbner V. Urwirbel und Neugliederung der Wirbelsaule. *Sitzungber Akad Wiss Wein.* 1889;III/101:235-260.
19. Bagnall KM, Higgins SJ, Sanders EJ. The contribution made by a single somite to the vertebral column: experimental evidence in support of resegmentation using the chick-quail chimera model. *Development.* 1988;103:69-85.
20. Ewan KB, Everett AW. Evidence for resegmentation in the formation of the vertebral column using the novel approach of retroviral-mediated gene transfer. *Exp Cell Res.* 1992;198:315-320.
21. Huang R, Zhi Q, Brand-Saberi B, et al. New experimental evidence for somite resegmentation. *Anat Embryol (Berl).* 2000;202:195-200.
22. Huang R, Zhi Q, Neubuser A, et al. Function of somite and somitocele cells in the formation of the vertebral motion segment in avian embryos. *Acta Anat (Basel).* 1996;155:231-241.
23. Monsoro-Burq AH, Duprez D, Watanabe Y, et al. The role of bone morphogenetic proteins in vertebral development. *Development.* 1996;122:3607-3616.
24. Skawina S, Litwin JA, Gorczyca J, et al. The architecture of internal blood vessels in human fetal vertebral bodies. *J Anat.* 1997;191:259-267.
25. Nolting D, Hansen BF, Keeling J, et al. Prenatal development of the normal human vertebral corpora in different segments of the spine. *Spine.* 1998;23:2268-2271.
26. Noback CR, Robertson CC. Sequence of appearance of ossification centers in the human skeleton during the first five prenatal months. *Am J Anat.* 1951;89:1-28.
27. Gotz W, Osmers R, Herken R. Localisation of extracellular matrix components in the embryonic human notochord and axial mesenchyme. *J Anat.* 1995;186:111-121.
28. Cohen MM Jr. TGF beta/Smad signaling system and its pathologic correlates. *Am J Med Genet A.* 2003;116A(1):1-10.
29. Fuhrhop SK, McElroy MJ, Dietz HC 3rd, MacCarrick GL, Sponseller PD. High prevalence of cervical deformity and instability requires surveillance in Loeys-Dietz syndrome. *J Bone Joint Surg Am.* 2015;97(5):411-419.
30. Luschka H. *Die Halbgelenke des Menshlichen Korpers.* Berlin: Reimer; 1858.
31. Malinski J. Histochemical demonstration of carbohydrates in human intervertebral discs during postnatal development. *Acta Histochem.* 1958;5:120-126.
32. Schwabe R. Untersuchungen uber die Ruckbildung der Bandscheiben im Menschlichen Kreuzbein. *Virchows Arch.* 1933;287:651-665.
33. Khorooshi MH, Hansen BF, Keeling J, et al. Prenatal localization of the dorsal root ganglion in different segments of the normal human vertebral column. *Spine.* 2001;26:1-5.
34. Bohmig R. Die Blutgefassversorg ung der Wirbelbandscheiben das Verhalten des intervertebralen Chordasegments. *Arch Klin Chir.* 1930;158:374-382.
35. Taylor JR, Twomney LT. The development of the human intervertebral disc. In: Ghosh P, ed. *The Biology of the Intervertebral Disc.* Boca Raton, FL: CRC Press; 1988.
36. Whalen JL, Parke WW, Mazur JM, et al. The intrinsic vasculature of developing vertebral end plates and the nutritive significance to the intervertebral disc. *J Pediatr Orthop.* 1985;5:403-410.
37. Misawa H, Ohtsuka K, Nakata K, et al. Embryological study of the spinal ligaments in human fetuses. *J Spinal Disord.* 1994;7:495-498.
38. Boszczyk AA, Boszczyk BM, Putz RV. Prenatal rotation of the lumbar spine and its relevance for the development of the zygapophyseal joints. *Spine.* 2002;27:1094-1101.
39. Sensenig EC. The early development of the human vertebral column. *Contrib Embryol.* 1957;33:21-51.
40. DeBeer GR. *The Development of the Vertebral Skull.* Oxford: Oxford University Press; 1937.
41. Sensenig EC. The origin of the vertebral column in the deer-mouse, *Peromyscus maniculatus rufinus. Anat Rec.* 1943;86:123-141.
42. O'Rahilly R, Meyer DB. The timing and sequence of events in the development of the vertebral column during the embryonic period proper. *Anat Embryol (Berl).* 1979;157:167-176.
43. David KM, McLachlan JC, Aiton JF, et al. Cartilaginous development of the human craniovertebral junction as visualized by a new three-dimensional computer reconstruction technique. *J Anat.* 1998;192:269-277.
44. Muller F, O'Rahilly R. Occipitocervical segmentation in staged human embryos. *J Anat.* 1994;185:251-258.
45. Akobo S, Rizk E, Loukas M, et al. The odontoid process: a comprehensive review of its anatomy, embryology, and variations. *Childs Nerv Syst.* 2015;31(11):2025-2034.
46. Vijayasaradhi M, Phaniraj GL, Kumar BL. Anteverted odontoid: a rare congenital bony anomaly of craniovertebral junction. *Neurol India.* 2010;58(3):490-492.
47. Cesmebasi A, Loukas M, Hogan E, et al. The Chiari malformations: a review with emphasis on anatomical traits. *Clin Anat.* 2015;28(2):184-194.
48. Lang J. *Clinical Anatomy of the Head.* Berlin: Springer-Verlag; 1983.
49. Toro I, Szepe L. Untersuchungen uber die Frage der Assimilation und Manifestation des Atlas. *Z Anat Entwickl.* 1942;111:186-200.
50. Hadley LA. Atlanto-occipital fusion, ossiculum terminale and occipital vertebra as related to basilar impression with neurological symptoms. *Am J Roentgenol Radium Ther.* 1948;59:511-524.
51. Inglemark BE. Uber das Craniovertebrale Grenzgebiet beim Menschen. *Acta Anat Suppl.* 1947;VI:1-116.
52. Bergman E. *Die Lehre von den Kopfverletzungen (cited by Lang J).* Stuttgart: Enke; 1880.
53. Putz VR. Zur Manifestation der hypochordalen Spangen im cranio-vertebralen Grenzebiet beim Menschen. *Anat Anz.* 1975;137:65-74.
54. Bateson W. *Materials for the Study of Variation Treated with the Especial Regards to Discontinuity in the Origin of Species.* London: Macmillan; 1894.
55. McGinnis W, Garber RL, Wirz J, et al. A homologous protein-coding sequence in *Drosophila* homeotic genes and its conservation in other metazoans. *Cell.* 1984;37: 403-408.
56. Bennett D. The T-locus of the mouse. *Cell.* 1975;6:441-454.
57. Check W. First data for human developmental genes. *JAMA.* 1977;238:2253-2254.
58. Keynes RJ, Stern CD. Mechanisms of vertebrate segmentation. *Development.* 1988;103:413-429.
59. Kaushal SP. Sacral ribs. *Int Surg.* 1977;62:37-38.

CHAPTER 2 Applied Anatomy of the Spine

Christopher M. Bono
Amandeep Bhalla
Steven R. Garfin

The spine is a segmental column of similar formed bones that constitutes the major subcranial part of the axial skeleton. Its individual elements are united by a series of intervertebral articulations that form a flexible, although neuroprotective, support to the trunk and limbs. The spinal column typically consists of 33 vertebrae. The mobile section of the spine comprises 7 cervical, 12 thoracic, and 5 lumbar vertebrae; 5 fused vertebrae form the inflexible sacrum that offers a relatively rigid connection to the innominate bones. Caudad to the sacrum, four or five irregular ossicles compose the coccyx.

Vertebrae

The movements of the spine involve 97 diarthroses (i.e., synovial joints, having substantial motion) and an even greater number of amphiarthroses (i.e., fibrocartilaginous joints, having less motion). The individual vertebrae bear multiple processes and surface markings that indicate the attachments of the numerous ligaments that stabilize these articulations. Despite an appreciable degree of regional variation of these characteristics, the embryologically homologous segmental origin of the spine provides a basic uniformity so that a single generalized description can be applied to the basic morphology of all but the most superior and inferior elements.

The typical vertebra consists of two major components: a roughly cylindrical ventral mass of mostly trabecularized cancellous bone, called the *body,* and a denser, more cortical posterior structure, called the *dorsal vertebral arch*. The vertebral bodies vary considerably in size and sectional contour but exhibit no salient processes or unique external features other than the facets for rib articulation in the thoracic region. In contrast, the vertebral arch has a more complex structure. It is attached to the dorsolateral aspects of the body by two stout pillars, called the *pedicles*. These are united dorsally by a pair of arched flat laminae that are surmounted in the midline by a dorsal projection, called the *spinous process*. The pedicles, laminae, and dorsum of the body form the vertebral foramen, a complete osseous ring that encloses the spinal cord.

The transverse processes and the superior and inferior articular processes are found near the junction of the pedicles and the laminae. The transverse processes extend laterally from the sides of the vertebral arches, and because all vertebrae are phyletically and ontogenetically associated with some form of costal element, they either articulate with or incorporate a rib component. In the thoracic spine, the costal process persists as a rib proper. In the cervical spine, the costal process becomes the anterior part of the transverse process that encloses the vertebral artery foramen, and in the lumbar spine it becomes the mature transverse process; the immature posterior (neural arch) component becomes the mammillary process.

The articular processes (zygapophyses) form the paired diarthrodial articulations (facet joints) between the vertebral arches. The superior processes (prezygapophyses) always bear an articulating facet, whose surface is directed dorsally to some degree, whereas the complementary inferior articulating processes (postzygapophyses) direct their articulating surfaces ventrally. Variously shaped bony prominences (mammillary processes or parapophyses) may be found lateral to the articular processes and serve in the multiple origins and insertions of the spinal muscles.

The superoinferior dimensions of the pedicles are roughly half that of their corresponding body, so that in their lateral aspect the pedicles and their articulating processes form the superior and inferior vertebral notches. Because the base of the pedicle arises superiorly from the dorsum of the body, particularly in the lumbar spine, the inferior vertebral notch appears more deeply incised. In the articulated spine, the opposing superior and inferior notches form the intervertebral foramina that transmit the neural and vascular structures between the corresponding levels of the spinal cord and their developmentally related body segments.

Pars Interarticularis

The pars interarticularis defines the parts of the arch that lie between the superior and inferior articular facets of all subatlantal movable vertebral elements (Fig. 2.1). The term *pars interarticularis* arose to designate that area of the arch that is most stressed by translational movement between adjacent

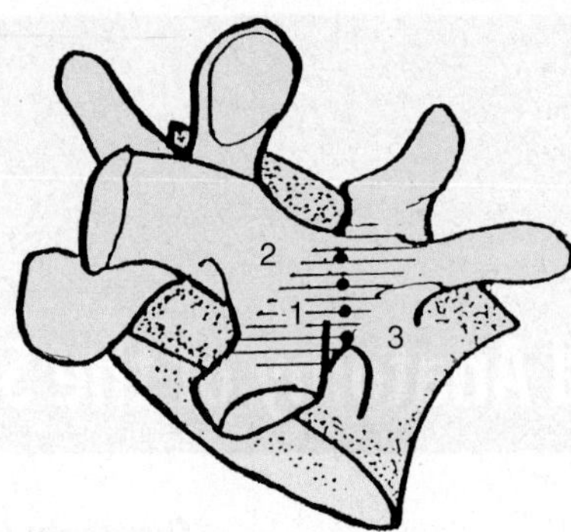

FIG. 2.1 Rendering of the oblique dorsal view of the L5 vertebra showing the parts of the vertebral arch: (*1*) pars interarticularis as the *cross-hatched area,* (*2*) pars laminalis, and (*3*) pars pedicularis. *Dotted line* indicates the most frequent site of mechanical failure of the pars interarticularis.

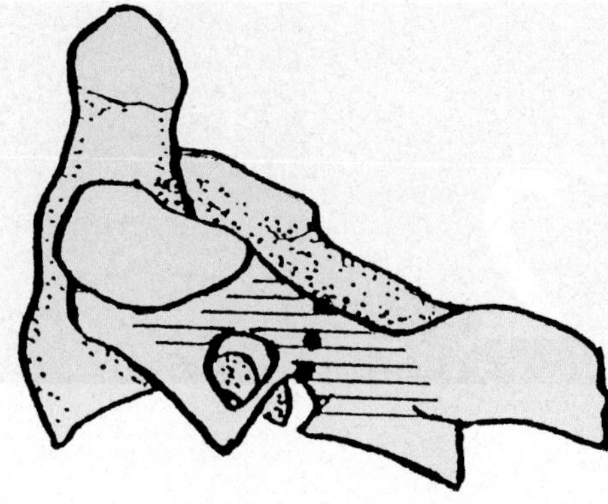

FIG. 2.2 Depiction of lateral view of C2 (axis) vertebra. The offset relationship of the superior facet to the inferior facet elongates the pars interarticularis (*cross-hatched area*). *Dotted line* indicates the most frequent site of failure in upper cervical hyperextension injury (hangman's fracture).

segments, particularly in the second cervical and fifth lumbar vertebrae, which are susceptible to traumatic and stress fractures in this region (i.e., hangman's fracture of C2 and isthmic spondylolysis of L5).[1] In sequential alternation with the intervertebral facet joints, it roofs the lateral recesses of the spinal canal and contributes to the dorsal margins of the intervertebral foramina. In the subcervical vertebrae, it also provides the dorsal part of the base of the transverse process.

Biomechanical forces on the pars interarticularis place it in a position to receive the shearing stresses that occur when translational (spondylolisthetic) forces tend to displace, in a dorsoventral plane, the superior articular processes with respect to their inferior counterparts on the same vertebra. The usual site of failure in the pars interarticularis permits the superior articular facets, pedicles, and vertebral body to be ventrally displaced as a unit, while the inferior articular facets remain attached to the dorsal arch components. These tend to retain their articular relationships with the superior facets of the next lower vertebra.

In the case of the second cervical vertebra (axis) there is a unique anterior relationship of its superior articular facets with the more posteriorly positioned inferior processes that elongates the C2 pars interarticularis. As this offset area receives the greatest leverage between the "cervicocranium" and the lower cervical spine, the indicated line in the illustration in Fig. 2.2 shows the common site of mechanical failure in hyperextension injuries to the upper cervical spine.

In the case of the lumbar vertebrae, the pars interarticularis has been subdivided further. McCulloch and Transfeldt[2] referred to the "lateral buttress," which they believed offered particular structural support to the intervening structures. They described it as the bony bridge that connects the superolateral edge of the inferior facet to the junction of the transverse process and the pedicle. In a follow-up anatomic study, Weiner and colleagues[3] measured the surface area of the lateral buttress in human cadaveric lumbar spines. They found the greatest areas (about 80 mm^2) from L1 to L3, whereas area averaged 50 mm^2 at L4 and only 15 mm^2 at L5. These investigators thought that the broadness of the buttress in the upper lumbar spine can obscure or confuse landmarks for placement of pedicle screws, and its relative thinness (or nonexistence) in the lower lumbar spine can be a predisposing factor to stress fractures or iatrogenic injury to the pars interarticularis. Cadaveric study of L5 pedicle morphology in patients with L5-S1 isthmic spondylolisthesis has shown greater L5 pedicle length compared to that of unaffected subjects, which increases with age.[4]

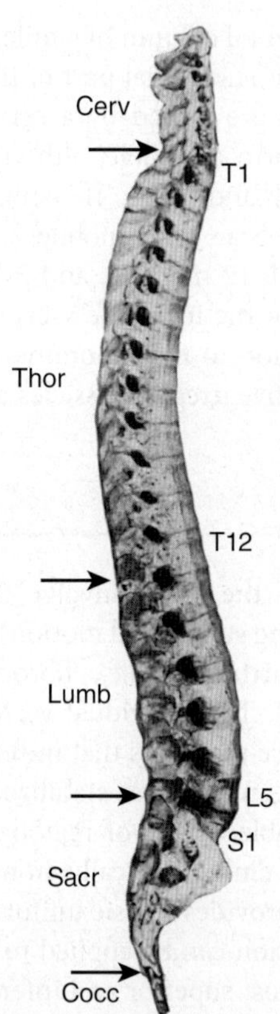

FIG. 2.3 Lateral view of dried preparation of the spine with anterior longitudinal and supraspinous ligaments intact.

Regional Characteristics

Although the 24 vertebrae of the presacral spine are divided into three distinct groups (Fig. 2.3), in which the individual members may be recognized by one or two uniquely regional features, there is a gradual craniocaudal progression of morphologic changes. The vertebrae found above and below the point of regional demarcation are transitional and bear some of the characteristics of both areas. There may be variations in the number of vertebrae, particularly with adolescent idiopathic scoliosis, where up to 10% of individuals can have atypical number of thoracic or lumbar vertebrae.[5]

Cervical Vertebrae

Of the seven cervical vertebrae, the first two (Fig. 2.4A–D) and the last require special notation, but the third to the sixth are fairly uniform, and a common description suffices (Fig. 2.4E–F). Because the cervical vertebrae bear the least weight, their bodies are relatively small and thin with respect to the size of the vertebral arch and vertebral foramen. In addition, their diameter is greater transversely than in the anteroposterior direction. The lateral edges of the superior surface of each body are sharply turned upward to form the uncinate processes that are characteristic of the cervical region. The most obvious diagnostic feature of the cervical vertebrae is the transverse foramina that perforate the transverse processes and transmit the vertebral arteries. The anterior part of the transverse processes represents fused costal elements that arise from the sides of the body. The lateral extremities of the transverse processes bear two projections, the anterior and posterior tubercles. The former serve as origins of anterior cervical muscles; the latter provide origins and insertions for posterior cervical muscles. A deep groove between the upper aspects of the tubercles holds the cervical spinal nerves.

The cervical pedicles connect the posterior vertebral arch to the vertebral body. Anatomic studies have shown that the cervical pedicle height ranges from 5.1 to 9.5 mm, and width ranges from 3 to 7.5 mm.[6,7] The pedicle is angled medially between 90 and 110 degrees.[7]

The superior and inferior articular processes appear as obliquely sectioned surfaces of short cylinders of bone that, when united with the adjacent vertebrae, form two osseous shafts posterolateral to the stacked vertebral bodies. The

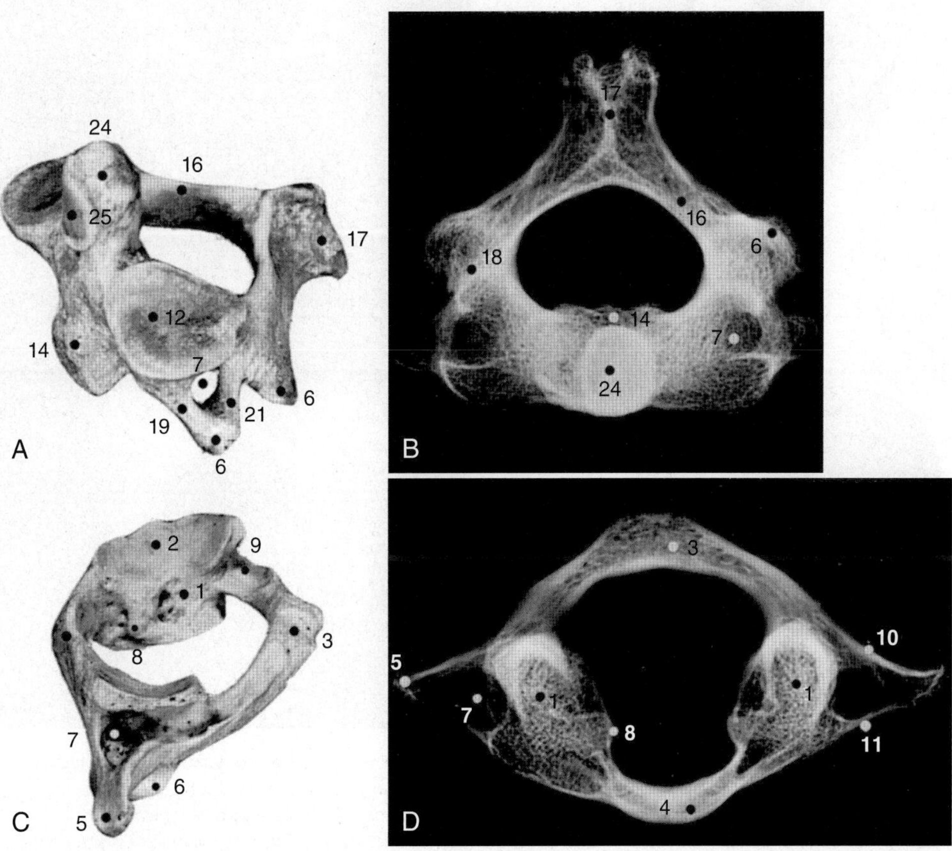

FIG. 2.4 Atlas, axis, and a typical vertebra of each region are illustrated photographically and radiographically. The following numerical key is applicable to all subdivisions of this figure. (A) Oblique view of atlas. (B) Ventral radiographic view of atlas. (C) Oblique view of axis. (D) Vertical radiographic view of axis. *1,* Lateral mass of atlas. *2,* Superior articulating process. *3,* Posterior arch. *4,* Anterior arch. *5,* Transverse process. *6,* Inferior articulating process. *7,* Transverse foramen. *8,* Alar tubercle. *9,* Groove for vertebral artery.*10,* Neural arch element of transverse process. *11,* Costal element of transverse process. *12,* Superior articulating process. *13,* Pedicle. *14,* Body. *15,* Uncinate process. *16,* Lamina. *17,* Spinous process. *18,* Articular pillar. *19,* Anterior tubercle of transverse process. *20,* Neural sulcus. *21,* Posterior tubercle of transverse process. *22,* Superior demifacet for head of rib. *23,* Inferior demifacet for head of rib. *24,* Odontoid process. *25,* Articular facet for anterior arch of atlas.

Continued

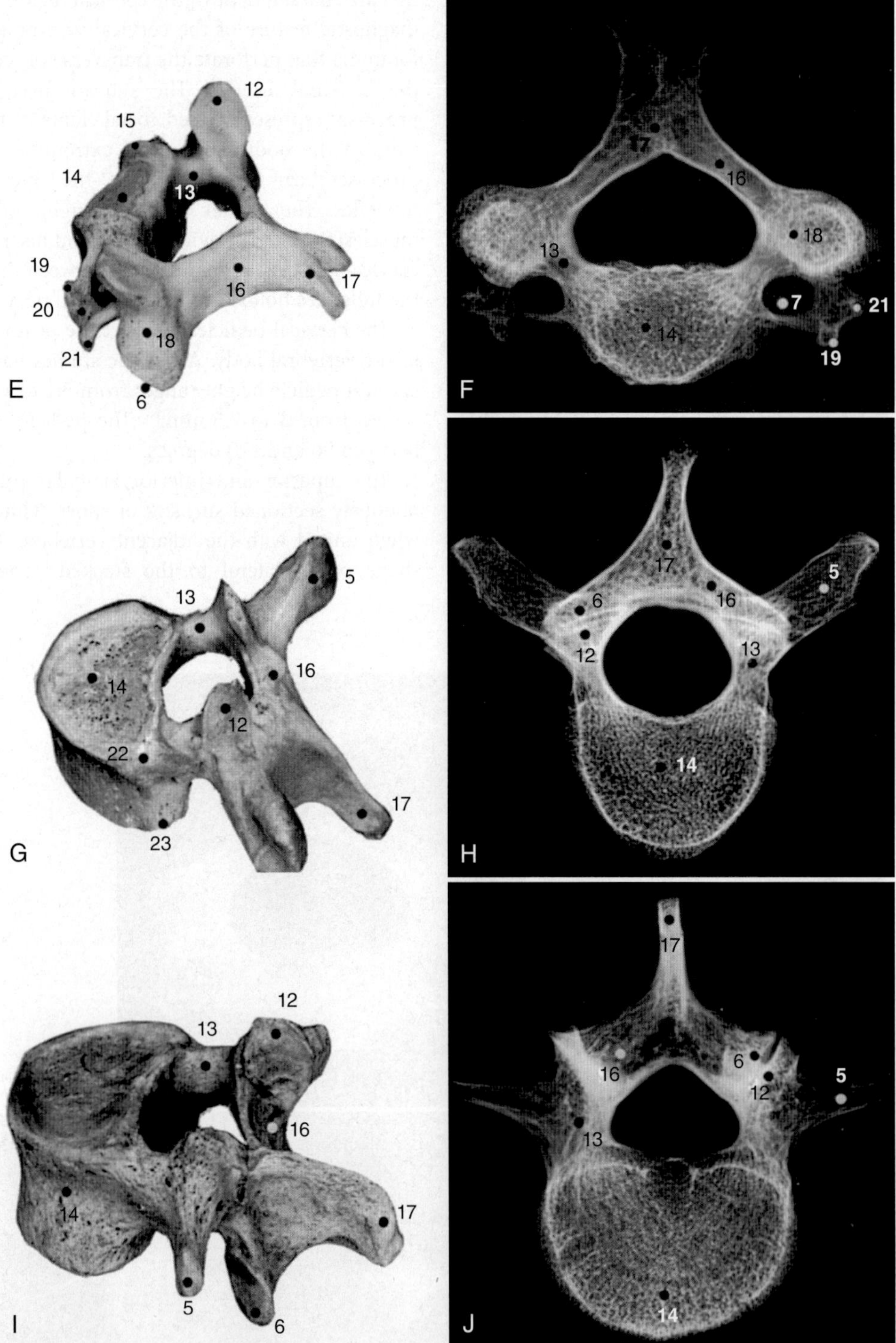

FIG. 2.4, cont'd (E) Oblique view of typical (fourth) cervical vertebra. (F) Vertical radiographic view of typical cervical vertebra. (G) Oblique view of typical (fifth) thoracic vertebra. (H) Vertical radiographic view of thoracic vertebra. The plane of the articular facets would readily permit rotation. (I) Oblique view of typical (third) lumbar vertebra. (J) Vertical radiographic view of lumbar vertebra. The plane of the articular facets is situated to lock the lumbar vertebrae against rotation.

cervical vertebrae present a tripod of flexible columns for the support of the head. As in the upper cervical spine, the combination of the articular processes and the intervening bone is often referred to as the lateral mass in the subaxial region. It is a common site for screw insertion during internal fixation of the cervical spine.[8]

The laminae are narrow and have a thinner superior edge. At their mid-dorsal junction, they bear a bifid spinous process that receives the insertions of the semispinalis cervicis muscles. The height of the lamina of C4 is 10 to 11 mm, whereas the lamina thickness at C5 is about 2 mm.[9] The lamina is thickest at T2, where it measures an average of 5 mm.

Atlantoaxial Complex

The first two cervical vertebrae are structurally and developmentally different. Together, they form a complex articular system that permits the nutational (i.e., nodding) and rotational movements of the head. The first cervical vertebra, or atlas, is a bony ring consisting of an anterior and a posterior arch, which are connected by the two lateral masses. It has all the homologous features of a typical vertebra with the exception of the body. The lateral masses correspond to the combined pedicles and articular pillars of the lower cervical vertebrae, but the superior and inferior articular facets are concave. The superior articular surfaces face upward and internally to receive the occipital condyles of the skull, whereas the inferior articulating surfaces face downward and internally to rotate on the sloped "shoulders" of the axis. This slope helps prevent lateral translation while permitting rotation.

The posterior arch consists of modified laminae that are more round than flat in their sectional aspect and a posterior tubercle that represents an attenuated spinous process that gives origin to suboccipital muscles. Immediately behind the lateral masses on the superior surface of the posterior arch of C1, two smooth grooves house the vertebral arteries as they penetrate the posterior atlanto-occipital membrane. These arteries take a tortuous course from the transverse processes of the atlas, making an almost 90-degree turn medially as they exit the foramen and a subsequent 90-degree turn superiorly to enter the dura and subsequently the foramen magnum. The vertebral artery courses over the posterior ring of the atlas 10 to 15 mm from the midline in adults and, although the arteries are closer to the midline in the pediatric population, 97% are located at least 1 cm from the midline.[10] Dissection further lateral risks injury to these vessels.

The transverse foramen also houses a venous system. In an anatomic and radiologic study to characterize the venous system within the transverse foramen, Magro and colleagues[11] found ventral longitudinal veins that may also exist in a plexus arrangement. Anastomosis between the plexus transverse veins and vertebral veins can be present. An understanding of venous anatomy in the transverse foramen may help contextualize false-positive diagnoses of vertebral artery dissection from magnetic resonance angiography caused by slow flow vertebral veins.

The anterior arch forms a short bridge between the anterior aspects of the lateral masses. It bears an anterior tubercle that is the site of insertion of the longus colli muscle. On the posterior surface of the anterior arch, a semicircular depression marks the synovial articulation of the odontoid process. Internal tubercles on the adjacent lateral masses are the attachment sites of the transverse atlantal ligaments that hold the odontoid against this articular area. Cadaveric studies have shown that the right-sided tubercles tend to be of larger caliber and that the mean angle formed between both tubercles and the dental facet is 75 degrees.[12]

The second cervical vertebra, or axis, provides a bearing surface on which the atlas may rotate. Its most distinctive characteristic is the vertically projecting odontoid process that serves as a pivotal restraint against horizontal displacements of the atlas. This bony prominence represents the phyletically purloined centrum of the first cervical vertebra. It exhibits a slight constriction at its neck and an anterior facet for its articulation with the anterior arch of the atlas. Posteriorly, a groove in the neck of the odontoid marks the position of the strong transverse atlantal ligament.

The apex of the odontoid process is slightly pointed. It is the attachment site of the apical ligament. Posterior to the apex, two lateral roughened prominences indicate the attachments of the alar ligaments. These structures and the apical ligament connect the odontoid process to the base of the skull at the basion, the anterior aspect of the foramen magnum. The occipital attachments of the alar ligaments are on the medial surface of the occipital condyles, adjacent to the atlanto-occipital joints. Atlantal attachments of the alar ligaments have also been described, but these are more likely to be anatomic variants and not essential components of craniovertebral junction stability.[13] The superior articulating surfaces of the axis are convex and are directed laterally to receive the lateral masses of the atlas. The inferior articulating surfaces are typical of those of the cervical vertebrae and serve as the start of the articular columns. The transverse processes of the axis are directed downward. Anteriorly, the inferior aspect of the body of the axis forms a liplike process that descends over the first intervertebral disc and the body of the third cervical vertebra.

The seventh cervical vertebra is transitional. The inferior surface of its body is proportionately larger than the superior surface. It has a long, distinct spinous process that is usually easily palpable (the vertebra prominens). The superior and inferior articulating facets are more steeply inclined and presage the form of these structures in the thoracic region. Blunt transverse processes have heavy posterior struts and much lighter anterior struts that surround transverse foramina that are often bilaterally unequal and seldom pass the vertebral arteries. Frequently, one or both of the anterior struts realize their true potential as a costal element and develop into a cervical rib.

Thoracic Vertebrae

All 12 thoracic vertebrae support ribs and have facets for the diarthrodial articulations of these structures. The first and last four have specific peculiarities in the manner of costal articulations, but the second to the eighth are similar (Fig. 2.4G–H).

The body of a mid-thoracic vertebra is heart-shaped. Its length and width are roughly halfway between that of the cervical and lumbar bodies. Often a flattening of the left side of the body indicates its contact with the descending aorta. In the mid-thorax, the heads of the ribs form a joint that spans the intervertebral disc, so that the inferior lip of the body of one vertebra and the corresponding site of the superior lip of the infrajacent element share in the formation of a single articular facet for the costal capitulum. The typical thoracic vertebra bears two demifacets on each side of its body. The thoracic vertebral arch encloses a small, round vertebral foramen that would not admit the tip of an index finger, even when the specimen is from a large adult. This limited space for the spinal cord predisposes to severe spinal cord injury with minimal dimensional compromise.

Because the pedicles arise more superiorly on the dorsum of the body than they do in the cervical region, the inferior vertebral notch forms an even greater contribution to the intervertebral foramen. The pedicle height increases from T1 to T12, but the transverse pedicle width (which is more critical for transpedicular screw containment) does not follow this same craniocaudal pattern.[14] Cinotti and colleagues[15] found that the pedicles in the T4 to T8 region had the smallest transverse diameter. Scoles and colleagues[16] documented similar findings in 50 cadaveric human spines, with the smallest diameters measured at T3 to T6. On average, the transverse pedicle diameter at T3 is 3.4 mm in women and 3.9 mm in men. At T6, it averages 3 mm in women and 3.5 mm in men. At T1, however, the mean diameter is 6.4 mm in women and 7.3 mm in men. Lehman and colleagues described key morphologic characteristics to facilitate safe medial-lateral starting points for placement of thoracic pedicle screws.[17] The ventral lamina is an anatomically reproducible structure consistently located medial to the superior articular facet in the thoracic spine. They also noted the center of the pedicle lays 2 to 3 mm lateral to the midline of the superior articular facet.

The superior articular facets form a stout shelflike projection from the junction of the laminae and the pedicles. Their ovoid surfaces are slightly convex, are almost vertical, and are coronal in their plane of articulation. They face dorsally and slightly superolaterally, and in bilateral combination they present the segment of an arc whose center of radius lies at the anterior edge of the vertebral body. They permit a slight rotation around the axis of this radius. The inferior articular facets are borne by the inferior edges of the laminae. The geometry of their articular surfaces is complementary to the superior processes.

On the ventral side of the tip of the strong transverse processes, another concave facet receives the tuberculum of the rib whose capitulum articulates with the superior demifacet of the same vertebra. The spinous processes of the thoracic vertebrae are long and triangular in section. The spinous processes of the upper four thoracic vertebrae are more bladelike and are directed downward at an angle of about 40 degrees from the horizontal. The middle four thoracic spinous processes are longer but directed downward at an angle of 60 degrees, so that they completely overlap the adjacent lower segment. The lower four resemble the upper four in direction and shape.

The first thoracic vertebra has a complete facet on the side of its body for the capitulum of the first rib and an inferior demifacet for the capitulum of the second rib. The costal articulations of the 9th to 12th thoracic vertebrae are confined to the sides of the bodies of their respective segments. On the last two thoracic vertebrae, transitional characteristics are evident in the diminution of the transverse processes and their failure to buttress the last two ribs. Because the ribs are disconnected from the sternum, they are frequently referred to as "floating ribs."

Lumbar Vertebrae

The lumbar vertebrae are the lowest five vertebrae of the presacral column (see Fig. 2.4I–J). All their features are expressed in more massive proportions. They are easily distinguished from other regional elements by their lack of a transverse foramen or costal articular facets. The body is large, having a width greater than its anteroposterior diameter, and is slightly thicker anteriorly than posteriorly. All structures associated with the vertebral arch are blunt and stout. The thick pedicles are widely placed on the dorsolaterosuperior aspects of the body, and with their laminae they enclose a triangular vertebral foramen. Although the inferior vertebral notch is deeper than the superior, both make substantial contributions to the intervertebral foramen. The transverse processes are flat and winglike in the upper three lumbar segments, but in the fifth segment they are thick, rounded stumps. The fourth transverse process is usually the smallest.

Aside from their relative size, the lumbar vertebrae can be recognized by their articular processes. The superior pair arise in the usual manner from the junction of the pedicles and laminae, but their articular facets are concave and directed dorsomedially, so that they almost face each other. The inferior processes are extensions of the laminae that direct the articulating surfaces ventrolaterally and lock themselves between the superior facets of the next inferior vertebra in an almost mortise-and-tenon fashion. This arrangement restricts rotation and translation in the lumbar region. The lumbar segments also have pronounced mammillary processes, which are points of origin and insertion of the thick lower divisions of the deep paraspinal muscles.

Sacral Vertebrae

The sacrum consists of five fused vertebrae that form a single triangular complex of bone that supports the spine and forms the posterior part of the pelvis (Figs. 2.5 and 2.6). It is markedly curved and tilted backward, so that its first element articulates with the fifth lumbar vertebra at a pronounced angle (the sacrovertebral angle).

Close inspection of the flat, concave ventral surface and the rough, ridged convex dorsal surface reveals that, despite their fusion, all the homologous elements of typical vertebrae are still evident in the sacrum. The heavy, laterally projecting alae that bear the articular surfaces for articulation with the pelvis are fused anterior costal and posterior transverse processes of the first three sacral vertebrae. These lateral fusions require that separate dorsal and ventral foramina provide egress for the anterior and posterior divisions of the sacral nerves. The ventral four pairs of sacral foramina are larger than their dorsal counterparts because they must pass the thick sacral contributions to the sciatic nerve. The ventral surface of the sacrum is relatively smooth. There are four transverse ridges that mark the fusions of the vertebral bodies and enclose remnants of the intervertebral discs. Lateral to the bodies of the second, third, and fourth elements, the ridges of bone that

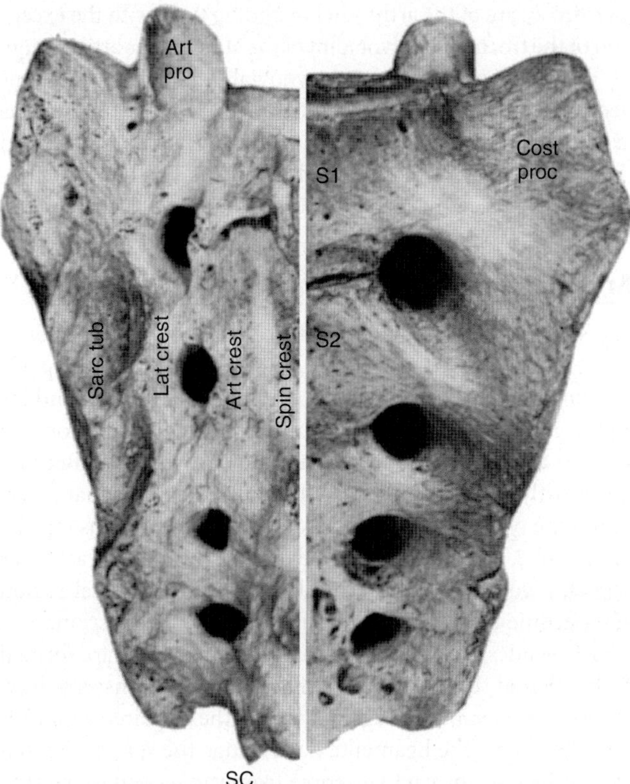

FIG. 2.5 Composite anteroposterior view of sacrum. The roughened crests on the dorsum (*left side*) indicate longitudinal fusions of vertebral arch structures. The articular process is directed backward to buttress the vertebral arch of the fifth lumbar vertebra. *Art crest,* articular crest; *Art pro,* articular process; *Cost proc,* costal process; *Lat crest,* lateral crest; *Sarc tub,* superior articulating tubercle; SC, sacral comua; *Spin crest,* spinous crest.

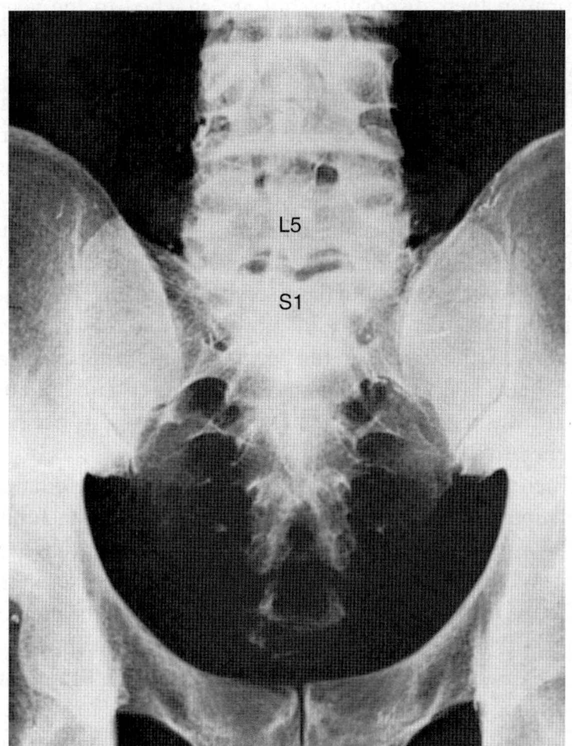

FIG. 2.6 Anterior radiographic view of lumbosacral and sacroiliac articulations. Load transfer from the lumbar spine to the iliac bones via the costal processes of the first and second sacral segments is obvious.

separate the anterior sacral foramina are quite prominent and give origin to the piriformis muscle.

The dorsal aspect of the sacrum is convex, rough, and conspicuously marked by five longitudinal ridges. The central one, the middle sacral crest, is formed by the fusion of the spinous processes of the sacral vertebrae. On either side, a sacral groove separates it from the medial sacral articular crest that represents the fused articular process. The superior ends of these crests form the functional superior articular processes of the first sacral vertebra, which articulate with the inferior processes of the fifth lumbar vertebra. They are very strong, and their facets are directed dorsally to resist the tendency of the fifth lumbar vertebra to be displaced forward. Inferiorly, the articular crests terminate as the sacral cornua, two rounded projections that bracket the inferior hiatus where it gives access to the sacral vertebral canal. More laterally, the lateral crests and sacral tuberosities form uneven elevations for the attachments of the dorsal sacroiliac ligaments.

The sacrum and its posterior ligaments lie ventral to the posterior iliac spines and form a deep depression that accommodates, and gives origin to, the inferior parts of the paraspinal muscles. The grooves between the central spinous crest and the articular crests are occupied by the origins of the multifidus muscles. Dorsal and lateral to these are attached the origins of the iliocostal and iliolumbar muscles.

Coccyx

The coccyx is usually composed of four vertebral rudiments, but one fewer or one greater than this number is not uncommon. The coccyx is the vestigial representation of the tail. The first coccygeal segment is larger than the succeeding members and resembles to some extent the inferior sacral element. It has an obvious body that articulates with the homologous component of the inferior sacrum, and it bears two cornua, which may be regarded as vestiges of superior articulating processes. The three inferior coccygeal members are most frequently fused and present a curved profile continuous with that of the sacrum. They incorporate the rudiments of a body and transverse processes but possess no components of the vertebral arch.

The coccyx contributes no supportive function to the spine. It serves as an origin for the gluteus maximus posteriorly and the muscles of the pelvic diaphragm anteriorly.

Arthrology of the Spine

The articulations of the spine include the three major types of joints: synarthroses, diarthroses, and amphiarthroses (Figs. 2.7 to 2.9). The *synarthroses* are found during development and the first decade of life. The best examples are the neurocentral joints of the immature spine, which are the two unions between the centers of ossification for the two halves of the vertebral arch and that of the centrum. Until they are obliterated during the 2nd decade, they possess a thin plate cartilage between the two apposed bony surfaces. Another example is

FIG. 2.7 (A) Anteroposterior radiograph of dried preparation of cervical and upper thoracic spine. Note greater relative thickness of cervical discs and more lateral disposition of cervical articular pillars. (B) Lateral view of preceding specimen. The normal curvatures did not survive the preparation, but the gradual increase in size of the bodies and the intervertebral foramina is well illustrated.

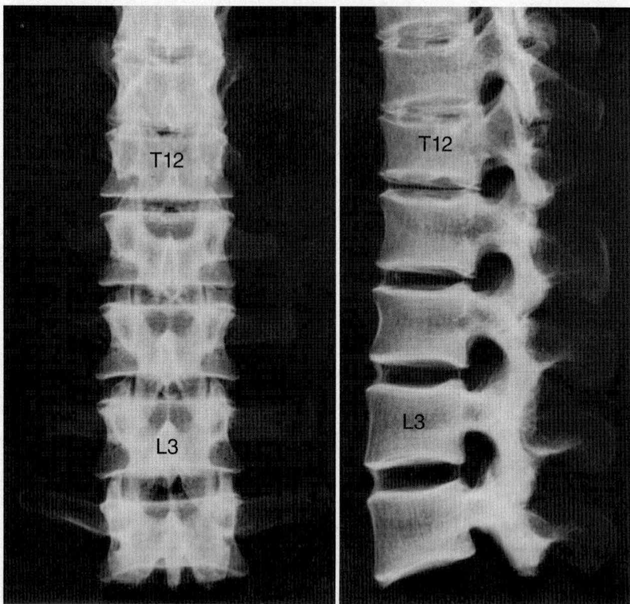

FIG. 2.8 Anteroposterior *(left)* and lateral *(right)* radiographs of lower thoracic and upper lumbar region of articulated dried preparation.

the early union between the articular processes of the sacral vertebrae, known as *ephemeral synchondroses*.

The *diarthroses* are true synovial joints, formed mostly by the facet joints and costovertebral joints, but also include the atlantoaxial and sacroiliac articulations. All the spinal diarthroses are of the arthrodial or gliding type, with the exception of the trochoid or pivot joint of the atlantodens articulation.

The *amphiarthroses* are nonsynovial, slightly movable connective tissue joints. They are of two types: the symphysis, as exemplified by the fibrocartilage of the intervertebral disc, and the syndesmosis, as represented by all the ligamentous connections between the adjacent bodies and the adjacent arches.

Articulations of the Vertebral Arches

The synovial facet joints formed by the articular processes of the vertebral arches possess a true joint capsule and are capable of a limited gliding articulation. The capsules are thin and lax and are attached to the bases of the engaging superior and inferior articulating processes of opposing vertebrae. Because it is mostly the plane of articulation of these joints that determines the types of motion characteristic of the various regions of the spine, it would be expected that the fibers of the articular capsules would be longest and loosest in the cervical region and become increasingly taut in an inferior progression.

The syndesmoses between the vertebral arches are formed by the paired sets of ligamenta flava, the intertransverse ligaments, the interspinous ligaments, and the unpaired supraspinous ligament. The ligamenta flava bridge the spaces between the laminae of adjacent vertebrae from the second cervical to the lumbosacral interval. The lateral extent of each half of a paired set begins around the bases of the articulating processes and can be traced medially where they nearly join in the midline. This longitudinal central deficiency serves to transmit small vessels and facilitates the passage of a needle during lumbar punctures. The fibers of the ligamenta flava are almost vertical in their disposition, but are attached to the ventral surface of the cephalad lamina and to the superior lip of the subjacent lamina.

This shinglelike arrangement conceals the true length of the ligaments because of the overlapping of the superior lamina. Their morphology is best appreciated from the ventral aspect as in Fig. 2.9B. The yellow elastic fibers that give the ligamenta flava their name maintain their elasticity even in embalmed specimens. It has been stated in some texts that the elasticity of the ligamenta flava serves to assist in the maintenance of the erect posture. A more probable reason for this property is simply to keep the ligament taut during extension, where any laxity would permit redundancy and infolding toward the ventrally related nervous structures, as occurs in degenerative lumbar spinal stenosis.

There are two separable layers of the ligamentum flavum, one superficial and one deep, that have distinct attachments to the inferior lamina.[18] The superficial component inserts at the classically described location along the posterosuperior aspect of the lamina. The deep component inserts along the anterosuperior surface of the lamina.[18] This attachment can have significance during surgical removal of the ligamentum flavum for exposure of the neural elements.

The intertransverse ligaments are fibrous connections between the transverse processes. They are difficult to distinguish from extensions of the tendinous insertions of the segmental muscles and in reality may be just that in some regions.

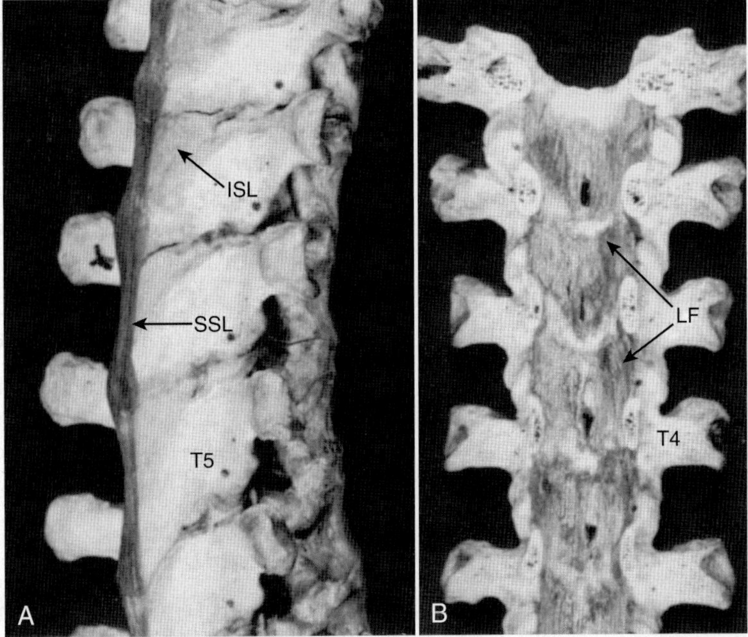

FIG. 2.9 (A) Dried preparation of thoracic vertebrae showing the supraspinous ligament (SSL) and interspinous ligaments (ISL). (B) Anterior view of upper thoracic vertebral arches showing the disposition of the ligamenta flava (LF).

They appear as a few tough, thin fibers between the cervical transverse processes, and in the thoracic area they blend with the intercostal ligaments. Being most distinct between the lumbar transverse processes, the intertransverse ligaments may be isolated here as membranous bands.

The interspinous ligaments (see Fig. 2.9A) are membranous sets of fibers that connect adjoining spinous processes. They are situated medial to the thin pairs of interspinal muscles that bridge the apices of the spine. The fibers of the ligaments are arranged obliquely as they connect the base of the superior spine with the superior ridge and apex of the next most inferior spinous process. These midline ligaments are found in pairs with a distinct dissectible cleft between them.

The supraspinous ligament (see Fig. 2.9A) is a continuous fibrous cord that runs along the apices of the spinous processes from the seventh cervical to the end of the sacral spinous crest. Similar to the longitudinal ligaments of the vertebra, the more superficial fibers of the ligament extend over several spinal segments, whereas the deeper, shorter fibers bridge only two or three segments. In the cervical region the supraspinous ligament assumes a distinctive character and a specific name, the *ligamentum nuchae.* This structure is bowstrung across the cervical lordosis from the external occipital protuberance to the spine of the seventh cervical vertebra. Its anterior border forms a sagittal fibrous sheet that divides the posterior nuchal muscles and attaches to the spinous processes of all cervical vertebrae. The ligamentum nuchae contains an abundance of elastic fibers. In quadrupeds, it forms a strong truss that supports the cantilevered position of the head.

Special Articulations

The atlanto-occipital articulation consists of the diarthrosis between the lateral masses of the atlas and the occipital condyles of the skull and the syndesmoses formed by the atlanto-occipital membranes. The articular capsules around the condyles are thin and loose and permit a gliding motion between the condylar convexity and the concavity of the lateral masses. The capsules blend laterally with ligaments that connect the transverse processes of the atlas with the jugular processes of the skull. Although the lateral ligaments and the capsules are sufficiently lax to permit nodding, they do not permit rotation.

The anterior atlanto-occipital membrane is a structural extension of the anterior longitudinal ligament that connects the forward rim of the foramen magnum, also known as the *basion,* to the anterior arch of the atlas and blends with the joint capsules laterally. It is dense, tough, and virtually cordlike in its central portion.

The posterior atlanto-occipital membrane is homologous to the ligamenta flava and unites the posterior arch of the atlas. It is deficient laterally where it arches over the groove on the superior surface of the arch. Through this aperture, the vertebral artery enters the neural canal to penetrate the dura. Occasionally, the free edge of this membrane is ossified to form a true bony foramen (called the *ponticulus posticus*) around the artery.

The median atlantoaxial articulation is a pivot (trochoid) joint (Figs. 2.10 and 2.11). The essential features of the articulation are the odontoid process (dens) of the axis and the internal surface of the anterior arch of the atlas. The opposition of the two bones is maintained by the thick, straplike transverse atlantal ligament. The ligament and the arch of the atlas have true synovial cavities intervening between them and the odontoid process. Alar expansions of the transverse ligament attach to tubercles on the lateral rims of the anterior foramen magnum, and a single, unpaired cord, the apical odontoid ligament, attaches the apex of the process to the

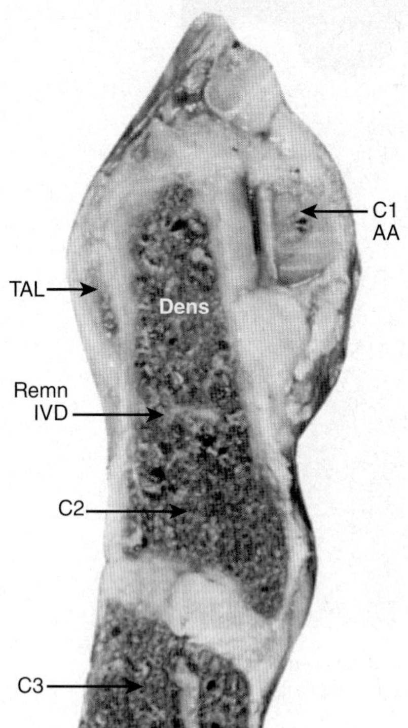

FIG. 2.10 Sagittal section through adult odontoid process showing articular relationships with anterior arch of the atlas (AA) and transverse atlantal ligament (TAL). Despite the fact this patient was older than 50 years, a cartilaginous remnant of the homologue of an intervertebral disc (Remn IVD) may be discerned. Radiologically, this might be confused with fracture or a nonunion status.

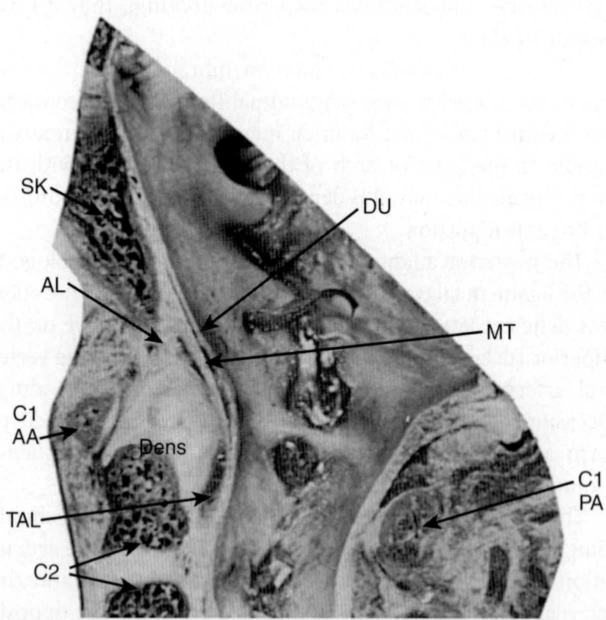

FIG. 2.11 Sagittal section through atlanto-occipital articulation of a 4-year-old child. The major ossification centers of the odontoid process are still separated from the body of C2 by a well-differentiated disc. The cartilaginous apex of the process shows a condensation marking the apical ossific center. C1 AA and C1 PA mark the anterior and posterior atlantal arches. The dura (DU) overlies the membrana tectoria (MT), which is a superior extension of the posterior longitudinal ligament. The transverse atlantal ligament (TAL) and apical ligament (AL) are also indicated. SK, skull.

basion. The entire joint is covered posteriorly by a cranial extension of the posterior longitudinal ligament, which is named *tectorial membrane* in this region. Because the atlas freely glides over the superior articulating facets of C2, the atlantoaxial pivot is essential for preventing horizontal displacements between C1 and C2. Fracture of the odontoid or, less likely, rupture of the transverse ligament produces a very unstable articulation.

Articulations of the Vertebral Bodies

The vertebral bodies are connected by the two forms of amphiarthroses. Symphyses are represented by the intervertebral discs, and syndesmoses are formed by the anterior and posterior longitudinal ligaments.

Intervertebral Disc

In view of the semiliquid nature of the nucleus pulposus and the vacuities that may be shown in the nucleus of aging specimens, von Luschka[19] attempted to classify the intervertebral disc as a diarthrosis, in which the vertebral chondral plates were the articular cartilages, the anulus provided the articular capsule, and the fluid and ephemeral spaces within the nucleus corresponded to the synovia and the joint cavity. Although the intervertebral disc forms a joint that should be classified in its own exclusive category because its development, structure, and function are generally different from those of any other joint, it most closely conforms to an amphiarthrosis of the symphysis type.

The intervertebral disc is the fibrocartilaginous complex that forms the articulation between the bodies of the vertebrae. Although it provides a very strong union, ensuring the degree of intervertebral fixation that is necessary for effective action and the protective alignment of the neural canal, the summation of the limited movements allowed by each disc imparts to the spinal column as a whole its characteristic mobility. The discs of the various spinal regions may differ considerably in size and in some detail, but they are basically identical in their structural organization. Each consists of two components: the internal semifluid mass, called the *nucleus pulposus,* and its laminar fibrous container, known as the *anulus fibrosus.*

Nucleus Pulposus

Typically, the nucleus pulposus occupies an eccentric position within the confines of the anulus, usually being closer to the posterior margin of the disc. Its most essential character becomes obvious in either transverse or sagittal preparations of the disc in which, as evidence of internal pressure, it bulges beyond the plane of section. Palpation of a dissected nucleus from a young adult shows that it responds as a viscid fluid under applied pressure, but it also exhibits considerable elastic rebound and assumes its original physical state on release. These properties may still be shown in the spine of a cadaver that has been embalmed for many months.

Histologic analysis provides a partial explanation for the characteristics of the nucleus. As the definitive remnant of the embryonic notochord, it is similarly composed of loose, delicate fibrous strands embedded in a gelatinous matrix. In the center of the mass, these fibers show no geometric preference in their arrangement but form a felted mesh of undulating bundles. Only the fibers that are in approximation to the vertebral chondral plates display a definite orientation. These approach the cartilage at an angle and become embedded in its substance to afford an attachment for the nucleus. Numerous cells are suspended in the fibrous network. Many of these are fusiform and resemble typical reticulocytes, but vacuolar and darkly nucleated chondrocytes are also interspersed in the matrix. Even in the absence of vascular elements, the profusion of cells should accentuate the fact that the nucleus pulposus is composed of vital tissue. There is no definite structural interface between the nucleus and the anulus. Rather, the composition of the two tissues blends imperceptibly.

Anulus Fibrosus

The anulus is a concentric series of fibrous lamellae that encase the nucleus and strongly unite the vertebral bodies (Fig. 2.12). The essential function of the nucleus is to resist and redistribute compressive forces within the spine, whereas one of the major functions of the anulus is to withstand tension, whether the tensile forces be from the horizontal extensions of the compressed nucleus, from the torsional stress of the column, or from the separation of the vertebral bodies on the convex side of a spinal flexure. Without optical aid, simple dissection

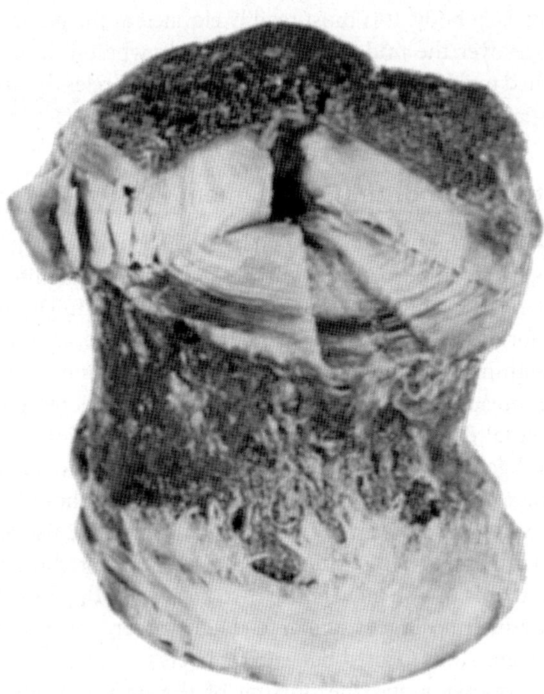

FIG. 2.12 A dissected third lumbar disc. Lamellar bands are still visible when the section is cut deep into bony apophyseal ring. A layer of spongiosa was left attached to the superior surface of the disc to show that only a thin chondral plate intervenes between the vascular trabeculae and the disc. The inward buckling of the lamellae near the cavity of the extirpated nuclear material is well shown. The specimen is from a 52-year-old man.

and discernment reveals how well the anulus is constructed for the performance of this function.

On horizontal section, it is noted that an individual lamella encircling the disc is composed of glistening fibers that run an oblique or spiral course in relation to the axis of the vertebral column. Because the disc presents a kidney-shaped or heart-shaped horizontal section, and the nucleus is displaced posteriorly, these lamellae are thinner and more closely packed between the nucleus and the dorsal aspect of the disc. The bands are stoutest and individually more distinct in the anterior third of the disc, and here when transected they may give the impression that they are of varying composition because every other ring presents a difference in color and elevation with reference to the plane of section. Teasing and inspection at an oblique angle shows in the freed lamellae, however, that this difference is due to an abrupt change in the direction of the fibers of adjacent rings. Previous descriptions of the anulus have claimed that the alternating appearance of the banding is the result of the interposition of a chondrous layer between each fibrous ring.[20] In reality, the alternations of glistening white lamellae with translucent rings result from differences in the incidence of light with regard to the direction of the fiber bundles. This repeated reversal of fiber arrangement within the anulus has implications in the biomechanics of the disc, which are discussed later.

The disposition of the lamellae on sagittal section is not consistently vertical. In the regions of the anulus approximating the nucleus pulposus, the first distinct bands curve inward, with their convexity facing the nuclear substance. As one follows the successive layers outward, a true vertical profile is assumed, but as the external laminae of the disc are approached, they may again become bowed, with their convexity facing the periphery of the disc.[21,22]

The attachment of the anulus to its respective vertebral bodies warrants particular mention. This attachment is best understood when a dried preparation of a thoracic or lumbar vertebra is examined first. In the adult, the articular surface of the body presents two aspects: a concave central depression that is quite porous and an elevated ring of compact bone that appears to be rolled over the edge of the vertebral body. Often a demarcating fissure falsely suggests that the ring is a true epiphysis of the body, but postnatal studies of ossification have indicated that it is a traction apophysis for the attachment of the anulus and associated longitudinal ligaments.[23]

In life, the depth of the central concavity is filled to the level of the marginal ring by the presence of a cribriform cartilaginous plate. In contrast to other articular surfaces, there is no closing plate of compact osseous material intervening between this cartilage and the cancellous medullary part of the bone. The trabeculations of the spongiosa blend into the internal face of the chondrous plate, whereas fibers from the nucleus and inner lamellae of the anulus penetrate its outer surface. As intimate as this union between the central disc and vertebra may appear, the outer bony ring affords the disc its firmest attachment because the stoutest external lamellar bands of fibers actually penetrate the ring as Sharpey fibers. Scraping the disc to the bone shows the concentric arrangements reflecting the different angles at which the fibers insert (see

Fig. 2.12). The fibers of the outermost ring of the anulus have the most extensive range of attachment. They extend beyond the confines of the disc and blend with the vertebral periosteum and the longitudinal ligaments.

Regional Variations of the Disc

The discs in aggregate make up approximately one-fourth of the length of the spinal column, exclusive of the sacrum and coccyx. Their degree of contribution is not uniform in the various regions. According to Aeby,[24] the discs provide more than one-fifth of the length of the cervical spine, approximately one-fifth of the length of the thoracic column, and approximately one-third of the length of the lumbar region.

The discs are smallest in the cervical spine. Their lateral extent is less than that of the corresponding vertebral body because of the uncinate processes (Fig. 2.13). Here, as in the lumbar region, they are wedge-shaped, the greatest width being anterior, producing lordosis. The thoracic discs are heart-shaped on section, with the nucleus pulposus being more centrally located than in the lumbar region. The thickness and the horizontal dimensions of the thoracic disc increase caudad with the corresponding increase in size of the vertebral bodies. The normal thoracic kyphosis results from a disparity between the anterior and posterior heights of the vertebral bodies because the discs are of uniform thickness. The lumbar discs are reniform and are relatively and absolutely the thickest in the spine. The progressive caudal increase in the degree of lumbar lordosis is due to the equivalent increase in the differential between the anterior and posterior thickness of the disc. In a study of lumbar disc morphology, Zhong and colleagues noted that disc length increased from upper to lower lumbar levels, although the L4–L5 disc, and the L5-S1 discs had similar lengths.[25] The L4–L5 nucleus pulposus height was tallest of the lumbar levels. The authors concluded that the geometry of the anulus fibrosus and nucleus pulposus show segment-dependent properties.

The cervical intervertebral discs have been a source of controversy because of the so-called joints of Luschka, or uncovertebral joints. These articular modifications are found on both sides of the cervical discs as oblique, cleftlike cavities between the superior surfaces of the uncinate processes and the corresponding lateral lips of the interior articular surface of the next superior vertebra. Because they initially appear in the latter part of the first decade and are not universally demonstrable in all cervical spines, or even in all subaxial discs of the same cervical spine, it is preferable to call them "accommodative joints" that have developed in response to the shearing stresses of the torsions of cervical mobility (see Fig. 2.13).

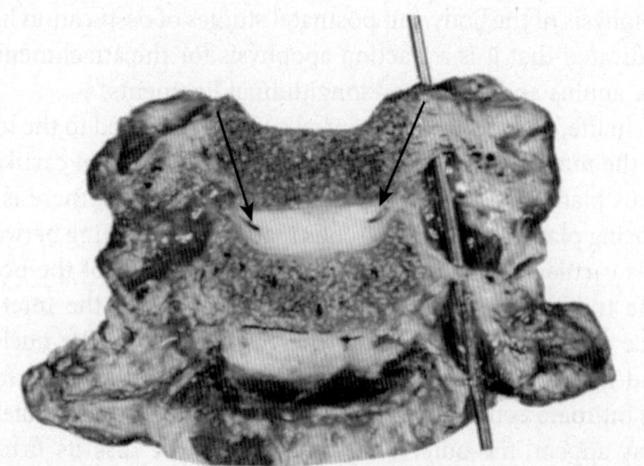

FIG. 2.13 Frontal section through fourth to fifth cervical vertebrae showing typical cervical disc and its joints of Luschka (*arrows*). A probe has been passed through the vertebral arterial canal to show its relationships to the uncovertebral joints.

Spinal Ligaments

Anterior Longitudinal Ligament

The anterior longitudinal ligament is a strong band of fibers that extends along the ventral surface of the spine from the skull to the sacrum. It is narrowest and cordlike in the upper cervical region, where it is attached to the atlas and axis and their intervening capsular membranes. It widens as it descends the column to the extent, in the lower lumbar region, of covering most of the anterolateral surfaces of the vertebral bodies and discs before it blends into the presacral fibers. The anterior longitudinal ligament is not uniform in its composition or manner of attachment. Its deepest fibers, which span only one intervertebral level, are covered by an intermediate layer that unites two or three vertebrae and a superficial stratum that may connect four or five levels. Where the ligament is adherent to the anterior surface of the vertebra, it also forms its periosteum. It is most firmly attached to the articular lip at the end of each body. It is most readily elevated at the point of its passage over the midsection of the discs, where it is loosely attached to the connective tissue band that encircles the anulus (Fig. 2.14).

Posterior Longitudinal Ligament

The posterior longitudinal ligament differs considerably from its anterior counterpart with respect to the clinical significance of its relationships to the intervertebral disc. Similar to the anterior ligament, it extends from the skull to the sacrum, but it is within the vertebral canal. Its central fiber bundles diminish in breadth as the size of the spinal column increases. The segmental denticulate configuration of the posterior longitudinal ligament is one of its most characteristic features. Between the pedicles, particularly in the lower thoracic and lumbar regions, it forms a thick band of connective tissue that is not adherent to the posterior surface of the vertebral body. Instead, it is bowstrung across the concavity of the dorsum of the body. The large vascular elements enter and leave the medullary sinus located beneath its fibers.

In approximating the dorsum of the disc, the posterior longitudinal ligament displays two strata of fibers. The superficial, longer strands form a distinct strong strap whose filaments bridge several vertebral elements. A second, deeper stratum spans only two vertebral articulations and forms lateral curving extensions of fibers that pass along the dorsum of the disc and out through the intervertebral foramen. These

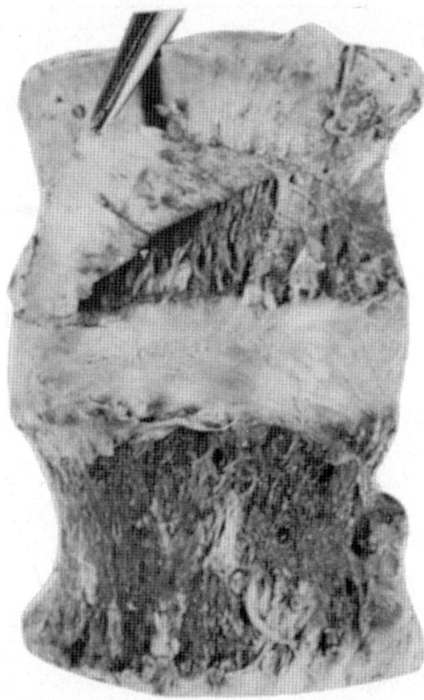

FIG. 2.14 Bodies of third and fourth lumbar vertebrae from a 58-year-old man. The spiral course of fibers of the outer lamellae is evident. The periosteal attachment of the reflected anterior longitudinal ligament is well shown, in addition to the delineation of the loosely attached area raised from the surface of the disc.

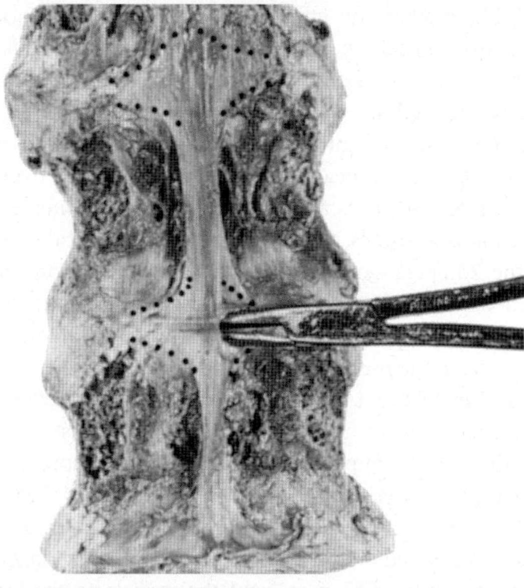

FIG. 2.15 Posterior longitudinal ligament traversing the bodies of third and fourth lumbar vertebrae. The central strap of long fibers can be seen passing over the hemostat. The lines of strong attachment of the fibers at the lateral expansions are indicated by the *black dots* as they outline the rhomboid area, where the fibers are readily dissected from the dorsal surface of the disc. In this case, the instrument was inserted into an actual fascial cleft, and the points show the weakest area of the lateral expansion.

deeper intervertebral expansions of the ligament have the most significant relationship with the disc.

These fibers are most firmly fixed at the margins of their lateral expansions. This produces a central rhomboidal area of loose attachment, or in some cases an actual fascial cleft of equivalent dimensions, on the dorsolateral aspect of the disc. At dissection, this characteristic may be readily shown by inserting a blunt probe beneath the intervertebral part of the longitudinal ligament and exploring the area to define the margins of the space where the fibers are strongly inserted (Fig. 2.15). This situation is particularly pertinent to problems involving dorsal or dorsolateral prolapse of the nucleus pulposus. With a dorsocentral protrusion of a semifluid mass, the strong midline strap of posterior longitudinal fibers tends to restrain the herniation. If an easily dissectible cleft offers a space for lateral expansion, however, the mass can extend to either side, dissecting the loose attachments.

Trabeculations of connective tissue bind the dura to the dorsal surface of the posterior longitudinal ligament. This attachment is firmest along the lateral edges. Numerous venous cross connections of the epidural sinuses pass between the dura and the ligament. The venous elements are the most ubiquitous structures among the components related to the vertebral articulations.

Although not frequently included in anatomic discussions of the spine, an additional structure travels deep to the posterior longitudinal ligament, extending laterally and posteriorly to surround the dura of the cauda equina. It has been termed the *peridural membrane,* first by Dommissee in 1975[26] and later by Wiltse.[27] The basivertebral veins cross the peridural membrane because it offers no obstruction to vascular communication between the intraosseous vessels of the vertebral body and the epidural space. Its possible clinical significance is that it may provide a containing membrane for herniated discs or hematomas, which may be noted on advanced imaging such as computed tomography (CT) or magnetic resonance imaging (MRI) as a delimiting barrier to the pathology.

Relationships of the Roots of the Spinal Nerves

The dorsal and ventral nerve roots pass through the subarachnoid space and converge to form the spinal nerve at approximately the level of its respective intervertebral foramen. Owing to the ascensus spinalis—the apparent cranial migration of the distal end of the spinal cord during development that actually arises from differential growth of the lower parts of the vertebral column—the course of the nerve roots becomes longer and more obliquely directed in the lower lumbar segments. In the cervical region, the nerve root and the spinal nerve are posteriorly related to the same corresponding intervertebral disc; in other words, the nerve root exits the spinal canal at the same level it branches from the spinal cord.

In the lumbar region, a different situation prevails. The nerve roots contributing to the cauda equina travel an almost vertical course over the dorsum of one intervertebral disc to exit with the spinal nerve of the foramen one segment lower. In the cervical and lumbar regions, dorsal or dorsolateral (i.e., paracentral) protrusions of disc material affect the descending rather than exiting nerve root. When the meningeal coverings (dura) blend with the epineurium, the nerve components become extrathecal. The actual point of this transition is variable but usually occurs in relation to the distal aspect of the dorsal root ganglion.

The nerve root is intimately related to the pedicle of the vertebra. Ugur and colleagues[28] found no distance between the upper cervical pedicles and their corresponding nerve roots in 20 cadaveric spines, whereas there was a slight distance in 4 of the 20 specimens in the lower cervical region. For all specimens, the distance from the nerve root to the inferior aspect of the upper pedicle ranged from 1 to 2.5 mm. The distance from the medial aspect of the pedicle to the dural sac ranged from 2.4 to 3.1 mm. A similar relationship between the thoracic nerve roots and pedicle exists.[29] The distance from the pedicle to the superior nerve root in the thoracic spine ranges from 1.5 to 6.7 mm, and the distance from the pedicle to the inferior nerve root, 0.8 to 6 mm. Ebraheim and colleagues[30] measured these distances in the lumbar spine, finding a mean distance of 1.5 mm from the pedicle to the inferior nerve root, 5.3 mm from the pedicle to the superior nerve root, and 1.5 mm from the medial pedicle wall to the dura.

Of particular interest is the distribution of epidural fat around and within the intervertebral foramen. This fat has a firm character and forms a mechanically supportive "bushing" for structures entering and leaving the spinal canal. A prominent extension of this fat body also follows the inferior and ventral surfaces of each lumbar nerve. It is interposed between the root and the external surfaces of the pedicle and vertebral body that define the inferior part of the intervertebral foramen. Its amelioration of the downward and ventral distraction of the nerve that accompanies the spine and lower limb motions is obvious. Histologically, it is composed of uniform cells that are contained within a fine membrane (perhaps the elusive peridural membrane).[31] There is no fibrous tissue in normal epidural fat and only tenuous attachments to the dura.

Intervertebral Foramen

The intervertebral foramen is the aperture that gives exit to the segmental spinal nerves and entrance to the vessels and nerve branches that supply the bone and soft tissues of the vertebral canal. It is superiorly and inferiorly bounded by the respective pedicles of the adjacent vertebrae. Its ventral and dorsal components involve the two major intervertebral articulations. The dorsum of the intervertebral disc, covered by the lateral expansion of the posterior longitudinal ligament, provides a large part of its ventral boundary, whereas the joint capsule of the articular facets and the ligamentum flavum contribute the major parts of its dorsal limitation. Along with the root, the remaining space is filled with loose areolar tissue and fat (Fig. 2.16).

However ample the overall dimensions of the intervertebral foramen may be, its elliptical nature is responsible for many of its relational problems. In the lumbar region, the vertical diameter of the foramen ranges from 12 to 19 mm; this undoubtedly accounts for the fact that a complete collapse of the disc may produce little or no evidence of nerve compression.

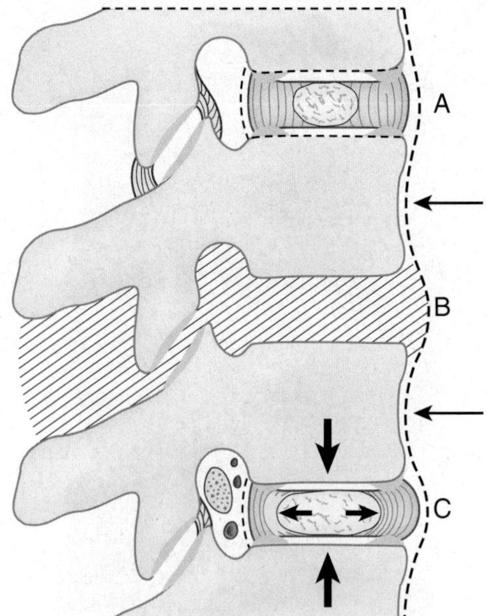

FIG. 2.16 Three aspects of the relational anatomy of the disc. *A* shows the topographic arrangement of the normal disc with the apophyseal ring and perforated chondral plate in relation to the nucleus pulposus and the anulus. *B* indicates the inclusions of the motor segment as originally described by Junghanns *(cross-hatched area)*. *Arrows* define the limits of the motor segment proposed here. *C* indicates the dissipation by the lateral thrust in a compressed disc. Related anatomy of the intervertebral foramen is also indicated. The two structures passing ventral to the spinal nerve are the sinuvertebral nerve and the artery. The other vessels are veins.

The sagittal diameter may be only 7 mm, however, making this dimension exquisitely sensitive to changes. Because the diameter of the fourth lumbar nerve can be just slightly less than 7 mm, the tolerance for pathologic alteration of the bony or connective tissue relationships is restricted.[32]

The existence of additional ligamentous elements in relation to the intervertebral foramen could limit further the space for the exiting spinal nerve. These structures, known as the *transforaminal ligaments,* are frequently found in the lumbar region.[33,34] The transforaminal ligaments are strong, unyielding cords of fibrous tissue that pass anteriorly from various parts of the neural arch to the body of the same or the adjacent vertebra and may be 5 mm wide. Grimes and colleagues[35] found these ligaments span from the nerve root itself. These investigators noted four different bands, the most significant of which spread from the nerve root to the anterior aspect of the facet capsule. Other bands spanned from the nerve root to the superior pedicle, the inferior pedicle, and the intervertebral disc anteriorly.

In the cervical spine, the space available for the exiting nerve root may be compromised by structures just lateral to the foramen. In 10 adult human cadaveric specimens, Alleyne and colleagues[36] found the dorsal root ganglia of the C3 to C6 spinal nerves to be slightly compressed by the ascending vertebral artery. This compression was most pronounced at the C5 level, which the authors suggested as a possible explanation for the greater susceptibility of this nerve to iatrogenic injury during procedures such as laminoplasty.

Lumbosacral Nerve Root Variations

Numerous anatomic variations in the relationships of the lumbosacral nerve roots can exist. These variations may help explain seemingly anatomically inconsistent neurologic findings with compressive disorders such as herniated discs or lateral stenosis.

The most common variation involves atypical origins, or foraminal exits, of individual lumbosacral roots. Although myelographic studies indicated only a 4% incidence of lumbosacral root anomalies, an anatomic study by Kadish and Simmons[37] reported an incidence of 14%. The L5-S1 level is the most commonly involved. Observations by these authors provided four types of variations: (1) intradural interconnections between roots at different levels, (2) anomalous levels of origin of nerve roots, (3) extradural connections between roots, and (4) extradural division of nerve roots. Furthermore, nerve roots may be conjoined, in which two adjacent roots share a common dural envelope as they leave the dural sac.[38] The bifurcation of conjoined roots can occur close to the intervening pedicle, creating a secondary axilla, which may be involved in the etiology of neuropathy. The L5-S1 segment is the most common for presence of a conjoined nerve root. Although the diagnosis of a conjoined nerve root is often made during surgery, clinical suspicion should be raised in a patient with a herniated disc with symptoms corresponding to two dermatomes.

A source of confusing neurologic findings may relate to the variant anatomy of the furcal nerve. The name *furcal nerve* has been applied to the fourth lumbar nerve because it exhibits a prominent bifurcation to contribute to the lumbar plexus (femoral and obturator nerves) and sacral plexus (lumbosacral trunk). Kikuchi and Hasue[39] found that it is often indefinite in its intradural affinities, frequently exhibiting two dorsal root ganglia that have distinct root sources at the conus medullaris. They proposed that when symptoms indicate the involvement of two levels, suspicion should be directed toward four possible causes: (1) two roots compressed by a single lesion, (2) the presence of two lesions, (3) the anomalous emergence of two roots through the same foramen, or (4) the existence of the peculiarly doubled components of the furcal nerve (Fig. 2.17).

Infrequently, variant "fixation" alters the expected sequences of nerve root exit. In a *prefixed* lumbosacral plexus, the furcal nerve (the division between the lumbar and sacral plexuses) exits through the third lumbar foramen, and the preceding and subsequent nerves exit one vertebral level higher than in the conventional distribution. Conversely, in the *postfixed* plexus, the furcal nerve exits the L5-S1 foramen, and the lumbosacral nerve sequence is all one level lower than usually described.[40]

Although Kadish and Simmons[37] noted that the existence of anomalous interconnections between nerve root levels dispels any notion of "absolute innervation," Parke and Watanabe[41] showed that there is a consistent system of intersegmental connections between the roots of the lumbosacral nerves. They described an epispinal system of motor axons

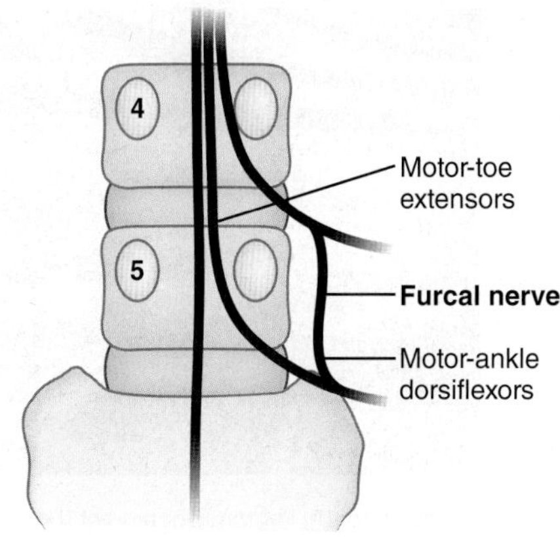

FIG. 2.17 Cross connection L4 and L5 nerve roots (spinal nerves) in the extraforaminal region through the furcal nerve. (Modified from McCulloch JA, Young PH. *Essentials of Spinal Microsurgery.* Philadelphia: Lippincott-Raven; 1998:390.)

that courses among the meningeal fibers of the conus medullaris and virtually ensheathes its ventral and lateral funiculi between the L2 and S2 levels. These nerve fibers apparently arise from motor neuron cells of the ventral horn gray matter and join spinal nerve roots caudal to their level of origin. In all the spinal cords studied, many of these axons commingled at the cord surface to form an irregular group of ectopic rootlets that could be visually traced to join conventional spinal nerve roots at one to several segments inferior to their original segmental level (Figs. 2.18 and 2.19). Occasionally, these ventral ectopic rootlets course dorsocaudad to join a dorsal (sensory) nerve root. Although the function and the clinical significance of this epispinal system of axons have yet to be explained, a given segmental level of motor nerve cells may contribute fibers not only to an adjacent segment, but also to nerve roots of multiple inferior levels.

An additional variant aspect of the lumbosacral nerve roots concerns the relative location of their dorsal root ganglia. Almost all anatomic illustrations depict the lumbosacral dorsal root ganglia in an intraforaminal position, the central part of the ganglion lying between the adjacent pedicles. Hasue and colleagues[42,43] found, however, that the lumbosacral dorsal root ganglia may also be positioned internal or external to their foramina. They designated the internal positions as *subarticular* or *sublaminar,* depending on their relationship to these structures roofing the spinal canal, and found that approximately one-third of the L4 and L5 ganglia are in the subarticular position. If the ganglion is subarticular, it is in the lateral recess and subject to the direct consequences of a lateral stenosis.

Innervation of the Spine

The distribution of the medial branches of the dorsal ramus of the spinal nerve to the external periosteum, facet joints, and ligamentous connections of the neural arches (and the general ramification of the "recurrent" sinuvertebral nerve, known as the nerve of Luschka or *ramus meningeus,* to structures related

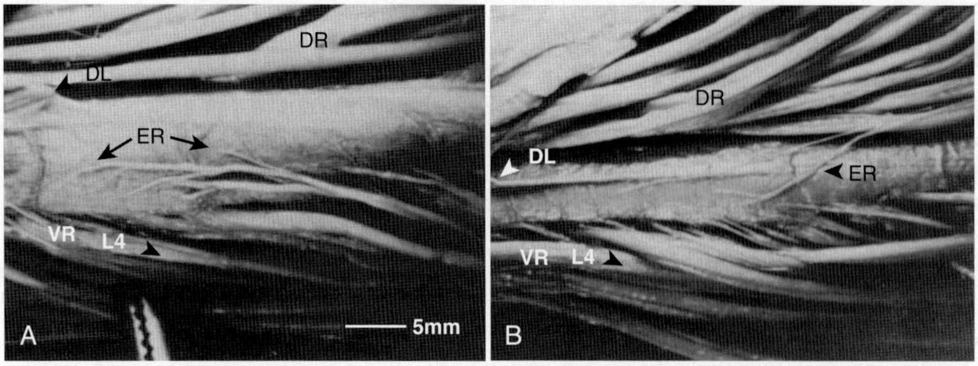

FIG. 2.18 (A) Photomicrograph of the lateral surface of human conus medullaris showing ectopic rootlets (ER) that receive axons from cells in the ventral horn nuclei. Note origin of some fibers at the level of L4 motor nuclei extends caudad to join S1 root. (B) Photomicrograph showing ER passing posteriorly to join a dorsal (sensory) nerve root (DR). DL, last denticulum of denticulate ligament; VR, ventral root.

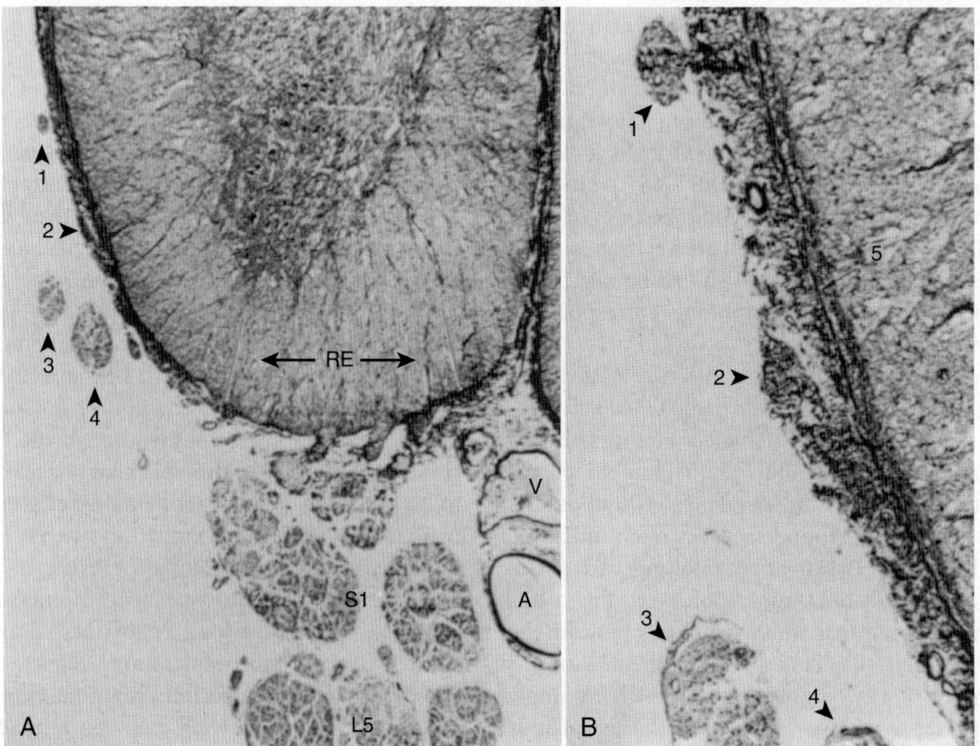

FIG. 2.19 Photomicrographs of a 5-μm cross section from the conus medullaris at the S1 level showing ectopic rootlets in various stages characteristic of their emergence from the ventrolateral surface of the cord. (A) Rootlets just appearing on the pial surface (*1, 2*) eventually join free rootlets (*3, 4*) that have originated from higher levels. The conventional roots of L5 and S1 nerves have emerged from the typical zone of rootlet emergence (RE). *A and V,* Anterior spinal artery and vein. (B) Higher power photomicrograph of (A) shows greater detail of rootlet emergence. The entire ventrolateral pia is intertwined with epispinal axons, of which only a few form ectopic rootlets. Dense circular band of pial straps (*5*) is characteristic of the region of the epispinal fibers. ([A], ×33. [B], ×133.) (From Parke WW, Watanabe R. Lumbosacral intersegmental epispinal axons and ectopic ventral nerve rootlets. *J Neurosurg.* 1967;67:269-277.)

to the spinal canal) has been known for more than a century. The recognition that degenerative disease of the intervertebral disc and its consequences is a major cause of low back pain has stimulated more inquiries, however.

Many investigations have attempted to delineate the origins, terminal ramifications, and nerve ending types of the sinuvertebral nerve, often with contradictory results. More comprehensive works[22,44-51] have agreed on the general source and composition of this nerve and have described it as variously branching from the distal pole of the dorsal root ganglion, the initial part of the spinal nerve, or the dorsal sections of the rami communicantes. It was recognized that a multiple origin is common, especially in the lumbar region, and small autonomic branches often have a separate course, entering the intervertebral foramen independently. The extent and complexity of the relationships of the sinuvertebral nerve within the spinal canal have engendered much argument, however, particularly concerning the segmental range of the individual nerve ramifications.

In illustrations based on dissections, Bogduk and colleagues[44] and Parke[52] agreed that each nerve supplies two intervertebral discs via superiorly and inferiorly directed branches—the inferiorly directed branch ramifying over the dorsum of the disc at the level of entry and the longer, superiorly directed branch coursing along the edge of the posterior longitudinal ligament to reach the disc of the next superior level (Fig. 2.20). Dissections identify mainly the larger ramifications. Smaller fibers are usually localized with staining techniques. Conventional methods of staining using silver or lipotrophic stains have given controversial results, however, because of a lack of specificity.

Groen and colleagues,[53] using a highly specific acetylcholinesterase staining method on large cleared sections of fetal human spines, resolved many conflicts concerning the ramifications of the nerves supplying spinal structures. They found that, in contrast to most previous reports, the human sinuvertebral nerves were almost exclusively derivatives of the rami communicantes close to their connections with the spinal nerves. These origins were fairly consistent throughout the length of the thoracolumbar sympathetic trunk, but in the cervical region they were also derived from the perivascular plexus of the vertebral artery.

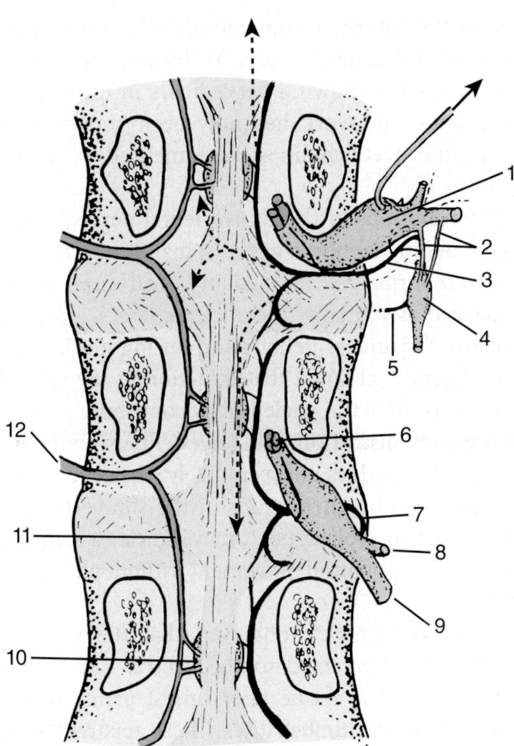

FIG. 2.20 Schema of major intraspinal distribution of dorsal central branches of segmental vertebromedullary arteries and distribution and source of the sinuvertebral nerves. The pattern of the nerve shown entering the superior foramen is derived from the data provided by Groen and colleagues.[53] *Dotted lines* show a composite of the variant ranges (*arrows* indicate two or more segments) and ramifications tabulated by these authors. The nerve entering the inferior foramen shows the extent and distribution described in previous reports. *1,* Dorsal root ganglion. *2,* Rami communicantes. *3,* Sinuvertebral nerve and its origin according to Groen and colleagues. *4,* Autonomic ganglion. *5,* Nerve to anterior longitudinal ligament. *6,* Spinal nerve roots. *7,* Sinuvertebral nerve arising from distal pole of ganglion (thought to be its most common source before report of Groen and colleagues). *8,* Dorsal primary ramus of spinal nerve. *9,* Ventral primary ramus of spinal nerve. *10,* Arteries entering basivertebral sinus to supply cancellous bone. *11,* Descending dorsal central branch of vertebromedullary (spinal) artery. *12,* Ventral branch of vertebromedullary artery.

Five sinuvertebral nerves have been observed passing into one intervertebral foramen. Typically, the group consists of one thick nerve (perhaps the one seen in most conventional dissections) and several fine fibers. The thick, or predominant, sinuvertebral nerve is often absent, however, in the upper cervical and sacral regions. The major sinuvertebral element enters the foramen ventral to the spinal ganglion and gives off some fine branches at this point. As the nerve enters the spinal canal, the major branch usually divides into rami that course in approximation to the distribution of the posterior central branches of the segmental artery, with a long ascending element and a shorter descending one. From these branches, one to three coiled rami supply the ventral dura.

The acetylcholinesterase technique used by Groen and colleagues[53] made it possible to delineate details of the plexus of the posterior longitudinal ligament. The work of these authors supports the idea that the posterior longitudinal ligament is highly innervated by an irregular plexiform distribution of fibers that have a greater density in the ligament expansions dorsal to the discs. These authors were able to note the primary direction, length, and "termination area" of the branches of a single segmental sinuvertebral nerve. They classified the variations of individual nerves as follows: (1) ascending one segment, (2) descending one segment, (3) dichotomizing toward one segment caudal and one segment cranial or horizontal, (4) ascending two or more segments, and (5) descending two or more segments (see Fig. 2.20). The existence of the latter two categories, although they are not as common as the others, shows that the sinuvertebral nerve can supply more than two adjacent segmental levels. A basis for the poor pain localization of an offending disc may be related to the generous distribution possible in the individual sinuvertebral nerve. The large totomounts treated with acetylcholinesterase also showed that the patterns of sinuvertebral nerve distribution to the posterior longitudinal ligament did not display significant regional variations apart from an expected pronounced diminution in the plexus density in the immovable lower sacral region.

The posterior longitudinal ligament is highly innervated with complex encapsulated nerve endings and numerous low-myelinated free nerve endings (Fig. 2.21). The lateral expansion of the posterior longitudinal ligament extends through the intervertebral foramen covering all the dorsal and most of the dorsolateral aspects of the disc. The elevation of this thin, highly innervated strap of connective tissue may provide a significant component of the pain manifest in acute disc protrusions.

The probable range of diverse functions of the sinuvertebral nerve may be indicated by the analysis of its cross-sectional composition. Stained preparations taken from a section near

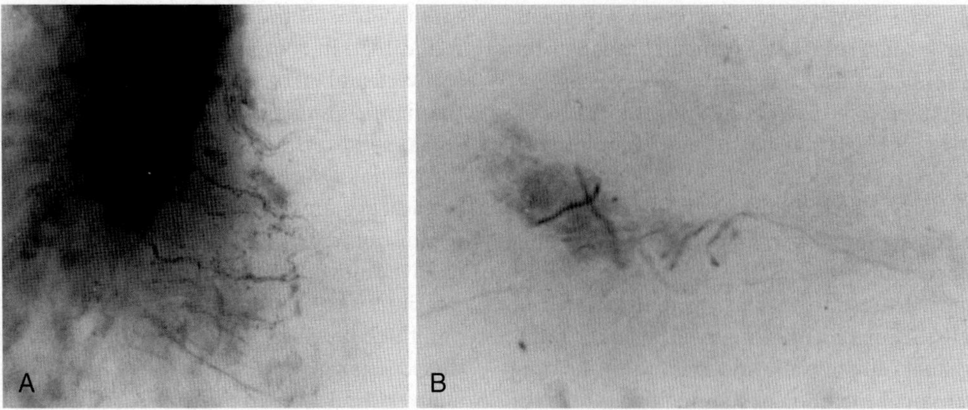

FIG. 2.21 Photomicrographs of nerve endings in posterior longitudinal ligament of a dog. (A) Section of ligament dorsal to a lumbar intervertebral disc. The dark area is the central strap of the ligament, and the light area is the thin lateral expansion over the dorsum of the disc. These fine nerve endings are characteristic of those in known nociceptors. (B) Complex nerve ending from posterior longitudinal ligament. This type of ending is believed to be a transducer of mechanical deformation for postural senses. (Methylene blue vital tissue stain: [A], ×300; [B], ×500.)

the nerve origin show many small myelinated fibers, although some myelin sheaths are greater than 10 μm in diameter.[54] Many of the smaller fibers are postganglionic efferents from the thoracolumbar autonomic ganglia that mediate the smooth muscle control of the various vascular elements within the spinal canal, and many of the larger fibers are involved in proprioceptive functions. Concerning the latter, Hirsch and colleagues[46,55] found numerous complex encapsulated nerve endings in the posterior longitudinal ligament (see Fig. 2.21B). It is assumed that these may be associated with the larger myelinated fibers whose postganglionic axons enter the cord to mediate postural reflexes because similar fibers in the cervical region of cats have been shown to be important in tonic neck reflexes.[56] It seems, however, that the smaller fibers making up the bulk of the sinuvertebral nerve are afferents, associated with simple, nonencapsulated, or "free" nerve endings that are generally regarded as nociceptive (see Fig. 2.21A).

The fact that the sinuvertebral nerve carries pain fibers has been amply shown by clinical and laboratory experimentation. Direct stimulation of tissues known to be served by the nerve elicits back pain in humans. Pedersen and colleagues[54] showed that stimulation of these tissues in decerebrate cats resulted in blood pressure and respiratory changes similar to those elicited by noxious stimuli to known pain receptors in other areas of the body.

Disagreement exists over whether the anulus itself is innervated and, if so, how extensively. The classic work of Hirsch and colleagues[55] claimed that nerve endings are only in the dorsal aspect of the most superficial layer of the anulus, and these presumably are from branches of the same nerve fibers that innervate the overlying expansions of the posterior longitudinal ligament.

Pedersen and colleagues,[54] Stilwell,[57] and Parke[52] have failed to show nerve endings in the anulus. Because the connective tissue structures intimately related to the disc show a profusion of nerve endings, Parke[52] assumed that their disruption could account for discogenic pain. Inappropriate methodology may account for the failure to show intradiscal nerves. Malinsky,[49] Bogduk and colleagues,[44,45] and Yoshizawa and colleagues[58] published accounts showing nerve fibers in the outer lamina of the anulus. This work has now been supported by the highly specific acetylcholinesterase method of Groen and colleagues.[53]

Most descriptions of the sinuvertebral nerve indicate that the major meningeal fibers to the spinal dura are distributed to its ventral surface.[59] The median dorsal dural surface has been regarded as virtually free of nerve fibers, a convenience that permits its painless penetration during needle puncture. Although Cyriax[60] claimed that irritation of the ventral dura during protrusion of the nucleus may contribute to discogenic pain, a sufficient distortion of the nerve fibers on the movable or unattached dura does not seem likely. The coiled configuration of these dural contributions of the sinuvertebral nerve, noted by Groen and colleagues,[61] may indicate a compensation to permit a degree of dural movement without placing traction on these nerves.

Parke and Watanabe[62] observed that the ventral lower lumbar dura is often fixed to the ventral canal surface by numerous connective tissue fibers, most firmly fixed at the margins of the lower lumbar discs. These apparently acquired adhesions are not to be confused with the ligaments of Hofmann, which are normal straps of tissue connecting the dura to the ventral canal surface that have been obliquely positioned by the developmental cranial traction of the dura and its contents. This observation has been supported by a series of dissections by Blikra,[63] who was seeking a rationale for lower lumbar intradural disc protrusions. His analysis showed that in some cases the dura may be sufficiently fixed to the ventral surface of the canal, particularly at the L4–L5 level, for protruding nucleus material to rupture the ventral dura. Parke and Watanabe,[62] by microscopic analysis of sections of the dura that had been forcibly freed from these adhesions overlying the fourth or fifth lumbar disc, showed disruption of the nerve fibers bound in the adhesion. In the numerous cases in which such adhesions are present, the forceful elevation of the dura by a disc protrusion may provide an adjunctive source of the discogenic pain.

Spinal Motion Segment

The inclusion of all articular tissue, the overlying spinal muscles, and the segmental contents of the vertebral canal and intervertebral foramen into a single functional and anatomic unit was first suggested by Junghanns.[64,65] Originally called the "motor" segment, this unit represents a useful concept that stresses the developmental and topographic interdependence between the fibrous structures that surround the intervertebral foramen and the functioning of the structures that pass through it. Although the 23 or 24 individual motion segments must be considered in relation to the spinal column as a whole, no congenital or acquired disorder of a single major component of a unit can exist without affecting first the functions of the other components of the same unit and then the functions of other levels of the spine.

Although Junghanns[64] defined the unit primarily in terms of the movable structures making up the intervertebral articulations, a logical, if not necessary, extension of the motion segment concept should include some aspect of the vertebral elements. DePalma and Rothman[66] included both adjacent vertebrae in their illustration of the unit, but depiction of the unit concept is improved by incorporating only the opposing superior and inferior halves of each vertebra, eliminating redundancy (see Fig. 2.16). In visualizing the motion segment unit as a musculoskeletal complex surrounding a corresponding level of nervous structures, it must be realized that the intervertebral disc and the facets are but two of the articulations involved. The interosseous fibrous connections that include the interspinous, intertransverse, costovertebral, and longitudinal ligaments and the ligamentum flavum are varieties of syndesmoses.

Nutrition of the Intervertebral Disc

Most descriptive accounts of the intervertebral disc dismiss the subject of its vascular nutrition with a brief mention of the general agreement that the normal adult disc is avascular. The demonstrable truth of this statement may give the impression that the substance of the disc is inert biologically. Experimental evidence has indicated that the normal disc tissue is quite vital and has a demonstrable rate of metabolic turnover.[67,68] In contrast to the nonvascular cartilage in the diarthroses, the cellular elements of the disc cannot receive the blood-borne nutrients through the mediation of the synovial fluid but must rely on a diffusional system with the vessels that lie adjacent to the disc. Diffusion is also the mechanism for removal of products of metabolism from the disc, such as lactic acid.[69]

The qualitative and quantitative aspects of the diffusional nutrition of the disc have been studied.[68-72] The peripheral vascular plexus of the anulus and the vessels adjacent to the hyaline cartilage of the bone-disc interface provide the two sources for the diffusion of metabolites into the disc. Although the interface shows an average permeability of 40%, there is a decreasing centrifugal gradient that starts with an 80% permeability at the center. Because diffusion is the major mechanism that carries small solutes through the disc matrix, the two main parameters affecting this flow are the *partition coefficient,* which defines the equilibrium between the solutes within the plasma and the solutes within the disc, and the *diffusion coefficient,* which characterizes the solute mobility.

The partition coefficient varies with the size and charge of the solute particle. Small uncharged solutes show a near-equilibrium between their plasma and intradiscal concentrations, but because the disc matrix has a predominantly negative charge, anionic solutes have a lower intradiscal concentration in relation to the plasma, whereas the reverse is true for positively charged solutes, whose intradiscal concentration is greater than that of the plasma. Because the range of these effects depends on the concentration of the fixed, negatively charged, larger molecular aggregates (proteoglycans), the partition coefficient is regionally variable within the disc matrix and especially pronounced in the inner annular lamellae and nucleus, where the concentration of proteoglycans is the highest.

Solute mobility (the diffusion coefficient) within the disc is slower than in the plasma because the presence of solids in the form of collagen and proteoglycans impedes diffusional progress. Without regard to charge, the diffusion coefficient within the disc is 40% to 60% of free diffusion within water, and mobility is greatest in the inner anulus and nucleus where the water concentrations are the highest.

Because of the regional differentials in the densities of the fixed charges within the disc, the two vascular sources for disc nutrition vary in their significance in the supply of certain solutes. With respect to the small uncharged particles, there is little difference in the transport potential of either the peripheral or the endplate vascular routes, but because of the greater collective negative charge within the central substances of the disc (from proteoglycans), the interface vasculature is a greater source of cationic solutes, whereas the anions would gain easier access through the peripheral vessels.

The effect of fluid "pumping" under changes in the load applied to the disc is minimal with respect to the transport of small solutes because the matrix has a low hydraulic permeability relative to their higher rates of diffusion. With regard to the larger solutes, however, the pumping may have a more substantial effect.

Metabolic turnover, as indicated by proteoglycan synthesis in discs in dogs, is variable according to age within the range of 2 to 3 years. It is roughly equivalent to that of articular cartilage. The central disc tissues have a low oxygen tension and a high concentration of lactic acid, indicating that the inner disc cell respiration is primarily anaerobic. Because this type of respiration is heavily dependent on glycolytic energy requirements, the interface vasculature must deliver the needed glucose to maintain the central disc cell viability.

Because this interface exchange is precariously dependent on the integrity of the fine vasculature subjacent to the cartilaginous endplate, any change from the optimal state occasioned by age-dependent vagaries in the intrinsic vertebral vasculature may partly explain the marked predisposition to degenerative changes characteristic of the aging disc. Calcification and sclerosis of the endplate decrease permeability and contact area with the disc space, further contributing to disc degeneration. MRI studies following the movement of contrast medium into the disc have demonstrated a decreased ability of a degenerated disc to accept solutes, both in speed and quantity.[69]

Blood Supply of the Vertebral Column

The descriptions and terminology of the nutritional vessels of the vertebrae vary considerably in anatomy texts. In general, the texts illustrate and discuss the vascularity of a typical thoracic or lumbar vertebra, with a lack of agreement on such basic issues as to whether the vertebral body does[73] or does not[74] receive an anterior supply. In addition, discussions of the vascularization of the atypical (craniocervical, cervical, and sacral) vertebral regions are either superficial or entirely lacking. Much of the information presented here is the result of a de novo investigation by Parke and colleagues,[77] and the terminology ascribed to the vessels is derived from a selection of what seem to be the most descriptive names previously used in the literature.[75-77]

Despite the fact that regional variations may at first seem to thwart the perception of a common pattern of vertebral vascularization, the homologous origin of all vertebral elements nevertheless provides a certain constancy. From a segmental artery, or its regional equivalent, each vertebra receives several sets of nutritional vessels, which consist of anterior central, posterior central, prelaminar, and postlaminar branches. The first and last of these are derived from vessels external to the vertebral column, whereas the posterior central and prelaminar branches are derived from spinal branches that enter the intervertebral foramina and supply the neural, meningeal, and epidural tissues as well. In the mid-spinal region, the internal arteries (i.e., the posterior central and prelaminar branches) provide the greater part of the blood supply to the body and vertebral arch, but reciprocal arrangements may occur, particularly in the cervical region.

This general pattern of the vasculature is best shown in the area between the second thoracic and fifth lumbar vertebrae, where the segments are associated with paired arteries that arise directly from the aorta (Fig. 2.22). Typically, each segmental artery leaves the posterior surface of the aorta and follows a dorsolateral course around the middle of the vertebral body. Near the transverse processes, it divides into a lateral (intercostal or lumbar) and a dorsal branch. The dorsal branch runs lateral to the intervertebral foramen and the articular processes as it continues backward between the transverse processes eventually to reach the spinal muscles. Because the segmental artery is closely applied to the anterolateral surface of the body, its first spinal derivatives are two or more anterior central branches that directly penetrate the cortical bone of the body and that may be traced radiologically into the spongiosa (Figs. 2.23 and 2.24). The same region of the segmental

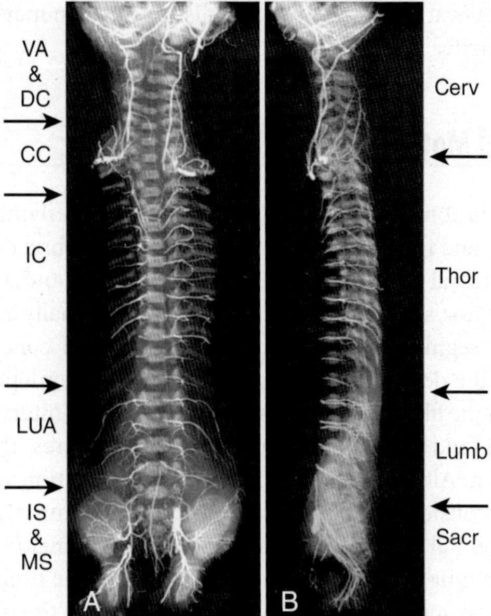

FIG. 2.22 (A) Anteroposterior and (B) lateral radiographs of spine of an 8-month fetus injected with finely divided barium sulfate. Traditional regional subdivisions of the spine are indicated on the *left*, and regional arteries that provide the segmental branches to the individual vertebrae are shown on the *right*. The upper cervical region is supplied by vertebral and deep cervical arteries (VA & DC), the lower cervical and upper two thoracic segments are supplied by the costocervical trunk (CC), and the remaining thoracic vertebrae receive intercostal vessels (IC). The lumbar arteries (LUA) supply their regional vertebrae, and the sacral segments are provided with branches from lateral sacral (LS) and middle sacral (MS) arteries.

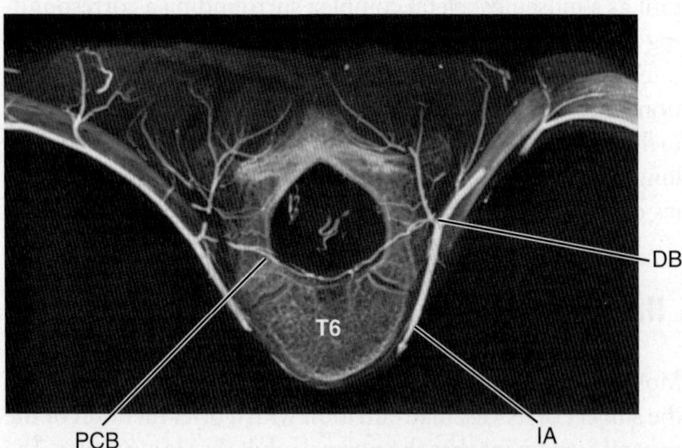

FIG. 2.23 Ventral radiograph of section through T6 of a specimen from a 6-year-old child injected with barium sulfate. The intercostal arteries (IA) give rise to dorsal branches (DB) that provide spinal branches to the vertebral canal and posterior branches to the arch and dorsal musculature. The posterior central branches (PCB) are well shown as they send vessels into the vertebral body. Fine anterior central and anterior laminar and posterior laminar vessels can be seen. Note the neurocentral synchondrosis.

artery also supplies longitudinal arteries to the anterior longitudinal ligament (Fig. 2.25).

After the segmental artery divides into its dorsal and lateral branches, the dorsal component passes lateral to the intervertebral foramen, where it gives off the spinal branch that provides the major vascularity to the bone and contents of the vertebral canal. This branch may enter the foramen as a

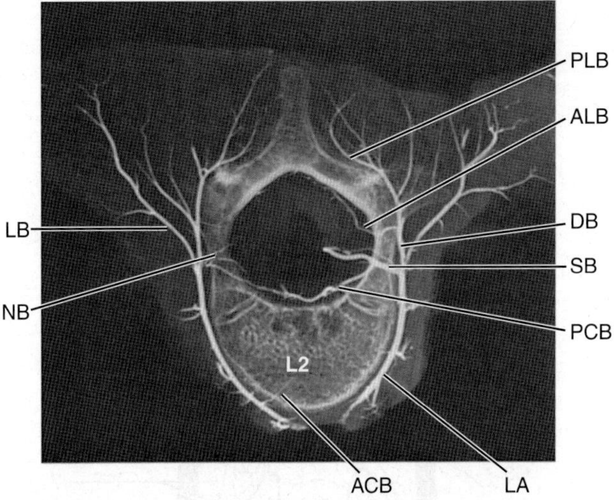

FIG. 2.24 Vertical radiograph of section through lumbar vertebra of a 6-year-old child. The vascularity of the lumbar vertebra may be regarded as the archetypal pattern from which other regions evolved variations. The segmental lumbar artery (LA) gives rise to numerous anterior central branches that penetrate the cortical bone of the body. The spinal branch (SB) sends prominent posterior central branches to the dorsum of the body, whereas the dorsal branch (DB) supplies the anterior (ALB) and posterior (PLB) laminar branches. Neural branches (NB) follow the nerve roots to the cord. In this section, the arteria radicularis magna is seen as a neural branch on the right side. ACB, anterior central branches; LB, lumbar branches; PCB, posterior central branches.

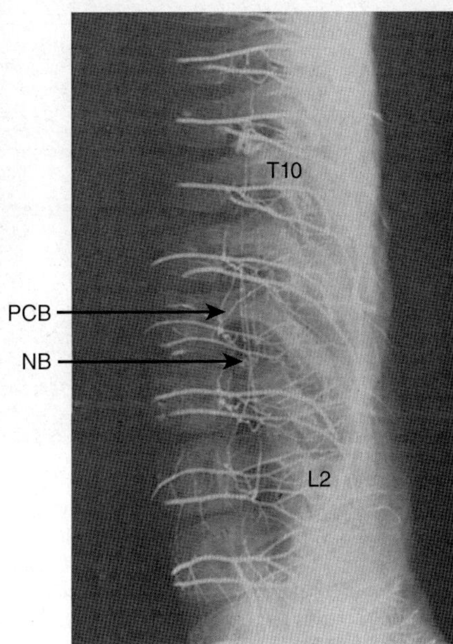

FIG. 2.25 Lateral view of lumbar vertebra shown in Fig. 2.24. Longitudinal anastomoses of posterior central branches (PCB) can be appreciated, and the disposition of neural branches (NB) is clarified. The lumbar arteries also supply small longitudinal branches to the anterior longitudinal ligament.

single vessel, or it may arise from the dorsal segmental branch as numerous independent rami. In either case, it ultimately divides into a triad of posterior central, prelaminar, and intermediate neural branches. The posterior central branch passes over the dorsolateral surface of the intervertebral disc and divides into a caudal and a cranial branch, which supply the two adjacent vertebral bodies.

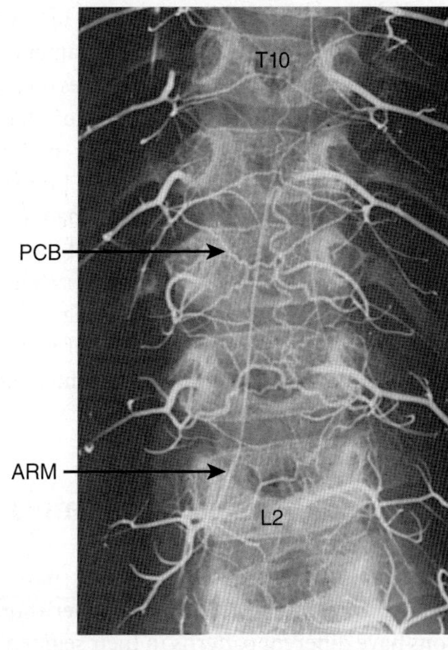

FIG. 2.26 Anteroposterior arteriogram of lower thoracic and upper lumbar vertebrae in a 6-year-old child. The interlocking anastomotic pattern formed by the posterior central branches (PCB) and the manner in which four branches converge over the center of the dorsum of the body of each vertebra are well shown. The arteria radicularis magna (ARM), which forms a major contribution to the anterior spinal artery of the cord, can be seen arising at L2.

Coursing in the same plane as the posterior longitudinal ligament, these branches vascularize the ligament and the related dura before entering the large concavity in the central dorsal surface of the vertebral body. The dorsum of each vertebral body is supplied by four arteries derived from two intervertebral levels. As these vessels tend to converge toward the dorsal central concavity, where they are cross-connected with their bilateral counterparts, their connections with other vertebral levels give the appearance of a series of rhomboid anastomotic loops (Fig. 2.26) that illustrate the extent of collateral supply to a single vertebra.

The prelaminar branch of the spinal artery follows the inner surface of the vertebral arch, giving fine penetrating nutrient branches to the laminae and ligamenta flava, while also supplying the regional epidural and dorsal tissue. The neural branches that enter the intervertebral foramen with the above-described vessels supply the pia-arachnoid complex and the spinal cord itself. In the fetus and the adult, the neural or radicular branches are not segmentally uniform in their size or occurrence. Although all spinal nerves receive fine twigs to their ganglia and roots, the major contributions to the cord are found at irregular intervals. Several larger radicular arteries may be discerned in the cervical and upper thoracic regions, but the largest, the arteria radicularis magna (artery of Adamkiewicz[76]), is an asymmetrical contribution from one of the upper lumbar, or lower thoracic, segmental arteries. It travels obliquely upward with a ventral spinal root to join the anterior spinal artery in the region of the conus medullaris. Radicular contributions to the dorsal spinal plexus may usually be distinguished by their more tortuous course (see Figs. 2.25 and 2.26).

After the dorsal branch of the segmental artery has provided the vessels to the intervertebral foramen, it passes between the transverse processes, where it gives off a fine spray of articular branches to the joint capsule of the articular processes. Immediately distal to this point, it divides into dorsal and medial branches; the larger, dorsal branch ramifies in the greater muscle mass of the erector spinae, whereas the medial branch follows the external contours of the lamina and the spinous process. This postlaminar artery supplies the musculature immediately overlying the lamina and sends fine nutrient branches into the bone. The largest of these branches penetrates the lamina through a nutrient foramen located just dorsomedial to the articular capsule.

Regional Variations in Spinal Vasculature

Only vertebrae that are related to the aorta have access to direct segmental branches. The cervical, upper thoracic, and sacral regions have different patterns in their segmental supply that affect to various extents the arrangements of the finer vessels. In an arteriogram of the entire fetal spine (see Fig. 2.22), it can be seen that the greater part of the cervical region is supplied by the vertebral arteries and the deep cervical arteries. An intermediate area that usually includes the lower two cervical and upper two thoracic vertebrae is supplied by costocervical branches of the subclavian artery that are of variable pattern and often bilaterally dissimilar. From T2 to L3, the typical segmental arrangement prevails, but in the sacral area lateral sacral branches of the hypogastric artery and middle sacral branches assume the function of supporting the nutritional vasculature to the vertebral elements.

Cervical Region

The general patterns of the arterial supply with respect to the typical cervical vertebrae are schematically represented in Figs. 2.27A and 2.28.[77] The vertebral arteries represent a lateral longitudinal fusion of the original segmental vessels and provide a ventrally coursing anterior central artery and a medially directed posterior central artery to each subaxial vertebral element. The anterior spinal plexus is best developed in the cervical region, where it exhibits a rectangular mesh of vessels in which the transverse members (anterior central arteries) run along the upper ventral edges of their respective intervertebral discs. The conspicuousness of this plexus reflects the fact that it also serves the cervical prevertebral musculature. The thyrocervical and costocervical trunks assist in the lower cervical region, and the upper cervical part of the plexus receives contributions from the ascending pharyngeal arteries (Fig. 2.29).

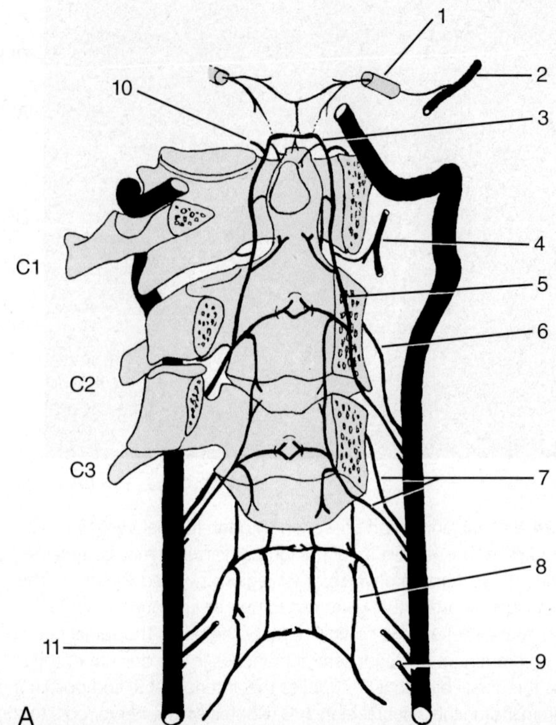

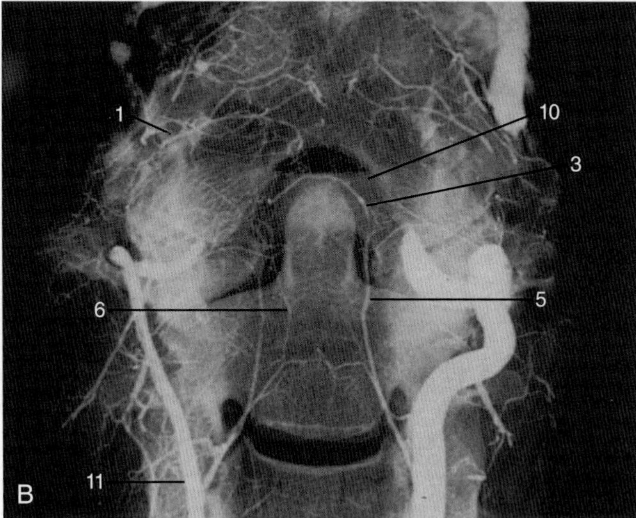

FIG. 2.27 (A) Schema of arterial supply to bodies of the upper cervical vertebrae and the odontoid process. Numerical designations apply to the same structures in (B). *1*, Hypoglossal canal passing meningeal artery. *2*, Occipital artery. *3*, Apical arcade of odontoid process. *4*, Ascending pharyngeal artery giving collateral branch beneath anterior arch of atlas. *5*, Posterior ascending artery. *6*, Anterior ascending artery. *7*, Precentral and postcentral arteries to typical cervical vertebral body. *8*, Anterior spinal plexus. *9*, Medullary branch of vertebral artery; radicular, prelaminar, and meningeal branches are also found at each level. *10*, Collateral to ascending pharyngeal artery passing rostral to anterior arch of atlas. *11*, Left vertebral artery.

Atlantoaxial Complex

With their complex phyletic and developmental history, the components of the atlantoaxial articulation display the most atypical vascular pattern of all the vertebrae. Although the odontoid process represents the definitive centrum of the first cervical vertebra, it develops and remains as a projecting process of the axis that is almost completely isolated from the rest of the atlas by synovial joint cavities. Its fixed position relative to the rotation of the atlas and the adjacent sections of the vertebral arteries prevents formation of major vascularization by direct branches at its corresponding segmental level.

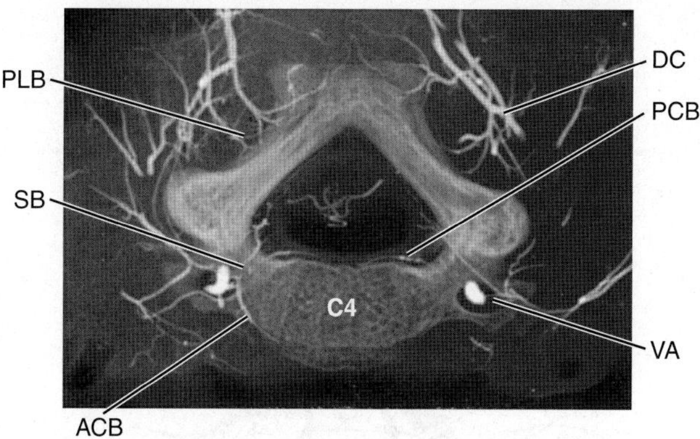

FIG. 2.28 Vertical radiograph of section through fourth cervical vertebra of a 6-year-old child, showing vascularity. The deep cervical artery (DC) provides the posterior laminar branches (PLB). Vertebral arteries show numerous anastomoses with other cervical arteries and send spinal branches (SB) that form posterior central branches (PCB) of the body and anterior lamina branches of the arch. Anterior central branches (ACB) may arise independently from the vertebral arteries (VA).

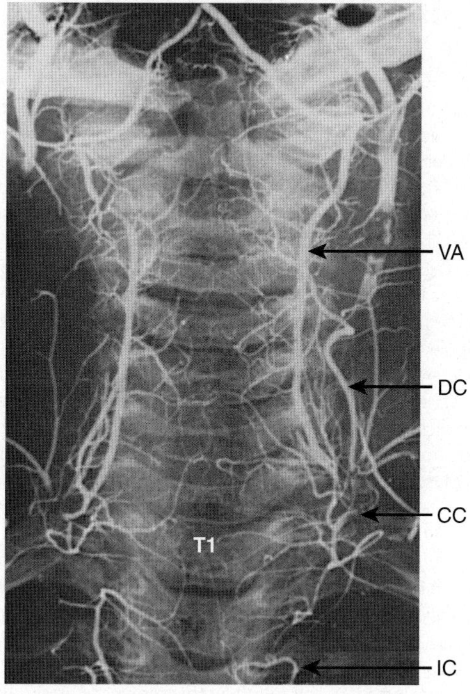

FIG. 2.29 Arteriogram of cervical and upper thoracic regions of the 6-year-old spine seen in Figs. 2.23 and 2.24. The vertebral artery (VA) and deep cervical branch (DC) of the costocervical trunk (CC) supply segmental branches to each vertebra. The costocervical artery also typically supplies T1 and T2, but in this case T2 receives a high intercostal (IC) branch on the left side.

One might assume that the nutrition of the dens would easily be accomplished by interosseous vessels derived from the spongiosa within the supporting body of the axis. It is axiomatic, however, that the vascular patterns of bones were developmentally established to supply the original ossification centers within the nonvascular cartilage matrices, and despite the eventual obliteration of the separating cartilage, the original patterns of vascularity generally prevail throughout life. The transient cartilaginous plate, which represents an incipient intervertebral disc between the atlas and axis, does not calcify until the latter half of the first decade and effectively prevents the development of any significant vascular communication between the axis centrum and the odontoid process. Occasionally, noncalcified remnants of this plate may persist in adults; although there may be a stable union between the two elements, a radiolucent area may suggest a fracture nonunion or a "false" os odontoideum.

In light of the foregoing facts, it was not unexpected that the investigations of Schiff and Parke[78] revealed that the odontoid process was supplied primarily by pairs of anterior and posterior central branches that coursed upward from the surfaces of the body of the axis and were derived from the vertebral arteries at the level of the foramen of the third cervical nerve. The posterior ascending arteries are the larger members of these two sets of vessels and usually arise independently from the posteromedial sides of their respective vertebral arteries. The individual artery enters the vertebral canal through the foramen between the second and third vertebrae and trifurcates on the dorsum of the axis body. The typical posterior central perforators course medially passing deep to the posterior longitudinal ligament (called the *tectorial membrane* in the craniocervical region) to penetrate into the spongiosa of the axis. A small descending branch anastomoses distally with vessels of the next lower segment.

The major part of the posterior ascending artery crosses the dorsal surface of the transverse ligament of the atlas about 1.5 mm lateral to the neck of the odontoid process (see Fig. 2.27). Dorsal to the alar ligament, it sends an anterior anastomotic branch over the cranial edge of this ligament to form collateral connections with the anterior ascending artery. The posterior ascending artery continues on a medial course to meet its opposite counterpart and forms the apical arcade that arches over the apex of the odontoid process.

The smaller anterior ascending arteries arise from the anteromedial aspect of the vertebral arteries and pass to the ventral surface of the axis body. Fine medial branches send perforators into the substance of the vertebral body and meet in a median anastomosis typical of the anterior central branches of the lower cervical region. The rostral continuance of the anterior ascending arteries brings them dorsal to the anterior arch of the atlas. Here each artery sends numerous fine perforators into the anterolateral surfaces of the neck of the odontoid process and terminates in a spray of vessels that supply the synovial capsule of the median atlantoaxial joint.

Fine branches from the anterior and posterior ascending arteries also assist in the nutrition of the syndesmotic relations of the atlantoaxial and craniovertebral articulations. The main blood supply to the atlanto-occipital joint is provided by a complex of vessels derived from the vertebral and occipital arteries.

Collateral vessels pass over and under the anterior arch of the atlas to anastomose with the apical arcade and ascending arteries.[79] These are derived from some component of the external carotid system. These vessels are branches of the ascending pharyngeal artery, which has a nearly ubiquitous distribution in the upper pharyngeal region and sends a branch along the inner aspect of the carotid sheath that, on reaching the base of the skull, becomes recurrent and descends deep to the prevertebral fascia to supply the upper prevertebral cervical muscles and anastomose with the anterior spinal plexus. Numerous small-bore vessels that descend from the rim of the foramen magnum to anastomose with the apical arcade are derivatives of a meningeal branch of the occipital artery that enters the skull through the hypoglossal canal (see Fig. 2.27). Its descending branches supply the periforaminal dura, the tectorial membrane and alar and apical ligaments, and the fine anastomoses to the arcade.

Sacroiliolumbar Arterial System

From the second thoracic vertebra to the fourth lumbar vertebra, the spine and its regionally related structures are supplied by pairs of segmental arteries that are direct branches of the aorta. Because the aorta terminates in a bifurcation ventral to the fourth lumbar vertebral body, the vertebrae and the associated tissues caudad to this point rely on an arterial complex derived mostly from the internal iliac (hypogastric) arteries. This "sacroiliolumbar system" consists of contributions from the fourth lumbar artery, the iliolumbar artery, and the middle and lateral sacral arteries.

With the increasing use of percutaneous approaches to the lower lumbar discs, this infra-aortic system of vessels has assumed some surgical significance, particularly because, in contrast to the conventional segmental supply to the more superior vertebrae, its major components are longitudinally related to the dorsolateral surfaces of the discs most frequently involved in these procedures.[79]

Fourth Lumbar Arteries

The peculiarities of the sacroiliolumbar system of arteries may best be understood if compared with the pattern of distribution of the typical aortic segmental branches. The ramifications of the fourth lumbar arteries were selected for this purpose because they not only exemplify the conventional segmental distribution, but often are involved in the nutrition of the next lower segments by variable contributions to the iliolumbar vessels. These vessels often may be twice the caliber of their more cephalad homologues because of a greater muscular and intersegmental distribution.

As depicted in Figs. 2.30 and 2.31, the distribution of the major ramifications is similar to that of the thoracic segmental vessels, with the exception of additional branches that supply the psoas and quadratus lumborum muscles. The lateral muscular branch (equivalent of the thoracic intercostals) may be quite large at the fourth lumbar level, where, in contrast to the other lumbar laterals, it passes anterior, rather than posterior, to the quadratus lumborum. It then continues to supply the lower posterolateral abdominal wall as it courses superior to the crest of the ilium. As can be seen in Fig. 2.30, it may be equivalent in size to the iliac branch of the iliolumbar artery. Its position superior to the crest indicates that it is more likely to be encountered by percutaneous instrumentation than the latter vessel.

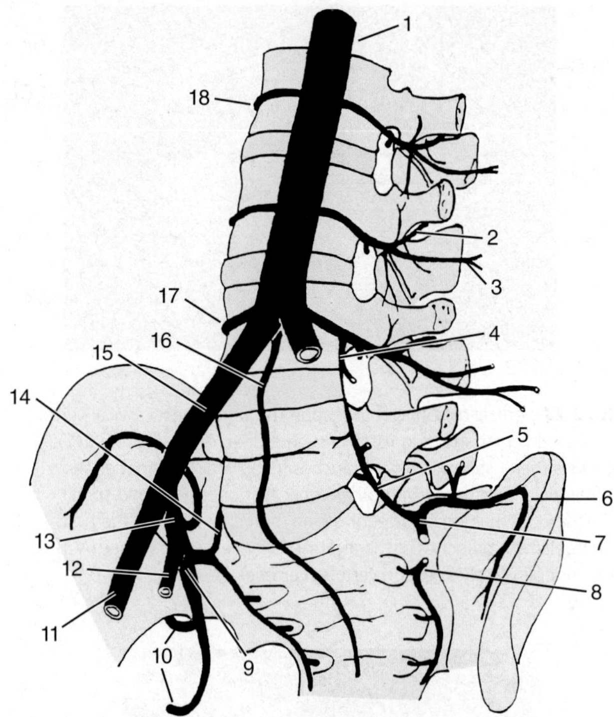

FIG. 2.30 Distribution and major variations of sacroiliolumbar system of arteries that supply the vertebrae and their associated structures inferior to the fourth lumbar vertebra. These patterns of the vessels were derived from radiographs of perinatal specimens and dissections of adults and drawn against a tracing of the lumbosacral region taken from a left anterior oblique radiograph of a man. The aorta lies to the left of center as it approaches the bifurcation ventral to the fourth lumbar vertebra. This schema shows the more frequent arrangement of the sacroiliolumbar system on the right side of the illustration, where the iliolumbar vessel (*7*) has a single origin from the dorsum of the posterior division of the (removed) internal iliac artery. The left side shows the common variation where the iliac artery and the lumbar artery (*14*) are derived separately. The middle sacral artery (*16*) is in its typical position, and the anastomotic contribution from the fourth lumbar artery (*4*) shows its most frequent form. *1,* Aorta. *2,* Musculocutaneous branch of third lumbar artery. *3,* Muscular branch to posterior abdominal wall. *4,* Anastomotic contribution of fourth lumbar artery to sacroiliolumbar system. *5,* Lumbar branch of iliolumbar artery. *6,* Iliac branch of iliolumbar artery. *7,* Iliolumbar artery. *8,* Left lateral sacral artery. *9,* Posterior division of internal iliac artery. *10,* Superior and inferior gluteal arteries. *11,* External iliac artery. *12,* Anterior (visceral) division of internal iliac artery. *13,* Internal iliac artery. *14,* Variant origin of lumbar branch of iliolumbar artery from lateral sacral artery. *15,* Common iliac artery. *16,* Middle sacral artery. *17,* Left fourth lumbar segmental artery. *18,* Left second lumbar segmental artery.

The dorsal musculocutaneous branch of the fourth lumbar artery is equivalent in distribution to other thoracolumbar segmental arteries. It usually has a medial branch that supplies the external aspects of the facet joints and neural arch components and the transversospinal group of muscles and a lateral branch to the transversocostal group of the erector spinae. The vertebromedullary (spinal) branches of the fourth lumbar artery are also similar to those of other segmental arteries (see Fig. 2.24). They are a group of vessels of variable caliber that may generally be sorted into three divisions: (1) the ventral periosteal and osseous branches that supply the posterior longitudinal ligament, the periosteum, and the

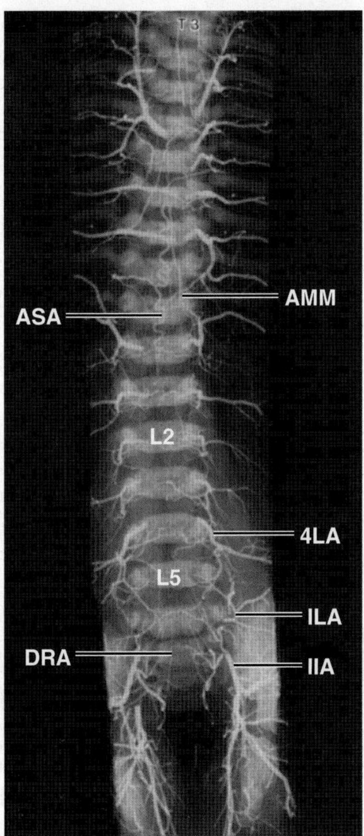

FIG. 2.31 Anteroposterior radiograph of spine from a perinatal cadaver injected with barium sulfate. The aorta and common iliac vessels have been removed before radiography. This specimen shows considerable variation between the two sides of the sacroiliolumbar system. On the *right,* a small lumbar branch and a descending branch from the fourth lumbar artery (4LA) enter the L5-S1 intervertebral foramen. On the *left,* there is no lumbar branch, and a descending branch of the L4 artery supplies all of the vessels to the L5-S1 foramen. The middle sacral artery is also absent, and other branches of the system supply its domain. The radicular branches of the vertebromedullary vessels supply the distal radicular arteries (DRA) and reveal the positions of the lower ends of the lumbosacral nerve roots. *AMM,* Arteria medullaris magna; *ASA,* anterior spinal artery; *IIA,* internal iliac artery; *ILA,* iliolumbar artery.

cancellous bone of the vertebral body; (2) the radiculomedullary division that provides the irregularly located medullary arteries of the cord and the constant distal radicular arteries to all the roots; and (3) the dorsal division that supplies fine articular branches to the deep aspects of the facet joints and the periosteum of the deep surfaces of the laminae and their associated ligaments. The first two divisions usually originate from a common branch of the segmental artery and enter the intervertebral foramen just rostral to their respective vertebral pedicle and ventral to the dorsal root ganglion, whereas the dorsal division arises from the musculocutaneous branch of the segmental artery and enters the foramen dorsal to the nerve components. All the vertebromedullary branches may provide fine branches to the spinal dura.

The aortic segmental arteries course around their respective vertebral body at its narrowest circumference and are positioned almost equidistant between the adjacent discs. These parts of the arterial distribution are relatively safe from instrumentation properly positioned to enter the discs.

A major peculiarity of the fourth lumbar artery is its proclivity toward providing a relatively large, caudally directed intersegmental branch that arises near the level of the intervertebral foramen and becomes reciprocally involved with the lumbar branch of the iliolumbar artery. When this latter vessel is small or absent, the descending branch of the fourth lumbar artery may be sufficiently large to provide the predominant nutritional system to two vertebral segments caudad to its origin (see Figs. 2.30 and 2.31).

Iliolumbar Artery

As opposed to the mostly visceral distribution of the anterior division of the internal iliac (hypogastric) artery, the posterior division is essentially a somatic artery giving rise to gluteal, iliolumbar, and lateral sacral branches. The iliolumbar artery most frequently is the first branch of this dorsal division. It is directed dorsosuperiorly, passing close to the ventrolateral surface of the first sacral vertebral segment. It courses superiorly, dorsal to the obturator nerve and ventral to the lumbosacral trunk. Lateral to the inferior margin of the L5-S1 disc, the iliolumbar artery usually divides into a laterally directed iliac artery and an ascending lumbar artery. The first of these crosses the sacroiliac joint to reach the iliac fossa of the pelvis, where it courses inferior to the iliac crest and usually deep to the muscle to provide muscular branches to the iliac muscle and articular twigs to the acetabulum and eventually anastomoses with the deep circumflex branch of the femoral artery.

The lumbar artery ascends posterolateral to the L5-S1 disc, still between the obturator nerve and the lumbosacral trunk, to provide the vertebromedullary vessels to the L5-S1 intervertebral foramen (Fig. 2.32; also see Figs. 2.30 and 2.31). In most cases, a branch of this vessel continues rostrally to anastomose with the descending branch of the fourth lumbar artery. The lumbar branch of the iliolumbar artery provides regional branches to the psoas and quadratus lumborum muscles.

Sacral Arteries

Lateral Sacral Arteries

Lateral sacral arteries usually form the second branch of the dorsal division of the internal iliac arteries and course down the pars lateralis on each side of the sacrum. Opposite the sacral foramina, they give off medial branches that dorsally enter the foramina. After providing the typical vertebromedullary derivatives, their dorsal muscular branches exit through the dorsal sacral foramina to supply the sacral origins of the erector spinae muscles.

Middle Sacral Artery

The middle sacral artery is an unpaired vessel that is the last branch of the aorta, usually derived from its dorsal median surface just above the carina of the bifurcation (Fig. 2.33; also see Fig. 2.30). It descends down the ventral surface of the anterior longitudinal ligament over the fourth and fifth lumbar

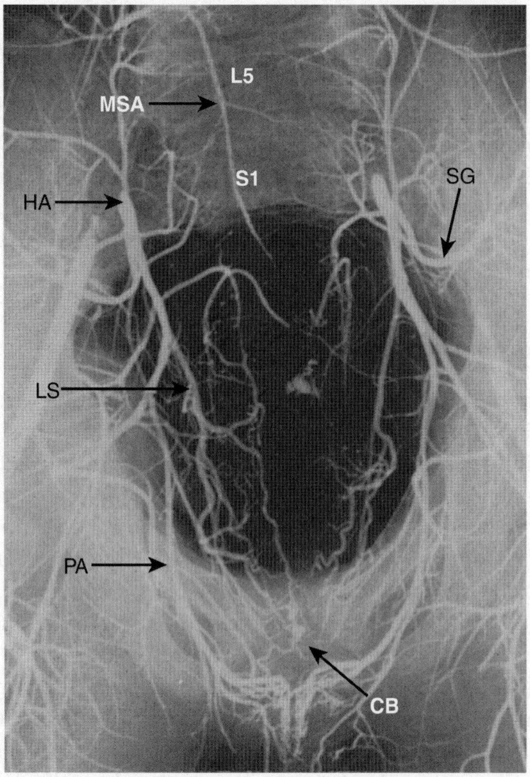

FIG. 2.32 Anteroposterior arteriogram of sacral region in a 7-year-old child. The lateral sacral arteries (LS) can be seen coming from the hypogastric vessels (HA). The middle sacral artery (MSA) is atypical in this specimen because it stops at S1. Just anterior to the coccyx, the coccygeal bodies (CB) are indicated as small knots of arteriovenous anastomoses. Pudendal arteries (PA) are well injected.

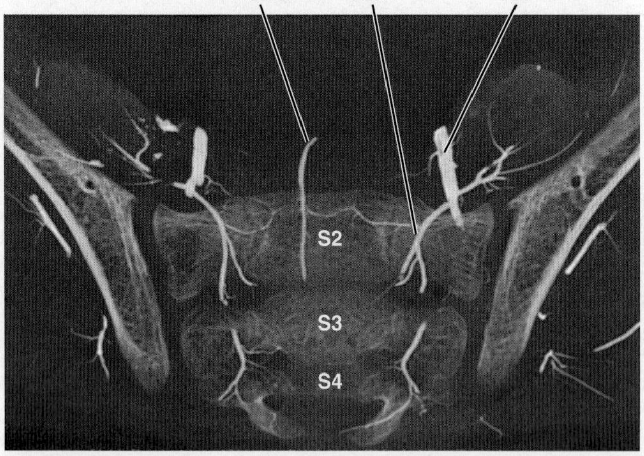

FIG. 2.33 Radiograph of horizontal section through sacroiliac joint. The natural curvature of the sacrum provided oblique sections through segments 2, 3, and 4. The hypogastric artery (HA) gives off the lateral sacral artery (LSA) that sends anastomotic branches to join the middle sacral artery (MSA); from these, the sacral segments receive the penetrating anterior central branches. The dorsal branches pass into the anterior sacral foramina to provide posterior, central, neural, and prelaminar branches. The dorsal branches leave through the posterior sacral foramina to supply the muscles and posterior laminar branches.

bodies and down the ventral sacrum to terminate at the sacrococcygeal junction in a vascular glomus (sacrococcygeal body) in tail-less mammals or continues ventral to the coccygeal (caudal) vertebrae in tailed mammals as the caudal artery. In humans, this is a variable vessel, being totally absent in some cases or replaced by a branch of one of the lateral sacral arteries. Where it is a significant component of the sacroiliolumbar system, its first lateral branches on the ventral surface of the fifth lumbar body may entirely replace this segment's contributions from the iliolumbar or fourth lumbar vessels and provide its osseous, muscular, and vertebromedullary requirements.

Where it is conspicuously present in the sacral region, the middle sacral artery may also contribute a vertebromedullary branch to each anterior sacral foramen. When it is absent, these ventral sacral territories are provided with segmental medial branches from the lateral sacral arteries.

Functional Significance

The sacroiliolumbar system, despite its complexity and seemingly endless combinations of reciprocal substitutions, supplies the lower lumbosacral elements of the spine and the inferior half of the lumbosacral spinal nerve roots (cauda equina) and the back musculature inferior to the L4 level. It is also a major contributor to the vasa nervorum of the lumbosacral plexus. The distal radicular arteries define the positions of the lumbosacral roots (see Fig. 2.25). Although significant medullary branches to the spinal cord are seldom found below L4, they do occur, and from the preceding descriptions it is obvious why the ligation of both internal iliac arteries during radical cystoprostatectomy can result in spinal cord ischemia.[80]

Venous System of the Vertebral Column

An external plexus and an internal plexus of veins are associated with the vertebral column. The distribution of the two systems roughly coincides with the areas served by the external and internal arterial supplies. The external venous plexus also consists of an anterior and a posterior set of veins. The small anterior external plexus is coextensive with the anterior central arteries and receives tributaries that perforate the anterior and lateral sides of the vertebral body.

The more extensive posterior external veins drain the regions supplied by posterior (muscular and postlaminar) branches of the segmental artery. The posterior external veins form an essentially paired system, which lies in the two vertebrocostal grooves, but has cross anastomoses between the spinous processes. It is a valveless venous complex that receives the draining segmental tributaries of the internal veins through the intervertebral foramina and communicates ultimately with the lumbar and intercostal tributaries of the caval and azygos system. The posterior external plexus becomes most extensive in the posterior nuchal region, where it receives the intraspinous tributaries via the vertebral veins and drains into the deep cervical and jugular veins.

The internal venous plexus is of more functional and anatomic interest. This plexus is essentially a series of irregular, valveless epidural sinuses that extend from the coccyx to the foramen magnum. Its channels are embedded in the epidural fat and are supported by a network of collagenous fibers, but their walls are so thin that their extent or configuration cannot be discerned by gross dissection. This latter property may account for the fact that the epidural venous sinuses have been periodically "rediscovered." The epidural vertebral veins were known to Vesalius and his contemporaries and were described and illustrated in the first part of the 19th century by Breschet.[81] Batson,[82] Clemens,[83] and others made the functional and pathologic significance of these vessels apparent (Fig. 2.34).

The plexus does not entwine the dura in a completely haphazard fashion but is arranged in a series of cross-connected expansions that produce anterior and posterior ladderlike configurations up the vertebral canal. The main anterior components of the epidural plexus consist of two continuous channels that course along the posterior surface of the vertebral bodies just medial to the pedicles. These channels expand medially to create cross anastomoses over the central dorsal area of each vertebral body and are thinnest where they overlie the intervertebral discs. When injected with a contrast medium, the main channels may appear as a segmental chain of rhomboid beads. Chaynes and colleagues[84] studied the internal venous plexus using silicon injection techniques. They found that anterior longitudinal veins were located in a "dehiscence" within the periosteum along the lateral aspect of the spinal canal and that veins of each side communicated with each other through a retrocorporeal vein. In the cervical spine, the retrocorporeal vein was found deep to the posterior longitudinal ligament, whereas it was superficial to the ligament in the thoracic and lumbar regions.

Where the main anterior sinuses cross connect, they receive the large unpaired basivertebral sinus that arises within the dorsal central concavity of the spongiosa and drains the intraosseous labyrinth of sinusoids. Regional visualization of the epidural plexus can be accomplished by introducing a radiopaque medium directly into the spongiosa or the cancellous bone of the spinous process (intraosseous venography).

The major external connections of the epidural plexus consist of the veins that pass through the intervertebral foramen and eventually empty into the segmentally available intercostal or lumbar veins (Fig. 2.35). Because these sinuses are valveless, one cannot refer accurately to directions of drainage and flow. The greatest functional significance of these vessels lies in their ability to pass blood in any direction according to the constantly shifting intraabdominal and intrathoracic pressures. Breschet[81] surmised that the epidural plexus served as a collateral route for the valveless caval and azygos systems. This ability has been shown by experimental ligation of either the superior vena cava or the inferior vena cava. In addition, the Queckenstedt maneuver, which tests the patency of the spinal subarachnoid space by compressing the jugular or intraabdominal veins, causes an increase in cerebrospinal fluid pressure through dural compression from the expansion of the collaterally loaded epidural plexus.

The plexus is evidently capable of passing large quantities of blood without developing varices. Clemens claimed that this feature was due to the intricate network of collagenous fibers that supports the thin walls of the sinuses. Also, passive

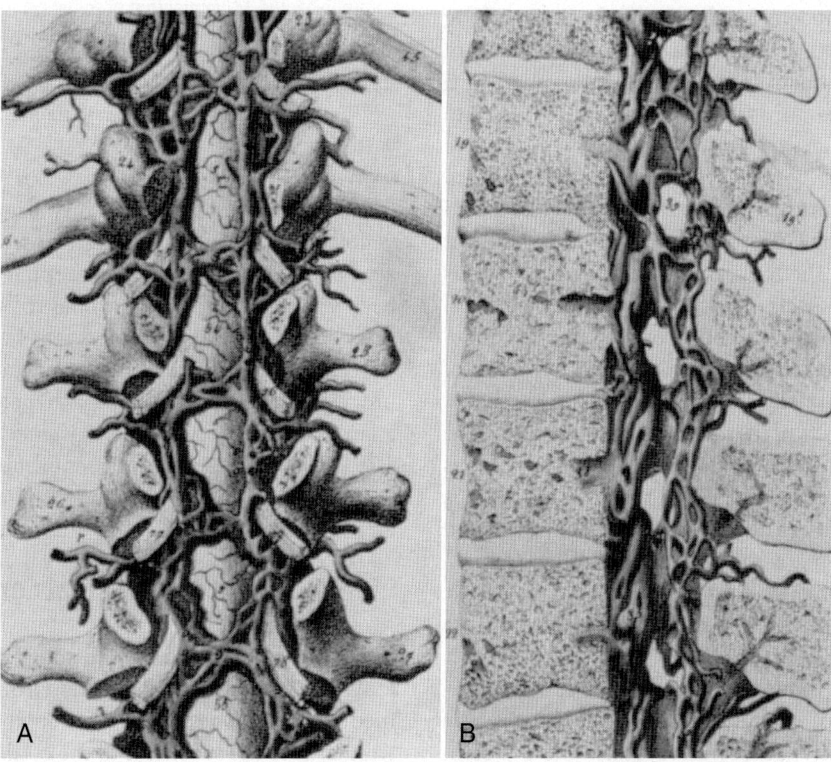

FIG. 2.34 (A) Posterior and (B) lateral illustrations of the spinal epidural venous plexus taken from hand-colored copies of Breschet's original work (ca. 1835). (Courtesy Scott Memorial Library, Jefferson Medical College.)

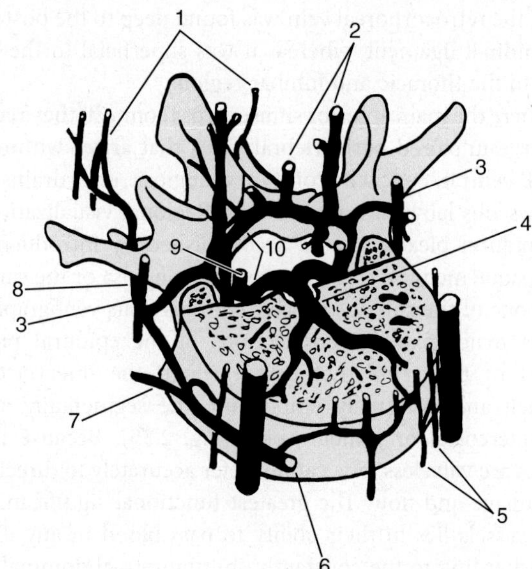

FIG. 2.35 Schema showing venous relationships of a lumbar vertebra. Engorgement and relative venous hypertension in the epidural vessels exacerbate neuroischemic conditions in the lumbosacral roots. *1,* Dorsal external vertebral plexus. *2,* Dorsal epidural plexus. *3,* Ascending lumbar veins. *4,* Basivertebral vein. *5,* Ventral external vertebral plexus. *6,* Lumbar segmental vein. *7,* Muscular vein from posterior abdominal wall. *8,* Circumferential channels (sinuses) of epidural plexus. *9,* ventral internal vertebral plexus. *10,* anterior and posterior longitudinal sinuses of internal vertebral plexus.

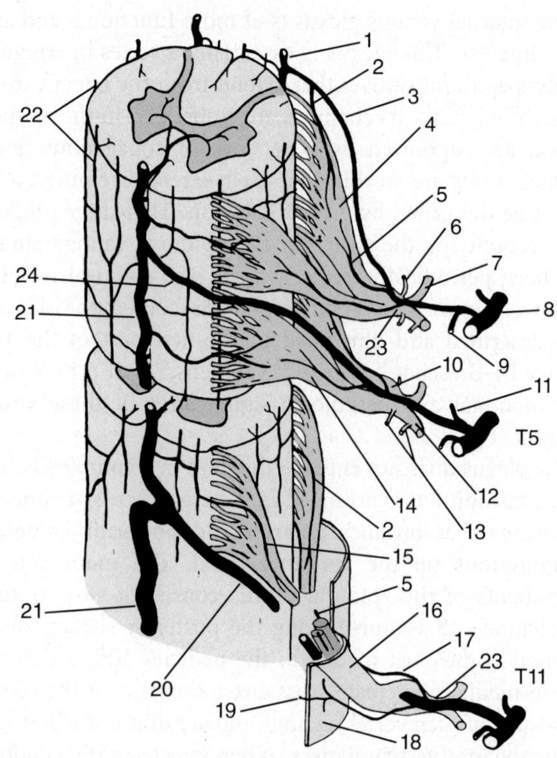

FIG. 2.36 Composite schema of blood supply to spinal cord and nerve roots showing two regions of the cord. Note the distinction between medullary arteries and true radicular arteries and that the medullary arteries usually run a course that is independent of the roots. *1,* Dorsolateral longitudinal artery. *2,* Proximal radicular artery (of dorsal root). *3,* Dorsal medullary artery. *4,* Dorsal root of thoracic spinal nerve. *5,* Distal radicular artery (of dorsal root). *6,* Sinuvertebral nerve. *7,* Dorsal ramus of spinal nerve. *8,* Segmental artery. *9,* Dorsal central artery. *10,* Dorsal root ganglion. *11,* Anterior laminar artery. *12,* Ventral ramus of spinal nerve. *13,* Rami communicantes. *14,* Ventral root of spinal nerve. *15,* Proximal radicular artery of ventral root. *16,* Periradicular theca of dura. *17,* Dorsal meningeal branch of vertebromedullary artery. *18,* Dura. *19,* Ventral meningeal plexus. *20,* Great ventral medullary artery (great "radicular" artery of Adamkiewicz). *21,* Anterior (ventral) spinal artery. *22,* Vasa corona of spinal cord. *23,* Spinal nerve. *24,* Ventral medullary artery of thoracic cord.

congestion of the spinal cord is prevented by minute valves in the radicular branches draining the spinal cord.[83] This latter fact is anatomically unique because valves exist nowhere else in the venous channels associated with the central nervous system. An ancillary function of the epidural plexus may be to act in a mechanical capacity as a hydraulic shock-absorbing sheath that helps buffer the spinal cord during movements of the vertebral column, similar to the epidural fat.

The vertebral sinuses are largest in the suboccipital and upper cervical region. Here they also receive numerous nerve endings from the sinuvertebral nerves and are associated with glomerular arteriovenous anastomoses, which suggests a possible baroceptive function.[85] The patency of these anastomoses is most easily shown in the fetus, in which arterial injections of a contrast medium may also fill the upper cervical epidural sinuses. Similarly, the coccygeal bodies of the same specimen pass the arterial injection directly into the epidural veins of the lower sacral region.

The detrimental aspects of the vertebral epidural veins have been well stated by Batson.[82] Retrograde flow from venous connections to the lower pelvic organs provides an obvious route of metastasis for pelvic neoplasms to the spine itself and to the regions of the trunk associated with valveless connections to the plexus. Batson[82] claimed that direct metastatic transfer can occur between the pelvic organs and the brain via the vertebral epidural route.

Another extraspinal-intraspinal venous connection implicated in the transfer of pathologic processes involves the pharyngovertebral veins.[86] These vessels constitute a system that drains the superior posterolateral regions of the nasopharynx and coalesces into two to several veins that penetrate the anterior atlanto-occipital membrane to discharge into the venous complex surrounding the median and lateral atlantoaxial joints. Because posterior pharyngeal infections have been linked with the atlantoaxial rotatory subluxations characteristic of Grisel syndrome,[87] it is believed that the pharyngovertebral veins are instrumental in transporting infectious processes that may produce a hyperemic relaxation of the atlantoaxial ligaments. The existence of this venous system also explains the ease in transfer of superior pharyngeal metastatic processes to the upper cervical epidural veins.

Blood Supply of the Spinal Cord

Throughout the length of the spinal cord, a system of three longitudinal vessels receives blood from the irregularly located medullary branches of the segmental spinal arteries and distributes it to the substance of the cord. This system consists of the single median ventral anterior spinal artery and two smaller dorsolateral spinal arteries (Fig. 2.36).

Anterior Spinal Artery

Despite its great functional significance, the anterior spinal artery remains one of the more inaccurately described and inadequately understood blood vessels. Derived from the fusion of bilateral pairs of ascending and descending anastomotic branches of the original segmental arteries of the developing spinal cord,[88] this median ventral pial vessel supplies approximately 80% of the intrinsic spinal cord vasculature. It is usually depicted in texts as a single continuous artery of nearly uniform caliber that extends from the medulla oblongata to the conus. The anterior spinal artery is actually a longitudinal series of functionally independent vessels that may show wide luminal variations and anatomic discontinuities.[88-90]

Although the investigations of Crock and Yoshizawa[75] have tended to minimize the significance of predominant regional feeders, many functionally oriented reports have claimed that the cord has three major arterial domains along its vertical axis: (1) the cervicothoracic region (C1–T3), (2) the mid-thoracic region (T3–T8), and (3) the thoracolumbar (including sacral cord) region (T8-conus). The reports have also claimed that these areas have little anastomotic exchange between their junctions (Fig. 2.37).

Brewer and colleagues[89] and Lazorthes and associates[90] maintained that a series of human anterior spinal arteries consistently show interruptions, or critically narrow zones, in the mid-thoracic region, and these influence the potential collateral blood flow along the longitudinal axis of the cord. It is not only the observed size of the vessel that is of physiologic significance, however. The existence of a marked autoregulatory control of the intrinsic spinal cord blood flow has been independently shown in many mammalian species.[32,91] Microscopic investigation[92] of sections of the descending and ascending contributions of the arteria medullaris magna (artery of Adamkiewicz, also known as the arteria radicularis magna) to the anterior spinal artery showed that these arteries, in addition to their well-developed circumferential muscle of the tunica media, also possess a layer of predominantly longitudinal intimal musculature. Located between the internal elastic lamina and the endothelium, this layer ranges in thickness from one-fifth to one-half of the tunica media (Fig. 2.38).

In following a series of cranial to caudal sections of the thoracolumbar anterior spinal artery, it was noted that the intimal muscle layer did not extend into any of its branches. At the mouth of the central (sulcal) arteries, which are the largest anterior spinal artery derivatives, the intimal musculature stops abruptly, often forming a liplike projection over the opening of the branch vessel, but no intimal muscle fibers extend into the central arteries. A sphincter-like thickening of the central artery tunica media, seen at the ostium of the vessels, indicates that this muscle layer has a greater contractile influence at this point (see Fig. 2.38). The intimal musculature, in addition to enhancing the luminal control of the anterior spinal artery, also is involved in controlling the blood flow into the central arteries. Where the intimal layer shows the liplike projections, successive serial sections indicate that contraction of the longitudinally disposed intimal muscle fibers forms an ellipsoidal buttonhole-shaped orifice whose long axis is parallel to that of the fiber orientation. Such an arrangement permits exquisite muscular control of the blood flow from the anterior spinal artery to its central artery branches.

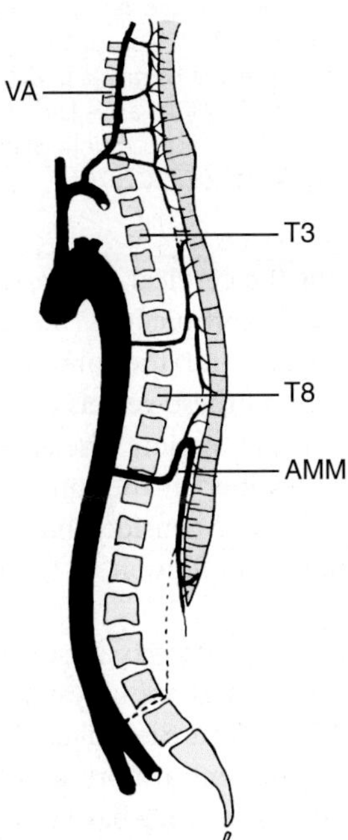

FIG. 2.37 Schema illustrating sources and relationships of medullary feeder arteries to the spine and the spinal cord. Anterior spinal artery (ASA) is shown to be formed by an anastomotic chain of ascending and descending branches of medullary feeders. Cervicothoracic, mid-thoracic, and thoracolumbar (includes sacral cord) regions are indicated, and their usual boundaries at vertebral levels T3 and T8 are shown. Medullary feeders range from 6 to 14, but the respective domains persist. *Dotted line* indicates frequent position of a smaller accessory medullary feeder to the thoracolumbar area. *AMM,* Arteria medullaris magna; *VA,* vertebral artery. (From Parke WW, Whalen JL, Bunger PC, et al. Intimal musculature of the lower anterior spinal artery. *Spine.* 1995;20:2074.)

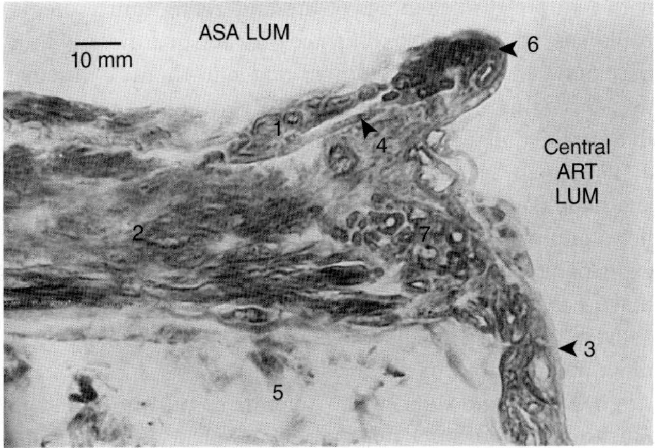

FIG. 2.38 High-power cross section of thoracolumbar anterior spinal artery (ASA) wall at junction with one side of a central artery. The intimal musculature (*1*) may extend as a liplike projection (*6*) over the central artery orifice. This muscle layer stops at this point and does not extend into branch vessels. A sphincter-like enlargement of the conventional circular muscle of the central artery (*7*) is indicated. Endothelium (*3*) and internal elastic lamina (*4*), tunica media (*2*), and adventitia-pia (*5*) are labeled. ART, artery; LUM, lumbar. (From Parke WW, Whalen JL, Bunger PC, et al: Intimal musculature of the lower anterior spinal artery. Spine 1995;20:2075.)

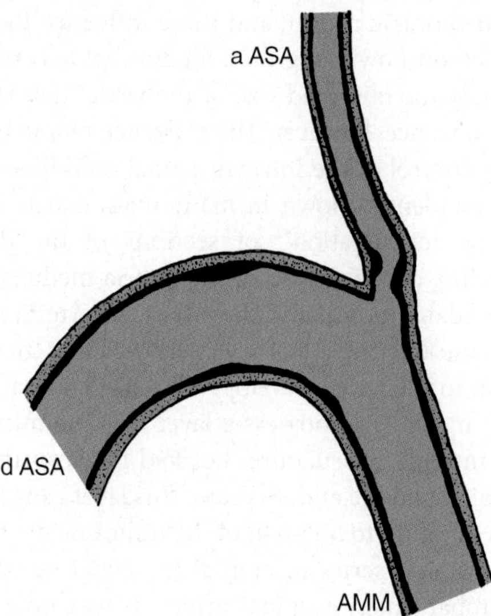

FIG. 2.39 Schema derived from sections of arteria medullaris magna (AMM)–anterior spinal artery (ASA) junction to show distribution of intimal musculature (*solid black*) in this region. Intimal cushions are shown guarding the orifice of the ascending ASA (a ASA) and a typical distribution is found in the arch of the descending ASA (d ASA). (From Parke WW, Whalen JL, Bunger PC, et al. Intimal musculature of the lower anterior spinal artery. *Spine.* 1995;20:2076.)

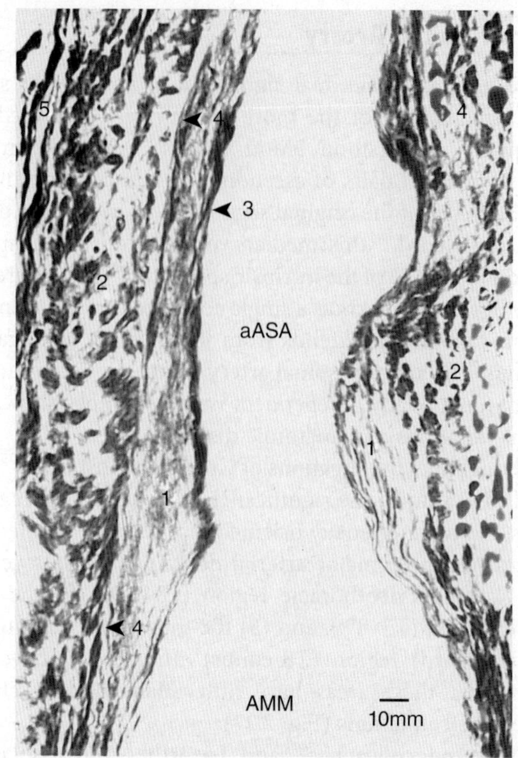

FIG. 2.40 Sagittal section through junction of arteria medullaris magna (AMM) arch and ascending anterior spinal artery (aASA) showing the intimal cushions guarding the aASA orifice (*1*). These may be reinforced by underlying enhancement of the circular fibers of the tunica media (*2*). Endothelium (*3*) and elastic lamina (*4*) are indicated. The longitudinal disposition of the intimal muscle fibers is apparent, particularly in the intimal cushion on the right side. The contraction of these muscular systems would dramatically alter the radius of the aASA lumen. *5,* Adventitia-pia. (From Parke WW, Whalen JL, Bunger PC, et al. Intimal musculature of the lower anterior spinal artery. *Spine.* 1995;20:2076.)

In addition to the fairly uniform layer of the intimal musculature throughout the walls of the examined sections of the thoracolumbar anterior spinal artery, serial sections cut through the arch-shaped junction of the arteria medullaris magna and the descending anterior spinal artery branches show that this intimal layer, in most cases, is organized into prominent intimal cushions. These muscular thickenings are erratically distributed along the lumen of the hairpin-shaped arterial arch and the initial segment of the ascending branch of the anterior spinal artery (Figs. 2.39 and 2.40). This latter location is of considerable interest because its prominent cushions, with reinforced thickenings of the underlying tunica media, could exert considerable influence over the quantity of blood flow between the thoracolumbar and mid-thoracic vascular domains. This intimal control system, when coupled with the intramedullary arteriovenous anastomoses (described in a subsequent section on intrinsic vascularity), provides an anatomic basis for the dramatic range of spinal cord blood flow autoregulation. The presence of the intimal cushions explains the often-noted failure of the arteria medullaris magna to supply adequately the mid-thoracic cord region above the arteria medullaris magna–anterior spinal artery junction during aortic cross clamping.

The ventral position of the anterior spinal artery and its nutritional importance may have consequence in spinal stenosis. Particularly in the lower cervical region, its compression by dorsal osteophytes and cartilaginous protrusions related to cervical disc degeneration may lead to the neurologically disastrous anterior spinal artery syndrome.[93] The medullary feeder arteries that supply the anterior spinal artery may arise from any spinal segmental artery. Studies by Dommissee[94] showed, however, that there are statistical preferences for certain segmental levels. There are usually three anterior medullary arteries for the cervical region, one or two for the thoracic region, and a conspicuous medullary vessel (the arteria medullaris magna) for the lumbosacral cord region. The levels of origin for all these vessels center around certain "average" locations in each region. The anterior spinal artery is usually of greatest caliber in the lumbosacral part of the cord, where it supplies the considerable tissue mass of the proximal cauda equina in addition to the lumbosacral cord intumescence.

The dorsolateral spinal arteries arise from the posterior inferior cerebellar vessels and are of lesser caliber and nutritional significance. They also are less likely to be longitudinally continuous and often present a more plexiform distribution over the dorsum of the cord. They have a greater frequency of smaller medullary sources.

The larger intradural spinal arteries are unusual in that, similar to the cerebral arteries, they have no significant vasa vasorum. In all other regions of the body, a vessel with an external diameter approaching 1 mm shows a fine vascular plexus (vasa vasorum) on its external surface that supplies nutrients to its outer layers of tissue. Because the cerebral and spinal vessels are bathed in the nutrient-rich cerebrospinal fluid, their external layers presumably derive metabolic exchange from this source.

Lateral Spinal Arteries of the Cervical Cord

The highest three to four segments of the cervical spinal cord receive blood from a unique pair of vessels, the lateral spinal arteries. Although, ontogenetically, these seem to be the most rostral expressions of the dorsolateral spinal arteries, they have a more extensive distribution and are without equivalents in other levels of the cord. They usually arise from the intradural parts of the vertebral arteries near the origins of the posterior inferior cerebellar arteries, or they may arise from the proximal sections of the posterior inferior cerebellar arteries themselves. Their typical course carries them anterior to the posterior roots of the cervical spinal nerves C1 to C4, dorsal to the denticulate ligaments, and parallel to the spinal components of the 11th cranial nerve. Their general distribution is to the dorsolateral and ventrolateral cord regions caudad to the olives.

Although these vessels were observed in the later 19th century, they were usually regarded as variants, and their functional significance was not appreciated. Lasjaunias and colleagues[95] compiled an extensive report on the variations and selective angiography of these important vessels.

Intrinsic Vascularity of the Spinal Cord

The tissues of the spinal cord are supplied by two systems of vessels that enter its substance. The first is a centripetal arrangement of arteries that supplies the superficial tracts of the ventral and lateral funiculi, all of the dorsal funiculus, and the extremities of the dorsal horns. They are radially penetrating branches of the vasa corona and the dorsolateral spinal arteries, which serve only a little more than one-fourth of the cord. The greater part of the cord and almost all of its gray matter is supplied by a second centrifugal system of vessels derived from the sulcal (or central) arteries.[96] These arteries are a repetitive series of branches derived from the dorsal aspect of the anterior spinal artery that penetrate the depths of the anterior median fissure. In the mid-sagittal plane, they form a close palisade of vessels that occur with a frequency of 3 to 8 arteries per 1 cm in the cervical region and 2 to 6 per 1 cm in the thoracic cord; they are densest in the lumbar region, where they number 5 to 12 per 1 cm of the anterior spinal artery. The average diameters of the sulcal arteries are greater in the cervical (0.21 mm) and lumbosacral (0.23 mm) regions than in the thoracic cord (0.14 mm).[97]

As these vessels approach the anterior commissure, most turn to either the right or the left and supply only the corresponding side of the cord.[14,73,98,99] This unilateral proclivity reflects their origins in the early embryonic stages when the anterior spinal arteries first condensed from a primitive plexus as a symmetrical pair of longitudinal vessels, each supplying its respective half of the cord. In subsequent development, these two vessels fused in the midline to form the definitive single median anterior spinal artery, but their sulcal branches retained their original unilateral affinities. Bilateral distributions occur in 9%, 7%, and 14% of the cervical, thoracic, and lumbar vessels.[97,100]

Although the sulcal arteries may give infrequent branches to the septomarginal white fibers as they extend into the median anterior fissure, their major distribution is derived after they enter the substance of the cord, just ventral to the anterior white commissure. Here the individual right and left arteries subdivide into dorsal and ventral branches. A group of ventral branches supplies the ventral horns and, through more radial extensions, provides vessels to Clarke column and the deeper fibers of the anterior and lateral funiculi. The smaller, more dorsal group of branches supplies the gray commissure and the ventral one-half to two-thirds of the dorsal horns. A few second-order or third-order branches form anastomotic arcades with their counterparts of adjacent sulcal artery territories. All these vessels provide the finer arterioles that eventually lead to the spinal capillary beds.

The greater metabolic requirements of the spinal gray matter, in contrast to the funicular tissue, are dramatically reflected in their relative capillary densities. Quantification of the microvascularity in the spinal cord has shown that the capillary density of the gray matter is four to five times as great as the white matter.[101] The capillary distribution within the gray matter is not homogeneous, however, and varies with the regional concentrations of the nuclei. The nuclei of the dorsal horn are fairly uniformly distributed. The ventral horn shows segmental nuclear clusters, which display distinct nerve cell groups.

As noted by Feeney and Watterson,[102] the capillary densities of the white and gray matter of the central nervous system are established at a level that is minimally requisite for the metabolic needs of the given tissue. This situation is in contrast to most other body tissues, which have a capillary "reserve" and normally function with only part of their capillary channels open, varying their intrinsic vascular resistance by dilation of the accessory channels. Nevertheless, despite the lack of this method of control, the spinal cord exhibits a remarkable range of blood flow autoregulation.[1,32,103] The intrinsic cord vasculature maintains a constant blood flow throughout a wide range of systemic blood pressure alterations, although each animal species has a definite upper and lower limit to the systemic blood pressure at which the regulation decompensates. Because transection of the upper cervical cord has no effect on this autoregulatory capacity, it may be assumed that this reflex is local and independent of autonomic nerve control.

Numerous third-order branches of the sulcal arteries communicate directly with veins through convoluted anastomoses. These vascular structures are located primarily in the area that divides the ventral two-thirds of the dorsal horn from the dorsal one-third and in the more central regions of the ventral horn. They show a paucity of contractile elements and instead exhibit an "epithelioid" type of media that seems capable of swelling and diminishing its thickness. Because this action could rapidly control the caliber of the anastomotic lumina in immediate response to local metabolic changes, these anastomotic convolutions may be the site of the reflex adjustment in the flow resistance of the spinal cord vasculature.[104]

Perhaps the most essential part of knowledge of the vascular supply of the spinal cord is awareness of the ranges of individual variability. The numerous successful surgical cases in which the arteria medullaris magna has been inadvertently interrupted without producing a disastrous spinal cord ischemia give the impression that an adequate collateral vascularity may protect the cord in most individuals when a single major artery is compromised. In procedures involving the interruption of blood flow in numerous consecutive segmental branches of the aorta, such as aortic cross clamping for abdominal vascular surgery, the maintenance of adequate spinal cord blood flow, particularly in the thoracic area, seems to depend more on the regional competence of the anterior spinal artery than on the number of collateral sources to the cord. Spinal cord injury after cross clamping without adjunctive vascular support has been reported to range from 15% to 25%, depending on the series of cases reviewed.[105,106] Proximal-to-distal aortic shunting may alleviate the undesirable hypertension in the aortic distribution proximal to the first clamp and the hypotension in the segments distal to the second clamp. The work of Molina and colleagues[105] on dogs indicated, however, that the shunt capacity should provide more than 60% of the baseline descending aortic flow and have a diameter greater than one-half of the descending aorta to be effective.

Of particular significance was the study by Svensson and colleagues[107] on the blood flow in the baboon spinal cord and its implications in aortic cross clamping. This animal was chosen because its spinal vascularity is similar to humans in that its anterior spinal artery is a continuous vessel without the occasional interruptions noted in some quadrupeds. This study indicated that in baboons, as in humans, the caliber of the anterior spinal artery is often critically narrowed where the thoracic anterior spinal artery joins the lumbar segment of this vessel at their common junction with the arteria medullaris magna. The functional implication is that the shunting of the cross-clamped aorta may help maintain an adequate flow in the lumbosacral sections of the cord but is of little help to the supply of the lower sections of the thoracic cord, owing to the marked discrepancy that usually exists between the anterior spinal artery diameters above and below the junction of the arteria medullaris magna.

In accordance with the hemodynamic principles of Poiseuille's equation, the resistance to blood flow upward from the arteria medullaris magna junction was more than 50 times greater than the flow resistance downward into the lumbosacral anterior spinal artery in the baboon. Because a series of direct measurements showed that this discrepancy in the anterior spinal artery diameters was even greater in humans, Svensson and colleagues[107] concluded that even the lowest segments of the thoracic cord were dependent on a blood flow from the superior end of the thoracic anterior spinal artery despite the shunting.

Intrinsic Venous Drainage of the Spinal Cord

Compared with the arterial anatomy, the structural and functional aspects of the venous drainage of the spinal cord have been relatively neglected. In contrast to other organ systems in which the equivalent orders of veins and arteries tend to course in a common vascular bundle, the veins of the central nervous system are generally less numerous than the arteries, they are larger than their corresponding efferent vessels, the larger branches may not show a pattern concurrent with the arterial distribution, and they are not accompanied by lymphatics.

The internal substance of the dorsal half of the cord drains by a centrifugal arrangement of intrinsic vessels that are tributaries, by way of a venous vasa corona, to a large median dorsal longitudinal spinal vein; the ventral half sends tributaries to sulcal veins that empty into a large median ventral longitudinal vein that runs parallel to the anterior spinal artery. Both of these longitudinal vessels are circumferentially connected by a prominent venous vasa corona. This entire system drains into the epidural venous plexus by medullary (previously called *radicular*) veins that are as infrequent in their distribution as the medullary arteries.[108] The proximal sections of the spinal nerve roots drain centripetally into the vasa corona and longitudinal veins of the cord and then to the epidural system via the medullary veins.

Vascularization of the Spinal Nerve Roots

Although it has been generally recognized that much of the pain consequent to degenerative changes in the spinal motion segment is associated with compression or tension on the spinal nerve roots, the mechanisms that initiate the actual nerve discharge have remained obscure. Because experimental studies on peripheral nerves and observations on numerous cases of neurogenic claudication have suggested that much of the pain may have a neuroischemic basis, investigations were undertaken to determine the nature of the intrinsic vascularity of the spinal nerve root and its response to localized compression or tension. The nerve roots had long been regarded as part of the peripheral nervous system and were viewed as histologically and vascularly similar to peripheral nerves. Consequently, research on the latter was often uncritically extrapolated to apply to the nerve roots.

The very long roots of the lumbosacral spinal nerves seemed to be particularly vulnerable because their vascularity was initially believed to be supplied only from their distal ends without the access to the frequent collateral support that is characteristic of peripheral nerves. Because the nerve root fasciculi do not have a strong connective tissue support, it also seemed that the fine vascularity they possessed would be at risk from the repeated tension and relaxation resulting from the flexion and extension of the spine. Parke and colleagues[109] and Parke and Watanabe[110] showed by vascular injection that the roots receive their arterial supply from both ends (Fig. 2.41; see Fig. 2.36), however, a fact physiologically confirmed by Yamamoto.[111]

The existence of many redundant coils along the branches of the true radicular arteries ameliorates the stresses that would result from the interfascicular movements that accompany the repeated stretch and relaxation. A significant finding was the occurrence of numerous, relatively large arteriovenous anastomoses throughout the length of the root (Fig. 2.42).

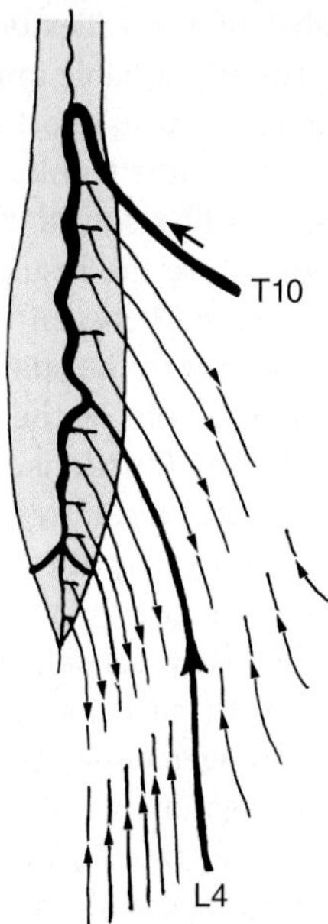

FIG. 2.41 Schema indicating directions of normal blood flow in cauda equina. The anterior spinal artery of the lumbosacral part of the cord is supplied by medullary arteries and supplies 75% at the cord substance and upper parts of the cauda equina via the proximal radicular arteries. This accounts for enlargement of the anterior spinal artery in the lumbosacral region.

These vascular cross connections apparently allow blood flow to be maintained in sections of the root above and below a point of compression. Of particular significance to root nutrition is the work of Rydevik and colleagues[111a] who, using isotopically labeled methylglucose, showed that approximately 50% of the root nutrition is derived from the ambient cerebrospinal fluid; this necessitates a gauzelike architecture of the radicular pia-arachnoid sheath (Fig. 2.43; see Fig. 2.42B).

A study by Watanabe and Parke[112,113] of chronically compressed roots indicated that the compressed segment is most likely metabolically deprived. It has been suggested that radicular pain is related to root ischemia because a reduction of oxygen intake in patients with neurogenic claudication exacerbates the symptoms.[114] The arterial side of the vasa radiculorum seems to be well compensated, however, and maintains a continuity despite severe chronic compression. Further study has indicated that the venous side of the radiculomedullary circulation is more vulnerable.[113] Because the roots are part of the central nervous system, the relationships of the arteries to the veins resemble those of the brain more than those of peripheral nerves. The radicular veins do not follow the arterial pattern. They are fewer in number and run a separate and usually deeper (more central) course. Being thin-walled, they are more liable to the spatial restrictions imposed by degenerative changes in the dimensions of the spinal canal and intervertebral foramina and show complete interruption in the chronically compressed root. The metabolically deprived, or inflamed, nerve root becomes hypersensitive to any mechanical deformation, and any additional insult to such a nerve may initiate ectopic impulses that produce pain.

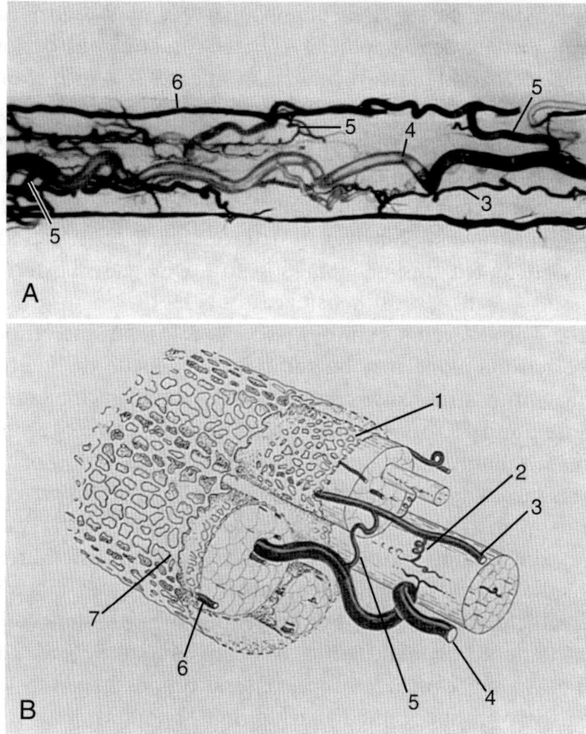

FIG. 2.42 (A) Low-power (×20) transillumination photomicrograph of midsection from part of L4 nerve root treated with hydrogen peroxide after vascular injection with latex–India ink but before clearing in a solution of tributyl-tricresyl phosphates. The peroxidases within the residual blood elements inflated the radicular veins (*4*) to provide a temporary contrast medium. Note the frequency of the large arteriovenous anastomoses (*5*) that permitted the latex–India ink to enter the veins. (B) Compilation showing structure of a typical lumbosacral nerve root derived from data obtained by injection studies and scanning electron microscopy (see Fig. 2.38). The gauzelike pia-arachnoid membranes permit the cerebrospinal fluid to percolate into nerve tissues and assist metabolic support. Numbers in (A) and (B) are common to equivalent structures. *1*, Fascicular pia. *2*, Interfascicular and intrafascicular arteries showing compensating coils to allow interfascicular movement. *3*, Longitudinal radicular artery. *4*, Large radicular vein (does not course with arteries). *5*, Arteriovenous anastomosis. *6*, Collateral radicular artery. *7*, Gauzelike pia-arachnoid that permits percolation of cerebrospinal fluid to assist in metabolic support.

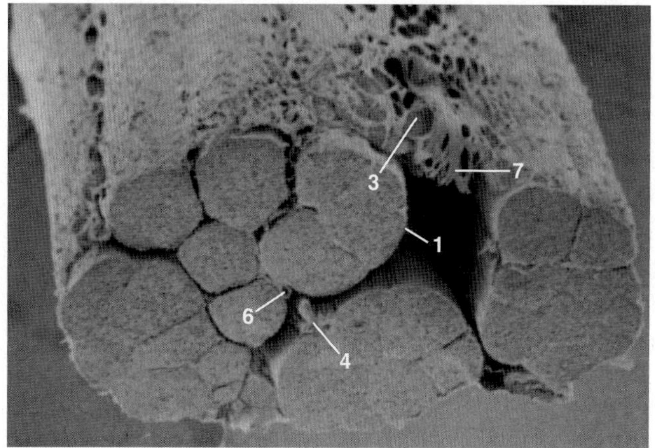

FIG. 2.43 Scanning electron photomicrograph of section of proximal part of L5 ventral nerve root. The gauzelike pia-arachnoid sheath is very evident. The numbers correspond to the structures labeled in Fig. 2.42.

Impedance of the radiculomedullary venous return can occur without topographically related venous constriction. The exacerbation of neurogenic pain in cases in which spinal stenosis has been associated with venous hypertension has been recorded by clinical investigators. LaBan[115] and LaBan and Wesolowski[116] noted that patients with diminished right-sided heart compliance and spinal stenosis may eventually exhibit neurogenic pain even in static or recumbent situations. They attributed this phenomenon to an increased external pressure on the already sensitized roots by the engorgement of the epidural venous sinuses (see Fig. 2.35), but the venous hypertension alone may be sufficient to impede the venous return from an already compromised radicular circulation. Madsen and Heros[117] showed that "arterialization" of spinal veins by abnormal arteriovenous shunts in the region of the conus medullaris exacerbates the neurogenic pain in patients with spinal stenosis. Their hypothesis suggested that a variable combination of increased mechanical constriction by dilated epidural veins and the direct increased resistance to the radicular circulation by the venous hypertension could contribute to the elicitation of pain. Aboulker and colleagues[118] also concluded that epidural venous hypertension alone may produce radicular symptoms or cord symptoms or both without adjunctive stenotic compression.

If the intrinsic circulation of the nerve root is impeded in either its arterial input or its venous outflow, the net effect seems to be the same: a neuroischemia of the compressed root segment that may enhance the generation of ectopic nerve impulses. A phenomenon that could be related to radicular venous stasis is the swelling of the disc-distorted nerve root that Takata and colleagues[119] showed in CT myelograms. This phenomenon is difficult to explain because extravasated fluids in the root tissues should have free access to the surrounding cerebrospinal fluid. Nevertheless, the fluid balance of the root tissues seems to be altered, particularly in the segment proximal to the level of the offending disc. The intricacies of the hemodynamic relationships responsible for this change remain unknown.

The role of the ubiquitous arteriovenous anastomosis in autoregulation of the intrinsic radicular vasculature also offers a fertile field for clinical investigations. Because these vascular shunts are mostly without contractile elements but seem instead to control their lumina by the thickening response of an epithelioid endothelium, they probably react to chemical changes in the blood within their lumina and can offer an immediate local reflex to alterations in the nerve root metabolism.

Functional Anatomy of the Spine

The biomechanics of the spine is a very complex and extensive subject. A comprehensive discussion is beyond the scope of this chapter, so the reader is directed to the work of White and Panjabi,[120] which is generally regarded as the major book in this field. Because an appreciation of the essential functional relationships of the spinal components does enhance an understanding of their anatomy, however, a brief overview follows.

The spine is capable of ventroflexion, extension, lateral flexion, and rotation. This remarkable universal mobility may seem at odds with the fact that its most essential function is to provide a firm support for the trunk and appendages. The apparent contradiction may be resolved when one realizes that the total ranges of motion are the result of a summation of limited movements permitted between the individual vertebrae and that the total length of the spine changes very little during its movements. The role of the musculature in the performance of the supportive functions cannot be minimized, as the disastrous scolioses that result from their unilateral loss in a few motor segment units may attest.

The degree and combination of the individual types of motion described earlier vary considerably in the different vertebral regions. Although all subaxial-presacral vertebrae are united in a tripod arrangement consisting of the intervertebral disc and the two zygapophyseal articulations, the relative size and shape of the former and the articular planes of the latter determine the range and types of motion that an individual set of intervertebral articulations contributes to the total mobility of the spine. In general, flexion is the most pronounced movement of the vertebral column as a whole. It requires an anterior compression of the intervertebral disc and a gliding separation of the articular facets, in which the inferior set of an individual vertebra tends to move upward and forward over the opposing superior set of the adjacent inferior vertebra. The movement is checked mainly by the posterior ligaments and epaxial muscles.

Extension tends to be a more limited motion, producing posterior compression of the disc, with the inferior articular process gliding posteriorly and downward over the superior set below. It is checked by the anterior longitudinal ligament and all ventral muscles that directly or indirectly flex the spine. Also, the laminae and spinous processes may sharply limit extension. Lateral flexion is accompanied by some degree of rotation. It involves a rocking of the bodies on their discs, with a sliding separation of the diarthroses on the convex side and an overriding of the diarthroses related to the concavity. The rotational component brings the anterior surface of the bodies toward the convexity of the flexure and the spinous processes toward its concavity. This phenomenon is well illustrated in a dried preparation of a scoliotic spine. Lateral flexion is checked by the intertransverse ligaments and the extensions of the ribs or their costal homologues.

Pure rotation is directly proportional to the relative thickness of the intervertebral disc and is mainly limited by the geometry of the planes of the diarthrodial surfaces. Although the architecture of the disc permits limited rotation between the bodies, it also serves to check this movement by its resistance to compression. The consecutive layers of the anulus fibrosus have their fibers arranged in an alternating helical fashion, and rotation in either direction can be accompanied only by increasing the angularity of the opposing fibers to the horizontal, which requires compression of the disc.

The entire vertebral column rotates approximately 90 degrees to either side of the sagittal plane, but most of this traversion is accomplished in the cervical and thoracic sections. It flexes nearly the same amount, using primarily the cervical and thoracic regions. Approximately 90 degrees of extension is permitted by the cervical and lumbar regions, whereas lateral flexion with rotation is allowed to 60 degrees to both sides, again primarily by the cervical and lumbar areas.

Specific Regional Considerations

The atlanto-occipital joints mostly permit flexion and extension with a limited lateral action, all being checked by the suboccipital musculature and the atlanto-occipital ligaments. The atlantoaxial articulations allow only rotation, the pivoted joint being stabilized and checked by the alar ligaments and the ligaments forming the capsules of the atlantoaxial diarthroses.

One-half of the rotational mobility of the entire cervical region takes place between the atlas and the axis, and the remainder is distributed among the joints of the subaxial vertebrae. The atlanto-occipital joint accounts for approximately half of the cervical flexion. The remaining 50% is not evenly distributed among the cervical vertebrae but is greater in the upper section.

The subaxial part of the cervical region shows the ranges of motion that are the most free of all the presacral vertebrae. The discs are quite thick in relation to the heights of the vertebral bodies and contribute about one-fourth of the height of this part of the column. In addition, a sagittal section shows the middle part of the cervical disc to be lenticular, so that the anteroinferior lips of the bodies are more capable of sliding slightly forward and overriding one another. The range of spinal flexion is greatest in the cervical region, and although the posterior nuchal ligaments and muscles may tend to resist this motion, it is ultimately checked by the chin coming to rest on the chest.

The cervical spine is normally carried in a moderately extended position and shows a median variation of 91 degrees between extension and flexion. Extension is checked by the anterior longitudinal ligament and the combined resistances of the anterior cervical musculature, fascia, and visceral structures, all three of which may be traumatized in hyperextension injuries.

Cervical lateral flexion is quite limited by the articular pillars and the intertransverse ligaments, and most lateral motion involves considerable rotation. The nearly horizontal position of the planes of the cervical articular facets provides good supportive strength to the articular pillars but increases the lateral rigidity, so that hyperextension injuries may be more disastrous if the head is rotated at the time of impact from the rear.

The mobility of the thoracic region is also not uniform throughout its length. Although the upper segments resemble the cervical vertebrae with respect to the size of the bodies and the discs, the ribs attached to the sternum greatly impair the ranges of motion. The circumferential arc of the plane of the articular facets shows that rotation is the movement least restricted by these structures.

Flexion and extension become freer in the lower thoracic region, where the discs and vertebral bodies progressively increase in size and the more mobile and less restrictive they become. The last few thoracic vertebrae are transitional with respect to the surfaces of the articular facets. These begin to turn more toward the sagittal plane and tend to limit rotation and permit greater extension.

The articulations of the lumbar region permit ventroflexion, lateral flexion, and extension, but the facets of the synovial joints lie in a ventromedial to dorsolateral plane that virtually locks them against rotation. This lumbar nonrotatory rigidity is a feature shared with most mammals and achieves its greatest manifestation in certain quadrupeds in which the inferior articulation fits like a cylindric tenon into the semicircular mortise of the corresponding superior process of the vertebra below. It provides a gliding action that permits the neural arches to separate or approximate each other only during extension and flexion. The morphology of the joints can be well appreciated in an appropriate cut of loin chop or T-bone steak.

The synovial articulations at the lumbosacral junctions are unique. In contrast to the more superior lumbar joints, the facets of the inferior articulating processes of the fifth lumbar vertebra face forward and slightly downward, to engage the reciprocally corresponding articular processes of the sacrum. Because of the position of these joint surfaces, a certain amount of rotation should be possible between the fifth lumbar segment and the sacrum, but the presence of the strong iliolumbar ligaments quite likely restricts much motion of this type.

The most essential function of the synovial lumbosacral articulations involves their role as buttresses against the forward and downward displacement of the fifth lumbar vertebra in relation to the sacrum. When one considers that each region of the spine has its own characteristic curvature, the tracing of the vertical line indicating the center of gravity shows that it intersects the column through the bodies of the transitional vertebrae. The normal cervical lordosis places most of the cervical vertebrae anterior to the center of gravity, and the compensating thoracic kyphosis places the thoracic vertebrae posterior to the center of gravity. The lumbar lordosis brings the middle lumbar vertebrae anterior to the line. The transitional vertebrae between each region intersect the center of gravity and seem to be the most unstable regions of the spine; this is emphasized by the fact that disc problems and fractures most frequently occur in the transitional vertebrae.

Because the sacrovertebral angle produces the most abrupt change of direction in the column, and the center of gravity, which passes through the fifth lumbar body, falls anterior to the sacrum, there is a marked tendency for the thick, wedge-shaped fifth lumbar disc to give way to the shearing vector that the lumbosacral angularity produces. The resulting condition, spondylolisthesis, most frequently reveals a deficiency in the laminae (spondylolysis) that fails to anchor the fifth vertebral body to the sacrum and allows its forward displacement. There has been considerable discussion as to whether spondylolysis is congenital or acquired, but the spondylolisthesis seldom occurs without the laminar deficiencies as a preceding condition.

Biomechanics of the Intervertebral Disc

It is axiomatic in mechanical engineering that a well-designed machine automatically reveals its function through the analysis of its structure. There are few instances in biologic circumstances in which this statement is more applicable than in the case of the intervertebral disc. Even when the disc is simply divided with a knife and examined grossly, it is apparent that one is dealing with an organ that is remarkably constructed simultaneously to alleviate shock and transmit forces from every conceivable combination of vectors. This appreciation of the functional competency of the disc increases as its structure is analyzed at the finer levels of organization.

The internal composition of the disc has evolved to withstand great stresses through the liquid and elastic properties of nucleus and anulus acting in combination. The nucleus is distorted by compression forces, but being liquid it is in itself incompressible. It serves to receive primarily vertical forces from the vertebral bodies and redistribute them radially in a horizontal plane. It is the distortion of the anulus by the internal pressure of the nucleus that gives the disc its compressibility, and its resilience makes possible the recovery from pressure.

Were the nucleus pulposus simply a cavity filled with water, it would momentarily act in the same capacity, but the ability to maintain the appropriate quantity of fluid during the continual compression and recovery cycle would be lacking. This ability to absorb and retain relatively large amounts of water is the unique property of the living tissue of the nucleus.[121] The essential compound involved in this process is a protein-polysaccharide gel, which through a high imbibition pressure binds nearly nine times its volume of water. It is apparent that the hydrophilia is not a form of biochemical bonding because a quantity of water can be expressed from the nucleus by prolonged mechanical pressure. This accounts for the diurnal decrease in the total length of the spine and its recovery in the supine position at night.

The anulus must receive the ultimate effects of most forces transmitted from one vertebral body to another. Because the major loading of the intervertebral disc is in the form of vertical compression, it may seem paradoxical that the anulus is best constructed to resist tension, but the nucleus transforms the vertical thrust into a radial pressure that is resisted by the tensile properties of the lamellae. Although the basic plan of alternating bands of fibers is one of the obvious sources of the tensile strength of the anulus, this arrangement is not uniform with respect to the directions of the fibers or the degrees of resistance and resilience encountered throughout the anulus. The fibers generally become longer, and the angle of their spiral course becomes more horizontal near the circumference of the disc because it is here that the shearing stresses of vertebral torsions would be most effective. Experimental analysis has also shown that various parts of the anulus do not respond equally to the same degree of tension, and the discrepancies were related to the plane of section and the location of the sample.[122] The anulus proved to have the greatest resistance and the greatest recovery in horizontal sections of the peripheral lamellae, whereas vertical and more medial sections were more distensible.

Because the spine acts as a flexible boom to the guidewire actions of the erector spinae muscles, it is essentially the fulcrum of a lever system of the first class, in which the loading has a considerable mechanical advantage. Pure vector analysis has indicated that a theoretical pressure of approximately three-fourths of a ton could be applied to a disc when 100 lb is lifted by the hands,[21] but this is considerably in excess of the actual pressures achieved. Increased intrathoracic and intra-abdominal pressures alleviate much of the fulcrum compression of the discs by effectively counteracting the load of the anterior lever arm.

The actual pressure variations occurring with postural changes have been recorded by inserting transducers into the third lumbar disc.[123,124] This procedure indicated that the internal disc pressure increases from approximately 100 kg in a standing position with the spine erect to 150 kg when the trunk is bent forward and to 220 kg when a 70-kg man lifts a 50-kg weight. It was particularly revealing that the pressure showed a considerable increase when the equivalent maneuvers were repeated in a sitting position, and the weight lifting ultimately created a pressure of 300 kg on the third lumbar disc.

The disc is also "preloaded." The inherent tensions of the intervertebral ligaments and the anulus exert a pressure of about 15 kg because this weight is required to restore the original thickness of the disc after the ligaments have been divided.[110] From a comparative standpoint, this preloading probably offers increased stability to the spine as a functional flexible rod. One is almost induced unconsciously to use teleologic thinking in terms of the vertical thrust resistance when regarding the structure of the disc. In perspective, however, the intervertebral disc shows a consistent morphology in all mammals, yet humans are the only species that truly stand erect. Although analysis of muscular action would most likely show that all mammalian discs must dissipate and transfer axial thrusts, the preloading would enhance the "beam strength" that is obviously necessary in the vertebral column of quadrupeds.

Acknowledgments

The authors acknowledge Wesley W. Parke, PhD (deceased), an original author of this chapter in previous editions who was responsible for much of the critical information included in this work.

The vascular studies presented in this chapter were supported by National Institutes of Health research grant HL-14035.

KEY REFERENCES

1. Bajwa NS, Toy JO, Ahn NU. L5 pedicle length is increased in subjects with spondylolysis: an anatomic study of 1072 cadavers. *Clin Orthop Relat Res*. 2012;470(11):3202-3206.
2. Goldstein RY, Sunde CD, Assaad P, et al. Location of the vertebral artery at C1 in children: how far out laterally can one safely dissect? *J Bone Joint Surg Am*. 2014;96(18):1552-1556.

3. Grunhagen T, Shirazi-Adl A, Fairbank JC, Urban JP. Intervertebral disk nutrition: a review of factors influencing concentrations of nutrients and metabolites. *Orthop Clin North Am.* 2011;42(4):465-477, vii.
4. Ibrahim DA, Myung KS, Skaggs DL. Ten percent of patients with adolescent idiopathic scoliosis have variations in the number of thoracic or lumbar vertebrae. *J Bone Joint Surg Am.* 2013;95(9):828-833.
5. Lehman RA Jr, Kang DG, Lenke LG, Gaume RE, Paik H. The ventral lamina and superior facet rule: a morphometric analysis for an ideal thoracic pedicle screw starting point. *Spine J.* 2014;14(1):137-144.
6. Magro E, Gentric JC, Talagas M, et al. Venous organization in the transverse foramen: dissection, histology, and magnetic resonance imaging. *J Neurosurg.* 2015;123(1):118-125.
7. Osmotherly PG, Rivett DA, Mercer SR. Revisiting the clinical anatomy of the alar ligaments. *Eur Spine J.* 2013;22(1):60-64.
8. Trimba R, Spivak JM, Bendo JA. Conjoined nerve roots of the lumbar spine. *Spine J.* 2012;12(6):515-524.
9. Tubbs RS, Wellons JC 3rd, Banks J, Blount JP, Oakes WJ. Quantitative anatomy of the transverse ligament tubercles. *J Neurosurg.* 2002;97(3 suppl):343-345.
10. Zhong W, Driscoll SJ, Wu M, et al. In vivo morphological features of human lumbar discs. *Medicine (Baltimore).* 2014;93(28):e333.

REFERENCES

1. Francis WR, Fielding JW. Traumatic spondylolisthesis of the axis. *Orthop Clin North Am.* 1978;9:1011-1027.
2. McCulloch JA, Transfeldt EE. *Macnab's Backache.* Baltimore: Williams & Wilkins; 1997.
3. Weiner BK, Walker M, Wiley W, et al. The lateral buttress: an anatomic feature of the lumbar pars interarticularis. *Spine.* 2002;27:E385-E387.
4. Bajwa NS, Toy JO, Ahn NU. L5 pedicle length is increased in subjects with spondylolysis: an anatomic study of 1072 cadavers. *Clin Orthop Relat Res.* 2012;470(11):3202-3206.
5. Ibrahim DA, Myung KS, Skaggs DL. Ten percent of patients with adolescent idiopathic scoliosis have variations in the number of thoracic or lumbar vertebrae. *J Bone Joint Surg Am.* 2013;95(9):828-833.
6. An HS, Wise JJ, Xu R. Anatomy of the cervicothoracic junction: a study of cadaveric dissection, cryomicrotomy and magnetic resonance imaging. *J Spinal Disord.* 1999;12:519-525.
7. Ebraheim NA, Xu R, Knight T, et al. Morphometric evaluation of lower cervical pedicle and its projection. *Spine.* 1997;22:1-6.
8. Pait TG, McAllister PV, Kaufman HH. Quadrant anatomy of the articular pillars (lateral cervical mass) of the cervical spine. *J Neurosurg.* 1995;82:1011-1014.
9. Xu R, Burgar A, Ebraheim NA, et al. The quantitative anatomy of the laminas of the spine. *Spine.* 1999;24:107-113.
10. Goldstein RY, Sunde CD, Assaad P, et al. Location of the vertebral artery at C1 in children: how far out laterally can one safely dissect? *J Bone Joint Surg Am.* 2014;96(18):1552-1556.
11. Magro E, Gentric JC, Talagas M, et al. Venous organization in the transverse foramen: dissection, histology, and magnetic resonance imaging. *J Neurosurg.* 2015;123(1):118-125.
12. Tubbs RS, Wellons JC 3rd, Banks J, Blount JP, Oakes WJ. Quantitative anatomy of the transverse ligament tubercles. *J Neurosurg.* 2002;97(3 suppl):343-345.
13. Osmotherly PG, Rivett DA, Mercer SR. Revisiting the clinical anatomy of the alar ligaments. *Eur Spine J.* 2013;22(1):60-64.
14. Chaynes P, Sol JC, Vaysse P, et al. Vertebral pedicle anatomy in relation to pedicle screw fixation: a cadaver study. *Spine.* 2001;23:85-90.
15. Cinotti G, Gumina S, Ripani M, et al. Pedicle instrumentation in the thoracic spine: a morphometric and cadaveric study for placement of screws. *Spine.* 1999;24:114-119.
16. Scoles PV, Linton AE, Latimer B, et al. Vertebral body and posterior element morphology: the normal spine in middle life. *Spine.* 1988;13:1082-1086.
17. Lehman RA Jr, Kang DG, Lenke LG, Gaume RE, Paik H. The ventral lamina and superior facet rule: a morphometric analysis for an ideal thoracic pedicle screw starting point. *Spine J.* 2014;14(1):137-144.
18. Olszewski AD, Yaszemski MJ, White AA. The anatomy of the human lumbar ligamentum flavum: new observations and their surgical implications. *Spine.* 1996;21:2307-2312.
19. von Luschka H. *Die Halbgelenke des Menschlichen Korpers.* Berlin: Karpess; 1858.
20. Beadle OA. *The Intervertebral Discs.* Special Report No. 160. London: Medical Research Council; 1931:6-9.
21. Bradford DL, Spurling RG. *The Intervertebral Disc.* Springfield, IL: Charles C Thomas; 1945.
22. Humzah MD, Soames RW. Human intervertebral disc: structure and function. *Anat Rec.* 1988;229:337-356.
23. Bick EM. The osteohistology of the normal human vertebra. *J Mt Sinai Hosp N Y.* 1952;19:490-527.
24. Aeby C. Die Alterverschiedenheiten der menschlichen Wirbelsaule. *Arch Anat Physiol (Anat Abst).* 1879;10:77.
25. Zhong W, Driscoll SJ, Wu M, et al. In vivo morphological features of human lumbar discs. *Medicine (Baltimore).* 2014;93(28):e333.
26. Dommissee G. Morphological aspects of the lumbar spine and lumbosacral regions. *Orthop Clin North Am.* 1975;6:163-175.
27. Wiltse LL. Anatomy of the extradural compartments of the lumbar spinal canal: peridural membrane and circumneural sheath. *Radiol Clin North Am.* 2000;38:1177-1206.
28. Ugur HC, Attar A, Uz A, et al. Surgical anatomic evaluation of the cervical pedicle and adjacent neural structures. *Neurosurgery.* 2000;47:1162-1168.
29. Ugur HC, Attar A, Uz A, et al. Thoracic pedicle: surgical anatomic evaluation and relations. *J Spinal Disord.* 2001;14:39-45.
30. Ebraheim NA, Xu R, Darwich M, et al. Anatomic relations between the lumbar pedicle and the adjacent neural structures. *Spine.* 1997;15:2338-2341.
31. Hogan Q, Toth J. Anatomy of the soft tissues of the spinal canal. *Reg Anesth Pain Med.* 1999;24:303-310.
32. Kobrine AI, Doyle DF, Rizzoli HV. Spinal cord blood flow as affected by changes in systemic arterial blood pressure. *J Neurosurg.* 1976;44:12-15.
33. Golub GS, Silverman B. Transforaminal ligaments of the lumbar spine. *J Bone Joint Surg Am.* 1969;51:947-956.
34. Park HK, Rudrappa S, Dujovny M, et al. Intervertebral foraminal ligaments of the lumbar spine: anatomy and biomechanics. *Childs Nerv Syst.* 2001;4-5:275-282.
35. Grimes PF, Massie JB, Garfin SR. Anatomic and biomechanical analysis of the lower lumbar foraminal ligaments. *Spine.* 2000;25:2009-2014.
36. Alleyne CH, Cawley CM, Barrow DL, et al. Microsurgical anatomy of the dorsal cervical nerve roots and the cervical dorsal root ganglion/ventral root complexes. *Surg Neurol.* 1998;50:213-218.

37. Kadish LJ, Simmons EH. Anomalies of the lumbosacral nerve roots. *J Bone Joint Surg Br.* 1984;66:411-416.
38. Trimba R, Spivak JM, Bendo JA. Conjoined nerve roots of the lumbar spine. *Spine J.* 2012;12(6):515-524.
39. Kikuchi S, Hasue M. Anatomic features of the furcal nerve and its clinical significance. *Spine.* 1986;11:1002-1007.
40. Piacsecka-Kacperska A, Gladykowska-Rzeczycka J. The sacral plexus in primates. *Folia Morphol (Warsz).* 1972;31:21-31.
41. Parke WW, Watanabe R. Lumbosacral intersegmental epispinal axons and ectopic ventral nerve rootlets. *J Neurosurg.* 1987;67:269-277.
42. Hasue M, Kunogi J, Konno S, et al. Classification by position of dorsal root ganglia in the lumbosacral region. *Spine.* 1989;14:1261-1264.
43. Kikuchi S, Hasue M. Combined contrast studies in lumbar spine diseases. *Spine.* 1988;13:1327-1331.
44. Bogduk N, Tynan W, Wilson AS. The nerve supply to the human lumbar intervertebral disc. *J Anat.* 1981;132:39-56.
45. Bogduk N, Windsor M, Inglis A. The innervation of the cervical intervertebral discs. *Spine.* 1988;13:2-8.
46. Hirsch C. Studies on mechanism of low back pain. *Acta Orthop Scand.* 1953;22:184-231.
47. Jung A, Brunschwig A. Recherches histologiques sur l'innervation des articulations et des corps vertebreaux. *Presse Med.* 1932;40:316-317.
48. Larmon AW. An anatomic study of the lumbosacral region in relation to low back pain and sciatica. *Ann Surg.* 1944;119:892.
49. Malinsky J. The ontogenetic development of nerve terminations in the intervertebral discs of man. *Acta Anat (Basel).* 1959;38:96-113.
50. Nade S, Bell S, Wyke BD. The innervation of the lumbar spine joints and its significance. *J Bone Joint Surg Br.* 1980;62:225-261.
51. Wiberg G. Back pain in relation to nerve supply of intervertebral disc. *Acta Orthop Scand.* 1949;19:211-221.
52. Parke WW. Applied anatomy of the spine. In: Rothman RH, Simeone FA, eds. *The Spine.* Philadelphia: WB Saunders; 1982:18-51.
53. Groen GJ, Baljet B, Drukker J. The nerves and nerve plexuses of the human vertebral column. *Am J Anat.* 1990;188:282-296.
54. Pedersen HE, Blunck CFJ, Gardner E. The anatomy of the lumbosacral posterior rami and meningeal branches of spinal nerves (sinuvertebral nerves). *J Bone Joint Surg Am.* 1956;38:377-391.
55. Hirsch C, Inglemark B, Miller M. The anatomical basis for low back pain. *Acta Orthop Scand.* 1963;33:1-17.
56. McCouch GP, During ID, Ling TH. Location of receptors for tonic reflexes. *J Neurophysiol.* 1951;14:191-195.
57. Stilwell DL. The nerve supply of the vertebral column and its associated structures in the monkey. *Anat Rec.* 1956;125:139-169.
58. Yoshizawa H, O'Brien JP, Thomas-Smith W, et al. The neuropathology of intervertebral discs removed for low back pain. *J Pathol.* 1980;132:95-104.
59. Kimmel DL. Innervation of the spinal dura and the dura of the posterior cranial fossa. *Neurology.* 1986;11:800-809.
60. Cyriax J. Dural pain. *Lancet.* 1978;1:919-921.
61. Groen GJ, Baljet B, Drukker J. The innervation of the spinal dura mater: anatomy and clinical implications. *Acta Neurochir (Wien).* 1988;92:39-46.
62. Parke WW, Watanabe R. Adhesions of the ventral lumbar dura: an adjunct source of discogenic pain? *Spine.* 1990;15:300-303.
63. Blikra G. Intradural herniated lumbar disc. *J Neurosurg.* 1969;31:676-679.
64. Junghanns H. Der Lumboscralwinkel. *Dtsch Z Chit.* 1929;213:332.
65. Schmorl G, Junghanns H. *The Human Spine in Health and Disease.* New York: Grune & Stratton; 1959.
66. DePalma AF, Rothman RH. *The Intervertebral Disc.* Philadelphia: WB Saunders; 1970.
67. Brown MD. *The Pathophysiology of the Intervertebral Disc: Anatomical, Physiological and Biomedical Considerations.* Philadelphia: Jefferson Medical College; 1969.
68. Maroudas A. Nutrition and metabolism of the intervertebral disc. In: Ghosh P, ed. *The Biology of the Intervertebral Disc.* Boca Raton, FL: CRC Press; 1988.
69. Grunhagen T, Shirazi-Adl A, Fairbank JC, Urban JP. Intervertebral disk nutrition: a review of factors influencing concentrations of nutrients and metabolites. *Orthop Clin North Am.* 2011;42(4):465-477, vii.
70. Holm S, Maroudas A, Urban JPG, et al. Nutrition of the intervertebral disc: an in vivo study of solute transport. *Clin Orthop.* 1977;129:104-114.
71. Holm S, Maroudas A, Urban JPG, et al. Nutrition of the intervertebral disc: solute transport and metabolism. *Connect Tissue Res.* 1981;8:101-110.
72. Maroudas A, Nachemson A, Stockwell RA, et al. Factors involved in the nutrition of human lumbar intervertebral disc: cellularity and diffusion of glucose in vitro. *J Anat.* 1975;120:113-130.
73. Ferguson WP. Some observations on the circulation in fetal and infant spines. *J Bone Joint Surg.* 1950;32:640-645.
74. Willis TA. Nutrient arteries of the vertebral bodies. *J Bone Joint Surg.* 1949;31:538-541.
75. Crock HV, Yoshizawa H. *The Blood Supply of the Vertebral Column and Spinal Cord in Man.* New York: Springer-Verlag; 1977.
76. Milen MT, Bloom DA, Culligan J, et al. Albert Adamkiewicz (1850-1921)—his artery and its significance for the retroperitoneal surgeon. *World J Urol.* 1999;17:168-170.
77. Parke WW. The vascular relations of the upper cervical vertebrae. *Orthop Clin North Am.* 1978;9:879-889.
78. Schiff DCM, Parke WW. The arterial supply of the odontoid process. *Anat Rec.* 1972;172:399-400.
79. Jasani V, Jaffray D. The anatomy of the iliolumbar vein: a cadaver study. *J Bone Joint Surg Br.* 2002;84:1046-1049.
80. Kaisary AV, Smith P. Spinal cord ischemia after ligation of both internal iliac arteries during radical cystoprostectomy. *Urology.* 1985;25:395-397.
81. Breschet G. *Essai sur les Veines der Rachis.* Paris: Mequigon-Morvith; 1819.
82. Batson OV. The function of the vertebral veins and their role in the spread of metastases. *Am Surg.* 1940;112:138-145.
83. Clemens HJ. *Die Venesysteme der Menschlichen Wirbelsaule.* Berlin: Walter de Gruyter; 1961.
84. Chaynes P, Verdie JC, Moscovici J, et al. Microsurgical anatomy of the internal vertebral venous plexuses. *Surg Radiol Anat.* 1998;20:47-51.
85. Parke WW, Valsamis MP. The ampulloglomerular organ: an unusual neurovascular complex in the suboccipital region. *Anat Rec.* 1967;159:193-198.
86. Parke WW, Rizzoli HV, Brown MD. The pharyngovertebral veins: an anatomic rationale for Grisel's syndrome. *J Bone Joint Surg Am.* 1984;66:568-574.

87. Wetzel FT, LaRocca H. Grisel's syndrome: a review. *Clin Orthop*. 1989;240:141-152.
88. Corbib JL. *Anatomie et Pathologie Arterielles de la Moelle*. Paris: Masson et Cie; 1961:787-796.
89. Brewer LA, Fosburg RG, Mulder GA, et al. Spinal cord complications following surgery for coarctation of the aorta. *J Thorac Cardiovasc Surg*. 1972;64:368-379.
90. Lazorthes G, Gouaze A, Zadeh JO, et al. Arterial vascularization of the spinal cord. *J Neurosurg*. 1971;35:253-262.
91. Marcus ML, Heistad DD, Ehrardt JC, et al. Regulation of total and regional spinal cord blood flow. *Circ Res*. 1977;41:128-134.
92. Parke WW, Whalen JL, Bunger PC, et al. Intimal musculature of the lower anterior spinal artery. *Spine*. 1995;20:2073-2079.
93. Parke WW. Correlative anatomy of cervical spondylotic myelopathy. *Spine*. 1988;13:831-837.
94. Dommissee GF. *The Arteries and Veins of the Human Spinal Cord From Birth*. Edinburgh: Churchill-Livingstone; 1975.
95. Lasjaunias P, Vallee B, Person H, et al. The lateral artery of the upper cervical spinal cord. *J Neurosurg*. 1985;63:235-241.
96. Gillilan LA. The arterial blood supply of the human spinal cord. *J Comp Neurol*. 1958;110:75-103.
97. Hassler O. Blood supply to human spinal cord. *Arch Neurol*. 1966;15:302-307.
98. Herren RY, Alexander L. Sulcal and intrinsic blood vessels of human spinal cord. *Arch Neurol Psychiatry*. 1939;41:678-683.
99. Kadyi H. *Über die Blutgefasse des menschlichen Ruckenmarkes: Nach einer im XV Bande der Denkschriften d. math-naturw. Cl. d. Akad. d. Wissensch. Krakau erschienen Morphology, aus dem Polnischen Ubersaatz vom Verfasser*. Lemberg: Grubrnowicz & Schmidt; 1889.
100. Turnbull IM, Brieg A, Hassler O. Blood supply of cervical spinal cord in man. *J Neurosurg*. 1966;24:951-965.
101. Ireland WP, Fletcher TF, Bingham C. Quantification of microvasculature in the canine spinal cord. *Anat Rec*. 1981;200:103-113.
102. Feeney JF, Watterson RL. The development of the vascular pattern within the walls of the central nervous system of the chick embryo. *J Morphol*. 1946;78:231-303.
103. Lobosky JM, Hitchon PW, Torner JC, et al. Spinal cord autoregulation in the sheep. *Curr Surg*. 1984;41:264-267.
104. Parke WW. Arteriovenous anastomoses in the spinal cord: probable role in blood flow autoregulation [abstract]. *Anat Rec*. 1989;223:87A.
105. Molina JE, Cogordon J, Einzig S, et al. Adequacy of ascending-descending aorta shunt during cross-clamping of the thoracic aorta for prevention of spinal cord injury. *J Thorac Cardiovasc Surg*. 1985;90:126-136.
106. Wadouh F, Arndt CF, Opperman E, et al. The mechanism of spinal cord injury after simple and double aortic cross-clamping. *J Thorac Cardiovasc Surg*. 1986;92:121-127.
107. Svensson LG, Rickards E, Coull A, et al. Relationship of spinal cord blood flow to vascular anatomy during thoracic aorta cross-clamping and shunting. *J Thorac Cardiovasc Surg*. 1986;91:71-78.
108. Gillilan LA. Veins of the spinal cord. *Neurology*. 1970;20:860-868.
109. Parke WW, Gammel K, Rothman RH. Arterial vascularization of the cauda equina. *J Bone Joint Surg Am*. 1981;63:53-62.
110. Parke WW, Watanabe R. The intrinsic vasculature of the lumbosacral spinal nerve roots. *Spine*. 1985;10:508-515.
111. Yamamoto H. Quantitative measurements of blood flow in cauda equina in spinal cords of monkeys by using radioactive microspheres. *J Jpn Coll Angiol*. 1982;22:35-42.
111a. Rydevik B, Holm S, Brown MD, et al. Diffusion from the cerebrospinal fluid as a nutritional pathway for spinal nerve roots. *Acta Physiol Scand*. 1990;138(2):247-248.
112. Watanabe R, Parke WW. The vascular and neural pathology of lumbosacral spinal stenosis. *J Neurosurg*. 1986;65:64-70.
113. Watanabe R, Parke WW. Structure of lumbosacral spinal nerve roots: anatomy and pathology in spinal stenosis. *J Clin Orthop Surg (Jpn)*. 1987;22:529-539.
114. Evans JG. Neurogenic intermittent claudication. *BMJ*. 1964;2:985-987.
115. LaBan MM. "Vesper's curse": night pain, the bane of Hypnos. *Arch Phys Med Rehabil*. 1984;65:501-504.
116. LaBan MM, Wesolowski DP. Night pain associated with diminished cardiopulmonary compliance. *Am J Phys Med Rehabil*. 1988;67:155-160.
117. Madsen JR, Heros RC. Spinal arteriovenous malformations and neurogenic claudication. *J Neurosurg*. 1988;68:793-797.
118. Aboulker J, Bar D, Marsault C, et al. L'hypertension veineuse intra-rachidienne par anomalies multiples du système cave: une cause majeure de souffrance médullaire. *Clin Obstet Gynecol*. 1977;103:1003-1015.
119. Takata K, Inoue S, Takashi K, et al. Swelling of the cauda equina in patients who have herniation of a lumbar disc. *J Bone Joint Surg Am*. 1988;70:361-368.
120. White A, Panjabi M. *Clinical Biomechanics of the Spine*. 2nd ed. Philadelphia: JB Lippincott; 1990.
121. Puschel J. Der Wassergehalt normaler and degenerierter Zwischenwirbelscheiben. *Beitr Pathol Anat*. 1930;84:123-130.
122. Galante JO. Tensile properties of the human lumbar annulus fibrosus. *Acta Orthop Scand*. 1967;100(suppl):1-91.
123. Nachemson A. The load on lumbar discs in different positions of the body. *Clin Orthop*. 1966;45:107-122.
124. Petter CK. Methods of measuring the pressure of intervertebral discs. *J Bone Joint Surg*. 1933;15:365.

SECTION I

CHAPTER 3 Skeletal Muscle: Architectural Design, Physiology, and Function

Samuel R. Ward
Anita Vasavada
Scott Delp
Richard L. Lieber

Spinal muscles generate movement of the spine and provide the stability needed to protect vital anatomic structures, in coordination with the rest of the neuromusculoskeletal system (vertebrae, tendons, ligaments, and the nervous system). For example, large movements of the head require appropriate muscle strength, vertebral geometry (e.g., facet joint orientation), ligament compliance, and neural control. Spinal muscles have been described as one of three subsystems (along with passive spinal column and neural control) that must work together to stabilize the spine.[1]

Spinal musculature dysfunction is hypothesized to be the cause of a variety of pathologic conditions, such as segmental instability, low back or neck pain, and degenerative disc syndromes. However, the mechanisms that relate muscle function (or dysfunction) to pathologic processes are unclear. Some factors that lead to pathologic processes may be elucidated by biomechanical analyses of spine kinematics along with the associated tissue strains and loads. Such analyses rely heavily on accurate knowledge of muscle forces, moment arms, and activation patterns to calculate loads and displacements, which is frequently unavailable for spinal muscles. Often, spinal muscles are ignored or overly simplified (e.g., modeled together as one muscle) because the anatomy of these muscles is considered too complex to represent realistically. However, the complex anatomy and architecture of spinal muscles profoundly influence their function; thus, this information must be incorporated into analyses in order to accurately predict the role of these muscles in spinal function and dysfunction.

In this chapter, an overview of skeletal muscle contractile properties is presented first. Then, a description of the important, and often neglected, principles of skeletal muscle architecture along with the ways that architecture determines muscle function are provided. In Chapter 4, specific information about the anatomy and architecture of the spinal musculature is provided, as well as information on the implications of spinal muscle anatomy and architecture for motor control, injury, and pain.

Cross-Bridge Cycle

The basic force-generating event in skeletal muscle is the cyclic formation of cross-bridges between the filamentous proteins actin and myosin. Most of our understanding of the mechanism of muscle contraction has come from excellent biochemical studies performed in the 1950s and the decades that followed.[2-4] It was during this period that methods for isolating specific muscle proteins were developed, together with methods for measuring their physicochemical and biochemical properties. In simple terms, biochemical experiments on muscle contractile proteins have shown that, during the cross-bridge cycle, actin (A) combines with myosin (M) and adenosine triphosphate (ATP) to produce force, adenosine diphosphate (ADP), and inorganic phosphate (P_i), which can be represented as a chemical reaction in this form:

$$A + M + ATP \rightarrow A + M + ADP + P_i + \text{Force} \qquad (\text{Eq. } 1)$$

It is obvious that if ATP is either not present or is rapidly depleted with the muscle cell, the number of A-M cross-bridges, and therefore force, will decrease. This is manifested in muscles as "fatigue." Importantly, many factors can cause ATP depletion and fatigue, which may predispose muscle tissue to injury.

Muscle Fiber Types

Overwhelming evidence indicates that skeletal muscle fibers are heterogeneous. In the early 1800s, it was observed that the gross appearance of different skeletal muscles ranged in color from pale white to deep red. In fact, one of the earliest classification schemes for muscle was based on color; thus, muscles were classified as "red" or "white" (Table 3.1). However, as experimental methods became more sophisticated, it became clear that numerous other differences existed between muscles. For example, certain muscles contract rapidly, whereas others contract more slowly; certain muscles maintain force for a

TABLE 3.1 Fiber Type Classification Schemes

Basis for Scheme	FIBER TYPE SPECTRUM			Reference
Metabolic	SO	FOG	FG	Peter et al., 1972[39]
Morphology and physiology	Slow red	Fast white	Fast white	Ranvier, 1873[40]
Z-line width	Red	Intermediate	White	Gauthier, 1969[41]
Histochemistry	III	II	I	Romanul, 1964[42]
Histochemistry	Type 1	Type 2A	Type 2B	Brooke and Kaiser, 1972[43]
M-band bridging pattern	Five bridges	Three inner, two faint outer bridges	Three bridges	Sjöström et al. 1982[44]
Immunohistochemistry	Type 1	Types 2A and 2X	Type 2B	Schiaffino et al., 1989[45]
Gene sequencing	Type 1	Types 2A and 2X	Type 2B	Schiaffino and Reggiani, 1993[46]

FG, fast glycolytic; FOG, fast oxidative glycolytic; SO, slow oxidative.

long period of time, whereas others fatigue rapidly; and certain muscles generate large forces, while others generate small forces. These functional properties led to descriptions of muscle as "fast twitch" or "slow twitch," and "fatigable" or "nonfatigable." In addition, with the advent of light microscopy and histochemistry, it became possible to classify individual fibers based on their appearance following a particular staining protocol. Unfortunately, many of these classification schemes did not correlate simply with muscle color. In fact, many of them did not correlate at all with one another. The main problem with fiber-type classification schemes is that the classified feature may correlate with one physiologic or biochemical property, but may have no relationship to others.

The current view of muscle fiber types is that skeletal-muscle fibers possess a wide spectrum of morphologic, contractile, and metabolic properties.[5] The appropriate view of any classification scheme, therefore, is that it is an artificial system superimposed on a continuum of properties for our convenience. Probably the most useful "fiber-typing" scheme is one that describes contractile speed and muscle oxidative capacity. There are a variety of ways to do this; several schemes are listed in Table 3.1. The most definitive method for typing human skeletal muscle (not necessary the most physiologic, but very consistent among labs) is to use the type of myosin heavy chain expressed in the fibers. One of the most convenient methods to type a muscle based on myosin heavy chains is to homogenize large-muscle biopsies and separate the myosin isoforms on protein gels.[6] Using this method, it is possible to identify the three fiber types in human muscle: types 1, 2A, and 2X (see Table 3.1). Although there are four human myosin heavy chain gene—type 1, type 2A, type 2X, and type 2B—only the former three are expressed.[7] This strange phenomenon can make it difficult to compare animal muscle studies with human muscle studies.

Fiber Type Distribution of Paraspinal Muscles

Since fiber types develop in response to functional demands, the fiber type of paraspinal and lumbar extensor muscles provides insight into their function and use patterns. It has been clearly shown that the paraspinal and lumbar extensor muscles are largely composed of type 1 and type 2A fibers. Thus, these muscles are predicted to be relatively slow contracting and fatigue resistant compared to most limb muscles. In fact, recent analysis of paraspinal muscles showed that multifidus, longissimus, and iliocostalis muscles comprised more than 60% type 1 muscle fibers[8]; this proportion is greater than many limb muscles, such as flexor digitorum profundus (35.5 ± 4.8%), triceps (42.4 ± 3.6%), brachioradialis (45.5 ± 6.4), or vastus lateralis (48.3 ± 9.5%), but approaching the values of other tonic, postural muscles such as soleus (88%).[9] Fiber-type distributions of different spinal muscles are described further in Chapter 4.

Muscle Injury

Injury to muscle fibers can occur as a result of trauma, disease, application of myotoxic agents (e.g., local anesthetics), inflammatory processes, or intense exercise. The degree to which muscle injury relates to low back pain or neck pain is unknown. However, muscle injury, and the pain that accompanies it, have been studied extensively. Skeletal-muscle injury and soreness frequently occur when a muscle is rapidly lengthened while it is activated. Active lengthening of muscle (also called eccentric contraction) has been used to study injuries in animals and humans for more than 30 years. Muscle pain accompanying eccentric exercise peaks 24 to 48 hours after the exercise bout. Several studies have reported that eccentric exercise results in a significant increase in serum creatine kinase levels 24 to 48 hours after the exercise bout[10,11] that may persist for 3 to 6 days, depending on the precise nature of the exercise. The appearance of creatine kinase in the serum is interpreted as a result of increased permeability, or breakdown of the muscle cell membrane surrounding the muscle cell.

Eccentric training of a specific muscle group prevents, or at least attenuates, the magnitude of muscle injury that occurs after eccentric exercise in that muscle group. However, general increased fitness does not prevent or reduce eccentric contraction-induced muscle injury.

Experimental studies of skeletal muscles directly subjected to eccentric exercise suggest that early mechanical events result in muscle injury.[12,13] For example, during cyclic eccentric exercise of the rabbit tibialis anterior, significant biomechanical changes were observed in the first 5 to 7 minutes of exercise.[14] Other studies have revealed structural disruption of the cytoskeleton within the fibers during these early time periods,[15,16] which may provide further insights into the damage mechanism.

Animal and human studies have provided evidence for selective damage of fast-fiber types after eccentric exercise.[17-19] In human studies, this damage was generally confined to the type 2 muscle fibers; but in animal studies, damage has been further localized to the fastest of the fast-fiber subtypes. Because these are also the most highly fatigable muscle fibers,[20] it has been speculated that the high degree of fatigability of these fibers may predispose them to injury. In fact, several clinical studies have proposed that the fatigability of spinal muscles may be a predisposing factor to injury. However, it is difficult to test this idea directly because of the many other differences between these fibers and other fiber types. Further studies are required to elucidate the basis for fiber type–specific injury to skeletal muscle and to document the relationship between spinal muscle injury and back and neck pain.

Muscle Architecture

While muscle fiber types are much more widely studied and reported (probably due to the ease with which fiber-type data can be obtained), muscle functional properties are much more highly determined by muscle architecture—the number and arrangement of muscle fibers relative to the axis of force generation.[21–23] Whereas muscle fiber size (which is directly proportional to force generation) is relatively consistent among muscles of different sizes, architectural differences between muscles are much more variable and much more strongly affect function. Thus, muscle architecture is a primary determinant of muscle function, and understanding this structure–function relationship is of great practical importance not only in clarifying the physiologic basis for production of force and movement but also in providing a scientific rationale for surgery or rehabilitation. Muscle architectural studies also guide electrode placement for electromyographic measures of muscle activity, explain the mechanical basis of muscle injury during movement, and aid in the interpretation of histologic specimens obtained from muscle biopsies.

Basic Architectural Definitions

The various types of architectural arrangement are as numerous as the muscles themselves. For discussion purposes, however, we present three general classes of muscle-fiber architecture. Muscles composed of fibers that extend parallel to the muscle's force-generating axis are described as having a parallel or longitudinal architecture (Fig. 3.1A). Muscles with fibers that are oriented at a single angle relative to the force-generating axis are described as having unipennate architecture (Fig. 3.1B). The angle between the fiber and force-generating axis has been measured at resting length in different mammalian muscles and varies from about 0 to 30 degrees. It becomes obvious when performing muscle dissections that most muscles fall into the third and most general category,

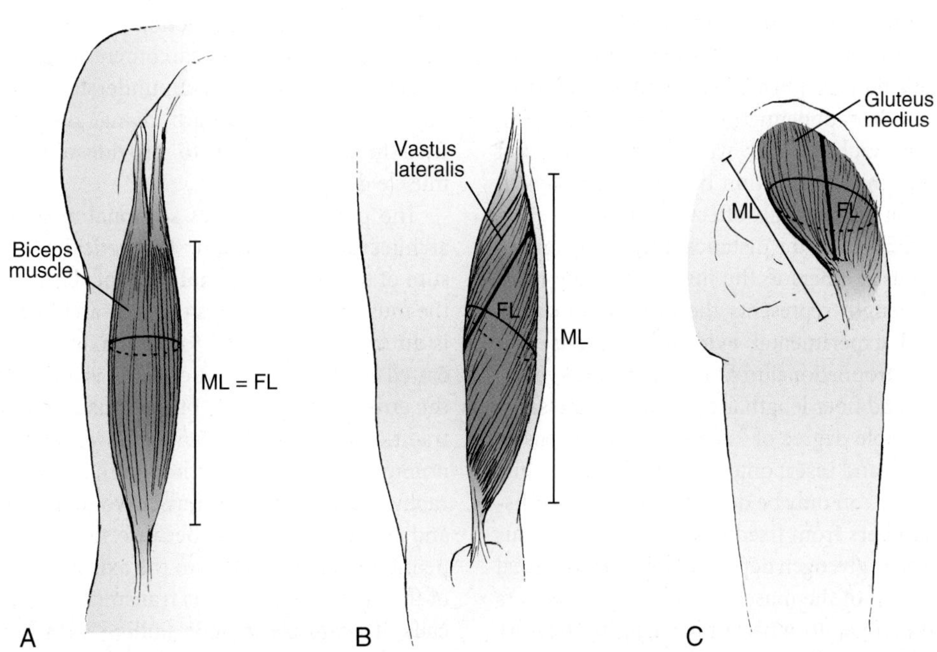

FIG. 3.1 Three general types of skeletal muscle architecture. (A) Longitudinal architecture in which muscle fibers run parallel to the muscle force-generating axis. A typical example is the biceps brachii. (B) Unipennate architecture in which muscle fibers run at a fixed angle relative to the muscle's force-generating axis. The vastus lateralis muscle is shown. (C) Multipennate architecture in which muscle fibers run at several angles relative to the muscle's force-generating axis. The gluteus medius muscle is shown. FL, fiber length; ML, muscle length.

multipennate muscles—muscles constructed of fibers that are oriented at several different angles relative to the axis of force generation (Fig. 3.1C). Obviously, these three designations are oversimplified, but they provide a vocabulary with which to describe muscle architecture. Because fibers may not be oriented along any of the classic anatomic axes, determination of muscle architecture is impossible from a single biopsy or even magnetic resonance imaging (MRI), computed tomography (CT), or ultrasonography, because these methods cannot account for the variations in fiber length and orientation that occur along the muscle length. Thus, other methods, which are described in some detail later, have been developed to characterize the architectural properties of skeletal muscle.

Experimental Determination of Skeletal Muscle Architecture

Quantitative studies of muscle architecture were pioneered by Gans and his colleagues,[23,24] who developed a precise methodology for defining muscle architecture based on microdissection of whole muscles. The parameters usually included in an architectural analysis are muscle length, fiber or fascicle length, pennation angle (i.e., the fiber angle relative to the axis of force generation), and physiologic cross-sectional area (PCSA). Typically, muscles are chemically fixed in formalin to maintain fiber integrity during dissection.

Pennation angle (θ) is measured by determining the average angle of the fibers relative to the axis of force generation. Usually only the pennation angle of fibers on the superficial muscle surface is measured, although pennation angles may vary from superficial to deep and also from proximal to distal. In fact, variation in pennation from superficial to deep fibers has been documented in several spinal muscles (see Chapter 4). Although more sophisticated methods could be developed for measurement of pennation angle (e.g., diffusion tensor imaging), it is doubtful they would provide a great deal more insight into muscle function because variations in pennation angle do not dramatically affect function.[23]

Muscle length is defined as "the distance from the origin of the most proximal muscle fibers to the insertion of the most distal fibers."[25] Fiber length represents the number of sarcomeres in series, and experimental evidence suggests that muscle fiber length is proportional to fiber contraction velocity.[24,26] Muscle length and fiber length are not always the same because there is a variable degree of "stagger" seen in muscle fibers as they arise from and insert onto tendon plates (see Fig. 3.1). Muscle fiber length can only be determined by microdissection of individual fibers from fixed tissues or by laborious identification of fibers by glycogen depletion followed by serial sections along the length of the muscle.[27] Unless investigators are explicit when they refer to muscle fiber length, they are probably referring to muscle fiber bundle length (also known as fascicle length) because it is extremely difficult to isolate intact fibers that run from origin to insertion, especially in mammalian tissue.[27,28] Experimental studies of mammalian muscle suggest that individual muscle fibers do not extend the entire muscle length and may not even extend the entire length of a fascicle.[27,28] Detailed studies of individual muscle fiber lengths have not been conducted in human spinal muscles, but studies in feline neck muscles illustrate that muscle fibers are often arranged in series, ending in tendinous inscriptions within the muscle or terminating intrafascicularly.[29,30] Although the terms fiber length and fascicle length are often used interchangeably, technically they are identical only if muscle fibers span the entire length of a fascicle. In muscle architecture studies, bundles consisting of 5 to 50 fibers are typically used to estimate fiber length, which may be reported as either fiber length or fascicle length.

The final and crucial experimental step required to perform architectural analysis of a whole muscle is to measure the sarcomere length within the isolated fibers. This is necessary to compensate for differences in muscle length that occur during fixation. In other words, to conclude that a muscle has "long fibers" one must ensure that it was not merely fixed in highly stretched position corresponding to a long sarcomere length. Similarly, muscles with "short fibers" must be further investigated to ensure that they were not simply fixed at a short sarcomere length. To permit such conclusions, fiber length measurements should be normalized to a constant sarcomere length. Fiber (or fascicle) lengths are usually normalized to the sarcomere length at which the sarcomere generates maximum force. This normalized fiber length is referred to as optimal fiber (or fascicle) length and provides a reference value that can be related back to the physiologic length if the relationship between muscle length and joint position is noted. Then, based on measured architectural parameters and joint properties, the relationship between sarcomere length and joint angle can be calculated. As an alternative to measurements in cadavers, sarcomere lengths can be measured in live humans using intraoperative laser diffraction[31] or less invasively with microendoscopy.[32,33] Because sarcomere length strongly influences muscle force generation, an understanding of the relationship between sarcomere length change and movement has been used in many studies to provide added understanding of muscle design.[31,34–37]

The physiologic cross-sectional area (PCSA) is the main architectural calculation. Theoretically, PCSA represents the sum of the cross-sectional areas of all the muscle fibers within the muscle, and thus it is the only architectural parameter that is directly proportional to the maximum tetanic tension generated by the muscle. The PCSA is almost never the same as the cross-sectional area of the muscle measured in any of the traditional anatomic planes, as would be obtained using a noninvasive imaging method such as MRI, CT, or ultrasonography. It is calculated as muscle volume divided by fiber length and has units of area. Because fibers may be oriented at a pennation angle relative to the axis of force generation, not all of the fiber tensile force is transmitted to the tendons. Specifically, if a muscle fiber is pulling with X units of force at a pennation angle θ relative to the muscle axis of force generation, only a component of muscle fiber force ($X \bullet \cos\theta$) will actually be transmitted along the muscle axis. Thus, the volume/length is often multiplied by cosineθ (pennation angle) to yield PCSA.

Mechanical Properties of Muscles With Different Architectures

As stated earlier, muscle force is proportional to PCSA and muscle velocity is proportional to fiber length. By stating that velocity is proportional to fiber length, it is implicit that the total excursion (active range) of a muscle is also proportional to fiber length. Thus, it is important to understand how these two architectural parameters, PCSA and fiber length, affect muscle function.

Comparison of Two Otherwise Identical Muscles With Different PCSAs

Suppose that two muscles have identical fiber lengths and pennation angles but one muscle has twice the mass (equivalent to saying that one muscle has twice the number of fibers, thus twice the PCSA). For the sake of simplicity, suppose that these two muscles have identical fiber-type distributions and that they generate the same force per unit area. The functional difference between these two muscles is shown in Fig. 3.2.

The muscle with twice the PCSA has an isometric length–tension curve with the same shape, but it is amplified upward by a factor of 2. Thus, the maximal tetanic tension (P_o) of the larger muscle will be twice that of the smaller muscle. Similarly, comparison of isotonic force-velocity curves indicates that the differences between muscles will simply be an upward shift in P_o for the larger muscle.

Comparison of Two Otherwise Identical Muscles With Different Fiber Lengths

For two muscles with identical PCSAs and pennation angles but different fiber lengths, the schematic in Fig. 3.3 demonstrates that the effect of increased fiber length is to increase muscle excursion and velocity. Peak force of the length–tension curves is identical between muscles, but the range of lengths over which the muscle generates active force is different. For the same reason that increased fiber length increases the active muscle range of the length–tension relationship, it also results in an increase in the muscle's maximum velocity (V_{max}).

Interplay of Muscle Architecture and Moment Arm

In addition to its architecture, the moment generated by a muscle is influenced by its moment arm. Moment arm, the

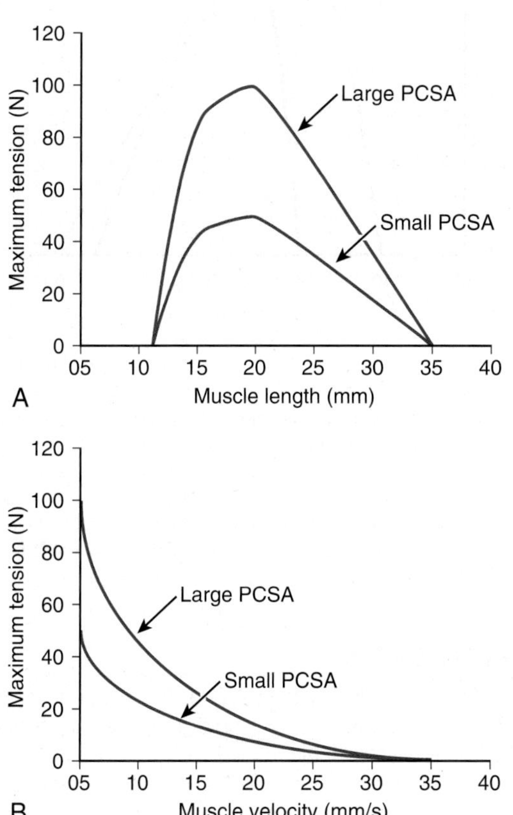

FIG. 3.2 Two muscles with different physiologic cross-sectional areas (PCSAs) but identical mass. (A) Comparison of isometric length–tension properties. (B) Comparison of isotonic force–velocity properties. The effect of increased PCSA with identical fiber length is to shift the absolute length–tension and force–velocity curves to higher values, but with retention of the same range and intrinsic shape.

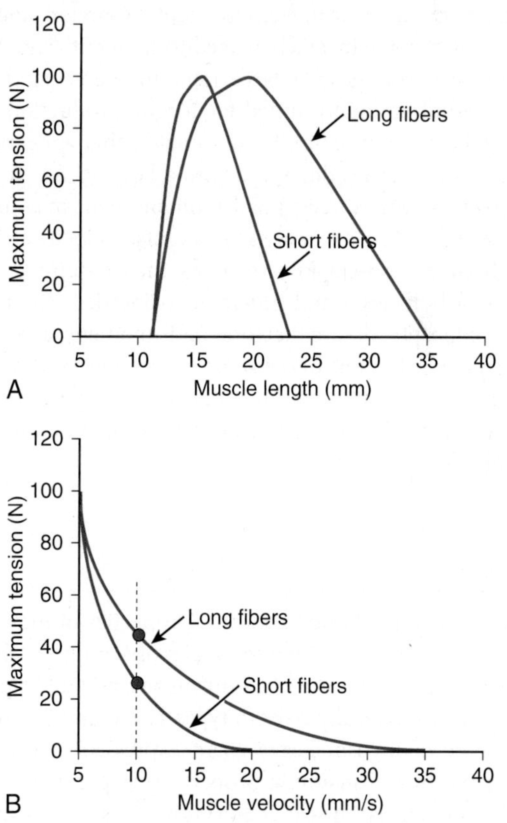

FIG. 3.3 Two muscles with different fiber lengths but identical physiologic cross-sectional areas. (A) Comparison of isometric length–tension properties. (B) Comparison of isotonic force–velocity properties. The effect of increased fiber length is to increase the absolute range of the length–tension curve and absolute velocity of the force–velocity curve, but with retention of the same peak force and intrinsic shape. The dotted vertical line in (B) demonstrates that, for an equivalent absolute velocity, the muscle with longer fibers will generate a greater force.

"mechanical advantage" of a muscle, is the distance from a muscle's line of action to the joint axis of rotation and is directly related to a muscle's change in length with joint rotation.[38] In other words, the amount of muscle fiber length change that occurs as a joint rotates—and, consequently, the range of joint angles over which the muscle develops active force—both depend on the muscle moment arm. This idea can be explained by comparing the situation in which two muscles with identical fiber lengths have different moment arms at a joint (Fig. 3.4). In the case in which the moment arm is greater, muscle fibers will change length much more for a given change in joint angle compared with a muscle with a shorter moment arm. As a result, the range of joint motion over which the muscle develops active force will be smaller for the muscle with the larger moment arm in spite of the fact that the muscular properties of both muscles are identical. The architectural design of a muscle and its placement in relation to skeletal geometry are both important determinants of its function. Although it is true that muscles with longer fibers can generate force over a greater range of lengths than muscles with shorter fibers (e.g., Fig. 3.3A), this does not necessarily indicate that muscles with longer fibers are associated with joints that have larger ranges of motion. Muscles that appear to be designed for speed based on their long fibers may not actually produce large joint velocities if they are placed in the skeleton with a very large moment arm, because joint excursion and joint angular velocity are inversely related to moment arm. A large moment arm results in a large joint moment, so that the muscle would be highly suited for torque production but at low angular velocities. Similarly, a muscle that appears to be designed for force production due to a large PCSA, if placed in a position with a very small moment arm, may actually produce high joint excursions or angular velocities. Differences between muscle–joint systems thus require complete analysis of both joint and muscular properties. These interrelated concepts of architecture and moment arm (gross anatomy) must be considered when examining the design and function of spinal muscles. This concept is fairly complex and it takes practice to become facile with such functional anatomic descriptions.

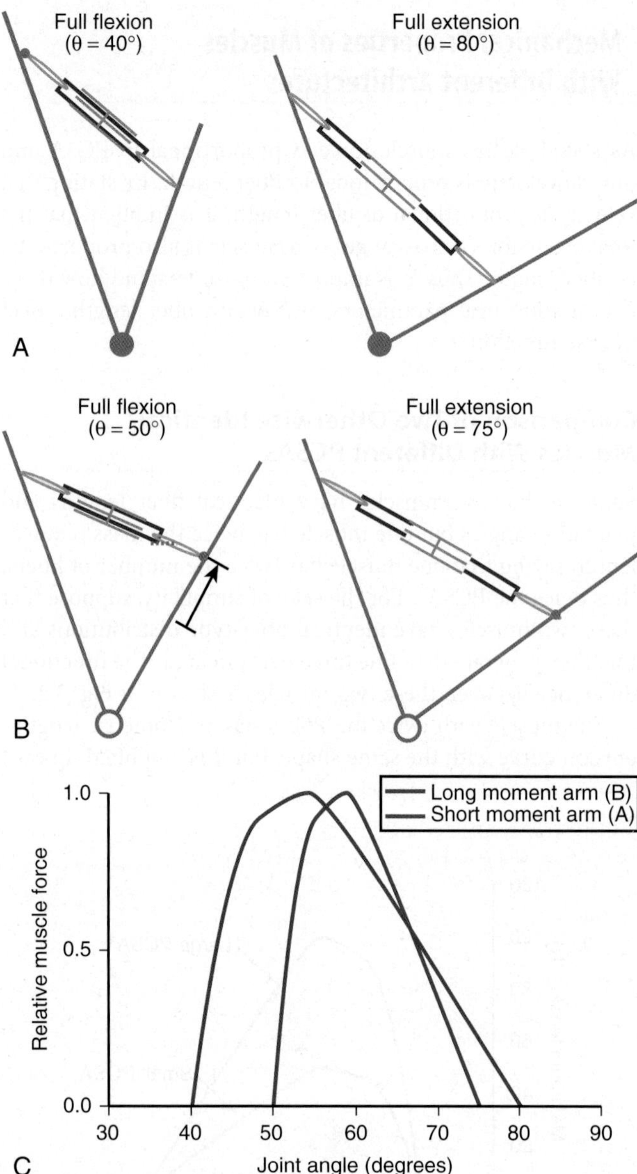

FIG. 3.4 Effect of changing moment arm on active range of motion (ROM). In this example, a schematic muscle (shown as a sarcomere in series with some tendon) is attached with two different moment arms. (A) 40 degrees range of motion for "normal" muscle (from 40 degrees to 80 degrees). (B) Moment arm increase results in a decrease in range of motion to 25 degrees muscle (from 50 degrees to 75 degrees). In (B), the active ROM is smaller since the moment arm is greater; therefore, more sarcomere length change occurs for a given angular rotation. (C) Comparison of force versus joint angle (ROM) for muscles with short or long moment arms.

Summary

In this chapter, the basic functional properties of muscle sarcomeres that generate force via the cross-bridge cycle were reviewed. Muscle fibers are heterogeneous, and descriptors of human muscle typically refer to types 1, 2A, and 2X, relating to the type of myosin heavy chain expressed in the fibers. Finally, the major anatomic property that predicts skeletal-muscle function is muscle architecture. This arrangement of muscle fibers and placement of the muscle in relation to skeletal geometry determines the moments generated at all joints—whether relatively simple, such as the elbow, or complex, such as intervertebral movement. Application of these concepts to the spine and spinal muscles is presented in more detail in Chapter 4.

KEY REFERENCES

1. Burke RE, Levine DN, Tsairis P, Zajac FE. Physiological types and histochemical profiles in motor units of the cat gastrocnemius. *J Physiol.* 1973;234:723-748.
This publication is the classic reference that describes the relationship between the anatomic, physiologic, and biochemical properties of the mammalian motor unit. This work helps to explain the orderly recruitment of motor neurons during normal movement.
2. Evans WJ, Meredith CN, Cannon JG, et al. Metabolic changes following eccentric exercise in trained and untrained men. *J Appl Physiol.* 1986;61:1864-1868.

This paper is one of the earliest demonstrations of the protective effect of training on muscle injury due to eccentric exercise. It is also a very clear demonstration of the delayed nature of the injury that occurs to muscle after eccentric exercise.

3. Fridén J, Sjöström M, Ekblom B. Myofibrillar damage following intense eccentric exercise in man. *Int J Sports Med.* 1983;4:170-176.
This paper is the seminal demonstration of cytoskeletal damage to muscle after eccentric exercise. It contains classic micrographs demonstrating the "Z-band streaming" that occurs when muscles are subjected to high-intensity exercise.

4. Gans C. Fiber architecture and muscle function. *Exercise Sport Sci Rev.* 1982;10(1):160-207.
This review highlights experimental work in mammalian muscle that led to the concept that muscle architecture dominates muscle function.

5. Warren GW, Hayes D, Lowe DA, Armstrong RB. Mechanical factors in the initiation of eccentric contraction-induced injury in rat soleus muscle. *J Physiol.* 1993;464:457-475.
This work represents a multiple regression experimental model that describes the relationship between muscle stress, muscle strain, and muscle strain rate as mechanical causal factors in muscle injury. A slow mammalian muscle is used as the experimental model, so applicability to human muscle is not yet clear.

REFERENCES

1. Panjabi MM. The stabilizing system of the spine. Part I. Function, dysfunction, adaptation, and enhancement. *J Spinal Disord.* 1992;5(4):383-389.
2. Hill AV. The mechanics of active muscle. *Proc R Soc Lond B Biol Sci.* 1953;141(902):104-117.
3. Hill AV. The efficiency of mechanical power development during muscular shortening and its relation to load. *Proc R Soc Lond B Biol Sci.* 1964;159:319-324.
4. Goldman YE. Kinetics of the actomyosin ATPase in muscle fibers. *Annu Rev Physiol.* 1987;49:637-654.
5. Schiaffino S, Reggiani C. Fiber types in mammalian skeletal muscles. *Physiol Rev.* 2011;91(4):1447-1531.
6. Talmadge RJ, Roy RR. Electrophoretic separation of rat skeletal muscle myosin heavy-chain isoforms. *J Appl Physiol.* 1993;75(5):2337-2340.
7. Smerdu V, Karsch-Mizrachi I, Campione M, Leinwand L, Schiaffino S. Type IIx myosin heavy chain transcripts are expressed in type IIb fibers of human skeletal muscle. *Am J Physiol.* 1994;267(6 Pt 1):C1723-C1728.
8. Regev GJ, Kim CW, Thacker BE, et al. Regional myosin heavy chain distribution in selected paraspinal muscles. *Spine.* 2010;35(13):1265-1270.
9. Johnson MA, Polgar J, Weightman D, Appleton D. Data on the distribution of fibre types in thirty-six human muscles. An autopsy study. *J Neurol Sci.* 1973;18(1):111-129.
10. Clarkson PM, Johnson J, Dextradeur D, et al. The relationships among isokinetic endurance, initial strength level, and fiber type. *Res Q Exerc Sport.* 1982;53(1):15-19.
11. Evans WJ, Meredith CN, Cannon JG, et al. Metabolic changes following eccentric exercise in trained and untrained men. *J Appl Physiol.* 1986;61(5):1864-1868.
12. Lieber RL, Friden J. Muscle damage is not a function of muscle force but active muscle strain. *J Appl Physiol.* 1993;74(2):520-526.
13. Warren G, Hayes D, Lowe D, Armstrong R. Mechanical factors in the initiation of eccentric contraction-induced injury in rat soleus muscle. *J Physiol.* 1993;464:457-475.
14. Lieber R, Woodburn T, Friden J. Muscle damage induced by eccentric contraction of 25% strain. *J Appl Physiol.* 1991;70(6):2498-2507.
15. Lieber RL, Schmitz MC, Mishra DK, Friden J. Contractile and cellular remodeling in rabbit skeletal muscle after cyclic eccentric contractions. *J Appl Physiol.* 1994;77(4):1926-1934.
16. Lieber R, Thornell L, Friden J. Muscle cytoskeletal disruption occurs within the first 15 minutes of cyclic eccentric contraction. *J Appl Physiol.* 1996;80(1):278-284.
17. Friden J. Changes in human skeletal muscle induced by long-term eccentric exercise. *Cell Tissue Res.* 1984;236(2):365-372.
18. Friden J, Sjostrom M, Ekblom B. Myofibrillar damage following intense eccentric exercise in man. *Int J Sports Med.* 1983;4(3):170-176.
19. Lieber RL, Friden J. Selective damage of fast glycolytic muscle fibres with eccentric contraction of the rabbit tibialis anterior. *Acta Physiol Scand.* 1988;133(4):587-588.
20. Burke RE, Levine DN, Tsairis P, Zajac FE 3rd. Physiological types and histochemical profiles in motor units of the cat gastrocnemius. *J Physiol.* 1973;234(3):723-748.
21. Gans C. Fiber architecture and muscle function. *Exerc Sport Sci Rev.* 1982;10:160-207.
22. Lieber RL, Friden J. Functional and clinical significance of skeletal muscle architecture. *Muscle Nerve.* 2000;23(11):1647-1666.
23. Gans C, Bock WJ. The functional significance of muscle architecture—a theoretical analysis. *Ergeb Anat Entwicklungsgesch.* 1965;38:115-142.
24. Gans C, de Vree F. Functional bases of fiber length and angulation in muscle. *J Morphol.* 1987;192(1):63-85.
25. Lieber RL. *Skeletal Muscle Structure and Function: Implications for Physical Therapy and Sports Medicine.* Baltimore: Williams & Wilkins; 1992.
26. Bodine SC, Roy RR, Meadows DA, et al. Architectural, histochemical, and contractile characteristics of a unique biarticular muscle: the cat semitendinosus. *J Neurophysiol.* 1982;48(1):192-201.
27. Ounjian M, Roy RR, Eldred E, et al. Physiological and developmental implications of motor unit anatomy. *J Neurobiol.* 1991;22(5):547-559.
28. Loeb GE, Pratt CA, Chanaud CM, Richmond FJ. Distribution and innervation of short, interdigitated muscle fibers in parallel-fibered muscles of the cat hindlimb. *J Morphol.* 1987;191(1):1-15.
29. Armstrong JB, Rose PK, Vanner S, Bakker GJ, Richmond FJ. Compartmentalization of motor units in the cat neck muscle, biventer cervicis. *J Neurophysiol.* 1988;60(1):30-45.
30. Richmond FJ, MacGillis DR, Scott DA. Muscle-fiber compartmentalization in cat splenius muscles. *J Neurophysiol.* 1985;53(4):868-885.
31. Lieber RL, Loren GJ, Friden J. In vivo measurement of human wrist extensor muscle sarcomere length changes. *J Neurophysiol.* 1994;71(3):874-881.
32. Llewellyn ME, Barretto RP, Delp SL, Schnitzer MJ. Minimally invasive high-speed imaging of sarcomere contractile dynamics in mice and humans. *Nature.* 2008;454(7205):784-788.

33. Cromie MJ, Sanchez GN, Schnitzer MJ, Delp SL. Sarcomere lengths in human extensor carpi radialis brevis measured by microendoscopy. *Muscle Nerve.* 2013;48(2):286-292.
34. Burkholder TJ, Lieber RL. Sarcomere length operating range of vertebrate muscles during movement. *J Exp Biol.* 2001;204(Pt 9):1529-1536.
35. Lieber RL, Ljung BO, Friden J. Intraoperative sarcomere length measurements reveal differential design of human wrist extensor muscles. *J Exp Biol.* 1997;200(Pt 1):19-25.
36. Rome LC, Sosnicki A, Choi IH. The influence of temperature on muscle function in the fast swimming scup. II. The mechanics of red muscle. *J Exp Biol.* 1992;163:281-295.
37. Rome LC, Sosnicki AA. Myofilament overlap in swimming carp. II. Sarcomere length changes during swimming. *Am J Physiol.* 1991;260(2 Pt 1):C289-C296.
38. An KN, Takahashi K, Harrigan TP, Chao EY. Determination of muscle orientations and moment arms. *J Biomech Eng.* 1984;106(3):280-282.
39. Peter JB, Barnard RJ, Edgerton VR, et al. Metabolic profiles on three fiber types of skeletal muscle in guinea pigs and rabbits. *Biochemistry (Mosc).* 1972;11:2627-2733.
40. Ranvier ML. Des muscles rouges et des muscles blancs chez les rongeurs. *C R Aca Sci.* 77:1030-1040.
41. Gauthier GF. On the relationship of ultrastructural and cytochemical features to color in mammalian skeletal muscle. *ZZellforsch Mikrosk Anat.* 1969;95:462-482.
42. Romanul FCA. Enzymes in muscle. 1. Histochemical and contractile properties in the cross innervated guinea pig soleus muscle. *Arch Neurol.* 1964;20:318-329.
43. Brooke MH, Kaiser KK. Muscle fiber types: how many and what kind? *Arch Neurol.* 1970;23:369-379.
44. Sjöström M, Kidman S, Henriksson-Larsen K, et al. Z- and M-band appearance in different histochemically defined types of human skeletal muscle fibers. *J Histochem Cytochem.* 1982;30:1-11.
45. Schiaffino S, Gorza L, Sartore S, et al. Three myosin heavy chain isoforms in type 2 skeletal muscle fibers. *J Muscle Res Cell Motil.* 1989;10:197-205.
46. Schiaffino S, Reggiani C. Molecular diversity of myofibrillar proteins: gene regulation and functional significance. *Physiol Rev.* 1996;76:371-423.

4 CHAPTER Spinal Musculature: Anatomy and Function

Anita Vasavada
Samuel R. Ward
Scott Delp
Richard L. Lieber

Anatomy and Architecture of Spinal Musculature

The architecture of spinal muscles is complex and dramatically different from the architecture of limb muscles. For example, instead of distinct tendinous attachments to bone, many spinal muscles have very little tendon at their ends, but have a complex arrangement of internal tendons and aponeuroses. Their attachments are generally broad, and many spinal muscles branch and have insertions at multiple vertebral levels. Some spinal muscles have short fascicles and high pennation, whereas others have long, parallel fascicles. All of these factors affect the force- and moment-generating capacity of muscles (as described in Chapter 3), which ultimately influences control of spinal movement and injury mechanisms.

Spinal muscles can be divided into intrinsic muscles, which connect vertebrae with each other or with the skull, and extrinsic muscles, which attach vertebrae to the limbs, shoulder girdle, ribcage, or pelvis. Embryologically, intrinsic muscles originate from the epimere and extrinsic muscles originate from the hypomere. Intrinsic muscles receive innervation from the dorsal rami of spinal nerves, whereas extrinsic muscles are innervated by the ventral rami of spinal nerves and generally have functions related more to the proximal portion of limbs or respiration.

Intrinsic Spinal Muscles in the Lumbar, Thoracic, or Cervical Spine

Intrinsic muscles of the spine are dominated by the erector spinae, a group of interdigitated muscles that span the entire length of the spine, from the sacrum and iliac crest to the skull. Another important group of muscles, the multifidus, are shorter and deeper, and are described in more detail later. In the thoracolumbar region, the erector spinae and multifidus muscles comprise the bulk of the spinal musculature. These two distinct functional units have large differences in innervation that probably result in significant functional differences,[1] although the detailed biomechanical function of these groups remains only partially elucidated.[2] Lying deep to the multifidus are even smaller muscles: the rotatores, interspinales, and intertransversarii. The cervical region is composed of other unique intrinsic muscles (described later).

The erector spinae are commonly considered to be composed of three muscles; from medial to lateral, they are the spinalis, longissimus, and iliocostalis. The anatomy and architecture of these muscles vary among different levels of the spine. Therefore, the words "lumborum," "thoracis," "cervicis," and/or "capitis" are often appended to the muscle name to describe the anatomy more accurately. Although there are varying definitions of the composition of the erector spinae, the study by MacIntosh and Bogduk[2] provides the most comprehensive descriptive anatomy of the lumbar erector spinae to date; Delp and colleagues[3] provided the first architectural measurements of these muscles. A description of the continuation of the erector spinae into the cervical region is discussed by Kamibayashi and Richmond.[4]

The spinalis muscle is the most medial division of the erector spinae. MacIntosh and Bogduk[2] describe the spinalis as mostly aponeurotic in the lumbar region, but Delp and colleagues[3] obtained architecture measurements from muscle fibers in the thoracic spinalis (Table 4.1). The spinalis is generally absent in the cervical region.

Caudad to rostrad, the longissimus consists of the longissimus thoracis, cervicis, and capitis. The longissimus thoracis is divided into lumbar and thoracic portions. The lumbar fascicles of the longissimus thoracis (longissimus thoracis pars lumborum) are composed of five bands that arise from the lumbar transverse processes and attach in a caudal fashion onto the iliac crest (Fig. 4.1A). Each band arising from vertebrae L1 to L4 is actually a small fusiform muscle that has an elongated and flattened caudal tendon of insertion. Bands from more rostral levels attach more medially on the iliac crest. The juxtaposition of these caudally located tendons forms the lumbar intermuscular aponeurosis. Fascicles of the thoracic component of longissimus thoracis (longissimus thoracis pars thoracis) arise from all thoracic transverse processes and most ribs, and attach to either lumbar spinous processes, the sacrum, or the ilium. These are long slender muscles with pronounced caudal tendons that juxtapose to

TABLE 4.1 Architectural Data of Rectus Abdominis and Lumbar Spine Muscles

Muscle	Musculotendon Length (cm)	Muscle Length (cm)	Fascicle Length (cm)	Pennation Angle (degrees)	Sarcomere Length (μm)	Optimal Fascicle Length (cm)	Muscle Fiber Mass (g)	PCSA (cm²)
Rectus abdominis	35.9 (1.9)	34.3 (2.7)	28.3 (3.6)	0 (0)	2.83 (0.28)	28 (4.2)	92.5 (30.5)	2.6 (0.9)
Quadratus lumborum (proximal)	11.7 (1.7)	10.7 (1.3)	7.3 (1.3)	7.4 (2.9)	2.39 (0.21)	8.5 (1.5)	13.3 (5.2)	1.6 (0.6)
Quadratus lumborum (distal)	9.3 (1.3)	8.1 (1.2)	4.7 (0.5)	7.4 (6.2)	2.37 (0.20)	5.6 (0.9)	7.3 (2.4)	1.2 (0.4)
Spinalis thoracis	24.7 (1.5)	18.2 (3.2)	5.2 (0.4)	16 (3.8)	2.26 (0.17)	6.4 (0.6)	10.2 (6)	1.6 (0.9)
Longissimus thoracis	42.6 (5.5)	34.7 (4.8)	9.6 (1.2)	12.6 (5.8)	2.31 (0.17)	11.7 (2.1)	73.4 (31)	5.9 (2.5)
Iliocostalis lumborum	43.8 (4.3)	33.1 (9)	12 (1.7)	13.8 (4.5)	2.37 (0.17)	14.2 (2.1)	60.9 (29.9)	4.1(1.9)
Multifidus	NA	NA	4.8 (1.7)	18.4 (4.2)	2.26 (0.18)	5.7 (1.8)	73 (12.4)	23.9 (8.4)

Values are mean (standard deviation).
NA, not applicable; PCSA, physiologic cross-sectional area.
Modified from Delp SL, Suryanarayanan S, Murray WM, et al. Architecture of the rectus abdominis, quadratus lumborum, and erector spine. *J Biomech* 2001;34:371–375; and Ward, SR, Kim CW, Eng CM, et al. Architectural analysis and intraoperative measurements demonstrate the unique design of the multifidus for lumbar spine stability. *J Bone Joint Surg Am.* 2009;91:176-185.

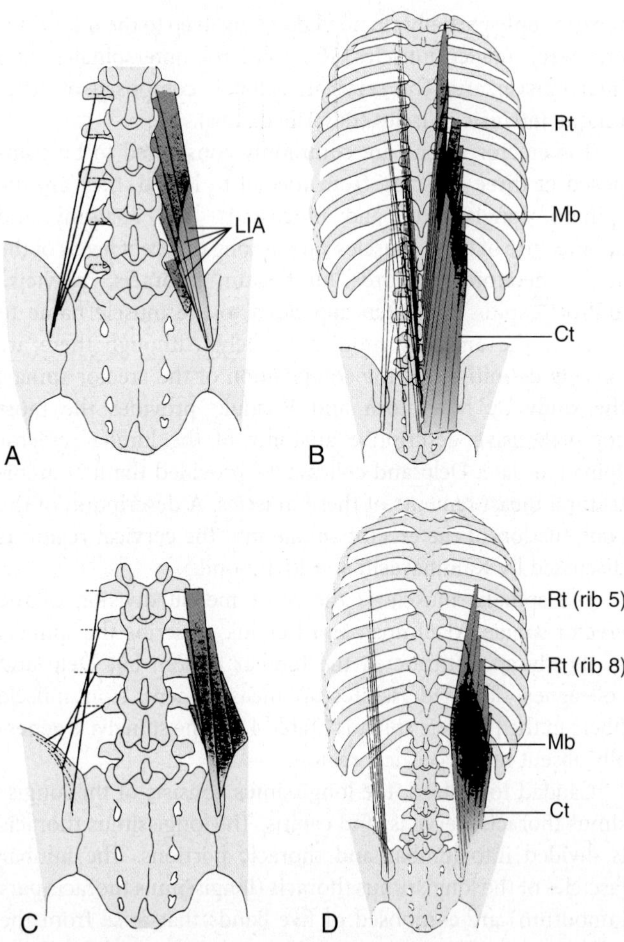

FIG. 4.1 Longissimus thoracis (medial division of erector spinae) schematic of (A) lumbar and (B) thoracic regions and iliocostalis lumborum (lateral division of erector spinae) schematic of (C) lumbar and (D) thoracic regions. Ct, caudal tendon; Mb, muscle belly; LIA, lumbar intermuscular aponeurosis; Rt, rostral tendon. (From Bogduk N. A reappraisal of the anatomy of the human lumbar erector spinae. *J Anat*, 1980;131:525-540; and MacIntosh JE, Bogduk N. The morphology of the lumbar erector spinae. *Spine.* 1987;12:658–668.)

form the strong erector spinae aponeurosis (see LIA and Ct in Fig. 4.1A–B), which bounds the lumbar paraspinal muscles dorsally. In the upper thoracic and cervical region, the longissimus cervicis connects transverse processes of thoracic and cervical vertebrae, whereas the longissimus capitis originates on transverse processes and inserts on the mastoid process of the skull (Fig. 4.2B).

The lumbar fascicles of the iliocostalis lumborum (iliocostalis lumborum pars lumborum) lie lateral to the longissimus thoracis muscles arising from the tip of the transverse processes of vertebrae L1 to L4 in the lumbar region, thus are composed of four small, broad bands (see Fig. 4.1C) that attach to the thoracolumbar fascia and the iliac crest. The thoracic fascicles of the iliocostalis lumborum (iliocostalis lumborum pars thoracis) arise from ribs and attach to the iliac spine and crest, forming the lateral part of the erector spinae aponeurosis. In contrast to the more medially located longissimus thoracis, the caudal tendons are less prominent, giving the iliocostalis lumborum a much more fleshy appearance. Caudad to rib 10, the iliocostalis lumborum and longissimus thoracis lie side by side, forming the erector spinae aponeurosis. Rostral to rib 9 or 10, the iliocostalis thoracis separates the iliocostalis lumborum and longissimus thoracis. In the upper thoracic and cervical region, the iliocostalis cervicis connects the ribs to the transverse processes of cervical vertebrae. MacIntosh and Bogduk measured muscle and tendon lengths in the thoracic portions of the longissimus thoracis and iliocostalis lumborum (Table 4.2).[2] Detailed architecture of the lumbar erector spinae, including muscle tendon and fascicle length, sarcomere lengths, and physiologic cross-sectional areas (PCSAs) have also been reported by Delp et al.[3] (see Table 4.1). They found that fascicle lengths were approximately 30% of muscle lengths in these muscles and that sarcomere lengths measured from cadavers in the supine position were generally shorter than the optimal length, which may imply that the erector spinae are capable of developing greater force in elongated positions (i.e., in flexion).[5] This muscle may thus be designed to restore spine extension from flexion. Although longissimus and iliocostalis may have different functions because of their medial-to-lateral anatomic locations, their fiber type distributions are similar, with approximately 60% type 1 fibers,[6] the slowest muscle fiber

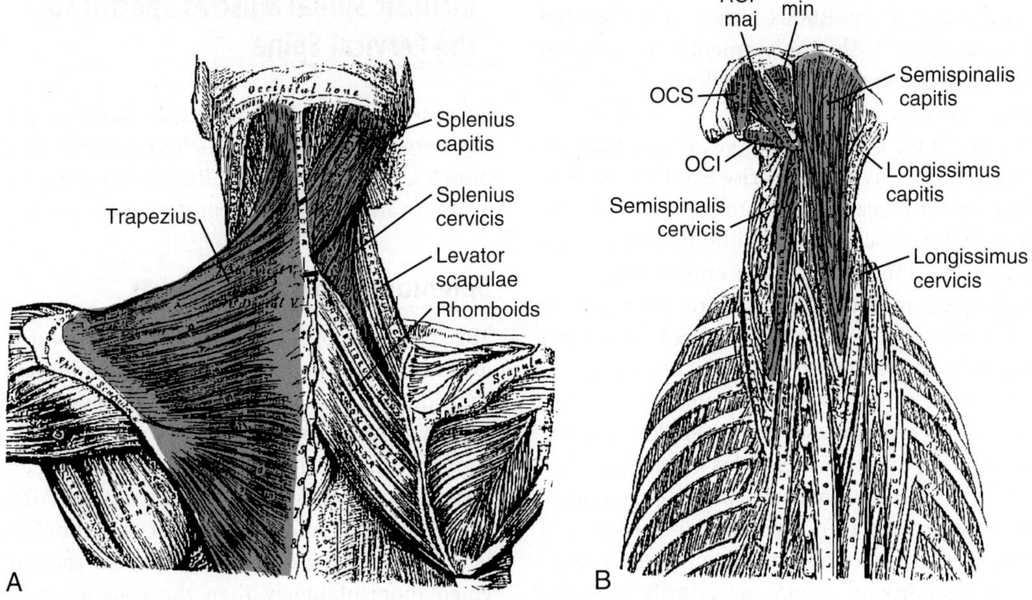

FIG. 4.2 Posterior view of neck muscles. (A) Left side shows the superficial muscle, the trapezius. Underneath the trapezius lie the splenius capitis, splenius cervicis, levator scapulae, and rhomboids. (B) Right side shows semispinalis capitis, longissimus capitis, and longissimus cervicis, which lie deep to splenius capitis. Left side shows semispinalis cervicis and the suboccipital muscles, which lie under semispinalis capitis. OCI, obliquus capitis inferior; OCS, obliquus capitis superior; RCP maj, rectus capitis posterior major; RCP min, rectus capitis posterior minor. (Modified from Gray H. *Gray's Anatomy.* New York, Gramercy Books, 1977.)

TABLE 4.2 Muscle and Tendon Length Data of Lumbar Erector Spinae

Muscle	Muscle Belly Length (cm)	Rostral Tendon Length (cm)	Caudal Tendon Length (cm)
Longissimus thoracis pars thoracis	9-12	3-4	Up to 24
Iliocostalis lumborum pars thoracis	10-13	12-15	18-19

From MacIntosh JE, Bogduk N. The morphology of the lumbar erector spinae. *Spine.* 1987;12:658–668.

type. The detailed anatomy of the erector spinae provided by MacIntosh and Bogduk[2] also provides important information for electromyographic studies. Because thoracic fascicles of the longissimus thoracis and iliocostalis lumborum lie over the lumbar fascicles, electrodes placed at lumbar vertebral levels may not represent activity of fascicles directly attached to lumbar vertebrae.

The lumbar multifidus muscles consist of multiple separate bands arising from each vertebral spinous process and lamina, and inserting from two to four segments below the level of origin (Fig. 4.3B). The shortest fascicle of each muscle inserts onto the mammillary process of the vertebra located two segments caudad, whereas longer, more superficial fascicles insert sequentially onto subsequent vertebrae three or more segments lower (see Fig. 4.3). Thus, the shortest band of the multifidus arising from L1 inserts on L3; subsequent bands insert sequentially on L4, L5, and the sacrum. Multifidus muscles arising from lower lumbar vertebrae consist of fewer fascicles because the number of vertebrae caudad to the origin decreases. Of note is the fact that all multifidus muscles that arise from a given level are innervated by the medial branch

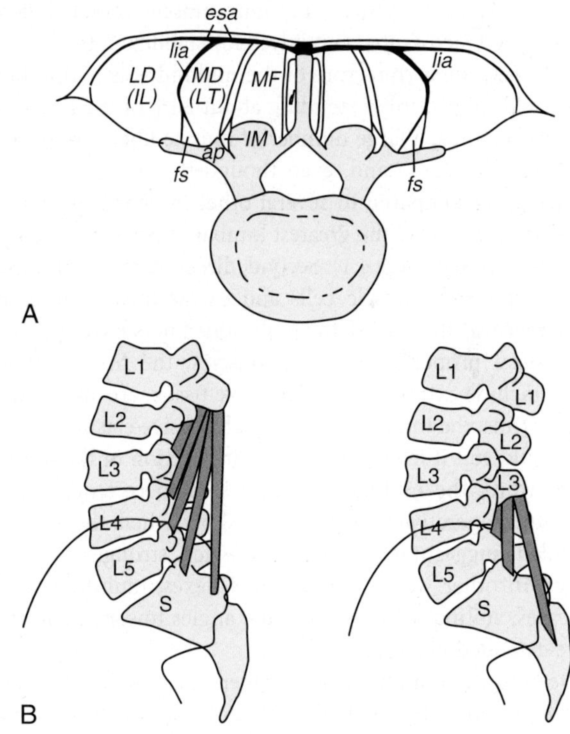

FIG. 4.3 Schematic arrangement of multifidus muscle in (A) cross-section and (B) longitudinal section. ap, accessory process; esa, erector spinae aponeurosis; fs, fat-filled space; I, interspinalis; IL, iliocostalis lumborum; IM, intertransversarii mediales; LD, lateral division; lia, lumbar intermuscular aponeurosis; MF, multifidus. (From Bogduk N. A reappraisal of the anatomy of the human lumbar erector spinae. *J Anat.* 1980;131:525–540.)

of the primary dorsal rami of the spinal nerve from a single segment (i.e., each band of multifidus muscle is innervated from a single dorsal ramus). This unisegmental innervation has implications for electromyography and diagnosis of zygapophyseal joint pain related to abnormal activity in multifidus. For instance, medial fibers of multifidus (i.e., those immediately lateral to a given spinous process) arise from the spinous process directly above, whereas those from higher levels will be more lateral, but all the fibers of the multifidus arising from a particular vertebra are innervated by the same nerve.[7]

In the cervical region, multifidus fascicles from the spinous processes and laminae of C2, C3, and C4 attach onto facet capsules of two adjacent vertebral articular processes from C4 to C7; fascicles from the spinous processes and laminae of C4 to C7 attach onto transverse processes of upper thoracic vertebrae.[8] The principal action of the multifidus is extension, but the multisegmental nature of the muscle as well as the complex three-dimensional orientation in the cranial-caudad and mediolateral directions renders this statement a gross oversimplification.[9] The multifidus is not necessarily a prime mover of the spine; rather, its function is likely to produce small vertebral stabilizations. Its fiber type distribution of approximately 60% type 1 fibers supports this postural role. In fact, similar fiber type distributions between multifidus and erector spinae muscles suggest similar functions for these two muscle groups.[6,10]

A recent study of the multifidus muscle revealed three major design factors that suit it well for stabilizing the lumbar spine.[5] First, the architecture of the multifidus is highly pennated, with fibers only extending about 20% of the length of the muscle. Thus, a large number of muscle fibers are packed into a small volume and, even though the multifidus has a smaller mass compared to several other lumbar extensors, it is predicted to create the greatest lumbar extension force by a factor of two (see Table 4.1). Second, direct mechanical testing of the multifidus muscle cells and extracellular connective tissue revealed that, while the multifidus fibers have the same mechanical properties as limb muscles, the fiber bundles, which include extracellular connective tissue, are about twice as stiff. Thus, the multifidus has a high passive elastic capacity that would suit it for passively resisting flexion of the lumbar spine. Third, the multifidus muscle sarcomere length, measured intraoperatively, is relatively short when the spine is extended, suggesting that the muscle gets stronger as it gets longer. In other words, as the spine flexes, multifidus force increases, suiting it to restore spine angles toward neutral or more extended positions.

Deep to the multifidus are smaller muscles that span one or two vertebral segments. The rotatores attach from caudal transverse processes to the base of rostral spines one or two segments away. Rotators are prominent in the thoracic region; although some authors claim that they exist in the lumbar region,[11,12] MacIntosh and Bogduk did not find any muscles deep to the lumbar multifidus.[7] Likewise, Anderson et al.[8] did not find rotatores in the cervical region. The interspinalis and intertransversarii (found in the lumbar and cervical regions) connect the spines and transverse processes, respectively, of adjacent vertebrae.

Intrinsic Spinal Muscles Specific to the Cervical Spine

Because of different functional demands in the cervical spine (e.g., large head movements), this region has additional intrinsic muscles. Kamibayashi and Richmond quantified neck muscle anatomy and architecture of the neck muscles (Table 4.3).[4]

Splenius Capitis and Cervicis

The splenius capitis originates at the spinous processes of the lower cervical and upper thoracic vertebrae and inserts on the skull near the mastoid process (see Fig. 4.2A). Contiguous, slightly deeper, and sometimes inseparable is the splenius cervicis, which originates on thoracic spinous processes and inserts on cervical transverse processes. Although both the splenius capitis and splenius cervicis function in extension, lateral bending, and axial rotation, the splenius capitis is oriented more obliquely than the splenius cervicis, providing more axial rotation capacity for movements of the skull relative to the vertebrae. The fascicle lengths of the splenius capitis and splenius cervicis are similar, but their muscle tendon lengths are not similar. This occurs because the splenius capitis has short aponeuroses, whereas the splenius cervicis has long aponeuroses (Fig. 4.4A).[4]

Semispinalis Capitis and Cervicis

The semispinalis capitis originates on the articular processes of the lower cervical vertebrae and transverse processes of the upper thoracic vertebrae, and inserts medially on the skull between the inferior and superior nuchal line (see Fig. 4.2B). The semispinalis capitis is characterized by complex patterns of internal tendon and tendinous inscriptions in the medial portion, whereas fascicles in the lateral portion are uninterrupted (see Fig. 4.4B).[4] The semispinalis cervicis (deep to the semispinalis capitis) originates on thoracic transverse processes and inserts on cervical spinous processes from C2 to C5, with the bulk of its mass inserting on C2.

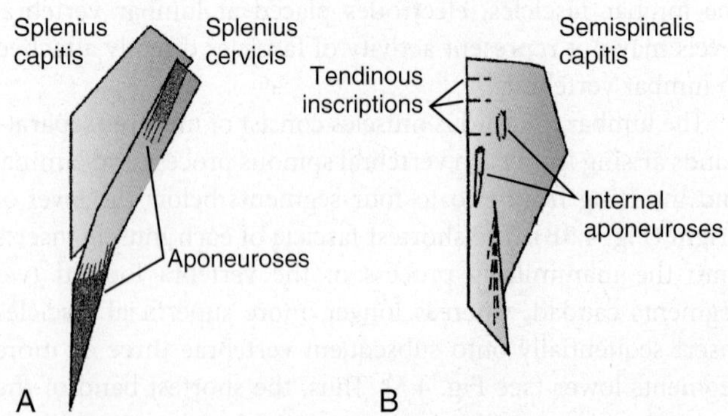

FIG. 4.4 Architecture of splenius capitis, splenius cervicis, and semispinalis capitis. (A) Splenius capitis and splenius cervicis. Note aponeuroses at both ends of splenius cervicis. (B) Semispinalis capitis. The medial portion is characterized by tendinous inscriptions and internal aponeuroses interrupting the fascicles. (Modified from Kamibayashi LK, Richmond FJR. Morphometry of human neck muscles. *Spine.* 1998;23:1314–1323.)

TABLE 4.3 Morphometric Parameters of Human Neck Muscles

Muscle	N	MASS (g)		Angle Range (degrees)	MUSCLE LENGTH (cm)		NF Length (cm), Mean (SD)	PCSA (cm^2)	
		Range	Mean (SD)		Range	Mean (SD)		Range	Mean (SD)
Sternocleidomastoideus	9	21–50.5	40.4 (9)	0–20	16.5–21.2	19 (1.6)	10.8 (0.9)	1.81–5.26	3.72 (0.91)
Clavotrapezius		10.7–27.1	18.7 (4.5)	0–30	9–14.8	12 (1.9)	8.4 (2.1)	1.25–2.94	1.96 (0.62)
Acromiotrapezius		68.6–128.4	103.5 (23.5)	0–10	10–14.5	12.6 (1.7)	9.2 (1.8)	7.99–15.26	10.77 (2.38)
Rhomboideus	9	18.8–58.3	40.9 (15.6)	0–5			7.2 (2)	1.76–9.93	5.84 (2.77)
Minor					6.5–12	8.7 (1.9)			
Major					5.3–13	8.2 (2.7)			
Rectus capitis posterior major	9	1.4–5.5	3.5 (1.2)	0–5	3–4.8		3.7 (0.7)	0.44–1.45	0.93 (0.33)
Rectus capitis posterior minor	9	0.6–1.6	1 (0.3)	0–5	2.6–3.1		1.9 (0.2)	0.28–0.83	0.50 (0.19)
Obliquus capitis superior	8	1–3.7	2.5 (0.9)	0–20	4.3–5.7		2.5 (0.5)	0.29–1.69	1.03 (0.46)
Obliquus capitis inferior	9	2.1–8.1	5.1 (1.8)	0–5	3.6–5.4	4.4 (0.6)	3.8 (0.8)	0.69–1.73	1.29 (0.54)
Longus capitis	7	2.4–5.6	3.7 (1.2)	0–10	7.8–11.1	9.2 (1.4)	3.8 (1)	0.54–1.63	0.92 (0.35)
Splenius	9	21.6–59.3	42.9 (13.8)	0–5			9.5 (2.3)	2.57–5.48	4.26 (1.04)
Capitis					9.5–15	12.3 (1.5)			
Cervicis					11.5–18.5	14.7 (2.3)			
Semispinalis capitis	9	21.3–55.8	38.5 (9.4)	0–20	13–20	11.7 (1.9)	6.8 (1.7)	3.93–7.32	5.40 (1.30)
Scalenus anterior	9	5.7–12.4	5.6 (3)	0–20	5.5–7.8	6.8 (0.9)	4.2 (1.3)	0.37–4.51	1.45 (1.23)
Scalenus medius	9	5.6–14.5	10.6 (3.0)	0–30	6.8–9.6	8.1 (1)	5 (0.8)	1.00–3.34	2.00 (0.73)
Scalenus posterior	9	4–23.5	10.6 (7.7)	0–20	7–10	8 (1.1)	6.2 (2.1)	0.59–3.15	1.55 (0.90)
Levator scapulae	8	16.5–38.9	24.6 (8.3)	0–5	13.2–17.5	15.1 (1.6)	11.3 (3.1)	1.39–3.24	2.18 (0.80)

Values in each column represent the range or average of individual values computed on specimen at one time.
NF Length, normalized fascicle length; PCSA, physiologic cross-sectional area; SD, standard deviation.
From Kamibayashi LK, Richmond FR. Morphometry of human neck muscles. *Spine.* 1998;23:1314-1323.

Longus Capitis and Colli

On the anterior side of the vertebral column, the longus capitis runs from the anterior surface of transverse processes to the baso-occiput (Fig. 4.5). Because it lies close to the vertebral bodies, it has only a small flexion moment arm; the superomedial orientation could provide ipsilateral rotation. Its counterpart, the longus colli, has a more complicated structure. Some fibers run vertically along the anterior vertebral bodies, other fibers run superolaterally from thoracic vertebral bodies to lower cervical transverse processes, and others run superomedially from transverse processes to the anterior vertebral bodies (see Fig. 4.5). Thus, although all parts of the longus colli have small flexion moment arms, the superomedial and superolateral portions would have ipsilateral and contralateral rotation moment arms, respectively. The longus capitis and colli are also characterized by an aponeurosis covering much of the superficial surface, from which fascicles have long tendons that attach to the vertebrae (Fig. 4.6).[4]

The longus capitis and longus colli were found to be composed of 50% type 1 fibers by number and 61% to 64% type 1 fibers by area.[13] Because of their small moment arms, their function is considered to be postural. The cross-sectional area of longus colli was found to be inversely correlated to cervical lordosis, suggesting a stabilizing function.[14]

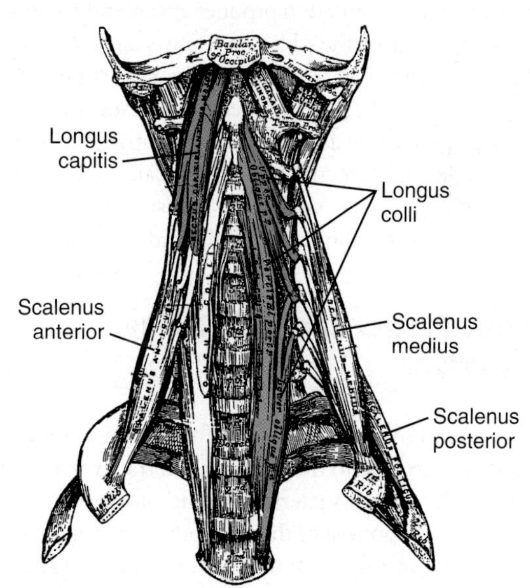

FIG. 4.5 Anterior view of deep neck muscles: longus capitis, longus colli, and scalenes. Note the three parts of longus colli: superior oblique, vertical, and inferior oblique. (Modified from Gray H. *Gray's Anatomy*. New York: Gramercy Books; 1977.)

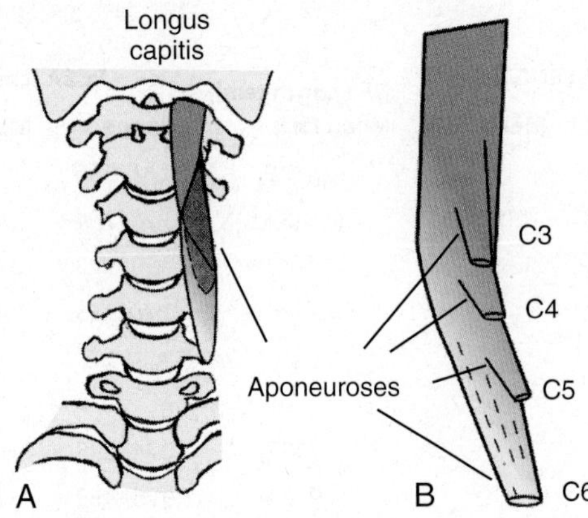

FIG. 4.6 Architecture of longus capitis. (A) Superficial surface, with long aponeurosis. (B) Deep surface, with individual tendons to lower cervical vertebrae. (Modified from Kamibayashi LK, Richmond FJR. Morphometry of human neck muscles. *Spine.* 1998;23:1314–1323.)

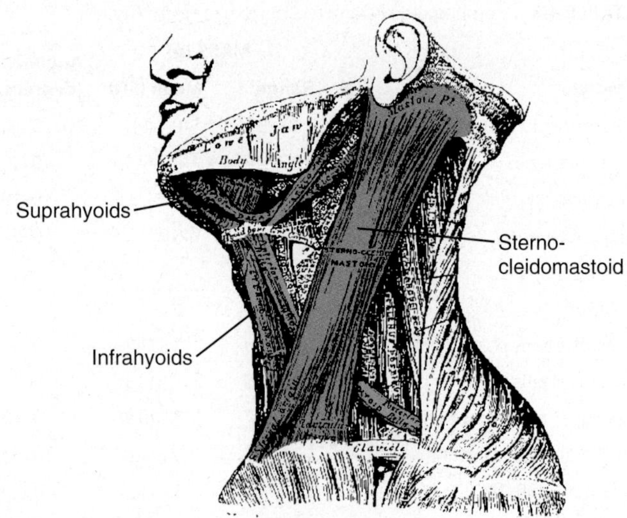

FIG. 4.7 Lateral view of sternocleidomastoid and hyoid muscles. (Modified from Gray H. *Gray's Anatomy.* New York: Gramercy Books; 1977.)

Suboccipital Muscles

The suboccipital muscles span the region between C2 and the skull (see Fig. 4.2B). The rectus capitis posterior major and minor connect the spinous processes of C2 and C1, respectively, with the skull. The obliquus capitis superior is oriented in a superoinferior direction between the transverse process of C1 and the skull, and the obliquus capitis inferior runs primarily mediolaterally from the spinous process of C2 to the transverse process of C1. All four of these muscles can contribute to extension of the head with respect to the neck. In addition, the rectus capitis posterior major and the obliquus capitis inferior are oriented to produce ipsilateral rotation, and the lateral location of the obliquus capitis superior implies a lateral bending function. The obliquus capitis superior has an internal tendon on the deep surface that causes some fascicles to have large pennation angles.[4] On the ventral side, the rectus capitis anterior and rectus capitis lateralis are very small muscles that connect the skull to C1, presumably with (small) moment arms for flexion and lateral bending, respectively.

Extrinsic Muscles Linking Vertebrae to the Pelvis

The quadratus lumborum attaches from the iliolumbar ligament and iliac crest onto the 12th rib and transverse processes of L1 to L4. It assists in lateral bending of the lumbar spine. The proximal component of the quadratus lumborum (i.e., the set of fascicles running from the iliac crest to the 12th rib and L1) has a larger moment arm for lateral flexion and has longer fascicles than the distal component of the muscle. Electromyographic evidence shows that the quadratus lumborum has a dominant role in spine stabilization.[15]

The psoas major attaches from the anterior surface of the transverse processes, the sides of vertebral bodies, and intervertebral discs of all lumbar vertebrae. Together with the iliacus, which arises from the ilium, they form the iliopsoas, which inserts on the lesser trochanter of the femur and is a major flexor of the thigh and trunk. Fascicles of the psoas generally have the same length, regardless of their level of origin. Thus, because of their attachments to a common tendon, bundles from higher levels are more tendinous, whereas the bundle from L5 remains fleshy until it joins the common tendon.[16] The psoas is the largest muscle in cross-section at the lower levels of the lumbar spine.[17] Biomechanical analysis shows that the psoas has the potential to laterally flex the lumbar spine, generate compressive forces that would increase stability, and create large anterior shear forces at L5 to S1.[18] However, if psoas were designed for lumbar spine motions, one would expect an architectural design consisting of longer fascicles attaching to more rostral segments because they would undergo larger excursion. The uniform fascicle lengths suggest that the psoas may actually be designed to flex the hip[19]; electromyographic studies confirm that its primary function is hip flexion.[20]

Extrinsic Muscles Linking Vertebrae or Skull to the Shoulder Girdle or Rib Cage

On the anterior and lateral surface of the neck, the sternocleidomastoid originates from the sternum and medial clavicle to attach on the skull at the mastoid process and superior nuchal line of the occiput (Fig. 4.7). Kamibayashi and Richmond[4] divided this muscle into three subvolumes: sternomastoid, cleidomastoid, and cleido-occipital. The fascicles on the superficial surface (sternomastoid and cleido-occipital portions) lie in parallel. However, the cleidomastoid portion on the deep surface, which runs from the clavicle to mastoid process, increases the proportion of muscle fascicles exerting force on the mastoid process (Fig. 4.8).[4] Superficial inspection of muscle architecture can neglect the arrangement of these deep fascicles, which would decrease the estimated moment-generating capacity of the sternocleidomastoid in

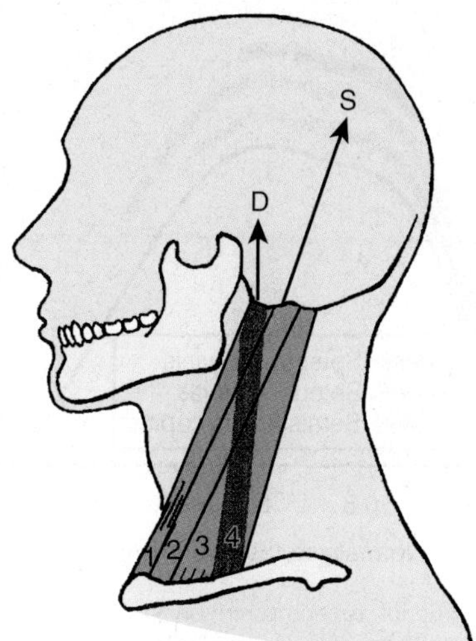

FIG. 4.8 Lines of action of sternocleidomastoid, including deep cleidomastoid portion. Arrows indicate differences in pulling direction of deep (D) and superficial (S) subvolumes. (Modified from Kamibayashi LK, Richmond FJR. Morphometry of human neck muscles. *Spine.* 1998;23:1314–1323.)

biomechanical models by more than 30%.[21] The sternocleidomastoid has moment arms for flexion, contralateral rotation, and lateral bending, and has been found to be active during movements in all three of these directions.

Also on the anterior surface of the neck, the infrahyoid muscles (sternohyoid, sternothyroid, thyrohyoid) link the hyoid bone, thyroid cartilage, and sternum, whereas the suprahyoid muscles (digastric, stylohyoid, mylohyoid, and geniohyoid) connect the hyoid bone to the mastoid process and mandible (see Fig. 4.7). The hyoid muscles are generally considered to maneuver the hyoid bone for deglutition and maintaining airway patency, but could potentially generate a neck flexion moment if the infrahyoid and suprahyoid muscles were activated in concert.

On the posterior surface of the neck, the trapezius is the most superficial muscle (see Fig. 4.2A). It can be divided into three segments: the rostral segment (also called clavotrapezius or trapezius pars descendens) runs from the lateral part of the clavicle to the occiput or ligamentum nuchae; the middle part (acromiotrapezius or pars transversa) runs nearly perpendicular to the midline at the lower cervical and upper thoracic levels from the lateral part of the scapular spine; and the caudal part (spinotrapezius or pars ascendens) attaches to spinous processes of T4 to T12 from the scapula. Its superficial position means that the trapezius has large moment arms for spine and head movements; however, its attachments to the scapula mean that shoulder movements also influence its function. Furthermore, the clavotrapezius (which attaches to the skull) has less than one-fifth of the mass of the acromiotrapezius,[4] indicating that the trapezius has less moment-generating potential for movements of the skull than generally believed.

Three other muscles connect the scapula to the cervical and thoracic vertebrae. The rhomboideus major and rhomboideus minor run from the medial border of the scapula to the midline at upper thoracic levels. Their major function is retraction of the scapula. The levator scapulae runs from the superior border of the scapula to the transverse processes of upper cervical vertebrae (see Fig. 4.2A). Like the trapezius, the functions of these muscles are related to movements of the shoulder.

The scalene muscles (scalenus anterior, medius, and posterior) run from the ribs to transverse processes of cervical vertebrae (see Fig. 4.5). Because of their lateral placement due to attachments to the ribs, the scalene muscles have substantial moment arms for cervical lateral bending; however, their main function is likely related to respiration. The scalene muscles were found to be composed of 52% to 72% type 1 fibers by number and 76% to 84% type 1 fibers by area. Although they are not postural muscles, the high percentage of type 1 fibers is likely related to their tonic function in respiration.[13] The serratus posterior superior and inferior also attach the vertebral column to the ribs. The serratus posterior superior arises from the lower part of ligamentum nuchae and the spines of the upper thoracic vertebrae, and attaches to ribs 2 to 5. The serratus posterior inferior originates from the spines of the lower thoracic and upper lumbar vertebrae, and attaches to ribs 9 to 12. These muscles function to elevate and depress the ribs, respectively.

The latissimus dorsi arises from the spinous processes of the lower six thoracic and upper two lumbar vertebrae, the thoracolumbar fascia, the iliac crest, and the lower ribs to insert on the humerus. The magnitudes of its potential force and moment on the lumbar spine and sacroiliac joint are small.[22] It is generally considered to move the arm, but if the upper limb were fixed, its activity could move the trunk (e.g., as in wheelchair transfers or crutch locomotion).

In summary, the spinal muscles are characterized by complex anatomy and architecture, and important biomechanical features are revealed when the architecture is studied in detail. However, the architecture of many spinal muscles, and its effects on function, remains to be determined.

Implications of Spinal Muscle Anatomy and Architecture for Motor Control

While the function of a muscle is dependent on muscle activity, neural control of a muscle is influenced by its architecture. Thus, architectural specialization of muscles means that the nervous system is not the only means available to modify muscular force and excursion. Although neural inputs can change muscle force, the effectiveness of neural input is altered by different muscle architectural features. In other words, nervous system commands are "interpreted" through the design of muscles to control posture and movement. Understanding both the biomechanics and neural control of spinal muscles, through models and experimental studies, is vital to understanding their role in pain and injury mechanisms.

Fascicle Length Changes With Posture

In the cervical spine, many extensor muscles undergo large length changes over the flexion–extension range of motion

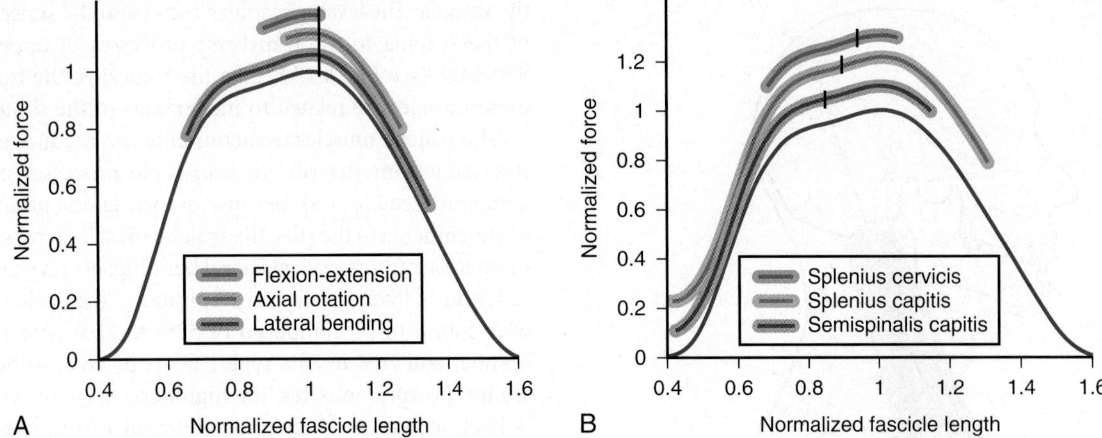

FIG. 4.9 Fascicle length excursions over the range of neck flexion–extension motion superimposed on a normalized muscle active force-length curve. (Modified from Vasavada A, Li S, Delp S. Influence of muscle morphometry and moment arms on the moment-generating capacity of human neck muscles. *Spine.* 1998;23:412–421.)

(ROM). A biomechanical model showed that the splenius capitis, semispinalis capitis, semispinalis cervicis, rectus capitis posterior major, and rectus capitis posterior minor all experience fascicle length changes greater than 70% of optimal length over the full ROM.[21] The change in fascicle length depends on both the optimal fascicle length of the muscle and the moment arm. For example, the splenius capitis and splenius cervicis have the same optimal fascicle length (see Table 4.3), but the splenius capitis has a much larger moment arm than the splenius cervicis. Thus, the splenius capitis undergoes larger fascicle length changes than the splenius cervicis over the same ROM (Fig. 4.9). On the other hand, the semispinalis capitis has shorter fascicle lengths but also a smaller moment arm than the splenius capitis. Thus, both the semispinalis capitis and splenius capitis experience similar large fascicle length excursions over the range of flexion–extension motion (see Fig. 4.9). In both muscles, fascicle lengths are extremely short in extended postures. This implies that the central nervous system must compensate for the associated decrease in force-generating potential by increasing activation or recruiting other extensors of the neck.

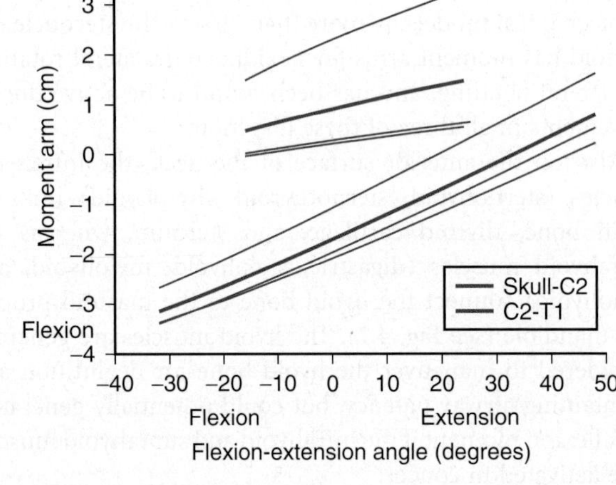

FIG. 4.10 Sternocleidomastoid flexion–extension moment arms. Light lines indicate individual subvolumes (sternomastoid, cleidomastoid, and cleido-occipital), and dark lines indicate a mass-weighted average. (Modified from Vasavada A, Li S, Delp S. Influence of muscle morphometry and moment arms on the moment-generating capacity of human neck muscles. *Spine.* 1998;23:412–421.)

Moment Arm Changes With Posture

Different parts of a muscle may have different moment arms, and the magnitude (and in some cases, direction) of these moment arms changes with posture. Furthermore, muscles that cross multiple joints (as most spinal muscles do) may have different mechanical functions at different joints. A biomechanical model of the neck muscles[21] demonstrated that the moment arm of sternocleidomastoid varies dramatically for flexion–extension movements (Fig. 4.10). For motions of the upper cervical joints, the cleido-occipital segment of the sternocleidomastoid actually has an extension moment arm that increases in extended postures (see Fig. 4.10); the other two subvolumes of sternocleidomastoid (which attach to the mastoid process) have very small moment arms. During flexion of the lower cervical joints, the flexion moment arm of the sternocleidomastoid increases. These results indicate that the function of sternocleidomastoid depends highly on posture and the joints about which movement occurs. Furthermore, the change in sternocleidomastoid flexion moment arm in the lower cervical region indicates a destabilizing effect, because it potentially increases the flexion moment-generating capacity of the muscle in flexed postures.

The same model[21] also showed that for axial rotation of the upper cervical region, many muscles have moment arms that vary by 2 to 3 cm but remain in the same direction throughout the ROM (e.g., sternocleidomastoid, splenius capitis; Fig. 4.11). For other muscles, the direction of moment arm changes with axial rotation. At the neutral position, the right rectus capitis posterior major has a right rotation moment arm; its magnitude

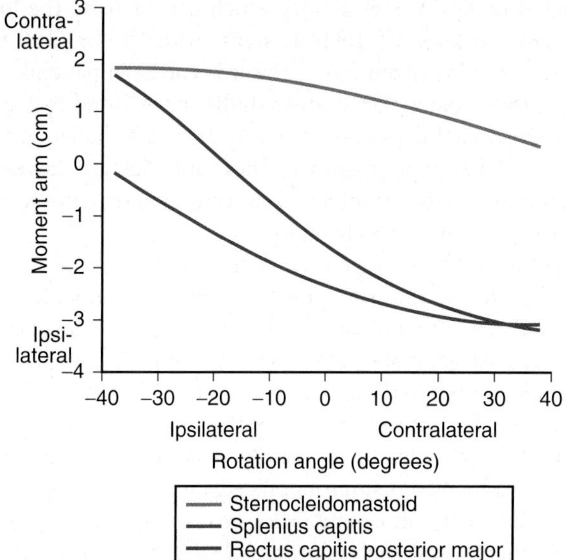

FIG. 4.11 Axial rotation moment arms for the upper cervical region. (Modified from Vasavada A, Li S, Delp S. Influence of muscle morphometry and moment arms on the moment-generating capacity of human neck muscles. *Spine*. 1998;23:412–421.)

increases in left rotated postures. However, when the head is rotated to the right, the moment arm decreases in magnitude and eventually changes to a left rotation moment arm. These results indicate that the rectus capitis posterior major has an axial rotation moment arm appropriate to restore the head to neutral posture from the most rotated head positions. The moment arms of other muscles, such as the semispinalis capitis and longissimus capitis, show the same pattern, although their moment arms are smaller. The implication of these findings is that the moment arm provides a "self-stabilizing" function to assist the central nervous system in maintaining neutrally rotated (i.e., eyes forward) head posture. This function is particularly relevant in the upper cervical region, because most axial rotation occurs between C1 and C2.

In the lumbar spine, posture also changes the mechanical function of erector spine muscles. McGill and associates[23] measured the fiber angles of longissimus thoracic and iliocostalis lumborum with the lumbar spine in neutral and fully flexed using high-resolution ultrasound. They found that flexion changes the line of action of these muscles, decreasing their capacity to resist anterior shear forces. This finding is important because anterior shear loads are related to the risk of back injury.[24]

Implications of Spinal Muscle Anatomy and Architecture for Injury and Pain

There are at least three ways in which spinal muscles may be implicated in mechanisms of injury and pain. First, the muscle itself may be injured from eccentric contraction, as described in Chapter 3. This may occur during an imposed movement (particularly one in which the kinematics are abnormal). Second, muscle forces may alter the load distribution within anatomic structures that have been clinically linked to pain. Third, muscle activity can alter spinal stiffness and kinematics, which would indirectly affect soft-tissue loads and strains. The relationship between muscles and injury can be elucidated by biomechanical models, the validity of which depends on accurate modeling of anatomy and architecture.

Muscle Injury Resulting From Eccentric Contraction

As noted in Chapter 3, rapid lengthening of muscle is an important mechanism of muscle injury. An example of potential muscle injury due to imposed lengthening occurs during whiplash. During the retraction phase of whiplash injury, when the head translates rearward with respect to the torso, the sternocleidomastoid muscle can experience lengthening strains of 5% to 10% while it is active.[25,26] During the rebound phase of whiplash injury, when the head translates forward with respect to the torso, the splenius capitis and semispinalis capitis muscles can experience lengthening strains of 10% to 20%. These predictions of muscle strains, based on a biomechanical model that incorporates muscle architecture,[21] are above thresholds for strain that causes injury to active-lengthening muscle.[27–29]

Muscles Altering Load Distribution in Other Anatomic Structures

Because muscles are oriented primarily vertically, their activation produces axial compression of the spine. The compressive loads on the discs and facet joints are a function of muscle force, moment arm, and activation. When the detailed anatomy of the lumbar erector spinae was included in a biomechanical model,[30] the predicted disc compression and shear loads were reduced compared with a lumped extensor "muscle equivalent" commonly used in many models. This study highlights the importance of creating an accurate representation of muscle anatomy in biomechanical models.

Compressive loads may severely alter tissue loads, particularly if abnormal vertebral kinematics occur. For example, the synovial fold of the facet joint may become impinged during the abnormal kinematics that occur during whiplash.[31] Muscles may also contribute to injury by directly loading passive structures. For instance, the cervical multifidus has direct attachments to facet capsular ligaments[8,32]; the combined loading from joint motion and muscle forces may lead to subcatastrophic injuries in facet capsular ligaments. These observations are important because the cervical facet joints and capsular ligaments have been clinically isolated as a source of neck pain.[33]

Muscle Effects on Spinal Stiffness and Stability

It has long been recognized that muscles are necessary for spinal stability. However, it is unclear which muscles contribute most to spinal stability; this question has been addressed in several theoretical and experimental studies. Crisco and Panjabi[34] examined the role of gross muscle anatomy (e.g., the number of joints crossed by a muscle) in lateral stabilization of the lumbar spine using a mathematical model. They calculated minimal muscle stiffness necessary for spinal stability and found that muscles spanning only one vertebral body required the highest stiffness (i.e., activation) for stability, whereas those muscles that spanned the largest number of vertebrae were most efficient (required the least activation). Efficient stabilization (less muscle activation) is important because it implies lower disc loads. Electromyographically driven modeling by Cholewicki and McGill[35] suggested that large muscles may provide the bulk of stiffness to the spinal column, as suggested by Crisco and Panjabi,[34] but that the activity of short intrinsic muscles was also necessary to maintain stability. In fact, biomechanical models have shown that buckling (loss of stability) can occur from a temporary reduction in activation to one or more intersegmental muscles.[35] Presumably, small intrinsic muscles are better suited to stabilize displacements at a single joint with a minimum increase in joint loads at other levels. Similarly, Winters and associates used both computer and physical models of the cervical spine to demonstrate that activating only large, long muscles resulted in instability, especially around the upright posture.[36,37] The authors also concluded that activation of deep muscles was necessary for spinal stability. These types of analyses demonstrate the importance of both gross anatomy and architecture of spinal muscles on spinal stability. However, many important questions remain, such as the effect of muscle fatigue on spinal stability and the best muscle activation patterns for stability in the prevention and rehabilitation of low back and neck pain.

Muscle fatigue has been implicated in low back and neck pain[38]; the mechanism may be related to altered loads in other structures, decreased spinal stability, accumulation of metabolites, or involvement of peripheral and central mediation of pain. Patients with neck pain or cervical radiculopathy demonstrate altered neck muscle endurance and myoelectric evidence of fatigue.[39,40] In patients with pain, as well as healthy subjects, fatigue can lead to differences in neuromuscular control, including altered activation patterns or flexion–relaxation, which can increase the loads in passive tissues.[39,41] There is some evidence for fiber type transformations (from type 1 toward type 2) in patients with back or neck pain,[42,43] but other studies have found that spine musculoskeletal disorders are not related to a change in fiber type.[44,45] Fiber type studies in these muscles are extremely difficult due to their complex architectural design and limited ability to perform muscle biopsies.

Although the average architectural features of the major muscles in the lumbar spine have been documented (see earlier discussion and associated tables), there is an increasing need to generate patient-specific architectural data for diagnostic purposes, surgical planning, and musculoskeletal modeling. Recent advances in MRI and image processing allow these muscles to be rapidly visualized and quantified in three dimensions in an unprecedented fashion previously impossible with ultrasound, MRI, or CT scanning (Fig. 4.12). Additionally, these tools allow muscle tissue to be fractionated into contractile and fat compartments, which is extremely relevant clinically, as "muscle quality" appears to be an important feature in the lumbar spine and other joint systems subjected to chronic disease. As can be seen in Fig. 4.13, the fraction of muscle contained within "normal" muscle boundaries can be substantially lower than anticipated. Further, fatty infiltration is found in neck muscles in cases of whiplash injury with poor functional recovery[46] and the amount decreases with exercise[47]; disc injury is associated with increased adipose and connective tissue in lumbar multifidus, and a decrease in adipose tissue on biopsy was associated with positive outcome after surgery.[48] Last, in Chapter 3 we discussed the need for (and difficulty of) quantifying muscle fiber or fascicle lengths in individual patients. Magnetic resonance diffusion tensor imaging (MR-DTI) now allows fascicle length estimates on a subject-by-subject basis (Fig. 4.14). However, it is important to note that these are nonnormalized fascicle (not fiber) lengths; thus, they cannot be used to predict muscle excursion or velocity, nor can they be used to calculate PCSA. Future developments in methods to measure sarcomere length are required to make these normalizations. Nevertheless, these are emerging scientific tools that should be considered in clinical and scientific work as they are more rigorously validated.

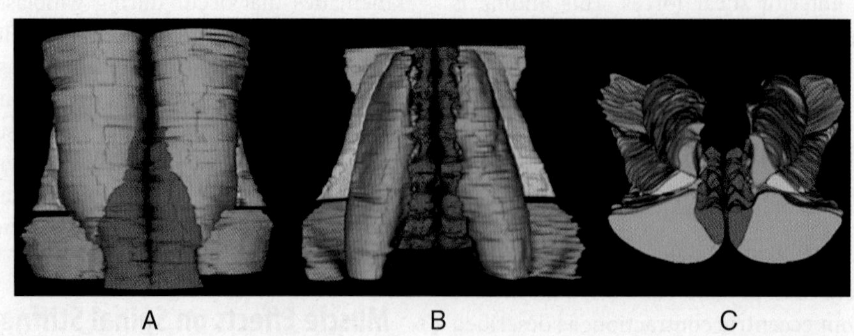

FIG. 4.12 Magnetic resonance imaging–based, patient-specific three-dimensional lumbar spine muscle volumes view from (A) posterior, (B) anterior, and (C) inferior. Multifidus *(red)*, erector spinae *(blue)*, quadratus lumborum *(yellow)*, and psoas *(green)* are easily visualized.

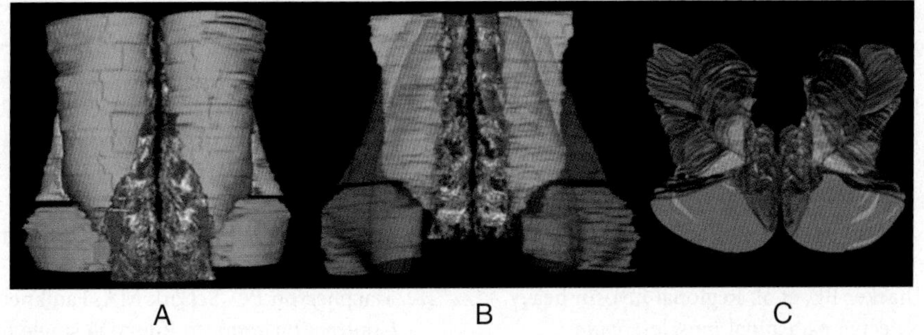

FIG. 4.13 Magnetic resonance imaging–based, patient-specific three-dimensional lumbar spine muscle volume fractions (muscles in colors and fat in white) view from (A) posterior, (B) anterior, and (C) inferior. Multifidus *(red)*, erector spinae *(blue)*, quadratus lumborum *(yellow)*, and psoas *(green)* are easily visualized and quantified.

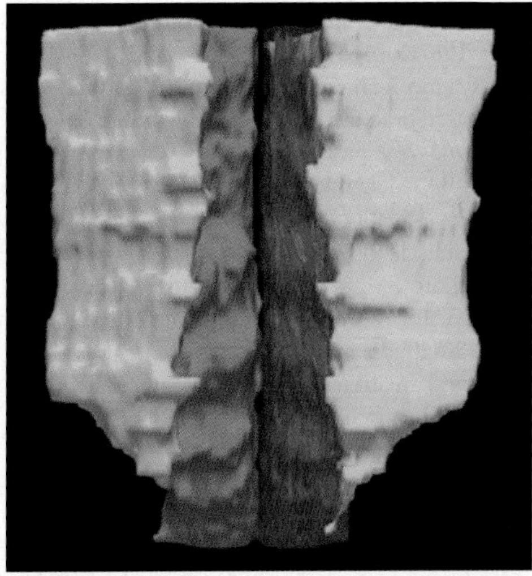

FIG. 4.14 Magnetic resonance diffusion tensor imaging (MR-DTI) can be used to generate tractography maps of individual muscles. Based on imaging resolution, these tracts likely represent muscle fascicles (or larger), but the diffusion properties themselves are heavily influenced by muscle fiber geometry. In this example, a posterior view of three-dimensional muscle volumes demonstrates bilateral erector spinae *(blue)* and multifidus muscles *(red)*. The right multifidus muscle has MR-DTI tractography results superimposed on the multifidus muscle volume depicting fascicle orientations and lengths.

Summary

Muscular architecture is an important, and often overlooked, determinant of muscle function. Because muscle architecture interacts with the skeletal and nervous systems in complex ways, all of these factors must be examined together to fully understand the biomechanical function of a muscle and its contribution to any pain or injury mechanisms. Detailed anatomic and architectural studies have yielded insights into spinal muscle functions, but the architecture of many spinal muscles remains to be examined. These data are necessary for accurate biomechanical models, which must be used in conjunction with experimental studies to elucidate the function of spinal muscles and their role in pathologic processes of the spine. This information can ultimately be used to develop improved prevention and rehabilitation strategies.

KEY REFERENCES

1. Macintosh JE, Bogduk N. The biomechanics of the lumbar multifidus. *Clin Biomech (Bristol, Avon)*. 1986;1:205-213.
2. MacIntosh JE, Bogduk N. The morphology of the lumbar erector spinae. *Spine*. 1987;12:658-668.
3. MacIntosh JE, Valencia F, Bogduk N, Munro RR. The morphology of the human lumbar multifidus. *Clin Biomech (Bristol, Avon)*. 1986;1:196-204.
   This series of papers describes the complex but highly reproducible anatomy of the lumbar and thoracic spine musculature. Progressing from superficial to deep and thoracic to lumbar, the extraordinary level of organization of this musculature is clearly apparent.
4. Kamibayashi LK, Richmond FJR. Morphometry of human neck muscles. *Spine*. 1998;23:1314-1323.
   This paper represents the first quantitative study of muscle architecture in the cervical spine. The work highlights unique architectural features of the neck muscles and provides data for comparative studies and the development of biomechanical models.
5. Cholewicki J, McGill SM. Mechanical stability of the in vivo lumbar spine: implications for injury and chronic low back pain. *Clin Biomech (Bristol, Avon)*. 1996;11(1):1-15.
   This paper combines a detailed anatomic model of the lumbar musculature with passive tissue properties, cross-bridge modeling, and electromyography to estimate muscle forces and spine stability. The authors relate spine stability to potential mechanisms of low back injury and pain.
6. Ward SR, Kim CW, Eng CM, et al. Architectural analysis and intraoperative measurements demonstrate the unique design of the multifidus muscle for lumbar spine stability. *J Bone Joint Surg Am*. 2009;91(1):176-185.
   This paper combined architectural measurements from cadaver specimens, in vivo intraoperative sarcomere length measurements in flexed and extended postures, and passive mechanical property measurements from biopsy. The results highlight the high force-generating capacity of multifidus in flexed lumbar spine positions, indicating a design for spine stabilization.

REFERENCES

1. Kalimo H, Rantanen J, Viljanen T, Einola S. Lumbar muscles: structure and function. *Ann Med*. 1989;21(5):353-359.
2. Macintosh JE, Bogduk N. 1987 Volvo award in basic science. The morphology of the lumbar erector spinae. *Spine*. 1987;12(7):658-668.

3. Delp SL, Suryanarayanan S, Murray WM, Uhlir J, Triolo RJ. Architecture of the rectus abdominis, quadratus lumborum, and erector spinae. *J Biomech.* 2001;34(3):371-375.
4. Kamibayashi LK, Richmond FJ. Morphometry of human neck muscles. *Spine.* 1998;23(12):1314-1323.
5. Ward SR, Kim CW, Eng CM, et al. Architectural analysis and intraoperative measurements demonstrate the unique design of the multifidus muscle for lumbar spine stability. *J Bone Joint Surg Am.* 2009;91(1):176-185.
6. Regev GJ, Kim CW, Thacker BE, et al. Regional myosin heavy chain distribution in selected paraspinal muscles. *Spine.* 2010;35(13):1265-1270.
7. Macintosh JE, Valencia F, Bogduk N, Munro RR. The morphology of the human lumbar multifidus. *Clin Biomech (Bristol, Avon).* 1986;1(4):196-204.
8. Anderson JS, Hsu AW, Vasavada AN. Morphology, architecture, and biomechanics of human cervical multifidus. *Spine.* 2005;30(4):E86-E91.
9. Macintosh JE, Bogduk N. The biomechanics of the lumbar multifidus. *Clin Biomech (Bristol, Avon).* 1986;1(4):205-213.
10. Thorstensson A, Carlson H. Fibre types in human lumbar back muscles. *Acta Physiol Scand.* 1987;131(2):195-202.
11. Donisch EW, Basmajian JV. Electromyography of deep back muscles in man. *Am J Anat.* 1972;133(1):25-36.
12. Gray H. *Gray's Anatomy.* New York: Gramercy Books; 1977.
13. Cornwall J, Kennedy E. Fiber types of the anterior and lateral cervical muscles in elderly males. *Eur Spine J.* 2015;24(9):1986-1991.
14. Mayoux-Benhamou MA, Revel M, Vallee C, et al. Longus colli has a postural function on cervical curvature. *Surg Radiol Anat.* 1994;16(4):367-371.
15. McGill S, Juker D, Kropf P. Quantitative intramuscular myoelectric activity of quadratus lumborum during a wide variety of tasks. *Clin Biomech (Bristol, Avon).* 1996;11(3):170-172.
16. Bogduk N, Pearcy M, Hadfield G. Anatomy and biomechanics of psoas major. *Clin Biomech (Bristol, Avon).* 1992;7(2):109-119.
17. McGill SM, Patt N, Norman RW. Measurement of the trunk musculature of active males using CT scan radiography: implications for force and moment generating capacity about the L4/L5 joint. *J Biomech.* 1988;21(4):329-341.
18. Santaguida PL, McGill SM. The psoas major muscle: a three-dimensional geometric study. *J Biomech.* 1995;28(3):339-345.
19. Gans C, Bock WJ. The functional significance of muscle architecture—a theoretical analysis. *Ergeb Anat Entwicklungsgesch.* 1965;38:115-142.
20. Juker D, McGill S, Kropf P, Steffen T. Quantitative intramuscular myoelectric activity of lumbar portions of psoas and the abdominal wall during a wide variety of tasks. *Med Sci Sports Exerc.* 1998;30(2):301-310.
21. Vasavada AN, Li S, Delp SL. Influence of muscle morphometry and moment arms on the moment-generating capacity of human neck muscles. *Spine.* 1998;23(4):412-422.
22. Bogduk N, Johnson G, Spalding D. The morphology and biomechanics of latissimus dorsi. *Clin Biomech (Bristol, Avon).* 1998;13(6):377-385.
23. McGill SM, Hughson RL, Parks K. Changes in lumbar lordosis modify the role of the extensor muscles. *Clin Biomech (Bristol, Avon).* 2000;15(10):777-780.
24. Norman R, Wells R, Neumann P, et al. A comparison of peak vs cumulative physical work exposure risk factors for the reporting of low back pain in the automotive industry. *Clin Biomech (Bristol, Avon).* 1998;13(8):561-573.
25. Brault JR, Siegmund GP, Wheeler JB. Cervical muscle response during whiplash: evidence of a lengthening muscle contraction. *Clin Biomech (Bristol, Avon).* 2000;15(6):426-435.
26. Vasavada AN, Brault JR, Siegmund GP. Musculotendon and fascicle strains in anterior and posterior neck muscles during whiplash injury. *Spine.* 2007;32(7):756-765.
27. Lieber RL, Friden J. Muscle damage is not a function of muscle force but active muscle strain. *J Appl Physiol.* 1993;74(2):520-526.
28. Macpherson PC, Schork MA, Faulkner JA. Contraction-induced injury to single fiber segments from fast and slow muscles of rats by single stretches. *Am J Physiol.* 1996;271(5 Pt 1):C1438-C1446.
29. Patel TJ, Das R, Friden J, Lutz GJ, Lieber RL. Sarcomere strain and heterogeneity correlate with injury to frog skeletal muscle fiber bundles. *J Appl Physiol.* 2004;97(5):1803-1813.
30. McGill SM, Norman RW. Effects of an anatomically detailed erector spinae model on L4/L5 disc compression and shear. *J Biomech.* 1987;20(6):591-600.
31. Kaneoka K, Ono K, Inami S, Hayashi K. Motion analysis of cervical vertebrae during whiplash loading. *Spine.* 1999;24(8):763-769.
32. Winkelstein BA, McLendon RE, Barbir A, Myers BS. An anatomical investigation of the human cervical facet capsule, quantifying muscle insertion area. *J Anat.* 2001;198(Pt 4):455-461.
33. Barnsley L, Lord SM, Wallis BJ, Bogduk N. The prevalence of chronic cervical zygapophysial joint pain after whiplash. *Spine.* 1995;20(1):20-25, discussion 26.
34. Crisco JJ 3rd, Panjabi MM. The intersegmental and multisegmental muscles of the lumbar spine. A biomechanical model comparing lateral stabilizing potential. *Spine.* 1991;16(7):793-799.
35. Cholewicki J, McGill SM. Mechanical stability of the in vivo lumbar spine: implications for injury and chronic low back pain. *Clin Biomech (Bristol, Avon).* 1996;11(1):1-15.
36. Daru K. *Computer Simulation and Static Analysis of the Human Head, Neck and Upper Torso.* Tempe, AZ: Arizona State University; 1989.
37. Winters JM, Peles JD. Neck muscle activity and 3-D head kinematics during quasi-static and dynamic tracking movements. In: Winters JM, Woo SL-Y, eds. *Multiple Muscle Systems: Biomechanics and Movement Organization.* New York: Springer-Verlag; 1990. Multiple Muscle Systems: Biomechanics and Movement Organization.
38. Hamberg-van Reenen HH, Ariens GA, Blatter BM, et al. Physical capacity in relation to low back, neck, or shoulder pain in a working population. *Occup Environ Med.* 2006;63(6):371-377.
39. Zabihhosseinian M, Holmes MW, Ferguson B, Murphy B. Neck muscle fatigue alters the cervical flexion relaxation ratio in sub-clinical neck pain patients. *Clin Biomech (Bristol, Avon).* 2015;30(5):397-404.
40. Halvorsen M, Abbott A, Peolsson A, Dedering A. Endurance and fatigue characteristics in the neck muscles during sub-maximal isometric test in patients with cervical radiculopathy. *Eur Spine J.* 2014;23(3):590-598.
41. Nimbarte AD, Zreiqat MM, Chowdhury SK. Cervical flexion-relaxation response to neck muscle fatigue in males and females. *J Electromyogr Kinesiol.* 2014;24(6):965-971.
42. Uhlig Y, Weber BR, Grob D, Muntener M. Fiber composition and fiber transformations in neck muscles of patients with dysfunction of the cervical spine. *J Orthop Res.* 1995;13(2):240-249.

43. Mazis N, Papachristou DJ, Zouboulis P, et al. The effect of different physical activity levels on muscle fiber size and type distribution of lumbar multifidus. A biopsy study on low back pain patient groups and healthy control subjects. *Eur J Phys Rehabil Med.* 2009;45(4):459-467.
44. Brown SH, Gregory DE, Carr JA, et al. ISSLS prize winner: Adaptations to the multifidus muscle in response to experimentally induced intervertebral disc degeneration. *Spine.* 2011;36(21):1728-1736.
45. Crossman K, Mahon M, Watson PJ, Oldham JA, Cooper RG. Chronic low back pain-associated paraspinal muscle dysfunction is not the result of a constitutionally determined "adverse" fiber-type composition. *Spine.* 2004;29(6):628-634.
46. Elliott JM, Courtney DM, Rademaker A, et al. The rapid and progressive degeneration of the cervical multifidus in whiplash: an MRI study of fatty infiltration. *Spine.* 2015;40(12): E694-E700.
47. O'Leary S, Jull G, Van Wyk L, Pedler A, Elliott J. Morphological changes in the cervical muscles of women with chronic whiplash can be modified with exercise—a pilot study. *Muscle Nerve.* 2015;52(5):772-779.
48. Rantanen J, Hurme M, Falck B, et al. The lumbar multifidus muscle five years after surgery for a lumbar intervertebral disc herniation. *Spine.* 1993;18(5):568-574.

5 CHAPTER The Intervertebral Disc: Normal, Aging, and Pathologic

Adam S. Olsen
James D. Kang
Nam Vo
Gwendolyn Sowa

The intervertebral disc is a structure interposed between the bodies of the vertebral column that acts as the shock absorber of the spine, transmitting compressive loads between bony segments. Its structure is generally fibrocartilaginous, consisting of several anatomic segments with distinct functional importance in both the native and pathologic spine. Degeneration of the disc is thought to be the leading cause of low back pain worldwide and is associated with multiple other conditions, such as spinal stenosis, herniated nucleus pulposus, and deformity.[1] Throughout the human life span, intervertebral discs undergo progressive but highly variable degeneration, often beginning in early life.[1,2]

This chapter discusses the basic structure of the intervertebral disc and surrounding tissues, followed by a review of the degenerative cascade leading to intervertebral disc degeneration (IDD) as well as clinical consequences. Despite the ubiquity of IDD and its association to low back pain, the exact mechanisms of discogenic low back pain IDD are not well defined. What has been established is that the process is multifactorial, involving a complex interaction of genetics, aging, mechanics, and environment biology.

Normal Disc

Disc Anatomy

The intervertebral disc is composed of three main structures: the cartilaginous endplates (CEP), the central nucleus pulposus (NP), and the peripherally located anulus fibrosus (AF) (Fig. 5.1).

Cartilaginous Endplates

The endplates are cartilaginous structures that serve as the superior and inferior margins of the intervertebral disc. In early life, the endplates are analogous to epiphyseal plates elsewhere in the body, and serve as the growth centers of the intervertebral bodies.[3] Similar to epiphyses elsewhere, the hyaline cartilage of the endplate initially occupies a significant portion of the disc. As aging occurs, this cartilage layer thins, and by adulthood consists of about a 1-mm-thick layer of avascular tissue composed of rounded chondrocytes and type II collagen.[4] Cartilaginous endplates (along with surrounding subchondral bone) do undergo some degree of elastic deformation during loading, but their contribution to the shock-absorptive properties of the disc is minimal. Instead, the endplates functionally allow force transmission along the vertebral axis via the discs and act as semipermeable barriers for nutrient and waste exchange.

Nucleus Pulposus

The nucleus lies between adjacent endplates and forms the gel-like core of the disc. The nucleus consists of a proteoglycan and water matrix held together by an irregular network of collagen type II and elastin fibers. Proteoglycans have numerous highly anionic glycosaminoglycan (GAG) side chains (i.e., chondroitin sulfate and keratan sulfate), which attract countercations and allow the NP to imbibe water. This composition is similar to articular cartilage, and the ability of the matrix to imbibe and release water in relation to applied stresses allows the disc to cushion against compressive loads. The primary proteoglycan is aggrecan; the high concentration of this hydrophilic molecule provides the osmotic properties needed to resist compression.[5]

Cells in the NP are initially notochordal, but their numbers decline after birth and eventually become undetectable at about age 4 to 10 years in humans.[6] The NP is gradually replaced during growth by smaller and rounded cells resembling the chondrocytes of articular cartilage.[7] These chondrocyte-like cells synthesize mostly proteoglycans and collagen type II in response to changes in hydrostatic pressure. These cells are also able to survive in the hypoxic environment of the intervertebral disc and contain inducible hypoxia-responsive transcription factors.[8] The NP functions as a shock absorber, acting in essence as a pressurized, deformable sphere that dissipates compressive forces to the AF and the adjacent vertebral bodies. As compressive forces on the spine increase, hydrostatic pressure within the nucleus pushes outward from its center in all directions.

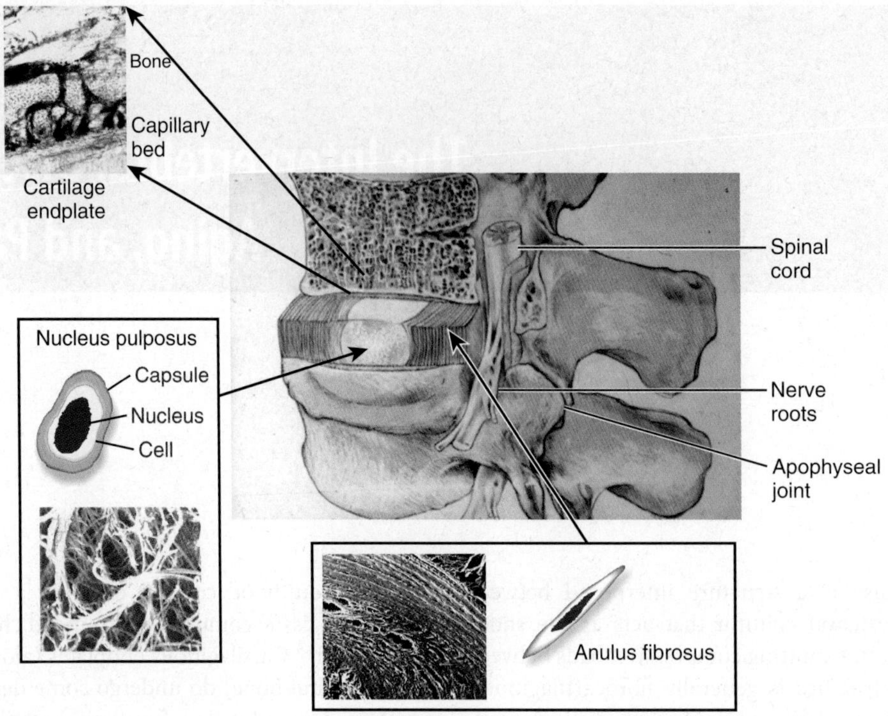

FIG. 5.1 The intervertebral disc is a pivotal part of the spinal column; its properties influence behavior of adjacent tissues. There is great variation in matrix organization, composition, and cell morphology and activity in different regions of the disc.

Anulus Fibrosus

The AF surrounds the NP and is composed of approximately 20 concentric rings (lamellae) of highly organized collagen fibers, primarily collagen type I. The collagen fibers are oriented approximately 60 degrees to the vertical axis of the spine and run parallel within each lamella but perpendicular between adjacent lamellae, allowing for maximal tensile strength.[9] Individual lamellae are connected to one another by radially oriented elastin fibers, which account for approximately 2% of the anulus' dry weight. A network of bridging tissues that span multiple lamellae, containing both elastic and vascular elements, has also been described.[10] Fibers of the outer anulus attach to the periphery of the vertebral bodies, whereas inner fibers pass from one endplate to another. Cells in the anulus are found between lamellae, arranged in parallel to the collagen fibers. Outer anulus cells are thin, elongated, and phenotypically similar to fibroblasts, whereas cells of the innermost anulus are more spheroid, similar to articular chondrocytes.[1,11] The anulus contains the NP and maintains its pressurization under compressive loads. The tensile properties of the anulus allow the nucleus to recover its original shape and position when the compressive load is reduced.

Blood Supply, Nutrition, and Innervation

Blood Supply

In early fetal life, vascular channels traverse the endplates, but they diminish in size starting at birth until complete disappearance by approximately 5 years of age. In adults, the blood supply of the disc arises from two capillary plexuses. One plexus penetrates 1 to 2 mm into the outer anulus, supplying only the periphery of the anulus. The other capillary plexus begins in the vertebral body and penetrates the subchondral bone (see Fig. 5.1), terminating in capillary loops at the bone-cartilage junction.[12] The density of this capillary network varies in location across the endplate, being greatest in the center and lowest at the periphery. Although blood flow to the disc is minimal, it may not be entirely passive as muscarinic receptors have been identified on the disc periphery, which may influence perfusion.[13] Cells in the center of the human adult lumbar NP are 8 mm from the nearest blood source, making the disc one of the largest avascular structures in the body.

Nutrition

The limited vascularity of the intervertebral disc has important physiologic implications—mainly that nutrition depends almost entirely on diffusion (Fig. 5.2).[14–16] The nutritional environment of the cells varies throughout the disc because of its size and architectural makeup, with cells in the NP being 6 to 8 mm from the nearest blood vessel. Small molecules necessary to maintain cellular function (i.e., glucose and oxygen) readily leave vertebral capillaries and diffuse across the thin cartilaginous endplate and the outermost layers of the anulus into the disc extracellular matrix (ECM). Concentration gradients of glucose, oxygen, and other nutrients and metabolites exist across the disc, regulated by the rates of nutrient supply and consumption as well as the net negative charge of the NP produced by high proteoglycan concentration. The low

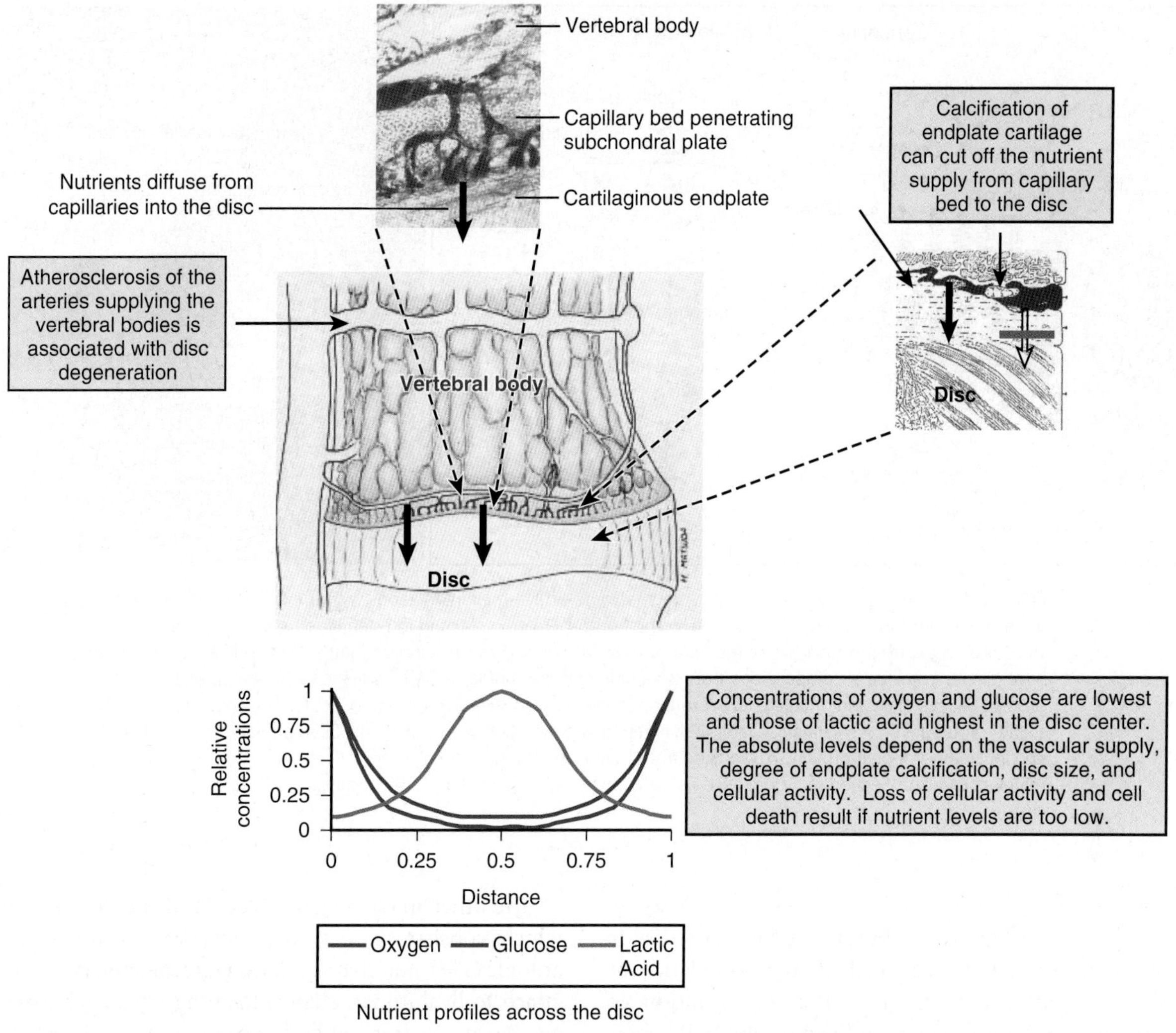

FIG. 5.2 Schematic view of routes for nutrient transport into avascular disc and resulting nutrient profiles. The diagram also shows possible regions of disturbance. (Modified from Crock HV, Goldwasser M, Yoshizawa H. Vascular anatomy related to the intervertebral disc. In: Ghosh P, ed. *Biology of the Intervertebral Disc*. Boca Raton, FL: CRC Press; 1991:109–133.)

oxygen tension in the nucleus leads to anaerobic metabolism (i.e., glycolysis), resulting in a high concentration of lactic acid and a lower pH in the nucleus compared with the periphery of the disc.[16] Metabolic byproducts, such as lactic acid, diffuse from the disc in the opposite direction of glucose entry.

Innervation

Under normal conditions, only the outer 1 to 2 mm of the AF is innervated in nondegenerated human discs; the majority of these fibers are sympathetic perivascular nerves. A small number of mechanoreceptors are also reported in the outer several AF lamellae, likely providing some level of proprioceptive feedback.[17] The sources of this innervation are variable, but include plexuses contained in both the anterior longitudinal and posterior longitudinal ligaments; these nerves have been found to contain various substances, such as neuropeptide Y, substance P, acetylcholinesterase, and others.[18] The remainder of the anulus and nucleus are uniquely avascular and lacking neurons under normal, nondegenerated conditions. Several studies have described further nerve ingrowth into degenerated lumbar discs, however, which is discussed later in this chapter.

Disc Composition

The function of the intervertebral disc depends greatly on the properties of its ECM. The ECM provides the biomechanical properties and acts to regulate the extracellular fluid composition and the rate at which nutrients and metabolites are exchanged. The ECM consists of a complex network of macromolecules whose composition varies in different regions of the disc (Fig. 5.3).[4,19] ECM macromolecules are synthesized and maintained by a small population of cells (~9000 cells/mm^3 in the anulus and ~5000 cells/mm^3 in the nucleus) occupying less than 1% of the disc volume.[4] Disc cells also produce a complex array of cytokines, growth factors, and proteases to maintain equilibrium between the rates of synthesis and degradation of ECM components.[20,21]

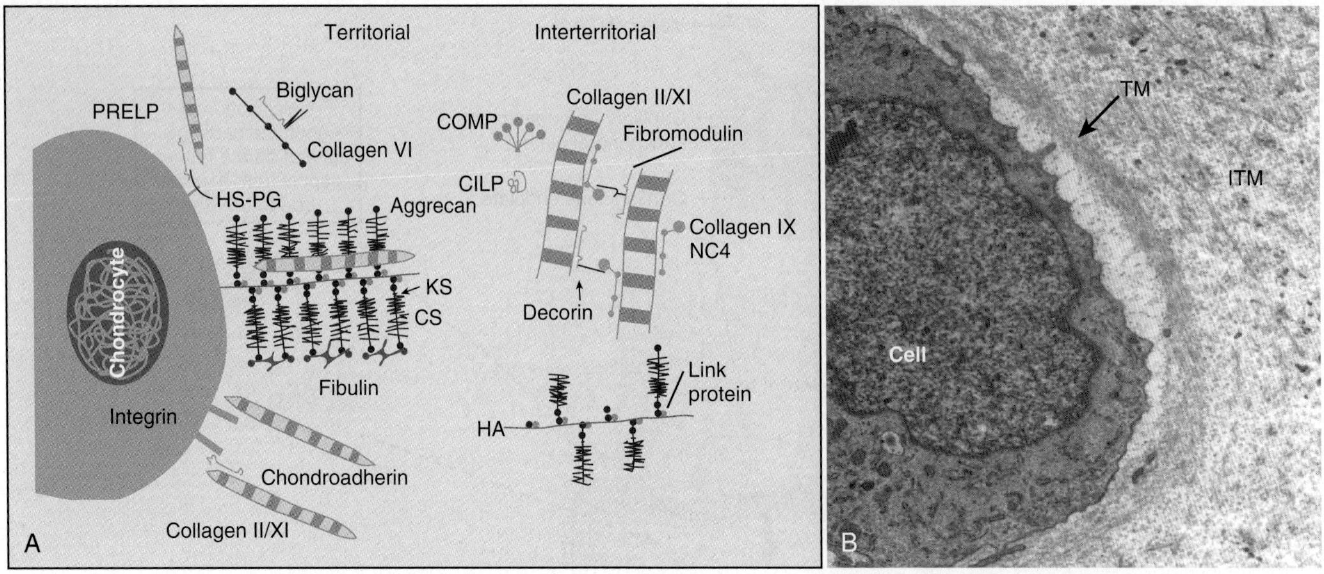

FIG. 5.3 (A) Schematic view of different matrix macromolecules, their interactions with the cell and with other matrix molecules, and their distribution within the territorial matrix (TM) and interterritorial matrix (ITM). (B) Transmission electron micrograph of section through disc cell and its surrounding matrix. TM and ITM not only have different molecular compositions, but also a different morphology. COMP, cartilage oligomeric matrix protein; CILP, cartilage intermediate layer protein; CS, chondroitin sulfate; HA, hyaluronan; HS-PG, heparan sulfate-proteoglycan; KS, keratan sulfate; NC4, N-terminal noncollagenous domain 4; PRELP, proline/arginine-rich end leucine-rich repeat protein. (A, Modified from Heinegard D, Aspberg A, Morgelin M, et al. Extracellular matrix of cartilage. Section for Connective Tissue Biology, University of Lund, 2003. Available at http://www.cmb.lu.se/ctb.)

Water

The major component by weight of the intervertebral disc is water; its concentration is regulated by the abundance of proteoglycan aggregates in the disc. The concentration of water varies with age, location within the disc, and body position.[22] The NP is most highly hydrated, and the water concentration can be as high as 90% in an infant, declining to approximately 80% in nondegenerated young adult discs.[23] The water content of the anulus is lower than the nucleus, declining to 65% in the outer anulus in adult discs.

Water content varies with load, leading to diurnal changes in disc hydration.[24] During the diurnal cycle, 25% of the disc's water can be lost and regained in young lumbar discs.[25] Some water is expelled from the disc during the day because of the increased forces of body weight and muscle contractions; it is reimbibed at night when the compressive forces are removed. This diurnal cycle results in changes in disc height and affects the disc's mechanical properties.

Macromolecules

Collagen is one major macromolecular component of the disc. The collagen content of the disc is highest in the outer anulus, and the dry weight decreases significantly in the nucleus of adult discs.[26] The concentration of collagen type I is highest in the outer anulus and decreases going toward the nucleus.[26] Collagen type II follows the opposite gradient, with the highest concentration located in the nucleus. Along with collagen types I and II, the ECM contains many other minor collagens, including types III, V, VI, IX, and XI.

The other major macromolecule of the disc is aggrecan,[27] which consists of a protein core with approximately 100 anionic GAG side chains. Many aggrecan molecules covalently attach to hyaluronan chains, forming large aggregates. These aggregates are trapped by the surrounding collagen network, imparting a net negative charge to the ECM. The interstitial water contains an excess of cations, which is directly related to the concentration of negative charge (i.e., GAG concentration). The high concentration of cations imparts a high osmotic pressure in the nucleus. Changes in proteoglycan concentration and GAG concentration lead to changes in osmotic pressure, affecting the ability of the disc to maintain hydration and turgor when loaded.[27]

In addition to collagens and aggrecan, the disc contains lower concentrations of numerous other macromolecules,[14] including elastin, the smaller proteoglycans decorin and fibromodulin, cartilage oligomeric matrix protein, and cartilage intermediate layer protein. These molecules function either structurally or biomechanically and are important for normal disc function.

Intervertebral Disc Degeneration

Degeneration

IDD is defined as an aberrant, cell-mediated response to progressive damage, with combined structural failure and accelerated or advanced signs of aging. These proposed definitions also suggest that structurally intact discs with accelerated age-related changes be classified as *early degenerative discs*, whereas the term *degenerative disc disease* should be applied if the disc is also painful.[28]

Although the exact mechanism of disc degeneration has not been determined, it is known to involve a complex interaction of factors, including ECM macromolecule changes, decreased water content, altered enzyme activity, decreased endplate permeability, impaired metabolite transport, structural failure, and cell senescence and death. These biologic and biomechanical factors cause extensive histomorphologic changes of the disc, leading to disorganization of the anulus, solidification of the nucleus, and thinning and calcification of the cartilaginous endplates. Recently, it has also been suggested that several general types of degeneration may exist—namely, endplate driven and anulus driven—that potentially affect different areas of the spine at different ages.[29]

Matrix Macromolecule Changes

The most physiologically important changes of disc degeneration start in the nucleus.[23] Early changes include increased proteolytic degradation of aggrecan and other aggregating proteoglycans coupled with an increased concentration of nonaggregating proteoglycans. The accumulation of degraded proteoglycans further impairs diffusion of nutrients and oxygen through the disc. A change in the proportions of the GAGs chondroitan sulfate, heparan sulfate, and keratan sulfate also occurs, with increasing amounts of heparan sulfate and keratan sulfate as degeneration progresses. These changes diminish the hydroscopic properties of the ECM further, resulting in decreased water content and decreased ability to imbibe water. Loss of proteoglycans and hydration leads to decreased swelling pressure[27] and loss of disc height. The changes result in altered responses to applied biomechanical loads, ultimately leading to the structural features of degeneration.

Intervertebral disc degeneration also results in disorganization and destruction of the collagen network.[30] As the overall proteoglycan and water content decreases, there is a corresponding increase in collagen content. Collagen type I replaces collagen type II in the inner anulus and nucleus, and there is a tendency for collagen type I fibrils throughout the disc to become coarser. The highly organized collagen fiber arrangements of the anulus are also disrupted, and collagen and elastin networks become more disorganized. When the collagen network has been damaged, disc biomechanics are markedly altered, and the potential for structural damage increases.

Increased levels of proinflammatory cytokines lead to increased production of proteinases, causing breakdown of collagens such as types VI, IX, and X. Collagen type IX is degraded in the pericellular microenvironment, allowing for local alteration of this microenvironment during degeneration. With disc degeneration, collagen type IX decreases similarly to collagen type II, implying advanced stages of degeneration and fibrosis of the nucleus. The synthesis of collagen type VI, a matrix protein with relatively low cross-linking, increases as degeneration progresses and functions to hold proliferating cells together.

The overall ECM content in the nucleus is a well-controlled equilibrium between degradative and synthetic pathways involving numerous proteins. In disc degeneration, there is an imbalance between degradative and synthetic pathways whereby the latter overtake the former with a predominance of catabolic enzyme activity. Proteinases of the matrix metalloproteinase (MMP) and "a disintegrin and metalloproteinase with thrombospondin motifs" (ADAMTS) families cleave proteoglycans, collagens, and other macromolecules and have been implicated in the breakdown of the ECM.[31] The degradative enzymes MMP-3 and MMP-13 (also known as stromelysin-1 and collagenase 3, respectively) have been found at increased levels in degenerated human discs.

The regulation of MMP and ADAMTS production and ECM macromolecule production is achieved by numerous cytokines and growth factors. Of particular importance in disc ECM homeostasis are members of the interleukin (IL) family (catabolism) and transforming growth factor-β (anabolism) superfamily.[32,33] Mediators of inflammation such as nitric oxide and prostaglandin E_2 and the cytokines IL-1 and IL-6 are found at increased levels in degenerated discs.[32–34] The synthetic capabilities of nucleus cells are unable to sustain appropriate levels of aggrecan and collagen production in the face of this increased catabolism, which contributes to further degeneration of the disc.

Cellular Changes

It has long been recognized that there is a gradual progressive loss of cells during disc degeneration,[35] leading to further loss of the ECM due to synthesis deficiency. An increasing body of literature has shown that apoptosis, or programmed cell death, and cellular senescence may be responsible for many of the features of degeneration.[36–38] More recent literature has also shown an increase in lacunae containing cell clusters,[39,40] possibly causing an overall increased number of cells at the site of injury. This increased cell proliferation may be an attempt to offset the progressive destruction and loss of the ECM. One reason for increased cellularity may be the focal increase in nutrient supply owing to the ingrowth of blood vessels in degenerating discs, as discussed elsewhere in this chapter.

Cell clusters have been discovered in areas adjacent to the newly formed blood vessels within degenerated discs. Cells in these areas have access to nutrient supply and growth factors, and undergo proliferation. The cellular changes in degenerated discs resemble osteoarthritis, in which remodeling of the pericellular microenvironment with chondrocyte proliferation and cluster formation have also been found. Ultimately, cellular attempts at repair become ineffective as disc degeneration progresses due to the abnormal local mechanical environment of the cells.

Structural Changes

As disc hydration decreases, the distinction between anulus and nucleus becomes less defined and disc height decreases (Fig. 5.4).[41] In later stages, gross tissue changes become

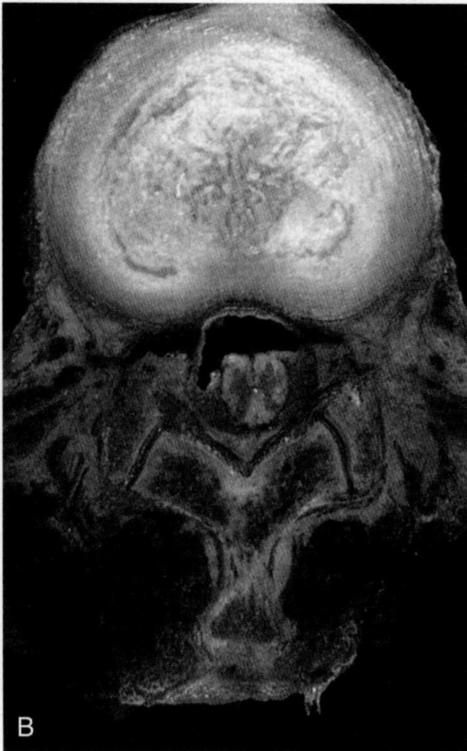

FIG. 5.4 Transverse sections of lumbar discs and apophyseal joints showing decrease in nucleus hydration, loss of demarcation between anulus and nucleus with age, and appearance of circumferential fissures by the third decade. (A) Adolescent. (B) At age 28 years. (Courtesy Bullough PG, Vigorita VJ. *Bullough's and Vigorita's Atlas of Orthopaedic Pathology*. Baltimore, MD: University Park Press–Gower Medical Publishing; 1995.)

increasingly apparent, including loss of lamellae organization, fissuring of the anulus,[42] and discoloration and solidification of the nucleus.[35,43] Radial and circumferential annular tears are often evident, sometimes extending to the disc periphery.[42] These changes are accompanied by ingrowth of nerves and blood vessels into the disc, as well as deposition of granulation tissue and calcification within the endplates. Endplate sclerosis is thought to impede nutrient transport to the disc by occluding both nutrient channels and blood vessels. These structural changes ultimately lead to altered, abnormal biomechanical properties of the disc. Damage to one area of the disc increases load bearing by adjacent tissues, making it more likely for damage to spread throughout the disc eventually. While a healthy intervertebral disc equalizes pressure within it, the decreased shock-absorbing capacity of the decompressed nucleus leads to high compressive stresses in the anulus.[44] Other gross morphologic changes of degeneration include disc bulging, disc space narrowing, endplate irregularities, and osteophyte formation.

Neovascularization and Sensory Nerve Innervation

As stated previously, the disc is largely avascular in adults with blood vessels normally restricted to only the outermost layers of the anulus. Likewise, only the outer 1 to 2 mm of the anulus is innervated in the normal human disc. The ingrowth of blood vessels and sensory nerves is an important feature of degenerated discs and seems to be associated with pain.[45] Ingrowth of capillaries may be facilitated by the loss of hydrostatic pressure in the inner regions of the disc, which would normally collapse small vessels. These newly formed microvessels release neurotrophic growth factors, such as nerve growth factor, allowing the ingrowth of small, nonmyelinated nerve fibers.[46–48] It has been hypothesized that discogenic pain arises because these nociceptive nerve fibers grow into areas of the disc that previously had no neurons.

Etiology of Intervertebral Disc Degeneration

Multiple risk factors have been hypothesized as the underlying cause, including aging, genetic predisposition, mechanical overload, and numerous environmental factors. Biomechanical studies have shown that excessive mechanical loading causes disruption of disc structure, including endplate defects, fissures, bulging, disc prolapse, and annular collapse.[49] Further experiments have confirmed that structural damage precipitates a cascade of cell-mediated responses, leading to further damage. Although mechanical loading may precipitate degeneration, the most important cause may be age-related biologic processes that impair the healing response and/or weaken the disc before structural damage. However, recent studies have shown that low-impact, cyclic loading increases trans-endplate nutrient diffusion in both healthy and degenerated discs, suggesting a complex interaction of host and environmental factors.[50] The combined effects of aging, unfavorable genetics, altered nutrition and metabolite transport, and excessive or repetitive loading all have been implicated in contributing to the process of degeneration.

Aging

The incidence of intervertebral disc degeneration increases with age and is most common in the lumbar spine.[51,52] Human intervertebral discs undergo very early aging and degeneration, resulting in histomorphologic and functional changes (Fig. 5.5).[41] Endplate permeability and vascular supply decrease throughout growth and aging, leading to altered metabolite transport.[41] Proteoglycans begin to fragment during childhood, and the overall proteoglycan content decreases with age, especially in the nucleus. There is a corresponding increase in collagen content, with collagen type I fibers replacing collagen type II fibers in the inner anulus and nucleus. In addition, reduced matrix turnover in older discs enables collagen fibrils to become increasingly cross-linked,[53] leading to retention of damaged fibers and reduced tissue strength. Synthesis of ECM components decreases steadily throughout life, which is partly attributable to decreased cell density, although synthesis rates per cell also decrease.

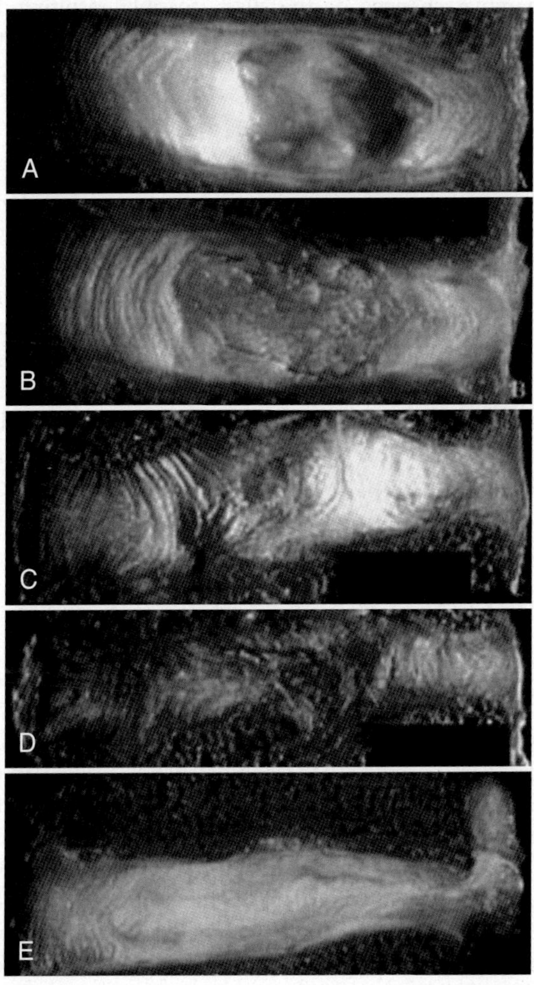

FIG. 5.5 Cadaveric lumbar intervertebral discs sectioned in midsagittal plane (anterior on left). (A) Young disc (35-year-old man). (B) Mature disc (47-year-old man). (C) Disrupted young disc (31-year-old man). Note endplate damage and inward collapse of inner anulus. (D) Severely disrupted young disc (31-year-old man). Note collapse of disc height. (E) Disc induced to prolapse in the laboratory (40-year-old man). Some nucleus pulposus has herniated through radial fissure in posterior anulus (right). (From Adams MA, Bogduk N, Burton K, et al. *The Biomechanics of Back Pain.* Edinburgh: Churchill Livingstone; 2002.)

In infants, the nucleus contains approximately 90% water and appears translucent.[23] The disc dehydrates slowly with aging, with water content of the nucleus declining to around 80% in young adults.[41] The nucleus also accumulates yellow pigmentation and becomes less distinguishable from the surrounding anulus.[23,41] As the disc water content decreases, the nucleus becomes smaller and decompressed, often condensing into several fibrous lumps. Dehydration of the nucleus leads to altered biomechanical properties of the disc, forcing the anulus to act as a fibrous solid to resist compression directly. The proteoglycan content of the anulus also decreases with aging, and the anulus becomes stiffer and weaker, resisting compressive loads in a haphazard manner.

Aging also causes progressive changes in disc nutrient supply and ECM composition. These changes decrease tissue strength and alter cell metabolism.[54] The alterations of proteoglycans and GAGs, decreased hydration, and changes in collagen distribution and cross-linking make the disc physically more vulnerable to injury. Age-related alteration to the vascular supply to the disc has been hypothesized as a primary initiator of age-dependent IDD. However, experimental endplate damage leads to degeneration[35] despite enhanced metabolite transport into the disc, suggesting that structural damage more strongly influences the degenerative process. Inadequate nutrition likely predisposes the disc to degeneration by compromising its ability to respond to increased loading or injury.

Genetic Predisposition

Genetic predisposition has been suggested as the greatest risk factor for disc degeneration, accounting for approximately 50% to 70% of the variability in identical twin studies.[55–57] Individual gene polymorphisms associated with disc degeneration include aggrecan,[57] cartilage intermediate layer protein,[57] collagen type IX,[58,59] MMP-3,[60] and vitamin D receptor.[61,62] The products of these genes alter the ECM composition, decrease tissue strength, impair regenerative capability, and undoubtedly influence disc cell function. There has also been recent attention to the roles of microRNA molecules, 18-22 nucleotide posttranslational regulatory elements, in intervertebral disc generation, but their roles have yet to be established.[62] Age-related disc degeneration develops after many decades, however, and preferentially affects the lumbar spine. Since unfavorable genetic predisposition is present throughout the life span, this suggests that genetic inheritance and polymorphic variations in susceptibility genes predispose the disc toward degeneration, but further insults such as excessive loading, structural damage, and other aging changes are necessary to trigger the cascade of degenerative events.

Nutrition

The failure of nutrient supply is hypothesized to be a primary cause of disc degeneration.[63] In vitro studies demonstrate that the metabolic activity of disc cells is sensitive to extracellular oxygen and pH, with matrix synthesis rates decreasing at acidic pH and low oxygen concentrations.[64,65] A decrease in glucose supply or altered pH could negatively affect the ability of disc cells to synthesize and maintain the ECM, ultimately leading to disc degeneration.

A relationship between loss of cell viability and a decrease in nutrient transport in scoliotic discs has been found,[66] and there is evidence that nutrient transport is affected in disc degeneration in vivo.[67,68] Likewise, the transport of solutes from bone to disc was significantly lower in degenerated discs compared with normal discs as measured by in vitro studies.[63] Other factors affecting the blood supply to the vertebral body that may lead to an increased incidence of disc degeneration include atherosclerosis,[69,70] sickle cell anemia, caisson disease (decompression sickness), and Gaucher disease. In addition, calcification of the cartilaginous endplates can cause decreased nutritional supply even if the blood supply remains undisturbed, as seen in scoliotic discs.[63,71] All of this evidence supports the hypothesis that a decrease in nutrient supply ultimately leads to degeneration of the disc.

Environmental Factors

Environmental risk factors hypothesized to influence disc degeneration include heavy or repetitive mechanical loading (i.e., occupational physical loading and whole-body vibration),[56,72] obesity, and cigarette smoking.[73] Heavy physical loading, particularly related to occupation, was previously suspected to be a major risk factor for degeneration and commonly viewed as a "wear and tear" phenomenon. However, results of identical twin studies on physical loading specific to occupation or sport suggest that repetitive physical loading plays a relatively minor role in disc degeneration.[72]

Obesity has often been implicated as a risk factor for degeneration, but epidemiologic studies have reported mixed findings. More recently, obesity was found to be a risk factor for marked reduction of the NP magnetic resonance imaging (MRI) signal intensity of lumbar discs. The mechanism by which obesity contributes to degeneration is thought to be a combination of mechanical and systemic factors. Some authors suggest that atherosclerosis and cardiovascular disease associated with obesity parallel atherosclerosis of the spinal vessels, with decreased blood and nutrient supply leading to increased risk of degeneration.

The only chemical exposure associated with disc degeneration is cigarette smoking, which explains only 2% of the variance in lumbar disc MRI changes between identical twins with highly discordant lifetime exposures. In other studies of monozygotic twins in whom the mean of co-twin discordance was less, no significant association between disc degeneration and cigarette smoking was found. Cigarette smoke is presumed to alter blood flow to disc capillaries and nutrient transport, possibly as a result of the presence of muscarinic receptors in blood vessels of the vertebral endplate.[74]

Facet Joints, Ligaments, and Vertebral Bodies

No discussion of intervertebral disc degeneration would be complete without consideration of the other elements of the spine. Degeneration of the spine has an impact not only on the disc, but also the surrounding structures, such as the facet joints, ligaments, and vertebral bodies. Degenerative changes are thought to occur simultaneously or close in time in each of these components, altering the ability of the spine to respond to normal physiologic loads. In addition, degeneration of the surrounding nondisc structures may cause pain and reduced mobility of the spine.

Facet Joints

Degeneration of the facet joints resembles osteoarthritic changes occurring at other synovial joints, starting with synovitis and progressing to articular cartilage loss, capsular redundancy, and eventually degenerative spondylolisthesis. Hypertrophic osteophytes at the joint margins and periarticular fibrosis can also result in reduced mobility and pain at the facet joint. Osteoarthritis of the facet joints parallels degenerative changes of the disc, possibly resulting from abnormal loading and narrowing of the disc in the early stages of degeneration.[75]

Ligaments

The anterior longitudinal ligament and posterior longitudinal ligament contribute to the overall stability of the spine. The strong anterior longitudinal ligament buttresses the anulus anteriorly, whereas the posterior longitudinal ligament offers only weak reinforcement to the posterior anulus. Information regarding degenerative changes of these ligaments is minimal, but the anterior longitudinal ligament and the posterior longitudinal ligament become more redundant as disc height decreases, and ossification occurs in later stages. These changes may contribute to pain and reduced mobility of the spine.

Vertebral Bodies

Osteoarthritic changes of the vertebral body are also associated with intervertebral disc degeneration.[76] The cartilaginous endplates are normally the weakest structure under compressive loads, and thinning and calcification with aging further compromise endplate strength. The endplates accumulate trabecular microdamage and undergo remodeling in response to altered loads, and the nucleus bulges into the vertebral body as degeneration progresses. Endplate damage decompresses the nucleus further, and loss of disc height transfers forces onto the anulus, causing it to bulge into the nucleus.[49,76] The nucleus may eventually herniate through a damaged endplate; subsequent calcification of the herniated nucleus is called a Schmorl node. The loss of disc height and annular laxity leads to formation of osteophytes at the vertebral body margins, decreased separation of the posterior neural arches, and eventual bony ankylosis (Fig. 5.6).

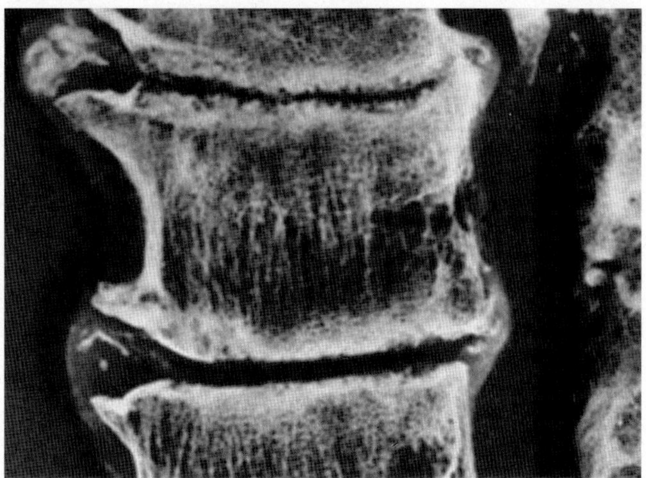

FIG. 5.6 Radiograph of old cadaveric lumbar spine (anterior on left). Radiograph depicts how severe disc narrowing can be associated with vertebral osteophytes, sclerosis of vertebral endplates, and selective loss of horizontal trabeculae from the vertebral body. (From Adams MA, Bogduk N, Burton K, et al. *The Biomechanics of Back Pain*. Edinburgh: Churchill Livingstone; 2002.)

REFERENCES

1. Buckwalter JA. Aging and degeneration of the human intervertebral disc. *Spine*. 1995;20:1307-1314.
2. Miller JA, Schmatz C, Schultz AB. Lumbar disc degeneration: correlation with age, sex, and spine level in 600 autopsy specimens. *Spine*. 1988;13:173-178.
3. Bernick S, Cailliet R. Vertebral end-plate changes with aging of human vertebrae. *Spine*. 1982;7:97-102.
4. Maroudas A, Stockwell RA, Nachemson A, et al. Factors involved in the nutrition of the human lumbar intervertebral disc: cellularity and diffusion of glucose in vitro. *J Anat*. 1975;120(Pt 1):113-130.
5. Watanabe H, Yamada Y, Kimata K. Roles of aggrecan, a large chondroitin sulfate proteoglycan, in cartilage structure and function. *J Biochem*. 1998;124:687-693.
6. Pazzaglia UE, Salisbury JR, Byers PD. Development and involution of the notochord in the human spine. *J R Soc Med*. 1989;82:413-415.
7. Sive JI, Baird P, Jeziorsk M, et al. Expression of chondrocyte markers by cells of normal and degenerate intervertebral discs. *Mol Pathol*. 2002;55:91-97.
8. Rajpurohit R, Risbud MV, Ducheyne P, et al. Phenotypic characteristics of the nucleus pulposus: expression of hypoxia inducing factor -1, glucose transporter-1, and MMP-2. *Cell Tissue Res*. 2002;308:401-407.
9. Inoue H. Three-dimensional architecture of lumbar intervertebral discs. *Spine*. 1981;6:139-146.
10. Yu J, Schollum ML, Wade KR, et al. A detailed examination of the elastic network leads to a new understanding of annulus fibrosus organization. *Spine*. 2015;40(15):1149-1157.
11. Errington RJ, Puustjarvi K, White IR, et al. Characterisation of cytoplasm-filled processes in cells of the intervertebral disc. *J Anat*. 1998;192(Pt 3):369-378.
12. Urban JP, Holm S, Maroudas A. Diffusion of small solutes into the intervertebral disc: an in vivo study. *Biorheology*. 1978;15:203-221.
13. Wallace AL, Wyatt BC, McCarthy ID, et al. Humoral regulation of blood flow in the vertebral endplate. *Spine*. 1994;19:1234-1238.
14. Holm S, Maroudas A, Urban JP, et al. Nutrition of the intervertebral disc: solute transport and metabolism. *Connect Tissue Res*. 1981;8:101-119.
15. Ferguson SJ, Ito K, Nolte LP. Fluid flow and convective transport of solutes within the intervertebral disc. *J Biomech*. 2004;37:213-221.
16. Urban JP, Smith S, Fairbank JC. Nutrition of the intervertebral disc. *Spine*. 2004;29:2700-2709.
17. Roberts S, Urban JP, Evans H, et al. Transport properties of the human cartilage endplate in relation to its composition and calcification. *Spine*. 1996;21:415-420.
18. Roberts S, Menage J, Urban JP. Biochemical and structural properties of the cartilage end-plate and its relation to the intervertebral disc. *Spine*. 1989;14:166-174.
19. Palmgren T, Gronblad M, Virri J, et al. An immunohistochemical study of nerve structures in the annulus fibrosus of human normal intervertebral discs. *Spine*. 1999;23(20):2075-2079.
20. Feng H, Danfelter M, Strömqvist B, et al. Extracellular matrix in disc degeneration. *J Bone Joint Surg Am*. 2006;88(suppl 2):25-29.
21. Roberts S, Caterson B, Menage J, et al. Matrix metalloproteinases and aggrecanase: their role in disorders of the human intervertebral disc. *Spine*. 2000;25:3005-3013.
22. Melrose J, Ghosh P, Taylor TK. Neutral proteinases of the human intervertebral disc. *Biochim Biophys Acta*. 1987;923:483-495.
23. Antoniou J, Steffen T, Nelson F, et al. The human lumbar intervertebral disc: evidence for changes in the biosynthesis and denaturation of the extracellular matrix with growth, maturation, ageing, and degeneration. *J Clin Invest*. 1996;98:996-1003.
24. Nachemson A, Elfstrom G. Intravital dynamic pressure measurements in lumbar discs: a study of common movements, maneuvers and exercises. *Scand J Rehabil Med Suppl*. 1970;1:1-40.
25. Boos N, Wallin A, Gbedegbegnon T, et al. Quantitative MR imaging of lumbar intervertebral disks and vertebral bodies: influence of diurnal water content variations. *Radiology*. 1993;188:351-354.
26. Eyre DR, Muir H. Quantitative analysis of types I and II collagens in human intervertebral discs at various ages. *Biochim Biophys Acta*. 1977;492:29-42.
27. Urban JP, McMullin JF. Swelling pressure of the intervertebral disc: influence of proteoglycan and collagen contents. *Biorheology*. 1985;22:145-157.
28. Adams MA, Dolan P. Intervertebral disc degeneration: evidence for two distinct phenotypes. *J Anat*. 2012;221: 497-506.
29. Le Maitre CL, Pockert A, Buttle DJ, et al. Matrix synthesis and degradation in human intervertebral disc degeneration. *Biochem Soc Trans*. 2007;35(Pt 4):652-655.
30. Le Maitre CL, Freemont AJ, Hoyland JA. Localization of degradative enzymes and their inhibitors in the degenerate human intervertebral disc. *J Pathol*. 2004;204:47-54.
31. Kang JD, Georgescu HI, McIntyre-Larkin L, et al. Herniated lumbar intervertebral discs spontaneously produce matrix metalloproteinases, nitric oxide, interleukin-6, and prostaglandin E2. *Spine*. 1996;21:271-277.

32. Kang JD, Stefanovic-Racic M, McIntyre LA, et al. Toward a biochemical understanding of human intervertebral disc degeneration and herniation: contributions of nitric oxide, interleukins, prostaglandin E2, and matrix metalloproteinases. *Spine.* 1997;22:1065-1073.
33. Le Maitre CL, Freemont AJ, Hoyland JA. The role of interleukin-1 in the pathogenesis of human intervertebral disc degeneration. *Arthritis Res Ther.* 2005;7:R732-R745.
34. Singh K, Masuda K, Thonar EJ, et al. Age-related change in the extracellular matrix of nucleus pulposus and annulus fibrosus of the human intervertebral disc. *Spine.* 2009;34(1):10-16.
35. Gruber HE, Hanley EN Jr. Analysis of aging and degeneration of the human intervertebral disc: comparison of surgical specimens with normal controls. *Spine.* 1998;23:751-757.
36. Trout JJ, Buckwalter JA, Moore KC. Ultrastructure of the human intervertebral disc: II. Cells of the nucleus pulposus. *Anat Rec.* 1982;204:307-314.
37. Zhao CQ, Wang LM, Jiang LS, et al. The cell biology of intervertebral disc aging and degeneration. *Ageing Res Rev.* 2007;6:247-261.
38. Le Maitre CL, Freemont AJ, Hoyland JA. Accelerated cellular senescence in degenerate intervertebral discs: a possible role in the pathogenesis of intervertebral disc degeneration. *Arthritis Res Ther.* 2007;9(3):R45.
39. Johnson WE, Eisenstein SM, Roberts S. Cell cluster formation in degenerate lumbar intervertebral discs is associated with increased disc cell proliferation. *Connect Tissue Res.* 2001;42:197-207.
40. Osti OL, Vernon-Roberts B, Fraser RD. 1990 Volvo Award in experimental studies. Annulus tears and intervertebral disc degeneration: an experimental study using an animal model. *Spine.* 1990;15:762-767.
41. Boos N, Weissbach S, Rohrbach H, et al. Classification of age-related changes in lumbar intervertebral discs. *Spine.* 2002;27:2631-2644.
42. Thompson JP, Pearce RH, Schechter MT, et al. Preliminary evaluation of a scheme for grading the gross morphology of the human intervertebral disc. *Spine.* 1990;15:411-415.
43. Holm S, Holm AK, Ekström L, et al. Experimental disc degeneration due to endplate injury. *J Spinal Disord Tech.* 2004;17:64-71.
44. Roberts S, Eisenstein SM, Menage J, et al. Mechanoreceptors in intervertebral discs: morphology, distribution, and neuropeptides. *Spine.* 1995;20:2645-2651.
45. Freemont AJ, Peacock TE, Goupille P, et al. Nerve ingrowth into diseased intervertebral disc in chronic back pain. *Lancet.* 1997;350:178-181.
46. Freemont AJ, Watkins A, Le Maitre C, et al. Nerve growth factor expression and innervation of the painful intervertebral disc. *J Pathol.* 2002;197:286-292.
47. Kauppila LI. Ingrowth of blood vessels in disc degeneration: angiographic and histological studies of cadaveric spines. *J Bone Joint Surg Am.* 1995;77:26-31.
48. Luoma K, Riihimäki H, Luukkonen R, et al. Low back pain in relation to lumbar disc degeneration. *Spine.* 2000;25: 487-492.
49. Gullbrand SE, Peterson J, Mastropolo R, et al. Low rate loading-induced convection enhances net transport into the intervertebral disc in vivo. *Spine J.* 2015;15(5):1028-1033.
50. Battié MC, Videman T, Gibbons LE, et al. Determinants of lumbar disc degeneration: a study relating lifetime exposures and magnetic resonance imaging findings in identical twins. *Spine.* 1995;20:2601-2612.
51. Videman T, Battié MC, Gill K, et al. Magnetic resonance imaging findings and their relationships in the thoracic and lumbar spine: insights into the etiopathogenesis of spinal degeneration. *Spine.* 1995;20:928-935.
52. Adams MA, Freeman BJ, Morrison HP, et al. Mechanical initiation of intervertebral disc degeneration. *Spine.* 2000;25:1625-1636.
53. Duance VC, Crean JK, Sims TJ, et al. Changes in collagen cross-linking in degenerative disc disease and scoliosis. *Spine.* 1998;23:2545-2551.
54. Vo NV, Hartman RA, Patil PR, et al. Molecular mechanisms of biological aging in intervertebral discs. *J Orthop Res.* 2016;34(8):1289-1306.
55. Battie MC, Videman T, Parent E. Lumbar disc degeneration: epidemiology and genetic influences. *Spine.* 2004;29:2679-2690.
56. Sambrook PN, MacGregor AJ, Spector TD. Genetic influences on cervical and lumbar disc degeneration: a magnetic resonance imaging study in twins. *Arthritis Rheum.* 1999;42:366-372.
57. Kawaguchi Y, Osada R, Kanamori M, et al. Association between an aggrecan gene polymorphism and lumbar disc degeneration. *Spine.* 1999;24:2456-2460.
58. Paassilta P, Lohiniva J, Göring HH, et al. Identification of a novel common genetic risk factor for lumbar disk disease. *JAMA.* 2001;285:1843-1849.
59. Takahashi M, Haro H, Wakabayashi Y, et al. The association of degeneration of the intervertebral disc with 5a/6a polymorphism in the promoter of the human matrix metalloproteinase-3 gene. *J Bone Joint Surg Br.* 2001;83:491-495.
60. Kawaguchi Y, Kanamori M, Ishihara H, et al. The association of lumbar disc disease with vitamin-D receptor gene polymorphism. *J Bone Joint Surg Am.* 2002;84:2022-2028.
61. Li Z, Yu X, Shen J, et al. MicroRNA in intervertebral disc degeneration. *Cell Prolif.* 2015;48(3):278-283.
62. Nachemson A, Lewin T, Maroudas A, et al. In vitro diffusion of dye through the end-plates and the annulus fibrosus of human lumbar inter-vertebral discs. *Acta Orthop Scand.* 1970;41:589-607.
63. Ishihara H, Urban JP. Effects of low oxygen concentrations and metabolic inhibitors on proteoglycan and protein synthesis rates in the intervertebral disc. *J Orthop Res.* 1999;17: 829-835.
64. Ohshima H, Urban JP. The effect of lactate and pH on proteoglycan and protein synthesis rates in the intervertebral disc. *Spine.* 1992;17:1079-1082.
65. Urban MR, Fairbank JC, Bibby SR, et al. Intervertebral disc composition in neuromuscular scoliosis: changes in cell density and glycosaminoglycan concentration at the curve apex. *Spine.* 2001;26:610-617.
66. Bartels EM, Fairbank JC, Winlove CP, et al. Oxygen and lactate concentrations measured in vivo in the intervertebral discs of patients with scoliosis and back pain. *Spine.* 1998;23:1-7.
67. Rajasekaran S, Babu JN, Arun R, et al. ISSLS prize winner. A study of diffusion in human lumbar discs: a serial magnetic resonance imaging study documenting the influence of the endplate on diffusion in normal and degenerate discs. *Spine.* 2004;29:2654-2667.
68. Kauppila LI. Prevalence of stenotic changes in arteries supplying the lumbar spine: a postmortem angiographic study on 140 subjects. *Ann Rheum Dis.* 1997;56:591-595.
69. Kauppila LI, McAlindon T, Evans S, et al. Disc degeneration/ back pain and calcification of the abdominal aorta: a 25-year

follow-up study in Framingham. *Spine*. 1997;22:1642-1647, discussion 1648-1649.
70. Roberts S, Urban JP, Evans H, et al. Transport properties of the human cartilage endplate in relation to its composition and calcification. *Spine*. 1996;21:415-420.
71. Videman T, Sarna S, Battié MC, et al. The long-term effects of physical loading and exercise lifestyles on back-related symptoms, disability, and spinal pathology among men. *Spine*. 1995;20:699-709.
72. Wang D, Nasto LA, Roughley P, et al. Spine degeneration in a murine model of chronic human tobacco smokers. *Osteoarthritis Cartilage*. 2012;20(8):896-905.
73. Boden SD, Riew KD, Yamaguchi K, et al. Orientation of the lumbar facet joints: association with degenerative disc disease. *J Bone Joint Surg Am*. 1996;78:403-411.
74. Battié MC, Videman T, Gill K, et al. Smoking and lumbar intervertebral disc degeneration: an MRI study of identical twins. *Spine*. 1991;16:1015-1021.
75. Simpson EK, Parkinson IH, Manthey B, et al. Intervertebral disc disorganization is related to trabecular bone architecture in the lumbar spine. *J Bone Miner Res*. 2001;16:681-687.
76. Vernon-Roberts B, Pirie CJ. Healing trabecular microfractures in the bodies of lumbar vertebrae. *Ann Rheum Dis*. 1973;32:406-412.

CHAPTER 6 Biomechanics of the Spinal Motion Segment

William S. Marras
Prasath Mageswaran
Safdar N. Khan
Ehud Mendel

In biomechanics, information from the biologic sciences and engineering mechanics is integrated for the purpose of analyzing and quantifying the function of and forces occurring on tissue under various conditions. With an understanding of the natural behavior mechanics of the spinal motion segment, it can be possible to better understand the limitations of the system and the conditions under which tissue damage occurs and subsequent pain would be likely. Biomechanical assessments provide a quantitative means by which to accomplish this goal.

From a biomechanical standpoint, the spine accomplishes three major functions.[1] First, the spine provides a structure by which loads can be transmitted through the body. Second, the spine permits motion in multidimensional space. Third, the spine provides a structure to protect elements of the nervous system (spinal cord). To appreciate the ability of the spine to accomplish these functions, we need to understand the natural movements of the spine and its ability to withstand forces or loads that are transmitted through its structure.

With these goals in mind, this chapter (1) considers the physical characteristics of the spinal tissues that could influence function, (2) assesses the motion characteristics (kinematics) of the different portions of the spine, and (3) summarizes the ability of the spine to withstand forces that it is supporting (load tolerance). Collectively, this chapter shows, from a biomechanical perspective, how the spine functions and how it breaks down. Box 6.1 is a glossary of terms to facilitate better understanding of the content of this chapter.

Assessing the Biomechanics of the Spinal Motion Segment

Ideally, it would be desirable to measure directly the forces imposed on the various tissues within the spine. With current technology, invasive measures would be required, however, to understand the loading imposed on the various spinal tissues. Such invasive measures would disrupt the tissues of interest and would most likely alter the very factors that one is attempting to measure. Direct biomechanical measurements of the spine in vivo are rare and currently difficult in humans. Much of the biomechanical information about the human spinal motion segment is based on in vitro studies. This information must be considered with caution because the properties of the spine derived from cadaveric studies are understood to be different in many respects from those of a live individual.

An alternative to direct measurement of spine tissue loading is the prediction of tissue loads based on in silico or biomechanical models. A biomechanical model is a conceptual representation and prediction of how the forces within the biomechanical system interact ultimately to impose force on a particular tissue of interest. Biomechanical analyses assume that the body behaves according to the laws of newtonian mechanics that must govern the distribution of forces within the musculoskeletal system. The object of interest in spinal biomechanics is a precise quantitative assessment of the movement behavior and mechanical loading occurring within the tissue of the musculoskeletal system. Biomechanical modeling permits estimation of the direction and magnitude of forces acting on the spinal motion segment and allows estimation of when natural motion tolerances have been exceeded and when damage or degeneration would be expected to occur. Biomechanical assessments help one understand potential pathways of low back disorders and can potentially help surgeons understand how contemplated surgical interventions might affect the health of the spine.

Ultimately, biomechanical assessments are intended to determine how much loading of the tissues within the spinal motion segment is too much loading. This high degree of precision and quantification is the characteristic that distinguishes biomechanical analyses from other types of analyses.

Physical Charcteristics of the Spine Structures

The spine is composed of four types of vertebrae classified according to their regional location along the spinal column—cervical, thoracic, lumbar, and sacral. There are 7 cervical vertebrae, 12 thoracic vertebrae, and 5 lumbar vertebrae. In addition, the sacrum consists of five immobile— or

BOX 6.1 Glossary

Acceleration. The rate of change of velocity. In body angular motion, defined in degrees per second.

Acute trauma. Load applied to a structure with enough force to result in damage in one application.

Axis of rotation. The point about which two vertebrae move relative to one another.

Bending. Load applied to a structure at a point where it is not directly supported, causing it to deform.

Biomechanical model. A theoretical representation of how forces behave and interact in a biomechanical system.

Cortical bone. Compact bone forming a protective outer shell for a bone. It has high resistance to bending and torsion, and provides strength where bending would be undesirable.

Cancellous bone. Inner portion of bone containing a spongy matrix. Forms the interior scaffolding of the structure and helps maintain bone shape during force application.

Central coordinate system. A reference system that defines the positions and motions of the body in space.

Compression. Force that pushes together the materials of a structure.

Contact pressure. The force per unit area distributed over a contact area.

Coupling. Movements in which one motion is accompanied by the motion in a different plane.

Cumulative trauma. Repetitive load applied to a structure that weakens the structure and results in damage.

Degree of freedom. The number of directions and motions in which a body is able to move.

Dynamics. The study of forces applied to a structure in motion.

Force. An action that changes the state of rest or motion of a body.

Kinematics. The study of the motion of a structure that considers position, velocity, and acceleration without taking into account the force that produces the motion.

Kinetics. The study of the relationship between the force acting on a body and the change in motion produced

Load. The application of force or moment (torque) to a structure.

Loading cycle. The number of repetitions of a load application.

Local coordinate system. A reference system that defines the positions and motions of vertebrae relative to one another.

Microfracture. Small cracks in a structure.

Moment. A force applied about an axis. A force multiplied by a distance. Also known as *torque.*

Neutral zone. The amount of displacement between the neutral position of the vertebrae and point at which resistance to physiologic motion is experienced.

Pressure. Force per unit area.

Range of motion. The two points that define the extremes of physiologic motion.

Rotations. Movement about a point, as when bending.

Shear. A force applied parallel to the surface upon which it acts.

Stability. The ability of a system to respond to a perturbation and reestablish a state of equilibrium.

Statics. The study of forces occurring within a structure when they are not in motion.

Strain. The change in unit length or angle of a material that is subjected to load.

Stress. A measure of the intensity of force represented in force per unit area.

Tolerance. The point at which a structure can no longer resist a load without suffering damage.

Torsion. A twisting load applied about the long axis of a structure.

Translations. Straight line movements in any direction.

Velocity. The rate of change of position. In angular body motion, defined in degrees per second.

"fused"—vertebrae, and the coccyx (often referred to as the tailbone) is a fusion of four coccygeal vertebrae at the base of the spine. Each vertebra is referenced according to a nomenclature system in which the spine region (e.g., cervical, thoracic) is followed by a numbering system that refers to the vertical position of the vertebral body along the spine (beginning with the vertebra closest to the head) (e.g., first cervical vertebra, or C1). Disc levels are referenced relative to the vertebral levels surrounding the disc. The lowest lumbar vertebra (fifth lumbar vertebra, or L5) is adjacent to the first sacral vertebra (S1), and the disc between these vertebrae is referred to as L5–S1.

The shape of the vertebrae changes from level to level in the spine. The vertebral body shape and the orientation of the posterior elements change. In particular, the orientation of the bony structures that compose the posterior elements change in their shapes and contact angles. These subtle changes permit or restrict motions in different directions along the human spine.

Several physiologic curves are also characteristic of the upright spine (Fig. 6.1A). The curves within the cervical and lumbar regions of the spine are referred to as *cervical lordosis* and *lumbar lordosis,* whereas the thoracic and sacral curves are referred to as *thoracic kyphosis* and *sacral kyphosis* because these curves bow in the opposite direction of the lordotic curves. These curves work collectively to accommodate pelvic orientation under different conditions. When sitting, the pelvis rotates backward and the lumbar curve flattens. When the pelvis is rotated forward, the lumbar curve is accentuated. Collectively, the spinal curves balance each other and form a stable system that maintains the center of gravity in a balanced state. However, this normal balance can change with age and a number of other factors such as degeneration, osteoporosis, and trauma.

The "building blocks" of the spine are the spinal motion segments (Fig. 6.1B), also known as the *functional spinal unit.* This unit consists of two vertebrae and the disc in between them. This unit represents the central focus of biomechanical functioning and clinical assessment. This chapter explores the spinal motion segment from a biomechanical perspective with the intent of understanding the significance of features that may influence status.

Support Structures

The spine is constructed of a series of vertebral bones that are stacked on one another to form the spinal column that runs from the pelvis to the head. A vertebral bone, or vertebra, is shown in Fig. 6.2. The large, round portion of the bone is the vertebral body, which is the major load-bearing structure of the spinal column. The outer portion of this bone is composed of a thin, yet very strong, layer of cortical bone. Cortical bone, also known as *compact bone,* forms a protective outer shell, has a high resistance to bending and torsion, and provides strength in situations in which bending would be undesirable. The inner portion of the bone consists of a spongy matrix of

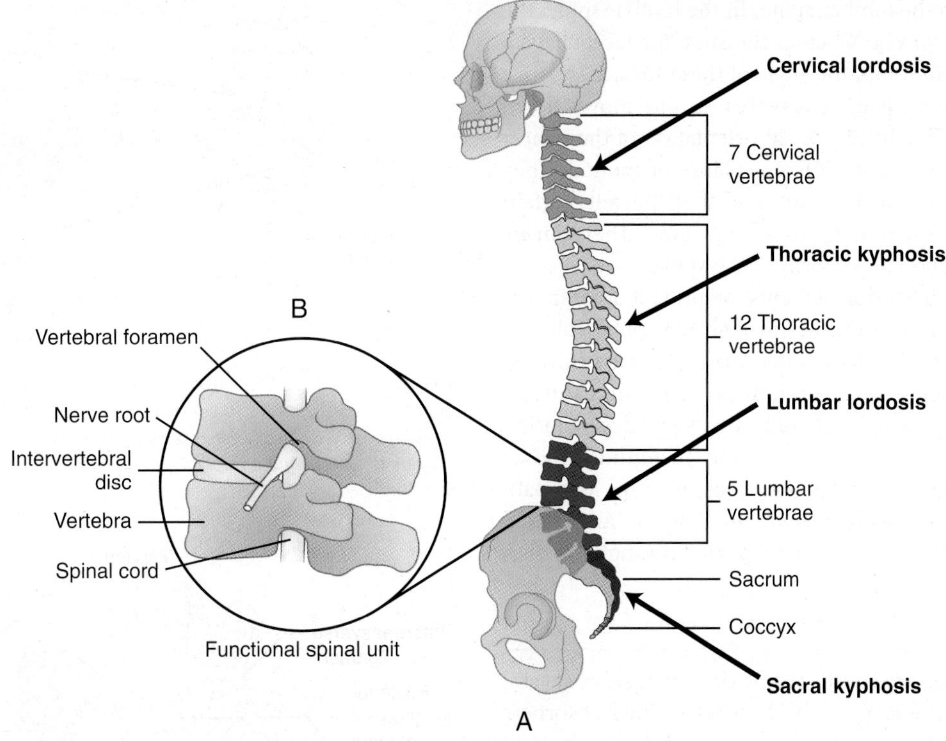

FIG. 6.1 (A) Arrangement of the vertebral bones and spinal curves and (B) a functional spinal unit or spinal motion segment. (Modified from Marras WS. *The Working Back: A Systems View.* Hoboken, NJ: John Wiley & Sons; 2008.)

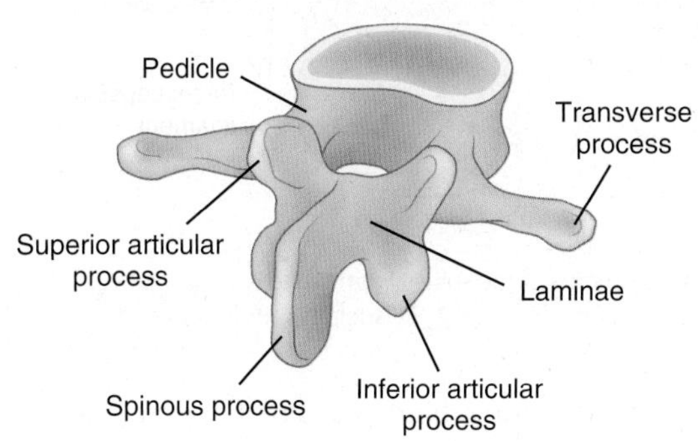

FIG. 6.2 Lumbar vertebra and its posterior elements. (Modified from Marras WS. *The Working Back: A Systems View.* Hoboken, NJ: John Wiley & Sons; 2008.)

cancellous bone. This type of bone is less dense and more elastic than cortical bone. Cancellous bone forms the interior scaffolding of the structure and helps the bone to maintain its shape despite compressive forces. This structure is composed of bundles of short and parallel strands of bone fused together.

The bony structures that constitute the posterior elements form a protective channel, or tunnel, for the spinal cord and nerves (see Fig. 6.1B). The biomechanical role of the posterior elements is to control the position of the vertebral bodies. These elements provide attachment points for muscles to control the position of the vertebra and supply lever arms to provide the system with mechanical advantage. In addition, these structures control motion and provide mechanical "stops" to prevent excessive movement of the vertebral body. A significant portion of the mechanical load is borne by the posterior elements, relieving the disc of excessive loading.

As shown in Fig. 6.2, toward the top of the posterior surface of each vertebra are pedicles. The pedicles provide a robust support structure (a type of pillar) to transmit force between the posterior elements and the vertebral body. Projecting out from each pedicle are the lamina structures that come together at the midline of the body and form a neural arch. This arch is a strong structure that provides protection to the spinal cord in the form of a channel (vertebral foramen).

Emanating out from the junction of the two laminae at the midline of the body is a bony protrusion called the *spinous process.* Projecting laterally on each side of the structure at the junction of the pedicle and the laminae is another bony structure called the *transverse process.* These processes provide muscle attachment surfaces and mechanical advantage for control of the spinal column.

Two sets of articulating surfaces are also present in the posterior elements. Projecting out from each of the cephalic lateral corners of the lamina is a bony extension called the *superior articular process.* A portion of this surface is covered by articular cartilage. Emanating from the caudal lateral corner of the lamina on each side are the *inferior articular processes.* The superior articular process from the lower vertebra interacts with the inferior articular process of the vertebra above it to form a synovial joint known as the *zygapophyseal joint.* This joint is also referred to as the *facet joint.* The inclination of the facet joint changes from the cervical spine to the thoracic spine to the lumbar spine. This joint is defined as a plane surface in the cervical and thoracic joints, but becomes a curved surface in the lumbar spine. In the lumbar spine, the inferior facets are convex, whereas the superior facets have a concave shape. In addition, the angle of these surfaces relative to the sagittal plane changes (increases) as one moves down the lumbar spine. The differences in orientation of these facet joints restrict movement in different planes of motion. They serve an important function in that they permit certain motions and limit other motions of the spine. They can be thought of as the guidance system of the spine.

Collectively, the posterior elements can provide a significant load path for the forces running through the spinal column. Approximately one-third of a spinal load is carried through the posterior elements in the upright posture. The nature of the load transmission can be altered when spine degeneration occurs by altering the vector of force and magnitude of force transmitted through these posterior elements. This load path can be disengaged, however, when the spine is in a flexed posture, and the load can be entirely passed through the disc.

Disc

The vertebral bodies are connected by discs that serve several biomechanical purposes. First, the discs act as shock absorbers between the vertebrae, absorbing a portion of the mechanical forces transmitted through the spine. Second, they can transmit a portion of the mechanical load between vertebrae. Third, the discs are able to permit and govern motion between the vertebral bodies. Functionally, the discs are intended to provide a separation between consecutive vertebrae. This separation provides space between vertebrae so that the vertebral bodies can independently change their orientation and execute bending movements. With this arrangement, a pliable and deformable spinal structure is possible.

The disc consists of two distinct portions, each of which is associated with a distinct mechanical function. The outer portion of the disc, called the *anulus fibrosus* (AF), consists of alternating layers of fibers that are oriented at a 60- to 65-degree angle relative to the vertical. The AF consists of about 10 to 20 concentric, circumferential sheets of collagen called *lamellae* that are nestled together around the periphery of the disc (Fig. 6.3). The lamellae are stiff and can withstand significant compression loading. Given the collagenous nature of these lamellae, they are pliable and can also permit bending of the spinal column. If the structure were to buckle, however, it would lose its stiffness and would be unable to support compression. The second portion of the disc—the nucleus pulposus (NP)—is designed to overcome this potential problem.

Within the AF is a gelatinous core, the just-mentioned nucleus pulposus (see Fig. 6.3). When compressed, this core expands radially and places the AF in tension, providing stiffness. The integrity of the system changes throughout the day. The disc absorbs water while one is recumbent, which makes the system stiffer than when one is upright. Conversely, when one is upright, water is squeezed out of the disc, and the structure becomes more lax.

Finally, the endplate is located at the intersection of the disc and the vertebral body. The endplates are composed of cartilage and cover the superior and inferior portions of the disc. These structures bind the disc fibers to the vertebral bones and play a significant role in disc nutritional transport.

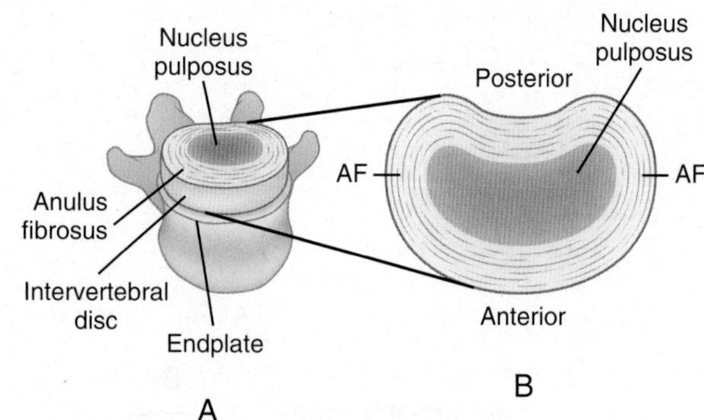

FIG. 6.3 (A) Disc, vertebral endplate, and vertebral body. (B) Construction of intervertebral disc. AF, anulus fibrosus. (Modified from Marras WS. *The Working Back: A Systems View*. Hoboken, NJ: John Wiley & Sons; 2008; and Bogduk N. *Clinical Anatomy of the Lumbar Spine and Sacrum*, ed 4. Edinburgh: Elsevier; 2005.)

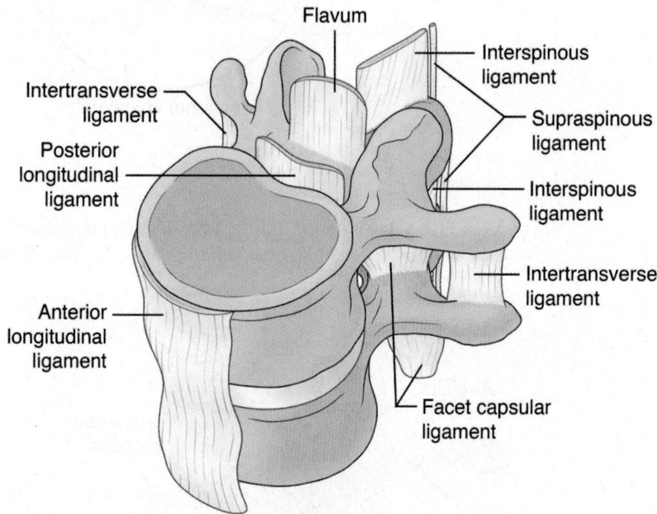

FIG. 6.4 Ligaments of the spine. (From White AA III, Panjabi MM. *Clinical Biomechanics of the Spine*, ed 2. Philadelphia: JB Lippincott; 1990.)

Spinal Ligaments

The spinal ligaments play a significant role from a biomechanical standpoint. Ligaments are most effective in supporting loads in the direction in which their fibers run. They support loads under tension and can buckle under compression. These structures can store energy and act much like a rubber band in that they can provide resistance to loads by developing tension.

The ligaments play three roles in biomechanics. First, they permit motion and help orient the vertebrae without muscle recruitment. Second, ligaments protect the spinal cord by restricting spinal motion segment movement to within specific ranges. Third, they absorb energy and protect the spinal cord during rapid motions.

The spinal ligaments are shown in Fig. 6.4. The arrangement of these structures provides support for the spine in different dimensions of loading. Because support is offered in the different directions of motion, these structures provide stability when the spinal system is intact.

Coordinate System and Force/Movement Definitions

A biomechanical assessment of the spine is concerned with the analysis of movements and forces developing within the spine as it is exposed to activities of daily living (ADLs) and other work or environmental conditions. Movements or motions are compared with the natural limits of movement, and forces imposed on a tissue (also called *tissue loading*) are compared with tissue tolerances (magnitude of load at which damage occurs). To describe movement and force transmission through tissue accurately, it is necessary to describe precisely direction of movement and direction and magnitude of the force application on the tissue. Direction is defined relative to a coordinate system or reference frame. The central (global) coordinate system of the body is shown in Fig. 6.5. The origin or center of this coordinate system is located at the base of the spine. Fig. 6.5 describes the coordinate system (used in this chapter) as a traditional three-dimensional cartesian coordinate system with three mutually perpendicular axes oriented with a vertical *z* axis. Some references have adopted the International Society of Biomechanics (ISB) coordinate convention, in which the *y* axis is defined as the vertical axis.

All movements of the spine are described relative to the origin of the central coordinate system. Flexion and extension are typically described in the sagittal plane, lateral bending occurs in the coronal plane, and twisting occurs along the horizontal or transverse plane. Most activities are combinations of movements in these planes.

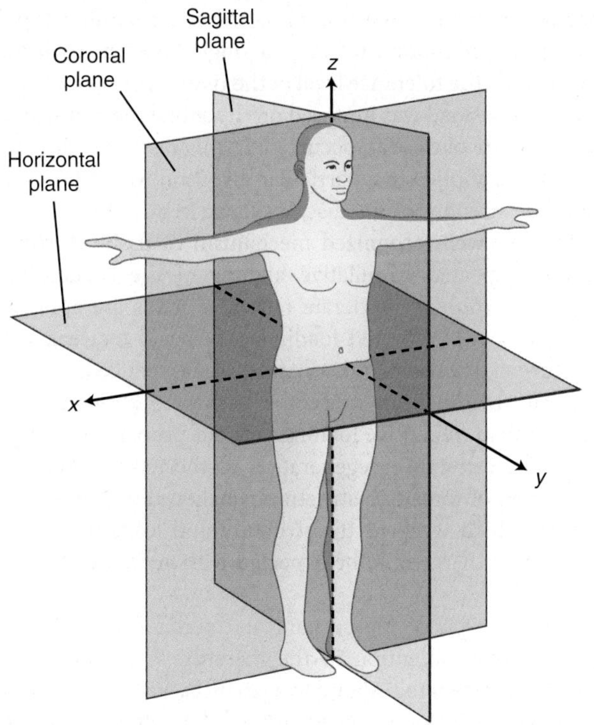

FIG. 6.5 Central or global coordinate system for the body.

Within the spinal motion segment or functional spinal unit, a local coordinate system can also be defined. The convention that defines this local coordinate system is shown in Fig. 6.6. Movement of the spinal motion segments is defined relative to the subjacent vertebrae. Movements of the motion segment can be either translations (indicating straight line movements in any direction) or rotations (indicating movement around a point, as when bending).

Fig. 6.6 indicates that forces and moments (torques) can develop along each dimension of the reference frame. Forces along the *z* dimension are either compression or tension depending on whether they compress the spinal motions segment or pull on the tissues. These are typically the forces of concern when lifting an object in the sagittal plane. Two types of shear forces are also of concern when evaluating the biomechanics of the spine. Anteroposterior shear force describes the forward or backward force in the *y* axis that can result from pushing or pulling activities. The lateral shear forces refer to the sideways forces acting along the *x* axis and represent the forces that develop in the spinal motion segment when pushing an object to the side of the body.

Compression of the disc causes pressure within the NP in all directions; this pressure places the AF under tension. As shown in Fig. 6.7, the nucleus pressure can lead to deformation near the center of the endplate with this form of loading.

Fig. 6.8 illustrates how shear, torsion, and tension influence the fibers of the anulus. Shear forces tense the fibers in the direction of movement and relax the fibers in the opposite direction. Similarly, torsion or twisting tenses the fibers that are lengthened by the movement and relaxes the remaining fibers. This differential of force among the fibers is believed to result in tissue damage. Finally, lengthening of the spine places the fibers under tension. This action increases the force on all the fibers regardless of their orientation.

Bending moments refer to forces acting around an axis, as seen in Fig. 6.6. The curved arrows in this figure show the direction in which moments act around a spinal segment. A bending moment can be defined around the *x* axis, resulting in a movement in the sagittal plane (forward bending moment), or it can be defined around the *y* axis, indicating a sideways or lateral bend. In either of these situations, the moment or torque around the central axis defines the loading of the segment. Twisting of the spine can result when forces are applied around the *z* axis of the spine. This situation results in what is typically referred to as a *torsional moment.*

The forces and moments can be defined around each vertebra along the spine, resulting in a very large number of forces and moments and numerous degrees of freedom. For practical purposes, the forces and moment are typically defined in most situations around one particular vertebra or disc (e.g., L5–S1) depending on the purpose of the study.

Movements between vertebral bodies can also be coupled. Coupling refers to the motion relationship of one vertebra around an axis relative to another vertebra around a different axis. In other words, coupling refers to the motion in different planes that occurs simultaneously. The spine can bend forward and twist at the same time—this is a coupled motion.

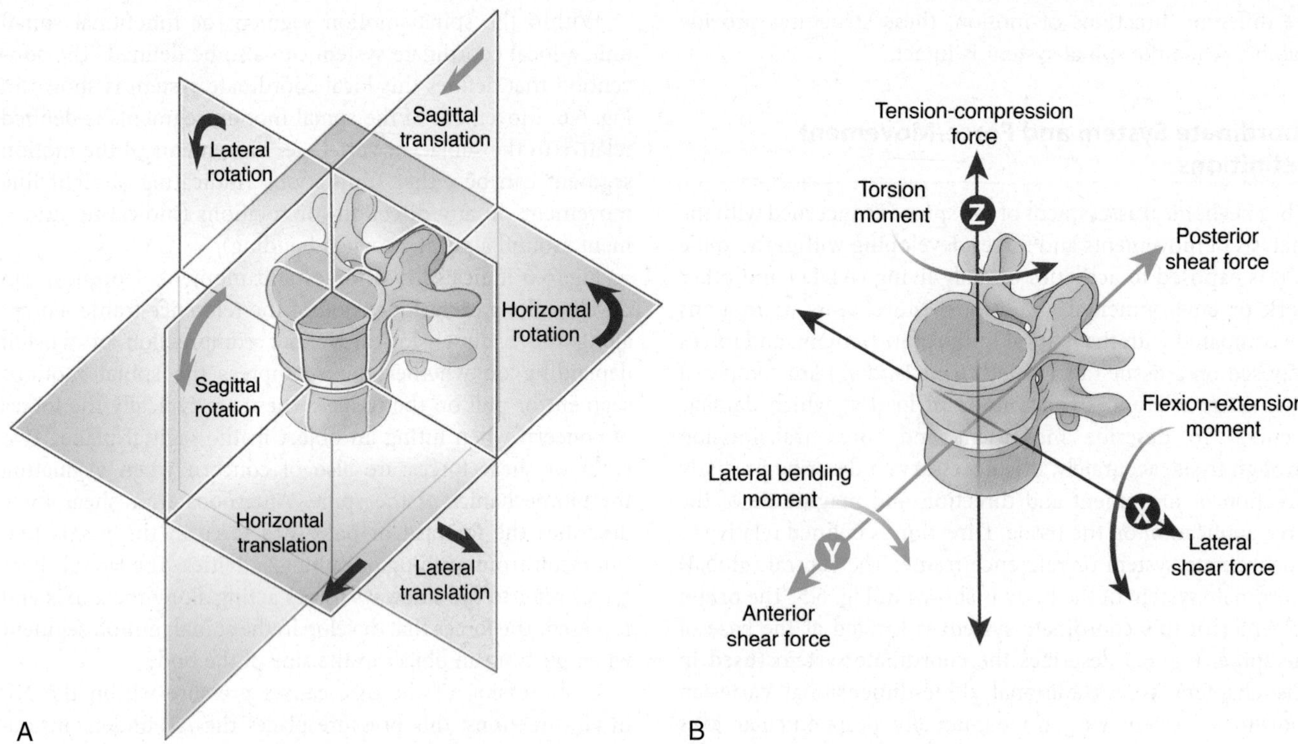

FIG. 6.6 (A) Spinal motion segment planes and directions of motion and (B) biomechanical coordinate system and direction of forces and moments. Motions and forces are described relative to this coordinate system. (Reproduced with permission from Bogduk N. *Clinical Anatomy of the Lumbar Spine and Sacrum*. 4th ed. Edinburgh: Elsevier, 2005.)

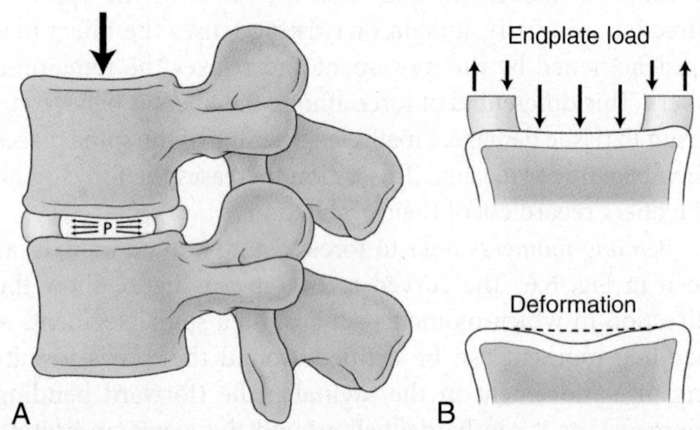

FIG. 6.7 (A) Compression of disc leading to increased pressure in the disc nucleus. (B) Increased nucleus pressure causes endplate loading and deformation. (From White AA III, Panjabi MM. *Clinical Biomechanics of the Spine*, ed 2. Philadelphia: JB Lippincott; 1990.)

The amount of displacement between the neutral position of the vertebra and the point at which resistance to physiologic motion is experienced is referred to as a *neutral zone*.[2] Neutral zones can be defined for translational and rotational movements. The neutral zone can be described for each of 6 degrees of freedom.

Tissue Load Characteristics

The forces represented in Fig. 6.6 define the direction of load application and the magnitude of the force. The nature and temporal characteristics of the loading situation also define the probability that the load application will result in tissue damage. It is believed that tissue damage can result from several different "types" of trauma to the tissue. Each type of trauma is believed to be associated with very different tolerance levels. First, acute trauma is the most familiar type of loading. *Acute trauma* refers to a single application of force that exceeds the tolerance level of the tissue. This would be the case if a large load was imposed on the spinal motion segment and a rupture of the disc occurred. In this case, the magnitude of the force applied in a particular direction would far exceed the tissue strength of the disc, resulting in a rupture.

Another well-recognized mechanism of tissue disruption involves repeated cumulative loading of the tissues. With *cumulative trauma*, moderate repetitive loads are applied to the tissues; this repeated loading is believed to weaken the structure so that the tolerance of the tissue is reduced. Although moderate loading can cause the tissues to strengthen and adapt to load, repetitive loading without proper rest (adaptation) time can cause degeneration of the tissues. Repetitive application of force to a structure is believed to cause microtrauma, which weakens the structure and leads to failure at lower levels than would be expected with an acute trauma to the tissue.

A third type of biomechanical trauma (instability) has received much attention in the literature.[3–8] Stability is the ability of a system to respond to a perturbation and reestablish a state of equilibrium.[2] *Instability* of the spine refers to the abnormal displacement of the spine under physiologic loading.

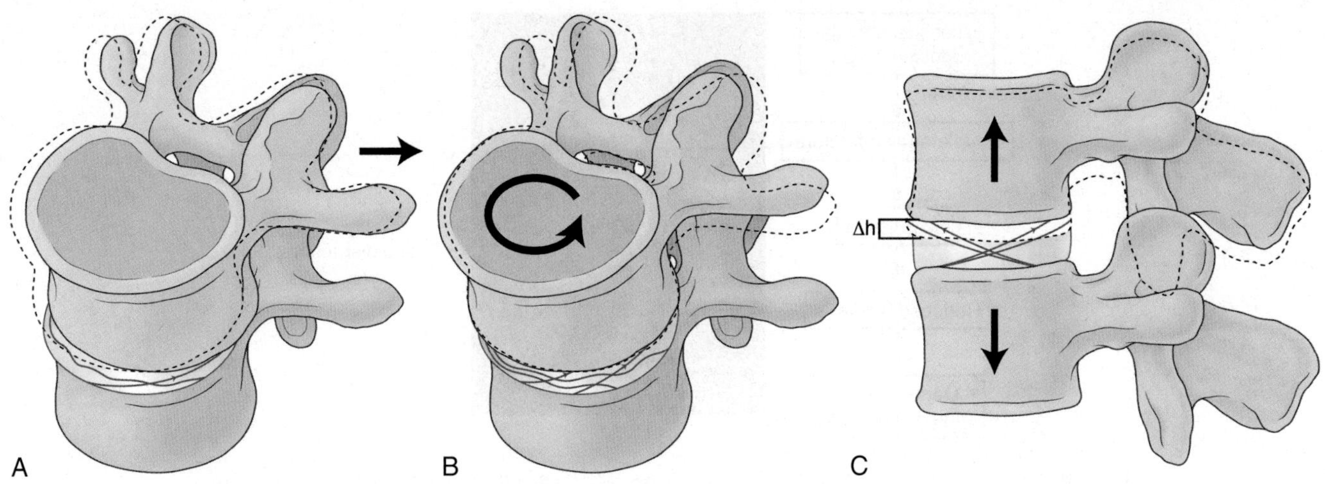

FIG. 6.8 The effects of shear (A), torsion (B), and tension (C) on the fibers of the anulus fibrosus. (From Adams MA, Bogduk N, Burton AK, et al. *The Biomechanics of Back Pain*, ed 2. Edinburgh: Elsevier; 2013.)

The abnormal displacement can occur in translation or rotation, but most likely would be some combination of these two types of motions. These abnormal motions are often small in magnitude, but the displacement may be enough to stimulate pain in sensitive tissue. Stability is significant because it is often the initiator of tissue damage when the system is out of alignment or when the musculoskeletal system overcompensates for a perturbation.[2] When the supporting musculature cannot offer adequate stability to a joint (owing to improper muscle recruitment, fatigue, structure laxity, or weakness), the structure may move abnormally and result in sudden and unexpected force applications on a tissue. This type of trauma is similar to the acute trauma pathway but is initiated by a miscalculation of the muscle recruitment pattern. Instability can also be secondary to trauma, developing over time in cases of degeneration and cancer.

Mechanical Degeneration: Tissues at Risk

Many tissues in the spinal motion segment can be influenced by structure loading. These tissues include bones, discs, ligaments, tendons, and nerves. Tissue loading can result in a disruption of tissue integrity. Bones can be cracked or broken, disc endplates can sustain microfractures, the disc can bulge or rupture, muscle can experience fiber tears, and blood flow to the tissues can be disrupted. All of these events are believed to be capable of initiating a sequence or cascade of events leading to back pain. The tolerance of many of these structures within the spine is reviewed in detail in this chapter.

Clinicians are beginning to understand that low back disorders can occur before tissue damage. Biochemical studies have shown that these types of tissue insults can result in an upregulation of proinflammatory cytokines. This upregulation may result in tissue inflammation at much lower levels of load than would occur under normal conditions. This inflammation makes nociceptive tissues more sensitive to pain and may initiate back pain.[9]

Much attention in spine biomechanics and clinical care has been focused on the intervertebral disc because disc disruption has been associated with pain. Over the past several decades, clinicians have also begun to understand how spine loading can initiate the degeneration process within the disc. To appreciate this process, the system behavior of the disc, vertebral body, and endplate must be considered in response to cumulative trauma. The disc receives no direct blood supply for nourishment. It relies heavily on nutrient flow and diffusion from surrounding vascularized tissue for disc viability. The nourishment is transported from the vertebral body through the endplate to the disc. The endplate is very thin (about 1 mm thick) and facilitates nutrient transport to the disc.

When endplate loading exceeds its tolerance limit, microfractures can occur in the structure. Microfracture of the endplate itself usually does not initiate pain because few pain receptors reside within the disc and endplate. Repeated microfracture of this vertebral endplate can lead to the formation of scar tissue and calcification, which can interfere with nutrient flow to the disc fibers. Because scar tissue is thicker and denser than endplate tissue, the scar tissue interferes with nutrient delivery to the disc. This reduced nutrient flow can lead to atrophy and weakening of the disc fibers and disc degeneration. Because the disc has relatively few nociceptors except at the outer layers, this degenerative process is usually not noticed by the individual until the disc is weakened to the point at which bulging or rupture occurs, and surrounding tissues that are rich in nociceptors are stimulated. Fig. 6.9 illustrates this sequence of events that are believed to lead to disc degeneration and potential tissue damage, such as herniation.[9]

The literature also provides some evidence that excessive motion within the spinal segment can lead to degeneration. Excessive motion at a joint is believed to increase the cumulative trauma on the spinal structures and potentially initiate either tissue degeneration or an upregulation of proinflammatory cytokines. This has become apparent in studies that have examined the degeneration of segments adjacent to spinal fusions.[10] If two spinal levels are fused, trunk motion usually results in exacerbated movement, especially at the facet joints within spinal levels adjacent to the fusion. One study noted

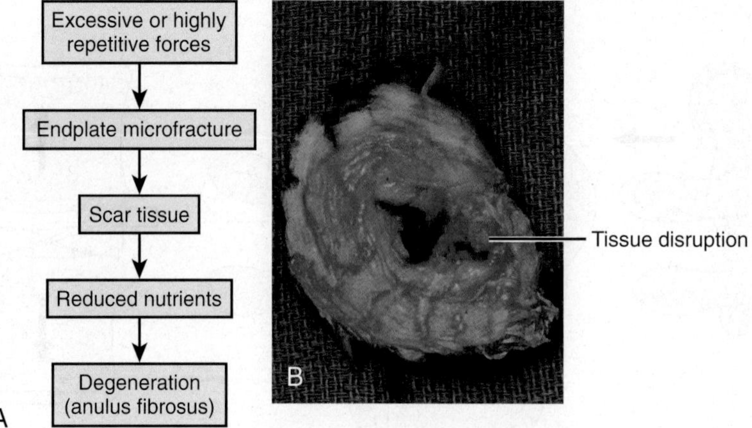

FIG. 6.9 (A) Sequence of events associated with cumulative or repeated trauma leading to disc degeneration. (B) Herniated disc showing disruptions to the anulus fibrosus. (B, Courtesy Ehud Mendel.)

hypertrophic degenerative arthritis of the facet joints in motion segments adjacent to a fusion typically following a symptom-free period (8.5 years, on average).[10] Another study found significant evidence of degeneration at levels adjacent to a fusion with the rate of symptomatic degeneration at the adjacent segment warranting either decompression or arthrodesis to be 16.4% at 5 years after fusion and 36.1% at 10 years after the surgery.[11] In addition, more recent studies examining artificial discs have reported facet arthrosis.[12] Facet load forces have been shown to depend on artificial disc placement and the subsequent load transferred to the facets.[13]

The application of damaging compressive forces on the vertebral body can result in several different types of failures of vertebrae. The failure characteristics have been described in the literature[14] and are shown graphically in Fig. 6.10. This figure indicates that seven types of failures are typically seen as a result of compression. These consist of stellate fracture, step fracture, intrusion fracture (with Schmorl's nodes), depression of the endplate, Y-shaped fracture, edge fracture, and transverse fracture.

Many of these fractures suggest weakness of the endplate. This weakness is a result of the thinness of the endplate necessary for nutrient transport to the disc. These fractures are believed to result from the NP of the adjacent disc bulging into the vertebra.[15] Clinically, vertebral body fractures that occur purely from axial compression are classified as type A based on the AOSpine classification system.[16] Fig. 6.11 shows four common subtypes of type A fractures.

In Vitro Spine Biomechanics

Motion Characteristics (Kinematics) of the Spinal Motion Segments

The typical ranges of motion (ROMs) associated with cervical, thoracic, and lumbar motion segments have been well described in the literature[4] and are summarized in Table 6.1. A graphic estimate of spinal segment ROM associated with the entire spine is presented in Fig. 6.12.[2] Table 6.1 shows the vast differences in motion capacity for the various vertebrae as a function of the spine region and the vertebral level. Each region of the spine allows or limits motion in a particular motion direction compared with other regions of the spine. This information shows that, in the sagittal plane, the most ROM occurs in the cervical spine followed by the lumbar spine. Laterally directed motions, although much smaller in magnitude than motions in the sagittal plane, occur freely in the cervical spine, with much less movement available in the thoracic and lumbar spine. Finally, very little axial rotation is possible in the lumbar spine, with most motion occurring in the thoracic vertebrae except for C1–C2.

Collectively, the body of work described in Table 6.1 and Fig. 6.12 represents the summary of expected movement characteristics derived in vitro. To the extent that in vitro characteristics are indicative of in vivo characteristics, they can provide a baseline for movement expectations for the various vertebrae along the spinal column.

It is also possible that abnormal movement of the motion segment can indicate disc damage. Studies have also shown that tears in the AF change the movement characteristics of the motion segments. Specifically, tears in the anulus increase the amount of motion in the motion segment when torque is applied to the segment.[17]

Axis of Rotation

To understand and describe better how motion occurs among vertebrae, an axis (or center) of rotation is often defined. When bones move relative to one another in a single plane, there is a point around which the object rotates. If a hypothetical line is extended from the constant point within a vertebra, the point at which these two lines meet when the vertebra moves between two different positions is called the *instantaneous axis of rotation*. This concept can be extended to three-dimensional space; however, identifying the axis of rotation becomes more complex. Understanding of the axis of rotation helps one understand how kinematics are altered because of degeneration or surgical intervention. Identification of this point also has implications for how forces are transmitted through the spine.

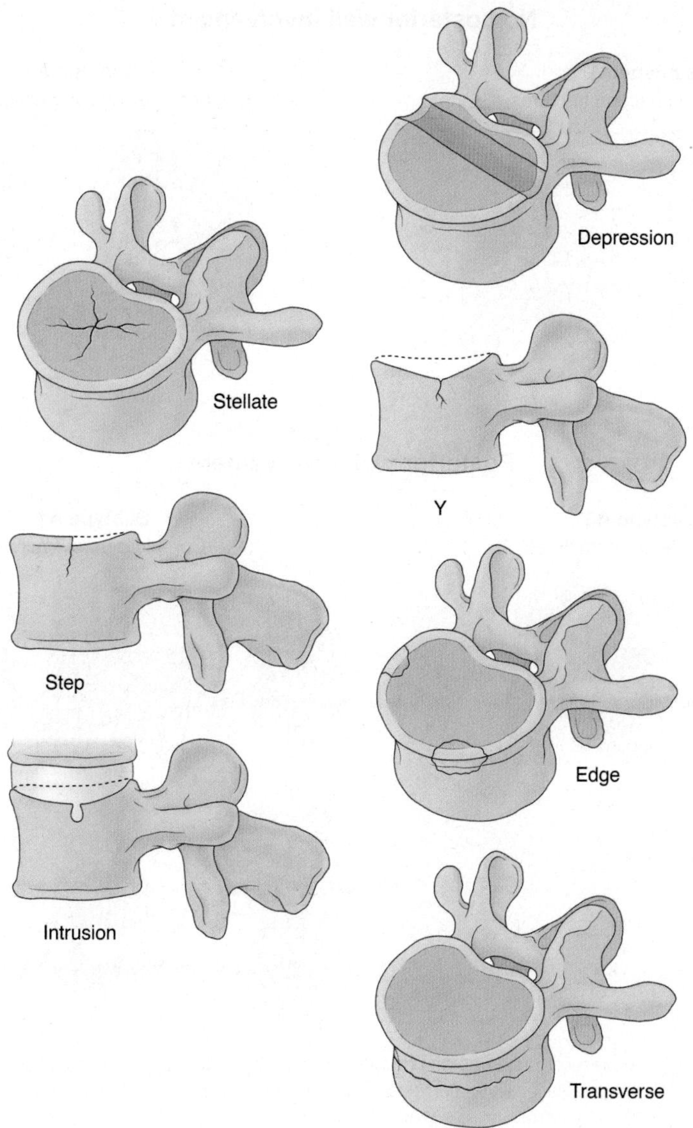

FIG. 6.10 Seven types of fractures identified by Brinkmann and colleagues.[14] (From Adams MA, Bogduk N, Burton AK, et al. *The Biomechanics of Back Pain*, ed 2. Edinburgh: Elsevier; 2013.)

Relative movement of a vertebra can be divided into translational movement (sliding motions) and rotational movement. During physiologic movements, the components of compression force and bending moment acting on the spine vary, along with the translational and bending movements. This action results in a varying axis of rotation position. The axis of rotation is defined as a "locus," or path, that the axis of rotation takes.[18]

During sagittal and frontal plane motions, the axis of rotation in the cervical spine is believed to be located in the anterior portion of the subjacent vertebra.[2] Coupling also occurs with cervical motions, however. In the thoracic spine, loads applied during flexion and extension motions result in an axis of rotation located at the inferior endplate of the lower vertebra. This axis of rotation moves farther down the vertebra when posterior shear force occurs during extension motions.[2] During flexion and extension motions, the axis of rotation occurs in the superior endplate of the inferior vertebra of the spinal motion segment.

During sagittal plane bending, the axis of rotation varies according to whether forward or backward bending is occurring. Because much of the flexion and extension in the sagittal plane occurs in the lumbar spine, much of the interest in the axis of rotation has also been focused on the lumbar spine. The superior vertebra translates anteriorly and posteriorly relative to the inferior vertebra as the vertebral body rotates around the nucleus. After degeneration of the disc, the axis of rotation can change dramatically,[19] resulting in marked changes in spine loading. Under these degenerative conditions, the axis of rotation has been reported to migrate toward the zygapophyseal joint during extension motions.[20] During flexion, the axis of rotation seems to move and is dependent on coupling patterns during the flexion movement.

During lateral motions, the axis of rotation in the lumbar spine lies at the opposite side of the disc from the direction of motion. In other words, when bending to the right, the left side of the disc is where the axis of rotation is located.[2]

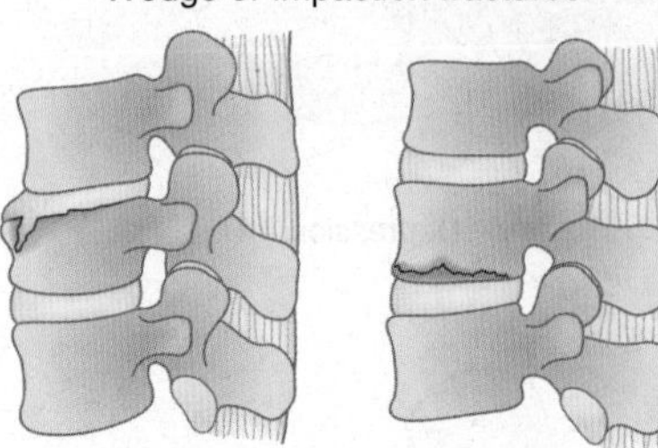

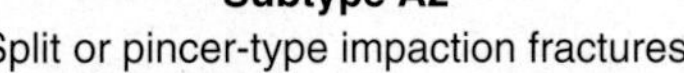

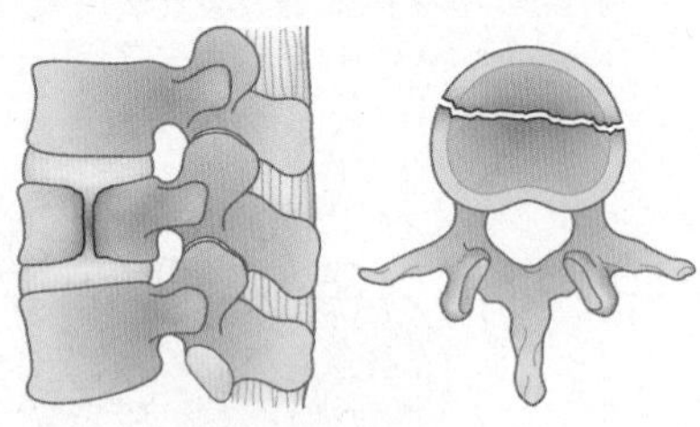

FIG. 6.11 Type A compression fractures based on the AOSpine Classification. (From Reinhold M, Audige L, Schnake KJ, et al. AO spine injury classification system: a revision proposal for the thoracic and lumbar spine. *Eur Spine J*. 2013;22[10]:2184-2201.)

The axis of rotation for axial (torsion) movements has been difficult to locate. This axis of rotation is believed to lie within the posterior AF when exposed to torque.[21] Even small axial motion can create compression at one facet surface and tension at the opposite facet surface.[5] With disc degeneration, the axis of rotation becomes far less apparent, however, in the lumbar spine.[4] Under degenerative conditions, the locus of the axis of rotation has been reported to be significantly spread out over an extended area.[21]

Collectively, the literature has described the locations of the axis of rotation for various "normal" motions. It is apparent, however, that these axes change dramatically with degeneration, and should be factored in when considering load bearing through the spine and motion profiles.

Motion Coupling

A significant amount of coupling has been observed along the spinal column. Coupling is a function of the geometric characteristics of specific vertebrae, limitations in tissue properties of the disc and ligaments, and spine curvature. Movements are considered coupled when one motion is accompanied by motion in a different plane.[2] The motion in the primary, or intended, plane of movement is referred to as the *main motion*; the accompanying motions are referred to as *coupled motions*.

Because coupling can have profound implications on the transmission of forces through the spine, it is important that the nature of coupling in the different regions of the spine be understood. From a clinical perspective, coupling is important in understanding the impact of various pathologies, such as scoliosis and different types of spine trauma. In addition, an appreciation for coupling is important for understanding the impact of surgical interventions, such as the impact of fusion.

Coupling is most common in the cervical and lumbar spine, but can also occur in the thoracic spine. Coupling in the cervical and lumbar spine involves axial rotation coupled with lateral bending. Lumbar motion can involve cross-coupling in all three rotation directions. Motions in the lumbar spine are rarely unaccompanied by coupled movements. Coupled motions of the lumbar spine vary as a function of the spine level and a function of spine posture.[2]

Coupling patterns within the spine differ depending on the region of the spine. The cervical spine exhibits a striking degree of coupling in that lateral bending of the head is

TABLE 6.1 Limits and Representative Values of Ranges of Rotation for Cervical, Thoracic, and Lumbar Spine

Interspace	COMBINED FLEXION-EXTENSION (± *Y*-AXIS ROTATION) Limits of Ranges (Degrees)	Representative Angle (Degrees)	ONE SIDE LATERAL BENDING (*X*-AXIS ROTATION) Limits of Ranges (Degrees)	Representative Angle (Degrees)	ONE SIDE AXIAL ROTATION (*Z*-AXIS ROTATION) Limits of Ranges (Degrees)	Representative Angle (Degrees)
C0–C1		25		5		5
C1–C2		20		5		40
Middle						
C2–C3	5–16	10	11–20	10	0–10	3
C3–C4	7–26	15	9–15	11	3–10	7
C4–C5	13–29	20	0–16	11	1–12	7
Lower						
C5–C6	13–29	20	0–16	8	2–12	7
C6–C7	6–26	17	0–17	7	2–10	6
C7-T1	4–7	9	0–17	4	0–7	2
T1–T2	3–5	4	5	5	14	9
T2–T3	3–5	4	5–7	6	4–12	8
T3–T4	2–5	4	3–7	5	5–11	8
T4–T5	2–5	4	5–6	6	5–11	8
T5–T6	3–5	4	5–6	6	5–11	8
T6–T7	2–7	5	6	6	4–11	7
T7–T8	3–8	6	3–8	6	4–11	7
T8–T9	3–8	6	4–7	6	6–7	6
T9–T10	3–8	6	4–7	6	3–5	4
T10–T11	4–14	9	3–10	7	2–3	2
T11–T12	6–20	12	4–13	9	2–3	2
T12–L1	6–20	12	5–10	8	2–3	2
L1–L2	5–16	12	3–8	6	1–3	2
L2–L3	8–18	14	3–10	6	1–3	2
L3–L4	6–17	15	4–12	8	1–3	2
L4–L5	9–21	16	3–9	6	1–3	2
L5–S1	10–24	17	2–6	3	0–2	1

From White AA III, Panjabi MM. *Clinical Biomechanics of the Spine*, ed 2. Philadelphia: JB Lippincott; 1990.

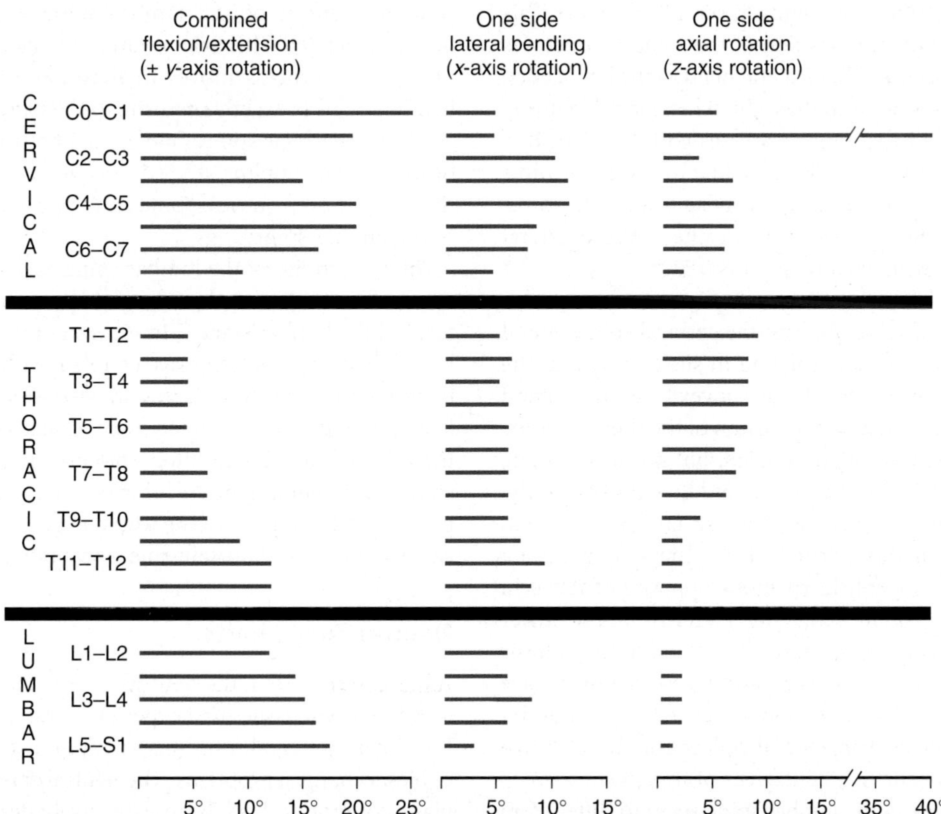

FIG. 6.12 Composite estimate of representative values for ranges of motion at different levels of the spine in sagittal, lateral, and transverse planes of the body. (From White AA III, Panjabi MM. *Clinical Biomechanics of the Spine*, ed 2. Philadelphia: JB Lippincott; 1990.)

TABLE 6.2 Coupled Motions of the Lumbar Spine

Primary Movement and Level	AXIAL ROTATION, DEGREES (+ TO LEFT)		FLEXION-EXTENSION, DEGREES (+ FLEXION)		LATERAL FLEXION, DEGREES (+ TO LEFT)	
	Mean	**Range**	**Mean**	**Range**	**Mean**	**Range**
Right Rotation						
L1	−1	−2 to 1	0	−3 to 3	3	−1 to 5
L2	−1	−2 to 1	0	−2 to 2	4	1 to 9
L3	−1	−3 to 1	0	−2 to 2	3	1 to 6
L4	−1	−2 to 1	0	−9 to 6	1	−3 to 3
L5	−1	−2 to 1	0	−5 to 3	−2	−7 to 0
Left Rotation						
L1	1	−1 to 1	0	−4 to 4	−3	−7 to −1
L2	1	−1 to 1	0	−4 to 4	−3	−5 to 0
L3	2	0 to 1	0	−3 to 2	−3	−6 to 0
L4	2	0 to 1	0	−7 to 2	−2	−5 to 1
L5	0	−2 to 1	0	−5 to 3	1	0 to 2
Right Lateral Flexion						
L1	0	−3 to 1	−2	−5 to 1	−5	−8 to −2
L2	1	−1 to 1	−1	−3 to 1	−5	−8 to −4
L3	1	−1 to 1	−1	−3 to 1	−5	−11 to 2
L4	1	0 to 1	0	−1 to 4	−3	−5 to 1
L5	0	−1 to 1	2	−3 to 8	0	−2 to 3
Left Lateral Flexion						
L1	0	−2 to 1	−2	−9 to 0	6	4 to 10
L2	−1	−3 to 1	−3	−4 to −1	6	2 to 10
L3	−1	−4 to 1	−2	−4 to 3	6	−3 to 8
L4	−1	−4 to 1	−1	−4 to 2	3	−3 to 6
L5	−2	−3 to 1	0	−5 to 5	−3	−6 to 1

(From Adams MA, Bogduk N, Burton AK, et al. *The Biomechanics of Back Pain,* ed 2. Edinburgh: Elsevier, 2006.)

accompanied by significant amounts of cervical rotation. This is evident by observing the position of the spinous processes as lateral bending occurs. When lateral bend to the left occurs, the spinous processes point to the right; when lateral bending to the right occurs, the spinous processes go to the left. It is generally thought that the angle of incline of the facet joints in the sagittal plane increases from the head toward the lower spine.[2] Generally, the average ratio of the coupled lateral bending compared with axial rotation is 0.51.[22]

The coupling of lateral bending and spine rotation can also occur in the thoracic spine. As with the cervical spine, lateral bending is coupled with axial rotation in such a way that the spinous process moves toward the convexity of the lateral curve. The vertebrae in the upper portion of the thoracic spine have motions that are strongly coupled, but not to the same degree as in the cervical spine. In the middle segments of the thoracic spine, the coupling motions are far less apparent. Coupled motions in this portion of the thoracic spine are inconsistent and can result in rotations opposite of those in the upper thoracic spine. Coupling patterns in the lower portion of the thoracic spine are weak. Although the patterns of coupling between axial rotation and lateral bending have been described in the literature, most likely owing to a desire to understand scoliosis, Panjabi and colleagues[23] have shown that coupling can occur in all 6 degrees of freedom.

Coupling patterns in the lumbar spine seem to differ from those of the cervical and thoracic spine. The most dominant coupling pattern of the lumbar spine seems to be lateral bending coupled with axial rotation (Table 6.2).[24] In this case, the spinous process moves in the same direction as lateral bending. This is exactly opposite to the pattern in the cervical and upper thoracic spine. One group of researchers[25] reported, however, that coupling at L5–S1 occurs in a fashion similar to that of the lower cervical spine and opposite to that of the rest of the lumbar spine.

In vivo studies of the lumbar spine have shown the importance of muscular involvement in determining coupling patterns of the lumbar spine.[25] In vitro studies have reported that lateral bending motion was coupled with flexion motions between L1 and L3, whereas in vivo studies reported that lateral motions are coupled with extension movements in these vertebrae. In addition, biomechanical analyses have shown that coupling in the lumbar spine can be influenced by posture of the spine.[25,26] One would expect that muscle control can also play an important role in coupling patterns.

Neutral Zone Limits

As discussed earlier, the neutral zone is important for understanding when tissues first experience resistance to movement. Low intersegmental resistance to motion can be an indication of biomechanical problems. The neutral zones for the different planes of motion have been extensively described by Panjabi and colleagues.[27-29] Table 6.3 shows estimates for the neutral

TABLE 6.3 Average Neutral Zone (Degrees of Motion) for Different Spinal Motion Segments in Different Motion Planes

Vertebral Segments	Flexion-Extension	Lateral Bending	Axial Rotation
C0–C1	1.1	1.6	1.5
C1–C2	3.2	1.2	29.6
C3–C6	4.9	4	3.8
C7–T1 and T11–T1	1.5	2.2	1.2
L1–L2 and L3–L4	1.5	1.6	0.7
L5–S1	3	1.8	0.4

From White AA III, Panjabi MM. *Clinical Biomechanics of the Spine*, ed 2. Philadelphia: JB Lippincott; 1990.

zones for rotary motions as a function of the plane of motion and the spine level.[2] For the most part, the neutral zone is limited in range except for certain vertebrae in certain axes of rotation. From a clinical perspective, one must be sensitive to the fact that normal and abnormal neutral zones can be very different for different vertebrae.

A large neutral zone can be an indication of several biomechanical factors. First, the neutral zone has been observed to increase with age.[30] Second, a larger-than-expected neutral zone can indicate injury to the tissue.[31] Third, some clinicians contend that low resistance to movement is an indication of clinical instability.[32] There are several reasons to consider carefully the range of movement within the neutral zone.

Load Tolerance of the Spinal Motion Segments

The precise tolerance characteristics of human spinal tissues—such as muscles, ligaments, tendons, and bones—loaded under various conditions have been difficult to establish. Structure tolerances have been observed to vary greatly even under similar loading conditions because of their dependence on many factors, such as strain rate (rate of loading), age of the structure, frequency of loading, physiologic influences, heredity, conditioning, and other unknown factors. In addition, it has been impossible to measure these tolerances under in vivo conditions. Many of the estimates of tissue tolerance have been derived from various animal or theoretical constructs.

Tolerance data limits have been derived primarily from cadaveric tissue. The obvious compromise in this approach is that in vitro tissue when tested does not have the ability to adapt or recover (and potentially increase tolerance) as does a live human. The material properties of cadaveric tissue vary depending on the manner in which the specimen was prepared for testing. At least one study suggests that living tissue failure might occur at magnitudes below those observed in cadaveric specimens.[33]

Muscle and Tendon Strain

Muscle has the lowest tolerance among the tissues of the spine. The ultimate strength of a muscle has been estimated at 32 MPa.[34] Muscle often ruptures before a (healthy) tendon.[35] Tendon stress has been estimated to be between 60 MPa and 100 MPa.[34,35] There seems to be a safety margin between the muscle failure point and the failure point of the tendon by a factor of about twofold[35] to threefold.[34]

Ligament and Bone Tolerance

Ultimate ligament stress has been estimated at approximately 20 MPa. The ultimate stress of bone has been found to depend on the direction of loading. Bone tolerance can range from 51 MPa in transverse tension to 190 MPa in longitudinal compression.

A temporal component to ligament recovery has also been reported. One study found that ligaments required extended periods to regain structural integrity. During the recovery period, compensatory muscle activities have been observed.[36–43] Recovery time has been observed to be several times the loading duration.

Because the spinal ligaments often are the structure that protects the spinal system, it is important to appreciate the failure limits of the various spinal ligaments; these are shown in Table 6.4. Note that the load tolerance of these ligaments and the deformation characteristics of the ligaments vary markedly according to the region of the spine and the specific ligament involved. Generally, the lower the level of the spinal ligament, the greater is the tolerance of the ligament. There are notable exceptions to this trend, however. Spinal ligaments are viscoelastic and can increase their length under load. They can be responsible for an increase in the neutral zone; excessive movement can also initiate muscle activities intended to regain stability.[36,44]

Contact Force Tolerance

Contemporary logic suggests that pain secondary to biomechanical loading of the spine may result from direct stimulation to the facet joints, pressure on the anulus, or pressure on the longitudinal ligaments.[9] At these sites, inflammatory responses and analgesic responses are thought to be involved in the development of pressure and pain. It is much more difficult to specify load tolerance thresholds for contact pressures because the body's individual responses to the imposed loads collectively define the pressure imposed on the spinal structure. The tolerance limits for these structures has not been well defined at this time.

Tolerance of Specific Spine Structures

The general structure tolerance, or failure, limits in response to loading of the lumbar spine have been well investigated. Table 6.5 provides a summary of these tolerances reported as a function of the nature of the loading for the spinal motion segment structures and the disc and vertebral body structures.[18]

Compression

The compression dimension of spine tolerance has been widely examined. Of all the structures in the spinal motion

TABLE 6.4 Failure Strength of Spinal Ligaments

	LOAD (N)		DEFORMATION (mm)		STRESS (MPa)		STRAIN (%)	
	Average	**Range**	**Average**	**Range**	**Average**	**Range**	**Average**	**Range**
Upper Cervical								
C0–C1								
Anterior atlanto-occipital membrane	233		18.9					
Posterior atlanto-occipital membrane	83		18.1					
C1–C2								
ALL	281	170–700	12.3					
Atlanto-axial membrane	113		8.7					
CL	157		11.4					
Transverse ligament	354							
C0–C2								
Apical	214		11.5					
Alar	286	215–357	14.1					
Vertical cruciate	436		25.2					
Tectorial membrane	76		11.9					
Lower Cervical								
ALL	111.5	47–176	8.95	4.2–13.7				
PLL	74.5	47–102	6.4	3.4–9.4				
LF	138.5	56–221	8.3	3.7–12.9				
CL	204	144–264	8.4	6.8–10				
ISL	35.5	26–45	7.35	5.5–9.2				
SSL	—		—					
Thoracic								
ALL	295.5	123–468	10.25	6.3–14.2				
PLL	106	74–138	5.25	3.2–7.3				
LF	200	135–265	8.65	6.3–11				
CL	168	63–273	6.75	3.9–9.6				
ISL	75.5	31–120	5.25	3.8–6.7				
SSL	319.5	101–538	14.1	7.2–21				
Lumbar								
ALL	450	390–510	15.2	7–20	11.6	2.4–21	36.5	16–57
PLL	324	264–384	5.1	4.2–7	11.5	2.9–20	26	8–44
LF	285	230–340	12.7	12–14.5	8.7	2.4–15	26	10–46
CL	222	160–284	11.3	9.8–12.8	7.6	7.6	12	12
ISL	125	120–130	13	7.4–17.8	3.2	1.8–4.6	13	13
SSL	150	100–200	25.9	22.1–28.1	5.4	2–8.7	32.5	26–39

From White AA III, Panjabi MM. *Clinical Biomechanics of the Spine*, ed 2. Philadelphia: JB Lippincott; 1990.
ALL, anterior longitudinal ligament; CL, capsular ligament; ISL, interspinous ligament; LF, ligamentum flavum; PLL, posterior longitudinal ligament; SSL, supraspinous ligament.

segment, the endplate is considered to be the "weak point of the system," or the structure with the lowest tolerance to force. Compression failure limits are a function of age, with older endplates failing at lower levels of force, and a function of gender, with female tolerances lower than male tolerances.[45,46] Fig. 6.13 shows a summary of the compression strength for much of the spine. The magnitude of force required for endplate tissue failure follows a normal distribution that ranges from 2000 to greater than 14,000 N. When compression forces increase on a spinal motion segment, the first signs of damage usually occur at the endplate or the trabeculae that support the endplate. The endplate must be a thin structure to serve its nutrition transport function. Because it is thin, it is also a very weak structure, however, and subject to early failure when load is applied.

Failure is believed to be initiated by the NP of the adjacent disc. This nucleus causes the endplate to bulge and compromise the vertebral body. The superior endplate is damaged more often than the lower endplate. In some cases, it is possible for a portion of the NP to make its way vertically through a herniation of the endplate into the bone.[18] This herniation can calcify and form a Schmorl node. Endplate fractures are difficult to detect via routine radiographs; however, magnetic resonance imaging (MRI) can indicate biologic (modic) changes that are characteristic of vertical displacement of the NP.[18]

When the endplate experiences excessive compressive load, the endplate can bulge into the vertebral body, increasing the volume available to the nucleus. This decompression of the nucleus means that it cannot resist compression well, and more of the load is borne by the AF. The anulus can become unstable and the lamellae can become compressed, and cannot be supported any longer by the nucleus. It is believed that this form of disc loading can result in internal derangement of the disc and potentially reverse bulging of the inner lamellae.

TABLE 6.5 Tolerance of Lumbar Motion Segment and Disc Structures as a Function Load and Motion Characteristics

	Failure Site	Average Tolerance
Motion Segments		
Compression	Endplate	5.2 (±1.8) kN all specimens 6.1 (±1.8) kN men (20–50 y)
Shear	Neural arch	2 kN
Flexion	Posterior ligaments	73 (±18) N-m with compressive load of 0.5–1 kN
Extension	Neural arch	26–45 N-m
Torsion	Neural arch	25–88 N-m
Flexion and compression	Disc or vertebra	5.4 kN
Disc Plus Vertebral Bodies		
Shear	Anulus	0.5 kN
Flexion	Posterior anulus	33(±13 N-m)
Torsion	Anulus	10–31 N-m

From Adams MA, Bogduk N, Burton AK, et al. *The Biomechanics of Back Pain*, ed 2. Edinburgh: Elsevier; 2013.

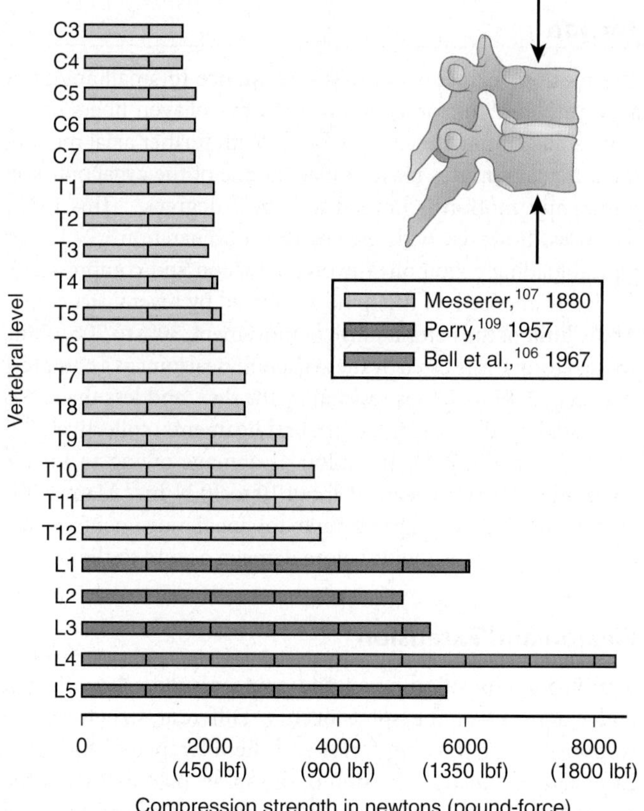

FIG. 6.13 Estimates of vertebral compression tolerance (strength) under slow load rates for the various vertebrae from C3 to L5.[106–108] (From White AA III, Panjabi MM. *Clinical Biomechanics of the Spine*, ed 2. Philadelphia: JB Lippincott; 1990.)

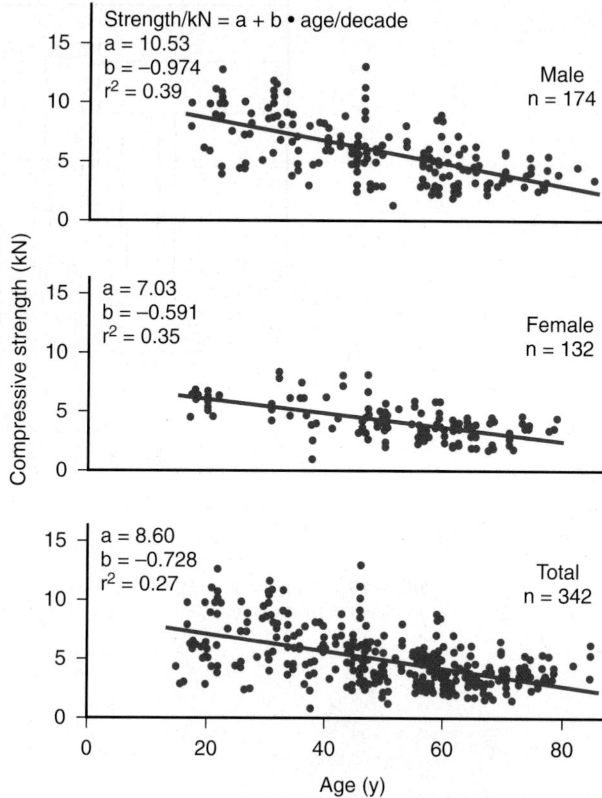

FIG. 6.14 Strength tolerance to static lumbar compression derived from the literature as a function of age and gender. (From Jager M, Luttmann A, Laurig W. Lumbar load during one-hand bricklaying. *Int J Indust Ergo.* 1991;8:261–277.)

As noted earlier, endplate tolerance seems to be a function of gender and age.[45,46] Tolerance estimates based on a review of the literature are shown in Fig. 6.14. Although great variability is evident, women generally have lower compression tolerance by an average of almost 2 kN compared with men. In addition, tolerance reduces significantly with age. Age influences endplate tolerance differently between men and women, however. The decrease in tolerance with age is nearly two times greater for men compared with women.[45,46] In addition, the strength of the vertebrae is nearly 0.8 kN lower than that of the disc.[46] Finally, strength increases as one moves down the lumbar spine by approximately 0.3 kN per lumbar level.[47]

Repetitive loading also seems to influence the tolerance to load of the motion segment. Fig. 6.15 shows how the number of load repetitions and the relative magnitude of the load collectively have a dramatic impact on probability of failure of the segment. As can be seen in this figure, when the relative load becomes greater, the chances of failure increase the risk significantly when the number of loading cycles increases.[48] Studies have also shown that, as the flexion angle increases, the number of cycles required for failure is dramatically reduced.[47,49]

Shear

The disc fibers and intervertebral ligaments are inadequately oriented to resist shear forces. Shear causes the disc to creep during repetitive loading.[50] Under many situations, the neural arch resists shear force, however. The articular process resists on average 2 kN of load before failure; however, this can range from 0.6 kN to 2.8 kN.[51] The specific point of load application can also greatly affect tolerance of the neural arch to shear. Fig. 6.16 shows how differing methods of shear force application can result in dramatically different neural arch load tolerances.[52,53]

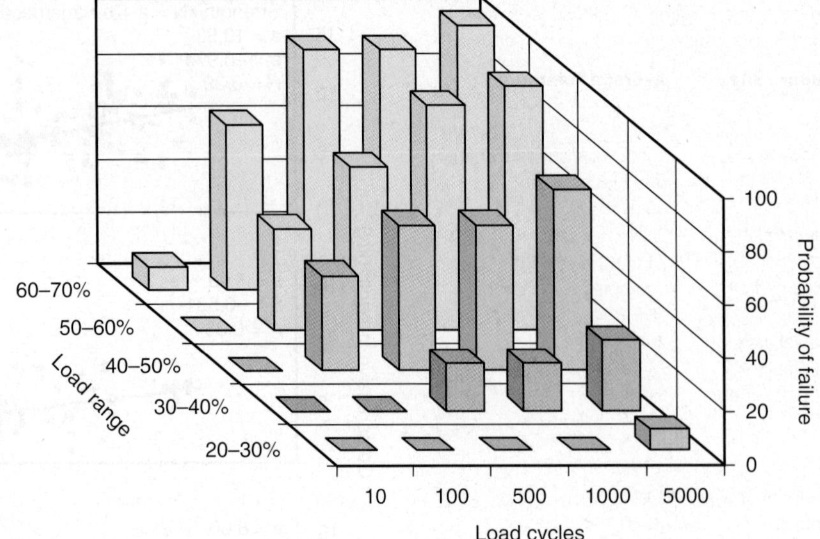

FIG. 6.15 Probability of vertebrae failure as a function of load magnitude and number of cycles of loading.[48] (Modified from Marras WS. *The Working Back: A Systems View*. Hoboken, NJ: John Wiley & Sons; 2008.)

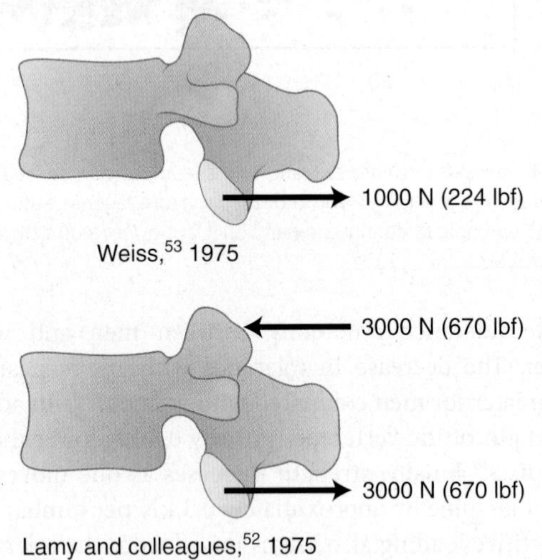

FIG. 6.16 Force tolerance of neural arch varies greatly as a function of shear force application method.[22,53] (From White AA III, Panjabi MM. *Clinical Biomechanics of the Spine*, ed 2. Philadelphia: JB Lippincott; 1990.)

Repetitive shear loading can also reduce the tolerance to 380 N.[51] Some authors have concluded that the limit at which shear begins to increase risk is 750 to 1000 N,[54–56] although this is also known to vary according to load rate.[57,58] In addition, studies have reported failure occurring at the pars under these conditions. Fig. 6.17 shows a summary of results of ultimate shear strength of human cadaveric lumbar spines obtained from in vitro studies.[59] Gallagher and Marras conducted a Weibull analysis on shear failure data of human cadaveric lumbar spines and recommended a maximum permissible shear limit of 1000 N for occasional exposure to shear loading (≤100 loadings/day) during occupational tasks. However, for activities resulting in more frequent shear loadings (100–1000 loadings/day), they recommended a shear limit of 700 N.[59]

Torsion

The motion segments offer little resistance to small angles of axial rotation. Torsion is first resisted by collagen fibers in the anulus that simply stretch slightly.[18,60] With further axial motion, the articular surfaces make contact at one of the zygapophyseal joints, and motion is limited to 1 or 2 degrees.[21] This ROM increases, however, with greater disc degeneration.[61–63] Under typical loading conditions (involving torsion and compression), the loads imposed on the spine are shared by several structures. At the limit of the natural range of movement, 30% to 70% of the applied torque is resisted by the zygapophyseal joint as a compressive load, 20% to 50% is resisted by the disc, and less than 15% is resisted by all of the intervertebral ligaments, collectively.[18,21]

The lower limit for initiation of damage owing to torque application seems to begin at about 10 to 30 N-m.[21] Many clinicians believe that damage owing to torsional movements occurs at the zygapophyseal joint before damage occurs to the discs.[18]

Flexion and Extension

Significant repositioning of the spine results when flexion and extension of the spine occurs. Different structures are responsible for resisting force, and the tolerance of the spine can change. During extension of the spine, 60% to 70% of the applied load is resisted by the neural arch. Studies have reported damage resulting from 3 to 8 degrees of extension under bending moments of 28 to 45 N-m.[64,65] Resistance to extension is offered by the disc and the anterior longitudinal ligament.[18] Of particular concern is the risk of the anulus bulging into the vertebral canal and compromising canal space.

It is hypothesized that the zygapophyseal joint would be the structure damaged first owing to extension. However, it is also believed that the interspinous ligament may be at risk because it would be compressed by opposing spinous processes. Rapid load rates, possibly resulting from athletic endeavors, are also thought potentially to increase risk.

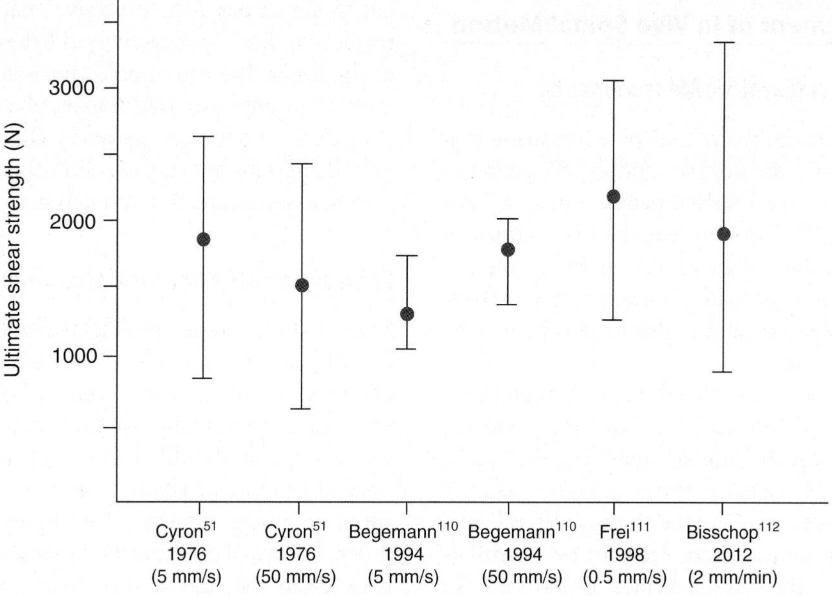

FIG. 6.17 Summary of in vitro studies measuring the ultimate shear stress of human lumbar segments (error bars represent the range of shear tolerance values). (From Gallagher S, Marras WS. Tolerance of the lumbar spine to shear: a review and recommended exposure limits. *Clin Biomech [Bristol, Avon]*. 2012;27[10]:973-978.)

Flexion can lead to injury when imposed moments reach 50 to 80 N-m.[66–68] Damage occurs when the spinal motion segment reaches 5 to 9 degrees per motion segment in the upper lumbar spine and 10 to 16 degrees per segment in the lower lumbar spine. The first structures to sustain damage are the interspinous and supraspinous ligaments.[68] During complex motions involving flexion and lateral bending, the capsular ligaments can also be compromised. The final tissue to fail is the outer posterior AF. In isolation (without the ligaments), the disc can fail when flexed at 18 degrees with an application of 15 to 50 N-m of load.[69] As with most structures, load rate also plays a role in tolerance. Resistance to flexion can increase by more than 10% when rapid motions (10 seconds) are compared with slow motions (1 second).[70] Static postures seem to reduce resistance to bending by very large amounts, probably owing to the interrelationship between the ligamentous system and muscular control.[38]

Lateral Motion

Less has been reported about the tolerance associated with lateral bending moment exposure. Some studies have reported that a lateral bending moment of 10 N-m results in 4 to 6 degrees of lateral bending in the lumbar spine, with most of the resistance occurring at the disc.[62,71] If the disc experiences degeneration, the ROM is greatly reduced to 3 to 4 degrees, however, practically eliminating the neutral zone.[62]

In Vivo Spine Biomechanics

Overview

Our fundamental knowledge of spine biomechanics has been primarily gained through in vitro studies on animal and human cadaveric models in laboratories. However, the value of these biomechanical results increases significantly only when it can be directly correlated to clinical outcomes.[72,73] Intuitively and experientially, we know that there are several limitations associated with in vitro studies—such as specimen integrity, lack of complex neuromuscular control, and proprioceptive and nociceptive inputs—that all play a significant role in producing the natural, graceful, and efficient motion of the spine. Of particular clinical significance is the understanding of pain-modulated motion, which is an in vivo phenomenon. Several studies have explored this complex phenomenon in symptomatic individuals with low back disorders and found significant modifications to their kinematics due to underlying pathology and pain when compared to asymptomatic individuals.[74–76] Unfortunately, current in vitro testing methods are unable to replicate pain-modulated kinematics, estimate pain, or determine the impact of altered kinematics due to pain avoidance on the overall mechanical response of the spine and potential injury risk or damage. This creates a substantial impetus for improving our understanding of the mechanical behavior of the spine under in vivo conditions and developing strategies to better translate biomechanical parameters from benchtop to bedside.

To address these limitations, over the past 15 years, several researchers have developed tools to enhance our understanding of in vivo spine biomechanics using advanced medical imaging, motion-capture systems, and efficient numerical techniques to help provide clinically measurable biomechanical metrics. These tools have the potential to help determine accurate in vivo spinal motions in three-dimensional (3D) load exposures, provide insights into mechanisms of spinal injury and pathology, and facilitate overall assessment of treatment outcomes, design of novel spinal implants, and improve current prevention and rehabilitation strategies. The following sections highlight key areas of research on in vivo spine biomechanics.

Quantitative Assessment of in Vivo Spinal Motion

Overall Spine Kinematics (Extrinsic Measurements)

To appreciate the differences involved in spine impairment, it is important to understand the normal motion or kinematics of the spine. It has been observed that people with low back pain move more slowly.[74,75,77] Motion reduction is assumed to be a result of the "guarding" that occurs in an attempt to minimize the stimulation of pain-producing nociceptors. Abnormal coupling of movement has also been shown to be associated with low back pain.[76]

Spine kinematic profiles associated with asymptomatic individuals and people with low back pain have been reported in the literature at least for the lumbar spine. Fig. 6.18 summarizes how trunk ROM, velocity, and acceleration change as a function of low back pain in the sagittal, lateral, and transverse planes of the body. There seem to be no differences in ROM between the low back pain group and the asymptomatic group. Significant differences are apparent, however, when trunk velocity and acceleration are considered. This seems to be the case in all motion planes of the body. More recent studies have shown that kinematic ability can be used to document the extent of a low back disorder.[74,77] These differences in velocity and acceleration are believed to be a result of protective "guarding" employed by patients with low back pain through the excessive coactive recruitment of the trunk muscles. This coactivity is believed to slow the motions of the torso. The use of objective quantitative biomechanical metrics to augment traditional subjective measures such as pain questionnaires or Oswestry Disability Index (ODI) may provide new insights during clinical evaluation and potentially improve overall treatment outcomes.

Spine Kinematics (Intrinsic Measurements)

Several studies have investigated noninvasive techniques to quantify normal in vivo spinal kinematics to aid in the clinical diagnosis of spinal impairments and instability.[27,78–81] A majority of these studies relied on static planar radiographs to assess in vivo spinal ROM.[27,82] Fig. 6.19 illustrates the estimated normal movement characteristics of the lumbar spine measured in living subjects. This figure indicates significantly different normal movements, particularly in flexion-extension, between in vivo and in vitro observations.[18,27] Fig. 6.20 highlights this difference between the in vitro and in vivo observations in the sagittal plane.[27]

There is a general overestimation of extension movement range in vitro and a general underestimation of flexion range in vitro. In addition, significant differences can be seen between levels between the two states. It should be noted that the measurements from these studies were from static

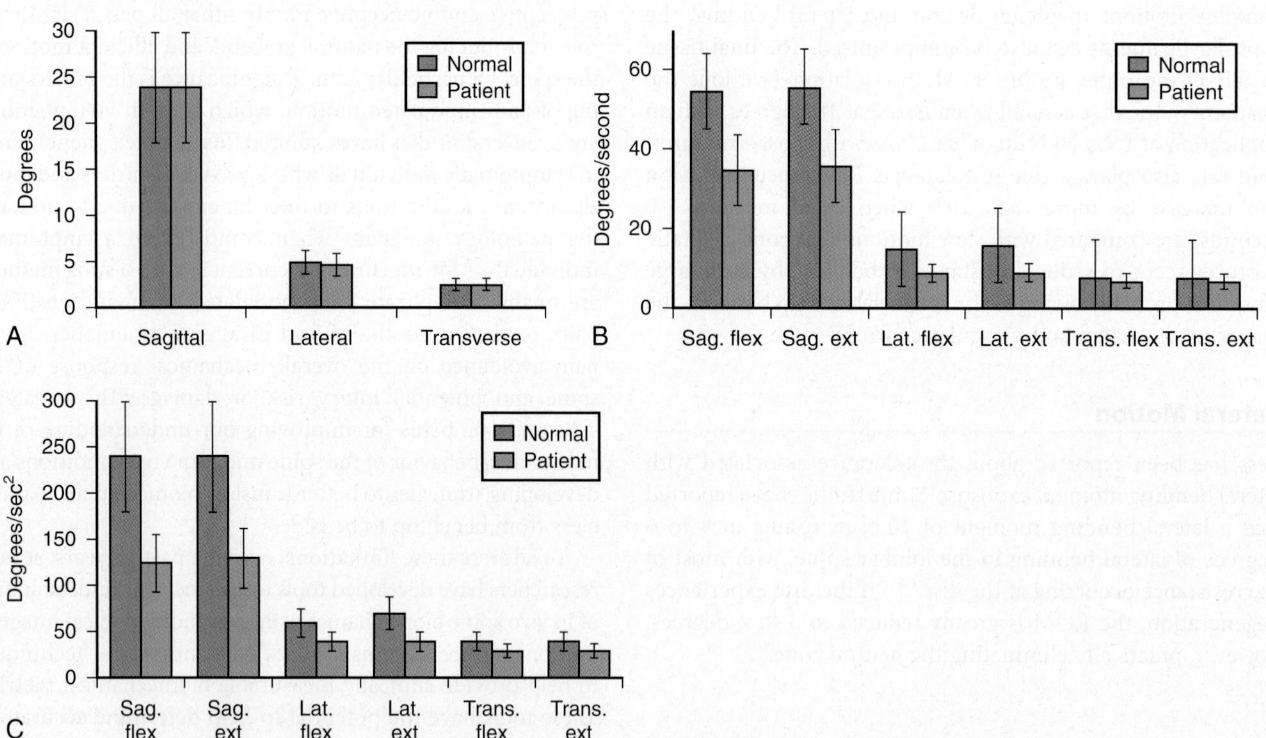

FIG. 6.18 (A) Spine range of motion characteristics (mean and standard deviation [SD]) associated with asymptomatic patients versus patients with low back pain in sagittal, lateral, and transverse planes of the body. (B) Spine velocity characteristics (mean and SD) associated with asymptomatic patients versus patients with low back pain in sagittal, lateral, and transverse planes of the body. (C) Spine acceleration characteristics (mean and SD) associated with asymptomatic patients versus patients with low back pain in sagittal, lateral, and transverse planes of the body.

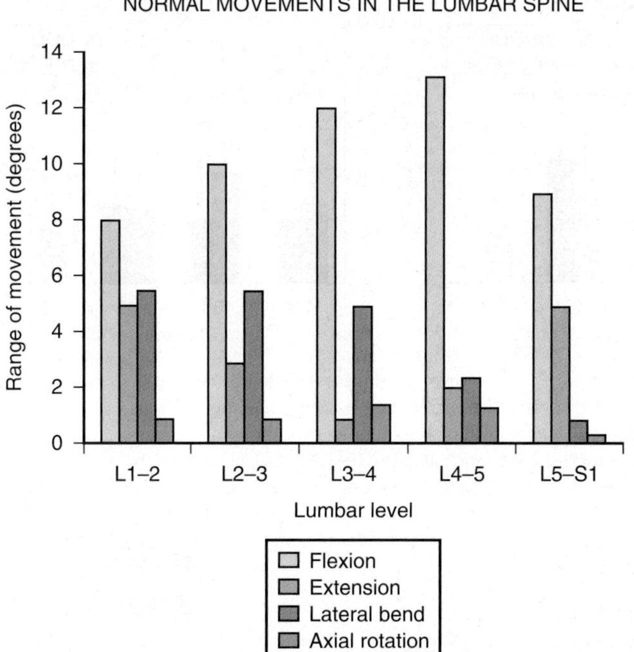

FIG. 6.19 Ranges of motion in lumbar spine during flexion, extension, lateral bending, and rotation.[25,27] (From Adams MA, Bogduk N, Burton AK, et al. *The Biomechanics of Back Pain*, ed 2. Edinburgh: Elsevier; 2013.)

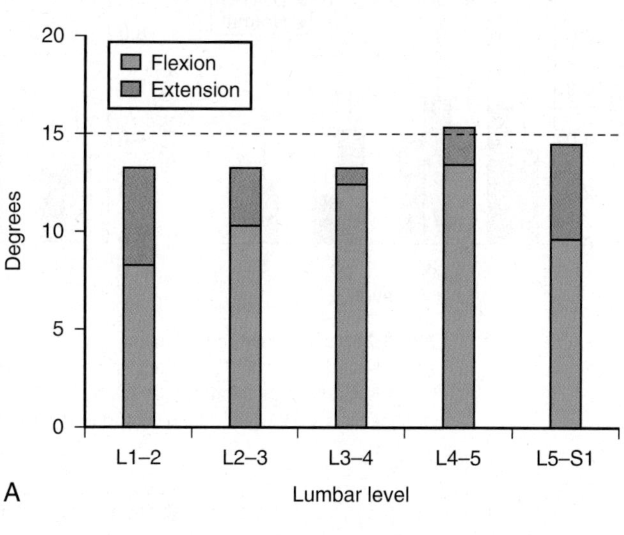

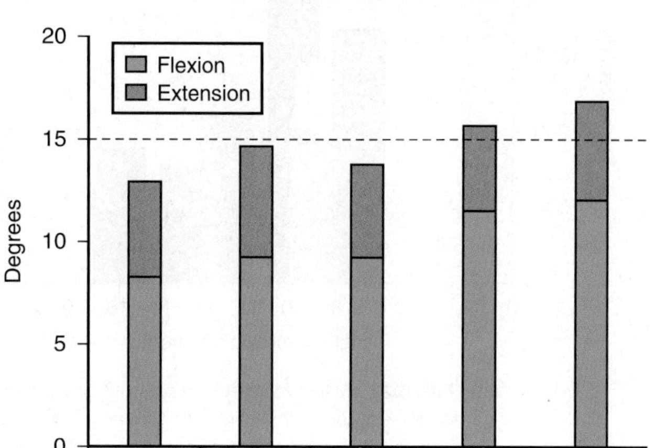

FIG. 6.20 Range of flexion and extension motion in lumbar spine measured (A) in vivo and (B) in vitro.[18,27] (From Adams MA, Bogduk N, Burton AK, et al. *The Biomechanics of Back Pain*, ed 2. Edinburgh: Elsevier; 2013.)

two-dimensional (2D) positions; thus, there are several inherent limitations with these measurements, such as kinematic differences between static and dynamic motions, inaccuracies in measurements using radiographs, and inability to measure multiplanar motion.[83–85]

Recent advances in imaging technologies have helped to address the limitations of static 2D measurements and have facilitated 3D dynamic motions of the spine to be measured in vivo with high accuracy and precision using a system of synchronized biplanar radiographs.[78–81] 3D person-specific spine models developed from computed tomography or MRI can be directly matched to the biplane radiographs, and segmental kinematics can be determined in real time. Using this technique, one study reported that, for healthy subjects, the upper vertebrae in the lumbar spine had larger ROMs than the lower vertebrae during functional flexion-extension. However, during lateral bending, the lower vertebrae showed higher motion than the upper vertebrae. They also found no significant difference between levels during axial rotation motion.[80] A subsequent study on patients with degenerative disc disease (DDD) found significant differences in spinal kinematics between patients and healthy controls, especially at L3–L4. They found that L3–L4 showed the largest ROM in patients in all planes of motion.[81] Fig. 6.21 shows the results of in vivo spinal rotations during dynamic functional motion of patients with DDD and healthy controls.

Adjacent-level degeneration is a common occurrence clinically following a fusion surgery; however, its etiology is unclear and controversial. Several in vitro studies have shown that there is a significant increase in adjacent-level kinematics following fusion; however, the findings of these studies are based on assumptions and testing protocols that are not necessarily true under in vivo conditions.[86] A group investigating in vivo segmental kinematics using dynamic biplanar radiography recently showed that cervical spine patients followed 1 year postoperatively after a fusion surgery at C5–C6 showed no increase in adjacent-level motions, contrary to the findings of in vitro studies.[78,79] Rather, they observed that, during flexion-extension, a redistribution of adjacent-level motion occurred with more extension motion, less flexion occurring at segments rostral to the fusion, and more posterior translations rostral and caudal to the fusion. These differences in motion may be attributed to iatrogenic factors such as alteration in neutral sagittal alignment and disruption of the anterior longitudinal ligament during fusion.[79] It appears also that, under in vivo conditions, overall ROM of the entire spine actually decreases after fusion.[87]

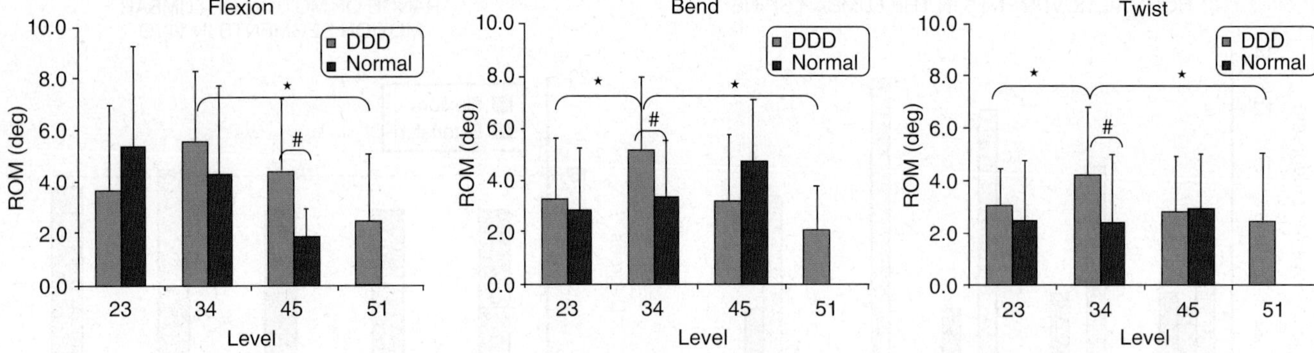

FIG. 6.21 Range of motion (ROM) of vertebral levels of patients with degenerative disc disease (DDD) and normal healthy controls. *Significant difference within group; #Significant difference between normal healthy controls and patients. (From Passias PG, Wang S. Kozanek M, et al. Segmental lumbar rotation in patients with discogenic low back pain during functional weight-bearing activities. *J Bone Joint Surg Am*. 2011;93[1]:29-37.)

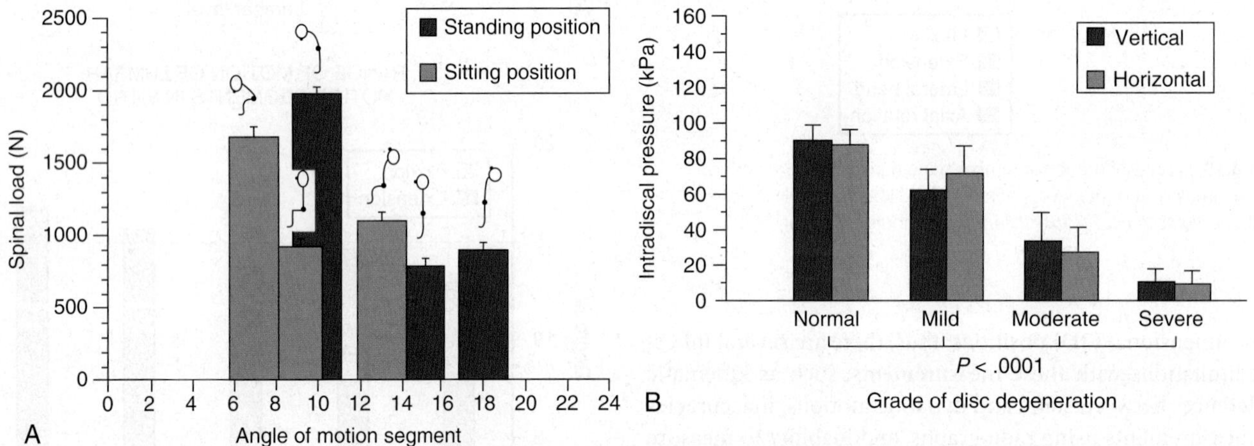

FIG. 6.22 (A) In vivo intradiscal pressure at different postures. (B) Intradiscal pressure variation with progression of disc degeneration. (From Sato K, Kikuchi S, Yonezawa T. In vivo intradiscal pressure measurement in healthy individuals and in patients with ongoing back problems. *Spine*. 1999;24[23]:2468-2474.)

Quantitative Assessment of in Vivo Spinal Loading

Accurate in vivo measurement of internal spinal loads requires placement of a measuring device or sensor invasively into the region of interest. This would not only pose ethical concerns, but there is potential risk associated with the implantation of load sensors in living subjects. Due to these factors, there are only a few documented studies that have investigated in vivo spinal loads. The earliest attempt at quantifying in vivo compressive loads was conducted by Nachemson in 1964, who measured intradiscal pressures using a needle-mounted pressure gauge.[88,89] Similar attempts were made again by two other groups in 1999.[90,91] The results from these studies can be summarized as follows: the lowest compressive loads were seen when lying down (144–250 N), standing upright showed loads of 500 to 800 N, and sitting erect was 700 to 996 N.[88–91] These studies also showed that both forward and backward bending caused an increase in spinal loads. Fig. 6.22A shows intradiscal pressures measured in vivo from different postures. One of these studies also compared intradiscal pressure (horizontal and vertical pressures based on orientation of pressure gauge) with respect to progression of disc degeneration, and found a significant reduction in pressure with grade of degeneration. Fig. 6.22B shows reduction in intradiscal pressure with disc degeneration.[91]

Rohlmann and colleagues implanted telemeterized vertebral body replacements (VBRs) on five patients with L1 or L3 compression fractures and measured the spinal loads in their anterior spinal column. Using this setup, they investigated the effect of locomotion on spinal loads and found that walking caused significantly higher loads than standing.[92] They also found that ascending stairs caused higher loads than descending (Fig. 6.23).

They also conducted a longitudinal study and observed 10 everyday activities that caused significant increases in spinal loads.[93] Fig. 6.24 shows 10 activities that caused the highest increase in spinal loads (compression and shear forces) for five patients. They observed large individual variations in loads for the various activities.

In Silico Modeling in the Spine

The structural architecture of the human spine exhibits a hierarchical organization spanning from the whole system level (macroscale), to the organ, tissue, and cellular levels

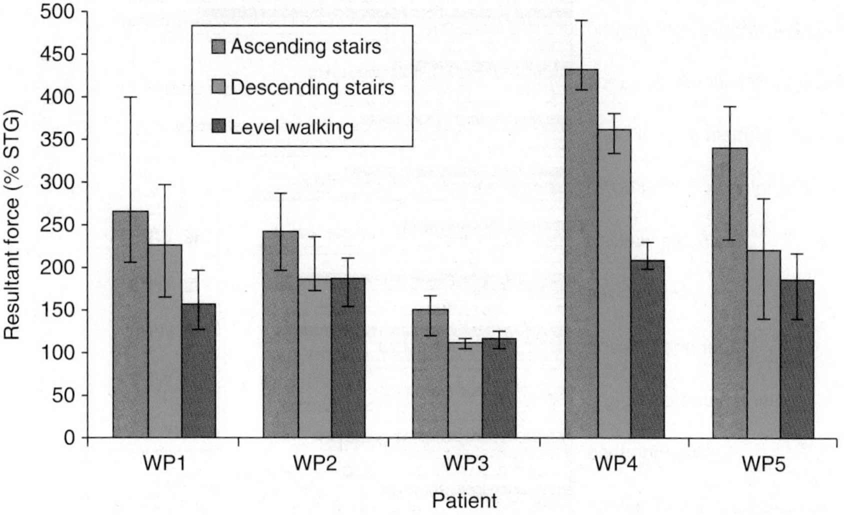

FIG. 6.23 Comparison of peak resultant forces while ascending stairs, descending stairs, and level walking normalized to standing.[92] STG, percentage relative to standing. (From Rohlmann A, Pohl D, Bender A, et al. Activities of everyday life with high spinal loads. *PloS One*. 2014;9[5].)

(microscale). Within this complex organization, there is a network of biologic and mechanical interactions between the different levels that dictates overall biomechanical responses of the spine. Unfortunately, it is extremely difficult to obtain biomechanical parameters, such as internal stress and strain distributions, especially at lower spatial scales (cellular). This knowledge would improve our understanding of the complex micromechanical environments in relation to normal structure–function relationships as well as the underlying mechanisms behind structural and functional breakdown due to disease.

In silico models, more commonly known as computational or biomechanical models, are seeing an increased utilization in spine-related research for investigating complex mechanobiologic phenomena. These models provide a viable and practical alternative to relate the physical and material characteristics of the spine to its mechanical function. Using advanced numerical and imaging techniques, detailed anatomic and material representations of each hierarchical level (macroscale to microscale) can be developed and used for biomechanical evaluations.[94,95] This multiscale approach enables whole body level simulations of spinal kinematics to be used to predict spinal loads within each segment, and then quantify tissue- and cellular-level stresses and strains. These models have the flexibility of precisely controlling a variety of parameters, then observing the effects of these changes on the biomechanical response of the modeled structures. They provide a unique platform to complement in vitro and in vivo experimental techniques.[96–100]

Within the spine, there are several areas of application for in silico models; for instance, mechanical loads are believed to play a major role in the initiation of degenerative changes in the disc. However, the underlying mechanisms by which onset of damage occurs is not well understood.[18,101,102] It is not clear how whole body level mechanical loads translate to deformations at the cellular levels that lead to localized damage and the onset of a degenerative cascade. Using in silico models, we can now begin to explore these complex mechanical relationships across spatial and temporal scales. It also paves the way for the exploration of various other mechanobiologic scenarios, such as age-related degeneration, effect of endplate microfractures, nutrient transport, and tissue remodeling and repair. This whole systems approach to predict the impact of spinal loads on the mechanical behavior of the spine would provide invaluable information for the development of appropriate preventive and therapeutic strategies against back injury.

Clinically, in silico models demonstrate a great potential to aid clinicians in the management of complex spinal ailments. Patient-specific computational models can be developed for use in presurgical planning and evaluation, and an optimized therapy can be implemented for the patient. These models can also be used for conducting comparative analysis of spinal implants.[99,100,103,104] In essence, an in silico model can serve as a valuable, cost-effective tool for the modification of existing implants or the design of new spinal implants aimed at stabilizing and/or preserving motion. Spinal stability following a surgical intervention on an individual can be simulated and evaluated, providing the clinician with valuable insight and quantifiable metrics to help guide the decision-making process prior to actual implementation of desired course of treatment. Knapik and colleagues investigated the biomechanical consequences of a total artificial disc replacement (TDR) at L5–S1 under various simulated dynamic loading conditions obtained from real-life task performance, such as forward bending and lifting of different weights (9.5 and 19 kg).[105] Fig. 6.25 shows mechanical stress distribution following a TDR.[105] Their study found a significant increase in spinal loads between intact and TDR at insertion level (Fig. 6.26). They also found that motion increased in all three planes (sagittal, lateral, and twisting) at insertion level. Fig. 6.27 shows sagittal motion across lumbar levels as a function of intact, TDR, and external loading. Their model was able to effectively show in detail the biomechanical trade-offs with TDR specific to that subject's spine under realistic loading conditions.

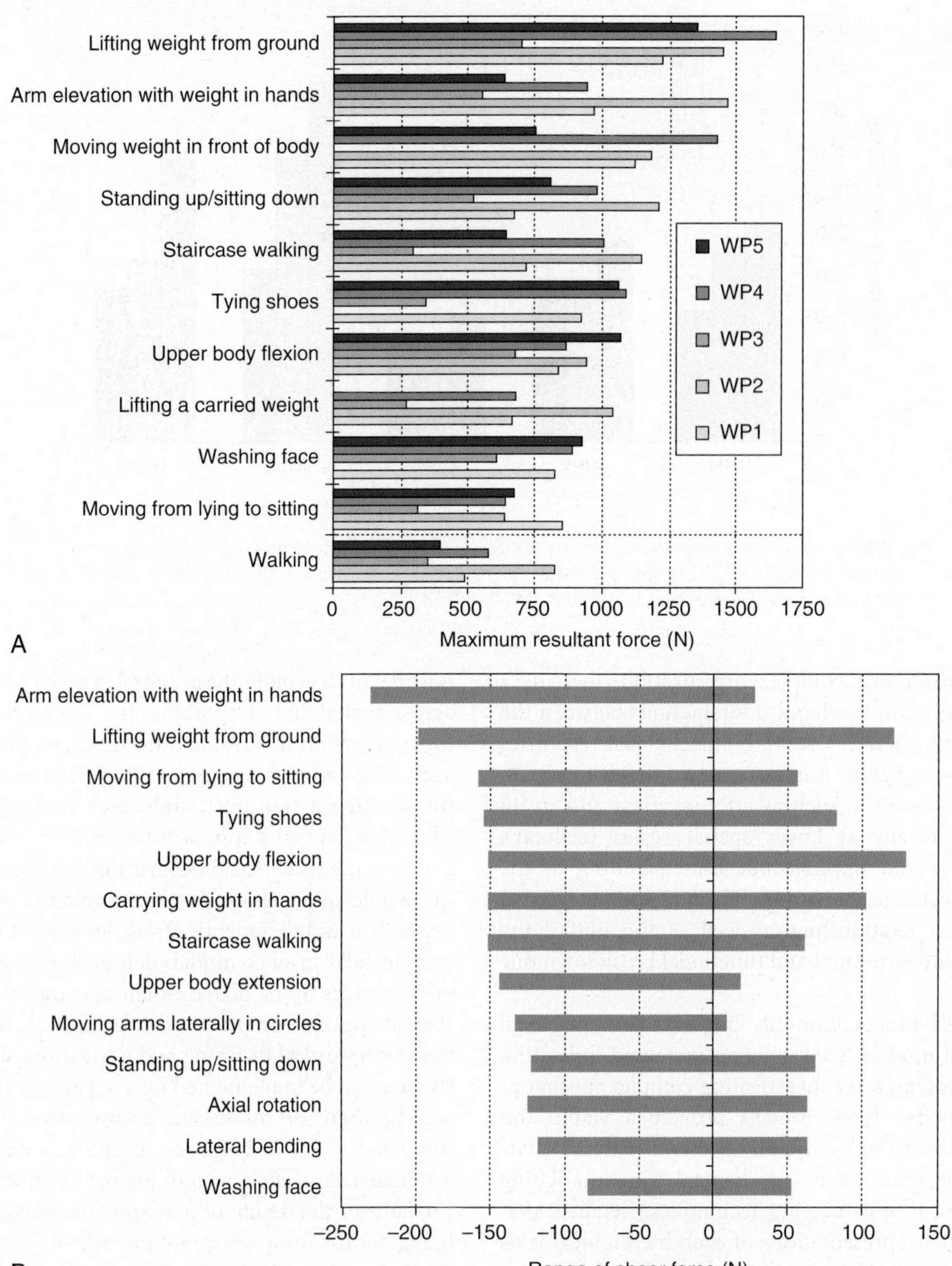

FIG. 6.24 (A) Ten activities with highest compressive forces. (B) Anterior (positive) and posterior (negative) shear forces for the 10 activities.[93] WP, patient label. (From Rohlmann A, Dreischarf M, Zander T, et al. Loads on a vertebral body replacement during locomotion measured in vivo. *Gait Posture*. 2014;39[2]:750-755.)

The System

As can be seen through this review, the spine performs several important functions: it transmits force, allows motion, and protects the spinal cord. Although these functions have been considered independently here, it is important to develop an appreciation for the systematic nature of these spine functions. Although these functions have been described independently, they interact in such a way that the inability to perform one of these functions can also affect the ability to perform other functions.

If the disc becomes compromised in its mechanical integrity, and disc space is reduced, it can alter the load transmission between vertebrae. With less disc space, more of the load may be transmitted through the posterior elements; this repeated loading may change the biochemical behavior of the system. This change may result in an upregulation of proinflammatory biochemical activity and increased pain transmission. Similarly, reduced disc space height may alter the motion characteristics of the spinal motion segments. With less disc space, the stability of the joint can be compromised, and the contact points of the posterior elements can be altered.

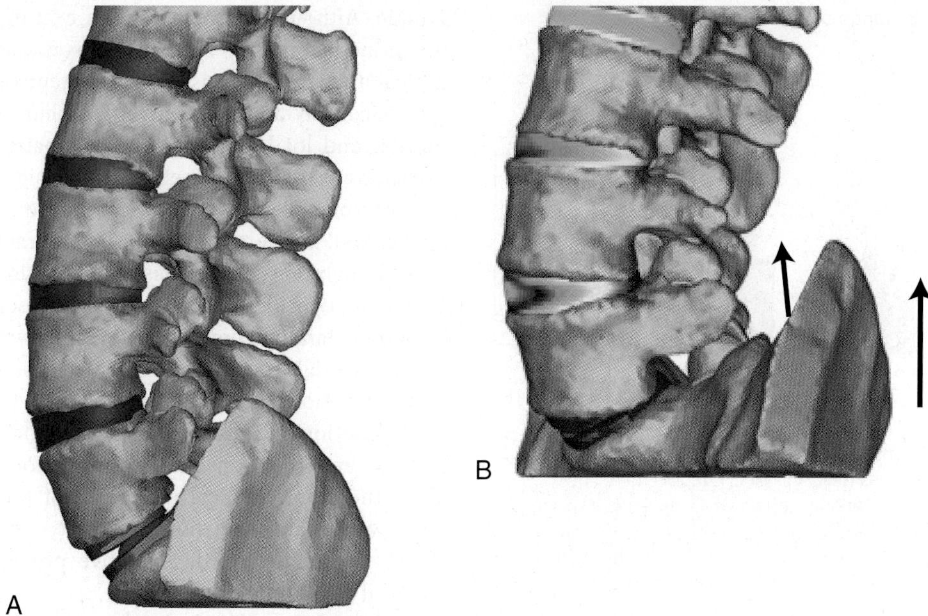

FIG. 6.25 (A) Sagittal view of computational model and (B) stress distributions following total artificial disc placement at L5–S1. (From Knapik GG, Mendel E, Marras WS. Use of a personalized hybrid biomechanical model to assess change in lumbar spine function with a TDR compared to an intact spine. *Eur Spine J.* 2012;21[suppl 5]:S641-S652.)

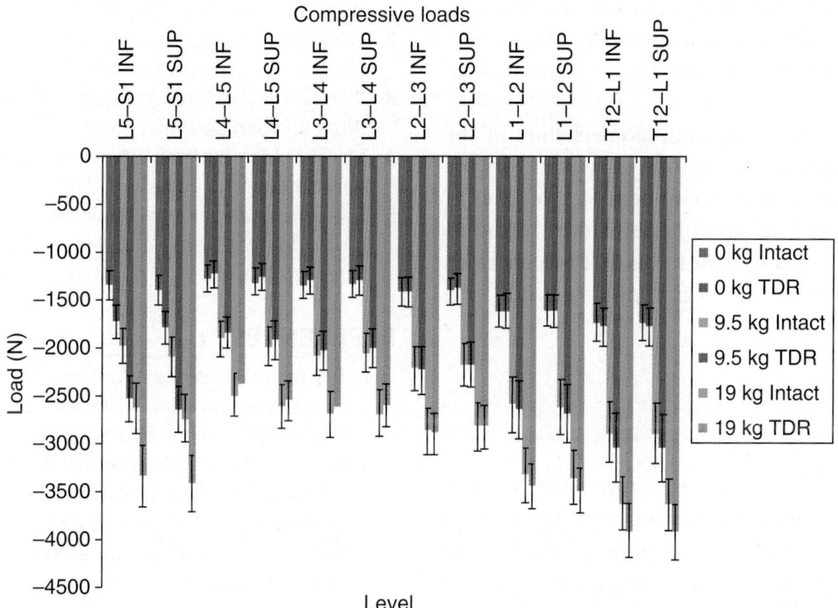

FIG. 6.26 Average of the peak compression loads on the lumbar spine endplates as a function of intact spine versus total artificial disc replacement (TDR) spine and external loading condition (bending while unloaded 0 kg, lifting 9.5 kg, lifting 19 kg). INF, inferior; SUP, superior. (From Knapik GG, Mendel E, Marras WS. Use of a personalized hybrid biomechanical model to assess change in lumbar spine function with a TDR compared to an intact spine. *Eur Spine J.* 2012;21[suppl 5]:S641-S652.)

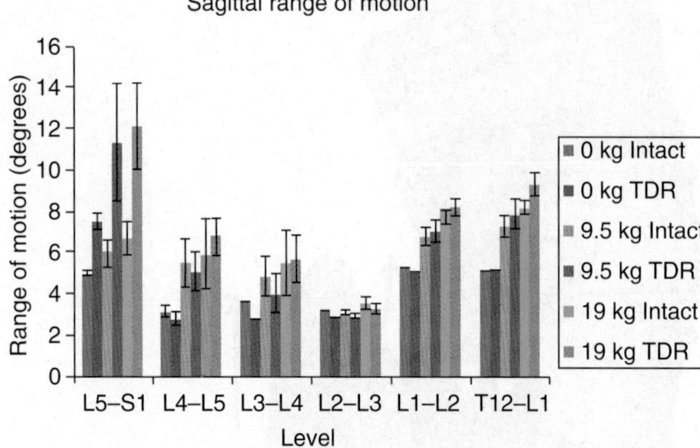

FIG. 6.27 Mean sagittal plane range of motion at each lumbar level as a function of intact spine versus total artificial disc replacement (TDR) spine and external loading condition (bending while unloaded 0 kg, lifting 9.5 kg, lifting 19 kg). (From Knapik GG, Mendel E, Marras WS. Use of a personalized hybrid biomechanical model to assess change in lumbar spine function with a TDR compared to an intact spine. *Eur Spine J.* 2012;21[suppl 5]:S641-S652.)

This alteration could change the kinematic signature of the spine.

Finally, a narrowed disc space could compromise the protection of the nerve root because there is less space for the nerve root to pass through the intervertebral foramen. A compromise of the disc could lead to load transmission irregularities, instability, motion restrictions, and a compromise of the nerve root. This is just one example of how interrelated the components of the spine are from a biomechanical perspective.

As can be seen from this discussion, biomechanics of the spine not only can influence the various dimensions of the biomechanical system, but it also can influence the biochemical behavior of the system. Because biomechanical considerations provide an understanding of the forces that are generated on the system, some authors are beginning to consider the spine as a mechanobiologic system.

Summary

By nature, the spine is a complex structure that provides protection for the spinal cord and a structure to support loads in numerous postures and positions. In addition, the healthy spine limits physiologic movement to conditions that protect the structures of the spine. With trauma and degeneration, the spine loses its ability to achieve these functions adequately.

Biomechanics provides a means to characterize and assess the status of the spine quantitatively and precisely. Quantification provides a rationale for one to determine "how much is too much" exposure to the physical conditions that might damage the spinal system. This chapter has systematically summarized and characterized the capacity of the spinal motion segments in terms of kinematic capacity and load tolerance.

The spinal structures themselves are physiologically unique, and have evolved in such a manner that their functions are unique. Although this chapter has examined the capacity of the individual motion segments, this evaluation should make it clear that the spine is truly a system of components that act collectively and interactively to achieve the functions of motion and load support. The kinematic and load support capacities of the motion segment vary significantly as a function of spinal level, direction of motion, direction of load application, and temporal exposure characteristics.

Although presented as basic information, this information should be considered the fundamental scientific foundation for understanding how the spine functions, how disorders and pain might occur in the spine, how exposure to ADLs and occupational conditions might affect the spine status, and what functions need to be restored clinically. Biomechanical features and function change throughout life. Aging alone alters the biomechanical properties of the spine. It has also been well established, however, that various exposures can greatly accelerate the degenerative process and the biomechanical functioning of the spine.

As knowledge of the spine increases, it is clear that a biomechanical foundation is essential for prevention and treatment of spinal disorders. A better understanding of spine function can be achieved through a better quantification of physical attributes, yielding improved sensitivity and specificity of functional understanding and interventions.

KEY REFERENCES

1. Adams MA, Bogduk N, Burton AK, Dolan P. *The Biomechanics of Back Pain.* Edinburgh: Elsevier; 2013.
2. White AA 3rd, Panjabi MM. *Clinical Biomechanics of the Spine.* Philadelphia: Lippincott-Raven; 1990.
3. Marras WS. *The Working Back: A Systems View.* Hoboken, NJ: John Wiley and Sons; 2008.
4. McGill S. *Ultimate Back Fitness and Performance.* Waterloo, Canada: Wabuno Publishers; 2004.
5. National Research Council & Institute of Medicine [NRC-IOM]. *Musculoskeletal Disorders and the Workplace: Low Back and Upper Extremities.* Washington, DC: National Academy Press; 2001.

REFERENCES

1. Bernhardt M, White AA, Panjabi MM. Biomechanical considerations of spinal stability. In: Herkowitz HN, Garfin SR, Eismont FJ, eds. *Rothman-Simeone The Spine.* Philadelphia: WB Saunders; 2006.
2. White AA, Panjabi MM. *Clinical Biomechanics of the Spine.* Philadelphia: Lippincott-Raven; 1990.
3. Quint U, Wilke HJ, Shirazi-Adl A, et al. Importance of the intersegmental trunk muscles for the stability of the lumbar spine: a biomechanical study in vitro. *Spine.* 1998;23:1937-1945.
4. Cholewicki J, McGill S. Mechanical stability of the in vivo lumbar spine: implications of injury and chronic low back pain. *Clin Biomech (Bristol, Avon).* 1996;11:1-15.
5. Farfan HF, Gracovetsky S. The nature of instability. *Spine.* 1984;9:714-719.
6. Granata KP, Marras WS. Cost-benefit of muscle cocontraction in protecting against spinal instability. *Spine.* 2000;25:1398-1404.
7. Panjabi MM. Clinical spinal instability and low back pain. *J Electromyogr Kinesiol.* 2003;13:371-379.

8. Reeves NP, Narendra KS, Cholewicki J. Spine stability: the six blind men and the elephant. *Clin Biomech (Bristol, Avon)*. 2007;22:266-274.
9. Marras WS. *The Working Back: A Systems View*. Hoboken, NJ: John Wiley & Sons; 2008.
10. Lee CK. Accelerated degeneration of the segment adjacent to a lumbar fusion. *Spine*. 1988;13:375-377.
11. Ghiselli G, Wang JC, Bhatia NN, et al. Adjacent segment degeneration in the lumbar spine. *J Bone Joint Surg Am*. 2004;86:1497-1503.
12. van Ooij A, Oner FC, Verbout AJ. Complications of artificial disc replacement: a report of 27 patients with the SB Charite disc. *J Spinal Disord Tech*. 2003;16:369-383.
13. Dooris AP, Goel VK, Grosland NM, et al. Load-sharing between anterior and posterior elements in a lumbar motion segment implanted with an artificial disc. *Spine*. 2001;26:E122-E129.
14. Brinkmann P, Biggermann M, Hilweg D. Prediction of the compressive strength of human lumbar vertebrae. *Clin Biomech (Bristol, Avon)*. 1989;4:S1-S27.
15. Yoganandan N, Larson SJ, Gallagher M, et al. Correlation of microtrauma in the lumbar spine with intraosseous pressures. *Spine*. 1994;19:435-440.
16. Reinhold M, Audigé L, Schnake KJ, et al. AO spine injury classification system: a revision proposal for the thoracic and lumbar spine. *Eur Spine J*. 2013;22(10):2184-2201.
17. Haughton VM, Schmidt TA, Keele K, et al. Flexibility of lumbar spinal motion segments correlated to type of tears in the annulus fibrosus. *J Neurosurg*. 2000;92:81-86.
18. Adams MA, Bogduk N, Burton AK, et al. *The Biomechanics of Back Pain*. Edinburgh: Churchill Livingstone; 2013.
19. Gertzbein SD, et al. Centrode patterns and segmental instability in degenerative disc disease. *Spine*. 1985;10:257-261.
20. Zhao F, Pollintine P, Hole BD, et al. Discogenic origins of spinal instability. *Spine*. 2005;30:2621-2630.
21. Adams MA, Hutton WC. The relevance of torsion to the mechanical derangement of the lumbar spine. *Spine*. 1981;6:241-248.
22. Moroney SP, Schultz AB, Miller JA, et al. Load-displacement properties of lower cervical spine motion segments. *J Biomech*. 1988;21:769-779.
23. Panjabi MM, Brand RA, White AA. Three-dimensional flexibility and stiffness properties of the human thoracic spine. *J Biomech*. 1976;9:185-192.
24. Bogduk N. *Clinical Anatomy of the Lumbar Spine and Sacrum*. Edinburgh: Churchill Livingstone; 2005.
25. Pearcy MJ, Tibrewal SB. Axial rotation and lateral bending in the normal lumbar spine measured by three-dimensional radiography. *Spine*. 1984;9:582-587.
26. Cholewicki J, Crisco JJ, Oxland TR, et al. Effects of posture and structure on three-dimensional coupled rotations in the lumbar spine: a biomechanical analysis. *Spine*. 1996;21:2421-2428.
27. Pearcy M, Portek I, Shepherd J. Three-dimensional x-ray analysis of normal movement in the lumbar spine. *Spine*. 1984;9:294-297.
28. Panjabi M, et al. Three-dimensional movements of the upper cervical spine. *Spine*. 1988;13:726-730.
29. Yamamoto I, Panjabi MM, Crisco T, et al. Three-dimensional movements of the whole lumbar spine and lumbosacral joint. *Spine*. 1989;14:1256-1260.
30. Mimura M, et al. Disc degeneration affects the multidirectional flexibility of the lumbar spine. *Spine*. 1994;19:1371-1380.
31. Oxland TR, Panjabi MM. The onset and progression of spinal injury: a demonstration of neutral zone sensitivity. *J Biomech*. 1992;25:1165-1172.
32. Panjabi MM. The stabilizing system of the spine. Part II: neutral zone and instability hypothesis. *J Spinal Disord*. 1992;5:390-396.
33. Yoganandan N. Biomechanical identification of injury to an intervertebral joint. *Clin Biomech (Bristol, Avon)*. 1986;1:149.
34. Hoy MG, Zajac FE, Gordon ME. A musculoskeletal model of the human lower extremity: the effect of muscle, tendon, and moment arm on the moment-angle relationship of musculotendon actuators at the hip, knee, and ankle. *J Biomech*. 1990;23:157-169.
35. Nordin M, Frankel V. *Basic Biomechanics of the Musculoskeletal System*. Philadelphia: Lea & Febiger; 1989.
36. Solomonow M. Ligaments: a source of work-related musculoskeletal disorders. *J Electromyogr Kinesiol*. 2004;14:49-60.
37. Solomonow M, Zhou BH, Baratta RV, et al. Biomechanics of increased exposure to lumbar injury caused by cyclic loading. Part 1: loss of reflexive muscular stabilization. *Spine*. 1999;24:2426-2434.
38. Solomonow M, Zhou BH, Harris M, et al. The ligamento-muscular stabilizing system of the spine. *Spine*. 1998;23:2552-2562.
39. Stubbs M, et al. Ligamento-muscular protective reflex in the lumbar spine of the feline. *J Electromyogr Kinesiol*. 1998;8:197-204.
40. Gedalia U, et al. Biomechanics of increased exposure to lumbar injury caused by cyclic loading. Part 2: recovery of reflexive muscular stability with rest. *Spine*. 1999;24:2461-2467.
41. Wang JL, Parnianpour M, Shirazi-Adl A, et al. Viscoelastic finite-element analysis of a lumbar motion segment in combined compression and sagittal flexion: effect of loading rate. *Spine*. 2000;25:310-318.
42. Solomonow M, Zhou B, Baratta RV, et al. Neuromuscular disorders associated with static lumbar flexion: a feline model. *J Electromyogr Kinesiol*. 2002;12:81-90.
43. Solomonow M, et al. Biexponential recovery model of lumbar viscoelastic laxity and reflexive muscular activity after prolonged cyclic loading. *Clin Biomech (Bristol, Avon)*. 2000;15:167-175.
44. Solomonow M, Eversull E, He Zhou B, et al. Neuromuscular neutral zones associated with viscoelastic hysteresis during cyclic lumbar flexion. *Spine*. 2001;26:E314-E324.
45. Jager M, Luttmann A. Compressive strength of lumbar spine elements related to age, gender, and other influences. *J Electromyogr Kinesiol*. 1991;1:291-294.
46. Jager M, Luttmann A, Laurig W. Lumbar load during one-hand bricklaying. *Int J Indust Ergo*. 1991;8: 261-277.
47. Gallagher S, Marras WS, Litsky AS, et al. Torso flexion loads and the fatigue failure of human lumbosacral motion segments. *Spine*. 2005;30:2265-2273.
48. Brinkmann P, Biggermann M, Hilweg D. Fatigue fracture of human lumbar vertebrae. *Clin Biomech (Bristol, Avon)*. 1988;3:S1-S23.
49. Gallagher S, Marras WS, Litsky AS, et al. An exploratory study of loading and morphometric factors associated with specific failure modes in fatigue testing of lumbar motion segments. *Clin Biomech (Bristol, Avon)*. 2006;21:228-234.

SECTION I

50. Cyron BM, Hutton WC. The behaviour of the lumbar intervertebral disc under repetitive forces. *Int Orthop.* 1981;5:203-207.
51. Cyron BM, Hutton WC, Troup JD. Spondylolytic fractures. *J Bone Joint Surg Br.* 1976;58:462-466.
52. Lamy C, Bazergui A, Kraus H, et al. The strength of the neural arch and the etiology of spondylolysis. *Orthop Clin North Am.* 1975;6:215-231.
53. Weiss EB. Stress at the lumbosacral junction. *Orthop Clin North Am.* 1975;66:83.
54. McGill S. *Low Back Disorders: Evidence-Based Prevention and Rehabilitation.* Champaign, IL: Human Kinetics; 2002.
55. Marras WS. Occupational low back disorder causation and control. *Ergonomics.* 2000;43:880-902.
56. National Research Council & Institute of Medicine [NRC-IOM]. *Musculoskeletal Disorders and the Workplace: Low Back and Upper Extremities.* Washington, DC: National Academy Press; 2001.
57. Yingling VR, McGill SM. Anterior shear of spinal motion segments: kinematics, kinetics, and resultant injuries observed in a porcine model. *Spine.* 1999;24:1882-1889.
58. Yingling VR, McGill SM. Mechanical properties and failure mechanics of the spine under posterior shear load: observations from a porcine model. *J Spinal Disord.* 1999;12(6):501-508.
59. Gallagher S, Marras WS. Tolerance of the lumbar spine to shear: a review and recommended exposure limits. *Clin Biomech (Bristol, Avon).* 2012;27(10):973-978.
60. Adams MA, Dolan P. Spine biomechanics. *J Biomech.* 2005;38:1972-1983.
61. Oxland TR, Crisco JJ, Panjabi MM, et al. The effect of injury on rotational coupling at the lumbosacral joint: a biomechanical investigation. *Spine.* 1992;17:74-80.
62. Oxland TR, et al. The relative importance of vertebral bone density and disc degeneration in spinal flexibility and interbody implant performance: an in vitro study. *Spine.* 1996;21:2558-2569.
63. Oxland TR, Grant JP, Dvorak MF, et al. Effects of endplate removal on the structural properties of the lower lumbar vertebral bodies. *Spine.* 2003;28:771-777.
64. Adams MA, Dolan P, Hutton WC. The lumbar spine in backward bending. *Spine.* 1988;13:1019-1026.
65. Green TP, Allvey JC, Adams MA. Spondylolysis: bending of the inferior articular processes of lumbar vertebrae during simulated spinal movements. *Spine.* 1994;19:2683-2691.
66. Adams MA, Dolan P. A technique for quantifying the bending moment acting on the lumbar spine in vivo. *J Biomech.* 1991;24:117-126.
67. Adams MA, Hutton WC. The effect of posture on diffusion into lumbar intervertebral discs. *J Anat.* 1986;147:121-134.
68. Adams MA, Hutton WC, Stott JR. The resistance to flexion of the lumbar intervertebral joint. *Spine.* 1980;5:245-253.
69. Adams MA, Green TP, Dolan P. The strength in anterior bending of lumbar intervertebral discs. *Spine.* 1994;19:2197-2203.
70. Adams MA, Dolan P. Time-dependent changes in the lumbar spine's resistance to bending. *Clin Biomech (Bristol, Avon).* 1996;11:194-200.
71. Peng B, et al. Possible pathogenesis of painful intervertebral disc degeneration. *Spine.* 2006;31:560-566.
72. Benzel EC, Kayanja M, Fleischman A, Roy S. Spine biomechanics: fundamentals and future. *Clin Neurosurg.* 2006;53:98-105.
73. Cheng B, Goel V. Foreword, Biomechanics Special Issue. *Int J Spine Surg.* 2015;9:31.
74. Marras WS, et al. The classification of anatomic- and symptom-based low back disorders using motion measure models. *Spine.* 1995;20:2531-2546.
75. Marras WS, Wongsam PE. Flexibility and velocity of the normal and impaired lumbar spine. *Arch Phys Med Rehabil.* 1986;67:213-217.
76. Stokes IA, Wilder DG, Frymoyer JW, et al. 1980 Volvo award in clinical sciences. Assessment of patients with low-back pain by biplanar radiographic measurement of intervertebral motion. *Spine.* 1981;6:233-240.
77. Marras WS, et al. The quantification of low back disorder using motion measures: methodology and validation. *Spine.* 1999;24:2091-2100.
78. Anderst WJ, Donaldson WF 3rd, Lee JY, Kang JD. Cervical motion segment percent contributions to flexion-extension during continuous functional movement in control subjects and arthrodesis patients. *Spine.* 2013;38(9):E533-E539.
79. Anderst WJ, Lee JY, Donaldson WF 3rd, Kang JD. Six-degrees-of-freedom cervical spine range of motion during dynamic flexion-extension after single-level anterior arthrodesis: comparison with asymptomatic control subjects. *J Bone Joint Surg Am.* 2013;95(6):497-506.
80. Li G, Wang S, Passias P, et al. Segmental in vivo vertebral motion during functional human lumbar spine activities. *Eur Spine J.* 2009;18(7):1013-1021.
81. Passias PG, Wang S, Kozanek M, et al. Segmental lumbar rotation in patients with discogenic low back pain during functional weight-bearing activities. *J Bone Joint Surg Am.* 2011;93(1):29-37.
82. Adams MA, Dolan P. Recent advances in lumbar spinal mechanics and their clinical significance. *Clin Biomech (Bristol, Avon).* 1995;10(1):3-19.
83. Anderst W. Narrative review of the in vivo mechanics of the cervical spine after anterior arthrodesis as revealed by dynamic biplane radiography. *J Orthop Res.* 2016;34(1):22-30.
84. Panjabi M, Chang D, Dvorák J. An analysis of errors in kinematic parameters associated with in vivo functional radiographs. *Spine.* 1992;17(2):200-205.
85. Inoue N, Espinoza Orías AA. Biomechanics of intervertebral disk degeneration. *Orthop Clin North Am.* 2011;42(4):487-499.
86. Volkheimer D, Malakoutian M, Oxland TR, Wilke HJ. Limitations of current in vitro test protocols for investigation of instrumented adjacent segment biomechanics: critical analysis of the literature. *Eur Spine J.* 2015;24(9):1882-1892.
87. Malakoutian M, Volkheimer D, Street J, et al. Do in vivo kinematic studies provide insight into adjacent segment degeneration? A qualitative systematic literature review. *Eur Spine J.* 2015;24(9):1865-1881.
88. Nachemson A, Morris JM. In vivo measurements of intradiscal pressure discometry, a method for the determination of pressure in the lower lumbar discs. *J Bone Joint Surg Am.* 1964;46:1077-1092.
89. Nachemson A. The load on lumbar disks in different positions of the body. *Clin Orthop Relat Res.* 1966;45:107-122.

90. Wilke HJ, Neef P, Caimi M, Hoogland T, Claes LE. New in vivo measurements of pressures in the intervertebral disc in daily life. *Spine*. 1999;24(8):755-762.
91. Sato K, Kikuchi S, Yonezawa T. In vivo intradiscal pressure measurement in healthy individuals and in patients with ongoing back problems. *Spine*. 1999;24(23):2468-2474.
92. Rohlmann A, Pohl D, Bender A, et al. Activities of everyday life with high spinal loads. *PLoS One*. 2014;9(5).
93. Rohlmann A, Dreischarf M, Zander T, Graichen F, Bergmann G. Loads on a vertebral body replacement during locomotion measured in vivo. *Gait Posture*. 2014;39(2):750-755.
94. Tawhai M, Bischoff J, Einstein D, et al. Multiscale modeling in computational biomechanics. *IEEE Eng Med Biol Mag*. 2009;28(3):41-49.
95. Erdemir A, Bennetts C, Davis S, Reddy A, Sibole S. Multiscale cartilage biomechanics: technical challenges in realizing a high-throughput modelling and simulation workflow. *Interface Focus*. 2015;5(2).
96. Freutel M, Schmidt H, Dürselen L, Ignatius A, Galbusera F. Finite element modeling of soft tissues: material models, tissue interaction and challenges. *Clin Biomech (Bristol, Avon)*. 2014;29(4):363-372.
97. Fagan MJ, Julian S, Mohsen AM. Finite element analysis in spine research. *Proc Inst Mech Eng H*. 2002;216(5):281-298.
98. Schmidt H, Heuer F, Drumm J, et al. Application of a calibration method provides more realistic results for a finite element model of a lumbar spinal segment. *Clin Biomech (Bristol, Avon)*. 2007;22(4):377-384.
99. Schmidt H, Heuer F, Wilke HJ. Which axial and bending stiffnesses of posterior implants are required to design a flexible lumbar stabilization system? *J Biomech*. 2009;42(1):48-54.
100. Rohlmann A, Mann A, Zander T, Bergmann G. Effect of an artificial disc on lumbar spine biomechanics: a probabilistic finite element study. *Eur Spine J*. 2009;18(1):89-97.
101. Adams MA, Freeman BJ, Morrison HP, Nelson IW, Dolan P. Mechanical initiation of intervertebral disc degeneration. *Spine*. 2000;25(13):1625-1636.
102. Adams MA. Basic science of spinal degeneration. *Surgery (Oxford)*. 2012;30(7):347-350.
103. Aubin CE, Petit Y, Stokes IA, et al. Biomechanical modeling of posterior instrumentation of the scoliotic spine. *Comput Methods Biomech Biomed Engin*. 2003;6(1):27-32.
104. Faizan A, Goel VK, Garfin SR, et al. Do design variations in the artificial disc influence cervical spine biomechanics? A finite element investigation. *Eur Spine J*. 2012;21 (suppl 5):S653-S662.
105. Knapik GG, Mendel E, Marras WS. Use of a personalized hybrid biomechanical model to assess change in lumbar spine function with a TDR compared to an intact spine. *Eur Spine J*. 2012;21(suppl 5):S641-S652.
106. Bell GH, Dunbar O, Beck JS, et al. Variations in strength of vertebrae with age and their relation to osteoporosis. *Calcif Tissue Res*. 1967;1:75-86.
107. Messerer O. *Uber Elasticitat and Festigkeit der Meuschlichen Knochen*. Stutgart: J.G. Cottaschen Buch-handling; 1880.
108. Perry O. *Encyclopedia of Medical Radiology*. New York: Springer Verlag; 1974.
109. Perry O. Fracture of the vertebral end-plate in the lumbar spine. *Acta Orthop Scand*. 1957;25(suppl).
110. Begeman PC, Visarius H, et al. Viscoelastic shear responses of the cadaver and hybrid III lumbar response. Presented at the 38th Stapp Car Crash Conference, Ft. Lauderdale, FL; 1994.
111. Frei H, Oxland TR, Nolte LP. Thoracolumbar spine mechanics contrasted under compression and shear loading. *J Orthop Res*. 2002;20:1333-1338.
112. Bisschop A, Mullender MD, Kingma I, et al. The impact of bone mineral density and disc degeneration on shear strength and stiffness of the lumbar spine following laminectomy. *Eur Spine J*. 2012;21:530-536.

7 CHAPTER Nerve Root Pain in Disc Herniation and Spinal Stenosis

Robert R. Myers
Björn Rydevik
Kjell Olmarker
Shinichi Kikuchi

The clinical symptoms associated with lumbar disc herniation and spinal stenosis are attributed to pathophysiologic changes in spinal nerve roots. Recent research has defined the basic pathophysiologic events at the tissue, cellular, or subcellular levels in relationship to the pathogenesis of sciatica and nerve root pain. This chapter reviews the current knowledge about these mechanisms and discusses these mechanisms in relation to the clinical features of lumbar disc herniation and spinal stenosis.

Nerve root pain is typically radiating in nature and usually related to a specific nerve root or adjacent roots. It is associated with pathologic changes and nerve dysfunction and may be present in motor and sensory modalities, producing motor weakness and sensory disturbances. These changes are tightly linked through mechanisms that are discussed in this chapter.

Two specific mechanisms at the "tissue level" may be defined: (1) mechanical deformation of the nerve roots and (2) biologic or biochemical activity of the disc tissue causing neuroinflammation of nerve roots.

Mechanical Effects on Nerve Roots

Enclosed by the vertebral bones, the spinal nerve roots are relatively well protected from external trauma, although somewhat more susceptible to injury than peripheral nerves. In 1934, Mixter and Barr[1] described that intervertebral discs can rupture and cause mechanical compression of the nerve roots, leading to sciatica. However, there has been moderate research interest in the past regarding nerve root compression. Gelfan and Tarlov[2] in 1956 and Sharpless[3] in 1975 performed some initial experiments on the effects of compression on nerve impulse conduction and showed that nerve roots were more susceptible to compression than peripheral nerves. Interest in nerve root pathophysiology has increased more recently, and numerous studies are reviewed here.

In 1991, a model was presented that allowed for experimental, graded compression of cauda equina nerve roots at known pressure levels.[4] In this model, the cauda equina of pigs was compressed by an inflatable balloon fixed to the spine (Fig. 7.1). The cauda equina could also be observed through the translucent balloon. This model made it possible to study the flow in the intrinsic nerve root blood vessels at various pressure levels.[5] The average occlusion pressure for the arterioles was found to be slightly below and directly related to the systolic blood pressure. The blood flow in the capillary networks was intimately dependent on the blood flow of the adjacent venules. This finding corroborates the assumption that venular stasis may induce capillary stasis and changes in the microcirculation of the nerve tissue, which has been suggested as one mechanism in carpal tunnel syndrome.[6] The mean occlusion pressures for the venules showed large variations; however, a pressure of 5 to 10 mm Hg was found to be sufficient for inducing venular occlusion.

Because the nutrition of the nerve root is affected by ischemia, a compression-induced impairment of the vasculature may be one mechanism for nerve root dysfunction. The nerve roots also have a considerable nutritional supply via diffusion from the cerebrospinal fluid.[7] To assess the compression-induced effects on the total contribution to the nerve roots, an experiment was performed in which ^{3}H-labeled methylglucose was allowed to be transported to the nerve tissue in the compressed segment via the blood vessels and via the cerebrospinal fluid diffusion after systemic injection.[8] The results showed that no compensatory mechanism from cerebrospinal fluid diffusion could be expected at low pressure levels. On the contrary, 10 mm Hg compression was sufficient to induce a 20% to 30% reduction of the transport of methylglucose to the nerve roots.

It is known from experimental studies on peripheral nerves that compression may also induce an increase in vascular permeability, leading to intraneural edema formation.[9] Such edema may increase the endoneurial fluid pressure, which impairs the endoneurial capillary blood flow and nutrition of the nerve roots.[10] Because the edema usually persists for some time after the removal of a compressive agent, edema may negatively affect the nerve root for a longer period than the compression itself. The presence of intraneural edema is also

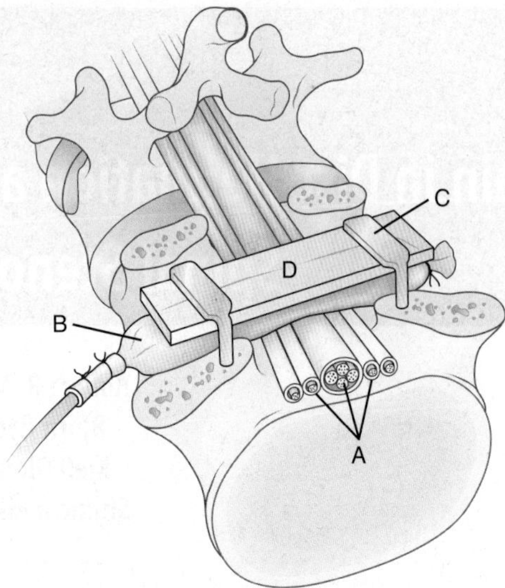

FIG. 7.1 Schematic of an experimental nerve root compression model. Cauda equina *(A)* is compressed by an inflatable balloon *(B)* that is fixed to the spine by two L-shaped pins *(C)* and Plexiglas plate *(D)*. (From Olmarker K, Holm S, Rosenqvist A-L, et al. Experimental nerve root compression: a model of acute, graded compression of the porcine cauda equina and an analysis of neural and vascular anatomy. *Spine [Phila Pa 1976]*. 1991;16:61-69.)

related to subsequent formation of intraneural fibrosis,[11] a neuroinflammatory response that is seen in some patients with nerve compression disorders.

Nerve root compression directly affects nerve conduction.[12,13] Our data show that the sensory fibers are slightly more susceptible to compression than the motor fibers.[13,14]

One factor that has not been fully recognized in compression trauma of nerve tissue is the onset rate of the compression. The onset rate (i.e., the time from compression start until full compression) may vary clinically from fractions of seconds in traumatic conditions to months or years in association with degenerative processes.

A rapid-onset rate of less than 1 second has been found to induce more pronounced pathophysiologic dysfunction. For the rapid-onset compression, which is likely to be more closely related to spine trauma or disc herniation than to spinal stenosis, it has been seen that a pressure of 600 mm Hg maintained only for 1 second is sufficient to induce a gradual impairment of nerve conduction during the 2 hours studied after the compression was ended.[15] In the case of spinal stenosis, the rate may be a great deal slower, and pain or nerve dysfunction may not be seen until after considerable ischemic injury.

Chronic Experimental Nerve Root Compression

To mimic various clinical situations, compression must be applied for long periods. In clinical syndromes with nerve root compression, the onset time may be quite slow and the duration may be quite long. A gradual development of degenerative changes that induce spinal stenosis leads to an onset time that can be many years. It is difficult to mimic such a situation in an experimental model. Chronic models should induce a controlled compression with a slow-onset time that is easily reproducible.

Delamarter and colleagues[16] introduced a model on the dog cauda equina in which they applied a constricting plastic band that was left in place for various times. The band was tightened around the thecal sac to induce a 25%, 50%, or 75% reduction of the cross-sectional area. The data indicated that structural and functional changes were proportional to the degree of constriction.

To induce a slower onset and more controlled compression, Cornefjord and colleagues[17] used a constrictor to compress the nerve roots in the pig. The constrictor consisted of an outer metal shell that on the inside was covered with a material called *ameroid* that expands when in contact with fluids. Because of the metal shell, the ameroid expands inward with a maximum of expansion after 2 weeks, resulting in a compression of a nerve root placed in the central opening of the constrictor. Compression of the first sacral nerve root in the pig resulted in a significant reduction of nerve conduction velocity and axonal injuries.[17] It has also been found that there is an increase in substance P in the nerve root and the dorsal root ganglion after such compression.[18] Substance P is a neurotransmitter that is related to pain transmission.

One important aspect in clinical nerve root compression conditions is that the compression level is probably unstable and varies as the result of changes in posture and movements.[19,20] In 1995, Konno and colleagues[21] introduced a model in which the pressure could be changed after some time of initial chronic compression. An inflatable balloon was introduced under the lamina of the seventh lumbar vertebra in the dog. By inflating the balloon at a known pressure slowly over 1 hour with a viscous substance that would harden in the balloon, compression of the cauda equina could be induced with a known initial pressure level. The compression was verified by myelography. Because the balloon under the lamina was composed of a twin set of balloons, the second balloon component could be connected to a compressed air device and could be used to add compression to the already chronically compressed cauda equina.

Acute nerve root compression experiments have established critical pressure levels for interference with various physiologic parameters in the spinal nerve roots. Studies on chronic compression may provide knowledge that would be more applicable to the clinical situation.

Spinal Stenosis: Experimental-Clinical Correlation

Patients with double or multiple levels of spinal stenosis may have more pronounced symptoms than patients with stenosis only at one level.[22] The mechanism for the difference between single and double compression may not simply be based on the fact that the nerve impulses have to pass more than one compression zone at double-level compression. There may also be a mechanism based on the local vascular anatomy of the nerve roots. In contrast to peripheral nerves, there are no regional nutritive arteries from surrounding structures to the intraneural vascular system in spinal nerve roots.[23-25] Compression at two levels might induce a nutritionally impaired region between the two compression sites. In this way the segment affected by the compression would be widened. Data from a study on the nutritional transport to the nerve tissue in double-level compression showed that there is a reduction of this transport to the uncompressed nerve segment located between the two compression balloons that was similar to the reduction within the two compression sites.[26] Thus, there is experimental evidence that the nutrition to the nerve segment located between two compression sites in nerve roots is severely impaired, although this nerve segment itself is uncompressed.

If nerve compression is of an extremely low onset rate, as in spinal stenosis, there may be an adaptation of the nerve tissue to the applied pressure. In cadaveric experiments, Schönström and colleagues[27] found that when a hose clamp was tightened around a human cadaveric cauda equina specimen there was a critical cross-sectional area of the dural sac when the first signs of pressure increase among nerve roots were recorded by a catheter placed in the compression zone. This cross-sectional area was approximately 75 mm^2, which was also found to correlate with a corresponding measurement on computed tomography (CT) in patients with spinal stenosis.[28] When the hose clamp was tightened further, the pressure increased. Owing to creep phenomena in the nerve tissue, the pressure decreased with time, however. When the pressure did not normalize within 10 minutes, the "sustained size" was registered and was found to be in the range of 45 to 50 mm^2.[27] This study indicates that even in acute compression there is an adaptation of the nerve tissue to the applied pressure. From a longer perspective, this probably means that the nerve may also be reorganized in its microstructural elements, which would result in a nerve with a smaller diameter. Under such circumstances, with gradually decreasing nerve diameter, the pressure acting on the nerve would be reduced to some degree.

There is a correlation between the experimental animal observations regarding critical pressures for functional and nutritional changes in nerve roots under compression and the measurements of pressure levels among nerve roots in human cadaveric lumbar spines after experimental constriction of the dural sac.

Epidural pressure measurements have been performed, evaluating the relationship between epidural pressure and posture.[20] It was found that the local epidural pressure at the stenotic level was low in lying and sitting postures and high in standing postures. Pressure was increased with extension but decreased with flexion of the spine. The highest epidural pressure, 117 mm Hg, was found in standing with extension. Measurements have also been reported regarding changes in epidural pressure during walking in patients with lumbar spinal stenosis.[29] The pressure changed during walking with a wave pattern of increasing and decreasing changes. Such observations correlate with the previously mentioned experimental observations regarding intermittent cauda equina compression.[19]

Mechanical Nerve Root Deformation and Pain

Some experimental observations indicate that mechanical nerve root deformation per se may induce impulses that cause pain. Howe and colleagues[30] found that mechanical stimulation of nerve roots or peripheral nerves resulted in nerve impulses of short duration and that these impulses were prolonged if the nerve tissue had been exposed to mechanical irritation by a chromic gut ligature for 2 to 4 weeks. Corresponding results were obtained in an in vitro system using rabbit nerve roots.[31] In this setup, it was also evident that the dorsal root ganglion was more susceptible to mechanical stimulation than the nerve roots. The dorsal root ganglion has elicited special interest in this regard, and an increase in the level of neurotransmitters related to pain transmission has been found in the dorsal root ganglion in response to whole-body vibration of rabbits.[32] A similar increase has been seen in the dorsal root ganglion and nerve root after local constriction of the same nerve root.[18] In vivo models of pain behavior have shown that mechanical nerve deformation superimposed on inflammation is painful, whereas either factor alone might not cause severe pain.[31-34] The magnitude of nerve root compression pressure (measured intraoperatively) correlates with neurologic deficit but not with degree of straight-leg raising test.

Neuropathologic Changes and Pain

There is considerable research evidence regarding the relationship of pain to neuropathologic changes.[35] Much of what is known has been studied in relationship to mechanical and inflammatory injury of the sciatic nerve in the rat. Entrapment of a peripheral nerve produces pathologic change in proportion to the degree of compression and its duration,[36] as is known to be the case for nerve root compression. In an electron microscopic study,[36] minor degrees of nerve compression were associated with ischemic injury to Schwann cells, resulting in their necrosis and in demyelination. Severe nerve compression was associated with injury to the axon, resulting in wallerian degeneration.

Subsequent experiments established the relationship of pain to these forms of neuropathologic change.[37] These studies established that mild levels of ischemia producing demyelination were generally not painful, whereas severe ischemia-producing wallerian degeneration resulted in hyperalgesia. The pathology of the chronic constriction injury model of neuropathic pain is based on this relationship and the added insult of inflammation caused by the chromic gut ligatures used to compress the nerve.[38] It is now recognized that the cytokine-driven processes of wallerian degeneration are the dominant neuropathologic factors linking nerve injury and pain[37,39,40] and that the degree and extent of wallerian degeneration relate directly to the magnitude and duration of hyperalgesia.[41]

Biologic and Biochemical Effects on Nerve Roots

The clinical picture of sciatica with a characteristic distribution of pain and nerve dysfunction in the absence of herniated disc material at radiologic examination and at surgery has indicated that mechanical nerve root compression may not be the only factor that is responsible for sciatic pain. In 1984 it was suggested that the disc tissue per se may have some injurious properties.[42] It was later confirmed experimentally that local epidural application of autologous nucleus pulposus in the absence of mechanical deformation induces significant changes in structure and function of the adjacent nerve roots.[43]

Biologic Effects of Nucleus Pulposus

In 1993, Olmarker and colleagues[43] published a study that showed that autologous nucleus pulposus can induce a reduction in nerve conduction velocity and light microscopic structural changes in a pig cauda equina model of nerve root injury. These axonal changes had a focal distribution, however, and the quantity of injured axons was too low to be responsible for the significant neurophysiologic dysfunction observed. A follow-up study of areas of the nerve roots exposed to nucleus pulposus that appeared to be normal by light microscopy revealed that there were significant injuries of Schwann cells with vacuolization and disintegration of Schmidt-Lanterman incisures (Fig. 7.2).[44] Schmidt-Lanterman incisures are essential for the normal exchange of ions between the axon and the surrounding tissues. An injury to this structure would be likely to interfere with the normal impulse conduction properties of the axons, although these models' changes may not fully explain the neurophysiologic dysfunction observed.

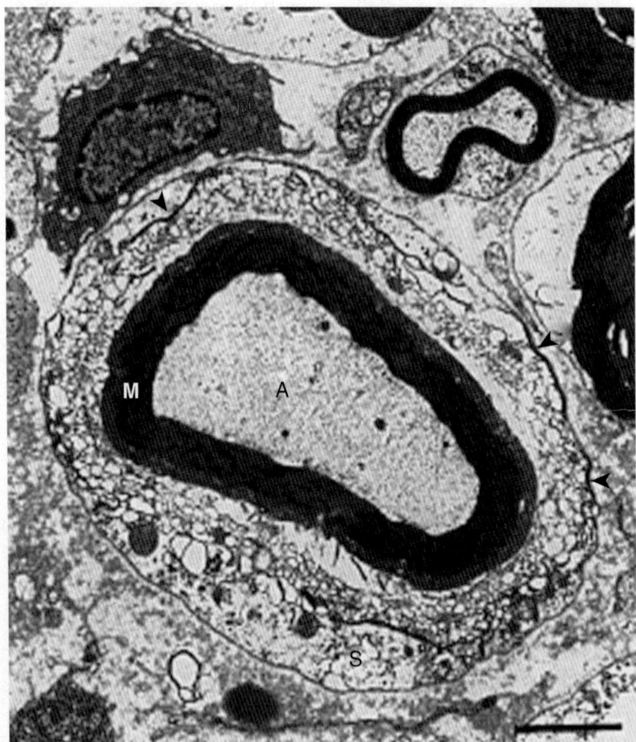

FIG. 7.2 Seven days after application of nucleus pulposus. Myelinated nerve fiber with prominent vesicular swelling of Schmidt-Lanterman incisure. Note mononuclear cell (*red M*) in close contact with nerve fiber. *Arrowheads* indicate myelin sheath layers outside Schmidt-Lanterman incisure. *A*, well-preserved axon; *white M*, myelin sheath; *S*, outer Schwann cell cytoplasm. (*Bar* = 2.5 μm.) (From Olmarker K, Nordborg C, Larsson K, et al. Ultrastructural changes in spinal nerve roots induced by autologous nucleus pulposus. *Spine [Phila Pa 1976]*. 1996;21:411-414.)

The pathophysiologic potential of the nucleus pulposus was emphasized further in an experiment using a dog model in which it was seen that a surgical incision of the anulus fibrosus, with minimal leakage of nucleus pulposus, was enough to induce significant changes in structure and function of the adjacent nerve root.[45] It has also been seen that epidural application of the autologous nucleus pulposus within 2 hours induces an intraneural edema[46,47] that leads to a reduction of the intraneural blood flow.[47] Histologic changes of the nerve roots are present after 3 hours,[48] and a subsequent reduction of the nerve conduction velocity starts 3 to 24 hours after application.[43,48] The nucleus pulposus may also interfere with the nutrition to the intraspinal nerve tissue. After application to the dorsal root ganglion, it was found that the intraneural blood flow was dramatically decreased and that there was a simultaneous increase of the tissue fluid pressure.[47]

Methylprednisolone reduces the pathophysiologic events of the nucleus pulposus–induced nerve root injury if given within 24 hours. To establish if the presence of autologous nucleus pulposus could initiate a leukotactic response from the surrounding tissues, a study was initiated that assessed the potential inflammatogenic properties of the nucleus pulposus.[49] Autologous nucleus pulposus and autologous retroperitoneal fat were placed in separate perforated titanium chambers and placed subcutaneously, together with a sham chamber, in the pig. The number of leukocytes was assessed 7 days later for the chambers. The nucleus pulposus–containing chambers had a number of leukocytes that exceeded the two others by 150%. In another experiment, autologous nucleus pulposus and muscle were placed in Gore-Tex tubes subcutaneously in rabbits.[50] After 2 weeks, there was an accumulation of macrophages and T-helper and T-suppresser cells in the tube with nucleus pulposus that persisted the full observation time of 4 weeks.

Kawakami and colleagues[51] showed that neuropathic pain in an experimental setting seems to be mediated by infiltrating leukocytes, a finding consistent with the previous observations of neuroimmunologic inflammatory changes and pain.[52] In rats made leukopenic by using nitrogen mustard, the pain response was absent after application of nucleus pulposus, whereas normal rats with nucleus pulposus application displayed a pathologic response to stimulation. The same group also showed that inhibition of cyclooxygenase-2 might reduce nucleus pulposus–induced pain behavior.[53] Taken together, these data further support the impression that autologous nucleus pulposus may elicit inflammatory reactions when outside the intervertebral disc space and that such reactions may not be restricted to resorption of the herniated tissue but also may be intimately involved in the pathophysiology of sciatica.

Nucleus Pulposus and Sciatic Pain

Pain is much more difficult to assess than nerve conduction in controlled experimental studies. The available literature indicates that pain may be induced by both mechanical factors and nucleus pulposus–mediated factors. The role of the nucleus pulposus in this context is interesting in view of patients with obvious symptoms of disc herniation but with no visible herniation at radiologic examination or surgery.[54,55] The potential of nucleus pulposus material to induce pain has also been indicated in clinical studies that showed that non-contained herniations (the nucleus pulposus was in contact with the epidural space) were much more painful and had a more pronounced straight-leg raising test result than contained herniations.[56-58]

Studies on rats using pain behavior assessment indicated that the nucleus pulposus is involved in pain production. Pain behavior in this context refers to response thresholds to thermal and mechanical stimulation. The role of the various anatomic components of the nerve root complex for the production of spinal pain was further elucidated by Cavanaugh and colleagues[31] and Weinstein and colleagues.[32] Other studies[33] suggest a dose-response relationship between pain behavior and the amount of nucleus pulposus material in the epidural space. The combination of nucleus pulposus herniation and mechanical injury produces pain.[33] This observation is consistent with the neuropathologic understanding of pain and the consequences of combined mechanical and inflammatory injury to nerve fibers that are superimposed to increase the number of fibers injured and the corresponding increase in proinflammatory cytokines.[40,41]

These experimental studies on pain behavior suggest that the presence of nucleus pulposus has sensitized the nerve tissue. Minor compression of peripheral nerves is not painful, and touching of a normal nerve root during local anesthesia is not painful.[59] Touching of a nerve root exposed to a disc herniation often reproduces the sciatic pain, however.[59] Although the combination of a mechanical component and the presence of nucleus pulposus seems to be a prerequisite to produce changes in the in vivo situation, more recent neurophysiologic studies have shown that the mere application of nucleus pulposus may induce increased neuronal pain transmission.[60]

The spinal dura mater is known to contain nerve endings, and stimulation of the dura has been suggested as a mechanism for sciatic pain.[42,59,61,62] Irritation or stimulation of the dura as one important factor for sciatica is an interesting theory that could explain many clinical features. One may assume that the dura is segmentally innervated, the sensory nerves travel in a caudal-lateral direction, and the dura is drained to the corresponding nerve root by the nerve of Luschka.[63] Stimulation of the dura at a point where dorsolateral disc herniations appear (*1* in Fig. 7.3) might be recorded by the corresponding nerve root. At this location, the irritation may spread medially to the contralateral segment, producing bilateral symptoms, or laterally, producing symptoms from levels above. Similarly, a lateral disc herniation (*2* in Fig. 7.3) could produce symptoms in the lower level.

If the pain of the straight-leg raising test is the result of dura irritation owing to friction to the herniated mass, one may consider the phenomenon of crossed straight-leg raising to be based on simultaneous stimulation of the contralateral dura. Such a "radiculitis" or "local meningitis" probably could be regarded as similar to peritonitis. When there is peritonitis, there is usually a reflectory muscle contraction present over the affected area. An analogue for this local meningitis could be the reflectory ipsilateral contraction of the spinal muscles, producing the "sciatic scoliosis" or lateral bending of the spine at the level of herniation.

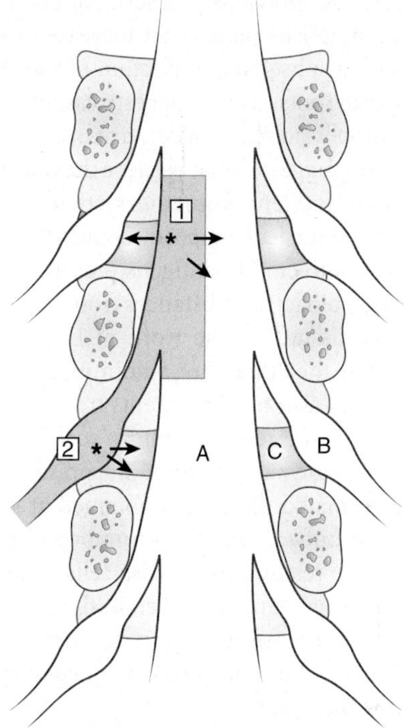

FIG. 7.3 Suggested area of innervation by one recurrent sinuvertebral nerve (nerve of Luschka). Disc herniation at location 1 may be recorded by the same nerve and by the nearby innervation areas, laterally and contralaterally, as indicated by *arrows*. At location 2, lateral disc herniation of disc one level below may affect same nerve root but also root one level below, located medial to this root, as indicated by *arrows*. *A*, Thecal sac; *B*, dorsal root ganglion; *C*, intervertebral disc. (From Olmarker K. The experimental basis of sciatica. *J Orthop Sci.* 1996;1:230-242.)

Other Consequences of Herniated Nucleus Pulposus

Histologic observations have indicated that nerve root changes caused by nucleus pulposus are focal and mainly found in the center of the nerve roots, resembling a mononeuritis simplex that is induced by nerve infarction secondary to embolism of the intraneural vessels.[43,44] Particularly in view of the work of Jayson and colleagues[64,65] indicating an impairment of the venous outflow from the nerve roots owing to periradicular vascular changes, one must consider vascular impairment as one factor.

The inflammatory components of nucleus pulposus may be involved in vascular and rheologic phenomena, such as coagulation, and may be involved in nerve root vascular embolism. It has been observed that the presence of nucleus pulposus may induce thrombus formation in microvessels.[49] Inflammatory mediators may also exert a direct effect on the myelin sheaths, as indicated by an electron microscopic study of nerve roots exposed to autologous nucleus pulposus in the pig.[44] There were significant injuries of Schwann cells with vacuolization and disintegration of Schmidt-Lanterman incisures, which closely resembles the injury pattern of inflammatory nerve disease.[66,67] As previously described, epidural application of nucleus pulposus induces an increase of the vascular permeability and a subsequent reduction of the blood flow in the adjacent nerve roots, which suggests vascular impairment as being of pathophysiologic importance.

It has also been suggested that because the nucleus pulposus is avascular and "hidden" from the systemic circulation, a presentation of the nucleus pulposus could result in an autoimmune reaction directed to antigens present in the nucleus pulposus and that bioactive substances from this reaction may injure the nerve tissue.[68-75] The work of Li and colleagues[76] has demonstrated that there are autoimmune reactions not only to the disc but also to components from the nerve tissue that are released as the result of injury, such as basic myelin proteins. Another study also assessed the presence of immune complexes in herniated disc tissue obtained at surgery as an indicator of immunoactivation.[77] Immunoglobulin G (IgG) was found in close relation to the disc cells in herniated disc material. No IgG was found, however, in the residual disc that was evacuated at the time of surgery. No immune complexes were found in control disc material obtained at spine surgery for other causes than pain.

Chemical Components of Nucleus Pulposus

The nucleus pulposus is composed mainly of proteoglycans, collagen, and cells.[78,79] The proteoglycan component has gained the most attention and has been suggested to have a direct irritating effect on nerve tissue.[74,80,81] Neither the collagen nor the cells have previously been suggested to be of pathophysiologic importance. More recent studies of the cells of the nucleus pulposus have shown, however, that these cells are capable of producing metalloproteinases such as collagenase or gelatinase and interleukin (IL)-6 and prostaglandin E_2 and do so spontaneously in culture.

Substances such as IgG, hydrogen ions, nitric oxide, and phospholipase A_2 have also been suggested to be responsible for the pathophysiologic reactions.[74,82-86] Another substance produced by the disc cells that has similar pathophysiologic effects as nucleus pulposus is tumor necrosis factor (TNF)-α.[87]

Cytokines as Mediators of Nerve Dysfunction and Pain

TNF is known to be a regulatory proinflammatory cytokine that has specific biologic effects and the ability to upregulate and act synergistically with other cytokines such as IL-1β and IL-6.[88-90] Immediately after nerve injury, TNF is released and upregulated by Schwann cells at the site of nerve injury[91]; this is followed by release and upregulation of TNF in many other endoneurial cells, including endothelial cells, fibroblasts, and mast cells. This local production of TNF is the stimulus that results in macrophage attraction to the injury site,[39] which contributes massively to the concentration of proinflammatory cytokines in the injured tissue. Several studies have shown that blocking TNF production or delaying the invasion of macrophages to the site of nerve injury results in reduced or delayed neuropathologic change and reduced hyperalgesia.[52,92]

TNF is known to induce axonal and myelin injury similar to that observed after nucleus pulposus application,[93-99] intravascular coagulation,[100-102] and increased vascular permeability.[102] TNF is also known to be neurotoxic[96,98,103,104] and to induce painful behavioral changes[93,105] and ectopic nerve activity when applied locally.[94,104] TNF is sequestered in a membrane-bound form and is activated after shedding by certain enzymes. Matrix metalloproteinases (MMPs) are particularly important in this regard. MMP-9 and MMP-2 are upregulated immediately after a nerve injury.[106] MMPs process the inactive, membrane-bound form of TNF and its receptors to the biologically active form and are directly associated with breakdown of the blood-brain and blood-nerve barriers. MMP-9 and TNF receptors are also retrogradely transported from the site of nerve injury to the corresponding dorsal root ganglion and spinal cord,[107] where they may have a direct role in gene regulation. This may relate to the observation that cell membranes of disc cells are sufficient to mediate the nucleus pulposus–induced effects.

TNF induces activation of endothelial adhesion molecules such as intercellular and vascular cell adhesion molecules, adhering circulating immune cells to the vessel walls (Fig. 7.4).[88,108,109] As a consequence of the TNF-induced increased vascular permeability, these cells migrate into the endoneurial space where the axons are located. The cells release their content of TNF and other cytokines, which may induce accumulation of ion channels locally in the axonal membranes.[110-112] The channels may allow for an increased passage of sodium and potassium, which may result in spontaneous discharges and in discharges of ectopic impulses after mechanical stimulation. TNF by itself can cause spontaneous electrical activity in A-delta and C nociceptors.[104] Such discharges, whether they come from a pain fiber or a nerve fiber transmitting other sensory information, are interpreted as pain by the brain.

Previous studies have also indicated that local application of nucleus pulposus may disintegrate the myelin sheath[42,43]; this is also a known effect of TNF.[113] This injury could also contribute to the formation of ectopic impulses and to the sensitization to mechanical stimulus. Experimental and clinical studies have shown that nerve root compression and disc herniation can induce increased concentrations of neurofilament in the cerebrospinal fluid.[114,115] Increased levels of serum antibodies against one or more nervous system–associated glycosphingolipids have been shown in patients with sciatica and disc herniation, indicating a possible autoimmune response.[116]

More recent work regarding molecular events in the pathophysiology of neuropathic pain has suggested a potential role of TNF for inducing allodynia.[94,117,118] TNF may mediate the formation of allodynia in the dorsal root ganglion and at the spinal cord level because of its local upregulation, which occurs via a positive feedback loop caused by TNF itself. This cycle seems to be broken by a direct effect of TNF on the upregulation of antiinflammatory cytokines such as IL-10, which eventually leads to a reduction of TNF and the physiologic balance of proinflammatory and antiinflammatory cytokines. Such regulation seems to be induced by mechanical

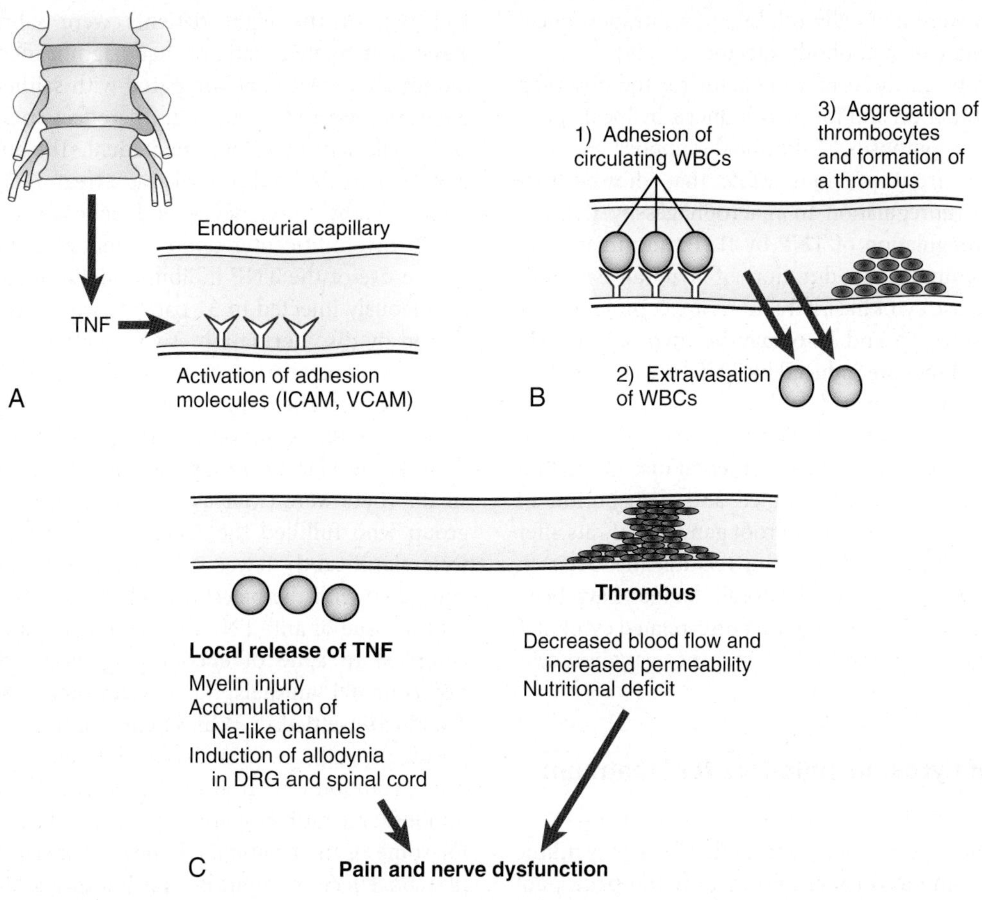

FIG. 7.4 Suggested mechanism of action for tumor necrosis factor (TNF). (A) TNF from cells of herniated nucleus pulposus enters endoneurial capillaries and activates endothelial adhesion molecules. (B) Circulating white blood cells (WBCs) adhere to vessel walls (*1*) and extravasate from capillaries out among axons owing to TNF-induced increase in vascular permeability (*2*). TNF also induces accumulation of thrombocytes that form intravascular thrombus (*3*). (C) There is local release of TNF from extravasated WBCs among axons that induce myelin injury, accumulation of sodium channels, and allodynia in the dorsal root ganglion (DRG) and at the spinal cord level. Thrombus, together with edema owing to increased permeability, induces nutritional deficit in the nerve root. Local effects of TNF and nutritional deficit may induce pain and nerve dysfunction. CAM, cell adhesion molecule; VCAM, vascular cell adhesion molecule. (From Olmarker K, Myers R, Kikuchi S, et al. Pathophysiology of nerve root pain in disc herniation and spinal stenosis. In: Herkowitz H, Dvorak J, Bell G, et al, eds. *The Lumbar Spine.* 3rd ed. Philadelphia: Lippincott Williams & Wilkins; 2004:11-30.)

injury to peripheral parts of the axons and by a direct effect of TNF exposure and further enhances the impression that TNF may be an important mediator of neuropathic pain. TNF is a potent activator of cells; because it is retrogradely transported from the site of nerve injury to the dorsal root ganglion and spinal cord, it may be this proinflammatory stimulus that activates central glia and neurons.[107]

Apart from directly affecting the endoneurially located axons, TNF may also indirectly interfere with the axons by compromising the nutritional transport. TNF can induce intravascular coagulation after local application[119]; this reduces the local blood flow in the intraneural capillaries.[54]

TNF was found in disc cells and there is evidence that elevated levels of TNF and its receptor, TNFR1. In herniated lumbar discs correlated with the chronicity of postoperative sciatic pain.[120] Specific TNF inhibitors, such as a monoclonal antibody to TNF (infliximab) and a soluble TNF receptor (etanercept) can inhibit pathophysiologic dysfunction. It has been shown that infliximab may attenuate immunoreactivity of brain-derived neurotrophic factor and may prevent neurologic and histologic changes in dorsal root ganglion in rats after experimental disc herniation.[121] More recent studies reinforce the potential utility of cytokine inhibition in treating the inflammatory hyperalgesia induced by nucleus pulposus[122] and spinal nerve injury.[123]

Application of certain cytokines to intraspinal nerves may also increase the somatosensory neural response.[124] Discharges from wide-dynamic-range neurons after stimulation of a receptor field of a dorsal root ganglion exposed to nucleus pulposus increased significantly after application. This increase may be related to the sensitization of the sensory system caused by proinflammatory cytokines and the production of low-grade spontaneous electrophysiologic activity in nociceptors by TNF,[104] which by itself is an important factor that contributes to sensitization. Administering an antibody specific for TNF efficiently inhibited this effect. An in vivo study assessing changes in spontaneous behavior clearly showed that changes induced by the combined action of mechanical deformation and disc incision were markedly inhibited by intraperitoneal injection of a monoclonal antibody specific for TNF.[55]

TNF seems to be an important mediator for the observed effects on nerve function and for pain induced by local application of nucleus pulposus. Additional support for this hypothesis comes from previous work that showed that blockade of TNF upregulation in macrophages by thalidomide[92] and downregulation of TNF by IL-10 administration reduced the magnitude and duration of hyperalgesia after nerve injury. Because cytokine interactions are complex, other cytokines such as IL-1β and IL-6 may be involved as well. Because these cytokines are induced by TNF, as well as inducing TNF, their role is complex.

The possible role of brain-derived neurotrophic factor in nerve root pathophysiology and experimental disc herniation has been analyzed.[125] The appearance and distribution of macrophages and TNF in the dorsal root ganglion of rats after experimental disc herniation and the relationship between nerve growth factor and pain behavioral changes have been described.[126] It has also been shown that disc-related cytokines can inhibit axonal outgrowth from dorsal root ganglion cells in vitro.[127]

Clinical Use of Cytokine Inhibitors for Treatment of Sciatica

On the basis of the experimental findings that TNF may mimic nucleus pulposus–induced nerve dysfunction and pain, pilot clinical trials regarding the possible use of TNF inhibition for the treatment of sciatica were initiated. Karppinen and colleagues[128] administered a monoclonal antibody specific for TNF (infliximab [Remicade]) to 10 volunteers waiting for surgery for radiologically verified disc herniations with severe sciatica. In this open-label study, infliximab reduced pain assessed by visual analog scale by 50% at 1 hour after infusion. After 2 weeks, 60% of the patients were pain free. At 3 months after the single infusion, 90% were pain free. No adverse drug reactions were noted, and no patients required surgery. A 1-year follow-up[129] of the 10 patients treated with infliximab showed that the beneficial effect of a single infusion of 3 mg/kg of infliximab for disc herniation–induced sciatica was sustained in most patients. The authors also noted that infliximab did not seem to interfere with spontaneous resorption of disc herniations.

Genevay and colleagues[130] administered a TNF inhibitor in the form of a soluble TNF receptor (etanercept [Enbrel]) by three subcutaneous injections to 10 patients with severe sciatica. The patients had a 70% reduction of leg pain assessed by visual analog scale 10 days after starting the treatment. At 6 weeks, the reduction was 83%. The results were statistically significantly better than for 10 patients treated with three intravenous injections of methylprednisolone.

In one randomized study published by Cohen and colleagues,[131] treatment of sciatica by local epidural injections of the TNF inhibitor etanercept was effective. The investigators randomly assigned 24 patients with subacute radiculopathy into three groups each consisting of eight patients. The patients in each group received either 2, 4, or 6 mg on two occasions, and two of the eight patients were saline controls. All etanercept-treated patients had significant improvement 1 month after treatment compared with saline-treated patients regarding leg and back pain. The effects persisted 6 months after treatment in all but one patient. The authors concluded that "etanercept holds promise as a treatment for lumbosacral radiculopathy."[131] Genevay and colleagues[132] published the results of a multicenter, double-blind, placebo-controlled trial on the use of the TNF inhibitor adalimumab (Humira) subcutaneously injected in 31 patients with severe, acute sciatica caused by disc herniation. Two injections were given 7 days apart; 30 control patients received placebo injections in the same manner. The results showed that there was a significantly more favorable evolution of leg pain in the adalimumab group than in the placebo group, but the effect size was relatively small. There were twice as many patients in the adalimumab group who fulfilled the criteria for "responders," and there were significantly fewer surgical discectomies in this group compared with the placebo-treated controls.

The issue of anti-TNF therapy for human sciatica remains complex. In spite of encouraging basic science studies in experimental animals, its efficacy and utility in humans remains unsettled.[133] While there continues to be reports of positive results in animals and humans,[134] a second multicenter, randomized trial by Cohen et al.[135] of 84 adults with lumbosacral radiculopathy revealed only a short-term relief for some of their patients. Issues of experimental design and placebo effects complicate the interpretation of the results. Indeed, this point is emphasized by Williams et al.,[119] who performed a systematic review and meta-analysis of biologic treatments targeting TNF-α for sciatica and concluded that there was insufficient evidence to recommend these agents when treating sciatica. They concluded, however, that additional studies are warranted.

Taken together, these observations indicate a potential clinical effect of TNF inhibition in the treatment of sciatica. It is unconfirmed although provocative that early treatment with TNF inhibition seems superior to late antiinflammatory treatment by nonsteroidal antiinflammatory drugs, methylprednisolone, or even morphine in many patients. We suggest that it is more efficient to target the responsible mediators of neuropathic pain early and directly before additional dysfunction occurs than to treat a patient with conventional antiinflammatory drugs after the neuropathic pain state has fully developed. Sciatica has a neuropathic pain component, and nonspecific antiinflammatory medication and morphine are less efficient in such conditions. Further studies must be undertaken, however, before any definite conclusions regarding the efficacy of anti-TNF therapy for the treatment of sciatica may be drawn.

Summary

The pathophysiology of sciatica is complex, with numerous substances and mechanisms acting at various levels of the neural axis. These mechanisms have attracted attention of basic scientists, and numerous studies looking into neuroimmunologic events have provided important insights into the pathophysiologic mechanisms of the human disease state. The intervertebral disc has certain biologic effects that contribute directly to these pathophysiologic processes. Epidural application of nucleus pulposus induces structural and functional changes that relate closely to sciatica. The nucleus pulposus also sensitizes nerve roots, producing a painful condition. These experimental observations correlate with the clinical impression that preoperative touching of nerve roots that have been exposed to disc herniation under local anesthesia reproduces the sciatic pain and that surgical removal of the mechanical compression of the nerve root often relieves symptoms.

The biologic substance of importance in the pathogenesis of painful radiculopathy seems clearly at this stage of understanding to be TNF-α. The activation and upregulation of this ubiquitous proinflammatory cytokine produces acute pain and neuropathologic changes associated with chronic pain states. TNF stimulates fibroblast scar formation in a vicious cycle whereby the local presence of TNF stimulates other cells to upregulate this cytokine. Initiation of this cycle by the leakage of TNF from herniated nucleus pulposus produces a cascade of tissue injury, scar formation, and local pain. Superimposition of mechanical injury to the nerve root in this environment exacerbates the neural immune insult, causing macrophage-mediated wallerian degeneration with significant increases in TNF concentrations. We suggest that these combined events explain the problem of sciatica. Although the pathophysiology of sciatica is far more complex than one might first suspect, future research is certain to reveal substances and mechanisms of importance to the induction of symptoms in sciatica, and such research would provide a basis for improved diagnosis and treatment of this common disorder.

KEY REFERENCES

1. Mixter WJ, Barr JS. Rupture of the intervertebral disc with involvement of the spinal canal. *N Engl J Med.* 1934;211:210-215.
   This article is about the discovery of the herniated disc.
2. Olmarker K, Rydevik B, Nordborg C. Autologous nucleus pulposus induces neurophysiologic and histologic changes in porcine cauda equina nerve roots. *Spine.* 1993;18:1425-1432.
   This study demonstrated the injurious effects of autologous nucleus pulposus.
3. Kawakami M, Weinstein JN, Chatani K, et al. Experimental lumbar radiculopathy. Behavioral and histologic changes in a model of radicular pain after spinal nerve root irritation with chromic gut ligatures in the rat. *Spine.* 1994;19:1795-1802.
   This early study examined nerve root pain in an experimental model.
4. Olmarker K, Myers RR. Pathogenesis of sciatic pain: role of herniated nucleus pulposus and deformation of spinal nerve root and dorsal root ganglion. *Pain.* 1998;78:99-105.
   This study was the first to examine nerve root pain induced by nucleus pulposus in an autologous system.
5. Olmarker K, Larsson K. Tumor necrosis factor alpha and nucleus-pulposus-induced nerve root injury. *Spine.* 1998;23:2538-2544.
   This study linked a specific molecule to the pathophysiology of sciatica.
6. Williams NH, Lewis R, Din NU, et al. A systematic review and meta-analysis of biologic treatments targeting tumor necrosis factor alpha for sciatica. *Eur Spine J.* 2013;22:1921-1935.
   This review article summarizes current concepts regarding anti-TNF therapy for sciatica.

REFERENCES

1. Mixter WJ, Barr JS. Rupture of the intervertebral disc with involvement of the spinal canal. *N Engl J Med.* 1934;211:210-215.
2. Gelfan S, Tarlov IM. Physiology of spinal cord, nerve root and peripheral nerve compression. *Am J Physiol.* 1956;185:217-229.
3. Sharpless SK. Susceptibility of spinal nerve roots to compression block: the research status of spinal manipulative therapy. In: Goldstein M, ed. *NIH Workshop: NINCDS Monograph.* 1975:155-161.
4. Olmarker K, Holm S, Rosenqvist AL, et al. Experimental nerve root compression: a model of acute, graded compression of the porcine cauda equina and an analysis of neural and vascular anatomy. *Spine.* 1991;16:61-69.
5. Olmarker K, Rydevik B, Holm S, et al. Effects of experimental graded compression on blood flow in spinal nerve roots: a vital microscopic study on the porcine cauda equina. *J Orthop Res.* 1989;7:817-823.
6. Sunderland S. The nerve lesion in the carpal tunnel. *J Neurol Neurosurg Psychiatry.* 1976;39:615-626.
7. Rydevik B, Holm S, Brown MD, et al. Diffusion from the cerebrospinal fluid as a nutritional pathway for spinal nerve roots. *Acta Physiol Scand.* 1990;138:247-248.
8. Olmarker K, Rydevik B, Hansson T, et al. Compression-induced changes of the nutritional supply to the porcine cauda equina. *J Spinal Disord.* 1990;3:25-29.
9. Rydevik B, Lundborg G. Permeability of intraneural microvessels and perineurium following acute, graded experimental nerve compression. *Scand J Plast Reconstr Surg.* 1977;11:179-187.
10. Myers RR, Murakami H, Powell HC. Reduced nerve blood flow in edematous neuropathies: a biomechanical mechanism. *Microvasc Res.* 1986;32:145-151.
11. Rydevik B, Lundborg G, Nordborg C. Intraneural tissue reactions induced by internal neurolysis: an experimental study on the blood-nerve barrier, connective tissues and nerve fibres of rabbit tibial nerve. *Scand J Plast Reconstr Surg.* 1976;10:3-8.
12. Garfin SR, Cohen MS, Massie JB, et al. Nerve-roots of the cauda equina: the effect of hypotension and acute graded compression on function. *J Bone Joint Surg Am.* 1990;72:1185-1192.
13. Pedowitz RA, Garfin SR, Massie JB, et al. Effects of magnitude and duration of compression on spinal nerve root conduction. *Spine.* 1992;17:194-199.
14. Rydevik BL, Pedowitz RA, Hargens AR, et al. Effects of acute, graded compression on spinal nerve root function and structure: an experimental study of the pig cauda equina. *Spine.* 1991;16:487-493.
15. Olmarker K, Lind B, Holm S, et al. Continued compression increases impairment of impulse propagation in experimental compression of the porcine cauda equina. *Neuroorthopaedics.* 1991;11:75-81.
16. Delamarter RB, Bohlman HH, Dodge LD, et al. Experimental lumbar spinal stenosis: analysis of the cortical evoked potentials, microvasculature, and histopathology. *J Bone Joint Surg Am.* 1990;72:110-120.

17. Cornefjord M, Sato K, Olmarker K, et al. A model for chronic nerve root compression studies: presentation of a porcine model for controlled, slow-onset compression with analyses of anatomic aspects, compression onset rate, and morphologic and neurophysiologic effects. *Spine*. 1997;22:946-957.
18. Cornefjord M, Olmarker K, Farley DB, et al. Neuropeptide changes in compressed spinal nerve roots. *Spine*. 1995;20:670-673.
19. Konno S, Olmarker K, Byrod G, et al. Intermittent cauda equina compression: an experimental study of the porcine cauda equina with analyses of nerve impulse conduction properties. *Spine*. 1995;20:1223-1226.
20. Takahashi K, Miyazaki T, Takino T, et al. Epidural pressure measurements: relationship between epidural pressure and posture in patients with lumbar spinal stenosis. *Spine*. 1995;20:650-653.
21. Konno S, Yabuki S, Sato K, et al. A model for acute, chronic, and delayed graded compression of the dog cauda equina: presentation of the gross, microscopic, and vascular anatomy of the dog cauda equina and accuracy in pressure transmission of the compression model. *Spine*. 1995;20:2758-2764.
22. Porter RW, Ward D. Cauda equina dysfunction: the significance of two-level pathology. *Spine*. 1992;17:9-15.
23. Lundborg G. Structure and function of the intraneural microvessels as related to trauma, edema formation, and nerve function. *J Bone Joint Surg Am*. 1975;57:938-948.
24. Parke WW, Watanabe R. The intrinsic vasculature of the lumbosacral spinal nerve roots. *Spine*. 1985;10:508-515.
25. Petterson CA, Olsson Y. Blood supply of spinal nerve roots: an experimental study in the rat. *Acta Neuropathol (Berl)*. 1989;78:455-461.
26. Cornefjord M, Takahashi K, Matsui Y, et al. Impairment of nutritional transport at double-level cauda equina compression: an experimental study. *Neuroorthopaedics*. 1992;11:107-112.
27. Schönström N, Bolender NF, Spengler DM, et al. Pressure changes within the cauda equina following constriction of the dural sac: an in vitro experimental study. *Spine*. 1984;9:604-607.
28. Schönström NS, Bolender NF, Spengler DM. The pathomorphology of spinal stenosis as seen on CT scans of the lumbar spine. *Spine*. 1985;10:806-811.
29. Takahashi K, Kagechika K, Takino T, et al. Changes in epidural pressure during walking in patients with lumbar spinal stenosis. *Spine*. 1995;20:2746-2749.
30. Howe JF, Loeser JD, Calvin WH. Mechanosensitivity of dorsal root ganglia and chronically injured axons: a physiological basis for the radicular pain of nerve root compression. *Pain*. 1977;3:25-41.
31. Cavanaugh JM, Ozaktay AC, Yamashita T, et al. Mechanisms of low back pain: a neurophysiologic and neuroanatomic study. *Clin Orthop Relat Res*. 1997;335:166-180.
32. Weinstein J, Pope M, Schmidt R, et al. Neuropharmacologic effects of vibration on the dorsal root ganglion: an animal model. *Spine*. 1988;13:521-525.
33. Omarker K, Myers RR. Pathogenesis of sciatic pain: role of herniated nucleus pulposus and deformation of spinal nerve root and dorsal root ganglion. *Pain*. 1998;78:99-105.
34. Olmarker K, Nutu M, Storkson R. Changes in spontaneous behavior in rats exposed to experimental disc herniation are blocked by selective TNF-alpha inhibition. *Spine*. 2003;28:1635-1641.
35. Myers R, Shubayev VI, Campana WM. Neuropathology of painful neuropathies. In: Sommer C, ed. *Pain in Peripheral Nerve Disease*. Basel: Karger; 2001:8-30.
36. Powell HC, Myers RR. Pathology of experimental nerve compression. *Lab Invest*. 1986;55:91-100.
37. Myers RR, Yamamoto T, Yaksh TL, et al. The role of focal nerve ischemia and wallerian degeneration in peripheral nerve injury producing hyperesthesia. *Anesthesiology*. 1993;78:308-316.
38. Sommer C, Galbraith JA, Heckman HM, et al. Pathology of experimental compression neuropathy producing hyperesthesia. *J Neuropathol Exp Neurol*. 1993;52:223-233.
39. Stoll G, Jander S, Myers RR. Degeneration and regeneration of the peripheral nervous system: from Augustus Waller's observations to neuroinflammation. *J Peripher Nerv Syst*. 2002;7:13-27.
40. Myers R, Wagner R, Sorkin LS. Hyperalgesic action of cytokines on peripheral nerves. In: Watkins LR, Maier SF, eds. *Cytokines and Pain*. Basel: Birkhäuser Verlag; 1999:133-157.
41. Myers RR, Heckman HM, Powell HC. Axonal viability and the persistence of thermal hyperalgesia after partial freeze lesions of nerve. *J Neurol Sci*. 1996;139:28-38.
42. Rydevik B, Brown MD, Lundborg G. Pathoanatomy and pathophysiology of nerve root compression. *Spine*. 1984; 9:7-15.
43. Olmarker K, Rydevik B, Nordborg C. Autologous nucleus pulposus induces neurophysiologic and histologic changes in porcine cauda equina nerve roots. *Spine*. 1993;18: 1425-1432.
44. Olmarker K, Nordborg C, Larsson K, et al. Ultrastructural changes in spinal nerve roots induced by autologous nucleus pulposus. *Spine*. 1996;21:411-414.
45. Kayama S, Konno S, Olmarker K, et al. Incision of the anulus fibrosus induces nerve root morphologic, vascular, and functional changes: an experimental study. *Spine*. 1996;21:2539-2543.
46. Byrod G, Otani K, Brisby H, et al. Methylprednisolone reduces the early vascular permeability increase in spinal nerve roots induced by epidural nucleus pulposus application. *J Orthop Res*. 2000;18:983-987.
47. Yabuki S, Kikuchi S, Olmarker K, et al. Acute effects of nucleus pulposus on blood flow and endoneurial fluid pressure in rat dorsal root ganglia. *Spine*. 1998;23:2517-2523.
48. Byrod G, Rydevik B, Nordborg C, et al. Early effects of nucleus pulposus application on spinal nerve root morphology and function. *Eur Spine J*. 1998;7:445-449.
49. Olmarker K, Blomquist J, Stromberg J, et al. Inflammatogenic properties of nucleus pulposus. *Spine*. 1995;20:665-669.
50. Takino T, Takahashi K, Miyazaki T, et al. *Immunoreactivity of Nucleus Pulposus*. 1995 Presented at International Society for the Study of the Lumbar Spine, Helsinki, Finland.
51. Kawakami M, Tamaki T, Matsumoto T, et al. Role of leukocytes in radicular pain secondary to herniated nucleus pulposus. *Clin Orthop Relat Res*. 2000;376:268-277.
52. Myers RR, Heckman HM, Rodriguez M. Reduced hyperalgesia in nerve-injured WLD mice: relationship to nerve fiber phagocytosis, axonal degeneration, and regeneration in normal mice. *Exp Neurol*. 1996;141: 94-101.
53. Kawakami M, Matsumoto T, Hashizume H, et al. Epidural injection of cyclooxygenase-2 inhibitor attenuates pain-related behavior following application of nucleus pulposus to the nerve root in the rat. *J Orthop Res*. 2002;20:376-381.

54. Macnab I. Negative disc exploration: an analysis of the causes of nerve-root involvement in sixty-eight patients. *J Bone Joint Surg Am*. 1971;53:891-903.
55. Crock HV. Observations on the management of failed spinal operations. *J Bone Joint Surg Br*. 1976;58:193-199.
56. Jonsson B, Stromqvist B. Clinical appearance of contained and noncontained lumbar disc herniation. *J Spinal Disord*. 1996;9:32-38.
57. Ito T, Takano Y, Yuasa N. Types of lumbar herniated disc and clinical course. *Spine*. 2001;26:648-651.
58. Nygaard OP, Mellgren SI, Osterud B. The inflammatory properties of contained and noncontained lumbar disc herniation. *Spine*. 1997;22:2484-2488.
59. Kuslich SD, Ulstrom CL, Michael CJ. The tissue origin of low back pain and sciatica: a report of pain response to tissue stimulation during operations on the lumbar spine using local anesthesia. *Orthop Clin North Am*. 1991;22:181-187.
60. Anzai H, Hamba M, Onda A, et al. Epidural application of nucleus pulposus enhances nociresponses of rat dorsal horn neurons. *Spine*. 2002;27:E50-E55.
61. Olmarker K, Rydevik B. Pathophysiology of sciatica. *Orthop Clin North Am*. 1991;22:223-234.
62. El-Mahdi MA, Abdel Latif FY, Janko M. The spinal nerve root "innervation," and a new concept of the clinicopathological interrelations in back pain and sciatica. *Neurochirurgia (Stuttg)*. 1981;24:137-141.
63. Edgar MA, Nundy S. Innervation of the spinal dura. *J Neurol Neurosurg Psychiatry*. 1966;29:530-534.
64. Hoyland JA, Freemont AJ, Jayson MI. Intervertebral foramen venous obstruction: a cause of periradicular fibrosis? *Spine*. 1989;14:558-568.
65. Cooper RG, Freemont AJ, Hoyland JA, et al. Herniated intervertebral disc-associated periradicular fibrosis and vascular abnormalities occur without inflammatory cell infiltration. *Spine*. 1995;20:591-598.
66. Dalcanto MC, Wisniewski HM, Johnson AB, et al. Vesicular disruption of myelin in autoimmune demyelination. *J Neurol Sci*. 1975;24:313-319.
67. Hahn AF, Gilbert JJ, Feasby TE. Passive transfer of demyelination by experimental allergic neuritis serum. *Acta Neuropathol (Berl)*. 1980;49:169-176.
68. Bisla RS, Marchisello PJ, Lockshin MD, et al. Auto-immunological basis of disk degeneration. *Clin Orthop Relat Res*. 1976;121:205-211.
69. Bobechko WP, Hirsch C. Auto-immune response to nucleus pulposus in the rabbit. *J Bone Joint Surg Br*. 1965;47:574-580.
70. Gertzbein SD, Tile M, Gross A, Falk R. Autoimmunity in degenerative disc disease of the lumbar spine. *Orthop Clin North Am*. 1975;6:67-73.
71. Gertzbein SD. Degenerative disk disease of the lumbar spine: immunological implications. *Clin Orthop Relat Res*. 1977;129:68-71.
72. Gertzbein SD, Tait JH, Devlin SR. The stimulation of lymphocytes by nucleus pulposus in patients with degenerative disk disease of the lumbar spine. *Clin Orthop Relat Res*. 1977;123:149-154.
73. LaRocca H. New horizons in research on disc disease. *Orthop Clin North Am*. 1971;2:521-531.
74. Naylor A. The biophysical and biochemical aspects of intervertebral disc herniation and degeneration. *Ann R Coll Surg Engl*. 1962;31:91-114.
75. Geiss A, Larsson K, Rydevik B, et al. Autoimmune properties of nucleus pulposus: an experimental study in pigs. *Spine*. 2007;32:168-173.
76. Liu H, Shiryaev SA, Chernov AV, et al. Immunodominant fragments of myelin basic protein initiate T cell-dependent pain. *J Neuroinflammation*. 2012;9:119.
77. Satoh K, Konno S, Nishiyama K, et al. Presence and distribution of antigen-antibody complexes in the herniated nucleus pulposus. *Spine*. 1999;24:1980-1984.
78. Bayliss MT, Johnstone B. Biochemistry of the intervertebral disc. In: Jayson MIV, ed. *The Lumbar Spine and Back Pain*. Edinburgh: Churchill-Livingstone; 1992:111-131.
79. Eyre D, Benya P, Buckwalter J. Intervertebral disc. In: Frymoyer JW, Gordon SL, eds. *New Perspectives on Low Back Pain*. Rosemont, IL: American Academy of Orthopaedic Surgeons; 1988:149-207.
80. Marshall LL, Trethewie ER. Chemical irritation of nerve-root in disc prolapse. *Lancet*. 1973;2:320.
81. Marshall LL, Trethewie ER, Curtain CC. Chemical radiculitis: a clinical, physiological and immunological study. *Clin Orthop Relat Res*. 1977;129:61-67.
82. Brisby H, Byrod G, Olmarker K, et al. Nitric oxide as a mediator of nucleus pulposus-induced effects on spinal nerve roots. *J Orthop Res*. 2000;18:815-820.
83. Diamant B, Karlsson J, Nachemson A. Correlation between lactate levels and pH in discs of patients with lumbar rhizopathies. *Experientia*. 1968;24:1195-1196.
84. Nachemson A. Intradiscal measurements of pH in patients with lumbar rhizopathies. *Acta Orthop Scand*. 1969;40:23-42.
85. Pennington JB, McCarron RF, Laros GS. Identification of IgG in the canine intervertebral disc. *Spine*. 1988;13:909-912.
86. Saal JS, Franson RC, Dobrow R, et al. High levels of inflammatory phospholipase A2 activity in lumbar disc herniations. *Spine*. 1990;15:674-678.
87. Olmarker K, Larsson K. Tumor necrosis factor alpha and nucleus-pulposus-induced nerve root injury. *Spine*. 1998;23:2538-2544.
88. McHale JF, Harari OA, Marshall D, et al. TNF-alpha and IL-1 sequentially induce endothelial ICAM-1 and VCAM-1 expression in MRL/lpr lupus-prone mice. *J Immunol*. 1999;163:3993-4000.
89. McGee DW, Bamberg T, Vitkus SJ, et al. A synergistic relationship between TNF-alpha, IL-1 beta, and TGF-beta 1 on IL-6 secretion by the IEC-6 intestinal epithelial cell line. *Immunology*. 1995;86:6-11.
90. Satomi N, Haranaka K, Kunii O. Research on the production site of tumor necrosis factor (TNF). *Jpn J Exp Med*. 1981;51:317-322.
91. Wagner R, Myers RR. Schwann cells produce tumor necrosis factor alpha: expression in injured and non-injured nerves. *Neuroscience*. 1996;73:625-629.
92. Sommer C, Marziniak M, Myers RR. The effect of thalidomide treatment on vascular pathology and hyperalgesia caused by chronic constriction injury of rat nerve. *Pain*. 1998;74:83-91.
93. Wagner R, Myers RR. Endoneurial injection of TNF-alpha produces neuropathic pain behaviors. *Neuroreport*. 1996;7:2897-2901.
94. Igarashi T, Kikuchi S, Shubayev V, et al. Exogenous tumor necrosis factor-alpha mimics nucleus pulposus-induced neuropathology: molecular, histologic, and behavioral comparisons in rats. *Spine*. 2000;25:2975-2980.

95. Liberski PP, Yanagihara R, Nerurkar V, et al. Further ultrastructural studies of lesions produced in the optic nerve by tumor necrosis factor alpha (TNF-alpha): a comparison with experimental Creutzfeldt-Jakob disease. *Acta Neurobiol Exp (Wars)*. 1994;54:209-218.
96. Madigan MC, Sadun AA, Rao NS, et al. Tumor necrosis factor-alpha (TNF-alpha)-induced optic neuropathy in rabbits. *Neurol Res*. 1996;18:176-184.
97. Redford EJ, Hall SM, Smith KJ. Vascular changes and demyelination induced by the intraneural injection of tumour necrosis factor. *Brain*. 1995;118(Pt 4):869-878.
98. Selmaj K, Raine CS. Tumor necrosis factor mediates myelin damage in organotypic cultures of nervous tissue. *Ann N Y Acad Sci*. 1988;540:568-570.
99. Stoll G, Jung S, Jander S, et al. Tumor necrosis factor-alpha in immune-mediated demyelination and wallerian degeneration of the rat peripheral nervous system. *J Neuroimmunol*. 1993;45:175-182.
100. Nawroth P, Handley D, Matsueda G, et al. Tumor necrosis factor/cachectin-induced intravascular fibrin formation in meth A fibrosarcomas. *J Exp Med*. 1988;168: 637-647.
101. van der Poll T, Jansen PM, Van Zee KJ, et al. Tumor necrosis factor-alpha induces activation of coagulation and fibrinolysis in baboons through an exclusive effect on the p55 receptor. *Blood*. 1996;88:922-927.
102. Watts ME, Arnold S, Chaplin DJ. Changes in coagulation and permeability properties of human endothelial cells in vitro induced by TNF-alpha or 5,6 MeXAA. *Br J Cancer*. 1996;74(suppl 27):S164-S167.
103. Viviani B, Corsini E, Galli CL, et al. Glia increase degeneration of hippocampal neurons through release of tumor necrosis factor-alpha. *Toxicol Appl Pharmacol*. 1998;150:271-276.
104. Sorkin LS, Xiao WH, Wagner R, et al. Tumour necrosis factor-alpha induces ectopic activity in nociceptive primary afferent fibres. *Neuroscience*. 1997;81:255-262.
105. Sommer C, Schmidt C, George A, et al. A metalloprotease-inhibitor reduces pain associated behavior in mice with experimental neuropathy. *Neurosci Lett*. 1997;237:45-48.
106. Shubayev VI, Myers RR. Upregulation and interaction of TNFalpha and gelatinases A and B in painful peripheral nerve injury. *Brain Res*. 2000;855:83-89.
107. Shubayev VI, Myers RR. Axonal transport of TNF-alpha in painful neuropathy: distribution of ligand tracer and TNF receptors. *J Neuroimmunol*. 2001;114:48-56.
108. Mattila P, Majuri ML, Mattila PS, et al. TNF alpha-induced expression of endothelial adhesion molecules, ICAM-1 and VCAM-1, is linked to protein kinase C activation. *Scand J Immunol*. 1992;36:159-165.
109. Pober JS. Effects of tumour necrosis factor and related cytokines on vascular endothelial cells. *Ciba Found Symp*. 1987;131:170-184.
110. Kagan BL, Baldwin RL, Munoz D, et al. Formation of ion-permeable channels by tumor necrosis factor-alpha. *Science*. 1992;255:1427-1430.
111. Baldwin RL, Stolowitz ML, Hood L, et al. Structural changes of tumor necrosis factor alpha associated with membrane insertion and channel formation. *Proc Natl Acad Sci USA*. 1996;93:1021-1026.
112. Wei Y, Babilonia E, Pedraza PL, et al. Acute application of TNF stimulates apical 70-pS K+ channels in the thick ascending limb of rat kidney. *Am J Physiol Renal Physiol*. 2003;285:F491-F497.
113. Selmaj K, Raine CS, Cross AH. Anti-tumor necrosis factor therapy abrogates autoimmune demyelination. *Ann Neurol*. 1991;30:694-700.
114. Brisby H, Olmarker K, Rosengren L, et al. Markers of nerve tissue injury in the cerebrospinal fluid in patients with lumbar disc herniation and sciatica. *Spine*. 1999;24:742-746.
115. Cornefjord M, Nyberg F, Rosengren L, et al. Cerebrospinal fluid biomarkers in experimental spinal nerve root injury. *Spine*. 2004;29:1862-1868.
116. Brisby H, Balague F, Schafer D, et al. Glycosphingolipid antibodies in serum in patients with sciatica. *Spine*. 2002;27:380-386.
117. Schafers M, Svensson CI, Sommer C, et al. Tumor necrosis factor-alpha induces mechanical allodynia after spinal nerve ligation by activation of p38 MAPK in primary sensory neurons. *J Neurosci*. 2003;23:2517-2521.
118. DeLeo JA, Rutkowski MD, Stalder AK, et al. Transgenic expression of TNF by astrocytes increases mechanical allodynia in a mouse neuropathy model. *Neuroreport*. 2000;11:599-602.
119. Williams NH, Lewis R, Din NU, et al. A systematic review and meta-analysis of biological treatments targeting tumor necrosis factor alpha for sciatica. *Eur Spine J*. 2013;22:1921-1935.
120. Andrade P, Hoogland G, Teernstra OP, et al. Elevated levels of tumor necrosis factor-alpha and TNFR1 in recurrent herniated lumbar discs correlate with chronicity of postoperative sciatic pain. *Spine J*. 2016;16:243-251.
121. Onda A, Murata Y, Rydevik B, et al. Infliximab attenuates immunoreactivity of brain-derived neurotrophic factor in a rat model of herniated nucleus pulposus. *Spine*. 2004;29:1857-1861.
122. deSouza Grava AL, Ferrari LF, Defino HL. Cytokine inhibition and time-related influence of inflammatory stimuli on the hyperalgesia induced by the nucleus pulposus. *Eur Spine J*. 2012;537-545.
123. Andrade P, Hoogland G, Del Rosario JS, et al. Tumor necrosis factor-alpha inhibitors alleviation of experimental induced neuropathic pain is associated with modulation of TNF receptor expression. *J Neurosci Res*. 2014;92: 1490-1498.
124. Aoki Y, Rydevik B, Kikuchi S, et al. Local application of disc-related cytokines on spinal nerve roots. *Spine*. 2002;27:1614-1617.
125. Onda A, Murata Y, Rydevik B, et al. Immunoreactivity of brain-derived neurotrophic factor in rat dorsal root ganglion and spinal cord dorsal horn following exposure to herniated nucleus pulposus. *Neurosci Lett*. 2003;352:49-52.
126. Onda A, Murata Y, Rydevik B, et al. Nerve growth factor content in dorsal root ganglion as related to changes in pain behavior in a rat model of experimental lumbar disc herniation. *Spine*. 2005;30:188-193.
127. Larsson K, Rydevik B, Olmarker K. Disc related cytokines inhibit axonal outgrowth from dorsal root ganglion cells in vitro. *Spine*. 2005;30:621-624.
128. Karppinen J, Korhonen T, Malmivaara A, et al. Tumor necrosis factor-alpha monoclonal antibody, infliximab, used to manage severe sciatica. *Spine*. 2003;28:750-753.
129. Korhonen T, Karppinen J, Malmivaara A, et al. Efficacy of infliximab for disc herniation-induced sciatica: one-year follow-up. *Spine*. 2004;29:2115-2119.

130. Genevay S, Stingelin S, Gabay C. Efficacy of etanercept in the treatment of acute severe sciatica. *Ann Rheum Dis.* 2004;63:1120-1123.
131. Cohen SP, Bogduk N, Dragovich A, et al. Randomized, double-blind, placebo-controlled, dose-response, and preclinical safety of transforaminal epidural etanercept for the treatment of sciatica. *Anesthesiology.* 2009;110:1116-1126.
132. Genevay S, Viatte S, Finck A, et al. Adalimumab in severe and acute sciatica: a multicentre, randomised, double-blind, placebo controlled trial. *Arthritis Rheum.* 2010;62(8):2339-2346.
133. Cooper RG, Freemont AJ. TNF-alpha blockade for herniated intervertebral disc-induced sciatica: a way forward at last? [editorial]. *Rheumatology.* 2004;43:119-121.
134. Freeman BJC, Ludbrook GL, Hall S, et al. Randomized, double-blind, placebo-controlled, trial of transforaminal epidural etanercept for the treatment of symptomatic lumbar disc herniation. *Spine.* 2013;38:1986-1994.
135. Cohen SP, White RL, Kurihara C, et al. Epidural steroids, etanercept, or saline in subacute sciatica: a multicenter, randomized trial. *Ann Intern Med.* 2012;156:551-559.

8 CHAPTER Basic Concepts in Genetics and Intervertebral Disc Degeneration and Scoliosis

Jason Pui Yin Cheung
Kenneth M.C. Cheung

Introduction to Genetics

Genetics has a growing role in the field of clinical medicine. Genes are the fundamental make-up of any organism; thus, understanding what genes and environmental factors contribute to certain disease traits/phenotypes are of interest. By identifying the mutations in the genes that lead to disease, focused management such as early detection, targeted therapies, or even disease prevention can be developed.

With genome sequencing and public access to the electronically compiled genome data, the Human Genome Project allows scientists to identify genes of interest at particular locations in the genome. This can allow researchers to use a certain DNA sequence of a particular gene as an initial reference sequence to carry out mutation screening and permit rapid identification of genetic markers within or adjacent to genes of interest. This database of DNA reference sequences can also help design primers that bind to a certain sequence of the genome. The available data allow studies regarding expression patterns in different tissues and sequence variations between subjects such as single nucleotide polymorphisms (SNPs).

Many genetic disorders have already been identified and stored in the Online Mendelian Inheritance in Man (OMIM) database. The pattern of how genetic information is passed through subsequent generations is based on the Mendelian laws of inheritance. Using modern technology, potential genetic variants that predispose to disease can be determined. For spine surgeons, disc degeneration and scoliosis are two of the most sought after conditions in terms of genetic background. Both conditions are likely influenced by multiple genes and various environmental factors. This chapter aims to provide clinicians with a basic concept of genetics with regard to the terminology and principles, with a specific focus on disc degeneration and scoliosis. Readers may be able to equip themselves with a general understanding and thereby the ability to follow novel literature regarding advances in genetics.

Chromosomes and DNA

Before discussing genetics and how to determine genetic variations, concepts of chromosomes, DNA, and polymorphisms need to be understood. Any single human genome is comprised of 22 pairs of homologous chromosomes with an additional pair of sex chromosomes inherited from parents. A full set of chromosomes is also known as diploid and a half set is known as haploid. Chromosomes are made up of DNA, which is a nucleic acid that carries genetic material. DNA contains a super-phosphate with nitrogenous bases. The nitrogenous bases include base pairs of adenine (A) and guanine (G)—purines—and cytosine (C) and thymine (T)—pyrimidines. Each molecule of DNA is comprised of two nucleotide chains that are coiled in a clockwise fashion to form the double helix. These chains have two ends, called the 5′ and 3′ ends, and the two nucleotide chains run in opposite directions, either from 5′ to 3′ or from 3′ to 5′. Base pairings in these chains are obligatory A:T and G:C.

The main function of these nucleic acids is coding protein synthesis. The basic architecture of proteins is comprised of amino acids, and the order of sequence in which amino acids are encoded judge the way the resulting protein is formed and functions. These proteins are encoded by DNA, and therefore by its gene. DNA is double stranded, whereas ribonucleic acid (RNA) is single stranded. In addition to this difference, uracil (U) replaces T in RNA sequences. Exons are sequences of DNA that contain coding information, whereas introns are noncoding sequences. DNA is used as a template to create RNA in a process known as transcription. As any set of three base pairs form the codes for an amino acid, the transcribed messenger RNA (mRNA) encodes the information for a certain protein with a specific amino acid sequence that is imprinted by a certain gene. Through the transcription process, the DNA strands separate and act as the template for the enzyme RNA polymerase II to synthesize nucleotides in the opposite direction of the DNA template (5′ to 3′ matched to 3′ to 5′). This process will include all introns and exons. Despite being a noncoding region, introns have regulatory functions during transcription. Introns are eventually removed after splicing; the remaining exons form mature mRNA.

The next stage in protein synthesis is known as translation, which occurs in the cell cytoplasm. The mRNA attaches to a ribosome; each ribosome moves along the mRNA to form a matching transfer RNA (tRNA), which will contribute its specific amino acid to a growing protein chain until it reaches a stop codon. Proteins are important for normal bodily functions, as they regulate different mechanisms both intracellularly and extracellularly.

Genetic Variations

Despite having pairs of chromosomes, there are variations in sequencing that distinguish between chromosomes. Variants on the same location of paired chromosomes are known as alleles. They may be homozygous, meaning the same, or heterozygous, meaning different. Small variations can exist in individual nucleotides. Larger variations include microsatellites, deletions, insertions, and copy number variations (CNVs). All variations can cause significant alteration of the protein structure, thus gene expression and possibly disease manifestation. However, these genetic variants can be manipulated into a genetic marker for identifying their location on the DNA sequence. These markers are important for studying the causative relationship between a genetic variant and an inherited disease.

SNPs are particularly of interest, as they are commonly used for genetic analysis. They are also commonly found throughout the genome, comprising up to 90% of the genetic variants. They are 1-base pair (bp) substitutions of DNA sequences that can occur anywhere in the genome. On average, a SNP may be observed in every set of 300 nucleotides; thus, there are approximately 10 million SNPs found in the entire human genome.

Microsatellites or variable number of tandem repeats refer to repeating short nucleotide sequences. Due to the variable number of repeats in different chromosomes, it is a useful marker for identifying different people. Deletion or insertion of one or more base changes may lead to significant changes in DNA sequences, thus causing missing or extra amino acids in any protein chain. A complete change in protein sequence may result from more than 3 bp of sequence addition or loss. These usually cause serious genetic diseases. CNV refers to large structural variations in DNA sequences. The "copy number" refers to the number of duplications that occur. CNV involves duplications of large segments of a certain chromosome that alters one or more genes. Inversions may also occur as a result of reversal in a segment of chromosome, which may cause complex genetic diseases.

Mutations and Polymorphisms

Mutations result from permanent damages to DNA or replication errors. The effects are variable: from fatal to only mildly detrimental. If fatal, these mutations will not be inherited, thus are very rarely found in the population. For mild cases, individuals are likely to reproduce and encourage the mutation to be inherited, leading to an increase in prevalence in the general population. Rare variants are more commonly researched, as they are more likely to have positive findings in genetic research and usually are associated with more clinically relevant diseases. They are defined as variants with a minor allele frequency (MAF) of less than 1%. Polymorphisms are defined as MAF greater than 1%; among these, MAF greater than 5% are common variants and those from 1% to 5% are low-frequency variants. Polymorphisms rarely cause significant external effects despite changes in the gene sequence.

Terminology and Types of Disease

Genotype is the definition of the status of two alleles or actual denotation of the genetic data. In contrast, *phenotype* is the observable expression of the subjects' traits. Differences in genotypes contributed by polymorphisms lead to phenotypical variations between individuals. Expression can exist at the molecular level in the form of protein expression or can be more clinically notable, such as height differences and symptoms. As the clinical expression of the disease relies heavily on the genotype, being able to phenotype a disease carefully is very important for any genetic analysis. Not all genotypical differences may manifest clinically, however, as this relies on penetrance. Incomplete penetrance may not result in disease, as the genotype is not fully expressed clinically. These cases are considered to be complex genetic disorders in which environmental factors must interact with the susceptibility genes before developing disease. Many orthopedic conditions—such as osteoarthritis, disc degeneration, and even scoliosis—are types of complex genetic disorders. This is in contrast to Mendelian diseases, which are simpler but rarer forms of disease caused by single gene mutations.[1,2] Usually, these are severe diseases, such as osteogenesis imperfecta. Mendelian diseases are usually predictable in inheritance patterns.

For complex disorders, meticulous qualitative and quantitative phenotyping is important to classify disease severity.[3] For example, in disc degeneration, most phenotyping relies on magnetic resonance imaging (MRI) which is used to assess the disc's hydration status, any bulging discs or herniation, and Schmorl's nodes or endplate irregularities. Qualitatively, whether there is disc degeneration is evaluated. However, quantitative evaluation is more important in these complex disorders, as the phenotype may alter in severity and over time, such as with the degenerative process. On the MRI, Schneiderman's and Pfirrmann's grading describe the signal intensity of the nucleus pulposus on T2-weighted MRI. Schneiderman's grading describes the signal intensity of the nucleus pulposus by four grades (grade 0 indicating a normal disc and grade 3 indicating hypointensity with disc space narrowing).[4] Pfirrmann's classification evaluates the homogeneity of disc structure, signal intensity, distinction of nucleus pulposus and anulus fibrosus, and disc height by five grades (grade 0 indicating a homogeneous disc structure, hyperintense signal, and normal disc height with grade 5 indicating inhomogeneous disc structure, hypointense signal, loss of distinction between nucleus pulposus and anulus fibrosus, and collapsed disc space).[5]

Gene Mapping

Gene mapping must be performed prior to claiming that a disease is caused by a certain gene. Accurate mapping helps us understand the etiology and pathogenesis, and identifies genes that may be manipulated into targeted therapies. The method for gene mapping works differently for Mendelian versus complex diseases. In Mendelian diseases, due to the rarity of the contributing gene variations, most are identified by studying affected families. Family genetics allow visualization of the mode of inheritance, and can help locate the position of the genetic variant. Although there are limitations in this analysis because family members are exposed to similar environmental factors and may mask some real genetic factors, examining monozygotic (identical) twins may help analysis for purely genetic disorders since they should both have disease. However, if both monozygotic and dizygotic (non-identical) twins both have similar disease rate (concordance rate), then it is likely that shared environmental factors are the major factor instead. In complex genetic diseases, there is contribution from multiple genes; with their complex interactions with the environment, special mapping designs are required. For family-based designs, linkage analysis will be used. For population-based designs, association analysis or biologically relevant candidate gene analysis are used.

Linkage Analysis

Preferably, linkage analysis has the greatest yield with large families and multiple affected members. Genotyping for microsatellite markers is performed to locate disease genes that are nearby (Fig. 8.1). The premise of linkage analysis is that recombination is less likely to occur between the disease gene and the designated genetic marker since their positions are nearby, allowing "linkage" of the disease gene with the marker. In other words, affected members of the same family are likely to pass on this region of the genome with the disease gene. If sufficient microsatellite markers are available to cover the whole genome, linkage analysis can help locate the diseased gene even if it is unknown at the outset. However, this is dependent on the distance between the disease gene and marker. With a large distance, it is likely that recombination may have occurred in between. Thus, the rate of recombination can help calculate the distance between the diseased gene and marker used. In general, a 1% recombination rate (θ) is represented as 1 centimorgan (cM) apart or approximately 1 million bp distance.[6,7]

One of the main tests used is the parametric linkage analysis, in which the test hypothesis (true linkage of the diseased gene to the marker) is tested against the null hypothesis (no linkage). Sequential recombination rates are performed to compare the likelihood of either hypothesis. This is known as likelihood ratio or odds. Using a logarithm to base 10 of this ratio, the logarithm of odds (LOD) score can be calculated. The highest LOD score represents the likely distance between the disease gene and marker.[8] LOD is an important parameter to decide whether a finding is significant or not; a score of 3.3 is required to achieve genome-wide significance.[9] This LOD score can be strengthened by combining results from different studies with the same disease model.

With linkage analysis, prior knowledge of the position of the disease gene is unnecessary since it can be determined by linkage with microsatellite markers. Thus, it is most useful in diseases in which only a small number of genes are involved. The main limitation is its inability to detect common alleles without a strong influence on the disease. Therefore, in common conditions with multiple gene and environmental contributions, such as disc degeneration, association studies are preferred.

Association Studies

Population-based gene association studies aim to identify alleles associated with a single trait across the population. Although it is similar to linkage analysis, in that it identifies a disease gene in subjects with a common ancestry (population based instead of family based), it assumes that the "linkage" distance between the marker and disease gene of interest is extremely close so that recombination over generations would not affect its position. Thus, positive association represents that a particular disease gene is overexpressed in diseased individuals as well as underexpressed in normal subjects.

Association studies can be classified as either direct or indirect.[10] Direct association studies target the variants that have functional effects, which leads to disease. Although successful identification of a predisposing allele shows powerful association, the chance of positive identification is low. In indirect association studies, the association between the marker and disease gene is targeted. This association relies on the concept of linkage disequilibrium (LD), that is, because

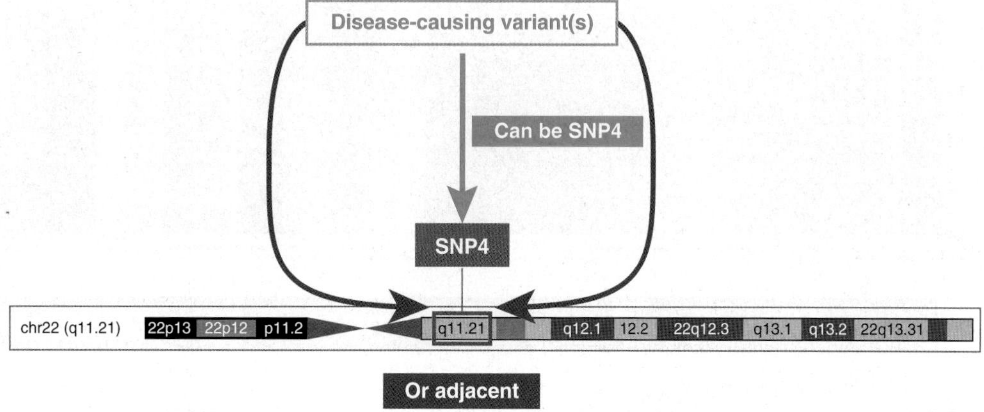

FIG. 8.1 SNP4 is the disease-causing variant. In linkage analysis, markers nearby (or adjacent in this figure) to the disease variant can be easily picked up, as recombination is unlikely to have occurred in between.

markers are near the disease gene, they are associated and thus lead to higher frequency of disease than expected. Identifying this marker will suggest that a disease-causing variant is nearby, helping to narrow down the search for the disease gene.

Association studies can be conducted via a candidate-gene or genome-wide association type of approach. Candidate-gene approaches utilize possible disease genes that are previously identified or are in relation to the disease pathway and directly screen the individuals for these disease genes using markers, which are usually selected SNPs. Genome-wide association studies (Fig. 8.2) adopt a similar principle as candidate-gene studies, but, rather than testing for possible single genes, a SNP mapping of the entire genome is performed. All possible SNPs are tested for association with the disease by comparing the frequencies of occurrence between cases and controls. Conventionally, the threshold for genomewide significance is 5×10^{-8}. Technological advancements with the addition of DNA genechips allow for this scale of study.[11] The cost and time spent to perform these studies are now much more reasonable.

Newer Technologies

With the advancement in sequencing technologies,[12] whole human genome or whole exon (1%–2% of the human genome)

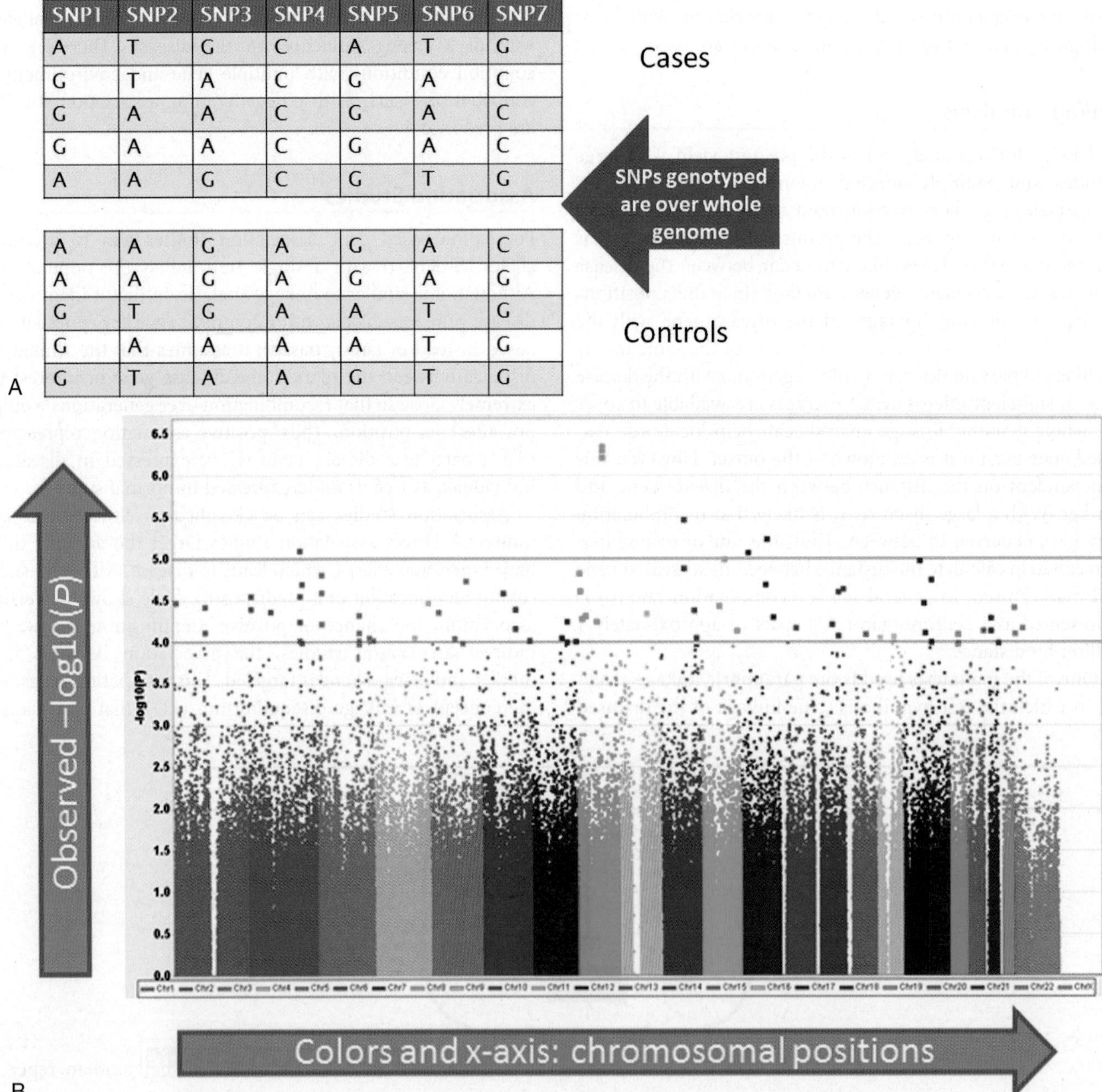

SNP1	SNP2	SNP3	SNP4	SNP5	SNP6	SNP7
A	T	G	C	A	T	G
G	T	A	C	G	A	C
G	A	A	C	G	A	C
G	A	A	C	G	A	C
A	A	G	C	G	T	G
A	A	G	A	G	A	C
A	A	G	A	G	A	G
G	T	G	A	A	T	G
G	A	A	A	A	T	G
G	T	A	A	G	T	G

FIG. 8.2 (A) Genome-wide association studies pick up all single nucleotide polymorphisms (SNPs) between cases and controls. (B) Manhattan plots are used to define which SNPs are significant by logarithm to base 10 of the observed *P* value.

sequencing is becoming more affordable and feasible. This allows assessing of all DNA variations in the genome, such as CNVs instead of only SNPs or microsatellites. Exome sequencing is used for sequencing the protein-coding genes in a genome. Thus, only the DNA that encodes for proteins is sequenced. This technique is a simpler approach to rare variants. Since diseases are caused by these rare variants, targeting the protein coding sequence usually has a high yield for identifying the causative variants. Because of this, an understanding of the clinical implication of the disease and the protein sequence that is defective is required. This is in contrast to whole-genome sequencing, which determines the entire DNA sequence of an individual's genome. More than 95% of the genome is thus genotyped, allowing information on the individual's genetic susceptibility to diseases to be generated. Despite its wide coverage and reduced cost with technological advancements, it is still comparably the most expensive sequencing technique.

Interpretation of Results

Using association studies, possible significant results may be generated in the form of direct or indirect association or false-positive results. Direct association indicates that the genotyped polymorphisms are the true causal genetic variant leading to disease. Indirect association indicates that the polymorphisms are in LD with the true variant. A false-positive result is usually due to population stratification, suggesting that differences in allele frequency exist between subpopulations of the subject population, indicating that these individuals are of a different ancestry.

As with all statistical analysis, genetic testing to determine whether variants are associated with disease susceptibility requires certain *P* values. The null hypothesis with regard to *P* value is the possibility of no association in genotype distribution between cases and controls. Similarly, this hypothesis of no association is rejected with a $P < .05$. Special tests may be adopted in candidate-gene or genome-wide association studies since all variants undergo study. Increased false-positive rates exist with increased hypothesis testing. Bonferroni correction is one of the most common approaches[13] in these studies. The corrected statistical significance level is 1/n times what is expected from only one variant testing. Therefore, the significance threshold is 0.05 divided by the number of markers under testing.

Disc Degeneration Genetics

There has been a gradual shift in understanding of disc degeneration from purely a reaction to aging and prolonged mechanical load to a more complex interaction between genetics (Table 8.1) and environmental factors.[14] Earlier studies suggest contributions of age, gender, occupation, cigarette smoking, and increased height and weight.[15] Using familial studies, several genetic variants have suggested this relationship, as young patients may also develop disc degeneration.[16,17] In addition, a familial link can be generated due to similarities (26%–72%) found between identical twin pairs.[18] With analysis of monozygotic twins, up to 61% of the genetic variance can be explained by familial aggregation with only limited (16%) contribution by age and mechanical loading.[19] Subsequent twin studies suggest that 74% of disc degeneration is heritable after adjustment for age, body weight and height, smoking, occupation, and degree of physical exercise.[20]

As compared to spine deformity, in which the phenotype is clear, disc degeneration is overall more subjective for diagnosis (Fig. 8.3). There is a wide range of symptoms, severity, and presentations, with particularly complex MRI features including loss of nucleus pulposus signal intensity, disc herniation and bulging, endplate irregularities and Schmorl's nodes, osteophyte formation, and disc space narrowing, Modic changes, and high-intensity zones. Some very young individuals may develop severe disc degeneration, while some of the elderly may have normal discs. Clinical presentation is especially variable as not all individuals with "black" discs develop back pain.

Despite evidence of heritability suggested by studies of twins, limited validation studies exist for the identified common variants. Considering the substantial population with disc degeneration, causality is still unclear with many unknown common variants still requiring identification. Most of the current studies focus around candidate-gene analysis with common SNPs. However, there is an increasing interest in rare variants due to their role in complex diseases.

Via linkage study, a novel susceptible variant in carbohydrate sulfotransferase 3 (*CHST3*) is found to be associated with early-onset disc degeneration.[21] This is accomplished by genotyping candidate regions on chromosomes 1, 5, 8, 10, and 20. A follow-up epigenetics study detected a reduction in expression of *CHST3* mRNA in intervertebral disc cells of individuals carrying the A allele of the SNP rs4148941. By understanding the biologic pathways leading to the disc degeneration phenotype, probable candidate genes can be used to identify possible disease variants. The extracellular matrix is an integral part of the disc architecture; thus, genes encoding structural proteins including collagen and aggrecan are good candidate genes to analyze with regard to disc degeneration.

The vitamin-D receptor (*VDR*) has been most commonly replicated in different population cohorts, thus is the most robust of all associated genes under study. A Finnish twin study[22] first identified *TaqI* and *FokI* polymorphisms manifesting as reduced signal intensity of the disc on MRI. *TaqI* has been replicated in a Japanese cohort[23] and a Chinese population-based study.[24] The next stage of functional validation has yet to be performed, however. The expression of this variant is likely extracellular matrix alterations.[25]

The gene *ACAN* encodes aggrecan, which is responsible for maintaining disc hydration as it is the major proteoglycan contributing to the cartilage and nucleus pulposus structure of the intervertebral disc. Variable number tandem repeats in *ACAN* is associated with disc degeneration in a young Japanese cohort,[26] which has been replicated in the Han Chinese,[27] Korean,[28] and Turkish[29] populations. A greater risk of symptoms has been observed in smokers (odds ratio [OR]

TABLE 8.1 Genetic Variants for Disc Degeneration

Gene	Protein	Cohort/Study Population Size (N)	Variant	Reference
ACAN	Aggrecan	Japanese (64) Chinese (132) Korean (104) Turkish (100)	Variable number tandem repeats	26 27 28 29
ASPN	Asporin	Japanese (1353) Chinese (1055)	D14 allele	3
CHST3	Carbohydrate sulfotransferase 3	Japanese (23,136) Chinese (6088) Finnish (6069)	rs4148941	21
CILP	Cartilage intermediate layer protein	Finnish (538)	rs2073711	46
COL11A1	Type XI collagen	Japanese (1852)	rs1676486	30
COL1A1, COL1A2	Type I collagen	Dutch (517)	rs1800012	35
COL9A2	Type IX collagen	Finnish (966) Chinese (804)	Trp2	31 32
COL9A3	Type IX collagen	Finnish (492)	Trp3	33
GDF5	Growth differentiation factor	Northern European (5259)	rs143383	38
IL6	Interleukin 6	Finnish (538)	rs1800795 rs1800797	46
MMP1	Matrix metalloproteinase-1	Chinese (691)	−1607 promoter (G to D allele)	40
MMP2	Matrix metalloproteinase-2	Chinese (480)	−1306 promoter (T to C allele)	41
MMP3	Matrix metalloproteinase-3	Japanese (109)	MMP-3 promoter (5A5A and 5A6A)	42
MMP9	Matrix metalloproteinase-9	Chinese (859)	−1562 promoter (C to T allele)	43
PARK2	Parkin (E3 ubiquitin ligase)	Northern European (4600)	rs926849	47
SKT	Sickle tail	Japanese (1758) Finnish (538)	rs16924573	45 46
THB2	Thrombospondin-2	Japanese (1743)	rs9406328	44
VDR	Vitamin D receptor	Finnish (85 twins) Japanese (205) Chinese (804)	TaqI, FokI TaqI TaqI	22 23 24

= 4.5), suggesting further interactions with environmental factors.

Collagen is another structural protein that has been commonly studied. Type XI collagen encoded by *COL11A1* (SNP: rs1676486; T-allele) has been suggested in a Japanese study to be associated with disc herniation and sciatica due to destabilizing mRNA.[30] Trp2 allele is a rare mutation of *COL9A2* (type IX collagen) and is suggested to be a disease-causing mutation in a Finnish family linkage study.[31] This association is replicated in the Chinese population, in which its frequency is even higher.[32] Trp3 is another variant suggested to be causative in a Finnish population,[33] but is not replicated in the Chinese[32] or Southern European[34] cohorts. *COL1A1* and *COL1A2* are two genes encoding collagen type I, and a SNP (rs1800012) is identified to be associated with disc degeneration.[35] However, no large-scale study has replicated these results.

Other degeneration phenotypes, such as osteoarthritis, may have similar variants as disc degeneration. For example, associations with the gene *ASPN* (Asporin) have been observed in Asian cohorts.[3] Asporin is an extracellular matrix protein that contributes to knee osteoarthritis. Growth differentiation factor (*GDF5*) is also a commonly used candidate gene for osteoarthritis[36] as it is important for joint formation,[37] but has also been shown to lead to disc degeneration. A SNP (rs143383) is related to disc space narrowing and osteophyte formation.[38] In a meta-analysis with regard to rs143383, a significant association can be detected among women for this phenotype.[38]

Matrix metalloproteinases (MMPs) are important proteins that are expressed in intervertebral discs. Thus, MMPs have increased enzymatic activity and increased expression in degenerated disc cells.[39] *MMP1*, *MMP2*, *MMP3*, and *MMP9* have been linked to disc degeneration. In a cohort of Southern Chinese subjects, the significance of the *MMP1* variant is found only in subjects older than 40 years.[40] A significant SNP located at the promoter region of *MMP2* is associated with severe disc degeneration.[41] Polymorphisms of *MMP3* may lead to the onset and progression of disc degeneration.[42] Finally, for *MMP9*, a SNP at the promoter region may also be associated with disc degeneration.[43] All of these findings are in Asian cohorts and have yet to be replicated in other ethnicities.

Thrombospondin-2 genes (*THBS2*) have also been studied in Japanese cohorts as possible candidate genes. A significant

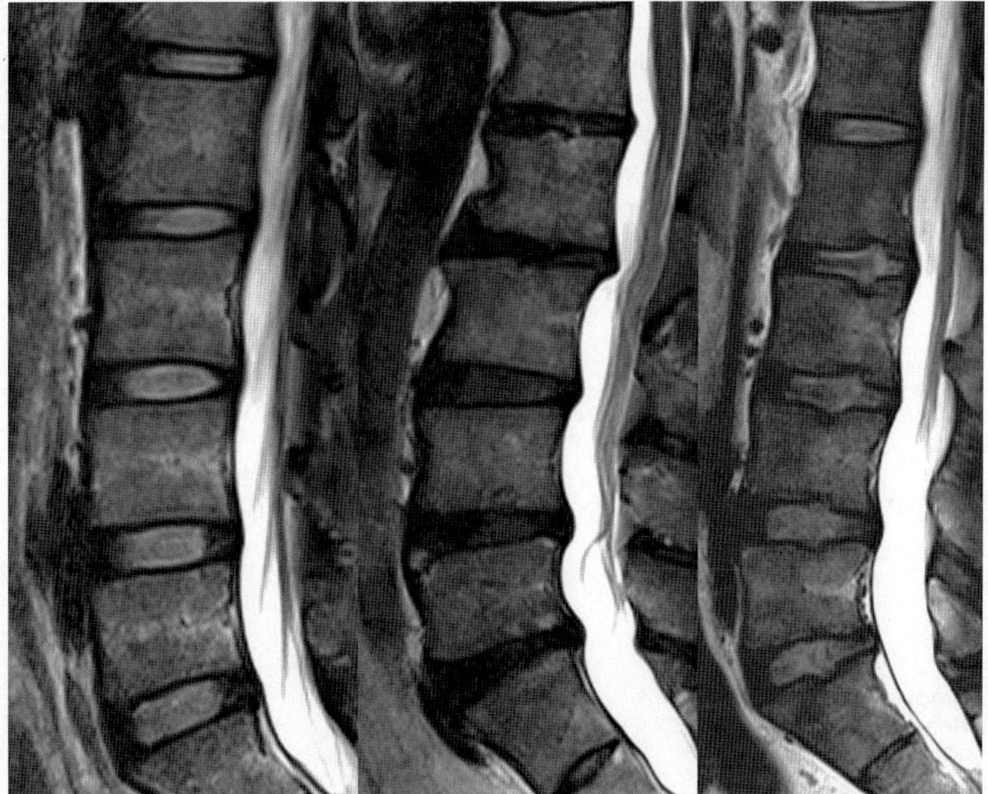

FIG. 8.3 Importance and variations in phenotypes observed in disc degeneration. The left T2-weighted magnetic resonance image (MRI) shows a relatively normal phenotype with signal intensity of the nucleus pulposus. The center MRI shows multiple discs with loss of signal intensity and disc height, bulging and high-intensity zone anteriorly at L4–L5. The right MRI shows discs with normal signal intensities but multiple endplate irregularities and Schmorl's nodes.

SNP (rs9406328) has been proposed[44] to be related to regulation of *MMP* expression in the disc. The combined effects of *THBS2* and *MMP9* variants amounts to an OR of 3.3 for disc degeneration.[44]

Sickle tail (*SKT*) gene polymorphisms have been analyzed in a Japanese cohort.[45] Here, a significant SNP (rs16924573) observed has been replicated in the Finnish population.[46] The risk of lost signal intensity at the nucleus pulposus and the *SKT* SNP has been established (OR = 0.27 [95% CI, 0.07–0.96], $P = .024$).[46] However, further functional studies of this relationship are required.

A recent large-scale (4600 subjects) genome-wide association study of a Northern European cohort suggests that the SNP (rs926849) of the *PARK2* gene ($P = 2.8 \times 10^{-8}$) is also associated with disc degeneration.[47] Polymorphisms have also been found for *CILP* (rs2073711) and *IL6* (rs1800795 and rs1800797) genes via association study.[46]

From the summary of genetic studies with regard to lumbar disc degeneration, many genes have been reported, but just a few have been replicated with different cohorts and ethnicities. A systematic review of disc degeneration association studies[14] suggests that most of the reported studies have only a weak level of evidence. It is thus likely that cross-cohort validations are required in subsequent studies to raise the significance of reported results.

Scoliosis Genetics

Early-Onset Scoliosis and Congenital Scoliosis

Early-onset scoliosis (EOS), according to the Scoliosis Research Society, is a lateral curvature of the spine that is diagnosed before the age of 10. Thus, any diagnoses can fall under this category including neuromuscular, syndromic, congenital, and idiopathic scoliosis. With regard to idiopathic scoliosis, both infantile (ages 0–3 years) and juvenile (ages 4–10 years) idiopathic scoliosis are considered EOS. Due to the variable presentations of EOS, little evidence is available in regard to their inheritance. For idiopathic scoliosis, subjects that are younger commonly are boys as compared to older age groups, in which girls are more commonly affected.[48] Older-onset scoliosis, in particular, has a higher incidence among relatives.

The occurrence of congenital scoliosis is usually sporadic, with an incidence of 0.5 to 1 per 1000 live births.[49,50] Its etiology is likely to be multifactorial, with contributions from both genetic and environmental factors. Vertebral anomalies may arise from the fetal development with mothers exposed to environmental factors such as hypoxia, hyperthermia, carbon monoxide, and alcohol exposure.[51] Gestational hypoxia, in particular, has been shown to potentiate abnormal fibroblast

TABLE 8.2 Genetic Variants for Congenital Scoliosis

Gene	Function	Cohort/Study Population (N)	Variant/Location	Reference
JAG1	Notch signaling pathway	United States (4 families)	Chromosome 20p12	58
PAX1		United States (48)	Chromosomes 20, 21	64
DLL3		United States (50)	Chromosome 19	63
		United Kingdom (3 families)	Chromosome 19q13.1-q13.3	57
TBX6	T-box 6	China (254)	rs2289292 rs3809624	62

TABLE 8.3 Genetic Variants for Adolescent Idiopathic Scoliosis

Linkage		Cohort/Study Population (N)		Reference
Chromosomes 6p,10q,18q		United States (1 family)		72
Chromosome 19p13.3		Chinese (7 families)		73
Chromosome X		United States (202 families)		75
Chromosomes 5p13, 13q13, 13q32		United States (7 families)		76
Chromosome 17p11		Italy (1 family)		77
Chromosomes 9q31.2-q34.2, 17q25.3-qtel		United States (10 families)		78
Gene	**Protein**	**Cohort/Study Population (N)**	**Variant/Location**	**Reference**
CHD7	Chromodomain-helicase-DNA-binding protein 7 (also associated with CHARGE syndrome)	France (10) United States (52 families)	Intron 2 Exons 2–4 Chromosome 8q12	79 80
MATN1	Matrilin 1, cartilage matrix protein	Italy (81 families)	Chromosome 1p35	81
MTNR1b	Melatonin receptor 1B	Chinese (1465)	rs4753426	82
Xbal	Estrogen receptor	Japanese (304) Chinese (376)	Chromosome X	85 86
CHL1	Neural cell adhesion molecule L1-like protein (Robo3 related)	United States (419 families)	rs1400180 rs10510181	89
LBX1	Ladybird homeobox 1	Japanese (1376 families) ICSG (6 Asian, 3 non-Asian cohorts)	rs11190870	90 93
GPR126	G protein–coupled receptor 126	Japanese (1819 cases)	rs6570507	94

ICSG, International Consortium for Scoliosis Genetics.

growth factor (FGF) signaling in mice, which thus develop congenital scoliosis.[52]

The phenotype of congenital scoliosis includes vertebral and rib malformation caused by failure of segmentation or formation in utero. Overall, the genetic understanding (Table 8.2) of this condition is still limited, with only a few significant association studies performed. Complex interactions between the signaling pathways such as *FGF*, *Wnt*, and *Notch*, occur in the embryo to form vertebral bodies from somites.[53] Various notch pathway genes. including *MESP2*,[54] *LFNG*,[55] and *HES7*,[56] have been identified to trigger normal somite segmentation and vertebral development in mice. Any mutation in these genes alters the pathway of vertebral development and may lead to anomalies. The association is more complex in humans due to the less predictable vertebral and rib malformations. Several gene variants of the *Notch* pathway have been identified in spondylocostal dysostosis[57] and Alagille syndrome.[58,59] However, the actual gene and protein mechanisms responsible for the phenotype representation are still unknown; thus, these mutations may not be the sole contributory element. Via animal studies, several human candidate genes from the *Wnt*, *FGF*, and *Notch* signaling pathways have been identified.[49,60] *PAX1*, *DLL3*, and *TBX6* are candidate genes that have been studied using association analysis.[61–65] One study on Han Chinese subjects comparing patients with congenital scoliosis with normal spines yielded two SNPs of the *TBX6* gene (rs2289292 and rs3809624) to be in strong LD (LOD = 57.48), suggesting that these rare variants play important roles in the development of congenital scoliosis.[62]

Adolescent Idiopathic Scoliosis

As compared to EOS, adolescent idiopathic scoliosis (AIS) involves patients older than 10 years of age. AIS usually involves girls and with right-sided thoracic involvement instead of the opposite in early-onset idiopathic scoliosis. It is the most common pediatric spinal deformity, affecting 2% to 3% of children.[66] There is an adequate sampling for genetic studies (Table 8.3) as shown by more research in this area as compared to EOS. Original twin studies supported a genetic etiology in AIS.[48,67] Within AIS families, the disease characteristic may differ and may not affect every generation.

Similar to other spinal deformities, it is a complex trait that likely involves more than one gene.

In a further assessment of AIS family history, one study found that 97% of AIS patients have familial origins.[68] The genes that contribute to AIS are likely to exist with different types of expression and penetrance, which explains why some subjects have more florid phenotypes than others despite sharing a similar gene pool. This suggests that only up to 30% male and 50% female carriers of the disease variant develop more pronounced scoliosis.[69]

Based on family studies, linkage analysis and association studies are conducted to identify the disease susceptibility genes. Previous reviews on familial AIS genetics have been published[70,71] with identification of significant linkage regions specifically located on chromosomes 6, 10, and 18. Large family genetics showed the highest LOD score on chromosome 18.[72] This prompted further study into AIS families, which found a plethora of susceptibility areas in the genome that might give rise to scoliosis. Some found linkage areas with a LOD score of 3.63 on chromosome 19p13.3.[73] This region was verified in a subset of families with probands having Cobb angles of 30 degrees or greater.[74] Others reported the X chromosome with a maximum LOD score of 1.69[75] and specifically kyphoscoliosis to be associated with linkage at chromosomes 5 and 13.[76] Other positive findings were observed with marker D17S799 (LOD 3.20) in a three-generation Italian family,[77] and linkage at marker D9S2157 of chromosome 9q (LOD 3.64) and at marker AAT095 of chromosome 17q (LOD 4.08) in the British population.[78]

Overlap of genes associated with congenital abnormalities is also observed in AIS subjects. The *CHD7* gene has been found to be associated with CHARGE syndrome during gene mapping.[79] The *CHD7* gene is known to be expressed in undifferentiated neuroepithelium and in neural crest mesenchymal cells. It is found in the dorsal root ganglia, cranial nerves, auditory area, pituitary area, nasal tissues, and neural retina near the end of the first trimester. Gao et al.[80] identified an A to G SNP in intron 2 of the *CHD7* gene that disrupted a transcription factor binding site associated with late-onset idiopathic scoliosis. Resequencing of the *CHD7* gene verified potential functional polymorphisms that may disrupt this transcription factor binding site, suggesting an etiologic overlap between CHARGE syndrome and idiopathic scoliosis.[80]

Using genome-wide association studies, several genes have been identified as potential susceptibility genes. An allele of a microsatellite marker in the *MATN1* gene is overtransmitted from parents to affected probands, suggesting a link to familial idiopathic scoliosis.[81] Using a chicken pinealectomy model, melatonin deficiency is observed as a possible disease mechanism for AIS. The melatonin receptor 1B (*MTNR1B*) has also been identified as a possible candidate gene in a study on Chinese AIS subjects.[82] A "C-C" genotype with a promoter SNP (rs4753426) significantly increases the risk of AIS (OR, 1.29). These results, however, are not verified in Japanese and Hungarian cohorts.[83,84] The *XbaI* polymorphism of the gene encoding the estrogen receptor has been linked to curve severity.[85] Although this association is observed in a Chinese dataset,[86] this has not been replicated in other studies.[87]

Several contributing variants have been detected by linkage analysis. However, detecting disease genes related to AIS remains limited. Complex genetic disorders such as AIS are expected to be associated with multiple gene variants with only moderate effects of each. In view of this, linkage analysis may be limited in detection of all genes, and association studies may have better success.[88] In addition to larger sample sizes to obtain significant findings, identified disease genes require verification in other populations and ethnicities.

Using genome-wide association studies, several recent findings are worth mentioning. The SNPs (rs10510181) near the *CHL1* gene[89] and (rs11190870) near the *LBX1* gene[90] have been identified and replicated in the Chinese population.[91,92] Several Asian and non-Asian cohorts have also verified rs11190870 in a meta-analysis and yielded *P* values of 1.22×10^{-43} for both genders and 2.94×10^{-48} for females.[93] This is the first susceptibility locus for AIS that is replicated in several populations. A third significant SNP (rs6570507) has also been detected in a Japanese population to exist in the *GPR126* (encoding G protein–coupled receptor 126) gene, which has been replicated in Chinese and European cohorts.[94] These SNPs are suggested to have ORs of 1.2 to 1.4 for AIS susceptibility. These association studies are now the go-to method for identifying gene variants; further studies are expected to be generated in a similar manner.

Conclusions and the Future

This chapter is an introduction into the field of genetics. It acts as a basic guideline for clinicians to understand the genetic jargon and available evidence with regard to genetic susceptibility genes identified for disc degeneration and scoliosis. Numerous genetic studies have been carried out to locate susceptibility genes responsible for development of lumbar disc degeneration and scoliosis. As both are complex diseases, studies have identified multiple gene interactions as well as different risk patterns according to exposure to environmental factors such as aging and smoking for disc degeneration. With increasing demand and interest for higher-level genetic studies, the advancement of genotyping and sequencing technologies have followed suit, with the more complex and stronger association studies and exome-sequencing methods.

Due to these advances, better understanding of complex disorders is possible.[95] However, there are still significant limitations in our current understanding. Very few of the susceptible genes are replicated, and many of their functions are unknown. Before functional studies can be performed by testing gene knockout in animal models, larger sample sizes with cross-validation of different cohorts are necessary to have a more accurate evaluation of possible genetic variants to avoid testing incorrect and false-positive polymorphisms. Thus, multicenter and multiethnic genetic studies with international collaborations are inevitable to produce results of higher significance. To ensure standardization among research groups, phenotypes should be defined properly with good reliability of assessment. In addition to the study phenotypes, gene–gene and gene–environmental interactions must be assessed and accounted for during analysis. This is a necessary process for all complex genetic diseases.

KEY REFERENCES

1. Song YQ, Karasugi T, Cheung KM, et al. Lumbar disc degeneration is linked to a carbohydrate sulfotransferase 3 variant. *J Clin Invest.* 2013;123(11):4909-4917.
2. Cheung KM, Chan D, Karppinen J, et al. Association of the Taq I allele in vitamin D receptor with degenerative disc disease and disc bulge in a Chinese population. *Spine.* 2006;31(10):1143-1148.
3. Williams FM, Bansal AT, van Meurs JB, et al. Novel genetic variants associated with lumbar disc degeneration in northern Europeans: a meta-analysis of 4600 subjects. *Ann Rheum Dis.* 2013;72(7):1141-1148.
4. Takahashi Y, Kou I, Takahashi A, et al. A genome-wide association study identifies common variants near LBX1 associated with adolescent idiopathic scoliosis. *Nat Genet.* 2011;43(12):1237-1240.
5. Londono D, Kou I, Johnson TA, et al. A meta-analysis identifies adolescent idiopathic scoliosis association with LBX1 locus in multiple ethnic groups. *J Med Genet.* 2014;51(6):401-406.
6. Kou I, Takahashi Y, Johnson TA, et al. Genetic variants in GPR126 are associated with adolescent idiopathic scoliosis. *Nat Genet.* 2013;45(6):676-679.

REFERENCES

1. Pritchard JK, Cox NJ. The allelic architecture of human disease genes: common disease-common variant…or not? *Hum Mol Genet.* 2002;11(20):2417-2423.
2. Pagon RA. Genetic testing for disease susceptibilities: consequences for genetic counseling. *Trends Mol Med.* 2002;8(6):306-307.
3. Song YQ, Cheung KM, Ho DW, et al. Association of the asporin D14 allele with lumbar-disc degeneration in Asians. *Am J Hum Genet.* 2008;82(3):744-747.
4. Schneiderman G, Flannigan B, Kingston S, et al. Magnetic resonance imaging in the diagnosis of disc degeneration: correlation with discography. *Spine.* 1987;12(3):276-281.
5. Pfirrmann CW, Metzdorf A, Zanetti M, et al. Magnetic resonance classification of lumbar intervertebral disc degeneration. *Spine.* 2001;26(17):1873-1878.
6. Ott J. *Analysis of Human Genetic Linkage.* Baltimore: Johns Hopkins University Press; 1999.
7. Sham P. *Statistics in Human Genetics.* London: Arnold; 1998.
8. Morton NE. Sequential tests for the detection of linkage. *Am J Hum Genet.* 1955;7(3):277-318.
9. Lander E, Kruglyak L. Genetic dissection of complex traits: guidelines for interpreting and reporting linkage results. *Nat Genet.* 1995;11(3):241-247.
10. Cordell HJ, Clayton DG. Genetic association studies. *Lancet.* 2005;366(9491):1121-1131.
11. Peters T, Sedlmeier R. Current methods for high-throughput detection of novel DNA polymorphisms. *Drug Discov Today Technol.* 2006;3(2):123-129.
12. Koboldt DC, Steinberg KM, Larson DE, et al. The next-generation sequencing revolution and its impact on genomics. *Cell.* 2013;155(1):27-38.
13. Bland JM, Altman DG. Multiple significance tests: the Bonferroni method. *BMJ.* 1995;310(6973):170.
14. Eskola PJ, Lemmela S, Kjaer P, et al. Genetic association studies in lumbar disc degeneration: a systematic review. *PLoS ONE.* 2012;7(11):e49995.
15. Hassett G, Hart DJ, Manek NJ, et al. Risk factors for progression of lumbar spine disc degeneration: the Chingford Study. *Arthritis Rheum.* 2003;48(11):3112-3117.
16. Varlotta GP, Brown MD, Kelsey JL, et al. Familial predisposition for herniation of a lumbar disc in patients who are less than twenty-one years old. *J Bone Joint Surg Am.* 1991;73(1):124-128.
17. Matsui H, Terahata N, Tsuji H, et al. Familial predisposition and clustering for juvenile lumbar disc herniation. *Spine.* 1992;17(11):1323-1328.
18. Battie MC, Haynor DR, Fisher LD, et al. Similarities in degenerative findings on magnetic resonance images of the lumbar spines of identical twins. *J Bone Joint Surg Am.* 1995;77(11):1662-1670.
19. Battie MC, Videman T, Gibbons LE, et al. 1995 Volvo Award in clinical sciences. Determinants of lumbar disc degeneration. A study relating lifetime exposures and magnetic resonance imaging findings in identical twins. *Spine.* 1995;20(24):2601-2612.
20. Sambrook PN, MacGregor AJ, Spector TD. Genetic influences on cervical and lumbar disc degeneration: a magnetic resonance imaging study in twins. *Arthritis Rheum.* 1999;42(2):366-372.
21. Song YQ, Karasugi T, Cheung KM, et al. Lumbar disc degeneration is linked to a carbohydrate sulfotransferase 3 variant. *J Clin Invest.* 2013;123(11):4909-4917.
22. Videman T, Leppavuori J, Kaprio J, et al. Intragenic polymorphisms of the vitamin D receptor gene associated with intervertebral disc degeneration. *Spine.* 1998;23(23): 2477-2485.
23. Kawaguchi Y, Kanamori M, Ishihara H, et al. The association of lumbar disc disease with vitamin-D receptor gene polymorphism. *J Bone Joint Surg Am.* 2002;84-A(11):2022-2028.
24. Cheung KM, Chan D, Karppinen J, et al. Association of the Taq I allele in vitamin D receptor with degenerative disc disease and disc bulge in a Chinese population. *Spine.* 2006;31(10):1143-1148.
25. Fernandes I, Hampson G, Cahours X, et al. Abnormal sulfate metabolism in vitamin D-deficient rats. *J Clin Invest.* 1997;100(9):2196-2203.
26. Doege KJ, Coulter SN, Meek LM, et al. A human-specific polymorphism in the coding region of the aggrecan gene. Variable number of tandem repeats produce a range of core protein sizes in the general population. *J Biol Chem.* 1997;272(21):13974-13979.
27. Cong L, Pang H, Xuan D, et al. The interaction between aggrecan gene *VNTR* polymorphism and cigarette smoking in predicting incident symptomatic intervertebral disc degeneration. *Connect Tissue Res.* 2010;51(5):397-403.
28. Kim NK, Shin DA, Han IB, et al. The association of aggrecan gene polymorphism with the risk of intervertebral disc degeneration. *Acta Neurochir (Wien).* 2011;153(1):129-133.
29. Eser O, Eser B, Cosar M, et al. Short aggrecan gene repetitive alleles associated with lumbar degenerative disc disease in Turkish patients. *Genet Mol Res.* 2011;10(3):1923-1930.
30. Mio F, Chiba K, Hirose Y, et al. A functional polymorphism in *COL11A1*, which encodes the alpha 1 chain of type XI collagen, is associated with susceptibility to lumbar disc herniation. *Am J Hum Genet.* 2007;81(6):1271-1277.
31. Annunen S, Paassilta P, Lohiniva J, et al. An allele of *COL9A2* associated with intervertebral disc disease. *Science.* 1999;285(5426):409-412.

32. Jim JJ, Noponen-Hietala N, Cheung KM, et al. The TRP2 allele of *COL9A2* is an age-dependent risk factor for the development and severity of intervertebral disc degeneration. *Spine*. 2005;30(24):2735-2742.
33. Paassilta P, Lohiniva J, Goring HH, et al. Identification of a novel common genetic risk factor for lumbar disk disease. *JAMA*. 2001;285(14):1843-1849.
34. Kales SN, Linos A, Chatzis C, et al. The role of collagen IX tryptophan polymorphisms in symptomatic intervertebral disc disease in Southern European patients. *Spine*. 2004;29(11):1266-1270.
35. Pluijm SM, van Essen HW, Bravenboer N, et al. Collagen type I alpha1 Sp1 polymorphism, osteoporosis, and intervertebral disc degeneration in older men and women. *Ann Rheum Dis*. 2004;63(1):71-77.
36. Miyamoto Y, Mabuchi A, Shi D, et al. A functional polymorphism in the 5' UTR of GDF5 is associated with susceptibility to osteoarthritis. *Nat Genet*. 2007;39(4): 529-533.
37. Francis-West PH, Abdelfattah A, Chen P, et al. Mechanisms of GDF-5 action during skeletal development. *Development*. 1999;126(6):1305-1315.
38. Williams FM, Popham M, Hart DJ, et al. GDF5 single-nucleotide polymorphism rs143383 is associated with lumbar disc degeneration in Northern European women. *Arthritis Rheum*. 2011;63(3):708-712.
39. Bachmeier BE, Nerlich A, Mittermaier N, et al. Matrix metalloproteinase expression levels suggest distinct enzyme roles during lumbar disc herniation and degeneration. *Eur Spine J*. 2009;18(11):1573-1586.
40. Song YQ, Ho DW, Karppinen J, et al. Association between promoter -1607 polymorphism of MMP1 and lumbar disc disease in Southern Chinese. *BMC Med Genet*. 2008; 9:38.
41. Dong DM, Yao M, Liu B, et al. Association between the -1306C/T polymorphism of matrix metalloproteinase-2 gene and lumbar disc disease in Chinese young adults. *Eur Spine J*. 2007;16(11):1958-1961.
42. Takahashi M, Haro H, Wakabayashi Y, et al. The association of degeneration of the intervertebral disc with 5a/6a polymorphism in the promoter of the human matrix metalloproteinase-3 gene. *J Bone Joint Surg Br*. 2001;83(4):491-495.
43. Sun ZM, Miao L, Zhang YG, et al. Association between the -1562 C/T polymorphism of matrix metalloproteinase-9 gene and lumbar disc disease in the young adult population in North China. *Connect Tissue Res*. 2009;50(3):181-185.
44. Hirose Y, Chiba K, Karasugi T, et al. A functional polymorphism in *THBS2* that affects alternative splicing and MMP binding is associated with lumbar-disc herniation. *Am J Hum Genet*. 2008;82(5):1122-1129.
45. Karasugi T, Semba K, Hirose Y, et al. Association of the tag SNPs in the human *SKT* gene (KIAA1217) with lumbar disc herniation. *J Bone Miner Res*. 2009;24(9):1537-1543.
46. Kelempisioti A, Eskola PJ, Okuloff A, et al. Genetic susceptibility of intervertebral disc degeneration among young Finnish adults. *BMC Med Genet*. 2011;12:153.
47. Williams FM, Bansal AT, van Meurs JB, et al. Novel genetic variants associated with lumbar disc degeneration in northern Europeans: a meta-analysis of 4600 subjects. *Ann Rheum Dis*. 2013;72(7):1141-1148.
48. Wynne-Davies R. Familial (idiopathic) scoliosis. A family survey. *J Bone Joint Surg Br*. 1968;50(1):24-30.
49. Giampietro PF, Blank RD, Raggio CL, et al. Congenital and idiopathic scoliosis: clinical and genetic aspects. *Clin Med Res*. 2003;1(2):125-136.
50. Shands AR Jr, Eisberg HB. The incidence of scoliosis in the state of Delaware; a study of 50,000 minifilms of the chest made during a survey for tuberculosis. *J Bone Joint Surg Am*. 1955;37-A(6):1243-1249.
51. Ingalls TH, Curley FJ. Principles governing the genesis of congenital malformations induced in mice by hypoxia. *N Engl J Med*. 1957;257(23):1121-1127.
52. Sparrow DB, Chapman G, Smith AJ, et al. A mechanism for gene-environment interaction in the etiology of congenital scoliosis. *Cell*. 2012;149(2):295-306.
53. Pourquie O. Vertebrate segmentation: from cyclic gene networks to scoliosis. *Cell*. 2011;145(5):650-663.
54. Whittock NV, Sparrow DB, Wouters MA, et al. Mutated *MESP2* causes spondylocostal dysostosis in humans. *Am J Hum Genet*. 2004;74(6):1249-1254.
55. Sparrow DB, Chapman G, Wouters MA, et al. Mutation of the LUNATIC FRINGE gene in humans causes spondylocostal dysostosis with a severe vertebral phenotype. *Am J Hum Genet*. 2006;78(1):28-37.
56. Sparrow DB, Sillence D, Wouters MA, et al. Two novel missense mutations in HAIRY-AND-ENHANCER-OF-SPLIT-7 in a family with spondylocostal dysostosis. *Eur J Hum Genet*. 2010;18(6):674-679.
57. Bulman MP, Kusumi K, Frayling TM, et al. Mutations in the human delta homologue, DLL3, cause axial skeletal defects in spondylocostal dysostosis. *Nat Genet*. 2000;24(4): 438-441.
58. Li L, Krantz ID, Deng Y, et al. Alagille syndrome is caused by mutations in human Jagged1, which encodes a ligand for Notch1. *Nat Genet*. 1997;16(3):243-251.
59. Oda T, Elkahloun AG, Pike BL, et al. Mutations in the human Jagged1 gene are responsible for Alagille syndrome. *Nat Genet*. 1997;16(3):235-242.
60. Giampietro PF. Genetic aspects of congenital and idiopathic scoliosis. *Scientifica (Cairo)*. 2012;2012:152365.
61. Erol B, Tracy MR, Dormans JP, et al. Congenital scoliosis and vertebral malformations: characterization of segmental defects for genetic analysis. *J Pediatr Orthop*. 2004;24(6): 674-682.
62. Fei Q, Wu Z, Wang H, et al. The association analysis of TBX6 polymorphism with susceptibility to congenital scoliosis in a Chinese Han population. *Spine*. 2010;35(9):983-988.
63. Giampietro PF, Raggio CL, Reynolds C, et al. *DLL3* as a candidate gene for vertebral malformations. *Am J Med Genet A*. 2006;140(22):2447-2453.
64. Giampietro PF, Raggio CL, Reynolds CE, et al. An analysis of *PAX1* in the development of vertebral malformations. *Clin Genet*. 2005;68(5):448-453.
65. Maisenbacher MK, Han JS, O'Brien ML, et al. Molecular analysis of congenital scoliosis: a candidate gene approach. *Hum Genet*. 2005;116(5):416-419.
66. Weinstein SL. Natural history. *Spine*. 1999;24(24):2592-2600.
67. Andersen MO, Thomsen K, Kyvik KO. Adolescent idiopathic scoliosis in twins: a population-based survey. *Spine*. 2007;32(8):927-930.
68. Ogilvie JW, Braun J, Argyle V, et al. The search for idiopathic scoliosis genes. *Spine*. 2006;31(6):679-681.
69. Axenovich TI, Zaidman AM, Zorkoltseva IV, et al. Segregation analysis of idiopathic scoliosis: demonstration of a major gene effect. *Am J Med Genet*. 1999;86(4):389-394.

70. Cheung KM, Wang T, Qiu GX, et al. Recent advances in the aetiology of adolescent idiopathic scoliosis. *Int Orthop*. 2008;32(6):729-734.
71. Miller NH. Genetics of familial idiopathic scoliosis. *Clin Orthop Relat Res*. 2007;462:6-10.
72. Wise CA, Barnes R, Gillum J, et al. Localization of susceptibility to familial idiopathic scoliosis. *Spine*. 2000;25(18):2372-2380.
73. Chan V, Fong GC, Luk KD, et al. A genetic locus for adolescent idiopathic scoliosis linked to chromosome 19p13.3. *Am J Hum Genet*. 2002;71(2):401-406.
74. Alden KJ, Marosy B, Nzegwu N, et al. Idiopathic scoliosis: identification of candidate regions on chromosome 19p13. *Spine*. 2006;31(16):1815-1819.
75. Justice CM, Miller NH, Marosy B, et al. Familial idiopathic scoliosis: evidence of an X-linked susceptibility locus. *Spine*. 2003;28(6):589-594.
76. Miller NH, Marosy B, Justice CM, et al. Linkage analysis of genetic loci for kyphoscoliosis on chromosomes 5p13, 13q13.3, and 13q32. *Am J Med Genet A*. 2006;140(10):1059-1068.
77. Salehi LB, Mangino M, De Serio S, et al. Assignment of a locus for autosomal dominant idiopathic scoliosis (IS) to human chromosome 17p11. *Hum Genet*. 2002;111(4-5):401-404.
78. Ocaka L, Zhao C, Reed JA, et al. Assignment of two loci for autosomal dominant adolescent idiopathic scoliosis to chromosomes 9q31.2-q34.2 and 17q25.3-qtel. *J Med Genet*. 2008;45(2):87-92.
79. Sanlaville D, Etchevers HC, Gonzales M, et al. Phenotypic spectrum of CHARGE syndrome in fetuses with CHD7 truncating mutations correlates with expression during human development. *J Med Genet*. 2006;43(3):211-217.
80. Gao X, Gordon D, Zhang D, et al. CHD7 gene polymorphisms are associated with susceptibility to idiopathic scoliosis. *Am J Hum Genet*. 2007;80(5):957-965.
81. Montanaro L, Parisini P, Greggi T, et al. Evidence of a linkage between matrilin-1 gene (*MATN1*) and idiopathic scoliosis. *Scoliosis*. 2006;1:21.
82. Qiu XS, Tang NL, Yeung HY, et al. Melatonin receptor 1B (*MTNR1B*) gene polymorphism is associated with the occurrence of adolescent idiopathic scoliosis. *Spine*. 2007;32(16):1748-1753.
83. Morocz M, Czibula A, Grozer ZB, et al. Association study of *BMP4*, IL6, Leptin, MMP3, and *MTNR1B* gene promoter polymorphisms and adolescent idiopathic scoliosis. *Spine*. 2011;36(2):E123-E130.
84. Takahashi Y, Matsumoto M, Karasugi T, et al. Lack of association between adolescent idiopathic scoliosis and previously reported single nucleotide polymorphisms in *MATN1*, *MTNR1B*, *TPH1*, and *IGF1* in a Japanese population. *J Orthop Res*. 2011;29(7):1055-1058.
85. Inoue M, Minami S, Nakata Y, et al. Association between estrogen receptor gene polymorphisms and curve severity of idiopathic scoliosis. *Spine*. 2002;27(21):2357-2362.
86. Wu J, Qiu Y, Zhang L, et al. Association of estrogen receptor gene polymorphisms with susceptibility to adolescent idiopathic scoliosis. *Spine*. 2006;31(10):1131-1136.
87. Tang NL, Yeung HY, Lee KM, et al. A relook into the association of the estrogen receptor [alpha] gene (PvuII, XbaI) and adolescent idiopathic scoliosis: a study of 540 Chinese cases. *Spine*. 2006;31(21):2463-2468.
88. Freely associating. *Nat Genet*. 1999;22(1):1-2.
89. Sharma S, Gao X, Londono D, et al. Genome-wide association studies of adolescent idiopathic scoliosis suggest candidate susceptibility genes. *Hum Mol Genet*. 2011;20(7):1456-1466.
90. Takahashi Y, Kou I, Takahashi A, et al. A genome-wide association study identifies common variants near LBX1 associated with adolescent idiopathic scoliosis. *Nat Genet*. 2011;43(12):1237-1240.
91. Fan YH, Song YQ, Chan D, et al. SNP rs11190870 near LBX1 is associated with adolescent idiopathic scoliosis in southern Chinese. *J Hum Genet*. 2012;57(4):244-246.
92. Gao W, Peng Y, Liang G, et al. Association between common variants near LBX1 and adolescent idiopathic scoliosis replicated in the Chinese Han population. *PLoS ONE*. 2013;8(1):e53234.
93. Londono D, Kou I, Johnson TA, et al. A meta-analysis identifies adolescent idiopathic scoliosis association with LBX1 locus in multiple ethnic groups. *J Med Genet*. 2014;51(6):401-406.
94. Kou I, Takahashi Y, Johnson TA, et al. Genetic variants in GPR126 are associated with adolescent idiopathic scoliosis. *Nat Genet*. 2013;45(6):676-679.
95. Chan WC, Sze KL, Samartzis D, et al. Structure and biology of the intervertebral disk in health and disease. *Orthop Clin North Am*. 2011;42(4):447-464, vii.

9 CHAPTER Twin Studies: Elucidating Genetic and Environmental Influences

Michele C. Battié
Jaakko Kaprio

For the latter half of the 20th century, problems with back pain and degenerative conditions were thought to be primarily a result of excessive loading and the cumulative effects of physical demands on the back. Thus, injury and "wear-and-tear" models were commonly used to explain degenerative conditions and back pain.[1] Accordingly, prevention focused on ergonomic interventions, education in proper lifting and other strategies aimed at decreasing daily loading of the spine, particularly through workplace safety and health initiatives.[2] However, over the past few decades, a dramatic shift has occurred away from this view such that degenerative conditions, such as disc degeneration and lumbar spinal stenosis, are now thought to be substantially driven by genetic factors.[3,4] While environmental factors are also important, exposure to heavy materials handling and other physical demands that were once believed to be the primary risk factors appear to have relatively modest effects overall. Twin studies have been major contributors to this shift in how common degenerative spinal conditions are viewed.

This chapter briefly reviews some of the highlights of what has been learned about common degenerative conditions through twin studies. Many examples come from the Twin Spine Study, a research program spanning more than 2 decades utilizing the Finnish Twin Cohort,[3] and projects utilizing the TwinsUK registry,[5] which have been long-standing contributors in the area. Chapter 8 focuses specifically on genotypes suspected of influencing risk of various common spinal disorders and the biologic mechanisms through which they may act. This chapter concentrates on the contribution of twin studies to elucidating overall genetic versus environmental influences.

Twin Studies

Many traits, conditions, and diseases run in families; therefore, family history is often assessed in the work-up of a patient. However, families share not only genes but also many aspects of the environment (here defined very broadly as all nongenetic influences, be they physical, chemical or microbiologic agents, lifestyle factors, or psychosocial influences). These nongenetic environmental influences are more important during the time that family members share a common household, that is, during childhood and adolescence, but these influences can be maintained either socially or even through epigenetic mechanisms. If we study nuclear families (parents and children), we can observe familial aggregation but cannot be confident in ascribing where it arises from—is it common genes, shared exposures and experiences, or both? Naturally, there may be opportunities to conduct experiments (in animal models) or even interventions/field trials in humans to resolve this, but for many putative causes of disease, such experimentation is not possible logistically or ethically.

One approach to provide more insight into the relative role of genetics versus environment is the study of twins. Two types of twinning exist. First, monozygotic (MZ; early division of the zygote into two individuals) twins share the same genomic sequence and hence are genetically identical, thus often called identical twins. However, external influences act in them in utero and postnatally; thus, they can be and are to some degree phenotypically different from one another. Dizygotic (DZ) twinning arises from the release and fertilization of two eggs. DZ twins are genetically full siblings and often called nonidentical, or fraternal, twins. Both twinning types result in a twin pregnancy with birth of the two individuals at the same time.

For more than 100 years, the realization of two types of twins has led to comparison of the similarity of MZ versus DZ twins to provide information about the contribution of genetic factors. If MZ and DZ twin pairs are overall more similar than two individuals chosen at random from the same population, this result, like those from other types of family studies, is evidence for familial aggregation and familial influences on the trait being studied. If there is no difference in the average similarity of MZ versus DZ cotwins, this speaks to primarily nongenetic family influences giving rise to familial resemblance and suggests the absence of genetic influences. If there are genetic influences, then MZ twins would be expected to resemble each other for the trait in question more than DZ twins, as MZ twins share the same genomic sequence and DZ twins share only 50% of their segregating genes, on average.

For a trait that is due to multiple genes, each of quite small effect, the similarity of MZ twins is expected to be twice that of DZ twins. If assessed as correlations, the expected genetic correlation of MZ pairs is unity (1) and that of DZ twins is 0.5. This has been found to be the case for multiple traits, a prime example of this being height. Such effects are additive across all contributing loci and each risk allele contributes equally in both heterozygotes (i.e., carrying one risk allele) and homozygotes (carrying two risk alleles having twice the effect size compared to heterozygotes). This source of variation in the phenotype is known as additive genetic variance (A). Extensive reviews of twin study designs and modeling approaches are available elsewhere.[6,7]

Genetic effects may also be due to dominance, that is, the sum of all nonlinear effects of alleles at a locus, in which the heterozygote phenotype value deviates from the midvalue predicted from the two homozygotes. The genetic correlation reflecting dominance effects is unity in MZ but only 0.25 in DZ pairs; this gives rise to genetic variance due to dominance (D). Finally, there may be gene-gene interactions or epistasis affecting phenotypes.

Nongenetic variance in a trait is divided into that shared by the twin siblings, that is, those experiences and exposures that make them similar, termed environmental effects in common (C) and those that are not shared; that is, unique to each twin (E). These are distinguished by whether the effects of the experiences and exposures are shared and have equal effects on both twins, not by the actual environmental factor. Thus, if both twins exercise extensively and that has effects on back pain, for example, that will create common (C) effects on back pain, but if only one twin does so, this will result in a contribution to unique environmental effects (E).

Based on these expectations, it is possible to model data from MZ and DZ twin pairs, to derive estimates of the relative contribution of genetics, and thus estimate the heritability of a trait. The latter is defined as the proportion of total variance for a trait accounted for by genetic factors, typically additive (A), but sometimes the overall genetic variance A+D. Of note is that A effects are transmitted from one generation to the next, but D effects are not. The current statistical approaches to modeling permit evaluation of which models best account for the observed variance in a trait, providing the best statistical fit. Thus, we can evaluate which of several models fits the data when a single trait is looked at. The simplest model is unique environment only (E), thus rejecting all evidence for familial effects. As measurement error and random effects are part of E, E is included in all more complex models. An AE model would specify that the pattern of twin similarity in MZ and DZ models fits a polygenic additive model, with no shared environmental effects (C) and no genetic effects due to dominance (D). Alternative models CE, ACE, and ADE can also be specified and tested. By comparing the fit of two models, such as ACE and AE, one can decide whether shared environment (C) effects are statistically compelling. The broad sense heritability or overall genetic influences from both A and D will be primarily reported from the so-called "classic twin studies" included in this chapter.

The statistical models and software to run such models have developed greatly in the past 30 years. At present, many types of multivariate and longitudinal models based on twin data are possible. Multivariate models permit answering questions about the degree of shared genetic or environmental effects across related traits. Such an example is our analysis of the genetic correlation of back pain and MRI-assessed disc degeneration.[8] Likewise, the longitudinal stability and change of genetic effects can be assessed. In other words, are the same genetic effects present in disc degeneration when assessed 10 years later, as the participants have aged? While genes do not change in structure over time, their expression and activity do, resulting in possible novel genetic effects as people develop and age. Finally, these models permit assessment of gene-environment interactions, asking whether a known exposure modifies the impact of genetic variation. An example is the well-replicated finding that physical activity buffers the impact of genes on obesity; among sedentary persons, genes account for a much larger fraction of variance in body mass index (BMI) than among physically active persons. This observation from twin studies[9] has now been extensively corroborated using measured genotypes associated with BMI.[9a] These designs have not yet been extensively used in back pain studies.

All of the aforementioned models target primarily the estimation of familial aggregation and the contribution of genetic and shared environmental effects. There is a massive twin literature on this topic summarized in a recent review article.[10] Nearly all studied traits have some degree of genetic influence.

When studying the association of a putative risk factor or exposure on an outcome, such as back pain, the association may be causal, that is, implying that reducing the risk factor would lead to a reduction in back pain. Alternatively, it can be due to confounding. Measurement of known confounders and adjustment for them in statistical models has been the standard approach in observational epidemiology, be they cohort or case-control studies. However, not all confounders are known or measureable. Genetic factors underlying back pain, as shown by the studies in this chapter, may be shared with genetic effects on the risk factor. Thus, the association of smoking with disc degeneration may be causal (and there are plausible biologic explanations for that) or it may be accounted for by confounders, known and unknown. As smoking itself is, in part, heritable and genes for various aspects of smoking behavior have been identified,[11] there is potential for confounding due to shared genes.

Study designs that adjust for genetic variation made possible by the study of twins are exposure-discordant and matched case-control designs to study nongenetic effects. As MZ twins share the same genomic sequence, all differences between the twins arise from nongenetic causes. If we can identify twin pairs in which one smokes and the other does not (exposure discordant), then a test of the causal hypothesis of the association between smoking and back pain would be to study back pain in a sufficiently large number of such pairs discordant for smoking. If the MZ cotwins who are smokers have significantly more back pain than their cotwins who do not smoke, strong evidence would be provided to support a causal hypothesis. The design controls for genetic background and for sex and age effects as well as the exposures that both twins have shared (such as numerous childhood and adolescent exposures from their common childhood home). Matched case-control designs have also been used for the study of environmental influences on back pain, selecting pairs in which one cotwin has back pain and the other is "pain free."

Critical Importance of Phenotype

It is the observable trait (e.g., lumbar spinal stenosis, disc narrowing, and chronic low back pain), referred to as the phenotype, that we are trying to better understand through whatever genetic or other research is being conducted. Thus, a clear, well-conceptualized case definition is critical, yet often neglected. Inadequate phenotype definitions or descriptions can lead to an incorrect interpretation of results and inability to replicate findings. This problem became very apparent when a simple literature search was performed to identify gene association studies of "disc disease."[29] Definitions of phenotypes under the rubric of "lumbar disc disease" varied greatly, ranging from "discogenic sciatica" with severe, unilateral pain radiating from the back to below the knee to a loss of disc signal observed on magnetic resonance imaging (MRI) regardless of back pain history. Phenotypes of "degenerative disc disease" also lacked consistency in the underlying concept, varying from observations of disc signal loss, narrowing or bulging irrespective of history of back symptoms, to a diagnosis of degenerative disc disease for chronic low back pain for which spine surgery was planned.[29] Such widely varying, disparate phenotype definitions reveal underdeveloped clinical concepts (e.g., degenerative disc disease) that are the root of much miscommunication and misunderstanding. This problem is receiving long overdue attention; there are several international groups currently working toward consensus of broad underlying concepts and associated phenotype definitions of prevalent spinal conditions to create a common language to move the field forward. Furthermore, agreement on phenotype definitions would greatly facilitate the search for associated gene variants, as very large subject samples are needed, typically requiring meta-analyses across studies to confidently identify associated genes.

Phenotype measurement accuracy and precision are also important in all studies, including twin studies, as inaccurate measurements dilute or mask true associations. A couple of examples of this come from twin studies. For example, with respect to smoking, when nicotine intake was of interest and the associated phenotype was defined as the reported number of cigarettes smoked per day, the most strongly associated single nucleotide polymorphism within a cluster of three nicotinic acetylcholine receptor genes accounted for only 1% of the variance in nicotine intake. However, the variance explained by the single nucleotide polymorphism increased nearly fivefold when the phenotype was defined using cotinine, a more accurate biomarker of nicotine intake.[12] Some discrepant findings related to the heritability of disc degeneration, as indicated by disc signal loss on MRI, may have their roots in a similar problem. When defined by a four-point qualitative score, disc signal loss was not found to be heritable in a classic twin study of English and Australian women.[13] However, when using a more precise quantitative, continuous MRI measure of disc signal, disc desiccation was found to be substantially heritable (30%–54%) in a classic twin study of Finnish men.[14]

SECTION I

Genetic Versus Environmental Influences on Lumbar Degenerative and Pathoanatomic Findings

Disc Degeneration

High suspicions of substantial genetic influences are often raised when traits are observed to be much more similar within family members than would be expected by chance. Such was the case for disc degeneration. While there had been a number of previous case reports documenting high degrees of similarity in disc degeneration within family members, it was two studies of independent samples of Finnish male monozygotic twins in 1995, one with 20 pairs and the other 116 pairs, which provided strong evidence of familial aggregation suggesting that disc degeneration may be much more genetically determined than previously thought (Fig. 9.1).[15] Not only were the lumbar spines of the cotwins morphologically similar, as might have been expected, they were also similar in terms of the degree, type, and location of qualitatively assessed degenerative findings (e.g., disc signal loss, narrowing, and bulging) on MRI. The suspicion that the similarities observed may have been largely due to genetic influences rather than shared environmental influences was heightened as exposures to the main suspected environmental risk factors explained very little of the variance in disc degeneration or the high degree of cotwin similarities.

Later, *heritability,* or the proportion of population variance in a trait or disease accounted for by interindividual genetic variation, was estimated for various disc degeneration phenotypes using a classic twin study design and genetic influences were confirmed to be high. In a classic twin study involving primarily English and Australian women (326 twin pairs) reported in 1999, Sambrook et al. found that approximately 75% of the variance in disc degeneration—defined as a summary score of disc signal loss, bulging, disc narrowing, and osteophyte formation—was explained by genetic influences.[13] A later study of a sample of 300 pairs of monozygotic and dizygotic adult male Finnish twins investigated genetic influences on disc signal, bulging, and narrowing and found less dramatic but substantial heritability estimates of 29% to 54% depending on the particular phenotype.[14]

Findings from the latter study also included multivariate analyses to examine shared genetic influences between traits. The findings suggested that disc signal, bulging, and narrowing have primarily shared genetic influences, with lumbar disc bulging and narrowing nearly fully sharing their genetic influences (genetic correlations >0.90). However, degenerative findings at upper and lower lumbar levels have important independent genetic effects. Thus, it may be wise to consider lumbar level when defining phenotypes for gene mapping of

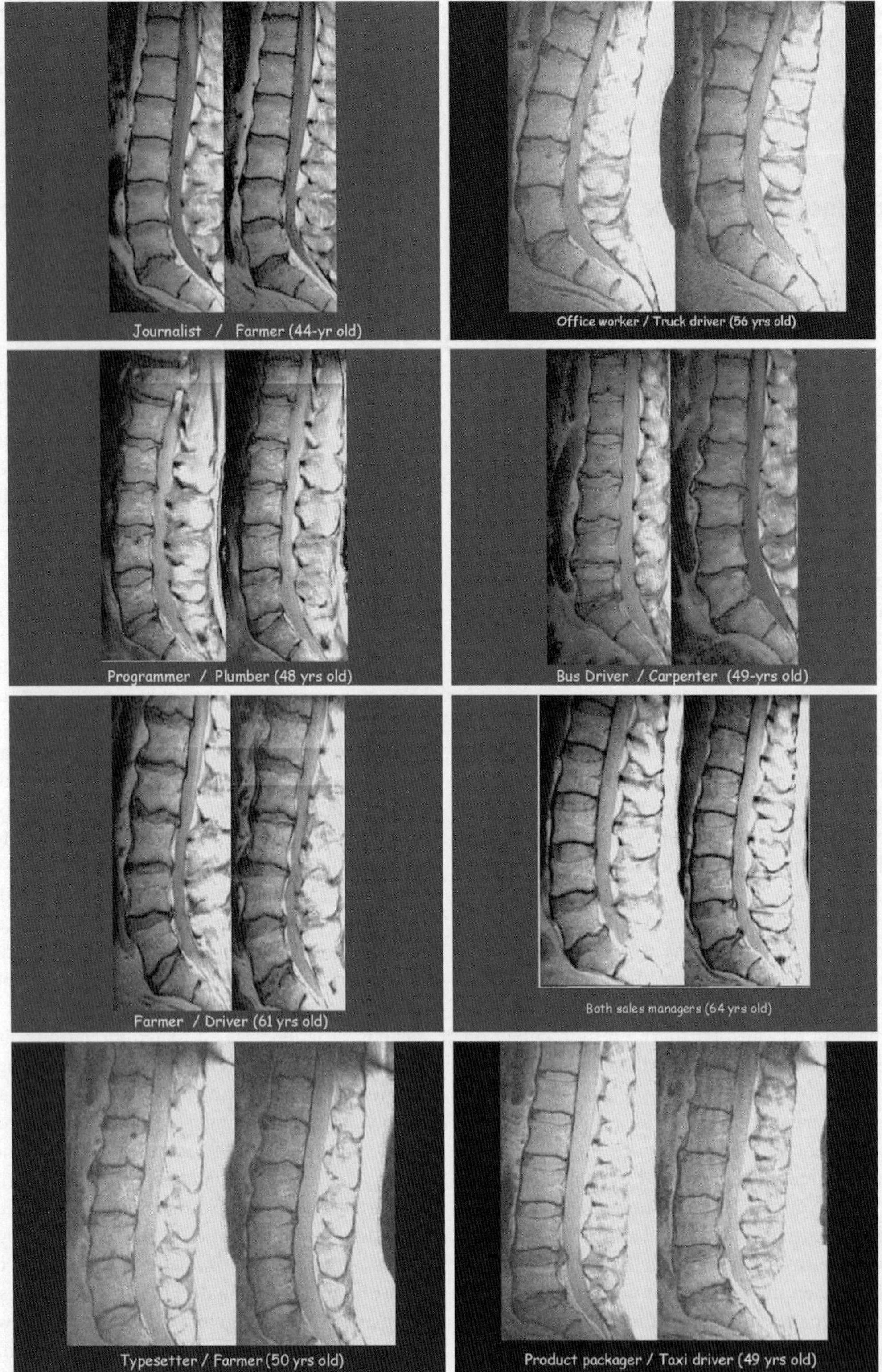

FIG. 9.1 A high degree of similarities in disc degeneration and endplate defects or irregularities was noted between twin siblings, often despite high discordance in lifetime occupational loading histories. (From Battié MC, Videman T, Kaprio J, et al. The Twin Spine Study: contributions to a changing view of disc degeneration. *Spine J.* 2009;9(1):47–59.)

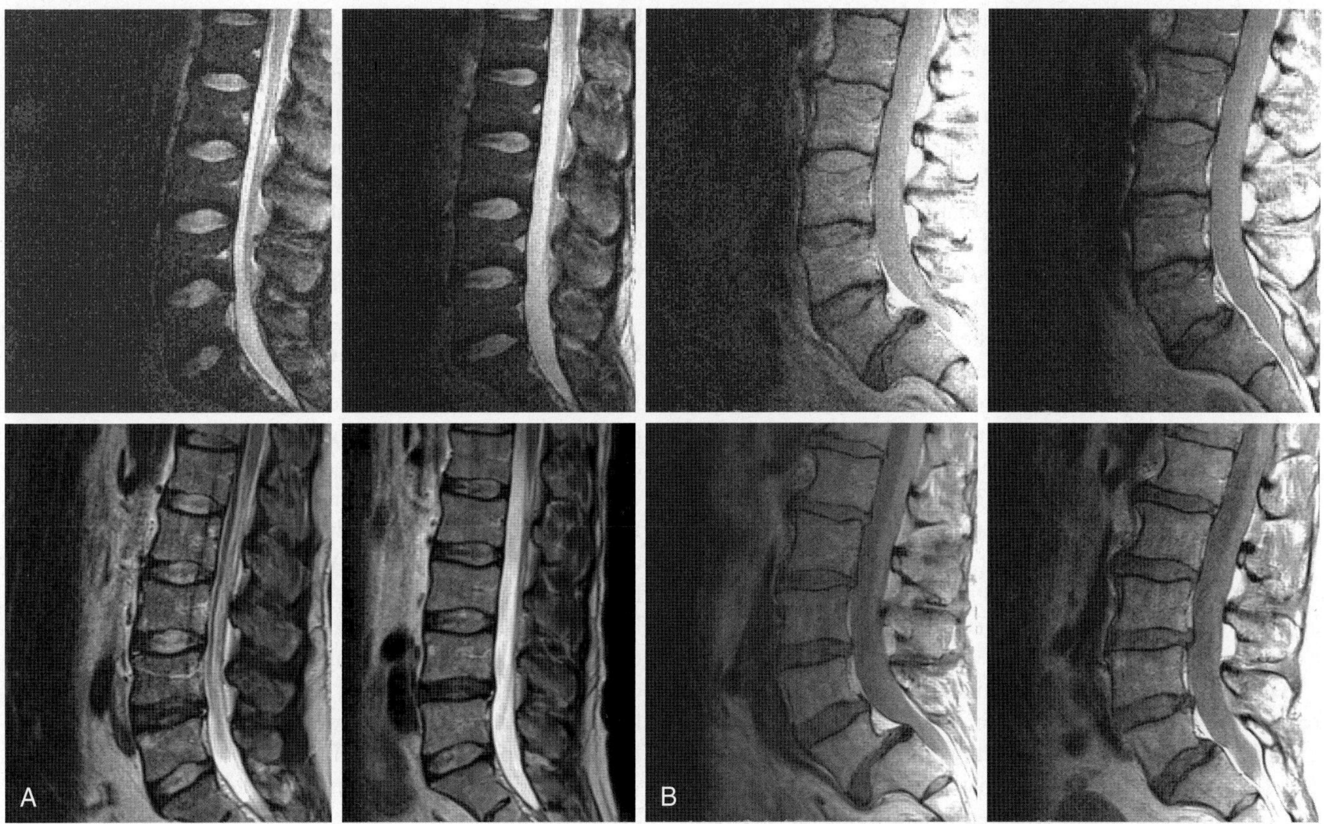

FIG. 9.2 (A) *Top,* Images from a pair of 51-year-old male monozygotic twins from the Twin Spine Study; *bottom,* images of the same pair 15 years later. (B) *Top,* Images from a pair of 36-year-old male monozygotic twins; *bottom,* images of the same pair 15 years later.

disc degeneration and related pathology or, at least, to consider upper and lower lumbar levels separately.[14]

Not surprisingly, as disc degeneration is substantially genetically determined when studied in cross-sectional studies, the rate or progression of degenerative findings (disc signal loss, bulging) assessed longitudinally has also demonstrated familial aggregation and genetic influences (Fig. 9.2).[16–18] Yet, it is interesting that familial aggregation explained 56% of the variance in progression of disc narrowing in 75 MZ male twin pairs,[16] whereas no heritability was found for the progression of disc narrowing in a classic twin study of 234 pairs of primarily female MZ and DZ twins.[18] The contrasting findings are curious, as it seems unlikely that the high degree of familial aggregation for disc narrowing found in the male MZ twins would be entirely explained by shared environmental influences. While heritability of progression is notable, the identification of stark variations in the development of degenerative and pathoanatomic findings between MZ cotwins may offer unique opportunities for exploration of possible environmental and behavioral influences.

When considering overall genetic influences, it should be kept in mind that heritability of a trait in a population is not necessarily static. For example, if important influential environmental and behavioral exposures change over time and explain more or less of the population variance in a trait, all else being equal, there will be inverse variations in the heritability of the trait. In addition, heritability of a trait may vary by gender and age. For example, findings from the previously mentioned twin study of disc degeneration progression in women suggested that genetic influences on progression of disc bulging were only clear under the age of 50 years.[18] While heritability is an important concept related to the overall magnitude of genetic versus environmental influences on a trait at the population level, it must be recognized that there is a highly complex interplay between genetic and environmental factors, as seen in epigenetics and gene expression, for example.

Beyond heritability estimates, classic twin studies with multivariate analyses have allowed the examination of shared genetic influences between phenotypes to test hypotheses regarding shared etiologies or possible pathways of genetic influences on clinical phenotypes. For example, a couple of studies have investigated disc degeneration as one pathway through which genes may influence back pain reporting.[19,20] Both studies identified shared genetic influences between disc degeneration and back pain phenotypes. In one study, significant genetic correlations were observed for disc degeneration (narrowing) and hospitalization due to back problems, duration of worst back pain episode, and presence of disabling back pain over the prior year, but only a minority of the genetic variance of the pain phenotypes examined was explained by genetic influences in common with disc degeneration.[20] Both studies found that while disc degeneration may be one pathway through which genes influence back pain phenotypes, it would appear to account for only a small portion of genetic influences on back pain problems at the population level.

The role of disc degeneration in lumbar range of motion and lordosis has also been investigated in twin studies using multivariate analyses. Findings from the Finnish Twin Spine Study (300 male pairs) suggested that lumbar flexion was predominantly influenced by genetic factors (64%) and extension to a lesser extent (39%).[20] Following an earlier observation of an association between lesser lumbar range of motion and greater disc degeneration after adjusting for age,[21] correlations between the genetic components of the phenotypes were examined. The genetic correlations of lumbar extension and the disc degeneration phenotypes of disc bulging and disc narrowing demonstrated shared genetic influences (r = −0.38 to −0.43, respectively).[20] Thus, one pathway through which genetic influences appear to affect lumbar extension is through degenerative changes of the spinal motion segment as seen through disc bulging and narrowing, which explained approximately one-fifth of the genetic influences on lumbar extension.

Lumbar lordosis has also been shown to be largely genetically determined in a classic twin study of women from the TwinsUK registry, with a heritability estimate of 59% based on 123 twin pairs. While multivariate analyses were not conducted to look specifically at shared genetic influences between lordosis and disc degeneration, more disc degeneration—as indicated by a summary score of disc signal, bulging, narrowing, and anterior osteophytes—was found to be strongly associated with less lordosis.[22]

Modic Changes

Modic changes are signal variations at the endplate extending into the vertebral body as seen on MRI,[23] which have been associated with disc degeneration and back pain.[24,25] Modic changes are classified into three types. Type 1 is thought to reflect edema and is demonstrated by decreased signal on T1-weighted MR images and increased signal on T2-weighted images; type 2, fatty degeneration demonstrated by increased signal on both T1- and T2-weighted images; and type 3, endplate sclerosis with decreased signal on both T1- and T2-weighted images.

A twin study of mostly women from the TwinsUK registry suggests that Modic changes are primarily environmentally determined, with overall genetic influences on their presence estimated at 30%. However, as only T2-weighted images were available in the study, the presence of type 1 and type 2 Modic changes could not be differentiated.[24] Given that Modic changes are associated with disc degeneration, it could be informative to investigate shared genetic and other influences to gain insights into the causal pathways and mechanisms of these phenotypes.

The TwinsUK registry study also found that when both Modic changes and a summary disc degeneration variable—including disc signal, narrowing, and osteophytes—was considered in multivariable analysis, only disc degeneration remained in the model explaining "having ever experienced back pain disability lasting more than one day."[24] Yet our preliminary analyses utilizing the Twin Spine Study cohort as a population-based sample of Finnish men suggest that while correlated, both disc degeneration and Modic changes have modest independent contributions to explaining back pain depending on the back pain phenotype. More research is needed to understand the relationships of Modic changes, disc degeneration, and back pain, with careful attention given to the particular case definitions or phenotypes of each.

Schmorl's Nodes and Endplate Defects

Endplate defects have attracted attention recently as another possible condition or pathology underlying back pain. There appear to be several distinct endplate lesion or defect types, which vary in their association with back pain.[26,27] From visual inspection of the osseous endplates of a large cadaveric study, defects were categorized by Wang et al. as Schmorl's nodes, fractures, erosions, and calcification.[26,27] Unfortunately, challenges in adequately visualizing the endplate on MRI and other clinical imaging modalities create difficulties in both detecting and characterizing endplate defects, but this will likely improve as imaging technologies continue to develop. Presently, given prior and current limitations, endplate defects visualized on MRI are often lumped into the category of Schmorl's nodes.

In another study using the TwinsUK data from over 250 twin pairs, Schmorl's nodes were found to be common in middle-aged women and highly genetic, as indicated by a heritability estimate of 70%.[28] Furthermore, the endplate defects labeled as Schmorl's nodes were associated with disc degeneration and back pain. However, in multivariable analyses, once disc degeneration was in the model, no independent association of Schmorl's nodes with the back pain phenotype remained. Thus, the association of the endplate defects with back pain appeared to be through their association with disc degeneration. A clearer understanding of the interrelationship of endplate defects, disc degeneration, and back pain may require improved imaging and careful attention to the specific definitions of the imaging and pain phenotypes.

Lumbar Spinal Stenosis

Lumbar spinal stenosis is an increasingly common clinical syndrome responsible for chronic pain and disability in older adults. It is considered to be primarily a degenerative condition, but through an investigation of 299 twin pairs in the Finnish Twin Spine study, the pathoanatomic component was found to be *highly* genetic.[29] The heritability of lumbar spinal stenosis was estimated at 67% when assessed from the clinical perspective of an experienced spine surgeon using a standard qualitative rating scheme for MRI. When dural sac cross-sectional area was measured quantitatively across lumbar levels at the narrowest point at each disc, the heritability estimate was even higher (81%).

In the sample of Finnish male twins, spinal stenosis as measured at the narrowest point of the spinal canal at the disc level was explained from the best-fitting model by additive and dominance genetic influences as well as unique environmental effects, whereas the mean anteroposterior diameter of the bony canal, as measured along the length of the vertebral body, had a particularly strong dominance genetic component, suggesting an influence of one or more major genes or important gene–gene interactions. If this is truly the case and is not due to chance fluctuation, there may be implications for the search for influential genes with substantial effects. However, even with a relatively large sample of 598 twins, the study was underpowered to definitively distinguish additive and dominance genetic effects simultaneously.

Disc degeneration as measured through disc bulging and stature as a measure of bone size and development were investigated as possible pathways through which genes may be influencing spinal stenosis. Remarkably, additive genetic influences on dural sac cross-sectional area (measured at the disc level) were fully shared with those of disc bulging, while dominance genetic influences were completely independent. This suggests the presence of a set of gene variants with effects that are additive to each other and usually small and another set of gene variants with specific effects that tend to interact with each other, creating larger effects. Consistent with earlier research (other than on achrondroplasia) revealing low correlations of bony lumbar vertebral canal size and vertebral body size or stature, skeletal size or development as depicted through standing height had no genetic association with dural sac cross-sectional area.[29]

Another interesting finding from the Finnish twin study was that the heritability across lumbar levels differed depending on the particular stenosis phenotype used. The genetic contribution to the variance in qualitatively assessed lumbar spinal stenosis differed significantly by lumbar level, being less at the lower than upper lumbar levels. Yet, heritability estimates were similarly high across all lumbar levels for dural sac cross-sectional area measured quantitatively. This difference in heritability by spinal level between the surgeon's qualitative assessments and the quantitative measurements suggest that the spine surgeon's assessments may be taking other factors into account in determining stenosis beyond dural sac cross-sectional area, which are more affected by environmental influences in the lower than upper lumbar levels.

While a narrow canal, either central or foraminal, is an essential aspect of the clinical diagnosis of spinal stenosis, findings on imaging are generally poorly correlated with symptoms and disability. Thus, it cannot be assumed that the heritability estimates for the pathoanatomic aspects of spinal stenosis will generalize to the clinical syndrome. Furthermore, there are likely to be mediators (e.g., neurovascular or inflammatory factors) that cause symptoms to manifest in the presence of a narrow canal, which may have their own sets of genetic and environmental influences.

Genetic Versus Environmental Influences on Back Pain

Back pain phenotypes, while very important, present many research challenges. Among them are the subjective nature of reported back pain, measuring symptoms that are often transient and of varying intensity when present, and inaccurate recall. Furthermore, there are no universally accepted case definitions for back pain that have been consistently used across twin and other studies, making it difficult to compare study results and conduct meta-analyses.

Despite the challenges, there have been approximately a dozen twin studies of the heritability of back pain, defined in a variety of ways, coming primarily from developed countries of Northern Europe and Scandinavia.[19,20,30–37] Several years ago Nielsen et al.[38] conducted a review of twin studies of pain, which investigated back and neck pain separately from other pain conditions. While they found widely varying heritability estimates ranging from 0% to 68%, when studies of children and the elderly were excluded, estimates were less disparate in the remaining studies of adults. The related meta-analysis of back pain studies yielded an overall heritability estimate of 34% (95% confidence interval, 30–39%). There was also a tendency noted for greater heritability for case definitions involving more severe back pain problems.[20,34]

In the aforementioned review, widespread pain and the diagnosis of fibromyalgia, which often includes back pain, had a somewhat higher heritability estimate of around 50% based on available studies.[38] Concordant with a higher genetic influence on widespread pain compared to single-site musculoskeletal pain, a Swedish twin study found a higher heritability estimate for concurrent back and neck pain (60%) than for either when present alone (24–30%).[35] However, there have been conflicting findings. Heritability estimates for neck, thoracic, and lumbar pain experienced separately or altogether were similar (32–39%) in a large sample (>15,000) of Danish twins, with lower estimates for various combinations of pain affecting any two spinal regions.[32]

Pain comorbidity is common in cases of back pain problems and raises questions about shared genetic or environmental influences, which can be investigated through twin studies. A few studies from the TwinsUK registry have investigated shared genetic influences between back pain and pain at other musculoskeletal sites and chronic widespread pain.[37,39] Both studies, using different analytic approaches, supported substantial shared genetic influences between the pain phenotypes. The authors reported that 39% of the variance in chronic widespread pain and 70% of the variance in low back pain interfering with daily activities due to genetic influences was attributable to shared genetic effects and that roughly 40% and 67% of the residual variation was caused by shared environmental influences affecting both pain syndromes.[39] Moderate to high genetic correlations for pain in different spinal regions (neck, thoracic, and lumbar) have also been found in a large Danish twin study (>15,000).[32] The possibility of largely shared influential gene variants, as well as environmental factors, between back pain and musculoskeletal pain at various body sites and chronic widespread pain has important implications. Such findings may point to systemic pain mediators (e.g., inflammatory and neurologic) or differences in pain processing, rather than purely local factors (e.g., disc degeneration) driving pain, which could inform the search for important causal factors and mechanisms that are needed to develop more effective preventive and therapeutic interventions.

Specific Environmental and Behavioral Influences on Disc Degeneration and Back Pain

Exposure-Discordant Twin Studies of Disc Degeneration

When twin studies were first used in the early 1990s to study the etiology of common spinal conditions, the main suspected risk factors for disc degeneration, pathology, and so-called degenerative disc disease were heavy physical loading (typically occupational), exposure to motorized vehicles and associated whole-body vibration, and cigarette smoking. Effects of height, weight, and genetics were unclear.[40] However, there was much conflicting evidence and uncertainty related to whether or not these factors did indeed affect the disc, as there were concerns about inadequate control of potentially confounding factors in the available epidemiologic literature. This motivated a series of studies using exposure-discordant MZ twins selected from the Finnish Twin Cohort to examine each of the suspected factors.[3] As discussed earlier in this chapter, well-designed, exposure-discordant MZ twin studies provide an exceptionally high degree of control of confounding factors, particularly since genetic influences on disc degeneration are substantial.

The first study of this type related to spinal conditions was of the effects of long-term cigarette smoking on disc degeneration (disc signal, bulging, and narrowing).[41] Findings from the study of 20 MZ twin pairs with an average smoking discordance of 32 pack-years revealed greater disc degeneration in smokers as compared to their nonsmoking cotwins. Also, the difference was present across spinal levels, supporting a mechanism acting systemically. While degeneration was clearly higher in smoking than nonsmoking cotwins (mean, 18%), smoking only explained 2% of the variance in disc degeneration in the study sample. In addition to providing evidence of smoking effects, the study demonstrated the efficiency of the exposure-discordant twin study design in investigating environmental and behavioral influences on spinal conditions of multifactorial etiology.

Subsequently, the same design has been used to study the effects of driving and associated whole-body vibration,[42] heavy physical workload,[3] excessive body weight,[43] recalled trauma or injury to the back,[44] and various types of exercise on disc degeneration in men.[45] The studies of heavy physical loading were remarkable in that despite extreme, long-term contrasts in physical workload between cotwins, related differences between cotwins in disc degeneration (e.g., signal, bulging, narrowing) were modest or equivocal. This was also the case for cotwins who had maintained highly discordant body weight[43] or were discordant in recalled history of back trauma or injury.[44] In 12 twin pairs, in which cotwins had an average contrast of 2300 versus 200 hours of weightlifting exercise, there was only slightly more degeneration seen in the mid- to lower thoracic region in the weightlifters as compared to their MZ cotwins. A difference was not observed in the lumbar region.[45] These findings suggest that routinely performed heavy occupational and leisure physical activities have a relatively minor effect on disc degeneration. Finally, our study of 45 pairs of MZ twins grossly discordant for exposure to driving and associated whole-body vibration revealed no tendency for greater disc degeneration in the drivers, even when considering a range of phenotypes of lumbar degeneration.[42] Collectively, the studies provided strong evidence raising doubts about whether the main previously suspected environmental risk factors were really important causative factors in disc degeneration.

Cohort and Matched Case-Control Studies of Back Pain

There have been several exposure-discordant twin studies of various back pain phenotypes embedded in larger twin cohort studies of back pain, such as an investigation of incident low back pain in 1387 elderly Danes, including 86 pairs that were discordant for occasional strenuous activity at baseline.[46] The more active elderly twins had significantly lower risk of developing low back pain of both shorter and longer duration over the following 2 years. We will likely see many more twin studies of back pain using similar combined study designs, as in just the past year combined cohort and case-control designs have been reported investigating the effects of educational attainment,[47] obesity and body fat distribution,[48] and depression.[49]

Summary

Twin studies have been major contributors to the shift away from the long-standing injury or wear-and-tear model of degenerative spinal conditions, in which exposure to heavy occupational and other physical loading factors were viewed as the major determinants. Following consistent evidence from so-called "classic" twin studies, it is now recognized that spinal function, degenerative conditions, pathology, and pain have important genetic influences. As a result, twin studies have been transformative in changing the research agenda for common spinal disorders.

Furthermore, a combination of cohort, exposure-discordant, and matched case-control twin studies are helping elucidate the effects of suspected environmental factors and have persuasively demonstrated that some factors once thought to have major effects on spinal degeneration (e.g., routine, heavy physical loading) have much more modest influences. Yet, environmental factors are clearly important, particularly for back pain phenotypes, although the specific factors with major effects remain elusive. Twin studies examining gene–environment interactions, which have not yet been widely utilized in degenerative and other spinal conditions, may shed light on such factors and the complex interplay between genetic and environmental factors that surely exists. Finally, much more attention needs to be given to phenotype definition to enhance the success of future twin and other studies of common spinal disorders.

KEY REFERENCES

1. Battié MC, Videman T, Levälahti E, Gill K, Kaprio J. Genetic and environmental effects on disc degeneration by phenotype and spinal level: a multivariate twin study. *Spine*. 2008;33(25): 2801-2808.
2. Battié MC, Videman T, Kaprio J, et al. The Twin Spine Study: contributions to a changing view of disc degeneration. *Spine J*. 2009;9(1):47-59.
3. Malkin I, Williams FM, LaChance G, et al. Low back and common widespread pain share common genetic determinants. *Ann Hum Genet*. 2014;78(5):357-366.
4. Nielsen CS, Knudsen GP, Steingrímsdóttir ÓA. Twin studies of pain. *Clin Genet*. 2012;82(4):331-340.
5. van Dongen J, Slagboom PE, Draisma HH, Martin NG, Boomsma DI. The continuing value of twin studies in the omics era. *Nat Rev Genet*. 2012;13(9):640-653.
6. Williams FM, Popham M, Sambrook PN, et al. Progression of lumbar disc degeneration over a decade: a heritability study. *Ann Rheum Dis*. 2011;70(7):1203-1207.

REFERENCES

1. Videman T, Battié MC. The influence of occupation on lumbar degeneration. *Spine*. 1999;24(11):1164-1168.
2. Chaffin DB. Manual materials handling and the biomechanical basis for prevention of low-back pain in industry—an overview. *Am Ind Hyg Assoc J*. 1987;48(12):989-996.
3. Battié MC, Videman T, Kaprio J, et al. The Twin Spine Study: contributions to a changing view of disc degeneration. *Spine J*. 2009;9(1):47-59.
4. Ikegawa S. The genetics of common degenerative skeletal disorders: osteoarthritis and degenerative disc disease. *Annu Rev Genomics Hum Genet*. 2013;14:245-256.
5. Spector TD, Williams FM. The UK Adult Twin Registry (TwinsUK). *Twin Res Hum Genet*. 2006;9(6):899-906.
6. Boomsma D, Busjahn A, Peltonen L. Classical twin studies and beyond. *Nat Rev Genet*. 2002;3(11):872-882.
7. van Dongen J, Slagboom PE, Draisma HH, Martin NG, Boomsma DI. The continuing value of twin studies in the omics era. *Nat Rev Genet*. 2012;13(9):640-653.
8. Battié MC, Levalahti E, Videman T, Burton K, Kaprio J. Heritability of lumbar flexibility and the role of disc degeneration and body weight. *J Appl Physiol*. 2008;104(2): 379-385.
9. Mustelin L, Silventoinen K, Pietiläinen K, Rissanen A, Kaprio J. Physical activity reduces the influence of genetic effects on BMI and waist circumference: a study in young adult twins. *Int J Obes (Lond)*. 2009;33(1):29-36.

9a. Kilpeläinen TO, Qi L, Brage S, et al. Physical activity attenuates the influence of FTO variants on obesity risk: a meta-analysis of 218,166 adults and 19,268 children. *PLoS Med*. 2011;8(11):e1001116.

10. Polderman TJ, Benyamin B, de Leeuw CA, et al. Meta-analysis of the heritability of human traits based on fifty years of twin studies. *Nat Genet*. 2015;47(7):702-709.
11. Loukola A, Hällfors J, Korhonen T, Kaprio J. Genetics and smoking. *Curr Addict Rep*. 2014;1(1):75-82.
12. Keskitalo K, Broms U, Heliovaara M, et al. Association of serum cotinine level with a cluster of three nicotinic acetylcholine receptor genes (CHRNA3/CHRNA5/ CHRNB4) on chromosome 15. *Hum Mol Genet*. 2009;18(20):4007-4012.
13. Sambrook PN, MacGregor AJ, Spector TD. Genetic influences on cervical and lumbar disc degeneration: a magnetic resonance imaging study in twins. *Arthritis Rheum*. 1999;42(2):366-372.
14. Battié MC, Videman T, Levälahti E, Gill K, Kaprio J. Genetic and environmental effects on disc degeneration by phenotype and spinal level: a multivariate twin study. *Spine*. 2008;33(25):2801-2808.
15. Battié MC, Haynor DR, Fisher LD, et al. Similarities in degenerative findings on magnetic resonance images of the lumbar spines of identical twins. *J Bone Joint Surg Am*. 1995;77(11):1662-1670.
16. Videman T, Battié MC, Ripatti S, et al. Determinants of the progression in lumbar degeneration: a 5-year follow-up study of adult male monozygotic twins. *Spine*. 2006;31(6):671-678.
17. Videman T, Battié MC, Parent E, et al. Progression and determinants of quantitative magnetic resonance imaging measures of lumbar disc degeneration: a five-year follow-up of adult male monozygotic twins. *Spine*. 2008;33(13):1484-1490.
18. Williams FM, Popham M, Sambrook PN, et al. Progression of lumbar disc degeneration over a decade: a heritability study. *Ann Rheum Dis*. 2011;70(7):1203-1207.
19. Livshits G, Popham M, Malkin I, et al. Lumbar disc degeneration and genetic factors are the main risk factors for low back pain in women: the UK Twin Spine Study. *Ann Rheum Dis*. 2011;70(10):1740-1745.
20. Battié MC, Videman T, Levalahti E, Gill K, Kaprio J. Heritability of low back pain and the role of disc degeneration. *Pain*. 2007;131(3):272-280.
21. Burton AK, Battié MC, Gibbons L, Videman T, Tillotson KM. Lumbar disc degeneration and sagittal flexibility. *J Spinal Disord*. 1996;9(5):418-424.
22. Stone MA, Osei-Bordom DC, Inman RD, et al. Heritability of spinal curvature and its relationship to disc degeneration and bone mineral density in female adult twins. *Eur Spine J*. 2015;24(11):2387-2394.
23. Modic MT, Masaryk TJ, Ross JS, Carter JR. Imaging of degenerative disk disease. *Radiology*. 1988;168:177-186.
24. Määttä JH, Kraatari M, Wolber L, et al. Vertebral endplate change as a feature of intervertebral disc degeneration: a heritability study. *Eur Spine J*. 2014;23(9):1856-1862.
25. Brinjikji W, Diehn FE, Jarvik JG, et al. MRI findings of disc degeneration are more prevalent in adults with low back pain than in asymptomatic controls: a systematic review and meta-analysis. *AJNR Am J Neuroradiol*. 2015;36(12):2394-2399.
26. Wang Y, Videman T, Battié MC. Modic changes: prevalence, distribution patterns, and association with age in white men. *Spine J*. 2012;12(5):411-416.
27. Wang Y, Videman T, Battié MC. Lumbar vertebral endplate lesions: prevalence, classification, and association with age. *Spine*. 2012;37(17):1432-1439.
28. Williams FM, Manek NJ, Sambrook PN, Spector TD, Macgregor AJ. Schmorl's nodes: common, highly heritable, and related to lumbar disc disease. *Arthritis Rheum*. 2007;57(5):855-860.
29. Battié MC, Lazáry A, Fairbank J, et al. Disc degeneration-related clinical phenotypes. *Eur Spine J*. 2014;23(suppl 3):S305-S314.
30. El-Metwally A, Mikkelsson M, Ståhl M, et al. Genetic and environmental influences on non-specific low back pain in children: a twin study. *Eur Spine J*. 2008;17(4):502-508.
31. Hartvigsen J, Petersen HC, Frederiksen H, Christensen K. Small effect of genetic factors on neck pain in old age: a study of 2,108 Danish twins 70 years of age and older. *Spine*. 2005;30(2):206-208.

32. Hartvigsen J, Nielsen J, Kyvik KO, et al. Heritability of spinal pain and consequences of spinal pain: a comprehensive genetic epidemiologic analysis using a population-based sample of 15,328 twins ages 20-71 years. *Arthritis Rheum.* 2009;61(10):1343-1351.
33. Hestbaek L, Iachine IA, Leboeuf-Yde C, Kyvik KO, Manniche C. Heredity of low back pain in a young population: a classical twin study. *Twin Res.* 2004;7(1):16-26.
34. MacGregor AJ, Andrew T, Sambrook PN, Spector TD. Structural, psychological, and genetic influences on low back and neck pain: a study of adult female twins. *Arthritis Rheum.* 2004;51(2):160-167.
35. Nyman T, Mulder M, Iliadou A, Svartengren M, Wiktorin C. High heritability for concurrent low back and neck-shoulder pain: a study of twins. *Spine.* 2011;36(22):E1469-E1476.
36. Reichborn-Kjennerud T, Stoltenberg C, Tambs K, et al. Back-neck pain and symptoms of anxiety and depression: a population-based twin study. *Psychol Med.* 2002;32(6):1009-1020.
37. Williams FM, Spector TD, MacGregor AJ. Pain reporting at different body sites is explained by a single underlying genetic factor. *Rheumatology (Oxford).* 2010;49(9):1753-1755.
38. Nielsen CS, Knudsen GP, Steingrímsdóttir ÓA. Twin studies of pain. *Clin Genet.* 2012;82(4):331-340.
39. Malkin I, Williams FM, LaChance G, et al. Low back and common widespread pain share common genetic determinants. *Ann Hum Genet.* 2014;78(5):357-366.
40. Frymoyer JW. Lumbar disk disease: epidemiology. *Instr Course Lect.* 1992;41:217-223.
41. Battié MC, Videman T, Gill K, et al. 1991 Volvo Award in clinical sciences. Smoking and lumbar intervertebral disc degeneration: an MRI study of identical twins. *Spine.* 1991;16(9):1015-1021.
42. Battié MC, Videman T, Gibbons LE, et al. Occupational driving and lumbar disc degeneration: a case-control study. *Lancet.* 2002;360(9343):1369-1374.
43. Videman T, Gibbons LE, Kaprio J, Battié MC. Challenging the cumulative injury model: positive effects of greater body mass on disc degeneration. *Spine J.* 2010;10(1):26-31.
44. Hancock MJ, Battie MC, Videman T, Gibbons L. The role of back injury or trauma in lumbar disc degeneration: an exposure-discordant twin study. *Spine.* 2010;35(21): 1925-1929.
45. Videman T, Battié MC, Gibbons LE, et al. Lifetime exercise and disk degeneration: an MRI study of monozygotic twins. *Med Sci Sports Exerc.* 1997;29(10):1350-1356.
46. Hartvigsen J, Christensen K. Active lifestyle protects against incident low back pain in seniors: a population-based 2-year prospective study of 1387 Danish twins aged 70-100 years. *Spine.* 2007;32(1):76-81.
47. Zadro JR, Shirley D, Pinheiro MB, et al. Does educational attainment increase the risk of low back pain when genetics is considered? A population based study of Spanish twins. *Spine J.* 2016;17(4):518-530.
48. Dario AB, Ferreira ML, Refshauge K, et al. Are obesity and body fat distribution associated with low back pain in women? A population-based study of 1128 Spanish twins. *Eur Spine J.* 2016;25(4):1188-1195.
49. Pinheiro MB, Ferreira ML, Refshauge K, et al. Symptoms of depression and risk of low back pain: a prospective co-twin study. *Clin J Pain.* 2016;[Epub ahead of print].

CHAPTER 10 Outcomes Research for Spinal Disorders

Dipak B. Ramkumar
Adam M. Pearson
Kevin Spratt
James N. Weinstein

Need for Outcomes Research

Outcomes research can be defined simply as "the measurement of the value of a particular course of therapy."[1] It is based on the principle that every clinical intervention produces a change in the health status of a patient that can be measured. The motivation for outcomes research varies depending on one's perspective, but all parties involved in health care have a vested interest in defining outcomes related to medical interventions. Health care providers have a responsibility to provide the highest level of care to their patients, which can be done only if the best treatment for a given condition has been determined through research. Patients need to be well informed about their prognosis, treatment options, and expected outcomes associated with each treatment option so that they can make an appropriate decision with their physician. Private and government payers have the right to demand evidence that the interventions for which they are paying yield improvement in the health of the patients they cover.

The United States has the highest gross domestic product (GDP) in the world and spends a higher proportion of its GDP on health care than any other country in the world, with little evidence to suggest that the level of public health is better than other developed countries.[2,3] Wennberg and Gittelsohn[4] developed the method of small area analysis in which variations in practice patterns, spending, and outcomes could be compared across hospital referral regions. They showed markedly different rates of hospital use between Boston, Massachusetts, and New Haven, Connecticut, for conditions without defined treatment protocols such as back pain, with no discernible differences in outcomes.[5] Using the technique of small area analysis, Fisher and colleagues[6,7] studied the relationship between Medicare expenditures and outcomes in hospital referral regions across the United States, and found no relationship between the level of health care spending and outcomes. The substantial geographic variation in rates of lumbar surgery in the Medicare population was documented by Weinstein and colleagues (Fig. 10.1).[8] These studies have shown that practice patterns vary substantially across different regions, indicating that the "best" practice for many conditions is unknown. The wide variation in the rates of health care use suggests that many regions are not practicing in the optimal zone of use, resulting in "unwarranted" variation due to either "supply-sensitive," "preference-sensitive," or "effective" care, indicating that health services are likely underused in some regions and overused in others.[9–13]

In the past, health care providers have assumed that increased use of health care services was associated with higher-quality outcomes, a relationship that is shown by the upward-sloping portion of the curve shown in Fig. 10.2. Economists have theorized, however, that eventually this curve flattens out such that additional expenditures yield increasingly fewer benefits until there is no marginal benefit (law of diminishing marginal returns).[14] Although it has not been explicitly shown, it is possible that the curve eventually starts sloping downward, indicating that outcomes worsen with increasing use. Such a phenomenon could occur if patients were being inappropriately selected for treatment from which they were unlikely to benefit, but might still experience treatment side effects. The Maine Lumbar Spine Study suggested that such a down-sloping portion of the curve might exist, as outcomes for lumbar intervertebral disc herniation and spinal stenosis were worst in the regions where the rates of surgery were the greatest.[15,16]

Given the wide variation in practice across all of medicine, and spine surgery in particular, policymakers have demanded that the research community perform outcome studies to determine the best practices for treating various conditions. In 2007, a Medicare Evidence Development and Coverage Advisory Committee (MedCAC) questioned the role of fusion for degenerative lumbar conditions in patients older than 65 years and suggested that Medicare could discontinue reimbursement for the procedure unless it could be shown to be effective.[17] In response, Glassman and colleagues[18] analyzed their results of lumbar fusion in this population and found that older patients had equivalent or better outcomes compared with younger patients. Although it is unclear how these data will be acted on, the MedCAC study and response to it

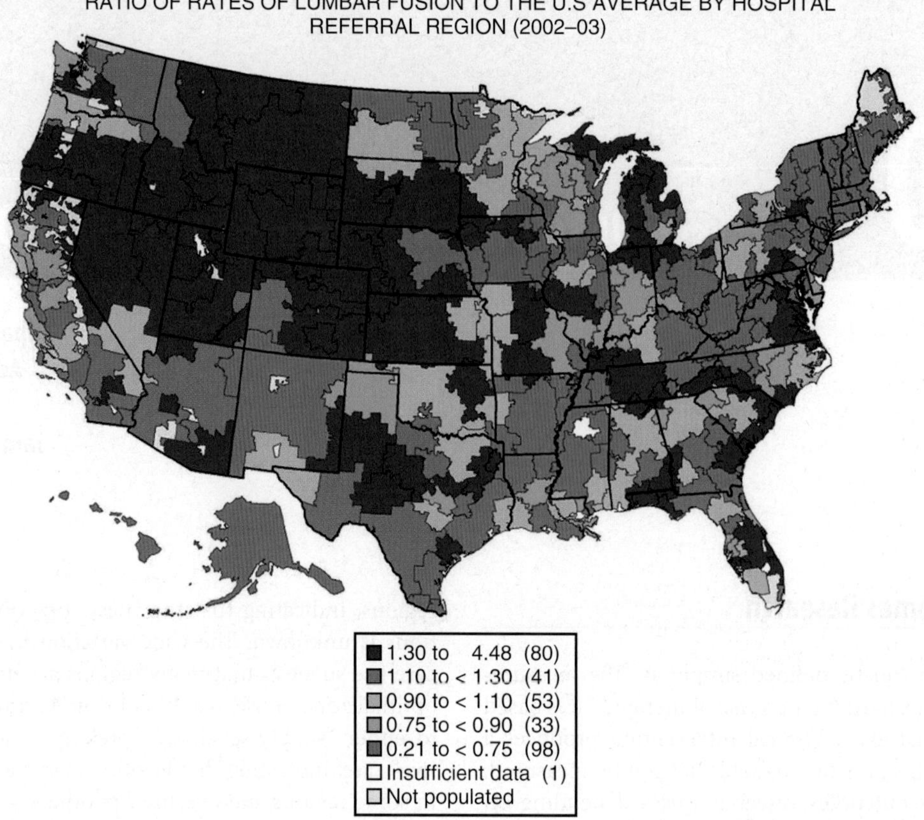

FIG. 10.1 Rates of lumbar fusion in hospital referral regions across the United States in 2002–2003, normalized to average rate. (From Weinstein JN, Lurie JD, Olson PR, et al. United States' trends and regional variations in lumbar spine surgery: 1992–2003. *Spine*. 2006;31:2707–2714.)

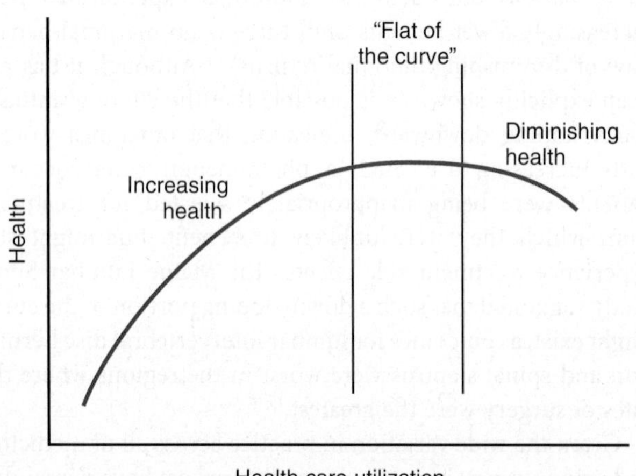

FIG. 10.2 Theoretical relationship between health and resource use. At low levels of use, health increases with use. As use increases, the marginal return decreases until there is no marginal return ("flat of the curve"). In some cases, increasing use could lead to further worse health outcomes.

provide an example of how researchers can respond effectively to policymakers who are looking for evidence to justify health care expenditures. As part of the 2009 economic stimulus package and, more recently, the Affordable Care Act, more than 1 billion dollars has been allocated for comparative-effectiveness health research, suggesting that outcomes and cost-effectiveness research are likely to play an increasingly important role in guiding health policy. This chapter introduces the spine surgeon to some methods of outcomes research, including outcomes measurement, study design, and cost-effectiveness analysis.

Measuring Outcomes in Spinal Disorders

One of the first principles of science is that something must be measured, and a cornerstone of outcomes research is that any change in health status is measurable. Measuring subjective qualities such as pain and function, two important outcomes in patients with spinal disorders, can be quite challenging, however. In the classic literature, outcomes were often physiologic (e.g., motor function), radiographic (e.g., fusion), or subjectively defined by the treating physician (e.g., "poor," "fair," or "good").[19,20] Over the last 30 years, clinical studies have adopted patient-based outcome measures. Outcome measures can be classified as global measures of health (SF-36 Health Survey,[21] EuroQoL[22] Sickness Impact Profile [SIP],[23] and Patient Reported Outcomes Measurement Information System [PROMIS])[24,25] or condition-specific measures (Oswestry Disability Index [ODI],[26] Roland-Morris Disability Questionnaire [RDQ]).[27] High-quality outcome measures need to be practical, precise (reliable), accurate (valid), and responsive.[28]

Practical surveys are of an acceptable length and include easily answered questions so that patients are willing and able to complete them. *Precision*, or reliability, refers to the reproducibility of a survey—will a patient in the same state of health score the same on the outcome measure on different occasions? *Validity* is the ability of the survey to measure the quality that it aims to measure. Assessing the validity of a tool often requires multiple approaches. The score on a new instrument can be compared with a "gold standard" outcome measure to assess its convergent validity. Additionally, the ability of the measure to discriminate between patients in different health states can be evaluated to determine its discriminate validity. Ironically, "face" validity, the concept that the instrument appears to be measuring what it is designed to measure, is fundamental to instrument development and often the weakest form of validity evidence. This is especially true when the group that designed the instrument is evaluating its face validity. Responsive outcome measures are able to detect health status changes in an individual patient before and after successful treatment of low back pain.

In the medical literature, it is commonly held that many of the well-known generic and back-specific outcome measures have been shown to be practical, precise, valid, and responsive, and thus can be considered "validated" outcome measures.[29] From a psychometric perspective, much of this evidence is post-hoc, however, meaning that the instrument's validity is based on its use in a study in which the results showed that one group improved more than another by some statistically significant amount. By this logic, the fact that the tool "worked" (i.e., allowed for a statistically significant difference to be observed) is taken as de facto evidence that (1) the tool is practical because the patients completed it, (2) the tool is reliable because a significant difference between groups was observed, (3) the tool is valid because the goal of the instrument is to document the magnitude of an outcome that was expected to be different for the various treatment groups, and (4) the tool is responsive because the difference in outcomes was detectable. Subsequent studies use these same tools, often for different populations, justifying their use because the instrument has been "validated" in a previous study.

The Spine Patient Outcomes Research Trial (SPORT) intervertebral discs herniation (IDH) study serves as a good example to examine the selection of outcome measures. The primary outcome measures were the SF-36 bodily pain and physical function scales and the ODI (American Academy of Orthopaedic Surgeons MODEMS version). Secondary outcome measures included work status, satisfaction, and the Sciatica Bothersomeness Index.[30] The distinction between the primary and secondary outcome measures was that the study was powered to detect a prespecified difference in the primary outcome measures (i.e., a 10-point difference on the SF-36 scales or ODI), whereas the secondary outcome measures did not factor into the power analysis. As has been recommended, SPORT included a generic (SF-36) and condition-specific (ODI) primary outcome measure.[31] Given the extensive use of the SF-36, ODI, and RDQ in the spine literature, we examine these questionnaires in greater detail.

The SF-36 is among the most commonly used generic health questionnaires, and has been extensively validated across many medical conditions.[32] It consists of 36 questions and can be completed in less than 10 minutes. Responses are scored on eight nonoverlapping scales (physical functioning, role–physical, bodily pain, general health, vitality, social functioning, role–emotional, and mental health), which are summarized as a physical and mental component summary score. All scales range from 0 to 100 (lower scores represent worse symptoms), with the component summary scores transformed to have means of 50 and standard deviations of 10. In looking at the specific scales used in SPORT, the physical function scale is based on ratings of activity limitation (e.g., carrying groceries, climbing stairs, walking), and the bodily pain scale is based on two questions about the severity of pain and the degree to which pain interferes with work. At baseline, the patients in the SPORT IDH randomized controlled trial (RCT) had a mean baseline physical function score of 39.4 (age-adjusted and sex-adjusted norm of 89) and bodily pain score of 26.9 (age-adjusted and sex-adjusted norm of 81), suggesting that they were markedly affected by their disc herniation.

PROMIS is a psychometrically validated, dynamic survey that utilizes patient responses to questions to produce quantitative values to ascertain a patient's state of well-being or suffering.[24,25,33,34] PROMIS aims to improve the quality and precision of measurement of patient-reported outcomes through the utilization of item response theory.[35,36] Item response theory (IRT) is a psychometric method commonly used in education testing. It has recently been expanded to health outcomes research. IRT is fundamentally based on statistical models, which produce calibrations associated with answers to specific questions.[35,36] These calibrations are then processed through computer software in order to select the most informative follow-up question to an initial question, allowing the content of the survey to adapt to the patient's responses to previous questions.[35,36] The PROMIS initiative began in 2004; through continued support from the National Institutes of Health, it has now developed three major instrument types—short forms, profiles, and computer adaptive tests (CATs)—measuring physical, mental, and social health, which have been used across a variety of chronic conditions.[24,25,33,34,37] Short forms are a fixed set of items administered in its entirety. These metrics usually include 4 to 10 items per domain. For instance, the Physical Functioning item bank is comprised of 124 items and has a 10-item short form comprised of a subset of those items. These 10-item short forms have become increasingly popular in the literature for a wide variety of chronic conditions.[37] Recently, Hung et al.[38] reviewed the psychometric properties of the PROMIS Physical item bank and noted that the survey adequately addressed outcomes of patients with spinal disorders with excellent reliability, minimal ceiling/floor effect, and limited item bias. All PROMIS instruments utilize a T-score, for which the mean is 50 and the standard deviation is 10. For most domains, the mean of 50 references the United States general population. In all cases, a high score reflects more of a domain. For instance, a higher score on a physical functioning measure indicates better physical functioning and thus better health, whereas a higher score in fatigue indicates greater fatigue and, likely, poorer health. In utilizing the T-score metric, the PROMIS-10 physical function short form and the PROMIS-13 CAT fatigue short form were found to have greater precision across a broader range of the respective domains than the SF-36.[39–42] Thus, although still a relatively new entrant, utilization of PROMIS metrics is becoming more popular in the research community and will likely become increasingly common in the spine literature.

The ODI was designed specifically for use in a back pain clinic. It asks one question about the intensity of pain and nine questions about the degree to which pain limits specific activities (i.e., lifting, walking, traveling). Scores can range from 0 to 100, with higher scores indicating more severe disability. The mean score among "normals" is about 10, with mean scores in the 30s for patients with neurogenic claudication and 40s for patients with metastatic disease.[43] In the SPORT IDH RCT, the average baseline ODI score was 46.9, indicating substantial pain-related disability.[44] The ODI has been extensively validated and used in the spine literature, and has been recommended to be used as a back pain–specific questionnaire (the RDQ is the other outcome measure recommended for this purpose).[43]

The RDQ is a 24-item survey developed from the 136-item SIP, with the phrase "because of my back" added to the end of the SIP statements to focus the survey on back-related problems.[27,43] The questions focus primarily on function and pain, with only one question asking about the psychological effects of back pain and none inquiring about social function. Each question is a statement about the effect of back pain on function on the day the survey is taken (i.e., walking, bending, sitting, lying down, dressing, sleeping, self-care), with which the respondent must agree or disagree. The number of positive responses is the score (0–24), with median scores of 11 in a population with back pain presenting to a primary care clinic.[45] The RDQ has been shown to be valid and responsive, although reproducibility has been difficult to show because it refers to symptoms only over a 24-hour period. In comparing the RDQ and the ODI, it has been suggested that the RDQ may be better able to detect changes in function in patients with a mild to moderate degree of disability, whereas the ODI may be better suited to patients with a more severe degree of disability.[43]

Experts have recommended using global health and back-specific outcomes questionnaires.[46] The SF-36 or EuroQoL are recommended for measuring global health in spine patients, whereas the ODI or RDQ are the recommended back-specific instruments. In addition to these formal outcome measures, measuring work status and overall satisfaction with treatment is recommended.

Importance of Study Design in Outcomes Research

The goal of any outcomes research study is to measure results from a study sample and extrapolate those results to understand health outcomes in the real world. The results of research studies are highly dependent on the details of study design, however. Reviewing three RCTs comparing lumbar fusion with nonoperative treatment for chronic low back pain reveals one study that showed a clear advantage for surgery,[47] one that showed only a minor benefit to surgery,[47] and one that reported no benefit for surgery.[48] How can three RCTs asking the same essential question come to three contradictory conclusions? The answer may reflect differences in research methods and details of study design. In designing or evaluating a research study, one must consider the research question, the target population and study sample, the interventions being compared, the outcome measures employed, and the specific study design.

A well-posed research question is the foundation of the entire research project. No elaborate study methodology, new data collection technique, or statistical expertise can make up for a poorly chosen research question. For this reason, sufficient time and energy should be devoted to developing, critically evaluating, and refining the research question. In evaluating the results of a study, one must determine what question was really answered because it may be different than what was suggested by the authors.

When the research question has been specified, the next step is to define the target population and study sample. The *target population* is the group of people to whom the results of the study should be generalizable, whereas the *study sample* is the group of patients actually available for study.[49] The target population is defined by the inclusion and exclusion criteria. There is an inherent struggle between having inclusion and exclusion criteria that are very restrictive yet provide a homogeneous study population (i.e., 34-year-old women with left-sided posterolateral L4–L5 disc extrusions and extensor hallucis longus weakness) and criteria that are less restrictive and yield a more diverse study population (i.e., anyone with a disk herniation). More restrictive studies can specifically evaluate the effect of treatment on specific patient subgroups, whereas less restrictive studies are inherently more generalizable. Defining subgroups that have different outcomes is important to determine the best treatment for individual patients, although it is not usually possible to perform separate trials for each subgroup.[50] Understanding the actual target population is essential to interpreting and acting on the findings of a study.

Most clinical studies evaluate the effect of an intervention on an outcome.[51] Similar to the study participants and outcome measures, the intervention also needs to be clearly defined. The intervention for the control or comparative group also needs to be specified. Differences in the experimental and control interventions may explain some of the differences among the aforementioned studies comparing fusion with nonoperative treatment for the treatment of chronic low back pain. Fritzell and colleagues[47] compared three types of fusion techniques with nonspecific physical therapy and showed a clear benefit to fusion. In contrast, Brox and colleagues[48] compared instrumented posterolateral fusion with a very specific program of cognitive therapy and 3 weeks of intensive physical therapy, and reported no differences in results. These two studies did not compare the same interventions, which may be one reason for the discrepant results.

The specific study design used by a research project can have profound effects on the interpretation of the results. Each study design has inherent advantages and disadvantages that must be weighed when planning an investigation. Although the RCT is considered the gold standard of clinical research designs, it is often the case that mounting an RCT before the preliminary case series, case-control, and cohort studies have been performed would be counterproductive. The high cost in terms of researcher and clinical time often greatly outweighs the results obtained from a poorly planned RCT. Before launching a large RCT, observational pilot studies should be performed to generate hypotheses and reveal challenges (e.g., adequate assessment, compliance with treatment, treatment harms and side effects) that are difficult to anticipate. A unique aspect of the study design of SPORT was its concurrent use of an RCT and observational cohort study that allowed patients to choose enrollment in the randomized or observational arms.[52]

Understanding Threats to Study Validity

In general, threats to study validity have been classified as internal and external (Table 10.1). *Internal validity* is related to the validity of the conclusions of a study within the study sample—was the observed difference between the treatment groups real? *External validity* refers to whether the findings of the study can be generalized to populations and settings outside of the study sample—would the difference observed in the trial be observed in the real world?

Clinical studies generally aim to determine if a specific intervention results in a certain outcome. Although a study may show an association between an intervention and an outcome, this association may be spurious (i.e., the association exists in the study but not in the real world), or the association may not represent a cause-effect relationship (i.e., the intervention was associated with but was not the cause of the observed outcome). The two main causes of spurious associations are chance (random measurement errors) and bias.[53] Confounding is another threat to validity that can obscure the cause-effect relationship between the intervention and outcome being studied. Different types of study designs are prone to different types of inferential errors, which are discussed in detail when each study design is considered.

Chance

When an association is observed between an intervention and an outcome, it is possible that this observation is due to chance rather than to the intervention causing the outcome. Fritzell and colleagues[47] reported that fusion for chronic back pain reduced ODI scores by 11 points, whereas nonoperative treatment resulted in only a 2-point decrease. Although surgery effectiveness may have been responsible for the difference, it is also possible that surgery had no beneficial effect and that the observed differences were due to chance alone. Statistical tests are used to evaluate the possibility that an observed relationship between an intervention and outcome was due to chance. In the case of the study by Fritzell and colleagues,[47] statistical testing showed a statistically significant difference ($P = .015$), indicating that the association between surgery and symptom improvement was probably real. Details about the theories underlying probability testing are beyond the scope of this chapter, and can be found in standard biostatistics textbooks.[54]

TABLE 10.1 Internal and External Validity Threats

Internal Validity Threats	External Validity Threats
History: Specific events occurring between first and second assessment in addition to experimental variable	Selection bias: To the extent that patients presenting at study sites are not representative of patients in general
Maturation: Processes within patient operating as a function of time (e.g., favorable natural history)	Reactive or interactive effects: Screening process (informed consent, extra attention, additional procedures to identify inclusion/exclusion criteria) is not done with nonstudy patients
Testing: Effects that testing itself has on subsequent scores	Reactive effects of experimental procedures: Just being in a study may affect patient responses
Instrumentation: Changes in obtained measurements owing to changes in instrument calibration, observers, or raters	Multiple treatment effects: When treatments have multiple components (i.e., surgery, postsurgical rehabilitation) or when patient has multiple treatments (e.g., nonoperative treatment followed by surgery), possible effects of former treatment on latter may influence efficacy
Statistical regression: Lack of reliability in tools, which is especially problematic when patients are selected on basis of extreme scores	
Selection: Biases resulting from differential selection of patients into treatment arms	
Patient attrition: Differential loss of patients from treatment groups (e.g., loss to follow-up, crossover)	
Interactions of above effects: Interactions among above variables may have effects that are mistakenly attributed to treatment	

Bias

Bias is the other major cause of spurious associations. Bias has been defined as "the non-random-systematic error in the design or conduct of a study."[51] Although numerous types of biases have been identified, most bias is related to patient selection, treatment, attrition, and outcome detection. If the patients enrolled in a study differ from the target population, an association observed in the study may not exist in the target population. If the patients who enrolled in the SPORT IDH RCT had less severe symptoms than the target population, the benefit of surgery could be underestimated if the treatment effect is less among this group. Performance bias exists when patients are treated differently in ways other than the intervention being studied, with a "cointervention" being the true driver of the association. If patients undergoing discectomy were more likely to be treated with long-term narcotics postoperatively, the association observed between surgery and outcome could actually be due to narcotics.

Attrition bias results when patients drop out of a study in a nonrandom manner that is associated with the group assignment. If patients who failed nonoperative treatment dropped out of the study to receive surgical treatment elsewhere, the outcomes for the nonoperative patients remaining in the study would be spuriously inflated. Bias in outcome detection can occur if outcome assessors are nonsystematic in their evaluation of patients and tend to change their procedures depending on the assigned treatment. Generally, if the outcomes assessor is not blinded to the treatment received, the assessor is liable to be biased (consciously or not) in his or her assessment. Similarly, patients who are not blinded to their treatment may also be biased in self-reported outcomes.

Bias tends to be insidious; investigators should attempt to prevent it in the planning stages and detect it during the analysis. Efforts should be made to ensure that the patients enrolling in the study are similar to the target population to eliminate selection bias. Blinding can eliminate many forms of bias related to treatment and outcomes assessment because patients cannot be treated or assessed differently if the patient and the assessor are unaware of the treatment assignment. Blinding (shams) can often be difficult, however, or potentially unethical in surgical studies.[55] The best way to combat attrition bias is to limit attrition through aggressive efforts to ensure follow-up. After a study has been completed, the authors should consider the role that bias could have played in their findings and address these limitations transparently.

Confounding

Confounders are variables that are associated with the exposure (i.e., the intervention) and affect the outcome (Fig. 10.3). If patients undergoing discectomy are less likely to be depressed than patients undergoing nonoperative treatment, and depression is associated with worse outcomes, the relationship between treatment and outcome is confounded by depression.

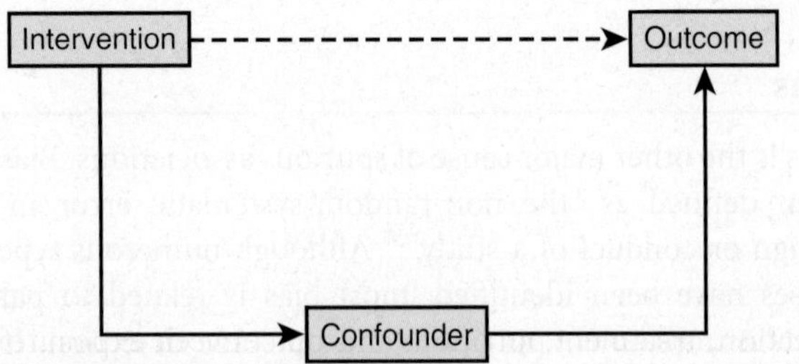

FIG. 10.3 Relationship between intervention, outcome, and a confounder. Although there may be an association between the intervention and the outcome, there may be a third variable, or confounder, that is associated with the intervention but is the actual cause of the outcome observed.

Although the association between better outcomes with surgery is real (i.e., greater than would be expected by chance) in this case, the true cause of the difference may be the better psychological state of the surgical patients rather than the surgery itself. The only way to eliminate confounding is to ensure that the treatment groups are equivalent. True equivalence is never achievable, however, given the vast number of potential differences in patients. The best method to minimize group differences is to randomize in the case of clinical trials, or use methods such as specification or matching in the case of observational studies.

Depending on the nature of the particular study, randomization might be simple (i.e., each subject has an equal chance of being placed in any of the available treatments) or stratified on specific variables of interest given the context of the problem. It is common to stratify patients by gender and age group, ensuring that the various treatment groups are "reasonably" equivalent with respect to these factors before randomly assigning these subgroups to treatment. Randomization does not ensure equivalence for any given finite sample, however. With small samples (≤20), randomization often can fail to produce reasonably equivalent groups. If an investigator randomizes 20 patients, 10 males (M) and 10 females (F), and defines a "fair" split of males to females as 6M4F, 5M5F, or 4M6F, this result is likely to occur 82.1% of the time. More extreme splits occur 17.9% of the time. Thus, with smaller sample sizes, stratified randomization should be considered. Confounding can be a major threat to the validity of observational studies. Strategies to eliminate confounding in observational studies can be used in either the design or the analysis phase; however, potential confounders must be anticipated and measured to be addressed.[53] Specification and matching are techniques that can be used when designing the study. *Specification* involves stipulating a certain level of the confounder as an inclusion criterion. In an observational study comparing discectomy with nonoperative treatment, the investigator could specify that only patients without depression be included to eliminate depression as a potential confounder. The disadvantage of this strategy would be that the results would apply only to patients without depression. Attempting to use this strategy for many confounders would soon become quite limiting. *Matching* is another technique that is often used in case-control studies, in which a control is found for each case that is matched on numerous potential confounders. Although this approach can eliminate the effects of confounding, it also makes it impossible to evaluate the association between potential confounders and the outcome. In addition, matching can be difficult and require a large sample of potential controls to match successfully on many variables.

Analytic techniques are used more commonly than design techniques to address potential confounding. The most straightforward approach is a stratified analysis with a stratum defined for each level of confounder. If many confounders and their interactions are being considered, the individual strata soon contain too few subjects, however, to make meaningful estimates. The most common statistical method used to control for potential confounders is adjustment using multiple regression. The details of multiple regression analysis and analysis of covariance are beyond the scope of this chapter; readers should consult a standard biostatistics textbook for further information.[54]

Randomized Controlled Trials

The gold standard for evaluating the effect of an intervention on an outcome is the prospective, double-blinded RCT. Most providers are familiar with the basic design of an RCT: a group of patients that have met selection criteria are randomly assigned to either the intervention or the control treatment and followed prospectively to compare outcomes between the two groups (Fig. 10.4). The main advantage to an RCT is that successful randomization minimizes baseline differences between the two groups. To the extent that randomization is successful, the potential for confounding by either measured or unmeasured variables is reduced. As mentioned previously, successful blinding of study participants and investigators should eliminate the effects of observer, detection, and performance biases. The double-blinded RCT is the design that most convincingly shows the cause-effect relationship between an intervention and an outcome because it provides the best defenses against confounding and bias.

RCTs can have substantial limitations and disadvantages. They tend to be prospective studies with large sample sizes, and can be very expensive and time-consuming to perform. By design, they usually address only one primary research question. The generalizability of the study can be limited if the patients who are willing to be randomly assigned are markedly different from the target population. The effects of potentially harmful exposures cannot easily be studied ethically using an experimental design, although some trials involving cessation of exposures presumed to be harmful may be possible. Studies of certain interventions, especially surgery, are difficult to blind, and RCTs that are not blinded are subject to observer, detection, and performance biases. Prospective trials in which definitive treatment is not performed at the time of randomization are potentially subject to crossover between treatment groups.

To maintain the benefits of randomization, results should be analyzed using an intention-to-treat (ITT) analysis. An ITT analysis compares the outcomes between the groups based on the treatment assigned rather than actual treatment received. Patients who cross over are analyzed as part of their assigned treatment group despite receiving the alternate treatment. Crossover typically results in an underestimation of the treatment effect of the intervention. Researchers studying treatments in which crossover is likely, such as surgical versus nonoperative care in patients with back pain, are encouraged to develop recruitment, consent, and treatment procedures to minimize crossover, within the obvious constraint that patients ultimately have the right to change their course of treatment. Finally, RCTs are also subject to attrition bias if patients are lost to follow-up.

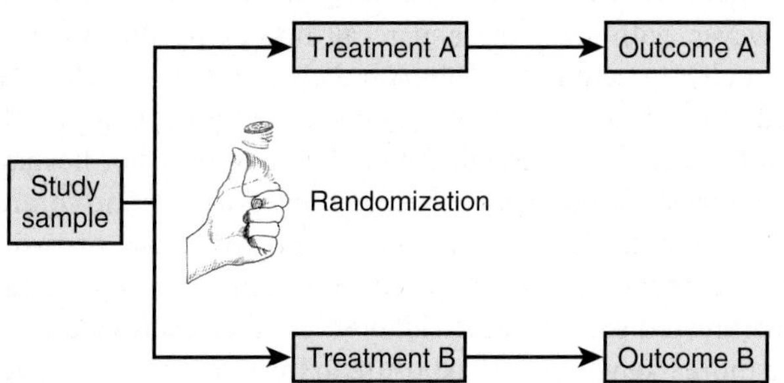

FIG. 10.4 Basic design of randomized controlled trial. Study sample is randomized to different treatments, and outcomes are prospectively determined.

To illustrate how these principles affect the interpretation of an RCT, we consider how these issues apply to the SPORT IDH RCT. Data from this study revealed that there were no significant differences between the surgery and nonoperative groups at baseline on more than 25 variables, suggesting that randomization was effective.[44] Given that patients were randomly assigned to either surgery or nonoperative treatment, blinding was considered inappropriate because it would have required a sham surgery with significant risks.[52,53] As such, the possibility of treatment and detection bias must be considered. Greater than 80% of patients in both groups completed the 1-year follow-up, although follow-up decreased to around 75% in both groups at 2 years. The role of attrition bias should be considered for the 2-year data.

The most striking aspect of the SPORT IDH RCT was the high rate of crossover between the treatment groups in both directions, attributable to the elective nature of the procedure and the generous period allowed per protocol for receiving assigned surgery. In the first 2 years of follow-up, 40% of patients assigned to surgery did not have surgery, and 45% of patients assigned to nonoperative treatment did have surgery.[44] As a result, the surgery and nonoperative groups ended up receiving nearly the same treatment, and the ITT analysis revealed no significant differences on the primary outcome measures. Given the high rate of crossover, the ITT analysis alone does not allow strong conclusions to be made based on the RCT.

Observational Cohort Studies

The key difference between randomized and observational studies is that the determination of treatment is not randomized in the case of observational studies. Thus, in an observational study evaluating an intervention, the patient and physician determine the patient's treatment. The study groups are defined by the presence or absence of an exposure or intervention, and the outcomes are compared (Fig. 10.5). Cohort studies can be prospective or retrospective, but the group assignment is determined by the presence or absence of the exposure in both cases. The main advantage of a cohort study is that the temporal relationship between exposure and outcome is known, making it unlikely that the outcome was actually the cause of the exposure (this is known as "effect-cause"). This type of study may also have better generalizability to the target population because the patient treatment is

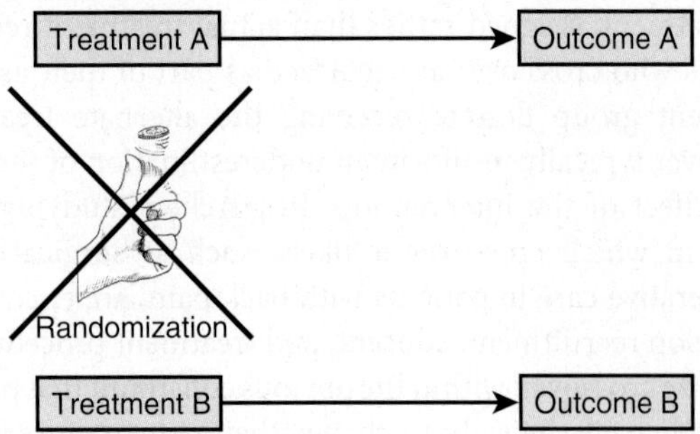

FIG. 10.5 Basic design of observational cohort study. Treatment is chosen by patient and physician rather than through randomization. Study groups are defined by treatment, and outcomes are compared. Cohort studies can be prospective or retrospective.

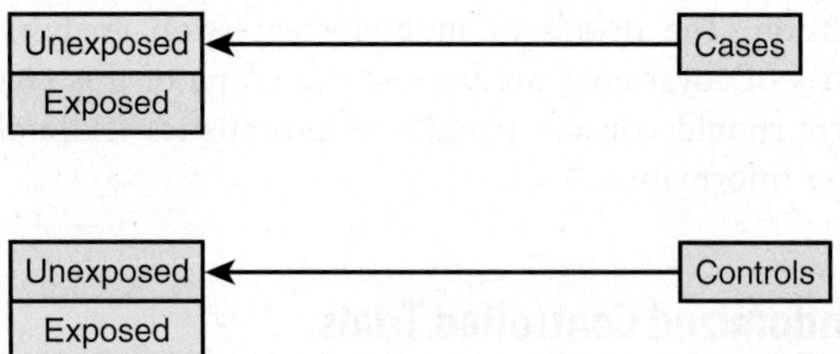

FIG. 10.6 Basic design of case-control study. Study groups are determined by outcomes; patients with a particular outcome are cases, whereas patients without the outcome are controls. This study design looks retrospectively to determine if there is a difference in rate of exposure to a particular variable between cases and controls.

determined in the same manner as for a nonstudy patient. Prospective observational cohort studies are also a very powerful design when randomization is impossible or unethical (i.e., studying a harmful exposure).

Observational studies have many potential disadvantages. Because randomization and blinding are impossible in an observational design, confounding and bias must be taken into account. The two groups being compared often have important baseline differences, some of which can be responsible for confounding. Confounding can be addressed through design-phase and analysis-phase techniques, both of which have been discussed previously. The lack of blinding makes treatment and detection bias possible, and these issues are much more difficult to address. Blinding is often impossible in RCTs comparing surgery with nonoperative treatment, however; thus, the RCT does not always offer an advantage in this regard. Prospective cohort studies tend to require large numbers of patients and can take many years to perform. On the other hand, retrospective cohort studies tend to be much less resource intensive, but evaluation of the exposures and outcomes is limited by what was recorded in the medical record.

Comparison of the SPORT IDH RCT[44] and observational cohort study[56] helps to illustrate the differences in the two study designs. Whereas the ITT analysis of the RCT showed no significant differences between the surgery and nonoperative groups on the primary outcome measures at 2 years, the observational study (and the as-treated analysis of the RCT) showed clinically and statistically significant advantages for surgery on all outcome measures. How should these differences be interpreted? Longitudinal regression was used in the observational analysis to account for potential confounding and attrition related to the baseline variables that were measured. Such an analysis cannot control for potential confounding by unmeasured variables, however. Baseline differences on unmeasured variables could act as confounders and be responsible for some of the differences observed between the surgery and nonoperative groups. Similar to the RCT, the lack of blinding in the observational study limits the control of observer/performance biases. Attrition rates were lower in the observational cohort than the RCT (<20% for both groups at 2 years); thus, the potential for attrition bias is less. Given these considerations, are the results of the observational study valid?

In 2000, Benson and Hartz[57] compared findings between modern randomized and observational studies on various medical questions and found that the results were similar for most studies. In the two instances in which there were different findings between the study designs, the RCTs reported a greater treatment effect than the observational studies. These findings strongly support the validity of well-designed observational studies. Although confounding by unmeasured variables and bias may have resulted in some overstatement or understatement of the treatment effect of surgery for IDH in SPORT, with the numerous potential confounders measured and used to adjust the analysis and the strong effects observed, it seems likely that there was a benefit to surgery.

Case-Control Studies

The case-control study is another commonly used observational design, although it has not been used frequently in the spine literature. In this study design, the groups are defined by their outcomes, and the rates of exposure are compared between the two groups (Fig. 10.6). Typically, cases are identified, a matching control group is assembled, and the rates of exposure to the risk factor of interest are compared between the two groups. The main advantage of a case-control study is its ability to assess risk factors for a rare outcome with a relatively small group of cases in a retrospective fashion. Additionally, the retrospective approach and the ability to examine a large number of predictor variables also makes case-control studies useful for hypothesis generation.

There are many potential pitfalls with case-control studies, however, with sampling and recall bias being the two most difficult to overcome.[58] *Sampling bias* results when the cases and controls are not drawn from the same population. This can be controlled through the use of clinic-based or hospital-based controls, population-based samples of cases and controls (i.e., through disease registries), through the use of two or more control groups, or through the technique of matching, as discussed previously. *Recall bias* can also result when cases are more likely to report exposure to the risk factor of interest, based on their knowledge of the outcome. Recall bias can be minimized through the use of data recorded prior to the onset of the outcome or through the use of blinding.

An interesting feature of case-control studies includes their ability to be "nested" within a defined cohort. This is referred to as a nested case-control or nested case-cohort design. Here, the cohort has typically been assembled for another purpose and, as such, has previously stored images, specimens, and other data, or has been assembled de novo to answer the research question. The investigator would typically measure the outcome variable in this cohort to distinguish cases from controls, and then measure the predictor variables in the banked specimens and images. This allows for comparison of risk factors in the cases and controls. The main advantage of this subtype of case-control study design is that it is especially useful for minimizing costly measurements on serum and other specimens (since these will only have to be conducted on all the cases and a sample of the controls, instead of the entire cohort). Additionally, this design also preserves the advantages of cohort studies that result from collecting predictor variables prior to the occurrence of the outcome.

Although case-control studies have rarely been used in the spine literature, a hypothetical example would be the comparison of the rate of exposure to nonsteroidal antiinflammatory drugs (NSAIDs) between patients with a lumbar pseudarthrosis (the cases) and patients with a successful fusion (controls). This approach might prove useful in evaluating the hypothesis that NSAID use might affect the likelihood of successful fusion. Sampling bias (e.g., differential rates of smoking, diabetes, and other risk factors for nonunion between the cases and controls) and recall bias (patients with pseudarthroses might be more likely to report exposure to NSAIDs) would have to be taken into account.

Case Series

Case series are reports of outcomes for patients undergoing a treatment without any control group. The spine literature is replete with this type of study. No inferential conclusions can be made from case series because there is no control group with which to compare outcomes. Case series should be based on a consecutive series of patients to avoid selection bias in which the investigator includes only patients with desirable outcomes. These studies are useful for hypothesis generating or reporting outcomes on rare conditions. They should not be used to develop treatment guidelines because they lack a control group and do not allow for the assessment of effectiveness of a treatment.

Levels of Evidence

Investigators have created a hierarchy of study designs based on the quality of causal inference that one can make with each study design (Fig. 10.7). Well-controlled RCTs and meta-analyses of such studies are at the pinnacle of the hierarchy. These studies have been labeled level I evidence.[59] Observational cohort studies or RCTs with methodologic shortcomings are level II evidence. Case-control studies are considered level III evidence. Descriptive studies such as case

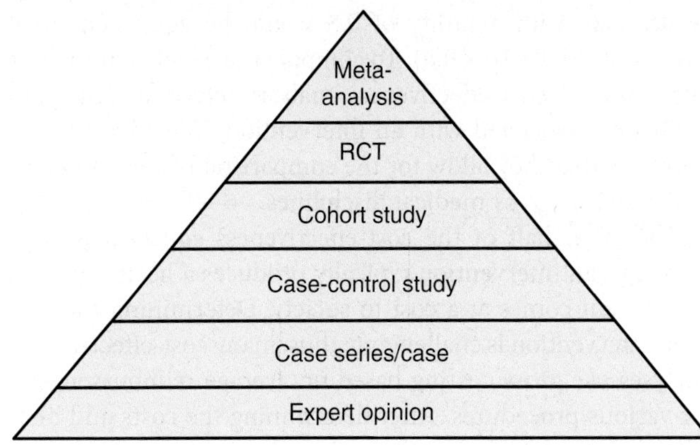

FIG. 10.7 Hierarchy of research designs in evidence-based medicine.

series and case reports are level IV evidence. Expert opinion is considered level V evidence. As shown by the SPORT IDH RCT, all questions are not best answered with a randomized design. In addition, when modern observational studies are compared with RCTs, it has been shown that they do not usually overstate the treatment effect of an intervention.[57,60] Whereas the hierarchy of evidence is useful for comparing study designs in general, the merits of each individual study should be assessed, and high-quality, observational studies should not be discounted.

Cost-Effectiveness Analysis

Given the ever-increasing costs of health care, policymakers have recommended that medical interventions be evaluated for their cost-effectiveness.[61] Cost-effectiveness analysis aims to determine the cost to society for the incremental health benefit derived from an intervention that is more costly than an alternative, less effective treatment. Although an RCT can show the efficacy of a treatment, further economic analysis can be performed alongside the RCT to evaluate how much society must pay for the treatment effect. To compare the cost-effectiveness of a wide variety of treatments across many medical specialties, a universal scale of health must be used to measure preference for health outcomes. In cost-effectiveness analysis, the *quality-adjusted life-year* (QALY), which combines length and quality of life in a single number, is the recommended measure of health benefit.

To estimate QALYs, a *utility*, which is a numeric preference rating of health ranging from 0 (equivalent to death) to 1 (perfect health) is used to value the health states associated with a treatment. Classically, utilities have been derived using techniques such as the time trade-off, which essentially determines how much time in a state of suboptimal health people would be willing to trade for a lesser amount of time in perfect health.[61] More recently, techniques have been developed to determine utilities based on standard questionnaires such as the SF-36.[62] QALYs are determined by multiplying utility for each health state by the length of time in each health state and summing up over time. For example, 2 years spent in a poor health state with a utility of 0.5 followed by 10 years in a good health state with a utility of 0.8 would be equivalent to 9 QALYs ($2 \times 0.5 + 10 \times 0.8$). To compare the benefits of various interventions, cost-effectiveness analysis determines the gain in QALYs associated with an intervention. The advantage of QALYs is that they allow for the comparison of very different health states across medical disciplines.

The other half of the cost-effectiveness equation is cost. Although an intervention typically produces a health benefit, that benefit comes at a cost to society. Determining the cost of an intervention is challenging; thus, many cost-effectiveness analyses use gross costing based on average reimbursements for various procedures. After determining the costs and benefits associated with an intervention, these must be compared with another treatment. This is done by determining the *incremental cost-effectiveness ratio* (ICER). The ICER is defined as the difference in cost between two treatments divided by the difference in utility. Tosteson and colleagues[63] reported that discectomy resulted in a gain of 0.21 QALYs compared with nonoperative treatment at an additional cost of $14,137, which yielded an ICER of $67,319/QALY ($14,137/0.21 QALY). Traditionally, an ICER of $50,000/QALY has been used as a cost-effectiveness threshold because this was the ICER for hemodialysis, an intervention for which society has decided to pay.[64] More recently, some authors have suggested that $100,000/QALY is a more realistic cost-effectiveness threshold because many frequently used interventions fall in the $50,000 to $100,000/QALY range.[63,65,66]

Theoretically, cost-effectiveness analysis should allow societies to maximize the value of their health care expenditures; the United Kingdom has set ICER thresholds to determine which services should be provided by their National Health Service.[67] There is little evidence, however, that health care systems, including systems that currently ration care, have been consistently using cost-effectiveness analysis to guide rational treatment guidelines.[68] As health care spending comes under greater scrutiny and decisions regarding which treatments to provide are made, evaluating the cost-effectiveness of an intervention will be essential.

Future of Outcomes Research: Patient-Specific Recommendations

Since the prior edition of this textbook, the quality of spine outcomes research has improved markedly alongside a more sophisticated understanding of the issues surrounding outcomes research within the spine community. A study of spine-related clinical trials published in 2007 reported that 60% were performed and reported in an acceptable fashion, a result that is better than seen in a general orthopaedic journal.[69] Although this percentage is likely an improvement from years prior, there is further work to be done on the quality of the spine literature. The 4-year and 8-year outcome data from the SPORT IDH study, the largest scale outcomes research study ever performed in the field of spinal disorders, have been published more recently.[70,71] Although this and most large-scale trials are able to determine the treatment effect of an intervention for the "average" patient, it can be difficult to apply the results to clinical practice, in which no patient is "average."

In the case of IDH, there are clearly patients who fail surgical treatment and others who are very successful with nonoperative treatment. Blind application of the results of SPORT to all patients who met the inclusion criteria (symptoms lasting at least 6 weeks, the presence of neurologic findings, and imaging consistent with their symptoms) would result in surgery for all such patients. Although this approach would result in greater clinical improvement than nonoperative treatment, on average, surgery would be performed on some patients who would have improved to an acceptable, and even to a greater, degree with nonoperative treatment. Other patients would fail to improve with surgery and perhaps experience an additional decrease in their quality of life.

To avoid unnecessary surgery on these two groups of patients, models that take individual characteristics and values into account when predicting outcomes are needed. When sufficiently powerful models are developed, individual baseline characteristics, physical findings, and results from imaging studies can be entered into such models to determine the likelihood of success with surgery or nonoperative treatment. Individual patient values should also be considered in defining success and assigning utilities to the various possible outcomes. Such an approach represents the true integration of evidence-based medicine with shared decision making at the level of the individual patient and should be the next step in spine outcomes research.

KEY POINTS

1. With constantly increasing health care costs, policymakers are demanding outcomes research to show the effectiveness of treatments, especially in fields that require expensive technology, such as spine surgery.
2. There is substantial geographic variation in the rates of spine surgery across the United States, indicating that further research is needed to determine which patients are served best with surgery.
3. Chance, bias, and confounding all threaten the validity of conclusions based on clinical research and need to be addressed in study design and data analysis.
4. RCTs can yield the highest level of evidence, although many surgical questions are not amenable to this type of study design. In these cases, well-designed observational studies may be more appropriate.
5. Cost-effectiveness analysis will become more important as decisions need to be made about the use of scarce health care resources.

KEY REFERENCES

1. Fisher ES, Wennberg DE, Stukel TA, et al. The implications of regional variations in Medicare spending. Part 2: health outcomes and satisfaction with care. *Ann Intern Med.* 2003;138:288-298.
   This study showed wide variation in Medicare spending across hospital referral regions with no measurable improvement in outcomes in areas with the highest levels of spending.
2. Weinstein JN, Lurie JD, Olson PR, et al. United States' trends and regional variations in lumbar spine surgery: 1992-2003. *Spine.* 2006;31:2707-2714.

This small area analysis showed the increase in the rate of lumbar fusion in the Medicare population throughout the 1990s and the wide geographic variation in fusion rates in this population.

3. Bombardier C. Outcome assessments in the evaluation of treatment of spinal disorders. Introduction. *Spine.* 2000;25:3097-3099.
This article reviews the differences between different outcome measures used in the spine literature and introduces an issue dedicated to this topic.
4. Kocher MS, Zurakowski D. Clinical epidemiology and biostatistics: a primer for orthopaedic surgeons. *J Bone Joint Surg Am.* 2004;86:607-620.
This is a good review of basic epidemiology and biostatistics as they apply to orthopedics.
5. Benson K, Hartz AJ. A comparison of observational studies and randomized, controlled trials. *N Engl J Med.* 2000;342:1878-1886.
This article convincingly shows that well-designed observational trials yield similar results to randomized controlled trials.

REFERENCES

1. *Webster's New World Medical Dictionary.* 3rd ed. Hoboken, NJ: Wiley Publishing; 2008.
2. Musgrove P, Zeramdini R, Carrin G. Basic patterns in national health expenditure. *Bull World Health Organ.* 2002;80:134-142.
3. Wilkinson RG, Pickett KE. Income inequality and population health: a review and explanation of the evidence. *Soc Sci Med.* 2006;62:1768-1784.
4. Wennberg JE, Gittelsohn A. Health care delivery in Maine, I: patterns of use of common surgical procedures. *J Maine Med Assoc.* 1975;66:123-130, 149.
5. Wennberg JE, Freeman JL, Culp WJ. Are hospital services rationed in New Haven or over-utilised in Boston? *Lancet.* 1987;1:1185-1189.
6. Fisher ES, Wennberg DE, Stukel TA, et al. The implications of regional variations in Medicare spending. Part 1: the content, quality, and accessibility of care. *Ann Intern Med.* 2003;138:273-287.
7. Fisher ES, Wennberg DE, Stukel TA, et al. The implications of regional variations in Medicare spending. Part 2: health outcomes and satisfaction with care. *Ann Intern Med.* 2003;138:288-298.
8. Weinstein JN, Lurie JD, Olson PR, et al. United States' trends and regional variations in lumbar spine surgery: 1992-2003. *Spine.* 2006;31:2707-2714.
9. Fisher ES, Wennberg JE. Health care quality, geographic variations, and the challenge of supply-sensitive care. *Perspect Biol Med.* 2003;46(1):69-79.
10. Wennberg DE, Wennberg JE. Addressing variations: is there hope for the future. *Health Aff (Millwood).* 2003;10.
11. Wennberg JE. Unwarranted variations in healthcare delivery: implications for academic medical centres. *BMJ.* 2002;325(7370):961.
12. Wennberg JE. Practice variations and health care reform: connecting the dots. *Health Aff.* 2004;23:VAR-140.
13. Wennberg JE. Time to tackle unwarranted variations in practice. *BMJ.* 2011;342.
14. Fuchs VR. More variation in use of care, more flat-of-the-curve medicine. *Health Aff.* 2004;VAR104-VAR107.
15. Atlas SJ, Deyo RA, Keller RB, et al. The Maine Lumbar Spine Study, Part II: 1-year outcomes of surgical and nonsurgical management of sciatica. *Spine.* 1996;21:1777-1786.
16. Atlas SJ, Deyo RA, Keller RB, et al. The Maine Lumbar Spine Study, Part III: 1-year outcomes of surgical and nonsurgical management of lumbar spinal stenosis. *Spine.* 1996;21:1787-1795.
17. Schafer J, O'Connor D, Feinglass S, et al. Medicare Evidence Development and Coverage Advisory Committee Meeting on lumbar fusion surgery for treatment of chronic back pain from degenerative disc disease. *Spine.* 2007;32:2403-2404.
18. Glassman SD, Polly DW, Bono C, et al. *Outcome of lumbar fusion in patients over 65 years old.* Presented at American Academy of Orthopaedic Surgeons Annual Meeting, Las Vegas, NV, 2009.
19. Bombardier C. Outcome assessments in the evaluation of treatment of spinal disorders. Introduction. *Spine.* 2000;25:3097-3099.
20. Weber H. Lumbar disc herniation: a controlled, prospective study with ten years of observation. *Spine.* 1983;8:131-140.
21. Ware JE Jr, Sherbourne CD. The MOS 36-item short-form health survey (SF-36): I. Conceptual framework and item selection. *Med Care.* 1992;30:473-483.
22. Brooks R. EuroQol: the current state of play. *Health Policy (New York).* 1996;37:53-72.
23. Bergner M, Bobbitt RA, Carter WB, et al. The Sickness Impact Profile: development and final revision of a health status measure. *Med Care.* 1981;19:787-805.
24. Cella D, Yount S, Rothrock N, et al. The Patient-Reported Outcomes Measurement Information System (PROMIS): progress of an NIH Roadmap cooperative group during its first two years. *Med Care.* 2007;45(5 suppl 1):S3.
25. Reeve BB, Hays RD, Bjorner JB, et al. Psychometric evaluation and calibration of health-related quality of life item banks: plans for the Patient-Reported Outcomes Measurement Information System (PROMIS). *Med Care.* 2007;45(5):S22-S31.
26. Fairbank JC, Couper J, Davies JB, et al. The Oswestry low back pain disability questionnaire. *Physiotherapy.* 1980;66:271-273.
27. Roland M, Morris R. A study of the natural history of back pain. Part I: development of a reliable and sensitive measure of disability in low-back pain. *Spine.* 1983;8:141-144.
28. Lurie J. A review of generic health status measures in patients with low back pain. *Spine.* 2000;25:3125-3129.
29. Zanoli G, Stromqvist B, Padua R, et al. Lessons learned searching for a HRQoL instrument to assess the results of treatment in persons with lumbar disorders. *Spine.* 2000;25:3178-3185.
30. Atlas SJ, Deyo RA, Patrick DL, et al. The Quebec Task Force Classification for Spinal Disorders and the severity, treatment, and outcomes of sciatica and lumbar spinal stenosis. *Spine.* 1996;21:2885-2892.
31. Deyo RA, Battie M, Beurskens AJ, et al. Outcome measures for low back pain research: a proposal for standardized use. *Spine.* 1998;23:2003-2013.
32. Ware JE Jr. SF-36 health survey update. *Spine.* 2000;25:3130-3139.
33. Ader DN. Developing the patient-reported outcomes measurement information system (PROMIS). *Med Care.* 2007;45(5):S1-S2.
34. DeWalt DA, Rothrock N, Yount S, Stone AA. Evaluation of item candidates: the PROMIS qualitative item review. *Med Care.* 2007;45(5 suppl 1):S12.
35. Wainer H, Dorans NJ, Flaugher R, Green BF, Mislevy RJ. *Computerized Adaptive Testing: A Primer.* Abingdon-on-Thames, UK: Routledge; 2000.
36. van der Linden WJ, Hambleton RK. *Handbook of Modern Item Response Theory.* Berlin: Springer Science & Business Media; 2013.

SECTION I

37. Rothrock NE, Hays RD, Spritzer K, et al. Relative to the general US population, chronic diseases are associated with poorer health-related quality of life as measured by the Patient-Reported Outcomes Measurement Information System (PROMIS). *J Clin Epidemiol.* 2010;63(11): 1195-1204.
38. Hung M, Hon SD, Franklin JD, et al. Psychometric properties of the PROMIS physical function item bank in patients with spinal disorders. *Spine.* 2014;39(2):158-163.
39. Rose M, Bjorner JB, Becker J, Fries J, Ware J. Evaluation of a preliminary physical function item bank supported the expected advantages of the Patient-Reported Outcomes Measurement Information System (PROMIS). *J Clin Epidemiol.* 2008;61(1):17-33.
40. Garcia SF, Cella D, Clauser SB, et al. Standardizing patient-reported outcomes assessment in cancer clinical trials: a patient-reported outcomes measurement information system initiative. *J Clin Oncol.* 2007;25(32):5106-5112.
41. Fries JF, Krishnan E, Rose M, Lingala B, Bruce B. Improved responsiveness and reduced sample size requirements of PROMIS physical function scales with item response theory. *Arthritis Res Ther.* 2011;13(5):R147.
42. Fries J, Bruce B, Cella D. The promise of PROMIS: using item response theory to improve assessment of patient-reported outcomes. *Clin Exp Rheumatol.* 2005;23(5):S53.
43. Roland M, Fairbank J. The Roland-Morris Disability Questionnaire and the Oswestry Disability Questionnaire. *Spine.* 2000;25:3115-3124.
44. Weinstein JN, Tosteson TD, Lurie JD, et al. Surgical vs nonoperative treatment for lumbar disk herniation. The Spine Patient Outcomes Research Trial (SPORT): a randomized trial. *JAMA.* 2006;296:2441-2450.
45. Roland M, Morris R. A study of the natural history of low-back pain. Part II: development of guidelines for trials of treatment in primary care. *Spine.* 1983;8:145-150.
46. Kopec JA. Measuring functional outcomes in persons with back pain: a review of back-specific questionnaires. *Spine.* 2000;25:3110-3114.
47. Fritzell P, Hagg O, Wessberg P, et al. 2001 Volvo Award Winner in Clinical Studies. Lumbar fusion versus nonsurgical treatment for chronic low back pain: a multicenter randomized controlled trial from the Swedish Lumbar Spine Study Group. *Spine.* 2001;26:2521-2534.
48. Brox JI, Sorensen R, Friis A, et al. Randomized clinical trial of lumbar instrumented fusion and cognitive intervention and exercises in patients with chronic low back pain and disc degeneration. *Spine.* 2003;28:1913-1921.
49. Hulley SB, Newman TB, Cummings SR. Choosing the study subjects: specification, sampling, and recruitment. In: *Designing Clinical Research.* 2nd ed. Philadelphia: Lippincott Williams & Wilkins; 2001:25-35.
50. Spratt K. Statistical relevance. In: Garfin S, Abitbolet J, eds. *Orthopaedic Knowledge Update: Spine.* Rosemont, IL: American Academy of Orthopaedic Surgeons; 2002:497-505.
51. Kocher MS, Zurakowski D. Clinical epidemiology and biostatistics: a primer for orthopaedic surgeons. *J Bone Joint Surg Am.* 2004;86:607-620.
52. Birkmeyer NJ, Weinstein JN, Tosteson AN, et al. Design of the Spine Patient Outcomes Research Trial (SPORT). *Spine.* 2002;27:1361-1372.
53. Newman TB, Browner WS, Hulley SB. Enhancing causal inference in observational studies. In: *Designing Clinical Research.* 2nd ed. Philadelphia: Lippincott Williams & Wilkins; 2001:125-137.
54. Dawson B, Trapp RG. *Basic and Clinical Biostatistics.* 4th ed. New York: McGraw-Hill; 2004.
55. Flum DR. Interpreting surgical trials with subjective outcomes: avoiding UnSPORTsmanlike conduct. *JAMA.* 2006;296:2483-2485.
56. Weinstein JN, Lurie JD, Tosteson TD, et al. Surgical vs nonoperative treatment for lumbar disk herniation: the Spine Patient Outcomes Research Trial (SPORT) observational cohort. *JAMA.* 2006;296:2451-2459.
57. Benson K, Hartz AJ. A comparison of observational studies and randomized, controlled trials. *N Engl J Med.* 2000;342:1878-1886.
58. Newman TB, Browner WS, Cummings SR, et al. Designing an observational study: cross-sectional and case-control studies. In: *Designing Clinical Research.* 2nd ed. Philadelphia: Lippincott Williams & Wilkins; 2001:107-123.
59. Brighton B, Bhandari M, Tornetta P 3rd, et al. Hierarchy of evidence: from case reports to randomized controlled trials. *Clin Orthop Relat Res.* 2003;413:19-24.
60. Concato J, Shah N, Horwitz RI. Randomized, controlled trials, observational studies, and the hierarchy of research designs. *N Engl J Med.* 2000;342:1887-1892.
61. Gold MG, Siegel JE, Russell LB, et al. *Cost-Effectiveness in Health and Medicine.* New York: Oxford University Press; 1996.
62. Brazier J, Roberts J, Deverill M. The estimation of a preference-based measure of health from the SF-36. *J Health Econ.* 2002;21:271-292.
63. Tosteson AN, Skinner JS, Tosteson TD, et al. The cost effectiveness of surgical versus nonoperative treatment for lumbar disc herniation over two years: evidence from the Spine Patient Outcomes Research Trial (SPORT). *Spine.* 2008;33:2108-2115.
64. Winkelmayer WC, Weinstein MC, Mittleman MA, et al. Health economic evaluations: the special case of end-stage renal disease treatment. *Med Decis Making.* 2002;22:417-430.
65. Laupacis A, Feeny D, Detsky AS, et al. How attractive does a new technology have to be to warrant adoption and utilization? Tentative guidelines for using clinical and economic evaluations. *Can Med Assoc J.* 1992;146:473-481.
66. Tosteson AN, Lurie JD, Tosteson TD, et al. Surgical treatment of spinal stenosis with and without degenerative spondylolisthesis: cost-effectiveness after 2 years. *Ann Intern Med.* 2008;149:845-853.
67. Rawlins MD, Culyer AJ. National Institute for Clinical Excellence and its value judgments. *BMJ.* 2004;329:224-227.
68. Appleby J, Devlin N, Parkin D, et al. Searching for cost effectiveness thresholds in the NHS. *Health Policy.* 2009;91:239-245.
69. Dodwell E, Fischer CG, Reilly CW, et al. *A quality assessment of randomized controlled trials in the spine literature.* Presented at American Academy of Orthopaedic Surgeons Annual Meeting, Las Vegas, NV, 2009.
70. Weinstein JN, Lurie JD, Tosteson TD, et al. Surgical versus nonoperative treatment for lumbar disc herniation: four-year results for the Spine Patient Outcomes Research Trial (SPORT). *Spine.* 2008;33:2789-2800.
71. Lurie JD, Tosteson TD, Tosteson AN, et al. Surgical versus non-operative treatment for lumbar disc herniation: eight-year results for the Spine Patient Outcomes Research Trial (SPORT). *Spine.* 2014;39(1):3.

CHAPTER 11 Finite Element Analysis

Emily Walsh
M. Saeid Asadollahi
Raj Nangunoori
Jie Zheng
Daniel Cook
Boyle C. Cheng
Vijay K. Goel

Introduction

Computational and numeric methods have been used to assess the biomechanical behaviors of biologic systems. The advent and continuous development of powerful computing systems in addition to improvement of the emerging computational packages in computer-aided engineering (CAE) with enhanced modeling features have enabled scientists to develop more rigorous models of biologic systems to predict the behavior of these systems under different biologic conditions. In orthopaedic biomechanics, the latest advances in medical imaging technologies have helped researchers obtain a better resolution of geometric and anthropometric specifications of individual organs in the human body, including micro-scale computational models of the knee, hip, spine, and bone itself.

In addition to ethical considerations, the practical difficulties, restrictions, and cost involved in experimental in vitro and in vivo studies highlight the utility of computational models as complementary tools for studies in orthopaedic biomechanics.

The future challenge will be how to apply these approaches to those areas of science that are not yet considered and how to further improve present generation models to better simulate the couplings and nonlinearities that occur in physical incidents.

One of the most applicable approaches used in biomechanical studies is finite element analysis (FEA), in which the object or system is represented by a geometrically similar model consisting of multiple linked representations of discrete regions. The basic idea for the finite element (FE) method originated from advances made in aircraft structural analysis in the 1940s. Since then, the FE method has become a powerful tool for the numeric solution to a wide range of engineering problems. In this method of analysis, a complex region defining a continuum is broken into simple geometric shapes called finite elements. Material properties and governing relationships are assigned to the elements. With the advances in computational power and computer-aided drawing (CAD) systems, complex problems can now be solved with relative ease. Specialized FE method software—such as Abaqus (Simulia), ANSYS, COMSOL Multiphysics, and others—provides linear, nonlinear, static, and dynamic solutions to many industrial problems.

In general, FEA includes three main steps: preprocessing, analysis, and postprocessing. Preprocessing is the first step in FEA, in which an FE model of the structure is created. Most FEA packages require a topological description of the structure's geometric features as input, which can be in one-, two-, or three-dimensional (3D) form, representing line, surface, or structural elements, respectively. However, 3D models are used in most cases. Design files, CAD models, and preexisting digital scans can be imported into an FEA environment to be utilized for an FEA. Once the FE geometric model is developed, a meshing procedure is used to define and divide the model into small discrete elements. An FE model is defined by creation of a mesh network, which includes the geometric arrangement of elements and nodes. When the FE model is created, the material properties are assigned to the individual parts, and proper interactions and constraints are defined between interacting part and surfaces. Finally, the boundary conditions and loads are assigned to the model.

The next step is analysis, which solves the model to converge for solutions within the predefined boundary, load conditions, and constraints. To better simulate the physical conditions of the problem, different types of analysis, such as static or dynamic (time-dependent) simulation, can be considered. In static simulation, the inputs and outputs are independent of time and the system is solved to balance the load and boundary conditions. In dynamic simulation, time can affect the input and output parameters and the behavior of the model varies over the time. Examples of dynamic simulations are dynamic loading, impact, and long-term creep (or wear).

Once the simulation is finished, postprocessing of the data can be performed using visualization tools. The analysis outputs can be in the form of nodal outputs, including

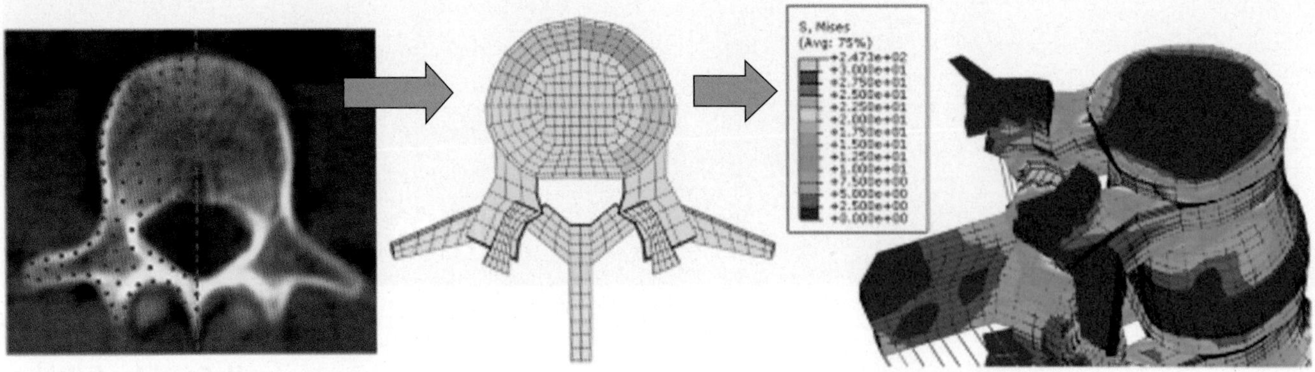

FIG. 11.1 Steps of creating the finite element (FE) model of spine. The computed tomographic images are used to develop a grid at each transverse plane. The coordinates of the nodes are imported to the FE package, and the elements are created. The material properties are defined for individual elements; the loads, boundary conditions, and constraints are defined as the last step in modeling. The model is run and various FE outputs, such as stresses and nodal displacements, are calculated for sections of interest.

displacement at each node and element outputs, such as stresses and strains (Fig. 11.1).

Finite Element Modeling of the Spine

Low Back Pain

The human spine is a complex structure that supports the upper trunk weight and external loads applied to the human body. The spine column also protects the delicate spinal cord and provides adequate flexibility and stiffness to perform various daily activities. The stability of the ligamentous spine is significantly reduced in vivo due to absence of muscles.[1]

Low back pain (LBP) is one of the common musculoskeletal disorders that affects the functionality of the spine. While there are many causes of back pain, the most prevalent causes are muscle strain, degenerative disc disease, spinal stenosis, disc herniation, facet hypertrophy, isthmic spondylolisthesis, degenerative spondylolisthesis, or (rarely) a spinal tumor.

In the United States, LBP is one of the major reasons for disability for people younger than 45 years. More than 80% of Americans suffer from LBP at some point in life. According to an estimate, LBP costs between $100 and $200 billion annually, two-thirds of which is a result of decreased wages and productivity.[1] Thus, there is a need to study the origin of pain associated with the lumbar spine and search for simple, cost-effective, and safe treatment options. While there are a number of avenues that researchers are pursing in this direction, the role of mechanical factors in back disorders is significant. Thus, it is prudent to undertake biomechanical studies of the spine in various conditions: intact-normal, degenerated, surgery, and then "stabilization" of some sort. These issues have been investigated using cadaver models, animal models, and numeric tools. This chapter focuses on the application of numeric approaches in understanding the biomechanics of the human spine, especially the analyses of spinal implants.

The human spine is composed of highly specific tissues and structures, which together provide an extensive range of motion (ROM) and considerable load-carrying capacity.

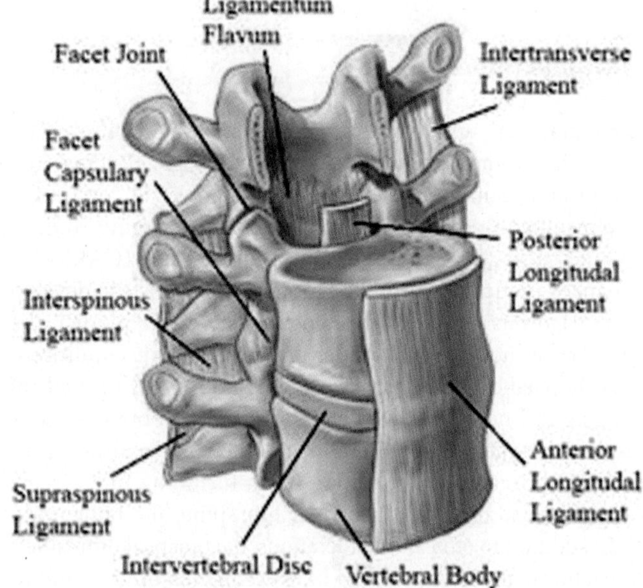

FIG. 11.2 A motion segment in the lumbar spine.

Alteration of the form of these structures with increasing age, injury, or any other reason can have a profound influence on the quality of life. Low back pain is generally associated with degenerative changes occurring in the spine. Mechanical property changes resulting from degeneration are likely contributors to lumbar spine instability that may lead to other pathologies. This instability may be accelerated by injuries or deformities.[2] Vertebral body degeneration and ligament degeneration are degenerative diseases that can occur with age.[3] The intervertebral disc and two facet joints form a three-joint complex and share the majority of the load on the spine.[4] Due to this, degenerative changes of the spine can be initiated as disc degeneration or facet joint osteoarthritis.[5]

In a spine segment (Fig. 11.2), the intervertebral disc and facet joints are the main load-bearing structures in the spine, and thus are most susceptible to mechanical wear and tear. Back pain arising from degenerative disease could be discogenic or may be directly due to diseased facet joints. The advanced stage of disc degeneration or facet degeneration may call for replacement surgery to achieve spinal stability and symptom relief. Disc arthroplasty and facet joint replacement technologies aim to restore the normal kinematics of the spine by acting as load-bearing devices.[5] Surgery for these devices is highly invasive. Replacing either the disc or the facet joint would be considered a partial joint replacement. As load-bearing structures, there is also a possibility of wear of the device, leading to osteolysis. There is a lack of literature on the kinematic effect of these replacement technologies on the remaining structures of motion segments.

Many cadaveric and experimental studies have been formulated to compare the biomechanical behavior of the intact spine versus the injured or implanted spine. Motion across the segments as well as disc pressure measurements and facet loads have been quantified. However, there are many factors that come into play, such as specimen variability and errors involved in experimental testing. In addition, prototyping of many implants at once is not physically easy. Currently, mathematical models are being widely used to quantify forces and moments acting on the lumbar spine during various activities in life. They can be used to quantify stresses at any area and thus point to the area where a fracture might occur. Almost all results seen in experimental testing can be quantified by mathematical modeling. Hence, the use of a mathematical method such as the FE method is justified for the study of the lumbar spine.

Because of the difficulty in analyzing the spine as a whole, it has been divided into a number of regions (e.g., cervical, thoracic, lumbar), and each area has been analyzed separately in different studies. For example, numerous studies of the lumbar spine have applied the FE models of the entire ligamentous lumbosacral spine (LI–S1) or individual lumbar functional spinal units (FSUs; each functional unit consists of two adjacent vertebrae with connecting ligaments and intervertebral disc) to investigate the biomechanical behavior of the spine.

Some of the previous FE models of the lumbar spine have studied only the response of the motion segments, neglecting posterior elements,[6] while the others did the entire motion segment with posterior elements[7] or multimotion segments or the whole ligamentous lumbosacral spine.[8] It is crucial to bear in mind that the simplifications made in the development of the model—such as in geometry, material definitions, load and boundary conditions, and so on—will directly affect the accuracy of predictions.[9]

Once the FE model is developed, it must be validated with relevant in vivo and in vitro test data. The model to be validated should replicate the crucial features and characteristics of the real specimen in order to be able to be compared to experimental data that may help in fine-tuning the FE model. For components such as ligaments, the experimental test data are required to define the true mechanical behavior as well as failure modes and hysteresis characteristics of the corresponding element in the model. All these will enhance the precision of the FE simulations and outputs and will make them comparable with real behavior of the spine.

There are some specific considerations that should be taken into account in FE modeling of the spine in order to make the FE prediction reliable under a specific loading or motion condition. Following are some of these characteristics[10]:

- The geometry of specific features should match the real case, in which the shape of the construct affects the biomechanical outputs; examples are geometry of discs at different levels with the proper boundary profile in the sagittal plane and the proper simulation of the anterior/posterior disc height and the angle between vertebral endplates at each segment.
- The correct simulation of the lordosis angle due to its main role in the stability of the spine under loads and load sharing across the segments.
- The geometry of the posterior bone and partitioning of the bony elements into cancellous and cortical with proper thickness of cortical bone across the vertebrae.
- Proper definition of the element types for specific features, such as ligaments, which can be defined either by two-dimensional (2D) truss or beam elements connecting to nodes of the model with correct moment arm with respect to the center of the segment. Ligaments can be modeled either as a bundle with appropriate cross-section or as a combination of individual truss elements with cross-section of unity.
- The geometry of the facet articulations with their gap distance and likely asymmetry.
- Contact pattern between the articulating surfaces of facets as a finite large-displacement contact problem with proper sliding (with or without friction) and normal (soft or hard) behavior.
- The disc should be modeled as a nonhomogeneous composite structure, including an amorphous matrix (protoglycan and water) reinforced by collagenous fibers. Proper element types should be used for each area of the disc, that is, the nucleus can be modeled with noncompressible fluid elements, while the anulus can be modeled with solid elastic elements with fibers at proper angles by considering the radial variation of the collagenous fibers' mechanical properties and volume fracture.
- In case a nonstatic simulation—such as dynamic loading, impact, long-term creep and wear—is being considered, the time-dependent behavior of elements and materials needs to be specified.
- The definition of loads and boundary conditions for example, if the study of kinematics of L3–S1 spine is of interest, S1 is fixed in all degrees of freedom and the compressive loads and bending moments are applied at L3 level.

Modeling of the Lumbar Spine

The first intact FE model of the ligamentous lumbar spine that was developed consisted of two motion segments (L3–L5).[11] The geometric data for the L3–L4 motion segment were acquired from 1.5-mm thick computed tomography (CT) scans (transverse slices) of a cadaveric ligamentous spine specimen. Radiographs and dual-energy x-ray absorptiometry (DEXA) were used to ensure that no osseous abnormalities existed with the specimen and that the bone quality was good. Each region was then divided into several quadrilaterally shaped elements. The four nodes characterizing a particular element were digitized to obtain their X and Z coordinates with respect to the global axes system. The Y coordinate equaled the depth of the corresponding transverse slice on the CT film. The transverse cross-sectional shape of an intact normal specimen is symmetric about the midsagittal plane. Thus, only one-half of the model was digitized; the other half was simulated as a reflection of the first half automatically by the FE software. The coordinate data of elements from different cross-sections were then assembled to generate three-dimensional meshes. The midtransverse plane of the L3–L4 disc was horizontal. A lordotic curve of approximately 9 degrees was simulated at the L4–L5 level of the FE model, based on the anthropometric data. The model validation study was undertaken by Kong.[12]

Then, the L5–S1 disc and the S1 vertebral body were added to the existing L3–L5 model to construct an L3–S1 segment. A total lordotic curve of approximately 27 degrees was simulated across the L3–S1 level with the mid-L3–L4 disc kept horizontal. The concluding L3–S1 model has a total of 27,540 elements and 32,946 nodes (Fig. 11.3). The number of elements and the material properties of the intact L3–S1 model are presented in Table 11.1.

Vertebral Body and Posterior Bone

The vertebral body and posterior bony regions were defined using three-dimensional solid continuum hexagonal elements with eight nodes, each possessing six degrees of freedom. The vertebral bodies were modeled as a cancellous (porous) bone core surrounded by a 0.5-mm thick cortical (dense) bone shell. The appropriate isotropic material properties were defined for the respective regions (see Table 11.1).

Intervertebral Disc

The intervertebral disc was modeled as the anulus fibrosus and nucleus pulposus. The anulus fibrosus was modeled as a composite solid ground substance, reinforced with embedded fibers. The ground substance was made up of 3D solid hexagonal elements. The REBAR option (Abaqus) was used to define the fibers, which were oriented at alternating angles ±30 degrees to the horizontal. The "no compression" option was used for the REBAR elements such that they could transmit

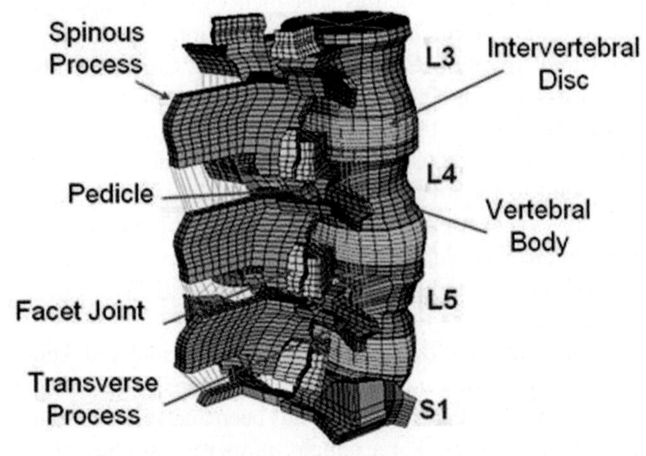

FIG. 11.3 Finite element model of the ligamentous L3–S1 segment.

TABLE 11.1 Element Types and Material Properties for the Intact L3–S1 Finite Element Spine Model

Element Set	Elements (n)	Element Type	Young's Modulus (MPa)	Poisson's Ratio	Cross-Sectional Area (mm²)
Bony Regions					
Vertebral cortical bone	3312	C3D8	12,000	0.30	
Vertebral cancellous	10,608	C3D8	100	0.20	
Posterior cortical bone	3632	C3D8	12,000	0.30	
Posterior cancellous	1834	C3D8	100	0.20	
Intervertebral Disc					
Anulus (ground)	5376	C3D8	1.2	0.45	
Anulus fibers	2685	REBAR	357.5–550	0.30	0.00601–0.00884
Nucleus pulposus	1920	C3D8	1.0	0.4999	
Joints					
Apophyseal joints	216	GAPUNI	Softened, 12,000		
Ligaments					
Anterior longitudinal	216	T3D2	7.8 (<12%), 20.0 (>12%)	0.30	74
Posterior longitudinal	144	T3D2	10.0 (<11%), 20.0 (>11%)	0.30	14.4
Intertransverse	30	T3D2	10.0 (<18%), 58.7 (>18%)	0.30	1.8
Ligamentum flavum	21	T3D2	15.0 (<6.2%),19.5 (>6.2%)	0.30	40
Interspinous	21	T3D2	9.8 (<14%), 12.0 (>14%)	0.30	40
Supraspinous	9	T3D2	8.8 (<20%), 15.0 (>20%)	0.30	30
Capsular	84	T3D2	8.48 (<25%), 32.9 (>25%)	0.30	34

GAPUNI, two-node unidirectional gap element.
From Dooris A. *Experimental and Theoretical Investigations Into the Effects of Artificial Disc Implantation.* Doctoral dissertation. Iowa City: University of Iowa; 2001.

only tension; also, the fiber thickness and stiffness increased in the radial direction. An overall collagenous fiber content of 16% of the annular volume was distributed in the anulus.

The nucleus pulposus was modeled with C3D8 hexagonal elements. Isotropic material property with a stiffness of 1 MPa and near incompressibility simulated with a Poisson's v = 0.4999 was assigned to the nucleus to simulate its hydrostatic characteristics.

Apophyseal (Facet) Joint

Simulation of the facet joints is crucial for the spine model since it drastically affects the outcome of the analysis. In this model, the facet joints were simulated using 20 three-dimensional gap elements (GAPUNI). The facets were oriented at an inclination of 72 degrees from the horizontal plane. An initial gap of 0.5 mm was specified between these elements. Force is transmitted by using the Abaqus "softened contact," which exponentially adjusts the force transfer as the gap is closed. At full closure, the joint assumes the same stiffness as the posterior bone (Fig. 11.4).

Ligaments

All seven major ligaments—interspinous, supraspinous, intertransverse, capsular, posterior longitudinal, anterior longitudinal, and ligamentum flavum—were simulated in the model. The ligaments were modeled using three-dimensional two-node truss elements (T3D2). Hypoelastic material properties were assigned to each of these ligaments, allowing a "neutral zone" to be incorporated in which the ligament provided little stability under minimally applied external loads. The hypoelastic material definition was given by specifying varying Young's modulus and Poisson's ratio along with the strain invariants at the specified strain rate. The material properties of ligaments were taken from the literature, including our own experimental data.[13] The defining elements were aligned along the respective ligament fiber orientation. Although the ligamentum flavum and the longitudinal ligaments experience a prestress at rest, all ligaments were assumed to be unstressed initially. Modeling the ligaments causes nonlinearity in kinematics of the spine model (see Fig. 11.3).

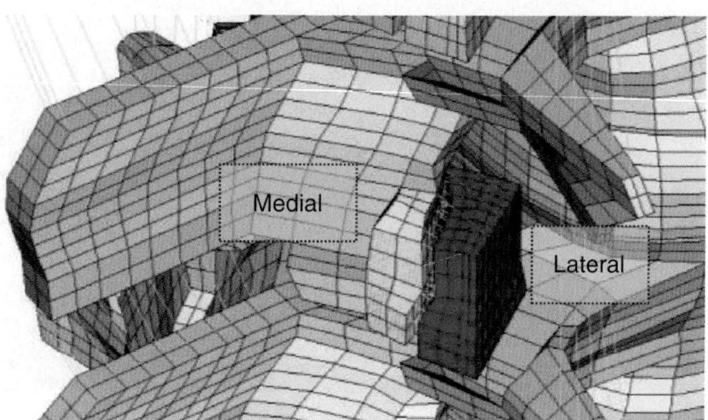

FIG. 11.4 Facet joint in the finite element model of the L3–S1 spine.

The entire process of developing the FE models of the spine has been simplified due to the advances in technology.

The reconstruction of soft tissue and hard tissue geometry from magnetic resonance imaging (MRI) and CT scans is completed through the use of Mimics v15.0 (Materialise). MRI is capable of imaging both hard and soft tissue (vertebrae and intervertebral discs) through manual segmenting. CT scans are capable of autosegmenting hard bone tissue but are difficult to use for reconstruction of soft tissue. The segmented geometry is exported in the form of a standard triangle language (STL) surface file. These files (especially manually segmented geometries) are not smooth and require further processing.

Surface processing of the reconstructed geometry is conducted in Geomagic Studio 2014. This software is a reverse-engineering software that provides surface geometry modifications. After importing the geometry, there are various functions that allow the surface to be precisely smoothed and edited. The smoothing is utilized to be able to achieve uniform meshes that are critical for achieving accurate and stable FE solutions. The editing that is conducted is used to adjust the overlapping surfaces to satisfy the requirements of the FE analysis software.

The prepared surface geometry is then imported into HyperMesh 14.0 (Altair) to create the three-dimensional meshes. These meshes are created such that they have optimal Jacobian and aspect ratios. Multiple mesh densities are created of each body to then perform mesh convergence. Mesh convergence is used to show that the solution of the FE problem is independent of mesh density. This method allows us to utilize accurate mesh with the lowest possible computational expense.

The converged mesh is then imported into Abaqus 6.14 (Simulia), and constructed. The construction of the model consists of assigning material properties to all geometries. Abaqus has the capability of assigning a variety of material types and constitutive models to accurately simulate the linear elastic, plastic, and hyperelastic properties of bones, implants, and soft tissue. Interactions are then generated to tie surfaces together, such as the vertebral endplate to the intervertebral disc. Interactions are also used to generate contact definitions, such as the articulation between a cage and endplate, to accurately simulate the contact force, contact area, stress, displacement, and so on. The appropriate one-dimensional elements are then added to the model to represent the small soft-tissue restraints that are not able to be reconstructed through MRI or CT data. Loading and boundary conditions are then applied to simulate various clinically relevant conditions. The outputs of the model are ROM, stress, strain, force, and contact mechanics in all of the reconstructed and instrumented geometries. Complex subroutines are available to simulate growth and deformities of the spine. Last, both static and dynamic loading scenarios are available to fully capture all studies of interest.

Validation of the Lumbar Model

Formulating an FE model for a biologic system often involves making justifiable assumptions. Validation of an FE model is essential in order to indicate whether the model predictions are similar to the experimental predictions. Previous biomechanical studies using the intact two-segment FE model were validated with experimental in vitro studies.[12,14–17]

Axial compressive preload acts as the major component of the in vivo preload. The exact degree and magnitude of the net preload relies on the degree of lumbar lordosis and the posture of the individual during physiologic loading. Axial compressive preload affects the load displacement characteristics of the joint.[4] The model was subjected to an axial preload of 400 N as a follower load since it is physiologic. In addition to the axial preload, motion was predicted for all six degrees of freedom with a moment of 10 Nm. Schultz et al.[12] have reported the load-displacement properties in all principal directions with a compressive preload of 400 N. The compressive preload of 400 N was maintained while moments (4.7 Nm and 10 Nm) about the three principal axes were applied individually. Table 11.2 provides a comparison of the model predictions in response to bending and torsional moments compared to those reported by Schultz et al.[12] The predicted facet loads were compared with Yang and King,[17a] Shirazi-Adl and Drouin,[17b] and Kim.[15] Radial disc bulge predictions at L4–L5, measured at the disc mid-height, were compared to previous experimental and analytic results. In response to the compressive preload, the mean lateral disc bulge was 0.12 mm for a 400 N load. Although these values are somewhat low, the values were in the range reported by Dooris et al.[7] Ligament strains were predicted in response to an axial compressive load of 400 N, coupled with bending moments of 5 and 10 Nm about the three principal axes. The trends seen were close to the in vitro work reported by Panjabi et al.[17]

TABLE 11.2 Comparison of Intact L3–L5 and L3–S1 Finite Element Predictions and Results From Schultz et al.[12]

	L3/5 FE Model Predictions	L3/S1 FE Model Predictions	In Vitro Results
Rotation (Degrees) From 4.7 Nm Moment + 400 N Compression			
Flexion	L3–L4: 3.29 L4–L5: 3.36	L3–L4: 3.20 L4–L5: 3.32 L5–S1: 4.45	5.13 ± 1.86
Extension	L3–L4: 1.84 L4–L5: 1.62	L3–L4: 1.67 L4–L5: 1.40 L5–S1: 0.59	2.12 ± 0.98
Right lateral bending	L3–L4: 2.33 L4–L5: 2.31	L3–L4: 2.32 L4–L5: 2.13 L5–S1: 1.63	4.47 ± 1.63
Left lateral bending	L3–L4: 2.33 L4–L5: 2.31	L3–L4: 2.32 L4–L5: 2.13 L5–S1: 1.63	4.32 ± 1.47
Right axial rotation	L3–L4: 1.28 L4–L5: 1.25	L3–L4: 1.34 L4–L5: 1.20 L5–S1: 1.00	0.69 ± 0.33
Rotation (Degrees) From 10.6 Nm Moment + 400 N Compression			
Flexion	L3–L4: 5.32 L4–L5: 5.08	L3–L4: 5.19 L4–L5: 5.00 L5–S1: 6.45	5.51 ± 1.00
Extension	L3–L4: 3.45 L4–L5: 3.35	L3–L4: 3.83 L4–L5: 3.80 L5–S1: 3.72	2.99 ± 1.02
Right lateral bending	L3–L4: 5.13 L4–L5: 5.18	L3–L4: 5.15 L4–L5: 4.91 L5–S1: 3.73	5.64 ± 1.22
Left lateral bending	L3–L4: 5.13 L4–L5: 5.18	L3–L4: 5.15 L4–L5: 4.91 L5–S1: 3.73	4.90 ± 0.79
Right axial rotation	L3–L4: 2.98 L4–L5: 2.75	L3–L4: 3.17 L4–L5: 2.97 L5–S1: 2.56	1.50 ± 0.67

Finite element model predictions fall within one standard deviation of in vitro results.

The FE solutions are dependent on the mesh refinement. Using a large number of elements is known to reduce error, and the mesh should be refined until a stage is reached at which the results from the current refinement iteration are similar to the results obtained by the previous refinement iterations. Such a mesh would be an optimized mesh, which enables the model to predict correct results. Further refinement beyond this point can theoretically induce more errors. Thus, the mesh of the L3–L5 FE model was further refined and the L5–S1 segment was added. The results between the L3–L5 model and L5–S1 model exhibited a strong correlation (see Table 11.2).

To further validate the L3–S1 model, a cadaveric study was undertaken recently. The study involved comparing experimentally predicted load-displacement behavior using the Optotrak with FE model predictions.[18] Five fresh ligamentous lumbar L1–S1 spine specimens were used for the experimental tests. Specimens were potted in a rigid base secured to the sacrum and a loading frame likewise was secured to the L1 vertebral body. To determine the load-displacement behavior of the specimen, a set of three light-emitting diodes (LEDs) was attached to each vertebral body (Fig. 11.5). The Optotrak motion measuring system (Northern Digital Inc.) was used to track the spatial location of the LED markers secured rigidly to the vertebral bodies, including the base, during the load-displacement evaluation. The specimen was loaded to a maximum of 9 Nm in all six degrees of freedom. The intact FE model was also subjected to similar loading of 9 Nm as the cadaveric testing. The angular displacement data for the

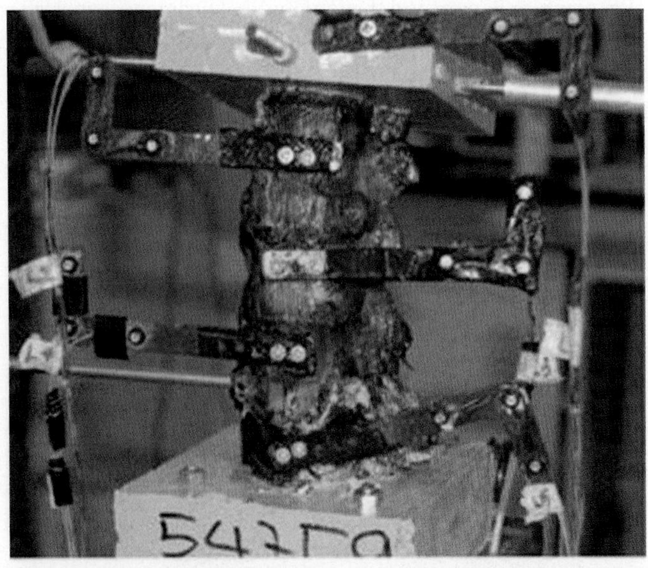

FIG. 11.5 The ligamentous L1–S1 segment with light-emitting diodes, used to predict angular displacements.

experimental testing and the FE model were compared across L3–S1, L3–L4, L4–L5, and L5–S1 segments. It was found that the FE model predicted angular displacements across the segments falling within one standard deviation of the experimental data (Fig. 11.6).

Finite Element Model of the Cervical Spine

A full cervical spine (C1–C7) computational model was developed that involved the following steps.

CADAVERIC AND FE MODEL COMPARISON

Intact flexion (cadaveric)
Intact flexion (FE model)
Intact extension (cadaveric)
Intact extension (FE model)
Flexion
Extension
Angular displacement (degrees)
L3-S1
L3-L4
L4-L5
L5-S1
A
Spinal segment

CADAVERIC AND FE MODEL COMPARISON

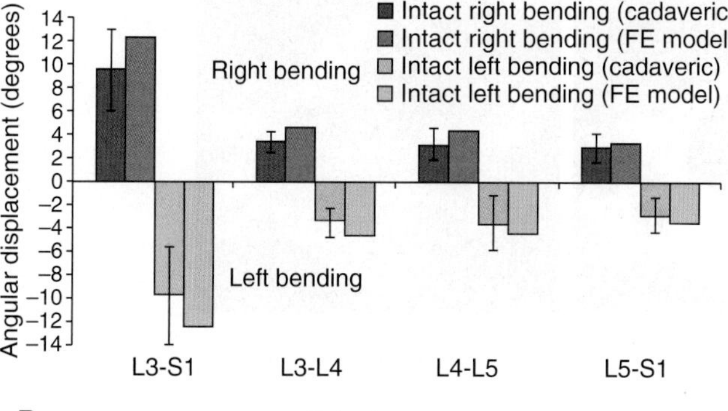

B
Spinal segment

CADAVERIC AND FE MODEL COMPARISON

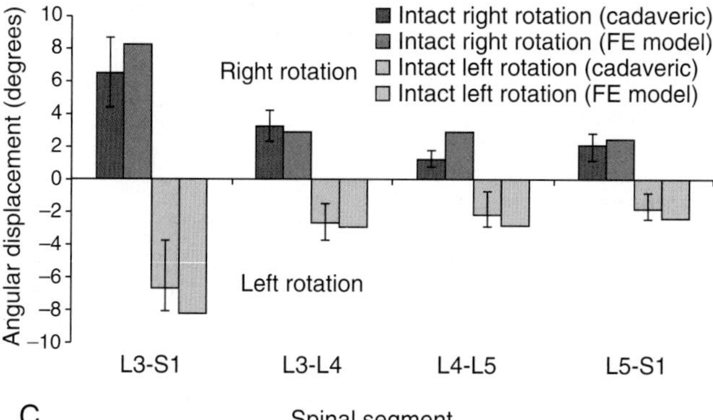

C
Spinal segment

FIG. 11.6 (A) Comparison of the experimental and finite element (FE) model results for flexion and extension in response to a 9-Nm pure moment. (B) Experimental and FE model results are compared in left and right bending in response to a 9-Nm pure moment. (C) Experimental and FE model results are compared in left and right rotation in response to a 9 Nm pure moment.

Conversion of CT and MRI Scans to 3D Solid Model

To construct the geometry of the cervical spine, CT scan images of a woman (25 years old) without any abnormalities with 1-mm slice thickness were obtained from the radiography department of University of Toledo Medical School. Mimics 13.1 software package (Materialise) was used to construct the required 3D structures. For the CT images obtained, bone contrasting and thresholding procedures were done to each bone part, and related masks were developed. Then, by utilizing the region growing tool, the initial geometry was developed (Fig. 11.7). Smoothing, wrapping, and filtering functions were executed to obtain good-quality geometry. A similar procedure was followed to obtain 3D structures of five intervertebral discs (C23, C34, C45, C56, and C67) from MRI scans.

Meshing

Each individual 3D structure was imported into the Iowa FE Mesh software for creating the mesh structure. A series of building blocks was constructed around the 3D structure, assigned a desired mesh density, and projected onto the surface representation, creating a 3D FE model. Finally, the mesh quality module in the software was used to evaluate, and thus develop, the high-quality mesh for the model. Fig. 11.8 shows the meshing procedure for C3 vertebra.

Finite Element Analysis (Using Abaqus Version 6.11)

Abaqus software was used for the FEA. Meshed parts were imported into this software for FEA. Ligament insertion points and material properties of all of the soft and hard tissues were extracted from literature.[18a] Finally, assembling all of these parts and assigning their respective material properties developed the three-dimensional nonlinear full cervical spine FE model.

The intact model contained 217,366 nodes and 181,336 elements. The global coordinate system of the model (X, Y, and Z) was oriented in such a way that the positive Y is from anterior to posterior of the spine, positive X is from right to left of the spine, and positive Z is from bottom to top of the spine.

Vertebral Body and Posterior Bone

Similar to the lumbar model, the cervical vertebral body consists of a thin cortical shell (0.5 mm of thickness) surrounding a softer cancellous core. The posterior region was assigned attributes, which lay between those of the cortical and cancellous regions. Three-dimensional, isoparametric solid elements (C3D8) were used to define the osseous geometry.

Facet Joints

A contact formulation was used to define the contact pattern between articulating surfaces in facet joints with an initial gap of 0.5 mm based on CT imaging and dissection procedures. The contact was defined with an exponentially increasing modulus as the gap distance between the inferior and superior facets decreased, simulating the presence of cartilage in the facet region. The facets were oriented at approximately 45

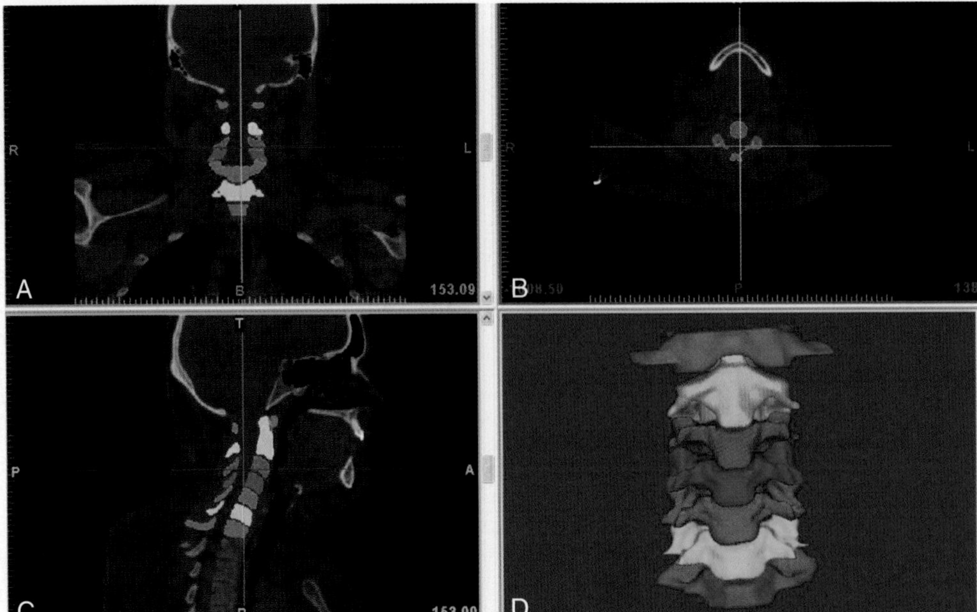

FIG. 11.7 Visualization module of Mimics version 13.1 (Materialise). (A–C) Frontal, axial, and sagittal scan views, respectively, in which bone contrasting, thresholding, and masking were performed for the computed tomographic slices. (D) Three-dimensional structures developed by performing the smoothing and filtering options.

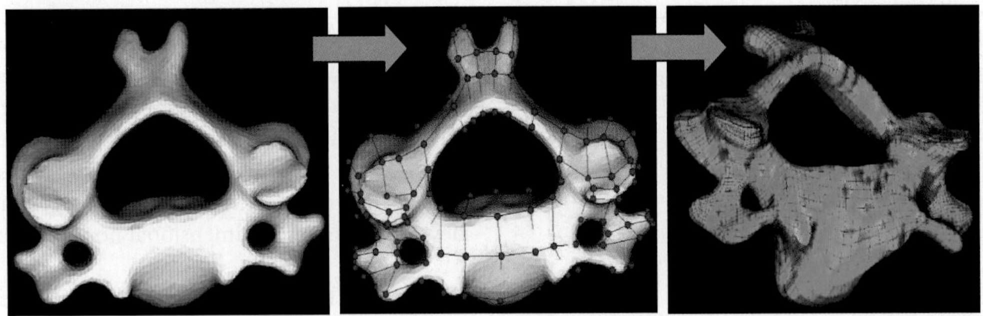

FIG. 11.8 Meshing procedure for the C3 vertebra. The left image depicts the three-dimensional C3 vertebra, the center image shows the constructed building blocks, and the right image depicts the meshed vertebra, respectively.

degrees from the horizontal plane, with some variation in the sagittal plane alignment, according to CT geometry. The facets were also of varying curvatures from right to left sides, indicating the possibility of varying contact during right or left loading modalities from the right to left facets.

Intervertebral Disc and Luschka's Joints

The anulus fibrosus was modeled as a composite configuration in which a series of fibers simulating the lamellae of the disc were embedded in a ground substance surrounding a more gelatinous nucleus region. Each layer of ground substance contained two alternating layers of fibers arranged at ±65 degrees from the transverse plane, with an overall fiber content of 20% of the annular volume assumed. REBAR element type with no-compression option was used to define the fibers. Brick elements were used to model ground substance and the nucleus pulposis was defined as incompressible fluid.

Luschka's joints were modeled as well in the cervical discs. These were simulated around the area of the uncinate processes and the anulus horizontal layers around the uncinate processes.

Ligaments

The ligaments of the lower cervical spine that were modeled include the anterior longitudinal ligament (ALL), posterior longitudinal ligament (PLL), interspinous ligament (ISL), ligamentum flavum (LF), and the capsular ligaments (CAPs). The alar ligament (AL), transverse ligament (TL), anterior and posterior atlantoaxial ligaments (AT-AX, PAT-AX) were modeled for the upper cervical spine. The ligaments were modeled using three-dimensional truss elements with hypoelastic material behavior.

Fig. 11.9 shows a 3D view of an FE model of the C1–C7 spine and all its components. Material properties and

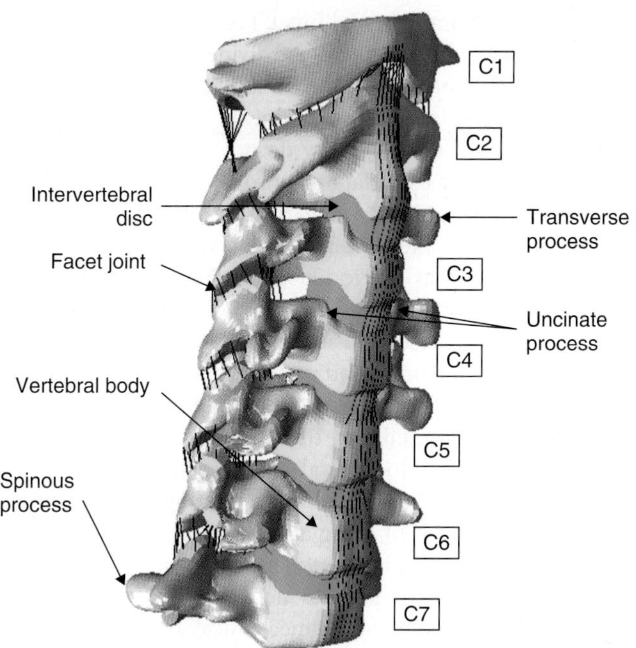

FIG. 11.9 Finite element model of the ligamentous C1–C7 cervical spine.

TABLE 11.3 Element Types and Material Properties for Finite Element Model of Intact C1–C7 Cervical Spine

Element Group Name	Element Type	Young's Modulus (MPa)	Poisson's Ratio	Cross-sectional Area (mm^2)
Cortical bone	C3D8	10,000	0.3	–
Cancellous bone	C3D8	450	0.25	–
Posterior bone	C3D8	3500	0.25	–
Anulus ground substance	C3D8	4.2	0.25	–
Anulus fibers	REBAR	–	0.45	–
Nucleus pulposus	C3D8H	1	0.4999	–
ALL	T3D2	15 (<12%) 30 (>12%)	0.3	33.0
PLL	T3D2	10 (<12%) 20 (>12%)	0.3	33.0
LF	T3D2	7 (<12%) 30 (>12%)	0.3	50.1
ISL	T3D2	5(<25%) 10 (>25%)	0.3	13.0
CAP	T3D2	15 (20-40%) 30 (>40%)	0.3	46.6
TL	T3D2	20	0.3	18.0
AL	T3D2	3.0(<17%) 8.5(>17%)	0.3	22.0
AT-AX	T3D2	0.2(<17%) 1.25 (>17%)	0.3	5.0
PAT-AX	T3D2	6.0(<17%) 10.0 (>17%)	0.3	5.0

AL, alar ligament; ALL, anterior longitudinal ligament; AT-AX, anterior atlantoaxial ligament; CAP, capsular ligament; ISL, interspinous ligament; LF, ligamentum flavum; PAT-AX, posterior atlantoaxial ligament; PLL, posterior longitudinal ligament; TL, transverse ligament.

cross-sectional areas used in defining the various entities in the C1–C7 model are summarized in Table 11.3. These were chosen based on values published in the literature and were assumed to be homogeneous and isotropic.[7]

Application of the Finite Element Model of the Spine

One of the main advantages of FE modeling of the spine is its extensive application in simulating the effects of various trauma and spinal disorders on the biomechanics of the spine. Numerous studies have simulated different spinal injuries and compared various biomechanical parameters, such as angular motion and stress distribution across degenerated and adjacent segments, between intact and injured spine models. The outcomes of such analysis have well served engineers in coming up with innovative ideas and solutions in the design of suitable implants to address the pain and restore to normal the biomechanics of the damaged segment. Implants are useful in treatment of spinal injuries when conservative therapies fail to reduce the pain and restore the patient to a normal daily routine. Invasive surgeries aim to remove the pain-causing structures, stabilize the segment, and correct bone failure due to trauma or disease.

Once the FE model of the intact spine is created, it can be easily modified to simulate different injuries by various techniques, such as removing certain elements (e.g., facetectomy, laminectomy), changing the material properties (e.g., laxity in ligaments), or modifying the geometry (disc herniation and degeneration).

For example, spinal stenosis is a progressive degenerative condition that occurs when the articulating facet joints become arthritic and no longer provide necessary stability to the spine. The arthritic facets become inflamed and osteophytic (produce bony spurs), resulting in irritation and impingement of nearby nerves, leading to clinical symptoms. The current nonconservative treatment for spinal stenosis is surgical decompression and spinal fusion with instrumentation to achieve spinal stability and symptom relief. Decompression is a surgical procedure, which is performed to alleviate pain caused by pinched nerves (neural impingement). The surgical procedure for decompression includes removal of part of the lamina (laminectomy), spinous process, facets (facetectomy), ligaments, and/or sometimes part of the intervertebral disc (microdiscectomy).

Although clinical studies have shown that decompression surgery enhances neurologic recovery, pain relief, and mobility, significant destabilization of the spinal motion segment is seen after decompression, especially if the facet joint is removed.

Addition of a posterior fusion system, including pedicle screws interconnected with a rigid rod, is a common procedure to restore the stability of the affected segment.

Though fusion is able to restabilize the implanted segment, it can result in accelerated degeneration of the adjacent motion segment and morbidity from muscle stripping. Fig. 11.8 shows an L3–S1 model of the spine with a fusion system at the L4–L5 level.

Clinical Application of the Finite Element Models of the Spine

FE analysis has become a cost-effective and efficient means to predict the biomechanics of the spine under physiologic and pathologic conditions. While useful, the model is not without limitations due to the constraints of a biologic system and its associated properties being modeled by a digital representation. The material properties of the ligaments (supraspinous, interspinous, ligamentum flavum, and so on) were obtained from the literature, while the intervertebral disc was modeled as a homogeneous composite ground substance. It can be inferred that the data used to generate the models can be thought of as an "average" of the normal population, just as reference ranges are for determining the upper and lower threshold of certain markers in routine bloodwork.

FE models are based on a number of assumptions, such as the fact that the generated models should apply equally to all members of a population. In clinical practice, this does not often hold true. Just as individual patients may have variations in their spine anatomy, the rate of degeneration and the impact of degenerative processes may vary from patient to patient, making generalizations about the "best" treatment for a particular type of spinal pathology far from simple. Often in clinical practice, patients with a similar degree of degenerative pathology may have widely different clinical manifestations or, in some cases, may be completely asymptomatic. The challenge in making decisions with patients in regard to their pathology rests on the ability of the clinician to integrate biomechanical data derived from FE models, the radiographic data, and the patient's clinical symptoms. Thus, it becomes important to not use computational models alone to determine the appropriate treatment for an individual patient. Additionally, the patients that are seen in practice often are far down the degenerative cascade, at which point surgery may only temporarily alleviate their symptoms before their recurrence due to scarring, nociceptor hypersensitivity, and/or further degeneration.

Another limitation of an FE model is that the stability of the ligamentous spine is less than a spine in vivo due to absence of the muscles and ligaments. The load-bearing qualities and structural support afforded by the muscles and ligaments have been shown to vary greatly, and are influenced by the age and quality of bone, the rate of loading, as well as other physiologic and hereditary characteristics that cannot be modeled by current computational techniques. In addition, there have been observations that cadaveric models may show different biomechanical properties based on preparation, and that the in vivo tissue failure properties may be lower than that predicted by FE models.[19] The importance of the musculature and ligaments and their contribution to spinal stability is emphasized by the recent surge of interest in minimally invasive techniques for arthrodesis that minimize muscle dissection.

Currently, FE models are limited in their ability to evaluate the spine as a whole, and are instead divided into regions (cervical, thoracic, lumbar) to facilitate analysis of their mechanical properties. By isolating these segments and subjecting them to biomechanical analysis, they do not address global spinal parameters, such as sagittal and coronal balance, which have become increasingly important in treating spinal pathology. In addition, the spine's relationship to the pelvis and pelvic parameters—such as pelvic tilt, pelvic incidence, and sacral slope—are currently not addressed by FE models but are used increasingly by surgeons in making treatment decisions that impact clinical outcomes and patient satisfaction.

Because FE models are typically based on a specific subject or an ideal average subject, there is concern regarding the applicability of FEA to clinical practice. Many studies have been conducted with the goal of accounting for intersubject variability as a result of aging and anatomic deformities. For example, patient-specific FE models have been constructed to investigate the risk of femoral neck fracture,[20] account for intersubject variability of biomechanical factors in animal studies,[21] and to support the interpretation of clinical results in follow-up studies. Reggiani et al. reported a preliminary validation of patient-specific FE models with regard to predicting the subject-specific primary stability of cementless implants during preoperative planning.[22]

Although a need remains for a validated model that accounts for injury, deformity, or disease, more recent studies have demonstrated the usefulness of coupling FEA with patient-specific information from clinical CT scans to mechanistically simulate bone failure. This approach has been validated by numerous groups for the spine and hip, and clinically has been shown to be significantly associated with incident and prevalent fracture in multiple cohorts. A study conducted by Kopperdahl et al. has further demonstrated clinical integration of FEA through its use of FEA-based vertebral strength assessments and vertebral trabecular bone mineral density (BMD) to predict incident vertebral fractures in women.[23]

The International Society for Clinical Densitometry (ISCD) has recently developed new official positions for the clinical use of quantitative CT (QCT)-based FEA of the spine and hip, specifically with regard to the management of osteoporosis in adults. According to the ISCD, QCT-based FEA can be used to assess fracture risk, initiate pharmacologic treatment of low vertebral and femoral strength, as well as monitor age- and treatment-related changes to bone strength.[24]

Perhaps the most important application of FE models in the spine is their utility in creating medical devices that are intended to arrest the degenerative cascade. In current clinical practice, a significant proportion of spine procedures are centered around removing offending pathology (laminectomy, facetectomy, corpectomy, and so on) and fusing the levels of interest using implants such as rods and pedicle screws. Over time, the inflammatory cascade that promotes healing fuses the operated levels while placing stress on the adjacent motion segment. While, in many cases, the patient's preoperative symptoms may temporarily improve, symptom recurrence and/or exacerbation in the future is not uncommon due to accelerating the degenerative cascade in the adjacent level. The existence of conditions such as "failed back surgery syndrome" (FBSS) and patient dissatisfaction after repeat fusion surgery suggest that the data used to create implants and to perform spine surgery are limited in their ability to truly predict the surgical solution that is ideal for a particular patient. Importantly, the data used to generate FE models is from cadaveric spine specimens that have not undergone fusion surgery, making predictions about the rate of degeneration or adjacent-level disease approximations at best.

These developments highlight the advantages of FEA and advance the goal of bringing FEA closer to clinical application. As FE models evolve, the ability to evaluate the spine as a whole, incorporation of global spinal alignment parameters, and including elements such as spinal musculature and ligaments may aid in increasingly accurate predictions of the spine in vivo. It should also be noted that current FE models are based on static imaging and do not incorporate dynamic radiographs (flexion, extension, and lateral bending), which also prove to be important in surgical decision making.

More recently, nonfusion-based spinal implants are being used as an alternative to stabilizing the spine after decompression. Unlike fusion, nonfusion stabilizing systems allow for angular motion, shear stability, and adjusting to the instant axis of rotation of the motion segment during movement. Fig. 11.9 shows the L3–S1 spine implanted with a posterior dynamic stabilizer system (PDS; Disc Motion Technologies). The implant was placed at L4–L5 following the surgical procedure of total facetectomy at L4–L5. The PDS consisted of a pair of metallic (chrome-cobalt) sliding parts (male and female) connected to the spine by titanium pedicle screws at each side.

To simulate the physiologic loading condition on the spine, once the implanted model was created, both implanted and intact models were loaded with 400 N of compressive follower preload plus 10 Nm of moment to simulate flexion, extension, left/right bending, and left/right rotation. Various biomechanical parameters such as motions, intradiscal pressure, and facet loads were compared between the intact and implanted model (Fig. 11.10).

The intervertebral artificial disc is another example of spinal implants recently proposed as a treatment for the degenerated disc. Unlike fusion systems, the total disc replacement (TDR) promises to address facet pain, mimic the motion of the intact spine, and avoid degeneration at the adjacent segment. There are various designs available for discs. Some require an anterior surgical approach for replacement as opposed to others that are placed from the posterior side of the spine. Fig. 11.11 shows a posterior disc system (Disc Motion Technologies), including a pair of cobalt-chrome sliding parts. This disc is placed into the spine following the surgical removal of the facets at the operative level. Since the facets are removed, the spine is restabilized by the addition of a PDS system as previously discussed. The combination of PDS and disc is a 360-degree motion system that is able to restore the motion of the operated segment back to normal. To assess the biomechanics of the implanted spine, FEA was

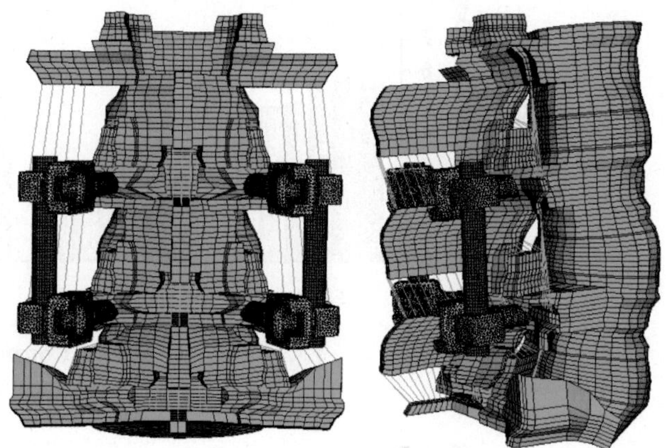

FIG. 11.10 Fusion system at the L4–L5 level of the lumbar spine.

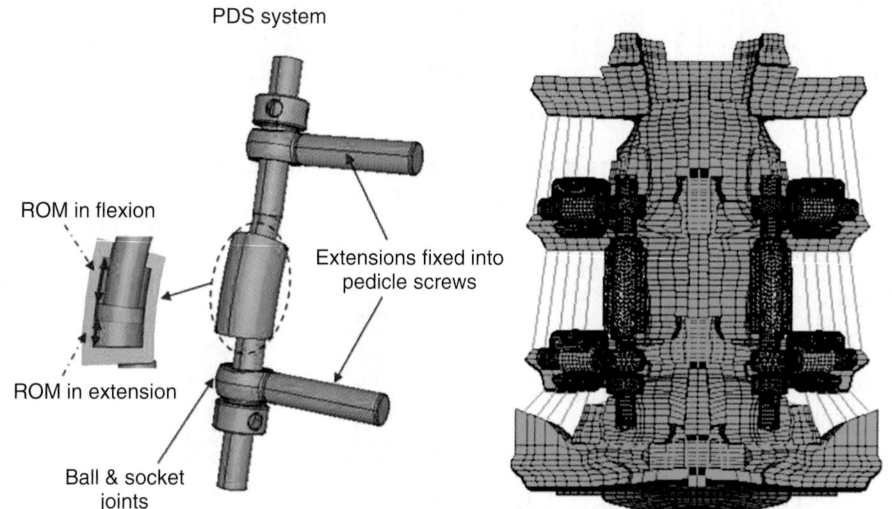

FIG. 11.11 The L3–S1 spine implanted with a posterior dynamic stabilizer system at L4–L5. *ROM*, range of motion; *PDS*, posterior dynamic stabilizer.

SECTION I

used, and motion, intradiscal pressure, and facet loads across segments were calculated and compared between intact and implanted models (Figs. 11.10–11.12).

Conclusion

In addition to its most obvious and time-tested uses, such as the evaluation of early-stage prototypes, FEA is a useful tool in the evaluation of the biomechanical effect of various surgical interventions, including a range of implants—from those that are designed for fusion to motion preservation devices. FEA aids in predicting the behavior of such implants in the long term by means of evaluating some crucial mechanical factors, such as wear and fatigue.

Studies in biomechanics of the spine have shown that FEA and in vitro cadaveric testing are complementary techniques,

Posterior
artificial disc

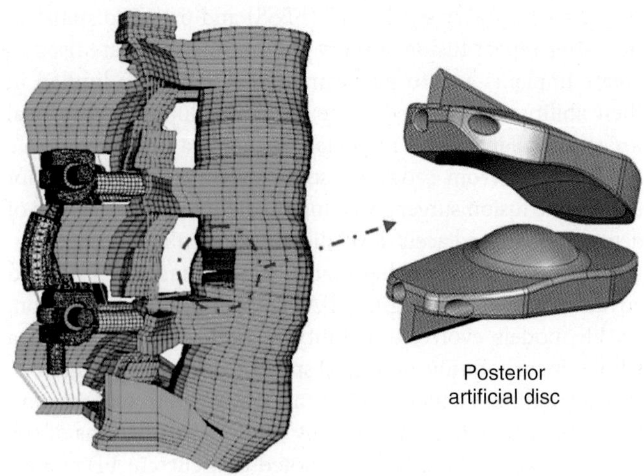

FIG. 11.12 The L3–S1 spine implanted with a posterior dynamic stabilizer and artificial disc at L4–L5.

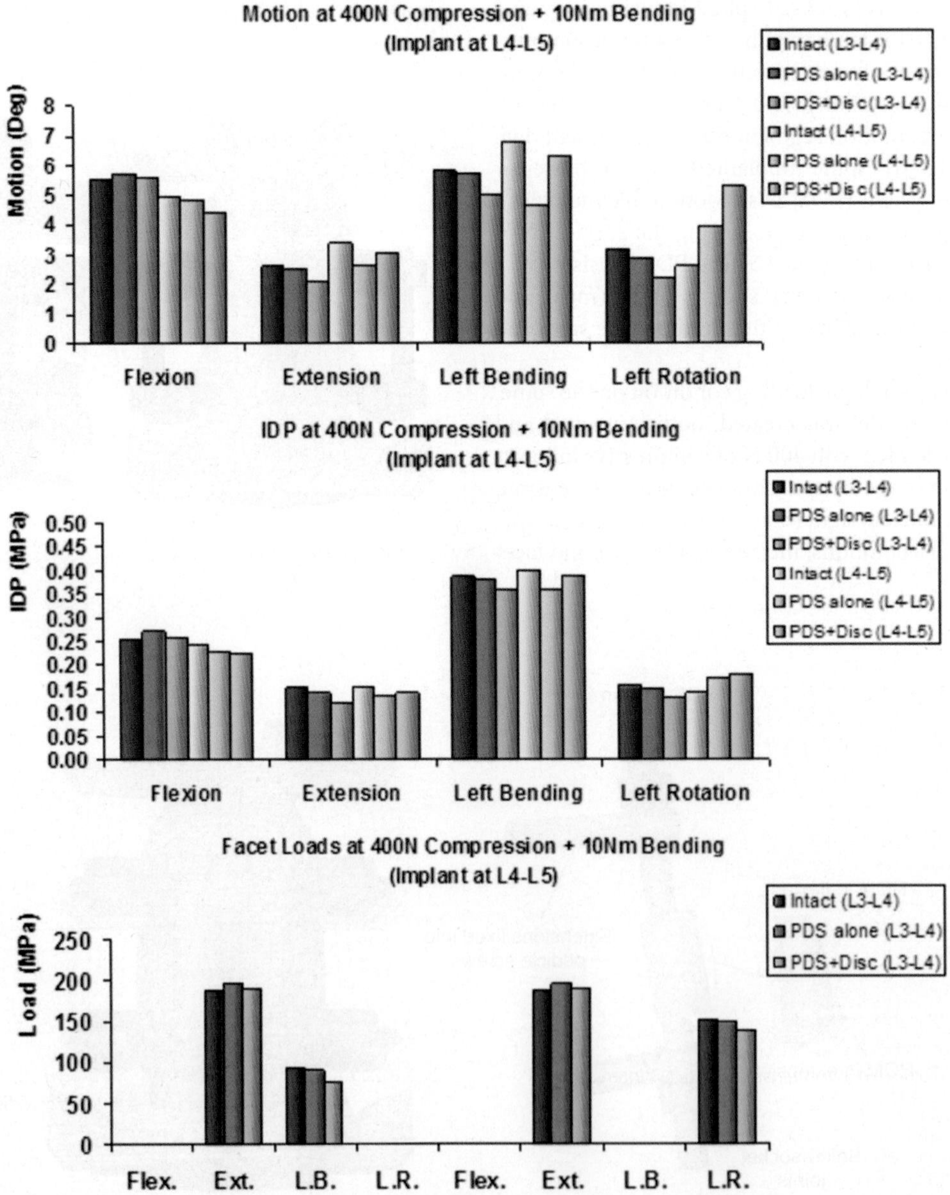

Motion at 400N Compression + 10Nm Bending
(Implant at L4-L5)
Motion (Deg)
0
1
2
3
4
5
6
7
8
Flexion
Extension
Left Bending
Left Rotation
Intact (L3-L4)
PDS alone (L3-L4)
PDS+Disc (L3-L4)
Intact (L4-L5)
PDS alone (L4-L5)
PDS+Disc (L4-L5)
IDP at 400N Compression + 10Nm Bending
(Implant at L4-L5)
IDP (MPa)
0.00
0.05
0.10
0.15
0.20
0.25
0.30
0.35
0.40
0.45
0.50
Flexion
Extension
Left Bending
Left Rotation
Intact (L3-L4)
PDS alone (L3-L4)
PDS+Disc (L3-L4)
Intact (L4-L5)
PDS alone (L4-L5)
PDS+Disc (L4-L5)
Facet Loads at 400N Compression + 10Nm Bending
(Implant at L4-L5)
Load (MPa)
0
50
100
150
200
250
Flex.
Ext.
L.B.
L.R.
Flex.
Ext.
L.B.
L.R.
Intact (L3-L4)
PDS alone (L3-L4)
PDS+Disc (L3-L4)

FIG. 11.13 Motion, intradiscal pressure, and facet loads across segments for intact and implanted models. *Ext.*, extension; *Flex.*, flexion; *L.B.*, left bending; *L.R.*, left rotation.

and thus are well suited to characterize the complex biomechanical behavior of the spine and its anatomic structures, including internal stresses/strains of the intervertebral disc, facet joints, and any ligaments of interest. However, like cadaver investigations, FE models have several limitations. For example, they do not account for variations in the geometry of the specimens, such as facet orientation and material properties that vary from specimen to specimen. But, for a given model geometry, the predicted data are in reasonable agreement with the results from the in vitro investigations. Thus, the use of an experimentally validated FE model can provide very useful information for many clinical questions being raised by the use of spinal implants.

One of the most far-reaching and interesting questions for which FEA may be able to provide some insight is in the nature of adjacent-level degeneration. Because the FE method provides the means for simulation of changes in motion and loads over time along with the effects of surgical intervention and changes in geometry and material properties due to degeneration, highly advanced, dynamic models of the spine may be able to replicate the progression of degeneration following surgical intervention and compare it to the natural course of the disease. While this will require considerable advancement in FE modeling techniques, it is perhaps the most promising means of answering the age-old question of whether adjacent-segment degeneration is actually attributable to surgical intervention or solely the manifestation of the underlying disease.

KEY REFERENCES

1. Mimura M, Panjabi MM, Oxland TR, et al. Disc degeneration affects the multidirectional flexibility of the lumbar spine. *Spine*. 1994;19(12):1371-1380.
The authors were able to show that in flexion-extension, the range of motion decreased and neutral zone ratio increased with degeneration. In axial rotation, neutral zone and neutral zone ratio increased with degeneration. In lateral bending, the range of motion significantly decreased and the neutral zone ratio increased with degeneration. In all three loading directions, the neutral zone ratio increased, indicating greater joint laxity with degeneration.
2. Dooris AP, Goel VK, Grosland NM, Gilbertson LG, Wilder DG. Load-sharing between anterior and posterior elements in a lumbar motion segment implanted with an artificial disc. *Spine (Philadelphia, Pa 1976)*. 2001;26(6):122-129.
The authors showed that by altering placement of the artificial disc in the anteroposterior direction, the motion-segment flexural stiffness and posterior load-sharing can be altered, even if the specific disc replacement design has no inherent rotational stiffness.
3. Dreischarf M, Zander T, Shirazi-Adl A, et al. Comparison of eight published static finite element models of the intact lumbar spine: predictive power of models improves when combined together. *J Biomech*. 2014;47(8):1757-1766.
Eight well-established finite element models of the lumbar spine (L1–L5) of different research centers were subjected to loading and compared to in vitro and in vivo measurements for intervertebral rotations, disc pressures, and facet joint forces. In pure moment loading, L1–L5 rotations, facet joint forces, and disc pressures fell within report ranges of in vitro motion with similar median values. The authors were able to conclude that the pooled median of various model results can be used as an improved predictive tool over the results of a single model alone.
4. Rohlmann A, Zander T, Schmidt H, Wilke HJ, Bergmann G. Analysis of the influence of disc degeneration on the mechanical behaviour of a lumbar motion segment using the finite element method. *J Biomech*. 2006;39(13):2484-2490.
The authors were able to demonstrate marked differences in intervetebral motion in a finite element model of the degenerative lumbar spine that closely mimics the reported in vitro behavior as a function of degeneration. The mildly degenerated segment showed an increase in motion in all loading cases with further degeneration resulting in decreases in motion.

REFERENCES

1. Freburger JK, Holmes GM, Agans RP, et al. The rising prevalence of chronic low back pain. *Arch Intern Med*. 2009;169(3):251-258.
2. Mimura M, Panjabi MM, Oxland TR, et al. Disc degeneration affects the multidirectional flexibility of the lumbar spine. *Spine*. 1994;19(12):1371-1380.
3. Brennan JJ, Lauryssen C. Current indications for posterior lumbar interbody fusions. *Semin Neurosurg*. 2000;11(2).
4. White AA, Panjabi MM. *Clinical Biomechanics of the Spine*. 2nd ed. Philadelphia: JB Lippincott Co.; 1978.
5. Sengupta DK. Dynamic stabilization devices in the treatment of low back pain. *Neurol India*. 2005;53(4):466-474.
6. Rohlmann A, Zander T, Schmidt H, Wilke HJ, Bergmann G. Analysis of the influence of disc degeneration on the mechanical behaviour of a lumbar motion segment using the finite element method. *J Biomech*. 2006;39(13):2484-2490.
7. Dooris AP, Goel VK, Grosland NM, Gilbertson LG, Wilder DG. Load-sharing between anterior and posterior elements in a lumbar motion segment implanted with an artificial disc. *Spine (Phila, Pa 1976)*. 2001;26(6):122-129.
8. Guan Y, Yoganandan N, Zhang J, et al. Validation of a clinical finite element model of the human lumbosacral spine. *Med Biol Eng Comput*. 2006;44(8):633-641.
9. Dreischarf M, Zander T, Shirazi-Adl A, et al. Comparison of eight published static finite element models of the intact lumbar spine: predictive power of models improves when combined together. *J Biomech*. 2014;47(8):1757-1766.
10. Momeni Shahraki N, Fatemi A, Agarwal A, Goel VK. Failure criteria for prediction of clinically relevant damage of annulus fibrosus. *iMedPub, Spine Res*. 2015;1(1:7).
11. Kim YE. *Analytical investigation of ligamentous lumbar spine biomechanics* (dissertation). Iowa City, IA: University of Iowa; 1988.
12. Schultz AB, et al. Mechanical properties of human spine motion segment part I: responses in flexion, extension, lateral bending, and torsion. *J Biomech Eng*. 1979;101:46-52.
13. Lindsey DP, Kiapour A, Yervy S, Goel VK. Sacroiliac joint fusion minimally affects adjacent lumbar segment motion: a finite element study. *Int J Spine Surg*. 2015;13:9-64.
14. Agarwal A, Zakeri A, Agarwal AK, Jayaswal A, Goel VK. Distraction magnitude and frequency affects the outcome in juvenile idiopathic patients with growth rods: finite element study using a representative scoliotic spine model. *Spine J*. 2015;15(8):1848-1855.
15. Grosland N. *Biomechanics of interbody fusion cages: a theoretical and experimental investigation* (dissertation). Iowa City, IA: University of Iowa; 1997.
16. Goel VK, Monroe BT, Gilbertson LG, Brinckmann P. Interlaminar shear stresses and laminae separation in a disc: finite element analysis of the L3-L4 motion segment subjected to axial compressive loads. *Spine*. 1995;20(6):689-698.

17. Khandha A. *A Parametric Evaluation of the Biomechanics of Lower Lumbar Spine After Fusion Surgery* (thesis). Toledo, OH: University of Toledo; 2004.

17a. Yang KH, King AI. Mechanism of facet load transmission as a hypothesis for low-back pain. *Spine.* 1984;9:557-565.

17b. Shirazi-Adl A, Drouin G. Load-bearing role of facets in a lumbar segment under sagittal plane loadings. *J Biomech.* 1987;20:601-613.

18. Panjabi MM, Goel VK, Walter SD, Schick S. Errors in the center and angle of rotation of a joint: an experimental study. *J Biomech Eng.* 1982;104(3):232-237.

18a. Dooris A. *Experimental and theoretical investigations into the effects of artificial disc implantation on the lumbar spine (dissertation).* Iowa City, IA: University of Iowa; 2001.

19. Zhu R, Rohlmann A. Discrepancies in anthropometric parameters between different models affect intervertebral rotations when loading finite element models with muscle forces from inverse static analyses. *Biomed Tech (Berl).* 2014;59(3):197-202.

20. Schileo E, Taddei F, Cristofolini L, Viceconti M. Subject-specific finite element models implementing a maximum principal strain criterion are able to estimate failure risk and fracture location on human femurs tested in vitro. *J Biomech.* 2008;41(2):356-367.

21. Viceconti M, Davinelli M, Taddei F, Cappello A. Automatic generation of accurate subject-specific bone finite element models to be used in clinical studies. *J Biomech.* 2004;37(10):1597-1605.

22. Reggiani B, Cristofolini L, Varini E, Viceconti M. Predicting the subject-specific primary stability of cementless implants during pre-operative planning: preliminary validation of subject-specific finite-element models. *J Biomech.* 2007;40:2552-2558.

23. Kopperdahl DL, Aspelund T, Hoffmann PF, et al. Assessment of incident spine and hip fractures in women and men using finite element analysis of CT scans. *J Bone Miner Res.* 2014;29(3):570-580.

24. Zysset P, Qin L, Lang T, et al. Clinical use of quantitative computed tomography-based finite element analysis of the hip and spine in the management of osteoporosis in adults: the 2015 ISCD official positions. Part II. *J Clin Densitom.* 2015;18(3):359-392.

SECTION II

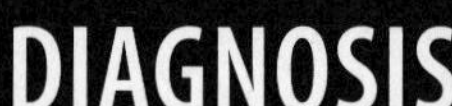

12 CHAPTER Patient History and Physical Examination: Cervical, Thoracic, and Lumbar

Christopher J. Standaert
Stanley A. Herring
J. David Sinclair

Caring for patients with spine disorders can be extremely challenging for clinicians because of the complexities of spinal anatomy and pathophysiology as well as the multifactorial nature of pain. Despite extensive advances in imaging of and interventions for the spine, a massive medical and social problem related to spinal pain and disability remains. To address the needs of patients with spine disorders and to select appropriate patients for whom specific care may be beneficial, clinicians need to identify the true nature of a patient's problem. Frequently, the patient's problem may extend well beyond any anatomic derangement that can be identified on imaging studies and involve numerous psychosocial factors in the patient's life. Through the history and physical examination, clinicians are able to identify not only the physical manifestations of a spine disorder but also the root causes of a patient's distress, suffering, and disability, all of which ultimately need to be addressed if a successful outcome is to be achieved.

A thorough history and physical examination of a patient with a spine disorder has several aims. From a strictly medical perspective, the examiner must be aware of the full medical context of the patient's complaints and how the complaints may relate to the overall health of the patient. It is imperative to ascertain the presence of an emergent medical problem promptly and to identify patients who need more urgent (or emergent) assessment and care. Clinicians must also identify any secondary medical issues that may directly affect the care of spine-related problems or may be associated with broader health concerns. In a more focused sense, the history and physical examination should allow an examiner to identify relevant spine problems that have led to the issue for which the patient is seeking care (e.g., the source of pain or neurologic loss, anatomic derangements). The history and physical examination also allow the practitioner to understand the level of function and impairment that is associated with the patient's presentation.

Moving beyond the strictly medical context, identification of the factors associated with the patient's pain and disability that pose the dominant barriers to optimal functional recovery is an important goal of the history and physical examination. To decide on the appropriate intervention for a patient, it is imperative to understand what exactly is being treated. Despite all the attention paid to pain, frequently the patient's sense of suffering is the real problem, particularly in patients with chronic pain. The only way to identify the issues behind the presentation of many patients is by asking the right questions. This chapter addresses relevant issues in the history and physical examination in patients with spine disorders, particularly as these issues relate to the assessment of patients seen commonly in clinical practice, and provides information on how to identify patients at risk for ongoing pain despite what seems to be appropriate care for their structural problems.

Differential Diagnosis

The differential diagnosis of spinal pain or related symptoms is enormous when considered in a general sense. Numerous anatomic structures may be associated with pain, multiple local or systemic disease processes can affect the spine, and numerous non–spine-related structures or conditions can result in back or neck pain or mimic syndromes related to spine disorders.[1–5] In addition, numerous psychosocial factors can produce ongoing pain and disability. The ability to process all of the available possibilities and to develop a relatively short list of diagnostic options depends heavily on the ability to obtain a thorough history and physical examination. It is helpful to begin with an understanding of structures in the spine that can be associated with pain and their patterns of pain referral.

From an anatomic perspective, a structure must be innervated to cause pain. In the spine, the list of discrete anatomic structures with sensory innervation (i.e., potential pain generators) includes muscles, tendons, ligaments, fascia, anulus of the intervertebral discs, bone, zygapophyseal joints, dura mater, nerve roots and dorsal root ganglia, and vascular elements.[1,2] All structures of common embryologic segmental origin tend to refer pain in very similar patterns, and the pattern of pain is determined by the nerve supply to the structure.[1] The end result is that there is substantial overlap between the referral patterns for anatomic structures of the same spinal level, such as intervertebral discs and zygapophyseal joints, and dermatomal, myotomal, and sclerotomal referral patterns at many spinal levels (Fig. 12.1). The location

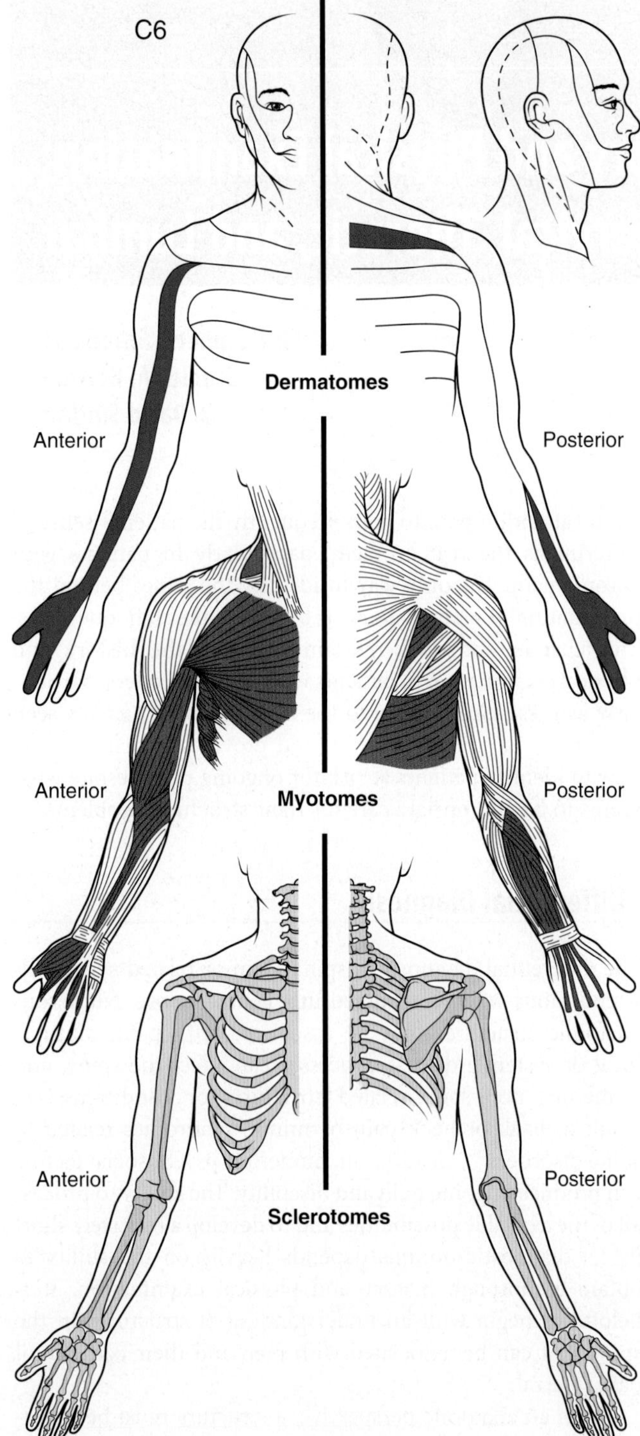

FIG. 12.1 Dermatome, myotome, and sclerotome of C6 level showing substantial overlap in distribution. (From Bland JH. *Disorders of the Cervical Spine: Diagnosis and Medical Management*. 2nd ed. Philadelphia: WB Saunders; 1994.)

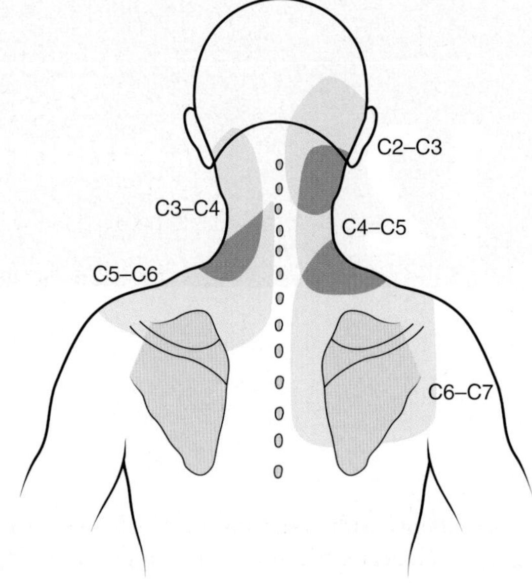

FIG. 12.2 Map of characteristic areas of pain referred from the cervical zygapophyseal joints (C2–C3 to C6–C7). (From Dwyer A, Aprill C, Bogduk N. Cervical zygapophyseal joint pain patterns I: a study in normal volunteers. *Spine*. 1990;15:453–457.)

of pain or radiating symptoms can often be a useful feature in the identification of an affected spinal level, although the location of pain alone does not indicate which particular anatomic structure is the source of the specific symptom.

The zygapophyseal joints are one of the best-studied structures in terms of pain referral patterns and relative prevalence in patients with spinal pain. In the cervical spine, the pattern of pain distribution from the stimulation of specific zygapophyseal joints has been described (Fig. 12.2).[6] Those results were subsequently validated in a study of patients with cervical complaints based on pain distribution and response to diagnostic blocks.[7] Another study using a double-block protocol on patients with persisting symptoms after whiplash injury found that the prevalence of C2–C3 zygapophyseal joint pain in patients with headache was 50%; in patients without C2–C3 zygapophyseal joint pain, the prevalence of symptoms related to the lower cervical zygapophyseal joints was 49%.[8] Although there is far less clinical information on pain associated with thoracic zygapophyseal joints, a similar map of referral patterns has been identified (Fig. 12.3).[9]

In the lumbar spine, there has also been a great deal of attention directed to the zygapophyseal joints as potential sources of pain, although the relative frequency with which they seem to be primary pain generators is less than for cervical zygapophyseal joints causing pain in patients with chronic whiplash. A more recent study noted a 15% overall prevalence of zygapophyseal pain in a group of 176 patients with chronic low back pain using a diagnostic double-block protocol.[10] Although pain associated with lumbar zygapophyseal joints is generally described as occurring with lumbar extension and rotation, the authors of that study did not find any consistent clinical features that were associated with the presence of a positive diagnostic response to injections.[10] Stimulation of lumbar zygapophyseal joints can result in either local axial or, far less frequently, radiating pain, and pain referral patterns have been documented.[11]

Multiple authors have addressed the distribution of pain associated with intervertebral discs. Cloward[12] first described cervical discography and noted that pain that seemed to be emanating from irritation of the anulus resulted in radiating pain into the thoracic or scapular regions in distinct patterns

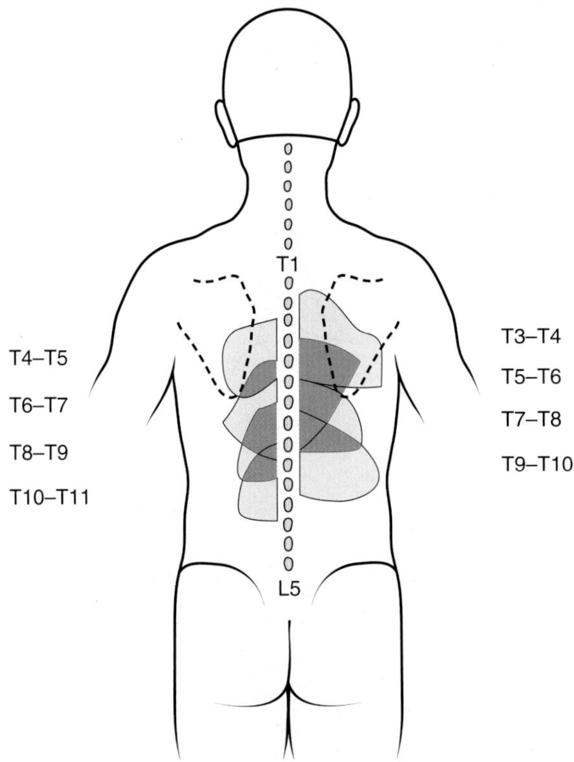

FIG. 12.3 Map of characteristic areas of pain referred from thoracic zygapophyseal joints (T3–T4 to T10–T11). (From Dreyfuss P, Tibiletti C, Dreyer S. Thoracic zygapophyseal joint pain patterns: a study in normal volunteers. *Spine*. 1994;19:807–811.)

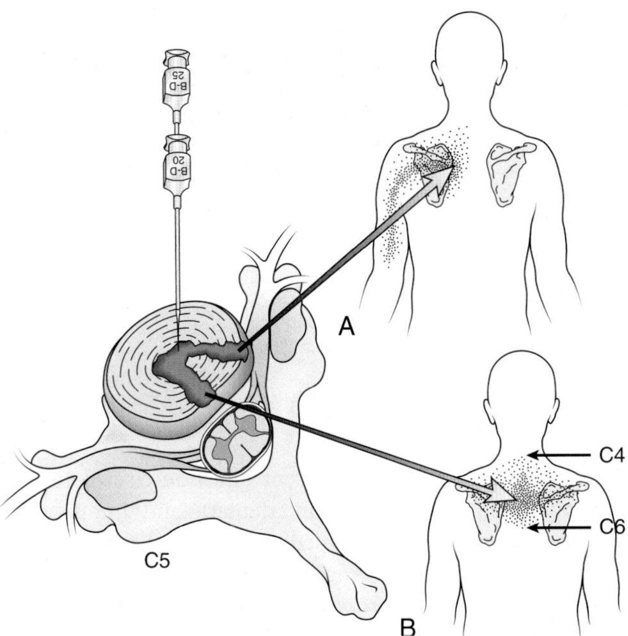

FIG. 12.4 Pain referral pattern from (A) posterolateral and (B) central discs. (From Cloward RB. Cervical discography: a contribution to the etiology and mechanism of neck, shoulder and arm pain. *Ann Surg*. 1959;150:1052–1064.)

(Fig. 12.4). Similar findings were more recently described by others.[13] As mentioned previously, pain referral patterns are similar to patterns noted for cervical zygapophyseal joints, with the level of spine pathology, rather than the actual structure involved, affecting the pain referral pattern.

Other pain referral patterns that should be recognized by all physicians treating patients with spine disorders include patterns related to neurologic injury. These patterns are discussed further later in the section on the neurologic examination, but identifying the dermatomal pattern of pain is central to the assessment of individuals with potential nerve root pathology (Fig. 12.5). Nerve root symptoms include paresthesias, burning, hyperalgesia, aching, analgesia, or pain. The ability to identify a dermatomal pattern to the symptoms can help localize the area of spine involvement.

The clinical utility of pain provocation is uncertain because there are inherent problems with this approach owing to the complex nature of pain perception.[1,14–18] The identification of a "pain generator" in individuals with chronic spinal pain can be difficult. In contrast to cutaneous sensation, nociceptive signals from deep somatic structures—such as joint capsules, fascia, and periosteum—are carried by relatively few primary afferent fibers, resulting in only vague localization of pain.[16] Additionally, there is the issue of convergence, in which a single dorsal horn cell may receive synaptic input from afferent fibers that innervate many structures and can result in multiple structures producing similar patterns of pain perception. This convergence makes it extremely difficult to validate a single entity as the cause of an individual's pain because the stimulation of any one of numerous structures may result in identical perceptions of pain.[16] These issues become even more complex when additional potential neurologic and psychological changes that can occur with chronic pain are involved.

Biomedical Factors and the Medical History

It is essential to obtain a thorough and appropriate medical history from patients presenting with spine disorders or related complaints. The identification of potentially serious problems is one of the most important functions of obtaining a good medical history. Ideally, the medical history also should help the clinician establish a reasonable differential diagnosis that can direct further diagnostic or therapeutic steps. Given the scope and complexities of spine disorders, it can be useful to break down some aspects of the clinical presentation into broad categories. This categorization may allow clinicians to focus their thought process and subsequent efforts more effectively. Useful categories to consider relate to the presence or absence of radiating pain and specific demographic factors. The following categories can help in obtaining a concise medical history.

Red Flags: What Not to Miss

It is essential to identify all conditions that pose a substantial, imminent risk for further harm to the patient. Many authors have identified specific red flags in the history of patients with low back complaints that indicate the presence of such a condition; these include infection, tumor, fracture, cauda equina injury, and progressive neurologic injury, such as motor loss or myelopathy (Table 12.1).[19–22] Red flags for the

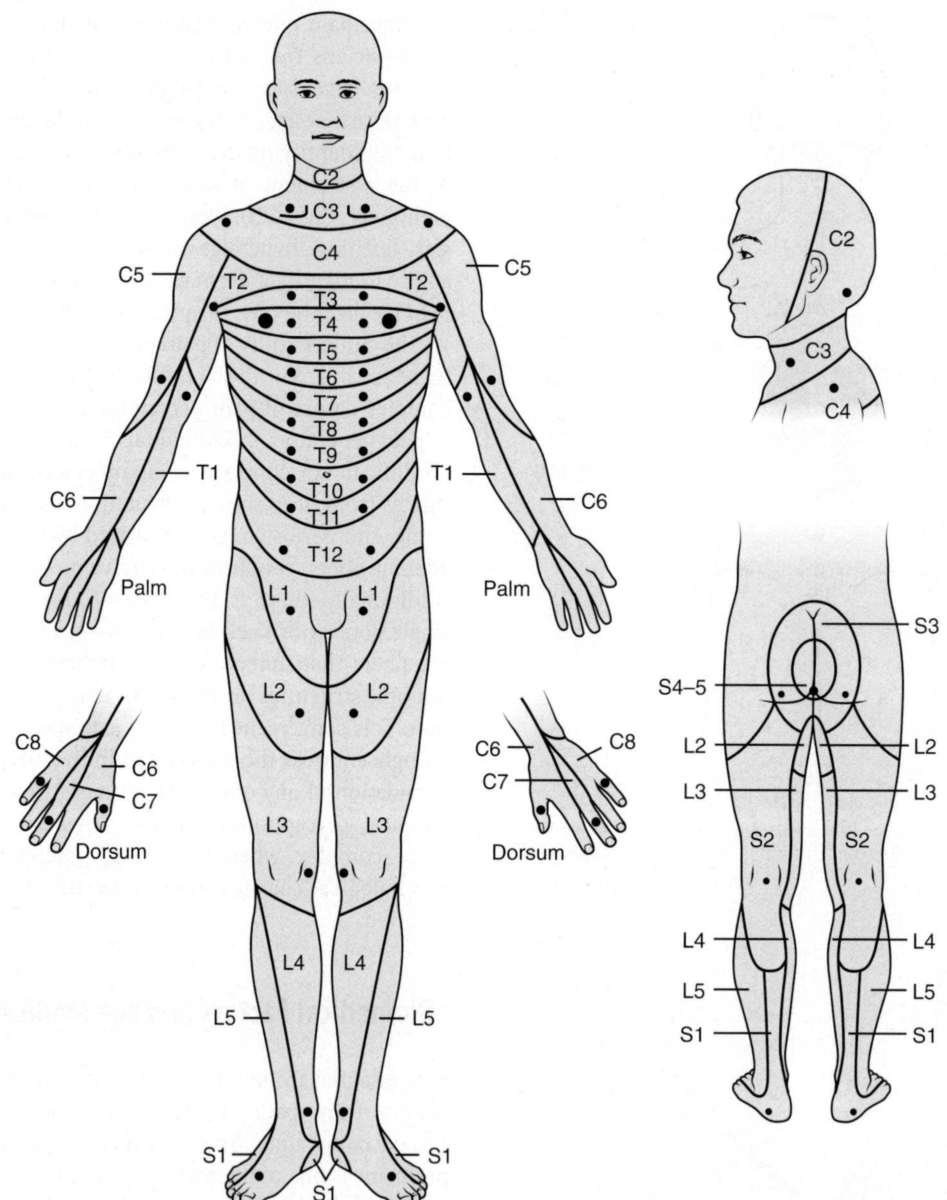

FIG. 12.5 Dermatomal distribution and key sensory points. (From American Spinal Injury Association. *International Standards for Neurological Classification of Spinal Cord Injury [reprint].* Chicago: American Spinal Injury Association; 2008.)

possibility of *cancer* include age older than 50 years, previous cancer history, unexplained weight loss, pain not relieved by bed rest, duration of pain for more than 1 month, and failure of conservative therapy after 1 month.[22] Although widely used clinically, systematic reviews have found limited data to support the use of any individual red flags in the identification of patients with malignancy, with a Cochrane review noting particularly high false-positive rates for factors such as insidious onset of pain, persistence of pain for greater than 1 month, and age greater than 50 years.[23,24] A history of malignancy seems to exhibit the strongest posttest probability for detecting spinal malignancy.[24]

Spine infections—including discitis, osteomyelitis, and epidural abscess—are usually blood-borne from other regions.[22] Important risk factors for infection include the use of illicit intravenous drugs, active or recent infection elsewhere (e.g., urinary tract, pulmonary, skin, dental), and immunosuppression (owing to either medications or illness affecting the immune system).[19,22] Additional risk factors for infection include diabetes and history of tuberculosis or exposure to a region endemic for tuberculosis.

The risk of *fracture* is elevated in patients older than 50 years, particularly patients older than 70 years.[22] Patients with a history of corticosteroid use or known osteopenia or osteoporosis are also at increased risk for fracture. A study of 669 patients greater than 55 years of age presenting to their primary physician identified four patients (1%) with malignancy and 33 (5%) with a fracture, 30 of which were associated with osteoporosis.[25] Trauma, osteoporosis, pain greater than 7 out of 10, and thoracic pain were all associated

TABLE 12.1 "Red Flags": Emergent or Urgent Medical Conditions That Need to Be Identified Promptly in All Patients Presenting With Possible Issues Related to the Spine

Symptom or Finding	Possible Significance
History of cancer	Cancer
Unexplained weight loss	
Age >50 y	
Failure to respond to >1 mo of conservative care	
Duration of pain >1 mo	
No pain relief with bed rest	
Night pain	
History of smoking	
Known osteopenia or osteoporosis	Fracture
History of corticosteroid use	
Age >50 y	
DISH or ankylosing spondylitis	
Trauma (major in younger individual, minor in older individual)	
Fever	Infection
Illicit use of intravenous or percutaneously injected drugs	
Recent or known infection	
Immunosuppressive illness	
Use of immunosuppressive medications	
Tuberculosis exposure	
Progressive weakness in limbs	Cauda equina or spinal cord injury
Progressive balance deficit or loss of coordination	
Bowel or bladder dysfunction or urinary retention	
Sexual dysfunction	
Numbness or paresthesias in perineum or saddle anesthesia	
Significant weakness of major muscle group or progressive motor loss in limb	Severe or progressive radiculopathy

DISH, diffuse idiopathic skeletal hyperostosis.

with the identification of a fracture, with a history of trauma having the strongest predictive value.[25] Trauma and fracture risk are discussed further elsewhere in this book.

Significant *neurologic* injuries include cauda equina syndrome, progressive radiculopathy, or myelopathy. Cauda equina syndrome should be considered in a patient with saddle anesthesia; bowel, bladder, or sexual dysfunction; or significant lower extremity pain and weakness, particularly if bilateral.[19,22] Progressive neurologic loss from nerve root compression is an indication for urgent surgical intervention, thus needs to be identified promptly. Myelopathy can present in various ways, including hand paresthesias or decreased fine motor control; lower extremity weakness or gait instability; sensory alterations in the trunk or extremities; or changes in bowel, bladder, or sexual function.[26]

Historical Features of the Presenting Complaint

Specifying the exact nature of the patient's chief complaint and provocative and palliative factors is an extremely important part of the diagnostic assessment. The examiner must identify the nature, onset, duration, and course of the primary complaint; history of previous injury; character and distribution of symptoms; prior diagnostic testing and treatment; other circumstances surrounding an injury (e.g., perceived fault, the presence of workers' compensation or litigation status); and the degree of pain and disability perceived by the patient. All of these factors are important in establishing an appropriate differential diagnosis and identifying some of the potential barriers to recovery.

Axial Versus Radicular Pain

The distinction between axial and radicular pain is fundamental in assessing a patient with a potentially neurogenic problem. *Axial* pain in the cervical, thoracic, or lumbar region suggests a different etiology, evaluation, diagnosis, and potentially treatment than radicular pain. For all levels of the spine, pathology involving the musculotendinous and ligamentous structures, zygapophyseal joints, vertebrae, and anulus of the intervertebral discs tends to cause axial pain. Other structures in the cervical and thoracic regions that can result in axial pain include soft tissue structures in the neck; vascular structures (e.g., aorta or carotid arteries); portions of the brachial plexus, such as the long thoracic or suprascapular nerves; the proximal portion of the ribs; costovertebral or costotransverse articulations; various structures within the shoulder; and various visceral structures, including the pancreas, gallbladder, lung and pleura, and stomach or duodenum (Fig. 12.6).

Radicular pain radiating into the upper extremities generally has a different etiology. If related to spine pathology, radicular pain implies neural compression from many potential causes, including disc herniation, spinal canal or neuroforaminal stenosis, or intrinsic disease of the spinal cord or nerve roots (e.g., herpes zoster). Radicular pain in the thoracic region can result in a bandlike distribution on one or both sides of the chest wall or abdominal region. Additional structures that can result in radiating upper extremity pain include peripheral nerves, such as the median nerve (e.g., carpal tunnel syndrome); ulnar nerve; portions of the brachial plexus (e.g., lower trunk plexopathies related to true neurogenic thoracic outlet syndrome or a Pancoast tumor); vascular structures; the shoulder; the heart; and musculotendinous, ligamentous, or bony structures in the upper extremities.

For the lumbar spine, the hip and pelvic structures must be considered as potential sources of low back, buttocks, or posterolateral hip pain. Particular sources of low back or buttock pain related to the bony pelvis include the sacroiliac joints, the sacrum (e.g., stress fractures), the ilia, and the hip joints. Other structures and processes that can result in low back pain include the kidneys and ureters; the pancreas; gastric ulcers; vascular abnormalities (e.g., aortic aneurysm); and retroperitoneal processes such as hematoma, endometriosis, or lymphadenopathy associated with malignancy.[27]

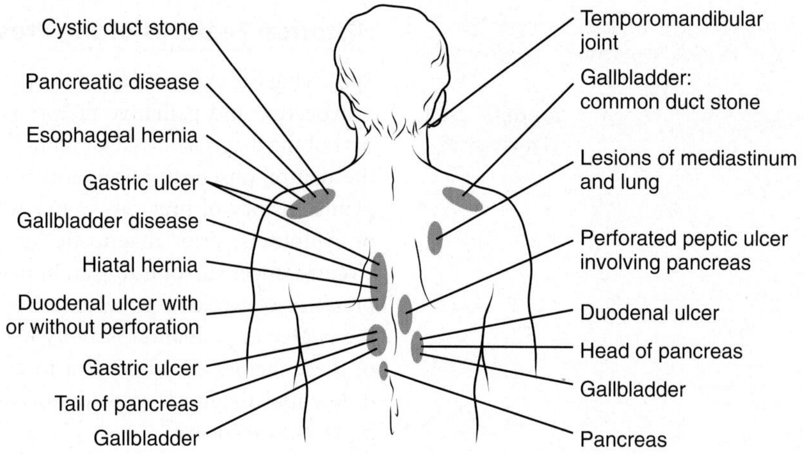

FIG. 12.6 Posterior referral sites from distant visceral or somatic structures. (From Nakano KK. Neck pain. In: Kelley WN, Harris ED Jr., Ruddy S, et al, eds. *Textbook of Rheumatology*. 4th ed. Philadelphia: WB Saunders; 1993.)

As with upper extremity pain, lower extremity radicular pain often has different etiologies and generally implies involvement of the lumbosacral nerve roots, the conus medullaris, or the spinal cord. The lumbar zygapophyseal joints and the sacroiliac joints also may occasionally be associated with radicular leg pain.[11,28] Distal lower extremity symptoms also may arise from intraarticular hip pathology; greater trochanteric bursitis; vascular pathology (e.g., vascular claudication); peripheral nerve injuries; compartment syndrome; local musculotendinous, ligamentous, or bony structures; and pelvic causes, such as endometriosis. Whatever the cause, the presence of leg pain with low back pain appears to increase the overall severity of the clinical state. Compared with those who have axial lumbar pain alone, patients with associated radicular pain experience a lower quality of life, require more resources, and have higher levels of pain and disability.[29] Given this, efforts to identify and appropriately treat the cause of leg symptoms have particular importance.

Patient Demographics

Demographic characteristics—such as age, gender, educational background, occupation, and cultural milieu—are important factors that must be considered in the history of a patient with a spine problem. Age is a primary determinant in establishing a differential diagnosis. Different spine problems appear at different frequencies at different ages. The social and psychological issues of individuals can also be quite distinct at different ages.

Growth and development have a profound impact on the approach to various processes, such as spondylolisthesis, scoliosis, and Scheuermann kyphosis. In contrast to the adult spine, the developing bony spine is relatively more prone to injury than some soft tissue structures. In a study by Micheli and Wood,[30] 47% of adolescents presenting to a pediatric sports medicine clinic were diagnosed with spondylolysis and only 11% had disc abnormalities compared with 48% of adults presenting to a low back pain clinic who were thought to have disc pathology. Generally, symptomatic isthmic spondylolysis is almost entirely seen in older children, adolescents, or young adults, and the rate of pars defects identified in the general population does not change substantially between the ages of 20 and 80 years.[31,32] Although 50% or more of children may be affected by low back pain by age 15 years,[33,34] significant spinal pain in children is uncommon and should raise concern for the presence of serious medical pathology.[35,36] Infection, neoplasm, rheumatologic conditions such as ankylosing spondylitis and juvenile rheumatoid arthritis, and other non-spine sources of pain may be more common in children and adolescents than in adults.[35,36]

In adults, the frequency of certain spine conditions varies by age group. Disc herniations are most frequent during the 4th and 5th decades, although they can affect individuals in their 50s and 60s or children and young adults.[37] Degenerative spinal stenosis and degenerative spondylolisthesis tend to present later in life. As mentioned previously, some medical conditions, including ankylosing spondylitis, spondylitis associated with inflammatory bowel disease, and tumors such as osteoid osteoma and osteoblastoma, tend to manifest in younger adults (20s and 30s). Other conditions—such as osteoporosis, polymyalgia rheumatica, metastatic cancer, or multiple myeloma—tend to occur in older adults (40s and 50s or older; Fig. 12.7).[3,38]

Gender is a factor in many spine pathologies. Osteoporosis is more common in women than in men, and osteoporotic fractures are more common in women. Neck pain also has been noted to be more prevalent in women than in men.[39,40] Rheumatoid arthritis, polymyalgia rheumatica, and endocrine disorders also tend to occur more frequently in women.[38] Spondyloarthropathies, infections, and various spine tumors—such as multiple myeloma, lymphoma, osteoblastoma, and eosinophilic granuloma—occur more frequently in men.

Demographic factors—such as race, ethnicity, and cultural milieu—may also play a role in the prevalence of some spine disorders, but are less well studied. Whites tend to have higher rates of osteoporosis than some other races, and metabolic conditions such as Gaucher disease can be associated with certain ethnic groups.[3] Whites have a higher rate of spondylolysis than African Americans.[31] The prevalence of low back pain also varies in different parts of the world, with

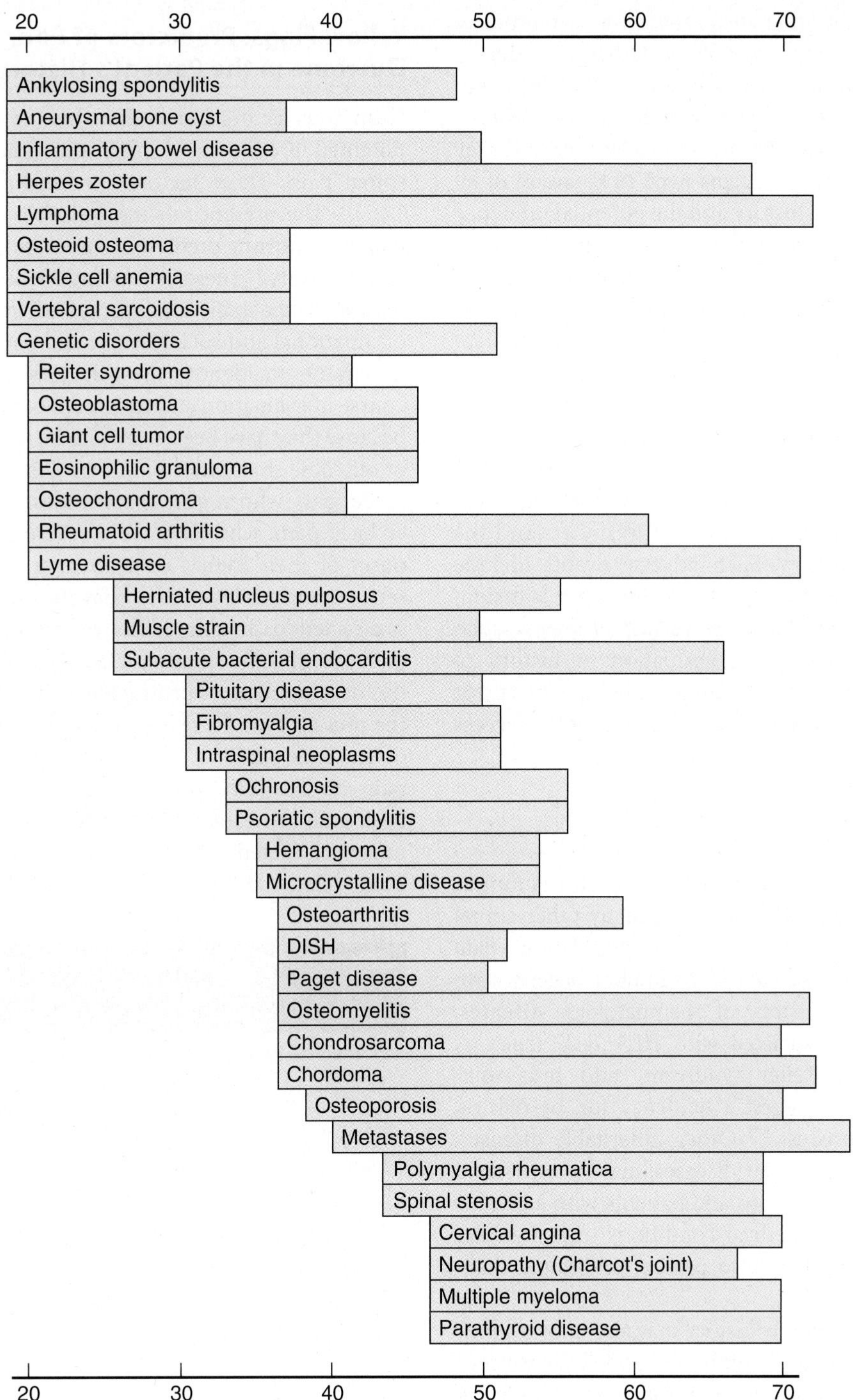

FIG. 12.7 Age at peak incidence of neck pain associated with various disorders. DISH, diffuse idiopathic skeletal hyperostosis. (From Borenstein DG, Wiesel SW, Boden SD. *Neck Pain: Medical Diagnosis and Comprehensive Management*. Philadelphia, WB Saunders; 1996.)

industrialized regions reporting a higher prevalence of low back complaints than rural, low-income areas.[41] Pain perception, disability, and other effects of pain on individuals vary widely and depend on many cultural and social factors.

Past Medical History

In addition to identifying prior surgical procedures, it is important to identify all past and current medical conditions because many medical problems can be associated with spine issues and can affect care of a patient with a spine disorder. As noted previously, a history of cancer, recent infection, or disease processes that affect the immune system or may require immunosuppressive medications can be associated with significant spine problems. Other medical conditions—such as osteoporosis, ankylosing spondylitis, and diffuse idiopathic skeletal hyperostosis—may place patients at increased risk for spine fracture.[42] Some congenital or genetic syndromes, such as Marfan syndrome and Down syndrome, can be associated with spine anomalies that must be identified. Vascular disease, such as vascular claudication or aortic aneurysm, can produce symptoms that mimic spine pathology. Other disorders—including cardiac or pulmonary disease, renal disorders, skin conditions, gastric ulcers, diabetes, and hepatic disorder—may have an impact on potential treatment options and may preclude certain therapies. Clinicians need to be aware of all facets of a patient's medical history and the potential influence that medical issues may have on the care of the patient.

An additional aspect that must be considered in a patient with a spine disorder is a history of prior injury. Previous spine problems, trauma, and surgery may have important implications for the care of the patient. Details about the type and severity of injury and the type of treatment (including surgery), as well as the patient's response to it, are important historical features. Whenever possible, prior operative reports should be obtained. Short-term and long-term problems potentially can develop after surgery, and it is important to understand the nature of any prior surgery. Such adverse events include adjacent-segment degeneration or instability after a fusion, epidural fibrosis, infection, hardware-related problems, such as loosening, and recurrent disc herniation. A history of multiple or prolonged periods of pain or disability after prior treatments should raise concerns about the chances for success with future treatments.

Family History

The family history is a necessary component of a complete medical history. Although back pain and many other spinal conditions are common in the general population, data suggest possible genetic risk factors for lumbar degenerative disc disease.[43] A family history of rheumatologic diseases, particularly conditions associated with *HLA B-27* (such as ankylosing spondylitis, Reiter syndrome, and inflammatory bowel disease) can suggest a tendency for, or risk of, developing a similar process.[3,44] Other inheritable diseases, including certain neuromuscular diseases, may be associated with progressive spinal deformity, and patients with a genetic predisposition for certain medical conditions (e.g., vascular disease, specific cancers) may also present additional diagnostic considerations.

Obtaining a thorough family history may also allow a clinician to understand potentially complicated or delicate psychosocial aspects of a patient's life. Identifying significant disability in a family member or altered family dynamics from a spine issue may provide useful insight into a patient's expectations, fears, or other psychological features that could have a strong bearing on outcome. By asking about family members and parents, one can begin to understand the nature of family dynamics that may be influencing the presentation of a patient with spinal pain. A history of abuse, the presence of a disruptive home environment, and a history of poor parenting or alcoholism in the family may have a significant future impact on the psychological makeup of an individual. Anger, unmet dependency needs, and problems with trust in authority figures are some of the issues that could result in chronic pain issues. Probing these issues in taking a family history may provide valuable insight into potential barriers to recovery.

Yellow Flags: Predictors of Poor Outcome in the Patient's History

Numerous factors in a patient's history have been identified as potential predictors of poor outcome in the treatment of spinal pain. These factors are known as yellow flags (Box 12.1).[45] The presence of more than one of these factors in a patient is a strong predictor of poor outcome and chronic pain and disability.[45] These yellow flags include issues related to the nature of the patient's injury and general medical health, occupational and social issues, and psychological factors. It is imperative to identify these factors, if present, early in the course of evaluation and treatment of patients with spinal pain because they have been shown to be more powerful predictors of outcome than other biomedical issues.[44–48]

Patients who report more widespread symptoms of neck or back pain, who have more severe pain or disability at the onset of their injury, or who have higher rates of concurrent comorbidities tend to have a higher risk of developing protracted pain complaints or disability.[47–50] For low back pain specifically, dominant medical factors associated with the development of protracted pain or disability seem to be the presence of severe leg pain and a history of prior episodes of low back pain.[47,49,51] In the setting of whiplash, more severe pain or disability, the immediate onset of neck pain, low back pain or headache, and a history of neck pain all predict more protracted problems after the injury, as do less strictly event-related factors, such as a high level of catastrophizing

BOX 12.1 Yellow Flags: Potential Predictors of Poor Outcomes or Persisting Pain and Disability, Particularly When More Than One Is Present

Biomedical Factors

Widespread pain
High levels of comorbidity
Prior episodes of spinal pain (particularly if associated with disability)
Severe radiating limb pain
Poor sleep

Occupational Factors

Poor job satisfaction
Perceived poor-quality work environment
Absence of light-duty alternatives
Short time at current position
Low level of education
Physically demanding work
Extensive time off from work

Psychosocial or Cognitive Factors

Fear-avoidance beliefs
Catastrophizing
Passive coping style
Depression
Anxiety
Somatization
Psychological distress
History of abuse
Self-perceived poor health
Social withdrawal
History of substance abuse

From Gaunt AM. Caring for patients who have acute and subacute low back pain. *CME Bull.* 2008;7:1–7.

and a low educational level (less than a secondary education). Interestingly, accident-related details, including a rear-end mechanism and accident severity, are not predictive of worse outcomes.[52] Some distinct occupational factors that have been shown to be related to the development of chronic pain include heavy physical workload, unavailability of light duties on return to work, perceived poor working environment or job dissatisfaction, a low level of education, and a short time of employment on the job.[47–49,51,53] The amount of time off work from an injury also has a negative correlation with return to work rates.[54,55]

As noted previously, psychological factors seem to play a substantial role in the development of chronic spinal pain. In a review on this topic, Linton[46] noted that psychological variables are clearly linked to the transition from acute to chronic pain and generally have a stronger impact on chronicity than medical or biomechanical factors. Pertinent emotional factors cited include depression, anxiety, distress, and self-perceived poor health. Cognitive and behavioral factors also apparently play a key role in the development of a chronic pain state; these include a passive coping style, catastrophizing, and fear-avoidance beliefs (beliefs that certain activities should be avoided owing to fear of injury). A history of sexual or physical abuse also may be related to chronic pain and disability.[46] A systematic review of psychosocial factors found that psychological distress, depressed mood, and somatization were associated with the transition to chronic low back pain.[56]

Despite the high prevalence of psychopathology in patients with chronic pain, there does not seem to be a premorbid "pain-prone" personality; the depressive features of chronic spinal pain generally seem to arise more as a consequence, rather than a cause, of the pain state.[46,57,58] One study did identify premorbid depression, however, as an independent, robust risk factor for the onset of an episode of troublesome neck or low back pain.[59]

From a strictly surgical perspective, the outcomes of lumbar surgical procedures are influenced by numerous factors completely unrelated to the anatomy or pathophysiology of the spine. The results of lumbar discography are influenced by psychosocial variables to such a large degree that there are concerns about the validity of the procedure.[15] Factors identified as predictors of poor outcome from surgical intervention in the lumbar spine include low level of education, low income at the time of injury, the presence of pending litigation, the presence of an industrial injury, anxiety, neuroticism, and depression.[60–65] Surgical outcomes have also been found to be worse in geographic regions with higher rates of surgical intervention.[66] From a clinical standpoint, it is important to identify predictors of poor outcome or chronicity to provide appropriate care to address these issues and to *avoid* invasive care that is highly unlikely to be helpful and could contribute to the perpetuation of chronic pain and disability.

Obtaining a Psychosocial History

Obtaining information necessary for successful decisions about care requires the spine specialist to evaluate a patient with chronic pain differently from a patient with an acute injury. It is particularly true in treating the patient with chronic pain that the foundation for good decision making is having a good knowledge of the *person* with a back disorder; the spine itself is less important. In other words, it is more important to know about the patient who has the disease than to know about the disease the patient has. This is well borne out in the data presented earlier on prognostic and predictive factors, which generally have much more to do with the psychological state or approach of the affected individual than they do with the actual injury.

It is dangerous to assume that a patient's presenting symptoms are solely the result of the injury that led to the consultation. Patients in whom disability greatly exceeds that expected on the basis of objective findings have been shown to be much more likely to have encountered childhood abuse and conflict, parental job stress, or a difficult divorce. Pain is an experience that is influenced by everything that is currently occurring in the life of the patient. Equally or sometimes more important is everything that has gone on in the patient's life in the past. In a study of more than 25,000 subjects in 14 countries, the World Health Organization found that physical disability is more closely associated with psychological factors than with medical diagnosis.[67] Regardless of the presence of anatomic pathology, it is important to understand that a family member, a stressful circumstance, regular use of opioid analgesics, money issues related to compensation or litigation, and other factors can contribute to a patient's ongoing pain and disability. This comment should not be construed as indicating that the pain is "all in the patient's head," and it is not intended to suggest that the patient is malingering or that the patient's pain is invalid or trivial. Pain and the disability it may produce are complex and multidimensional.

It has been estimated that approximately 50% of patients with chronic pain in rehabilitation and family practice settings have a personality disorder, as documented through structured interviews and psychological testing.[68] Thorough evaluation of patients with back pain needs to include some form of psychological testing because psychological factors play a critical role in patient recovery from illness or injury and the response to surgery or other medical interventions. Ignoring either the physical or the psychological components of pain in diagnosis and treatment is a prescription for failure, disappointment, and dissatisfaction. Several psychological test instruments are available for this purpose.

Additional Assessment Tools

Although there is no substitute for a concise, yet thorough, history, there are some tools that can improve efficiency. Preprinted questionnaires can be used to obtain details of a patient's history. Including some questions about the psychological issues noted previously can facilitate the efficient acquisition of a large pool of information. Other vehicles—such as pain drawings, pain scales, and functional outcome measures—can also be used.

Pain drawings have been used since the 1940s, and research into their significance has provided mixed results.[69] Although there are data supporting an association between psychological distress and widespread, nonanatomic markings on the pain drawing, there is contradictory evidence in other studies. Data are also contradictory on the usefulness of pain drawings in predicting surgical outcomes.[69] Pain drawings have been assessed using various means and have been shown to have relatively high repeatability.[69,70] Although the presence of widespread or nonanatomic patterns of pain on these drawings may be of some use in identifying pain intensity and the presence of depression or psychological distress, one systematic review did not find evidence to support their use as a formal psychological assessment tool (Fig. 12.8).[69,71,72]

A variety of pain scales may be used in patient assessment. Various visual analog scales have been reported. The Million Visual Analog Scale has been shown to have good reliability,

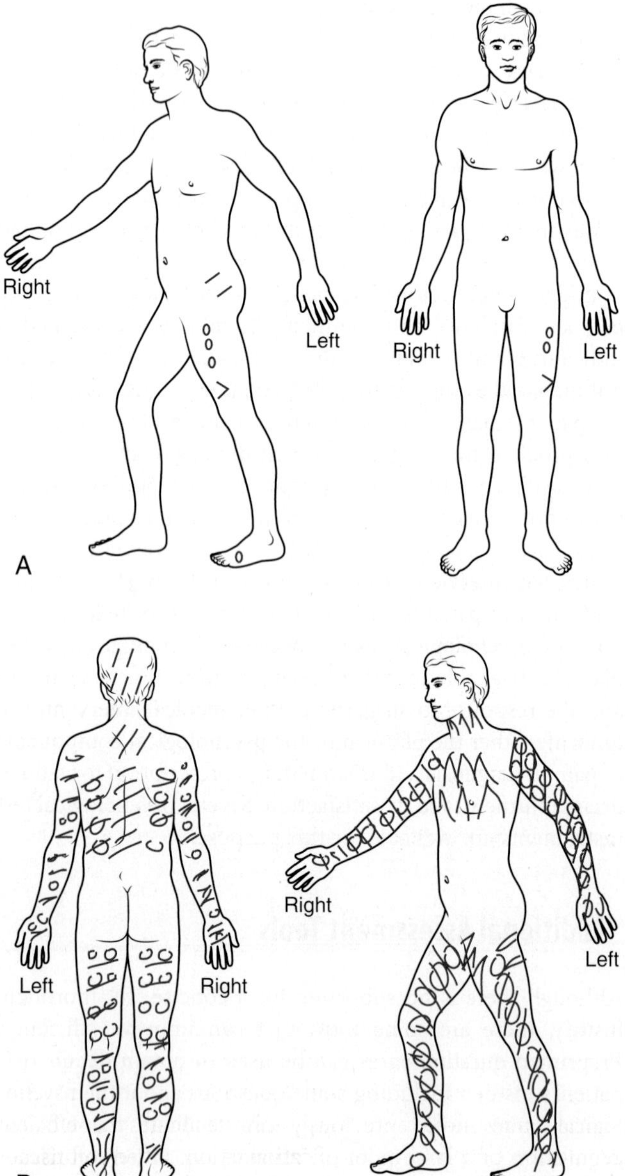

FIG. 12.8 Pain drawings by patients. (A) The patient had radiating pain in an L3 pattern related to intraforaminal disc herniation at L3–L4. (B) The patient had long-standing, widespread pain in nonanatomic distribution.

validity, and responsiveness.[73] The McGill Pain Questionnaire has also been widely used and is well validated. This questionnaire provides a quantitative assessment using numerous descriptors of pain over three separate domains that are identified by the test taker and scored.[73] Other scales identifying the "bothersomeness" of pain and the bodily pain item in the Medical Outcomes Study 36-item Short Form Health Survey (SF-36) have also been applied in the assessment of patients with spine disorders.[74]

Numerous functional scales exist, including the Oswestry Low Back Pain Disability Questionnaire, the modified Roland scale, the Neck Disability Index, the Sickness Impact Profile and the related Disability Questionnaire, and the SF-36.[73–77] The Oswestry questionnaire, which uses self-rated functional impairment in numerous activities of daily living, has been shown to be valid and responsive, and is generally easy to administer and score.[73,75] The modified Roland scale, which consists of 24 "yes" or "no" questions regarding the functional impact of back pain, was originally derived from the Sickness Impact Profile, has been well validated, has a high responsiveness, and is very easy to score.[73,74]

Several brief psychological scales are also useful. The presence of fear-avoidance beliefs and catastrophizing are particularly important in the development and maintenance of chronic pain and disability. The Fear-Avoidance Beliefs Questionnaire[78] and the Pain Catastrophizing Scale[79] are validated assessment tools that can be used to quantify these factors.

The Battery for Health Improvement-2 is a self-report multiple-choice instrument designed for assessment of medical patients. It is intended to provide one source of clinical hypotheses that professionals can use to explore the interrelationships between a patient's psychological and medical conditions. The information can be particularly useful in helping to determine factors that may be influencing an inexplicable delay in recovery of an injured patient. The Opioid Risk Tool is clinically relevant and easily employed during the interview.[80]

The Patient-Reported Outcomes Measurement Instrumentation System (PROMIS) is a set of publicly available measures to evaluate patient-reported outcomes through the assessment of physical, social, and emotional health. There is a wide range of measures that have been developed and validated, including a number for pain, emotional distress, alcohol use, and other issues that may be related to chronic spinal pain. There are several composite scales available, including the PROMIS-29, which covers the domains of anxiety, depression, fatigue, pain interference, physical function, sleep, and social functioning.[81] The PROMIS measures have been studied in a vast array of medical conditions, and are likely to play an important role in research and clinical care in the chronic pain population.

Physical Examination

After obtaining a complete history, a focused examination can be performed to establish a baseline functional and neurologic assessment, identify pertinent positive and negative findings that can help narrow the differential diagnosis, and define further issues that may need to be addressed through additional testing. Although a thorough discussion is beyond the scope of this chapter, appropriate portions of a general medical examination need to be included in the assessment of a spinal patient depending on the nature of the presenting issues. Neurologic and orthopaedic examinations of varying degree and complexity are also necessary. This chapter follows a more focused approach to the examination of the spine with a discussion of basic neurologic assessment and relevant provocative maneuvers appropriate to a patient's presenting problem.

Observation

The physical examination starts with observation, which begins when the physician first sees the patient. Movement patterns, preferred postures, inconsistencies, and gait abnormalities should be noted by the clinician and staff members throughout the patient's visit. This observation needs to be done casually during office or facility interactions and during the medical history, then in a more formal manner during the examination. Formal observation should include an examination from the feet to the head. Trunk and appendicular alignment should be noted, paying particular attention to hip and knee alignment. The spine should be assessed for alterations from normal alignment or resting curvature, including scoliosis, kyphosis, alterations in lumbar or cervical lordosis, a lumbar shift, and head and neck alignment with the trunk. Symmetry of shoulder height and scapular positioning should also be noted.

Gait assessment can be done after initial observation, looking specifically for gait patterns suggestive of neurologic deficits, such as a steppage gait associated with footdrop or a wide-based gait suggestive of proprioceptive, cerebellar, or myelopathic pathology. Gait can be tested further by tandem gait testing (heel-to-toe walking). Balance can be assessed by simple observation and performing a single-leg stance with various postural challenges (e.g., crouching on one leg). If a patient has an antalgic gait (i.e., shortened stance phase of the gait cycle), consideration should be given to a musculoskeletal problem involving the hips, knees, or foot and ankle. Generally, patients with a lumbar radiculopathy do not exhibit an antalgic gait pattern.

Spine range of motion (ROM) should be assessed for all relevant spine segments. There is debate as to what constitutes "normal" range of spine motion and the significance of any perceived restriction of motion. In the lumbar spine, ROM has been variably reported by using inclinometry, measuring the distance from the fingertips to the floor, assessing segmental motion, measuring dynamic motion, measuring motion with the pelvis restrained, radiographic measurement, and using variations of the Schober test (measuring the change in distance between a mark over the S1 spinous process and one made 10 cm above this in standing that occurs between standing and flexion).[82–85]

The value of ROM measurements is questionable, however, because some data do indicate that there is no consistent relationship between ROM and physical or functional impairment in subjects with chronic low back pain.[83] ROM generally seems to decline with age, further complicating attempts at establishing normative data.[82] Gross lumbar motions generally include motion from the hips and lower extremities, and any lateral flexion or rotation involves coupled motion at multiple levels, making it difficult to assess these reliably. It is important to examine hip motion, however, because painful and restricted hip motion, particularly in flexion with internal rotation, that mimics the patient's usual pain would generally implicate the hip as a source of pain.

Despite these substantial limitations, it is still important to assess active spine motion in flexion, extension, rotation, and lateral flexion. Along with absolute degrees of movement, the examiner can assess symmetry of motion, preferred movement patterns, pain or symptom reproduction associated with motion, the relative contributions of associated body segments to motion (e.g., hips), motor control, and inconsistencies between movement noted on formal examination and that seen during casual observation or while the patient is otherwise distracted. Generally, patient motion should be assessed actively within the patient's range of comfort. There is little or no role for passive ROM because this adds little to the clinical assessment and may place the patient at risk for further injury.[38]

For cervical and thoracic complaints, it is also important to assess shoulder and scapular motion. Shoulder ROM can be assessed actively by flexion and abduction along with passive motion of the glenohumeral joint. Scapular position at rest and with various arm positions can reveal abnormal movement patterns and may indicate problems with scapulothoracic function, other shoulder joint complex disorders, or neurologic injury affecting the parascapular musculature (e.g., a long thoracic or spinal accessory nerve injury). Scapulothoracic dysfunction of various kinds may also be a source of pain in patients with thoracic complaints.[86] Reproduction of a patient's shoulder region pain by passive shoulder motion, particularly if it is restricted, would generally implicate the shoulder rather than the neck as the source of pain. Patients with a cervical radiculopathy obtain relief with ipsilateral shoulder abduction (the shoulder abduction relief maneuver); patients with intrinsic shoulder pathology often have reproduction of pain with shoulder abduction.

Observation should also include looking for atrophy, edema, vasomotor changes, skin lesions, limb or joint deformity, contracture, and other signs that may have an impact on a patient's care.

Palpation

The relevant areas of the patient's spine and related structures should be palpated with the patient standing or, when appropriate, in side-lying or prone position. Palpation may aid in the localization of the patient's symptoms, the identification of an injured structure, or the identification of associated soft tissue or bony abnormalities. It should be noted whether tenderness is elicited in the midline or to either side of the midline, potentially differentiating between spinal pain and pain from an adjacent soft tissue source.[38] Localized tenderness should be distinguished from diffuse tenderness, the latter being less consistent with a focal injury.

In the cervical spine, palpation should include the occipital region; the anterior neck; the clavicular, supraclavicular, and scapular regions; and the areas of the associated cervicothoracic musculature.[38] In the thoracic region, palpation should also extend across the posterior ribs to identify focal bony tenderness that may suggest rib pathology rather than spine pathology. Pain with palpation or percussion of the costovertebral angle may suggest renal pathology.[87] Spondylolisthesis can frequently be appreciated by a palpable step-off of the spinous processes in the lumbar spine. In the lumbar region, palpation should include not only the lumbar spine but also the iliac crests, sacrum, sacroiliac joints, ischial tuberosities, proximal hamstring, and greater trochanteric areas, as indicated, to assess for the possibility of contributing problems from these regions. Trochanteric pain may mimic pain from a spine etiology.

Clinicians need to recognize that the ability to accurately identify a spinal level by palpation is quite limited. Multiple studies have confirmed high rates of inaccuracy with manual palpation, which raises concerns for the manual identification of structural problems and for the precise placement of medical instruments for spinal interventions.[88,89]

Neurologic Examination

As with the general medical examination, the neurologic examination may cover a wide range of factors, depending on the particular presenting problem. The most common neurologic manifestations of spine pathology generally involve the spinal nerve roots or the spinal cord, resulting in radicular or myelopathic findings on examination. The symptoms resulting from spine pathology may frequently overlap, however, with symptoms of various peripheral nerve processes, central nervous system disease, or anterior horn cell disease. An examiner needs to be aware of the clinical presentations and neurologic findings associated with these disorders. A full discussion of all relevant examination techniques and neurologic pathology is beyond the scope of this chapter, but can be found in general neurology texts. This section focuses on findings more directly related to spine pathology.

A thorough understanding of dermatomal patterns is essential for all clinicians examining spine patients. As a reference, the key sensory points identified by the American Spinal Injury Association[90] can be helpful in assessing or screening patients with spine pathology (see Fig. 12.5). Soft-touch and pin-prick sensation can be assessed well in most patients; the examiner should distinguish between a dermatomal distribution suggesting nerve root pathology, a stocking or stocking-and-glove distribution suggesting peripheral polyneuropathy, multiple nerve distribution suggesting alternative peripheral nerve pathology, or a nonorganic distribution. Proprioception, vibration, position sense, and temperature sensation may also be tested, particularly when there is concern for a spinal cord or central nervous system process or a peripheral neuropathy.

Motor examination consists of several parts, including strength, tone, coordination, muscle bulk, and involuntary movements.[87] Strength is the modality most generally assessed by clinicians, but all portions of the motor examination may be important in some patients with spine disorders. Involuntary movements may be noted in patients with cervical dystonia or in various neurologic diseases that may affect function, such as Parkinson disease. The presence or absence of focal muscle atrophy should be noted in all patients. The mere presence of focal atrophy implies neurologic injury or disease, and the distribution of atrophic muscles can be helpful in defining the type of pathology present. Fasciculations associated with atrophic muscles imply the presence of lower motor neuron injury. Muscle tone can be affected by many neurologic processes. Reduced tone suggests lower motor neuron involvement, whereas increased tone or spasticity is seen with upper motor neuron disease. Coordination may be disrupted by numerous pathways, generally involving the cerebellum or its pathways, but weakness, proprioceptive loss, and cognitive disturbance may also affect motor performance on tests of coordination. Clinical methods to assess coordination include rapid alternating hand and foot movements and finger-to-nose testing.[87]

Strength testing is generally done isometrically, but sometimes weakness can be better appreciated through dynamic or repetitive movements that address endurance (e.g., multiple single-leg toe raises to assess plantar flexor strength). It is essential to be aware of key muscle groups by myotome and the peripheral nerve origin of those muscles. Important muscle groups and motions associated with cervical and lumbar myotomes are as follows:

C5—elbow flexors, shoulder abductors and external rotators
C6—elbow flexors, wrist extensors and pronators, shoulder external rotators
C7—elbow extensors, wrist pronators
C8—extension of index finger, finger abduction and flexion, abduction of thumb
T1—finger abduction
L2—hip flexion
L3—hip flexion, hip adduction, knee extension
L4—knee extension, ankle dorsiflexion
L5—ankle dorsiflexion, great toe extension, ankle eversion, hip abduction and internal rotation
S1—ankle plantar flexion, toe flexion

Strength is generally graded on a scale of 0 to 5 as follows:[87]

5—active movement against full resistance (normal strength)
4—active movement against gravity and some resistance
3—active movement against gravity
2—active movement with gravity eliminated
1—trace movement or barely detectable contraction
0—no muscular contraction identified

Active movement is generally meant to imply joint motion through the full available ROM. For some muscle groups, patients can often have significant loss of strength that is not detectable by providing manual resistance with the examiner's arms; thus, other test maneuvers may be necessary to identify more subtle weakness. Examples of such maneuvers would be having the patient do a partial squat or arise from sitting without using the upper extremities to assess for weakness in the knee extensors. The Beevor sign (in which the umbilicus moves craniad during contraction of the abdominal muscles with supine neck flexion) indicates weakness of the lower abdominal muscles.[26]

Reflex testing can further aid in the localization of neurologic injury and help distinguish upper motor neuron from lower neuron disease. In lower motor neuron injuries, deep tendon reflexes of affected regions are generally reduced, whereas they are brisk in upper motor neuron injuries. The Babinski response to appropriate plantar stimulation, Hoffman sign in the hand, and clonus all can indicate the presence of upper motor neuron injury. As with other physical examination findings, the sensitivity and specificity of these findings are limited for any particular condition. In a study assessing the prevalence of physical examination findings in cervical myelopathy treated surgically, it was noted that 21% of the patients had no myelopathic findings on examination. Of the findings just mentioned, the Hoffman sign was the most sensitive (59%), whereas the Babinski response had very low sensitivity (13%) but was highly specific.[91] Various other reflexes—including abdominal, cremasteric, and palmomental—can also be used as part of the neurologic examination when appropriate.

Although a neurologic injury often manifests as either an upper or a lower motor neuron lesion, it can also manifest with a mixed pattern of upper and lower motor neuron features, as can be seen with amyotrophic lateral sclerosis. The segmental distribution of commonly tested deep tendon reflexes is as follows[87]:

Biceps reflex—C5, C6
Brachioradialis reflex—C5, C6
Triceps reflex—C6, C7
Patellar tendon reflex—L2, L3, L4
Medial hamstring reflex—L5, S1
Ankle jerk reflex (Achilles tendon)—S1

For the most part, the sensitivity and specificity of isolated tests for sensation, strength, and reflexes are relatively limited in the assessment of spine conditions, particularly when any one single test is considered.[22,85,92] There may be more utility in combining a variety of findings across multiple modalities, especially when the findings are consistently reproducible. The degree of consistency between examination findings, history, imaging results, and self-reported levels of pain and disability for affected patients should always be considered when clinical decisions on care are made.

Special Tests and Provocative Maneuvers

In addition to the standard examination techniques described earlier, various provocative maneuvers and other tests have been used to aid in the diagnosis of patients with spine conditions. The sensitivity and specificity of many of these tests are either unclear or suboptimal, but a working knowledge of their applicability is useful in the diagnosis and management of patients with spine conditions.

The *Lhermitte sign,* although more technically a symptom, is the presence of an electric shock–type sensation radiating into the limbs with cervical flexion. Although first described in a patient with multiple sclerosis, this sign is associated with various spinal cord lesions.[26,38] If elicited with neck flexion, this sign should raise concern for the presence of a cervical cord lesion. If elicited with trunk flexion, this may indicate a thoracic cord lesion.[26]

The *Spurling maneuver* is a test for cervical nerve root compression or irritation. A positive test is elicited by extending, rotating, and laterally bending the head to one side with reproduction of radicular pain into the affected ipsilateral extremity.[26,38] One study comparing the Spurling maneuver with the results of electrodiagnostic testing found that the maneuver had poor sensitivity (30%) but good specificity (93%) in the diagnosis of electrodiagnostically confirmed cervical radiculopathy.[93]

The *Valsalva maneuver* is performed by having a patient hold his or her breath and bear down. A reproduction of the patient's radicular symptoms or spinal pain with this maneuver is believed to indicate a space-occupying lesion, such as a disc herniation, in the spinal canal.[26,38]

Dural tension signs are frequently used to assess lumbar spine pathology. Many different maneuvers have been described. A supine *straight-leg raise* is performed by elevating the leg with knee extended and assessing for the reproduction of pain into the leg. The test is considered positive if pain occurs between 30 degrees and 70 degrees of elevation because no true change in tension on the nerve roots is believed to occur outside of this range.[3,85] Variations on this test include the *Lasègue sign* or *Bragard sign,* which involves raising the leg to the point of symptom reproduction and then lowering the leg slightly and dorsiflexing the foot passively; a positive test results in reproduction of the patient's radiating leg pain.[3,94] Other variants include internally rotating the leg to increase "dural tension," raising the leg with knee flexed and then slowly extending the knee to the point of reproduction of leg pain (also sometimes referred to as the *Lasègue sign*), and either relieving pain by flexing the already extended knee at the point of symptom reproduction or eliciting pain by pressing on the popliteal fossa of the elevated leg with the knee partially flexed (both varyingly called the *bowstring sign*).[3,85,92,94]

Additional tests include the *crossed straight-leg raise,* in which symptoms are reproduced in the symptomatic leg by performing a supine straight-leg raise on the contralateral leg, and the *femoral nerve stretch test* or *reverse straight-leg raise,* in which the patient is prone and the knee is passively flexed, with a positive test reproducing pain into the anterior thigh. A positive straight-leg raise test and its variations indicates tension on the lower lumbar roots and upper sacral root (L4, L5, and S1 nerve roots). A positive femoral nerve stretch test is the equivalent tension sign for the upper lumbar (L2–L4) nerve roots.[3,85,92]

Numerous studies have looked at the sensitivity and specificity of some of these maneuvers. As might be surmised by the varying descriptions and terminology, there are some difficulties with consistency in the literature. Overall, the ipsilateral straight-leg raise test has a good sensitivity of 72% to 97% but a poorer specificity of 11% to 66%.[92] The crossed straight-leg raise test is less sensitive (23–42%) but more specific (85–100%) than the ipsilateral straight-leg raise.[85,92]

Tests proposed for assessing the sacroiliac joint include the *Gillet, Patrick,* and *Gaenslen tests.* Although the sacroiliac joint can be a source of pain, the diagnosis of "sacroiliac joint dysfunction" is debated as a true pathologic entity. Dreyfuss and colleagues[28] studied numerous supposedly diagnostic tests for this condition, including the Gillet, Patrick, and Gaenslen tests, and compared the responses on these test maneuvers with the results of fluoroscopically guided sacroiliac joint blocks. They found that no historical feature, none of the diagnostic tests performed, and no combination of these tests showed any significant and reliable diagnostic value.

Nonorganic Signs

Chronic pain behavior is often believed to display common physical examination findings suggesting symptom magnification and psychological distress, possibly an expression of suffering.[95,96] Waddell and colleagues[95] defined and studied a group of five findings on physical examination, commonly known as *Waddell signs.* These findings consist of a superficial or nonanatomic distribution of tenderness; a nonanatomic motor or sensory impairment (regional disturbance); excessive verbalization of pain or gesturing (overreaction); production of pain complaints by tests that simulate only a specific movement, such as low back pain that occurs with axial loading on the crown of the head (simulation); and inconsistent reports of pain when the same movement is performed in different positions, such as a straight-leg raise in a seated versus supine position (distraction).[95]

The presence of three or more of these signs indicates a nonorganic component to an individual's pain complaints. The presence of Waddell signs does not mean, however, that there is no significant organic pathology present or that the patient is malingering; objective clinical signs may be present as well. Although some studies have found these maneuvers to be reproducible, an evidence-based review by Fishbain and colleagues[97] noted that these findings do not correlate with psychological distress or secondary gain, and they do not discriminate nonorganic from organic problems. They are associated with poorer treatment outcomes and higher pain levels. Although these maneuvers may be useful, the clinician should be wary of placing too much emphasis on any one part of the physical examination.

Additional Orthopaedic Assessment

Depending on the area of the spine involved, it is frequently important to cover additional areas of the orthopaedic examination. As was previously mentioned, examination of the shoulder complex is often necessary in evaluating the cervical and thoracic spine. Following the concept of the *kinetic chain,* it is also often helpful to assess multiple other joint structures and movement patterns from the feet up through the trunk to the neck, depending on the individual patient's situation.[98] For the lumbar spine, examination of the hip is also generally important, although examination of more distal lower extremity structures and more cranial regions of the spine and upper extremities may be necessary as well. Because other conditions—such as carpal tunnel syndrome, ulnar neuropathy, brachial plexopathy, peroneal neuropathy, and femoral nerve injury (among others)—can masquerade as radiculopathies, examination for these entities is also often indicated. As noted previously, an appropriate history can help greatly in defining the scope of examination necessary to evaluate a particular patient.

There is a large body of literature on manual orthopaedic examination.[99,100] These techniques generally are poorly validated and of uncertain correlation to some of the more "objective" findings noted earlier. A systematic review of the literature on the reliability of palpatory examination maneuvers found that most procedures have moderate or strong evidence for low reliability.[101] The authors noted that "a consistent finding from work in this field is the generally low reliability of palpation-based assessment."[101] These techniques may be helpful in certain treatment paradigms, however, and they may be more useful when symptom response with repeated movements is considered.[101] Another systematic review assessed the literature on chiropractic tests of the lumbar spine and found insufficient evidence on the reliability and validity of these tests to support their clinical role.[102]

Risk Stratification

Distinct from the idea of the evaluation of an individual patient is the concept of risk stratification within a population. Within the clinical array of patients with spinal disorders, there are clearly those who will require more extensive care and/or be at risk for particularly poor outcomes. There is increasing interest in applying screening mechanisms across a population to help identify those patients with a poor prognosis for recovery or in need of more intensive or multidisciplinary care. This type of assessment may be incorporated into a patient's initial evaluation. An example of such a screening approach is the STarT Back tool.[103] Consistent with the data noted earlier on prognostic factors for those with spinal pain, the STarT Back questionnaire consists of nine questions addressing the bothersomeness of pain, the presence of leg pain or concurrent neck symptoms, and the presence of fear avoidance or other generally detrimental belief systems regarding pain.[104] The intent is to separate patients with more limited symptom complexes and better coping skills who will likely do well with standard treatments from those who may require more advanced or complex interventions in order to improve outcomes. In the primary study of the STarT Back tool, the researchers developed and implemented a psychologically driven physical therapy program for the more at-risk population, finding improvements in outcomes for those treated based on risk stratification from those managed without any such tool. They also found that primary care providers did a relatively poor job of appropriately identifying the physical therapy needs of patients without using the questionnaire.[103] The broader applicability of this tool is currently under study, but this type of work highlights the potential benefits of stratifying patients for treatment. This may become an important component of the medical history for patients with spinal disorders.

Summary

The history and physical examination of a spine patient is a complex undertaking. The nature of the patient's presenting complaints and relevant aspects of the history have a strong bearing on the nature and extent of assessment required. Clinicians caring for patients with spine disorders need to be aware of all of the issues that may affect the presentation of a patient and how these issues can affect the delivery of care. As noted previously, it is of paramount importance to realize that the person presenting with the spine problem is the primary concern, and the spine problem is only secondary. Only by speaking with and directly examining a patient can clinicians truly understand the nature of the problem that they are being asked to address.

KEY POINTS

1. A thorough and appropriate history and physical examination are essential in the assessment of patients with spine disorders to identify the physical manifestations of a spine disorder and the root causes of the patient's distress, suffering, and disability.
2. It is crucial to identify red flags and yellow flags in a patient's clinical presentation. Red flags are factors suggestive of the presence of an urgent or emergent medical issue (e.g., infection, tumor, fracture, cauda equina injury, progressive neurologic loss). Yellow flags are factors associated with poor outcomes and persisting pain and disability.
3. The medical history can be used to narrow down the differential diagnosis and direct further diagnostic efforts through physical examination and other tools.
4. The value of isolated findings on physical examination is limited, although physical examination findings become much more significant in the context of correlating history and imaging.
5. Despite the importance of a thorough medical history, clinicians need to realize that psychosocial factors are a more important predictor of outcome in patients with spinal pain than biomedical factors.

KEY REFERENCES

1. Bogduk N. The anatomy and pathophysiology of neck pain. *Phys Med Rehabil Clin N Am*. 2003;14:455-472.
   This is a concise overview of some important issues in assessing patients with neck pain.
2. Henschke N, Maher CG, Ostelo RWJG, et al. Red flags to screen for malignancy in patients with low-back pain. *Cochrane Database Syst Rev*. 2013;(2):CD008686.
   An overview of the existing evidence on the use of red flags.
3. Linton SJ. A review of psychosocial risk factors in back and neck pain. *Spine*. 2000;25:1148-1156.
   This is a useful and well-executed review of the role of psychosocial risk factors in the development of chronic spinal pain.
4. http://www.healthmeasures.net/explore-measurement-systems/promis.
   This is the website for the Patient-Reported Outcomes Measurement Instrumentation System, a publically available set of outcome tools for a variety of health conditions, including pain, developed by the National Institutes of Health.
5. Solomon J, Nadler SF, Press J. Physical examination of the lumbar spine. In: Malanga G, Nadler SF, eds. *Musculoskeletal Physical Examination: An Evidence-Based Approach*. Philadelphia: Hanley & Belfus; 2006:189-226.
   This is one of many useful chapters in a well-prepared text assessing the literature on musculoskeletal physical examination.
6. Hill JC, Whitehurst DGT, Lewis M, et al. Comparison of Stratified Primary Care Management for Low Back Pain with Current Best Practice (STarT Back): a randomised controlled trial. *Lancet*. 2011;378:1560-1571.
   Article on the STarT Back screening tool to assist in the treatment stratification of patients with low back pain.

REFERENCES

1. Bogduk N. The anatomy and pathophysiology of neck pain. *Phys Med Rehabil Clin N Am*. 2003;14:455-472.
2. Bogduk N. *Clinical Anatomy of the Lumbar Spine and Sacrum*. 3rd ed. New York: Churchill-Livingstone; 1997.
3. Borenstein DG, Wiesel SW. *Low Back Pain: Medical Diagnosis and Comprehensive Management*. Philadelphia: WB Saunders; 1989.
4. Liss H, Liss D, Pavell J. History and past medical history. In: Cole AJ, Herring SA, eds. *The Low Back Pain Handbook*. 2nd ed. Philadelphia: Hanley & Belfus; 2003:49-67.
5. Weinstein SM, Herring SA, Standaert CJ. Low back pain. In: Delisa JA, Gans BM, Walsh NE, eds. *Physical Medicine and Rehabilitation: Principles and Practice*. 4th ed. Philadelphia: Lippincott-Williams & Wilkins; 2005:653-678.
6. Dwyer A, Aprill C, Bogduk N. Cervical zygapophyseal joint pain patterns I: a study in normal volunteers. *Spine*. 1990;15:453-457.
7. Aprill C, Dwyer A, Bogdul N. Cervical zygapophyseal joint pain patterns II: a clinical evaluation. *Spine*. 1990;15:458-461.
8. Lord SM, Barnsley L, Wallis BJ, et al. Chronic cervical zygapophyseal joint pain after whiplash: a placebo-controlled prevalence study. *Spine*. 1996;21:1737-1745.
9. Dreyfuss P, Tibiletti C, Dreyer S. Thoracic zygapophyseal joint pain patterns: a study in normal volunteers. *Spine*. 1994;19:807-811.
10. Schwarzer AC, Aprill CN, Derby R, et al. Clinical features of patients with pain stemming from the lumbar zygapophysial joints: is the lumbar facet syndrome a clinical entity? *Spine*. 1994;19:1132-1137.
11. Marks R. Distribution of pain provoked from lumbar facet joints and related structures during diagnostic spinal infiltration. *Pain*. 1989;39:37-40.
12. Cloward RB. Cervical discography: a contribution to the etiology and mechanism of neck, shoulder and arm pain. *Ann Surg*. 1959;150:1052-1064.
13. Grubb SA, Kelly CK. Cervical discography: clinical implications from 12 years of experience. *Spine*. 2000;25:1382-1389.
14. Campbell JN. Nerve lesions and the generation of pain. *Muscle Nerve*. 2001;24:1261-1273.
15. Carragee EJ, Alamin TF. Discography: a review. *Spine J*. 2001;1:364-372.
16. Hogan Q. Back pain: beguiling physiology (and politics). *Reg Anesth*. 1997;22:395-399.
17. Sinclair JD. Chronic noncancer pain basics for the primary care physician. *Primary Care Rep*. 2002;8:63-73.
18. Sheather-Reid RB, Cohen ML. Psychophysiological evidence for a neuropathic component of chronic neck pain. *Pain*. 1998;75:341-347.

19. Agency for Health Care Policy and Research. *Acute Low Back Problems in Adults: Assessment and Treatment.* Washington, DC: US Department of Health and Human Services; 1994.
20. Akuthota V, Willick SE, Harden RN. The adult spine: a practical approach to low back pain. In: Rucker KS, Cole AJ, Weinstein SM, eds. *Low Back Pain: A Symptom-Based Approach to Diagnosis and Treatment.* Boston: Butterworth-Heinemann; 2001:15-41.
21. Carragee EJ, Hannibal M. Diagnostic evaluation of low back pain. *Orthop Clin North Am.* 2004;35:7-16.
22. Deyo RA, Rainville J, Kent DL. What can the history and physical examination tell us about low back pain? *JAMA.* 1992;268:760-765.
23. Henschke N, Maher CG, Ostelo RWJG, et al. Red flags to screen for malignancy in patients with low-back pain. *Cochrane Database Syst Rev.* 2013;(2):CD008686.
24. Downie A, Williams CM, Henschke N, et al. Red flags to screen for malignancy and fracture in patients with low back pain: systematic review. *BMJ.* 2013;347:f7095.
25. Enthoven WTM, Geuze J, Scheele J, et al. Prevalence and "red flags" regarding specified causes of back pain in older adults presenting in general practice. *Phys Ther.* 2016;96:305-312.
26. Bland JH. *Disorders of the Cervical Spine: Diagnosis and Medical Management.* 2nd ed. Philadelphia: WB Saunders; 1994.
27. Mazanec D. Pseudospine pain: conditions that mimic spine pain. In: Cole AJ, Herring SA, eds. *The Low Back Pain Handbook.* 2nd ed. Philadelphia: Hanley & Belfus; 2003:117-131.
28. Dreyfuss P, Michaelsen M, Pauza K, et al. The value of medical history and physical examination in diagnosing sacroiliac joint pain. *Spine.* 1996;21:2594-2602.
29. Konstantinou K, Hider SL, Jordan JL, et al. The impact of low back-related leg pain on outcomes as compared with low back pain alone. A systematic review of the literature. *Clin J Pain.* 2013;29:644-654.
30. Micheli LJ, Wood R. Back pain in young athletes: significant differences from adults in causes and patterns. *Arch Pediatr Adolesc Med.* 1995;149:15-18.
31. Roche MA, Rowe GG. The incidence of separate neural arch and coincident bone variations: a survey of 4,200 skeletons. *Anat Rec.* 1951;109:233-252.
32. Standaert CJ, Herring SA. Spondylolysis: a critical review. *Br J Sports Med.* 2000;34:415-422.
33. Burton AK, Clarke RD, McClune TD, et al. The natural history of low back pain in adolescents. *Spine.* 1996;21:2323-2328.
34. Kovacs FM, Gestoso M, Gil del Real MT, et al. Risk factors for non-specific low back pain in schoolchildren and their parents: a population based study. *Pain.* 2003;103:259-268.
35. Andersen SJ. Adolescent lumbar spine disorders. In: Rucker KS, Cole AJ, Weinstein SM, eds. *Low Back Pain: A Symptom-based Approach to Diagnosis and Treatment.* Boston: Butterworth-Heinemann; 2001:3-14.
36. Hosalkar H, Dormans J. Back pain in children requires extensive workup. *Biomechanics.* 2003;10:51-58.
37. Malanga GA, Nadler SF, Ageson T. Epidemiology. In: Cole AJ, Herring SA, eds. *The Low Back Pain Handbook.* 2nd ed. Philadelphia: Hanley & Belfus; 2003:1-7.
38. Borenstein DG, Wiesel SW, Boden SD. *Neck Pain: Medical Diagnosis and Comprehensive Management.* Philadelphia: WB Saunders; 1996.
39. Bovim G, Schrader H, Sand T. Neck pain in the general population. *Spine.* 1994;19:1307-1309.
40. Makela M, Heliovaara M, Sievers K, et al. Prevalence, determinants, and consequences of chronic neck pain in Finland. *Am J Epidemiol.* 1991;134:1356-1367.
41. Volinn E. The epidemiology of low back pain in the rest of the world: a review of surveys in low- and middle-income countries. *Spine.* 1997;22:1747-1754.
42. Belanger TA, Rowe DE. Diffuse idiopathic skeletal hyperostosis: musculoskeletal manifestations. *J Am Acad Orthop Surg.* 2001;9:258-267.
43. Paassilta P, Lohiniva J, Goring HH, et al. Identification of a novel common genetic risk factor for lumbar disk disease. *JAMA.* 2001;285:1843-1849.
44. Canoso JJ. *Rheumatology in Primary Care.* Philadelphia: WB Saunders; 1997.
45. Gaunt AM. Caring for patients who have acute and subacute low back pain. *CME Bull.* 2008;7:1-7.
46. Linton SJ. A review of psychosocial risk factors in back and neck pain. *Spine.* 2000;25:1148-1156.
47. Valat JP, Goupille P, Vedere V. Low back pain: risk factors for chronicity. *Rev Rheum [Engl Ed].* 1997;64:189-194.
48. van der Giezen AM, Bouter LM, Nijhuis FJN. Prediction of return-to-work of low back pain patients sicklisted 3-4 months. *Pain.* 2000;87:285-294.
49. Fransen M, Woodward M, Norton R, et al. Risk factors associated with the transition from acute to chronic occupational back pain. *Spine.* 2002;27:92-98.
50. Radanov BP, Sturzenegger M. The effect of accident mechanisms and initial findings on the long-term outcome of whiplash injury. *J Musculoskelet Pain.* 1996;4:47-59.
51. McIntosh G, Frank J, Hogg-Johnson S, et al. Prognostic factors for time receiving workers' compensation benefits in a cohort of patients with low back pain. *Spine.* 2000;25:147-157.
52. Walton DM, Macdermid JC, Giorgianni AA, et al. Risk factors for persistent problems following acute whiplash injury: update of a systematic review and meta-analysis. *J Orthop Sports Phys Ther.* 2013;43:31-43.
53. Krause N, Ragland DR, Greiner BA, et al. Physical workload and ergonomic factors associated with prevalence of back and neck pain in urban transit operators. *Spine.* 1997;22:2117-2126.
54. McGill CM. Industrial back problems: a control program. *J Occup Med.* 1968;10:174-178.
55. Waddell G. Epidemiology: a new clinical model for the treatment of low back pain. In: Weinstein JN, Wiesel SW, eds. *The Lumbar Spine: The International Society for the Study of the Lumbar Spine.* Philadelphia: Saunders; 1990:38-56.
56. Pincus T, Burton AK, Vogel S, et al. A systematic review of psychosocial factors as predictors of chronicity/disability in prospective cohorts of low back pain. *Spine.* 2002;27:E109-E120.
57. Gatchel RJ, Polatin PB, Mayer TG. The dominant role of psychosocial risk factors in the development of chronic low back pain disability. *Spine.* 1995;20:2702-2709.
58. Wallis BJ, Lord SM, Bogduk N. Resolution of psychological distress of whiplash patients following treatment by radiofrequency neurotomy: a randomized, double-blind, placebo-controlled trial. *Pain.* 1997;73:15-22.
59. Carroll LJ, Cassidy JD, Cote P. Depression as a risk factor for onset of an episode of troublesome neck and low back pain. *Pain.* 2004;107:134-139.

60. Chaichana KL, Mukherjee D, Adogwa O, et al. Correlation of preoperative depression and somatic perception scales with postoperative disability and quality of life after lumbar discectomy. *J Neurosurg Spine*. 2011;14:261-267.
61. Daubs MD, Norvell DC, McGuire R, et al. Fusion versus nonoperative care for chronic low back pain. Do psychological factors affect outcomes? *Spine*. 2011;36:S96-S109.
62. DeBerard MS, Masters KS, Colledge AL, et al. Outcomes of posterolateral lumbar fusion in Utah patients receiving workers' compensation: a retrospective cohort study. *Spine*. 2001;26:738-747.
63. Junge A, Dvorak J, Ahrens S. Predictors of bad and good outcomes of lumbar disc surgery: a prospective clinical study with recommendations for screening to avoid bad outcomes. *Spine*. 1995;20:460-468.
64. Loupasis GA, Stamos K, Katonis PG, et al. Seven to 20-year outcome of lumbar discectomy. *Spine*. 1999;24:2313-2317.
65. Pappas CTE, Harrington T, Sonntag VK. Outcome analysis in 654 surgically treated lumbar disc herniations. *Neurosurgery*. 1992;30:862-866.
66. Keller RB, Atlas SJ, Soule DN, et al. Relationship between rates and outcomes of operative treatment for lumbar disc herniation and spinal stenosis. *J Bone Joint Surg Am*. 1999;81:752-762.
67. Fishbain DA, Goldberg M, Meagher BR, et al. Male and female chronic pain patients categorized by DSM-III psychiatric diagnostic criteria. *Pain*. 1986;26:181-197.
68. Ormel J, VonKorff M, Ustun TB, et al. Common mental disorders and disability across cultures: results from the WHO Collaborative Study on Psychological Problems in General Health Care. *JAMA*. 1994;272:1741-1748.
69. Hagg O, Fritzell P, Hedlund R, et al. Pain-drawing does not predict the outcome of fusion surgery for chronic low-back pain: a report from the Swedish Lumbar Spine Study. *Eur Spine J*. 2003;12:2-11.
70. Ohnmeiss DD. Repeatability of pain drawings in a low back pain population. *Spine*. 2000;25:980-988.
71. Dahl B, Gehrchen PM, Kiaer T, et al. Nonorganic pain drawings are associated with low psychological scores on the preoperative SF-36 questionnaire in patients with chronic low back pain. *Eur Spine J*. 2001;10:211-214.
72. Carnes D, Ashbey D, Underwood M. A systematic review of pain drawing literature: should pain drawings be used for psychologic screening? *Clin J Pain*. 2006;22:449-457.
73. Gatchel RJ, ed. *Compendium of Outcome Instruments for Assessment and Research of Spinal Disorders*. La Grange, IL: North American Spine Society; 2001.
74. Patrick DL, Deyo RA, Atlas SJ, et al. Assessing health-related quality of life in patients with sciatica. *Spine*. 1995;20:1899-1908.
75. Fairbank JCT, Couper J, Davies JB, et al. The Oswestry low back pain disability questionnaire. *Physiotherapy*. 1980;66:271-273.
76. Millard RW. A critical review of questionnaires for assessing pain-related disability. *J Occup Rehabil*. 1991;1:289-302.
77. Vernon H, Mior S. The neck disability index: a study of reliability and validity. *J Manipulative Physiol Ther*. 1991;14:409-415.
78. Waddell G, Newton M, Henderson I, et al. A fear-avoidance beliefs questionnaire (FABQ) and the role of fear-avoidance beliefs in chronic back pain and disability. *Pain*. 1993;52:157-168.
79. Sullivan MJL, Bishop SR, Pivik J. The pain catastrophizing scale: development and validation. *Psychol Assess*. 1995;7:524-532.
80. Webster LR, Webster RM. Predicting aberrant behaviours in opioid treated patients: preliminary validation of the opioid risk tool. *Pain Med*. 2005;6:432-442.
81. Health Measures. *PROMIS: Patient-Reported Outcomes Measurement Information System*. Available at: http://www.healthmeasures.net/explore-measurement-systems/promis.
82. McGregor AH, McCarthy ID, Hughes SP. Motion characteristics of the lumbar spine in the normal population. *Spine*. 1995;20:2421-2428.
83. Nattrass CL, Nitschke JE, Disler PB, et al. Lumbar spine range of motion as a measure of physical and functional impairment: an investigation of validity. *Clin Rehabil*. 1999;13:211-218.
84. Ng JKF, Kippers V, Richardson CA, et al. Range of motion and lordosis of the lumbar spine: reliability and measurement of normative values. *Spine*. 2001;26:53-60.
85. Solomon J, Nadler SF, Press J. Physical examination of the lumbar spine. In: Malanga G, Nadler SF, eds. *Musculoskeletal Physical Examination: An Evidence-based Approach*. Philadelphia: Hanley & Belfus; 2006:189-226.
86. Burkhart SS, Morgan CD, Kibler WB. The disabled throwing shoulder: spectrum of pathology, part III: the SICK scapula, scapular dyskinesis, the kinetic chain, and rehabilitation. *Arthroscopy*. 2003;19:641-661.
87. Bates B. *A Guide to Physical Examination and History Taking*. 5th ed. Philadelphia: JB Lippincott; 1991.
88. Merz O, Wolf U, Robert M, et al. Validity of palpation techniques for the identification of the spinous process L5. *Man Ther*. 2013;18:333-338.
89. Tanaka K, Irikoma S, Kokubo S. Identification of the lumbar interspinous spaces by palpation and verified by x-rays. *Rev Bras Anestesiol*. 2013;63:245-248.
90. American Spinal Injury Association. *International Standards for Neurological Classification of Spinal Cord Injury* [reprint]. Chicago: American Spinal Injury Association; 2008.
91. Rhee JM, Heflin JA, Hamasaki T, et al. Prevalence of physical signs in cervical myelopathy: a prospective, controlled study. *Spine*. 2009;34:890-895.
92. Andersson GBJ, Deyo RA. History and physical examination in patients with herniated lumbar discs. *Spine*. 1996;21:10S-18S.
93. Tong HC, Haig AJ, Yamakawa K. The Spurling test and cervical radiculopathy. *Spine*. 2002;27:156-159.
94. Supik LF, Broom MJ. Sciatic tension signs and lumbar disc herniation. *Spine*. 1994;19:1066-1069.
95. Waddell G, McCulloch JA, Kummel E, et al. Nonorganic physical signs in low-back pain. *Spine*. 1980;5:117-125.
96. Maruta T, Goldman S, Chan CW, et al. Waddell's nonorganic signs and Minnesota Multiphasic Personality Inventory profiles in patients with chronic low back pain. *Spine*. 1997;22:72-75.
97. Fishbain DA, Cole B, Cutler RB, et al. A structured evidence-based review on the meaning of nonorganic physical signs: Waddell signs. *Pain Med*. 2003;4:141-181.
98. Kibler WB. Determining the extent of the functional deficit. In: Kibler WB, Herring SA, Press JM, et al., eds. *Functional Rehabilitation of Sports and Musculoskeletal Injuries*. Gaithersburg, MD: Aspen; 1998:1-8.

99. Basmajian JV, Nyberg R, eds. *Rational Manual Therapies.* Baltimore: Williams & Wilkins; 1993.
100. Brieve GP. *Mobilization of the Spine.* 4th ed. New York: Churchill-Livingstone; 1984.
101. May S, Littlewood C, Bishop A. Reliability of procedures used in the physical examination of non-specific low back pain: a systematic review. *Aust J Physiother.* 2006;52:91-102.
102. Hestbaek L, Leboeuf-Yde C. Are chiropractic tests for the lumbo-pelvic spine reliable and valid? A systematic critical literature review. *J Manipulative Physiol Ther.* 2000;23:258-275.
103. Hill JC, Whitehurst DGT, Lewis M, et al. Comparison of Stratified Primary Care Management for Low Back Pain with Current Best Practice (STarT Back): a randomised controlled trial. *Lancet.* 2011;378:1560-1571.
104. Maina CJ, Sowdena G, Hill JC, et al. Integrating physical and psychological approaches to treatment in low back pain: the development and content of the STarT Back trial's high-risk' intervention. *Physiotherapy.* 2012;98:110-116.

CHAPTER 13 Spine Imaging

Todd M. Emch
Jeffrey S. Ross
Gordon R. Bell

Multiple imaging methods with tremendous technologic complexity and sophistication can be used to evaluate spinal pathology. Magnetic resonance imaging (MRI) quickly emerged as the study of choice for many disorders of the spine, with computed tomography (CT) continuing to play a key role, bolstered by newer innovations such as helical scanning and multidetector arrays allowing isotropic voxels and multiplanar reformatting without loss of resolution. This chapter reviews the basic imaging approaches to the spine and their usefulness, both in specific disease states, and in the context of the anatomic categories of spine pathology (extradural, intradural extramedullary, and intramedullary).

Modalities

Radiographs

Routine plain films are universally available and inexpensive, but are limited by an inability to directly visualize neural structures and nerve root or cord compression. Ionizing radiation is used to obtain the radiographic image, which despite the relatively fast time of acquisition, can still be susceptible to motion.[1] Radiographs can be used for evaluation of alignment, status of hardware in the postoperative patient, intraoperative localization, and motion with flexion-extension views.

Radiographs can visualize osseous structures and surrounding soft tissues (i.e., extradural pathology). A routine examination of the spine includes frontal or anteroposterior and lateral views, with additional views such as oblique or flexion-extension also available.[2]

Orthogonal conventional radiography is the first line of evaluation in an instrumented postoperative patient, and plain radiographs are usually obtained at 6 weeks and 3, 6, and 12 months postoperatively.[3] Regardless of which fusion approach is taken, the presence or absence of demonstrable motion or evidence of hardware failure or loosening is a key factor in the evaluation. In the case of posterolateral fusion, arthrodesis is deemed successful if follow-up radiographs show continuity in the fusion mass between the cephalad and the caudal transverse processes. Instrumented interbody fusion is considered fused if any of the following is present:

1. Increased or maintained bony density within the cage implant because of the presence of mature bony trabeculae bridging the interbody space
2. Absence of a halo or a periprosthetic lucency around the implant
3. A sclerotic line between the cage and the vertebral bone because of bone remodeling and new bone formation
4. Resorption of anterior vertebral traction spurs or the presence of bone graft anterior to an intervertebral implant (sentinel sign)
5. Lack of motion on flexion-extension views

Pseudarthrosis or failure of fusion is indicated by progressive loss of disc height, vertebral displacement, broken or loose hardware, and loss of position of the implant or resorption of the bone graft. Flexion and extension views are useful for assessing stability or functional fusion, but the central x-ray beam should pass through the same area in both views.[4]

Myelography

Myelography involves instillation of the contrast agent through either lumbar puncture (midline or oblique approaches) or lateral C1–C2 puncture with subsequent radiographic and CT imaging of the region of interest. The diagnosis of extradural neural compression by myelography is inferred indirectly by changes in the contour of normal contrast agent–filled thecal sac and root sleeves rather than by direct visualization of the lesion.[5] Expansion of the spinal cord (Fig. 13.1) can be visualized as well as intradural extramedullary lesions; however nonexpansile cord pathology cannot be detected with myelography.[6]

The major disadvantage of myelography is its invasive nature and lack of diagnostic specificity.[7] The use of less toxic second-generation, water-soluble nonionic agents has obviated the need for overnight hospitalization after the procedure. Routine postprocedural monitoring of 2 to 4 hours is usually sufficient. Multiple water-soluble agents are available that provide excellent contrast and lower rates of side effects, such as iohexol (Omnipaque) and iopamidol (Isovue).

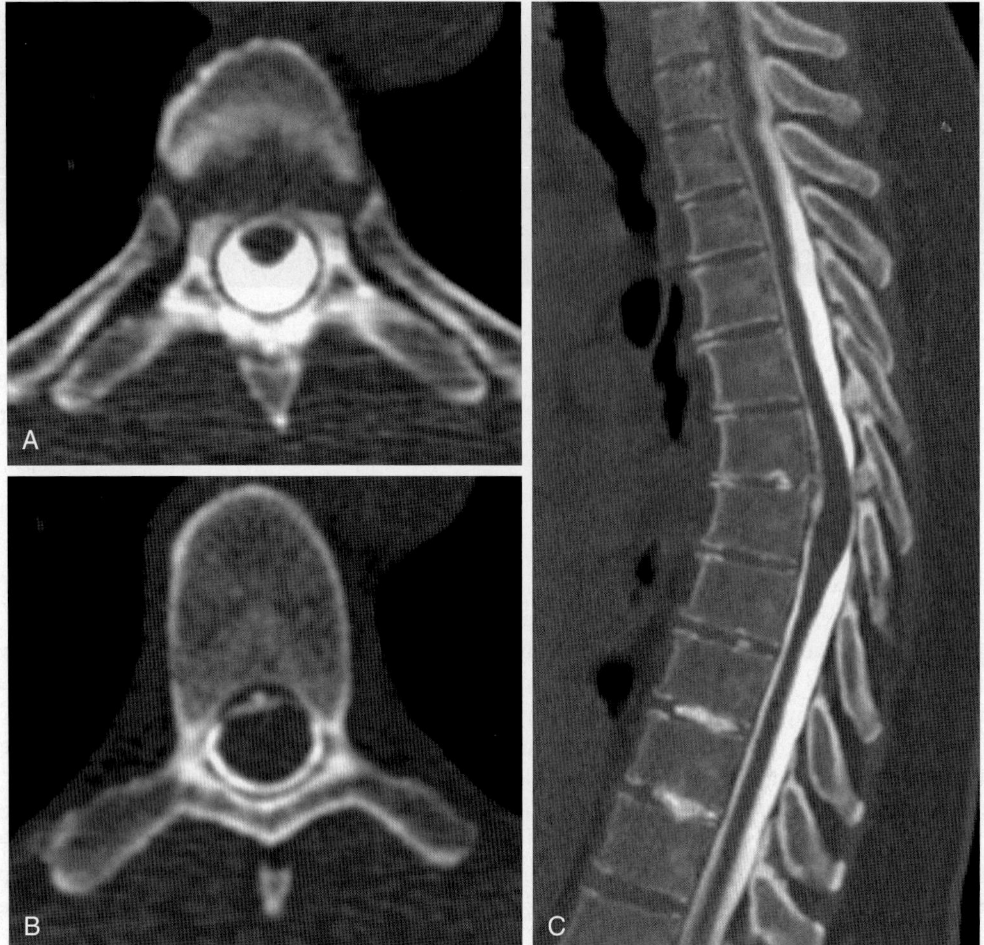

FIG. 13.1 Computed tomographic myelogram demonstrating an intramedullary mass lesion. (A) Axial image demonstrates normal diameter of the thoracic spinal cord. (B) Axial and (C) sagittal images demonstrate fusiform expansion of the mid-thoracic spinal cord in this patient with an ependymoma.

Current water-soluble agents are associated with less toxicity, and their absorption through the theca and arachnoid villi makes their removal unnecessary.[8] Newer nonionic water-soluble agents generally produce mild side effects, although significant adverse reactions can still rarely occur, such as hallucinations, confusion, or seizures. Considerations before myelography include obtaining screening laboratory tests such as platelets, prothrombin time/international normalized ratio, and partial thromboplastin time; medication history of the patients, especially metformin; psychiatric medications, which can lower seizure threshold; and anticoagulants.[9,10]

Computed Tomography

CT permits direct visualization of potential neural compressing structures and provides better visualization of lateral pathology, such as foraminal stenosis.[11-13] An important benefit from a surgical perspective is the ability of CT to distinguish neural compression due to soft tissue from compression from bone pathology.[12,14-16]

Disadvantages of CT include radiation exposure, the effects of partial volume averaging, streak artifacts in the cervical spine caused by the dense bone of the shoulder girdle, and changes in configuration of the spine that occur between successive motion segments.[17] Many of the limitations can be obviated by obtaining multiple thin sections (1.5 to 3 mm) with the gantry tilted to permit imaging parallel to the plane of the disc. Further accuracy is obtained by routinely imaging the spine by CT after the introduction of water-soluble contrast agents (intrathecal contrast medium–enhanced CT).

Reported accuracy rates for CT range from 72% to 91%.[7,12,14,15] Agreement rates between contrast medium–enhanced CT and myelography have been reported to range from 75% to 96%.[12,14] When a discrepancy exists between myelographic and CT findings, postcontrast CT is invariably the more accurate study (Fig. 13.2). Current multirow detector technology is now available that allows for extremely rapid thin-slice acquisitions over long body segments. With this technology, contiguous 3-mm slices can be obtained from L1 to S1 in less than 30 seconds. The acquisition of isotropic voxels allows for multiplanar reformation of the CT data with no loss in spatial resolution. Changes in the windowing and leveling of the images can change the focus onto either osseous structures or soft tissues.[1]

Magnetic Resonance Imaging

MRI can readily evaluate the extradural, intradural extramedullary, and intramedullary spaces and is also the only modality

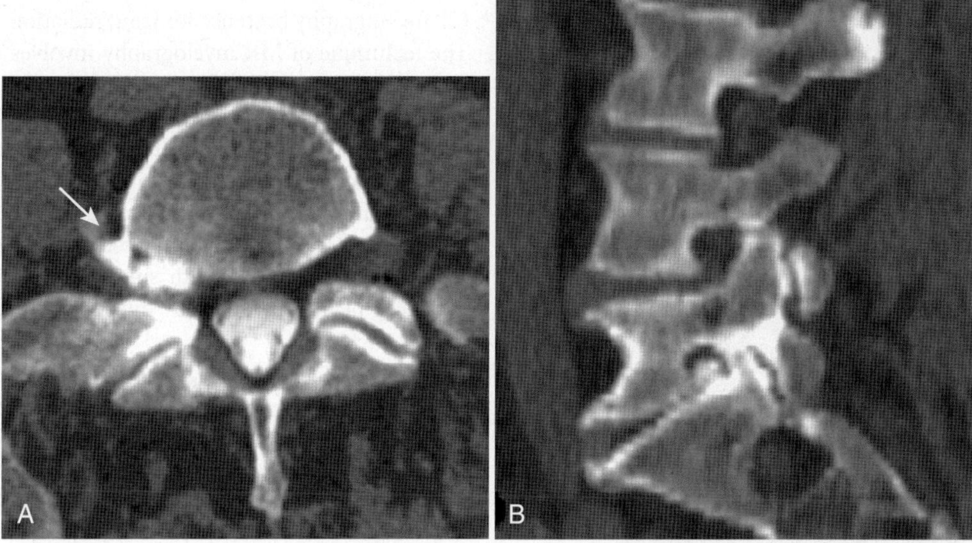

FIG. 13.2 Foraminal stenosis. (A) Axial computed tomographic (CT) scan after myelography shows severe right bony foraminal stenosis with no evidence of central stenosis or herniations (*arrow*). (B) Sagittal reformat of CT data also shows severe foraminal narrowing, in contrast to more normal superior foramen.

that can directly image bone marrow. Since the beginning of its clinical use in the early 1980s, MRI technology has progressed with improved quality and decreased examination times.[18-21]

Routine Magnetic Resonance Imaging

Pulse sequences that constitute a routine spine MR exam include axial gradient recalled echo or T2, T1, and sagittal T2, T1, and short-tau inversion recovery (STIR). Depending on the imaging indication T1-weighted images can also be obtained with gadolinium contrast agents, especially when there is a concern of infection or when there has been a history of spine surgery.[22-30] STIR has shown a high sensitivity for musculoskeletal pathology (Fig. 13.3).[31-33] STIR has been favorably compared with T1-weighted and T2-weighted fast spin-echo (FSE), conventional spin-echo, and fat-saturated FSE in the detection of vertebral metastatic disease.[34-36] STIR may also be used for intramedullary cord lesions. Each examination also includes a scout image that, depending on the type of image, can include much of the abdomen or chest in the field of view (Fig. 13.4).

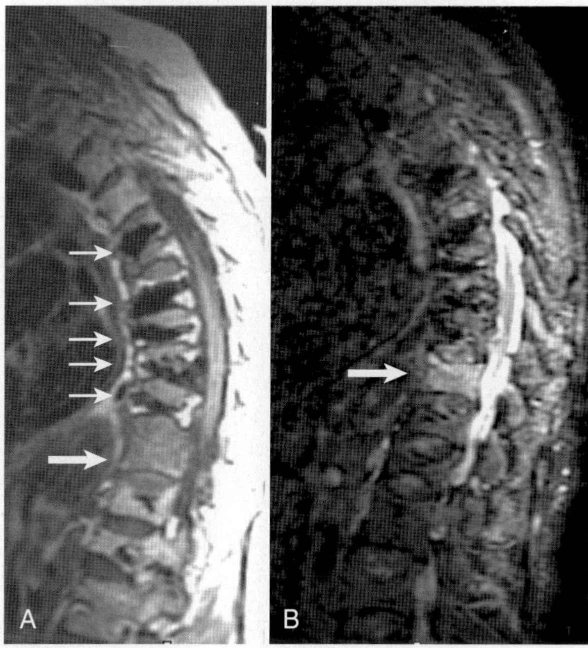

FIG. 13.3 Multiple osteoporotic compression fractures. (A) Sagittal T1-weighted magnetic resonance image through thoracic spine shows multiple collapsed bodies with central low signal reflecting prior vertebroplasties (*small arrows*). The marrow adjacent to methacrylate shows normal fatty signal intensity. (B) T12 body (*large arrow*) shows low signal on T1-weighted image and increased signal on sagittal short-tau inversion recovery image consistent with acute age.

Dynamic Magnetic Resonance Imaging

CT and MRI are typically obtained with the patient positioned supine. Radiographs can be more readily obtained with the patient standing or in flexion or extension. The rationale for MRI with patients in a sitting position, in flexion or extension, or with axial loading is that these positions are believed to be the positions in which the patient is the most symptomatic. In extension the lumbar spinal canal decreases, as does the cervical spinal canal (Fig. 13.5).[37-40] Axial loading has been shown to decrease the diameter of the lumbar spine.[41] In a study of 200 patients with symptoms of spinal stenosis who underwent MRI with axial loading, 20 showed a decreased diameter of the canal with axial loading. Of those 20 patients, the plan of care was changed in five patients because of the added information of axial loading images.[42]

Magnetic Resonance Myelography

MR myelography can be obtained for evaluation for cerebrospinal fluid (CSF) leak in conditions such as intracranial

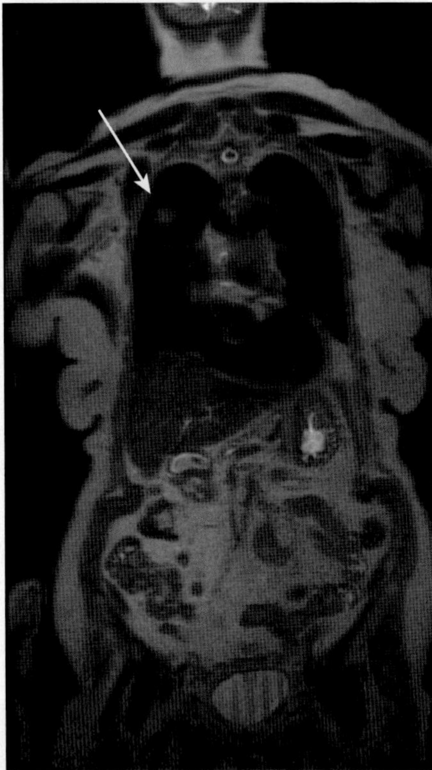

FIG. 13.4 Half-Fourier acquisition single-shot turbo spin-echo scout image obtained during a routine lumbar spine examination demonstrates an unsuspected right upper lobe lung mass *(arrow)*, a possible malignancy.

hypotension. Radionuclide cisternography and conventional CT myelography both use ionizing radiation and are invasive. The technique of MR myelography involves the use of heavy T2-weighted sequences[43] and can readily identify paravertebral fluid collections or spinal diverticuli. Sensitivities for radionuclide cisternography, CT myelography, and MR myelography have been reported to be 55%, 67%, and 86%, respectively.[44-46] Additionally, there has been use of intrathecal gadolinium, although off-label and not approved by the US Food and Drug Administration (FDA), with subsequent MRI that has been shown to be advantageous by multiple authors.[47,48]

Magnetic Resonance Neurography

For evaluation of the peripheral nerves, MRI using T1-weighted images and fat-saturated T2 or STIR images can be used to evaluate for neoplasm (Fig. 13.6), entrapment, or nerve injury.[49] Severity of nerve injury can be evaluated from mild injury (neurapraxia) where there is mild nerve enlargement and T2 hyperintensity to complete nerve transection where the separation of the nerve can be visualized.[49] MR neurography is also useful for evaluation of diffuse peripheral nerve lesions such as neurofibromatosis or the inflammatory or hereditary neuropathies.[50]

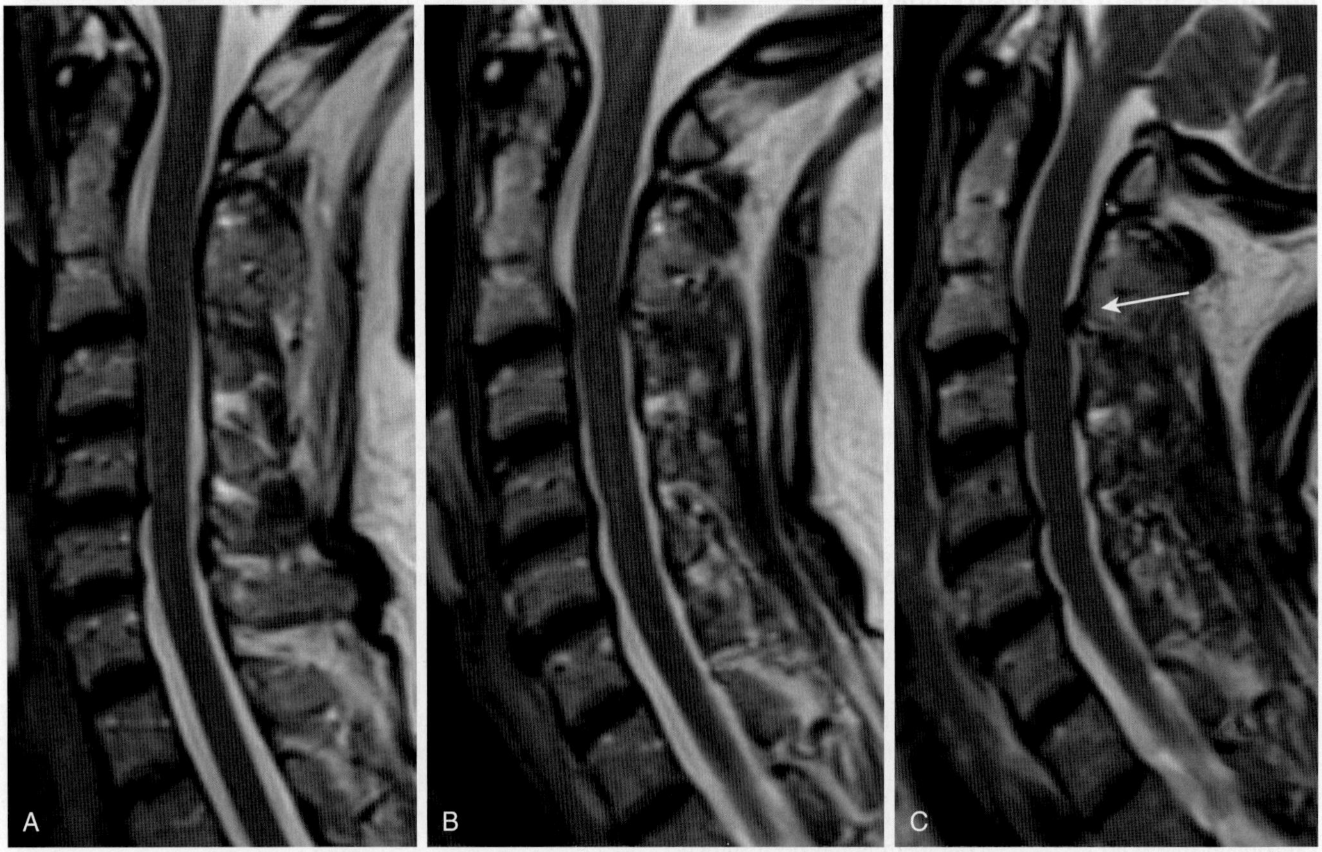

FIG. 13.5 Sagittal T2-weighted images of the cervical spine demonstrate developmental fusion of C2 and C3 vertebral bodies. Images are obtained in (A) flexion, (B) neutral, and (C) extension. There is ligamentous buckling with extension resulting in more profound canal compromise *(arrow)* compared with neutral and flexion positioning.

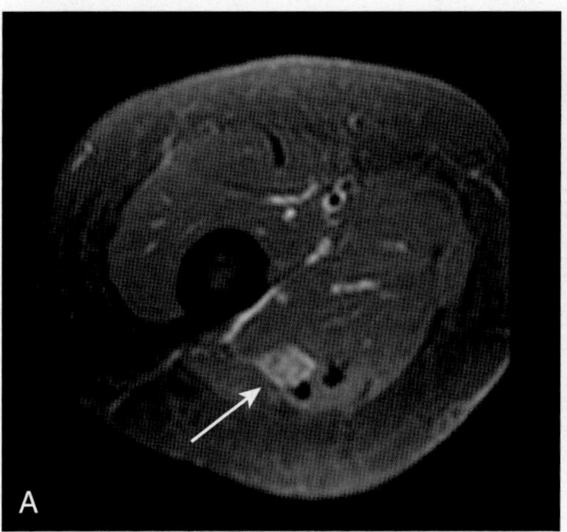

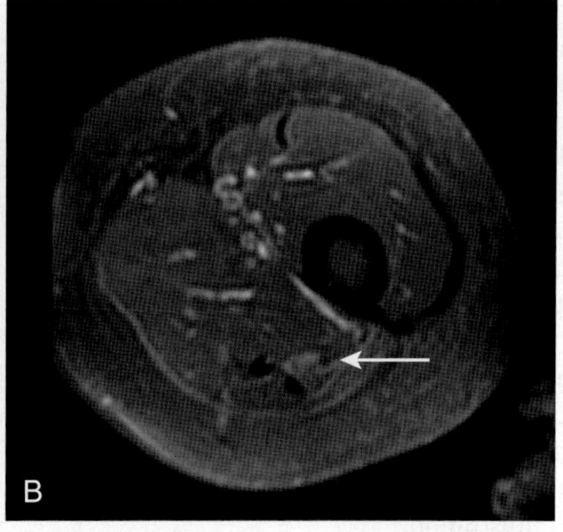

FIG. 13.6 (A) Axial fat-saturated contrast-enhanced T1-weighted images demonstrate asymmetric enlargement and enhancement of the right sciatic nerve *(arrow)*, representing neoplastic infiltration in this patient with leukemia. (B) Normal sciatic nerve for comparison *(arrow)*.

Diffusion-Weighted Imaging

Diffusion-weighted imaging (DWI) is routinely used for brain imaging. However, its use for spine imaging is not routine secondary to multiple technical limitations, including motion artifact and the relatively small size of the spinal cord.[51] Similar caveats apply to diffusion tensor imaging (DTI), in which the diffusivity of water molecules can imply the course of white matter tracts.[52]

DWI of the spine can be applied to the vertebral bodies as well as the spinal cord. Multiple studies have been performed looking at the ability to discriminate benign versus pathologic compression fractures based on DWI; however, the results have been conflicting.[53-57] Evaluation of spinal cord neoplasm or ischemia using DWI has also been described.[58]

DTI of the spine is also fraught with technical difficulties. Applications in regard to suspected neoplasm include both lesion characterization and evaluation of the lesion's margins for surgical planning purposes.[59,60] In cases of cord compression DTI has demonstrated cord injury that is not accompanied by T2-weighted signal abnormalities.[61] In addition, DTI has been shown to be more sensitive than T2-weighted imaging for evaluation of spinal cord inflammation.[62]

Cerebrospinal Fluid Flow Imaging

CSF imaging demonstrates biphasic pulsatile CSF flow with caudal systolic and cranial diastolic flow. Applications include Chiari malformations or evaluation of spinal cord syrinx cavities or tethered cord.[63-66]

Magnetic Resonance Spectroscopy

^{1}H-MR spectroscopy (MRS) uses a conventional MR machine to evaluate metabolites in an area of interest and has been extensively used with brain imaging. MRS for spinal imaging is met with extensive technical challenges, including motion, small size of the spinal cord, distance of the spinal cord from surface coils, and the inherent composition of the immediately surrounding soft tissues and osseous structures, which can result in distortion of the magnetic field.[67] Clinical applications include demyelination[68] and neoplasm.[69]

Magnetic Resonance Imaging Safety and Patient Issues

The specific and important aspects of MRI safety (including patient exposure to the magnetic field and gadolinium-based contrast media) are widely available on multiple websites, and the interested reader is referred to them for detailed answers (e.g., www.MRIsafety.com). Certain implants or metallic foreign bodies can increase in temperature or move, potentially leading to patient harm—hence the need for all patients to fill out a safety screening form before placement in the MRI machine.[70] Recently MRI-compatible pacemakers, although with some stipulations, have been developed.[71]

Bleicher and colleagues[72] found a serious complication rate of approximately 0.03% of gadolinium contrast agents when reviewing records of more than 23,000 patients, attesting to the overall favorable safety profile of gadolinium contrast agents. However, there are two important issues: gadolinium deposition in patients with normal renal function and nephrogenic systemic fibrosis (NSF).

In 2014 Kanda and colleagues[73] correlated a dose-dependent T1 hyperintensity in certain structures intracranially in patients with a history of gadolinium administration. McDonald and coworkers[74] confirmed the presence of gadolinium in the globus pallidus, pons, dentate nucleus, and thalamus in autopsy specimens of 13 patients with normal renal function who all underwent a minimum of four gadolinium contrast-enhanced examinations. Whether the intracranial accumulation of gadolinium is harmful is not clear at this point.[75]

NSF, previously called nephrogenic fibrosing dermopathy, is a systemic disorder of widespread fibrosis that has been tied to prior administration of gadolinium-based contrast agents in the setting of renal disease. The incidence of NSF in the setting of severe renal dysfunction is approximately 1% to 7% after exposure to gadolinium-based contrast material. The FDA has asked manufacturers to include a new boxed warning on the product labeling of all gadolinium-based contrast agents used to enhance the quality of MRI. The warning states that patients with severe kidney insufficiency who receive gadolinium-based agents are at risk for developing NSF, a debilitating and potentially fatal disease.[76,77] Also, patients just before or just after liver transplantation and patients with chronic liver disease are at risk for developing NSF if they are experiencing kidney insufficiency of any severity. The risk of a patient developing NSF may be minimized by the following steps[76,78-81]:

1. Identify patients with a glomerular filtration rate less than 30 mL/min/1.73 m^2 as at risk.
2. Administer contrast medium to a patient at risk for developing NSF only when the expected benefit clearly outweighs the risk of administration.
3. Perform unenhanced MRI first with proper monitoring so that unnecessary contrast medium administration is avoided.
4. Use the lowest dose of gadolinium-based contrast medium that is feasible for the examination.

Spinal Angiography

Spinal angiography is extremely useful for spinal vascular malformations for the delineation of the vascular supply and for therapeutic treatment.[82,83] Spinal angiography is also used in the pretherapeutic workup of suspected vascular neoplasms involving the vertebral bodies, posterior elements, and spinal canal and is coupled with preoperative or palliative embolization. Spinal angiography should address three areas for the surgeon or interventionalist: (1) the exact location and configuration of the lesion, (2) vascularity of the lesion, including feeding and draining vessels, and (3) regional vascular anatomy.[84]

Spinal vascular malformations are a very heterogeneous group of lesions that have had a wide variety of classification schemes applied to them. One common classification system is from Anson and Spetzler,[85] who classified them as types 1 to 4:

Type 1: spinal dural arteriovenous fistula between the dural branch of the spinal ramus of the radicular artery and intradural medullary vein

Type 2: spinal cord arteriovenous malformation with shunting across an interposed vascular nidus (intramedullary glomus malformation)

Type 3: complex spinal arteriovenous malformation with metameric extension (juvenile malformation)

Type 4: direct arteriovenous fistula (intradural perimedullary fistula)

The most common spinal vascular lesion is a dural arteriovenous fistula (Fig. 13.7). These lesions are thought to be acquired and are particularly present in the thoracic and lower lumbar spine. Spinal dural arteriovenous fistulas are more common in men. There is often a delay from symptom onset to time of diagnosis, averaging 27 months. Clinical findings include weakness (55%), a progressive clinical course (100%), and myelopathy on examination (84%). In the spine, nidus of the fistula is most often located between T6 and T12 or in the sacrum. In 1977, Kendall and Logue[86] definitively identified the site of the arteriovenous shunting within the root sleeve. The symptoms are a result of intramedullary edema and ischemia secondary to increased venous backpressure within the varicose coronal veins. Gilbertson and colleagues[87] and Masaryk and colleagues[88] identified increased signal intensity on T2-weighted images within the cord as the most sensitive imaging finding in spinal dural fistula.

Although imaging, in particular MRI, has become a mainstay for the evaluation of vascular malformations, spinal angiography remains a crucial technique for precise definition of the type of lesion, the overall morphology, the flow characteristics, and the identification of specific feeding vessels.[89] Arterial and delayed venous imaging may be necessary to appreciate fully the venous drainage of the vascular pathology, particularly in arteriovenous malformations and dural fistulas. Arterial films allow examination of abnormal blush or arteriovenous shunting. The normal vascular supply to the cord, in particular the artery of Adamkiewicz, should be defined. In addition to the usual general complications of angiography, embolization to the anterior spinal artery could occur after angiography, which may lead to an ascending paralysis. In general complications are rare, given the small catheters used, nonionic contrast medium, and an improved speed of the examination with digital subtraction angiography.

Technologic advances have allowed high-resolution, high-contrast discrimination MR or CT imaging for evaluation of the spinal arteries, with the goal of minimizing the need for conventional catheter angiography for identification of spinal vascular disease.[90-92] The size of the anterior spinal artery (0.2 to 0.8 mm) and the close approximation of the spinal veins necessitate a sophisticated MRI sequence with bolus gadolinium–based intravenous contrast medium administration. Although various techniques may be used, the three main requirements are a large field of view, high spatial resolution, and high temporal resolution.

In a series of 34 patients, Mull and colleagues[92] showed that contrast-enhanced spinal MR angiography (MRA) could reliably detect or exclude spinal cord arteriovenous abnormalities with a 100% predictive value. The main arterial feeder can be reliably defined by MRA, but small secondary feeders may be missed. The main reasons for obtaining MRA would be for primary identification of a vascular abnormality and to pinpoint the likely site of a feeder for conventional catheter angiography. CT angiography can also define normal and abnormal spinal vasculature.[93,94] The technique requires a multidetector row CT scanner (generally 16) and 1-mm section thickness.

Discography

Discography was originally conceived as a morphologic study of disc herniation but then morphed into a useful but limited test relying on pain provocation through disc pressurization.[95,96] Although discography can accurately define disc degeneration, this procedure is now seen as a physiologic evaluation of the disc consisting of volumetric, manometric, radiographic, and pain provocative challenge.[97,98] This procedure remains quite

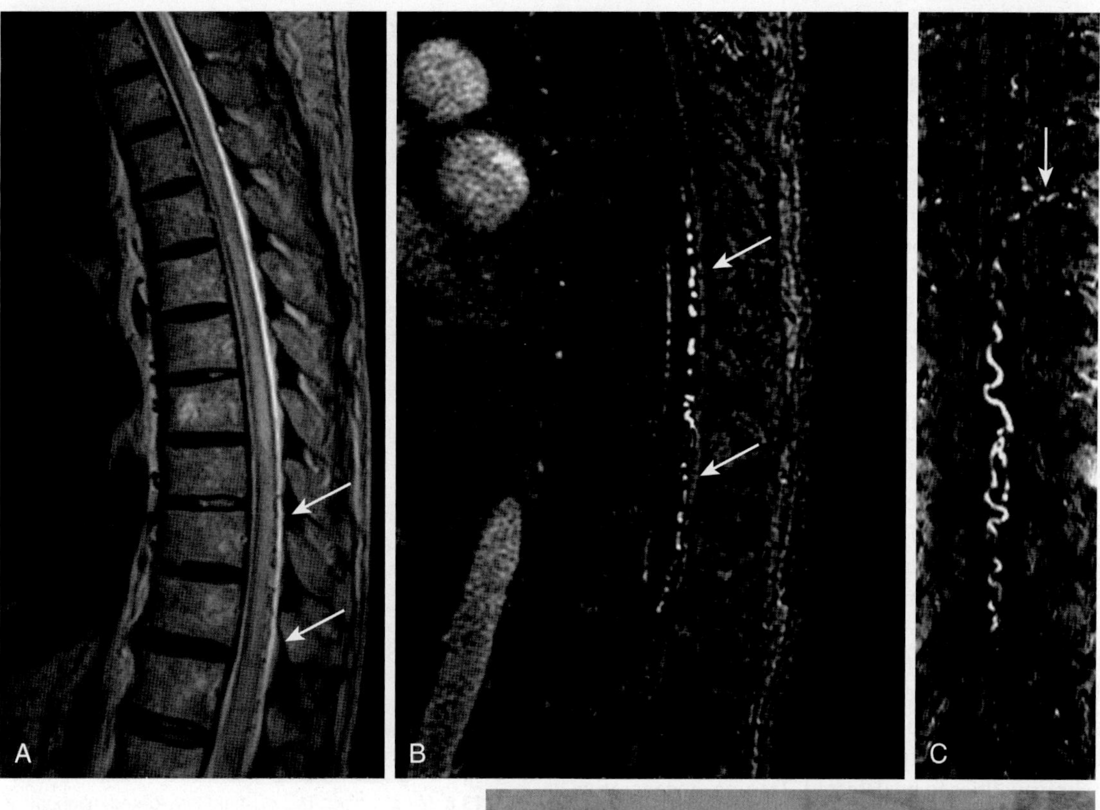

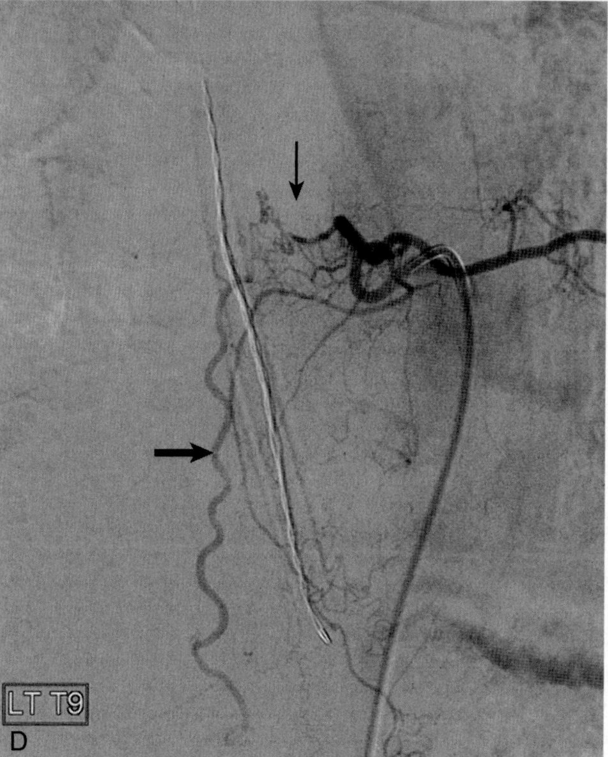

FIG. 13.7 Dural fistula. (A) Sagittal T2-weighted magnetic resonance (MR) image shows diffuse abnormal increased signal from the central aspect of thoracic cord, sparing a small rind of peripheral cord. There are faint serpentine areas of flow void along the dorsal aspect of the thoracic cord (*arrows*). (B) Single slice from a three-dimensional gradient-echo dynamic enhanced MR angiogram shows multiple dilated intradural vessels primarily along the dorsal surface of the cord (*arrows*). (C) Coronal reformat of MR angiogram shows dorsal enlarged vessels and small nidus of vessels on the left at T9 (*arrow*). (D) Anteroposterior view of a spinal angiogram at the left T9 intercostal level shows a fistula at the foraminal level (*arrow*), with shunting to intraspinal dilated veins (*large arrow*).

controversial; it has enthusiastic supporters and detractors and has generated a voluminous literature. Some authors see discography as helpful in identifying internal disc disruption and in verifying painful disc levels before surgery (particularly fusion), whereas others see it as unproven and of questionable benefit.[99-106]

Discography is an invasive procedure and is not performed as a screening technique. Discography is most accurate when the diagnosis of discogenic pain is probable based on appropriate history, physical examination, and imaging.[96] This test is always limited in sensitivity and specificity owing to the subjective report of pain type and location by the patient. According to Tehranzadeh and others,[107-109] indications for discography include the following:

1. Negative MRI, CT, or myelography findings with equivocal findings for disc disease

2. Cases with positive MRI, CT, or myelography findings with disc disease at multiple levels
3. Presence of equivocal MRI, CT, or myelography findings
4. Recurrent back pain in postsurgical patients with difficulty in evaluating scar versus disc
5. Cases of failed back surgery to evaluate painful pseudarthrosis or symptomatic disc
6. Evaluation of spinal fusion disc above or below the fusion level
7. Therapeutic injection of corticosteroid or anesthetic into the disc itself

Nuclear Medicine Examinations

Nuclear medicine examinations commonly performed for spine imaging include bone scintigraphy using technetium 99m (^{99m}Tc) and 18F-fluorodeoxyglucose positron emission tomography (PET) imaging. Other radiotracers are also available, including somatostatin analogs, that are useful with neuroendocrine tumors and meningiomas.[110]

For evaluation of metastatic disease, bone scans image osteoblastic activity and are less useful for aggressive lytic metastases. Sensitivity and specificity range from 62% to 100% and 78% to 100%, respectively. Bone scans require a 5% to 10% change for abnormalities to be detected. Trauma, degenerative changes, infection, and other conditions can also show uptake on bone scans.[111,112] PET imaging measures metabolic uptake and is more sensitive for lytic rather than sclerotic metastatic disease.[111,113,114] Similar to bone scans, PET imaging can show uptake in nonneoplastic conditions such as inflammation, infection, or degenerative change.[115]

Radionuclides most commonly used for detecting inflammatory changes of the spine are ^{99m}Tc phosphate complexes, gallium (^{67}Ga) citrate, and indium-111 (^{111}In)–labeled white blood cells. Although scintigraphy with ^{99m}Tc and ^{67}Ga compounds is sensitive to infection, it is also nonspecific. Healing fractures, degenerative arthritis, sterile inflammatory reactions, tumors, and loosened prosthetic devices can show increased uptake.[116-118] ^{111}In has several advantages compared with other radionuclides, including higher target-to-background ratios, better image quality (compared with ^{67}Ga), and more intense uptake by abscesses. Its main disadvantage is its accumulation within any inflammatory lesion, whether infectious or not.[119] The radionuclide study also takes hours to days to perform.

Imaging Artifacts

Artifacts invariably occur during spine imaging and can either obscure or simulate pathology. Stainless steel implants are known to generate substantial metal artifact with MRI and CT. On CT, metal causes severe x-ray attenuation (missing data) in selected planes. These missing data or hollow projections cause classic "starburst" or streak artifacts during image reconstruction. The resulting distortions often render these studies useless. Materials with lower x-ray attenuation coefficients (plastic, titanium, tantalum, stainless steel, cobalt chrome) produce fewer distortions. Metal composition, mass, orientation, and position of the implant in the body all are important factors that determine the magnitude of image artifact. Titanium wires exhibit the least artifact on CT and MRI compared with cobalt chrome or stainless steel.

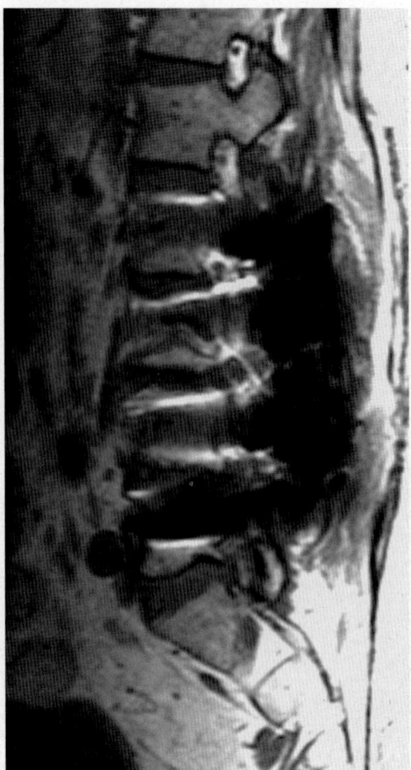

FIG. 13.8 Metal artifact. This sagittal T1-weighted magnetic resonance image is severely degraded by fixation hardware (four-level pedicle screws) that does not allow adequate evaluation of the neural foramen.

MRI studies may be severely compromised in the presence of spinal instrumentation, and there can be potential safety and biologic considerations (Fig. 13.8). Many strategies can reduce susceptibility artifacts on MRI, including the use of spin-echo techniques, especially FSE variants over gradient echo; larger fields of view; higher readout bandwidths; smaller voxel sizes; and appropriate geometric orientation of the frequency-encoded direction in relationship to metallic objects (Fig. 13.9).[120,121] Additional MR artifacts can be present, such as motion artifact (Fig. 13.10), flow-related artifact, chemical shift, Gibb's artifact, and aliasing or wrap-around artifact.[122]

Pathology

When interpreting a radiographic examination of the spine, the first step is to identify the abnormality and then arrive at a diagnosis or reasonable differential diagnosis. One of the most critical pieces of imaging information regarding spinal pathology used in forming a differential diagnosis involves determination of whether the lesion is intramedullary, intradural extramedullary, or extradural.

Degenerative Disc Disease

The morphologic findings of degenerative disc are well documented and demonstrated, especially with MRI. There are,

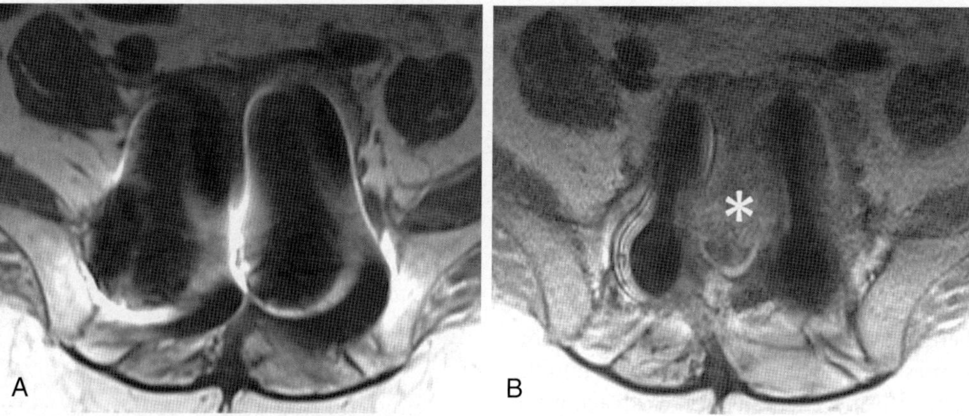

FIG. 13.9 (A) Extensive artifact from posterior instrumentation in this T1-weighted image obscures evaluation of the spinal canal. (B) T1-weighted image with contrast and metal reduction technique demonstrates improved evaluation of the canal with epidural extension of disease *(asterisk)*.

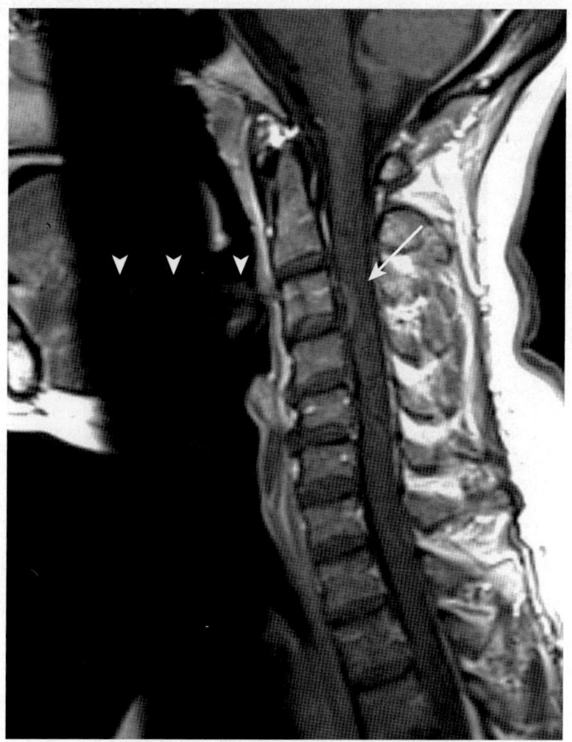

FIG. 13.10 Sagittal contrast-enhanced T1-weighted image of the cervical spine demonstrates apparent signal abnormality/enhancement of the cord at level of C3 *(arrow)*. However, this is motion artifact from swallowing/epiglottis movement with a similar morphologic abnormality tracking outside the cervical spinal cord (arrowheads) conforming to the shape of the epiglottis.

however, many factors to consider before imaging patients who present with uncomplicated low back pain, including that the findings of degenerative disc disease are common in asymptomatic individuals, degenerative disc disease has a favorable natural history, and there is a potential impact on clinical decision making.[123]

The presence of degenerative changes within the cervical and lumbar spine has been shown to be age related and equally present in asymptomatic and symptomatic individuals.[124,125] By the fifth decade of life, 25% of asymptomatic patients have degenerative changes in the intervertebral disc spaces. By the seventh decade, 75% have degenerative changes.[126] Myelograms performed in patients without symptoms revealed abnormalities in 24% of the exams,[124] and MR exams in patients without symptoms demonstrated normal exams in only 36% of cases.[127]

Overall, the natural history of low back pain is favorable, with most patients experiencing improvement within 4 weeks regardless of whether they are imaged.[128,129] Over time, disc herniations can improve or decrease in size and new extrusions can occur after the onset of original symptoms.[130-132]

Multiple studies have shown that imaging in cases of uncomplicated low back pain does not positively affect patient management and that imaging can actually be harmful. Studies of radiographic evaluations have shown that there is little effect on patient management.[133,134] Treatment and diagnosis were not different in patients who were not imaged as opposed to patients who underwent advanced imaging.[135] When comparing patients with low back pain receiving either radiographs or an abbreviated MR imaging protocol, there was no advantage to the MR imaging group.[136] Gillan et al. found no treatment difference between imaging versus no imaging in patients with low back pain.[135] Imaging for low back pain can be associated with potential harm, including radiation exposure if CT imaging is used,[137] potential for increased rates of spine surgery,[138-140] and the potential for patients to have a lesser sense of well-being.[141]

Multiple authors suggest that an imaging study is indicated in the evaluation of a patient with sciatica when (1) true radicular symptoms are present, (2) there is objective evidence of nerve root irritation on physical examination (i.e., positive straight-leg raise test), and (3) the patient has not responded to "conservative management" of 4 to 6 weeks' duration.[142-144] Earlier imaging is considered appropriate if clinical features raise concern regarding malignant or infectious causes or if neurologic findings worsen during observation. These recommendations are based on several studies of successful nonoperative treatment of sciatica.[145-150] Imaging is recommended only for the remaining minority of patients with persistent signs and symptoms who are believed to be surgical candidates or in whom diagnostic uncertainty remains. In the 2009 American College of Radiology appropriateness criteria for imaging patients with low back pain, imaging patients was noted to be inappropriate if the following were absent: trauma in patients older than 50 years of age, unexplained fever or weight loss, immunosuppression, history of cancer or intravenous drug use, steroid use, age greater than 70 years, progressive neurologic symptoms or loss of function, or symptoms being present for longer than 6 weeks.[151]

Intervertebral Disc

Because of its inherent contrast sensitivity, MRI reveals morphologic abnormalities well and also provides insight into the biochemical changes of the degenerating disc. With aging and degeneration, there is gradual narrowing of the disc space and loss of the normal high intradiscal signal intensity on T2-weighted images. The latter is believed to be secondary to changes in proteoglycan composition within the disc rather than to absolute changes in water content.[152] As degeneration progresses, small fluid-filled fissures or cracks may develop that manifest as intradiscal areas of linear high signal on T2-weighted images.[153-155] Gas and calcification can also develop within a degenerating disc.

Fissures (tears) of the anulus fibrosus can also be visualized with MRI. They appear as small areas of increased signal on T2-weighted images and can enhance after contrast agent administration, presumably secondary to the ingrowth of granulation tissue into the fissure as a consequence of healing.[156] Three types of anular fissures have been described, depending on their orientation relative to the concentric anular fibers.[157] The high frequency of anular fissures seen in association with large disc bulges challenges the concept that the anulus fibrosus is intact in bulging discs but ruptured in herniated discs. The clinical significance of anular fissures is unknown. In patients without nerve root compression, back pain may be secondary to irritation of the nerve endings in the peripheral anulus either from scar tissue within an anular fissure or from a disc herniation; this is referred to as *discogenic pain.* Although this concept is often used to ascribe clinical significance to these lesions, many asymptomatic patients harbor anular fissures.

There is no universally accepted classification system describing degenerative disc disease. A multispecialty task force released recommendations for disc nomenclature spanning the orthopedic, neurosurgical, and radiologic communities.[158] This group has defined a *protrusion* as a herniation that maintains contact with the disc of origin by a bridge as wide as, or wider than, any diameter of the displaced material (Fig. 13.11). An *extruded* disc is a larger herniation in which the diameter of the disc material beyond the interspace is wider than the bridge, if any, that connects it to the disc of origin (Fig. 13.12). A *sequestered (free)* disc fragment is an extrusion that is no longer contiguous with the parent disc. It may reside either anterior or posterior to the posterior longitudinal ligament or rarely may be intradural (Figs. 13.13 and 13.14). A free fragment may be located at the disc level or may migrate superiorly or inferiorly, often lateralized by the thin, sagittally oriented midline septum seen in the lower anterior epidural space.

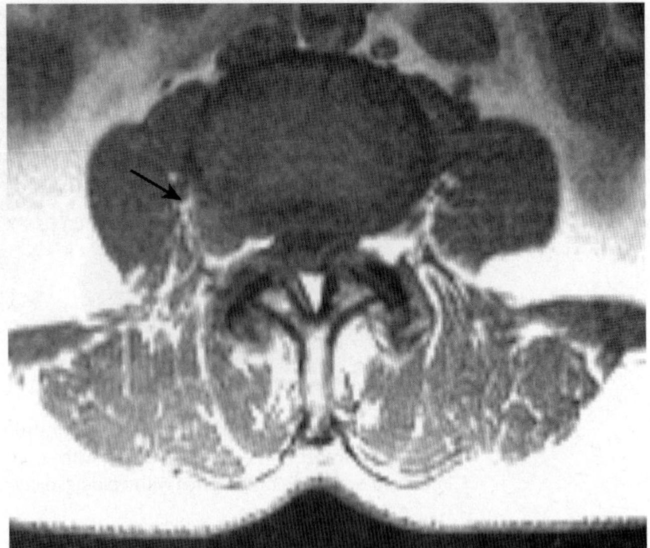

FIG. 13.11 Lateral disc herniation. Axial T1-weighted magnetic resonance image shows well-defined right lateral herniation with no thecal sac compromise *(arrow).*

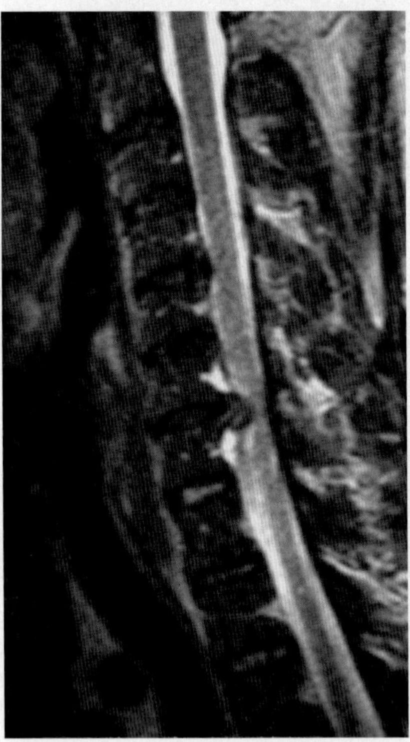

FIG. 13.12 Cervical disc extrusion. Sagittal T2-weighted magnetic resonance image shows large disc extrusion at C6–C7 severely effacing the anterior thecal sac and cord. Signal intensity of the cord is normal.

Degenerative Endplate Changes

In addition to these observed changes within the degenerating disc, vertebral marrow signal abnormalities adjacent to the degenerating disc are common.[159] Type 1 endplate change manifests as decreased marrow signal paralleling the endplates on T1-weighted images and increased signal on T2-weighted images. These changes reflect replacement of normal fatty marrow with fibrovascular marrow, which has greater water

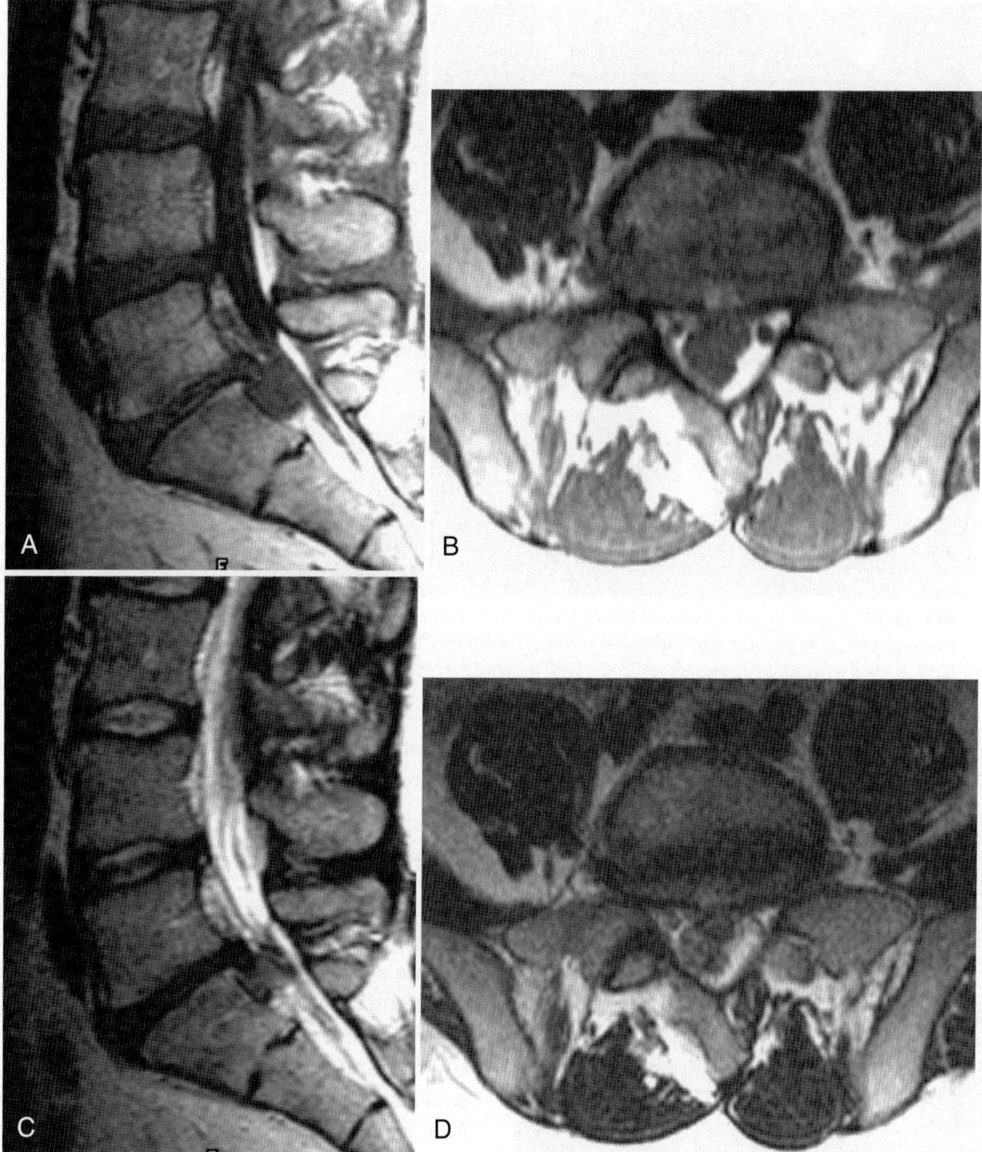

FIG. 13.13 Disc extrusion with free fragment. (A) Sagittal and (B) axial T1-weighted magnetic resonance images show a large central extrusion at L5–S1 extending dorsally and inferiorly, suggesting a free fragment. There is severe effacement of caudal thecal sac. (C) Sagittal and (D) axial T2-weighted images show extrusion as intermediate signal and confirm mass effect on sac.

content. Type 2 endplate changes are slightly more common than type 1 changes, showing increased signal on T1-weighted images and isointense to slightly increased signal on T2-weighted images. Histologically, these changes correlate with fatty marrow replacement. These changes may be preceded by type 1 changes, and often these changes exist in combination at the same level or different levels. Type 3 endplate changes show decreased marrow signal on T1-weighted and T2-weighted images, a finding that correlates with endplate sclerosis seen radiographically.[159]

Recent researchers have suggested that type 1 endplate changes can be secondary to a low-grade infection,[160,161] with one study showing that patients with type 1 endplate changes treated with antibiotics showed improvement over the placebo group.[162]

Lumbar Stenosis

As an anatomic entity, spinal stenosis refers to narrowing of the central spinal canal, neural foramina, or lateral recesses. Most commonly, it is acquired secondary to degenerative disease of the intervertebral disc or facets or both, although developmentally shortened pedicles are an important component of symptomatic spinal stenosis in patients with otherwise mild degenerative changes (Figs. 13.15 and 13.16).[163] Before the development of MRI, plain films and CT were used to diagnose spinal stenosis by measuring the dimensions of the bony canal. At present, such measurements are not commonly performed. These measurements do not take into account the normal anatomic variation between patients or the role of the disc and ligamentum flavum in spinal stenosis and are inaccurate predictors of clinical symptoms. MRI accurately depicts

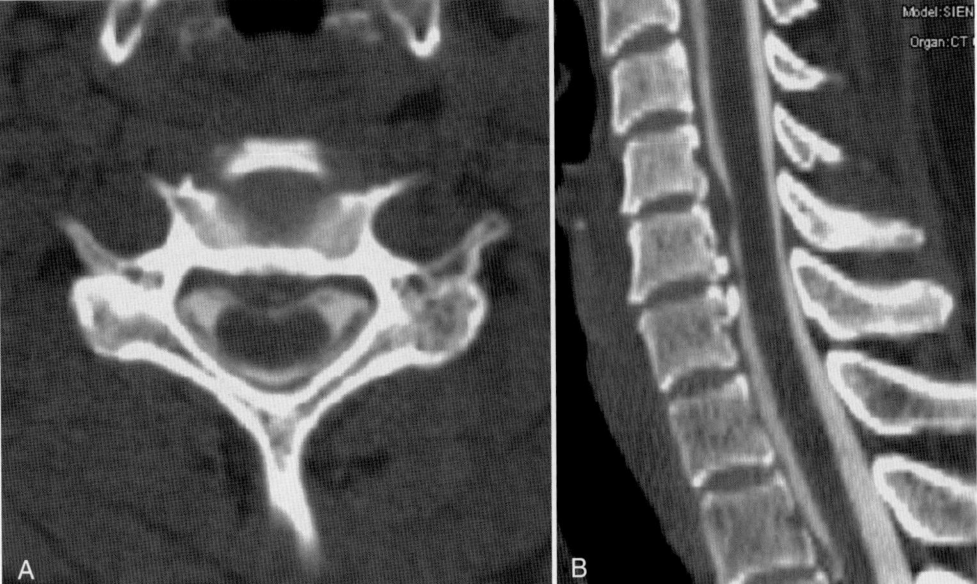

FIG. 13.14 Cervical disc herniation. (A) Axial computed tomographic scan and (B) sagittal reformat after myelography show well-defined extradural lesion at C4–C5 effacing the anterior thecal sac and touching the cord. A small osteophyte is present at C5–C6 with no cord compromise.

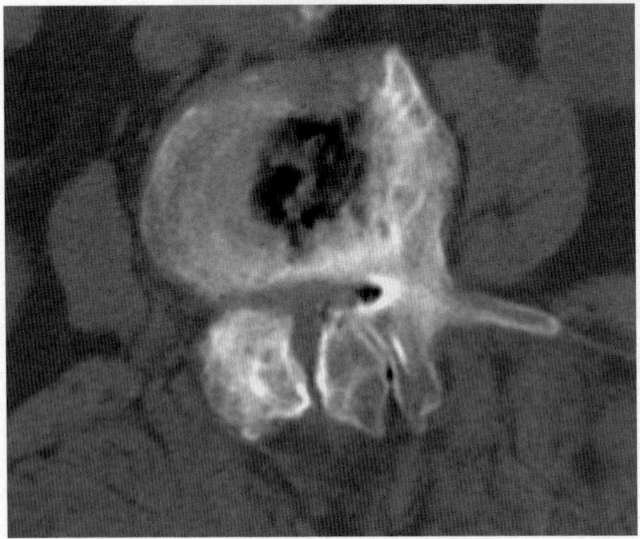

FIG. 13.15 Lumbar canal stenosis. Axial computed tomographic scan at L4–L5 shows marked bony central canal stenosis with mild anterior osteophyte and marked facet hypertrophic degenerative change. The disc is degenerated with vacuum phenomenon.

the degree and cause of thecal sac narrowing in patients with central canal stenosis. Such narrowing is most commonly due to bony and ligamentous hypertrophy.

In addition to central canal stenosis, stenosis of the lateral recess is an important cause of lower extremity pain and paresthesias. The lateral recess is bordered anteriorly by the posterior aspect of the vertebral body and disc, laterally by the pedicle, and posteriorly by the superior articular facet. The root sleeve within the lateral recess is often compressed by bony hypertrophy of the superior facet, often in combination with disc bulging and osteophyte along the anterior border of the lateral recess. Lateral recess pathology can clinically mimic disc herniation. MRI allows differentiation between central and lateral recess stenosis and provides important information for presurgical planning.[164]

Facet Disease

Degenerative disease of the facet joints typically occurs in combination with degenerative disc disease, although facet disease alone may be responsible for symptoms of back pain and radiculopathy. As with any synovial-lined joint, facet joints are susceptible to the development of joint space loss, subchondral sclerosis and cyst formation, osteophytosis, and subluxation. Because of the richly innervated synovium and joint capsule, these changes alone can be a source of pain, or alternatively they can contribute to nerve root impingement by causing spinal stenosis or foraminal compromise. On MRI, degenerated facets appear hypertrophied, sclerotic, and irregular. Enlarged ligamentum flavum is commonly present. Facet degeneration can lead to the formation of synovial cysts that can compress the thecal sac and roots from a posterior direction. Synovial cysts are best depicted on axial images and appear as posterolateral epidural masses adjacent to a degenerated facet, most commonly at the L4–L5 level. Synovial cysts have variable signal characteristics secondary to varying cyst fluid composition and associated hemorrhage, calcification, or gas within the cyst (Fig. 13.17).[165] A peripheral hypointense rim on T2-weighted images related to calcification may be seen. Intravenous contrast medium is useful in suspected cases to define better the lesion and its relationship to the adjacent facet joint and thecal sac.

Instability

The most frequently seen alignment abnormality is spondylolisthesis, which is defined as ventral slippage of a vertebra relative to the vertebrae below. The two most common causes of

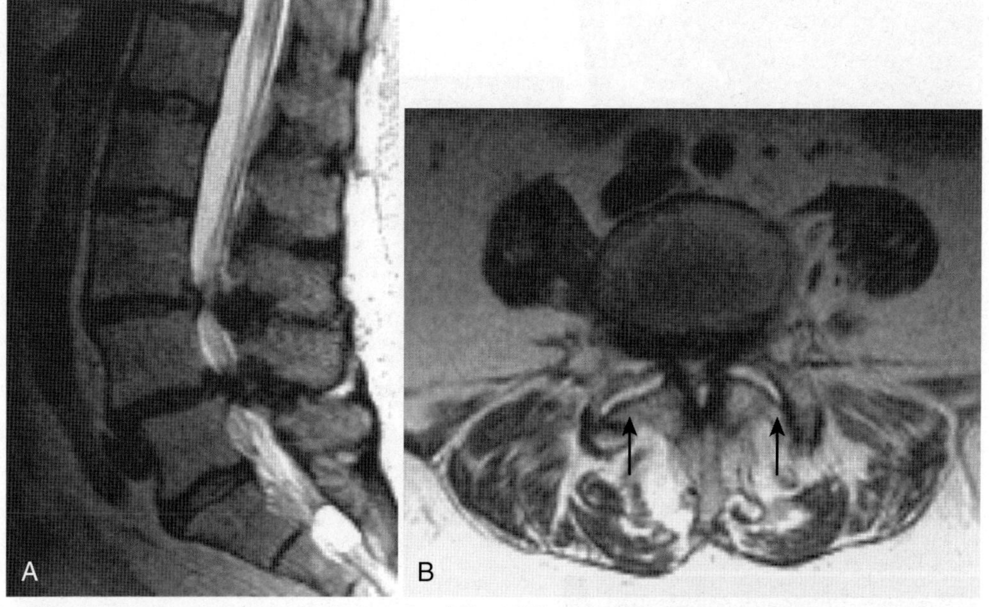

FIG. 13.16 Lumbar canal stenosis. (A) Sagittal and (B) axial T2-weighted magnetic resonance images show severe central canal stenosis at L3–L4 and L4–L5 with marked compression of the thecal sac owing to anterior bulge of the anulus fibrosus and facet hypertrophic degenerative change. There are small bilateral facet effusions *(arrows)*.

spondylolisthesis are bilateral defects in the pars interarticularis (isthmic spondylolisthesis) and facet disease (degenerative spondylolisthesis). The degenerative variety is the most common in older adults.

Because of its ability to obtain direct sagittal images free of overlapping structures and patient rotation, MRI is an accurate method of diagnosing spondylolisthesis. MRI is nearly always performed with the patient supine, however. In that position, a vertebra with subluxation can be normally aligned. A more accurate method of detecting listhesis is by weight-bearing lateral lumbar radiographs. The detection of spondylolysis (pars interarticularis defect without ventral slippage) by MRI can be problematic, and it is generally agreed that plain films and CT are more reliable for its diagnosis. Because MRI is being increasingly used as the first and only imaging modality in evaluating patients with low back pain and radicular symptoms, many cases of spondylolysis are imaged without the benefit of correlative plain films or CT studies.[166] Using MRI, sagittal T1-weighted images are best for showing the pars interarticularis owing to their higher signal-to-noise ratio, the depiction of the pars marrow as hyperintense, and the minimal obliquity of the pars in this imaging plane (Fig. 13.18). If the pars appears normal (i.e., contiguous normal marrow signal), one can be certain that it is intact.[167]

Cervical Radiculopathy and Myelopathy

Various studies have shown that canal size is reduced in patients with cervical spondylotic myelopathy. The normal diameter of the canal from C3 to C7 is approximately 17 mm and can be decreased to 12 mm or less in cervical spondylotic myelopathy. The size that is associated with myelopathy has ranged, however, from less than 10 mm up to 14 mm. Additionally, myelopathic symptoms tend to occur when the canal cross-sectional area is less than 60 mm^2. The ratio of the anteroposterior canal diameter to the vertebral body diameter has been used to assess cervical stenosis. This Pavlov ratio (sometimes referred to as the Torg ratio) is normal if it is 1 or greater.[168] A ratio of 0.8 or less is considered abnormal. As a ratio, however, it can be abnormal not only because of an abnormally small canal diameter (small numerator), but also because of an abnormally large vertebral body (large denominator). This ratio method also does not take into account the size of the spinal cord itself. As an isolated tool, this method is of historical interest only and is useless in evaluating cervical spinal cord compression.

Takahashi and colleagues and others have described areas of increased signal intensity on T2-weighted images within the cervical cord owing to extradural compression, which variously reflects myelomalacia, gliosis, and demyelination and edema (Fig. 13.19).[169] Patients who show areas of abnormal signal within the cord tend to have a worse clinical condition than patients with normal cord signal intensity. These abnormal signal changes can disappear or diminish after surgery to relieve the cord compression.

Postoperative Imaging

Causes of early and delayed failure of surgery are listed in Boxes 13.1 and 13.2. Caution must be used in interpretation of CT, CT myelography, and MRI within the first 6 weeks after surgery owing to the large amount of tissue disruption and edema that may be present producing mass effect on the anterior thecal sac, even in the absence of any clinical symptoms. MRI may be used in the immediate postoperative period for a

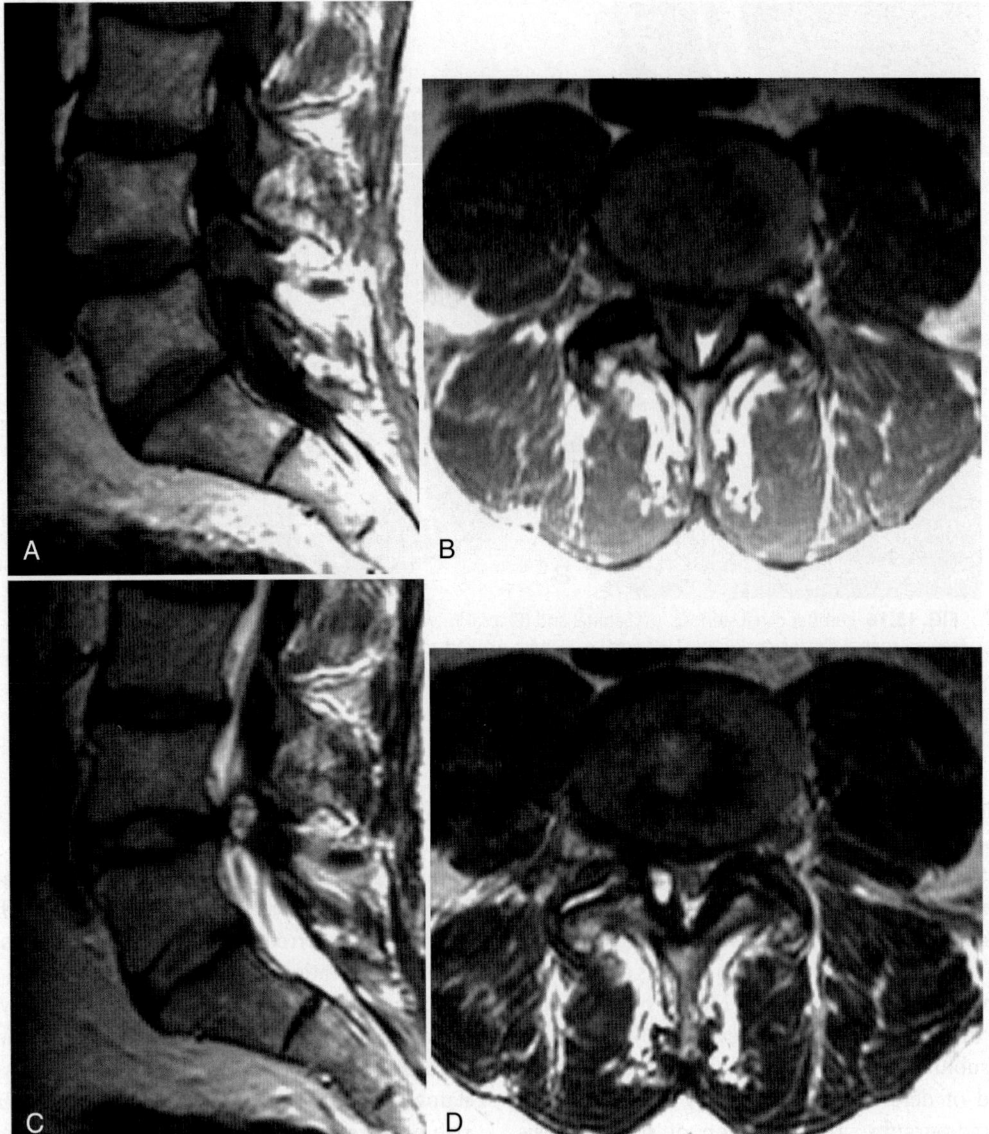

FIG. 13.17 Synovial cyst. (A) Sagittal and (B) axial T1-weighted magnetic resonance images show mass with central low signal centered on the right anterior facet that effaces the right dorsal aspect of the thecal sac. (C) Sagittal and (D) axial T2-weighted images show central high signal of fluid consistent with synovial cyst.

BOX 13.1 Technical Causes of Early Spine Surgery Failure

Hematoma
Infection
Inadequate decompression of bony foraminal or central stenosis
Insufficient removal of herniation
Neural trauma
Unrecognized free disc fragment
Wrong level surgery

BOX 13.2 Technical Causes of Delayed Recurrence of Low Back Pain or Radiculopathy

Arachnoiditis
Epidural fibrosis
Facet arthropathy with foraminal stenosis
Instability
New or recurrent herniation
Pseudomeningocele
Central canal stenosis
Infection

more gross view of the thecal sac and epidural space, to exclude significant postoperative hemorrhage, pseudomeningocele, or disc space infection at the laminectomy site. CT myelography is also a direct way to define a pseudomeningocele and to image the spine when hardware is present (Fig. 13.20).

Small fluid collections are commonly seen in the posterior tissues after laminectomy. The signal intensities can vary depending on whether the collections are serous (follow CSF signal intensity) or serosanguineous (increased signal on T1-weighted images owing to hemoglobin breakdown products). The distinction between small postoperative fluid collections and infected collections cannot be made by MRI morphology or signal intensity. Acute hemorrhage typically shows isointense to increased signal in the epidural space on T1-weighted images and should show diminished signal on gradient-echo or T2-weighted images. Very acute blood collections may be isointense, however, on T1-weighted and T2-weighted images (Fig. 13.21).

Aside from the various options for instrumentation that are available, different types of bone graft materials are available, some with ramifications when imaging.[170] Bone morphogenic protein (BMP) can produce imaging findings that can be misinterpreted as infection, including prevertebral soft tissue swelling and vertebral body endplate resorption, although these findings typically resolve by 6 months.[171-173]

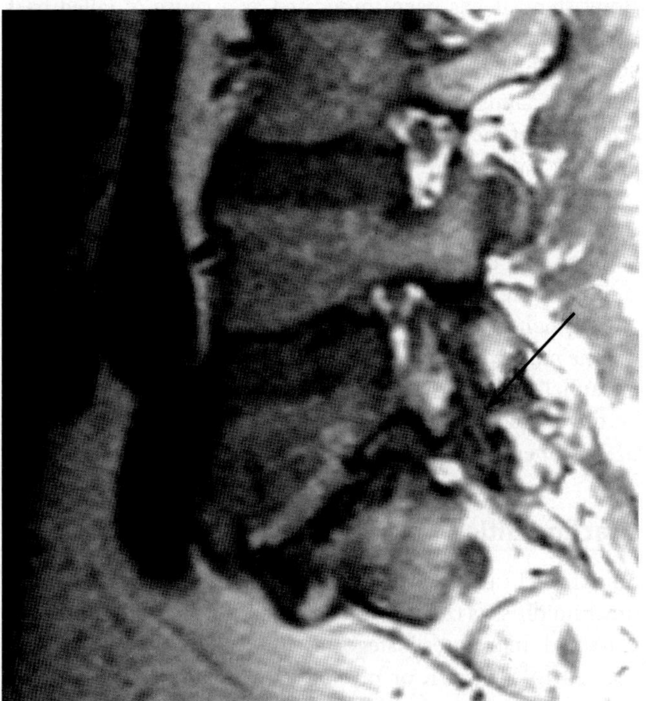

FIG. 13.18 Spondylolysis. Sagittal T1-weighted magnetic resonance image shows disruption of cortical margin of pars interarticularis *(arrow)* at L5–S1 consistent with spondylolysis. There is severe foraminal stenosis at L5–S1.

Epidural Fibrosis and Disc Herniations

The use of contrast medium–enhanced MRI in the evaluation of scar versus disc has been examined by several authors, with reported accuracy rates of 96% to 100% for distinguishing scar from disc.[174] Lumbar epidural fibrosis (scar) is a replacement of the normal epidural fat with postoperative fibrotic tissue, which is capable of binding the dura and nerve roots to the surrounding structures anteriorly and posteriorly. Epidural fibrosis is seen to enhance consistently immediately after injection of contrast material (Fig. 13.22). This enhancement occurs regardless of the time since surgery. Disc material does not enhance on the early postinjection images owing to its lack of vascularity (Fig. 13.23). In cases with a mixture of scar and disc material, scar enhances but the disc material does not enhance on early postinjection images.

Selective fat suppression on T1-weighted images has been used in the evaluation of postoperative patients. Georgy et al.[175] examined 25 patients with recurrent pain after lumbar disc surgery with MRI to evaluate the usefulness of gadolinium-enhanced fat suppression imaging in patients with failed back surgery. The addition of fat suppression to enhanced T1-weighted images improved the visualization of enhancing scar in all cases, helped distinguish scar from recurrent herniated disc, and showed more clearly the relationship of scar to the nerve

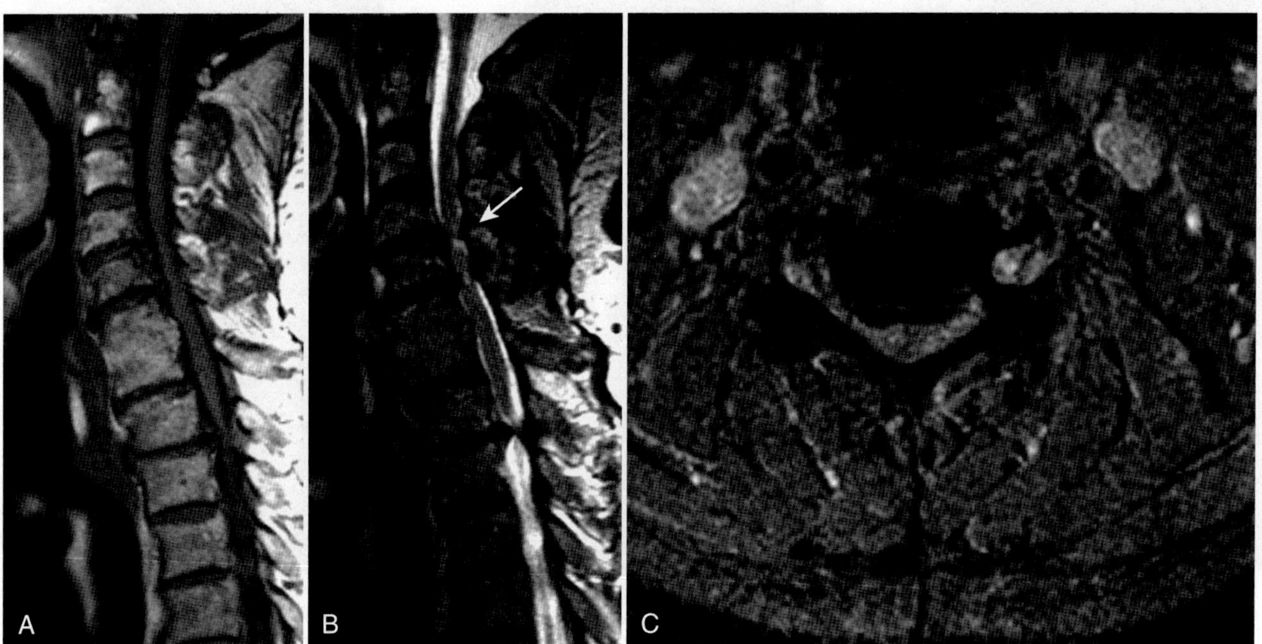

FIG. 13.19 Cervical spondylosis. (A) Sagittal T1- and (B) T2-weighted magnetic resonance images show solid fusion at C6–C7 level with a small osteophyte. There is severe central stenosis of the disc and osteophyte complex and posterior ligamentous hypertrophy at C4–C5, C5–C6, and T1–T2 levels. There is myelomalacia within the cord seen as high signal intensity on the T2-weighted image at C4–C5 *(arrow)*. (C) Axial gradient-echo image at C4–C5 confirms severity of central stenosis owing to broad-based disc and osteophyte.

roots and thecal sac. Overall there are conflicting data as to whether epidural scar is associated or causative of symptoms following back surgery. The presence of scar did not correlate with symptoms in a study of 40 patients.[176] When epidural scar is present in symptomatic patients undergoing reoperation, it is associated with a poor outcome.[177] Others suggest that psychosocial factors rather than the presence of epidural scar correlate better with symptoms.[178]

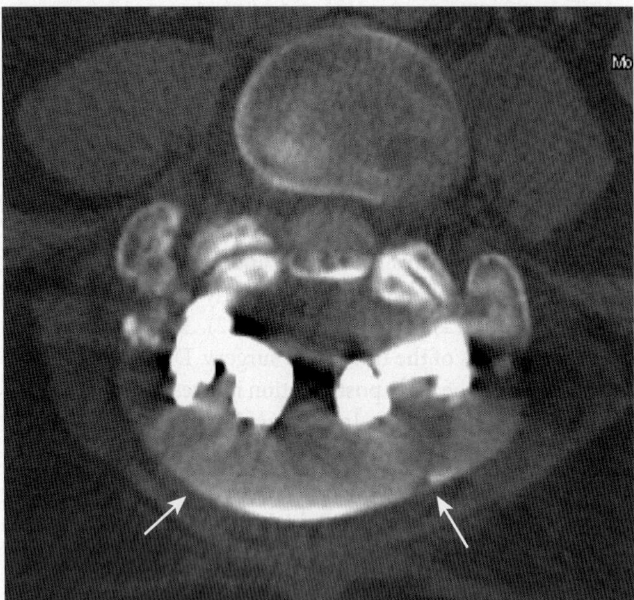

FIG. 13.20 Pseudomeningocele. Axial computed tomographic scan after myelography shows metal artifact from prior pedicle screw fixation. There is pooling of contrast medium around and dorsal to the hardware owing to a large pseudomeningocele (*arrows*).

Stenosis

Bony stenosis has been implicated as a cause of failed back surgery in 60% of cases. Various mechanisms can lead to stenotic changes in the canal or foramina. Their significance may vary, and many of these stenoses are not symptomatic. Examples of mechanisms are as follows:

1. Bony overgrowth after facetectomy may compromise a lateral recess.
2. After posterior fusion, there may be late overgrowth of bone into the posterior or lateral canals.
3. After anterior fusion, bone may extend into the canal or foramen.
4. The narrowing of the interspace after discectomy may allow sufficient facet overriding to produce a decreased size of the lateral recesses or foramina.
5. Postoperative spondylolisthesis can produce focal stenosis.

Arachnoiditis

Spinal MRI can identify the various characteristics of lumbar arachnoiditis, as can CT and myelography.[179-181] These may be classified into three categories or patterns, which can be applied to MRI, CT, or myelography, although a mixture of patterns can occur in any one patient.[182]

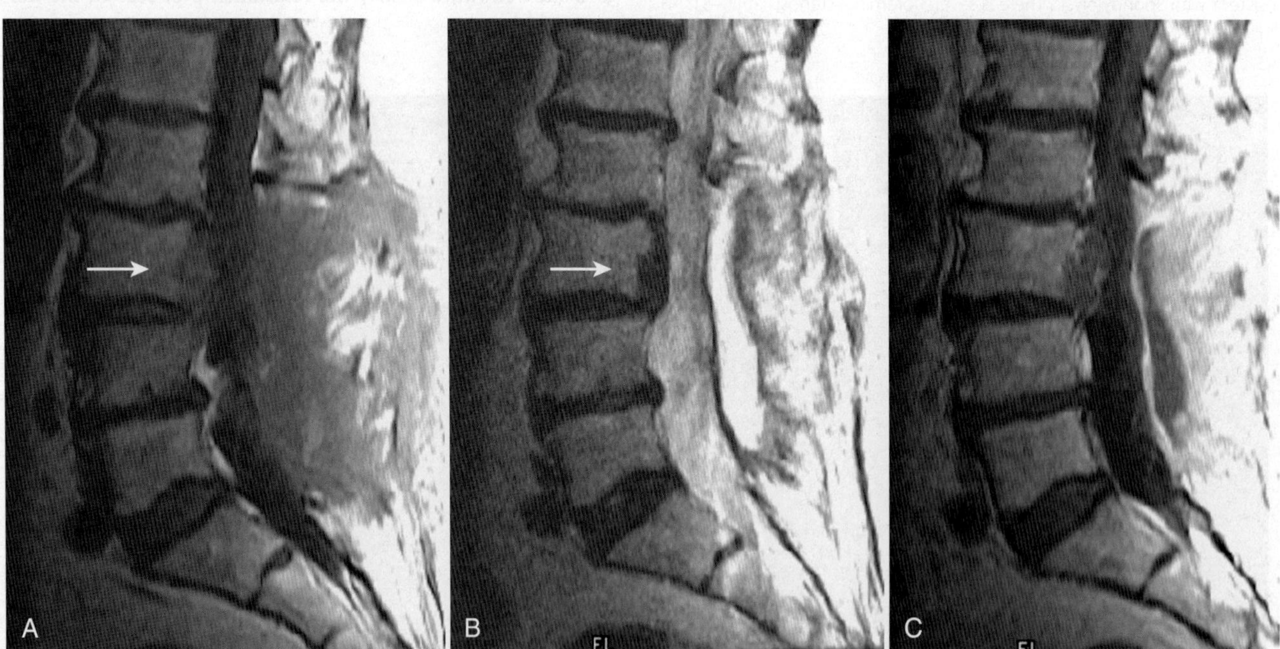

FIG. 13.21 Recurrent herniation mimicking blood. This patient underwent multilevel laminectomy and L3–L4 discectomy 3 weeks before examination. (A) Sagittal T1-weighted magnetic resonance image shows vague anterior epidural mass at L3 and extensive postoperative changes in dorsal epidural soft tissues. (B) Sagittal T2-weighted image shows L3 epidural mass to be of low signal, with effacement of anterior thecal sac. (C) After contrast administration, sagittal T1-weighted image shows slight peripheral enhancement. Differential diagnosis included acute blood (deoxyhemoglobin) and large recurrent herniation. Because of homogeneity of low signal and contiguity with disc space at L3–L4, recurrent herniation was favored. A large herniation was found at reoperation.

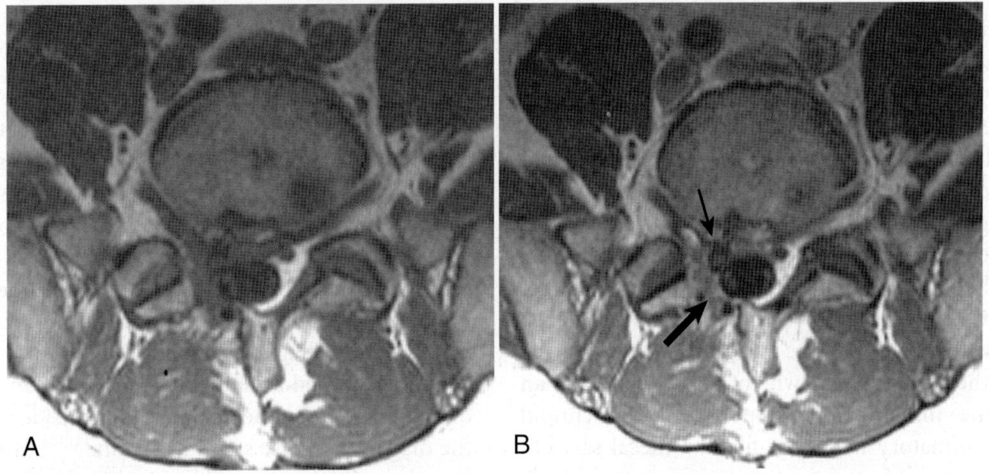

FIG. 13.22 Postoperative epidural scar. Axial T1-weighted magnetic resonance images (A) before and (B) after contrast administration show diffuse enhancement of tissue surrounding the right lateral aspect of the thecal sac *(large arrow)* and exiting the right S1 root *(small arrow)*.

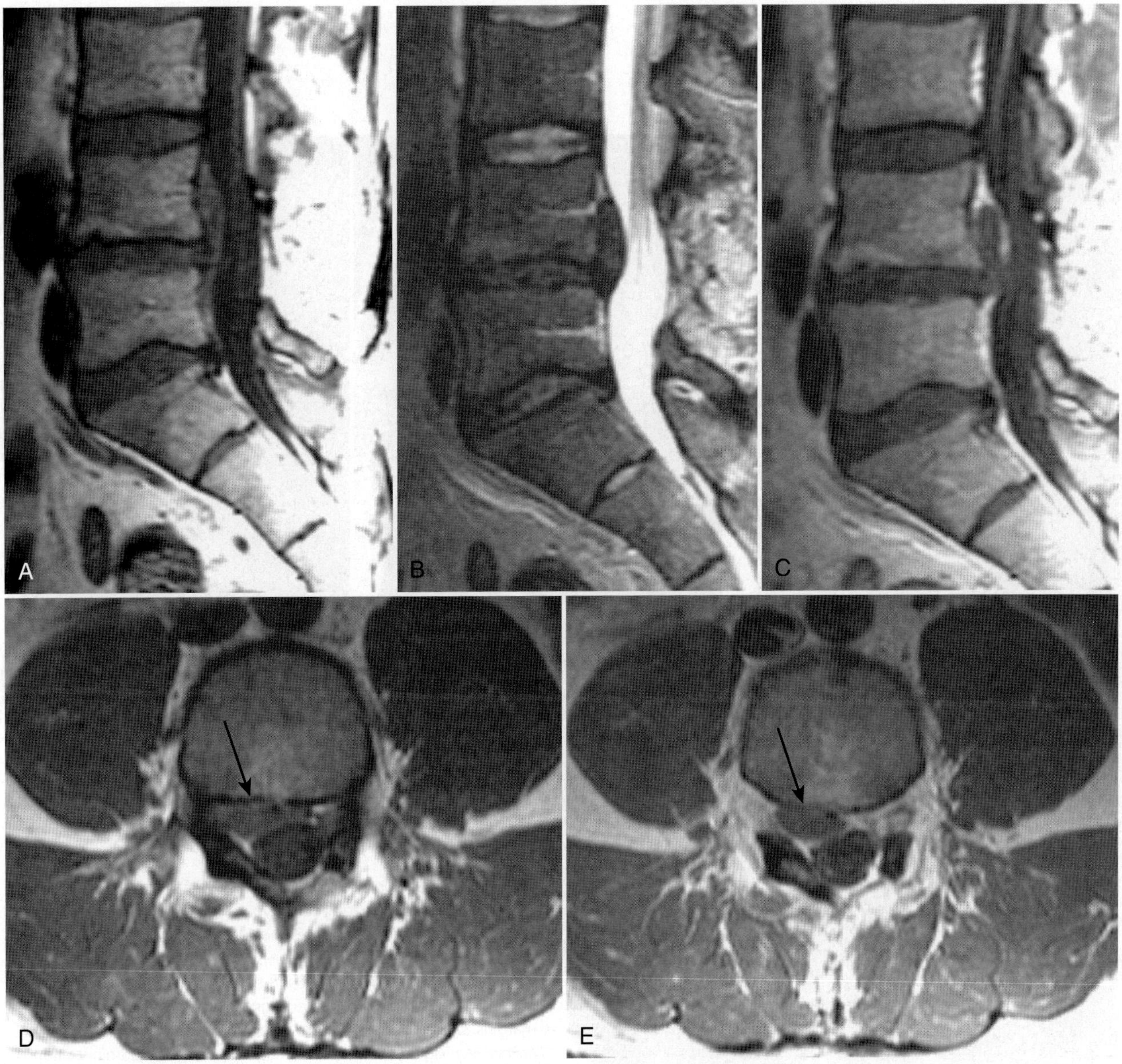

FIG. 13.23 Recurrent herniation. (A) Sagittal T1-weighted magnetic resonance image shows large anterior epidural mass extending dorsal to L4 body from L4–L5 disc space. The patient previously underwent L4 laminectomy and discectomy. (B) Sagittal T2-weighted image shows a large disc extrusion migrating superiorly from the disc space level, reflecting free fragment. (C) After contrast medium administration, sagittal T1-weighted image shows typical peripheral enhancement of large herniation. Axial T1-weighted images (D) before and (E) after contrast administration show peripheral enhancement of the disc component at mid-L4 level *(arrow)*.

The first pattern is central adhesion of the nerve roots within the thecal sac into a central clump of soft tissue signal. Instead of showing their normal feathery pattern, the nerve roots are clumped into one or more cords. This pattern is most easily identified on axial CT myelography or T1-weighted MRI. The second pattern is adhesion of the nerve roots to the meninges, giving rise to an "empty thecal sac" sign. On MRI, only the homogeneous signal of the CSF is present within the thecal sac, and the nerve roots are peripherally attached to the meninges. On CT myelography, only the high-attenuation contrast agent within the thecal sac is visualized, without the nerve roots. In the third pattern, which can be viewed as an end stage of the inflammatory response, the arachnoid becomes an inflammatory mass that fills the thecal sac. On myelography, this type of arachnoiditis gives rise to a block, with an irregular "candle dripping" appearance. MRI shows a nonspecific soft tissue mass, as does CT myelography.

Infection

Infection should be considered in the differential diagnosis for back pain even though it is an uncommon disorder (1% of all cases of osteomyelitis). When infection is considered, accurate imaging is a necessary prelude for microbiologic diagnosis or surgical drainage. Because abnormalities that appear on plain radiographs usually take days to weeks to become apparent, radionuclide studies and MRI have been the primary imaging modalities for diagnosis of vertebral osteomyelitis.

CT has played a minor diagnostic role in cases with bony or soft tissue components and is not considered a mainstay for the diagnosis of disc space infection.[183,184] MRI is more sensitive than either plain films or CT for detecting vertebral osteomyelitis, and it approaches or equals the sensitivity of radionuclide studies (Figs. 13.24 and 13.25).[185,186]

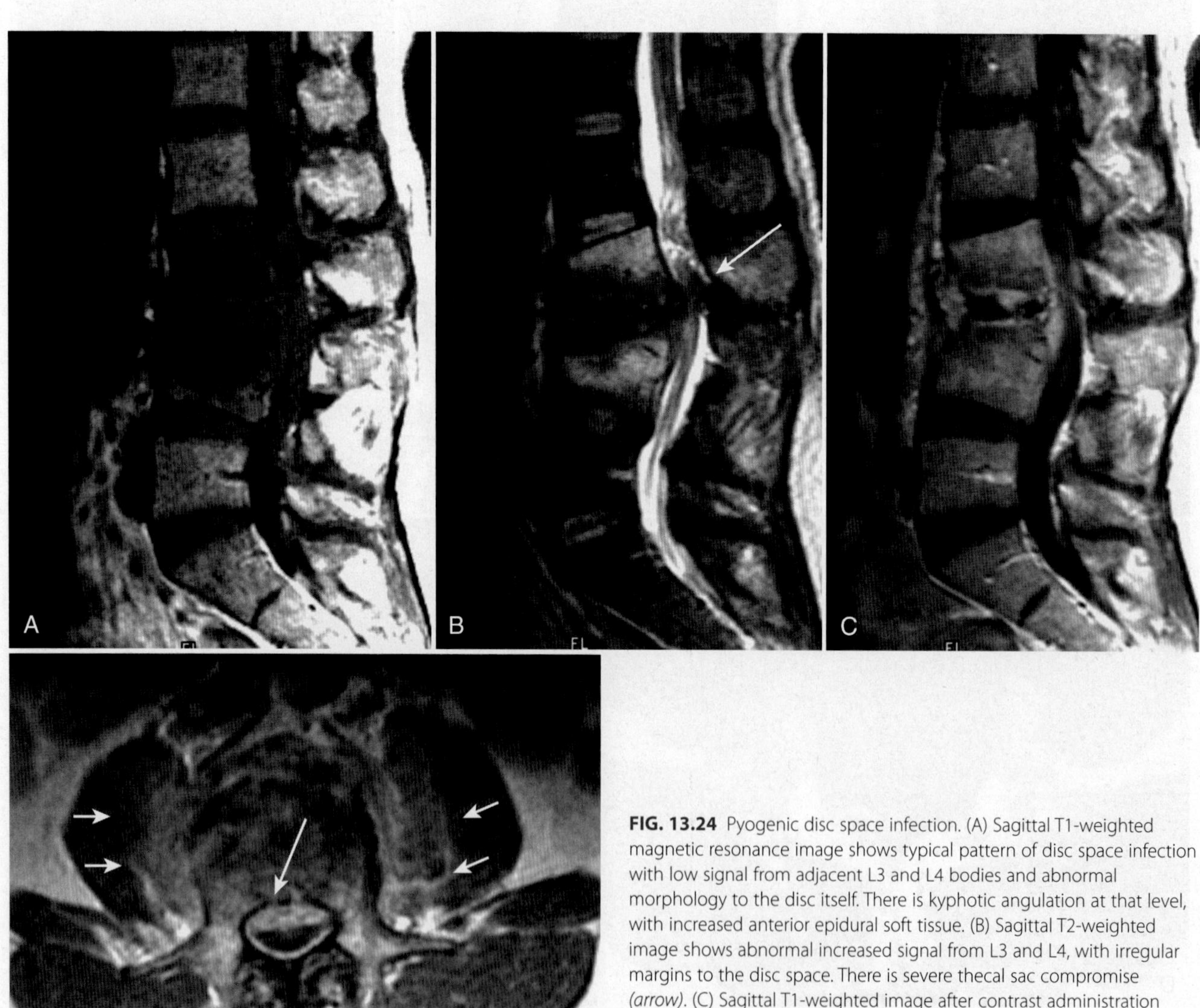

FIG. 13.24 Pyogenic disc space infection. (A) Sagittal T1-weighted magnetic resonance image shows typical pattern of disc space infection with low signal from adjacent L3 and L4 bodies and abnormal morphology to the disc itself. There is kyphotic angulation at that level, with increased anterior epidural soft tissue. (B) Sagittal T2-weighted image shows abnormal increased signal from L3 and L4, with irregular margins to the disc space. There is severe thecal sac compromise *(arrow)*. (C) Sagittal T1-weighted image after contrast administration shows marked enhancement of vertebral bodies, disc space, and epidural phlegmon. (D) Degree of thecal sac compromise (*large arrow*) and diffuse paravertebral extension of inflammatory process (*small arrows*) are shown on axial T1-weighted image.

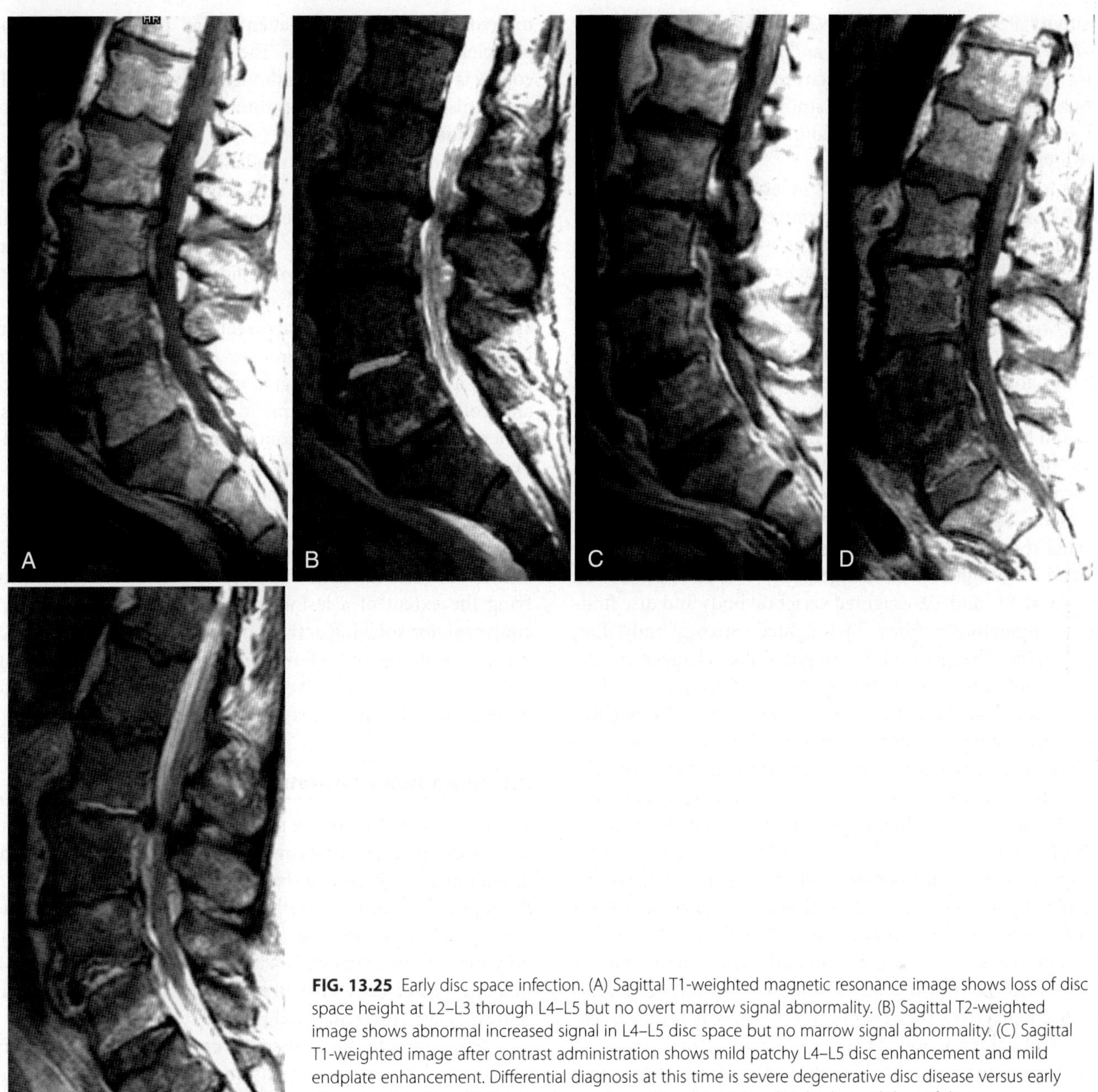

FIG. 13.25 Early disc space infection. (A) Sagittal T1-weighted magnetic resonance image shows loss of disc space height at L2–L3 through L4–L5 but no overt marrow signal abnormality. (B) Sagittal T2-weighted image shows abnormal increased signal in L4–L5 disc space but no marrow signal abnormality. (C) Sagittal T1-weighted image after contrast administration shows mild patchy L4–L5 disc enhancement and mild endplate enhancement. Differential diagnosis at this time is severe degenerative disc disease versus early disc space infection. (D) Grossly abnormal signal involving L4 and L5 bodies with loss of disc margin was visible 5 weeks later on T1-weighted image. (E) L4–L5 disc now shows more marked increased signal on T2-weighted image.

It is imperative to obtain both T1- and T2-weighted images in the sagittal plane for optimal sensitivity to detect disease. The T1-weighted spin-echo image allows detection of the increased water content or marrow fluid seen with inflammatory exudate or edema. Similar to most pathologic processes, disc space infection or vertebral osteomyelitis results in increased signal intensity on T2-weighted images. The diagnostic specificity of MRI is provided by the signal intensity changes on T1- and T2-weighted images and by the anatomic pattern of disease involvement and the appropriate clinical situation.

On T2-weighted images, the normal intervertebral disc usually shows increased signal intensity within its central portion that is bisected by a thin horizontal line of decreased signal, termed the *intranuclear cleft*. After the age of 30 years, the cleft is almost a constant feature of normal intervertebral discs. Disc space infections on MRI typically produce confluent decreased signal intensity of the adjacent vertebral bodies and the involved intervertebral disc space on T1-weighted images compared with the normal vertebral body marrow. A poorly defined endplate margin exists between the disc and adjacent vertebral bodies. T2-weighted images show increased signal intensity of the vertebral bodies adjacent to the involved disc and an abnormal morphology and increased signal intensity from the disc itself, with absence of the normal intranuclear cleft. These MRI findings are much more typical of pyogenic than of tuberculous osteomyelitis.[187] In a comparative study of patients with suspected vertebral osteomyelitis, MRI had a sensitivity of 96%, a specificity of 92%, and an overall accuracy of 94%.[185] Scintigraphy with ^{67}Ga and ^{99m}Tc bone scintigraphy had a sensitivity of 90%, specificity of 100%, and accuracy of 94% when combined. In this study, MRI was as accurate and sensitive as radionuclide scanning for the detection of osteomyelitis.

Dagirmanjian and colleagues[188] investigated the sensitivity of MRI findings for vertebral osteomyelitis. They considered the "classic" MRI changes of vertebral osteomyelitis to include decreased signal of disc and adjacent vertebral bodies on T1-weighted images, increased nonanatomic signal of the disc on T2-weighted images, increased signal of the adjacent vertebral bodies on T2-weighted images, and enhancement of the disc and adjacent vertebral bodies. These investigators found 95% of disc space infection levels had typical T1-weighted vertebral body changes, and 90% had increased nonanatomic signal of the disc on T2-weighted images. Only 54% of the abnormal levels showed increased signal of the vertebral bodies on T2-weighted images, however. Although 84% of patients showed the typical T1-weighted vertebral body and T1- and T2-weighted disc changes, only 49% of cases showed the typical T1- and T2-weighted vertebral body and disc findings as originally described. T1-weighted vertebral body, disc, and endplate changes and T2-weighted disc changes are the most reliable findings of disc space infection and vertebral osteomyelitis. In the initial stages of vertebral osteomyelitis, when the disc space is not yet involved, it may be difficult to exclude neoplastic disease or compression fracture from the differential diagnosis using only MRI. Follow-up studies are usually necessary to define the nature of the lesion further.

Boden and colleagues[189] suggested that in the postoperative spine the triad of intervertebral disc space enhancement, anular enhancement, and vertebral body enhancement leads to the diagnosis of disc space infection, with the appropriate laboratory findings, such as an elevated sedimentation rate. A group of normal postoperative patients, however, has anulus enhancement (at the surgical site), intervertebral disc enhancement, and vertebral endplate enhancement without evidence of disc space infection. In these cases, the intervertebral disc enhancement is typically seen as thin bands paralleling the adjacent endplates, and the vertebral body enhancement is associated with type 1 degenerative endplate changes. This pattern should be distinguished from the amorphous enhancement seen within the intervertebral disc with disc space infection.

Staphylococcus aureus is the organism most commonly associated with vertebral osteomyelitis and epidural abscess, accounting for approximately 60% of the cases (Fig. 13.26). *S. aureus* is ubiquitous, tends to form abscesses, and can infect compromised and normal hosts. Other gram-positive cocci account for approximately 13% of cases, and gram-negative organisms account for approximately 15%. Clinical acute symptoms classically include back pain, fever, obtundation in severe cases, and neurologic deficits. Chronic cases may have less pain and no elevated temperature. Rankin and Flothow[190] described the classic clinical course of epidural abscess in four stages: spinal ache, root pain, weakness, and paralysis. Acute deterioration from spinal epidural abscess remains unpredictable, however. Patients may present with abrupt paraplegia and anesthesia. The cause for this precipitous course is unknown, but it is thought to be related to a vascular mechanism (e.g., epidural thrombosis and thrombophlebitis, venous infarction).[191,192]

The primary diagnostic modality in the evaluation of epidural abscess is MRI. MRI is as sensitive as CT myelography for diagnosing epidural infection, but it also allows the exclusion of other entities, such as herniation, syrinx, tumor, and cord infarction.[193,194] MRI of epidural abscess shows a soft tissue mass in the epidural space with tapered edges and an associated mass effect on the thecal sac and cord. The epidural masses are usually isointense to the cord on T1-weighted images and of increased signal on T2-weighted images. Post and colleagues[195,196] recommended that in ambiguous cases either CT myelography or contrast medium–enhanced MRI is necessary for full elucidation of the abscess (Fig. 13.27).

The patterns of MRI contrast medium enhancement of epidural abscess include (1) diffuse and homogeneous, (2) heterogeneous, and (3) thin peripheral. Post and colleagues[196] found that enhancement was a very useful adjunct for identifying the extent of a lesion when the plain MR image was equivocal, for showing activity of an infection, and for directing needle biopsy and follow-up treatment. Successful therapy should cause a progressive decrease in enhancement of the paraspinal soft tissues, disc, and vertebral bodies.[197]

Intramedullary Lesions

Diagnostic considerations of pathology involving the intramedullary space include neoplasm, vascular malformation, syrinx, granulomatous disease, inflammation, or demyelination.[198-200] Radiographs without intrathecal contrast have no value for nonexpansile cord pathology, with late findings of cord neoplasm only inferred by canal expansion or osseous destruction. MR imaging can directly visualize the cord and can characterize nonexpansile cord abnormalities.

The imaging findings of spinal cord neoplasm most commonly include cord expansion, syrinx formation, and enhancement. For low-grade nonenhancing neoplasms there is typically cord expansion.[201,202] When faced with a nonexpansile T2 or STIR hyperintense spinal cord, distribution of signal abnormalities, enhancement, blood degradation byproducts, and its behavior over time (if available) are all useful factors to consider when arriving at an appropriate differential diagnosis. Transverse myelitis tends to involve longer segments of the cord as opposed to multiple sclerosis, which tends to be patchy and involves the dorsal or lateral aspects of the cord. Enhancement should typically resolve by 2 months when present with multiple sclerosis (Fig. 13.28). Spinal cord infarct can involve the ventral gray matter centrally within the spinal cord; subacute combined degeneration has a more posterior distribution.[200]

Neoplasms

The most common intramedullary neoplasms are *gliomas,* principally astrocytomas and ependymomas. *Ependymomas*

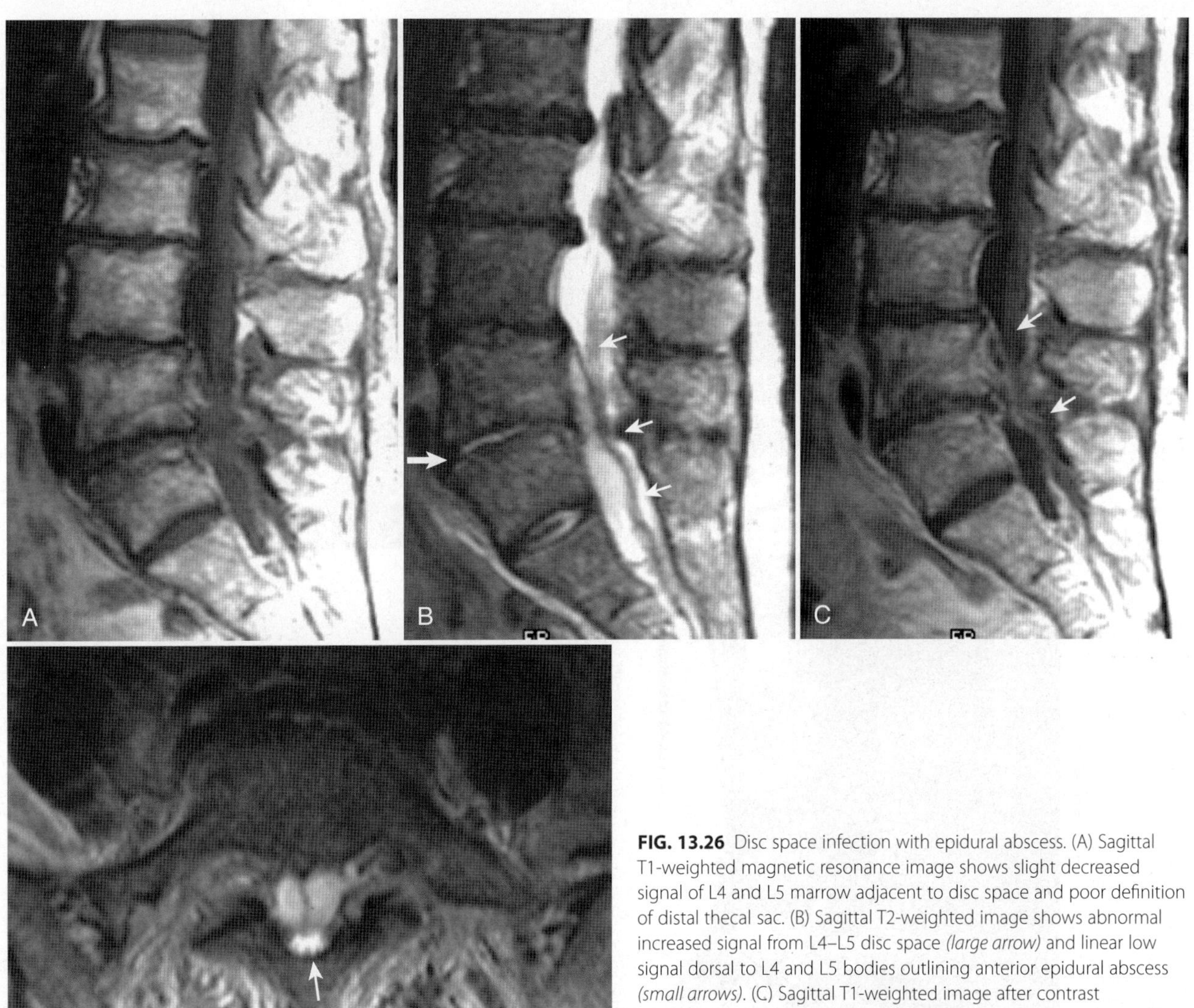

FIG. 13.26 Disc space infection with epidural abscess. (A) Sagittal T1-weighted magnetic resonance image shows slight decreased signal of L4 and L5 marrow adjacent to disc space and poor definition of distal thecal sac. (B) Sagittal T2-weighted image shows abnormal increased signal from L4–L5 disc space *(large arrow)* and linear low signal dorsal to L4 and L5 bodies outlining anterior epidural abscess *(small arrows)*. (C) Sagittal T1-weighted image after contrast administration better defines margins of epidural abscess *(arrows)* by enhancing margin extending inferiorly toward S1 level. Slight abnormal enhancement is present within the disc itself. (D) Axial T2-weighted image shows loculated abscess as foci of high signal, displacing caudal thecal sac dorsally *(arrow)*.

are cited as the most frequent intramedullary tumors in adults (Fig. 13.29). Although ependymomas may involve any portion of the cord, they most commonly involve the conus medullaris and filum terminale and are the most common primary tumor of the lower spinal cord. Patients with these tumors present in the fourth to fifth decades of life, often with back pain.[203,204] A typical appearance is an intradural extramedullary mass involving the filum terminale and cauda equina, although it can appear as fusiform enlargement of the cord itself.[205] Cervical intramedullary tumors may be seen in patients with neurofibromatosis type 2 (Fig. 13.30). These tumors typically enhance and may have intratumoral cysts. The myxopapillary subtype is particularly common in the lumbosacral region, typically appearing as a large, intensely enhancing mass spanning several vertebral levels. In most cases, the tumors appear as intradural extramedullary lesions because of their bulky exophytic growth, which fills the spinal canal. Overall signal intensities are nonspecific, but because of their highly vascular nature, ependymomas often show areas of T2-weighted shortening secondary to the presence of hemosiderin and ferritin, which is strongly suggestive of the diagnosis.[206] They also may manifest as subarachnoid hemorrhage.[207]

Intramedullary astrocytomas constitute 6% to 8% of primary spine tumors, with a peak incidence in the third to fourth decades of life. Astrocytomas produce focal enlargement and occasionally exophytic growth involving the cord. Of these tumors, 75% to 92% are relatively benign, such as grades 1 and 2. Imaging shows fusiform enlargement of the cord over several segments, whereas T2-weighted MRI shows increased signal intensity reflecting tumor and edematous cord. Cysts are often associated with these intramedullary tumors. These cysts may be benign, syringomyelic type of cavities, or actual cysts associated with the tumor.

Hemangioblastomas are unusual cord tumors and typically manifest in the third to fourth decades of life. They are frequently multiple and seen in association with von

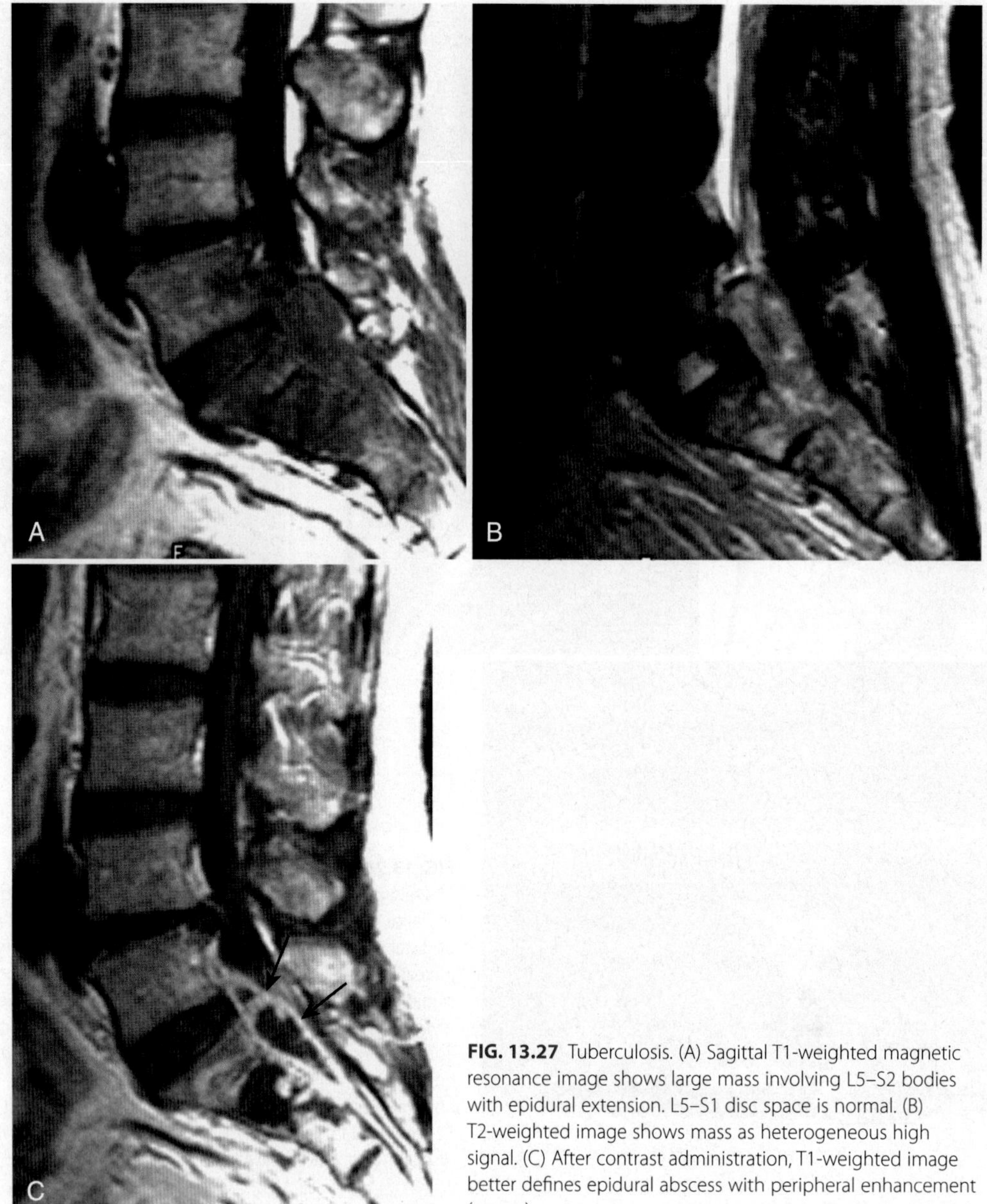

FIG. 13.27 Tuberculosis. (A) Sagittal T1-weighted magnetic resonance image shows large mass involving L5–S2 bodies with epidural extension. L5–S1 disc space is normal. (B) T2-weighted image shows mass as heterogeneous high signal. (C) After contrast administration, T1-weighted image better defines epidural abscess with peripheral enhancement (*arrows*).

Hippel–Lindau disease.[208-213] These lesions most often manifest as dorsal intramedullary masses containing a nodule that enhances, although these vary by the amount of cyst component and solid component. There may be extensive widening of the cord, showing increased signal intensity on T2-weighted images related to cord edema and extending several segments away from the nidus itself.

Occasionally, metastatic disease may manifest as an intramedullary enhancing mass. Carcinoma of the lung and breast is the most common, with melanoma, lymphoma, and renal cell carcinoma also reported.[214,215] Spread of intracranial neoplasms such as ependymoma and glioma may also seed the leptomeninges and produce direct involvement of the cord.[216-218]

Benign intramedullary tumors are uncommon, but *cavernous angiomas* (cavernous malformations) can occur in the cord with typical signal characteristics of speckled increased and decreased signal on T1-weighted images and evidence of hemosiderin deposition on T2-weighted images (Fig. 13.31).

Inflammation

The various causes of inflammatory myelopathies include multiple sclerosis, postviral demyelinating disease, viral infection, pyogenic infection, and granulomatous disease. The archetypal inflammatory lesion is *multiple sclerosis* (Fig. 13.32). The spinal cord is the site of much clinical involvement in patients with multiple sclerosis; however, imaging of the spinal cord has always been subordinate to brain imaging in radiologic investigations of multiple sclerosis. Because some of the clinical disease activity in multiple sclerosis is related to the spinal cord, it is important to correlate cord disease with clinical activity to gain further insights into the nature of disability in these patients and to correlate objective

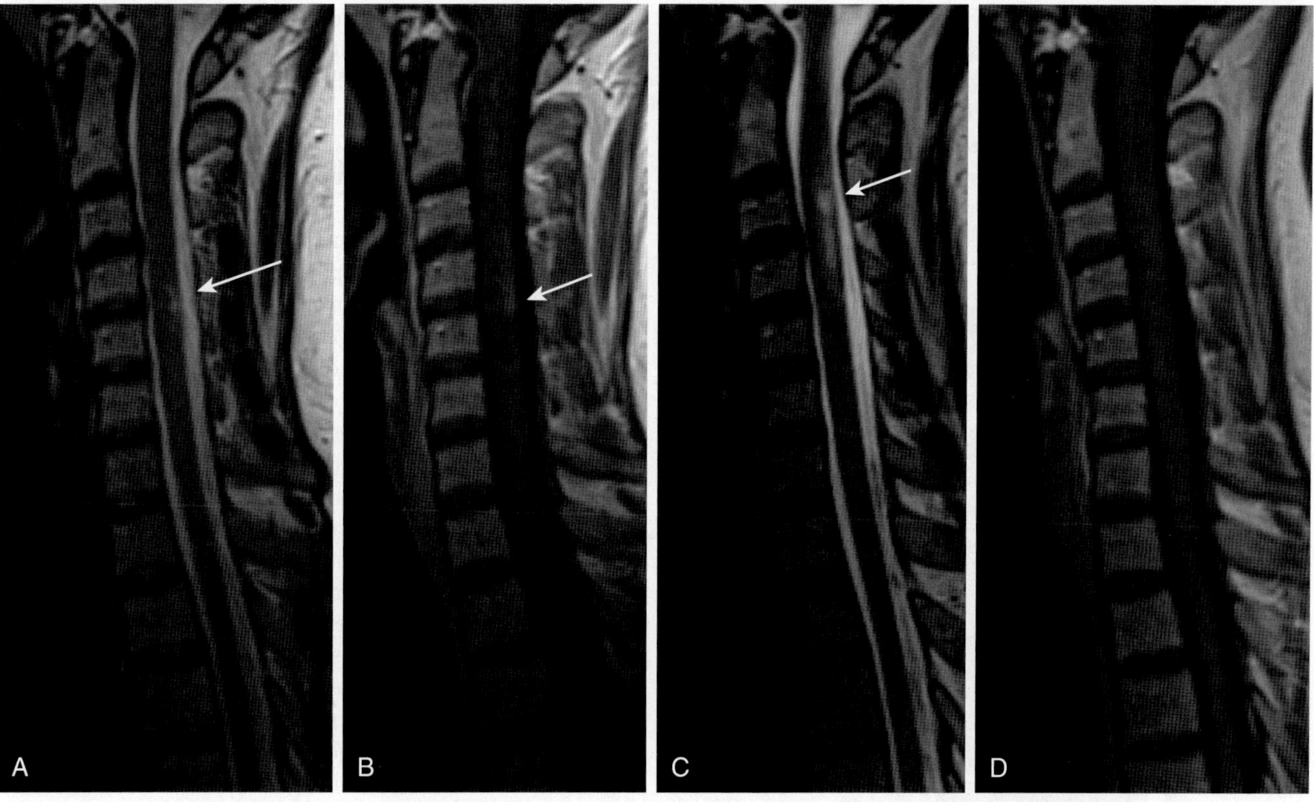

FIG. 13.28 Follow-up imaging is valuable when evaluating lesion behavior over time. (A) Sagittal T2-weighted magnetic resonance image and (B) sagittal T1-weighted contrast-enhanced image demonstrate cord signal abnormality and enhancement *(arrow)*. Follow-up imaging obtained 1 year later demonstrates (C) progression of T2 signal abnormality *(arrow)* and (D) resolution of the enhancement. Findings are consistent with demyelination.

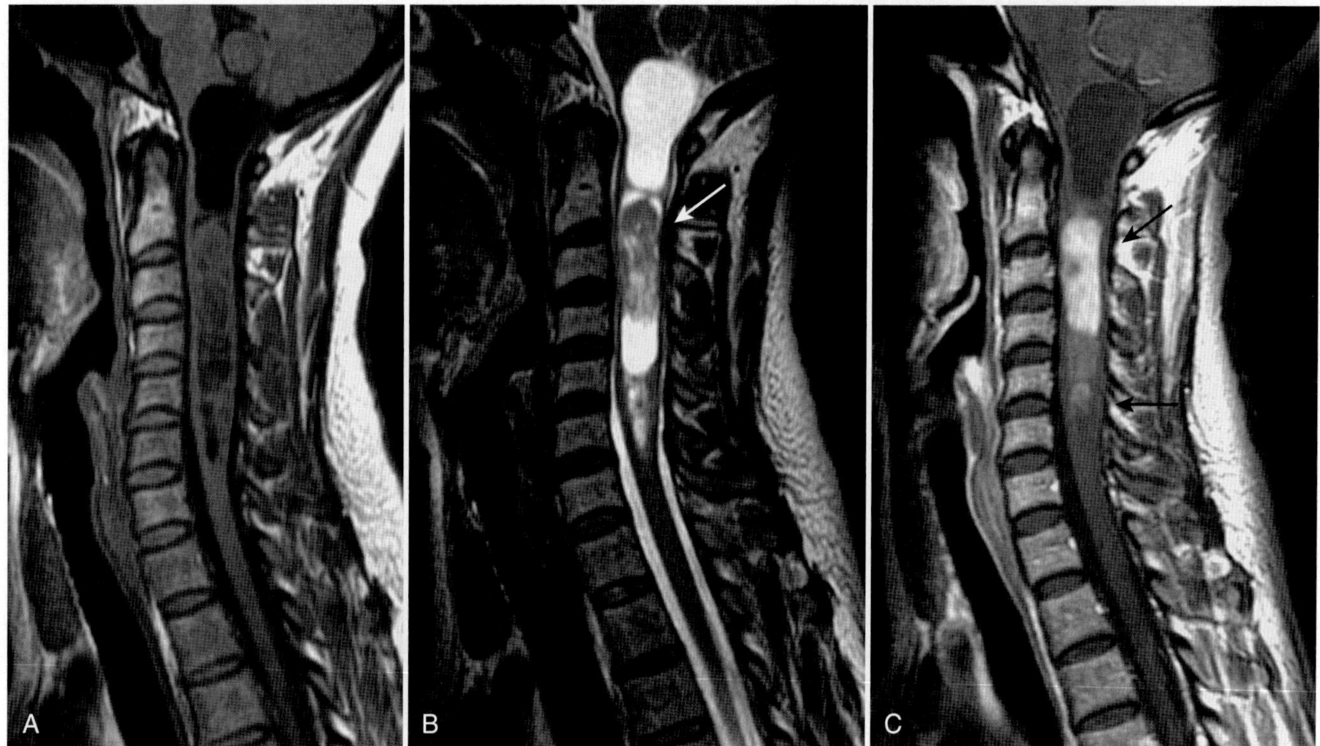

FIG. 13.29 Ependymoma. (A) Sagittal T1-weighted magnetic resonance image shows large cystic and solid intramedullary mass within the cervical cord. A tumor-associated cyst extends to the medulla. (B) Sagittal T2-weighted image shows central solid component *(arrow)* with cephalad and caudad cystic components. (C) Sagittal T1-weighted image after contrast administration shows large enhancing solid component extending down to C5–C6 *(black arrows)*.

improvements in brain and cord lesion burden with changes in clinical disability scoring. Most focal plaques are less than two vertebral body lengths in size, occupy less than half the cross-sectional diameter of the cord, and are characteristically peripherally located with respect to a transverse, cross-sectional reference. Of spinal cord multiple sclerosis lesions, 60% to 75% are present in the cervical region, and more than half of multiple sclerosis patients with cord plaques have multiple plaques. Of patients with cord plaques, 90% have intracranial multiple sclerosis plaques.[200,219,220]

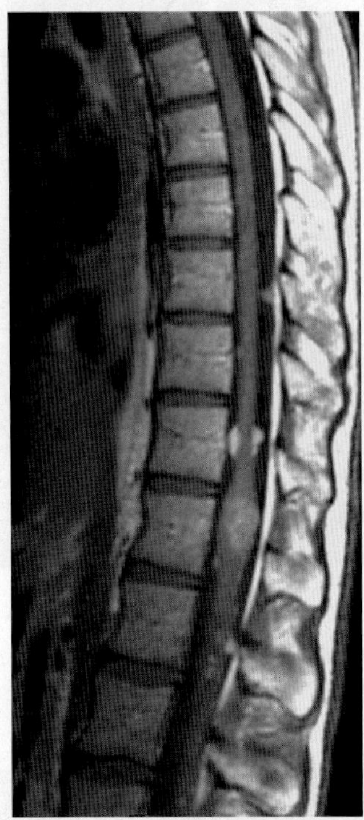

FIG. 13.30 Ependymoma in a patient with neurofibromatosis type 2. Sagittal T1-weighted magnetic resonance image after contrast administration shows multiple intradural extramedullary enhancing masses (schwannomas or meningiomas), combined with a less intensely enhancing mass within the conus (ependymoma).

Intradural Extramedullary Lesions

Intradural extramedullary neoplasms constitute the largest single group of primary spine neoplasms, accounting for approximately 55% of all primary spine tumors. Most of these tumors are benign, with *nerve sheath tumors* and *meningiomas* representing the most common lesions.[218] *Nerve sheath tumors* are the most common intraspinal tumors and are divided histologically into two types: *schwannomas* (i.e., neuromas, neurinomas, and neurilemmomas) and *neurofibromas* (Fig. 13.33). Solitary schwannomas constitute most intraspinal nerve sheath tumors, whereas neurofibromas are almost always associated with neurofibromatosis type 1. Patients with neurofibromatosis type 2 more commonly have multiple schwannomas rather than neurofibromas, however.[221] Isolated nerve sheath tumors can arise anywhere in the spine.[222]

Nerve sheath tumors are easily recognized on MRI as typically isolated, well-circumscribed, solid masses of soft tissue signal intensity on T1-weighted images surrounded by low signal CSF. On T2-weighted images, they are of variable signal intensity. Schwannomas are more vascular and include cystic degeneration, necrosis, and hemorrhage more commonly than neurofibromas. Various local osseous changes, consisting mainly of smooth bony remodeling or foraminal enlargement, are common. Enhancement is almost always present, but the pattern is variable.

Meningiomas most commonly occur in the thoracic spine.[223] As is the case intracranially, there is a female sex predilection, and these lesions occur in a slightly older age group than nerve sheath tumors. Most are entirely intradural and typically are isointense to the neural elements on T1- and

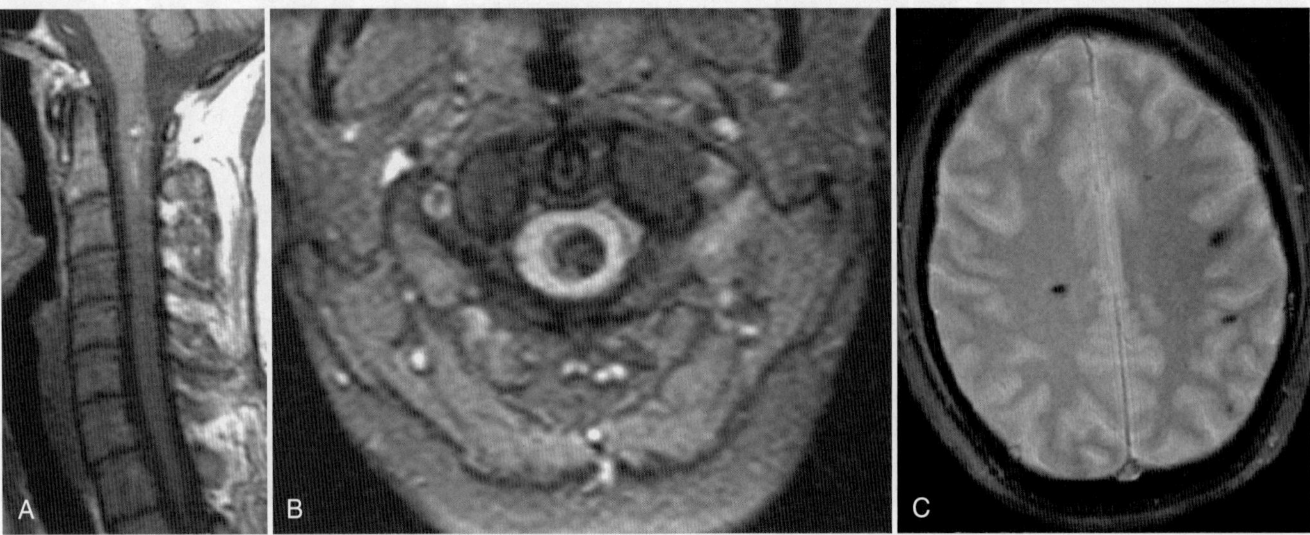

FIG. 13.31 Cavernous angioma. (A) Sagittal T1-weighted magnetic resonance image shows linear focus of high signal reflecting hemorrhage within the cord at C2 level. (B) Axial gradient-echo image confirms blood as focal low signal within substance of cord. (C) Axial gradient-echo image through the brain shows multiple areas of low signal *(dark spots)* reflecting hemosiderin deposition owing to multiple cavernous angiomas.

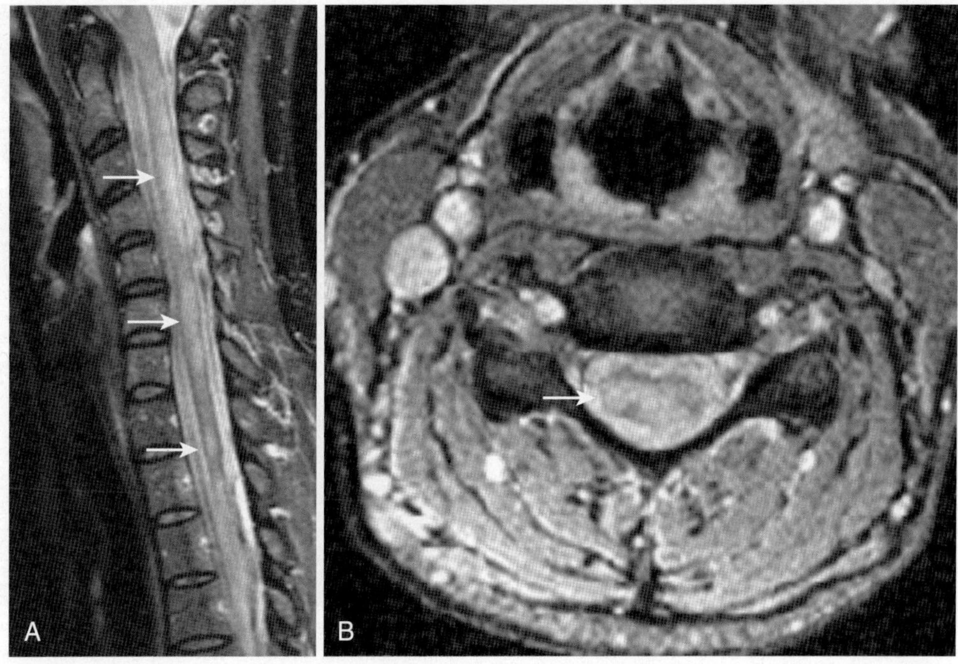

FIG. 13.32 Short-tau inversion recovery imaging for intramedullary inflammatory disease. (A) Sagittal and (B) axial images show multiple foci of abnormal increased signal throughout the cervical cord without expansion, reflecting demyelinating disease *(arrows)*.

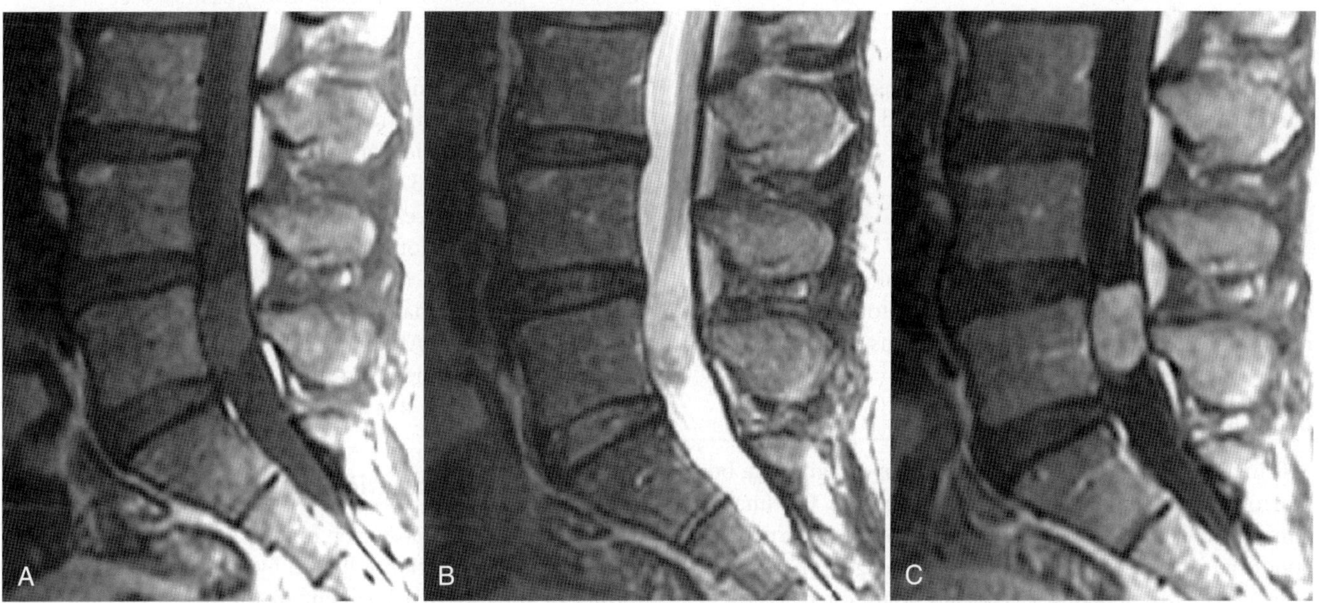

FIG. 13.33 Schwannoma. (A) Sagittal T1-weighted, (B) T2-weighted, and (C) T1-weighted enhanced magnetic resonance images show a round, intensely enhancing intradural mass at the L4 level, displacing the adjacent cauda equina.

T2-weighted images. Meningiomas enhance intensely after gadolinium–diethylenetetramine-pentaacetic acid (DTPA) administration, which may allow demonstration of the typical broad dural base.[224,225]

The last category of intradural extramedullary lesions is the so-called *leptomeningeal* pattern, which includes leptomeningeal metastatic disease, inflammation, and benign granulomatous processes such as sarcoid and tuberculosis (Fig. 13.34).[226] The list of tumors that may seed the CSF is long, but the most common types are cranial ependymomas, glioblastomas, and medulloblastomas (especially in pediatric patients). Additional malignancies that can spread less commonly are ependymoma, pineoblastoma, germinoma, and retinoblastoma. Lesions outside the central nervous system that are capable of spreading along the leptomeninges include carcinoma of the lung and breast, lymphoma, leukemia, and melanoma. Administration of contrast material with T1-weighted images is mandatory and shows a linear and nodular enhancement pattern along the leptomeninges. The overall sensitivity of MRI examinations is low in patients with

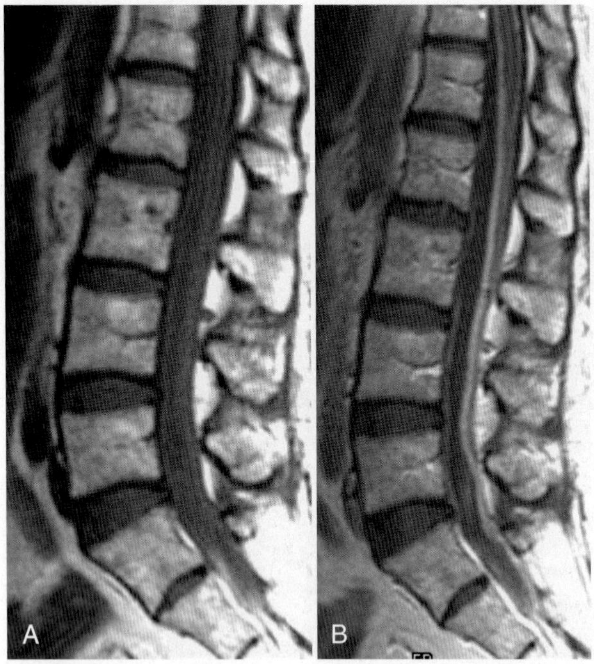

FIG. 13.34 Leptomeningeal enhancement. Sagittal T1-weighted magnetic resonance images (A) before and (B) after contrast administration show extensive leptomeningeal enhancement of cauda equina and distal cord surface in a patient with *Staphylococcus aureus* meningitis.

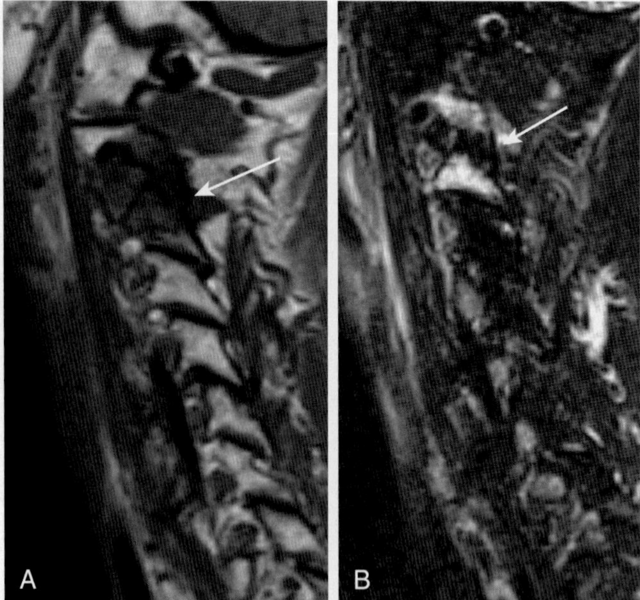

FIG. 13.35 In general, most pathologic marrow (neoplastic, degenerative, or infectious) demonstrates water signal intensity. However, distribution of the signal abnormality can be helpful in arriving at a differential diagnosis. (A) Sagittal T1-weighted image and (B) sagittal short-tau inversion recovery (STIR) image demonstrates abnormal low T1 signal intensity and STIR hyperintensity centered about the C2–C3 facet joint *(arrow)*, which is degenerative or inflammatory in nature rather than neoplastic.

proven histologic evidence of neoplastic seeding, so examination of the CSF remains the gold standard.

Extradural Lesions

Pathology that can involve the extradural space can include degenerative disc disease, epidural hematoma or abscess, or neoplasm extending from adjacent osseous structures.[227]

Bone Marrow Imaging

MR imaging is the preferred modality for imaging the bone marrow when compared with radiographs or CT imaging, although CT imaging can demonstrate osseous destruction or abnormal increased attenuation. Pathologic or abnormal marrow on MR imaging is typically manifested as low T1 signal intensity and T2 or STIR hyperintensity. Distribution of the marrow abnormalities is helpful, as abnormal marrow centered about a joint or articulating surface can be degenerative or inflammatory in nature rather than neoplastic (Fig. 13.35). Complete marrow replacement by low T1 signal intensity can be seen with both metastatic disease and red marrow replacement in patients with anemia.[228] CT imaging can demonstrate the matrix of a lesion (increased attenuation when osteogenic, ground glass for fibrous lesions, or anular calcifications in cartilaginous lesions). Lesions with sclerotic borders tend to be less aggressive compared with lesions with ill-defined or poor margins.[229]

Primary and secondary tumors to the extradural space are well evaluated by MRI and CT (Fig. 13.36). *Metastatic disease* to the spine is the most common type of extradural tumor. Because of its high contrast sensitivity and spatial resolution, MRI is the examination of choice in the detection of osseous metastases (Figs. 13.37 and 13.38).[230,231] Because many metastatic tumors enhance, the routine use of contrast medium–enhanced studies alone is not recommended because the distinction between metastases and normal marrow fat is diminished, occasionally to the point of masking even large lesions (Fig. 13.39). Although diffuse osseous metastases can appear as homogeneous, diffuse, low marrow signal on T1-weighted images, this appearance is not specific.

Ossification of Posterior Longitudinal Ligament

Ossification of the posterior longitudinal ligament (OPLL) begins with calcification followed by frank ossification of the posterior longitudinal ligament in the upper cervical spine (C3–C4 or C4–C5). It may progress inferiorly to the upper thoracic spine (Figs. 13.40 and 13.41).[232] Patients tend to present in the sixth decade of life, are generally older than typical patients with disc disease, and are younger than patients with cervical spondylosis. Presenting complaints include neck pain, dysesthesias, and upper and lower extremity weakness. CT findings often show the bony pathology better than MRI. Hirabayashi and Satomi[233] divided OPLL into four types based on CT: (1) *continuous* OPLL extends between vertebral bodies and crosses multiple disc spaces (27% of cases), (2) *segmental* OPLL is limited to the posterior vertebral body margins (39% of cases), (3) *mixed* OPLL is continuous and segmental (29% of cases), and (4) the remaining 5% of OPLL is restricted to the disc space level.

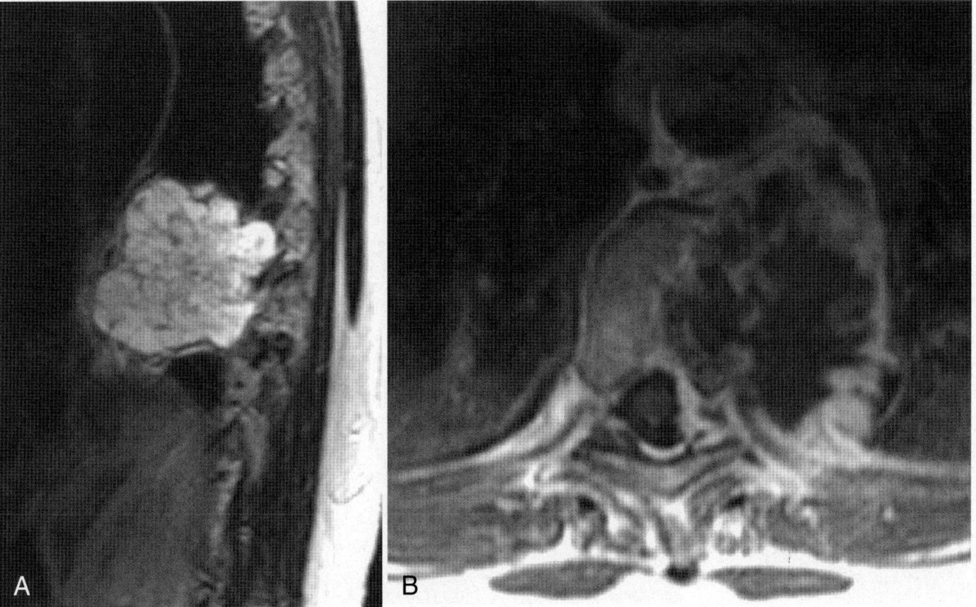

FIG. 13.36 Chondroblastic osteosarcoma. (A) Sagittal T2-weighted magnetic resonance image shows large paraspinal mass with well-defined margins and heterogeneous internal signal typical of cartilaginous lesions, including chordoma. (B) Axial T1-weighted image after contrast administration shows a large, irregularly enhancing mass involving the left lateral aspect of the thoracic body with extension into the paravertebral region. There is left lateral epidural extension of tumor with mild mass effect on the cord.

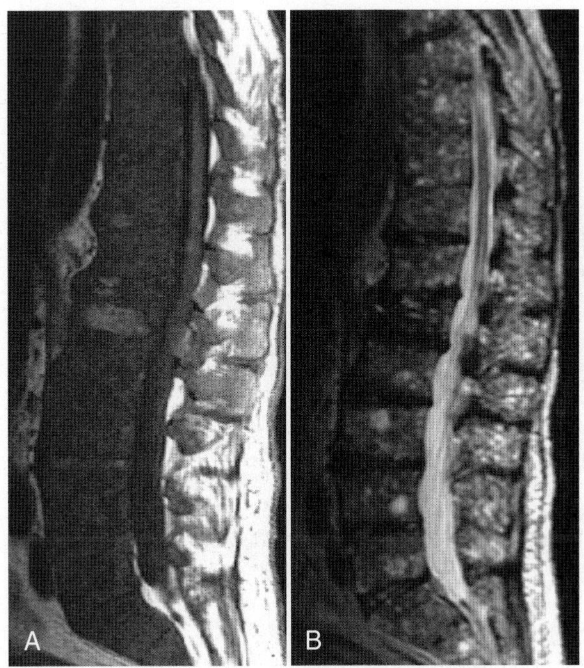

FIG. 13.37 Multiple myeloma. (A) Sagittal T1-weighted magnetic resonance image shows markedly diminished signal from all the visualized marrow of thoracolumbar spine. There is severe compression deformity at L1. (B) Sagittal T2-weighted image shows typical "salt and pepper" pattern of multiple myeloma. No epidural tumor is identified.

Circumferential compression of the cord may result from combined OPLL and ossification of the ligamentum flavum. In continuous OPLL, MRI shows a thick band of decreased signal on T1- and T2-weighted images. The segmental type is more difficult to discern on MRI and shows a thin area of decreased signal intensity, without signal from within the ossification region.

Spinal Cysts

Various investigators,[234-236] including Nabors and colleagues,[235] have clarified the confusing array of terms for spinal meningeal cysts. *Spinal meningeal cysts* are congenital diverticula of the dural sac, root sheaths, or arachnoid that may be classified into three major groups. The first group includes extradural cysts without spinal nerve roots (type I), the second includes extradural cysts with spinal nerve roots (type II), and the third includes intradural cysts (type III) (Fig. 13.42). Type I are diverticula that maintain contact with the thecal sac by a narrow ostium. Type I cysts include extradural cysts, pouches, and diverticula and the so-called *occult intrasacral meningoceles*. Sacral type I cysts are found in adults and are connected to the tip of the caudal thecal sac by a pedicle. Type II meningeal cysts with contained nerve roots are extradural lesions previously called *Tarlov cysts, perineural cysts,* or *nerve root diverticula*. These are generally seen as multiple incidental lesions but are occasionally associated with radiculopathy or incontinence. Type III meningeal cysts are intradural lesions most commonly found on the posterior subarachnoid space and have been called *arachnoid diverticula* or *arachnoid cysts*. These are lined by a single layer of normal arachnoid cells and filled with CSF.

Trauma

Studies have shown that if strict criteria are followed, patients who arrive at the emergency department with a collar in place can be clinically evaluated as to whether plain films are required.[237,238] Patients with cervical fractures typically have

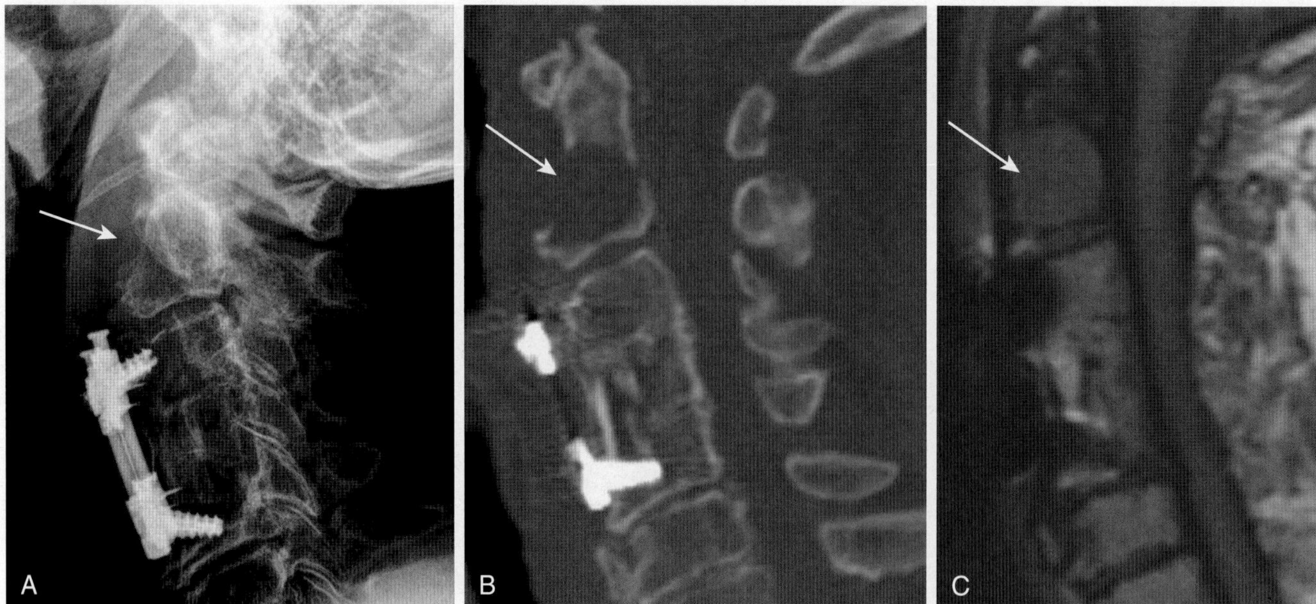

FIG. 13.38 Metastatic disease. (A) Lateral radiograph of the cervical spine demonstrates subtle cortical irregularity *(arrow)*, which is much more apparent on (B) computed tomographic and (C) magnetic resonance imaging *(arrows)*.

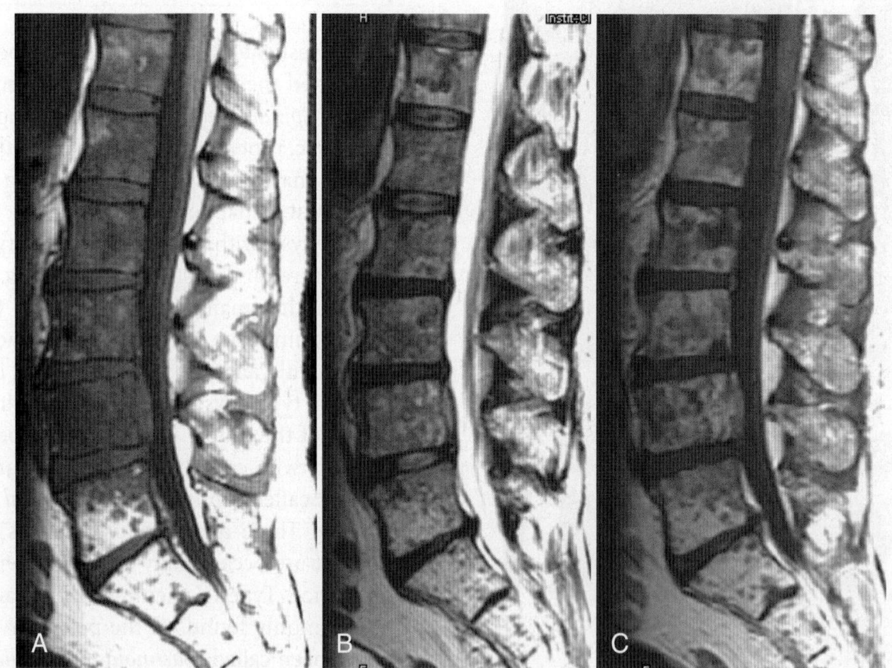

FIG. 13.39 Diffuse metastatic disease. (A) Sagittal T1-weighted magnetic resonance image shows diffuse abnormal decreased marrow signal from L4 through L1 bodies. There is residual fatty marrow replacement involving L5 and the sacrum from prior radiation therapy. There is mild anterior epidural extension of tumor at L4. (B) T2-weighted image shows mass effect of epidural tumor but tends to minimize marrow signal abnormality. (C) After contrast material is administered, T1-weighted image shows less marrow abnormality owing to enhancing tumor mimicking fatty marrow signal.

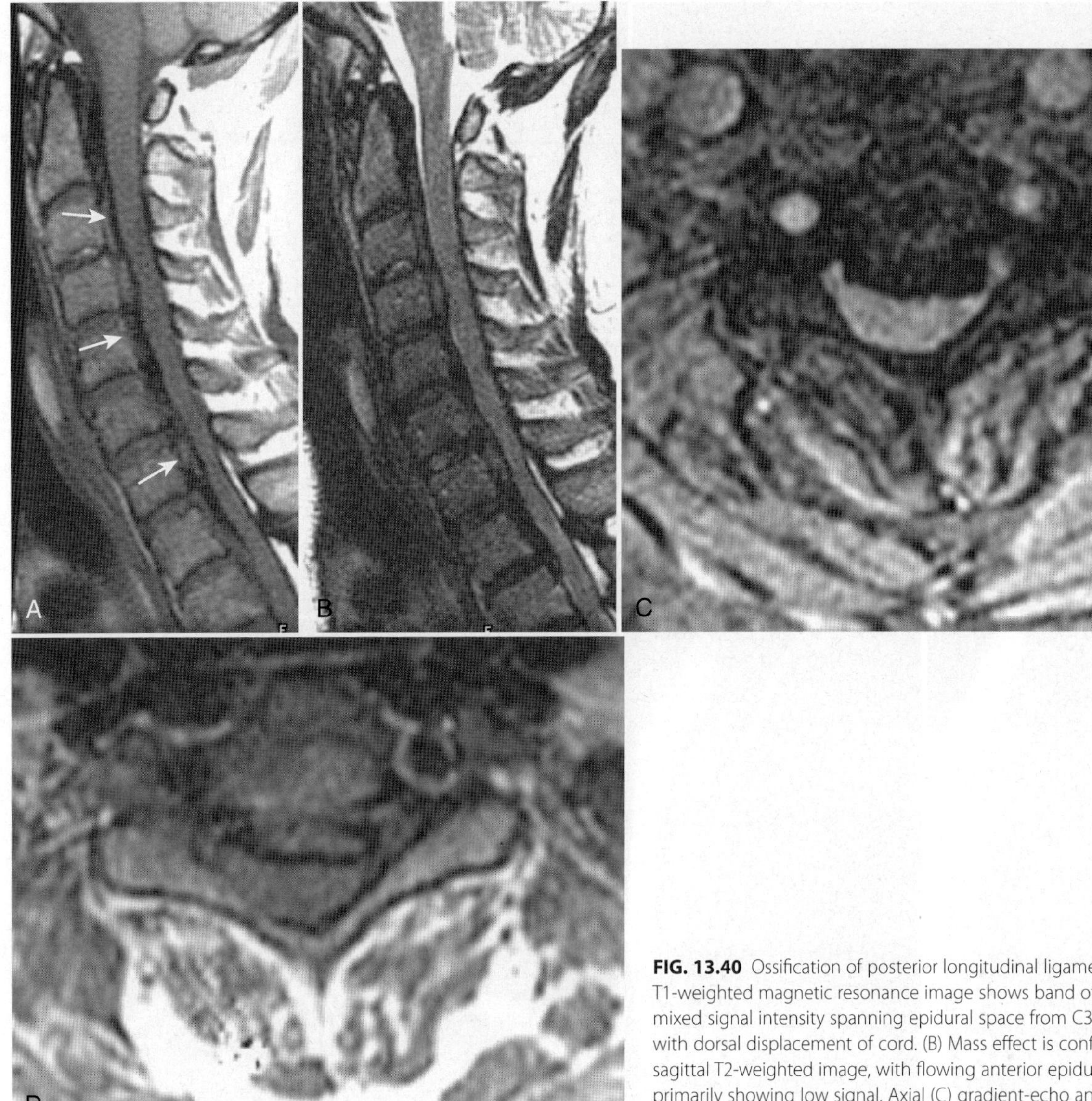

FIG. 13.40 Ossification of posterior longitudinal ligament. (A) Sagittal T1-weighted magnetic resonance image shows band of abnormal mixed signal intensity spanning epidural space from C3–T1 *(arrows)*, with dorsal displacement of cord. (B) Mass effect is confirmed on sagittal T2-weighted image, with flowing anterior epidural mass primarily showing low signal. Axial (C) gradient-echo and (D) T1-weighted images show mass severely effacing cord.

at least one of the following: intoxication, neck tenderness, altered level of consciousness, or a painful injury elsewhere. Indications for CT in evaluation of the cervical spine include further evaluation of known or questionable fracture on plain films and evaluation of areas inadequately seen on plain films.[239,240] Techniques vary from institution to institution, but slice thickness is generally 1.5 to 2 mm, sagittal and coronal reformats, soft tissue and bone windows, with no intravenous contrast material. The sensitivity of CT to detect fracture is 78% to 100%.[241,242] CT is particularly useful in diagnosing posterior element (laminar) fractures. The use of spiral thin-section techniques (1 to 1.5 mm) with multiplanar reformats should enable sensitivity approaching 100%. Most institutions use CT as the primary screening study in patients with multiple areas of trauma, bypassing plain films.[243,244] When imaging the cervical spine with radiographs, the average time to complete the examination approaches 22 minutes as opposed to an average time of 12 minutes with CT imaging.[245,246] Plain films with flexion and extension can be of use in defining instability in patients with persistent pain or soft tissue swelling without a definite fracture on the initial plain film evaluation.

MRI allows direct visualization of cord abnormalities, which cannot be identified by any other imaging modality. MRI can define intramedullary hematoma, intramedullary edema and contusion, disc herniations, ligamentous injury, and epidural hemorrhage (Fig. 13.43).[247-250] Hemorrhage within the first week is seen as low signal on T2-weighted images related to deoxyhemoglobin. Contusion without hemorrhage is identified as high signal on T2-weighted images and as isointense or decreased signal on T1-weighted images. Ligamentous disruption is seen as loss of the usual low signal from the anterior and posterior longitudinal ligaments, with increased signal on T2-weighted images in the adjacent tissues.[251,252]

The most common area of traumatic involvement in the lumbar spine is the thoracolumbar junction, which acts as a fulcrum for spine motion and is susceptible to unstable

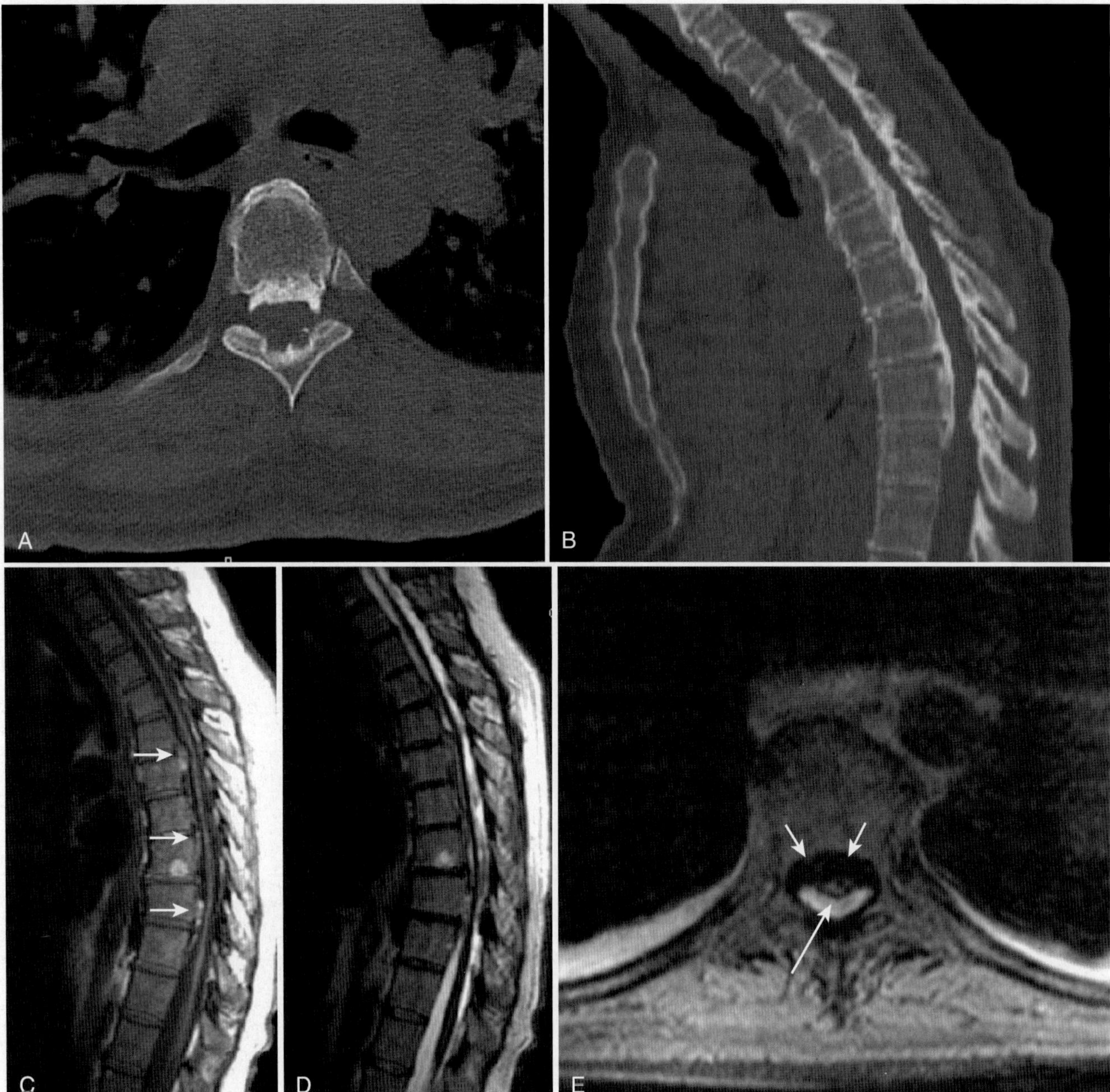

FIG. 13.41 Thoracic ossification of posterior longitudinal ligament. (A) Axial computed tomographic (CT) scan and (B) sagittal reformat show large flowing bony mass encompassing the anterior epidural space throughout the mid-thoracic spine. Sagittal (C) T1-weighted and (D) T2-weighted magnetic resonance (MR) images are more difficult to interpret without CT guidance because the heterogeneous anterior epidural signal could reflect blood or fatty marrow (*arrows*). MR images do show the degree of mass effect on the thecal sac and cord. (E) On axial gradient-echo image, the cord is atrophic and there is diffuse hemosiderosis of the cord surface seen as linear low signal *(long arrow)*, with ossification of the posterior longitudinal ligament mass of very low signal within anterior epidural space *(short arrows)*. There are small bilateral pleural effusions.

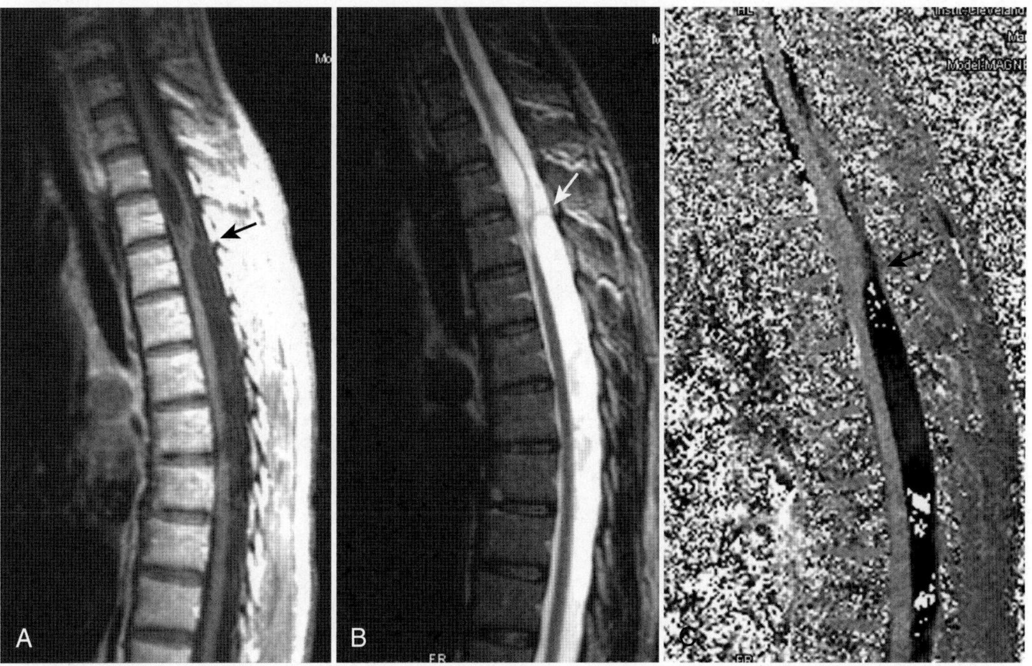

FIG. 13.42 Arachnoid cyst and syrinx. (A) Sagittal T1-weighted magnetic resonance image through the thoracic spine shows a ventrally displaced cord with abruptly expanding dorsal margin at T4 level *(arrow)*, with a small syrinx seen as linear low signal within the cord. (B) Sagittal T2-weighted image shows a thin line of low signal at the cephalad margin of the dorsally expanded cerebrospinal fluid (CSF) space *(arrow)* with a "windsock" pattern reflecting an arachnoid cyst margin. (C) Single sagittal image from a cine CSF flow series is encoded to show upward motion as dark areas. This technique outlines the abrupt change in CSF flow pattern at the top of the cyst *(arrow)*.

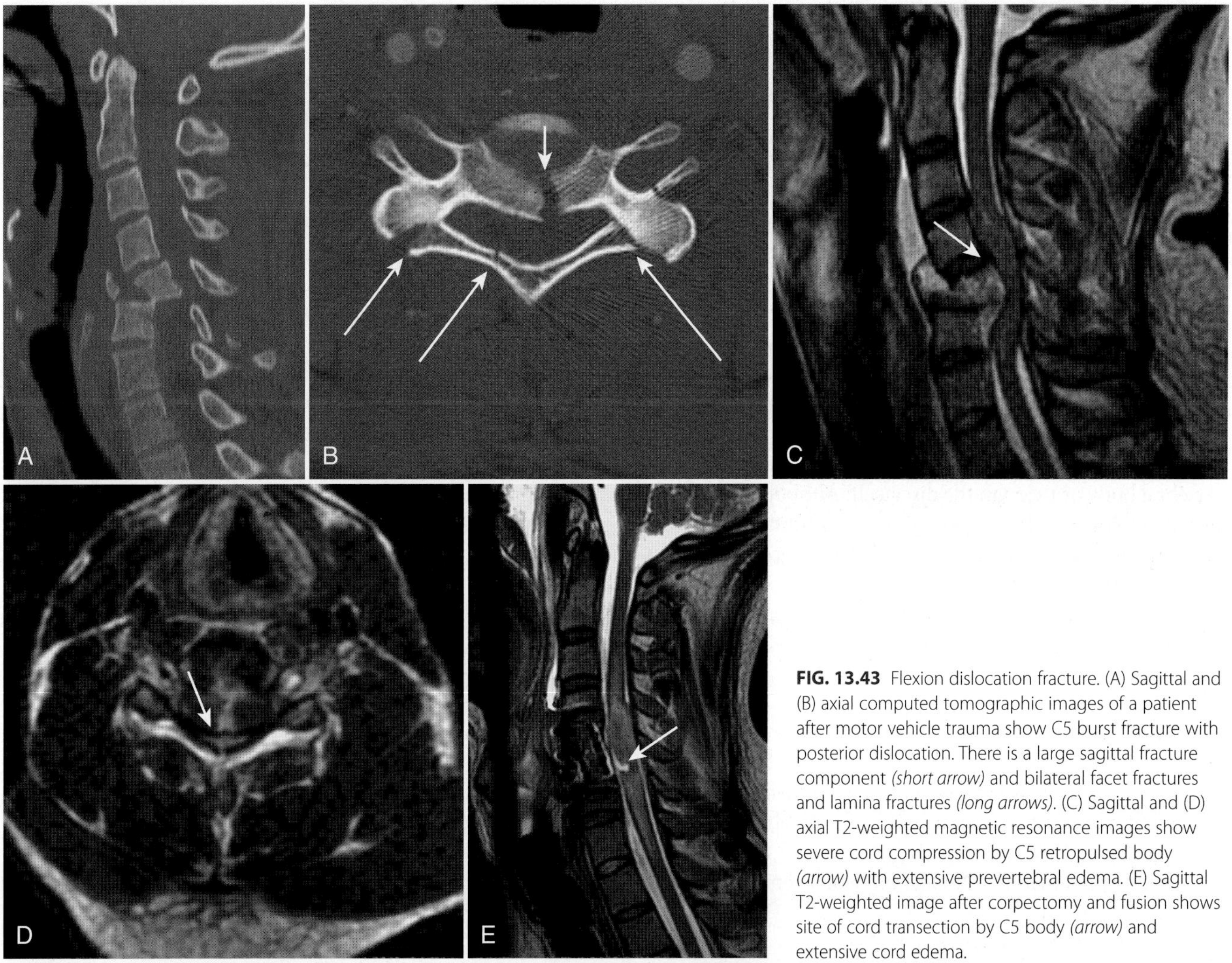

FIG. 13.43 Flexion dislocation fracture. (A) Sagittal and (B) axial computed tomographic images of a patient after motor vehicle trauma show C5 burst fracture with posterior dislocation. There is a large sagittal fracture component *(short arrow)* and bilateral facet fractures and lamina fractures *(long arrows)*. (C) Sagittal and (D) axial T2-weighted magnetic resonance images show severe cord compression by C5 retropulsed body *(arrow)* with extensive prevertebral edema. (E) Sagittal T2-weighted image after corpectomy and fusion shows site of cord transection by C5 body *(arrow)* and extensive cord edema.

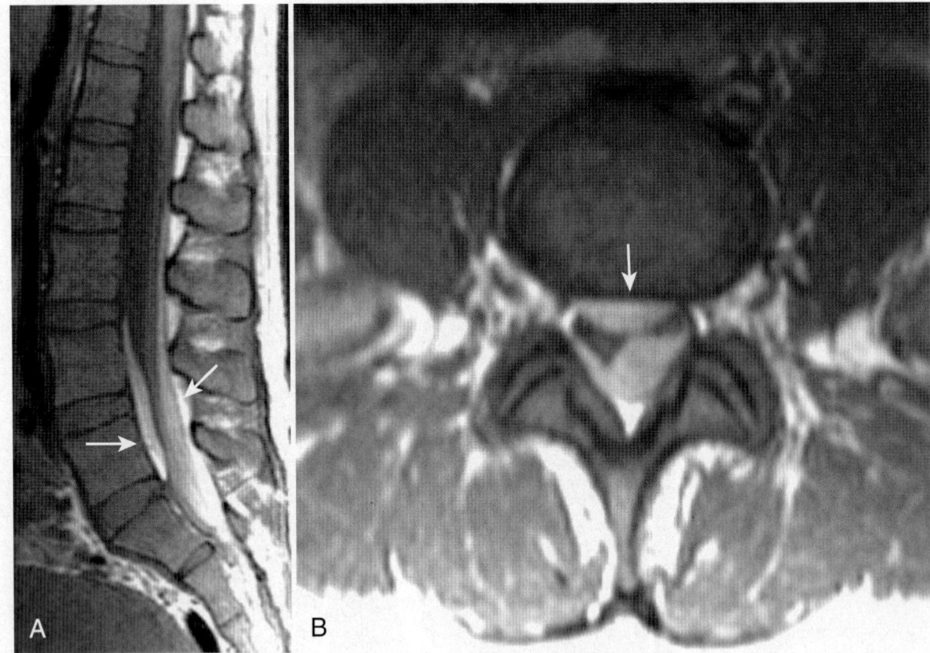

FIG. 13.44 Subdural hemorrhage. (A) Sagittal and (B) axial T1-weighted magnetic resonance images show high signal blood along dural margin from L3 to S1 *(arrows)*. Axial image shows that the exterior margin of blood is delimited by dura, so it must be either subarachnoid or subdural in location. Loculation on the axial view is typical for a subdural location.

traumatic injury. The thick, sagittally oriented lumbar facets minimize rotational injury, but flexion and axial loading injuries often occur. The forces may combine to produce flexion-compression injuries or the so-called *burst fracture*. Burst fractures are notable for instability and a predisposition for displacing fracture fragments posteriorly and causing spinal cord compression.[253,254] CT remains the method of choice for the detection of retropulsed bony fragments and for the demonstration of fractures of the posterior elements.[255] In trauma patients when CT imaging of the chest, abdomen, and pelvis is obtained, the existing image data set can be processed to evaluate the spine, negating the need for additional image acquisition and resultant radiation exposure.[256]

A hyperflexion injury occurring in the lumbar spine is the seat belt or Chance fracture, which is associated with rapid deceleration motor vehicle accidents. This type of trauma produces a horizontal fracture through anterior and posterior elements.[257,258] The anterior component may be through the vertebral body or through the disc itself. Although CT is more sensitive than MRI for detecting bony abnormalities, MRI is often superior for evaluating soft tissue structures. In particular, the spinal ligaments show focal discontinuity on T1-weighted images and areas of increased signal intensity on T2-weighted images.

Hemorrhage

Epidural spinal hematomas occur most frequently in elderly adults but can occur at any age.[259-261] Epidural spinal hematomas are broadly classified into two groups: nonspontaneous and spontaneous. Nonspontaneous epidural spinal hematomas may result from spinal taps, spinal anesthesia, trauma, pregnancy, bleeding diathesis, anticoagulant therapy, spinal hemangiomas, vascular malformations, hypertension, and neoplasms. The history can often be revealing, yet these tumors commonly occur merely from an episode of sneezing, bending, voiding, turning in bed, or other mild trauma. Epidural spinal hematomas can be localized or can spread anywhere along the spinal column. Blood more commonly accumulates posterolaterally.

Subdural hemorrhage is capable of producing severe and irreversible neurologic deficits, and acute surgical intervention may be needed. Spinal subdural hematomas can have a typical configuration (Fig. 13.44A).[262,263] As opposed to epi dural hematomas, which tend to be capped by fat, subdural hematomas are located within the thecal sac and are separate from the adjacent extradural fat, the vertebral bodies, and the posterior elements. Axial images are useful in defining the epidural fat surrounding the thecal sac as well as the blood relating to the interior of the sac with subdural hematomas. These may be loculated anteriorly and posteriorly within the thecal sac. The loculation can take the form of a "Mercedes Benz sign," showing a trefoil configuration (Fig. 13.44B).

KEY POINTS

1. Metal artifact on MRI can be reduced with use of FSE, larger fields of view, higher readout bandwidths, smaller voxel sizes, and appropriate geometric orientation of the frequency-encoded direction in relationship to the metal.
2. The most common spinal vascular lesion is the dural fistula, and the most sensitive MRI finding is increased signal on T2-weighted images within the cord.

3. The most critical imaging information regarding spinal neoplasms used in forming a differential diagnosis involves determining whether the lesion is intramedullary, intradural extramedullary, or extradural.
4. CT remains the method of choice for detecting retropulsed bony fragments and for showing fractures of the posterior elements.
5. MRI is useful in the immediate postoperative period for evaluating fluid collections including hemorrhage and for showing mass effect on the thecal sac, cord, and cauda equina but not for defining residual disc material.
6. Paravertebral enhancement on fat-suppressed axial T1-weighted images is very helpful in defining early disc space infection.
7. The apparent size of neural foramina on axial gradient MR images is critically dependent on the sequence echo time; longer echo times give susceptibility artifact, which may give the false appearance of stenosis.
8. Synovial cysts are very difficult to identify on T1-weighted images and require T2-weighted images or intravenous contrast medium enhancement, or both, for definition.
9. Early disc space infection and degenerative disc disease with type 1 endplate change can be indistinguishable by MRI alone.
10. Acute spinal hemorrhage may show no characteristics of "blood" on MRI owing to the lack of susceptibility effect of oxyhemoglobin.
11. OPLL may be missed on T1-weighted images by merging into the low signal of CSF.
12. Use of contrast medium may mask spinal bony metastatic disease by causing the enhancing tumor signal to match that of adjacent normal fatty marrow.

KEY REFERENCES

1. Fardon DF, Milette PC. Nomenclature and classification of lumbar disc pathology: recommendations of the combined task forces of the North American Spine Society, American Society of Spine Radiology, and American Society of Neuroradiology. *Spine.* 2001;26:E93-E113.
   This is a must-read for standardization of this Tower of Babel.
2. Mehta RC, Marks MP, Hinks RS, et al. MR evaluation of vertebral metastases: T1-weighted, short-inversion-time inversion recovery, fast spin-echo, and inversion-recovery fast spin-echo sequences. *AJNR Am J Neuroradiol.* 1995;16:281-288.
   T1-weighted images, FSE, and fat-saturated FSE are superior for detecting epidural metastatic disease.
3. Modic MT, Feiglin DH, Piraino DW, et al. Vertebral osteomyelitis: assessment using MR. *Radiology.* 1985;157:157-166.
   This classic definition of MRI changes still applies today.
4. Nabors MW, Pait TG, Byrd EB, et al. Updated assessment and current classification of spinal meningeal cysts. *J Neurosurg.* 1988;68:366-377.
   A cogent classification of a confusing area is presented.
5. Russell EJ. Cervical disk disease. *Radiology.* 1990;177:313-325.
   The author provides an excellent summary of a broad subject.

REFERENCES

1. Bushberg JT. *The Essential Physics of Medical Imaging.* 3rd ed. Philadelphia: Lippincott Williams & Wilkins; 2012.
2. Bontrager KL, Lampignano JP, Bontrager KL. *Bontrager's Handbook of Radiographic Positioning and Techniques.* 7th ed. Philadelphia: Elsevier; 2010.
3. Slone RM, McEnery KW, Bridwell KH, Montgomery WJ. Principles and imaging of spinal instrumentation. *Radiol Clin North Am.* 1995;33(2):189-211.
4. Hanley SD, Gun MT, Osti O, Shanahan EM. Radiology of intervertebral cages in spinal surgery. *Clin Radiol.* 1999;54(4):201-206.
5. Bell GRMM. *Radiology of the Lumbar Spine.* 3rd ed. Philadelphia: WB Saunders; 1992.
6. Jacobeus HC. On insufflation of air into the spinal canal for diagnostic purposes in cases of the spinal cord. *Acta Med Scand.* 1921;21:555-560.
7. Modic MT, Ross JS, Masaryk TJ. Imaging of degenerative disease of the cervical spine. *Clin Orthop Relat Res.* 1989;239: 109-120.
8. Olsen NK, Madsen HH, Eriksen FB, Svare U, Zeeberg I. Intracranial iohexol-distribution following cervical myelography, postmyelographic registration of adverse effects, psychometric assessment and electroencephalographic recording. *Acta Neurol Scand.* 1990;82(5):321-328.
9. Layton KF, Kallmes DF, Horlocker TT. Recommendations for anticoagulated patients undergoing image-guided spinal procedures. *AJNR Am J Neuroradiol.* 2006;27(3):468-470.
10. Sandow BA, Donnal JF. Myelography complications and current practice patterns. *AJR Am J Roentgenol.* 2005;185(3): 768-771.
11. Jahnke RW, Hart BL. Cervical stenosis, spondylosis, and herniated disc disease. *Radiol Clin North Am.* 1991;29(4): 777-791.
12. Landman JA, Hoffman JC Jr, Braun IF, Barrow DL. Value of computed tomographic myelography in the recognition of cervical herniated disk. *AJNR Am J Neuroradiol.* 1984;5(4):391-394.
13. Simon JE, Lukin RR. Diskogenic disease of the cervical spine. *Semin Roentgenol.* 1988;23(2):118-124.
14. Nakagawa H, Okumura T, Sugiyama T, Iwata K. Discrepancy between metrizamide CT and myelography in diagnosis of cervical disk protrusions. *AJNR Am J Neuroradiol.* 1983;4(3): 604-606.
15. Sobel DF, Barkovich AJ, Munderloh SH. Metrizamide myelography and postmyelographic computed tomography: comparative adequacy in the cervical spine. *AJNR Am J Neuroradiol.* 1984;5(4):385-390.
16. Vassilouthis J, Kalovithouris A, Papandreou A, Tegos S. The symptomatic incompetent cervical intervertebral disc. *Neurosurgery.* 1989;25(2):232-239.
17. Dorwart RH, LaMasters DL. Applications of computed tomographic scanning of the cervical spine. *Orthop Clin North Am.* 1985;16(3):381-393.
18. Edelman RR, Shoukimas GM, Stark DD, et al. High-resolution surface-coil imaging of lumbar disk disease. *AJR Am J Roentgenol.* 1985;144(6):1123-1129.
19. Hoeffner EG, Mukherji SK, Srinivasan A, Quint DJ. Neuroradiology back to the future: spine imaging. *AJNR Am J Neuroradiol.* 2012;33(6):999-1006.
20. Modic MT, Pavlicek W, Weinstein MA, et al. Magnetic resonance imaging of intervertebral disk disease. Clinical and pulse sequence considerations. *Radiology.* 1984;152(1):103-111.
21. Norman D, Mills CM, Brant-Zawadzki M, et al. Magnetic resonance imaging of the spinal cord and canal: potentials and limitations. *AJR Am J Roentgenol.* 1983;141(6): 1147-1152.
22. Filippi M, Yousry T, Baratti C, et al. Quantitative assessment of MRI lesion load in multiple sclerosis. A comparison of conventional spin-echo with fast fluid-attenuated inversion recovery. *Brain.* 1996;119(Pt 4):1349-1355.

23. Finelli DA, Hurst GC, Karaman BA, et al. Use of magnetization transfer for improved contrast on gradient-echo MR images of the cervical spine. *Radiology*. 1994;193(1): 165-171.
24. Kidd D, Thorpe JW, Thompson AJ, et al. Spinal cord MRI using multi-array coils and fast spin echo. II. Findings in multiple sclerosis. *Neurology*. 1993;43(12):2632-2637.
25. Lycklama a Nijeholt GJ, Barkhof F, Castelijns JA, et al. Comparison of two MR sequences for the detection of multiple sclerosis lesions in the spinal cord. *AJNR Am J Neuroradiol*. 1996;17(8):1533-1538.
26. Rocca MA, Mastronardo G, Horsfield MA, et al. Comparison of three MR sequences for the detection of cervical cord lesions in patients with multiple sclerosis. *AJNR Am J Neuroradiol*. 1999;20(9):1710-1716.
27. Ross JS, Ruggieri P, Tkach J, et al. Lumbar degenerative disk disease: prospective comparison of conventional T2-weighted spin-echo imaging and T2-weighted rapid acquisition relaxation-enhanced imaging. *AJNR Am J Neuroradiol*. 1993;14(5):1215-1223.
28. Sze G, Kawamura Y, Negishi C, et al. Fast spin-echo MR imaging of the cervical spine: influence of echo train length and echo spacing on image contrast and quality. *AJNR Am J Neuroradiol*. 1993;14(5):1203-1213.
29. Tartaglino LM, Friedman DP, Flanders AE, et al. Multiple sclerosis in the spinal cord: MR appearance and correlation with clinical parameters. *Radiology*. 1995;195(3):725-732.
30. Thorpe JW, Halpin SF, MacManus DG, et al. A comparison between fast and conventional spin-echo in the detection of multiple sclerosis lesions. *Neuroradiology*. 1994;36(5):388-392.
31. Dwyer AJ, Frank JA, Sank VJ, et al. Short-tau inversion-recovery pulse sequence: analysis and initial experience in cancer imaging. *Radiology*. 1988;168(3):827-836.
32. Mehta RC, Marks MP, Hinks RS, Glover GH, Enzmann DR. MR evaluation of vertebral metastases: T1-weighted, short-inversion-time inversion recovery, fast spin-echo, and inversion-recovery fast spin-echo sequences. *AJNR Am J Neuroradiol*. 1995;16(2):281-288.
33. Weinberger E, Shaw DW, White KS, et al. Nontraumatic pediatric musculoskeletal MR imaging: comparison of conventional and fast-spin-echo short inversion time inversion-recovery technique. *Radiology*. 1995;194(3):721-726.
34. Baker LL, Goodman SB, Perkash I, Lane B, Enzmann DR. Benign versus pathologic compression fractures of vertebral bodies: assessment with conventional spin-echo, chemical-shift, and STIR MR imaging. *Radiology*. 1990;174(2): 495-502.
35. Hilfiker P, Zanetti M, Debatin JF, McKinnon G, Hodler J. Fast spin-echo inversion-recovery imaging versus fast T2-weighted spin-echo imaging in bone marrow abnormalities. *Invest Radiol*. 1995;30(2):110-114.
36. Jones KM, Schwartz RB, Mantello MT, et al. Fast spin-echo MR in the detection of vertebral metastases: comparison of three sequences. *AJNR Am J Neuroradiol*. 1994;15(3):401-407.
37. Danielson B, Willen J. Axially loaded magnetic resonance image of the lumbar spine in asymptomatic individuals. *Spine*. 2001;26(23):2601-2606.
38. Fujiwara A, An HS, Lim TH, Haughton VM. Morphologic changes in the lumbar intervertebral foramen due to flexion-extension, lateral bending, and axial rotation: an in vitro anatomic and biomechanical study. *Spine*. 2001;26(8):876-882.
39. Kitagawa T, Fujiwara A, Kobayashi N, et al. Morphologic changes in the cervical neural foramen due to flexion and extension: in vivo imaging study. *Spine*. 2004;29(24): 2821-2825.
40. Schmid MR, Stucki G, Duewell S, et al. Changes in cross-sectional measurements of the spinal canal and intervertebral foramina as a function of body position: in vivo studies on an open-configuration MR system. *AJR Am J Roentgenol*. 1999;172(4):1095-1102.
41. Kanno H, Endo T, Ozawa H, et al. Axial loading during magnetic resonance imaging in patients with lumbar spinal canal stenosis: does it reproduce the positional change of the dural sac detected by upright myelography? *Spine*. 2012;37(16):E985-E992.
42. Hiwatashi A, Danielson B, Moritani T, et al. Axial loading during MR imaging can influence treatment decision for symptomatic spinal stenosis. *AJNR Am J Neuroradiol*. 2004;25(2):170-174.
43. Algin O, Turkbey B. Intrathecal gadolinium-enhanced MR cisternography: a comprehensive review. *AJNR Am J Neuroradiol*. 2013;34(1):14-22.
44. Albayram S, Kilic F, Ozer H, et al. Gadolinium-enhanced MR cisternography to evaluate dural leaks in intracranial hypotension syndrome. *AJNR Am J Neuroradiol*. 2008;29(1): 116-121.
45. Algin O, Taskapilioglu O, Zan E, Hakyemez B, Karaoglanoglu M. Detection of CSF leaks with magnetic resonance imaging in intracranial hypotension syndrome. *J Neuroradiol*. 2011; 38(3):175-177.
46. Mokri B. Spontaneous cerebrospinal fluid leaks: from intracranial hypotension to cerebrospinal fluid hypovolemia—evolution of a concept. *Mayo Clin Proc*. 1999;74(11):1113-1123.
47. Chazen JL, Talbott JF, Lantos JE, Dillon WP. MR myelography for identification of spinal CSF leak in spontaneous intracranial hypotension. *AJNR Am J Neuroradiol*. 2014;35(10):2007-2012.
48. Yoo HM, Kim SJ, Choi CG, et al. Detection of CSF leak in spinal CSF leak syndrome using MR myelography: correlation with radioisotope cisternography. *AJNR Am J Neuroradiol*. 2008;29(4):649-654.
49. Chhabra A, Andreisek G, Soldatos T, et al. MR neurography: past, present, and future. *AJR Am J Roentgenol*. 2011;197(3):583-591.
50. Thawait SK, Chaudhry V, Thawait GK, et al. High-resolution MR neurography of diffuse peripheral nerve lesions. *AJNR Am J Neuroradiol*. 2011;32(8):1365-1372.
51. Ducreux D, Fillard P, Facon D, et al. Diffusion tensor magnetic resonance imaging and fiber tracking in spinal cord lesions: current and future indications. *Neuroimaging Clin N Am*. 2007;17(1):137-147.
52. Kim TH, Zollinger L, Shi XF, et al. Quantification of diffusivities of the human cervical spinal cord using a 2D single-shot interleaved multisection inner volume diffusion-weighted echo-planar imaging technique. *AJNR Am J Neuroradiol*. 2010;31(4):682-687.
53. Baur A, Dietrich O, Reiser M. Diffusion-weighted imaging of bone marrow: current status. *Eur Radiol*. 2003;13(7): 1699-1708.
54. Baur A, Stabler A, Bruning R, et al. Diffusion-weighted MR imaging of bone marrow: differentiation of benign versus pathologic compression fractures. *Radiology*. 1998;207(2): 349-356.
55. Castillo M. Diffusion-weighted imaging of the spine: is it reliable? *AJNR Am J Neuroradiol*. 2003;24(6):1251-1253.

56. Luboldt W, Kufer R, Blumstein N, et al. Prostate carcinoma: diffusion-weighted imaging as potential alternative to conventional MR and 11C-choline PET/CT for detection of bone metastases. *Radiology*. 2008;249(3):1017-1025.
57. Takenaka D, Ohno Y, Matsumoto K, et al. Detection of bone metastases in non-small cell lung cancer patients: comparison of whole-body diffusion-weighted imaging (DWI), whole-body MR imaging without and with DWI, whole-body FDG-PET/CT, and bone scintigraphy. *J Magn Reson Imaging*. 2009;30(2):298-308.
58. Bammer R, Fazekas F, Augustin M, et al. Diffusion-weighted MR imaging of the spinal cord. *AJNR Am J Neuroradiol*. 2000;21(3):587-591.
59. Ducreux D, Lepeintre JF, Fillard P, et al. MR diffusion tensor imaging and fiber tracking in 5 spinal cord astrocytomas. *AJNR Am J Neuroradiol*. 2006;27(1):214-216.
60. Setzer M, Murtagh RD, Murtagh FR, et al. Diffusion tensor imaging tractography in patients with intramedullary tumors: comparison with intraoperative findings and value for prediction of tumor resectability. *J Neurosurg Spine*. 2010;13(3):371-380.
61. Facon D, Ozanne A, Fillard P, et al. MR diffusion tensor imaging and fiber tracking in spinal cord compression. *AJNR Am J Neuroradiol*. 2005;26(6):1587-1594.
62. Renoux J, Facon D, Fillard P, et al. MR diffusion tensor imaging and fiber tracking in inflammatory diseases of the spinal cord. *AJNR Am J Neuroradiol*. 2006;27(9):1947-1951.
63. Levy LM. MR imaging of cerebrospinal fluid flow and spinal cord motion in neurologic disorders of the spine. *Magn Reson Imaging Clin N Am*. 1999;7(3):573-587.
64. Mauer UM, Freude G, Danz B, Kunz U. Cardiac-gated phase-contrast magnetic resonance imaging of cerebrospinal fluid flow in the diagnosis of idiopathic syringomyelia. *Neurosurgery*. 2008;63(6):1139-1144.
65. Quigley MF, Iskandar B, Quigley ME, Nicosia M, Haughton V. Cerebrospinal fluid flow in foramen magnum: temporal and spatial patterns at MR imaging in volunteers and in patients with Chiari I malformation. *Radiology*. 2004;232(1):229-236.
66. Rubin JB, Enzmann DR, Wright A. CSF-gated MR imaging of the spine: theory and clinical implementation. *Radiology*. 1987;163(3):784-792.
67. Hock A, Henning A, Boesiger P, Kollias SS. (1)H-MR spectroscopy in the human spinal cord. *AJNR Am J Neuroradiol*. 2013;34(9):1682-1689.
68. Blamire AM, Cader S, Lee M, Palace J, Matthews PM. Axonal damage in the spinal cord of multiple sclerosis patients detected by magnetic resonance spectroscopy. *Magn Reson Med*. 2007;58(5):880-885.
69. Kim YG, Choi GH, Kim DH, et al. In vivo proton magnetic resonance spectroscopy of human spinal mass lesions. *J Spinal Disord Tech*. 2004;17(5):405-411.
70. Shellock FG, Spinazzi A. MRI safety update 2008. Part 2: screening patients for MRI. *AJR Am J Roentgenol*. 2008;191(4):1140-1149.
71. Colletti PM, Shinbane JS, Shellock FG. "MR-conditional" pacemakers: the radiologist's role in multidisciplinary management. *AJR Am J Roentgenol*. 2011;197(3):W457-W459.
72. Bleicher AG, Kanal E. Assessment of adverse reaction rates to a newly approved MRI contrast agent: review of 23,553 administrations of gadobenate dimeglumine. *AJR Am J Roentgenol*. 2008;191(6):W307-W311.
73. Kanda T, Ishii K, Kawaguchi H, Kitajima K, Takenaka D. High signal intensity in the dentate nucleus and globus pallidus on unenhanced T1-weighted MR images: relationship with increasing cumulative dose of a gadolinium-based contrast material. *Radiology*. 2014;270(3):834-841.
74. McDonald RJ, McDonald JS, Kallmes DF, et al. Intracranial gadolinium deposition after contrast-enhanced MR imaging. *Radiology*. 2015;275(3):772-782.
75. Kanal E, Tweedle MF. Residual or retained gadolinium: practical implications for radiologists and our patients. *Radiology*. 2015;275(3):630-634.
76. Shellock FG, Spinazzi A. MRI safety update 2008. Part 1: MRI contrast agents and nephrogenic systemic fibrosis. *AJR Am J Roentgenol*. 2008;191(4):1129-1139.
77. Thomsen HS. Nephrogenic systemic fibrosis: a serious late adverse reaction to gadodiamide. *Eur Radiol*. 2006;16(12): 2619-2621.
78. Broome DR, Girguis MS, Baron PW, et al. Gadodiamide-associated nephrogenic systemic fibrosis: why radiologists should be concerned. *AJR Am J Roentgenol*. 2007;188(2):586-592.
79. Kuo PH, Kanal E, Abu-Alfa AK, Cowper SE. Gadolinium-based MR contrast agents and nephrogenic systemic fibrosis. *Radiology*. 2007;242(3):647-649.
80. Prince MR, Zhang H, Morris M, et al. Incidence of nephrogenic systemic fibrosis at two large medical centers. *Radiology*. 2008;248(3):807-816.
81. Sadowski EA, Bennett LK, Chan MR, et al. Nephrogenic systemic fibrosis: risk factors and incidence estimation. *Radiology*. 2007;243(1):148-157.
82. Choi IS, Berenstein A. Surgical neuroangiography of the spine and spinal cord. *Radiol Clin North Am*. 1988;26(5): 1131-1141.
83. Di Chiro G, Wener L. Angiography of the spinal cord. A review of contemporary techniques and applications. *J Neurosurg*. 1973;39(1):1-29.
84. Nelson PK, Setton A, Berenstein A. Vertebrospinal angiography in the evaluation of vertebral and spinal cord disease. *Neuroimaging Clin N Am*. 1996;6(3):589-605.
85. Anson JA, Spetzler RF. Interventional neuroradiology for spinal pathology. *Clin Neurosurg*. 1992;39:388-417.
86. Kendall BE, Logue V. Spinal epidural angiomatous malformations draining into intrathecal veins. *Neuroradiology*. 1977;13(4):181-189.
87. Gilbertson JR, Miller GM, Goldman MS, Marsh WR. Spinal dural arteriovenous fistulas: MR and myelographic findings. *AJNR Am J Neuroradiol*. 1995;16(10):2049-2057.
88. Masaryk TJ, Ross JS, Modic MT, et al. Radiculomeningeal vascular malformations of the spine: MR imaging. *Radiology*. 1987;164(3):845-849.
89. Merland JJ, Riche MC, Chiras J. Intraspinal extramedullary arteriovenous fistulae draining into the medullary veins. *J Neuroradiol*. 1980;7(4):271-320.
90. Backes WH, Nijenhuis RJ. Advances in spinal cord MR angiography. *AJNR Am J Neuroradiol*. 2008;29(4):619-631.
91. Bowen BC, Fraser K, Kochan JP, et al. Spinal dural arteriovenous fistulas: evaluation with MR angiography. *AJNR Am J Neuroradiol*. 1995;16(10):2029-2043.
92. Mull M, Nijenhuis RJ, Backes WH, et al. Value and limitations of contrast-enhanced MR angiography in spinal arteriovenous malformations and dural arteriovenous fistulas. *AJNR Am J Neuroradiol*. 2007;28(7):1249-1258.
93. Lai PH, Weng MJ, Lee KW, Pan HB. Multidetector CT angiography in diagnosing type I and type IVA spinal vascular malformations. *AJNR Am J Neuroradiol*. 2006;27(4):813-817.

94. Yoshioka K, Niinuma H, Ohira A, et al. MR angiography and CT angiography of the artery of Adamkiewicz: noninvasive preoperative assessment of thoracoabdominal aortic aneurysm. *Radiographics.* 2003;23(5):1215-1225.
95. Guyer RD, Ohnmeiss DD. Lumbar discography. Position statement from the North American Spine Society Diagnostic and Therapeutic Committee. *Spine.* 1995;20(18):2048-2059.
96. Saal JS. General principles of diagnostic testing as related to painful lumbar spine disorders: a critical appraisal of current diagnostic techniques. *Spine.* 2002;27(22):2538-2545.
97. Bernard TN Jr. Don't discard diskography. *Radiology.* 1987;162(1 Pt 1):285.
98. Milette PC, Fontaine S, Lepanto L, Cardinal E, Breton G. Differentiating lumbar disc protrusions, disc bulges, and discs with normal contour but abnormal signal intensity. Magnetic resonance imaging with discographic correlations. *Spine.* 1999;24(1):44-53.
99. Bernard TN Jr. Repeat lumbar spine surgery. Factors influencing outcome. *Spine.* 1993;18(15):2196-2200.
100. Bogduk N, Modic MT. Lumbar discography. *Spine.* 1996; 21(3):402-404.
101. Holt EP Jr. The question of lumbar discography. *J Bone Joint Surg Am.* 1968;50(4):720-726.
102. Modic MT. Diskography: science and the ad hoc hypothesis. *AJNR Am J Neuroradiol.* 2000;21(2):241-242.
103. Mooney V. Lumbar discography. *Spine.* 1996;21(12):1479.
104. Simmons JW, Aprill CN, Dwyer AP, Brodsky AE. A reassessment of Holt's data on: "The question of lumbar discography." *Clin Orthop Relat Res.* 1988;237:120-124.
105. Smith SE, Darden BV, Rhyne AL, Wood KE. Outcome of unoperated discogram-positive low back pain. *Spine.* 1995;20(18):1997-2000.
106. Walsh TR, Weinstein JN, Spratt KF, et al. Lumbar discography in normal subjects. A controlled, prospective study. *J Bone Joint Surg.* 1990;72(7):1081-1088.
107. Bosacco SJ. Lumbar discography: redefining its role with intradiscal therapy. *Orthopedics.* 1986;9(3):399-401.
108. Simmons JW, McMillin JN, Emery SF, Kimmich SJ. Intradiscal steroids. A prospective double-blind clinical trial. *Spine.* 1992;17(6 suppl):S172-S175.
109. Tehranzadeh J. Discography 2000. *Radiol Clin North Am.* 1998;36(3):463-495.
110. Whiteman ML, Serafini AN, Telischi FF, Civantos FJ, Falcone S. ^{111}In octreotide scintigraphy in the evaluation of head and neck lesions. *AJNR Am J Neuroradiol.* 1997;18(6):1073-1080.
111. Even-Sapir E. Imaging of malignant bone involvement by morphologic, scintigraphic, and hybrid modalities. *J Nucl Med.* 2005;46(8):1356-1367.
112. Thrall JH, Ellis BI. Skeletal metastases. *Radiol Clin North Am.* 1987;25(6):1155-1170.
113. Cook GJ, Fogelman I. Skeletal metastases from breast cancer: imaging with nuclear medicine. *Semin Nucl Med.* 1999;29(1):69-79.
114. Cook GJ, Houston S, Rubens R, Maisey MN, Fogelman I. Detection of bone metastases in breast cancer by 18FDG PET: differing metabolic activity in osteoblastic and osteolytic lesions. *J Clin Oncol.* 1998;16(10):3375-3379.
115. Metser U, Miller E, Lerman H, Even-Sapir E. Benign nonphysiologic lesions with increased 18F-FDG uptake on PET/CT: characterization and incidence. *AJR Am J Roentgenol.* 2007;189(5):1203-1210.
116. Gelman MI, Coleman RE, Stevens PM, Davey BW. Radiography, radionuclide imaging, and arthrography in the evaluation of total hip and knee replacement. *Radiology.* 1978;128(3):677-682.
117. Lisbona R, Rosenthal L. Observations on the sequential use of Tc99-m phosphate complex and Ga-67 imaging in osteomyelitis, cellulitis, and septic arthritis. *Radiology.* 1977;123:123-129.
118. Weiss PE, Mall JC, Hoffer PB, et al. 99mTc-methylene diphosphonate bone imaging in the evaluation of total hip prostheses. *Radiology.* 1979;133(3 Pt 1):727-729.
119. McAfee JG, Samin A. In-111 labeled leukocytes: a review of problems in image interpretation. *Radiology.* 1985;155(1):221-229.
120. Frazzini VI, Kagetsu NJ, Johnson CE, Destian S. Internally stabilized spine: optimal choice of frequency-encoding gradient direction during MR imaging minimizes susceptibility artifact from titanium vertebral body screws. *Radiology.* 1997;204(1):268-272.
121. Lazik A, Landgraeber S, Schulte P, et al. Usefulness of metal artifact reduction with WARP technique at 1.5 and 3T MRI in imaging metal-on-metal hip resurfacings. *Skeletal Radiol.* 2015;44(7):941-951.
122. Zhuo J, Gullapalli RP. AAPM/RSNA physics tutorial for residents: MR artifacts, safety, and quality control. *Radiographics.* 2006;26(1):275-297.
123. Chou R, Deyo RA, Jarvik JG. Appropriate use of lumbar imaging for evaluation of low back pain. *Radiol Clin North Am.* 2012;50(4):569-585.
124. Hitselberger WE, Witten RM. Abnormal myelograms in asymptomatic patients. *J Neurosurg.* 1968;28(3):204-206.
125. Brinjikji W, Luetmer PH, Comstock B, et al. Systematic literature review of imaging features of spinal degeneration in asymptomatic populations. *AJNR Am J Neuroradiol.* 2015;36(4):811-816.
126. Boden SD, Davis DO, Dina TS, Patronas NJ, Wiesel SW. Abnormal magnetic-resonance scans of the lumbar spine in asymptomatic subjects. A prospective investigation. *J Bone Joint Surg.* 1990;72(3):403-408.
127. Jensen MC, Brant-Zawadzki MN, Obuchowski N, et al. Magnetic resonance imaging of the lumbar spine in people without back pain. *N Engl J Med.* 1994;331(2):69-73.
128. Pengel LH, Herbert RD, Maher CG, Refshauge KM. Acute low back pain: systematic review of its prognosis. *BMJ.* 2003;327(7410):323.
129. Vroomen PC, de Krom MC, Knottnerus JA. Predicting the outcome of sciatica at short-term follow-up. *Br J Gen Pract.* 2002;52(475):119-123.
130. Modic MT, Obuchowski NA, Ross JS, et al. Acute low back pain and radiculopathy: MR imaging findings and their prognostic role and effect on outcome. *Radiology.* 2005;237(2): 597-604.
131. Modic MT, Ross JS, Obuchowski NA, et al. Contrast-enhanced MR imaging in acute lumbar radiculopathy: a pilot study of the natural history. *Radiology.* 1995;195(2):429-435.
132. Saal JA, Saal JS, Herzog RJ. The natural history of lumbar intervertebral disc extrusions treated nonoperatively. *Spine.* 1990;15(7):683-686.
133. Halpin SF, Yeoman L, Dundas DD. Radiographic examination of the lumbar spine in a community hospital: an audit of current practice. *BMJ.* 1991;303(6806):813-815.
134. Rockey PH, Tompkins RK, Wood RW, Wolcott BW. The usefulness of x-ray examinations in the evaluation of patients with back pain. *J Fam Pract.* 1978;7(3):455-465.

135. Gillan MG, Gilbert FJ, Andrew JE, et al. Influence of imaging on clinical decision making in the treatment of lower back pain. *Radiology*. 2001;220(2):393-399.
136. Jarvik JG, Hollingworth W, Martin B, et al. Rapid magnetic resonance imaging vs radiographs for patients with low back pain: a randomized controlled trial. *JAMA*. 2003;289(21):2810-2818.
137. Fazel R, Krumholz HM, Wang Y, et al. Exposure to low-dose ionizing radiation from medical imaging procedures. *N Engl J Med*. 2009;361(9):849-857.
138. Errico TJ, Fardon DF, Lowell TD. Open discectomy as treatment for herniated nucleus pulposus of the lumbar spine. *Spine*. 1995;20(16):1829-1833.
139. Keller RB, Atlas SJ, Soule DN, Singer DE, Deyo RA. Relationship between rates and outcomes of operative treatment for lumbar disc herniation and spinal stenosis. *J Bone Joint Surg*. 1999;81(6):752-762.
140. Lurie JD, Birkmeyer NJ, Weinstein JN. Rates of advanced spinal imaging and spine surgery. *Spine*. 2003;28(6):616-620.
141. Ash LM, Modic MT, Obuchowski NA, et al. Effects of diagnostic information, per se, on patient outcomes in acute radiculopathy and low back pain. *AJNR Am J Neuroradiol*. 2008;29(6):1098-1103.
142. Deyo RA, Bigos SJ, Maravilla KR. Diagnostic imaging procedures for the lumbar spine. *Ann Intern Med*. 1989; 111(11):865-867.
143. Fager CA. Identification and management of radiculopathy. *Neurosurg Clin N Am*. 1993;4(1):1-12.
144. Long DM. Decision making in lumbar disc disease. *Clin Neurosurg*. 1992;39:36-51.
145. Bell GR, Rothman RH. The conservative treatment of sciatica. *Spine*. 1984;9(1):54-56.
146. Bozzao A, Gallucci M, Masciocchi C, et al. Lumbar disk herniation: MR imaging assessment of natural history in patients treated without surgery. *Radiology*. 1992;185(1): 135-141.
147. Bush K, Cowan N, Katz DE, Gishen P. The natural history of sciatica associated with disc pathology. A prospective study with clinical and independent radiologic follow-up. *Spine*. 1992;17(10):1205-1212.
148. Cowan NC, Bush K, Katz DE, Gishen P. The natural history of sciatica: a prospective radiological study. *Clin Radiol*. 1992;46(1):7-12.
149. Delauche-Cavallier MC, Budet C, Laredo JD, et al. Lumbar disc herniation. Computed tomography scan changes after conservative treatment of nerve root compression. *Spine*. 1992;17(8):927-933.
150. Saal JA, Saal JS. Nonoperative treatment of herniated lumbar intervertebral disc with radiculopathy. An outcome study. *Spine*. 1989;14(4):431-437.
151. Davis PC, Wippold FJ 2nd, Brunberg JA, et al. ACR Appropriateness criteria on low back pain. *J Am Coll Radiol*. 2009;6(6):401-407.
152. Majors A, McDevitt C, Sigalis I, Modic MT *A correlative analysis of T2, ADC and MT ratio with water, hydroxyproline and GAG content in excised intervertebral disk*. In: Transactions of the Orthopaedic Research Society Annual Meeting, New Orleans: 1994:116-120.
153. Coventry MB. Anatomy of the intervertebral disk. *Clin Orthop Relat Res*. 1969;67:9-15.
154. Sether LA, Yu S, Haughton VM, Fischer ME. Intervertebral disk: normal age-related changes in MR signal intensity. *Radiology*. 1990;177(2):385-388.
155. Yuh WT, Marsh EE 3rd, Wang AK, et al. MR imaging of spinal cord and vertebral body infarction. *AJNR Am J Neuroradiol*. 1992;13(1):145-154.
156. Ross JS, Modic MT, Masaryk TJ. Tears of the anulus fibrosus: assessment with Gd-DTPA-enhanced MR imaging. *AJNR Am J Neuroradiol*. 1989;10(6):1251-1254.
157. Yu SW, Sether LA, Ho PS, Wagner M, Haughton VM. Tears of the anulus fibrosus: correlation between MR and pathologic findings in cadavers. *AJNR Am J Neuroradiol*. 1988;9(2):367-370.
158. Fardon DF, Milette PC. Nomenclature and classification of lumbar disc pathology. Recommendations of the Combined Task Forces of the North American Spine Society, American Society of Spine Radiology, and American Society of Neuroradiology. *Spine*. 2001;26(5):E93-E113.
159. Modic MT, Steinberg PM, Ross JS, Masaryk TJ, Carter JR. Degenerative disk disease: assessment of changes in vertebral body marrow with MR imaging. *Radiology*. 1988;166(1 Pt 1): 193-199.
160. Albert HB, Lambert P, Rollason J, et al. Does nuclear tissue infected with bacteria following disc herniations lead to Modic changes in the adjacent vertebrae? *Eur Spine J*. 2013;22(4):690-696.
161. Stirling A, Worthington T, Rafiq M, Lambert PA, Elliott TS. Association between sciatica and *Propionibacterium acnes*. *Lancet*. 2001;357(9273):2024-2025.
162. Albert HB, Sorensen JS, Christensen BS, Manniche C. Antibiotic treatment in patients with chronic low back pain and vertebral bone edema (Modic type 1 changes): a double-blind randomized clinical controlled trial of efficacy. *Eur Spine J*. 2013;22(4):697-707.
163. Amundsen T, Weber H, Lilleas F, et al. Lumbar spinal stenosis. Clinical and radiologic features. *Spine*. 1995;20(10): 1178-1186.
164. Bartynski WS, Lin L. Lumbar root compression in the lateral recess: MR imaging, conventional myelography, and CT myelography comparison with surgical confirmation. *AJNR Am J Neuroradiol*. 2003;24(3):348-360.
165. Silbergleit R, Gebarski SS, Brunberg JA, McGillicudy J, Blaivas M. Lumbar synovial cysts: correlation of myelographic, CT, MR, and pathologic findings. *AJNR Am J Neuroradiol*. 1990;11(4):777-779.
166. Ulmer JL, Elster AD, Mathews VP, King JC. Distinction between degenerative and isthmic spondylolisthesis on sagittal MR images: importance of increased anteroposterior diameter of the spinal canal ("wide canal sign"). *AJR Am J Roentgenol*. 1994;163(2):411-416.
167. Jinkins JR, Matthes JC, Sener RN, Venkatappan S, Rauch R. Spondylolysis, spondylolisthesis, and associated nerve root entrapment in the lumbosacral spine: MR evaluation. *AJR Am J Roentgenol*. 1992;159(4):799-803.
168. Pavlov H, Torg JS, Robie B, Jahre C. Cervical spinal stenosis: determination with vertebral body ratio method. *Radiology*. 1987;164(3):771-775.
169. Takahashi M, Yamashita Y, Sakamoto Y, Kojima R. Chronic cervical cord compression: clinical significance of increased signal intensity on MR images. *Radiology*. 1989;173(1):219-224.
170. Agarwal R, Williams K, Umscheid CA, Welch WC. Osteoinductive bone graft substitutes for lumbar fusion: a systematic review. *J Neurosurg Spine*. 2009;11(6):729-740.
171. Helgeson MD, Lehman RA Jr, Patzkowski JC, et al. Adjacent vertebral body osteolysis with bone morphogenetic protein

use in transforaminal lumbar interbody fusion. *Spine J.* 2011;11(6):507-510.

172. Sethi A, Craig J, Bartol S, et al. Radiographic and CT evaluation of recombinant human bone morphogenetic protein-2-assisted spinal interbody fusion. *AJR Am J Roentgenol.* 2011;197(1):W128-W133.
173. Vaidya R, Sethi A, Bartol S, et al. Complications in the use of rhBMP-2 in PEEK cages for interbody spinal fusions. *J Spinal Disord Tech.* 2008;21(8):557-562.
174. Hueftle MG, Modic MT, Ross JS, et al. Lumbar spine: postoperative MR imaging with Gd-DTPA. *Radiology.* 1988;167(3):817-824.
175. Georgy BA, Hesselink JR, Middleton MS. Fat-suppression contrast-enhanced MRI in the failed back surgery syndrome: a prospective study. *Neuroradiology.* 1995;37(1):51-57.
176. Cervellini P, Curri D, Volpin L, et al. Computed tomography of epidural fibrosis after discectomy: a comparison between symptomatic and asymptomatic patients. *Neurosurgery.* 1988;23(6):710-713.
177. Ross JS, Robertson JT, Frederickson RC, et al. Association between peridural scar and recurrent radicular pain after lumbar discectomy: magnetic resonance evaluation. ADCON-L European Study Group. *Neurosurgery.* 1996;38(4):855-861.
178. Coskun E, Suzer T, Topuz O, et al. Relationships between epidural fibrosis, pain, disability, and psychological factors after lumbar disc surgery. *Eur Spine J.* 2000;9(3):218-223.
179. Burton CV. Causes of failure of surgery on the lumbar spine: ten-year follow-up. *Mt Sinai J Med.* 1991;58(2):183-187.
180. Djukic S, Genant HK, Helms CA, Holt RG. Magnetic resonance imaging of the postoperative lumbar spine. *Radiol Clin North Am.* 1990;28(2):341-360.
181. Johnson CE, Sze G. Benign lumbar arachnoiditis: MR imaging with gadopentetate dimeglumine. *AJNR Am J Neuroradiol.* 1990;11(4):763-770.
182. Ross JS, Masaryk TJ, Modic MT, et al. MR imaging of lumbar arachnoiditis. *AJR Am J Roentgenol.* 1987;149(5):1025-1032.
183. Golimbu C, Firooznia H, Rafii M. CT of osteomyelitis of the spine. *AJR Am J Roentgenol.* 1984;142(1):159-163.
184. Jeffrey RB, Callen PW, Federle MP. Computed tomography of psoas abscesses. *J Comput Assist Tomogr.* 1980;4(5):639-641.
185. Modic MT, Feiglin DH, Piraino DW, et al. Vertebral osteomyelitis: assessment using MR. *Radiology.* 1985;157(1):157-166.
186. Modic MT, Weinstein MA, Pavlicek W, et al. Nuclear magnetic resonance imaging of the spine. *Radiology.* 1983;148(3):757-762.
187. de Roos A, van Persijn van Meerten EL, Bloem JL, Bluemm RG. MRI of tuberculous spondylitis. *AJR Am J Roentgenol.* 1986;147(1):79-82.
188. Dagirmanjian A, Schils J, McHenry M, Modic MT. MR imaging of vertebral osteomyelitis revisited. *AJR Am J Roentgenol.* 1996;167(6):1539-1543.
189. Boden SD, Davis DO, Dina TS, Sunner JL, Wiesel SW. Postoperative diskitis: distinguishing early MR imaging findings from normal postoperative disk space changes. *Radiology.* 1992;184(3):765-771.
190. Rankin RM, Flothow PG. Pyogenic infection of the spinal epidural space. *West J Surg Obstet Gynecol.* 1946;54:320-323.
191. Baker AS, Ojemann RG, Swartz MN, Richardson EP Jr. Spinal epidural abscess. *N Engl J Med.* 1975;293(10):463-468.
192. Browder J, Meyers R. Pyogenic infections of the spinal epidural space. *Surgery.* 1941;10:296-308.
193. Angtuaco EJ, McConnell JR, Chadduck WM, Flanigan S. MR imaging of spinal epidural sepsis. *AJR Am J Roentgenol.* 1987;149(6):1249-1253.
194. Tins BJ, Cassar-Pullicino VN, Lalam RK. Magnetic resonance imaging of spinal infection. *Top Magn Reson Imaging.* 2007;18(3):213-222.
195. Post MJ, Quencer RM, Montalvo BM, et al. Spinal infection: evaluation with MR imaging and intraoperative US. *Radiology.* 1988;169(3):765-771.
196. Post MJ, Sze G, Quencer RM, et al. Gadolinium-enhanced MR in spinal infection. *J Comput Assist Tomogr.* 1990;14(5):721-729.
197. Kowalski TJ, Layton KF, Berbari EF, et al. Follow-up MR imaging in patients with pyogenic spine infections: lack of correlation with clinical features. *AJNR Am J Neuroradiol.* 2007;28(4):693-699.
198. Bowen BC, Pattany PM. Vascular anatomy and disorders of the lumbar spine and spinal cord. *Magn Reson Imaging Clin N Am.* 1999;7(3):555-571.
199. Krings T, Lasjaunias PL, Hans FJ, et al. Imaging in spinal vascular disease. *Neuroimaging Clin N Am.* 2007;17(1):57-72.
200. Thurnher MM, Cartes-Zumelzu F, Mueller-Mang C. Demyelinating and infectious diseases of the spinal cord. *Neuroimaging Clin N Am.* 2007;17(1):37-55.
201. Koeller KK, Rosenblum RS, Morrison AL. Neoplasms of the spinal cord and filum terminale: radiologic-pathologic correlation. *Radiographics.* 2000;20(6):1721-1749.
202. White JB, Miller GM, Layton KF, Krauss WE. Nonenhancing tumors of the spinal cord. *J Neurosurg Spine.* 2007;7(4):403-407.
203. Kahan H, Sklar EM, Post MJ, Bruce JH. MR characteristics of histopathologic subtypes of spinal ependymoma. *AJNR Am J Neuroradiol.* 1996;17(1):143-150.
204. Rawlings CE 3rd, Giangaspero F, Burger PC, Bullard DE. Ependymomas: a clinicopathologic study. *Surg Neurol.* 1988;29(4):271-281.
205. Wippold FJ 2nd, Smirniotopoulos JG, Moran CJ, Suojanen JN, Vollmer DG. MR imaging of myxopapillary ependymoma: findings and value to determine extent of tumor and its relation to intraspinal structures. *AJR Am J Roentgenol.* 1995;165(5):1263-1267.
206. Nemoto Y, Inoue Y, Tashiro T, et al. Intramedullary spinal cord tumors: significance of associated hemorrhage at MR imaging. *Radiology.* 1992;182(3):793-796.
207. Shen WC, Ho YJ, Lee SK, Lee KR. Ependymoma of the cauda equina presenting with subarachnoid hemorrhage. *AJNR Am J Neuroradiol.* 1993;14(2):399-400.
208. Choyke PL, Glenn GM, Walther MM, et al. von Hippel-Lindau disease: genetic, clinical, and imaging features. *Radiology.* 1995;194(3):629-642.
209. Ho VB, Smirniotopoulos JG, Murphy FM, Rushing EJ. Radiologic-pathologic correlation: hemangioblastoma. *AJNR Am J Neuroradiol.* 1992;13(5):1343-1352.
210. Hoff DJ, Tampieri D, Just N. Imaging of spinal cord hemangioblastomas. *Can Assoc Radiol J.* 1993;44(5): 377-383.
211. Murota T, Symon L. Surgical management of hemangioblastoma of the spinal cord: a report of 18 cases. *Neurosurgery.* 1989;25(5):699-707.
212. Sze G, Krol G, Zimmerman RD, Deck MD. Intramedullary disease of the spine: diagnosis using gadolinium-DTPA-enhanced MR imaging. *AJR Am J Roentgenol.* 1988;151(6):1193-1204.

213. Yu JS, Short MP, Schumacher J, Chapman PH. Harsh GR 4th. Intramedullary hemorrhage in spinal cord hemangioblastoma. Report of two cases. *J Neurosurg.* 1994;81(6):937-940.
214. Tognetti F, Lanzino G, Calbucci F. Metastases of the spinal cord from remote neoplasms. Study of five cases. *Surg Neurol.* 1988;30(3):220-227.
215. Winkelman MD, Adelstein DJ, Karlins NL. Intramedullary spinal cord metastasis. Diagnostic and therapeutic considerations. *Arch Neurol.* 1987;44(5):526-531.
216. DeAngelis LM. Current diagnosis and treatment of leptomeningeal metastasis. *J Neurooncol.* 1998;38(2-3):245-252.
217. Hamilton MG, Tranmer BI, Hagen NA. Supratentorial glioblastoma with spinal cord intramedullary metastasis. *Can J Neurol Sci.* 1993;20(1):65-68.
218. McCormick PC, Post KD, Stein BM. Intradural extramedullary tumors in adults. *Neurosurg Clin N Am.* 1990;1(3):591-608.
219. Stankiewicz JM, Neema M, Alsop DC, et al. Spinal cord lesions and clinical status in multiple sclerosis: A 1.5 T and 3 T MRI study. *J Neurol Sci.* 2009;279(1-2):99-105.
220. Bourgouin PM, Lesage J, Fontaine S, et al. A pattern approach to the differential diagnosis of intramedullary spinal cord lesions on MR imaging. *AJR Am J Roentgenol.* 1998;170(6):1645-1649.
221. Halliday AL, Sobel RA, Martuza RL. Benign spinal nerve sheath tumors: their occurrence sporadically and in neurofibromatosis types 1 and 2. *J Neurosurg.* 1991;74(2): 248-253.
222. Egelhoff JC, Bates DJ, Ross JS, Rothner AD, Cohen BH. Spinal MR findings in neurofibromatosis types 1 and 2. *AJNR Am J Neuroradiol.* 1992;13(4):1071-1077.
223. Levy WJ Jr, Bay J, Dohn D. Spinal cord meningioma. *J Neurosurg.* 1982;57(6):804-812.
224. Roux FX, Nataf F, Pinaudeau M, et al. Intraspinal meningiomas: review of 54 cases with discussion of poor prognosis factors and modern therapeutic management. *Surg Neurol.* 1996;46(5):458-463.
225. Sevick RJ. Cervical spine tumors. *Neuroimaging Clin N Am.* 1995;5(3):385-400.
226. Yousem DM, Patrone PM, Grossman RI. Leptomeningeal metastases: MR evaluation. *J Comput Assist Tomogr.* 1990;14(2):255-261.
227. Shapiro JHOM, Jacobson HG. Differential diagnosis of intradural (extramedullary) and extradural spinal canal tumors. *Radiology.* 1961;76:718-732.
228. Hanrahan CJ, Shah LM. MRI of spinal bone marrow. Part 2: T1-weighted imaging-based differential diagnosis. *AJR Am J Roentgenol.* 2011;197(6):1309-1321.
229. Rodallec MH, Feydy A, Larousserie F, et al. Diagnostic imaging of solitary tumors of the spine: what to do and say. *Radiographics.* 2008;28(4):1019-1041.
230. Carmody RF, Yang PJ, Seeley GW, et al. Spinal cord compression due to metastatic disease: diagnosis with MR imaging versus myelography. *Radiology.* 1989;173(1): 225-229.
231. Chimelli L. Tumors and tumorlike lesions of the spine and spinal cord. *Neuroimaging Clin N Am.* 2001;11(1):79-110.
232. Epstein N. Diagnosis and surgical management of cervical ossification of the posterior longitudinal ligament. *Spine J.* 2002;2(6):436-449.
233. Hirabayashi K, Satomi K. Operative procedure and results of expansive open-door laminoplasty. *Spine.* 1988;13(7): 870-876.
234. Kronborg O. Extradural spinal cysts. A literature survey and a case of multiple extradural cysts. *Dan Med Bull.* 1967;14(1):46-48.
235. Nabors MW, Pait TG, Byrd EB, et al. Updated assessment and current classification of spinal meningeal cysts. *J Neurosurg.* 1988;68(3):366-377.
236. Rothman RH, Jacobs SR, Appleman W. Spinal extradural cysts. A report of five cases. *Clin Orthop Relat Res.* 1970;71: 186-192.
237. Hoffman JR, Schriger DL, Mower W, Luo JS, Zucker M. Low-risk criteria for cervical-spine radiography in blunt trauma: a prospective study. *Ann Emerg Med.* 1992;21(12):1454-1460.
238. Roberge RJ, Wears RC, Kelly M, et al. Selective application of cervical spine radiography in alert victims of blunt trauma: a prospective study. *J Trauma.* 1988;28(6):784-788.
239. Cornelius RS, Leach JL. Imaging evaluation of cervical spine trauma. *Neuroimaging Clin N Am.* 1995;5(3):451-463.
240. Schwartz ED, Flanders AE. *Spinal Trauma: Imaging, Diagnosis, and Management.* Philadelphia: Lippincott Williams & Wilkins; 2007.
241. Kaye JJ, Nance EP Jr. Cervical spine trauma. *Orthop Clin North Am.* 1990;21(3):449-462.
242. Schleehauf K, Ross SE, Civil ID, Schwab CW. Computed tomography in the initial evaluation of the cervical spine. *Ann Emerg Med.* 1989;18(8):815-817.
243. Kirshenbaum KJ, Nadimpalli SR, Fantus R, Cavallino RP. Unsuspected upper cervical spine fractures associated with significant head trauma: role of CT. *J Emerg Med.* 1990;8(2):183-198.
244. Lindsey RW, Diliberti TC, Doherty BJ, Watson AB. Efficacy of radiographic evaluation of the cervical spine in emergency situations. *South Med J.* 1993;86(11):1253-1255.
245. Daffner RH. Cervical radiography for trauma patients: a time-effective technique? *AJR Am J Roentgenol.* 2000;175(5): 1309-1311.
246. Daffner RH. Helical CT of the cervical spine for trauma patients: a time study. *AJR Am J Roentgenol.* 2001;177(3): 677-679.
247. Davis SJ, Teresi LM, Bradley WG Jr, Ziemba MA, Bloze AE. Cervical spine hyperextension injuries: MR findings. *Radiology.* 1991;180(1):245-251.
248. Flanders AE, Spettell CM, Tartaglino LM, Friedman DP, Herbison GJ. Forecasting motor recovery after cervical spinal cord injury: value of MR imaging. *Radiology.* 1996;201(3): 649-655.
249. Kulkarni MV, Bondurant FJ, Rose SL, Narayana PA. 1.5 tesla magnetic resonance imaging of acute spinal trauma. *Radiographics.* 1988;8(6):1059-1082.
250. Schaefer DM, Flanders AE, Osterholm JL, Northrup BE. Prognostic significance of magnetic resonance imaging in the acute phase of cervical spine injury. *J Neurosurg.* 1992;76(2):218-223.
251. Hall AJ, Wagle VG, Raycroft J, Goldman RL, Butler AR. Magnetic resonance imaging in cervical spine trauma. *J Trauma.* 1993;34(1):21-26.
252. Silberstein M, Tress BM, Hennessy O. Prevertebral swelling in cervical spine injury: identification of ligament injury with magnetic resonance imaging. *Clin Radiol.* 1992;46(5): 318-323.
253. Holdsworth F. Fractures, dislocations, and fracture-dislocations of the spine. *J Bone Joint Surg.* 1970;52(8):1534-1551.

254. Roab R. International classification of spine injuries. *Paraplegia.* 1972;10:78.
255. Tarr RW, Drolshagen LF, Kerner TC, et al. MR imaging of recent spinal trauma. *J Comput Assist Tomogr.* 1987;11(3):412-417.
256. Sheridan R, Peralta R, Rhea J, Ptak T, Novelline R. Reformatted visceral protocol helical computed tomographic scanning allows conventional radiographs of the thoracic and lumbar spine to be eliminated in the evaluation of blunt trauma patients. *J Trauma.* 2003;55(4):665-669.
257. Chance GQ. Note on a type of flexion fracture of the spine. *Br J Radiol.* 1948;21(249):452.
258. Smith WS, Kaufer H. Patterns and mechanisms of lumbar injuries associated with lap seat belts. *J Bone Joint Surg.* 1969;51(2):239-254.
259. Avrahami E, Tadmor R, Ram Z, Feibel M, Itzhak Y. MR demonstration of spontaneous acute epidural hematoma of the thoracic spine. *Neuroradiology.* 1989;31(1):89-92.
260. Beatty RM, Winston KR. Spontaneous cervical epidural hematoma. A consideration of etiology. *J Neurosurg.* 1984; 61(1):143-148.
261. Foo D, Rossier AB. Preoperative neurological status in predicting surgical outcome of spinal epidural hematomas. *Surg Neurol.* 1981;15(5):389-401.
262. Johnson PJ, Hahn F, McConnell J, Graham EG, Leibrock LG. The importance of MRI findings for the diagnosis of nontraumatic lumbar subacute subdural haematomas. *Acta Neurochir (Wien).* 1991;113(3-4):186-188.
263. Levy JM. Spontaneous lumbar subdural hematoma. *AJNR Am J Neuroradiol.* 1990;11(4):780-781.

CHAPTER 14 Electrodiagnostic Examination

Jinny Tavee

The electrodiagnostic examination is comprised of two parts: the nerve conduction studies (NCSs) and the needle electrode examination (NEE). Together, they assess the peripheral sensory and motor nervous system. *Sensory* NCSs assess the integrity of dorsal root ganglion (DRG) cells (usually residing within the intervertebral foramina), their axonal projections within mixed sensory and motor nerve trunks, and arborizations into individual nerve fibers innervating sensory organs subserving primarily vibration and proprioception. *Motor* NCSs assess the integrity of anterior horn cells (in the anterior region of the spinal cord), their axonal projections within pure motor or mixed nerve trunks, arborizations into individual motor nerve fibers, the neuromuscular junctions, and attached muscle fibers.

The electrodiagnostic examination is best conceptualized as an extension of the neurologic examination of the peripheral nervous system. In the setting of abnormalities identified in the neurologic history and examination, the electrodiagnostic examination can be valuable in (1) confirming the clinical impression, (2) investigating the presence of other conditions in the differential diagnosis, and (3) localizing the precise site of a focal nerve trunk lesion not clearly defined on clinical examination.

The electrodiagnostic examination can discriminate between the two main types of pathologic responses that can affect nerve fibers: axon loss (neurotmesis and axonotmesis) and demyelinating conduction block (neurapraxia). In cases of axon loss, the electrodiagnostic examination has the potential of discriminating acute, subacute, and chronic nerve lesions. It can identify early evidence of reinnervation and can quantitatively track the reinnervation process over weeks to months. In the setting of diffuse signs and symptoms, the electrodiagnostic examination can discriminate among generalized sensory and motor polyneuropathy, myopathy, and diffuse motor axon loss processes, such as motor neuron disease.

A well-executed electrodiagnostic examination can confirm or refute the presumptive diagnosis and can provide a screening assessment for other peripheral nerve and muscle conditions that could reasonably be the cause of the patient's symptoms. In that way, the electrodiagnostic examination should be thought of as an electrodiagnostic consultation and not solely a test to rule in a specific diagnosis. Qualified electrodiagnostic consultants usually are board certified in electrodiagnosis, clinical neurophysiology, or neuromuscular medicine, having completed an approved training program and having shown competence by examination. The electrodiagnostic examination must be interpreted by the individual performing the study, because there is no single machine-generated tracing (as would be the case for an electrocardiogram or electroencephalogram) that can be interpreted simply by reviewing data collected elsewhere.

Pathophysiology

The clinical practice of electrodiagnosis is based on numerous precepts that are derived from the pathophysiology of nerve and muscle function. These provide the basic principles that define the clinical utility and limits of this procedure.

Regardless of etiology, most focal nerve lesions—including lesions at the root level—result in either *axon loss* or *demyelination*. Axon loss produces nerve transmission failure along the affected fibers; focal demyelination causes either conduction block or conduction slowing at the lesion site, depending on its severity. One fundamental difference between these two types of lesions is that focal demyelination remains localized and does not materially affect the segments of the axon proximal or distal to the lesion. In contrast, an axon-loss lesion results in wallerian degeneration, which eventually involves the entire course of the nerve affected.

Because axon loss and demyelinating conduction block stop nerve impulse transmission across the lesion site rather than merely slowing it, both can result in clinical weakness and sensory abnormalities whenever they affect a sufficient number of motor and sensory axons. However, demyelinating conduction slowing does not affect muscle strength. This is because all of the nerve impulses ultimately reach their destination, although slightly later in time than they normally would.[1]

The electrodiagnostic examination assesses the integrity of large sensory and motor nerve fibers, but not small fibers, as the electrical fields that they generate are too small to reach the recording electrodes in routine studies. For this reason, pain alone cannot be assessed because that sensory modality is mediated through small C-type nerve fibers. When pain is associated with large nerve fiber dysfunction, such as weakness, electrodiagnostic testing is more valuable.

General Concepts of Electrodiagnostic Examination

Nerve Conduction Studies

NCSs are the first component of the electrodiagnostic examination. During the NCS, a peripheral nerve is stimulated, resulting in an electrical response generated directly by the nerve itself (as with a sensory response) or the muscle that it innervates (as with a motor response). The duration and intensity of the stimulus are gradually increased until a maximal response is generated. These responses are recorded using surface electrodes placed over the skin and then analyzed. During each study, valuable information is produced regarding the number of functioning nerve fibers, the speed of conduction along those fibers, and their relative rates of conduction.

Three basic types of NCS are available: motor, sensory, and mixed (Fig. 14.1). Motor and sensory NCSs are generally performed on every patient. Mixed NCSs are typically used in the evaluation of specific disorders, such as carpal tunnel syndrome, and are of limited value in the evaluation of spine-related nerve pathology. NCS protocols vary depending on the diagnosis in question, and can be tailored to help exclude other diagnoses in the differential. Most electrodiagnostic laboratories have a routine protocol for a general study of the upper extremity (Table 14.1) and lower extremity (Table 14.2).

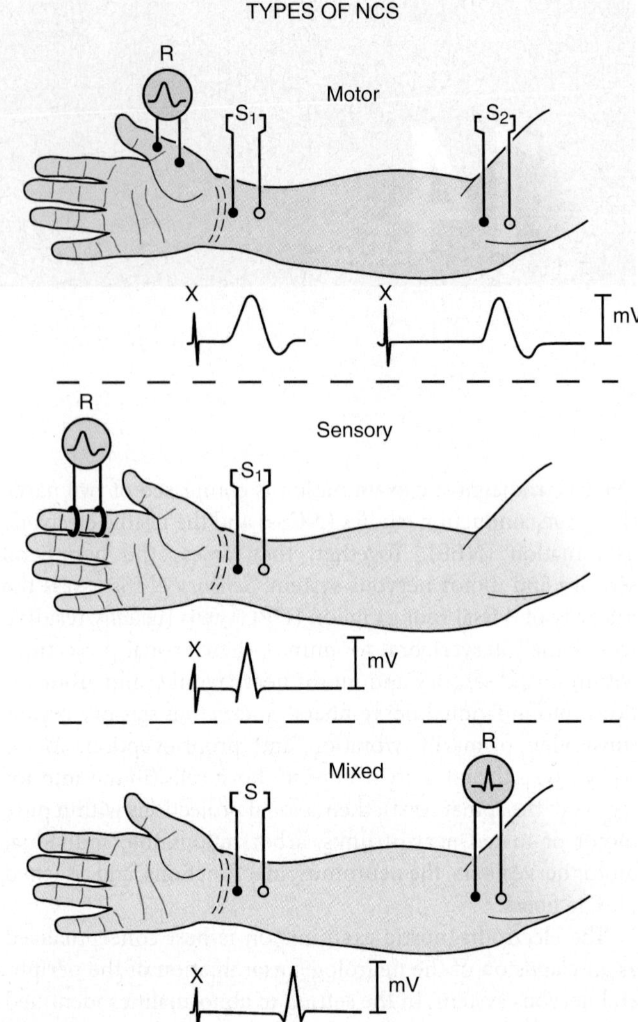

FIG. 14.1 Three basic types of nerve conduction studies: motor, sensory, and mixed (S_1 and S_2 are stimulation sites, R is the recording site, and X overlies the shock artifact.) (Modified from Isle M, Krauss G, Levin K, et al. Electromyography/Electroencephalography. Redford, WA: Spacelabs Medical; 1993:4.)

Motor Nerve Conduction Studies

For motor NCSs, the recording electrode is placed over the muscle belly, and the reference electrode is affixed over the tendon. The nerve supplying that muscle is stimulated; the resulting motor nerve response is a compound muscle action potential (CMAP), a biphasic waveform that represents summated muscle fiber action potentials (Fig. 14.2). In routine

TABLE 14.1 Nerve Conduction Studies in the Upper Limb

Motor	Sensory
Standard	
Median: thenar (C8, **T1**)	Median: index (C6, **C7**)
Ulnar: hypothenar (**C8**, T1)	Ulnar: fifth (C8)
Nonstandard	
Ulnar: first dorsal interosseous (C8, T1)	Median: thumb (C6)
Radial: extensor indicis proprius (C8)	Median: middle (C7)
Radial: brachioradialis (**C5, C6**)	Ulnar: hand dorsum (C8)
Musculocutaneous: biceps (C5, **C6**)	Radial: thumb base (**C6, C7**)
Axillary: deltoid (**C5**, C6)	Lateral antebrachial cutaneous: forearm (C6)
	Medial antebrachial cutaneous: forearm (T1)

The nerve being studied is listed first, followed by the recording site, then the root innervation (motor) or derivation (sensory). **Bolded** root provides major innervation.

TABLE 14.2 Nerve Conduction Studies in the Lower Limb

Motor	Sensory
Standard	
Peroneal: extensor digitorum brevis (L5–S1)	Sural: lateral ankle (S1)
Tibial: abductor hallucis (S1)	
Nonstandard	
Peroneal: tibialis anterior (L5)	Superficial peroneal sensory: dorsum ankle (L5)
Tibial: abductor digiti quinti pedis (S1)	Saphenous: medial ankle (L4)[b]
Tibial: gastrocnemii (S1)[a]	Lateral femoral cutaneous: lateral thigh (L3, L4)[b]
Femoral: quadriceps (L3, L4)	

The nerve being studied is listed first, followed by the recording site, then the root innervation (motor) or derivation (sensory).

[a]M component of H response.

[b]Studies are technically difficult to perform.

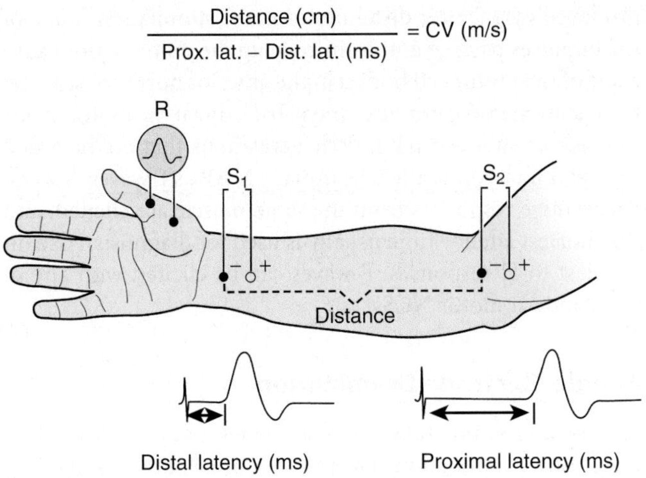

$$\frac{\text{Distance (cm)}}{\text{Prox. lat.} - \text{Dist. lat. (ms)}} = \text{CV (m/s)}$$

Distal latency (ms) Proximal latency (ms)

FIG. 14.2 Various components of the motor nerve conduction study assessing the median nerve. Dist. lat., distal latency; Prox. lat., proximal latency. (Modified from Isle M, Krauss G, Levin K, et al. Electromyography/Electroencephalography. Redford, WA: Spacelabs Medical; 1993:40.)

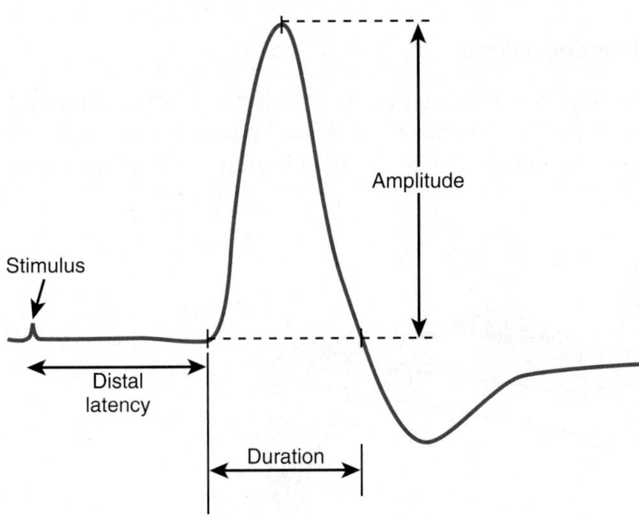

FIG. 14.3 Compound muscle action potential. Distal latency is measured from the stimulus to onset of the negative response. Amplitude is measured from the baseline to the negative peak.

motor NCSs, small muscles of the hand and feet serve as recording muscles; the nerves supplying them are stimulated at two separate points along their course. For the upper extremity, the wrist (distal) and elbow (proximal) are used as stimulation sites. For the lower extremity, the ankle (distal) and knee (proximal) are used as stimulation sites.

Numerous parameters are assessed with each CMAP obtained, including amplitude, latency, and conduction velocity (Fig. 14.3). The CMAP *amplitude* represents the number of nerve fibers that responded to the stimulus and are capable of conducting impulses to the recorded muscle.[1,2] It is measured from baseline to negative peak (negative being up) and reported in millivolts. The *latency* is the time interval between the instant that the nerve was stimulated and the onset of the CMAP, and is reported in milliseconds. The *conduction velocity* is the speed of transmission over the fastest

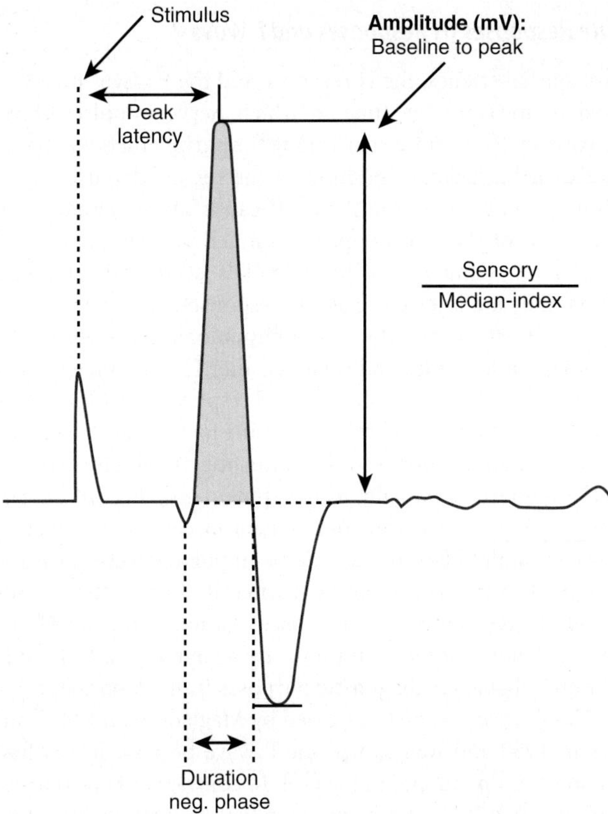

FIG. 14.4 Sensory nerve action potential. Peak latency is measured to the onset of the negative phase. Amplitude is measured from the baseline to the negative peak.

conducting nerve fibers assessed and is reported in meters per second. Conduction velocities are calculated by dividing the distance traveled along a nerve segment (as determined by surface measurements) by the latency difference between the responses to proximal and distal stimulation. Normal conduction velocity in the upper limb is greater than 50 m/s; in the lower limb, it is greater than 40 m/s.

Sensory Nerve Conduction Studies

For sensory NCSs, a sensory nerve or the sensory component of a mixed nerve is stimulated at one point with recording electrodes placed distally, usually on the fingers or on the ankle with routine studies. This stimulation results in a sensory nerve action potential (SNAP), which is a biphasic or triphasic waveform that represents summated nerve action potentials. In contrast to CMAPs, which are generated by motor units and are measured in millivolts, SNAPs are generated directly by the nerve fibers. SNAPs are 100 times smaller and are measured in microvolts. Generally, only two sensory NCS measurements are reported: (1) the *amplitude,* which is the height of the response measured from baseline to negative peak and represents the number of sensory axons that depolarize; and (2) the *peak latency,* which is the time interval between the moment that the nerve was stimulated and the negative peak of the response, reported in milliseconds (Fig. 14.4).[1]

Late Responses (H Responses and F Waves)

Two special studies, the H response and the F wave, are NCSs used to measure the time in which nerve impulses travel proximally to the spinal cord along the peripheral nerve trunk and then back down the limb to the recorded muscle after distal stimulation of the nerve. Because the potentials seen with both of these techniques are much delayed after nerve stimulation compared with potentials seen with standard NCSs, they are referred to as late responses.

The *H response* is the electrophysiologic correlate of the Achilles tendon reflex and is named after Hoffmann, who first described it in 1918. To obtain the H response, the tibial nerve is stimulated in the popliteal fossa using low voltage to activate sensory fibers (as opposed to motor fibers), which carry the nerve impulse proximally to the spinal cord (Fig. 14.5). The fibers synapse there with motor neuron cells to complete a monosynaptic reflex arc. The nerve impulse travels down the motor efferent nerve to the gastrocnemius, where the recording electrode captures the response. Although the amplitude and the latency of the H response are analyzed, the amplitude is more reliable for diagnostic purposes in my laboratory.

The *F wave* was first described by Magladery and McDougall in 1950 and was named the F wave because it was first recorded from muscles in the foot. In contrast to H responses, F waves are not a component of a reflex arc because the nerve impulses recorded travel only along motor axons. F waves are produced when, after distal motor nerve stimulation, some of the impulses passing antidromically up the motor axons cause a few of the motor cell bodies in the anterior horns to backfire; the resulting nerve impulses travel back down the motor axons to produce submaximal muscle activations that are recorded several milliseconds after the initial CMAP as F waves. Several consecutive responses from the same muscle are elicited, and the shortest latency time usually is used for diagnosis. Also, in contrast to H responses, F waves can be elicited with any of the standard motor NCSs.

Needle Electrode Examination

NEE is the second and oldest component of the basic electrodiagnostic examination. During this procedure, a recording needle electrode is inserted into various muscles, and the electrical activity being generated in them is evaluated on a visual and audio display system via a differential amplifier. NEE records activity in muscle (1) at rest during needle insertion, (2) at rest without needle movement, and (3) during voluntary muscle activation.

Insertional Phase

During the *insertional phase,* the electrical activity resulting from needle movement in a relaxed muscle is evaluated. In a normal muscle, each needle insertion and advancement

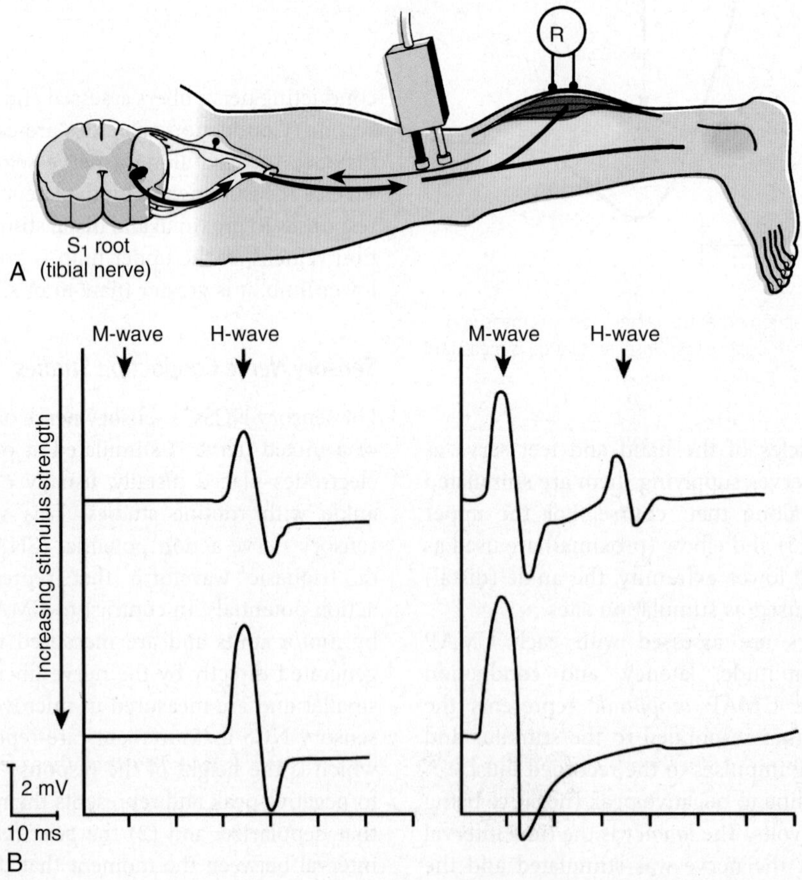

FIG. 14.5 Standard lower limb H response. (A) With minimal stimulus strength, only the H wave is elicited. (B) As stimulation strength increases, the M wave appears and becomes progressively larger, while the H wave progressively loses amplitude.

injures a few individual muscle fibers, which generate a small burst of electrical potentials called *insertional activity*. These electrical potentials prove that the needle electrode is in a viable muscle because they are not seen if it is in subcutaneous tissue, fat, or severely fibrotic muscle. In the context of peripheral nerve fiber lesions, if the NEE is performed on a partially denervated muscle a few days before spontaneous fibrillation potentials appear (discussed later), the insertional activity is abnormal in that unsustained trains of insertional positive sharp waves are seen.

At-Rest Phase

During the *at-rest phase,* electrical silence ordinarily is noted. With neuromuscular pathology, various types of spontaneous activity may be discernible. Only three of these are relevant to spine-related nerve disease: fibrillation potentials, fasciculation potentials, and complex repetitive discharges.[2–4]

Fibrillation potentials are spontaneous, usually regularly firing action potentials of individual muscle fibers. Although nonspecific in that they can be seen with neuropathic and myopathic disorders, their presence indicates denervation. Fibrillation potentials typically appear in the form of a biphasic spike if the tip of the recording needle electrode is near the denervated muscle fiber. Alternatively, they may appear as a positive sharp wave if the needle has injured the abnormal muscle fiber. In the setting of nerve lesions, fibrillation potentials are not present at the onset of motor axon loss. Instead, they are first seen 14 to 35 days after axon degeneration has been initiated; the most widely cited average time is 21 days. When established, fibrillation potentials persist until the denervated muscle fibers generating them either reinnervate or degenerate for lack of a nerve supply. The latter usually occurs 18 to 24 months after the initial nerve fiber injury.

Fibrillation potentials are the most reliable and objective manifestation of active or recent motor axon loss. They can be neither produced nor abolished voluntarily by the patient. They are very sensitive indicators of such loss because the degeneration of a single motor axon can result in hundreds of individual muscle fibers fibrillating within a given muscle, depending on the innervation ratio of the latter. Fibrillation potentials objectively can show that motor axon loss has occurred when the lesion is far too mild in degree to produce clinical muscle weakness, atrophy, or loss of CMAP amplitude on motor NCS.[3] Showing fibrillation potentials in a myotome distribution has been the principal method of identifying root lesions in the electrodiagnostic laboratory for more than half a century.[5,6]

Fasciculation potentials are spontaneous action potentials of an individual motor unit. Unlike fibrillation potentials, they are indicative of motor unit *irritation* rather than denervation; only intact motor unit potentials (MUPs) can generate them. They are encountered far less often than fibrillation potentials, being restricted essentially to radiculopathies, anterior horn cell disorders, radiation-induced plexopathies, a few entrapment neuropathies, polyneuropathies, and, most often, the syndrome of generalized benign fasciculations.

Complex repetitive discharges are produced when a single muscle fiber is depolarized and that depolarization is spread by ephaptic transmission to adjacent muscle fibers, which reactivate the initial muscle fiber. A recurrent cycle of firing is established. These potentials have a bizarre configuration and fire at high frequency. For many years, they were known as *bizarre high-frequency discharges*. Although they are abnormal, they are nonspecific, being seen with neuropathic and myopathic disorders. Generally, they appear when there is grouped atrophy (i.e., denervation, reinnervation, and subsequent denervation) and are evidence of chronicity. Although these potentials are not helpful in localization, they are frequently encountered on NEE of the cervical paraspinal muscles in patients with chronic cervical root lesions.[3]

SECTION II

Activation Phase

After the muscle is evaluated at rest, the patient is asked to contract the muscle. This contraction results in the generation of MUPs, which represent the summated electrical activity produced by contracting muscle fibers of a single motor unit. MUPs are assessed in regard to their recruitment pattern and appearance.

Recruitment

Recruitment of MUPs refers to the orderly increase in number and firing rate of activated motor units as force is increased during contraction of muscle. On initial activation of the muscle with minimal force, a single motor unit fires at its basal rate of 5 to 10 Hz. As the force is increased, additional units are recruited, and the firing rate gradually increases by 5 Hz with each additional unit—up to 20 to 30 Hz. With progressively increasing force, spatial and temporal recruitment occurs, resulting in a full interference pattern in which the screen is obscured by the firing patterns of several MUPs.

Reduced MUP recruitment, also known as a *neurogenic MUP firing pattern,* is observed whenever numerous motor units in the muscle being sampled cannot be activated on maximal effort because either conduction block or axon loss affects their axons. The fewer MUPs seen on maximal effort, the weaker the muscle is clinically. MUPs that are capable of firing are noted to do so in decreased numbers and often faster than their basal firing rate of 5 to 10 Hz.[3,7] The rapid rate of firing of the still functioning motor units is important because, similar to fibrillation potentials, it is unequivocal evidence of involuntary interruption of motor axon impulse transmission. Conversely, if the muscle was weak because of an upper motor neuron lesion or because voluntary effort was simply submaximal (e.g., because of malingering or pain on activation), incomplete MUP activation would be seen—that is, MUPs would fire in equally decreased numbers but at a *slow to moderate rate.*

Morphology

The amplitude, duration, and configuration of MUPs are important morphologic characteristics that are assessed during the activation phase. Together, these features reflect the number and size of muscle fibers within a motor unit and their ability to fire in synchrony. Patient age, technical details (e.g., filter setting, type of needle used), and the specific muscle being examined are some of the factors that affect the appearance of MUPs. Based on quantitative analyses, normal ranges for MUP morphology are available for comparison, which vary depending on the patient age and proximity of the muscle to the trunk. A normal MUP has a triphasic waveform appearance.

With chronic nerve lesions, the process of reinnervation of denervated muscle fibers can occur as the result of regeneration of the nerve trunk from the point of nerve transection or (when the nerve transection is not total) by collateral nerve branch sprouting from remaining intact nerve fibers close to the denervated muscle fibers. The latter process is much faster because nerve fiber regeneration occurs at the rate of about 1 mm/day. On NEE, manifestations of reinnervation include resolution of fibrillation potentials; return of activation of motor unit action potentials with voluntary muscle contraction; and appearance of polyphasic, enlarged (so-called neurogenic) motor unit action potentials, reflecting the increased number of muscle fibers attached to surviving nerve fibers owing to collateral sprouting.

Chronic neurogenic MUP changes generally develop about 4 to 6 months after an axon loss injury has occurred because it takes this much time for such configurational remodeling to occur. After chronic neurogenic MUP changes develop, they can persist indefinitely. With many remote, proximal neurogenic lesions (e.g., radiculopathies and, particularly, poliomyelitis), they are the sole electrical residuals detected during the entire electrodiagnostic examination.[3,7,8]

Electrodiagnostic Findings in Radiculopathy

The electrodiagnostic examination has been used to assess patients with possible radiculopathies for more than 50 years. Root lesions were one of the first focal peripheral nerve fiber disorders for which the diagnostic utility of NEE was shown.[5,6] For many years, lumbosacral radiculopathies were the most common reason for referral to the electrodiagnostic laboratory.[9,10] Although several other electrodiagnostic procedures have been introduced over the past half-century, NEE remains the mainstay for diagnosing radiculopathies. The amplitudes of motor NCS are also helpful when root damage is severe, extensive, or both.[8,9]

Radiculopathies are most commonly caused by nerve root compression secondary to degenerative spine changes, disc herniation, or rupture. The type of nerve pathology at the lesion site depends on the nature of the injury and degree of nerve compression. When the injury results in significant motor axon loss, NEE shows numerous abnormalities, including the presence of fibrillation potentials in corresponding myotomes. Demyelinating conduction block may also be inferred by findings on the electrodiagnostic examination. In many cases of nerve root disease, the electrodiagnostic examination can provide invaluable information regarding localization, severity, age of the lesion, and nerve pathophysiology.

Nerve Conduction Studies

Routine Studies

Axon loss occurs when the axon is disconnected from its cell body. The motor cell body (anterior horn cell) resides in the anterior zone of the spinal cord; the sensory cell body (DRG) resides outside the spinal cord, either within individual intervertebral foramina or within the spinal canal (intradural and intraarachnoid) (Fig. 14.6). A disc protrusion causing severe compression of a motor and sensory nerve root within the spinal canal disconnects the anterior horn cell from its motor axon, but if the DRG is distal to the point of compression, the extraspinal sensory axons remain connected to their DRG and do not undergo degeneration (see Fig. 14.6). In that setting, motor NCSs show amplitude loss, but sensory NCSs are normal despite marked clinical sensory impairment with few exceptions.

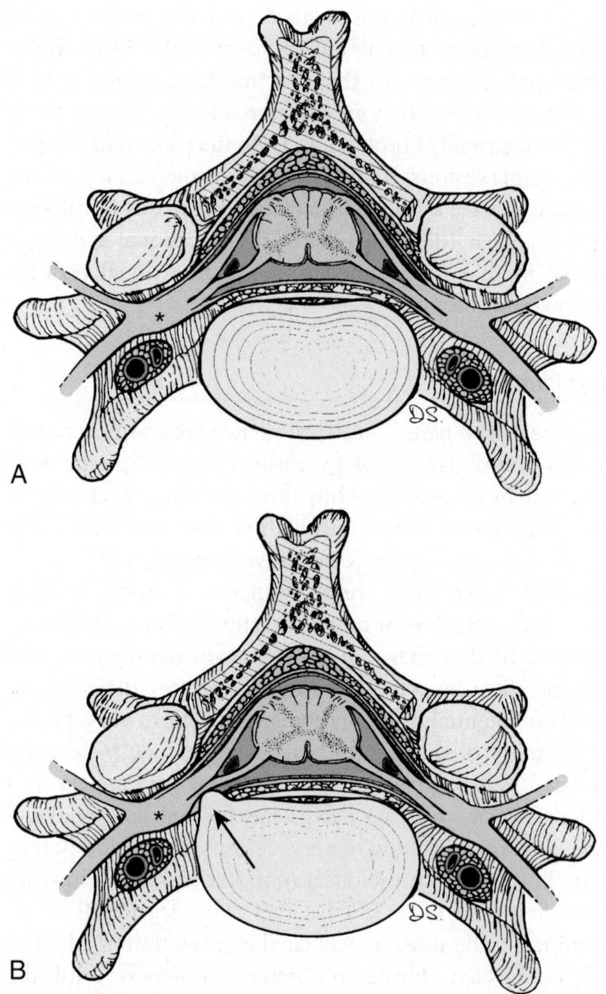

FIG. 14.6 Cross-sectional views of cervical region, showing (A) relationship of dorsal root ganglia (*asterisk*) to surrounding structures and (B) usual site of disc herniation (*arrow*). Preganglionic sensory root fibers usually are compromised.

One exception is seen with nerve root pathology that extends beyond the intraspinal canal. A mass lesion (e.g., meningioma) or infiltrative process (e.g., malignancy, inflammatory cause, or infection) that progresses distally along the nerve root to involve the DRG can result in decreased SNAP amplitudes. The other exception is when the DRG resides inside the intraspinal canal, proximal to the intervertebral foramina; this has been found to occur in the lumbosacral region. Based on cadaveric, radiographic, and magnetic resonance imaging (MRI) studies, 3% of L3 and L4 DRG are intraspinal, about 11% to 38% of L5 DRG are intraspinal, and 71% of S1 DRG are intraspinal.[11] As a result, root lesions in the lower spine, particularly lesions involving the L5 root, can affect the corresponding SNAP amplitude, which in the case of an L5 lesion is the superficial peroneal SNAP (discussed later). SNAP peak latency and nerve conduction velocity are never involved in radiculopathy, however.

The CMAP amplitude is the only portion of motor NCS that may be significantly affected in radiculopathy. Because it is a measure of the number of viable, conducting nerve fibers, the CMAP amplitude can be decreased with severe motor axon-loss lesions. The ulnar CMAP amplitude would be reduced in a severe C8 radiculopathy. In chronic lesions, reinnervation changes, such as collateral sprouting, can contribute to the CMAP amplitude and may lead to normal or near-normal values over time.

In many cases, motor NCSs remain relatively unaffected in radiculopathies for two reasons. First, most radiculopathies result in only partial nerve injuries. For the CMAP amplitude to be significantly reduced on motor NCS, about half of the motor axons within the peripheral nerve trunk need to be lost or injured. Second, the myotomes of the affected nerve root must be accessible to stimulation and recording. The ulnar-innervated hand muscles may be examined for a C8 radiculopathy, and the biceps and deltoids are available for assessing a C5 radiculopathy. Muscles innervated by C6 and C7 nerve roots cannot be reliably examined with routine motor NCSs, however, owing to technical factors and overlap in innervation.

Late Responses

Although the H response and F wave are theoretically helpful in the evaluation of the damaged proximal nerve root segment, there are technical limitations to each procedure that can hamper their utility in the evaluation of a radiculopathy.[7,9] Because the H response is elicited by stimulating the tibial nerve in the popliteal fossa while recording from the gastrocnemius/soleus muscle group, as described previously, it is highly sensitive and very useful in the evaluation of S1 radiculopathy. In axon loss lesions affecting the S1 nerve root, the amplitude may be either reduced or absent. The normal value of the H amplitude, as defined by my electrodiagnostic laboratory, is 1 mV, with abnormal values being either less than 1 mV or reduced by 50% compared with the contralateral response. Additionally, the H response may become abnormal at the onset of nerve root injury and remain so until the injury is resolved or may remain abnormal despite resolution of clinical symptoms.[7]

A major limitation of the H responses is that they are frequently absent bilaterally in patients older than 60 years, in patients with polyneuropathies, and in patients who have had lumbar laminectomies even when the S1 roots reportedly were not within the operative field. Also, when the H responses are abnormal, they do not localize to the S1 root because the lesion could be at many other points along the extended neural pathway that the impulses traverse (e.g., S1 spinal cord segment, sacral plexus, sciatic nerve, and proximal tibial nerve). When H responses are abnormal, they remain so indefinitely in many cases.[8,9]

Despite these limiting and confounding factors, H responses are very helpful in the evaluation of a possible lumbosacral radiculopathy because they are seldom normal with S1 root lesions. Part of their high sensitivity may be because, in contrast to all other constituents of the electrodiagnostic examination, they evaluate the preganglionic components of the S1 sensory root fibers.[8,9] Although most electrodiagnostic physicians agree on the value of H responses, they disagree regarding which component (amplitude or latency) of the H response is likely to be abnormal.[9,12–14]

Ideally, F waves should be able to detect demyelinating conduction slowing along the motor fibers at the root level.[9,15,16] However, this is not the case in practical application. They are often normal in unequivocal cases of radiculopathy, and even when abnormal, they do not provide any additional information because the abnormalities are already clearly seen on NEE.[4,7] Therefore, F waves are of no significant value in the evaluation of root lesions.

Needle Electrode Examination

Because NCSs and the late responses generally are normal with isolated root lesions (except for the H response with S1 radiculopathies), NEE usually is the sole component of the electrodiagnostic examination that is beneficial in detecting a radiculopathy. The diagnosis depends on finding abnormalities on NEE in a root or *myotome* (all the muscles that receive innervation from a single spinal cord segment or root). These abnormalities include insertional positive sharp waves, fibrillation potentials, a reduced or neurogenic recruitment of motor units, and changes in the motor unit morphology (e.g., increased duration, amplitude, and polyphasia).

The most widely used criterion for diagnosing radiculopathies by NEE is that abnormalities should be found in two, and preferably more, limb muscles innervated by the same root but different peripheral nerves. In addition, muscles in the limb not innervated by the damaged root, but rather by the roots contiguous to it, should appear normal. For instance, a patient with a C7 radiculopathy should have fibrillation potentials or other signs of denervation in the triceps (radial nerve) and pronator teres (median nerve), but not the abductor digiti minimi or deltoid muscles. Needle electromyography (EMG) not only should be tailored to the clinical question and the patient's symptoms, but it also should include a comprehensive survey of a sufficient number of muscles (proximal and distal when possible) to make a reliable diagnosis of a radiculopathy.

Numerous myotome charts derived from radiographic, cadaveric, and electrodiagnostic studies have been established to help guide the electrodiagnostic physician in choosing the best muscles to examine for each patient (Figs. 14.7 through 14.9). A radiculopathy screen in my laboratory consists of an examination of at least seven muscles, including the paraspinals, to help with localization in the upper extremity (Table 14.3) and lower extremity (Table 14.4). The presence of fibrillation potentials in the paraspinals is typically indicative of an

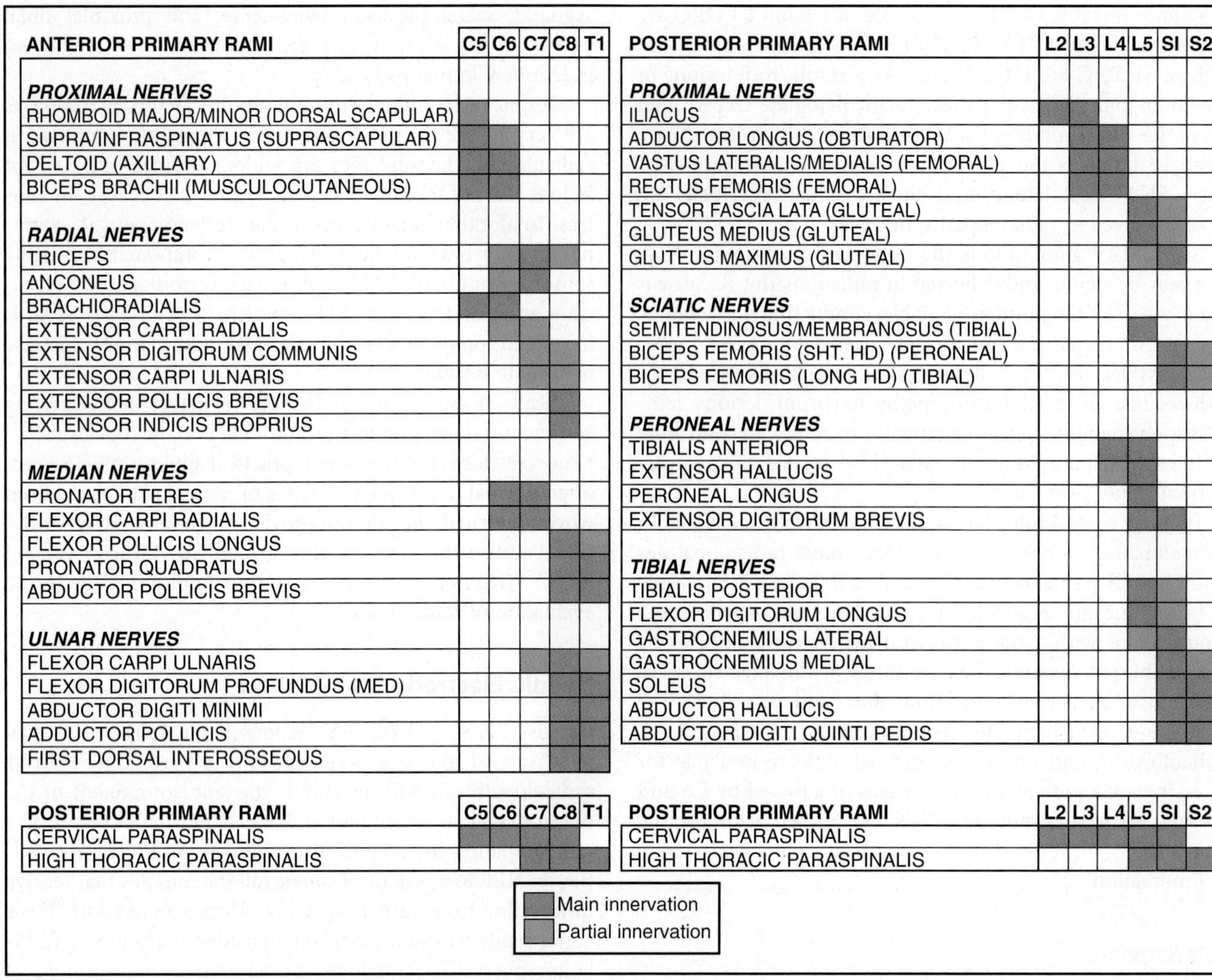

ANTERIOR PRIMARY RAMI	C5	C6	C7	C8	T1
PROXIMAL NERVES					
RHOMBOID MAJOR/MINOR (DORSAL SCAPULAR)					
SUPRA/INFRASPINATUS (SUPRASCAPULAR)					
DELTOID (AXILLARY)					
BICEPS BRACHII (MUSCULOCUTANEOUS)					
RADIAL NERVES					
TRICEPS					
ANCONEUS					
BRACHIORADIALIS					
EXTENSOR CARPI RADIALIS					
EXTENSOR DIGITORUM COMMUNIS					
EXTENSOR CARPI ULNARIS					
EXTENSOR POLLICIS BREVIS					
EXTENSOR INDICIS PROPRIUS					
MEDIAN NERVES					
PRONATOR TERES					
FLEXOR CARPI RADIALIS					
FLEXOR POLLICIS LONGUS					
PRONATOR QUADRATUS					
ABDUCTOR POLLICIS BREVIS					
ULNAR NERVES					
FLEXOR CARPI ULNARIS					
FLEXOR DIGITORUM PROFUNDUS (MED)					
ABDUCTOR DIGITI MINIMI					
ADDUCTOR POLLICIS					
FIRST DORSAL INTEROSSEOUS					

POSTERIOR PRIMARY RAMI	C5	C6	C7	C8	T1
CERVICAL PARASPINALIS					
HIGH THORACIC PARASPINALIS					

POSTERIOR PRIMARY RAMI	L2	L3	L4	L5	SI	S2
PROXIMAL NERVES						
ILIACUS						
ADDUCTOR LONGUS (OBTURATOR)						
VASTUS LATERALIS/MEDIALIS (FEMORAL)						
RECTUS FEMORIS (FEMORAL)						
TENSOR FASCIA LATA (GLUTEAL)						
GLUTEUS MEDIUS (GLUTEAL)						
GLUTEUS MAXIMUS (GLUTEAL)						
SCIATIC NERVES						
SEMITENDINOSUS/MEMBRANOSUS (TIBIAL)						
BICEPS FEMORIS (SHT. HD) (PERONEAL)						
BICEPS FEMORIS (LONG HD) (TIBIAL)						
PERONEAL NERVES						
TIBIALIS ANTERIOR						
EXTENSOR HALLUCIS						
PERONEAL LONGUS						
EXTENSOR DIGITORUM BREVIS						
TIBIAL NERVES						
TIBIALIS POSTERIOR						
FLEXOR DIGITORUM LONGUS						
GASTROCNEMIUS LATERAL						
GASTROCNEMIUS MEDIAL						
SOLEUS						
ABDUCTOR HALLUCIS						
ABDUCTOR DIGITI QUINTI PEDIS						

POSTERIOR PRIMARY RAMI	L2	L3	L4	L5	SI	S2
CERVICAL PARASPINALIS						
HIGH THORACIC PARASPINALIS						

Main innervation
Partial innervation

FIG. 14.7 Traditional myotome chart. (From Wilbourn AJ, Aminoff MF. Radiculopathies. In Brown WF, Bolton CF, eds. *Clinical Electromyography*. 2nd ed. Boston: Butterworth-Heinemann; 1993:192.)

TABLE 14.3 Screening Needle Electrode Examination for the Arm

Muscle	Root Level	Nerve Trunk
First dorsal interosseous	C8	Ulnar
Extensor indicis proprius	C8	Posterior interosseous (radial)
Flexor pollicis longus	C8	Anterior interosseous (median)
Pronator teres	C6–C7	Median
Triceps	C6–C7	Radial
Biceps	C5–C6	Musculocutaneous
Deltoids	C5–C6	Axillary
C7 paraspinal	Overlap	

TABLE 14.4 Screening Needle Electrode Examination for the Leg

Muscle	Root Level	Nerve Trunk
Abductor hallucis	S1	Tibial
Medial gastrocnemius	S1	Tibial
Biceps femoris (short head)	S1	Peroneal
Extensor digitorum brevis	L5–S1	Peroneal
Flexor digitorum longus	L5	Tibial
Gluteus medius	L5	Superior gluteal
Tibialis anterior	L4–L5	Peroneal
Rectus femoris	L2–L4	Femoral
S1 paraspinal	Overlap	

axon-loss lesion localized to or near the intraspinal canal, excluding the possibility of a plexopathy or more distal lesion. Paraspinal fibrillation potentials are most valuable for the support of radiculopathy when they are present at only one or two contiguous segmental levels and absent at levels above, below, and contralaterally.

Many limitations can reduce the value of the paraspinal examination. First, there is overlapping innervation of most paraspinals, which prevents accurate localization of fibrillation potentials to one specific segment or root. Second, even in proven radiculopathies, fibrillation potentials may be absent owing to reinnervation or sampling error. Third, paraspinal fibrillation potentials may be seen in diabetic patients, in patients with a prior history of spine surgery, or in some asymptomatic elderly patients. Finally, paraspinal denervation

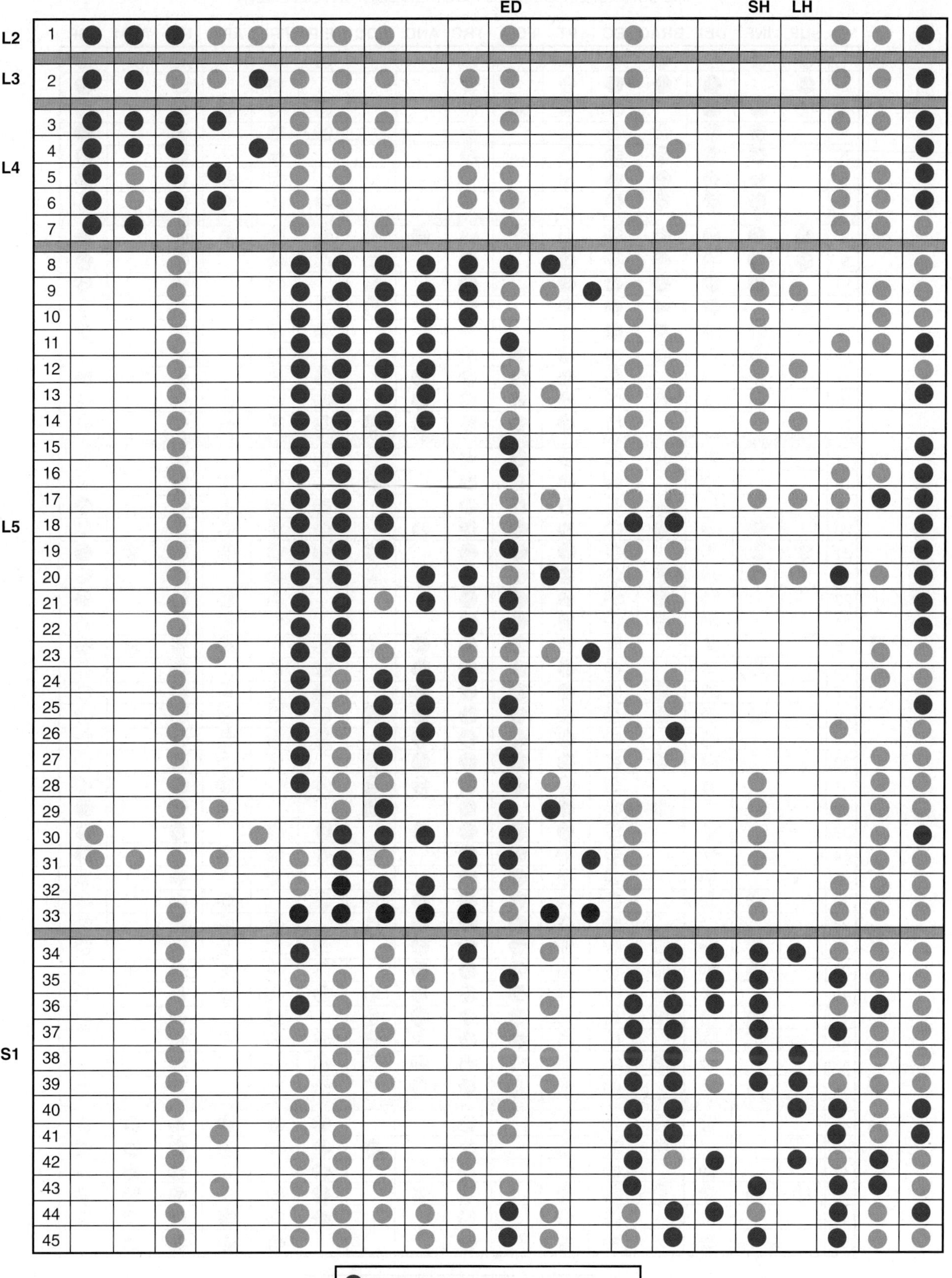

FIG. 14.8 Lower limb myotome chart. Needle electrode examination results grouped by surgically defined root level of involvement. Numbers in the left column represent patients. *Blue circle,* positive waves or fibrillation, with or without neurogenic recruitment and motor unit changes; *red circle,* neurogenic recruitment changes only; *green circle,* normal examination. (From Tsao BE, Levin KH, Bodner RA. Comparison of surgical and electrodiagnostic findings in single root lumbosacral radiculopathies. *Muscle Nerve.* 2003;27:61.)

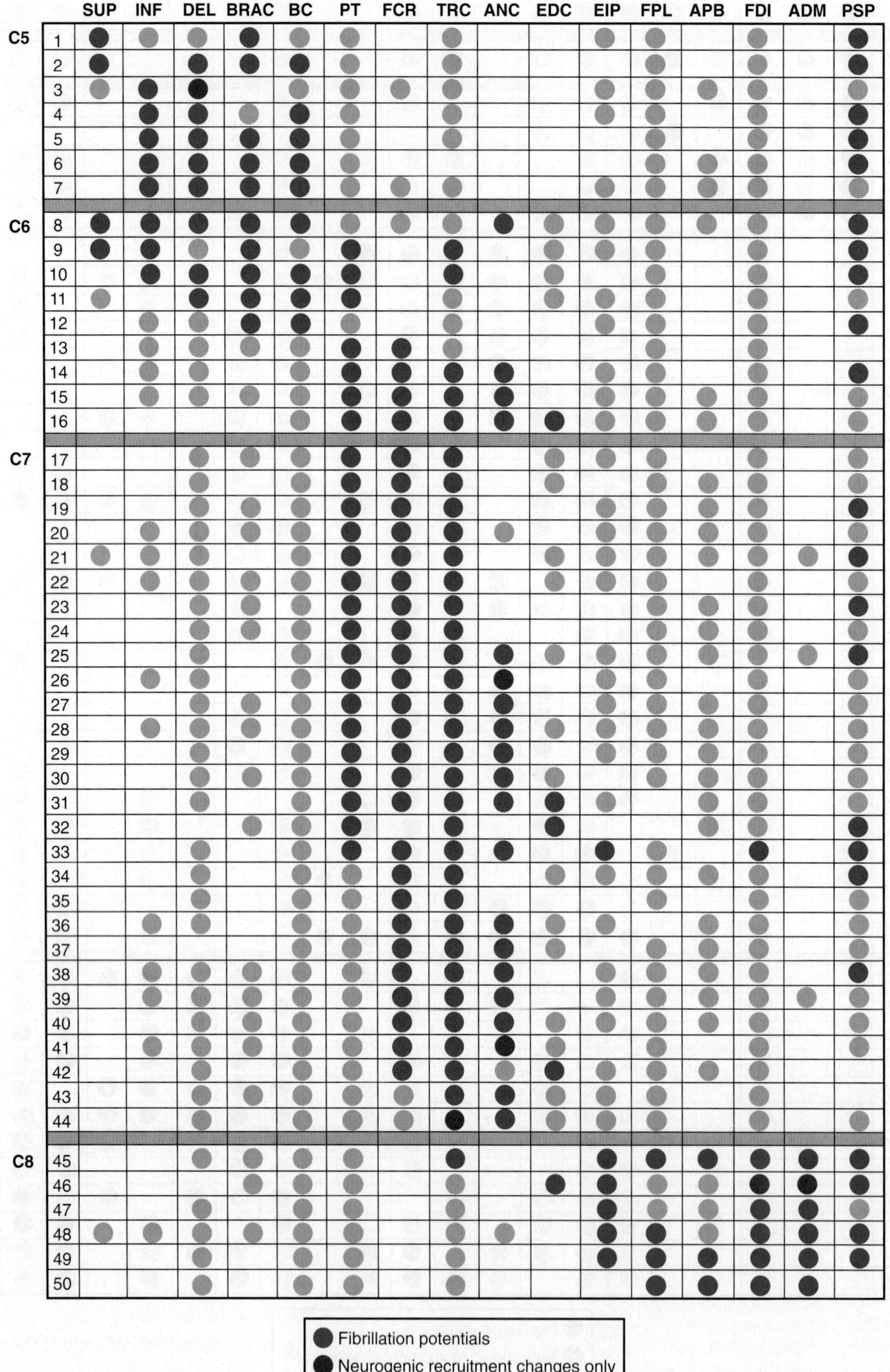

FIG. 14.9 Upper limb myotome chart. Needle electrode examination results grouped by surgically defined root level of involvement. Numbers in the left column represent patients. *Blue circle,* positive waves or fibrillation, with or without neurogenic recruitment and motor unit changes; *red circle,* neurogenic recruitment changes only; *green circle,* normal examination. (From Levin KH, Maggiano HJ, Wilbourn AJ. Cervical radiculopathies: comparison of surgical and EMG localization of single-root lesions. *Neurology.* 1996;46:1023.)

BOX 14.1 Appropriate Timing of the Electrodiagnostic Examination

- When aiming for a single comprehensive study, reliable interpretations can be made from nerve conduction studies (NCSs) and needle electrode examination (NEE) obtained any time after 3 wk from onset of symptoms.
- For earliest possible information about an axon-loss lesion, reliable interpretations can be made from NCSs obtained after 10 days from onset of symptoms.
- For earliest possible information about a demyelinating conduction block lesion (neurapraxia), such as might be the case for perioperative peroneal or ulnar neuropathy owing to positioning on the operating table, reliable interpretations can be made from NCSs obtained any time after onset of symptoms
- In the setting of preexisting symptoms of peripheral nerve disease, such as diabetic polyneuropathy, it is reasonable to consider baseline electrodiagnostic examination (NCS and NEE) immediately after the onset of new symptoms of a potential iatrogenic cause. This study is to assess the nature of preexisting abnormalities before acute changes from new symptoms are visible on electrodiagnostic examination. This is especially useful if a medicolegal issue may arise from new symptoms, because it would be valuable to differentiate preexisting nerve pathology from any procedure-related changes. A second study is necessary when sufficient time has elapsed to assess a new lesion.

is not specific to radiculopathy and is seen in other disorders, including diseases of the muscle (e.g., inflammatory myopathy) and the anterior horn cell (e.g., amyotrophic lateral sclerosis). Nonetheless, NEE of the paraspinal muscles is an integral portion of the electrodiagnostic examination and should be routinely performed in all patients with suspected nerve root disease.

The timing of needle EMG is also crucial. Fibrillation potentials do not appear in a denervated muscle until 2 to 3 weeks after the onset of the initial injury and in some patients may require 4 to 6 weeks to develop.[11] Consequently, the findings on NEE performed earlier than 3 weeks after onset of a radiculopathy are likely to be false-negative or, at best, indeterminate, even if subsequently they would be positive for a root lesion. It is optimal to wait at least 3 weeks after the onset of symptoms before performing NEE. Guidelines that help the clinician decide the best timing of a study to obtain maximal information are provided in Box 14.1. These are based on the neurophysiologic concepts of axon loss as described in Box 14.2.

Determining Duration of Radiculopathy: Acute Versus Chronic

Information regarding the duration of a radiculopathy is often derived by findings on NEE. Whenever evidence of an isolated compressive root disorder of recent onset is detected on the electrodiagnostic examination, the typical combination of findings is as follows: (1) motor NCSs are normal (unless the degree of axon loss is severe); (2) sensory NCSs are normal; (3) with S1 root involvement, the H response usually is abnormal; and (4) NEE discloses fibrillation potentials in several muscles that are innervated by the compromised root unaccompanied by changes in the size and configuration of the MUP.

BOX 14.2 Timing of Nerve Pathology: Neurophysiologic Concepts

- After transection of the motor nerve trunk, nerve conduction response amplitude from electrical stimulation distal to the transection point decreases from day 3 through days 5 to 8 after transection. For sensory nerve fibers, response amplitude decreases progressively from day 5 through days 9 to 11, coinciding with evolution of wallerian degeneration of nerve fibers. For this reason, identifying maximum axon loss cannot be assessed by nerve conduction studies until at least 11 days have elapsed since the date of nerve injury or onset of symptoms.
- As Wallerian degeneration of the motor nerve fiber reaches completion, the attached muscle fiber becomes denervated, leading to breakdown of the neuromuscular junction. Over 2 to 3 weeks, membrane changes occur along the muscle fiber, resulting in spontaneous, continuous action potential propagation along the muscle fiber, recognized during needle electrode examination (NEE) as fibrillation potentials. About 3 weeks must elapse after an acute axon-loss event before fibrillation potentials can be reliably visualized on NEE.
- The process of reinnervation of denervated muscle fibers can occur as the result of regeneration of the nerve trunk from the point of the nerve transection, or (when nerve transection is not total) by the collateral nerve branch sprouting from the remaining intact nerve fibers close to the denervated muscle fibers. The latter process is much faster because nerve fiber regeneration occurs at rate of about 1 mm/day. On NEE, manifestations of reinnervation include resolution of fibrillation potentials, return of activation of motor unit action potentials with voluntary muscle contraction, and the appearance of polyphasic motor unit potential changes.

In contrast, when chronic neurogenic MUP changes (polyphasic configuration with increased duration and amplitude) are the prominent finding on NEE with only a few fibrillation potentials, the lesion is likely to be chronic. When the chronic neurogenic MUP changes are limited to distal muscles within a myotome in the absence of fibrillation potentials, the radiculopathy is likely to be static and remote.

Finally, when fibrillation potentials and chronic neurogenic MUP changes are found in a myotome distribution, the diagnostic possibilities include a chronic, progressive radiculopathy or an acute root lesion superimposed on a remote lesion. The latter possibility is the more likely choice if fibrillation potentials are found in proximal muscles (e.g., the glutei and hamstrings with L5 or S1 root lesions), in addition to more distal muscles in the same myotome.[7–9]

When the previous factors are considered, it is apparent that whenever the classic NEE presentation of a radiculopathy is encountered—fibrillation potentials in most or all of the muscles constituting the myotome—the root lesion in question usually is of more recent onset, and motor root axon loss has been substantial. Whenever other circumstances prevail, as is far more commonly the case, fibrillation potentials usually are found in only some, if any, of the muscles of the myotome. They are typically seen in the more distal muscles. Fibrillation potentials generally are important only if they are present; their absence in any specific muscle does not exclude the diagnosis.[8,9]

Determining Severity of Radiculopathy

The severity of a nerve root lesion is based on motor NCSs and NEE. The degree of reduced MUP recruitment seen on

NEE correlates with the degree of muscle weakness and, in combination with the CMAP amplitude reduction (in muscles that can be assessed with NCS), the degree of axon loss. The amount of fibrillation potentials seen in a muscle is a subjective measure and does not correlate as well with the degree of axon loss.

Electrodiagnostic Findings at Specific Root Levels

Cervical Radiculopathy

Lesions of the cervical nerve roots account for 36% of all radiculopathies.[9] In clinical and radiographic studies, the most common root affected is at the C7 level (70% of the time) followed by C6 (19% to 25%), C8 (4% to 10%), and C5 (2%).[9,16–18] The electrodiagnostic examination presentations with C5 radiculopathies are typically manifested as abnormalities in the spinati, deltoid, biceps, and brachioradialis muscles. NCSs are typically unhelpful because proximal muscles are not assessed during routine studies, although the biceps and deltoid muscles are amenable to NCS and may show reduced CMAP amplitudes when axon loss is sufficiently severe.

C6 radiculopathies do not have a single, discrete appearance. Rather, they have two very different ones, which imitate those of C5 and C7 root lesions. Manifestations of C5 root lesions may also be seen with some C6 radiculopathies.[19] C7 lesions are diagnosed by the presence of abnormalities in some muscles innervated by radial and median nerves: the triceps and anconeus (radial) and the pronator teres and flexor carpi radialis (median). As stated before, NEE abnormalities sometimes are seen in the same combination of upper limb muscles with C6 root lesions as well.

In contrast, C8 radiculopathies have a very characteristic electrodiagnostic presentation, manifesting as abnormalities in ulnar-innervated muscles, the extensor indicis proprius, and the flexor pollicis longus.[19] Nonetheless, they can sometimes be confused with combined axon-loss lesions of the posterior interosseous nerve and the ulnar nerve whenever the ipsilateral ulnar SNAP is of low amplitude or cannot be elicited (e.g., because of advanced age or a coexisting polyneuropathy). For uncertain reasons, the axon loss that occurs with many C8 radiculopathies is exceptionally severe, so much so that the CMAPs recorded from the ulnar nerve–innervated hand muscles, particularly the hypothenar, are low in amplitude. Some of these patients never regain normal hand strength.

Differential Diagnoses

Findings on NEE of cervical radiculopathies can look identical to brachial plexopathies (Table 14.5). In particular, lesions affecting the C5 and C6 roots may resemble upper trunk plexus lesions, whereas lesions of the C8 and T1 roots can mimic lower trunk lesions. There are two critical parameters on the electrodiagnostic examination that can discern the two types of lesions. The first parameter is NEE findings in the paraspinals. With nerve root lesions, the paraspinal muscles show fibrillation potentials but are spared in a lesion of the brachial plexus. The second parameter is the assessment of the SNAPs. In radiculopathies, the lesion is located within the intraspinal canal and proximal to the DRG, which results in normal SNAPs. In plexopathies, the lesion is distal to the DRG, producing reduced amplitude or absent SNAPs.

TABLE 14.5 Disorders Commonly Confused With Compressive Radiculopathies

Roots	Entity
Cervical	
C5, C6	Upper trunk brachial plexopathy Neuralgic amyotrophy Axillary/suprascapular neuropathies Motor neuron disease Rotator cuff tear
C6, C7	Carpal tunnel syndrome
C8, T1	Lower trunk brachial plexopathy Ulnar neuropathy Motor neuron disease
Thoracic	
T1	Neurogenic thoracic outlet syndrome
Lumbosacral	
L2–L4	Diabetic amyotrophy Lumbar plexopathy Femoral neuropathy
L5	Sacral plexopathy Peroneal neuropathy Motor neuron disease
S1, S2	Sacral plexopathy Sciatic neuropathy Tibial neuropathy
Bilateral (L5), S1, S2	Polyneuropathy

Clinically, this second parameter is especially important when distinguishing a radiculopathy from neuralgic amyotrophy, which commonly affects proximal shoulder girdle muscles (e.g., the spinati and the deltoids) derived from C5 and C6 roots. Abnormally reduced or absent SNAP amplitudes of the lateral antebrachial cutaneous sensory nerve and median sensory branch recording from the thumb and index finger point to a plexus lesion.

Likewise, carpal tunnel syndrome can resemble C6 and C7 radiculopathies clinically but are easily distinguished by the presence of abnormalities seen in the triceps and pronator teres and other muscles proximal to the hand or outside of the median nerve territory. In contrast, C8 radiculopathies may be difficult to discern from an ulnar mononeuropathy, especially in the setting of partial lesions in which the ulnar SNAP is unaffected. Finding abnormalities in C8-innervated radial muscles is important in this setting. Finally, unless a rotator cuff injury results in entrapment of a nerve innervating proximal muscles located in the shoulder girdle (e.g., suprascapular nerve), the electrodiagnostic examination would show no abnormalities.

Thoracic Radiculopathy

Radiculopathies in this region are difficult to assess by electrodiagnostic examination because there are relatively few muscles in each myotome, and only some of them can be sampled. With suspected thoracic radiculopathies, only the paraspinal and abdominal muscles are sampled routinely; the intercostal muscles are typically not studied for fear of entering the pleural space. Generally, if NEE abnormalities are seen, no attempt is made to identify a specific root lesion. Instead, the localization is limited to upper thoracic, midthoracic, or lower thoracic root involvement. Most patients found to have thoracic radiculopathies have diabetes mellitus, and the pathology is probably root infarction or ischemia rather than compression. In any case, these radiculopathies often produce very severe axon loss and frequently apparently involve two or more adjacent roots.[9,20,21] T1 radiculopathies are quite rare and typically produce changes only in the lateral thenar muscles.[22]

Differential Diagnoses

Although neurogenic thoracic outlet syndrome may technically be considered an extraspinal radiculopathy affecting the T1 nerve root and to a lesser extent C8, it has classically been categorized as a lower trunk brachial plexopathy (see Table 14.5). The preferential involvement of the T1 nerve root leads to prominent abnormalities of the abductor pollicis brevis muscle and the medial antebrachial cutaneous sensory response, both of which are heavily innervated by T1. In contrast, the ulnar-innervated segments, which are predominantly innervated by C8, are sometimes spared or only mildly affected. Abnormalities in the abductor pollicis brevis are evident on motor NCS (manifested as decreased CMAP amplitude) and NEE (fibrillation potentials or neurogenic recruitment pattern), whereas the medial antebrachial cutaneous SNAP is reduced or absent. The latter abnormality is helpful in distinguishing this syndrome from a typical T1 radiculopathy.

Lumbosacral Radiculopathy

Nerve root lesions are most commonly seen in the lumbosacral spine—more than two-thirds of all radiculopathies occur in this region.[7] In contrast to lesions involving the cervical roots, it is difficult sometimes to localize lumbosacral radiculopathies accurately to a vertebral level with the electrodiagnostic examination. This difficulty is primarily due to anatomic reasons. Given their long intraspinal course, lumbosacral nerve roots may be injured anywhere along their tract from the T12–L1 vertebral level where they are formed, down through the canal into the cauda equina, and the site where they exit from their respective foramina. The L5 nerve root can be compressed by a central disc herniation at the L3–L4 level, a posterolateral disc herniation at the L4–L5 level, or foraminal stenosis at the L5–S1 level. Additionally, when nerves are affected at the level of the cauda equina where the fibers are compact, a single lesion in this location can result in injury to multiple roots bilaterally. It is important to perform comparison NEE of the contralateral limb when any abnormalities are seen to exclude the possibility of subclinical nerve root involvement.

L2, L3, and L4 radiculopathies are generally considered together because of the myotome overlap of the thigh muscles and the paucity of muscles that are innervated solely by one individual nerve root. Localization of an L2 root lesion is difficult because only the iliacus muscle may show abnormalities on NEE. Lesions at these levels typically produce denervation changes in the quadriceps, thigh adductors, and iliacus. With L4 lesions, abnormalities may also be seen in the tibialis anterior occasionally.

The most common lumbosacral radiculopathies involve the L5 and S1 roots. Lesions of these two roots are most amenable to recognition on electrodiagnostic examination. In addition, the L5 nerve root is the most common single radiculopathy seen.[3] L5 radiculopathies produce abnormalities in the tibialis anterior, flexor digitorum longus, and posterior tibialis in greater than 75% of surgically proven cases.[23] In a more recent study, 100% of patients with L5 radiculopathies, which were also surgically proven, showed abnormalities in the peroneus longus and tensor fascia lata.[24] Changes may also be seen in the extensor digitorum brevis, gluteus medius, and semitendinosus.

An exception to the rule that SNAPs are not affected in radiculopathies has been found to occur with some L5 root lesions. As stated before, SNAPs are typically spared in radiculopathies because the lesion is situated proximal to sensory cell bodies (DRG), which lie in the intervertebral foramina *outside* of the intraspinal canal. However, at the level of the lumbosacral spine, the DRG is sometimes found proximal to the intervertebral foramina *within* the intraspinal canal, leaving them vulnerable to injury from a herniated disc or other degenerative spine condition. Based on cadaveric, radiographic, and MRI studies, 3% of L3 and L4 DRG are intraspinal, 11% to 38% of L5 DRG are intraspinal, and up to 71% of S1 DRG are intraspinal.[24–26] Thus, in some cases, the L5 nerve root may be affected distal to the DRG, resulting in an abnormal superficial peroneal SNAP. In one retrospective study, six patients with clinical and radiographic evidence of an L5 radiculopathy were found to have reduced amplitude of the ipsilateral superficial peroneal SNAP along with denervation changes in the L5 myotome.[27] This condition has not been found with S1 nerve root lesions, in which the sural SNAP remains normal despite the higher percentage of DRG located within the intraspinal canal.

S1 radiculopathies are the second most common root lesion encountered. Needle EMG may show abnormalities in the gastrocnemii, abductor hallucis, abductor digit quinti pedis, glutei, and biceps femoris short head. In addition, the H response is either absent or reduced in amplitude.

Differential Diagnoses

As seen in the cervical spine, it is often difficult to clinically distinguish lesions of the lumbosacral nerve roots from lesions of the lumbar and sacral plexuses (see Table 14.5). L2–L4 radiculopathies can look identical to lumbar plexopathies, whereas L5–S1 nerve root lesions closely resemble lesions of the sacral plexus. In both cases, the combination of fibrillation potentials in the lumbosacral paraspinals and preserved sensory nerve conduction responses (lateral femoral cutaneous and saphenous SNAPs for L2–L4 lesions and sural and superficial peroneal SNAPs for L5–S1 lesions) points to the diagnosis of radiculopathy.

A major limitation is encountered when SNAPs are absent bilaterally. In the workup of a lesion in the lumbar plexus versus an L2–L4 nerve root lesion, the sensory nerve conduction responses are not consistently obtainable from a technical standpoint, even in normal individuals. Likewise, in the evaluation of a sacral plexus versus an L5–S1 lesion, SNAPs may be absent in elderly patients or patients with a history of a polyneuropathy. In both instances, the diagnosis rests on a single crucial finding: the absence or presence of denervation in the paraspinals. This finding in itself is unreliable, as noted earlier, in that paraspinal fibrillation potentials may be present rarely in normal individuals older than 60 years, in patients with a history of prior spine surgery, and in patients with diabetes. Denervation changes may be absent because of early reinnervation or sampling error. As a result, in patients with bilaterally absent SNAPs (owing to technical or other reasons), the final electrodiagnostic impression may be inconclusive.

For similar reasons, bilateral S1 radiculopathies, particularly when chronic, may be confused with distal axon-loss polyneuropathies. In younger patients (<60 years old), an absent sural response combined with abnormalities seen in the intrinsic foot muscles on NEE typically indicates the presence of a polyneuropathy rather than S1 radiculopathy.

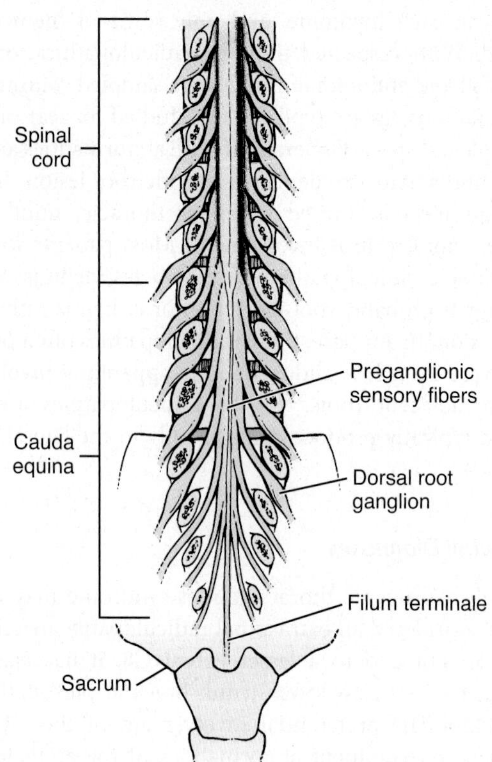

FIG. 14.10 Coronal view of inferior spinal cord, cauda equina, and surrounding structures. Dorsal root ganglia are located in the intervertebral foramina so that all the sensory fibers composing the cauda equina are "preganglionic." Axon-loss lesion of cauda equina generally has no effect on lower limb sensory nerve conduction studies, regardless of its severity.

Electrodiagnostic Findings of Other Spine-Related Disorders

Cauda Equina Syndrome

Multiple lumbosacral radiculopathies are encountered with some frequency. Typically, the involvement is bilateral and often asymmetric.[10,20] Most of these lesions are attributable to midline lumbar disc protrusions or lumbar canal stenosis. Characteristically, S1 and S2 roots, being the most medial of the roots supplying the lower limbs, are affected. In many patients, more extensive lumbosacral root involvement occurs; a common combination is bilateral S1 and S2 root compromise accompanied by unilateral or bilateral L5 root involvement.

The electrodiagnostic findings most commonly seen consist of a mixture of low-amplitude CMAPs and normal SNAPs on NCS, along with fibrillation potentials and MUP dropout on needle EMG (Fig. 14.10). On NEE, the abnormalities often are more severe in muscles located distal to the knees. With some substantial lesions of recent onset, they are just as prominent in the more proximal muscles. Whenever the disorder is subacute or chronic, fibrillation potentials usually are accompanied by chronic neurogenic MUP changes. Low lumbar or high sacral paraspinal fibrillation potentials often are found bilaterally with more acute lesions, but are undetectable with many chronic ones. Typically, the H responses cannot be elicited, and even the M components of the H responses, recorded from the gastrocnemius/soleus muscles, are quite low in amplitude.

Lumbar Canal Stenosis

Lumbar canal stenosis has no single characteristic electrodiagnostic presentation. Rather, the findings are extremely variable, depending on the degree of axon loss affecting the lumbosacral motor roots. At one extreme are patients who experience only intermittent, short-lived symptoms that often can be relieved completely by various maneuvers (e.g., sitting, flexing at the waist). In these patients, the electrodiagnostic examination often is completely normal. At the opposite end of the spectrum are patients who have substantial cauda equina lesions with severe, bilateral, fixed motor and sensory deficits. These lesions produce the electrodiagnostic presentation described previously.

Between these two extremes are numerous different electrodiagnostic patterns: (1) two or more radiculopathies, far more often bilateral than strictly unilateral; (2) a single radiculopathy, typically S1, that is sometimes detected in the less symptomatic or asymptomatic limb; (3) unilateral or bilateral absent H responses alone; (4) NEE changes restricted to just one or two limb muscles, most commonly those innervated by the S1 roots; or (5) fibrillation potentials limited to the paraspinal muscles.[9,19]

Myelopathy

The effect that a focal myelopathy has on the electrodiagnostic examination depends principally on whether the anterior horn cells or their existing fibers are compromised at the level of the lesion. If only the descending corticospinal tracts of the spinal cord are affected (upper motor neuron lesion), the only abnormality found on the electrodiagnostic examination concerns the MUP firing pattern of muscles receiving innervation from spinal cord segments caudal to the lesion. In these muscles, the MUPs show no or incomplete activation (i.e., they fire in decreased numbers at a slow to moderate rate).

In contrast, if the anterior horn cells or the intramedullary fibers derived from them are involved, the electrodiagnostic findings are those of a focal intraspinal canal lesion that is characteristically bilateral, but often asymmetric. How prominent the electrodiagnostic changes are with such focal disorders depends mainly on where the lesions are located along the spinal cord. Lesions situated in C5–T1 segments and L4–S2 segments produce substantial abnormalities on motor NCSs and NEE, and generally are readily recognized as intraspinal canal lesions. All such disorders result in low-amplitude CMAPs or CMAPs that cannot be elicited and normal SNAPs on NCS, accompanied by fibrillation potentials, MUP dropout, and, depending on lesion duration, chronic neurogenic MUP changes on needle EMG. Conversely, lesions involving T2 through L3 segments result only in NEE changes (i.e., motor NCSs using various limb muscles as recording sites are normal). Finally, lesions involving the upper cervical cord segments (C1–C4) have essentially no electrodiagnostic manifestations because that region of the spinal cord cannot be assessed.[27]

Postlaminectomy Electrodiagnostic Findings

Electrodiagnostic examinations are obtained frequently on patients who have undergone neck or back surgery. The specific diagnostic benefit derived from such assessments varies considerably, depending on the reason for referral and the time that has elapsed since operation. Overall, such postoperative studies are of limited value, however, unless they are obtained after very remote surgery to diagnose a recent-onset lesion. In the immediate postoperative period (first 10–14 days after surgery), the electrodiagnostic examination can reveal preexisting abnormalities because any NEE changes observed during that period, with the exception of a reduced MUP recruitment, are caused by a lesion that predated the operation.

During the early postoperative period (3 weeks to 3–4 months after surgery), the electrodiagnostic examination is of considerable benefit in assessing patients with postoperative weakness, principally because a normal CMAP amplitude recorded from a weak muscle (e.g., the tibialis anterior, resulting in footdrop) 7 or more days after onset of symptoms virtually excludes motor axon loss as the cause. The remaining possibilities include a proximal conduction block (neurapraxia), an upper motor neuron lesion, or hysteria or malingering. In the rare patient who develops nonorganic weakness postoperatively, the electrodiagnostic examination can prove that the symptoms are not the result of significant nerve fiber damage.

The electrodiagnostic examination usually cannot answer reliably the early postoperative question: "Was the root adequately decompressed?" Axon loss features of radiculopathy persist for weeks to months or indefinitely. Even an electrodiagnostic examination performed 2 to 3 months postoperatively is not likely to show significant improvement compared with a preoperative study. An exception is radiculopathy resulting from conduction block at the root level, which may resolve rapidly after the pressure is relieved. With an S1 radiculopathy, an H response that could not be elicited preoperatively may reappear in the early postoperative period. Similarly, on NEE, reduced MUP recruitment (and clinical weakness) could resolve rapidly in the affected muscles postoperatively.

An electrodiagnostic examination can be valuable in identifying root damage as the cause of new or worsening weakness in the postoperative period. The extent, amount, and distribution of fibrillation potentials provide information when compared with the preoperative study.

Cervical Root Avulsion

Root avulsions, which are usually restricted to the cervical region, differ from the typical single compressive radiculopathy principally in the degree of axon loss that results. Because the entire motor supply from one or both roots innervating the particular muscle has been disrupted, that muscle is severely or totally denervated. If it is used as a recorded muscle during motor NCS, the CMAP obtained is of very low amplitude, if it can be elicited. Similarly, during needle EMG of that muscle, fibrillation potentials are abundant, and MUPs are either absent or, if present, quite sparse and show reduced recruitment. Sensory NCS responses derived from the same roots are normal because the sensory roots are interrupted proximal to their DRG. Fibrillation potentials are often not found in the appropriate paraspinal muscles in patients with cervical avulsion injuries; thus, their absence does not exclude this diagnosis.[9]

Acknowledgments

I acknowledge the late Dr. Asa J. Wilbourn for his contributions to the original version of this chapter.

KEY POINTS

1. The electrodiagnostic examination is an essential tool in the evaluation of radiculopathy. When performed by an experienced electrodiagnostic consultant, the electrodiagnostic examination can confirm the diagnosis and determine the localization, lesion duration, and severity.
2. The electrodiagnostic examination assesses the integrity of large sensory and motor nerve fibers, but not small fibers, such as small C-type fibers that mediate pain. Therefore, pain alone cannot be assessed by electrodiagnostic testing. Electrodiagnostic testing is more valuable when pain is associated with large nerve fiber dysfunction, such as weakness.
3. For a comprehensive study, the electrodiagnostic examination should be performed at least 3 weeks after the onset of symptoms.

4. The most widely used criterion for diagnosing radiculopathies by NEE is that abnormalities (e.g., fibrillation potentials or neurogenic MUP changes) should be found in at least two limb muscles within the same myotome that is innervated by different peripheral nerves.
5. Sensory nerve conduction responses are typically normal in radiculopathy owing to the location of the DRG outside of the intraspinal canal, distal to the site of the nerve lesion. In contrast, amplitudes of the motor NCS may be decreased when root damage is severe, extensive, or both.

KEY REFERENCES

1. Wilbourn AJ, Aminoff MJ. AAEM Minimonograph #32: the electrodiagnostic examination in patients with radiculopathies. *Muscle Nerve.* 1998;21:1612-1631.
   This review article describes and critically analyzes the various neurophysiologic techniques used in assessment of radiculopathy and details the findings with root lesions at various levels.
2. Wilbourn AJ. Nerve conduction studies: types, components, abnormalities, and value in localization. *Neurol Clin.* 2002;20:305-338.
   This article reviews the types of pathophysiology manifested by focal nerve fiber lesions and what effect each has on NCS; it also describes the types of localization possible with the electrodiagnostic examination and the major sources of error.
3. Shea PA, Woods WW, Werden DH. Electromyography in diagnosis of nerve root compression syndrome. *Arch Neurol Psychiatry.* 1950;64:93-104.
4. Woods WW, Shea PA. The value of electromyography in neurology and neurosurgery. *J Neurosurg.* 1951;8:595-607.
   Key References 3 and 4 were the first to discuss the methodology used for diagnosing radiculopathies in the clinical EMG laboratory (which is still used currently).
5. Yoss RE, Corbin KB, MacCarty CS, et al. Significance of symptoms and signs in localization of involved root in cervical disc protrusion. *Neurology.* 1957;7:673-683.
   This unique article remains the best source regarding the specific symptoms and clinical findings with lesions of each of the cervical roots (C5 through C8).

REFERENCES

1. Wilbourn AJ. Nerve conduction studies: types, components, abnormalities, and value in localization. *Neurol Clin.* 2002;20:305-338.
2. Preston DC, Shapiro BE. *Electromyography and Neuromuscular Disorders.* Boston: Butterworth-Heinemann; 1998.
3. Wilbourn AJ, Ferrante MA. Clinical electromyography. In: Joynt RJ, Greggs RC, eds. *Baker's Clinical Neurology on CD-ROM.* Philadelphia: Lippincott Williams & Wilkins; 2000.
4. Dimitru D, Amato AA, Awarts MJ. *Electrodiagnostic Medicine.* 2nd ed. Philadelphia: Hanley & Belfus; 2002.
5. Shea PA, Woods WW, Werden DH. Electromyography in diagnosis of nerve root compression syndrome. *Arch Neurol Psychiatry.* 1950;64:93-104.
6. Woods WW, Shea PA. The value of electromyography in neurology and neurosurgery. *J Neurosurg.* 1951;8:595-607.
7. Wilbourn AJ, Aminoff MJ. Radiculopathies. In: Brown WF, Bolton CF, eds. *Clinical Electromyography.* 2nd ed. Boston: Butterworth-Heinemann; 1993:177-209.
8. Wilbourn AJ. The value and limitations of the electromyographic examination in the diagnosis of lumbosacral radiculopathy. In: Hardy RW, ed. *Lumbar Disc Disease.* New York: Raven Press; 1982:65-109.
9. Wilbourn AJ, Aminoff MJ. AAEM Minimonograph #32: the electrodiagnostic examination in patients with radiculopathies. *Muscle Nerve.* 1998;21:1612-1631.
10. Raynor EM, Kleiner-Fisman G, Nardin RA. Lumbosacral and thoracic radiculopathies. In: Kitirji B, Kaminski HJ, Preston DC, et al., eds. *Neuromuscular Disorders in Clinical Practice.* Boston: Butterworth-Heinemann; 2002:859-883.
11. Levin KH. Radiculopathy. In: Levin KH, Luders HO, eds. *Comprehensive Clinical Neurophysiology.* Philadelphia: WB Saunders; 2000:189-200.
12. Johnson EW. Electrodiagnosis of radiculopathy. In: Johnson EW, ed. *Practical Electromyography.* 2nd ed. Baltimore: Williams & Wilkins; 1988:229-245.
13. Braddom RI, Johnson EW. Standardization of "H" reflex and diagnostic use in S1 radiculopathies. *Arch Phys Med Rehabil.* 1974;55:161-164.
14. Schuchmann J. H-reflex latency in radiculopathy. *Arch Phys Med Rehabil.* 1978;59:185-187.
15. Eisen A, Schomer D, Melmad C. An electrophysiological method for examining lumbosacral root compression. *Can J Neurol Sci.* 1977;4:117-123.
16. Fisher MN, Shidve AJ, Terxera C, et al. The F response—a clinically useful physiological parameter for the evaluation of radicular injury. *Electromyogr Clin Neurophysiol.* 1979;19: 65-75.
17. Yoss RE, Corbin KB, MacCarty CS, et al. Significance of symptoms and signs in localization of involved root in cervical disc protrusion. *Neurology.* 1957;7:673-683.
18. Marinacci AA. A correlation between operative findings in cervical herniated disc with the EMGs and opaque myelograms. *EMG.* 1966;6:5-20.
19. Levin KH, Maggiano HJ, Wilbourn AJ. Cervical radiculopathies: comparison of surgical and EMG localization of single-root lesions. *Neurology.* 1996;46:1022-1025.
20. Wilbourn AJ. The electrodiagnostic examination. In: Herkowitz HN, Garfin SR, Barlderston RA, et al., eds. *The Spine.* 4th ed. Philadelphia: WB Saunders; 1999:135-150.
21. Wilbourn AJ. Diabetic neuropathies. In: Brown WF, Bolton CF, eds. *Clinical Electromyography.* 2nd ed. Boston: Butterworth-Heinemann; 1993:447-515.
22. Levin KH. Neurological manifestations of compressive radiculopathy of the first thoracic root. *Neurology.* 1999;53:1149-1151.
23. Bodner RA, Levin KH, Wilbourn AJ. Lumbosacral radiculopathies: comparison of surgical and EMG localization. *Muscle Nerve.* 1995;18:1071.
24. Tsao BE, Levin KH, Bodner RA. Comparison of surgical and electrodiagnostic findings in single root lumbosacral radiculopathies. *Muscle Nerve.* 2003;27:60-64.
25. Hamanishi C, Tanaka S. Dorsal root ganglia in the lumbosacral region observed from the axial view of MIR. *Spine.* 1993;18:1753-1756.
26. Sato K, Kikuchi S. An anatomic study of foraminal nerve root lesions in the lumbar spine. *Spine.* 1993;18:2246-2251.
27. Levin KH. L5 radiculopathy with reduced superficial peroneal sensory responses: intraspinal and extraspinal causes. *Muscle Nerve.* 1998;21:3-7.

CHAPTER 15 Intraoperative Neurophysiologic Monitoring of the Spine

Dileep R. Nair
Ajay Gupta

The primary objective in intraoperative neurophysiologic monitoring is to identify and prevent the development of a new neurologic deficit or worsening of a preexisting neurologic injury to a patient who is undergoing surgery. The aim of most spinal cord monitoring is to prevent intraoperative injury that results in irreversible paraplegia or quadriplegia. Due to the inability of performing a neurologic examination in an anesthetized patient, intraoperative neurophysiologic monitoring is used to determine the patient's neurologic status during surgery. By evaluating the responses produced by the patient's nervous system to a variety of stimulation, the integrity of that neural pathway can be monitored. These recordings are started prior to surgery, referred to as baseline recordings, then continued throughout the surgery. Any significant changes or fluctuations from these baseline values are then used to determine whether any significant neurologic injury has occurred. With this strategy, the patient's own responses serve as the control for the detection of any abnormalities that may occur during the surgery. The term *significant change* is used in reference to the degree of changes seen in the neurophysiologic recordings. Changes termed *significant* have been shown to correlate well with intraoperative injury to the nervous system. However, it is also possible that some of these significant changes may also arise from other changes in physiologic parameters, anesthetic parameters, or possibly technical issues. It is then up to the intraoperative neurophysiologic monitoring team to determine whether the significant changes noted in the neurophysiologic responses are truly related to the surgical procedure at hand. The challenge to the intraoperative neurophysiologist and the monitoring team is to alert the surgeon of these changes as early as possible and to evaluate and rule out various technical and nonsurgical causes that may also affect the responses being recorded.

Key to the success of intraoperative neurophysiologic monitoring is a good understanding of the capabilities and limitations of the neurophysiologic tests being monitored. These limitations should be understood not only by the intraoperative neurophysiologist but also by the anesthesiologist and surgeon. For seamless integration of intraoperative neurophysiologic monitoring into the intraoperative team, a good working relationship among the intraoperative neurophysiology team, anesthesiologist, and surgeon is imperative. This allows for rapid communication between teams and a quick resolution of issues, thus optimizing the benefits of intraoperative neurophysiologic monitoring for the patient.

One of the first issues to address when planning for intraoperative neurophysiologic monitoring is to determine the types of neurophysiologic tests to perform on a particular patient undergoing surgery. This is accomplished by understanding the type of surgery the patient will undergo, the types of intraoperative injuries that may occur, and the mechanisms of how these injuries occur in surgery. By planning ahead with these issues in mind, the team can also attempt to anticipate the type of changes that could occur as well the risky periods during surgery when these changes would be likely. Ideally, they would prospectively plan for interventions to reduce intraoperative neurologic injury.

Intraoperative Monitoring of the Spinal Cord

Somatosensory-evoked potential (SEP) monitoring has been used for many years to monitor spinal function intraoperatively during a variety of surgeries involving the spine (e.g., corrective surgery for scoliosis or other congenital deformities, removal of intraspinal tumors or arteriovenous malformations). This monitoring modality has been shown to reduce the incidence of neurologic damage in large-scale studies of experienced monitoring teams.[1] SEPs only monitor sensory transmission through the dorsal column pathways. In other words, this modality does not provide a direct measure of motor function. In addition, it is important to be aware that the dorsal columns receive their blood supply from the posterior spinal arteries, whereas the anterior spinal arteries supply the motor pathways. Therefore ischemic damage to the spinal cord from an anterior spinal artery may go undetectable with SEP monitoring.[2,3] Therefore a significant change in SEP monitoring might mandate further assessment of the patient's motor function by waking the patient up during surgery to evaluate leg and arm motor function (the "wake-up test"). The disadvantages of this strategy include the lack of online intraoperative motor function assessment as well as the anesthesia risks associated with performing the wake-up test. An alternative is monitoring the motor pathway through the recording of motor-evoked potentials (MEPs).

MEP monitoring has been performed in the past by directly relying on stimulation of the spinal cord.[4] Spinal cord stimulation can be done with the use of epidural electrodes inserted after a laminectomy or by percutaneous intraspinous needle electrodes. The epidural electrodes are invasive and often require placment by a skilled anesthesiologist. Percutaneous intraspinous needles are difficult to place accurately and thus may not achieve adequate or consistent stimulation of the spinal cord. In addition, there is the question of whether MEPs generated through spinal cord stimulation arise solely from propagation through the motor pathway or if multiple pathways are involved in their generation.[5,6] There are reports of MEP monitoring in which spinal cord stimulation resulted in no significant intraoperative changes but yet a postoperative neurologic motor deficits occurred (so-called *false-negative result*).[7] It has been suggested that motor cortex stimulation with transcranial electrical stimulation would provide a more reliable methodology for monitoring the motor pathways. This technique has become a routine modality in spinal cord monitoring along with SEPs.

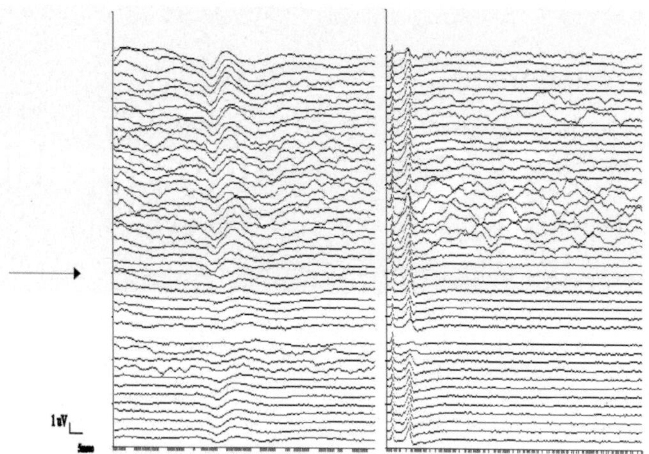

FIG. 15.1 Significant amplitude change in cortical response due to ischemic etiology. The stack on the left shows the leg cortical response; the stack on the right shows the popliteal fossa response. Both were obtained after left posterior tibial stimulation. The baseline responses are shown at the top of the stack and the end of monitoring is shown at the bottom of the stack. A drop in the leg cortical amplitude can be appreciated at the point depicted by the *arrow*. Note the popliteal fossa responses are intact during this time. There is a return of the response by the end of surgery seen at the bottom of the stack. This change was attributed to an ischemic change to the cord with the retractor placed over the left iliac artery. The responses returned when the retractor was adjusted away from the artery.

Somatosensory-Evoked Potential Monitoring

The use of SEPs in intraoperative monitoring of complex spine surgeries began in the early 1970s.[8] Although SEP monitoring primarily evaluates the integrity of the posterior columns, it is often used to give an overall assessment of the spinal cord based on the assumption that many intraoperative mechanisms of injury affect the spinal cord diffusely. An example of such an injury is spine distraction during scoliosis surgery. In addition, ischemic injury may initially result in a more diffuse dysfunction of the spinal cord that could be detected by SEPs (Fig. 15.1). SEP responses are thought to pass through both large fiber somatosensory pathways of the dorsal column as well as possibly the anterior spinothalamic tract. This may be another reason why anterior spinal artery ischemia could be detected by this technique.

Generators of the Somatosensory-Evoked Potential Responses

The cortical response for the lower extremity is called the P37 potential. The generator of this response arises from the primary somatosensory cortex of the leg, which is located in the mesial parietal cortex. The cortical response for the upper extremity, which is generated from the primary somatosensory cortex of the hand, is called the N20 potential (Fig. 15.2). Two important characteristics of these waveforms include (1) amplitude, which is recorded in microvolts and determined by either a baseline to peak or peak to trough measure of the waveform, and (2) latency, which is recorded in milliseconds and is the time interval from the stimulus to the occurrence of the potential. An amplitude change from the initial baseline measure to a decrease of more than 50% is often termed a significant change in SEP amplitude.[9] Significant latency changes in SEP monitoring consist of a 10% prolongation beyond the baseline latency value (Table 15.1).[10] Although these deviations from the baseline measures are thought to be significant, they should be interpreted with caution, taking into account various factors that include the evolution of the changes (e.g., a trend toward worsening is an ominous sign) and various other intraoperative factors that include length of the surgery, type of anesthetic agent, and temperature effects. It is also important to remember that significant latency and amplitude changes can occur in isolation. It is quite common to see a significant amplitude change without any associated latency changes. The most significant change is a complete loss of the cortical potential.

TABLE 15.1 Significant Changes in Different Monitoring Modalities

Type of Study	Significant Changes	Highly Significant Changes
Somatosensory-evoked potentials	Amplitude <50%; latency >10%	Complete loss of amplitude
Motor-evoked potentials	Increase threshold voltage >50–100 V	Complete loss of amplitude
Pedicle screw stimulation	Current intensity <7–10 mA	

Another measurement made in posterior tibial or peroneal nerve SEP monitoring is the popliteal fossa (PF) potential. This is a nerve action potential that is recorded as the impulses pass under the popliteal fossa in the peripheral nervous system. This measurement ensures that an adequate stimulus has been applied. If the PF response is absent in addition to an absent leg cortical (P37) response, the changes seen may

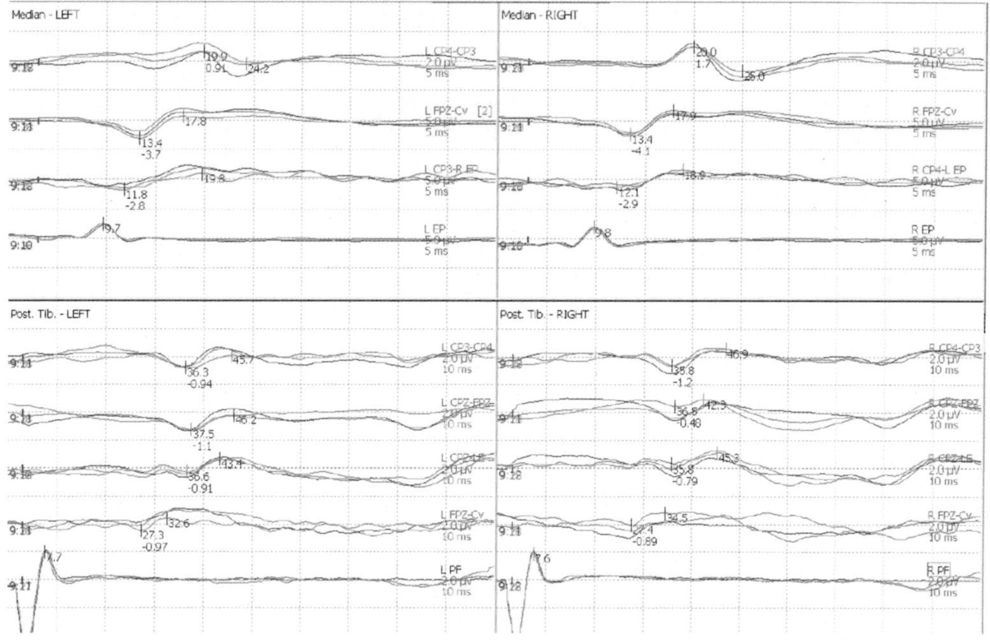

FIG. 15.2 Typical morphology of the cortical generators of median nerve and posterior tibial nerve somatosensory-evoked potential (SEP) waveforms are shown. Note that the display time is different between the two modalities. Median nerve SEP is shown in a 5 ms per division display and posterior tibial nerve SEP is shown in a 10 ms per division display.

not be a result of a lesion at the level of the spinal cord. In this case, the change may be either technical (e.g., the stimulating needles may have dislodged) or the leg may be ischemic (e.g., in the case of femoral artery catheterization during thoracoabdominal aneurysm surgery or direct compression of the peripheral nerve) (Fig. 15.3).

Another posterior tibial stimulation SEP response that can be monitored is the P31/N34 complex, often termed the *subcortical response,* because the generator for these responses is at the level of medulla and midbrain. These responses are relatively more resistant to the effects of anesthesia compared with the cortical P37 response (see Fig. 15.2). The same is true for the subcortical potentials from median nerve stimulation (P14/N18) potential. In pediatric cases, the subcortical potentials may also be better formed and more easily monitored than cortical responses. Some of this effect may be the result of the variation of myelination in the younger age groups and more significant effects of anesthetics on these patients. Moreover, these differences from the adult morphology can persist into the early teenage years. Other factors affecting the responses include core body temperature changes. It is not uncommon for the core body temperature to change more than 1°C. The cooling affects the limbs disproportionately to the core body temperature, which can result in slowing of conduction.

Motor-Evoked Potential Monitoring

A variety of methods have been used to monitor spinal motor pathways during surgery, as mentioned earlier. Most of these methods involve recording of electromyographic (EMG) readings from appropriate muscles in response to stimulation of a motor pathway rostral to the operative site. The difference among the various methods is the nature of the stimulation. There are three basic categories of stimulation: rostral spinal stimulation, transcranial magnetic stimulation, and transcranial electrical stimulation (TCES). Magnetic stimulation is effective in nonanesthetized patients for motor pathways evaluation, but the suppression of cortical responsiveness under anesthesia (mainly inhalational anesthetics) renders this method less effective for surgical use. In addition, the equipment used for magnetic stimulation is expensive, bulky, and has a tendency to overheat.

Noninvasive stimulation of the brain using TCES was first reported in 1980.[11] Soon after, single-pulse TCES was used in monitoring motor pathways.[12-17] Because of the effects of general anesthesia, single-pulse stimulation was found to be less reliable in recording MEPs.[18-22] With the introduction of the multipulse technique for motor pathway monitoring, reliable and robust MEP recording can now be obtained in most patients using specific general anesthesia protocols.[23-27] Multipulse techniques require that neuromuscular blockade not be used during this part of the monitoring. Occasionally the use of partial neuromuscular blockade may still allow for TCES moniotring.[28] This method reportedly achieves more reliable stimulation of the motor cortex intraoperatively and is more resilient to the effects of general anesthesia.

The methodology of MEP monitoring has been revolutionized by the use of multipulse TCES. Previous methods for MEP recording used a variety of stimulation and recording techniques. Spinally elicited neurogenic responses were used and were putatively stated to be a result of activation of the motor pathways in the spinal cord. Recent evidence has suggested that these spinally elicited neurogenic responses are

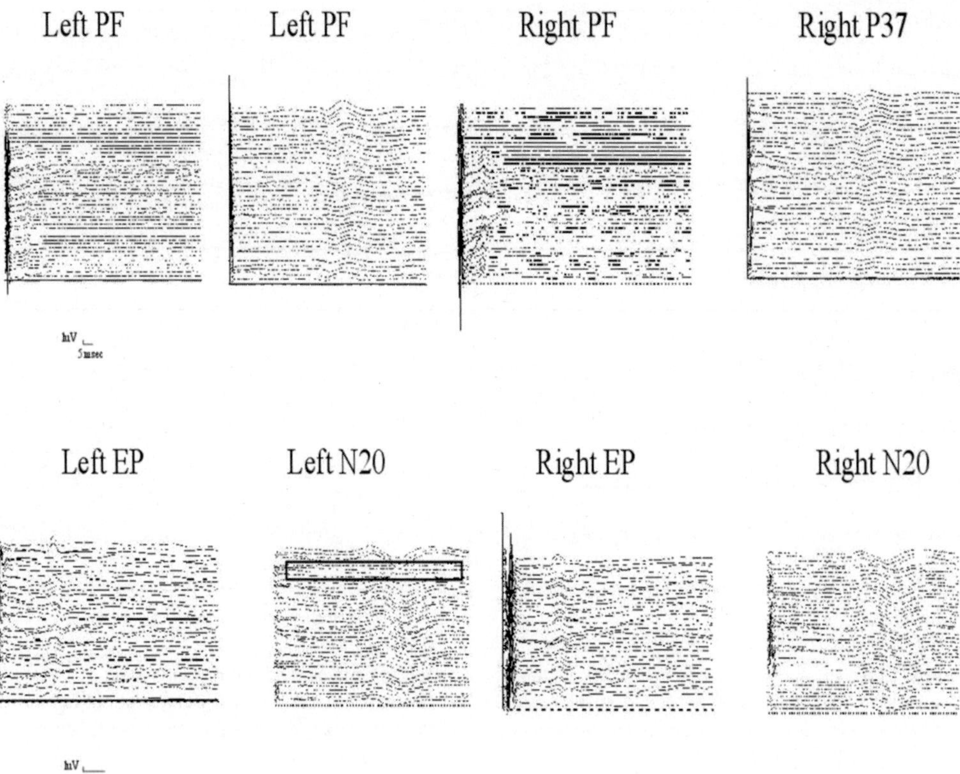

FIG. 15.3 Significant change in left N20 cortical amplitude due to arm positioning and nonsignificant latency prolongation of all cortical responses due to anesthetic effect. The top row of stacks shows popliteal fossa (PF) and leg cortical (P37) responses from the posterior tibial stimulation, first from left-side stimulation and then right-side stimulation. The bottom row of stacks shows Erb's point (EP) and arm cortical (N20) response from median nerve stimulation, with the left side shown first followed by right-side stimulation. There is a drop in the left N20 amplitude (the *rectangular box*). At this point there is also a loss of the left EP response. This change was attributed to left arm malposition. When the left arm was repositioned, the response returned to baseline. Also noticeable in all the leg and arm cortical responses from both left and right sides is mild prolongation of latencies in the stacks, but these latencies all returned to baseline by the end of surgery. These changes are likely from an anesthetic effect because they are bilateral, affecting both the arm and left responses in a spine operation, which was performed at the L3–S1 level.

generated through activation of the sensory pathways and retrograde activation of the alpha motor neurons. In a collision experiment using stimulation of the spinal cord followed by stimulation of the posterior tibial nerve at various interstimulus intervals, the neurogenic responses were abolished, suggesting that the potentials were colliding in the spinal cord.[6]

At the beginning of TCES-MEP monitoring, threshold voltages for each side of the body and amplitudes of MEPs are calculated.[23] The motor cortex on the side of the brain receiving the anodal stimulus is typically the first region to activate at the lowest stimulus threshold. The initial current used is typically 100 V, with a train of stimuli delivered to the cortex. Following stimulation, a MEP response is monitored in the muscles contralateral to the side receiving the anodal stimulus. If no response is seen, the voltage is typically increased by 50-V increments and the process is repeated until an MEP response is seen in all the muscles contralateral to the anodal stimulus. This voltage is called the *threshold voltage* for that side. The highest amplitude of the myogenic response below the level of surgery is also noted. Typically, amplitude measures for myogenic responses are best recorded as the area-under-the-curve measurements or simply documented as either presence or absence of the myogenic response. This procedure is repeated after reversing the anodal-cathodal configuration using a switch box. The voltage used for TCES-MEP recordings typically does not exceed 500 V. Note that the anticipated latency of the EMG responses ranges from 20 to 40 ms or more depending on the patient's height, owing to the conduction time in the descending motor pathways. Latency values have not always been found to be reliable indicators of significant change in TCES monitoring in clinical practice. Another advantage of the multipulse technique is that it requires no averaging. A train of pulses elicits a clear response of sufficient amplitude, which requires no averaging.

Two different methods of recordings can be used. In myogenic MEPs, responses can be recorded directly from the muscle (either a surface electrode or needle electrodes placed within the muscle). In spinal cord MEPs, responses may be recorded directly from the spinal cord with use of an epidural catheter electrode that records a direct D wave and a volley of indirect I waves. Using single-pulse TCES, recording both D and I waves is frequently required, meaning a D wave could be recorded when a myogenic MEP is not yet seen. This is because a series of D and I waves is required for

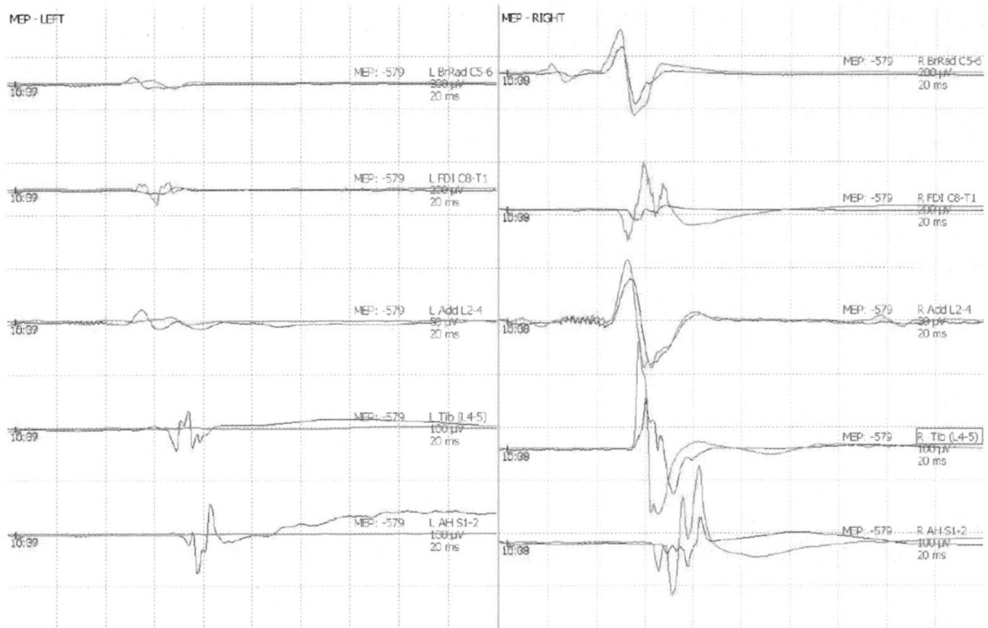

FIG. 15.4 Significant change in transcranial electrical motor-evoked potential (MEP) response during spinal instrumentation. The figure shows transcranial MEP responses from the left and right muscle groups. The traces in red represent the responses at baseline (at the beginning of surgery). The first two muscle groups on each side of the figure represent upper extremity MEP response from the brachioradialis (BrRad) and first dorsal interosseous (FDI). The lower three traces on each side represent the responses from the lower extremities on each side of the body: adductors of the thigh (Add), tibialis anterior (Tib), and adductor hallucis (AH). The green traces represent the most recent acquisition and show the change from baseline over the left lower extremity muscle groups. Notice the MEP responses of the left tibialis anterior and adductor hallucis are absent, whereas they are preserved in the left upper extremity and adductor of the thigh as well as both lower and upper extremity of the right side of the body. This is consistent with injury to the left lower lumbar and sacral nerve roots (L5, S1, S2).

the alpha motor neurons to generate a myogenic response. The spinal recorded responses can also be recorded with full muscle relaxation, whereas myogenic responses require either no or very little muscle relaxation, even with the multipulse technique.

Determining significant changes during the course of surgery typically is most reliable if there is an absolute loss of myogenic responses to stimulation (Fig. 15.4). Some authors have also suggested that amplitude drops of MEP to 25% of baseline amplitude values are predictive of motor pathway impairments.[29] Significant changes can also be determined by a change of voltage required to obtain MEPs of greater than 50 V beyond baseline thresholds used in obtaining MEPs at the beginning of monitoring (see Table 15.1).[30]

Clinical Use of Intraoperative Monitoring

SEPs have become a useful modality in monitoring scoliosis surgery and have been shown to reduce the risk of neurologic deficits, especially when used by surgeons experienced in neurophysiologic monitoring. The occurrence of definite neurologic deficits in the presence of unchanged SEP recordings has been estimated to be approximately 0.063%.[31] Intraoperative neurophysiology can play both a neuroprotective (through the detection of early changes) and an educational role during surgery.[32] Surgeons who use intraoperative neurophysiologic monitoring over time may begin to understand which specific surgical techniques have a higher propensity for damaging the neurologic system. In this way surgeons may find methods to avoid the use of high-risk techniques.

Many surgeons have found that TCES-evoked MEP monitoring during spinal surgery is a safe and reliable method of monitoring corticospinal tract activity and is indispensable for these surgeries.[33] There has been no evidence that TCES has resulted in the development of new-onset epilepsy or brain damage. There are some risks associated with TCES monitoring, including tongue or lip laceration and, rarely, mandibular fractures. The use of a soft bite block may prevent these injuries. Relative contraindications include epilepsy, cortical lesions, convexity skull deficits, raised intracranial pressure, cardiac disease, intracranial electrodes or shunts, cardiac pacemakers, and other implantable biomedical devices.[34]

A study that looked at the reproducibility of various monitoring methods during scoliosis surgery found that MEPs could be obtained in 80% of patients compared with SEPs, which could be obtained in 93% of patients.[35] In spinal surgery, MEPs obtained from upper and lower extremities were consistently recorded in 22 patients with multipulse stimulation using trains of 3 to 6 pulses separated by 2 ms, with responses measuring more than 100 µV in all but one patient. These responses persisted with nitrous oxide concentration of up to 74%. One patient had loss of responses from one lower limb in which increased weakness was noted for a few days after surgery; in three patients there was an increase in weakness or spasticity without any accompanying intraoperative MEP changes.[36] In another study,[37] MEPs during TCES were reproducibly recorded during spinal surgery in 40 patients with partial neuromuscular blockade. In two patients there were some significant changes in the motor potentials that correlated with postoperative neurologic deficits. No postoperative neurologic deficits were observed in nine patients in whom MEP amplitudes decreased to less than 20% of baseline values.[37]

TCES-induced MEPs have been used to monitor cases of intramedullary spinal cord tumor resection. In 32 consecutive patients, MEPs were elicited in 19 patients before myelotomy, and three of these patients had MEP amplitude decrease below 50% from baseline, all of whom had postoperative neurologic deficits.[38]

In a review of 160 patients undergoing scoliosis surgery, a combination of SEP and transcranial MEP monitoring was successfully recorded in 81% of the patients, with changes seen in 5% of monitored cases that was reversible after taking appropriate surgical corrective measures. None of these patients had new postoperative deficits or worsening of preexisting deficits. This combination of techniques was considered safe, reliable, and accurate and made the wake-up test unnecessary.[39]

Use of TCES-evoked MEPs has been relatively easily accomplished with an anesthetic combination of narcotic drip accompanied by nitrous oxide. The use of isoflurane in addition to this combination resulted in a tendency for deterioration of amplitude of the MEP responses.[40] MEPs elicited by TCES are more feasible with total intravenous anesthesia compared with balanced anesthesia using nitrous oxide, isoflurane, and fentanyl. Some of the suppressant effects of balanced anesthesia can be overcome with higher stimulation intensities and repetitive stimulation.[41]

Pedicle Screw Stimulation

Intraoperative assessment during pedicle screw insertion can be used to avoid nerve root trauma from a misdirected screw. The integrity of the pedicle screw placement can be assessed by its direct electrical stimulation with simultaneous myogenic response recordings from the appropriate myotomes. Using a direct monopolar nerve stimulator, with serial increments of the level of current intensity from 1 to 20 mA, triggered EMG recordings can be performed (Fig. 15.5). Absence of a myogenic response up to 10 mA is thought to be indicative of an intact pedicle. The presence of a pedicle breach is suspected by a stimulation-induced myogenic response below 7 to 10 mA (see Table 15.1).[7]

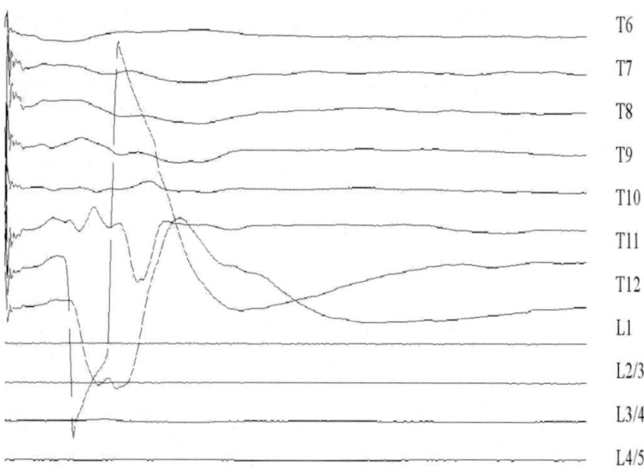

FIG. 15.5 Nonsignificant triggered electromyographic (EMG) response with pedicle screw stimulation. Pedicle screw stimulation of the T12 screw shows threshold of triggered EMG response at an intensity of 12 mA.

Summary

Intraoperative neurophysiologic monitoring of the spinal cord can be used to help detect the early occurrence of neurophysiologic changes, thereby allowing corrective action to reduce the incidence of neurologic injury to patients undergoing spine surgery. In our opinion, the most important aspects of successful intraoperative monitoring include the following:

1. Availability of the right equipment to allow multimodality recordings (e.g., combinations of EMG, SEP, and/or MEPs)
2. Presence of a highly skilled and experienced technical and neurophysiologic team that will ensure for optimal technical recordings and accurate interpretation of any changes that may occur
3. Rapid communication between the neurophysiologic team and the surgical/anesthesia teams
4. A knowledge of both the functional anatomy of the structures to be monitored and the limitations of the techniques to be used

The combination of different monitoring techniques, such as SEP and transcranial MEP monitoring, has enabled better interpretations of the neurologic status of the spinal cord. The newer techniques of MEPs with TCES have gained widespread acceptance as a standard clinical intraoperative neurophysiologic application. MEPs have allowed for a more accurate assessment and interpretation of the functional status of the motor pathways at various levels of the neuraxis.

PEARLS

1. One key to the success of intraoperative neurophysiologic monitoring is a good understanding of the capabilities and limitations of the neurophysiologic tests being monitored.
2. One of the first issues to address when planning for intraoperative neurophysiologic monitoring is to determine the types of neurophysiologic tests to perform on a particular patient undergoing surgery.
3. SEPs only monitor sensory transmission through the dorsal column pathways; they do not provide a direct measure of motor function.
4. In SEP monitoring an amplitude drop of greater than 50% and latency prolongation of more than 10% are considered significant. The most significant change is a complete loss of the cortical potential.
5. MEP monitoring is a more direct technique that evaluates the motor pathway. Motor cortex stimulation with TCES provides a more reliable methodology for monitoring the motor pathways.

PITFALLS

1. Significant changes in SEP monitoring can involve significant latency and amplitude changes that can occur in isolation.
2. If there is an absence of the peripheral response in SEP monitoring, a technical cause to the change must be ruled out.
3. There has been recent evidence to suggest that these spinally elicited neurogenic responses are generated through activation of the sensory pathways and retrograde activation of the alpha motor neurons.
4. Latency values have not always been found to be reliable indicators of significant change in TCES monitoring in clinical practice.
5. The use of inhalational agents has a tendency to deteriorate MEP amplitudes.

KEY POINTS

1. The aim of most spinal cord monitoring is to prevent intraoperative injury that results in irreversible paraplegia or quadriplegia. Due to the inability to perform a neurologic examination in an anesthetized patient, intraoperative neurophysiologic monitoring is used to determine the patient's neurologic status during surgery.
2. The term *significant change* is used in reference to the degree of changes seen in the neurophysiologic recordings. Changes termed *significant* have been shown to correlate well with intraoperative injury to the nervous system.
3. SEP monitoring has been used for many years to monitor spinal function intraoperatively during a variety of surgeries involving the spine, such as corrective surgery for scoliosis or other congenital deformities and removal of intraspinal tumors or arteriovenous malformations. SEPs only monitor sensory transmission through the dorsal column pathways.
4. A variety of methods have been used to monitor spinal motor pathways during surgery. The methodology of MEP monitoring has been revolutionized by the utilization of multipulse TCES. Two different methods of recording MEPs can be used. In myogenic MEPs, responses can be recorded directly from the muscle. The second method involves recording responses directly from the spinal cord with use of an epidural catheter electrode that records a direct D wave and a volley of indirect I waves.
5. A combination of SEP and transcranial MEP monitoring can be used to successfully monitor the spinal cord. This combination of techniques is considered safe, reliable, and accurate and may obviate the need for the wake-up test.
6. Intraoperative assessment during pedicle screw insertion can be used to minimize the risk of nerve root trauma from a misdirected screw. The integrity of pedicle screw placement can be assessed by directly stimulating the screw and by simultaneously recording myogenic responses from the appropriate myotomes.

KEY REFERENCES

1. Nuwer MR, Dawson EG, Carlson LG, et al. Somatosensory evoked potential spinal cord monitoring reduces neurologic deficits after scoliosis surgery: results of a large multicenter survey. *Electroencephalogr Clin Neurophysiol.* 1995;96:6-11.
2. Toleikis JR, Skelly JP, Carlvin AO, Burkus JK. Spinally elicited peripheral nerve responses are sensory rather than motor. *Clin Neurophysiol.* 2000;111:736-742.
3. Calancie B, Harris W, Broton JG, et al. "Threshold-level" multipulse transcranial electrical stimulation of motor cortex for intraoperative monitoring of spinal motor tracts: description of method and comparison to somatosensory evoked potential monitoring. *J Neurosurg.* 1998;88:457-470.
4. Deletis V, Sala F. The role of intraoperative neurophysiology in the protection or documentation of surgically induced injury to the spinal cord. *Ann N Y Acad Sci.* 2001;939:137-144.
5. MacDonal DB. Safety of intraoperative transcranial electrical stimulation motor evoked potential monitoring. *J Clin Neurophysiol.* 2002;19(5):416-429.

REFERENCES

1. Nuwer MR, Dawson EG, Carlson LG, et al. Somatosensory evoked potential spinal cord monitoring reduces neurologic deficits after scoliosis surgery: results of a large multicenter survey. *Electroencephalogr Clin Neurophysiol.* 1995; 96:6-11.
2. Lesser RP, Raudzens P, Luders H, et al. Postoperative neurological deficits may occur despite unchanged intraoperative somatosensory evoked potentials. *Ann Neurol.* 1986;19:22-25.
3. Zornow MH, Grafe MR, Tybor C, Swenson MR. Preservation of evoked potentials in a case of anterior spinal artery syndrome. *Electroencephalogr Clin Neurophysiol.* 1990;77: 137-139.
4. Lueders H, Gurd A, Hahn J, et al. A new technique for intraoperative monitoring of spinal cord function: multichannel recording of spinal cord and subcortical evoked potentials. *Spine.* 1982;7:110-115.
5. Su CF, Haghighi SS, Oro JJ, Gaines RW. "Backfiring" in spinal cord monitoring: high thoracic spinal cord stimulation evokes sciatic response by antidromic sensory pathway conduction, not motor tract conduction. *Spine.* 1992;17:504-508.
6. Toleikis JR, Skelly JP, Carlvin AO, Burkus JK. Spinally elicited peripheral nerve responses are sensory rather than motor. *Clin Neurophysiol.* 2000;111:736-742.
7. Minahan RE, Sepkuty JP, Lesser RP, et al. Anterior spinal cord injury with preserved neurogenic "motor" evoked potentials. *Clin Neurophysiol.* 2001;112:1442-1450.
8. Nash CL Jr, Lorig RA, Schatzinger LA, Brown RH. Spinal cord monitoring during operative treatment of the spine. *Clin Orthop.* 1977;126:100-105.
9. Jones SJ, Edgar MA, Ransford AO. Sensory nerve conduction in the human spinal cord: epidural recordings made during scoliosis surgery. *J Neurol Neurosurg Psychiatry.* 1982;45: 446-451.
10. Nuwer MR, Daube J, Fischer C, et al. Neuromonitoring during surgery. Report of an IFCN Committee. *Electroencephalogr Clin Neurophysiol.* 1993;87:263-276.
11. Merton PA, Morton HB. Stimulation of the cerebral cortex in the intact human subject. *Nature.* 1980;285:227.
12. Agnew WF, McCreery DB. Considerations for safety in the use of extracranial stimulation for motor evoked potentials. *Neurosurgery.* 1987;20:143-147.
13. Amassian VE, Cracco RQ. Human cerebral cortical responses to contralateral transcranial stimulation. *Neurosurgery.* 1987; 20:148-155.
14. Amassian VE, Stewart M, Quirk GJ, Rosenthal JL. Physiological basis of motor effects of a transient stimulus to cerebral cortex. *Neurosurgery.* 1987;20:74-93.
15. Cracco RQ. Evaluation of conduction in central motor pathways: techniques, pathophysiology, and clinical interpretation. *Neurosurgery.* 1987;20:199-203.
16. Cracco RQ, Amassian VE, Maccabee PJ, Cracco JB. Comparison of human transcallosal responses evoked by magnetic coil and electrical stimulation. *Electroencephalogr Clin Neurophysiol.* 1989;74:417-424.

17. Day BL, Rothwell JC, Thompson PD, et al. Motor cortex stimulation in intact man: II. Multiple descending volleys. *Brain*. 1987;110:1191-1209.
18. Jellinek D, Jewkes D, Symon L. Noninvasive intraoperative monitoring of motor evoked potentials under propofol anesthesia: effects of spinal surgery on the amplitude and latency of motor evoked potentials. *Neurosurgery*. 1991;29:551-557.
19. Jellinek D, Platt M, Jewkes D, Symon L. Effects of nitrous oxide on motor evoked potentials recorded from skeletal muscle in patients under total anesthesia with intravenously administered propofol. *Neurosurgery*. 1991;29:558-562.
20. Kalkman CJ, Drummond JC, Ribberink AA. Low concentrations of isoflurane abolish motor evoked responses to transcranial electrical stimulation during nitrous oxide/opioid anesthesia in humans. *Anesth Analg*. 1991;73:410-415.
21. Hicks R, Burke D, Stephen J, et al. Corticospinal volleys evoked by electrical stimulation of human motor cortex after withdrawal of volatile anesthetics. *J Physiol*. 1992;456: 393-404.
22. Hicks RG, Woodforth IJ, Crawford MR, et al. Some effects of isoflurane on I waves of the motor evoked potential. *Br J Anaesth*. 1992;69:130-136.
23. Calancie B, Harris W, Broton JG, et al. "Threshold-level" multipulse transcranial electrical stimulation of motor cortex for intraoperative monitoring of spinal motor tracts: description of method and comparison to somatosensory evoked potential monitoring. *J Neurosurg*. 1998;88:457-470.
24. Jones SJ, Harrison R, Koh KF, et al. Motor evoked potential monitoring during spinal surgery: responses of distal limb muscles to transcranial cortical stimulation with pulse trains. *Electroencephalogr Clin Neurophysiol*. 1996;100:375-383.
25. Rodi Z, Deletis V, Morota N, Vodusek DB. Motor evoked potentials during brain surgery. *Pflugers Arch*. 1996;431:R291-R292.
26. van Dongen EP, ter Beek HT, Schepens MA, et al. Effect of nitrous oxide on myogenic motor potentials evoked by a six pulse train of transcranial electrical stimuli: a possible monitor for aortic surgery. *Br J Anaesth*. 1999;82:323-328.
27. van Dongen EP, ter Beek HT, Schepens MA, et al. The influence of nitrous oxide to supplement fentanyl/low-dose propofol anesthesia on transcranial myogenic motor-evoked potentials during thoracic aortic surgery. *J Cardiothorac Vasc Anesth*. 1999;13:30-34.
28. van Dongen EP, ter Beek HT, Schepens MA, et al. Within-patient variability of myogenic motor-evoked potentials to multipulse transcranial electrical stimulation during two levels of partial neuromuscular blockade in aortic surgery. *Anesth Analg*. 1999;88:22-27.
29. Meylaerts SA, Jacobs MJ, van Iterson V, et al. Comparison of transcranial motor evoked potentials and somatosensory evoked potentials during thoracoabdominal aortic aneurysm repair. *Ann Surg*. 1999;230:742-749.
30. Calancie B, Harris W, Broton JG, et al. "Threshold-level" multipulse transcranial electrical stimulation of motor cortex for intraoperative monitoring of spinal motor tracts: description of method and comparison to somatosensory evoked potential monitoring. *J Neurosurg*. 1998;88:457-470.
31. Nuwer MR, Dawson EG, Carlson LG, et al. Somatosensory evoked potential spinal cord monitoring reduces neurologic deficits after scoliosis surgery: results of a large multicenter survey. *Electroencephalogr Clin Neurophysiol*. 1995;96:6-11.
32. Deletis V, Sala F. The role of intraoperative neurophysiology in the protection or documentation of surgically induced injury to the spinal cord. *Ann N Y Acad Sci*. 2001;939:137-144.
33. Cioni B, Meglio M, Rossi GF. Intraoperative motor evoked potentials monitoring in spinal neurosurgery. *Arch Ital Biol*. 1999;137:115-126.
34. MacDonal DB. Safety of intraoperative transcranial electrical stimulation motor evoked potential monitoring. *J Clin Neurophysiol*. 2002;19(5):416-429.
35. Luk KD, Hu Y, Wong YW, Cheung KM. Evaluation of various evoked potential techniques for spinal cord monitoring during scoliosis surgery. *Spine*. 2001;26:1772-1777.
36. Jones SJ, Harrison R, Koh KF, et al. Motor evoked potential monitoring during spinal surgery: responses of distal limb muscles to transcranial cortical stimulation with pulse trains. *Electroencephalogr Clin Neurophysiol*. 1996;100:375-383.
37. Lang EW, Beutler AS, Chesnut RM, et al. Myogenic motor-evoked potential monitoring using partial neuromuscular blockade in surgery of the spine. *Spine*. 1996;21:1676-1686.
38. Morota N, Deletis V, Constantini S, et al. The role of motor evoked potentials during surgery for intramedullary spinal cord tumors. *Neurosurgery*. 1997;41:1327-1336.
39. Stephen JP, Sullivan MR, Hicks RG, et al. Cotrel-Dubousset instrumentation in children using simultaneous motor and somatosensory evoked potential monitoring. *Spine*. 1996;21:2450-2457.
40. Calancie B, Klose KJ, Baier S, Green BA. Isoflurane-induced attenuation of motor evoked potentials caused by electrical motor cortex stimulation during surgery. *J Neurosurg*. 1991; 74:897-904.
41. Pechstein U, Nadstawek J, Zentner J, Schramm J. Isoflurane plus nitrous oxide versus propofol for recording of motor evoked potentials after high frequency repetitive electrical stimulation. *Electroencephalogr Clin Neurophysiol*. 1998;108:175-181.

SECTION II

CHAPTER 16 Targeting Pain Generators

Richard Derby
Lee Wolfer
Zachary McCormick

Spinal pain is very common, exacting a significant toll for the individual and society. Spine pain with a significant recurrence has lifetime prevalence estimated between 24% and 80%,[1,2] an annual prevalence of 15% to 45%, and a point prevalence of 18% to 30%.[3,4] Low back pain and neck pain are the first and fourth most common reason for disability among adults in the United States,[1,2,5] and both low back and neck pain rank within the top five reasons worldwide.[6] Chronic low back pain alone has been estimated to account for more than $100 billion in health care expenditure per year.[7] The prevalence of individuals seeking care for low back pain has increased significantly since the early 1990s. From 1992 to 2006, the prevalence of patients presenting with chronic impairing low back pain increased from 4% to 10%.[8] Targeting pain generators through precision diagnostic methods is the first step toward appropriate and effective treatments for chronic spinal pain.

Much of the epidemiologic data on low back pain are nonspecific, meaning that a cause cannot be found in most cases. Despite evidence to the contrary in the 21st century, these older, inaccurate epidemiologic studies continue to be quoted by current authors. One of the oldest epidemiologic studies commonly quoted was published more than 40 years ago by Dillane and colleagues[8] and was based on a retrospective practice audit of data gathered more than *50 years ago*. Dillane and colleagues[8] reported that they could not detect a cause for low back pain in approximately 80% of female and 90% of male patients with acute back syndrome. These authors did not report the use of any radiographic studies and apparently relied solely on history and physical examination.[9] They diagnosed approximately 11% of male patients and approximately 4% of female patients with low back "strain." Until more recently, the only tools to diagnose the etiology of low back pain have been history, physical examination, and sometimes radiographs or computed tomography (CT).

In 1982, Nachemson[10] reviewed the literature on chronic low back pain. In perhaps the most frequently quoted epidemiologic study on the cause of chronic low back pain, he reported that in only 15% of cases could a pathoanatomic explanation be found for patients with chronic low back pain (>3 months). As stated in the study, "probably very little can be done at our present state of ignorance to treat these patients and to improve their natural histories."[10] Low back pain is a symptom, not a diagnosis, in the same way that abdominal pain is a symptom and not a diagnosis. In acute cases of low back pain, this nonspecific diagnosis usually suffices because most cases of acute, first-time low back pain resolve with minimal intervention. However, when low back pain becomes chronic, recurrent, and disabling, the clinician must diagnose the source of the pain so that an appropriate treatment plan may be devised.

When a source of pain is not obvious, diagnosis often depends on who makes the diagnosis and sets the reference standards by which the diagnosis is "proven." Who is right? For that matter, can anyone reliably diagnose the cause of chronic benign spinal pain? Many authors argue that chronic benign spinal pain is largely due to exaggerated functional complaints and irreversible central nervous system sensitization,[11] making pain self-perpetuating and diagnosis all but impossible. These contentions are not often supported by primary studies,[12] however, and authors and clinicians question this diagnosis.[13,14]

Interventionalists developed and refined precision, fluoroscopically guided diagnostic interventional spine procedures in the 1980s and 1990s[15] to diagnose and treat nonspecific spinal pain more effectively. Fluoroscopically guided block procedures are now considered the reference standard to confirm a tissue diagnosis.[16] Out of the previous era of "ignorance," many diagnostic protocols have been validated and standardized.[17,18] Using the results of precision-guided diagnostic procedures, surgeons identify spinal segments for fusion at various stages of the degenerative cascade.[19] Most surgeons still depend on an accurate diagnosis of a specific pain generator to select appropriate therapy[20] because surgical results for chronic benign pain syndromes without a reversible anatomic cause are generally poor.[21]

The debate continues regarding diagnostic injections as new research emerges, along with better treatment options. Spinal pain is a complex interaction of many biopsychosocial factors. Chronic spinal pain may originate from one or more spinal levels and different anatomic structures in the anterior, middle, and posterior columns. Spinal pain also varies over time. Pain can be caused by abnormal mechanical stress on normal tissue affected by structural deformity, normal mechanical stress on injured tissues, minor stress on chronically inflamed and sensitized tissues, damaged nerves, and a varying combination of all of these. Chronic pain causes a greater or lesser degree of central sensitization and—together with a multitude of functional factors, including the requirement for copious amounts of opiates—often makes accurate diagnosis difficult. Nevertheless, it can be argued that most chronic axial spinal pain is due to accumulated repetitive strain or low-grade trauma,[22] acute injuries to the major underlying structures and their supporting ligaments, or both. Ongoing stimulation from these peripheral structures to a greater or lesser extent maintains a state of peripheral and central sensitization. In time, adaptive responses within the posterior, middle, and anterior columns may attenuate, exacerbate, or cause new sources of pain.

Despite this complexity, specific tissue pain generators can be hypothesized based on history, physical examination, imaging studies, and response to directed treatment. Interventional procedures are used to test the hypothesis that pain is related to a structural abnormality hypothesized by clinical and imaging findings. (The word *hypothesis* is used loosely here; arguably, one can only confirm a *clinical impression* using diagnostic blocks. A hypothesis is confirmed using a study protocol that can show approximately <5% probability that the findings are due to chance.) Foremost, interventional procedures are perhaps best used to refute one's hypothesis that a particular structure is painful. That is, diagnosis is made through the process of systematically excluding various tissue causes of axial and extremity pain in the posterior, middle, and anterior columns.[21]

This chapter presents primarily evidence-based standards and some expert opinions for confirming or refuting one's hypothesis that a particular structure, structures, or segments are a source of spinal pain.[17] A discussion of pain resulting from "red flag" conditions, such as fracture, tumor, infection, systemic diseases, or referred from nonspinal structures, is not included; likewise, "yellow flag" conditions (psychosocial factors) are not discussed in detail. Evaluation of the anterior column using provocative discography is discussed elsewhere; the discussion in this chapter is focused on diagnosis of pain originating from the posterior and middle columns, in particular, pain originating from the zygapophyseal joint and sacroiliac joint in the posterior column and from the nerve root, dorsal root ganglion, and dura in the middle column. The diagnostic use of injection procedures is explored but not their therapeutic value other than the diagnostic value of response or nonresponse to treatment. Finally, and most important, this chapter is not a systematic review. The interested reader is referred to numerous systematic reviews on the diagnostic value of spine injections.[3,17,18,22–28]

Diagnostic Analgesic Injections as Reference Standard

The belief that chronic benign spinal pain is difficult to diagnose is supported by the low specificity and sensitivity of the history, physical examination, and various imaging modalities as the reference standard for diagnosing chronic benign spinal pain[12,29,30] and a bias that chronic pain is to a greater rather than lesser extent a neuropathic process with central sensitization.[21] If one uses interventional diagnosis with precision fluoroscopically guided procedures as a reference standard for identifying pain, however, one can arrive at a tissue diagnosis in approximately 70% to 80% of cases.[31,32] Which approach is right? Truth usually lies somewhere in between.

The primary treating physician or consultant needs to formulate the diagnosis based on the available information and must be prepared to defend the diagnosis to contracted physician reviewers. Understanding the strengths and weaknesses of diagnostic analgesic data may help the practitioner decide whether the risk-to-benefit ratio of obtaining such information is appropriate for any given circumstance. Perhaps more important, the process of investigation itself may lead to a better understanding of the patient's capacity to respond appropriately to a technically successful surgical or interventional procedure.

The rationale for zygapophyseal joint blocks is based on the anatomic fact that the innervation of zygapophyseal joints (medial branches) is known and that zygapophyseal joints are capable of causing pain.[17] Local anesthetic blocks rely on the specificity of anesthetizing a single or limited number of structures or nerves and on the patient's capacity to distinguish clearly a reduction in preblock pain after anesthetizing one or more structures. Injection of a limited volume of local anesthetic into a zygapophyseal joint or its nerve supply is relatively specific for anesthetizing a joint and its capsule. Similarly, local anesthetic injected into the disc should anesthetize nociceptors within radial annular fissures that communicate with the nucleus. When anesthetizing the nerve root within the middle column, the block is less specific for axial pain relief because several structures may be partially blocked (e.g., dorsal root ganglion, ventral rami, sinuvertebral nerve, posterior longitudinal ligament).

Anesthetizing a structure does not reveal the cause of pain; anesthetizing the nerve supply simply relieves pain. This is an important concept. The cause of pain should dictate the type of treatment, and the treatment is only as good or bad as its success in eliminating or modulating the cause. If the cause of pain in the case of a specific zygapophyseal joint is synovial inflammation, one would expect short-term to intermediate pain relief after the intraarticular injection of corticosteroids. If a patient's pain is due to mechanical or neuropathic causes, there is no reason that corticosteroids would be effective other than the expected duration of the local anesthetic. There is no reason that there should be longer-term pain relief except for the expected rate of placebo response or reported pain relief secondary to spontaneous pain regression.[33] That is, relief of pain during the local anesthetic phase does not distinguish irreversible neuropathic pain from reversible nociceptive pain. In the case of chronic radicular pain, significant relief of pain for several weeks after the injection of corticosteroids would suggest that there is a reversible structural cause.[34]

Testing Protocols for Diagnostic Injections

As essential as precision technique is in the performance of diagnostic blocks, so is standardized assessment. Standardized diagnostic block evaluation sheets should be filled out for each patient; detailed postprocedure assessment protocols and sample evaluation instruments are available in the Spine Intervention Society Practice Guidelines.[18] Preprocedural and postprocedural evaluation should be performed by unbiased personnel and checked by the physician. It is recommended that the patient fill out a body pain diagram with pain scores (visual analog scale [VAS]) before and after the procedure. Additionally, the patient should rate current pain levels with various movements (e.g., lumbar flexion, extension, side-bending, sitting, and standing).

Evaluation after the procedure includes VAS scores with the same positions and maneuvers and a subjective report of percent relief of pain. The patient's narrative response should corroborate with VAS score, and any discrepancies should be explained. With medial branch blocks, relief of pain may vary according to the mass of drug reaching the nerve, and one may not reliably achieve a long-acting block; however, relief for less than 1 hour is unconvincing. In the case of selective nerve root blocks, it is often useful to have the patient distinguish between axial, proximal (shoulder or buttock), and extremity pain, the caveat being that a diagnostic block may not significantly reduce axial pain, but that does not mean that the block was unsuccessful. Some patients also need to be counseled to ignore injection site pain. Specific provoking maneuvers should be evaluated, such as the Spurling test for cervical radiculopathy and three or more sacroiliac joint provocative maneuvers before and after the procedure. Ideally, the patient would be tested at approximately 15 minutes after a lidocaine block and approximately 30 minutes after a bupivacaine block. Additional evaluations at 1 and 2 hours after block are useful but may depend on availability of staff.

The patient may be sent home with a pain diary to keep for 6 to 8 hours after the procedure. For any diagnostic injection, a patient should have at least approximately 5/10 intensity of pain to be able to judge the degree of relief reliably. A subject should have at least 50% relief for a positive response to be considered; at least 70% relief is more convincing. In regard to selective nerve root blocks, no more than two levels should be checked on one session. Depending on the importance of refuting or confirming whether a particular nerve is symptomatic, one may choose to inject the most probable source of pain or a level that it is hoped can be proven nonpainful.

A common problem encountered when attempting to identify the etiologic structure of pain with a diagnostic injection occurs when the nature of pain is intermittent or determined by prolonged activity. For example, a patient may experience significant symptoms late in the day or after an hour of prolonged standing or sitting. If this patient were to present to the office for a diagnostic block early in the morning, pain may not be present, clouding the ability of the patient to report relief (or lack thereof) after a diagnostic block procedure. If such is the case, the patient may be asked to perform provocative maneuvers that typically incite pain prior to the diagnostic block procedure. Repeated or sustained extension and rotation movements may be useful in these situations for posterior structures such as zygapophyseal joints or spinal nerve root–mediated pain related to central canal or neural foraminal stenosis; repeated flexion maneuvers may be helpful to incite spinal nerve root pain of presumed discogenic etiology. These maneuvers can then be repeated after the block procedure, and the patient is queried as to the relative reduction of pain with these movements compared to preblock testing. Alternatively, the patient can be rescheduled with instructions to perform activities (i.e., prolonged standing, walking, or sitting) that typically provoke pain and also to stop taking analgesic medications prior to the appointment for diagnostic blocks. If a patient's pain varies by time of day, the block procedure may be scheduled to accommodate this pattern, and if pain typically peaks well after clinic hours, a longer-acting local anesthetic (i.e., bupivacaine) should be used. Particularly in such situations, patients must be instructed to keep thorough pain diaries for the 6 to 8 hours following the diagnostic block procedure.

Confounding Factors

Sedation

An important, potentially confounding factor when performing diagnostic blocks concerns the use of sedation. Logically, one would assume that administration of opiates and sedatives before a diagnostic block would increase the false-positive rate; however, Manchikanti and colleagues[35] found that this proportion of patients was relatively small and that there was no difference with use of saline, opiate, or sedative. In a randomized study of 60 patients, these authors titrated medication to relaxation using saline, midazolam, or fentanyl. They found that only 50% of patients receiving sodium were relaxed, whereas 100% of patients receiving either fentanyl or midazolam were relaxed. In all groups, 10% of the patients reported greater than 80% pain relief with active motion testing. Even so, typically, one limits or omits sedation before a diagnostic injection, however. If the patient is anxious or especially if the patient routinely takes significant doses of opiates and may be in early opiate withdrawal owing to NPO status, the patient could be sedated and tested after the administration of a judicious dose of opiate.

Biopsychosocial Factors

More recently, authors have reiterated the importance of shifting the concept of "backache." Kikuchi[36] recommended changing the term *spinal disorder* to *biopsychosocial pain syndrome* and the term *morphologic abnormality* to *mechanical, functional disorder*. According to Kikuchi,[36] morphologic and structural abnormalities do not always explain all of a patient's pain, and chronic backache should not be seen as an isolated spinal disease. A significant amount of scholarship has been devoted to enumerating the psychosocial factors associated with spinal pain. In a classic study comparing workers with symptomatic disc herniation (requiring surgery) versus asymptomatic workers, significant differences were found in three areas: presence of nerve root compromise, psychosocial factors (depression, anxiety, marital status, self-control), and work perception (satisfaction, job loss, occupational stress, intensity of concentration).[37] Of the risk factors, two of three were functional, not morphologic.

We agree with this model and acknowledge that psychosocial factors have a significant impact on spinal pain; we also acknowledge the importance of treating the "bio" component of the *biopsychosocial syndrome*. Today's spine specialists readily acknowledge that patients often benefit from a multidisciplinary approach to treatment. Research continues to investigate the best way to treat patients with chronic spinal pain and significant psychosocial comorbidities.

Although the long-term results of treatment for chronic axial back pain may be influenced by various psychosocial factors,[38,39] the possible effect of psychosocial factors in determining the patient's tested perception of pain and functional improvement with treatment does not indicate that the diagnosis was incorrect. In many cases, when a "biologic" pain generator can be correctly identified and treated, the psychosocial distress resolves. If it is true that psychological variables determine whether a patient admits relief on various testing instruments, does the evidence of physiologic distress noted on test scores reverse when the patient's chronic pain is relieved?

Wallis and colleagues[40] studied 17 patients after whiplash injury with a single symptomatic cervical zygapophyseal joint who were enrolled in a randomized controlled trial of percutaneous radiofrequency neurotomy. At 3 months after the procedure, all patients whose pain was relieved had complete resolution of preoperative psychological distress; in contrast, all but one of the patients who did not experience pain relief continued to experience psychological distress. Manchikanti and colleagues[41] found no correlation between somatization disorder and inappropriate Waddell signs and symptoms to response in pain relief after a comparative double-block protocol for diagnosing zygapophyseal joint pain. Derby and colleagues[42] found no difference in response to pressure-controlled disc stimulation between patients with abnormal psychometric Distress Risk Assessment Method scores and asymptomatic volunteers.

Posterior Compartment: Zygapophyseal Joint and Sacroiliac Joint

The zygapophyseal joint and sacroiliac joint are the two primary structures within the posterior compartment that are sources of chronic spinal pain. In addition, hip and shoulder pain may cause symptoms similar to spinal structures and localized injections into these joints with preblock and postblock active examination can help differentiate hip and shoulder pain from spinal pain. Although soft tissues may be painful, for the purpose and brevity of this chapter, these structures are considered a secondary source of pain in most chronic spinal conditions.

Zygapophyseal Joint

Each spinal segment is composed of a three-joint complex: the intervertebral discs and two posterolateral zygapophyseal joints.[41] The word *apophysis* is Greek, meaning an "offshoot" or a "bony protuberance."[43] Anatomically, the zygapophyseal joint is an outgrowth of the vertebral body. The zygapophyseal joints are formed by the articulation of the inferior articular process of one vertebra with the superior articular process of the inferior vertebra. Zygapophyseal joints have classic synovial joint features: hyaline cartilage surfaces, a synovial membrane, and a surrounding joint capsule.[44] Zygapophyseal joints have varied morphology and function based on their location within the spine. Although the intervertebral disc is loaded primarily in flexion, the zygapophyseal joints are loaded in extension and lumbar rotation.[45,46] The orientation of the zygapophyseal joint varies based on the requirements of regional spine function. Lumbar zygapophyseal joints are situated sagittally to limit axial rotation and to allow flexion and extension, whereas the cervical and thoracic zygapophyseal joints are oriented coronally to limit shearing forces on the disc. Innervation is via the medial branches of the dorsal ramus in most locations.

Pathophysiology of Zygapophyseal Joint Pain

Traumatic injury to lumbar and cervical zygapophyseal joints is common and probably occurs to a lesser extent to the thoracic joints consistent with the relative degree of load bearing in extension at these levels. In the setting of trauma, there is a clear pathophysiologic difference between zygapophyseal joints and nontraumatic controls. Zygapophyseal joint sections from autopsy specimens of individuals with a past history of trauma but dying of natural causes show significant age-related, gender-related, and trauma-related changes in the bone, cartilage, and soft tissues, including subchondral sclerosis, fibrillation and splitting of cartilage, and cartilage length differences, versus subjects with no history of trauma.[47] Histologic sections of the lumbar zygapophyseal joints of mostly motor vehicle accident victims revealed fractures of the superior articular process, central infarctions of the subchondral bone plate, and capsule tears, including the ligamentum flavum.[48,49] Most tissue sections (77%) show soft tissue injuries, and approximately 30% (11 of 33) show fractures and infarctions. Sections from the cervical spine in trauma victims show similar injuries to the zygapophyseal joint articular cartilage and annular lesions in the intervertebral discs and cartilaginous endplates (Fig. 16.1).[50] In the lumbar and cervical spines, lesions were found exclusively in the trauma patients and in none of the patients in the control group.[47,50,51]

Many of these pathoanatomic findings are occult on routine radiographs, CT scan, and magnetic resonance imaging (MRI) but may be the cause of ongoing neck pain in survivors of motor vehicle accidents or other significant trauma. In a small study with short-term follow-up (approximately 3 months), Eisenstein and Parry[52] examined zygapophyseal joints in 12 patients who underwent successful fusion for zygapophyseal joint–mediated pain (diagnosed by provocation arthrography, intraarticular blocks, and negative discography) versus controls and found histologic changes similar to changes of chondromalacia patellae and osteoarthritis of large joints. The most frequent finding was focal full-thickness cartilage

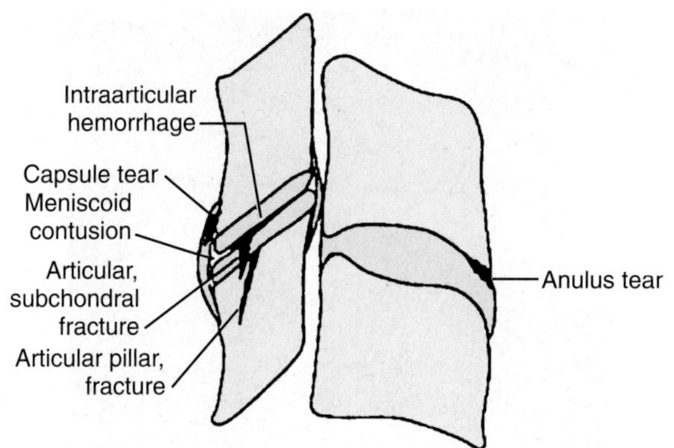

FIG. 16.1 Postmortem studies of motor vehicle victims reveal the following sites of injury; many of these injuries may not be visible on routine MRI. (From Bogduk N, McGuirk B. *Management of Acute and Chronic Neck Pain: An Evidence-Based Approach*. Philadelphia, PA: Elsevier; 2006.)

necrosis or loss of cartilage with exposure of subchondral bone; osteophyte formation was absent in all specimens.[52] Degenerative histologic findings alone do not make a definitive diagnosis of zygapophyseal joint syndrome, however. Ziv and colleagues[53] reported a high proportion of coarsely fibrillated and/or ulcerated zygapophyseal joints in fresh cadaveric spines from young adults (30–50 years old); such degeneration remains constant throughout adulthood.

Traumatic and repetitive injury leading to painful "facet (zygapophyseal joint) arthritis"[49] may cause pain because zygapophyseal joints and their capsules are heavily innervated structures subject to high stress and strain during spinal loading.[54] Joints comprise free and encapsulated nerve endings containing substance P and calcitonin gene-related peptide.[55–57] Substance P, calcitonin gene-related peptide, and immunoreactive sensory and autonomic nerves are found in zygapophyseal joint synovial membranes.[58] Zygapophyseal joint capsules contain low-threshold mechanoreceptors, mechanically sensitive nociceptors, and silent nociceptors.[59] These low-threshold and high-threshold mechanoreceptors fire when the joint capsule is stretched or compressed; their firing can be suppressed by injected lidocaine and hydrocortisone.[60] In animal models, induced inflammation decreases the threshold of nerves within the joint capsules and causes elevated baseline discharge rates.[60] In animal models of knee arthritis, acute inflammation sensitizes fine articular afferents, which become active at rest and respond more vigorously to routine painless joint range of motion.[61]

Excessive stretching damages the zygapophyseal joint capsules and causes axonal swelling, retraction balls, and inflammation.[59] The result is hyperexcitability and spontaneous firing, which are synonymous with neuropathic pain. Capsular injury during a whiplash injury may cause persistent neck pain secondary to chronic capsular overstretching. Animal studies suggest that zygapophyseal joint capsule strains comparable to strains previously reported for whiplash kinematics and subcatastrophic failures of this ligament activate nociceptors within the capsule.[62–66] In addition, chronic capsular loading in animals may cause central inflammation, resulting in mechanical hyperalgesia and, in some cases, centrally maintained pain.[57,64,67,68]

Animal studies showing central sensitization are consistent with the widespread hypersensitivity documented in whiplash patients. Although focal sensitization to mechanical stimuli may be found 3 months after whiplash injury, which mostly resolves by 6 months, some patients develop persistent pain with symptoms that are consistent with chronic neuropathic pain.[69] Patients with persistent pain at approximately 6 months show signs of more widespread hyperalgesia[70] and hypersensitivity to cutaneous and muscular stimulation in the neck and lower limb consistent with central hypersensitivity.[11,71]

If chronic pain originating from injury to the zygapophyseal joints is due to capsular stretch and maintained by central hypersensitivity, local anesthetic with or without corticosteroid should suppress nociceptive input for the duration of the local anesthetic effect and, in some cases (e.g., similar to a sympathetically maintained pain state), for days to weeks.[72] If most of a patient's pain is due to mechanical and central causes, there would be no reason why local anesthetic and corticosteroid would be more effective than local anesthetic alone.[73–75] Former and latter logical outcomes are supported in prospective and randomized controlled trials,[75] although alleviating pain with medial branch blocks was shown in one study to relieve pain for an average of several months.[76,77]

Decreasing peripheral input 6 months or longer by heat ablation of medial branches relieves pain[78,79]; the pain typically returns within the expected time it takes for the medial branches to regenerate. Such prolonged relief of pain, if accompanied by resolution of widespread hypersensitivity, would imply that central hypersensitivity is reversible when the peripheral source of input is interrupted. That is, if there is a concern that persistent central hypersensitivity would lead to failure of a proposed localized or segmental stabilization procedure, resolution of widespread and local hypersensitivity after medial branch neurotomy might predict that decrease in nociceptive input by surgical stabilization would be successful. Zygapophyseal joint pain often occurs at more than one segment, however; adjacent or skipped level sources of zygapophyseal joint pain must be identified, especially when considering surgical fusion or arthroplasty.

When cadaveric lumbar spines are anteriorly fixated at one level, motion is transferred to adjacent segments, causing increased capsular stretch in the adjacent zygapophyseal joints.[80] In extension, cervical arthroplasty models exhibit significant increases of zygapophyseal joint force at the treated level. In the fusion model, the zygapophyseal joint forces decrease at the treated segment and increase at the adjacent segment.[81] Failure to recognize symptomatic pathology at an adjacent level or the same level may lead to early or late return of pain. This is not a failure of the diagnostic blocks; it is a failure to obtain a thorough diagnosis.

Rationale for Control Blocks in Diagnostic Zygapophyseal Joint Intraarticular and Medial Branch Blocks

Can a diagnosis of zygapophyseal joint syndrome be made without injections? The diagnosis of zygapophyseal joint pain is typically hypothesized based on clinical findings and imaging studies. Most clinicians rely on a variety of criteria, such as localized unilateral pain that is worse in extension, pain worse in the morning and better with gentle movement, concordant pain provoked with palpation approximately 1 cm lateral to the midline over the zygapophyseal joints, and imaging studies showing signs of zygapophyseal joint degeneration. A "facet (zygapophyseal joint) syndrome"[82] diagnosed by clinical findings alone has not been substantiated; rather, a reference standard of pain relief after placebo-controlled anesthetic blocks is necessary.[25,29,83] The current best evidence has not found any individual clinical finding or cluster of findings that can predict response to the reference standard of pain relief after local anesthetic block of the medial branches or intraarticular zygapophyseal joint block.

The purpose of diagnostic zygapophyseal joint blocks is to establish the diagnosis or rule it out, similar to a liver biopsy of a suspicious lesion. Diagnostic zygapophyseal joint blocks are a tertiary intervention in patients with chronic pain that has not resolved with time and conservative care. The current standard for the diagnosis of zygapophyseal joint–mediated pain is the use of controlled differential (double) blocks to confirm or refute one's hypothesis that the zygapophyseal joint is a pain generator. Because of the high false-positive rates of single diagnostic blocks, a single block does not constitute a diagnosis, and control blocks are essential to decrease the incidence of false-positive responses.[84] The reported false-positive rate of a single diagnostic block ranges from 17% to 63%.[85] In a retrospective review of 438 patients using a double-block paradigm requiring 80% relief, the false-positive rates for a single diagnostic block were 45%, 42%, and 45% for the cervical, thoracic, and lumbar regions, respectively.[85]

Although Cohen and colleagues[86] showed that treatment results after medial branch neurotomies were not changed by requiring a placebo control, the current published standard of interventional societies requires a confirmatory block before making a diagnosis of zygapophyseal joint–mediated pain.[17] The best-studied double-block protocol requires a difference in pain relief that is of concordant duration to the duration of action of the local anesthetic used to anesthetize the medial branch nerves—typically, greater than 2 to 3 hours for lidocaine and 4 to 6 hours for bupivacaine.[87,88] Because the goal is to have a placebo control and because consent and patient compliance issues hinder using a saline block control, one may argue that any prior diagnostic injection in which the patient reports no relief is a valid control block, especially because the patient and the physician were anticipating relief. Because many insurance companies in the United States no longer authorize or consider double blocks medically necessary, the occurrence of a previous "negative" block evaluation could be the negative control.

When the treatment is relatively benign, convincing relief with physician and staff testing after zygapophyseal joint or medial branch injections in an older patient with clinical symptoms consistent with zygapophyseal joint pain may not justify confirmatory injections.[86,89] A young patient who has little or no zygapophyseal joint abnormalities, who is on a significant dose of narcotics, and who reports less-than-convincing

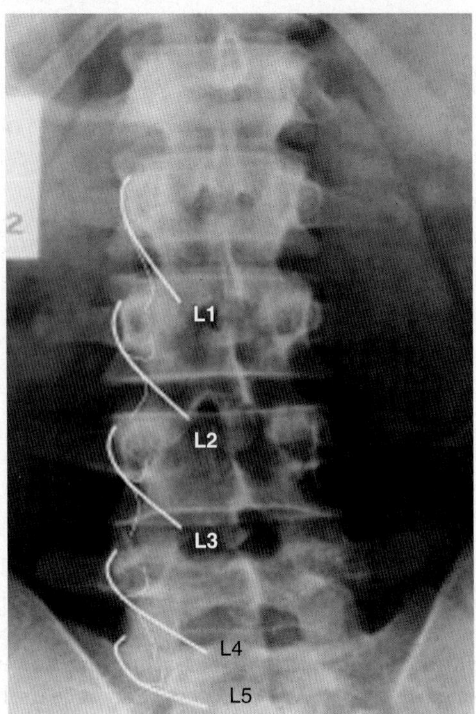

FIG. 16.2 Anteroposterior radiograph of the lumbar spine showing course of medial branches of L1–L4 dorsal rami, L5 dorsal ramus, and their articular branches to lumbar zygapophyseal joints. Medial branches are blocked at the junction of the superior articular process and transverse process. (From Bogduk N, ed. *Practice Guidelines for Spinal Diagnostic and Treatment Procedures*. San Francisco, CA: International Spine Intervention Society; 2004.)

approximately 80% relief should undergo a second confirmatory injection before considering interventional or surgical treatment based on the block results.

The rationale for how many levels and which levels to test is being debated. Levels are typically chosen based on known pain referral patterns, prevalence studies, and localized manual palpation. Using a comparative double-block control, Manchukonda and colleagues[85] found that, most often, two joints were symptomatic in the lumbar spine and three adjacent joints were symptomatic in the thoracic and cervical spine. The most logistically efficient and least costly method is to rule out zygapophyseal joint pain globally on the side or sides of the patient's pain and at the proximity of approximately two to three adjacent levels. One would inject (in the case of lumbar spine) the L2, L3, and L4 medial branch nerves and the dorsal ramus of the L5 nerve root in order to block the L3–L4, L4–L5, and L5–S1 zygapophyseal joints (Fig. 16.2 shows medial branch anatomy of the lumbar spine; Fig. 16.3 shows a lumbar medial branch block). If no relief occurred, there was no evidence that the higher joints were involved, and if one is confident that the zygapophyseal joints were denervated, one can eliminate zygapophyseal joint pain from the diagnosis. If the result is positive, one can perform more selected denervation on a confirmatory injection. Although this could be argued to be the most efficient method, many third-party payers in the United States limit injections to two levels per session.

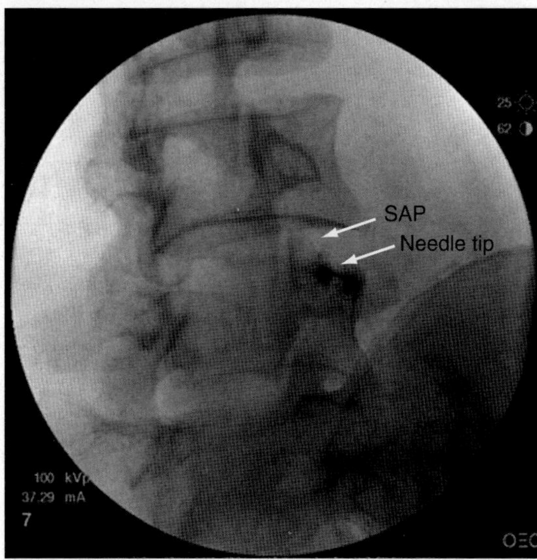

FIG. 16.3 Oblique view of right L4 medial branch block. A 3.5-inch, 25-gauge needle is placed at the junction of the L5 superior articular process and transverse process. A total of 0.5 mL of contrast dye is injected along the medial branch. SAP, superior articular process. (Courtesy Richard Derby, MD.)

Diagnostic Accuracy

The features of a test that indicate its diagnostic accuracy are sensitivity and specificity. From these measures, the false-positive and false-negative rates and predictive value can be derived. *Sensitivity* refers to the ability of the test to identify correctly patients with the disease. Several factors that affect sensitivity should be discussed. Vessels accompany the medial branch as they course around the waist of the superior articular pillar, and injecting local anesthetic into a vessel rather than around the nerve may cause a false-negative response.

Kaplan and colleagues[90] reported that medial branch blocks may fail because of venous uptake. Venous uptake occurred in 7 of 20 (35%) medial branch blocks. If venous uptake was encountered, repositioning of the needle resulted in joint anesthesia only 50% of the time. When venous uptake was encountered, the subjects were brought back for a later injection. These findings stress the importance of using contrast medium for medial branch blocks and carefully observing the flow pattern. Kaplan and colleagues[90] also found that in 11% of cases they were unable to anesthetize the joint, even in the absence of venous uptake. Medial branch blocks in the lumbar spine would have an 11% false-negative rate. This may have been due to anomalous or collateral zygapophyseal joint innervation or insufficient volume of local anesthetic reaching the target nerve, which may be shielded by an ossified mamalloaccessory ligament. This occurs in approximately 10% of patients.[91,92]

Rarely discussed is the consistency with which one may expect a longer duration of action of bupivacaine versus lidocaine. Although bupivacaine has a longer duration of action than lidocaine, the mass of drug reaching the nerve is the most important variable, and one cannot guarantee that the same amount will be available on consecutive sessions. In addition, most patients are not kept in the recovery area for the duration of local anesthetic to be evaluated, and the duration depends on a patient's self-reporting, which may or may not be consistent between injections. Lord and colleagues[88] showed that, using a double-block comparative standard, 65% of patients failed to recognize the difference in duration of pain relief but did accurately distinguish a separate placebo-controlled block with saline. This underscores the importance of instructing the patient to keep a diligent pain diary for the 6 to 8 hours following diagnostic blocks and then to report this information the following day in order to minimize recall bias.

The crucial factors for specificity of the diagnosis of zygapophyseal joint pain are accurate targeting of the intended structure under fluoroscopy, confirmed by contrast medium, and the delivery of the appropriate volume of local anesthetic. Intraarticular joint blocks are specific, unless there is a medial capsular tear or injection of excessive volumes (>1 mL injected into a lumbar zygapophyseal joint or 0.3 mL injected into a cervical zygapophyseal joint), which may rupture the capsule and spread medially into the epidural space.[93,94] Many early studies of zygapophyseal joint intraarticular blocks used 2 to 8 mL per injection. When reviewing negative studies regarding zygapophyseal joint injections and the systematic reviews that still quote these studies, the discerning reader should check the total volume of injectant used.[94,95] Destouet and colleagues[94] found that volumes of injectant of 0.5 to 1.5 mL commonly ruptured the superior recess of the capsule and extravasated. In later studies, Destouet and colleagues[94] aspirated the 0.5 to 1.5 mL of contrast dye before adding local anesthetic and steroid. Cadaveric studies performed with variable volumes of methylene blue injected into the zygapophyseal joint (1–4 mL) showed that the dye extended not as expected into the paraspinal tissues but rather into the epidural space and around the spinal nerves.[96] Moran and colleagues[96] described the zygapophyseal joint capsule as thick dorsally, whereas anteriorly the zygapophyseal joint synovial membrane is contiguous with the ligamentum flavum and the adipose tissue in the superior recess is in direct contact with the adipose tissue around the spinal nerve. Clearly, extravasation of local anesthetic through the anterior aspect of the zygapophyseal joint capsule and subsequent anesthesia of potential pain generators outside of the zygapophyseal joint—such as the adjacent spinal nerve root, posterior longitudinal ligament, or sinuvertebral nerve—can potentially affect the diagnostic specificity of the block procedure.

In contrast, randomized controlled studies validate the specificity of medial branch blocks for relief of zygapophyseal joint–mediated pain.[97] To maintain the specificity of medial branch block, a low volume of local anesthetic is used to anesthetize a specific cervical[97] or lumbar medial branch.[90,93] If volumes greater than 0.5 mL are used, the close proximity of the lumbar lateral and intermediate branch to the medial branch potentially might increase false-positive rates by blocking paraspinal soft tissues (ligaments or muscles or both).[22,98] In addition, volumes greater than 0.5 mL on the superior edge of the lumbar transverse process may spread onto the dorsal and ventral spinal nerves.[37] Decreasing input into the central nervous system by anesthetizing any structure or nerve could relieve pain by decreasing or modulating central input. Although this is a probable confounding factor, the reference typically cited is the study by North and colleagues,[99] which reported an unacceptably high false-positive rate for diagnostic blocks in patients with low back pain. The conclusion reached by that author group was that diagnostic blocks had limited specificity. Their protocol clearly lacked diagnostic specificity, however. They used an excessive 3 mL volume of bupivacaine for the medial branch blocks. Because 0.5 mL of local anesthetic placed too close to the superior edge flows onto the exiting root, the reported decrease in sciatic pain was more likely due to anesthetizing the spinal nerve and not a false-positive effect of neuromodulation.[93]

Because patients in the study by North and colleagues[99] reported an average relief of 75% to 80% after anesthetizing the sciatic nerve, operators must be aware that blocking this nerve anywhere along its course may result in the report of pain relief. As previously mentioned, relief of pain for the duration of the local anesthetic effect cannot distinguish between reversible inflammatory or compressive causes of pain and nonreversible neuropathic causes of pain.

Although North and colleagues[99] found that 3 mL of local anesthetic placed into muscles at several levels has relatively minimal effect on sciatic pain, some authors question whether anesthetizing the needle track increases false-positive responses.[22] Patients probably report more pain relief when the needle track is anesthetized. Rather than a false-positive response, one would expect better pain relief when patients are not experiencing lingering needle-related pain at the same time as pain relief resulting from anesthetizing the zygapophyseal joints.

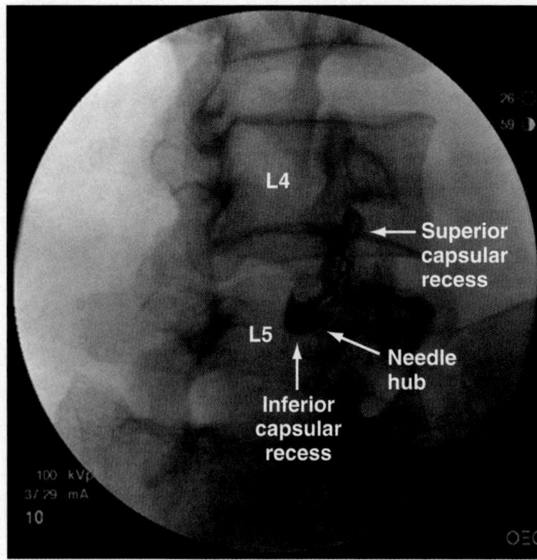

FIG. 16.4 Right L4–L5 zygapophyseal joint intraarticular injection. Note the filling of the superior and inferior subcapsular capsular recesses with contrast dye (*arrow*). The needle hub partially overlies the inferior capsular recess. (Courtesy Richard Derby, MD.)

Lumbar Spine: Zygapophyseal Joint Syndrome

History

In 1911, Goldthwait[100] reported that zygapophyseal joint asymmetry could cause lumbago, sciatica, and paraplegia. Ghormley[101] first coined the term *zygapophyseal joint syndrome* as a cause of referred pain and the sciatica resulting from direct nerve root compression by the zygapophyseal joint. Badgley[102] first described the zygapophyseal joint as an independent source of referred pain in greater detail. Mooney and Robertson[82] described "facet (zygapophyseal joint) syndrome" referral patterns by injection of hypertonic saline into the lumbar zygapophyseal joints of patients with positive diagnostic blocks. Subsequently, Mooney and Robertson[82] were the first to use radiographically guided intraarticular injections with local anesthetic and corticosteroid. They reported complete pain relief in approximately one-fifth of patients presenting with low back and leg pain. Dreyfuss and colleagues[93] were the first to describe an effective lumbar medial branch block technique. Using this technique, Kaplan and colleagues[90] showed that pain resulting from zygapophyseal joint capsular distention could be successfully blocked in approximately 90% of cases by medial branch anesthesia with 2% lidocaine versus saline.

Lumbar Zygapophyseal Joint Pain

Lumbar zygapophyseal joint pain is common and seems to become more prevalent as patients age and as the duration of chronic back pain increases. The prevalence is directly inversely correlated, however, to the stringency of the reference standard. Prevalence studies consistently find the zygapophyseal joint as a common source of pain, but diagnosis using a single anesthetic block has a potential high placebo rate versus a double-block comparative control requiring a longer duration of relief after lidocaine versus bupivacaine.

Studies reporting the prevalence of zygapophyseal joint pain report figures ranging from 15% to 52%. In 1994, Schwarzer and colleagues[103] established the prevalence of zygapophyseal joint pain using a double-block comparative protocol in 96 patients with a mean age of 38 years and mean duration of low back pain of 16 months mostly secondary to work-related injuries and trauma presenting to two tertiary US clinics. (Fig. 16.4 shows a lumbar intraarticular zygapophyseal joint block.) These authors found that the combination of discogenic pain and zygapophyseal joint pain is uncommon. In a group of 176 patients, 47% had initial relief with a screening lidocaine block, but only 15% had 50% or greater relief with a confirmatory block.

Manchikanti and colleagues,[104] also using a double-block protocol but requiring 75% pain relief and a differential response, reported an even higher initial response of 81 of 120 (67.5%) to lidocaine medial branch blocks and a much greater percentage (45%) of the total reporting longer 75% relief after confirmatory bupivacaine medial branch blocks. This patient group was older than Schwarzer's group, however, with a mean age of 47 years and with a longer mean duration of low back pain of 47 months. The false-positive rate for one block was 41%. In a later study, Manchikanti and colleagues[105] revised the prevalence of zygapophyseal joint pain downward from 45% to 27% (95% confidence interval [95% CI], 22–32%). Schwarzer and colleagues[106] studied an older group of patients with a mean age of 57 years referred to an Australian rheumatology clinic with low back pain for an average of 7 years. A diagnosis of zygapophyseal joint pain was made in 40% (95% CI, 27–53%). Requiring 90% relief of original pain, the prevalence was 32%; requiring 100% relief, the prevalence was 11%. Manchikanti and colleagues[105] reported an even higher prevalence of 52% zygapophyseal joint pain in a group of patients 65 years old or older.

No consistent history, physical examination, or imaging findings correlated to positive block responses have been found. In the early 1980s, uncontrolled single, variable injectant volume, intraarticular zygapophyseal joint injections were used as the reference standard for identifying lumbar zygapophyseal joint pain; these authors reported correlations with various history or physical examination findings.[52,107] Some studies[108,109] reported that a cluster of five of seven features (*Revel criteria*) could predict a 75% decrease in pain after a single intraarticular block. The seven items in the cluster are age older than 65 years, pain well relieved by recumbency, no exacerbation of pain with coughing and sneezing, no exacerbation of pain with forward flexion, no exacerbation of pain with extension, no exacerbation of pain with rising from flexion, and no exacerbation of pain with the extension-rotation test. Subsequent well-conducted studies did not replicate these studies.[32,110] As mentioned, most of these earlier studies used single medial branch blocks, which have been reported to have 25% and 38% false-positive rates for the diagnosis of zygapophyseal joint pain.[111,112]

Newer studies of clinical correlations refined the technique with an appropriate injectant volume and a confirmatory double-block paradigm with either a second intraarticular injection or a medial branch confirmatory injection with bupivacaine lasting longer than the pain relief after a prior lidocaine block[30,96,106,111,113–115] These studies did not find any clinical correlates with history or physical examination. In particular, extension and rotation were not predictive of response. A systematic review of all published studies comparing clinical outcome after local anesthetic blocks and clinical signs and symptoms found no consistent clinical features with a high specificity.[12] The review found several clinical features with a high sensitivity, however, which may be cautiously used to *exclude* the diagnosis of zygapophyseal joint–mediated pain. These features include pain not increased with cough, pain not relieved with recumbency, and pain that can be centralized.[50] There are no consistent reproducible history or physical examination criteria that predict a positive response to a zygapophyseal joint block. History and physical examination are better at ruling out zygapophyseal joint–mediated pain than diagnosing zygapophyseal joint pain.

The current best evidence also shows that radiologic imaging, with a few more recent exceptions, does not correlate with response to zygapophyseal joint blocks. Conflicting evidence that radiologic imaging may predict outcome from uncontrolled lumbar zygapophyseal joint blocks may be partially due to lack of rigor in the reference standard used to define a positive response in earlier studies.[22] In 1979, Carrera[115] reported that 73% (n = 63) of patients describing pain relief after uncontrolled intraarticular injection of 2 to 4 mL of local anesthetic had CT evidence of lumbar zygapophyseal joint disease versus 13% who had no evidence of disease. It is well accepted, however, that injectant volume should not exceed 1 mL; otherwise, the injection loses specificity, with a leak/extravasation of local anesthetic and potential contact with the adjacent spinal nerve root or other possible pain generators located outside of the zygapophyseal joint, as described earlier.[96]

A large study by Jackson and colleague[116] of 390 patients found no relationship between imaging and pain relief after uncontrolled intraarticular lumbar zygapophyseal joint injections. Supporting the findings by Jackson and colleagues,[116] Schwarzer and colleagues,[106] in the only study using placebo-controlled injection, found no correlation between CT findings and a positive response comparing local anesthetic with saline blocks in 63 patients when more stringent criteria of controlled injections were used as the reference standard. Similarly, Cohen and colleagues[117] found no relationship in 192 patients between MRI findings of zygapophyseal joint hypertrophy or degeneration and response to medial branch neurotomies based on positive response to a single medial branch block. Kawaguchi and colleagues[118] likewise found no significant relationship between low back pain symptoms and radiographic abnormalities in a group of 106 patients with rheumatoid arthritis.

The intriguing bright spot on the horizon is the finding that where MRI or single photon emission computed tomography (SPECT) shows imaging findings consistent with either "inflammation" or "edema," a stronger correlation emerges (Fig. 16.5). Although not confirming the diagnosis of zygapophyseal joint pain with a reference standard, Friedrich and colleagues[119] more recently found that an estimated 14% (21 of 145) of patients with low back pain had MRI evidence of zygapophyseal joint edema, and follow-up MRI scan showed "almost perfect" agreement between change in pain and a reduction in intensity of edema on sagittal short-tau

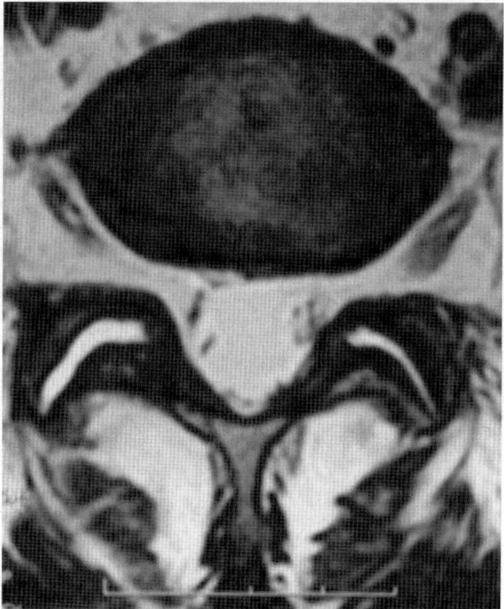

FIG. 16.5 L5–S1 axial T2-weighted magnetic resonance image showing zygapophyseal edema (right greater than left), suggestive of instability. In the upright weight-bearing position, anterolisthesis was noted; in the unloaded supine position, anterolisthesis reduced and zygapophyseal joints are gapped and filled with fluid. (Courtesy Richard Derby, MD.)

inversion recovery images. Radionuclide bone scintigraphy detects bone areas with synovial changes (inflammation or hyperemia) or increased osteoblast activity and degenerative regions with a high degree of remodeling. Osteophytes in the process of growing show a high degree of bone scan activity. As mentioned earlier, a positive lumbar SPECT scan predicts a statistically significant reduction in pain after zygapophyseal joint blocks.[33]

Zygapophyseal Joint Pain Referral Maps

Pain referral patterns have been studied using stimulation of patients during provocative diagnostic injections[120] by injection of hypertonic solutions into normal and abnormal subjects[121] or by electrical stimulation of medial branches.[120,121] Most studies showed distinct but overlapping referral areas; it is likely that the pain referral patterns obtained in normal volunteers are smaller because of less sensitization. There are also limits to the referral maps; Mooney and Robertson[121] reported on lumbar zygapophyseal joint referral maps in normal volunteers and subjects with a positive diagnostic zygapophyseal joint block (Fig. 16.6). Under fluoroscopic guidance, they injected contrast dye (unspecified volume) followed by 3 to 5 mL of hypertonic saline. Some of the distal extremity pain seen in the diagrams may be due to excessive volume of saline with irritation of the sciatic nerve roots. Given the lack of sensitivity and specificity of history, physical examination, and imaging and until more research is performed with finite injectant volumes (in patients with confirmed dual positive blocks), these referral maps can be used as a starting point to guide selection of levels to be injected.

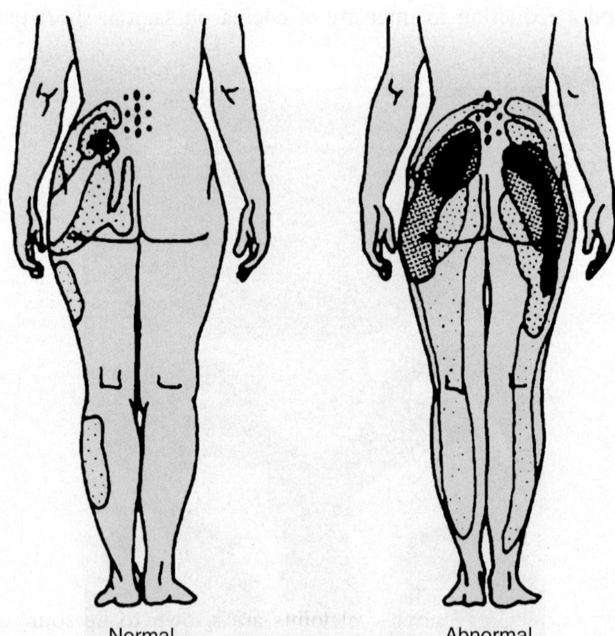

FIG. 16.6 Pain referral patterns for asymptomatic (normal) and symptomatic (abnormal) subjects obtained by intraarticular zygapophyseal joint injection of contrast dye followed by 3 to 5 mL of hypertonic saline. (From Mooney V, Robertson J. The facet syndrome. *Clin Orthop Relat Res.* 1976;115:149–156.)

Predictive Value

How useful are diagnostic zygapophyseal joint injections? The predictive value of any spinal diagnostic test directly varies with the rigorousness of test standards and the inherent ability of that treatment to alleviate the source of pain without creating new sources unrelated to the original cause or causes. A positive test is valuable if it can guide treatment and obtain better outcomes than not using the diagnostic test at all. A systematic review of the evidence for treatment of zygapophyseal joint pain is beyond the scope of this chapter; however, a case is made for the therapeutic utility of zygapophyseal joint blocks.

Historically, lacking robust studies, guideline and systematic review articles have been relegated to quoting studies with methodologic flaws as implied evidence that one need not diagnose zygapophyseal joint–mediated pain before surgery.[24,98] There is no reason that a variable amount of relief after uncontrolled, variable volume, intraarticular zygapophyseal joint blocks should predict fusion outcomes using surgical fusion techniques from the 1980s in a group of patients being operated on for various unknown or unstated reasons. Jackson[122] correlated relief after spinal fusion in 36 patients from 1980 to 1988 to results of a single intraarticular zygapophyseal joint injection with 1.5 mL of local anesthetic and an unknown volume of contrast dye. Of the patients, 85% had "some improvement" with an average relief after injection of 29%. The authors found no relationship between fusion surgery performed for unstated reasons and a "favorable response" to zygapophyseal joint injection. The surgeries were presumably performed not because the authors believed the patients' symptoms were due to their zygapophyseal joints. The surgical results based on their "mean pain and functional assessment scores" also seemed to improve by significantly less than 50%, suggesting poor patient selection.

An important historical study, published by Esses and Moro in 1993,[123] is often quoted to refute the therapeutic utility of zygapophyseal joint blocks; however, it warrants a careful, critical review. These authors concluded that single intraarticular diagnostic zygapophyseal joint injections "should not be used in determining treatment because they are not predictive of either surgical or nonsurgical success." This study had significant methodologic shortcomings, which limit the validity of the authors' conclusions. First, the study was retrospective, with patients surveyed by telephone approximately 5 years after surgery. Second, 1.5 mL of local anesthetic was injected into the zygapophyseal joints, and no mention is made of the volume of contrast dye needed to confirm needle position; the injections likely were nonspecific because of zygapophyseal joint capsule rupture from excessive volume (>1.5 mL). Third, the patient population was markedly heterogeneous, with significant confounding factors: an average duration of back pain of 8 years and approximately 40% of patients with a history of prior surgeries, including failed fusions. More than 50% of patients underwent three-level, four-level, or five-level fusions, which are known to have a worse outcome than single-level or two-level fusions. Fourth, of the 82 patients who underwent surgery, 36 (44%) had 0%

relief from zygapophyseal joint injections. Almost half of the patients undergoing surgery had no relief from diagnostic blocks. Eight of 19 (42%) of the patients with complete relief after zygapophyseal joint injections declined surgery, leaving only 11 of 82 (13%) patients who underwent surgery who had 100% relief from zygapophyseal joint blocks. The remaining 35 of 82 patients (43%) had "partial but significant relief" (the exact percentage relief is not reported). Fifth, 30 of 82 (37%) patients had prior surgeries (laminectomy, discectomy, and fusion). It is well known that patients with failed back surgery syndrome often fare poorly with repeat surgery. Also, during the 1980s, diagnosis of the etiology of failed back surgery syndrome was elusive and might not be corrected by a posterior arthrodesis. For failed back surgery syndrome, zygapophyseal joint pain comprises only 3% of cases; the most common diagnoses are foraminal stenosis (25–29%), painful disc (20–22%), pseudarthrosis (14%), neuropathic pain (10%), recurrent disc herniation (7–12%), and sacroiliac joint pain (2%).[124]

Next, Esses and Moro[123] did not match the surgery to specific zygapophyseal joint levels blocked. Patients had either one-level or two-level zygapophyseal joint blocks, yet the following posterior fusions were performed: 20 single-level; three two-level; 10 three-level; four four-level; and 12 five-level or greater, including thoracic spine (wherein zygapophyseal joints were never blocked). Finally, significant questions arise regarding the efficacy of the surgical intervention because there was no significant difference between surgical and nonsurgical outcomes. As reported, only approximately one-third of patients in either the surgical or the nonsurgical group had a good outcome. Because of methodologic flaws and limitations of the Esses and Moro study,[123] zygapophyseal joint intraarticular injections cannot be impugned as either predictive or nonpredictive of surgical success.

In another observational study, Lovely and Rastogi[125] required a "positive response" to intraarticular injection of greater than 70% relief after bupivacaine zygapophyseal joint block for 6 hours and required a confirmatory response on two subsequent injections. Of 28 patients, 23 had a good to excellent outcome after fusion surgery; however, large volumes of 3 to 5 mL were used during the blocks, making interpretation difficult. At present, there is no research regarding the utility of cervical or thoracic zygapophyseal joint blocks as presurgical screening tests.

By comparison, when a specific treatment is directed at a cause of pain originating from the zygapophyseal joint, accurate diagnostic testing does matter. In a more recent study, researchers reported that when a putative inflammatory cause of lumbar zygapophyseal joint pain was confirmed using a positive SPECT scan, a positive response (a significant reduction in pain) was clearly predicted with intraarticular and pericapsular steroids at 1 and 3 months compared with subjects with negative scans or routine care.[33]

In contrast to diagnostic intraarticular zygapophyseal joint injections, evidence supports the use of diagnostic medial branch nerve blocks (MBBs) as the criterion standard to diagnose zygapophyseal mediated pain.[17,126] Using controlled blocks and progressively stringent pain relief requirements for a positive block incrementally decreases the potential false-positive rate and improves results for a well-validated treatment for zygapophyseal joint pain, medial branch neurotomy.[17,126–128]

Most consensus standards for diagnosis of zygapophyseal-mediated pain require at a minimum 70% to 80% reported pain relief for the duration of the local anesthetic obtained in two separate sessions.[17,126] In particular, Dreyfuss and colleagues,[129] studied patients who obtained greater than or equal to 80% relief from MBBs selected to undergo lumbar radiofrequency neurotomy. At 12 months, 60% of the patients obtained at least 90% relief of pain, and 87% obtained at least 60% relief. Dreyfuss and colleagues[129] concluded that lumbar medial branch neurotomy is an effective means of reducing pain in patients carefully selected on the basis of controlled diagnostic blocks. A high-quality study randomized controlled trial evaluating radiofrequency neurotomy in patients with chronic low back pain[130] used three positive blocks in the inclusion criteria and a "sham radiofrequency" procedure for comparison; statistically significant reduction in pain and improvement in various quality-of-life variables were obtained. In another study, when the diagnosis is confirmed by relief of pain for greater than 3 months after medial branch neurotomies, repeat neurotomies are successful in greater than 75% in the lumbar and cervical spine.[131,132] More recently, Derby et al. used percent pain relief following MBB in 10% increments, finding a statistically favorable outcome for medial branch neurotomy using an MBB protocol requiring 70% or greater reported pain relief for the duration of the local anesthetic recorded on two separate sessions (double-block protocol).[127] Using a single-session protocol, 80% or greater report of pain relief predicted favorable medial branch neurotomy outcome, albeit less favorable than the two-session protocol.[127,133]

In regard to newer surgical treatments, the development and perfection of procedures such as minimally invasive zygapophyseal joint fusions or various types of total and subtotal arthroplasties require accurate diagnosis along with stringent criteria for success. The many confounding variables and often-reported weak results of current spinal fusion and arthroplasty techniques make disproving these results relatively easy. The diagnosis of zygapophyseal joint pain employing strict double-block or placebo-controlled standards should perhaps be used to restrain a surgeon from offering a circumferential (360 or 280 degrees) segmental fusion or arthroplasty. The failure to confirm zygapophyseal joint pain is perhaps even more important because doing so leaves other sources of pain that may be better suited to a particular surgical technique or limits the number of levels needing stabilization.

Cervical Spine Zygapophyseal Joint Syndrome

History

The cervical zygapophyseal joints are known to be sources of persistent chronic pain and central sensitization.[134,135] In 1940, Hadden[136] described pain from zygapophyseal joints causing headache. In the 1970s, Macnab[137] described pain arising from the zygapophyseal joints after whiplash injury. Bogduk and Marsland[138] devised a technique to block the third occipital nerve, which relieved neck pain and headache stemming from the C2–C3 zygapophyseal joint in 70% of patients. Headache arising from C0–C1 or C1–C2 joints has also been described.[139,140] Bogduk and Marsland[141] were also the first to describe medial branch blocks for all cervical spine levels. They studied patients presenting with idiopathic neck pain and reported that medial branch block and intraarticular blocks provided complete, temporary relief of pain for 70% of patients.

Cervical Zygapophyseal Joint Pain

Based on the confirmatory block paradigm, the cervical zygapophyseal joints are a common source of chronic neck pain; the prevalence of cervical zygapophyseal joint syndrome is greater than the prevalence of lumbar zygapophyseal joint syndrome. Cervical discogenic pain shares referral patterns with zygapophyseal joint pain, but it is far less common.[142] Based on comparative blocks of cervical zygapophyseal joints causing chronic neck pain with either associated headache or shoulder pain, the C2–C3 (36%) and C5–C6 zygapophyseal joints (35%) were the most common pain generators.[143] After whiplash injury, level I prospective clinical studies provide evidence that zygapophyseal joints are the most common source of chronic pain.[144,145] Cervicogenic headache stemming from the C2–C3 zygapophyseal joint after whiplash has a 53% prevalence.[144]

Often neglected are C0–C1 and C1–C2 joints in evaluation of upper neck pain and headache. Dreyfuss and colleagues[139] studied the referral patterns for the atlantoaxial and lateral atlantoaxial joints. In 2002, Aprill and colleagues[146] failed to confirm the null hypothesis that lateral atlantoaxial joints are *not* a common source of occipital headache. These investigators found that of 34 patients presenting with symptoms and signs of atlantoaxial joint pain, 21 obtained complete relief of headache after diagnostic injection of local anesthetic. Pain referral patterns have been defined in C2–C3 through C7–T1 zygapophyseal joints (Fig. 16.7).[147] Innervation of the cervical zygapophyseal joints is well described (Fig. 16.8).[147] The cervical zygapophyseal joints can be blocked either by MBBs or with intraarticular injections (Fig. 16.9).

Prevalence rates for neck pain originating from cervical zygapophyseal joints range from 36% to 60%. The false-positive rate for a single, uncontrolled block is 27% (95% CI, 15–38%).[148] The following prevalence rates (mean [95% CI]) are reported from studies using either a double-block or a triple-block paradigm (normal saline as a placebo): 54% (95% CI, 40–68%),[144] 36% (95% CI, 27–45%),[149] 60% (95% CI, 33–64%),[145] and 60% (95% CI, 50–70%).[150] Manchikanti and colleagues[151] restudied the prevalence of cervical zygapophyseal joint pain in a larger group of patients and found a similar 55% (95% CI, 49–61%) prevalence. In a study by Manchikanti's group in 2007,[85] of 438 patients requiring 80% relief of pain for 2-hour duration with lidocaine and 3-hour duration with bupivacaine, a 39% prevalence of zygapophyseal joint–mediated pain was demonstrated. Corroborating the high prevalence of cervical zygapophyseal joint pain, Yin and Bogduk[186] in a private practice clinic audit found a 55% prevalence of cervical zygapophyseal joint–mediated neck pain using a strict double-block comparative protocol. In a recent well-executed prospective outcome study, MacVicar et al.[152] further corroborated the diagnostic value of diagnostic MBBs. His study found that 100% pain relief following rigorously evaluated comparative MBBs predicted that between 61% to 74% of patients will obtain 80% or greater pain relief following cervical medial branch neurotomies for an average of 17 to 20 months after the primary procedure and an average of 15 months after repeat procedures.[152]

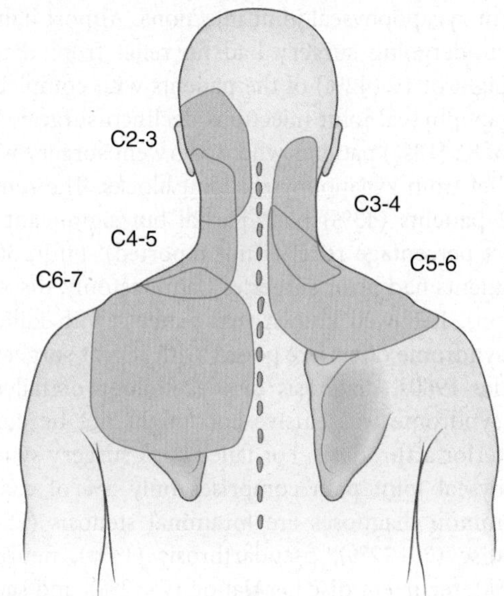

FIG. 16.7 Patterns of referred pain from cervical zygapophyseal joints in normal volunteers (From Dwyer A, Aprill C, Bogduk N. Cervical zygapophyseal joint pain patterns. Part 1: a study in normal volunteers. *Spine.* 1990;15:453–457.)

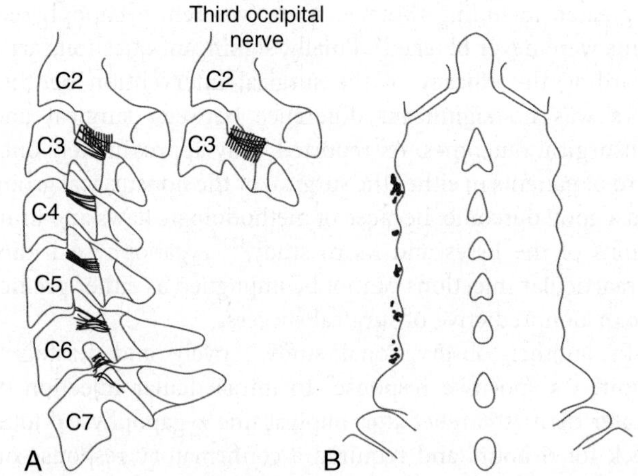

FIG. 16.8 (A) Lateral view of cervical spine showing variable locations of medial branches. At C3, the location of the C3 deep medial branch is shown. The *inset* shows the location of the third occipital nerve. The *shaded area* shows where the C3 deep branches and third occipital nerve overlap. The C5 medial branch is located in the middle of the articular pillar; at C6 and C7, medial branches are located progressively higher. (B) Anteroposterior view of the cervical medial branches. (From Bogduk N, ed. *Practice Guidelines for Spinal Diagnostic and Treatment Procedures.* San Francisco: International Spine Intervention Society; 2004.)

Similar to lumbar zygapophyseal joint pain, there are no high-quality studies showing a particular set of clinical features that can predict results of diagnostic cervical zygapophyseal joint blocks or MBBs.[153] With diagnosis by MBBs, one exceptionally skilled manipulative therapist was able to identify all 15 subjects with diagnostic block–proven symptomatic zygapophyseal joints and specify the correct symptomatic segment. None of the five patients with asymptomatic joints was misdiagnosed as having symptomatic zygapophyseal joints.[154] A later follow-up study by the same group failed to confirm the apparent high specificity and sensitivity, however, and reported a high sensitivity but low specificity and concluded that manual examination of the cervical spine lacks validity for the diagnosis of cervical zygapophyseal joint pain. In the study by Aprill and colleagues[146] of C1–C2 zygapophyseal joint pain as a source of occipital headache, only 60% of the patients shared clinical criteria that predicted a positive response to the block.

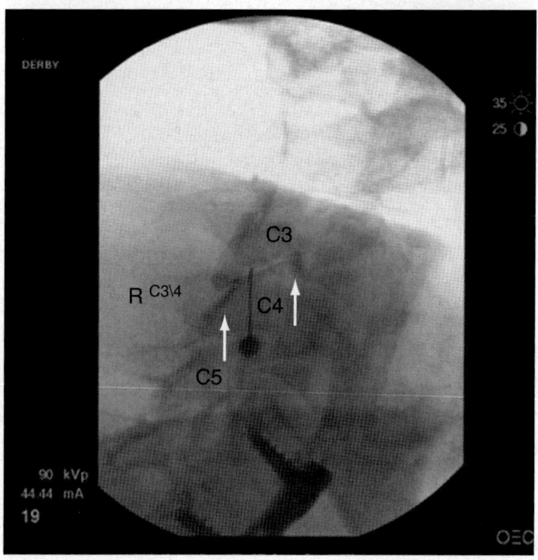

FIG. 16.9 Lateral fluoroscopic view of a C3–C4 zygapophyseal joint injection using a 3.5-inch, 25-gauge needle. Note contrast dye in posterior and anterior capsular folds (*arrows*). (Courtesy Richard Derby, MD.)

Advanced imaging has not been correlated with positive responses to diagnostic blocks. Hechelhammer and colleagues[155] found no relationship between short-term pain relief after cervical intraarticular and pericapsular injection of local anesthetic and corticosteroid and the degree of osteoarthritis graded on a CT scan.

Thoracic Spine

The prevalence of patients who complain of chronic upper back or mid-back pain ranges from 3% to 22%.[32,156,157] One survey study of 35- to 45-year-old patients estimated the prevalence of thoracic pain to be 15%.[158] Thoracic zygapophyseal joint pain referral patterns have been reported (Fig. 16.10).[159,160] Thoracic medial branch anatomy has also been described (Fig. 16.11).[161] However, it must be acknowledged that a "thoracic zygapophyseal joint syndrome" has not been described in detail relative to the cervical and lumbar zygapophyseal joint syndromes outlined earlier. Given the relative lack of mobility in the sagittal plane (i.e., flexion and extension) at the thoracic zygapophyseal joints due to their relatively coronal orientation, less loading stress occurs at these levels

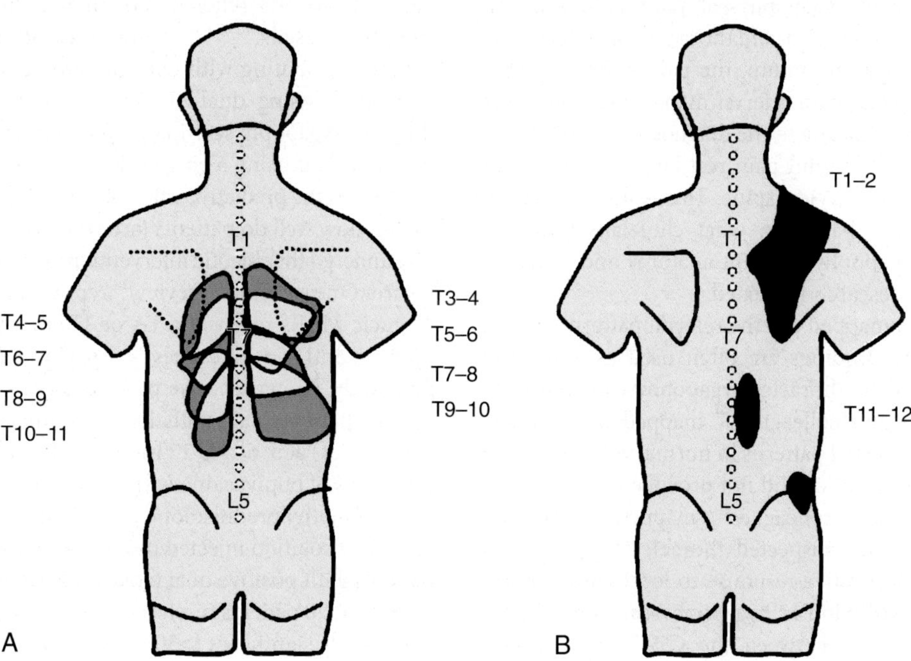

FIG. 16.10 Maps of referred pain patterns in segments indicated. (A) Based on Dreyfuss et al.[139] in normal volunteers. (B) Based on Fukui et al.[160] in patients with single positive zygapophyseal joint block. (From Bogduk N, ed. *Practice Guidelines for Spinal Diagnostic and Treatment Procedures.* San Francisco: International Spine Intervention Society; 2004.)

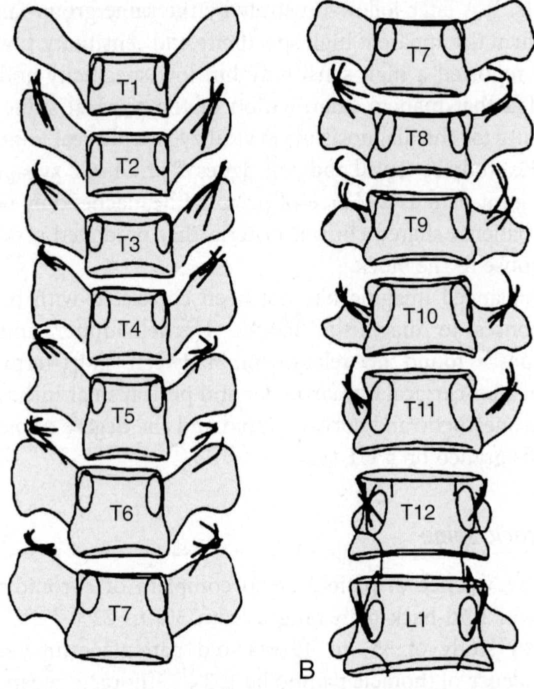

FIG. 16.11 (A–B) Composite sketch of work by Chua and Bogduk[161] with radiographs of cadaveric thoracic spines. Medial branches of thoracic dorsal rami marked with wires to depict location with respect to transverse processes. Note middle thoracic levels, where medial branches are within intertransverse space versus crossing transverse process. (From Bogduk N, ed. *Practice Guidelines for Spinal Diagnostic and Treatment Procedures*. San Francisco: International Spine Intervention Society; 2004.)

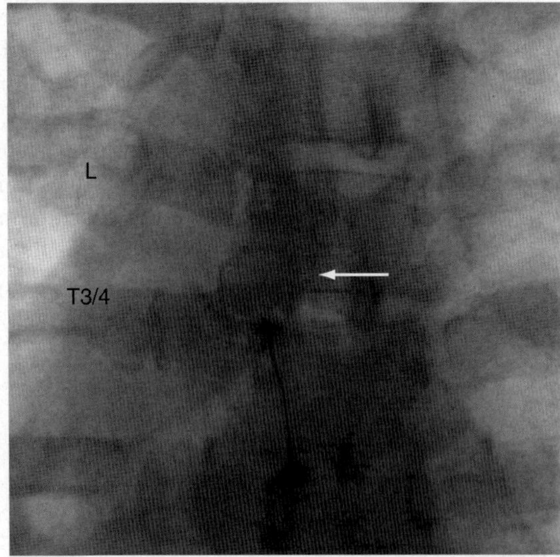

FIG. 16.12 Left T3–T4 zygapophyseal joint intraarticular injection. Note circular zygapophyseal joint arthrogram (*arrow*). (Courtesy Richard Derby, MD.)

relative to the cervical and lumbar zygapophyseal joints during extension movements and postures.[162,163]

There are no pathognomonic clinical or radiographic findings by which thoracic zygapophyseal joint pain may be diagnosed.[164] As with the cervical and thoracic spine, diagnosis is by suspicion and, at a minimum, the pain pattern should correlate with established pain referral maps.[147] The methods that physicians apply clinically to the diagnosis and treatment of thoracic zygapophyseal joint pain rest largely on research done in the lumbar and cervical spine. This is not an entirely unreasonable approach based on what clinicians know in general regarding zygapophyseal joint anatomy and innervation; however, more research is needed.

Investigators have mapped out the referral patterns for the thoracic joints. These findings are often used as a starting point to select which thoracic zygapophyseal joints to block.[159,160] Dreyfuss and colleagues[159] mapped out thoracic zygapophyseal joint referral patterns in normal volunteers and found that capsular distention did not provoke pain in 27.5% of volunteers. Fukui and colleagues[160] mapped out referral patterns in patients with suspected thoracic zygapophyseal joint pain who had a positive response to local anesthetic in C7–T1 to T2–T3 and T11–T12 zygapophyseal joints. There was considerable overlap between the C7–T1 and T2–T3 thoracic joints; thus, pain maps from these joints are not considered reliable enough to identify the symptomatic segmental level. Dreyfuss and colleagues[159] studied nine asymptomatic volunteers who underwent 40 provocative thoracic zygapophyseal joint injections from T3–T4 to T10–T11. Referral patterns were consistently unilateral. The area of the most intense pain for segments from T2–T3 to T11–T12 was one level inferior and lateral. Significant overlap occurred over three to five levels. The researchers found that needle position can be confirmed with 0.1 to 0.3 mL of contrast dye, and adequate blocks can be achieved with a volume of 0.5 to 0.6 mL. Normally, thoracic zygapophyseal joints cannot hold more than 0.75 mL (Fig. 16.12 shows a typical thoracic zygapophyseal joint block).[17]

One research group has performed the three studies in the literature using a controlled, double-block paradigm, requiring 75% to 80% relief based on the duration of the local anesthetic used.[105,165,166] Combining all three studies with patients presenting with chronic middle or upper spinal pain (n = 183), using dual blocks obtains a 40% prevalence of thoracic zygapophyseal joint syndrome, with a false-positive rate of 42% if using a single-block paradigm.[28]

What is the predictive value of a positive dual block? In other words, how well do patients fare who have positive dual blocks and undergo therapeutic intervention? Research is limited in this regard. One systematic review[28] reported that only therapeutic thoracic MBBs received a 1A or 1B/strong recommendation. Manchikanti and colleagues[167,168] performed two studies. In the first study, 55 consecutive patients were studied; greater than 70% of patients had statistically significant relief (defined as >50% relief) at 3, 6, and 12 months. Most patients received four injections of bupivacaine with or without 1 mL of Sarapin and 1 mg of methylprednisolone per milliliter of solution with 1 to 1.5 mL of solution injected per nerve. In the second study of 48 patients with positive dual blocks, 24 patients received bupivacaine, and 20 patients received bupivacaine plus betamethasone. Statistically significant (>50%) pain relief was reported in both groups at all time points up to 1 year. In the systematic review of radiofrequency neurotomy, only two studies were on thoracic medial branch neurotomy; however, both were of low quality and failed to meet inclusion criteria for the review because of lack of diagnosis by controlled blocks, small patient sample, and other methodologic shortcomings.[28] More research is needed in regard to diagnosis and treatment of thoracic pain so that the evidence can be graded and systematically reviewed, the caveat being that a lack of evidence is not equivalent to no evidence.

Summary

Chronic disabling spinal pain in a patient suggestive of "facet (zygapophyseal joint) syndrome" that is unresponsive to usual care may be considered for diagnostic comparative MBBs, with low-volume MBBs favored due to superior evidence for diagnostic specificity. The levels to be investigated are typically chosen by pain referral patterns described by the patient, which are correlated with validated zygapophyseal joint pain referral patterns. Upper neck pain and headache are most commonly caused by the C2–C3 zygapophyseal joint, and neck pain with shoulder girdle pain is most commonly caused by the C5–C6 zygapophyseal joint. The clinician should not neglect the C0–C1 and C1–C2 articulations as potential pain generators, in which case diagnostic intraarticular blocks would be used to help confirm or refute the diagnosis. Evaluation of the exact level of thoracic zygapophyseal joint pain can be more challenging because pain may be referred over more than three segments. Lumbar zygapophyseal joint referral patterns are also reported in the literature; zygapophyseal joint pain may be localized or referred to the buttocks and lower extremity.

Although comparative double blocks are considered the reference standard for diagnosis, routine history, physical examination, radiographs, and advanced imaging should be obtained for completeness. The clinician often finds elements that rule out zygapophyseal joint syndrome and are more suggestive of disc pathology, radiculopathy, or "red flag" conditions that require different diagnostic and treatment methods. There are also cases in which a history of trauma, particularly whiplash, is highly suggestive of pain of zygapophyseal joint origin, with a known greater than 50% prevalence in the cervical spine. Certain specific imaging findings, if present, also may suggest zygapophyseal joint syndrome, such as a positive SPECT scan, approximately 2 mm edema on axial MRI of lumbar zygapophyseal joints, or a single zygapophyseal joint with markedly deforming arthropathy compared with other joints.

With regard to testing protocol, whether to perform MBBs, intraarticular zygapophyseal joint injections, or both varies depending on the situation and preference of the physician. If one is confirming zygapophyseal joint–mediated pain in preparation for possible medial branch neurotomy, one could argue that MBB should be the method of choice due to improved specificity. If radiofrequency denervation of the zygapophyseal joint is not planned or SPECT scan imaging shows edema, intraarticular block is reasonable. In the case of C0–C1 and C1–C2, intraarticular injections are the only practical method of diagnosing zygapophyseal joint pain.

As noted earlier, preprocedural and postprocedural evaluation should be performed by unbiased personnel and checked by the physician using standardized instruments. Evaluation after the procedure includes VAS of standard provocative maneuvers and positions, as well as a report of subjective percent relief of pain. Ideally, the patient would be tested at approximately 30 minutes after lidocaine block and approximately 40 to 60 minutes after bupivacaine block. Ideally, a pain diary over the 6 to 8 hours following the block procedure is recorded by the patient and then reported the following day in order to decrease recall bias. However, retesting at 2 to 3 hours postinjection is a more reliable protocol. A subject should have at least 70% to 80% relief for a positive response to be considered; at least 80% relief is more convincing. Usually, two to three levels are evaluated per session. Depending on the importance of refuting or confirming whether a particular zygapophyseal joint is symptomatic, one may select fewer joints if needed.

Several technical parameters must be met to obtain useful diagnostic information. Diagnostic volumes must be appropriate. Contrast medium will confirm accurate target identification. For intraarticular zygapophyseal joint blocks, injection volumes should be limited to 0.3 mL, 0.75 mL, and 1 mL in the cervical, thoracic, and lumbar spine, respectively. For MBBs, needle position may be confirmed with injection of a small volume (0.3–0.5 mL) of contrast dye and the same volume of local anesthetic. The interventionalist should observe for venous uptake or undesirable flow patterns. If there is venous uptake, there is only a 50% chance of successfully anesthetizing the joint; thus, the interventionalist may consider bringing the patient back at a later date or interpreting the results of the block accordingly.

Infection may occur after any interventional procedure. Various infections are reported after zygapophyseal joint injections, including paraspinal abscess,[169] zygapophyseal joint abscess,[170] osteomyelitis,[171] and epidural abscess.[172] In addition to infections, subdural injections or injection into the spinal cord may occur. A case of transient tetraplegia[173] was reported during a cervical zygapophyseal joint injection performed without fluoroscopy and most likely was an accidental subdural injection of local anesthetic. Even when using fluoroscopy, there is a risk of accidental subdural injection or potential spinal cord injection. The danger is especially real when performing cervical intraarticular injection using a lateral technique. Using this technique, the needle is passed laterally using a lateral fluoroscopy view. If the anteroposterior view is not periodically checked, one may not recognize passage of the needle through the zygapophyseal joint and dura and then into the cord. In a thin individual, the cord may be reached with a 1-inch needle. Keeping the needle directly over the inferior or superior zygapophyseal joint and touching the bone before entering the joint helps the interventionalist avoid accidentally entering the spinal canal.

Sacroiliac Joint

With the gradual acceptance of local anesthetic block relief after fluoroscopy-guided sacroiliac joint blocks as the reference standard for diagnosis, there is a renewed interest in the sacroiliac joint as a legitimate source of chronic pain.[26] The degree of impact on health is the same as that of radiculopathy, as evidenced by statistically similar scores in health-related quality-of-life testing instruments between patients with a diagnosis of sacroiliac joint pain and patients with a diagnosis of radiculopathy.[161]

Similar to zygapophyseal joint and discogenic pain, the diagnosis of sacroiliac joint pain depends on the reference standard used (and the particular population studied) to confirm the diagnosis. Society guidelines most often require a placebo control or differential blockade with 50% to 90% relief.[3,147,174] Typically, a differential duration of reported pain relief of lidocaine (approximately 2–3 hours) compared with bupivacaine (approximately 4–6 hours) is required. Although concordant provocation of pain during joint arthrography has been used as an additional requirement, the high percentage of asymptomatic patients reporting pain during sacroiliac joint injection implies that provocation has a high false-positive potential. Currently, using the dual-block paradigm, the best estimates of prevalence of sacroiliac joint–mediated pain in patients with low back symptoms range from 10% to 38%, but the lower end of this range is likely most accurate.[175,176] For single, uncontrolled sacroiliac joint injections, the false-positive rate is 20% to 54%.[177–181]

Pathophysiology

The sacroiliac joint has long been recognized as a synovial, fluid-filled diarthrodial joint between the sacrum and ilia with thick, 6-mm sacral cartilage and thinner, approximately 1-mm iliac cartilage (Fig. 16.13). The joint is auricular or C-shaped, with the convex side of the "C" facing anteriorly and inferiorly (Fig. 16.14).[182] Although the anterior portion is no more than a thickened capsule, the posterior capsule blends into the extensive, thick posterior ligamentous structures, which bind the sacrum to the spine and bilaterally to the ilia. After puberty, the iliac surface develops a convex ridge and the sacral surface develops a corresponding concave depression. These articular surfaces allow slight movement between the contiguous bony surfaces.

Although early in life gliding motions in all directions are permitted, by the middle of the second decade of life, the joints develop prominent ridges centrally along the entire length of the iliac surface and a corresponding groove along the sacral surface. Bowen and Cassidy[182] believed that this interdigitation of the joint surfaces restricts motion to a sagittal rotation or posterosuperior-anteroinferior "nodding" along the crest of the interdigitations. The motion is complex, however, and usually limited to less than 4 degrees of rotation and less than 1.6 mm of translation. Significant motion occurs only after severing the interosseous ligament.[183] It is unclear whether a type or degree of sacroiliac joint motion causes pain in older individuals. Beyond the sixth decade, cadaveric specimens commonly show a central region of ossification of the interosseous sacroiliac ligament and the presence of ridges and depressions, which likely result in little to no movement of the sacroiliac joint in these older individuals.[184] Although there is restriction by periarticular osteophyte formation, intraarticular bony ankylosis appears rare.[182]

Several investigators have studied the innervation of the sacroiliac joint. Nakagawa[185] reported innervation from the ventral rami of L4 and L5; the superior gluteal nerve; and the dorsal rami of L5, S1, and S2. An anatomic dissection of the innervation of the sacroiliac joint was performed by Yin and colleagues[186] for the purpose of defining the exact position of the nerves for "sensory stimulation–guided sacroiliac joint radiofrequency neurotomy." These authors dissected cadavers and placed small-gauge wires adjacent to the lateral branch nerves entering the joint and over the dorsal sacrum to the dorsal sacral foramen from S1 to S3. In 1988, Willard[187] reported dissection of 10 cadavers, which revealed that the S1 and S2 lateral branches provide the primary innervation of the sacroiliac joint and associated dorsal ligaments. An occasional contribution was found by S3 but not S4. Predominant

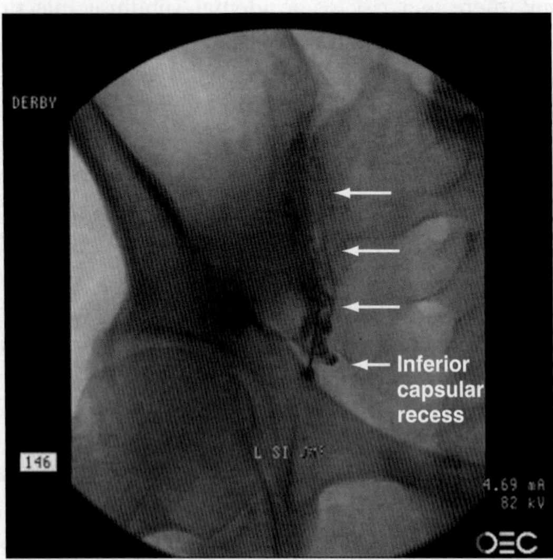

FIG. 16.13 Anteroposterior view of left sacroiliac joint injection. Note contrast dye filling the capsule, including the inferior capsular recess (*arrows*). (Courtesy Richard Derby, MD.)

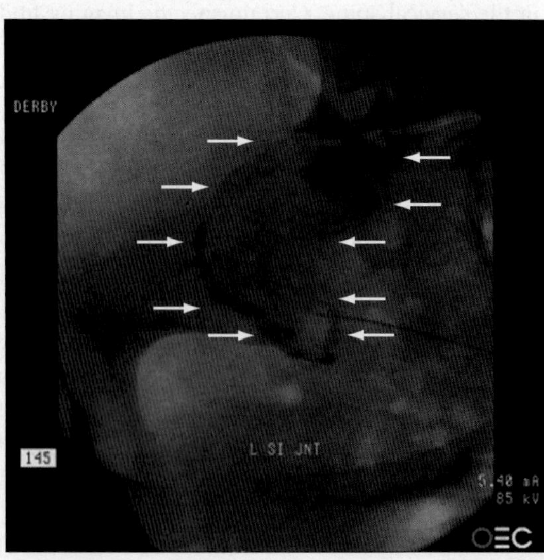

FIG. 16.14 Lateral view of sacroiliac joint injection. Note contrast dye filling the joint space. Also, note the C shape of the joint facing anteriorly (*arrows*). (Courtesy Richard Derby, MD.)

innervation from lateral branches of S1 was also reported by Grob and colleagues.[188] These authors found that dorsal nerves derived from S1–S4 exclusively innervated the sacroiliac joint and associated ligaments. Nerves were distributed to superficial and deep dorsal sacroiliac ligaments and to the sacrotuberous and sacrospinous ligaments. Emerging from the sacral foramen, the nerves course laterally, sandwiched between superficial and deep portions of the sacroiliac ligaments. There is a great variability in the location and number of lateral branch nerves side to side and between individuals.[186] Due to this variability, the current standard for blocking the posterior sacroiliac joint as associated dorsal ligaments is to block the L5 dorsal ramus and S1–S3 lateral branches using a multisite, multidepth technique described by Dreyfuss and colleagues.[189]

Berthelot and colleagues[190] used the term *sacroiliac joint lato-sensu* to describe pain from the sacroiliac joint that may be emanating from adjoining ligaments rather than simply the synovial joint. These ligaments include the iliolumbar ligaments, dorsal and ventral sacroiliac ligaments, and sacrospinous and sacrotuberous ligaments. The prevalence of pain originating from these structures has received little formal study, and there is no validated technique to diagnose ligamentous pain. Nevertheless, sacroiliac joint ligamentous pain is proclaimed as a frequent primary source of low back and buttock pain by orthopaedists.[191] More important, a negative response to a sacroiliac joint injection does not mean that pain does not originate from the iliolumbar ligament and sacroiliac joint ligaments. A more recent histologic study found calcitonin gene-related peptide and substance P immunoreactive nerve fibers in the normal sacroiliac joint anterior capsular ligament and interosseous ligament. The authors of the study opined that diagnostic infiltration techniques for sacroiliac joint pain should employ extraarticular and intraarticular approaches.[192]

In contrast to the zygapophyseal joints, the sacroiliac joint supporting ligaments are thick, and intraarticularly injected local anesthetic may not adequately diffuse into the sacroiliac ligaments. Using a single or comparative block protocol, one can investigate sacroiliac joint ligaments by fluoroscopically guided injections of local anesthetics into the ligaments. Ligamentous injections have not undergone rigorous academic inquiry, however, and because the injections are rarely or poorly reimbursed by third-party payers and treatment of ligamentous laxity typically involves unreimbursed "prolotherapy," there is little incentive for expensive investigations. The information is important, however, and differential pain arising from the sacroiliac joint versus sacroiliac joint ligaments is reported.

In a comparative study, Murakami and colleagues[193] performed periarticular injections in 25 patients and intraarticular injections in another 25 patients. Periarticular injections relieved, on average, 92% pain in 100% of the injected patients compared with only 9 of 25 patients receiving intraarticular injections. All 16 patients not receiving relief by intraarticular injections were improved after periarticular injections. The presence of other structural abnormalities does not rule out the sacroiliac joint as a primary source of pain. Weksler and colleagues[194] studied 55 patients with herniated discs with axial and referred leg pain, without objective neurologic deficits but with positive sacroiliac provocation tests. Using intraarticular injection of local anesthetic as the reference standard, the mean baseline VAS pain score decreased 30 minutes after injection, from 7.8 to 1.3. In 46 patients 8 weeks after injection, VAS scores ranged from 0 to 3.

The question of whether fusion surgery leads to increased stress on the sacroiliac joint and may be a cause of failed back surgery syndrome was first raised by Frymoyer and colleagues,[195] although their method of assessing sacroiliac joint pathology yielded a negative result. In 1978, Frymoyer and colleagues[195] evaluated patients with radiographs (no diagnostic blocks) 10 years after posterior fusion versus postdiscectomy and found no significant difference in radiographic abnormalities; they opined that sacroiliac pain was "noncontributory" to persistent low back pain after surgery. In their subject population, they believed that the graft donor site was a more common pain generator. Fusion to the sacrum might be expected to stress the sacroiliac joints and lead to late failures or to early failures owing to undiagnosed sacroiliac joint pain. Ha and colleagues[196] prospectively examined 37 patients undergoing posterolateral lumbar and lumbosacral fusions; 22 patients had a floating fusion, and 10 patients had a lumbosacral fusion. CT scans of the sacroiliac joint were performed before surgery and at 2 weeks, 1 year, and 5 years after surgery and compared with 34 matched controls. The incidence of sacroiliac joint degeneration was 75% in the fusion group versus 38.2% in the control group and greater in patients fused to the sacrum. Both groups reported significant improvements in VAS and Oswestry Disability Index scores, and there was no difference in scores between the two groups.

More recent research has shown that the sacroiliac joint can be a significant source of pain after fusion. Biomechanical models seem to support these conclusions. Ivanov and colleagues[197] performed a finite-element study with lumbosacral models and fusion constructs and found that fusion to the sacrum increased motion and stresses at the sacroiliac joint. Cadaveric studies show that disruption of the ventral band of the iliolumbar ligament significantly increases sacroiliac joint mobility.[198] Ebraheim and colleagues[199] evaluated the prevalence of sacroiliac joint disruption by CT scan in 24 patients after fusion with persistent "donor site pain" after posterior superior iliac crest graft harvesting. They found a high prevalence of persistent sacroiliac joint pain in patients with inner-table disruption. Patients with violation of the synovial portion of the sacroiliac joint had severe degenerative changes on CT versus mild to moderate degeneration with inner-table disruption only. It seems that the original hypothesis by Frymoyer and colleagues[195] that sacroiliac joint dysfunction was the cause of donor site pain may have been correct.

What is the evidence for using diagnostic blocks as the reference standard? Diagnosis of sacroiliac joint pain has been reported by researchers using single and dual blocks; with these methods, prevalence rates of sacroiliac joint pain after lumbar fusion range from 27% to 35%. Maigne and Planchon[200] studied 40 patients after fusion with continued pain using 75% pain relief after a single sacroiliac joint intraarticular injection as the gold standard. They reported a 35% rate of positive blocks. The only characteristic that distinguished the positive from the negative responders was a different distribution of postoperative pain compared with preoperative pain. A pain-free interval of 3 months after surgery was significant; however, increased uptake in the sacroiliac joint on bone scintigraphy or posterior iliac bone graft harvesting was not significant.

Katz and colleagues[201] studied 34 patients after lumbosacral fusion with continued pain thought to be due to the sacroiliac joint with intraarticular injections of local anesthetic and corticosteroids. Eleven patients (32%) had greater than 75% pain relief with local anesthetic and a minimum of 10 days of continued pain relief (with steroid) and were considered to have definite sacroiliac joint pain. Another 10 patients (29%) had greater than 75% relief with local anesthetic but no long-term relief. There was no correlation between the donor site and pain side. Irwin and colleagues[177] used dual comparative sacroiliac joint blocks as the reference standard to define sacroiliac joint pain and found that the 27% of positive responders tended to be older. They found no statistical relationship between age, body mass index, and gender.

Diagnostic Accuracy of Clinical History and Physical Examination for Sacroiliac Pain

The diagnostic utility of history and accepted sacroiliac joint physical examination tests was first rigorously examined by Dreyfuss and colleagues in 1996.[202] Their study was designed to determine if any single or combination of 12 history and physical examination findings could predict intraarticular sacroiliac joint pain as judged against a single positive intraarticular sacroiliac joint block with greater than 90% pain relief. In 85 patients, there were 45 positive blocks. None of the 12 physical examination tests, the presence of 5 to 12 positive tests, or any combination of these 12 tests correlated with the presence of sacroiliac joint pain. One important historical feature was notable, however: only 2 of 45 patients drew pain above the L5 level, suggesting that pain below L5 is more likely to be of sacroiliac joint origin. Maigne and colleagues[176] reached a similar conclusion using dual comparative blocks: no single provocation test reached statistical significance in the 10 patients (18.5%) who had temporary pain relief on the confirmatory injection.

Although no single provocative maneuver has been shown to be of diagnostic value, using the dual-block paradigm, several studies have obtained highly acceptable sensitivity (85–91%) and specificity (78–79%) rates by combining three or more sacroiliac joint pain provocation tests for diagnosis by physical examination.[12,178,179,181,203] There is some slight variation in the tests used by various authors but, in summary, they include the following provocation tests: thigh thrust, distraction test, Gaenslen test, Patrick sign, compression test, midline sacral thrust test, and heel drop test. Specificity increased to 87% if the patient's pain did not centralize or could not be made to move toward the spinal midline (which is typical of discogenic pain).[204] When three or more provocation tests (distraction, compression, thigh thrust, Patrick sign, Gaenslen test) are negative, the likelihood of sacroiliac joint pain is very low (6–15%); when all provocation tests are negative, the sacroiliac joint was never the source of pain.[178,179,181,204]

With regard to pain referral maps, Slipman and colleagues[205] and Dreyfuss and colleagues[202] concluded that of all alleged signs of sacroiliac joint pain, maximum pain below L5 coupled with pointing to the posterior superior iliac spine or tenderness just medial to the posterior superior iliac spine (sacral sulcus tenderness) has the highest positive predictive value of 60% of true sacroiliac joint–mediated pain; if these do not exist, the likelihood of sacroiliac joint pain is less than 10%. It must be noted that sacroiliac joint pain can refer into various aspects of the lower extremity, with 94% of patients reporting buttock pain, 48% reporting thigh pain, and 28% reporting lower leg pain (Fig. 16.15).[175,176,206] However, referral to the lower extremity may not always be reliably distinguished from other pain sources (e.g., S1 radiculopathy).[175,207]

Last, although pain referral patterns between responders and nonresponders are similar, Fortin and colleagues[208] described an area of pain approximately 3 × 10 cm just inferior to the posterior superior iliac spine that was common in all subjects with sacroiliac joint pain. More recently, Murakami and colleagues[209] studied the specificity and sensitivity of the "Fortin" point with periarticular injections. Labeled the *one finger test,* 18 of 38 patients pointed to a location of pain at the posterior superior iliac spine or within 2 cm of the posterior superior iliac spine, which had a positive response to periarticular sacroiliac joint block. The authors recommended that sacroiliac joint pain should be considered in patients who can point to their pain using one finger in the vicinity of the posterior superior iliac spine.

Systematic reviews report various conclusions regarding the specificity of the physical examination and sacroiliac joint

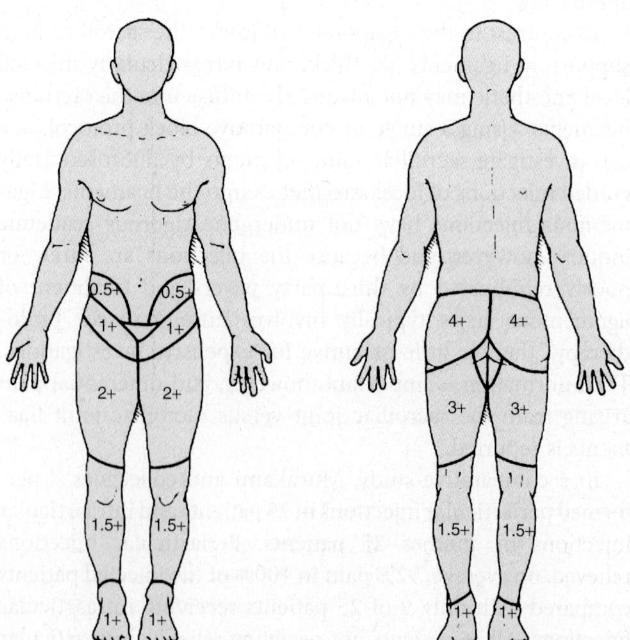

FIG. 16.15 Density of referral zones for sacroiliac joint pain. 0.5+ is the least common referral zone; 4+ is the most common referral zone. (From Dreyfuss P, Dreyer S. Sacroiliac joint pain. *J Am Acad Orthop Surg.* 2004;12:255–265.)

block to diagnose sacroiliac joint pain based on the authors' assessment of the diagnostic accuracy of sacroiliac joint blocks. The review by Berthelot and colleagues[190] concluded that sacroiliac joint blocks and sacroiliac joint maneuvers were unreliable for diagnosing sacroiliac joint pain. In contrast, Hansen and colleagues[210] concluded in their review that there was moderate evidence for the specificity and validity of diagnostic sacroiliac joint injection and limited evidence for the accuracy of provocative maneuvers. Using a comparative double-block reference standard, the most recent meta-analysis and systematic review concluded that the pooled data of the thigh thrust test, compression test, and three or more positive stress tests showed discriminative power for diagnosing sacroiliac joint pain.[211]

Diagnostic Accuracy of Imaging

No imaging studies consistently provide findings that are helpful to diagnose primary sacroiliac joint pain. CT, MRI, and bone scan are done predominantly to exclude other causes of pain rather than to diagnose mechanical sacroiliac joint pain. Among patients referred to a low back pain clinic with a variety of pathologies, Hodge and Bessette[212] found a high percentage (75%) of patients with sacroiliac joint arthritis shown on CT scan. Although these authors did not confirm the diagnosis with sacroiliac joint injections, they opined that sacroiliac joint arthritis should be considered a possible diagnosis.

There is limited diagnostic value of CT scan in mechanical sacroiliac joint disease as defined by pain relief after sacroiliac joint blocks under CT scan guidance. Comparing the CT scans of patients diagnosed with sacroiliac joint pain using image-guided analgesic sacroiliac joint blocks with a matched control group of asymptomatic patients, Elgafy and colleagues[213] reported that an abnormal sacroiliac joint CT scan had a sensitivity of 57% and a specificity of 69% for identifying sacroiliac joint pain. Although sacroiliac joint scintigraphy can detect early sacroiliitis,[214] stress fractures, infection, and tumors, the sensitivity of bone scans for detecting mechanical sacroiliac joint pain is poor (range, 12–46%),[215,216] Patients with a positive bone scan are likely to have mechanical or arthritic sacroiliac joint pain with a reported specificity of 90% to 100%.[205,217]

Diagnostic Accuracy of Sacroiliac Joint Injections

In a recent prospective case series of 1408 patients undergoing dual-session sacroiliac joint blocks, the authors found that the first sacroiliac joint block will be confirmed by the confirmatory injection in 87% of cases.[218] However, the current recommended standard for diagnosing sacroiliac joint pain is pain relief after dual controlled sacroiliac joint injections, owing to the high false-positive rate of single blocks reported in prior publications[17,177] When blocking the sacroiliac joint or lateral branches of the sacroiliac joint, imaging guidance must be used. The success of "blind" intraarticular injection is only 22%.[219] A positive response should include approximately 70% to 80% relief for 1 to 2 hours of relief after a lidocaine block and 3 to 4 hours of relief after a confirmatory block with bupivacaine. Although the reference standard is reasonable, there are several caveats for the diagnosis of mechanical pain originating within the sacroiliac joint. Patients may exhibit extraarticular or periarticular sacroiliac joint pain or perhaps both. As noted earlier, Murakami and colleagues[193] relieved a significant amount of sacroiliac joint pain with periarticular injections. In a retrospective review of 120 patients, subjects who received intraarticular and periarticular injections had superior pain relief compared with subjects receiving intraarticular injections alone.[220]

False-positive results may occur secondary to leak of local anesthetic through capsular tears, which may be present even in asymptomatic individuals. Extracapsular flow is present in 61% of sacroiliac joint intraarticular injections in patients.[221] Of sacroiliac joint intraarticular injections, 27% show extravasation that communicates with nearby neural structures, including dorsal sacral foramina extravasation, superior recess extravasation at the sacral ala level to the fifth lumbar epiradicular sheath, and ventral extravasation to the lumbosacral plexus.[221] Patients who have postblock extremity numbness are usually considered to have a leak, and the block is typically repeated at a different session. In such cases, it may also be reasonable to use multisite, multidepth blocks of the L5 dorsal ramus and S1–S3 lateral branches in order to avoid anesthesia of confounding anterior structures.

More important is the potentially significant false-negative response rate because of a failure to anesthetize extracapsular pain sources mentioned previously. Block of the sacroiliac joint dorsal innervations may offer a solution because the block would potentially denervate intraarticular and extraarticular pain sources. Because the sacroiliac joint and ligaments are innervated, similar to the zygapophyseal joint, the joint and capsules are regarded as the same structure. In contrast to the zygapophyseal joint, the sacroiliac joint is surrounded by thick supporting ligaments, and intraarticular injected local anesthetic may not anesthetize the ligaments.

Dreyfuss and colleagues[207] used a double-blind randomized controlled trial to assess ability of single-site, single-depth L5 dorsal ramus and S1–S3 lateral branch blocks to anesthetize the sacroiliac joint in 19 volunteers, using sacroiliac joint fluid distraction before and after blocks to determine effectiveness. The authors reported that only 40% of the volunteers did not feel distention after the blocks. The poor results prompted a cadaveric study of multisite,[189] multidepth blocks to anesthetize the joint. L5 dorsal ramus block was performed at the standard location of the S1 superior articular process and the sacral ala; S1–S2 lateral branches were blocked (right side) at these clock positions—2:30, 4:00, and 5:30; and S3 lateral branch was blocked at the right 2:30 and 4:00 positions. The lateral branch blocks were performed 8 to 10 mm lateral to the posterior sacral foramen. A 0.2 mL volume of green dye was injected on the dorsal sacral plate, and an additional 0.2 mL was injected 2 to 3 mm above the sacral plate.

Dissection revealed that the S1–S3 lateral branch nerves were stained in 91% (31 of 34) of cases. Employing the same protocol on 20 volunteer subjects using intraosseous ligament probing and capsular distention, Dreyfuss and colleagues[189] found that 86% of the sham local anesthetic injection subjects retained the ability to feel capsular distention, leading the authors to conclude that lateral branch blocks do not reliably block the intraarticular portion of the joint and that intraarticular blocks do not reliably block the extraarticular ligaments. One may conclude that to evaluate fully intraarticular and extraarticular pain sources, dorsal ramus and lateral branch blocks and intraarticular injections should be done. The caveat is that the nerve blocks were successful in 70% of cases, leaving a potential 30% false-negative cases. Injecting larger volumes or injecting the ligaments directly may potentially reduce the false-negative results with the risk of increasing false-positive results secondary to leak of local anesthetic through the posterior foramen.

Predictive Value

Surgical fusion outcomes for mechanical sacroiliac joint pain are reported for only a few small case series audits of initial outcomes after several "new" techniques for fusing the sacroiliac joint.[222–225] Published case series use pain relief after image-guided analgesic sacroiliac joint injections as the reference standard for diagnosing sacroiliac joint pain. Although Schutz and Grob[223] reported an 82% unacceptable outcome after bilateral sacroiliac joint fusion in 17 patients based on results from sacroiliac joint anesthetic block, three other studies using novel techniques reported more favorable results for mostly unilateral fusions. Al-Khayer and colleagues[224] reported an approximate 50% decrease in VAS and a 14-point decrease in Oswestry Disability Index in nine patients at 2 years after percutaneous sacroiliac joint arthrodesis using a Hollow Modular Anchorage screw (Aesculap). Using percutaneously inserted fusion cages and bone morphogenetic protein, Wise and Dall[222] reported an average back pain VAS improvement of 4.9 and leg pain VAS improvement of 2.4 in 13 patients at 6 months. Finally, Ziran and colleagues,[225] using CT-guided sacroiliac joint blocks as a reference standard, percutaneously fused 17 patients with recalcitrant sacroiliac joint pain and found a statistically significant correlation ($P < .02$) between final postoperative pain scores and preinjection as well as postinjection pain scores.

Evidence is limited to a small body of literature, including mostly observational studies assessing the outcome of various treatments for sacroiliac joint pain. Cohen and colleagues[226] performed a randomized sham-controlled trial, selecting patients for various types of radiofrequency neurotomy of the L4 medial branch, L5 dorsal branch, and S1–S3 lateral branches using the reference standard of a single sacroiliac joint intraarticular block with greater than or equal to 75% relief of pain for 2 hours after injection of 2 mL of bupivacaine. Of 18 patients, 13 obtained satisfactory relief of pain with average scores reduced by 60%, 50%, and 57% at 1 month, 3 months, and 6 months, respectively. Only two patients in the placebo group obtained relief; pain scores of the placebo subjects were unchanged from baseline. Yin and colleagues[186] used dual injection into the sacroiliac joint intraosseous ligament to diagnose sacroiliac joint pain. Of patients, 64% reported a minimum of 60% subjective pain relief for a minimum of 6 months after sensory stimulation–guided sacral lateral branch radiofrequency neurotomy. The remainder of this clinical outcome literature is reviewed elsewhere.[227]

Summary

Sacroiliac joint pain is a significant cause of chronic low back pain that is diagnosable and treatable with precision injection techniques. The prevalence of sacroiliac joint pain, based on a dual differential block protocol, ranges from 10% to 38%; for single, uncontrolled blocks, the false-positive rate is 54%.[177–181] The sacroiliac joint as a pain generator is no longer disputed. Current research also suggests that the sacroiliac joint is a significant source of persistent pain after lumbar fusion and may be a cause of graft donor site pain.[199–201] Although motion is limited and complex, the joint is known to rotate less than 4 degrees and to translate less than 1.6 mm. Anatomic studies have elucidated the innervation to the joint, with most practitioners directing diagnostic and therapeutic interventions to the L5 dorsal ramus and S1–S3 lateral branches.[185,187] Sacroiliac joint pain is now thought to emanate from the joint itself but also from extraarticular dorsal ligamentous sources. Interventionalists are just beginning to diagnose and treat putative extraarticular pain generators.

In contrast to the history and physical examination for zygapophyseal joint pain, certain diagnostic features for sacroiliac joint pain have been validated by controlled blocks. Maximal pain below L5 coupled with pointing to the posterior superior iliac spine has a predictive value of 60%.[202,205] Although no single physical examination test has been shown to be of satisfactory diagnostic value in isolation, using the dual-block paradigm, several studies have shown high sensitivity (85–91%) and specificity (78–79%) for accurately identifying the sacroiliac joint as the source of pain by combining three or more provocative maneuvers.[179,181] Specificity increases to 87% if the patient's pain cannot be centralized.[204] Diagnostic imaging of sacroiliac joint pain has not been shown to be helpful other than excluding nonmechanical causes of sacroiliac joint pain. The sensitivity of bone scans for detecting sacroiliac joint pain is poor (range 12–46%).[215,217] CT scan of the sacrum in a patient with persistent low back or buttock pain after lumbar fusion may be useful, particularly if the synovial joint has been violated. In these patients, severe degenerative changes were found on CT scan.[199]

The current standard for diagnosis of sacroiliac joint pain is approximately 70% relief of pain for 1 to 2 hours after lidocaine block and 3 to 4 hours after bupivacaine block. Total volume should be limited to 1.5 mL. The interventionalist should carefully study the joint arthrogram for any evidence of extravasation via the dorsal sacral foramina, superior joint recess and fifth lumbar epiradicular sheath, or ventral capsule to the lumbosacral plexus because this can cause false-positive responses. Not all patients obtain relief from intraarticular joint injections, and extraarticular sources of pain must be evaluated as well. Other techniques for diagnosis and treatment of the sacroiliac joint include targeting the L5 dorsal ramus and S1–S3 lateral branches.

If pain persists, new techniques have also been described for blocking the interosseous sacral ligaments.[220] Regarding the predictive value of diagnostic sacroiliac joint injection for sacroiliac joint arthrodesis, some case studies show poor results for arthrodesis; other studies using novel techniques report better results.[222–225] Evidence exists for the effectiveness of neurotomy of sacroiliac joint lateral branches after diagnostic block.[227] Other researchers have also shown promising results with periarticular blockade.[193]

Middle Compartment: Selective Nerve Root Blocks

Radicular Pain and the Role of Selective Nerve Root Blocks

Patients with clinically significant radicular pain unresponsive to conservative care and medications may be offered a therapeutic injection, including local anesthetic and corticosteroids. The injection can be performed using an interlaminar, transforaminal, or combined approach and can be performed at all suspected levels using volumes of injectant that cover all suspected symptomatic levels. If the patient has convincing pain relief for 1 week or longer, it is likely that the cause of pain is reversible and secondary to inflammation.[34] More important, if the patient reports minimal or very short-term relief of extremity pain, the pain has been present for greater than 1 year, and the offending pathology is unconvincing, the pain may be neuropathic or referred somatic pain.[34] If pain relief is satisfactory and lasts several weeks or longer, one may use additional therapeutic injections to facilitate conservative care, and there may be no need to proceed with exactly identifying the symptomatic level. When pain recurs or is poorly responsive to therapeutic injections and the clinical and imaging studies are inconclusive or indicate more than one potential pain level, diagnostic transforaminal injections may be considered. Box 16.1 summarizes indications for diagnostic selective nerve root blocks.

Despite the growing sophistication of modern imaging, the source of extremity pain is not always clearly apparent. Extremity pain may also be referred from the hip, buttock, or shoulder secondary to intrinsic pathology in these structures. Radicular pain can be secondary to entrapment by bone, ligament, or disc or result from leakage of noxious cytokines from either the disc or an inflamed zygapophyseal joint without evidence of compression. *Segmental instability*, albeit difficult to detect or prove, may cause repetitive dynamic irritation of the dorsal root ganglion leading to chronic dorsal root ganglion hypersensitivity. Advanced MRI often shows multilevel degenerative pathology, abnormalities on the side opposite the patient's symptoms, or abnormalities that are asymptomatic.[228–230] Except for the most profound structural abnormalities, MRI provides morphologic information only; correlations must be made with clinical presentation in order to establish the significance of imaging findings.[231] Confounding the diagnosis further, pain patterns may not follow classic referral distributions.[232,233]

Before considering surgical interventions, one should have a clear diagnosis with concordant imaging studies that show a surgically correctable lesion compressing the spinal nerve root, dorsal root ganglion, or ventral ramus. Pain referral patterns and physical examination findings should also be consistent with the suspected level of pathology. Most single-level entrapments are obvious. If not, further diagnostic information may be considered, such as selective nerve root blocks. Some interventionalists and surgeons still find myelography useful because MRI may miss a sequestered fragment or the MRI cuts may not be fine enough to detect the pathologic lesion.

Selective injection of local anesthetic around the spinal nerve within or near the intervertebral foramen has long been used to help surgeons confirm or refute a hypothesis that a particular spinal nerve root is the source of pain. Selective nerve root blocks are distinguished from transforaminal epidural steroid injections. With a selective nerve root block, a small volume of contrast medium, approximately 0.5 mL, is injected with the goal of outlining the exiting spinal nerve and ventral and dorsal roots (Figs. 16.16 to 16.18); then, the same volume of local anesthetic is injected such that epidural flow

BOX 16.1 Indications for diagnostic selective nerve root blocks

1. Patients with radicular pain without localizing signs to indicate which level is involved
2. Patients without obvious nerve root entrapment on high-quality imaging studies
3. Patients with chronic radicular pain present for ≥1 year, resistant to usual care and being considered for surgery
4. Patients with persistent pain after surgery or status following multiple surgeries
5. Patients with radicular symptoms in more than one distribution with multilevel structure impingement
6. Patients with atypical extremity pain
7. Nondiagnostic or conflicting results of imaging studies, discography, or electromyography

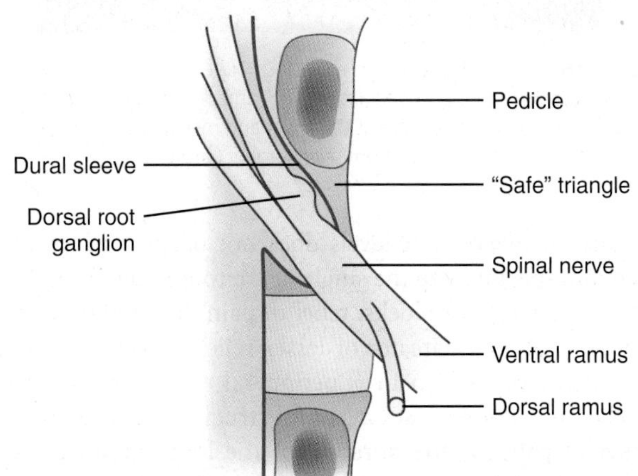

FIG. 16.16 Spinal nerve within the intervertebral foramen. The spinal nerve is a short segmental structure that quickly divides into ventral and dorsal rami. A selective nerve root block places local anesthetic no further than the 6 o'clock position on the pedicle. (From Bogduk N, Aprill C, Derby R. Epidural steroid injections. In: White AH, ed. *Spine Care. Vol. 1: Diagnosis and Conservative Treatment*. St. Louis: Mosby; 1995:322–343.)

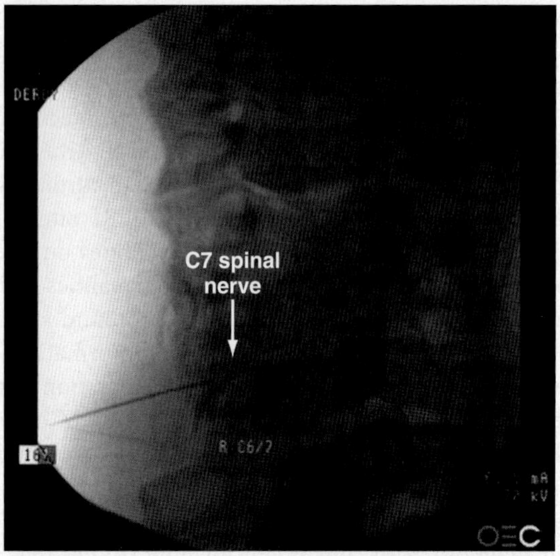

FIG. 16.17 Anteroposterior view of a right C7 selective nerve root block (*arrow*). The C7 nerve root is outlined by contrast dye and is located in the C6–C7 foramen. A 1.5-inch, 25-gauge needle was used to inject 0.3 mL of contrast dye. There is no spread of contrast dye around the pedicle and into the epidural space. (Courtesy Richard Derby, MD.)

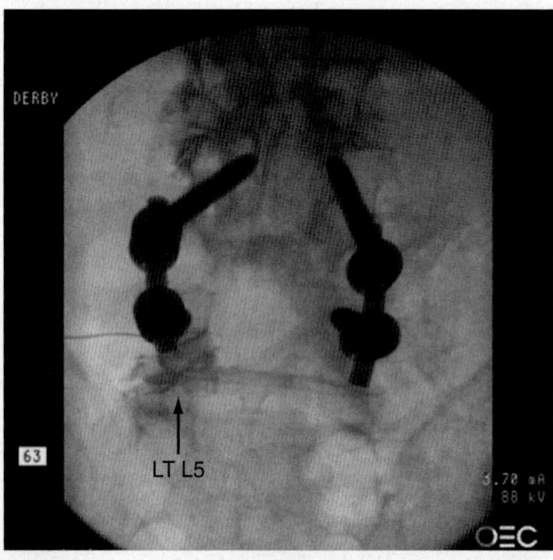

FIG. 16.18 Left L5 selective nerve root block. Note how 0.5 mL of injected contrast dye surrounds and outlines the root and dorsal root ganglion. There is a cutoff of contrast dye at the lower and medial border of the pedicle because of scar tissue from prior surgery (*arrow*).

to adjacent nerve root levels does not occur[234] in order to maintain specificity to the single nerve root in question. With selective nerve root blocks, relief of pain does not determine the cause of pain. Greater or lesser relief of pain may occur even if the cause of pain is peripheral entrapment or if the blocked nerve innervates a painful structure, such as the hip. Relief of pain for the duration of the local anesthetic may occur even if the root has irreversible damage.

History

Spine surgeons began using diagnostic root blocks in the late 1960s to help locate sources of radicular pain not well visualized with myelography.[233,235–238] Provocation of symptoms, pattern of the neurogram, and relief of pain were used to identify hidden pathology that was later confirmed or refuted during surgical exploration. A high degree of correlation was found between "positive" blocks and surgical findings. In addition, some early studies began reporting the surgical outcome based on selective nerve root block findings.[236] The routine use of CT and MRI improved the identification of structural causes of root compression, and some surgeons began using root blocks in difficult cases in which provocation and relief of pain helped to determine the operated level.[239–242] Surgeons noted that although MRI and CT improved visualization of pathology, imaging did not correlate with cause of pain and it did not correlate the abnormal anatomy with actual symptoms.[239]

Structural confirmation of suspected pathology and subsequent pain relief after surgery were reported in mostly retrospective case series. These studies also reported that selective nerve root blocks were better able to identify a symptomatic root compared with CT and MRI in "difficult" cases.[231,240,241,243,244] Of particular note was a finding that although outcome of patients diagnosed with various nerve root entrapment syndromes was excellent, patients diagnosed with scarring or arachnoiditis had very poor outcomes.[239,241] All studies reported "successful" surgery to a greater or lesser extent in approximately 90% to 95% of patients following pain relief after selective nerve injections if patients having prior surgery, scarring, and arachnoiditis were excluded. In the two studies that evaluated surgical outcome on patients with less than approximately 95% relief after injection, surgical results were modest to poor.[239,243]

In an observational study in 1971, Macnab[235] analyzed the causes of nerve root involvement in 68 patients who had undergone a "negative exploration" for presumed radicular pain caused by a herniated disc. Various pathologies were described, including migration of a disc fragment into the intervertebral foramen, nerve root kinking by the pedicle, articular process impingement, and extraforaminal lateral disc herniation. In the case of pedicular kinking, Macnab[235] described a technique of placing a 25-gauge needle into the intervertebral foramen and injecting 0.5 to 1 mL of oil-soluble contrast material. The provocation of concordant pain by striking the nerve with the needle, the characteristic contrast outline of the "kinked" nerve root within the foramen, and subsequent relief of pain after injection of 1 mL of 2% lidocaine were used to establish the diagnosis and led to "excellent results" in the six studied patients. Macnab[235] also described two patients with an undiscovered extraforaminal lateral disc herniation who underwent successful operation after relief of pain with a selective nerve root block. Likewise, Schutz and colleagues[237] in 1973 described the use of selective root blocks in 23 patients. In 13 of 15 patients who underwent surgery, the positive results of the selective nerve root blocks were confirmed.

Using a selective nerve root block technique similar to Macnab, Tajima and colleagues[238] in 1977 described various contrast patterns after injection of 2 mL of water-soluble contrast media, including cutoff patterns of contrast flow within the foramen and lateral recess indicating stenosis or block by a herniated disc. Provocation and pain relief after injection of 3 mL of 1% lidocaine confirmed the diagnosis, which was later proven during surgical exploration in this small case series. Kikuchi and colleagues[233] published a larger case series comprised of 332 patients in 1984, in which they performed nerve root infiltration in all patients and correlated the resulting neurogram with anatomic findings of cadaveric dissections. In most patients, pain was relieved by injection at a single level. The cadaveric studies revealed the following causes of atypical pain: congenital or acquired abnormalities of nerve and nerve roots, sensory rootlets communicating with adjacent nerves, conjoined nerves, and the common occurrence of the nerve exiting much more commonly at the L4 than L5 level and giving branches to the lumbosacral trunk and femoral and obturator nerves. Kikuchi and colleagues[233] also described the descent of the vertebral pedicle associated with disc collapse, degenerative changes of the articular zygapophyseal joint, and compression of the nerve at different sites.

Krempen and Smith[236] in 1974 were the first to report surgical outcomes based on provocation and pain relief after injection of the nerve root with 1 mL of 1% lidocaine. They also described and included radiographs of neurogram patterns of extraforaminal disc herniations, pedicle kinking, articular process impingement, and scar tissue. These authors used the injections to diagnose pain in 21 patients with prior lumbar laminectomies and commented that most patients were able to pinpoint the level of the lesion to either of two injected levels. Of the 16 operated patients, three had excellent results, nine had good results, and four had moderate results. The technique involved inserting an 18-gauge spinal needle 4 cm above the transverse process and approximately 6 cm from midline, directed downward and medially to strike the nerve. In the 1980s, Haueisen and colleagues[244] used Krempen and Smith's technique of spinal nerve injections to diagnose pain in difficult-to-diagnose patients, including 57% who had previous lumbar surgery. Of 63 operated patients, Haueisen and colleagues[244] confirmed compression of the suspected nerve root in 93% of the cases; at an average follow-up of 20 months, 73% of patients had no pain, slight pain, or some pain. Myelography and electromyelography aided in correct diagnosis of the lesion in only 24% and 38% of the cases.

Dooley and colleagues[239] used provocation and relief of pain after selective nerve root block to review retrospectively the results of 63 patients undergoing operations based on positive pain reproduction and pain relief after injection of 1 mL of 1% lidocaine correlated with surgical findings and outcome. The authors presented results according to whether the patients had full or incomplete pain relief and whether pain was reproduced. Of patients with reproduction and full pain relief, 45 of 46 had an anatomic diagnosis made at the time of surgery. Eight patients had herniated nucleus pulposus and all were relieved of leg pain at follow-up. At follow-up, 17 patients had bony entrapment and 14 (82%) were asymptomatic. Only one of 11 patients found to have arachnoiditis was pain free at follow-up, although five of seven patients found to have periradicular adhesions but without intraneural scarring were asymptomatic at follow-up. Patients with reproduction but incomplete relief included one patient who was diabetic with probable neuropathy causing failed surgery; the other three patients had pathology at other levels, and only one of the three had a satisfactory surgical outcome. In patients who had no reproduction and incomplete relief, only five of 14 cases were relieved of symptoms, and the authors recommended that patients with this group of responses should undergo careful reevaluation.

In 1988, Jonsson and colleagues[245] reported total relief of pain in 51% of patients undergoing diagnostic lumbar "root anesthesia" in 100 cases of sciatic pain with normal findings on myelography, CT, or MRI. The patients experiencing pain relief underwent surgical root decompression with short-term surgical outcome comparable to conventional surgery in more obvious cases.

In 1990, Stanley and colleagues[240] likewise reported outcomes based on response to injection in which they included only positive and negative responses. Positive responses required pain provocation and relief of pain with 1 mL of 1% lidocaine; a negative response was defined as nonconcordant pain provocation immediately and only partial relief or no relief of pain after the expected duration of onset of lidocaine. At least two roots were studied in each patient. Of 20 patients with positive responses, 19 underwent operation, and Stanley and colleagues[240] found that "nerve root infiltration" identified the symptomatic level in 18 of 19 cases. CT scan and myelogram identified the correct level in only 14 of 19 cases and 12 of 19 cases, respectively.

In 1989, Herron[241] reported the use of spinal nerve root blocks with pain provocation immediately and pain relief after 1 mL of 0.5% bupivacaine. A positive response included reproduction of pain and at least 75% pain relief. Herron[241] divided outcomes into good, fair, and poor. A good outcome was defined as 75% pain relief and return to previous work status with minimal medications and minimal or no restrictions of physical activities. In the previously unoperated disc herniation group, 15 of 18 patients had good results, and three had fair results. In nine patients, the imaging studies were positive at two levels, but surgery was performed only at one symptomatic level identified with a root block. There were seven good results and two fair results. In patients with previous unoperated spinal stenosis, 19% had a poor outcome versus 52% poor outcomes in patients with prior stenosis surgery. Herron[241] noted that in most patients with radiculopathy, selective nerve root blocks are not needed because the level was readily apparent on clinical examination and imaging studies; however, root blocks were useful for patients with equivocal findings, previous surgery, and multilevel structural pathology.

Porter and colleagues[242] used CT-guided root blocks, employing a two-needle technique to place an inner needle adjacent to the target nerve. In contrast to previous authors, these authors did not include provocation and injected 1.5 mL of 0.5% bupivacaine. Porter and colleagues[242] reported that, of the 18 patients undergoing surgery, 78% had a good outcome; two patients had unsuccessful surgeries.

The study in 2005 by Sasso and colleagues[243] is the most comprehensive, albeit retrospective, evaluation of the value of selective nerve root injections to predict lumbar and cervical surgical outcomes. These authors studied 101 patients culled from an institutional database from 1996 to 1999. Injections were performed by placing the needle tip just below the superior pedicle without intentional pain provocation. Additionally, a stimulating electrode to locate the needle close to the exiting nerve was employed. A neurogram was obtained, and a volume of 0.5 to 0.75 mL of 2% lidocaine was injected with the requirement of greater than 95% pain relief during postblock provocative testing in order to be considered "positive." Confirmatory injections were performed when pain relief was rated as 80% to 95%. Surgical follow-up occurred at a mean of 16 months, with 18 patients undergoing cervical surgery and 83 patients undergoing lumbar surgery. Of patients with positive selective nerve root injections, 91% had a good surgical outcome defined as a follow-up VAS of 2 or less and a positive patient satisfaction score. In 10 patients with negative selective nerve root injections, only 60% obtained a good surgical outcome. Patients undergoing surgery at a level with a positive block were 9.1 times more likely to have good outcomes than patients who had surgery at negative selective nerve root injection levels. When the findings between selective nerve root injection and MRI differed (n = 20), surgery at a level consistent with the selective nerve root injection was more strongly associated with a good surgical outcome than surgery based on MRI. For selective nerve root injection, the positive predictive value was 91.2% with a negative predictive value of 40% compared with 88.4% positive predictive value of MRI. Subgroup analysis of lumbar and cervical results was not reported.

Finally, Derby and colleagues[34] in 1992 reported the correlation between immediate leg pain relief after lumbar block and 1-year surgical outcomes. The authors segregated 78 patients undergoing epidural injections with a minimum of 80% immediate postblock leg pain relief into two dichotomous groups: patients with 50% or greater subjective leg pain relief lasting for 1 week or longer and patients with duration of extremity pain lasting 1 year or longer. Regardless of immediate pain relief, 85% of patients who had pain for less than 1 year had a positive surgical result defined as 50% or greater pain relief at 1 year. More important, 95% of the patients who did not respond to the block had a poor surgical outcome. Derby and colleagues[34] opined that the poor outcome might be explained in some cases by an inadequate structural correction, inadequate stabilization, or functional reasons, but most failures probably represented irreversible changes in the neural structures. Although unstudied, thus unconfirmed, the results by Derby and colleagues[34] are consistent with findings reported by Kumar and colleagues[246] that outcome after spinal cord stimulation in patients with failed back surgery syndrome was superior to revision surgery.

Diagnostic Accuracy of Selective Nerve Root Blocks

Diagnostic accuracy and ultimately utility depend on the degree to which a selective nerve root block relieves pain caused by any lesion within the nerve at or distal to the injection site. A greater or lesser degree of pain relief caused by a lesion affecting the nerve proximal to the injection site should also be taken into account when determining value.[99] Ideally, blocking an unaffected nerve would not relieve any pain. The degree to which these goals are accomplished constitutes the diagnostic accuracy as measured by sensitivity, specificity, and predictive value. Understanding these variables guides the clinician in terms of either accepting or discarding the block results or whether even to consider obtaining the information.

To study the diagnostic accuracy, one would select cases of acute or subacute monoradiculopathy caused by an obvious single-level lesion verified by imaging studies, intraoperative findings, and relief after surgical intervention. The most common gold standard lesion would be L4–L5 paracentral herniation irritating the traversing L5 root.[243] Blinding the patient, the symptomatic root and presumably at least one unaffected root would be blocked at different sessions, and the data would be prospectively collected. The lesion would be confirmed at surgery and by postsurgical pain relief.

Although many prior studies retrospectively studied the ability of provocation and relief of pain to predict structural nerve entrapment and surgical outcome, only two studies examined injections performed on symptomatic roots and presumed asymptomatic roots with the expressed goal of defining sensitivity and specificity, and both studied only the value of lumbar injections.[247,248] From these two studies, particularly the more recent study by Yeom and colleagues,[247] one may estimate the diagnostic value of lumbar diagnostic root blocks. An additional study evaluated the effect of needle tip position on the accuracy of selective nerve root block (with lack of epidural spread), and found that a needle tip position lateral to the middle third of the pedicle produced an accurate contrast pattern in 92% of cases, which fell to 70% when the needle was advanced beyond the lateral third of the pedicle[249]

Assessment of Effect

Only the study by Yeom and colleagues[247] determined the optimal cutoff level in the percent relief of pain reported by a patient after a procedure needed to qualify for a positive response. Using receiver operator curves, these authors chose a cutoff of 70% subjective relief of pain after a lumbar transforaminal block as the best value to provide optimal accuracy but stated that this level could be adjusted depending on the importance of avoiding false-negative versus false-positive results.

We recommend adjusting the cutoff criteria between 50% and 90% depending on the importance of avoiding false-negative versus false-positive blocks. In our opinion, it is probably best not to treat results as a dichotomous variable but rather as a data point that is more or less likely to indicate the root is a source of pain. If a discrete cutoff is required, 70% is a good compromise. One might also consider requiring a similar degree in change of VAS improvement or, if inconsistent with the patient's subjective report of pain relief, asking the patient why the discrepancy exists or performing a confirmatory injection. The patient often reports a global relief of pain, whereas diagnostically one is interested only in the degree of pain relief of the particular extremity distribution being evaluated. Relief or nonrelief of axial pain is important information but not pertinent to the location of the patient's extremity pain and to surgical outcomes.

Although provocation of concordant pain was frequently used in the past and perhaps is useful information, more recent studies use techniques to avoid creating pain during injection.[243,247] Pain referral patterns obtained by electrical stimulation may be considered as supplementary proof or nonproof.[243]

Sensitivity

The most likely causes of low sensitivity or a high rate of false-negative injections are inadequate blocks owing to poor spread around the root, failure to reach the pathologic site, dilutional effects with inadequate mass of anesthetic reaching the root, or poor diffusion because of scarring.[247] van Akkerveeken[248] found 100% sensitivity in 46 patients using 0.2 to 0.5 mL of 0.5% bupivacaine (with provocation) and reported 100% pain relief at 1 hour. Yeom and colleagues,[247] using 1 mL of 2% lidocaine without considering provocation, calculated a lower sensitivity of 57% (27 of 47) in all patients, increasing to 71% (25 of 35) when injections with inadequate spread were excluded. The causes of the inadequate blocks were spread of injectant into adjacent tissues in 4 of 10 patients, block by large disc herniation in 4 of 10 patients, and intraepiradicular sheath injection in 2 of 10 patients. Although Yeom and colleagues[247] had no explanation in the remaining 10 cases, these false-negative results might be explained by a paracentral herniated disc, which, although affecting primarily the traversing root, may also cause chemical irritation of the exiting root.

In addition, Dooley and colleagues[239] found that the most common reason for typical pain provocation during lumbar block with incomplete pain relief is multilevel pathology. The most probable cause in obvious cases is an inadequate block performed at a location distal to the structural entrapment. Diagnostic injections are often performed in patients with long-standing chronic pain and patients with prior surgery who may have intraneural and extraneural scarring. In such cases, local anesthetic may not penetrate the nerve effectively, and incomplete relief would be expected. Using a more concentrated anesthetic or an anesthetic that preferentially blocks nociceptors (e.g., bupivacaine) may reduce these false-negative responses.

Specificity

Because surgery is often less effective in patients with equivocal structural pathology, in patients with atypical, long-standing pain or prior surgery, one would ideally want to have minimal or no pain relief after the block of an asymptomatic root. van Akkerveeken[248] used a 0.2- to 0.5-mL volume of 0.5% bupivacaine and required 100% pain relief for 1 hour. He reported a specificity of "around" 90%.[248] In the lumbar spine, using 1 mL of 2% lidocaine and a cutoff value of greater than or equal to 70% pain relief, Yeom and colleagues[247] calculated 86% (50 of 58) specificity, which increased to 91% (43 of 47) specificity after excluding seven patients with overflow of local anesthetic. Although this overflow was thought to be a probable cause of false-positive blocks in 4 of 11 cases, 7 of 11 cases were true negatives, indicating that the estimated overflow when using 1 mL is about 20% (10 of 47) and with a potentially clinically observable effect in less than 10%.

Furman and colleagues[234] showed that even after injecting only 0.5 mL, the contrast pattern indicated nonselective flow in 30% of lumbar injections. The mass of drug overflowing at these low volumes may not be significant and is consistent with van Akkerveeken's higher, approximately 90% specificity. North and colleagues[99] reported an average 50% relief of sciatic pain when blocking the medial branches at several levels using a 3-mL volume, which would spread into the neuroforamen and epidural space, making the putative medial branch block nonspecific.[93] Nevertheless, sensory pathway convergence may be an alternative explanation of less than 50% pain relief in some cases, and a nonspecific "placebo" response may explain some or most false-positive responses.

Predictive Value

Many, mostly retrospective, observational studies describe in variable levels of detail the predictive value of lumbar spinal nerve root blocks. One retrospective study included the surgical predictive value of cervical and lumbar spinal nerve root injections.[243] Another prospective, diagnostic cervical selective root block study compared the diagnostic value of imaging with the short-term surgical predictive value of the test.[243] No studies to date support the use of diagnostic thoracic selective root injections, although this is primarily because the thoracic spine is not often studied because of the low prevalence of herniated thoracic discs.

In the only prospective outcome study, van Akkerveeken,[248] in his doctoral thesis, presented a series of studies correlating the value of selective root blocks to diagnosis of various lumbar entrapment syndromes and later summarized the data in a journal publication in 1993. A positive response was provocation of concordant pain and "disappearance" of leg pain after 0.2 to 0.5 mL of 0.5% bupivacaine. He studied patients with radiologic signs of nerve root entrapment but without localizing neurologic signs who subsequently underwent surgical decompression. Excluding the patients who had positive blocks and refused surgery, van Akkerveeken[248] reported a positive predictive value of 95% with a 95% confidence interval of 77% to 100%.

Technical Considerations and Potential Pitfalls

Techniques used by diagnostic lumbar studies place a needle varying in size from 22-gauge to 25-gauge into the foramen. Although older studies located the root by producing paresthesias,[233,235,238,239,241,242,244] more recent studies use a standard Spine Intervention Society technique of placing the needle tip just below the pedicle at the approximate 6 o'clock position viewed in and oblique plane (approximately 25–35 degrees) without purposefully provoking pain.[17,147] The transforaminal lumbar technique used by Macnab in the 1960s is similar to the current technique and the technique often used by many longer-term interventionalists, including the senior author (R.D.).[34,250] The needle is first advanced to contact the transverse process beginning approximately 6 cm from the midline, parallel to the transverse process and at an angle of approximately 30 degrees. The needle is advanced into the foramen at a position that would be approximately 6 o'clock below the pedicle.[235,239]

Another older described selective nerve root block technique used in the lumbar spine begins with needle insertion approximately 6 cm from the midline and approximately 2 to 3 cm above the transverse process with needle advancement into the foramen at a cephalad-caudad angle to contact the ventral root at approximately the midpoint between the upper and lower pedicles and slightly lateral to the foramen.[233,238,244] A stimulating electrode can also be used to verify close proximity of the needle tip to the nerve.[243] Although this technique has been referred to as a selective nerve root block, it is actually a selective ventral ramus block or, if the dorsal root ganglion is outside the foramen, additionally a dorsal root ganglion block. A standard needle, blunt tip needle, or a polytef (Teflon)-coated (e.g., approximately 3.5-inch, 22-gauge) radiofrequency needle may be used to position the needle tip within approximately 1 to 2 mm of the nerve, which in many cases is adjacent to the dorsal root ganglion. If a stimulating needle is used, observing motor stimulation at 2 Hz and approximately 2 V helps position the needle, and pain referral patterns can be noted using sensory stimulation at 50 Hz at approximately 0.2 to 0.5 V. Using live fluoroscopic monitoring, a volume of contrast medium equal to that used for local anesthesia is injected. The presence or absence of axial, buttock–hip, and extremity provocation and the location of contrast dye when provocation occurs should be recorded (e.g., within the foramen or more proximal or distal to the foramen). The pattern and extent of contrast flow is recorded via digital copy. Flow of contrast dye should show a negative outline of the dorsal root ganglion, spinal nerve, and ventral ramus. If spread of contrast dye is clearly outside the foramen and does not surround the nerve, the needle can be repositioned and reinjected.

All prior lumbar studies except one[242] used approximately 1 mL of contrast dye to outline the nerve. Most studies and guidelines recommend visualizing contrast spread using live fluoroscopy during injection. In the cervical spine, some authors advocate observing contrast flow in an anteroposterior view using digital subtraction fluoroscopy to better recognize potential injection into an artery coursing medially toward the spinal cord.[251,252]

Some prior studies used a volume varying from 0.3 to 0.5 mL of 0.5% bupivacaine[248] to 1.5 mL of 0.5% bupivacaine in the lumbar spine,[242] but most injected 1 mL of either 1% or 2% lidocaine. In the only diagnostic article that evaluated cervical injections, Sasso and colleagues[243] used 0.5 to 0.75 mL of 2% lidocaine but varied volume depending on the observed contrast dye distribution. No studies have evaluated the diagnostic value of thoracic injections.

We recommend limiting the volume to 0.5 to 1 mL in the lumbar spine and 0.3 to 0.5 mL in cervical and thoracic spine. Although many prior studies used 1% to 2% lidocaine, we recommend a higher concentration to ensure adequate block.[243,247] At a minimum, 2% lidocaine should be used; however, an equal combination of 4% lidocaine and 0.5% bupivacaine can be used. The volume can be adjusted between the lower and upper limit depending on the contrast flow pattern. Higher concentrations must, however, be used with caution as seizure is a reported complication of local anesthetic injection in the cervical transforaminal space using a subpedicular approach.[253]

Pitfalls regarding selective nerve root blocks include complications of the procedure. Although complications after transforaminal injections are mostly minor,[254–256] there are growing concerns regarding the safety of cervical transforaminal injections[257,258] and to a lesser extent thoracic and lumbar injections based on published and unpublished cases of neurologic damage after the injection of local anesthetic and corticosteroids into the neuroforamen.[259–263] Reported and unreported complications all involve the use of particulate corticosteroids that are alleged to have been injected into the vertebral or radicular artery. Some unpublished legal cases are, however, consistent with direct injection into the cord. Although legal cases claim that injury was secondary to injection of particulate corticosteroids into a lumbar or thoracic radicular artery, to our knowledge, there has been no reported case of neurologic damage secondary to arterial injection using nonparticulate corticosteroids. Nonparticulate corticosteroids are now recommended when performing cervical transforaminal injections.[264] Furthermore, as studies[265,266] show little difference in therapeutic efficacy between particulate and nonparticulate steroids, there is a growing consensus for the use of nonparticulate steroids for all transforaminal injections. On the other hand, if steroid is not added to the injectate for selective nerve root block, there should be no risk of spinal cord infarction due to intravascular injection of local anesthetic. Direct spinal cord injection is rare and in cervical transforaminal injections is likely preventable by using a shorter needle, always advancing the needle over bone (superior articular process), checking an anteroposterior fluoroscopy view before injection, and titrating patient sedation appropriately.

Although current techniques strive to avoid contacting the nerve, contact does occasionally occur, and probing for paresthesias was a common technique in the past. Lasting effects are probably uncommon, and none of the prior reviewed diagnostic block studies reported any complications. Injecting local anesthetic or contrast dye directly into the dorsal root ganglion, nerve, or epiradicular sheath may cause a flare in pain, however, lasting several days to several weeks.[247] Permanent injury is probably rare and to our knowledge unreported.

A needle placed too far medially can pierce the nerve root sleeve surrounded by the dura contiguous with the subarachnoid space. Injection may cause a high spinal block, which may necessitate resuscitation if injected in the cervical spine and may potentially lead to some degree of cord or root irritation secondary to added preservatives if depot steroids are injected. Puncture of the dura may also cause a low-pressure cerebrospinal fluid headache, which usually resolves spontaneously or can be treated with a routine blood patch. Slipman and colleagues[232] reported a case of recalcitrant headache cured after transforaminal blood patch. Infection may occur, but is rare. If the patient has a foraminal disc protrusion, inadvertently passing a needle into the disc may occasionally occur and could lead to a disc space infection.[267] If the operator knows that disc injection has occurred, use of a small amount of intradiscal and intravenous antibiotics may be considered (as would be the routine with discography).

Confounding Factors

Blocking the exiting spinal nerve anesthetizes several important neural elements. Receiving branches from the sympathetic system, the sinuvertebral nerve emerges lateral to the foramen and courses back through the foramen to innervate the posterior longitudinal ligament, the disc anulus at that level and one or two levels above. The sinuvertebral nerve can also innervate the contralateral side. In addition, lateral to the dorsal root ganglion, the dorsal root branches innervate posterior structures, including branches to the zygapophyseal joint at the same level and level below as well as the interspinous and supraspinous ligaments. Relief of pain may be due to anesthesia of these structures, which are not typically considered. Additionally, the furcal nerve, which typically exits the L4 foramen, is a separate nerve with its own dorsal root ganglion; it sends branches to the lumbosacral trunk, femoral, and obturator nerves. Irritation of this nerve causes seemingly aberrant pain distribution to the hip, groin, and inner thigh.

Summary

When pain recurs or is poorly responsive to therapeutic injections and the clinical and imaging studies are inconclusive or indicate more than one potential pain level, diagnostic transforaminal injections may be considered. As with all diagnostic spine injections, preprocedural and postprocedural evaluation should be performed with a standardized protocol by unbiased personnel and confirmation by the physician. Using the same testing protocol, the patient is tested at approximately 20 to 40 minutes after block with lidocaine and approximately 40 to 60 minutes after block with bupivacaine or ropivacaine. Additional testing at 1 to 3 hours postblock may help reduce both false-positive and false-negative results. The block should last for 2 hours if lidocaine is used and about 2 to 4 hours if bupivacaine or ropivacaine is used. If the pain relief is less than 70%, one can return the patient to the interventional suite and block one more additional suspected level. Diagnostic injection should be performed using one of the standard transforaminal approaches, preferably performed by an experienced interventionalist or surgeon. The patient should be no more than lightly sedated or sedated with a low dose of propofol that has a very short half-life.

A low volume of a concentrated anesthetic solution should be used that is limited to 0.3 mL or less in the cervical spine, 0.5 mL or less in the thoracic spine, and 1 mL or less in the lumbar spine.[234] One might consider using an equal mixture of 1% and 4% lidocaine or 0.5% bupivacaine. If performing a therapeutic injection, 0.5 mL of nonparticulate corticosteroid (e.g., 5 mg dexamethasone) may be injected in the cervical and thoracic spine approximately 1 to 2 minutes after local anesthetic injection, and either nonparticulate or a longer-acting depot preparation may be injected in the lumbar spine (e.g., approximately 20 mg of triamcinolone acetonide or 5–10 mg of betamethasone).

The immediate results and patients' longer-term pain relief are used to counsel them on their chances of obtaining relief of extremity pain after a surgical procedure. Patients who have immediate pain relief after one-level block of approximately 70% or greater and pain less than 1 year's duration have an 85% or greater chance of a satisfactory result.[239,240,243,247,248,250] If the patient has had prior surgery, one might want to lower the patient's expectation from 85% to perhaps approximately 70% or less depending on how convincing the structural pathology appears on MRI or CT.[241,244] Patients who have unconvincing structural pathology, radicular pain greater than 1 year's duration, relief of less than approximately 70% of pain after block, less than approximately 1 week of therapeutic pain relief, and especially evidence of intraradicular or extraradicular scarring should be referred for possible spinal cord stimulation or other nonoperative treatment.[34,239,241,247,248]

Patients with clear structural nerve entrapment with radicular pain less than approximately 1 year's duration, with no immediate or delayed longer-duration relief, may be offered surgery, but the patient should be counseled that there is an approximately 60% chance of a good outcome.[243] If the duration of the patient's pain is greater than 1 year, perhaps the patient should be told that there is an approximately 60% chance of having partial pain relief but that the pain relief would likely be less than 50%.[34,243] Even if the same patient with more chronic radicular pain had immediate pain relief but no longer-term relief, and especially if there was suspected neuropathic pain and a prior surgery, the patient should be counseled that the chances of a good outcome are no greater than approximately 50%.[241] Finally, we emphasize that relief of pain does not determine the cause of the pain, and if a patient's spinal nerve root pain is neuropathic, decompression with or without stabilization would most likely not provide satisfactory relief of pain.[268]

PEARLS AND PITFALLS

1. Much is learned during the process of diagnosis, especially if the process includes unpleasant diagnostic interventional procedures.
2. Diagnosis is the process of elimination. Patients should be counseled that negative responses are useful and important information.
3. Beware of patients with chronic pain without convincing structural pathology who consistently complain that they are no better or worse after appropriate therapeutic interventional procedures. Your reconstructive spine surgery may suffer the same fate.
4. Indeterminate and negative diagnostic block results are more common than clearly positive results.

5. Chronic spinal pain is often caused by structures in different columns and levels. Treating one source of pain often unmasks pain from a different source. Failure to relieve other sources of pain does not necessarily mean one's surgery failed, but the possibility of failure due to other sources is best identified before surgery.
6. When the diagnosis is not obvious and most of the pain is axial and referred extremity pain, consider first evaluating the posterior elements. Blocking the medial and/or lateral branches of the dorsal ramus will denervate most structures in the posterior column.
7. Do not neglect to rule out shoulder and hip pathology.
8. Convincing relief of pain for several weeks or longer is consistent with a reversible cause of pain.
9. Fusing to a painful sacroiliac joint is best avoided. Investigate and discuss the possibility before surgery rather than after.
10. Chronic dynamic irritation of neuraxial structures can cause buttock and axial pain in addition to referred extremity pain. Relief of axial pain following selective epidural block(s) that lasts several weeks or longer is consistent with pain due to static or dynamic stenosis. If in doubt, diagnosis can be confirmed by a *negative* response to medial branch block and a *negative* response to pressure-controlled discography, analgesic discography, or both.

KEY POINTS

1. Image-guided, precision injections (with local anesthetic and a dual-block paradigm) are the current reference standard for diagnosis of chronic spinal pain emanating from the middle and posterior column. Current research shows that history, physical examination, and advanced imaging findings have insufficient sensitivity and specificity for identifying the pain generator. Ideally, as with sacroiliac pain, the reference standard will evolve to include validated and accurate historical and physical examination features; however, with radicular pain and zygapophyseal joint pain, this is not yet the case.
2. Diagnostic injections are typically reserved as a tertiary intervention for patients with chronic, disabling spinal pain that is nonresponsive to conservative care and for patients with atypical presentations in whom the history, physical examination, and electrodiagnostic and imaging studies are unrevealing or nondiagnostic.
3. During a diagnostic block, relief of pain is more convincing than provocation of pain. The standard for percent relief is, at a minimum, greater than 50%; however, greater than 70% is more convincing.
4. Patients with psychosocial distress can have legitimate pain. Often, the psychosocial distress resolves with appropriate diagnosis and treatment of the pain generator.
5. Negative diagnostic blocks also provide useful information. A negative response suggests alternate explanations: first, the structure evaluated may not be the source of pain and therefore additional structures must be evaluated. Lack of relief may also be due to the development of irreversible local damage (e.g., intraneural fibrosis) or neuropathic pain with significant peripheral and central sensitization.
6. If rigorous technical and procedural performance standards are adhered to, the response to diagnostic blocks has been shown to predict good to excellent surgical and interventional treatment outcomes. Fair or poor response to diagnostic blocks can be used to counsel patients appropriately in terms of surgical outcomes.

KEY REFERENCES

1. Hancock MJ, Maher CG, Latimer J, et al. Systematic review of tests to identify the disc, SIJ or facet joint as the source of low back pain. *Eur Spine J.* 2007;16:1539-1550.
   This is a systematic review of the evidence for identifying the source of chronic low back pain.
2. Cohen SP, Raja SN. Pathogenesis, diagnosis, and treatment of lumbar zygapophysial (facet) joint pain. *Anesthesiology.* 2007; 106:591-614.
   This article provides a comprehensive review of zygapophyseal joint anatomy, biomechanics, and function as well as a systematic review of diagnosis and treatment of zygapophyseal joint pain.
3. Manchukonda R, Manchikanti KN, Cash KA, et al. Facet joint pain in chronic spinal pain: an evaluation of prevalence and false-positive rate of diagnostic blocks. *J Spinal Disord Tech.* 2007;20:539-545.
   This study of prevalence of facet joint pain based on dual-block paradigm reported a high false-positive rate with single diagnostic blocks.
4. Dreyfuss P, Dreyer SJ, Cole A, et al. Sacroiliac pain. *J Am Acad Orthop Surg.* 2004;12:255-265.
   This excellent review of the anatomy, pathophysiology, history, physical examination, and imaging findings associated with sacroiliac joint pain discusses the standards for diagnosis of sacroiliac joint pain with controlled blocks and treatment.
5. Bogduk N, ed. *Practice Guidelines: Spinal Diagnostic and Treatment Procedures.* 2nd ed. San Francisco: International Spine Intervention Society; 2013.
   State-of-the-art guidelines for the performance of diagnostic and therapeutic spinal injections are presented.

REFERENCES

1. Hoy D, March L, Brooks P, et al. The global burden of low back pain: estimates from the Global Burden of Disease 2010 study. *Ann Rheum Dis.* 2014;73(6):968-974.
2. Hoy D, March L, Woolf A, et al. The global burden of neck pain: estimates from the Global Burden of Disease 2010 study. *Ann Rheum Dis.* 2014;73(7):1309-1315.
3. Boswell MV, Trescot AM, Datta S, et al. Interventional techniques: evidence-based practice guidelines in the management of chronic spinal pain. *Pain Physician.* 2007; 10(1):7-111.
4. Fejer R, Ruhe A. What is the prevalence of musculoskeletal problems in the elderly population in developed countries? A systematic critical literature review. *Chiropr Man Therap.* 2012;20(1):31.
5. US Burden of Disease Collaborators. The state of US health, 1999-2010: burden of diseases, injuries, and risk factors. *JAMA.* 2013;310:591-608.
6. GBD 2013 DALYs and HALE Collaborators, Murray CJ, et al. Global, regional, and national disability-adjusted life years (DALYs) for 306 diseases and injuries and healthy life expectancy (HALE) for 188 countries, 1990-2013: quantifying the epidemiological transition. *Lancet.* 2015;386(10009): 2145-2191.
7. Mafi JN, McCarthy EP, Davis RB, Landon BE. Worsening trends in the management and treatment of back pain. *JAMA Intern Med.* 2013;173(17):1573-1581.
8. Freburger JK, Holmes GM, Agans RP, et al. The rising prevalence of chronic low back pain. *Arch Intern Med.* 2009;169(3):251-258.
9. Dillane JB, Fry J, Kalton G. Acute back syndrome—a study from general practice. *Br Med J.* 1966;2(5505):82-84.

10. Nachemson A. The natural course of low back pain. In: White A, Gordon SL, eds. *Symposium on Idiopathic Low Back Pain.* St Louis: Mosby; 1982:46-51.
11. Sheather-Reid RB, Cohen ML. Psychophysical evidence for a neuropathic component of chronic neck pain. *Pain.* 1998;75(2-3):341-347.
12. Hancock MJ, Maher CG, Latimer J, et al. Systematic review of tests to identify the disc, SIJ or facet joint as the source of low back pain. *Eur Spine J.* 2007;16(10):1539-1550.
13. Fritz JM, George S. The use of a classification approach to identify subgroups of patients with acute low back pain. Interrater reliability and short-term treatment outcomes. *Spine.* 2000;25(1):106-114.
14. Kent P, Keating J. Do primary-care clinicians think that nonspecific low back pain is one condition? *Spine.* 2004;29(9):1022-1031.
15. Derby R. Diagnostic block procedures: use in pain localization. In: White AH, ed. *Spine: State of the Art Reviews, Failed Back Surgery Syndrome.* Philadelphia: Hanley & Belfus; 1986:47-64.
16. DePalma MJ, Ketchum JM, Saullo T. What is the source of chronic low back pain and does age play a role? *Pain Med.* 2011;12(2):224-233.
17. Bogduk N. *Practice Guidelines for Spinal Diagnostic and Treatment Procedures.* 2nd ed. San Francisco: International Spine Intervention Society; 2013.
18. Boswell MV, Colson JD, Sehgal N, Dunbar EE, Epter R. A systematic review of therapeutic facet joint interventions in chronic spinal pain. *Pain Physician.* 2007;10(1):229-253.
19. Boden S, Wiesel S, Law E, Rothman R. *The Aging Spine.* Philadelphia: WB Saunders; 1991.
20. Berven S, Tay BB, Colman W, Hu SS. The lumbar zygapophyseal (facet) joints: a role in the pathogenesis of spinal pain syndromes and degenerative spondylolisthesis. *Semin Neurol.* 2002;22(2):187-196.
21. Wetzel FT. Chronic benign cervical pain syndromes: surgical considerations. *Spine.* 1992;17(10 suppl):S367-S374.
22. Cohen SP, Raja SN. Pathogenesis, diagnosis, and treatment of lumbar zygapophysial (facet) joint pain. *Anesthesiology.* 2007;106(3):591-614.
23. Cohen SP. Sacroiliac joint pain: a comprehensive review of anatomy, diagnosis, and treatment. *Anesth Analg.* 2005;101(5):1440-1453.
24. Resnick DK, Choudhri TF, Dailey AT, et al. Guidelines for the performance of fusion procedures for degenerative disease of the lumbar spine. Part 13: injection therapies, low-back pain, and lumbar fusion. *J Neurosurg Spine.* 2005;2(6):707-715.
25. Boswell MV, Singh V, Staats PS, Hirsch JA. Accuracy of precision diagnostic blocks in the diagnosis of chronic spinal pain of facet or zygapophysial joint origin. *Pain Physician.* 2003;6(4):449-456.
26. Dreyfuss P, Dreyer SJ, Cole A, Mayo K. Sacroiliac joint pain. *J Am Acad Orthop Surg.* 2004;12(4):255-265.
27. Datta S, Lee M, Falco FJ, Bryce DA, Hayek SM. Systematic assessment of diagnostic accuracy and therapeutic utility of lumbar facet joint interventions. *Pain Physician.* 2009;12(2): 437-460.
28. Atluri S, Datta S, Falco FJ, Lee M. Systematic review of diagnostic utility and therapeutic effectiveness of thoracic facet joint interventions. *Pain Physician.* 2008;11(5): 611-629.
29. Sehgal N, Dunbar EE, Shah RV, Colson J. Systematic review of diagnostic utility of facet (zygapophysial) joint injections in chronic spinal pain: an update. *Pain Physician.* 2007;10(1):213-228.
30. Manchikanti L, Pampati V, Fellows B, Baha AG. The inability of the clinical picture to characterize pain from facet joints. *Pain Physician.* 2000;3(2):158-166.
31. Yin W, Bogduk N. The nature of neck pain in a private pain clinic in the United States. *Pain Med.* 2008;9(2): 196-203.
32. Manchikanti L, Pampati V, Rivera J, et al. Role of facet joints in chronic low back pain in the elderly: a controlled comparative prevalence study. *Pain Pract.* 2001;1(4):332-337.
33. Pneumaticos SG, Chatziioannou SN, Hipp JA, Moore WH, Esses SI. Low back pain: prediction of short-term outcome of facet joint injection with bone scintigraphy. *Radiology.* 2006;238(2):693-698.
34. Derby R, Kine G, Saal JA, et al. Response to steroid and duration of radicular pain as predictors of surgical outcome. *Spine.* 1992;17(6 suppl):S176-S183.
35. Manchikanti L, Boswell MV, Manchukonda R, Cash KA, Giordano J. Influence of prior opioid exposure on diagnostic facet joint nerve blocks. *J Opioid Manag.* 2008;4(6):351-360.
36. Kikuchi S. New concept for backache: biopsychosocial pain syndrome. *Eur Spine J.* 2008;17(suppl 4):421-427.
37. Boos N, Rieder R, Schade V, et al. The diagnostic accuracy of magnetic resonance imaging, work perception, and psychosocial factors in identifying symptomatic disc herniations. *Spine.* 1995;20(24):2613-2625.
38. Lilius G, Laasonen EM, Myllynen P, Harilainen A, Gronlund G. Lumbar facet joint syndrome. A randomised clinical trial. *J Bone Joint Surg Br.* 1989;71(4):681-684.
39. Lilius G, Harilainen A, Laasonen EM, Myllynen P. Chronic unilateral low-back pain. Predictors of outcome of facet joint injections. *Spine.* 1990;15(8):780-782.
40. Wallis BJ, Lord SM, Bogduk N. Resolution of psychological distress of whiplash patients following treatment by radiofrequency neurotomy: a randomised, double-blind, placebo-controlled trial. *Pain.* 1997;73(1):15-22.
41. Kirkaldy-Willis WH, Farfan HF. Instability of the lumbar spine. *Clin Orthop Relat Res.* 1982;165:110-123.
42. Derby R, Lee S-H, Chen Y, et al. The influence of psychologic factors on diskography in patients with chronic axial low back pain. *Arch Phys Med Rehabil.* 2008;89(7):1300-1304.
43. Wikipedia. *Apophysis.* https://en.wikipedia.org/wiki/Apophysis.
44. Bogduk N. *Clinical Anatomy of the Lumbar Spine.* 4th ed. London: Elsevier; 2005.
45. Andersson GB, Ortengren R, Nachemson A. Intradiskal pressure, intra-abdominal pressure and myoelectric back muscle activity related to posture and loading. *Clin Orthop Relat Res.* 1977;129:156-164.
46. Adams MA, Hutton WC. The mechanical function of the lumbar apophyseal joints. *Spine.* 1983;8(3):327-330.
47. Uhrenholt L, Hauge E, Charles AV, Gregersen M. Degenerative and traumatic changes in the lower cervical spine facet joints. *Scand J Rheumatol.* 2008;37(5):375-384.
48. Taylor JR, Twomey LT, Corker M. Bone and soft tissue injuries in post-mortem lumbar spines. *Paraplegia.* 1990; 28(2):119-129.
49. Twomey LT, Taylor JR, Taylor MM. Unsuspected damage to lumbar zygapophyseal (facet) joints after motor-vehicle accidents. *Med J Aust.* 1989;151(4):210-212, 215-217.
50. Taylor JR, Twomey LT. Acute injuries to cervical joints: an autopsy study of neck sprain. *Spine.* 1993;18(9):1115-1122.

51. Uhrenholt L, Grunnet-Nilsson N, Hartvigsen J. Cervical spine lesions after road traffic accidents: a systematic review. *Spine.* 2002;27(17):1934-1941.
52. Eisenstein SM, Parry CR. The lumbar facet arthrosis syndrome: clinical presentation and articular surface changes. *J Bone Joint Surg Br.* 1987;69(1):3-7.
53. Ziv I, Maroudas C, Robin G, Maroudas A. Human facet cartilage: swelling and some physicochemical characteristics as a function of age. Part 2: age changes in some biophysical parameters of human facet joint cartilage. *Spine.* 1993;18(1):136-146.
54. Kallakuri S, Singh A, Chen C, Cavanaugh JM. Demonstration of substance P, calcitonin gene-related peptide, and protein gene product 9.5 containing nerve fibers in human cervical facet joint capsules. *Spine.* 2004;29(11):1182-1186.
55. Giles LG, Taylor JR. Innervation of lumbar zygapophyseal joint synovial folds. *Acta Orthop Scand.* 1987;58(1):43-46.
56. Giles LG, Taylor JR. Human zygapophyseal joint capsule and synovial fold innervation. *Br J Rheumatol.* 1987;26(2):93-98.
57. Kallakuri S, Singh A, Lu Y, et al. Tensile stretching of cervical facet joint capsule and related axonal changes. *Eur Spine J.* 2008;17(4):556-563.
58. Ahmed M, Bjurholm A, Kreicbergs A, Schultzberg M. Sensory and autonomic innervation of the facet joint in the rat lumbar spine. *Spine.* 1993;18(14):2121-2126.
59. Cavanaugh JM, Lu Y, Chen C, Kallakuri S. Pain generation in lumbar and cervical facet joints. *J Bone Joint Surg Am.* 2006;88(suppl 2):63-67.
60. Cavanaugh JM, Ozaktay AC, Yamashita HT, King AI. Lumbar facet pain: biomechanics, neuroanatomy and neurophysiology. *J Biomech.* 1996;29(9):1117-1129.
61. Schaible HG, Schmidt RF. Effects of an experimental arthritis on the sensory properties of fine articular afferent units. *J Neurophysiol.* 1985;54(5):1109-1122.
62. Lu Y, Chen C, Kallakuri S, Patwardhan A, Cavanaugh JM. Neural response of cervical facet joint capsule to stretch: a study of whiplash pain mechanism. *Stapp Car Crash J.* 2005;49:49-65.
63. Lu Y, Chen C, Kallakuri S, Patwardhan A, Cavanaugh JM. Neurophysiological and biomechanical characterization of goat cervical facet joint capsules. *J Orthop Res.* 2005;23(4):779-787.
64. Lee KE, Davis MB, Winkelstein BA. Capsular ligament involvement in the development of mechanical hyperalgesia after facet joint loading: behavioral and inflammatory outcomes in a rodent model of pain. *J Neurotrauma.* 2008;25(11):1383-1393.
65. Lee KE, Davis MB, Mejilla RM, Winkelstein BA. In vivo cervical facet capsule distraction: mechanical implications for whiplash and neck pain. *Stapp Car Crash J.* 2004;48: 373-395.
66. Winkelstein BA, Santos DG. An intact facet capsular ligament modulates behavioral sensitivity and spinal glial activation produced by cervical facet joint tension. *Spine.* 2008;33(8):856-862.
67. Woolf CJ. Evidence for a central component of post-injury pain hypersensitivity. *Nature.* 1983;306(5944):686-688.
68. Quinn KP, Lee KE, Ahaghotu CC, Winkelstein BA. Structural changes in the cervical facet capsular ligament: potential contributions to pain following subfailure loading. *Stapp Car Crash J.* 2007;51:169-187.
69. Kasch H, Stengaard-Pedersen K, Arendt-Nielsen L, Staehelin Jensen T. Pain thresholds and tenderness in neck and head following acute whiplash injury: a prospective study. *Cephalalgia.* 2001;21(3):189-197.
70. Sterling M, Jull G, Vicenzino B, Kenardy J. Sensory hypersensitivity occurs soon after whiplash injury and is associated with poor recovery. *Pain.* 2003;104(3):509-517.
71. Curatolo M, Petersen-Felix S, Arendt-Nielsen L, et al. Central hypersensitivity in chronic pain after whiplash injury. *Clin J Pain.* 2001;17(4):306-315.
72. Manchikanti L, Manchikanti KN, Manchukonda R, et al. Evaluation of lumbar facet joint nerve blocks in the management of chronic low back pain: preliminary report of a randomized, double-blind controlled trial: clinical trial NCT00355914. *Pain Physician.* 2007;10(3):425-440.
73. Bogduk N. A narrative review of intra-articular corticosteroid injections for low back pain. *Pain Med.* 2005;6(4):287-296.
74. Barnsley L, Lord SM, Wallis BJ, Bogduk N. Lack of effect of intraarticular corticosteroids for chronic pain in the cervical zygapophyseal joints. *N Engl J Med.* 1994;330(15):1047-1050.
75. Carette S, Marcoux S, Truchon R, et al. A controlled trial of corticosteroid injections into facet joints for chronic low back pain. *N Engl J Med.* 1991;325(14):1002-1007.
76. Manchikanti L, Singh V, Falco FJ, Cash KM, Fellows B. Cervical medial branch blocks for chronic cervical facet joint pain: a randomized, double-blind, controlled trial with one-year follow-up. *Spine.* 2008;33(17):1813-1820.
77. Manchikanti L, Singh V, Falco FJ, Cash KA, Pampati V. Lumbar facet joint nerve blocks in managing chronic facet joint pain: one-year follow-up of a randomized, double-blind controlled trial: clinical trial NCT00355914. *Pain Physician.* 2008;11(2):121-132.
78. Smuck M, Crisostomo RA, Trivedi K, Agrawal D. Success of initial and repeated medial branch neurotomy for zygapophysial joint pain: a systematic review. *PM R.* 2012;4(9):686-692.
79. MacVicar J, Borowczyk JM, MacVicar AM, Loughnan BM, Bogduk N. Lumbar medial branch radiofrequency neurotomy in New Zealand. *Pain Med.* 2013;14(5):639-645.
80. Little JS, Ianuzzi A, Chiu JB, Baitner A, Khalsa PS. Human lumbar facet joint capsule strains: II. Alteration of strains subsequent to anterior interbody fixation. *Spine J.* 2004;4(2):153-162.
81. Chang UK, Kim DH, Lee MC, et al. Changes in adjacent-level disc pressure and facet joint force after cervical arthroplasty compared with cervical discectomy and fusion. *J Neurosurg Spine.* 2007;7(1):33-39.
82. Mooney V, Robertson J. The facet syndrome. *Clin Orthop Relat Res.* 1976;115:149-156.
83. Sehgal N, Shah RV, McKenzie-Brown AM, Everett CR. Diagnostic utility of facet (zygapophysial) joint injections in chronic spinal pain: a systematic review of evidence. *Pain Physician.* 2005;8(2):211-224.
84. Bogduk N. Evidence-informed management of chronic low back pain with facet injections and radiofrequency neurotomy. *Spine J.* 2008;8(1):56-64.
85. Manchukonda R, Manchikanti KN, Cash KA, Pampati V, Manchikanti L. Facet joint pain in chronic spinal pain: an evaluation of prevalence and false-positive rate of diagnostic blocks. *J Spinal Disord Tech.* 2007;20(7):539-545.
86. Cohen S, Stojanovic M, Crooks M, et al. Lumbar zygapophysial (facet) joint radiofrequency denervation success as a function of pain relief during diagnostic medial branch blocks: a multicenter analysis. *Spine J.* 2008;8(3): 498-504.

87. Barnsley L, Lord S, Bogduk N. Comparative local anaesthetic blocks in the diagnosis of cervical zygapophysial joint pain. *Pain*. 1993;55(1):99-106.
88. Lord SM, Barnsley L, Bogduk N. The utility of comparative local anesthetic blocks versus placebo-controlled blocks for the diagnosis of cervical zygapophysial joint pain. *Clin J Pain*. 1995;11(3):208-213.
89. McCormick ZL, Marshall B, Walker J, McCarthy R, Walega DR. Long-term function, pain and medication use outcomes of radiofrequency ablation for lumbar facet syndrome. *Int J Anesth Anesth*. 2015;2(2).
90. Kaplan M, Dreyfuss P, Halbrook B, Bogduk N. The ability of lumbar medial branch blocks to anesthetize the zygapophysial joint: a physiologic challenge. *Spine (Phila Pa 1976)*. 1998;23(17):1847-1852.
91. Mahato NK. Mamillo-accessory notch and foramen: distribution patterns and correlation with superior lumbar facet structure. *Morphologie*. 2014;98(323):176-181.
92. Bogduk N. The lumbar mamillo-accessory ligament. Its anatomical and neurosurgical significance. *Spine*. 1981;6(2): 162-167.
93. Dreyfuss P, Schwarzer AC, Lau P, Bogduk N. Specificity of lumbar medial branch and L5 dorsal ramus blocks. A computed tomography study. *Spine*. 1997;22(8):895-902.
94. Destouet JM, Gilula LA, Murphy WA, Monsees B. Lumbar facet joint injection: indication, technique, clinical correlation, and preliminary results. *Radiology*. 1982;145(2):321-325.
95. Carrera GF. Lumbar facet joint injection in low back pain and sciatica: description of technique. *Radiology*. 1980;137(3):661-664.
96. Moran R, O'Connell D, Walsh MG. The diagnostic value of facet joint injections. *Spine*. 1988;13(12):1407-1410.
97. Barnsley L, Bogduk N. Medial branch blocks are specific for the diagnosis of cervical zygapophyseal joint pain. *Reg Anesth*. 1993;18(6):343-350.
98. Cohen SP, Hurley RW. The ability of diagnostic spinal injections to predict surgical outcomes. *Anesth Analg*. 2007;105(6):1756-1775.
99. North RB, Kidd DH, Zahurak M, Piantadosi S. Specificity of diagnostic nerve blocks: a prospective, randomized study of sciatica due to lumbosacral spine disease. *Pain*. 1996;65(1):77-85.
100. Goldthwait J. The lumbosacral articulation: an explanation of many cases of lumbago, sciatica and paraplegia. *Boston Med Surg J*. 1911;164:356-372.
101. Ghormley R. Low back pain with special reference to the articular facets, with presentation of an operative procedure. *JAMA*. 1933;101:1773-1777.
102. Badgley CE. Pain of spinal origin. *J Mich State Med Soc*. 1947;46(7):812.
103. Schwarzer AC, Aprill CN, Derby R, et al. The relative contributions of the disc and zygapophyseal joint in chronic low back pain. *Spine*. 1994;19(7):801-806.
104. Manchikanti L, Pampati V, Fellows B, Bakhit CE. Prevalence of lumbar facet joint pain in chronic low back pain. *Pain Physician*. 1999;2(3):59-64.
105. Manchikanti L, Boswell MV, Singh V, et al. Prevalence of facet joint pain in chronic spinal pain of cervical, thoracic, and lumbar regions. *BMC Musculoskelet Disord*. 2004;5:15.
106. Schwarzer AC, Wang SC, Bogduk N, McNaught PJ, Laurent R. Prevalence and clinical features of lumbar zygapophysial joint pain: a study in an Australian population with chronic low back pain. *Ann Rheum Dis*. 1995;54(2):100-106.
107. Fairbank JC, Park WM, McCall IW, O'Brien JP. Apophyseal injection of local anesthetic as a diagnostic aid in primary low-back pain syndromes. *Spine*. 1981;6(6):598-605.
108. Revel ME, Listrat VM, Chevalier XJ, et al. Facet joint block for low back pain: identifying predictors of a good response. *Arch Phys Med Rehabil*. 1992;73(9):824-828.
109. Revel M, Poiraudeau S, Auleley GR, et al. Capacity of the clinical picture to characterize low back pain relieved by facet joint anesthesia. Proposed criteria to identify patients with painful facet joints. *Spine*. 1998;23(18):1972-1976.
110. Laslett M, Oberg B, Aprill CN, McDonald B. Zygapophysial joint blocks in chronic low back pain: a test of Revel's model as a screening test. *BMC Musculoskelet Disord*. 2004;5:43.
111. Schwarzer AC, Aprill CN, Derby R, et al. The false-positive rate of uncontrolled diagnostic blocks of the lumbar zygapophysial joints. *Pain*. 1994;58(2):195-200.
112. Manchikanti L, Pampati V, Fellows B, Bakhit CE. The diagnostic validity and therapeutic value of lumbar facet joint nerve blocks with or without adjuvant agents. *Curr Rev Pain*. 2000;4(5):337-344.
113. Schwarzer AC, Derby R, Aprill CN, et al. Pain from the lumbar zygapophysial joints: a test of two models. *J Spinal Disord*. 1994;7(4):331-336.
114. Anand S, Butt MS. Patients' response to facet joint injection. *Acta Orthop Belg*. 2007;73(2):230-233.
115. Carrera GF. Lumbar facet arthrography and injection in low back pain. *Wis Med J*. 1979;78(12):35-37.
116. Jackson RP, Jacobs RR, Montesano PX. Facet joint injection in low-back pain. A prospective statistical study. *Spine*. 1988;13(9):966-971.
117. Cohen SP, Hurley RW, Christo PJ, et al. Clinical predictors of success and failure for lumbar facet radiofrequency denervation. *Clin J Pain*. 2007;23(1):45-52.
118. Kawaguchi Y, Matsuno H, Kanamori M, et al. Radiologic findings of the lumbar spine in patients with rheumatoid arthritis, and a review of pathologic mechanisms. *J Spinal Disord Tech*. 2003;16(1):38-43.
119. Friedrich KM, Nemec S, Peloschek P, et al. The prevalence of lumbar facet joint edema in patients with low back pain. *Skeletal Radiol*. 2007;36(8):755-760.
120. Windsor RE, King FJ, Roman SJ, et al. Electrical stimulation induced lumbar medial branch referral patterns. *Pain Physician*. 2002;5(4):347-353.
121. Mooney V, Robertson J. The facet syndrome. *Clin Orthop Relat Res*. 1976;115:149-156.
122. Jackson RP. The facet syndrome: myth or reality? *Clin Orthop Relat Res*. 1992;279:110-121.
123. Esses SI, Moro JK. The value of facet joint blocks in patient selection for lumbar fusion. *Spine*. 1993;18(2):185-190.
124. Schofferman J, Reynolds J, Herzog R, et al. Failed back surgery: etiology and diagnostic evaluation. *Spine J*. 2003;3(5):400-403.
125. Lovely TJ, Rastogi P. The value of provocative facet blocking as a predictor of success in lumbar spine fusion. *J Spinal Disord*. 1997;10(6):512-517.
126. Falco FJ, Manchikanti L, Datta S, et al. An update of the systematic assessment of the diagnostic accuracy of lumbar facet joint nerve blocks. *Pain Physician*. 2012;15(6): E869-E907.
127. Derby R, Melnik I, Lee JE, Lee SH. Correlation of lumbar medial branch neurotomy results with diagnostic medial branch block cutoff values to optimize therapeutic outcome. *Pain Med*. 2012;13(12):1533-1546.

128. Derby R, Melnik I, Choi J, Lee JE. Indications for repeat diagnostic medial branch nerve blocks following a failed first medial branch nerve block. *Pain Physician*. 2013;16(5): 479-488.
129. Dreyfuss P, Halbrook B, Pauza K, et al. Efficacy and validity of radiofrequency neurotomy for chronic lumbar zygapophysial joint pain. *Spine (Phila Pa 1976)*. 2000;25(10):1270-1277.
130. Nath S, Nath C, Pettersson K. Percutaneous lumbar zygapophysial (facet) joint neurotomy using radiofrequency current, in the management of chronic low back pain: a randomized double-blind trial. *Spine (Phila Pa 1976)*. 2008; 33(12):1291-1297.
131. Husted DS, Orton D, Schofferman J, Kine G. Effectiveness of repeated radiofrequency neurotomy for cervical facet joint pain. *J Spinal Disord Tech*. 2008;21(6):406-408.
132. Schofferman J, Kine G. Effectiveness of repeated radiofrequency neurotomy for lumbar facet pain. *Spine (Phila Pa 1976)*. 2004;29(21):2471-2473.
133. Derby R, Melnik I, Lee JE, Lee SH. Cost comparisons of various diagnostic medial branch block protocols and medial branch neurotomy in a private practice setting. *Pain Med*. 2013;14(3):378-391.
134. Crosby ND, Gilliland TM, Winkelstein BA. Early afferent activity from the facet joint after painful trauma to its capsule potentiates neuronal excitability and glutamate signaling in the spinal cord. *Pain*. 2014;155(9):1878-1887.
135. Crosby ND, Weisshaar CL, Winkelstein BA. Spinal neuronal plasticity is evident within 1 day after a painful cervical facet joint injury. *Neurosci Lett*. 2013;542:102-106.
136. Hadden S. Neurologic headache and facial pain. *Arch Neurol*. 1940;43:405.
137. Macnab I. The whiplash syndrome. *Clin Neurosurg*. 1973;20: 232-241.
138. Bogduk N, Marsland A. On the concept of third occipital headache. *J Neurol Neurosurg Psychiatry*. 1986;49(7):775-780.
139. Dreyfuss P, Michaelsen M, Fletcher D. Atlanto-occipital and lateral atlanto-axial joint pain patterns. *Spine*. 1994;19(10):1125-1131.
140. Dreyfuss P, Rogers J, Dreyer S, Fletcher D. Atlanto-occipital joint pain: a report of three cases and description of an intraarticular joint block technique. *Reg Anesth*. 1994;19(5):344-351.
141. Bogduk N, Marsland A. The cervical zygapophysial joints as a source of neck pain. *Spine*. 1988;13(6):610-617.
142. Bogduk N, Aprill C. On the nature of neck pain, discography and cervical zygapophysial joint blocks. *Pain*. 1993;54(2):213-217.
143. Cooper G, Bailey B, Bogduk N. Cervical zygapophysial joint pain maps. *Pain Med*. 2007;8(4):344-353.
144. Barnsley L, Lord SM, Wallis BJ, Bogduk N. The prevalence of chronic cervical zygapophysial joint pain after whiplash. *Spine*. 1995;20(1):20-25.
145. Lord SM, Barnsley L, Wallis BJ, Bogduk N. Chronic cervical zygapophysial joint pain after whiplash: a placebo-controlled prevalence study. *Spine*. 1996;21(15):1737-1744.
146. Aprill C, Axinn MJ, Bogduk N. Occipital headaches stemming from the lateral atlanto-axial (C1-2) joint. *Cephalalgia*. 2002; 22(1):15-22.
147. Bogduk N. *Practice Guidelines for Spinal Diagnostic and Treatment Procedures*. San Francisco: International Spine Intervention Society; 2004.
148. Barnsley L, Lord S, Wallis B, Bogduk N. False-positive rates of cervical zygapophysial joint blocks. *Clin J Pain*. 1993;9(2): 124-130.
149. Speldewinde GC, Bashford GM, Davidson IR. Diagnostic cervical zygapophyseal joint blocks for chronic cervical pain. *Med J Aust*. 2001;174(4):174-176.
150. Manchikanti L, Singh V, Rivera J, Pampati V. Prevalence of cervical facet joint pain in chronic neck pain. *Pain Physician*. 2002;5(3):243-249.
151. Manchikanti L, Boswell MV, Singh V, et al. Prevalence of facet joint pain in chronic spinal pain of cervical, thoracic, and lumbar regions. *BMC Musculoskelet Disord*. 2004;5:15.
152. MacVicar J, Borowczyk JM, Macvicar AM, Loughnan BM, Bogduk N. Cervical medial branch radiofrequency neurotomy in New Zealand. *Pain Med*. 2012;13(5):647-654.
153. Kirpalani D, Mitra R. Cervical facet joint dysfunction: a review. *Arch Phys Med Rehabil*. 2008;89(4):770-774.
154. Jull G, Bogduk N, Marsland A. The accuracy of manual diagnosis for cervical zygapophysial joint pain syndromes. *Med J Aust*. 1988;148(5):233-236.
155. Hechelhammer L, Pfirrmann CW, Zanetti M, et al. Imaging findings predicting the outcome of cervical facet joint blocks. *Eur Radiol*. 2007;17(4):959-964.
156. Manchikanti L, Pampati V. Research designs in interventional pain management: is randomization superior, desirable or essential? *Pain Physician*. 2002;5(3):275-284.
157. Stolker RJ, Vervest AC, Groen GJ. Percutaneous facet denervation in chronic thoracic spinal pain. *Acta Neurochir (Wien)*. 1993;122(1-2):82-90.
158. Linton SJ, Hellsing AL, Hallden K. A population-based study of spinal pain among 35-45-year-old individuals. Prevalence, sick leave, and health care use. *Spine*. 1998;23(13):1457-1463.
159. Dreyfuss P, Tibiletti C, Dreyer SJ. Thoracic zygapophyseal joint pain patterns: a study in normal volunteers. *Spine*. 1994;19(7):807-811.
160. Fukui S, Ohseto K, Shiotani M. Patterns of pain induced by distending the thoracic zygapophyseal joints. *Reg Anesth*. 1997;22(4):332-336.
161. Chua WH, Bogduk N. The surgical anatomy of thoracic facet denervation. *Acta Neurochir (Wien)*. 1995;136(3-4):140-144.
162. Stemper BD, Yoganandan N, Pintar FA, Maiman DJ. The relationship between lower neck shear force and facet joint kinematics during automotive rear impacts. *Clin Anat*. 2011; 24(3):319-326.
163. Oda I, Abumi K, Lu D, Shono Y, Kaneda K. Biomechanical role of the posterior elements, costovertebral joints, and rib cage in the stability of the thoracic spine. *Spine*. 1996;21(12):1423-1429.
164. Dreyfuss P, Tibiletti C, Dreyer S, et al. Thoracic zygapophyseal joint pain: a review and description of an intra-articular block technique. *Pain Digest*. 1994;4:46-54.
165. Manchikanti L, Singh V, Pampati V, Beyer CD, Damron KS. Evaluation of the prevalence of facet joint pain in chronic thoracic pain. *Pain Physician*. 2002;5(4):354-359.
166. Manchukonda R, Manchikanti KN, Cash KA, Pampati V, Manchikanti L. Facet joint pain in chronic spinal pain: an evaluation of prevalence and false-positive rate of diagnostic blocks. *J Spinal Disord Tech*. 2007;20(7):539-545.
167. Manchikanti L, Manchikanti KN, Manchukonda R, Pampati V, Cash KA. Evaluation of therapeutic thoracic medial branch block effectiveness in chronic thoracic pain: a prospective outcome study with minimum 1-year follow up. *Pain Physician*. 2006;9(2):97-105.
168. Manchikanti L, Singh V, Falco FJ, Cash KA, Pampati V. Effectiveness of thoracic medial branch blocks in managing chronic pain: a preliminary report of a

randomized, double-blind controlled trial. *Pain Physician.* 2008;11(4):491-504.

169. Cook NJ, Hanrahan P, Song S. Paraspinal abscess following facet joint injection. *Clin Rheumatol.* 1999;18(1):52-53.
170. Coscia MF, Trammell TR. Pyogenic lumbar facet joint arthritis with intradural extension: a case report. *J Spinal Disord Tech.* 2002;15(6):526-528.
171. Arun R, Al-Nammari SS, Mehdian SM. Multilevel vertebral osteomyelitis and facet joint infection following epidural catheterisation. *Acta Orthop Belg.* 2007;73(5):665-669.
172. Alcock E, Regaard A, Browne J. Facet joint injection: a rare form cause of epidural abscess formation. *Pain.* 2003;103(1-2):209-210.
173. Heckmann JG, Maihöfner C, Lanz S, Rauch C, Neundörfer B. Transient tetraplegia after cervical facet joint injection for chronic neck pain administered without imaging guidance. *Clin Neurol Neurosurg.* 2006;108(7):709-711.
174. Rupert MP, Lee M, Manchikanti L, Datta S, Cohen SP. Evaluation of sacroiliac joint interventions: a systematic appraisal of the literature. *Pain Physician.* 2009;12(2):399-418.
175. Schwarzer AC, Aprill CN, Bogduk N. The sacroiliac joint in chronic low back pain. *Spine.* 1995;20(1):31-37.
176. Maigne JY, Aivaliklis A, Pfefer F. Results of sacroiliac joint double block and value of sacroiliac pain provocation tests in 54 patients with low back pain. *Spine.* 1996;21(16): 1889-1892.
177. Irwin RW, Watson T, Minick RP, Ambrosius WT. Age, body mass index, and gender differences in sacroiliac joint pathology. *Am J Phys Med Rehabil.* 2007;86(1):37-44.
178. Laslett M, Aprill CN, McDonald B, Young SB. Diagnosis of sacroiliac joint pain: validity of individual provocation tests and composites of tests. *Man Ther.* 2005;10(3):207-218.
179. Laslett M, Young SB, Aprill CN, McDonald B. Diagnosing painful sacroiliac joints: a validity study of a McKenzie evaluation and sacroiliac provocation tests. *Aust J Physiother.* 2003;49(2):89-97.
180. Manchikanti L, Singh V, Pampati V, et al. Evaluation of the relative contributions of various structures in chronic low back pain. *Pain Physician.* 2001;4(4):308-316.
181. van der Wurff P, Buijs EJ, Groen GJ. A multitest regimen of pain provocation tests as an aid to reduce unnecessary minimally invasive sacroiliac joint procedures. *Arch Phys Med Rehabil.* 2006;87(1):10-14.
182. Bowen V, Cassidy JD. Macroscopic and microscopic anatomy of the sacroiliac joint from embryonic life until the eighth decade. *Spine.* 1981;6(6):620-628.
183. Simonian PT, Routt ML Jr, Harrington RM, Tencer AF. Anterior versus posterior provisional fixation in the unstable pelvis: a biomechanical comparison. *Clin Orthop Relat Res.* 1995;310:245-251.
184. Rosatelli AL, Agur AM, Chhaya S. Anatomy of the interosseous region of the sacroiliac joint. *J Orthop Sports Phys Ther.* 2006;36(4):200-208.
185. Nakagawa T. Study on the distribution of nerve filaments over the iliosacral joint and its adjacent region in the Japanese. *Nippon Seikeigeka Gakkai Zasshi.* 1966;40:419-430.
186. Yin W, Willard F, Carreiro J, Dreyfuss P. Sensory stimulation-guided sacroiliac joint radiofrequency neurotomy: technique based on neuroanatomy of the dorsal sacral plexus. *Spine.* 2003;28(20):2419-2425.
187. Willard F. *S1-S4 Dorsal Rami and Divisions.* Presented at Third World Conference on Low Back and Pelvic Pain. Vienna, 1988.
188. Grob KR, Neuhuber WL, Kissling RO. [Innervation of the sacroiliac joint of the human]. *Z Rheumatol.* 1995;54(2):117-122.
189. Dreyfuss P, Henning T, Malladi N, Goldstein B, Bogduk N. The ability of multi-site, multi-depth sacral lateral branch blocks to anesthetize the sacroiliac joint complex. *Pain Med.* 2009;10(4):679-688.
190. Berthelot JM, Labat JJ, Le Goff B, Gouin F, Maugars Y. Provocative sacroiliac joint maneuvers and sacroiliac joint block are unreliable for diagnosing sacroiliac joint pain. *Joint Bone Spine.* 2006;73(1):17-23.
191. Dorman T. *Diagnosis and Injection Techniques in Orthopedic Medicine.* Baltimore: Williams & Wilkins; 1999.
192. Szadek KM, Hoogland PV, Zuurmond WW, de Lange JJ, Perez RS. Nociceptive nerve fibers in the sacroiliac joint in humans. *Reg Anesth Pain Med.* 2008;33(1):36-43.
193. Murakami E, Tanaka Y, Aizawa T, Ishizuka M, Kokubun S. Effect of periarticular and intraarticular lidocaine injections for sacroiliac joint pain: prospective comparative study. *J Orthop Sci.* 2007;12(3):274-280.
194. Weksler N, Velan GJ, Semionov M, et al. The role of sacroiliac joint dysfunction in the genesis of low back pain: the obvious is not always right. *Arch Orthop Trauma Surg.* 2007;127(10):885-888.
195. Frymoyer JW, Howe J, Kuhlmann D. The long-term effects of spinal fusion on the sacroiliac joints and ilium. *Clin Orthop Relat Res.* 1978;134:196-201.
196. Ha KY, Lee JS, Kim KW. Degeneration of sacroiliac joint after instrumented lumbar or lumbosacral fusion: a prospective cohort study over five-year follow-up. *Spine.* 2008;33(11): 1192-1198.
197. Ivanov AA, Kiapour A, Ebraheim NA, Goel V. Lumbar fusion leads to increases in angular motion and stress across sacroiliac joint: a finite element study. *Spine.* 2009;34(5): E162-E169.
198. Pool-Goudzwaard A, Hoek van Dijke G, Mulder P, et al. The iliolumbar ligament: its influence on stability of the sacroiliac joint. *Clin Biomech (Bristol, Avon).* 2003;18:99-105.
199. Ebraheim NA, Elgafy H, Semaan HB. Computed tomographic findings in patients with persistent sacroiliac pain after posterior iliac graft harvesting. *Spine.* 2000;25(16):2047-2051.
200. Maigne JY, Planchon CA. Sacroiliac joint pain after lumbar fusion: a study with anesthetic blocks. *Eur Spine J.* 2005;14(7):654-658.
201. Katz V, Schofferman J, Reynolds J. The sacroiliac joint: a potential cause of pain after lumbar fusion to the sacrum. *J Spinal Disord Tech.* 2003;16(1):96-99.
202. Dreyfuss P, Michaelsen M, Pauza K, McLarty J, Bogduk N. The value of medical history and physical examination in diagnosing sacroiliac joint pain. *Spine.* 1996;21(22): 2594-2602.
203. Young S, Aprill C, Laslett M. Correlation of clinical examination characteristics with three sources of chronic low back pain. *Spine J.* 2003;3(6):460-465.
204. Laslett M. Evidence-based diagnosis and treatment of the painful sacroiliac joint. *J Man Manip Ther.* 2008;16(3): 142-152.
205. Slipman CW, Sterenfeld EB, Chou LH, Herzog R, Vresilovic E. The predictive value of provocative sacroiliac joint stress maneuvers in the diagnosis of sacroiliac joint syndrome. *Arch Phys Med Rehabil.* 1998;79(3):288-292.
206. Slipman CW, Jackson HB, Lipetz JS, et al. Sacroiliac joint pain referral zones. *Arch Phys Med Rehabil.* 2000;81(3):334-338.

207. Dreyfuss P, Snyder BD, Park K, et al. The ability of single site, single depth sacral lateral branch blocks to anesthetize the sacroiliac joint complex. *Pain Med.* 2008;9(7): 844-850.
208. Fortin JD, Dwyer AP, West S, Pier J. Sacroiliac joint: pain referral maps upon applying a new injection/arthrography technique. Part I: asymptomatic volunteers. *Spine.* 1994;19(13):1475-1482.
209. Murakami E, Aizawa T, Noguchi K, et al. Diagram specific to sacroiliac joint pain site indicated by one-finger test. *J Orthop Sci.* 2008;13(6):492-497.
210. Hansen H, McKenzie-Brown A, Cohen S, et al. Sacroiliac joint interventions: a systematic review. *Pain Physician.* 2007;10(1):165-184.
211. Szadek KM, van der Wurff P, van Tulder MW, Zuurmond WW, Perez RS. Diagnostic validity of criteria for sacroiliac joint pain: a systematic review. *J Pain.* 2009;10(4):354-368.
212. Hodge JC, Bessette B. The incidence of sacroiliac joint disease in patients with low-back pain. *Can Assoc Radiol J.* 1999;50(5):321-323.
213. Elgafy H, Semaan HB, Ebraheim NA, Coombs RJ. Computed tomography findings in patients with sacroiliac pain. *Clin Orthop Relat Res.* 2001;382:112-118.
214. Kacar G, Kacar C, Karayalcin B, et al. Quantitative sacroiliac joint scintigraphy in normal subjects and patients with sacroiliitis. *Ann Nucl Med.* 1998;12(3):169-173.
215. Slipman CW, Sterenfeld EB, Chou LH, Herzog R, Vresilovic E. The value of radionuclide imaging in the diagnosis of sacroiliac joint syndrome. *Spine.* 1996;21(19):2251-2254.
216. Maigne JY, Boulahdour H, Chatellier G. Value of quantitative radionuclide bone scanning in the diagnosis of sacroiliac joint syndrome in 32 patients with low back pain. *Eur Spine J.* 1998;7(4):328-331.
217. Maigne JY, Boulahdour H, Chatellier G. Value of quantitative radionuclide bone scanning in the diagnosis of sacroiliac joint syndrome in 32 patients with low back pain. *Eur Spine J.* 1998;7(4):328-331.
218. Mitchell B, MacPhail T, Vivian D, Verrills P, Barnard A. Diagnostic sacroiliac joint injections: is a control block necessary? *Surgical Sci.* 2015;6:273-281.
219. Rosenberg JM, Quint TJ, de Rosayro AM. Computerized tomographic localization of clinically guided sacroiliac joint injections. *Clin J Pain.* 2000;16(1):18-21.
220. Borowsky CD, Fagen G. Sources of sacroiliac region pain: insights gained from a study comparing standard intra-articular injection with a technique combining intra- and peri-articular injection. *Arch Phys Med Rehabil.* 2008;89(11):2048-2056.
221. Fortin JD, Washington WJ, Falco FJ. Three pathways between the sacroiliac joint and neural structures. *AJNR Am J Neuroradiol.* 1999;20(8):1429-1434.
222. Wise CL, Dall BE. Minimally invasive sacroiliac arthrodesis: outcomes of a new technique. *J Spinal Disord Tech.* 2008; 21(8):579-584.
223. Schutz U, Grob D. Poor outcome following bilateral sacroiliac joint fusion for degenerative sacroiliac joint syndrome. *Acta Orthop Belg.* 2006;72(3):296-308.
224. Al-Khayer A, Hegarty J, Hahn D, Grevitt MP. Percutaneous sacroiliac joint arthrodesis: a novel technique. *J Spinal Disord Tech.* 2008;21(5):359-363.
225. Ziran BH, Heckman D, Smith WR. CT-guided stabilization for chronic sacroiliac pain: a preliminary report. *J Trauma.* 2007;63(1):90-96.
226. Cohen SP, Hurley RW, Buckenmaier CC 3rd, et al. Randomized placebo-controlled study evaluating lateral branch radiofrequency denervation for sacroiliac joint pain. *Anesthesiology.* 2008;109(2):279-288.
227. King W, Ahmed SU, Baisden J, et al. Diagnosis and treatment of posterior sacroiliac complex pain: a systematic review with comprehensive analysis of the published data. *Pain Med.* 2015;16(2):257-265.
228. Benzel EC, Hart BL, Ball PA, et al. Magnetic resonance imaging for the evaluation of patients with occult cervical spine injury. *J Neurosurg.* 1996;85(5):824-829.
229. Lehto IJ, Tertti MO, Komu ME, et al. Age-related MRI changes at 0.1 T in cervical discs in asymptomatic subjects. *Neuroradiology.* 1994;36(1):49-53.
230. Siivola SM, Levoska S, Tervonen O, et al. MRI changes of cervical spine in asymptomatic and symptomatic young adults. *Eur Spine J.* 2002;11(4):358-363.
231. Anderberg L, Annertz M, Brandt L, Saveland H. Selective diagnostic cervical nerve root block–correlation with clinical symptoms and MRI-pathology. *Acta Neurochir (Wien).* 2004;146(6):559-565.
232. Slipman CW, Plastaras CT, Palmitier RA, Huston CW, Sterenfeld EB. Symptom provocation of fluoroscopically guided cervical nerve root stimulation. Are dynatomal maps identical to dermatomal maps? *Spine.* 1998;23(20):2235-2242.
233. Kikuchi S, Hasue M, Nishiyama K, Ito T. Anatomic and clinical studies of radicular symptoms. *Spine.* 1984;9(1):23-30.
234. Furman MB, Lee TS, Mehta A, Simon JI, Cano WG. Contrast flow selectivity during transforaminal lumbosacral epidural steroid injections. *Pain Physician.* 2008;11(6):855-861.
235. Macnab I. Negative disc exploration. An analysis of the causes of nerve-root involvement in sixty-eight patients. *J Bone Joint Surg Am.* 1971;53A(5):891-903.
236. Krempen JF, Smith BS. Nerve-root injection: a method for evaluating the etiology of sciatica. *J Bone Joint Surg Am.* 1974;56(7):1435-1444.
237. Schutz H, Lougheed WM, Wortzman G, Awerbuck BG. Intervertebral nerve-root in the investigation of chronic lumbar disc disease. *Can J Surg.* 1973;16(3):217-221.
238. Tajima T, Furukawa K, Kuramochi E. Selective lumbosacral radiculography and block. *Spine.* 1980;5(1):68-77.
239. Dooley JF, McBroom RJ, Taguchi T, Macnab I. Nerve root infiltration in the diagnosis of radicular pain. *Spine.* 1988;13(1):79-83.
240. Stanley D, McLaren MI, Euinton HA, Getty CJ. A prospective study of nerve root infiltration in the diagnosis of sciatica. A comparison with radiculography, computed tomography, and operative findings. *Spine.* 1990;15(6):540-543.
241. Herron LD. Selective nerve root block in patient selection for lumbar surgery: surgical results. *J Spinal Disord.* 1989;2(2):75-79.
242. Porter DG, Valentine AR, Bradford R. A retrospective study to assess the results of CT-directed peri-neural root infiltration in a cohort of 56 patients with low back pain and sciatica. *Br J Neurosurg.* 1999;13(3):290-293.
243. Sasso RC, Macadaeg K, Nordmann D, Smith M. Selective nerve root injections can predict surgical outcome for lumbar and cervical radiculopathy: comparison to magnetic resonance imaging. *J Spinal Disord Tech.* 2005;18(6):471-478.
244. Haueisen DC, Smith BS, Myers SR, Pryce ML. The diagnostic accuracy of spinal nerve injection studies. Their role in the evaluation of recurrent sciatica. *Clin Orthop Relat Res.* 1985;198:179-183.

245. Jonsson B, Stromqvist B, Annertz M, Holtas S, Sunden G. Diagnostic lumbar nerve root block. *J Spinal Disord.* 1988;1(3):232-235.
246. Kumar K, Taylor RS, Jacques L, et al. Spinal cord stimulation versus conventional medical management for neuropathic pain: a multicentre randomised controlled trial in patients with failed back surgery syndrome. *Pain.* 2007;132(1-2):179-188.
247. Yeom JS, Lee JW, Park KW, et al. Value of diagnostic lumbar selective nerve root block: a prospective controlled study. *AJNR Am J Neuroradiol.* 2008;29(5):1017-1023.
248. van Akkerveeken PF. The diagnostic value of nerve root sheath infiltration. *Acta Orthop Scand Suppl.* 1993;251:61-63.
249. Irwin A, Khan AL, Fender D, Sanderson PL, Gibson MJ. The role of needle tip position on the accuracy of diagnostic selective nerve root blocks in spinal deformity. *Eur Spine J.* 2014;23(suppl 1):S33-S39.
250. White AH, Derby R, Wynne G. Epidural injections for the diagnosis and treatment of low-back pain. *Spine.* 1980;5(1):78-86.
251. Jasper JF. Role of digital subtraction fluoroscopic imaging in detecting intravascular injections. *Pain Physician.* 2003; 6(3):369-372.
252. Baker R, Dreyfuss P, Mercer S, Bogduk N. Cervical transforaminal injection of corticosteroids into a radicular artery: a possible mechanism for spinal cord injury. *Pain.* 2003;103(1-2):211-215.
253. Chung SG. Convulsion caused by a lidocaine test in cervical transforaminal epidural steroid injection. *PM R.* 2011;3(7):674-677.
254. Derby R, Lee S-H, Kim B-J, Chen Y, Seo K. Complications following cervical epidural steroid injections by expert interventionalists in 2003. *Pain Physician.* 2004;7(4):445-449.
255. Pobiel RS, Schellhas KP, Eklund JA, et al. Selective cervical nerve root blockade: prospective study of immediate and longer term complications. *AJNR Am J Neuroradiol.* 2009;30(3):507-511.
256. Huston CW, Slipman CW, Garvin C. Complications and side effects of cervical and lumbosacral selective nerve root injections. *Arch Phys Med Rehabil.* 2005;86(2):277-283.
257. Scanlon GC, Moeller-Bertram T, Romanowsky SM, Wallace MS. Cervical transforaminal epidural steroid injections: more dangerous than we think? *Spine.* 2007;32(11):1249-1256.
258. Provenzano DA, Fanciullo G. Cervical transforaminal epidural steroid injections: should we be performing them? *Reg Anesth Pain Med.* 2007;32(2):168; author reply 169-170.
259. Lee JH, Lee JK, Seo BR, et al. Spinal cord injury produced by direct damage during cervical transforaminal epidural injection. *Reg Anesth Pain Med.* 2008;33(4):377-379.
260. Ruppen W, Hugli R, Reuss S, Aeschbach A, Urwyler A. Neurological symptoms after cervical transforaminal injection with steroids in a patient with hypoplasia of the vertebral artery. *Acta Anaesthesiol Scand.* 2008;52(1):165-166.
261. Muro K, O'Shaughnessy B, Ganju A. Infarction of the cervical spinal cord following multilevel transforaminal epidural steroid injection: case report and review of the literature. *J Spinal Cord Med.* 2007;30(4):385-388.
262. Suresh S, Berman J, Connell DA. Cerebellar and brainstem infarction as a complication of CT-guided transforaminal cervical nerve root block. *Skeletal Radiol.* 2007;36(5):449-452.
263. Tiso RL, Cutler T, Catania JA, Whalen K. Adverse central nervous system sequelae after selective transforaminal block: the role of corticosteroids. *Spine J.* 2004;4(4):468-474.
264. Derby R, Lee SH, Date ES, Lee JH, Lee CH. Size and aggregation of corticosteroids used for epidural injections. *Pain Med.* 2008;9(2):227-234.
265. Kennedy DJ, Plastaras C, Casey E, et al. Comparative effectiveness of lumbar transforaminal epidural steroid injections with particulate versus nonparticulate corticosteroids for lumbar radicular pain due to intervertebral disc herniation: a prospective, randomized, double-blind trial. *Pain Med.* 2014;15(4):548-555.
266. El-Yahchouchi C, Geske JR, Carter RE, et al. The noninferiority of the nonparticulate steroid dexamethasone vs the particulate steroids betamethasone and triamcinolone in lumbar transforaminal epidural steroid injections. *Pain Med.* 2013;14(11):1650-1657.
267. Hooten WM, Mizerak A, Carns PE, Huntoon MA. Discitis after lumbar epidural corticosteroid injection: a case report and analysis of the case report literature. *Pain Med.* 2006;7(1):46-51.
268. North RB, Kidd DH, Campbell JN, Long DM. Dorsal root ganglionectomy for failed back surgery syndrome: a 5-year follow-up study. *J Neurosurg.* 1991;74(2):236-242.

CHAPTER 17 Discography

Eugene Carragee
Michael Stauff

Provocative discography is a diagnostic test sometimes used to evaluate the disc as a potential source of persistent back and neck pain syndromes. In its simplest form, provocative discography is an injection into the nucleus of an intervertebral disc; the test result is determined by the pain response to this injection. If the injection reproduces the patient's usual pain, some authors have proposed that the "cause" of the axial pain syndrome can be ascribed to that disc—that is, *primary discogenic pain*.

In 1948, Lindblom[1] originally reported discography as a method to identify herniated discs in the lumbar spine by injecting contrast medium into the disc and following the outline of contrast medium into the spinal canal. It was noted as only a secondary consideration of the test that reproduction of the patient's usual sciatica sometimes occurred during the disc injection. It was observed later that back pain was sometimes reproduced during the injection as opposed to sciatica. Eventually, some clinicians began using the test to evaluate discs as the source of axial pain in patients without radicular symptoms.

Since the early use of discography, it has been unclear whether reproduction of pain with injection indicated that the injected disc is the true primary source of clinical back pain, or whether the injection had simulated the usual pain in an artificial manner. Over time, attempts have been made to determine the specificity of the test and to refine the technique to reduce the risk of false-positive or false-negative results. Currently, this test remains highly controversial. Even the staunchest proponents of the procedure state that "discography is a test that is easily abused."[2] Assessment of provocative discography as a basic diagnostic test has found fundamental problems with test reliability (i.e., does the test give the same result on repeated testing?) and validity (i.e., does the test prove what it purports to prove?). Also, it has not been shown that using the test improves the outcomes in patients receiving the test compared with patients not receiving the test. More recently, the long-term safety of disc puncture and injection has also been questioned. This chapter discusses the rationale, technique, utility, and clinical effects of provocative discography when used in patients with primary axial pain syndromes.

Clinical Context

Back and neck pain are very common, and in most cases determining the "cause" of a specific episode of back or neck pain is unimportant because these symptoms frequently resolve in a short time or do not seriously interfere with function.[1] Provocative discography may be described as representing a *tertiary diagnostic* evaluation, which should be considered only in a select group of patients.

A *primary diagnostic* evaluation usually involves screening for serious underlying disease ("red flags") by history and physical examination aimed at detecting systemic disease, spinal deformity, and neurologic loss. In most patients, these examinations are negative, and nonspecific treatment alone is recommended. In a patient who does not recover good function in 6 to 12 weeks, a *secondary diagnostic* survey may be indicated. This follow-up evaluation should identify serious psychosocial barriers to recovery ("yellow flags") and definitively rule out serious conditions that may result in neurologic injury; structural failure; or progression of a visceral disease, systemic infection, or malignant process. Diagnostic tests for serious structural disease, including blood tests and imaging studies, have become so sensitive that these serious conditions are usually identified in the early stages.

Establishing a more specific pathoanatomic diagnosis than "nonspecific back pain syndrome" or "persistent back pain illness" becomes important only if specific therapy directed to common age-related structural changes is considered because of continued serious symptoms and functional loss. At this point, if the primary and secondary evaluations have revealed neither serious structural pathology nor significant confounding psychosocial or neurophysiologic factors, a tertiary diagnostic evaluation may be undertaken. This evaluation may occasionally uncover a clear degenerative cause of symptoms, such as unstable spondylolisthesis or progressive degenerative deformity, such as degenerative scoliosis.

The most common structural degenerative changes (e.g., loss of disc height, loss of nuclear signal, minor facet arthrosis, anular fissures) may be very difficult to reconcile with the severity of apparent symptoms and pain behavior, however, because many people with minimal or no spinal symptoms have similar mild degenerative findings. The question is why do individuals with such benign findings sometimes report severe and persistent pain and impairment? The rationale of provocative discography in the tertiary evaluation is to separate anatomic spinal changes causing serious primary pain illnesses from similarly appearing common degenerative changes that do not cause serious illness. As this chapter shows, it is unclear that this goal is routinely achievable with provocative discography.

Discography Technique

Discography is performed using local anesthetic and mild sedation. The objective is percutaneous injection of a nonirritating radiopaque dye, under fluoroscopic guidance, into one or more intervertebral discs. The technique involves using a long, fine-gauge needle to penetrate the nucleus from a posterolateral approach in the thoracolumbar spine and anterolaterally in the cervical spine. In the lumbar spine, the needle passes posterior to the exiting nerve root and anterolateral to the traversing root. Sometimes a bend of the needle or introducer is required to place the needle accurately, especially at L5–S1.

The passage of the needle in skilled hands should be quick and atraumatic. When the position is verified in two planes using fluoroscopy, the dye is slowly injected into the nucleus of several lumbar discs with the patient blinded to the timing and site of injection. The spread of the dye in the disc is noted on the images, and the patient's response to the injection is documented. The patient is queried at each injection or at random intervals as to whether or not the procedure is painful and is asked to rate the pain against a standardized scale (e.g., 0–5, 0–10, none to unbearable). If the injection is painful, the patient is asked to describe the discomfort provoked qualitatively. The injection is usually rated as exactly the same as, similar to (concordant), or dissimilar to the patient's usual back or neck pain.

Criteria for Positive Test

In an effort to improve the specificity of discography in diagnosing so-called discogenic pain, some investigators have used additional criteria beyond pain reproduction on injection. The criteria for establishing a positive discogram are controversial. The primary criteria for a "positive" disc injection are pain of "significant" intensity on disc injections (usually defined as ≥6 out of 10 pain scale) and a reported similarity of that pain to the patient's usual, clinical discomfort (concordant pain). Walsh and colleagues proposed these basic criteria in their experimental work in 1990.[3] In this study, "significant pain" was defined as 3 out of 5 (or 6 out of 10) on an arbitrary pain thermometer. "Bad pain" was defined as 3 out of 5 pain, and "moderate pain" was described as 2 out of 5 pain. The authors did not stringently define concordance of pain reproduction. Some investigators have proposed additional and sometimes idiosyncratic criteria for positive injections (Table 17.1).

Pain Generator Concept and Provocative Discography

The diagnosis made by a "positive provocative discogram" should indicate that the disc identified is the primary or only cause of the patient's back pain illness, or the *pain generator*. The idea of a pain generator, however, has proven to be problematic. In a patient with persistent symptoms and a secondary workup with only degenerative findings, the task of identifying a specific isolated pain generator can be formidable. Most patients have multiple findings of disc changes and facet arthrosis, often at multiple levels. To determine which degenerative finding is associated with a patient's severe axial back pain can be difficult. Many people have occasional back or neck ache with common activities or episodic axial pain without impairment. The question is not whether any previous or possible future back or neck pain may be coming from a certain spinal structure because it may be assumed that most people with degenerative change of the axial skeleton may have occasional discomfort from several sites alone or at the same time.

The pertinent question is whether or not a suspected local anatomic structure (e.g., disc, facet, sacroiliac joint) is causing serious, disabling axial pain illness or is only a minor contributor to a generalized pain-sensitivity syndrome (e.g., fibromyalgia), a central pain-processing syndrome, an overuse syndrome related to posture or activity, or other conditions. It is hoped that some diagnostic test can identify whether or not a specific *local* spinal pathoanatomic structure adequately explains the severity of clinical symptoms. As a matter of practical definition, for a pathoanatomic diagnosis to be clinically relevant requires that the identified pain generator not only be capable of causing some discomfort under any circumstances (e.g., puncture and injection of a disc) but also that this structure is a primary independent cause of the patient's apparent severe illness.

When only degenerative changes are found, it is controversial that a discrete local pain generator can be identified as the cause of serious back pain illness. Some clinicians believe that serious axial pain and disability can be so multifactorial (mechanical, psychological, social, and neurophysiologic contributors) that it is unreasonable to expect specific diagnostic studies to confirm an anatomic "diagnosis" for axial pain illness in every patient.[4–6] Even if a pain generator is suspected, it is unclear how this can be reliably confirmed as the cause of the patient's perceived pain, impairment, and disability in the face of complex social, emotional, and neurophysiologic confounders.

Other clinicians believe that identifying a pain generator is central to spine evaluations because it meets patients' expectations and leads to an optimal treatment that focuses on an anatomic structure. In this model, social issues such as disability, litigation, psychological distress, and pain intolerance are believed to be *secondary* issues to the structural pathology.[1,7–13] These clinicians generally believe that although the history and physical examination may be helpful in suggesting serious underlying pathology, such as infection and tumor,

TABLE 17.1 Suggested Criteria for Positive Provocative Discographic Injection

Test Criteria for Positive Result	Positive Test Threshold	Comments
Pain response (intensity)	≥6/10 or 3/5 "Bad" pain or worse on pain thermometer ≥7/10	Subjective and arbitrary scale. No data on reliability. Data on validity in small groups of asymptomatic subjects without psychosocial comorbidity are good (specificity >90%). Data in several studies of subjects with increased psychosocial or chronic pain comorbidity indicate validity in these subgroups is poor (specificity 20–60%).
Qualitative pain assessment (concordant pain)	"Concordant pain" usually including "similar" but not exact pain "Exact" pain only	Subjective response. Data on reliability are unknown. Data on validity in small study of experimental nondiscogenic low back pain indicate that validity is questionable.
Anular disruption	Dye must show fissure to or through outer anulus	Tested only in clinical studies without follow-up to confirm outcome or other gold standard. Radiologic reliability best with computed tomography scan after disc injection compared with radiograph alone. Validity of additional criteria as confirming true-positive test unknown; positive injection in discs without anular disruption more common in psychologically disturbed subjects.
Control disc injections	"Negative" injection (minimal or discordant pain) required adjacent to proposed "positive" disc "Normal" injection (i.e., no pain) Some authors insist that adjacent "control disc" must also have grade 3 anular fissure, which is "relatively painless" at equal or higher pressures than "positive disc"	Injections in morphologically normal discs seem to be reliably negative even in subjects with serious psychological distress and no back pain. Reliability in other disc morphology unknown. Validity of this additional criterion as confirming true-positive test unknown.
Demonstration of pain behavior	Facial expressions of pain must be observed to confirm verbal pain report	Reliability and validity of this criterion as confirming true-positive test unknown.
Pressure-controlled injection	Disc injections should be classified into low (<15 or <20 psi) or high (>50 psi) pressures at time of significant pain response; responses at pressures in between are indeterminate	Small outcomes series suggest that low-pressure sensitive discs are better treated with interbody fusion techniques. Reliability and validity unknown.
Volume-controlled injections	"Excessive volume" or speed to injection invalidates injection	Unvalidated concept based on anecdotal evidence. Primary data unavailable to analyze.
Maximum one or two positive disc injections	More than one or two positive disc injections invalidates study (all are indeterminate)	Assumption is made that generalized hyperalgesic effect may lead to multiple positive discs around single pain generator.
Quantify pain tolerance by response to buffered anesthetic injection	Subjects with poor pain tolerance may not be "ideal" candidates for discography; needs to be detected	It is unclear that pain tolerance to intradermal anesthetic injection is valid test to determine "pain tolerance" in patients with long-standing axial pain.
Needles should be inserted from asymptomatic or least symptomatic side	Theoretically may decrease confusion between injection and insertion pain	Some data suggest this is not an important technique. No gold standard confirmation was applied.
Any positive disc injection must be repeated with similar outcomes before accepting result as "positive"	Intraprocedure reliability test	No data available on whether this improved or decreased test accuracy.

these methods are not helpful in determining the true pain generator among many degenerative structures.

Diagnostic Injections and Modulation of Pain Perception in Axial Pain Syndromes

Provocative discography relies on a patient's subjective perception and report of pain after a progressive pressurization injection of a disc. Alternatively, a disc may be injected with an anesthetic agent with subsequent documentation of the patient's subjective pain relief after activities that usually provoke pain. These diagnostic injections seek to identify a primary pain generator by provocative testing (stimulating a potential site of pain, as in discography) or by temporary local anesthetic relief. These are subjective tests of pain perception and are subject to the effects of volitional and neurophysiologic modulation at multiple points along the neuraxis. Many common factors are known to have potential dampening or amplifying effects on the perception of back and neck pain. These factors must be considered when evaluating the validity of diagnoses determined by diagnostic injections.[14–19]

Adjacent Tissue Injury

Injury to adjacent tissues may increase the perception of pain in surrounding structures by a local *hyperalgesic effect*. This is a well-known phenomenon that occurs with any tissue damage; it may amplify pain perception by increasing local inflammatory processes with secondary neurologic sensitization in areas not directly injured, such as the area surrounding a burn or a fracture that is sensitive but without any thermal or mechanical injury. This is an important phenomenon in patients with low back pain and significant disease at one or more levels, which may sensitize the adjacent segments to provocative testing (e.g., a spine that has undergone multiple operations).[14,20]

Local Anesthetic

Local anesthetic injections may decrease the perception of pain at a local site. This is the specific, active effect used in diagnostic blocks. This decrease in pain perception can also be a source of confounding effects if the exact placement of the agent is not well controlled. In addition to this direct local effect, a nonspecific placebo effect and a neurophysiologic modulation effect may occur. A relevant example is the effect of local anesthetic blockade on the perception of painful stimulus along the neuraxis proximal to the injection. A local anesthetic injection in the lower extremity may be perceived as relieving sciatica owing to disc herniation.[21] This is not a placebo effect (i.e., the phenomenon is seen only with an active anesthetic agent) but rather an effect on neuromodulation. This effect is important in diagnostic anesthetic blockade as a source of false-positive and false-negative findings.[22]

Tissue Injury and Nociception in Adjacent or Same Sclerotome

Tissue injury having the same or adjacent sclerotomal afferents as lower spinal elements may increase pain sensitivity at any given site. This effect is thought to be due to physiologic and anatomic changes at the level of the dorsal root ganglion or spinal cord ascending tracts. In animal models, single afferent neurons from a dorsal root ganglion may innervate three adjacent discs and a wide range of adjacent structures. This effect is important in considering the specificity of discography at sites of similar embryonic derivation to a known pathologic structure (e.g., nonunion, spondylolisthesis, painful iliac crest bone graft site). The confounding effect of this phenomenon in discography has been experimentally and empirically shown (discussed later).[14,23]

Chronic Pain Syndromes

Chronic pain syndromes may complicate the evaluation of low back pain. Chronic pain from regional sites that are near the lumbar spine (chronic pelvic pain, irritable bowel syndrome, failed hip arthroplasty) or distant to the lumbar spine (chronic neck pain, chronic headache, temporomandibular joint syndrome) may increase pain sensitivity at lower spinal elements. This effect may be regional or global and may be related to neurophysiologic changes at multiple levels along the neuraxis. Preexisting chronic pain syndromes are also associated with depression, narcotic use, and habituation, which have independent pain perception effects. This effect has been shown to have an impact on the pain intensity from discography in experimental subjects.[14,23]

Narcotic Analgesia and Habituation

Narcotic medications act at multiple levels to decrease pain sensitivity thresholds, intensity, and affective response. Administration of a narcotic medication may act as a common confounder for diagnostic techniques that require accurate feedback of pain perception from a patient.[14,24,25] Chronic narcotic habituation may act to decrease pain tolerance in the absence of increased narcotic intake. Narcotic habituation decreases endogenous abilities to modulate peripheral nociceptive input. This effect is multifactorial. Chronic narcotic habituation is also associated with depression and sleep disturbances.

Depression, Anxiety, and Somatic Distress

Clinical depression, anxiety disorders, and increased somatic awareness may be seen as predisposing factors to chronic low back pain syndromes or reactions to the pain and disability of chronic low back pain illness, or both. In either event, psychological distress usually decreases the pain threshold perception and increases perceived pain intensity and affective response.[5,24,26] These effects are likely due to central neurochemical changes and systemic effects and have been shown to affect pain responses in discographic evaluation.

Social Imperatives

Overriding social imperatives may result in a decreased pain perception or a dissociation of pain perception and functional loss. A decreased pain perception or even an absence of pain perception despite injury can be seen during some short-term stressful events, such as in accident victims, soldiers in combat, or individuals in certain training environments. Even over long periods, social and cultural factors reinforce low pain-perception reporting and muted or absent pain behaviors.

Social Disincentive

Secondary gain issues may exaggerate pain responses of all types. When the intensity of pain behavior and report is correlated with a real or perceived social benefit or monetary compensation, the reported pain perception and pain behavior may be increased. This situation can have direct effects on provocative testing (e.g., discography) and the need for a specific anatomic diagnosis to establish social validity of an ongoing "sick role." A real-world example of social disincentive exists in patients who have sustained a work-related injury that requires an extended course of evaluation and treatment.

Summary

When considering the diagnostic certainty of a possible pain generator in chronic axial pain illness, it is necessary to view the aforementioned confounding factors for contribution to the illness behavior observed (Table 17.2). An injured soldier with facial trauma, after narcotic administration and in the heat of combat, may mask the perception of a significant low back pain injury that otherwise could be clearly symptomatic. In this case, a bona fide local pain generator results in little pain perception. Conversely, a very minor nociceptive input (common backache) from a disc can be amplified in the case of a patient with multiple chronic pain syndromes, narcotic habituation, depression, and compensation issues (social disincentives). In this case, a common mild backache pain generator is amplified to become a catastrophic illness.

Evidence for Validity and Usefulness of Provocative Discography

Sackett and Haynes have described the criteria for an evidence-based evaluation of diagnostic test validity.[27] Four phases of scientific scrutiny and evidence in discography research are shown in Table 17.3. These phases of evidence progress from the simple comparison of testing in subjects known to have

TABLE 17.2 Neurophysiologic Factors Influencing Result of Diagnostic Injections

Modulator of Diagnostic Injection Effect	Type of Effect on Pain Perception at Site of Injection	Diagnostic Effect
Adjacent tissue injury	Increased regional pain perception	Decreased specificity in provocative injection
Local anesthetic	Decreased pain perception at depot site and sometimes in sclerotomal or referral pattern	Decreased specificity in provocative injection
Tissue injury in adjacent or same sclerotome	Increased regional pain perception	Decreased specificity in provocative injection
Chronic pain syndrome	Increased generalized pain perception	Decreased specificity in provocative injection
Narcotic analgesia	Decreased generalized pain perception and affective response	Decreased sensitivity and increased specificity of provocative injections
Narcotic habituation	Increased pain perception and exaggerated affective response	Decreased specificity in provocative injection
Depression, anxiety, and somatic distress	Decreased generalized pain perception and unpredictable affective response	Decreased specificity in provocative injection
Social imperatives	Decreased pain perception, suppressed affective response	Decreased sensitivity and increased specificity of provocative injections
Social disincentives	Specific increased pain reporting and demonstration of pain behavior	Decreased specificity in provocative injection

TABLE 17.3 Four Phases of Evidence-Based Criteria for Evaluation Diagnostic Tests

Phase of Study	Strategy	Discography Evidence
Phase I	Diagnostic test compared in subjects with index disease vs. results in complete normals (experimental setting)	Few painful disc injections in completely normal asymptomatic subjects (e.g., normal psychometric testing, normal disc morphology, no chronic pain issues, no compensation issues) Examples: Walsh et al., 1990[3]; Carragee et al., 2000[16]
Phase II	Evaluation of range of test results in subjects with disease (establishes positive result guidelines) compared with known normals	Wide range of pain reactions to injections in asymptomatic subjects depending on psychological status, disc morphology, chronic pain issues, compensation issues. Wide overlap between asymptomatic subjects and patients with presumed discogenic pain. Examples: Carragee et al., 2000[16]; O'Neill and Kurgansky, 2004[23]; Carragee et al., 2006[38]
Phase III	Diagnostic test applied in clinical subjects likely to have disease (clinical setting of test application in subjects with similar presentation, signs, symptoms, and risk factors)	Poor validity testing subjects with persistent low back pain with known nondiscogenic pain syndromes (e.g., iliac crest pain) or asymptomatic disc pathology (i.e., previous disc surgery). PPV approximately 50% in ideal patient, PPV <50% in typical discography patient (outcome findings). Examples: Carragee et al., 1999[15]; Carragee et al., 2000[35]; Derby et al., 2005[36]; Carragee et al., 2002[37]; Carragee et al., 2006[43]
Phase IV	Does having the diagnostic test result improve outcomes compared with management without test result (controlled trial)?	Little to no evidence of provocative discography improving outcomes compared with modern diagnostic techniques.[40] Substantial evidence provocative discography is worse than anesthetic injection alone.[42] Substantial evidence discography may worsen outcomes in certain at-risk groups.[44–46]

Data from Sackett D, Haynes R. Evidence base of clinical diagnosis: The architecture of diagnostic research. *BMJ*. 2002;324:539–541.
PPV, positive predictive value.

a disease with subjects who are completely normal without any signs, symptoms, or morbidity associated with the disease (phase I) to the blinded study of a diagnostic test in determining outcomes in actual clinical therapeutic intervention (phase IV).

An example of a phase I diagnostic study is the classic study of discography by Walsh and colleagues[3] in asymptomatic healthy young men without significant degenerative disease or comorbidities associated with chronic low back pain illness (e.g., depression, chronic pain behavior, compensation issues). Discography seemed to perform well in this phase I study, with little pain provocation in the subjects with a lack of disease (one of 10 subjects [10%; 95% confidence interval, 0–40%] had pain intensity rated "bad"). In phase II and III studies, comparing subjects without low back pain illness but with significant comorbidities, discography did not perform as well.[15,16]

Generally, there has been limited high-quality evidence supporting provocative disc injections. Despite the limited evidence, some authors believe that primary discogenic pain is the most common cause of chronic low back pain illness.[12,13,28,29] As is shown subsequently, a major constraint in this research has been a failure to use a bona fide gold standard for primary discogenic pain causing low back pain illness against which investigators document that the diagnosis suggested by discography is correct.

Validity of Discography

Discography purports to diagnose the presence or absence of a disc lesion responsible for the syndrome of chronic low back pain illness caused by primary discogenic pain. There is no commonly used gold standard or criterion to determine who actually has chronic low back pain illness from primary discogenic pain. There are well-accepted standards, however, for who does not—someone with no evidence of significant low back pain. Similarly, someone with new pain resulting from another process (pelvic fracture) does not have "chronic low back pain illness caused by primary discogenic pain." Provocative discography can be assessed by the results of disc injections in subjects who definitively do not have chronic low back pain illness caused by primary discogenic pain.

Alternatively, a patient's response to treatment may be considered a surrogate gold standard if the treatment definitively removes the pain generator (the disc) and adjustments can be made for surgical and nonspecific limitations of the treatment. The following section describes a series of clinical and experimental studies that have attempted to define the specificity of discography in different at-risk subgroups.

Specificity of Positive Discography: Testing on Subjects With No Axial Pain History

Careful technique and the standardization of discography were believed by many discographers to have reduced the false-positive rate to a negligible level in experienced hands. In 1990, Walsh and colleagues[3] performed a carefully controlled set of discographic lumbar injections in 10 paid volunteers, all asymptomatic young men (mean age, 22 years) with little disc degeneration. Of 30 discs injected in this asymptomatic group, five produced "minimum" pain (16.7%), two produced "moderate" pain (6.7%), and one produced "bad" pain (3.3%). Based on these data, the authors believed that the risk of false-positive injections was very low. This study is frequently, and incorrectly, cited to confirm a 0% false-positive rate.

In 1997, a review of one discography practice[26] found cases that seemed to be clinically apparent false-positive cases. These injections were believed to meet full criteria for discogenic pain, with concordant, painful injections and negative control injections. Clinical follow-up revealed other causes of the patients' back pain illness, however, including spinal tumor, sacroiliac joint disease, and emotional problems. Block and colleagues[30] related abnormal Minnesota Multiphasic Personality Inventory (MMPI) testing and Ohnmeiss and colleagues[31] related abnormal pain drawings with "nonorganic" features, suggesting possible false-positive discographic injections. Other authors performed thoracic[32] and cervical[33] injections in subjects asymptomatic for pain in those areas. Significantly painful injections were found to occur in approximately 30% of these volunteers.

Following the Walsh protocol, Carragee and colleagues[16] examined 30 volunteer subjects with no history of low back pain who were recruited to undergo a physical examination, magnetic resonance imaging (MRI), psychometric testing, and provocative discography. The results showed that little pain was elicited by injection of any anatomically normal disc. Discs with advanced degenerative anular fissuring with dye leakage to the outer (innervated) anular margins were more commonly painful after discography than less degenerative or normal discs. The intensity of the pain reported by the subjects with anular disruption was predicted by the presence of chronic nonlumbar pain and abnormal psychological scores. Only 10% of subjects without any other pain processes had a positive disc injection by the Walsh criteria, but 50% of subjects with nonlumbar chronic pain had at least one positive disc injection.

The interaction between pending compensation claims and discographic pain was also significant in this select group of volunteers. Of the 10 subjects with positive injections, 8 had contested workers' compensation or personal injury claims, with resulting litigation. Conversely, of 9 subjects with disputed litigation claims, 8 had positive injections ($P < .0001$).[16] It was not found, however, that all subjects involved in previous work injury claims had similar rates of positive disc injection. A history of an uncontested claim from a past compensation injury and no pending legal action did not predict significant pain on disc injection. Given that no subject in this study stood to have any secondary gain from positive discography, the increased pain reporting in subjects with unrelated but contested compensation claims is intriguing. It is possible that the effect of the prolonged social turmoil associated with a litigation dispute has the effect of diminishing one's resilience to irritative stimuli. Another explanation could be that persons with abnormally low pain tolerance are more likely to have a legal dispute regarding the significance and damages associated with previous minor injury.

Discographic Injections in Previously Operated Discs

Provocative discography is frequently used to evaluate persistent or recurrent low back pain syndromes in patients who have had a posterior discectomy. The validity of interpreting painful injections after herniation is unknown despite its common usage. Heggeness and colleagues[34] reported on 83 postdiscectomy patients and found that 72% had a positive concordant pain response on injection of the previously operated disc. This study did not address the possibility of false-positive injections. All positive injections were assumed to be true-positive injections for identifying the source of the patient's pain.

Using the same methodology developed by Walsh and colleagues,[3] a large study of discography in asymptomatic patients after discectomy for sciatica was performed.[35] Painful disc injections were frequently seen in the asymptomatic postdiscectomy group. As in previous studies, a higher rate of painful injections was seen in patients with abnormal psychological profiles.

Validity of Concordance Report

Provocative discography is considered positive only when the injection elicits the patient's usual pain in quality and in location. The reliability of the test would be substantially supported *if* patients could identify the quality of pain coming from a particular disc and differentially compare that sensation with their usual pain. It is unclear to what extent similar neurologic and behavioral factors may influence the results in provocative discography. It is possible that the disc stimulation in discography may also provoke a "concordant" pain response without actually having located a true pain source. As discussed earlier, there have been reported cases of individuals undergoing discography who were diagnosed as having discogenic pain as the source of their illness on the basis of positive concordant disc injections, but who were subsequently shown to have nonspinal sources for their pain.[26]

This issue was investigated using an experimental model to determine the response to disc injection in patients known to have nonspinal back pain.[15] Subjects were recruited to participate in this study if they had no history of back pain and were scheduled to undergo posterior iliac crest bone graft harvesting for nonspinal problems, including appendicular fracture nonunions or bone tumors. Most of these patients experienced low back and buttock pain from bone grafting for several months postoperatively; this pain was in a similar distribution to what is normally considered discogenic lumbar pain. Discography was performed several months after bone graft harvesting; subjects were asked to compare the quality and location of the disc injection pain with their usual iliac crest pain.

Eight volunteer subjects were studied using the same protocol as the Walsh and colleagues study.[3] All subjects had some disc degeneration on MRI, and 24 of the discs were injected. Of the 14 disc injections causing some pain response, five were believed to be "different" (nonconcordant) pains (35.7%), seven were "similar" (50%), and two were "exact" pain reproductions (14.3%). The presence of anular disruption was correlated with concordant pain reproduction ($P < .05$). Of 10 discs with anular tears, injection of seven elicited "similar" or "exact" pain reproduction to the pain at iliac crest bone graft harvest sites. By the strict criteria for positive discography, four of the eight patients (50%) had positive injections: The pain on a single disc injection was "bad" or "very bad," and the pain quality was noted to be exact or similar to the usual discomfort. All subjects had a negative control disc. All positive disc injections had anular fissures. Half of the positive disc injections occurred at low pressures (< 20 psi).[15]

Discography in Subjects With Minimal Low Back Symptoms

The ability of a test such as discography to discriminate a true pain generator disc responsible for causing serious disabling low back pain illness from another disc that causes only trivial or clinically inconsequential backache is critical to the test's validity in clinical practice. Derby and colleagues[36] performed discography in a group of 16 subjects with occasional or minimal low back pain, none of whom required current medical care or were experiencing disability because of low back pain. Of the 16 subjects, five (31%) had a pain response of 5 out of 10 or greater, and two (12.5%) had a pain response of 6 out of 10 or greater. The subjects with more frequent benign low back pain had more painful injections. None of these subjects had abnormal psychological profiles, compensation issues, or chronic pain syndromes or had significant secondary gain motivation to underreport pain. In this study, there were significant confounding methodologic issues that made the results open to criticism. These issues include using the investigators' employees and staff as the subjects of the study.

In another study, the Stanford group performed experimental discography on 25 volunteer subjects with no clinical back pain illness; these volunteers had persistent low backache unassociated with any physical restrictions that was not bad enough to seek medical care.[37] All subjects had normal psychological profiles, but half had other chronic pain syndromes that are risk factors for positive injections. In 36% of these subjects with common backache, discographic injection of one or more discs was significantly painful and concordant. All positive discs had anular disruption, and all had negative control discs. By the usual proposed criteria, these were positive disc injections for clinically significant discogenic pain illness. Discs sensitive to low-pressure injections were found in 28% of subjects.

Pressure-Sensitive Injections and Discography Validity

In some cases, dye injected at low pressures may cause significant pain. Derby and colleagues[9] labeled these "chemically" sensitive discs as opposed to discs that are painful only on injection with high pressures. These authors theorized that "chemically" sensitive discs are painful because of the exposure of anular nerve endings or nearby neural structures to the

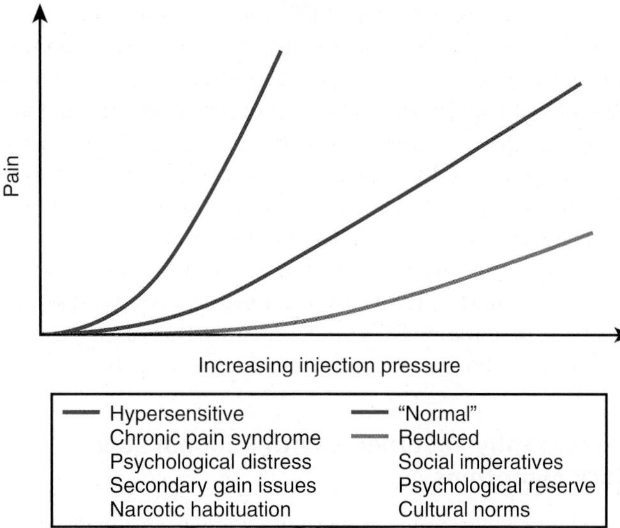

FIG. 17.1 Hypothetical responses to pressurization of degenerative disc depending on pain sensitivity and reporting biases of the patient.

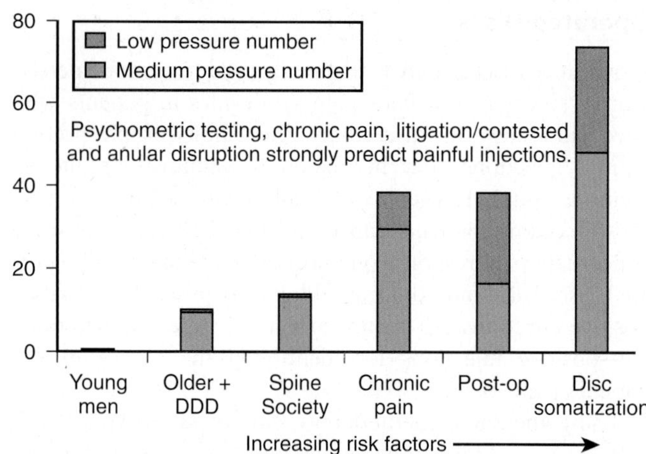

FIG. 17.2 Discography testing in asymptomatic subjects with varying risk factors. Proportion of painful disc injections and painful injections at low pressures seems to increase with increasing risk factors. DDD, degenerative disc disease; LBP, low back pain; Post-op, postoperative. (Data from references 15, 20, 29, and 36.)

leakage of irritating substances. It is postulated that this pain is incited by chemical leakage from the disc during daily activities. Some theorize that the disc injections simulate this chemical leakage. Low-pressure–positive discs are arbitrarily defined as discs found to be painful at pressures less than 15 or 22 psi greater than opening pressures.[9,23] Derby and colleagues[9] postulated further that disc injections eliciting pain at higher pressures (> 50 psi), called "mechanically" sensitive discs, physically distend the anulus and simulate mechanical loading. In these discs, it is presumed that a mechanical deformation of the anulus is the inciting painful event.

The use of pressure measurements has been postulated as a means to decrease the risk of false-positive injections. This assertion would be true if injections were rarely, if ever, positive at low pressures in subjects without true low back pain illness. Previous neurophysiologic considerations suggest that a pain and pressure profile for a given disc lesion may depend on individual pain sensitivity and local pain processes not related to the disc. Hypothetically, the pain and pressure profile may be depicted as shown in Fig. 17.1. The presence of the factors enumerated in Table 17.2 thought to have a desensitizing effect would move the curve down and to the right, whereas factors that increase pain sensitivity may move the pain and pressure curve up and to the left.

Experimental work has corroborated this hypothetical pain response. Discographic injections have been performed with pressure measurements in asymptomatic or minimally symptomatic volunteers.[3,16,35–37] Fig. 17.2 shows the proportion of painful injections at low pressures in volunteers with varying risk factors for increased pain sensitization. It seems from these and other data[38] that low-pressure injections are more likely positive in subjects with some type of chronic pain state, psychological distress, and, presumably, a generalized sensitization to irritable stimuli. An increased perception of pain at low-pressure injections seems to affect the pain response even when the chronic pain state is not in the low back region.

Evidence That Discography in Clinical Practice May Improve Outcomes

Many case series report that provocative discography is helpful in management of patients with chronic low back pain illness. These are uncontrolled studies, however, and the relationship of discography findings to clinical outcome after surgery is speculative. When encountered, good outcomes may be the result of nonspecific effects, natural history of the condition independent of diagnosis or treatment, scrupulous patient selection, or confounding findings on standard imaging studies. In a retrospective literature review, Cohen and Hurley[39] compared outcomes of spinal fusions in studies that included patients who had preoperative discography versus those who did not have preoperative discography. The outcomes were not significantly different.

In the era before routine MRI use, Colhoun and colleagues[40] retrospectively compared a series of fusions planned with and without preoperative discography. In this study on patients having surgery in the 1970s and early 1980s, there were no preoperative dynamic radiographs, MRI, or computed tomography (CT). The authors reported better results in the discography group. The two groups were not similar at baseline, however, and the authors did not examine or account for potential biases. One important bias in the study population is the fact that some patients had preoperative discography, whereas some did not. In the era before contemporary imaging techniques, this study suggested that discography might assist in the evaluation of patients before surgery. Even if this conclusion was true, this paradigm is currently unusual given the widespread availability of advanced imaging modalities in modern medicine.

Madan and colleagues[41] did a retrospective review of consecutive patients undergoing spinal fusion performed by the same surgeons, with and without preoperative discography. The two groups seemed well matched for demographic, psychometric, and radiographic features. At a minimum of 2-year

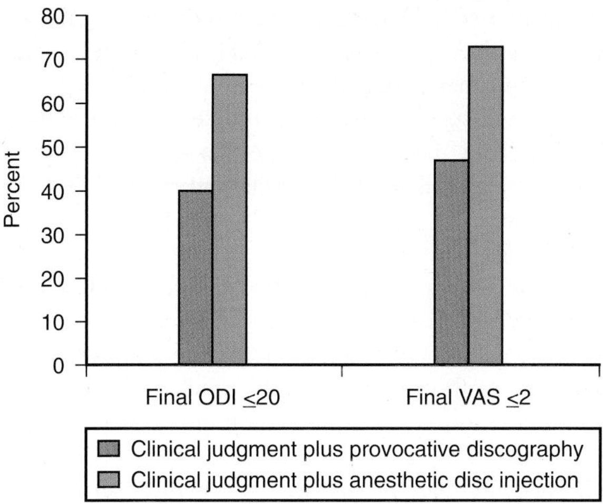

FIG. 17.3 Randomized clinical trial by Ohtori and colleagues comparing the proportion of good outcomes for pain and function after single-level spinal fusion in patients selected by best clinical judgment and provocative discography with best clinical judgment plus anesthetic disc injection. These were best-case scenario subjects in many respects: no worker's compensation cases, no road traffic accident litigation cases, no high somatic distress cases, no depression cases, all selected by very experienced spinal surgeons in Japan. Outcomes are clearly inferior when discography is used to select patients for fusion. ODI, Oswestry Disability Index, VAS, visual analog scale. (Data from Ohtori S, Kinoshita T, Yamashita M, et al: Results of surgery for discogenic low back pain: a randomized study using discography versus discoblock for diagnosis. *Spine*. 2009;34:1345–1348.)

follow-up, there was no significant difference in outcome between the two groups. The addition of discography to radiographs and MRI did not improve outcomes compared with radiographs and MRI alone.

A more recent randomized clinical trial compared outcomes of subjects having single-level fusion based on preoperative evaluation using provocative discography with subjects having an anesthetic disc injection.[42] In many ways, these subjects were the best-case scenarios given the lack of psychological distress, depression, workers' compensation cases, or traffic accident litigants. The discography was performed using low-pressure injections. The outcomes in the discography group were uniformly worse than the group using an anesthetic block to diagnose discogenic pain (Fig. 17.3). Despite the number of different studies on provocative discography, a phase IV evaluation (based on evidence-based criteria as described by Sackett and Haynes[27]) of discography has not been performed to date (see Table 17.3).

Clinical Outcome as a Gold Standard in Provocative Discography

From the evidence reviewed in this chapter, discography has been shown to be frequently positive in asymptomatic subjects and in subjects with pelvic pain owing to iliac crest harvesting. It has also been shown to be frequently fully concordant in subjects with clinically insignificant backache. These findings suggest that there is limited experimental evidence to support the premise that discography can accurately identify clinically significant lesions responsible for a patient's chronic low back pain illness. Direct assessment of a positive test against an accepted gold standard, confirming a true-positive result, has not been performed.

A common empirical gold standard would involve comparing the test results with clinical surgical outcomes, assuming that an excellent clinical outcome would confirm a true-positive test. There is concern, however, that an excellent clinical result may overestimate the number of true-positive results because of a placebo or nonspecific effect of spinal fusion or other intervention. There is also concern that clinical outcomes may underestimate the number of true-positive tests because the ability to achieve outstanding results is limited by patient-specific variables (psychological distress or social issues preventing recovery despite surgical cure of the lesion). Other concerns include results tempered by operative morbidity or technical limitations, which, in the best of cases, cannot achieve 100% success in the ideal situation of an accurate diagnosis.

An attempt was made to control these variables (patient-specific variables and operative comorbidities) in a prospective controlled study of spinal fusion for presumed diagnoses of unstable spondylolisthesis versus discogenic pain diagnosed by discography. Identical operative techniques were used, and patients had no psychosocial comorbidities.[43] Both groups included only highly selected patients with 6 to 18 months of severe low back pain, normal psychological testing, no previous or concomitant pain syndromes, and no workers' compensation or personal injury claims. All patients had either positive discography at one level only and at low pressures (< 20 psi) or unstable spondylolisthesis by strict radiographic criteria. All patients were working full time before their low back problem, and no patient was taking daily narcotic medications.

Both groups underwent an anterior spinal fusion with posterior instrumentation and fusion. Two years after surgery, only 27% of patients in the discography group met stringent criteria for clinical success compared with 71% of the spondylolisthesis group. Success was defined as full return to work and recreational activities, pain scores on a visual analog pain scale less than 2, Oswestry Disability Index score less than 15, and no daily medications for back pain. Even using less rigorous outcome measures, 43% of the discography group compared with 91% of the spondylolisthesis group reported at least moderate improvement. Even after controlling for operative morbidity, the maximum proportion of true-positive discograms in a best-case scenario (i.e., assuming normal psychometric testing, no other chronic pain history, no compensation issues or litigation, and single-level degeneration) was 40% to 60%, with a false-positive rate of approximately 50%.

For less "ideal" patients, provocative discography may be an extremely poor tool to select appropriate operative candidates. Freeman and colleagues,[44] used CT and provocative discography to select a wide range of typical low back pain subjects for an intradiscal electrothermal therapy trial, including patients with psychometric distress and compensation claims. These investigators found no improvement compared with control subjects. In a similarly designed trial, Pauza and colleagues[45] reported only slightly better outcomes even though they excluded patients with psychological abnormality, workers' compensation claims, or litigation claims.

SECTION II

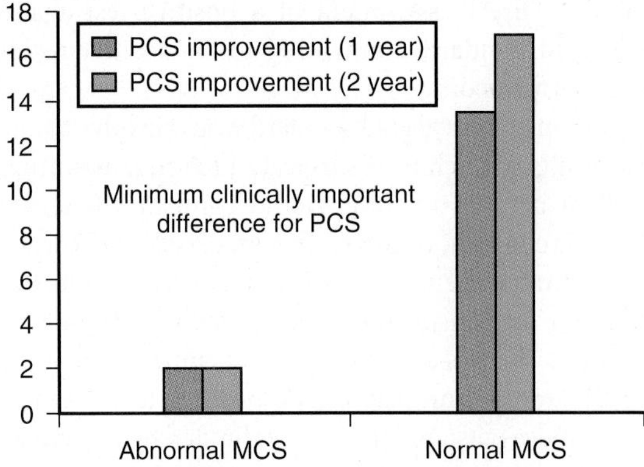

FIG. 17.4 Outcomes of spinal fusion when discography was used in patient selection. Subjects with a positive discogram in the setting of abnormal mental component scores (MCS) in the 36-Item Short Form Health Survey were highly unlikely to improve or reach even minimum clinically important change in physical outcomes. In contrast, subjects with more normalized mental component scores had significantly better improvement in outcomes ($P < .005$). In this study, positive provocative discography result in clinical subset of psychologically distressed patients seems to select patients unlikely to improve with surgical treatment. PCS, pain catastrophizing scale.

Even more striking, Derby and colleagues[46] found such poor outcomes for spinal fusion after provocative discography in patients with abnormal mental component scores on the 36-Item Short Form Health Survey that the discography seemed to *preselect* patients who were extremely unlikely to have a satisfactory outcome. These results, illustrated in Fig. 17.4, may be substantially worse than using alternative patient selection strategies without discography (e.g., radiographs, MRI, patient interview, or psychological screening).

Complications

Although there are many potential complications of any invasive procedure, several potential complications of discography warrant specific discussion:

1. *Infection*: There is a small but definite risk of discitis after percutaneous puncture and injection. The absolute risk is difficult to calculate, but modern methods likely limit this risk to much less than 1%. Double-needle techniques for insertion, less irritating dye, and intravenous or injectable antibiotics all have been postulated to decrease the infection risk.
2. *Prolonged pain episode*: Occasionally, patients may experience a prolonged episode of pain after a disc injection. One reason given for this phenomenon is the hypothetical displacement of fibrous repair over anular fissures owing to disc pressurization.[2] Other work has shown that 40% of subjects with psychological distress at the time of injection can have markedly increased back pain for 1 year after discography. This effect was not seen in subjects with normal psychological profiles.[47]
3. *Misleading diagnosis resulting in inappropriate or ineffective invasive treatments*: As discussed previously, subjects with one or more risk factors for false-positive testing may be misdiagnosed as having primary discogenic pain as the cause of their persistent low back pain illness. Patients with abnormal psychometric testing undergoing surgery based on this test are extremely unlikely to have substantial benefit from disc-directed interventions (see Fig. 17.4) and are exposed to the hazards and morbidity of these procedures.[46]
4. *Accelerated disc degeneration*: In animal models, disc puncture with a needle has provided a reliable model to initiate rapid disc injury with structural changes similar in some respects to naturally occurring disc degeneration. Working with a large animal model, Korecki and colleagues[48] showed that relatively minor disruption in the disc from even a 25-gauge needle puncture injury had "immediate and progressive mechanical and biologic consequences with important implications for the use of discography…." Similarly, Nassr and colleagues[49] showed that needle puncture in cervical discs during cervical spinal surgery localization radiographs was apparently associated with a threefold risk of rapid disc degeneration. Carragee and colleagues[50] performed a prospective, matched-cohort study of disc degeneration progression over 10 years with and without baseline discography. The investigators performed a protocol MRI and L3–L4, L4–L5, and L5–S1 provocative discography at baseline in 75 subjects without serious low back pain illness. The investigators enrolled a matched group at the same time and performed the same protocol MRI examination. Subjects were followed for 10 years. At 7 to 10 years after baseline assessment, eligible discography and control subjects underwent another protocol MRI examination. MRI examinations were scored for qualitative findings (Pfirrmann grade, herniations, endplate changes, and high-intensity zone). Loss of disc height and loss of disc signal were measured by quantitative methods (Fig. 17.5). The investigators found that modern discography techniques with small-gauge needle and limited pressurization resulted in accelerated disc degeneration, disc herniation, loss of disc height and signal, and development of reactive endplate changes compared with matched controls. The clinical follow-up of these patients demonstrated even more concerning findings in the study subjects through 10 years.[51] Despite some attrition related to a 10-year study, 110 of 150 subjects were available for all interval assessments. In these subjects, there was a statistically significant increase in the number of medical visits, lumbar CT/MRI tests, and lumbar spine surgery in the cohort exposed to provocative discography compared to the control cohort (Fig. 17.6). These data suggest that lumbar provocative discography leads to an increased risk of harm to exposed subjects.

Conclusions Regarding Provocative Discography

As for most diagnostic tests, the usefulness of discography is affected by the characteristics of the population being studied. As a provocative test depending on the subjective reporting of

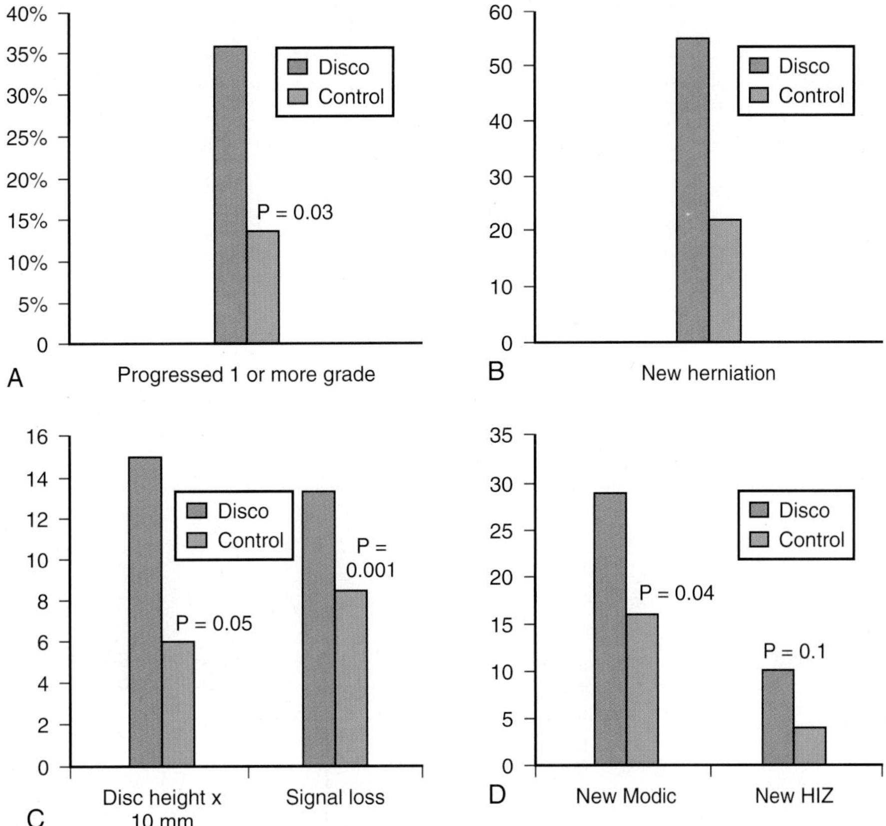

FIG. 17.5 Progression of disc degeneration in matched cohorts of subjects, discography (Disco) versus nondiscography controls. Baseline versus 10-year follow-up magnetic resonance imaging studies were compared for (A) progression of Pfirrmann grade, (B) development of new disc herniations, (C) loss of disc height and nuclear signal, and (D) development of new Modic findings or high-intensity zones (HIZ). In all parameters, degeneration was greater in discography group. (Data from Carragee EJ, Don AS, Hurwitz EL, et al: Does discography cause accelerated progression of degeneration changes in the lumbar disc: a ten-year matched cohort study. *Spine.* 2009;34:2338–2345.)

pain with injection, the central factors influencing reliability and validity of discography have to do with the neurophysiologic, psychological, and social factors that affect pain perception and expression. In the subset of patients without significant confounding factors, the test may be more likely to identify accurately a local pain generator as a primary cause of disabling axial pain illness. In subjects with significant psychosocial risk factors or confounding neurophysiologic factors, even the theoretical basis of the test is in doubt. Finally, the ability of the test to improve clinical outcomes has not been proven, and studies so far have been disappointing. Serious risks of accelerated disc degeneration are also suspected after disc puncture/injection and more recent clinical data have corroborated this concern. The risk and benefits of this procedure must be carefully weighed.

PEARLS

1. Patient selection for discography is of primary importance in determining the accuracy and utility of the test.
2. Results need to be interpreted in the context of the patient's entire medical history, including other chronic pain issues.
3. It is extremely unlikely that a disc with a negative injection, normal morphology, and no pain with the injection would be a primary cause of serious low back pain illness.
4. In the best-case scenario of a patient with no known risk factors for a false-positive test, the positive predictive value of the test is not greater than 50%.
5. Most low back pain syndromes are multifactorial.

PITFALLS

1. During injection, it is important to avoid high-pressure injections (> 100 psi) because these may cause gross mechanical motion of the segment or injure the endplate directly.
2. In patients with psychological distress, disputed compensation claims, or multiple chronic pain syndromes, the reported pain responses to disc injection have not been shown to be reliable or valid.
3. There is clear risk of accelerated disc degeneration with discographic injections and this disc degeneration may lead to clinically significant sequelae.
4. Disc injections in patients with psychological distress may result in an increase in back pain for weeks or months.

KEY POINTS

1. Provocative discography is a diagnostic test that may identify primary "discogenic" pain if present in psychologically normal patients without confounding pain or compensation issues.
2. Patient responses to disc injection are subjective and strongly influenced by pain sensitivity and reporting variables, including

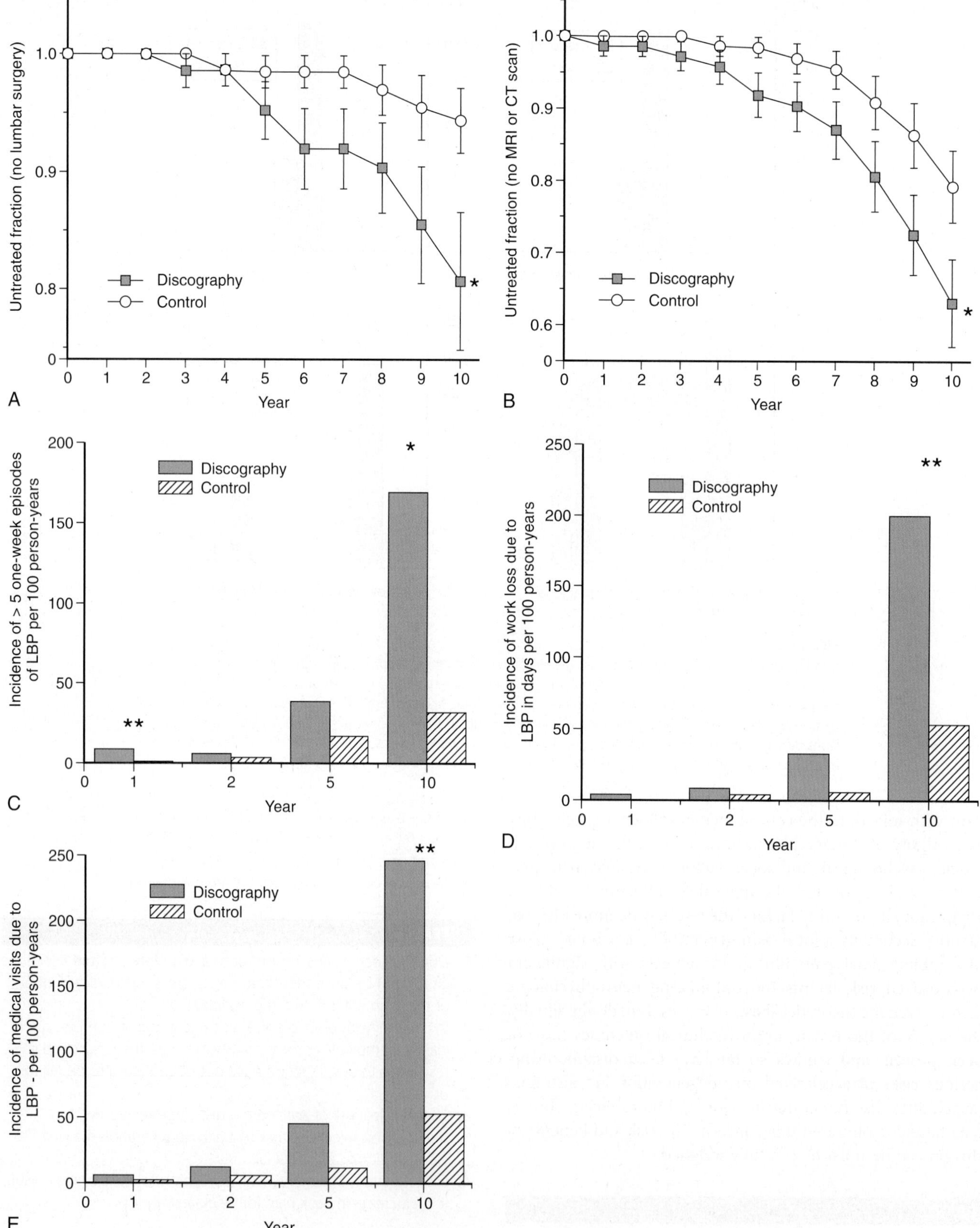

FIG. 17.6 The comparative incidence of clinical variables in patients exposed to lumbar provocative discography and controls over 10 years. Asterisks indicate statistically significant difference. (A) Surgery-free survivorship ($P = .016$). (B) Imaging-free survivorship ($P = .044$). (C) Serious low back pain episodes (**$P = .008$ and *$P = .016$). (D) Work loss ($P = .009$). (E) Medical visits for low back pain ($P = .002$). CT, computed tomography; LBP, low back pain; MRI, magnetic resonance imaging.

psychological factors, chronic pain behavior, regional or central pain syndromes, and compensation issues.

3. Provocative discography has not been proven to improve outcomes of treatment for low back pain syndromes. In patients with emotional distress issues or compensation issues, there is some evidence that using discography may result in poorer outcomes and inappropriate invasive procedures.
4. Risks of provocative discography include false and misleading diagnoses in patients with high pain-sensitive risk factors, increased axial pain for weeks or months after injection, pyogenic discitis, and accelerated disc degeneration after long-term follow-up.

KEY REFERENCES

1. Sackett D, Haynes R. Evidence base of clinical diagnosis: the architecture of diagnostic research. *BMJ*. 2002;324:539-541.
This article defines the necessary conditions to establish validity and clinical usefulness of a diagnostic test. The gold standard necessary to compare diagnostic test results is of prime importance, as is a careful assessment of the study population. These conditions are problematic in the evaluation of provocative discography.
2. Carragee EJ, Tanner CM, Yang B, et al. False-positive findings on lumbar discography: reliability of subjective concordance assessment during provocative disc injection. *Spine*. 1999;24:2542-2547.
This study looks at the reliability of the concordance response during discography. The authors found that volunteer subjects with known pelvic area pain cannot reliably distinguish the sensation coming from a pelvic pain generator from the sensation caused by the injection of an asymptomatic disc. The implications for validity of provocative injections are discussed.
3. Ohtori S, Kinoshita T, Yamashita M, et al. Results of surgery for discogenic low back pain: a randomized study using discography versus discoblock for diagnosis. *Spine*. 2009;34:1345-1348.
The authors performed a randomized clinical trial comparing outcomes of subjects having single-level fusion based on an evaluation using provocative discography with subjects having an anesthetic disc injection. These were in some respects best-case scenario subjects (no psychological distress, no depression, no worker's compensation cases, and no traffic accident litigants). The discography was performed using low-pressure injections. The outcomes in the discography group (reported pain, function, pain medications) were uniformly worse than the group using an anesthetic block to determine fusion.
4. Carragee EJ, Don AS, Hurwitz EJ, et al. Does discography cause accelerated progression of degeneration changes in the lumbar disc: a ten-year matched cohort study. *Spine*. 2009;34:2338-2345.
Matched asymptomatic cohorts with and without baseline pressure-limited provocative discography were followed with a detailed MRI protocol compared against baseline MRI findings. The discography group had greater progression of disc degeneration scores, more new disc herniations, greater loss of disc height, and greater loss of disc signal compared with the control group. In the discography cohort, new disc herniations were disproportionately found near the puncture site.
5. Chou R, Loesser JD, Owens DK. Interventional therapies, surgery, and interdisciplinary rehabilitation for low back pain: an evidence-based clinical practice guideline from the American Pain Society. *Spine*. 2009;34:1066-1077.
In a comprehensive multidisciplinary review, the authors concluded: "In patients with chronic nonradicular low back pain, provocative discography is not recommended as a procedure for diagnosing discogenic low back pain (strong recommendation, moderate-quality evidence)."

REFERENCES

1. Lindblom L. Diagnostic puncture of intervertebral disks in sciatica. *Acta Orthop Scand*. 1948;17:231-239.
2. Derby R, Guyer R, Lee S-H, et al. The rational use and limitations of provocative discography. International Spine Intervention Society 13th annual meeting, New York. *ISIS Newsletter*. 2004;5:6-20.
3. Walsh T, Weinstein J, Spratt K, et al. Lumbar discography in normal subjects: a controlled prospective study. *J Bone Joint Surg Am*. 1990;72:1081-1088.
4. Allan DB, Waddell G. An historical perspective on low back pain and disability. *Acta Orthop Scand Suppl*. 1989;234:1-23.
5. Burton A. Spine update: back injury and work loss: biomechanical and psychosocial influences. *Spine*. 1997;22:2575-2580.
6. Burton A, Tillotson K, Main C, et al. Psychosocial predictors of outcome in acute and subacute low back trouble. *Spine*. 1995;20:722-728.
7. Aprill C, Bogduk N. High-intensity zone: a diagnostic sign of painful lumbar disc on magnetic resonance imaging. *Br J Radiol*. 1992;65:361-369.
8. Crock H. Internal disc disruption. *Med J Aust*. 1970;1:983-990.
9. Derby R, Howard MW, Grant JM, et al. The ability of pressure-controlled discography to predict surgical and nonsurgical outcomes. *Spine*. 1999;24:364-371.
10. O'Neill C, Derby R, Kanderes L. Precision injection techniques for diagnosis and treatment of lumbar disc disease. *Semin Spine Surg*. 1999;11:104-118.
11. Schwarzer A, Aprill C, Derby R, et al. The prevalence and clinical features of internal disc disruption in patients with chronic LBP. *Spine*. 1995;20:1878-1883.
12. Schwarzer A, Aprill C, Fortin J, et al. The relative contribution of the zygapophyseal joint in chronic low back pain. *Spine*. 1994;19:801-806.
13. Schwarzer A, Bogduk N. The prevalence and clinical features of internal disk disruption in patients with low back pain [letter]. *Spine*. 1996;21:776.
14. Siddle P, Cousins M. Spinal pain mechanisms. *Spine*. 1997;22: 98-104.
15. Carragee EJ, Tanner CM, Yang B, et al. False-positive findings on lumbar discography: reliability of subjective concordance assessment during provocative disc injection. *Spine*. 1999;24:2542-2547.
16. Carragee EJ, Tanner CM, Khurana S, et al. The rates of false-positive lumbar discography in select patients without low back symptoms. *Spine*. 2000;25:1373-1380.
17. Gracely R, Dubner R, McGrath P. Narcotic analgesia: fentanyl reduces the intensity but not the unpleasantness of painful tooth pulp stimulation. *Science*. 1979;203:1261-1263.
18. Lenz F, Gracely R, Romanoski A, et al. Stimulation in the somatosensory thalamus can reproduce both the affective and sensory dimensions of previously experienced pain. *Nat Med*. 1995;1:910-913.
19. Lenz FA, Gracely RH, Hope EJ, et al. The sensation of angina can be evoked by stimulation of the human thalamus. *Pain*. 1994;59:119-125.
20. Saal JSM. General principles of diagnostic testing as related to painful lumbar spine disorders—a critical appraisal of current diagnostic techniques. *Spine*. 2002;27:2538-2545.
21. Carragee EJ. Psychological screening in the surgical treatment of lumbar disc herniation. *Clin J Pain*. 2001;17:215-219.
22. North R, Kidd D, Zahurak M, et al. Specificity of diagnostic nerve blocks: a prospective, randomized study of sciatica due to lumbosacral spine disease. *Pain*. 1996;65:77-85.

23. O'Neill C, Kurgansky M. Subgroups of positive discs on discography. *Spine*. 2004;29:2134-2139.
24. Handwerker HO, Kobal G. Psychophysiology of experimentally induced pain. *Physiol Rev*. 1993;73:639-671.
25. Rhudy JL, Meagher MW. Fear and anxiety: divergent effects on human pain thresholds. *Pain*. 2000;84:65-75.
26. Carragee E, Tanner C, Vittum D, et al. *Positive provocative discography as a misleading finding in the evaluation of low back pain*. Proceedings of the North American Spine Society, 1997, p 388.
27. Sackett D, Haynes R. Evidence base of clinical diagnosis: the architecture of diagnostic research. *BMJ*. 2002;324:539-541.
28. Schwarzer A, Wang S, Bogduk N, et al. Prevalence and clinical features of lumbar zygapophysial joint pain: a study in an Australian population with chronic low back pain. *Ann Rheum Dis*. 1995;54:100-106.
29. Schwarzer AC, Aprill CN, Derby R, et al. The false-positive rate of uncontrolled diagnostic blocks of the lumbar zygapophysial joints. *Pain*. 1994;58:195-200.
30. Block A, Vanharanta H, Ohnmeiss D, et al. Discographic pain report: influence of psychological factors. *Spine*. 1996;21:334-338.
31. Ohnmeiss DD, Vanharanta H, Guyer RD. The association between pain drawings and computed tomographic/discographic pain responses. *Spine*. 1995;20:729-733.
32. Schellhas KP, Pollei SR, Dorwart RH. Thoracic discography: a safe and reliable technique. *Spine*. 1994;19:2103-2109.
33. Nordin M, Carragee EJ, Hogg-Johnson S, et al. Assessment of neck pain and its associated disorders. Results of the Bone and Joint Decade 2000-2010 Task Force on Neck Pain and Its Associated Disorders. *Spine*. 2008;33:S101-S122.
34. Heggeness MH, Watters WC III, Gray PM Jr. Discography of lumbar discs after surgical treatment for disc herniation. *Spine*. 1997;22:1606-1609.
35. Carragee EJ, Chen Y, Tanner CM, et al. Provocative discography in patients after limited lumbar discectomy: a controlled, randomized study of pain response in symptomatic and asymptomatic subjects. *Spine*. 2000;25:3065-3071.
36. Derby R, Kim B-J, Lee S-H, et al. Comparison of discographic findings in asymptomatic subject discs and the negative discs of chronic LBP patients: can discography distinguish asymptomatic discs among morphologically abnormal discs? *Spine J*. 2005;5:389-394.
37. Carragee EJ, Alamin TF, Miller J, et al. Provocative discography in volunteer subjects with mild persistent low back pain. *Spine J*. 2002;2:25-34.
38. Carragee EJ, Alamin TF, Parmar V, et al. Low pressure positive discography in subjects asymptomatic of significant LBP illness. *Spine*. 2006;31:505-509.
39. Cohen SP, Hurley RW. The ability of diagnostic spinal injections to predict surgical outcomes. *Anesth Analg*. 2007;105:1756-1775.
40. Colhoun E, McCall IW, Williams L, et al. Provocation discography as a guide to planning operations on the spine. *J Bone Joint Surg Br*. 1988;70:267-271.
41. Madan S, Gundanna M, Harley JM, et al. Does provocative discography screening of discogenic back pain improve surgical outcome? *J Spinal Disord Tech*. 2002;15:245-251.
42. Ohtori S, Kinoshita T, Yamashita M, et al. Results of surgery for discogenic low back pain: a randomized study using discography versus discoblock for diagnosis. *Spine*. 2009;34:1345-1348.
43. Carragee EJ, Lincoln T, Parmar VS, et al. A gold standard evaluation of the "discogenic pain" diagnosis as determined by provocative discography. *Spine*. 2006;31:2115-2123.
44. Freeman BJ, Fraser RD, Cain CM, et al. A randomized, double-blind, controlled trial: intradiscal electrothermal therapy versus placebo for the treatment of chronic discogenic low back pain. *Spine*. 2005;30:2369-2377.
45. Pauza KJ, Howell S, Dreyfuss P, et al. A randomized, placebo-controlled trial of intradiscal electrothermal therapy for the treatment of discogenic low back pain. *Spine*. 2004;4:27-35.
46. Derby R, Lettice JJ, Kula TA, et al. Single-level lumbar fusion in chronic discogenic low-back pain: psychological and emotional status as a predictor of outcome measured using the 36-item Short Form. *J Neurosurg Spine*. 2005;3:255-261.
47. Carragee EJ, Chen Y, Tanner CM, et al. Can discography cause long-term back symptoms in previously asymptomatic subjects? *Spine*. 2000;25:1803-1808.
48. Korecki CL, Costi JJ, Iatridis JC. Needle puncture injury affects intervertebral disc mechanics and biology in an organ culture model. *Spine*. 2008;33:235-241.
49. Nassr A, Lee JY, Bashir RS, et al. Does incorrect level needle localization during anterior cervical discectomy and fusion lead to accelerated disc degeneration? *Spine*. 2009;34:189-192.
50. Carragee EJ, Don AS, Hurwitz EL, et al. Does discography cause accelerated progression of degeneration changes in the lumbar disc: a ten-year matched cohort study. *Spine*. 2009;34:2338-2345.
51. Cuellar JM, Stauff MP, Herzog RJ, et al. Does provocative discography cause clinically important injury to the lumbar intervertebral disc? A 10-year matched cohort study. *Spine J*. 2016;16(3):273-280.

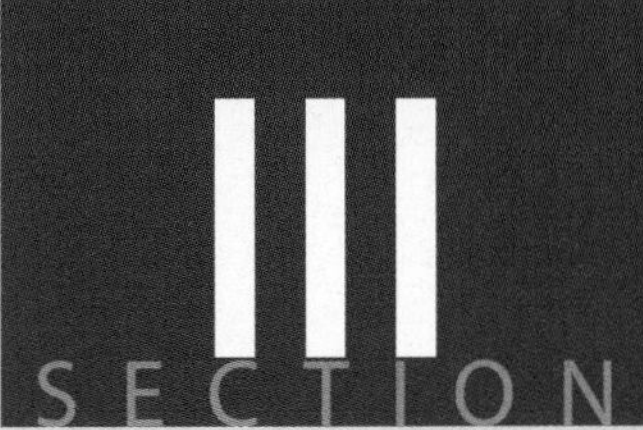

SURGICAL ANATOMY AND APPROACHES

SECTION III

CHAPTER 18 Cervical Spine: Surgical Approaches

Hamid Hassanzadeh
Varun Puvanesarajah
Howard S. An

The cervical spine is a complex structure with many sensitive anatomic elements. Successful surgical manipulation of the cervical spine requires an in-depth understanding of how vascular, neural, and musculoskeletal elements interweave in order to prevent dire complications. This chapter first examines the anatomy of the cervical spine, focusing on surface anatomy, osseous anatomy, bony articulations, ligaments, intervertebral discs, neurovascular structures, musculature, and triangles of the cervical spine. In the second section, the applied surgical anatomy is explored, with descriptions of both anterior and posterior approaches to the cervical spine.

Surgical Anatomy

Surface Anatomy and Skin

Surface landmarks are the key to successful localization of specific vertebral levels. For example, prominent musculoskeletal structures—namely, the hyoid bone, thyroid cartilage, and cricoid cartilage—delineate C3, C4, and C6, respectively.[1] The transverse processes can generally be palpated, with the transverse process of the atlas prominently featured anterior and inferior to the mastoid process. The Chassaignac tubercle, the anterior prominence of the transverse process of C6, is another important landmark that can be palpated. When palpating in a cranial-to-caudal direction along the posterior midline, the spinous process of the second vertebra is the first bony prominence that can be felt. Due to the natural lordosis of the cervical spine, the next palpable spinous process is typically of the sixth or seventh vertebra, with the seventh vertebra being particularly prominent.

When considering anterior approaches, surgical incisions should fall in line with skin creases to facilitate healing and prevent more noticeable scarring. In the lower neck, skin creases are transverse. Moving cranially, skin creases become more oblique in orientation. Skin on the front of the neck is generally softer, more mobile, and well vascularized, in contrast to skin on the back of the neck. As such, the typical longitudinal midline skin incision used on the posterior neck results in increased scar formation because of trapezius muscle tension.

Osseous Anatomy and Bony Articulation

The cervical spine comprises the first seven vertebrae in the spinal column. The bony anatomy and articulations of the upper cervical spine (occiput–C1–C2) are unique and distinct from the remaining lower five cervical vertebrae (C3–C7).

The atlas, or C1, is a ringlike structure lacking a body and a spinous process. It consists of two thick lateral masses plus an anterior and posterior arch. The longus colli muscle and anterior longitudinal ligament attach to the anterior tubercle of the atlas, whereas the posterior tubercle serves as the bony attachments for the rectus minor muscle and suboccipital membrane. The superior and inferior oblique muscles attach to the large transverse processes. The vertebral artery passes through the foramen transversarium located within the transverse process and courses posteriorly within a sulcus on the superior aspect of the posterior arch of the atlas. In 15% of the population, the sulcus for the vertebral artery can be completely covered by an anomalous ossification, which has been called the *ponticulus posticus* and may have surgical implications when identifying anatomic landmarks for bony fixation of C1.[2]

The axis, or C2, is characterized by an odontoid process, or dens, that projects upward anteriorly, articulating with the posterior aspect of the anterior arch of the atlas as a synovial joint. At its narrowest portion, at the base of the dens, the coronal and sagittal plane diameters are 8 to 10 mm and 10 to 11 mm.[3,4] Posteriorly, the axis has a large lamina and a bifid spinous process, which serve as attachments for the rectus major and inferior oblique muscles. The zone between the lamina and the lateral mass of the axis is indistinct, and posteriorly the neural arch connects to the body by large pedicles that are 8 mm wide and 10 mm long.[5] Lying directly anterolateral to the pedicle is the vertebral artery, which runs through the foramen transversarium. The pedicle of the axis projects 30 degrees medially and 20 degrees superiorly from a posterior-to-anterior direction.[4]

The bony articulations of the upper cervical spine (occiput–C1–C2) are unique and warrant special attention (Fig. 18.1). The atlanto-occipital articulation is a shallow ball-and-socket joint allowing for considerable motion mostly in flexion, extension, and lateral bending. The greatest degree of flexion

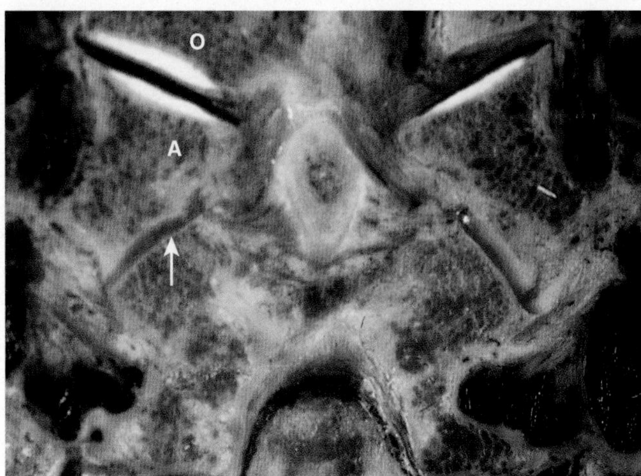

FIG. 18.1 Coronal cryomicrotome section of the upper cervical spine. Note articulation between occiput (O) and atlas (A). The atlantoaxial joint is identified by the arrow.

and extension of any cervical articulation occurs at this level (25 degrees).[6] Lateral displacement is minimized because the lateral wall of the cup-shaped articulation of the atlas is higher than the medial wall. The superior articular surface of the atlas projects cephalad and medially, articulating with the occipital condyle, which projects caudad and laterally. Conversely, the inferior articular surface of the atlas projects caudad and medially and articulates with the laterally projecting superior facet of the axis. As a result of this bony configuration, axial loads on the atlas tend to result in horizontal displacement of the lateral masses.[7]

The atlantoaxial articulation provides about 50% of rotatory motion of the cervical spine.[6,8] The transverse ligament, which spans across the arch of the atlas, holds the odontoid process against the anterior arch of the atlas, creating a pivot joint with a synovial membrane and capsular ligaments anteriorly and posteriorly to the dens. This transverse ligament is the principal stabilizing structure for the atlantoaxial articulation and averages 21.9 mm in length.[9] The transverse ligament has superior and inferior extensions, which form the cruciform ligament of the atlas, connecting it to the anterior edge of the foramen magnum and posterior aspect of the C2 body. To allow more rotatory motion, the inferior facets of the atlas are flatter and more circular than the superior facets, and face inferiorly to articulate with the axis.

The lower cervical vertebrae are morphologically similar and increase in dimension as they proceed inferiorly from C3 to C6, with C7 as the transitional vertebra into the thoracic spine. The vertebral bodies are small and oval, with the mediolateral diameter greater than the anteroposterior diameter.

The inferior surface of the vertebral body is convex in the coronal plane and concave in the sagittal plane, with the anterior lip occasionally overlapping the inferior vertebra.[9] Conversely, the superior surface of the vertebral body is convex or straight in the sagittal plane and concave in the coronal plane, creating projections on either side of the lateral superior surface, called the *uncus,* or hook. These processes project upward and conform to small grooves in the inferolateral border of the cephalad vertebra, forming the uncovertebral joints, or joints of Luschka. The width and depth of the vertebral surfaces average 17 mm and 15 mm from C2 to C6 and increase to about 20 mm and 17 mm at C7. Vertebral heights on the posterior wall in the mid-sagittal plane range from 11 to 13 mm.[10]

The pedicles project posterolaterally from the vertebral body and join the lamina to form the vertebral arch. From C3 to C7, the angulation of the pedicles varies from 8 degrees below to 11 degrees above the transverse plane, and decreases from 45 degrees to 30 degrees in relation to the sagittal plane.[10] The width and height of the pedicles increase slightly in size from C3 to C7, and average diameters are 5 to 6 mm and 7 mm. The lateral wall of the pedicle is thinner than the medial wall and should be taken into consideration if attempts at pedicle fixation are considered in this region.[11–13]

At the junction of the pedicle and lamina, the anterior tubercle of the transverse process projects laterally and is connected to the posterior tubercle by the costotransverse lamella (bar), creating the foramen transversarium. Passing through the foramen transversarium is the vertebral artery and venous system.

In the lower cervical spine, the neural foramina are bounded anteriorly by the uncinate process, the posterolateral aspect of the intervertebral disc, and the inferior portion of the vertebral body; posteriorly by the facet joint and superior articular process of the vertebral body below; and superiorly and inferiorly by adjacent pedicles. Vertebral notches located on the superior and inferior aspect of each pedicle contribute to the size of the neural foramina, which are 9 to 12 mm in height, 4 to 6 mm in width, and 4 to 6 mm in length, and are aligned 45 degrees to the sagittal plane.[14,15] They can be visualized radiographically with oblique views, with the right neural foramina outlined on the left posterior oblique view and the left neural foramina outlined on the right posterior oblique view.

The spinal canal is triangular and at all levels in the cervical spine is significantly greater in the medial-to-lateral dimension than in the anterior-to-posterior dimension. The cross-sectional area of the spinal canal is largest at C2 and smallest at C7, with a sagittal diameter of about 23 mm at C1 and 20 mm at C2, decreasing to 17 to 18 mm at C3–C6 and to 15 mm at C7.[8] This is one reason that the passage of sublaminar wires is safer in the upper cervical spine than in the lower cervical spine.

The lateral mass, an important structure for posterior cervical plate-screw systems, forms at the junction of the lamina and the pedicle and gives rise to the superior and inferior articular processes. These processes project upward and downward and are angled approximately 45 degrees cephalad from the transverse plane, gradually assuming a more vertical position as they descend into the thoracic region (Fig. 18.2). The articular process of the superior facet faces posteriorly, whereas the inferior facet of the upper vertebra faces anteriorly; the facets oppose one another to form a zygapophyseal joint. The facet joints are true diarthrodial

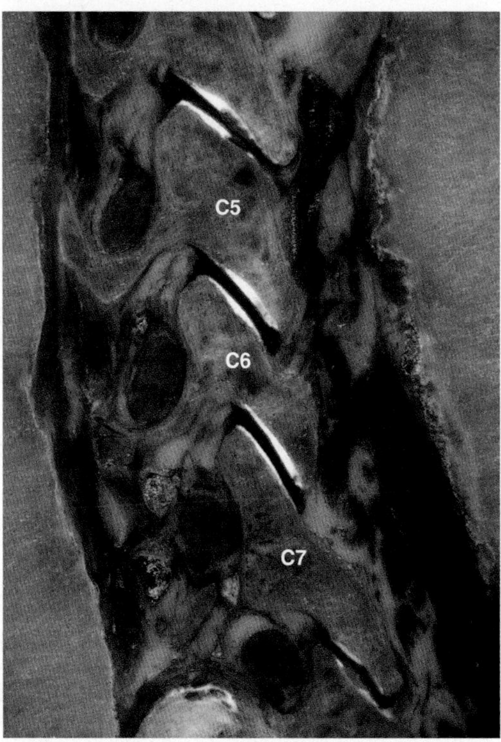

FIG. 18.2 Parasagittal cryomicrotome section of facet joints. The lateral mass of C7 is more elongated from superior to inferior and thinner from anterior to posterior. The facet joint angle is roughly 45 degrees from the transverse plane and assumes a more vertical position distally.

joints, with articular cartilage and menisci surrounded by a fibrous capsule lined by a synovial membrane. The interfacet distances are relatively constant between levels, with individual variations ranging from 9 to 16 mm (average, 13 mm).[5,16]

Posteriorly, the spinous processes project inferiorly and are bifid from C3 to C6; the C7 spinous process is large and not bifid, and is often called the *vertebra prominens*. The junction between the spinous process and lamina, the spinolaminar line, is an important anatomic landmark during spinous process wiring. Inadvertent penetration of the wire anterior to this line may result in spinal cord impingement.

The cervicothoracic junction is a transition region, with C7 having similar anatomic characteristics as T1 and T2. The dimensions of the vertebral body and the sizes of the transverse processes and spinous processes are larger at C6 and C7. Additionally, dimensions of the spinal canal decrease at C6 and C7, representing a distinct transition to the thoracic region. The articulating facet joint between C7 and T1 resembles the thoracic facet joint, and the lateral mass of C7 is thinner than that of upper levels. Morphologic characteristics of pedicles of C7, T1, and T2 were obtained with respect to diameters, depths, and medial angulations. Inner diameters of the pedicles at C7, T1, and T2 from medial to lateral plane averaged 5.2, 6.3, and 5.5 mm. Medial angulations were 34, 30, and 26 degrees at C7, T1, and T2, respectively.[10,17] These morphologic characteristics should be remembered when performing transpedicular procedures in the cervicothoracic region.

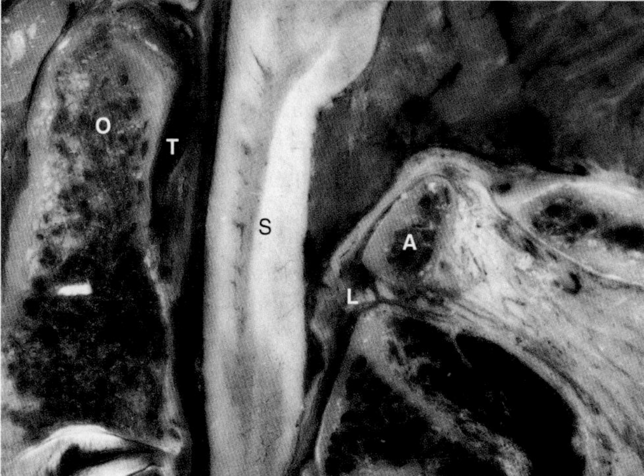

FIG. 18.3 Midsagittal microtome section at the upper cervical spine. The transverse ligament (T) acts as a stabilizer of the atlantoaxial joint by helping to restrain the odontoid (O) from posterior translation. The spinal cord (S), ligamentum flavum (L), and posterior arch of atlas (A) are also identified.

Ligaments

In addition to the bony anatomy, the ligamentous attachments provide support to the cervical spine and associated articulations. In the atlanto-occipital complex, two membranous attachments, the anterior and posterior atlanto-occipital membranes, connect the anterior and posterior arch of C1 to the margins of the foramen magnum. The anterior atlanto-occipital membrane is the superior continuation of the anterior longitudinal ligament, whereas the posterior membrane is the superior continuation of the ligamentum flavum.

The transverse ligament is the major stabilizer of the atlantoaxial complex (Fig. 18.3). It attaches laterally to tubercles located on the posterior aspect of the anterior arch of C1, where it blends with the lateral mass. Secondary stabilizers include the thick alar ligament, which arises from the sides of the dens to the medial aspects of the condyles of the occipital bone, and the apical ligament, which arises from the apex of the dens to the anterior edge of the foramen magnum. In some individuals, an anterior atlantodental ligament exists connecting the base of the dens to the anterior arch of the atlas.[18] The tectorial membrane, the superior continuation of the posterior longitudinal ligament, covers the dens and all the occipitoaxial ligaments and extends from the posterior body of C2 to the basilar portion of the occipital bone and the anterior aspect of the foramen magnum.

The bodies of the lower cervical vertebrae (C3–C7) are connected by two longitudinal ligaments and the intervertebral discs. The anterior longitudinal ligament is a strong band that attaches from the skull, as the anterior atlanto-occipital membrane, and continues caudad over the entire length of the spine down to the sacrum. The anterior longitudinal ligament is thinner and more closely attached at the intervertebral disc margins than at the anterior vertebral surfaces.[19] The anterior longitudinal ligament also sweeps around and envelops the lateral aspect of the vertebral bodies under the longus colli muscle, and the lateral extension is continuous with the deep layer of the posterior longitudinal ligament in the region of the intervertebral foramina.

The posterior longitudinal ligament, lying within the vertebral canal on the posterior aspect of the vertebral body and intervertebral disc, is wider in the upper cervical spine than the lower cervical spine.[19] Superiorly, it is continuous with the tectorial membrane; as it descends, it widens over the intervertebral discs and narrows behind each vertebral body. The posterior longitudinal ligament supplies additional strength and stability to the posteromedial fibers of the anulus. There is an area of relative weakness in the posterolateral corners of the disc, however, at the junction of the posterior longitudinal ligament and uncinate process. As a result, it is the site of most cervical disc herniations.[20] According to Hayashi and colleagues,[21] the posterior longitudinal ligament is double-layered, and the deep layer sends fibers to the anulus fibrosus and continues laterally to the region of the intervertebral foramina. The superficial or more dorsal layer of the posterior longitudinal ligament is adjacent to the dura mater and continues as a connective tissue membrane, which envelops the dura mater, nerve roots, and vertebral artery, suggesting that this membrane may serve as a protective barrier.

The ligamentum flavum of the cervical spine attaches to the anterior surface of the lamina above and to the superior margin of the lamina below and extends laterally to the articular processes, contributing to the boundary of the intervertebral foramen. The ligamentum flavum consists primarily of elastic fibers, whose numbers lessen with aging, resulting in anterior buckling that can contribute to symptoms of spinal cord compression. A gap in the midline of the ligamentum flavum allows for the exit of veins.

The interspinous ligament of the cervical spine is thin and less well developed than in the lumbar region. It attaches in an oblique orientation from the posterosuperior aspect to the anteroinferior aspect of the spinous process. There is no separate supraspinous ligament in the cervical region. The ligamentum nuchae, a fibroelastic septum, is the superior continuation of the supraspinous ligament of the thoracolumbar spine and extends from the external occipital protuberance to C7.

Intervertebral Discs

Intervertebral discs are present between all vertebrae except at the atlantoaxial level. Each intervertebral disc is an avascular structure that consists of the nucleus pulposus at the interior of the disc, the outer anulus fibrosus, and the cartilaginous endplates adjacent to the vertebral surfaces. The nucleus pulposus functions as a shock absorber, and the anulus fibrosus maintains the stability of the motion segment. With increasing age, the margin between the nucleus pulposus and anulus fibrosus becomes less distinct. Often, by age 50 years, the nucleus pulposus has become a fibrocartilaginous mass similar to the inner zone of the anulus fibrosus.[22]

The anulus has an outer collagenous layer, in which the fibers are arranged in oblique layers of lamellae. The outermost fibers of the anulus fibrosus are contiguous with the anterior and posterior longitudinal ligaments and are firmly attached to the adjacent vertebral endplates. The fibers of the lamella run perpendicular to the fibers of the adjacent lamella. The collagen fibers in the posterior portion of the disc run more vertical than oblique; this may account for the relative frequency of radial tears seen clinically. The discs are shaped to conform to the surface of the bodies; the superior surface of the disc is concave, and the inferior surface of the disc is correspondingly convex in the coronal plane. The discs are also slightly thicker anteriorly than posteriorly, which contributes to the lordotic posture of the cervical spine. The cervical intervertebral discs allow some translational movement in the sagittal plane, but the uncinate processes resist lateral movement. The uncinate process, located in the posterolateral aspect of the disc, also helps prevent disc herniations in this area. Degeneration of the anulus fibrosus (Fig. 18.4) in the cervical region is similar to the lumbar region in that concentric, transverse, and radial tears of the anulus occur, and the radial tear in the posterior aspect of the disc may be more clinically significant.

The cartilaginous endplate is a layer of hyaline cartilage resting on the subchondral bone and serves as a barrier between the pressure of the nucleus pulposus and the adjacent vertebral bodies. This cartilage is a growth plate and responsible for endochondral ossification during growth (Fig. 18.5). The cartilaginous endplates also allow the insertion of the inner fibers of the anulus fibrosus and the diffusion of nutrients from the subchondral bone to the disc.

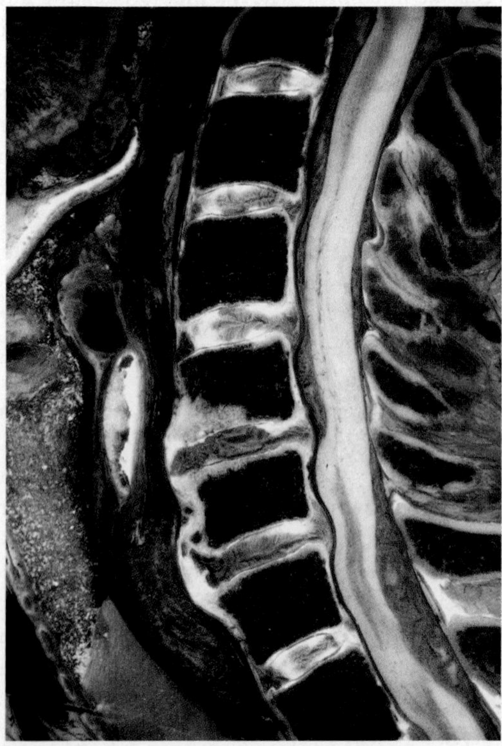

FIG. 18.4 Midsagittal cryomicrotome section of a degenerative cervical spine showing degeneration of anulus fibrosus and herniation of nucleus pulposus posteriorly with impingement of the spinal cord.

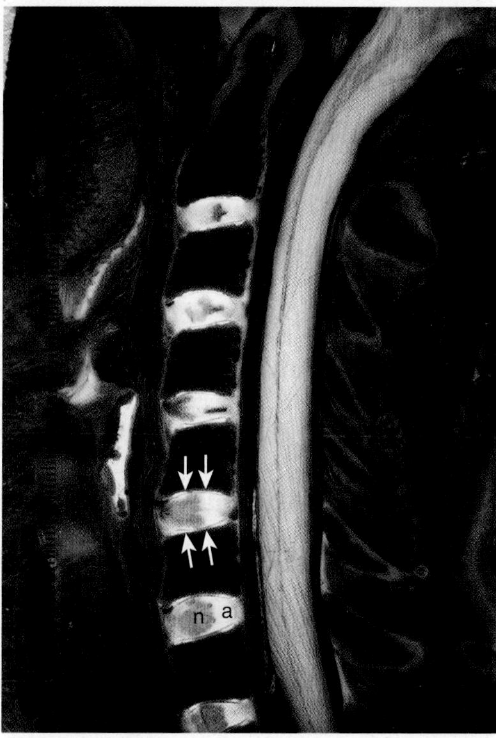

FIG. 18.5 Midsagittal microtome section of the cervical spine showing nucleus pulposus (n) and outer anulus fibrosus (a) of the intervertebral disc. Arrows identify a cartilaginous endplate.

Neural Elements

The cervical cord emerges from the foramen magnum as a continuation of the medulla oblongata. There is considerable variation in size of the spinal cord; however, in general, owing to the increased nerve supply to the upper limbs, the cervical cord enlarges from C3 and becomes maximal at C6. Maximal transverse diameters of 13 to 14 mm have been reported,[23] with transverse areas ranging from 58.3 ± 6.7 mm^3 at C6[24] to 85.8 ± 7.2 mm^3 at C4–C5.[25]

The spinal cord includes the outer white matter and the inner gray matter. The white matter of the spinal cord contains nerve fibers and glia, and is divided into the posterior, lateral, and anterior columns. The posterior column includes the fasciculus cuneatus laterally and fasciculus gracilis medially, mediating proprioceptive, vibratory, and tactile sensations. The lateral column contains the descending motor lateral corticospinal and lateral spinothalamic fasciculi. The anterior funiculus contains the ascending anterior spinothalamic tract and other descending tracts. The lateral spinothalamic tracts cross through the ventral commissure to the contralateral side of the cord, conveying pain and temperature sensations. The anterior spinothalamic tract conveys the crude touch sensation.

The gray matter of the spinal cord contains cell bodies of efferent and internuncial neurons. The somatosensory neurons are located in the posterior horn, and the somatomotor neurons are found in the anterior horn of the gray matter. The visceral center of the gray matter is found in the intermediolateral horn. In the center of the spinal cord is the central ependymal canal for the passage of cerebrospinal fluid.

The spinal cord is covered by the pia mater, which is the outer lining of the cord, and transparent arachnoid membrane that contains the cerebrospinal fluid. The dura mater is the outer covering of the spinal cord, which becomes the inner layer of the cranial dura at the level of the foramen magnum. The cervical cord is anchored to the dura by the dentate ligaments that project laterally from the lateral side of the cord to the arachnoid and dura at points midway between exiting spinal nerves. By suspending the spinal cord in the cerebrospinal fluid, the dentate ligaments cushion and protect the cord, while minimizing the movement of the cord during range of motion (ROM). The epidural space contains fat, internal vertebral venous plexus, and loose connective tissue. This venous plexus may be involved in spreading infection or neoplasm. There is a potential space between the dura and the arachnoid, and the subarachnoid space is between the arachnoid and the pia. The subarachnoid space contains the cerebrospinal fluid (CSF), spinal blood vessels, and nerve rootlets from the spinal cord.

The dorsal sensory rootlets enter the cord through the lateral longitudinal sulcus, and the ventral motor rootlets exit the cord through the ventral lateral sulcus. The six or eight rootlets at each level leave the spinal cord laterally to lie in the lateral subarachnoid space bathed in the CSF. The rootlets join to form the dorsal and ventral root, which together enter a narrow sleeve of arachnoid and pass through the dura to become a nerve root at each level. The cervical nerve roots that form from the ventral and dorsal nerve rootlet extend anterolaterally at a 45-degree angle to the coronal plane and inferiorly at about 10 degrees to the axial plane.[15] The nerve roots enter the intervertebral foramina by passing directly laterally from the spinal canal adjacent to the corresponding disc and over the top of the corresponding pedicle. The anterior root lies anteroinferiorly adjacent to the uncovertebral joint; the posterior root is close to the superior articular process. The nerve root is positioned at the tip of the superior articular process in the medial aspect of the neural foramen; it courses more inferiorly to position over the pedicle in the lateral aspect of the neural foramen (Fig. 18.6).

The roots occupy about one-third of the foraminal space in the normal spine but much more in the degenerative spine. The roots are located in the inferior half of the neural foramen normally, but the nerve roots occupy a more cranial part of the foramina, and the size of the foramen is diminished if the neck is fully extended.[26] The upper half of the neural foramen contains fat and small veins.[27] The nerve root is enlarged in the distal aspect of the intervertebral foramen, and the dorsal root ganglion is located just distal to the foramen.[28] The dorsal root ganglion is located between the vertebral artery and a small concavity in the superior articular process. Just distal to the ganglion and outside the intervertebral foramen, the anterior and posterior roots join to form the spinal nerve. The spinal nerve divides into dorsal and ventral primary rami branches.

The gray rami from the sympathetic cervical ganglion join the ventral primary rami. There are interconnections between gray rami, the perivascular plexus around the vertebral artery, and the sympathetic trunk, all of which give contributions

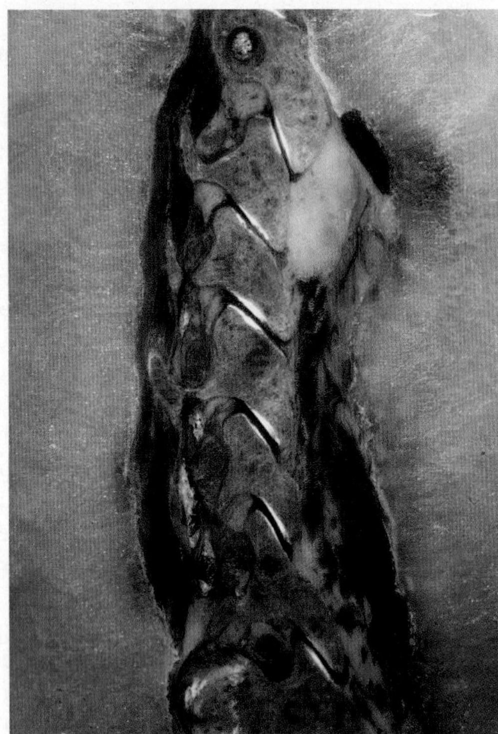

FIG. 18.6 Parasagittal cryomicrotome section of the lateral aspect of the neural foramen shows a nerve root coursing more inferiorly lying over a pedicle as it begins to exit the foramen.

to the ventral nerve plexus to innervate the anterior longitudinal ligament, outer anulus fibrosus, and anterior vertebral body.[29,30] The dorsal nerve plexus receives contributions from the sinuvertebral nerves, which originate from the gray rami and perivascular plexus of the vertebral artery. The dorsal nerve plexus innervates the posterior longitudinal ligament, and the sinuvertebral nerves give branches to the posterior part of the anulus and the ventral part of the dura. The sinuvertebral nerves innervate two or more discs or motion segments.

The first cervical nerve or suboccipital nerve exits the vertebral canal above the posterior arch of the atlas and posteromedial to the lateral mass, and lies between the vertebral artery and the posterior arch. The posterior primary ramus of the first cervical nerve enters the suboccipital triangle and sends motor fibers to the deep muscles. The anterior primary ramus of the first cervical nerve forms a loop with the second anterior primary ramus and sends fibers to the hypoglossal nerve. The cervical plexus receives fibers from anterior primary rami of C1–C4. The cervical plexus is located opposite C1–C3, ventral and lateral to the levator scapulae and middle scalene muscles. The cervical plexus has distributions to the skin and muscles, such as the rectus capitis anterior and lateralis, longus capitis and cervicis, levator scapulae, and middle scalene. The cervical plexus forms loops and branches to supply the sternocleidomastoid and trapezius muscles. It has communications with the hypoglossal nerve from C1 and C2, and leaves this trunk as the superior root of the *ansa cervicalis*, which is a nerve loop that is formed with the inferior root from C2 and C3.

The second cervical nerve lies on the lamina of the axis posterior to the lateral mass; the posterior primary ramus or the greater occipital nerve pierces the trapezius about 2 cm below the external occipital protuberance and 2 to 4 cm from the midline. Trauma or irritation to any of the three terminal nerves (the greater and lesser occipital nerve and the greater auricular nerve) can produce pain, headache, or hyperesthesia in their dermal distribution over the occiput and around the ear.

Cutaneous branches of the posterior primary rami of C2–C5 are consistently present in the skin of the nuchal region; the largest cutaneous nerve in this region is the greater occipital nerve. The lesser occipital nerve is a branch from the anterior cervical plexus, running upward and lateral to the greater occipital nerve. The posterior primary ramus of C3, or the third occipital nerve, pierces the trapezius more inferiorly and about 1 cm medial from the midline. The cervical nerve exits over the pedicle that bears the same number except the C8 cervical nerve lies between the C7 and T1 vertebrae. The posterior primary rami of cervical nerves send motor fibers to the deep muscles and sensory fibers to the skin, but the first cervical nerve has no cutaneous branches. The anterior primary rami of C1–C4 form the cervical plexus, and the rami of C5–T1 form the brachial plexus.

Vascular Structures

The major blood supply of the cervical cord and cervical spine is the vertebral artery. Variations of the course of the vertebral artery have been reported.[31] In most cases, the vertebral artery originates from the first part of the subclavian artery and begins its ascent behind the common carotid artery between the longus colli and the anterior scalene. In the lower cervical spine, the vertebral arteries are crossed by the inferior thyroid artery and on the left by the thoracic duct. The vertebral arteries course anterior to the ventral rami of the seventh and eighth cervical nerves and the C7 transverse process before entering the C6 transverse foramen, where they ascend within the transverse foramen of C6–C2.

The surgeon should remember that the vertebral artery is located lateral to the uncinate process and in line with the middle one-third of the vertebral body just anterior to the nerve root. During anterior exposure of the vertebral body and intervertebral discs, too far lateral dissection on the inferior half of the vertebral body and uncovertebral joints would endanger the vertebral artery and spinal nerve around the intervertebral foramen. The vertebral artery may also be involved in patients with severe cervical spondylosis when it may be impinged by the osteophyte. At the level of the atlas, the artery winds posteromedially around the lateral mass and over the posterior arch of the atlas before passing through the posterior atlanto-occipital membrane into the foramen magnum, joining the other vertebral artery to form the basilar artery.

In the foramen magnum region, the vertebral artery gives branches anteriorly that join to form the single anterior spinal artery, whereas the paired posterior spinal arteries are branches from the posterior inferior cerebellar arteries. The anterior and posterior spinal arteries are the major blood supplies of the spinal cord. The posterior spinal arteries give rise to plexiform channels that are arranged transversely on the dorsum of the cord. The anterior spinal artery supplies most of the spinal cord, except the posterior columns.[32] The spinal cord also receives blood supplies from radicular arteries or medullary feeders from the vertebral arteries and ascending cervical arteries.[32] The segmental arteries that are branches of the vertebral artery are present at each level to supply the vertebrae and surrounding tissues, but only a few segmental vessels give rise to radicular arteries or medullary feeders to the spinal cord. These vessels have a variable distribution, but medullary feeders are more commonly present at C6 and C3 from the left and C5 and T1 from the right.[19]

Venous blood returns from the cord through three veins posteriorly and three veins anteriorly. The venous system within the spinal canal consists of valveless sinuses in the epidural space. The venous plexus is most apparent anteriorly just medial to the pedicles over the mid-portion of the vertebral bodies and anastomoses with the veins from the opposite side and with the basivertebral sinus, which is located in the space between the posterior longitudinal ligament and the posterior aspect of the vertebral body.

Musculature

The musculature of the cervical spine can be grouped into the anterolateral and posterior muscle groups. The anterolateral muscles of the neck include the platysma muscle, sternocleidomastoid muscle, hyoid muscles, strap muscles of the larynx, scalene muscles, longus colli muscle, and longus capitis muscle. The posterior musculature is subdivided into superficial, intermediate, and deep muscle groups.[33]

The platysma is a thin muscle underneath the subcutaneous tissue that spans from the deltoid and upper pectoral fascia and crosses over the clavicle and passes obliquely upward and medially to insert to the mandible, muscles of the lip, and skin of the lower part of the face. The platysma depresses the lower jaw and the lip, and tenses and ridges the skin of the neck.

The sternocleidomastoid originates from the sternum and the medial clavicle to the mastoid process and the lateral half of the superior nuchal line of the occipital bone. The second cervical nerve and the spinal accessory nerve innervate the sternocleidomastoid, which functions to draw the head toward the ipsilateral shoulder and rotate it and point the chin craniad toward the contralateral side. The sternocleidomastoid muscles together flex the head and raise the thorax when the head is fixed.

Muscles that attach to the hyoid bone include the digastric, stylohyoid, mylohyoid, geniohyoid, and omohyoid muscles; the strap muscles of the larynx include the sternohyoid and sternothyroid muscles. These muscles do not control the cervical spine but are important in controlling the movement of the hyoid and larynx, and are important landmarks in the anterior approach to the cervical spine.

The longus colli and longus capitis are the prevertebral muscles of the neck. The longus colli spans from C1 to T3 and extends laterally to attach to the anterior tubercles of the transverse processes of C3–C6. The longus capitis originates from the anterior tubercles of the transverse processes of C3–C6 and attaches on the inferior surface of the basilar part of the occipital bone. Underneath the longus capitis, the rectus capitis anterior spans from the lateral mass of the atlas to the base of the occipital bone. The rectus capitis lateralis runs laterally from the transverse process of the atlas to the inferior surface of the jugular process of the occipital bone.

The scalenus anterior originates from the anterior tubercles of the transverse processes of C3–C6 and inserts on the first rib. The scalenus medius originates from the posterior tubercles of the transverse processes of C2–C7 and inserts on the first rib. A vascular impingement of the subclavian artery may occur as it runs between the scalenus anterior and scalenus medius, as seen in the thoracic outlet syndrome. The scalenus posterior originates from the posterior tubercles of the transverse processes of C4–C6 and inserts on the second rib.

The posterior muscles of the neck are divided into superficial, intermediate, and deep groups.[33] The most superficial muscle is the trapezius, which originates from the external occipital protuberance and the medial nuchal line of C7–T12 spinous processes and inserts on the spine of the scapula, the acromion, and the lateral aspect of the clavicle. The trapezius is innervated by the 11th cranial nerve and functions to extend the head. The intermediate muscles beneath the trapezius muscle are the splenius capitis and splenius cervicis, which originate from the spinous processes of the lower cervical and upper thoracic spines and insert on the transverse processes of the upper cervical spine and the mastoid process. In the deep layer, the erector spinal muscles continue into the cervical region, which includes the iliocostalis laterally; the longissimus cervicis and longissimus capitis centrally; and the spinalis cervicis, semispinalis capitis, and semispinalis cervicis medially. Beneath the semispinalis muscles lie the multifidus from C4–C7 and rotatores muscles, which cross only one segment from the transverse processes to the spinous processes.

In the upper cervical spine, suboccipital muscles attach at the occiput to the second vertebra. The rectus capitis posterior major originates from the C2 spinous process and inserts to the inferior nuchal line of the occiput, and the rectus capitis posterior minor originates from the posterior tubercle of the atlas and inserts to the occiput. The obliquus capitis inferior originates from the C2 spinous process and inserts on the transverse process of the atlas, and the obliquus capitis superior originates from the transverse process of the atlas and inserts on the occiput between the superior and inferior nuchal lines. Most posterior muscles are involved in producing extension of the neck and head, and some muscles produce rotation and lateral flexion. The posterior deep muscles are innervated by the posterior primary rami, and the blood supply is by the deep cervical vessels.

Fascial Layers

The key to understanding the anterior approach to the cervical spine lies in recognizing the fascial layers of the neck, which invest the muscles and viscera and separate them into different compartments.[20] Anteriorly, the cervical fascia is divided into one superficial and four deep layers. The superficial fascia contains fat and areolar tissue, including the platysma muscle, external jugular vein, and cutaneous sensory nerves. The deep cervical fascia, including the outer investing layer of deep fascia, middle cervical fascia, and prevertebral fascia, compartmentalizes the structures deep to the superficial fascia. The superficial layer of the deep fascia extends from the trapezius muscle over the posterior triangle and splits to enclose the sternocleidomastoid muscle. The middle layers of the deep cervical fascia enclose the strap muscles and omohyoid and extend as far laterally as the scapula. The deeper middle layer is the visceral fascia that surrounds the thyroid gland, larynx, trachea, pharynx, and esophagus. The alar fascia spreads behind the esophagus and surrounds the carotid sheath structures laterally. The carotid sheath encloses the carotid artery, internal jugular vein, and vagus nerve. The deepest layer of the deep fascia is the prevertebral fascia, which covers the scaleni muscles, longus colli muscles, and anterior longitudinal ligament.

Understanding these fascial planes also helps localize the source of cervical infections. Abscesses originating from either the vertebral body or the intervertebral disc generally start in the midline, whereas abscesses that are pharyngeal in origin tend to occur lateral to the midline. This is because the prevertebral fascia and alar fascia are fused laterally over the transverse processes, but not in the midline. If this infection breaks through the prevertebral fascia, it can spread inferiorly between the alar fascia and prevertebral fascia into the posterior mediastinum. With pharyngeal infections, the opposite occurs because the visceral fascia and alar fascia are fused in the midline; these abscesses tend to occur laterally, on either side of the midline.

Triangles of the Neck

The cervical region is divided into two anatomic compartments, the anterior and posterior triangles, by the sternocleidomastoid. The anterior triangle is formed by the midline anteriorly, the anterior border of the sternocleidomastoid posteriorly, and the inferior border of the mandible superiorly. The posterior triangle is bound anteriorly by the posterior border of the sternocleidomastoid, posteriorly by the anterior border of the trapezius, and inferiorly by the middle third of the clavicle. Understanding the structures within the triangles and their complex relationship helps the surgeon to learn these important landmarks during surgical approaches to the neck.[6]

The anterior triangle is subdivided further into the digastric (submandibular), carotid, and muscular triangles. The digastric triangle, so called because it is bound by the two bellies of the digastric muscle as well as the inferior border of the mandible, contains the submandibular gland; facial artery and vein; mylohyoid artery and nerve; and, posteriorly, a portion of the parotid gland and external carotid artery. Lying deeper in the digastric triangle is the internal carotid artery, jugular vein, and glossopharyngeal and vagus nerves. The carotid and muscular triangles are separated by the superior belly of the omohyoid muscle. The carotid triangle contains the carotid artery and its bifurcation; the superior thyroid, lingual, and facial branches of the external carotid artery; and the internal jugular vein. It also contains the ansa cervicalis; portions of cranial nerves X, XI, and XII; and the larynx, pharynx, and superior laryngeal nerve.

The posterior triangle is subdivided into the occipital and supraclavicular triangles by the inferior belly of the omohyoid muscle. The posterior triangle contains the accessory nerve, the brachial plexus, the third part of the subclavian artery, the dorsal scapular nerve, the long thoracic nerve, the nerve to the subclavius, the suprascapular nerve, and the transverse cervical artery.[19]

The brachial plexus travels behind the inferior belly of the omohyoid, crossing between the anterior and middle scalene muscles and over the first rib and beneath the clavicle. Its location in the posterior triangle can be identified by drawing a line from the posterior margin of the sternocleidomastoid at the level of the cricoid cartilage to the midpoint of the clavicle. The accessory nerve lies on the levator scapula on the floor of the posterior triangle. Emerging from behind the posterior border of the sternocleidomastoid muscle are the lesser occipital, greater auricular, and supraclavicular nerves. The subclavian artery lies inferior to the inferior belly of the omohyoid in the subclavian triangle and courses behind the anterior scalene laterally toward the border of the first rib.

Surgical Approaches

Although surgical approaches to the cervical spine are well described in the literature, certain approaches are more commonly used than others. A decision to use a particular approach should take into account the site of the pathologic process, the health of the patient, and the skill and comfort level of the surgeon with that specific exposure. An understanding of the advantages and limitations of each surgical exposure can help improve patient outcome and reduce complications. In this section, anterior and posterior operative approaches from the occiput to the cervicothoracic junction are described with their associated complications.

Anterior Approaches to Upper Cervical Spine

The complex anatomy of the upper neck makes adequate and safe exposure of the upper cervical spine challenging. The two main techniques are transoral and retropharyngeal exposures. If necessary, both techniques can be combined with a mandibulotomy or dislocation of the temporomandibular joint to gain additional local exposure.

The transoral approach provides anterior exposure to the atlantoaxial complex. Inferior exposure down to C3–C4 can be obtained with the addition of a lip-splitting approach with mandibulotomy, whereas superior exposure up to the clivus of the occiput can be obtained by splitting the uvula, soft palate, and posterior pharyngeal wall.[34,35] If necessary, a portion of the hard palate can also be cut with a rongeur. Thoughtful placement of a self-retaining retractor system also facilitates exposure by retraction of the hard and soft palate and tongue.

Several variations to the retropharyngeal exposure have been described, which can be divided into anteromedial and anterolateral approaches depending on the relationship of the dissection to the carotid sheath.[36–38] The anteromedial retropharyngeal approach uses the interval medial (anterior) to the carotid sheath, whereas the anterolateral approach uses the plane lateral (posterior) to the carotid sheath. In both cases, a thorough understanding of the local anatomy is imperative. For right-handed surgeons, the approach is typically from the patient's right side. At this level, above C5, the recurrent laryngeal nerve has already crossed the surgical field from lateral to medial and runs safely within the tracheoesophageal groove.

Transoral Technique

The transoral technique requires broad-spectrum antibiotic administration prior to incision. Antibiotics should cover both gram-positive and gram-negative bacteria.[39] It is further recommended to continue antibiotics for 3 days following surgery. Care must be exercised during this approach to stay in the midline and develop full-thickness pharyngomucosal flaps. A vertical incision is made through the posterior pharyngeal mucosa, the constrictors, and the longus colli muscle with the anterior arch of the atlas as the landmark. The incision should be directly down to bone. In total, the incision should be 3 to 5 cm in length, with its midpoint approximately 1 cm caudal to the anterior tubercle of C1. After adequate superior and inferior exposure is obtained, subperiosteal lateral dissection is done to expose the medial edge of the C1–C2 facet joint and can extend as far laterally as the lateral masses. Dissection beyond the lateral edge of the C1–C2 facet risks injury to the vertebral artery, which usually lies at a minimum of 20 mm from the midline.[40]

In a pure transoral approach, exposure is limited by the interdental distance and the degree of neck extension. Recommended interdental distances to allow an appropriate surgical corridor should be at least 25 mm. Associated pathologies, including temporomandibular joint stiffness, cervical kyphosis, and basilar invagination, can hinder the surgical approach. Use of a Mayfield retractor and a roll beneath the shoulder blades can allow appropriate neck hyperextension to facilitate the approach. The addition of a mandibulotomy can further increase exposure. The mandibulotomy is achieved with a midline incision of the lower lip around the chin in a C-shaped fashion and then straight down to the hyoid bone to expose the mandible subperiosteally.[41] Titanium plates are then fit for later closure; screw holes should be drilled before the actual osteotomy is performed, as this all decreases the risk of postoperative malocclusion. The mandible is then osteotomized between the central incisors, without overt removal of an incisor. Another incision is then made to divide the inferior mouth mucosa, with the incision falling between the submaxillary duct orifices and beneath the tongue. The divided mandible is then retracted laterally. If the decision is made to split the tongue as well, this should be done in the midline, with care taken not to injure the epiglottis.[41]

Complications

Reported results with this exposure are variable. Although access to the upper cervical vertebra through this approach is relatively direct, the potential for significant morbidity and mortality exists owing to the risk of infection by pharyngeal flora, the confined working area, and the lack of extensile exposure.[42] Complications can be minimized with careful patient selection and proper surgical technique.

Infection is a frequently reported complication with the transoral approach,[43] particularly with extensive resections and use of bone graft. Direct contamination and septic encephalomeningitis can occur through direct exposure or opening of the dura. In a series reported by Fang and Ong[43] in six patients who underwent extensive vertebral body resection and bone grafting, four developed wound infections, and one developed encephalomeningitis. In a separate study of 10 patients in whom the transoral approach was used to treat irreducible craniovertebral junction anomalies, one patient had a retropharyngeal infection, which was ultimately treated with saline irrigation, reclosure, and antibiotics.[44] Using perioperative antibiotics, limiting the use of bone graft when possible, and minimizing the exposure and resection can help decrease these risks. The use of a nasogastric tube postoperatively for 5 days until evidence of mucosal healing may decrease wound contamination.

Difficulty with wound closure may also occur. In the Lee et al series,[44] two patients were noted to have wound dehiscence that required resuturing. Dehiscence is a particular risk if the incision extends down to C3, where the overlying tissues can be thin and intimately adherent to the underlying vertebral body. Difficulty with wound closure can also occur if bone grafting is excessive or placed improperly. This difficulty can be managed by ensuring that the grafts are recessed beyond the anterior margin of the vertebral body or by creating lateral flaps to help provide additional tissue length to assist in coverage.

Vascular complications are also an inherent risk of this procedure. Venous hemorrhage from epidural veins can typically be controlled with the use of cellulose and cottonoid patties. Arterial hemorrhage owing to injury to the vertebral artery or its branches can be more problematic. Excessive or uncontrolled bleeding can occur if the dissection is not performed subperiosteally or strays too lateral into the vertebral arteries. Life-threatening hemorrhage or basilar artery ischemia can result, especially in elderly patients. Tamponade of the bleeding with hemostatic agents and bone wax may result in a false aneurysm or late bleeding, requiring urgent surgery or balloon embolization.[40] Uncontrolled bleeding often requires emergent balloon embolization or immediate surgical exposure of the vertebral artery in the foramen transversarium for ligation.

After surgery, the airway remains at risk from edema, hemorrhage, or continued drainage. Due to this risk, some patients may require endotracheal (ET) tube retention for a full day following surgery. ET tube retention is often determined by assessment of soft tissue swelling on postoperative lateral cervical radiographs. A nasogastric tube is also placed and retained for 5 to 7 days to prevent reflux.[45] Careful intraoperative placement of retractors to ensure that the tongue and lips are not trapped and the application of topical hydrocortisone can help decrease postoperative oropharyngeal edema. If a tongue-splitting approach is planned, a tracheotomy should be considered.

Anteromedial Retropharyngeal Technique

Described by deAndrade and McNab in 1969[37] and later by McAfee and colleagues in 1987,[36] the anteromedial retropharyngeal approach is the superior extension of the anteromedial approach to the lower cervical spine, as described by Southwick and Robinson.[46] Similar to the anteromedial approach to the lower cervical spine, familiarity with the fascial planes is vital to understanding the approach. These planes include (1) the superficial fascia containing the platysma; (2) the superficial layer of the deep fascia extending from the sternocleidomastoid anteriorly and enclosing the trapezius posteriorly; (3) the middle layer of the deep fascia covering the strap muscles and omohyoid and visceral fascia surrounding the thyroid gland, larynx, trachea, pharynx, and esophagus; and (4) the deep layer of the cervical fascia, which includes the alar fascia connecting the two carotid sheaths laterally and fusing in the midline to the visceral fascia and the prevertebral fascia covering the scaleni and longus colli muscles and the anterior longitudinal ligament (Fig. 18.7).

A transverse submandibular incision is used in this approach, extending from the mastoid process and extending to the midline at the level of the hyoid. To complete a T-shaped incision, the opening is extended along the anterior aspect of the sternocleidomastoid muscle (Fig. 18.8A). The platysma and the superficial layer of the deep cervical fascia are divided in line with the incision to expose the anterior border of the sternocleidomastoid (Fig. 18.8B). With the help of a nerve stimulator, the marginal mandibular branch of the facial nerve (cranial nerve VII) is isolated and protected. Because the branches of the mandibular nerve are superficial to the lateral crossing veins, ligating the retromandibular vein as it joins the internal jugular vein and keeping the dissection deep and inferior to the vein during the exposure help protect the superficial branch of the facial nerve.

Next, the superficial layer of the deep cervical fascia is incised anterior to the sternocleidomastoid, and the carotid sheath is identified by palpating for the carotid pulse. The digastric lymph nodes and submandibular gland are resected, and the salivary duct is sutured to prevent a fistula. The stylohyoid and digastric muscle are identified and ligated to help mobilize the hyoid bone to improve exposure. Injury to the facial nerve may occur with excessive superior traction of the stylohyoid muscle. The nerve stimulator is used to identify and completely mobilize the hypoglossal nerve, which is retracted superiorly.

The retropharyngeal space is entered by using blunt dissection to develop the plane between the carotid sheath laterally and the visceral fascia containing the larynx and pharynx medially. Exposure can be improved by sequentially ligating tethering branches of the carotid artery and jugular vein, which may include the superior thyroid artery and vein, lingual artery and vein, ascending pharyngeal artery and vein, and facial artery and vein (Fig. 18.8C). The superior laryngeal nerve is identified, protected, and mobilized as it travels from its origin near the nodose ganglion into the larynx.

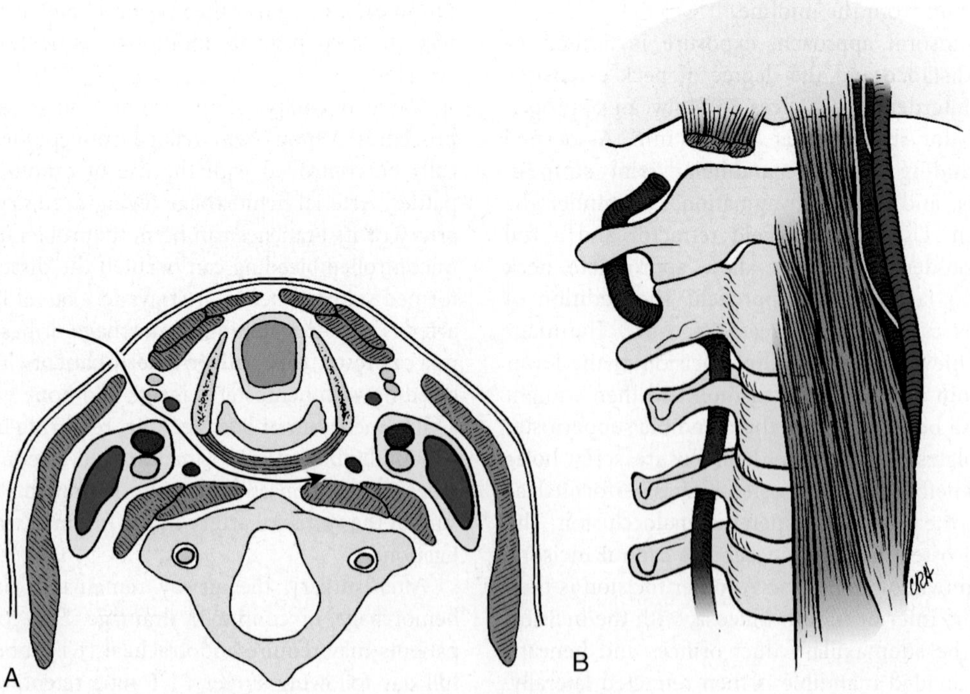

FIG. 18.7 Anteromedial approach to the upper cervical spine. (A) Dissection is done through a retropharyngeal approach as an extension of the Southwick-Robinson approach to the lower cervical spine. (B) The longus colli muscle is retracted to expose the anterior tubercle of the atlas and body of axis.

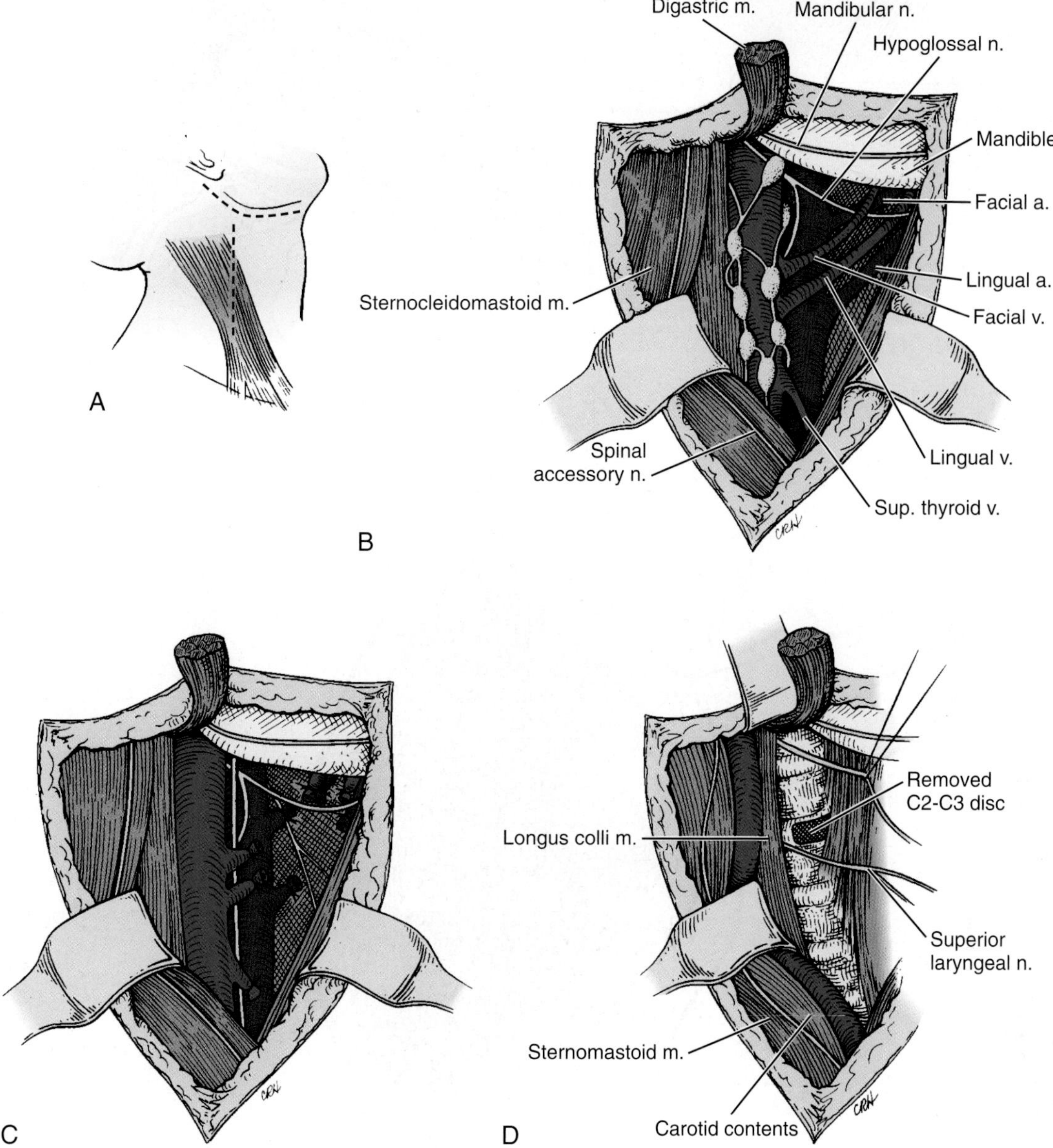

FIG. 18.8 (A) Right-sided submandibular transverse incision. (B) The anterior border of the sternocleidomastoid muscle is mobilized, and the digastric tendon is divided. The submandibular salivary gland and jugular digastric lymph nodes are resected. The hypoglossal nerve is identified and mobilized. (C) The carotid sheath is opened, and the arterial and venous branches are ligated. (D) The superior laryngeal nerve is identified and protected.

The prevertebral fascia overlying the vertebral body, intervertebral disc, and longus colli are now visible (Fig. 18.8D). The two longus colli converge in the midline on the anterior tubercle of the atlas. Because the hypoglossal, glossopharyngeal, vagus, and accessory nerves and the internal carotid artery and jugular vein are tethered to the occiput as they exit their respective foramina, they can be injured with vigorous retraction or greater than 2 cm lateral dissection from the midline. Additionally, excess anterior retraction of the pharynx can result in injury to the pharyngeal and laryngeal branches of the vagus nerve. At this point, a midline incision over the basiocciput, atlas, and axis can be performed, and the anterior longitudinal ligament and longus colli muscle can be dissected subperiosteally to obtain lateral exposure to the cervical spine.

Anterolateral Retropharyngeal Technique

Described by Whitesides and Kelly,[47] the anterolateral retropharyngeal approach provides exposure of the upper cervical spine by partially transecting the sternocleidomastoid and proceeding laterally and posterior to the carotid sheath (Fig. 18.9). As a result, the major branches of the external carotid and laryngeal nerves are not disturbed. Although this exposure allows for distal extension to include T1, its superior extension is limited to the ring of the atlas. Because the internal carotid artery; jugular vein; and vagus, accessory, and hypoglossal nerves are tethered to the skull, adequate retraction necessary to expose the basiocciput would result in injury to these structures.

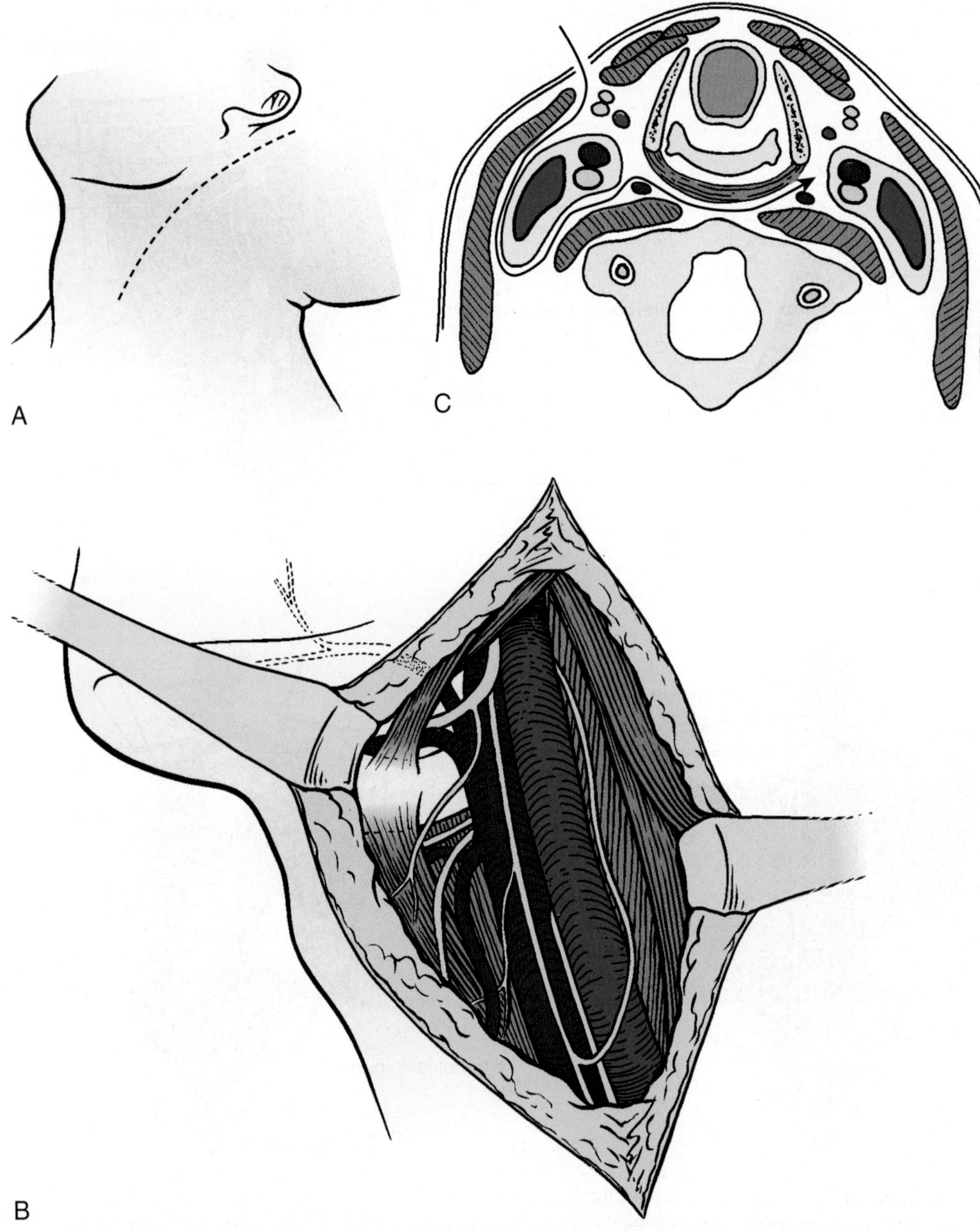

FIG. 18.9 Anterolateral retropharyngeal approach. (A) A skin incision is made from the mastoid along the anterior aspect of the sternocleidomastoid. (B) This approach involves dissection anterior to the sternocleidomastoid but posterior to the carotid sheath. (C) Neurovascular structures that are encountered in this approach include the carotid contents and branches, superior laryngeal nerves, hypoglossal nerve, and ansa cervicalis.

A longitudinal skin incision is made from the mastoid extending distally and anteriorly along the anterior aspect of the sternocleidomastoid muscle. The external jugular vein is identified and ligated, and the greater auricular nerve running parallel to the external jugular vein is spared if possible. The sternocleidomastoid now is prominent; if only a limited exposure (C1–C2) is required, consideration can be given to preserving the sternocleidomastoid. In most cases, the sternocleidomastoid and splenius capitis muscles are detached from the mastoid, leaving a fascial edge for later repair. The spinal accessory nerve enters the sternocleidomastoid approximately 3 cm distal to the mastoid tip, which should be identified and protected.[47]

Next, one can proceed laterally and posterior to the carotid sheath and dissect it free from the sternocleidomastoid. The carotid contents are retracted along with the hypoglossal nerve anteriorly and the sternocleidomastoid muscle and accessory nerve posteriorly. The plane between the alar and prevertebral fascia is developed with blunt dissection to expose the transverse processes and anterior aspect of C1–C3. The most pronounced bony prominence laterally is the transverse process of C1. Although the basiocciput, clivus, and sphenoid may be palpated through this approach, they are poorly visualized.

When the appropriate level is identified, a midline longitudinal incision is made in the middle of the vertebral body, and the ligament and overlying muscles are dissected subperiosteally and laterally. Alternatively, if more lateral exposure is needed, the longus colli and capitis muscles can be separated from their bony insertion on the transverse process and retracted anteriorly. This provides direct exposure to the nerve roots, transverse processes, and vertebral artery, but disturbs the sympathetic rami communicantes and may cause Horner syndrome.

Complications

Complications common to the anterolateral and anteromedial retropharyngeal approaches include airway obstruction, hemorrhage, and nerve injury. Airway obstruction and difficulty swallowing secondary to hematoma or edema of the pharynx and larynx can be an immediate life-threatening complication. Typically, nasotracheal intubation is adequate; however, a tracheostomy can be considered either preoperatively or postoperatively for airway management if this complication is expected or encountered. Hemorrhage from the carotid artery, jugular vein, or their branches can occur and can be difficult to control.

Laryngeal and pharyngeal dysfunction can result from retraction of the laryngeal nerves. Patients should be advised preoperatively to expect difficulty with phonation and swallowing, especially in the early postoperative course. Problems can persist if the external branch of the superior laryngeal nerve is sacrificed or transected. In three of five cases reported by deAndrade and McNab,[37] persistent postoperative hoarseness, laryngeal fatigue, and inability to produce high tones persisted. Nerve injury to the spinal accessory nerve can occur, particularly with the anterolateral retropharyngeal approach. Care should be taken to identify and protect this nerve intraoperatively as iatrogenic damage can result in weakness of the sternocleidomastoid and trapezius muscles postoperatively.

Anterior Exposure of Lower Cervical Spine

Similar to approaches to the upper cervical spine, anterior exposures to the lower cervical spine can be divided into anterolateral and anteromedial approaches based on their relationship to the carotid sheath. First described by Southwick and Robinson,[46] the anteromedial approach employs the interval between the sternocleidomastoid laterally and the strap muscles and tracheoesophageal complex medially and is used in most cases. In special circumstances, the anterolateral approach described by Henry[48] and Hogson[49] may be used. Hogson[49] described an approach to the lower cervical spine in which dissection was done posterior to the carotid sheath to expose the anterior and lateral aspects. Verbiest[50] described a modification of the original approach for the exposure of the vertebral artery. Dissection anterior to the carotid sheath, as in the anteromedial Smith-Robinson technique, provides more lateral exposure to the cervical spine and may be better in cases in which the lesion is localized more laterally or if the vertebral artery must be exposed. The spinal nerve can also be identified posterior to the vertebral artery (Fig. 18.10).

To minimize injury to the recurrent laryngeal nerve, the cervical spine is often approached from the left, particularly at the C6–T1 region. Although a right-handed surgeon may prefer the right-sided approach, the recurrent laryngeal nerve is at greater risk of injury because it may leave the carotid sheath at a higher level on the right side. The hyoid bone overlies the third vertebra, the thyroid cartilage overlies the C4–C5 intervertebral disc space, and the cricoid ring is at the C6 vertebra (Fig. 18.11).[6] In many cases, when the neck is in

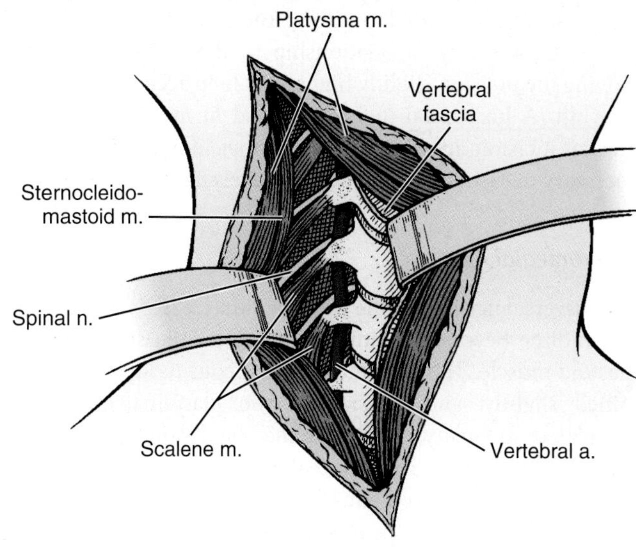

FIG. 18.10 Verbiest's approach. The sternocleidomastoid and carotid sheath are identified and retracted laterally, and visceral structures are retracted medially. The anterior tubercle of the transverse process is identified by palpation. Muscular insertions of the longus colli, longus capitis, and anterior scalene are dissected sharply to the bone, and the anterior tubercle is cleared of soft tissues. The costotransverse lamellae can be resected to provide exposure to the vertebral artery and spinal nerve lying posteriorly.

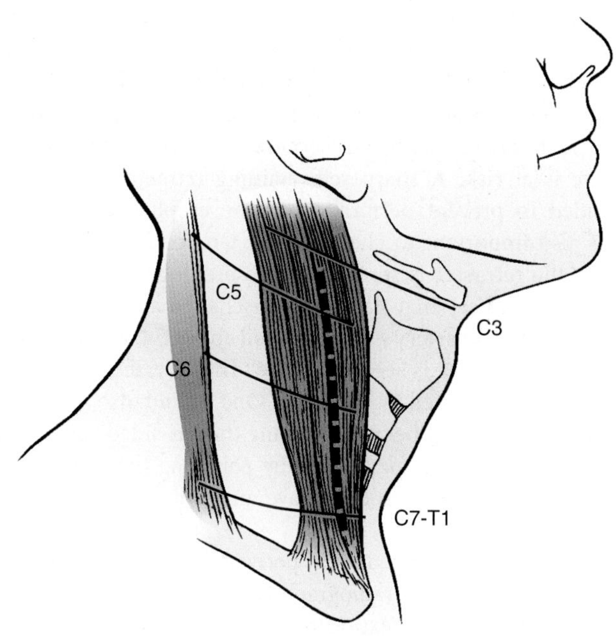

FIG. 18.11 Surface anatomy can help identify the approximate level of vertebral bodies in the cervical spine. The hyoid bone overlies C3, thyroid cartilage overlies C5, the cricoid ring is at C6, and the supraclavicular level is in the C7–T1 region.

a significantly extended position, these landmarks may be displaced inferiorly in relationship to the vertebral bodies; moving the incision slightly higher can help accommodate for the shift. A horizontal incision is used in most cases, but a vertical incision anterior to the sternocleidomastoid may be necessary in cases in which multiple levels need to be exposed.

Anteromedial Approach

A transverse incision in line with the skin crease is made from the midline beyond the anterior aspect of the sternocleidomastoid muscle. The skin and subcutaneous tissue are undermined slightly, and division of the platysma muscle is completed. The platysma muscle may be divided either horizontally or vertically. Retraction of the divided muscle exposes the sternocleidomastoid muscle laterally and strap muscles medially. The anterior and external jugular veins may be encountered and can be ligated to improve exposure. The deep cervical fascia is divided between the sternocleidomastoid muscle and strap muscles, and blunt finger dissection is done through the pretracheal fascia while palpating and retracting the carotid sheath laterally.

A self-retaining retractor is positioned to expose the prevertebral fascia and longus colli muscles. One must be careful not to enter the carotid sheath laterally to avoid injury to the carotid artery, internal jugular vein, or vagus nerve. Great caution should also be exercised medially because the strap muscles surround the thyroid gland, trachea, and esophagus. The surgical dissection should not enter the plane between the trachea and esophagus because the recurrent laryngeal nerve is at risk. A sharp self-retaining retractor should be avoided to prevent perforation of the esophagus medially. It is also important to check for the temporal arterial pulse when the retractor is spread because prolonged occlusion of the carotid artery may cause brain ischemia and stroke. The superior thyroid artery is encountered above C4, and the inferior thyroid artery is seen below C6. These vessels should be identified and ligated as necessary. One should also be aware of the thoracic duct below C7 during the left-sided approach. Further dissection is performed by palpating the prominent disc margins ("hills") and concave anterior vertebral bodies ("valleys").

A hemostat is clamped to the perivertebral fascia to localize the level, and a lateral radiograph is taken. When the correct level is confirmed, the exposure is completed by dividing the pretracheal fascia and anterior longitudinal ligament in the midline to minimize bleeding and prevent injury to the sympathetic chain and subperiosteal mobilization of the longus colli laterally. Too vigorous lateral dissection may damage the vertebral artery or nerve roots, especially at the level of the intervertebral disc space.[20] At the level of the vertebral body, the anterior aspect of the foramen transversarium offers some protection to the vertebral artery.

Anterolateral Approach

By performing the dissection posterior to the carotid sheath, the anterolateral approach avoids the thyroid vessel, vagus nerve, and superior laryngeal nerve, and provides access to the anterior and lateral aspect of the cervical spine. Superior extension of this approach allows access to the upper cervical spine as described by Whitesides and Kelly[47] (see "Anterolateral Retropharyngeal Technique"). A transverse or oblique skin incision is made from the right side. The subcutaneous tissue and the platysma muscle are divided, and the branches of the external jugular vein are ligated, but the cutaneous nerves should be protected if possible. The posterior border of the sternocleidomastoid muscle is identified; blunt dissection should follow the fat pad through the posterior triangle of the cervical spine. The dissection should stay anterior to the anterior scalene muscle and anterior to the anterior tubercle of the transverse process to avoid injuries to the vertebral artery or nerve root. If retraction of the sternocleidomastoid muscle is difficult, the posterior third and the omohyoid muscle can be divided to enhance exposure. The cervical sympathetic plexus on the lateral aspect of the prevertebral musculature should be identified and protected. The prevertebral fascia and longus colli muscle are incised in the midline for subperiosteal exposure of the cervical spine. After palpation of the anterior tubercle of the transverse process, the anterior tubercle can be removed to gain access to the vertebral artery and venous plexus.

Complications

The most devastating complication is neurologic deterioration. Most spinal cord or nerve root injuries are associated with technical mishaps. In myelopathic patients, attention should be paid to proper positioning of the neck, fiberoptic nasotracheal awake intubation, and intraoperative monitoring of the spinal cord function. Utmost care should be taken when removing osteophytes and disc material in the lateral corner near the uncovertebral joint to avoid nerve root injury. If removal of the posterior longitudinal ligament or osteophytes is necessary because of perforating disc fragments or large osteophytes, an operating microscope should be used. If neurologic complications are discovered postoperatively, one should administer dexamethasone and obtain a lateral radiograph to determine the position of the bone graft. Computed tomography (CT) or magnetic resonance imaging (MRI) may be valuable in determining hematoma or cord contusion. If hematoma or bone graft is suspected to be the cause of postoperative myelopathy, expeditious re-exploration is required.

Airway obstruction after extubation may occur in the postoperative period. One must be certain that the patient can exchange air before extubation. In cases in which multiple vertebrectomy has been performed with retraction of soft tissues for a prolonged period, intubation should continue for a few days until retropharyngeal edema subsides. Corticosteroids may be used to decrease edema in these cases. Postoperatively, a patient who underwent a prolonged operation for decompression of the spinal cord should be intubated for 2 to 3 days until retropharyngeal edema subsides. Corticosteroids may decrease severe edema in the postoperative period. Airway obstruction and difficulty with swallowing because of retropharyngeal edema may require reintubation or tracheostomy.

Serious bleeding complications after anterior cervical surgery are rare, but hematoma-related wound complications are common, with an incidence of 5.6% in one series.[51] Arterial bleeding from the superior or inferior thyroid artery can be prevented by careful identification and ligation during surgery. Care should be taken not to dissect too far laterally because the vertebral artery is in danger along with the nerve roots. Tears on the vertebral artery should be repaired by direct exposure of the vessel in the foramen rather than merely packing the bleeding site. Injuries to the carotid artery or internal jugular vein are exceedingly rare. A hematoma rarely may be responsible for airway obstruction or spinal cord compression. The patient should have the head elevated in the immediate postoperative period because the source of bleeding is frequently venous. Meticulous hemostasis and placement of a drain should be routine to prevent these complications.

Esophageal perforation is a rare but serious complication of anterior cervical spine fusion, occurring in about 1 of 500 procedures. Sharp retractors must be avoided, and gentle handling of the medial soft structures is mandatory. In revision cases, the use of a nasogastric tube may help identify the esophagus intraoperatively. If perforation is suspected during surgery, methylene blue can be injected for better visualization. The perforation is frequently not recognized until the patient develops an abscess, tracheoesophageal fistula, or mediastinitis in the postoperative period.[52] The usual treatment consists of intravenous antibiotics, nasogastric feeding, drainage, débridement, and repair. Early consultation with head and neck surgeons is recommended.

Minor hoarseness or sore throat after anterior cervical fusion may be due to edema or endotracheal intubation, and occurs in nearly half of the patients. Recurrent laryngeal nerve palsy may be the cause of persistent hoarseness in a few patients, however. As many as 11% of patients may experience some degree of recurrent laryngeal nerve palsy following anterior cervical spine surgery,[53] with permanent hoarseness occurring in 2% to 4% of patients.[54] The superior laryngeal nerve is a branch of the inferior ganglion of the vagus nerve, and travels along with the superior thyroid artery to innervate the cricothyroid muscle. Damage to this nerve may result in hoarseness, but often produces symptoms such as easy fatiguing of the voice. The inferior laryngeal nerve is a recurrent branch of the vagus nerve that innervates all laryngeal muscles except the cricothyroid.

On the left side, the recurrent laryngeal nerve loops under the arch of the aorta and is protected in the left tracheoesophageal groove. On the right side, the recurrent nerve travels around the subclavian artery, passing dorsomedial to the side of the trachea and esophagus. It is vulnerable as it passes from the subclavian artery to the right tracheoesophageal groove. The recurrent laryngeal nerve should be located when working from C6 downward. The best guideline to its location is the inferior thyroid artery. The nerve usually enters the tracheoesophageal groove where the inferior thyroid artery enters the lower pole of the thyroid. It is also more common for the right inferior laryngeal nerve to be nonrecurrent where it travels directly from the vagus nerve and carotid sheath to the larynx. The incidence of nonrecurrent laryngeal nerve on the right side can be as high as 2.7%.[55]

If hoarseness persists for more than 6 weeks after anterior cervical surgery, laryngoscopy should be done to evaluate the vocal cord and laryngeal muscles. Treatment of the inferior laryngeal nerve should include waiting at least 6 months for spontaneous recovery of function to occur. Further treatment or surgery by the otolaryngologist may be necessary in persistent cases.

Injury to the sympathetic chain may result in Horner syndrome. The cervical sympathetic chain lies on the anterior surface of the longus colli muscles posterior to the carotid sheath. Subperiosteal dissection is important to prevent damage to these nerves. Horner syndrome is usually temporary but may be permanent in some cases. The incidence of permanent Horner syndrome is less than 1%. Ophthalmologic consultation may be needed for treatment of ptosis.

Anterior Approach to Cervicothoracic Junction

Anterior approaches to the cervicothoracic junction are challenging because of the proximity of the great vessels and overlying sternum and clavicle (Fig. 18.12). Three main approaches have been described to address access in this region: the modified anterior approach, the sternal-splitting approach, and the transthoracic approach.[56-58] Each approach has its own advantages and disadvantages, thus should be chosen accordingly. Theoretically, the modified anterior approach can provide visualization and access to the anterior spinal structures from C4 to T4, but requires resection of the medial clavicle and sternoclavicular joint. Similarly, the sternal-splitting approach, when combined with the anteromedial approach to the neck, offers access from C4 to T4 through retraction of the great vessels. Although the transthoracic approach provides adequate exposure to the upper thoracic spine, access to the cervical spine is limited to C7 at best. Given inherent accessibility challenges, multiple algorithms dependent on imaging and demographic variables have been developed to assess accessibility.[59,60]

Modified Anterior Approach

The patient is positioned supine on the operating table with a bump between the scapula. Typically, an angled incision is used for this approach. The transverse limb is made 2 cm proximal to and parallel to the left clavicle extending from the midline to the lateral border of the sternocleidomastoid. The transverse limb is generally left sided, as the left recurrent laryngeal nerve has a less variable path.[61] The vertical limb runs from the medial aspect of the transverse incision and extends just distally past the manubriosternal junction. The platysma is divided in line with the skin incision and undermined proximally and distally to mobilize the muscle. In some instances, the superficial veins and external jugular vein are mobilized. However, they may need to be cauterized as necessary for exposure.

The strap muscles and sternocleidomastoid are dissected and divided subperiosteally off the medial clavicle and

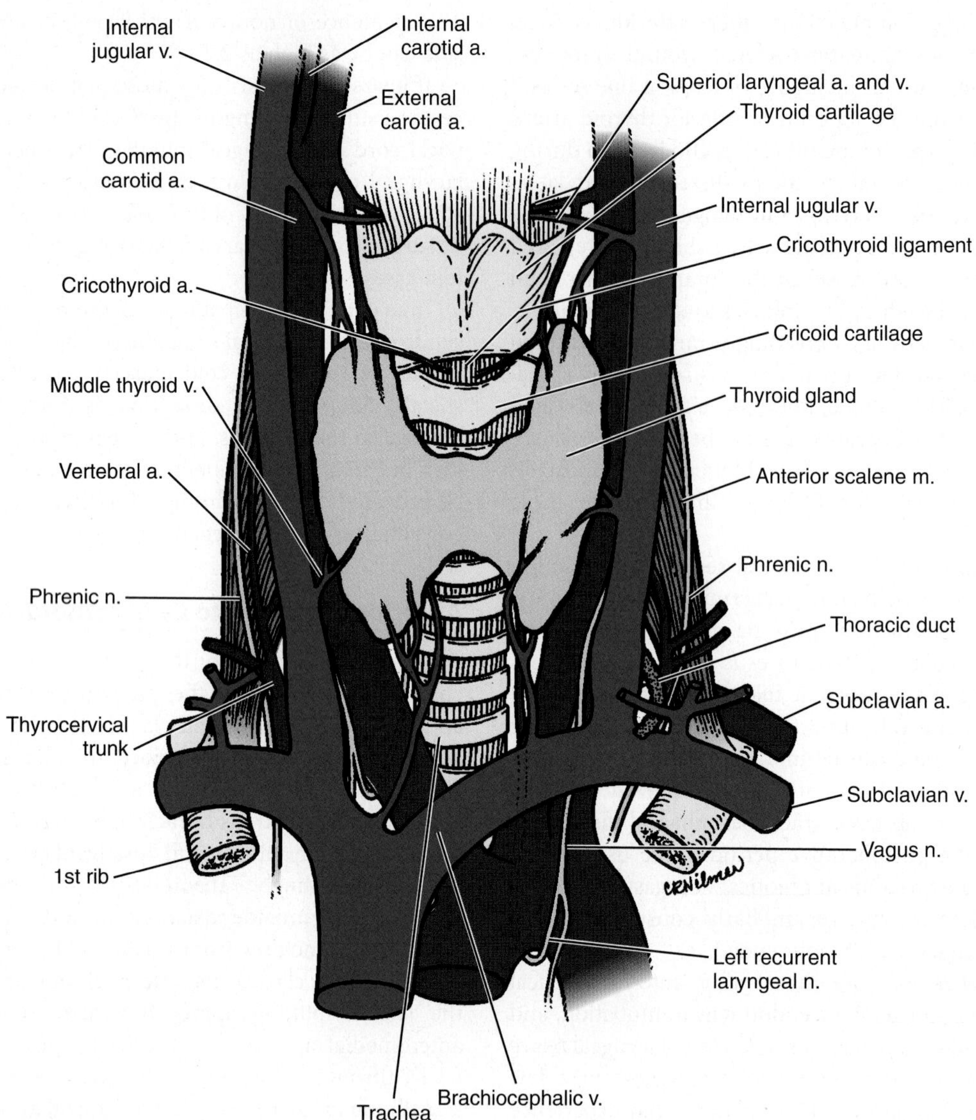

FIG. 18.12 Anterior access to the cervicothoracic junction is complicated by proximity of the great vessels and associated neural structures.

manubrium, and retracted proximally. With care taken to avoid the subclavian vein, the clavicle is osteotomized at the junction of the middle and medial third and disarticulated from the manubrium with division of the first costal cartilage. In some cases, the inferior thyroid vein may lie medially in the surgical field and require ligation for exposure.

Next, the interval is developed between the carotid sheath laterally and the strap muscles, esophagus, and trachea medially. The recurrent laryngeal nerve muscle must be identified from the right-sided approach, whereas the thoracic duct must be protected and spared with the left-sided approach. At this level, the recurrent laryngeal nerve already lies safely within the tracheoesophageal groove with a left-sided approach.

With the use of hand-held retractors, the cervicothoracic junction can now be accessed by carefully mobilizing the esophagus, trachea, and right brachiocephalic artery and vein toward the patient's right, while the left carotid sheath and brachiocephalic and subclavian veins are retracted to the left. The prevertebral fascia overlying the anterior aspect of the vertebrae from C4 to T4 can now be visualized.

Sternal-Splitting Approach

Combined with the anteromedial approach to the cervical spine, the sternal-splitting approach provides access to the cervicothoracic junction from C4 to T4, particularly in obese or muscular patients. A vertical skin incision is made anterior to the left sternocleidomastoid muscle and extended along the midline from the suprasternal notch proximally to the xiphoid process distally. Proximally, after division of the platysma muscle and superficial cervical fascia, blunt dissection is performed between the laterally situated carotid sheath and medial visceral structures. Distally, the subcutaneous soft tissue over the sternum is divided in line with the skin incision, and the retrosternal space is developed with blunt finger dissection. This helps reflect the parietal pleura from the posterior surface of the sternum and costal cartilage. The sternum is cut longitudinally with an oscillating saw. The inferior thyroid vein located just proximal to the suprasternal notch must be avoided. A self-retainer is inserted to split the sternum.

Blunt dissection is performed from the cranial toward the caudal portion until the left brachiocephalic vein is exposed. As in the modified anterior approach to the cervicothoracic junction, the esophagus, trachea, left carotid sheath, left subclavian artery, and brachiocephalic vein are retracted to the patient's left, whereas the esophagus, trachea, and right brachiocephalic artery and vein are mobilized to the right. The prevertebral fascia can now be divided in the midline to provide access to the C4–T4 vertebral bodies.

Transthoracic Approach

With the patient in the left lateral decubitus position, the right chest is prepared and draped. The bony prominences are padded accordingly, and a left roll is placed in the axilla to prevent neurovascular compromise to the left upper extremity. A right-sided approach is preferred because of the location of the great vessels and heart in the left-sided approach. A standard thoracotomy centered on the third rib provides access to the upper thoracic vertebra, but exposure to the low cervical region is restricted. A first or second rib level entry does not improve access because these ribs are much shorter, and the scapula interferes posteriorly.

The incision is made beginning at the anterior axillary line and extending posteriorly to the lateral border of the paraspinal muscles. The scapula is retracted laterally by dividing the trapezius and latissimus dorsi muscles. The subscapular space is developed with blunt dissection, and the third rib is identified by counting down from the thoracic inlet.

While protecting the intercostal neurovascular bundle, the appropriate rib is subperiosteally dissected out and resected anteriorly and posteriorly as far as possible. A rib spreader is inserted, and the lung is retracted anteriorly. The parietal pleura is incised overlying the vertebral artery, making sure to identify the segmental vessels.

Complications

Postoperative weakness secondary to weakness of the shoulder girdle musculature from the joint resection can occur. The thoracic duct should be identified if approached from the left. If damaged, the thoracic duct should be doubly ligated proximally and distally to prevent chylothorax. Great caution should be taken to avoid injuries to the sympathetic nerves, the cupola of the pleura at the level of T1, the great vessels, and the thoracic duct, which passes into the left venous angle between the subclavian artery and the common carotid artery. Potential complications of this approach include restriction of scapular movement and paralysis of intercostal muscles owing to the muscle-splitting aspects of this dissection. We recommend use of this approach in older patients and perhaps in patients with malignant conditions.

Posterior Approaches

Posterior exposures to the cervical spine are among the safest and most used exposures for management of cervical spine disorders, allowing direct access to the posterior elements from the occiput to the thoracic spine.[6,62] The particular anatomy of the upper cervical spine and the transitional anatomy of the cervicothoracic junction should also be understood when approaching these regions posteriorly.

Posterior Approach to Upper Cervical Spine

The posterior approach to the upper cervical spine grants exquisite access to the posterior elements of the occiput, atlas, and axis, allowing for easy atlantoaxial and occipitocervical decompression and fusion. The exposure begins with a midline incision extending from the inion to the C4 spinous process, an incision length that can be tailored depending on the treated pathology. The incision should fall along an internervous plane in the midline that separates the muscles from the segmental innervation supplied by the right and left posterior rami of the cervical nerves. Staying in the midline, within the avascular plane of the ligamentum nuchae minimizes bleeding and the risk of injury to surrounding muscle tissue and neurovascular structures, while providing a stout tissue layer for tissue closure at the end of the case. This principle is especially important in the cervical spine as the posterior cervical musculature is particularly vascular.

If the location of pathology is at the occipitocervical junction, that is, in the case of basilar impression, fracture of the odontoid with C1 fracture, or tumor, bone landmarks can be used to determine the appropriate level. The external occipital protuberance and the spinous process of C2 can typically be easily palpated, with the incision made from the inion caudad approximately 8 cm. As discussed earlier, the dissection is continued through the ligamentum nuchae, and the paraspinal muscles are stripped from C3 to the occiput. The surgeon should be cautious when dissecting at the inferior edge of the foramen magnum because uncontrollable bleeding from a group of veins present in this location may be encountered. Sharp subperiosteal dissection of the external occipital protuberance and lamina is performed, and care is taken to protect the vertebral arteries at the lateral border of the atlas. With a fine curet or an elevator, the posterior atlanto-occipital ligament can be separated from the posterior lip of the foramen magnum if necessary.

The greater occipital nerve (C2) and the third occipital nerve cross the field and course laterally in the paracervical muscles. Subperiosteal dissection and avoidance of vigorous *lateral* dissection should prevent injury to these nerves. If occipital fixation is required, the inion is thickest at its prominence near the ridge, and the passage of wires is possible without violating both tables of the occiput. If screw fixation is being used, bicortical purchase is recommended for the occiput, and screw lengths of typically 10 to 12 mm can be accepted in this region.[63]

If access to the posterior elements of C1–C2 is necessary, the incision can be extended inferiorly. Palpation of the large

C2 spinous process and the posterior C1 ring confirms the correct level. The posterior arch of the atlas is deeper anteriorly than the occiput and C2 spinous process, and the facet joint of C1–C2 lies about 2.5 cm anterior to the C2–C3 joint. A large broad elevator is used to dissect the posterior paracervical muscles from the arches of C1 and C2, and caution should be taken to avoid plunging instruments into the spinal canal. A small curet can be helpful to remove the muscular attachments on the bifid spinous process of C2 while stabilizing the arch of C2. Capsular ligaments of the facets should be preserved to maintain stability.

The passage of sublaminar wires at the C1–C2 level is common because the spinal canal at this level is capacious, but passage at lower cervical levels is associated with increased risk of neurologic injury. The removal of the atlantoaxial ligament or atlanto-occipital membrane is not required except for laminectomy cases. Careful separation of the membrane or ligament from the bone is all that is usually needed to pass sublaminar wires. This separation can be performed with a small-angled curet or a small Freer elevator. Slight head flexion can also help by opening the space between the ring of C1 and the occiput. The mean thickness of the posterior ring is 8 mm, and the cortical bone is thin.[64] Great care must be taken not to fracture the posterior ring of C1 while dissecting the ligamentum flavum.

An additional technique to expose the lateral aspect of C1 or C2 is to elevate the periosteum with a small Freer elevator. This allows the vertebral artery to be protected at the lateral aspect of the C1 arch. Lateral dissection should not exceed greater than 1.5 cm from the midline in an adult and 1 cm in a child due to risk of injury to the vertebral artery.[65,66] The vertebral artery courses over the arch of the atlas and pierces the lateral angle of the posterior atlanto-occipital membrane, although preoperative imaging should be obtained to evaluate the course of the vertebral artery and rule out anomalous vascular anatomy.

Brief consideration is given here to the regional anatomy for the C1–C2 transarticular screw fixation (Magerl) technique,[67–69] C1 lateral mass and C2 pedicle screw (Harms) technique,[69,70] and C2 translaminar screw.[69,71] A thin-cut CT scan with sagittal reconstructions and/or MRI imaging are necessary to fully track vertebral artery course and structure. This imaging is especially important to obtain in rheumatoid patients in whom an anomalous or enlarged foramen transversarium is common, which may place the vertebral arteries at increased risk with this technique. Attention should be paid to the presence of a ponticulus posticus, an anomalous ossification overlying the vertebral artery as it runs in the superior sulcus of C1, which can occur in 15% of the population. Regardless of the technique used, the intraoperative use of anteroposterior and lateral fluoroscopy can inform screw inclination in the coronal and parasagittal plane.

Because of the amount of cephalad angulation required to place the C1–C2 transarticular screw, subperiosteal exposure should extend down to C4.[65] The main landmark is the medial part of the isthmus of the axis, which can be visualized directly by subperiosteal dissection of the C2 lamina proceeding along the bony contour around the spinal canal until the maximum width in the coronal plane is reached. A Kirschner wire (K-wire) can be used to retract the soft tissues containing the greater occipital nerve and accompanying the venous plexus. The point of entry can be approximated as 3 mm cranial to the C2–C3 facet joint and 3 mm medial to the lateral border of the C2 inferior facet. The drilling for the screw is strictly sagittal and extends through the pars interarticularis, before perforating the atlantoaxial joint approximately in the posteromedial part entering the lateral mass of the atlas.[72] Lateral drill excursion should be avoided to prevent additional risk of injury to the vertebral arteries.

In the case of placement of a C1 lateral mass screw, the C1–C2 joint is the key anatomic landmark to be identified.[70] This identification can be facilitated by caudal retraction of the C2 nerve, which exposes the posterior aspect of the lateral mass of C1.[69] Subperiosteal dissection must be carried out on the inferior edge of the posterior arch of C1. The starting point of the C1 lateral mass screw lies directly in the midportion in the lateral mass. Often, a small emissary vein is located at this point. The C2 pedicle screw is identified by delineating the medial border of the isthmus and pars of the axis, as in the C1–C2 transarticular screw. However, the trajectory of the C2 pedicle screw is more medial and follows the path of the pedicle, as would be expected.[69,70]

Technical challenges associated with the C1–C2 transarticular screw and C2 pedicle screw placement led to the development of the C2 translaminar screw. Use of this screw is possible because of the predictably large size of the C2 lamina combined with the fact that the use of this screw eliminates the possibility for vertebral artery injury.[69,71] The starting point is identified as the junction of the C2 spinous process and the lamina, and the trajectory of the screw parallels the down slope of the dorsal aspect of the contralateral lamina. Care should be taken not to breach the ventral aspect of the lamina, resulting in placement of the screw within the spinal canal and to ensure that the C2–C3 facet joint is not violated by placement of a screw that is too long.[71]

Posterior Approach to Lower Cervical Spine

A reverse Trendelenburg position minimizes venous bleeding and reduces CSF pressure (Fig. 18.13). The posterior approach uses a longitudinal midline incision that extends above and below the segments required for the procedure. This extension of the skin and subcutaneous tissues is necessary because the skin of the posterior neck is less mobile and thicker for retraction. The skin is incised sharply, and electrocautery is used to incise the ligamentum nuchae in the midline. With a wide, flat periosteal elevator such as a Cobb, the dissection is carried subperiosteally down the spinous processes. Inadvertent penetration of instruments into the spinal canal can be minimized by examining preoperative films for evidence of spina bifida and other bony defects and by realizing that, in the cervical spine, the laminae do not override each other as much as in the thoracic spine, resulting in wider interlaminar spaces. Care should be taken to stay subperiosteal because the bifid nature of the spinous processes may result in a bulbous expanse, and the dissection may err into the paraspinal musculature. A superficial plexus of

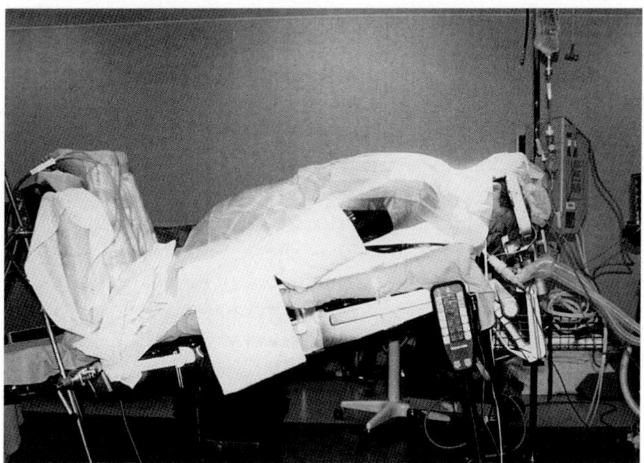

FIG. 18.13 Standard prone positioning for posterior cervical procedures. The reverse Trendelenburg position minimizes venous bleeding and reduces cerebrospinal fluid pressure.

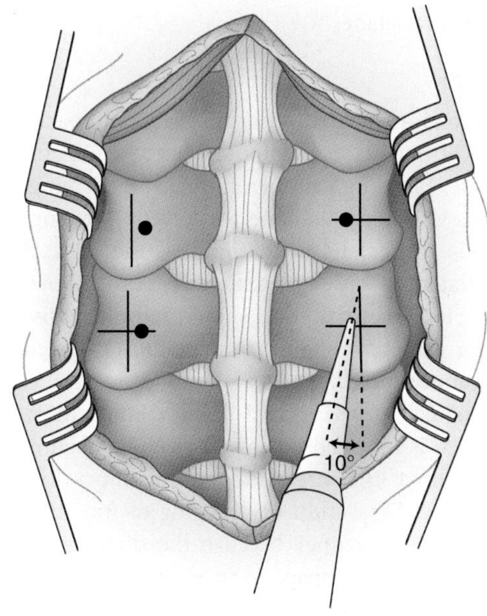

FIG. 18.14 The Roy-Camille technique for lateral mass screws. The entry point is at or near the anatomic center of the lateral mass and directed 10 degrees laterally.

veins may be encountered, which should be cauterized as needed. In general, subperiosteal dissection should be performed in a caudal-to-cephalad direction to minimize bleeding.

Subperiosteal dissection of muscles is performed to expose the spinous processes, lamina, lateral mass, and facet joints. Dissection should extend laterally to the medial third of the facet joint, with preservation of the capsule unless a fusion is planned. Extreme caution is needed during the exposure of the lamina and the interlaminar space to prevent dural tear and CSF leakage. Care should be taken at the lateral edge of the joint because the nerve root and vertebral artery lie anterior to the spinolamellar membrane of the adjoining transverse processes. Vigorous decortication or stripping may damage the thin bone and subsequently the nerve root and vertebral artery. The segmental artery at the lateral edge of the facet joints may be cauterized as it exits between the transverse processes. Various retractors may be used to facilitate exposure. For fusion cases, one should expose only the levels to be fused because creeping fusion extension is common. Supplementation of the fusion with posterior lateral mass plating may obviate the need for a halo vest postoperatively.

First popularized by Roy-Camille and colleagues,[73] placement of posterior cervical screws requires a thorough understanding of the lateral mass anatomy to minimize injury to associated neurovascular structures. Different entry points and screw orientations have been recommended. In the original description by Roy-Camille and colleagues,[73] the entry point was the center of the lateral mass, with the screw angled 10 degrees laterally (Fig. 18.14), whereas Magerl recommended the drilling angle to be 25 degrees laterally and 45 degrees superiorly. An and colleagues[5] found that, by orienting the screw 15 degrees cephalad and 30 degrees laterally with an entry point 1 mm medial to the anatomic center of the lateral mass, the facet joint and nerve root are avoided.

Posterior Approach to Cervicothoracic Junction

Lesions of the cervicothoracic junction are generally anterior, for which extensive anterior approaches with or without posterior fixation are usually required. Lesions that may require posterior stabilization include lesions resulting from tumors, trauma, postlaminectomy instability, or infection. If the posterior elements are intact, the simple triple-wiring procedure can be done for a short fusion, or rods may be used for a longer fusion, using a standard posterior approach.

Pedicle screw fixation is an alternative technique if the posterior elements are deficient. The transpedicular technique at the cervicothoracic junction is an exacting procedure with very little margin for error. Through cadaveric studies, the pedicle landmarks and anatomic characteristics of the cervicothoracic region were found. A standard posterior approach is used with the dissection performed to expose the lateral mass and to the tips of the transverse processes of the upper thoracic vertebrae. The facet joint to be fused is cleaned of its capsule, and the articular margins are identified. The entry point of the pedicle lies at the intersection of a horizontal line at the midportion of the transverse processes and a vertical line at the lamina–transverse process junction. This pedicle entrance point is 1 mm inferior to the facet joint and the middle point from the medial to the lateral margins of the facet joint. The outer cortex is decorticated at this point with a small bur, and a small Penfield elevator or straight curet is used to probe bluntly and enter the pedicle. A 2.5-mm drill may be used to enter the pedicle when it is identified. Medial angulation is required for entry of the pedicle into the vertebral body. Medial angulation has been observed to vary between individuals, thus it must be measured preoperatively in preparation for surgery. An et al. most recently reported that medial angulation averages 35.85 degrees at C7, 31.65 degrees at T1, and 23.35 degrees at T2.[74] Compared with the pedicles of the lumbar spine, the superoinferior diameter of the thoracic pedicles at the cervicothoracic junction is greater than its mediolateral diameter, which leaves little margin for error in the mediolateral plane.[74]

Complications

Complications associated with posterior approaches to the upper and lower cervical spine are uncommon but can be catastrophic. Bleeding can be minimized by staying subperiosteal and within the midline to prevent entering into the paraspinous musculature. The arch of the atlas should be dissected laterally only approximately 1.5 cm because the vertebral artery is at risk. One should minimize dissecting at the inferior edge of the foramen magnum to prevent uncontrollable venous bleeding.

Neurologic injury is a devastating complication of spine surgery. Care is required during passage of sublaminar wires or application of the screws to prevent injury to the brain or spinal cord. Dissection on the ring of the atlas must be done in a gentle manner because the direct pressure may result in fracture or slippage of an instrument into the spinal canal. A thorough understanding of the size, orientation, and relationship of the pedicles and lateral masses to surrounding neurovascular structures is imperative before the use of spinal instrumentation is undertaken. Posterior fusion without decompressive laminectomy tends to compress the spinal canal.

PEARLS

1. The anterior tubercle of the transverse process of C6 is an important palpable surface landmark for anterior cervical approaches.
2. The key to understanding the anterior approach to the cervical spine lies in recognizing the various investing fascial layers of the neck.
3. Placement of the deep retractors anteriorly should be deep to the longus colli to reduce the risk of injury to the sympathetic chain.
4. Posteriorly, the first bony prominence palpated inferior to the occiput is the spinous process of C2.
5. Reformatted fine-cut CT scans of the cervical spine help to improve understanding of the bony anatomy.

PITFALLS

1. The variable course of the vertebral artery as it ascends through the cervical spine places it at risk for injury during the anterior and posterior cervical approach.
2. The incorrect approach may be chosen without careful preoperative imaging review.
3. Increased rates of injury to surrounding structures may be observed if a modified anterior approach to the cervical spine is not used.
4. Increased bleeding is likely with dissection away from the midline that is not subperiosteal.
5. Airway obstruction after extubation may occur in the postoperative period after anterior and posterior cervical procedures.

KEY POINTS

1. Understanding the surgical anatomy of the cervical spine requires knowledge of the bony, ligamentous, muscular, and neurovascular anatomy of the neck and the complex relationship these structures have to one another.
2. The surgical approach selected should take into account the site of the pathologic process, the health of the patient, and the skill and comfort level of the surgeon with each particular exposure.
3. Understanding the advantages and limitation of each surgical exposure improves patient outcome and reduces complications.
4. Anatomic and surgical considerations at the occipitocervical and cervicothoracic junction are particularly challenging and should be thoroughly understood before approaching pathologic processes in these regions.
5. Complications of the cervical spine are infrequent but potentially devastating; careful preoperative planning, precise surgical technique, and a high index of suspicion should be maintained to minimize and identify complications.

KEY REFERENCES

1. An HS, Cotler JM, eds. *Spinal Instrumentation*. 2nd ed. Philadelphia: Lippincott Williams & Wilkins; 1990.
This text compiles the knowledge of multiple contributing authors to provide valuable information on surgical indications, principles, and techniques of new and classic spinal instrumentation.
2. Graham JJ. Complications of cervical spine surgery: a five-year report on a survey of the membership of the Cervical Spine Research Society by the Morbidity and Mortality Committee. *Spine*. 1989;14:1046.
A compilation of annual reports collected, at the time, by the newly formed Morbidity and Mortality Committee headed by Graham, this article analyzed 5 years of data submitted to the Cervical Spine Research Society from its members.
3. Heller JG, Pedlow FX. Anatomy of the cervical spine. In: Clark CR, ed. *The Cervical Spine*. 3rd ed. Philadelphia: Lippincott-Raven; 1998:3-36.
Edited and reviewed by the Cervical Spine Research Society Editorial Committee, this chapter provides the pertinent anatomy necessary to understand the complex relationship of the structures in the cervical spine.
4. Miller MD, Chhabra AB, Hurwitz SR, et al., eds. *Orthopaedic Surgical Approaches*. Philadelphia: Elsevier; 2008:211-329.
This updated text of orthopaedic exposures not only focuses on applied surgical anatomy and intraoperative photographs, but also provides valuable insight into patient positioning, bony and topical landmarks, and planes of surgical dissection.
5. Southwick WO, Robinson RA. Surgical approaches to the vertebral bodies in the cervical and lumbar regions. *J Bone Joint Surg Am*. 1957;39:631-644.
This article provides the original description of the classic anteromedial approach to the cervical spine that popularized anterior cervical surgery.

REFERENCES

1. Albert TJ. Anterior, middle, and lower cervical exposures. In: Albert TJ, Balderston RA, Northrup BE, eds. *Surgical Approaches to the Spine*. Philadelphia: WB Saunders; 1997:9-24.
2. Young JP, Young PH, Ackermann MJ, Anderson PA, Riew KD. The ponticulus posticus: implications for screw insertion into the first cervical lateral mass. *J Bone Joint Surg Am*. 2005; 87(11):2495-2498.
3. Schaffler MB, Alson MD, Heller JG, et al. Morphology of the dens. *Spine*. 1992;17:738-743.
4. Xu R, Naduad MC, Ebraheim NA, et al. Morphology of the second cervical vertebra and the posterior projection of the cervical pedicle axis. *Spine*. 1995;20:259-263.

5. An H, Gordin R, Renner K. Anatomic considerations for plate-screw fixation of the cervical spine. *Spine*. 1991;16(suppl): S548-S551.
6. Johnson RM, Murphy MJ, Southwick WO, et al. Surgical approaches to the spine: function and surgical anatomy of the neck. In: Herkowitz HN, Garfin SR, Balderston RA, eds. *Rothman-Simeone the Spine*. 4th ed. Philadelphia: WB Saunders; 1999:1463-1571.
7. Jefferson G. Fracture of atlas vertebra: report of four cases and review of those previously reported. *Br J Surg*. 1920; 7:407.
8. An HS. Anatomy of the spine. In: An HS, ed. *Principles and Techniques of Spine Surgery*. Philadelphia: Lippincott Williams & Wilkins; 1998:1-30.
9. Heller JG, Pedlow FX. Anatomy of the cervical spine. In: Clark CR, ed. *The Cervical Spine*. 3rd ed. Philadelphia: Lippincott-Raven; 1998:3-36.
10. Panjabi MM, Duranceau J, Goel V, et al. Cervical human vertebrae: quantitative three-dimensional anatomy of the middle and lower regions. *Spine*. 1993;16:861-874.
11. Karaikovic EE, Kunakornsawat S, Daubs MD, et al. Surgical anatomy of the cervical pedicles: landmarks for posterior cervical pedicle entrance localization. *J Spinal Disord*. 2000;13:63-72.
12. Karaikovic EE, Yingsakmongkol W, Gaines RW Jr. Accuracy of cervical pedicle screw placement using the funnel technique. *Spine*. 2001;26:2456-2462.
13. Karaikovic EE, Yingsakmongko LW, Griffiths HJ, et al. Possible complications of anterior perforation of the vertebral body using cervical pedicle screws. *J Spinal Disord Tech*. 2002;15:75-78.
14. Czervionke LF, Daniels DL, Ho PSP, et al. Cervical neural foramina: correlative anatomic and MR imaging study. *AJNR Am J Neuroradiol*. 1988;169:753-759.
15. Daniels DL, Hyde JS, Kneeland JB, et al. The cervical nerves and foramina: local-coil MR imaging. *AJNR Am J Neuroradiol*. 1986;7:129-133.
16. Aebi M, Thalgott JS, Webb JK. Stabilization techniques: lower cervical spine. In: Aebi M, Thalgott JS, Webb JK, eds. *AO/ASIF Principles in Spine Surgery*. New York: Springer; 1998:54-79.
17. Ebraheim NA, Xu R, Knight T, et al. Morphometric evaluation of the lower cervical pedicle and its projection. *Spine*. 1997;22:1-6.
18. Dvorak JPM. Functional anatomy of the alar ligaments. *Spine*. 1987;12:183-189.
19. Parke WW, Sherk HH. Normal adult anatomy. In: Sherk HH, Dunn EJ, Eismont FJ, eds. *The Cervical Spine*. Philadelphia: JB Lippincott; 1988:11-32.
20. An HS. Anatomy of the cervical spine. In: An HS, Simpson MJ, eds. *Surgery of the Cervical Spine*. London: Martin Dunitz; 1994:1-40.
21. Hayashi K, Yabuki T, Kurokawa T, et al. The anterior and posterior longitudinal ligaments of the lower cervical spine. *J Anat*. 1977;124:633-636.
22. Bland JH, Boushey DR. Anatomy and physiology of the cervical spine. *Semin Arthritis Rheum*. 1990;20:1-20.
23. Lang J. *Clinical Anatomy of the Cervical Spine*. New York: Thieme; 1993.
24. Kameyama T, Hashizume Y, Ando T, et al. Morphometry of the normal cadaveric cervical spinal cord. *Spine*. 1994;19:2077-2081.
25. Okada Y, Ikata T, Katoh S, et al. Morphologic analysis of the cervical spinal cord, dural tube and spinal canal by magnetic resonance imaging in normal adults and patients with cervical spondylotic myelopathy. *Spine*. 1994;19:2231-2235.
26. Rauschning W. Anatomy and pathology of the cervical spine. In: Frymoyer JW, ed. *The Adult Spine*. New York: Raven Press; 1991:907-929.
27. Flannigan BD, Lufkin RB, McGlade C, et al. MR imaging of the cervical spine: neurovascular anatomy. *AJR Am J Roentgenol*. 1987;148:785-790.
28. Pech P, Daniels DL, Williams AL, et al. The cervical neural foramina: correlation of microtomy and CT anatomy. *Radiology*. 1985;155:143-146.
29. Bogduk N. The clinical anatomy of the cervical dorsal rami. *Spine*. 1982;7:319-320.
30. Gerbrand JG, Baljet B, Drukker J. Nerves and nerve plexuses of the human vertebral column. *Am J Anat*. 1990;188: 282-296.
31. Rickenbacher J, Landolt AM, Theiler K. *Applied Anatomy of the Back*. Berlin: Springer-Verlag; 1982.
32. Dommisse GF. The blood supply of the spinal cord. *J Bone Joint Surg Br*. 1974;56:225.
33. Hoppenfeld S, deBoer P. The spine. In: Hoppenfeld S, deBoer P, eds. *Surgical Exposures in Orthopaedics: The Anatomic Approach*. 2nd ed. Philadelphia: JB Lippincott; 1994:215-301.
34. Arbit E, Patterson RH Jr. Combined transoral and median labiomandibular glossotomy approach to the upper cervical spine. *Neurosurgery*. 1981;8:672-674.
35. Ashraf J, Crockard HA. Transoral fusion for high cervical fractures. *J Bone Joint Surg Br*. 1990;72:76.
36. McAfee PC, Bohlman HH, Riley LH III, et al. The anterior retropharyngeal approach to the upper part of the cervical spine. *J Bone Joint Surg Am*. 1987;69:1371.
37. deAndrade J, McNab I. Anterior occipitocervical fusion using extrapharyngeal approach. *J Bone Joint Surg Am*. 1969;51:1621.
38. Whitesides TE, McDonald P. Lateral retropharyngeal approach to the upper cervical spine. *Orthop Clin North Am*. 1978;9:115.
39. Henn JS, Lee MC, Rhoton ALJ. Transoral approach to craniocervical junction and upper cervical spine. In: Kim DH, Henn JS, Vaccaro AR, et al., eds. *Surgical Anatomy & Techniques to the Spine*. Philadelphia: Saunders Elsevier; 2006:3-32.
40. Mendoza N, Crockard HA. Anterior transoral procedures. In: An HS, Riley LH III, eds. *An Atlas of Surgery of the Spine*. Philadelphia: Lippincott-Raven; 1998:55-69.
41. Rosen MR, Keane WM, Rosen D. Anterior upper cervical exposures. In: Albert TJ, Balderston RA, Northrup BE, eds. *Surgical Approaches to the Spine*. Philadelphia: WB Saunders; 1997:25-52.
42. Menezes AH. Complications of surgery at the craniovertebral junction: avoidance and management. *Pediatr Neurosurg*. 1992;17:254.
43. Fang H, Ong G. Direct anterior approach to the upper cervical spine. *J Bone Joint Surg Am*. 1962;44:1588-1604.
44. Lee SH, Park K, Kong DS, Kim ES, Eoh W. Long-term follow up of transoral anterior decompression and posterior fusion for irreducible bony compression of the craniovertebral junction. *J Clin Neurosci*. 2010;17(4):455-459.
45. Cheung KM, Mak KC, Luk KD. Anterior approach to cervical spine. *Spine*. 2012;37(5):E297-E302.
46. Southwick WO, Robinson RA. Surgical approaches to the vertebral bodies in the cervical and lumbar regions. *J Bone Joint Surg Am*. 1957;39:631-644.
47. Whitesides TE, Kelly RP. Lateral approach to the upper cervical spine for anterior fusion. *South Med J*. 1966;59:879.

48. Henry AK. *Extensile Exposure.* Baltimore: Williams & Wilkins; 1959:53.
49. Hogson AR. An approach to the cervical spine (C3-C7). *Clin Orthop.* 1965;39:129.
50. Verbiest H. Anterolateral operations for fractures and dislocations in the middle and lower parts of the cervical spine. *J Bone Joint Surg Am.* 1969;51A:1489-1530.
51. Fountas KN, Kapsalaki EZ, Nikolakakos LG, et al. Anterior cervical discectomy and fusion associated complications. *Spine.* 2007;32(21):2310-2317.
52. Whitehill R. Late esophageal perforation from an autogenous bone graft: report of a case. *J Bone Joint Surg Am.* 1985;67:644-645.
53. Heeneman H. Vocal cord paralysis following approaches to the anterior cervical spine. *Laryngoscope.* 1973;83(1):17-21.
54. Jung A, Schramm J. How to reduce recurrent laryngeal nerve palsy in anterior cervical spine surgery: a prospective observational study. *Neurosurgery.* 2010;67(1):10-15.
55. Donatini G, Carnaille B, Dionigi G. Increased detection of non-recurrent inferior laryngeal nerve (NRLN) during thyroid surgery using systematic intraoperative neuromonitoring (IONM). *World J Surg.* 2013;37(1):91-93.
56. Kurz LT, Herkowitz HN. Anterior exposures of the cervicothoracic junction and upper thoracic spine. In: Albert TJ, Balderston RA, Northrup BE, eds. *Surgical Approaches to the Spine.* Philadelphia: WB Saunders; 1997:61-80.
57. Sundaresan N, Shah J, Foley KM, et al. An anterior surgical approach to the upper thoracic vertebrae. *J Neurosurg.* 1984;61:686-690.
58. Vaccaro AR, An HS. Anterior exposures of the cervicothoracic junction. In: An HS, Riley LH III, eds. *An Atlas of Surgery of the Spine.* Philadelphia: Martin Dunitz; 1998:113-130.
59. Mai HT, Mitchell SM, Jenkins TJ, et al. Accessibility of the cervicothoracic junction through an anterior approach: an MRI-based algorithm. *Spine.* 2016;41:69-73.
60. Cho W, Buchowski JM, Park Y, et al. Surgical approach to the cervicothoracic junction: can a standard Smith-Robinson approach be utilized? *J Spinal Disord Tech.* 2012;25(5):264-267.
61. Capener N. The evolution of lateral rhachotomy. *J Bone Joint Surg Br.* 1954;36:173-179.
62. Andreshak TG, An HS. Posterior cervical exposures. In: Albert TJ, Balderston RA, Northrup BE, eds. *Surgical Approaches to the Spine.* Philadelphia: WB Saunders; 1997:81-114.
63. Winter RB, Lonstein JW, Denis F, et al. Posterior upper cervical procedures. In: Winter RB, Lonstein JW, Denis F, et al., eds. *Atlas of Spine Surgery.* Philadelphia: WB Saunders; 1995:19-33.
64. Doherty B, Heggeness MH. The quantitative anatomy of the atlas. *Spine.* 1994;19:2497-2500.
65. An H, Xu R. Posterior cervical spine procedures. In: An H, Riley L III, eds. *An Atlas of Surgery of the Spine.* Philadelphia: Lippincott-Raven; 1998:13-14.
66. Ebraheim N, Xu R, Ahmad M, et al. The quantitative anatomy of the vertebral artery groove of the atlas and its relation to the posterior atlantoaxial approach. *Spine.* 1998;23:320-323.
67. Magerl F, Seemann P. Stable posterior fusion of the atlas and axis by transarticular screw fixation. In: Kehr P, Weidner A, eds. *Cervical Spine.* New York: Springer-Verlag; 1987:322.
68. Grob D, Crisco J, Panjabi MM, et al. Biomechanical evaluation of four different posterior atlantoaxial fixation techniques. *Spine.* 1991;17:480-490.
69. Shen FH. Spine. In: Miller MD, Chhabra AB, Hurwitz SR, et al., eds. *Orthopaedic Surgical Approaches.* Philadelphia: WB Saunders; 2008:211-329.
70. Harms J, Melcher RP. Posterior C1-C2 fusion with polyaxial screw and rod fixation. *Spine.* 2001;26:2467-2471.
71. Wright NM. Posterior C2 fixation using bilateral, crossing C2 laminar screws. *J Spinal Disord Tech.* 2004;17:158-162.
72. Grob D, An HS. Posterior occipital and C1/C2 instrumentation. In: An HS, Cotler JS, eds. *Spinal Instrumentation.* 2nd ed. Philadelphia: Lippincott Williams & Wilkins; 1999:191-201.
73. Roy-Camille RR, Sailant G, Mazel C. Internal fixation of the unstable cervical spine by posterior osteosynthesis with plate and screws. In: Cervical Spine Research Society, ed. *The Cervical Spine.* 2nd ed. Philadelphia: JB Lippincott; 1989:390-404.
74. An HS, Wise JJ, Xu R. Anatomy of the cervicothoracic junction: a study of cadaveric dissection, cryomicrotomy, and magnetic resonance imaging. *J Spinal Disord.* 1999;12(6):519-525.

CHAPTER 19 Anatomy of the Anterior Cervicothoracic Spine

Kenneth A. Hood
Shyam Shridharani

The cervicothoracic spine corresponds to the region just superior to the mediastinum and extends into the sternum and T4–T5 intervertebral disc space. In this region, knowledge of the vascular and neural anatomy is of utmost importance. The left brachiocephalic vein is found posterior to the upper sternum and lies directly posterior to the thymus gland. The right and left brachiocephalic veins merge behind the right first intercostal space to form the superior vena cava. The superior vena cava drains into the right atrium behind the third costal cartilage.

The recurrent laryngeal nerve is a branch of the vagus nerve that supplies the intrinsic muscles of the larynx with the exception of the cricothyroid muscles. Injury to this nerve can result in dysphonia and dysphagia. The left recurrent laryngeal nerve can be found emerging from the vagus nerve anterior to the arch of the aorta between T1 and T3. The phrenic nerve can also be found in this region, anterior to the arch of the aorta (Fig. 19.1). From there, its course is noted to predictably travel in the tracheoesophageal groove. The right recurrent laryngeal nerve, on the other hand, branches off the vagus nerve in the upper cervical region and loops around the right subclavian artery. It can also course anteriorly behind the thyroid before entering the tracheoesophageal groove.

Given the important function of the recurrent laryngeal nerve, there has been much debate as to whether a left- or right-sided approach is safer, minimizing risk to the nerve. In their classic work, Tew and Mayfield report the asymmetric course between the right and left recurrent laryngeal nerves.[1] According to their work, the left recurrent laryngeal nerve takes a longer, more predictable, protected course around the arch of the aorta. Because of this, they believed that a left-sided approach minimized the risk of injury to the recurrent laryngeal nerve. Other work has reported no statistical difference between nerve injury rates and side of approach.[2] Overall, for anterior surgery, the reported incidence of dysphonia ranges from 2% to 30%, and the incidence of dysphagia ranges from 28% to 57%.[3]

Another important neural structure in the anterior cervicothoracic spine is the phrenic nerve. The phrenic nerve innervates the diaphragm. It courses anterior to the pulmonary hilum before reaching the diaphragm.

Last, mention should be made of the thoracic duct, which is the largest lymphatic vessel in the body. It typically starts at the level of the twelfth thoracic vertebra and enters the thorax through the aortic opening of the diaphragm between the aorta and azygos vein. In the mediastinum, it is located on the left side behind the arch of the aorta and ascends between the left subclavian artery and the esophagus, and drains at the angle of junction of the left subclavian vein and left internal jugular vein.

Surgical Approaches to the Anterior Thoracic Spine

Low Anterior Cervical and High Transsternal Approach

The cervicothoracic junction is a biomechanical transition zone between the lordotic cervical spine and the kyphotic thoracic spine. This approach allows for exposure of the lower cervical spine and upper thoracic spine, from C7 to T4. A successful approach to this region requires navigation through numerous important neurovascular structures. Indications for this approach include infectious, traumatic, and neoplastic processes that require decompression and fusion or corpectomy.

The patient is positioned supine on a radiolucent table. A towel roll or bump is placed between the scapulae, allowing for gentle neck and shoulder extension. The arms are padded and tucked at the sides. The shoulders are gently taped downward and the neck is turned slightly away from the approach side, allowing for improved access and fluoroscopic visualization. The shoulders should not be overaggressively taped, as this can cause a traction injury to the brachial plexus. The table can be positioned in slight Trendelenberg to minimize venous engorgement and pooling.

As previously mentioned, there is controversy as to which side the approach should be performed. Classically, a left-sided approach is performed as the recurrent laryngeal nerve is thought to follow a more predictable course in the tracheoesophageal groove, minimizing risk of injury.

After standard sterile preparation and drape, a skin incision is made from the anterior border of the sternocleidomastoid to the sternal notch (Fig. 19.2A). For cases requiring full exposure, from C7 to T4, the vertical limb of the incision can

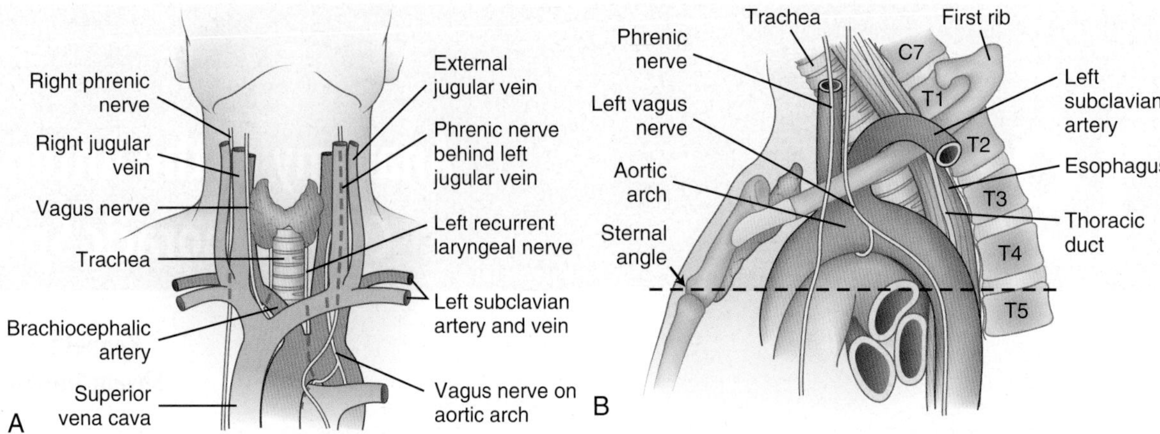

FIG. 19.1 (A) Anteroposterior view of cervicothoracic junction. (B) Lateral view of cervicothoracic junction.

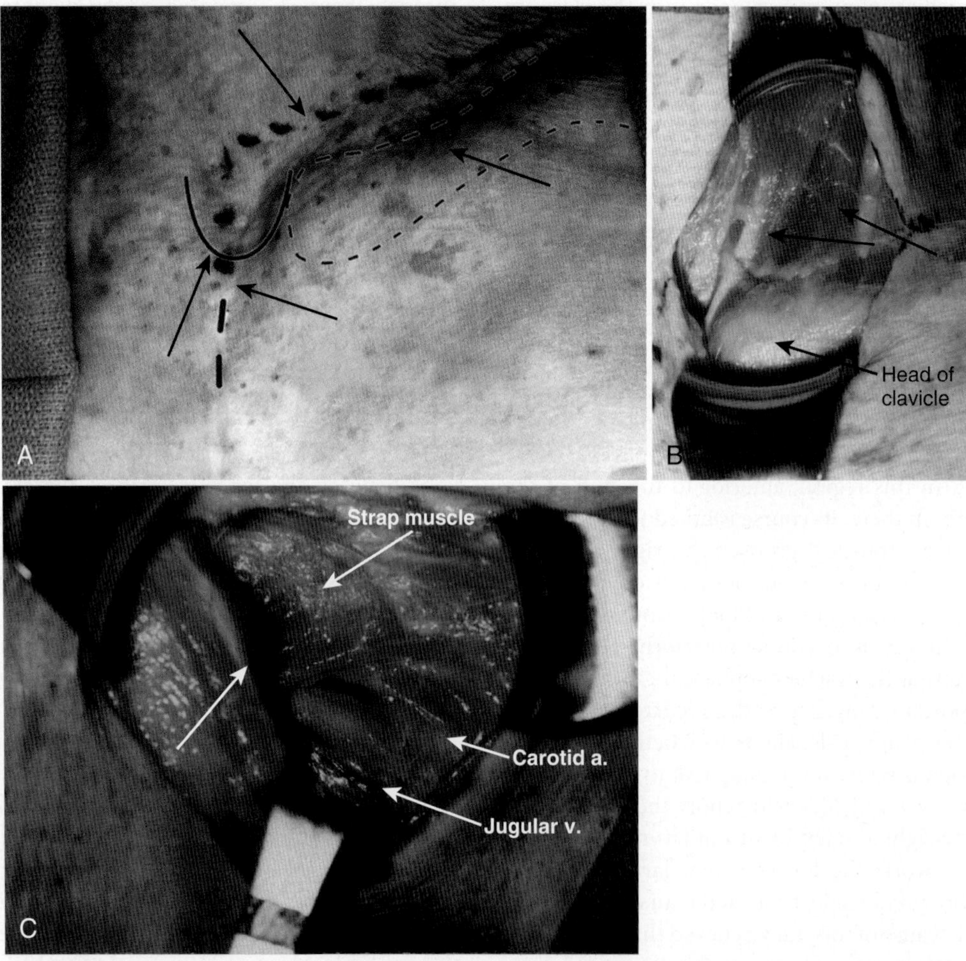

FIG. 19.2 (A) Inverted L-shaped incision for cervicothoracic junction. Midsternal extension of incision can be extended further vertically for more exposure distally. (B) Insertion of sternocleidomastoid muscle into clavicular head. (C) Sternocleidomastoid muscle retracted laterally revealing underlying strap muscle. Carotid sheath and jugular vein should be mobilized laterally as well.

be carried inferiorly over the middle of the manubrium to the level of the third costal cartilage. Subcutaneous dissection is performed down to the platysma. Once the platysma is well defined, it is carefully split in a longitudinal fashion. One should avoid injuring the underlying jugular veins, but they can be sacrificed if they hinder the approach.

Next, the sternocleidomastoid and strap muscles are identified at their insertion onto the clavicle (Figs. 19.2B–C). The clavicular and manubrial heads of the sternocleidomastoid are elevated proximal and lateral in a subperiosteal manner. The strap muscles are similarly elevated medially. Subperiosteal exposure should be undertaken until the ipsilateral half of the manubrium and junction of the medial and middle third of the clavicle are exposed.

The clavicle is cut at the junction of the medial and middle third with an osteotome or oscillating saw. Care should be taken to ensure that the underlying neurovascular structures are protected during this process. Once free laterally, the clavicle is gently lifted up and disarticulated from the manubrium.

For greater distal exposure, a sternal splitting approach can be performed. This involves splitting the manubrium down the midline to the level of exposure required. Retrosternal adipose tissue and the thymus are retracted and protected. The sternum is then exposed subperiosteally. The manubrium is subsequently split with an oscillating or Gigli saw. The inferior thyroid vessels can be ligated if necessary and the left innominate vein is retracted caudally or ligated (if necessary). Care should be taken not to injure the thoracic duct, which is located left of the esophagus starting at T4 as it ascends to its junction with the left internal jugular vein and subclavian vein.

The remainder of the dissection is similar to the Smith-Robinson approach. The interval between the trachea and esophagus medially and the carotid sheath laterally is identified and developed. When placing retractors it should be ensured that they are safely placed to avoid injury to the recurrent laryngeal nerve, which lies in the tracheoesophageal groove. The right brachiocephalic artery can be taken to the right along with the trachea and esophagus. The left brachiocephalic and subclavian veins are retracted inferiorly and to the left. The longus colli muscles on either side of the spine are identified and the prevertebral fascia is spread with a Kittner, exposing the anterior thoracic spine.

Transpleural Transthoracic Third Rib Resection

An alternative approach to the low anterior cervical high transsternal approach is the transpleural transthoracic third rib resection. This approach allows excellent exposure of the anterolateral thoracic spine from T1 to T4. The indications for this approach are similar. The drawbacks to this approach include the need for mobilization of the scapula and violating of the chest wall musculature and pleural space.

For this approach, a double-lumen endotracheal tube should be placed by anesthesia to allow for isolated lung deflation on the approach side. The patient is positioned in the lateral decubitus position with the approach side up. The knees and elbows are gently flexed and the arms are abducted. An axillary roll is placed and all bony prominences are padded. The patient can be secured to the table via bolsters or a beanbag. The approach-side arm can be supported by stacked pillows/towels or an arm holder. The area of prep and drape is demarcated from the shoulder to above the iliac crest (cephalad-caudad) and from the midline of the spine posteriorly to the umbilicus anteriorly (posterior-anterior).

The incision is carried from the paraspinous area at approximately T1 distally along the medial border of the scapula to the seventh rib (Fig. 19.3). It is then carried laterally and anteriorly toward the costal cartilage of the third

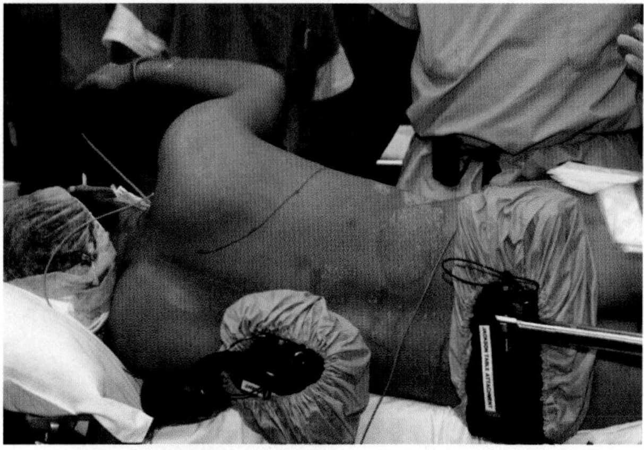

FIG. 19.3 Patient is positioned in lateral position on a Jackson spinal table with incision marked for a high transthoracic approach. (From Le HN, Kim DH. Anterolateral transthoracic approaches to the cervicothoracic junction [transaxillary approach, transpleural transthoracic third rib resection approach]. In: Kim DH, ed. *Surgical Anatomy and Techniques to the Spine*. Philadelphia: Elsevier; 2006.)

rib. The trapezius and latissimus dorsi are divided, and the scapula is retracted cephalad and medially (Fig. 19.4). The third rib is identified. It should be kept in mind that the second rib is typically the easiest rib to palpate, as it is elevated relative to the surrounding ribs. The first rib sits medial to the second rib.[4]

The approach-side lung is now selectively deflated. The third rib is skeletonized in a subperiosteal manner (Fig. 19.5). Anteriorly, this can be performed with Bovie electrocautery and curettes. A Doyen is a great tool for performing posterior subperiosteal dissection around the rib while protecting the underlying neurovascular bundle (Fig. 19.6). The third rib is cut as far anteriorly and posteriorly as possible and can be used for bone graft (Fig. 19.7). The third rib bed—consisting of the periosteum, endothoracic fascia, and parietal pleura—is transected, allowing entrance into the thoracic cavity (Fig. 19.8). A chest spreader can be placed along with a second retractor at a right angle to allow for maximum visualization. The lung is retracted and protected with a malleable retractor and moist lap sponge (Fig. 19.9).

The aorta, spine, parietal pleura, veins, and sympathetic plexus are identified. Next, the parietal pleura is gently incised in a longitudinal fashion over the indicated disc space. This area is relatively avascular as compared to directly over the vertebral body. The vertebral body is then exposed and the intercostal arteries and veins are ligated and cut. Exposure can be extended as necessary (Fig. 19.10).

Closure for this approach is as follows. The parietal pleura is repaired, if feasible. Lung reexpansion is then performed. The ribs are reapproximated with heavy nonabsorbable suture or wire in figure-of-eight fashion utilizing a rib reapproximator. Care should be taken not to injure the neurovascular bundle of the caudad rib being reapproximated when using the rib reapproximator. The lung should also be protected during this process. Last, a chest tube is placed through a separate incision at the level of the ninth intercostal space and set to water seal.

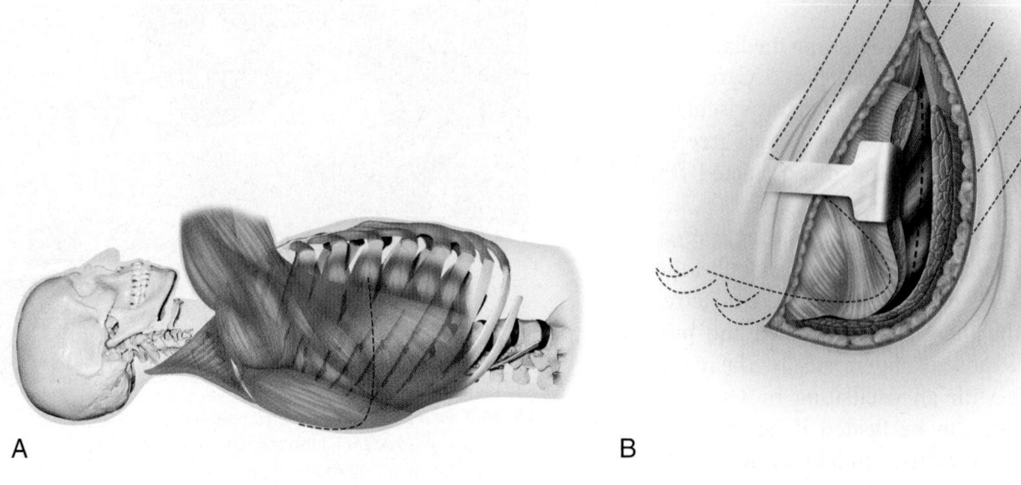

FIG. 19.4 Muscular exposure. (A) Note the relationship of the periscapular muscular anatomy. (B) Retracting or detaching the latissimus muscle will reveal the underlying upper thoracic ribs and the attachments of the serratus anterior muscles. (From Le HN, Kim DH. Anterolateral transthoracic approaches to the cervicothoracic junction [transaxillary approach, transpleural transthoracic third rib resection approach]. In: Kim DH, ed. *Surgical Anatomy and Techniques to the Spine*. Philadelphia: Elsevier; 2006.)

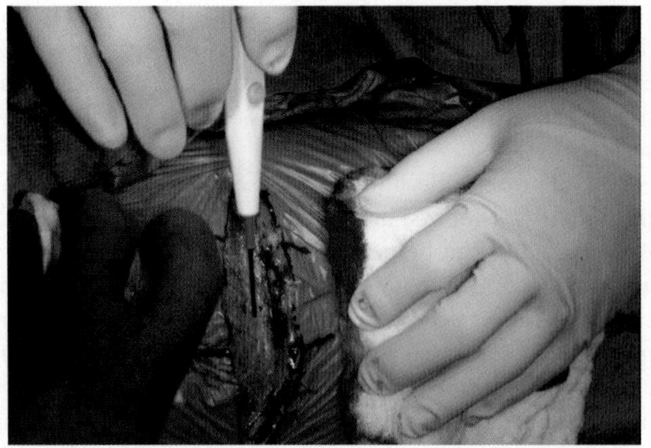

FIG. 19.5 Rib dissection can be exposed with use of cautery and subperiosteal dissection. (From Le HN, Kim DH. Anterolateral transthoracic approaches to the cervicothoracic junction [transaxillary approach, transpleural transthoracic third rib resection approach]. In: Kim DH, ed. *Surgical Anatomy and Techniques to the Spine*. Philadelphia: Elsevier; 2006.)

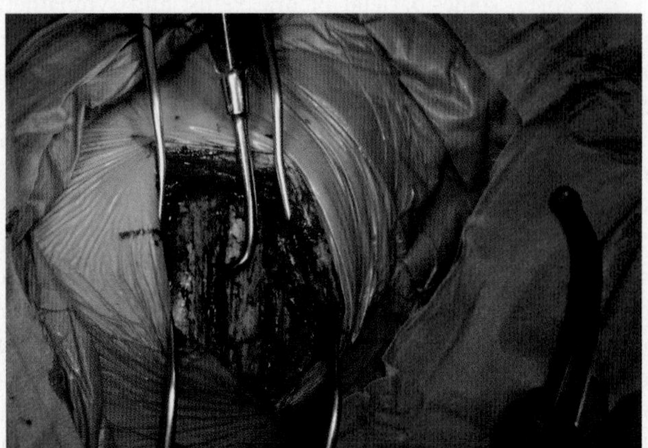

FIG. 19.6 A posterior subperiosteal dissection of the third rib is performed using a doyen. (From Le HN, Kim DH. Anterolateral transthoracic approaches to the cervicothoracic junction [transaxillary approach, transpleural transthoracic third rib resection approach]. In: Kim DH, ed. *Surgical Anatomy and Techniques to the Spine*. Philadelphia: Elsevier; 2006.)

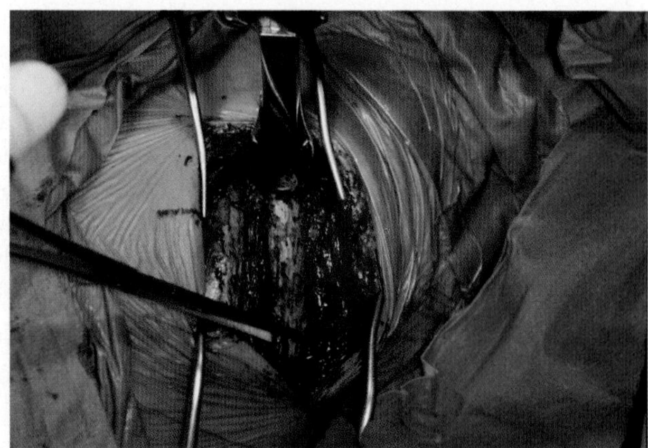

FIG. 19.7 Third rib is resected using a rib cutter as far anteriorly and posteriorly as possible. (From Le HN, Kim DH. Anterolateral transthoracic approaches to the cervicothoracic junction [transaxillary approach, transpleural transthoracic third rib resection approach]. In: Kim DH, ed. *Surgical Anatomy and Techniques to the Spine*. Philadelphia: Elsevier; 2006.)

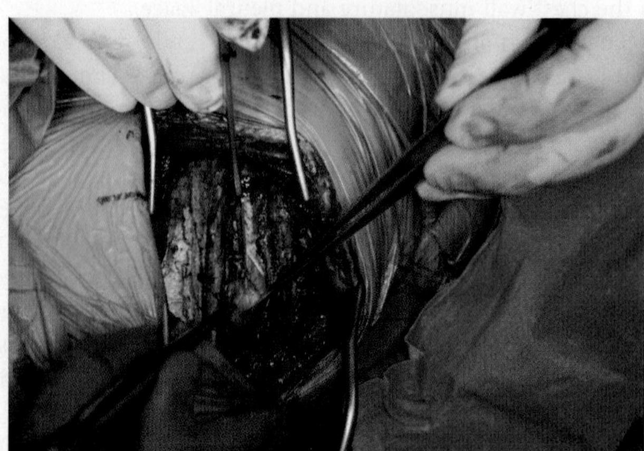

FIG. 19.8 Third rib bed consisting of periosteum, endothoracic fascia, and parietal pleura is identified and transected to enter the thoracic cavity. (From Le HN, Kim DH. Anterolateral transthoracic approaches to the cervicothoracic junction [transaxillary approach, transpleural transthoracic third rib resection approach]. In: Kim DH, ed. *Surgical Anatomy and Techniques to the Spine*. Philadelphia: Elsevier; 2006.)

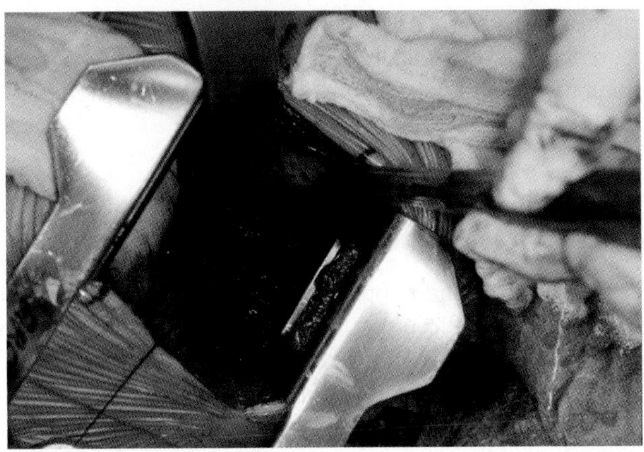

FIG. 19.9 Operative exposure. A chest spreader can then be inserted and opened after rib resection. (From Le HN, Kim DH. Anterolateral transthoracic approaches to the cervicothoracic junction [transaxillary approach, transpleural transthoracic third rib resection approach]. In: Kim DH, ed. *Surgical Anatomy and Techniques to the Spine*. Philadelphia: Elsevier; 2006.)

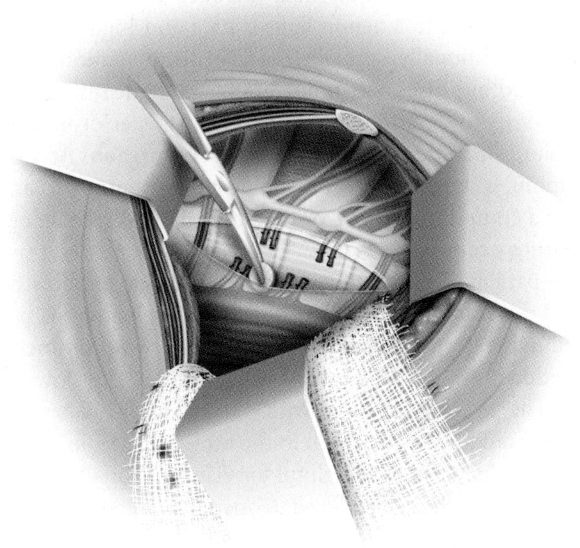

FIG. 19.10 Appropriate intercostal arteries and veins are dissected, ligated, and cut. (From Le HN, Kim DH. Anterolateral transthoracic approaches to the cervicothoracic junction [transaxillary approach, transpleural transthoracic third rib resection approach]. In: Kim DH, ed. *Surgical Anatomy and Techniques to the Spine*. Philadelphia: Elsevier; 2006.)

Thoracotomy (Anterior) Approach to the Thoracic Spine

The transthoracic approach offers extensile exposure of the anterior vertebral bodies from T6 to T12.[4] The benefits of this approach include excellent access to the anterior column and less risk of direct injury to the neural elements. Indications for this approach include treatment of vertebral osteomyelitis, resection of the vertebral body for tumors and trauma, deformity correction, and decompression of the anterior thoracic spine. Despite this, the transthoracic approach is rarely used secondary to the advent of posterior-based approaches that allow the surgeon to use the same procedures with less morbidity and risk.

The patient is intubated by anesthesia using a double-lumen endotracheal tube with lung isolation.[5] This will allow for selective lung deflation based on the approach side. The patient is then placed in the lateral decubitus position with the head in neutral position and an axillary roll or pad placed underneath the downside axilla to protect the brachial plexus. The arms are slightly abducted and the elbows slightly flexed. The downside leg is slightly flexed at the hip and the knee; the upside leg is slightly extended and adducted to allow for soft tissue tension, which aids in opening the intercostal space. All bony prominences must be well padded. The patient is secured in the lateral decubitus position via a beanbag or padded bolsters (Fig. 19.11A).

Although the approach can be made from the left or right side, the right side is preferred if the approach is to be made above T10, as it avoids manipulation of the aorta. If the approach is for access from T10 and caudad, a left-sided approach is preferred since the liver elevates the diaphragm on the right side in this region.

Localization of the operative level is then performed with the aid of fluoroscopy and palpation. The rib to be resected should correspond to two levels above the operative vertebral body level given the oblique nature of the rib. Once this is confirmed, the rib is marked from the posterior angle of the rib to the anterior margin.

The skin and subcutaneous tissues are incised with a No. 10 blade scalpel (Fig. 19.11B). Further dissection is carried out with Bovie electrocautery. The latissimus dorsi is identified and incised in line with the skin in an incision over the course of the rib. After completing dissection through the latissimus dorsi, the posterior margin of the serratus anterior is encountered and incised in a similar fashion. At this point, the rib should be visible. Subperiosteal dissection is then performed, skeletonizing the superficial surface of the rib without violating the inferior margin since this is where the neurovascular bundle runs. The intercostal muscles are then bluntly released from the superior and inferior margins of the rib using an Alexander Farabeuf periosteotome. Tissue attachments to the undersurface of the rib are then carefully released in a subperiosteal fashion without violating the parietal pleura using a Doyen dissector. The rib is then cut with a rib cutter at the costotransverse junction posteriorly and the costal margin anteriorly. Sharp bony edges at the margins of resection are smoothed with a bone rasp. Bony bleeding is controlled with bone wax. The resected rib can be saved and used for bone graft.

Following rib resection, the appropriate lung corresponding to the operative side is selectively deflated. The pleural cavity is then entered with Metzenbaum scissors. Rib spreaders can be placed at right angles to aid in visualization. A malleable retractor padded with moist lap sponges can be used to further retract and protect the deflated lung. One of the major complications associated with this approach is microatelectasis. In order to help prevent this, the lung can be periodically reinflated by the anesthesiologist.

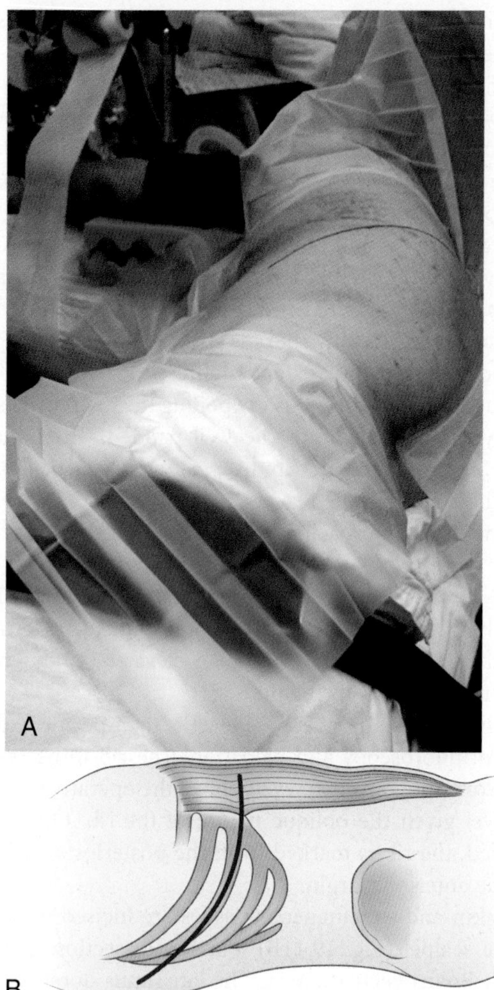

FIG. 19.11 (A) The patient is placed in the lateral decubitus position. The arms are abducted and elbows are slightly flexed in a position of comfort, using blankets or pillows to hold the position. (B) The thoracotomy incision is centered over the rib to be resected. The incision is drawn from the posterior angle of the corresponding rib and following its curvature anteriorly. Typically, the numbered rib that is resected is considered to be two levels above the expected working level.

The parietal pleura is incised longitudinally over the pertinent disc space with atraumatic pickups and Metzenbaum scissors. The parietal pleura is retracted laterally. Underlying segmental vessels that interfere with access are carefully dissected and ligated with several vascular clips or 2-0 silk ties. Ligation should be performed away from the aorta in order to minimize the risk of loosening of the clips or ties. Further cephalad or caudad exposure is gained by further longitudinal release of the parietal pleura and ligation of segmental vessels. It is important not to tie off more segmental vessels than necessary, as blood supply to the spinal cord from these vessels is variable and may result in inadvertent cord ischemia. In an animal model, it has been shown that ligation of bilateral segmental arteries at 4 or greater consecutive levels can produce ischemic cord dysfunction.[6]

Upon completion of the procedure, the parietal pleura is repaired and the lung is reinflated. A chest tube is then placed through the ninth intercostal space. The ribs are then reapproximated using a rib approximator and the interval is secured in place with heavy nonabsorbable suture. Routine subcutaneous and skin closure is then performed and a sterile dressing is placed.

Endoscopic Anterior Approach to the Thoracic Spine

The benefits of an endoscopic approach to the anterior thoracic spine include reduced postoperative pain levels, hastened recovery, and minimization of common complications associated with open thoracotomy approaches.[7,8] The indications for this approach are the same as those of an open thoracotomy approach: traumatic, degenerative, infectious, and neoplastic etiologies requiring access to the anterior vertebral body and disc space. Contraindications to the endoscopic approach include patients with cardiopulmonary insufficiency, acute posttraumatic respiratory failure, or coagulopathy. A relative contraindication is a patient with previous surgical interventions or infectious diseases of the lung, as the patient may have excessive adhesions.[9]

For this approach, equipment includes a 30-degree endoscope connected to a xenon light source and high-definition camera. Additionally, specially made instrumentation for soft tissue handling, disc space preparation, and bone resection are required. Consideration should be given to performing this procedure in conjunction with a thoracic surgeon. At a bare minimum, a thoracic surgeon should be on standby to assist should a complication arise or the need to convert to an open procedure occurs.

The patient is intubated with a double-lumen endotracheal tube to allow for selective lung deflation. The patient is positioned in the lateral decubitus position. All bony prominences are padded. An axillary roll is placed under the downside axilla. The patient is secured with a beanbag or bolsters. The patient should be secured well to the table since table rotation of up to 15 degrees can be helpful for visualization intraoperatively. The table should be flexed to open the intercostal spaces.

The level of interest is marked on the lateral thoracic wall utilizing a lateral fluoroscopic image (in reference to the patient's body). There are several described working portal configurations.[10] Traditionally, two to three working portals and two additional portals are used. The working portal is marked directly above the lesion in line with the posterior axillary line. The portal for the endoscope is marked cranial to the working portal approximately 2 intercostal spaces in line with the midaxillary line. The portal sites for suction and retraction are placed anterior to these portals[9] (Fig. 19.12).

The ipsilateral lung is deflated and a 1-inch oblique incision is made over the site of the superior endoscope portal. This portal hole is always created first, as it minimizes risk to the liver, diaphragm, and spleen. The approach is made using a minithoracotomy technique and the chest cavity is entered with a blunt clamp or thoracoscopic introducer. Entry should be made on the superior portion of the rib in order to avoid the neurovascular bundle on the undersurface of the rib.

A 10-mm, 30-degree rigid scope is inserted through a 10-mm trocar at this portal site. The remaining portals are

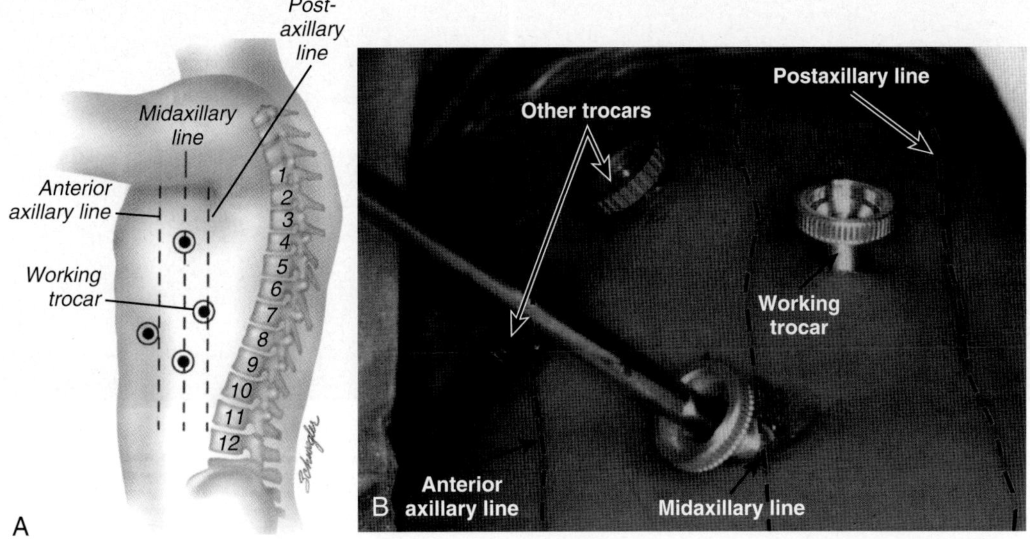

FIG. 19.12 (A) Diagram of trocar positions for T7–T8 pathology. (B) Actual trocar positions.

placed under direct thoracoscopic visualization. At this point, the patient can be rotated up to 15 degrees anteriorly and placed in the Trendelenberg position for work in the lower thoracic spine or reverse Trendelenberg for work in the upper thoracic spine. This allows the lung to fall away from the surgical field.

Diagnostic thoracoscopy is performed and the target level is identified. The ribs can be counted internally by a blunt palpation with a grasping instrument to confirm the appropriate surgical level. Once the appropriate level is identified, a 20-gauge needle or Kirschner wire (K-wire) is placed percutaneously into the disc space and confirmed with a fluoroscopic image.

With the appropriate surgical level confirmed, the parietal pleura over this level is cut over the rib head with cautery. The free edge of the pleura is then grasped and released cephalad and caudad with a hook dissector to expose the operative level(s). If access to the vertebral body is necessary, the segmental vessels need to be clipped and ligated.

If vertebral body work is necessary, the rib head is exposed and the costovertebral ligaments are released. The rib is then cut 2 to 3 cm from its attachment to the spine using a burr or Kerrison rongeur and the rib head is removed. Removal of the rib head allows for clear visualization of the disc, pedicle, and posterior vertebral margin. Resection of the superior vertebral body and pedicle allows for exposure of the exiting nerve root and spinal canal.

At the end of the procedure, hemostasis should be achieved. Tears involving the visceral pleura should be repaired. A chest tube is placed through the inferiormost portal, secured with 2-0 silk ties to the skin, and placed on a water seal. The lung is reinflated under direct visualization and a radiograph is obtained to ensure full lung reexpansion. The fascia and skin of each portal is closed in a layered fashion.

Postoperatively, serial chest radiographs are obtained until it is felt that they can be safely discontinued. The chest tube can be discontinued once output is less than 150 mL over a 24-hour period and no air leak is present.

Anterior Anatomy of the Thoracolumbar Junction

The thoracolumbar junction spans from T10 to L2. It is the transition zone between the rigid kyphotic thoracic spine and the mobile lumbar spine. Because of this transition, the thoracolumbar spine is predisposed to a high proportion of trauma.[11]

Across the thoracolumbar junction, the aorta lies to the left of the midline; the azygos vein, splanchnic nerves, and thoracic duct lie to the right of midline. In the thoracolumbar spine, the segmental arteries run horizontally from the aorta toward their respective vertebral body.

The diaphragm is the dome-shaped structure of muscle and fibrous tissues that separates the thoracic cavity from the abdomen. The diaphragm is made up of two main parts: the clover-shaped central tendon and a peripheral muscular portion that attaches to the chest wall. The sternal portion of the diaphragm is made up of two small muscular segments that attach to the posterior aspect of the xiphoid process. The costal portion of the diaphragm is made up of several wide muscle segments whose origins are found on the internal surface of the inferior six ribs and costal cartilages. The lumbar portion of the diaphragm attaches to the spine at L1 through the left and right crura, which blend with the anterior longitudinal ligament. Additional spine attachments come from the medial and lateral arcuate ligaments. The medial arcuate ligaments arise from the crura and bridge the psoas muscle, inserting onto the transverse processes of L1. The lateral arcuate ligament arises from the L1 transverse process, bridges the quadratus lumborum, and attaches to the twelfth rib.

Anterior Approach to the Thoracolumbar Spine

The indications for anterior approach to the thoracolumbar spine include traumatic, infectious, and malignant etiologies between T10 and L2. Additionally, this approach can be employed for deformity correction as well as to treat pseudoarthrosis.

Similar to thoracotomy approaches, a double-lumen endotracheal tube should be used to allow for selective lung

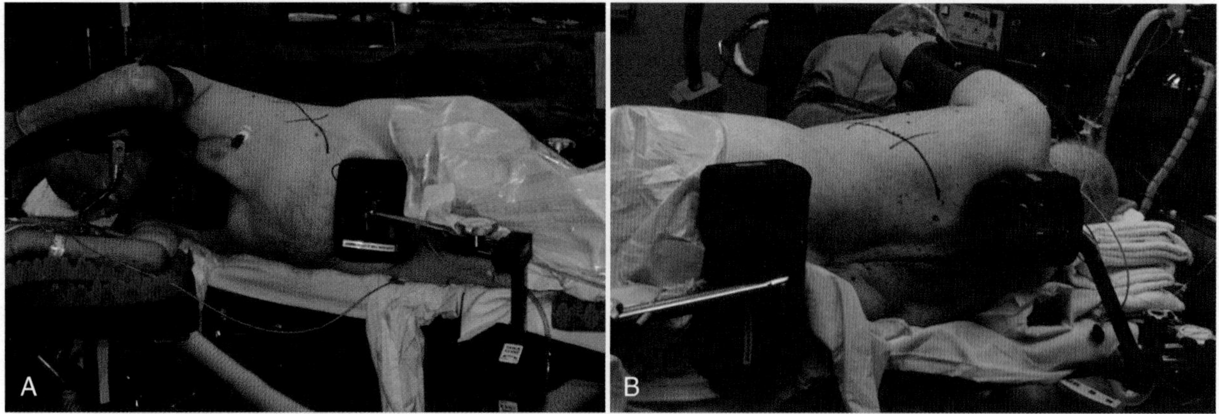

FIG. 19.13 Left-sided lateral approach positioning. (From Thongtrangan I, Le HN, Park J, Kim DH. Thoracolumbar and lumbar spines. In: Kim DH, ed. *Surgical Anatomy and Techniques to the Spine*. Philadelphia: Elsevier; 2006.)

deflation. A nasogastric tube should also be in place. The patient is positioned in the lateral decubitus position with the approach side up. A left-side approach offers the advantage of avoiding the need to mobilize the thin-walled vena cava as well as risking a view obscured by the liver. If the vena cava is injured, it can bleed profusely and can be very difficult to repair. Sometimes, however, a right-sided approach is necessary as dictated by the surgical pathology, such as in the case of treating the apex of a scoliotic curve.[12]

After placing the patient in the lateral decubitus position with the operative approach side up, the patient can be secured with a beanbag or bolsters. All bony prominences about the lower extremities should be padded. An axillary roll is placed. The down leg is straightened; the top leg is flexed and slightly externally rotated to help relax the psoas muscle. Pillows can be placed between the legs to aid in positioning. The arms are abducted and slightly flexed at the elbow. The upside arm can be supported by an arm holder, pillows, or blankets. The patient is further secured to the table by placing tape over the hip and shoulder or upper chest. Care should be taken to avoid placing the tape directly over the breast and nipple. Fluoroscopy is then used to mark the operative levels and incision. Typically, the ninth, tenth, eleventh, or twelfth rib is selected, depending on the exposure required. The skin incision is marked from the posterior angle of the corresponding rib anteriorly along its course and ending distally at a level just lateral to the pubic symphysis. The length of the incision can be altered depending on the exposure necessary (Fig. 19.13).

Standard sterile prep and drape is performed. A No. 10 blade scalpel is used to make the skin incision over the aforementioned distribution. Subcutaneous dissection is performed with Bovie electrocautery. The latissimus dorsi and external oblique are split with cautery in a layered fashion. The rib is superficially exposed posteriorly from the costotransverse junction anteriorly to the costal margin. Next, the rib is dissected in a subperiosteal manner. When working on the undersurface of the rib, a Doyen can be helpful. Care should be taken to avoid injuring the underlying neurovascular bundle and parietal pleura.

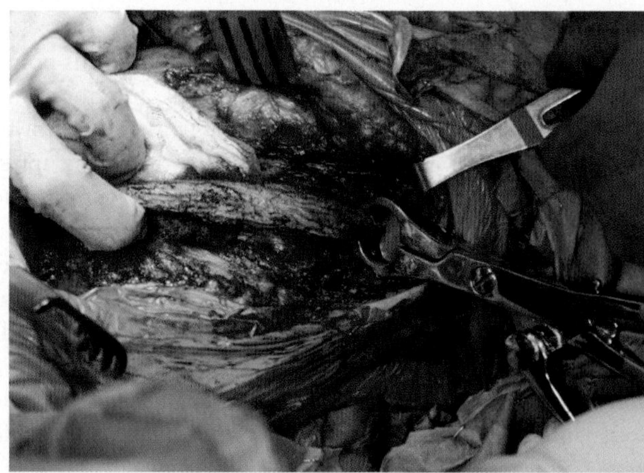

FIG. 19.14 A rib cutter is used to cut the tenth rib to expose the pleura underneath. (From Thongtrangan I, Le HN, Park J, Kim DH. Thoracolumbar and lumbar spines. In: Kim DH, ed. *Surgical Anatomy and Techniques to the Spine*. Philadelphia: Elsevier; 2006.)

The rib is cut anteriorly at the costal margin and posteriorly at the costotransverse junction. The resected rib can be saved and used for bone graft (Fig. 19.14). Bleeding from the cut edges is controlled with bone wax.

After rib resection, the lung is selectively deflated on the approach side. The pleura is identified and protected by splitting the undersurface of the costal cartilage anteriorly (Fig. 19.15). The retroperitoneal space is entered through the split costal cartilage (Fig. 19.16). If the twelfth rib is being resected, the diaphragm attaches superiorly and the transverse abdominis attaches inferiorly. The diaphragm can be retracted superiorly and the transverse abdominis inferiorly, allowing entrance into the retroperitoneum. The peritoneum is bluntly swept off the diaphragm and abdominal muscles (Fig. 19.17). If necessary for exposure, the external oblique, internal oblique, and transverse abdominis muscles are incised.

With the rib resected and the peritoneum safely swept away, a rib retractor is placed. A malleable retractor covered with a moist lap sponge is then placed to further protect the

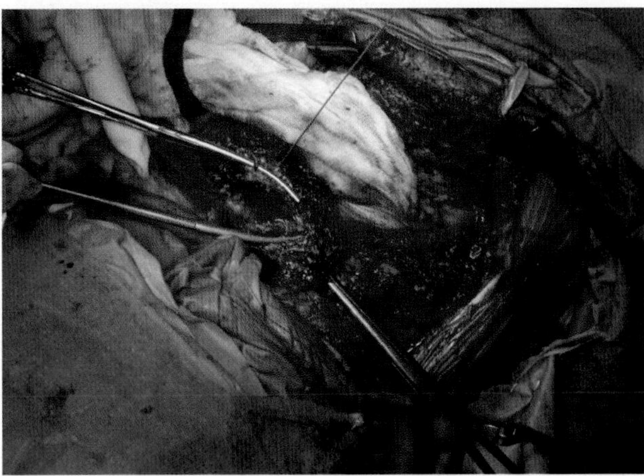

FIG. 19.15 The costal cartilage is split and serves as a landmark for closure. Careful dissection underneath the split cartilage will expose the peritoneal fat, which will lead to the retroperitoneal space. (From Thongtrangan I, Le HN, Park J, Kim DH. Thoracolumbar and lumbar spines. In: Kim DH, ed. *Surgical Anatomy and Techniques to the Spine*. Philadelphia: Elsevier; 2006.)

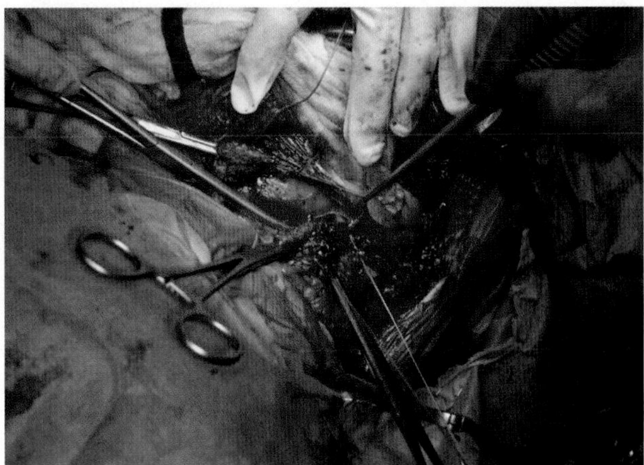

FIG. 19.16 The split costal cartilage is tagged temporarily. The retroperitoneal fat is identified. (From Thongtrangan I, Le HN, Park J, Kim DH. Thoracolumbar and lumbar spines. In: Kim DH, ed. *Surgical Anatomy and Techniques to the Spine*. Philadelphia: Elsevier; 2006.)

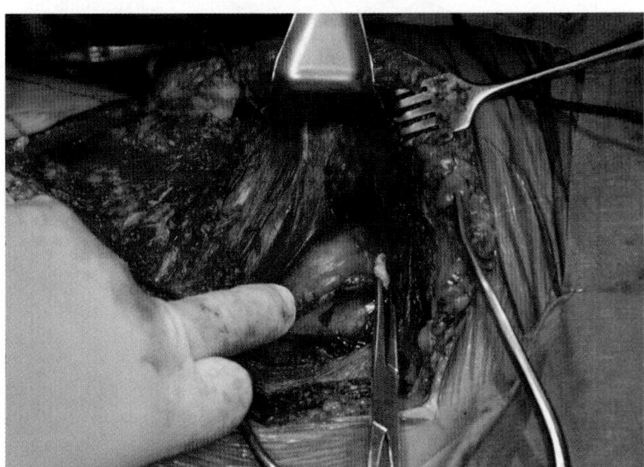

FIG. 19.17 The retroperitoneal space is entered by pushing the peritoneal fat along with the peritoneal content toward the midline. (From Thongtrangan I, Le HN, Park J, Kim DH. Thoracolumbar and lumbar spines. In: Kim DH, ed. *Surgical Anatomy and Techniques to the Spine*. Philadelphia: Elsevier; 2006.)

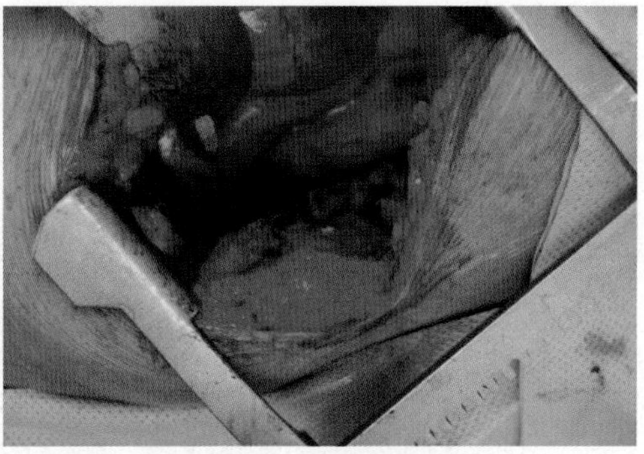

FIG. 19.18 A rib spreader can be used to provide retraction for entry into chest cavity. The lung is further protected with a malleable retractor shielded with a sponge.

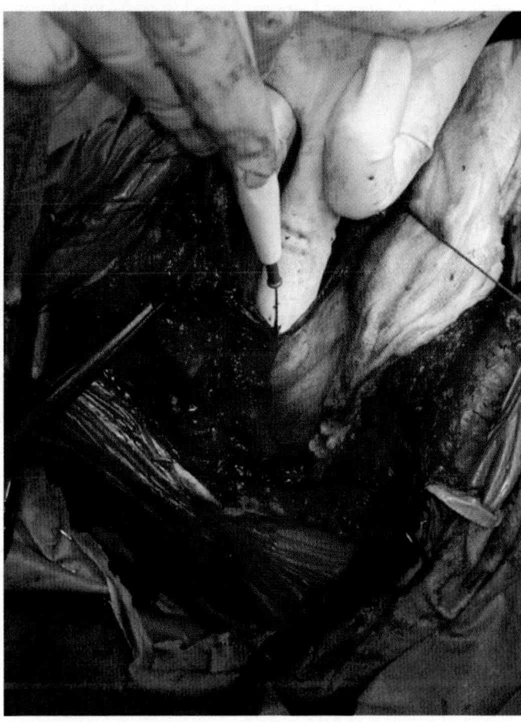

FIG. 19.19 The diaphragm is carefully cut peripherally. (From Thongtrangan I, Le HN, Park J, Kim DH. Thoracolumbar and lumbar spines. In: Kim DH, ed. *Surgical Anatomy and Techniques to the Spine*. Philadelphia: Elsevier; 2006.)

lung. A second retractor placed perpendicular to the first retractor can be placed for improved visualization, if necessary (Fig. 19.18).

The thoracoabdominal cavity is entered and the peritoneum is carefully swept off the psoas and undersurface of the diaphragm. The diaphragm, which should be clearly delineated at this point, is incised circumferentially to release it (Fig. 19.19). A cuff of muscle 1 cm in size should be left and tagged for reapproximation at the end of the case (Fig. 19.20). The crus can be taken down from its attachment at L1 if access to T12 and L1 vertebral bodies is necessary.

For access to the thoracic spine, the parietal pleura is incised, exposing the vertebral body. The intercostal vessels are tied and ligated in order to mobilize the major blood vessels to allow access to the vertebral body of interest. They

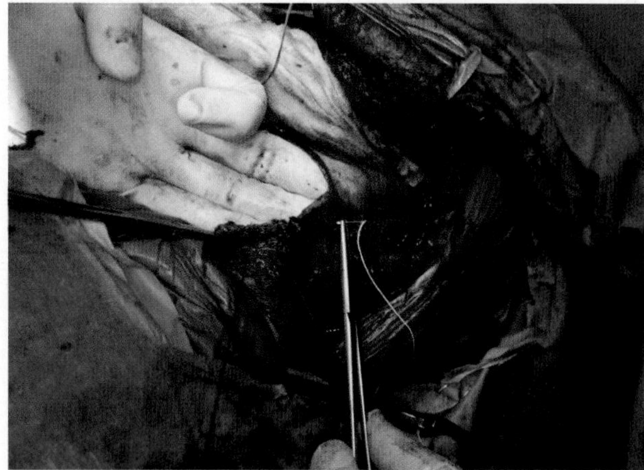

FIG. 19.20 Temporary tagged sutures are used while cutting the diaphragm, which will serve as a landmark for closure. (From Thongtrangan I, Le HN, Park J, Kim DH. Thoracolumbar and lumbar spines. In: Kim DH, ed. *Surgical Anatomy and Techniques to the Spine*. Philadelphia: Elsevier; 2006.)

should be tied and ligated greater than 1 cm from their respective foramen. Care should be taken not to injure the sympathetic plexus, which is in close proximity to the intercostal vessels. If mobilization of the psoas muscle is required in the lumbar spine for exposure, it should be done subperiosteally to avoid injuring the lumbar plexus.

A layered closure for this approach should be performed. The previously tagged diaphragm attachments are repaired with nonabsorbable heavy suture. The parietal pleura is repaired, if possible. The abdominal muscles are repaired in a layered fashion. Lung reexpansion is performed. A chest tube can be placed, if necessary. Care should be taken to ensure that the junction of the diaphragm and abdominal musculature is securely reapproximated to prevent hernia formation.

Posterior Anatomy of the Thoracic Spine

The posterior thoracic spine is covered by a superficial, intermediate, and deep muscle layer (Fig. 19.21). The superficial layer consists of the trapezius and latissimus dorsi muscles. Deep to these muscles, but still considered part of the superficial layer, are the rhomboid major and minor muscles. All of the superficial muscles are innervated by peripheral nerves. The intermediate layer is comprised of the serratus posterior inferior and superior muscles. These muscles are innervated by the anterior rami of the thoracic nerves. Deepest of all, the erector spinae muscles are found (semispinalis, multifidus, and rotatores muscles; see Fig. 19.21). The erector spinae muscles are innervated by the posterior rami of the thoracic nerves. The fascia invests the erector spinae muscles dorsally and ventrally. The dorsal layer constitutes the thoracodorsal fascia. Laterally, the thoracodorsal fascia blends with the aponeurosis of the transverse abdominis muscle; caudally it attaches to the iliac crest and lateral crest of the sacrum.[10] Posterior thoracic spine approaches typically exploit planes that avoid direct injury to the nerves that innervate the posterior musculature.

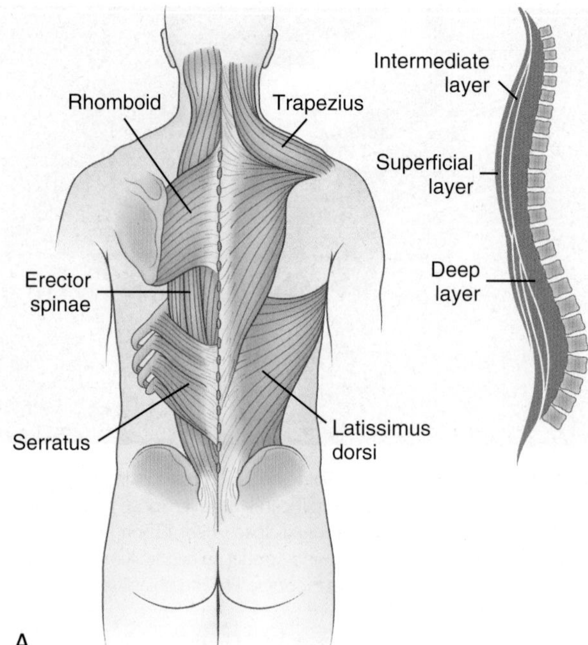

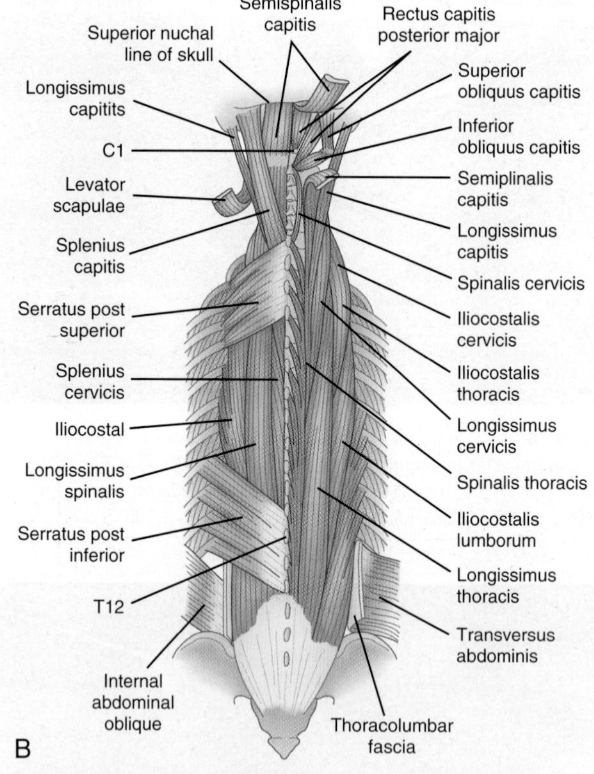

FIG. 19.21 (A) Muscles of the thoracic spine. (B) Intermediate and deep muscles of the thoracic spine. (B, From An HS. *Principles and Techniques of Thoracic Surgery*. Baltimore: Williams & Wilkins; 1998.)

The ligamentous structures of the thoracic spine from dorsal (superficial) to ventral (deep) are the supraspinous ligament, interspinous ligament, ligamentum flavum, posterior longitudinal ligament, and anterior longitudinal ligament (Fig. 19.22). The supraspinous ligament attaches the tips of the spinous processes. The interspinous ligament attaches the spinous process to the adjacent spinous processes with obliquely oriented fibers. The ligamentum flavum runs from

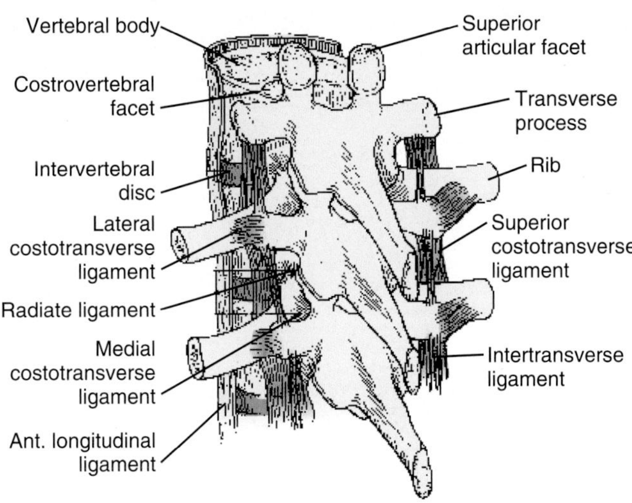

FIG. 19.22 Ligaments of the thoracic spine. (From An HS. *Principles and Techniques of Thoracic Surgery*. Baltimore: Williams & Wilkins; 1998.)

the undersurface of the trailing margin of the cephalad vertebra and inserts on the top portion of the caudad lamina. Of all the ligamentous structures supporting the thoracic spine, the ligamentum flavum is the strongest and most robust. It provides extension support to the adjacent vertebrae. The posterior longitudinal ligament runs along the dorsal aspect of the vertebrae and intervertebral discs and the anterior longitudinal ligament runs ventrally.

The thoracic vertebrae are made up of the vertebral body, pedicles, superior and inferior articular facet, transverse costal facet, pars interarticularis, lamina, and spinous process. There are 12 thoracic vertebral bodies. Vertebral body size sequentially decreases from T1 to T3, then sequentially increases to T12.[13] The spinous processes in the thoracic spine project posteroinferiorly with the tip of the spinous process overlying the preceding vertebral body.

The thoracic ribs articulate with the thoracic vertebral bodies via the transverse costal facet starting at T1. The first rib articulates only with T1. Ribs 1 through 7 have direct attachments to the sternum, thus are referred to as true ribs. Ribs 8 through 10 connect via costal cartilage to the rib above and are called false ribs. Ribs 11 and 12 are floating ribs, and have no attachment point other than to their corresponding vertebral body.[13] The rib heads of ribs 1 through 10 overlie the adjoining intervertebral disc space via two types of articulations: the costovertebral articulation and the costotransverse articulation. The costovertebral articulation is between the rib head and the vertebral body. This articulation is stabilized by the articular capsule, radiate ligament, and intraarticular ligaments. The costotransverse articulation is between the neck and tubercle of the rib and the transverse process.

The facet joints of the thoracic spine have a unique orientation. They are oriented in a more coronal plane and undergo transition from T1 to T12. At T1, the superior facet faces up and back, whereas the inferior facet faces down and forward. Progressing caudad, the superior facet transitions to facing up, back, and slightly lateral. The inferior facet faces down, forward, and more medial. This orientation allows for some rotation. The superior facet contains articular cartilage on its dorsal surface; the inferior facet has articular cartilage on its ventral surface. The pars interarticularis is the portion of bone that connects the superior and inferior articular processes.

Since the advent of pedicle screw fixation and its current widespread use for posterior instrumentation, understanding the anatomy of the thoracic pedicle has become paramount. The pedicle of each vertebral body is located at the base of each facet (Fig. 19.23). There have been numerous studies looking at the morphology of the thoracic pedicles.[14–19] Projecting from their respective vertebrae, thoracic pedicles angle posteriorly and laterally. Moving from cephalad (T1) to caudad (T12), the pedicle aims successively less medially (see Fig. 19.23). The superoinferior pedicle diameter is larger than the mediolateral diameter.[3] The smallest pedicle diameter (medial to lateral) is typically found at T4. In terms of strength, the medial pedicle wall is two to three times stronger than the lateral wall.[14]

The transverse process is found at the junction of the pars interarticularis and facet. The associated nerve root is anterior and superior to the transverse process. The associated dorsal rami are found anteroinferiorly.[1] Protecting the underlying nerve root is an intertransverse aponeurosis.

Posterior Approaches to the Thoracic Spine

The posterior-based approaches to the thoracic spine are the workhorse approaches for a majority of pathologies, including degenerative, traumatic, infectious, and neoplastic conditions. Slight variations in approach allow the surgeon access to midline, lateral, dorsal, and ventral aspects of the spinal column while avoiding associated morbidity with thoracotomy approaches.

Posterior Approach for Decompressive Laminectomy and Fusion

After successful induction of anesthesia, the patient is placed in the prone position. Either a Jackson frame or regular operating room bed with chest rolls is ideal. This allows the abdomen to rest free of pressure, decreasing venous engorgement of the epidural venous plexus, which helps minimize blood loss. Localization is then performed with the aid of fluoroscopy and palpable landmarks. The superior border of the scapula corresponds to T3, the inferior angle of the scapula corresponds to T7, and the most prominent spinous process corresponds to C7. Fluoroscopic visualization of the upper thoracic region can prove difficult secondary to overlap from the shoulders. A combination of anteroposterior (AP) and lateral fluoroscopy should be used to ensure that the appropriate surgical level(s) is marked. The skin is then marked in the midline, directly over the spinous process from the cephalad to caudad surgical level.

A No. 10 blade scalpel is used to incise the skin in this distribution. Subcutaneous dissection is performed with Bovie electrocautery. Subperiosteal dissection is then undertaken by separating the muscular attachments from the spinous process and lamina. Subperiosteal dissection helps minimize blood

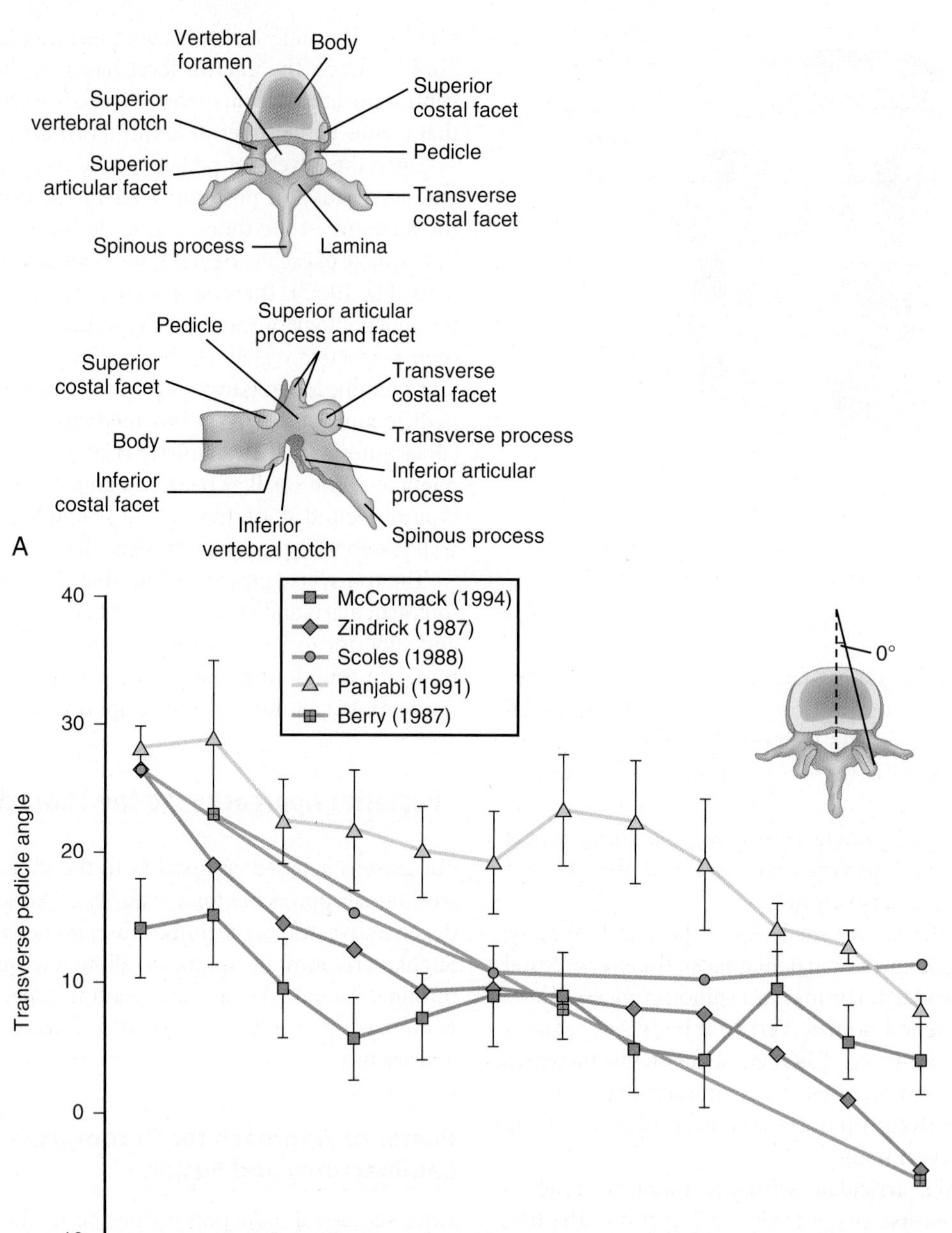

FIG. 19.23 (A) Osseous structure of the thoracic spine and thoracic vertebra. (B) Transverse pedicle angles found in five different studies. (A, From Netter FH. *Atlas of Human Anatomy*. 2nd ed. Philadelphia: Elsevier; 1998. B, From McCormack BM, Benzel EC, Adams MS, et al. Anatomy of the thoracic pedicle. *Neurosurgery*. 1995;37: 303-308.)

loss. Superficially, in the upper thoracic spine, the rhomboid and trapezius muscle attachments are encountered. In the lower thoracic spine, the latissimus dorsi attachments are encountered. Deep to these superficial attachments are the erector spinae and transversospinal muscle attachments. The muscles are retracted laterally and self-retaining retractors are placed.

When performing laminectomy alone, the lateral margins of the lamina and pars interarticularis are exposed while being sure to avoid violating the facet joint capsule. Violating the facet joint capsule when performing wide laminectomy can lead to iatrogenic instability.[20] Care should be taken when exposing the lateral margins of the pars interarticularis and facet joints, as unnecessary bleeding can result.

The next step is performing the laminectomy. There are several ways to accomplish laminectomy in the thoracic spine. A gentle, relatively atraumatic technique that minimizes pressure on the thoracic cord is to use a high-speed burr to create a trough on both sides of the lamina at the junction of the lamina and corresponding facet joint. To complete the troughs, No. 1 and No. 2 Kerrison rongeurs are used. Care should be taken to avoid violating the underlying dura during this process. Once the troughs are complete, the lamina is gently lifted and underlying ligamentum flavum and adhesions are gently released from the undersurface of the caudad margin of the lamina. Using a combination of curettes, No. 1 and No. 2 Kerrison rongeurs, the laminectomy is completed. Further decompression, including partial medial facetectomy and foraminotomy, is performed depending on the degree of decompression necessary.

After ensuring hemostasis has been achieved, the wound is closed in standard fashion.

Transpedicular Approach

The posterior transpedicular approach was first described by Patterson and Arbit in 1978 for approaching thoracic disc herniations.[21] As the approach has gained popularity, its indications have expanded to include tumor, infectious, and traumatic etiologies. The approach can be performed unilaterally or bilaterally depending on the need for isolated access to the posterolateral aspect of the vertebral body and disc space on one side versus the need for bilateral access, as in the case of tumors affecting both nerve roots or for complete discectomy.

A unilateral transpedicular approach is less destabilizing than a bilateral transpedicular approach. However, the bilateral transpedicular approach can allow one to perform near-circumferential decompression, such as in the case of extensive tumor involvement or if there is a need for complete discectomy. In fact, this approach can be used to perform circumferential decompression and vertebrectomy.[22,23] If bilateral transpedicular approaches are being performed, serious consideration should be given to stabilization to prevent iatrogenic instability and deformity.

After intubation, the patient is placed in the prone position on a Jackson table or radiolucent table with chest rolls. Image intensification is then used to mark the surgical levels. Standard sterile prep and drape is performed.

A midline incision is then made over the surgical level(s) being addressed. Subperiosteal dissection is performed laterally until the lamina and facet joint of the level to be treated is exposed. This is undertaken bilaterally if bilateral transpedicular approaches are being used.

The pedicle overlying the disc herniation or level to be treated is identified. For a thoracic disc herniation, the caudal pedicle is adjacent to the intervertebral disc (i.e., the T9–T10 disc is adjacent to the T10 pedicle). To help further identify the pedicle, spinal cord and affected nerve root laminectomy can be performed prior to pedicle removal. Once the pedicle is identified, it is entered with a high-speed burr and the central, cancellous portion is removed to the depth of the pedicle vertebral body junction. Intraoperative fluoroscopy can be useful for this portion of the procedure to help safely guide the surgeon down the pedicle as well as aid in depth of resection. After removal of the cancellous portion of the pedicle has been achieved, the remaining cortical wall is taken down with either a pituitary rongeur or down-biting curettes. In the classical approach, only the medial and superior borders of the pedicle are resected, but the entire pedicle can be taken down if necessary. Decompression is then performed in a lateral to medial trajectory, with care taken to avoid injuring the spinal cord and nerve root (Fig. 19.24).

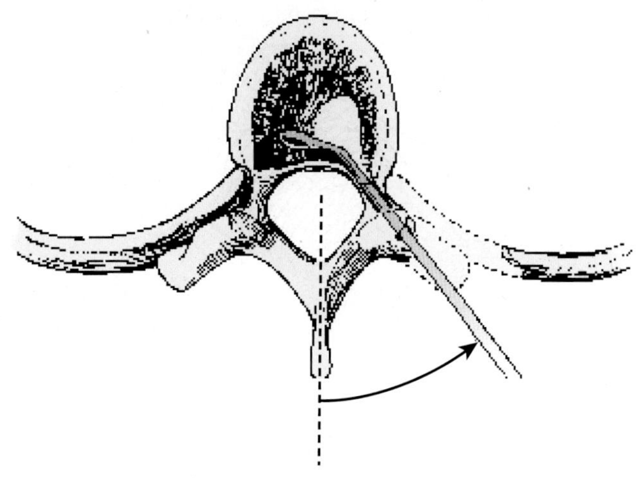

FIG. 19.24 The transpedicular approach.

Costotransversectomy

First described in 1894 by Menard, the costotransversectomy approach was originally created for the treatment of spinal abscess.[24] Since its first description, many variations and alternate indications have been established. The approach allows near-circumferential access to the anterior thoracic spine while avoiding the potential morbidity associated with an anterior approach. Additionally, this approach allows for single-stage surgery, with the ability to decompress and stabilize simultaneously. Current indications include thoracic disc herniations, fractures, tumor, infection, and deformity.[25]

Traditionally, the patient is placed in the prone position on a Jackson table or radiolucent table with chest rolls. Alternatively, the patient can be placed in a semiprone or modified lateral decubitus position. The table should allow circumferential fluoroscopic visualization of the surgical level. Having the ability to airplane the table can help aid in visualization.

Fluoroscopy is used to help mark the skin incision at the appropriate surgical level(s). Sterile prep and drape is performed. Attention should be given to ensuring that wide draping is achieved, as this approach involves partial rib exposure.

There are several incision variations that can be used. Ultimately, the decision regarding which incision to use depends on the indication for the procedure and whether or not laminectomy and/or instrumentation is required. Traditionally, a curvilinear incision approximately 8 cm lateral to the spinous process of the surgical level that is 10 to 13 cm in length has been described (Fig. 19.25). [4] Since most procedures involve scenarios requiring simultaneous laminectomy and/or stabilization, the following technique is described from a midline posterior approach.

Using the previously described standard posterior approach to the thoracic spine, subperiosteal dissection is performed exposing the lamina and transverse process. Further lateral dissection is carried posteriorly and laterally along the corresponding rib approximately 6 to 8 cm depending on the extent of exposure required. The transverse process and rib

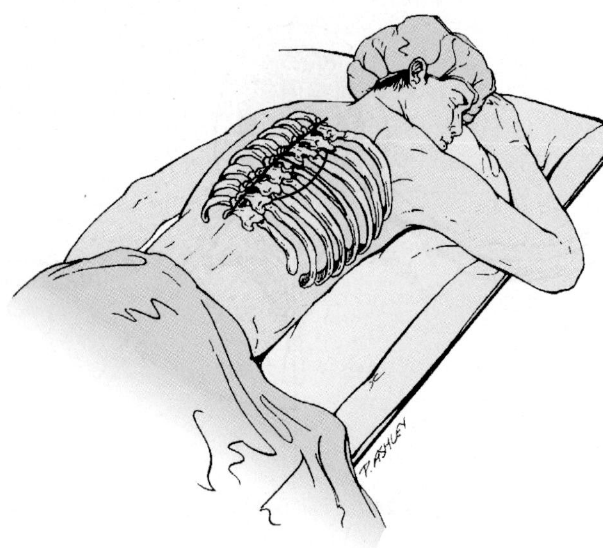

FIG. 19.25 A median or paramedian incision may be made straight or curved centered over the desired vertebral level. Traditionally, a curvilinear incision about 8 cm lateral to the intended spinous process and 10 cm to 13 cm long has been used.

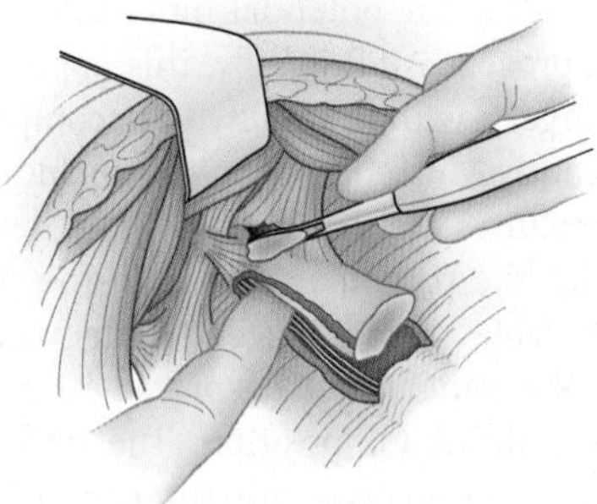

FIG. 19.26 The rib and its arthrodial junction can now be disarticulated. A subperiosteal dissection is done along the pedicle and upper and lower vertebral body to separate the pleura from the vertebral wall.

are then dissected circumferentially using a periosteal elevator, rib dissector, or curettes. Great care should be taken to avoid violating the underlying pleura and the neurovascular bundle, which travels on the underside of the rib. Once entirely skeletonized, the rib is cut laterally with a rib cutter or large Kerrison rongeur. The rib is then gently lifted up and away from the underlying pleura and neurovascular bundle, and disarticulated from the costovertebral joint attachment with Bovie electrocautery or curettes, removing the rib en bloc (Fig. 19.26). If a fusion is being performed, the rib can be used for bone graft. The corresponding transverse process can also be resected for further visualization of the pedicle and lateral vertebral body. Bone bleeding is controlled with bone wax.

Next, the lateral pedicle wall is identified and careful subperiosteal dissection is performed along the lateral aspect of the vertebral body with a Cobb elevator while protecting the underlying pleura. Dissection is carried ventral until the anterior margin of the vertebral body is reached. A malleable retractor is then placed to create a working window and protect the underlying pleura and vascular structures (Fig. 19.27).

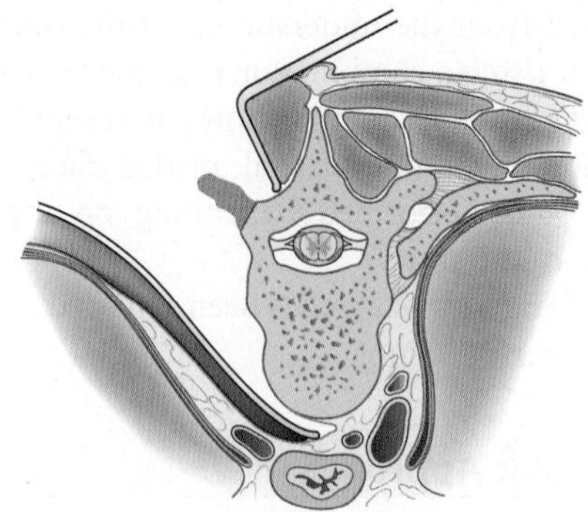

FIG. 19.27 A subperiosteal dissection is done along the pedicle and upper and lower vertebral body to separate the pleura from the vertebral wall.

Lateral Extracavitary Approach

The lateral extracavitary approach was developed by Larson and colleagues at the University of Wisconsin in 1976, after expanding on the work of Menard and Capener.[26] This approach is an expansion of the costotransversectomy approach, allowing for greater exposure and visualization of the ventral thecal sac. The indications for this approach include tumors, infection, trauma, and treatment of thoracic disc disease.[27] This approach can be utilized throughout the entire thoracic spine. Similar to the costotransversectomy, it is a versatile approach that avoids the need for formal thoracotomy.

The patient is placed in the prone position on a Jackson table or radiolucent surgical bed with chest rolls. The patient should be secured to the table to allow for bed rotation of 20 to 30 degrees if necessary.

Once positioned, localization for the skin incision is performed with the aid of the fluoroscope. The patient should be draped widely to allow for formal thoracotomy, if necessary.

After prep and drape, a midline incision centered over the spinous process of the level of interest is made. The superficial and deep fascia to trapezius and latissimus dorsi are incised. Depending on surgeon preference, the incision can be carried laterally in hockey stick fashion 8 cm if a wider exposure is needed. In the lower thoracic spine, the fibers of the trapezius are close to the transverse process of the rib. A plane is now established to expose the lateral margin of the paraspinal muscles. Working lateral to medial, the paraspinal muscles are elevated subperiosteally and retracted. Similar to the costotransversectomy approach, the rib of interest is skeletonized utilizing the subperiosteal technique while being careful not to damage the underlying parietal pleura. The transverse process of the rib and the lamina on the operative side are similarly exposed. The transverse process is removed. If more exposure is required, the cephalad rib can be similarly exposed, allowing for even greater visualization.

The rib is cut laterally with a rib cutter or large Kerrison rongeurs. As opposed to the limited rib resection with

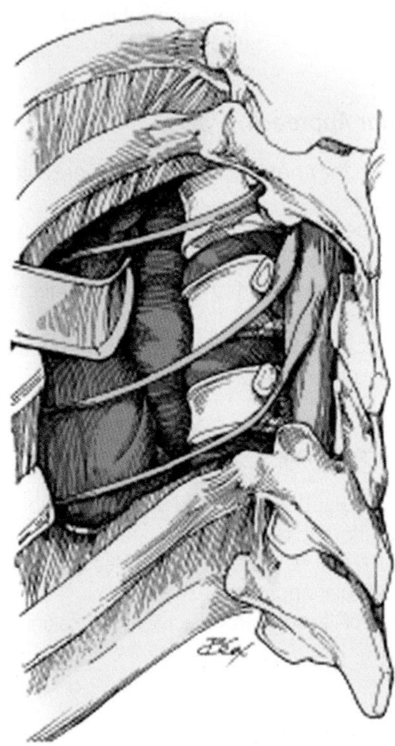

FIG. 19.28 When posterolateral structures of the transverse process and pedicle have been removed, exposure should be adequate for discectomy.

costotransversectomy, approximately 12 cm of rib can be resected with the lateral extracavitary approach. Once cut laterally, it is gently lifted off the underlying parietal pleura and detached medially from its vertebral body and costal attachments.

The neurovascular bundle is visualized and traced back to the neural foramen, allowing for identification of the corresponding pedicle. The pedicle is now very carefully taken down with a high-speed burr or rongeur while not violating the underlying dura.

Upon complete pedicle and transverse process resection, good visualization of the disc space should be achievable (Fig. 19.28). Depending on the indication for the approach, discectomy is then performed followed by corpectomy.

Corpectomy can be performed from pedicle to pedicle with a combination of curettes, high-speed burr, and pituitary rongeur. Great caution should be exercised during corpectomy to avoid injuring the ventral dura and spinal cord. To improve visualization, the bed can be rotated 20 to 30 degrees away from the operating surgeon. Additionally, a thin shell of posterior vertebral body cortex can be left behind until central and ventral corpectomy has been completed. This remaining shell of bone can then be carefully removed, pushing it away from the ventral dura.

After completion of the corpectomy, the corpectomy cage and/or graft is placed and positioning confirmed with fluoroscopy. If posterior pedicle screw and rod stabilization is to be performed, a separate, standard, midline fascial incision and approach is performed medial to the paraspinal muscles, elevating them in a subperiosteal manner.

Upon completion of corpectomy and stabilization, the pleura is examined for any breaches. If a breach is identified, it is repaired. If the breach is considered significant, chest tube placement may be necessary.[28]

Minimally Invasive Approaches to the Thoracic and Thoracolumbar Spine

Recent advances in techniques have led to the development of minimally invasive approaches to the thoracic and thoracolumbar spine that exploit the same tissue planes as traditional open procedures but achieve access through smaller incisions and less tissue disruption. Potential benefits of minimally invasive approaches include less postoperative pain, quicker recovery, and avoiding complications and morbidities associated with larger open procedures. Early results are promising, with complication rates ranging from 4.8% to 13.5%.[28,29] That being said, they can be technically demanding and, if complications do arise, they can be difficult to manage through the small access site.

Minimally invasive lateral approaches to the thoracic spine have been described.[29,30] Similar techniques have been applied to traumatic fractures requiring corpectomy.[31] The patient is positioned in the true lateral decubitus position similar to thoracotomy approaches. A transthoracic or retropleural approach can be utilized. For the transthoracic approach, a 3- to 4-cm oblique incision paralleling and between the ribs of interest is made. The intercostal muscles and parietal pleura are incised in line with the skin incision, allowing entry into the thoracic cavity. Depending on the exposure required, a portion of the rib can be resected. Care should be taken to avoid injuring the neurovascular bundle that lies on the undersurface of the rib.

If a retropleural approach is utilized, a 6-cm oblique incision following the course of the rib is made in the midaxillary line. Approximately 5 cm of rib is then carefully subperiosteally dissected and resected, with care taken not to violate the parietal pleura or neurovascular bundle. The plane between the endothoracic fascia and parietal pleura is developed and the pleura mobilized anteriorly until the lateral side of the vertebral body, pedicle, and disc space are exposed. If a left-sided approach is performed, the aorta and hemizygos vein are retracted anteriorly with the pleura. An expandable retractor system is then placed, protecting the surrounding structures and allowing focal access to the surgical pathology. Standard surgical techniques are employed. For corpectomies, an expandable cage can be utilized.

KEY POINTS

Low Anterior Cervical and High Transsternal Approach

1. The plane between the midline esophagus and airway and the carotid sheath laterally is utilized with this approach.
2. A left-sided approach should be considered given the predictable course of the recurrent laryngeal nerve on this side.
3. Turning the head away from the approach side and gently taping the shoulders downward will improve access and fluoroscopic visualization.

Transpleural Transthoracic Third Rib Approach

1. A double-lumen endotracheal tube should be used to allow for selective lung deflation.
2. The first rib sits medial and recessed to the second rib. The second rib is typically the highest palpable rib.
3. The parietal pleura should be entered over the relatively avascular disc space as opposed to directly over the vertebral body in order to avoid inadvertent injury to the intercostal vessels.
4. A chest tube should be placed at the end of the case.

Thoracotomy (Anterior) Approach to the Thoracic Spine

1. A right-sided approach should be considered above T10 to avoid having to manipulate the aorta. Below T10, a left-sided approach should be considered to avoid working around the liver.
2. Ligation of the segmental vessels should be performed away from the aorta to minimize the risk of the ties or clips loosening.
3. The parietal pleura should be entered over the relatively avascular disc space as opposed to directly over the vertebral body in order to avoid inadvertent injury to the intercostal vessels.
4. A double-lumen endotracheal tube should be used to allow for selective lung deflation.

Endoscopic Anterior Approach to the Thoracic Spine

1. A double-lumen endotracheal tube should be used to allow for selective lung deflation.
2. The initial trocar is placed using blunt dissection on the superior margin of the intervening rib, avoiding damage to the neurovascular bundle on the undersurface of the rib. Subsequent trocars are placed under direct thoracoscopic visualization.
3. A chest tube should be placed through the inferiormost trocar site.
4. A chest radiograph should be obtained at the end of the case prior to complete closure to ensure full reexpansion of the lung.

Anterior Approach to the Thoracolumbar Spine

1. A double-lumen endotracheal tube should be used to allow for selective lung deflation.
2. The peritoneum is bluntly released from the diaphragm and abdominal musculature.
3. Care should be taken to avoid injuring the sympathetic chain in the thoracic cavity and the lumbar plexus in the abdominal cavity.
4. Special attention should be given to closure at the junction of the diaphragm and abdominal musculature to avoid hernia formation.

Posterior Approach for Decompressive Laminectomy and Fusion

1. Subperiosteal dissection is employed to minimize bleeding.
2. A high speed burr is used to create bilateral troughs at the junction of the lamina and facet joints for the laminectomy. The troughs are completed with small Kerrison rongeurs, and the lamina is carefully and gently removed in its entirety. This minimizes pressure on the spinal cord.

Transpedicular Approach

1. This approach may not be ideal for decompression of central pathology.
2. Care should be taken not to retract the spinal cord. If necessary, additional bone should be resected for visualization.
3. Turning the bed away from the operating surgeon can aid with ventral visualization.
4. Pedicle entry and takedown should be performed under fluoroscopic guidance to aid in proper trajectory and depth.

Costotransversectomy

1. The neurovascular bundle on the undersurface of the rib is protected during rib resection.
2. This approach utilizes a more lateral trajectory as compared to the transpedicular approach.
3. Additional visualization can be achieved by taking down an adjacent rib.

Lateral Extracavitary Approach

1. This approach is similar to a costotransversectomy approach. However, a large portion of the rib is resected, providing additional exposure.
2. The ventral dura can be protected during corpectomy by leaving a thin shell of dorsal vertebral body behind until central and anterior portions of the corpectomy are complete. This remnant shell can then be gently pushed away from the dura into the corpectomy cavity and removed safely.
3. Improved central and contralateral visualization can be achieved by rotating the bed away from the operating surgeon 20 to 30 degrees.
4. Any violation of the parietal pleura should be repaired, if possible. Consideration should be given to placing a chest tube.

Minimally Invasive Approaches

1. A transthoracic or retropleural approach can be performed through a minimally invasive approach.
2. Early results of minimally invasive lateral approaches to the thoracic and thoracolumbar spine are promising.
3. One should be prepared to convert to a traditional open technique should a complication arise or minimally invasive access is not achievable.

KEY REFERENCES

1. Tew JM Jr, Mayfield FH. Complications of surgery of the anterior cervical spine. *Clin Neurosurg*. 1976;23:424-434.
2. Kothe R, O'Holleran JD, Liu W, et al. Internal architecture of the thoracic pedicle: an anatomic study. *Spine*. 1996;21: 264-270.
3. Patterson RH Jr, Arbit E. A surgical approach through the pedicle to protruded thoracic disks. *J Neurosurg*. 1978;48: 768-772.
4. Benzel EC. The lateral extracavitary approach to the spine using the three quarter prone position. *J Neurosurg*. 1989;71: 837-841.

REFERENCES

1. Tew JM Jr, Mayfield FH. Complications of surgery of the anterior cervical spine. *Clin Neurosurg*. 1976;23:424-434.
2. Kilburg C, Sullivan HG, Mathiason MA. Effect of approach side during anterior cervical discectomy and fusion on the incidence of recurrent laryngeal nerve injury. *J Neurosurg Spine*. 2006;4:273-277.
3. Daniels AH, Riew KD, Yoo JU, et al. Adverse events associated with anterior cervical spine surgery. *J Am Acad Orthop Surg*. 2008;16:729-738.
4. Hoppenfeld S, DeBoer P, Buckley R, et al. *Surgical Exposures in Orthopedics: The Anatomic Approach*. Philadelphia: JB Lippincott; 2009.
5. Campos JH. Lung isolation techniques. *Anesthesiol Clin North Am*. 2001;19:455-474.
6. Fujimaki Y, Kawahara N, Tomita K, et al. How many ligations of bilateral segmental arteries cause ischemic spinal cord dysfunction? An experimental study using a dog model. *Spine*. 2006;31(21):E781-E789.
7. Landreneau RJ, Hazelrigg SR, Mack MJ, et al. Postoperative pain related morbidity: video-assisted thoracic surgery versus thoracotomy. *Ann Thorac Surg*. 1993;56:1285-1289.
8. Hazelrigg SR, Landreneau RJ, Boley TM, et al. The effect of muscle-sparing versus standard posterolateral thoracotomy on pulmonary function, muscle strength, and postoperative pain. *J Thorac Cardiovasc Surg*. 1991;101:394-400.
9. Wang JC. *Advanced Reconstruction: Spine*. Rosemont, IL: American Association of Orthopaedic Surgeons; 2011.
10. Kim DH. *Surgical Anatomy and Techniques to the Spine*. Philadelphia: WB Saunders; 2006.
11. Whang PG, Vaccaro AR. Thoracolumbar fracture: posterior instrumentation using distraction and ligamentotaxis reduction. *J Am Acad Orthop Surg*. 2007;15:695-701.
12. Kirkpatrick JS. Thoracolumbar fracture management: anterior approach. *J Am Acad Orthop Surg*. 2003;11:355-363.
13. Magee DJ. *Orthopedic Physical Assessment*. 4th ed. Philadelphia.: Saunders; 2002.
14. Kothe R, O'Holleran JD, Liu W, et al. Internal architecture of the thoracic pedicle: an anatomic study. *Spine*. 1996;21:264-270.
15. Banta CJ 2nd, King AG, Dabezies EJ, et al. Measurement of effective pedicle diameter in the human spine. *Orthopedics*. 1989;12:939-942.
16. Berry JL, Moran JM, Berg WS, et al. A morphometric study of the human lumbar and selected thoracic vertebrae. *Spine*. 1987;12:362-367.
17. Krag MH, Weaver DL, Beynonn BD, et al. Morphometry of the thoracic and lumbar spine related to transpedicular screw placement for surgical spine fixation. *Spine*. 1988; 13:27-32.
18. Panjabi MM, Takata K, Goel V, et al. Thoracic human vertebrae: quantitative three-dimensional anatomy. *Spine*. 1991;16:888-901.
19. Zindrick MR, Wiltse LL, Doornik A, et al. Analysis of the morphometric characteristics of the thoracic and lumbar pedicles. *Spine*. 1987;12:160-166.
20. Oda I, Abumi K, Cunningham BW, Kaneda K, McAfee PC. An in vitro human cadaveric study investigating the biomechanical properties of the thoracic spine. *Spine*. 2002;27(3):E64-E70.
21. Patterson RH Jr, Arbit E. A surgical approach through the pedicle to protruded thoracic disks. *J Neurosurg*. 1978;48: 768-772.
22. Metcalfe S, Gbejuade H, Patel NR. The posterior transpedicular approach for circumferential decompression and instrumented stabilization with titanium cage vertebrectomy reconstruction for spinal tumors: consecutive case series of 50 patients. *Spine*. 2012;37(16):1375-1383.
23. Wong ML, Lau HC, Kaye AH. A modified posterolateral transpedicular approach to thoracolumbar corpectomy with nerve preservation and bilateral cage reconstruction. *J Clin Neurosci*. 2014;21(6):988-992.
24. Campbell WC, Edmonson AS, Crenshaw AH. Infections of the spine. In: *Campbell's Operative Orthopaedics*. 13th ed. St. Louis: Elsevier; 2017.
25. Daubs M, Fernandez ML. The costotransversectomy approach for vertebrectomy. In: Wang JC, ed. *Advanced Reconstruction: Spine*. Rosemont, IL: American Academy of Orthopaedic Surgeons; 2011:243-249.
26. Lifshutz J, Lidar Z, Maiman D. Evolution of the lateral extracavitary approach to the spine. *Neurosurg Focus*. 2004;16:E12.
27. Benzel EC. The lateral extracavitary approach to the spine using the three quarter prone position. *J Neurosurg*. 1989;71:837-841.
28. Vacarro AR. *Fractures of the Cervical, Thoracic and Lumbar Spine*. New York: Marcel Dekker; 2003.
29. Uribe JS, Dakwar E, Le TV, et al. Minimally invasive surgery treatment for thoracic spine tumor removal. *Spine*. 2010;35(26):347-354.
30. Serak J, Vanni S, Levi AD. The extreme lateral approach for the treatment of thoracic and lumbar vertebral body metastasis. *J Neurosurg Sci*. 2015. Epub ahead of print.
31. Smith WD, Dakwar E, Le TV, et al. Minimally invasive surgery for traumatic spinal pathologies. *Spine*. 2010;35(26):338-346.

CHAPTER 20 Lateral and Posterior Approaches to the Lumbosacral Spine

Yu-Po Lee
Saif Aldeen Farhan
Nitin N. Bhatia

Selection of Approach to the Lumbar Spine

Once the decision has been made to operate, the surgeon must choose the best procedure and approach. When considering the options in the lumbar spine, many factors must be taken into account. First is the location of the pathology. Disease or deformity that primarily involves the vertebral bodies may be most easily approached through the abdomen or flank. The posterior elements are most easily approached through a posterior, midline incision. Second, the morbidity of each approach must fit the risk tolerance of each individual patient. For example, it may be preferable to avoid an anterior approach in a young male who has pathology at L5–S1 to avoid the risk of retrograde ejaculation.[1–3] With the advent of minimally invasive techniques, decreasing overall morbidity from tissue dissection must be weighed against more complete visualization that the more traditional open approaches provide. Chapter 21 discusses lateral and posterior approaches to the lumbar spine and their pros and cons.

Minimally Invasive Lateral Approach to the Spine

The concept of minimally invasive spine surgery is attractive to both patients and surgeons alike. Decreased postoperative pain, shorter hospital stay, and quicker return to activities support the use of minimally invasive techniques whenever possible.[4–8] One such technique is lateral access to the spine.[9] This can be used for multilevel interbody fusions to correct kyphoscoliosis, for interbody support when treating adjacent segment degeneration or multilevel fusions, or to drain a psoas abscess (Fig. 20.1). With this approach, access to the spine from T7 down to L4–L5 is possible. However, L4–L5 is often difficult to reach due to a high-riding iliac crest, and a lateral interbody fusion at this level is controversial at this time. The means to accessing L5–S1 laterally has not been developed.

Technique

Once the patient has been intubated and prophylactic antibiotics given, the patient is placed in the lateral decubitus position. When correcting a kyphoscoliosis, it is often easier to perform the lateral approach on the side of the concavity. When planning to perform a lateral interbody fusion, we advise studying the preoperative anteroposterior (AP) and lateral radiographs and the axial magnetic resonance images (MRIs) to determine if this procedure is feasible. The AP and lateral radiographs will show if the iliac crests are too high (see Figs. 20.1A–B). The axial MRI should also be evaluated to see where the nerves are preoperatively (Fig. 20.2). If the nerve is in the middle of the disc space, the surgeon may attempt to approach from the other side or plan for a different procedure.

The table should be flexed slightly to increase the distance between the iliac crest and the rib cage, and the patient secured with tape over the greater trochanter and chest wall (Fig. 20.3). Care should be taken not to flex the table too much, as that may put increased strain on the psoas and lumbar plexus. The leg on top should also be flexed, abducted with pillows, and externally rotated to relax the psoas. A cross-table AP should be taken and the table should be rotated to place the patient in a true AP position (Fig. 20.4A). A corresponding lateral fluoroscopic image should also be taken to verify that access to the disc space is possible (Fig. 20.4B). Minor adjustments should be made to the table to obtain a true lateral.

Once the patient has been prepped and draped, start with the lateral image. A radiopaque marker is placed over the center of the affected disc space (Fig. 20.5). Once this point has been identified, a mark is made. Through this mark, a small incision will be made for insertion of the dilators and an expandable retractor, which will provide access to the lateral spine. A second mark is made posterior to this first mark at the border between the erector spinae muscles and the abdominal obliques (Fig. 20.6). At this second mark, a transverse incision about 2 cm long is made to accommodate the surgeon's index finger. Finger dissection is used down to the lumbodorsal fascia. A clamp, or scissors, can be used to spread the fascia and muscle fibers and provide entry into the retroperitoneal space. Once an opening is created, the index finger is used to sweep the peritoneum anteriorly and to palpate the psoas muscle (Fig. 20.7AB). Sweep the index finger inferiorly to feel the inner table of the iliac crest (if in the lower lumbar spine) to verify that you are in the abdominal cavity.

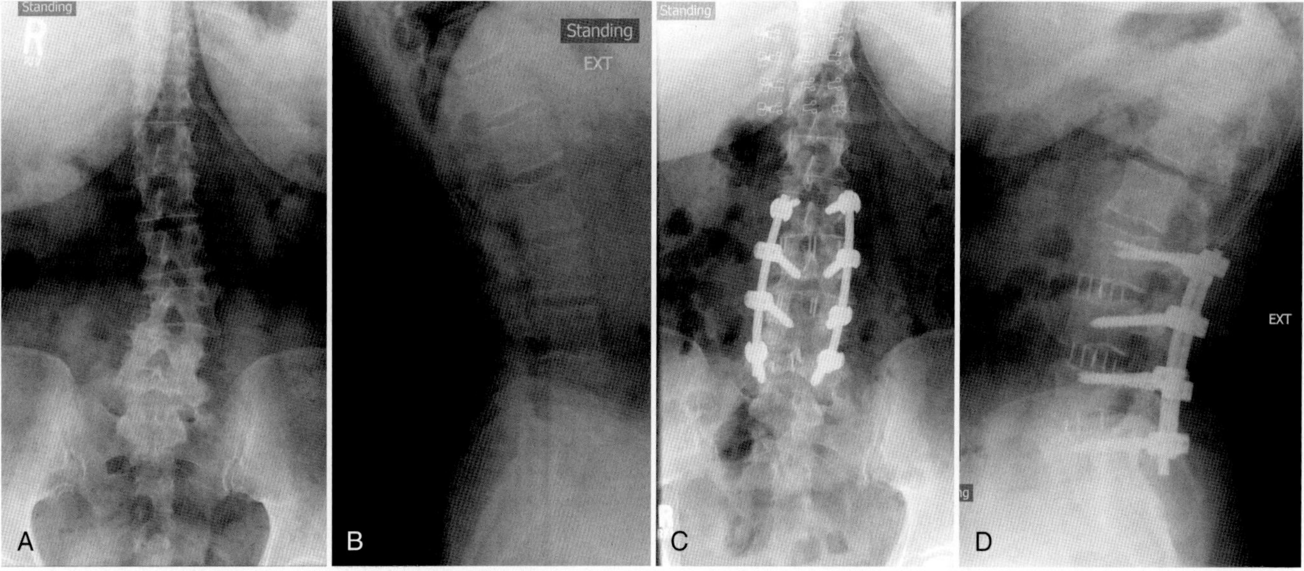

FIG. 20.1 (A–B) Anteroposterior and lateral radiographs of a 71-year-old woman with degenerative scoliosis. (C–D) Anteroposterior and lateral radiographs after L3–L4 and L4–L5 lateral interbody fusions and minimally invasive transforaminal lumbar interbody fusion at L5–S1.

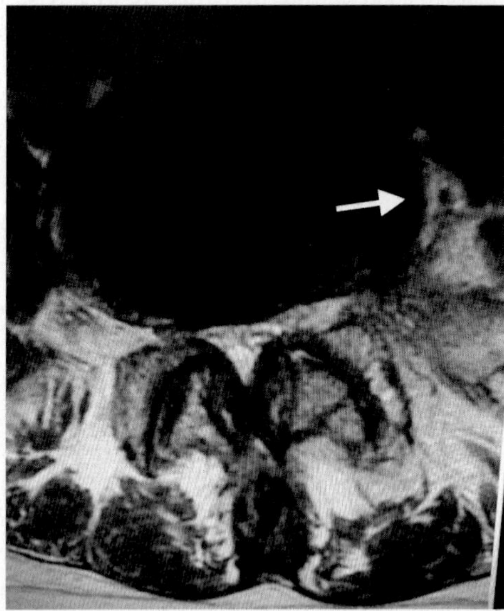

FIG. 20.2 Axial magnetic resonance image showing nerve roots in the axial plane. *Arrow* is pointing to the ventral nerve root. In this case, the surgeon may wish to approach from the right side to avoid the nerve root here.

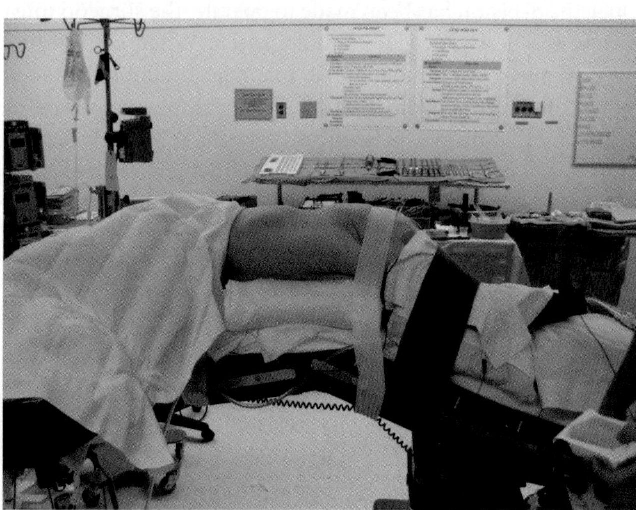

FIG. 20.3 Patient placed in right lateral decubitus position with table flexed to increase the distance between his ribs and iliac crest.

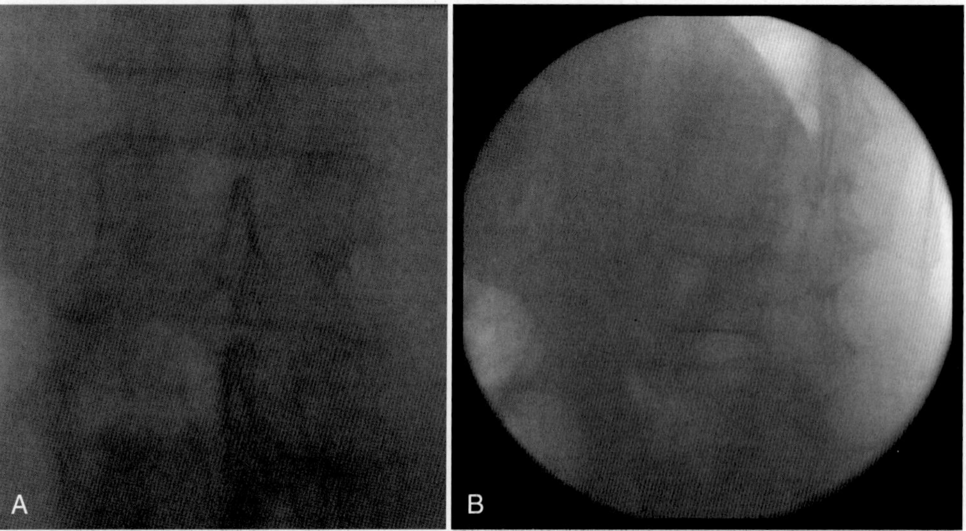

FIG. 20.4 (A) Cross-table anteroposterior (AP) position showing a true AP view. The endplates are parallel and the spinous process is midline. (B) Corresponding lateral fluoroscopic image showing parallel endplates and superimposed pedicles.

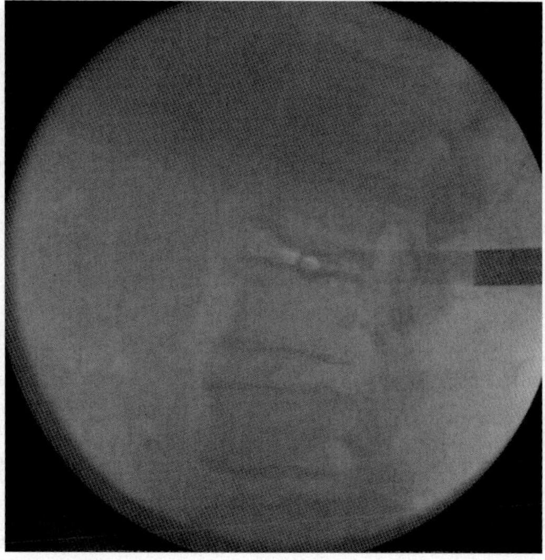

FIG. 20.5 Fluoroscopic image showing center positioning over the disc space. A mark is made on the skin here.

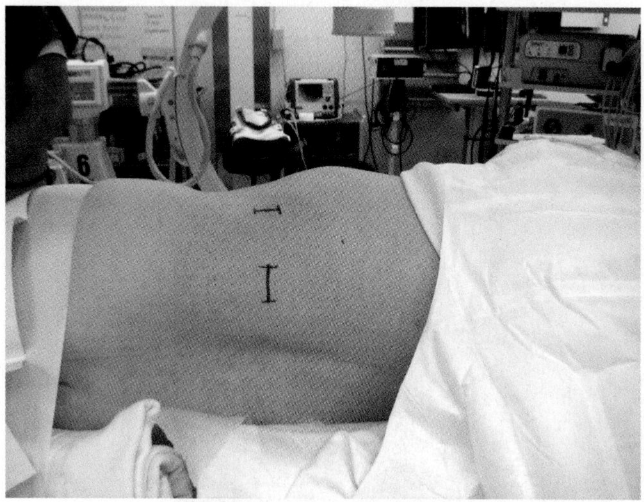

FIG. 20.6 Two-incision technique shown with lateral and posterolateral marks. The posterolateral incision is made about the length of the surgeon's index finger away from the lateral incision. From this mark, the surgeon should also measure the distance to the spine to make sure to be able to reach the psoas from this incision.

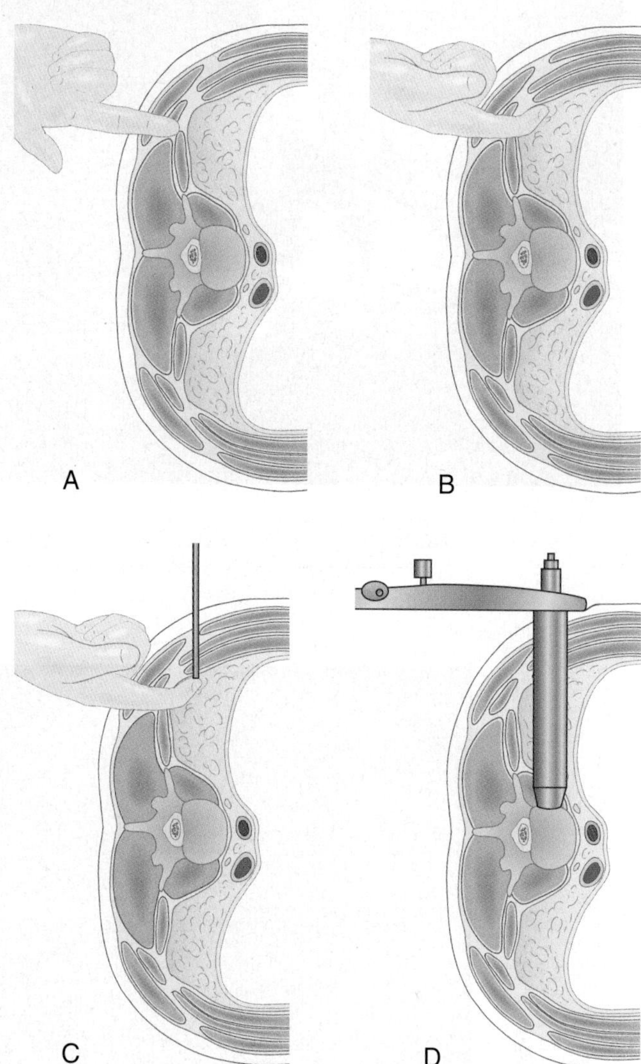

FIG. 20.7 (A–B) The surgeon uses digital palpation to sweep the abdominal contents anteriorly and create a cavity in the retroperitoneal space. (C) The index finger guides the initial dilator down to the psoas. (D) Once the initial dilator is secured in place with a K-wire, larger dilators are used to spread the psoas under neuromonitoring, and a retractor is placed over the dilators.

Once the psoas is identified, the index finger is swept up to the previously made direct lateral mark. A 2-cm incision is made and the external and internal oblique muscles and the transverses abdominis muscles are split; dilators are placed through this opening. The index finger, which is already in the retroperitoneal space, guides the initial dilator onto the psoas (Fig. 20.7C). The fibers of the psoas are then split with the dilator, using neuromonitoring as a safety measure, if desired. A lateral radiograph should be taken to verify the central position of the dilator at the desired disc space. Once the position of the initial dilator is secured by placing a Kirschner wire (K-wire) through the dilator and into the disc space, larger dilators are used to spread the psoas under neuromonitoring. Then, an expandable retractor is placed over the dilators (Fig. 20.7D). Once the retractor is secured to the table, the dilators are removed to provide lateral access to the disc (Figs. 20.8). A neuromonitoring probe can be used to check for any nerves that may be crossing the working window of the retractor. If a nerve is detected, the K-wire should be repositioned away from the nerve and the psoas redilated. If this fails, conversion to another means of interbody fusion should be considered, as repeated positioning of the retractor, or pressure on the nerve, could result in postoperative paresthesias or palsies.

AP and lateral radiographs should be taken at this point to verify that the retractor is docked on the disc space and that the retractor is positioned over the center of the disc. Once appropriate positioning has been confirmed, the retractor should be secured in place. A lateral discectomy is then performed in standard fashion with shavers, curettes, and rasps. Care must be taken not to violate the endplates because much of the correction from a lateral interbody fusion is based

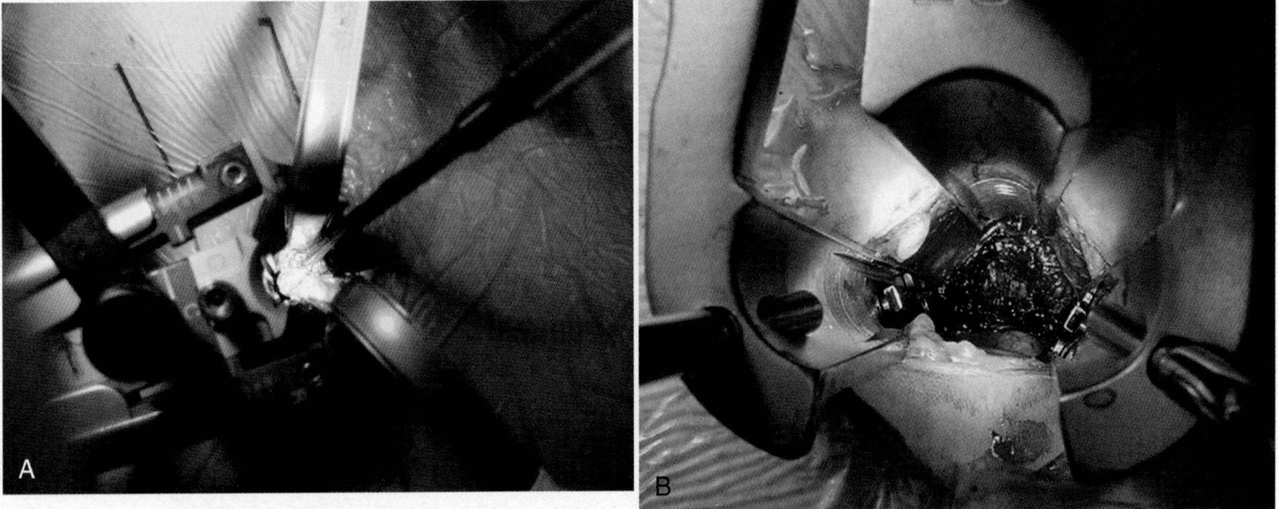

FIG. 20.8 (A) Once the retractor is deployed, soft tissue over the disc space must be cleared away. Use a probe to detect any nerves that may cross the field. (B) The disc can be visualized after the psoas muscle has been cleared from the field of view.

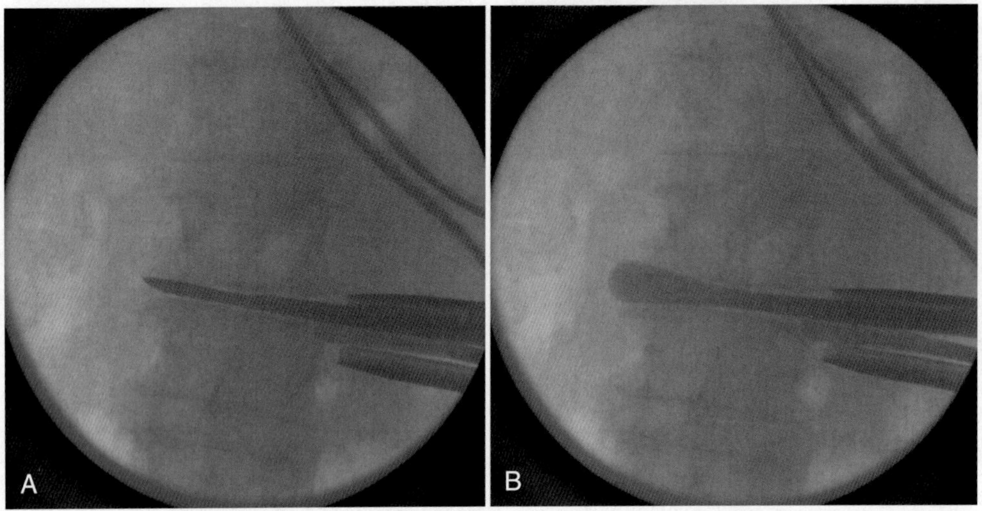

FIG. 20.9 (A) A Cobb elevator is used to release the contralateral anulus. This aids in the coronal correction of the deformity. (B) Rotating the Cobb elevator 90 degrees will further release the contralateral anulus.

on distraction and a compromised endplate will allow the endplate to subside. A Cobb elevator should be used to release the contralateral anulus (Fig. 20.9). Releasing the contralateral anulus loosens the spine in the coronal plane and aids in the correction of coronal plane deformities. Sizers and trials are then used to determine the optimal implant size (Fig. 20.10). The implant is then filled with the surgeon's graft or fusion enhancer of choice and impacted across (Fig. 20.11). The wound is then closed in layers. No drains are typically necessary.

Complications

Since minimally invasive lateral access to the spine is a relatively new procedure, publications regarding the efficacy and complication rates are sparse. Numbness in the lateral thigh and psoas weakness have been noted by some physicians; however, the rate still remains unknown.[10–12] To minimize this risk, open the retractor just enough to perform the lateral discectomy. Exuberant deployment of the retractor may place undue pressure on the nerve roots and/or the psoas itself. Limiting the amount of time that the retractor is open is also advised to decrease the length of time that the nerves are under pressure. In addition, neuromonitoring is advised to decrease the possibility of nerve injury.

Injury to the bowel and vessels have also been reported.[13] It is recommended that this procedure be done at a facility where a general or vascular surgeon is available. One method to decrease the rate of bowel or vascular injury is to place the initial dilator under direct visualization. After the lateral incision has been made, the retractor can be passed down to the psoas. Then, the initial dilator is placed through the psoas under direct visualization.

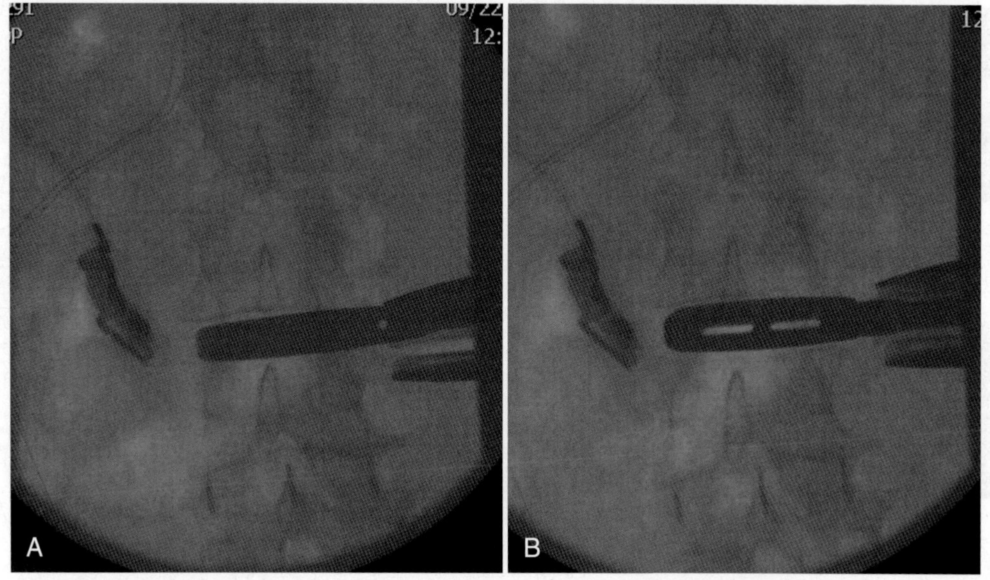

FIG. 20.10 Trialing of the disc space with a (A) paddle trial and (B) implant trial.

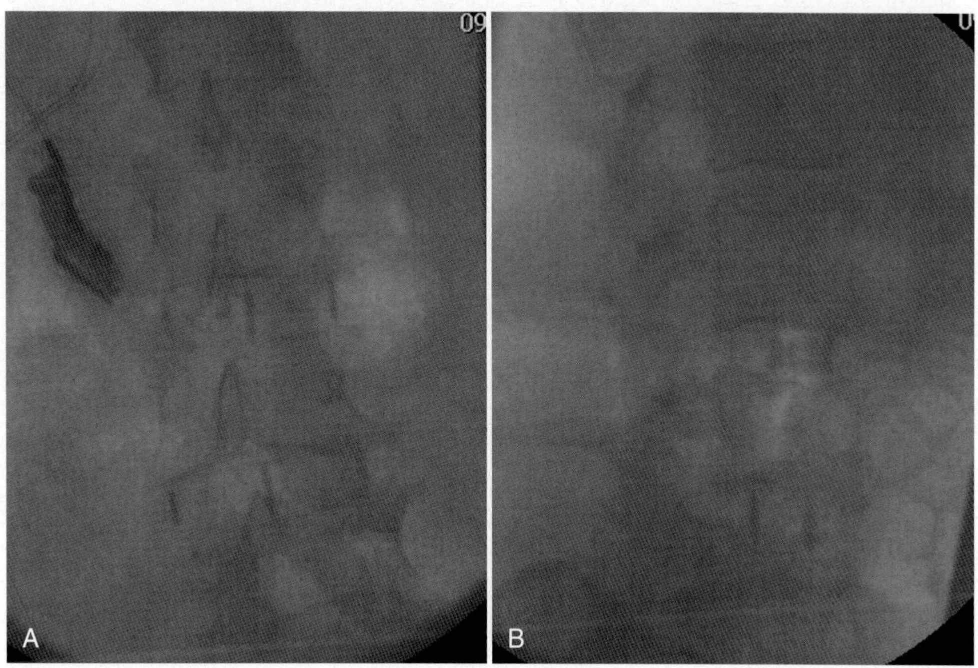

FIG. 20.11 Final (A) anteroposterior and (B) lateral radiographs after two-level lateral interbody fusion.

Posterior Approach to the Lumbar Spine

The posterior approach through a midline, longitudinal incision is the most common approach to the lumbar spine. It provides direct access to the spinous processes, laminae, facets, and even the pedicles, as well as lateral aspects of the vertebral bodies at all levels of the lumbar spine. The pedicle starting holes and transverse processes can be reached by dissecting and retracting the paraspinal muscles laterally. Through this approach, it is possible to perform most of the spine procedures currently practiced today, including microdiscectomies, laminectomies, and most fusion procedures. The posterior aspect of the vertebral body and disc space over the lower lumbar levels can be reached following laminectomy by retracting the dura; however, the exposure is limited.

It is important to bear in mind that anatomic variations exist among individuals, which must be taken into account when planning surgery. The intercrestal line typically crosses at L4–L5; however, this is not a rigid anatomic finding. A lateral radiograph will show where the intercrestal line is. Also, lumbarization or sacralization of the last vertebral segment can confuse the surgeon when localizing the level of pathology. Additionally, a spina bifida occulta or an unusually wide interlaminar space may exist. To avoid inadvertent injury to the dura or nerve roots with a Bovie or periosteal elevator during the exposure, the surgeon should study radiographs prior to surgery to look for these abnormalities.

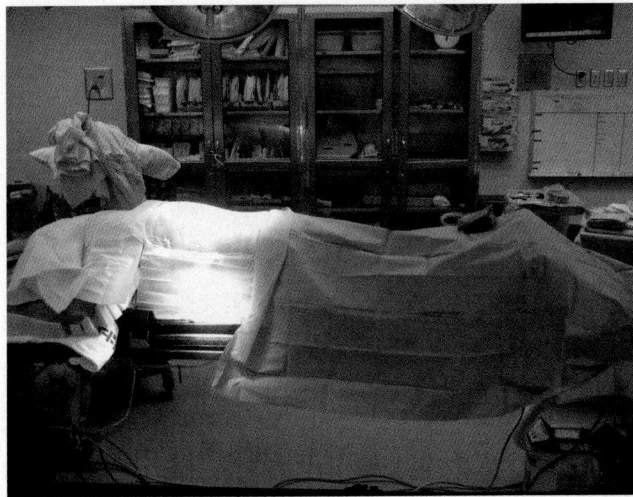

FIG. 20.12 Patient in standard prone position. Note how the area beneath the patient is cleared of wires to accommodate imaging.

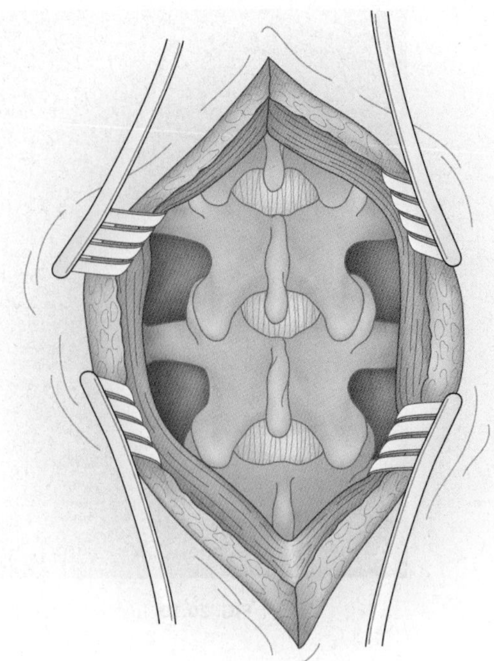

FIG. 20.13 Exposure of the lumbar spine.

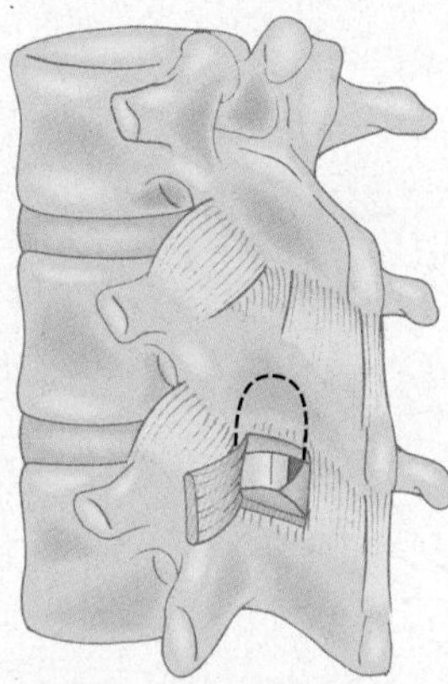

FIG. 20.14 Removal of the ligamentum flavum. (From Benzel E. *Spine Surgery: Techniques, Complication Avoidance, and Management*. Philadelphia: Churchill Livingstone; 2004.)

Technique

Position the patient prone to allow the abdomen to hang free of pressure (Fig. 20.12). This will reduce venous plexus filling around the cauda equina by permitting the venous plexus to drain directly into the inferior vena cava. Also, the anesthesiologist should check the patient's eyes and the surgeon and nurses should assess the bony prominences to ensure that they are well padded. If a microdiscectomy or decompression is to be performed, flexing the lumbar spine on a Wilson frame or similar table is recommended to open up the interspinous spaces. If a fusion is also to be performed, placing the patient on a Jackson table is recommended to maintain the lumbar lordosis. A solution containing epinephrine in a 1:500,000 concentration may be injected into the subcuticular tissues and muscles to decrease blood loss.

A midline incision is made between the spinous processes of the levels to be exposed, and the erector spinae and multifidus muscles are dissected from the bony elements (spinous processes, interspinous ligaments, laminae, facet joints, and transverse processes) as needed for the levels that must be visualized, using electrocautery or sharp dissection (Fig. 20.13). The paraspinal muscles should be elevated subperiosteally to minimize blood loss. Care should be taken not to injure the facet joint capsules and interspinous ligaments in areas where motion will be expected following the operation. If the transverse processes must be reached, continue dissecting down the lateral side of the facet joints and onto the transverse process itself. Close to the facet joints and the pars interarticularis are the vessels supplying the paraspinal muscles segmentally.

If these vessels are cut, they can bleed vigorously. Cauterization is necessary to stop these bleeders. The posterior primary rami of the lumbar nerves run with these vessels.

In order to perform a decompression or a discectomy, it may be necessary to remove the ligamentum flavum. The superficial ligamentum flavum blends laterally into the facet joint capsule. Use a forward-angled or small straight curette to detach the superficial and deep layers of the ligamentum flavum from the caudal edge of the cephalad lamina. Sweep the curette medial to lateral and advance the curette with each successive sweep to detach the ligamentum flavum from the lamina. The ligamentum flavum typically inserts over the caudal 50% of the undersurface of the lamina. Place a small, angled elevator under the ligamentum flavum to lift it off the dura and protect the latter. A Kerrison rongeur, pituitary rongeur, or knife can be used to remove the ligamentum flavum. The epidural fat, the dura, the nerve root, and the epidural veins can be seen once the ligamentum flavum has been removed (Fig. 20.14).

If a discectomy or exploration of the disc space is required, it can typically be performed through this opening. Removal of a portion of the lamina (laminotomy) may need to be done to adequately access the disc space. A Penfield 4 can then be used to help mobilize the traversing nerve root and a nerve root retractor can be used to gently retract the nerve roots

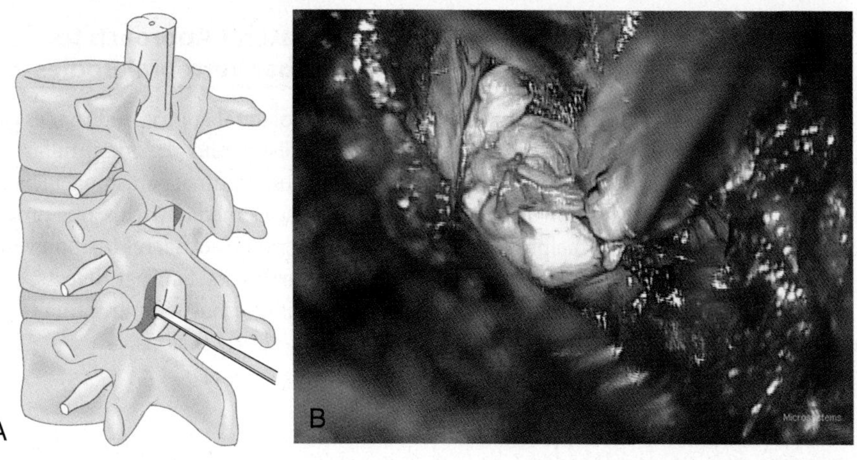

FIG. 20.15 (A) Exposure of the lumbar disc by retracting the thecal sac medially. (B) View of microdiscectomy under a microscope. The thecal sac is retracted medially by a nerve root retractor. ((A, From Benzel E. *Spine Surgery: Techniques, Complication Avoidance, and Management.* Philadelphia: Churchill Livingstone; 2004.)

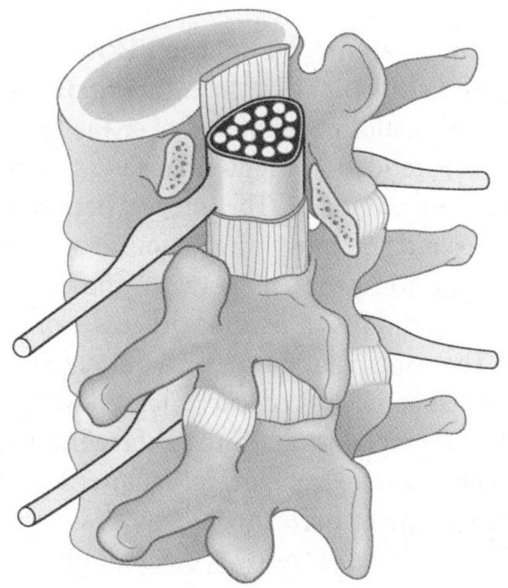

FIG. 20.16 Structures relative to the pedicle.

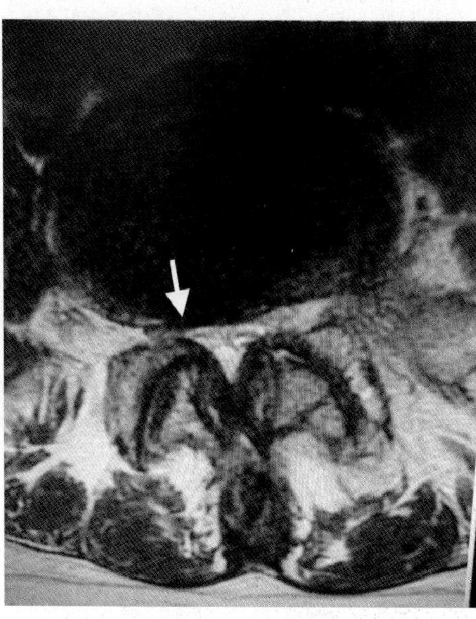

FIG. 20.17 Axial magnetic resonance image of the lumbar spine. The *arrow* is pointing to the lateral recess.

medially (Fig. 20.15). Care must be used not to retract too vigorously to avoid too much tension on the exiting nerve root. Bleeding from the epidural veins commonly occurs. Hemostasis can be obtained with bipolar cautery and/or the use of cottonoids, Surgicel, and thrombin-soaked Gelfoam. Cottonoids can be placed in the cephalad and caudal extremes of the exposure to collapse the vessels and provide a working window. The key to intracanal anatomy is the pedicle (Fig. 20.16). The disc space is just cephalad to the pedicle, and the intervertebral foramen above the pedicle accommodates the exiting nerve root. The traversing nerve root lies just medial to the pedicle and exits the intervertebral foramen caudally. The disc space can be found by retracting the traversing nerve root medially and exploring the space above the pedicle. Feel for the disc space with a Penfield 4. It should be a raised, white, soft structure.

If a total laminectomy is needed to decompress or expose the dura and nerve roots, remove the fascia entirely from the tip of the spinous process bilaterally. Dissect the muscles off of the spinous processes and lamina subperiosteally and take care to protect the facet joints. The pars interarticularis must be exposed fully to avoid transecting it during the decompression. A rongeur can be used to remove the spinous processes. The laminectomy may be performed many ways. A high-speed burr may be used to thin the lamina down to a thin cortical shell over the dura and then removed with a Kerrison rongeur. Alternatively, the tip of a rongeur may be inserted under the caudal edge of the cephalad lamina to remove the lamina. Use the rongeur to cut from the underside in an upward direction. This will lessen the chance of catching dura. A Kerrison rongeur can be used to complete the laminectomy near the pars and the cephalad edge. To adequately decompress the nerve roots, the lateral recesses and intervertebral foramen must also be explored (Fig. 20.17). A Woodson elevator or dural guide may be used to gently compress the dura and expose the lateral recesses. This will expose the ligamentum flavum in the lateral recess and intervertebral foramen. This ligamentum flavum should be removed to perform an adequate decompression. The medial aspect of the caudal pedicle marks the medial border of the intervertebral foramen. Often, osteophytes from the facet joints compress the exiting nerve root. Care must be taken when removing these osteophytes to avoid injury to the exiting nerve root and to avoid iatrogenic instability caused by too much removal of the facet joint. Typically, removal of less than 50% of the facet joint will preserve its stability. This may necessitate the use of a 1- or 2-mm Kerrison rongeur. The use of curved Kerrison rongeurs can be helpful here. Bearing in mind that the facet joints are oriented sagittal in the lumbar spine, cutting the undersurface of the facet joint provides a greater means of decompressing the nerve roots while preserving the overall stability of the joint.

With the advent of pedicle screw fixation for the lumbar vertebrae, there are now several additional anatomic relationships that are of importance at the level of the posterior bony elements. The location of the pedicles is identified by anatomic landmarks and by radiography or image-intensification fluoroscopy in the operating room.

In the lumbar region, the center of the pedicles is usually at the inferolateral edge of the facet joint, on an imaginary transverse line bisecting the transverse processes (Fig. 20.18). However, if there is severe facet arthrosis, the lateral edge of the facet joint may be lateral to the true pedicle entry site. In these cases, also refer to the pars interarticularis. The lateral border of the pars typically corresponds to the medial border of the pedicle. In the lumbar region, from this point, one may use a pedicle finder, with a 20-degree medial inclination at L5, 10 degrees at L4, 5 degrees at L3 and L2, and no inclination at L1 (Fig. 20.19). One may follow the progress of the pedicle finder by feeling inside the pedicle with a pedicle feeler and by checking with the image intensifier or by radiographs. In the lateral view, the probe/marker should be parallel to the disc space.

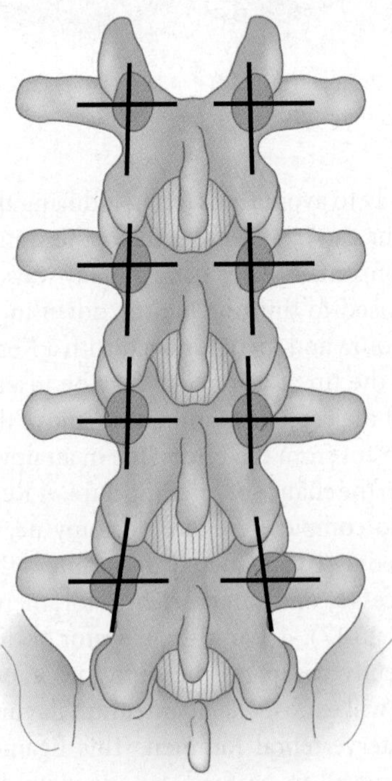

FIG. 20.18 Pedicle entry points.

Posterolateral Approach to the Lumbar Vertebral Bodies

The posterolateral approach provides direct access to the transverse processes and the mammillary processes of the facets through a longitudinal paraspinal incision, retracting the erector spinae muscles medially. This area provides an excellent bed for posterolateral lumbosacral fusion even in the face of preexisting pseudarthrosis, laminar defects, or spondylolisthesis. This approach is the basis for minimally invasive transforaminal lumbar interbody fusions.

Technique

General endotracheal anesthesia is recommended for this procedure. The patient is placed on the operating table in the prone position with chest rolls on either side of the thorax to protect ventilation or on a radiolucent table with chest and hip pads.

A longitudinal paramedian incision is made at the lateral border of the erector spinae muscles (approximately 2 fingerbreadths from the midline) centered over the level of interest. The incision is extended to the lumbar fascia, and the erector spinae muscles are identified. The interval between the erector spinae muscles and the multifidus is found after opening the fascia, and dissection proceeds between these muscles down to the facet joints and the transverse processes of the vertebrae (Fig. 20.20). The paraspinal muscles are retracted medially, the transverse process at the desired level is tagged with a radiopaque marker, and radiographs are made to confirm the vertebral level. For a minimally invasive transforaminal interbody fusion, this exposure is adequate to perform a decompression and fusion.

If access to the vertebral body is desired, the dissection can be carried further anteriorly. The transverse process is divided with an osteotome and is retracted laterally with its musculotendinous attachments. The vertebral pedicle is palpated, and the lumbar nerves are identified and protected as they leave their foramina above and below the pedicle (Fig. 20.21). The psoas muscle is carefully separated from the vertebra using a

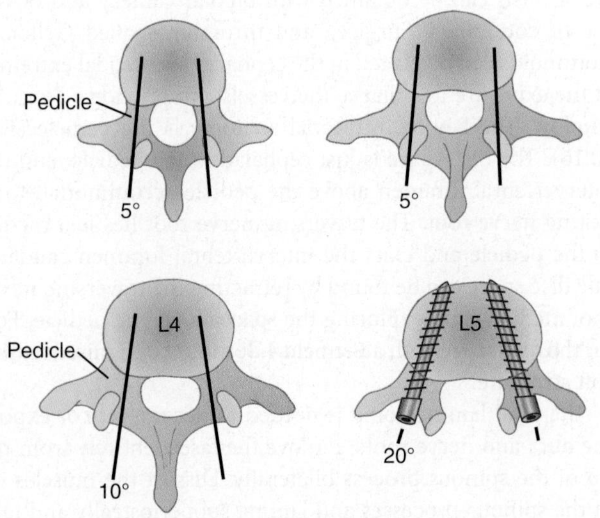

FIG. 20.19 Transaxial position of the pedicle screws.

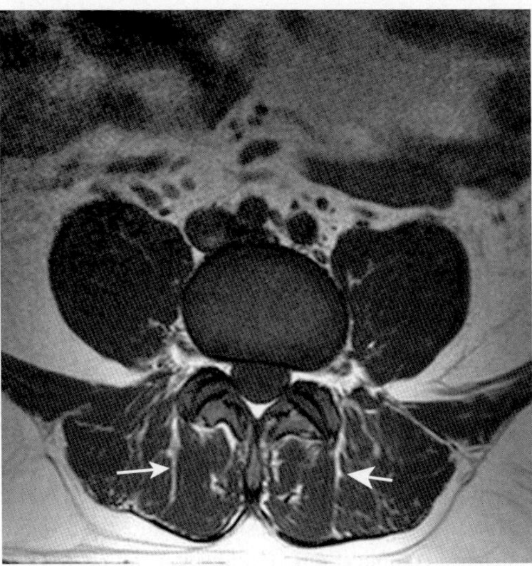

FIG. 20.20 Cross-section of the lumbar spine and paraspinal structures at the level of the third lumbar vertebra. The arrows point to the interval between the erector spinae muscles and the multifidus.

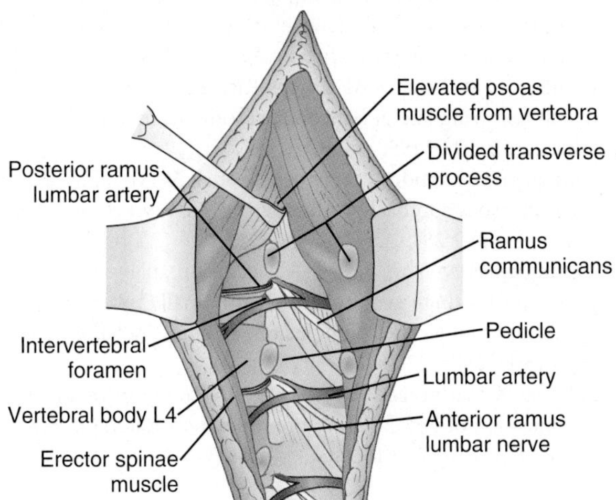

FIG. 20.21 Lumbar vertebrae as viewed from the posterolateral approach. The dissection proceeds directly anterior to the stump of the transverse process, along the pedicle of the vertebral body in front. Note the lumbar segmental vessels draped over the waist or midportion of the vertebral bodies. By dissecting directly anterior to the pedicles, one can avoid these vessels as well as the lumbar nerves leaving the neural foramina below the pedicles.

periosteal elevator. The lumbar vessels lie on the waist or midportion of the vertebral body posterior to the psoas muscle and should be separated from the body during this portion of the dissection. They may be clamped and cauterized, if necessary. An opening may be made in the lateral aspect of the vertebral body anterior to the pedicle, using a curette or drill (Fig. 20.22). The lesion may be identified grossly at this time, but should be verified radiographically with a curette placed within the lesion. Through this approach, specimens may be obtained from the lateral, central, or anterior aspect of the vertebral body or pedicle. The lesion may be curetted, and small chips of cancellous bone graft may be installed to stimulate osteogenesis within a sterile defect. The wound is

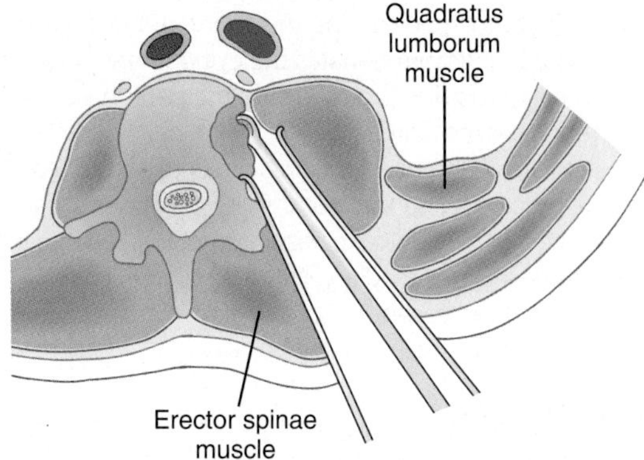

FIG. 20.22 Posterolateral approach to the lumbar vertebrae, lateral to the erector spinae muscle mass and behind the psoas. The transverse process is divided and retracted laterally with its musculotendinous insertions to gain access to the lateral aspect of the vertebral body.

copiously irrigated with saline and inspected for hemorrhage. The margins are allowed to fall together, and the lumbar fascia is closed with interrupted sutures. The skin is repaired, and the patient is nursed with some form of external spinal support, depending on the postoperative stability of the spine.

PEARLS

1. For lateral interbody fusions, it is often easier to adjust the table to get the perfect AP and lateral, and just have the C-arm rotate between 0 degrees and 90 degrees.
2. For lateral interbody fusions, take frequent images to ensure good position. Since you are using a smaller incision and thus see less, you must rely on imaging more to make sure that you are in the right position.
3. For lateral interbody fusions, study the MRI preoperatively to get an idea of where the nerves are. If the neuromonitor shows that the nerve is in the field, be prepared to convert to another form of interbody fusion.
4. To adequately decompress the nerve roots, the lateral recesses and intervertebral foramen must also be explored.

PITFALLS

1. For lateral interbody fusions, aggressive deployment of the retractor or repeated passes with the initial dilator may injure the nerve.
2. For lumbar decompressions, be careful about removing too much of the pars or facet joints to avoid iatrogenic instability.
3. When placing pedicle screws, if there is severe facet arthrosis, the lateral edge of the facet joint may be lateral to the true pedicle entry site.

KEY POINTS

1. Lateral interbody fusion is a good technique for correction of degenerative scoliosis, multilevel fusions, or adjacent segment degeneration. This can be done in a minimally invasive fashion that will improve recovery while maximizing results.
2. Since the lateral approach to the spine requires traversing the psoas, neuromonitoring is required to decrease the risk of nerve injury. Also, since the incision is smaller and less tissue dissection is done, there is a greater reliance on imaging.
3. The posterior approach to the lumbar spine is commonly used for microdiscectomies and lumbar decompressions.

4. The key to intracanal anatomy is the pedicle. The disc space is just cephalad to the pedicle, and the intervertebral foramen above the pedicle accommodates the exiting nerve root. The traversing nerve root lies just medial to the pedicle and exits the intervertebral foramen caudally.
5. The posterolateral approach provides direct access to the transverse processes and the mammillary processes of the facets through a longitudinal paraspinal incision, retracting the erector spinae muscles medially. This is a muscle-splitting approach and is the basis for minimally invasive transforaminal lumbar interbody fusions.

KEY REFERENCES

1. Bateman DK, Millhouse PW, Shahi N, et al. Anterior lumbar spine surgery: a systematic review and meta-analysis of associated complications. *Spine J.* 2015;15(5):1118-1132.
2. Rodgers WB, Gerber EJ, Patterson JR. Intraoperative and early postoperative complications in extreme lateral interbody fusion (XLIF): an analysis of 600 cases. *Spine.* 2011;36(1):26-32.
3. Isaacs RE, Hyde J, Goodrich JA, et al. A prospective, nonrandomized, multicenter evaluation of extreme lateral interbody fusion for the treatment of adult degenerative scoliosis: perioperative outcomes and complications. *Spine.* 2010;35(suppl 26):S322-S330.
4. Alimi M, Hofstetter CP, Cong GT, et al. Radiological and clinical outcomes following extreme lateral interbody fusion. *J Neurosurg Spine.* 2014;20(6):623-635.
5. Patel AA, Zfass-Mendez M, Lebwohl NH, et al. Minimally Invasive versus open lumbar fusion: a comparison of blood loss, surgical complications, and hospital course. *Iowa Orthop J.* 2015;35:130-134.
6. Ozgur BM, Aryan HE, Pimenta L, et al. Extreme Lateral Interbody Fusion (XLIF): a novel surgical technique for anterior lumbar interbody fusion. *Spine J.* 2006;6(4):435-443.

REFERENCES

1. Bateman DK, Millhouse PW, Shahi N, et al. Anterior lumbar spine surgery: a systematic review and meta-analysis of associated complications. *Spine J.* 2015;15(5):1118-1132.
2. Lindley EM, McBeth ZL, Henry SE, et al. Retrograde ejaculation after anterior lumbar spine surgery. *Spine.* 2012;37(20):1785-1789.
3. Jarrett CD, Heller JG, Tsai L. Anterior exposure of the lumbar spine with and without an "access surgeon": morbidity analysis of 265 consecutive cases. *J Spinal Disord Tech.* 2009;22(8):559-564.
4. Rodgers WB, Gerber EJ, Patterson JR. Intraoperative and early postoperative complications in extreme lateral interbody fusion (XLIF): an analysis of 600 cases. *Spine.* 2011;36(1):26-32.
5. Isaacs RE, Hyde J, Goodrich JA, et al. A prospective, nonrandomized, multicenter evaluation of extreme lateral interbody fusion for the treatment of adult degenerative scoliosis: perioperative outcomes and complications. *Spine.* 2010;35(suppl 26):S322-S330.
6. Alimi M, Hofstetter CP, Cong GT, et al. Radiological and clinical outcomes following extreme lateral interbody fusion. *J Neurosurg Spine.* 2014;20(6):623-635.
7. Patel AA, Zfass-Mendez M, Lebwohl NH, et al. Minimally invasive versus open lumbar fusion: a comparison of blood loss, surgical complications, and hospital course. *Iowa Orthop J.* 2015;35:130-134.
8. Phan K, Rao PJ, Kam AC, et al. Minimally invasive versus open transforaminal lumbar interbody fusion for treatment of degenerative lumbar disease: systematic review and meta-analysis. *Eur Spine J.* 2015;24(5):1017-1030.
9. Ozgur BM, Aryan HE, Pimenta L, et al. Extreme Lateral Interbody Fusion (XLIF): a novel surgical technique for anterior lumbar interbody fusion. *Spine J.* 2006;6(4):435-443.
10. Pumberger M, Hughes AP, Huang RR, et al. Neurologic deficit following lateral lumbar interbody fusion. *Eur Spine J.* 2012;21(6):1192-1199.
11. Houten JK, Alexandre LC, Nasser R, et al. Nerve injury during the transpsoas approach for lumbar fusion. *J Neurosurg Spine.* 2011;15(3):280-284.
12. Cummock MD, Vanni S, Levi AD, et al. An analysis of postoperative thigh symptoms after minimally invasive transpsoas lumbar interbody fusion. *J Neurosurg Spine.* 2011;15:11-18.
13. Balsano M, Carlucci S, Ose M, et al. A case report of a rare complication of bowel perforation in extreme lateral interbody fusion. *Eur Spine J.* 2015;24(suppl 3):405-408.

CHAPTER 21 Lateral Lumbar Interbody Fusion

Sina Pourtaheri
R. Todd Allen
John Attenello
Steven R. Garfin

History

A variety of approaches to the interbody space exist to surgically manage pathologies of the lumbar spine.[1] The advantage of interbody fusions over posterolateral fusions are superiority in fusion rates as well as segmental coronal and sagittal correction.[2–4] Open anterolateral thoracolumbar approaches have been associated with vascular/bowel injury, abdominal hernia, ileus, and retrograde ejaculation.[5] However, the minimally invasive lateral retroperitoneal transpsoas approach has minimized these approach-related complications.[6,7] Open posterior approaches are associated with significant infection rates, blood loss, operative time, length of hospital stay, prolonged recovery, and delayed return to work due to procedural morbidity.[8]

Following instrumentation advances in visualization, lighting technology, and specialized surgical instruments fit for smaller incisions, minimally invasive surgery (MIS) became progressively more popular. After Obenchain et al. described a laparoscopic approach to anterior lumbar interbody fusion (ALIF) in 1991, MIS techniques to the spine began to rapidly evolve.[6,9] Pimenta has been given credit for being the creator of the minimally invasive lateral retroperitoneal transpsoas approach for lateral lumbar interbody fusions (LLIFs) in 2001.[6] However, Harmon described the approach in 1963.[10,11] MIS approaches such as LLIFs were developed for several reasons, including the ability to meet increasing patient demands and expectations for shorter hospital stays, earlier return to work, improved cosmesis, and decreased postoperative pain.[12–14] Last, LLIFs can be used for any condition that requires access to the interbody space from the mid to upper thoracic spine (e.g., T6, occasionally T5) through L4–L5. The lateral approach is possibly best suited for levels L2 to L4 due to anatomic considerations (the 12th rib and iliac crest).

Indications

Absolute indication for interbody fusion (ALIF, posterior lumbar interbody fusion [PLIF], transforaminal lumbar interbody fusion [TLIF], LLIF) is the treatment of pseudarthrosis.[12,15–17] Relative indications are foraminal height loss, coronal tilt/lateral-listhesis, flatback, and long adult thoracolumbar fusions.[12,15–17] Interbody fusions provide superior fusion rates over posterolateral fusions due to the mechanical and biologic advantage of the interbody space.[18–24] The interbody space is under compression and load sharing while having a large surface area.[18–24] However, the posterolateral space is under tension, has muscle creep, and has limited surface area.[18–24] Therefore, interbody fusion is indicated for pseudarthrosis following posterolateral fusion. Furthermore, multilevel posterolateral lumbar fusions have significantly high pseudarthrosis rates compared to interbody fusions.[25,26] Therefore, multilevel fusions have a relative indication for interbody fusion.

Advantages

LLIF and ALIF have superior fusion rates over TLIF due to mechanical and biologic factors: a more thorough discectomy and large surface area of graft extending to the apophyseal ring bilaterally.[18–24] In regard to foraminal height restoration and indirect decompression, ALIF, TLIF, and LLIF provide significant height restoration compared to posterolateral fusion, with LLIF and ALIF providing superior height restoration.[27–35] In regard to coronal tilt and lateral-listhesis, LLIF and TLIF are superior to ALIF and posterolateral fusions.[36–41] In regard to lumbar lordosis, ALIF and LLIF are superior to TLIF.[36,42,43] In regard to morbidity, ALIF and LLIF provide shorter operative time, decreased blood loss, shorter length of stay, and shorter time to return to work compared to open TLIF.[12,44,45] Furthermore, LLIFs minimize ileus-related issues compared to ALIF.[41,46–48] Last, LLIF allows for the option of an anterior column reconstruction or release (ACR), which can achieve similar lordosis correction as pedicle subtraction osteotomy.[49,50] One caveat is that ACRs require a mobile disc and are not applicable for fixed sagittal imbalance.

Contraindications

L5–S1 interspace is a relative contraindication to LLIF since the iliac wing precludes access to the disc space. L4–L5 may also occasionally be obstructed by the iliac crest and a lumbarized sacrum has been described as a relative contraindication to this approach.[51] The more caudal levels carry a higher risk of injury to iliac vasculature and lumbar plexus because the lumbar plexus begins to course more anteriorly and the iliac vasculature more laterally.[41] In most cases, access to L5–S1 is limited by a high lateral ilium, anterior course of the neural elements over the lateral disc at that level, and/or the vasculature. Uncommonly, L5–S1 may be approached when the intercrestal line transects the mid to lower L5 body or the L5–S1 disc. Rostrally, the 12th rib may obstruct access from T12 to L2, which may require rib excision or manipulation.

Other contraindications to LLIF include bilateral retroperitoneal scarring from prior approaches (e.g., nephrectomy, retroperitoneal abscess and subsequent scarring), high-grade spondylolisthesis, and pregnancy.[47,52,53] In high-grade spondylolisthesis, the more anterior exiting nerve root is horizontalized and creates difficulty in the placement of even the smallest interbody graft.

LLIF may also be potentially contraindicated if direct decompression is required, such as with congenital stenosis, large posterior osteophytes, severe facet hypertrophy with lateral recess stenosis, sequestered disc, and radiculopathy that persists in flexion.[27]

Special consideration should be taken with stand-alone LLIF without posterior instrumentation since lateral fixation alone may not provide sufficient stabilization.[54] Stand-alone LLIF may be contraindicated at levels under high biomechanical stress such as isthmic spondylolisthesis, osteoporosis, or adjacent fusion.[54] Levels at the apex of deformity or associated pars fracture may require posterior instrumentation.[54]

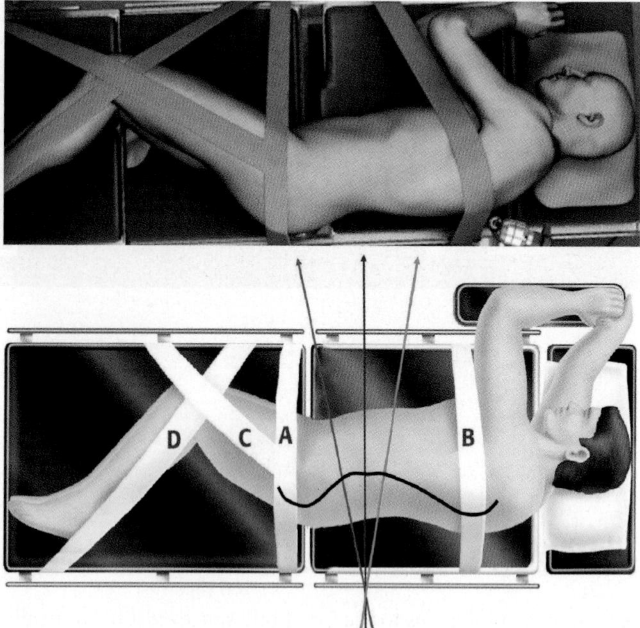

FIG. 21.1 Lateral decubitus positioning for lateral lumbar interbody fusion to minimize upper and lower extremity neurapraxia and proper taping technique of the iliac crest *(A)*, chest *(B)*, greater trochanter *(C)*, and leg *(D)* to secure the patient to the operating room bed.

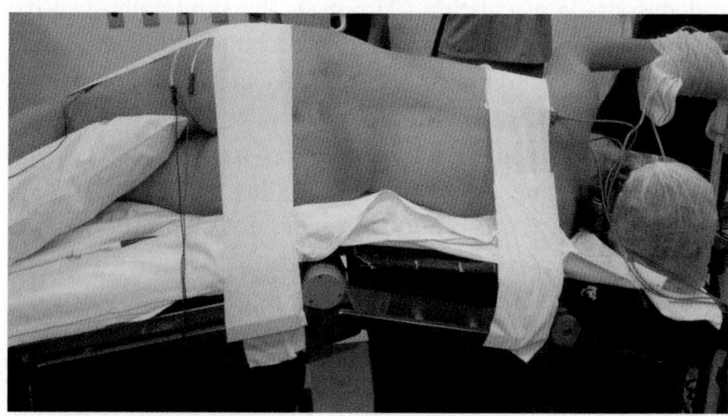

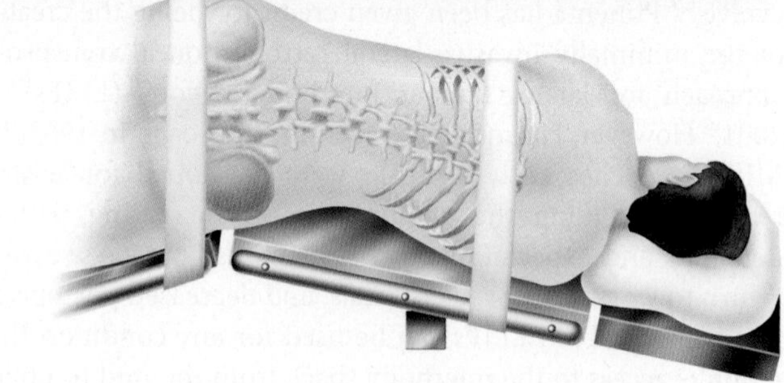

FIG. 21.2 Breaking of the operating room bed to position the iliac crest away for L4–L5 access and even L5–S1 with angled instruments.

Technique

LLIF is a lateral approach to the intervertebral disc space and/or vertebral body through a less invasive (or minimally invasive), retroperitoneal-transpsoas approach. The patient is positioned in the lateral decubitus position, typically left side up, with axillary roll in place and moderate-sized "sticky" rolls for anterior and posterior stabilization (Fig. 21.1). Patients are taped carefully; at times, the table may be bent to level the iliac crest away from the disc space. Orthogonal, anteroposterior, and then lateral fluoroscopic images are taken (Fig. 21.2). The vertebral bodies and disc spaces are marked superficially on the skin under fluoroscopy to determine the appropriate direct lateral incision. A second, posterolateral, 1.5- to 2.0-cm incision is made just above the pelvis within one fingerbreadth length from the direct lateral incision (Fig. 21.3). The trajectory of this posterolateral incision is lateral to the paraspinal muscles and medial to the oblique muscles in an avascular plane to enter the retroperitoneal space (see Fig. 21.3). The posterolateral incision allows the surgeon to enter the retroperitoneal space safely from a posterior approach by starting behind the transverse process and marching anteriorly to the psoas (see Fig. 21.3). The purpose of this incision is to avoid entering into the peritoneum when going from the direct lateral approach, thus preventing an inadvertent bowel injury. Once your finger is on the psoas, bring the index finger to the deep surface of the oblique muscles to determine the safe trajectory of the direct lateral approach (Fig. 21.4). With the lateral skin incision marking, center it over where you palpate your finger in the retroperitoneal space. Develop the lateral approach dissection to the external oblique muscle. Again, check the trajectory through the oblique muscles by bringing your finger in the retroperitoneal space to the psoas;

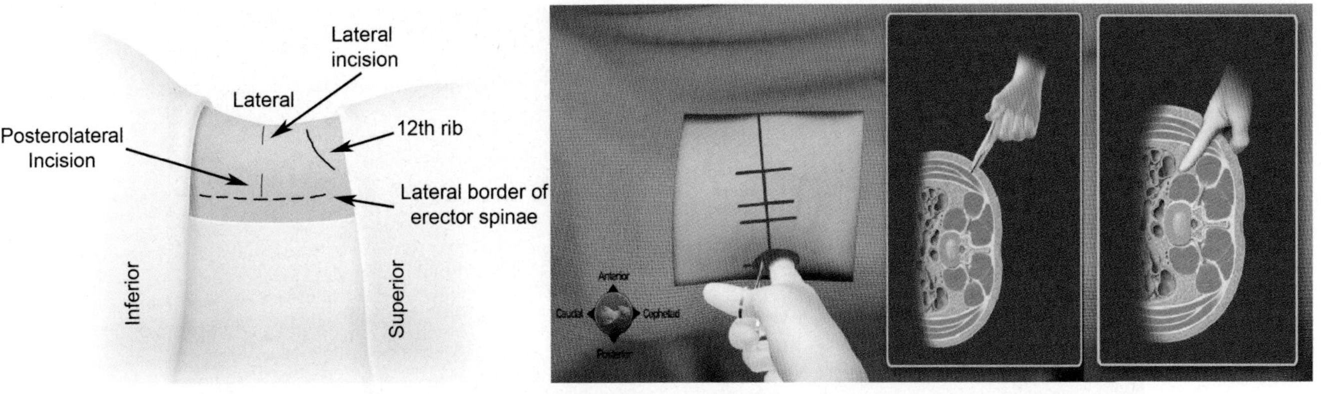

FIG. 21.3 The posterolateral incision allows for a safe trajectory with the direct lateral approach through the retroperitoneal space to prevent bowel injury.

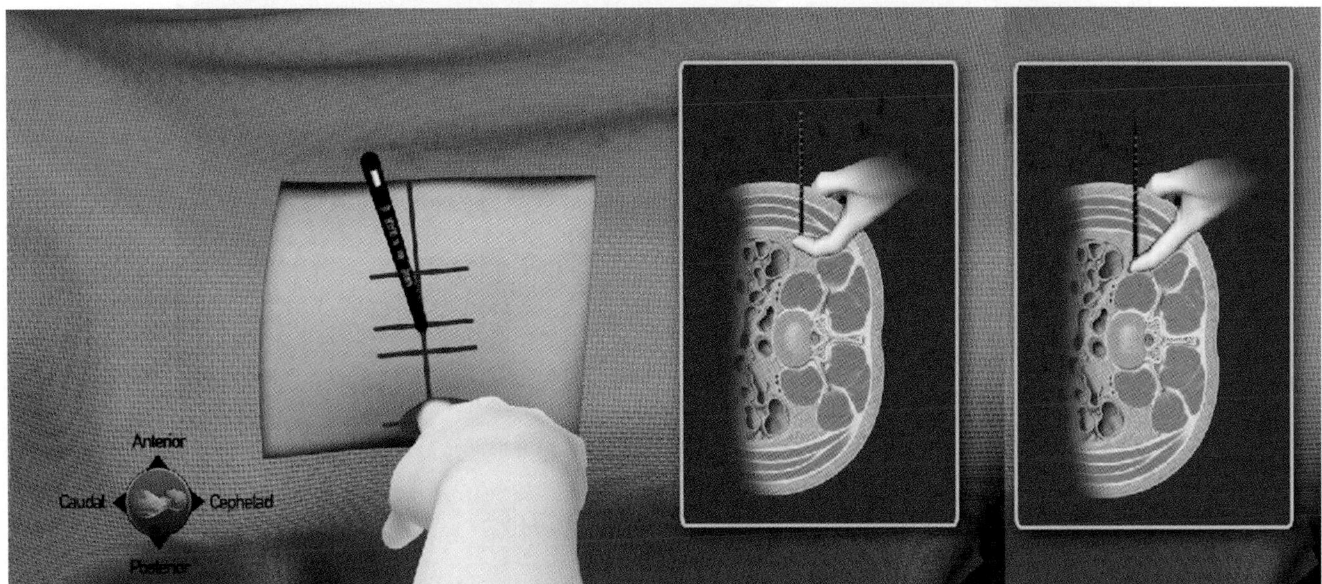

FIG. 21.4 From the posterolateral incision, palpate the psoas and bring the index finger to the undersurface of the abdominal wall to guide the trajectory of the initial dilator safely away from the bowel.

then, go directly vertical from there to the undersurface of the oblique muscle (see Fig. 21.4). Allow your finger to sweep the retroperitoneal fat anteriorly for a safer corridor. Blunt dissection through the oblique muscles and transverse abdominal fascia is made with two Kocher clamps at the same time. The Kocher clamps spread in opposite directions of each other to develop the plane through the muscles in line with their fibers to avoid segmental innervation disruption of the muscles and subsequent pseudohernia. Through this passage hole, place the first dilator (see Fig. 21.4). Let the finger from the posterolateral incision localize the midpoint of the psoas and feel the peak of the disc space (Fig. 21.5). Dock the dilator on this spot and obtain a lateral radiograph to determine that you are at the correct level and centered on the posterior 40% of the disc space (Fig. 21.6). Now, stimulate the dilator and rotate it in all directions to determine proximity of the lumbar plexus (Fig. 21.7). Pass a guidewire through the dilator to anchor the dilator to the disc space (Fig. 21.8). Place larger dilators sequentially. With each dilator, stimulate in all directions to determine the proximity of the lumbar plexus (Fig. 21.9).[6] Slide the retractor

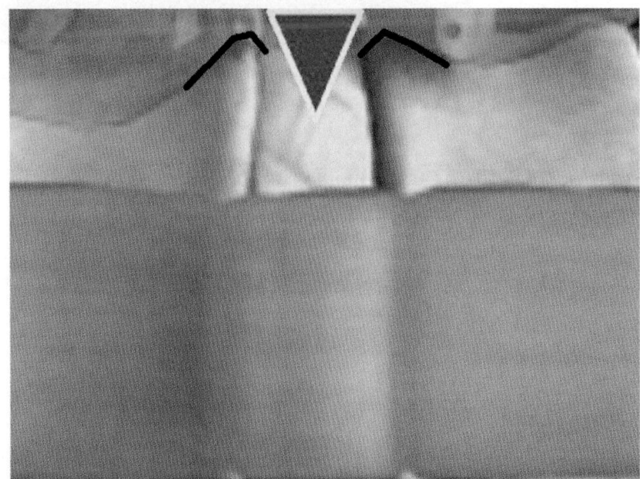

FIG. 21.5 On palpation, the disc space is the peak compared to the valley of the vertebral body.

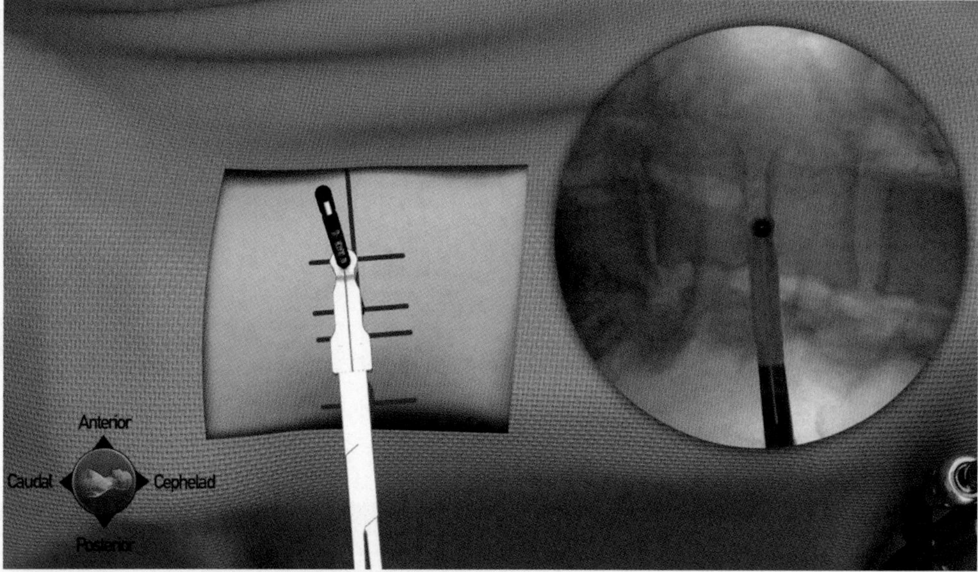

FIG. 21.6 Dock the dilator on the posterior 40% of the disc space in the lateral plane to get access to the anterior 60% of the disc space.

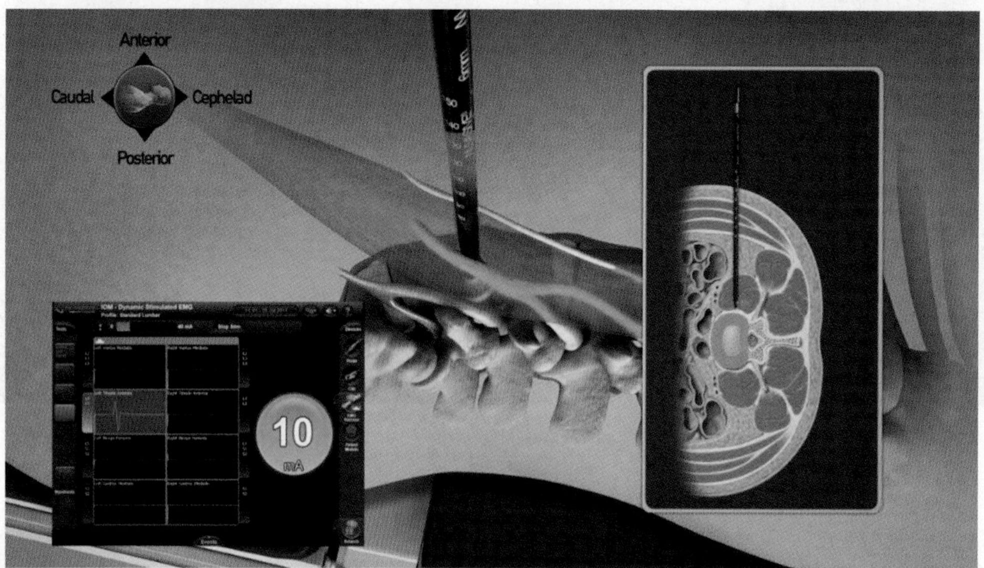

FIG. 21.7 Rotate the dilator 360 degrees while stimulating to ensure that the lumbar plexus is a safe distance from the dilator in all directions.

over the final dilator and obtain an anteroposterior radiograph to determine whether the retractor is centered over the disc with regard to cranial-caudal orientation (Fig. 21.10). Open the anteroposterior retractor blades, which will translate the anterior blade anteriorly toward the anterior longitudinal ligament to give access to the anterior 60% of the disc space (Fig. 21.11). Pivot the up-down retractor blades, which will slide the top and bottom blades cranially and caudally over the disc space and lateral osteophytes, respectively, for complete access to the disc (Fig. 21.12). Turn on the light source. Obtain an anteroposterior radiograph to establish that the up-down blades have passed the osteophytic lateral edges of the vertebral body, above and below the disc space, therefore avoiding inadvertent endplate fractures (see Fig. 21.10). At this point, it is optional to pass the shim into the disc to anchor the retractor firmly into the disc space (Fig. 21.13). Remove the guidewire. It is recommended at this point to take the nerve probe to find the lumbar plexus and determine if the anterior and posterior blades are a safe distance from it. Perform the annulotomy. Through the annulotomy, place the Cobb retractor directed toward the inferior endplate to release the anulus from it (Fig. 21.14). Perform this under lateral fluoroscopy to avoid injury to the endplate. Take the Cobb retractor to the contralateral side and rotate it 90 degrees to distract the contralateral anulus (see Fig. 21.14). Perform the same task with the Cobb retractor angled toward the superior endplate. The disc material is then removed via a combination of blunt dilators, shavers, ring curette, and pituitary (Fig. 21.15). Place a trial cage and obtain anteroposterior and lateral images to determine the correct size for lordosis, coronal tilt, and lateral-listhesis correction,

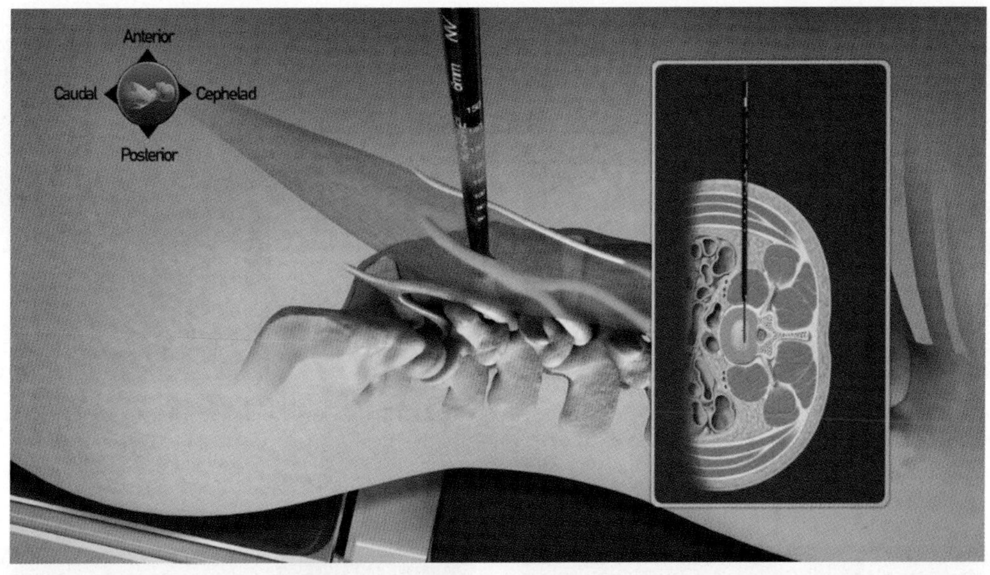

FIG. 21.8 Anchor the dilator to the disc space with a guide wire when the position has been determined as safe and adequate for the discectomy.

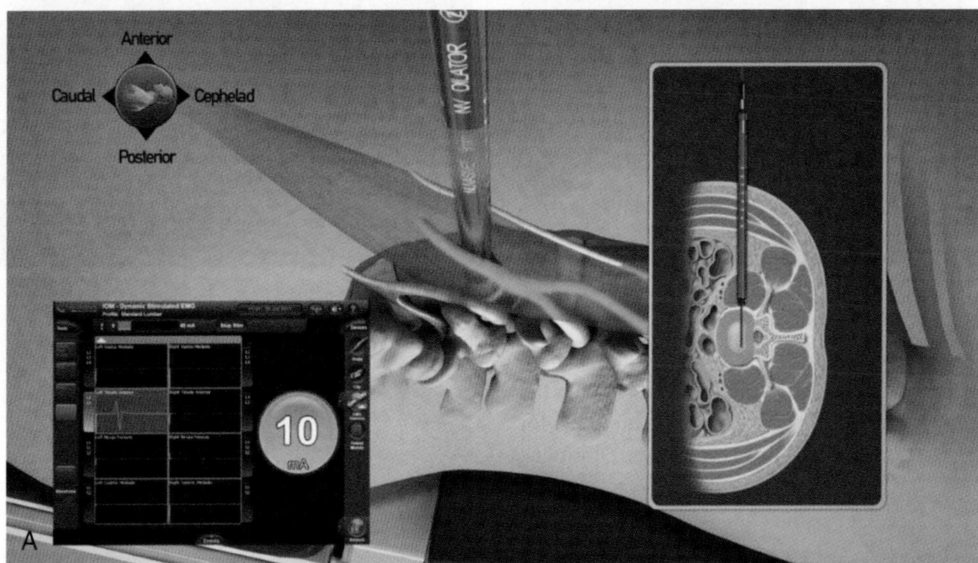

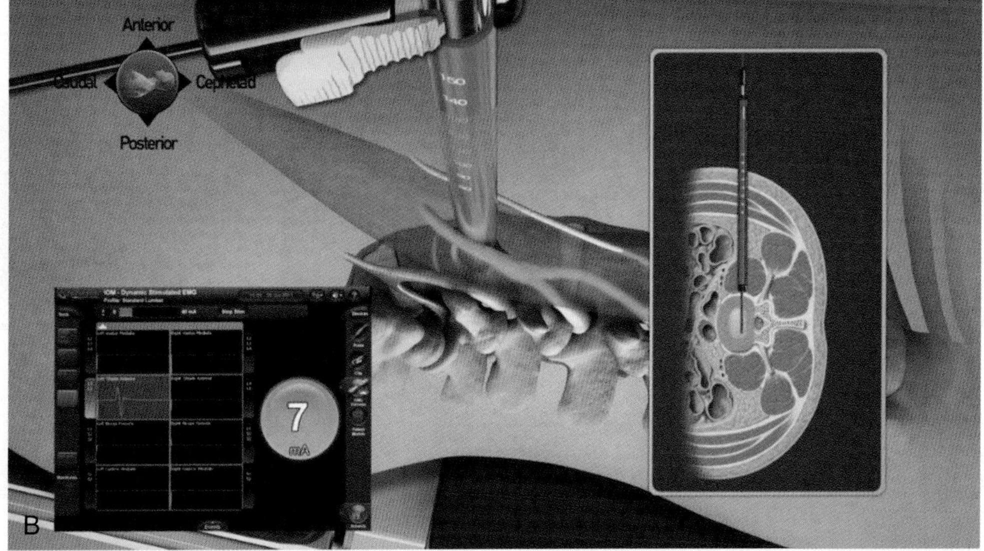

FIG. 21.9 Sequentially dilate to larger sizes while stimulating each time to confirm safety of the corridor to the disc space.

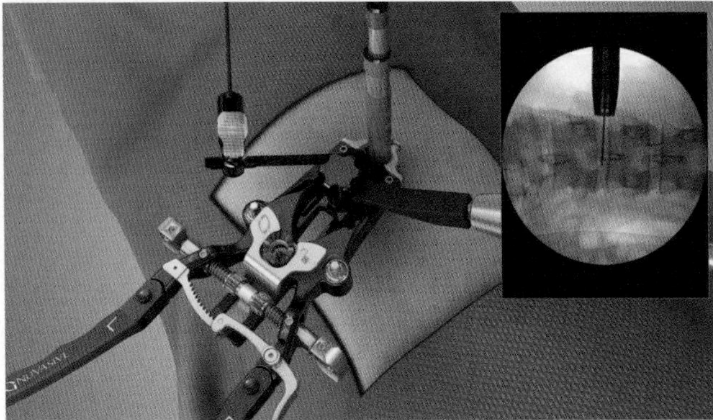

FIG. 21.10 After sliding the retractor over the final dilator, obtain a radiograph to confirm that the cranial and caudal blades are centered over the disc space to prevent inadvertent entry and/or fracture of the endplates.

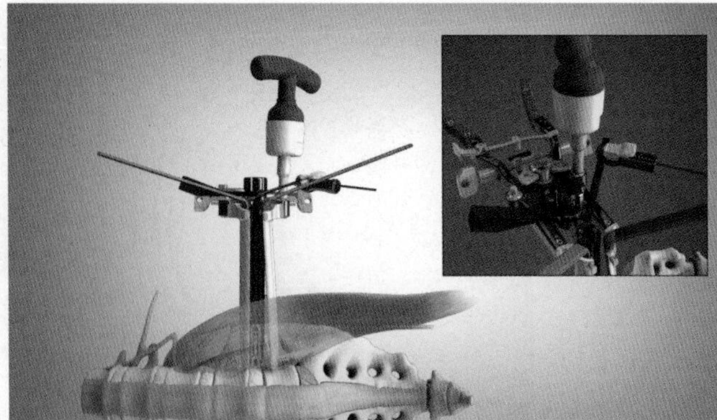

FIG. 21.12 The cranial and caudal retractor blades can be pivoted to get over the lateral osteophytes overlying the disc space.

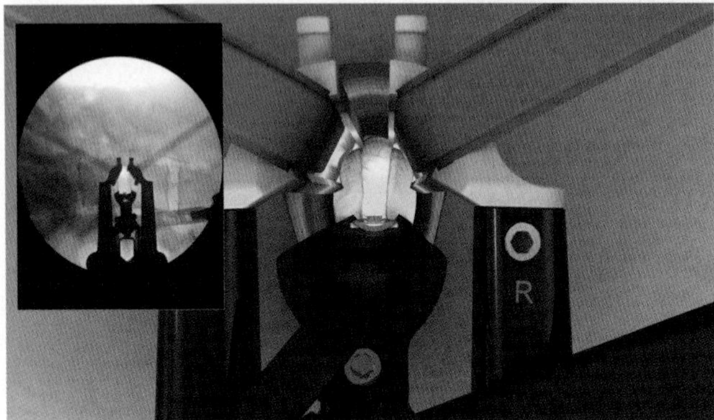

FIG. 21.11 Open the retractor anteriorly to give access to the disc space.

as well as foraminal height restoration (Fig. 21.16). Place the final graft, packed with the surgeon's preferred biologic for bone growth, with the assistance of shims to prevent endplate strain and/or fracture (Fig. 21.17).

Anatomic Considerations

Lumbar Plexus

A thorough understanding of the regional anatomy is essential to avoid complications with the lateral approach. The close proximity of the lumbar plexus poses a risk for permanent and disabling nerve injury, manifested by weakness or radiculopathy. Meticulous examination of the preoperative magnetic resonance imaging (MRI) for relation of the lumbar plexus to the disc space, use of real-time neuromonitoring and biplanar fluoroscopy, and careful dissection of the iliopsoas can aid in a safe approach.

Multiple studies have attempted to map out the relationship of the lumbar plexus within the psoas and identify safe corridors or "safe zones" for accessing each disc space to avoid injury to the plexus and the genitofemoral nerve.[55] An early cadaveric study by Moro et al. examined the lumbar plexus through axial cuts of the lumbar spine and determined the safe zone for the lateral retroperitoneal approach, excluding the genitofemoral nerve, for L4–L5 and above.[55] A cadaveric study

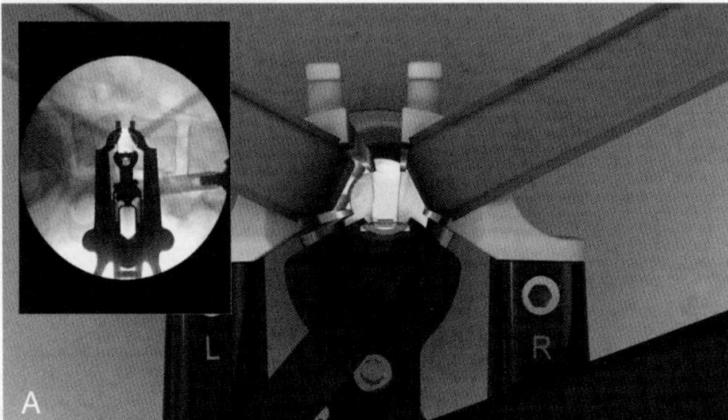

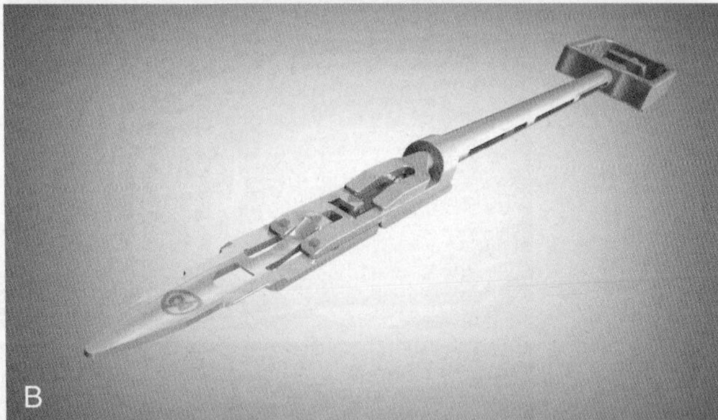

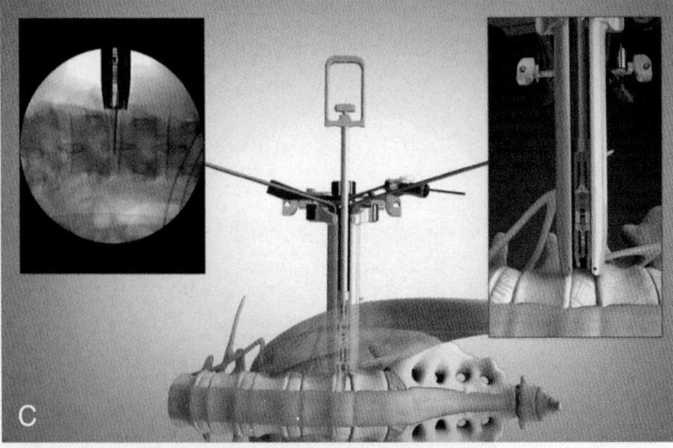

FIG. 21.13 Placement of the shim anchors the retractor to the disc space. (A) Shim in the lateral view. (B) Shim blade inserter. (C) Removal of wire in the disc space after anchoring of the shim into the disc to further stabilize the retractor to the disc space.

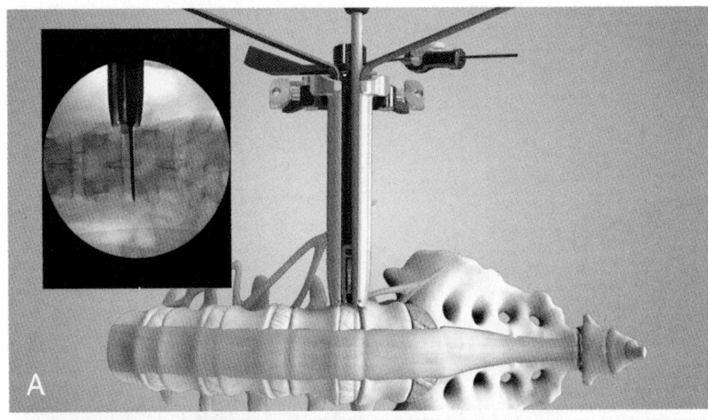

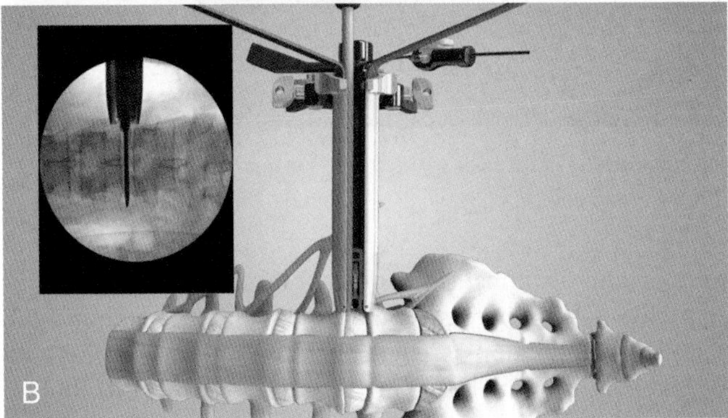

FIG. 21.14 Release the anulus from the endplate with a Cobb retractor and advance through the contralateral anulus in a controlled fashion to release it while avoiding a contralateral plexus injury.

by Benglis et al. demonstrated that the lumbar plexus lies on the dorsal surface of the psoas at a cleft between transverse process and vertebral body and there is a general trend toward progressive dorsal to ventral migration as the psoas descends from L1 to L5, with the L4–L5 disc space being most vulnerable to nerve injury.[56] Park et al. showed the transpsoas exiting nerve roots to be a relatively safe distance from the center of the intervertebral disc space with the exception of a few anatomic variants.[57]

In a 2010 cadaveric study, Uribe et al.[55] further examined the relationship of the lumbar plexus to the disc space, in which the authors separated the vertebral body into four zones on the sagittal plane, each representing a quarter of the distance across the body (Fig. 21.18).[58] In their anatomic study, the safe zone for levels L1–L2, L2–L3, and L3–L4 were at the middle posterior quarter of the vertebral body (zone III) and for L4–L5 at the midpoint of the vertebral body (junction of zones II and III).[55,58] The genitofemoral nerve was found to be at risk at zone II when it moves ventrally at L2–L3 and then ventrally at zone I as it migrates caudally.[55]

Although safe zones are useful guidelines, heterogeneity exists in the relationship between the lumbar plexus and the psoas. Meticulous preoperative planning, judicious dissection without excessive pressure or manipulation of the psoas, direct visualization of the surgical field, and the use of electrophysiologic monitoring are essential for success.

Immediately after incision, caution should be taken when splitting the lateral abdominal musculature to avoid injury to the L1 branches of the iliohypogastric and ilioinguinal nerves (encountered between the internal and external obliques) as

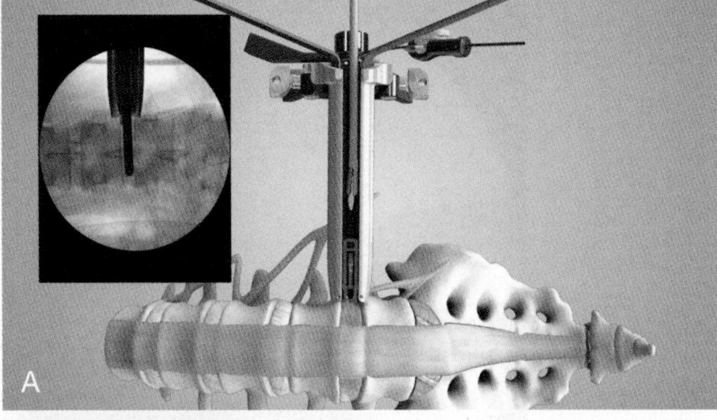

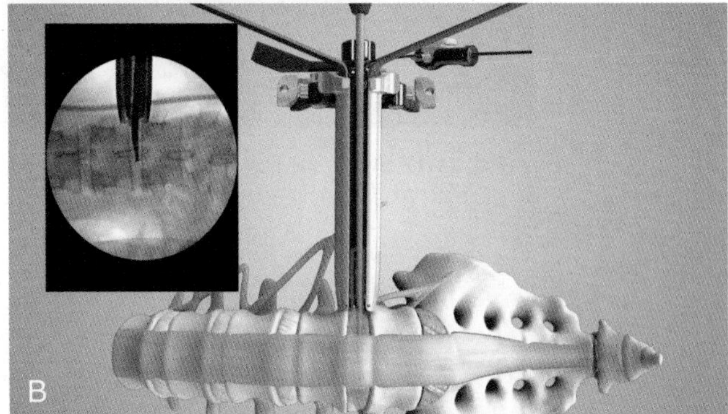

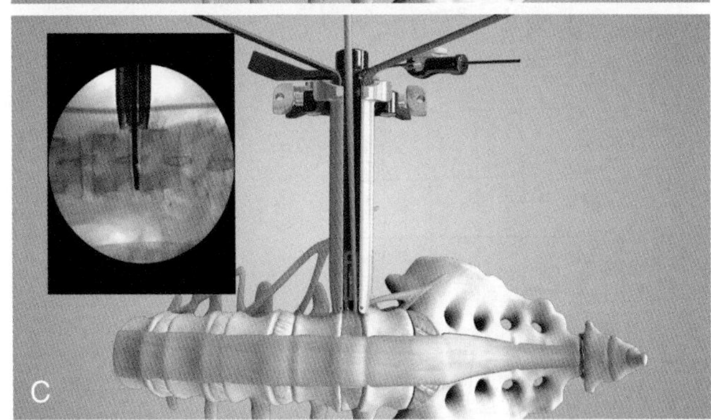

FIG. 21.15 Complete a thorough discectomy and endplate preparation to enhance the biologic environment for a fusion.

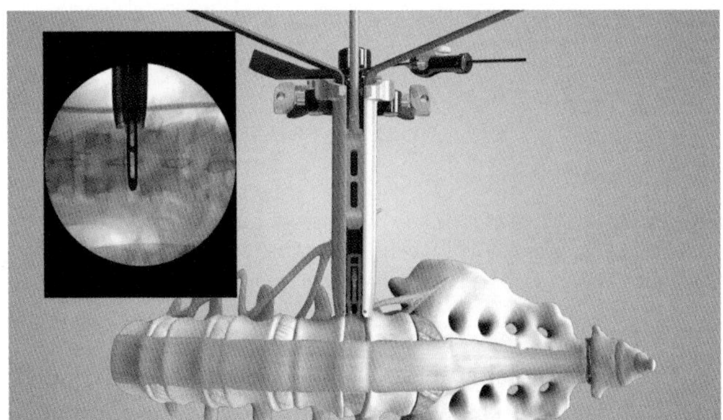

FIG. 21.16 Trial for the proper graft height and lordotic angle to optimize lordosis and/or coronal correction while providing enough foraminal height for an indirect decompression.

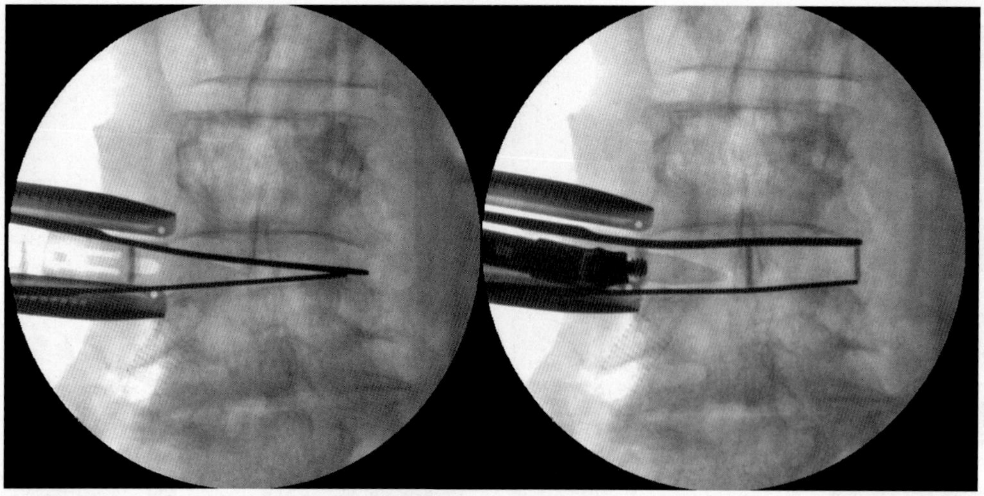

FIG. 21.17 Impact the final graft over shims to provide smooth translation of the graft to the contralateral side while preventing strain and/or fracture of the endplates.

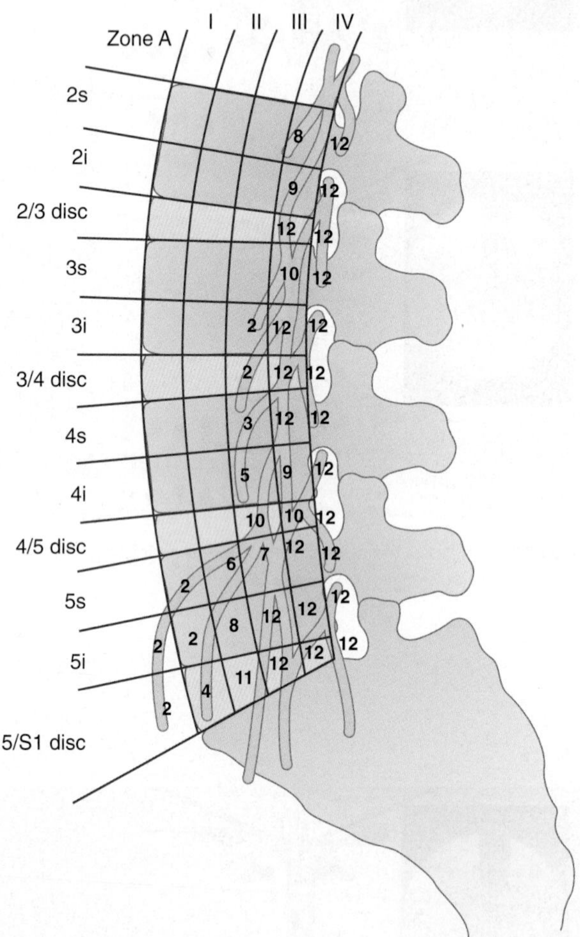

FIG. 21.18 Safe zone and the four quadrants of the disc space. (From Arnold PM, Anderson KK, McGuire RA Jr. The lateral transpsoas approach to the lumbar and thoracic spine: a review. *Surg Neurol Int.* 2012;3:S198–S215.)

well as for "pseudohernia" prevention related to denervation of the oblique muscles and resultant paresis of the abdominal wall as described by Dakwar et al.[59] After development of the retroperitoneal plane by finger dissection, careful dissection of the iliopsoas must be performed to avoid injury to the muscle and its intrinsic motor branches with dilators or retractor positioning/tension. Additionally, the amount and duration of retraction used and operative time per level should be taken into consideration in order to decrease the likelihood of traction injury to nerves.[60]

Advanced imaging should be evaluated for neurovascular anatomy and its course with respect to the psoas and operative level. Use of axial MRI (Fig. 21.19) to evaluate the size of the psoas, rotation of the vertebral bodies, neurovascular anatomy, and how the lumbosacral plexus migrates within the psoas from proximal to distal is especially helpful in surgical planning.[12,61] A large psoas may present challenges to safe transpsoas entry, as can the location of the 11th or 12th rib during access to the upper lumbar spine, alerting the surgeon to the need for rib resection or use of an intercostal approach.

Our preference is to minimize "breaking" of the table to a degree that is necessary to access the operative level(s). The tension of the psoas is assessed by palpation in every procedure to minimize excessive traction of the lumbar plexus. If breaking the table is required for lateral disc space access, we have found that "unbreaking" the table after only the inner dilator and wire are in can substantially decrease psoas tension while maintaining safe access with little anatomic distortion.

Real-time, directionally stimulated neuromonitoring is employed intraoperatively to determine the proximity of the exiting and traversing neural elements. The genitofemoral nerve, most commonly seen at the L3–L4 lumbar level within the more superficial dissection plane, should be directly visualized and requires special attention because it is primarily a sensory nerve and not detected by triggered or free-run electromyography.[60]

Vascular Anatomy

The retroperitoneal space houses the great vessels, including the aorta, inferior vena cava, and common iliacs. Vascular anatomy should be well visualized and carefully evaluated on preoperative MRI. Regev et al. found that the highest risk of injury to the retroperitoneal vessels was at L4–L5 due to the

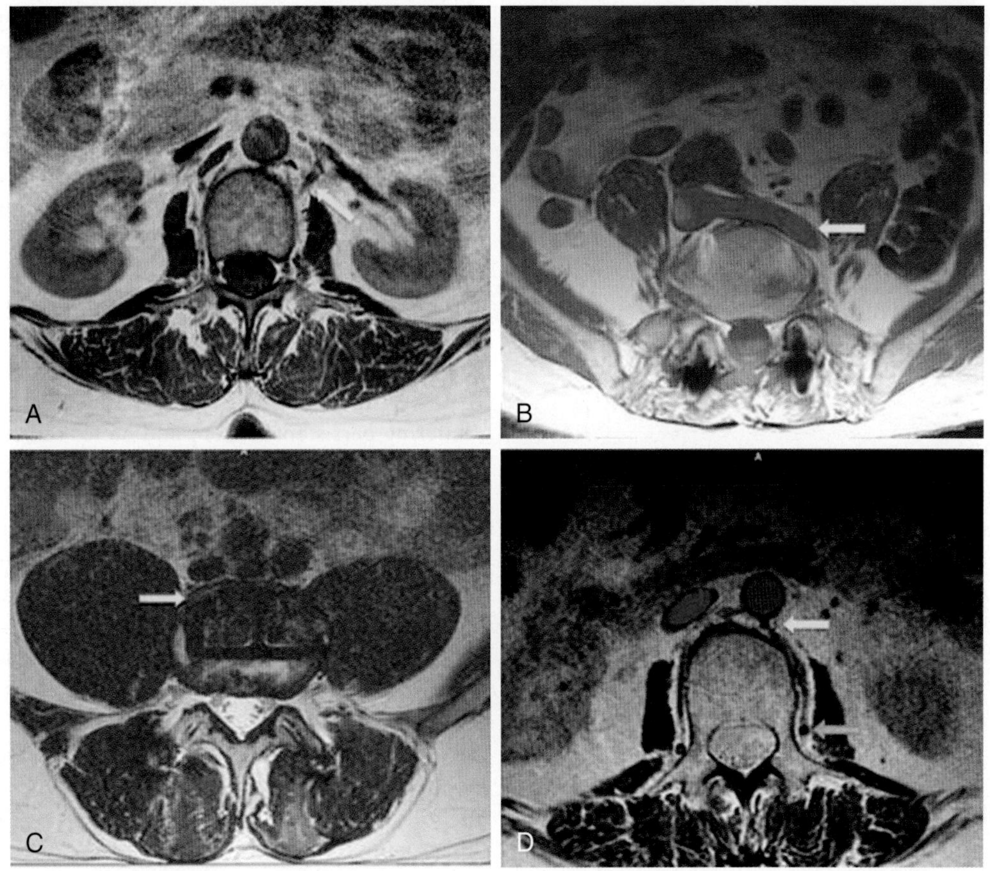

FIG. 21.19 (A) Axial T1 magnetic resonance image (MRI) of the lumbar spine showing anastomosis between the renal and segmental vessels in close proximity to the L1–L2 disc space (*arrow*). *Red area*, abdominal aorta. (B) Axial T1-weighted MRI of the lumbar spine at the L5 level showing the left common iliac vein. *Blue area*, inferior vena cava. *Yellow arrow*, left common iliac vein. (C) Axial T2-weighted MRI of the lumbar spine at the L3–L4 level. *Yellow arrow*, lateral lumbar interbody fusion cage. Note the close proximity of the cage and the great vessels. (D) Axial T2-weighted MRI of the lumbar spine. *Red area*, abdominal aorta. *Blue area*, inferior vena cava. *Yellow arrow*, lumbar arteries branching off the aorta. *Red arrow*, proximal vessel of lumbar arteries anastomosis. (From Alkadhim M, Zoccali C, Abbasifard S, et al. The surgical vascular anatomy of the minimally invasive lateral lumbar interbody approach: a cadaveric and radiographic analysis. *Eur Spine J*. 2015;24[Suppl 7]:906–911.)

more posterior location of the retroperitoneal vessels.[62] Furthermore, the risk of vasculature injury is further increased with rotatory deformities.[62] Rare contralateral injuries to vasculature can also occur; therefore, particular care should be taken with the use of instruments when dissecting across the disc space and when inserting the interbody graft.[63,64]

High Iliac Crest/Lumbosacral Junction

During preoperative evaluation, standing anteroposterior lumbar radiographs should be scrutinized for access to the operative level, with particular attention to the height of the lateral iliac crest and angle required for accessing L4–L5. Positioning the patient in a true lateral decubitus position with lateral bending (see Fig. 21.1) of the torso can increase the distance between the iliac crest and ribs. However, this must be weighed against the increased tension and traction placed on the psoas and lumbar plexus.[60,65] In most cases, access to L5–S1 is limited by a high lateral ilium, anterior course of the neural elements pulled directly across the lateral disc, and/or the vasculature, precluding safe access. Uncommonly, L5–S1 may be approached when the intercrestal line transects the mid to lower L5 body or the L5–S1 disc space. Angled instruments are also an option to improve access.

Scoliosis

Special consideration must be made in scoliosis patients. Identify abnormal displacement of vascular structures with severe rotational deformity and approaching from the convex side because the approach angle is more rostral. Preoperative planning with identifying the lumbar plexus, iliac vein and artery, aorta, and inferior vena cava on MRI is important to determine which side is safer to approach (see Fig. 21.19).[56,66,67]

Thoracolumbar Junction

Rostrally, the 12th rib may obstruct access from T12 to L2, which may require excision or manipulation. Partial rib resection can be commonly performed in thoracolumbar approaches with little morbidity. Another technique to improve access is to place a bump or roll under the contralateral flank to help increase the distance between the 12th rib and iliac crest (see Fig. 21.2).[6]

A retrodiaphragm approach can be done by partial rib resection and using the rib posteriorly as a guide to the disc space and as a plane to retract the diaphragm anteriorly. Care should be taken not to injure the diaphragm. Sometimes a transdiaphragm approach is required for the thoracolumbar junction since the diaphragm cannot be mobilized sufficiently to gain access to the disc. With significant diaphragm dissection, the diaphragm should be repaired prior to closure.

Thoracic Spine

Partial rib resection can be commonly performed in anterolateral thoracic approaches with little morbidity. Several other techniques to minimize rib resection or preserve this anatomy have been utilized, including performing LLIF in between ribs. If that technique is performed, expansion of the lateral access retractor should be minimized to prevent prolonged compression of the neural elements on the rib underside for risk of postoperative radicular/rib pain.

Complications

Although the minimally invasive nature of LLIF avoids many serious approach-related risks of the anterior and posterior techniques, there exists a significant risk of neurologic injury. The most common and well-documented complication is lumbar plexus nerve root injury from either direct compression, laceration, or traction while traversing the psoas or through prolonged retraction.[12,13,47,59,65,68,69] In the largest series of LLIF cases, Rodgers et al. reported a 0.66% incidence of transient hip flexor weakness that occurred only when approaching the L4–L5 level and a 6.2% overall complication rate.[12] These authors contend that approach-related complication rates of LLIF are lower than the traditional open approaches, including posterolateral lumbar fusion, PLIF, TLIF, and ALIF. However, it should be noted that these rates are significantly lower than other smaller series reported in the literature. Moller et al. found in their series of 53 patients that 36% of patients experienced subjective hip flexor weakness, 23% experienced thigh numbness, and 25% experienced thigh pain.[13] Hip flexion weakness resolved in 84% at 6 months, with most patients returning to baseline at 8 weeks; 69% and 75% of patients with thigh numbness and pain, respectively, returned to baseline at 6 months and with many reporting improvement at 8 weeks. Cummock et al. observed thigh pain and numbness in 39% and 42.4% of 59 patients, respectively, and nearly half resolved at 3 months and 90% resolved at 1 year.[70] Pumberger et al. reviewed 235 patients who underwent LLIF and found sensory deficits in 1.6% of patients, psoas motor deficit in 1.6%, and lumbar plexus deficit in 2.9% at 12 months follow-up.[71]

Transient hip flexor weakness and pain that occurs in the absence of sensory deficits is thought to be due to splitting of the psoas muscle fibers rather than a neurapraxia. Weakness is typically transient and resolves within 3 months.[46] Longer duration of retraction has been suggested to predict postoperative weakness.[46] If a nerve injury is suspected, electrodiagnostic studies have been recommended at 6 weeks and 3 months postoperatively. If no clinical recovery is observed, some surgeons perform a limited electromyographic test monthly over the subsequent 3 months to evaluate for reinnervation.[65]

Although rare, permanent or disabling nerve injury may occur. Knight et al. reported two cases of L4 nerve injury in their study of 58 patients.[69] The incidence appears to be higher in scoliosis patients, with Tormenti et al. reporting five of eight patients treated with LLIF for adult degenerative scoliosis suffering persistent sensory and motor radiculopathy.[37]

The incidence of lumbar plexus nerve root injuries varies widely, in part due to inconsistency in the literature regarding diagnosis and evaluation. Ahmadian et al. therefore developed a diagnostic standardization of and classification for postoperative nerve injuries seen with LLIFs that correspond to sensory dermatomal zones.[65]

The retroperitoneal nature of the approach also exposes thoracoabdominal structures to potential injury that can be significant. Reported complications include bowel perforation,[37,72] incisional hernias,[12,59] pleural effusions,[37] kidney lacerations,[47] retrocapsular hematoma,[73] abdominal wall paresis,[59,74] and pseudohernia.[59,74] Each case of bowel perforation required emergent exploratory laparotomy with resection of bowel. When operating in the thoracolumbar spine, the pleural space can be violated, leading to pleural effusion and requiring careful intraoperative evaluation to evaluate whether a chest tube is needed.

The most common implant-related complication is symptomatic graft subsidence, which can lead to pseudarthrosis, back and/or leg pain, adjacent vertebral body fractures, or neurologic complications. Rodgers et al. reported 3 cases of subsidence in 600 patients that required reoperation due to adjacent vertebra fracture, graft fracture, and screw penetration of the endplate.[12] Other authors have reported early subsidence with stand-alone LLIFs due to excessive motion that resolved after posterior instrumentation was performed.[27] Karikari et al. reported a 16.7% incidence of subsidence in a series of patients older than 70 years of age who underwent LLIF for degenerative conditions.[17] Excessive motion and osteoporotic bone are the common etiologies for graft subsidence, but "overstuffing" the interbody space and endplate perforation can be precursors to subsidence. Consideration for supplemental posterior instrumentation should be made that includes patient's bone mineral density. The risk of subsidence is theoretically lower with the use of wider LLIF cages with larger surface contact area and greater distribution of force throughout the apophyseal ring.[27]

Outcomes

The minimally invasive lateral approach for interbody fusion has shown promise in minimizing approach-related morbidity by minimizing surgical dissection and soft tissue trauma with shorter operating room time, shorter hospital stay, and decreased blood loss while maintaining equivalent or improved clinical and radiographic outcomes compared to traditional open anterior or posterior approaches.[12–14]

In 2013, Ahmadian et al. reported in a series of 31 patients who underwent LLIF for grade I or grade II spondylolisthesis that there was significant reduction in anterolisthesis, with 27 of 31 achieving complete reduction of the spondylolisthesis.[65] At 6 months, all patients had clinical and radiographic evidence of fusion on computed tomography (CT) and plain radiographs as well as significant improvements in Oswestry Disability Index (ODI), visual analog scale (VAS), and Short Form-36 scores.

The lateral approach has been shown to be a feasible operative treatment for adjacent-segment degeneration. In a prospective series of 100 patients who underwent LLIF for adjacent-segment degeneration, Rodgers et al. reported significant improvement in VAS pain scores (from 8.6 to 2.8), low complication rate (9%), and evidence of radiographic and clinical fusion at 6 months.[47] The benefit of utilizing an alternative lateral approach avoids the technically challenging task and increased risk of complications with reoperation through the prior anterior or posterior scar.[46]

With obese patients, the lateral approach has been suggested to be a favorable alternative. In a comparative series of 313 obese and nonobese patients who underwent LLIF for degenerative conditions, Rodgers et al. found no greater incidence of complication.[75] This finding is not seen with traditional open anterior or posterior fusion approaches in which body habitus presents a technical challenge and has been shown to increase rates of infection and other complications.[76]

The use of LLIF for deformity correction in adult degenerative scoliosis (ADS) has been shown to result in lower complication rates, shorter operative times, and less blood loss with equal or better clinical and radiographic outcomes when compared to traditional open anterior or posterior approaches.[12,27,40,47,73,77,78] This is particularly relevant to the elderly patient population that suffers from ADS given that they frequently have coexisting osteoporosis and multiple comorbidities that put them at higher risk for pseudarthrosis, hardware failure, and other complications with multilevel deformity correction.[79,80] Complication rates of up to 66% have been reported.[81] Charosky et al. reported a 39% complication rate with 20% requiring reoperation in 306 patients undergoing primary ADS treatment by traditional anterior, posterior, or combined approaches.[82] Daubs et al. reported a 37% complication rate, with 20% major complications in patients over 60 years.[83] In a large prospective series of 107 patients who underwent LLIF for ADS, Phillips et al. demonstrated significant improvements in clinical and radiographic outcomes at 24 months with a lower incidence of complications (24%, with half being minor complications).[47] The lower rate is likely attributed to the lateral approach avoiding mobilization of abdominal viscera and great vessels or dissection of the posterior musculature.[47] Perioperative morbidity is also decreased by the minimally invasive nature of the lateral approach, which minimizes surgical morbidity and allows for early ambulation and shorter hospital stay.[12–14] Although minor complications of hip flexor weakness and thigh pain have been reported, most are transient and resolved by 6 months.[13]

Coronal deformity correction achieved with LLIF for ADS has been reported to be similar to that achieved by traditional approaches. Wang and Mummaneni reported a mean coronal correction of 20 degrees (63%) in 23 patients with a solid fusion at all interbody levels.[39] Anand et al.[73] reported a 15-degree correction (68%) in 28 patients, all of whom fused and maintained their correction at 12 months. Acosta et al.[13] reported an 11.7-degree correction (55%) in eight patients. Tormenti et al.[37] reported a 70% curve correction in eight patients. Phillips et al.[46] reported a 7.4-degree (35%) correction in 107 patients, with greater correction seen with posterior instrumentation. In comparison, in a systematic review of 49 publications on ADS deformity correction, mean postoperative coronal correction was 40.7%.[84] Anand et al. also reported significant improvements in VAS and ODI scores with no major complications.[73] Uribe et al. demonstrated that deformity corrections in a series of 39 ADS patients were all maintained with ongoing improvement in VAS pain scores up to 3 years postoperatively.[49] Dakwar et al. reported that all 25 adult deformities in their series maintained correction at 2 years, achieved fusion on CT and plain radiographs, and experienced significant improvement in VAS and ODI scores with only minor complications.[85] Ozgur et al. reported excellent clinical and radiographic results equal to or superior to traditional approaches with no major complications in their 62 patients.[16] Wang and Mummaneni also encountered no intraoperative complications.[39] Pimenta et al. and Benglis et al. independently found significant deformity correction with significant mid- to long-term clinical outcomes in their individual series of ADS patients who underwent LLIF.[86,87]

The anterior column fusion rates achieved with LLIF are equivalent or greater than traditional approaches such as ALIF, for which 92% to 97% have evidence of fusion on CT at 12 months.[88] A 96% fusion rate by CT and over 90% patient response of "satisfied or very satisfied" was reported by Rodgers et al. at 12-month follow-up in a series of 66 patients who underwent LLIF of 88 levels.[89] Similarly, Ozgur et al. reported radiographic evidence of fusion after LLIF for degenerative disease in 91% of 62 patients with 113 levels, and significant improvement in VAS and ODI scores at 24 months.[16] This high rate of fusion is consistent with a low incidence of revisions for pseudarthrosis. Phillips et al.[46] observed a 2% rate of revision for pseudarthrosis, which is superior to rates of 0% to 19%[90-94] reported for anterior and/or posterior approaches.

Indications for the MIS lateral approach have expanded to the thoracolumbar junction, including corpectomy and reconstruction. Addressing anterior column pathology in the thoracic spine is technically challenging and a thoracotomy can lead to poor pulmonary function postoperatively, with major complications reported in up to 12% of patients.[95] Khan et al. followed a series of 25 patients who underwent an MIS lateral approach for corpectomy and observed shorter operative times, decreased blood loss, decreased use of blood products, shorter postoperative time to extubation, and significant pain relief compared to a standard open corpectomy.[96] The benefit is attributed to the minimally invasive nature of the approach and the absence of prolonged lung deflation. Karikari et al.[17] reported a series of 22 patients who underwent LLIF for thoracolumbar disease, including degeneration, tumor, adjacent-segment disease, disc herniation, and infection. They observed that 95.5% of patients achieved a substantial clinical benefit and demonstrated evidence of fusion at 6 months postoperatively. Although deformity correction was less pronounced than with the traditional open thoracolumbar approach, no major complications occurred. The MIS lateral approach to the thoracolumbar spine may be a well-suited safe alternative for elderly patients or those with significant comorbidities, and in multiple other settings including trauma, infection, tumor, and corpectomies for canal decompression for a variety of pathologies.

In regard to costs, Lucio et al. performed a cost analysis for two-level LLIF and two-level PLIF for degenerative lumbar disease; they showed a cost saving of $2825.37 (10.4%) per patient in the early perioperative period with LLIF.[97] The costs were calculated from the index procedure, transfusions, reoperations, and residual events, which were defined by hospital readmissions, emergency department visits, postoperative rehabilitation, and additional diagnostics. These authors also reported shorter hospital stay and decreased blood loss in the LLIF group.

Summary

LLIF has evolved over decades into a safe and common procedure. LLIFs provide superior fusion rates compared to other fusion options. LLIFs provide indirect decompression of foraminal, lateral recess, and central stenosis. With osteoporosis, LLIF allows load sharing over a large footprint on the apophyseal ring and decreases osteoporotic-related hardware complications. Preoperative MRI evaluation is imperative to identify the neurovascular anatomy to prevent vascular and lumbar plexus injuries. LLIFs provide significant coronal and sagittal correction in ADS compared to traditional open procedures. Anterior column reconstruction through the lateral approach provides equivalent sagittal plane correction as pedicle subtraction osteotomy with significantly less blood loss. LLIFs meet the demand for earlier postoperative recovery and return to work. Lateral interbody fusions limit infection rates compared to open posterior fusions with the obese population. Last, minimally invasive lateral interbody fusion is cost-effective and provides health care savings compared to other lumbar fusion options.

KEY REFERENCES

1. Ozgur BM, Aryan HE, Pimenta L, Taylor WR. Extreme Lateral Interbody Fusion (XLIF): a novel surgical technique for anterior lumbar interbody fusion. *Spine*. 2006;6:435-443.
2. Rodgers WB, Gerber EJ, Patterson J. Intraoperative and early postoperative complications in extreme lateral interbody fusion: an analysis of 600 cases. *Spine*. 2011;36:26-32.
3. Oliveira L, Marchi L, Coutinho E, Pimenta L. A radiographic assessment of the ability of the extreme lateral interbody fusion procedure to indirectly decompress the neural elements. *Spine*. 2010;35:S331-S337.
4. Phillips FM, Isaacs RE, Rodgers WB, et al. Adult degenerative scoliosis treated with XLIF: clinical and radiographical results of a prospective multicenter study with 24-month follow-up. *Spine*. 2013;38:1853-1861.
5. Isaacs RE, Hyde J, Goodrich JA, Rodgers WB, Phillips FM. A prospective, nonrandomized, multicenter evaluation of extreme lateral interbody fusion for the treatment of adult degenerative scoliosis: perioperative outcomes and complications. *Spine*. 2010;35:S322-S330.
6. Benglis DM, Vanni S, Levi AD. An anatomical study of the lumbosacral plexus as related to the minimally invasive transpsoas approach to the lumbar spine. *J Neurosurg Spine*. 2009;10:139-144.
7. Davis TT, Bae HW, Mok JM, Rasouli A, Delamarter RB. Lumbar plexus anatomy within the psoas muscle: implications for the transpsoas lateral approach to the L4-L5 disc. *J Bone Joint Surg Am*. 2011;93:1482-1487.

REFERENCES

1. Nachemson A, Zdeblick TA, O'Brien JP. Lumbar disc disease with discogenic pain. What surgical treatment is most effective? *Spine*. 1996;21:1835-1838.
2. Liu X, Wang Y, Qiu G, Weng X, Yu B. A systematic review with meta-analysis of posterior interbody fusion versus posterolateral fusion in lumbar spondylolisthesis. *Eur Spine J*. 2014;23:43-56.
3. Zhang Q, Yuan Z, Zhou M, et al. A comparison of posterior lumbar interbody fusion and transforaminal lumbar interbody fusion: a literature review and meta-analysis. *BMC Musculoskelet Disord*. 2014;15:367.
4. Liu XY, Wang YP, Qiu GX, Weng XS, Yu B. Meta-analysis of circumferential fusion versus posterolateral fusion in lumbar spondylolisthesis. *J Spinal Disord Tech*. 2014;27:E282-E293.
5. Kim YB, Lenke LG, Kim YJ, et al. The morbidity of an anterior thoracolumbar approach: adult spinal deformity patients with greater than five-year follow-up. *Spine*. 2009;34:822-826.
6. Ozgur BM, Aryan HE, Pimenta L, Taylor WR. Extreme Lateral Interbody Fusion (XLIF): a novel surgical technique for anterior lumbar interbody fusion. *Spine*. 2006;6:435-443.
7. Peterson MD. Complications avoidance in extreme lateral interbody fusion (XLIF): video lecture. *Eur Spine J*. 2015;24(suppl 3):439-440.
8. Pateder DB, Gonzales RA, Kebaish KM, et al. Short-term mortality and its association with independent risk factors in adult spinal deformity surgery. *Spine*. 2008;33:1224-1228.
9. Obenchain TG. Laparoscopic lumbar discectomy: case report. *J Laparoendosc Surg*. 1991;1:145-149.
10. Harmon PH. Anterior excision and vertebral body fusion operation for intervertebral disk syndromes of the lower lumbar spine: three-to five-year results in 244 cases. *Clin Orthop Relat Res*. 1963;26:107-127.
11. Harmon PH. Anterior disc excision and fusion of the lumbar vertebral bodies. A review of diagnostic level testing, with operative results in more than seven hundred cases. *J Int Coll Surg*. 1963;40:572-586.
12. Rodgers WB, Gerber EJ, Patterson J. Intraoperative and early postoperative complications in extreme lateral interbody fusion: an analysis of 600 cases. *Spine*. 2011;36:26-32.
13. Moller DJ, Slimack NP, Acosta FL Jr, et al. Minimally invasive lateral lumbar interbody fusion and transpsoas approach-related morbidity. *Neurosurg Focus*. 2011;31:E4.

14. Patel AA, Zfass-Mendez M, Lebwohl NH, et al. Minimally invasive versus open lumbar fusion: a comparison of blood loss, surgical complications, and hospital course. *Iowa Orthop J.* 2015;35:130-134.
15. Brau SA. Mini-open approach to the spine for anterior lumbar interbody fusion: description of the procedure, results and complications. *Spine J.* 2002;2:216-223.
16. Ozgur BM, Agarwal V, Nail E, Pimenta L. Two-year clinical and radiographic success of minimally invasive lateral transpsoas approach for the treatment of degenerative lumbar conditions. *SAS J.* 2010;4:41-46.
17. Karikari IO, Nimjee SM, Hardin CA, et al. Extreme lateral interbody fusion approach for isolated thoracic and thoracolumbar spine diseases: initial clinical experience and early outcomes. *J Spinal Disord Tech.* 2011;24:368-375.
18. Delecrin J, Aguado E, NGuyen JM, et al. Influence of local environment on incorporation of ceramic for lumbar fusion. Comparison of laminar and intertransverse sites in a canine model. *Spine.* 1997;22:1683-1689.
19. Johnston CE 2nd, Ashman RB, Baird AM, Allard RN. Effect of spinal construct stiffness on early fusion mass incorporation. Experimental study. *Spine.* 1990;15:908-912.
20. Johnston CE 2nd, Welch RD, Baker KJ, Ashman RB. Effect of spinal construct stiffness on short segment fusion mass incorporation. *Spine.* 1995;20:2400-2407.
21. Nagel DA, Kramers PC, Rahn BA, Cordey J, Perren SM. A paradigm of delayed union and nonunion in the lumbosacral joint. A study of motion and bone grafting of the lumbosacral spine in sheep. *Spine.* 1991;16:553-559.
22. Boden SD, Schimandle JH, Hutton WC. An experimental lumbar intertransverse process spinal fusion model. Radiographic, histologic, and biomechanical healing characteristics. *Spine.* 1995;20:412-420.
23. Li H, Zou X, Laursen M, et al. The influence of intervertebral disc tissue on anterior spinal interbody fusion: an experimental study on pigs. *Eur Spine J.* 2002;11:476-481.
24. Thomas I, Kirkaldy-Willis WH, Singh S, Paine KW. Experimental spinal fusion in guinea pigs and dogs: the effect of immobilization. *Clin Orthop Relat Res.* 1975;112:363-375.
25. Fritzell P, Hagg O, Wessberg P, Nordwall A, Swedish Lumbar Spine Study Group. Chronic low back pain and fusion: a comparison of three surgical techniques: a prospective multicenter randomized study from the Swedish Lumbar Spine Study Group. *Spine.* 2002;27:1131-1141.
26. Lee CS, Hwang CJ, Lee DH, Kim YT, Lee HS. Fusion rates of instrumented lumbar spinal arthrodesis according to surgical approach: a systematic review of randomized trials. *Clin Orthop Surg.* 2011;3:39-47.
27. Oliveira L, Marchi L, Coutinho E, Pimenta L. A radiographic assessment of the ability of the extreme lateral interbody fusion procedure to indirectly decompress the neural elements. *Spine.* 2010;35:S331-S337.
28. Park SJ, Lee CS, Chung SS, et al. The ideal cage position for achieving both indirect neural decompression and segmental angle restoration in lateral lumbar interbody fusion (LLIF). *Clin Spine Surg.* 2017;30(6):E784-E790.
29. Peddada K, Elder BD, Ishida W, et al. Clinical outcomes following sublaminar decompression and instrumented fusion for lumbar degenerative spinal pathology. *J Clin Neurosci.* 2016;30:98-104.
30. Alimi M, Hofstetter CP, Tsiouris AJ, Elowitz E, Hartl R. Extreme lateral interbody fusion for unilateral symptomatic vertical foraminal stenosis. *Eur Spine J.* 2015;24(suppl 3):346-352.
31. Cho PG, Park SH, Kim KN, et al. A morphometric analysis of contralateral neural foramen in TLIF. *Eur Spine J.* 2015;24:783-790.
32. Iwata T, Miyamoto K, Hioki A, et al. Morphologic changes in contralateral lumbar foramen in unilateral cantilever transforaminal lumbar interbody fusion using kidney-type intervertebral spacers. *J Spinal Disord Tech.* 2015;28:E270-E276.
33. Hsieh PC, Koski TR, O'Shaughnessy BA, et al. Anterior lumbar interbody fusion in comparison with transforaminal lumbar interbody fusion: implications for the restoration of foraminal height, local disc angle, lumbar lordosis, and sagittal balance. *J Neurosurg Spine.* 2007;7:379-386.
34. Phan K, Thayaparan GK, Mobbs RJ. Anterior lumbar interbody fusion versus transforaminal lumbar interbody fusion—systematic review and meta-analysis. *Br J Neurosurg.* 2015;29:705-711.
35. Crandall DG, Revella J. Transforaminal lumbar interbody fusion versus anterior lumbar interbody fusion as an adjunct to posterior instrumented correction of degenerative lumbar scoliosis: three year clinical and radiographic outcomes. *Spine.* 2009;34:2126-2133.
36. Dorward IG, Lenke LG, Bridwell KH, et al. Transforaminal versus anterior lumbar interbody fusion in long deformity constructs: a matched cohort analysis. *Spine.* 2013;38:E755-E762.
37. Tormenti MJ, Maserati MB, Bonfield CM, Okonkwo DO, Kanter AS. Complications and radiographic correction in adult scoliosis following combined transpsoas extreme lateral interbody fusion and posterior pedicle screw instrumentation. *Neurosurg Focus.* 2010;28:E7.
38. Anand N, Baron EM, Thaiyananthan G, Khalsa K, Goldstein TB. Minimally invasive multilevel percutaneous correction and fusion for adult lumbar degenerative scoliosis: a technique and feasibility study. *J Spinal Disord Tech.* 2008;21:459-467.
39. Wang MY, Mummaneni PV. Minimally invasive surgery for thoracolumbar spinal deformity: initial clinical experience with clinical and radiographic outcomes. *Neurosurg Focus.* 2010;28:E9.
40. Khajavi K, Shen AY. Two-year radiographic and clinical outcomes of a minimally invasive, lateral, transpsoas approach for anterior lumbar interbody fusion in the treatment of adult degenerative scoliosis. *Eur Spine J.* 2014;23:1215-1223.
41. Mobbs RJ, Phan K, Malham G, Seex K, Rao PJ. Lumbar interbody fusion: techniques, indications and comparison of interbody fusion options including PLIF, TLIF, MI-TLIF, OLIF/ATP, LLIF and ALIF. *J Spine Surg.* 2015;1:2-18.
42. Watkins RGt, Hanna R, Chang D, Watkins RG 3rd. Sagittal alignment after lumbar interbody fusion: comparing anterior, lateral, and transforaminal approaches. *J Spinal Disord Tech.* 2014;27:253-256.
43. Kim CH, Chung CK, Park SB, Yang SH, Kim JH. A change in lumbar sagittal alignment after single-level anterior lumbar interbody fusion for lumbar degenerative spondylolisthesis with normal sagittal balance. *Clin Spine Surg.* 2016. Epub ahead of print.
44. Lee SH, Choi WG, Lim SR, Kang HY, Shin SW. Minimally invasive anterior lumbar interbody fusion followed by percutaneous pedicle screw fixation for isthmic spondylolisthesis. *Spine J.* 2004;4:644-649.
45. Lu VM, Kerezoudis P, Gilder HE, et al. Minimally invasive surgery versus open surgery spinal fusion for spondylolisthesis: a systematic review and meta-analysis. *Spine.* 2017;42:E177-E185.

46. Phillips FM, Isaacs RE, Rodgers WB, et al. Adult degenerative scoliosis treated with XLIF: clinical and radiographical results of a prospective multicenter study with 24-month follow-up. *Spine*. 2013;38:1853-1861.
47. Isaacs RE, Hyde J, Goodrich JA, Rodgers WB, Phillips FM. A prospective, nonrandomized, multicenter evaluation of extreme lateral interbody fusion for the treatment of adult degenerative scoliosis: perioperative outcomes and complications. *Spine*. 2010;35:S322-S330.
48. Mobbs RJ, Sivabalan P, Li J. Minimally invasive surgery compared to open spinal fusion for the treatment of degenerative lumbar spine pathologies. *J Clin Neurosci*. 2012;19:829-835.
49. Manwaring JC, Bach K, Ahmadian AA, et al. Management of sagittal balance in adult spinal deformity with minimally invasive anterolateral lumbar interbody fusion: a preliminary radiographic study. *J Neurosurg Spine*. 2014;20:515-522.
50. Saigal R, Mundis GM Jr, Eastlack R, et al. Anterior column realignment (ACR) in adult sagittal deformity correction: technique and review of the literature. *Spine*. 2016;41(suppl 8):S66-S73.
51. Smith WD, Youssef JA, Christian G, Serrano S, Hyde JA. Lumbarized sacrum as a relative contraindication for lateral transpsoas interbody fusion at L5-6. *J Spinal Disord Tech*. 2012;25:285-291.
52. McAfee PC, Shucosky E, Chotikul L, et al. Multilevel extreme lateral interbody fusion (XLIF) and osteotomies for 3-dimensional severe deformity: 25 consecutive cases. *Int J Spine Surg*. 2013;7:e8-e19.
53. Youssef JA, McAfee PC, Patty CA, et al. Minimally invasive surgery: lateral approach interbody fusion: results and review. *Spine*. 2010;35:S302-S311.
54. Malham GM, Ellis NJ, Parker RM, et al. Maintenance of segmental lordosis and disc height in standalone and instrumented extreme lateral interbody fusion (XLIF). *Clin Spine Surg*. 2017;30(2):E90-E98.
55. Moro T, Kikuchi S, Konno S, Yaginuma H. An anatomic study of the lumbar plexus with respect to retroperitoneal endoscopic surgery. *Spine*. 2003;28:423-428.
56. Benglis DM, Vanni S, Levi AD. An anatomical study of the lumbosacral plexus as related to the minimally invasive transpsoas approach to the lumbar spine. *J Neurosurg Spine*. 2009;10:139-144.
57. Davis TT, Bae HW, Mok JM, Rasouli A, Delamarter RB. Lumbar plexus anatomy within the psoas muscle: implications for the transpsoas lateral approach to the L4-L5 disc. *J Bone Joint Surg Am*. 2011;93:1482-1487.
58. Arnold PM, Anderson KK, McGuire RA Jr. The lateral transpsoas approach to the lumbar and thoracic spine: a review. *Surg Neurol Int*. 2012;3:S198-S215.
59. Dakwar E, Le TV, Baaj AA, et al. Abdominal wall paresis as a complication of minimally invasive lateral transpsoas interbody fusion. *Neurosurg Focus*. 2011;31:E18.
60. Uribe JS, Isaacs RE, Youssef JA, et al. Can triggered electromyography monitoring throughout retraction predict postoperative symptomatic neuropraxia after XLIF? Results from a prospective multicenter trial. *Eur Spine J*. 2015;24(suppl 3):378-385.
61. Buric J. Relationship between psoas muscle dimensions and postoperative thigh pain. A possible preoperative evaluation factor. *Int J Spine Surg*. 2015;9:27.
62. Regev GJ, Chen L, Dhawan M, et al. Morphometric analysis of the ventral nerve roots and retroperitoneal vessels with respect to the minimally invasive lateral approach in normal and deformed spines. *Spine*. 2009;34:1330-1335.
63. Papanastassiou ID, Eleraky M, Vrionis FD. Contralateral femoral nerve compression: an unrecognized complication after extreme lateral interbody fusion (XLIF). *J Clin Neurosci*. 2011;18:149-151.
64. Assina R, Majmundar NJ, Herschman Y, Heary RF. First report of major vascular injury due to lateral transpsoas approach leading to fatality. *J Neurosurg Spine*. 2014;21:794-798.
65. Ahmadian A, Verma S, Mundis GM Jr, et al. Minimally invasive lateral retroperitoneal transpsoas interbody fusion for L4-5 spondylolisthesis: clinical outcomes. *J Neurosurg Spine*. 2013;19:314-320.
66. He L, Kang Z, Tang WJ, Rong LM. A MRI study of lumbar plexus with respect to the lateral transpsoas approach to the lumbar spine. *Eur Spine J*. 2015;24:2538-2545.
67. Alkadhim M, Zoccali C, Abbasifard S, et al. The surgical vascular anatomy of the minimally invasive lateral lumbar interbody approach: a cadaveric and radiographic analysis. *Eur Spine J*. 2015;24(suppl 7):906-911.
68. Kotwal S, Kawaguchi S, Lebl D, et al. Minimally invasive lateral lumbar interbody fusion: clinical and radiographic outcome at a minimum 2-year follow-up. *J Spinal Disord Tech*. 2015;28:119-125.
69. Knight RQ, Schwaegler P, Hanscom D, Roh J. Direct lateral lumbar interbody fusion for degenerative conditions: early complication profile. *J Spinal Disord Tech*. 2009;22:34-37.
70. Cummock MD, Vanni S, Levi AD, Yu Y, Wang MY. An analysis of postoperative thigh symptoms after minimally invasive transpsoas lumbar interbody fusion. *J Neurosurg Spine*. 2011;15:11-18.
71. Pumberger M, Hughes AP, Huang RR, et al. Neurologic deficit following lateral lumbar interbody fusion. *Eur Spine J*. 2012;21:1192-1199.
72. Malham GM, Ellis NJ, Parker RM, Seex KA. Clinical outcome and fusion rates after the first 30 extreme lateral interbody fusions. *ScientificWorldJournal*. 2012;2012:246989.
73. Anand N, Rosemann R, Khalsa B, Baron EM. Mid-term to long-term clinical and functional outcomes of minimally invasive correction and fusion for adults with scoliosis. *Neurosurg Focus*. 2010;28:E6.
74. Cahill KS, Martinez JL, Wang MY, Vanni S, Levi AD. Motor nerve injuries following the minimally invasive lateral transpsoas approach. *J Neurosurg Spine*. 2012;17:227-231.
75. Rodgers WB, Cox CS, Gerber EJ. Early complications of extreme lateral interbody fusion in the obese. *J Spinal Disord Tech*. 2010;23:393-397.
76. Vaidya R, Carp J, Bartol S, et al. Lumbar spine fusion in obese and morbidly obese patients. *Spine*. 2009;34:495-500.
77. Dangelmajer S, Zadnik PL, Rodriguez ST, Gokaslan ZL, Sciubba DM. Minimally invasive spine surgery for adult degenerative lumbar scoliosis. *Neurosurg Focus*. 2014;36:E7.
78. Phan K, Huo YR, Hogan JA, et al. Minimally invasive surgery in adult degenerative scoliosis: a systematic review and meta-analysis of decompression, anterior/lateral and posterior lumbar approaches. *J Spine Surg*. 2016;2:89-104.
79. Carreon LY, Puno RM, Dimar JR 2nd, Glassman SD, Johnson JR. Perioperative complications of posterior lumbar decompression and arthrodesis in older adults. *J Bone Joint Surg Am*. 2003;85-A:2089-2092.
80. Raffo CS, Lauerman WC. Predicting morbidity and mortality of lumbar spine arthrodesis in patients in their ninth decade. *Spine*. 2006;31:99-103.

81. Fujita T, Kostuik JP, Huckell CB, Sieber AN. Complications of spinal fusion in adult patients more than 60 years of age. *Orthop Clin North Am.* 1998;29:669-678.
82. Charosky S, Guigui P, Blamoutier A, et al. Complications and risk factors of primary adult scoliosis surgery: a multicenter study of 306 patients. *Spine.* 2012;37:693-700.
83. Daubs MD, Lenke LG, Bridwell KH, et al. Decompression alone versus decompression with limited fusion for treatment of degenerative lumbar scoliosis in the elderly patient. *Evid Based Spine Care J.* 2012;3:27-32.
84. Campbell PG, Malone J, Yadla S, et al. Early complications related to approach in thoracic and lumbar spine surgery: a single center prospective study. *World Neurosurg.* 2010;73:395-401.
85. Dakwar E, Cardona RF, Smith DA, Uribe JS. Early outcomes and safety of the minimally invasive, lateral retroperitoneal transpsoas approach for adult degenerative scoliosis. *Neurosurg Focus.* 2010;28:E8.
86. Castro C, Oliveira L, Amaral R, Marchi L, Pimenta L. Is the lateral transpsoas approach feasible for the treatment of adult degenerative scoliosis? *Clin Orthop Relat Res.* 2014;472:1776-1783.
87. Benglis DM, Elhammady MS, Levi AD, Vanni S. Minimally invasive anterolateral approaches for the treatment of back pain and adult degenerative deformity. *Neurosurgery.* 2008;63:191-196.
88. Burkus JKTE, Kitchel SH, et al. Clinical and radiographic outcomes of anterior lumbar interbody fusion using recombinant human bone morphogenetic protein-2. *Spine.* 2002;27:2396-2408.
89. Rodgers WB, Gerber EJ, Rodgers JA. Clinical and radiographic outcomes of extreme lateral approach to interbody fusion with beta-tricalcium phosphate and hydroxyapatite composite for lumbar degenerative conditions. *Int J Spine Surg.* 2012;6:24-28.
90. Pateder DB, Kebaish KM, Cascio BM, et al. Posterior only versus combined anterior and posterior approaches to lumbar scoliosis in adults: a radiographic analysis. *Spine.* 2007;32:1551-1554.
91. Maeda T, Buchowski JM, Kim YJ, Mishiro T, Bridwell KH. Long adult spinal deformity fusion to the sacrum using rhBMP-2 versus autogenous iliac crest bone graft. *Spine.* 2009;34:2205-2212.
92. Scheufler KM, Cyron D, Dohmen H, Eckardt A. Less invasive surgical correction of adult degenerative scoliosis, part I: technique and radiographic results. *Neurosurgery.* 2010;67:696-710.
93. Wu CH, Wong CB, Chen LH, et al. Instrumented posterior lumbar interbody fusion for patients with degenerative lumbar scoliosis. *J Spinal Disord Tech.* 2008;21:310-315.
94. Emami A, Deviren V, Berven S, et al. Outcome and complications of long fusions to the sacrum in adult spine deformity: Luque-Galveston, combined iliac and sacral screws, and sacral fixation. *Spine.* 2002;27:776-786.
95. Landreneau RJ, Hazelrigg SR, Mack MJ, et al. Postoperative pain-related morbidity: video-assisted thoracic surgery versus thoracotomy. *Ann Thorac Surg.* 1993;56:1285-1289.
96. Khan SN, Cha T, Hoskins JA, Pelton M, Singh K. Minimally invasive thoracolumbar corpectomy and reconstruction. *Orthopedics.* 2012;35:e74-e79.
97. Lucio JC, Vanconia RB, Deluzio KJ, et al. Economics of less invasive spinal surgery: an analysis of hospital cost differences between open and minimally invasive instrumented spinal fusion procedures during the perioperative period. *Risk Manag Healthc Policy.* 2012;5:65-74.

22 CHAPTER Anatomy, Nonoperative Results, Preoperative Injections, and Prescriptions

Jeffrey L. Chen
Timothy J. Furnish
Mark S. Wallace

The literature for spinal injections is rife with small studies of limited quality. There are multiple difficulties with the research on invasive pain therapies. First has been a lack of funding for large-scale, high-quality, randomized controlled trials (RCTs). This is partially due to the fact that there are no device or pharmaceutical companies with a vested interest in funding research on these therapies. Second, pain is, by definition, a subjective experience. As with studies of therapies for psychological disorders, there is a significant and growing placebo effect in pain studies, which confounds the ability of studies to show a significant response over placebo.[1] Alternatively, the natural course for many patients with new-onset spinal pain from disc herniation or other causes is to improve. Injection therapies that do show improvement over time may, in part, reflect the natural healing process and overrepresent the effects of these interventions. Third, there is substantial variability in the way that trials of some of these therapies have been conducted. Some of the earlier trials of interlaminar and caudal epidural steroid injections were done before fluoroscopy and epidural contrast were routinely used. Comparing these blind injections to the current standard of practice is problematic. For many interventional pain procedures, the bulk of the studies performed have been observational, retrospective, or otherwise of limited quality. Last, many studies that purport to be placebo controlled have compared an active treatment to something less than clearly a sham treatment. For example, some studies have compared epidural steroids to steroids given via another route. Other studies have compared epidural injections to local anesthetic injections. There is some evidence that simply injecting saline or other solutions into the epidural space has a therapeutic effect.[2] Thus, the selection of a reasonable sham for double-blind trials has been problematic and even RCTs with epidural saline as a control may underestimate the effects of such interventions.

Anatomic Considerations in Spinal Pain

In order for a spinal structure to transmit painful impulses into the central nervous system (CNS), the structure must be innervated with nociceptors. There are numerous structures within the spine that are capable of transmitting pain when diseased. Often, more than one structure can be diseased and transmit pain, making it challenging to identify the pain generator. Spinal injections can be useful, both diagnostically and therapeutically, in the treatment of spine pain. However, they should follow a careful history, physical examination, and diagnostics tests. An understanding of the anatomy and innervation of the spine is critical when utilizing spinal injections for diagnosis and treatment.

The innervation of the spine is complex, as both the sensory and sympathetic nervous systems contribute to pain pathways. The posterior aspect of vertebrae and discs as well as all structures posterior to the vertebrae (i.e., neural foramen, facets, and so on) are innervated segmentally from each spinal root. However, since the sensory innervation of the anterior and lateral portion of the vertebrae and discs travels via the sympathetic nervous system, only the thoracic spinal nerves and upper two lumbar spinal nerves transmit sensory fibers segmentally into the spinal cord. The anterior cervical spine and lower anterior lumbar spine transmit sensory fibers through the first 2 to 3 thoracic nerve roots and upper lumbar nerve roots, respectively.

Zygapophyseal Joint (Facet Joint)

The facet joints are true diarthrodial joints with a rich nerve supply transmitting both nociception and mechanoreception.[3] The synovial membrane of the facet joints is rich in free nerve endings associated with painful sensation.[4] In addition, morphologic studies on human[5–8] facet joints support the role of the facet joint in low back pain. A recent study in degenerative human facet joints and facet joint capsular tissue harvested at the time of surgery showed an upregulation in inflammatory cytokines and neuropeptides (nerve growth factor) that can sensitize and activate nociceptors.[9]

The pain patterns that result from facet joint pathology have been described by several investigators. Because these joints are deep structures, there is a higher ratio of C fiber to A-delta fiber innervation. This results in poorly localized pain with a wide referral pain pattern from the ipsilateral lumbar area to the ipsilateral posterior thigh. These referral patterns may result in secondary zones of reflex muscle spasm and resultant trigger points.

All facet joints are innervated segmentally by a medial branch of the posterior ramus of the nerve root. However, segmental innervation differs between the cervical, thoracic, and lumbar spines. The cervical facet joint receives innervation from one level above and below, with the medial branch located along the waist of the articular process above and below the joint articulation. For example, the C3–C4 facet joint is innervated by the C3 and C4 medial branches. The C2–C3 facet joint receives innervation from the third occipital nerve as it courses across the anterior lateral portion of this joint as well as innervation from the C3 medial branch. The thoracic facet joint medial branch travels superior to the tip of the transverse process and courses proximally over the pedicle to reach the joint capsule. Lumbar facets are supplied by a medial branch at the corresponding level and a branch from one level above. For example, the L4–L5 facet joint is innervated by the L3 and L4 medial branch. The L5–S1 facet joint is innervated by the L4 and L5 medial branches as well as a branch from the posterior rami of S1.

Sacroiliac Joint

As with the facet joint, there has been controversy on the sacroiliac (SI) joint as a cause of low back pain. Like the facet joints, the SI joint is richly innervated with both free nerve endings and mechanoreceptors. The innervation has been extensively described and supports this joint as a pain-sensitive structure.[10,11] Most of the innervation of the SI joint is supplied dorsally from L4–S4 nerve roots, which results in the bulk of the innervation occurring in the dorsal segment of the joint.[12]

Pain from the SI joint is usually referred to the buttocks, groin, posterior thigh, and occasionally, below the knee.[13–15] Because of the anatomic location of the SI joint, this structure is difficult to examine, and many of the provocative tests can result in false-positives and intertester differences.[16,17]

Intervertebral Disc

It is clear that the outer one-third of the intervertebral disc (ID) is well innervated; however, there is controversy regarding whether this is a pain-producing structure.[18–20] There is little, if any, controversy over the role that a herniated disc plays in producing radicular pain; however, controversy arises over isolated disc pathology without nerve compression as a cause of axial low back pain. Nerve endings capable of transmitting pain impulses are abundant in the outer one-third of the anulus fibrosus in both the cervical disc[21] and the lumbar disc.[22] In addition, nerves within the ID contain neuropeptides that are involved in pain transmission.[23] Injuries in the anulus fibrosus may result in pain while the external appearance of the disc remains normal and before nerve roots are affected.[24]

The referral pattern of pain originating solely from the disc is similar to that produced by facet joint pain.[25] The pain from diseased intervertebral discs may not arise directly from the disc, but rather from other structures that develop abnormal stresses as a result of the diseased disc.[26] Other structures surrounding the disc are known to have pain fibers (e.g., facet joints, anterior and posterior longitudinal ligaments).

Ligaments of the Spine

There are many ligamentous structures in the spine that are innervated with free nerve endings. However, there is variability in the density of this innervation. Of all of the ligamentous structures, the posterior longitudinal ligament appears to be the most heavily innervated with free nerve endings[27,28] and the ligamentum flavum the least innervated.[29] Degenerative changes within these ligaments may result in sensitization of free nerve endings, leading to chronic pain. In addition, the close proximity of the anterior and posterior longitudinal ligament to the discs makes the structures susceptible to exposure to the disc contents in the event of disc rupture. The disc contents may induce an inflammatory process in these ligaments, leading to pain.

Nerve Root

The nerve root is innervated by the sinuvertebral nerve, which branches from the segmental nerve and travels backward into the neural foramen. The arachnoidal covering of the nerve root is heavily innervated and a source of pain. Mechanical compression or irritation of these structures can lead to pain in the extremities that is associated with neurologic changes. The nerve root may be stimulated mechanically by disc herniation, osteophyte formation, foraminal narrowing due to degenerative disc disease, or tumor invasion. In addition, it has been postulated that both the disc contents and the facet joint contents may induce an arachnoiditis; however, Haughton et al.[30] showed this only to be true for the disc contents.

Cervical Spine Injections

Cervical epidural steroid injections have been performed from both an interlaminar and transforaminal approach. All epidural injections carry a small risk of complications. However, the cervical transforaminal approach, more than other spinal locations or approaches, has been associated with rare but significant complications, including spinal cord injury, stroke, and death.[31–33]

The majority of studies of cervical epidural injections have utilized the interlaminar approach. In two recent reviews of cervical epidural steroid injections, seven RCTs for the treatment of axial or radicular pain of cervical spinal origin were evaluated.[34,35] Only three of the seven studies were performed using fluoroscopy. Of the studies for cervical radicular pain, only one study made use of fluoroscopic guidance. All of the studies showed significant pain improvement but no differences between epidural steroid treatment and active-control groups, with the exception of one study, which used an intramuscular injection of steroid as the control group. The remaining studies compared epidural steroids versus other substances (mostly local anesthetics) injected epidurally.

The literature regarding the treatment of acute and chronic pain conditions is increasingly focused on multimodal therapies. Patients who undergo treatment with multiple modalities or combinations of pharmaceutical and

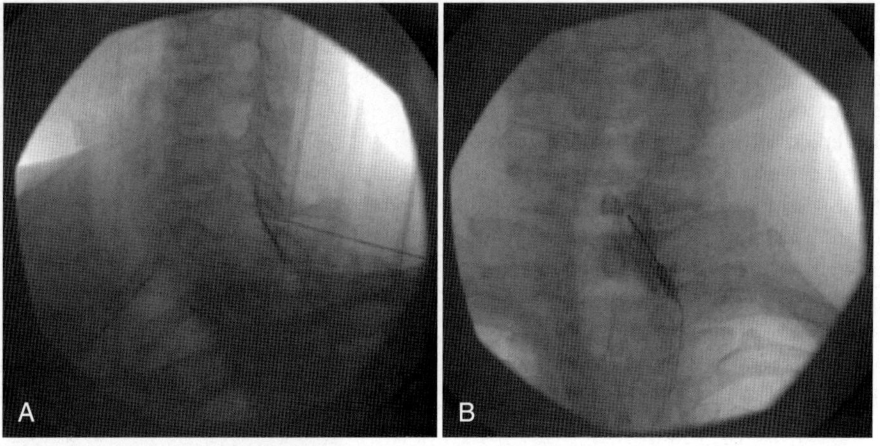

FIG. 22.1 Cervical epidural steroid injection. (A) Contralateral oblique view showing contrast medium in the cervical epidural space. (B) Anteroposterior view showing contrast medium highlighting epidural fat with needle entry at the right C7–T1 level.

nonpharmaceutical treatments fare better than those receiving a single-modality treatment. A recent multicenter RCT of cervical epidural steroid injections (CESIs) for the treatment of cervical radiculopathy showed greater benefits for multimodal therapy over more limited therapy.[36] A total of 169 subjects were randomized to physical therapy plus gabapentin, cervical epidural steroid injections alone, or a combination of physical therapy, gabapentin, and CESIs. All three groups showed significant improvement in arm pain at follow-up. However, the magnitude of improvement was significantly greater for the multimodal group than the physical therapy or epidural-alone groups. The conservative therapy group fared the worst.

Procedure: Cervical Interlaminar Epidural Steroid Injection

The patient is placed in a prone position. The patient is prepped and draped in the usual sterile fashion. A fluoroscopic image is taken in the anteroposterior (AP) direction and a 5- to 10-degree cephalad tilt of the C-arm may be required to open the C7–T1 space. The C7–T1 level is selected because the epidural space is widest and there is a higher chance of an intact ligament, both making a safer injection. The C6–C7 space may be occasionally used, but it is not recommended that the injection be performed above C6 as the cervical enlargement of the spinal cord, thin ligament, and small epidural space increase risk of injury. A pointer is then placed over the superior edge of the lamina of the inferior vertebral level of the target, at the ipsilateral side of the pain complaint for a paramedian approach. (An alternative method is the trajectory view, to follow.) A skin wheal is performed and the area is anesthetized with lidocaine 1%. A Tuohy needle is then inserted coaxial to the radiographic beam and advanced until contacting the lamina. The needle is then walked off the lamina superiorly and advanced into the ligamentum flavum. The stylet is removed, and a loss of resistance (LOR) syringe is then placed on the hub of the needle. At this stage, a contralateral oblique 50-degree C-arm view is recommended to watch needle depth. Continuous light pressure is applied with one hand to the LOR syringe, and the needle is advanced with the other hand. Once LOR is obtained, the LOR syringe is removed. In the contralateral oblique view, the needle tip should be advanced just ventral to the spinolaminar line. When using a paramedian approach, a lateral view is not appropriate, as it will not give an adequate view of needle depth just below the ipsilateral lamina. Iohexol (Omnipaque 240) is injected slowly to confirm proper spread of the contrast medium within the epidural space, also confirming that there is no evidence of intrathecal spread or intravascular runoff. About 3 mL of injectate mix of steroid, and normal saline with or without anesthetic is then performed.[37–39] An alternative method is the trajectory view, in which the needle trajectory is directed toward the interlaminar space without any intent of contacting lamina; a 50-degree contralateral oblique C-arm view is required to watch needle depth, prior to advancing the needle into the epidural space[38] (Fig. 22.1).

Transforaminal epidural steroid injections (TFESIs) and selective nerve root blocks have been promoted as a more targeted modality for treatment or diagnostic purposes. However, there are no randomized, double-blind trials of cervical transforaminal ESIs or comparative studies between transforaminal and interlaminar ESIs. In a review of fluoroscopically guided transforaminal CESIs, Engel et al.[40] reported on six observational studies totaling 357 patients who underwent fluoroscopically guided cervical TFESIs for radicular pain. Of these subjects, 180 (50%) obtained at least a 50% reduction of arm pain. Of the six studies, four had a positive outcome—at least 50% of subjects achieving significant improvement. One of these studies was halted early due to published reports of complications with cervical TFESI.[41] Two of the six studies of cervical TFESIs also reported on progression to surgery. In a study of 70 subjects by Lin in 2006, 44 of the 70 subjects had significant and sustained improvement such that they did not proceed to surgery.[42] However, in a study of 21 subjects with cervical radiculopathy by Kolstad in 2005, only 5 of the 21 had improvement sufficient to prevent progression to surgery.[41]

There have been at least 23 reports of serious complications after cervical TFESI.[36] These have included cerebral injuries with cortical blindness, spinal cord infarcts, vertebral artery occlusion, cerebral and cerebellar infarcts, spinal cord injury, grand mal seizure, and epidural hematomas, among others. There are also reports of adverse events following cervical interlaminar ESIs, but many of these are minor and transient.[32] There have been a small number of direct spinal cord injuries, but in all of these cases, the injections were performed in heavily sedated patients.[32] The use of heavy sedation for spinal injection procedures, especially in the cervical region, is discouraged for this reason.[43] There is growing consensus that transforaminal injections in the cervical region pose a significantly higher risk than interlaminar epidurals and perhaps should be avoided.[2,44]

Cervical selective nerve root blocks have been promoted as a diagnostic test to aid in planning surgical treatment of cervical radiculopathy. However, scant evidence exists for the diagnostic utility of cervical selective nerve root blocks. In a review of the literature on selective nerve root blocks, only one study was found that evaluated cervical injections.[45] In this study, 30 patients with unilateral cervical radiculopathy and more than one level of pathology on magnetic resonance imaging (MRI) underwent diagnostic selective nerve blocks.[46] Correlation between positive selective nerve block and clinical determination of nerve root level from neurologic deficits was only 28%. Correlation with the most severe pathology on MRI was 60%. Given the limited evidence and potential risks, there is little to support the use of cervical diagnostic nerve root blocks for surgical planning.

Procedure: Cervical Transforaminal Epidural Steroid Injection

The patient is placed in a supine position. The appropriate vertebral level is identified under the posteroanterior (PA) view, and the C-arm is tilted until the superior endplate is squared, and the spinous process is midline to the level that is targeted. The fluoroscope is then tilted ipsilaterally to about 45 degrees or until the targeted foramen comes into complete view. A pointer is then placed over the intervertebral foramen at the dorsal and posterior aspect. The skin is anesthetized. A straight short-bevel needle is then advanced toward the target. A PA view is then obtained, and the needle can be advanced, but not past the midline of the lateral mass in order to minimize the potential for dural or spinal cord puncture. Iohexol (Omnipaque 240) is then injected under live fluoroscopy to confirm contrast spread medially around the pedicle, and inferiolaterally along the exiting spinal nerve, without vascular runoff. It has been suggested that use of digital subtraction angiography (DSA) has a greater accuracy in detecting intravascular injection. Lee et al.[47] showed that, of 87 lumbar TFESIs, 20 cases of intravascular injection were detected with DSA. Only 12 of these cases were detected with contrast injection under standard fluoroscopy. In a study of 177 cervical TFESIs in 134 patients, Mclean et al.[48] detected intravascular injection in 18% with real-time fluoroscopy versus 32.8% with DSA. About 1 to 2 mL of injectate mix of dexamethasone and normal saline with or without anesthetic is then performed.[49,50] All other steroids should be avoided due to the risk of neurologic damage. In a rat study of four different steroid preparations (both soluble and nonsoluble), dexamethasone was the only one that did not result in serious neurologic injury after carotid artery injection.[51] The general consensus is that DSA is not required when using dexamethasone. However, DSA should be strongly considered if a particulate steroid is used under special circumstances (Fig. 22.2).

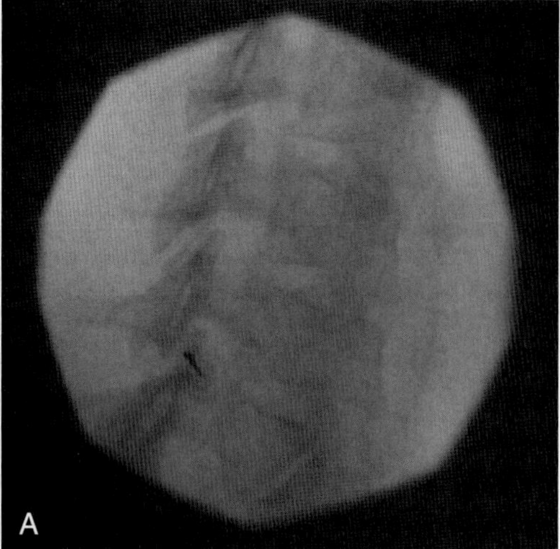

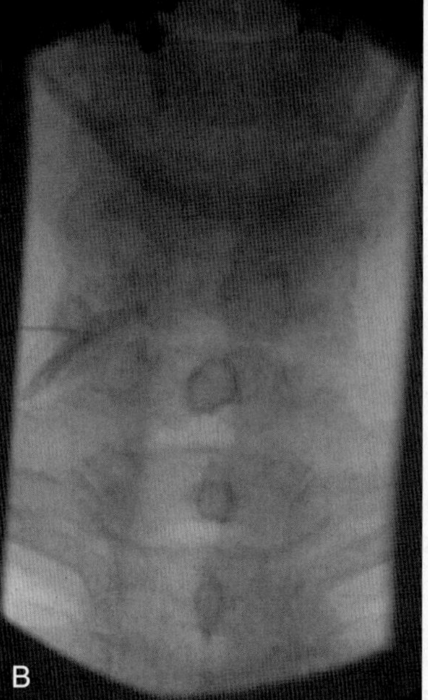

FIG. 22.2 Cervical transforaminal epidural steroid injection. (A) Oblique view of a C6–C7 intervertebral foramen aligned with the needle coaxial to the target point. (B) Posteroanterior view showing the contrast medium filling the foramen, extending peripherally along the ventral ramus, and to the epidural space.

Pain from the cervical facet joints has been reported to account for between 36% and 67% of patients with chronic neck pain.[52,53] Cervical facet-mediated pain is routinely treated with ablation of the medial branch nerves. Unlike in the lumbar region, there is limited literature on the use of intraarticular steroid injections into the cervical facet joints. Only one randomized trial exists that compared intraarticular injection of steroid to local anesthetic.[54] Both groups obtained relief lasting only days, with no difference between groups. Two observational studies of cervical facet intraarticular steroid injections showed short-term benefit.[55,56]

There is one high-quality RCT of cervical medial branch radiofrequency ablation (RFA) after controlled diagnostic blocks.[57] In this small study by Lord, 24 patients were randomized to sham or RFA. The median time to return of pain was 284 days in the treatment group and 8 days in the sham group. Nonrandomized prospective studies have also found both short-term and long-term benefit from cervical RFA of the medial branch nerves, while two larger retrospective studies found no benefit.[52,53]

Procedure: Cervical Medial Branch Blocks and Radiofrequency Ablation

Cervical medial branch blocks (MBB) are typically performed as a diagnostic technique to determine whether the patient's neck pain is secondary to a facet joint pathology and to determine if the patient is a candidate for RFA. Prior to considering MBB and RFA the pain should have been present for at least 3 months, and the patient needs to have not responded to conservative therapy. The goal of the procedure is to inject anesthetic at the paravertebral facet joint nerves or the medial branches.

Each facet joint is supplied by two medial branches of the dorsal rami. In the cervical spine, two levels must be anesthetized for each joint. For example, the C3 and C4 MBB is performed to obtain information about the C3–C4 facet joint, and the C4 and C5 MBB is performed to obtain information regarding the C4–C5 facet joint.

For the diagnostic cervical MBB, the patient is usually placed in a prone position. The patient is prepped and draped in the usual sterile fashion. The skin and soft tissues are anesthetized with lidocaine 1%. At each level from a lateral direction, a 1.25- to 1.5-inch needle—or from a posterior position, a spinal needle—is inserted under frontal, lateral, and oblique fluoroscopic projections with the needle tip advanced to contact the centroid of the lateral articular pillar at each respective level. Aspiration of each needle must be negative for blood, cerebrospinal fluid, or paresthesia prior to injection. The nerve blocks are then performed by injecting bupivacaine 0.5%, 0.25 mL through each needle.

If the patient exhibits greater than 50% improvement of index pain with 0.25 mL of local anesthetic for at least 3 hours, this is considered a positive diagnostic block. The patient may then proceed to a therapeutic procedure, such as RFA.

RFA is performed with the same set-up and targets as the MBB, except the needle tip should be placed parallel to the nerve. The RF lesion is an oval-shaped lesion that is circumferentially around the shaft of the active tip; thus, an ideal position of the tip is parallel to the targeted nerve.[58]

From a posterior approach at each level, a 22-gauge, 100-mm RF cannula needle with a 10-mm active tip is inserted percutaneously to the radiographic target with the needle tip parallel to the periosteum of the lateral articular pillar. Alternatively, from a lateral approach, a 20-gauge, 50-mm RF cannula needle with a 5-mm active tip is inserted percutaneously to the radiographic target at the center of the lateral mass. The RF probes are then placed through the cannula. Needle placement is confirmed radiographically and with neurologic stimulation. Axial sensory perception threshold using 50-Hz sensory stimulation is achieved at 0.5 V or less at each level. Extremity motor stimulation at 2 Hz is negative at a minimum of 1.5 V, or 2 to 3 times the sensory threshold at each level. Motor stimulation is positive for multifidus stimulation. The paravertebral facet joint nerve blockade is performed by injection of lidocaine 2%, 0.5 mL per level prior to treatment. Each nerve is then treated at 80°C in continuous RF mode for 90 seconds. The needle can be rotated and treated again.[57,59,60] Next, paravertebral facet joint nerve blockade is performed by injection of bupivacaine 0.5%, 0.25 mL. If steroid is mixed with the bupivacaine, it is recommended that dexamethasone be used for reasons described earlier under the risk of intraarterial injection of particulate steroid. The deep cervical artery is at risk of penetration and can communicate with the spinal radicular arteries (Fig. 22.3).

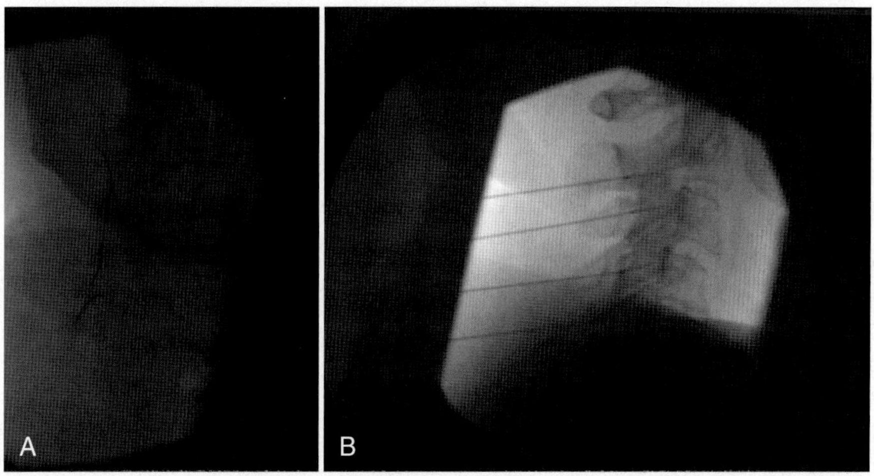

FIG. 22.3 Cervical medial branch block/radiofrequency (RF) ablation. (A) Anteroposterior view showing RF needles placed at the left spine lateral to the articular pillars. (B) Lateral view with the electrodes in the proper position over the left cervical third occipital, third, fourth, and fifth articular pillars.

Lumbar Spine Injections

Lumbar epidural steroid injections have been used for years as a treatment for axial or radicular pain of spinal origin. Lumbar ESIs are often used as an intermediate or conservative treatment measure before considering surgery. In a meta-analysis, Bicket et al. evaluated the effect of lumbar epidural steroid injections for preventing surgery for lumbar radiculopathy.[61] They identified 22 studies of lumbar ESIs that were RCTs and also reported subject progression to surgery. They found that fewer patients in the groups who had received ESIs went on to have surgery in both the short term and long term, but the effect fell short of statistical significance. However, only one of the included studies specifically sought to determine the effect of ESIs on surgery as a primary outcome measure. This study by Riew et al. found that significantly fewer patients who received ESIs (8 out of 28 [28.6%]) compared to epidural bupivacaine alone (18 out of 27 [66.7%]) underwent surgery at 13 to 28 months of follow-up.[62]

Therapeutic epidural steroid injections have been used for the treatment of pain from spinal stenosis, discogenic pain, and lumbar radiculopathy. Radiculopathy from lumbar disc herniation remains the primary indication for ESIs. In a review of fluoroscopically guided lumbar interlaminar ESIs, 5 out of 8 randomized controlled trials showed positive short-term pain relief.[63] In a separate review of 4 randomized trials of transforaminal ESIs for lumbar radiculopathy, all showed positive short-term improvement and 2 of 4 showed longer-term improvement.[64] In his study of 160 patients with unilateral radiculopathy, Karppinen found that, for contained herniations, a transforaminal ESI prevented progression to surgery but provided no relief in herniations with extrusion.[65]

Axial low back and leg pain from lumbar spinal stenosis has also been treated with epidural steroid injections. The use of epidural steroid injections for lumbar stenosis has recently been mired in some controversy. While lumbar decompression is considered the gold standard therapy for lumbar spinal stenosis, not all patients are acceptable surgical candidates. In an RCT that received wide reporting in the lay press, Friedly et al.[66] reported no difference for epidural steroid injections when compared to epidural lidocaine injections at 6 weeks and concluded that ESIs were ineffective for lumbar spinal stenosis. However, this study has been criticized for using relatively low volumes of injectate, inclusion of patients with acute low back pain, and the injection of an active drug, lidocaine, as an inactive control.[67] While the steroid group had significant improvement compared to lidocaine at 3 weeks for both of the primary outcome measures, Roland-Morris Disability Questionnaire (RMDQ) score and leg pain, there was no statistical difference at 6 weeks. However, both the lidocaine and steroid groups had substantial percentages (nearly 50%) of subjects achieving more than 30% relief of leg pain compared to baseline and 38% in both groups reported more than 50% relief of leg pain. In a meta-analysis of epidural steroid injections compared to epidural injections of nonsteroid solutions and injections of solutions outside of the epidural space, Bicket et al.[2] concluded that epidural injections of any solution appear to confer therapeutic benefit and the use of epidural nonsteroid solution injections as a "placebo" control may be misleading. In a systematic review of RCTs of ESIs for lumbar stenosis, Manchikanti[68] concluded that interlaminar and caudal injections of either local anesthetic with steroid or local anesthetic alone provided short- and long-term benefit for back and leg pain.

Procedure: Lumbar Interlaminar Epidural Steroid Injection

For this procedure, the patient is placed in a prone position. The patient is prepped and draped in the usual sterile fashion. A fluoroscopic image is taken in the AP direction and the endplates at the level of planned entry are lined up, most commonly at L5–S1. A pointer is then placed over the superior edge of the lamina of the inferior vertebral level of the target, at the ipsilateral side of the pain for a paramedian approach. (As with a cervical epidural steroid injection, an alternative method for the lumbar epidural steroid injection is the trajectory view, in which the needle trajectory is directly toward the interlaminar space; a 45-degree contralateral oblique C-arm view is required to watch needle depth if the lamina is not going to be contacted prior to advancing the needle into the epidural space). A skin wheal is performed and the area is anesthetized with lidocaine 1%. A Tuohy needle is then inserted coaxial to the radiographic beam and advanced until contacting the lamina. The needle is then walked off the lamina superiorly and advanced anteriorly to the ligamentum flavum. The stylet is removed, and a LOR syringe is then placed on the hub of the needle. Continuous light pressure is applied with one hand to the LOR syringe, and the needle is advanced. At this stage, a contralateral oblique 50-degree C-arm view is recommended to watch needle depth. Once LOR is obtained, the LOR syringe is removed. In the contralateral oblique view, the needle tip should be advanced just ventral to the spinolaminar line. Iohexol (Omnipaque 240) is injected slowly to confirm proper spread of the contrast medium within the epidural space, also confirming that there is no evidence of intrathecal spread or intravascular runoff. When using a paramedian approach, a lateral view is not appropriate, as it will not give an adequate view of needle depth just below the ipsilateral lamina. If using a midline approach, a lateral view is appropriate to monitor needle depth. About 5 mL of injectate mix of steroid and normal saline with or without anesthetic is then performed[38,69,70] (Fig. 22.4).

Procedure: Caudal Epidural Steroid Injection

The patient is placed in a prone position with a pillow under the abdomen, and the legs slightly abducted with internal rotation. The patient is prepped and draped in the usual sterile fashion. The sacral cornu may be palpated to determine the approximation of the sacral hiatus. A pointer is placed over the sacral hiatus at around a 45-degree angle using a lateral fluoroscopic projection to assist in identifying the sacral hiatus. The skin is then anesthetized with lidocaine 1%, and

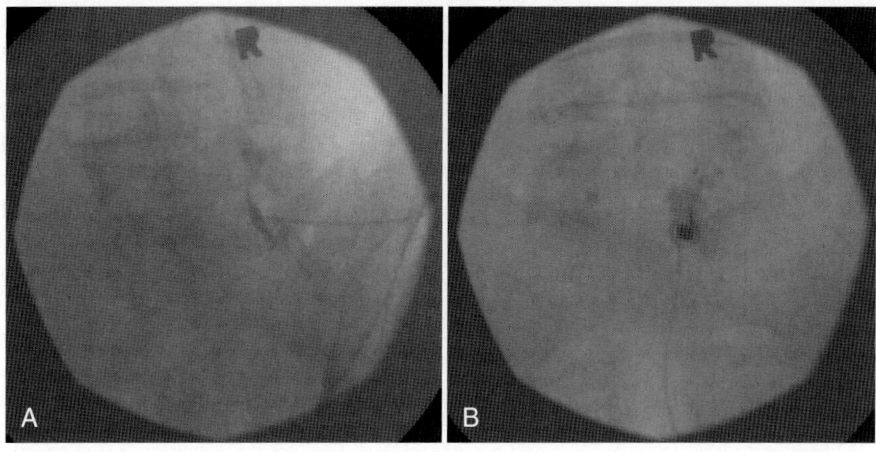

FIG. 22.4 Lumbar epidural steroid injection. (A) Contralateral oblique view showing contrast medium in the lumbar epidural space. (B) Anteroposterior view showing contrast medium highlighting epidural fat with the needle at right L5–S1 level.

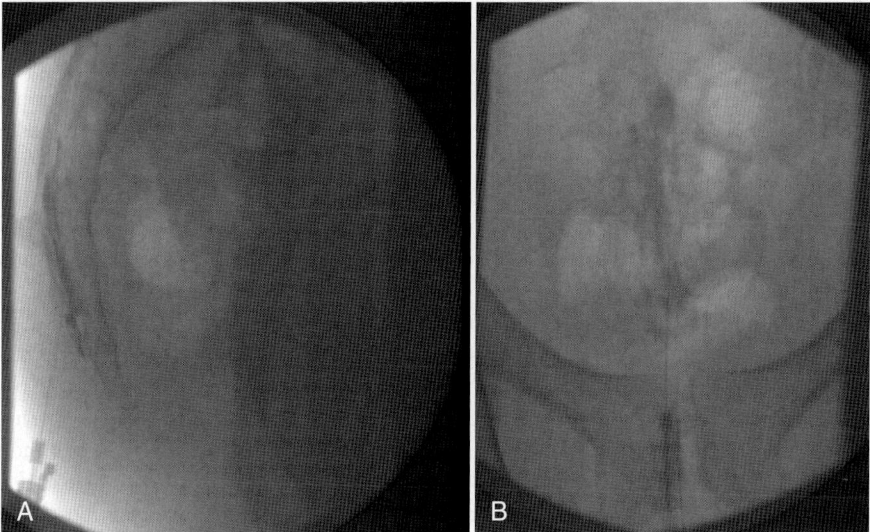

FIG. 22.5 Caudal epidural steroid injection. (A) Lateral view showing a 25-gauge needle in the caudal epidural space with contrast medium flowing superiorly in the epidural space. (B) Anteroposterior view showing contrast medium highlighting caudal epidural fat.

a 27-gauge, 1.25-inch needle, or longer needle if needed, is inserted into position through the sacral hiatus. The needle is advanced midline, and kept inferior to S3 to avoid dural puncture. After negative needle aspiration, contrast is then injected to demonstrate epidural spread in both a lateral and AP projection. Live AP fluoroscopic imaging is then obtained highlighting epidural fat, and cephalad contrast spread without vascular runoff. The usual volume of 5 to 10 mL of injectate mix of steroid and normal saline with or without anesthetic is then performed[71–73] (Fig. 22.5).

The use of diagnostic selective nerve root blocks to identify a particular spinal nerve level in the lumbar region has significantly more evidence than in the cervical region. In his review of these blocks, Datta[45] found moderate evidence for the efficacy of selective nerve blocks as a diagnostic tool in radicular pain. However, there are significant variables that may confound the results of these injections. First, there may be confusion between the interventional pain physician and spine surgeon regarding what type of block is being performed and for what purpose. Some physicians will use the terms *transforaminal* and *selective nerve block* interchangeably. The goal of a truly selective nerve block is to place the needle tip just outside of the foramen and inject a low volume of local anesthetic alone in order to block a single nerve root. Improper placement of the needle tip into the foramen, injection of steroid along with local anesthetic, or use of a larger volume of injectate may negate the diagnostic utility of the injection. In one study, 0.5 mL of local anesthetic and iohexol resulted in epidural spread in 47% of L4 blocks and 28% of L5 blocks.[74] The sensitivity and specificity of nerve root blocks for predicting surgical outcome ranges from 45% to 100% in the various studies. There may be a role for the use of selective nerve blocks when there is clinical evidence of radiculopathy but inconclusive imaging studies. However, surgeons should consider the subjective nature of these blocks as a diagnostic test when evaluating their results.

Procedure: Lumbar Transforaminal Epidural Steroid Injection

There are different approaches for this procedure, including the supraneural (subpedicular) approach and infraneural (retrodiscal) approach. The supraneural approach is the traditional method and most commonly used among pain practitioners, and is described here. All of the risks and precautions described for cervical TFESIs should be considered for lumbar TFESIs.

The patient is placed in a prone position. The appropriate vertebral level is identified, and the fluoroscope is angled cephalocaudad until the superior endplate is squared, and mediolaterally until the spinous process is midline between the pedicles. The C-arm is then tilted ipsilaterally to between 15 and 25 degrees, until the superior articular process projects over the lateral third of the vertebral body. A pointer is then placed under the 6 o'clock position of the pedicle, adjacent to the pars interarticularis. A spinal needle is then advanced coaxial to the fluoroscopic image to the target. A lateral fluoroscopic view is then obtained, and the needle is advanced to the cephalad third of the intervertebral foramen and midway anteriorly into the neural foramen, to potentially avoid vascular structures. At this point, the C-arm is moved to an AP position and the needle position is confirmed to have not passed the midpedicular line to minimize the potential of dural puncture. Iohexol (Omnipaque 240) is then injected under live fluoroscopy. Ideal epidural contrast spread should be medially and cephalad around the pedicle, and inferior along the exiting spinal nerve, without vascular runoff or intrathecal spread. About 1 to 2 mL of an injectate mix of dexamethasone and normal saline with or without preservative-free local anesthetic is then performed.[75,76]

The lumbar TFESI can be performed at the L5–S1 and S1 levels with slight variation. At L5–S1, the iliac crest may obscure the view, and the C-arm may require a larger degree of cephalocaudal tilt.[77] For S1, the C-arm is adjusted to optimize visualization of the dorsal S1 foramen, just inferior to the S1 pedicle, with the target more medial within the foramen. The lateral view is used to confirm needle depth.[78]

The technique for a selective nerve root block is similar to what is described earlier for the TFESI, however, with final needle position more lateral and inferior. As the goal for a selective nerve root block is an anesthetic block to the exiting spinal nerve, ideal contrast spread is inferior along the exiting spinal nerve, without medial epidural spread. To be selective, a nerve root block should be performed extraforaminally, distal to the division of the ventral and dorsal rami and with low volumes of local anesthetic—no more than 0.5 mL[79] (Fig. 22.6).

In the lumbar region, the facet joints have been implicated as a source of axial low back pain in 15% to 45% of patients.[52] Diagnostic physical examination maneuvers and radiographic studies are unreliable in diagnosing facet-mediated pain. The use of controlled diagnostic medial branch nerve blocks is considered the most reliable means of diagnosing pain arising from the facet joints. Additionally, a positive response to two comparative local anesthetic diagnostic blocks significantly increases the likelihood of a robust response to radiofrequency ablation treatments compared to a single diagnostic block.[52] In their review of RFA for lumbar facet pain, Manchekanti et al. evaluated four randomized, sham controlled trials of RFA for lumbar facet mediated pain.[80] Three showed positive results for both short-term (<6 months) and long-term (>6 months) pain relief. Additionally, they found three other randomized, active controlled trials and 10 observational studies with positive results. In one representative study by van Kleef, success was defined as a more than 2-point reduction in visual analogue pain scale and more than 50% reduction in Oswestry Disability Index.[81] Patients were assessed at

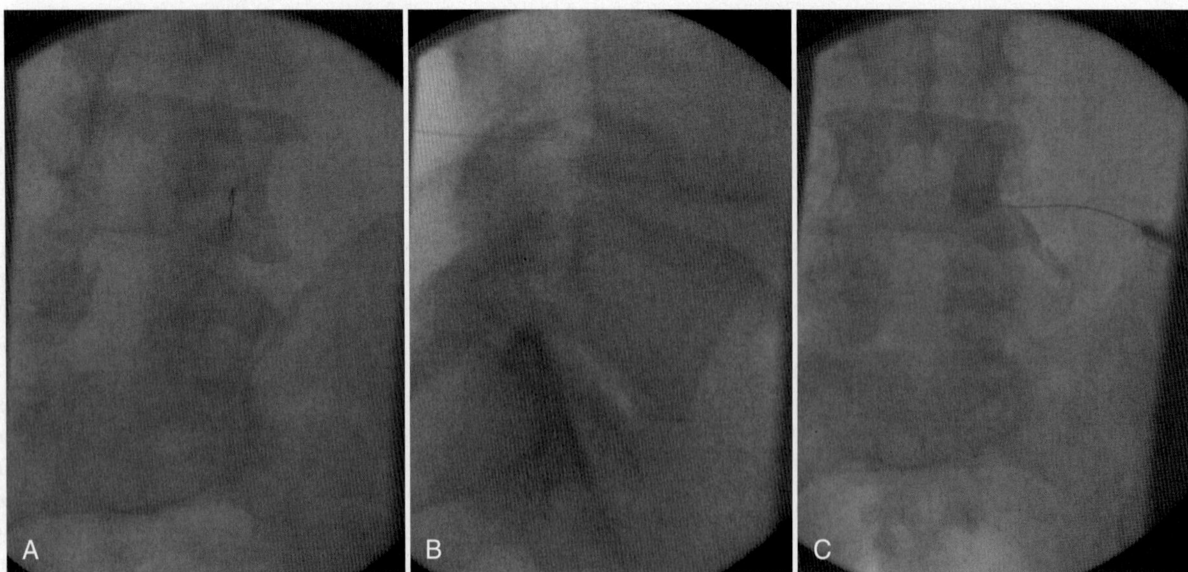

FIG. 22.6 Lumbar transforaminal epidural steroid injection. (A) Oblique radiograph of the spinal needle placed below the L5 pedicle. (B) Lateral radiograph showing the spinal needle in the upper third of the L5–S1 neural foramen. (C) Anteroposterior radiograph showing contrast medium highlighting the exiting nerve root.

2, 3, 6, and 12 months; the treatment group had significantly greater improvement at all time points.

There have been a handful of observational and retrospective studies of intraarticular injection of local anesthetic and steroids.[82] Most of the studies found greater than 50% of patients obtained initial and immediate relief and some short-term but not long-term benefit. There is no well-done, randomized, placebo-controlled trial of intraarticular facet injections.

Procedure: Lumbar Zygapophyseal Joint Injections (Facet Joint)

The patient is placed in a prone position. The patient is prepped and draped in the usual sterile fashion. The C-arm is positioned in the AP direction, and is given a 5- to 15-degree ipsilateral tilt until the facet joint space is identified clearly. The target is the middle to upper half of the joint space at the medial or lateral side of the joint. Osteophytic formation may affect the superior articular process more than the inferior articular process, making the lateral portion of the joint more difficult to enter. The medial border of the joint may be better suited in these cases. Special attention is paid to the L5–S1 facet joint, as the iliac crest can be superimposed, and may require more cephalad tilt. The skin is then anesthetized, and a spinal needle is then inserted and advanced coaxial to the radiographic beam until it enters the joint. At this point, more than one oblique angle, or lateral image, can be checked to confirm the needle tip within the joint space. Injection of iohexol (Omnipaque 240) shows joint space and capsular spread. Due to the small volume of the facet joint, a volume of no more than 1 to 1.5 mL per level of injectate mix of steroid and anesthetic is then performed[83–85] (Fig. 22.7).

Procedure: Lumbar Medial Branch Blocks and Radiofrequency Ablation

Lumbar MBBs are typically performed for two reasons. The first is to obtain diagnostic information as to whether the patient's axial back pain is secondary to facet-mediated pain from lumbar spondylosis. The second reason is to determine if the patient is a candidate for RFA. Prior to considering MBB and RFA, the pain should have been present for at least 3 months, and the patient needs to have not responded to conservative therapy. The goal of the procedure is to inject anesthetic at the paravertebral facet joint nerves or the medial branches.

Each facet joint is supplied by two medial branches of the dorsal rami. In the lumbar spine, two levels must be anesthetized for each joint. At the lowest joint, L5–S1, the L4 medial branch and the L5 dorsal ramus must be blocked. As the most common severe lumbar spondylosis occurs at the L4–L5 and L5–S1 joints, the most common MBB procedures are performed at the L3, L4, and L5 medial branches.

For the diagnostic lumbar MBB, the patient is placed in a prone position. The patient is prepped and draped in the usual sterile fashion. A fluoroscopic image is taken in the AP direction and the endplates at the level of proposed entry are lined up. Next, the fluoroscope is rotated ipsilaterally 10 to 20 degrees until the junction of the superior articular process and transverse process is clearly visible, with the circular projection of the pedicle outlining this junction. The skin and soft tissues are anesthetized with lidocaine 1% at each site.

To block the lumbar medial branch nerves, a spinal needle is inserted percutaneously and advanced under fluoroscopic guidance using dorsal, lateral, and oblique projections to its radiographic target. For each of the lumbar levels, the tip of the needle should be placed at the junction of the superior articular process and the transverse process. The L5 posterior

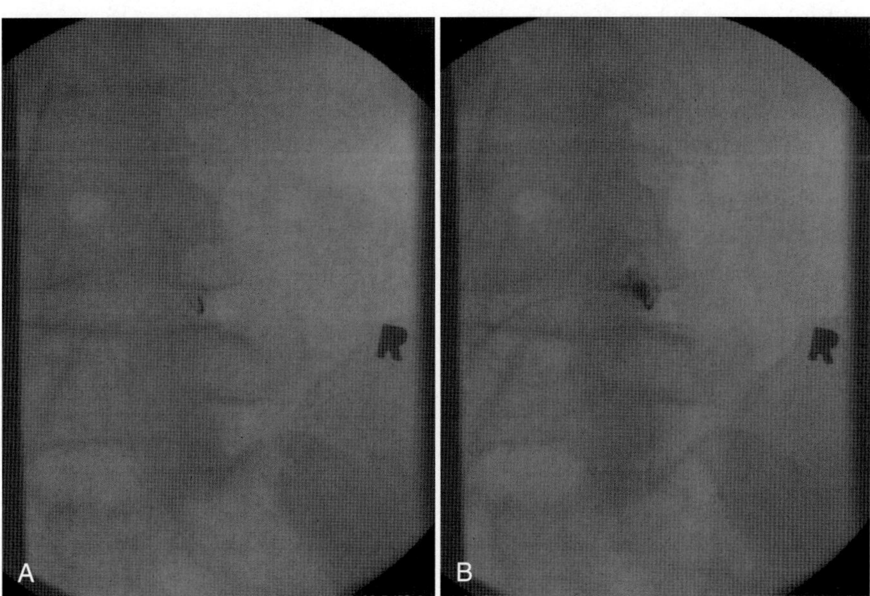

FIG. 22.7 Lumbar facet joint injection. (A) Oblique radiograph with the tip of the spinal needle placed in the right L4–L5 facet joint. (B) Oblique radiograph with contrast spread at the right L4–L5 facet joint.

SECTION III

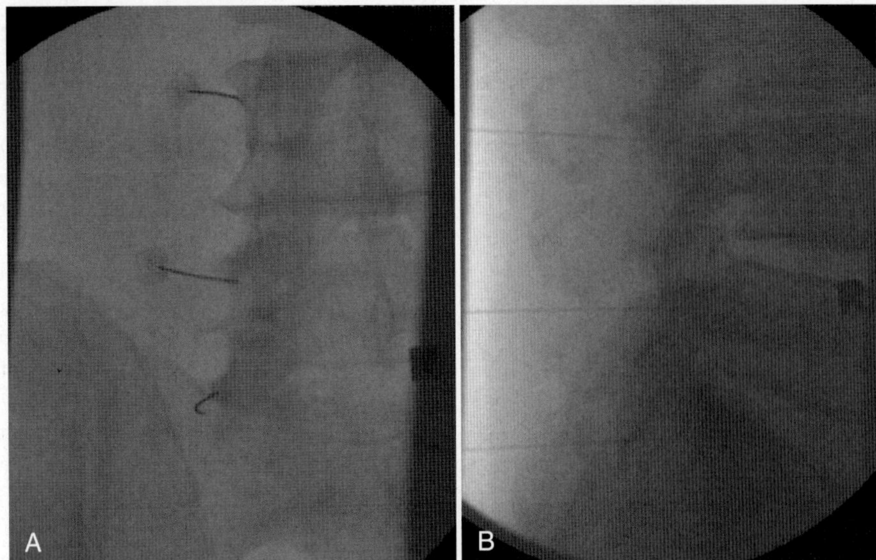

FIG. 22.8 Lumbar medial branch block/radiofrequency ablation. (A) Anteroposterior radiograph showing needles placed at the target of the left L3, L4, and L5 medial branches. (B) Lateral radiograph showing appropriate placement of the needles.

rami are blocked at the junction of the sacral ala just lateral to the articular process. At the sacral levels, the needle is placed at the lateral border of the respective sacral foramen. Next, paravertebral facet joint nerve blockade is performed by injection of bupivacaine 0.5% or lidocaine 2%, 0.5 mL of anesthetic at each level.

A patient exhibiting greater than 50% improvement of axial low back pain with 0.5 mL of local anesthetic for at least 3 hours may be a candidate for RFA. The purpose of RFA of the paravertebral facet joint nerves is to provide prolonged symptomatic pain relief.

For lumbar RFA, the patient is once again placed in the prone position, and prepped and draped in the usual sterile fashion. A fluoroscopic image is taken in the AP direction and the endplates at the level of proposed entry are lined up. The skin and soft tissues are anesthetized with lidocaine 1% at each site.

A 20- or 22-gauge, 10-cm RFA needle is inserted percutaneously and advanced under fluoroscopic guidance using dorsal, lateral, and oblique projections to its radiographic target, as described earlier in the MBB section. The difference in technique is that the needle tip should be placed parallel to the nerve. As described in the cervical section, the RF causes an oval circumferential shaped lesion around the shaft of the active tip; thus, an ideal position of the tip is parallel to the targeted nerve.[58] The RF probes are then placed through the cannula. In addition to fluoroscopic confirmation, neurologic stimulation is undertaken with both motor and sensory testing. Axial sensory perception threshold using 50-Hz sensory stimulation is achieved at 0.5 V or less at each level. Extremity motor stimulation at 2 Hz is shown to be negative at a minimum of 1.5 V, or 2 to 3 times the sensory threshold at each level, and motor stimulation is positive for multifidus stimulation, without movement of the buttock or leg muscles. Paravertebral facet joint nerve blockade is performed by injection of lidocaine 2%, 0.5 mL per level before treatment. After nerve block is achieved, each nerve is then treated at 80°C in continuous RF mode, for 90 seconds. The needle can be rotated and treated again.[86–90] Finally, paravertebral facet joint nerve blockade is performed by injection of bupivacaine 0.5%, 0.5 mL at each level (Fig. 22.8).

The SI joint has long been an acknowledged source of low back pain. Diagnosis of the SI joint as the source of pain remains a challenge as the diagnostic examination maneuvers for SI joint pain lack specificity. Based on a combination of multiple examination maneuvers and diagnostic nerve blocks, the prevalence of SI joint dysfunction in unilateral low back pain has been estimated at 15% to 25%.[91] There are many physical examination tests that have been advocated for diagnosing SI joint pain. Two of the most common are the Patrick's (FABERS) test and Gaenslen's test. Two studies have shown an improvement in specificity to 79% and 85% when three or more examination tests are positive.[92,93] Imaging study findings are poorly correlated with injection-confirmed SI joint pain.[91,94] The International Association for the Study of Pain (IASP) criteria for diagnosing SI joint pain mandates that the pain should be alleviated by the intraarticular injection of local anesthetics.[95] However, even this diagnostic technique has its limits. Intraarticular injection of the SI joint is one of the most challenging spinal injection procedures. There are several factors that may confound the diagnostic utility of an SI joint injection. The SI joint space is small; thus, local anesthetics injected may extravasate and block other anatomic structures such as muscles, ligaments, or lumbosacral nerve roots, resulting in false positives. Failure to get local anesthetic spread within the joint may result in a false negative.[91,94] All of these factors require consideration while attempting to diagnose pain from the SI joint.

Nonsurgical SI joint pain procedural interventions are limited to the injection of steroids and local anesthetics or radiofrequency treatment of the nerves supplying the joint. The injection of steroids and local anesthetics for treatment of SI joint pain has often been assumed to require the intraarticular injection of the medication. However, the periarticular muscular and ligamentous connections are complex, and may also be a source of pain.[96] A retrospective study of 120 patients found that the combination of intraarticular and extraarticular injection provided better pain relief than intraarticular alone.[97] In randomized controlled studies, the periarticular injection of local anesthetic and steroids has provided short-term relief. There have been several studies of intraarticular injection of steroids, most of which have found at least short-term benefit.[91] However, two separate systematic reviews of SI joint pain found that the quality of these studies was too poor to grade the evidence or assessed the evidence to be limited.[96,98] A more recent systematic review of SI joint diagnosis and treatment graded the evidence as moderate.[99]

The treatment of SI joint pain with radiofrequency ablation has limited evidence through mostly observational studies, with pain improvement lasting up to a year.[96,98] In a small randomized, placebo-controlled trial of cooled-radiofrequency (cooled-RF) ablation versus sham ablation, the treatment group had significant relief compared to baseline at 1, 3, and 6 months.[100] Additionally, 11 of those who received the sham treatment crossed over to cooled-RF treatment and exhibited similar pain relief results to the initial treatment group. An additional sham-controlled study of cooled-RF found similar results.[101] Studies for conventional radiofrequency have been more limited and mostly observational, with a couple of randomized studies comparing cooled-RF to conventional RF. In one of those studies, Cheng et al. found that both provided greater than 50% pain relief for 3 to 6 months, with no significant difference between the treatments.[102] Last, there is one study of pulsed-radiofrequency neuromodulation of the lateral branch nerves for SI joint pain. In this study by Vallejo et al., 22 patients with SI joint pain confirmed with diagnostic blocks underwent pulsed-radiofrequency of the L4 medial branch, L5 posterior rami, and S1 and S2 lateral branch nerves; 73% achieved at least 50% pain relief at 6 to 9 weeks.[103] The percentage with significant improvement dropped to 32% at 17 to 32 weeks.

Procedure: Sacroiliac Joint Injection

The patient is placed in a prone position, and prepped and draped in the usual sterile fashion. The C-arm is positioned in the AP direction, and the posterior inferior SI joint is identified. At this point, the practitioner may use a combination of either cephalad versus caudal or ipsilateral versus contralateral oblique to increase the lucency of the target, which is located about 1 to 2 cm superior to the inferior aspect to the joint, at the medial side of the joint. The skin is then anesthetized with lidocaine 1%; a spinal needle is then directly coaxial to target. The needle is then walked into the joint, with a medial to lateral trajectory. Iohexol (Omnipaque 240) is injected to confirm proper spread of the contrast medium within the joint space, also confirming that there is no intravascular runoff. A lateral view should be checked to confirm that needle placement is ventral to the posterior sacrum but is not advanced too far ventrally through the joint into the viscera. No more than 1.5 to 2 mL of injectate mix of steroid and local anesthetic is then performed.[15,98,104] (Fig. 22.9).

Summary

This chapter has discussed the etiology of joint, disc, ligamentous, and nerve root pain and how each contributes to the complexity of the pain experience. In general, evidence for spinal injections is rather limited and high-quality gold standard studies are few. Diagnostic and therapeutic spinal injections must be performed in conjunction with a good history, physical examination, and appropriate diagnostic workup. There are complications with any procedure, and the risks and benefits must be weighed before proceeding. Given reports of serious complications in the cervical spine with spinal cord injury and vascular infarcts, cervical TFESI should be avoided, and cervical interlaminar epidurals performed instead. There is also an increased risk from transforaminal epidural steroid injections in the lumbar spine, but significantly lower than seen in the cervical spine. Therefore, TFESI, lumbar interlaminar epidural steroid injection, and CESI

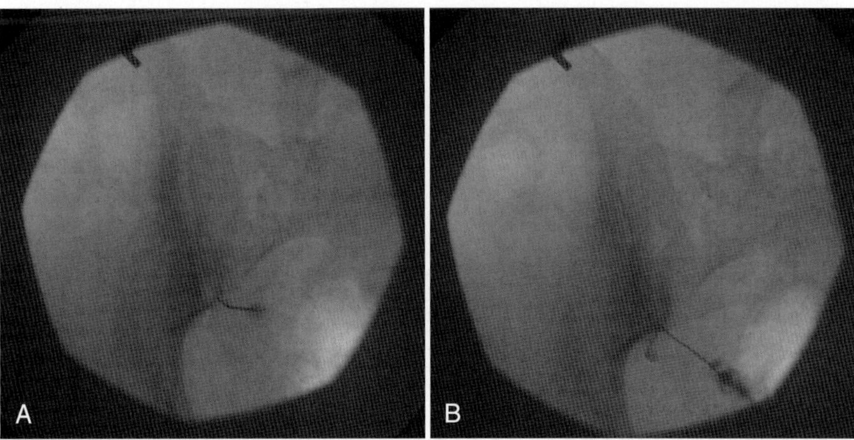

FIG. 22.9 Sacroiliac joint injection. (A) Anteroposterior radiograph showing the left sacroiliac joint. (B) Anteroposterior radiograph showing contrast spread in the left sacroiliac joint with superior and lateral flow, highlighting the joint space.

are routinely performed to help treat radicular symptoms or symptoms of central stenosis. For axial pain, diagnostic medial branch blocks must be performed before treating with RFA. In the lumbar spine, there is also the option of direct zygapophyseal joint or facet joint injections. Finally, the SI joint should also be considered as a common reason for low back pain, and SI joint injections or RFA may be considered.

REFERENCES

1. Tuttle AH, Tohyama S, Ramsay T, et al. Increasing placebo responses over time in U.S. clinical trials of neuropathic pain. *Pain*. 2015;156:2616-2626.
2. Bicket MC, Gupta A, Brown CH 4th, Cohen SP. Epidural injections for spinal pain: a systematic review and meta-analysis evaluating the "control" injections in randomized controlled trials. *Anesthesiology*. 2013;119(4):907-931.
3. Yamashita T, Cavanaugh JM, el-Bohy AA, Getchell TV, King AI. Mechanosensitive afferent units in the lumbar facet joint. *J Bone Joint Surg Am*. 1990;72(6):865-870.
4. Edgar MA, Ghadially JA. Innervation of the lumbar spine. *Clin Orthop Relat Res*. 1976;115:35-41.
5. Ashton IK, Ashton BA, Gibson SJ, et al. Morphological basis for back pain: the demonstration of nerve fibers and neuropeptides in the lumbar facet joint capsule but not in ligamentum flavum. *J Orthop Res*. 1992;10(1):72-78.
6. Beaman DN, Graziano GP, Glover RA, Wojtys EM, Chang V. Substance P innervation of lumbar spine facet joints. *Spine*. 1993;18(8):1044-1049.
7. Giles LG. Pathoanatomic studies and clinical significance of lumbosacral zygapophyseal (facet) joints. *J Manipulative Physiol Ther*. 1992;15(1):36-40.
8. Videman T, Nurminen M, Troup JD. Lumbar spinal pathology in cadaveric material in relation to history of back pain, occupation, and physical loading. *Spine*. 1990;15(8):728-740.
9. Kim JS, Ali MH, Wydra F, et al. Characterization of degenerative human facet joints and facet joint capsular tissues. *Osteoarthritis Cartilage*. 2014;23(12):2242-2251.
10. Bogduk N. The innervation of the lumbar spine. *Spine*. 1983;8(3):286-293.
11. Ikeda R. Innervation of the sacroiliac joint. Macroscopical and histological studies. *Nihon Ika Daigaku Zasshi*. 1991;58(5):587-596.
12. Grob KR, Neuhuber WL, Kissling RO. Innervation of the sacroiliac joint of the human. *Z Rheumatol*. 1995;54(2):117-122.
13. Fortin JD, Dwyer AP, West S, Pier J. Sacroiliac joint: pain referral maps upon applying a new injection/arthrography technique. Part I: asymptomatic volunteers. *Spine*. 1994;19(13):1475-1482.
14. Fortin JD, Aprill CN, Ponthieux B, Pier J. Sacroiliac joint: pain referral maps upon applying a new injection/arthrography technique. Part II: clinical evaluation. *Spine*. 1994;19(13):1483-1489.
15. Schwarzer AC, Aprill CN, Bogduk N. The sacroiliac joint in chronic low back pain. *Spine*. 1995;20(1):31-37.
16. Dreyfuss P, Dryer S, Griffin J, Hoffman J, Walsh N. Positive sacroiliac screening tests in asymptomatic adults. *Spine*. 1994;19(10):1138-1143.
17. Potter NA, Rothstein JM. Intertester reliability for selected clinical tests of the sacroiliac joint. *Phys Ther*. 1985;65(11):1671-1675.
18. Esses SI, et al. The diskography dilemma. *APS J*. 1994;3(3): 155-156.
19. Aprill C, Bogduk N. High-intensity zone: a diagnostic sign of painful lumbar disc on magnetic resonance imaging. *Br J Radiol*. 1992;65(773):361-369.
20. Guyer RD, Ohnmeiss DD. Lumbar discography. Position statement from the North American Spine Society Diagnostic and Therapeutic Committee. *Spine*. 1995;20(18): 2048-2059.
21. Bogduk N, Windsor M, Inglis A. The innervation of the cervical intervertebral discs. *Spine*. 1988;13(1):2-8.
22. Coppes MH, Marani E, Thomeer RT, Groen GJ. Innervation of "painful" lumbar discs. *Spine*. 1997;22(20):2342-2350.
23. Weinstein J, Claverie W, Gibson S. The pain of discography. *Spine*. 1988;13(12):1344-1348.
24. Freemont AJ, Peacock TE, Goupille P, et al. Nerve ingrowth into diseased intervertebral disc in chronic back pain. *Lancet*. 1997;350(9072):178-181.
25. Feinstein B, Langton JN, Jameson RM, Schiller F. Experiments on pain referred from deep somatic tissues. *J Bone Joint Surg Am*. 1954;36-A:981-997.
26. Loeser J, Bigos S, Fordyce W. Low back pain. In: Bonica J, ed. *The Management of Pain*. Philadelphia: Lea & Febiger; 1990:1448-1483.
27. Grönblad M, Weinstein JN, Santavirta S. Immunohistochemical observations on spinal tissue innervation. A review of hypothetical mechanisms of back pain. *Acta Orthop Scand*. 1991;62(6):614-622.
28. Pionchon H, Tommasi M, Pialat J, et al. Study of the innervation of the spinal ligaments at the lumbar level. *Bull Assoc Anat*. 1986;70(210):63-67.
29. Rhalmi S, Yahia LH, Newman N, Isler M. Immunohistochemical study of nerves in lumbar spine ligaments. *Spine*. 1993;18(2):264-267.
30. Haughton VM, Nguyen CM, Ho KC. The etiology of focal spinal arachnoiditis. An experimental study. *Spine*. 1993;18(9):1193-1198.
31. Scanlon GC, Moeller-Bertram T, Romanowsky SM, Wallace MS. Cervical transforaminal epidural steroid injections: more dangerous than we think? *Spine*. 2007;32(11): 1249-1256.
32. Stout A. Epidural steroid injections for cervical radiculopathy. *Phys Med Rehabil Clin N Am*. 2011;22(1):149-159.
33. Abbasi A, Malhotra G, Malanga G, Elovic EP, Kahn S. Complications of interlaminar cervical epidural steroid injections: a review of the literature. *Spine*. 2007;32: 2144-2151.
34. Manchikanti L, Nampiaparampil DE, Candido KD, et al. Do cervical epidural injections provide long-term relief in neck and upper extremity pain? A systematic review. *Pain Physician*. 2015;18(1):39-60.
35. Diwan S, Manchikanti L, Benyamin RM, et al. Effectiveness of cervical epidural injections in the management of chronic neck and upper extremity pain. *Pain Physician*. 2012;15(4):E405-E434.
36. Cohen SP, Hayek S, Semenov Y, et al. Epidural steroid injections, conservative treatment, or combination treatment for cervical radicular pain: a multicenter, randomized, comparative-effectiveness study. *Anesthesiology*. 2014;121(5):1045-1055.
37. Lieberman R, Dreyfuss P, Baker R, et al. Fluoroscopically guided interlaminar cervical epidural injections. *Arch Phys Med Rehabil*. 2003;84(10):1568-1569.

38. Furman M, Jasper NR, Lin HW. Fluoroscopic contralateral oblique view in interlaminar interventions: a technical note. *Pain Med (United States)*. 2012;13(11):1389-1396.
39. Landers MH, Dreyfuss P, Bogduk N. On the geometry of fluoroscopy views for cervical interlaminar epidural injections. *Pain Med*. 2012;13(1):58-65.
40. Engel A, King W, Macvicar J. The effectiveness and risks of fluoroscopically guided cervical transforaminal injections of steroids: a systematic review with comprehensive analysis of the published data. *Pain Med (United States)*. 2014;15(3):386-402.
41. Kolstad F, Leivseth G, Nygaard OP. Transforaminal steroid injections in the treatment of cervical radiculopathy. A prospective outcome study. *Acta Neurochir (Wien)*. 2005;147(10):1065-1070.
42. Lin EL, Lieu V, Halevi L, Shamie AN, Wang JC. Cervical epidural steroid injections for symptomatic disc herniations. *J Spinal Disord Tech*. 2006;19(3):183-186.
43. Hodges SD, Castleberg RL, Miller T, Ward R, Thornburg C. Cervical epidural steroid injection with intrinsic spinal cord damage. Two case reports. *Spine*. 1998;23(19):2137-2142.
44. Manchikanti L, Falco FJE, Diwan S, Hirsch JA, Smith HS. Cervical radicular pain: the role of interlaminar and transforaminal epidural injections. *Curr Pain Headache Rep*. 2014;18(1).
45. Datta S, Everett CR, Trescot AM, et al. An updated systematic review of the diagnostic utility of selective nerve root blocks. *Pain Physician*. 2007;10(1):113-128.
46. Anderberg L, Annertz M, Rydholm U, Brandt L, Säveland H. Selective diagnostic nerve root block for the evaluation of radicular pain in the multilevel degenerated cervical spine. *Eur Spine J*. 2006;15(6):794-801.
47. Lee MH, Yang KS, Kim YH, et al. Accuracy of live fluoroscopy to detect intravascular injection during lumbar transforaminal epidural injections. *Korean J Pain*. 2010;23(1):18-23.
48. McLean JP, Sigler JD, Plastaras CT, Garvan CW, Rittenberg JD. The rate of detection of intravascular injection in cervical transforaminal epidural steroid injections with and without digital subtraction angiography. *PM R*. 2009;1(7):636-642.
49. Dreyfuss P, Baker R, Bogduk N. Comparative effectiveness of cervical transforaminal injections with particulate and nonparticulate corticosteroid preparations for cervical radicular pain. *Pain Med*. 2006;7(3):237-242.
50. Windsor RE, Storm S, Sugar R, Nagula D. Cervical transforaminal injection: review of the literature, complications, and a suggested technique. *Pain Physician*. 2003;6(4):457-465.
51. Dawley JD, Moeller-Bertram T, Wallace MS, Patel PM. Intra-arterial injection in the rat brain: evaluation of steroids used for transforaminal epidurals. *Spine*. 2009;34(16):1638-1643.
52. Boswell MV, Trescot AM, Datta S, et al. Interventional techniques: evidence-based practice guidelines in the management of chronic spinal pain. *Pain Physician*. 2007;10(1):7-111.
53. Falco FJ, Erhart S, Wargo BW, et al. Systematic review of diagnostic utility and therapeutic effectiveness of cervical facet joint interventions. *Pain Physician*. 2009;12(2): 323-344.
54. Barnsley L, Lord SM, Wallis BJ, Bogduk N. Lack of effect of intraarticular corticosteroids for chronic pain in the cervical zygapophyseal joints. *N Engl J Med*. 1994;330(15):1047-1050.
55. Kim KH, Choi SH, Kim TK, et al. Cervical facet joint injections in the neck and shoulder pain. *J Korean Med Sci*. 2005;20(4):659-662.
56. Folman Y, Livshitz A, Shabat S, Gepstein R. Relief of chronic cervical pain after selective blockade of zygapophyseal joint. *Harefuah*. 2004;143(5):339-341, 391.
57. Lord SM, Barnsley L, Wallis BJ, McDonald GJ, Bogduk N. Percutaneous radio-frequency neurotomy for chronic cervical zygapophyseal-joint pain. *N Engl J Med*. 1996;335(23):1721-1726.
58. Bogduk N, Macintosh J, Marsland A. Technical limitations to the efficacy of radiofrequency neurotomy for spinal pain. *Neurosurgery*. 1987;20(4):529-535.
59. Manchikanti L, Singh V, Falco FJE, Cash KA, Fellows B. Comparative outcomes of a 2-year follow-up of cervical medial branch blocks in management of chronic neck pain: a randomized, double-blind controlled trial. *Pain Physician*. 2010;13(5):437-450.
60. Barnsley L, Bogduk N. Medial branch blocks are specific for the diagnosis of cervical zygapophyseal joint pain. *Reg Anesth*. 1993;18(6):343-350.
61. Bicket MC, Horowitz JM, Benzon HT, Cohen SP. Epidural injections in prevention of surgery for spinal pain: systematic review and meta-analysis of randomized controlled trials. *Spine J*. 2015;15(2):348-362.
62. Riew KD, Yin Y, Gilula L, et al. The effect of nerve-root injections on the need for operative treatment of lumbar radicular pain. A prospective, randomized, controlled, double-blind study. *J Bone Joint Surg Am*. 2000;82-A(11):1589-1593.
63. Benyamin RM, Manchikanti L, Parr AT, et al. The effectiveness of lumbar interlaminar epidural injections in managing chronic low back and lower extremity pain. *Pain Physician*. 2012;15(4):E363-E404.
64. Buenaventura RM, Datta S, Abdi S, Smith HS. Systematic review of therapeutic lumbar transforaminal epidural steroid injections. *Pain Physician*. 2009;12(1):233-251.
65. Karppinen J, Malmivaara A, Kurunlahti M, et al. Periradicular infiltration for sciatica: a randomized controlled trial.[see comment]. *Spine*. 2001;26(9):1059-1067.
66. Friedly JL, Comstock BA, Turner JA, et al. A randomized trial of epidural glucocorticoid injections for spinal stenosis. *N Engl J Med*. 2014;371(1):11-21.
67. Manchikanti L, Candido KD, Kaye AD, et al. Randomized trial of epidural injections for spinal stenosis published in the *New England Journal of Medicine:* further confusion without clarification. *Pain Physician*. 2014;17(4):E475-E487.
68. Manchikanti L, Kaye AD, Manchikanti K, et al. Efficacy of epidural injections in the treatment of lumbar central spinal stenosis: a systematic review. *Anesthesiol Pain Med*. 2015;5(1):e23139.
69. Parr AT, Diwan S, Abdi S. Lumbar interlaminar epidural injections in managing chronic low back and lower extremity pain: a systematic review. *Pain Physician*. 2009;12(1): 163-188.
70. Davidoff S, Furman M. Lumbar interlaminar epidural steroid injection, paramedian approach. In: Furman M, Lee T, Berkwits L, eds. *Atlas of Image-Guided Spinal Procedures*. Elsevier; 2013:111-117.
71. Botwin K, Brown LA, Fishman M, Rao S. Fluoroscopically guided caudal epidural steroid injections in degenerative lumbar spine stenosis. *Pain Physician*. 2007;10(4): 547-558.

72. Manchikanti L, Cash KA, Pampati V, McManus CD, Damron KS. Evaluation of fluoroscopically guided caudal epidural injections. *Pain Physician.* 2004;7(1):81-92.
73. Willis R. Caudal epidural blockade. In: Cousins M, Bridenbaugh P, eds. *Neural Blockade in Clinical Anesthesia and Management of Pain.* 2nd ed. Lippincott; 1988:361-383.
74. Wolff AP, Groen GJ, Wilder-Smith OHG, et al. Do diagnostic segmental nerve root blocks in chronic low back pain patients with radiation to the leg lack distinct sensory effects? A preliminary study. *Br J Anaesth.* 2006;96(2):253-258.
75. Botwin K, Natalicchio J, Brown LA. Epidurography contrast patterns with fluoroscopic guided lumbar transforaminal epidural injections: a prospective evaluation. *Pain Physician.* 2004;7(2):211-215.
76. Furman MB, Lee TS, Mehta A, Simon JI, Cano WG. Contrast flow selectivity during transforaminal lumbosacral epidural steroid injections. *Pain Physician.* 2008;11(6):855-861.
77. Ra IH, Min WK. Optimal angle of needle insertion for fluoroscopy-guided transforaminal epidural injection of L5. *Pain Pract.* 2014;15(5):393-399.
78. Stone J, Berkwitz L, Furman MB, Berkwits L, Furman MB. S1 transforaminal epidural steroid injection. In: Furman M, Lee T, Berkwits L, eds. *Atlas of Image-Guided Spinal Procedures.* Elsevier; 2013:87-92.
79. Gajraj NM. Selective nerve root blocks for low back pain and radiculopathy. *Reg Anesth Pain Med.* 2004;29(3):243-256.
80. Manchikanti L, Abdi S, Atluri S, et al. An update of comprehensive evidence-based guidelines for interventional techniques in chronic spinal pain. Part II: guidance and recommendations. *Pain Physician.* 2013;16(2 suppl):S49-S283.
81. van Kleef M, Barendse GA, Kessels A, et al. Randomized trial of radiofrequency lumbar facet denervation for chronic low back pain. *Spine.* 1999;24(18):1937-1942.
82. Boswell MV, Colson JD, Sehgal N, Dunbar EE, Epter R. A systematic review of therapeutic facet joint interventions in chronic spinal pain. *Pain Physician.* 2007;10(1):229-253.
83. Revel ME, Listrat VM, Chevalier XJ, et al. Facet joint block for low back pain: identifying predictors of a good response. *Arch Phys Med Rehabil.* 1992;73(9):824-828.
84. Dreyfuss P, Dreyer S, Vaccaro A. Lumbar zygapophysial (facet) joint injections. *Spine J.* 2003;3(3 suppl):S50-59.
85. Moran R, O'Connell D, Walsh MG. The diagnostic value of facet joint injections. *Spine.* 1988;13(12):1407-1410.
86. Cohen SP, Raja SN. Pathogenesis, diagnosis, and treatment of lumbar zygapophysial (facet) joint pain. *Anesthesiology.* 2007;106(3):591-614.
87. Cohen SP, Stojanovic MP, Crooks M, et al. Lumbar zygapophysial (facet) joint radiofrequency denervation success as a function of pain relief during diagnostic medial branch blocks: a multicenter analysis. *Spine J.* 2008;8(3):498-504.
88. Dreyfuss P, Halbrook B, Pauza K, et al. Efficacy and validity of radiofrequency neurotomy for chronic lumbar zygapophysial joint pain. *Spine.* 2000;25(10):1270-1277.
89. Gofeld M, Faclier G. Radiofrequency denervation of the lumbar zygapophysial joints: targeting the best practice. *Pain Med.* 2008;9(2):204-211.
90. Nath S, Nath CA, Pettersson K. Percutaneous lumbar zygapophysial (facet) joint neurotomy using radiofrequency current, in the management of chronic low back pain: a randomized double-blind trial. *Spine.* 2008;33(12):1291-1298.
91. Cohen SP. Sacroiliac joint pain: a comprehensive review of anatomy, diagnosis and treatment. *Anesth Analg.* 2005;101(5):1440-1453.
92. Laslett M, Aprill CN, McDonald B, Young SB. Diagnosis of sacroiliac joint pain: validity of individual provocation tests and composites of tests. *Man Ther.* 2005;10(3):207-218.
93. Van Der Wurff P, Buijs EJ, Groen GJ. A multitest regimen of pain provocation tests as an aid to reduce unnecessary minimally invasive sacroiliac joint procedures. *Arch Phys Med Rehabil.* 2006;87(1):10-14.
94. Vanelderen P, Szadek K, Cohen SP, et al. Sacroiliac joint pain. *Pain Pract.* 2010;10(5):470-478.
95. Merskey H, Bogduk N, eds. *Classification of Chronic Pain: Descriptions of Chronic Pain Syndromes and Definitions of Pain Terms.* 2nd ed. Seattle, WA: IASP Press; 1994. http://www.iasp-pain.org/files/Content/ContentFolders/Publications2/FreeBooks/Classification-of-Chronic-Pain.pdf.
96. Rupert MP, Lee M, Manchikanti L, Datta S, Cohen SP. Evaluation of sacroiliac joint interventions: a systematic appraisal of the literature. *Pain Physician.* 2009;12(2):399-418.
97. Borowsky CD, Fagen G. Sources of sacroiliac region pain: insights gained from a study comparing standard intra-articular injection with a technique combining intra- and peri-articular injection. *Arch Phys Med Rehabil.* 2008;89(11):2048-2056.
98. Hansen HC, McKenzie-Brown AM, Cohen SP, et al. Sacroiliac joint interventions: a systematic review. *Pain Physician.* 2007;10(1):165-184.
99. Kennedy DJ, Engel A, Kreiner DS, Nampiaparampil D. Fluoroscopically guided diagnostic and therapeutic intra-articular sacroiliac joint injections: a systematic review. *Pain Med.* 2015;16(8):1500-1518.
100. Cohen SP, Hurley RW, Buckenmaier CC, et al. Randomized placebo-controlled study evaluating lateral branch radiofrequency denervation for sacroiliac joint pain. *Anesthesiology.* 2008;109(2):279-288.
101. Patel N, Gross A, Brown L, Gekht G. A randomized, placebo-controlled study to assess the efficacy of lateral branch neurotomy for chronic sacroiliac joint pain. *Pain Med.* 2012;13(3):383-398.
102. Cheng J, Pope JE, Dalton JE, Cheng O, Bensitel A. Comparative outcomes of cooled versus traditional radiofrequency ablation of the lateral branches for sacroiliac joint pain. *Clin J Pain.* 2013;29(2):132-137.
103. Vallejo R, Benyamin RM, Kramer J, Stanton G, Joseph NJ. Pulsed radiofrequency denervation for the treatment of sacroiliac joint syndrome. *Pain Med.* 2006;7(5):429-434.
104. Fortin JD, Washington WJ, Falco FJE. Three pathways between the sacroiliac joint and neural structures. *AJNR Am J Neuroradiol.* 1999;20(8):1429-1434.

SECTION III

CHAPTER 23 Sacroiliac Joint Pain: Pathophysiology and Diagnosis

Alexandra Schwartz
Vinko Zlomislic
W. Carlton Reckling*
Daniel Cher*

Introduction

Low back pain remains a significant burden on the health care system, representing a source of approximately 12 million physician office visits per year in the United States. It is among the leading causes of disability, accounting for expenditures in excess of $80 billion every year.[1–3] Surgical management of low back pain is known to result in variable success rates, suggesting that the etiology of back pain is complex, often multifactorial, and frequently not clearly known or that treatments provided (or their execution) inadequately address pain generators.

Sacroiliac joint (SIJ) pain is a difficult problem with marked impact on quality of life[4] that is becoming increasingly recognized for its contribution to low back pain. In certain circumstances, SIJ pain may present as an isolated condition. However, in many scenarios, the SIJ represents one of many factors contributing to axial back pain and its various referral patterns. Studies have shown that sacroiliac pathology may either present in association with, or contribute directly to, the etiology of back pain in 15% to 30% of cases.[5–9] The SIJ is often overlooked as a contributing source of back pain. Maintaining an index of suspicion—and a thorough understanding of the relevant anatomy, biomechanics, and clinical presentation involved in SIJ-mediated pain—are required for accurate diagnosis. This chapter presents a comprehensive review of SIJ pathology and diagnostic algorithms as well as current surgical and nonsurgical treatment options and techniques.

Background

Successful management of low back pain requires recognition and appropriate management of the pain source. Studies have shown that the cause of low back pain may not only have variable lumbar origins but may also be a manifestation of hip or SIJ etiology. In a review of over 1200 cases, 44% of individuals presenting with low back pain had findings consistent with lesser-recognized diagnoses such as SIJ and posterior facet syndromes.[6] An additional 33% of patients in their cohort had concordant SIJ symptoms in addition to lumbar stenosis or spondylolisthesis. Further work has shown that of patients presenting to spine clinics for back pain, only 65% have a singular pain generator localized to the spine and 15% to 30% have pain that involves the SIJ to some degree.[5–9]

Adjacent-segment degeneration in instrumented lumbar or lumbosacral fusion is well documented. Not surprisingly, adjacent-segment degeneration of the SIJ also occurs. In a prospective cohort, the rate of radiographic findings consistent with SIJ degeneration was nearly double in patients who had undergone posterior spinal fusion compared to age-matched nonfusion controls followed over a 5-year period.[10] Finite element analysis simulating the effects of lumbar fusion has demonstrated increased forces transmitted across the SIJ that could precipitate degeneration[11]; angular motion and stress were increased along the articular surface following a lumbosacral fusion. A three-level lumbar fusion may result in up to 30% incidence of SIJ degeneration over about 4 years.[12]

Anatomy

The SIJ is the largest axial joint in the human body, with an average surface area of approximately 17.5 cm^2.[13–15] Appreciation of the complex anatomy is critical to making a diagnosis of SIJ dysfunction. As first described in 1864, the SIJ is characterized as a true synovial joint[16] despite the fact that over 70% of its surface area is comprised of capsular and ligamentous structures. A thick layer of hyaline cartilage covers the sacral side of the SIJ. The thinner covering of the iliac surface, though commonly described as fibrocartilage, contains chondrocytes with type II collagen, making this surface a variant of hyaline cartilage.[17] These surface differences may increase the likelihood of SIJ degeneration.[18]

The SIJ undergoes significant morphologic changes throughout life. Development is complete by early adulthood, with formation of an auricular or C-shaped articular joint

*Dr. Reckling and Dr. Cher are employees of SI-Bone, a medical device company.

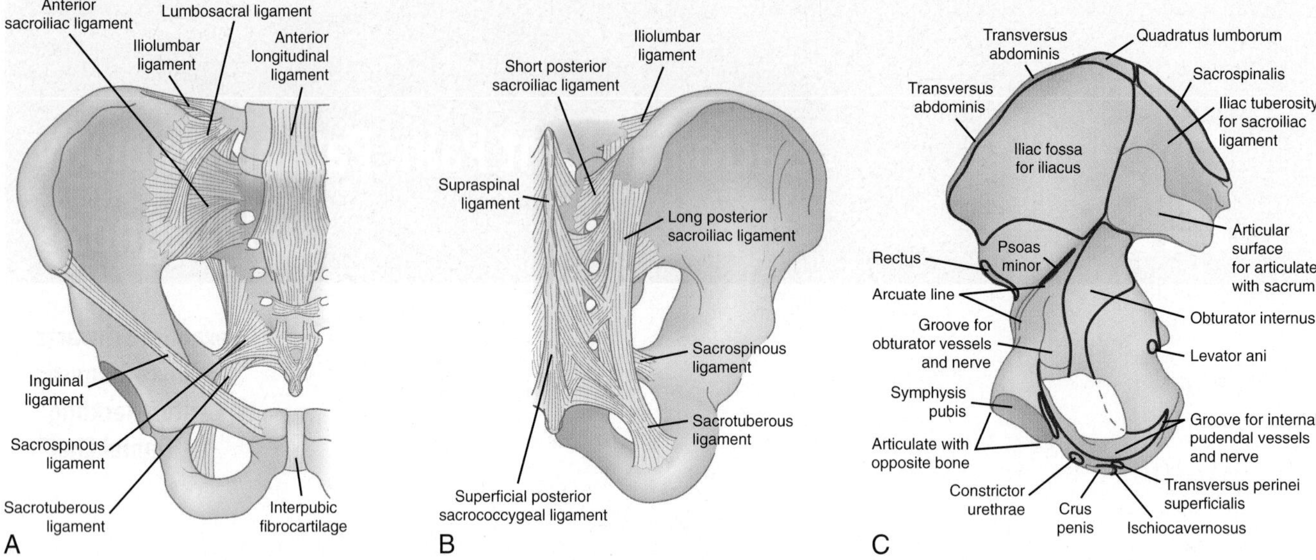

FIG. 23.1 Anatomy of the sacroiliac joint. (A) Anterior ligamentous and capsular structures. (B) Posterior ligamentous and capsular structures. (C) En face view of ilium depicting auricular nature of sacral articulation.

whose final anatomic orientation varies substantially across individuals (Fig. 23.1). Degenerative changes are common over the course of adulthood and have a predilection for the iliac side of the joint first, followed by sacral involvement. It should be stressed, however, that nonspecific degeneration is common, with more than two-thirds of asymptomatic older adults showing radiographic changes consistent with SIJ degeneration.[19]

The SIJ capsule is primarily located in the anterior third of the joint and has a distinct synovial membrane, lined by a thin capsule and overlying ligament that are confluent with the iliolumbar ligament. There is no synovial membrane posteriorly. The interosseous ligament and the dorsal ligaments, which function as a tension band, form a functional dorsal capsule of the SIJ. The sacrospinous and sacrotuberous ligaments contribute to this dorsal capsule (see Fig. 23.1). Additional stabilization is provided by the dynamic function of the gluteus maximus and gluteus medius, erector spinae, biceps femoris, psoas, and piriformis muscles, as well as the lumbodorsal fascia.[14] These structures allow indirect transfer of regional muscle forces to the SIJ and, in many cases, have expansions that invest with the posterior sacroiliac ligament structures. The structural integrity of the capsular and ligamentous structures is at least partly gender specific, with hormonally induced increased laxity in females, allowing for additional necessary motion during parturition.[20–22]

The sacrum is considered the keystone of the pelvis. It is the most caudal component of the vertebral column and provides the transition from the spinal axis to the pelvis. It is critical in the transfer of load from the lower extremities and pelvis to the lumbar spine. The SIJ is six times stronger in lateral compression than the lumbar spine, but fails at one-twentieth the axial load and one-half the shear force.[23] A common misconception is that the SIJ is static. However, current research has shown an average of 2 to 4 degrees of motion in the sagittal plane and smaller amounts of motion in the other planes.[24–26] The primary joint motion is nutation, which refers to a rocking forward of the sacrum relative to the ilium, and counternutation (rocking backward). With nutation of the sacrum, there is concurrent lateral translation of the ilium. Interestingly, the degree of SIJ motion does not correlate with the presence of SIJ pain.[20]

In a series of lectures from 1860 through 1862, John Hilton observed that a nerve that both crosses a joint and innervates the muscles crossing and acting on a joint also innervates the joint.[27] The complexity and ambiguity of SIJ innervation is in part based on Hilton's law. Various macroscopic, histologic, and immunohistochemical studies have demonstrated that the SIJ is highly innervated, with multiple nociceptors and mechanoreceptors present.[28] The synovium and capsule contain unmyelinated nerve endings for pain and temperature. The nerve supply to the posterior joint originates from either L4 to S3 root dorsal rami branches or independent contributions from the L3 and S4 nerve roots.[29,30] The anterior joint similarly has significant variability, with innervation supplied by the ventral rami from L2 to S2 roots.[13] Additional animal studies have evaluated the various pain thresholds of the nociceptive fields involving innervations of the lumbar facet articulations, SIJs, and lumbar disc. Pain sensitivity measured as mechanical threshold was 70 g for the SIJ, which was significantly greater than the lumbar facet (6 g), and less than the lumbar disc (241 g).[31,32]

Relevant surrounding neurologic anatomy consists of the L5 ventral ramus and lumbosacral plexus, which cross the cephalad portion of the SIJ approximately 2 cm distal to the pelvic brim.[33] The L5 root then courses along the anterior aspect of the sacral ala. The S1 ventral ramus crosses the SIJ more caudally, near the inferior aspect of the joint.

Pathology

SIJ dysfunction, a term commonly used to describe pain and disability related to poor functioning of the SIJ, has multiple

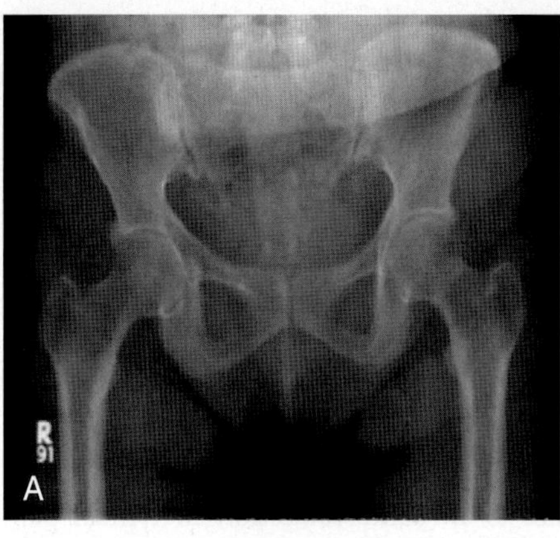

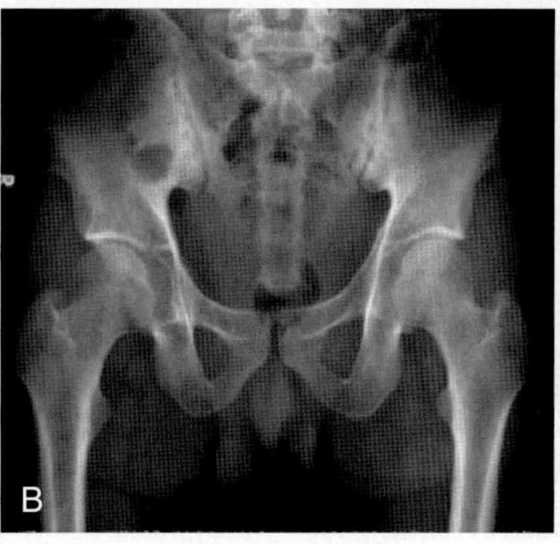

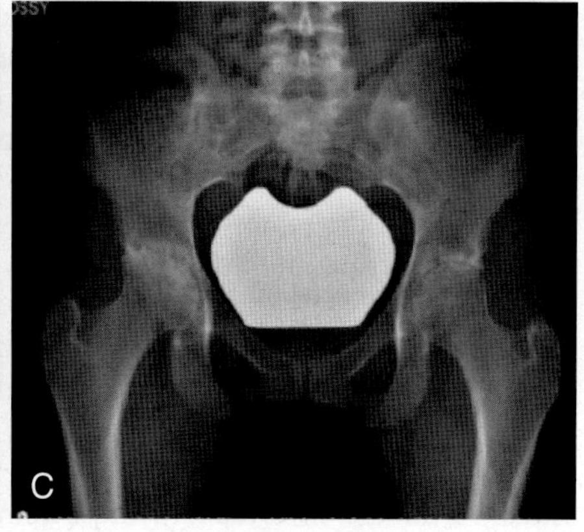

FIG. 23.2 (A) Degenerative changes within the sacroiliac joint (SIJ) with dense sclerosis and osteophytes. (B) Inflammatory changes in the SIJ with bilateral erosive sacroiliitis. (C) Complete fusion of the SIJ.

etiologies. SIJ dysfunction may result from capsular or synovial disruption, ligamentous tension, altered joint mobility and stress, microfracture, or disruption in the myofascial kinetic chain. Pathology may be categorized as either intra- or extraarticular. Common causes of intraarticular pathology include infection, inflammation, and degenerative or inflammatory arthritis. The most common infectious organisms include *Staphylococcus*, *Pseudomonas*, *Cryptococcus*, and *Mycobacterium* and should be suspected in intravenous drug use, endocarditis, or posttraumatic situations.[14] Degenerative changes occur over the course of decades and are related to repeated microtrauma, ultimately presenting as a progression of joint sclerosis on imaging studies (Fig. 23.2). Far more rarely, unilateral or bilateral sacroiliitis can be an early symptom in the seronegative and HLA-B27–associated spondyloarthropathies, occurring in individuals diagnosed with ankylosing spondylitis. There is a strong male predilection for the inflammatory spondyloarthropathies and the association with HLA-B27 supports an immune-mediated etiology that is characterized by more erosive changes on radiographs (see Fig. 23.2). These cases must be identified and distinguished from degenerative changes so that they can be referred for the appropriate nonsurgical management.[34]

Extraarticular pathology, often posttraumatic, may be attributable to ligamentous injury, myofascial pain, and fractures. The underlying causes are myriad, including leg-length discrepancy, gait abnormalities, prolonged exercise, athletic injuries, and prolonged lifting and bending.[13] In a retrospective study of 54 patients with injection-confirmed SIJ pain, trauma was the cause in 44% of cases, 35% were idiopathic, and 21% were due to repeated stress.[35] The most common traumatic events were categorized as motor vehicle accidents followed by falls. In young adults, major trauma resulting in SIJ disruption is most common, with lateral compression injuries more likely to result in later development of SIJ dysfunction.[36] Cumulative microtrauma from overzealous activity and repetitive loading, microfracture, and ligamentous or capsular injuries may also commonly cause insidious onset of SIJ pain.

Additional common causes of SIJ pathology may arise from iatrogenic injury due to overaggressive iliac crest graft harvest that inadvertently violates the SIJ or damages the iliolumbar ligament.[37] Increasingly recognized in females, hormonal changes during the final trimester of pregnancy may induce hypermobility of the SIJ that predisposes it and surrounding ligaments to additional injury, resulting in chronic pain and instability. There is evidence that a prior history of lumbar fusion contributes to biomechanical and anatomic alteration of the SIJ.[10,11] Metabolic diseases such as calcium pyrophosphate crystal deposition disease, gout, hyperparathyroidism, and renal osteodystrophy may potentiate early inflammation and degeneration.[14] Although primary sacroiliac tumors are rare, bony metastasis to the pelvis ranks second only behind spinal metastasis and must be ruled out.

Diagnosis

Although often perceived as challenging, diagnosis of the SIJ as a pain generator is possible through a combination of history, physical examination, and diagnostic SIJ block. The importance of the clinical examination may be a "paradigm shift" for surgeons who rely primarily on imaging for orthopedic diagnoses, as imaging plays little role in the diagnosis of SIJ pain. Because SIJ pain referral patterns vary and can overlap with those of other pathologic conditions, the SIJ should be kept in mind when evaluating patients with chronic low back, buttocks, and hip pain.

Clinical History

Patients with SIJ complaints may present with a constellation of variable, and sometimes inconsistent, pain complaints in the lumbosacral region. Pain is usually off-center below L5 in the area of the posterior superior iliac spine (PSIS), with radiation into the buttocks, or, less commonly, into the groin. Pain in the legs above the knee is relatively common; pain below the knee is less commonly reported. Patients with SIJ dysfunction commonly point to an area just medial to and inferior to the PSIS (the insertion of the long dorsal ligament), which is deemed a positive Fortin finger test.[38]

Patients frequently report pseudoradicular pain, numbness, tingling, and weakness in the distribution of the L5 and S1 nerve roots. However, physical examination typically demonstrates no true neurologic deficit. SIJ arthrography has shown a high proportion of patients with anatomic connections along the dorsum of the SIJ underneath the ligaments between the SIJ and the S1 neuroforamen or S1 nerve root.[39] Likewise, an anatomic connection is frequently demonstrated between the anterior SIJ capsule and the L5 nerve root/lumbar plexus. Finally, the same segmental spinal nerves innervate a variety of structures in the low back, pelvis, and proximal legs, and potentially can cause pain referral patterns from these structures due to convergent sensory pathways. Together, these anatomic findings may explain pseudoradicular pain in patients with SIJ dysfunction.

Typical complaints include pain with activities that preferentially load the involved SIJ, most commonly sitting for prolonged periods, rolling over in bed, sleeping on the affected side, passing over road bumps while driving, or getting in and out of a car or chair. Activities that offload the affected SIJ typically lessen SIJ pain. In prospective studies of patients undergoing surgical intervention, subjects reported the common occurrence of radiating leg pain, groin pain, pain worse with sitting (especially on the affected side), rising, walking, and climbing stairs. Pain occurs during the stance phase of gait. However, no specific aspect of the patient history is considered diagnostic of SIJ pain.

Physical Examination

Physical examination of the SIJ focuses on provocative maneuvers (Table 23.1) that stress the SIJ. A maneuver is considered positive if the test reproduces the patient's pain. Interrater reliability of physical examination maneuvers is high for most tests.[40] No single test is perfectly correlated with results from diagnostic SIJ block (considered the reference standard); however, meta-analysis has shown that the occurrence of three or more positive physical examination tests has a high predictive value for a positive diagnostic SIJ block.[41] Another test, used more commonly in Europe, is the active straight-leg raise test. In this test, the supine patient is asked to rate the difficulty of actively raising the leg 20 cm off the examining table. This test is commonly positive in women with peripartum pelvic pain attributed to the SIJ.[42] In one study of minimally invasive SIJ fusion (SIJF), the active straight-leg raise test improved in patients undergoing fusion but remained at baseline levels in patients undergoing nonsurgical treatment.[43]

Role of Imaging

Imaging is considered an important part of diagnosis of autoimmune sacroiliitis, being part of the New York Criteria for this condition.[44] Whether MRI is best for detecting early autoimmune disease is still being debated.[45] However, in the more common setting of suspected SIJ dysfunction due to osteoarthritis or joint disruption, imaging—including plain radiography and scintigraphic scans—has not been found to be useful.[46] Signs of osteoarthritis degeneration (sclerosis, osteophytes, vacuum phenomenon, subchondral cysts) on CT scan are common in patients without suspected SIJ pain.[19] While findings suggestive of osteoarthritis have been reported as somewhat more common in patients with suspected SIJ pain than an age-matched cohort, sensitivity and specificity of CT findings were low.[47] In summary, no finding on radiography or CT scan has been shown to be diagnostic of SIJ pain. Imaging, especially plain radiographs and cross-sectional imaging, is therefore primarily used during diagnosis to rule out inflammatory SIJ arthropathy or other hip or spine conditions.

Diagnostic Injection

As in most pain conditions, there is no gold standard for diagnosis of SIJ pain. The accepted reference standard for diagnosis of SIJ pain is an acute reduction in typical pain in response to a fluoroscopically or CT-guided diagnostic intraarticular joint injection with a combination of radiographic contrast and local anesthetic, that is, an SIJ block (Fig. 23.3). Several aspects of SIJ block remain to be optimized: Are one or two blocks required? Which anesthetic should be used? Should nonresponse to a control injection (e.g., saline) be required? What threshold for acute decrease in pain is most appropriate? While steroids are commonly used in combination with local anesthetic, does subacute response to steroids aid in diagnosis? Despite these questions, it is well accepted that blind SIJ injections are unacceptable; SIJ injections must be performed under imaging guidance in order to confirm intraarticular entry and spread in the anterior and lower two-thirds of the SIJ.[15] Extravasation outside the joint suggests the potential for nonspecific responses, though this has not been proven. Injection volumes are typically about 1 to 2 mL; larger volumes may promote leakage and nonspecificity. Even with image guidance, various studies have demonstrated a significant number of false-positive and false-negative results,[48] though one study suggests that SIJ block is more accurate than previously reported.[49] False-positives may result from placebo effect, extravasation of local anesthetic to surrounding structures, or convergence of pain referral patterns. Conversely, false-negative results may be attributed to failure of local anesthetic to reach symptomatic regions of the SIJ, particularly the most anterior and cephalad areas or in the presence of extraarticular pain sources. In the absence of a gold standard for diagnosis, all such injection studies remain of questionable validity.

Extraarticular SIJ blocks, which focus on anesthetizing lateral branches of sacral nerve roots, are often used to screen for SIJ-mediated pain potentially responsive to radiofrequency ablation. In one study, extraarticular blocks at multiple depths were able to mask pain due to probing the interosseous and posterior sacroiliac ligaments but not pain elicited by distending the joint itself.[50] The study suggests not only dual innervation of the SIJ complex but also the probability of extraarticular pain generators.

Summary

SIJ pain is a common but often overlooked cause of low back pain. Diagnosis is based on a combination of history, physical examination tests that stress the SIJ and reproduce typical pain,

TABLE 23.1 Physical Examination Tests for Sacroiliac Joint Pain

Test	Description	Example
Distraction	The patient lies supine and is asked to place the forearm behind the lumbar spine to support the natural lordosis. A pillow is placed under the patient's knees. The examiner places his or her hands on the anterior and medial aspects of both of the patient's anterior superior iliac spines (ASISs) with arms crossed. A slow and steady increasing pressure is placed through the arms and held.	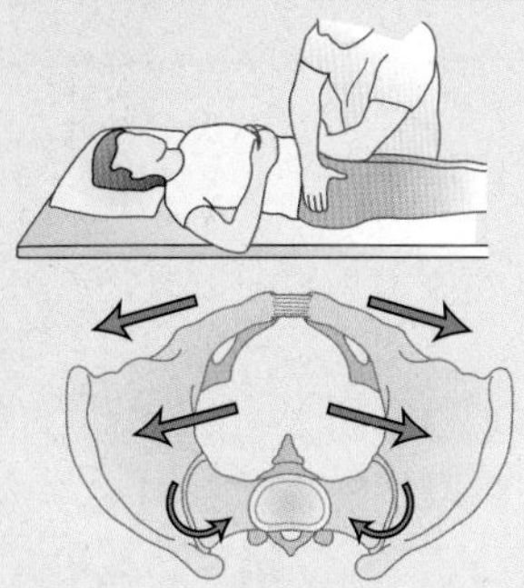
Compression	The patient is placed in a side-lying position, facing away from the examiner, with a pillow between the knees. The examiner places a downward pressure through the lateral aspect of the patient's top-side ASIS and pelvis, anterior to the greater trochanter.	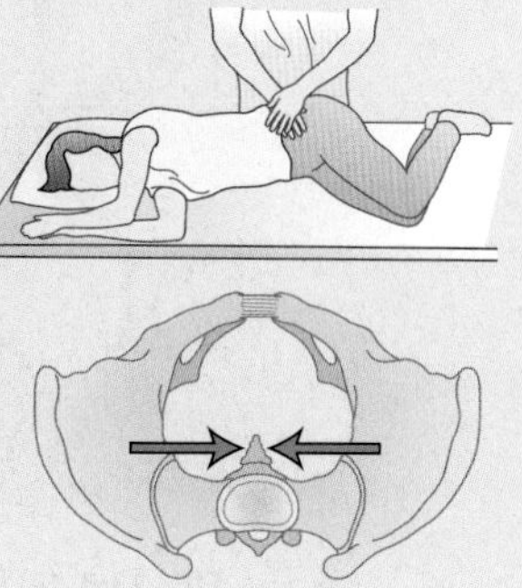
FABER (Patrick test)	The patient lies supine as the examiner crosses the same-side foot over the opposite-side thigh. A force is steadily increased through the knee of the patient, exaggerating the motion of hip *f*lexion, *ab*duction, and *e*xternal *r*otation (FABER). The pelvis is stabilized at the opposite ASIS with the hand of the examiner.	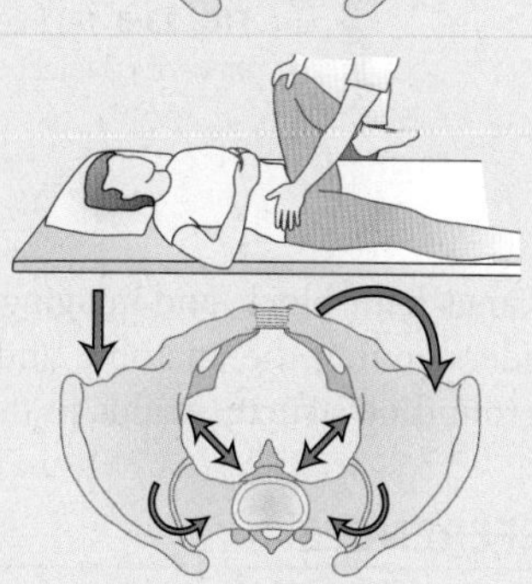
Thigh thrust	The patient lies supine, with one hip flexed to 90 degrees. The examiner stands on the same side as the flexed leg. The examiner provides either a quick thrust or a steady increasing pressure through the line of the femur. The pelvis is stabilized at the opposite ASIS with the hand of the examiner.	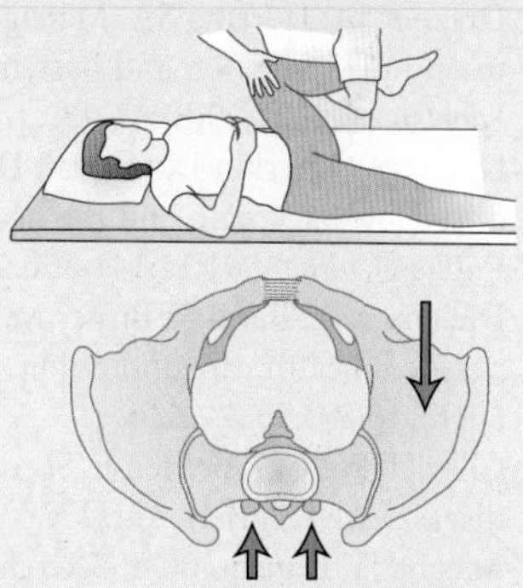
Gaenslen's	The patient lies supine with the near-side leg hanging off the table. The patient is asked to hold the opposite-side knee into flexion. The examiner applies an extension force to the near-side thigh and a flexion force to the opposite knee. The patient assists with opposite-side hip flexion. This is performed bilaterally.	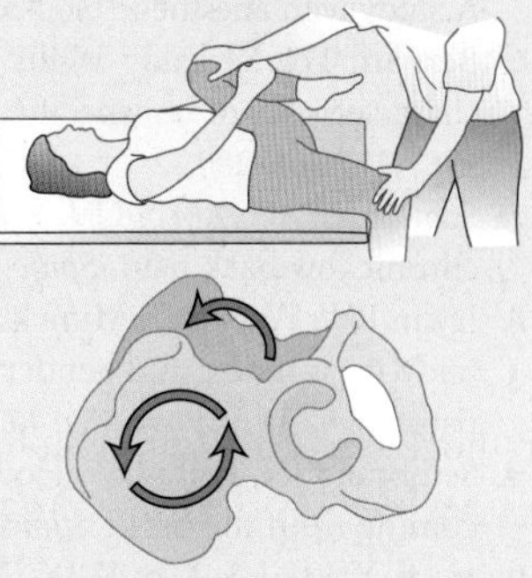

A combination of three positive tests has a high predictive value for a positive sacroiliac joint block.

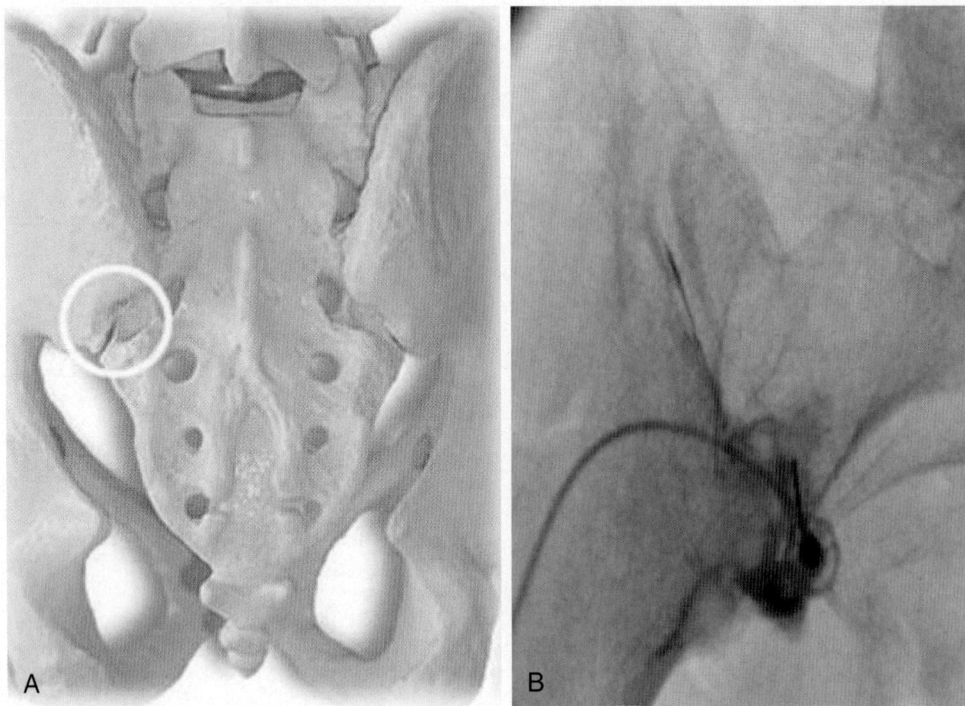

FIG. 23.3 (A) Inferior pole of sacroiliac joint (SIJ), entry point for an intraarticular SIJ injection. (B) Fluoroscopic view of SIJ injection with contrast in joint.

SIJ anesthetic block, and imaging to rule out other conditions. Understanding the anatomy and function of the SIJ and its surrounding structures aids in the diagnosis of the condition.

REFERENCES

1. Drezner JA, Herring SA. Managing low-back pain: steps to optimize function and hasten return to activity. *Phys Sportsmed.* 2001;29(8):37-43.
2. Deyo RA, Cherkin D, Conrad D, Volinn E. Cost, controversy, crisis: low back pain and the health of the public. *Annu Rev Public Health.* 1991;12:141-156.
3. Dieleman JL, Baral R, Birger M, et al. US spending on personal health care and public health, 1996-2013. *JAMA.* 2016;316(24):2627-2646.
4. Cher D, Polly D, Berven S. Sacroiliac joint pain: burden of disease. *Med Devices Auckl NZ.* 2014;7:73-81.
5. Maigne JY, Planchon CA. Sacroiliac joint pain after lumbar fusion. A study with anesthetic blocks. *Eur Spine J.* 2005;14(7):654-658.
6. Bernard TN, Kirkaldy-Willis WH. Recognizing specific characteristics of nonspecific low back pain. *Clin Orthop.* 1987;217:266-280.
7. Schwarzer AC, Aprill CN, Bogduk N. The sacroiliac joint in chronic low back pain. *Spine.* 1995;20(1):31-37.
8. Irwin RW, Watson T, Minick RP, Ambrosius WT. Age, body mass index, and gender differences in sacroiliac joint pathology. *Am J Phys Med Rehabil.* 2007;86(1):37-44.
9. Sembrano JN, Polly DW. How often is low back pain not coming from the back? *Spine.* 2009;34(1):E27-E32.
10. Ha K-Y, Lee J-S, Kim K-W. Degeneration of sacroiliac joint after instrumented lumbar or lumbosacral fusion: a prospective cohort study over five-year follow-up. *Spine.* 2008;33(11):1192-1198.
11. Ivanov AA, Kiapour A, Ebraheim NA, Goel V. Lumbar fusion leads to increases in angular motion and stress across sacroiliac joint: a finite element study. *Spine.* 2009;34(5):E162-E169.
12. Unoki E, Abe E, Murai H, Kobayashi T, Abe T. Fusion of multiple segments can increase the incidence of sacroiliac joint pain after lumbar or lumbosacral fusion. *Spine.* 2016;41(12):999-1005.
13. Cohen SP. Sacroiliac joint pain: a comprehensive review of anatomy, diagnosis, and treatment. *Anesth Analg.* 2005;101(5):1440-1453.
14. Dreyfuss P, Dreyer SJ, Cole A, Mayo K. Sacroiliac joint pain. *J Am Acad Orthop Surg.* 2004;12(4):255-265.
15. Rana SH, Farjoodi P, Haloman S, et al. Anatomic evaluation of the sacroiliac joint: a radiographic study with implications for procedures. *Pain Physician.* 2015;18(6):583-592.
16. Vanelderen P, Szadek K, Cohen SP, et al. Sacroiliac joint pain. *Pain Pract.* 2010;10(5):470-478.
17. Vleeming A, Schuenke MD, Masi AT, et al. The sacroiliac joint: an overview of its anatomy, function and potential clinical implications. *J Anat.* 2012;221(6):537-567.
18. Bowen V, Cassidy JD. Macroscopic and microscopic anatomy of the sacroiliac joint from embryonic life until the eighth decade. *Spine.* 1981;6(6):620-628.
19. Eno J-J, Boone C, Bellino M, Bishop J. The prevalence of sacroiliac joint degeneration in asymptomatic adults. *J Bone Joint Surg Am.* 2015;97(11):932-936.
20. Kibsgård TJ, Røise O, Sturesson B, Röhrl SM, Stuge B. Radiostereometric analysis of movement in the sacroiliac joint during a single-leg stance in patients with long-lasting pelvic girdle pain. *Clin Biomech (Bristol, Avon).* 2014;29(4):406-411.
21. Sturesson B, Uden A, Vleeming A. A radiostereometric analysis of the movements of the sacroiliac joints in the reciprocal straddle position. *Spine.* 2000;25(2):214-217.

22. Sturesson B, Uden A, Vleeming A. A radiostereometric analysis of movements of the sacroiliac joints during the standing hip flexion test. *Spine*. 2000;25(3):364-368.
23. Miller JA, Schultz AB, Andersson GB. Load-displacement behavior of sacroiliac joints. *J Orthop Res Off Publ Orthop Res Soc*. 1987;5(1):92-101.
24. Weisl H. The movements of the sacroiliac joint. *Acta Anat (Basel)*. 1955;23(1):80-91.
25. Sturesson B, Selvik G, Uden A. Movements of the sacroiliac joints. A roentgenstereophotogrammetric analysis. *Acta Orthop Scand Suppl*. 1988;59(suppl 227):89.
26. Vleeming A, van Wingerden JP, Dijkstra PF, et al. Mobility in the sacroiliac joints in the elderly: a kinematic and radiologic study. *Clin Biomech (Bristol, Avon)*. 1992;7(1):170-176.
27. Hilton J. The classic: on rest and pain: lecture XIV. *Clin Orthop*. 2009;467(9):2208-2214.
28. Vilensky JA, O'Connor BL, Fortin JD, et al. Histologic analysis of neural elements in the human sacroiliac joint. *Spine*. 2002;27(11):1202-1207.
29. Bernard TN Jr, Cassidy JD. The sacroiliac joint syndrome: pathophysiology, diagnosis, and management. In: Frymoyer JW, ed. *The Adult Spine: Principles and Practice*. 2nd ed. Philadelphia: Lippincott-Raven; 1997:2343-2366.
30. Murata Y, Takahashi K, Yamagata M, et al. Sensory innervation of the sacroiliac joint in rats. *Spine*. 2000;25(16):2015-2019.
31. Yamashita T, Minaki Y, Oota I, Yokogushi K, Ishii S. Mechanosensitive afferent units in the lumbar intervertebral disc and adjacent muscle. *Spine*. 1993;18(15):2252-2256.
32. Minaki Y, Yamashita T, Ishii S. An electrophysiological study on the mechanoreceptors in the lumbar spine and adjacent tissues. *Neurol Orthop*. 1996;20:23-35.
33. Ebraheim NA, Lu J, Biyani A, Huntoon M, Yeasting RA. The relationship of lumbosacral plexus to the sacrum and the sacroiliac joint. *Am J Orthop (Belle Mead NJ)*. 1997;26(2):105-110.
34. O'Shea FD, Boyle E, Salonen DC, et al. Inflammatory and degenerative sacroiliac joint disease in a primary back pain cohort. *Arthritis Care Res*. 2010;62(4):447-454.
35. Chou LH, Slipman CW, Bhagia SM, et al. Inciting events initiating injection-proven sacroiliac joint syndrome. *Pain Med (Malden Mass)*. 2004;5(1):26-32.
36. Pohlemann T, Tscherne H, Baumgärtel F, et al. [Pelvic fractures: epidemiology, therapy and long-term outcome. Overview of the multicenter study of the Pelvis Study Group]. *Unfallchirurg*. 1996;99(3):160-167.
37. Ebraheim NA, Ramineni SK, Alla SR, Ebraheim M. Sacroiliac joint fusion with fibular bone graft in patients with failed percutaneous iliosacral screw fixation. *J Trauma*. 2010;69(5):1226-1229.
38. Fortin JD, Falco FJ. The Fortin finger test: an indicator of sacroiliac pain. *Am J Orthop (Belle Mead NJ)*. 1997;26(7):477-480.
39. Fortin JD, Washington WJ, Falco FJ. Three pathways between the sacroiliac joint and neural structures. *AJNR Am J Neuroradiol*. 1999;20(8):1429-1434.
40. Laslett M, Williams M. The reliability of selected pain provocation tests for sacroiliac joint pathology. *Spine*. 1994;19(11):1243-1249.
41. Szadek KM, van der Wurff P, van Tulder MW, Zuurmond WW, Perez RSGM. Diagnostic validity of criteria for sacroiliac joint pain: a systematic review. *J Pain*. 2009;10(4):354-368.
42. Mens JMA, Huis in 't Veld YH, Pool-Goudzwaard A. The active straight leg raise test in lumbopelvic pain during pregnancy. *Man Ther*. 2012;17(4):364-368.
43. Sturesson B, Kools D, Pflugmacher R, et al. Six-month outcomes from a randomized controlled trial of minimally invasive SI joint fusion with triangular titanium implants vs. conservative management. *Eur Spine J*. 2017;26(3):708-719.
44. van der Linden S, Valkenburg HA, Cats A. Evaluation of diagnostic criteria for ankylosing spondylitis. A proposal for modification of the New York criteria. *Arthritis Rheum*. 1984;27(4):361-368.
45. Weber U, Jurik AG, Lambert RGW, Maksymowych WP. Imaging in spondyloarthritis: controversies in recognition of early disease. *Curr Rheumatol Rep*. 2016;18(9):58.
46. Slipman CW, Sterenfeld EB, Chou LH, Herzog R, Vresilovic E. The value of radionuclide imaging in the diagnosis of sacroiliac joint syndrome. *Spine*. 1996;21(19):2251-2254.
47. Elgafy H, Semaan HB, Ebraheim NA, Coombs RJ. Computed tomography findings in patients with sacroiliac pain. *Clin Orthop*. 2001;382:112-118.
48. Simopoulos TT, Manchikanti L, Singh V, et al. A systematic evaluation of prevalence and diagnostic accuracy of sacroiliac joint interventions. *Pain Physician*. 2012;15(3):E305-E344.
49. Mitchell B, MacPhail T, Vivian D, Verrills P, Barnard A. Diagnostic sacroiliac joint injections: is a control block necessary? *Surg Sci*. 2015;06(07):273.
50. Dreyfuss P, Henning T, Malladi N, Goldstein B, Bogduk N. The ability of multi-site, multi-depth sacral lateral branch blocks to anesthetize the sacroiliac joint complex. *Pain Med*. 2009;10(4):679-688.

24 CHAPTER Outcomes of Nonsurgical and Surgical Treatment of Chronic Sacroiliac Joint Pain

Alexandra Schwartz
Vinko Zlomislic
W. Carlton Reckling*
Daniel Cher*

Nonsurgical and surgical treatments for sacroiliac joint (SIJ) pain have been the subject of intermittent study since the early 1900s. Multiple treatments of several modalities are commonly provided, although published high-quality studies supporting safety and efficacy are often lacking. Published high-quality literature on minimally invasive SIJ fusion is growing.

Nonsurgical Treatment

Multiple nonsurgical treatment options exist for the management of SIJ pain, with limited evidence to support successful treatment.

Medication Management

Medications such as opioids and nonsteroidal anti-inflammatory drugs may be useful for acute pain control. Newer agents, including immunomodulators and protease inhibitors, have shown success in management of inflammatory spondyloarthropathy but play no role in the more common degenerative and disruption-based SIJ syndromes. Moreover, no medical treatment has been shown to alter the course of SIJ pain due to degenerative sacroiliitis or SIJ disruption. As with other chronic pain syndromes, opioid abuse remains a significant concern.

Physical Therapy

Physical therapy for nonautoimmune SIJ pain is commonly employed. The goals of therapy are to identify underlying functional deficits and provide improved flexibility and strengthening of stabilizing trunk muscles, often in combination with direct joint manipulation, while also training the patient to avoid activities that exacerbate symptoms. In spite of trials that have shown some benefit with manual therapy and stabilizing exercises,[1–3] no high-quality studies determining the impact of physical therapy on SIJ pain related to osteoarthritic degeneration or SIJ disruption have been published. While physical therapy remains a reasonable nonsurgical option and is used as part of the standard management algorithm, evidence of effectiveness is modest at best and whether it is cost-effective is not known. Anecdotally, failure of physical therapy in treatment of SIJ pain is common.

Pelvic Bracing

Bracing with a pelvic belt, used in pregnancy-related pelvic pain,[4,5] has also been described in the nonsurgical treatment of SIJ dysfunction,[6,7] but no high-quality evidence exists to support its use.

Sacroiliac Joint Injection

Intraarticular and periarticular injections have been employed in the treatment of SIJ pain, with therapeutic effects related to the (as yet undocumented) anesthetic and steroid phases of relief. Intraarticular SI injections are increasingly performed in the United States,[8] but there is no high-quality evidence to support their use. In a blinded randomized trial of periarticular steroid injections, women with pelvic pain after pregnancy attributed to SIJ pain had improved pain levels, disability, 6-minute walk test, and isometric trunk extensor test results at 4 weeks after infiltration of 20 mg of triamcinolone around (but not into) the SIJ compared to after saline placebo.[9] Two small blinded randomized trials from a single group in Finland showed improvement in SIJ symptoms at 1 month after periarticular steroid infiltration compared to lidocaine injections.[10,11] No high-quality study has shown long-term benefit from periarticular steroids.

Radiofrequency Ablation

Radiofrequency (RF) ablation has also been employed to provide pain relief through denervation of the SIJ. Two high-quality blinded trials have shown short-term (1 or 3 months)

**Dr. Reckling and Dr. Cher are employees of SI-Bone, a medical device company.

pain relief after RF ablation of lateral branches of sacral nerve roots.[12,13] In these trials, patients were screened using diagnostic periarticular local anesthetic blocks. A 12-month follow-up in one randomized trial showed moderate pain relief.[14,14a,14b] No high-quality evidence demonstrates long-term pain relief after RF ablation of the lateral branches of sacral nerve roots. The major shortcoming involving percutaneous RF ablation is that the ventral aspect of the joint cannot be addressed. Furthermore, due to complex innervation patterns, many of the nerves ablated during these procedures target other surrounding structures. Finally, much of the innervation of the SIJ is inaccessible to the RF probe. This may contribute to the relatively high rates of return of SIJ pain following RF ablation.

Surgical Treatment

In appropriately selected patients who have failed nonsurgical treatment, surgical management may be considered, with the treatment of choice being SIJ arthrodesis. Goals of SIJF are acute stabilization of the SIJ with hardware and long-term stabilization via biologic fusion. Stabilization and fusion of the SIJ may allow the spine-pelvis-hip complex to function more normally, which can contribute to reduction in pain and improvement of overall function.

Open Surgery

Initially described with a dorsal approach in 1908,[15] subsequent detailed descriptions of lateral-based SIJF were described in the 1920s.[16,17] Since then, scattered case series have demonstrated variably successful results following open SIJF.[18–26]

Access to the SIJ may involve either an anterior, posterior, or lateral approach. The anterior surgical technique utilizes a standard ilioinguinal approach during which the interval between the external oblique and gluteal fascia is developed and the iliacus is elevated from the iliac fossa allowing exposure of the SIJ. The joint is then curetted and fusion is achieved with placement of bone graft, with plate and screw fixation (Fig. 24.1A). The anterior approach affords access to the articular SIJ, especially to the anterior and cranial aspects, as well as preservation of the primary posterior ligamentous stabilizers.[21]

Several posterior-based SIJF techniques have been described, though the posterior approach offers only limited access to the SIJ articular surfaces. Posterior approaches range from simple onlay grafting of the dorsal sacrum and adjacent ilium followed by cast immobilization,[27] debridement and grafting of the dorsal ligamentous portion of the SIJ,[26,28] and debridement and grafting of the articular SIJ, which requires removal of a portion of the overlying posterior iliac crest.[29] Various types of fixation have been described in conjunction with posterior SIJ fusion, including screws placed laterally from ilium to sacrum,[30] screws in the ilium and sacrum dorsally with a rod spanning the SIJ,[23] and hybrid fixation with a plate dorsally and screws laterally.[20,31] Alternatively, a modified Smith-Petersen approach may be carried out to access the SIJ from a lateral approach.[16] This involves removing a rectangular or cylindrical core of ilium (across the joint), allowing exposure, decortication, and grafting of the SIJ. The bony core is then impacted back in so that the thicker iliac component sits across the joint for a fusion, which may or may not include supplemental screw fixation (Fig. 24.1B).[32,33]

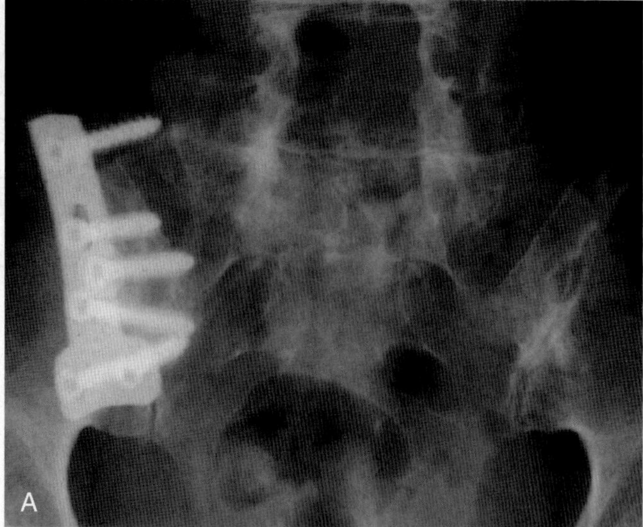

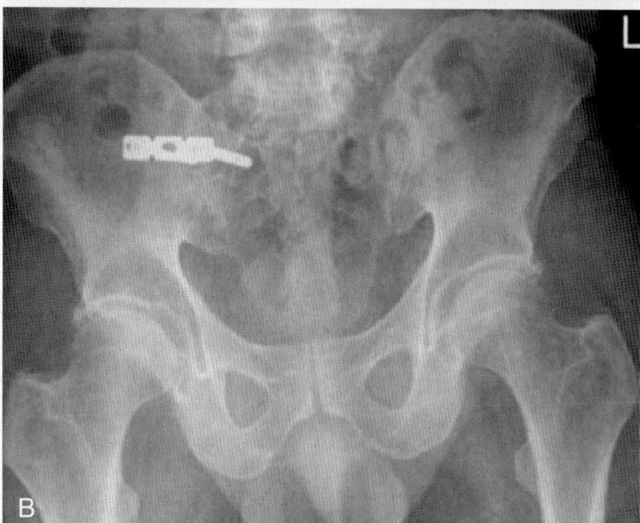

FIG. 24.1 Anteroposterior plain radiographs of the pelvis. (A) Use of T-plate to achieve arthrodesis of the sacroiliac joint using a modified Smith-Petersen approach. (B) Three-hole reconstruction plate spanning the sacroiliac joint following anterior ilioinguinal approach.

Open SIJF is marred by long operative times, high blood loss, long hospital stays, and significant patient morbidity—including infection, prolonged recovery times, and pseudarthrosis.[34] In addition, numerous complications have been reported for open approaches, including injury to the erector spinae muscle insertions, iatrogenic injury to the dorsal sensory nerve roots, sacral plexus, and internal iliac vessels. The most effective method for open SIJF remains unknown, as no comparative studies have been published. Nonetheless, given the historical context of limited surgical technology in use at the time, open SIJF resulted in modest rates of patient improvement along with radiographic fusion rates near 70%. Overall, approximately 60% of patients have indicated they would choose to have the surgery again.[21] However, with the advent of minimally invasive approaches, interest in open fusion has waned and the open technique is now used primarily in the setting of acute trauma or revision surgery.[35]

Minimally Invasive Surgery

Recent advances in surgical technology, along with a progression toward minimally invasive surgical (MIS) techniques, have resulted in the development and commercial availability of several devices used in MIS SIJF. Minimally invasive SIJF is predicated on a thorough understanding of the anatomy of the pelvis, including bony architecture as well as the position of the neurovascular structures. Appropriate imaging (including pelvic anteroposterior, inlet, and outlet views, and, if possible, computed tomography [CT] scan) must be obtained and studied preoperatively. Images should be reviewed, with particular attention paid to the possibility of a dysmorphic sacrum, which may significantly alter, or decrease, the safe zone for implant placement.

Three approaches similar to those used in open SIJF have been described for MIS SIJF. First, an *anterior approach* with endoscopic placement of a fusion cage has been described.[25] Second, two reports describe a *dorsal approach* with placement of fusion cages into the ligamentous portion of the joint. In one report, a hollow threaded fusion cage was used, with modest improvements.[36] In a second report, a fusion cage filled with recombinant human bone morphogenetic protein-2 was used, with somewhat larger improvements.[31] As of late 2016, no devices placed via the posterior approach are US Food and Drug Administration cleared/approved for SIJF.

The most commonly reported technique for MIS SIJF is the *lateral transarticular approach*, which was derived in part from modifications of the Smith-Petersen technique.[16] In this approach, devices are placed across the SIJ from lateral to medial under fluoroscopic guidance or navigational control.

Outcomes From Minimally Invasive Sacroiliac Joint Fusion

Although several devices are cleared by the Food and Drug Administration for lateral transarticular SIJF, the majority of the published clinical literature for this approach reports use of porous triangular titanium implants (iFuse Implant System, SI-Bone). Three prospective multicenter clinical trials, including two randomized clinical trials, report successful outcomes with use of these implants. A US prospective, multicenter randomized controlled trial (INSITE; n = 148) compared minimally invasive SIJF using triangular titanium implants to nonoperative care.[37] Nonsurgical care consisted of medication management, physical therapy, SIJ steroid injections and RF ablation of lateral branches of sacral nerve roots, administered according to patient needs. Success—a composite of pain reduction, absence of serious adverse events or neurologic worsening, and absence of repeat surgery—occurred in 82% in the SIJF group and 26% of in the nonsurgical group ($P <$ .0001). By month 24, 82% received substantial clinical benefit (Glassman criteria[38]) in visual analog scale SIJ pain score and 66% had received substantial clinical benefit in Oswestry Disability Index (ODI) score. In the nonsurgical group, these proportions were less than 10% with nonsurgical treatment only. Parallel changes were seen for EuroQOL-5D and Short Form-36 quality-of-life surveys, with larger changes in the surgery group at 6 months compared to nonsurgical treatment. The rate of adverse events related to SIJF was low. Three subjects assigned to SIJF underwent revision surgery within the 24-month follow-up period.

In a second prospective, multicenter randomized controlled trial conducted in Europe (iMIA; n = 103), patients with SIJ dysfunction were assigned to either MIS SIJF using titanium implants or conservative management.[39] At 6 months, mean low back pain improved by 43.3 points in the SIJF group and 5.7 points in the conservative management group (difference of 38.1 points; $P < .0001$). Mean ODI improved by 26 points in the SIJF group and 6 points in the nonsurgical group ($P <$ .0001). Other outcomes, such as active straight leg raise test,[40] EuroQOL-5D-3L, walking distance and satisfaction, were statistically superior in the fusion group. The frequency of adverse events did not differ between groups. One case of postoperative nerve impingement occurred in the surgical group. Twelve-month outcomes were sustained.[41]

Positive results from both randomized trials are supported by a large prospective, multicenter, single-arm clinical trial conducted in the United States (SIFI; n = 172).[42] In this study, patients (mean age, 51 years; 70% women) had SIJ pain for 5 years prior to SIJF, on average. Visual analog scale SIJ pain levels improved from close to 80 at baseline (0–100 scale) to 31 at 24 months. Large improvements were seen in ODI and two quality-of-life measures (SF-36 and EuroQOL-5D). Also observed was a decrease in opioid use for back pain from 76% at baseline to 55% at 24 months. A total of 4.7% of subjects underwent a revision surgery during follow-up. The study showed a high rate of bony apposition to implants on both sides of the SIJ, with modest 1-year fusion rates.

A pooled analysis of all three prospective porous triangular titanium implant studies (Fig. 24.2) showed high degrees of homogeneity across trials and statistically significant but clinically unimportant predictors of success (smoking and baseline opioid use).[43]

In addition to prospective studies, retrospective case series show positive outcomes after SIJF with porous titanium implants.[44–53] Of these case series, notable studies include those with 3-year,[53] 4-year,[52] and 5-year[44] follow-up. In the latter study, 5-year joint fusion rates were high.[44] Three studies[34,54,55] comparing open and MIS SIJF substantiated the potential benefits of the MIS approach, including one study[55] showing less blood loss, shorter operative times, and shorter hospital stays as well as improved pain levels at 1 and 2 years in the MIS approach.

In a comparative long-term case series from Spain, a minority of patients with diagnosed SIJ dysfunction were able to undergo MIS SIJF using triangular titanium implants or RF ablation; the remainder were, due to insurance noncoverage, forced to undergo continued conservative management. Patients in the SIJF group showed marked, immediate, and sustained reductions in SIJ pain and disability scores (ODI), along with a profound decrease in opioid use (63% at baseline

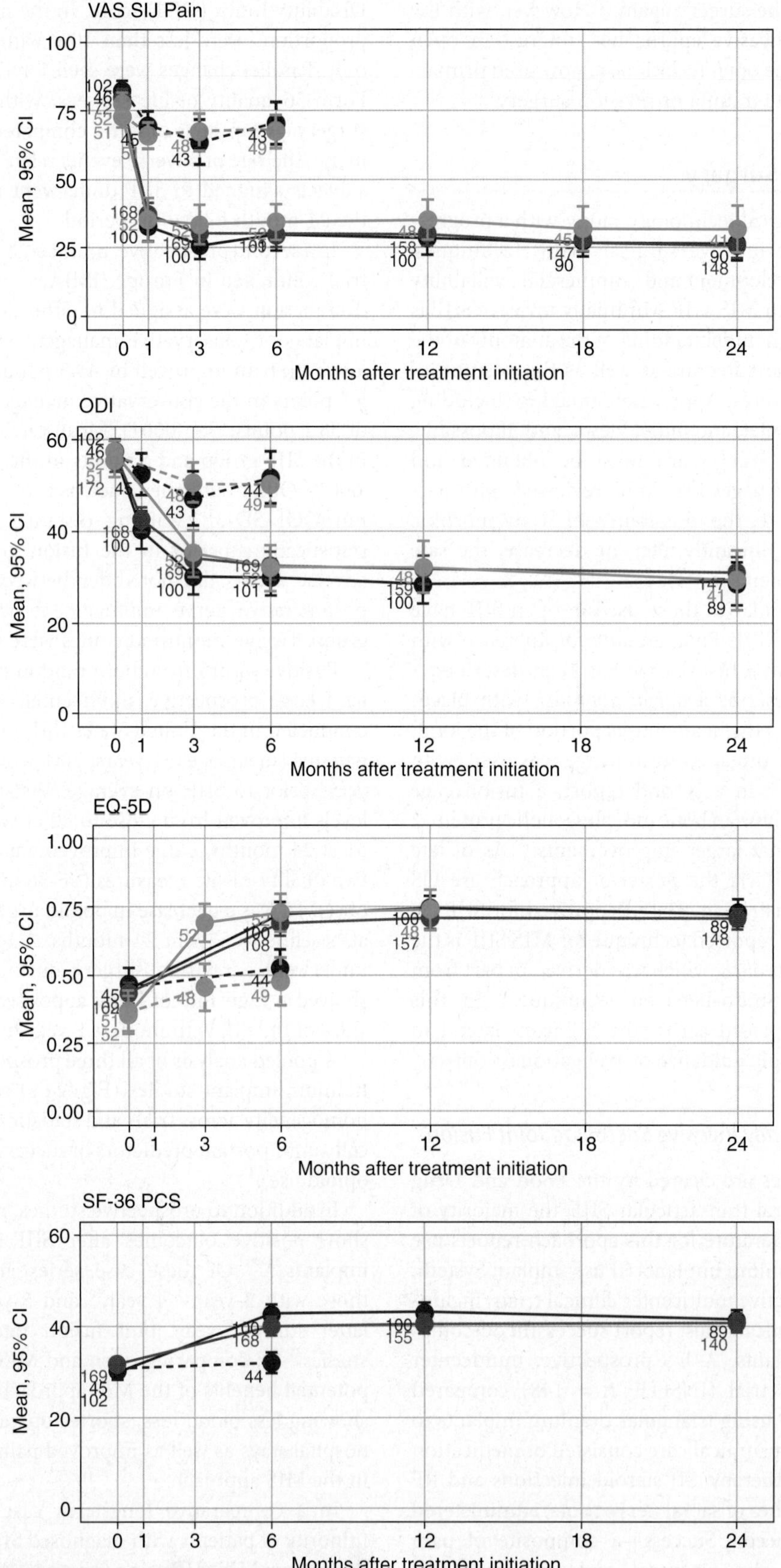

FIG. 24.2 Improvement in sacroiliac joint (SIJ) pain as measured using a visual analog scale (VAS), Oswestry Disability Index (ODI), EQ-5D time tradeoff index, and Short Form-36 physical component summary (PCS) in three prospective trials, including two randomized trials, of sacroiliac joint (SIJ) fusion. CI, confidence interval.

to 7% at last follow-up). In contrast, patients who underwent either RF ablation or conservative management showed worsening of pain and disability scores, increased opioid use, and worsened job status at last follow-up.[56] CT scans in one study showed a modest rate of bridging bone at 1 year[42] and a high rate at 5 years.[44]

Data supporting other commercially available SIJF systems include two small retrospective case series using hollow modular anchor screws,[57,58] one case series in which a minority of patients were treated with the Samba screw,[59] one case series with the Zyga screw,[60] and one single-center prospective study using SI-LOK (Globus).[61] These studies were neither blinded nor randomized; the degree to which outcomes from randomized trials of the triangular titanium implant pertain to screw-based systems is not known and no ongoing comparative studies are in progress. A comparative case series suggests that screw loosening may be more common than loosening of triangular titanium implants.[62]

Complications From Minimally Invasive Surgical Sacroiliac Joint Fusion

Complications of MIS SIJF fall into four categories: (1) device breakage, which has been reported with some systems, but not iFuse implants; (2) standard local operative complications; (3) implant malposition resulting in neuropathic pain due to irritation of the L5 or S1 nerve roots by the distal tip of the misplaced implant; and (4) implants placed insufficiently into the sacrum, resulting in continued or recurrent pain. In prospective trials, local surgical complications did not appear to occur more commonly than after other procedures. Implant malposition causing acute neuropathic pain occurred in about 1% of subjects in prospective clinical trials of triangular titanium implants and at a similar rate in a postmarket surveillance study.[63] In most cases with implant malposition causing new-onset neuropathic pain, pain resolves with repositioning of the implant(s). Failure to place devices sufficiently into the sacrum causes inadequate SIJ stabilization, which may result in either lack of improvement of SIJ pain or pain recurrence. Long-term revision rates after SIJF with triangular titanium implants appear to be low,[64] especially in comparison to some lumbar spine surgeries.[65,66] In some cases, such failures are associated with radiolucencies around the implants due presumably to persistent micromotion. Though not documented, placement of implants under CT guidance may help to improve implant placement accuracy.

Minimally Invasive Surgical Fusion Technique

MIS sacroiliac fusion is done with the patient in the prone position on a radiolucent table. Rolls are placed under the patient's chest. Care is taken to pad all bony prominences, and sequential compression devices are placed on both lower extremities. The arms are placed in an abducted and externally rotated position, rather than adducted at the patient's side, to allow for lateral fluoroscopic imaging. Biplanar fluoroscopy may be used. If two C-arms are used, one is positioned in the anteroposterior plane and one is placed in the lateral plane. If one C-arm is used, it is helpful to mark both positions of the C-arm base on the floor, as well as the various angles of inlet and outlet positions on the machine with tape. Adjust the table height such that no changes need to be made intraoperatively to obtain a good lateral sacral view. When using a single C-arm, it is positioned opposite the surgical site.

The ability to obtain proper imaging views must be ensured before initiation of surgery and should be performed before prepping and draping the patient. Several factors can interfere with the ability to visualize appropriate bony landmarks, including bowel gas, patient habitus, and prior lumbosacral instrumentation. Consideration of preoperative bowel prep should be given to improve visualization if needed. The inlet view is deemed ideal when all sacral bodies are overlapped. The outlet view is best when the S2 foramina are seen immediately cephalad and adjacent to the superior aspect of the superior pubic rami. The ideal sacral lateral view is seen when the greater sciatic notches are perfectly overlapped. The sacral lateral view is critical to understanding the sacral alar slope. The alar slope is best estimated by the iliac cortical density (ICD) and delineates the anterior extent of the "safe zone" if the implant is posterior and caudal to it.[67] Care must be taken in patients with a dysmorphic sacrum (Fig. 24.3), in which the sacral alar cortical bone limit is not represented by the ICD. Due to the more acute slope of the sacral ala, the sacral alar cortical line is cephalad and anterior to the ICD.

The affected gluteal region is prepped and draped in the usual sterile fashion. Draping should extend from midline to the greater trochanter, and from the gluteal crease to proximal to the iliac crest. A timeout procedure is performed.

Various methods have been described to place percutaneous fusion devices. Depending on the system chosen by the surgeon, this may involve a cannula through which one

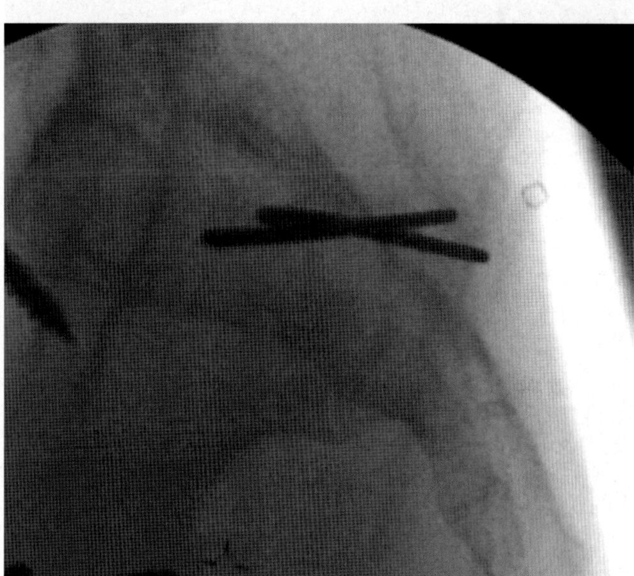

FIG. 24.3 The greater sciatic notches are overlapped, indicating an adequate lateral view. The sacral alar cortical bone limit is not represented by the iliac cortical density, due to the more acute slope of the sacral ala. The sacral alar cortical line is cephalad and anterior to the iliac cortical density.

can accomplish a technique to debride the sacroiliac joint (SImmetry; Zyga Technology), or a percutaneous technique using cannulated wires, broaches, and triangular titanium-coated implants without debriding the chondral surfaces (iFuse Implant System; SI-Bone). The goal of the latter is to create stability by bony growth onto the implant, not necessarily bone growth across the SI joint, though anecdotally this has been observed. Various reports describe other implants used for such minimally invasive, fluoroscopically placed implants.

For the triangular titanium-coated implant system, typically three implants are inserted. A 2-cm incision is first made in line with the midsagittal sacrum. Blunt percutaneous dissection is then carried out to the lateral ilium. The first cannulated guide wire placed should be the most cephalad wire. The goal is to center the guide pin between the S1 foramen and superior endplate of the sacrum on the outlet view while maintaining the guide pin parallel to the superior endplate of S1 (Fig. 24.4). On the inlet view, the guide pin should be aimed from slightly posterior to anterior, care being taken not to violate the sacral canal or exit the front of the sacrum (Fig. 24.5). To avoid the L5 nerve root, which drapes across the anterior sacrum just medial to the sacroiliac joint, the guide pin should be distal to the ICD. The pin should be parallel to the S1 endplate and aim from posterior to anterior on the lateral view (Fig. 24.6). Sequential drilling, broaching, measuring, and ultimately placing the implant are then carried out. Care should be taken to avoid migration of the guide pin. A parallel drill guide is then used to facilitate placement of additional caudal implants, in similar fashion, ensuring that each ends lateral to the sacral foramina (Figs. 24.7 and 24.8).

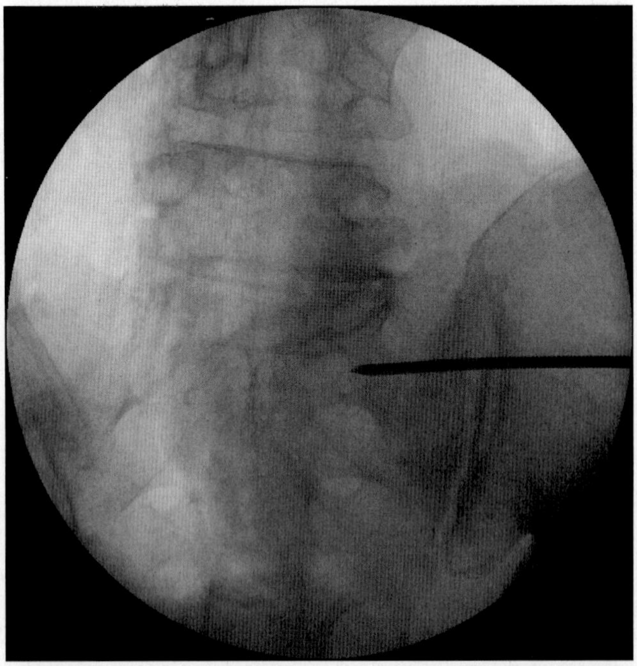

FIG. 24.4 In this outlet view, the guide pin is located between the S1 foramen and superior endplate of the sacrum and is parallel to the superior endplate of S1.

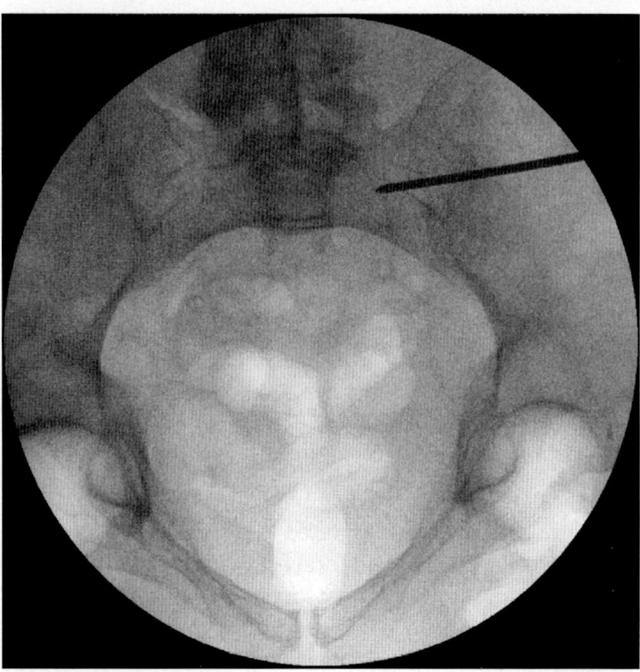

FIG. 24.5 On this inlet view, the guide pin is aimed from slightly posterior to anterior with care being taken not to violate the sacral canal or exit the front of the sacrum.

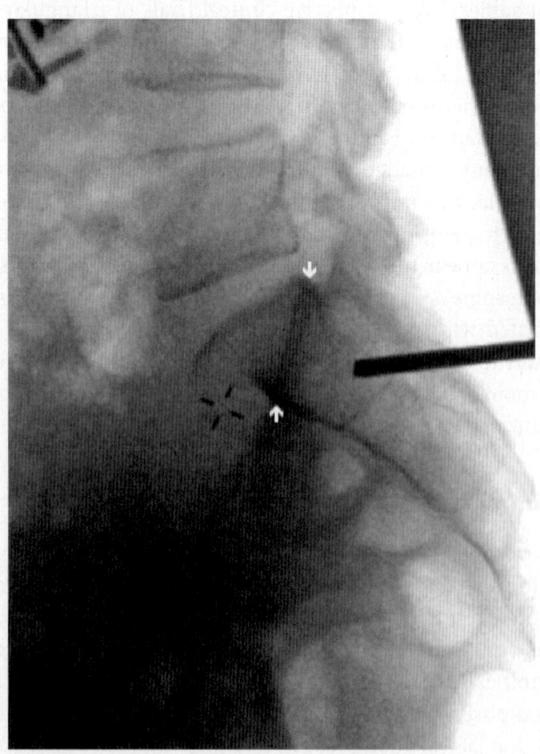

FIG. 24.6 Sacral lateral view demonstrating guide pin caudal to iliac cortical density (*arrowheads*).

Summary

SIJ pathology is a common cause of low back pain and often presents in the setting of degenerative lumbar disease. Accurate diagnosis seems limited by lack of interest in the

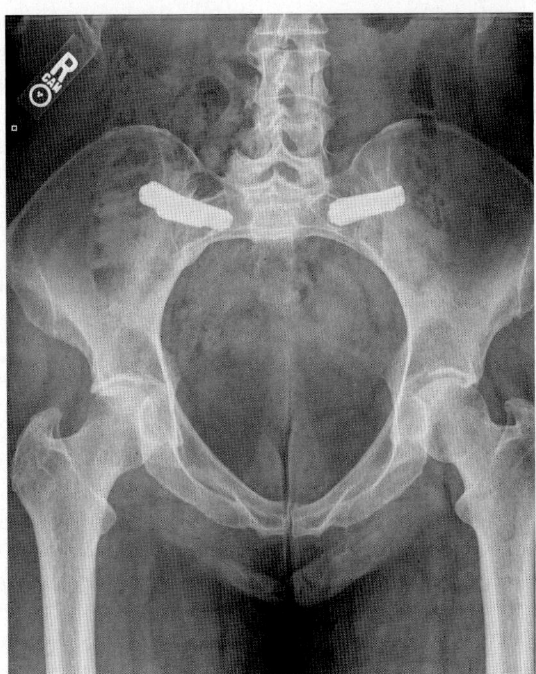

FIG. 24.7 Postoperative inlet view.

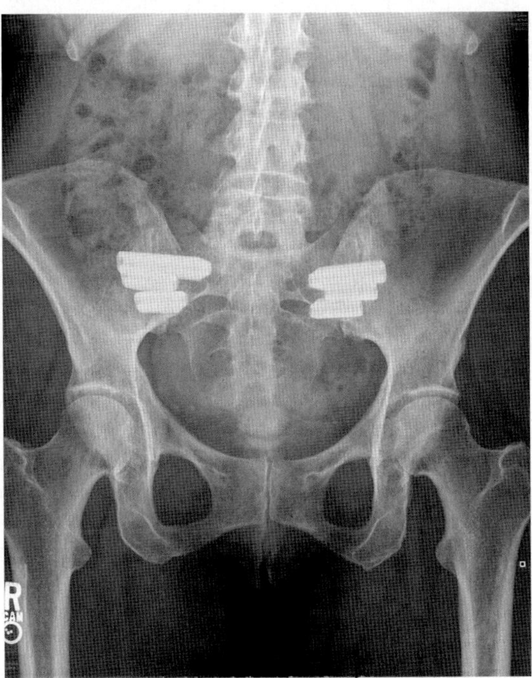

FIG. 24.8 Postoperative anteroposterior view.

condition as well as the perceived unreliability of diagnosis. The fact that high-quality randomized trials have shown that patients with this condition can be diagnosed and treated with high levels of efficacy using multiple endpoint types argues against diagnostic unreliability. Provocative examination of the SIJ and positive responses to image-guided injections are necessary to confirm the SIJ as the pain source. Once SIJ etiology is established, multiple modes of treatment exist. While evidence for nonsurgical treatment is limited, conservative management with physical therapy and/or injections may be effective for many patients. For those who remain symptomatic, MIS SIJF is an effective option in reducing pain and disability and improving quality of life. Currently, strong literature support is available only for porous triangular titanium implants. The clinical utility of other devices available for MIS SIJF, which have different designs, placement, and fusion strategies, is less well understood and the applicability of evidence from published randomized trials of triangular titanium implants to these other devices is unclear. Procedure success requires careful attention to technical and anatomic factors, including sacral bony and neurovascular anatomy. The likelihood of positive outcomes is increased with careful patient selection and accurate device placement fully across the SIJ.

REFERENCES

1. Stuge B, Laerum E, Kirkesola G, Vøllestad N. The efficacy of a treatment program focusing on specific stabilizing exercises for pelvic girdle pain after pregnancy: a randomized controlled trial. *Spine*. 2004;29(4):351-359.
2. Mens JM, Snijders CJ, Stam HJ. Diagonal trunk muscle exercises in peripartum pelvic pain: a randomized clinical trial. *Phys Ther*. 2000;80(12):1164-1173.
3. Visser LH, Woudenberg NP, de Bont J, et al. Treatment of the sacroiliac joint in patients with leg pain: a randomized-controlled trial. *Eur Spine J*. 2013;22(10):2310-2317.
4. Flack NA, Hay-Smith EJC, Stringer MD, Gray AR, Woodley SJ. Adherence, tolerance and effectiveness of two different pelvic support belts as a treatment for pregnancy-related symphyseal pain—a pilot randomized trial. *BMC Pregnancy Childbirth*. 2015;15:36.
5. Nilsson-Wikmar L, Holm K, Oijerstedt R, Harms-Ringdahl K. Effect of three different physical therapy treatments on pain and activity in pregnant women with pelvic girdle pain: a randomized clinical trial with 3, 6, and 12 months follow-up postpartum. *Spine*. 2005;30(8):850-856.
6. Hammer N, Möbius R, Schleifenbaum S, et al. Pelvic belt effects on health outcomes and functional parameters of patients with sacroiliac joint pain. *PLoS One*. 2015;10(8): e0136375.
7. Jung H-S, Jeon H-S, Oh D-W, Kwon O-Y. Effect of the pelvic compression belt on the hip extensor activation patterns of sacroiliac joint pain patients during one-leg standing: a pilot study. *Man Ther*. 2013;18(2):143-148.
8. Manchikanti L, Hansen H, Pampati V, Falco FJE. Utilization and growth patterns of sacroiliac joint injections from 2000 to 2011 in the Medicare population. *Pain Physician*. 2013;16(4): E379-E390.
9. Torstensson T, Lindgren A, Kristiansson P. Improved function in women with persistent pregnancy-related pelvic pain after a single corticosteroid injection to the ischiadic spine: a randomized double-blind controlled trial. *Physiother Theory Pract*. 2013;29(5):371-378.
10. Luukkainen R, Nissilä M, Asikainen E, et al. Periarticular corticosteroid treatment of the sacroiliac joint in patients with seronegative spondylarthropathy. *Clin Exp Rheumatol*. 1999;17(1):88-90.
11. Luukkainen RK, Wennerstrand PV, Kautiainen HH, Sanila MT, Asikainen EL. Efficacy of periarticular corticosteroid treatment of the sacroiliac joint in non-spondylarthropathic patients with

chronic low back pain in the region of the sacroiliac joint. *Clin Exp Rheumatol.* 2002;20(1):52-54.

12. Patel N, Gross A, Brown L, Gekht G. A randomized, placebo-controlled study to assess the efficacy of lateral branch neurotomy for chronic sacroiliac joint pain. *Pain Med.* 2012;13(3):383-398.
13. Cohen SP, Hurley RW, Buckenmaier CC, et al. Randomized placebo-controlled study evaluating lateral branch radiofrequency denervation for sacroiliac joint pain. *Anesthesiology.* 2008;109(2):279-288.
14. Patel N. Twelve-month follow-up of a randomized trial assessing cooled radiofrequency denervation as a treatment for sacroiliac region pain. *Pain Pract.* 2016;16(2):154-167.

14a. van Tilburg CWJ, Schuurmans FA, Stronks DL, et al. Randomized sham-controlled double-blind multicenter clinical trial to ascertain the effect of percutaneous radiofrequency treatment for sacroiliac joint pain: three-month results. *Clin J Pain.* 2016. [Epub before print].

14b. Juchs JNS, Maas ET, Ostelo RWJG, et al. Effect of radiofrequency denervation on pain intensity among patients with chronic low back pain: the MINT randomized clinical trials. *JAMA.* 2017;318(1):68-81.

15. Painter CF. Excision of the os innominatum. Arthrodesis of the sacro-iliac synchrondrosis. *Boston Med Surg J.* 1908;159(7):205-208.
16. Smith-Petersen MN. Arthrodesis of the sacroiliac joint. A new method of approach. *J Bone Joint Surg.* 1921;3(8):400-405.
17. Smith-Petersen MN, Rogers WA. End-result study of arthrodesis of the sacro-iliac joint for arthritis—traumatic and non-traumatic. *J Bone Joint Surg.* 1926;8(1):118-136.
18. McGuire RA, Chen Z, Donahoe K. Dual fibular allograft dowel technique for sacroiliac joint arthrodesis. *Evid Based Spine Care J.* 2012;3(3):21-28.
19. Kibsgard TJ, Roise O, Stuge B, Sudmann E. Pelvic joint fusions in patients with chronic pelvic girdle pain: a 23-year follow-up. *Eur Spine J.* 2013;22(4):871-877.
20. Schütz U, Grob D. Poor outcome following bilateral sacroiliac joint fusion for degenerative sacroiliac joint syndrome. *Acta Orthop Belg.* 2006;72(3):296-308.
21. Buchowski JM, Kebaish KM, Sinkov V, et al. Functional and radiographic outcome of sacroiliac arthrodesis for the disorders of the sacroiliac joint. *Spine J.* 2005;5(5):520-528.
22. Giannikas KA, Khan AM, Karski MT, Maxwell HA. Sacroiliac joint fusion for chronic pain: a simple technique avoiding the use of metalwork. *Eur Spine J.* 2004;13(3):253-256.
23. Belanger TA, Dall BE. Sacroiliac arthrodesis using a posterior midline fascial splitting approach and pedicle screw instrumentation: a new technique. *J Spinal Disord.* 2001;14(2):118-124.
24. Berthelot JM, Gouin F, Glemarec J, Maugars Y, Prost A. Possible use of arthrodesis for intractable sacroiliitis in spondylarthropathy: report of two cases. *Spine.* 2001;26(20):2297-2299.
25. Guner G, Gurer S, Elmali N, Ertem K. Anterior sacroiliac fusion: a new video-assisted endoscopic technique. *Surg Laparosc Endosc.* 1998;8(3):233-236.
26. Waisbrod H, Krainick JU, Gerbershagen HU. Sacroiliac joint arthrodesis for chronic lower back pain. *Arch Für Orthop Unf-Chir.* 1987;106(4):238-240.
27. Campbell WC. An operation for extra-articular fusion of the sacro-iliac joint. *Surg Gynecol Obstet.* 1927;45:218-219.
28. Mitchell JI. Surgical treatment of affections of the lumbo-sacral and sacroiliac joints. *Surgery.* 1938;4(1):33-43.
29. Graham Smith A. *Arthrodesis of the sacroiliac joint using pedicle screw fixation and bone morphogenetic protein for chronic sprain causing disabling pain.* Presented at the North American Spine Society Annual Meeting, Hawaii, 2009.
30. Keating JG, Avillar MD, Price M. Sacroiliac joint arthrodesis in selected patients with low back pain. In: Vleeming A, Mooney V, Snijders CJ, Stoeckart R, eds. *Movement, Stability, and Low Back Pain: The Essential Role of the Pelvis.* New York: Churchill Livingstone; 1997:573-586.
31. Wise CL, Dall BE. Minimally invasive sacroiliac arthrodesis: outcomes of a new technique. *J Spinal Disord Tech.* 2008;21(8): 579-584.
32. Moore MR. Surgical treatment of chronic painful sacroiliac joint dysfunction. In: Vleeming A, Mooney V, Snijders CJ, Stoeckart R, eds. *Movement, Stability, and Low Back Pain: The Essential Role of the Pelvis.* New York: Churchill Livingstone; 1997:563-572.
33. Kurica K. A prospective study of sacroiliac joint arthrodesis with one to six year patient follow-up. In: *The Second Interdisciplinary World Congress on Low Back Pain in Relation to the Sacro-Iliac Joint.* San Diego, CA: 1995.
34. Ledonio CGT, Polly DW, Swiontkowski MF. Minimally invasive versus open sacroiliac joint fusion: are they similarly safe and effective? *Clin Orthop.* 2014;472(6):1831-1838.
35. Lorio MP, Polly DW Jr, Ninkovic I, et al. Utilization of minimally invasive surgical approach for sacroiliac joint fusion in surgeon population of ISASS and SMISS membership. *Open Orthop J.* 2014;8:1-6.
36. Endres S, Ludwig E. Outcome of distraction interference arthrodesis of the sacroiliac joint for sacroiliac arthritis. *Indian J Orthop.* 2013;47(5):437-442.
37. Polly DW, Swofford J, Whang PG, et al. Two-year outcomes from a randomized controlled trial of minimally invasive sacroiliac joint fusion vs. non-surgical management for sacroiliac joint dysfunction. *Int J Spine Surg.* 2016;10:28.
38. Glassman SD, Copay AG, Berven SH, et al. Defining substantial clinical benefit following lumbar spine arthrodesis. *J Bone Joint Surg.* 2008;90(9):1839-1847.
39. Sturesson B, Kools D, Pflugmacher R, et al. Six-month outcomes from a randomized controlled trial of minimally invasive SI joint fusion with triangular titanium implants vs. conservative management. *Eur Spine J.* 2016;26(3):708-719.
40. Mens JM, Vleeming A, Snijders CJ, Koes BW, Stam HJ. Reliability and validity of the active straight leg raise test in posterior pelvic pain since pregnancy. *Spine.* 2001;26(10):1167-1171.
41. Dengler J, Kools D, Pflugmacher R, et al. Low back pain originating from the sacroiliac joint—1 year results from a randomized controlled trial of conservative management vs. minimally invasive surgical treatment. *Pain Physician.* In press.
42. Duhon BS, Bitan F, Lockstadt H, et al. Triangular titanium implants for minimally invasive sacroiliac joint fusion: 2-year follow-up from a prospective multicenter trial. *Int J Spine Surg.* 2016;10:13.
43. Dengler J, Duhon B, Whang P, et al. Predictors of outcome in conservative and minimally invasive surgical management of pain originating from the sacroiliac joint: a pooled analysis. *Spine.* 2017. [Epub ahead of print].
44. Rudolf L, Capobianco R. Five-year clinical and radiographic outcomes after minimally invasive sacroiliac joint fusion using triangular implants. *Open Orthop J.* 2014;8:375-383.
45. Rudolf L. Sacroiliac joint arthrodesis—MIS technique with titanium implants: report of the first 50 patients and outcomes. *Open Orthop J.* 2012;6:495-502.

46. Sachs D, Capobianco R. One year successful outcomes for novel sacroiliac joint arthrodesis system. *Ann Surg Innov Res.* 2012;6(1):13.
47. Sachs D, Capobianco R. Minimally invasive sacroiliac joint fusion: one-year outcomes in 40 patients. *Adv Orthop.* 2013;2013:536128.
48. Cummings J Jr, Capobianco RA. Minimally invasive sacroiliac joint fusion: one-year outcomes in 18 patients. *Ann Surg Innov Res.* 2013;7(1):12.
49. Gaetani P, Miotti D, Risso A, et al. Percutaneous arthrodesis of sacro-iliac joint: a pilot study. *J Neurosurg Sci.* 2013;57(4): 297-301.
50. Schroeder JE, Cunningham ME, Ross T, Boachie-Adjei O. Early results of sacro-iliac joint fixation following long fusion to the sacrum in adult spine deformity. *HSS J.* 2013;10(1):30-35.
51. Sachs D, Capobianco R, Cher D, et al. One-year outcomes after minimally invasive sacroiliac joint fusion with a series of triangular implants: a multicenter, patient-level analysis. *Med Devices (Auckl).* 2014;7:299-304.
52. Vanaclocha-Vanaclocha V, Verdú-López F, Sánchez-Pardo M, et al. Minimally invasive sacroiliac joint arthrodesis: experience in a prospective series with 24 patients. *J Spine.* 2014;3:185.
53. Sachs D, Kovalsky D, Redmond A, et al. Durable intermediate-to long-term outcomes after minimally invasive transiliac sacroiliac joint fusion using triangular titanium implants. *Med Devices (Auckl).* 2016;9:213-222.
54. Ledonio CGT, Polly DW Jr, Swiontkowski M, Cummings JT. Comparative effectiveness of open versus minimally invasive sacroiliac joint fusion. *Med Devices (Auckl).* 2014;7:187-193.
55. Smith AG, Capobianco R, Cher D, et al. Open versus minimally invasive sacroiliac joint fusion: a multi-center comparison of perioperative measures and clinical outcomes. *Ann Surg Innov Res.* 2013;7(1):14.
56. Vanaclocha V, Herrera JM, Sáiz-Sapena N, Rivera-Paz M, Verdú-López F. Minimally invasive sacroiliac joint fusion, radiofrequency denervation, and conservative management for sacroiliac joint pain: 6-year comparative case series. *Neurosurgery.* 2017. [Epub ahead of print].
57. Al-Khayer A, Hegarty J, Hahn D, Grevitt MP. Percutaneous sacroiliac joint arthrodesis: a novel technique. *J Spinal Disord Tech.* 2008;21(5):359-363.
58. Khurana A, Guha AR, Mohanty K, Ahuja S. Percutaneous fusion of the sacroiliac joint with hollow modular anchorage screws: clinical and radiological outcome. *J Bone Joint Surg Br.* 2009;91(5):627-631.
59. Kancherla VK, McGowan SM, Audley BN, Sokunbi G, Puccio ST. Patient reported outcomes from sacroiliac joint fusion. *Asian Spine J.* 2017;11(1):120-126.
60. Kube RA, Muir JM. Sacroiliac joint fusion: one year clinical and radiographic results following minimally invasive sacroiliac joint fusion surgery. *Open Orthop J.* 2016;10(1):30.
61. Rappoport LH, Luna IY, Joshua G. Minimally invasive sacroiliac joint fusion using a novel hydroxyapatite-coated screw: preliminary 1-year clinical and radiographic results of a 2-year prospective study. *World Neurosurg.* 2017;101:493-497.
62. Spain K, Holt T. Surgical revision after sacroiliac joint fixation or fusion. *Int J Spine Surg.* 2017;11:5.
63. Miller L, Reckling WC, Block JE. Analysis of postmarket complaints database for the iFuse SI Joint Fusion System: a minimally invasive treatment for degenerative sacroiliitis and sacroiliac joint disruption. *Med Devices (Auckl).* 2013;6: 77-84.
64. Cher DJ, Reckling WC, Capobianco RA. Implant survivorship analysis after minimally invasive sacroiliac joint fusion using the iFuse Implant System. *Med Devices (Auckl).* 2015;8:485-492.
65. Martin BI, Mirza SK, Comstock BA, et al. Reoperation rates following lumbar spine surgery and the influence of spinal fusion procedures. *Spine.* 2007;32(3):382-387.
66. Martin BI, Mirza SK, Flum DR, et al. Repeat surgery after lumbar decompression for herniated disc: the quality implications of hospital and surgeon variation. *Spine J.* 2012;12(2):89-97.
67. Routt ML Jr, Simonian PT, Agnew SG, Mann FA. Radiographic recognition of the sacral alar slope for optimal placement of iliosacral screws: a cadaveric and clinical study. *J Orthop Trauma.* 1996;10:171-177.

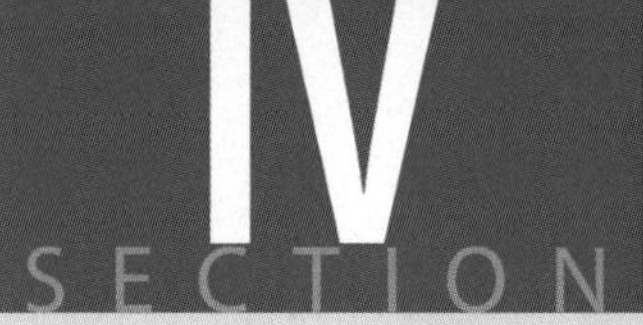

SECTION IV

PEDIATRICS

CHAPTER 25 Back Pain in Children and Adolescents

Lori A. Karol
Lauren LaMont
Megan Mignemi

Introduction

The prevalence of back pain in children and adolescents is rising.[1-3] While it is assumed that pediatric back pain is rare, more than 50% of children note episodes of back pain by 15 years of age.[4-7] In 2001, it was reported that, although 39% of teenagers complain of low back pain, few actually present for medical evaluation.[8] While the incidence of back pain in adolescents was previously reported to be around 18% to 30%,[9-11] a recent Danish study reported an 86% incidence of self-reported back pain in a prospective cohort study of 1348 students ages 11 to 13 years, which increased to 89% at 2-year follow-up.[12]

As complaints of back pain in young adults continue to rise, the classically held belief that back pain in children and adolescents is due to serious pathology is no longer thought to be true.[13] In 1985, Hensinger found a specific diagnosis in 84% of children presenting for treatment of back pain.[14] In a more recent analysis, however, Yang and colleagues found that over 80% of adolescents had no identifiable etiology for their back pain within 1 year of presenting to a physician.[3] In this cohort, the most common etiology of back pain in ages 10 to 19 years was muscle strain or sprain. A similar study of patients screened by single photon emission computed tomography (SPECT) scans found a cause for back pain in only 22% of 217 children.[15] Based on this, it is up to the evaluating surgeon to identify which children are most likely to have an underlying musculoskeletal condition and require a comprehensive evaluation to identify the etiology of their back pain.

Studies suggest that back pain in younger children is more worrisome, while adolescent pain is more likely to pattern after adult complaints, especially when the complaint is chronic.[16] The thought that a pathologic abnormality can nearly always be identified as the cause of the symptoms is evolving as more studies demonstrate fewer pathologic findings.[16,17] As children reach adolescence, diagnostic imaging is less likely to yield a diagnosis.[18] As the radiologic armamentarium grows, the treating physician has more choices in the evaluation of these patients, yet every child who presents to the physician does not need to undergo a comprehensive workup. Therefore, a complete understanding of the potential causes of back pain will enable treating physicians to properly evaluate the pediatric patient who complains of back pain.

History

The initial step in distinguishing which children require symptomatic treatment from those who merit a complete radiographic evaluation is obtaining a detailed history. The characteristics of the pain are most helpful. Acute pain following trauma is seen with fractures, disc herniations, and apophyseal ring separations. Insidious pain without a specific antecedent event is characteristic of developmental conditions such as Scheuermann kyphosis and benign neoplasms. However, in adolescent patients, pain without a specific event may also be attributable to mechanical back pain, as is seen in adults with similar complaints. Recurrent pain associated with athletics and relieved by rest leads to suspicion of overuse injuries, such as spondylolysis, or may also be mechanical in nature. Unremitting pain, especially if it is worse at night or wakes the child from sleep, is most worrisome, as this type of pain can be seen in malignancies and infection.[19,20]

The location of the pain is very helpful in narrowing down the differential diagnosis. Localized bony pain may indicate either benign or malignant neoplasms. Lumbar pain may be produced by spondylolysis or spondylolisthesis, while pain in the thoracic area may be due to Scheuermann kyphosis. It is important to note whether pain in each region is bony tenderness elicited while palpating spinous processes or paraspinal soreness, which may point more to muscle strain or mechanical pain. When pain radiates into either the buttocks or legs, there is concern for a disc herniation, apophyseal fracture, and spinal cord or vertebral tumors. As with all examinations, when pain radiates down into the leg or groin, it is important to rule out hip pathology, especially in the adolescent female, who may suffer from unrecognized hip dysplasia.

The presence or absence of constitutional symptoms is useful in deciding the potential severity of the underlying condition. Fever in a child with acute back pain points to an infectious or neoplastic etiology. It is important to question the parents about malaise, anorexia, and the presence of a rash or abnormal bruising, as back pain can be the presenting complaint in children with leukemia. These concerns call for more emergent blood work and imaging to confirm the diagnosis.

Next, a detailed neurologic history must be obtained. The presence of numbness, weakness, decreased ability to walk, and changes in coordination require prompt imaging of the spinal cord. Questioning the patient and parents as to how much these neurologic symptoms have altered activity level can also be helpful to determine their severity. The treating physician should ask specifically about changes in bowel or bladder function, as adolescents are hesitant to admit to these symptoms.

The patient's age is also very helpful in directing the evaluation of back pain. Back pain in children younger than 4 years is usually due to either infection or malignancy. A history of fever, limp, and malaise should be sought, and an immediate diagnostic evaluation should be performed. Children in the first decade of life commonly present with discitis and/or osteomyelitis and malignant neoplasms, but also may present with benign conditions such as eosinophilic granuloma.[20] Patients older than 10 years are most likely to have back pain secondary to trauma or overuse, resulting in spondylolysis, disc herniations, or apophyseal fractures.[21] Scheuermann kyphosis typically presents in adolescence. Patients older than 10 years are also more likely to have pain attributable to overuse, strain, or mechanical low back pain without abnormal imaging.[3] While more common in younger children, teenagers can present with malignancies. Thus, the evaluating physician should weigh the relative frequency of conditions based on age, but always remain cautious.

A family history should be taken regarding back pain. Adolescents with ill-defined pain, no constitutional symptoms, no history of excessive athletic activity, no anatomically consistent neurologic complaints, and a positive family history often do not have a musculoskeletal etiology for their pain.[5,20] Psychosomatic pain does occur in this age group, but remains a diagnosis of exclusion. History of sleep habits, school performance, changes in weight, mood, and mental health problems can also help identify patients in whom pain is associated with a psychiatric diagnosis that at times may require urgent referral.

Finally, a complete review of systems should be obtained. Back pain associated with menses is rarely orthopaedic in nature. Flank pain may be renal in origin. A recent study showed that 5% of children presenting to an emergency department for evaluation of back pain had urinary tract infections.[22]

Physical Examination

The general appearance of the child should be noted. If the child appears systemically ill, immediate evaluation for infection or malignancy is warranted. Whether the child can walk and the characteristics of the child's gait are important, as the inability to walk can be due to infection or spinal cord compromise. Specific gait abnormalities, such as increased posterior pelvic tilt and decreased hip flexion, may be seen in spondylolisthesis. Examination of the skin for dysraphic lesions, such as hairy patches or deep sinuses, as well as for café-au-lait spots, is also required. Palpation of the spine can identify the location of the pathologic abnormality.

The spine should be inspected for sagittal and coronal alignment. The Adams forward bend test identifies patients with scoliosis, but the presence of scoliosis is more likely to be a symptom of underlying pathology rather than a cause of pain. Trunk lean and decompensation may indicate such pathology as benign or malignant neoplasms, or irritating lesions such as herniated discs. Stiffness of the spine should be noted. Thoracic kyphosis typically increases and lumbar lordosis reverses as a child bends forward. In the presence of significant pain, the child will not allow the spine to move, and will bend the knees to touch the floor rather than flex the spine. Pain with hyperextension of the spine is often seen in patients with spondylolysis and is often worsened with one-legged hyperextension on the affected side if unilateral. This can be further exacerbated by twisting during hyperextension. The Lasegue sign is nearly always positive in patients with herniated discs or fractured apophyses. The straight-leg raise is also diminished in patients with tight hamstrings due to spondylolisthesis, and popliteal angles will also be increased.

Next, a thorough neurologic examination is critical in the evaluation of the child with back pain. Motor and sensory function and deep tendon reflexes should be tested. Long tract signs, such as clonus and the Babinski reflex, must be evaluated to rule out spinal cord compression or abnormality. The abdominal reflex is tested by lightly stroking the four quadrants around the umbilicus in the supine child. While an absent abdominal reflex is not abnormal, an asymmetric response may indicate spinal cord abnormalities.

Diagnostic Studies

With the information obtained from the history and physical, a focused approach to diagnostic studies can be taken. If the patient is aged 10 years or younger, has had pain for 2 months or longer, has night pain, had traumatic injury, or if there are constitutional symptoms, standard radiographs of the spine should be obtained at once. If the patient is older, the pain is of short duration with no major traumatic event, and the physical examination is completely normal, the patient may be observed for a short period of time. Most patients fall between these two groups; thus, the extent of the radiographic evaluation should be decided on an individual basis.

Radiographs

Plain radiographs are the best screening examination for the child with back pain.[19,23] Anteroposterior (AP) and lateral views of the spine should be obtained without pelvic shielding, as the shield hides the sacrum, sacroiliac (SI) joints, and pelvis. The physician should carefully examine the films for alignment, disc space narrowing, endplate irregularities, and lytic or blastic lesions. Each pedicle should be identified on the AP view. If a question of a lesion arises, a focused coned-down view taken with the patient supine provides better bony detail.

The lateral film should be reviewed for the presence of spondylolysis or spondylolisthesis. As on the AP view, if there is a question of lysis on the lateral view, a spot lateral of the lumbosacral junction better visualizes the pars interarticularis. Oblique views of the lumbosacral spine can also show the lysis; however, recent studies demonstrate that, in the majority of cases, oblique films do not improve the rate of diagnosis of spondylolysis.[18]

The identification of scoliosis on screening films of a child with back pain should not lead to the conclusion that the curve is the cause of the pain. Although up to 33% of adolescents diagnosed with scoliosis complain of some back pain, it is usually located over the rib prominence and is rarely a presenting complaint.[23] The apex of the curve should be carefully inspected for bony lesions in the child with painful scoliosis.

Bone Scan

If plain radiographs are normal, the neurologic examination is normal, but the symptoms of the patient are suggestive of bony pathology, a triphasic technetium bone scan is recommended. Scintigraphy is a highly sensitive but nonspecific tool to localize bony processes. Infection, most benign and malignant bony lesions, and stress fractures will have increased bone turnover, which is visualized as increased tracer uptake on scintigraphic images. Pinhole collimation is helpful in localizing the increased uptake. The study should include the SI joints and pelvis, as pathology in these areas often presents as back pain.

SPECT scanning combines the physiology of a bone scan with the ability to precisely localize lesions within the vertebra, similar to a CT scan. Increased uptake can be seen in the posterior elements in stress fractures; therefore, SPECT is particularly helpful in diagnosing spondylolysis.[24–27] A recent study of children younger than 10 years with back pain found SPECT to be highly sensitive for identifying injury to the pars.[28] Another study of 100 patients aged 2 to 18 years presenting with low back pain found that a negative SPECT scan was most helpful in ruling out an organic cause for back pain of less than 6 weeks' duration.[29]

Computed Tomography

Computed tomography (CT) provides the best imaging of the vertebral anatomy. It is not used as a screening tool, but it is useful when a lesion is seen on plain radiography or when plain radiography is negative but bone scintigraphy shows increased uptake. It can be used to assess the status of the pars interarticularis in patients with spondylolysis or to better delineate the extent of bony tumors. Although bone lesions can be seen on magnetic resonance imaging (MRI), surrounding edema may overestimate the extent of skeletal involvement.

Magnetic Resonance Imaging

MRI is used to image the neural axis in all children who have an abnormal neurologic examination. MRI is able to identify spinal neoplasms, cord abnormalities such as syringomyelia and tethers, discitis, and herniated discs, among other conditions. Auerbach and coworkers[29] recommend MRI as the best imaging modality for patients with low back pain of greater than 6 weeks' duration. In support of this, a recent study of pediatric patients found the incidence of abnormal pathology on MRI to be 34% in patients with constant pain, night pain, radicular pain, and abnormal neurologic examination.[30]

Laboratory Tests

Laboratory tests should be obtained at presentation in all young children with back pain and those with night pain, fever, malaise, or easy bruising. A complete blood count with differential should be obtained. The peripheral smear should be ordered to look for abnormal cell lines consistent with leukemia. The erythrocyte sedimentation rate and C-reactive protein should also routinely be studied because they are elevated in infection and malignancy. Urinalysis should be used to screen for renal conditions.

Differential Diagnosis

Muscle Strain

A very common cause of back pain, especially in athletic adolescents, is muscular strain, which can be up to 3 to 5 times more prevalent in elite athletes.[31] Pain can often be attributed to changes in amount and level of training, ill-fitting equipment, or poor technique. Poor strength of the back extensor and abdominal musculature, as well as tight hamstrings and hip flexor muscles, may be found in patients with muscular strain.[32] Absence of concerning history, such as night pain or radicular pain, and relation to activity can be helpful in excluding other more concerning diagnoses.

Treatment consisting of temporary activity modification, application of ice in the acute phase and heat later for spasm, in combination with nonsteroidal antiinflammatory drugs (NSAIDs), is often sufficient for most young adults. In patients who have failed these measures, a home physical therapy program for core and back strengthening, as well as hamstring stretching, may be prescribed. Important in the counseling of these patients is the emphasis that without regularly performing these exercises, there will be no significant improvement in pain. Return to activity is based on resolution of symptoms while continuing a core strengthening program as part of athletic training.

Disc Herniation

Intervertebral disc herniation occasionally occurs in older children and teens. The onset of symptoms is usually related to acute or repetitive trauma.[33] Of affected patients, 82% complain of back pain with radiation into the legs.[34] This radicular

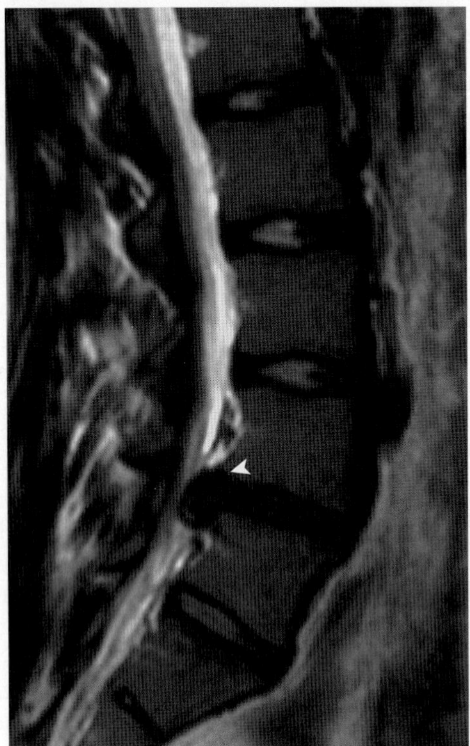

FIG. 25.1 Magnetic resonance image of a 16-year-old female with back and right leg pain demonstrates a herniated L4–L5 disc *(arrowhead)*.

pain is exacerbated by activity and relieved by rest. As in the adult population, the pain is worsened by sneezing, coughing, or straining. Recent studies have demonstrated a higher incidence of disc herniation in female patients and support that leg pain is the most common presenting complaint.[35]

Physical examination reveals decreased spinal flexibility, with inability to touch the toes. On bending toward the floor, the patient often lists to one side. The straight-leg raise test (Lasegue sign) is positive in 85% of children with herniated discs, while objective neurologic findings—such as absent reflexes, motor weakness, and decreased sensation—are less common in pediatric patients than in adults.[36] Hamstring tightness is often present and has been found to persist even after treatment of disc hernation.[37]

Radiographs are generally normal, although if sufficiently symptomatic, films may show an olisthetic scoliosis or trunk lean away from the side of herniation. There is an increased incidence of concomitant spinal abnormalities in patients with herniated discs. In particular, congenital spinal stenosis is frequently seen. Other findings include transitional vertebrae or spondylolisthesis.[38]

Disc herniation is seen best on MRI (Fig. 25.1). The involved disc is readily appreciated, and other processes that might produce sciatica, such as epidural abscess and spinal cord tumor, can be ruled out.[20] Herniation of the disc can be differentiated from an avulsed vertebral apophysis on either MRI or CT scan. Correlation of the MRI findings with the history and clinical examination is necessary, as mild disc bulging can exist as a normal variant.

Treatment is initially conservative, consisting of antiinflammatory medication and bed rest. Prolonged nonoperative management may lead to persistent pain, however; if the patient does not respond to symptomatic treatment, disc excision should be offered.[36] More urgent surgical intervention is indicated when a progressive neurologic deficit develops. Short-term results are very encouraging, with 95% good and excellent results and nearly universal resolution of back and leg pain.[36] Long-term follow-up, however, shows a deterioration in results, with a 24% reoperation rate after 30 years.[39] Outcome studies demonstrate that patients treated with discectomy as adolescents function better than adults following the same surgery.[40] Surgical technique is similar to that in adult patients.

Apophyseal Ring Fracture/Slipped Vertebral Apophysis

The apophyseal ring fracture, also known as a slipped vertebral apophysis, occurs in adolescents and young adults prior to fusion of the vertebral body to the cartilaginous ring apophysis. The etiology is either acute trauma resulting in rapid flexion and axial compression, or cumulative microtrauma. The fracture typically develops at the junction of the posteroinferior vertebral body and the cartilaginous ring apophysis, with posterior displacement of the fragment into the spinal canal.[41] CT can demonstrate the size and location of the bony fragment, with large central fragments being both most common and most likely to result in significant pain if left untreated.[42]

The symptoms are very similar to those of a herniated disc, with the sudden onset of severe back pain radiating into the leg. Physical examination will show a positive straight-leg raise test, but, as is the case with disc herniations, neurologic signs are infrequently present.

The diagnosis is made radiographically. High-quality lateral radiographs may show an arc-shaped rim of cartilage, cartilage with attached underlying bone, or a small triangular bony fragment lying posterior to the vertebral body. The fragment is best visualized on CT scan.[41] The levels most frequently injured are L4 or S1. Treatment is surgical excision of the avulsed fragment.

Vertebral Fractures

Pediatric patients with spine fractures present with back pain. If the energy of injury is sufficient enough that fracture is possible, radiographs should be obtained at once. When compression fractures are seen in children without high-energy trauma, an immediate evaluation should be performed for underlying malignancy. When patients have undergone high-energy trauma and fracture has been ruled out, however, the patient still complains of severe back pain, MRI may be indicated to rule out ligamentous injury, which can lead to instability in one or more of the spinal columns, especially in younger children.[43]

Developmental Disorders

Spondylolysis and Spondylolisthesis

Spondylolysis refers to a stress fracture of the pars interarticularis, occurring predominantly in the lower lumbar spine. The most frequent level is L5, followed by L4. It is extremely rare to have more than one vertebral level involved. Spondylolysis is bilateral in 80% of cases, and unilateral in 20%, although in certain athlete groups unilateral spondylolysis is more prevalent.[44]

Up to 50% of young athletes presenting for evaluation of back pain have injuries to the pars interarticularis.[45] The mechanism of injury is repetitive microtrauma in hyperextension, overloading the pars interarticularis and over time leading to stress fracture. Sports linked to a high incidence of spondylolysis are gymnastics, diving, ballet, and football. Gymnasts and football linemen have a fourfold increase in incidence of spondylolysis compared with the general pediatric population.[46]

Symptoms consist of low back pain, which is exacerbated by athletic activity and at least partly relieved by rest. The pain is present in the lower back, but can radiate into the legs.

Physical examination may reveal hamstring tightness and loss of normal lumbar mobility. The ability to bend forward to the floor may be diminished. In hyperflexible patients (e.g., gymnasts and ballerinas), motion may appear normal. The patient is usually tender to palpation about the lumbar spine. Hyperextension usually reproduces the back pain, and axial rotation in hyperextension exacerbates that pain.

Lateral radiographs may show lysis across the pars interarticularis, and oblique radiographs can be helpful in less obvious cases (Fig. 25.2). The appearance of a collar on the "Scottie dog" suggests stress fracture. Often, plain radiographs are nondiagnostic. In these cases, scintigraphy can reveal increased tracer uptake at the involved level. The use of the SPECT scan is particularly helpful in localizing increased uptake in the pars interarticularis[25,26,47] (Fig. 25.3). A specific scintigraphic pattern, seen as a triangle of increased signal with increased uptake in the pedicles, has been described.[48] Positive bone scans and SPECT imaging are generally seen in the prefracture state and in relatively acute injuries.[49] The bone scan may not be "hot" in chronic spondylolysis.[26]

MRI has also been used to diagnose spondylolysis, but false-positive scans do occur.[50] Better bony definition of the fracture is obtained using CT scans. Additionally, CT is superior to MRI in the assessment of incomplete fractures and in establishing healing in patients with spondylolysis.[51] The pars is best imaged by using a reverse gantry angle and obtaining thin slices on the CT.[52]

Spondylolysis and spondylolisthesis can produce scoliosis. Curves due to these conditions are usually described as olisthetic, are associated with oblique take-off of the spine from the pelvis, are small in degree, and have little rotation. Spondylolysis and spondylolisthesis occur in patients with idiopathic scoliosis more frequently than in the general population but are usually asymptomatic.

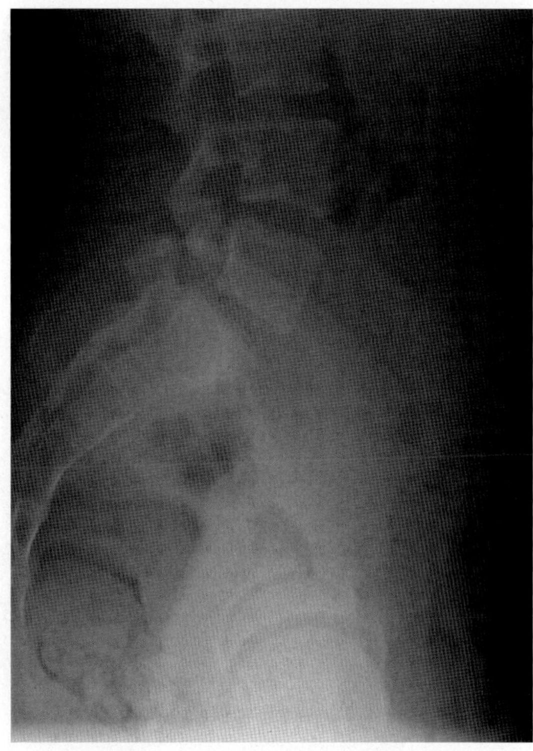

FIG. 25.2 Lateral radiograph of the lumbar spine shows spondylolysis of L5 in a 16-year-old volleyball player.

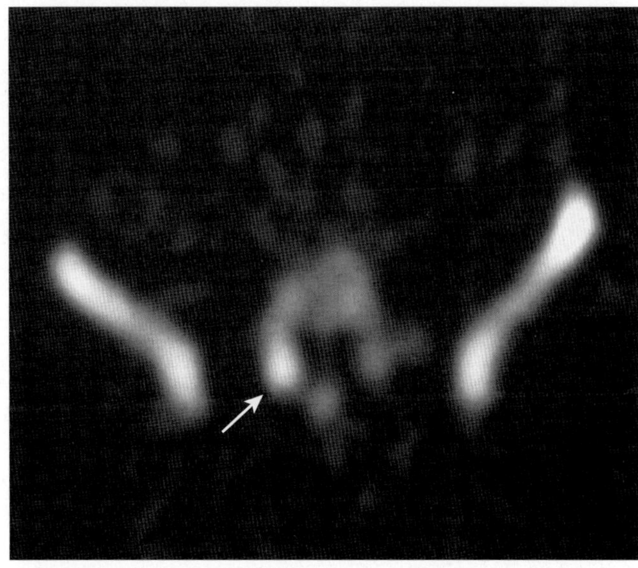

FIG. 25.3 Increased uptake in the pars interarticularis *(arrow)* of an adolescent ballerina with spondylolysis.

Treatment of spondylolysis is initially nonoperative and first involves modifying the patient's level of athletic activity.[53] Cessation of sport until the resolution of symptoms is combined with a concomitant exercise program to stretch the hamstrings and strengthen the paraspinal and abdominal musculature. Resumption of activities is gradual. Modification of the patient's technique or training should be made to minimize recurrent fractures. Use of an antilordotic lumbar orthosis increases the success of nonoperative treatment,

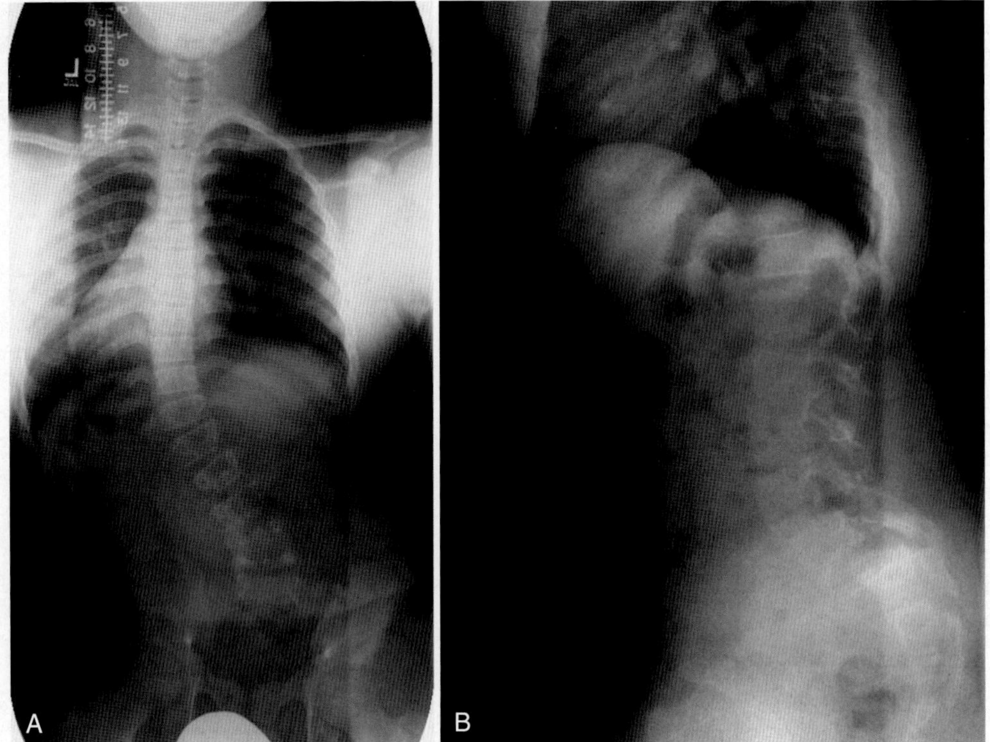

FIG. 25.4 (A) Scoliosis in a 13-year-old male with low back and leg pain of 6 months' duration. (B) Lateral radiograph shows spondylolisthesis at L5–S1.

particularly in patients with acute injuries and "hot" bone scans.[54,55] A recent study found resolution of symptoms following bracing correlated with initial increased activity on SPECT scans and decreased uptake on follow-up scans, while SPECT scans for patients whose pain did not improve showed no significant decrease in activity following bracing.[56] The overall success rate of nonoperative treatment ranges from 73% to 100%.[55] A recent multicenter study of 436 children and adolescents with CT-proven spondylolysis found 95% excellent results and 100% return to sport without surgery following 3 months of cessation of activity with use of a thoracolumbar orthosis.[57] Patients who have normal radiographs but are found to have a stress reaction without fracture on further imaging are highly likely to improve (and not progress to radiographic fracture) with conservative treatment.[58,59] Surgery is typically reserved for the few patients whose symptoms are refractory to 6 months of conservative measures and whose pain recurs with activity following initial nonoperative success.[60]

Spondylolisthesis is a related condition in which anterior slippage of a vertebral body occurs on the more distal vertebra. Most often it is due to bilateral spondylolysis, with the portion of the vertebra anterior to the pars fracture slipping anteriorly. Dysplastic spondylolisthesis occurs in teens who have an elongated but intact pars interarticularis, which allows for the anterior translation without pars fracture.[61]

Patients with spondylolisthesis often present with complaints of low back pain. The pain may radiate into the legs. Physical findings mimic those of spondylolysis, with the addition of a possible palpable step-off at the area of listhesis. In severe spondylolisthesis, the buttocks may appear "heart shaped." If there is significant hamstring tightness, gait alterations are seen where the teen appears to be shuffling with posterior pelvic tilt. Patients may have a painful, or olisthetic, scoliosis (Fig. 25.4).

Plain radiographs establish the diagnosis. The slip is easily seen on a spot lateral radiograph of the lumbosacral junction, and the severity of the spondylolisthesis can be classified as the percentage of forward translation of L5 on the sacrum. Abnormal kyphosis is also seen as the cephalad vertebra tips forward on the caudal segment. A characteristic finding on the AP radiograph, which is the appearance of "Napoleon's hat," can be seen as L5 moves forward on the sacrum and is seen in a nearly axial view.

Treatment is initially conservative in mild spondylolisthesis, and surgical as the magnitude of the slip increases. Surgical treatment of high-grade spondylolisthesis is recommended, but preferred techniques vary among surgeons and reduction remains controversial.[62]

Scheuermann Kyphosis

Scheuermann kyphosis is a developmental condition occurring in adolescence characterized by increased thoracic kyphosis accompanied by lumbar hyperlordosis. Males are affected slightly more frequently than females.

Presenting symptoms are those of back pain, which is usually located at the apex of the thoracic kyphosis, and also may be present in the lower lumbar spine. The pain is usually described as aching in nature, does not wake the patient from sleep, and does not radiate. It is exacerbated by vigorous activity and prolonged sitting. The severity of the back pain is variable, with some patients denying significant symptoms and instead presenting for evaluation of poor posture. Neurologic symptoms are highly unusual.

Physical examination of the patient with Scheuermann disease shows increased thoracic kyphosis, which is most notable on forward bending, in which the apex appears to protrude posteriorly. The deformity is usually fairly rigid, and does not disappear with hyperextension. There may be concomitant hamstring tightness, with inability to touch the floor with the fingertips.

The diagnosis is made radiographically (Fig. 25.5). Criteria for the diagnosis of Scheuermann disease have been outlined by Sorenson as:

1. three contiguous vertebral bodies with greater than 5 degrees of anterior wedging
2. abnormal disc narrowing
3. endplate irregularities
4. Schmorl nodes, defined as disc herniations into the vertebral bodies

The vast majority of patients with Scheuermann disease can be managed nonoperatively.[63] Physical therapy exercises and nonsteroidal medication can be helpful in relieving symptoms. The role of bracing is controversial. Patients with significant remaining spinal growth may benefit from orthotic treatment because it has been proposed that correction of deformity may be achieved in compliant patients.[64] The Milwaukee brace is the orthosis of choice for the treatment of Scheuermann disease.[65] Surgical correction of deformity and fusion is reserved for patients with severe kyphosis measuring greater than 75 degrees, those whose symptoms are refractory to conservative measures, and those who have significant cosmetic concerns.[66]

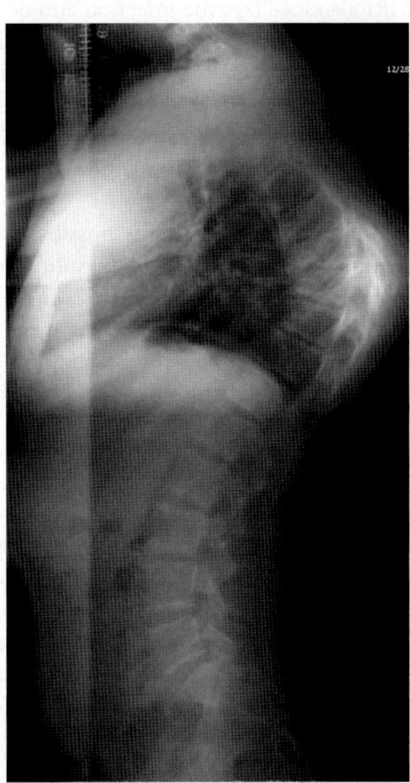

FIG. 25.5 Anterior wedging of the thoracic spine in a 15-year-old male with Scheuermann kyphosis.

Lumbar Scheuermann Disease

Lumbar Scheuermann disease is a less common variant in which increased kyphosis and endplate changes are seen in the lumbar spine.[67] It also occurs most frequently in adolescence, with overuse believed to be the cause. Microfractures occur in the vertebral endplates, resulting in low back pain. Radiographs reveal endplate irregularities and disc space narrowing, anterior Schmorl nodes, and possible anterior wedging of the affected vertebrae, leading to loss of lumbar lordosis. Radiographs may also show associated spondylolysis or scoliosis.[27,68] The radiographic appearance of vertebral changes and disc space narrowing may resemble infection or tumor. Scintigraphy may reveal mildly increased uptake at one or two vertebral levels.[27] MRI shows signal change and dehydration in the lumbar discs, with further disc deterioration occurring over time.[69] Treatment is symptomatic, and pain is usually ameliorated with modification of activity or use of an orthosis.

Idiopathic Scoliosis

The majority of patients who have idiopathic scoliosis do not complain of back pain, but symptoms are not as uncommon as previously thought. In a study by Ramirez and coworkers,[23] 32% of 2442 children believed to have idiopathic curves complained of some degree of back pain. The most common factor associated with a positive diagnosis on further evaluation were left-sided thoracic curves, which were associated with spinal cord abnormalities. Plain radiographs were found to be sufficient in the evaluation of typical curves if the neurologic examination was normal. Careful inspection of the apex of the deformity and at the lumbosacral junction (for spondylolysis and spondylolisthesis) will occasionally yield a cause for both the pain and the scoliosis (see Fig. 25.4). In the absence of neurologic findings on physical examination, MRI was not helpful. A recent study did show that MRI was useful in identifying neural axis abnormalities in 6% of 104 patients. Back pain and early age of onset of scoliosis were present in those with MRI abnormalities.[70]

Syringomyelia

Syringomyelia is defined as cystic dilation of the central canal of the spinal cord. The dilation of the cord leads to abnormalities in the neurologic pathways that transmit pain and temperature. While not always symptomatic, patients may complain of pain. There is a predisposition toward left thoracic scoliosis in patients with syringomyelia.[71] Physical findings include scoliosis, foot deformities such as cavus, decreased sensation, and asymmetric abdominal reflexes. The syrinx is clearly imaged on MRI. Treatment is neurosurgical decompression, although controversy exists regarding the size of syrinx that requires surgery.

Tethered Spinal Cord

Low back pain may be the presenting complaint in children with tethered spinal cords. The cord normally terminates at the L1–L2 level. Persistence of the cord more distally implies tethering. Physical findings may include foot deformity, spasticity, or weakness. Often, radiographs will show coexistent congenital vertebral abnormalities. The diagnosis is made on MRI, in which the filum may appear thickened or the conus visualized at L3 or distal. Treatment of the symptomatic tethered cord is surgical release, which is typically performed by a neurosurgeon.

Idiopathic Juvenile Osteoporosis

Idiopathic juvenile osteoporosis is a rare disease that usually affects children in the first 2 decades of life. Presenting symptoms include back and leg pain due to compression fractures and pain during weight bearing.[72,73] Radiographic findings include vertebral wedging due to compression fractures with mildly increased kyphosis. Bone mineral density is decreased, but metabolic laboratory values are normal. The differential diagnosis includes leukemia. Orthotic management of back pain is usually sufficient. Medical management should be under the supervision of a pediatric rheumatologist. The disease is self-limiting, and symptoms resolve during puberty.[74]

Infectious and Inflammatory Etiologies

Discitis

Discitis is defined as a presumed bacterial infection of the intervertebral disc space. It is the most common cause of back pain in the young child. The incidence of discitis is greatest in children aged 5 years and younger, though it can occur in older children.[75] The etiology is believed to be infectious. In the immature child, blood vessels traverse the vertebral endplates and terminate in the nucleus pulposus. Therefore, in young children the disc is vascular, which allows for seeding of bacteria into the disc space.[76–78] Presenting complaints vary, but include back pain, refusal to walk, limping, and abdominal pain. The child usually is systemically ill; therefore, the patient often presents to the emergency department. Approximately half will have fever on presentation.

Physical examination reveals spinal stiffness, and often the spine is held in a flexed position. If asked to retrieve a toy from the floor, the child with discitis will squat by bending the knees rather than bend the spine. Young children may exhibit Gower's sign when rising from the floor, using their upper extremities to push up on the legs as a strategy to minimize lumbar motion. Tenderness in palpation of the affected area can be present.

Radiographic findings are usually minimal at the time of presentation. Subtle disc space narrowing and paraspinal soft tissue swelling on the lateral view are the first radiographic changes (Fig. 25.6). Over time, endplate irregularities are seen. Because plain radiographs are usually normal at the time of presentation, further imaging is required. Technetium bone

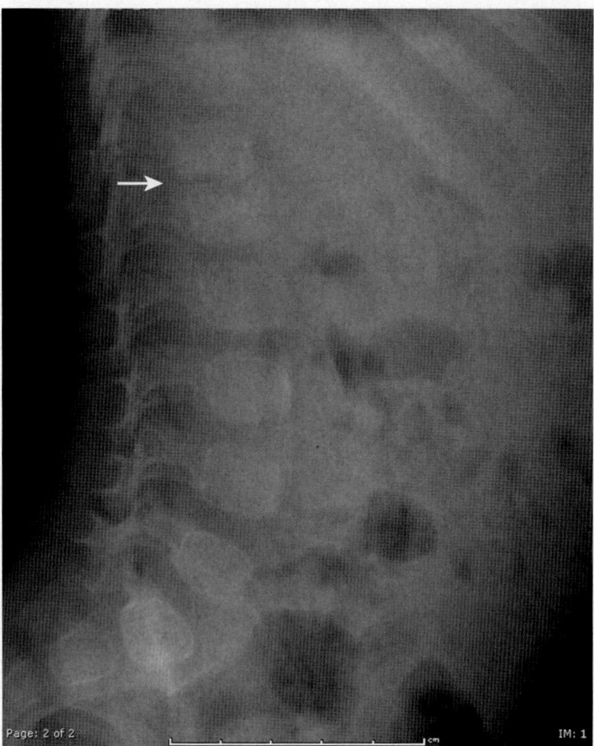

FIG. 25.6 Disc space narrowing *(arrow)* and endplate irregularities in a child with T11–T12 discitis.

scans show increased uptake on both sides of the affected disc space (Fig. 25.7A). Bone scans are positive in 74% to 100% of children with discitis[79,80] and can lead to earlier diagnosis and treatment. MRI also localizes the infection and delineates the extent of soft tissue involvement (Fig. 25.7B). In patients who are refractory to treatment, MRI is useful in assessing whether a soft tissue abscess is present.[81] MRI shows decreased signal on T1-weighted images and increased signal on T2 images. If an abscess is present, there is peripheral enhancement with the administration of gadolinium.[82]

The evaluation of the child with possible discitis also includes obtaining laboratory studies. Elevation of the sedimentation rate and C-reactive protein are seen in more than 90% of children with discitis.[20] The white blood cell count may be elevated but is less reliable.[76] Blood cultures should be obtained and are positive in more than 50% of children with discitis.[80]

In the past, the treatment of discitis was controversial, but now there is agreement that discitis represents a bacterial infection and should be treated with antibiotics.[76,81,83] Cultures of the intervertebral disc are positive in 60% of children, with *Staphylococcus aureus* the most common organism. A recent study of disc space cultures showed that *S. aureus* was cultured in 55% and *Kingella kingae* in 27% of children with discitis.[84] Because of the preponderance of *S. aureus*, and the fact that 40% of cultures from the disc space remain negative, routine aspiration of the affected disc is not recommended.[83] If the patient fails to improve quickly with antistaphylococcal antibiotics, then fine-needle aspiration under CT guidance can be useful.[85] Although administration of a second-generation

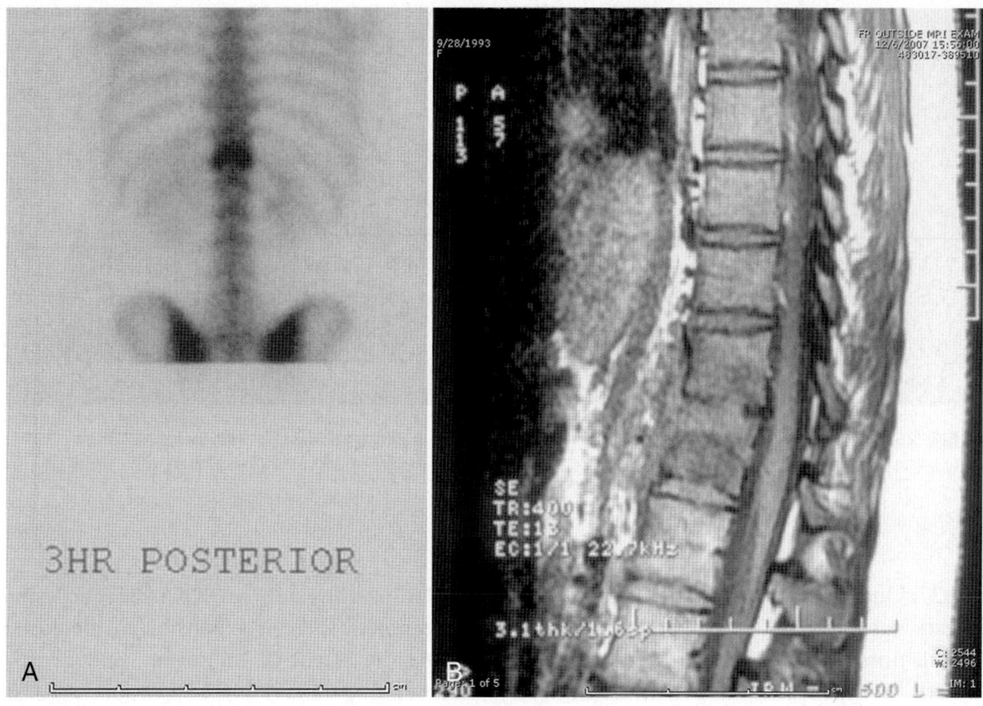

FIG. 25.7 (A) Bone scan in a child with discitis shows increased uptake. (B) Magnetic resonance image reveals destruction of the disc space, erosion of endplates, and vertebral involvement.

cephalosporin for 3 weeks has been recommended,[83] epidemiologic trends in antibiotic resistance may alter which antibiotic should be chosen. Surgical biopsy and debridement are reserved for patients who do not respond to medical management, have a neurologic deficit, have an abscess on MRI, or whose diagnosis is in question.

The outcome of pediatric discitis is favorable. Ten-year radiographic follow-up has shown narrowed disc space (60% of children) or bony ankylosis (40%), but kyphosis is rare and generally mild and patients are pain free.[86]

Disc space infection in children younger than 1 year is usually very aggressive and requires immediate diagnosis and treatment. Infants are often septic at presentation. Residual kyphosis following eradication of the infection has been described.[87]

Vertebral Osteomyelitis

The distinction between discitis and osteomyelitis in children is blurred. It is believed that osteomyelitis is a continuation of discitis,[77] with the two entities representing a condition called *infectious spondylitis*. Osteomyelitis produces more notable vertebral body radiographic changes. Again, *S. aureus* is the most common organism.[78]

Opportunistic infections may also affect the vertebral column, especially in immunocompromised patients such as those with malignancies or who have had organ transplants. Fungal infections such as coccidioidomycosis are rare but must be kept in mind in endemic regions.[88]

Tuberculosis is increasing in frequency and is seen most commonly in children from endemic regions. Symptoms include fever, malaise, weight loss, and night sweats. Neurologic findings occur more frequently in tuberculosis than in discitis.[89] Radiographic changes are more advanced in children with tuberculous spondylitis, and consist of bony destruction of the vertebral body, kyphosis, soft tissue abscesses, and soft tissue calcifications. CT scan findings include erosions with calcification, and intraspinous, paravertebral, and epidural abscesses.[90,91] A chest radiograph shows evidence of tuberculosis in 67% of children with tuberculous infection of the spine.[90] The purified protein derivative test is usually positive, except in the immunologically challenged child, in whom it remains nonreactive. Pathologic examination of tissue from fine-needle aspiration of the affected bone yields a positive diagnosis in 83% of children and teens[92] and shows epithelioid giant cells and caseous necrosis or tubercle bacilli. Polymerase chain reaction has been used for faster identification of the organism.

Ankylosing Spondylitis and Rheumatologic Conditions

Ankylosing spondylitis is a rheumatologic condition characterized by loss of spinal mobility. It may present in adolescence as back pain. It occurs more frequently in males than in females. Physical findings include loss of lumbar flexibility so that lordosis does not reverse on forward flexion, increased kyphosis, and limited chest expansion with inspiration. Plain radiographs may reveal sclerosis, narrowing, or fusion of the SI joints. MRI has been shown to be superior to bone scan in identifying inflammation of the SI joint.[93,94] Laboratory evaluation of patients with ankylosing spondylitis shows a high

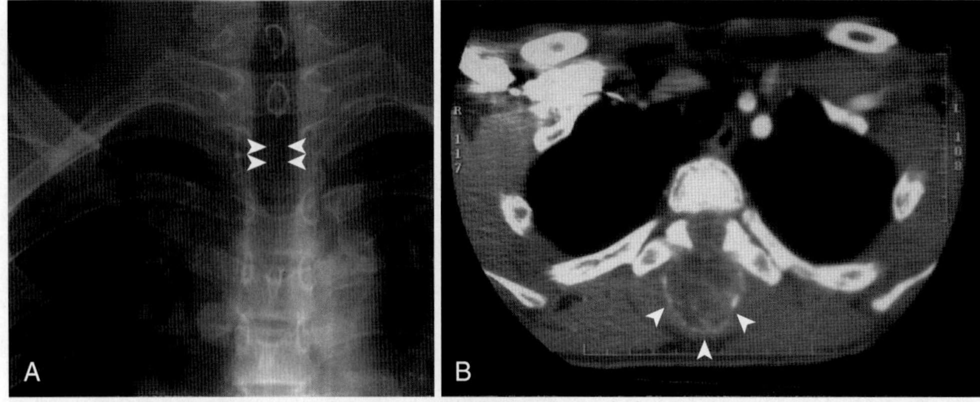

FIG. 25.8 (A) Anteroposterior radiograph of the thoracic spine of a 16-year-old male with lower extremity weakness and loss of bladder function shows absence of the spinous process at T2 *(arrowheads)*. (B) Computed tomographic scan delineates the extent of the aneurysmal bone cyst of the posterior elements of T2 *(arrowheads)*.

incidence of HLA-B27. Onset of ankylosing spondylitis prior to the age of 16 years has been linked to worse functional outcomes than in adult-onset patients.[95] Other rheumatologic conditions linked with back pain include polymyositis, dermatomyositis, and inflammatory bowel disease.

Hematologic Conditions

Sickle Cell Anemia

In a recent study of pediatric patients presenting to a Canadian emergency department for the evaluation of back pain, 13% were found to have sickle cell anemia.[22] The spine has been reported as the second most common site for pain crisis in these patients, second only to the knee. Anemia is present in 86%.[96] Physical examination reveals tenderness to palpation. Treatment is pain management and admission to the hematology service.

β-Thalassemia may also produce pain crises that affect the spine. Up to 25% of patients with thalassemia complained of low back pain in a recent study.[97]

Neoplasms

Aneurysmal Bone Cysts

Aneurysmal bone cysts (ABCs) are nonmalignant expansile lytic lesions of bone characterized by their vascularity. Although not malignant tumors, they can be locally aggressive. Their etiology remains unclear, and a few familial cases have been identified.[98] Approximately 15% of ABCs affect the spinal column, with a predilection for the posterior elements. If of sufficient size, the lesion may extend into the anterior column.[99,100] A large multicenter series of spinal aneurysmal bone cysts documented that 30% were located in the cervical spine, 30% in the thoracic spine, and 40% in the lumbar spine.[101]

Symptoms consist of back pain that can result from the lesion itself, or from an associated pathologic fracture. Neurologic compromise is unusual.

Radiographs show an expansile lytic lesion with a "bubbly" appearance. There is expansion of the cortex. CT scans best define the extent of the lesion, and reveal the thin rim of surrounding bone (Fig. 25.8). On occasion, sacral lesions have been shown to affect more than one vertebral level.[102]

Treatment of ABCs is surgical curettage with bone grafting.[103] Due to the vascularity of the cysts, preoperative embolization is very helpful in reducing intraoperative blood loss and therefore improving visualization.[104–106] Spinal cord monitoring during embolization has been advocated to avoid vascular injury to the spinal cord.[107] Scheduling the surgical resection shortly following embolization is necessary to prevent revascularization of the lesion prior to curettage. When resection of the lesion leads to mechanical instability, simultaneous fusion is recommended.[108] There is a 10% to 14% recurrence rate following curettage and grafting for spinal ABCs. A four-step surgical program—consisting of curettage, use of a high-speed burr, electrocautery, and bone grafting, with stabilization via short posterior fusion with instrumentation as needed—has been recently proposed, with all patients free from disease at follow-up.[109]

Repeat embolizations as well as radionuclide ablation have been used to definitively treat spinal ABCs in limited cases.[106] Repeat embolization has been advocated in patients who do not have neurologic findings or pathologic fracture, for whom the diagnosis is certain, or in patients whose lesions have recurred.[110]

Osteoid Osteoma

Osteoid osteomas are the most common benign spinal tumor occurring in children, with presentation occurring in the second decade of life. They typically are located in the posterior elements of the spine. Osteoid osteomas produce back pain that is worse at night, and ameliorated by aspirin or nonsteroidal medication.

Physical examination reveals decreased spinal flexibility. Often, the patient will stand with a list. The neurologic examination is generally normal.

Plain radiographs are usually insufficient to make the diagnosis, but an olisthetic scoliosis might be apparent. When scoliosis is present, the lesion is usually located in the concavity of the apex of the curve.[111] Bone scan is positive, with distinct increased uptake seen (Fig. 25.9). CT scans provide the best imaging of osteoid osteomas, with a small radiolucent nidus and surrounding sclerosis and new bone apparent (Fig. 25.10). MRI shows increased signal intensity in the muscles and surrounding bone.[112] The MRI appearance, as well as the tendency for enhancement in the soft tissues near the lesion, may lead the physician to suspect a malignant tumor.[113]

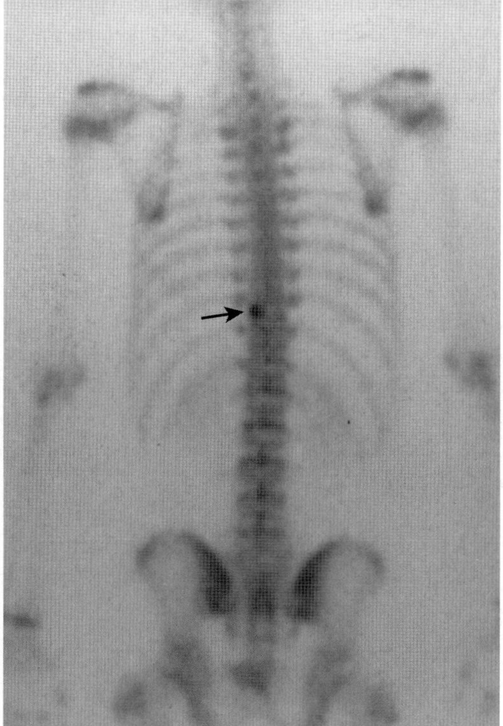

FIG. 25.9 Bone scan of a 15-year-old male with a 2-year history of back pain shows increased uptake at T10 *(arrow)*.

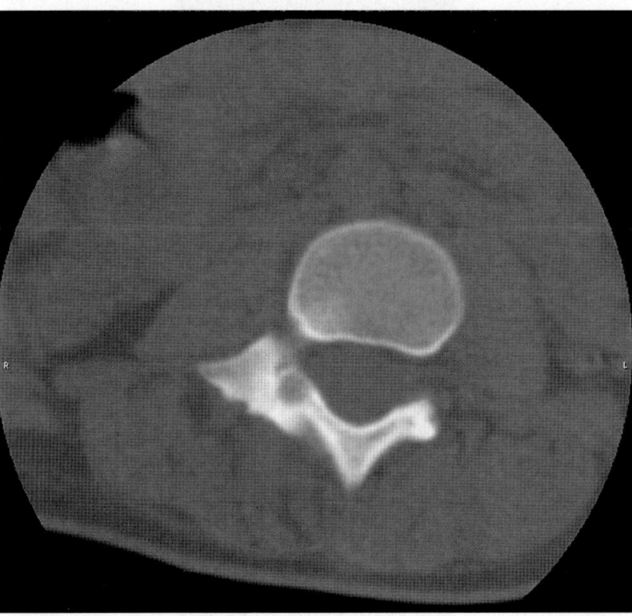

FIG. 25.10 Computed tomographic scan shows a radiolucent nidus with surrounding bony sclerosis in an 11-year-old with back pain due to an osteoid osteoma.

Long-term administration of NSAIDs can provide pain relief in a small group of patients with spinal osteoid osteomas; thus, a trial of nonsurgical treatment is warranted. Usually, symptoms are sufficient to merit surgical removal of the nidus, which typically results in immediate relief of pain. Intraoperative CT imaging has been used to better target the nidus and therefore minimize bony resection.[114] Newer treatments are under investigation, including percutaneous CT-guided burring of the nidus and thermocoagulation.[115,116] When scoliosis has been long-standing, persistence of the deformity is possible following successful removal of the osteoid osteoma.

Osteoblastoma

Although osteoblastoma is a less common benign lesion of the spine, 40% of osteoblastomas are located in the vertebrae. They also are located in the posterior elements of the spine, but because they are by definition larger than osteoid osteomas, they often extend anteriorly into the vertebral bodies.[117] The primary symptom of osteoblastoma is back pain, which is usually less severe than in osteoid osteoma. Neurologic abnormalities may result based simply on the size of the lesion and its encroachment on the spinal canal or neural foramina.[112]

The lesion can be usually seen on plain radiographs, but CT scans are invaluable in assessing the size and extent of the osteoblastoma. As in osteoid osteoma, the MRI in osteoblastoma can overestimate the extent and aggressiveness of the lesion.[118] Plain radiographs also reveal scoliosis in approximately 40% of affected patients.[111]

Treatment is surgical removal of the lesion, with fusion as needed to address instability based on the size of resection. Recurrence occurs in 10% of osteoblastomas.

Eosinophilic Granuloma/Langerhans Cell Histiocytosis

Eosinophilic granuloma, also known as Langerhans cell histiocytosis (LCH) or histiocytosis X, is a peculiar condition of childhood typified by the development of lytic lesions of bone. The lesions may occur singly or affect multiple areas of the skeleton, including the spine. When the condition is associated with systemic involvement, it is known as Hand-Schuller-Christian disease or the more severe Letterer-Siwe disease. LCH has a higher incidence in males. The average age at diagnosis is 6 years, with the majority of patients in their first decade of life.[119]

Vertebral lesions in LCH occur in 10% to 17% of affected children. The patients may present with back pain or a limp. On occasion, neurologic signs can be present.

Radiographs show lytic lesions within the vertebral body or, more rarely, the posterior elements. Larger lesions lead to collapse of the vertebral body, which can be either symmetric or asymmetric (Fig. 25.11). Although vertebra plana (also known as coin-on-end appearance) is the classically described spinal lesion in LCH, it has been reported that only 40% of children with LCH and vertebral lesions have vertebra plana.[120] Skeletal surveys often result in the identification of other sites of involvement, which supports the diagnosis. Typical sites of involvement include the skull, the pelvis, and the diaphysis of the long bones. Bone scan is positive in 90% of children with LCH.[121]

The differential diagnosis includes leukemia, infection, and other malignant tumors, such as Ewing sarcoma.[122] If the radiographic appearance is atypical and other peripheral skeletal lesions are not identified, a surgical biopsy of the spinal lesion is warranted. Pathologic specimens show clonal proliferation of Langerhans-type histiocytes, eosinophils, and giant cells.[123]

Most patients with LCH experience spontaneous resolution of their disease. Because the condition appears to be self-limiting, the indications for treatment are few. Back pain due to a unifocal spinal lesion can usually be relieved by rest and the use of orthoses.[119,123] Patients with neurologic compromise may be treated with low-dose radiation therapy or surgical debridement of the lesion and stabilization.[121,124] Radiation therapy has fallen out of favor as treatment for LCH of the spine due to the potential for secondary malignancies. Multifocal disease, particularly when associated with systemic involvement, is treated with chemotherapy.[125]

The long-term outcome of LCH in the absence of systemic disease is very good. Recurrence of disease is not seen in children.[125,126] Over time, improvement in vertebral body height is seen, although complete restoration to normal is unusual.[127,128]

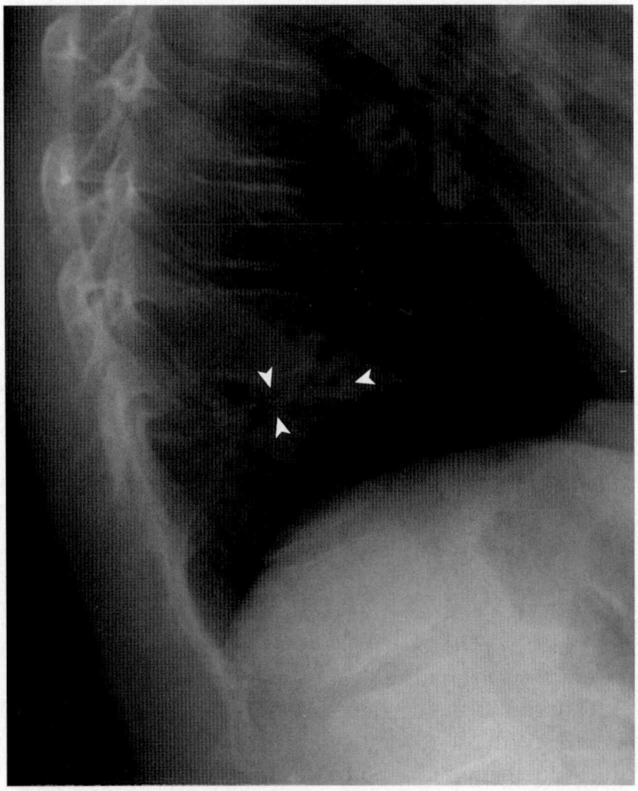

Malignant Tumors

Leukemia

Leukemia is the most common pediatric malignancy that produces back pain. Many children first present to the orthopaedic surgeon; reports indicate that 6% to 25% of children with acute leukemia present initially with back pain.[129,130] Many of these children are initially misdiagnosed; thus, the orthopaedic surgeon must have a high level of suspicion to properly evaluate this population.[131] The history may reveal symptoms of pallor, fatigue, loss of appetite, or fever. The parent should be questioned about a history of bruising or abnormal bleeding.

Radiographic findings are not always initially present but include generalized osteopenia, vertebral compression fractures, and metaphyseal leukemic lines. Of children with acute lymphoblastic leukemia, 7% have vertebral compression fractures[130,132] (Fig. 25.12).

The diagnosis can usually be made on laboratory examination, with abnormalities seen in any or all of the three cell lines, that is, anemia, thrombocytopenia, and leukopenia. The sedimentation rate is usually elevated. Of children with leukemia, 10% or more will initially have normal automated counts.[132,133] Inspection of the peripheral smear will reveal the diagnosis in some of these children.

Chemotherapy under the direction of pediatric oncology is the treatment of choice. Spinal bracing can be prescribed to relieve back pain and prevent further compression fractures.

FIG. 25.11 Lateral radiograph of a 12-year-old male with vertebra plana of T11 consistent with eosinophilic granuloma *(arrowheads)*. Back pain resolved with conservative treatment.

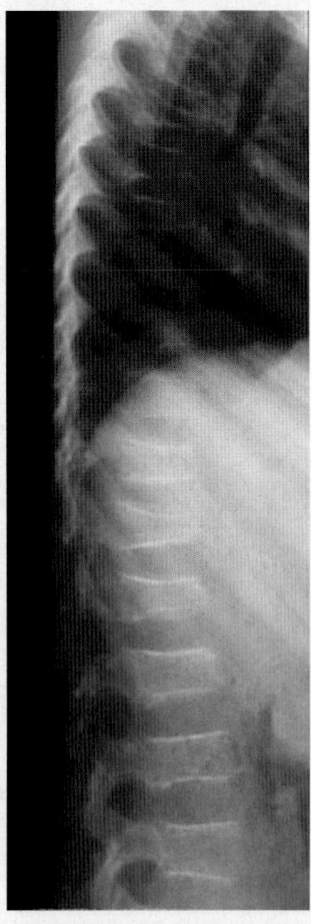

FIG. 25.12 Osteopenia and multiple compression fractures in a child presenting with back pain due to leukemia.

Vertebral Malignant Tumors

Malignant tumors of the spine cause significant back pain in over 50% of children at the time of diagnosis.[134] Although rare, they must remain in the differential diagnosis of pediatric back pain. Pain may radiate into the legs, resembling the symptoms of a herniated disc. While patients with disc herniation are in their second decade of life, children with spinal or spinal cord tumors may be younger. Neurologic deficits and reflex changes are uncommon in disc herniation but frequent in tumors.[135]

Vertebral tumors include Ewing sarcoma and osteosarcoma.[136] Osteosarcoma rarely affects the spine.[137] Radiographs are variable, with osteolytic, osteoblastic, and mixed appearances possible. CT and MRI are used to stage the tumor. Treatment is difficult.

Up to 10% of Ewing sarcomas occur in the spine, with the sacrum the most frequent site.[138] The average age at presentation is 13.3 years.[139] Symptoms consist of relentless back pain. Neurologic deficits are present in 58% of patients with spinal Ewing tumors.[140] Radiographs may show an expansile lytic lesion with variable vertebral collapse. Cases of Ewing sarcoma that radiographically resemble vertebra plana have been reported, leading to the misdiagnosis of eosinophilic granuloma.[140] MRI delineates the extent of the lesion and its accompanying soft tissue mass.

Spinal Metastasis

Neuroblastoma is the most frequent tumor to metastasize to the spine in children.[141] In a recent study of 29 malignant spine tumors, neuroblastoma represented one-third of all cases.[134] Radiographs usually show diffuse vertebral involvement. The thoracic spine is most frequently involved. An elevation of urinary normetanephrine may help diagnosis.[138] Other tumors that involve the spine include rhabdomyosarcoma, Wilms tumor, and primary neuroectodermal tumors.[142]

Spinal Cord Tumors

Common spinal cord tumors in children are astrocytomas and ependymomas. The onset of symptoms is indolent. Neurologic signs such as deterioration of gait, delay in motor skills, and loss of bladder control raise suspicion.[143–145] Back pain is usually present, leading to initial referral to the orthopaedic surgeon in 31% to 58% of patients who are eventually diagnosed with spinal cord tumors.[143,144] Physical examination reveals motor deficits, clonus, and possibly scoliosis. There may be limitation of spinal flexibility. Radiographs can show changes due to pressure or expansion of the tumor, including absence or thinning of the pedicle or widening of the intervertebral foramina. Spinal cord tumors are best seen on MRI.

Although uncommon, neurofibromas in children and adolescents with neurofibromatosis can undergo malignant degeneration into neurofibrosarcoma. Back pain in a patient with neurofibromatosis should be evaluated.

Nonorthopaedic Causes of Pain

Intraabdominal processes such as inflammatory bowel disease, hydronephrosis, ovarian cysts, endometriosis, and urinary tract infections can produce back pain. Pain due to these conditions is not exacerbated by activity and tends to be more intense at night. Pediatric referral should be made when nonmusculoskeletal causes are suspected.

Psychosomatic Pain (Conversion Reaction)

As discussed in the beginning of this chapter, there are children in whom an organic etiology for back pain cannot be found despite thorough evaluation. Back pain can be influenced by psychosocial factors that alter the patient's perception of pain and the effect of pain on everyday life. Psychosomatic pain remains a diagnosis of exclusion. It is more prevalent in adolescence, particularly in those teens whose family members have a history of similar back pain. A detailed social history often reveals problems at home or school, often resulting in anxiety and depression. Treatment is difficult but includes intervention by a psychologist and physical therapy. Recent studies show that up to 71% of children and adolescents who have negative diagnostic evaluations for back pain continue to have pain at an average of 4.4 years of follow-up.[19] Even 8 years after initial evaluation, 62% of 58 patients were still symptomatic.[146]

KEY POINTS

Use of Diagnostic Tests

Radiograph: History of significant trauma; night pain, fever or inability to walk; age 8 years or younger; duration of pain greater than 2 months

Bone scan: Negative plain radiograph with normal neurologic examination, persistent pain, history of athletic overuse

CT scan: Positive plain radiograph or bone scan

MRI: Abnormal neurologic examination, painful scoliosis in patient younger than 8 years, painful left thoracic scoliosis

Laboratory tests: Night pain, fever, age younger than 8 years, constant pain

Likely Diagnoses Based on Age

Younger than 5 years: Tumor, discitis

Age 5 to 10 years: LCH, discitis, tumor/leukemia

Age 10 to 18 years: Musculoskeletal back pain, lumbar Scheuermann disease, herniated disc or apophysis, spondylolysis, osteoid osteoma, tumor/leukemia

REFERENCES

1. Aartun E, Hartvigsen J, Wedderkopp N, Hestbaek L. Spinal pain in adolescents: prevalence, incidence, and course: a school-based two-year prospective cohort study in 1,300 Danes aged 11-13. *BMC Musculoskelet Disord.* 2014; 15(1):187.

2. Jeffries LJ, Milanese SF, Grimmer-Somers KA. Epidemiology of adolescent spinal pain: a systematic overview of the research literature. *Spine*. 2007;32(23):2630-2637.
3. Yang S, Werner BC, Singla A, Abel MF. Low back pain in adolescents: a 1-year analysis of eventual diagnoses. *J Pediatr Orthop*. 2015. Epub ahead of print.
4. Burton AK, Clarke RD, McClune TD, Tillotson KM. The natural history of low back pain in adolescents. *Spine*. 1996;21(20):2323-2328.
5. Balagué F, Skovron ML, Nordin M, et al. Low back pain in schoolchildren. A study of familial and psychological factors. *Spine*. 1995;20(11):1265-1270.
6. Harreby M, Nygaard B, Jessen T, et al. Risk factors for low back pain in a cohort of 1389 Danish school children: an epidemiologic study. *Eur Spine J*. 1999;8(6):444-450.
7. Olsen TL, Anderson RL, Dearwater SR, et al. The epidemiology of low back pain in an adolescent population. *Am J Public Health*. 1992;82(4):606-608.
8. Wedderkopp N, Leboeuf-Yde C, Andersen LB, Froberg K, Hansen HS. Back pain reporting pattern in a Danish population-based sample of children and adolescents. *Spine*. 2001;26(17):1879-1883.
9. Stanford EA, Chambers CT, Biesanz JC, Chen E. The frequency, trajectories and predictors of adolescent recurrent pain: a population-based approach. *Pain*. 2008;138(1):11-21.
10. King S, Chambers CT, Huguet A, et al. The epidemiology of chronic pain in children and adolescents revisited: a systematic review. *Pain*. 2011;152(12):2729-2738.
11. Olsen TL, Anderson RL, Dearwater SR, et al. The epidemiology of low back pain in an adolescent population. *Am J Public Health*. 1992;82(4):606-608.
12. Aartun E, Hartvigsen J, Wedderkopp N, Hestbaek L. Spinal pain in adolescents: prevalence, incidence, and course: a school-based two-year prospective cohort study in 1,300 Danes aged 11-13. *BMC Musculoskelet Disord*. 2014; 15(1):187.
13. Turner PG, Green JH, Galasko CS. Back pain in childhood. *Spine*. 1989;14(8):812-814.
14. Hensinger RN. Back pain in children. In: Bradford DS, Hensinger RN, eds. *The Pediatric Spine*. New York: Thieme; 1985:41.
15. Feldman DS, Straight JJ, Badra MI, Mohaideen A, Madan SS. Evaluation of an algorithmic approach to pediatric back pain. *J Pediatr Orthop*. 2006;26(3):353-357.
16. Combs JA, Caskey PM. Back pain in children and adolescents: a retrospective review of 648 patients. *South Med J*. 1997;90(8):789-792.
17. Kandwal P, Vijayaraghavan G, Goswami A, Jayaswal A. Back pain in children—how sinister? *Indian J Pediatr*. 2016;83: 834-843.
18. Miller R, Beck NA, Sampson NR, et al. Imaging modalities for low back pain in children: a review of spondylosis and undiagnosed mechanical back pain. *J Pediatr Orthop*. 2013;33(3):282-288.
19. Feldman DS, Hedden DM, Wright JG. The use of bone scan to investigate back pain in children and adolescents. *J Pediatr Orthop*. 2000;20(6):790-795.
20. Ginsburg G, Bassett G. Back pain in children and adolescents: evaluation and differential diagnosis. *J Am Acad Orthop Surg*. 1997;5(2):67-78.
21. Micheli LJ, Wood R. Back pain in young athletes. Significant differences from adults in causes and patterns. *Arch Pediatr Adolesc Med*. 1995;149(1):15-18.
22. Selbst SM, Lavelle JM, Soyupak SK, Markowitz RI. Back pain in children who present to the emergency department. *Clin Pediatr (Phila)*. 1999;38(7):401-406.
23. Ramirez N, Johnston CE, Browne RH. The prevalence of back pain in children who have idiopathic scoliosis. *J Bone Joint Surg Am*. 1997;79(3):364-368.
24. Bellah RD, Summerville DA, Treves ST, Micheli LJ. Low-back pain in adolescent athletes: detection of stress injury to the pars interarticularis with SPECT. *Radiology*. 1991;180(2):509-512.
25. Bodner RJ, Heyman S, Drummond DS, Gregg JR. The use of single photon emission computed tomography (SPECT) in the diagnosis of low-back pain in young patients. *Spine*. 1988;13(10):1155-1160.
26. Lusins JO, Elting JJ, Cicoria AD, Goldsmith SJ. SPECT evaluation of lumbar spondylolysis and spondylolisthesis. *Spine*. 1994;19(5):608-612.
27. Mandell GA, Morales RW, Harcke HT, Bowen JR. Bone scintigraphy in patients with atypical lumbar Scheuermann disease. *J Pediatr Orthop*. 1993;13(5):622-627.
28. Spencer HT, Sokol LO, Glotzbecker MP, et al. Detection of pars injury by SPECT in patients younger than age 10 with low back pain. *J Pediatr Orthop*. 2013;33(4): 383-388.
29. Auerbach JD, Ahn J, Zgonis MH, et al. Streamlining the evaluation of low back pain in children. *Clin Orthop Relat Res*. 2008;466(8):1971-1977.
30. Ramirez N, Flynn JM, Hill BW, et al. Evaluation of a systematic approach to pediatric back pain: the utility of magnetic resonance imaging. *J Pediatr Orthop*. 2015;35(1):28-32.
31. van Hilst J, Hilgersom NFJ, Kuilman MC, Kuijer PP, Frings-Dresen MHW. Low back pain in young elite field hockey players, football players and speed skaters: prevalence and risk factors. *J Back Musculoskelet Rehabil*. 2015;28(1):67-73.
32. Harvey J, Tanner S. Low back pain in young athletes. A practical approach. *Sports Med*. 1991;12(6):394-406.
33. Grobler LJ, Simmons EH, Barrington TW. Intervertebral disc herniation in the adolescent. *Spine*. 1979;4(3):267-278.
34. Parisini P, Di Silvestre M, Greggi T, Miglietta A, Paderni S. Lumbar disc excision in children and adolescents. *Spine*. 2001;26(18):1997-2000.
35. Frino J, McCarthy RE, Sparks CY, McCullough FL. Trends in adolescent lumbar disk herniation. *J Pediatr Orthop*. 2006;26(5):579-581.
36. DeLuca PF, Mason DE, Weiand R, Howard R, Bassett GS. Excision of herniated nucleus pulposus in children and adolescents. *J Pediatr Orthop*. 1994;14(3):318-322.
37. Zhu Q, Gu R, Yang X, et al. Adolescent lumbar disc herniation and hamstring tightness: review of 16 cases. *Spine*. 2006;31(16):1810-1814.
38. Epstein JA, Epstein NE, Marc J, Rosenthal AD, Lavine LS. Lumbar intervertebral disk herniation in teenage children: recognition and management of associated anomalies. *Spine*. 1984;9(4):427-432.
39. Luukkonen M, Partanen K, Vapalahti M. Lumbar disc herniations in children: a long-term clinical and magnetic resonance imaging follow-up study. *Br J Neurosurg*. 1997;11(4):280-285.
40. Durham SR, Sun PP, Sutton LN. Surgically treated lumbar disc disease in the pediatric population: an outcome study. *J Neurosurg*. 2000;92(suppl 1):1-6.

41. Takata K, Inoue S, Takahashi K, Ohtsuka Y. Fracture of the posterior margin of a lumbar vertebral body. *J Bone Joint Surg Am*. 1988;70(4):589-594.
42. Chang C-H, Lee Z-L, Chen W-J, Tan C-F, Chen L-H. Clinical significance of ring apophysis fracture in adolescent lumbar disc herniation. *Spine*. 2008;33(16):1750-1754.
43. Knox JB, Schneider JE, Cage JM, Wimberly RL, Riccio AI. Spine trauma in very young children: a retrospective study of 206 patients presenting to a level 1 pediatric trauma center. *J Pediatr Orthop*. 2014;34(7):698-702.
44. Scheepers MS, Streak Gomersall J, Munn Z. The effectiveness of surgical versus conservative treatment for symptomatic unilateral spondylolysis of the lumbar spine in athletes: a systematic review. *JBI Database System Rev Implement Rep*. 2015;13(3):137-173.
45. Sassmannshausen G, Smith BG. Back pain in the young athlete. *Clin Sports Med*. 2002;21(1):121-132.
46. Jackson DW, Wiltse LL, Cirincoine RJ. Spondylolysis in the female gymnast. *Clin Orthop Relat Res*. 1976;117:68-73.
47. Lawrence JP, Greene HS, Grauer JN. Back pain in athletes. *J Am Acad Orthop Surg*. 2006;14(13):726-735.
48. Van der Wall H, Storey G, Magnussen J, et al. Distinguishing scintigraphic features of spondylolysis. *J Pediatr Orthop*. 2002;22(3):308-311.
49. Dutton JA, Hughes SP, Peters AM. SPECT in the management of patients with back pain and spondylolysis. *Clin Nucl Med*. 2000;25(2):93-96.
50. Yamane T, Yoshida T, Mimatsu K. Early diagnosis of lumbar spondylolysis by MRI. *J Bone Joint Surg Br*. 1993;75(5):764-768.
51. Campbell RSD, Grainger AJ, Hide IG, Papastefanou S, Greenough CG. Juvenile spondylolysis: a comparative analysis of CT, SPECT and MRI. *Skeletal Radiol*. 2005;34(2):63-73.
52. Harvey CJ, Richenberg JL, Saifuddin A, Wolman RL. The radiological investigation of lumbar spondylolysis. *Clin Radiol*. 1998;53(10):723-728.
53. Smith JA, Hu SS. Management of spondylolysis and spondylolisthesis in the pediatric and adolescent population. *Orthop Clin North Am*. 1999;30(3):487-499–ix.
54. d'Hemecourt PA, Zurakowski D, Kriemler S, Micheli LJ. Spondylolysis: returning the athlete to sports participation with brace treatment. *Orthopedics*. 2002;25(6):653-657.
55. Morita T, Ikata T, Katoh S, Miyake R. Lumbar spondylolysis in children and adolescents. *J Bone Joint Surg Br*. 1995;77(4):620-625.
56. Anderson K, Sarwark JF, Conway JJ, Logue ES, Schafer MF. Quantitative assessment with SPECT imaging of stress injuries of the pars interarticularis and response to bracing. *J Pediatr Orthop*. 2000;20(1):28-33.
57. Kurd MF, Patel D, Norton R, et al. Nonoperative treatment of symptomatic spondylolysis. *J Spinal Disord Tech*. 2007;20(8):560-564.
58. Sys J, Michielsen J, Bracke P, Martens M, Verstreken J. Nonoperative treatment of active spondylolysis in elite athletes with normal X-ray findings: literature review and results of conservative treatment. *Eur Spine J*. 2001;10(6):498-504.
59. Takemitsu M, Rassi El G, Woratanarat P, Shah SA. Low back pain in pediatric athletes with unilateral tracer uptake at the pars interarticularis on single photon emission computed tomography. *Spine*. 2006;31(8):909-914.
60. Cavalier R, Herman MJ, Cheung EV, Pizzutillo PD. Spondylolysis and spondylolisthesis in children and adolescents: I. Diagnosis, natural history, and nonsurgical management. *J Am Acad Orthop Surg*. 2006;14(7):417-424.
61. Lonstein JE. Spondylolisthesis in children. Cause, natural history, and management. *Spine*. 1999;24(24):2640-2648.
62. Cheung EV, Herman MJ, Cavalier R, Pizzutillo PD. Spondylolysis and spondylolisthesis in children and adolescents: II. Surgical management. *J Am Acad Orthop Surg*. 2006;14(8):488-498.
63. Tribus CB. Scheuermann's kyphosis in adolescents and adults: diagnosis and management. *J Am Acad Orthop Surg*. 1998;6(1):36-43.
64. Pizzutillo PD. Nonsurgical treatment of kyphosis. *Instr Course Lect*. 2004;53:485-491.
65. Sachs B, Bradford D, Winter R, et al. Scheuermann kyphosis. Follow-up of Milwaukee-brace treatment. *J Bone Joint Surg Am*. 1987;69(1):50-57.
66. Lowe TG. Scheuermann's disease. *Orthop Clin North Am*. 1999;30(3):475-487.
67. Blumenthal SL, Roach J, Herring JA. Lumbar Scheuermann's. A clinical series and classification. *Spine*. 1987;12(9):929-932.
68. Ogilvie JW, Sherman J. Spondylolysis in Scheuermann's disease. *Spine*. 1987;12(3):251-253.
69. Heithoff KB, Gundry CR, Burton CV, Winter RB. Juvenile discogenic disease. *Spine*. 1994;19(3):335-340.
70. Benli IT, Uzümcügil O, Aydin E, et al. Magnetic resonance imaging abnormalities of neural axis in Lenke type 1 idiopathic scoliosis. *Spine*. 2006;31(16):1828-1833.
71. Akhtar OH, Rowe DE. Syringomyelia-associated scoliosis with and without the Chiari I malformation. *J Am Acad Orthop Surg*. 2008;16(7):407-417.
72. Dimar JR, Campbell M, Glassman SD, Puno RM, Johnson JR. Idiopathic juvenile osteoporosis. An unusual cause of back pain in an adolescent. *Am J Orthop*. 1995;24(11):865-869.
73. Smith R. Idiopathic juvenile osteoporosis: experience of twenty-one patients. *Br J Rheumatol*. 1995;34(1):68-77.
74. Tortolani PJ, McCarthy EF, Sponseller PD. Bone mineral density deficiency in children. *J Am Acad Orthop Surg*. 2002;10(1):57-66.
75. Early SD, Kay RM, Tolo VT. Childhood diskitis. *J Am Acad Orthop Surg*. 2003;11(6):413-420.
76. Ring D, Johnston CE, Wenger DR. Pyogenic infectious spondylitis in children: the convergence of discitis and vertebral osteomyelitis. *J Pediatr Orthop*. 1995;15(5):652-660.
77. Song KS, Ogden JA, Ganey T, Guidera KJ. Contiguous discitis and osteomyelitis in children. *J Pediatr Orthop*. 1997;17(4):470-477.
78. Tay BK-B, Deckey J, Hu SS. Spinal infections. *J Am Acad Orthop Surg*. 2002;10(3):188-197.
79. Crawford AH, Kucharzyk DW, Ruda R, Smitherman HC. Diskitis in children. *Clin Orthop Relat Res*. 1991;266:70-79.
80. Wenger DR, Bobechko WP, Gilday DL. The spectrum of intervertebral disc-space infection in children. *J Bone Joint Surg Am*. 1978;60(1):100-108.
81. Ring D, Wenger DR. Magnetic resonance-imaging scans in discitis. Sequential studies in a child who needed operative drainage: a case report. *J Bone Joint Surg Am*. 1994;76(4):596-601.
82. Lac du P, Panuel M, Devred P, Bollini G, Padovani J. MRI of disc space infection in infants and children. Report of 12 cases. *Pediatr Radiol*. 1990;20(3):175-178.
83. Glazer PA, Hu SS. Pediatric spinal infections. *Orthop Clin North Am*. 1996;27(1):111-123.

84. Garron E, Viehweger E, Launay F, et al. Nontuberculous spondylodiscitis in children. *J Pediatr Orthop.* 2002;22(3):321-328.
85. Hoffer FA, Strand RD, Gebhardt MC. Percutaneous biopsy of pyogenic infection of the spine in children. *J Pediatr Orthop.* 1988;8(4):442-444.
86. Kayser R, Mahlfeld K, Greulich M, Grasshoff H. Spondylodiscitis in childhood: results of a long-term study. *Spine.* 2005;30(3):318-323.
87. Eismont FJ, Bohlman HH, Soni PL, Goldberg VM, Freehafer AA. Vertebral osteomyelitis in infants. *J Bone Joint Surg Br.* 1982;64(1):32-35.
88. Wrobel CJ, Chappell ET, Taylor W. Clinical presentation, radiological findings, and treatment results of coccidioidomycosis involving the spine: report on 23 cases. *J Neurosurg.* 2001;95(suppl 1):33-39.
89. Mushkin AY, Kovalenko KN. Neurological complications of spinal tuberculosis in children. *Int Orthop.* 1999;23(4):210-212.
90. Magnus KG, Hoffman EB. Pyogenic spondylitis and early tuberculous spondylitis in children: differential diagnosis with standard radiographs and computed tomography. *J Pediatr Orthop.* 2000;20(4):539-543.
91. Morris BS, Varma R, Garg A, Awasthi M, Maheshwari M. Multifocal musculoskeletal tuberculosis in children: appearances on computed tomography. *Skeletal Radiol.* 2002;31(1):1-8.
92. Francis IM, Das DK, Luthra UK, et al. Value of radiologically guided fine needle aspiration cytology (FNAC) in the diagnosis of spinal tuberculosis: a study of 29 cases. *Cytopathology.* 1999;10(6):390-401.
93. Blum U, Buitrago-Tellez C, Mundinger A, et al. Magnetic resonance imaging (MRI) for detection of active sacroiliitis–a prospective study comparing conventional radiography, scintigraphy, and contrast enhanced MRI. *J Rheumatol.* 1996;23(12):2107-2115.
94. Kurugoglu S, Kanberoglu K, Kanberoglu A, Mihmanli I, Cokyuksel O. MRI appearances of inflammatory vertebral osteitis in early ankylosing spondylitis. *Pediatr Radiol.* 2002;32(3):191-194.
95. Stone M, Warren RW, Bruckel J, et al. Juvenile-onset ankylosing spondylitis is associated with worse functional outcomes than adult-onset ankylosing spondylitis. *Arthritis Rheum.* 2005;53(3):445-451.
96. Roger E, Letts M. Sickle cell disease of the spine in children. *Can J Surg.* 1999;42(4):289-292.
97. Onur O, Sivri A, Gümrük F, Altay C. Beta thalassaemia: a report of 20 children. *Clin Rheumatol.* 1999;18(1):42-44.
98. DiCaprio MR, Murphy MJ, Camp RL. Aneurysmal bone cyst of the spine with familial incidence. *Spine.* 2000;25(12):1589-1592.
99. Hay MC, Paterson D, Taylor TK. Aneurysmal bone cysts of the spine. *J Bone Joint Surg Br.* 1978;60-B(3):406-411.
100. Vergel De Dios AM, Bond JR, Shives TC, McLeod RA, Unni KK. Aneurysmal bone cyst. A clinicopathologic study of 238 cases. *Cancer.* 1992;69(12):2921-2931.
101. Cottalorda J, Kohler R, Sales de Gauzy J, et al. Epidemiology of aneurysmal bone cyst in children: a multicenter study and literature review. *J Pediatr Orthop B.* 2004;13(6):389-394.
102. Papagelopoulos PJ, Choudhury SN, Frassica FJ, et al. Treatment of aneurysmal bone cysts of the pelvis and sacrum. *J Bone Joint Surg Am.* 2001;83-A(11):1674-1681.
103. Papagelopoulos PJ, Currier BL, Shaughnessy WJ, et al. Aneurysmal bone cyst of the spine. Management and outcome. *Spine.* 1998;23(5):621-628.
104. De Cristofaro R, Biagini R, Boriani S, et al. Selective arterial embolization in the treatment of aneurysmal bone cyst and angioma of bone. *Skeletal Radiol.* 1992;21(8): 523-527.
105. de Kleuver M, van der Heul RO, Veraart BE. Aneurysmal bone cyst of the spine: 31 cases and the importance of the surgical approach. *J Pediatr Orthop B.* 1998;7(4):286-292.
106. DeRosa GP, Graziano GP, Scott J. Arterial embolization of aneurysmal bone cyst of the lumbar spine. A report of two cases. *J Bone Joint Surg Am.* 1990;72(5):777-780.
107. Berenstein A, Young W, Ransohoff J, Benjamin V, Merkin H. Somatosensory evoked potentials during spinal angiography and therapeutic transvascular embolization. *J Neurosurg.* 1984;60(4):777-785.
108. Ozaki T, Halm H, Hillmann A, Blasius S, Winkelmann W. Aneurysmal bone cysts of the spine. *Arch Orthop Trauma Surg.* 1999;119(3-4):159-162.
109. Garg S, Mehta S, Dormans JP. Modern surgical treatment of primary aneurysmal bone cyst of the spine in children and adolescents. *J Pediatr Orthop.* 2005;25(3):387-392.
110. Boriani S, De Iure F, Campanacci L, et al. Aneurysmal bone cyst of the mobile spine: report on 41 cases. *Spine.* 2001;26(1):27-35.
111. Saifuddin A, White J, Sherazi Z, et al. Osteoid osteoma and osteoblastoma of the spine. Factors associated with the presence of scoliosis. *Spine.* 1998;23(1):47-53.
112. Ozaki T, Liljenqvist U, Hillmann A, et al. Osteoid osteoma and osteoblastoma of the spine: experiences with 22 patients. *Clin Orthop Relat Res.* 2002;397:394-402.
113. Lefton DR, Torrisi JM, Haller JO. Vertebral osteoid osteoma masquerading as a malignant bone or soft-tissue tumor on MRI. *Pediatr Radiol.* 2001;31(2):72-75.
114. Rajasekaran S, Kamath V, Shetty AP. Intraoperative Iso-C three-dimensional navigation in excision of spinal osteoid osteomas. *Spine.* 2008;33(1):E25-E29.
115. Baunin C, Puget C, Assoun J, et al. Percutaneous resection of osteoid osteoma under CT guidance in eight children. *Pediatr Radiol.* 1994;24(3):185-188.
116. Cové JA, Taminiau AH, Obermann WR, Vanderschueren GM. Osteoid osteoma of the spine treated with percutaneous computed tomography-guided thermocoagulation. *Spine.* 2000;25(10):1283-1286.
117. Boriani S, Capanna R, Donati D, et al. Osteoblastoma of the spine. *Clin Orthop Relat Res.* 1992;278:37-45.
118. Shaikh MI, Saifuddin A, Pringle J, Natali C, Sherazi Z. Spinal osteoblastoma: CT and MR imaging with pathological correlation. *Skeletal Radiol.* 1999;28(1):33-40.
119. Levine MJ, McGuire KJ, McGowan KL, Flynn JM. Assessment of the test characteristics of C-reactive protein for septic arthritis in children. *J Pediatr Orthop.* 2003;23(3):373-377.
120. Floman Y, Bar-On E, Mosheiff R, et al. Eosinophilic granuloma of the spine. *J Pediatr Orthop B.* 1997;6(4): 260-265.
121. Ghanem I, Tolo VT, D'Ambra P. Malogalowkin MH. Langerhans cell histiocytosis of bone in children and adolescents. *J Pediatr Orthop.* 2003;23(1):124-130.
122. Papagelopoulos PJ, Currier BL, Galanis E, et al. Vertebra plana caused by primary Ewing sarcoma: case report and review of the literature. *J Spinal Disord Tech.* 2002;15(3):252-257.

123. Willman CL, Busque L, Griffith BB, et al. Langerhans'-cell histiocytosis (histiocytosis X)–a clonal proliferative disease. *N Engl J Med*. 1994;331(3):154-160.
124. Yeom JS, Lee CK, Shin HY, et al. Langerhans' cell histiocytosis of the spine. Analysis of twenty-three cases. *Spine*. 1999;24(16):1740-1749.
125. Garg S, Mehta S, Dormans JP. Langerhans cell histiocytosis of the spine in children. Long-term follow-up. *J Bone Joint Surg Am*. 2004;86-A(8):1740-1750.
126. Plasschaert F, Craig C, Bell R, et al. Eosinophilic granuloma. A different behaviour in children than in adults. *J Bone Joint Surg Br*. 2002;84(6):870-872.
127. Mammano S, Candiotto S, Balsano M. Cast and brace treatment of eosinophilic granuloma of the spine: long-term follow-up. *J Pediatr Orthop*. 1997;17(6):821-827.
128. Raab P, Hohmann F, Kühl J, Krauspe R. Vertebral remodeling in eosinophilic granuloma of the spine. A long-term follow-up. *Spine*. 1998;23(12):1351-1354.
129. Rogalsky RJ, Black GB, Reed MH. Orthopaedic manifestations of leukemia in children. *J Bone Joint Surg Am*. 1986;68(4):494-501.
130. Kobayashi D, Satsuma S, Kamegaya M, et al. Musculoskeletal conditions of acute leukemia and malignant lymphoma in children. *J Pediatr Orthop B*. 2005;14(3):156-161.
131. Santangelo JR, Thomson JD. Childhood leukemia presenting with back pain and vertebral compression fractures. *Am J Orthop*. 1999;28(4):257-260.
132. Meehan PL, Viroslav S, Schmitt EW. Vertebral collapse in childhood leukemia. *J Pediatr Orthop*. 1995;15(5):592-595.
133. Kayser R, Mahlfeld K, Nebelung W, Grasshoff H. Vertebral collapse and normal peripheral blood cell count at the onset of acute lymphatic leukemia in childhood. *J Pediatr Orthop B*. 2000;9(1):55-57.
134. Conrad EU, Olszewski AD, Berger M, Powell E, Bruckner J. Pediatric spine tumors with spinal cord compromise. *J Pediatr Orthop*. 1992;12(4):454-460.
135. Martínez-Lage JF, Martínez Robledo A, López F, Poza M. Disc protrusion in the child. Particular features and comparison with neoplasms. *Childs Nerv Syst*. 1997;13(4):201-207.
136. Garg S, Dormans JP. Tumors and tumor-like conditions of the spine in children. *J Am Acad Orthop Surg*. 2005;13(6):372-381.
137. Shives TC, Dahlin DC, Sim FH, Pritchard DJ, Earle JD. Osteosarcoma of the spine. *J Bone Joint Surg Am*. 1986;68(5):660-668.
138. Dormans JP, Moroz L. Infection and tumors of the spine in children. *J Bone Joint Surg Am*. 2007;89(suppl 1):79-97.
139. Venkateswaran L, Rodriguez-Galindo C, Merchant TE, et al. Primary Ewing tumor of the vertebrae: clinical characteristics, prognostic factors, and outcome. *Med Pediatr Oncol*. 2001;37(1):30-35.
140. Grubb MR, Currier BL, Pritchard DJ, Ebersold MJ. Primary Ewing's sarcoma of the spine. *Spine*. 1994;19(3):309-313.
141. Leeson MC, Makley JT, Carter JR. Metastatic skeletal disease in the pediatric population. *J Pediatr Orthop*. 1985;5(3):261-267.
142. Lam CH, Nagib MG. Nonteratomatous tumors in the pediatric sacral region. *Spine*. 2002;27(11):E284-E287.
143. Parker AP, Robinson RO, Bullock P. Difficulties in diagnosing intrinsic spinal cord tumours. *Arch Dis Child*. 1996;75(3):204-207.
144. Peña M, Galasko CS, Barrie JL. Delay in diagnosis of intradural spinal tumors. *Spine*. 1992;17(9):1110-1116.
145. Newton HB, Newton CL, Gatens C, Hebert R, Pack R. Spinal cord tumors: review of etiology, diagnosis, and multidisciplinary approach to treatment. *Cancer Pract*. 1995;3(4):207-218.
146. Mirovsky Y, Jakim I, Halperin N, Lev L. Non-specific back pain in children and adolescents: a prospective study until maturity. *J Pediatr Orthop B*. 2002;11(4):275-278.

CHAPTER 26 Congenital Scoliosis

Alexandra Miller Dunham
Paul D. Sponseller

Congenital scoliosis is a three-dimensional deformity of the spine that is directly due to congenitally anomalous vertebral development. This results in an imbalance of the longitudinal growth of the spine, which is most typically progressive in nature. By definition, this is different from neuromuscular scoliosis, in which deformity is secondary to myoneural causes, and idiopathic scoliosis, the cause of which is unknown.

Some cases of congenital scoliosis cause such minor deformity that they remain undetected; thus, the true incidence in the general population remains difficult to determine. However, current estimates suggest that approximately one in 1000 persons is affected.[1,2]

The familial incidence in the congenital scoliosis population is estimated between 1% and 5%, suggesting that most cases appear to be sporadic.[3–6] The male/female ratio for congenital scoliosis is 1 : 1.4.[7–9]

To fully understand the management of congenital scoliosis, one must first appreciate the foundation of how the deformity develops in utero. This discussion encompasses embryology as it relates to the bony etiology of deformity and associated differences, a classification system that aids in understanding growth potential, the natural history of curve progression, assessment of the patient, various imaging modalities and their unique utility, and, finally, treatment modalities.

Embryology

Congenital scoliosis is accurately described as altered embryologic development of the spine. Depending on which step of development is altered, spine morphology will be differently impacted. The bony malformations that cause congenital scoliosis typically occur during the fourth through sixth weeks of gestation. This timing is of particular importance, as it explains why patients with congenital scoliosis often have additional associated anomalies, which likely develop during the same intrauterine time period as other organ systems are similarly developing.

Normal Development

In the process of somitogenesis, paired paraxial mesoderms on either side of the notochord condense to form somites. Each somite further differentiates into a ventral sclerotome and a dorsolateral dermomyotome. During the fourth week of gestation, cells from each sclerotome migrate ventrally to fully engulf the notochord. The cranial half of one sclerotome and the caudal half of the adjacent sclerotome fuse, each contributing a portion of cells to the development of a single vertebra. Thus, a single vertebra results from the proper formation and migration of cells from two somite levels (Fig. 26.1). The ventrally migrated cells of the sclerotome will go on to form the vertebral body, and the dorsal portion of the sclerotome will form the vertebral arch as well as costal processes.[10]

Ossification begins during the sixth week of gestation from three primary ossification centers: one in the body (or centrum, formed by early fusion of two centers) and one in each half of the vertebral arch. During the sixth week of development, mesenchymal cells between cranial and caudal parts of the original sclerotome fill the space between two vertebral bodies to contribute to formation of the intervertebral structures.[11]

Somitogenesis relies on the oscillatory expression of several genes and gene products, some of which have been elucidated. Principal gene networks influence *Notch, Wnt,* and *FGF* pathway targets.[12–15] The networks responsible for putative segmentation appear to be regulated by cell-autonomous oscillations between permissive and nonpermissive states in a consistently timed manner, so much so that somitogenesis is said to be coordinated by a "clock-and-wave" mechanism[16,17] (Fig. 26.2). One of the many key outputs of the clock mechanism is the interval production of *MESP2* transcription factor, which has been implicated in the formation of somite boundaries and the rostrocaudal development of the sclerotome.[18,19]

Associated Anomalies

Because the development of the spine coincides with the development of many other organ systems, associated anomalies occur in 30% to 60% of children with congenital spine malformations. Many associated anomalies are part of the VATER association. The acronym includes various deficiencies: vertebral defects (V), anal atresia (A), tracheoesophageal fistula (TE), radial limb reduction, and renal defects (R). The acronym VATER was modified in 1975 to VACTERLS by adding cardiac defect (C) and limb defect (L)[20–22] and single umbilical artery (S; Fig. 26.3). The most common anomalies involve the spinal cord, the genitourinary tract, and the cardiac system. Intraspinal anomalies include problems such as tethered cord, diastematomyelia, syringomyelia/Chiari malformations, and intradural lipomas (present in up to 35% of patients with congenital scoliosis). The most common genitourinary defects are horseshoe kidney, renal aplasia, ectopic kidney, duplication, reflux, and hypospadias (present in up to 20% of patients with congenital scoliosis). Congenital heart defects range from the more common atrial and ventricular septal defects to the more complex tetralogy of Fallot, transposition of the great vessels (present in up to 25% of patients with congenital scoliosis).[23,24]

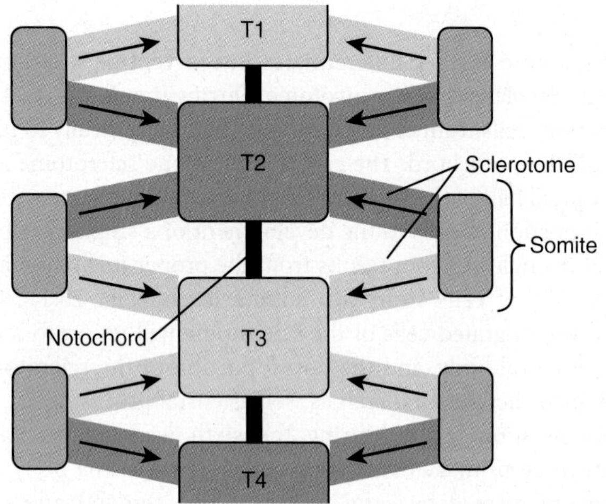

FIG. 26.1 Each vertebra is formed by a part of four somites.

Genetic Etiology

Mutations in downstream components and targets of the Notch signaling pathway contribute to observed congenital vertebral malformation phenotypes in humans,[25] which are mirrored in mouse models. Specifically, genetic mapping has enabled the identification of three forms of spondylocostal dysostosis (SCD): mutations of *DLL3*[26–29] to *SCD1, MESP2* to *SCD2,*[30–32] and *LFNG* to *SCD3.*

Alagille syndrome is an autosomal dominant condition characterized by bile duct, heart, eye, kidney, pancreas, and facial anomalies, as well as butterfly vertebral anomalies.[33,34] Vertebral anomalies are observed in 22% to 87% of patients with Alagille syndrome. Mutations in *JAG1* have been identified in approximately 70% of patients with Alagille syndrome.[35] Additionally, mutations in Notch2 have been observed, especially in those with severe renal anomalies.[36]

Congenital vertebral anomalies are also found with a high incidence in Klippel-Feil syndrome, which is characterized by the combination of cervical fusion, limited neck range of motion, short neck, and low hairline.[37] Various genetic anomalies have been reported to occur in association with Klippel-Feil syndrome including *SLIT3, FBXW11, DUSP1, FGF18, DC-UbP,* and *CDCA2.*[25,38]

Additionally, congenital scoliosis has been associated with Sprengel deformity, Mayer-Rokitansky-Küster-Hauser syndrome, Jarcho-Levin syndrome, Goldenhar syndrome, Genoa syndrome,[39–42] and many others.

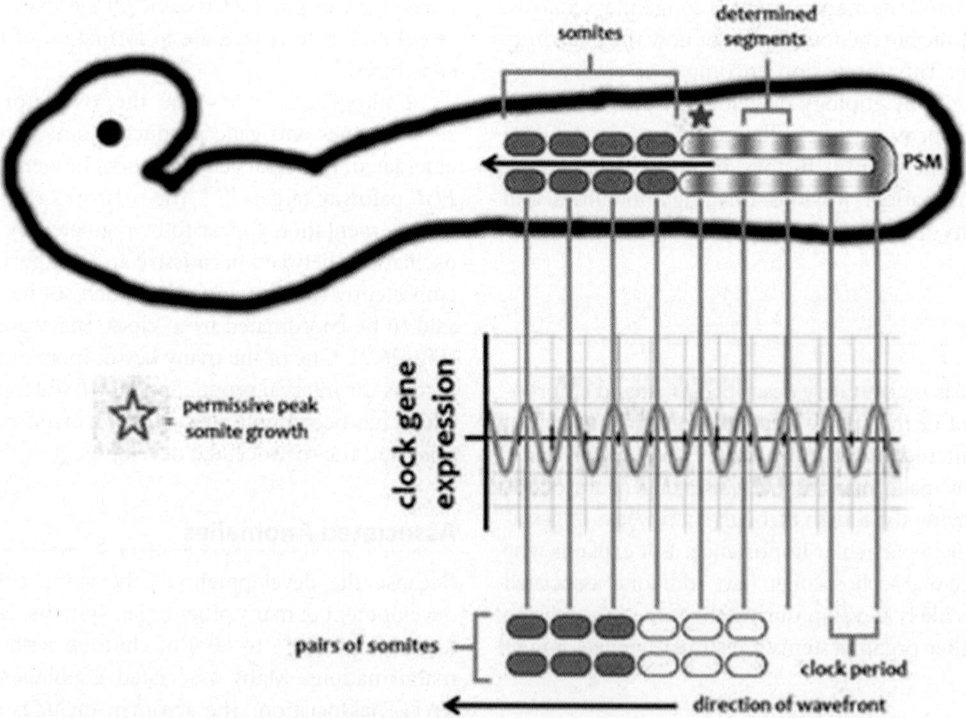

FIG. 26.2 Illustration of "clock-and-wave" mechanism of somitogenesis segmentation. Oscillatory gene expressions allow the development of "permissive peaks," leading to somite formation. Shorter clock periods lead to shorter somites and shorter intersomite spacing. PSM, presomitic mesoderm.

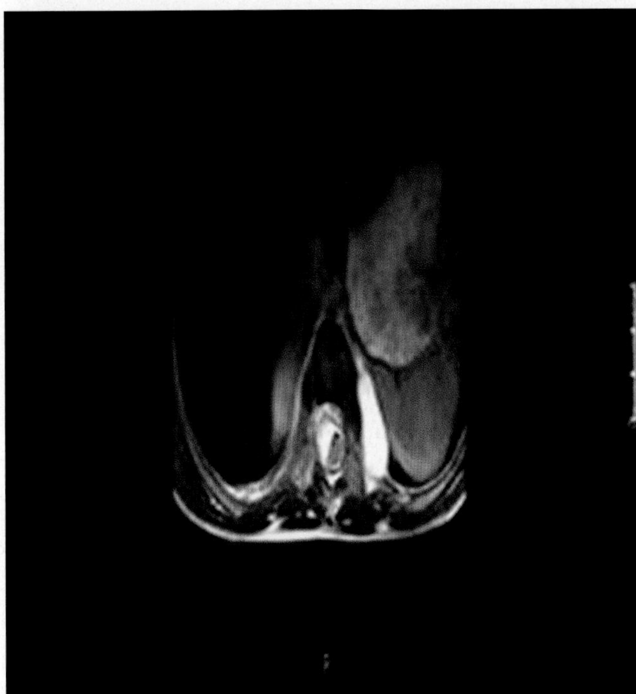

FIG. 26.3 Computed tomographic image of a 6-year-old child with congenital scoliosis who also has epidural lipoma and neurenteric cyst at T12.

Environmental Etiology

Growing evidence continues to suggest that congenital scoliosis is not strictly a genetically caused anomaly. Studies in mice suggest that maternal exposure to medications or toxins, such as carbon monoxide, alcohol, boric acid, and/or valproic acid, may cause congenital scoliosis.[43–48] Aberrations in the developmental milieu have also been associated with vertebral malformations consistent with congenital scoliosis such as hyperglycemia, hypoxia, and hyperthermia.[45,49–51] The causative mechanism underlying the carbon monoxide effect on vertebral anomalies remains vague. However, maternal acute exposure to carbon monoxide during embryo somitogenesis may act via gene mutation from the resulting hypoxia or directly by disruption of the cartilaginous spine.

The interplay between genetics and environmental factors is complex. Epigenetic factors in the development of congenital vertebral malformations are a possible pursuit.[52] The observation that increased DNA methylation can alter the phenotypic expression of tail kinks in the axin-fused mouse (AxinFu) supports an epigenetic contribution to congenital scoliosis.[43,53] The literature continues to grow in elucidating the multiple factors of pathogenesis of congenital vertebral malformations.

Classification

Two basic types of vertebral anomalies occur: failures of formation and failures of segmentation.[54-57] These anomalies can occur as a solitary malformation or in conjunction with additional vertebral malformations, adding complexity to the resulting deformity with each additional malformation.

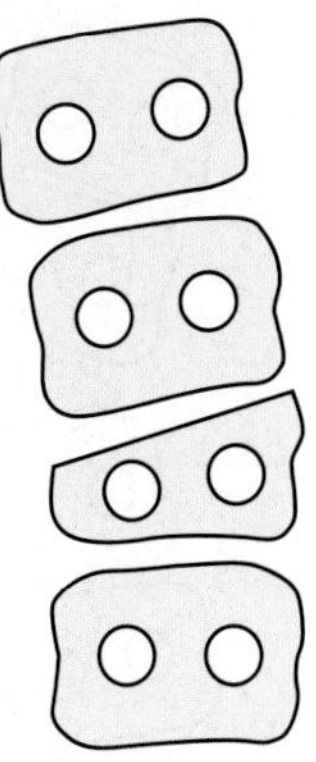

FIG. 26.4 Wedge vertebrae due to a mild form of unilateral vertebral failure of formation. Vertebral height is asymmetrical on the right and left sides.

As in other types of scoliosis, compensatory curves also develop.

Failures of Formation

Failures of formation (type I deformity) exist along a broad spectrum and have multiple subtypes characterized by longitudinal growth potential. Formation deformity can be partial, which causes wedged vertebrae with intact pedicles, or complete, which causes hemivertebrae with a unilateral pedicle (Fig. 26.4). Vertebral growth typically is provided by apophyses on both the superior and inferior endplate of each vertebra. In vertebrae affected by failure of formation, the apophyses may be disrupted, thus affecting growth and lending a natural method to the subtyping of type I deformity.

- *Fully segmented*: Both the superior and inferior endplates of the affected vertebrae have growth potential, with disc space both above and below. Adjacent vertebrae are normal.
- *Semisegmented*: Either the superior or inferior endplate of the affected vertebrae has growth potential, with normal disc space with the adjacent vertebrae; the other end is fused to the adjacent vertebrae with an intervening thin, fibrous lamellar tissue (Fig. 26.5).
- *Nonsegmented*: Neither the superior nor inferior endplate of the affected vertebrae has growth potential. Both endplates are fused to the adjacent vertebrae and the interval disc space is replaced by fibrous lamellar tissue (see Fig. 26.5).
- *Incarcerated*: Both the superior and inferior endplates of the affected vertebrae have growth potential; however, the affected vertebra is bound within the lateral margins of the adjacent vertebrae, and the adjacent vertebrae compensate for the deformity by expanding their growth potential. This results in the affected vertebrae appearing "carved into" the adjacent levels (see Fig. 26.5).

Failures of Segmentation

Failure of segmentation (type II deformity) is associated with derangements of the segmentation phase of somitogenesis. Improper segmentation occurs along a spectrum from a partial failure resulting in a partially segmented vertebra,

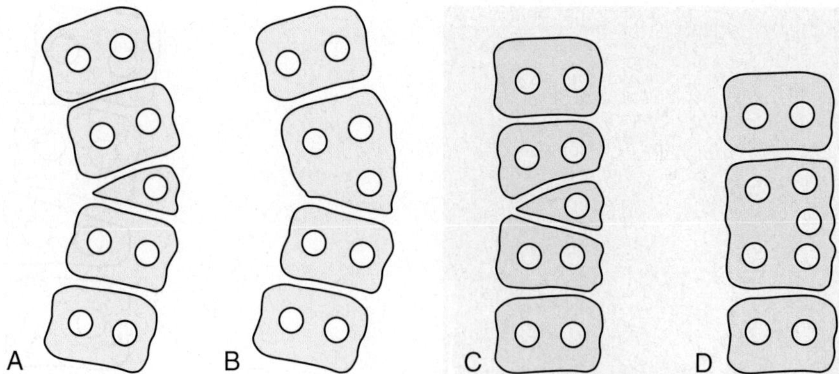

FIG. 26.5 Hemivertebrae, classified according to growth potential. (A) Segmented hemivertebra. (B) Semisegmented hemivertebra. (C) Incarcerated hemivertebra. (D) Nonsegmented hemivertebra.

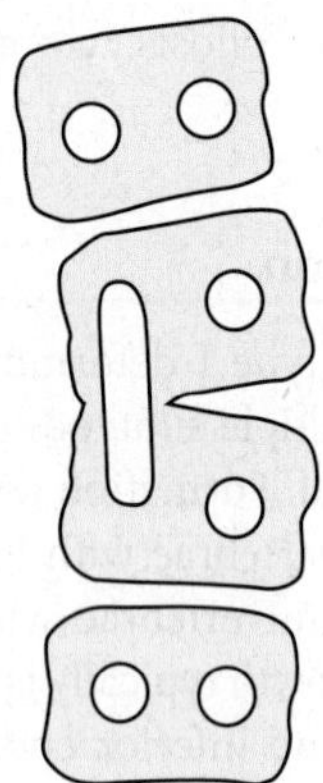

FIG. 26.6 Congenital unilateral bar. Partial fusion between two vertebrae prevents longitudinal growth on its side.

causing a bar, or complete failure resulting in a complete absence of intervening space between vertebrae, causing a block vertebra. A congenital bar can be anterior, posterior, lateral, or mixed. Depending on the position of the bar, a different deformity may develop as the patient grows (Fig. 26.6). As with other bar malformations in the body, the bony vertebral bar resulting from a partial failure in segmentation will restrict growth in the same plane of direction as the bar.

Mixed Deformity

Vertebral anomalies often exist in conjunction—failures of formation and failures of segmentation frequently coexist as mixed deformity (type III deformity). Occasionally, anomalies are found on several levels. For example, unilateral bar with contralateral fully segmented hemivertebra is a type III deformity and has the most rapid progression of curvature among the deformities (Fig. 26.7).

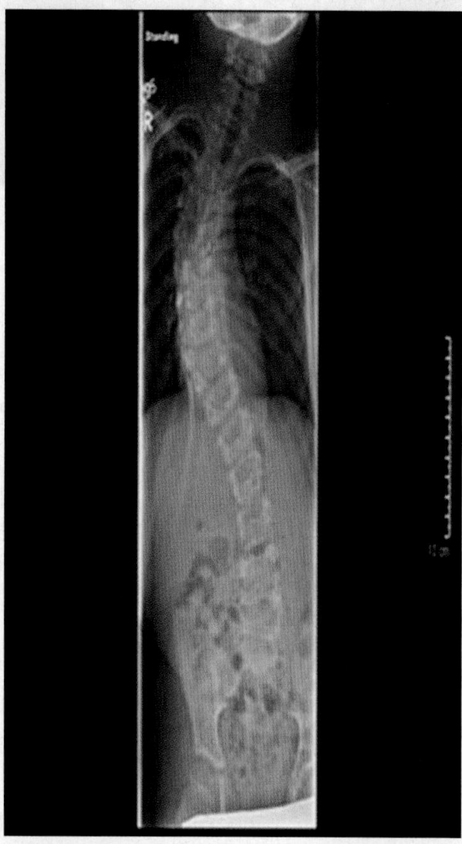

FIG. 26.7 Radiograph of 9-year-old child with congenital scoliosis of mixed pattern, including multiple hemivertebrae, both incarcerated and nonincarcerated, and fused pedicles and ribs on the left at T9–T10.

Natural History

Congenital scoliosis, as with other types of scoliosis, progresses in the majority of patients during periods of rapid growth. Given that deformities of congenital scoliosis are by definition present at birth, they are subject to the intense growth of early childhood—progression is most rapid in the first 3 years of life. Multiple reviews have shown that, statistically, 25% of curves do not progress, 25% progress minimally, while 50% progress significantly and require treatment[58–61] (Fig. 26.8). Without any treatment, 85% of patients with congenital scoliosis will have a curve greater than 45 degrees by maturity.[56] The potential for the increase in curvature is dependent on the imbalances of growth potential (Fig. 26.9). The natural history of congenital scoliosis relates to the type of deformity, location, number and span of deformities, initial severity of the scoliosis, and the global growth potential balance between each side of the spine. Analysis of these factors will allow the

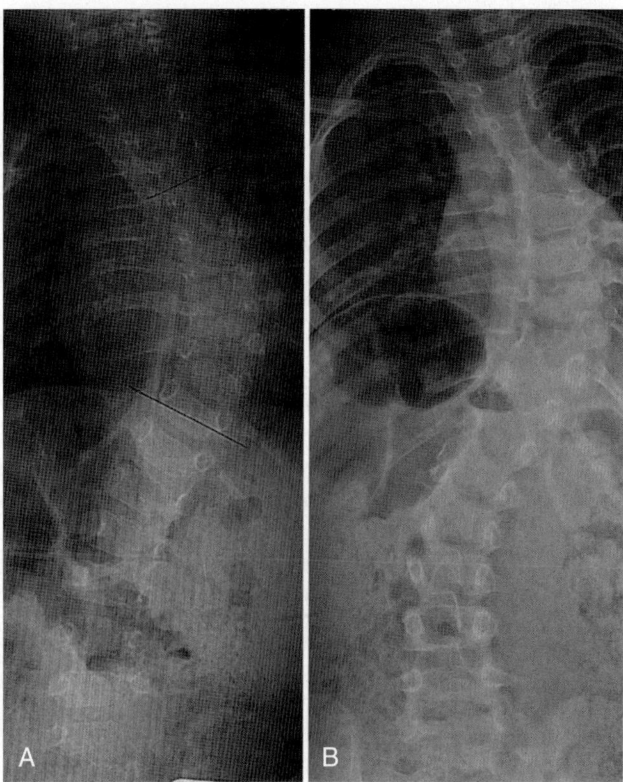

FIG. 26.8 Radiographs of congenital scoliosis with VACTERLS association (vertebral defects, anal atresia, cardiac defects, tracheoesophageal fistula, renal anomalies, and limb abnormalities) managed by observation since birth. Right thoracic curve and compensatory lumbar curve remain relatively unchanged from birth at (A) age 1 year and (B) age 8 years.

surgeon to determine the most appropriate treatment at the proper time.

Location

The most deforming anomalies tend to be those at the cervicothoracic or lumbosacral junction. Both types of deformity (formation and segmentation) may be lateral, causing scoliosis; dorsal, causing lordosis; ventral, causing kyphosis[62]; or a combination of these positions. Posterolateral positioning of a hemivertebra may cause kyphoscoliosis; anterolateral may cause kyphoscoliosis.[62] Furthermore, if the anterior part of the vertebra is deficient while the dorsal part is not malformed, kyphoscoliosis, especially in the lumbar spine, is common.[58,62]

Progression of Curvature by Deformity Type and Location

The spectrum of vertebral deformities associated with congenital scoliosis is associated with different growth potentials. In general, curves with fully segmented hemivertebrae have a greater capacity for continued growth potential and therefore greater risk for progression of curvature, whereas vertebrae whose apophysis is blocked are at minimal risk. Complex combinations of deformity contribute to a more pronounced spine imbalance and are associated with the greatest risk for curve progression.

For example, complete block vertebrae (complete type II deformity) or nonsegmented hemivertebrae are blocked

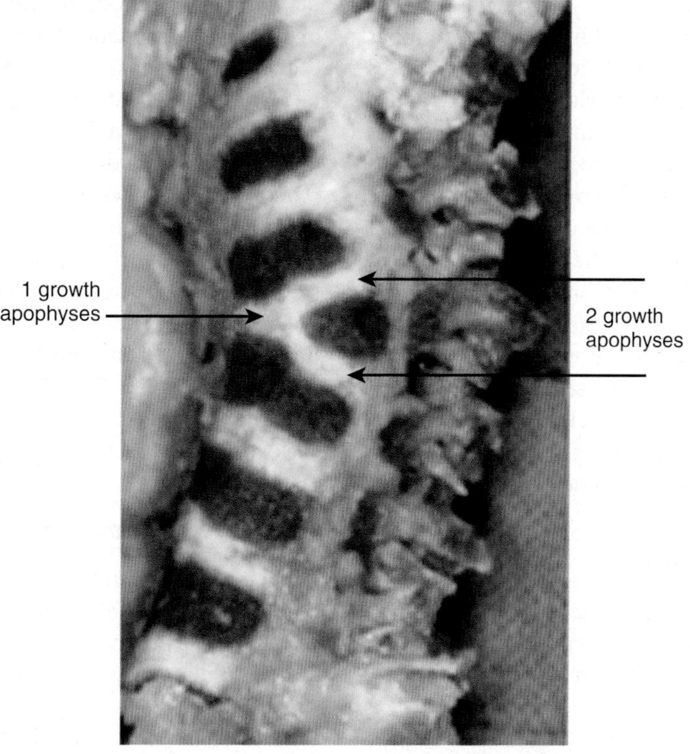

FIG. 26.9 Hemivertebra forcing spine into a curve. There are two growth apophyses on the hemivertebra side and only one on the other side, leading toward worsening during growth.

on both the superior and inferior apophysis. Therefore, the longitudinal growth potential is very small, and tends not to cause progressive scoliosis. Block vertebrae usually occur in multiple sites along the spine and are associated with a small potential for growth and a slow rate of progression (<1 degree per year[56,58,63]). Nonsegmented hemivertebrae demonstrate a similar rate of progression since they are also limited in their growth potential by being fused to the adjacent vertebrae. Incarcerated hemivertebrae also do not cause progressive scoliosis. When wedge vertebrae are located in the lower thoracic or thoracolumbar regions, the deformity demonstrates a relatively low rate of progression of 1 to 2 degrees per year.[56,58,63]

The location and number of hemivertebrae deformities along the spine affect the rate of curve progression. Specifically, the upper thoracic hemivertebrae tend to progress on average 1 to 2 degrees per year before puberty, then 2 to 2.5 degrees during the pubertal growth spurt. However, when the deformity is present in the lower thoracic spine, curves demonstrate a more rapid progression of 2 degrees per year before puberty and 2.5 to 3 degrees per year during the pubertal growth spurt. Furthermore, when located in the thoracolumbar spine, the rate of progression is again much more rapid—2 to 2.5 degrees per year before puberty and about 3.5 degrees per year during puberty. The more rapid progression and caudal location result in substantial trunk imbalance compared to other locations of curvature.[56,58,63]

Similarly, the span and location along the spine of a unilateral unsegmented bar greatly affect the natural development of the resultant curve. When located in the upper thoracic spine, the rate of progression averages 2 degrees per year before puberty and 4 degrees afterward. For deformity located within the lower thoracic area, curvature progression is 5 degrees per year before puberty and 6.5 degrees per year during puberty. Again, deformities with an apex located in the thoracolumbar area demonstrate the highest rate of deterioration—curves typically increase 6 degrees per year prior to puberty and 9 degrees per year after. Curves in the lumbar area progress about 5 degrees per year both before and after puberty.[56,58,63]

The most progressive anomaly is a convex, fully segmented hemivertebra associated with a concave unilateral bar. There is no growth potential on the side of the bar, but the side of the spine with the segmented hemivertebra continues to grow. Therefore, the spine is imbalanced, resulting in highly progressive curves. These types of disorders occur more frequently in the thoracic spine and are the most severe of all scoliosis disorders. They demonstrate rapid deterioration of up to 14 degrees per year prior to puberty, resulting in trunk shortening, limb-length discrepancy, and frank cosmetic deformity.[56,58,63]

Effects on Thoracic Contents

Congenital defects in the ribs and vertebrae often occur in conjunction. Rib fusion in the setting of scoliosis may constrict the thoracic contents during a crucial developmental period, and ultimately compromise pulmonary development. This occurs because alveolar development mostly takes place before 5 years of age and early restriction of the respiratory physiology effectively causes restrictive lung disease.[64–66] As the patient grows, the patient's thorax becomes unable to support normal respiration, a condition termed thoracic insufficiency syndrome (TIS). TIS can be assessed both clinically by respiratory rate and the thumb excursion test, by specific tests such as pulmonary function tests, and radiographically by plain radiographs and computed tomography (CT) volumetric studies.[67] Early fusion of scoliotic deformity before age 9 years, especially in patients requiring more than four levels of fusion and those with proximal fusions, also puts patients at risk for the development of restrictive pulmonary disease.[68,69] Additionally, compared with healthy peers, congenital scoliosis patients who were treated with extensive early spinal fusion demonstrate decreased pulmonary function test values in forced vital capacity, forced expiratory volume, vital capacity, and total lung capacity, and lower quality-of-life scores at 6.9 years' follow-up. Compared to congenital scoliosis patients who were fused in nonthoracic areas, patients treated with thoracic spinal fusion have reported shorter spinal height, more pain, and lower pulmonary functioning.[70] The increased appreciation of the need to preserve pulmonary function and to allow maximum spinal height has spurred the development of growth-preserving surgical alternatives to spinal fusion, including growing rods, guided growth, epiphysiodesis, and distraction thoracoplasty.

Assessment of Patient

Physical Examination

The physical examination of a patient with congenital scoliosis is guided by the knowledge of a high frequency of other structural and neural anomalies. Maternal, perinatal history, and developmental milestones must be fully explored. Presence of a dimple, nevi, hemangiomas, or hairy patches and/or any other cutaneous mark on the back should be noted. The sagittal plane balance and coronal balance, shoulder malalignment, as well as any deviation of head and trunk from the center of the pelvis should be checked. Due to the connection of scoliosis with Klippel-Feil syndrome, the cervical spine should be especially examined, including range of neck motion. In addition, it is critical to assess and document the neurologic status, including strength, reflexes, presence of atrophy, and the existence of latent ataxia or myelopathy. Flexibility of the deformity, gait, trunk shortening, and limb-length inequality should be checked. Pain, if present, should be localized and quantified. The examiner should search for other anomalies of the extremities (particularly radial malformation).

Associated Anomalies

Patients with congenital scoliosis have an increased incidence of other systemic differences including but not limited to respiratory, cardiac, renal, gastrointestinal, and neurologic systems. Pulmonary function tests, echocardiogram, and renal duplex may add to the overall case preparation. Often, the renal system is visualized on spinal magnetic resonance imaging (MRI), obviating the need for an additional study.[71] Collaboration with other specialties and with the patient's

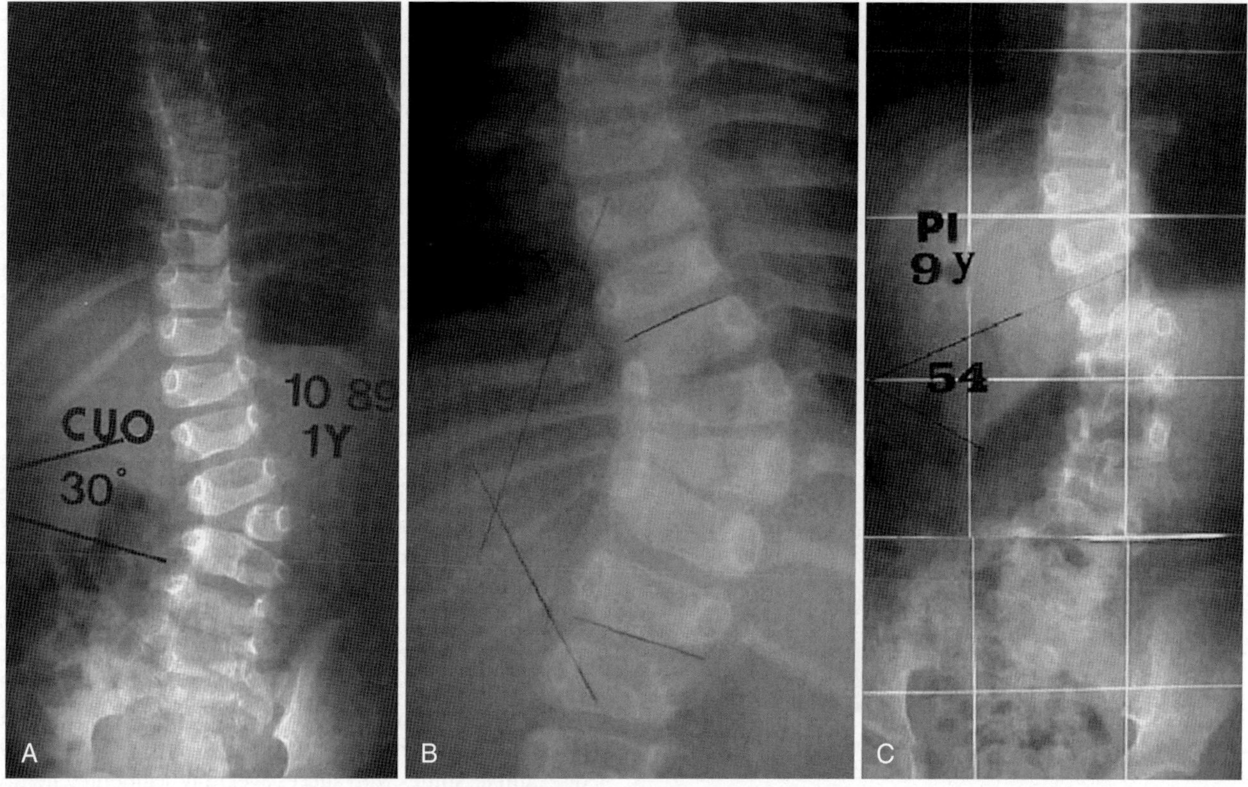

FIG. 26.10 It is easier to analyze a (A) segmented hemivertebra or a (B) unilateral bar when radiographs are taken prior to 4 years of age. (C) Lumbar segmented hemivertebra in a 9-year-old child.

primary care provider will serve to prepare the surgical team and optimize the patient for surgery.

Imaging

Preoperative CT scans define the anatomy and posterior element deficiencies. MRIs can exclude associated conditions of the spine, craniocervical junction, and viscera.

Radiographs

Plain radiographs remain the standard for the diagnosis and classification of congenital scoliosis and measuring curve magnitude and progression. Ideally, radiographs are obtained prior to 4 years of age (Fig. 26.10). After this time period, it may be difficult to fully appreciate the deformity because vertebrae are more ossified, especially in the areas of fusion or bars. Radiographs that were taken earlier—such as chest, abdominal, or renal radiographs—can provide valuable information to the orthopaedic surgeon about early development. Subtle findings—such as the presence and spacing of pedicles as well as fused, atretic, or absent ribs—provide clues about underlying deformity.

Standard anteroposterior and lateral films allow one to check the type and the location of deficiency, to measure the spine curvature, and to assess the pedicle width. However, studies have shown that, even in the hands of an expert, congenital scoliosis curves measured by the Cobb angle on traditional radiographs are difficult to reliably measure. Irregular landmarks and irregular numbering/positioning of vertebrae increase intraobserver and interobserver measurement error up to 10 degrees. Comparing current radiographs with prior radiographs reduces this error.[72–74] Since compensatory curves involve normally formed vertebrae, they are more reproducibly measured and can serve as a marker for progression of the congenital curvature. If a compensatory curve has not progressed, it is less likely that significant progression has occurred in a congenital curve.

Computed Tomography

Intraobserver reliability of measuring Cobb angles from plain radiographs is low in congenital scoliosis, with up to 10 degrees of measurement error; interobserver reliability demonstrates a greater measurement error.[74] Accurate and reliable reporting of curves as the patient matures through time is especially difficult. Furthermore, plain radiographs cannot demonstrate the spatial relationship of each structure of the vertebrae and the three-dimensional component of congenital scoliosis is difficult to appreciate. CT with three-dimensional reconstruction can be used to more completely and more consistently identify spinal abnormalities, especially posterior element deficiencies, in complex cases (Fig. 26.11). Spatial disposition of the affected vertebrae and the balance of deformity can be better classified. CT and three-dimensional reconstruction aid in the evaluation of the thorax and the lung and highlight thoracic wall deformities, including: rib synostoses, rib hypoplasia or agenesis, intracanal protrusions through the radicular foramina, and evaluation of TIS.[75,76]

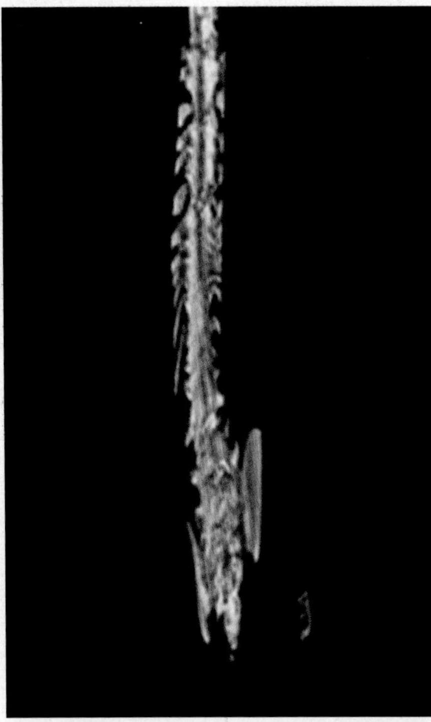

FIG. 26.11 Computed tomographic image with three-dimensional reconstruction allows the surgeon to more fully appreciate complex spine abnormalities.

Magnetic Resonance Imaging

Intraspinal anomalies are often associated with congenital scoliosis. Careful physical examination can suggest underlying spinal dysraphism.[38,77] MRI demonstrates intraspinal anomalies in 30% to 41% of cases.[78–80] Congenital scoliosis patients with cervical and thoracic hemivertebrae tend to have more intraspinal abnormalities than those with lumbar hemivertebrae.[81] The most common anomalies reported are tethered cord, syringomyelia, and diastematomyelia. MRI is indicated to assess congenital scoliosis because of three factors:

1. Intraspinal anomalies are encountered in about one-third of cases of congenital scoliosis.[81] Some may require neurosurgical treatment for their own sake (e.g., a large syrinx), whereas others may require neurosurgical collaboration if corrective orthopaedic surgery is planned (e.g., diastematomyelia).
2. Normal neurologic exam does not rule out malformations of the neuraxis.[79,80]
3. MRI of the spine will also typically demonstrate the presence or absence of renal anomalies, which may or may not capture evaluation of genitourinary anomalies.[71]

In practice, given the need for general anesthesia to obtain MRI in young children, it should be ordered when there is a concerning examination finding and/or prior to surgical procedure.

Treatment

Those malformations that present a very low progression rate should be periodically evaluated for possible progression. However, about 50% of congenital scoliosis cases require surgical treatment.[58–61] Correction of deformity should occur early in congenital scoliosis, which allows the correction of the fewest vertebrae possible and protection against continued, severe structural spine decompensation.[82–84]

Congenital vertebral anomalies require close clinical monitoring at periodic intervals during growth. Consistent observation allows for assessment of the evolution of spinal curves. In complex malformations, early treatment is often more straightforward and safer.

Nonoperative

Contrary to idiopathic scoliosis, nonoperative treatment has little value in congenital scoliosis. Only a small number of cases, characterized by long and flexible curves, may be temporized by bracing to slow the progression of the curvatures.[58,85,86] However, these curves will eventually decompensate to the degree requiring surgical management. In general, carefully monitoring every 4 to 6 months with regular examination and radiographic evaluation is prudent in curves measuring up to 40 degrees.[87] However, other factors—including deformity personality, pulmonary, cardiac, or neurologic function—may require earlier surgical intervention. For example, spines with successive, fully segmented hemivertebrae concomitant with additional severe deformities of the rib cage, therefore causing TIS, may undergo surgical intervention earlier regardless of the Cobb's angle.[87]

Operative

Without any treatment, 85% of patients with congenital scoliosis will have a curve greater than 45 degrees by maturity.[56] Congenital scoliosis progresses because the growth potential of the spine is imbalanced. Early recognition of curves with a poor prognosis is crucial to prevent severe curve progression and possible neurologic complications. The advent of pediatric-specific implants has minimized the problem of implant prominence in young children and has been shown to be safe from a neurologic standpoint.[83] Motor- and sensory-evoked potential monitoring is recommended whenever possible. There is an increased risk of a perioperative neurologic injury when baseline monitoring cannot be established.[88] Furthermore, postoperative monitoring and thorough documentation of neurologic functioning is important because paraplegia after deformity surgery may present in a delayed fashion, especially in the first 72 hours.[89,90]

Indications for surgery depend on many factors, including the nature of the vertebral anomaly as well as its location and span, the curve magnitude and its flexibility, the patient's age, and the presence of other deformities. The aim of surgery is fourfold: (1) achieve a straight spine, with or without deformity reduction; (2) restore a physiologic sagittal profile while maintaining flexibility; (3) limit curve progression; and (4) preserve normal spinal growth as much as possible by fusing only a short segment. Seven major operations have been described: posterior spine fusion, combined anterior and posterior spine fusion, convex hemiepiphyseodesis, hemivertebra excision, vertebral column resection, osteotomies, and guided growth progression.

Posterior Spine Fusion

Posterior fusion is among the "simplest" and "safest" techniques, but is not without its limitations or complications.[91] Ideal candidates for posterior fusion are those with small, relatively short curves who otherwise have limited growth potential in the anterior spine. In general, curves no greater than 25 degrees that are limited to no greater than five vertebrae may be considered.[87]

Selection of these curves minimizes the risk of the crankshaft phenomenon[92] that can be seen if the anterior spinal growth is still active. The crankshaft phenomenon occurs when growth remaining increases the curve. Additionally, lordosis in the proposed region of fusion is a contraindication to posterior fusion because anterior growth will worsen lordosis. A review of 54 congenital scoliosis patients reported a 15% crankshaft incidence in patients undergoing posterior fusion before the age of 10 years, especially those with surgery at an early age and greater than 50-degree curves.[92]

Posterior spinal fusion may cause significant issues as the child continues to age. In a large meta-analysis review of patients with early-onset scoliosis, congenital scoliosis, and infantile scoliosis who underwent posterior spinal fusion for presumed definitive fusion in early childhood, revision surgery has been required in 24% to 39% of cases.[93] Additionally, restrictive pulmonary disease occurs in many of these patients,[93] although it should be noted that nonoperative management and continued curve progression are also likely to have negative effects on pulmonary function.[94] Patients 1 to 4 years old are best suited for this procedure. Posterior fusion can be considered a prophylactic procedure.

Imaging the spine prior to exposure is useful because the area of deformity is often difficult to localize by inspection and palpation alone. During exposure, failure to recognize the potentially complex posterior laminar defects can lead to neurologic injury. After exposure of the posterior elements, the spine should again be imaged to confirm that the targeted deformity, which may have anterior components, aligns with posterior elements. Some deformities, particularly anterior bars or malaligned hemivertebrae, have anterior elements that do not correspond to the logical posterior elements. Due to difficult localization of the deformity, there is a risk of extending the fusion past the originally planned surgery. Fusion must include all vertebrae involved in the congenital curve and should extend laterally to the transverse processes. Successful fusion is achieved by thorough facet resection, decortication, and placement of abundant bone graft. Posterior instrumentation can be used safely in the pediatric patient to decrease the risk of pseudarthrosis. Of course, posterior elements may be deformed, with fused or missing laminae, or thin pedicles that do not lend themselves well to instrumentation. With advancing age, typically by the age of 2 years, instrumentation becomes feasible. A postoperative cast or a rigid brace is then required for 2 to 3 months to achieve fusion and curve correction.

Combined Anterior and Posterior Spine Fusion

While the posterior-only approach has shortcomings due to the risk of anterior growth, the combined anterior and posterior fusion can more effectively prevent progression.[84] The main indications for a combined anterior and posterior fusion are a deformity with significant anterior and posterior growth potential. For example, a unilateral bar with a contralateral hemivertebra would be appropriate for a combined anterior and posterior spine fusion.

Performing an anterior approach allows for discectomy and removal of the vertebral endplates, which augments spine flexibility and the potential for deformity correction. Unlike the posterior-only fusion, the combined approach, or even anterior only, is appropriate for lordotic curves. The combined fusion may decrease the rate of pseudarthrosis, decrease the crankshaft phenomenon, and can also be augmented by instrumentation. Anterior bone graft is typically placed for fusion. Depending on surgeon preference and the location of the deformity, the anterior procedure may be performed either through an anterior, open technique, thoracoscopically,[95] or through a posterior approach. Accessing the anterior vertebrae via a posterior approach is most feasible at the thoracolumbar junction via retropleural dissection, especially if the surgeon is able to take advantage of a kyphotic element.

Convex Hemiepiphysiodesis

The concept of convex hemiepiphysiodesis is the same as that commonly employed for deformity of growing long bones. The surgeon is able to take advantage of this and spare the patient intraoperative destabilization or growth arrest of the whole fused spine segment, with convex growth arrest. Convex hemiepiphysiodesis slows convex-side growth while the concave curve still grows, allowing for safe and relatively controlled progressive deformity correction.[96] Thus, failures of segmentation with little or no growth potential cannot be successfully treated this way. Ideal candidates for convex hemiepiphysiodesis are young enough that growth will allow for significant correction, a curve less than 70 degrees, have six or fewer involved vertebrae, and demonstrate significant concave growth potential.[97] Patients should be 6 years old or younger because spinal growth is two-thirds complete by this age.[98] Traditionally, pathologic congenital kyphosis or lordosis has been a contraindication for this procedure.[99] For example, an appropriate deformity for this treatment may be a single or multiple hemivertebrae in a patient 6 years old or younger.

Convex hemiepiphysiodesis typically requires an anterior and posterior exposure; however, posterior-only methods are feasible. The traditional combined anteroposterior approach allows for the removal of the convex portion of discs and vertebral endplates and fusion of this convex portion with bone graft via the anterior approach; removal of the unilateral facet joints and fusion is completed via the posterior exposure. Traditional convex hemiepiphysiodesis without instrumentation typically yields modest curve correction, on the order of 0 to 15 degrees by maturity; some patients achieve only an arrest of progression.[100] Much of the correction with convex growth arrest seems to be achieved acutely at the time of the initial procedure, which is then attempted to be maintained with postoperative immobilization.

As with the other treatments, instrumentation can be used to achieve better intraoperative correction—convex posterior compression is typically utilized with good results in convex growth arrest.[101,102] Early follow-up analysis of 11 patients with long, sweeping congenital curves (involving multiple anomalous vertebrae) who underwent this method of concave posterior distraction in convex instrumented hemiepiphysiodesis yields encouraging results. A posterior-only instrumented convex growth arrest with pedicle screws at each segment on the convex side may obviate the need for anterior surgery. A collection of 13 patients treated with the posterior-only convex growth arrest procedure described earlier demonstrated that the procedure is safe and that curves improved by 5 degrees or greater in nine patients, while two patients' curves remained the same.[103]

Hemivertebra Excision

Hemivertebra excision is preferred in cases in which a hemivertebra causes progressive curve and deformity with truncal imbalance. In contrast to fusion and convex epiphysiodesis, hemivertebra excision acutely corrects the curve and corrects for truncal imbalance. Excision of the hemivertebra is recommended if the curve progresses significantly. Instrumented hemivertebra excision provides the highest degree of correction, particularly if carried out before 3 years of age.[104] Hemivertebra excision is ideal for a fully segmented hemivertebra at the apex of the curve in the thoracolumbar junction, lumbar spine, or lumbar sacral spine, and with a fixed lateral translation of the trunk. Cervicothoracic or cervical hemivertebra excision has been reported but is a more complex procedure due to the vertebral artery.[105] Hemivertebrae may be resected by an anteroposterior or posterior procedure only.

The combined anterior and posterior excision of the hemivertebra allows for the circumferential exposure of the spine and complete excision of the adjacent discs. Anterior and posterior exposure can be achieved either by sequential procedures under a single anesthetic or when performed simultaneously.[106,107] After excision, the unstable spine is then stabilized with anterior and/or posterior instrumentation typically by utilizing an anterior structural graft, which is useful on the concave side to maintain a normal sagittal contour. Instrumentation may then be used both anteriorly and posteriorly to apply compression and to further stabilize the spine. The need for postoperative immobilization is determined by the surgeon's impression of spinal stability (Fig. 26.12).

Similar to convex hemiepiphysiodesis, hemivertebra excision can also be accomplished via a single posterior approach due to advances in imaging and monitoring.[108–111] The ideal indication for a posterior-only approach is a hemivertebra located at the thoracolumbar junction or in the lumbar spine, with some associated kyphosis.[62] The posterior-only approach is stabilized with segmental transpedicular instrumentation after excision.[111,112] Clinical experience has shown that pedicle screws even in young children do not cause spinal stenosis. If needed, hooks can augment the screws.

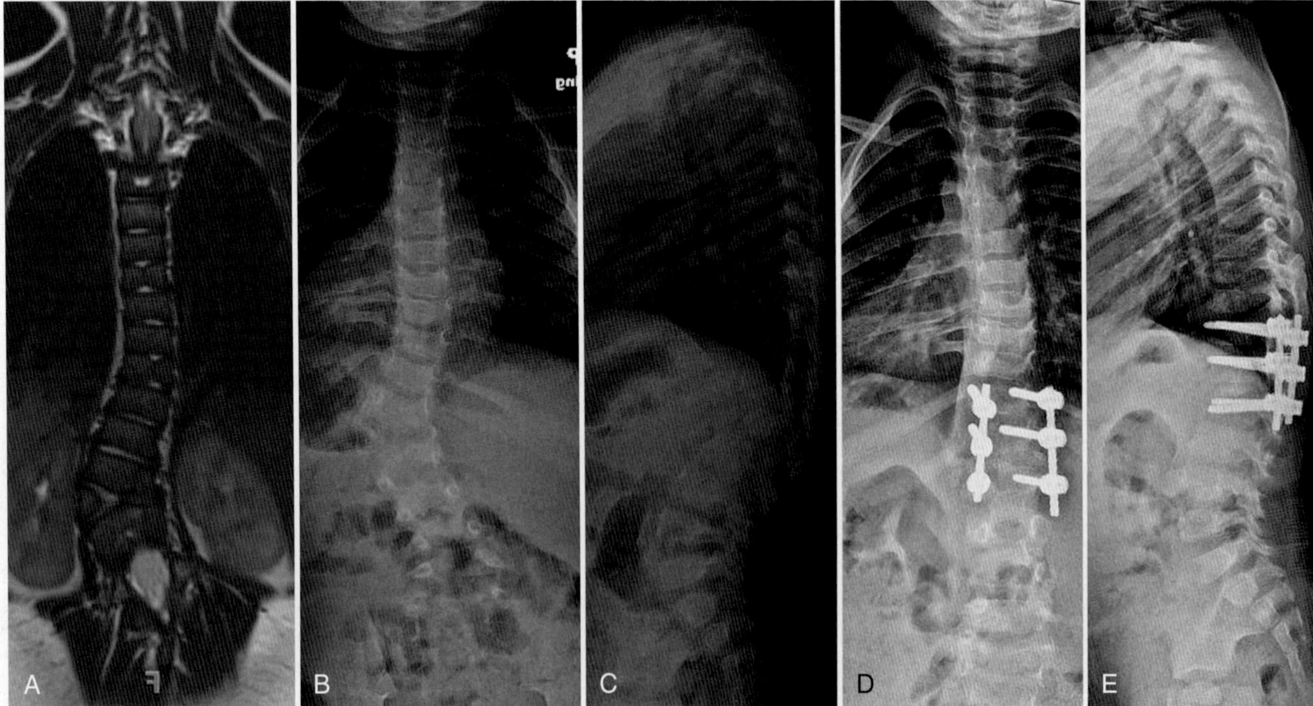

FIG. 26.12 (A–C) Radiographs of a 2-year-old boy with progressive kyphoscoliosis at the level of the L1 hemivertebra. (D–E) The patient underwent hemivertebra resection and anterior and posterior spinal fusion with posterior spinal instrumentation. He was placed in a cast and maintained good correction postoperatively.

Osteotomies

Complex curves with multiple fusions, prior instrumentation, and significant trunk imbalance may justify multiple anterior and posterior osteotomies to allow for spinal mobilization. Patients undergoing osteotomies should have preoperative imaging of the entire spine to rule out intraspinal anomalies in the canal. After osteotomies are created, correction of the curve may be achieved at the same stage. Complex deformity correction may incorporate osteotomies with other types of procedures. Multiple concave rib osteotomies add flexibility. It can be considered as an alternative in the treatment of rigid congenital curves involving more than three levels or multiple curves separated by at least two segments that would otherwise require multiple vertebral resections.

Vertebral Column Resection

Vertebral column resection (VCR) describes the complete resection of vertebral segments using either combined anterior and posterior approaches or a posterior-only approach, which enables significant three-dimensional deformity correction.[113,114] This technique may be applied to correct moderate to severe spinal deformities, including those with large rigid curves, fixed trunk translation, or asymmetry between the length of the convex and concave column of the deformity. VCR carries significant risk of neurologic injury[114–116] (Fig. 26.13). This high risk is partially secondary to the severe nature of the deformity eligible for VCR and partially due to the resulting instability from segmental resection and instrumentation.

Rigid instrumentation that controls the spinal column above and below the resection area must be performed in VCR procedures. Instrumentation is imperative for preventing and treating the very real risk of spinal subluxation. Anterior structural graft can be used on the concave side of the construct to maintain a normal sagittal contour. Similarly, a posterior structural graft, preferably from the patient's rib, can be used to cover a laminectomy defect.[115,116] Releases are also typically performed at the apex of scoliosis or kyphoscoliosis deformities to facilitate pedicle screw placement.

Guided Growth Procedures

In a young patient with progressive deformity, growing rods provide progressive correction of the curve and the expansion of the thorax. This is especially of value for congenital spine deformities with concomitant rib fusions, which lead to restrictive pulmonary disease and/or TIS. In general, guided growth procedures should be considered as an alternative to long spinal fusion. An important consideration to discuss with the patient and family is the commitment to undergoing multiple surgical spinal procedures, typically every 6 months. Among the potential complications are drift of the spinal anchors, infection, postoperative pain, device fracture due to stress fatigue, brachial plexus palsy, and neurologic injury.[117,118]

Dual growing rods lengthened at 6-month intervals were shown to achieve greater curve correction and allow for greater spinal growth when compared to single growing rods.[119] In patients with spondylocostal dysostosis, vertical expandable prosthetic titanium rib guided growth has more marked impact on curve progression and chest wall development:

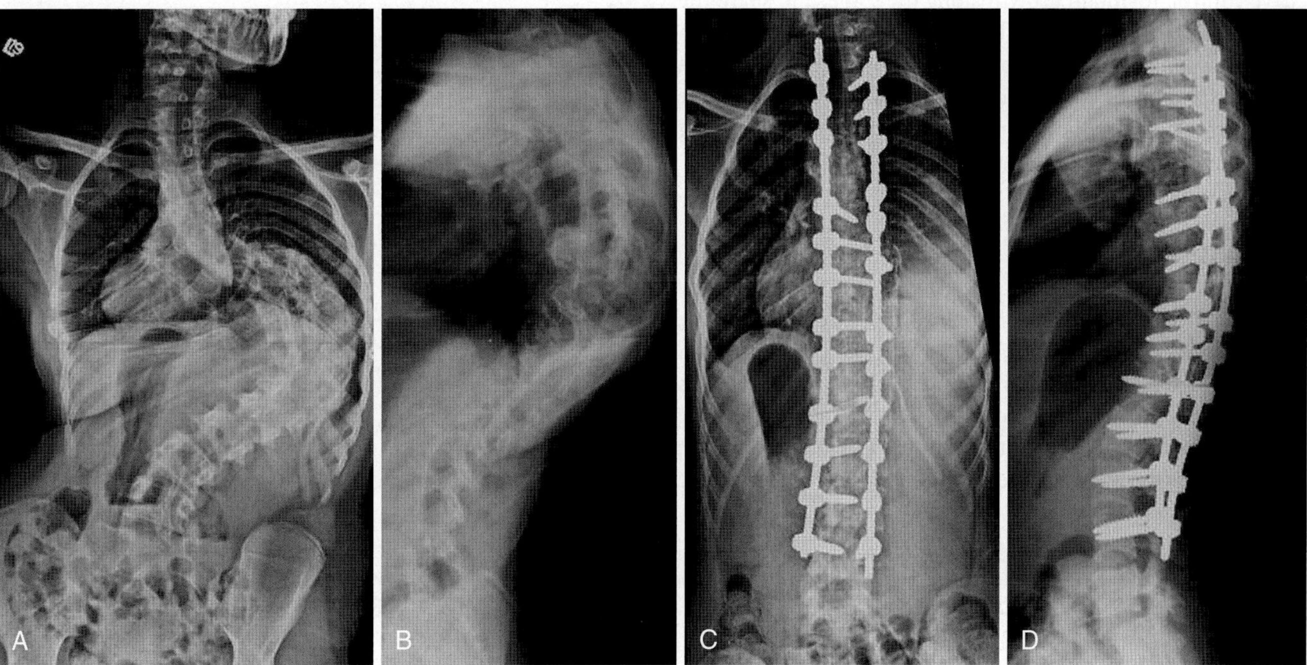

FIG. 26.13 (A–B) Radiographs of severe congenital scoliosis measuring 120 degrees in a 15-year-old girl. (C–D) The patient underwent posterior spinal fusion instrumentation, right vertebral column resection, and multiple discectomies.

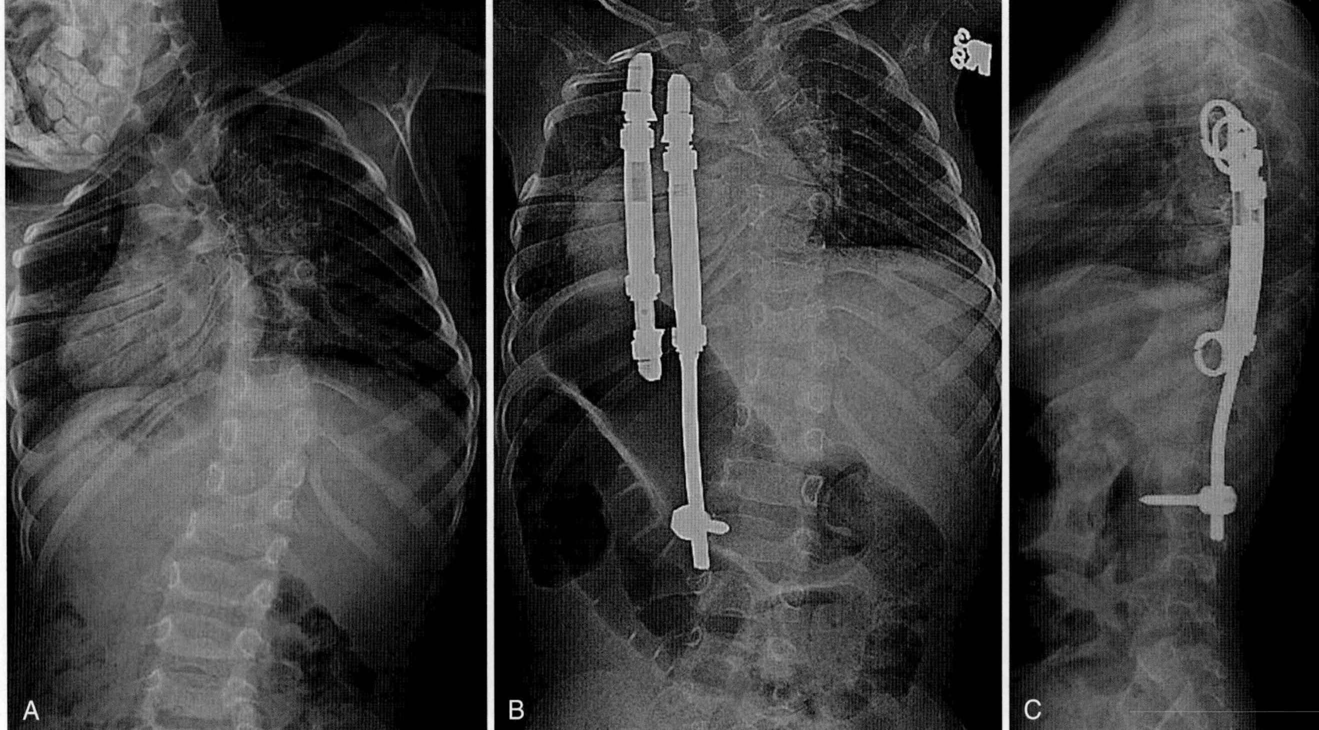

FIG. 26.14 (A) Radiograph of severe chest deformity associated with congenital scoliosis and multiple rib fusions in a symptomatic 4-year-old child. (B–C) The patient underwent multiple rib osteotomies with the use of vertical expandable prosthetic titanium rib anchored from rib to rib and from rib to spine.

increases in thoracic height and width and improvement in the Cobb angle (Fig. 26.14).

Magnetic controlled growing rods (MCGRs) continue to expand the possibilities for guided growth procedures. Rather than continued reoperation with exchange of implants, as is needed with conventional growing rods, MCGRs can facilitate curve control, maintain growth along the spine, and spare the patient multiple reoperations by using nonsurgical distraction methods. Preliminary data on MCGRs are promising both from a safety and efficacy standpoint.[120,121] Long-term outcome studies are needed to better inform surgical decision making regarding the use of guided growth procedures.

Conclusion

Congenital scoliosis presents immense variation in deformity, impact, and treatment options. Not all cases benefit from surgery. Regular examination will make clear which patterns require intervention. Advances in growth-friendly surgery have provided many other options for treatment. Advances in imaging, monitoring, and operative techniques will make the treatment as safe as possible.

KEY POINTS

1. Assessment of vertebral anomalies is best in early childhood.
2. Progressive deformation is due to imbalance in spine growth. Some vertebral anomalies do not lead to imbalance and are not likely to produce deformity.
3. Bracing has almost no effect on congenital spine curves.
4. Surgery should be performed as early as is practical to prevent secondary structural changes.
5. All patients with congenital scoliosis should be evaluated for genitourinary anomalies. They should also undergo panspinal MRI if significant progression occurs or if surgery is indicated.
6. The first available film should be analyzed and used for subsequent comparisons.
7. The measurement error for congenital scoliosis is greater than idiopathic (approximately 10 degrees).
8. Neurologic risk of spine surgery is higher for congenital scoliosis than other types.
9. Congenital anomalies of the posterior elements do not often correlate with anomalies of the bodies and may require three-dimensional CT to previsualize.
10. The surgeon should be aware of midline laminar defects when using a posterior exposure.

KEY REFERENCES

1. Loder RT, Urquhart A, Steen H, et al. Variability in Cobb angle measurements in children with congenital scoliosis. *J Bone Joint Surg Br*. 1995;77:768-770.
The measurement variation in congenital scoliosis was found to be 19 degrees in this study.
2. McMaster MJ, Ohtsuka K. The natural history of congenital scoliosis: a study of two hundred and fifty-one patients. *J Bone Joint Surg Am*. 1982;64:1128-1147.
This article defined the progression risk and the differences between patterns of anomalies and levels of the spine.
3. Ruf M, Harms J. Hemivertebra resection by a posterior approach: innovative operative technique and first results. *Spine*. 2002;27:1116-1123.
This article revolutionized the treatment of hemivertebrae by showing the safety of a posterior approach.

4. Giampietro PF, Dunwoodie SL, Kusumi K, et al. Progress in the understanding of the genetic etiology of vertebral segmentation disorders in humans. *Ann N Y Acad Sci.* 2009;1151:38-67.
This is an excellent review of advances in the understanding of the genetic and environmental factors that contribute to vertebral development.

5. Campbell RM Jr, Smith MD, Mayes TC, et al. The characteristics of thoracic insufficiency syndrome associated with fused ribs and congenital scoliosis. *J Bone Joint Surg Am.* 2003;85:399-408.
This article characterizes thoracic insufficiency syndrome, which has led to the development of guided-growth procedures in the treatment of congenital scoliosis.

REFERENCES

1. Shands AR Jr, Bundens WD. Congenital deformities of the spine: an analysis of the roentgenograms of 700 children. *Bull Hosp Jt Dis.* 1956;17:110-133.
2. Giampietro PF, Blank RD, Raggio CL, et al. Congenital and idiopathic scoliosis: clinical and genetic aspects. *Clin Med Res.* 2003;1:125-136.
3. Shahcheraghi GH, Hobbi MH. Patterns and progression in congenital scoliosis. *J Pediatr Orthop.* 1999;19(6):766-775.
4. Purkiss SB, Driscoll B, Cole WG, Alman B. Idiopathic scoliosis in families of children with congenital scoliosis. *Clin Orthop Relat Res.* 2002;401:27-31.
5. Winter RB. Congenital scoliosis. *Orthop Clin North Am.* 1988;19(2):395-408.
6. Wynne-Davies R. Congenital vertebral anomalies: aetiology and relationship to spina bifida cystica. *J Med Genet.* 1975; 12(3):280-288.
7. Bulent E, Tracy MR, Dormans JP, et al. Congenital scoliosis and vertebral malformations: characterization of segmental defects for genetic analysis. *J Pediatr Orthop.* 2004;24:674-682.
8. Campbell RM Jr, Hell-Vocke AK. Growth of the thoracic spine in congenital scoliosis after expansion thoracoplasty. *J Bone Joint Surg Am.* 2003;85-A(3):409-420.
9. Hedequist D, Emans J. Congenital scoliosis: a review and update. *J Pediatr Orthop.* 2007;27(1):106-116.
10. Larsen WJ, Sherman LS, Potter SS, Scott WJ. The fourth week. In: Larsen WJ, ed. *Human Embryology.* 3rd ed. New York: Churchill Livingstone; 2001:79-112.
11. Sadler TW, Langman J. Skeletal system. In: Sadler TW, ed. *Langman's Medical Embryology.* 8th ed. Philadelphia: Lippincott Williams & Wilkins; 2000.
12. Dequeant M, Pourquie O. Segmental patterning of the vertebrate embryonic axis. *Nat Rev Genet.* 2008;9:370-382.
13. Pourquie O, Kusumi K. When body segmentation goes wrong. *Clin Genet.* 2001;60:409-416.
14. Turnpenny PD, Alman B, Cornier AS, et al. Abnormal vertebral segmentation and the notch signaling pathway in man. *Dev Dyn.* 2007;236(6):1456-1474.
15. Vonk FJ, Richardson MK. Developmental biology: serpent clocks tick faster. *Nature.* 2008;454:282-283.
16. William DA, Saitta B, Gibson JD, et al. Identification of oscillatory genes in somitogenesis from functional genomic analysis of a human mesenchymal stem cell model. *Dev Biol.* 2007;305(1):172-186.
17. Aulehla A, Wehrle C, Brand-Saberi B, et al. Wnt3a plays a major role in the segmentation clock controlling somitogenesis. *Dev Cell.* 2003;4(3):395-406.
18. Morimoto M, Takahashi Y, Endo M, et al. The MESP2 transcription factor establishes segmental borders by suppressing Notch activity. *Nature.* 2005;435:354-359.
19. Takahashi Y, Koizumi K, Takagi A, et al. MESP2 initiates somite segmentation through the Notch signaling pathway. *Nat Genet.* 2000;25:390-396.
20. Quan L, Smith DW. The VATER association. Vertebral defects, anal atresia, T-E fistula with esophageal atresia, radial and renal dysplasia: a spectrum of associated defects. *J Pediatr.* 1973;82(1):104-107.
21. Nora AH, Nora JJ. A syndrome of multiple congenital anomalies associated with teratogenic exposure. *Arch Environ Health.* 1975;30(1):17-21.
22. Botto L, Khouy M, Mastroiacovo P, et al. The spectrum of congenital anomalies of the VATER association: an international study. *Am J Med Genet.* 1997;71:8-15.
23. Prahinski JR, Polly DW Jr, McHale KA, et al. Occult intraspinal anomalies in congenital scoliosis. *J Pediatr Orthop.* 2000;20:59-63.
24. Basu PS, Elsebaie H, Noordeen MH. Congenital spinal deformity: a comprehensive assessment at presentation. *Spine.* 2002;27(20):2255-2259.
25. Giampietro PF, Dunwoodie SL, Kusumi K, et al. Progress in the understanding of the genetic etiology of vertebral segmentation disorders in humans. *Ann N Y Acad Sci.* 2009; 1151:38-67.
26. Gruneberg H. Genetical studies on the skeleton of the mouse XIX: pudgy. *Genet Res.* 1961;2:384-393.
27. Dunwoodie SL, Clements M, Sparrow DB, et al. Axial skeletal defects caused by mutation in the spondylocostal dysplasia/pudgy gene DLL3 are associated with disruption of the segmentation clock within the presomitic mesoderm. *Development.* 2002;129:1795-1806.
28. Kusumi K, Sun ES, Kerrebrock AW, et al. The mouse pudgy mutation disrupts delta homologue DLL3 and initiation of early somite boundaries. *Nat Genet.* 1998;19:274-278.
29. Bulman M, Kusumi K, Frayling T, et al. Mutations in the human Delta homologue, DLL3, cause axial skeletal defects in spondylocostal dysostosis. *Nat Genet.* 2000;4: 438-441.
30. Yasuhiko Y, Haraguchi S, Kitajima S, et al. Tbx6-mediated Notch signaling controls somite-specific MESP2 expression. *Proc Natl Acad Sci USA.* 2006;103:3651-3656.
31. Whittock NV, Sparrow DB, Wouters MA, et al. Mutated MESP2 causes spondylocostal dysostosis in humans. *Am J Hum Genet.* 2004;74:1249-1254.
32. Saga Y, Hata N, Koseki H, et al. MESP2: a novel mouse gene expressed in the presegmented mesoderm and essential for segmentation initiation. *Genes Dev.* 1997;11:1827-1839.
33. Emerick KM, Rand EB, Goldmuntz E, et al. Features of Alagille syndrome in 92 patients: frequency and relation to prognosis. *Hepatology.* 1999;29:822-829.
34. Kamath BM, Loomes KM, Oakey RJ, et al. Facial features in Alagille syndrome: specific or cholestasis facies? *Am J Med Genet.* 2002;112:163-170.
35. Colliton RP, Bason L, Lu FM, et al. Mutation analysis of Jagged1 (JAG1) in Alagille syndrome patients. *Hum Mutat.* 2001;17:151-152.
36. McDaniell R, Warthen DM, Sanchez-Lara PA, et al. NOTCH2 mutations cause Alagille syndrome, a heterogeneous disorder of the notch signaling pathway. *Am J Hum Genet.* 2006;79:169-173.
37. Chaumien JP, Rigault P, Maroteaux P, Padovani JP, Touzet P. [The so-called Klippel-Feil syndrome and its orthopaedic incidences]. *Rev Chir Orthop Reparatrice Appar Mot.* 1990;76(1):30-38.

38. Winter RB, Moe JH, Lonstein JE. The incidence of Klippel-Feil syndrome in patients with congenital scoliosis and kyphosis. *Spine*. 1984;9(4):363-366.
39. Fisher K, Esham RH, Thorneycroft I. Scoliosis associated with typical Mayer- Rokitansky-Kuster-Hauser syndrome. *South Med J*. 2000;93(2):243-246.
40. Lapunzina P, Musante G, Pedraza A, Prudent L, Gadow E. Semilobar holoprosencephaly, coronal craniosynostosis, and multiple congenital anomalies: a severe expression of the Genoa syndrome or a newly recognized syndrome? *Am J Med Genet*. 2001;102(3):258-260.
41. Larson AR, Josephson KD, Pauli RM, Opitz JM, Williams MS. Klippel-Feil anomaly with Sprengel anomaly, omovertebral bone, thumb abnormalities, and flexion-crease changes: novel association or syndrome? *Am J Med Genet*. 2001;101(2):158-162.
42. Mooney JF 3rd, Emans JB. Progressive kyphosis and neurologic compromise complicating spondylothoracic dysplasia in infancy (Jarcho-Levin syndrome). *Spine*. 1995;20(17):1938-1942.
43. Giampietro PF, Raggio CL, Blank RD, et al. Clinical, genetic and environmental factors associated with congenital vertebral malformations. *Molecular Syndromology*. 2013;4(1-2):94-105.
44. Li Z, Yu X, Shen J. Environmental aspects of congenital scoliosis. *Environ Sci Pollut Res Int*. 2015;22(8):5751-5755.
45. Holmes LB. Vertebral anomalies: hemivertebrae. In: *Common Malformations*. New York: Oxford University Press; 2012:283-289.
46. Farley FA, Hall J, Goldstein SA. Characteristics of congenital scoliosis in a mouse model. *J Pediatr Orthop*. 2006;26:341-346.
47. Loder RT, Hernandez MJ, Lerner AL, et al. The induction of congenital spinal deformities in mice by maternal carbon monoxide exposure. *J Pediatr Orthop*. 2000;20:662-666.
48. Wide K, Winbladh B, Kallen B. Major malformations in infants exposed to antiepileptic drugs in utero, with emphasis on carbamazepine and valproic acid: a nation-wide, population-based register study. *Acta Paediatr*. 2004;93:174-176.
49. Alexander PG, Tuan RS. Role of environmental factors in axial skeletal dysmorphogenesis. *Birth Defects Res C Embryo Today*. 2010;90(2):118-132.
50. Bennett GD. Hyperthermia: malformations to chaperones. *Birth Defects Res B Dev Reprod Toxicol*. 2010;89(4):279-288.
51. Aberg A, Westbom L, Kallen B. Congenital malformations among infants whose mothers had gestational diabetes or preexisting diabetes. *Early Hum Dev*. 2001;61:85-95.
52. Sparrow DB, Chapman G, Smith AJ, et al. A mechanism for gene-environment interaction in the etiology of congenital scoliosis. *Cell*. 2012;149(2):295-306.
53. Waterland RA, Dolinoy DC, Lin JR, et al. Maternal methyl supplements increase offspring DNA methylation at Axin Fused. *Genesis*. 2006;44:401-406.
54. Winter RB, Moe JH, Eilers VE. Congenital scoliosis: a study of 234 patients treated and untreated. *J Bone Joint Surg Am*. 1968;50(1):1-47.
55. Winter RB. Congenital spinal deformity. In: Lonstein JE, Bradford DS, Winter RB, Ogilvie JW, eds. *Moe's Textbook of Scoliosis and Other Spinal Deformities*. Philadelphia.: Saunders; 1995:3.
56. McMaster M, Ohtsuka K. The natural history of congenital scoliosis: a study of 251 patients. *J Bone Joint Surg Am*. 1982;64A:1128-1147.
57. Jaskwhich D, Ali RM, Patel TC, Green DW. Congenital scoliosis. *Curr Opin Pediatr*. 2000;12(1):61-66.
58. Kaspiris A, Grivas TB, Weiss HR, Turnbull D. Surgical and conservative treatment of patients with congenital scoliosis: a search for long-term results. *Scoliosis*. 2011;6:12.
59. Arlet V, Odent T, Aebi M. Congenital scoliosis. *Eur Spine J*. 2003;12:456-463.
60. Hensinger RN. Congenital scoliosis: aetiology and associations. *Spine*. 2009;34(17):1745-1750.
61. Batra S, Ahuja S. Congenital scoliosis: management and future directions. *Acta Orthop Belg*. 2008;74(2):147-160.
62. Hedequist D, Emans J. Congenital scoliosis. a review and update. *J Pediatr Orthop*. 2007;27(1):106-116.
63. Marks DS, Qaimkhani SA. The natural history of congenital scoliosis and kyphosis. *Spine*. 2009;34(17):1751-1755.
64. Davies G, Reid L. Effect of scoliosis on growth of alveoli and pulmonary arteries and on right ventricle. *Arch Dis Child*. 1971;46:623-632.
65. Muirhead A, Conner AN. The assessment of lung function in children with scoliosis. *J Bone Joint Surg Am*. 1985;67:699-702.
66. DiMeglio A. Growth of the spine before age 5 years. *J Pediatr Orthop B*. 1993;1:102-108.
67. Vitale MG, Matsumoto H, Bye MR, et al. A retrospective cohort study of pulmonary function, radiographic measures, and quality of life in children with congenital scoliosis: an evaluation of patient outcomes after early spinal fusion. *Spine*. 2008;33(11):1242-1249.
68. Campbell RM Jr, Smith MD, Mayes TC, et al. The characteristics of thoracic insufficiency syndrome associated with fused ribs and congenital scoliosis. *J Bone Joint Surg Am*. 2003;85-A(3):399-408.
69. Karol LA, Johnston C, Mladenov K, et al. Pulmonary function following early thoracic fusion in non-neuromuscular scoliosis. *J Bone Joint Surg Am*. 2008;90(6):1272-1281.
70. Vitale MG, Matsumoto H, Bye MR, et al. A retrospective cohort study of pulmonary function, radiographic measures, and quality of life in children with congenital scoliosis: an evaluation of patient outcomes after early spinal fusion. *Spine*. 2008;33(11):1242-1249.
71. Riccio AI, Guille JT, Grissom L, Figueroa TE. Magnetic resonance imaging of renal abnormalities in patients with congenital osseous anomalies of the spine. *J Bone Joint Surg Am*. 2007;89(11):2456-2459.
72. Cobb JR. *Outline for the Study of Scoliosis. Instructional Course Lectures*. Vol. 5. Ann Arbor, MI: American Academy of Orthopaedic Surgeons; 1948:261-275.
73. Facanha-Filho FA, Winter RB, Lonstein JE, et al. Measurement accuracy in congenital scoliosis. *J Bone Joint Surg Am*. 2001;83-A(1):42-45.
74. Loder RT, Urquhart A, Steen H, et al. Variability in Cobb angle measurements in children with congenital scoliosis. *J Bone Joint Surg Br*. 1995;77(5):768-770.
75. Newton PO, Hahn GW, Fricka KB, Wenger DR. Utility of three-dimensional and multiplanar reformatted computed tomography for evaluation of pediatric congenital spine abnormalities. *Spine*. 2002;27(8):844-850.
76. Kawakami N, Tsuji T, Imagama S, et al. Classification of congenital scoliosis and kyphosis: a new approach to the three-dimensional classification for progressive vertebral anomalies requiring operative treatment. *Spine*. 2009;34(17):1756-1765.
77. Blake NS, Lynch AS, Dowling FE. Spinal cord abnormalities in congenital scoliosis. *Ann Radiol (Paris)*. 1986;29(3-4):377-379.

78. Bradford DS, Heithoff KB, Cohen M. Intraspinal abnormalities and congenital spine deformities: a radiographic and MRI study. *J Pediatr Orthop*. 1991;11(1):36-41.
79. Prahinski JR, Polly DW Jr, McHale KA, Ellenbogen RG. Occult intraspinal anomalies in congenital scoliosis. *J Pediatr Orthop*. 2000;20(1):59-63.
80. Suh SW, Sarwark JF, Vora A, Huang BK. Evaluating congenital spine deformities for intraspinal anomalies with magnetic resonance imaging. *J Pediatr Orthop*. 2001;21(4):525-531.
81. Basu PS, Elsebaie H, Noordeen MHH. Congenital spinal deformity: a comprehensive assessment at presentation. *Spine*. 2002;27(20):2255-2259.
82. Klemme WR, Polly DW Jr, Orchowski JR. Hemivertebral excision for congenital scoliosis in very young children. *J Pediatr Orthop*. 2001;21(6):761-764.
83. Hedequist DJ, Hall JE, Emans JB. The safety and efficacy of spinal instrumentation in children with congenital spine deformities. *Spine*. 2004;29(18):2081-2086.
84. McMaster MJ, Singh H. The surgical management of congenital kyphosis and kyphoscoliosis. *Spine*. 2001;26(19):2146-2154.
85. Weiss HR. Congenital scoliosis: presentation of three severe cases treated conservatively. *Stud Health Technol Inform*. 2008;140:310-313.
86. Cheneau J, Grivas TB, Engels G, Fritsch HS. Wedged vertebrae normalization in congenital scoliosis due to application of external forces by brace. *Scoliosis*. 2007;2 (suppl 1):S29.
87. Burnei G, Gavriliu S, Vlad C, et al. Congenital scoliosis: an up-to-date. *J Med Life*. 2015;8(3):388-397.
88. Thuet ED, Padberg AM, Raynor BL, et al. Increased risk of postoperative neurologic deficit for spinal surgery patients with unobtainable intraoperative evoked potential data. *Spine*. 2005;30:2094-2103.
89. Mooney JF III, Bernstein R, Hennrikus WL Jr, et al. Neurologic risk management in scoliosis surgery. *J Pediatr Orthop*. 2002;22:683-689.
90. Moroz P, Emans JB, Hedequist DJ, et al. *Outcomes of major peri-operative neurologic complications in paediatric spine deformity [paper 60]*. Presented at Scoliosis Research Society Annual Meeting; September 10-13, 2003; Quebec City, Canada.
91. Hedequist DJ. Instrumentation and fusion for congenital spine deformities. *Spine*. 2009;34(17):1783-1790.
92. Kesling KL, Lonstein JE, Denis F, et al. The crankshaft phenomenon after posterior spinal arthrodesis for congenital scoliosis: a review of 54 patients. *Spine*. 2003;28(3):267-271.
93. Karol LA. Early definitive spinal fusion in young children: what we have learned. *Clin Orthop Relat Res*. 2011;469(5):1323-1329.
94. Bowen RE, Scaduto AA, Banuelos S. Does early thoracic fusion exacerbate preexisting restrictive lung disease in congenital scoliosis patients? *J Pediatr Orthop*. 2008;28(5): 506-511.
95. Newton PO, White KK, Faro F, et al. The success of thoracoscopic anterior fusion in a consecutive series of 112 pediatric spinal deformity cases. *Spine*. 2005;30:392-398.
96. Demirkiran G, Yilmaz G, Kaymaz B, et al. Safety and efficacy of instrumented convex growth arrest in treatment of congenital scoliosis. *J Pediatr Orthop*. 2014;34(3):275-281.
97. Winter RB, Lonstein JE, Denis F, Sta-Ana de la Rosa H. Convex growth arrest for progressive congenital scoliosis due to hemivertebrae. *J Pediatr Orthop*. 1988;8(6):633-638.
98. Dimeglio A, Bonnel F. Growth of the spine. In: Raimondi AJ, ed. *The Pediatric Spine. Principles of Pediatric Neurosurgery*. Vol. 39. Springer Verlag; 1989.
99. Cil A, Yazici M, Alanay A, et al. The course of sagittal plane abnormality in the patients with congenital scoliosis managed with convex growth arrest. *Spine*. 2004;29(5):547-552.
100. Thompson AG, Marks DS, Sayampanathan SR, et al. Long-term results of combined anterior and posterior convex epiphysiodesis for congenital scoliosis due to hemivertebrae. *Spine*. 1995;20:1380-1385.
101. Shono Y, Abumi K, Kaneda K. One-stage posterior hemivertebra resection and correction using segmental posterior instrumentation. *Spine*. 2001;26(7):752-757.
102. Cheung KM, Zhang JG, Lu DS, K Luk KD, Y Leong JC. Ten-year follow-up study of lower thoracic hemivertebrae treated by convex fusion and concave distraction. *Spine*. 2002;27(7):748-753.
103. Demirkiran G, Yilmaz G, Kaymaz B, et al. Safety and efficacy of instrumented convex growth arrest in treatment of congenital scoliosis. *J Pediatr Orthop*. 2014;34(3): 275-281.
104. Repko M, Krbec M, Burda J, et al. [Simple bony fusion or instrumented hemivertebra excision in the surgical treatment of congenital scoliosis]. *Acta Chir Orthop Traumatol Cech*. 2008;75(3):180-184.
105. Ruf M, Jensen R, Harms J. Hemivertebra resection in the cervical spine. *Spine*. 2005;30(4):380-385.
106. Bollini G, Docquier PL, Viehweger E, et al. Lumbar hemivertebra resection. *J Bone Joint Surg Am*. 2006;88:1043-1052.
107. Hedequist DJ, Hall JE, Emans JB. Hemivertebra excision in children via simultaneous anterior and posterior exposures. *J Pediatr Orthop*. 2005;25:60-63.
108. Nakamura H, Matsuda H, Konishi S, Yamano Y. Single-stage excision of hemivertebrae via the posterior approach alone for congenital spine deformity: follow-up period longer than ten years. *Spine*. 2002;27(1):110-115.
109. Ruf M, Harms J. Hemivertebra resection by a posterior approach: innovative operative technique and first results. *Spine*. 2002;27(10):1116-1123.
110. Shimode M, Kojima T, Sowa K. Spinal wedge osteotomy by a single posterior approach for correction of severe and rigid kyphosis or kyphoscoliosis. *Spine*. 2002;27:2260-2267.
111. Ruf M, Harms J. Posterior hemivertebra resection with transpedicular instrumentation: early correction in children aged 1 to 6 years. *Spine*. 2003;28(18):2132-2138.
112. Shono Y, Abumi K, Kaneda K. One-stage posterior hemivertebra resection and correction using segmental posterior instrumentation. *Spine*. 2001;26:752-757.
113. Bradford DS. Vertebral column resection. *Orthop Trans*. 1987;11:502.
114. Suk SI, Kim JH, Kim WJ, et al. Posterior vertebral column resection for severe spinal deformities. *Spine*. 2002;27(21):2374-2382.
115. Lenke LG, Sides BA, Koester LA, Hensley M, Blanke KM. Vertebral column resection for the treatment of severe spinal deformity. *Clin Orthop Relat Res*. 2010;468(3):687-699.
116. Lenke LG, O'Leary PT, Bridwell KH, et al. Posterior vertebral column resection for severe pediatric deformity: minimum two-year follow-up of thirty-five consecutive patients. *Spine*. 2009;34(20):2213-2221.
117. Dayer R1, Ceroni D, Lascombes P. Treatment of congenital thoracic scoliosis with associated rib fusions using VEPTR

expansion thoracostomy: a surgical technique. *Eur Spine J.* 2014;23(suppl 4):S424-S431.

118. Parnell SE, Effmann EL, Song K, et al. Vertical expandable prosthetic titanium rib (VEPTR): a review of indications, normal radiographic appearance and complications. *Pediatr Radiol.* 2015;45(4):606-616.
119. Campbell RM Jr, Smith MD, Hell-Vocke AK. Expansion thoracoplasty: the surgical technique of opening-wedge thoracostomy. Surgical technique. *J Bone Joint Surg Am.* 2004;86-A(suppl 1):51-64.
120. Heydar AM, Sirazi S, Bezer M. Magnetic controlled growing rods as a treatment of early onset scoliosis: early results with two patients. *Spine.* 2016;41(22):E1336-E1342.
121. Yılmaz B, Ekşi MŞ, Işik S, et al. Magnetically controlled growing rod in early-onset scoliosis: a minimum of 2-year follow-up. *Pediatr Neurosurg.* 2016;51(6):292-296.

27 CHAPTER Idiopathic Scoliosis

Lawrence G. Lenke
Fernando E. Silva
Ronald A. Lehman Jr

Idiopathic scoliosis is the most common cause of spinal deformity in pediatric patients, encompassing 80% of all scoliosis. Because its etiology is not known, it is a diagnosis of exclusion—other causes such as congenital, syndromic, neuromuscular, and positional (leg-length discrepancy) must be ruled out. The radiographic diagnosis requires a coronal plane angle, measured by the Cobb method, of 10 degrees or greater. Patients with curves less than 10 degrees are considered to have spinal asymmetry.[1,2] Ponseti and Friedman[3] first described early-onset scoliosis in 1950. Later, Dickson[4] expanded further on that concept and proposed that idiopathic scoliosis be divided into early (0–5 years old) and late onset (>5 years old), based on spinal growth velocity noted in these two age groups. Currently, idiopathic scoliosis is divided into four categories based on the age of onset: infantile (birth to 2 years + 11 months), juvenile (3–9 years + 11 months), adolescent (10–17 years + 11 months), and adult (18 years and older).[5] Treatments include close observation, bracing, and surgical intervention. Patient safety is imperative and is achieved by appropriate training, careful patient selection, and adherence to the principles of deformity surgery. Advanced technology and procedures have improved surgical treatment, with the ultimate goals being patient safety, satisfaction, motion preservation, and choosing the optimal fusion levels to prevent the need for further surgical intervention.

Epidemiology

Infantile and juvenile scoliosis are less prevalent than adolescent idiopathic scoliosis. Infantile idiopathic scoliosis is more common in Europe, constituting less than 1% of idiopathic scoliosis cases in the United States. Typically, these are left-sided thoracic curves, often occurring among boys. Recent reviews suggest that there might be a decline in its incidence.[6] In contrast, juvenile cases are typically diagnosed at age 5 years in boys and 7 years in girls, accounting for about 10% to 20% of idiopathic scoliosis cases.[3] Additionally, juvenile cases occur predominantly in girls; however, between 3 and 6 years of age, there seems to be a similar distribution between boys and girls, only to become predominant again in girls after age 6 years. The curve patterns closely resemble those of adolescents. Adolescent idiopathic scoliosis (AIS) is the most prevalent type. Among adolescents, the prevalence of 10-degree curves is less than 3%, with about 5% of curves showing a progression of greater than 30 degrees.[4] This prevalence decreases as a function of curve magnitude, however, to about 0.3% to 0.5% and 0.1% in curves measuring 20 degrees and 40 degrees, respectively.[7] The prevalence of curves greater than 10 degrees is higher among girls, with a 4:1 ratio of girls to boys, increasing to 9:1 when curves reach an operative range of about 40 to 50 degrees.[8]

Etiology

Despite decades of research, the specific cause of idiopathic scoliosis remains elusive and likely multifactorial. Possible causes of infantile idiopathic scoliosis include intrauterine molding or postnatal pressure on the spinal column from supine positioning during sleep. Other etiologies that have been considered in idiopathic scoliosis include dysfunction in proprioception to maldevelopment in central pattern generators in the spinal cord, connective tissue disorders, hormonal issues, and muscle/structural changes.[9-12] The literature suggests, however, that in the observed deformation of the spine, the unique mechanics of the fully erect posture, which is exclusive to humans, as well as genetics, both play important roles in its development and progression. Kouwenhoven and Castelein[13] concluded that many factors may play a role in the initiation and progression of AIS at a certain age. The growth spurt noted among adolescents seems to play a role in progression because, as the spine grows, there seems to be a mechanical influence as a critical buckling load is reached. Reports in the literature continue to strongly suggest a genetic link.[14]

Genetics

It is widely accepted that genetics plays a major role in idiopathic scoliosis. In 2008, Kulkarni and colleagues[15] mapped a developmentally critical *CHD* gene to 15q26.1 and, together with *CHD7*, suggested a possible role of *CHD2* in the embryonic development of the spine. In efforts to map out the gene(s) responsible for idiopathic scoliosis, Gao and colleagues[16] reported the first gene (*CHD7*) in the 8q12 locus to be associated with a familial idiopathic scoliosis. However, Tilley and colleagues failed to replicate Gao's findings.[17] In contrast, Takahashi et al. detected a strong association between AIS and rs11190870 near LBX1, noting that this was associated with both susceptibility and curve progression of AIS.[18] Hua et al. corroborated the latter findings as they reported on the strong association between AIS and rs11190870 near LBX1 in a Japanese group with AIS.[19] In terms of inheritance, the prevalence is 11% among first-degree relatives, 2.4% among second-degree relatives, and 1.4% among third-degree relatives.[20] Concordance among monozygotic and dizygotic twins has been reported to range from 73% to 92% and 36% to 63%, respectively.[21,22] Anderson and colleagues[23] published a population-based study taken from the Danish Twin Registry in which 46,418 twins were registered. From the 34,944 respondents, the concordance rate for monozygotic twins was 13% versus 0% for dizygotic twins. Gurnett and colleagues[24] published a report of a single multigenerational family in which AIS and pectus excavatum segregated as an autosomal dominant condition. Through linkage analysis, the investigators identified a genetic locus for the two conditions on chromosome 18q. Hence, even though the exact genetic and hereditary basis of scoliosis remains elusive, several chromosomes appear to play a role. Furthermore, its mode of inheritance remains unclear as both autosomal recessive, autosomal dominant with variable penetrance, and X-linked dominant modes of inheritance have been reported.

Natural History

About 90% of infantile curves show spontaneous resolution, especially among infants who are younger than 1 year at diagnosis.[6,25] Curves that typically progress are double curves with a thoracic component. Insight into curve progression can be obtained from the rib-vertebral angle difference (RVAD) and "phase of the rib head."[26] To calculate the RVAD, a line is drawn perpendicular to the *apical* vertebral endplate, another line is drawn from the mid-neck to the mid-head of the corresponding rib; the angle formed by the intersection of these lines is the rib vertebral angle or RVA. For calculating the RVAD, the angle on the other side of the same vertebra is calculated as well. The difference between the values of the RVAs on the concave and convex sides of the curve is the RVAD. In terms of phase of the rib head, if the head and neck of the *convex* rib of the vertebral body at the apex of the curve does not overlap the vertebral body, it is termed *phase I*; if it does overlap, it is termed *phase II*. It is unnecessary to calculate the RVAD when a curve is noted to be a phase II type, as those are almost certain to progress. Curves with RVAD greater than 20 degrees or phase II angles are very likely to progress.

Although juvenile scoliosis curves less than 25 degrees can also spontaneously resolve, about 70% of juvenile curve types tend to progress, with 50% requiring bracing and 50% surgical treatment. These curves tend to progress if idiopathic scoliosis is diagnosed before age 6 years and/or if they have a Cobb angle of greater than 30 degrees. Here, the RVAD has not proven to be a useful predictor of curve progression.

Many factors influence the natural history of AIS. Growth potential, skeletal maturity, curve magnitude, and location are important considerations when assessing progression of AIS. Family history, gender, and rotation do not seem to influence progression. Peak height growth seems to correlate best with, and is a better predictor of, progression than skeletal maturity. In terms of biomechanical influences, this likely is secondary to attaining a critical vertebral column height, which leads to a critical buckling load and greater bending moments with eventual curve progression. In girls, peak height growth seems to occur 6 to 12 months before the onset of menarche. In boys, peak height growth seems to correlate with the closure of the triradiate cartilage. Larger or double curves tend to progress more than smaller or single curves. Additionally, curves can progress *after* skeletal maturity; thoracic curves greater than 50 degrees and thoracolumbar/lumbar (TL/L) curves greater than 40 degrees can progress on average 1 degree per year.[27,28]

Evaluation

History and Physical Examination

A complete history, including any family history of scoliosis, is obtained and a physical examination is performed. With infantile and juvenile cases, in particular, a thorough prenatal, birth, and developmental history is obtained. In the adolescent, the growth spurt history is noted. Length of time postmenarche is an indication of potential growth remaining. A girl grows fastest one year *before* onset of menarche and usually finishes growing 2 years *after* its onset. Voice changes in boys are noted as well, because when such change has begun, the growth spurt is in its most intense phase. When the voice has acquired adult characteristics, the growth rate has started to decelerate. The duration of voice change varies between less than 1 year to more than 3 years. This information is imperative in determining peak growth velocity and as predictors of growth potential and its implications on possible curve progression.[29] Symptoms of pain and/or weakness and how the patient perceives her or his appearance relative to the deformity are especially important with AIS.[30] During the examination, height, weight, and age (years plus months since last birthday) are recorded. The head is examined with special attention to torticollis and plagiocephaly, given its higher incidence with infantile scoliosis. Possible conditions and anomalies that might be present include buccal and palatal anomalies, café-au-lait spots, and midline dimples or hair patches, or both, over the lumbodorsal spine, which can be important clinical clues to the presence of intraspinal pathology. Limb laxity is also checked and, when present, genetic counseling is requested. Trunk shift, a clinical correlate of curve rotation, is evaluated as the patient stands with the hips and knees fully extended. The relationship of the patient's head to the pelvis is also noted in evaluating the overall coronal and sagittal balance. Any shoulder, breast, or pelvic asymmetry is noted.[31] Curve rotation is assessed by performing an Adams forward-bend test and is quantified with a scoliometer. This is of critical importance when considering a selective thoracic fusion. This assessment is modified in infants by laying the patient on the examiner's knee, which also helps in assessing the rigidity of the curve, an important factor in terms of prognostication. Alternatively, a sitting forward-bend test can be performed. The latter maneuver can also help assess for plagiocephaly and developmental hip dysplasia, especially in infants. Leg-length discrepancy and pelvic obliquity are also evaluated.[32] When leg-length discrepancy is the likely cause of the deformity, a shoe lift is used to reevaluate the patient to determine if the curve corrects. A thorough neurologic examination includes all cranial nerves, motor strength, reflexes (including abdominal reflexes, often associated with Chiari malformations), sensory modalities, and gait.[33] Finally, other possible causes of scoliosis—such as congenital, syndromic, and neuromuscular types, as well as infection, neoplasms, and spondylolisthesis—must also be ruled out.

Radiographic Evaluation

Initial posteroanterior and lateral 36- × 14-inch standing long cassette views are obtained. Coronal and sagittal Cobb angles are measured.[2] Curves greater than 20 degrees in infants and children; any neurologic symptoms present in patients with idiopathic scoliosis; and left-sided, sharp angular, or irregular curve patterns require further investigation, including screening with total spine magnetic resonance imaging.[34,35] When anomalies of the nervous system are present on magnetic resonance imaging, a pediatric neurosurgical consultation is indicated.[36,37] In advanced curves when surgery is planned, supine, side-bending, and push-prone films are obtained for curve classification and to assess curve flexibility.

Classification Systems

Currently, there are no accepted formal curve classification systems for infantile or juvenile scoliosis. However, utilizing formal consensus-building methods, surgeons experienced in treating early-onset scoliosis (EOS) have developed a novel classification system for EOS, with all core components demonstrating substantial to excellent interobserver reliability. This classification system will likely serve as a foundation to guide ongoing research efforts and standardize communication in the clinical setting.[38] Similarly, in their effort to develop a classification system for juvenile scoliosis, Lenke et al. have modified the initial Lenke classification for AIS. This basically follows all the tenets of the AIS classification, but uses the C7 plumb line and the central sacral vertical line (CSVL) to decide on whether the minor thoracic or thoracolumbar curves are structural or not, respectively. The proximal thoracic curve's structural character is assessed by the relationship of the first rib to the main thoracic curve. Although such classification has not gained wide use, it attests to the authors' desire to continue to contribute to the treatment of deformity patients.[39]

The first treatment-based AIS classification was developed in 1983 by King and colleagues.[40] Based on a series of 405 patients with AIS, their uniplanar system analyzed thoracic curves only in the coronal plane. This system allowed for surgical planning and helped in assessing whether or not a King II curve could be selectively fused.[41] Interobserver and intraobserver reliability of this traditional thoracic classification system has proven to be fair at best.[42,43] Additionally, coronal decompensation has been reported after King II selective fusions, leading Lenke et al. to develop stricter criteria for selective thoracic fusions.

Lenke and colleagues[44] developed a comprehensive, practical classification system in 2001 that analyzes the coronal and sagittal planes (Fig. 27.1). It includes not only thoracic curves, but also TL/L curve patterns. Its interobserver and intraobserver reliability has been demonstrated.[42,43] Its definition of the structural characteristics of the proximal thoracic curve has been deemed reliable, leading to shorter proximal fusions when that curve is nonstructural.[45] It also allows a stricter evaluation of a curve's structural nature, permitting a more objective analysis of when a given curve can tolerate a selective fusion leading to a balanced outcome.[46,47] The latter is clinically significant, as one of the most important principles in preventing postoperative decompensation is proper identification of curve patterns, including which curves can tolerate a selective fusion.[41,48] This three-tiered classification combines a curve type (1 through 6) with coronal lumbar (A, B, or C) and sagittal thoracic (–, N, or +) modifiers to produce a triad comprehensive curve classification (e.g., 1A–).

Recent advances based on the Lenke classification system have led to the tentative inclusion of a third modifier: the last touched vertebra (TV). The TV is the most cephalad TL/L vertebra, T12–L5, of the lowest *structural* curve that is touched by the CSVL. In curve types 3 to 6, the TV is the most cephalad vertebra (T12–L5) touched by the CSVL *below the apex* of the structural TL/L curve, whether that curve is included in the fusion or not. Such a modifier aids in a more thorough evaluation of the Lenke curve classification (e.g., 5CN–L3, where L3 is the TV of the lowest *structural* curve), and serves as a landmark for the objective selection of the lowest instrumented vertebra (LIV) in Lenke 1A curves as well as selective thoracic fusions. Identification of the TV and comparison with the selected LIV also helps in postoperative curve analysis, assessment of distal fusion length, and overall evaluation of the surgical treatment of AIS.[49,50] If the LIV is the preoperative TV, then the TV to LIV relationship is (0); if the LIV is one level cephalad to the TV, then it is (–1); and (+1) when the LIV is one level caudal to the preoperative TV.

Three-Dimensional Classification

Scoliosis is a known three-dimensional deformity, and although the Lenke classification system takes into account the coronal and sagittal planes, it does not account for the axial or transverse planes of the deformity. A task force of the Scoliosis Research Society continues to work on developing a clinically useful three-dimensional analysis to aid in further defining the classification of scoliosis. The key factor in a

THE LENKE CLASSIFICATION SYSTEM FOR AIS

Curve type	Proximal thoracic	Main thoracic	Thoracolumbar/lumbar	Descripition
1	Nonstructural	Structural*	Nonstructural	Main thoracic (MT)
2	Structural†	Structural*	Nonstructural	Double thoracic (DT)
3	Nonstructural	Structural*	Structural†	Double major (DM)
4	Structural†	Structural§	Structural§	Triple major (TM)
5	Nonstructural	Nonstructural	Structural*	Thoracolumbar/lumbar (TL/L)
6	Nonstructural	Structural†	Structural*	Thoracolumbar/lumbar-main thoracic (TL/L-MT)

*Major curve: largest Cobb measurment, always structural; †Minor curve: remaining structural curves; §Type 4 - MT or TL/L can be the major curve

STRUCTURAL CRITERIA
(Minor curves)

Proximal thoracic	– Side bending Cobb ≥25° – T2–T5 Kyphosis ≥+20°
Main thoracic	– Side bending Cobb ≥25° – T10–L2 Kyphosis ≥+20°
Thoracolumbar/lumbar	– Side bending Cobb ≥25° – T10–L2 Kyphosis ≥+20°

LOCATION OF APEX
(SRS definition)

CURVE	APEX
Thoracic	T2 to T11/12 disc
Thoracolumbar	T12/L1
Lumbar	L1/2 disc to L4

MODIFIERS

Lumbar coronal modifier	Center sacral vertical line to lumbar apex
A	Between pedicles
B	Touches apical body(ies)
C	Completely medial

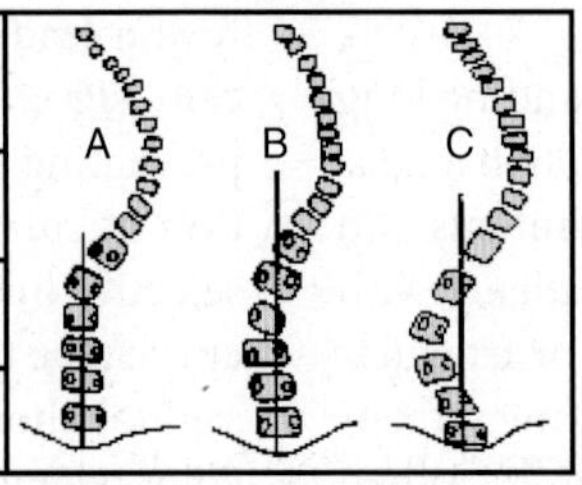

A B C

Thoracic sagittal profile T5-T12	
Modifier	Cobb angle
– (Hypo)	<10°
N (Normal)	10°–40°
+ (Hyper)	>40°

Curve type (1–6) + Lumbar coronal modifier (A. B, C) + Thoracic sagittal modifier (–, N, +) =
Curve classification (e.g. 1B+): ______

FIG. 27.1 Lenke adolescent idiopathic scoliosis (AIS) classification system schematic.

three-dimensional assessment is the plane of maximum curvature, which is the three-dimensional deformity that occurs as the spine translates and rotates out of the normal sagittal profile in scoliotic deformities. This work is expected to provide further understanding so that three-dimensional analysis and classification will become a standard for all scoliosis surgeons.[1,51]

Treatment Options

Three fundamental treatment options exist for idiopathic scoliosis: observation, casting/bracing, and surgery. These treatment modalities are based on the natural history of idiopathic scoliosis or the potential or probability of curve progression.[1,52] However, other modalities have been proposed to slow or halt curve progression, such as electrical stimulation and physical therapy. Yet, none of these modalities has been scientifically proven to be a viable alternative in the treatment of scoliosis.[53] Romano et al. noted that there is a lack of high-quality evidence to recommend the use of scoliosis-specific exercises for AIS, although a very low-quality study suggested that these exercises may be more effective than electrostimulation, traction, and postural training to avoid scoliosis progression.[54] Better-quality research needs to be conducted before the use of scoliosis-specific exercises can be recommended in clinical practice. Similarly, Mordecai et al. concluded from their extensive literature search that there is poor-quality evidence supporting the use of exercise therapy in the treatment of AIS.[55]

Observation

Up to 90% of infantile curves have been known to resolve spontaneously, but they can progress.[56] Deciphering which infantile curves will progress can be guided by the RVAD and the relationship of the apical rib head to the vertebral body, as previously noted.[27] Infants with curves less than 30 degrees and RVAD less than 20 degrees and juveniles with curves less than 20 degrees should be followed clinically and radiographically every 3 to 6 months. Adolescent idiopathic patients with curves less than 25 degrees are also followed clinically and radiographically every 3 to 6 months. Brace treatment is started for curve progression.

Bracing and Casting

Bracing[57] is the nonoperative treatment of choice in *small but progressive* scoliosis in growing children and adolescents. In about 75% of cases, bracing can control the curve and avoid progression, rendering the curve small enough so that the risk of progression after growth is unlikely.[53] In a younger child whose growth potential remains a significant issue, bracing allows curve control and continued growth until the patient requires eventual operative treatment should curve progression ensue.

With infantile cases, serial Mehta casting (derotational type) or a thoracolumbar orthosis are appropriate treatments in flexible curves, Cobb angles greater than 30 degrees, RVAD greater than 20 degrees, and curves with a phase II vertebral-rib relationship. Bracing alone can be employed where there is incomplete correction with Mehta casting. Bracing and casting of these patients comes with potential consequences, however, that include pulmonary restriction, which can have future ramifications.[58,59] Yet, Sanders and colleagues[60] found serial casting to be beneficial in the treatment of infantile scoliosis. They reported that curves less than 60 degrees often fully corrected in infants if casting was started before age 20 months.

Juveniles with curves 20 to 50 degrees are candidates for bracing. Here, the intent is *to prevent curve progression* and not so much attain correction. These patients are essentially braced 16 to 23 hours a day until the completion of skeletal growth or until they become surgical candidates. Patients with thoracic hypokyphosis should not be braced.

In adolescents with curves between 20 and 30 degrees, bracing is started if a curve progresses greater than or equal to 5 degrees or more in two consecutive visits or greater than or equal to 10 degrees in one visit. Bracing is usually started after the first office visit if the patient is skeletally immature (Risser ≤2) and presents with a 25- to 40-degree curve. This treatment modality is effective only for flexible curves and, as with the juvenile type, the goal is *to stop progression* versus curve correction. Male, obese, and noncompliant patients, as well as those with poor in-brace correction and hypokyphotic curves, are less likely to benefit from bracing. Patients must wear their brace 16 to 23 hours a day until the completion of skeletal growth or until they become surgical candidates. Bracing is deemed successful if there is less than 5 degrees progression at brace discontinuation (skeletal maturity). Conversely, if the curve progresses to greater than 60 degrees after brace discontinuation and/or if there is absolute progression to greater than 45 degrees at or prior to discontinuation, the patient is considered to have failed bracing treatment.

Several brace options exist. Deciding which brace to use depends on the apex of the curve and physician preference. Curves with an apex above T6 would likely require the use of a Milwaukee (cervicothoracolumbosacral orthosis).[61] Conversely, curves with apices at T7 or below and above L2 do well in a Boston underarm thoracolumbosacral orthosis. These braces are more socially acceptable due to lack of a cervical extension. The Charleston bending brace is an option if the child is noncompliant to wearing the brace during the day. Although the efficacy of a brace seems to depend on the length of time the brace is worn,[62] this brace is typically worn at night, and some studies have shown its efficacy.[63,64] Modifications to the standard thoracolumbosacral orthosis include variations of the Chêneau brace (Jacques Chêneau) and the SpineCor dynamic brace (SpineCorporation). The Chêneau 2000 orthosis allows for a greater amount of initial correction by using a hypercorrected mold and pads, which provide derotational forces.[65] This brace is the first that uses the theory of expansion to allow for active correction by respiratory movements.[66] The SpineCor[67] and TrIAC (Boston Brace International) are nonrigid braces. They work by using straps, which correspond to a specific correcting movement depending on the curve pattern, producing a progressive positional change, dynamic curve correction, and appropriate muscle balance. When bracing is initiated and pad placement is deemed appropriate, patient follow-up occurs every 4 to 6 months, with in-brace radiographic evaluation and appropriate fitting adjustments made when necessary.

Operative Intervention

Operative intervention is usually recommended for patients whose curves progress despite nonoperative management.[67] In infants, operative intervention is controversial. It is occasionally performed in infants with thoracic curves greater than 45 degrees, TL/L curves greater than 40 degrees, or those who fail Mehta casting or bracing. Juveniles are typically more prone to curve progression and are more likely to require operative intervention, particularly with curves greater than 50 degrees. Other patients who are likely to benefit from operative intervention are skeletally immature patients with AIS with a greater than 40- to 45-degree curve and mature patients with curves greater than 50 degrees.[27]

Surgical Techniques

Anterior-only, posterior-only, and circumferential procedures remain the mainstay of surgical treatment options.[68] However, the prevalence of anterior-only and circumferential procedures has declined with a concomitant development of surgical technologies permitting successful posterior-only procedures. Surgeons are now aware that early intervention with a definitive anteroposterior fusion for progressive infantile and juvenile curves leads to loss of trunk height development, which can lead to chest wall and lung underdevelopment.[69,70] This problem has promoted innovative techniques to try to control progressive curves surgically without definitive fusion, including epiphysiodesis,[71,72] dual growing rod placement (Fig. 27.2),[73] intervertebral stapling (Fig. 27.3),[74,75] spinal tethering (Fig. 27.4),[76,77] and the vertical expandable prosthetic titanium rib (VEPTR),[78] with the last used more in progressive EOS, in which rib and chest wall deformities can be quite severe. In those cases, Cobb angles greater than 45 degrees and failed Mehta casting or bracing are operative indications, with fusion as close to skeletal maturity as possible. Among juveniles, fusionless techniques are also indicated in small children with

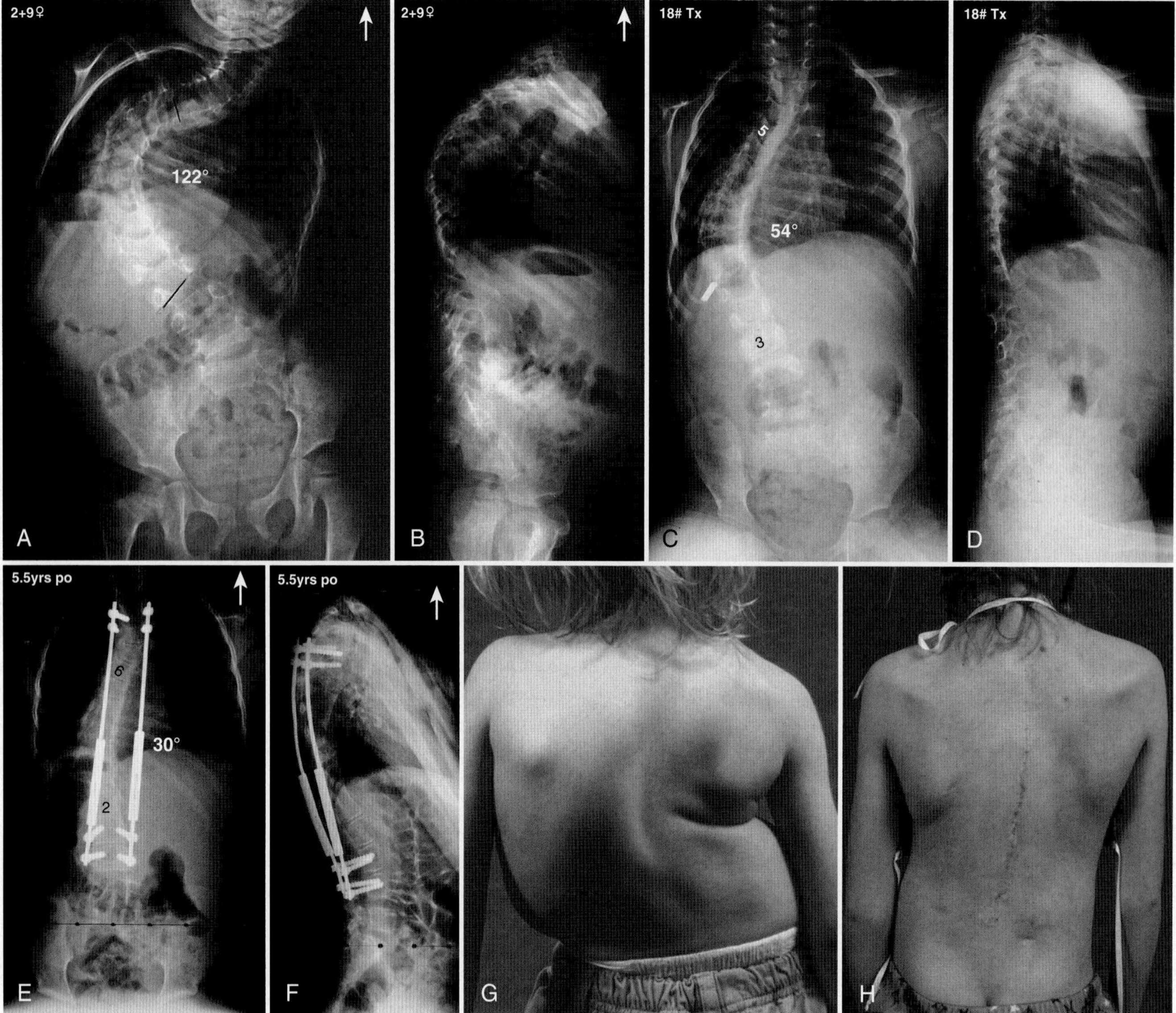

FIG. 27.2 (A–B) Radiographs of a girl, age 2 years + 9 months, who presented with severe infantile-onset idiopathic scoliosis. Her left thoracic curve measured 122 degrees. (C–D) She was placed in halo-gravity traction and underwent a short apical anterior release and fusion, and was prepared for a growing rod construct. (E–F) She had a dual-rod, pedicle screw growing rod construct placed. At 5 years + 6 months after initiation of growing rod treatment, she continues to be lengthened with overall good coronal and sagittal balance and acceptable lung fields. (G–H) Preoperative and latest postoperative clinical images show maintenance of trunk alignment and growth.

curves greater than 40 to 50 degrees with significant growth potential, allowing continued spinal growth over unfused segments, until a definitive fusion can be performed *close to or at* skeletal maturity. Anteroposterior fusions are reserved for younger patients with curves greater than 50 degrees with a potential to crankshaft or for very severe curves. Anterior-only instrumentation and fusions are indicated for TL/L curves greater than 40 to 50 degrees with a normal sagittal profile. Posterior-only fusions are performed for curves greater than 50 degrees as well as double major curves, when the child has grown closer to skeletal maturity, or even in those who are skeletally immature with the use of segmental pedicle screws and adequate fusion levels that will prevent the adding on phenomenon.

Many surgeons today still prefer to perform an anterior approach in younger patients when there is risk of crankshaft development and especially for thoracolumbar and lumbar major curves. However, with the introduction of pedicle screws, a posterior approach has shown numerous benefits over an anterior procedure, such as better maintenance of the obtained correction, more powerful corrective forces, three-column control, and often obviating the need for anterior releases and thoracoplasties.[79–85] In addition, a posterior approach avoids the negative consequences of chest cage disruption and pulmonary compromise that can result from an open anterior approach[86,87] (Fig. 27.5). Yet, according to a 2010 study by Tis and colleagues,[88] with the advances in anterior instrumentation, surgeons theoretically should see

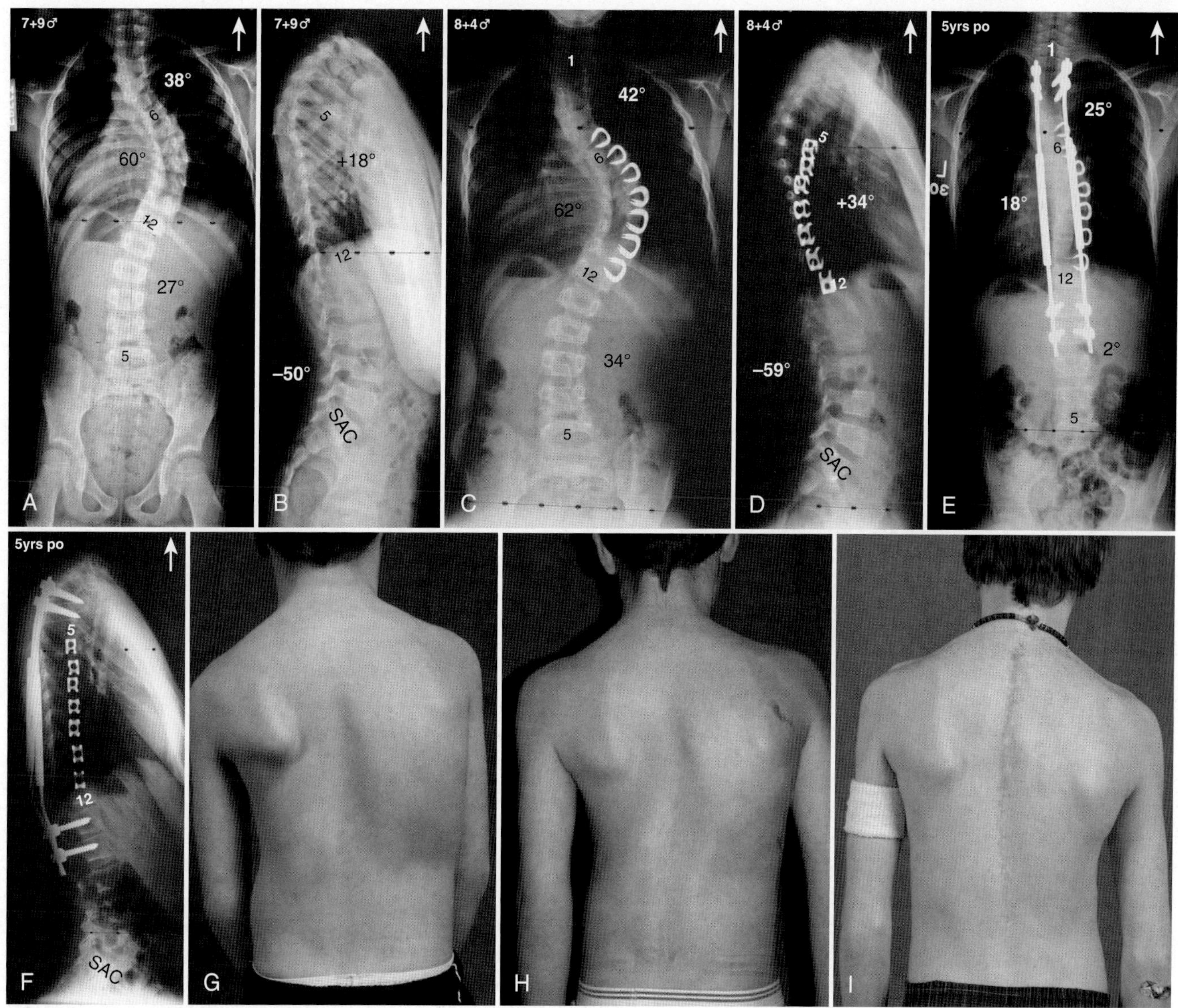

FIG. 27.3 (A–B) Radiographs of a boy, age 7 years + 9 months, who presented with progressive juvenile-onset right thoracic idiopathic scoliosis. His main thoracic curve measured 60 degrees and was progressive despite bracing. (C–D) He had anterior thoracic stapling performed but had slow progression of his deformity with growth. (E–F) A posterior dual screw-rod growing construct was placed. Five years after insertion, his deformity correction has been maintained to 18 degrees in the main thoracic curve with a good sagittal profile. (G–I) Clinical images before surgery, status post-stapling, and 5 years status post–growing rod construct show improvement of truncal deformation.

a reduction in the rate of rod breakage, pseudarthrosis, and sagittal decompensation, and obtain improved correction rates. These authors concluded that open anterior spinal fusion surgery is a safe method for the treatment of thoracic AIS. At 5-year follow-up, they reported good coronal and sagittal correction of the main thoracic and compensatory TL/L curves, but they also reported that pulmonary function was mildly decreased as with any procedure in which a thoracotomy is performed. Tis and colleagues also concluded that in skeletally immature patients, an open anterior spinal fusion can increase kyphosis; however, newer techniques used in their series seemed to limit progressive kyphosis, which has been noted in previously published reports.[89]

Adolescent curves can typically be surgically treated via an anterior or posterior approach (or both) with instrumentation and fusion.[88] Thoracoscopic procedures have shown advantages over open anterior thoracotomy procedures. Kishan and colleagues[90] showed that anterior thoracoscopy had fewer adverse effects on pulmonary function. Sucato and colleagues[91] found that adding a thoracoscopic release performed in the prone position to a posterior instrumentation and fusion offered the advantages of minimally invasive surgery and did not require repositioning to perform the posterior procedure. In addition, when double-lung ventilation is used, acute pulmonary complications are significantly reduced. A significant learning curve is required, however, and these techniques have diminished in popularity owing to the proliferation of pedicle screw constructs.

During surgical planning, determination of proximal and distal fusion levels is paramount because choosing incorrect

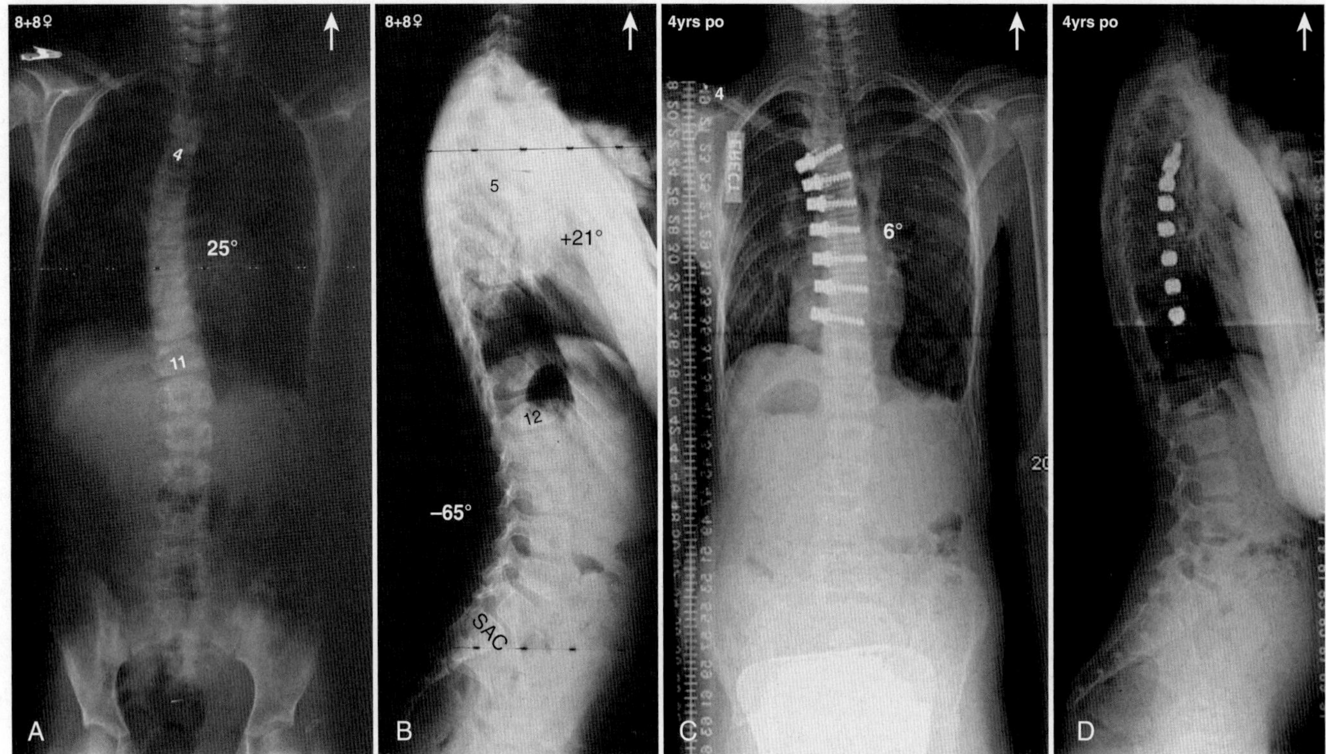

FIG. 27.4 (A–B) Radiographs of a girl age 8 years + 8 months who presented with progressive left thoracic scoliosis. She had a positive family history of scoliosis, with her mother requiring scoliosis fusion as a child. Her left thoracic curve progressed to 25 degrees with a normal sagittal profile. (C–D) She was treated with a single left thoracic mobile tether, with slow progressive correction of her deformity to 6 degrees with a normal sagittal profile 4 years after treatment. She had only one surgery and did not wear a brace postoperatively.

levels is the main reason for postoperative decompensation.[31,92] *Adding on* is another phenomenon that can result if a fusion is stopped "short." Suk and colleagues[93] reported 5-year results of 203 patients in which they found that adding on occurred in 17 patients who were fused, on average, two levels short of the neutral vertebra.

Upper and Lower Instrumented Vertebra Selection

With anterior-only approaches, fusion levels typically extend from end-to-end vertebrae, as measured with the Cobb technique. Short fusions above and below the apex, depending on whether the apex is a disc or a vertebra, have been advocated for flexible thoracolumbar curves.[9] In this technique, if the apex is a vertebral body, the discs above and below the apex are included in the fusion. If the apex is a disc, the two discs above and below the apex are included in the fusion. Brodner et al.[94] predicted fusion levels based on the supine-pull ("stretch") films, ensuring that a thorough release is performed to obtain a bone-on-bone fusion. Anterior structural grafts have been used to counter the kyphogenesis associated with anterior instrumentation.[88]

With posterior approaches, the selection of the upper instrumented vertebra is based on clinical and radiographic shoulder height, size, and stiffness of the proximal thoracic (PT) curve, hyperkyphosis of the upper thoracic region and amount of main thoracic curve correction planned (dynamic criteria). In general, when the left shoulder is elevated, the PT curve is structural and/or kyphotic (T2–T5 >20 degrees) and marked correction is planned (apical translation), T2 is a wise choice for the upper instrumented vertebra in this scenario. When the shoulders are level and the PT curve is close to being structural and/or mildly kyphotic (T2–T5 >10 degrees and <20 degrees), with marked correction planned, T3 is an appropriate choice. Finally, T4 or T5 is a wise choice when the right shoulder is elevated and the PT curve is nonstructural and not kyphotic.

Selection of the lower instrumented vertebra (LIV) requires identification of the end, neutral, and stable vertebra (SV) of the distal structural curve to be included in the fusion.[95] A safe place to end the fusion is the SV; however, the Lenke classification and current correction techniques employing pedicle fixation and derotation maneuvers allow for shorter distal fusion levels (Fig. 27.6). As noted earlier, in addition to all Lenke 1A curves, in selective thoracic fusions of Lenke 1C and 2C curves, the TV can be the LIV if it is proximal to the stable vertebra. With possible selective thoracic fusion of Lenke 3C and 4C curves, the TV is still going to be below the apex of the structural TL/L curve even when that curve is not included in the fusion. Similarly, with nonselective thoracic fusions, as well as Lenke 5C and 6C curves, the LIV can be cephalad to the SV provided that the intended LIV touches the CSVL, does not have significant rotation (Nash-Moe grade ≤1.5), and the disc below is parallel or closed on the convexity and the apex of the TL/L curve is L1 or the L1–L2 disc, *not* L2.

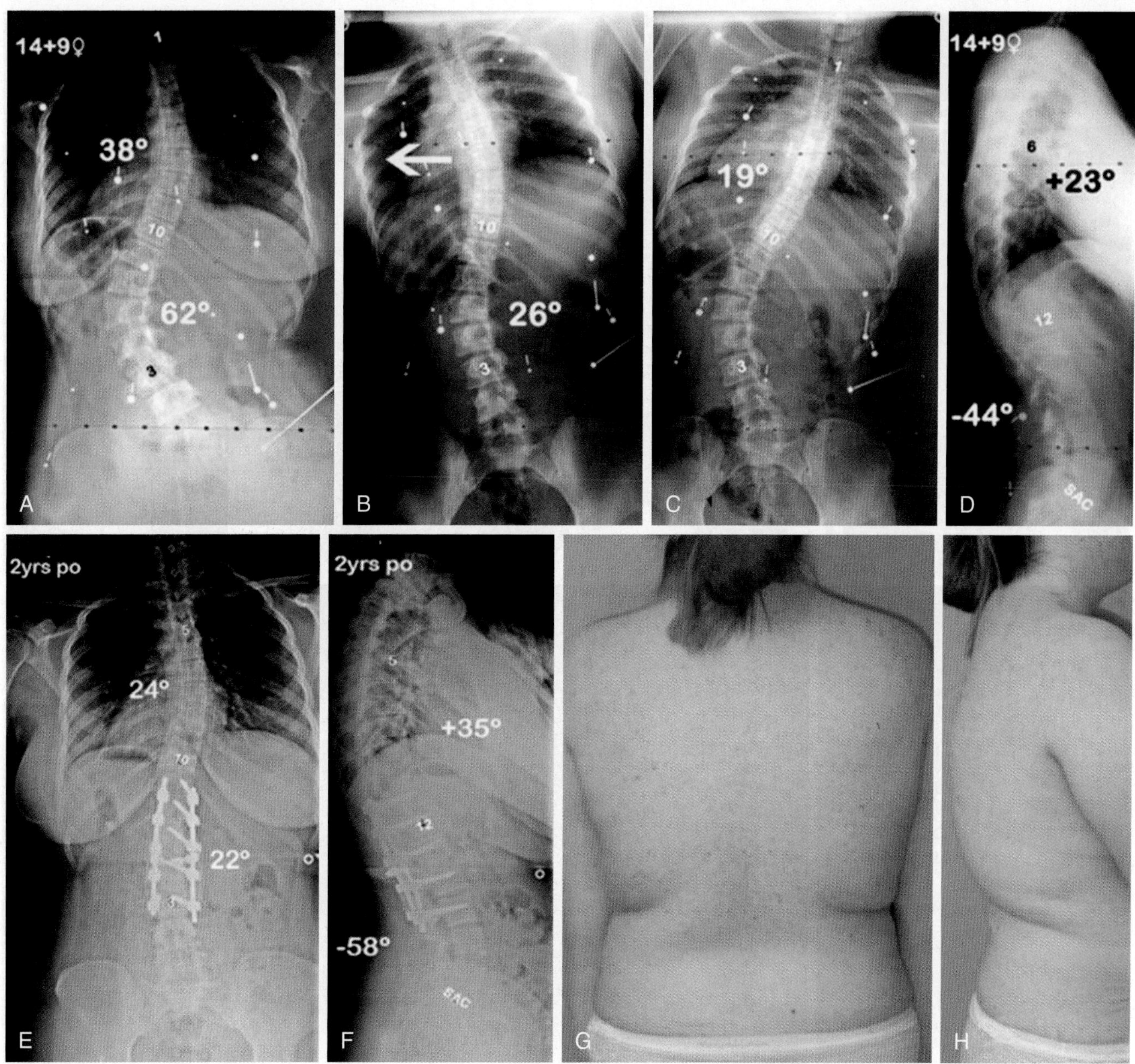

FIG. 27.5 (A–D) Radiographs of a female, age 14 years + 9 months, with a Lenke 5CN curve. She was treated with a posterior-only approach. (E–H) Note postoperative balanced spine and excellent clinical results.

In placing thoracic screws, it is essential to follow sequential steps at every screw placement.[79,80] With small pedicles, time should be taken to expand the pedicle to accommodate a screw.[96] Alternatively, parapedicular screw placement is a safe possibility.[97] Although we advocate the use of pedicle screws whenever possible, when employing hook-and-rod segmental instrumentation, it is imperative to reverse hook orientation where the discs are reversed in orientation to maintain coronal and sagittal balance.[98] We also advocate selective thoracic fusions whenever feasible.

Selective Fusions

The term *selective fusion* refers to minor structural thoracic or lumbar curves that cross the midline, but are not included in the fusion. That is, they are left untreated. Similarly, rare situations arise when one considers fusing nonstructural, secondary curves for the sake of cosmesis, spinal balance, or both.

The Lenke classification system provides an objective way to decide when to perform selective fusions in patients with AIS, especially with type C curve patterns, including Lenke 1 and 2C, and possibly Lenke 3C and 4C types.[47,92] Selective fusions of the latter types are achieved by having stricter criteria that define the *structural characteristics* of individual curves, leading to an objective analysis that helps in choosing which curves can be selectively fused without ensuing clinical imbalance.[43,44,99,100] Clinical assessment of the deformity cannot be overemphasized because it plays as important a role as the radiographic assessment when deciding whether to perform a selective fusion. Hence, the analysis of whether or not to proceed with a selective thoracic fusion (STF) begins

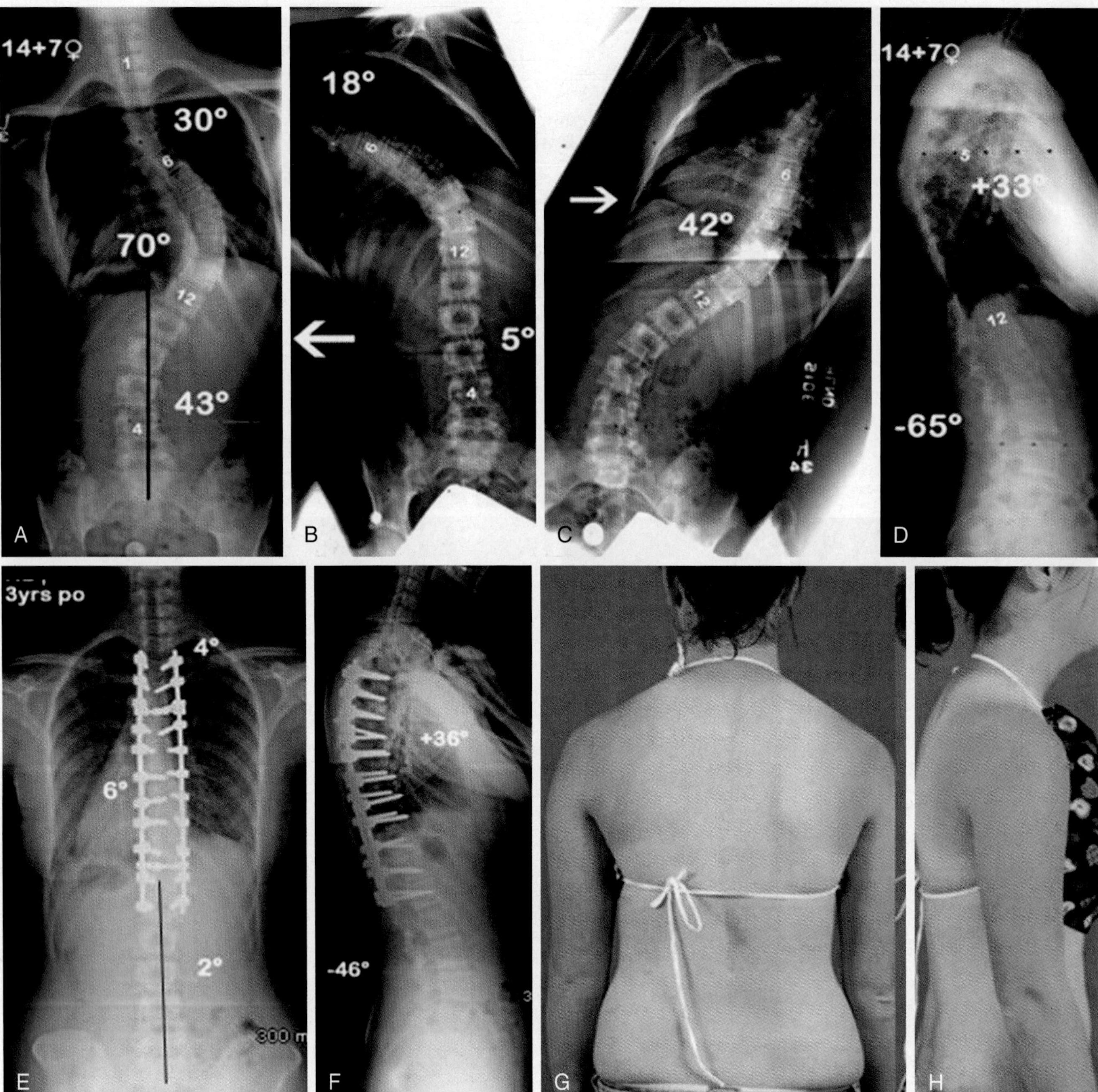

FIG. 27.6 (A–D) Radiographs of a female, age 14 years + 7 months, with a Lenke 1BN/L1 curve. She was treated by posterior-only approach, T3–L1 (0). (E–H) Note postoperative balanced spine with spontaneous lumbar correction from B to A modifier and excellent clinical results.

with the clinical assessment of the patient's deformity as well as skeletal maturity.[41,43,92] The magnitude of the thoracic and lumbar prominences are evaluated in order to decide if the patient is willing to accept a moderate lumbar hump when contemplating an STF. Next, the radiographic analysis entails comparing the relative Cobb angle measurements and apical vertebral rotation and translation ratios of the thoracic and TL/L curves.[48,49] Also, *one cannot overlook the thoracolumbar sagittal profile* because this can lead to curve misclassification and incorrect operative management; that is, proceeding with an STF in a curve pattern when selective fusion might not be recommended. In terms of operative management, attention must be paid to the degree of tilt left on the LIV when carrying out an STF; this is guided by the lumbar modifier to allow for harmonious balance of the unfused structural lumbar curve.

A rough estimate of the degree of tilt to be left on the LIV is equal to the remaining tilt on a preoperative supine film. This tilt is further assessed with intraoperative full-spine radiographs.[99] Again, this is imperative in allowing for accommodation of the structural component of the lumbar curve, especially with selective fusions.[47] The lower endplate of the

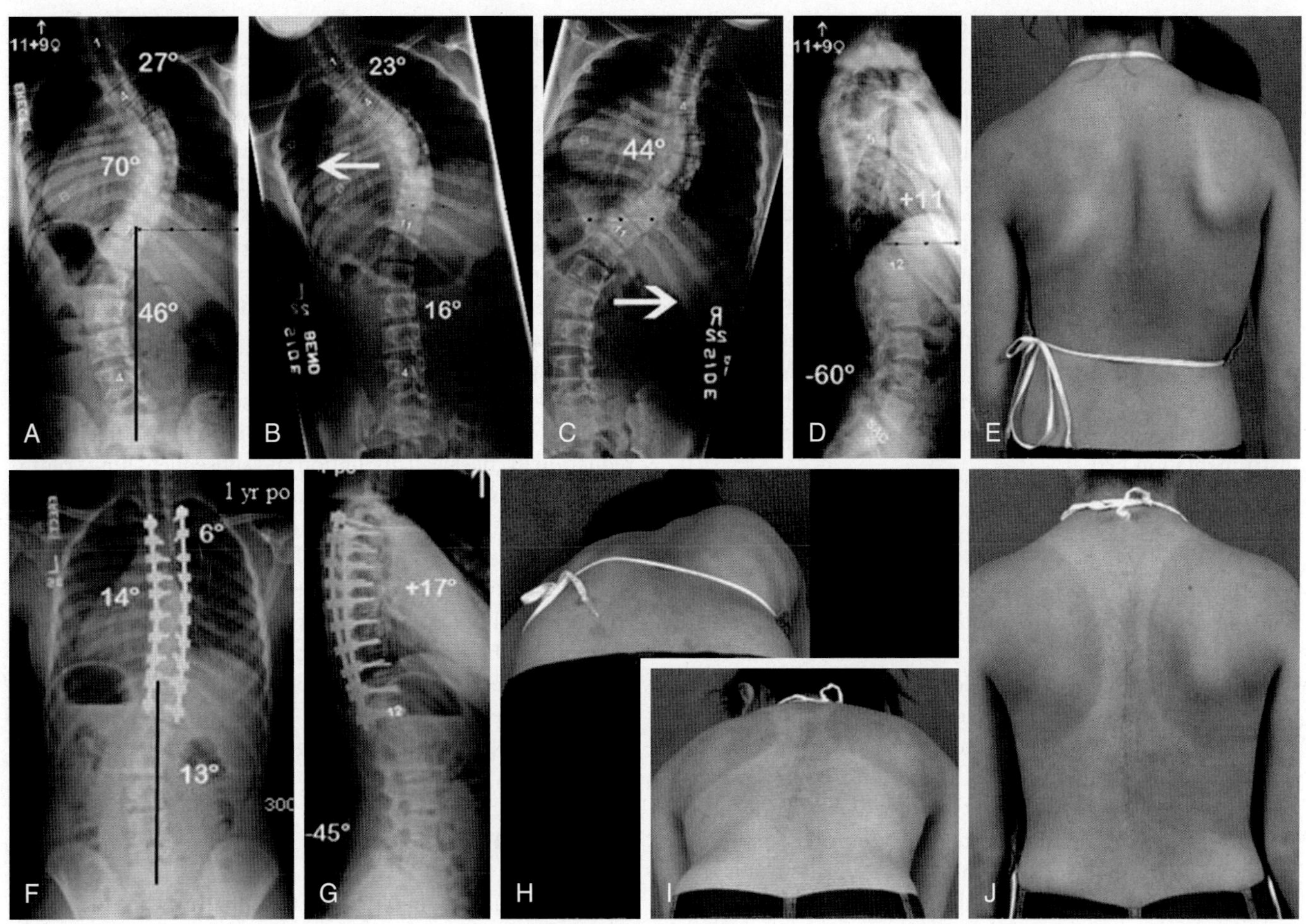

FIG. 27.7 (A–D) Radiographs of a girl, age 11 years + 9 months, with progressive right thoracic compensatory left lumbar scoliosis. Her main thoracic curve progressed to 70 degrees, and her compensatory 46-degree curve decreased on side bending to 16—a 1CN/T12 classification. (F–G) She underwent a selective thoracic fusion, T3–T12 (0) with a pedicle screw construct, with nicely matched 14-degree thoracic and 13-degree lumbar scoliotic curves 1 year postoperatively with spontaneous lumbar correction from modifier C to B and adequate sagittal balance. Preoperative and postoperative clinical images show improved truncal correction on upright (E, J) and forward bend (H, I) views.

LIV should be horizontal for type A lumbar modifier curves, a mild tilt should be left on type B curves, and an appropriate degree of tilt should be left on the LIV for type C curves (Fig. 27.7).

Selective anterior fusions of major TL/L curves associated with minor and partially structural thoracic curves in Lenke 5C and 6C curves can also be considered.[92] The analysis here parallels that of a thoracic STF. Additionally, the thoracic curve should be less than 50 degrees, bend out to 20 degrees or less, the TL/L-to-thoracic Cobb ratio should be 1.25 or greater, and the triradiate cartilages should be closed.[46] However, such selective fusions should *not* be undertaken when shoulder depression ipsilateral to the TL/L curve exists, the patient is highly skeletally immature, or a clinically unacceptable thoracic hump is present. To prevent decompensation, if the lumbar curve bends out more than the thoracic curve does, the lumbar curve should not be overcorrected because the thoracic curve likely would not compensate to achieve postoperative balance.[91] One study showed an average spontaneous correction of 14 degrees or 36% improvement of the thoracic curve when a selective TL/L fusion was performed.[47]

Adjuncts to Correction

Direct Vertebral Rotation

In the past, curves greater than 75 degrees, curves that do not correct below 50 degrees, and curves needing a thoracoplasty have required anterior releases. With the use of modern techniques of multisegmental pedicle screw fixation and the addition of direct vertebral rotation (DVR) techniques, safe and effective procedures demonstrating greater coronal and sagittal realignment along with acceptable cosmesis without the need for an anterior procedure have been reported.[101-103] Additionally, in the thoracic region, DVR helps derotate the spine and significantly decreases the rib prominence. Care must be taken to use stiffer rods, prebent in the sagittal profile, to prevent inducing hypokyphosis in the thoracic spine. DVR also helps to obtain better three-dimensional correction in the

TL/L component of Lenke double major curves and to minimize the LIV tilt angle.[101]

A DVR is performed only if screw placement is adequate, if the thoracic spine is not overly lordotic or kyphotic, and when there is a clinically significant thoracic or lumbar prominence. The DVR technique necessitates accurate placement of pedicle screws at the apex of the deformity and the three levels at the proximal and distal ends of the fusion. When the thoracic spine has a (+) sagittal modifier, per the Lenke classification, a DVR maneuver is not performed because increased kyphosis places considerable strain on the proximal screws unless appropriate releases via posterior column osteotomies are performed. Otherwise, the coronal and sagittal deformities are addressed simultaneously by convex rod instrumentation first.

Osteotomies

Several osteotomy choices are available to correct sagittal, coronal, and multiplanar deformities associated with previously fused or more severe idiopathic scoliosis curves, including posterior column osteotomies (Ponté, Smith-Petersen), pedicle subtraction osteotomy, and vertebral column resection (VCR). A Smith-Petersen osteotomy classically refers to an osteotomy performed through a previous lumbar fusion mass, whereas a Ponté osteotomy refers to a posteriorly based thoracic osteotomy through a previously unfused spine. We prefer the term posterior column osteotomy, as it avoids this prevalent confusion. Like sagittal imbalance, coronal imbalance can be classified as type A or B. In type A, the shoulders and pelvis are tilted in the opposite direction, whereas in type B, they tilt in the same direction.[104,105] Typically, single-plane type A deformities can be addressed with one pedicle subtraction osteotomy (PSO); multiple or asymmetrical pedicle subtraction osteotomies can be used when dealing with stiff or kyphoscoliotic cases. Simple trigonometric calculations at the vertebral body where the osteotomy is going to be performed permit precise determination of the angle of bony resection required for global balance.[106] Type B deformities likely require a VCR.

VCRs can be performed via a combined anterior and posterior approach (i.e., circumferentially) or from a posterior-only approach (Fig. 27.8).[107] Compromised pulmonary function lends consideration, however, to performing a posterior-only approach. The surgeon must balance the potential pulmonary compromise of the patient with the understanding that the extracavitary approach (i.e., posterior only) requires a higher level of surgical expertise and is technically more demanding.[108,109] As with all surgical procedures, adherence to safety is the most important principle, and if the surgeon is uncomfortable with a particular approach or technique, a referral should be made.[110] Nevertheless, this correction modality is appropriate in the setting of congenital cases, multiplanar or stiff kyphoscoliotic curves, curves previously fused circumferentially, and cases of global imbalance. In the last-mentioned situation, attention must be paid to the direction of the shoulder and pelvic tilt imbalance (see Fig. 27.8).

Minimally Invasive Techniques

Minimally invasive spine surgery is a popular concept that uses imaging, retraction, and implant technologies to help surgeons locate the exact area on which they are to operate. This type of procedure is done through incisions less than 1 inch long, minimizing damage to surrounding muscles and other tissues, which rapidly increases the healing and reduces recovery time. It also uses technology to perform the surgery more efficiently. One example is a video-assisted thoracoscopic procedure. According to Newton and colleagues,[111] this procedure can be used for an anterior thoracic release or to achieve deformity correction via rod-screw constructs. Given the small incisions and the muscle-splitting technique used, a reduction in chest wall disruption and subsequent lung volume decrease, as is the case with an open thoracotomy approach, was noted. This procedure offers comparable curve correction and a faster return to presurgical function.[90,91] However, with advances in instrumentation as mentioned previously and the enhanced ability to perform a direct vertebral derotation with posterior pedicle screw constructs, the use of video-assisted thoracoscopic instrumentation procedures has declined substantially. The decision between an anterior and a posterior approach is based purely on surgeon preference at this point.

Postoperative Care

Patients are usually observed in the intensive care unit overnight. Sitting and standing with assistance is permitted, and physical therapy is usually started on the first postoperative day. When stable, patients are transferred to the regular floor. As bowel function returns and patients are able to tolerate clear fluids, routine intravenous narcotics are replaced with oral narcotics as needed. Typically, no postoperative bracing is used. When patients are ambulatory, the urinary catheter is removed. On postoperative day 3, the drains are discontinued along with prophylactic antibiotics. After discharge, usually on postoperative day 4 or 5, patients may start to slowly resume activities.

Complications

Complications can occur during any of the treatment stages—preoperative, intraoperative, or postoperative.[112,113] At the preoperative stage, inappropriate curve classification and inadequate surgical planning can lead to inappropriate surgical decisions. Thus, it is essential to ensure that when performing a selective fusion, the clinical exam is considered and appropriate structural curve criteria are met.[92] Choosing inappropriate fusion levels can also be included in the category of preoperative complications.[114]

Intraoperative complications most commonly result from technical errors, including instrumentation misplacement. Hooks that do not hug the lamina or misplaced pedicle screws can lead to devastating complications, including spinal cord insults. Overcorrection of curves and, conversely, inadequate

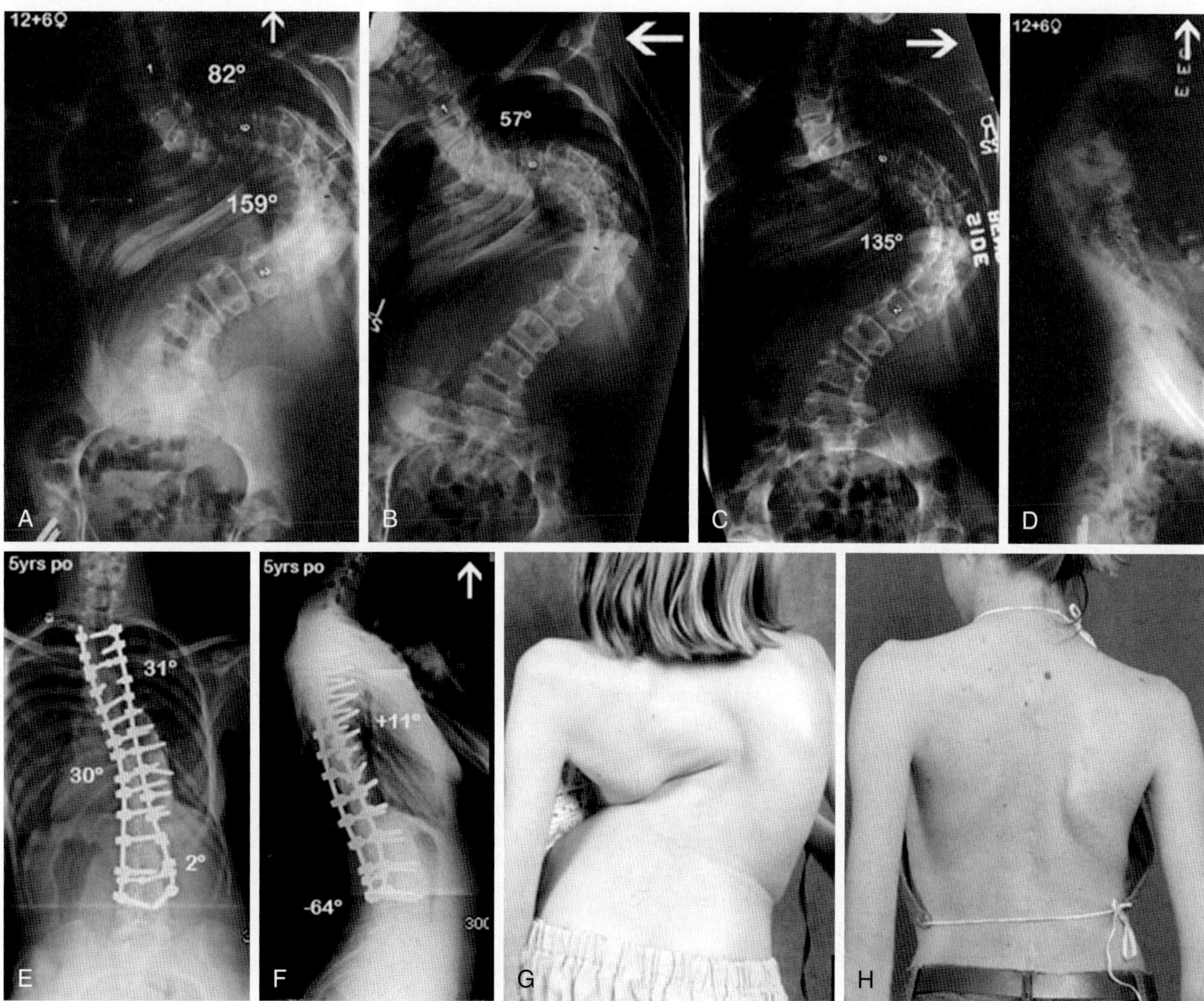

FIG. 27.8 (A–D) Radiographs of a girl, age 12 years + 6 months, with a severe progressive right thoracic scoliosis. Her curve progressed to 159 degrees bending to only 135 degrees. (E–F) She underwent a posterior single-level vertebrectomy and T2–L4 fusion with pedicle screw construct with marked correction of her coronal plane deformity at 5 years postoperatively. (G–H) Preoperative and postoperative clinical photographs show her much improved clinical appearance.

releases, leading to an unbalanced spine, account for other types of intraoperative complications. Inappropriate decortication, inadequate bone graft material, and the use of bulky crosslinks can result in a higher rate of pseudarthrosis.

Intraoperative neurophysiologic monitoring with somatosensory evoked potentials, motor evoked potentials, and/or descending neurogenic evoked potentials help alert the surgeon to any impending intraoperative spinal cord neurologic deficit.[115,116] These deficits typically occur from spinal cord distraction, overcorrection, vascular compromise, or, rarely, directly from instrumentation. If intraoperative neurophysiologic monitoring declines past warning criteria, the surgeon should implement a course of action that includes ensuring that the irrigation being used is of adequate temperature, keeping mean arterial blood pressure elevated at a minimum greater than 80 to 90 mm Hg, and reversing instrumentation or spinal correction to the prewarning criteria state. If intraoperative neurophysiologic monitoring data do not return to baseline within a reasonable time, a wake-up test should also be performed to assess true neurologic function. In addition to adhering to the proven sequential technique of freehand screw placement, pedicle screw stimulation provides an added safety measure.[79,80] Judicious use of intraoperative imaging can also be employed, especially with significant deformities.

Postoperative complications can arise from delayed consequences of technical errors, neurovascular compromise, medical comorbidities, and wound infections. Although perioperative antibiotics are commonly used, when wound infections do occur, they generally are treated aggressively with wound irrigation and debridement. Instrumentation well seated on the spine is always left in place; however, the decision to remove or maintain the bone graft is defined by the individual case and surgeon preference. Removal of the instrumentation can lead to loss of curve correction and decompensation.[117] Additionally, at final closure, powder antibiotics can be placed inside the wound (deep and superficial to the fascia), and long-term parenteral antibiotics are provided based on the results of intraoperative wound cultures and sensitivities. With delayed or late infections, the instrumentation is initially removed and later usually replaced because the deformity can progress as the fusion mass is subject to repeated bending forces.[117,118] Also, the fusion mass is inspected further, and any pseudarthrosis noted is repaired at the reinstrumentation stage.

Summary

Understanding and treatment of spinal deformities has broadened; however, idiopathic scoliosis remains a diagnosis of exclusion. With advances in genetic mapping of idiopathic scoliosis, better understanding of the etiology and incidence of the disease is promising. It is hoped that better understanding will bring earlier identification, more insight into curve progression risk, and treatments of the condition without the need for major surgery of severe curves. Technological advances—including the advent of pedicle screw instrumentation, better derotation equipment, and osteotomy techniques—have significantly improved spinal surgeons' ability to treat more rigid curves while obtaining better correction and maintaining safety.

Possible treatment modalities include close observation, bracing, and surgical intervention. The Lenke classification of AIS allows for the identification of appropriate fusion levels and choice of selective fusions, which are imperative for optimal surgical management. Although all curves can be approached posteriorly, one can employ an anterior approach in selected Lenke 1 curve patterns, Lenke 6CN curves, and many Lenke 5CN curves. Selective fusions should be performed whenever possible, and critical curve analysis should be performed preoperatively with all available objective modalities. Direct vertebral rotation offers improved thoracic correction and a decreased need for thoracoplasty. Complex, decompensated, large, rigid curves and curves previously fused may require osteotomies to achieve the desired correction. Some pitfalls of scoliosis surgery, such as decompensation and adding on of a fused curve, can be avoided when these principles are applied.

One must be mindful of the lessons of the past in understanding the assessment and management of spinal deformity. Spinal surgeons constantly must strive for improvements in surgical technique that lead to shorter, selective fusions and a balanced spine with maximum possible correction. These improvements can include less invasive approaches while not forgetting the basic principles of curve identification and fusion techniques. The ultimate goal should be correction of the curve without fusion of unnecessary vertebrae, allowing for continued spinal motion. Safety for patients is of the utmost importance and is achieved by appropriate training, careful patient selection, and adherence to the principles of deformity surgery.

PEARLS AND PITFALLS

1. Bracing of the juvenile idiopathic or skeletally immature adolescent idiopathic patient is still a viable option for those with curves between 25 degrees and 45 degrees. Brace compliance, the fit of the orthosis, and the number of hours of brace wear per day are critical components to success, along with the genetic predisposition toward curve progression.
2. It is important to determine the flexibility of the spinal deformity. Therefore, preoperative radiographic assessment should include not only upright radiographs, but also side-bending, supine, push-prone, traction (if applicable), and hyperextension (for hyperkyphosis) radiographs, alone or in combination.
3. Proper classification of AIS curves preoperatively will aid in the regions of the spine to be fused. One must remember to include the thoracolumbar sagittal profile in preoperative planning to prevent misclassification and incorrect surgical management.
4. It is critical to examine shoulder symmetry clinically and radiographically, the PT curve (stiffness and sagittal profile), and degree of MT curve correction when selecting proximal fusion levels in idiopathic scoliosis patients to obtain optimal shoulder balance after surgery.
5. Distal fusion levels are determined by the relationship among the end, neutral, and stable vertebrae of the distal structural curve to be fused, along with the TV in relation to the position of those vertebrae to the CSVL. Most commonly, the distal fusion level will be one level above stable if that level is fairly neutral and the vertebra is at least "touched" by the CSVL on the upright coronal film (the TV rule), does not have much rotation, and the disc below is parallel or closed on the convexity.
6. Satisfactory clinical and radiographic results can be achieved with selective thoracic fusions of properly selected lumbar C modifier curves.
7. The use of anterior procedures and circumferential surgery for AIS has markedly decreased since 2000, with the predominant use of posterior-only surgery with spinal osteotomies as needed for adequate three-dimensional correction. Disadvantages such as chest cage disruption (including suboptimal pulmonary function), risk of implants abutting the major vessels, and the ability to treat only a single curve at a time have limited these approaches over time.
8. The use of posterior instrumentation and fusion with or without various forms of spinal osteotomies has become the mainstay for the surgical management of pediatric and adult idiopathic scoliosis deformities. All curve patterns can be managed by surgeons familiar with the classic midline posterior approach.
9. Surgical outcomes are based on radiographic parameters and clinical assessments, such as scoliometer measurements and shoulder height, as well as patient-reported outcome questionnaires.
10. The use of segmental pedicle screw fixation for the posterior treatment of pediatric and adult idiopathic scoliosis curves has become the primary instrumentation construct. In addition, thorough bone grafting with a combination of autogenous bone, allograft bone, and/or the use of osteobiologics, especially in the adult population, has become routine at many centers throughout North America.
11. Optimal surgical outcomes in the treatment of idiopathic scoliosis deformities include proper patient selection, exacting surgical technique, and a well-balanced spinal alignment with minimal to no complications.

KEY POINTS

1. Patient evaluation skills and highly specialized technical skills are essential for the scoliosis surgeon.
2. Anterior approaches are possible, but all curves can be addressed posteriorly.
3. Selective fusions should always be considered when appropriate.
4. Adjuncts to posterior correction possibly can help obviate more extensive approaches.
5. Be careful in choosing appropriate fusion levels and leaving an appropriate tilt on the LIV when performing a selective fusion.
6. Avoidance and treatment of complications in the preoperative, intraoperative, and postoperative periods is important.
7. Some form of spinal cord monitoring is mandatory for all scoliosis corrective procedures.

KEY REFERENCES

1. Lenke LG, Betz RR, Bridwell KH, et al. Intraobserver and interobserver reliability of the classification of thoracic adolescent idiopathic scoliosis. *J Bone Joint Surg Am*. 1998;80:1097-1106.
   This study showed poor to fair reliability of the King classification of adolescent idiopathic scoliosis, questioning its usefulness as an accurate system.
2. Lenke LG, Betz RR, Harms J, et al. Adolescent idiopathic scoliosis: a new classification to determine extent of spinal arthrodesis. *J Bone Joint Surg Am*. 2001;83:1169-1181.
   This new two-dimensional treatment-based AIS classification system was found to have good to excellent reliability and allows classification of all adolescent idiopathic scoliosis curves.
3. Lenke LG, Betz RR, Clements D, et al. Curve prevalence of a new classification of operative adolescent idiopathic scoliosis: does classification correlate with treatment? *Spine*. 2002;27:604-611.
   Of 606 consecutive AIS cases classified by the Lenke et al system, type 1 main thoracic curves were the most common (51%), and 90% of curves were fused as predicted by the system.
4. Sanders AE, Baumann R, Brown H, et al. Selective anterior fusion of thoracolumbar/lumbar curves in adolescents: When can the associated thoracic curve be left unfused? *Spine*. 2003;28:706-713.
   Of 49 patients with AIS who underwent an anterior selective thoracic fusion, 43 had satisfactory results based on the preoperative thoracolumbar/lumbar-to-thoracic ratio of 1.25 or greater.
5. Edwards CC II, Lenke LG, Peelle M, et al. Selective thoracic fusion for adolescent idiopathic scoliosis with C modifier lumbar curves: 2- to 16- year radiographic and clinical results. *Spine*. 2004;29:536-546.
   Satisfactory results were achieved with selective thoracic fusion of properly selected C modifier lumbar curves with under-correction of the instrumented thoracic curve (36%) to match the spontaneous correction of the lumbar curve (34%).

REFERENCES

1. Bunnell WP. The natural history of idiopathic scoliosis before skeletal maturity. *Spine*. 1986;1:773-776.
2. Cobb JR. Outline for the study of scoliosis. *Instr Course Lect*. 1948;5:261-275.
3. Ponseti IV, Friedman B. Prognosis in idiopathic scoliosis. *J Bone Joint Surg Am*. 1950;32:381-395.
4. Dickson RA. Conservative treatment for idiopathic scoliosis. *J Bone Joint Surg Br*. 1985;67:176-181.
5. James JI. Idiopathic scoliosis: the prognosis, diagnosis, and operative indications related to curve patterns and the age at onset. *J Bone Joint Surg Br*. 1954;36:36-49.
6. Fernandes P, Weinstein SL. Natural history of early onset scoliosis. *J Bone Joint Surg Am*. 2007;89(suppl 1):21-33.
7. Kane WJ, Moe JH. A scoliosis-prevalence survey in Minnesota. *Clin Orthop Relat Res*. 1970;69:216-218.
8. Pring ME, Wenger DR. Adolescent deformity. In: Bono CM, Garfin SR, eds. *Spine Orthopedic Surgery Essentials*. Philadelphia: Lippincott Williams & Wilkins; 2004:163-164.
9. Moreau A, Wang DS, Forget S, et al. Melatonin signaling dysfunction in adolescent idiopathic scoliosis. *Spine*. 2004;29:1772-1781.
10. Azeddine B, Letellier K, Wang da S, et al. Molecular determinants of melatonin signaling dysfunction in adolescent idiopathic scoliosis. *Clin Orthop Relat Res*. 2007;462:45-52.
11. Yamamoto H. *A postural dysequilibrium as an etiological factor in idiopathic scoliosis [abstract O]*. In Programs and Abstracts of the 17th Annual Meeting of the Scoliosis Research Society, Denver, 1982, p 52.
12. Machida M, Dubousset J, Imamura Y, et al. An experimental study in chickens for the pathogenesis of idiopathic scoliosis. *Spine*. 1993;18:1609-1615.
13. De Seze M, Cugy E. Pathogenesis of idiopathic scoliosis: a review. *Ann Phys Rehabil Med*. 2012;55(2):128-138.
14. Kouwenhoven JW, Castelein RM. The pathogenesis of adolescent idiopathic scoliosis: review of the literature. *Spine*. 2008;33:2989-2998.
15. Kulkarni S, Nagarajan P, Wall J, et al. Disruption of chromodomain helicase DNA binding protein 2 (CHD2) causes scoliosis. *Am J Med Genet*. 2008;146A:1117-1127.
16. Gao X, Gordon D, Zhang D, et al. CHD7 gene polymorphisms are associated with susceptibility to idiopathic scoliosis. *Am J Hum Genet*. 2007;80:957-965.
17. Tilley MK, Justice CM, Swindle K, et al. CHD gene polymorphisms and familial idiopathic scoliosis. *Spine*. 2013;32(22):E1432-E1436.
18. Takahashi Y, Kou I, Takahashi A, et al. A genome-wide association study identifies common variants near LBX1 associated with adolescent idiopathic scoliosis. *Nat Genet*. 2011;43:1237-1240.
19. Hua J, Xusheng Q, Jin D, et al. Association of rs11190870 near LBX1 with adolescent idiopathic Scoliosis susceptibility in a Han Chinese population. *Eur Spine J*. 2013;22(2):282-286.
20. Risser JC, Norquist DM, Cockrell BR Jr, et al. The effect of posterior spine fusion on the growing spine. *Clin Orthop Relat Res*. 1966;46:127-139.
21. Carr AJ. Adolescent idiopathic scoliosis in identical twins. *J Bone Joint Surg Br*. 1990;72:1077.
22. Kesling LK, Reinker KA. Scoliosis in twins: a meta-analysis of the literature and report of six cases. *Spine*. 1997;22:2009-2014.
23. Anderson MO, Thomsen K, Kyvik KO. Adolescent idiopathic scoliosis in twins: a population-based survey. *Spine*. 2007;32:927-930.
24. Gurnett CA, Alaee F, Bowcock A, et al. Genetic linkage localizes an adolescent idiopathic scoliosis and pectus excavatum gene to 18q. *Spine*. 2009;4:E94-E100.
25. Diedrich O, von Strempel A, Scholz M, et al. Long-term observation and management of resolving infantile idiopathic scoliosis: a 25-year follow-up. *J Bone Joint Surg Br*. 2002;84:1030-1035.

SECTION IV

26. Mehta MH. The rib-vertebra angle in the early diagnosis between resolving and progressive infantile scoliosis. *J Bone Joint Surg Br.* 1972;54:230-243.
27. Weinstein SL, Ponseti IV. Curve progression in idiopathic scoliosis. *J Bone Joint Surg Am.* 1983;65:447-455.
28. Weinstein SL, Zavala DC, Ponseti IV. Idiopathic scoliosis: long-term follow-up and prognosis in untreated patients. *J Bone Joint Surg Am.* 1981;63:702-712.
29. Hägg U, Taranger J. Menarche and voice change as indicators of the pubertal growth spurt. *Acta Odontol Scand.* 1980;38(3):179-186.
30. Lonstein JE. Patient evaluation. In: Bradford DS, Lonstein JE, Moe JH, et al., eds. *Moe's Textbook of Scoliosis and Other Spinal Deformities.* 2nd ed. Philadelphia: WB Saunders; 1987:47-88.
31. Li M, Gu S, Ni J, et al. Shoulder balance after surgery in patients with Lenke type 2 scoliosis corrected with the segmental pedicle screw technique. *J Neurosurg Spine.* 2009;10:214-219.
32. Winter RB, Pinto WC. Pelvic obliquity: its causes and treatment. *Spine.* 1986;11(3):225-234.
33. Muhonen MG, Menezes AH, Sawin PD, et al. Scoliosis in pediatric Chiari malformations without myelodysplasia. *J Neurosurg.* 1992;77:69-77.
34. Dobbs MB, Lenke LG, Szymanski DA, et al. Prevalence of neural axis abnormalities in patients with infantile scoliosis. *J Bone Joint Surg Am.* 2002;84:2230-2234.
35. Gupta P, Lenke LG, Bridwell KH. Incidence of neural axis abnormalities in infantile and juvenile patients with spinal deformity: Is a magnetic resonance image screening necessary? *Spine.* 1998;23:206-210.
36. Whitaker C, Schoenecker PL, Lenke LG. Hyperkyphosis as an indicator of syringomyelia in idiopathic scoliosis. *Spine.* 2003;28(1):E16-E20.
37. Godzik J, et al. Relationship of syrinx size and tonsillar descent to spinal deformity in Chiari malformation type I with associated syringomyelia. *J Neurosurg Pediatr.* 2014;13:368-374.
38. Williams BA, Matsumoto H, McCalla DJ, et al. Development and initial validation of the classification of early-onset scoliosis (C-EOS). *J Bone Joint Surg Am.* 2014;96(16):1359-1367.
39. Lenke LG, Dobbs MB. Management of juvenile idiopathic scoliosis. *J Bone Joint Surg Am.* 2007;89:55-63.
40. King HA, Moe JH, Bradford DS, et al. The selection of fusion levels in thoracic idiopathic scoliosis. *J Bone Joint Surg Am.* 1983;65:1302-1313.
41. Lenke LG, Bridwell KH, Baldus C, et al. Preventing decompensation in King type II curves treated with Cotrel-Dubousset instrumentation: strict guidelines for selective thoracic fusion. *Spine.* 1992;17:274S-281S.
42. Schroeder TM, Blanke KM, Vaughan V, et al. *Validation of radiographic software to determine Lenke classification [abstract 54].* In Programs and Abstracts of the 40th Annual Meeting of the Scoliosis Research Society, Miami, 2005, p 93.
43. Lenke LG, Betz RR, Bridwell KH, et al. Intraobserver and interobserver reliability of the classification of thoracic adolescent idiopathic scoliosis. *J Bone Joint Surg Am.* 1998;80:1097-1106.
44. Lenke LG, Betz RR, Harms J, et al. Adolescent idiopathic scoliosis: a new classification to determine extent of spinal arthrodesis. *J Bone Joint Surg Am.* 2001;3:1169-1181.
45. Cil A, Pekmezci M, Yazici M, et al. *The validity of Lenke's criteria for defining structural proximal thoracic curves in patients with adolescent idiopathic scoliosis [abstract 74].* In Programs and Abstracts of the 40th Annual Meeting of the Scoliosis Research Society, Miami, 2005, p 120.
46. Sanders AE, Baumann R, Brown H, et al. Selective anterior fusion of thoracolumbar/lumbar curves in adolescents: When can the associated thoracic curve be left unfused? *Spine.* 2003;28:706-713.
47. Edwards CC 2nd, Lenke LG, Peelle M, et al. Selective thoracic fusion for adolescent idiopathic scoliosis with C modifier lumbar curves: 2- to 16- year radiographic and clinical results. *Spine.* 2004;29:536-546.
48. Lenke LG, Bridwell KH. *Achieving coronal balance using Cotrel-Dubousset instrumentation (C-D.I.).* In the 8th Proceedings of the International Congress on Cotrel-Dubousset Instrumentation. Montpellier, Sauramps Medical, 1991, pp 27-32.
49. Lenke LG, Kuklo TR, Sucato DJ, et al. *Comparison of the lower-end vertebra (LEV) to the lowest instrumented vertebra (LIV) in adolescent idiopathic scoliosis: a role for the addition of an LEV modifier to the Lenke classification system [abstract 131].* In Programs and Abstracts of the 13th International Meeting on Advanced Spine Techniques (IMAST), Athens, 2006, p 121.
50. Lenke LG, Newton PO, Lehman RA, et al. *Radiographic results of selecting the touched vertebra as the lowest instrumented vertebra in Lenke 1A AIS curves at a minimum five-year follow up.* Podium presentation 5. Scoliosis Research Society 49th Annual Meeting, Anchorage, AK, September 11-13, 2014.
51. Sangole A, Aubin CE, Labelle H, et al. The central hip vertical axis (CHVA): a reference axis for the Scoliosis Research Society three-dimensional classification of idiopathic scoliosis. *Spine.* 2010;35(12):E530-E534.
52. Nachemson AL, Peterson LE. Effectiveness of treatment with a brace in girls who have adolescent idiopathic scoliosis: a prospective, controlled study based on data from the Brace Study of the Scoliosis Research Society. *J Bone Joint Surg Am.* 1995;77:815-822.
53. Stone B, Beekman C, Hall V, et al. The effect of an exercise program on change in curve in adolescents with minimal idiopathic scoliosis: a preliminary study. *Phys Ther.* 1979;59:759-763.
54. Romano M1, Minozzi S, Zaina F, et al. Exercises for adolescent idiopathic scoliosis: a Cochrane systematic review. *Spine.* 2013;38(14):E883-E889.
55. Mordecai SC, Dabke HV. Efficacy of exercise therapy for the treatment of adolescent idiopathic scoliosis: a review of the literature. *Eur Spine J.* 2012;21(3):382-389.
56. Weinstein SL. Idiopathic scoliosis: natural history. *Spine.* 1986;11:780-783.
57. Fayssoux RS, Cho RH, Herman MJ. A history of bracing for idiopathic scoliosis in North America. *Clin Orthop Relat Res.* 2010;468:654-664.
58. Kennedy JD, Robertson CF, Olinsky A, et al. Pulmonary restrictive effect of bracing in mild idiopathic scoliosis. *Thorax.* 1987;42:959-961.
59. Katsaris G, Loukos A, Valavanis J, et al. The immediate effect of a Boston brace on lung volumes and pulmonary compliance in mild adolescent idiopathic scoliosis. *Eur Spine J.* 1999;8:2-7.
60. Sanders JO, D'Astous J, Fitzgerald M, et al. Derotational casting for progressive infantile scoliosis. *J Pediatr Orthop.* 2009;29:581-587.

61. Blount WP, Schmidt AC, Keever ED, et al. The Milwaukee brace in the operative treatment of scoliosis. *J Bone Joint Surg Am*. 1958;40:511-525.
62. Price CT, Scott DS, Reed FR Jr, et al. Nighttime bracing for adolescent idiopathic scoliosis with the Charleston bending brace: long-term follow-up. *J Pediatr Orthop*. 1997;17:703-707.
63. Trivedi JM, Thomson JD. Results of Charleston bracing in skeletally immature patients with idiopathic scoliosis. *J Pediatr Orthop*. 2001;21:277-280.
64. Clin J, Aubin CE, Parent S, et al. A biomechanical study of the Charleston brace for the treatment of scoliosis. *Spine*. 2010;35:E940-E947.
65. Kotwicki T, Chêneau J. Biomechanical action of a correction brace of thoracic idiopathic scoliosis: Chêneau 2000 orthosis. *Disabil Rehabil Assist Technol*. 2008;3:146-153.
66. Rigo M, Negrini S, Weiss H, et al. SOSORT consensus paper on brace action: TLSO biomechanics of correction (investigating the rationale for force vector selection). *Scoliosis*. 2006;1:11.
67. Szwed A, Kolban M, Jaloszewski M. Results of SpineCor dynamic bracing for idiopathic scoliosis. *Ortop Traumatol Rehabil*. 2009;11:427-432.
68. Maruyama T, Takeshita K. Surgical treatment of scoliosis: a review of techniques currently applied. *Scoliosis*. 2008;18:6.
69. Dobbs MB, Weinstein SL. Infantile and juvenile scoliosis. *Orthop Clin North Am*. 1999;30:331-341.
70. Lenke LG, Dobbs MB. Management of juvenile idiopathic scoliosis. *J Bone Joint Surg Am*. 2007;89(suppl 1):55-63.
71. Marks DS, Iqbal MJ, Thompson AG, et al. Convex spinal epiphysiodesis in the management of progressive infantile idiopathic scoliosis. *Spine*. 1996;21:1884-1888.
72. Bylski-Austrow DI, Wall EJ, Glos DL, et al. Spinal hemiepiphysiodesis decreased the sizes of vertebral growth plate hypertrophic zone and cells. *J Bone Joint Surg Am*. 2009;91:854-893.
73. Akbarnia BA, Marks DS, Boachie-Adjei O, et al. Dual growing rod technique for the treatment of progressive early-onset scoliosis: a multicenter study. *Spine*. 2005;30(17 suppl):S46-S57.
74. Betz RR, Kim J, D'Andrea LP, et al. An innovative technique of vertebral body stapling for the treatment of patients with adolescent idiopathic scoliosis: a feasibility, safety, and utility study. *Spine*. 2003;28:S255-S265.
75. Betz RR, Ranade A, Samdani AF, et al. Vertebral body stapling: a fusionless treatment option for a growing child with moderate idiopathic scoliosis. *Spine*. 2010;35:169-176.
76. Newton PO, Upasani VV, Farnsworth CL, et al. Spinal growth modulation with use of a tether in an immature porcine model. *J Bone Joint Surg Am*. 2008;90:2695-2706.
77. Crawford CH III, Lenke LG. Growth modulation by means of anterior tethering resulting in progressive correction of juvenile idiopathic scoliosis: a case report. *J Bone Joint Surg Am*. 2010;92:202-209.
78. Thompson GH, Akbarnia BA, Campbell RM Jr. Growing rod techniques in early-onset scoliosis. *J Pediatr Orthop*. 2007;27:354-361.
79. Lenke LG, Rinella A, Kim Y. Freehand thoracic pedicle screw placement. *Semin Spine Surg*. 2002;14:48-57.
80. Kim YJ, Lenke LG, Bridwell KH, et al. Free hand pedicle screw placement in the thoracic spine: Is it safe? *Spine*. 2004;29:333-341.
81. Good CR, Lenke LG, O'Leary PT, et al. Can posterior-only surgery provide similar radiographic and clinical results as combined anterior (thoracotomy/thoracoabdominal)/posterior approaches for adult scoliosis? *Spine*. 2010;35:210-218.
82. Kioschos HC, Asher MA, Lark RG, et al. Overpowering the crankshaft mechanism: the effect of posterior spinal fusion with and without stiff transpedicular fixation on anterior spinal column growth in immature canines. *Spine*. 1996;21:1168-1173.
83. Burton DC, Asher MA, Lai SM. Scoliosis correction maintenance in skeletally immature patients with idiopathic scoliosis: Is anterior fusion really necessary? *Spine*. 2000;25:61-68.
84. Suk SI, Kim JH, Cho KJ, et al. Is anterior release necessary in severe scoliosis treated by posterior segmental pedicle screw fixation? *Eur Spine J*. 2007;16:1359-1365.
85. Dobbs MB, Lenke LG, Kim YJ, et al. Anterior/posterior spinal instrumentation versus posterior instrumentation alone for the treatment of adolescent idiopathic scoliotic curves more than 90°. *Spine*. 2006;31:2386-2391.
86. Kim YJ, Lenke LG, Bridwell KH, et al. Pulmonary function in adolescent idiopathic scoliosis relative to the surgical procedure. *J Bone Joint Surg Am*. 2005;87:1534-1541.
87. Lonner BS, Auerbach JD, Estreicher MB, et al. Pulmonary function changes after various anterior approaches in the treatment of adolescent idiopathic scoliosis. *J Spinal Disord Tech*. 2009;22:551-558.
88. Tis JE, O'Brien MF, Newton PO, et al. Adolescent idiopathic scoliosis treated with open instrumented anterior spinal fusion: five-year follow-up. *Spine*. 2010;35:64-70.
89. Geck MJ, Rinella A, Hawthorne D, et al. Comparison of surgical treatment in Lenke 5C adolescent idiopathic scoliosis: anterior dual rod versus posterior pedicle fixation surgery: a comparison of two practices. *Spine*. 2009;34:1942-1951.
90. Kishan S, Bastrom T, Betz RR, et al. Thoracoscopic scoliosis surgery affects pulmonary function less than thoracotomy at 2 years postsurgery. *Spine*. 2007;32:453-458.
91. Sucato DJ, Erken YH, Davis S, et al. Prone thoracoscopic release does not adversely affect pulmonary function when added to a posterior spinal fusion for severe deformity. *Spine*. 2009;34:771-778.
92. Bridwell KH, Lenke LG. Prevention and treatment of decompensation: When can levels be saved and selective fusion be performed in idiopathic scoliosis? *Spine State Art Rev*. 1994;8:643-658.
93. Suk SI, Lee SM, Chung ER, et al. Selective thoracic fusion with segmental pedicle screw fixation in the treatment of thoracic idiopathic scoliosis: more than 5-year follow-up. *Spine*. 2005;30:1602-1609.
94. Brodner W, Mun Yue W, Möller HB, et al. Short segment bone-on-bone instrumentation for single curve idiopathic scoliosis. *Spine*. 2003;28:S224-S233.
95. O'Brien MF, Kuklo TR, Blanke KM, et al., eds. *Radiographic Measurement Manual*. Memphis, TN: Medtronic Sofamor Danek; 2004.
96. Rinella A, Cahill P, Ghanayem A, et al. *Thoracic pedicle expansion after pedicle screw placement in a pediatric cadaveric spine: A biomechanical analysis [abstract 35]*. In Programs and Abstracts of the 39th Annual Meeting of the Scoliosis Research Society, Argentina, 2004, p 70.
97. Watanabe K, Lenke LG, Matsumoto M, et al. A novel pedicle channel classification describing osseous anatomy: How many thoracic scoliotic pedicles have cancellous channels? *Spine*. 2010;35(20):1836-1842.

98. Bridwell KH, McAllister JW, Betz RR, et al. Coronal decompensation produced by Cotrel-Dubousset "derotation" maneuver for idiopathic right thoracic scoliosis. *Spine.* 1991;16:769-777.
99. Lehman RA Jr, Lenke LG, Helgeson MD, et al. Do intraoperative radiographs in scoliosis surgery reflect radiographic result? *Clin Orthop Relat Res.* 2010;468: 679-686.
100. Donaldson S, Stephens D, Howard A, et al. Surgical decision making in adolescent idiopathic scoliosis. *Spine.* 2007;32:1526-1532.
101. Keeler KA, Lehman RA, Lenke LG, et al. *Direct vertebral rotation (DVR) in the treatment of thoracolumbar/lumbar adolescent idiopathic scoliosis (AIS): can it optimize correction when fusing to L3? [abstract 137].* In Programs and Abstracts of the 15th International Meeting on Advanced Spine Techniques, Hong Kong, 2008, p 215.
102. Lee SM, Suk SI, Chung ER. Direct vertebral rotation: a new technique of three-dimensional deformity correction with segmental pedicle screw fixation in adolescent idiopathic scoliosis. *Spine.* 2004;29:343-349.
103. Kadoury S, Cheriet F, Beauséjour M, et al. A three-dimensional retrospective analysis of the evolution of spinal instrumentation for the correction of adolescent idiopathic scoliosis. *Eur Spine J.* 2009;18:23-37.
104. Bridwell KH. Adult spinal deformity revision surgery. In: Heary RF, Albert TJ, eds. *Spinal Deformity: The Essentials.* New York: Thieme; 2007:240-248.
105. Booth KC, Bridwell KH, Lenke LG, et al. Complications and predictive factors for the successful treatment of flatback deformity (fixed sagittal balance). *Spine.* 1999;24: 1712-1720.
106. Ondra SL, Marzouk S, Koski T, et al. Mathematical calculation of pedicle subtraction osteotomy size to allow precision correction of fixed sagittal deformity. *Spine.* 2006;31:E973-E979.
107. Bradford DS, Tribus CB. Vertebral column resection for the treatment of rigid coronal decompensation. *Spine.* 1997;22:1590-1599.
108. Lenke LG, O'Leary PT, Bridwell KH, et al. Posterior vertebral column resection for severe pediatric deformity: minimum two-year follow-up of thirty-five consecutive patients. *Spine.* 2009;34:2213-2221.
109. Lenke LG, Sides BA, Koester LA, et al. Vertebral column resection for the treatment of severe spinal deformity. *Clin Orthop Relat Res.* 2010;468:687-699.
110. Lenke LG, Ogilvie JG, Mumamenni P, Silva FE. *Safety measures and operative planning in the treatment of spinal deformities. Scoliosis Research Society, E-Text,* 2013.
111. Newton PO, Marks M, Faro F, et al. Use of video-assisted thoracoscopic surgery to reduce perioperative morbidity in scoliosis surgery. *Spine.* 2003;28:S249-S254.
112. Lykissas MG, Crawford AH, Jain VV. Complications of surgical treatment of pediatric spinal deformities. *Orthop Clin North Am.* 2013;44(3):357-370.
113. Lenke LG, Bridwell KH, Erickson MA, et al. *Prospective radiographic and clinical outcomes and complications of 756 consecutive operative adolescent idiopathic scoliosis patients [abstract 3].* In Programs and Abstracts of the 44th Annual Meeting of the Scoliosis Research Society, San Antonio, TX, 2009, p 39.
114. Trobisch PD, Ducoffe AR, Lonner BS, Errico TJ. Choosing fusion levels in adolescent idiopathic scoliosis. *J Am Acad Orthop Surg.* 2013;21(9):519-528.
115. Padberg AM, Wilson-Holden TJ, Lenke LG, et al. Somatosensory- and motor-evoked potential monitoring without a wake-up test during idiopathic scoliosis surgery: an accepted standard of care. *Spine.* 1998;23:1392-1400.
116. Cho SK, Lenke LG, Bolon SM, et al. Can intraoperative spinal cord monitoring reliably help prevent paraplegia during posterior vertebral column resection surgery? *Spine Deform.* 2015;3:73-81.
117. Potter BK, Kirk KL, Shah SA, et al. Loss of coronal correction following instrumentation removal in adolescent idiopathic scoliosis. *Spine.* 2006;31:67-72.
118. Luhmann SJ, Lenke LG, Bridwell KH, et al. Revision surgery after primary spine fusion for idiopathic scoliosis. *Spine.* 2009;34:2191-2197.

SECTION IV

CHAPTER 28 Neuromuscular Scoliosis

Peter O. Newton
Pawel P. Jankowski
Burt Yaszay
Dennis R. Wenger
Scott J. Mubarak

General Principles

Neuromuscular disorders commonly lead to spinal deformities that are some of the most challenging treatment dilemmas addressed by spine surgeons. Despite the various conditions that fall in this category, neuromuscular disorders involve neurologic or muscular deficiencies that produce progressive multiplanar skeletal deformities. Common features of neuromuscular scoliosis include the following:

Large curves early in life: Early neuromuscular insult predisposes patients to rapidly progressive scoliosis.

Stiff curves: These patients are more likely to develop stiff curves because of the early onset of neuromuscular deficiency, resulting in limited mobility and secondary contractures.

Progressive curves: As in idiopathic scoliosis, the potential for curve progression is greatest during rapid growth and with loss of ambulation. Increasing weakness or persistent muscle imbalance around the spine in patients with neuromuscular disorders can cause progression of scoliosis independent of growth, however.

Long curves: Less severely affected individuals may have an S-shaped curve with well-balanced double curves. Long C-shaped curves are more likely in severely affected patients with resultant sitting imbalance.

Pelvic obliquity: Lower extremity contractures and imbalanced spinal deformity cause pelvic obliquity, which may impair comfortable sitting for these patients.

Sagittal plane deformity: Gravity and muscular deficiency can also lead to sagittal plane deformity, including thoracic or lumbar hyperkyphosis or lumbar hyperlordosis.

Patients with neuromuscular disorders are challenging because of the complexity of their deformity and fragility of their overall health; they are best treated by an experienced surgeon with support from a multidisciplinary team.

Classification

The classification of neuromuscular scoliosis can be based on the underlying disorder: neurologic (e.g., cerebral palsy) or muscular (e.g., muscular dystrophy). Neurologic deficiencies can be broken down further into upper motor neuron dysfunction, as seen in myelomeningocele, or lower motor neuron dysfunction, as seen in spinal muscular atrophy (SMA).

Natural History and Associated Complications

Neuromuscular scoliosis generally begins early in life, is often rapidly progressive, and causes significant morbidity. Some patients are capable of ambulation, although many lose their ability to walk early in life or never achieve ambulatory status at all. The use of a wheelchair affords these patients educational and social opportunities that enrich their lives. Spinal deformity can impair comfortable sitting and dramatically reduce the individual's quality of life. Unbalanced curves and significant pelvic obliquity make wheelchair positioning difficult and may cause uneven distribution of weight that may lead to pressure sores (Fig. 28.1). Prominences created by the convexity of a curve may result in skin breakdown; creases within the concavity of the trunk deformity are susceptible to skin maceration and infection (Fig. 28.2). Majd and colleagues[1] showed a correlation between deformity size, functional decline, and decubitus. Large rigid curves restrict lung volume and impair respiration in patients who often already have limited pulmonary capacity. Treatment of neuromuscular scoliosis can also help the caretakers of these patients, improving the ease of transfers, positioning, feeding, and hygiene. The ultimate goal of treatment of patients with neuromuscular scoliosis is the maintenance of as much independence and function as possible. When patients with neuromuscular scoliosis lose the ability to sit comfortably, their quality of life is dramatically decreased. The natural history for a given patient is largely determined by the specific underlying neuromuscular condition and the degree of involvement.

Treatment Principles

The basic principles of observing or bracing smaller, flexible curves and surgically fusing larger, more rigid curves

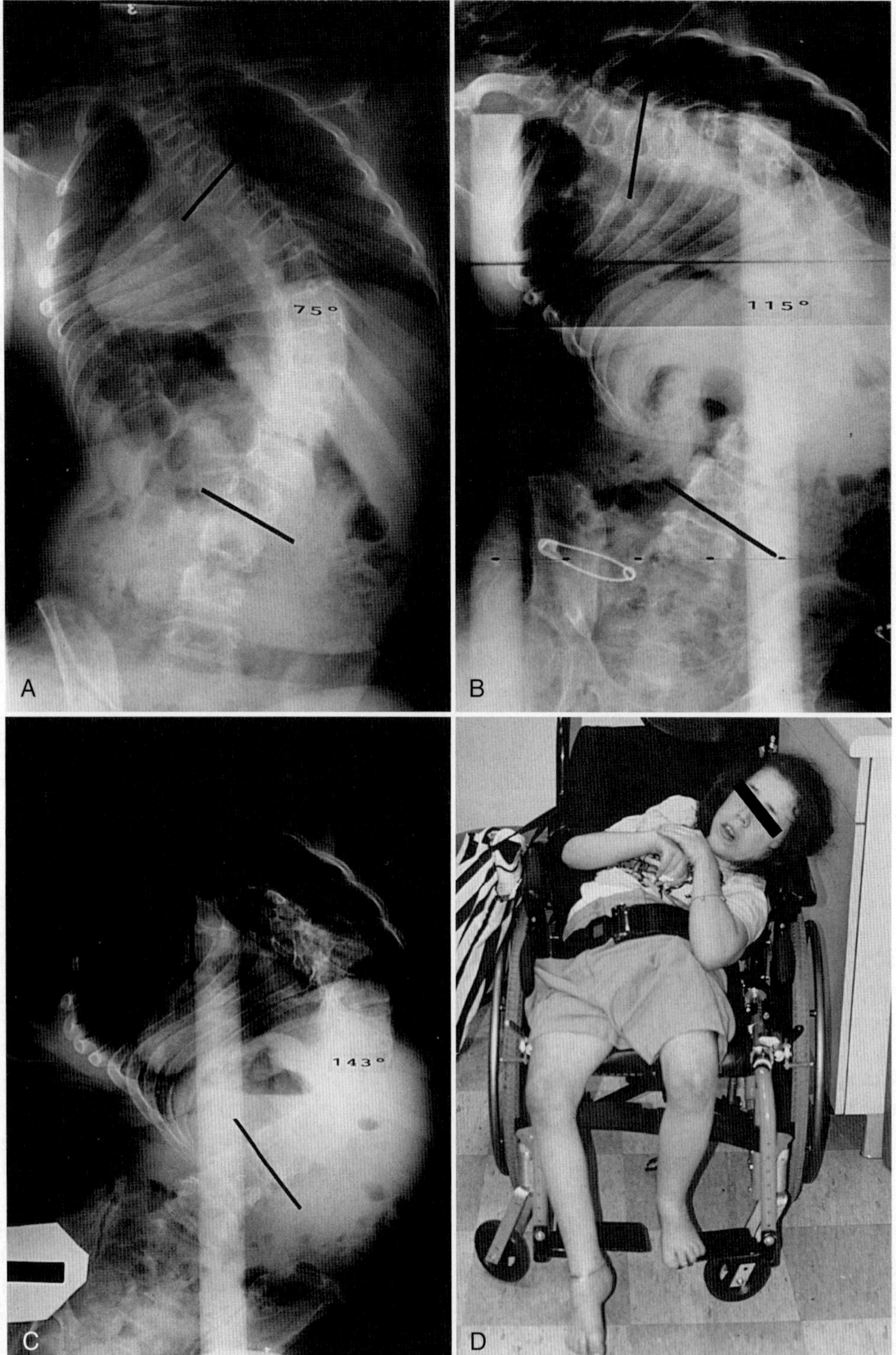

FIG. 28.1 Progression of scoliosis after skeletal maturity in a patient with cerebral palsy. (A) At age 15, curve measures 75 degrees. (B) At age 18, curve measures 115 degrees. (C) At age 23, curve measures 143 degrees. (D) The patient is unable to be comfortably positioned in her wheelchair.

in adolescent idiopathic scoliosis apply to the treatment of neuromuscular scoliosis, although with less aggressive parameters. Observation alone is employed until curves begin to cause functional impairment. Bracing can be a temporizing measure, used primarily to provide sitting support while the patient grows. Eventually, many of these patients require surgical stabilization with a spinal instrumentation and fusion procedure.

Nonoperative Treatment

Medical Treatment

Spinal Muscular Atrophy

Before the 1990s, there was no clear molecular target for SMA diseases. As a result, various medications were tried in an

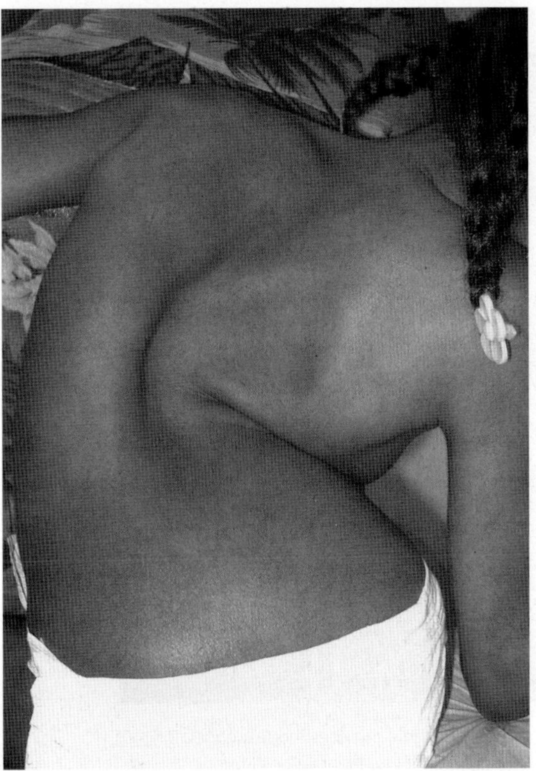

FIG. 28.2 Severe spinal deformity can lead to skin maceration on concave side of curvature and pressure sores on convex side.

off-label fashion that found different degrees of success in other diseases causing muscle weakness, such as amyotrophic lateral sclerosis. Randomized placebo-controlled trials have been conducted to investigate the efficacy of several medical treatments for SMA, including creatine, phenylbutyrate, gabapentin, and thyrotropin-releasing hormone.[2–5] None of these compounds has proven to be an efficacious drug treatment for SMA.[2] The discovery of the survival of motor neuron (SMN) gene has resulted in the development of animal models to test new therapies. The main objective of these therapies is to increase the expression of the SMN protein. These RNA-based molecule therapies along with gene therapy have shown promise in animal models and are currently in the preclinical testing phase.[6] However, as of yet these therapies have not been effective in human trials.

Cerebral Palsy

Several medical therapies have been investigated for the treatment of spasticity in patients with cerebral palsy (CP). Botulinum toxin has gained a growing acceptance as a treatment of upper and lower limb spasticity. Initial reviews of the literature by the Cochrane Collaboration and others yielded inconclusive evidence that could neither confirm nor deny the efficacy of botulinum toxin in the treatment of spasticity.[7] Inclusion of more recent randomized controlled trials (RCTs) into the analysis has provided evidence that supports the use of botulinum toxin to provide a time-limited benefit to decrease muscle tone in children with upper and lower limb spasticity associated with CP.[8] In a study of 16 children with CP, botulinum toxin A injections into the gastrocnemius muscle decreased spasticity and improved ankle range of motion (ROM), pattern of walking, and reduced energy consumption, providing improvement in function. The evidence trend is in favor of using this therapy to reduce spasticity early in the management of CP, although there is little evidence that this has a role in preventing or treating scoliosis.

Intrathecal baclofen is a well-established treatment that has been shown to provide significant benefits in controlling spasticity in patients with CP. Intrathecal baclofen has been shown to reduce the need for orthopaedic lower extremity procedures and the rate of postoperative complications associated with these procedures.[9] Concerns have been raised, however, regarding its impact on the progression of scoliosis in patients with spastic quadriplegia. In a retrospective review, Ginsburg and Lauder[10] found a six-fold increase in the rate of scoliosis curve progression at 2-year follow-up in a group of 19 quadriplegic CP patients with spasticity. Caird and colleagues[11] showed a significantly higher rate of complications associated with posterior spinal fusion and instrumentation in a group of 20 CP patients with spasticity with intrathecal baclofen pumps compared with a matched control group. This study was limited by its relatively small sample size and lack of a control group. Shilt and colleagues[12] found no difference in curve progression at 3-year follow-up between 50 CP patients treated with intrathecal baclofen and 50 matched control CP patients. In a review of the literature, Scannell and Yaszay suggested that no conclusive evidence exists to support the hypothesis that intrathecal baclofen pumps lead to worsening of the scoliosis in CP patients.[13] Therefore, based on the current evidence, no significant conclusions can be drawn about the impact of intrathecal baclofen pumps on the progression or treatment of spinal deformity in patients with CP. Baclofen can provide significant relief of spasticity, and this evidence must be considered in the context of any potential side effects.

Duchenne Muscular Dystrophy

Advances in general care, glucocorticoid treatment, noninvasive ventilatory support, cardiomyopathy management, and scoliosis management have significantly changed the course of Duchenne muscular dystrophy (DMD). Survival into adulthood is now a realistic expectation for many patients who receive optimal treatment.[13] Although gene-based and cellular-based therapies are currently under development for the treatment of DMD, the efficacy of glucocorticoid steroids has been evaluated by several randomized controlled trials. In their Cochrane review and meta-analysis, Manzur and colleagues[14,15] concluded that there is evidence that muscle function and strength are improved in the short term (6 months to 2 years) with corticosteroid therapy. The authors based their conclusion on six RCTs and observed that the most effective prednisolone dose seemed to be 0.75 mg/kg per day, given daily.[14] Markham and colleagues[16] showed that glucocorticoid therapy provides the added benefit of retarding the anticipated development of ventricular dysfunction if begun before ventricular dysfunction in their series of 14 DMD patients treated with steroids compared with 23 DMD

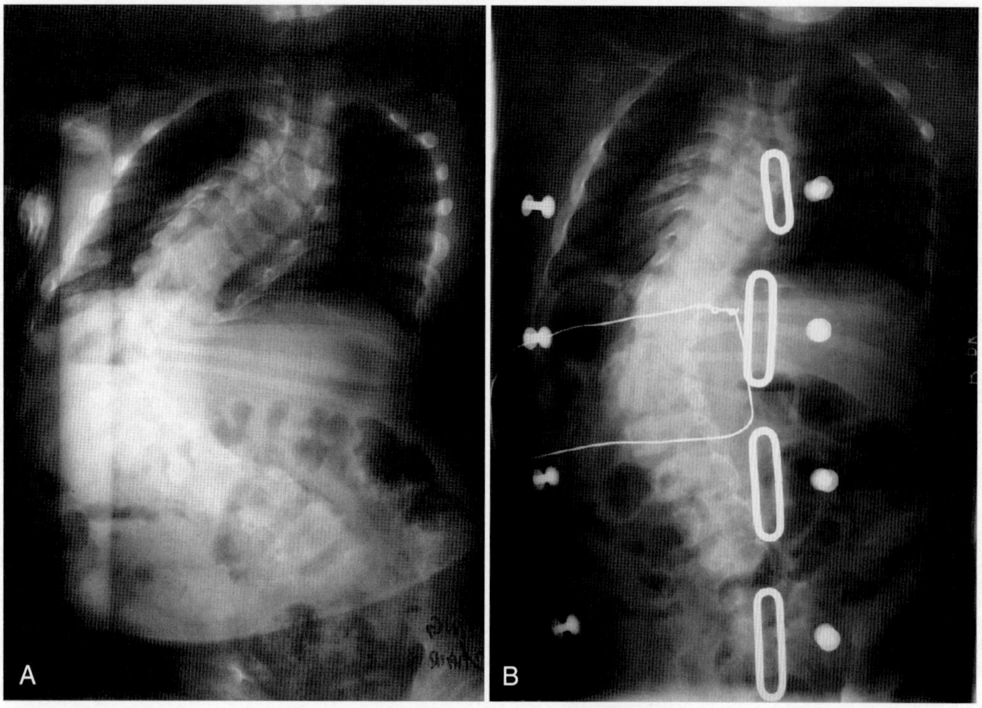

A B

FIG. 28.3 Bracing in neuromuscular scoliosis is often poorly tolerated. Although it provides modest correction, as shown in these radiographs, rigid bracing may lead to excessive skin pressure in patients who cannot actively pull away from the brace.

patients treated without steroids. Shapiro and colleagues[17] evaluated 85 DMD patients who were not receiving steroids, finding that 97% had progression of their scoliosis of more than 10 degrees after becoming wheelchair dependent, regardless of age. Based on their findings, Shapiro et al.[17] advocated for spinal fusion in the majority of patients after the curve had progressed beyond 20 degrees and who were not on steroid therapy to avoid future cardiac and pulmonary complications. Conversely, Lebel et al.[18] found a reduced incidence of scoliosis development and need for spinal fusion in patients treated with long-term glucocorticoids.

Genetic and Family Counseling

Because of the complexity of the medical and psychosocial issues associated with neuromuscular disorders and spinal deformity, care needs to be coordinated with a multidisciplinary team. The primary care physician should be well informed of all orthopaedic issues and play a central role in managing care. Psychosocial support for patients and parents is also vital. Patient advocacy groups have proven to be very useful in helping families cope with the illness and associated surgical care. Physicians may wish to provide information regarding clinical trials or refer families to clinical trial websites (www.clinicaltrials.gov provides a current listing of open clinical trials). Patients and parents may need to be referred for genetic counseling to confirm the patient's diagnosis and aid in family planning.

Bracing

Bracing is a controversial treatment method in idiopathic and neuromuscular scoliosis. Bracing in neuromuscular scoliosis may be used for postural support, although there is limited evidence of its efficacy in limiting curve progression (Fig. 28.3). The etiology of the patient's scoliosis and the patient's muscle tone have an impact on the practicality of brace treatment. Patients with spastic disorders generally do not tolerate rigid brace treatment, whereas patients with flaccid paresis are more apt to be compliant with brace treatment. The type of orthoses may play a role in the outcome of the treatment.

Kotwicki and colleagues[19] followed 45 nonambulatory patients with neuromuscular scoliosis treated with a suspension trunk orthosis (STO) and found that the STO slowed curve progression in 23 patients. The STO construction functions contrary to the classic thoracolumbosacral orthosis (TLSO), with the STO not resting against the patient's pelvis but rather directly against the seat. The evidence supporting STO use to prevent curve progression is limited, however, and skin intolerance found in 36 patients complicates its clinical practicality. Although there is limited research on the results of the STO brace, there are numerous studies investigating the TLSO brace. In a study of 15 patients, Shoham and colleagues[20] found that a TLSO reduced scoliotic deformity and pelvic obliquity leading to reduced sitting pressure. These results are contrary to other studies reported in the literature. In a study of 23 patients, Miller and colleagues[21] followed 23 patients with CP who wore a rigid Wilmington TLSO for an average of 67 months and concluded that the bracing did not slow progression of their deformity. Olafsson and colleagues[22] followed 90 patients with various neuromuscular conditions treated with a soft Boston orthosis for an average of 3 years after brace treatment. They concluded that brace wear was indicated only in a limited subset of patients—ambulatory patients with hypotonia and short thoracolumbar curves (<40

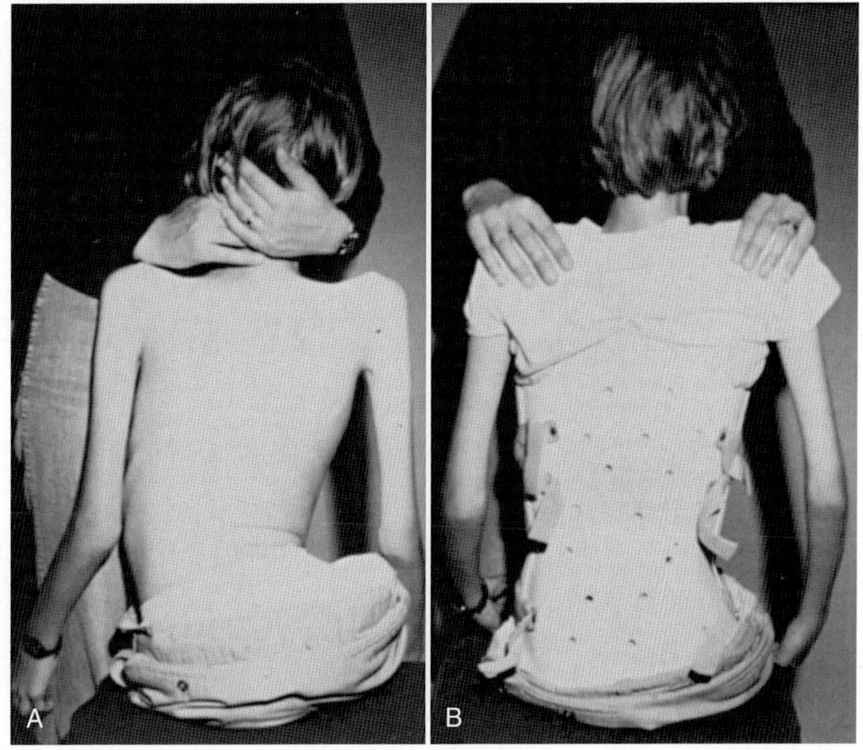

FIG. 28.4 Soft total-contact thoracolumbosacral orthosis in an older child. Less rigid forms of bracing are better tolerated but do not seem to alter the natural history of curve progression.

degrees). In all other patients, brace wear was ineffectual in altering progression but did provide assistance in sitting.

Patients with neuromuscular scoliosis may lack sensate skin to feel pressure from the brace or the muscular control to pull away from the sides of the brace. These patients rarely tolerate the rigid braces often used in idiopathic scoliosis. Patients tend to tolerate soft TLSOs designed to provide improved sitting stability and head and trunk control, while limiting discomfort and skin breakdown (Fig. 28.4).[23]

The impact of the orthosis on pulmonary function is another important factor to consider when contemplating a TLSO for patients with neuromuscular scoliosis. The effect of bracing on pulmonary dysfunction seems to depend on the level of muscle spasticity. Flaccid patients are more amenable to rigid bracing, although this bracing may significantly decrease chest expansion, leading to compromised pulmonary function.[24] Patients with spasticity seem to be more amenable to soft bracing, which does not seem to compromise pulmonary function,[24] although this bracing has been shown only to enhance seating comfort.[21] Olafsson and colleagues[22] and Bunnell and MacEwen[25] suggested that a subset of patients with minimum deformity and muscle hypotonia or mild spasticity may experience slowing of curve progression by bracing without a negative impact on pulmonary function.

Other factors to evaluate when choosing orthotic treatment for neuromuscular scoliosis include ease of application and obstructions. A bivalved brace may be easier for a caregiver to place, although it cannot provide as much corrective strength as a single-opening brace. Winter and Carlson[26] found the two-piece bivalved brace to be a useful support in children with myelomeningocele and SMA. Patients with a stoma or gastrostomy tube require modification of the brace to accommodate these features. Nakamura et al[27] described their preliminary results on 52 patients with neuromuscular scoliosis who were treated with a dynamic spinal brace (DSB), which is a novel three-point support brace. Many of the patients in the study were not surgical candidates due to significant surgical risk factors. Although the authors found that the brace could not prevent the progression of scoliosis, it was effective in maintaining sitting stability and function in neuromuscular patients. Furthermore, no patients needed to discontinue the brace during the study period due to complications. In summary, the study showed that the DSB could be a useful tool in patients who are poor surgical candidates with long C-shaped curves in the early stages of their scoliosis.

Wheelchair modifications can aid in providing a more comfortable seating position for patients with spinal deformity. Modular seating systems can be configured for optimal support of an individual patient (Fig. 28.5). A biomechanical evaluation of seating insert configurations by Holmes and colleagues[28] concluded that three-point force application provides significant sitting support and static correction of scoliosis. Patients with more severe deformity may benefit from custom-molded seatbacks, although these items are expensive, and younger patients may outgrow them quickly.

Operative Treatment

The timing for operative treatment is influenced by curve severity, underlying neuromuscular pathology, and other

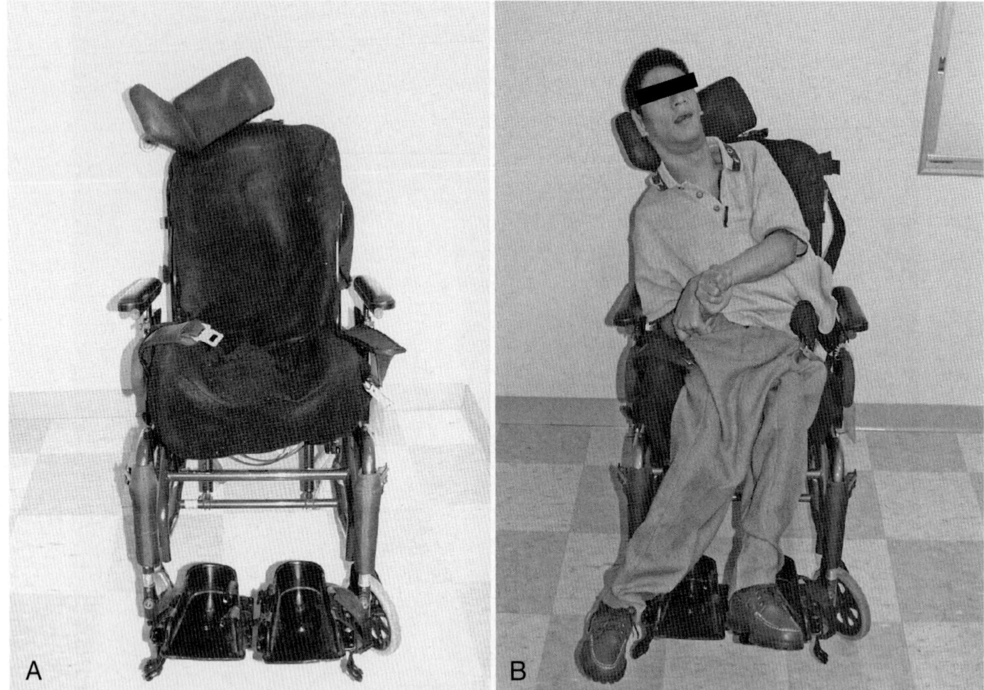

FIG. 28.5 Wheelchair systems can provide sitting support for patients who are not good candidates for bracing. Custom-molded seatbacks can be made to accommodate substantial spinal deformities.

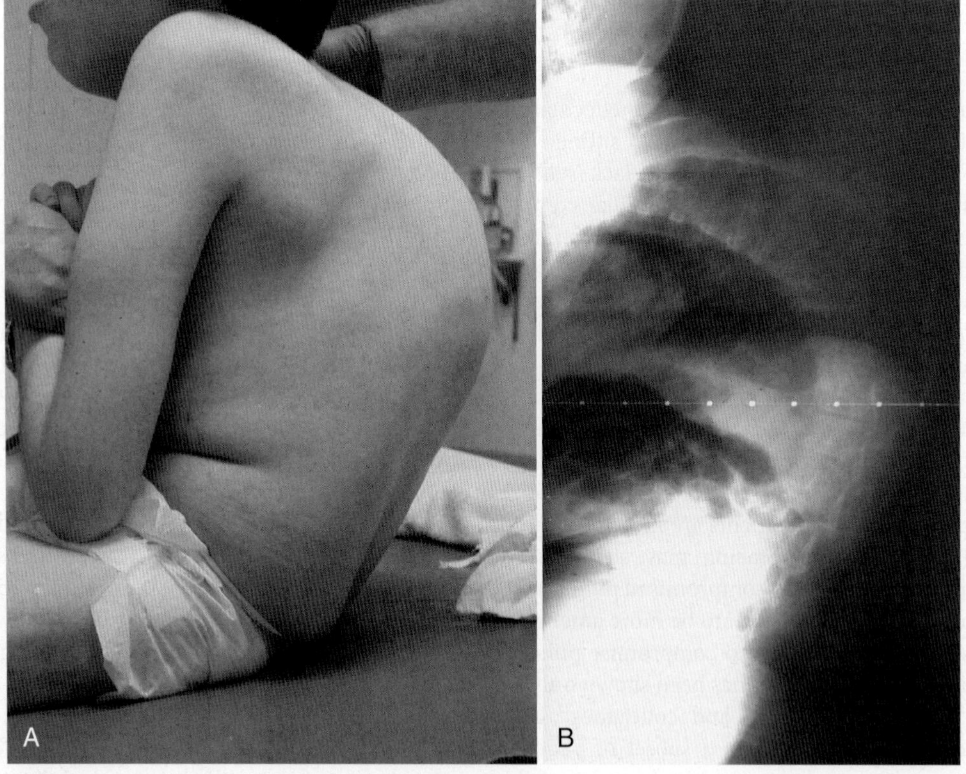

FIG. 28.6 (A) Clinical photograph and (B) lateral radiograph of a child with severe kyphosis that impedes balanced sitting.

factors. The curve severity guidelines are loosely based on, but less aggressive than, the guidelines used in idiopathic scoliosis. Fusion should be considered as coronal deformity approaches 40 to 60 degrees. DMD may be an important exception to this concept: surgery has been advocated when the deformity reaches 20 to 40 degrees because of pulmonary considerations.[29] Patients with severely limited respiratory function have been shown to have good outcomes in spinal surgery, however. The sagittal profile is another important consideration because lordotic and kyphotic deformities can also impair sitting balance and pulmonary capacity (Fig. 28.6). Other factors that play a role in the decision to operate include patient age, nutritional status, cardiac function, curve progression, patient comorbidities, and family and caretaker support.

The benefit of scoliosis surgery in this population is a topic of much debate. Many of these patients are poor operative candidates and risk much undergoing involved corrective surgery. Preoperatively, patients may have compromised pulmonary function, limited cardiac capacity, poor bone stock, and high risk for aspiration, which put them in danger of intraoperative or postoperative complications. Correction of large deformities requires extensive exposures and long procedures that can lead to blood loss greater than one to two patient blood volumes. Although many patients already have neurologic compromise, they are still at risk for further compromise because of intraoperative spinal column manipulation. More powerful instrumentation systems have led to less postoperative decompensation and pseudarthrosis; however, there remains a considerable risk of curve progression, sometimes necessitating revision surgery.[30-32]

Despite the risk of surgery, the benefits of corrective scoliosis surgery for many of these patients are substantial. Halting or slowing curve progression has a positive impact on the functional ability, comfort, and overall quality of life of these patients. Lonstein and Akbarnia[33] reported that more than 50% of patients treated had functional improvement after surgery. In a study of 79 patients with total body spastic CP, Comstock and colleagues[31] found that 85% of caretakers surveyed were satisfied with the surgery, reporting improved comfort, sitting ability, and cosmesis for the patients. Bridwell and colleagues[30] found similar trends in a study of 54 patients with neuromuscular disorders with all caretakers reporting benefit from the surgery, specifically in the areas of ease of patient care, skin breakdown, patient comfort, pulmonary complications, and quality of life. Askin and colleagues[34] evaluated 20 patients with neuromuscular scoliosis preoperatively and 6, 12, and 24 months after corrective spinal surgery. The authors noted decreased physical ability at the 6-month time point followed by a return to preoperative function by 12 months, and concluded that scoliosis surgery in these patients can stabilize, but not improve, function. However, 75% of patients or caregivers were extremely pleased with the cosmetic results of the surgery. Although most of these patients have deteriorating courses, the correction of spinal deformity seems to improve their function and quality of life.

Although these positive results make a strong case for spine surgery in patients with neuromuscular scoliosis, several review studies have been unable to show a clear benefit of surgical intervention for the patient. Mercado and colleagues[35] evaluated 198 publications and graded their results on the concept of Grades of Recommendation introduced in the *Journal of Bone and Joint Surgery*.[36] These authors concluded that the current literature shows that there is poor-quality evidence that spinal fusion improves the quality of life in patients with CP or DMD.[35] In a 2015 updated Cochrane Collaboration review by Cheuk and colleagues[37] that reviewed 49 relevant studies, they found that no relevant randomized controlled clinical trials were available to sufficiently evaluate the effectiveness of scoliosis surgery in DMD patients. Therefore, no evidence-based recommendations could be made. Although the practicality of conducting an RCT of this nature is questionable, the literature does not provide sufficient evidence to support the role of spinal surgical treatment in patients with neuromuscular scoliosis. It is recommended that the decision for surgical intervention be made based on the needs of the individual patient in consultation with the multidisciplinary neuromuscular care team.

The goal of treatment is preservation of function, which may entail maintaining ambulatory status, maintaining sitting without upper extremity support, or simply allowing assisted comfortable sitting. The decision to operate on a patient with neuromuscular scoliosis is a highly individualized process that should involve a frank and open discussion with the family and patient about the risks and expectations of such a procedure.

Preoperative Considerations

Neurologic

Many patients with neuromuscular scoliosis are on long-term antiseizure therapy, which has some important operative ramifications. Antiepileptic medications such as phenytoin and valproate have been linked to decreased bone turnover and decreased intestinal absorption of calcium, resulting in osteopenia, which may affect implant fixation and should be considered in the selection of construct components.[38,39] A study by Kumandas and colleagues[40] that analyzed 88 prepubertal ambulatory epileptic patients divided into two treatment groups over the course of 2 years on carbamazepine or valproic acid found bone mineral density (BMD) to be adversely affected. The BMD in the lumbar spine was significantly reduced in patients taking carbamezapine or valproic acid compared to the age- and sex-matched control group. According to the authors, carbamazepine and valproic acid therapy results in a hyperparathyroid state and altered vitamin D metabolism associated with reduced BMD. It is well known that antiepileptic drugs (AEDs) adversely affect the coagulation system. Drugs such as carbamazepine, phenytoin, and valproic acid can result in thrombocytopenia.[41] Valproic acid and gabapentin in previous studies have shown to cause acquired von Willebrand disease type 1, hypofibrinogenemia, decreased factor XIII, and abnormal platelet function.[42] Koenig and colleagues[43] showed that 47% of patients receiving valproic acid had abnormal thromboelastographs (TEGs). However, other studies have shown that patients on valproic acid are not at increased risk of bleeding complications at surgery. Manohar and colleagues[44] showed in a study of 84 children undergoing craniotomy for resection of seizure focus or hemispherectomy that none of the cohort showed significantly abnormal prothrombin time, activated partial thromboplastin time, or platelet count preoperatively. A total of 38% of the study patients received allogenic blood transfusions; 4.7% showed clinically significant coagulopathy intraoperatively and postoperatively. However, prospective clinical studies are needed that evaluate platelet function and coagulation problems to confirm if indeed AEDs pose little or significant intraoperative bleeding risks.

Pulmonary

Patients with neuromuscular disorders are prone to pulmonary complications, necessitating a thorough preoperative pulmonary assessment. Poor upper airway tone and anatomic deviations can lead to increased risk of airway obstruction during and after surgery. These patients are at high risk for aspiration because of poor oropharyngeal tone and coordination; not only can chronic aspiration lead to pulmonary fibrosis, but acute aspiration can result in perioperative aspiration pneumonia. Patients may require a dietary change, placement of a gastrostomy tube, or a Nissen fundoplication with gastrostomy tube placement to control this aspiration tendency before undergoing spinal surgery. Reactive airway disease is common in these patients and may necessitate the use of preoperative bronchodilators and inhaled steroids. In addition, these patients may have chronic hypoventilation with carbon dioxide retention and poor oxygenation.

Full pulmonary assessment should be conducted by a pulmonologist and include a chest radiograph, arterial blood gases, and pulmonary function tests if the patient's developmental age is at least 4 years old. Vital capacity that exceeds 500 mL and peak expiratory flow greater than 180 mL/min are associated with decreased perioperative pulmonary complications. Although surgery may be considered in appropriately selected patients with preexisting respiratory failure, Chambers et al.[45] and Gill and colleagues[46] showed that patients with a forced vital capacity (FVC) of 20% of predicted value can safely be operated on for deformity correction. This prospective observational study followed eight patients on noninvasive night ventilation for respiratory failure 48 months after surgery and found that all patients recovered well with no major complications.

As a follow-up study to that of Gill et al., Chong and colleagues[47] evaluated the prognostic value of preoperative pulmonary function tests (PFTs) for postoperative pulmonary complications and the operability despite significantly decreased FVC (<30%) in flaccid neuromuscular scoliosis. A total of 74 patients stratified into three groups (<30% FVC, 30–50% FVC, and >50% FVC) were evaluated. They found no statistical difference between groups in the number of complications. If a patient cannot be assessed with formal pulmonary function tests, other signs of ventilatory capacity must be used, including crying, laughing, and other vocalizations.[48-50]

Proper nutritional balance is crucial for successful surgical outcomes in patients with neuromuscular scoliosis. Many patients are malnourished secondary to a combination of reflux, low calorie intake, and high metabolic demand from frequent illness. Malnourished patients are more prone to perioperative complications such as wound dehiscence, wound infection, and pulmonary complications. Conversely, older patients may be obese, presenting further operative complications associated with their body habitus. Nutritional status should be assessed preoperatively with albumin and total blood lymphocyte levels. Albumin should be greater than 3.5 g/L, and total lymphocyte count should be greater than 1.5 g/L.[50] In a study of 44 patients, Jevsevar and Karlin[51] found that patients had a lower incidence of postoperative infections if they met these criteria.

A prospective randomized control study of total parenteral nutrition (TPN) for long spinal deformity, performed by Lapp and colleagues[52] on 46 patients who underwent same-day or staged procedures to evaluate the effect on complications and recovery from postoperative malnutrition, showed TPN to be safe. There was a trend toward faster recovery to nutritional baseline in patients receiving TPN versus those who did not.

Gastrointestinal

Because patients with neuromuscular scoliosis are prone to gastrointestinal dysmotility, they are at risk for a postoperative ileus, requiring aggressive hydration, maximized nutritional status, and a rigid daily toilet regimen. In addition, some patients are very thin, and supine positioning and the acute straightening of their deformity put them at risk for superior mesenteric artery syndrome with obstruction of the duodenum. Although less common since the advent of segmental instrumentation and decreased use of casting, this prolonged obstruction carries significant morbidity; identifying at-risk patients and maintaining a high index of suspicion when encountering protracted vomiting is essential.

Cardiovascular

Patients may have cardiac problems secondary to their deformity and other cardiac issues that are comorbidities of the primary disorder. Thoracic cage deformity resulting from scoliosis can cause hypoventilation and subsequent increased pulmonary vascular resistance; this increased vascular resistance can cause right ventricular hypertrophy and eventually cor pulmonale. Patients with DMD may have cardiomyopathy and arrhythmias. The complications associated with arrhythmias may be alleviated with glucocorticoid steroid treatment.[14] Patients with myotonic dystrophy may also have cardiac arrhythmias. Left ventricular hypertrophy can be associated with Friedreich ataxia.

Hematologic

Studies have shown that patients with neuromuscular scoliosis have greater blood loss than patients with idiopathic scoliosis undergoing similar procedures. In this neuromuscular group, the underlying disorder plays a major role in determining the extent of blood loss. In a review article, Shapiro and Sethna[53] found that patients with DMD had the greatest mean levels of blood loss. Much of this difference is due to the requirement for larger fusions in patients with neuromuscular scoliosis, although osteopenia in these patients may also play a role.[54,55] Preparation for major blood loss, sometimes exceeding 200% of a patient's blood volume, is essential.[48] Often, these patients have already had major surgery, and previous blood loss experience can be used as a guideline for preoperative preparation. Patients should have partial thromboplastin time, prothrombin time, and platelet function evaluated as a part of their preoperative blood work. A more aggressive coagulopathy workup should be conducted if the patient has previously shown a tendency toward excessive blood loss.

For a posterior procedure, 2 to 4 units of packed red blood cells is generally sufficient; however, the addition of a kyphectomy or an anterior procedure may increase this requirement. Intraoperative blood work may confirm a dilutional coagulopathy, necessitating the use of fresh frozen plasma, platelets, or cryoprecipitate to correct this imbalance.

Several pharmacologic agents have been under investigation for their efficacy in reducing blood loss during surgery. Aprotinin, tranexamic acid (TXA), and aminocaproic acid have also been investigated to determine their effect on blood loss in spinal surgery. Aprotinin, a serine protease inhibitor, was shown to reduce blood loss in adults, but its production was halted in 2007 by the US Food and Drug Administration (FDA) because of concerns of higher mortality rates after its use in cardiac surgery.

A prospective, double-blinded, placebo control study of 40 pediatric patients[56] found that TXA administration significantly reduced perioperative blood transfusions. These results have been supported by a meta-analysis by Gill and colleagues,[57] which found that TXA and aminocaproic acid are effective in minimizing blood loss and transfusion in patients undergoing spine surgery. A multicenter retrospective review of a prospectively collected database of 84 consecutive enrolled patients with CP who underwent posterior spinal fusion and instrumentation showed that the use of antifibrinolytic agents (AFs) significantly reduced the estimated blood loss (EBL) intraoperatively without adverse effects.[58] However, the investigators could not demonstrate a significant difference between total transfusion requirements between patients who received AF agents and those who did not except for cell salvage transfusion. The study showed that patients who received TXA had significantly less EBL compared with patients who did not.[58]

A prospective, randomized, double-blind comparative study performed on 125 patients with adolescent idiopathic scoliosis by Verma and colleagues showed that TXA and epsilon-aminocaproic acid (EACA) reduced operative blood loss but not transfusion rate compared to control subjects.[59] As in the study by Dhawale et al,[58] the investigators showed that TXA was more effective in reducing total blood loss and postoperative drainage compared to EACA. Furthermore, the authors recommended maintaining the mean arterial pressure (MAP) greater than 75 during the exposure to utilize the maximize benefit.[59] The side effects for TXA and aminocaproic acid are minor but should be discussed with the patient before using these agents. The surgeon and the anesthesiologist should familiarize themselves with these agents and make a collaborative decision on their use based on the needs and concerns of the individual patient.

Radiographic Assessment

Patients should have preoperative anteroposterior and lateral films taken of the entire spine, preferably in an upright (sitting or standing) position. For assessment of skeletal maturity, a separate anteroposterior radiograph of the pelvis should be considered because scoliosis films often truncate the anatomy necessary to determine skeletal maturity. To assess spinal flexibility, supine bending films or traction films are used. Accurate measurements of the coronal Cobb angle, sagittal Cobb angle, and pelvic obliquity are crucial for complete preoperative planning and postoperative evaluations. In a more recent analysis of the interobserver and intraobserver variability of radiographic measurements of patients with neuromuscular scoliosis, Gupta and colleagues[60] found that neuromuscular radiographs can be reliably analyzed with the use of the coronal Cobb angle. Patients who may have congenital spinal anomalies or spinal tethering, such as patients with myelomeningocele, should undergo MRI to evaluate the neural elements fully before surgery. CT may also be useful in some patients with severe deformity or in patients with a congenital malformation of the vertebrae.

History of Instrumentation in Neuromuscular Scoliosis

In 1942, Haas[61] published one of the first references to surgical intervention in neuromuscular scoliosis: a case report describing muscle and fascial transfers to obtain complete and permanent correction in one patient. With the introduction of the Harrington rod in 1962, use of this instrumentation with fusion of the spine in patients with neuromuscular scoliosis became the standard. Series using only Harrington rods and posterior spinal fusion have been associated with high incidences of pseudarthrosis (19–40%), moderate initial correction (20–57%), and loss of correction ranging from 14% to 28%.[33,62] After Harrington rod instrumentation, most patients required bed rest and bracing or casting for up to 1 year.

The introduction of segmental spinal instrumentation by Luque[63] in 1976 led to major advances in the biomechanical stability and correction of these very deformed spines (Fig. 28.7). Several studies revealed that Luque segmental sublaminar wire fixation had fewer complications than Harrington instrumentation and was stable enough so that most patients required no brace or cast postoperatively.[62,64,65] Using the Luque method, the only patients with CP requiring postoperative bracing may be patients with athetosis or poor fixation because of severe osteopenia. This is a tremendous advantage because postoperative casting carries the potential for skin and pulmonary complications. Because of these attributes, the Luque technique became the standard method for posterior spinal instrumentation in patients with neuromuscular spinal deformities.

Contouring Luque spinal rods after the technique introduced by Allen and Ferguson[66] (Galveston technique) allowed the rods to be fixed to the pelvis, providing surgeons with a more effective method of controlling pelvic obliquity. Bell, Moseley, and Koreska developed the unit rod, a precontoured U-shaped rod that includes the Galveston portion for pelvic fixation (Fig. 28.8). Studies of patient outcomes with unit rod fixation have revealed excellent correction and maintenance of correction.[66-69] Bulman and colleagues[70] compared the unit rod with double Luque rods and reported superior correction of sagittal and coronal alignment and pelvic obliquity with the unit rod constructs. Tsirikos and colleagues[71] evaluated 287 children treated with unit rod instrumentation to the pelvis

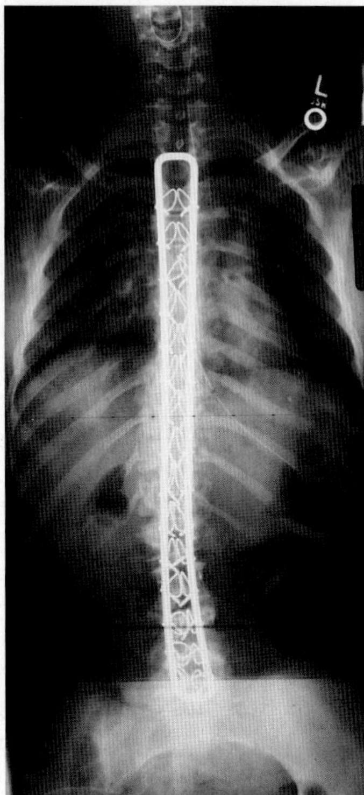

FIG. 28.7 The one-piece Luque "box" modification of the original double Luque rod technique is a more rigid construct.

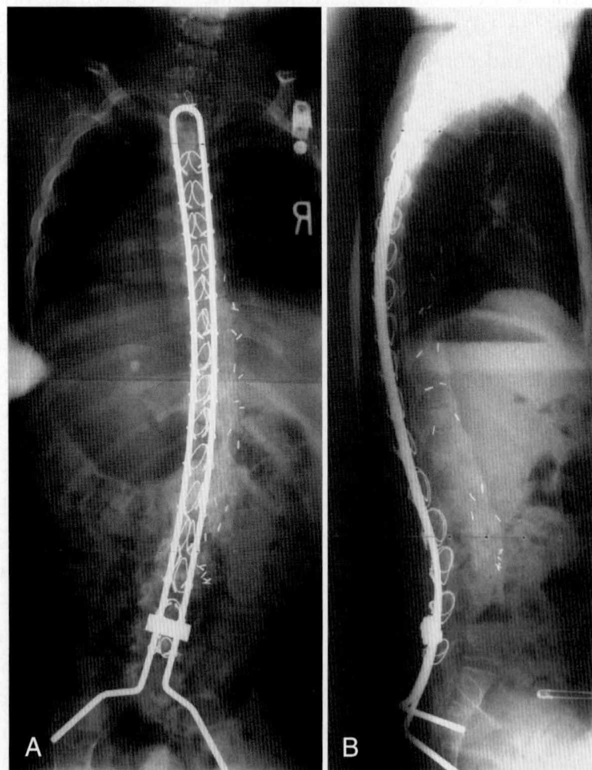

FIG. 28.8 Unit rod, as shown in a patient with cerebral palsy, provides a method for obtaining fixation to the pelvis and correction of pelvic obliquity.

with 2-year follow-up and concluded that it offers the advantages of good correction of deformity and pelvic obliquity, a low complication rate, and a 96% caretakers' survey satisfaction rate. Unit rod instrumentation has also been shown to have good results in ambulatory patients, with excellent deformity correction and preservation of ambulatory function at 2.9-year follow-up in 24 patients.[72] Additionally, biomechanical studies have shown that the addition of an L5 pedicle screw increases the construct stiffness and the strength-reducing complications associated with the loss of fixation.[73]

Through a desire to achieve similar correction as the unit rod construct, without the need for pelvic fixation, the U-rod was investigated by McCall and Hayes.[74] This rod is an outgrowth of the unit rod concept except that the rod terminates in pedicle screws at the L5 level, relying on the iliolumbar ligaments to achieve correction of the pelvic obliquity. In their comparison study of 30 patients with unit rod instrumentation and sacral fusion and 25 patients with U-rod instrumentation and L5 fusion, McCall and Hayes[74] found that the U-rod provided comparable correction of scoliosis and pelvic obliquity in curves with less than 15 degrees L5 tilt at 4 years of follow-up. Regardless of whether the precontoured unit rod or double Luque rods are used, segmental sublaminar wire instrumentation provides simple, inexpensive, and fairly powerful correction of coronal plane deformity. Segmental sublaminar wire instrumentation has limitations in the maintenance of sagittal plane alignment, however, because the sublaminar wiring fails to fix spinal length and the vertebrae can slide along the smooth rod construct, particularly during trunk flexion (Fig. 28.9A).

Multihook segmental systems, such as Cotrel-Dubousset (CD) and Isola, have also been shown to be efficacious in patients with neuromuscular scoliosis.[75-77] The comparative efficacy of these two different constructs is inconclusive. In a study of 47 patients with neuromuscular scoliosis, Yazici and colleagues[78] concluded that the Isola instrumentation combined with Galveston pelvic fixation provided correction and maintenance of pelvic obliquity superior to Luque-Galveston, unit rod, or CD instrumentation. The results of this study are in contrast to the work of Wimmer and colleagues,[77] who found that there was no difference between Luque-Galveston and Isola instrumentation in radiographic outcomes, patient satisfaction, or complication rate.

In some circumstances, a hybrid system with a combination of hooks, pedicle screws, and sublaminar wires may provide optimal fixation with maximal correction. A biomechanical study conducted at the authors' institution showed that the addition of bilateral L1 pedicle screws to a Luque-Galveston construct on a cadaveric axial skeleton increased construct stiffness by greater than 60%. The addition of selective hooks or screws or both to an otherwise sublaminar wire construct allows use of compressive and distractive force to address the coronal and the sagittal deformities. Additionally, proximal fixation with sublaminar wires compromises the ligaments above, making junctional kyphosis more likely. Hooks (transverse process) or pedicle screws or both may limit this complication in kyphotic patients at greatest risk. Pedicle screw fixation has become the standard at many

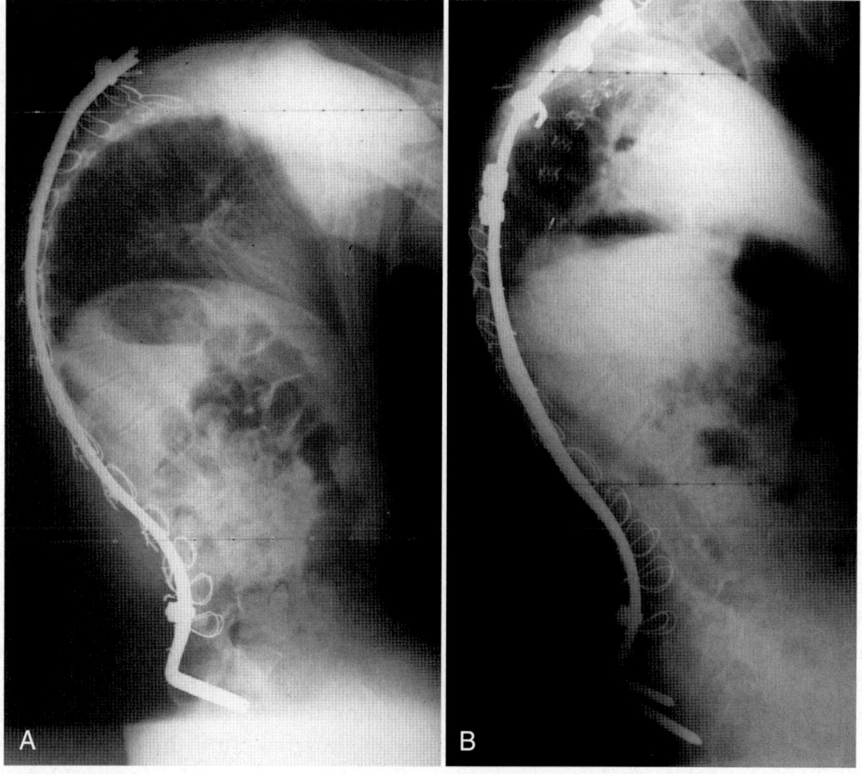

FIG. 28.9 (A) Failure of proximal sublaminar wiring in this construct resulted in increased kyphosis and prominent hardware, necessitating revision surgery 3 years after primary procedure. (B) After proximal revision, the patient developed pullout of the Galveston portion of his construct. This clinical course emphasizes that fixation challenges are present in patients with neuromuscular deformity, particular hyperkyphosis.

centers for nearly all forms of spinal deformity, although there are synthetic bands now available that can be utilized in a sublaminar fashion similar to Luque wires.

Pelvic and Sacral Fixation

Severe pelvic obliquity secondary to unbalanced scoliotic curves and lower extremity contractures is common and progressive in patients with neuromuscular scoliosis. A solid spinal fusion to the pelvis aids in sitting comfort and balance[79]; however, achieving this goal can be troublesome (see Fig. 28.9B). Controlling the motion across the lumbosacral joint requires secure fixation to the pelvis to prevent a pseudarthrosis.

Various systems have been proposed to provide fixation to the pelvis. The Galveston technique was the first advancement to improve fusion rates and clinical success in long fusions to the sacrum.[60,66] When paired with either contoured Luque rods or unit rods, it provides powerful coronal correction of pelvic obliquity. This technique places greater forces, however, on the lumbrosacral junction, and proper contouring of the rods may be difficult. The initial concern regarding the association between radiolucency around the screw tips ("windshield wiper" sign) and an increased incidence of complications is of little clinical significance (Fig. 28.10).[79-81] Although a biomechanical evaluation of the Galveston technique by Sink and colleagues[32] showed that this construct creates a long lever

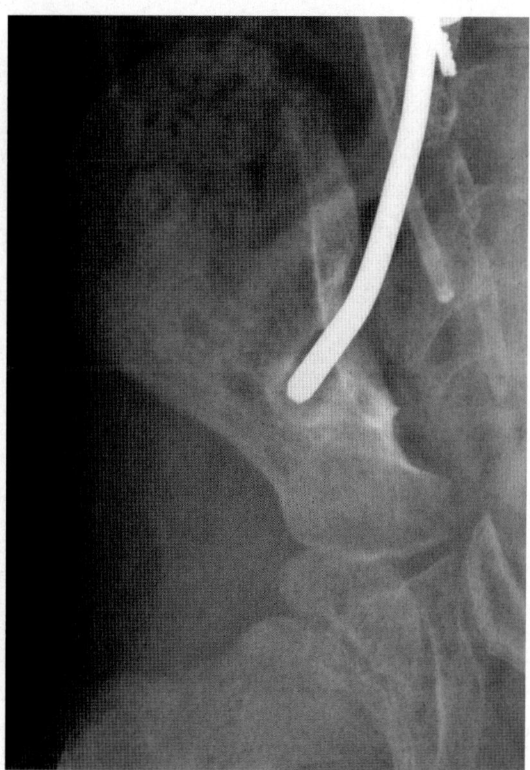

FIG. 28.10 Radiolucency around rod tip in ilium ("windshield wiper" effect) suggests lumbosacral pseudarthrosis, which may remain asymptomatic and resolve spontaneously.

arm that places considerable cantilever forces at the lumbrosacral junction, these forces lead to a high incidence of proximal fixation pullout and distal migration of Galveston rods. The rods also require three-dimensional bending, which makes it difficult to contour the rod properly.[82]

Other systems of sacropelvic fixation use an "S" bend,[83] which hooks distally over the sacral alae, while the more proximal portion is secured to the lumbar spine at L4 or above with a pedicle screw or infralaminar hook. Reviewing the results of 67 patients, McCarthy and colleagues[83] found that this technique had decreased operative time compared with Galveston fixation and achieved excellent clinical results, although in 2 of the 67 constructs, there was migration of the rods into the pelvis. Other techniques of rod contouring to fix to the pelvis include the Warner-Fackler and McCall techniques, both commonly used in the treatment of myelomeningocele-associated kyphosis, in which posterior elements of the lumbar or sacral spine may be absent. In the Warner-Fackler technique,[84] Luque rods are bent to 90 degrees in two places at the distal end, allowing the rods to pass through the S1 foramina and lever against the front of the sacrum to provide sagittal correction (Fig. 28.11). In a slight variation of this technique, McCall[85] described bending Luque rods to 20 to 40 degrees, passing them through the S1 foramina and bending the protruding portion according to the contour of the anterior sacrum. In 16 myelomeningocele patients with hyperkyphosis, McCall[85] found satisfactory correction and maintenance of correction after 5 years of follow-up.

Improvement on the Galveston concept has been the focus of many clinical studies.[83,86-88] The use of S1 screws alone was investigated, but bone quality is generally not substantial enough for successful use in patients with neuromuscular scoliosis. Early and colleagues[86] compared the biomechanical properties of Galveston sacropelvic fixation versus Colorado II sacropelvic plates using S1 screws, S2 alar screws, and iliac screws, and found that both methods provided similar construct stiffness with the Colorado II plate limiting L5–S1 motion in flexion-extension. These authors found that addition of a pair of L1 screws increased the construct stiffness by approximately 50% in both fixation techniques.

The use of iliac screw fixation has become a subject of several more recent articles because of its ease of implantation, avoiding the complex lumbosacral three-dimensional Galveston rod contouring. Clinical and biomechanical studies have shown an improved fusion rate and high pullout strengths after the use of iliac screws for caudad lumbosacral fixation.[87,88] In a review of 50 patients treated with one or two bilateral iliac screws, Phillips and colleagues[89] concluded that iliac screws provide a safe and effective means to treat neuromuscular scoliosis at 21 months of follow-up. These authors also noted that two screws in each iliac wing provided a more stable fixation with fewer implant-related complications than using a single screw. In a direct comparison of 20 patients with Galveston rod fixation versus 20 patients with iliac screw fixation, Peelle and colleagues[90] found that both techniques offer similar pelvic fixation with the iliac screw construct, allowing additional screw fixation points to the sacrum and lower lumbar vertebrae. The long-term impact of these screws on the sacroiliac joint was investigated in 67 adult patients by

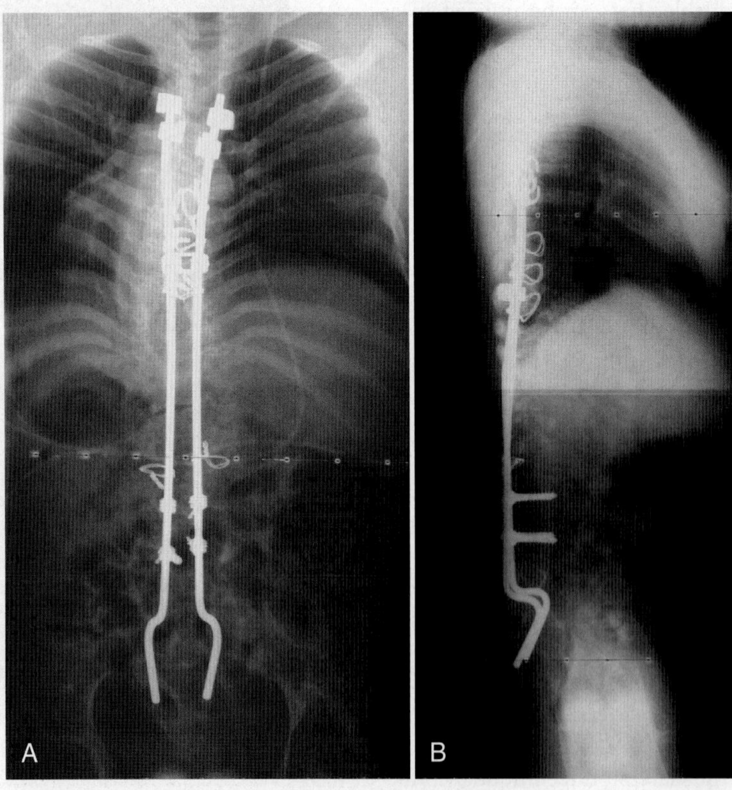

FIG. 28.11 Warner-Fackler method of pelvic fixation used after kyphectomy in a patient with myelodysplasia.

Tsuchiya and colleagues[88]; no evidence of degeneration was observed at 5- to 10-year follow-up.

Although iliac screws provide a promising alternative to Galveston fixation, several studies have shown difficulty with implant prominence causing skin irritation.[91] Peelle and colleagues[90] did not observe this complication in their patient series, however, because they countersunk the screws below the superficial portion of the posterior iliac crest. The patient's body habitus must be considered when selecting the means of sacropelvic fixation.

A lower profile method of iliac fixation has been developed by Kebaish[92] and Whitaker and colleagues[93] that starts in the sacral ala lateral to the S1 foramen and traverses the sacroiliac joint before entering the iliac wing. This has proven a useful method for limiting implant prominence (Fig. 28.12).

A retrospective study by Funk et al.[94] looking at patients treated with posterior spinal fusion to the pelvis for neuromuscular scoliosis with minimum 1-year follow-up in 80 patients showed advantages in favor of rigid spinopelvic instrumentation. In this study, the authors defined rigid instrumentation as consisting of at least 50% pedicle screw fixation with iliac or sacral alar iliac screw pelvic fixation. The correction of deformity at final follow-up was significantly greater when measuring Cobb angle and pelvic obliquity in the group of patients treated with rigid instrumentation. The pseudarthrosis rate was 5% in the rigid group and 22% in the nonrigid treated group.[94]

When patients with neuromuscular scoliosis are instrumented because of the severe obliquity of the pelvis, intraoperative halofemoral traction may also be beneficial. Previous studies on this traction technique have been described for patients with idiopathic and congenital scoliosis. In nonambulatory patients with neuromuscular scoliosis, surgeons have relied on rods or screws inserted into the iliac wings by a cantilever method to level the pelvis. This method has the potential to weaken the bone-construct connection in patients with poor bone stock. In a study of 20 nonambulatory patients with neuromuscular scoliosis with halofemoral traction and 20 matched patients without halofemoral traction, Takeshita and colleagues[95] found that halofemoral traction provided significantly improved lumbar curve and pelvic obliquity correction at 2-year follow-up. These authors had no associated perioperative complications with this technique, and found that unilateral femoral traction with corresponding halo traction was able to level the pelvis to an acceptable position before the surgery was begun. However, when a significant hip flexion contracture exists, traction results in an increase in lumbar lordosis that may be undesirable.

Some authors have argued that the pelvis can be left unfused in patients with slight pelvic obliquity, mild contractures, and little pelvic deformity in the sagittal plane, whereas others have argued that an ambulatory patient should never be fused to the pelvis.[92-94] McCall and colleagues[74] advocated that patients with less than 15 degrees of L5 tilt should be considered for a fusion to L5. These authors believed that this fusion allows greater mobility and improves the patients' ability to carry out activities of daily living (ADLs). Other studies promote fusion to the pelvis in all patients regardless of ambulatory status. A study by Tsirikos and colleagues[71] of

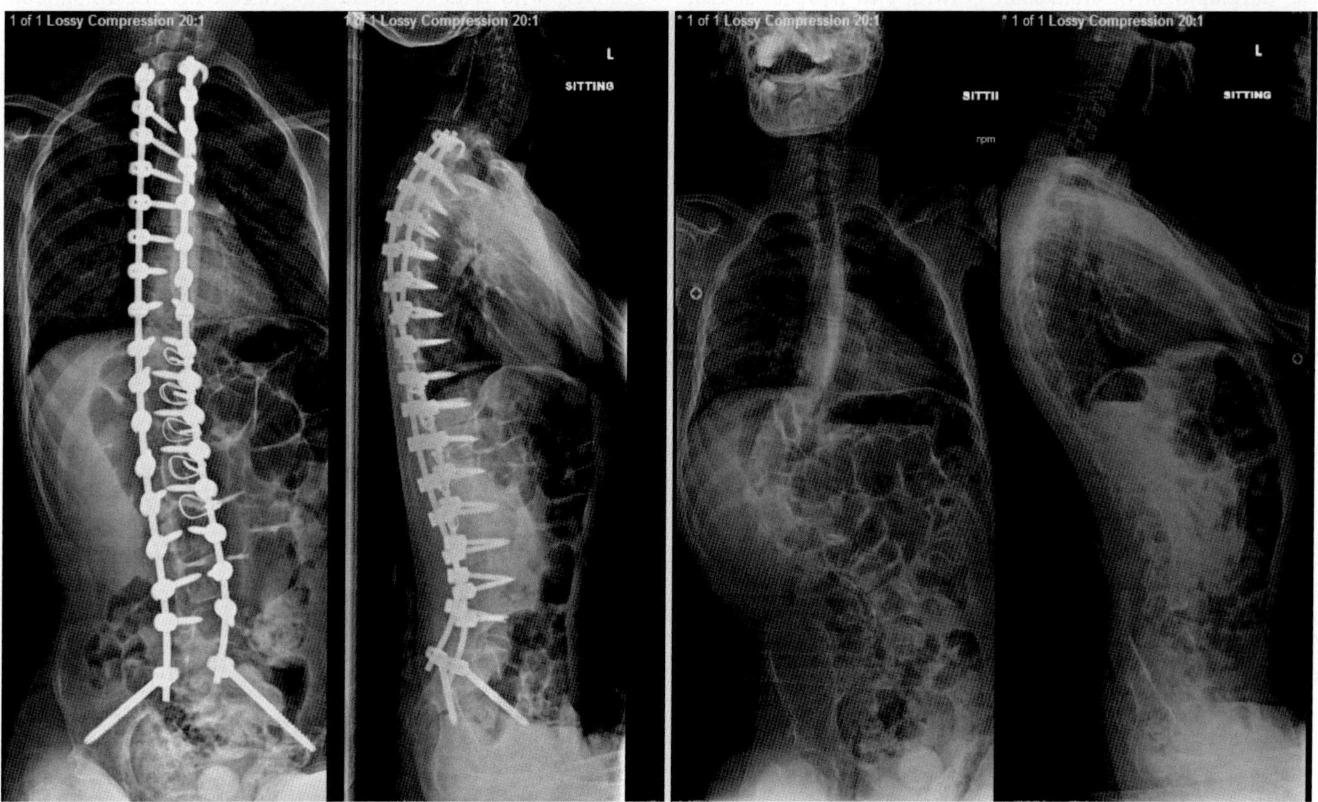

FIG. 28.12 A 12-yea-old with neuromuscular scoliosis status post T2 to pelvis with sacral-alar-iliac screw technique.

ambulatory CP patients with severe pelvic obliquity who were treated with fusion to the pelvis by Luque-Galveston instrumentation found that 23 of 24 patients maintained their ambulatory status. Given the progressive nature of this deformity and the fragility of these patients as operative candidates, the authors generally recommend including the pelvis in the fusion mass for most neuromuscular deformities.

Growing rod (GR) constructs connected to the pelvis in the neuromuscular population have become more common over the past decade. Sponseller and colleagues[96] analyzed the outcomes and complications unique to GR systems with the pelvis as the distal anchor point. The records of 36 patients from the Growing Spine database were analyzed with diagnoses including SMA, CP, multifocal motor neuropathy (MMN), congenital, arthrogryposis, and syndromic deformity with follow-up greater than 2 years. They found that GRs anchored to the pelvis can be used to safely and effectively correct pelvic obliquity, with dual iliac fixation providing the best correction. Iliac screws performed significantly better at correcting Cobb angle and pelvic obliquity when compared to sacral fixation.[97]

Anterior Spinal Release and Fusion

Indications

The addition of an anterior procedure can assist in the correction of neuromuscular spinal deformity and may be justified in several situations (Fig. 28.13). Anterior release and fusion has generally been indicated in patients with rigid scoliosis, patients with rigid kyphosis, immature patients at risk for the development of crankshaft growth, and patients at risk for pseudarthrosis owing to incompetent posterior elements (myelomeningocele or severe osteopenia).[93] In assessing the rigidity of the deformity, traction and supine bending films are useful but may underrepresent the available flexibility. An anterior release of a large rigid curve increases the overall spine mobility and makes the posterior correction easier with a relatively high fusion rate. In a study by Newton and colleagues,[98] the fusion rate achieved with anterior release combined with posterior corrective instrumentation and fusion was found to be comparable between adolescent patients with neuromuscular scoliosis and idiopathic scoliosis at 3-year follow-up. Keeler and colleagues[99] performed a comparative study in 52 patients who underwent intraoperative halofemoral traction. Twenty six patients underwent posterior spinal fusion (PSF) only for spastic neurmuscular scoliosis and were matched against an equal numbered cohort that underwent an anteroposterior spinal fusion (A/PSF) with no demographic or preoperative radiographic differences between the two groups. The study revealed that PSF-only surgery provides excellent curve correction and spinal balance with no statistical differences in terms of the final thoracolumbar/lumbar curve Cobb angle, percentage of correction of the thoracolumbar/lumbar Cobb angle, pelvic obliquity, C7 plumb line, and the center sacral vertical line at 2-year follow-up compared to A/PSF.[96] The patients who underwent PSF only had significantly reduced operative time, lower EBL, and lower frequency of postoperative pulmonary complications.[99] On the other hand, Auerback and colleagues[100] determined that CP patients with rigid and large major curves benefited more from an anterior release combined with a posterior fusion versus a posterior fusion alone. They compared 19 patients who had larger major curves, greater pelvic obliquity, and more rigid curves preoperatively who underwent anterior release against 42 patients with more flexible curves who underwent posterior fusion only. Correction of pelvic obliquity was similar in both groups.

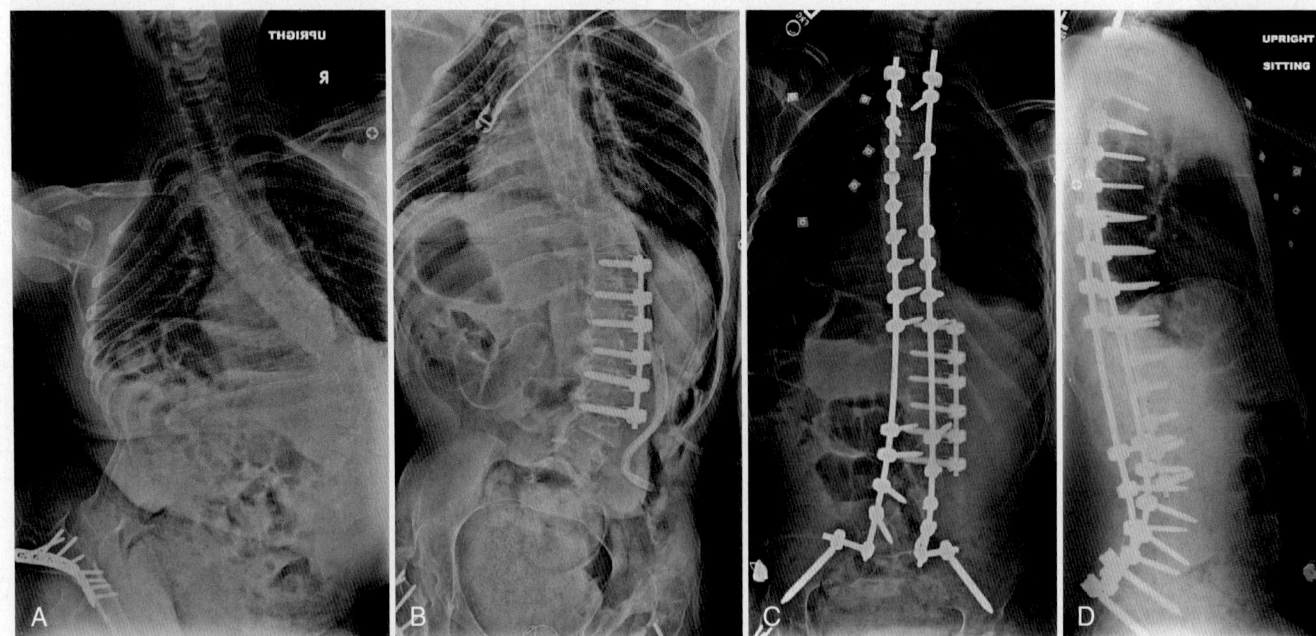

FIG. 28.13 (A) This severe thoracolumbar curve has a preoperative Cobb angle of 136 degrees. (B) Because of inflexibility, anterior disc excision and anterior instrumentation were used as the first stage of this procedure. (C–D) Posterior instrumentation T2 to pelvis was used in this quadriplegic patient with spasticity.

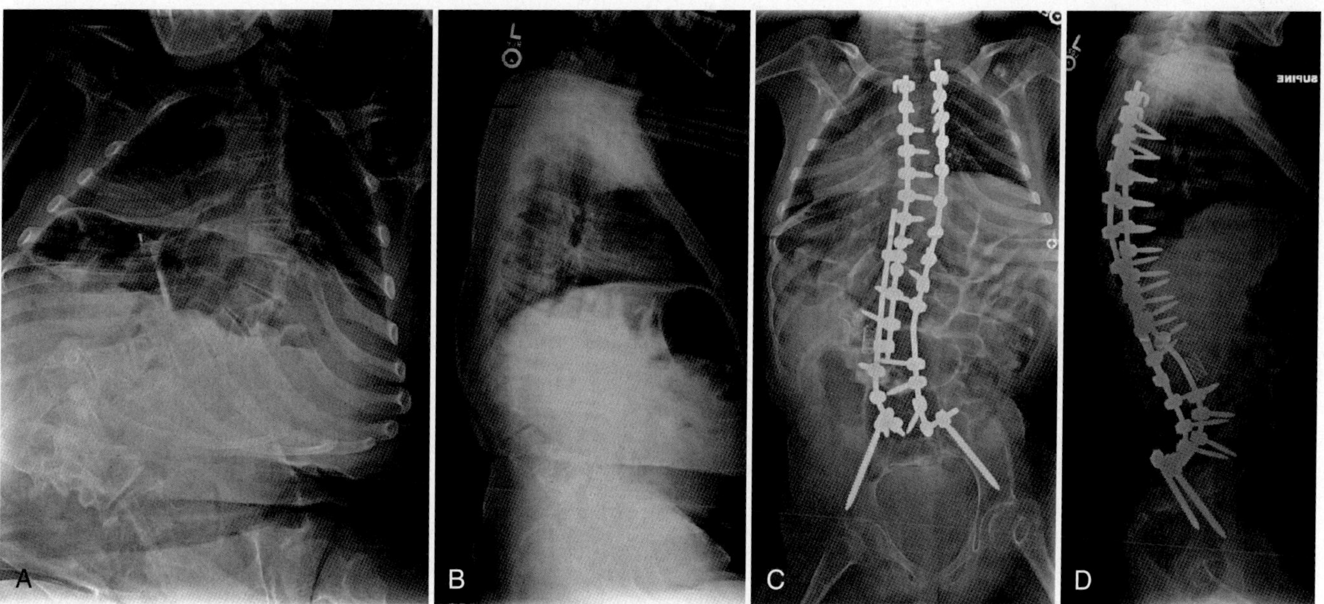

FIG. 28.14 (A–B) A severe 140-degree lumbar curve was upsetting wheelchair sitting balance in a quadriplegic patient with spasticity. (C–D) This curve was treated with a staged procedure. Anterior release did not provide sufficient flexibility, and anterior L1 and L2 corpectomy was performed. This procedure was followed by T2 to pelvis posterior instrumentation with completion of L1 and L2 corpectomy posteriorly.

While no significant difference was noted in the percentage of correction in the coronal and sagittal plane in the group, those with more rigid curves who underwent anterior release tended to have a greater percentage of correction compared to their preoperative bending films.[100]

Anterior instrumentation and spinal fusion alone and in combination with posterior instrumentation have also been shown to be successful techniques in a subset of patients with neuromuscular scoliosis. Our current algorithm indicates an anterior procedure for "severe" curves (most often thoracolumbar). If a near-complete correction of the major curve can be predicted with anterior instrumentation after an aggressive multilevel discectomy, a single-rod anterior system is included. If the curve remains rigid after an anterior release, the anterior instrumentation is skipped, and either an apical vertebrectomy is performed or the correction is achieved after posterior osteotomies (Fig. 28.14). It is important to avoid "locking in" a poor correction with anterior instrumentation in rigid curves. The goals of achieving a level pelvis and balanced spine must be weighed against the added morbidity of an anterior release or instrumentation procedures, or both.

In skeletally immature patients with idiopathic scoliosis, anterior release and fusion reduces anterior overgrowth that results in crankshaft deformity; however, whether this principle can be applied in neuromuscular scoliosis is controversial. In a study of 50 skeletally immature patients with neuromuscular scoliosis treated with posterior instrumentation only, Smucker and Miller[101] noted no significant curve progression at an average of 4 years of follow-up. In contrast, Comstock and colleagues,[31] after review of 60 skeletally immature patients with CP who underwent surgical scoliosis correction, concluded that skeletally immature patients have the best correction and long-term outcomes when treated with anterior and posterior procedures.

Instrumentation

The indications for anterior instrumentation have been a subject of investigation more recently. Several studies have shown that anterior instrumentation alone provides acceptable correction without the need for posterior instrumentation in selected short flexible curves that do not include the pelvis or have less than 15 degrees of pelvic obliquity.[102,103] Some studies advocate anterior release followed by posterior instrumentation, whereas others find indications for anterior disc excision and anterior instrumentation before proceeding posteriorly. Anterior instrumentation provides a very powerful means of addressing coronal plane deformities, and in many cases simplifies the posterior instrumentation across the levels instrumented anteriorly.

The present options for maximal deformity correction include anterior instrumentation followed by relatively simple posterior fixation versus anterior release and posterior fixation with greater use of posterior osteotomies. The first option also has the advantage of allowing an indefinite time between stages if required. Ultimately, the decision to include an anterior procedure (release or instrumentation) is multifactorial and depends on the experience of the surgeon, the overall health of the patient, and the characteristics of the deformity.

Intraoperative Considerations

Patient Positioning

The patient is positioned for anterior surgery with the apex of the deformity centered over the table break in a nearly lateral position. Flexing the table improves exposure, as does leaning the patient back toward the surgeon. If anterior instrumentation is planned, a direct lateral position is preferred. Posterior surgery is generally performed on a spinal frame; this allows the abdomen to hang free, decreasing the pressure on the vena cava and epidural venous system. This position limits problematic epidural blood loss, particularly when a laminotomy for posterior release and sublaminar wire passage are required at several levels. In a smaller patient, chest rolls may suffice for prone positioning.

Spinal Cord Monitoring

Multimodality monitoring is a useful tool in children with neuromuscular scoliosis. Although patients with true paralysis and myelomeningocele do not benefit from this observation, the use of spinal cord monitoring is helpful for other patients to protect existing extremity function. Current evidence supports the use of transcranial motor evoked potentials (TcMEPs), somatosensory spinal evoked potentials, and H-reflex potentials in spinal cord monitoring.[97,98] TcMEPs provide useful data on the motor function and vascular status of the spinal cord, whereas somatosensory spinal evoked potentials provide information on the integrity of the sensory pathways of the dorsal columns. TcMEP monitoring has become a vital component of spinal cord monitoring. In a study of 1121 consecutive patients with adolescent idiopathic scoliosis undergoing spine surgery, Schwartz and colleagues[105] concluded that TcMEP monitoring is the most effective means to detect evolving spinal cord injury. TcMEPs monitor the anterior horn motor neurons, whose high metabolic rate is especially vulnerable to ischemic injury.[106]

Salem and colleagues[106] determined that TcMEPs do not increase the likelihood of triggering intraoperative or postoperative seizures and are not associated with deterioration in the seizure control of patients afflicted with epilepsy prior to scoliosis surgery. Because of the complexity and associated hematologic issues of patients with neuromuscular scoliosis, multimodal spinal cord monitoring is highly recommended.

Surgical correction of scoliosis in patients with CP has a higher morbidity associated with it compared to adolescent scoliosis.[107,108] Reames et al.[107] showed that surgical correction of neuromuscular scoliosis had the highest rate of complications (17.9%) when compared with correction of congenital scoliosis (10.6%) and adolescent idiopathic scoliosis (AIS) (6.3%). The complication rate with surgical correction of neuromuscular scoliosis is 1.1% compared to 0.8% for AIS. Difficulties with obtaining baseline intraoperative neuromonitoring (IONM) signals with neurologic deficits such as CP is well documented. Mo and colleagues[108] analyzed the IONM data of 206 children with neuroanatomic malformations such as hydrocephalus, encephalomalacia, and periventricular leukomalacia. From their analysis, they found that patients with these neuroanatomic malformations are significantly at risk of having unobtainable IONM signals, in particular TcMEPs. They recommend, if possible, to review all cranial imaging studies prior to scoliosis correction to help with predicting IONM outcomes.[108]

Blood Conservation

Antifibrinolytic agents, hypotensive anesthesia, Cell Saver, subperiosteal dissection, and electrocautery all can reduce blood loss. If an anterior approach is selected, unilateral ligation of the segmental vessels can be performed without significant risk of ischemia of the neural elements. Several studies have concluded that unilateral ligation carries no risk of causing neurologic compromise. Some authors recommend spinal cord monitoring during temporary (10–15 minutes) clamping of the segmental vessels before division.[109-111] Periodic intraoperative coagulation panels should also be used to detect a dilutional coagulopathy, which ideally can be treated with early use of fresh frozen plasma, cryoprecipitate, and platelets before disseminated intravascular coagulopathy (DIC) develops. The hematologic status of CP patients should be monitored very closely because they typically have increased bleeding that starts earlier in a procedure despite a normal coagulation profile.[112]

Bone Graft

In patients with neuromuscular scoliosis, the autologous iliac crest bone graft is often of poor quality and limited quantity. Also, harvesting may interfere with the placement of pelvic instrumentation. Because these patients need a significant volume of graft given the extent of fusion, supplemental graft in the form of freeze-dried or frozen cancellous allogeneic bone is almost always necessary to supplement local bone graft (facets, spinous process). Although allograft is generally regarded as safe and reliable for fusion augmentation in these patients,[78] evaluation by Sponseller and colleagues[113] of 210 patients with neuromuscular scoliosis revealed an increased risk of infection with the use of allograft. Glotzbecker and colleagues[114] performed a systematic literature review to analyze the risk factors and preventive strategies for surgical site infection (SSI) following spine surgery in the pediatric population, finding good evidence from their review to indicate that ceramic bone substitute did not increase the risk of SSI when compared with autograft. However, there is poor-quality evidence to determine whether allograft increases SSI risk following scoliosis surgery in the pediatric age group.[114] In a study by Yazici and Asher,[115] the rate of pseudarthrosis in patients with neuromuscular scoliosis undergoing surgery with allograft was 2.5%.

Timing of Combined Procedures

The evidence for performing staged versus same-day anterior and posterior procedures is unclear. In a study of 45 patients who underwent combined anterior and posterior surgery, Tsirikos and colleagues[116] found that same-day procedures were associated with longer operative time, greater blood loss, and a higher incidence of medical and technical complications. These results were in contrast to a study by Mohamad and colleagues,[117] who found no difference between single-stage and staged surgical procedures in their review of 175 patients with neuromuscular scoliosis. Further studies on staging combined procedures have focused on the use of traction and defining the curve characteristics that would be most appropriate for a staged procedure. For large, rigid curves, the use of staged surgery with anterior release and halopelvic traction as the first stage and posterior instrumentation and fusion as the second stage was investigated by Yamin and colleagues.[118] These authors concluded that patients whose Cobb angle was greater than 80 degrees and flexibility was less than 20% should be treated with this method. Yamin and colleagues[118] also recommended that patients whose spine flexibility was less than 10% with a Cobb angle that remained greater than 70 degrees after the first-stage anterior release and halopelvic traction should undergo pedicle subtraction osteotomies in the second-stage surgery.

It is important to anticipate the need for a staged procedure because unplanned staged procedures have a higher complication rate than planned staged procedures.[117] Given the evidence, the authors recommend planning a staged procedure in larger patients with severe deformity or a history of large-volume blood loss in previous surgeries or both. Despite careful planning, hemodynamic instability may force unplanned staging. Blood loss in the posterior procedure tends to be two to three times the blood loss during the anterior procedure; if the surgeon encounters anterior blood loss greater than half the patient's blood volume, a staged procedure should be considered.

Anterior Surgical Approaches

Transthoracic Approach

The standard approach to the thoracic spine is via an open thoracotomy performed on the convexity of the scoliosis. The rib one to two levels above the most cephalad vertebral body to be approached should be removed. The spine can be exposed over approximately six levels between T4 and L1 with this approach. The superficial dissection is in line with the rib, dividing the serratus anterior and latissimus dorsi muscles. The rib is stripped subperiosteally and removed as far posteriorly as possible. With a rib-spreading retractor in place, the parietal pleura is opened longitudinally along the spine. The segmental vessels may be clamped and ligated or maintained, based on the required exposure.

Thoracoscopic Approach

In the thoracic spine, thoracoscopy is an option instead of open thoracotomy. Video-assisted thoracic surgery allows exposure of the entire thoracic spine through three to five intercostal portals. The thoracoscopic approach is less invasive, sparing the chest wall musculature. Investigation has shown that there is less perioperative pulmonary dysfunction associated with this approach in adolescent patients with idiopathic scoliosis. This assertion is supported by Newton and colleagues,[119] who found that comparable correction rates and pulmonary function are present at 5-year follow-up in adolescent patients with idiopathic scoliosis. Although the benefits in adolescent patients with idiopathic scoliosis have been well described, the potential benefits in respiratory function remain unclear in patients with neuromuscular scoliosis.

In a study of perioperative complications after surgical correction in 175 patients with neuromuscular scoliosis, Mohamad and colleagues[117] discussed no positive or negative correlations associated with video-assisted thoracic surgery and pulmonary function. Given this lack of evidence and the technical demands of this technique, the benefits of this procedure must be weighed in the context of the experience of the surgeon and possible complications. Mastery of this less invasive approach may prove to be a valuable tool in treating these fragile patients, however.

Thoracoabdominal Approach

When exposure of the thoracolumbar junction is required, the thoracoabdominal approach extends a thoracotomy incision distally. This extended incision allows exposure from the lower thoracic spine to the sacrum. The diaphragm is detached from the chest wall, which may have pulmonary consequences in patients with limited pulmonary reserve. The thoracotomy approach is combined with a retroperitoneal exposure of the lumbar spine. The diaphragm is divided near the chest wall circumferentially to its origin on the spine at L1.

Retroperitoneal Lumbar Approach

The retroperitoneal approach to the lumbar spine provides exposure from L1 to the sacrum, but placement of instrumentation above L2 often requires a thoracoabdominal exposure. The incision is in line with the 12th rib, curving to parallel the rectus abdominis inferiorly. The three abdominal muscle layers are divided, taking care to identify the translucent layer of peritoneum. The plane between the transversus abdominis and the peritoneum is developed posteriorly. The psoas muscle is reflected posteriorly, exposing the spine. Inferiorly, the iliac vessels and commonly a large iliolumbar vein require careful dissection. The L5–S1 disc can be exposed either by elevating the iliac vessels or by working between the bifurcation anteriorly.

Vertical Expandable Prosthetic Titanium Rib

The vertical expandable prosthetic titanium rib (VEPTR) has gained attention more recently for its role in the correction of early-onset scoliosis (EOS) and congenital spinal deformities.[120] Hell and colleagues[121] investigated the efficacy of VEPTR in 15 children, 6 of whom were diagnosed with neuromuscular scoliosis. These authors concluded that this technique was safe, effective, and improved sitting ability and cosmesis. These results were supported by a preliminary investigation by Latalski and colleagues, who found that VEPTR considerably improved respiratory capacity in two patients with congenital spinal deformity and one patient with neuromuscular scoliosis.[122]

Neuromuscular patients with pelvic obliquity can be treated with GR constructs anchored to the pelvis to help correct the obliquity. Sponseller and colleagues[96] analyzed the records of 36 patients from the Growing Spine Study Group database with neuromuscular disorders and found that GRs anchored to the pelvis with dual iliac fixation provided the best correction of the patient's pelvic obliquity.

Akabarnia and Emans[123] described that the best indication for VEPTR in EOS is thoracogenic scoliosis or multiple fused ribs in association with congenital scoliosis. This is compared to GRs, which are indicated in the setting of a progressive deformity in a normally segmented deformity such as infantile idiopathic scoliosis not controlled by bracing or casting. They also describe various complications associated with GR and VEPTR devices. Among the possible complications of VEPTR devices is proximal fixation failure. Neuromuscular scoliosis curves exert a high stress on VEPTR devices due to their rigidity. The high-tensile stress forces on the VEPTR devices caused by the coronal and sagittal demands of the curves can lead to proximal fixation failure. Park and colleagues[124] showed that neuromuscular patients with increased major curve angle and normokyphosis or hyperkyphosis had a high correlation with rapid VEPTR anchor failure. Neuromuscular scoliosis curves exhibit high stress on VEPTR devices due to the rigidness of the curves. Furthermore, the increased coronal and sagittal curves result in a high-tensile stress level on VEPTR devices, which leads to complications associated with growing spine surgery. Although initial results show promise, the clinical application of the VEPTR in neuromuscular scoliosis remains a subject that requires further study. The Shilla method[119] and others designed to guide growth posteriorly have also been utilized by some in the very young neuromuscular patients. Hybrid methods of limited fusion and some form of growth guidance/maintenance remain an option in these most challenging cases (Fig. 28.15).

Postoperative Care

Intensive Care Unit

Patients with neuromuscular scoliosis who have undergone extensive spinal surgery are best managed immediately postoperatively in an intensive care unit (ICU) setting. Ventilatory support is often needed for 24 to 48 hours or more. An intensivist accustomed to caring for these children is invaluable in the early postoperative course.

Bracing

Postoperative bracing is usually not required if the bone quality is sufficient to provide secure implant fixation. In difficult cases, a molded orthosis may be needed; it should be molded after the surgery if significant deformity correction is anticipated. After kyphosis correction, an orthosis may be helpful for reducing the stress on the proximal posterior fixation points.

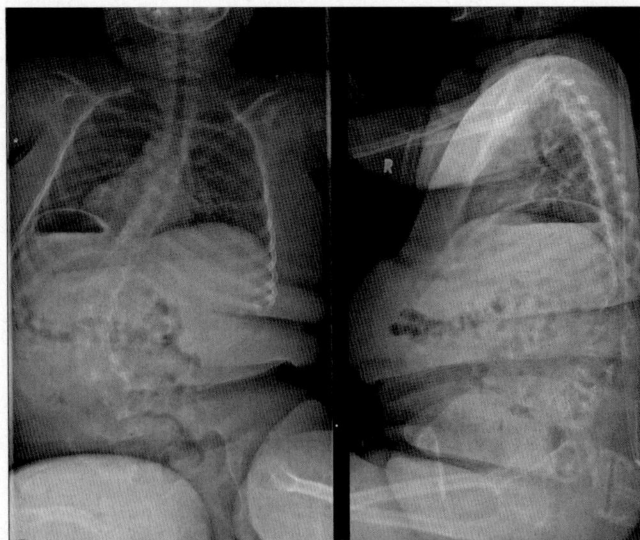

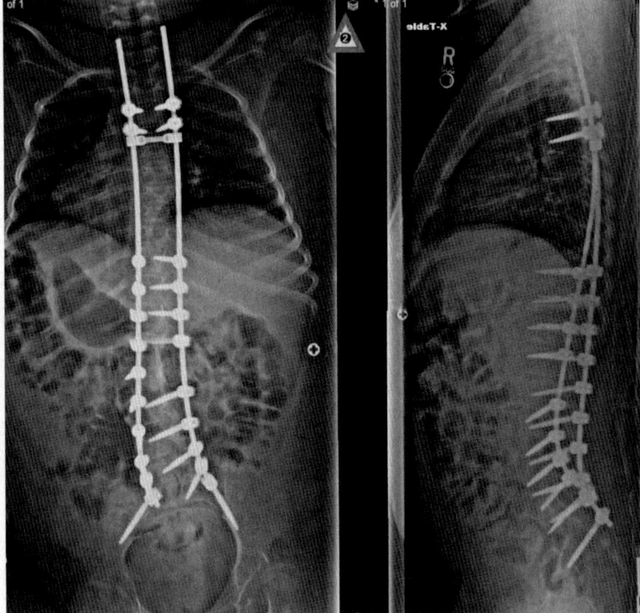

FIG. 28.15 An 8-year-old with spinal muscle atrophy status post T2 to T3 Shilla procedure and T10 to pelvis posterior spinal fusion.

Complications

The surgical treatment of neuromuscular scoliosis has been shown to have a higher complication rate compared with surgical treatment of idiopathic scoliosis. In the largest study to date of perioperative complications associated with neuromuscular scoliosis surgery, Mohamad and colleagues[117] reported their complication rate to be 33% in 175 patients. These results are consistent with previous studies that found the complication rate to range from 24% to 75%.[80,81,126,127] The factors that are associated with perioperative complications include a history of seizures, unplanned staged surgical procedures, and increased blood loss.[128] Pulmonary issues have been found to be the most prevalent complication of spinal surgery in these patients, thus should be closely monitored by the multidisciplinary care team.

Wound Infections

The rate of wound infections in this type of surgery is higher than in surgery for adolescent idiopathic scoliosis, ranging from 8% to 15% in the literature. Superficial wound infections are more common than deep wound infections, and require close monitoring because they can quickly progress in patients with neuromuscular disorders. Wound infection is also more common in nonambulatory patients with severe involvement, and tends to involve multiple gram-negative organisms. A higher rate of wound infection has also been found in patients with sacropelvic fixation with a trend toward a higher rate of deep wound infection.[117]

Croft et al. found in their analysis of 598 patients, 22 of which had SSIs, that patients with neuromuscular scoliosis and a weight-for-age at the 95th percentile or higher were at significantly higher risk for SSI.[129] Their results supported the findings of earlier studies by Allesia et al.[129a] and Mackenzie et al.[129b] The authors also found that use of allograft alone (or in combination with autografts or synthetic grafts) and increased blood loss were significantly correlated with SSI. Prevention of SSIs in this patient population is the goal, with one study showing that the incidence of deep wound infection may be reduced in patients with neuromuscular disease undergoing spine surgery by using an antibiotic-loaded bone graft. In a study of 220 children with CP treated with unit rod instrumentation, Borkhuu and colleagues[130] found that the use of gentamicin-impregnated bone graft decreased the incidence of deep wound infection by 11% compared with patients who received bone graft without antibiotics. However, when Mikhael et al.[131] analyzed the effects of gamma irradiation, they found that irradiated bone allograft did not decrease the rate of culture-positive infection following spinal fusion compared to nonirradiated allograft and autograft at 1 year.

In patients with neuromuscular disease, a high index of suspicion must still be maintained, and any suspected infection must be aspirated from deep and superficial layers. A wound infection requires débridement and closure over drains with broad-spectrum antibiotics. Vacuum-assisted closure for deep infections has shown good results, with an ease of use and a marked reduction in the need for hardware removal.[132] When a wound has been infected, the risk for pseudarthrosis increases.[115,126]

Respiratory Complications

Given the baseline susceptibility of patients with neuromuscular disorders to respiratory complications and the chest wall insult and immobilization associated with scoliosis correction, respiratory complications are common in the postoperative period; the reported incidence ranges from 9% to 22%. These complications include pneumonia, pleural effusion, and atelectasis that may require prolonged intubation.[80,81,127] A preoperative consultation with a pulmonologist to maximize the patient's pulmonary health and aggressive care in the ICU help to reduce the incidence of problems; however, caregivers and patients should be warned that permanent ventilator dependence is a possible sequela of surgery for some patients.

Urinary Tract Infections

The incidence reported in the literature of urinary tract infections (UTIs) in patients with neuromuscular scoliosis is 9% to 22%. Expeditious removal of a urinary catheter inserted for the procedure and adequate hydration may reduce the risk of UTI. Patients with myelomeningocele often have chronic colonization of bacteria in their bladder. Perioperative prophylactic antibiotics should address these organisms.[8,81,126,127]

Cerebral Palsy

An estimated 25,000 children are diagnosed with CP each year. With this huge volume of patients, CP has replaced polio as the prototypic neuromuscular disorder. CP is caused by a static upper motor neuron lesion that interferes with the developing motor system. This lesion is usually caused by an anoxic insult in the perinatal period; however, child abuse in young infants is another common cause of brain injury that can lead to CP.

Scoliosis in Cerebral Palsy

Scoliosis is common in CP, with a 25% incidence of spinal deformity in all CP patients. The incidence and degree of deformity correlate with the amount of neurologic deficit and ambulatory status. In a study of 272 institutionalized patients, the highest prevalence of scoliosis was found in the most severely affected patients with 75% of spastic quadriplegic and 68% of spastic diplegic patients having at least 10 degrees of spinal deformity. In this study, 44% of patients who could ambulate independently, 54% of patients who could ambulate with assistance, 61% of patients who could sit independently, 75% of patients who could sit with assistance, and 76% of bedridden patients had significant deformity. Although these numbers may be inflated by the fact that the study population was composed entirely of institutionalized patients, they still reveal a trend of increased deformity with increased spasticity and decreased independent mobility.[135,136]

The development of scoliosis in CP patients is thought to result partly from persistent primitive reflex patterns and asymmetrical tone in the paraspinous and intercostal muscles. Pelvic obliquity from contractures around the hip plays a role in scoliosis development; however, it is often difficult to isolate this as a contributing factor because pelvic obliquity, hip contractures, and scoliosis often develop simultaneously. Placing patients with a weak trunk and total body involvement into artificial upright sitting positions without appropriate spinal support may encourage gravity-related kyphosis and scoliosis. This suspicion was raised by Madigan and Wallace[136] when they found a 75% incidence of scoliosis in a predominantly institutionalized population comprising "prop sitters" but only a 25% incidence in a population of quadriplegics with spasticity in which prop sitting was not pursued.

Scoliosis in CP has been classified into four categories based on curve pattern (single vs double) and the presence or absence of pelvic obliquity. Long C curves with pelvic obliquity generally occur in more severely involved nonambulatory patients with spasticity. S curves occur more frequently in sitting or walking patients with little spasticity. S curves seem to be more idiopathic in nature, often without associated pelvic obliquity.[33] Patients with severe involvement and a developmental level less than 6 months seldom attain independent sitting balance. Lack of neuromuscular control prevents proper alignment of the head; these patients do not develop compensatory curves to bring the shoulders and head over the pelvis.

Curve progression is related to these risk factors and quadriplegia, poor functional status, and a single thoracolumbar curve.[1,137,138] As in idiopathic scoliosis, risk of progression is also related to curve magnitude and to the amount of remaining spinal growth. Because progression of spinal deformity begins at the onset of the neuromuscular condition, patients with CP have a much longer time to progress and have the potential for developing larger curves than patients with adolescent idiopathic scoliosis. This period of potential curve progression is prolonged further because these patients often maintain open growth plates into their late teens or early 20s. In adults, Thometz and Simon[138] found that larger curves progress faster than smaller curves; they noted curve progression of 0.8 degree per year in curves less than 50 degrees and 1.4 degrees per year in curves greater than 50 degrees. Even patients who have completed growth are at risk for scoliosis progression.

Treatment Options

Bracing

The natural history of scoliosis in children with CP is early onset with a flexible spine deformity between 3 and 10 years of age with a relatively fast progression to a rigid structural curve.[137] Most of the articles in the literature do not support the use of bracing. Bracing can function as a temporizing measure, however, in patients with early-onset, flexible scoliosis or in patients with contraindications for surgery.[19] CP patients with spasticity have poor tolerance for bracing because of the spasticity of their limbs inhibiting brace application, the incidence of skin pressure irritation, and sometimes increasing respiratory problems.[19,21] A soft brace may be used owing to the lack of practicality of dynamic bracing, although it becomes mainly a sitting support rather than a treatment modality. For patients who cannot tolerate bracing, wheelchair seating systems can facilitate upright posture and allow patients to participate in more activities with greater social interaction.

Surgical Management

Various techniques and instrumentation exist for surgical scoliosis correction in CP patients. In patients with hypotonia, a thoracolumbar or lumbar curve that does not extend to the pelvis, and a pelvic obliquity less than 15 degrees, fusion to L5 without sacropelvic fixation may occasionally be appropriate.[71] For most CP patients with spinal deformity, an extensive posterior fusion with instrumentation from the upper thoracic level (T1 or T2) to the pelvis is indicated. The most common instrumentation systems used have been the combination of Luque wires and a unit rod or two Galveston rods. Luque-Galveston constructs may be modified with iliac screw fixation to aid in the ease of insertion and to provide safe, reliable correction.[88,89] Several studies have shown the efficacy of these methods in CP patients. Boachie-Adjei and colleagues[127] retrospectively reviewed 45 patients treated with Luque-Galveston constructs and found 53% correction of scoliosis and 50% correction of pelvic obliquity. The correction was maintained at an average of 3 years of follow-up despite a 6.5% pseudarthrosis rate. Benson and colleagues[126] reported on a cohort of 50 patients also treated with Luque-Galveston instrumentation who showed a 65% scoliosis correction rate with maintenance of correction at 40 months of follow-up. Only one patient in this series had a pseudarthrosis (2%).

Other studies have reported successful correction using the unit rod system in CP patients. Bulman and colleagues[70] compared 15 patients instrumented with Luque-Galveston constructs to 15 patients with unit rod instrumentation and concluded that the unit rod provided significantly improved correction and maintenance of correction of both scoliosis and pelvic obliquity at 2 years after surgery. Although the power of this study is limited by its small size and short follow-up, the findings are echoed in the results of other studies. Westerlund and colleagues[139] reported 66% scoliosis correction and 75% pelvic obliquity correction that was maintained at an average of 5 years' follow-up. Tsirikos and colleagues[116] retrospectively reviewed 287 CP patients treated with unit rod instrumentation and found a 68% correction of scoliosis and 71% correction in pelvic obliquity at 2-year follow-up.

More recently, there has been a trend toward using more hooks and screws in neuromuscular constructs. Segmental screw fixation common in idiopathic scoliosis may result in improved fixation with a reduced complication rate.[140]

Teli et al.[141] analyzed 60 patients with CP with a minimum 2-year follow-up who were treated with segmental third-generation CD instrumentation and showed an average correction of coronal deformity of 60% and pelvic obliquity of 40%. In their study, 26 patients received anteroposterior surgeries and 34 had posterior-only procedures, noting that correction of the scoliosis was similar in both groups. However, correction of pelvic obliquity was improved in patients who underwent an anterior release. Significant complications affected 13.5% of patients and included loosening of implants, deep tissue infection, and pseudarthrosis.[141]

Despite the recent trend away from anterior approaches, in patients with very rigid curves, an anterior release is a powerful technique that can help correction of these challenging curves. Auerbach and colleagues[100] assessed whether posterior-only fusion would be sufficient for correcting large curves in CP patients. They compared 19 patients who underwent anterior release with larger major curves, greater pelvic obliquity, and more rigid curves preoperatively against 42 patients with more flexible curves who had posterioe-only fusion. Correction of pelvic obliquity was similar in both groups.[100]

Surgical correction of scoliosis and pelvic obliquity may also be improved with the use of intraoperative traction. In a comparison study of patients with and without asymmetrical intraoperative halopelvic traction, Vialle and colleagues[142] concluded that intraoperative traction resulted in reduced anesthetic duration and improved correction of scoliosis and pelvic obliquity. These results are supported by Takeshita and colleagues,[95] who found that halofemoral traction improved scoliosis and pelvic obliquity surgical correction in nonambulatory patients with neuromuscular disorders.

Keeler and colleagues[99] found that PSF-only surgery provides excellent curve correction and spinal balance with no statistical differences in terms of the final thoracolumbar/lumbar curve Cobb angle, percentage of correction of the thoracolumbar/lumbar Cobb angle, pelvic obliquity, C7 plumb line, and the center sacral vertical line at 2-year follow-up compared to A/PSF in patients with spastic neuromuscular scoliosis. The patients who underwent PSF only had significantly reduced operating room time, lower EBL, and lower frequency of postoperative pulmonary complications.

Sagittal plane deformities are also common problems in CP patients with scoliosis and require a different approach than that required for coronal plane deformities. Lumbar hyperlordosis and thoracic hyperkyphosis can impair sitting balance and comfort. Hyperkyphosis can be exacerbated by pelvic obliquity and gravity in a patient who sits propped up unsupported and is associated with an increased incidence of instrumentation pullout and failure.[32] Sagittal plane kyphotic deformities require treatment similar to treatment of the deformity in Scheuermann disease with or without an anterior release and a hybrid system of hooks and pedicle screws to apply segmental compression across the kyphotic segments.

Authors' Recommendations

For gravity-dependent mild scoliosis or hypotonic kyphosis in children younger than 10 years, the authors recommend a Plastizote body jacket. This body jacket supports the spine, assists head control, and is well tolerated by the patient. The orthosis usually lasts more than 2 years before it is outgrown. For more rigid curves, between 30 degrees and 50 degrees, or in less rapidly growing patients older than 12 years, a rigid total-contact orthosis may be tried. Although less well tolerated, a total-contact orthosis provides better correction and may delay the need for surgery by providing greater sitting support.

As discussed earlier, defining the precise indications for surgical intervention in patients with scoliosis and CP is difficult. The authors recommend that surgery be considered when scoliosis greater than 50 to 70 degrees exists, taking into consideration the patient's functional, mental, and general health status. The decision to proceed with surgery of this magnitude requires a thoughtful analysis and discussion with the family and caregivers. If Luque instrumentation is used posteriorly, when possible, 5.5- to 6.35-mm rods and a combination of infralaminar hooks, pedicle screws, and double 16- to 18-gauge wires should be used to maximize correction and rigidity. Smaller diameter rods (4.5–4.75 mm) should be used only in very small patients for fear of rod breakage. Anterior fusion should be considered in patients with rigid curves greater than 60 to 80 degrees, in skeletally immature patients, or in patients with fixed pelvic obliquity. In severe curves with marked pelvic obliquity, the correction of the pelvic obliquity and the certainty of permanent correction are often enhanced by the addition of anterior lumbar instrumentation.

The use of pedicle screws and aggressive posterior osteotomies has reduced the use of anterior surgery for some patients. For the most flexible cases, an all-posterior hybrid construct is appropriated; we prefer pelvic fixation with iliac bolts over Galveston rods. If the curve is more rigid, Ponte-type osteotomies are added, and the density of pedicle screws is increased. Patients with curves that do not correct to less than 70 degrees on side bending are considered for an anterior procedure, most often at the thoracolumbar junction. If, after complete disc excision (including the posterior longitudinal ligament), the spine is now flexible enough for near-complete correction, the correction is achieved with an anterior rod system. If the spine remains rigid after discectomy, performing an apical vertebral excision is considered. In either case, an anterior rod is avoided when residual rigidity remains, and the correction is achieved with posterior instrumentation.

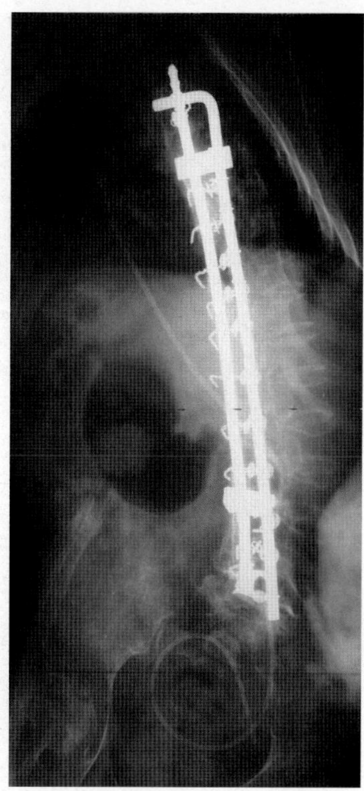

FIG. 28.16 This patient with cerebral palsy presented at age 17 years with Harrington-Luque instrumentation from T4 to L4 done 5 years previously. At presentation, the patient had 85-degree, C-shaped scoliosis with marked pelvic obliquity, rotational deformity, and resultant sitting difficulties. In most nonambulatory patients who have adequate spinal length, fusion to pelvis is recommended to avoid this dilemma.

All CP patients with limited ambulatory capacity should be fused inferiorly to include the pelvis, even if their pelvic obliquity is correctable, because of the potential for increased obliquity owing to persistent muscle imbalances (Fig. 28.16). Most patients do not require postoperative immobilization. In patients with poor bone stock or a motion disorder undergoing fusion to the pelvis, a brace is considered for 3 to 6 months after surgery.

Myelodysplasia

Myelodysplasia is characterized by a persistent open neural arch owing to failed proliferation of neuroectodermal cells in early embryonic development and has been associated with maternal hyperthermia and folate deficiency. The spinal deformity comes from a congenital malformation of levels at the defect, often resulting in a regional hyperkyphosis, and from the muscle imbalance around the spine distal to the lesion (Fig. 28.17).

Scoliosis in Myelodysplasia

The incidence of scoliosis in patients with myelodysplasia (spina bifida) varies in the literature from 52% to 90%.[143,144] In

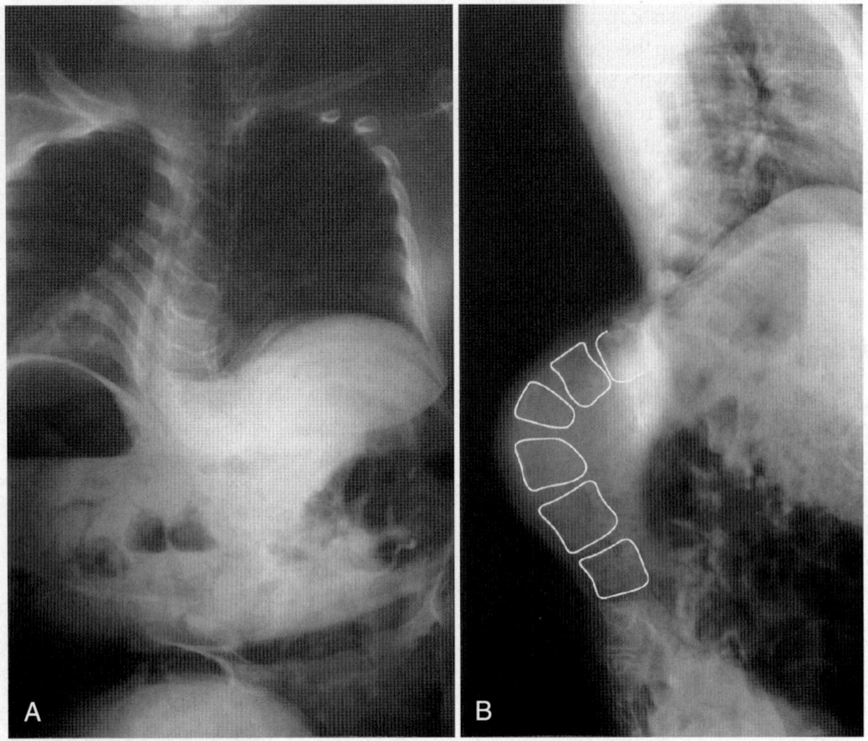

FIG. 28.17 Severe progressive kyphosis in a patient with thoracic-level myelomeningocele caused skin breakdown problems and difficulty with self-catheterization before she underwent kyphectomy and instrumentation (see Fig. 28.11).

a more recent study of 141 patients by Trivedi and colleagues,[144] the authors defined scoliosis in myelodysplasia as curvature greater than 20 degrees and concluded that new curvature could develop as late as 15 years of age. In this cohort of patients, 89% of patients with the last intact laminar arch located in the thoracic region had scoliosis, whereas 44% and 12% had scoliosis if their last intact laminar arch was in the upper and lower lumbar regions. From this trend, Trivedi and colleagues[144] concluded that the last intact laminar arch was the most useful early predictor of scoliosis risk, although ambulatory status and clinical motor levels were also useful predictors.

Myelodysplastic spine is one of the most difficult treatment dilemmas in scoliosis management. These patients present with congenital malformations (Fig. 28.18), often in the form of severe kyphosis preventing comfortable sitting and causing skin breakdown that may necessitate separate and early intervention. The risk of deformity from weak, spastic paraspinal musculature and asymmetrical hip contractures remains, often requiring more definitive surgical correction in the preteen or teen years. Surgical correction for myelodysplasia presents unique problems because of the absent posterior elements, increasing the dependence on anterior fusion and fixation. In addition, the posterior approach for surgical correction traverses the poor-quality skin and scar tissue that results from the defect and the early neurosurgical repair (Fig. 28.19).

There may be an association between myelodysplasia patients with a tethered spinal cord and rapidly progressive scoliosis.[145] Most of these patients have some variation of cord tethering as a residuum of the defect and its neurosurgical closure. The neural tube closure defect needs to be neurosurgically repaired between 24 and 72 hours after birth to avoid risk of infection.[146] The surgical repair, however, frequently later leads to tethering of the spinal cord at the repair site in as many as 70% of patients with myelomeningocele.[147] In patients with unexpected rapid curve progression or increased trunk spasticity (hypertonicity), a tethered cord with or without syringomyelia should be considered. Studies such as MRI or myelography may help define the anatomy; however, the literature does not support a causal relationship between scoliosis and Chiari malformation or syringomyelia.[145] Thoughtful teamwork with a neuroradiologist, neurologist, and neurosurgeon helps clarify these issues.

Jankowski and colleagues[148] in a single institution analysis over a 10-year period identified 15 pediatric patients with intraspinal pathology who had scoliosis and received neurosurgical intervention. Diseases of the neural axis in the studied population consisted of Chiari I malformation (CM I), Chiari II malformation (CM II), tethered cord syndrome (TCS), and syringomyelia. The authors found that for patients with preoperative Cobb angles less than 30 degrees and without CM II, neurosurgical intervention may prevent scoliosis curve progression irrespective of the intraspinal pathology. Patients with CM II are at a higher risk of curve progression and undergoing fusion compared to patients with CM I, TCS, or syringomyelia. The authors recommended, in patients with a preoperative Cobb angle less than 30 degrees and without CM II, neurosurgical intervention followed by a period of monitoring of the scoliosis for progression. For patients with CM II, the authors recommended close radiographic monitoring

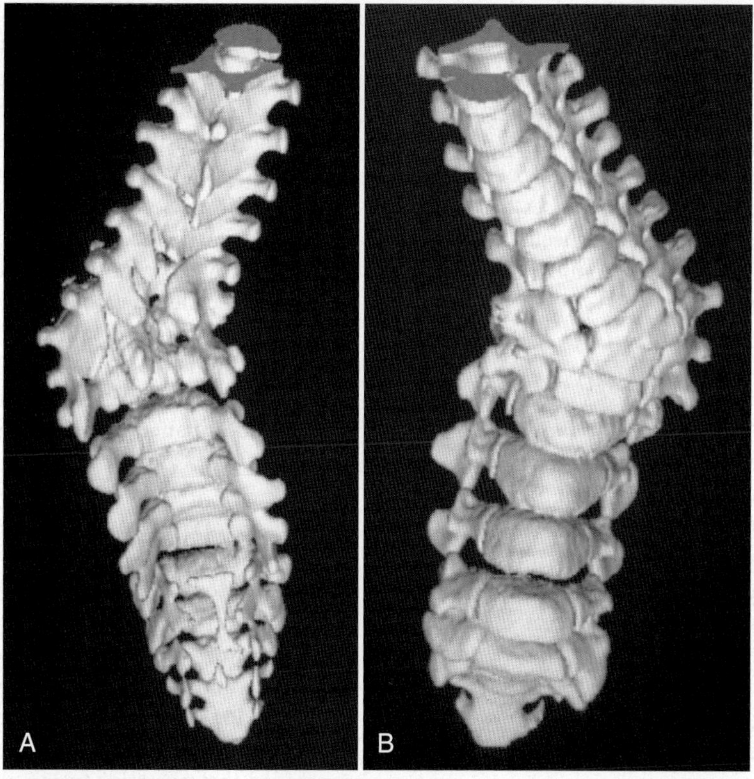

FIG. 28.18 Three-dimensional computed tomographic scan shows absence of posterior elements and congenital vertebral anomalies that make myelomeningocele spinal deformities challenging treatment dilemmas.

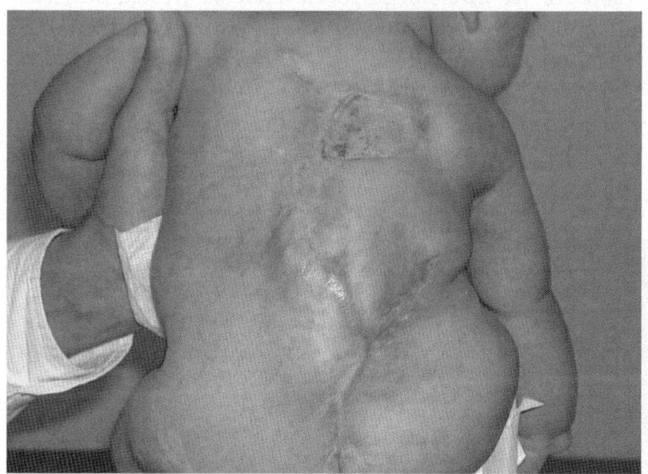

FIG. 28.19 An infant with severe scarring from original neurosurgical closure of spinal defect.

for curve progression with awareness of the high rate of scoliosis progression and eventual need for spinal fusion.

Surgical release of a tethered cord may help in scoliosis stabilization, maintenance of motor function, and decreased back pain.[149] Pierz and colleagues[150] evaluated 21 cases of detethering, however, and concluded that improvement or stabilization of scoliosis after detethering is less likely in patients with curves greater than 40 degrees or thoracic level defects, or both.

Chern and colleagues[151] analyzed 45 consecutive patients with tight film terminale who underwent tethered cord release. Of the 14 patients who presented with scoliosis prior to surgery, 7 had worsening of their curve deformity, in 5 the curve stabilized, and 2 had improvement after tethered cord surgery. The authors were able to conclude that patients who presented with a Cobb angle greater than 35 degrees were most likely to observe progression of their coronal deformity following tethered cord release.[148,151]

There has been an attempt to establish which curve characteristics might serve as predictive factors to aid in determining whether a curve's coronal deformity will progress or stabilize, albeit with inconclusive results.

Given the high incidence of scoliosis and the tendency for rapid progression in these patients, annual follow-up evaluations with posteroanterior and lateral radiographs should closely track coronal and sagittal spinal deformity, hip contractures, and trunk spasticity.

Treatment Options

Bracing

Bracing in myelodysplasia is even more difficult and less successful than in other neuromuscular disorders. Studies show that braces offered as a temporizing measure rarely yield effective curve control. Although Muller and Nordwall,[152] after evaluating 21 myelodysplasia patients treated with bracing, concluded that deformity progression can be halted in patients with curves less than 45 degrees, a more recent study by Olafsson and colleagues[22] reviewed outcomes in 20 patients and reported a successful outcome in only 20%

of patients. Bracing is difficult in these patients because of pressure sores, especially prevalent over kyphotic deformities at the level of the neurologic defect. Obesity, poor-quality and insensate skin, decreased vital capacity, and obstructing stomal bags also contribute to the difficulty of brace wear in these patients. In the study by Olafsson and colleagues,[22] half of the patients stopped wearing their braces because of discomfort. Custom-molded or modular wheelchair inserts offer another temporizing measure for comfortable upright posture until surgery is conducted.

Surgical Management

Definitive surgical management need only be delayed until patients reach 10 to 12 years of age because growth hormone deficiency limits their growth, and truncal height has reached its maximum around this time. Indications for operative management are similar to the indications for other neuromuscular disorders, although a curve that is rapidly progressive in a patient with myelodysplasia may be treated earlier at 40 to 50 degrees. Because a significant hip flexion–abduction contracture can produce lumbar lordosis and scoliosis, the hip contracture should be surgically released before any attempt at surgical correction of the spine.

Anterior Fusion

As previously discussed, anterior fusion is very important in myelodysplasia because the anterior spine provides a large surface for bony fusion in the lumbar spine, in contrast to the deficient posterior elements at these levels. A thoracoabdominal retroperitoneal approach from the convex side of the curve and division of the diaphragm allows anterior disc excision and bone grafting; this may be combined with posterior instrumentation to provide curve correction in select patients (Fig. 28.20). Use of anterior instrumentation alone has a specific role in the treatment of myelodysplasia scoliosis. In a study of 14 myelodysplasia patients treated with a Texas Scottish Rite Hospital anterior construct alone, Sponseller and colleagues[153] concluded that anterior instrumentation was successful in a select group of patients with thoracolumbar curves less than 75 degrees, compensatory curves less than 40 degrees, no hyperkyphosis, and no syrinx in the spinal cord. Basobas and colleagues[154] found excellent surgical correction and maintenance with an anterior instrumentation and fusion procedure in their study of 11 myelodysplasia patients at 5-year follow-up. In patients with a lumbar curve and fixed pelvic obliquity, anterior instrumentation provides a powerful means of correcting the deformity (Fig. 28.21).

Posterior Fusion

Although essential to a solid fusion in most myelodysplasia patients, the posterior procedure is difficult because of the poor quality of overlying tissue, decreased paraspinal muscle vascularity, and missing posterior elements. Posterior fusion in combination with anterior fusion is recommended by several authors. In a study of 50 patients, Banit and colleagues[155] concluded that posterior fusion alone yielded a much higher pseudarthrosis rate of 16% than rates reported for anterior and posterior fusion combined. Parsch and colleagues[156] reviewed results of 54 myelomeningocele patients treated surgically and also concluded that anterior and posterior instrumented fusion resulted in the best correction and lowest complication rate.

Luque or unit rods with sublaminar wiring can be used in segments of the spine in which the posterior elements are intact, although supplementation with screws and hooks

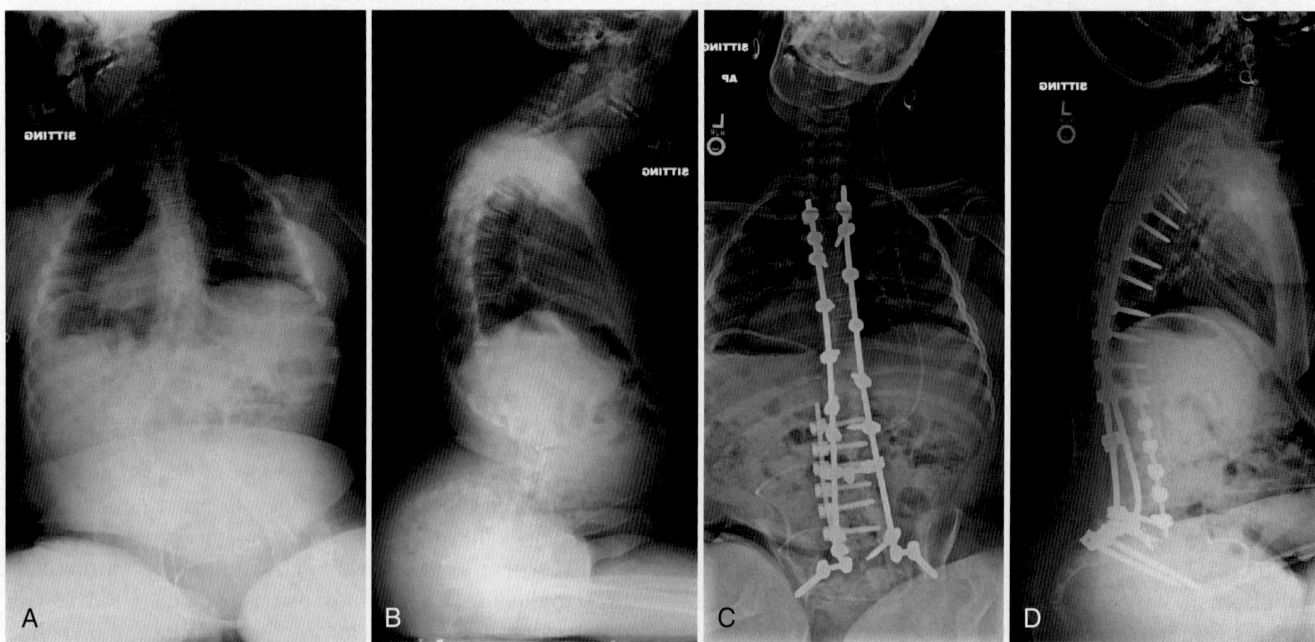

FIG. 28.20 (A–B) This young patient with myelodysplasia presented with 80 degrees of scoliosis and severe lordosis. (C–D) Severe lordosis was treated with anterior instrumentation from T12 to L5, followed by posterior instrumentation from T3 to the pelvis.

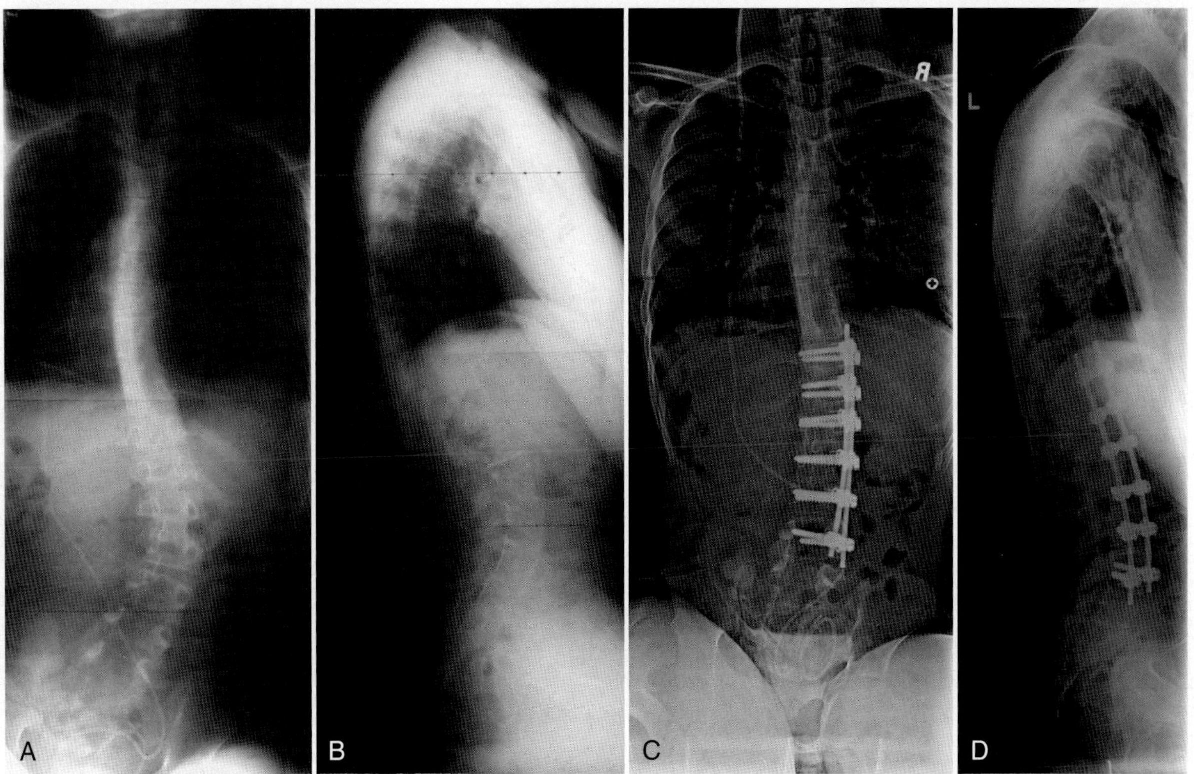

FIG. 28.21 Idiopathic-like lumbar or thoracolumbar curves in patients with myelomeningocele may be successfully treated with anterior instrumentation only.

increases construct stability. In regions in which the posterior elements are missing, pedicle screws are stronger, although the atypical anatomy makes accurate screw placement difficult. In addition, pedicle screws may be prominent, particularly in a kyphotic region because the lateral bony columns are often subcutaneous.

Fusion to the Pelvis

There is considerable controversy over whether the pelvis should be included in the fusion mass. Lindseth and colleagues[157] contended that this is necessary only if there is a component of kyphosis in the lumbar spine or if pelvic obliquity is greater than 15 degrees. They noted an increased incidence of ischial ulcers in patients left with residual pelvic obliquity and fusion to the pelvis probably because the rigid, long, curved segment prevents easy shifting of weight between ischial tuberosities. A prospective evaluation of 11 myelomeningocele patients treated with anterior and posterior instrumented fusion to the lumbar spine revealed good correction of coronal and sagittal plane deformities with fair maintenance of correction. From this experience, the authors of the study concluded that, with the advent of more stable segmental instrumentation, the pelvis could be spared to allow more lumbosacral mobility and to avoid the morbidities associated with pelvic fusion.[158] Similar results have been found in a select group of myelodysplasia patients with anterior-only instrumentation and fusion where pelvic obliquity can be corrected without pelvic fixation.[154]

The most predictable approach from the standpoint of the spinal deformity is fusion to the pelvis. In patients with limited activity, the authors recommend fusion to the pelvis to ensure a straight spine over a level pelvis. In ambulatory or very active patients who play recreational activities, such as wheelchair basketball, the pelvis may be spared with the knowledge that a later revision may be required.

Various options are available for instrumentation to the pelvis. The Galveston modification of Luque rods is a commonly used system, although it may not provide as much stability as the Warner-Fackler modification in correcting kyphosis. As previously described, the Warner-Fackler method involves two 90-degree bends in the distal end of a Luque rod, allowing the rod to pass through the S1 foramina and lever against the anterior aspect of the sacrum (see Fig. 28.11).[84] In a small series of nine patients treated with kyphectomy and this method of pelvic fixation, Thomsen and colleagues[159] reported excellent correction and maintenance of kyphosis correction at an average of 28 months of follow-up. The authors described two instances of complications (loss of rod connection and migration), both at about 32 months after surgery, and concluded that this technique, although effective, should be limited to patients weighing less than 30 kg. McCall described a similar technique with Luque rods passed through the S1 foramina and bent once to 20 to 40 degrees depending on sacral inclination. In his series of 16 patients, McCall[85] reported good correction of kyphosis and excellent maintenance after 57 months of follow-up. Iliac screw fixation has also been shown to afford equivalent maintenance of pelvic obliquity and scoliosis correction compared with the Galveston technique.[83,84]

True fusion to the pelvis (to the wing of the ilium rather than just to the sacrum) can be achieved by suturing the

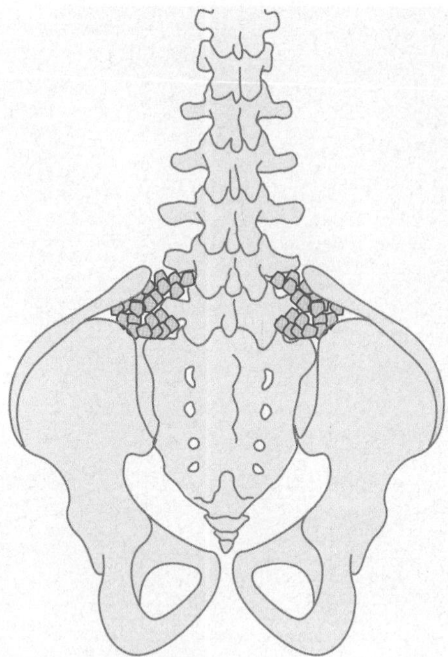

FIG. 28.22 This bone grafting technique increases the chance of stable fusion by including the wing of the ilium and the sacrum.

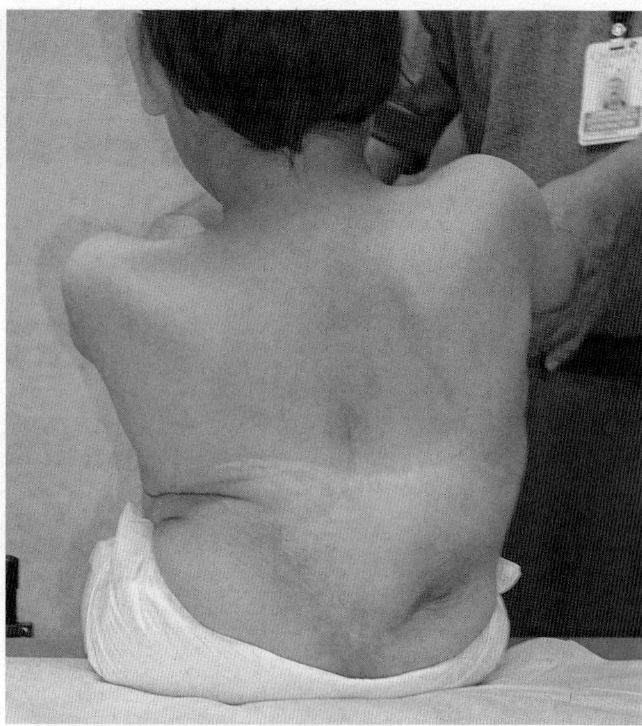

FIG. 28.23 Lumbar gibbus on a patient with thoracic-level myelomeningocele caused sitting difficulties and loss of trunk height before he underwent kyphectomy and spinal fusion.

detached iliac crest apophysis to the transverse process of the spine at L3 or L4 and filling the created triangle with bone graft (Fig. 28.22). Pseudarthrosis is common in fusions to the pelvis, and the authors still advise a conservative immobilization protocol.

Major and minor complications are more common in myelomeningocele patients than in other patients with neuromuscular scoliosis. Reports of the incidence of wound infections range from 19% to 43%.[160] Many patients have minor complications, such as urinary tract infections or minor wound dehiscence. Major complications, including massive blood loss and instrumentation failure, are more common in myelomeningocele scoliosis than in idiopathic scoliosis or other neuromuscular conditions.[155,160] Pseudarthrosis rates range from 16% to 50% in the literature.[155,161] In addition, the proximity of procedures to the dural sac and the abnormal anatomy increase the risk of shunt compromise and failure. By attending to detail and applying all that is currently known about myelomeningocele scoliosis surgery (careful anterior and posterior fusion, segmental attachment, cautious remobilization), the major complication rate can be reduced to 15% or less.

Kyphosis Treatment

As already noted, bracing is extremely difficult in the severe kyphosis associated with myelomeningocele. Kyphosis is relentlessly progressive (3–8 degrees per year) and can become pathologic in 20% of patients. Because surgical correction is complex and difficult, many children are left untreated and seem to function reasonably well, although skin breakdown over the kyphosis, pressure on abdominal contents, and loss of trunk height remain problems. Indications for surgery include progressive kyphosis, skin breakdown over the kyphosis, respiratory compromise, and concern regarding the effect of severe trunk shortening (Fig. 28.23).[85,162]

Kyphosis in myelomeningocele can be corrected, but intraoperative or perioperative death is frequent enough to give pause to all who treat this disorder. Death can occur from uncontrolled bleeding or problems with cerebrospinal fluid (CSF) dynamics. The advent of segmental spinal instrumentation has made kyphectomy with fusion at least moderately predictable. The segmental attachment must extend well into the thoracic spine to control the large sagittal plane bending moments.

Basic principles include a long midline posterior approach with exposure of five or six levels of normal closed laminae proximally and distal exposure down to the midsacral level. The sac and cord are retracted or resected, with care being taken to repair the dura slightly distal to and separate from the cord transection to avoid tying off the central canal and disturbing CSF dynamics.[163] In most cases, retracting the scarred thecal sac allows sufficient exposure.[162] The spine is prepared for segmental attachment by passing laminar wires or hooks through all normal laminae proximally. The distal segments can be attached by pedicle screw fixation or by screws placed directly into the vertebral bodies. Because the bleeding encountered with osteotomy may force a rapid finish, complete preparation is essential for a successful instrumentation.

The vertebral bodies making up the cranial two-thirds of the kyphosis are excised, allowing one to "fold in" the remaining proximal and distal spinal segments (Fig. 28.24). Care must be taken when the vertebrectomy is performed because the kidneys may be present in the concavity of the deformity and may sustain inadvertent injury. Often, ribs 10 to 12 must

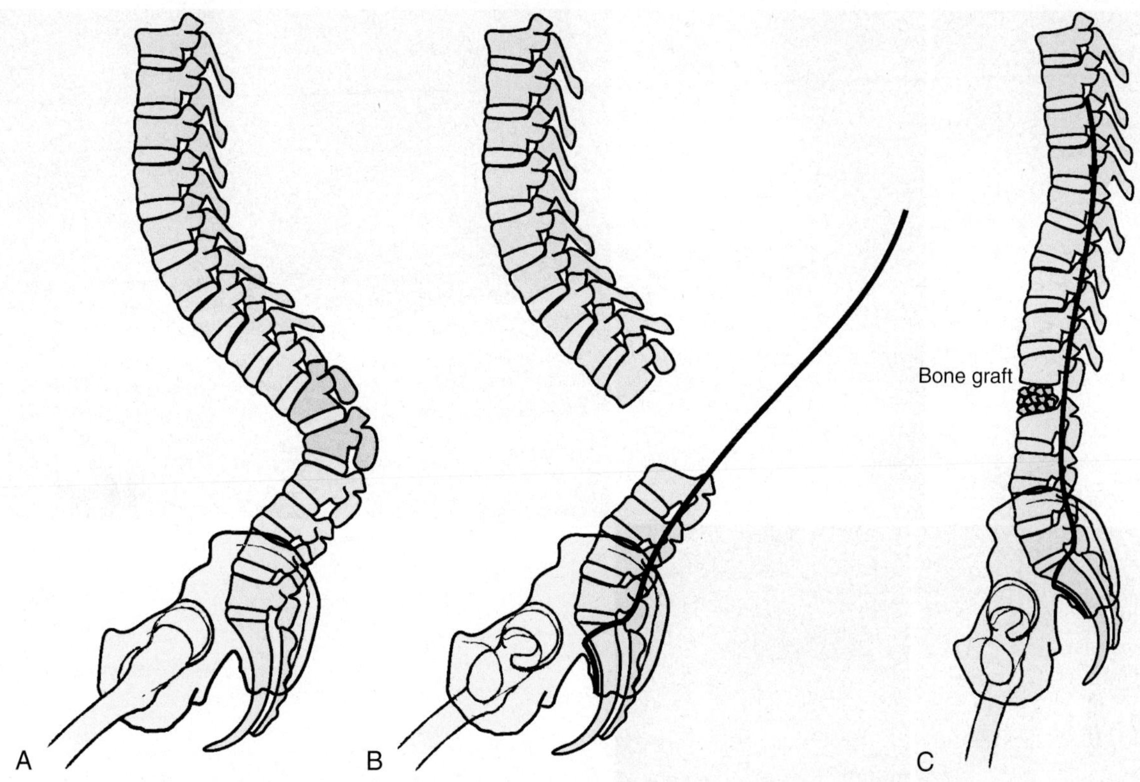

FIG. 28.24 Sagittal diagram describing sequence for performing kyphectomy. (A) The spine is exposed, the dural sac is tied off or retracted, and the kyphotic segment of the spine is excised. (B) To improve mobility of remaining segments, discs can be excised, and the lower two to three pairs of ribs can be sectioned from their origins. (C) Two segments of the spine are "folded inward," bone grafted (from the excised segments), and wired to previously contoured rods.

be transected bilaterally to free the proximal segment enough so that the spine folds inward. The rods are positioned posterior to the infolded segments and secured in place. Posterolaterally placed polyaxial screws may be used to augment wiring and provide greater construct rigidity (Fig. 28.25). In a study of seven myelomeningocele patients, Kocaoglu and colleagues[164] found that the addition of polyaxial screws provided greater correction capacity and a low instrumentation profile in patients with a kyphectomy and Luque instrumentation. The excised vertebrae provide adequate bone graft, applied anteriorly and posteriorly.

Spinal Muscular Atrophy

Affecting 1 in 11,000 newborns, SMA is a fairly common autosomal recessive disorder that is characterized by varying degrees of degeneration of the anterior horn cells, resulting in a symmetrical muscle paralysis of the trunk and proximal musculature. The etiology of SMA has been linked to an autosomal-recessive disorder resulting from a homozygous deletion or mutation of the *SMN1* gene on the 5q13 chromosome. All patients with SMA lack a functioning *SMN1* gene, making them dependent on their *SMN2* gene in order to produce the SMN protein. The severity of the disease is inversely correlated to the *SMN2* gene copy number.[6] Absence or deficiency of this inhibitory protein allows increased motor neuron death that leads to progressive muscle paralysis, eventually causing respiratory insufficiency and scoliosis (Fig. 28.26).[148] Although there are more severe forms, 80% of patients live to adulthood and achieve sitting balance.[165]

Spinal Muscular Atrophy Types

SMA is broken down into three types. First described in the 1890s, type I is also known as Werdnig-Hoffman disease or acute infantile SMA. In this form, children are born with a normal appearance but by 6 months begin to show signs of muscle weakness with poor head control, absent reflexes, and respiratory insufficiency, which is the cause of death by 2 to 3 years of age.[166] Children with type II SMA—the chronic infantile or Dubowitz form—experience the onset of muscle weakness between 6 and 19 months of age but do not have the same severity of symptoms. They attain sitting balance but rarely are able to walk independently. Although respiratory impairment is not as severe as in type I, respiratory complications are common. Type III SMA is also called the chronic juvenile form of the disease or Kugelberg-Welander syndrome and is characterized by onset after 2 years with milder impairment. Most children develop the ability to walk at some time, although many lose this ability around puberty.[167]

Scoliosis in Spinal Muscular Atrophy

The natural history of scoliosis in SMA depends on whether the patient has type I, II, or III. However, these types represent

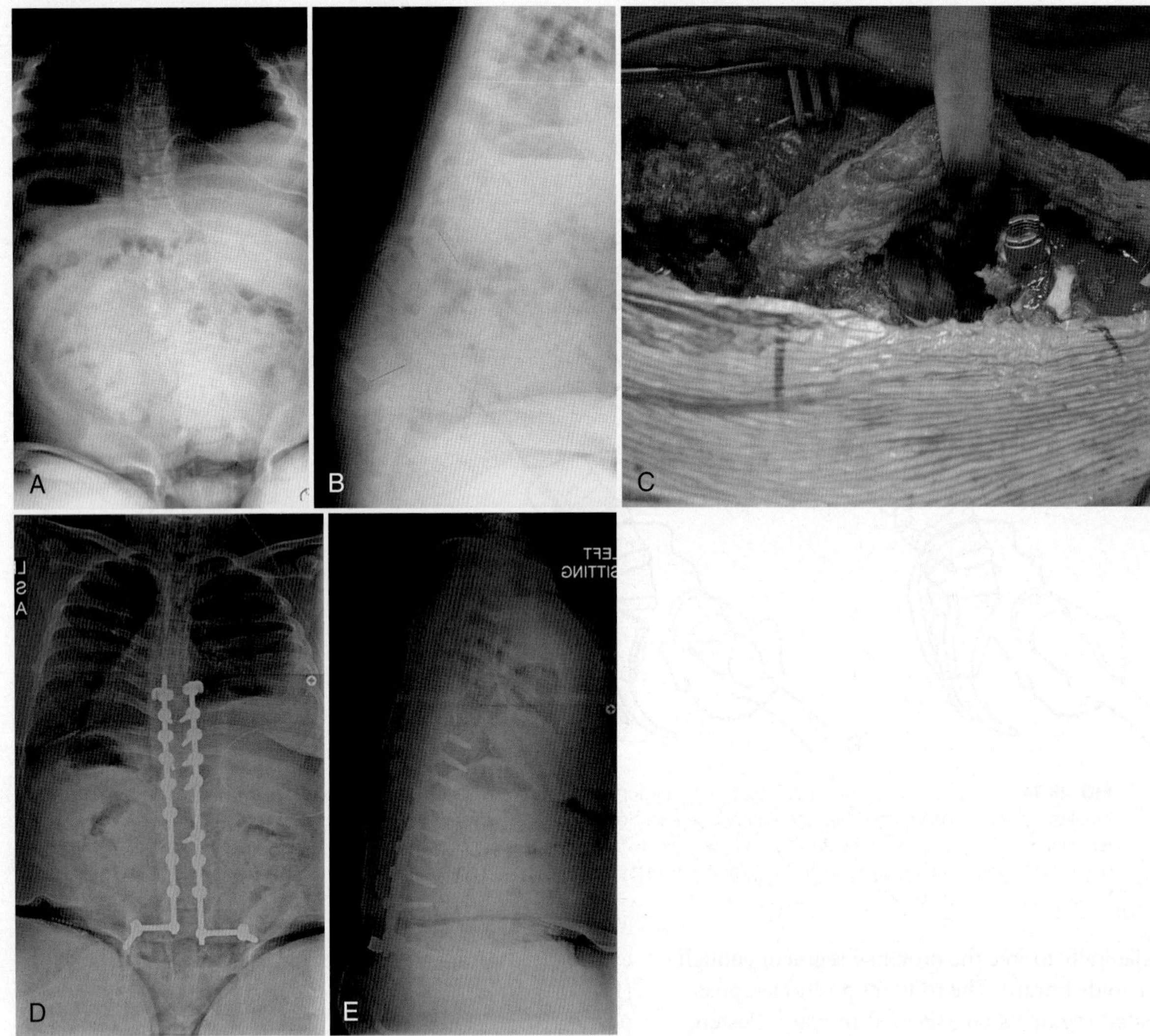

FIG. 28.25 (A–B) A young patient with spina bifida was missing posterior elements from T11 to the sacrum with 103-degree focal lumbar kyphosis with no associated scoliosis. (C) Kyphectomy was performed with excision of L2 and L3 vertebrae. (D–E) Posterior instrumentation and fusion were used from T7 to the pelvis.

a spectrum of disease, and the distinctions between types may not be absolute. One should be guarded in making unqualified predictions of prognosis based on type.

All patients with type I SMA develop curves greater than 15 degrees. Surgical intervention is not warranted in these patients because of their short life span; a body jacket provides good support for balanced and comfortable sitting. Patients with type II also develop curves greater than 15 degrees, although the onset of spinal deformity occurs later, between 2 and 4 years of age. Most of these patients do not ambulate and are likely to experience rapidly progressive scoliosis. The prevalence of spinal deformity in type III patients is varied, but it typically develops in about half of patients.[168] Some of these patients are independent walkers and more likely to escape spinal deformity.[166,169,170]

Scoliosis in SMA tends to progress. In 52 cases of SMA, Granata and colleagues[171] found an increase in curve magnitude of 8 degrees per year, despite brace use. They likewise showed a significant increase in curve progression when a patient with mild involvement stopped walking. In 13 nonwalking SMA patients, these investigators found a 3-degree per year curve progression. Walking patients with mild involvement showed only a 0.6-degree per year progression. The curve most often seen with SMA is a C-shaped thoracolumbar curve. Kyphosis can also be seen with these spinal deformities, but is typically not severe.

Treatment Options

Bracing

As with other neuromuscular diseases, bracing is mainly a temporizing measure to aid in sitting while patients attain more trunk height and vertebral size before surgical intervention. The effectiveness of bracing depends on the type of SMA, the severity of the deformity, and the remaining growth of the patient. Early studies reported delay of progression in a limited subset of patients with milder forms of SMA.[166,170] No studies have documented correction of deformity with dynamic bracing, however, because many patients do not

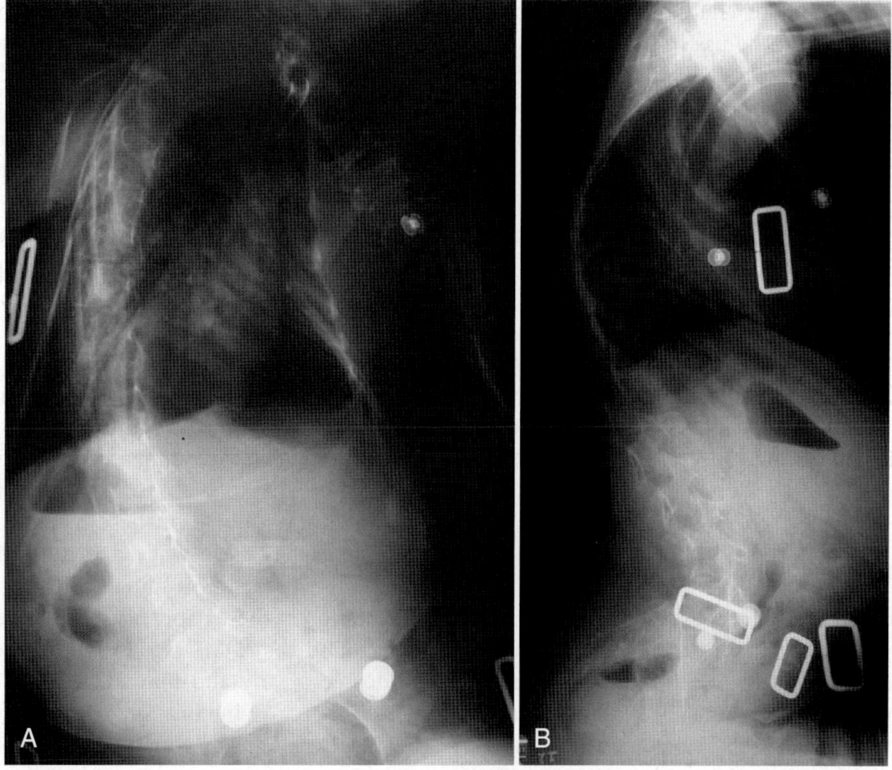

FIG. 28.26 This patient's bell-shaped thoracic cage, characteristic of spinal muscular atrophy, has been compromised further by severe scoliosis.

have the muscular control to pull away from the sides of the brace. The evidence for brace application is still inconclusive because no current studies stratify their results based on age and SMA type. When bracing is elected to provide support for comfortable, balanced sitting before or in lieu of surgery, pulmonary function must also be considered. SMA patients are abdominal breathers because the disease affects intercostal muscle and diaphragmatic function. Because bracing significantly restricts abdominal movement and tidal volume, pretreatment pulmonary function should be a consideration in choosing this treatment modality.[167]

Surgical Management

Several studies have supported the use of segmental instrumentation to the pelvis for the definitive management of scoliosis in SMA. Brown and colleagues[172] evaluated 40 patients with SMA who were treated with posterior fusions and concluded that there were fewer complications and better maintenance of correction with Luque instrumentation compared with Harrington instrumentation. A study by Bentley and colleagues[173] reported a 51% surgical correction rate of coronal deformity in 33 SMA patients with good maintenance of correction. Fusion should be performed before the patient's curve becomes too stiff; periodic bending films and examinations are important for the timing of fusion.

Spinal fusion almost always results in a loss of function. Evaluating 40 patients with preoperative and postoperative functional and strength testing, Furumasu and colleagues[174] found that the straight but rigid spine was not always an immediate advantage to patients. The increased length of the spine creates a longer lever arm against which weakened proximal muscles have to work. These investigators reported an increased use of assistive devices, such as mobile arm supports, reachers, and lapboards. In this study, stronger patients were still able to maintain function, but weaker patients lacked the strength and flexibility to move their trunk in daily activities. Other studies have also noted a postoperative loss of function[70,164,175,176]; Aprin and colleagues[176] noted increased preservation of preoperative function in 22 patients who underwent preoperative and postoperative physical therapy. Spinal fusion does not stabilize pulmonary function. In a study of eight patients—4 with SMA type II and 4 with SMA type III—Chng and colleagues[177] reported a continued decline in pulmonary function at 44 months after spinal fusion and instrumentation. These authors noted that this decline was less marked than the natural history of SMA and that it was most likely secondary to the progressive neuromuscular weakness of the disease.

Ultimately, spinal fusion limits the progressive decline in spinal deformity and pulmonary function that characterizes SMA. A straight spine over a level pelvis allows comfortable sitting and the use of upper extremities in daily functions, and is undoubtedly a great benefit to these patients. The timing of fusion should be an individual decision that takes into account the patient's comfort, functional status, and overall health. As with DMD, fusion needs to be performed before pulmonary function has declined to a level at which pulmonary complications are prohibitive. In the past decade, the treatment of collapsing scoliosis experienced in children with severe and intermediate forms of childhood SMA (types I and II) has been aided through the use of GRs. Early fusion in these patients has been demonstrated to limit trunk height and inhibit lung growth, exacerbating the pulmonary difficulties associated with SMA. GRs provide for continued trunk growth and lung growth, while at the same time controlling the spinal deformity. McElroy et al,[178] from analysis of a multicenter database, reported 15 nonambulatory patients with SMA treated with GRs and was able to show improvement in the deformity of the major curve, spinal growth (T1 to S1), and lung volumes with reasonable operative morbidity. However, GRs could not halt rib collapse in these patients. Further studies will be needed with greater patient cohorts to fully determine how effective and helpful GRs can be in treating patients with this debilitating subtype of neuromuscular scoliosis.

Our Recommendations

We use bracing in early flexible curves as soon as progression is documented. The goal in bracing is to temporize, allowing the child to achieve as much sitting height as possible. Spinal fusion may be delayed until approximately 10 to 12 years of age, unless the curve is uncontrollable by bracing and is greater than 40 degrees. Surgical intervention with posterior spinal instrumentation and fusion to the pelvis is the method of choice. In very young Risser 0 patients, anterior fusion without division of the diaphragm rarely may be considered to prevent the crankshaft phenomenon, but must be weighed against the pulmonary risk. Most patients are treated by posterior-only methods, particularly if pedicle screws can be inserted.

Duchenne Muscular Dystrophy

The most common hereditary neuromuscular condition, DMD is a sex-linked recessive disorder that affects 1 in 3500 boys. A deficiency of the muscle cell membrane stabilization protein dystrophin results in cell membrane leakage and gradual deterioration with fatty infiltration.[179] These patients typically present with progressive muscle weakness at 3 to 5 years of age. DMD patients are young boys with delayed onset of walking, a wide-based gait, a wide-based stance with pronounced lordosis, and pseudohypertrophy of the calves. Gower sign of DMD is a characteristic way in which these patients rise up from the floor using all four limbs to get into a "bear position" and then pushing off of their thighs with their upper extremities to force hip extension and right the trunk. In this manner, these children overcome their proximal muscle weakness. Elevated creatine kinase level (5000 to 15,000 U/L) is a good screening test. Definitive diagnosis is established by either a genetic analysis or a muscle biopsy specimen revealing decreased levels or absence of dystrophin.[180-182]

The clinical course of these patients is fairly predictable. Patients usually use a wheelchair full-time by 10 to 12 years of age. The incidence of spinal deformity and rate of scoliosis progression in these patients are controversial. Several studies have found that DMD scoliosis increases at a rate of 15 to 30 degrees yearly and may exceed 100 degrees if untreated (Fig. 28.27).[183-186] In contrast, a 10-year retrospective study of 123 DMD patients by Kinali and colleagues[187] found a highly variable rate of the presence and the progression of scoliosis in children with DMD. Despite this inconsistency, skeletally immature patients with a Cobb angle progression to greater than 20 degrees generally continue to progress. The association of the severity of spinal deformity and decline in pulmonary function has been well described. Respiratory failure generally leads to death in the late teens or early 20s, although advances in treatment have improved prognosis.[188]

Scoliosis in Duchenne Muscular Dystrophy

More than any other form of neuromuscular disorder, pulmonary function and life expectancy are directly correlated with spinal deformity. FVC begins to decline at the age that

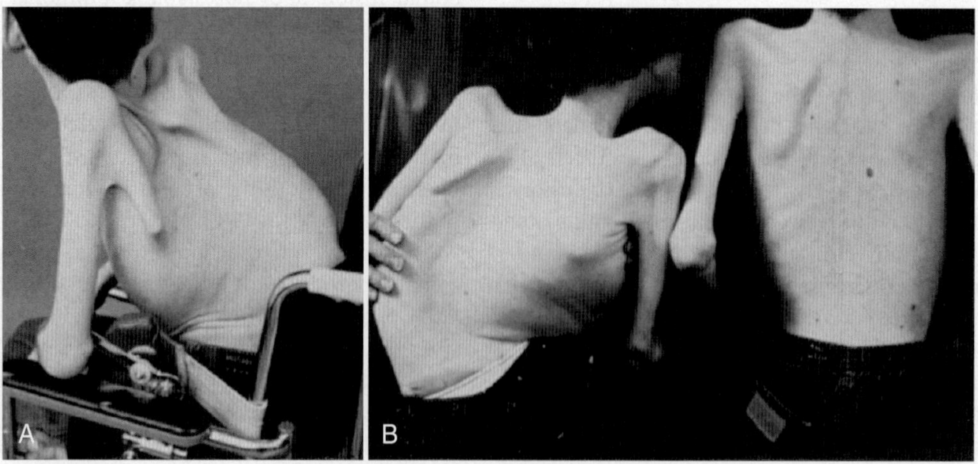

FIG. 28.27 Two brothers with severe scoliosis secondary to muscular dystrophy. (B) The younger boy underwent a successful posterior spinal instrumentation and fusion, achieving good sitting balance. (A) His older brother had already lost too much pulmonary function to tolerate surgery. He is unable to sit well, even with support.

patients stop standing. From that time, the restrictive effects of thoracic cage deformity and loss of respiratory muscle function cause pulmonary function to decline 4% for each 10 degrees of deformity and each year of age (Fig. 28.28).[175] Smith and colleagues[186] reviewed the natural history of DMD in 51 boys and found that the rate of progression of scoliosis was inversely related to the age of death. Although most studies have failed to identify a protective role of spinal surgery on pulmonary function,[187-189] Galasko and colleagues[190] reported a stabilization of pulmonary function at 3-year follow-up. They compared 32 patients who underwent spinal fusion and 23 patients who refused surgery. The FVC remained stable for 3 years postoperatively in the fused group compared with an 8% per year average decline in patients not operated on. Although the impact of spinal surgery on pulmonary function is unknown, the relationship between pulmonary decline and progression of scoliosis has been shown by Kennedy and colleagues[189] to be 3% to 5% per year. When scoliosis progression has reached 20 to 30 degrees, many authors recommend surgery (Fig. 28.29).[29,191,192] Glucocorticoid treatment seems to be affecting the natural history of this condition, but it is unclear how the surgical indications for spinal fusion should be modified.

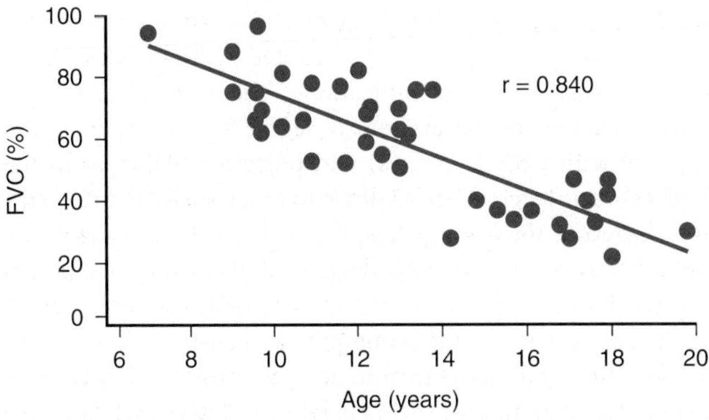

FIG. 28.28 Percentage of forced vital capacity (FVC) vs age in patients with Duchenne muscular dystrophy. FVC percentage was found to be the parameter of pulmonary function that most strongly correlated with age and thoracic Cobb angle measurement. (From Kurz LT, Mubarak SJ, Schultz P, et al. Correlation of scoliosis and pulmonary function in Duchenne muscular dystrophy. *J Pediatr Orthop.* 1983;3:347.)

Treatment Options

The preoperative evaluation of DMD patients must take into account other comorbidities of their disease. Pulmonary function testing should be done before surgery to assess the severity of preoperative respiratory compromise. Although more recent studies have reported successful spinal surgery at FVC of less than 35%,[193] previous work associated this lowered FVC value with increased postoperative morbidity.[192] Similar to the progressive decline in pulmonary function over time, the severity of cardiac dysfunction also increases with age. DMD patients are likely to develop cardiomyopathy and arrhythmias in the second decade of life, and an electrocardiogram, a chest radiograph, and an echocardiogram should be done to screen for cardiac problems. Despite the fact that many of these patients are obese, they should be evaluated for malnutrition because wound healing complications and increased infection rates have been reported.[194] DMD is also associated with a tendency for increased blood loss caused by

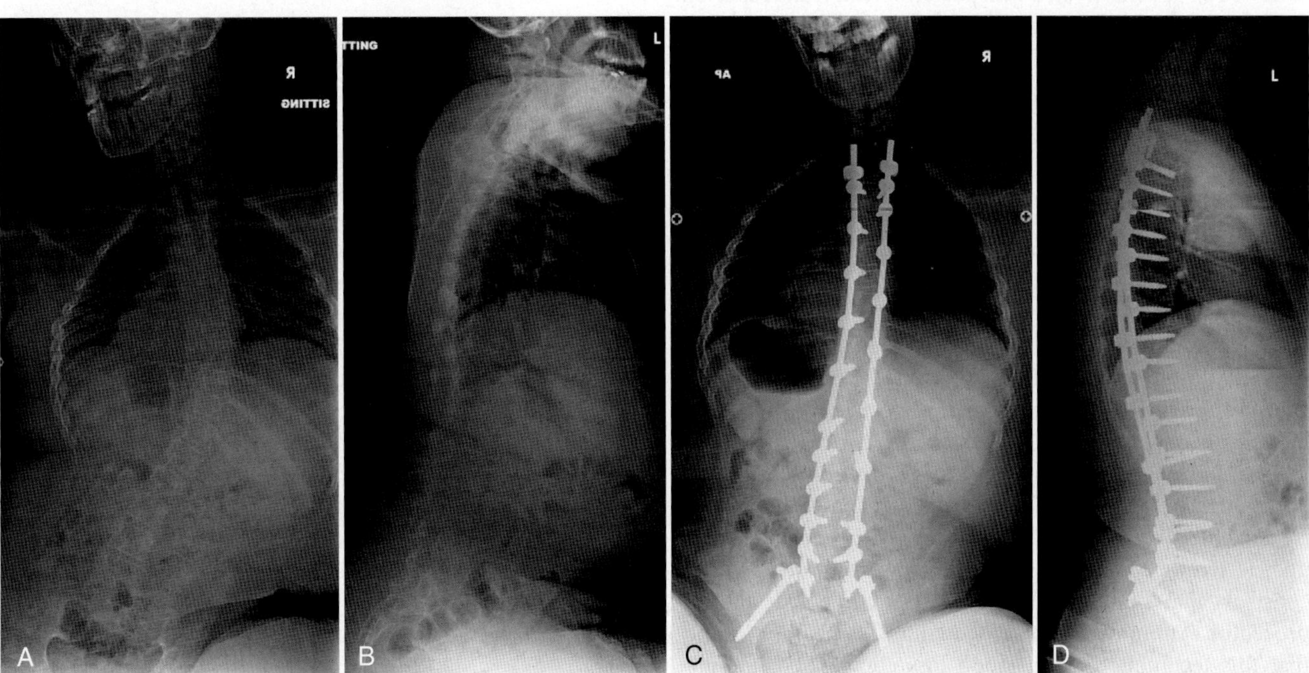

FIG. 28.29 Preoperatively, this boy with Duchenne muscular dystrophy had 20 degrees of scoliosis and 30 degrees of thoracolumbar region kyphosis. He underwent posterior instrumentation and fusion from T3 to L5 at age 13 years to retard further progression of spinal deformity. Treating the patient early allowed stopping short of the pelvis.

poor vasoconstrictive function owing to a lack of dystrophin in vessel smooth muscle; preparation for major operative blood loss should be made.[195] Additionally, patients with dystrophic myopathies have an increased risk of malignant hyperthermia.[196]

Surgical Management

Long fusions from T2 to either L5 or the pelvis are recommended. The distal extent of the fusion has been an area of much research and remains a controversial subject. Mubarak and colleagues[192] determined that instrumentation and fusion to L5 was effective in mild deformities with pelvic obliquity less than 15 degrees at 34-month follow-up. Sengupta and colleagues[197] found similar results in their review of posterior fusions in 50 patients, and concluded that fusion to L5 with pedicle screw instrumentation is adequate if done soon after patients lose walking ability. These results were supported further by McCall and Hayes,[74] who found that fusion to L5 was a viable alternative to fusion to the pelvis in patients with less than 15 degrees of L5 tilt.

Takaso and colleagues[198] supported the argument that the caudal extent of the fusion in DMD patients can be stopped at L5 if the degree of L5 tilt is less than 15 degrees.

Given the limitations of a minimal curve size and pelvic obliquity, fusion to the pelvis is the most common method of spinal fixation in DMD patients. Luque rods with the Galveston technique of pelvic fixation is a well-studied technique that offers acceptable results. Brook and colleagues[199] reviewed results of Luque and Luque-Galveston instrumentation in 17 patients and found an average of 63% correction as well as good maintenance of correction. Bentley and colleagues[173] reviewed 64 patients treated with posterior fusion and reported a 47% correction rate with good maintenance of correction. The authors recommended fusion to T4, stating that the lower level of fusion allows more freedom of movement for feeding and upper extremity use. Unit rods have also been evaluated in DMD patients and provide acceptable results; however, placement of the rods into the iliac wings makes this technique challenging.[199] The Dunn-McCarthy technique with S-shaped rods looped over the sacral alae has been shown to provide good results in DMD patients. This technique has gained popularity because of its dependable fixation in patients with osteopenia and ease of placement in the kyphotic lumbar spine that is often seen in DMD patients.[83,191]

More recent advances in segmental pedicle screw fixation have resulted in their promotion as an alternative to more traditional hook-wire and Galveston pelvic fixation techniques. Hahn and colleagues[200] reported results of 20 DMD patients treated with pedicle screw–alone fixation and concluded that pedicle screws combined with iliac screws provided a stable construct that eliminated the need for a combined anterior procedure at minimum 2-year follow-up. These authors found that this technique limited blood loss compared with sublaminar wiring, had no implant loosening, and allowed early mobilization, resulting in no pulmonary complications. These findings were supported by Mehta and colleagues,[201] who reported their cohort of 36 patients with DMD instrumented from upper thoracic level to L5 or the pelvis if the pelvic tilt was 15 degrees or greater (10 patients), unlike the study performed by Hahn et al.,[200] who instrumented the pelvis regardless of the pelvic tilt. All patients in the group were able to achieve a balanced sitting posture and a significantly improved lumbar lordosis. Also, the patients who underwent pelvic fixation had a significantly improved pelvic tilt following surgery compared to preoperative measurements.[201] Pedicle screw fixation with a free-hand technique has been shown to be as safe and accurate as in other conditions.[202]

Our Recommendations

In patients with DMD, spinal fusion is performed when curves reach 20 degrees and FVC is greater than 40%. Preoperative FVC of less than 30% to 35% is correlated with a high incidence of major respiratory complications. The surgical technique recommended by the authors is segmental instrumentation (mainly with pedicle screws) and posterior fusion from the high thoracic level (T2 or T3 down to L5). Usually, the ICU stay is 2 days, and the average hospital stay is 8 days. If the pelvic obliquity is greater than 10 degrees or the scoliosis curve is greater than 40 degrees, the authors consider instrumentation to the pelvis to correct this obliquity and ensure a level pelvis. The ultimate goal in the treatment of deformity in DMD is the maintenance of upright sitting balance and maximal pain-free function. Many of the authors' patients are now older than 20 years with an upright posture, minimal wheelchair difficulties, and improved quality of life.

Rett Syndrome

Rett syndrome is a developmental disorder of unknown etiology that occurs in 1 in 20,000 females. The syndrome is linked to a mutation in the *MeCP2* gene located on the X chromosome, which encodes a deacetylator that regulates the transcription of certain genes. Patients appear normal at birth but begin the stepwise deterioration characteristic of Rett syndrome. The syndrome has four stages. In the first stage, generally occurring when patients are 6 to 18 months of age, signs of the syndrome include developmental stagnation, slowed head and brain growth, and generalized hypotonia. From approximately age 1 to 3 years, patients begin to regress developmentally and exhibit autism-like symptoms. In the third stage, between ages 2 and 10 years, patients have seizures, exhibit ataxia, exhibit mental retardation, and perform stereotypical gestures such as repetitive hand wringing. During this phase, scoliosis and spasticity can be seen. In the fourth stage, patients exhibit upper and lower motor neuron signs with increased rigidity and muscle wasting. Scoliosis is most likely to develop in this final stage (Fig. 28.30).[203]

Scoliosis in Rett Syndrome

The incidence of scoliosis increases as patients get older: 8% of girls with Rett syndrome have scoliosis at age 5, 40% have it by age 11, and 80% have it by age 20. The deformity can be

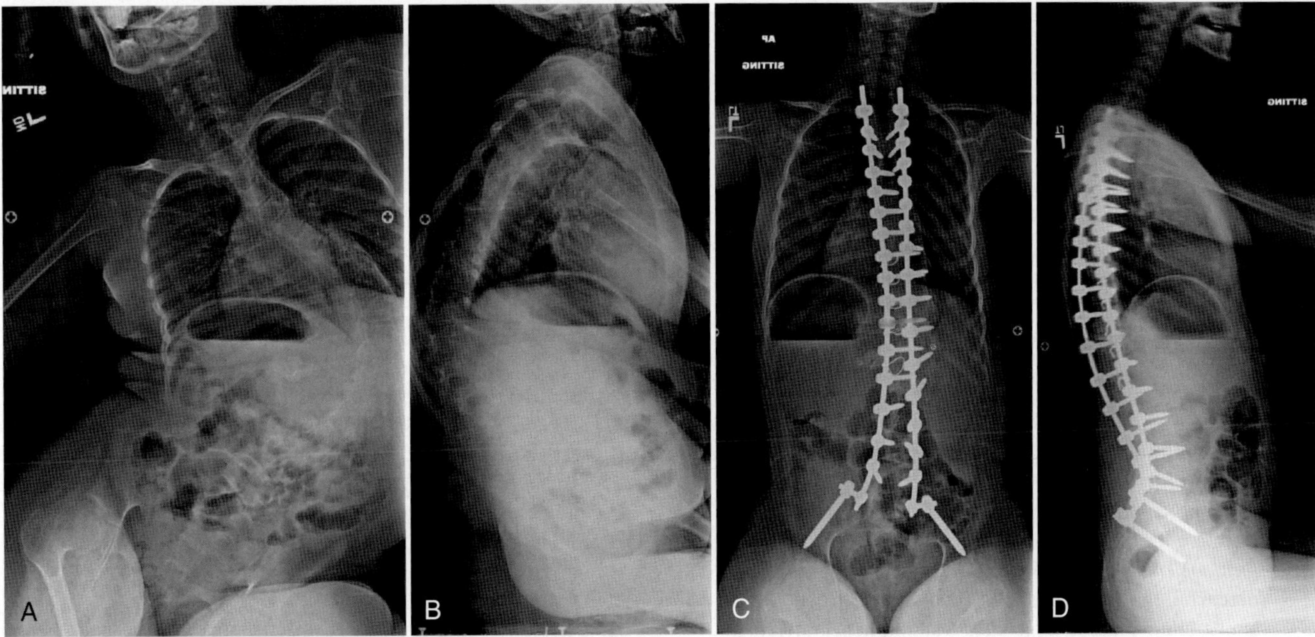

FIG. 28.30 A 9-year-old girl with Rett syndrome had 80 degrees of spinal deformity, despite bracing. Because her triradiate cartilage remained open, she underwent anterior thoracoscopic release and posterior instrumentation from T2 to the pelvis.

rapidly progressive; Lidstrom and colleagues[204] reported on 78 patients with Rett syndrome and reported progression rates of 20 to 41 degrees per year in the 10 most severe cases. Because scoliosis in Rett syndrome has this potential for progression, yearly evaluation of the spine should be conducted after the age of 5 years.[205]

The treatment for Rett syndrome is similar to treatment for CP. Bracing has a limited role in treatment, although it may provide support for comfortable sitting until surgery is performed.[206] As with CP, the authors recommend that if sitting comfort and balance become compromised, treatment with segmental instrumentation is indicated. Spinal surgery is indicated when the curve exceeds 40 degrees. Long-term outcome of surgery in patients with Rett syndrome has shown good results. In a prospective study of 23 girls with Rett syndrome and neuromuscular scoliosis, Larsson and colleagues[207] found improved seating position and patient satisfaction at 6-year follow-up. These authors reported that all patients who could walk preoperatively maintained ambulation postoperatively. They also noted that patients and parents reported an overall improvement in well-being with better sitting posture and improved breathing. As with all patients with neuromuscular disorders who undergo scoliosis surgery, spinal cord monitoring is advocated.[208]

PEARLS

1. Neuromuscular spinal deformities are often complex, multiplanar, and rigid.
2. Segmental instrumentation reduces the risk of progression. Hooks and screws add to construct rigidity compared with sublaminar wires alone.
3. Hyperkyphosis increases the risk of implant failure or junctional kyphosis, or both. Segmental posterior compression instrumentation reduces this risk.

PITFALLS

1. Blood loss should be anticipated. The surgeon should minimize blood loss during exposure and consider use of a pharmacologic agent to reduce blood loss during surgery. Transfusion should be done early, and clotting factors should be replaced (fresh frozen plasma) before coagulopathy develops.
2. The surgeon needs to be aware of infrapelvic causes of obliquity, such as hip contracture.
3. Preoperative nutritional supplementation, often via a gastrostomy tube with fundoplication, should be considered.
4. Postoperative intensive care unit support is crucial to negotiating major spinal surgery safely in these medically compromised patients.

KEY REFERENCES

1. Park HY, Matsumoto H, Feinberg N, et al. The Classification for Early-Onset Scoliosis (C-EOS) correlates with the speed of vertical expandable prosthetic titanium rib (VEPTR) proximal anchor failure. *J Pediatr Orthop*. 2015;[Epub ahead of print].
Growing rods have been employed over the past decade in neuromuscular scoliosis patients. In this article Park and colleagues describe outcomes and limitations of VEPTR technology in neuromuscular scoliosis.
2. Teli MGA, Pasquale C, Vincitorio F, Lovi A, Grava G, Brayda-Bruno M. Spinal fusion with Cotrel-Dubousset Instrumentation for neuropathic scoliosis in patients with cerebral palsy. *Spine*. 2006;31(14):E441-E447.
This article provides the outcomes of third-generation Cotrel-Dubousset segmental instrumentation in neuromuscular scoliosis patients.
3. Auerback JD, Spiegel DA, Zgonis MH, et al. The correction of pelvic obliquity in patients with cerebral palsy and neuromuscular scoliosis: is there a benefit of anterior release prior to posterior spinal arthrodesis? *Spine*. 2009;34(21):E766-E774.

This article describes how there still can be a role for anterior surgery in neuromuscular scoliosis patients with very rigid curves.

4. Trivedi J, Thomson JD, Slakey JB, et al. Clinical and radiographic predictors of scoliosis in patients with myelomeningocele. *J Bone Joint Surg Am.* 2002;84:1389-1394.
The risk of scoliosis in patients with myelodysplasia is substantial. This article presents the correlation with the level of paralysis.

5. McCarthy RE, McCullough FL. Shilla growth guidance for early-onset scoliosis: results after a minimum of five years of follow-up. *J Bone Joint Surg Am.* 2015;97(19):1578-1584.
The Shilla growth guidance method can also be applied in certain cases of young neuromuscular patients.

REFERENCES

1. Majd ME, Muldowny DS, Holt RT. Natural history of scoliosis in the institutionalized adult cerebral palsy population. *Spine.* 1997;22:1461-1466.
2. Wadman RI, Bosboom WM, van der Pol Wl, et al. Drug treatment for spinal muscular atrophy types II and III. *Cochrane Database Syst Rev.* 2012;(4):CD006282.
3. Mercuri E, Bertini E, Messina S, et al. Randomized, double-blind, placebo-controlled trial of phenylbutyrate in spinal muscular atrophy. *Neurology.* 2007;68:51-55.
4. Miller RG, Moore DH, Dronsky V, et al. A placebo-controlled trial of gabapentin in spinal muscular atrophy. *J Neurol Sci.* 2001;191:127-131.
5. Tzeng AC, Cheng J, Fryczynski H, et al. A study of thyrotropin-releasing hormone for the treatment of spinal muscular atrophy: A preliminary report. *Am J Phys Med Rehabil.* 2000;79:435-440.
6. Kolb SJ, Kissel JT. Spinal muscular atrophy. *Neurol Clin.* 2015;33:831-846.
7. Ade-Hall RA, Moore AP. Botulinum toxin type A in the treatment of lower limb spasticity in cerebral palsy. *Cochrane Database Syst Rev.* 2000;(2):CD001408.
8. Lukban MB, Rosales RL, Dressler D. Effectiveness of botulinum toxin A for upper and lower limb spasticity in children with cerebral palsy: a summary of evidence. *J Neural Transm.* 2009;116:319-331.
9. Gerszten PC, Albright AL, Johnstone GF. Intrathecal baclofen infusion and subsequent orthopedic surgery in patients with spastic cerebral palsy. *J Neurosurg.* 1998;88:1009-1013.
10. Ginsburg GM, Lauder AJ. Progression of scoliosis in patients with spastic quadriplegia after the insertion of an intrathecal baclofen pump. *Spine.* 2007;32:2745-2750.
11. Caird MS, Palanca AA, Garton H, et al. Outcomes of posterior spinal fusion and instrumentation in patients with continuous intrathecal baclofen infusion pumps. *Spine.* 2008;33:E94-E99.
12. Shilt JS, Lai LP, Cabrera MN, et al. The impact of intrathecal baclofen on the natural history of scoliosis in cerebral palsy. *J Pediatr Orthop.* 2008;28:684-687.
13. Scannell B, Yaszay B. Scoliosis, spinal fusion, intrathecal baclofen pump implantation. *Phys Med Rehabil Clin N Am.* 2015;26(1):79-88.
14. Manzur AY, Kinali M, Muntoni F. Update on the management of Duchenne muscular dystrophy. *Arch Dis Child.* 2008;93:986-990.
15. Manzur AY, Kuntzer T, Pike M, et al. Glucocorticoid corticosteroids for Duchenne muscular dystrophy. *Cochrane Database Syst Rev.* 2008;(1):CD003725.
16. Markham LW, Kinnett K, Wong BL, et al. Corticosteroid treatment retards development of ventricular dysfunction in Duchenne muscular dystrophy. *Neuromuscul Disord.* 2008;18:365-370.
17. Shapiro F, Zurakowski D, Bui T, Darras BT. Progression of spinal deformity in wheelchair-dependent patients with Duchenne muscular dystrophy who are not treated with steroids. *Bone Joint J.* 2014;96-B:100-105.
18. Lebel DE, Corston JA, McAdam LC, Biggar WD, Alman BA. Glucocorticoid treatment for the prevention of scoliosis in children with Duchenne muscular dystrophy: long-term follow-up. *J Bone Joint Surg Am.* 2013;95(12):1057-1061.
19. Kotwicki T, Durmala J, Czubak J. Bracing for neuromuscular scoliosis: orthosis construction to improve the patient's function. *Disabil Rehabil Assist Technol.* 2008;3:161-169.
20. Shoham Y, Meyer S, Katz-Leurer M, et al. The influence of seat adjustment and a thoraco-lumbar-sacral orthosis on the distribution of body-seat pressure in children with scoliosis and pelvic obliquity. *Disabil Rehabil.* 2004;26:21-26.
21. Miller A, Temple T, Miller F. Impact of orthoses on the rate of scoliosis progression in children with cerebral palsy. *J Pediatr Orthop.* 1996;16:332-335.
22. Olafsson Y, Saraste H, Al-Dabbagh Z. Brace treatment in neuromuscular spine deformity. *J Pediatr Orthop.* 1999;19:376-379.
23. Letts M, Rathbone D, Yamashita T, et al. Soft Boston orthosis in management of neuromuscular scoliosis: a preliminary report. *J Pediatr Orthop.* 1992;12:470-474.
24. Berven S, Bradford DS. Neuromuscular scoliosis: causes of deformity and principles for evaluation and management. *Semin Neurol.* 2002;22:167-178.
25. Bunnell WP, MacEwen GD. Non-operative treatment of scoliosis in cerebral palsy: preliminary report on the use of a plastic jacket. *Dev Med Child Neurol.* 1977;19:45-49.
26. Winter RB, Carlson JM. Modern orthotics for spinal deformities. *Clin Orthop Relat Res.* 1977;126:74-86.
27. Nakamura N, Uesugi M, Inaba Y, et al. Use of dynamic spinal brace in the management of neuromuscular scoliosis: a preliminary report. *J Pediatr Orthop B.* 2014;23(3):291-298.
28. Holmes KJ, Michael SM, Thorpe SL, et al. Management of scoliosis with special seating for the non-ambulant spastic cerebral palsy population—a biomechanical study. *Clin Biomech (Bristol, Avon).* 2003;18:480-487.
29. Sussman M. Duchenne muscular dystrophy. *J Am Acad Orthop Surg.* 2002;10:138-151.
30. Bridwell KH, Baldus C, Iffrig TM, et al. Process measures and patient/parent evaluation of surgical management of spinal deformities in patients with progressive flaccid neuromuscular scoliosis (Duchenne's muscular dystrophy and spinal muscular atrophy). *Spine.* 1999;24:1300-1309.
31. Comstock CP, Leach J, Wenger DR. Scoliosis in total-body-involvement cerebral palsy: analysis of surgical treatment and patient and caregiver satisfaction. *Spine.* 1998;23:1412-1424.
32. Sink EL, Newton PO, Mubarak SJ, et al. Maintenance of sagittal plane alignment after surgical correction of spinal deformity in patients with cerebral palsy. *Spine.* 2003;28:1396-1403.
33. Lonstein JE, Akbarnia A. Operative treatment of spinal deformities in patients with cerebral palsy or mental retardation: an analysis of one hundred and seven cases. *J Bone Joint Surg Am.* 1983;65:43-55.

34. Askin GN, Hallett R, Hare N, et al. The outcome of scoliosis surgery in the severely physically handicapped child: an objective and subjective assessment. *Spine.* 1997;22:44-50.
35. Mercado E, Alman B, Wright JG. Does spinal fusion influence quality of life in neuromuscular scoliosis? *Spine.* 2007;32:S120-S125.
36. Wright JG, Einhorn TA, Heckman JD. Grades of recommendation. *J Bone Joint Surg Am.* 2005;87:1909-1910.
37. Cheuk DK, Wong V, Wraige E, Baxter P, Cole A. Surgery for scoliosis in Duchenne muscular dystrophy. *Chochrane Database Syst Rev.* 2015;10:CD005375.
38. Farhat G, Yamout B, Mikati MA, et al. Effect of antiepileptic drugs on bone density in ambulatory patients. *Neurology.* 2002;58:1348-1353.
39. Sheth RD, Wesolowski CA, Jacob JC, et al. Effect of carbamazepine and valproate on bone mineral density. *J Pediatr.* 1995;127:256-262.
40. Kumandas S, Koklu E, Gumus H, et al. Effect of carabamezapine and valproic acid on bone mineral density, IGF-I and IGFBP-3. *J Pediatr Endocrinol Metab.* 2006;19(4):529-534.
41. Finsterer J, Pelzl G, Hess B. Severe, isolated thrombocytopenia under polytherapy with carbamazepine and valproate. *Psychiatry Clin Neurosci.* 2001;55:423-426.
42. Gerstner T, Teich M, Bell N, et al. Valproate-associated coagulopathies are frequent and variable in children. *Epilepsia.* 2006;47:1136-1143.
43. Koenig S, Koeni T, Keller A, et al. High incidence of vaproate-induced coagulation disorders in children receiving valproic acid: a prospective study. *Blood Coagul Fibrinolysis.* 2008;19:375-382.
44. Manohar C, Avitsian R, Lozano S, Gonzalez-Martinez J, Cata JP. The effect of anti epileptic drugs on coagulation and bleeding in the preoperative period of epilepsy surgery: the Cleveland Clinic experience. *J Clin Neurosci.* 2011;18(9):1180-1184.
45. Chambers HG, Weinstein CH, Mubarak SJ, et al. The effect of valproic acid on blood loss in patients with cerebral palsy. *J Pediatr Orthop.* 1999;19:792-795.
46. Gill I, Eagle M, Mehta JS, et al. Correction of neuromuscular scoliosis in patients with preexisting respiratory failure. *Spine.* 2006;31:2478-2483.
47. Chong HS, Moon ES, Park JO, et al. Value of preoperative pulmonary function test in flaccid neuromuscular scoliosis surgery. *Spine.* 2011;36(21):E1391-E1394.
48. Pruijs JE, van Tol MJ, van Kesteren RG, et al. Neuromuscular scoliosis: clinical evaluation pre- and postoperative. *J Pediatr Orthop B.* 2000;9:217-220.
49. Soudon P, Hody JL, Bellen P. Preoperative cardiopulmonary assessment in the child with neuromuscular scoliosis. *J Pediatr Orthop B.* 2000;9:229-233.
50. Winter S. Preoperative assessment of the child with neuromuscular scoliosis. *Orthop Clin North Am.* 1994;25:239-245.
51. Jevsevar DS, Karlin LI. The relationship between preoperative nutritional status and complications after an operation for scoliosis in patients who have cerebral palsy. *J Bone Joint Surg Am.* 1993;75:880-884.
52. Lapp MA, Bridwell KH, Lenke LG, et al. Prospective randomization of parenteral hyperalimentation for long fusions with spinal deformity; its effect on complications and recovery from postoperative malnutrition. *Spine.* 2001;26(7):809-817.
53. Shapiro F, Sethna N. Blood loss in pediatric spine surgery. *Eur Spine J.* 2004;13(suppl 1):S6-S17.
54. Kannan S, Meert KL, Mooney JF, et al. Bleeding and coagulation changes during spinal fusion surgery: a comparison of neuromuscular and idiopathic scoliosis patients. *Pediatr Crit Care Med.* 2002;3:364-369.
55. Meert KL, Kannan S, Mooney JF. Predictors of red cell transfusion in children and adolescents undergoing spinal fusion surgery. *Spine.* 2002;27:2137-2142.
56. Neilipovitz DT, Murto K, Hall L, et al. A randomized trial of tranexamic acid to reduce blood transfusion for scoliosis surgery. *Anesth Analg.* 2001;93:82-87.
57. Gill JB, Chin Y, Levin A, et al. The use of antifibrinolytic agents in spine surgery: a meta-analysis. *J Bone Joint Surg Am.* 2008;90:2399-2407.
58. Dhawale AA, Shah SA, Sponseller PD, et al. Are antifibrinolytics helpful in decreasing blood loss and transfusions during spinal fusion surgery in children with cerebral palsy scoliosis? *Spine.* 2012;37(9):E549-E555.
59. Verma K, Errico T, Diefenback C, et al. The relative efficacy of antifibrinolytics in adolescent idiopathic scoliosis: a prospective randomized trial. *J Bone Joint Surg Am.* 2014;96(10):e80.
60. Gupta MC, Wijesekera S, Sossan A, et al. Reliability of radiographic parameters in neuromuscular scoliosis. *Spine.* 2007;32:691-695.
61. Haas S. Spastic scoliosis and obliquity of the pelvis. *J Bone Joint Surg.* 1942;24:774-780.
62. Sullivan JA, Conner SB. Comparison of Harrington instrumentation and segmental spinal instrumentation in the management of neuromuscular spinal deformity. *Spine.* 1982;7:299-304.
63. Luque ER. Segmental spinal instrumentation for correction of scoliosis. *Clin Orthop Relat Res.* 1982;163:192-198.
64. Herring JA, Wenger DR. Segmental spinal instrumentation: a preliminary report of 40 consecutive cases. *Spine.* 1982;7:285-298.
65. Taddonio RF. Segmental spinal instrumentation in the management of neuromuscular spinal deformity. *Spine.* 1982;7:305-311.
66. Allen BL Jr, Ferguson RL. The Galveston technique for L rod instrumentation of the scoliotic spine. *Spine.* 1982;7:276-284.
67. Gupta MC, Wijeseka S, Sossan A, et al. Reliability of radiographic parameters in neuromuscular scoliosis. *Spine.* 2007;32:691-695.
68. Bell DF, Moseley CF, Koreska J. Unit rod segmental spinal instrumentation in the management of patients with progressive neuromuscular spinal deformity. *Spine.* 1989;14:1301-1307.
69. Dias RC, Miller F, Dabney K, et al. Surgical correction of spinal deformity using a unit rod in children with cerebral palsy. *J Pediatr Orthop.* 1996;16:734-740.
70. Bulman WA, Dormans JP, Ecker ML, et al. Posterior spinal fusion for scoliosis in patients with cerebral palsy: a comparison of Luque rod and Unit Rod instrumentation. *J Pediatr Orthop.* 1996;16:314-323.
71. Tsirikos AI, Lipton G, Chang WN, et al. Surgical correction of scoliosis in pediatric patients with cerebral palsy using the unit rod instrumentation. *Spine.* 2008;33:1133-1140.
72. Tsirikos AI, Chang WN, Shah SA, et al. Preserving ambulatory potential in pediatric patients with cerebral palsy who undergo spinal fusion using unit rod instrumentation. *Spine.* 2003;28:480-483.

73. Erickson MA, Oliver T, Baldini T, et al. Biomechanical assessment of conventional unit rod fixation versus a unit rod pedicle screw construct: a human cadaver study. *Spine.* 2004;29:1314-1319.
74. McCall RE, Hayes B. Long-term outcome in neuromuscular scoliosis fused only to lumbar 5. *Spine.* 2005;30:2056-2060.
75. Guidera KJ, Hooten J, Weatherly W, et al. Cotrel-Dubousset instrumentation: results in 52 patients. *Spine.* 1993;18:427-431.
76. Neustadt JB, Shufflebarger HL, Cammisa FP. Spinal fusions to the pelvis augmented by Cotrel-Dubousset instrumentation for neuromuscular scoliosis. *J Pediatr Orthop.* 1992;12:465-469.
77. Wimmer C, Wallnofer P, Walochnik N, et al. Comparative evaluation of Luque and Isola instrumentation for treatment of neuromuscular scoliosis. *Clin Orthop Relat Res.* 2005;439:181-192.
78. Yazici M, Asher MA, Hardacker JW. The safety and efficacy of Isola-Galveston instrumentation and arthrodesis in the treatment of neuromuscular spinal deformities. *J Bone Joint Surg Am.* 2000;82:524-543.
79. Pritchett JW. The untreated unstable hip in severe cerebral palsy. *Clin Orthop Relat Res.* 1983;173:169-172.
80. Broom MJ, Banta JV, Renshaw TS. Spinal fusion augmented by Luque-rod segmental instrumentation for neuromuscular scoliosis. *J Bone Joint Surg Am.* 1989;71:32-44.
81. Gau YL, Lonstein JE, Winter RB, et al. Luque-Galveston procedure for correction and stabilization of neuromuscular scoliosis and pelvic obliquity: a review of 68 patients. *J Spinal Disord.* 1991;4:399-410.
82. Allen BL Jr, Ferguson RL. The Galveston technique of pelvic fixation with L-rod instrumentation of the spine. *Spine.* 1984;9:388-394.
83. McCarthy RE, Bruffett WL, McCullough FL. S rod fixation to the sacrum in patients with neuromuscular spinal deformities. *Clin Orthop Relat Res.* 1999;364:26-31.
84. Warner WC Jr, Fackler CD. Comparison of two instrumentation techniques in treatment of lumbar kyphosis in myelodysplasia. *J Pediatr Orthop.* 1993;13:704-708.
85. McCall RE. Modified Luque instrumentation after myelomeningocele kyphectomy. *Spine.* 1998;23:1406-1411.
86. Early S, Mahar A, Oka R, et al. Biomechanical comparison of lumbosacral fixation using Luque-Galveston and Colorado II sacropelvic fixation: advantage of using locked proximal fixation. *Spine.* 2005;30:1396-1401.
87. Schwend RM, Sluyters R, Najdzionek J. The pylon concept of pelvic anchorage for spinal instrumentation in the human cadaver. *Spine.* 2003;28:542-547.
88. Tsuchiya K, Bridwell KH, Kuklo TR, et al. Minimum 5-year analysis of L5-S1 fusion using sacropelvic fixation (bilateral S1 and iliac screws) for spinal deformity. *Spine.* 2006;31:303-308.
89. Phillips JH, Gutheil JP, Knapp DR Jr. Iliac screw fixation in neuromuscular scoliosis. *Spine.* 2007;32:1566-1570.
90. Peelle MW, Lenke LG, Bridwell KH, et al. Comparison of pelvic fixation techniques in neuromuscular spinal deformity correction: Galveston rod versus iliac and lumbosacral screws. *Spine.* 2006;31:2392-2398.
91. Stevens DB, Beard C. Segmental spinal instrumentation for neuromuscular spinal deformity. *Clin Orthop Relat Res.* 1989;242:164-168.
92. Kebaish KM. Sacropelvic fixation: techniques and complications. *Spine.* 2010;35(25):2245-2251.
93. Whitaker C, Burton DC, Asher M. Treatment of selected neuromuscular patients with posterior instrumentation and arthrodesis ending with lumbar pedicle screw anchorage. *Spine.* 2000;25:2312-2318.
94. Funk S, Lovejoy S, Mencio G, Martus J. Rigid instrumentation for neuromuscular scoliosis improves deformity correction without increasing complications. *Spine.* 2015;41(1):46-52.
95. Takeshita K, Lenke LG, Bridwell KH, et al. Analysis of patients with nonambulatory neuromuscular scoliosis surgically treated to the pelvis with intraoperative halo-femoral traction. *Spine.* 2006;31:2381-2385.
96. Sponseller PD, Zimmerman RM, Ko PS, et al. Low profile pelvic fixation with the sacral alar iliac technique in the pediatric population improves results at two-year minimum follow-up. *Spine.* 2010;35(20):1887-1892.
97. Sponseller PD, Yang JS, Thompson GH, et al. Pelvic fixation of growing rods. *Spine.* 2009;34(16):1706-1710.
98. Newton PO, White KK, Faro F, et al. The success of thoracoscopic anterior fusion in a consecutive series of 112 pediatric spinal deformity cases. *Spine.* 2005;30:392-398.
99. Keeler KA, Lenke LG, Good CR, et al. Spinal fusion for spastic neuromuscular scoliosis. *Spine.* 2010;35(10):427-433.
100. Auerbach JD, Spiegel DA, Zgonis MH, et al. The correction of pelvic obliquity in patients with cerebral palsy and neuromuscular scoliosis: is there a benefit of anterior release prior to posterior spinal arthrodesis? *Spine.* 2009;34(21):E766-E774.
101. Smucker JD, Miller F. Crankshaft effect after posterior spinal fusion and unit rod instrumentation in children with cerebral palsy. *J Pediatr Orthop.* 2001;21:108-112.
102. de Haan P, Kalkman CJ, de Mol BA, et al. Efficacy of transcranial motor-evoked myogenic potentials to detect spinal cord ischemia during operations for thoracoabdominal aneurysms. *J Thorac Cardiovasc Surg.* 1997;113:87-100.
103. Tokala DP, Lam KS, Freeman BJ, et al. Is there a role for selective anterior instrumentation in neuromuscular scoliosis? *Eur Spine J.* 2007;16:91-96.
104. Deleted in review.
105. Schwartz DM, Auerbach JD, Dormans JP, et al. Neurophysiological detection of impending spinal cord injury during scoliosis surgery. *J Bone Joint Surg Am.* 2007;89:2440-2449.
106. Salem KM, Goodger L, Bowyer K, Shafafy M, Grevitt MP. Does transcranial stimulation for motor evoked potentials (TcMEP) worsen seizures in epileptic patients following spinal deformity surgery? *Eur Spine J.* 2016;10:3044-3048.
107. Reames DL, Smith JS, Fu KMG, et al. Complications in the surgical treatment of 19,360 cases of pediatric scoliosis: a review of the Scoliosis Research Society Morbidity and Mortality database. *Spine.* 2011;36:1484-1491.
108. Mo AZ, Asemota AO, Venkatesan A, et al. Why no signals? Cerebral anatomy predicts success of intraoperative neuromonitoring during correction of scoliosis secondary to cerebral palsy. *J Pediatr Orthop.* 2015;[Epub ahead of print].
109. Leung YL, Grevitt M, Henderson L, et al. Cord monitoring changes and segmental vessel ligation in the "at risk" cord during anterior spinal deformity surgery. *Spine.* 2005;30:1870-1874.
110. Tsirikos AI, Howitt SP, McMaster MJ. Segmental vessel ligation in patients undergoing surgery for anterior spinal deformity. *J Bone Joint Surg Br.* 2008;90:474-479.
111. Winter RB, Lonstein JE, Denis F, et al. Paraplegia resulting from vessel ligation. *Spine.* 1996;21:1232-1233.

112. Sarwark J, Sarwahi V. New strategies and decision making in the management of neuromuscular scoliosis. *Orthop Clin North Am*. 2007;38:485-496.
113. Sponseller PD, LaPorte DM, Hungerford MW, et al. Deep wound infections after neuromuscular scoliosis surgery: a multicenter study of risk factors and treatment outcomes. *Spine*. 2000;25:2461-2466.
114. Glotzbecker MP, Riedel MD, Vitale MG, et al. What's the evidence? Systematic literature review of risk factors and preventive strategies for surgical site infection following pediatric spine surgery. *J Pediatric Orthop*. 2013;33(5):479-487.
115. Yazici M, Asher MA. Freeze-dried allograft for posterior spinal fusion in patients with neuromuscular spinal deformities. *Spine*. 1997;22:1467-1471.
116. Tsirikos AI, Chang WN, Dabney KW, et al. Comparison of one-stage versus two-stage anteroposterior spinal fusion in pediatric patients with cerebral palsy and neuromuscular scoliosis. *Spine*. 2003;28:1300-1305.
117. Mohamad F, Parent S, Pawelek J, et al. Perioperative complications after surgical correction in neuromuscular scoliosis. *J Pediatr Orthop*. 2007;27:392-397.
118. Yamin S, Li L, Xing W, et al. Staged surgical treatment for severe and rigid scoliosis. *J Orthop Surg*. 2008;3:26.
119. Newton PO, Upasani VV, Lhamby J, et al. Surgical treatment of main thoracic scoliosis with thoracoscopic anterior instrumentation: a five-year follow-up study. *J Bone Joint Surg Am*. 2008;90:2077-2089.
120. Tobert DG, Vitale MG. Strategies for treating scoliosis in children with spinal muscular atrophy. *Am J Orthop (Belle Mead NJ)*. 2013;42(11):E99-E103.
121. Hell AK, Hefti F, Campbell RM Jr. [Treatment of congenital scoliosis with the vertical expandable prosthetic titanium rib implant]. *Orthopade*. 2004;33:911-918.
122. Latalski M, Fatyga M, Gregosiewicz A. The vertical expandable prosthetic titanium rib (VEPTR) in the treatment of scoliosis and thoracic deformities: preliminary report. *Orthop Traumatol Rehabil*. 2007;9:459-466.
123. Akbarnia BA, Emans JB. Complications of growth-sparing surgery in early onset scoliosis. *Spine*. 2010;35(25):2193-2204.
124. Park HY, Matsumoto H, Feinberg N, et al. The Classification for Early-onset Scoliosis (C-EOS) correlates with the speed of vertical expandable prosthetic titanium rib (VEPTR) proximal anchor failure. *J Pediatr Orthop*. 2015;[Epub ahead of print].
125. Deleted in review.
126. Benson ER, Thomson JD, Smith BG, et al. Results and morbidity in a consecutive series of patients undergoing spinal fusion for neuromuscular scoliosis. *Spine*. 1998;23:2308-2317.
127. Boachie-Adjei O, Lonstein JE, Winter RB, et al. Management of neuromuscular spinal deformities with Luque segmental instrumentation. *J Bone Joint Surg Am*. 1989;71:548-562.
128. Keeler KA, Lenke LG, Good CR, et al. Spinal fusion for spastic neuromuscular scoliosis. *Spine*. 2010;35(10):427-433.
129. Croft LD, Pottinger JM, Chiang HY, et al. Risk factors for surgical site infections after pediatric spine operations. *Spine*. 2015;40(2):E112-E119.
129a. Alessia S, Parsons D, Grant J, et al. Deep wound infection following pediatric scoliosis surgery: incidence and analysis of risk factors. *Can J Surg*. 2011;54:263-269.
129b. Mackenzie WGS, Matsumoto H, Williams B, et al. Surgical site infection following spinal instrumentation for scoliosis: a multicenter analysis of rates, risk factors, and pathogens. *J Bone Joint Surg Am*. 2013;95:800-806.
130. Borkhuu B, Borowski A, Shah SA, et al. Antibiotic-loaded allograft decreases the rate of acute deep wound infection after spinal fusion in cerebral palsy. *Spine*. 2008;33: 2300-2304.
131. Mikhael MM, Huddleston PM, Nassr A. Postoperative culture positive surgical site infections after the use of irradiated allograft, nonirradiated allograft, or autograft for spinal fusion. *Spine*. 2009;34(22):2466-2468.
132. Canavese F, Gupta S, Krajbich JI, et al. Vacuum-assisted closure for deep infection after spinal instrumentation for scoliosis. *J Bone Joint Surg Br*. 2008;90:377-381.
133. Deleted in review.
134. Deleted in review.
135. Kalen V, Conklin MM, Sherman FC. Untreated scoliosis in severe cerebral palsy. *J Pediatr Orthop*. 1992;12:337-340.
136. Madigan RR, Wallace SL. Scoliosis in the institutionalized cerebral palsy population. *Spine*. 1981;6:583-590.
137. Saito N, Ebara S, Ohotsuka K, et al. Natural history of scoliosis in spastic cerebral palsy. *Lancet*. 1998;351: 1687-1692.
138. Thometz JG, Simon SR. Progression of scoliosis after skeletal maturity in institutionalized adults who have cerebral palsy. *J Bone Joint Surg Am*. 1988;70:1290-1296.
139. Westerlund LE, Gill SS, Jarosz TS, et al. Posterior-only unit rod instrumentation and fusion for neuromuscular scoliosis. *Spine*. 2001;26:1984-1989.
140. Teli M, Elsebaie H, Biant L, et al. Neuromuscular scoliosis treated by segmental third-generation instrumented spinal fusion. *J Spinal Disord Tech*. 2005;18:430-438.
141. Teli MGA, Pasquale C, Vincitorio F, et al. Spinal fusion with Cotrel-Dubousset instrumentation for neuropathic scoliosis in patients with cerebral palsy. *Spine*. 2006;31(14):E441-E447.
142. Vialle R, Delecourt C, Morin C. Surgical treatment of scoliosis with pelvic obliquity in cerebral palsy: the influence of intraoperative traction. *Spine*. 2006;31:1461-1466.
143. Dunteman RC, Vankoski SJ, Dias LS. Internal derotation osteotomy of the tibia: pre- and postoperative gait analysis in persons with high sacral myelomeningocele. *J Pediatr Orthop*. 2000;20:623-628.
144. Trivedi J, Thomson JD, Slakey JB, et al. Clinical and radiographic predictors of scoliosis in patients with myelomeningocele. *J Bone Joint Surg Am*. 2002;84:1389-1394.
145. Dias MS. Neurosurgical causes of scoliosis in patients with myelomeningocele: an evidence-based literature review. *J Neurosurg*. 2005;103:24-35.
146. Greenberg MS. Developmental anomalies: myelomeningocele. In: Greenberg MS, ed. *Handbook of Neurosurgery*. New York: Thieme Publishers; 2010:249-250.
147. Osborn AG Chiari malformations. In: *Osborn's Brain*. Salt Lake City, UT: Amirsys Publishing Inc; 2013:1060-1069.
148. Jankowski PP, Bastrom T, Ciacci JD, et al. Intraspinal pathology associated with pediatric scoliosis: a ten-year review analyzing the effect of neurosurgery on scoliosis curve progression. *Spine*. 2016;41:1600-1605.
149. Sarwark JF, Weber DT, Gabrieli AP, et al. Tethered cord syndrome in low motor level children with myelomeningocele. *Pediatr Neurosurg*. 1996;25:295-301.
150. Pierz K, Banta J, Thomson J, et al. The effect of tethered cord release on scoliosis in myelomeningocele. *J Pediatr Orthop*. 2000;20:362-365.
151. Chern JJ, Dauser RC, Whitehead WE, et al. The effect of tethered cord release on coronal spinal balance in tight filum terminale. *Spine*. 2011;36:E944-E949.

152. Muller EB, Nordwall A. Brace treatment of scoliosis in children with myelomeningocele. *Spine*. 1994;19:151-155.
153. Sponseller PD, Young AT, Sarwark JF, et al. Anterior only fusion for scoliosis in patients with myelomeningocele. *Clin Orthop Relat Res*. 1999;364:117-124.
154. Basobas L, Mardjetko S, Hammerberg K, et al. Selective anterior fusion and instrumentation for the treatment of neuromuscular scoliosis. *Spine*. 2003;28:S245-S248.
155. Banit DM, Iwinski HJ Jr, Talwalkar V, et al. Posterior spinal fusion in paralytic scoliosis and myelomeningocele. *J Pediatr Orthop*. 2001;21:117-125.
156. Parsch D, Geiger F, Brocai DR, et al. Surgical management of paralytic scoliosis in myelomeningocele. *J Pediatr Orthop B*. 2001;10:10-17.
157. Lindseth RE, Dias LS, Drennan JC. Myelomeningocele. *Instr Course Lect*. 1991;40:271-291.
158. Wild A, Haak H, Kumar M, et al. Is sacral instrumentation mandatory to address pelvic obliquity in neuromuscular thoracolumbar scoliosis due to myelomeningocele? *Spine*. 2001;26:E325-E329.
159. Thomsen M, Lang RD, Carstens C. Results of kyphectomy with the technique of Warner and Fackler in children with myelodysplasia. *J Pediatr Orthop B*. 2000;9:143-147.
160. Geiger F, Parsch D, Carstens C. Complications of scoliosis surgery in children with myelomeningocele. *Eur Spine J*. 1999;8:22-26.
161. Ward WT, Wenger DR, Roach JW. Surgical correction of myelomeningocele scoliosis: a critical appraisal of various spinal instrumentation systems. *J Pediatr Orthop*. 1989;9:262-268.
162. Nolden MT, Sarwark JF, Vora A, et al. A kyphectomy technique with reduced perioperative morbidity for myelomeningocele kyphosis. *Spine*. 2002;27:1807-1813.
163. Ko AL, Song K, Ellenbogen RG, et al. Retrospective review of multilevel spinal fusion combined with spinal cord transection for treatment of kyphoscoliosis in pediatric myelomeningocele patients. *Spine*. 2007;32:2493-2501.
164. Kocaoglu B, Erol B, Akgulle H, et al. Combination of Luque instrumentation with polyaxial screws in the treatment of myelomeningocele kyphosis. *J Spinal Disord Tech*. 2008;21:199-204.
165. Dubowitz V. Benign infantile spinal muscular atrophy. *Dev Med Child Neurol*. 1974;16:672-675.
166. Evans GA, Drennan JC, Russman BS. Functional classification and orthopaedic management of spinal muscular atrophy. *J Bone Joint Surg Br*. 1981;63:516-522.
167. Tangsrud SE, Carlsen KC, Lund-Petersen I, et al. Lung function measurements in young children with spinal muscle atrophy: a cross sectional survey on the effect of position and bracing. *Arch Dis Child*. 2001;84:521-524.
168. Sucato DJ. Spine deformity in spinal muscular atrophy. *J Bone Joint Surg Am*. 2007;89(suppl 1):148-154.
169. Merlini L, Granata C, Bonfiglioli S, et al. Scoliosis in spinal muscular atrophy: natural history and management. *Dev Med Child Neurol*. 1989;31:501-508.
170. Schwentker EP, Gibson DA. The orthopaedic aspects of spinal muscular atrophy. *J Bone Joint Surg Am*. 1976;58:32-38.
171. Granata C, Merlini L, Magni E, et al. Spinal muscular atrophy: natural history and orthopaedic treatment of scoliosis. *Spine*. 1989;14:760-762.
172. Brown JC, Zeller JL, Swank SM, et al. Surgical and functional results of spine fusion in spinal muscular atrophy. *Spine*. 1989;14:763-770.
173. Bentley G, Haddad F, Bull TM, et al. The treatment of scoliosis in muscular dystrophy using modified Luque and Harrington-Luque instrumentation. *J Bone Joint Surg Br*. 2001;83:22-28.
174. Furumasu J, Swank SM, Brown JC, et al. Functional activities in spinal muscular atrophy patients after spinal fusion. *Spine*. 1989;14:771-775.
175. Phillips DP, Roye DP Jr, Farcy JP, et al. Surgical treatment of scoliosis in a spinal muscular atrophy population. *Spine*. 1990;15:942-945.
176. Aprin H, Bowen JR, MacEwen GD, et al. Spine fusion in patients with spinal muscular atrophy. *J Bone Joint Surg Am*. 1982;64:1179-1187.
177. Chng SY, Wong YQ, Hui JH, et al. Pulmonary function and scoliosis in children with spinal muscular atrophy types II and III. *J Paediatr Child Health*. 2003;39:673-676.
178. McElroy MJ, Shaner AC, Crawford TO, et al. Growing rods for scolioss in spinal muscular atrophy, structural effects, complications and hospital stays. *Spine*. 2011;36(16):1305-1311.
179. Miller F, Moseley CF, Koreska J, et al. Pulmonary function and scoliosis in Duchenne dystrophy. *J Pediatr Orthop*. 1988;8:133-137.
180. Ashton EJ, Yau SC, Deans ZC, et al. Simultaneous mutation scanning for gross deletions, duplications and point mutations in the DMD gene. *Eur J Hum Genet*. 2008;16:53-61.
181. Biggar WD, Klamut HJ, Demacio PC, et al. Duchenne muscular dystrophy: current knowledge, treatment, and future prospects. *Clin Orthop Relat Res*. 2002;401:88-106.
182. McDonald CM, Abresch RT, Carter GT, et al. Profiles of neuromuscular diseases: Duchenne muscular dystrophy. *Am J Phys Med Rehabil*. 1995;74:S70-S92.
183. Cambridge W, Drennan JC. Scoliosis associated with Duchenne muscular dystrophy. *J Pediatr Orthop*. 1987;7:436-440.
184. Miller F, Moseley CF, Koreska J. Spinal fusion in Duchenne muscular dystrophy. *Dev Med Child Neurol*. 1992;34:775-786.
185. Robin GC, Brief LP. Scoliosis in childhood muscular dystrophy. *J Bone Joint Surg Am*. 1971;53:466-476.
186. Smith AD, Koreska J, Moseley CF. Progression of scoliosis in Duchenne muscular dystrophy. *J Bone Joint Surg Am*. 1989;71:1066-1074.
187. Kinali M, Messina S, Mercuri E, et al. Management of scoliosis in Duchenne muscular dystrophy: a large 10-year retrospective study. *Dev Med Child Neurol*. 2006;48:513-518.
188. Kurz LT, Mubarak SJ, Schultz P, et al. Correlation of scoliosis and pulmonary function in Duchenne muscular dystrophy. *J Pediatr Orthop*. 1983;3:347-353.
189. Kennedy JD, Staples AJ, Brook PD, et al. Effect of spinal surgery on lung function in Duchenne muscular dystrophy. *Thorax*. 1995;50:1173-1178.
190. Galasko CS, Delaney C, Morris P. Spinal stabilisation in Duchenne muscular dystrophy. *J Bone Joint Surg Br*. 1992;74:210-214.
191. Karol LA. Scoliosis in patients with Duchenne muscular dystrophy. *J Bone Joint Surg Am*. 2007;89(suppl 1):155-162.
192. Mubarak SJ, Morin WD, Leach J. Spinal fusion in Duchenne muscular dystrophy—fixation and fusion to the sacropelvis? *J Pediatr Orthop*. 1993;13:752-757.
193. Harper CM, Ambler G, Edge G. The prognostic value of pre-operative predicted forced vital capacity in corrective spinal surgery for Duchenne's muscular dystrophy. *Anaesthesia*. 2004;59:1160-1162.

194. Ramirez N, Richards BS, Warren PD, et al. Complications after posterior spinal fusion in Duchenne's muscular dystrophy. *J Pediatr Orthop*. 1997;17:109-114.
195. Noordeen MH, Haddad FS, Muntoni F, et al. Blood loss in Duchenne muscular dystrophy: vascular smooth muscle dysfunction? *J Pediatr Orthop B*. 1999;8:212-215.
196. Flick RP, Gleich SJ, Herr MM, et al. The risk of malignant hyperthermia in children undergoing muscle biopsy for suspected neuromuscular disorder. *Paediatr Anaesth*. 2007;17:22-27.
197. Sengupta DK, Mehdian SH, McConnell JR, et al. Pelvic or lumbar fixation for the surgical management of scoliosis in Duchenne muscular dystrophy. *Spine*. 2002;27:2072-2079.
198. Takaso M, Nakazawa T, Imura T, et al. Can the caudal extent of fusion in the surgical treatment of scoliosis in Duchenne muscular dystrophy be stopped at lumbar 5? *Eur Spine J*. 2010;19(5):787-796.
199. Brook PD, Kennedy JD, Stern LM, et al. Spinal fusion in Duchenne's muscular dystrophy. *J Pediatr Orthop*. 1996;16:324-331.
200. Hahn F, Hauser D, Espinosa N, et al. Scoliosis correction with pedicle screws in Duchenne muscular dystrophy. *Eur Spine J*. 2008;17:255-261.
201. Mehta SS, Modi HN, Srinivasalu S, et al. Pedicle screw-only constructs with lumbar or pelvic fixation for spinal stabilization in patients with Duchenne muscular dystrophy. *J Spinal Disord Tech*. 2009;22(6):428-433.
202. Modi HN, Suh SW, Fernandez H, et al. Accuracy and safety of pedicle screw placement in neuromuscular scoliosis with free-hand technique. *Eur Spine J*. 2008;17:1686-1696.
203. Guidera KJ, Borrelli J Jr, Raney E, et al. Orthopaedic manifestations of Rett syndrome. *J Pediatr Orthop*. 1991;11:204-208.
204. Lidstrom J, Stokland E, Hagberg B. Scoliosis in Rett syndrome: clinical and biological aspects. *Spine*. 1994;19:1632-1635.
205. Bassett GS, Tolo VT. The incidence and natural history of scoliosis in Rett syndrome. *Dev Med Child Neurol*. 1990;32:963-966.
206. Keret D, Bassett GS, Bunnell WP, et al. Scoliosis in Rett syndrome. *J Pediatr Orthop*. 1988;8:138-142.
207. Larsson EL, Aaro S, Ahlinder P, et al. Long-term follow-up of functioning after spinal surgery in patients with Rett syndrome. *Eur Spine J*. 2009;18:506-511.
208. Master DL, Thompson GH, Poe-Kochert C, et al. Spinal cord monitoring for scoliosis surgery in Rett syndrome: can these patients be accurately monitored? *J Pediatr Orthop*. 2008;28:342-346.

CHAPTER 29

Thoracoscopic Approach for Spinal Conditions

SECTION IV

Peter O. Newton
Kuan Wen Wu
Burt Yaszay

Thoracoscopic Anterior Release and Fusion

Mack et al.[1] and Rosenthal et al.[2] first introduced video-assisted thoracoscopic surgery (VATS) as a therapeutic modality for various spinal disorders such as anterior release for deformities, discectomy, and vertebral body biopsy in the 1990s. VATS has since been widely developed to perform anterior thoracic or thoracolumbar reconstruction in cases of spinal tumors or fractures, drainage of vertebral abscess, and anterior instrumented fusion for the treatment of idiopathic scoliosis and other spinal deformities.[1-3] The goals of VATS are fundamentally the same as those of open surgery but is performed in a minimally invasive manner.

The adoption of thoracoscopic surgery in idiopathic scoliosis aims to improve the spinal alignment and balance in all planes comparable to that obtained with an open thoracotomy. In addition to idiopathic scoliosis, VATS has also been used to perform anterior spinal column release (discectomy) in scoliosis and kyphosis, as well as hemiepiphysiodeses or hemivertebrectomies in congenital scoliosis. As such, VATS may be executed alone or performed as an adjunct to posterior surgery.

The thoracoscopic approach potentially offers several advantages over an open anterior approach, including reduced postoperative pain, decreased intraoperative blood loss, lower pulmonary morbidity, access to multiple vertebral levels, and better cosmesis due to its less invasive nature. However, it is apparent that even after several series reported, VATS continues to be technically demanding and is associated with a significant learning curve. This may be the reason that VATS remains in limited use among spinal surgeons. Although the posterior approach continues to be the most familiar access for surgical treatment in the majority of spinal diseases, VATS may have an important role in a subset of spine patients.

Indications

Scoliosis

Anterior spinal surgery had been frequently used as a means for multiple discectomies and fusion in severe scoliosis or kyphosis, with the aim to bring greater curve flexibility and to prevent the "crankshaft" phenomenon in immature patients. Although no definite guidelines on the magnitude and flexibility of the spinal curvature necessary for anterior release have been established, it has been generally accepted that curves with a Cobb angle greater than 70 to 75 degrees and a bending correction lower than 50% are considered appropriate indications. When sufficient segmental mobility of the released vertebra has been achieved, posterior instrumentation and fusion is performed to make final correction of the deformity (Fig. 29.1).

In 2003, Lenke[4] reported the outcomes of adolescent idiopathic scoliosis (AIS) treated with a VATS anterior release and fusion followed by posterior instrumentation. The mean preoperative curve was 82 degrees (range, 41–125 degrees) and was corrected to a mean postoperative curve of 28 degrees (range, 5–60 degrees) resulting in a mean correction rate of 70%. In another consecutive series studied by Newton and coworkers,[5] 112 pediatric spinal deformity cases with an average preoperative curve of 80 degrees who underwent a combined anterior released fusion and posterior instrumentation surgery were found to have radiographic evidence of a solid anterior arthrodesis in 75% of the disc spaces. The scoliosis correction rate showed a nonsignificant difference between three diagnostic groups, though idiopathic scoliosis seemed to have a trend toward greater percent correction (67%) compared with patients with neuromuscular (52%) and other diagnoses (50%).

With the modern improvement on posterior spinal instrumentation techniques and increased popularity of Ponte osteotomies, more recent authors have started to question the necessity and indication of anterior release.[6,7] Suk et al.[6] found an average correction of 66% with posterior all-pedicle-screw instrumentation to treat severe scoliosis up to 110 degrees. Although modern pedicle screw constructs offer powerful correction, we still believe that thoracoscopic anterior release remains valuable to optimize coronal and axial plane correction and to improve sagittal alignment by increasing thoracic kyphosis in the most severe cases of scoliosis.[8]

Progressive scoliosis in children with open triradiate cartilage is known to be at risk for crankshaft deformity when

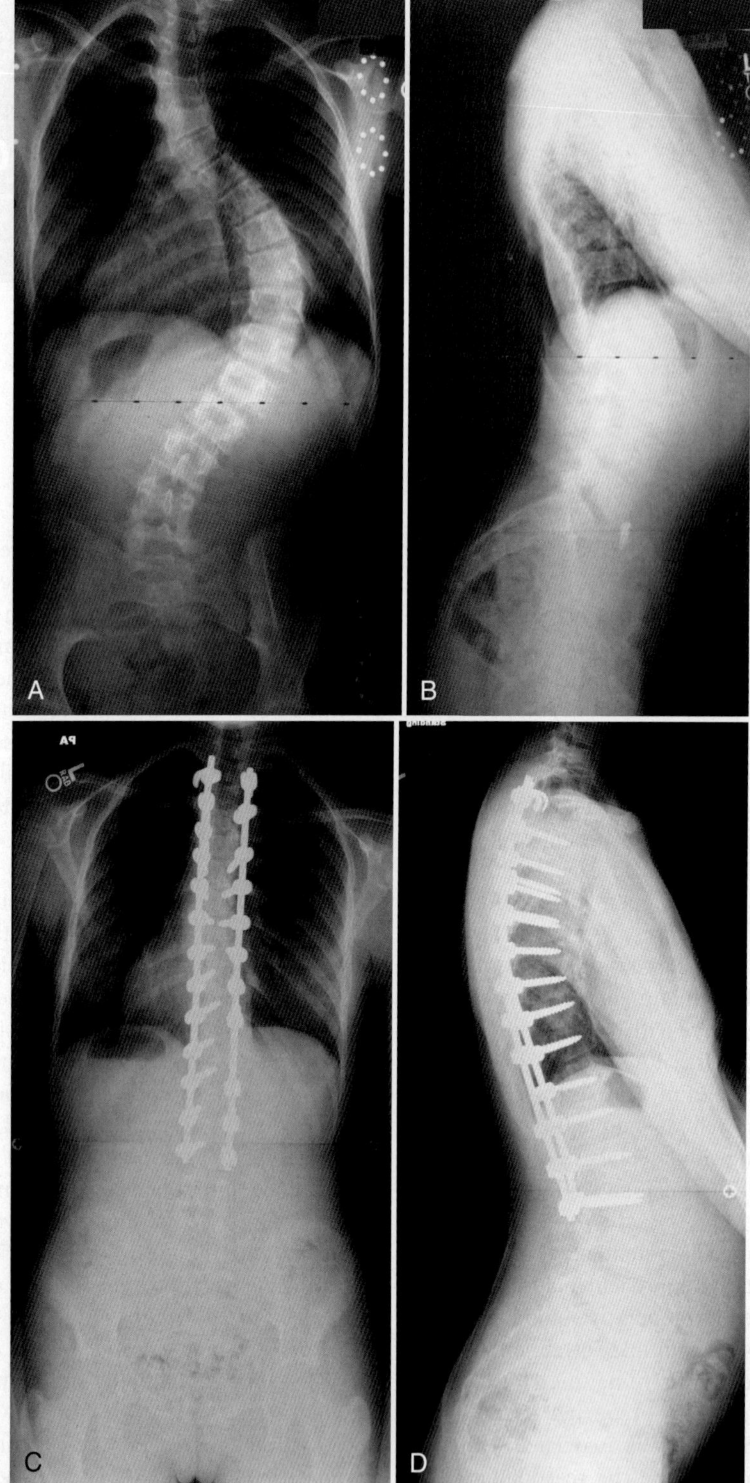

FIG. 29.1 Preoperative (A) posteroanterior and (B) lateral radiographs of large stiff curve. Postoperative (C) posteroanterior and (D) lateral radiographs. Thoracoscopic anterior spinal release and discectomy and combined posterior spinal instrumentation and fusion provide acceptable correction.

treated with a posterior fusion alone.[9] The phenomenon was more commonly encountered for children using hook and wire fixation, but less in those with modern pedicle screw instrumentation. Sarlak et al.[10] reported a 5-year follow-up series on seven idiopathic scoliosis children (average age, 7.4 years) who were treated with all-posterior–pedicle screw instrumentation. The authors found a 57% correction rate without evidence of crankshaft phenomenon in four patients. However, they also found a slight increase of curve angle in one patient and a significant increase in angle of trunk rotation (ATR), suggesting crankshaft phenomenon in two patients.[10] Given the lack of clear evidence on the appropriate treatment of these cases, thoracoscopic anterior fusion may be a viable option to limit anterior growth and prevent this late-presenting deformity in these youngest of patients.[11-14] Furthermore, the thoracoscopic procedure has been used in other diagnoses to prevent pseudarthrosis. Previous studies have suggested circumferential fusion with autogenous bone graft for certain syndromes, such as Marfan syndrome, neurofibromatosis, and prior spinal irradiation, because these conditions are susceptible to an increased risk of pseudarthrosis following posterior fusion alone.[5,8]

Kyphosis

Scheuermann kyphosis used to be a common indication for anterior spinal fusion and instrumentation.[15–17] Papagelopoulos et al.[18] and Sturm et al.[19] found that posterior fixation with hook or hybrid constructs alone did not yield adequate strength to maintain correction in patients with progressive kyphosis. Therefore, combined anterior and posterior approaches have been investigated to treat such kyphotic deformity. In a retrospective analysis of 32 patients with Scheuermann kyphosis, Lowe and Kasten[20] found that a combined approach resulted in a 51% correction of the deformity without major postoperative complications. Afterwards, Herrera-Soto et al.[21] specifically investigated the use of VATS in kyphosis patients and found similar benefits as those in scoliosis patients, including reduced blood loss and less morbidity, compared with open thoracotomy.

Given the benefits of modern posterior instrumentation, Lee et al.[16] performed a comparative study between the posterior thoracic segmental pedicle screw construct and a combined anteroposterior approach in a series of 39 patients. The authors found a similar correction rate between both techniques; however, they found increased complications in the combined technique group. In our institution, with the increasing utilization of Ponte osteotomies and improved spinal instrumentation and fixation techniques, we gradually undertook the posterior-only method and have limited indications for a combined anteroposterior approach to those with the severe rigid nonangular form of kyphosis.[8]

Congenital Deformity

Various operative methods have been used for management of congenital scoliosis, depending on the types of vertebral anomaly, location, associated conditions, and age of the patient. Even more of a concern in this younger group of patients than older children with AIS, reports have identified the crankshaft phenomenon, a progression of scoliotic deformity after a region of solid posterior arthrodesis, to be a particularly difficult problem with the surgical treatment of congenital deformity.[9] In a study with 12 years of follow-up in patients with congenital scoliosis, Kesling et al.[22] found that 15% of 54 patients who received a posterior-only arthrodesis subsequently developed a crankshaft deformity.

As a result of the unfavorable results with posterior-only surgery in the past, VATS has been advocated in the treatment of congenital scoliosis.[5,13,23] Anterior arthrodesis and growth-modifying hemiepiphysiodesis are both technically possible through an endoscopic approach. First introduced by Roaf,[24] hemiepiphysiodesis has been detailed more recently by Samdani and Storm,[25] who suggested that a convex anterior and posterior hemiepiphysiodesis is ideally performed on children older than 5 years with a short curve less than 40 degrees involving five or fewer vertebrae. In this combined hemiepiphysiodesis procedure, the convex halves of the discs were removed anteriorly, followed by a posterior arthrodesis and casting.[26] In addition, hemivertebrae at a lower thoracic level may occasionally be indicated for excision. In such a situation, performing a thoracoscopic surgery anterior hemivertebra excision is feasible in a combined-approach fashion. It should be noted that for children who are younger than 5 years who require anterior fusion over few levels of the spine, the benefit from a thoracoscopic approach may be limited. The use of VATS in these small patients must be considered on an individual basis.

Contraindications

As mentioned, the small size of the patient is a relative contraindication to thoracoscopy. Lung deflation is more difficult in these cases because standard-size double-lumen and bronchial blocking endotracheal tubes are too large. Another restriction is the markedly reduced working distance between the chest wall and the spine. In severe cases of scoliosis, the reduced distance limits the field of vision (in that the endoscope is too close to the spine to obtain any perspective) and the maneuverability of the working instruments. A minimum distance of 2 to 3 cm of working space between the rib cage and the spinal column is required to provide adequate visualization. If the distance is less than 2 cm, thoracoscopy is not advised. Body weight of less than 30 kg is a relative contraindication because the relative benefits of VATS seem to be reduced in small patients.[27]

Visualization of the surgical field is mandatory in all surgical approaches, and it may be compromised in VATS by incomplete deflation of the lung or pleural adhesions that preclude collapse away from the chest wall and spine. Pleural adhesions (Fig. 29.2) can be anticipated in patients with a history of prior ipsilateral thoracic surgery or significant

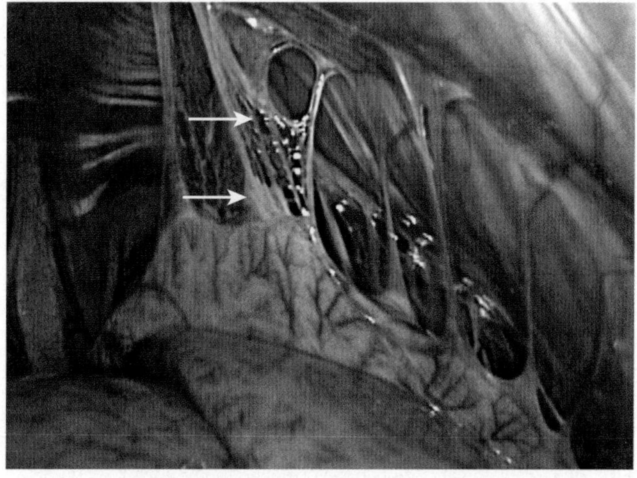

FIG. 29.2 Endoscopic view of pleural adhesions (*arrows*).

pulmonary infection, both of which may prevent the surgeon from safely using the thoracoscopic approach.

Surgical Technique

There are a number of special equipment needs for the safe performance of thoracoscopic surgery. High-quality endoscopes (10-mm diameter and 0-, 3-, and 45-degree angled optics), video camera, light source, and monitor have become standard in nearly all modern operating rooms. We prefer to have the surgeon and assistants stand anterior to the patient. An endoscopic suction-irrigation device, an ultrasonic dissector, and electrocautery are positioned at the head of the operating table. The operating table must be compatible with use of the image intensifier.

The patient is secured in a direct lateral position over an axillary roll with the convex side of the scoliosis up (Fig. 29.3). Some authors have suggested that prone positioning may be possible in select cases, which avoids the need to reposition the patient for the posterior procedure and allows anterior release and posterior instrumentation simultaneously.[28–30] Although the ability to convert to an open approach may be restricted, it has been shown that the prone position does not adversely affect postoperative pulmonary function.[31] This approach necessitates a more posterior portal placement strategy that may limit the anterior extent of spinal exposure and disc excision.

The role of the anesthesiologist is crucial in the success and safety of thoracoscopic surgery.[32] Spinal cord monitoring is advised using somatosensory and transcranial motor evoked potentials. Complete ipsilateral lung deflation is essential to prevent lung parenchymal injury from passing instruments and to allow visualization of the spine. Double-lumen endotracheal tubes are preferred in patients large enough (>45 kg) to accept these devices. In children (<45 kg), selective intubation of a single lung is often required as an alternative. A small balloon advanced into the main stem bronchus blocks ventilation to the lung on the operative side. In nearly all patients with normal preoperative pulmonary function, single-lung ventilation can be tolerated. The surgeon and anesthesiologist should be aware of the increased risk of developing postoperative mucous plugs as a result of single-lung ventilation.

After lung deflation, plastic tubular portals are established through the chest wall (Fig. 29.4). The orientation of these portals may vary depending on the pathology, although in most cases of deformity release and fusion, they are best placed in a linear relationship along the anterior axillary line. Owing to the site of diaphragm insertion, the inferior portals require a slightly more posterior placement to maintain an intrathoracic position. Initial exposure of the spine often requires gentle retraction of the lung, at least until it becomes completely atelectatic (Fig. 29.5). A fan retractor is often required early in the procedure before complete atelectasis of the lung has occurred. The vasculature, including the azygos vein and subclavian artery, is identified before the introduction of surgical instruments to prevent inadvertent injury (Fig. 29.6). The vertebral levels are selected by identifying the first rib partially hidden beneath the subclavian artery, counting down distally (Fig. 29.7) and confirming with a radiographic

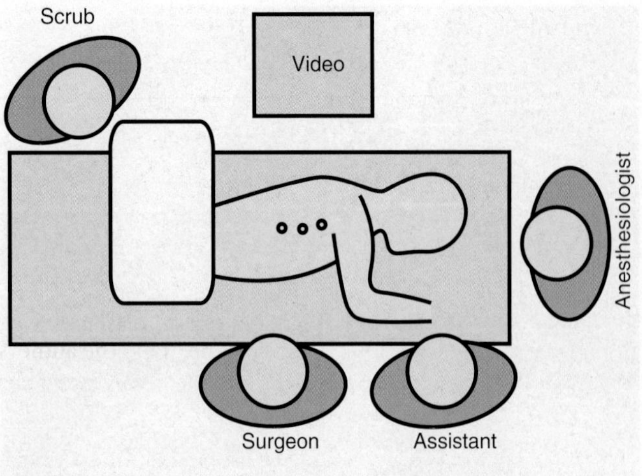

FIG. 29.3 Diagrammatic setup in the operating room shows position of surgeon, assistants, scrub nurse, and monitor for endoscopic surgery.

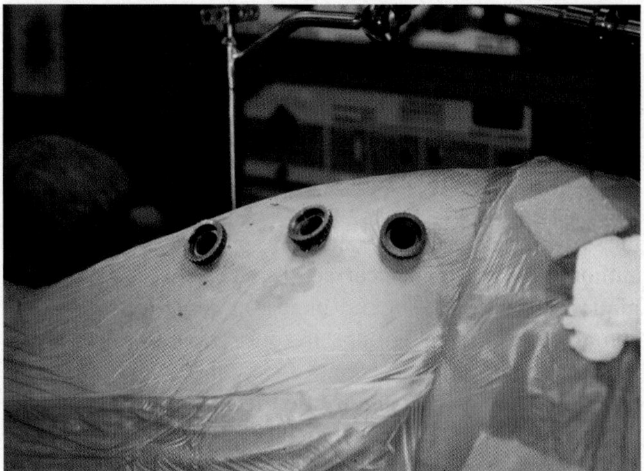

FIG. 29.4 Proper placement of portals is necessary for multilevel discectomies with the patient in the lateral position.

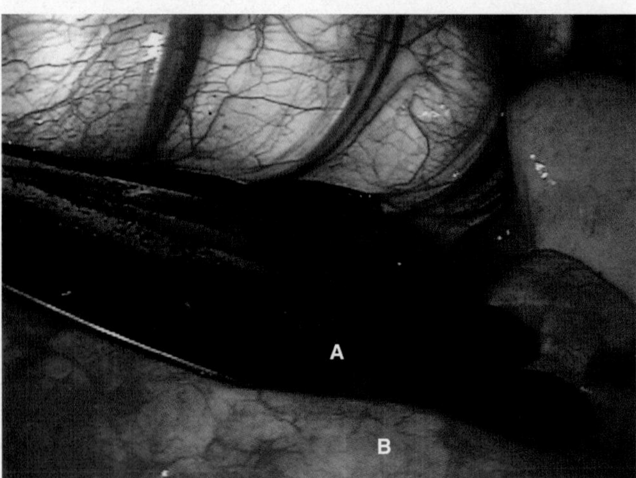

FIG. 29.5 Intraoperative endoscopic view of a fan retractor (*A*) placed on the lung (*B*) to aid in complete deflation.

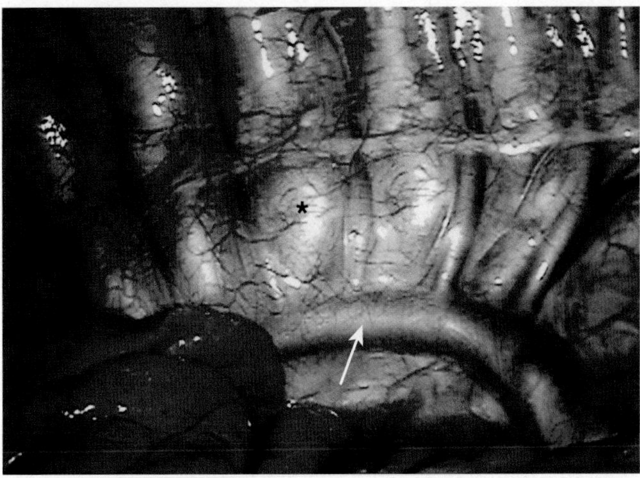

FIG. 29.6 Endoscopic view of the thoracic cavity shows the spine (*asterisk*), segmental vessels, azygos vein (*arrow*), and atelectatic lung.

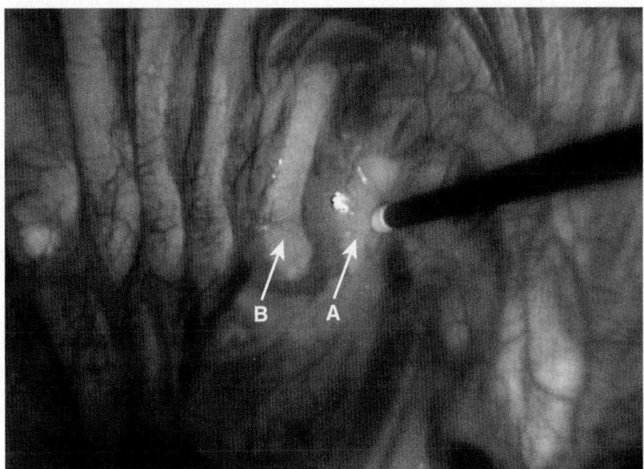

FIG. 29.7 A peanut dissector is used to palpate the first rib (*A*). The second rib (*B*) is most obvious.

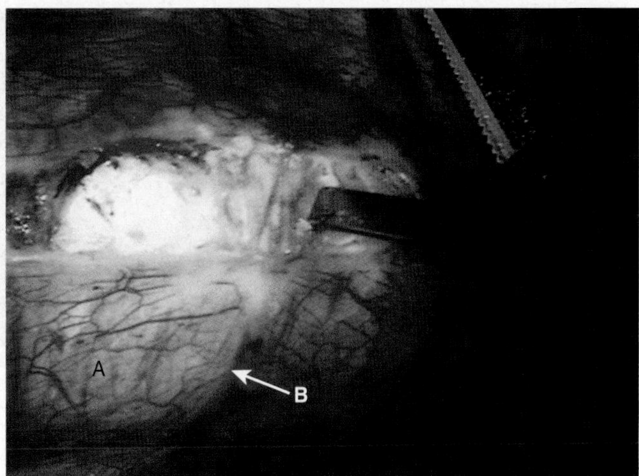

FIG. 29.8 After division of the pleura (*A*), HARMONIC laparoscopic coagulating shears (Ethicon) are applied to the segmental vessel (*B*).

marker. Division of the pleura overlying the spine may be performed either longitudinally, over the length of the spine to be fused, or transversely, at each disc space.

Treatment of the segmental vessels (Fig. 29.8) may be individualized with either division or preservation, depending on the needs of the case or preference of the surgeon. In most cases, we prefer a longitudinal pleural exposure with division of the segmental vessels using harmonic coagulation. Division of the segmental vessels allows greater anterior spinal exposure for more complete circumferential annular release. Blunt dissection of the pleura to the contralateral side of the spine is performed, exposing approximately 270 degrees of the disc perimeter. After division of the pleura, any remaining areolar tissue is divided, and packing sponges are used to create a space between the anterior spine and the pleura.

The accessible levels through thoracoscopy are T2–L1. Exposure of the T12–L1 disc and L1 vertebral body requires division of a small segment of the diaphragm insertion that can be accomplished by extending the pleural incision distally into the diaphragm. The proximal thoracic spine in the right chest is often covered by the confluence of the segmental veins, which may appear daunting at the T3 and T4 levels. With slow, cautious use of the ultrasonic devices, these vessels can be sealed and divided safely, exposing the upper thoracic spine. Disc excision techniques are similar to techniques used in open surgery. An annulotomy is performed with the electrocautery or ultrasonic scalpel. A rongeur is an excellent tool for most of the disc excision. Specially designed endoscopic rongeurs are available in extended lengths with various angles (straight, up, right, left) to reach the depths of each disc space (Fig. 29.9).

Awareness of the discectomy path is vital to avoid damage to the neural elements and to prevent excess bone excision that can cause increased bleeding and suboptimal visualization. An angled curette may also be used to remove residual endplate cartilage and expose the cancellous bony surface required for fusion. Bleeding from the bone can be limited by using the avascular plane of dissection between the cartilage endplate and the vertebral body in immature patients. The key to a comprehensive discectomy is optimal visualization deep into the disc space; this not only allows complete removal of all disc tissue, but also prevents injury to the posterior longitudinal ligament and neural elements.

When the discectomy is complete, either allogeneic cancellous or autogenous (rib or iliac crest) bone graft is placed into the disc space with an endoscopic tubular plunger (Fig. 29.10). The method and type of bone grafting also seems to be important to the success of arthrodesis. This may be crucial only in selected cases. However, all patients are at some risk for pseudarthrosis after posterior instrumentation and fusion procedures. In a study of 112 patients treated with an anterior release followed by posterior instrumentation, Newton et al.[5] compared the grade of arthrodesis between patients who received autogenous versus allogeneic bone graft. The authors found that the disc space was fused in 88% of the autograft group compared with 72% of the allograft group at 2-year follow-up.[5] If autograft is not available, either allograft bone or demineralized bone matrix may be used because they have been shown to result in similar fusion rates.[5,33]

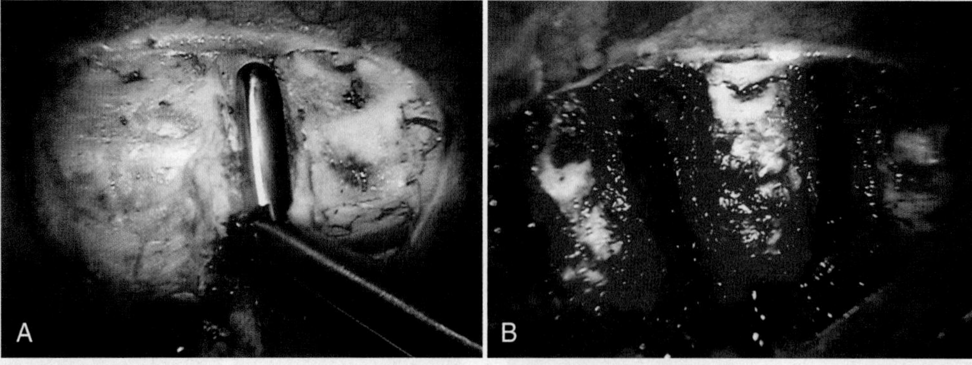

FIG. 29.9 (A) Discectomy can be done with a rongeur or curette or both, with complete removal of the anulus fibrosus, nucleus pulposus, and both endplates of cartilage. (B) Appearance after multilevel discectomies completed. Empty disc space can be temporarily packed with Surgicel for hemostasis control before application of bone graft.

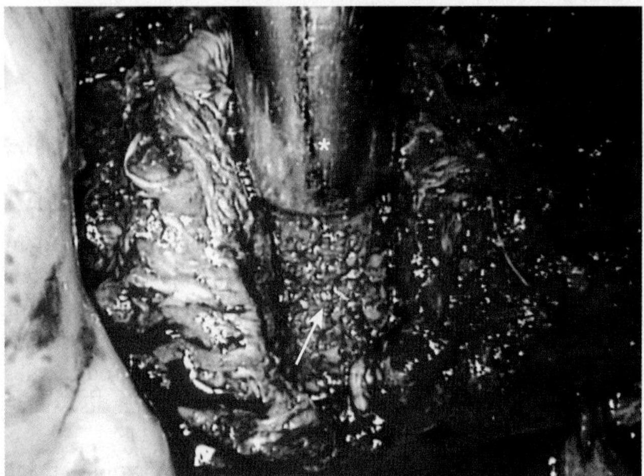

FIG. 29.10 Morcellized bone graft (*arrow*) is introduced into the disc space using a tubular plunger (*asterisk*).

Outcomes

Due to its minimally invasive character, thoracoscopic approach to the spine for an anterior release and fusion has several advantages over the more traditional open thoracotomy approach while achieving similar results in experienced hands. These advantages include less pulmonary morbidity, reduced recovery period, and improved cosmesis. However, the learning curve appears to be steep and operative times significantly longer when compared with open anterior or posterior technique.[14] Several studies have been conducted to evaluate the learning curve associated with VATS.[13,34,35] Newton et al.[13] found that there was a slight decrease in operative time throughout the course of the first 65 patients treated at their institution and concluded that VATS had a steep, but not prohibitive, learning curve. In a more recent study by Son-Hing and coworkers,[34] the learning curve was found to be short with appropriate training and resulted in an excision of a greater amount of disc tissue and a decrease in operative time, while providing similar curve correction to an open thoracotomy.

Several experimental studies have been done to analyze the extent of disc excision possible with thoracoscopic techniques. Biomechanical evaluations of the instability resulting from discectomy were equivalent between open and endoscopic approaches in various animal models.[35–38] The extent of endplate bony exposure has also been shown to be similar with the two approaches experimentally.[35,39]

The clinical results of VATS anterior release and fusion in patients with spinal deformity have been generally favorable but poorly controlled.[40] Although there was a trend in the use of this method during the 1990s, it has since declined in popularity with the widespread adoption of posterior segmental pedicle screw instrumentation. Luhmann et al.[6] and Suk et al.[7] investigated the severe and rigid scoliosis with a main thoracic curve between 70 degrees to 100 degrees and an average flexibility of 45%. Both authors concluded that posterior segmental pedicle screw fixation without anterior release in severe scoliosis had satisfactory deformity correction and prevented significant loss of curve correction. However, these studies did not address the extremely large and stiff deformities, such as curves more than 100 degrees and less than 25% flexibility. In a more recent study of 21 patients with an average preoperative Cobb angle greater than 110.5 degrees and flexibility of 13%, Yamin et al.[41] found a staged anteroposterior procedure to provide safe and effective treatment with a mean correction rate of 65.2%. These authors recommended that patients with a Cobb angle more than 80 degrees and flexibility less than 20% should be treated with a staged anterior release and posterior pedicle screw instrumentation with adjuvant halo-pelvic traction to gradually correct the deformity.[41] Despite recent studies calling the necessity of this technique into question for large and stiff curves, there is likely a subset of patients who continue to benefit from this procedure, particularly if a three-column osteotomy can be avoided.[6,7,41]

The time to perform VATS anterior release has ranged from 90 minutes to 4 hours, with a decrease in operative time as surgeons gain familiarity. The operative time per disc level excised averages 20 to 40 minutes in experienced hands.[13,34] The reported blood loss and chest tube drainage have been comparable to open procedures, with blood loss generally averaging less than 300 mL.[13,34,42,43] In cases of excessive blood loss, sometimes conversion to open surgery may be required. The incidence of major complications for either VATS or open thoracotomy is less than 1%.[13,34,44] The most common complications associated with VATS anterior release are pulmonary, such as atelectasis, pleural effusions, pneumothorax, and excessive chest tube drainage.[13,34,43,44] As with all anterior spinal surgery, these risks exist and must be minimized. There are few studies that compare the effect of variable surgical approaches to the thoracic spine on pulmonary function. Faro et al.[45] compared pulmonary function after an open surgery versus a VATS and found that pulmonary function recovered more quickly with VATS; this difference was maintained after 2 years of follow-up. A large series from Newton and coworkers[46] also showed that 2 years after anterior thoracic scoliosis correction, the VATS group was superior with regard to both absolute pulmonary function test volumes and percentage predicted values as compared with the open thoracotomy group that included a thoracoplasty. Although the instrumentation, techniques, and support for VATS continue to improve, proper training is essential to the success of this procedure.

Thoracoscopic Anterior Scoliosis Instrumentation

Anterior scoliosis instrumentation and fusion surgery has been recognized as an alternative to posterior surgery in isolated thoracic curves because it has the potential to save distal fusion levels, prevent crankshaft phenomenon, increase thoracic kyphosis restoration, and improve spontaneous correction of the unfused lumbar and cephalad thoracic curve.[5,44,47,48] Based on the principles of open thoracic anterior instrumentation, VATS anterior instrumentation has been developed to combine the advantages of the anterior approach and minimally invasive surgery simultaneously. Since the first thoracoscopic instrumented fusion of idiopathic scoliosis was accomplished in 1996, this technique has attracted considerable attention for the treatment of thoracic idiopathic scoliosis. Later, several authors also reported good scoliosis correction (mean, 55–65%) and cosmetic outcomes via this minimally invasive technique.[48–51] However, the superiority of VATS instrumented surgery over conventional surgery has not been clearly proven because of concerns with regard to implant failure, pseudarthrosis, and pulmonary complications. Furthermore, given the learning curve, VATS instrumentation has significantly longer operative times.[48,49]

Although the thoracoscopic approach was shown to have advantages over the open anterior approach because of less postoperative pain and pulmonary compromise, these advantages are less distinct compared with the current posterior techniques.[48,49] Thoracoscopic anterior instrumented fusion is an accepted alternative to treat spinal deformity. Nevertheless, careful patient selection and the potential benefits and risks must be balanced before such surgery.

Indications

Anterior instrumented fusion has been thought to allow greater restoration of sagittal alignment and might be beneficial for thoracic scoliosis with significant hypokyphosis. In general, AIS with a right single thoracic curve (Lenke type 1 curves) and those double-curve patterns in which only the thoracic component is structural can be considered for selective thoracoscopic anterior instrumented fusion (Fig. 29.11).[48,49] Ideal cases are relatively small to moderate magnitude and flexible curves requiring thoracic-only instrumentation between T4 and T12.[48–52] The upper limits of curve magnitude and rigidity for which the thoracoscopic approach can effectively be performed is unknown, although it is generally recommended to limit the procedure to patients with a structural scoliosis curve less than 70 degrees and thoracic kyphosis less than 40 degrees.[48,49] In fact, these cases are also candidates for a posterior all-pedicle-screw technique by current criteria. The decision relating to the best approach for each subject remains debatable and requires more substantial research.

Contraindications

The general contraindications for thoracoscopic instrumentation are similar to those described earlier for anterior release and fusion. The procedure is contraindicated if the patients have substantial restrictive lung disease, particularly in patients with marked hypokyphosis or pulmonary symptoms. Previous abscess, pneumonia, and ipsilateral thoracic surgery may result in extensive pleural adhesions that would obstruct thoracoscopic visualization. Additionally, large and stiff curves (scoliosis >70 degrees or thoracic bending >35 degrees) are relative contraindications. Patients with poor vertebral bone stock or insufficient vertebral size to accommodate the anterior screws are also inappropriate for this technique. Patients with a seizure disorder or mentally disabled patients who are unlikely to comply with postoperative instructions are poor candidates because of concerns about implant loosening with a single-rod construct. Since the visual field of thoracoscopy is limited from T4 to L1, secondary structural curves in the cephalad thoracic and thoracolumbar regions that might require instrumentation beyond these endpoints should be ruled out.[52–54]

Surgical Technique

The operating room setup and surgical instruments are similar to the VATS released procedure. The patient is held in a direct lateral decubitus position over an axillary roll with the convex side of the scoliosis up. After the patient has been properly positioned, a portable fluoroscopy unit is brought into position to ensure that adequate radiographic visualization is possible. Prior to preparation, fluoroscopy is used to plan the position of the skin incisions for thoracoport placement. The three posterior portals are placed in the posterior axillary line that allows screw placement in the posterior aspect of the vertebral bodies. Two or three vertebrae are accessible through each portal. One or two anterior portals are placed in the anterior axillary line to allow access to the discs for discectomy and for the scope as well as to assist in the application of spinal instrumentation.

After the portals are placed, a thorough discectomy and endplate preparation are performed as described previously for the VATS released fusion technique. Spinal instrumentation and curve correction is performed under the guidance of

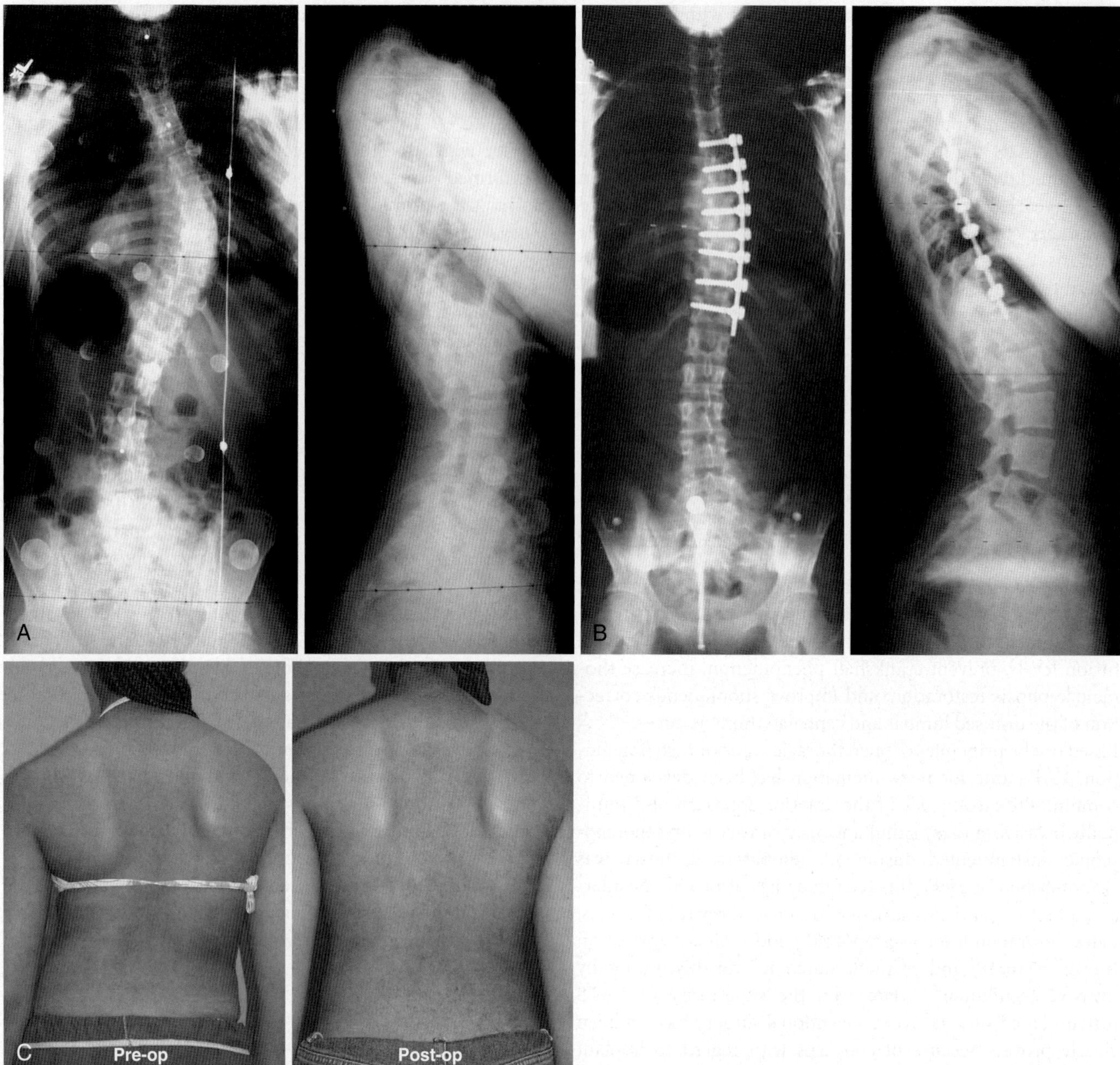

FIG. 29.11 (A) Preoperative posteroanterior and lateral radiographs of a patient with adolescent idiopathic scoliosis. (B) Postoperative posteroanterior and lateral radiographs after thoracoscopic instrumentation from T5 to T12 with correction of deformity. (C) Clinical appearance of the patient before and after thoracoscopic anterior instrumentation and fusion with excellent trunk balance and shoulder symmetry.

fluoroscopy and endoscopy. Either a single-rod or dual-rod system may be used depending on the size of the vertebrae, concerns for rod breakage, and experience of the surgeon. Single-rod systems offer a greater ease of implantation. However, biomechanical studies have suggested that dual-rod constructs are more stable than single-rod constructs.[55,56] The length of the cephalad-most screw is templated on the preoperative posteroanterior radiograph (usually 27.5 or 30 mm); this screw is placed first. A screw path is initiated with an awl and tap, with the entry site in the middle of the vertebral body just 1 to 2 mm anterior to the rib head and approximately 10 degrees of anterior angulation. Penetration of the far cortex greatly enhances the fixation and is mandatory at the proximal levels to reduce the risk of screw pullout. The posterior portals are adjusted to each interspace, allowing screws (typically 6 mm in diameter) to be placed at each desired level parallel to the superior and inferior endplates of the vertebra (Fig. 29.12). Care must be taken to avoid placing successive screws increasingly anterior in the vertebral body because this may negatively affect fixation and restoration of kyphosis. It also potentially places the aorta at increased risk of iatrogenic injury.[57] Although there have been concerns regarding vertebral body screws placed thoracoscopically, Qiu et al.[58] showed that there is no statistically significant difference in the accuracy of vertebral body screw placement in thoracoscopic versus mini-open thoracotomy approaches.

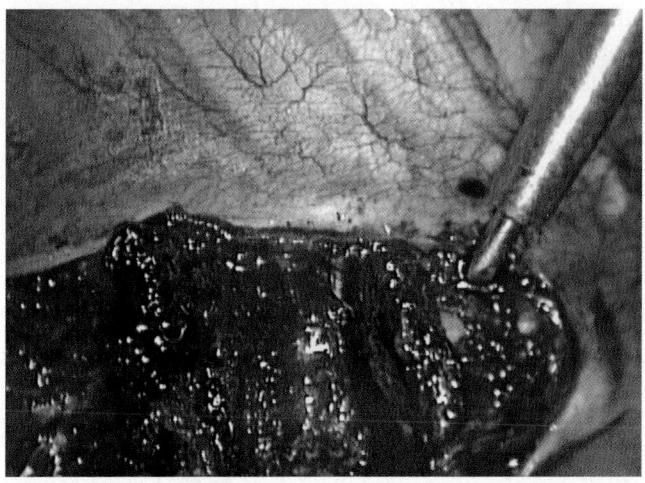

FIG. 29.12 Screws are placed along the path parallel to the endplates.

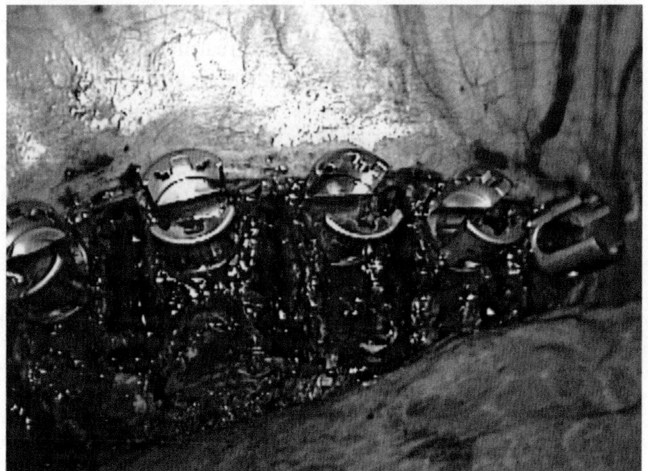

FIG. 29.13 Care must be taken in screw placement to ensure that screws are aligned to accept the rod.

After all the screws are placed (Fig. 29.13), the length of the rod is determined with a calibrated rod-measuring device. A rod of appropriate length is cut and contoured to the desired level of postoperative scoliosis and kyphosis. The rod is sequentially loaded into the screws and secured with locking nuts (Fig. 29.14). Fully seating the rod into the screws may be accomplished with either a rod pusher or the use of a reduction device. Several styles of compressors have been developed to compress between levels. This compression is an important component to the anterior correction of scoliosis but must be performed in a gentle manner, particularly at the upper levels, where screw fixation may be tenuous. Bone grafting is crucial to the success of this procedure. As previously mentioned in the section on thoracoscopic release, autogenous graft provides the optimal base for a solid fusion and is recommended.[5,33]

After completion of the instrumentation procedure, wound closure is initiated. An endoscopic suturing device is utilized to perform a running closure (2-0 suture) of the pleura. The chest is irrigated, and a chest tube is placed prior to closure of the skin incisions. The patient is instructed to wear a

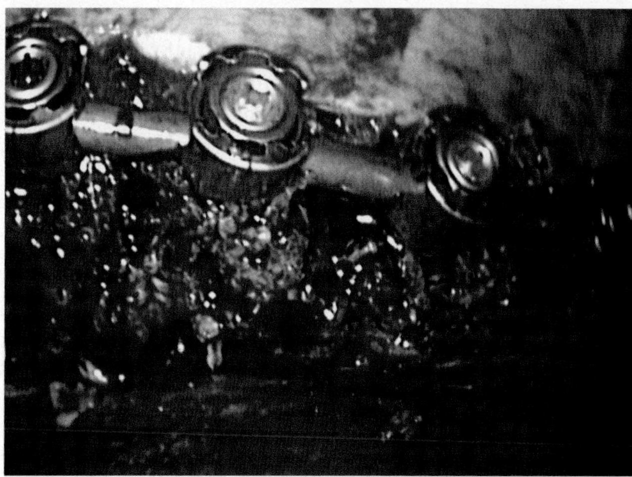

FIG. 29.14 Endoscopic view of a locked single-rod anterior screw and rod construct.

thoracolumbosacral orthosis when out of bed for 3 months postoperatively.

Outcomes

In 1998, Picetti et al.[59] were the first to report a clinical case of multilevel anterior scoliosis correction performed thoracoscopically. Early studies reported high rates of pseudarthrosis, implant failure, and loss of fixation.[54,60,61] After surgical experience grew, comparable results have been reported between thoracoscopic anterior procedures and open anterior and posterior techniques.[47–50,62] In a series of 45 patients with AIS, Norton et al.[3] found an overall curve correction of 87.3% (51.6 degrees preoperatively to 6.6 degrees postoperatively), an average hospital stay of 2.9 days, and a return to school after 2 to 4 weeks. Newton et al.[48,49] reported that radiographic findings, pulmonary function, and clinical measures remained stable between 2 and 5 years of follow-up in their series of 23 patients treated with VATS instrumented fusion. Both series found no significant loss of correction after an average 4.6-year (Norton series) and 5.3-year (Newton series) follow-up.

Although operative time is longer in VATS cases compared with an open anterior or posterior procedure, operative time does decrease with experience. Lonner et al.[62] reported a significant reduction in operative time from 6 hours in their first 28 cases to 4 hours and 30 minutes in the last 15 cases. Studies by Lonner et al.[14] and Wong et al.[63] compared VATS with standard posterior procedure and found a decrease in intraoperative blood loss and a reduced hospital stay in the Lonner study and a reduced intensive care unit stay in the Wong study. When pulmonary function is evaluated, VATS has been shown to result in better recovery of pulmonary function compared with open technique and similar return to function as in standard posterior technique.[14,45] Similarly, in regard to shoulder girdle function, Ritzman et al.[64] found that VATS was comparable to posterior instrumentation, which were both better than open anterior surgery. Further comparison by Lonner and coworkers[65] of the impact of VATS versus posterior spinal instrumentation and fusion on the patients' quality of life using the SRS-22 instrument revealed that patients who underwent VATS scored higher in the self-image, mental health, and total domains despite similar curve corrections.

In all of the aforementioned studies, VATS was compared with a mix of posterior spinal fusion instrumentation anchors (wires, hooks, screws). Although many of these past studies focused on the outcomes of thoracoscopic instrumentation compared with open anterior or posterior hybrid instrumentation, VATS has been directly compared more recently with posterior segmental pedicle screw constructs. Lonner et al.[47] performed a matched-pair analysis of 34 patients with AIS with single thoracic curves of approximately 50 degrees. The patients had equivalent radiographic results, patient-based clinical outcomes, and complication rates with the exception that the posterior thoracic pedicle screw group had a slightly better major curve correction (63.8% vs 57.3%). These authors concluded that VATS offers the advantages of reduced blood loss (371 vs 1018 mL), fewer total levels fused (5.9 vs. 8.9), and preservation of nearly one caudal fusion level. The disadvantages included increased operative time (325 vs 246 minutes) and slightly less improved pulmonary function. Similar findings were described by Lee et al.[66]; the VATS group had a relatively lower correction rate (66% vs 72%), longer operative time, and less blood loss compared to posterior all-pedicle-screw constructs. There was no difference at the last follow-up in terms of pain score and satisfaction between groups, but a loss of correction was significantly higher in the VATS group.[66]

The evidence supporting which AIS patients would be the best candidates for VATS is unclear. Since posterior pedicle screw instrumentation with Ponte osteotomies has gained popularity, the role of thoracoscopic surgery in the surgical treatment of AIS has been reduced.[66,67] The best indication today seems to be in selected patients who strongly desire minimally invasive surgery.

Treatment of Other Thoracic Spine Conditions

The thoracoscopic approach has been widely applied to thoracic and thoracolumbar reconstruction in cases of metastatic tumors, fractures, herniated discs, and infection. The clinical benefits compared with open thoracotomy include the following: (1) direct lesion visualization intraoperatively, (2) less postoperative pain, (3) reduced impairment of immediate postoperative pulmonary function, (4) shorter hospitalization, and (5) cosmetic advantages. The technical demands of treating these conditions may be greater; theoretically, however, any anterior lesion that causes compression of the spinal cord can be addressed with this technique.

Tumor

Of all spinal tumors, approximately 70% are located within the thoracic spine; 85% of these tumors predominantly invade the ventral vertebral body and anterior epidural space.[68,69] With the goals of decreasing pain, maintaining function, and decreasing tumor recurrence, vertebrectomy via posterior only or combined anterior and posterior approaches has been advocated by some surgical oncologists.[70–72] Patchell et al.[73] found that significantly more patients who underwent direct surgical decompression followed by radiation were capable of walking than patients who received radiotherapy alone. The advantages of the anterior approach is that it offers an extensive exposure for tumor resection with direct cord decompression, larger interbody reconstruction footprint and stabilization, and a lower rate of wound complications than posterior incisions.[69] Traditional open transthoracic approach is most commonly used. Nevertheless, it is associated with significant morbidity, yielding an opportunity for thoracoscopic techniques in select cases.[74]

Technologic advances in expandable interbody cages have made the wide resection of tumors and immediate stabilization of the spine possible through a VATS approach.[69,75] The minimally invasive nature substantially benefits these compromised patients, including reduced postoperative pain, shorter hospital stay, faster return to activity, and lower pulmonary complication rates.[69–75] Although data on large series are pending, VATS can be a valuable treatment modality for patients with a life expectancy greater than 8 to 12 months.

Apart from metastatic tumors, few studies report experience of VATS in the treatment of primary spinal tumors.[76,77] With the advent of navigation systems (NAVs) to guide the anatomic orientation and to define the tumor margin, the VATS-NAV combination may have the potential to achieve accurate spinal tumor localization and excision without unnecessary vertebral bony removal through a minimally invasive access approach.[78]

Trauma

The principles of surgical treatment in traumatic thoracic spinal injuries (e.g., compression fractures, burst fractures, Chance fractures, or dislocations) involve correction of alignment, decompression of the spinal canal, and stabilization. However, loss of kyphosis correction and chronic pain have been demonstrated in some patients treated with posterior instrumentation alone.[79] To address these pitfalls, additional ventral column stabilization and fusion may be of benefit in some cases.[80] Beisse et al.[81] reported 371 patients who underwent VATS anterior reconstruction and fusion with instrumentation for spinal trauma. The average duration of surgery was 6 hours, which gradually decreased to an average of 2.5 to 3 hours as the surgeons gained experience and skill. An 85% to 90% fusion rate was observed via the VATS technique; Beisse et al.[81] believed it was comparable with the posterior approach.

With the evolution of implant technologies and imaging tools, the use of VATS corpectomy followed by short segment percutaneous instrumentation has been described as an option in managing thoracic and thoracolumbar fractures.[82] Theoretically, the combination of two minimally invasive techniques can achieve the goals of anterior reconstruction and posterior stabilization while lessening the morbidities related to the open surgeries. Twenty-six patients with acute burst fracture were included in the series and 23 of 26 patients (88.5%) had radiographic fusion at 2 years follow-up. There was no case that required revision surgery due to metal failure, loosening, or adjacent segment problems.[82]

Thoracic Disc Herniation

Disc herniation has been estimated to occur in approximately 11% to 37 % of the population as diagnosed by magnetic resonance imaging (MRI) and postmyelographic CT scanning.[83] Despite a relatively low incidence of disc herniation in the thoracic spine compared with the cervical and lumbar spine regions, a symptomatic thoracic disc herniation may present with any combination of back pain, radiculopathy, and myelopathy from nerve root and/or spinal cord compression. Most patients resolve with nonoperative treatment, but for those with refractory radicular pain and progressive myelopathy, surgical intervention may be recommended. Current approaches for resection of symptomatic herniated thoracic disc include posterolateral and anterolateral (open thoracotomy or thoracoscopy). By convention, the posterolateral approach is most suitable for the small and lateral herniated disc, while an anterolateral approach is ideal for wide-based and central lesions.[84] With increased familiarity of VATS techniques and cumulative experience, favorable results and acceptable complication rates of VATS discectomy have been shown over the past decade.[85–89]

The endoscope provides a magnified view of the entire ventral surface of the spine and spinal cord. Excision of the rib head and herniated disc provides access to the spinal canal, which allows clear visualization to ensure adequate decompression. A systematic review of 12 articles reported complete resolution of symptoms in 79% of the patients and improvement but with residual symptoms in 10.2%. The overall complication rate was 24% with intercostal neuralgia (6%) as the most common, followed by atelectasis (2.8%).[90] The authors concluded that thoracoscopic discectomy was the best treatment in the single soft and centrally located disc between the T4 to T11 level because of its less invasive nature, whereas those with large calcified discs, likely dural adhesions, or multilevel involvement are preferably treated with open surgery.[90]

Infection

Spinal tuberculosis (Pott disease), accounting for 50% of the cases of extrapulmonary involvement, still remains a major health issue in both developed and developing countries. The hematogenous route is the most common pathway for vertebral inoculation. The thoracic spine is predominantly involved.[91] Although antituberculous drugs and bracing are the mainstays of treatment for spinal tuberculosis, they are not applicable for those with worsening neurologic deficit and spinal instability. The mass effect of paraspinal abscess and marked sagittal malalignment due to extensive anterior column destruction are responsible for direct and indirect compression of adjacent neural structures. Through the radical debridement of the necrotic bone debris and abscess drainage, surgical intervention aims to obtain tissue diagnosis confirmation, adequate neurologic decompression, and facilitate fusion with bone grafting. The conventional surgical method to decompress the tuberculous thoracic spine is either the anterolateral extrapleural or open transthoracic transpleural approach.[92] Both approaches are valuable methods for thorough decompression and graft implantation, but high morbidity (10% to 50%) and prolonged hospital stays have been reported.[93]

In the last 2 decades, some authors have suggested VATS as an alternative to treat tuberculous spine infections, reporting encouraging results.[92,94–97] The surgical goals—including decompression, bone grafting, and even screw/rod instrumentation—can be achieved with a VATS approach and provide the advantages of lower perioperative morbidity and early recovery due to minimally invasive access. The rate of neurologic recovery to ambulatory status in the available literature ranges from 82% to 95%, which was thought to be equivalent to the rates following open surgery.[92,94–97]

Although VATS was found to be an effective and reliable approach, there is a tendency for increased kyphosis postoperatively.[92,94,95] Sasani et al.[98] thus recommended the use of an iliac crest bone graft rather than a rib graft to bear more load over the anterior column, and none of their patients encountered the kyphotic deformity at the 2-year follow-up. Excluding inappropriate cases such as pleural adhesions and severe kyphotic instability, the minimally invasive anterior approach to treat spinal tuberculosis has shown promising results in many institutions if performed by experienced thoracoscopic surgeons.

Future of Thoracoscopic Spinal Surgery

The utilization of VATS in treating thoracic and upper lumbar spinal pathology continues to evolve since it appeared more than 25 years ago. It is currently used in a wide spectrum of therapeutic indications, including spinal deformities, thoracic disc herniation, spinal tumors, infections, and other pathologic processes if the lesion position is amenable to an anterolateral approach. Recent technologic advances, including topical hemostatic agents for controlling bleeding and modified bone graft materials for accelerating fusion, have improved the safety and efficiency of VATS fusion procedures. Successful incorporation with high-tech imaging systems, such as intraoperative navigation, has been useful in conjunction with the VATS technique to reinforce the location accuracy. Although VATS anterior instrumented fusion is losing its role in the surgical correction of AIS, the VATS instrumented technique may still be valuable in spinal growth modulation for juvenile idiopathic scoliosis. Gradual correction of a scoliotic deformity has been achieved with anterior vertebral growth modulation using a 4.5-mm-diameter polyethylene spinal tether, a procedure in which the VATS approach may be preferred.[99] Such cases are being undertaken in several centers (Fig. 29.15). This technique holds promise but remains relatively early in development. Presently, the implants are not approved by the US Food and Drug Administration for this indication, and long-term outcome studies are lacking.

When done well in properly selected patients, the VATS approach has clear advantages over open thoracotomy.

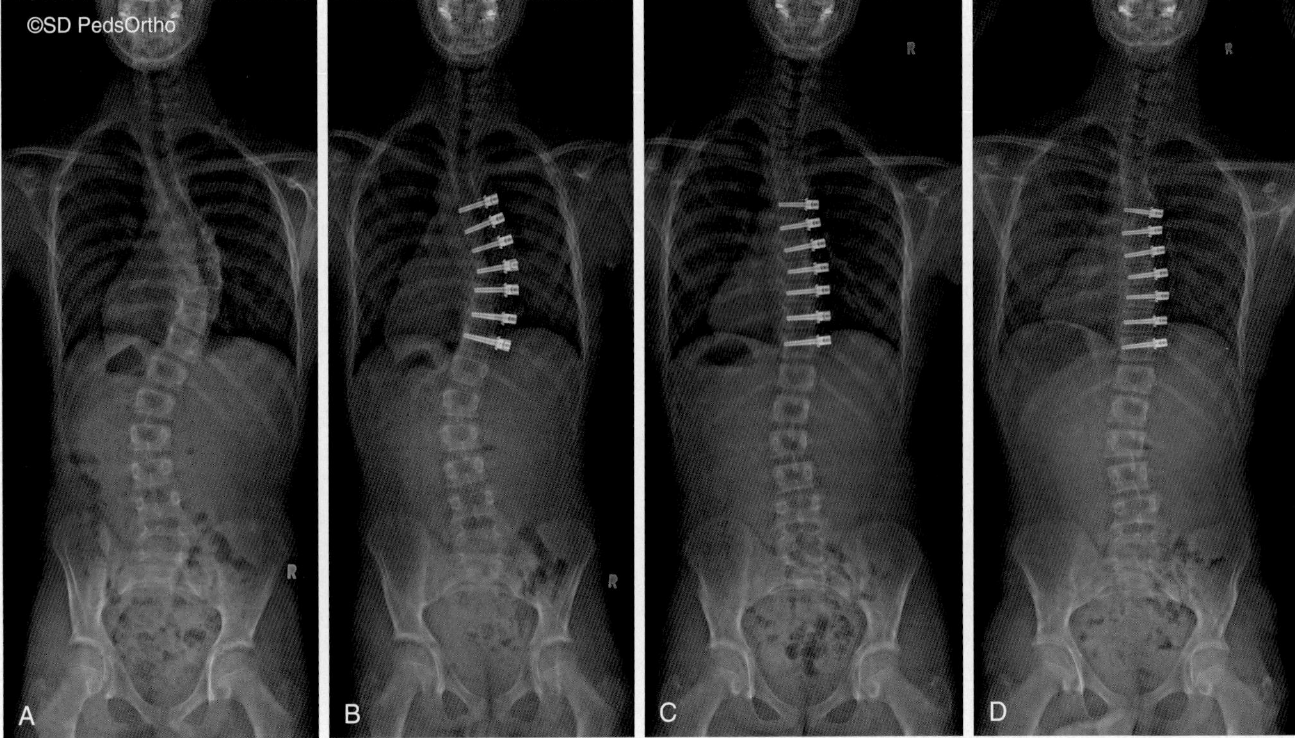

FIG. 29.15 A 13-year-old girl with adolescent idiopathic scoliosis Lenke 1a curve, showing Risser 0 and a T5–T12 Cobb angle of 53 degrees. She underwent spinal growth modulation surgery through anterior thoracoscopic instrumentation, then was tethered by a polyethylene flexible cord. (A) Preoperative posteroanterior (PA) standing radiograph. (B) PA standing radiograph immediately after surgery. (C) PA standing radiograph 2 years after surgery. (D) PA standing radiograph 3 years after surgery. The scoliotic curve continued improvement over time as the spine grew.

However, substantial experience and comprehensive judgment are required. Midterm reports show favorable outcomes using these techniques in a variety of spinal disorders, but further research remains to define which pathologies and patients are the optimal candidates for a VATS procedure.

PEARLS

1. Careful patient selection is the first step in reaching success with VATS.
2. Positioning of the patient is crucial; otherwise, the surgeon may be misled about spinal orientation and misplace instrumentation.
3. Portal placement should be optimized to facilitate the working range of the surgical instruments.
4. Adequate visualization can be obtained by complete lung deflation and meticulous hemostasis.
5. Surgeons should master anterior released discectomy and fusion before attempting to use fully endoscopic anterior instrumentation.

PITFALLS

1. Parenchymal lung injury can result from incomplete atelectasis.
2. Loss of perspective or orientation within the chest can be avoided by looking through the portal directly.
3. The surgeon can control bleeding from segmental vessels with a HARMONIC scalpel (Ethicon), bone bleeding with wax, and bleeding from epidural veins with bipolar cautery and topical hemostatic agents.
4. A mini-open approach should be a back-up plan to ensure safe completion of the procedure.
5. Pseudarthrosis can be avoided by performing a thorough discectomy and endplate excision. Complete autogenous bone grafting (if possible) is recommended.

KEY POINTS

1. Thoracoscopic spinal procedures are technically demanding.
2. Although performed through relatively small incisions, thoracoscopic surgeons must have substantial experience to perform similar procedures via a mini-open approach in properly selected cases.
3. Visualization is the key to performing surgery safely and effectively. This is critical in thoracoscopic surgery as well.
4. The addition of a current navigation-guided system with VATS assists in target localization and is potentially applicable for thoracic discectomy, spinal tumors, infection, and ossification of the posterior longitudinal ligament.

REFERENCES

1. Mack MJ, Regan JJ, Bobechko WP, et al. Application of thoracoscopy for diseases of the spine. *Ann Thorac Surg*. 1993;56:736-738.
2. Rosenthal D, Rosenthal R, de Simone A. Removal of a protruded thoracic disc using microsurgical endoscopy: a new technique. *Spine*. 1994;19:1087-1091.
3. Norton RP, Patel D, Kurd MF, et al. The use of thoracoscopy in the management of adolescent idiopathic scoliosis. *Spine*. 2007;32:2777-2785.
4. Lenke LG. Anterior endoscopic discectomy and fusion for adolescent idiopathic scoliosis. *Spine*. 2003;28(15 suppl):S36-S43.

5. Newton PO, White KK, Faro F, et al. The success of thoracoscopic anterior fusion in a consecutive series of 112 pediatric spinal deformity cases. *Spine*. 2005;30:392-398.
6. Luhmann SJ, Lenke LG, Kim YJ, et al. Thoracic adolescent idiopathic scoliosis curves between 70 degrees and 100 degrees: is anterior release necessary? *Spine*. 2005;30:2061-2067.
7. Suk SI, Kim JH, Cho KJ, et al. Is anterior release necessary in severe scoliosis treated by posterior segmental pedicle screw fixation? *Eur Spine J*. 2007;16:1359-1365.
8. Arunakul R, Peterson A, Bartley CE, et al. The 15-Year evolution of the thoracoscopic anterior release: does it still have a role? *Asian Spine J*. 2015;9(4):553-558.
9. Dubousset J, Herring JA, Shufflebarger H. The crankshaft phenomenon. *J Pediatr Orthop*. 1989;9:541-550.
10. Sarlak AY, Atmaca H, Buluc L, et al. Juvenile idiopathic scoliosis treated with posterior arthrodesis and segmental pedicle screw instrumentation before the age of 9 years: a 5-year follow-up. *Scoliosis*. 2009;4:1.
11. Lapinksy AS, Richards BS. Preventing the crankshaft phenomenon by combining anterior fusion with posterior instrumentation: does it work? *Spine*. 1995;20:1392-1398.
12. Gonzalez Barrios I, Fuentes Caparros S, Avila Jurado MM. Anterior thoracoscopic epiphysiodesis in the treatment of a crankshaft phenomenon. *Eur Spine J*. 1995;4:343-346.
13. Newton PO, Shea KG, Granlund KF. Defining the pediatric spinal thoracoscopy learning curve: sixty-five consecutive cases. *Spine*. 2000;25:1028-1035.
14. Lonner BS, Kondrachov D, Siddiqi F, et al. Thoracoscopic spinal fusion compared with posterior spinal fusion for the treatment of thoracic adolescent idiopathic scoliosis. *J Bone Joint Surg Am*. 2006;88:1022-1034.
15. Lowe TG, Line BG. Evidence based medicine: analysis of Scheuermann kyphosis. *Spine*. 2007;32(19 suppl):S115-S119.
16. Lee SS, Lenke LG, Kuklo TR, et al. Comparison of Scheuermann kyphosis correction by posterior-only thoracic pedicle screw fixation versus combined anterior/posterior fusion. *Spine*. 2006;31:2316-2321.
17. Bradford DS, Ahmed KB, Moe JH, et al. The surgical management of patients with Scheuermann's disease: a review of twenty-four cases managed by combined anterior and posterior spine fusion. *J Bone Joint Surg Am*. 1980;62:705-712.
18. Papagelopoulos PJ, Klassen RA, Peterson HA, et al. Surgical treatment of Scheuermann's disease with segmental compression instrumentation. *Clin Orthop Relat Res*. 2001;386:139-149.
19. Sturm PF, Dobson JC, Armstrong GW. The surgical management of Scheuermann's disease. *Spine*. 1993;18:685-691.
20. Lowe TG, Kasten MD. An analysis of sagittal curves and balance after Cotrel-Dubousset instrumentation for kyphosis secondary to Scheuermann's disease: a review of 32 patients. *Spine*. 1994;19:1680-1685.
21. Herrera-Soto JA, Parikh SN, Al-Sayyad MJ, et al. Experience with combined video-assisted thoracoscopic surgery (VATS) anterior spinal release and posterior spinal fusion in Scheuermann's kyphosis. *Spine*. 2005;30:2176-2181.
22. Kesling KL, Lonstein JE, Denis F, et al. The crankshaft phenomenon after posterior spinal arthrodesis for congenital scoliosis: a review of 54 patients. *Spine*. 2003;28:267-271.
23. Vitale MG, Matsumoto H, Bye MR, et al. A retrospective cohort study of pulmonary function, radiographic measures, and quality of life in children with congenital scoliosis: an evaluation of patient outcomes after early spinal fusion. *Spine*. 2008;33:1242-1249.
24. Roaf R. The treatment of progressive scoliosis by unilateral growth-arrest. *J Bone Joint Surg Br*. 1963;45:637-651.
25. Samdani AF, Storm PB. Other causes of pediatric deformity. *Neurosurg Clin North Am*. 2007;18:317-323.
26. Winter RB. The surgical treatment of congenital spine deformity: general principles and helpful hints. *Iowa Orthop J*. 1995;15:79-94.
27. Early SD, Newton PO, White KK, et al. The feasibility of anterior thoracoscopic spine surgery in children under 30 kilograms. *Spine*. 2002;27:2368-2373.
28. King AG, Mills TE, Loe WA Jr, et al. Video-assisted thoracoscopic surgery in the prone position. *Spine*. 2000;25:2403-2406.
29. Lieberman IH, Salo PT, Orr RD, et al. Prone position endoscopic transthoracic release with simultaneous posterior instrumentation for spinal deformity: a description of the technique. *Spine*. 2000;25:2251-2257.
30. Sucato DJ, Elerson E. A comparison between the prone and lateral position for performing a thoracoscopic anterior release and fusion for pediatric spinal deformity. *Spine*. 2003;28:2176-2180.
31. Sucato DJ, Erken YH, Davis S, et al. Prone thoracoscopic release does not adversely affect pulmonary function when added to a posterior spinal fusion for severe spine deformity. *Spine*. 2009;34:771-778.
32. Lischke V, Westphal K, Behne M, et al. Thoracoscopic microsurgical technique for vertebral surgery—anesthetic considerations. *Acta Anaesthesiol Scand*. 1998;42:1199-1204.
33. Weinzapfel B, Son-Hing JP, Armstrong DG, et al. Fusion rates after thoracoscopic release and bone graft substitutes in idiopathic scoliosis. *Spine*. 2008;33:1079-1083.
34. Son-Hing JP, Blakemore LC, Poe-Kochert C, et al. Video-assisted thoracoscopic surgery in idiopathic scoliosis: evaluation of the learning curve. *Spine*. 2007;32:703-707.
35. Zhang H, Sucato DJ, Hedequist DJ, et al. Histomorphometric assessment of thoracoscopically assisted anterior release in a porcine model: safety and completeness of disc discectomy with surgeon learning curve. *Spine*. 2007;32:188-192.
36. Connolly PJ, Ordway NR, Sacks T, et al. Video-assisted thoracic diskectomy and anterior release: a biomechanical analysis of an endoscopic technique. *Orthopedics*. 1999;22:923-926.
37. Wall EJ, Bylski-Austrow DI, Shelton FS, et al. Endoscopic discectomy increases thoracic spine flexibility as effectively as open discectomy: a mechanical study in a porcine model. *Spine*. 1998;23:9-15.
38. Newton PO, Cardelia JM, Farnsworth CL, et al. A biomechanical comparison of open and thoracoscopic anterior spinal release in a goat model. *Spine*. 1998;23:530-535.
39. Huntington CF, Murrell WD, Betz RR, et al. Comparison of thoracoscopic and open thoracic discectomy in a live ovine model for anterior spinal fusion. *Spine*. 1998;23:1699-1702.
40. Arlet V. Anterior thoracoscopic spine release in deformity surgery: a meta-analysis and review. *Eur Spine J*. 2000;9(suppl 1):S17-S23.
41. Yamin S, Li L, Xing W, et al. Staged surgical treatment for severe and rigid scoliosis. *J Orthop Surg*. 2008;3:26.
42. Krasna MJ, Jiao X, Eslami A, et al. Thoracoscopic approach for spine deformities. *J Am Coll Surg*. 2003;197:777-779.
43. Levin R, Matusz D, Hasharoni A, et al. Mini-open thoracoscopically assisted thoracotomy versus video-assisted thoracoscopic surgery for anterior release in thoracic scoliosis

and kyphosis: a comparison of operative and radiographic results. *Spine J*. 2005;5:632-638.
44. Upasani VV, Newton PO. Anterior and thoracoscopic scoliosis surgery for idiopathic scoliosis. *Orthop Clin North Am*. 2007;38:531-540, vi.
45. Faro FD, Marks MC, Newton PO, et al. Perioperative changes in pulmonary function after anterior scoliosis instrumentation: thoracoscopic versus open approaches. *Spine*. 2005;30:1058-1063.
46. Newton PO, Perry A, Bastrom TP, et al. Predictors of change in postoperative pulmonary function in adolescent idiopathic scoliosis: a prospective study of 254 patients. *Spine*. 2007;32:1875-1882.
47. Lonner BS, Auerbach JD, Estreicher M, et al. Video-assisted thoracoscopic spinal fusion compared with posterior spinal fusion with thoracic pedicle screws for thoracic adolescent idiopathic scoliosis. *J Bone Joint Surg Am*. 2009;91:398-408.
48. Newton PO, Upasani VV, Lhamby J, et al. Surgical treatment of main thoracic scoliosis with thoracoscopic anterior instrumentation: a five-year follow-up study. *J Bone Joint Surg Am*. 2008;90:2077-2089.
49. Newton PO, Parent S, Marks M, et al. Prospective evaluation of 50 consecutive scoliosis patients surgically treated with thoracoscopic anterior instrumentation. *Spine*. 2005;30(17 suppl):S100-S109.
50. Grewal H, Betz RR, D'Andrea LP, et al. A prospective comparison of thoracoscopic vs open anterior instrumentation and spinal fusion for idiopathic thoracic scoliosis in children. *J Pediatr Surg*. 2005;40:153-156, discussion 156-157.
51. Reddi V, Clarke DV Jr, Arlet V. Anterior thoracoscopic instrumentation in adolescent idiopathic scoliosis: a systematic review. *Spine*. 2008;33:1986-1994.
52. Lonner BS, Kondrachov D, Siddiqi F, et al. Thoracoscopic spinal fusion compared with posterior spinal fusion for the treatment of thoracic adolescent idiopathic scoliosis: surgical technique. *J Bone Joint Surg Am*. 2007;89(suppl 2 Pt 1):142-156.
53. Picetti GD, Pang D. Thoracoscopic techniques for the treatment of scoliosis. *Childs Nerv Syst*. 2004;20(11-12):802-810.
54. Picetti GD 3rd, Pang D, Bueff HU. Thoracoscopic techniques for the treatment of scoliosis: early results in procedure development. *Neurosurgery*. 2002;51:978-984, discussion 984.
55. Fricka KB, Mahar AT, Newton PO. Biomechanical analysis of anterior scoliosis instrumentation: differences between single and dual rod systems with and without interbody structural support. *Spine*. 2002;27:702-706.
56. Lowe TG, Enguidanos ST, Smith DA, et al. Single-rod versus dual-rod anterior instrumentation for idiopathic scoliosis: a biomechanical study. *Spine*. 2005;30:311-317.
57. Sucato DJ, Kassab F, Dempsey M. Analysis of screw placement relative to the aorta and spinal canal following anterior instrumentation for thoracic idiopathic scoliosis. *Spine*. 2004;29:554-559, discussion 559.
58. Qiu Y, Wang WJ, Wang B, et al. Accuracy of thoracic vertebral screw insertion in adolescent idiopathic scoliosis: a comparison between thoracoscopic and mini-open thoracotomy approaches. *Spine*. 2008;33:2637-2642.
59. Picetti G 3rd, Blackman RG, O'Neal K, et al. Anterior endoscopic correction and fusion of scoliosis. *Orthopedics*. 1998;21:1285-1287.
60. Picetti GD 3rd, Ertl JP, Bueff HU. Endoscopic instrumentation, correction, and fusion of idiopathic scoliosis. *Spine J*. 2001;1:190-197.
61. Sucato DJ. Thoracoscopic anterior instrumentation and fusion for idiopathic scoliosis. *J Am Acad Orthop Surg*. 2003;11:221-227.
62. Lonner BS, Scharf C, Antonacci D, et al. The learning curve associated with thoracoscopic spinal instrumentation. *Spine*. 2005;30:2835-2840.
63. Wong HK, Hee HT, Yu Z, et al. Results of thoracoscopic instrumented fusion versus conventional posterior instrumented fusion in adolescent idiopathic scoliosis undergoing selective thoracic fusion. *Spine*. 2004;29:2031-2038.
64. Ritzman TF, Upasani VV, Pawelek JB, et al. Return of shoulder girdle function after anterior versus posterior adolescent idiopathic scoliosis surgery. *Spine*. 2008;33:2228-2235.
65. Lonner BS, Auerbach JD, Estreicher M, et al. Video-assisted anterior thoracoscopic spinal fusion versus posterior spinal fusion: a comparative study utilizing the SRS-22 outcome instrument. *Spine*. 2009;34:193-198.
66. Lee CS, Park SJ, Chung SS, et al. A comparative study between thoracoscopic surgery and posterior surgery using all-pedicle-screw constructs in the treatment of adolescent idiopathic scoliosis. *J Spinal Disord Tech*. 2013;26:325-333.
67. Helenius I. Anterior surgery for adolescent idiopathic scoliosis. *J Child Orthop*. 2013;7:63-68.
68. Byrne TN, Borges LF, Loeffler JS. Metastatic epidural spinal cord compression: update on management. *Semin Oncol*. 2006;33:307-311.
69. Kan P, Schmidt MH. Minimally invasive thoracoscopic approach for anterior decompression and stabilization of metastatic spine disease. *Neurosurg Focus*. 2008;25:E8.
70. McLain R, Lieberman H. Controversy. endoscopic approaches to metastatic thoracic disease. *Spine*. 2000;25:1855-1858.
71. Konno S, Yabuki S, Kinoshita T, et al. Combined laminectomy and thoracoscopic resection of dumbbell–type thoracic cord tumor. *Spine*. 2001;26:E130-E134.
72. Sundaresan N, Rothman A, Manhart K, et al. Surgery for solitary metastases of the spine. *Spine*. 2002;27(16):1802-1806.
73. Patchell RA, Tibbs PA, Regine WF, et al. Direct decompressive surgical resection in the treatment of spinal cord compression caused by metastatic cancer: a randomised trial. *Lancet*. 2005;366:643-648.
74. Walsh GL, Gokaslan ZL, McCutcheon IE, et al. Anterior approaches to the thoracic spine in patients with cancer: indications and results. *Ann Thorac Surg*. 1997;64:1611-1618.
75. Dickman CA, Rosenthal D, Karahalios DG, et al. Thoracic vertebrectomy and reconstruction using a microsurgical thoracoscopic approach. *Neurosurgery*. 1996;38:279-293.
76. Mori K, Imai S, Saruhashi Y, et al. Thoracoscopic en bloc extirpation for subperiosteal osteoid osteoma of thoracic vertebral body: a rare variety and its therapeutic consideration. *Spine J*. 2011;11:e13-e18.
77. Gasbarrini A, Cappuccio M, Bandiera S, et al. Osteoid osteoma of the mobile spine: surgical outcomes in 81 patients. *Spine*. 2011;36:2089-2093.
78. Campos WK, Gasbarrini A, Boriani S. Osteoid osteoma of the mobile spine: surgical outcomes in 81 patients. *Clin Orthop Relat Res*. 2013;471(2):680-685.
79. McLain RF, Burkus JK, Benson DR. Segmental instrumentation for thoracic and thoracolumbar fractures: prospective analysis of construct survival and five-year follow-up. *Spine J*. 2001;1(5):310-323.

80. Pfeifer R, Pishnamaz M, Dombroski D, et al. Outcome after thoracoscopic ventral stabilisation of thoracic and lumbar spine fractures. *J Trauma Manag Outcomes*. 2012;6(1):10.
81. Beisse R, Muckley T, Schmidt MH, et al. Surgical technique and results of endoscopic anterior spinal canal decompression. *J Neurosurg Spine*. 2005;2:128-136.
82. Shawky A, Al-Sabrout AM, El-Meshtawy M, et al. Thoracoscopically assisted corpectomy and percutaneous transpedicular instrumentation in management of burst thoracic and thoracolumbar fractures. *Eur Spine J*. 2013;22(10):2211-2218.
83. Wait SD, Fox DJ Jr, Kenny KJ, et al. Thoracoscopic resection of symptomatic herniated thoracic discs: clinical results in 121 patients. *Spine*. 2012;37:35-40.
84. Han PP, Kenny K, Dickman CA. Thoracoscopic approaches to the thoracic spine: experience with 241 surgical procedures. *Neurosurgery*. 2002;51:S88-S95.
85. Rosenthal D. Endoscopic approaches to the thoracic spine. *Eur Spine J*. 2000;9:S8-S16.
86. Burke TG, Caputy AJ. Treatment of thoracic disc herniation: evolution toward the minimally invasive thoracoscopic technique. *Neurosurg Focus*. 2000;9:e9.
87. Lidar Z, Lifshutz J, Bhattacharjee S, et al. Minimally invasive, extracavitary approach for thoracic disc herniation: technical report and preliminary results. *Spine J*. 2006;6:157-163.
88. Anand N, Regan JJ. Video-assisted thoracoscopic surgery for thoracic disc disease: classification and outcome study of 100 consecutive cases with a 2-year minimum follow-up period. *Spine*. 2002;27:871-879.
89. Quint U, Bordon G, Preissl I, et al. Thoracoscopic treatment for single level symptomatic thoracic disc herniation: a prospective followed cohort study in a group of 167 consecutive cases. *Eur Spine J*. 2012;21:637-645.
90. Elhadi AM, Zehri AH, Zaidi HA, et al. Surgical efficacy of minimally invasive thoracic discectomy. *J Clin Neurosci*. 2015;22(11):1708-1713.
91. Ferrer MF, Torres LG, Ramirez OA, et al. Tuberculosis of the spine. A systematic review of case series. *Int Orthop*. 2012;36:221-231.
92. Singh R, Gogna P, Parshad S, et al. Video-assisted thoracic surgery for tubercular spondylitis. *Minim Invasive Surg*. 2014;2014:963497.
93. Ikard RW. Methods and complications of anterior exposure of the thoracic and lumbar spine. *Arch Surg*. 2006;141:1025-1034.
94. Huang TJ, Hsu RWW, Chen SH, et al. Video-assisted thoracoscopic surgery in managing tuberculous spondylitis. *Clin Orthop Relat Res*. 2000;379:143-153.
95. Jayaswal A, Upendra B, Ahmed A, et al. Video-assisted thoracoscopic anterior surgery for tuberculous spondylitis. *Clin Orthop Relat Res*. 2007;460:100-107.
96. Kapoor S, Kapoor S, Agrawal M, et al. Thoracoscopic decompression in Pott's spine and its long term follow-up. *Int Orthop*. 2012;36(2):331-337.
97. Kandwal P, Garg B, Upendra B, et al. Outcome of minimally invasive surgery in the management of tuberculous spondylitis. *Indian J Orthop*. 2012;46(2):159-164.
98. Sasani M, Ozer AF, Oktenoglu T, et al. Thoracoscopic surgical approaches for treating various thoracic spinal region diseases. *Turk Neurosurg*. 2010;20(3):373-381.
99. Crawford CH, Lenke LG. Growth modulation by means of anterior tethering resulting in progressive correction of juvenile idiopathic scoliosis: a case report. *J Bone Joint Surg Am*. 2010;92(1):202-209.

CHAPTER 30 Pediatric Kyphosis: Scheuermann Disease and Congenital Deformity

Steven S. Agabegi
Dinesh P. Thawrani
Alvin H. Crawford

The normal adult spine has four curves in the sagittal plane: cervical lordosis, thoracic kyphosis, lumbar lordosis, and sacrococcygeal kyphosis. In utero and at birth, there are two primary kyphotic curves in the thoracic spine and sacrococcygeal region. The lordotic curves in the cervical and lumbar spine are compensatory curves and develop as a child holds the head upright and begins to stand and walk.[1]

Lordotic curves are considered secondary and compensate for the degree of kyphosis in the primary curves to allow a balanced spine in the sagittal plane. There is great variability in defining the normal range of thoracic kyphosis. As measured by the Cobb method, the normal range of thoracic kyphosis is 20 to 45 degrees.[2,3] Normal kyphosis increases with age and is slightly greater in women.[3] Thoracic kyphosis is measured on a lateral radiograph using the Cobb method from the superior endplate of T2 to T5 depending on visibility to the inferior endplate of T12. The thoracolumbar junction is normally neutral or slightly lordotic (0–10 degrees of lordosis). Any degree of kyphosis at the thoracolumbar junction is considered abnormal. Lumbar lordosis is measured from the superior endplate of L1 to the superior endplate of S1, and normal values are 40 to 65 degrees.

The importance of achieving a neutral sagittal balance has been emphasized in recent years in the evaluation and treatment of various kyphotic deformities. The C7 plumb line, that is, the sagittal vertical axis (SVA) is a vertical line drawn from the midpoint of the C7 vertebral body. This should fall through the posterosuperior corner of the L5–S1 disc space. If it falls anterior to this point, there is positive sagittal balance; if it falls posterior to this point, there is negative sagittal balance. Jackson and McManus[4] reported values in asymptomatic adults with a mean sagittal vertical axis offset of 0.5 cm (±2.5 cm standard deviation). According to these data, offset greater than 2.5 cm anteriorly or posteriorly is considered beyond the normal range. A positive sagittal balance is poorly tolerated because intradiscal pressures increase in the lumbar spine and the posterior spinal musculature is placed at a mechanical disadvantage, leading to back pain.

Scheuermann Disease

In 1921, the Danish radiologist Scheuermann described a pathologic condition and distinguished it from passively correctable postural humpback when he noted the development of painful fixed kyphosis in 105 children.[5] Scheuermann likened the entity to the femoral head abnormality described by Calvé and Perthes, and named it *osteochondritis deformans juvenilis dorsi.* Several terms have been used in the past to describe this entity, including *kyphosis dorsalis juvenilis,* but *Scheuermann disease* and *Scheuermann kyphosis* are the most common.[6]

Scheuermann disease is the most common cause of severe thoracic kyphosis in adolescents, with a reported prevalence of 1% to 8%.[7–9] The prevalence is approximately equal in boys and girls. Approximately one-third of patients have concomitant scoliosis, which is usually mild.[10]

In 1964, Sorensen[11] defined the radiographic criteria that have now become widely accepted for diagnosing Scheuermann disease: anterior vertebral wedging greater than 5 degrees on three or more consecutive vertebrae or greater than 15 degrees combined over three vertebrae at the apex of the curve. Associated radiographic findings include endplate irregularities and Schmorl nodes (herniation of a disc into vertebral endplates). Schmorl nodes are not specific to Scheuermann disease and can be found in various conditions. Scheuermann disease is typically diagnosed at age 10 to 12 years. Sorensen's criteria are typically not present in patients younger than age 10 because the ring apophysis has not ossified before this age.

There are two curve patterns in Scheuermann disease. The thoracic type is most common, and its apex is located between T7 and T9 (Fig. 30.1). The thoracolumbar type has also been referred to as "atypical" Scheuermann disease; its apex is located between T10 and T12, and it is more likely to become symptomatic in adult life.[10] Vertebral endplate changes, Schmorl nodes, and disc space narrowing are much more common in the thoracolumbar form of Scheuermann disease.

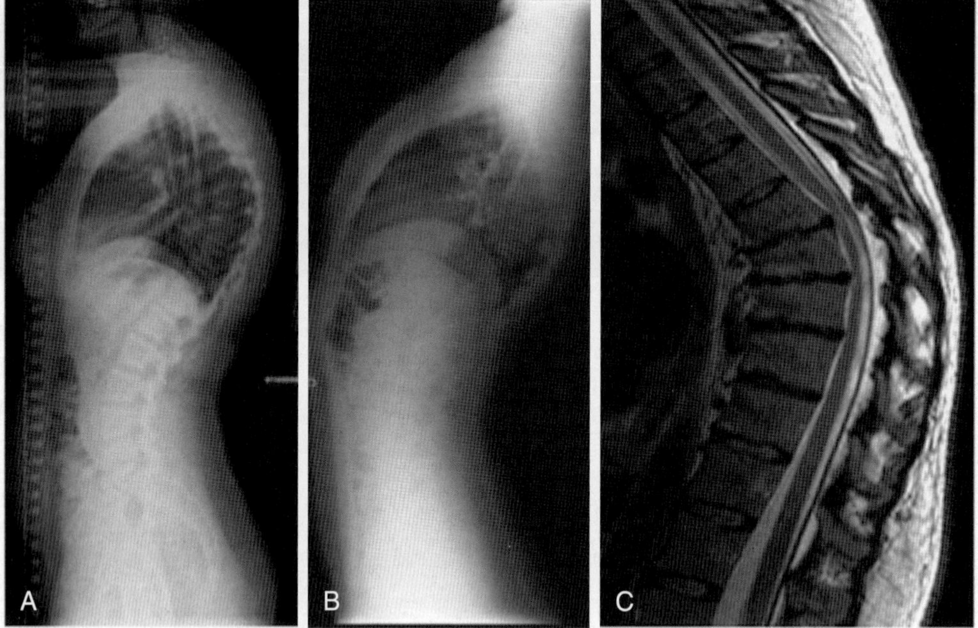

FIG. 30.1 (A) Standing lateral radiograph of a 15-year-old female with arms at a right angle illustrating typical thoracic Scheuermann kyphosis. (B) Supine cross-table hyperextension lateral radiograph. (C) Magnetic resonance imaging showing typical endplate changes at the midapical region with a bulging disc indenting the dural sleeve.

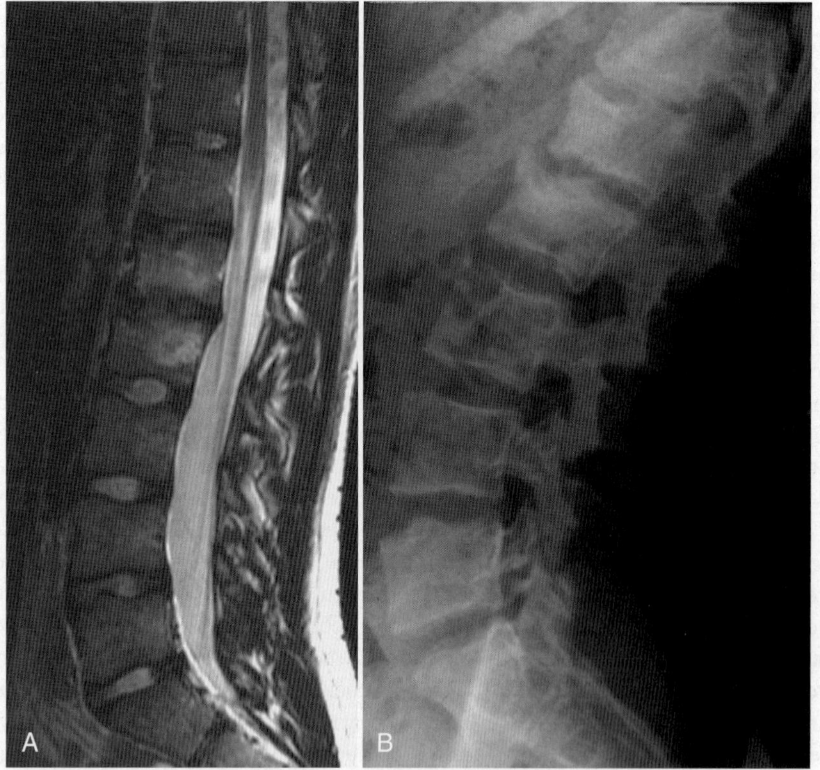

FIG. 30.2 A 16-year-old female with back pain and lumbar Scheuermann disease, with typical endplate changes at T12–L1 and L1–L2. (A) Sagittal cuts of lumbar spine magnetic resonance imaging. (B) Plain radiograph lateral view of lumbar spine.

Sorensen's criteria (three consecutive wedged vertebrae) are unnecessary to diagnose the thoracolumbar form of Scheuermann disease.

Lumbar Scheuermann disease is a distinct entity in which significant degenerative changes are present in the lumbar spine (typically L1–L4) without vertebral wedging or significant kyphotic deformity (Fig. 30.2). Schmorl nodes and endplate irregularities are common. Lumbar Scheuermann disease is more common in males, especially laborers who engage in heavy lifting activities.

Other causes of kyphosis include congenital kyphosis, postlaminectomy kyphosis, myelomeningocele, posttraumatic kyphosis, neuromuscular kyphosis, infections, tumors, and various metabolic conditions. The main differential diagnosis in patients with Scheuermann disease is postural kyphosis, that is, "juvenile roundback," in which the spine is flexible without structural vertebral wedging.

Etiology

Although the etiology of Scheuermann disease is unknown, several theories exist. Scheuermann's initial description suggested that the condition results from avascular necrosis of the vertebral ring apophyses, which leads to a premature growth arrest with resultant wedging of the anterior portion of the vertebral bodies, and mentioned that it resembled Legg-Calvé-Perthes disease of the hip.[5,6] Schmorl and Junghans[12] hypothesized that herniation of disc material into the vertebral body endplates occurred as a result of inherent weakening of the cartilaginous endplate, with resultant damage to the endplate causing growth disturbance and kyphosis. Schmorl nodes are not specific to kyphotic deformities, however, and are found in normal spines.

Genetic factors have also been proposed. An autosomal-dominant inheritance pattern with incomplete penetrance and variable expression in families with Scheuermann disease has been described.[13–15] Three cases of Scheuermann kyphosis in monozygotic twins have been reported in the English literature,[11,16,17] supporting the genetic etiology hypothesis.

Other etiologies of the deformity have been attributed to defective endplates, upright posture, juvenile osteoporosis, increased release of growth hormone, defective formation of collagen fibrils with subsequent weakening of vertebral endplates, strenuous manual labor, trauma, vitamin A deficiency, epiphysitis, poliomyelitis, prolonged sitting, and osteochondrosis.[18–23] Mechanical factors have also been proposed to play a role in pathogenesis, owing to partial reversal of vertebral wedging with brace treatment and thickening of the anterior longitudinal ligament.[10,24]

Clinical Evaluation

The clinical evaluation begins with a complete history and physical examination. The deformity is often attributed to poor posture in an adolescent, delaying diagnosis and treatment.[10] One should inquire about the onset of the deformity and the location of pain. If the patient has pain, it is usually mild and aggravated by prolonged sitting or exercise, and typically is near the apex of the kyphotic deformity.[10] Spondylolysis and spondylolisthesis have been noted with an increased incidence in patients with Scheuermann disease and can be a source of low back pain.[25] There is a 50% incidence of spondylolysis in Scheuermann kyphosis, presumably resulting from increased stress on the pars interarticularis in the lower lumbar spine as a result of hyperlordosis.[25] With significant deformity, the erector spinal musculature is placed at a mechanical disadvantage, which may also contribute to the pain that is common with this condition.

The Adams forward bending test is used to evaluate any deformity in the coronal plane. On the Adams test, the deformity of Scheuermann disease is sharply angulated compared with the harmonious curve of a postural kyphosis. The flexibility of the deformity should be assessed with a prone hyperextension maneuver. Typically, the kyphosis is fixed and remains visible with spine hyperextension, and patients cannot voluntarily correct the deformity.

Increased lumbar lordosis is often noted in these patients as compensation for the kyphotic deformity to maintain overall sagittal balance. It is important to assess coronal and sagittal balance. Lowe and Kasten[26] studied the sagittal contour of 24 patients with Scheuermann kyphosis and found that most patients with Scheuermann kyphosis have negative balance before surgery and slightly more negative balance after surgery. Lumbar hyperlordosis was reduced from an average of 75 degrees before surgery to 55 degrees after surgery.

Tightness and contracture of pectoral and hamstring muscles is common.[27] One should look for cutaneous lesions, foot deformities, or muscle contractures. These may signal an underlying neurologic problem. A complete neurologic examination should be performed. Although neurologic findings are rare in Scheuermann disease, spinal cord compression has been reported.[18,28–31] Causes of cord compression include thoracic disc herniation, dural cysts, or severe kyphosis.

Imaging Studies

Routine radiographs include standing posteroanterior and lateral 36-inch films. Sorensen's criterion (three consecutive wedged vertebrae of ≥5 degrees) is used as the diagnostic criterion. On the lateral view, the fists are placed in the supraclavicular fossa to visualize the upper thoracic spine better. Arm position has a tendency to displace the C7 plumb line. Patients with Scheuermann kyphosis typically have normal or negative sagittal balance, however. It is important to be consistent with the methods used when obtaining radiographs in the preoperative and postoperative periods. A supine hyperextension bolster lateral view is useful in assessing the flexibility of the deformity and can help differentiate it from postural kyphosis.[32] Other radiographic abnormalities that may be present—such as spondylolysis, scoliosis, disc space narrowing, and endplate irregularities—should be noted.

All patients with a rapidly progressive kyphosis, neurologic abnormalities, or any evidence of congenital kyphosis should undergo magnetic resonance imaging (MRI). One report showed transient paraparesis owing to thoracic spinal stenosis and recommended preoperative MRI in patients undergoing surgical correction.[33] Thoracic disc herniations are known to occur with increased frequency in patients with Scheuermann disease.[34,35] The issue of whether all surgical patients should undergo MRI preoperatively is controversial; our practice is to obtain MRI in all patients before surgery to rule out stenosis, disc herniation, or other pathologies. A retrospective study performed by Abul-Kasim et al. showed significantly higher spinal epidural lipomatosis at T7 level in patients with Scheuermann kyphosis as compared to a control group.[36] Further, degree of kyphosis in patients with Scheuermann kyphosis was correlated to the amount of epidural fat. These authors concluded that spine MRI should be routinely performed to screen each Scheuermann kyphosis patient to avoid impending neurologic injury during the surgery.[36]

Natural History

Several early studies suggested an ominous natural history for Scheuermann disease, with significant back pain, embarrassment about physical appearance, interference with social functioning, and cardiopulmonary failure.[11,37–41] Ponte and colleagues[37] showed in their series that all curves greater than 45 degrees in skeletally immature patients progressed during the adolescent growth spurt and continued to increase after age 30 years. Sorensen[11] reported a 50% incidence of pain during the adolescent growth spurt, and a high rate of pain was noted in patients with kyphosis greater than 60 degrees.[38] Other studies noted the often unremitting and incapacitating nature of the pain, progressive nature of the deformity, risk of cardiopulmonary failure, and unacceptable appearance of the deformity in untreated adults.[39–41] Aggressive surgical treatment was recommended to prevent these problems in the future.[41]

In 1993, Murray and colleagues[18] provided the first long-term follow-up study on the natural history of untreated Scheuermann disease in patients with an average age of 53 years and average kyphosis of 71 degrees. These investigators found that 64% of patients (compared with 15% of controls) reported back pain. The proportion of patients who had pain that interfered with their daily lives was not significantly different from control subjects, however. Their data suggested that, although patients with Scheuermann disease may have some functional limitations, they do not have major interference with their lives. Murray and colleagues[18] also found that their patients adapted reasonably well to this condition and recommended that surgical treatment should be carefully reviewed. Other reports have also suggested the generally benign natural history of this condition.[42–44]

The natural history is more favorable when the deformity is in the thoracic spine rather than the thoracolumbar spine. Back pain is more common in the latter. It is believed that thoracic kyphosis, compared with thoracolumbar kyphosis, has a lower incidence of progression because of the support provided by the surrounding rib cage.[45] When a thoracolumbar kyphosis exceeds 50 to 55 degrees, the deformity is readily apparent, especially in thin patients, and pain is common.[45] The thoracolumbar spine is typically neutral to slightly lordotic, and any degree of kyphosis may be clinically apparent. In adults, degenerative disc disease is frequently seen at the apical segments of the kyphosis and may be a source of back pain.[46,47]

Although progression of deformity can be rapid during the adolescent growth spurt, it is unknown whether the deformity would progress after skeletal maturity is reached. Thoracic curves greater than 80 degrees and thoracolumbar curves greater than 55 to 60 degrees may be at risk of progression after skeletal maturity, although the true incidence of progression is unknown.[10,45] If nonsurgical treatment is chosen for curves of this magnitude, periodic follow-up is recommended into adulthood.

Pulmonary failure secondary to severe deformity is very rare. Murray and colleagues[18] found that lung volume, lung mechanics, and diffusing capacity were not significantly affected and were normal in patients with curves less than 100 degrees. They found that as the deformity reaches 100 degrees, restrictive lung disease occurs more often when the curve apex is between T1 and T8.

Nonsurgical Treatment

Nonoperative treatment consists of observation, exercise, and physical therapy, or bracing and casting. As is the case with the management of all spinal deformities, diligent observation is the mainstay of nonoperative treatment. In a skeletally immature patient with a mild deformity, periodic observation every 6 months is recommended to document progression. Exercise and physical therapy are useful to treat associated back pain and to improve muscle tone and posture. There is no evidence that exercise improves the kyphotic deformity or reverses endplate changes. Adolescents with kyphosis less than 60 degrees are treated with a physical therapy and exercise program, with periodic radiographs until the patient is skeletally mature. Most adults with untreated Scheuermann disease respond well to a back exercise program if the kyphosis is not severe.

Applying a brace to a patient with Scheuermann kyphosis tends to be more challenging than applying one to a patient with idiopathic scoliosis. The apex of a typical thoracic Scheuermann kyphosis is usually at or above T8; a traditional thoracolumbosacral orthosis (TLSO) does not extend high enough to provide substantial corrective forces. The Milwaukee brace or serial hyperextension casts are the most effective in this regard but are poorly tolerated because of appearance issues. The Milwaukee brace is most effective in a skeletally immature patient with a flexible kyphosis greater than 55 to 60 degrees, who is highly motivated and has the appropriate body habitus. Patients with larger curves, patients with vertebral wedging greater than 10 degrees, and skeletally mature patients do not usually respond to bracing. An underarm TLSO is indicated when the apex of the curve is at or below T11, but in the senior author's experience (A.H.C.), relief of symptoms as opposed to correction is the main indication for a TLSO in these patients.

The use of the Milwaukee brace for the treatment of scoliosis was first reported by Blount and colleagues in 1958.[48] In 1959, Moe began treating Scheuermann kyphosis with the Milwaukee brace.[39] In 75 patients who completed treatment, the kyphosis improved by 40%, and the vertebral wedging improved by 42%. Bradford and colleagues[39] reported that factors that limited the amount of correction included kyphosis greater than 65 degrees, skeletal maturity, and vertebral wedging averaging more than 10 degrees. Sachs and colleagues[32] found that curves less than 74 degrees in skeletally immature patients can be successfully treated in a Milwaukee brace. They reported 120 patients with Scheuermann disease who were treated with the Milwaukee brace with more than 5 years of follow-up; 76 patients had improvement in kyphosis, 10 patients had no change in kyphosis, and 24 patients had worsening of deformity compared with initial studies.

One-third of patients with an initial kyphosis of 75 degrees or greater subsequently underwent surgery. Results showed that treatment with the Milwaukee brace consistently improved kyphosis by approximately 50% during the active phase of treatment, but some loss of correction occurred over time. The final result showed improvement in 69% of patients.

Gutowski and Renshaw[49] reported 75 patients treated with either a Milwaukee or Boston brace. For compliant patients, the average improvement in kyphosis was 27% in the Boston orthosis group and 35% in the Milwaukee orthosis group, despite the fact that patients in the former group were younger and had smaller, more flexible curves. Compliance with orthosis wearing was twice as likely with the Boston orthosis (61% compliance vs 29% compliance for the Milwaukee orthosis). Results in patients who wore their orthoses at least 16 hours per day were equal to results in patients with 23 hours of daily wear. The Boston brace provided satisfactory correction in curves less than 70 degrees and had better compliance. For larger curves, a Milwaukee brace was recommended.

Ponte and colleagues[37] reported on 1043 patients treated with casts for 8 to 16 months, followed by a Milwaukee brace and physical therapy until skeletal maturity. Patients had a mean initial curve of 57 degrees and at 3-year follow-up had a mean 62% wedge improvement and 40% curve correction.

Before considering brace treatment, a hyperextension cross-table lateral radiograph over a bolster (patient supine with the bolster at the apex of the deformity) is helpful to assess the potential efficacy of a brace. If the deformity is flexible, a brace may help. If the deformity is totally rigid, a brace is unlikely to be helpful, and casting may be better. A lateral radiograph in the brace should show correction of the kyphosis to within the normal range (<45 degrees).

If bracing is chosen, physical therapy should be initiated for trunk stabilization and postural exercises and to stretch the pectoral and hamstring muscles. The brace should be worn for 23 hours a day. To get a meaningful correction with brace treatment in Scheuermann disease, correction of the vertebral wedging deformity by bone remodeling is necessary. In contrast to scoliosis, in which bracing does not correct the curve, bracing in Scheuermann disease may help achieve some curve correction. After 12 to 18 months of bracing, partial reversal of anterior wedging of vertebral bodies is often noted.[10] Loss of correction can occur, however, after discontinuation of the brace. Montgomery and Hall[24] reported an average loss of correction of 15 degrees in 21 patients 18 months or more after they stopped wearing the brace. Brace treatment initially leads to some correction by opening the disc spaces, which close down again unless sufficient time is allowed to reverse the wedging of the vertebral bodies.

We consider a brace for curves of 55 to 70 degrees in skeletally immature patients (Risser 0 to 2) with the proper body habitus and motivation to wear a Milwaukee brace. A preliminary hyperextension plaster cast can be used to improve flexibility before application of a Milwaukee brace. We generally consider a brace or cast only if the deformity is flexible enough to allow at least 40% correction. In a skeletally immature patient with flexible deformities, we have developed the "four 6's" program, consisting of a hyperextension Risser cast for 6 weeks, Milwaukee brace for 6 months, weaning out of the brace for 6 weeks, and only sleeping in the brace for 6 months. This contract with teenage patients has resulted in improved compliance and satisfactory outcomes.

During bracing, follow-up radiographs are taken at 4- to 6-month intervals, and patients are followed to skeletal maturity. Patients and parents should expect a gradual loss of correction after the brace is discontinued.

Indications for Surgery

Surgical indications for patients with Scheuermann kyphosis are controversial because the true natural history of the disease with regard to curve progression has not been defined. Controversial issues are the importance of cosmesis, degree of pain and disability that warrants surgical intervention, and various opinions on the natural history of curves 65 to 80 degrees. These factors must be weighed against the risks of surgical intervention. Treatment decisions should be individualized after a thorough discussion with the patient and parents.

Despite controversy, generally accepted surgical indications include a progressive thoracic kyphosis greater than 75 to 80 degrees in a skeletally immature patient or severe thoracic hyperkyphosis associated with pain; thoracolumbar kyphosis exceeding 50 to 55 degrees that is associated with pain unresponsive to conservative treatment; progression of deformity despite bracing; and cosmetic deformity that the surgeon, patient, and family consider significant and unacceptable. Other factors to consider are patient age, location of the kyphosis, and extent to which the kyphosis is sharp and angular. If the apex is at the thoracolumbar junction, the deformity typically appears more significant clinically and is more likely to be disabling into adulthood because of the inability of the lumbar spine to compensate for the deformity. If the deformity is very sharp and angular, more consideration should be given to surgical treatment. Generally, pulmonary or neurologic compromise does not occur until the curve is greater than 100 degrees, and these are rarely indications for surgery.

Neurologic compromise is an indication for surgery, but it rarely occurs in Scheuermann disease. Cord compression may be due to disc herniation at the apex, severe kyphosis, and extradural cysts.[34] Similarly, pulmonary compromise is rare and does not occur until the curve is greater than 100 degrees.[7,18,41,44]

Surgical Treatment

The surgical options for Scheuermann disease include posterior-only correction and fusion, combined anterior and posterior fusion, and anterior-only procedures. Historically, the surgical treatment of Scheuermann disease consisted of apical anterior release and fusion followed by posterior fusion. This approach originated from work by Bradford and colleagues[50] in 1975, in which they found an unacceptably high rate of correction loss after posterior-only fusion with Harrington compression instrumentation. These investigators reported a 9% pseudarthrosis rate and 23% risk of instrumentation complications. In 1980, work from the same institution showed solid fusion and good maintenance of correction with anterior release and fusion followed by posterior compression instrumentation in 24 patients.[40]

The efficacy of combined anterior release and posterior fusion is well documented in the literature.[40,51–53] Anterior release traditionally has been recommended for patients with severe, rigid deformities that do not correct to less than 50 degrees on a hyperextension lateral radiograph. With the use of modern pedicle screw instrumentation and posterior osteotomies, the indications for performing an anterior release are less common, however, and even severe deformities are being successfully treated with a posterior-only approach.

The anterior release can be performed through an open thoracotomy or thoracoabdominal approach depending on the location of the apex of the deformity, or can be performed through a video-assisted thoracoscopic surgery (VATS) approach.[54,55] The senior author has achieved excellent results with simultaneous video-assisted thoracoscopic release and posterior fusion and instrumentation in the prone position (Figs. 30.3 and 30.4). The levels requiring anterior release typically include six to eight segments centered around the apex of the deformity. In general, vertebrae that fail to correct over hyperextension bolster radiographs are indicated for anterior release. The anterior longitudinal ligament and entire disc are removed, and the space is packed with fibular structural allograft bone. In very severe deformities, an intervening period of halofemoral traction may be considered between the anterior and posterior procedures.

Anterior release and fusion ensures that correction is reliably achieved and solid fusion is obtained. There is, however, the obvious morbidity of the additional operating time and reported complications, including hemothorax, pneumothorax, and pulmonary embolism.[7,51,56] There may be potential negative effects on pulmonary function, which may not return to baseline even at 2 years postoperatively.[57–59] Although anterior surgery has benefits in achieving correction of severe deformities, the additional surgery is not without consequence.

Over the last 3 decades, several studies have shown good results with posterior-only fusion and instrumentation with various constructs.[38,56,60–63] Speck and Chopin[38] found posterior-only fusion to be adequate in skeletally immature patients, but that combined anterior and posterior surgery is needed for skeletally mature patients.

In 1984, Ponte and colleagues[64] described shortening of the posterior column by employing multiple osteotomies and posterior compression instrumentation and fusion. The Ponte osteotomy (PO) is similar to the Smith-Petersen osteotomy except that it is performed at multiple levels in the thoracic spine (Figs. 30.5 and 30.6). Smith-Petersen's original osteotomy was in the lumbar spine, at one level, in patients with rheumatoid arthritis.[65] After Ponte's description in 1984,[64] this procedure did not gain popularity for many years, especially among North American surgeons, until pedicle screw instrumentation became popular in the thoracic spine. As pedicle screws became more widely used and the ability to obtain strong, three-column fixation in the spine became possible, several studies have documented successful results with posterior-only treatment of more severe deformities.[66–68]

The PO opens the anterior column (disc space), hinges on the middle column, and closes the posterior column by the amount that is removed posteriorly. Essentially, it is necessary to have a potentially open disc space to achieve correction

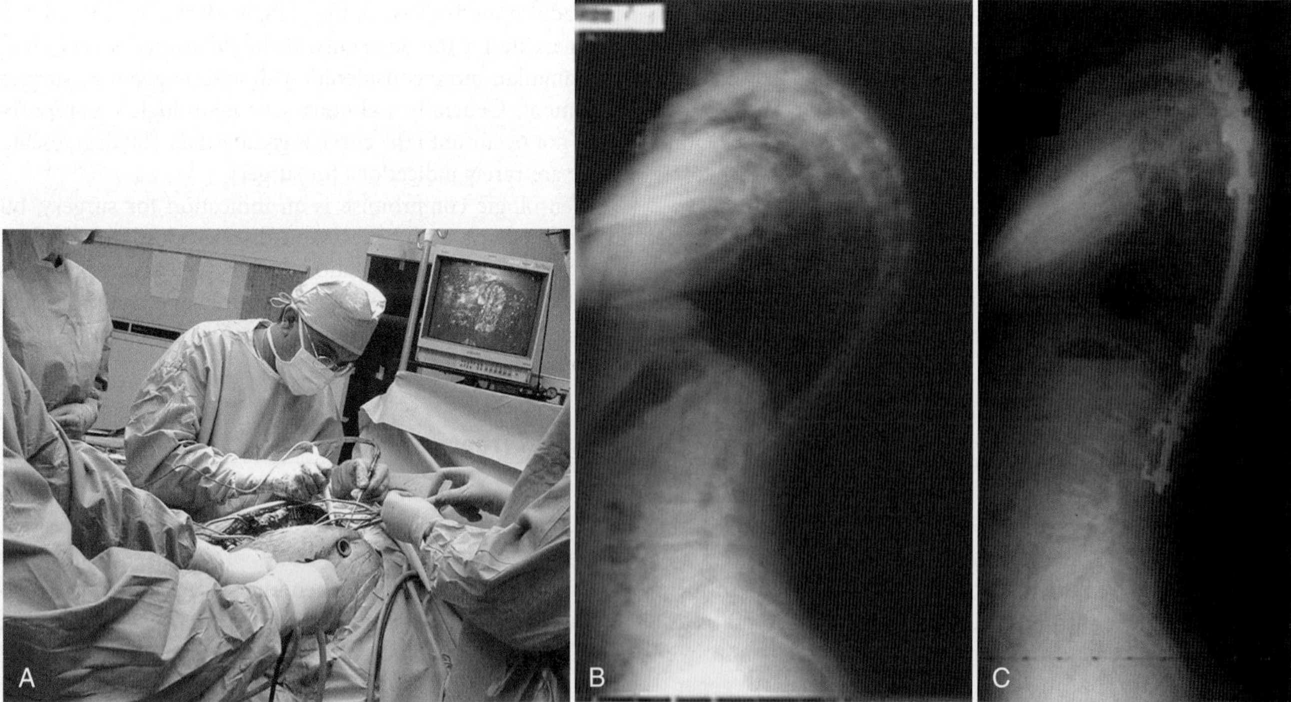

FIG. 30.3 A 17-year-old male underwent simultaneous prone video-assisted thoracoscopic surgery release and posterior spinal fusion with excellent correction of kyphosis. (A) Intraoperative image showing FlexiPort on patient's right side adjacent to midline surgical wound. The monitor at the top shows thoracic anatomy. (B) Preoperative and (C) postoperative lateral standing radiographs.

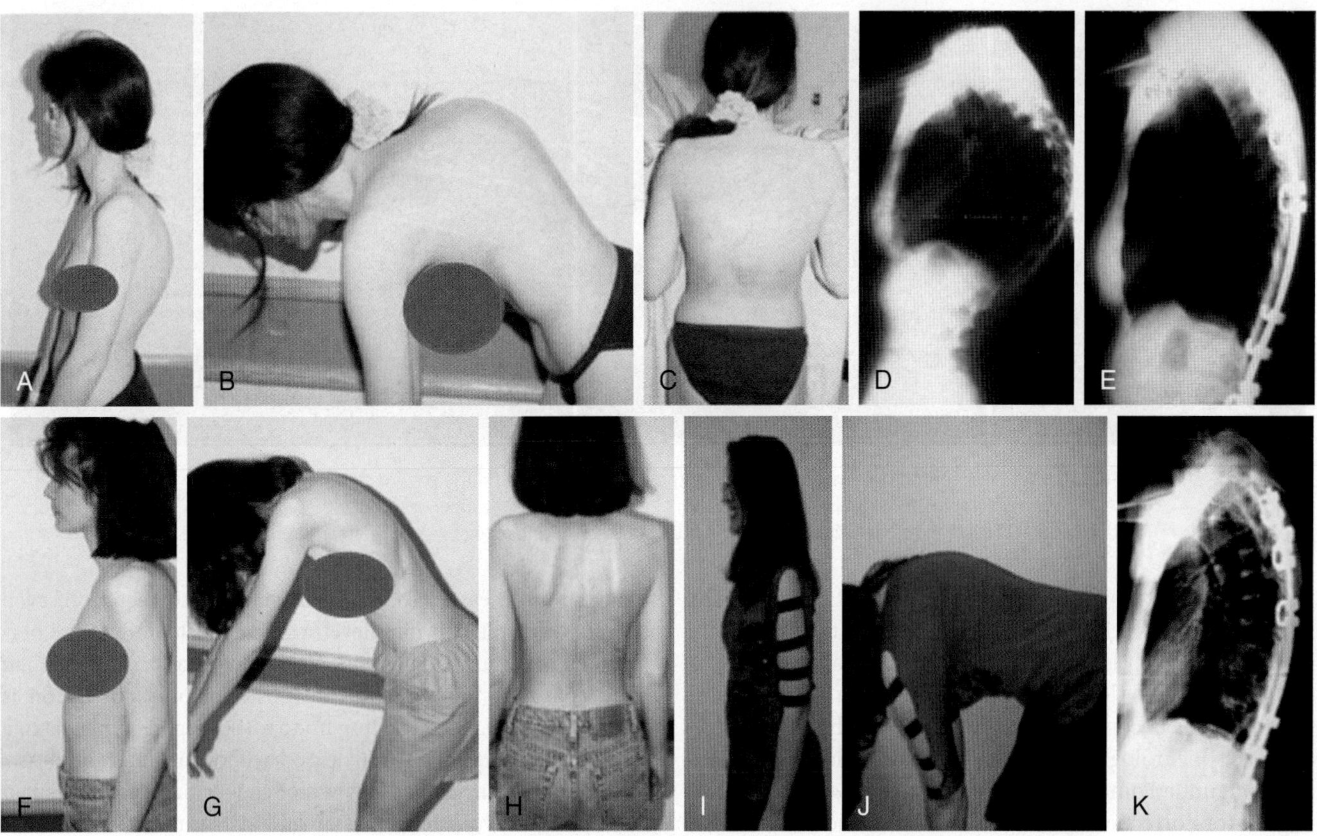

FIG. 30.4 (A–C) Preoperative clinical images of a 14-year-old female with Scheuermann kyphosis. (D) Preoperative standing lateral radiograph showing typical Scheuermann kyphosis. (E) One year postoperative standing lateral radiograph following video-assisted thoracoscopic surgery (VATS) along with posterior spinal fusion with instrumentation. (F–H) One year postoperative clinical pictures. (I–J) Twenty years postoperative clinical pictures. (K) Twenty years postoperative standing lateral radiograph illustrating fusion at the intervertebral disc spaces that were filled with allograft through VATS.

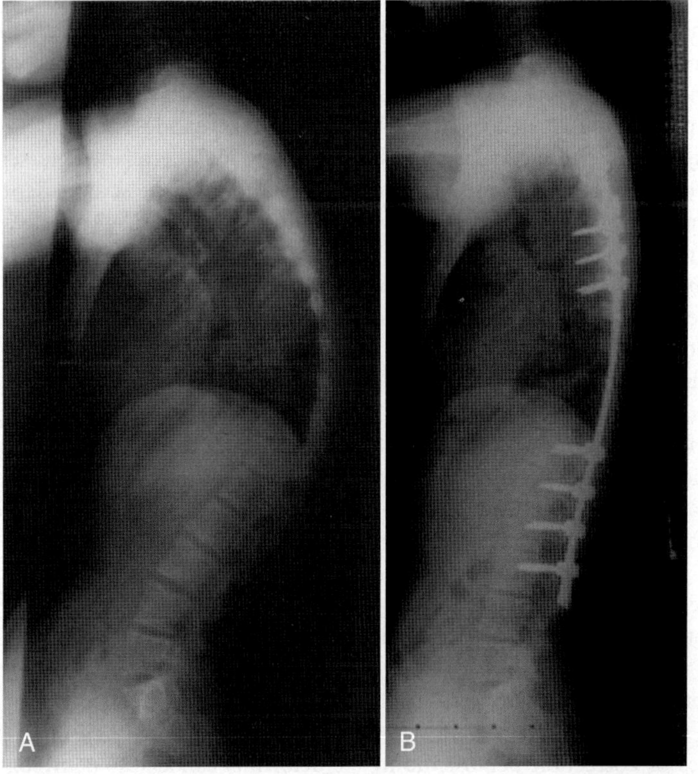

FIG. 30.5 A 15-year-old male with Scheuermann kyphosis, significant midback pain, and progression underwent posterior-only correction with multilevel Ponte osteotomies and pedicle screw instrumentation. (A) Preoperative and (B) postoperative standing lateral radiographs.

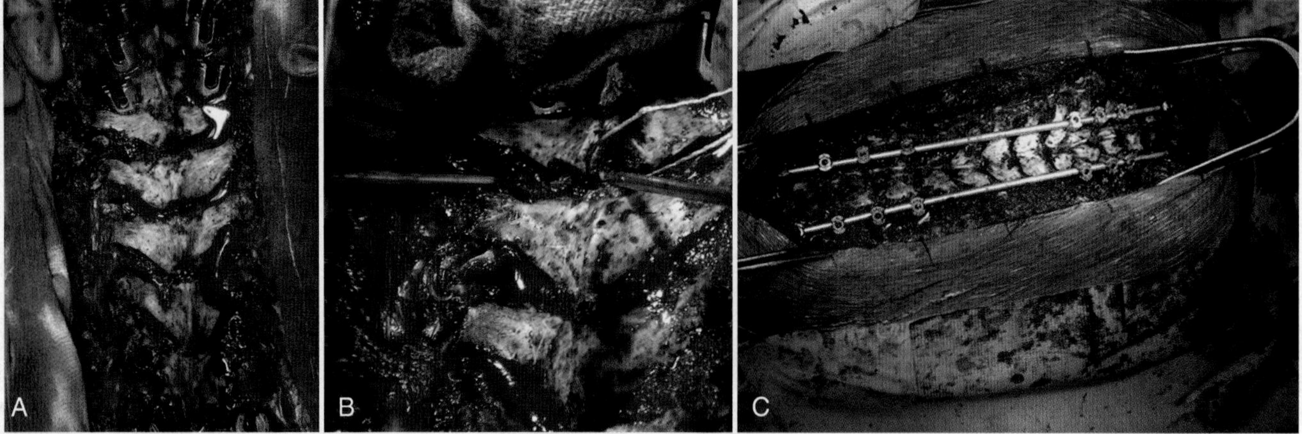

FIG. 30.6 Multiple Ponte osteotomies performed at the apex of the curve on the patient shown in Fig. 30.5. (A) Exposure of facet joints. (B) Excision of entire facet joint (inferior as well as superior articular process) and identification of nerve roots, as pointed out with a blunt instrument. (C) Intraoperative image after instrumentation.

with a PO. Critical review of radiographs of Scheuermann kyphosis patients will show that even discs at the apex of the curve or compromised in height have potential to open with a PO. The anterior longitudinal ligament in an unfused spine is not violated in common execution of a PO. This also reduces the risk of neurologic or anterior spinal vascular injury. Each segment undergoing PO can contribute between 5 and 15 degrees of correction. Multilevel PO is considered an ideal procedure for correcting Scheuermann kyphosis. However, there is no consensus regarding the number of levels or exact location where PO should ideally be performed. For example, Geck et al. reported performing osteotomies at each level of the intended instrumentation and fusion.[67] However, given that each level of PO contributes between 5 and 15 degrees of correction, we do not believe that PO is necessary at each level undergoing fusion. We routinely perform three to five levels of PO at the apex of the deformity, but this varies depending on the rigidity of the deformity and the angle of kyphosis. Emphasis should be given to performing a true PO in which the entire facet joint, including the superior articular process of the inferior vertebra, is completely removed and one can clearly visualize the underlying nerve roots on both sides. In addition to improving the degree of correction, removal of the superior articular process helps to avoid any impingement on the nerve roots during closure of the osteotomy. Care should also be taken to get a symmetrical opening at the osteotomy level on both sides to avoid any postoperative coronal plane deformity.

Lee and colleagues[68] compared posterior-only fusion (18 patients) with combined anterior-posterior fusion (21 patients) and found better correction and fewer complications in the posterior-only group at a mean 2-year follow-up. The anterior-posterior group did not have Ponte osteotomies, and hybrid hook and screw constructs were used, whereas the posterior-only group had Ponte osteotomies (in 67%) and had all-pedicle-screw constructs.

Geck and colleagues[67] obtained good correction in 17 patients, employing multiple osteotomies and pedicle screw fixation, averaging 9.3 degrees of correction per osteotomy across the apex. There is growing evidence that anterior release may be unnecessary to obtain satisfactory correction of even severe deformities if multilevel segmental osteotomies are performed in conjunction with pedicle screw fixation.[67–69] Hosman and colleagues[69] suggested that posterior-only correction is often adequate for correcting up to a 100-degree kyphosis to a physiologic range of 40 to 50 degrees without an anterior release.

In general, most patients with Scheuermann kyphosis can be managed by posterior fusion and instrumentation alone. A combined anterior-posterior procedure also has a longstanding successful track record. For very severe deformities (>100 degrees) that are rigid, an anterior release performed through an open or thoracoscopic approach is preferred to obtain some flexibility of the spine.

An alternative approach in the most severe and rigid deformities is either the eggshell decancellation procedure, also called vertebral column decancellation (VCD; Figs. 30.7 and 30.8) and/or vertebral column resection (VCR; Figs. 30.9 and 30.10) at the apical kyphotic segments.[70–72] VCD and VCR procedures are described later in this chapter. Instrumentation options include all pedicle screws or a hybrid construct of hooks and pedicle screws, depending on the preference of the surgeon. Successful results have been obtained regardless of the type of instrumentation. Behrbalk et al. found no differences in the efficiency in low- or high-density pedicle screw constructs.[73] We prefer to use pedicle screws bilaterally at most levels above and below the apex with correction achieved by cantilever forces and by compression. Shortening the posterior column is an important component of surgical treatment. Prebending the rods depending on the apical angle seen on hyperextension bolster films serves as a rough guideline on how much correction should be targeted.

Surgical Principles

Degree of Deformity Correction

Surgical treatment of Scheuermann kyphosis should aim to correct the thoracic kyphosis to the high-normal range of thoracic kyphosis (40–50 degrees). Overcorrection of a kyphotic deformity can lead to neurologic complications, postoperative sagittal malalignment, and proximal junctional kyphosis. The

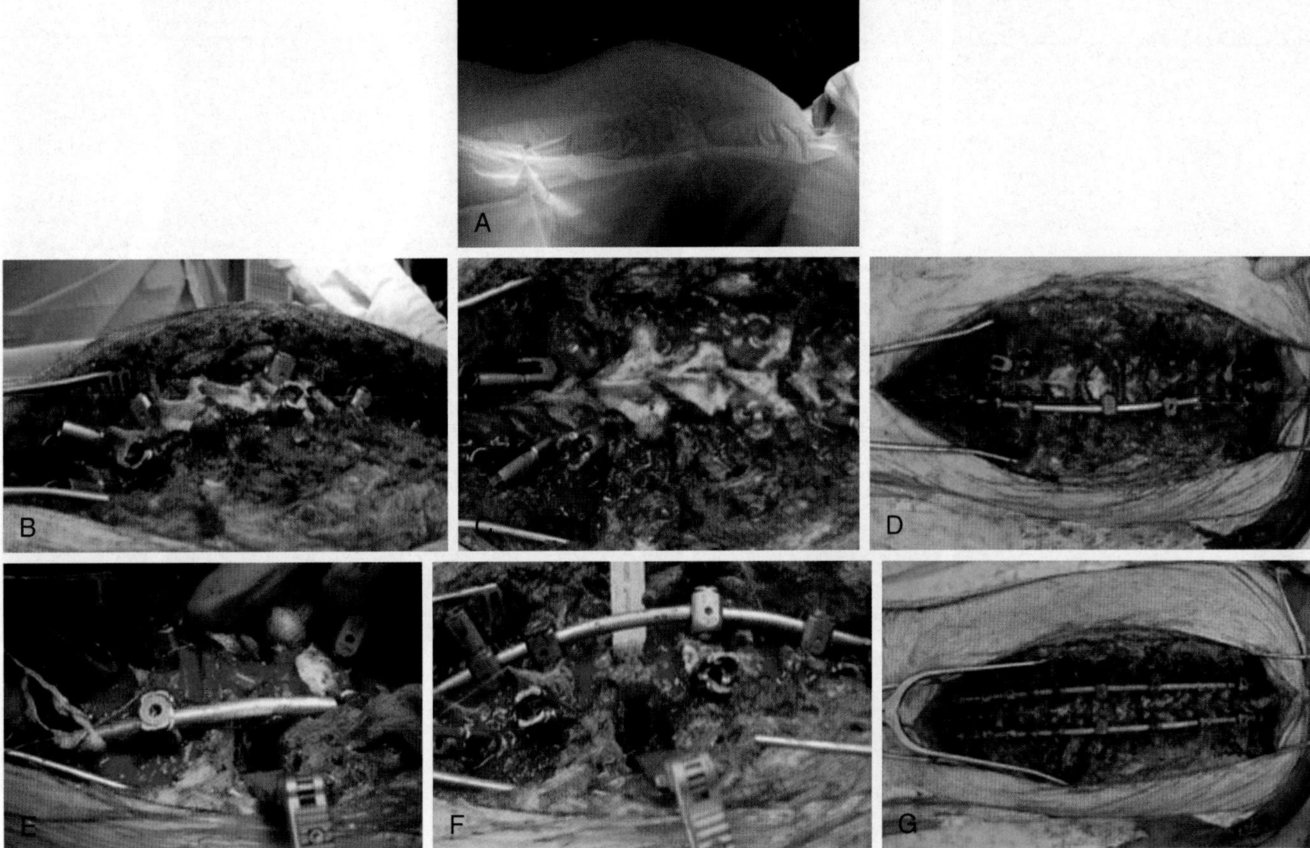

FIG. 30.7 (A) Cross-table lateral prone clinical image illustrating clinical kyphosis in a 16-year-old male. (B–C) Screw placed in apical vertebrae; note reduction screws in lumbar vertebrae and multiaxial in thoracic levels. (D) Single rod placed on one side to allow bony work from the other side. (E) Partial resection of the vertebral body (decancellation) under the curved temporary rod. (F) Complete decancellation of the apical vertebra showing spinal cord dorsally, bridging the gap. (G) Intraoperative image after instrumentation.

last condition may occur as a result of forces being transferred to the proximal junction after an aggressive corrective maneuver.[10,52,69] Lowe and Kasten[26] recommended that no more than 50% of the preoperative kyphosis be corrected and that the final kyphosis should never be less than 40 degrees. These authors also found that the negative sagittal balance is worsened postoperatively, which may predispose patients to junctional kyphosis.[26]

Selection of Fusion Levels

Proper selection of fusion levels is crucial to avoid complications related to junctional decompensation. The proximal extent of the fusion should be the proximal end vertebra in the measured kyphotic deformity.[7,26,56,74] There has been considerable debate regarding the optimal distal extent of the fusion. Traditionally, it has been suggested to extend the distal fusion level to the first lordotic disc beyond the end vertebra to minimize risk of junctional kyphosis.[26,61] Some authors have advocated inclusion of L1[20] or the inferior neutral vertebra, whereas others have advocated including L2 in the fusion. Poolman and colleagues[75] advocated the inclusion of the second lordotic disc below the kyphotic deformity. More recently, Cho and colleagues[76] emphasized the importance of the sagittal stable vertebra, defined as the most proximal vertebra touched by the posterior sacral vertical line. The posterior sacral vertical line is a line drawn vertically from the posterior-superior corner of the sacrum on the lateral upright radiograph. Cho and colleagues[76] found that distal junctional problems were more common when the fusion level was to the first lordotic vertebra rather than down to the sagittal stable vertebra. They recommended extending the distal end of the fusion to the vertebra that touches the posterior sacral vertical line. There is growing evidence to include sagittal stable vertebra in distal fusion to achieve a stable sagittal balance and prevent the distal junctional kyphosis.[77,78]

Spinopelvic Alignment

In the last decade, attention has been directed at the overall alignment of the spine in relation to the pelvis and lower extremities. For the assessment and reconstruction of global spinal alignment, several spinal and pelvic parameters can be measured on the lateral radiograph obtained in the standing position with the knees fully extended. Three commonly used pelvic parameters are pelvic tilt (PT), sacral slope, and pelvic incidence. PT is defined as an angle between the vertical line and a line through the midpoint of the sacral endplate to femoral head axis. PT is a major compensatory mechanism. When there is sagittal imbalance, pelvic retroversion is a

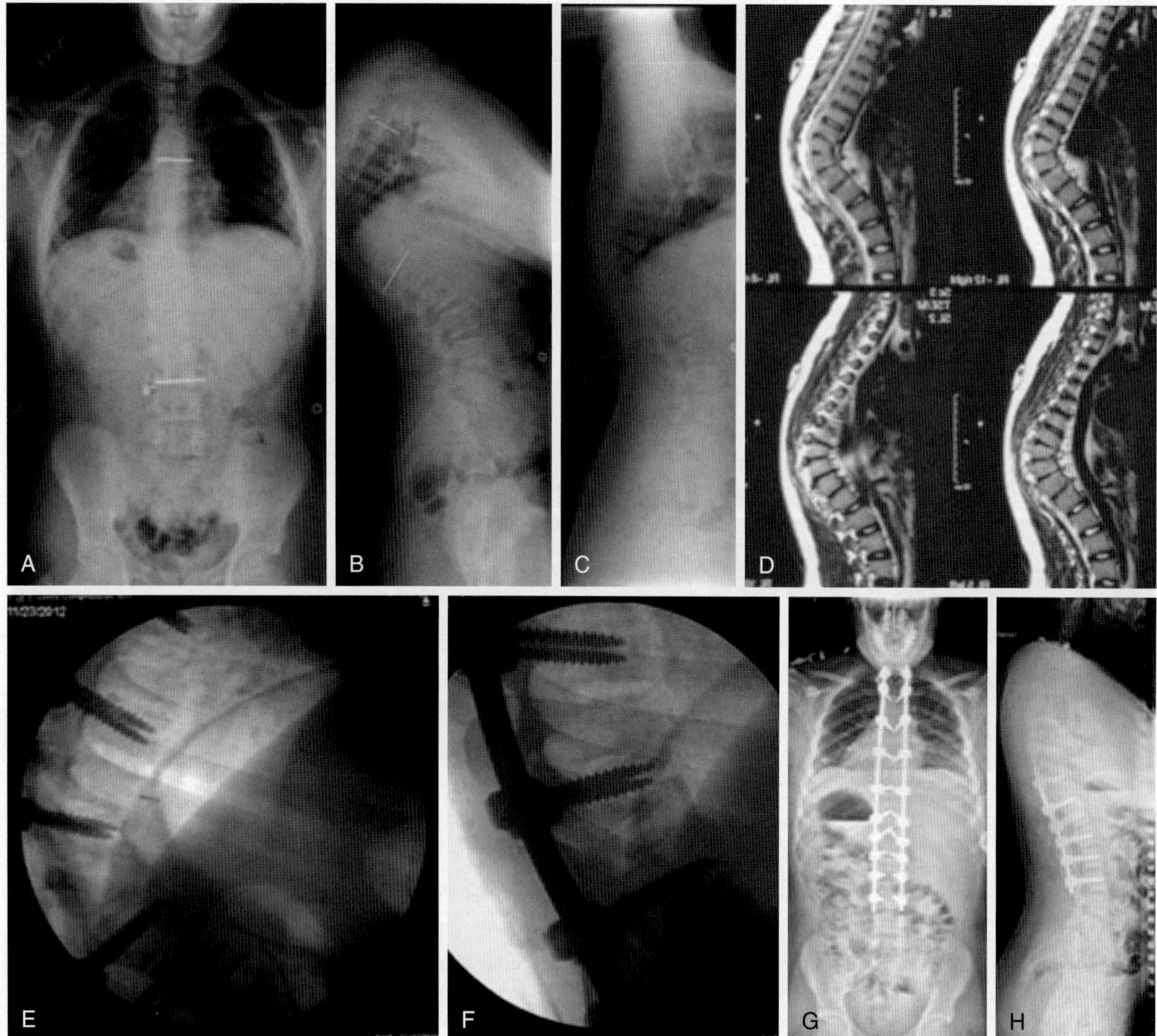

FIG. 30.8 (A) Standing posteroanterior radiograph of a 16-year-old male whose intraoperative images are shown in Fig. 30.7. (B) Standing lateral radiograph showing significant kyphosis. (C) Cross-table hyperextension lateral radiograph; note very little correction at the midapical region. (D) Sagittal magnetic resonance image showing bridging across the intervertebral spaces at the midapical region. (E) Intraoperative C-arm images showing lateral view following screw placement prior to the curve correction. (F) Intraoperative C-arm image showing lateral view following vertebral column decancellation and curve correction. (G, H) Standing posteroanterior and lateral radiographs 6 weeks postoperatively.

compensatory mechanism to improve sagittal balance. PT measures the degree of pelvic retroversion. Sacral slope (SS) is defined as the angle between the horizontal and sacral endplate. Pelvic incidence (PI) is defined as the angle between the line connecting the center of the femoral head axis to the center of the S1 endplate and the line perpendicular to the S1 endplate. PI is a stable anatomic parameter that is unique to each individual once maturity is achieved; it is constant and does not change with the position of the pelvis.

PI in patients with Scheuermann disease is lower than that reported for healthy adults and adolescents, and is not significantly different from PI reported for healthy children. Further, PI of patients with atypical Scheuermann disease is lower than PI of typical Scheuermann disease patients.[79] However, at this point, literature does not authenticate whether impaired spinopelvic parameters are the cause or result of Scheuermann disease. Nevertheless, in general, PI is the sum of PT and SS (PI = PT + SS).

Faldini et al. studied Scheuermann kyphosis patients who underwent posterior spinal fusion with PO and found that posterior spinal fusion for Scheuermann kyphosis significantly improved thoracic kyphosis and lumbar lordosis but did not affect the pelvic parameters.[80] In essence, while trying to achieve Scheuermann kyphosis correction, care should be taken to match the lumbar lordosis correction. As PI is constant for an individual and not going to change after surgery,

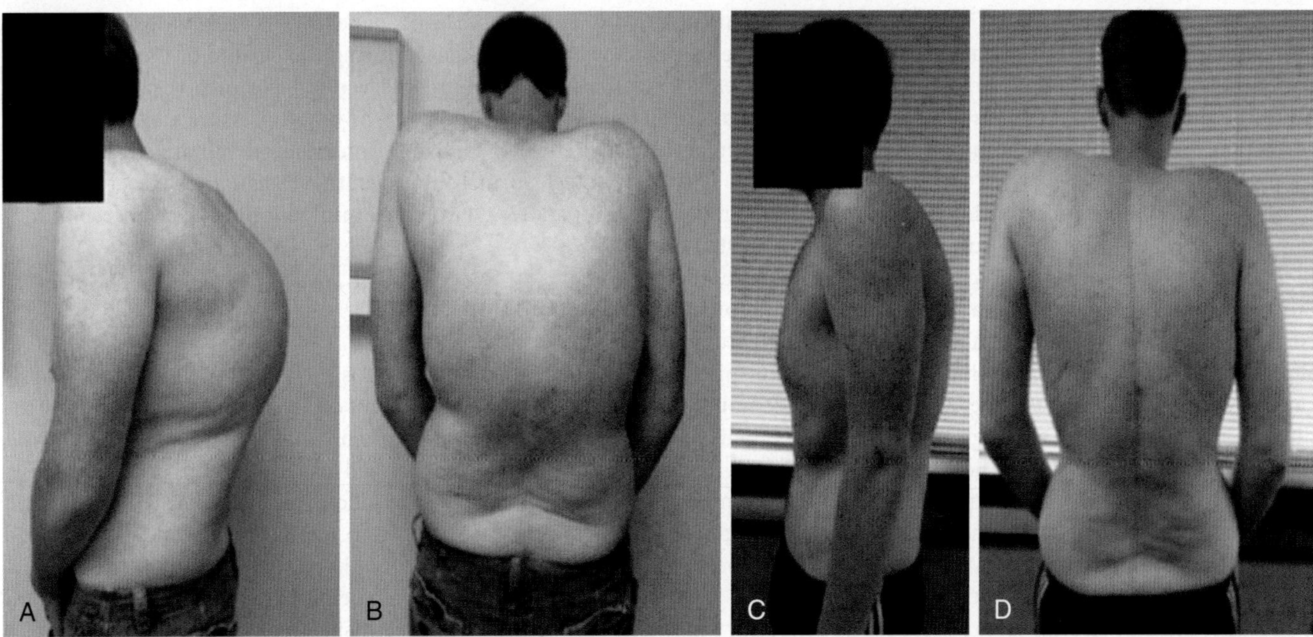

FIG. 30.9 (A–B) Preoperative clinical sagittal and coronal images of a 26-year-old male with significant Scheuermann kyphosis. (C–D) Postoperative clinical images showing curve correction.

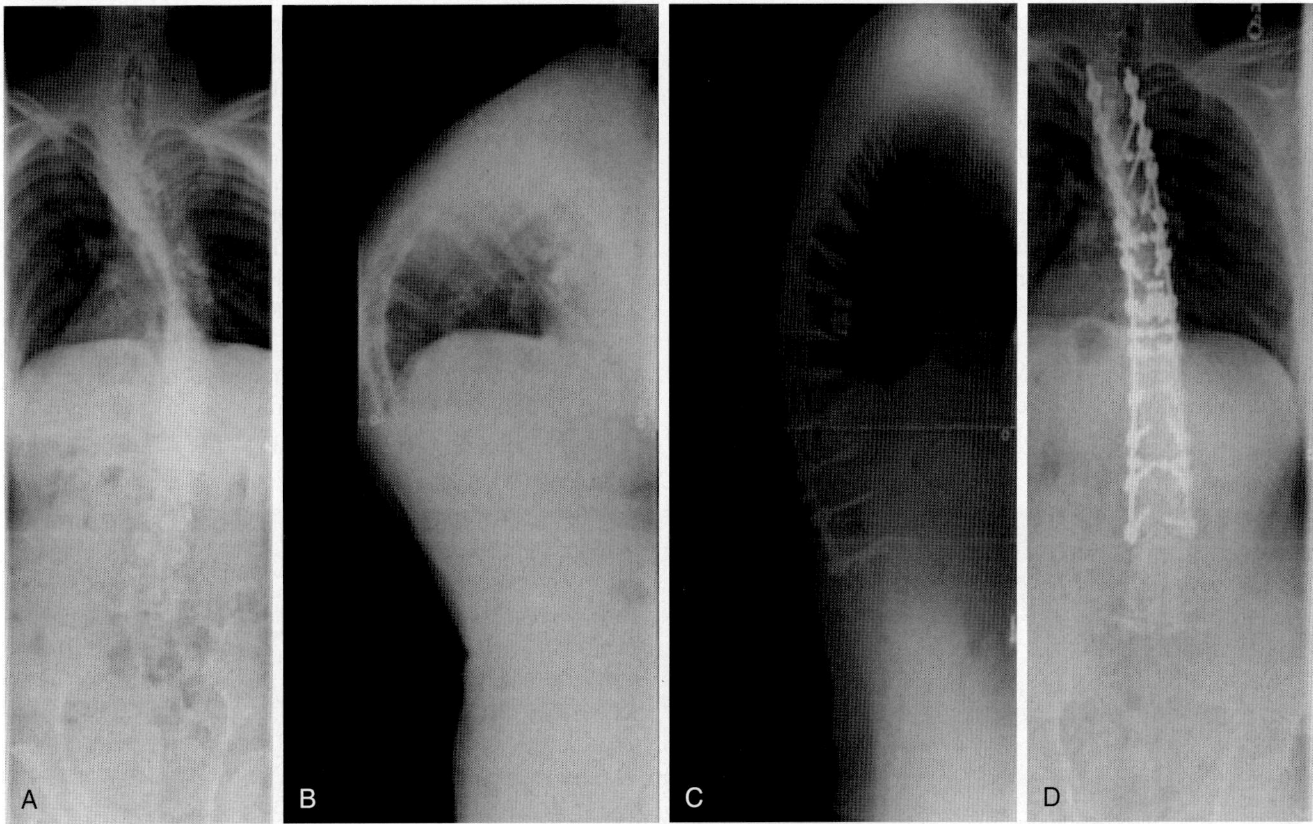

FIG. 30.10 (A–B) Standing posteroanterior and lateral radiographs of the patient shown in Fig. 30.9 illustrating more than 100-degree Scheuermann kyphosis. (C–D) Postoperative standing posteroanterior and lateral radiographs after vertebral column resection at T9 and posterior spinal fusion with instrumentation from T3 to L3.

any mismatch obtained by overcorrecting one over the other will lead to poor sagittal balance. Any suboptimal results will require compensatory actions from adjacent levels, leading to junctional problems or compensation by flexing hips or knees, which will lead to fatigue and discomfort.

Complications

The most worrisome complication of surgical treatment of Scheuermann disease is neurologic deficit. The 1999 Morbidity and Mortality Report of the Scoliosis Research Society reported the risk of neurologic injury during surgery for

Scheuermann disease to be 1 per 700 cases. Surgical treatment of kyphotic deformities is associated with a higher incidence of neurologic complications than treatment of coronal deformities because the spinal cord is lengthened anteriorly after correction, which may compromise its anterior vascular supply.[81]

Neurologic complications during deformity surgery can be caused by direct trauma to the neural elements (during instrumentation or osteotomies); stretch injury to the spinal cord during corrective maneuvers; or a vascular insult to the spinal cord, whether secondary to stretch or disruption of vascular supply or secondary to hypotension.[82–84] A preexisting spinal canal stenosis may increase the risk of neurologic injury during correction,[33] and although controversial, we believe that preoperative MRI should be obtained to rule out any compressive lesions. Overcorrection of a kyphotic deformity is hazardous to the neural elements because the spinal cord is lengthened; no more than a 50% correction (from preoperative kyphosis) should be attempted.

Distraction has been shown to induce spinal cord injury in feline studies by a reduction in cord perfusion.[85,86] Cantilever forces used during corrective maneuvers increase the length of the anterior column, which may have the same effect as distraction. Caution should be taken during correction, which should ideally be a gentle combination of cantilever forces and compressive forces to shorten the posterior column. We find the use of reduction pedicle screws at lumbar levels to be helpful in the correction maneuver.

Intraoperative neuromonitoring is an essential component of the surgery to lower the neurologic risks and safely execute the correction maneuver. Multimodality spinal cord monitoring with some type of motor tract assessment usually creates a safer, optimal intraoperative environment. Cheh et al. found a 35.7% true-positive rate of loss of intraoperative neurogenic mixed-evoked potential (NMEP) data sometime during the Scheuermann kyphosis correction surgery while concomitant somatosensory sensory-evoked potential (SSEP) remained within acceptable limits of baseline values.[81] Most of the cases showed loss of signals during the closure of the osteotomies. All patients had an intervention performed in the form of release of correction and/or blood pressure elevation. NMEP data returned following intervention ranging from 8 to 20 minutes. Normal intraoperative (Stagnara wake-up test) and postoperative neurologic examination results were reported.[81]

Junctional Kyphosis

Proximal junctional kyphosis (PJK) is defined as kyphosis measured from one segment cephalad to the upper end instrumented vertebra to the proximal instrumented vertebra, with an abnormal value defined as 10 degrees or greater (Fig. 30.11).[87] Similarly, distal junctional kyphosis (DJK) is defined as kyphosis measured from one segment caudal to the end instrumented vertebra to the distal instrumented vertebra, with abnormal value again being 10 degrees or more of kyphosis (Fig. 30.12).[87] In a retrospective multicenter review of 78 patients with Scheuermann kyphosis treated surgically, there was a 32% incidence of PJK and 5% incidence of DJK.[87] The investigators found that PJK was related to stopping the fusion caudal to the proximal end vertebra and is influenced by PI. DJK was always associated with fusion cephalad to the sagittal stable vertebra. Despite the high rate of PJK, the problem was clinically problematic or required reoperation in only 5.1% of cases.

Lowe and Kasten[26] reported a radiographic rate of PJK of 30%, ranging from 12 to 49 degrees and of DJK of 28%, ranging from 10 to 30 degrees. In their study, PJK was related to greater than 50% correction of the curve magnitude in 5 of 10 patients who developed PJK. PJK was also related to fusing short of (caudal to) the proximal Cobb end vertebrae by one or two levels. These authors recommended correcting kyphosis to no less than 40 degrees. Lonner et al. compared the combined anterior-posterior and posterior-only approaches

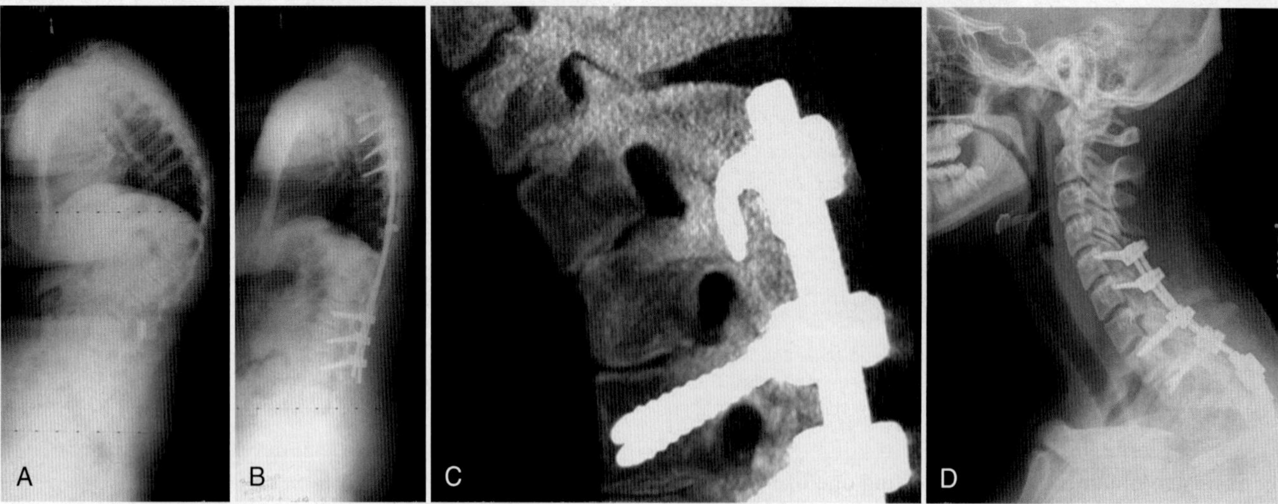

FIG. 30.11 An 18-year-old female noticed prominence of her neck 1 year postoperatively. She had developed proximal junctional kyphosis, which was revised with extension of fusion to the cervical spine. (A) Preoperative lateral standing radiograph. (B) Postoperative standing lateral radiograph. (C) Computed tomographic scan showing proximal junctional kyphosis. (D) Lateral radiographs of cervical spine showing extension of proximal fusion to C5.

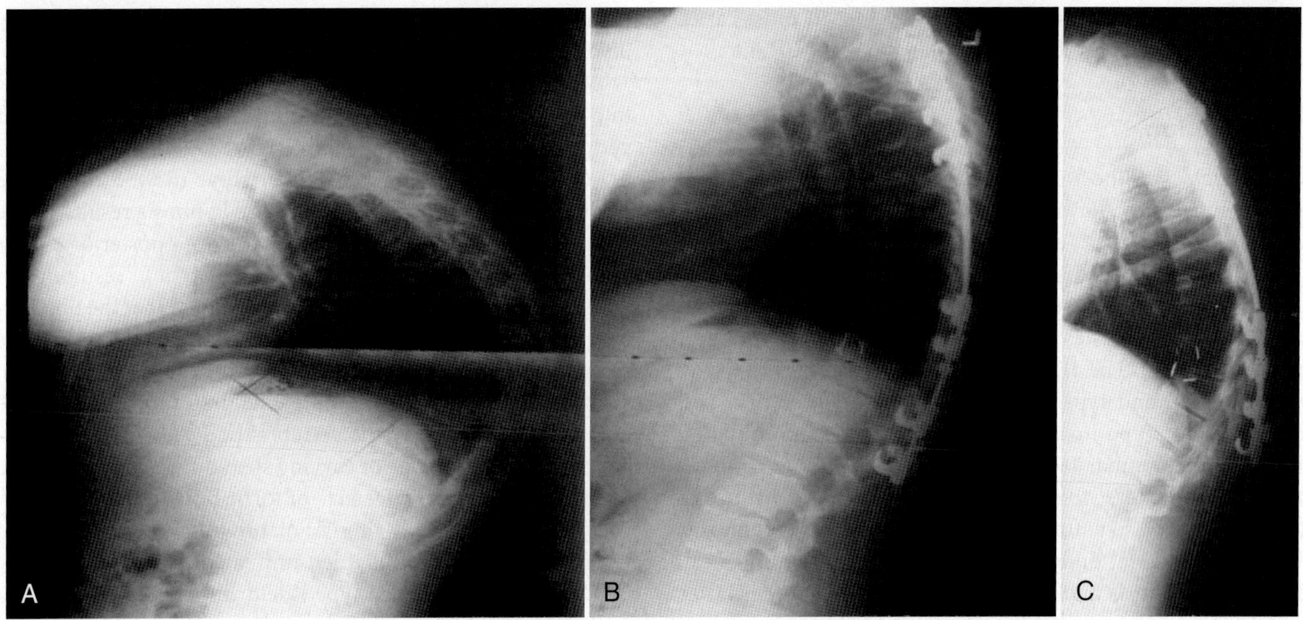

FIG. 30.12 A patient underwent surgical treatment of Scheuermann kyphosis and developed distal junctional kyphosis after surgery. This case illustrates the importance of extending fusion to the level that intersects the stable sagittal vertebra. (A) Preoperative standing lateral radiograph. (B) Immediate postoperative standing lateral radiograph. (C) Follow-up standing lateral radiograph showing distal junctional kyphosis.

and found no difference in the development of symptomatic PJK between the groups.[87]

Recent biomechanical studies showed that using transverse process hooks at the upper instrumented fusion level instead of pedicle screws provides a gradual transition from a rigid pedicle screw construct to the mobile normal adjacent spine.[88,89] Similarly, a finite element model study suggested that the use of a transition rod of lesser diameter at the proximal end of a long posterior spinal fusion construct minimizes the adjacent level abnormal pathomechanics, therefore possibly avoiding the development of PJK.[90]

To prevent PJK, we take the following precautions. (1) Always involve proximal end vertebra in fusion. Preoperative radiographic conditions when a proximal end vertebra is not clearly visualized, "best fit line" as was proposed by Denis et al.,[91] is recommended. (2) Preserve the interspinous and supraspinous ligament complex at the proximal two levels of the fusion that works as a tension band to minimize PJK. (3) We prefer to place transverse process hooks one level above the end instrumented vertebra for the gradual transition of forces to the adjacent level. In addition, the use of transverse process hooks requires less soft tissue dissection and produces less damage to the adjacent facet joint compared with pedicle screw insertion. (4) Aim to bring the curve correction into the upper normal physiologic range without overcorrecting the deformity. Do not do overcorrection.

Although earlier studies reported a high incidence of pseudarthrosis with a posterior-only procedure,[40,50] the use of modern instrumentation and techniques has resulted in a low rate of pseudarthrosis in adolescents. The tensile forces applied to a kyphotic deformity likely increase the incidence of pseudarthrosis in patients with Scheuermann disease as opposed to patients with idiopathic scoliosis, but this is unproven. Thorough preparation of the fusion bed with decortication and use of allograft bone is recommended. We do not use iliac crest autograft, but it is a viable option if other risk factors for pseudarthrosis exist.

Other reported complications include pulmonary embolus, pleural effusion, persistent back pain, instrumentation failure, and superior mesenteric artery syndrome.[9,26,50,53] Daniels and colleagues[92] reported a case of acute celiac artery occlusion resulting in necrosis of the stomach after combined anterior and posterior fusion with 50% correction of the curve.

Congenital Deformity

The first description of congenital kyphosis in the English language was by Greig[93] in 1916, who reported a 2-year-old child with a posterior hemivertebra. In 1932, Van Schrick[94] differentiated failure of vertebral body formation versus failure of segmentation as the cause of congenital kyphosis in four patients.

By definition, a vertebral anomaly is present at birth, but the clinical deformity may not manifest until much later. Congenital kyphosis develops prenatally as a result of growth deficits of the centrum occurring during the late stages of chondrification and ossification, leading to hypoplasia or aplasia of the vertebral body.[95,96] The defect is thought to be due to inadequate vascularization of the vertebral body during fetal development. Most vertebral malformations occur between days 20 and 30 of fetal development.[97]

Congenital kyphosis is less common than congenital scoliosis, but it is associated with a higher risk of neurologic compromise and progression of deformity if untreated.[98] Congenital kyphosis and kyphoscoliosis are not separate entities, but rather a spectrum of spinal deformities caused by vertebral anomalies. If one side of the vertebra is involved more than the other, concomitant scoliosis may develop. In most cases, the deformity involves the coronal plane to some extent.

Classification

Van Schrick[94] was the first to classify this condition into failure of vertebral body formation and failure of segmentation. Winter and colleagues[99] described three types in 1973 based on their classic review of 130 patients with kyphotic deformity of the spine owing to congenital vertebral anomalies. They classified the deformities as type I, congenital failure of vertebral body formation; type II, congenital failure of vertebral body segmentation; and type III, mixed failure of formation and segmentation. Type I was the most common, predominantly in the thoracolumbar region, followed by the upper thoracic region, and the least frequent in the lumbar spine. Failure of segmentation was symmetrical and produced pure kyphosis. Failure of vertebral body formation was often asymmetrical, producing scoliosis and kyphosis. In the series by McMaster and Singh,[100] 65% of patients had anterior failure of vertebral body formation, 20% had segmentation defects, 10% had mixed anomalies, and 5% could not be classified (Fig. 30.13).

Type I deformity is due to partial failure of vascularization of the cartilaginous centrum of the vertebral body.[100] These deformities are the most common type. The absence of two growth plates anteriorly with continued growth of posterior elements results in a sharp angular kyphosis and can lead to spinal cord compression. The prognosis is considerably worse than the unsegmented type (type II). The natural history involves relentless progression if untreated.

McMaster and Singh[100] further classified type I deformities into four patterns of malformations: posterolateral quadrant vertebra (35%), posterior hemivertebra (7%), butterfly vertebra (13%), and anterior wedged vertebrae (5%). If the failure of formation is purely anterior, a pure kyphosis results. More commonly, the defect is anterolateral with a posterior corner hemivertebra (posterolateral quadrant type), resulting in kyphoscoliosis. McMaster and Singh[100] noted that the posterolateral quadrant vertebra has the worst prognosis, progresses relentlessly, and has a high rate of spinal cord compression. This anomaly is due to a complete failure of formation of the anterolateral portion of the vertebral body, leaving a posterolateral fragment of bone of varying size attached to one pedicle and the neural arch.[100] Defects of formation are treated surgically because of the high risk of progression and potential neurologic complications if left untreated.

Dubousset[101] classified type I deformities into two types: a well-aligned spinal canal and a dislocated canal. Shapiro and Herring[102] and Zeller and colleagues[103] used the terms *congenital vertebral displacement* (Shapiro and Herring) and *congenital dislocated spine* (Zeller and colleagues) to describe deformities in which anterior and posterior elements were abnormal and there was posterior displacement of anomalous vertebrae. Zeller and colleagues[103] described the "step-off" sign as the loss of continuity of the posterior cortex of adjacent vertebral bodies as a half of a congenital dislocated spine.

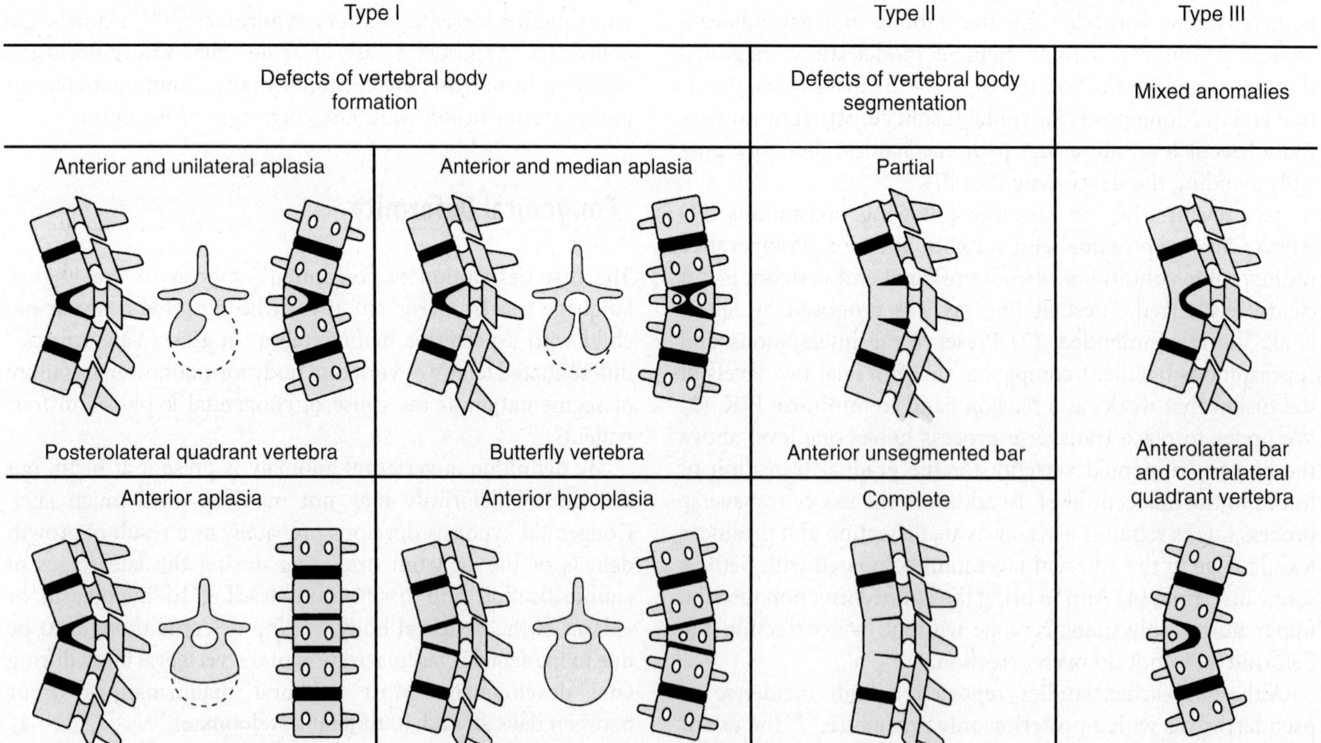

FIG. 30.13 Congenital kyphosis type I results from defects in vertebral body segmentation, and congenital kyphosis type III results from mixed anomalies. (From McMaster MJ, Singh H. Natural history of congenital kyphosis and kyphoscoliosis. *J Bone Joint Surg Am.* 1999;31:1369.)

Patients with type II deformity have a better prognosis in terms of rate of progression of deformity and neurologic complications. This deformity is secondary to bony metaplasia in the anterior portion of the anulus fibrosus, resulting in an anterior unsegmented bar.[100] There is no longitudinal growth, but posterior growth continues, resulting in a kyphotic deformity. The rate of progression is slow, and spinal cord compression does not occur.[100] McMaster and Singh[100] subdivided defects of vertebral body segmentation into partial (anterior unsegmented bar) or complete (block vertebrae) failure of segmentation.

Imaging Studies

In younger children, vertebral anomalies may be difficult to appreciate on plain films because of incomplete ossification. Computed tomography (CT) scans with three-dimensional reconstructions are useful for precisely defining the nature of the deformity. Flexion and extension lateral radiographs are useful to assess flexibility of the deformity. MRI is recommended preoperatively in all cases to rule out intraspinal anomalies, which can be present in 5% to 37% of patients with congenital kyphosis and scoliosis.[104,105] MRI is also useful in identifying cord compression or cord signal changes that may result from the angular kyphosis.

Clinical Evaluation

Numerous associated anomalies can accompany congenital spinal deformities, including renal and cardiopulmonary anomalies, chest deformities (pectus carinatum or excavatum), intraspinal anomalies (e.g., diastematomyelia, tethered cord, Arnold-Chiari malformation, syringomyelia). Proper workup of congenital deformities includes renal ultrasound, cardiac echocardiogram, and MRI of the brain and entire spine.

Progression can be insidious; thus, at each follow-up examination, the initial radiograph, previous radiograph, and present radiograph should be reviewed, using the same levels for comparison. Failure to recognize progression can lead to a severe deformity, requiring more extensive surgery with higher risks. During periods of rapid spinal growth (birth to 5 years and during the adolescent growth spurt), more frequent evaluation (every 6 months) is wise. During the "dormant" phase of growth (5 to 10 years), yearly evaluation is adequate. Even if the absolute magnitude of the kyphotic deformity is not increasing, its flexibility may worsen over time, which may be an indication for earlier surgery.

A complete neurologic examination is crucial. Before surgery, urodynamic testing should be considered in patients with large curves because it may detect subtle preexisting myelopathy in high-risk patients (especially young children).

Natural History

The natural history of congenital kyphosis depends on the type of deformity, age of the patient and amount of growth remaining, and location of the deformity. Winter and colleagues[99] found type I deformities to have the worst prognosis and to progress rapidly, followed by type III and type II. McMaster and Singh[100] found the most rapid progression to occur in type III deformities, followed by type I and II. The posterolateral quadrant vertebra has the worst prognosis.

Kyphosis resulting from defects of formation progresses an average of 7 degrees per year and is most rapid during the adolescent growth spurt.[99] Progression is most likely to occur during rapid periods of growth (birth to 3 years and adolescent growth spurt). Type II deformities progress an average of 5 degrees per year.[106] Progression rate is slower in type II deformities because bony bar formation of the anterior disc occurs later in childhood, and the growth discrepancy between the posterior and anterior elements is not as great as type I deformities.

Neurologic involvement and spinal cord compression occur primarily with anterior failure of vertebral body formation (type I or III) because of the acute angular kyphosis over a short segment. The rate of neurologic involvement has been estimated to be around 18%.[100] This rate would likely be much higher if all patients were untreated. Neurologic compromise is most common during the adolescent growth spurt, when progression is most rapid. The greatest risk of spinal cord compression occurs when the apex is at the midthoracic region (T4–T9) because this is a vascular watershed area. The onset of cord compression can occur at any age, but is most common during the adolescent growth spurt. All patients who develop neurologic deficit progress to paraplegia if left untreated.[100] Progressive neurologic deficit should be immediately treated surgically.

Type II deformities (failure of segmentation) produce a more rounded kyphosis compared with the angular gibbous deformity that occurs with failure of formation.[99,106] These deformities occur most often in the lower thoracic and thoracolumbar region. They are less likely to progress and rarely cause neurologic compromise because of the more gradual kyphosis that is spread out over several segments (as opposed to the sharp angular kyphosis of type I deformities).

Nonoperative Treatment

Nonoperative treatment in congenital kyphosis primarily consists of diligent observation to document progression of the deformity (Fig. 30.14). Bracing and casting are believed to be ineffective in congenital kyphosis.[99,107] Progression can be insidious, and radiographs may show small degrees of progression over months that may be deemed insignificant. However, over a 2- to 3-year time frame, the progression may be much more significant. At each follow-up evaluation, current radiographs should be compared with the initial radiographs to document progression more precisely. In all cases of congenital kyphoscoliosis, especially with type I deformities, it is crucial to obtain a posteroanterior radiograph and a lateral radiograph at each visit because the scoliosis may appear to be stable but the lateral view may show significant progression of the kyphosis owing to a hemivertebra. We refer to such a hemivertebra as a "snake in the grass" (Fig. 30.15).

The importance of observation was highlighted by a more recent report by Campos and colleagues,[108] who described

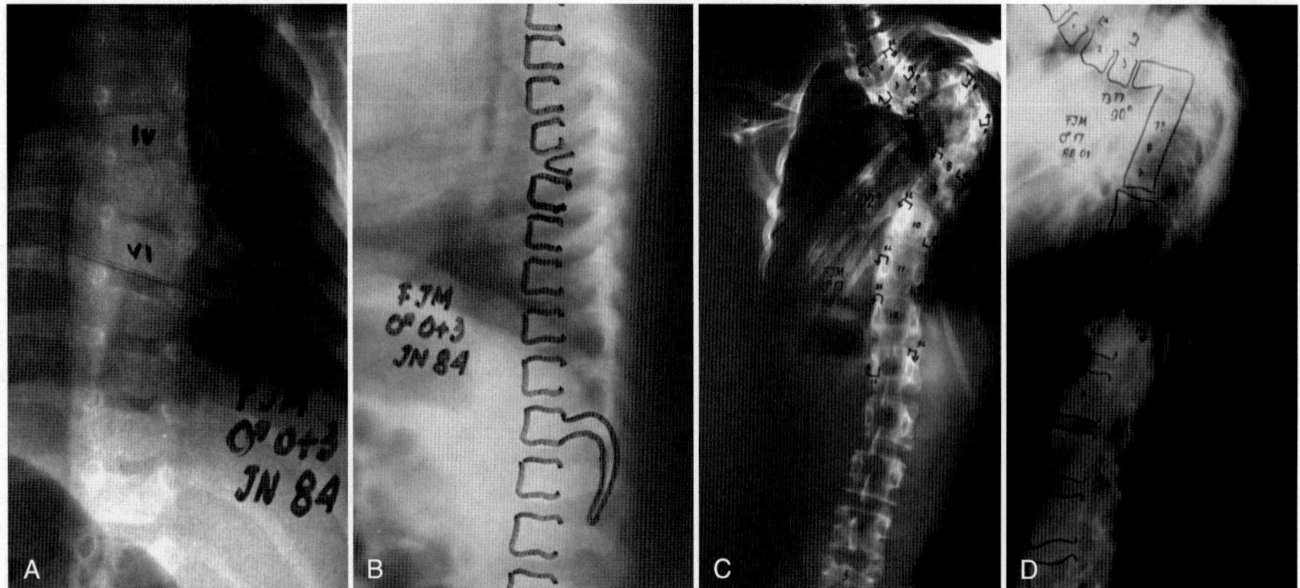

FIG. 30.14 T5 hemivertebra initially diagnosed at age 3 months. The patient was not followed up until age 17 years, when he became paraplegic and wheelchair dependent with severe spinal deformity. (A) Anteroposterior and (B) lateral radiographs of entire spine at 3 months of age. (C) Anteroposterior and (D) lateral radiographs of entire spine at 17 years of age. (Courtesy R. Maenza, MD, Italian Hospital, Buenos Aires, Argentina.)

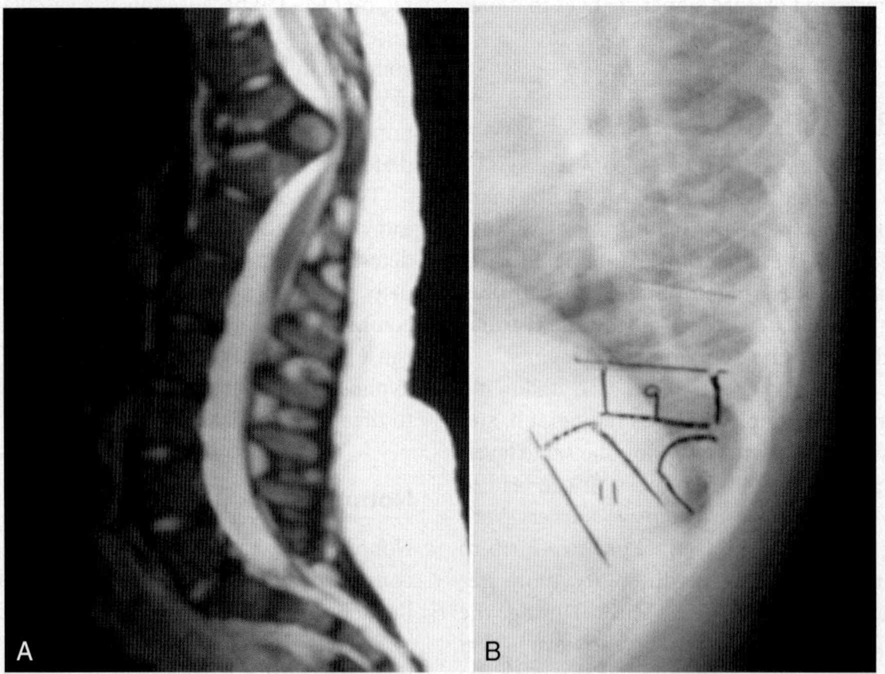

FIG. 30.15 Hemivertebra causing severe cord compression. This deformity is often not well appreciated on the posteroanterior view and can be missed if proper imaging is not performed. We refer to such a "hidden" anomaly on the posteroanterior view as a "snake in the grass." (A) Sagittal magnetic resonance cuts. (B) Lateral radiograph of spine.

seven patients with early thoracolumbar kyphosis associated with single lumbar vertebral hypoplasia, which appeared similar to a failure of formation (Fig. 30.16). All patients had spontaneous correction of alignment over time. In all seven patients, the anomaly was limited to one lumbar level (L1 or L2), and the defect was limited to the superior portion of the anterior half of the vertebral body without posterior malformations. The investigators recommended a brief period of observation to document progression versus spontaneous correction. If progression was documented or if the deformity persisted at age 3 years, further workup was recommended.

Surgical Treatment

The guiding principle of operative treatment of congenital kyphosis is early fusion to prevent severe deformity and to allow for some correction with growth.[98] If curves with a bad

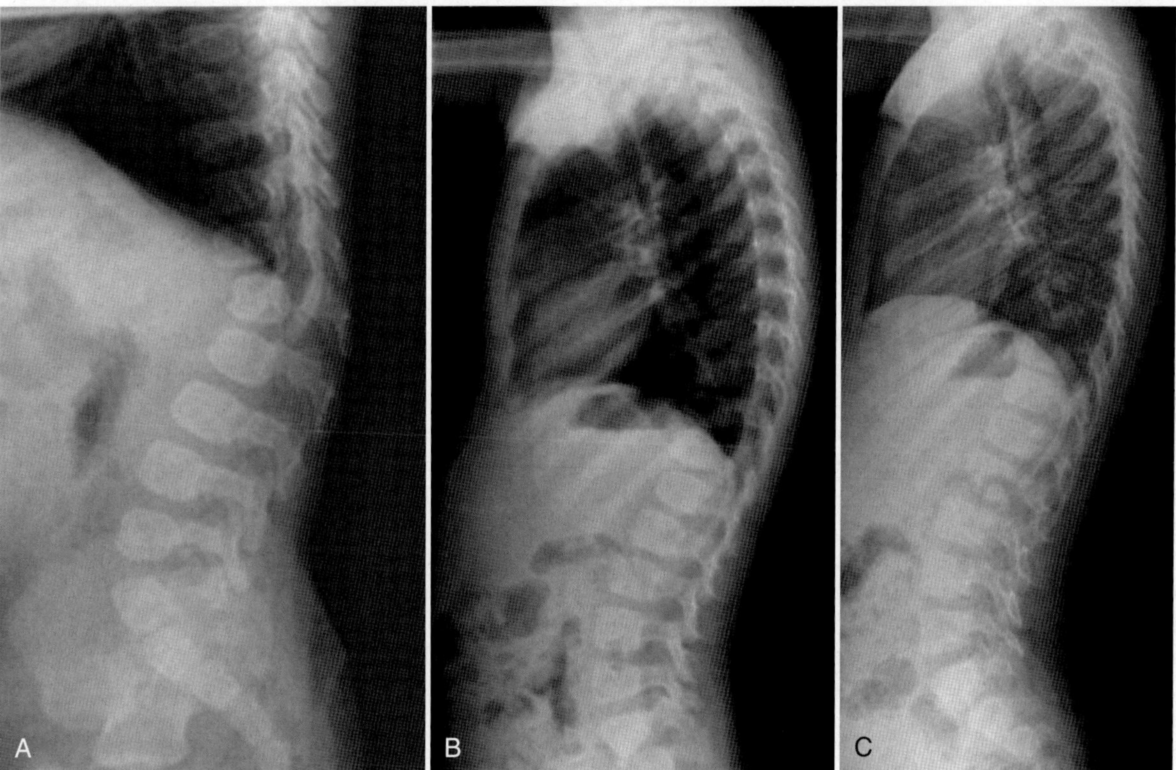

FIG. 30.16 A 6-month-old boy with wedging deformity of L1 vertebra, which spontaneously corrected over time. The patient was braced with a thoracolumbosacral orthosis. Lateral radiographs show deformity at (A) 6 months of age, (B) 3.5 years of age, and (C) 4.5 years of age. This case highlights the importance of diligent observation of all congenital deformities and performing surgery only if progression is documented.

prognosis are recognized at an early age, simple prophylactic surgical treatment can prevent progression and neurologic complications. The surgical treatment of congenital kyphosis can be challenging, and many factors must be considered when deciding on the operative plan, such as type of vertebral anomaly, patient age and amount of growth remaining, severity of deformity, and presence or absence of spinal cord compression or neurologic deficits, or both.[98]

All operations should be performed with spinal cord monitoring, including motor evoked potentials, somatosensory evoked potentials, and electromyography monitoring. Traction without anterior release is contraindicated because of the high incidence of neurologic complications.[99,109] Because of the rigidity of the kyphosis at the apex, traction primarily causes correction of the ends of the curve, which are more flexible. This correction lengthens the spine and pulls the spinal cord against the unforgiving apical bone, which may lead to more compression of the cord and resulting neurologic complications.

The treatment of type I deformities is almost always surgical because of the high risk of progression and neurologic sequelae if deformities are left untreated.

The presence of a posterolateral quadrant vertebra mandates early prophylactic surgical treatment before the child is 5 years of age and before the kyphosis is 50 degrees.[100] Traditionally, this treatment was best achieved by a posterior growth arrest procedure, which is essentially a posterior (convex) hemiepiphysiodesis. More recently, hemivertebra excision performed through an all-posterior approach has been used for these deformities, discussed later in this chapter. In situ fusion can be done with or without instrumentation, extending one level above to one level below the abnormal vertebra. If the deformity is less than 50 to 55 degrees, and there is growth potential anteriorly, creating a posterior tether allows some gradual correction in the presence of continuing anterior growth. This also eliminates the risk of spinal cord compression.

Early on, surgeons did not use instrumentation. Pseudarthrosis rates were relatively high and reexploration of the fusion mass was routinely recommended for this reason. Earlier reports recommended prolonged bed rest (up to 6 months) after surgery. The use of spinal instrumentation, specifically pedicle screw instrumentation, has been shown to be safe and effective in very young patients with congenital spinal deformities[110,111] and improves the fusion rate, making reexploration and prolonged bed rest unnecessary. We prefer to use allograft bone because fusion rates tend to be high in young patients. The fundamental principles of fusion surgery, including facet excision and thorough decortication, must be adhered to for optimal results. Postoperatively, we immobilize very young children in a brace, given their inability to restrict their activities.

The surgical treatment of older children (>5 years) with more severe deformities (>55–60 degrees) has traditionally been a combined anterior and posterior fusion. Several studies have documented the inefficacy of posterior fusion alone for these patients,[98,112,113] and a combined anterior and posterior fusion with or without instrumentation has been recommended.[24,99,109] Winter and colleagues[99] made this recommendation in a review of 94 patients in whom progressive congenital kyphosis had been treated after the age of 5 years. Some degree of vertebral resection is necessary to obtain satisfactory correction. McMaster and Singh[98] recommended anterior strut grafting and instrumented posterior fusion because of the substantial rate of pseudarthrosis and deformity progression with posterior fusion alone. Large curves place posterior fusion at a mechanical disadvantage in the absence of anterior fusion, leading to a high pseudarthrosis rate. Older children (>5 years) also lack sufficient spinal growth to produce an appreciable correction. Other studies have corroborated that posterior fusion alone, with or without instrumentation, is insufficient for a type I or type III kyphotic deformity greater than 50 degrees.[24,109] McMaster and Singh[98] recommended fusing the entire deformity in older patients with large curves (longer fusion than in younger patients with smaller curves).

The anterior and posterior procedures can be done in 1 day or can be staged, depending on the preference of the surgeon. The anterior procedure is done through a transthoracic, transthoracic-retroperitoneal, or purely retroperitoneal approach depending on the location of the deformity. When exposure is obtained, the segmental vessels are ligated, and periosteal flaps are created. The segmental vessels should be ligated as anteriorly as possible to avoid disruption of the collateral circulation, which lies closer to the foraminal regions. Complete discectomies are performed. Rib strut grafts are placed from end vertebra to end vertebra, creating slots in the vertebral bodies.

These studies were completed before pedicle screw instrumentation became widely used. The superior three-column fixation that is obtained with pedicle screws may obviate the need for an anterior surgery in many patients, even patients with severe deformities.

An alternative to early in situ posterior fusion for a hemivertebra is complete resection of the hemivertebra. Traditionally, hemivertebra excisions have been done through combined anterior and posterior exposures. More recent reports have shown this procedure to be safe and effective through a posterior-only approach,[114–116]; thus, this is our preference. Shono and colleagues[117] reported on one-stage posterior hemivertebra resection and fusion and instrumentation in 12 patients 8 to 24 years old with kyphoscoliosis. Satisfactory correction of the scoliosis (from 49 to 18 degrees) and the kyphosis (from 40 to 17 degrees) was obtained, without neurologic complications or pseudarthrosis. Ruf and Harms[110,114] described a similar approach in children 15 months old, mostly in congenital scoliosis, with successful outcomes. The location of a hemivertebra in congenital kyphosis or kyphoscoliosis (at the apex of kyphotic deformity) makes it amenable to resection from a posterior approach with visualization of the spinal cord during correction. This approach allows for correction and short-segment fusion without concern regarding continued growth of the anterior column that may lead to future progression or crankshaft phenomenon.

Patients with spinal cord compression and neurologic deficits require decompression of the spinal cord. This decompression can be done either from an anterior approach or posteriorly from a costotransversectomy approach. Laminectomies alone are contraindicated because the compression is from the ventral aspect of the cord, and laminectomies create further mechanical instability. If the deformity is severe and spinal cord compression exists, the apex of the deformity may be so far posterior that cord decompression may be more feasible from a posterior approach. In such cases, a vertebral body resection is performed through bilateral costotransversectomies or a transpedicular approach. After the body is resected, the spinal column is shortened in such cases to obtain some bony apposition anteriorly. In severe gibbous deformities, decompression is technically more feasible from a posterior approach. A cage can be inserted anteriorly if the deformity allows it.

With surgical treatment of kyphosis, some lengthening of spine usually results. The kyphotic apex is stiff; thus, the normal, flexible spine corrects and lengthens around a relatively fixed deformity. This can cause significant stress on the vascularity of the spinal cord. Every effort should be made to shorten the spine with correction.

A type II kyphosis does not require immediate surgical treatment unless the deformity is already sufficiently severe to require correction or the curve is shown to be progressive under observation.[98] If a type II deformity is detected early and has been noted to be progressive, but the curve is not severe and is within acceptable limits, a posterior fusion alone (one level above to one level below the congenital kyphosis) is sufficient to prevent further progression.[24,99,106,109] These deformities have no potential for anterior growth because of ossification of anterior disc spaces. For more severe curves, in which substantial correction is necessary, traditionally an anterior approach has been recommended to perform osteotomies of the unsegmented areas, discectomies and fusion, and posterior fusion and instrumentation.[106] All patients who undergo surgical treatment should be observed to skeletal maturity because adding on of additional vertebrae above and below the fused segment can occur during the adolescent growth spurt.

For relatively mild deformities, such as those from a wedge vertebra or failure of formation hemivertebra excision, a posterior column-shortening osteotomy, such as Ponte or pedicle subtraction, is sufficient. For severe, rigid deformities, three-column resection osteotomy, such as VCR, is often needed. Initially, VCR was performed through a combined anterior and posterior approach. To minimize the anterior approach–related morbidity, Suk et al.[116] described execution of VCR using the posterior-only approach. Lenke et al. then popularized posterior VCR with a comprehensive surgical technique.[70,72] The purpose of VCR is to circumferentially decompress the neural elements, correct the deformity, and do 360-degree fusion with instrumentation (see Figs. 30.9 and 30.10). It is a highly technically demanding procedure. Neurologic complications still remain the biggest challenge. The overall complication rate is reported to be as high as 59%.[71] The location of the apex of the deformity directly influences the neurologic complications. The thoracic (T6–T9) level apex carries higher intraoperative and postoperative risk for neurologic complications as compared to thoracolumbar or lumbar apex.[118] Several preoperative and intraoperative measures have been found helpful to minimize complications and optimize outcomes. A thorough understanding of the deformity with three-dimensional CT and/or with a three-dimensional spine model is an essential step in the preoperative planning. The nutritional optimization of the patient should be considered. During the procedure, sufficient height of anterior reconstruction, avoiding the sagittal translation of the upper and lower vertebrae, keeping a temporary rod in position at all times and intraoperative neuromonitoring, may help to improve the safety. Care should also be taken to control epidural bleeding and keeping the mean arterial blood pressure equal to or above 80 mm Hg during the correction maneuver to prevent neurologic complications.

An alternative to VCR for rigid, sharp complex deformities is the eggshell decancellation procedure, also called vertebral column decancellation (VCD).[119] The VCD technique does not require 360-degree exposure of the spinal cord; therefore, it reduces the instability-related complications, has low intraoperative blood loss, requires less surgical time, and causes less neurogenic complications. The decancellation of the vertebral body is executed through the pedicle in inside-to-outside order, reducing the exposure and damage to segmental vessels. VCD is a close-opening technique and the hinge of the correction is adjustable, often located at the junction of the anterior and middle column (see Figs. 30.7 and 30.8). The residual bone in the VCD technique may obviate the need for metal mesh needed in the VCR technique.[119–121] Although VCD is relatively safer than VCR, it still needs experience and high technical expertise to execute safely.[119]

Complications

Pseudarthrosis and Progressive Deformity

Techniques to obtain a solid fusion more reliably include combined anterior and posterior fusion, use of instrumentation, proper facet decortication, and use of autogenous bone graft. With use of modern spinal instrumentation and proper technique, pseudarthrosis rates are low in young children even with allograft and posterior-only fusion.[111,122] Pseudarthrosis typically leads to progression of the deformity; if any progression is noted in the postoperative period, reexploration of the fusion mass is recommended. For severe curves (>55–60 degrees), the most reliable means of avoiding these complications is by performing a combined anterior and posterior fusion.

Neurologic Complications

The rate of neurologic complications is higher in the surgical treatment of congenital kyphosis than other spinal deformities, especially in older patients with large deformities.[109] As mentioned previously, traction is contraindicated in the treatment of congenital kyphosis. Neurologic complications are more likely to occur if attempts are made to obtain maximum correction of the curve with use of instrumentation. Partial correction is preferable; the goal is to obtain a balanced spine in the coronal and sagittal planes, rather than maximal correction. Spinal cord monitoring is mandatory—the use of the wake-up test is recommended if the patient can cooperate.

PEARLS

1. Surgical correction of Scheuermann kyphosis can be accomplished in most cases by posterior-only fusion with multilevel POs. Complete removal of the inferior and superior facets and ligamentum flavum allows the posterior column to be shortened.
2. A combination of cantilever forces and compression is used to obtain correction in Scheuermann kyphosis. Intraoperative use of reduction screws in lumbar levels is often helpful.
3. MRI is recommended before surgical correction of Scheuermann kyphosis. The presence of stenosis or disc herniation may alter the operative plan.
4. In a very young child with congenital deformity, fusion should be as short as possible. In an adolescent patient, the entire deformity should be addressed.
5. Although bracing and casting are not very effective in congenital deformities, alternating with casting may be considered in a very young infant as a temporizing measure to allow further growth before surgery is performed.
6. Overcorrection of a kyphotic deformity can lead to neurologic injury because the spinal cord is lengthened. No more than 50% correction (from preoperative kyphosis) should be attempted.
7. Avoiding overcorrection, selection of proper fusion levels, and preservation of the supraspinous ligament at the proximal end of the construct have been found to be helpful to prevent a junctional kyphosis. The possibility of a junctional kyphosis should be discussed with the patient and family preoperatively.
8. All patients with congenital kyphosis require diligent observation. Not all patients experience progression, and early surgery in the absence of documented progression should be avoided.
9. In patients with congenital scoliosis, the lateral radiograph should be critically examined. The scoliosis may appear to be stable, but the kyphosis may be progressing.

KEY POINTS

1. The natural history of Scheuermann disease is generally benign, and most patients do not experience significant disability in adulthood.
2. A Milwaukee brace is recommended in skeletally immature patients with curves of 55 to 70 degrees.
3. Surgical indications include a progressive thoracic kyphosis greater than 75 to 80 degrees in a skeletally immature patient; thoracolumbar kyphosis exceeding 50 to 55 degrees that is associated with pain unresponsive to conservative treatment; progression of deformity despite bracing; or cosmetic deformity that the surgeon, patient, and family consider significant and unacceptable.
4. Patients diagnosed with congenital kyphosis should undergo MRI of the entire spine to rule out intraspinal anomalies.
5. Diligent periodic observation of all patients with congenital kyphosis is crucial; without such observation, severe deformities with neurologic sequelae may develop.
6. The natural history of congenital kyphosis, particularly type I deformities, is unfavorable. Insidious progression of the deformity can occur with growth, and surgery is recommended if progression is noted.
7. Goals of treatment are early fusion to prevent severe deformity, halt progression, and achieve head and trunk balance.
8. In a very young child, fusion should be as short as possible. The entire deformity should be addressed in adolescent patients.

9. Postoperatively, patients should be followed to skeletal maturity to ensure that progression of the primary or compensatory curves does not occur.

KEY REFERENCES

1. Winter RB, Moe JH. The results of spinal arthrodesis of congenital spinal deformities in patients younger than five years old. *J Bone Joint Surg Am.* 1982;64-A:419-432.
   The authors reviewed the results of spinal fusion for congenital deformity in 49 patients younger than 5 years.
2. Winter RB, Moe JH, Lonstein JE. The surgical treatment of congenital kyphosis: a review of 94 patients age 5 years or older with 2 years or more follow-up in 77 patients. *Spine.* 1985;10:224-231.
   The authors reviewed the results of spinal fusion for congenital kyphosis in 77 patients older than age 5.
3. Murray PM, Weinstein SL, Spratt KF. The natural history and long-term follow-up of Scheuermann's kyphosis. *J Bone Joint Surg Am.* 1993;75:236-248.
   This was the first long-term follow-up study on the natural history of Scheuermann disease.
4. McMaster MJ, Singh H. Natural history of congenital kyphosis and kyphoscoliosis. A study of one hundred and twelve patients. *J Bone Joint Surg Am.* 1999;81:1367-1383.
   The authors further classified type 1 deformities into four patterns of malformations. They noted that the posterolateral quadrant vertebra has the worst prognosis, progresses relentlessly, and has a high rate of spinal cord compression.
5. Lowe TG. Scheuermann's disease. *Orthop Clin North Am.* 1999;30:475-487.
   This review article discusses the natural history, diagnosis, and treatment of Scheuermann disease.
6. Campos MA, Fernandes P, Dolan LA, Weinstein SL. Infantile thoracolumbar kyphosis secondary to lumbar hypoplasia. *J Bone Joint Surg Am.* 2008;90:1726-1729.
   This is a report on seven patients with early thoracolumbar kyphosis with lumbar hypoplasia. All cases resolved without surgical treatment.

REFERENCES

1. Bernhardt M. Normal spinal anatomy: Normal sagittal plane alignment. In: Bridwell K, DeWald R, eds. *The Textbook of Spinal Surgery*. Vol. 1. 2nd ed. Philadelphia: Lippincott-Raven; 1997:185-191.
2. Bernhardt M, Bridwell KH. Segmental analysis of the sagittal plane alignment of the normal thoracic and lumbar spines and thoracolumbar junction. *Spine.* 1989;14(7):717-721.
3. Fon GT, Pitt MJ, Thies AC. Thoracic kyphosis: range in normal subjects. *AJR Am J Roentgenol.* 1980;134(5):979-983.
4. Jackson RP, McManus AC. Radiographic analysis of sagittal plane alignment and balance in standing volunteers and patients with low back pain matched for age, sex, and size. A prospective controlled clinical study. *Spine.* 1994;19:1611-1618.
5. Scheuermann H. Kyphosis dorsalis juvenilis. *Orthop Chir.* 1921;41:305.
6. Scheuermann H. The classic: kyphosis dorsalis juvenilis. *Clin Orthop Relat Res.* 1977;128:5-7.
7. Wenger DR, Frick SL. Scheuermann kyphosis. *Spine.* 1999;24(24):2630-2639.
8. Scoles PV, Latimer BM, DigIovanni BF, et al. Vertebral alterations in Scheuermann's kyphosis. *Spine.* 1991;16(5):509-515.
9. Tribus CB. Scheuermann's kyphosis in adolescents and adults: diagnosis and management. *J Am Acad Orthop Surg.* 1998;6(1):36-43.
10. Lowe TG. Scheuermann's disease. *Orthop Clin North Am.* 1999;30(3):475-487.
11. Sorensen K Scheuermann's juvenile kyhosis: clinical appearances, radiography, aetiology and prognosis. In: *Enjar Munksgaard Forlag Copenhagen*; Munksgaard: 1964.
12. Schmorl G, Junghans H. *Die Gesunde und Kranle Wirbel-seule in Roentgenbild.* Leipzig: Thieme Verlag; 1932.
13. McKenzie L, Sillence D. Familial Scheuermann disease: a genetic and linkage study. *J Med Genet.* 1992;29(1):41-45.
14. Nielsen OG, Pilgaard P. Two hereditary spinal diseases producing kyphosis during adolescence. *Acta Paediatr Scand.* 1987;76(1):133-136.
15. Findlay A, Conner AN, Connor JM. Dominant inheritance of Scheuermann's juvenile kyphosis. *J Med Genet.* 1989;26(6):400-403.
16. Carr AJ. Idiopathic thoracic kyphosis in identical twins. *J Bone Joint Surg Br.* 1990;72(1):144.
17. Graat HCA, van Rhijn LW, Schrander-Stumpel CTRM, van Ooij A. Classical Scheuermann disease in male monozygotic twins: further support for the genetic etiology hypothesis. *Spine.* 2002;27(22):E485-E487.
18. Murray PM, Weinstein SL, Spratt KF. The natural history and long-term follow-up of Scheuermann kyphosis. *J Bone Joint Surg Am.* 1993;75(2):236-248.
19. Ippolito E, Ponseti IV. Juvenile kyphosis: histological and histochemical studies. *J Bone Joint Surg Am.* 1981;63(2):175-182.
20. Ascani E, La Rosa G. Scheuermann kyphosis. In: Weinstein S, ed. *The Pediatric Spine: Principles and Practice.* New York: Raven Press; 1994:557-584.
21. Lambrinudi C. Adolescent and senile kyphosis. *Br Med J.* 1934;2(3852):800-820.
22. Lopez RA, Burke SW, Levine DB, Schneider R. Osteoporosis in Scheuermann's disease. *Spine.* 1988;13(10):1099-1103.
23. Bradford DS, Daher YH. Vascularised rib grafts for stabilisation of kyphosis. *J Bone Joint Surg Br.* 1986;68(3):357-361.
24. Montgomery SP, Hall JE. Congenital kyphosis. *Spine.* 1982;7(4):360-364.
25. Ogilvie JW, Sherman J. Spondylolysis in Scheuermann's disease. *Spine.* 1987;12(3):251-253.
26. Lowe TG, Kasten MD. An analysis of sagittal curves and balance after Cotrel-Dubousset instrumentation for kyphosis secondary to Scheuermann's disease. A review of 32 patients. *Spine.* 1994;19(15):1680-1685.
27. Somhegyi A, Ratko I. Hamstring tightness and Scheuermann's disease. Commentary. *Am J Phys Med Rehabil.* 1993;72(1):44.
28. Bhojraj SY, Dandawate AV. Progressive cord compression secondary to thoracic disc lesions in Scheuermann's kyphosis managed by posterolateral decompression, interbody fusion and pedicular fixation. A new approach to management of a rare clinical entity. *Eur Spine J.* 1994;3(2):66-69.
29. Klein DM, Weiss RL, Allen JE. Scheuermann's dorsal kyphosis and spinal cord compression: case report. *Neurosurgery.* 1986;18(5):628-631.
30. Lesoin F, Leys D, Rousseaux M, et al. Thoracic disk herniation and Scheuermann's disease. *Eur Neurol.* 1987;26(3):145-152.

31. Yablon JS, Kasdon DL, Levine H. Thoracic cord compression in Scheuermann's disease. *Spine*. 1988;13(8):896-898.
32. Sachs B, Bradford D, Winter R, et al. Scheuermann kyphosis. Follow-up of Milwaukee-brace treatment. *J Bone Joint Surg Am*. 1987;69(1):50-57.
33. Tribus CB. Transient paraparesis: a complication of the surgical management of Scheuermann's kyphosis secondary to thoracic stenosis. *Spine*. 2001;26(9):1086-1089.
34. Bradford DS, Garica A. Neurological complications in Scheuermann's disease. A case report and review of the literature. *J Bone Joint Surg Am*. 1969;51(3):567-572.
35. Chiu KY, Luk KD. Cord compression caused by multiple disc herniations and intraspinal cyst in Scheuermann's disease. *Spine*. 1995;20(9):1075-1079.
36. Abul-Kasim K, Schlenzka D, Selariu E, Ohlin A. Spinal epidural lipomatosis: a common imaging feature in Scheuermann disease. *J Spinal Disord Tech*. 2012;25(7):356-361.
37. Ponte A, Gebbia F, Eliseo F. Non-operative treatment of adolescent hyperkyphosis. *Orthop Trans*. 1985;9:185.
38. Speck GR, Chopin DC. The surgical treatment of Scheuermann's kyphosis. *J Bone Joint Surg Br*. 1986;68(2):189-193.
39. Bradford DS, Moe JH, Montalvo FJ, Winter RB. Scheuermann's kyphosis and roundback deformity. Results of Milwaukee brace treatment. *J Bone Joint Surg Am*. 1974;56(4):740-758.
40. Bradford DS, Ahmed KB, Moe JH, Winter RB, Lonstein JE. The surgical management of patients with Scheuermann's disease: a review of twenty-four cases managed by combined anterior and posterior spine fusion. *J Bone Joint Surg Am*. 1980;62(5):705-712.
41. Bradford DS. Vertebral osteochondrosis (Scheuermann's kyphosis). *Clin Orthop Relat Res*. 1981;158:83-90.
42. Travaglini F, Conte M. Progress in patologia vertebrate. *Cifosi*. 1982;5:163.
43. Travaglini F, Conte M. Untreated kyphosis: 25 years later. In: Gaggi A, ed. *Kyphosis*. Bologna: Italian Scoliosis Research Group; 1984.
44. Lowe TG. Scheuermann disease. *J Bone Joint Surg Am*. 1990;72(6):940-945.
45. Lowe TG. Kyphosis of the thoracic and thoracolumbar spine in the pediatric patient: surgical treatment. *Instr Course Lect*. 2004;53:493-500.
46. Harreby M, Neergaard K, Hesselsøe G, Kjer J. Are radiologic changes in the thoracic and lumbar spine of adolescents risk factors for low back pain in adults? A 25-year prospective cohort study of 640 school children. *Spine*. 1995;20(21):2298-2302.
47. Paajanen H, Alanen A, Erkintalo M, Salminen JJ, Katevuo K. Disc degeneration in Scheuermann disease. *Skeletal Radiol*. 1989;18(7):523-526.
48. Blount WP, Schmidt AC, Bidwell RG. Making the Milwaukee brace. *J Bone Joint Surg Am*. 1958;40-A(3):526-528.
49. Gutowski WT, Renshaw TS. Orthotic results in adolescent kyphosis. *Spine*. 1988;13(5):485-489.
50. Bradford DS, Moe JH, Montalvo FJ, Winter RB. Scheuermann's kyphosis. Results of surgical treatment by posterior spine arthrodesis in twenty-two patients. *J Bone Joint Surg Am*. 1975;57(4):439-448.
51. Herndon WA, Emans JB, Micheli LJ, Hall JE. Combined anterior and posterior fusion for Scheuermann's kyphosis. *Spine*. 1981;6(2):125-130.
52. Lowe TG. Double L-rod instrumentation in the treatment of severe kyphosis secondary to Scheuermann's disease. *Spine*. 1987;12(4):336-341.
53. Lim M, Green DW, Billinghurst JE, et al. Scheuermann kyphosis: safe and effective surgical treatment using multisegmental instrumentation. *Spine*. 2004;29(16):1789-1794.
54. Herrera-Soto JA, Parikh SN, Al-Sayyad MJ, Crawford AH. Experience with combined video-assisted thoracoscopic surgery (VATS) anterior spinal release and posterior spinal fusion in Scheuermann's kyphosis. *Spine*. 2005;30(19):2176-2181.
55. Yang C, Askin G, Yang S. Combined thoracoscopic anterior spinal release and posterior correction for Scheuermann's kyphosis. *Zhonghua Wai Ke Za Zhi*. 2004;42(21):1293-1295.
56. Papagelopoulos PJ, Klassen RA, Peterson HA, Dekutoski MB. Surgical treatment of Scheuermann's disease with segmental compression instrumentation. *Clin Orthop Relat Res*. 2001;386:139-149.
57. Vedantam R, Lenke LG, Bridwell KH, Haas J, Linville DA. A prospective evaluation of pulmonary function in patients with adolescent idiopathic scoliosis relative to the surgical approach used for spinal arthrodesis. *Spine*. 2000;25(1):82-90.
58. Graham EJ, Lenke LG, Lowe TG, et al. Prospective pulmonary function evaluation following open thoracotomy for anterior spinal fusion in adolescent idiopathic scoliosis. *Spine*. 2000;25(18):2319-2325.
59. Wong CA, Cole AA, Watson L, et al. Pulmonary function before and after anterior spinal surgery in adult idiopathic scoliosis. *Thorax*. 1996;51(5):534-536.
60. Taylor TC, Wenger DR, Stephen J, Gillespie R, Bobechko WP. Surgical management of thoracic kyphosis in adolescents. *J Bone Joint Surg Am*. 1979;61(4):496-503.
61. Sturm PF, Dobson JC, Armstrong GW. The surgical management of Scheuermann's disease. *Spine*. 1993;18(6):685-691.
62. Otsuka NY, Hall JE, Mah JY. Posterior fusion for Scheuermann's kyphosis. *Clin Orthop Relat Res*. 1990;251:134-139.
63. Johnston CE, Elerson E, Dagher G. Correction of adolescent hyperkyphosis with posterior-only threaded rod compression instrumentation: is anterior spinal fusion still necessary? *Spine*. 2005;30(13):1528-1534.
64. Ponte A, Vero B, Siccardi G. Surgical treatment of Scheuermann's hyperkyphosis. In: Winter RB, ed. *Progress in Spinal Pathology: Kyphosis*. Bologna: Aulo Gaggi; 1984:75-80.
65. Smith-Petersen MN, Larson CB, Aufranc OE. Osteotomy of the spine for correction of flexion deformity in rheumatoid arthritis. *Clin Orthop Relat Res*. 1969;66:6-9.
66. Ponte A. Posterior column shortening for Scheuermann's kyphosis. In: Haher T, Merola A, eds. *Surgical Techniques for the Spine*. New York: Thieme Verlag; 2003:107-113.
67. Geck MJ, Macagno A, Ponte A, Shufflebarger HL. The Ponte procedure: posterior only treatment of Scheuermann's kyphosis using segmental posterior shortening and pedicle screw instrumentation. *J Spinal Disord Tech*. 2007;20(8):586-593.
68. Lee SS, Lenke LG, Kuklo TR, et al. Comparison of Scheuermann kyphosis correction by posterior-only thoracic pedicle screw fixation versus combined anterior/posterior fusion. *Spine*. 2006;31(20):2316-2321.
69. Hosman AJ, Langeloo DD, de Kleuver M, et al. Analysis of the sagittal plane after surgical management for

Scheuermann's disease: a view on overcorrection and the use of an anterior release. *Spine*. 2002;27(2):167-175.

70. Lenke LG, Sides BA, Koester LA, Hensley M, Blanke KM. Vertebral column resection for the treatment of severe spinal deformity. *Clin Orthop Relat Res*. 2010;468(3):687-699.
71. Lenke LG, Newton PO, Sucato DJ, et al. Complications after 147 consecutive vertebral column resections for severe pediatric spinal deformity: a multicenter analysis. *Spine*. 2013;38(2):119-132.
72. Lenke LG, O'Leary PT, Bridwell KH, et al. Posterior vertebral column resection for severe pediatric deformity: minimum two-year follow-up of thirty-five consecutive patients. *Spine*. 2009;34(20):2213-2221.
73. Behrbalk E, Uri O, Parks RM, et al. Posterior-only correction of Scheuermann kyphosis using pedicle screws: economical optimization through screw density reduction. *Eur Spine J*. 2014;23(10):2203-2210.
74. de Jonge T, Illés T, Bellyei A. Surgical correction of Scheuermann's kyphosis. *Int Orthop*. 2001;25(2):70-73.
75. Poolman RW, Been HD, Ubags LH. Clinical outcome and radiographic results after operative treatment of Scheuermann's disease. *Eur Spine J*. 2002;11(6):561-569.
76. Cho K-J, Lenke LG, Bridwell KH, Kamiya M, Sides B. Selection of the optimal distal fusion level in posterior instrumentation and fusion for thoracic hyperkyphosis: the sagittal stable vertebra concept. *Spine*. 2009;34(8): 765-770.
77. Lundine K, Turner P, Johnson M. Thoracic hyperkyphosis: assessment of the distal fusion level. *Glob spine J*. 2012;2(2):65-70.
78. Mikhaylovskiy MV, Sorokin AN, Novikov VV, Vasyura AS. Selection of the optimal level of distal fixation for correction of Scheuermann's hyperkyphosis. *Folia Med (Plovdiv)*. 2015;57(1):29-36.
79. Tyrakowski M, Mardjetko S, Siemionow K. Radiographic spinopelvic parameters in skeletally mature patients with Scheuermann disease. *Spine*. 2014;39(18):E1080-E1085.
80. Faldini C, Traina F, Perna F, et al. Does surgery for Scheuermann kyphosis influence sagittal spinopelvic parameters? *Eur Spine J*. 2015;24(suppl 7):893-897.
81. Cheh G, Lenke LG, Padberg AM, et al. Loss of spinal cord monitoring signals in children during thoracic kyphosis correction with spinal osteotomy: why does it occur and what should you do? *Spine*. 2008;33(10):1093-1099.
82. Wilber RG, Thompson GH, Shaffer JW, Brown RH, Nash CL. Postoperative neurological deficits in segmental spinal instrumentation. A study using spinal cord monitoring. *J Bone Joint Surg Am*. 1984;66(8):1178-1187.
83. Winter RB. Neurologic safety in spinal deformity surgery. *Spine*. 1997;22(13):1527-1533.
84. Othman Z, Lenke LG, Bolon SM, Padberg A. Hypotension-induced loss of intraoperative monitoring data during surgical correction of Scheuermann kyphosis: a case report. *Spine*. 2004;29(12):E258-E265.
85. Dolan EJ, Transfeldt EE, Tator CH, Simmons EH, Hughes KF. The effect of spinal distraction on regional spinal cord blood flow in cats. *J Neurosurg*. 1980;53(6):756-764.
86. Yeoman PM, Gibson MJ, Hutchinson A, et al. Influence of induced hypotension and spinal distraction on feline spinal somatosensory evoked potentials. *Br J Anaesth*. 1989;63(3):315-320.
87. Lonner BS, Newton P, Betz R, et al. Operative management of Scheuermann's kyphosis in 78 patients: radiographic outcomes, complications, and technique. *Spine*. 2007;32(24):2644-2652.
88. Thawrani DP, Glos DL, Coombs MT, Bylski-Austrow DI, Sturm PF. Transverse process hooks at upper instrumented vertebra provide more gradual motion transition than pedicle screws. *Spine*. 2014;39(14):E826-E832.
89. Cammarata M, Aubin C-É, Wang X, Mac-Thiong J-M. Biomechanical risk factors for proximal junctional kyphosis: a detailed numerical analysis of surgical instrumentation variables. *Spine*. 2014;39(8):E500-E507.
90. Cahill PJ, Wang W, Asghar J, et al. The use of a transition rod may prevent proximal junctional kyphosis in the thoracic spine after scoliosis surgery: a finite element analysis. *Spine*. 2012;37(12):E687-E695.
91. Denis F, Sun EC, Winter RB. Incidence and risk factors for proximal and distal junctional kyphosis following surgical treatment for Scheuermann kyphosis: minimum five-year follow-up. *Spine*. 2009;34(20):E729-E734.
92. Daniels AH, Jurgensmeier D, McKee J, Harrison MW, d'Amato CR. Acute celiac artery compression syndrome after surgical correction of Scheuermann kyphosis. *Spine*. 2009;34(4):E149-E152.
93. Greig D. Congenital kyphosis. *Edinb Med J*. 1916;26:93.
94. Van Schrick F. Die angeborene kyphose. *Z Orthop Chir*. 1932;56:238-259.
95. Tsou PM. Embryology of congenital kyphosis. *Clin Orthop Relat Res*. 1977;128:18-25.
96. Tsou PM, Yau A, Hodgson AR. Embryogenesis and prenatal development of congenital vertebral anomalies and their classification. *Clin Orthop Relat Res*. 1980;152:211-231.
97. Rivard C, Narbaitz R, Uhthoff H. Congenital vertebral malformations: time of induction in human and mouse embryo. *Orthop Rev*. 1979;8(135).
98. McMaster MJ, Singh H. The surgical management of congenital kyphosis and kyphoscoliosis. *Spine*. 2001;26(19):2146-2155.
99. Winter RB, Moe JH, Wang JF. Congenital kyphosis. Its natural history and treatment as observed in a study of one hundred and thirty patients. *J Bone Joint Surg Am*. 1973;55(2):223-256.
100. McMaster MJ, Singh H. Natural history of congenital kyphosis and kyphoscoliosis. A study of one hundred and twelve patients. *J Bone Joint Surg Am*. 1999;81(10):1367-1383.
101. Dubousset J. Congenital kyphosis and lordosis. In: Weinstein S, ed. *The Pediatric Spine*. New York: Raven Press; 1994:245-258.
102. Shapiro J, Herring J. Congenital vertebral displacement. *J Bone Joint Surg Am*. 1993;75(5):656-662.
103. Zeller RD, Ghanem I, Dubousset J. The congenital dislocated spine. *Spine*. 1996;21(10):1235-1240.
104. Basu PS, Elsebaie H, Noordeen MHH. Congenital spinal deformity: a comprehensive assessment at presentation. *Spine*. 2002;27(20):2255-2259.
105. Suh SW, Sarwark JF, Vora A, Huang BK. Evaluating congenital spine deformities for intraspinal anomalies with magnetic resonance imaging. *J Pediatr Orthop*. 2001;21(4):525-531.
106. Mayfield JK, Winter RB, Bradford DS, Moe JH. Congenital kyphosis due to defects of anterior segmentation. *J Bone Joint Surg Am*. 1980;62(8):1291-1301.
107. James JI. Kyphoscoliosis. *J Bone Joint Surg Br*. 1955;37-B(3):414-426.
108. Campos MA, Fernandes P, Dolan LA, Weinstein SL. Infantile thoracolumbar kyphosis secondary to lumbar hypoplasia. *J Bone Joint Surg Am*. 2008;90(8):1726-1729.

109. Winter RB, Moe JH, Lonstein JE. The surgical treatment of congenital kyphosis. A review of 94 patients age 5 years or older, with 2 years or more follow-up in 77 patients. *Spine*. 1985;10(3):224-231.
110. Ruf M, Harms J. Pedicle screws in 1- and 2-year-old children: technique, complications, and effect on further growth. *Spine*. 2002;27(21):E460-E466.
111. Hedequist DJ, Hall JE, Emans JB. The safety and efficacy of spinal instrumentation in children with congenital spine deformities. *Spine*. 2004;29(18):2081-2086, discussion 2087.
112. Kim HW, Weinstein SL. Atypical congenital kyphosis. Report of two cases with long-term follow-up. *J Bone Joint Surg Br*. 1998;80(1):25-29.
113. Winter RB, Moe JH. The results of spinal arthrodesis for congenital spinal deformity in patients younger than five years old. *J Bone Joint Surg Am*. 1982;64(3):419-432.
114. Ruf M, Harms J. Posterior hemivertebra resection with transpedicular instrumentation: early correction in children aged 1 to 6 years. *Spine*. 2003;28(18):2132-2138.
115. Nakamura H, Matsuda H, Konishi S, Yamano Y. Single-stage excision of hemivertebrae via the posterior approach alone for congenital spine deformity: follow-up period longer than ten years. *Spine*. 2002;27(1):110-115.
116. Suk S-I, Kim J-H, Kim W-J, et al. Posterior vertebral column resection for severe spinal deformities. *Spine*. 2002;27(21):2374-2382.
117. Shono Y, Abumi K, Kaneda K. One-stage posterior hemivertebra resection and correction using segmental posterior instrumentation. *Spine*. 2001;26(7):752-757.
118. Sacramento-Domínguez C, Yagi M, Ayamga J, et al. Apex of deformity for three-column osteotomy. Does it matter in the occurrence of complications? *Spine J*. 2015;15(11):2351-2359.
119. Wang Y, Lenke LG. Vertebral column decancellation for the management of sharp angular spinal deformity. *Eur Spine J*. 2011;20(10):1703-1710.
120. Murrey DB, Brigham CD, Kiebzak GM, Finger F, Chewning SJ. Transpedicular decompression and pedicle subtraction osteotomy (eggshell procedure): a retrospective review of 59 patients. *Spine*. 2002;27(21):2338-2345.
121. Wang Y, Zhang Y, Zhang X, et al. A single posterior approach for multilevel modified vertebral column resection in adults with severe rigid congenital kyphoscoliosis: a retrospective study of 13 cases. *Eur Spine J*. 2008;17(3):361-372.
122. Kim YJ, Otsuka NY, Flynn JM, et al. Surgical treatment of congenital kyphosis. *Spine*. 2001;26(20):2251-2257.

CHAPTER 31 Spondylolysis and Spondylolisthesis

Suken A. Shah

Spondylolysis is defined as a defect in the pars interarticularis of the posterior vertebral arch and is a common cause of back pain and disability.[1] In addition, spondylolysis may lead to instability of the spinal column and result in anterior translation of the vertebral body relative to the level inferior to the defect. This translation in the setting of spondylolysis is termed *spondylolisthesis,* from the Greek roots, *spondylos,* meaning "vertebrae," and *olisthesis,* meaning "to slip."[2] Even in the absence of symptoms from the pars defects themselves, spondylolisthesis may lead to clinically significant radiculopathy and progressive neurologic deficits secondary to nerve root impingement. Both conditions vary in their presentations and require judicious application of conservative and surgical treatment strategies.

The clinical syndrome of spondylolisthesis was first described in 1782 by the Belgian obstetrician Herbiniaux[3] before an understanding of its pathophysiology. Herbiniaux reported a bony prominence anterior to the sacrum that created an impediment to vaginal delivery in a cohort of his patients. In 1853, the German physician Robert[4] reported on specific defects in the pars interarticularis; these defects were first labeled spondylolysis by Killian in 1854.[2] Killian[2] proposed that forces imposed by the body's weight caused subluxation of the lumbosacral facets and subsequent vertebral body subluxation. A short time later, in 1855, anatomic studies by Robert and Lambl revealed that a neural arch defect typically preceded the subluxation.[5] Robert freed the fifth lumbar vertebra successfully of surrounding soft tissue and showed that a neural arch defect was required for slippage to occur.[6]

In 1881, Neugebauer[7] detailed the clinical and anatomic manifestations of the deformity and suggested that lysis, elongation, and angulation of the pars interarticularis could lead to spondylolisthesis. In his travels through Europe in 1888, Neugebauer came across 10 specimens in which there was gross displacement of the fifth lumbar vertebra. He aptly termed this phenomenon *spondyloptosis,* from the Greek *ptosis,* meaning "falling off or down," to indicate a vertebra that is completely dislocated. Neugebauer initially attributed the deformity to traumatic injury; however, he later proposed that it was due to a congenital abnormality of neural arch ossification. This theory of abnormal ossification was questioned by Lane, who, in 1893, posited that spondylolisthesis was due to modification of the interarticular part of the fifth lumbar vertebra by pressure from the inferior facet of L4 superiorly and from the superior sacral process inferiorly.

Pathophysiology

As understanding of spondylolisthesis increased, classifications of common subtypes emerged. The most widely used classification system today was described by Wiltse.[8–11] This system represents a further development of the classification described by Newman and Stone,[12] who, in 1962, reported the long-term outcomes of 319 patients with spondylolisthesis. In their series, spondylolisthesis was classified in terms of radiographic appearance and proposed etiology.

Wiltse separated spondylolisthesis into five main groups (Table 31.1). Type I, also known as *congenital* or *dysplastic spondylolisthesis,* is secondary to a congenital defect of the superior sacral facet or the inferior L5 facet or both, with gradual anterior translation of the L5 vertebra. Type II, also known as *lytic* or *isthmic spondylolisthesis,* involves a defect in the isthmus or pars interarticularis. Type II is classified further into three subtypes. Type IIA represents a spondylolysis or a stress fracture of the pars region. Type IIB represents an intact but elongated pars caused by repeated stress and bony remodeling. Type IIC represents an acute traumatic fracture of the pars leading to anterolisthesis; this is the rarest of the subtypes. It is not the pars defect itself but the anterior translation that allows the lesion to be termed *spondylolisthesis.* Type III is degenerative in origin and is a disease of older adults that develops as a result of facet arthritis and remodeling. Such long-standing intersegmental instability can lead to either anterolisthesis or posterolisthesis. As the disease progresses, the articular processes may become more horizontally shaped, creating the potential for rotational deformity as well. Type IV is a posttraumatic disruption of posterior elements other than

TABLE 31.1 Spondylolisthesis Classification by Wiltse[18]

Type	Description
I	Congenital dysplastic
II	Isthmic: defect at pars interarticularis
IIA	Spondylolytic: stress fracture of pars interarticularis
IIB	Elongation of pars interarticularis
IIC	Acute or traumatic fracture of pars interarticularis
III	Degenerative: long-standing intersegmental instability
IV	Posttraumatic: defects of posterior elements (aside from pars interarticularis)
V	Pathologic

TABLE 31.2 Spondylolisthesis Classification by Marchetti and Bartolozzi[13]

Type	Features
Developmental	
High dysplastic	Interarticular lysis Elongation of pars interarticularis
Low dysplastic	Interarticular lysis Elongation of pars interarticularis
Acquired	
Traumatic	Acute or stress fracture
Postsurgical	Direct or indirect effect of surgery
Pathologic	Local or systemic pathology
Degenerative	Primary or secondary

the pars (as in type IIC). This disruption is a gradual event and not an acute fracture–dislocation, as seen in type IIC. Type V involves the destruction of the posterior elements in the setting of a pathologic process, such as malignancy, Paget disease, tuberculosis, or giant cell tumors. Additionally, an iatrogenic spondylolisthesis may occur after facetectomy.

Wiltse type I and type II constitute most cases, which are the focus of this chapter. Although the classification schemes described allow for the systematic study of these disparate disease entities, they are of no proven prognostic value in the prediction of deformity progression.

The extent to which spondylosis depends on genetic or developmental factors is controversial. In 1982, Marchetti and Bartolozzi[13] divided spondylolisthesis into developmental and acquired subtypes. Developmental etiologies included elongation of the pars, lytic lesions, and traumatic events, whereas acquired etiologies included iatrogenic, pathologic, and degenerative conditions. In 1994, a revised classification system subclassified the developmental group further into high or low dysplastic. In these two subgroups, the pars interarticularis was described as being either osteolytic or elongated. Traumatic lesions were incorporated into the acquired group and the iatrogenic etiology was relabeled as postsurgical (Table 31.2). Although developmental abnormalities of the posterior arch are typically insufficient to cause spondylolysis in the absence of other inciting factors, they may play a significant role in the predisposition to spondylolysis and subsequent spondylolisthesis.

A significant genetic predisposition is suggested by the observation that spondylolysis occurs in 15% to 70% of first-degree relatives of individuals with the disorder.[14-22] Spondylolisthesis also shows a strong familial association, with an incidence in first-degree or second-degree relatives of approximately 25% to 30%.[5,9,11,23] A radiographic study by Wynne-Davies and Scott[15] showed that dysplastic spondylolisthesis has a familial incidence of 33%, whereas the isthmic variant has a familial incidence of 15%. Compared with the incidence in the general population, this represents a fourfold and twofold increased familial risk in patients with dysplastic and isthmic spondylolisthesis, respectively. Wynne-Davies and Scott[15] suggested a multifactorial autosomal dominant pattern of inheritance with incomplete penetrance. Wiltse[22] suggested, however, that a cartilaginous defect in the vertebrae may be of autosomal recessive inheritance with varying expressivity. Additionally, the correlation between spina bifida occulta and spondylolisthesis strengthens the suggestion of a hereditary contribution.

In combination with developmental susceptibilities, certain activities are risk factors for spondylolysis because of the nature of the biomechanical stresses imparted on the pars interarticularis. Biomechanical analyses have shown that hyperextension and persistent lordosis increase shear stresses at the neural arch.[24–27] Wiltse and colleagues[28] hypothesized that most cases of isthmic spondylolysis should be considered fatigue fractures caused by repetitive load and stress as opposed to a single traumatic event, although a traumatic event may lead to completion of a fracture already in development. Farfan and colleagues[29] hypothesized that a single event leads to the initial microfracture in the pars, with fractures occurring as a result of repetitive overload. As a result of these biomechanical data, activities that involve hyperextension of the lumbar spine—such as gymnastics, weightlifting, diving, football, and volleyball—have been implicated as causative factors in the development of spondylolysis.[27,30–32]

Persistent lumbar lordosis may also increase susceptibility to spondylosis; Ogilvie and Sherman[14] reported a 50% prevalence of asymptomatic spondylolysis in patients with Scheuermann kyphosis. The tendency toward progression of slippage during adolescence and the observation that girls are several times more likely to have an increase in deformity are also suggestive of a hormonal role in the development of spondylolisthesis.[23]

Epidemiology

The exact prevalence of spondylolysis is uncertain because it is asymptomatic in a large proportion of patients. Reports regarding the prevalence of spondylolysis are based primarily on painful or symptomatic spondylolysis or cases associated with listhesis. The prevalence in whites has been reported as 3% to 6%, with a male-to-female ratio of 2 : 1.[33–35] Roche and Rowe[35] examined 4200 cadaveric specimens and found an overall prevalence of spondylolysis of 4.2%. Considerable ethnic variability exists in the prevalence of spondylolysis, with a lower prevalence in blacks (1.8%–2.4%) than in whites (5.6%).[36–39] The highest prevalence has been reported in the Eskimo population, with rates of 13% in adolescent patients and 54% in adults.[40] Although this prevalence may suggest a genetic predisposition, it has also been posited that Eskimos, who carry their infants in a papoose, place undue stress on the pars interarticularis.[36]

The reported incidence of isthmic spondylolisthesis ranges from 2.6% to 4.4%.[5,41–43] In the largest prospective radiographic study, Fredrickson and colleagues[41] evaluated 500 patients at age 6 years with a 20-year follow-up. A pars defect was appreciated in 4.4% of 6-year-old children. By age 12 years, 5.2% of the cohort was noted to have the defect (85% participation rate). This increased to 6% by age 18 years; however, most of the nonaffected patients had dropped out of the study (34% participation rate). Back pain had developed in only four of the patients, and one patient required an operative procedure to decompress a herniated disc at a level cephalad to the spondylolisthesis. Pars defects at L5 were noted to be bilateral in 78% of cases, with most of these progressing to spondylolisthesis. As a corollary to this study, Fredrickson and colleagues[41] also evaluated 500 newborns and found no evidence of spondylolysis or spondylolisthesis. The only reported case of a pars lesion in a newborn has been published by Borkow and Kleiger.[44] Isthmic spondylolisthesis is rare in children younger than 5 years old, with only a few reported cases.[43,45,46]

In spondylolysis, the pars interarticularis defect may be unilateral or bilateral. If the defect is bilateral, the chance of progression to listhesis is greater. The most common location of a spondylitic defect is L5 (85%)[47] and the defect may be observed as high as L2; multilevel defects are seen infrequently. Rarely, multiple defects may be seen at the same level. Ariyoshi and colleagues[48] reported a case of spondylolysis at three sites in L5 involving the bilateral pars interarticularis and the center of the right lamina.

The most common site of isthmic spondylolisthesis is at the L5–S1 level secondary to osteolysis at L5. Estimates show that this lesion is located at the L5 pars interarticularis in 90% of type II cases, at L4 in 5%, and in more cephalad vertebrae in the remaining 5% of cases.[11] Additionally, authors have reported spina bifida occulta at the same level in 30% of patients with pars lesions. The incidence of spina bifida associated with spondylolisthesis has been reported to range from 24% to 70%.[9,23,49,50] Age at presentation with isthmic spondylolisthesis follows a bimodal distribution. One peak occurs between the ages of 5 and 7 years, and the second occurs in the teenage years.[9,19,49,51] The incidence in athletes who subject themselves to excessive lumbar posturing, such as gymnasts, soccer players, pitchers, cricket bowlers, and divers, is higher than in the general population.[52–59]

In pediatric patients, dysplastic and isthmic are the most commonly encountered subtypes, with the latter representing 85% of the cases. As with spondylolysis, isthmic (type II) spondylolisthesis is two times more frequent in boys than girls.[35] Dysplastic spondylolisthesis, similar to its isthmic counterpart, is also most commonly found at the L5–S1 junction. The incidence is two times higher in girls[60,62] and, based on more recent published reports, it accounts for 14% to 21% of total cases.[61,62]

History and Physical Examination

Spondylolysis may be discovered incidentally or may manifest with low back pain typically in the teenage years.[63] In approximately half of cases, the onset of low back pain is associated with a history of trauma or an inciting event.[23,64,65] Usually, these patients complain of focal low back pain, only rarely radiating to the buttocks or posterior thigh, which becomes worse with activity or on hyperextension of the spine.[31,66–69] Lifting and weight bearing can exacerbate the pain, and a forced lumbar extension often intensifies the symptoms. Neurologic involvement is rare in isolated spondylolysis. Medical professionals who have little experience with spondylolysis often assume the defect to be a sequela of trauma requiring immediate immobilization and surgical intervention. In these cases, it is the responsibility of the spine surgeon to offer reassurance that imminent neurologic compromise is highly unlikely.[70,71]

Physical examination of the lumbar spine reveals focal tenderness in acute cases and mild discomfort in chronic cases. Patients maintain a full range of forward flexion (unless the hamstrings are tight) that is usually painless, but hyperextension movement leads to an exacerbation of symptoms, as does lateral bending or rotation. Other associated physical signs are an antalgic gait, increased lumbar lordosis, and hamstring tightness. A single-leg hyperextension test is used for the diagnosis and differentiation of unilateral spondylolysis from bilateral lysis. This test is performed by the patient bearing weight on one leg with the hip and knee of the other leg flexed while hyperextending the lumbar spine. This maneuver is performed on both sides; asymmetrical low back pain indicates unilateral spondylolysis. Bilateral lesions show symmetrical or asymmetrical pain with this maneuver.[72,73] The neurologic examination in isolated spondylolysis is generally normal, with radicular findings suggestive of foraminal stenosis owing to inflammation or instability.

Spondylolisthesis may manifest in a similar fashion but is also typically associated with hamstring tightness. This tightness manifests as a muscle spasm of the posterior thighs associated with a fixed flexion at the hip and knees. An increased popliteal angle is present on straight-leg raise. An increased popliteal angle is almost always observed universally, even in low-grade spondylolisthesis. Electromyographic and neurologic abnormalities are typically absent; this suggests that there is not a neurologic basis for the hamstring tightness but that it likely results from the patient's attempts to maintain global sagittal balance.[62,74] Other authors hypothesize that tightness results as a sequela of chronic nerve root irritation from the instability and micromotion of the involved segment.[74–77] Patients often ambulate and stand with increased flexion at the hips and knees, also known as the Phalen-Dickson sign.[75] This flexed posturing increases as the amount of slippage increases. The patient may also exhibit a shuffled or short-stepped gait.[77]

Patients with spondylolisthesis may initially present with focal neurologic deficits or radiculopathy, although this is uncommon. Bilateral radicular symptoms are more commonly observed than unilateral radiculopathy. Typically, the L5 root is involved, with pain radiating to the buttocks and posterior thigh or weakness of the extensor hallucis longus. Constant loading of the pars defects may hinder bony healing, resulting in a fibrous union that may be a persistent source of pain. Local expansion of fibrocartilaginous scar tissue within the area of the pars defect may cause nerve root compression. Tension on the nerve root also increases with progression of olisthesis, increasing further the likelihood of radicular symptoms with disease progression.[71] In higher-grade subluxations, traction of the cauda equina over the sacrum may exist. This traction may lead to signs and symptoms of cauda equina compression, such as perineal paresthesia, decreased sphincter tone, and urinary retention. Additionally, traction of the cauda is thought to create a reflex spasm of the hamstrings.[78,79]

Higher-grade spondylolisthesis results in a palpable step-off over the spinous processes. In isthmic spondylolisthesis, the step-off is typically found at the L4–L5 junction, as the neural arch of the L5 vertebra does not translate anteriorly with the body but remains within its geographic location in relation to the sacrum. In dysplastic spondylolisthesis, the neural arch is still attached to the vertebral body and slides anteriorly with the body, producing a palpable step-off that is typically appreciated at the lumbosacral junction. Lumbosacral kyphosis with a retroverted sacrum results in heart-shaped, flattened buttocks. In severe cases, the trunk appears grossly shortened, and the rib cage lies within close proximity to the iliac crests.

Scoliosis also may be associated with spondylolisthesis.[12,25,80–84] The incidence has been reported to be 60%. Scoliosis may result because of a combination of hamstring and paraspinal muscle spasm, rotational deformity, or truncal asymmetry. If scoliosis is secondary to spondylolisthesis (nonstructural), it usually resolves after treatment of the olisthesis. The patient may also have an adolescent idiopathic curve with a low-grade spondylolisthesis that was detected incidentally on radiographic evaluation.

Radiographic Evaluation

Many imaging modalities may be useful in the diagnosis and evaluation of spondylolisthesis. Radiographic evaluation of spondylolisthesis begins with plain radiographs, including lateral, anteroposterior, and oblique views.[85] The anteroposterior view should be angled 15 degrees to the inclination of the L5–S1 disc (Ferguson view). This view not only allows for visualization of the presence of sacral spinal bifida, but also evaluates the size of the lumbar transverse processes and height of the disc.

The defect in isthmic spondylolysis is visualized as lucency in the region of the pars interarticularis. The lucency is commonly described as having the appearance of a collar or a "broken neck on the Scotty dog" seen in lateral oblique radiographs. A spot lateral view is able to identify only 19% of pars defects,[33,86] whereas oblique lateral views can detect the pars defect in 84% of cases.[87] It is important to take right and left oblique views because pars defects may be unilateral in some cases, and the collar may be visible in only one projection.

Although oblique views are most sensitive in diagnosing spondylolysis, the lateral view is optimal for appreciating the degree of olisthesis in spondylolisthesis. The lateral view should be performed with the patient standing. Flexion-extension views may assess for the presence of associated instability. This subtle movement may be an important pain generator and is essential for further treatment planning. Additionally, these views show the extent of postural reduction of the lumbosacral angulation and translation that may be obtained without formal release.

Because the sensitivity of plain radiographs is limited, radionuclide (technetium-99m) bone imaging may be a good option in cases of suspected spondylolysis with negative plain radiographs. A bone scan identifies pars interarticularis stress fractures that can be missed in oblique radiographs because a stress reaction may be present without a bony defect. Patients who have had a recent trauma or performed strenuous activity and are symptomatic have a bone scan showing increased uptake in the spondylolytic area; however, patients with chronic low backache can have normal bone scans if the defect is chronic, is sclerotic, and has lost its blood supply. Single photon emission computed tomography (SPECT) is more sensitive and provides more details than plain radiographs and technetium bone scan.[88,89] A "hot" scan insinuates increased activity and the patient may benefit from orthotic immobilization, whereas a "cold" scan suggests a chronic lesion that is not metabolically active and is unlikely to respond to immobilization alone.[71]

Thin-cut axial computed tomography (CT) is highly accurate at visualizing osseous anatomy and is superior to plain radiography in its ability to show dysplastic facets and pars defects. CT may also be used after plain radiographs or bone scan to assess the healing potential of an identified pars defect.[90] In addition to showing spondylolysis accurately, CT may identify changes in the apophyseal joints associated with degenerative and reverse spondylolisthesis and can show minimal degrees of spondylolisthesis by the presence of a pseudo-bulging disc.[91]

Magnetic resonance imaging (MRI) is a highly sensitive imaging technique that allows for additional visualization of soft tissue and neural structures and is recommended in all cases associated with neurologic findings. MRI offers the distinct advantage of being able to image the spine in any plane without exposure to ionizing radiation. Sagittal thin slices (3-mm slice thickness for T1-weighted images and 4-mm slice thickness for T2-weighted images) are able to identify 95% of pars defects, with T1-weighted images being more sensitive than T2-weighted images.[92] In the early course of the disease, MRI helps in identifying the stress reaction at the pars interarticularis before the end-stage bony defect.[93,94] In more acute presentations in which plain radiographs may be negative, a fat saturation technique can be applied to minimize signal from fat and to bring out signal from fluid

TABLE 31.3 Meyerding Classification[a]

Grade	Percentage of Slippage (A/B)
0	0 (spondylolysis)
I	0–25%
II	25–50%
III	50–75%
IV	75–100%
V	Vertebral body completely displaced (spondyloptosis)

[a]Grades 0 and V were added later.

structures, such as bone edema. MRI also allows for evaluation of the spinal cord and its associated elements with greater anatomic detail and without the procedural risks associated with CT myelography. MRI may show the degree of impingement of neural elements by fibrous scar tissue at the spondylolytic defect. Additionally, involvement of adjacent discs should be evaluated because abnormal biomechanics can lead to early degenerative changes at adjacent levels.

The most commonly used radiographic grading system for spondylolisthesis is the one proposed by Meyerding in 1932.[95] The degree of slippage is measured as the percentage of distance the anteriorly translated vertebral body has moved forward. On the lateral radiograph, a line is drawn along the posterior sacral border. A line perpendicular to this is drawn at the superior part of the sacrum. The anterior translation or displacement of the inferior border of L5 as a proportion of the width of S1 is expressed as a percentage. The Meyerding classification grades increasing olistheses from I to IV (Table 31.3). Spondyloptosis, in which the fifth lumbar vertebra has slipped forward over 100% of the gliding plane past the sacral promontory, is referred to as grade V. Spondylolysis without olisthesis is referred to as grade 0.

Although the Meyerding classification system quantifies translational subluxation in the anteroposterior plane, it does not quantify the sagittal rotation of a vertebral body that may coexist in spondylolisthesis. This angular displacement is referred to as the *slip angle* and, as with the Meyerding grading system, the erect lateral radiograph is the basis for measurement. The slip angle is calculated by measuring the angle formed by the intersection of two lines: (1) a line perpendicular to the posterior cortex of the sacrum and (2) a line paralleling the inferior endplate of L5. In the normal spine, slip angle values should be close to zero. The slip angle quantifies the lumbosacral kyphosis and was shown by Boxall and colleagues[62] to be the most useful tool in determining the risk of the progression in a skeletally immature patient. A slip angle greater than 55 degrees is associated with a high probability and increased rate of progression.

Sacral inclination, or pelvic tilt, refers to the vertical position of the sacrum. It is the angle formed by the intersection of two lines: (1) a line perpendicular to the floor and (2) a line parallel to the posterior cortex of the sacrum. Normal values are greater than 30 degrees. With an increasing slip, lumbosacral kyphosis is increased and the sacrum is forced into a more vertical orientation, decreasing the pelvic tilt.

In 1983, Wiltse and Winter[96] proposed a classification that separated the tangential movement seen in low-grade slips (grades I and II) from the angular and tangential movement that was appreciated in high-grade slips (grade III or higher). The three measurements that were factored were degree of slip, vertebral wedging, and sacral rounding. These authors recommended that the forward displacement of the fifth lumbar vertebra in relation to the sacrum be measured as an actual percentage, as first described by Taillard[42] and later recommended by Laurent and Osterman.[97] It was stressed that even a small degree of progression should be measured, and this was not quantifiable on the Meyerding scale. Sacral tilt as described previously and sagittal rotation or slip angle were also used. The method for measuring slip angle, which Wiltse and Winter[96] termed *sagittal rotation,* was modified by measuring the angle formed by the intersection of two lines: (1) a line extending off the anterior cortex of the L5 vertebral body and (2) a line off the posterior border of the first sacral vertebra. Wiltse and Winter[96] believed the endplates of the L5 and S1 bodies to be unreliable osseous structures secondary to osseous hyperplasia.

Nonoperative Management

Treatment of spondylolysis mainly focuses on pain relief, core muscle strengthening, and restoration of full lumbar range of motion. Achieving these goals enables the patient to return to normal activity without any restrictions. Management of spondylolysis depends on the severity of the symptoms and level of activity. Initial conservative management in the form of activity restriction and bracing (for pain relief) relieves symptoms in patients with spondylolysis. It is likely that most lesions do not heal with bone but become a stable fibrous union that remains relatively asymptomatic.

In the pediatric population, nonoperative management of spondylolysis includes restriction of activity, rehabilitation with strengthening of the abdominal and paraspinal musculature, minimization of pelvic tilt, and perhaps antilordotic bracing.[98] Nonoperative management protocols also depend on several factors, such as disease involvement (spondylolysis vs. spondylolisthesis), level and laterality of the defect (unilateral vs. bilateral pars defects), duration since injury (acute vs. chronic), and age of the patient.[99] Many authors prefer to use a total-contact, low-profile polyethylene orthosis, which is designed to maintain an antilordotic posture and extends from just below the nipples to 1 inch above the greater trochanter. The brace is worn for 23 hours/day for a minimum of 3 to 6 months.[100] If clinical symptoms improve, the brace can be gradually weaned through a period of part-time wear.

Excellent clinical outcomes have been reported with a course of activity restriction and bracing that prevents repetitive hyperextension movements at the lumbar spine.[100–103] Good to excellent results with brace therapy have been shown in 80% of patients with grade 0 or I spondylolisthesis.[100,104,105] Bell and colleagues[104] showed prevention of increased slip angle and 100% reduction of pain in 28 patients with grade I or II spondylolisthesis after a mean brace treatment of 25 months. In a series of 82 symptomatic patients with various degrees of spondylolisthesis, Pizzutillo and Hummer[105] reported that nonoperative treatment of grade II or less was shown to relieve pain reliably in two-thirds of patients. A study by Steiner and Micheli[100] showed radiographic evidence of healing pars defects in 12 of 67 patients with spondylolysis or grade I spondylolisthesis after treatment in a modified Boston brace. Excellent or good results were achieved in 78%, with return to full activities. Patients with spondylolysis and grade I spondylolisthesis may return to full activity and sports with resolution of symptoms and documented lack of slip progression. Controversy exists regarding post-brace activity level for patients with grade II spondylolisthesis. The general consensus is that after successful brace treatment, a child with grade II spondylolisthesis may return to sports that do not involve hyperlordotic posturing.[18,26,27]

Patients with acute pars interarticularis fractures are best treated with immediate initiation of bracing for pain relief and restriction from athletic activity, with continued mobilization for activities of daily living. Anderson and colleagues[106] used clinical evaluation and SPECT imaging to compare the rate of response to early versus late initiation of bracing. In this study, patients with early bracing showed rapid relief of symptoms, a short bracing time, and rapid reduction of SPECT ratio. Patients showing a spondylolytic defect on plain radiography but whose bone scans were negative were determined to have inactive (terminal) spondylolytic defects, pseudarthrosis, or old unhealed fractures.[72,107] Athletes with low back pain and increased uptake on SPECT scan at the pars interarticularis but no defect on radiographs typically respond to a period of rest and active rehabilitation; very few athletes develop defects or persistent back pain.[108]

As the understanding of spinal biomechanics has progressed, Panjabi[109] posited the concept of specific training of lumbar muscles in chronic low back pain. According to his concept, specific training of muscles around the lumbar spine improves the dynamic stability and controls segmental spinal motion. The local muscular system that controls the lumbar spine consists of lumbar multifidus, internal oblique, and transverse abdominis.[109] A randomized trial by O'Sullivan of 44 patients who were treated with two different protocols showed that a specific strengthening program was more effective than generalized back strengthening exercises.[98] Along with exercises that target specific core muscle groups with the spine in neutral position, strengthening of hip flexors and hamstring stretching are important and recommended.[100,101,110]

Patients with low-grade dysplastic spondylolisthesis are less likely than patients with isthmic spondylolisthesis to respond to conservative measures,[5] but conservative therapy is still recommended as the initial modality. The importance of radiographic and neurologic follow-up should be stressed to these patients because they are at a higher risk for slip progression owing to facet hypoplasia. Radiographic follow-up is recommended at least annually until skeletal maturity and more frequently during peak height velocity before puberty. Documentation of slip percentage, angle, sacral inclination, wedging, and pelvic tilt is recommended as part of proper documentation of progression of the deformity.

Surgical Treatment

Surgical intervention is indicated for patients with persistent pain, progressive spondylolisthesis, or neurologic symptoms who fail conservative management. Treatment approach is influenced by the level of spinal maturity, degree of slippage, symptoms, the patient's activity level, and expected progression. In contrast to a comparable adult, an asymptomatic adolescent may be a candidate for surgical intervention because of expected progression of deformity in a high-grade slip, which may lead to mechanical and neurologic dysfunction. In a skeletally immature patient with slippage greater than 50% or a mature adolescent with a slip greater than 75%, operative intervention is recommended even if the patient is asymptomatic.[111-113] Surgical decompression is also indicated when a patient has neural compromise, with a radiculopathy or bowel or bladder dysfunction.[114–116]

Surgical treatment options may be broadly divided into two categories: direct repair of the pars defects versus arthrodesis of the involved segments to prevent slip progression with or without decompression of affected neural structures. Procedures for direct fixation of pars defects include the Buck technique,[117] Scott wiring,[118] and repair with an ipsilateral pedicle screw and hook.[119,120]

Fusion of the involved level has been widely advocated as treatment of symptomatic spondylolysis.[111,121] The long-term effects of fusion in a young patient must be considered, however, owing to the potential for adjacent-segment degeneration.[122,123] Based on their simulated lumbar fusion studies in cadavers, Weinhoffer and colleagues[124] concluded that increased intradiscal pressure at the level of fusion could lead to accelerated degeneration at the adjacent discs. Kinematic studies of adjacent vertebra after fusion have shown disc degeneration, increased stress at the facet joints, hypertrophy of the facets, and hypermobility at the adjacent level.[123,125,126] Based on these kinematic studies and the goal of preserving motion when possible, isolated repair of the pars interarticularis defect is the preferred treatment for symptomatic pars defects in patients with no slip or disc degeneration at that level and relief from the diagnostic injection. Fusion is an option if an attempt at pars repair is unsuccessful, the lamina is dysplastic, the defect is very large, or disc degeneration or listhesis is present. Some authors maintain that results for fusion are better at L5 because of the narrow lamina at L5 and the steep lordotic angle that may be present.[127]

To increase the probability of response to surgical treatment, Wu and colleagues[128] reported on the use of preoperative diagnostic pars injection at the site of the defect. In their series of 100 patients who had failed conservative management, the pain generator was confirmed by injecting 1.5 mL of bupivacaine (Marcaine) into the lytic area. Reproduction of similar pain and pain relief of at least 70% of the usual pain quality for more than 6 hours were considered as a positive response; these patients subsequently showed an excellent outcome after repair of the defect.[128]

Buck fusion is an open technique in which the fibrous tissue at the pars defect is identified, thoroughly debrided, and stabilized with a 4.5-mm stainless steel cortical screw in compression.[117] Buck[117] concluded that this technique was indicated only in cases in which the gap was smaller than 3 to 4 mm. Various studies showed 88% to 100% defect healing and satisfactory results with his technique.[129–131] Direct repair using a screw is a demanding procedure, however; owing to the narrowness of the lamina, a minimal displacement or malposition of the screw can lead to implant failure or complications such as nerve root irritation, injury to the posterior arch or dura, or pseudarthrosis.[132,133]

In the Scott technique, a stainless steel wire is looped from the transverse processes to the spinous process of the level involved and tightened in conjunction with local iliac crest bone graft.[118] This wire creates a tension band construct, placing the pars defect under compression, and holds the bone graft in place. Bradford and Iza[134] reported 80% good to excellent results and 90% radiographic healing of the defects. This technique requires greater surgical exposure, with extensive stripping of the muscles to expose the transverse process. Complications such as wire breakage are common with this technique. Salib and Pettine[135] modified this technique by passing a wire around the cortical screws introduced into both pedicles and tightening it beneath the spinous process. Biomechanical tests show that fixation of the wire to the pedicle screw does not increase the stiffness of the system.[136] Both cerclage techniques have good defect healing rates of 86% to 100%.[118,135,137,138] Songer and Rovin[139] modified this construct by replacing the wire with a cable tied up to a pedicle screw and then passed and wrapped around the contralateral lamina. This system provides solid fixation; the authors reported excellent outcome in five of seven patients and 100% solid union in all patients.

Morscher and colleagues[140] introduced a new technique to repair the pars defect with a laminar hook, which is loaded with compression by a spring placed against a screw threaded in the articular process. Healing rates with this technique range from 56% to 82%.[140–144] The major drawback of this procedure is screw penetration to the inferior articular process of the cephalad vertebra, which can lead to screw loosening or breakage.[145] Gillet and Petit[146] introduced the concept of the rod screw construct, in which the rod is firmly fixed to the spinous process, and published excellent outcomes in 6 of 10 patients.

Taddonio, using the Cotrel-Dubousset system, first introduced a repair using pedicle screw fixation.[146a] Tokuhashi and Matsuzaki[127] reported excellent outcomes with the Isola pediculolaminar system. Kakiuchi[147] reported similar results using the Texas Scottish Rite Hospital instrumentation system; with this technique, hooks are fixed at the lamina and connected with a rod to an ipsilateral pedicle screw after compression. Roca and colleagues[148] reported 92% excellent results with their new pedicle screw hook construct system in adolescents, but they have not recommended this technique for patients older than 20 years. Pellise and colleagues[149] advised 1-mm thin cuts to assess the pars anatomy, but 2.5-mm cuts help in assessing bone healing after direct repair in spondylolysis.

Our preferred technique for pars repair is to use minimal access tubes or retractors to obtain exposure of the pars defect and debride the fibrous tissue and hypertrophic nonunion with a burr and curettes to bleeding bone, but care must be taken not to enlarge the defect further and destabilize the segment. Iliac crest bone graft is placed into the defect and a cannulated laminar screw is placed percutaneously over a predrilled guidewire from the ipsilateral inferior lamina across the defect to engage the cortical bone of the pedicle or superior endplate for compression, avoiding the facet joint. Additional graft (or bone graft replacement) is placed over the defect, extending from the lamina to the junction of the transverse process. The patient is immobilized in a low-profile thoracolumbosacral orthosis for 12 weeks (hip joint locked with a leg extension for the first 6 weeks) and then progressed to rehabilitation. Healing is checked at 6 months and the patient is allowed to resume all sports.

For a pediatric patient with grade I or II spondylolisthesis, dysplastic spondylolisthesis at the lumbosacral junction, or a slip secondary to a defect of the L5 pars who has failed conservative treatment, posterior in situ fusion is recommended from L5 to S1. With the widespread use of pedicle screws and the myriad screw options that are available, numerous studies have been performed supporting the use of transpedicular fixation. Transpedicular fixation has been shown to increase the rate of fusion, and a positive correlation has been reported between successful fusion and clinical outcome.[150–156] Other series have not shown a statistically significant difference between instrumented and noninstrumented posterior fusions.[157,158] In one study of 10 patients in a cohort who had the working diagnosis of spondylolisthesis, 5 underwent instrumented fusion, 4 of whom achieved an excellent or good outcome, compared with 2 of 5 who underwent a noninstrumented fusion.[159]

Lenke and colleagues[160] performed noninstrumented in situ fusions in 56 pediatric patients with isthmic spondylolisthesis. Based on radiographic evidence, only 50% showed a solid fusion mass, whereas 33% showed radiographic changes highly unlikely or with no evidence of a fusion mass. Despite poor fusion rates, overall clinical improvement was noted in greater than 80% of the cohort with preoperative symptoms of back or leg pain or hamstring tightness. A trend for improved clinical outcome with increased rigidity of fixation has been noted.[151] Pedicle screw fixation systems have been shown to be mechanically superior to other fixation while allowing for the selective segmental force without extension to adjacent levels.[161] Additionally, the use of instrumentation obviates the need for postoperative casting in a compliant patient. If exposure of midline structures and decompression is not warranted, the paraspinal approach described by Wiltse and colleagues[11,162] is recommended because it avoids neural arch defects, minimizes soft tissue trauma, and improves visualization of posterolateral structures. It also helps maintain the position of the bone graft and may promote fusion. During surgical dissection, care must be taken to protect facets at levels cephalad to the proposed fusion because this may create instability or degeneration later on. Minimally invasive techniques are available.

The method of immobilization after an in situ posterior fusion ranges from bed rest to bilateral pantaloon spica casts for 6 months. Literature can be found to support either end of the spectrum.[112,163–169] Boxall and colleagues[62] and Sherman and colleagues[170] compared in situ patients who were immobilized in a cast or orthosis with patients who were treated with bed rest.[62,170] Each study showed no statistical difference in the fusion rate based on immobilization methods.

Decompression is warranted in patients with neurologic findings. Patients with low-grade spondylolisthesis generally do not have significant neurologic symptoms. In an adult patient with radiculopathy, it may be acceptable to perform only a decompressive procedure, as described in 1955 by Gill and colleagues.[114] The removal of loose posterior elements and cartilaginous tissue can increase vertebral column instability and further progression of deformity, however—an unacceptable risk in the pediatric spine.[171,172] Although a wide decompression may be warranted, it should be augmented with spinal fusion in a growing child.[114] Studies have also shown an increased risk of progression of deformity in patients with L5 laminectomy and posterior fusion versus patients with posterior fusion alone.[172–174]

Treatment of high-grade spondylolisthesis is a topic of great debate. Symptomatic patients with high-grade spondylolisthesis tend to fare poorer with nonoperative treatment compared with their counterparts with low-grade spondylolisthesis.[175] In high-grade spondylolisthesis, correction of the slip angle rather than the degree of anterior listhesis should be addressed. Although studies show that patients with greater than 50% of slippage may not have a poor nonoperative outcome,[176] fusion is the general treatment of choice among spinal surgeons. In determining the most appropriate procedure, one must take into account all presenting symptoms, neurologic function, radiographic findings, clinical deformity, patient's age, and the surgeon's experience.

As with low-grade spondylolisthesis, in situ fusion was a described treatment for pediatric patients with high-grade spondylolisthesis; however, cranial extension is recommended.[165] A Wiltse approach is suggested unless decompression is warranted. As reported by Pizzutillo and colleagues,[177] bone graft placement at the level of or anterior to the transverse processes extending to the sacral ala helps to ensure a large posterolateral fusion mass, which can effectively counteract shear forces at the lumbosacral junction. Allograft or autograft (or both) may be used, balancing the rate of successful fusion versus the potential for donor site pain and morbidity.[173,178–181]

Postoperative progression of deformity has been appreciated in patients and has been attributed to pseudarthrosis, lack of postoperative immobilization, lack of graft consolidation or maturation, or deterioration of the solid fusion mass. Progression has been appreciated in patients with a solid fusion mass, as evidenced by radiography. Patients with a greater preoperative deformity are at higher risk.[165,168,172,182,183] The advance of slippage is usually minor in these cases, and studies have shown that radiographic evidence of pseudarthrosis does not always lead to pain.[62,160,184] Studies with long-term follow-up of patients with high-grade spondylolisthesis show in situ fusion to be a viable solution in maintenance of symptom relief and prevention of degenerative arthrosis of mobile cephalad spinal segments.[163,185–187]

Grzegorzewski and Kumar[168] found no radiographic pseudarthrosis in 21 patients with high-grade spondylolisthesis treated with in situ fusion, postoperative immobilization in a pantaloon spica cast, and 4 months of bed rest. Although five patients showed evidence of slip progression, two of whom showed an increased slip angle within the first year, only four patients had symptoms of back pain after postoperative follow-up of almost 13 years. Overall reports show radiographic evidence of successful fusion to range from 71% to 100% and relief of back pain and neurologic symptoms to range from 74% to 100% in patients after in situ fusion.[1,165,170,175] Patients with high-grade spondylolisthesis who are at risk of developing pseudarthrosis require a wide decompression secondary to L5 radiculopathy or sacral root symptoms, and patients with excessive mobility at the L5–S1 junction require fusion with pedicle screw instrumentation. Patients with hypoplastic transverse processes, spina bifida, and sacral malformation are also at risk of pseudarthrosis.

Transsacral fusion using either a fibular graft or mesh cage has been shown more recently to be a viable treatment option. By providing an anterior column support and fusion bed, increased structural stability can be achieved. Smith and Bohlman[188] suggested a modification to posterolateral fusion to decrease the incidence of pseudarthrosis and progression of deformity. Eleven patients with high-grade spondylolisthesis were treated in a single-stage procedure involving spinal decompression, in situ posterolateral arthrodesis with autologous iliac crest graft, and anterior arthrodesis with a fibular graft inserted from the posterior approach. A cannulated drill was used to develop a transsacral osseous tunnel extending into the L5 vertebral body. A mid-diaphyseal fibular graft was harvested, trimmed, and inserted into this tunnel, acting as a dowel in the lumbosacral junction. Preoperative neurologic findings were sensory deficits in all but one patient and cauda equina syndrome in five patients. Six patients had prior spinal operations that had failed. The average duration of follow-up was 64 months, showing a solid fusion mass with complete or major neurologic recovery in all patients. Average time to solid fusion was 12 weeks.

In a patient with sagittal balance and high-grade spondylolisthesis, an in situ procedure or partial reduction can be performed, and a cage or fibular dowel can be inserted anteriorly from L5 into S1 or posteriorly with a retrograde direction from S1 into L5. Posterior insertion of the transvertebral cage or fibular graft is advantageous because it obviates the need for an anterior approach to the lumbosacral region, which has its own drawbacks. There is less blood loss and less risk of injury to great vessels. Because the entire procedure can be done with the patient in one position and with one incision, operative time is also greatly reduced. A partial reduction can be performed by use of concave rods, and fusion should be augmented with posterior instrumentation.

Mahmood and colleagues[189] presented a case series in which a transsacral mesh cage was used in lieu of a fibular strut graft. Partial reduction was accomplished with a pedicle screw curved-rod construct, after which an osseous tunnel was established and a transsacral cage impregnated with bone graft was inserted from a posterior approach. A distinct benefit of using a cage is increased biomechanical stability, as studies have shown fibular strut resorption, deformation, and even fracture.[189–191] Additionally, the use of a cage avoids potential donor site morbidity.[192,193] Average radiographic and clinical follow-up of these patients was 38 months, showing evidence of fusion and relief of symptoms.

There is no clear indication for when reduction of a high-grade spondylolisthesis is necessary as opposed to performing a fusion with mild correction of the slip angle. Many authors suggest that an in situ fusion or mild correction is indicated for patients who exhibit sagittal balance and acceptable slip angle. When considering reduction, improvement of slip angle should be the primary objective rather than improvement of grade of listhesis. In patients with a high-grade slip, a larger slip angle correlates with increased risk of progression of deformity.[74,76] Reduction of spondylolisthesis results in improved sagittal balance, improvement in cosmesis, and a biomechanically stable fusion mass. In addition, by reducing the deformity, canal stenosis is improved, and tension on nerve roots and the cauda equina is reduced. Improvement of overall sagittal alignment leads to improved posture, improved gait, and increased function. Reduction of spondylolisthesis in skeletally immature patients is recommended for patients with a high slip angle (>45 degrees), patients with severe sagittal imbalance, and patients who are at high risk of developing a pseudarthrosis with in situ fusion.[62,163,194]

Numerous methods of reduction have been described. The earliest reported reduction was published in 1936 by Jenkins,[195] who used longitudinal traction followed by anterior fusion; however, the reduction could not be maintained. Since his initial report, variations of Jenkins's described technique have been published.[163,185,196–206] Reduction techniques may be as minimally invasive as external casting after bone graft placement or as complex as staged procedures involving multiple posterior and anterior approaches.

Reduction with external casting is particularly beneficial in young patients, in whom pedicle screw fixation is not feasible. After an open procedure in which posterior elements are decorticated and bone graft is placed around the proposed fusion site, the surgical wound is closed. The patient is placed on an antilordotic frame or spica table with extension of the spine to reduce the lumbosacral kyphosis. The patient should be awake for this part of the procedure to report any changes in neurologic function. If this is impossible, the use of neuromonitoring may help in the neurologic assessment during the reduction. To hold the reduction, the spica cast should be extended to the trunk and incorporate at least one thigh. Burkus and colleagues[166] showed that the use of pantaloon spica cast immobilization led to a decrease in sagittal translation of more than 5% in three-quarters of patients treated with cast immobilization and a decrease in the slip angle of more than 5% in 58% of patients treated with cast immobilization. Of the patients who did not undergo cast immobilization, 45% had an increase in sagittal translation of more than 5% and 56% had an increase in slip angle of more than 5 degrees.

In patients in whom instrumentation can be placed, reduction followed by instrumentation for stability is recommended. Published procedures include halo-femoral or halo-pelvic traction and anteroposterior fusion followed by application of a pantaloon spica cast to apply anteriorly directed pressure.[163,200] Other authors have described anterior release with partial reduction and anterior interbody fusion,[207] intraoperative closed reduction followed by instrumented posterior fusion,[208] and a two-stage procedure with a posterior decompression and halo-skeletal traction followed by interbody fusion.[209] Drawbacks to these procedures included lengthy preoperative hospitalization for traction and lengthy postoperative immobilization in a cast. The study by Burkus and colleagues[166] compared patients treated with a pure in situ fusion with patients who underwent posterior fusion and were reduced postoperatively in a pantaloon spica cast. Reduction was found to be safe and fusion rates were noted to be higher in addition to less chance of late slip and slip angle progression in patients who were treated with a reduction.

Mehdian and Arun[211] published a three-stage procedure using a combined anterior and posterior approach performed in one operative sitting. In the first stage, a laminectomy of L5 is performed with wide decompression of the L4–S1 nerve roots. L5–S1 discectomy was performed next, followed by an osteotomy of the posterosuperior aspect of S1. The second stage consisted of a transperitoneal approach to the L5–S1 level, allowing removal of the anterior disc protrusion and associated thickened anulus fibrosus, effectively allowing posterior translation of the superior body. In the final stage, the patient is repositioned prone and instrumented from L4 to S1. Bilateral pedicle screws are initially placed at L4 and S1, and a reduction can be performed with the assistance of curved rods, after which bilateral L5 pedicle fixation points can be established. Cages may be inserted in the L5–S1 interspace to promote a solid arthrodesis.

Our preferred method for treating high-grade slips with significant lumbosacral kyphosis is postural reduction with positioning under anesthesia and a wide decompression of the L5 and S1 nerve roots bilaterally. The dysplastic L5–S1 disc is removed with a transforaminal approach, and the dome of the sacrum is osteotomized (sacroplasty) to facilitate gentle reduction. Reduction pedicle screws are used to reduce the slip gently, an interbody graft is placed, and the construct is compressed posteriorly to obtain lordosis.

Treatment of severe deformity, including spondyloptosis, can be challenging to the most experienced spine surgeon. The natural history of spondyloptosis is unclear because of its rarity and because it is frequently not reported separately from high-grade spondylolisthesis (grades III and IV). Most authors agree that in a symptomatic patient, benign neglect is not a viable option. The surgical management of spondyloptosis in children is variably documented in the literature. Some authors propose that posterior fusion in situ with or without decompression is a safe and reliable procedure,[168] whereas others suggest that reduction of the slipped vertebra may prevent some of the adverse sequelae of in situ fusion, which include nonunion, bending of the fusion mass, and persistent or increasing lumbosacral deformity.[191,211–214] Many investigators advocate a combined anterior and posterior fusion using instrumentation. An in situ circumferential fusion, as described by Smith and Bohlman,[188] has the lowest risk for iatrogenic nerve injury.

Resection of the L5 vertebra with reduction of L4 onto S1 was initially described by Gaines and Nichols in 1985.[215] The initial stage of the procedure involves an anterior L5 vertebrectomy, in which the L5 body is removed to the base of the pedicles. The second stage is performed through a midline posterior approach involving resection of the now loose L5 posterior elements, decompression, and instrumented reduction through transpedicular instrumentation of L4 onto S1.[214,215] Lehmer and colleagues[216] performed a retrospective review evaluating indications, techniques, results, and patient satisfaction. Of patients, 25% were found to require reoperation secondary to delayed union or instrumentation failure. Three-quarters were noted to have early postoperative neurologic deficits, more than half of which were present preoperatively, and most resolved. All three patients with preoperative cauda equina syndrome recovered postoperatively, and patient questionnaires revealed a high patient satisfaction rate.

As with other lumbar fusion surgery, the most common complication from an operative intervention is pseudarthrosis. Reported rates vary from 0% to 39%,[82,164,166,169,217] and pseudarthrosis occurs more frequently in fusions performed for lytic (type IIA) spondylolisthesis.[218] Radiographs often show lucency around pedicle screws, instrumentation failure, progression of slip angle, or increased vertebral displacement.

Reports exist of increase in spondylolisthesis even with an uninstrumented solid arthrodesis as shown radiographically.[8,62,106,168,169,177] In most of these reports, radiographs and not CT were used to assess fusion mass; many of these cases may have been pseudarthroses. Increased slip was reported in noninstrumented fusions, providing a sound argument for instrumented fusion.

As per the 2003 mortality and morbidity report of the Scoliosis Research Society, the incidence of neurologic complications with lytic spondylolisthesis surgery is 3.1%.[219] Radiculopathy is the most common surgical complication after reduction. Intraoperative manipulation can cause direct dural trauma, injuring multiple sacral and lumbar nerve roots and resulting in postoperative deficits. The L5 nerve roots are most commonly involved and reports show variable rates of resolution, with the highest risk associated with aggressive reductions of high-grade listhesis.[220–222]

Cauda equina syndrome is a potentially disastrous complication that can occur as a result of intraoperative technique, as a result of postoperative conditions, or with no apparent antecedent cause.[208,223–226] Schoenecker and colleagues[116] described 12 cases after in situ arthrodesis for grade III or grade IV L5–S1 spondylolisthesis. During the procedures, there was no evidence of compromise of the cauda equina. Of 12 patients, 5 showed complete recovery and 7 had permanent residual deficits manifested by bowel and bladder dysfunction. Although the exact etiology is unknown, it may be related to vascular phenomena, transient anterior displacement of L5 during the surgical exposure causing laminar impingement on the sacral dome, or a period of hyperextension during patient positioning.[226] With reduction of the deformity, the risk is far greater. If cauda equina syndrome is suspected, surgical decompression is imperative. Sacroplasty and resection of the adjacent disc or lamina of L5, or both, is recommended because it is thought to facilitate neurologic recovery.[116]

With surgical advances in technique and instrumentation, new biologic and mechanical fusion adjuvants, neuromonitoring, and advanced imaging, it is hoped that further reductions in complication rates may be achieved despite the risks inherent to these highly invasive procedures.

Summary

The treatment of patients with spondylolisthesis can be a challenge for the most experienced spinal specialists. With an increasing number of pediatric athletes and improvements in diagnostic imaging techniques, more patients with spondylolisthesis are presenting to the clinician's office. To address the patient's needs best, one first must establish a proper diagnosis, quantify the deformity, and understand properly the etiology of the disease and its risk of progression.

Most pediatric patients with low-grade slips can be treated effectively with nonoperative modalities such as immobilization, activity and sports restriction or modification, analgesia, and physical therapy. Severe spondylolisthesis in adolescents can be cosmetically and functionally debilitating and poses a challenge to the treating spinal surgeon. Management of high-grade spondylolisthesis often requires larger procedures with increased associated risks. In addition to fusion with or without instrumentation, reduction of the listhesis may be beneficial in certain high-grade lesions. With the increased risks and complexity of the reduction procedure, strict selection criteria must be applied to select proper surgical candidates. Improvement of the slip angle should be the primary objective in considering a patient for deformity reduction. Additionally, sagittal alignment and overall balance should be considered during the decision-making process. All risks must be thoroughly communicated to the patient and family before the decision is made to proceed with surgical intervention.

Acknowledgment

I thank Faisal Mahmood, K. Durga Nagraju, and Andrew J. Milby for their contributions to this chapter in previous editions of this text.

PEARLS

1. Spondylolysis is often discovered incidentally. In asymptomatic cases, patients may need no treatment other than monitoring for progression to spondylolisthesis.
2. Various surgical options have been described for direct fixation of the pars interarticularis in spondylosis and for decompression and fusion for spondylolisthesis. The risks and benefits of each of these options must be carefully considered before recommending surgical treatment.

PITFALL

1. Spondylolisthesis may be associated with neurologic findings attributable to canal stenosis or nerve root impingement. MRI is

recommended in cases with neurologic findings. Surgical intervention may be required even in asymptomatic cases if progressive translation is observed.

KEY POINTS

1. Spondylolysis is defined as a defect in the pars interarticularis and is likely multifactorial in etiology with activity-related, degenerative, and genetic components.
2. Spondylolysis is a common cause of back pain, particularly in young adults and athletes engaging in repetitive hyperextension activities.
3. Most cases of symptomatic spondylolysis respond to conservative management, including bracing, activity modification, and analgesia.
4. Spondylolisthesis is defined as the anterior translation of a superior vertebral body relative to an inferior vertebral body and may occur as a result of insufficiency of the pars interarticularis (isthmic spondylolisthesis), following spondylolysis, or in the absence of spondylolysis (degenerative spondylolisthesis).

KEY REFERENCES

1. Meyerding HW. Spondylolisthesis. *Surg Gynecol Obstet.* 1932;54:371-377.
   The first description of a systematic approach to the radiographic staging of spondylolisthesis.
2. Wiltse LL. The etiology of spondylolisthesis. *J Bone Joint Surg Am.* 1962;44-A:539-560.
   An early example from a series of works characterizing the disparate etiologies of spondylolisthesis.
3. Buck JE. Direct repair of the defect in spondylolisthesis: Preliminary report. *J Bone Joint Surg Br.* 1970;52:432-437.
   Description of operative technique for direct repair of defects in the pars interarticularis.
4. Fredrickson BE, Baker D, McHolick WJ, et al. The natural history of spondylolysis and spondylolisthesis. *J Bone Joint Surg Am.* 1984;66:699-707.
   An epidemiologic overview of spondylolysis and rates of radiographic progression to spondylolisthesis.
5. Bell DF, Ehrlich MG, Zaleske DJ. Brace treatment for symptomatic spondylolisthesis. *Clin Orthop Relat Res.* 1988;236:192-198.
   Clinical series showing good response to conservative treatment of symptomatic low-grade spondylolisthesis with antilordotic orthoses.
6. Panjabi MM. The stabilizing system of the spine: Part I. Function, dysfunction, adaptation, and enhancement. *J Spinal Disord.* 1992;5:383-389.
   A description of spinal biomechanics and the ramifications of spondylolisthesis.
7. Osterman K, Schlenzka D, Poussa M, et al. Isthmic spondylolisthesis in symptomatic and asymptomatic subjects, epidemiology, and natural history with special reference to disk abnormality and mode of treatment. *Clin Orthop Relat Res.* 1993;297:65-70.
   Retrospective analysis of 35 years of data on rates of slip progression, response to treatment, and indications for operative intervention in isthmic spondylolisthesis.
8. Lenke LG, Bridwell KH, Bullis D, et al. Results of in situ fusion for isthmic spondylolisthesis. *J Spinal Disord.* 1992;5:433-442.
   Series of noninstrumented fusions suggesting an incomplete correlation between fusion rates and symptomatic improvement.

REFERENCES

1. Bradford DS, Hu SS. Spondylolysis and spondylolisthesis. In: Weinstein SL, ed. *The Pediatric Spine: Principles and Practice.* New York: Raven Press; 1994:585-601.
2. Killian HF. *Schilderungen neuer beckenformen and ihres verhaltens im leben.* Mannheim: Verlag von Bassermann & Mathy; 1854.
3. Herbiniaux G. *Traite sur divers accouchemens labprieux, et sur polypes de la matrice.* Bruxelles: JL DeBoubers; 1782.
4. Robert C: *Eine cigenthumliche Angeborene lodose, Wahrscheinlich Bedingt durch eine Verschiebung des Korpers des letzen Lendenwirbels auf die Vordere fiache des ersten Kreuzbeinwirbels (spondylolisthesis killian) nebst Bemerkungen uber die Mechanic diser Bekenformation. Monatsschr Beburtskund Frauenkrankheiten, 2nd ed.* 1853, pp 429-432.
5. Ganju A. Isthmic spondylolisthesis. *Neurosurg Focus.* 2002;13:E1.
6. Newell RL. Spondylolysis: An historical review. *Spine.* 1995;20:1950-1956.
7. Neugebauer FL. Aetiologie der sogenannten Spondylolisthesis. *Arch Gynäkol.* 1882;20:133.
8. Wiltse L, Newman PH, Macnab I. Classification of spondylolysis and spondylolisthesis. *Clin Orthop Relat Res.* 1976;117:23-29.
9. Wiltse L, Rothman S. Spondylolithesis: Classification, diagnosis, and natural history. *Semin Spine Surg.* 1989;1:78-94.
10. Wiltse L, Rothman S. Spondylolisthesis: Classification, diagnosis, and natural history. *Semin Spine Surg.* 1993;5:264-280.
11. Wiltse L, Winter RB. Terminology and measurement of spondylolisthesis. *J Bone Joint Surg Am.* 1983;65:768-772.
12. Newman PH, Stone K. The etiology of spondylolisthesis: With a special investigation. *J Bone Joint Surg Br.* 1963;45:39-59.
13. Marchetti PG, Bartolozzi P. Classification of spondylolisthesis as a guidance for treatment. In: DeWald RL, Bridwell KH, eds. *The Textbook of Spinal Surgery.* Vol. 2. Philadelphia: Lippincott Wilkins & Williams; 1997:1211-1254.
14. Ogilvie JW, Sherman J. Spondylolysis in Scheuermann's disease. *Spine.* 1987;12:251-253.
15. Wynne-Davies R, Scott JH. Inheritance and spondylolisthesis: A radiographic family survey. *J Bone Joint Surg Br.* 1979;61:301-305.
16. Friberg S. Studies on spondylolisthesis. *Acta Chir Scand Suppl.* 1939;55.
17. Albanese M. Pizzutillo PD: Family study of spondylolysis and spondylolisthesis. *J Pediatr Orthop.* 1982;2:496-499.
18. Wiltse LL. Spondylolisthesis in children. *Clin Orthop Relat Res.* 1961;21:156-163.
19. Wiltse LL, Widell EH, Jackson DW. Fatigue fracture: The basic lesion in isthmic spondylolisthesis. *J Bone Joint Surg Am.* 1975;57:17-22.
20. Laurent LE. Spondylolisthesis. *Acta Orthop Scand.* 1958;35(suppl):1-45.
21. Shahriaree H, Sajadi K. Rooholamini SA: A family with spondylolisthesis. *J Bone Joint Surg Am.* 1979;61:1256-1258.
22. Wiltse LL. The etiology of spondylolisthesis. *J Bone Joint Surg Am.* 1962;44-A:539-560.
23. Newman PH. Degenerative spondylolisthesis. *Orthop Clin North Am.* 1975;6:197-199.
24. Dietrich M, Kurowski P. The importance of mechanical factors in the etiology of spondylolysis: A model analysis of loads and stresses in human lumbar spine. *Spine.* 1985;10:532-542.

25. Krenz J, Troup JD. The structure of the pars interarticularis of the lower lumbar vertebrae and its relation to the etiology of spondylolysis, with a report of a healing fracture in the neural arch of a fourth lumbar vertebra. *J Bone Joint Surg Br.* 1973;55:735-741.
26. Letts M, Smallman T, Afanasiev R, et al. Fracture of the pars interarticularis in adolescent athletes: A clinical-biomechanical analysis. *J Pediatr Orthop.* 1986;6:40-46.
27. Schulitz KP, Niethard FU. Strain on the interarticular stress distribution: Measurements regarding the development of spondylolysis. *Arch Orthop Trauma Surg.* 1980;96:197-202.
28. Wiltse LL, Widell EH Jr, Jackson DW. Fatigue fracture: The basic lesion is isthmic spondylolisthesis. *J Bone Joint Surg Am.* 1975;57:17-22.
29. Farfan HF, Osteria V, Lamy C. The mechanical etiology of spondylolysis and spondylolisthesis. *Clin Orthop Relat Res.* 1976;117:40-55.
30. Jackson DW, Wiltse LL, Cirincoine RJ. Spondylolysis in the female gymnast. *Clin Orthop Relat Res.* 1976;117:68-73.
31. Ciullo JV, Jackson DW. Pars interarticularis stress reaction, spondylolysis, and spondylolisthesis in gymnasts. *Clin Sports Med.* 1985;4:95-110.
32. Semon RL, Spengler D. Significance of lumbar spondylolysis in college football players. *Spine.* 1981;6:172-174.
33. Amato M, Totty WG, Gilula LA. Spondylolysis of the lumbar spine: Demonstration of defects and laminal fragmentation. *Radiology.* 1984;153:627-629.
34. Fredrickson BE, Baker D, McHolick WJ, et al. The natural history of spondylolysis and spondylolisthesis. *J Bone Joint Surg Am.* 1984;66:699-707.
35. Roche MB, Rowe GG. The incidence of separate neural arch and coincident bone variations: A summary. *J Bone Joint Surg Am.* 1952;34:491-494.
36. Yochum TR, et al. Natural history of spondylolysis and spondylolisthesis. In: Yochum TR, Rowe LJ, eds. *Essentials of Skeletal Radiology.* Baltimore: Williams & Wilkins; 1987:243-272.
37. Osterman K, Schlenzka D, Poussa M, et al. Isthmic spondylolisthesis in symptomatic and asymptomatic subjects, epidemiology, and natural history with special reference to disk abnormality and mode of treatment. *Clin Orthop Relat Res.* 1993;297:65-70.
38. Stewart T. The age incidence of neural arch defects in Alaskan natives, considered from the standpoint of etiology. *J Bone Joint Surg Am.* 1953;35:937.
39. Wong LC. Rehabilitation of a patient with a rare multi-level isthmic spondylolisthesis: A case report. *JCCA J Can Chiropr Assoc.* 2004;48:142-151.
40. Simper LB. Spondylolysis in Eskimo skeletons. *Acta Orthop Scand.* 1986;57:78-80.
41. Fredrickson B, Baker D, McHolick WJ, et al. The natural history of spondylolysis and spondylolisthesis. *J Bone Joint Surg Am.* 1984;66:699-707.
42. Taillard WF. Etiology of spondylolisthesis. *Clin Orthop Relat Res.* 1976;117:30-39.
43. Beguiristain JL, Díaz-de-Rada P. Spondylolisthesis in pre-school children. *J Pediatr Orthop.* 2004;13(4):225-230.
44. Borkow SE, Kleiger B. Spondylolisthesis in the newborn: A case report. *Clin Orthop Relat Res.* 1971;81:73-76.
45. Taillard WF. Etiology of spondylolisthesis. *Clin Orthop Relat Res.* 1976;117:30-39.
46. Turner RD, Bianco AJ Jr. Spondylolisthesis and spondylolysis in children and teen-agers. *J Bone Joint Surg Am.* 1971;53: 1298-1306.
47. Patel DR, Nelson TL. Sports injuries in adolescents. *Med Clin North Am.* 2000;84:983-1007.
48. Ariyoshi M, Nagata K, Sonoda K, et al. Spondylolysis at three sites in the same lumbar vertebra. *Int J Sports Med.* 1999;20:56-57.
49. Grobler LJ, Wiltse LL. Classification, non-operative, and operative treatment of spondylolisthesis. In: Frymoyer JW, Ducker TB, eds. *The Adult Spine: Principles and Practice.* Vol. 2. New York: Raven Press; 1991:1655-1704.
50. Saraste H. The etiology of spondylolysis: A retrospective radiographic study. *Acta Orthop Scand.* 1985;56:253-255.
51. Baker DR, McHollick W. Spondyloschisis and spondylolisthesis in children. *J Bone Joint Surg Am.* 1956;38:933-934.
52. Soler T, Calderon C. The prevalence of spondylolysis in the Spanish elite athlete. *Am J Sports Med.* 2000;28:57-62.
53. Wimberly RL, Lauerman WC. Spondylolisthesis in the athlete. *Clin Sports Med.* 2002;21:133-145.
54. Stinson JT. Spondylolysis and spondylolisthesis in the athlete. *Clin Sports Med.* 1993;12:517-528.
55. Standaert CJ. Spondylolysis in the adolescent athlete. *Clin J Sport Med.* 2002;12:119-122.
56. Lundin DA, Wiseman DB, Shaffrey CI. Spondylolysis and spondylolisthesis in the athlete. *Clin Neurosurg.* 2002;49:528-547.
57. Jackson DW, Wiltse LL, Cirincoine RJ. Spondylolysis in the female gymnast. *Clin Orthop Relat Res.* 1976;117:68-73.
58. Herman MJ, Pizzutillo PD, Cavalier R. Spondylolysis and spondylolisthesis in the child and adolescent athlete. *Orthop Clin North Am.* 2003;34:461-467.
59. MacDonald J, D'Hemecourt P. Back pain in the adolescent athlete. *Pediatr Ann.* 2007;36:703-712.
60. Wiltse L, Jackson DW. Treatment of spondylolisthesis and spondylolysis in children. *Clin Orthop Relat Res.* 1976;117:92-100.
61. Newman PH. Surgical treatment of spondylolisthesis in the adult. *Clin Orthop Relat Res.* 1976;117:106-111.
62. Boxall D, Bradford DS, Winter RB, et al. Management of severe spondylolisthesis in children. *J Bone Joint Surg Am.* 1979;61:479-495.
63. Arriaza BT. Spondylolysis in prehistoric human remains from Guam and its possible etiology. *Am J Phys Anthropol.* 1997;104:393-397.
64. El Rassi G, Takemitsu M, Woratanarat P, et al. Lumbar spondylolysis in pediatric and adolescent soccer players. *Am J Sports Med.* 2005;33:1688-1693.
65. Harvell JC Jr, Hanley EN Jr. Spondylolysis and spondylolisthesis. In: Pang D, ed. *Disorders of the Pediatric Spine.* New York: Raven Press; 1995:561-574.
66. Hambly MF, Wiltse LL, Peek RD. Spondylolisthesis. In: Watkins RG, Williams L, Lin P, et al., eds. *The Spine in Sports.* St Louis: Mosby; 1996:157-163.
67. Micheli LJ, Wood R. Back pain in young athletes: Significant differences from adults in causes and patterns. *Arch Pediatr Adolesc Med.* 1995;149:15-18.
68. Comstock CP, Carragee EJ, O'Sullivan GS. Spondylolisthesis in the young athlete. *Physician Sports Med.* 1994;22: 39-46.
69. Anderson S. Assessment and management of pediatric and adolescent patients with low back pain. *Phys Med Rehabil Clin North Am.* 1991;2:157-185.
70. Loman Y, Margulies JY, Nyska M, et al. Effect of major axial skeleton trauma on preexisting lumbosacral spondylolisthesis. *J Spinal Disord.* 1991;4:353-358.

71. Luhmann S, O'Brien MF, Lenke L. Spondylolysis and spondylolisthesis. In: Morrissy RT, Weinstein SL, eds. *Lovell and Winter's Pediatric Orthopaedics*. Vol. 2. 6th ed. Philadelphia: Lippincott Williams & Wilkins; 2006:839-870.
72. Weiker GG. Evaluation and treatment of common spine and trunk problems. *Clin Sports Med*. 1989;8:399-417.
73. Ralston S, Weir M. Suspecting lumbar spondylolysis in adolescent low back pain. *Clin Pediatr (Phila)*. 1998;37:287-293.
74. Barash HL, Galante JO, Lanthert CL, et al. Spondylolisthesis and tight hamstrings. *J Bone Joint Surg Am*. 1970;52:1319-1328.
75. Phalen GS, Dickson JA. Spondylolisthesis and tight hamstrings. *J Bone Joint Surg Am*. 1961;43:505-512.
76. Deyerle WM. Lumbar nerve-root irritation in children. *Clin Orthop Relat Res*. 1961;21:125.
77. Meyers LL, Dobson SR, Wiegand D, et al. Mechanical instability as a cause of gait disturbance in high-grade spondylolisthesis: A pre- and postoperative three-dimensional gait analysis. *J Pediatr Orthop*. 1999;19:672-676.
78. Guntz E, Schluter K. Dysplasia of the neural arch and its clinical manifestations (spondylolisthesis). *Clin Orthop Relat Res*. 1956;8:71-90.
79. Jones PH, Love JG. Tight filum terminale. *AMA Arch Surg*. 1956;73:556-566.
80. Libson E, Bloom RA, Shapiro Y. Scoliosis in young men with spondylolysis or spondylolisthesis: A comparative study in symptomatic and asymptomatic subjects. *Spine*. 1984;9:445-447.
81. Papagelopoulos PJ, Peterson HA, Ebersold MJ, et al. Spinal column deformity and instability after lumbar or thoracolumbar laminectomy for intraspinal tumors in children and young adults. *Spine*. 1997;22:442-451.
82. Seitsalo S, Osterman K, Poussa M. Scoliosis associated with lumbar spondylolisthesis: A clinical survey of 190 young patients. *Spine*. 1988;13:899-904.
83. Lindholm TS, Ragni P, Ylikoski M, et al. Lumbar isthmic spondylolisthesis in children and adolescents. *Spine*. 1990;15:1350-1355.
84. McCarroll JR, Miller JM, Bitter MA. Lumbar spondylolysis and spondylolisthesis in college football players. A prospective study. *Am J Sports Med*. 1986;14:404-406.
85. Lowe RW, Hayes TD, Kaye J, et al. Standing roentgenograms in spondylolisthesis. *Clin Orthop Relat Res*. 1976;117:80-84.
86. Libson E, Bloom RA, Dinari G. Symptomatic and asymptomatic spondylolysis and spondylolisthesis in young adults. *Int Orthop*. 1982;6:259-261.
87. Standaert CJ, Herring SA. Spondylolysis: A critical review. *Br J Sports Med*. 2000;34:415-422.
88. Bodner RJ, Heyman S, Drummond DS, et al. The use of single photon emission computed tomography (SPECT) in the diagnosis of low-back pain in young patients. *Spine*. 1988;13:1155-1160.
89. Bellah RD, Summerville DA, Treves ST, et al. Low-back pain in adolescent athletes: Detection of stress injury to the pars interarticularis with SPECT. *Radiology*. 1991;180:509-512.
90. Congeni J, McCulloch J, Swanson K. Lumbar spondylolysis: A study of natural progression in athletes. *Am J Sports Med*. 1997;25:248-253.
91. Teplick JG, Laffey PA, Berman A, et al. Diagnosis and evaluation of spondylolisthesis and/or spondylolysis on axial CT. *AJNR Am J Neuroradiol*. 1986;7:479-491.
92. Udeshi UL, Reeves D. Routine thin slice MRI effectively demonstrates the lumbar pars interarticularis. *Clin Radiol*. 1999;54:615-619.
93. Harvey CJ, Richenberg JL, Saifuddin A, et al. The radiological investigation of lumbar spondylolysis. *Clin Radiol*. 1998;53:723-728.
94. Yamane T, Yoshida T, Mimatsu K. Early diagnosis of lumbar spondylolysis by MRI. *J Bone Joint Surg Br*. 1993;75:764-768.
95. Meyerding HW. Spondylolisthesis. *Surg Gynecol Obstet*. 1932;54:371-377.
96. Wiltse LL, Winter RB. Terminology and measurement of spondylolisthesis. *J Bone Joint Surg Am*. 1983;65:768-772.
97. Laurent LE, Osterman K. Operative treatment of spondylolisthesis in young patients. *Clin Orthop Relat Res*. 1976;117:85-91.
98. O'Sullivan PB, Phyty GD, Twomey LT, et al. Evaluation of specific stabilizing exercise in the treatment of chronic low back pain with radiologic diagnosis of spondylolysis or spondylolisthesis. *Spine*. 1997;22:2959-2967.
99. Fujii K, Katoh S, Sairyo K, et al. Union of defects in the pars interarticularis of the lumbar spine in children and adolescents: The radiological outcome after conservative treatment. *J Bone Joint Surg Br*. 2004;86:225-231.
100. Steiner ME, Micheli LJ. Treatment of symptomatic spondylolysis and spondylolisthesis with the modified Boston brace. *Spine*. 1985;10:937-943.
101. Blanda J, Bethem D, Moats W, et al. Defects of pars interarticularis in athletes: A protocol for nonoperative treatment. *J Spinal Disord*. 1993;6:406-411.
102. Daniel JN, Polly DW Jr, Van Dam BE. A study of the efficacy of nonoperative treatment of presumed traumatic spondylolysis in a young patient population. *Mil Med*. 1995;160:553-555.
103. Morita T, Ikata T, Katoh S, et al. Lumbar spondylolysis in children and adolescents. *J Bone Joint Surg Br*. 1995;77:620-625.
104. Bell DF, Ehrlich MG, Zaleske DJ. Brace treatment for symptomatic spondylolisthesis. *Clin Orthop Relat Res*. 1988;236:192-198.
105. Pizzutillo PD, Hummer CD III. Nonoperative treatment of pain in adolescent spondylosis and spondylolisthesis. *J Pediatr Orthop*. 1989;9:538-540.
106. Anderson K, Sarwark JF, Conway JJ, et al. Quantitative assessment with SPECT imaging of stress injuries of the pars interarticularis and response to bracing. *J Pediatr Orthop*. 2000;20:28-33.
107. Dutton JA, Hughes SP, Peters AM. SPECT in the management of patients with back pain and spondylolysis. *Clin Nucl Med*. 2000;25:93-96.
108. Takemitsu M, El Rassi G, Woratanarat P, et al. Low back pain in pediatric athletes with unilateral tracer uptake at the pars interarticularis on single photon emission computed tomography. *Spine*. 2006;31:909-914.
109. Panjabi MM. The stabilizing system of the spine: Part I. Function, dysfunction, adaptation, and enhancement. *J Spinal Disord*. 1992;5:383-389.
110. Kurd MF, Patel D, Norton R, et al. Nonoperative treatment of symptomatic spondylolysis. *J Spinal Disord Tech*. 2007;20:560-564.
111. Hensinger RN. Spondylolysis and spondylolisthesis in children and adolescents. *J Bone Joint Surg Am*. 1989;71:1098-1107.

112. Harris IE, Weinstein SL. Long-term follow-up of patients with grade-III and IV spondylolisthesis: Treatment with and without posterior fusion. *J Bone Joint Surg Am.* 1987;69:960-969.
113. Bell DL, Ehrlich MG, Zaleske DJ. Brace treatment for symptomatic spondylolisthesis. *Clin Orthop Relat Res.* 1988;236:192-198.
114. Gill GG, Manning JG, White HL. Surgical treatment of spondylolisthesis without spine fusion: Excision of the loose lamina with decompression of the nerve roots. *J Bone Joint Surg Am.* 1955;37:493-520.
115. Gill GG. Long-term follow-up evaluation of a few patients with spondylolisthesis treated by excision of the loose lamina with decompression of the nerve roots without spinal fusion. *Clin Orthop Relat Res.* 1984;182:215-219.
116. Schoenecker P, Cole HO, Herring J, et al. Cauda equina syndrome after in situ arthrodesis for severe spondylolisthesis at the lumbosacral junction. *J Bone Joint Surg Am.* 1990;72:369-377.
117. Buck JE. Direct repair of the defect in spondylolisthesis: Preliminary report. *J Bone Joint Surg Br.* 1970;52:432-437.
118. Nicol RO, Scott JH. Lytic spondylolysis: Repair by wiring. *Spine.* 1986;11:1027-1030.
119. Ivanic GM, Pink TP, Achatz W, et al. Direct stabilization of lumbar spondylolysis with a hook screw: Mean 11-year follow-up period for 113 patients. *Spine.* 2003;28:255-259.
120. Lundin DA, Wiseman D, Ellenbogen RG, et al. Direct repair of the pars interarticularis for spondylolysis and spondylolisthesis. *Pediatr Neurosurg.* 2003;39:195-200.
121. Nachemson A. Repair of the spondylolisthetic defect and intertransverse fusion for young patients. *Clin Orthop Relat Res.* 1976;117:101-105.
122. Lehmann TR, Spratt KF, Tozzi JE, et al. Long-term follow-up of lower lumbar fusion patients. *Spine.* 1987;12:97-104.
123. Lee CK. Accelerated degeneration of the segment adjacent to a lumbar fusion. *Spine.* 1988;13:375-377.
124. Weinhoffer SL, Guyer RD, Herbert M, et al. Intradiscal pressure measurements above an instrumented fusion: A cadaveric study. *Spine.* 1995;20:526-531.
125. Axelsson P, Johnsson R, Stromqvist B. The spondylolytic vertebra and its adjacent segment: Mobility measured before and after posterolateral fusion. *Spine.* 1997;22:414-417.
126. Mihara H, Onari K, Cheng BC, et al. The biomechanical effects of spondylolysis and its treatment. *Spine.* 2003;28: 235-238.
127. Tokuhashi Y, Matsuzaki H. Repair of defects in spondylolysis by segmental pedicular screw hook fixation: A preliminary report. *Spine.* 1996;21:2041-2045.
128. Wu SS, Lee CH, Chen PQ. Operative repair of symptomatic spondylolysis following a positive response to diagnostic pars injection. *J Spinal Disord.* 1999;12:10-16.
129. Buck J. Further thoughts on direct repair of the defect in spondylolysis. *J Bone Joint Surg Br.* 1979;61:123.
130. Beckers L. Buck's operation for treatment of spondylolysis and spondylolisthesis. *Acta Orthop Belg.* 1986;52:819-823.
131. Buring K, Fredensborg N. Osteosynthesis of spondylolysis. *Acta Orthop Scand.* 1973;44:91-92.
132. Ebraheim NA, Xu R, Darwich M, et al. Anatomic relations between the lumbar pedicle and the adjacent neural structures. *Spine.* 1997;22:2338-2341.
133. Lu J, Ebraheim NA, Biyani A, et al. Screw placement in the lumbar vertebral isthmus. *Clin Orthop Relat Res.* 1997;338:227-230.
134. Bradford DS, Iza J. Repair of the defect in spondylolysis or minimal degrees of spondylolisthesis by segmental wire fixation and bone grafting. *Spine.* 1985;10:673-679.
135. Salib RM, Pettine KA. Modified repair of a defect in spondylolysis or minimal spondylolisthesis by pedicle screw, segmental wire fixation, and bone grafting. *Spine.* 1993;18:440-443.
136. Deguchi M, Rapoff AJ, Zdeblick TA. Biomechanical comparison of spondylolysis fixation techniques. *Spine.* 1999;24:328-333.
137. Johnson GV, Thompson AG. The Scott wiring technique for direct repair of lumbar spondylolysis. *J Bone Joint Surg Br.* 1992;74:426-430.
138. Hambly MF, Wiltse LL. A modification of the Scott wiring technique. *Spine.* 1994;19:354-356.
139. Songer MN, Rovin R. Repair of the pars interarticularis defect with a cable-screw construct: A preliminary report. *Spine.* 1998;23:263-269.
140. Morscher E, Gerber B, Fasel J. Surgical treatment of spondylolisthesis by bone grafting and direct stabilization of spondylolysis by means of a hook screw. *Arch Orthop Trauma Surg.* 1984;103:175-178.
141. Albassir A, Samson I, Hendricks L. [Treatment of painful spondylolysis using Morscher's hook]. *Acta Orthop Belg.* 1990;56:489-495.
142. Hefti F, Seelig W, Morscher E. Repair of lumbar spondylolysis with a hook-screw. *Int Orthop.* 1992;16:81-85.
143. Pavlovcic V. Surgical treatment of spondylolysis and spondylolisthesis with a hook screw. *Int Orthop.* 1994; 18:6-9.
144. Winter M, Jani L. Results of screw osteosynthesis in spondylolysis and low-grade spondylolisthesis. *Arch Orthop Trauma Surg.* 1989;108:96-99.
145. Sales de Gauzy J, Vadier F, Cahuzac JP. Repair of lumbar spondylolysis using Morscher material: 14 children followed for 1-5 years. *Acta Orthop Scand.* 2000;71:292-296.
146. Gillet P, Petit M. Direct repair of spondylolysis without spondylolisthesis, using a rod-screw construct and bone grafting of the pars defect. *Spine.* 1999;24:1252-1256.
146a. Taddonio RF Jr, McLachlan JE, D'Ambrosia RD. Spondylolysis: acute fracture versus congenital defect. *Orthopedics.* 1978;1(3):233-235.
147. Kakiuchi M. Repair of the defect in spondylolysis: Durable fixation with pedicle screws and laminar hooks. *J Bone Joint Surg Am.* 1997;79:818-825.
148. Roca J, Iborra M, Cavanilles-Walker JM, et al. Direct repair of spondylolysis using a new pedicle screw hook fixation: Clinical and CT-assessed study: an analysis of 19 patients. *J Spinal Disord Tech.* 2005;18(suppl):S82-S89.
149. Pellise F, Toribio J, Rivas A, et al. Clinical and CT scan evaluation after direct defect repair in spondylolysis using segmental pedicular screw hook fixation. *J Spinal Disord.* 1999;12:363-367.
150. Yuan HA, Garfin SR, Dickman CA, et al. A historical cohort study of pedicle screw fixation in thoracic, lumbar, and sacral spinal fusions. *Spine.* 1994;19(20 suppl):2279S-2296S.
151. Zdeblick TA. A prospective, randomized study of lumbar fusion: Preliminary results. *Spine.* 1993;18:983-991.
152. Bjarke Christensen F, Stender Hansen E, Laursen M, et al. Long-term functional outcome of pedicle screw instrumentation as a support for posterolateral spinal fusion: Randomized clinical study with a 5-year follow-up. *Spine.* 2002;27:1269-1277.

153. Deguchi M, Rapoff AJ, Zdeblick TA. Posterolateral fusion for isthmic spondylolisthesis in adults: Analysis of fusion rate and clinical results. *J Spinal Disord*. 1998;11:459-464.
154. Bono CM, Lee CK. Critical analysis of trends in fusion for degenerative disc disease over the past 20 years: Influence of technique on fusion rate and clinical outcome. *Spine*. 2004;29:455-463.
155. Chang P, Seow KH, Tan SK. Comparison of the results of spinal fusion for spondylolisthesis in patients who are instrumented with patients who are not. *Singapore Med J*. 1993;34:511-514.
156. Ricciardi JE, Pflueger PC, Isaza JE, et al. Transpedicular fixation for the treatment of isthmic spondylolisthesis in adults. *Spine*. 1995;20:1917-1922.
157. Moller H, Hedlund R. Surgery versus conservative management in adult isthmic spondylolisthesis—a prospective randomized study: Part 1. *Spine*. 2000;25:1711-1715.
158. Moller H, Hedlund R. Instrumented and noninstrumented posterolateral fusion in adult spondylolisthesis—a prospective randomized study: Part 2. *Spine*. 2000;25:1716-1721.
159. de Loubresse CG, Bon T, Deburge A, et al. Posterolateral fusion for radicular pain in isthmic spondylolisthesis. *Clin Orthop Relat Res*. 1996;323:194-201.
160. Lenke LG, Bridwell KH, Bullis D, et al. Results of in situ fusion for isthmic spondylolisthesis. *J Spinal Disord*. 1992;5:433-442.
161. Shirado O, Zdeblick TA, McAfee PC, et al. Biomechanical evaluation of methods of posterior stabilization of the spine and posterior lumbar interbody arthrodesis for lumbosacral isthmic spondylolisthesis: A calf-spine model. *J Bone Joint Surg Am*. 1991;73:518-526.
162. Wiltse LL, Bateman JG, Hutchinson RH, et al. The paraspinal sacrospinalis-splitting approach to the lumbar spine. *J Bone Joint Surg Am*. 1968;50:919-926.
163. Cheung EV, Herman MJ, Cavalier R, et al. Spondylolysis and spondylolisthesis in children and adolescents: II. Surgical management. *J Am Acad Orthop Surg*. 2006;14:488-498.
164. Hensinger RN, Lang JR, MacEwen GD. Surgical management of spondylolisthesis in children and adolescents. *Spine*. 1976;1:207-216.
165. Poussa M, Schlenzka D, Seitsalo S, et al. Surgical treatment of severe isthmic spondylolisthesis in adolescents: Reduction or fusion in situ. *Spine*. 1993;18:894-901.
166. Burkus JK, Lonstein JE, Winter RB, et al. Long-term evaluation of adolescents treated operatively for spondylolisthesis: A comparison of in situ arthrodesis only with in situ arthrodesis and reduction followed by immobilization in a cast. *J Bone Joint Surg Am*. 1992;74:693-704.
167. Bosworth DM, Fielding JW, Demarest L, et al. Spondylolisthesis: A critical review of a consecutive series of cases treated by arthrodesis. *J Bone Joint Surg Am*. 1955;37:767-786.
168. Grzegorzewski A, Kumar SJ. In situ posterolateral spine arthrodesis for grades III, IV, and V spondylolisthesis in children and adolescents. *J Pediatr Orthop*. 2000;20:506-511.
169. Newton PO, Johnston CE 2nd. Analysis and treatment of poor outcomes following in situ arthrodesis in adolescent spondylolisthesis. *J Pediatr Orthop*. 1997;17:754-761.
170. Sherman FC, Rosenthal RK, Hall JE. Spine fusion for spondylolysis and spondylolisthesis in children. *Spine*. 1979;4:59-66.
171. Wiltse LL, Jackson DW. Treatment of spondylolisthesis and spondylolysis in children. *Clin Orthop Relat Res*. 1976;117:92-100.
172. Seitsalo S, Osterman K, Hyvärinen H, et al. Severe spondylolisthesis in children and adolescents: A long-term review of fusion in situ. *J Bone Joint Surg Br*. 1990;72:259-265.
173. Al-Sayyad MJ, Abdulmajeed TM. Fracture of the anterior iliac crest following autogenous bone grafting. *Saudi Med J*. 2006;27:254-258.
174. Davis IS, Bailey RW. Spondylolisthesis: Long-term follow-up study of treatment with total laminectomy. *Clin Orthop Relat Res*. 1972;88:46-49.
175. Frennered AK, et al. Midterm follow-up of young patients fused in situ for spondylolisthesis. *Spine*. 1991;16:409-416.
176. Beutler WJ, Fredrickson BE, Murtland A, et al. The natural history of spondylolysis and spondylolisthesis: 45-year follow-up evaluation. *Spine*. 2003;28:1027-1035.
177. Pizzutillo PD, Mirenda W, MacEwen GD. Posterolateral fusion for spondylolisthesis in adolescence. *J Pediatr Orthop*. 1986;6:311-316.
178. Reference deleted in review.
179. Cricchio G, Lundgren S. Donor site morbidity in two different approaches to anterior iliac crest bone harvesting. *Clin Implant Dent Relat Res*. 2003;5:161-169.
180. Jenis LG, Banco RJ, Kwon B. A prospective study of autologous growth factors (AGF) in lumbar interbody fusion. *Spine*. 2006;6:14-20.
181. Seiler JG 3rd, Johnson J. Iliac crest autogenous bone grafting: Donor site complications. *J South Orthop Assoc*. 2000;9:91-97.
182. Silber JS, Anderson DG, Daffner SD, et al. Donor site morbidity after anterior iliac crest bone harvest for single-level anterior cervical discectomy and fusion. *Spine*. 2003;28:134-139.
183. Krenz J, Troup JD. The structure of the pars interarticularis of the lower lumbar vertebrae and its relation to the etiology of spondylolysis, with a report of a healing fracture in the neural arch of a fourth lumbar vertebra. *J Bone Joint Surg Br*. 1973;55:735-741.
184. Stanton RP, Meehan P, Lovell WW. Surgical fusion in childhood spondylolisthesis. *J Pediatr Orthop*. 1985;5:411-415.
185. Johnson JR, Kirwan EO. The long-term results of fusion in situ for severe spondylolisthesis. *J Bone Joint Surg Br*. 1983;65:43-46.
186. Ploumis A, Hantzidis P, Dimitriou C. High-grade dysplastic spondylolisthesis and spondyloptosis: Report of three cases with surgical treatment and review of the literature. *Acta Orthop Belg*. 2005;71:750-757.
187. Smith JA, Hu SS. Management of spondylolysis and spondylolisthesis in the pediatric and adolescent population. *Orthop Clin North Am*. 1999;30:487-499.
188. Smith MD, Bohlman HH. Spondylolisthesis treated by a single-stage operation combining decompression with in situ posterolateral and anterior fusion: An analysis of eleven patients who had long-term follow-up. *J Bone Joint Surg Am*. 1990;72:415-421.
189. Mahmood F, Emami A, Hwang K, et al.: *Trans-sacral mesh cage with partial reduction for treatment of high-grade spondylolisthesis*. Presented at the 13th International Meeting on Advanced Spinal Techniques, Hong Kong, 2008.
190. Roca J, Ubierna MT, Cáceres E, et al. One-stage decompression and posterolateral and interbody fusion for

severe spondylolisthesis: An analysis of 14 patients. *Spine.* 1999;24:709-714.

191. Smith JA, Deviren V, Berven S, et al. Clinical outcome of trans-sacral interbody fusion after partial reduction for high-grade L5-S1 spondylolisthesis. *Spine.* 2001;26: 2227-2234.
192. Bohlman HH, Cook SS. One-stage decompression and posterolateral and interbody fusion for lumbosacral spondyloptosis through a posterior approach: Report of two cases. *J Bone Joint Surg Am.* 1982;64:415-418.
193. Lee EH, Goh JC, Helm R, et al. Donor site morbidity following resection of the fibula. *J Bone Joint Surg Br.* 1990;72:129-131.
194. Youdas JW, Wood MB, Cahalan TD, et al. A quantitative analysis of donor site morbidity after vascularized fibula transfer. *J Orthop Res.* 1988;6:621-629.
195. Jenkins JA. Spondylolisthesis. *Br J Surg.* 1936;24:80-86.
196. Lenke LG, Bridwell KH. Evaluation and surgical treatment of high-grade isthmic dysplastic spondylolisthesis. *Instr Course Lect.* 2003;52:525-532.
197. Aota Y, Kumano K, Hirabayashi S, et al. Reduction of lumbar spondylolisthesis using a CDI pedicle screw system. *Arch Orthop Trauma Surg.* 1995;114:188-193.
198. Bell GR, Gurd AR, Orlowski JP, et al. The syndrome of inappropriate antidiuretic-hormone secretion following spinal fusion. *J Bone Joint Surg Am.* 1986;68:720-724.
199. Boachie-Adjei O, Do T, Rawlins BA. Partial lumbosacral kyphosis reduction, decompression, and posterior lumbosacral transfixation in high-grade isthmic spondylolisthesis: Clinical and radiographic results in six patients. *Spine.* 2002;27:E161-E168.
200. Bridwell KH. Surgical treatment of high-grade spondylolisthesis. *Neurosurg Clin N Am.* 2006;17:331-338.
201. Dubousset J. Treatment of spondylolysis and spondylolisthesis in children and adolescents. *Clin Orthop Relat Res.* 1997; 337:77-85.
202. Hu SS, Bradford DS, Transfeldt EE, et al. Reduction of high-grade spondylolisthesis using Edwards instrumentation. *Spine.* 1996;21:367-371.
203. Poussa M, Remes V, Lamberg T, et al. Treatment of severe spondylolisthesis in adolescence with reduction or fusion in situ: Long-term clinical, radiologic, and functional outcome. *Spine.* 2006;31:583-590.
204. Rengachary SS. Balabhandra R: Reduction of spondylolisthesis. *Neurosurg Focus.* 2002;13:E2.
205. Schwend RM, Waters PM, Hey LA, et al. Treatment of severe spondylolisthesis in children by reduction and L4-S4 posterior segmental hyperextension fixation. *J Pediatr Orthop.* 1992;12:703-711.
206. Weisskopf M, Ohnsorge JA, Wirtz DC, et al. [Reduction of spondylolisthesis by temporary adjacent segment distraction]. *Z Orthop Ihre Grenzgeb.* 2006;144:511-515.
207. Yan DL, Pei FX, Li J, et al. Comparative study of PILF and TLIF treatment in adult degenerative spondylolisthesis. *Eur Spine J.* 2008;17:1311-1316.
208. Muschik M, Zippel H, Perka C. Surgical management of severe spondylolisthesis in children and adolescents: Anterior fusion in situ versus anterior spondylodesis with posterior transpedicular instrumentation and reduction. *Spine.* 1997; 22:2036-2042.
209. Matthiass HH, Heine J. The surgical reduction of spondylolisthesis. *Clin Orthop Relat Res.* 1986;203:34-44.
210. Schoenecker PL, Cole HO, Herring JA, et al. Cauda equina syndrome after in situ arthrodesis for severe spondylolisthesis at the lumbosacral junction. *J Bone Joint Surg Am.* 1990;72: 369-377.
211. Mehdian S, Arun R. Reduction of severe adolescent isthmic spondylolisthesis: A new technique. *Spine.* 2005;30:E579-E584.
212. Al-Sebai MW, Al-Khawashki H. Spondyloptosis and multiple-level spondylolysis. *Eur Spine J.* 1999;8:75-77.
213. Ferris LR, Ho E, Leong JC. Lumbar spondyloptosis: A long term follow up of three cases. *Int Orthop.* 1990;14:139-143.
214. Hilibrand AS, Urquhart AG, Graziano GP, et al. Acute spondylolytic spondylolisthesis: Risk of progression and neurological complications. *J Bone Joint Surg Am.* 1995;77: 190-196.
215. Gaines RW, Nichols WK. Treatment of spondyloptosis by two stage L5 vertebrectomy and reduction of L4 onto S1. *Spine.* 1985;10:680-686.
216. Lehmer SM, Steffee AD, Gaines RW Jr. Treatment of L5-S1 spondyloptosis by staged L5 resection with reduction and fusion of L4 onto S1 (Gaines procedure). *Spine.* 1994;19:1916-1925.
217. Lamberg T, Remes V, Helenius I, et al. Uninstrumented in situ fusion for high-grade childhood and adolescent isthmic spondylolisthesis: Long-term outcome. *J Bone Joint Surg Am.* 2007;89:512-518.
218. Lee C, Dorcil J, Radomisli TE. Nonunion of the spine: A review. *Clin Orthop Relat Res.* 2004;419:71-75.
219. Montgomery D, *SRS Morbidity and Mortality Committee: Report of changing surgical treatment trends for spondylolisthesis.* Presented at Scoliosis Research Society Pre-Meeting Course, Quebec City, Quebec, 2003.
220. Albrecht S, Kleihues H, Gill C, et al. [Repositioning injuries of nerve root L5 after surgical treatment of high degree spondylolistheses and spondyloptosis—in vitro studies]. *Z Orthop Ihre Grenzgeb.* 1998;136:182-191.
221. Ogilvie JW. Complications in spondylolisthesis surgery. *Spine.* 2005;30(6 suppl):S97-S101.
222. Petraco DM, Spivak JM, Cappadona JG, et al. An anatomic evaluation of L5 nerve stretch in spondylolisthesis reduction. *Spine.* 1996;21:1133-1138.
223. DeWald RL, Faut MM, Taddonio RF, et al. Severe lumbosacral spondylolisthesis in adolescents and children: Reduction and staged circumferential fusion. *J Bone Joint Surg Am.* 1981;63:619-626.
224. Maurice HD, Morley TR. Cauda equina lesions following fusion in situ and decompressive laminectomy for severe spondylolisthesis: Four case reports. *Spine.* 1989;14: 214-216.
225. O'Brien JP, Mehdian H, Jaffray D. Reduction of severe lumbosacral spondylolisthesis: A report of 22 cases with a ten-year follow-up period. *Clin Orthop Relat Res.* 1994;300:64-69.
226. Ogilvie J. Complications in spondylolisthesis surgery. *Spine.* 2005;30:S97-S101.

SECTION IV

CHAPTER 32 Cervical, Thoracic, and Lumbar Spinal Trauma of the Immature Spine

Jesse E. Bible
J. Alex Sielatycki
Joon Yung Lee
Clinton J. Devin

Epidemiology

Spine injuries involve 1% to 5% of children admitted to trauma centers, making these injuries relatively uncommon in pediatric patients.[1,2] The true incidence may be higher given the challenges of obtaining a reliable examination and necessary images in children compared with adults.[1–3] A high index of suspicion is warranted in children with polytrauma, particularly those who have sustained a head injury given that 40% to 50% of children with a head injury also have a cervical spine injury.[3,4]

The cervical spine is most commonly involved in injuries in pediatric patients. The levels of cervical spine involvement and mechanisms vary with age. Due to a disproportionately larger head and inherent mobility, children younger than 8 years of age are more susceptible to upper cervical spine injuries. As the spine develops adult characteristics between the ages of 8 to 10 years, children older than this age more commonly sustain subaxial cervical spine injuries.[5] Similarly, thoracic and lumbar spine injuries also increase in incidence as children age and the spine takes on the biomechanical characteristics of an adult.[5]

Traffic-related incidents account for nearly one-third of all pediatric spine injuries; however, other mechanisms of injury are unique to particular age groups.[5] In neonates, birth trauma is the most common cause of spine injury, with an incidence of 1 in 60,000 live births.[6] Excessive distraction or hyperextension of the cervical spine is thought to be the mechanism, occurring in breach deliveries and large neonates.[7] Spinal cord injury should be considered in neonates with hypotonia or cardiopulmonary instability. In infants and young children, particular injuries should also raise suspicion for nonaccidental trauma, including avulsion fractures of the spinous processes or multilevel compression fractures in conjunction with rib fractures, long bone fractures, cutaneous lesions, and other characteristic injuries of abuse.[8,9] In older children and adolescents, sports-related injuries and diving accidents become more frequent.[5]

Developmental Anatomy and Biomechanics

Understanding the developmental anatomy allows identification of normal radiographic variants and synchondroses opposed to true pathology. The atlas (C1) and axis (C2) undergo unique development, whereas the subaxial cervical spine, thoracic spine, and lumbar spine follow a similar pattern of maturation. The atlas (C1) develops from three primary centers of ossification: the anterior arch and two neural arches[10] (Fig. 32.1). The two neural arches are visible at birth and develop into the lateral masses. The anterior arch is radiographically visible at birth in only 20% of infants; in the remaining infants, it ossifies over the subsequent year. Measuring the atlanto-dens interval (ADI) is therefore unreliable in infants younger than 1 year old. Posteriorly, the synchondrosis between the two neural arches closes by age 3 years, while the ossification between the anterior arch and the two neural arches occurs by age 7 years.[11]

The axis (C2) is formed by five primary centers of ossification. The odontoid process is formed by two parallel ossification centers that fuse in utero during the seventh fetal month. A secondary ossification center occurs at the tip of the odontoid, called the *os terminale,* arising between ages 3 and 6 years and fusing by age 12 years. The remaining three primary centers of ossification are the body and two neural arches. The body typically fuses with the odontoid by age 6 years, but this synchondrosis can persist until age 11 years (Fig. 32.2). The neural arches fuse anteriorly to the body by age 6 years and with each other posteriorly by age 3 years, similar to the atlas.

The subaxial cervical spine (C3–C7), thoracic spine, and lumbar spine all develop in a similar fashion. There are three primary ossification centers: the body and two neural arches. The neural arches typically fuse to the body anteriorly by age 6 years and to each other posteriorly by age 3 years. However, closure of the neurocentral synchondroses can remain incomplete until early adulthood, especially in the thoracic region.[12] Secondary centers of ossification can exist at the tips of the

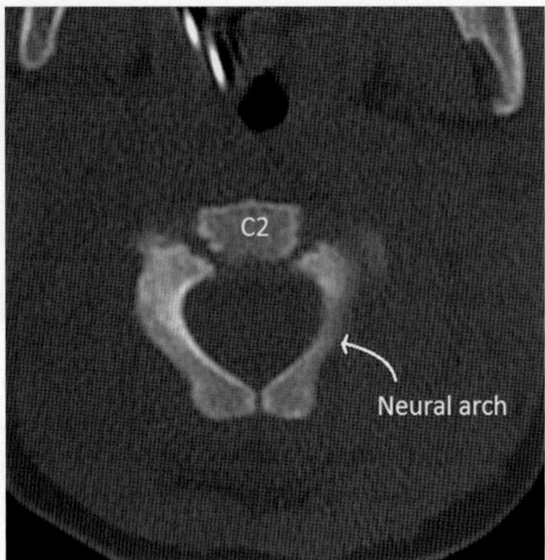

FIG. 32.1 Axial computed tomographic scan of C2 in an 18-month-old child demonstrating the ossification centers of the vertebral body and paired neural arches.

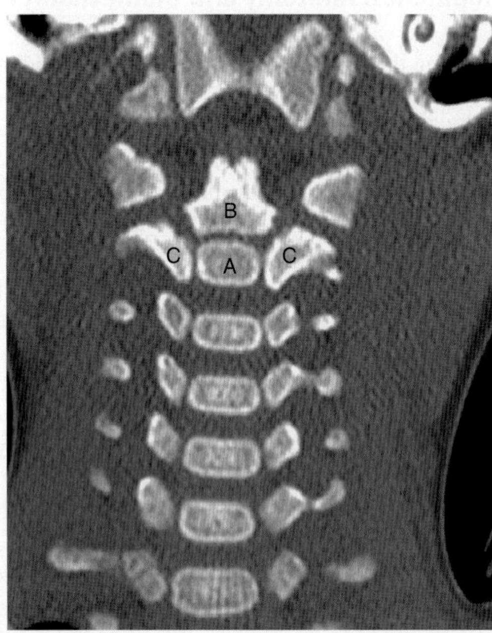

FIG. 32.2 Coronal computed tomographic reconstruction in the cervical spine of an 18-month-old child, showing the C2 body *(A)*, dens *(B)*, and neural arch *(C)* ossification centers.

transverse processes, spinous process, and superior and inferior aspects of the vertebral body. These areas ossify in early adulthood and can be mistaken as a fracture.[10,11] The vertebral bodies of the subaxial cervical, thoracic, and lumbar spine grow in height by endochondral ossification that progresses in posterior to anterior direction over time until the body takes on its characteristic rectangular shape by age 7 years. Until age 7, it is acceptable to have anterior wedging of the subaxial cervical vertebrae, which should not be confused with anterior compression fractures. This normal wedging can be most profound at C3.[13]

The spine typically assumes adult characteristics and size by ages 8 to 10 years. Therefore, spine injuries can typically be divided by age: younger or older than 8 years old. From birth until age 8 years, children are usually more susceptible to upper cervical spine injuries. In addition, it is more common for children in this younger age group to have a neurologic injury and subluxation or complete dislocation rather than a fracture, due to increased generalized laxity.[2,14–17] Proposed reasons for the increased incidence of upper cervical spine injuries in this younger age group are listed in Box 32–1. These unique characteristics, especially disproportionate head size, are important to keep in mind when transporting and evaluating a young child.

BOX 32.1 Risk Factors in Children <8 Years Old for Developing Upper Cervical Spine Injuries

Disproportionately large heads and weak neck muscles
Fulcrum of movement centered at C2–C3
Ligamentous and joint capsule laxity
Horizontal orientation facet joints
Increased cartilage/bone ratio with relative anterior wedging of vertebrae and incomplete ossification of odontoid process

Transport and Evaluation

Proper care of pediatric spine injuries begins at the scene of the accident. In a child with polytrauma, a spine injury must be assumed until proven otherwise, and all appropriate precautions and immobilization must be utilized. Children should be initially placed in a well-fitting cervical collar and immobilized on a spine board. Commercial collars often do not fit appropriately, preventing adequate immobilization. In this case, sandbags can be placed on each side of the head to prevent motion.

Herzenberg and colleagues[18] were the first to note that the transport of young children (< 8 years old) on a standard adult spine board tended to cause excessive flexion of the cervical spine. It was noted in all cases that the cervical spine was forced into relative kyphosis because of the disproportionately large head relative to the chest. This flexed position could potentially jeopardize the cervical cord if the mechanism of injury was a flexion force, which is often the case in motor vehicle accidents. To obtain a neutral position, Herzenberg and colleagues[18] recommended pediatric spine boards with a cutout for the occiput. Alternatively, a standard spine board can be used with a towel roll placed under the shoulders, allowing the head to drop into mild extension (Fig. 32.3). Several other studies have demonstrated that young children with suspected cervical spine injuries should be transported with relative chest elevation to allow for more anatomic alignment of the cervical spine. One should evaluate the child's cervical spine clinically after immobilization, looking from the side to ensure that the external auditory meatus is in line with the shoulder.[19,20]

Clinical evaluation of a child believed to have a spine injury is often hampered by an inability to obtain an accurate history and thorough physical examination. The clinician should have a heightened suspicion of spine injury in nonverbal children,

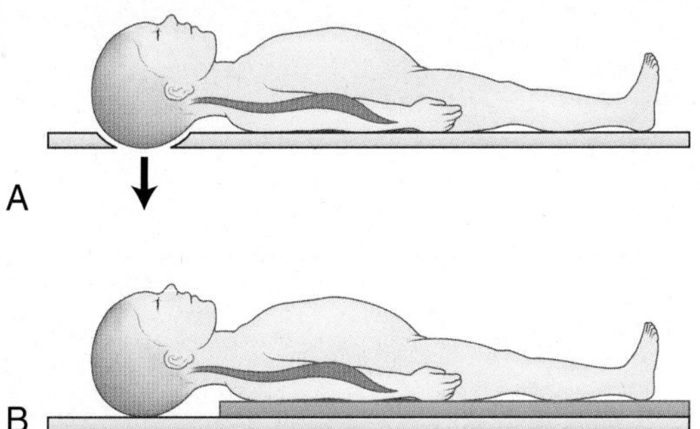

FIG. 32.3 The proportionally larger occiput in children requires a cutout from the spine board in emergency transportation. (From Herzenberg JE, Hensinger RN, Dedrick DK, et al. Emergency transport and position of young children who have an injury of the cervical spine: the standard backboard may be hazardous. *J Bone Joint Surg Am.* 1989;71:15–22.)

with a reported 23-fold increased likelihood of missing a cervical spine injury in this group.[21] The mechanism of injury should be taken into account when considering the likelihood of an occult spine injury. Additionally, the presence of associated injuries, including facial trauma, head injuries, thoracic wall injuries, and abdominal injuries, increases the likelihood of spine trauma.[22] Abdominal injuries, particularly injuries of the small bowel, are associated with flexion distraction injuries of the thoracolumbar spine.[23] Spinal injuries can occur at multiple levels, with noncontiguous fractures occurring in 16% of cases.[24]

For examination purposes, the cervical collar should be temporarily, carefully removed, with an assistant stabilizing the head and cervical spine during the log-roll maneuver. Cervical inline traction should be avoided in young children because of the increased risk of ligamentous and atlanto-occipital injuries. The entire spine is visually inspected and palpated for malalignment, asymmetry, interspinous widening, tenderness, abrasions, or other abnormalities. Careful spine precautions should be maintained until injury is ruled out.

A thorough baseline neurologic examination, as discussed in detail in other chapters, should be carefully documented. If a neurologic deficit is identified, frequent examinations should be performed to detect a change in the deficit. Throughout the sensory, motor, and reflex examination, the contralateral extremity should always be used as a comparison to detect subtle injuries. Also, given that an accurate examination can be difficult at times due to a child's age or altered mental status, close observation during other parts of a child's workup can be valuable, such as looking for withdrawal from painful stimuli or diaphragmatic breathing without assistance of accessary muscles.

Plain Radiography of the Cervical Spine

Imaging of the cervical spine should be performed if a child meets any of the following criteria (Box 32.2): (1) The child is nonverbal secondary to age or altered mental status, (2) intoxication is present, (3) a neurologic deficit (persistent or transient) is present, (4) neck pain is present, (5) there is a high-risk mechanism of injury, (6) physical signs of neck trauma or lap belt trauma are present, or (7) painful distracting injuries are present.[25] Additionally, unexplained cardiorespiratory instability can be an indication of a high cervical spine injury, and should be evaluated appropriately with imaging of the cervical spine.[26]

BOX 32.2 Criteria for Imaging the Cervical Spine in Pediatric Trauma

- Child is nonverbal (secondary to age or mental status)
- Intoxication is present
- Persistent or transient neurologic deficit
- Neck pain
- High-energy mechanism
- High-risk mechanism (i.e., fall onto head from a height)

The three-view cervical spine series may not be applicable in pediatric patients with polytrauma, but likely still has a role in patients without polytrauma. The supine lateral cervical radiograph has a reported sensitivity of 79% to 85% in pediatric patients.[27] This sensitivity is dependent on seeing all seven cervical vertebrae, including the occipitocervical and cervicothoracic junction. Lally and colleagues[28] found that all seven cervical vertebrae were seen in only 57% of children on the initial cervical spine series. The addition of the anteroposterior and open-mouth odontoid views increases the sensitivity to approximately 94% if ideal images can be obtained, although this can be extremely challenging in an uncooperative child.[29] Buhs and colleagues[30] showed that the open-mouth odontoid view did not provide additional information in children younger than 9 years that was not already appreciated on the anteroposterior and lateral views. In its place, these authors recommended use of computed tomography (CT) from the occiput to C2.

The use of flexion and extension radiographs during the initial evaluation has come into question. Ralston and colleagues[31] disputed the need for these dynamic studies in the acute setting. These investigators had blinded radiologists retrospectively review static and flexion-extension radiographs on 129 children. They found that if the static radiographs were normal, the flexion-extension views would reveal no abnormality. Additional studies have confirmed these findings and recommended against acute flexion-extension views.[32] Dynamic views may still be useful in evaluating for instability in the subacute outpatient setting after acute pain and muscle spasms have subsided.

Interpretation of the cervical spine series requires an understanding of the normal anatomy and the anatomic variants of the immature spine that can mimic trauma. Special attention should be given to the upper cervical spine, including the atlantoaxial and atlanto-occipital region given the propensity of injuries to this area in children and the subtle radiographic findings.[33] Several methods for evaluating the craniocervical junction using a lateral radiograph have been described. The "rule of twelves" is thought to be the most sensitive method (Fig. 32.4), whereby the distance between the basion and tip of the odontoid process should be 12 mm or less, and a line drawn parallel along the posterior aspect of the body of C2, including the odontoid, should come within

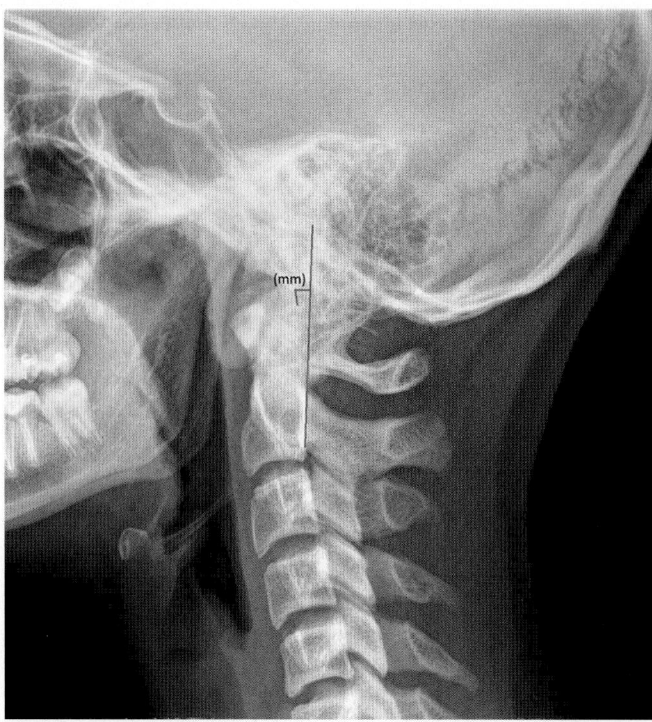

FIG. 32.4 Schematic illustrating the measurements required for the "rule of twelves" (*left*). Lateral radiograph of a teenager without a cervical spine injury with measurement lines superimposed (*right*).

12 mm of the basion. The former, tip of the odontoid to the basion distance, is unreliable in children younger than 13 years because of incomplete ossification of the odontoid. However, the line drawn parallel to the back of the C2 body and odontoid peg should be less than 12 mm from the basion.[24] Furthermore, a gap of more than 5 mm from the occipital condyle to the C1 facet articulation also represents a disruption of the occipitocervical junction.[34]

The atlantoaxial articulation is best evaluated with the atlantodens interval (ADI). In children, the normal ADI can be up to 5 mm. If the ADI exceeds 5 mm on lateral flexion and 4 mm on lateral extension, the transverse atlantal ligament is likely disrupted.[35] When the ADI exceeds 10 to 12 mm, the alar and apical ligaments have failed, with a high risk of cord compression.[36] The extent of cord compression at the atlantoaxial joint can be determined using Steel's rule of thirds,[37] which is based on dividing the inner diameter of the C1 ring into thirds. One-third of the space should be occupied by the odontoid, one-third by the spinal cord, and one-third by the space available for the cord. When the dens migrates posteriorly by greater than one-third of this space, the transverse ligament has been disrupted, and the spinal cord is likely being compressed.

Many normal anatomic variants should be recognized so as to not be confused with a "true" traumatic injury (Box 32.3). A normal finding on extension radiographs in 20% of children is overriding of the anterior arch of the atlas on the odontoid. This finding represents incomplete ossification of the dens.[38] Another common variant noted on cervical spine radiographs in an immature spine is pseudosubluxation of C2 on C3 and less commonly C3 on C4. Cattell and Filtzer[38] were the first to appreciate this normal finding in a study involving 160 pediatric patients with no history of cervical spine trauma. Pseudosubluxation can be differentiated from traumatic subluxation by evaluating the continuity of the spinolaminar line drawn along the posterior arch from C1–C3 (also known as the Swischuk line); with physiologic subluxation, this line should pass within 1 mm of the anterior cortex of the posterior arch of C2, while a distance greater than 1.5 mm should raise concern for injury (Fig. 32.5). On dynamic radiographs, 46% of children younger than 8 years showed 3 mm of anteroposterior motion of C2 on C3; 14% of children had radiographic pseudosubluxation of C3 on C4.[38,39] Based on this study and others, up to 4 mm of translation is considered normal.[6,31,38,40,41]

BOX 32.3 Common Radiographic Variants in Pediatric Spine Trauma

- Anterior wedging of vertebral bodies in children ≤7 y
- Pseudosubluxation of C2 on C3, or C3 on C4
- Lost cervical lordosis
- Atlanto-dens interval <5 mm on flexion views in children <8 y
- Persistent synchondrosis
- Increased rétropharyngeal space (≤7 mm) in the crying child
- Overriding of the anterior arch of the atlas on the odontoid

The absence of cervical lordosis on static lateral radiographs can be a normal finding in 14% of children up to age 16 years.[24] This normal variant can be differentiated from a more ominous sign of posterior ligamentous injury by assessing the posterior interspinous distance. Each interspinous distance should not be more than 1.5 times greater than the interspinous distance directly above and below a given level. The only exception to this rule is the C1–C2 interspinous distance, which can be

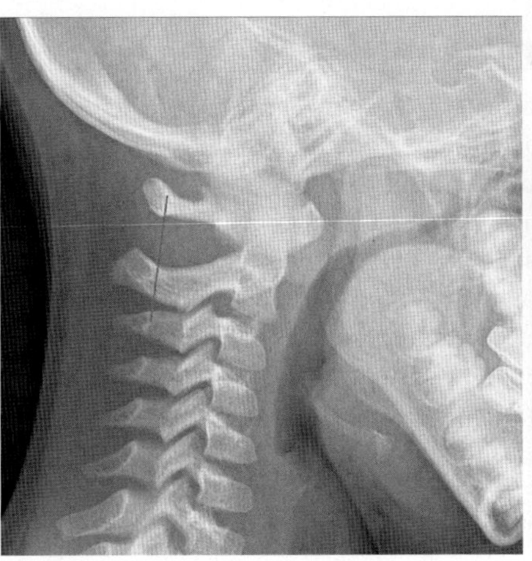
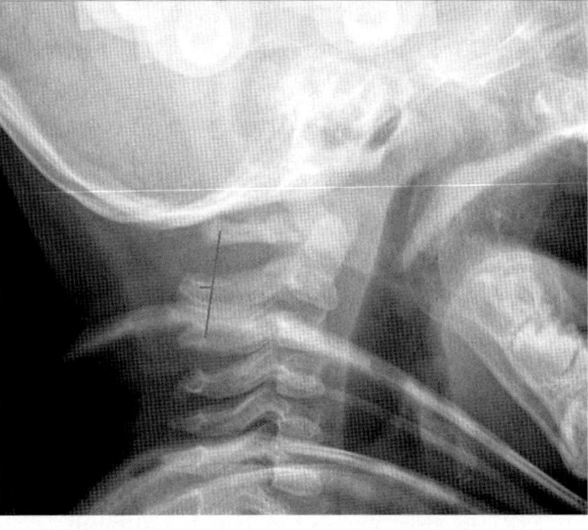

FIG. 32.5 Flexion radiograph of an uninjured cervical spine in a 6-year-old demonstrating pseudosubluxation and a congruent C1–C3 spinolaminar line (*left*). Upright radiograph in a 3-year-old child with traumatic subluxation of C2 on C3 (*right*).

greater than 1.5 times the distance of the level below. The increased mobility at this level is thought to be secondary to the stout posterior ligaments linking C1 to the occiput.[42,43]

Another challenge unique to the developing spine is differentiating a synchondrosis that has not yet ossified from a true fracture. A synchondrosis typically shows well-corticated sclerotic margins. Another helpful aid in differentiating a subtle fracture from a synchondrosis is evaluation of the prevertebral soft tissues. The retropharyngeal space at C2 should be less than 7 mm and the retrotracheal space at C6 should be less than 14 mm in children (as opposed to <22 mm in adults). In simplistic terms, the retropharyngeal space should be one-half the anteroposterior distance of a cervical vertebral body, and the retrotracheal space can be up to a full cervical vertebral body. The retropharyngeal soft tissue can be falsely increased with expiration, such as in a crying child.[44]

Computed Tomography and Magnetic Resonance Imaging of the Spine

The use of helical CT has replaced conventional radiography as the screening tool of choice for the adult cervical spine in the setting of blunt trauma.[45,46] CT of the chest, abdomen, and pelvis, originally targeted for evaluation of the thoracic and abdominal contents, has been shown to be very sensitive at screening for thoracolumbar spine injury. Multiple prospective studies have shown a higher sensitivity for CT (93–100%) compared with plain radiography (33–74%) with improved interobserver variability.[39,47-49] Thus, CT of the spine in high-energy trauma patients has been touted as the standard of care in the adult literature.[50] This information can potentially be extrapolated to pediatric patients, but further studies need to be performed before CT scans with sagittal and coronal reconstructions replace conventional radiography for thoracolumbar spine evaluation in children. As of 2007, the American College of Radiology Appropriateness Criteria advocates for plain radiographic imaging in children 14 years and under with suspected spinal trauma.[51] Additional studies advocate the judicious use of CT scan in children, with some recommending magnetic resonance imaging (MRI) over CT scan in children under 5 years with suspected spinal injury given the relatively high rate of ligamentous versus bony injury in the very young.[52,53] In 2001, Keenan et al. showed that adding CT of the cervical spine in the setting of head trauma decreased the occurrence of multiple additional radiographs, particularly when the patient was intubated.[54] In 2009, Rana et al. reported the sensitivity and specificity of CT to be 100% and 98%, respectively, as compared to plain radiographs showing sensitivity and specificity of 62% and 1.6%, respectively, in a review of 318 pediatric trauma patients.[55] Following practices in the adult population, the use of CT as a screening for spinal trauma in children continues to expand. Adelgais et al. found an increase in the use of CT of the cervical spine in pediatric trauma: from 2002 to 2011, use of cervical spine CT increased from 3.5% to 16.1% of traumas seen at pediatric trauma centers, and from 6.8% to 42% at general emergency departments.[56] Another study showed an increase in the proportion of pediatric fall patients receiving CT from 5.3% in 2001 to 16.6% in 2010. Cervical spine CT is the preferred screening method at our institution in the setting of high-energy trauma.

The increased radiation exposure and increased risk of thyroid cancer is of concern, particularly in the pediatric population. Studies have estimated that CT exposes patients to four times the radiation dose compared to plain radiographs.[57,58] Muchow et al.[59] calculated the radiation exposure to the thyroid after CT and estimated the median excess relative risk of thyroid cancer to be 13% in males and 25% in females for CT scan versus 0.24% in males and 0.5% in females after one radiograph. Based on this data, the increase in the absolute risk of thyroid cancer after CT in males is estimated to be 5.2 to 5.8 per 100,000 and 15.2 to 19 per 100,000 in females. Of note, radiation exposure from any particular CT scan is dependent on the specific scanner and imaging protocol used[60]; thus, advances in technology may allow radiation doses to decrease.

Whether the specificity and sensitivity of CT is sufficiently superior to radiography to justify the increased cost and radiation risk has not been firmly established. Studies in adult trauma have estimated the cost-effectiveness ratio (cost per quality-adjusted life-year [QALY]) of CT to range from $20,000 to $50,000/QALY in high-risk patients and up to $80,000/QALY in low-risk patients.[61] To our knowledge, there are no high-quality studies specifically investigating the cost-effectiveness ratio of spine CT in pediatric trauma. Analyses that also account for the added risk of cancer from radiation exposure are warranted in the pediatric trauma population. Based on available data, either CT or plain radiography may be used to screen for cervical spine injuries.

MRI is useful for evaluating a neurologic deficit and soft tissue involvement. MRI in this age group can be difficult because these young patients often need sedation to prevent movement during data acquisition. MRI should be obtained in patients with evidence of a persistent or transient neurologic deficit. A transient deficit can be an indication of a more serious ligamentous and neurologic injury, thus subsequent need for immobilization.[62]

MRI can also be especially helpful in clearing the cervical spine in obtunded patients. Frank and colleagues[63] showed the effectiveness of MRI at decreasing time to cervical spine clearance, length of time in the pediatric intensive care unit (ICU), and length of time in the hospital. In a meta-analysis of diagnostic imaging studies, Muchow et al.[59] advocate that a normal MRI is the gold standard for cervical spine clearance in obtunded trauma patients. In their meta-analysis, they identified five level I studies, inclusive of a total of 464 obtunded trauma patients with cervical spine MRIs at least 72 hours after admission. Patients with spinal cord injuries were excluded. Clinical follow-up awake examination and imaging was the gold standard comparison to MRI. There were zero false-negatives, yielding a negative predictive value of 100%; the positive predictive value was calculated at 90.2%. Thus, they concluded that a negative MRI can reliably be used to clear the cervical collar in obtunded patients. Also in this study, 97 (20.9%) of the 464 patients had abnormalities identified by MRI that were not seen on plain radiographs or CT; unfortunately, the nature of the injuries missed were not reported in any of the available studies. Of note, 15 of the 464 patients had spine injuries requiring surgical treatment, although all 15 of these injuries were also seen on CT or plain radiography. Thus, the literature suggests that MRI can be used to rule out cervical spine injury in the obtunded patient. There are case reports of spinal cord injuries in patients whose collar was "cleared" by a normal CT scan[64]; however, the incidence of significant spine injuries missed by CT or radiographs has not been firmly established. Fisher et al. performed a retrospective review of 277 patients, reporting that MRI detected an injury requiring intervention in 7 (3%) of patients with a negative CT scan.[65] Five of those 7 required longer-term use of a cervical collar, and 2 (0.7%) had injuries warranting surgical stabilization. Importantly, 4% of their patients had fracture seen on CT that were *not* seen on MRI, suggesting that both CT and MRI are needed to rule out a significant spine injury in obtunded patients.[66]

Spine Clearance

Early cervical spine clearance has multiple benefits as cervical collars have known complications. These include skin breakdown around the neck, dysphagia, pulmonary complications, and increased intracranial pressure.[40,67,68] After a cervical collar has been placed on a child, formal clearance must be obtained before it can be removed. Clinical clearance of the cervical spine has been evaluated using the National Emergency X-Radiography Utilization Study (NEXUS), which was originally developed for adults. NEXUS has been used as a decision-making instrument to determine the need for radiography. The criteria in adults for clinical clearance are absence of the following: neck pain, neurologic symptoms, distracting injuries, or altered mental status (owing to injury, age, or intoxication). If any one of these four criteria is present, the patient is considered to be high risk and must be radiographically cleared. If none of these criteria is present, the collar can be cleared without further imaging.

Application of NEXUS criteria in pediatric patients was studied in a prospective multicenter study. All 30 cervical spine injuries were placed correctly into the high-risk group, and, more important, no cervical spine injuries were noted in the low-risk group. Additionally, use of NEXUS criteria decreased pediatric cervical spine imaging by 20%.[69] These rules cannot be safely applied in children too young to cooperate with an examination, in children in the presence of a high-energy mechanism, or in children with associated injuries that heighten the suspicion of a spine injury. The Canadian C-spine rule (CCR) has gained popularity in the adult literature, showing a higher sensitivity than NEXUS (99.4% vs. 90.7%) and a higher specificity (45.1% vs. 36.8%).[70] According to the CCR, imaging is recommended if an adult patient is high risk (>65 years old, dangerous mechanism, or extremity paresthesias) and if the patient is unable to actively rotate the neck 45 degrees in each direction (tested only in low-risk patients).

In young children, however, the Canadian C-spine rule may not be as sensitive owing to potentially poor cooperation with exam or inability to communicate important symptoms.[71] The efficacy of the Canadian C-spine rule and NEXUS in young children was investigated by Ehrlich et al. in 2009. In a study of children 10 years and younger, the investigators retrospectively applied the NEXUS and CCR rules based on the initial history and physical, and compared these against the patients' imaging findings. With this method they reported that, if applied, the NEXUS had sensitivity of 43% and specificity of 96%, and the CCR showed a sensitivity of 86% and specificity of 94%.[72] We are not aware of any prospective studies specifically investigating clinical decision rules for spine imaging in young children.

It has been shown that an efficient, multidisciplinary approach can facilitate rapid clearance of the cervical spine, decreasing the average time to 7.5 hours in nonintubated patients and 19.4 hours in intubated patients.[25] This rapid clearance is dependent on a system that is safe and user-friendly enough to allow the primary admitting team to perform the clearance. Anderson and colleagues[73] evaluated

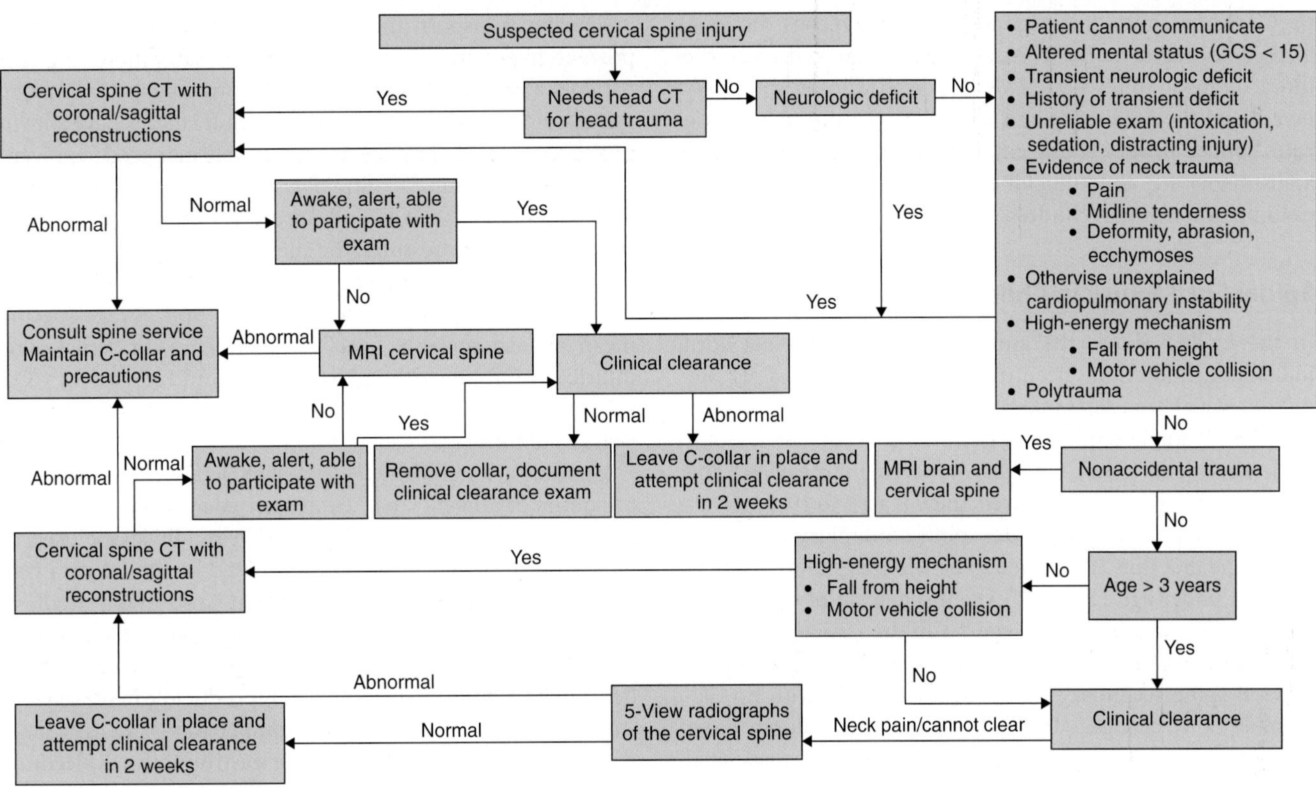

FIG. 32.6 Cervical spine clearance algorithm in pediatric trauma. CT, computed tomography; GCS, Glasgow Coma Scale; MRI, magnetic resonance imaging.

the percentage of cervical spines cleared by spine specialists before versus after the initiation of a clearance protocol, noting a 60% increase in spines cleared by nonspine physicians without any late injuries detected.

A spine clearance protocol should incorporate a thorough history and physical examination with judicious use of imaging modalities. If a low-risk/low-energy injury mechanism took place and there is cervical tenderness on examination, imaging should begin with plain anteroposterior and lateral radiographs. An open-mouth odontoid view should be obtained in children older than 8 years who have the ability to cooperate; otherwise, a CT scan from occiput to C2 should be performed. Children undergoing a CT scan to evaluate for head injury should have the cervical spine with reconstructions included. In the setting of high-risk/high-energy trauma, we recommend CT imaging as the screening tool of choice if a cervical spine injury is suspected. Children with no evidence of injury on plain radiography or CT scan who have persistent pain should remain in the cervical collar with later clearance in the clinic with dynamic radiographs. In the presence of a neurologic deficit or a history of a transient deficit before arrival, MRI of the entire spine should be obtained. If spinal cord injury without radiographic abnormality (SCIWORA) is suspected, the cervical collar should remain in place, spine precautions should be continued, and the patient should be admitted for observation to monitor for potential delayed neurologic deterioration.[74,75]

Clearing the cervical spine in an unconscious patient can be facilitated by a standard protocol. If the patient returns to a normal mental status, the protocol for a conscious patient can be used. There have been reports of delayed neurologic deterioration in patients with altered mental status and unrecognized ligamentous injury that subluxed on mobilization.[76] The two modalities available for evaluating ligamentous injury in an obtunded patient include fluoroscopic flexion-extension and MRI. Fluoroscopic flexion-extension examination can be labor intensive, and in an adult series it was difficult to visualize the cervicothoracic junction.[77] Because of these problems, MRI is superior for evaluating ligamentous injury. Fig. 32.6 presents a cervical spine clearance protocol in line with the best evidence available to date regarding collar clearance and cervical spine imaging.

MRI has been found to be most sensitive for detecting a ligamentous injury at postinjury day 2 or 3.[78] Stassen and colleagues[79] used MRI within their protocol at a level I adult trauma center for assisting in cervical spine clearance. All obtunded patients with a negative CT scan of the cervical spine underwent MRI on postinjury day 3 if they could not be clinically cleared. MRI allowed clearance of the cervical collar in 60% of subjects, and there was no delayed neurologic sequela. The remaining patients were treated in a cervical collar for 6 weeks without complication.

Equivocal MRI findings can be evaluated further with flexion-extension radiographs, or the physician can forgo further study and treat the patient with a collar for 6 weeks. At the termination of the 6-week period, the patient should undergo a flexion-extension series to ensure adequate healing. Expedient clearance of the thoracolumbar spine in a child with polytrauma is also very important to prevent skin breakdown, respiratory complications, and ileus. At our institution, the CT traumagram, with sagittal and coronal reconstructions, is used to augment the clinical examination and clear the thoracolumbar spine. Future work is needed to prospectively investigate the sensitivity and specificity of clinical decision rules applied in very young children. Such rules should make adjustments for the difficulties with history and physical examination in small children.[71]

Spinal Cord Injury in Children

In the United States, the annual incidence of spinal cord injuries in children has been reported at 19.9 injuries per one million, which translates into roughly 1400 spinal cord injuries per year.[2,80] Spinal cord injury most often occurs after motor vehicle accidents (56%), falls (14%), firearm injuries (9%), and sports injuries (7%).[80] In children, there is a 5% to 10% mortality rate during the first year after spinal cord injury, and death within the first year is reported to be five times more likely in children under age 11 years.[81] The mechanism of spinal cord injury differs depending on age.[24] Children younger than 8 years more often sustain spinal cord insult involving the upper cervical spine secondary to ligamentous injury with no discernible bony changes. This is in contrast to children older than 8 years who have spinal cord injuries with associated fractures secondary to biomechanics of the spine that more closely mirror those of an adult. A thorough neurologic examination should be performed to determine the level involved and whether the lesion is complete or incomplete. It is important to note whether there is sacral sparing as indicated by sensation at the anal mucocutaneous junction (S4–S5 dermatome) on the left and right side, ability to contract the anal sphincter voluntarily, and deep anal sensation. This sacral sparing indicates continuity of long tracts with improved likelihood for return of neurologic function.[82] As in adult injuries, the American Spinal Injury Association (ASIA) Impairment Scale is most frequently used in pediatric patients to provide a standardized description of injury.

Damage to the spinal cord has been categorized into primary and secondary injury. Primary injury occurs at the time of the trauma, leading to structural damage of the neural elements and supporting blood supply. This primary insult is irreversible. Secondary injury occurs within minutes of the trauma, setting off a cascade of events that result in ischemia, increased cell membrane permeability, pathologic electrolyte shift, edema, and production of free radicals.[83] This process continues to evolve over subsequent days, and medical and surgical strategies are directed at mitigating secondary injury. Current acute treatments of interest include support of spinal cord perfusion, intravenous corticosteroids, and early (versus delayed) decompression. Many pharmacologic therapies have been investigated for spinal cord injury, including corticosteroids, GM_1 ganglioside,[84] sodium channel blockers (Riluzole),[85] minocycline, Rho antagonists (Rho is a signaling molecule for myelin and extracellular matrix inhibitors of neural regeneration),[85] and mesenchymal stem cells.[86] There is no single "cure" for spinal cord injury, and the majority of the available treatment strategies remain investigational, with varying results.

During transport and initial evaluation, it is crucial to prevent hypotension and keep oxygen saturations high in patients suspected to have a spinal cord injury to optimize spinal cord perfusion.[87] Animal and adult studies have shown improved outcome in subjects aggressively managed to prevent spinal cord ischemia.[88–90] Strategies to this end include admitting patients to the ICU and accurately monitoring volume status and blood pressure. The mean arterial pressure should be maintained to promote spinal cord perfusion. At our institution, the pediatric trauma ICU utilizes age-specific mean arterial pressure goals for children with spinal cord injuries: age younger than 3 years = 60 mm Hg; 3 to 12 years = 70 mm Hg; 13 to 16 years = 75 mm Hg; and older than 16 years = 80 mm Hg.

Steroids are stabilizing agents; they act as a powerful anti-inflammatory agent that decreases edema and scavenges oxygen free radicals. High-dose methylprednisolone used to be administered to older children based on initial data collected in adults (National Acute Spinal Cord Injury Studies). However, controversy persists surrounding the efficacy of steroids in the setting of an acute spinal cord injury after neurologic improvements were not reproducible in subsequent studies. Additionally, significant complications are associated with high-dose steroids, including gastrointestinal bleeding, hyperglycemia, sepsis, wound complications, pneumonia, myopathy, and respiratory failure.[91,92] To date, we are aware of six randomized controlled trials investigating the use of intravenous methylprednisolone in the setting of spinal cord injury.[93–98] Despite these, no firm consensus has been established for the use of methylprednisolone in spinal cord injury; as such, this therapy can only be considered a treatment option. In 2013, the joint American Association of Neurological Surgeons/Congress of Neurological Surgeons recommended against the use of steroids altogether for treatment of spinal cord injury, stating that the evidence of potential harm outweighs the evidence of potential for benefit.[99] It should also be noted that studies of steroid treatment in the setting of spinal cord injury have not been stratified by injury level to distinguish between the effect of steroid use in cervical as compared with thoracic cord injuries. Additionally, to our knowledge, there are no high-quality randomized controlled trials investigating the use of steroids in pediatric spinal cord injury; thus, in this age group, the use of steroids is not evidence based at the time of this writing.[74]

The indications for early operative intervention for pediatric patients with spinal cord injury include radiographic confirmation of spinal cord compression in the setting of an incomplete injury or progressive deficit, an open spine injury, and a grossly unstable spine in patients who are neurologically intact. Studies have demonstrated improved neurologic recovery for adult patients undergoing early (<24 hours from injury) versus late (>48 hours from injury) decompression in the setting of a cervical spinal cord injury and continued compression.[100,101] This information can potentially be extrapolated to the pediatric population. However, to our knowledge, there have been no well-designed, prospective studies specifically in pediatric patients evaluating the effect and timing of decompression.[102]

Functional outcomes depend on the level of injury and whether it is complete or incomplete. Patients with injuries above C4 may be dependent on a respirator, and phrenic nerve pacemakers can be implanted. Patients with C3 lesions can shrug their shoulders and often have neck motion, permitting operation of equipment with sip/puff controls, voice activation, eyebrow or eye blink, and head or chin controls. Patients with C6 lesions are often able to propel a manual wheelchair with the assistance of fusions and tendon transfers. At least partial recovery after a complete spinal cord injury has been reported in 10% to 25% of patients.[24,87,103,104] In a series reported by Wang and colleagues,[105] 64% of patients showed at least partial recovery after spinal cord injury. Of patients with complete injuries, 25% eventually became ambulatory. Recovery was seen up to 1 year after injury.

Complications unique to pediatric patients with a spinal cord injury are susceptibility to development of posttraumatic deformity and growth arrest.[106] Causes can be divided into intrinsic, extrinsic, and iatrogenic factors. Intrinsic factors include injury to the vertebral apophyses, resulting in abnormal growth and change in biomechanics from altered shape of the vertebral body and loss of posterior ligamentous support. This change in biomechanics can alter the forces on the vertebral apophyses, exacerbating the deformity further.[107] Extrinsic factors include weak trunk muscles in the setting of gravity and spasticity with a contracture. Iatrogenic factors include improperly instrumented segments and use of a laminectomy without fusion. The risk of developing a deformity in the setting of a laminectomy without fusion is approximately 50%, with a much higher incidence in the cervical and thoracic spine.[108] Nonoperative treatment with a brace can help slow the progression of deformity, and can temporize the situation to allow the child maximum time to grow before undergoing a fusion.[109] Performing surgical correction and fusion needs to take into account remaining growth. An estimate of remaining growth can be determined by multiplying 0.7 mm times the number of segments fused times the number of years of remaining growth.[110]

Posterior fusion in young children has the added drawback of the crankshaft phenomenon. This phenomenon occurs with continued growth of the anterior column in the setting of a fused posterior column. With continued anterior growth, the apical vertebral body rotates, producing a scoliotic curve.[111] However, this is less of a problem now with the use of pedicle screw instrumentation, which theoretically captures all three spinal columns. The goals of surgery include halting progression, obtaining correction, and balancing the spine and pelvis to equalize sitting skin pressure. Indications include a scoliotic curve of greater than 40 degrees and kyphotic curves of greater than 60 degrees. Anterior release may be needed if the deformity is rigid, as shown on bending films. Including the sacrum in the fusion construct is recommended if pelvic obliquity exists.

Spinal Cord Injury Without Radiographic Abnormality (SCIWORA)

The biomechanical differences in the spine of children younger than 8 years place them at risk of a SCIWORA.[24] This entity was first described by Pang and Wilberger[112] in 1982 before the use of MRI. The term SCIWORA was developed to describe spinal cord injuries without overt vertebral column disruption, as displayed by conventional radiographs, CT scans, myelograms, and dynamic flexion-extension radiographs. SCIWORA excludes injuries secondary to penetrating trauma, secondary to electrical shock, secondary to obstetric complication, and in association with congenital anomalies. The incidence of SCIWORA in patients with spinal cord injury for ages birth to 17 years was reported to be 35% in earlier literature.[75] As MRI has become more widely used, the incidence of SCIWORA with spinal cord injuries is reported to be 3%.[5] This change likely reflects an improvement in imaging quality and the ability to detect subtle injuries previously missed, rather than a change in actual injury type. More recently, Bosch and colleagues[113] found that recurrent SCIWORA was an uncommon entity, which occurred only in low-energy, sports-related injuries, resulting in transient neurologic symptoms, with full recovery in all cases.

MRI is the study of choice for evaluation of patients suspected to have SCIWORA. On MRI, there are both extraneural soft tissue changes and intraneural changes. The changes seen on MRI are secondary to edema and methemoglobin, a processed form of hemoglobin. Edema is seen as isointense on T1 and hyperintense on T2; extracellular methemoglobin is seen as hyperintense on T1 and hyperintense on T2. MRI changes in the extraneural tissues can be detected within hours of injury because the blood is quickly metabolized into a form easily seen on MRI. Intraneural changes can take days to be detectable because of the delayed metabolism of a hemorrhage into a form visible on MRI.[114,115] It is recommended that MRI be obtained at the time of presentation to rule out a compressive lesion that needs to be surgically addressed and at 6 to 9 days after injury to improve detection of intraneural injuries related to SCIWORA.[75]

The recommended duration of immobilization in a brace has been somewhat controversial, with the concern for delayed neurologic deterioration or reinjury motivating the recommendation for a brace. A meta-analysis by Launay and colleagues[74] showed that patients immobilized for 8 weeks had a 17% chance of developing recurrent SCIWORA, whereas no patients immobilized for 12 weeks had recurrent SCIWORA develop.

Atlanto-Occipital Dislocation

Atlanto-occipital dislocations were previously thought to be rare injuries that were fatal and usually found on autopsy.[116,117] More recently, this injury has been identified more frequently with a higher survival rate, particularly among children. Increased survival is possibly due to faster response by emergency personnel, improved cervical immobilization, and faster diagnosis upon arrival to the emergency department.[117–122]

The atlanto-occipital joint is a condylar joint with minimal bony stability that is stabilized primarily by ligaments. In children, the occipital condyles are less cup shaped and the articulation is more horizontal, potentially explaining the higher incidence of dislocation among children compared with adults.[33,34,120] Ligamentous stability is provided primarily by the tectorial membrane, anterior longitudinal ligament, nuchal ligament, and paired alar ligaments.

Dislocation of the atlanto-occipital joint is usually due to a deceleration mechanism, such as a motor vehicle accident or pedestrian-vehicle accident, in which the head violently moves forward, causing separation of the condyles and the atlas. Diagnosing dislocation based on physical examination findings can be difficult because of varied presentation and concomitant traumatic brain injury. Neurologic function can range from a normal examination to flaccidity (early), absent deep tendon and sacral reflexes (early), poikilothermy, spasticity (late), urinary retention (late), priapism (late), and autonomic dysreflexia (late).

On lateral plain films, the "rule of twelves" should be remembered, looking at the dens-basion distance and distance from the basion to the line tangential to the dens posterior cortex. Additionally, the Powers ratio is the distance from the basion to the posterior aspect of the arch of the atlas divided by the distance from the anterior tubercle of the atlas to the rim of the foramen magnum, which is normally between 0.7 and 1, with a value greater than 1 indicating anterior atlanto-occipital dislocation.[123] The accuracy of these traditional radiographic criteria has been called into question, leading some to advocate using CT and MRI for diagnosis.[118,119,124] More recently, it has been suggested that a condyle–C1 interval of greater than 4 mm, as measured on a reformatted CT scan, is valuable in identifying atlanto-occipital dislocation.[124,125]

Although initial treatment of atlanto-occipital dislocation is immobilization in a halo or Minerva cast, most unstable injuries should be managed by posterior occipitoatlantal fusion with internal fixation. Wire fixation or fixation with a contoured rod and wires can be used from occiput to C1 to preserve C1–C2 motion. If the stability of the C1–C2 junction is questionable, fusion from occiput to C2, or C1 to C2, should be considered. Techniques have been developed to utilize occipital plates and lateral mass screw fixation to achieve successful fusion from the occiput to C2.[126] Harms described a technique for fusion of C1–C2 utilizing C1 lateral mass and C2 pedicle screws, with good fusion result.[127] This technique is considered a useful option for stabilization of the atlantoaxial complex, particularly in the setting of a fracture-dislocation when transarticular screws and wiring may not be an option due to subluxation of C1 on C2.

Fractures of the Atlas

A fracture of the ring of C1 is a rare injury in children that can occur when an axial load forces the occipital condyles into the lateral masses, resulting in fractures that involve the anterior and posterior rings (Jefferson fracture).[128–132] Children differ from adults because they can more often have plastic deformation of the ring and a single fracture with hinging on the contralateral synchondrosis. Instability exists when there is disruption of the transverse atlantal ligament. This disruption is determined on the anteroposterior cervical spine film (or coronal CT slice) by adding the overhang of the C1 lateral mass relative to the C2 lateral mass on the left and right sides. If the sum is greater than or equal to 8.1 mm on plain radiography or 6.9 mm on CT imaging, instability exists and should be treated with traction and a halo or Minerva cast. Cases with sums less than 7 mm can be treated with a well-fitting cervical orthosis.[132] Surgical stabilization of C1 fractures is rarely required in children[128,133]; if required, this can be accomplished with use of lateral mass screws in C1 and C2 connected by a cross link, as described by Tan et al.[134]

Atlantoaxial Instability

Instability at the level of C1–C2 can be secondary to traumatic ligamentous injury or chronic disease processes, including inflammatory diseases, malignancy, bone dysplasias, and congenital craniofacial malformations. An association with Down syndrome is well reported in the literature; there are other reports of atlantoaxial subluxation associated with Reiter syndrome, Larsen syndrome, juvenile rheumatoid arthritis, Morquio syndrome, and Kniest syndrome.[135–141] In traumatic atlantoaxial injury, the transverse atlantal ligament is disrupted, resulting in an increased ADI. The ADI is the distance as measured on a lateral cervical radiograph between the posterior aspect of the anterior ring of C1 and the anterior cortex of the dens. Active flexion views may be required to observe subluxation, and CT scans can show avulsion fractures at the insertions of the transverse ligament. In children, the upper limit for a normal distance is 4.5 mm; in adults, the upper limit is 3 mm. Acute rupture of the transverse ligament is rare in children.[142,143] Alternatively, the ligament itself may be intact, but can be avulsed from its attachment to C1. Surgical stabilization of C1–C2 after reduction in extension is generally recommended, followed by immobilization for 8 to 12 weeks in a halo brace, Minerva cast, or cervical orthosis. To document stability after treatment, flexion and extension views are recommended.

In Down syndrome, the frequency of atlantoaxial instability has been reported to approach 10% to 30% by adolescence.[136,144–147] Instability in patients with Down syndrome is attributed to laxity of the transverse ligament and C1–C2 joint capsules. Nearly 98% to 99% of patients are asymptomatic, but should be followed closely,[148–150] with some authors recommending yearly neurologic and dynamic radiographic examination.[151] Surgery is indicated in symptomatic and asymptomatic patients with an ADI greater than 10 mm or with less than 14 mm of space available for the spinal cord on lateral films.[152] There is a high reported surgical complication rate for these patients, including the risk of pseudarthrosis, wound infection/dehiscence, adjacent-level disease, and neurologic injury.[146,153]

Surgical fixation for atlantoaxial arthrodesis originated with posterior wire stabilization and structural bone grafting, as popularized by Gallie in 1939[154] and Brooks and Jenkins in 1978.[155] This technique requires the passage of wires into the spinal canal, with the potential risk of spinal cord injury.[156,157] Additionally, a wire construct often lacks sufficient stability[158,159] resulting in nonunion rates of 30% even with a halo

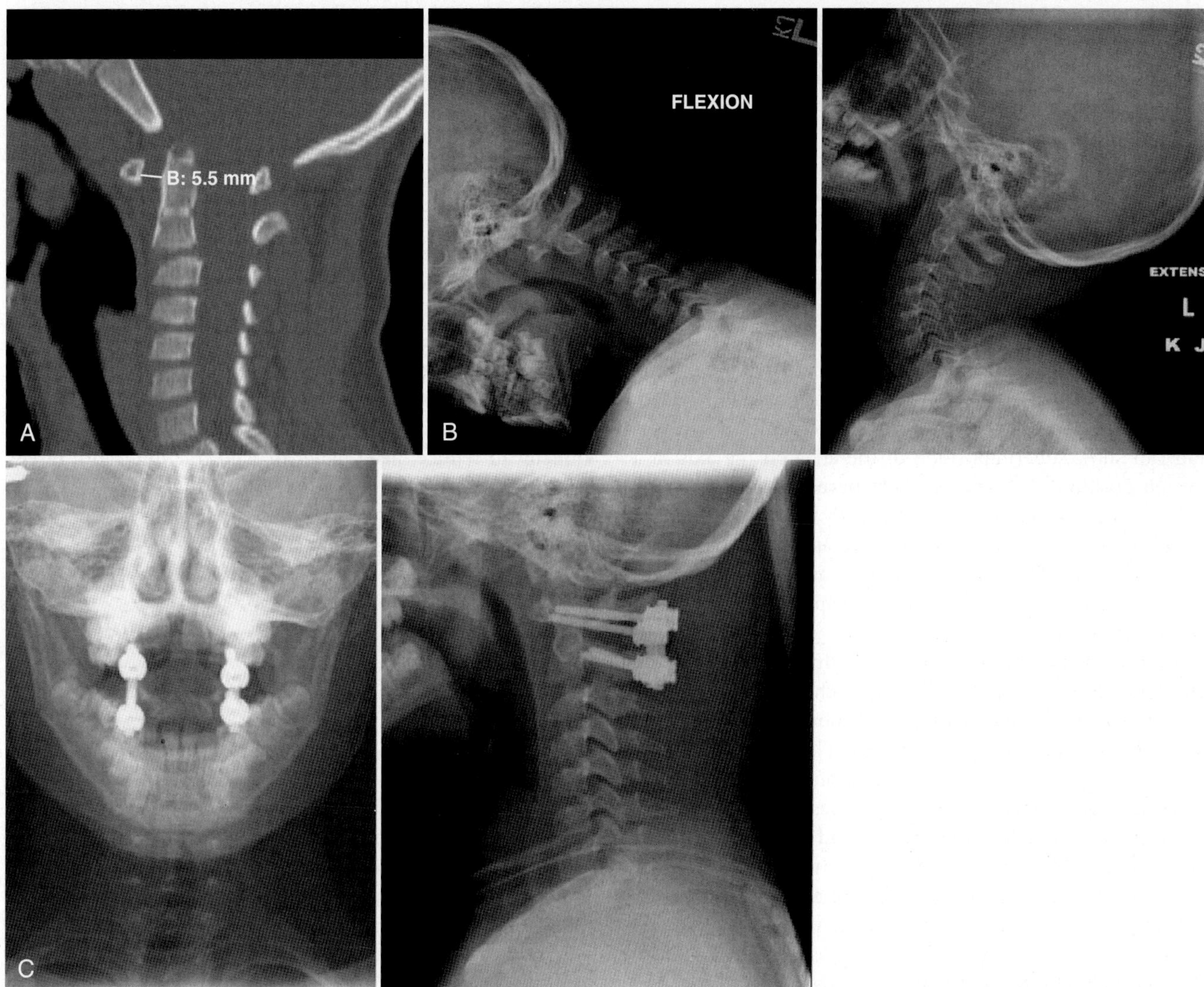

FIG. 32.7 Atlantoaxial subluxation. A 6-year-old boy was hit by a car. (A) A 5.5-mm atlanto-dens interval shown on lateral computed tomography reconstruction at the time of injury. (B) After 3 months of conservative treatment in a cervical collar, instability is shown on flexion and extension lateral cervical radiographs. (C) Postoperative radiographs after C1–C2 fusion.

vest postoperatively.[49,62,160–163] The C1–C2 posterior transarticular screw, or Magerl screw (1986), has a decreased rate of nonunion,[156,164–168] but carries the risk of injuring the vertebral artery.[169] Segmental C1–C2 fixation was introduced by Goel and Laheria in 1994[170] using a plate and lateral mass screws, and then by Harms and Melcher in 2001[127] using polyaxial C1 lateral mass screws and C2 pedicle screws with rod stabilization. This approach offers the distinct advantage of being able to insert the screws and then achieve the reduction compared with the Magerl screw technique, in which an anatomic reduction must be achieved before screw insertion. Fig. 32.7 shows a 6-year-old boy who had atlantoaxial subluxation.

Atlantoaxial Rotatory Subluxation

Atlantoaxial rotatory subluxation, also known as *atlantoaxial rotatory fixation,* if it has persisted for more than 3 months, is a frequent cause of torticollis in children. The most common etiologies are minor trauma and infection, although congenital and iatrogenic causes also exist. Patients present with neck pain, loss of cervical motion, and a "cock-robin" position, in which the head is tilted to one side and rotated to the contralateral side. In acute subluxations, movement is painful and accompanied by sternocleidomastoid spasms. In contrast to muscular torticollis, the sternocleidomastoid muscle is contracted on the same side to which the chin is rotated. This is likely due to a reactive muscle spasm attempting to reduce the subluxation. The child often has the ability to make the deformity worse, but cannot correct it. In fixed deformities, the pain subsides, but the lack of motion persists. Neurologic deficits are rare.[171]

The mechanism of injury is often trivial trauma, thus causing the diagnosis to be delayed.[172,173] The infectious etiology is known as Grisel syndrome and most commonly occurs after an upper respiratory tract infection, but can also occur after tonsillectomy, pharyngoplasty, or retropharyngeal abscess.[174] Because of the anastomoses between the veins and lymphatics draining the pharynx and periodontoid plexus, inflammation in the pharynx can lead to attenuation of the transverse ligament or synovium or both surrounding C1–C2, resulting in subluxation.

Radiographic examination can be challenging because of the difficulty in positioning a patient with torticollis.[175] On the anteroposterior and open-mouth odontoid views, the lateral masses appear different in size because one is rotated anteriorly and one posteriorly, and the distances from the lateral masses to the dens are asymmetrical. On lateral view, with the cassette placed parallel to the skull, the two halves of the posterior arch of C2 will not be superimposed, with the spinal canal appearing narrowed. Two-dimensional and three-dimensional CT scans have largely replaced cineradiography, and can show superimposition of the atlas on the axis in a rotated position.[176,177] Some authors have endorsed dynamic CT, in which 3-mm cuts are taken with the head in neutral position, then with left and right rotation.[178,179] Although improved sensitivity has been reported using this technique, the significantly increased radiation exposure undoubtedly lessens its utility.

Treatment options depend on the timing of injury and duration of symptoms,[180] with some children likely never receiving medical attention because of spontaneous reduction. Patients whose symptoms have persisted less than 1 week can be treated with a soft collar, antiinflammatories, and home exercises. If spontaneous reduction does not occur after a week, the patients should be put in head halter traction and bed rest, which usually relieves the symptoms if they have persisted less than 1 month. In cases of atlantoaxial rotatory subluxations that have endured more than 1 month, reduction with head halter traction is unlikely, due to secondary changes that have developed within the atlantoaxial joint and surrounding soft tissues.[181] Halo traction can then be attempted, as can be used with the halo, while applying a rotation to the right and left to assist the reduction. Documentation of the reduction should be performed by CT scan; then, the patient must remain in the collar or halo vest for 6 weeks. Recurrent subluxation should be treated with prompt cervical traction until reduction is achieved, followed by a 3-month course in a halo. If initial reduction is unable to be maintained, posterior fusion of C1–C2 is recommended. Additionally, fusion is recommended if the halo immobilization fails after 6 weeks, if the subluxation has been present for more than 3 months, or if the patient has instability or neurologic compromise.[182]

Odontoid Fractures

Odontoid fractures are one of the most common cervical spine fractures in children, reported to represent up to 75% of all cervical spine fractures owing to the large head/body size ratio.[183] In children, the most common mechanism is falling; in young adults, the mechanism is typically high-velocity trauma, such as motor vehicle accidents. Fractures of the odontoid in children typically occur through the synchondrosis, which is a cartilage line at the base of the odontoid. Fractures that reduce spontaneously can look like a Salter-Harris I injury or appear to be normal on plain films. CT scans with three-dimensional reconstructions can assist in identifying minimally displaced odontoid fractures,[184] and MRI can show bone and soft tissue edema around a minimally displaced fracture. Most odontoid fractures are displaced anteriorly with an intact anterior periosteal sleeve that can help stabilize the fracture when immobilized in extension, and encourage healing.[177,185–187] Treatment of displaced fractures is by closed reduction via an extension maneuver with immobilization in a halo cast or Minerva jacket for children younger than 3 years. Most fractures heal uneventfully after 6 to 8 weeks, at which time documentation of stability with flexion-extension views is recommended. In cases that are difficult to reduce, head halter or halo traction—and, rarely, manipulation under general anesthesia—is necessary. The need for surgical fixation is unusual, as there are excellent results from closed treatment.[188–190]

Os Odontoideum

Os odontoideum is an unsupported round ossicle that is separated from the body of the axis by a transverse gap. Some authors propose that os odontoideum is due to an unrecognized fracture that is distracted by the alar ligaments and results in nonunion,[37,171,191–199] whereas other authors suggest that it is congenital because of its association with congenital syndromes.[200–202] Presentation ranges from asymptomatic to frank myelopathy. Diagnosis can usually be made on routine radiographs, with lateral flexion-extension views showing the degree of displacement of C1 on C2. Measuring the distance between C1 and the ossicle is not helpful because they typically move together. Instead, one should evaluate the space available for the cord or the relationship of the body of the axis to the posterior aspect of the anterior arch of C1. More recently, investigators have suggested using dynamic (real-time) MRI to aid in diagnosis of instability.[203]

There is debate in the literature regarding management of patients with os odontoideum. Some authors advocate conservative management with yearly clinical and radiographic evaluation of patients with a stable os odontoideum.[192,204–206] There are reports, however, of decompensation and death in asymptomatic patients who have been followed conservatively.[192,207,208] Some surgeons favor surgical stabilization of patients with an os odontoideum due to the potential instability risk leading to catastrophic injuries.[206,208–211] Options include methods for C1–C2 arthrodesis, as already discussed.[211–213]

Hangman's Fracture

A hangman's fracture, or traumatic spondylolisthesis, is a fracture of the bilateral pars interarticularis of C2. This name derives from the fact that the fracture resembles the injury associated with a judicial hanging. Because the fracture fragments separate and decompress the cord, neurologic injury is unusual. Most of these injuries occur in children younger than 2 years, likely because of the large head size and poor muscle control. Radiographs often show anterior subluxation of C2 on C3, with lucency anterior to the pedicles of the axis. Persistent synchondroses of the axis have been reported that can be confused with hangman's fractures.[163,214–216] Treatment consists of immobilization for 8 to 12 weeks in a cervical orthosis, Minerva jacket, or halo. Pizzutillo and colleagues[217] reported healing in four of five children treated in a Minerva jacket or halo cast. If nonunion occurs, anterior or posterior arthrodesis can be considered for symptomatic patients.[182]

Lower Cervical (Subaxial) Spine Injuries

Traumatic injuries to the lower cervical spine (C3–C7) are rare in young children and infants, but are more common in adolescents and older children. Children younger than 9 years old account for only 22% to 31% of pediatric lower cervical spine injuries, whereas children older than 10 years account for 70% to 73%.[218] One should suspect a cervical spine injury if the patient is unconscious, has cervical rigidity, muscle guarding, neck pain, radicular pain, numbness, or neurologic deficits.[218] In infants, motor weakness and hypotonia should raise the suspicion of a cervical spine injury.

Compression Fractures

Compression fractures are the most common fracture in the pediatric lower cervical spine. Trauma causing flexion and axial loading leads to a loss of vertebral height. When evaluating a child, one must be careful not to mistake normal cervical wedging for a compression fracture. Ossification progresses in a posterior to anterior direction and remains incomplete until approximately age 8 years; thus, anterior wedging of the lower cervical spine until this age is considered normal. This wedging is usually most notable at the C3 vertebra.[219] Compression fractures are usually considered stable injuries and can be treated nonoperatively. With immobilization, these fractures normally heal in 3 to 6 weeks. Flexion and extension films should be obtained at 2 to 4 weeks to confirm stability and alignment of the fracture.

Facet Fractures and Dislocations

Facet fractures and dislocations are the second most common lower cervical spine injuries in children, and most commonly occur in adolescents.[182] Unilateral dislocations often affect the ipsilateral nerve root; bilateral dislocations affect the spinal cord.[220] The cartilaginous components are overlapped and locked, causing a "perched facet" on radiography, which indicates a true dislocation. Treatment for a unilateral dislocation is initially traction and reduction if the patient is awake and able to cooperate with an examination. The patient must be awake, cooperative, and able to provide a reliable examination in order for closed reduction to be done safely.[221] After reduction, surgical stabilization is typically needed. If the dislocation cannot be reduced, open reduction and arthrodesis is warranted. Similarly, bilateral facet fractures and dislocations are considered unstable; thus, reduction and stabilization is required.[182] Fig. 32.8 shows a 6-year-old girl with bilateral lumbar facet dislocations. If no disc herniation is present on MRI, either an anterior or posterior surgical approach can be used for reduction and stabilization of facet fracture-dislocations. The literature has not shown a clearly superior approach in terms of fusion rate, alignment, long-term complications, or neurologic recovery.[222] If a disc herniation is present, an anterior approach is preferable to allow direct removal of the impinging disc prior to reduction of the facet joints. In addition, the treating surgeon should assess the integrity of the posterior ligamentous complex (PLC) to determine whether an anterior-only procedure is adequate or whether a combined anteroposterior fusion is needed. In a cadaveric cervical corpectomy biomechanical study, anterior fixation with a static plate and cage adequately stabilized the injured level if the PLC was intact. If the PLC was sectioned, a combined anteroposterior approach was needed to achieve stability.[223]

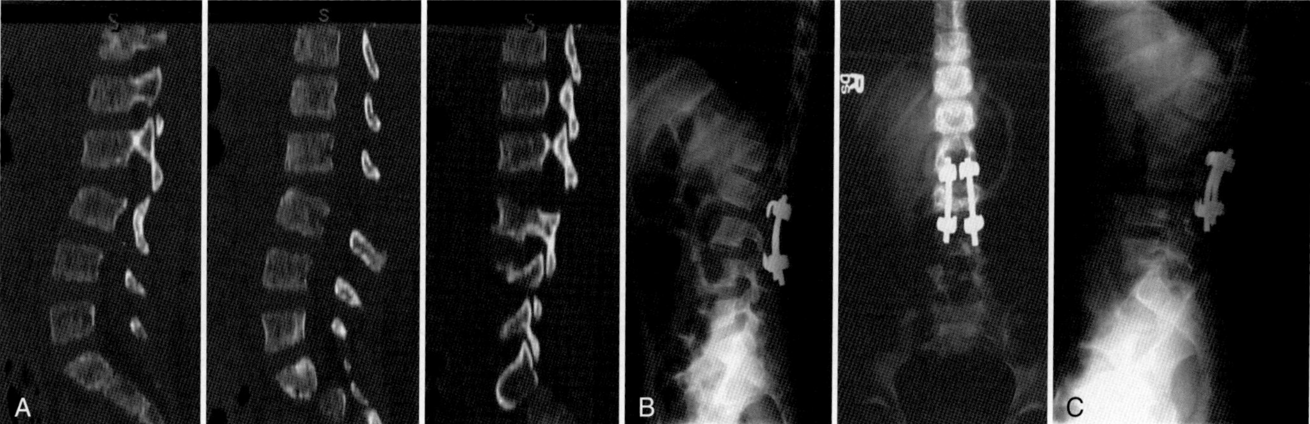

FIG. 32.8 Bilateral lumbar facet dislocation. A 6-year-old girl was in a motor vehicle accident. (A) Sagittal computed tomographic reconstructions show bilateral L2–L3 facet dislocations. (B) Postoperative image after L2–L3 fusion with pedicle hook instrumentation. (C) Image 3 years postoperatively.

Burst Fractures

Burst fractures in the subaxial spine are rare in pediatric patients. These injuries occur secondary to axial loading. Retropulsed fragments can compromise the spinal canal. CT is a useful modality in determining canal compromise and bony involvement. A burst fracture with no neurologic deficit and minimal spinal canal compromise can be treated by immobilization with a halo or rigid orthosis, depending on the level involved. If the patient has neurologic deficits due to significant canal compromise, surgical decompression and fixation is recommended. typically via anterior arthrodesis. This is one of the few instances in which anterior fusion is recommended in children because the need for stability outweighs the risk of developing a deformity secondary to destruction of the anterior growth plate. In older children and adolescents, anterior instrumentation can be used without as much risk of kyphotic deformity.[182] In cervical burst fractures that are more consistent with a flexion-distraction injury with posterior ligamentous disruption, an isolated posterior instrumented arthrodesis can be considered in those patients without active cord compression.

It is important to assess the integrity of the posterior ligamentous complex in the setting of burst fractures, as this can aid in determining whether the injury is stable or unstable.[224] Studies in the adult literature have shown that hyperintense signal on fat-suppressed T2-weighted MRI correlates with intraoperative confirmation of injury to the supraspinous ligament, interspinous ligament, and ligamentum flavum.[225] A detailed analysis by Vaccaro et al. reports the sensitivity of MRI in detecting PLC injury to range from 79% (facet capsule) to 90% (interspinous ligament).[226] More specific to the pediatric population, Sledge et al. also advocate MRI as a useful tool to assess the PLC in pediatric trauma based on a retrospective review of 19 MRI studies in children.[227]

Vertebral Growth Plate Fractures

In contrast to adults, lower cervical spine injuries in children can occur through the synchondrosis at the cartilaginous endplate. The primary ossification centers fuse by 7 to 8 years of age, but the secondary ossification centers can remain open until 25 years of age.[228] MRI can be used to assess the growth plate because it may be difficult to differentiate normal lucency of a synchondrosis from a traumatic lesion on radiography. Fracture of the synchondrosis can lead to anterior or posterior displacement of the endplate. Anterior displacement can be treated conservatively with a cervical orthosis until the fracture has healed. Posterior displacement of the endplate is treated with an anterior surgical approach to reduce the bony endplate, resulting in spinal decompression and alignment. The patient should remain in a cervical orthosis for 4 to 5 months.[229]

Pediatric Halo

Halo immobilization is often used in the treatment of pediatric cervical spine injuries, even in infants. Presized halos and vests are used in adults, which often work for adolescents. Prefabricated halos and vests are also available for children and infants, but because of the wide variability in size in children, custom vests and rings may be necessary. In some patients, CT can be helpful before pin placement to help determine bone structure. The pediatric skull is thickest anterolaterally and posterolaterally, and pins should be placed accordingly, with attention to the supraorbital and supratrochlear nerves.[230] The number of pins required varies with age. Children younger than 2 years require 8 to 10 pins, but by age 5 years, only 4 pins may be necessary.[220] Pins should be inserted perpendicular to the skull to improve pin-bone interface.[231] The amount of torque required during pin insertion decreases with age, with 2 to 4 inch-pounds required for younger children and standard torque of 6 to 8 inch-pounds in adolescents. There can be great variation in pressures with different torque wrenches, however, and they should be calibrated before any halo placement.[232] Pins should not be retightened at 48 hours in children. In adolescents, however, retightening can be performed at 48 hours.[182]

As in adults, complications are common with halo immobilizers in children. Dormans and colleagues[233] reported a complication rate of 68%, but noted that most complications were minor and all patients were able to wear the halo until fracture healing occurred. The most common complications include superficial pin tract infection and pin loosening. Serious, but less common, complications include dural penetration, supraorbital and supratrochlear nerve injury, pin scars, and deep pin infections.

Thoracolumbar Classification Systems

Thoracolumbar fractures in children are uncommon but can cause significant morbidity and mortality, requiring a high index of suspicion for these injuries. Two classification systems for thoracolumbar spine injuries are widely utilized: the Denis classification and the Thoracolumbar Injury Classification and Severity (TLICS) scale. These classification schemes are not specific to the immature pediatric spine; however, they are commonly extrapolated for use in pediatric spine trauma.[234] We are not aware of a classification scheme specific to thoracolumbar trauma in the immature skeleton, although recent studies have demonstrated that these classification systems have good reliability and validity in pediatric trauma.[235]

Denis[236] described a three-column classification system. The anterior column consists of the anterior ligament, anterior anulus fibrosus (AF), and anterior two-thirds of the vertebral body. The middle column contains the posterior longitudinal ligament, posterior AF, and posterior wall of the vertebral body. The posterior column comprises the supraspinous and interspinous ligaments, facet joint capsules, and ligamentum flavum. Denis[236] used this system to classify thoracolumbar injuries as compression fractures, burst fractures, flexion-distraction injuries, or fracture–dislocation injuries. He also classified the stability of these fractures based on the number of columns affected. If two or more columns failed, the fracture was considered unstable according to Denis.[236]

The Spine Trauma Study Group developed the TLICS scale. Although this classification system was developed in adult patients, recent studies have demonstrated reliability and validity of this system in pediatric trauma patients.[235] Three primary axes were identified to help analyze and manage fracture patterns: (1) injury morphology, (2) integrity of the posterior ligamentous complex, and (3) neurologic status. The three primary axes are divided further into subgroups. Morphology is determined from radiographs, MRI, and CT scan using one of three morphologic categories: (1) compression, which can be classified further with a burst component; (2) translation and rotation; and (3) distraction. The integrity of the posterior ligamentous complex is categorized as (1) intact, (2) disrupted, or (3) indeterminate. The neurologic status is categorized as intact, nerve root injury, complete spinal cord injury, or incomplete spinal cord injury. The TLICS score is based on these principles, and specific values are assigned to each subgroup with lesser point values for less severe injuries. These scores can help guide surgical treatment. Patients with a score of 3 or less are generally treated nonoperatively depending on the type of injury. Patients with a score of 5 or greater frequently require surgical fixation. Patients with a score of 4 fall in the intermediate zone, in which treatment is more ambiguous and up to the discretion of the surgeon.[219]

Compression Fractures

Compression fractures are the most common thoracolumbar fracture pattern.[182] The severity of the fracture is based on the percentage of height lost, but regardless of severity, these fractures are rarely associated with neurologic deficit. It is important to determine if the injury is acute or chronic because these injuries can commonly occur as a result of falls. Compression fractures are nearly always stable injuries, but one must be sure to examine the posterior soft tissues to rule out a flexion-distraction injury. Treatment options depend on whether the fracture is isolated or if contiguous fractures are present. Isolated compression fractures are best treated with an extension orthosis. These fractures usually heal in 4 to 6 weeks, but radiographs should be obtained to monitor alignment. Contiguous compression fractures can result in kyphosis. If kyphosis greater than 40 degrees is present, surgical treatment can be considered.[237] In the adult patient population, degree of kyphosis at the site of thoracolumbar compression fracture has not been shown to correlate with clinical outcomes in the setting of a normal neurologic exam.[224,238,239] In children, when kyphosis of 10 degrees or greater is seen on upright lateral radiographs, brace treatment has been shown to be more effective than no brace in terms of final alignment at skeletal maturity[240]; the clinical relevance of this finding has not been established. Finally, based on cadaveric studies, one must be careful to evaluate for injury to the PLC when 50% of the vertebral height is lost.[241]

Burst Fractures

Burst fractures involve, at a minimum, the anterior and middle columns.[236] These injuries are most common in the lower thoracic and upper lumbar region, due to this being the transition area from the stiff thoracic spine to the mobile lumbar spine. Spinal cord injury can occur with retropulsion of bony fragments at the thoracolumbar junction, resulting in conus medullaris or cauda equina syndromes. There have been few studies of burst fractures in immature patients. Most investigators believe that conservative treatment is warranted if the posterior ligament column is intact and there are no neurologic deficits. Treatment should include an extension molded cast or a thoracolumbosacral orthosis (TLSO). The goal is to allow the patient to maintain an upright position with ambulation while preventing progressive kyphosis and neurologic deficit.

If there is injury to the posterior ligamentous complex (PLC), surgical treatment may be used to protect the integrity of the spinal cord. Anterior and posterior approaches can be used.[238] The posterior approach is now more frequently utilized. The anterior approach allows direct canal decompression through corpectomy of the fractured vertebrae. When surgical stabilization of a burst fracture is deemed necessary, the surgeon should fuse as few motion segments as possible while still providing enough stability for healing and protection of the neural elements. Fig. 32.9 shows a 14-year-old boy with a lumbar burst fracture.

Chance Fractures

Chance fractures, or flexion-distraction injuries, are most often caused by lap belt injuries in motor vehicle accidents. With frontal impact, the lap belt causes the axis of rotation to be the anterior spine, causing distractive forces on the posterior spine and anterior vertebral compression. Owing to this mechanism, there is a high incidence of concurrent abdominal injury, which necessitates a thorough evaluation by a pediatric trauma specialist.[242] According to the Denis classification, this is a three-column injury and is unstable. The classic finding on radiography is an "empty facet" sign. The inferior articular process of the superior vertebrae is no longer in contact with the superior articular process of the inferior vertebrae, and the facet appears empty. Treatment of Chance fractures is based on severity of the injury. If only bony fractures are present, with no injury to the ligamentous complexes, a hyperextension cast can be used. If ligamentous disruption is present, surgical treatment is necessary. MRI should be performed to determine the integrity of the posterior ligamentous complex and guide management. Young children can be treated surgically with posterior wiring combined with a cast; older children and adolescents can undergo segmental fixation.[243] Fig. 32.10 shows a Chance fracture in a 5-year-old boy.

Fracture-Dislocations

Fracture-dislocations in the thoracolumbar spine are three-column injuries that are very unstable.[236] These injuries nearly always require surgical stabilization. If complete spinal cord injury is present, internal fixation is warranted because it may aid the rehabilitation process. Children younger than 10 years should undergo longer fusions to reduce the delayed development of paralytic scoliosis.[244,245]

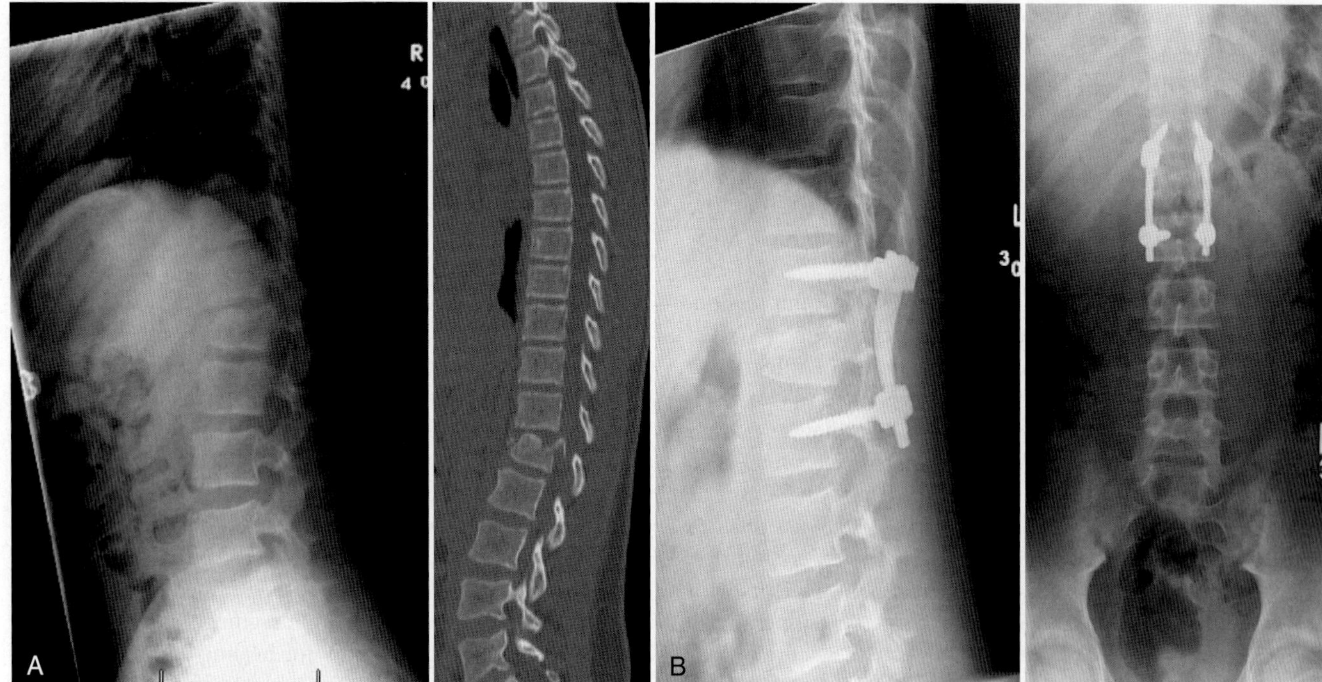

FIG. 32.9 Lumbar burst fracture. A 14-year-old boy was in a motor vehicle accident and had 50% retropulsion of the L1 vertebral body. (A) Lateral radiograph and sagittal computed tomographic reconstruction. (B) Postoperative result after decompression and fusion.

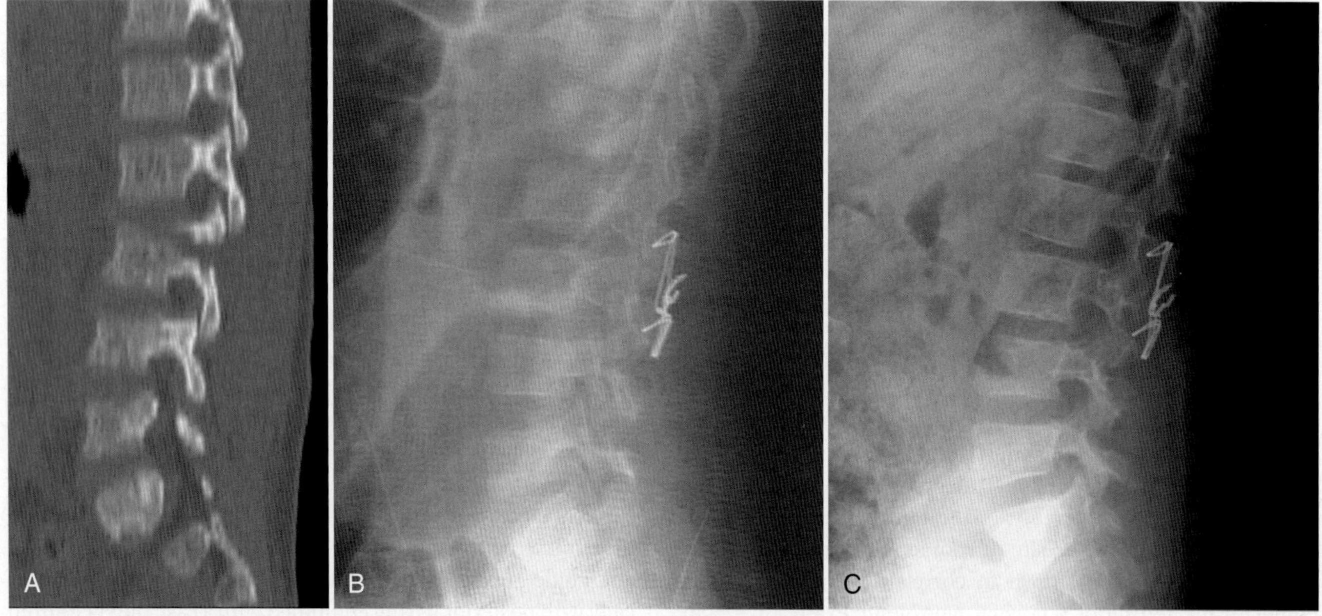

FIG. 32.10 Lumbar Chance fracture. A 5-year-old boy was restrained by a lap belt in a motor vehicle accident. (A) Sagittal computed tomographic reconstruction shows L2 Chance fracture. (B) Postoperative image after spinous process wiring. (C) Image 3 years postoperatively.

Limbus Fractures

Limbus fractures occur at the posterior vertebral endplate when disc material herniates between the unfused peripheral ring apophysis of the epiphyseal endplates and central cartilage (Fig. 32.11). These fractures often manifest as low back pain in adolescents and young adults, although they can be identified in older patients as well.[246] These lesions are usually located in the lower lumbar spine and appear on radiographs as a corner defect in the endplate and a wedge-shaped piece of bone posterior to the body or disc space. CT and MRI can help fully delineate the bony defect and disc injury. These injuries are less likely to resorb on their own and often require surgical decompression in symptomatic patients.

Depending on the size of the lesion, the disc (calcified or noncalcified) and bony fracture can be removed via an

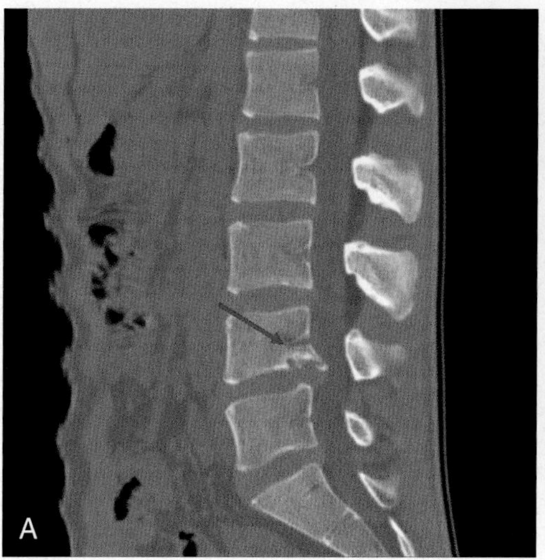

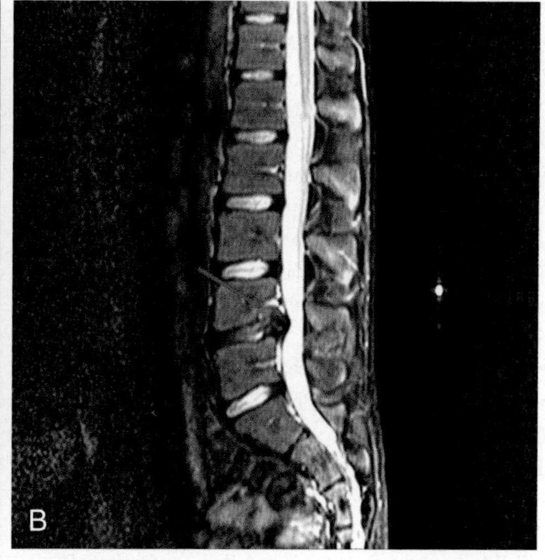

FIG. 32.11 (A) Computed tomographic and (B) magnetic resonance images showing a limbus fracture *(red arrow)* in a 17-year-old male with continued back pain 4 months after the initial injury.

extended laminotomy, hemilaminectomy, or laminectomy. In the absence of routine disc herniation, the discectomy can be performed in standard fashion, thus identifying the fracture as the endplate is exposed.[246]

KEY POINTS

1. Traumatic injury to the pediatric spine is relatively rare. Injuries in children younger than 8 years old typically affect the upper cervical spine because of the large head size; older children are more likely to sustain subaxial cervical spine injuries and thoracolumbar injuries as the spine takes on the biomechanical characteristics of an adult.
2. During transport, children younger than 4 years often require a cutout region for the occiput or elevation of the shoulders to accommodate the disproportionately large head and to keep the cervical spine in neutral alignment.
3. Spine imaging in an injured child should begin with a trauma radiographic series. Young children who cannot cooperate may require a CT scan from the occiput to C2. A CT traumagram—including sagittal and coronal reconstructions of the cervical, thoracic, and lumbar spine—is acceptable, and radiographs are not needed. MRI can be used to evaluate a neurologic deficit and determine if a ligamentous injury exists.
4. In spinal cord injury in pediatric patients, there is a susceptibility to development of posttraumatic deformity and growth arrest; surgical correction and fusion needs to take remaining growth into account.
5. Evaluation of cervical and lumbar trauma in children requires an understanding of developmental anatomy to differentiate trauma from age-appropriate findings. Evidence of soft tissue swelling and sharp edges at the suspected fracture are more indicative of trauma. Injuries that are unique to children include atlantoaxial rotatory instability, birth injuries, and limbus fractures. Generally, young children more often have ligamentous injuries; older children and adolescents have bony injuries as the spine takes on adult characteristics.

KEY REFERENCES

1. Herzenberg JE, Hensinger RN, Dedrick DK, et al. Emergency transport and positioning of young children who have an injury of the cervical spine: the standard backboard may be hazardous. *J Bone Joint Surg Am*. 1989;71:15-22.
   This article addresses the importance of accounting for the disproportionately large head in children during transport by using a backboard with an occipital cutout or elevating the shoulders.
2. Brown RL, Brunn MA, Garcia VF. Cervical spine injuries in children: a review of 103 patients treated consecutively at a level one pediatric trauma center. *J Pediatr Surg*. 2001;36:1107-1114.
   This article reports the increased prevalence of upper cervical spine injuries and SCIWORA in young children.
3. Bilston LE, Brown J. Pediatric spinal injury type and severity are age and mechanism dependent. *Spine*. 2007;32:2339-2347.
   This article shows that injury is age and mechanism dependent. Falls are the most common mechanism in children younger than 8 years old, minor neck injuries are more common in children older than 8 years, and sporting injuries are most common in older boys. Motor vehicle accidents cause the most serious spinal trauma in children.
4. Vaccaro AR, Lehman RA Jr, Hurlbert RJ, et al. A new classification of thoracolumbar injuries: the importance of injury morphology, the integrity of the posterior ligamentous complex, and neurologic status. *Spine*. 2005;30:2325-2333.
   The composite injury severity score derived from this classification system assigns 1 to 4 points to three critical components of an injury: integrity of the posterior ligamentous complex, injury morphology, and neurologic status. Fractures with scores of 3 points or less are considered nonoperative cases. Fractures with scores of 4 points can be considered for nonoperative or operative intervention. Fractures with scores of 5 or more points are considered surgical cases.
5. Mayfield JK, Erkkila JC, Winter RB. Spine deformity subsequent to acquired childhood spinal cord injury. *J Bone Joint Surg Am*. 1981;63:1401-1411.
   This article found that children who had spinal cord injury before the adolescent growth spurt were much more likely to have progressive spinal deformity than children who were injured after the growth spurt.

REFERENCES

1. Cirak B, Ziegfeld S, Knight VM, et al. Spinal injuries in children. *J Pediatr Surg*. 2004;39(4):607-612.

2. Kokoska ER, Keller MS, Rallo MC, Weber TR. Characteristics of pediatric cervical spine injuries. *J Pediatr Surg.* 2001;36(1):100-105.
3. d'Amato C. Pediatric spinal trauma: injuries in very young children. *Clin Orthop Relat Res.* 2005;432:34-40.
4. Givens TG, Polley KA, Smith GF, Hardin WD Jr. Pediatric cervical spine injury: a three-year experience. *J Trauma.* 1996;41(2):310-314.
5. Bilston LE, Brown J. Pediatric spinal injury type and severity are age and mechanism dependent. *Spine.* 2007;32(21):2339-2347.
6. Vogel LC. Unique management needs of pediatric spinal cord injury patients: etiology and pathophysiology. *J Spinal Cord Med.* 1997;20(1):10-13.
7. Leventhal HR. Birth injuries of the spinal cord. *J Pediatr.* 1960;56:447-453.
8. Ranjith RK, Mullett JH, Burke TE. Hangman's fracture caused by suspected child abuse. A case report. *J Pediatr Orthop B.* 2002;11(4):329-332.
9. Rooks VJ, Sisler C, Burton B. Cervical spine injury in child abuse: report of two cases. *Pediatr Radiol.* 1998;28(3): 193-195.
10. Bailey DK. The normal cervical spine in infants and children. *Radiology.* 1952;59(5):712-719.
11. Herman MJ, Pizzutillo PD. Cervical spine disorders in children. *Orthop Clin North Am.* 1999;30(3):457-466, ix.
12. Edelson JG, Nathan H. Stages in the natural history of the vertebral end-plates. *Spine.* 1988;13(1):21-26.
13. Lustrin ES, Karakas SP, Ortiz AO, et al. Pediatric cervical spine: normal anatomy, variants, and trauma. *Radiographics.* 2003;23(3):539-560.
14. Eleraky MA, Theodore N, Adams M, Rekate HL, Sonntag VK. Pediatric cervical spine injuries: report of 102 cases and review of the literature. *J Neurosurg.* 2000;92(1 suppl):12-17.
15. Finch GD, Barnes MJ. Major cervical spine injuries in children and adolescents. *J Pediatr Orthop.* 1998;18(6):811-814.
16. Nuckley DJ, Ching RP. Developmental biomechanics of the cervical spine: tension and compression. *J Biomech.* 2006;39(16):3045-3054.
17. Ouyang J, Zhu Q, Zhao W, et al. Biomechanical assessment of the pediatric cervical spine under bending and tensile loading. *Spine.* 2005;30(24):E716-E723.
18. Herzenberg JE, Hensinger RN, Dedrick DK, Phillips WA. Emergency transport and positioning of young children who have an injury of the cervical spine. The standard backboard may be hazardous. *J Bone Joint Surg Am.* 1989;71(1):15-22.
19. Curran C, Dietrich AM, Bowman MJ, et al. Pediatric cervical-spine immobilization: achieving neutral position? *J Trauma.* 1995;39(4):729-732.
20. Nypaver M, Treloar D. Neutral cervical spine positioning in children. *Ann Emerg Med.* 1994;23(2):208-211.
21. Laham JL, Cotcamp DH, Gibbons PA, Kahana MD, Crone KR. Isolated head injuries versus multiple trauma in pediatric patients: do the same indications for cervical spine evaluation apply? *Pediatr Neurosurg.* 1994;21(4):221-226.
22. Anderson PA, Rivara FP, Maier RV, Drake C. The epidemiology of seatbelt-associated injuries. *J Trauma.* 1991;31(1):60-67.
23. Slotkin JR, Lu Y, Wood KB. Thoracolumbar spinal trauma in children. *Neurosurg Clin N Am.* 2007;18(4):621-630.
24. Hadley MN, Zabramski JM, Browner CM, Rekate H, Sonntag VK. Pediatric spinal trauma. Review of 122 cases of spinal cord and vertebral column injuries. *J Neurosurg.* 1988;68(1):18-24.
25. Lee SL, Sena M, Greenholz SK, Fledderman M. A multidisciplinary approach to the development of a cervical spine clearance protocol: process, rationale, and initial results. *J Pediatr Surg.* 2003;38(3):358-362, discussion 358-362.
26. Hamilton MG, Myles ST. Pediatric spinal injury: review of 61 deaths. *J Neurosurg.* 1992;77(5):705-708.
27. Bonadio WA. Cervical spine trauma in children: part I. General concepts, normal anatomy, radiographic evaluation. *Am J Emerg Med.* 1993;11(2):158-165.
28. Lally KP, Senac M, Hardin WD Jr, et al. Utility of the cervical spine radiograph in pediatric trauma. *Am J Surg.* 1989;158(6):540-541, discussion 541-542.
29. Baker C, Kadish H, Schunk JE. Evaluation of pediatric cervical spine injuries. *Am J Emerg Med.* 1999;17(3): 230-234.
30. Buhs C, Cullen M, Klein M, Farmer D. The pediatric trauma C-spine: is the 'odontoid' view necessary? *J Pediatr Surg.* 2000;35(6):994-997.
31. Ralston ME, Chung K, Barnes PD, Emans JB, Schutzman SA. Role of flexion-extension radiographs in blunt pediatric cervical spine injury. *Acad Emerg Med.* 2001;8(3): 237-245.
32. Dwek JR, Chung CB. Radiography of cervical spine injury in children: are flexion-extension radiographs useful for acute trauma? *AJR Am J Roentgenol.* 2000;174(6): 1617-1619.
33. Bucholz RW, Burkhead WZ. The pathological anatomy of fatal atlanto-occipital dislocations. *J Bone Joint Surg Am.* 1979;61(2):248-250.
34. Kaufman RA, Carroll CD, Buncher CR. Atlantooccipital junction: standards for measurement in normal children. *AJNR Am J Neuroradiol.* 1987;8(6):995-999.
35. Roche C, Carty H. Spinal trauma in children. *Pediatr Radiol.* 2001;31(10):677-700.
36. Fielding JW, Cochran G, Lawsing JF 3rd, Hohl M. Tears of the transverse ligament of the atlas. A clinical and biomechanical study. *J Bone Joint Surg Am.* 1974;56(8):1683-1691.
37. Steel H. Anatomical and mechanical considerations of atlanto-axial articulations. *J Bone Joint Surg Am.* 1968;7:20.
38. Cattell HS, Filtzer DL. Pseudosubluxation and other normal variations in the cervical spine in children. A study of one hundred and sixty children. *J Bone Joint Surg Am.* 1965;47(7):1295-1309.
39. Sheridan R, Peralta R, Rhea J, Ptak T, Novelline R. Reformatted visceral protocol helical computed tomographic scanning allows conventional radiographs of the thoracic and lumbar spine to be eliminated in the evaluation of blunt trauma patients. *J Trauma.* 2003;55(4):665-669.
40. Stambolis V, Brady S, Klos D, et al. The effects of cervical bracing upon swallowing in young, normal, healthy volunteers. *Dysphagia.* 2003;18(1):39-45.
41. Shaw M, Burnett H, Wilson A, Chan O. Pseudosubluxation of C2 on C3 in polytraumatized children—Prevalence and significance. *Clin Radiol.* 1999;54(6):377-380.
42. Naidich JB, Naidich TP, Garfein C, Liebeskind AL, Hyman RA. The widened interspinous distance: a useful sign of anterior cervical dislocation in the supine frontal projection. *Radiology.* 1977;123(1):113-116.
43. Bonadio WA. Cervical spine trauma in children: part II. Mechanisms and manifestations of injury, therapeutic considerations. *Am J Emerg Med.* 1993;11(3):256-278.

44. Ardran GM, Kemp FH. The mechanism of changes in form of the cervical airway in infancy. *Med Radiogr Photogr.* 1968;44(2):26-38.
45. Grogan EL, Morris JA Jr, Dittus RS, et al. Cervical spine evaluation in urban trauma centers: lowering institutional costs and complications through helical CT scan. *J Am Coll Surg.* 2005;200(2):160-165.
46. Nunez DB Jr, Zuluaga A, Fuentes-Bernardo DA, Rivas LA, Becerra JL. Cervical spine trauma: how much more do we learn by routinely using helical CT? *Radiographics.* 1996;16(6):1307-1318.
47. Gestring ML, Gracias VH, Feliciano MA, et al. Evaluation of the lower spine after blunt trauma using abdominal computed tomographic scanning supplemented with lateral scanograms. *J Trauma.* 2002;53(1):9-14.
48. Hauser CJ, Visvikis G, Hinrichs C, et al. Prospective validation of computed tomographic screening of the thoracolumbar spine in trauma. *J Trauma.* 2003;55(2):228-234.
49. Wintermark M, Mouhsine E, Theumann N, et al. Thoracolumbar spine fractures in patients who have sustained severe trauma: depiction with multi-detector row CT. *Radiology.* 2003;227(3):681-689.
50. Antevil JL, Sise MJ, Sack DI, et al. Spiral computed tomography for the initial evaluation of spine trauma: a new standard of care? *J Trauma.* 2006;61(2):382-387.
51. Daffner RH, Hackney DB. ACR Appropriateness Criteria on suspected spine trauma. *J Am Coll Radiol.* 2007;4(11):762-775.
52. Booth TN. Cervical spine evaluation in pediatric trauma. *AJR Am J Roentgenol.* 2012;198(5):W417-W425.
53. Hutchings L, Willett K. Cervical spine clearance in pediatric trauma: a review of current literature. *J Trauma.* 2009;67(4):687-691.
54. Keenan HT, Hollingshead MC, Chung CJ, Ziglar MK. Using CT of the cervical spine for early evaluation of pediatric patients with head trauma. *AJR Am J Roentgenol.* 2001;177(6):1405-1409.
55. Rana AR, Drongowski R, Breckner G, Ehrlich PF. Traumatic cervical spine injuries: characteristics of missed injuries. *J Pediatr Surg.* 2009;44(1):151-155.
56. Adelgais KM, Browne L, Holsti M, et al. Cervical spine computed tomography utilization in pediatric trauma patients. *J Pediatr Surg.* 2014;49(2):333-337.
57. Huda W, Bissessur K. Effective dose equivalents, HE, in diagnostic radiology. *Med Phys.* 1990;17(6):998-1003.
58. Fearon T, Vucich J. Normalized pediatric organ-absorbed doses from CT examinations. *AJR Am J Roentgenol.* 1987;148(1):171-174.
59. Muchow RD, Egan KR, Peppler WW, Anderson PA. Theoretical increase of thyroid cancer induction from cervical spine multidetector computed tomography in pediatric trauma patients. *J Trauma Acute Care Surg.* 2012;72(2):403-409.
60. Marin D, Nelson RC, Schindera ST, et al. Low-tube-voltage, high-tube-current multidetector abdominal CT: improved image quality and decreased radiation dose with adaptive statistical iterative reconstruction algorithm—initial clinical experience 1. *Radiology.* 2009;254(1):145-153.
61. Blackmore CC, Ramsey SD, Mann FA, Deyo RA. Cervical spine screening with CT in trauma patients: a cost-effectiveness analysis. *Radiology.* 1999;212(1):117-125.
62. Brown RL, Brunn MA, Garcia VF. Cervical spine injuries in children: a review of 103 patients treated consecutively at a level 1 pediatric trauma center. *J Pediatr Surg.* 2001;36(8):1107-1114.
63. Frank JB, Lim CK, Flynn JM, Dormans JP. The efficacy of magnetic resonance imaging in pediatric cervical spine clearance. *Spine.* 2002;27(11):1176-1179.
64. Gebauer G, Osterman M, Harrop J, Vaccaro A. Spinal cord injury resulting from injury missed on CT scan: the danger of relying on CT alone for collar removal. *Clin Orthop Relat Res.* 2012;470(6):1652-1657.
65. Fisher BM, Cowles S, Matulich JR, et al. Is magnetic resonance imaging in addition to a computed tomographic scan necessary to identify clinically significant cervical spine injuries in obtunded blunt trauma patients? *Am J Surg.* 2013;206(6):987-993, discussion 993-994.
66. Muchow RD, Resnick DK, Abdel MP, Munoz A, Anderson PA. Magnetic resonance imaging (MRI) in the clearance of the cervical spine in blunt trauma: a meta-analysis. *J Trauma.* 2008;64(1):179-189.
67. Davis JW, Parks SN, Detlefs CL, et al. Clearing the cervical spine in obtunded patients: the use of dynamic fluoroscopy. *J Trauma.* 1995;39(3):435-438.
68. Kolb JC, Summers RL, Galli RL. Cervical collar-induced changes in intracranial pressure. *Am J Emerg Med.* 1999;17(2):135-137.
69. Viccellio P, Simon H, Pressman BD, et al. A prospective multicenter study of cervical spine injury in children. *Pediatrics.* 2001;108(2):E20.
70. Stiell IG, Clement CM, McKnight RD, et al. The Canadian C-spine rule versus the NEXUS low-risk criteria in patients with trauma. *N Engl J Med.* 2003;349(26):2510-2518.
71. Rozzelle CJ, Aarabi B, Dhall SS, et al. Management of pediatric cervical spine and spinal cord injuries. *Neurosurgery.* 2013;72(suppl 2):205-226.
72. Ehrlich PF, Wee C, Drongowski R, Rana AR. Canadian C-spine Rule and the National Emergency X-Radiography Utilization Low-Risk Criteria for C-spine radiography in young trauma patients. *J Pediatr Surg.* 2009;44(5):987-991.
73. Anderson RC, Scaife ER, Fenton SJ, et al. Cervical spine clearance after trauma in children. *J Neurosurg.* 2006;105 (5 suppl):361-364.
74. Launay F, Leet AI, Sponseller PD. Pediatric spinal cord injury without radiographic abnormality: a meta-analysis. *Clin Orthop Relat Res.* 2005;433:166-170.
75. Pang D. Spinal cord injury without radiographic abnormality in children, 2 decades later. *Neurosurgery.* 2004;55(6):1325-1342, discussion 1342-1343.
76. Levi AD, Hurlbert RJ, Anderson P, et al. Neurologic deterioration secondary to unrecognized spinal instability following trauma—a multicenter study. *Spine.* 2006;31(4):451-458.
77. Bolinger B, Shartz M, Marion D. Bedside fluoroscopic flexion and extension cervical spine radiographs for clearance of the cervical spine in comatose trauma patients. *J Trauma.* 2004;56(1):132-136.
78. Ajani AE, Cooper DJ, Scheinkestel CD, Laidlaw J, Tuxen DV. Optimal assessment of cervical spine trauma in critically ill patients: a prospective evaluation. *Anaesth Intensive Care.* 1998;26(5):487-491.
79. Stassen NA, Williams VA, Gestring ML, Cheng JD, Bankey PE. Magnetic resonance imaging in combination with helical computed tomography provides a safe and efficient method of cervical spine clearance in the obtunded trauma patient. *J Trauma.* 2006;60(1):171-177.

80. Vitale MG, Goss JM, Matsumoto H, Roye DP Jr. Epidemiology of pediatric spinal cord injury in the United States: years 1997 and 2000. *J Pediatr Orthop*. 2006;26(6):745-749.
81. Nitecki S, Moir CR. Predictive factors of the outcome of traumatic cervical spine fracture in children. *J Pediatr Surg*. 1994;29(11):1409-1411.
82. Marino RJ, Ditunno JF Jr, Donovan WH, Maynard F Jr. Neurologic recovery after traumatic spinal cord injury: data from the Model Spinal Cord Injury Systems. *Arch Phys Med Rehabil*. 1999;80(11):1391-1396.
83. Amar AP, Levy ML. Pathogenesis and pharmacological strategies for mitigating secondary damage in acute spinal cord injury. *Neurosurgery*. 1999;44(5):1027-1039.
84. Geisler FH, Dorsey FC, Coleman WP. Correction: recovery of motor function after spinal-cord injury–a randomized, placebo-controlled trial with GM-1 ganglioside. *N Engl J Med*. 1991;325(23):1659-1660.
85. Cadotte DW, Fehlings MG. Spinal cord injury: a systematic review of current treatment options. *Clin Orthop Relat Res*. 2011;469(3):732-741.
86. Oliveri RS, Bello S, Biering-Sorensen F. Mesenchymal stem cells improve locomotor recovery in traumatic spinal cord injury: systematic review with meta-analyses of rat models. *Neurobiol Dis*. 2014;62:338-353.
87. Zivin JA, DeGirolami U. Spinal cord infarction: a highly reproducible stroke model. *Stroke*. 1980;11(2):200-202.
88. Zach GA, Seiler W, Dollfus P. Treatment results of spinal cord injuries in the Swiss Paraplegic Centre of Basle. *Paraplegia*. 1976;14(1):58-65.
89. Vale FL, Burns J, Jackson AB, Hadley MN. Combined medical and surgical treatment after acute spinal cord injury: results of a prospective pilot study to assess the merits of aggressive medical resuscitation and blood pressure management. *J Neurosurg*. 1997;87(2):239-246.
90. Levi L, Wolf A, Belzberg H. Hemodynamic parameters in patients with acute cervical cord trauma: description, intervention, and prediction of outcome. *Neurosurgery*. 1993;33(6):1007-1016.
91. Galandiuk S, Raque G, Appel S, Polk HC Jr. The two-edged sword of large-dose steroids for spinal cord trauma. *Ann Surg*. 1993;218(4):419-425.
92. Ito Y, Sugimoto Y, Tomioka M, Kai N, Tanaka M. Does high dose methylprednisolone sodium succinate really improve neurological status in patient with acute cervical cord injury?: a prospective study about neurological recovery and early complications. *Spine*. 2009;34(20):2121-2124.
93. Bracken MB, Shepard MJ, Holford TR, et al. Administration of methylprednisolone for 24 or 48 hours or tirilazad mesylate for 48 hours in the treatment of acute spinal cord injury. Results of the Third National Acute Spinal Cord Injury Randomized Controlled Trial. National Acute Spinal Cord Injury Study. *JAMA*. 1997;277(20):1597-1604.
94. Bracken MB, Shepard MJ, Holford TR, et al. Methylprednisolone or tirilazad mesylate administration after acute spinal cord injury: 1-year follow up. Results of the third National Acute Spinal Cord Injury randomized controlled trial. *J Neurosurg*. 1998;89(5):699-706.
95. Pointillart V, Petitjean ME, Wiart L, et al. Pharmacological therapy of spinal cord injury during the acute phase. *Spinal Cord*. 2000;38(2):71-76.
96. Matsumoto T, Tamaki T, Kawakami M, et al. Early complications of high-dose methylprednisolone sodium succinate treatment in the follow-up of acute cervical spinal cord injury. *Spine*. 2001;26(4):426-430.
97. Otani K, Abe H, Kadoya S, et al. Beneficial effect of methylprednisolone sodium succinate in the treatment of acute spinal cord injury. *Sekitsui Sekizui J*. 1994;7(8):633-647.
98. Bracken MB, Collins WF, Freeman DF, et al. Efficacy of methylprednisolone in acute spinal cord injury. *JAMA*. 1984;251(1):45-52.
99. Hurlbert RJ, Hadley MN, Walters BC, et al. Pharmacological therapy for acute spinal cord injury. *Neurosurgery*. 2013;72(suppl 2):93-105.
100. Fehlings MG, Vaccaro A, Wilson JR, et al. Early versus delayed decompression for traumatic cervical spinal cord injury: results of the Surgical Timing in Acute Spinal Cord Injury Study (STASCIS). *PLoS One*. 2012;7(2):e32037.
101. Dvorak MF, Noonan VK, Fallah N, et al. The influence of time from injury to surgery on motor recovery and length of hospital stay in acute traumatic spinal cord injury: an observational Canadian cohort study. *J Neurotrauma*. 2015;32(9):645-654.
102. Fehlings MG, Perrin RG. The timing of surgical intervention in the treatment of spinal cord injury: a systematic review of recent clinical evidence. *Spine*. 2006;31(11 suppl): S28-S35.
103. Heary RF, Vaccaro AR, Mesa JJ, et al. Steroids and gunshot wounds to the spine. *Neurosurgery*. 1997;41(3):576-583.
104. Pang D, Pollack IF. Spinal cord injury without radiographic abnormality in children—the SCIWORA syndrome. *J Trauma*. 1989;29(5):654-664.
105. Wang MY, Hoh DJ, Leary SP, Griffith P, McComb JG. High rates of neurological improvement following severe traumatic pediatric spinal cord injury. *Spine*. 2004;29(13):1493-1497.
106. Pouliquen JC, Kassis B, Glorion C, Langlais J. Vertebral growth after thoracic or lumbar fracture of the spine in children. *J Pediatr Orthop*. 1997;17(1):115-120.
107. Vaccaro AR, Silber JS. Post-traumatic spinal deformity. *Spine*. 2001;26(24 suppl):S111-S118.
108. Yasuoka S, Peterson HA, MacCarty CS. Incidence of spinal column deformity after multilevel laminectomy in children and adults. *J Neurosurg*. 1982;57(4):441-445.
109. Mayfield JK, Erkkila JC, Winter RB. Spine deformity subsequent to acquired childhood spinal cord injury. *J Bone Joint Surg Am*. 1981;63(9):1401-1411.
110. Moe JH, Kharrat K, Winter RB, Cummine JL. Harrington instrumentation without fusion plus external orthotic support for the treatment of difficult curvature problems in young children. *Clin Orthop Relat Res*. 1984;185:35-45.
111. Dubousset J, Herring JA, Shufflebarger H. The crankshaft phenomenon. *J Pediatr Orthop*. 1989;9(5):541-550.
112. Pang D, Wilberger JE Jr. Spinal cord injury without radiographic abnormalities in children. *J Neurosurg*. 1982;57(1):114-129.
113. Bosch PP, Vogt MT, Ward WT. Pediatric spinal cord injury without radiographic abnormality (SCIWORA): the absence of occult instability and lack of indication for bracing. *Spine*. 2002;27(24):2788-2800.
114. Grabb PA, Pang D. Magnetic resonance imaging in the evaluation of spinal cord injury without radiographic abnormality in children. *Neurosurgery*. 1994;35(3): 406-414.
115. Flanders AE, Schaefer DM, Doan HT, et al. Acute cervical spine trauma: correlation of MR imaging findings with degree of neurologic deficit. *Radiology*. 1990;177(1):25-33.

116. Davis D, Bohlman H, Walker AE, Fisher R, Robinson R. The pathological findings in fatal craniospinal injuries. *J Neurosurg*. 1971;34(5):603-613.
117. Montane I, Eismont FJ, Green BA. Traumatic occipitoatlantal dislocation. *Spine*. 1991;16(2):112-116.
118. Farley FA, Graziano GP, Hensinger RN. Traumatic atlanto-occipital dislocation in a child. *Spine*. 1992;17(12):1539-1541.
119. Matava MJ, Whitesides TE Jr, Davis PC. Traumatic atlanto-occipital dislocation with survival. Serial computerized tomography as an aid to diagnosis and reduction: a report of three cases. *Spine*. 1993;18(13):1897-1903.
120. Papadopoulos SM, Dickman CA, Sonntag VK, Rekate HL, Spetzler RF. Traumatic atlantooccipital dislocation with survival. *Neurosurgery*. 1991;28(4):574-579.
121. Rockswold GL, Seljeskog EL. Traumatic atlantocranial dislocation with survival. *Minn Med*. 1979;62(3):151-152, 154.
122. Woodring JH, Selke AC Jr, Duff DE. Traumatic atlantooccipital dislocation with survival. *AJR Am J Roentgenol*. 1981;137(1):21-24.
123. Powers B, Miller MD, Kramer RS, Martinez S, Gehweiler JA Jr. Traumatic anterior atlanto-occipital dislocation. *Neurosurgery*. 1979;4(1):12-17.
124. Gerlock AJ Jr, Mirfakhraee M, Benzel EC. Computed tomography of traumatic atlantooccipital dislocation. *Neurosurgery*. 1983;13(3):316-319.
125. Theodore N, Aarabi B, Dhall SS, et al. The diagnosis and management of traumatic atlanto-occipital dislocation injuries. *Neurosurgery*. 2013;72(suppl 2):114-126.
126. Menendez JA, Wright NM. Techniques of posterior C1-C2 stabilization. *Neurosurgery*. 2007;60(1 Suppl 1): S103-S111.
127. Harms J, Melcher RP. Posterior C1-C2 fusion with polyaxial screw and rod fixation. *Spine*. 2001;26(22):2467-2471.
128. Judd DB, Liem LK, Petermann G. Pediatric atlas fracture: a case of fracture through a synchondrosis and review of the literature. *Neurosurgery*. 2000;46(4):991-994.
129. Jefferson G. Fracture of the atlas vertebra. Report of four cases, and a review of those previously recorded. *Br J Surg*. 1919;7(27):407-422.
130. Marlin AE, Williams GR, Lee JF. Jefferson fractures in children. Case report. *J Neurosurg*. 1983;58(2):277-279.
131. Mikawa Y, Watanabe R, Yamano Y, Ishii K. Fracture through a synchondrosis of the anterior arch of the atlas. *J Bone Joint Surg Br*. 1987;69(3):483.
132. Richards PG. Stable fractures of the atlas and axis in children. *J Neurol Neurosurg Psychiatry*. 1984;47(8):781-783.
133. Kesterson L, Benzel E, Orrison W, Coleman J. Evaluation and treatment of atlas burst fractures (Jefferson fractures). *J Neurosurg*. 1991;75(2):213-220.
134. Tan J, Li L, Sun G, et al. C1 lateral mass-C2 pedicle screws and crosslink compression fixation for unstable atlas fracture. *Spine*. 2009;34(23):2505-2509.
135. Greene KA, Dickman CA, Marciano FF, et al. Acute axis fractures. Analysis of management and outcome in 340 consecutive cases. *Spine*. 1997;22(16):1843-1852.
136. Burke SW, French HG, Roberts JM, et al. Chronic atlanto-axial instability in Down syndrome. *J Bone Joint Surg Am*. 1985;67(9):1356-1360.
137. Dawson EG, Smith L. Atlanto-axial subluxation in children due to vertebral anomalies. *J Bone Joint Surg Am*. 1979;61(4):582-587.
138. Hammerschlag W, Ziv I, Wald U, Robin GC, Floman Y. Cervical instability in an achondroplastic infant. *J Pediatr Orthop*. 1988;8(4):481-484.
139. Kobori M, Takahashi H, Mikawa Y. Atlanto-axial dislocation in Down's syndrome. Report of two cases requiring surgical correction. *Spine*. 1986;11(3):195-200.
140. Kransdorf MJ, Wehrle PA, Moser RP Jr. Atlantoaxial subluxation in Reiter's syndrome. A report of three cases and review of the literature. *Spine*. 1988;13(1):12-14.
141. Miz GS, Engler GL. Atlanto-axial subluxation in Larsen's syndrome. A case report. *Spine*. 1987;12(4):411-412.
142. McGrory BJ, Klassen RA, Chao EY, Staeheli JW, Weaver AL. Acute fractures and dislocations of the cervical spine in children and adolescents. *J Bone Joint Surg Am*. 1993;75(7):988-995.
143. Lui TN, Lee ST, Wong CW, et al. C1-C2 fracture-dislocations in children and adolescents. *J Trauma*. 1996;40(3):408-411.
144. Atlantoaxial instability in Down syndrome: subject review. American Academy of Pediatrics Committee on Sports Medicine and Fitness. *Pediatrics*. 1995;96(1 Pt 1):151-154.
145. Pueschel SM, Scola FH. Atlantoaxial instability in individuals with Down syndrome: epidemiologic, radiographic, and clinical studies. *Pediatrics*. 1987;80(4):555-560.
146. Segal LS, Drummond DS, Zanotti RM, Ecker ML, Mubarak SJ. Complications of posterior arthrodesis of the cervical spine in patients who have Down syndrome. *J Bone Joint Surg Am*. 1991;73(10):1547-1554.
147. Winell J, Burke SW. Sports participation of children with Down syndrome. *Orthop Clin North Am*. 2003;34(3): 439-443.
148. Pueschel SM, Scola FH, Tupper TB, Pezzullo JC. Skeletal anomalies of the upper cervical spine in children with Down syndrome. *J Pediatr Orthop*. 1990;10(5):607-611.
149. Cohen WI. Atlantoaxial instability. What's next? *Arch Pediatr Adolesc Med*. 1998;152(2):119-122.
150. Merrick J, Ezra E, Josef B, et al. Musculoskeletal problems in Down Syndrome European Paediatric Orthopaedic Society Survey: the Israeli sample. *J Pediatr Orthop B*. 2000;9(3):185-192.
151. Caird MS, Wills BP, Dormans JP. Down syndrome in children: the role of the orthopaedic surgeon. *J Am Acad Orthop Surg*. 2006;14(11):610-619.
152. Ferguson RL, Putney ME, Allen BL Jr. Comparison of neurologic deficits with atlanto-dens intervals in patients with Down syndrome. *J Spinal Disord*. 1997;10(3):246-252.
153. Sherk HH, Whitaker LA, Pasquariello PS. Facial malformations and spinal anomalies. A predictable relationship. *Spine*. 1982;7(6):526-531.
154. Gallie W. Fractures and dislocations of the cervical spine. *Am J Surg*. 1939;46(3):495-499.
155. Brooks AL, Jenkins EB. Atlanto-axial arthrodesis by the wedge compression method. *J Bone Joint Surg Am*. 1978;60(3):279-284.
156. Coyne TJ, Fehlings MG, Wallace MC, Bernstein M, Tator CH. C1-C2 posterior cervical fusion: long-term evaluation of results and efficacy. *Neurosurgery*. 1995;37(4):688-692, discussion 692-693.
157. Smith MD, Phillips WA, Hensinger RN. Complications of fusion to the upper cervical spine. *Spine*. 1991;16(7):702-705.
158. Crisco JJ 3rd, Panjabi MM, Oda T, Grob D, Dvorak J. Bone graft translation of four upper cervical spine fixation techniques in a cadaveric model. *J Orthop Res*. 1991;9(6):835-846.

159. Grob D, Crisco JJ 3rd, Panjabi MM, Wang P, Dvorak J. Biomechanical evaluation of four different posterior atlantoaxial fixation techniques. *Spine.* 1992;17(5):480-490.
160. Gerrelts BD, Petersen EU, Mabry J, Petersen SR. Delayed diagnosis of cervical spine injuries. *J Trauma.* 1991;31(12):1622-1626.
161. Hajek PD, Lipka J, Hartline P, Saha S, Albright JA. Biomechanical study of C1-C2 posterior arthrodesis techniques. *Spine.* 1993;18(2):173-177.
162. Naderi S, Crawford NR, Song GS, Sonntag VK, Dickman CA. Biomechanical comparison of C1-C2 posterior fixations. Cable, graft, and screw combinations. *Spine.* 1998;23(18):1946-1955, discussion 1955-1956.
163. Smith JT, Skinner SR, Shonnard NH. Persistent synchondrosis of the second cervical vertebra simulating a hangman's fracture in a child. Report of a case. *J Bone Joint Surg Am.* 1993;75(8):1228-1230.
164. Dickman CA, Sonntag VK. Surgical management of atlantoaxial nonunions. *J Neurosurg.* 1995;83(2):248-253.
165. Grob D, Magerl F. [Surgical stabilization of C1 and C2 fractures]. *Orthopade.* 1987;16(1):46-54.
166. Grob D, Jeanneret B, Aebi M, Markwalder TM. Atlanto-axial fusion with transarticular screw fixation. *J Bone Joint Surg Br.* 1991;73(6):972-976.
167. Jeanneret B, Magerl F. Primary posterior fusion C1/2 in odontoid fractures: indications, technique, and results of transarticular screw fixation. *J Spinal Disord.* 1992;5(4):464-475.
168. Stillerman CB, Wilson JA. Atlanto-axial stabilization with posterior transarticular screw fixation: technical description and report of 22 cases. *Neurosurgery.* 1993;32(6):948-954, discussion 954-955.
169. Madawi AA, Casey AT, Solanki GA, et al. Radiological and anatomical evaluation of the atlantoaxial transarticular screw fixation technique. *J Neurosurg.* 1997;86(6):961-968.
170. Goel A, Laheri V. Plate and screw fixation for atlanto-axial subluxation. *Acta Neurochir (Wien).* 1994;129(1-2):47-53.
171. Fielding JW, Hawkins R. Atlanto-axial rotatory fixation (fixed rotatory subluxation of the atlanto-axial joint). *J Bone Joint Surg Am.* 1977;59(1):37-44.
172. Coutts MB. Atlanto-epistropheal subluxations. *Arch Surg.* 1934;29(2):297-311.
173. Crook TB, Eynon CA. Traumatic atlantoaxial rotatory subluxation. *Emerg Med J.* 2005;22(9):671-672.
174. Wetzel FT, La Rocca H. Grisel's syndrome. *Clin Orthop Relat Res.* 1989;240:141-152.
175. Maheshwaran S, Sgouros S, Jeyapalan K, et al. Imaging of childhood torticollis due to atlanto-axial rotatory fixation. *Childs Nerv Syst.* 1995;11(12):667-671.
176. Geehr RB, Rothman SL, Kier EL. The role of computed tomography in the evaluation of upper cervical spine pathology. *Comput Tomogr.* 1978;2(2):79-97.
177. Scapinelli R. Three-dimensional computed tomography in infantile atlantoaxial rotatory fixation. *J Bone Joint Surg Br.* 1994;76(3):367-370.
178. Kowalski HM, Cohen WA, Cooper P, Wisoff JH. Pitfalls in the CT diagnosis of atlantoaxial rotary subluxation. *AJR Am J Roentgenol.* 1987;149(3):595-600.
179. Rinaldi I, Mullins WJ Jr, Delaney WF, Fitzer PM, Tornberg DN. Computerized tomographic demonstration of rotational atlanto-axial fixation. Case report. *J Neurosurg.* 1979;50(1):115-119.
180. Phillips WA, Hensinger RN. The management of rotatory atlanto-axial subluxation in children. *J Bone Joint Surg Am.* 1989;71(5):664-668.
181. Burkus JK, Deponte RJ. Chronic atlantoaxial rotatory fixation correction by cervical traction, manipulation, and bracing. *J Pediatr Orthop.* 1986;6(5):631-635.
182. Rockwood CA, Beaty JH, Kasser JR. *Rockwood and Wilkins' Fractures in Children.* Lippincott Williams & Wilkins; 2010.
183. Sherk HH. Fractures of the atlas and odontoid process. *Orthop Clin North Am.* 1978;9(4):973-984.
184. Sherburn EW, Day RA, Kaufman BA, Park TS. Subdental synchondrosis fracture in children: the value of 3-dimensional computerized tomography. *Pediatr Neurosurg.* 1996;25(5):256-259.
185. Apple JS, Kirks DR, Merten DF, Martinez S. Cervical spine fractures and dislocations in children. *Pediatr Radiol.* 1987;17(1):45-49.
186. Ries MD, Ray S. Posterior displacement of an odontoid fracture in a child. *Spine.* 1986;11(10):1043-1044.
187. Shaw BA, Murphy KM. Displaced odontoid fracture in a 9-month-old child. *Am J Emerg Med.* 1999;17(1):73-75.
188. Godard J, Hadji M, Raul JS. Odontoid fractures in the child with neurological injury. Direct anterior osteosynthesis with a cortico-spongious screw and literature review. *Childs Nerv Syst.* 1997;13(2):105-107.
189. Price E, Osmond CH. Fractured odontoid process with anterior dislocation. *J Bone Joint Surg Br.* 1960;42:2.
190. Schippers N, Konings P, Hassler W, Sommer B. Typical and atypical fractures of the odontoid process in young children. Report of two cases and a review of the literature. *Acta Neurochir (Wien).* 1996;138(5):524-530.
191. Fielding JW. Cineroentgenography of the normal cervical spine. *J Bone Joint Surg Am.* 1957;39-a(6):1280-1288.
192. Fielding JW, Hensinger RN, Hawkins RJ. Os odontoideum. *J Bone Joint Surg Am.* 1980;62(3):376-383.
193. Fielding JW, Stillwell WT, Chynn KY, Spyropoulos EC. Use of computed tomography for the diagnosis of atlanto-axial rotatory fixation. A case report. *J Bone Joint Surg Am.* 1978;60(8):1102-1104.
194. Hawkins R, Fielding J, Thompson W. Os odontoideum: congenital or acquired. A case report. *JBJS Case Connector.* 1976;(3):413-414.
195. Hukuda S, Ota H, Okabe N, Tazima K. Traumatic atlantoaxial dislocation causing os odontoideum in infants. *Spine.* 1980;5(3):207-210.
196. Kuhns LR, Loder RT, Farley FA, Hensinger RN. Nuchal cord changes in children with os odontoideum: evidence for associated trauma. *J Pediatr Orthop.* 1998;18(6):815-819.
197. Ricciardi JE, Kaufer H, Louis DS. Acquired os odontoideum following acute ligament injury. Report of a case. *J Bone Joint Surg Am.* 1976;58(3):410-412.
198. Stillwell WT, Fielding JW. Acquired os odontoideum. A case report. *Clin Orthop Relat Res.* 1978;135:71-73.
199. Verska JM, Anderson PA. Os odontoideum. A case report of one identical twin. *Spine.* 1997;22(6):706-709.
200. Giannestras NJ, Mayfield FH, Provencio FP, Maurer J. Congenital absence of the odontoid process. Case report. *J Bone Joint Surg Am.* 1964;46:839-843.

201. Sherk HH, Dawoud S. Congenital os odontoideum with Klippel-Feil anomaly and fatal atlanto-axial instability. Report of a case. *Spine*. 1981;6(1):42-45.
202. Wollin DG. The os odontoideum. Separate odontoid process. *J Bone Joint Surg Am*. 1963;45:1459-1471.
203. Hughes TB Jr, Richman JD, Rothfus WE. Diagnosis of os odontoideum using kinematic magnetic resonance imaging. A case report. *Spine*. 1999;24(7):715-718.
204. Clements WD, Mezue W, Mathew B. Os odontoideum—congenital or acquired? That's not the question. *Injury*. 1995;26(9):640-642.
205. Spierings E, Braakman R. The management of os odontoideum. Analysis of 37 cases. *J Bone Joint Surg Br*. 1982;64(4):422-428.
206. Dai L, Yuan W, Ni B, Jia L. Os odontoideum: etiology, diagnosis, and management. *Surg Neurol*. 2000;53(2): 106-108.
207. Michaels L, Prevost M, Crang D. Pathological changes in a case of os odontoideum (separate odontoid process). *J Bone Joint Surg*. 1969;51(5):965-972.
208. Klimo P Jr, Kan P, Rao G, Apfelbaum R, Brockmeyer D. Os odontoideum: presentation, diagnosis, and treatment in a series of 78 patients. *J Neurosurg Spine*. 2008;9(4):332-342.
209. Lowry DW, Pollack IF, Clyde B, Albright AL, Adelson PD. Upper cervical spine fusion in the pediatric population. *J Neurosurg*. 1997;87(5):671-676.
210. Taggard DA, Menezes AH, Ryken TC. Treatment of Down syndrome-associated craniovertebral junction abnormalities. *J Neurosurg*. 2000;93(2 suppl):205-213.
211. Wang J, Vokshoor A, Kim S, et al. Pediatric atlantoaxial instability: management with screw fixation. *Pediatr Neurosurg*. 1999;30(2):70-78.
212. Brockmeyer DL, York JE, Apfelbaum RI. Anatomical suitability of C1-2 transarticular screw placement in pediatric patients. *J Neurosurg Spine*. 2000;92(1):7-11.
213. Bach CM, Arbab D, Thaler M. Treatment strategies for severe C1–C2 luxation due to congenital os odontoideum causing tetraplegia. *Eur Spine J*. 2013;22(1):29-35.
214. Matthews LS, Vetter WL, Tolo VT. Cervical anomaly simulating hangman's fracture in a child. Case report. *J Bone Joint Surg Am*. 1982;64(2):299-300.
215. Nordstrom RE, Lahdenranta TV, Kaitila II, Laasonen EM. Familial spondylolisthesis of the axis vertebra. *J Bone Joint Surg Br*. 1986;68(5):704-706.
216. Williams JP 3rd, Baker DH, Miller WA. CT appearance of congenital defect resembling the Hangman's fracture. *Pediatr Radiol*. 1999;29(7):549-550.
217. Pizzutillo PD, Rocha EF, D'Astous J, Kling TF Jr, McCarthy RE. Bilateral fracture of the pedicle of the second cervical vertebra in the young child. *J Bone Joint Surg Am*. 1986;68(6):892-896.
218. Dogan S, Safavi-Abbasi S, Theodore N, et al. Pediatric subaxial cervical spine injuries: origins, management, and outcome in 51 patients. *Neurosurg Focus*. 2006;20(2):E1.
219. Rihn JA, Anderson DT, Harris E, et al. A review of the TLICS system: a novel, user-friendly thoracolumbar trauma classification system. *Acta Orthop*. 2008;79(4):461-466.
220. McCall T, Fassett D, Brockmeyer D. Cervical spine trauma in children: a review. *Neurosurg Focus*. 2006;20(2):E5.
221. Grant GA, Mirza SK, Chapman JR, et al. Risk of early closed reduction in cervical spine subluxation injuries. *J Neurosurg*. 1999;90(1 suppl):13-18.
222. Brodke DS, Anderson PA, Newell DW, Grady MS, Chapman JR. Comparison of anterior and posterior approaches in cervical spinal cord injuries. *J Spinal Disord Tech*. 2003;16(3):229-235.
223. Karam YR, Dahdaleh NS, Magnetta MJ, et al. Biomechanical comparison of anterior, posterior, and circumferential fixation after one-level anterior cervical corpectomy in the human cadaveric spine. *Spine*. 2011;36(7):E455-E460.
224. Vaccaro AR, Lehman RA Jr, Hurlbert RJ, et al. A new classification of thoracolumbar injuries: the importance of injury morphology, the integrity of the posterior ligamentous complex, and neurologic status. *Spine*. 2005;30(20): 2325-2333.
225. Lee HM, Kim HS, Kim DJ, et al. Reliability of magnetic resonance imaging in detecting posterior ligament complex injury in thoracolumbar spinal fractures. *Spine*. 2000;25(16):2079-2084.
226. Vaccaro AR, Rihn JA, Saravanja D, et al. Injury of the posterior ligamentous complex of the thoracolumbar spine: a prospective evaluation of the diagnostic accuracy of magnetic resonance imaging. *Spine*. 2009;34(23):E841-E847.
227. Sledge JB, Allred D, Hyman J. Use of magnetic resonance imaging in evaluating injuries to the pediatric thoracolumbar spine. *J Pediatr Orthop*. 2001;21(3):288-293.
228. Lawson JP, Ogden JA, Bucholz RW, Hughes SA. Physeal injuries of the cervical spine. *J Pediatr Orthop*. 1987;7(4):428-435.
229. Vialle R, Mary P, Schmider L, et al. Spinal fracture through the neurocentral synchondrosis in battered children: a report of three cases. *Spine*. 2006;31(11):E345-E349.
230. Garfin SR, Roux R, Botte MJ, Centeno R, Woo SL. Skull osteology as it affects halo pin placement in children. *J Pediatr Orthop*. 1986;6(4):434-436.
231. Copley LA, Dormans JP, Pepe MD, Tan V, Browne RH. Accuracy and reliability of torque wrenches used for halo application in children. *J Bone Joint Surg Am*. 2003;85-A(11):2199-2204.
232. Copley LA, Pepe MD, Tan V, Sheth N, Dormans JP. A comparison of various angles of halo pin insertion in an immature skull model. *Spine*. 1999;24(17):1777-1780.
233. Dormans JP, Criscitiello AA, Drummond DS, Davidson RS. Complications in children managed with immobilization in a halo vest. *J Bone Joint Surg Am*. 1995;77(9):1370-1373.
234. Sayama C, Chen T, Trost G, Jea A. A review of pediatric lumbar spine trauma. *Neurosurg Focus*. 2014;37(1):E6.
235. Savage JW, Moore TA, Arnold PM, et al. The reliability and validity of the thoracolumbar injury classification system in pediatric spine trauma. *Spine*. 2015;40(18):E1014-E1018.
236. Denis F. The three column spine and its significance in the classification of acute thoracolumbar spinal injuries. *Spine*. 1983;8(8):817-831.
237. Farcy JP, Weidenbaum M, Glassman SD. Sagittal index in management of thoracolumbar burst fractures. *Spine*. 1990;15(9):958-965.
238. Wood KB, Buttermann GR, Phukan R, et al. Operative compared with nonoperative treatment of a thoracolumbar burst fracture without neurological deficit: a prospective randomized study with follow-up at sixteen to twenty-two years. *J Bone Joint Surg Am*. 2015;97(1):3-9.
239. Wood KB, Li W, Lebl DS, Ploumis A. Management of thoracolumbar spine fractures. *Spine J*. 2014;14(1): 145-164.

240. Akbarnia BA. Pediatric spine fractures. *Orthop Clin North Am.* 1999;30(3):521-536, x.
241. Roaf R. A study of the mechanics of spinal injuries. *J Bone Joint Surg Br.* 1960;42(4):810-823.
242. Reid AB, Letts RM, Black GB. Pediatric Chance fractures: association with intra-abdominal injuries and seatbelt use. *J Trauma.* 1990;30(4):384-391.
243. Rumball K, Jarvis J. Seat-belt injuries of the spine in young children. *J Bone Joint Surg Br.* 1992;74(4):571-574.
244. Dearolf WW 3rd, Betz RR, Vogel LC, et al. Scoliosis in pediatric spinal cord-injured patients. *J Pediatr Orthop.* 1990;10(2):214-218.
245. Luque ER. Paralytic scoliosis in growing children. *Clin Orthop Relat Res.* 1982;163:202-209.
246. Epstein NE. Lumbar surgery for 56 limbus fractures emphasizing noncalcified type III lesions. *Spine.* 1992;17(12):1489-1496.

CHAPTER 33 The Immature Spine and Athletic Injuries

Jennifer J. Beck
Lyle J. Micheli

Most spine injuries in athletically active children and adolescents are chronic, resulting from repetitive demand on the immature spine during participation in sports. The most serious injuries are acute as a result of direct trauma. The age at which a child can be considered an athlete varies; a child may put on skis at 3 years old or begin to ride bulls at 10 years old (Fig. 33.1). Several sports—such as skiing, football, and horseback riding—involve increased risk of acute traumatic events, making spine fracture a significant concern when considering an adolescent athlete. Increase in pediatric involvement in nontraditional sports, such as cheerleading[1] and extreme sports,[2,3] have also increased sports-related injuries. In children, 32% of life-threatening injuries are sports related.[4] This chapter discusses the initial evaluation and on-field management of spine fractures; the complete treatment of spine fractures is covered elsewhere.

According to surveys of patients seen in sports medicine specialty clinics, the most common cause of back pain in adolescent athletes is stress fracture, or *spondylolysis*. Spine hyperextension and repeated twisting contribute to the high rate of spondylolysis seen in sports such as gymnastics, football, and weightlifting. The rate of spondylolysis in gymnasts is 20% compared with 5% to 6% in the general population.[5]

Less aggressive sports, such as golf, can also cause adolescent back pain and spine injury. The golf swing places significant torque on the spine and surrounding muscles, and can produce strains and sprains, which are minor injuries that interfere with performance. In all sports, appropriate strength training, routine stretching, and good technique are imperative for young athletes to avoid injury and to continue participation in sports throughout their lifetime.

The most effective technique in screening for serious disease is a good patient history; diagnosing spine injury is no exception. Although helpful, a radiograph is seldom definitive in diagnosing the cause of back pain. Radiography is imperative for diagnosis of an acute fracture, but back pain without a specific injury is usually treated on the basis of a careful history and a thorough physical examination.

Understanding the requirements of the particular sport and gaining knowledge of the training schedule of the athlete are important when performing the patient history. For example, a gymnast with no history of sudden trauma who practices 3 hours daily has a chronic stress that may account for the back pain. A young gymnast's developing spine, given insufficient recovery time, is highly susceptible to repetitive trauma.

Return to sport is a major goal for an athlete; the physician needs to be aware of the demands of the specific sport to determine when return to participation is reasonable. The physician should take heed of a young athlete who is reluctant to return to sport after an injury. Family dynamics often influence when a child is willing to resume activity.

Physical activity is the normal function of the musculoskeletal system. The American Academy of Orthopaedic Surgeons (AAOS) has encouraged physical activity as health promoting for all ages in its "Get Up, Get Out, Get Moving" program. The keys to maintaining a healthy spine are good nutrition and proper exercise. Good nutrition includes avoiding obesity and not smoking. Exercise programs should include strengthening for power and endurance, as well as stretching to improve joint range of motion (ROM) and muscle length.

Principles of Diagnosis

The initial treatment of low back pain usually begins without a specific diagnosis. A nonspecific diagnosis is satisfactory as long as the patient's condition improves. In contrast, the narrow area in which surgery offers reliable benefit to the patient requires a carefully determined, specific diagnosis. In children and adolescents, every attempt should be made to arrive at a specific diagnosis. Adults often have variable degrees of degenerative changes in the spine. In many such cases, treatment to restore ROM and strength of the spine and its associated structures is a first step.

History

A good patient history depends on effective patient-physician communication. When a patient presents with low back pain, the history is important to rule out serious diagnoses rather than leading to a definitive diagnosis. The physician brings knowledge of possible causes and treatments to the interview, and assembles a differential diagnosis. The patient wants to tell his or her story and brings knowledge of timelines and anecdotal details.

The term *interview* implies an interaction with the patient as opposed to the traditional notion of extracting information from the patient. When allowed to tell one's story, an adult patient takes an average of 90 seconds.[6] Adolescents tend to be more taciturn and talk less than the average adult. The average physician cuts off the patient with a question after 18 seconds because the physician has formed a differential diagnosis. Such interruption stops the flow of information, and often the patient is never permitted to relate pertinent facts.

The use of a visual pain scale facilitates consistent documentation. The patient's assessment of the intensity of the pain using a visual scale (Fig. 33.2) often stimulates a description of the circumstances that exacerbate or alleviate that pain. When making the differential diagnosis, the physician can classify the clinical syndrome into one of three categories: (1) nonmechanical back or leg pain (or both), (2) mechanical back or leg pain (or both), and (3) sciatica.

Warning signs for possible cancer include a history of cancer or constitutional symptoms, such as fever, weight loss, or night pain. Risk factors for infection include a history of recent bacterial infection, intravenous drug use, or an immunocompromised state. Patients with a spine cancer or spine infection often have pain that is not diminished by rest. Warning signs of possible spine fracture are major trauma (e.g., motor vehicle accident, blunt trauma, fall from a height), prolonged corticosteroid use, and osteoporosis. Symptoms suggestive of *cauda equina syndrome,* which requires urgent surgical consultation, include saddle anesthesia (found in 75% of patients); recent onset of bladder or bowel dysfunction (with urinary retention the most common symptom); and severe or progressive weakness of the lower extremities,[7] especially involving both lower extremities.

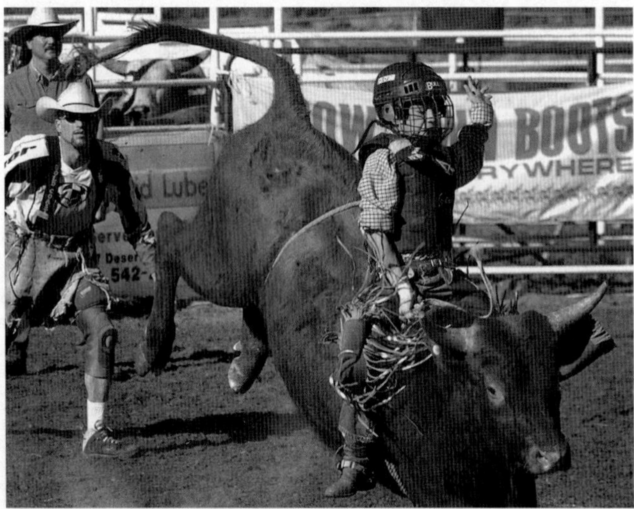

FIG. 33.1 This 10-year-old boy is following the traditions of ranch life in Colorado, where rodeo is a part of life. He won his first big belt buckle in competition at 8 years old.

There are several findings to note when ascertaining psychosocial contributions to nonorganic back pain, as follows[8]:

1. *Superficial nonanatomic tenderness.* Lightly pinching or rolling the skin should not affect the deep structures, which might cause true pain.
2. *Patient's response to positive stimulation, such as axial loading.* Lightly placing one's hand on top of the head should not significantly increase pressure in the low back.
3. *Distraction.* One should look for a significant difference in straight-leg raising ability in the seated versus supine position.
4. *Overreaction.* An overly loquacious patient or behavior disproportionate to the stimulus should be noted.
5. *Disturbances in sensation or distribution of pain or weakness that do not follow anatomic patterns.*

Symptoms and signs that suggest back pain from nonmechanical causes—such as subclinical pyelonephritis, kidney stones, or dissecting aneurysm—should also be considered.

Genetics

The wild card in the etiology of sciatic pain is genetics. Ala-Kokko[9] noted that scientific studies have identified specific versions of the genes encoding collagen, aggrecan, vitamin D receptor, and matrix metalloproteinase-3 that have significant associations with lumbar disc disease. Many other genes may also play a role in disc disease.[10–12] Although not a sports-related etiology, idiopathic adolescent scoliosis can be seen in adolescent athletes and is undergoing extensive research for genetic causes and predictors of curve progression.[13–15]

Physical Examination

The physical examination should take into consideration the three reasons for orthopaedic consultation: pain, deformity, and dysfunction. Although there is poor correlation between physical findings, symptoms, and treatment outcome, an examination of the patient's back is necessary. The purpose of physical examination is to confirm the impression gained from the history, if possible, and to look for surprises. Many obvious anatomic abnormalities can be visualized only when the patient's back is bare. The physical examination usually helps to exclude a serious disease rather than identify one. The

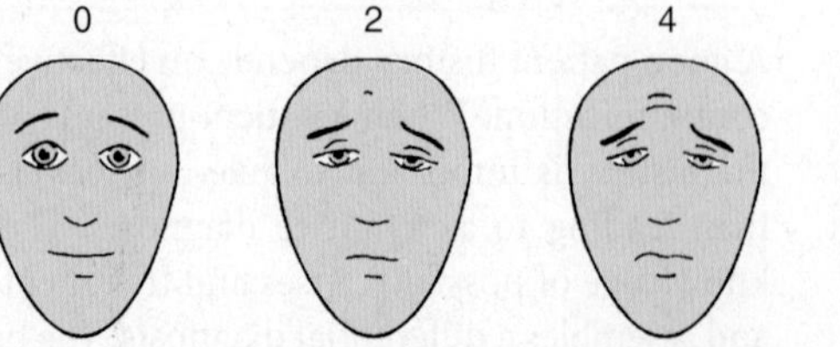

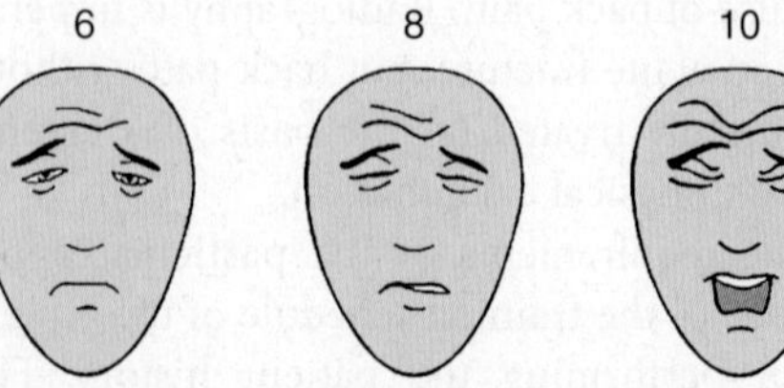

FIG. 33.2 Bieri faces. Drawings are neutral in terms of gender and ethnicity. The patient indicates a number that corresponds to his or her pain between 0 and 10.

three S's of an abnormal spine examination are apparent to observation: *spasm, scoliosis,* and *spondylolisthesis.*

Watching the patient move in flexion, extension, and rotation gives a visible assessment of pain. How a patient moves is as important to note as ROM. Whether the patient can bend to the knees, below the knees, or to the toes provides a rough measure of flexibility. Observing spinal rotation allows one to evaluate the facet joints.

After checking ROM and palpating for tenderness and muscle spasm, the physician should observe the rotational symmetry of the spine using the Adams forward-bend test and noting whether the pelvis is level. It is worthwhile to observe the effect of compression of the pelvis while the patient is lying on his or her back because this is a nonspecific test for sacroiliac joint disorders.

Observing standing posture in the coronal and sagittal planes is important to document evidence of deformity. Special tests, such as one-leg standing (the stork test) and compression tests for the neck (Spurling test), are indicated when one suspects spondylolysis or compression neuropathy. Anisomelia can be diagnosed by measuring limb lengths from the anterior superior iliac spine to the medial malleolus.

The neurologic examination requires close attention to detail and begins by having the patient heel walk and toe walk. Both functions demand strength, coordination, and cooperation one would expect from an athletic child. Testing deep tendon reflexes is important, especially if they are asymmetrical; testing the abdominal reflexes is essential to detecting hydromyelia.

The straight-leg raise test, or Lasègue sign, is a test for nerve root irritation or inflammation. A positive response is the reproduction of radicular pain. Pain on the opposite side or a positive cross straight-leg raise test is significant for diagnosis of a herniated disc. The straight-leg raise test can simultaneously provide evidence of sciatica and hamstring contracture.

Imaging

Modern imaging techniques, such as computed tomography (CT) and magnetic resonance imaging (MRI) permit accurate visualization of anatomic defects in the spine. Although both techniques are powerful diagnostic tools, the defects revealed by CT or MRI are not always causative with regard to the patient's pain. The literature is replete with cases in which anatomic defects are present on MRI or CT in completely asymptomatic patients.

The Cochrane group performed a meta-analysis of the literature and concluded that there is no correlation between radiographic changes and back pain.[16] Contrary to that opinion, researchers in Tokyo reported a study in which they correlated preparticipation spinal radiographs with the incidence of back pain and disability among young football players.[17] They followed 171 high school and 742 college football players over a 1-year period. High school players with spondylolysis had a higher incidence of low back pain (79.8%) than players with no radiographic abnormality (37.1%). College players with spondylolysis, disc space narrowing, and spinal instability had a higher incidence of low back pain (80.5%, 59.8%, and 53.5%, respectively) than players with normal radiographs (32.1%). College players with spondylolysis had a higher incidence of low back pain than players with disc space narrowing and spinal instability.

How can this incongruence of findings be explained? It is believed that asymptomatic abnormalities in the general population, particularly abnormalities seen with aging, may become symptomatic with vigorous physical activity. Abnormal spine radiographs in a young athlete should be considered a risk factor for injury.

Magnetic Resonance Imaging of the Spine

MRI technology takes advantage of the high hydrogen content of the molecules that make up biologic tissues. Hydrogen atoms have a specific "spin" property associated with them; that "spin" state can be altered in the presence of a strong magnetic field. Alterations in the "spin" properties of hydrogen atoms in biologic tissues can be detected by MRI technology, producing highly sensitive visual images.

Although MRI is a very sensitive and accurate assessment of spinal anatomy, it cannot distinguish between painful and painless structures in the spine. A patient may have severe back pain and MRI may reveal no abnormalities, or the converse may be true. It can be difficult for the physician to correlate MRI findings with the patient's signs and symptoms to make a clinical diagnosis. Typically, it is unnecessary to obtain MRI at the onset of spine-related pain because most cases of back and neck pain resolve within 2 to 12 weeks with proper conservative treatment. MRI is indicated when more aggressive treatments (e.g., injections or surgery) are contemplated.

Bone Scintigraphy (Bone Scan)

Bone scintigraphy (Bone scan) is not as specific as MRI or CT, but is very sensitive to changes in metabolic activity of bone. Increased metabolic activity is seen with inflammation, infection, and tissue proliferation owing to tumors such as osteoid osteoma. Bone scintigraphy uses a short-lived radioactive pharmaceutical agent to label specific tissues or structures, ultimately to visualize them via scintillation-mediated imaging. Gamma emissions from the radiopharmaceutical are detected by a gamma camera, converted to light photons, amplified with photomultiplier tubes, and digitized via computer to present a high-resolution (4–6 mm) two-dimensional image.

Single-Photon Emission Computed Tomography

With single-photon emission computed tomography (SPECT), gamma camera detectors rotate around the patient in small increments (usually 3- or 6-degree steps), and emission data are obtained from different plane angles. Computer algorithms break the image into pixels, each of which represents an approximately 6-mm area of the planar image. Pixel data are used to render clinically useful volumetric images. Auerbach[18] showed that SPECT exceeded MRI or plain radiography in accurately defining spondylolysis in a series of 100 children with significant back pain.

Principles of Treatment and Rehabilitation

Acute Treatment

When pain onset is acute and severe, bed rest may be necessary for 2 or 3 days for initial pain control. A longer period of bed rest quickly becomes counterproductive. The key to recovery is modified activity within a minimal range to start, followed by gentle progression of activity. The sooner the athlete begins a level of tolerated activity, the quicker and more effective is the recovery. Research and experience have dispelled the notion that prolonged absolute rest is beneficial for treatment of back pain.[19]

Nonsteroidal antiinflammatory drugs (NSAIDs) can be potent when given with muscle relaxants, but the duration of medication should be no longer than 10 days. Opioid administration is rarely necessary for more than a few days. Local anesthetic injections into the facet joints or into trigger points can be useful treatments that may help to diagnose disease related to the facet joint or fibromyalgia.

Passive physical therapy modalities such as ice, massage, or heat can be helpful in initial treatment, but the athlete needs to begin active rehabilitation and assume responsibility for his or her recovery. Strengthening should begin as soon as possible, and bracing should be minimized.

Bracing

Bracing may be effective if used intermittently and primarily as a tool for returning to activity.[20] The Cochrane Collaboration reported a meta-analysis on the use of braces for low back pain in 2000.[21] There was moderate evidence that lumbar supports are no more effective for primary prevention than other types of treatment or no intervention. The authors found no data promoting the effectiveness of lumbar supports for secondary prevention. This opinion is consistent with the generally held concept that passive treatment such as bracing should be limited to acute pain relief and that active rehabilitation is an early goal for return to participation in sports and prevention of future injury. Lumbar function assessed by self-reported and objective measures does not seem to worsen with short-term use of nonrigid, inelastic bracing for low back pain.[22]

Traction

Traction has historically been used to treat low back pain. Current thought remains disparate, however, regarding the therapeutic value of traction.[23] A 2013 Cochrane Review on traction for low back pain with or without sciatica found traction alone or in combination with other treatments has little to no value in low back pain treatment.[24]

Rehabilitation

The rehabilitation program consists of stages that encourages building a foundation of fundamentals and moving through increasingly difficult levels of activity. Physical rehabilitation should be designed to be sport specific and diagnosis specific. A gymnast with spondylolysis needs a program avoiding hyperextension while the bone is allowed to heal. As rehabilitation goals, the gymnast needs to stay active in the maneuvers that do not stress the back and to maintain general fitness.

Generally, rehabilitation begins with flexion and extension cycles to reduce joint stiffness and relax elastic structures. There should be minimal loading of the spine during this stage. Hip and knee ROM exercises are added next to offload the spine, followed by specific muscle training. Focus is first placed on the anterior abdominal muscles and maintaining the spine in neutral position, followed by lateral muscle exercises for side support of quadratus lumborum and abdominal wall muscles; finally, an extensor muscle program is added. Repetitions and movement duration should be closely monitored by the therapist.

Core Stabilization

A core stabilization program is based on the principle of coordinated muscle contraction. This contraction is done from a neutral, pain-free position. Finding and maintaining a pain-free position is fundamental to reestablishing isometric muscle control. Flexibility training should not be approached until strength has been regained.

Flexibility

Exercise programs that load the spine throughout ROM have poorer outcomes. Greater mobility is associated with poorer outcomes as well. ROM of the spine has little predictability for future low back pain. Programs emphasizing trunk stabilization with a neutral spine have had the most success.[25–27] These programs emphasize increasing ROM of the hips and knees.

Muscle Performance (Strength Versus Endurance)

The term *strength* is defined as the maximum force that a muscle can produce during a single exertion to create joint torque. The term *endurance* refers to the ability to maintain a force for a period of time. Muscle performance includes strength and endurance. The few studies available suggest that endurance has a much greater prophylactic value than strength.[28] The emphasis should be placed on endurance and should precede strengthening exercises in a gradual, progressive exercise program (i.e., longer duration, lower effort exercises).

Sport-Specific Exercise

The physical therapist, trainer, physician, and coach must collaborate in designing a sport-specific rehabilitation program. New exercises should closely simulate the sport. Progress should be slow enough to develop an awareness of muscle function. The buildup to maximum performance requires time and patience.

Deep Water Running and Swimming

Walking in a swimming pool is a gentle strengthening exercise for the back. Deep water running is excellent for treating athletes with back pain. The buoyancy of the water helps to unload the spine. Athletes run in the deep end of a swimming pool, normally with the aid of a flotation vest. Water is about 800 times denser than air; thus, resistance met during water running is greater than when running on land. Deep water running can help to maintain aerobic performance for 6 weeks in trained endurance athletes; sedentary individuals can appreciate significantly increased maximal oxygen uptake. During spine rehabilitation programs, deep water running can be used for maintenance training, but deep water running is not a substitute for conventional training.[29–31] Swimming is an excellent exercise for the back, but caution is advised for the novice. The swimming strokes can produce or exacerbate back injury if proper technique is not practiced.

Cycling

Although bicycling is generally considered a healthy form of non–weight-bearing, low-impact exercise, it is important to avoid prolonged flexion in a seated position. A more upright posture is easier on the intervertebral disc; thus, the upright mountain bike posture is preferred to the flexed racing bike posture. Avoiding the vibration of rough terrain is also logical, making stationary cycling a more reasonable option in the early stages of rehabilitation.

Program Guidelines

The following caveats should be considered when prescribing and monitoring any "return to sport" rehabilitation program[32]:

1. Low back exercises are most beneficial when performed daily.[33]
2. The "no pain, no gain" approach when exercising the spine may cause tissue damage associated with certain specific repeated movements.[34]
3. General exercise programs that include cardiovascular training (e.g., walking) have been shown to be effective for rehabilitation of individuals with low back pain and for injury prevention.[35]
4. Intervertebral discs are more hydrated early in the morning after rising from bed; it is unwise to perform full-range spinal motions (bending) shortly after rising.[36]
5. More repetitions of less-demanding exercises assist in the enhancement of endurance and strength. Evidence indicates that endurance has more protective value than strength, and strength gains should not be overemphasized at the expense of endurance.[37]
6. There is no such thing as an ideal set of exercises for all individuals. Although science at present cannot evaluate the optimal exercises for each situation, the combination of science and clinical experience should be used to select an exercise program.
7. Individuals need to be patient and stick with the program. Increased function and pain reduction may not occur for 3 months in some individuals.[37]

Education

Several studies have documented the value of patient education in the treatment of spine problems.[38] Education has been shown to be as valuable to the patient's recovery as physical therapy. In 2004, Frost and colleagues[38] measured the effectiveness of routine physical therapy compared with a single assessment session and advice from a physical therapist for patients with low back pain. They used a multicenter, randomized controlled trial in seven British National Health Service physiotherapy departments. These authors concluded that routine physical therapy was no more effective than a single assessment and advice session from a physiotherapist in treating low back pain.

In the physician's office, handouts are an excellent source of education and can be reference guides for the patient during rehabilitation activities (Table 33.1). Good preprinted handouts are available from multiple sources, such as the Krames (http://www.krames.com/) or the AAOS (http://www.aaos.org/) websites. Personalizing the handouts gives the athlete assurance in his or her provider's interest and commitment to the rehabilitation plan, as well as confidence in the treatment plan on leaving the office. With the availability of digital radiography, it is inexpensive to give the patient a copy of the patient's radiograph to take home. Being educated regarding the nature of the injury and being part of the rehabilitation team, not merely the subject, motivates the athlete, which can bring about speedier and more complete recovery.

Return to Play

For the athlete, returning to play is a central issue and may be measured in terms of games missed as opposed to return of

TABLE 33.1 Ways to Avoid Overuse Injuries

Use good technique.	An overhand pitch produces less strain than a side-arm pitch.
If it hurts, don't do it.	"No pain, no gain" is a poor concept. You feel the fatigue of a good workout, but you must recognize the pain of going beyond fatigue to injury.
Stop when fatigued.	Avoid the temptation of an extra repetition. Sprints are best done after a rest.
Increase duration gradually.	It takes time for the body to respond to increased demand and to strengthen.
Rest for a time after major increases.	It is better to alternate 3 hard days with an easy day, then rest for 2 days.
Quit when you are tired.	When you have exhausted the glycogen stored in your muscles, your technique falters and you are prone to injury.
Do preventive exercises.	Keep your body in balance by stretching to gain full range of motion and loosening contractures.
Remember your old injuries.	When you recall your old injuries, you can work to avoid repeating them.
Warm up slowly.	Use gentle stretching and gradually increasing effort to limber up muscles and deep breathing to stimulate the heart and lungs.

fitness. Generally, the athlete can return to play when there is no pain with sport-specific activities and when full ROM and strength has been recovered. There is no definitive test to measure when that point is reached. Gradual improvement in pain and progression in performing functional activities are predictive of a good prognosis.

Disorders and Treatment

Low Back Pain in Adolescent Athletes

Back pain in the pediatric and adolescent athlete has been well described in several recent articles.[39,40] Etiologies of pediatric back pain include spondylolysis, spondylolisthesis, posterior element overuse syndrome, sacroiliac joint irritation, atypical Scheuermann disease, and disc herniations. When a physician sees a child with back pain, the physician needs to rule out serious disorders, such as infection, tumors, cauda equina syndrome, and inflammatory spondyloarthropathies, then begin acute care, typically involving a rehabilitation program that allows the child to return to normal physical activity. Unlike adults, 90% of whom have no identifiable cause of their back pain, more than 50% of children with back pain were found to have an identifiable cause.[41] More recently, a study of 73 pediatric patients with low back pain resulted in 78% without identifiable cause after exhaustive workup.[42] Careful evaluation is important. An open-ended interview to hear the patient's story and expectations is the most valuable assessment instrument. Obtaining a detailed description of the pain is paramount.

The description of pain needs to include its location, duration, onset, and characteristic. If pain is associated with a particular activity or position, that information is helpful for diagnosis. Even with the most aggressive diagnostic workups and follow-ups, however, an organic cause for back pain in adolescents is found only about half of the time.

Lumbar spine pain or low back pain accounts for 5% to 8% of athletic injuries.[43] Injuries are often due to poor conditioning of the spine, poor biomechanics, or repetitive stresses placed on the spine by the nature of the sport. Overuse injuries from repeated lumbar hyperextension may be common in children participating in sports such as gymnastics, volleyball, and rowing. Evaluation of the sacroiliac joint should be completed, as nonoperative treatments result in significant improvement in 80% of cases.[44]

Historical studies show that the correct diagnosis of acute low back pain is established on the first visit only 2% of the time. After 6 weeks, the diagnostic accuracy increases to 15%, and it increases to 30% at 3 months.[45] The physician's initial visit is best used to rule out serious disorders, such as disc herniation or malignant disease. Although less than 1% of back pain complaints are related to serious spine pathology or require emergent treatment, such as neoplasm or cauda equina syndrome, it is important to exclude these conditions and reassure the patient accordingly.

Aggressive diagnostic workup may be deferred and implemented only for patients who do not improve within 3 or 4 weeks. Often, pain resolves without much treatment, and the athlete continues participation in sports. With severe or prolonged pain that prompts medical consultation, a diagnostic workup is appropriate for guiding the treatment.

Back pain that follows an acute injury is usually attributed to muscle strain. There is little scientific evidence showing muscle strain as a back pain generator, however, probably because pain produced by an injury cannot be differentiated to the various soft tissues of the back.[46] The pain may be localized or diffuse. The patient frequently relates that more stiffness occurred after a night's sleep. This type of back pain attributed to muscle strain tends to improve with time.

Growth is not linear, and as growth spurts occur, an imbalance between new length of bone and old length of muscles occurs. These contractures, whether of the hamstrings or other muscles adjacent to the spine, can produce limited motion and pain with athletic activities.

An adolescent with normal musculoskeletal structure may have back pain from poor standing and sitting posture. The typical profile is of lumbar hyperlordosis, thoracic hyperkyphosis, and contracted hamstrings. Radiographs are unnecessary to make the diagnosis or to institute a program of stretching and postural correction.

Mechanical backache secondary to poor posture is more common in sedentary children. Athletic children are less likely to report nonspecific back pain than their nonathletic counterparts. Children who do not walk to school and have a poor self-image of their health in general report more back pain. Multivariate analysis showed that the incidence of low back pain in adolescents is inversely related to time spent doing physical activity (e.g., regular walking or bicycling) and directly related to television or computer time.[47]

Posture and inactivity contribute to low back pain. The intervertebral discs have the highest fluid content in the morning, which influences the pressure generated on spinal tissues during flexion.[48] Avoidance of flexion after arising in the morning significantly reduces nonspecific back pain.[49]

Plain radiographs are indicated at the time of the first visit if there is a history of severe trauma, loss of neurologic function, or history of unexplained fevers or malignancy. For an adolescent athlete with a high-risk factor because of a repetitive hyperextension maneuver, oblique views are appropriate for evaluation of the pars interarticularis.

Spondylolysis

Spondylolysis is a stress fracture of the pars interarticularis. It is generally considered to be a low-risk fracture that may heal on its own. The fracture occurs most frequently at L5, followed by L4 and L3. Spondylolysis occurs in 5% to 6% of the general population.[1] The lesion is usually asymptomatic and appreciated only incidentally on a radiograph. Generally, no single traumatic event causes spondylolysis; rather, repetitive stress produces fatigue defects, and a single event may complete the fracture. These fractures may not develop bony union but develop fibrous nonunion or heal in an elongated state in a relatively high percentage of patients.[50]

The incidence of pars defects is greater in adolescent athletes than in the general population, and is a particular clinical problem for this population.[51] Sports that require repetitive hyperextension or extension combined with rotation—such as gymnastics, wrestling, and weightlifting—are more often associated with a stress fracture of the pars interarticularis. White female gymnasts experience a rate of spondylolysis (11%) five times that of the general white female population.[52] Certain participants in sports—such as diving, weightlifting, wrestling, and gymnastics—have disproportionately high rates of spondylolysis. A study of elite Spanish athletes showed the highest rates of spondylolysis in gymnasts and weightlifters followed by throwing athletes and rowers.[53] Other reports suggest that a wide variety of sports increase the risk of spondylolysis, including soccer, volleyball, and baseball.[54]

A major concern for patients with defects in the pars interarticularis is the progressive development of symptomatic spondylolisthesis. The incidence of progressive spondylolisthesis is low (3% to 10%), and mainly occurs during adolescence.[55,56] There is no known correlation between active sports participation and either the occurrence or the progression of spondylolisthesis.

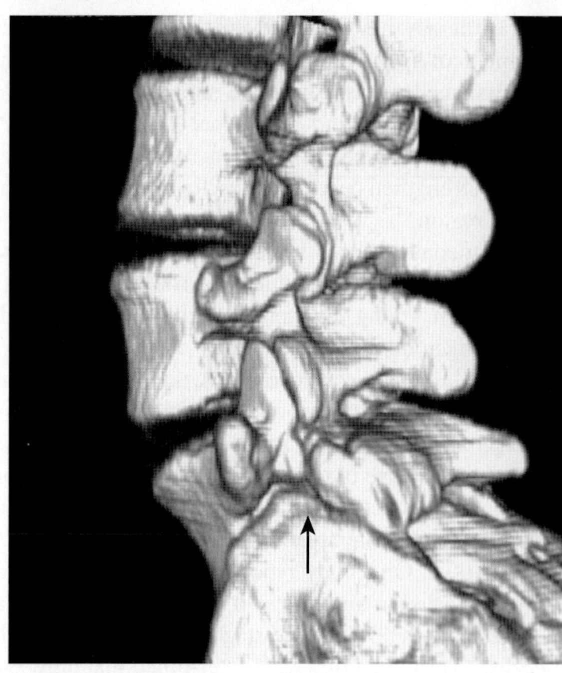

FIG. 33.3 Spondylolysis. Three-dimensional computed tomographic scan shows pars interarticularis defect (*arrow*).

Clinical Presentation

Pain may begin after acute injury, or there may be acute exacerbation of mild symptoms present for weeks or months. Lumbar spinal extension or rotation activities are particularly associated with the generation of symptomatic low back pain. Commonly, affected patients have a hyperlordotic posture and hamstring contractures. The classic test during physical examination is to have the patient stand on one leg and lean backward—the stork test. If the lesion is unilateral, the pain is most often produced by standing on the ipsilateral leg. This test is not definitive, but contributes to the diagnosis.

Spondylolysis is a bone lesion that, in most patients, does not produce a neurologic deficit. Any nerve root signs would suggest an alternative pathology, such as a herniated nucleus pulposus (HNP).

Diagnostic Imaging

Spondylolysis cannot be diagnosed by history and physical examination alone. The key to establishing the diagnosis of spondylolysis is visual confirmation of the pars lesion. The determination of a symptomatic spondylolytic lesion has become more sophisticated with the use of nuclear imaging, CT, and MRI.

A defect in the pars interarticularis is apparent in Fig. 33.3, which shows a three-dimensional CT scan. The classic description of this appearance on the oblique view radiograph is that of a collar on the "Scottie dog." Approximately 20% of the pars interarticularis lesions are seen only on the lateral oblique views, but no difference in sensitivity and specificity between anterior-posterior/lateral and anteroposterior/lateral/two obliques radiographs has been found.[57] Advanced imaging is often required to determine an accurate diagnosis.

MRI is typically used as the primary investigation for adolescents with back pain and suspected stress reactions of the pars interarticularis. MRI has been found to be 92% sensitive for detecting pars injuries, including stress reactions and stress fractures,[58] being especially useful in patients with negative CT who have stress reactions. SPECT use is limited by the high rate of false-positive and false-negative results, and by considerable ionizing radiation exposure.[59]

Bone scans have been found to be 94% sensitive and 100% specific for detecting skeletal abnormalities in pediatric patients with back pain.[60] For an adolescent with low back pain, normal radiographs, and a negative bone scan, spondylolysis is ruled out. Other causes should be investigated. MRI may be ordered under these circumstances to rule out disc pathology or other causes for pain in nonosseous tissues. Similarly, adolescents with back pain, positive radiographs, and negative bone scan warrant MRI to investigate further the basis for pain.

Treatment

Most patients with symptomatic spondylolysis do well with conservative treatment short term.[61] The main goals of treatment are amelioration of pain, return to activity, and the attainment of bony healing. Treatment modalities include rest, medication, and bracing, alone or in combination. Some pars interarticularis lesions heal with early care and bracing, particularly early-stage unilateral defects. Osseous healing is unnecessary to achieve an excellent clinical outcome with full return to activities, although attaining bony union, particularly in younger adolescents, should be the goal since the long-term outcome of unhealed spondylolysis is not known.

Activity restriction is important to limit pain. Running, jumping, and sport-specific activities that produced the pain should be eliminated for 4 to 6 weeks. Contact and collision sports are not allowed, and hyperextension activities should specifically be eliminated.

Physical therapy has been proven to be quite effective in the treatment of spondylolysis. Patients with a specific and carefully managed exercise program show significant reduction in pain intensity and functional disability levels.[62,63] Therapy should include exercises to increase hamstring flexibility and to strengthen deep core muscles in the abdomen and the lumbar region.[64]

Transcutaneous elective bone stimulation has received increased attention as an adjunct in promoting healing of spondylolysis in young athletes, though controlled studies have not yet been done.[65]

The role of bracing is controversial. A rigid brace is not uniformly used for the treatment of symptomatic spondylolysis. Many surgeons begin bracing immediately for spondylolysis, whereas others reserve bracing for patients who do not progress with their conservative program or who experience increasing pain. Chronicity of the lesion is important to healing potential. One study reports that 94% of early-stage defects were healed in an average of 3.2 months using a hard brace, whereas only 27% of late-stage defects were healed in 5.7 months.[66] Various studies have determined that only 9% to 15% of cases of symptomatic spondylolysis or grade 1 spondylolisthesis require surgery.[67–69] The indications for surgery are progressive slip, intractable pain, development of neurologic defects, and segmental instability associated with pain. Pain alone can be controlled by activity modification and medication, and is not an indication for surgery. Surgical treatment is directed at repairing the fracture in the pars interarticularis using bone grafting and internal fixation. Various techniques using wires and screws have been advocated. The technique by Chen and Lee,[70] using a pedicle screw and laminar hook, has the advantage of not violating the facet joints, while providing excellent stabilization for healing.

Return to Activity

When follow-up examination reveals no discomfort and pain is well controlled with ordinary daily activities, a low level of sports participation is appropriate. Return to sport can be achieved after 4 to 6 weeks of modified activity. Activity intensity can increase as tolerated. Continued therapy should focus on core strengthening, improvement in posture, and avoidance of hyperextension.

A case report of pediatric cervical spondylolysis showed that over 1.5 million children participate in American football without reported injury due to cervical spondylolysis; therefore, this pathology should not be a restriction to play.[71]

Preventing recurrence is a major goal of treatment. A maintenance fitness program should be included in any workout regimen that is prescribed. Any low back pain that is worsened by extension or twisting should prompt a reduction in activity and increased periods of rest. If these precautions are instituted at the first sign of symptoms, a long course of rest and rehabilitation may be avoided.

Spondylolisthesis

Spondylolisthesis occurs when there is a bilateral defect in the pars interarticularis and one vertebra slips forward relative to the vertebra beneath it. The incidence of spondylolisthesis in athletes is the same as in the general population. No substantiated criteria are available for predicting which cases of spondylolysis will progressively slip, resulting in spondylolisthesis. Patients with dysplastic posterior elements have a higher risk of slip progression. Radiographic studies have shown a strong correlation between slip progression and a more vertical inclination of the superior plate of S1.[72,73] Most cases of spondylolisthesis are mild, unlikely to progress, and cease to progress after growth is complete. With mild spondylolisthesis, there is no increased rate of disability and no reason to restrict participation in sports.

Isthmic spondylolisthesis is the type seen in young athletes, excluding the rare cases of congenital absence of facet joints. Bilateral stress fractures of the pars interarticularis are the distinguishing pathology of spondylolisthesis. The stress fractures are unusual in that they occur in young people and rarely heal spontaneously. The only suspected causative factor, other than familial predisposition, is minor or repetitive hyperextension.

Symptoms associated with spondylolisthesis are dull low back pain exacerbated by activity, particularly hyperextension and rotation. Sports requiring repetitive rotation and extension under load, such as gymnastics, football, wrestling, hockey, pole vaulting, diving, and throwing sports, have been incriminated as causative factors in multiple studies.[74,75] Typical of mechanical-type pain, rest tends to alleviate the pain.

During the examination, the findings of paravertebral muscle spasm, hamstring contractures, and limited flexibility may be dramatic. Kyphosis associated with severe grades of slip flattens the profile of the buttocks and creates a sagittal postural malalignment (Fig. 33.4). A step-off at the lumbosacral level may be palpable.

Weakness, loss of sensation, and a positive straight-leg raise test are usually absent, differentiating spondylolisthesis from a herniated disc. If radiculopathy is present, the L5 root is usually involved. Cauda equina syndrome has been reported in severe cases owing to nerve root stretch over the dome of the sacrum.[76]

The diagnosis is easily confirmed by a lateral radiograph of the lumbar spine. The severity of the slip is graded either by the quartile classification of Meyerding or, more commonly, as a percentage of displacement relative to the top of the sacrum. There is consensus that kyphosis is a more important measure of the deformity than displacement.[77] The slip angle and sacral inclination are used to describe the sagittal plane deformity.

The treatment of a young athlete with spondylolisthesis is based on the same principles as the population at large, but the desire of the individual to continue sports participation must be considered as well. The age of the patient, the severity and duration of pain, and the degree of deformity all must be considered when formulating a treatment plan. A young, minimally symptomatic patient with a less than 25% slip requires little restriction of activity, but should be monitored for progression. Initial flexion-extension lateral radiographs are useful for assessing instability. Serial lateral films at yearly intervals can document any progression of slipping, unless symptoms warrant more frequent follow-up. If the degree of

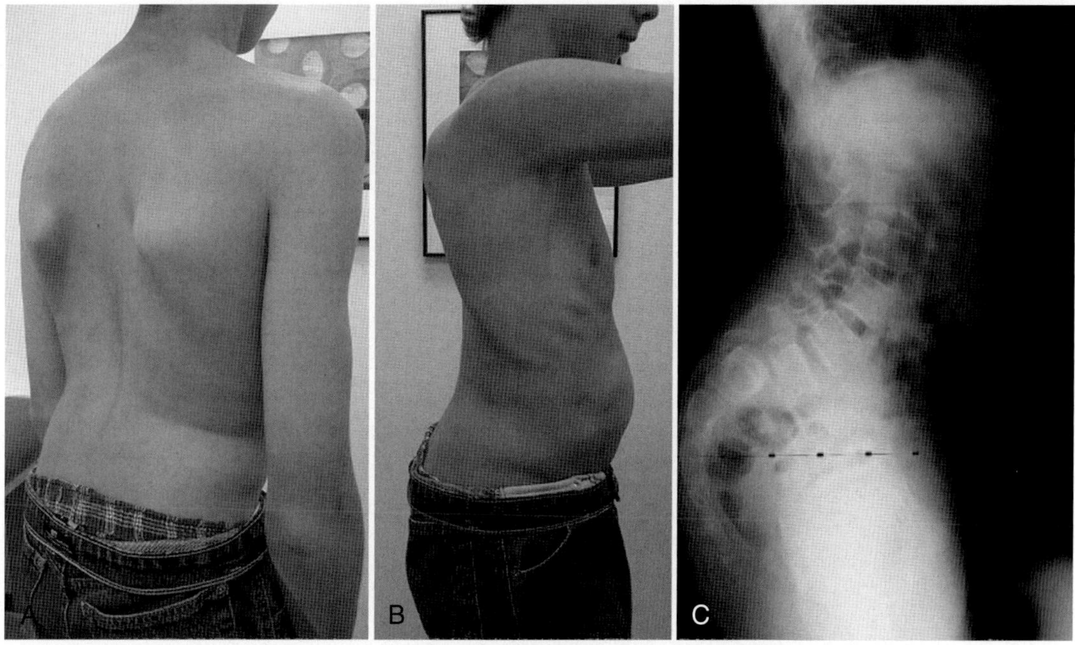

FIG. 33.4 Spondylolisthesis. (A) Paravertebral muscle spasm is striking. (B) Sagittal imbalance produced by severe slip made the clinical diagnosis evident. (C) Lateral radiograph showing the L5–S1 spondylolisthesis.

slip is 25% to 50%, the consensus is that the athlete should be restricted from collision sports, such as gymnastics and football. If the patient is truly asymptomatic, continued participation may be reasonable as a matter of judgment and cooperation.

Surgical stabilization is recommended for an immature patient with documented progression. Stabilization by spinal fusion is also recommended for slips greater than 50%, even if the patient is asymptomatic.

If the patient still has unremitting, disabling pain after a 6-month program of conservative treatment, certain surgical decisions are made: in situ fusion versus reduction, whether to perform decompression, whether to perform anterior and posterior fusion, and plus or minus bed rest. The debate over these issues remains. In situ fusion is the gold standard with well-documented long-term excellent outcomes.[78] Isolated removal of the laminar fragment, or Gill procedure, is contraindicated because further progression is common after that procedure.

Absolute indications for decompression are motor deficit and bowel or bladder dysfunction.[77] Some surgeons do not perform decompression even with motor or sensory signs because these signs tend to improve with a solid fusion.[79] Many surgeons perform a decompression at the time of fusion if weakness, sensory loss, or radicular pain is present, particularly in instances of severe slip. With severe degrees of slip, anterior fusion with or without reduction of the kyphotic deformity can be done using pedicle screw fixation and anterior interbody cages.

Although various methods for reduction of spondylolisthesis are advocated, many are associated with a significant rate of temporary or permanent nerve root damage. Reduction should be done only after wide decompression of the nerve roots, and significant nerve damage may still occur. Return to vigorous athletic participation is not guaranteed after surgery even if the fusion is solid. Most surgeons recommend against any but the least demanding of sports after such a major spine procedure. The decision regarding participation should be delayed until the outcome of surgery is clear.

Lumbar Scheuermann Disease (Juvenile Disc Disease)

The classic radiographic criteria for the diagnosis of Scheuermann disease is kyphosis of the thoracic spine with wedging of 15 or more degrees over three vertebrae.[80] Scheuermann disease is associated with endplate changes, such as irregularity of the apophyseal ring and Schmorl nodes due to defective endplate growth. The causes of Scheuermann disease, which has been attributed to juvenile osteoporosis, are controversial. This condition affects 0.4% to 8.3% of the general population and causes irregularities in ossification and endochondral growth in the thoracic spine in adolescents and young adults.[80] The disease leads to various pathologic changes at the junction of the vertebral body and the intervertebral disc, resulting in pronounced wedging of the vertebral bodies and progressive kyphosis in severe cases. According to various studies, it causes back pain in 20% to 60% of cases, and occasionally causes severe deformity of the spine.[80]

An increased frequency of radiologic abnormalities of the thoracolumbar spine has been reported among young athletes in various sports, such as soccer, gymnastics, waterski jumping, or wrestling, compared with nonathletes.[81–91] Although the origins of typical Scheuermann disease[91] have been a matter of controversy,[92] atypical Scheuermann disease is considered to be strongly associated with trauma or excessive loading of the spine, especially in the flexed posture and during growth spurts.[93] Axial compression forces apparently

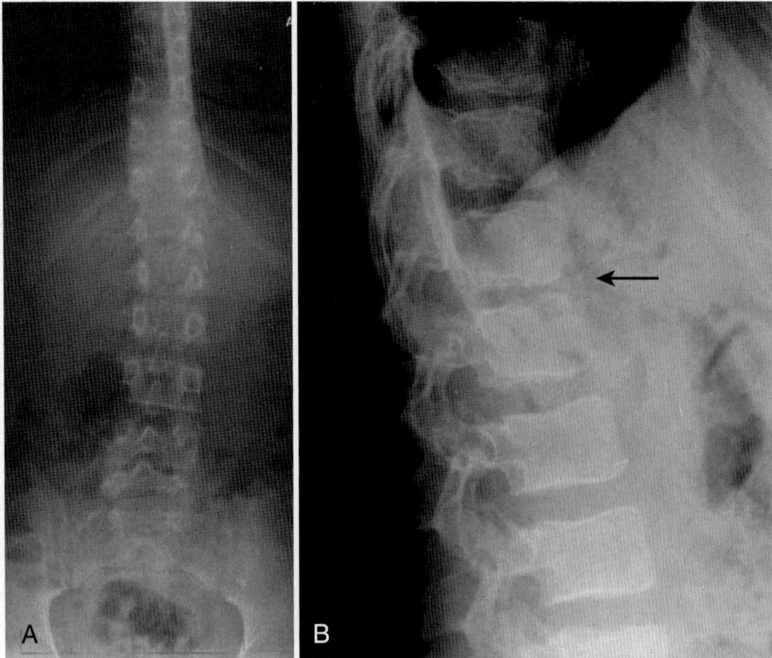

FIG. 33.5 Juvenile disc disease. This 14-year-old baseball player presented with pain localized to the upper lumbar level. (A) Anteroposterior radiograph shows irritative scoliosis. (B) Lateral radiograph shows endplate irregularity and erosion anteriorly at the L1–L2 level.

cause vertebral endplate bulging, whereas compression of the immature spine in flexion is considered to cause anterior intravertebral disc herniation (marginal Schmorl nodes).[92–95] Abnormalities of the vertebral ring apophysis are thought to be the result of failure in tension shear, analogous to Osgood-Schlatter avulsion at the knee (Fig. 33.5).[89]

In 1985, Greene and colleagues[92] described back pain and vertebral changes in the lumbar spine similar to changes seen in Scheuermann disease of the thoracic spine. These changes were accompanied by mechanical low back pain. In 1994, Heithoff and colleagues[96] saw similar changes on MRI and coined the term *juvenile discogenic disease*. Their group detected evidence of thoracolumbar Scheuermann disease and multilevel disc disease of the lower lumbar spine in 9% of the subjects studied. The patients ranged in age from 7 to 66 years, but most were young: slightly less than half of the patients were younger than 30 years; 9% were younger than 21 years. Males outnumbered females 3 : 1. Disc degeneration was found most frequently at the L5–S1 level, followed in order by L4–L5 and L3–L4. Of patients, 80% showed evidence of substantial degeneration at more than one lumbar level, and 53% had disc herniations involving at least one lower lumbar level.

Heithoff and colleagues[96] suspected that a substantial number of young adults have a combination of painful multilevel disc degeneration and lumbar spine changes typical of Scheuermann disease. In their view, both conditions may be caused by an underlying genetic defect in disc structure. It has been estimated that 80% of young patients requiring disc surgery have a genetic predisposition to disc degeneration.[96] Juvenile discogenic disease has been statistically associated with athletic activity and repetitive trauma. Most patients can be treated nonoperatively, but a subset has concurrent spinal stenosis, which may require decompression.[97]

Herniated Nucleus Pulposus

Acute disc herniation, or HNP, is relatively rare in children and adolescents compared with adults. Reports suggest that only 0.5% to 4% of surgically managed HNP occurs in patients younger than 18 years.[98–102] Despite the low incidence, approximately 10% of severe back pain in skeletally immature patients is due to disc herniation.[103,104] High-risk activities include weightlifting and collision sports, such as football.[104] HNP has also been associated with injuries sustained during gymnastics, basketball, baseball, and wrestling.[85] Nearly 95% of herniations occur from L4 to S1 and are fairly evenly distributed between L4–L5 and L5–S1.[105] The L3–L4 level is affected in only 5% of patients.[105]

The presenting symptoms of HNP in children differ from the symptoms seen in adults. The profile of an adolescent with HNP includes the presence of tension signs and sciatic scoliosis, without localizing neurologic signs. Most patients present with low back pain, with or without leg pain.[104,105] Associated leg pain is seen far less often than in adults (<20% of the time).[93] In children, the herniation is thought to be more central and the volume of extruded disc material less than in adults.[99,104] Actual rupture of the disc is rare in children.[106]

Physical examination often reveals an abnormal gait or scoliosis owing to paraspinal muscle spasm.[104,105] Nerve tension signs, such as a positive straight-leg raise test, are present in greater than 80% to 90% of patients, and the crossed-leg raise test is positive in more than 50%.[104,105,107] Objective motor

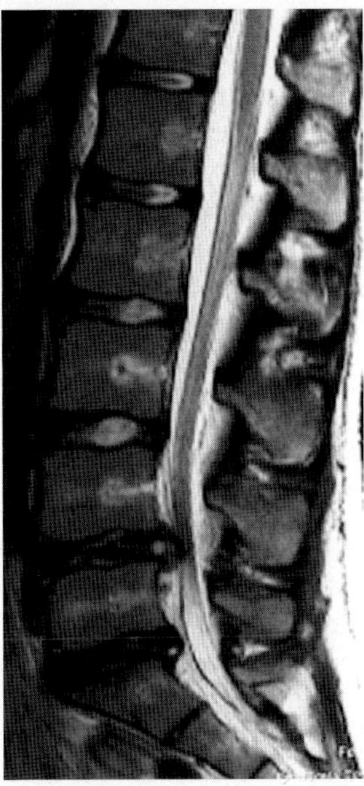

FIG. 33.6 Herniated nucleus pulposus. This 15-year-old wrestler has a black bulging disc at L4–L5 highlighted by a white dot on MRI. (Courtesy Charles Burton, MD.)

weakness may be present in 40%, with the extensor hallucis longus most commonly affected, and deep tendon reflexes at the knee and ankle are decreased in approximately 40% of patients.[105]

MRI is a very effective way to image the disc, spinal cord, and nerve roots. In addition, because of its noninvasive nature, it is a commonly used imaging technique. MRI has been shown to detect 100% of symptomatic herniations (Fig. 33.6).[108] Herniation is associated with endplate changes, with marrow signal intensity changes on MRI, and with increased cartilage in the material removed during surgery. There is a correlation of marrow signal intensity changes on MRI and the biology of the removed material. Avulsion-type disc herniation is common.[109] Occult spina bifida, extralumbar vertebrae, sacralization of the fifth lumbar vertebra, lateral recess stenosis, and spondylolisthesis have been associated with pediatric disc disease.[110]

Conservative treatment is as outlined for nonspecific low back pain. The literature suggests, however, that the overall outcomes of conservative treatment are generally poor. Recommendations suggest a 2- to 4-week trial of conservative management followed by surgical excision of the disc if symptoms have not resolved.[105]

Indications for surgical excision of the disc include persistent symptoms despite conservative management, cauda equina syndrome, progressive neurologic deficits, and reinjury.[104,105] Many authors have reported greater than 90% good to excellent results after surgical excision.[100,102,105,111] After surgical excision, low back pain and leg pain resolved within 3 weeks, and neurologic findings resolved after 3 months.[100] Reactive scoliosis almost always improves with successful treatment.[112] Long-term follow-up studies show excellent outcomes, including absence of pain and no activity limitations.[100,102,111] Satisfactory surgical outcomes may be seen for at least 10 years postoperatively, though may slightly deteriorate with time.[113]

Apophyseal Ring Fracture

Bone fragments at the posterior vertebral endplate have been given numerous names, such as posterior marginal node; limbus fracture; fracture of the vertebral rim, ring, or endplate; epiphyseal dislocation; and apophyseal ring fracture.[114] This condition is unique to adolescents,[104] and was first described by Skobowytsh-Okolot in 1962.[101,115] Endplate fracture was discovered in 20% of patients younger than 21 years and in 33% of patients younger than 17 years who were undergoing lumbar disc surgery.[116] The overall prevalence is only 0.07% of all patients of all ages undergoing disc surgery. There is a strong male predominance, with 85% of cases occurring in boys; 66% of cases are related to a traumatic event, such as weightlifting, heavy work, or sports injury.[101] Associations have also been found with Scheuermann disease[117] and lumbar disc herniations.[118]

Hyperextension of the lumbar spine[119] and rapid flexion together with axial compression to the vertebral column such as occurs with weightlifting are two proposed mechanisms of apophyseal ring injury.[101,104,120] The presenting symptoms of an apophyseal ring fracture are similar to the symptoms seen with HNP—back, buttock, and posterior thigh pain. Symptoms are worse with coughing, sneezing, sports, and prolonged sitting.[104] Pain may radiate down one or both legs. The straight-leg raise test is positive, and contralateral straight-leg raise is frequently positive. Paraspinal muscle spasm, lumbar tenderness, scoliosis, intermittent claudication, paraparesis, and cauda equina syndrome have been reported.[101,104]

Plain radiographs can be useful and show the avulsed fragment in approximately 40% of cases.[101,114] This fragment appears as an arcuate or wedge-shaped bone fragment posterior to the vertebral body or disc space. Alternatively, it can appear as a bony ridge on the posterior surface of the vertebral body. MRI may show a defect in the posterior vertebral rim. The fragment may be seen as a low signal area lying posteriorly, but can be difficult to distinguish from cortical bone and the posterior longitudinal ligament. MRI may be diagnostic in only 22% of cases.[114] CT is an excellent imaging study for these fractures because it can define the bony fragment, any associated disc prolapse, vertebral defect, and severity of any associated stenosis in approximately 75% of cases. CT should be considered if MRI fails to show an expected HNP or ring fracture.[114]

A trial of short-term rest, use of NSAIDs, and physical therapy is indicated. Physical therapy should focus on hamstring stretching, as persistent hamstring tightness has been found following conservative management in adolescent athletes.[121] If symptoms fail to resolve after 2 to 4 weeks or if there is progressive neurologic involvement or cauda equina syndrome, surgical excision of the fragment and any associated disc material should be performed.[104] Intervertebral fusion is controversial at this time due to lack of comparative, high-level studies.[122] Good to excellent results have been reported after surgical excision in nearly all pediatric cases of avulsed ring fracture.

Cervical Spine Injuries

Traumatic neck injuries in young athletes may be to bone, nerve, or soft tissue. These are increasingly common injuries. Recent data on American football suggests that 0.2/100,000 participants at the high school level and 2/100,000 participants per collegiate level are diagnosed with a cervical cord neurapraxia most commonly due to hyperflexion, during "spear tackling."[123] The order of incidence is as follows[124]:

1. Nerve root or brachial plexus neurapraxia (burners)
2. Cervical strains (muscular injury)
3. Disc injury with neck pain only
4. Cervical sprains (ligament injury)
5. Disc herniation with radicular symptoms
6. Transient spinal cord compression secondary to stenosis
7. Fractures

On-Field Examination

In an on-field examination, if a cervical spine injury is suspected, the physician or trainer should appreciate any spinal pain; altered perception of touch; numbness; and weakness in, or difficulty moving, the extremities. Any player with signs of head trauma, such as disturbed vision, headache, staggering gait, disorientation, or memory loss, should not participate further.

For an ambulatory athlete complaining of pain or spasm in the neck, the physician should localize the tenderness and evaluate for muscle spasm. The physician should evaluate neck ROM and perform a motor and sensory examination of the extremities. On failing the examination, the athlete should be removed from competition and immobilized in a cervical collar. Alarming signs associated with a cervical fracture are acute torticollis, resistance to any motion, and the patient using the hands to support the head. If the player is unconscious, the presumption is that a cervical spine injury exists, and the neck is immobilized. Any facemask should be removed, but the helmet should be left in place. The player should be immobilized before being moved. Players with persistent or severe pain should be given a prompt radiologic evaluation. Return to participation depends on complete resolution of symptoms and normal radiographs.

Field Treatment of Cervical Fractures

Fractures of the cervical spine are relatively rare. The on-field treatment protocol should be well rehearsed and efficient, however. The minimal equipment includes tools or instruments necessary to remove the facemask, a cervical collar, and a backboard. Such an extensive setup may be impractical, but the medical attendant is well advised to know what emergency medical services are available, such as a well-equipped ambulance. A cell phone or other communication capability should be available on the sideline. The key is advance planning.

Lifting an individual high enough to insert a backboard beneath requires a medical team chief who carefully links the head to the chest and six additional people to lift. If a team has not practiced or there are not six individuals immediately trained and available, the athlete should not be moved until there is adequate assistance to immobilize and transport him or her without incurring additional damage. Instructions for the prehospital care of a spinal cord injury on an athletic field are published online by an interdisciplinary task force.[125]

Prevention of Catastrophic Injuries to the Cervical Spine in Football

According to Cantu and Mueller[126] of the National Center for Catastrophic Sport Injury Research, prevention is related to teaching and enforcing good technique in blocking and tackling and the proper use of well-fitted equipment. Cantu and Mueller[126] noted, "The football helmet is not the cause of cervical spine injuries. Poorly executed tackling and blocking technique are the major problems." The neck should be kept upright, avoiding use of the helmet and facemask as the initial and primary contact point in blocking and tackling. Rules against spearing should be strongly enforced, and athletes should strengthen their necks for further protection in the event of a miss-hit. Cantu and Mueller[126–131] stated that being prepared for the treatment and transport of a player with a major spine injury can mean the difference between life and death. That means having a plan and practicing the teamwork necessary for a successful transport.

Return to Play Guidelines

Recent publications have focused on return to play guidelines after cervical spine injury though strong, evidence-based studies are lacking. General guidelines include resolution of symptoms, full ROM and normal or near-normal strength, but these are not unique to the cervical spine.[132] Based on expert opinions, return to sport should be based on radiographic findings as well.[133] Benign injuries, such as spinous process fractures, may be treated with immobilization and return to play once healed. Patients with more than three burners (see later) in a single season or recurrent transient quadriparesis should undergo evaluation and imaging to rule out stenosis or parenchymal injury prior to return to play. Patients who undergo cervical fusion of one or two segments may return to play after successful recovery. More complex injuries that require operative intervention of fusion of three or more levels are contraindicated for return to play.[134]

Cervical Peripheral Nerve Injuries

Burners

"Burners" (also known as "stingers") are common injuries to the neck in collision sports, such as football, hockey, or diving. A high percentage of football players, especially defensive players, experience burners during their playing career. Other sports in which burners occur include wrestling, backpacking, sledding, skiing, horseback riding, boxing, weightlifting, and climbing.

Burners are caused by either compression or distraction. An asymmetrical axial load on the neck causing compression in the neuroforamen can injure the peripheral nerve root. If the athlete falls directly on the shoulder and the head is distracted away from the shoulder, traction is applied to the nerve root and the brachial plexus. When the cervical spine is hyperextended, hyperflexed, or laterally flexed to the opposite side, the angle between the shoulder and neck is increased beyond the normal range, stretching the brachial plexus.

Symptoms are a severe burning or searing pain in the shoulder and arm associated with loss of sensation and weakness of the arm. The pain may be decreased by abducting the shoulder; this can be achieved by asking the athlete to place a hand on the top of the head. The Spurling maneuver is a provocative maneuver that reproduces the compression mechanism of injury. The patient's neck is extended, laterally flexed to the involved side, and rotated to the involved side with axial loading applied while in that position. The burning or searing pain is reproduced. Extension-compression mechanisms are most common, followed by brachial stretch and direct blow mechanisms.[135]

Burners are best prevented by enforcing the rules on spearing, by strengthening and conditioning the neck, and by proper use of good-quality protective equipment. Shoulder pads are protective equipment for the neck in football. An A-frame design to the shoulder pads brings lateral stability to the base of the neck, preventing lateral tilt while allowing rotation of the head, which occurs at C1–C2 (50%). The base of the shoulder pad needs to extend down well on the chest anteriorly and posteriorly to link the chest to the base of the neck. It is almost impossible to prevent extension of the head. The player needs to learn to block with the shoulder and keep the head down so that the opposing player is not contacted with a facemask or the helmet.

Initial treatment for this injury is removal from participation and rest, followed by strengthening exercises of the neck and, finally, careful stretching and restoration of ROM. Because the pain, paresthesias, and weakness typically last only a few seconds or minutes, these injuries fall into the Seddon classification of neurapraxia. Occasionally, athletes with more severe injuries experience a prolonged recovery period that may last hours to several weeks and may lead to a prolonged loss of time from competition.[136–143] Return to play criteria include full ROM of the neck associated with complete return of arm strength and sensation.

Burners may occur many times during the season, ranging from a transient nerve irritation without residual damage to a complete avulsion of the nerve root from the spinal cord with permanent deficit. Burners are symptoms of injury to either the brachial plexus or a nerve root, and must be evaluated systematically.

Quan and Bird[144] proposed a classification of peripheral nerve injuries that correlates well with electrodiagnostic studies and prognoses, based on earlier classifications by Seddon[145] and Sunderland.[146] This classification scheme is useful for diagnosis and advice in individual cases (Table 33.2).

TABLE 33.2 Quan and Bird Classification of Nerve Injury

Type of Injury	Mode of Recovery	Time to Recovery
Conduction block (neurapraxia)	Remyelination of focal segment involved	2–12 wk
Limited axonal loss	Collateral sprouting from surviving motor axons	2–6 mo
Intermediate axonal loss	Collateral sprouting and axonal regeneration from site of injury	2–6 mo
Severe axonal loss	Axonal regeneration	2–18 mo
Complete nerve discontinuity	No recovery without nerve grafting	2–18 mo

Data from Quan D, Bird SJ. Nerve conduction studies and electromyography in the evaluation of peripheral nerve injuries. *Univ Pa Orthop J.* 1999;12:45–51.

Cervical Stenosis

Congenital cervical stenosis is a risk factor for cervical spine injuries.[147] Two studies have analyzed the relationship of burners to cervical stenosis in college football players at the University of Iowa and Tulane University.[137,148] Burners were more common in players with spinal stenosis as defined by the Torg ratio, especially the occurrence of repeated episodes of neurapraxia. The Torg ratio is defined as the ratio of the spinal canal width to the width of the vertebral body at the same level, and is most narrow at C7. These studies suggest that a Torg ratio of 0.7 to 0.8 or lower is high risk. For players with cervical stenosis, the risk of burners is three times that of players without stenosis (Fig. 33.7).

Transient Spinal Cord Compression

Torg and colleagues[149] described the syndrome of transient quadriplegia, considered to represent a "neuropraxia of the cervical spinal cord." This syndrome includes bilateral upper extremity and lower extremity neurologic involvement with no associated fracture or dislocation. It usually resolves within 36 hours. The transient quadriplegia was associated with developmental spinal stenosis, either as an isolated entity or associated with congenital abnormalities, cervical instability, or intervertebral disc disease. The authors noted statistically significant spinal stenosis in all patients who incurred episodes of transient quadriparesis.[149,150] They also noted that there was "no evidence that the occurrence of neuropraxia of the cervical spinal cord predisposes an individual to permanent neurological injury."[149]

Fracture

Fracture of the Thoracolumbar Spine

Fracture or dislocation of the thoracolumbar spine is unusual. The typical mechanism is an axial load, as from a fall onto the buttocks from a height or at a relatively rapid speed. The injury is usually a relatively benign compression fracture occurring in the lower thoracic spine or at the thoracolumbar junction. Some compression fractures are not easily seen on plain radiographs (Fig. 33.8). When there is significant pain or tenderness using spot radiographs, CT or MRI can aid in identification and localization of the fracture. Any neurologic findings require special evaluation.

Treatment of spine fractures generally falls into two categories: closed and open. With closed treatment, the fracture is reduced if necessary, and the patient is immobilized in a body cast. Reduction is the primary technique for decompression of the spinal cord. If reduction is not required, the patient is fitted with a brace for comfort.

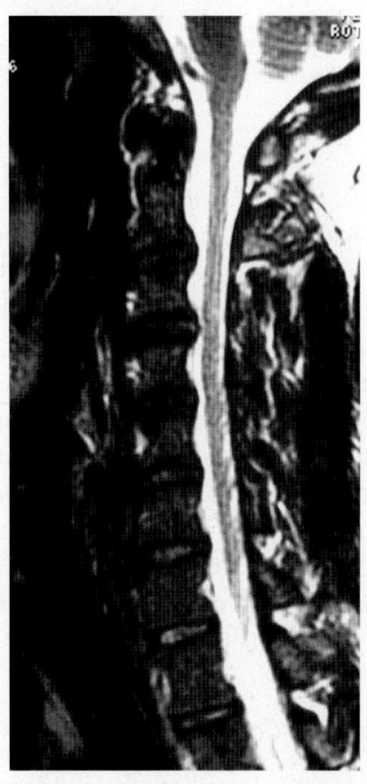

FIG. 33.7 Cervical stenosis. This young college football lineman has a Torg ratio of 0.4 and is at great risk in continuing the sport because of congenital spinal stenosis.

With open treatment, a surgical procedure is performed to reduce or secure severely displaced or unstable fractures. Open procedures are indicated when two or three of the pillars of the vertebral column are disrupted. Internal fixation is usually required. Pedicle screws and rods are the current devices used for posterior fixation. Anterior fixation with plates and screws is less common. Bone grafting to obtain spinal fusion and biologic long-term stabilization are the final parts of the procedure. Factors to consider when deciding when and if an athlete should return to play after spine fracture are healing, rehabilitation, risk of reinjury, and neurologic status.

Sacral Stress Fracture

Sacral stress fractures, more commonly seen in the intrapartum or postpartum period of pregnancy or elderly osteoporotic patients, also can occur in individuals participating in running sports, typically at an elite level. Large series studies are not available on this condition, and most literature consists of case reports. Pain is often localized to the low back and buttocks.[151] Diagnosis is made using plain radiographs and MRI or CT scan. Treatment includes a brief period of limited weight bearing followed by progressive mobilization, physical therapy, and return to sport in 1 to 2 months, after the pain has resolved. Addressing nutritional status and calcium/vitamin D intake are important in preventing repeat stress fractures.[152] Gait and running analysis can also be performed to assist in recovery and prevention.

Iliac Apophysitis

Apophyseal injuries are a unique injury in adolescent athletes, and are associated with skeletal immaturity and repetitive microtrauma. With iliac apophysis involvement, the patient usually presents with back pain localized to the iliac crest, which facilitates diagnosis. There is local tenderness, which is

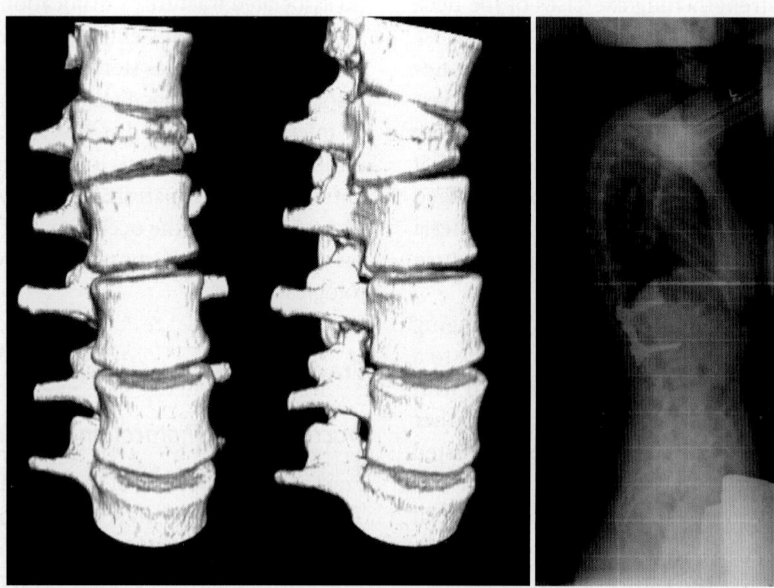

FIG. 33.8 Thoracolumbar fracture in a 16-year-old horsewoman. The fracture was aligned and stabilized by three-level fusion. Anatomic details are clear on this three-dimensional computed tomographic scan.

exacerbated by resisted lateral bending and extension. Radiographs are normal. The treatment is conservative for 3 to 6 weeks, during which time the pain predictably resolves. Bone stimulators have been successfully used in refractory cases.[153] Greater trochanter apophysitis has also been described in an adolescent athlete, whose radiographs showed a widened sclerotic apophysis. The patient had resolution of pain and symptoms after conservative management.[154]

The typical athlete affected is an adolescent runner. Clancy and Foltz[155] described a series of 21 young distance runners, in all of whom pain resolved with alteration of training and rest. As the apophysis closes at the end of growth, even the most recalcitrant cases resolve, similar to Osgood-Schlatter disease of the knee. There are a couple of case reports of avulsion of the apophysis in older teenagers that was surgically repaired, but this is rare.[156,157]

Tumor

Spine cancers in children are rare. Children 7 to 15 years old with spine infection or tumor tend to present with back, pelvic, or abdominal pain.[158] Intradural spinal metastasis pain is a characteristically cramping pain. The physician should take note of back pain that increases with recumbency and keeps the patient awake at night. Progressive pain is characteristic of tumors, not trauma-induced pain. The pain of cancer tends to be constant.

Neoplasia of the spine may originate in either the neural or the osseous elements. Most bony spine tumors of childhood are benign, but they usually cause pain or an irritative scoliosis (Fig. 33.9). Osteoid osteoma is a small, sclerotic, irritative lesion of the posterior spinal elements. The pain is worse at night, and is relieved by aspirin or other antiinflammatory drugs. Although the natural history is for spontaneous resolution of the pain over years, patients do not often tolerate long-term pain well.

Osteoblastoma is a larger version of the same process. Osteoid osteoma and osteoblastoma may manifest as stiffness or scoliosis with or without pain. The lesion may not be apparent on plain radiographs. Bone scan is intensely positive and an excellent first supplemental imaging study in children.

Eosinophilic granuloma in the spine produces a flattening of the vertebra, or *vertebra plana,* rarely with neurologic compromise. Some degree of vertebral regrowth occurs with time in this benign condition. Conservative treatment is indicated if the diagnosis is clear.

Bony malignancies are rare and include leukemia, Ewing sarcoma, and osteosarcoma in bone, and neuroblastoma or astrocytoma in the spinal cord. In the absence of actual bone destruction, these tumors may show subtle signs of pressure owing to their growth, such as separation or thinning of the pedicles or scoliosis.

Spinal cord tumors, such as astrocytoma or ependymoma, are more likely to manifest as extremity weakness, gait disturbance, or scoliosis. Precisely because they are rare, these serious lesions should always be kept in mind. MRI is the study of choice for diagnosis.

PEARLS

1. Back pain in an active adolescent athlete is due to spondylolysis until proven otherwise.
2. An open-ended history taken from the patient is the most cost-effective diagnostic tool and worth the time.

PITFALLS

1. Do not perform a cursory nonfocused history and examination for adolescent back pain.
2. Do not jump to surgery before implementing effective nonoperative treatment for back pain.

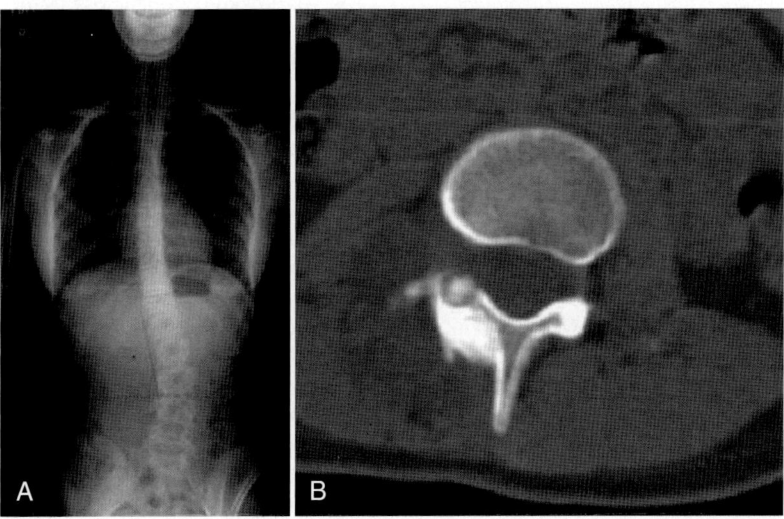

FIG. 33.9 Osteoid osteoma. Tumor did not show on magnetic resonance imaging done for this 14-year-old softball pitcher who presented with back pain and scoliosis. (A) The single-photon emission computed tomographic (CT) scan was hot at L3. (B) This computed tomographic scan clearly delineates pathologic lesion. Irritative scoliosis corrected spontaneously after the tumor was excised.

KEY POINTS

1. Most spine sports injuries in children are chronic injuries resulting from overuse rather than acute injuries secondary to direct trauma.
2. Encouraging the patient to relate his or her history by attentive listening is helpful in determining a differential diagnosis more quickly and accurately.
3. The most common cause of chronic back pain in adolescent athletes is stress fracture or spondylolysis.
4. Sports employing repeated hyperextension maneuvers, such as gymnastics, provide the mechanism for increased stress on the pars interarticularis, which is the site of spondylolysis.
5. Screening radiographs seldom augment a benign history in making a diagnosis. For patients who do not improve in 3 to 4 weeks, CT and MRI can be helpful for diagnosis.
6. Nonoperative treatment is effective for most back pain in children. Spondylolysis, spondylolisthesis, or the rare condition HNP may require operative treatment. Vigorous postoperative rehabilitation may return the athlete to sport.

KEY REFERENCES

1. Bono CM. Low back pain in athletes. *J Bone Joint Surg Am.* 2004;86:382-396.
   This review focuses on spondylolysis and degenerative lumbar disc disease as the major sources of chronic pain in athletes, while pointing out that most low back pain in athletes is due to self-limited sprains or strains. Although these injuries usually respond to nonoperative treatment, the author found direct repair of recalcitrant defects to be the usual course recommended in the literature. Whether the disc changes are worse than changes seen in the general population is debatable. The author advocates anterior interbody fusion for a patient who does not respond to a directed conservative program.
2. Brodke DS, Ritter SM. Nonoperative management of low back pain and lumbar disc degeneration. *J Bone Joint Surg Am.* 2004;86:1810-1818.
   This review article summarizes the treatment options for nonspecific low back pain, including bed rest, medications, physical therapy, manipulation, braces, and injections. The authors acknowledge that a specific pain generator should be sought and that scientific evidence is lacking to support any particular mode of treatment.
3. Ginsburg GM, Bassett GS. Back pain in children and adolescents: evaluation and differential diagnosis. *J Am Acad Orthop Surg.* 1997;5:67-78.
   The authors document the differential diagnosis for back pain in children to include spondylolysis, spondylolisthesis, Scheuermann kyphosis, disc herniations, infections, and tumors. They discuss the appropriate tests for early detection and treatment with a rationale for selecting the most appropriate study.
4. McGill SM. Low back exercises: evidence for improving exercise regimens. *Phys Ther.* 1998;78:754-765.
   This review article documents the biomechanical evidence from the laboratory that can be used to guide the scientific choice of an exercise program for back pain. The author recommends that an exercise program load tissues to strengthen them, while avoiding injury from overexertion. The relative importance of strength, flexibility, and endurance is explored. Specific exercises are described to enhance the stability of the back for rehabilitation and health maintenance.
5. Salminen JJ, Erkintalo MO, Pentti J, et al. Recurrent low back pain and early disc degeneration in the young. *Spine.* 1999;24:1316-1321.
   The authors studied a group of 14-year-old Finnish boys and girls prospectively who had chronic low back pain and compared them with a similar sample of 40 patients who were asymptomatic. The risk of reporting recurrent low back pain up to age 23 years was 16 times as high in the group with early degenerative disc findings. Significant changes included disc protrusion and Scheuermann-type changes on MRI of the lumbar spine.
6. Standaert CJ, Herring SA. Spondylolysis: a critical review. *Br J Sports Med.* 2000;34:415-422.
   The authors based their review on more than 125 articles addressing spondylolysis. They found no controlled clinical trials. Their conclusions were that isthmic spondylolysis is a fatigue fracture of the pars interarticularis, which is more often symptomatic in adolescent athletes. Treatment by activity modification and exercise is usually successful, with symptomatic relief occurring with or without healing of the skeletal defect. Multiple imaging studies have been recommended, and bracing was used in some studies. Rarely, surgery is indicated.

REFERENCES

1. Hardy I, McFaull S, Saint-Vill D. Neck and spine injuries in Canadian cheerleaders: an increasing trend. *J Pediatr Surg.* 2015;50:790-792.
2. Moroder P, Runer A, Hoffelner T, et al. A prospective study of snowkiting injuries. *Am J Sports Med.* 2011;39:1534-1540.
3. Daniels DJ, Clarke MJ, Puffer R, et al. High occurrence of head and spine injuries in the pediatric population following motocross accidents. *J Neurosurg Pediatr.* 2015;15:261-265.
4. Meehan WP, Mannix R. A substantial proportion of life-threatening injuries are sport-related. *Pediatr Emerg Care.* 2013;29:624-627.
5. Fredrickson B, Baker D, McHolick WJ, et al. The natural history of spondylolysis and spondylolisthesis. *J Bone Joint Surg Am.* 1984;66:699-707.
6. Langewitz W, Denz M, Keller A, et al. Spontaneous talking time at start of consultation in outpatient clinic: cohort study. *BMJ.* 2002;325:682-683.
7. Rydevik B. Neurophysiology of cauda equina compression. *Acta Orthop Scand Suppl.* 1993;251:52-55.
8. Waddell G, McCulloch JA, Kummel E, et al. Nonorganic physical signs in low-back pain. *Spine.* 1980;5:117-125.
9. Ala-Kokko L. Genetic risk factors for lumbar disc disease. *Ann Med.* 2002;34:42-47.
10. Solovieva S, Leino-Arjas P, Saarela J, et al. Possible association of interleukin 1 gene locus polymorphisms with low back pain. *Pain.* 2004;109:8-19.
11. Tolonen J, Gronblad M, Virri J, et al. Oncoprotein c-Fos and c-Jun immunopositive cells and cell clusters in herniated intervertebral disc tissue. *Eur Spine J.* 2002;11:452-458.
12. Wang YJ, Lu WJ, Shi Q, et al. Gene expression profile of degenerated cervical intervertebral disc tissues in rats. *Chin J Traumatol.* 2004;7:330-340.
13. Sharma S, et al. Genome-wide association studies of adolescent idiopathic scoliosis suggest candidate susceptibility genes. *Hum Mol Genet.* 2011;20:1456-1466.
14. Gorman K, Julien C, Moreau A. The genetic epidemiology of idiopathic scoliosis. *Eur Spine J.* 2012;21:1905-1919.
15. Ogilvie JW. Update on prognostic genetic testing in adolescent idiopathic scoliosis. *J Pediatr Orthop.* 2011;31:S46-S48.
16. Van Tulder MW, Assendelft WJ, Koes BW, et al. Spinal radiographic findings and nonspecific low back pain: a systematic review of observational studies. *Spine.* 1997;22:427-434.

17. Iwamoto J, Abe H, Tsukimura Y, et al. Relationship between radiographic abnormalities of lumbar spine and incidence of low back pain in high school and college football players: a prospective study. *Am J Sports Med.* 2004;32:781-786.
18. Auerbach JA. *Towards an Evidence-Based Approach for Imaging in Evaluation of Back Pain in Children.* Ottawa, Canada: Pediatric Orthopaedic Society of North America; 2005.
19. Brodke D, Ritter S. Nonoperative management of low back pain and lumbar disc degeneration. *J Bone Joint Surg Am.* 2004;86:1810-1818.
20. Aleksiev AR. Ten-year follow-up of strengthening versus flexibility exercises with or without abdominal bracing in recurrent low back pain. *Spine.* 2014;39:997-1003.
21. van Tulder MW, Jellema P, van Poppel MN, et al. Lumbar supports for prevention and treatment of low back pain. *Cochrane Database Syst Rev.* 2000;(3):CD001823.
22. Kawchuk GN, Edgecombe T, Wong A, Cojocaru A, Prasad N. A non-randomized clinical trial on the impact of non-rigid, inelastic corsets on spine function in low back pain participants and asymptomatic controls. *Spine J.* 2015. Epub ahead of print.
23. Ramos G, Martin W. Effects of vertebral axial decompression on intradiscal pressure. *J Neurosurg.* 1994;81:350-353.
24. Wegner I, Widyahening IS, van Tulder MW, et al. Traction for low-back pain with or without sciatica. *Cochrane Database Syst Rev.* 2013;(8):CD003010.
25. Saal JA, Saal JS. Nonoperative treatment of herniated lumbar intervertebral disc with radiculopathy: an outcome study. *Spine.* 1989;14:431-437.
26. Bridger RS, Orkin D, Henneberg M. A quantitative investigation of lumbar and pelvic postures in standing and sitting: interrelationships with body position and hip muscle length. *Int J Indust Ergonom.* 1992;9:235-244.
27. McGill SM, Norman RW. Low back biomechanics in industry in the prevention of injury. In: Grabiner M, ed. *Current Issues in Biomechanics.* Champaign, IL: Human Kinetics Publishers; 1992.
28. Alaranta H, Luoto S, Heliovaara M, et al. Static back endurance and the risk of low-back pain. *Clin Biomech (Bristol, Avon).* 1995;10:323-324.
29. Dowzer CN, Reilly T, Cable NT. Effects of deep and shallow water running on spinal shrinkage. *Br J Sports Med.* 1998;32:44-48.
30. Dowzer CN, Reilly T, Cable NT, et al. Maximal physiological responses to deep and shallow water running. *Ergonomics.* 1999;42:275-281.
31. Reilly T, Dowzer CN, Cable NT. The physiology of deep-water running. *J Sports Sci.* 2003;21:959-972.
32. McGill SM. Low back exercises: evidence for improving exercise regimens. *Phys Ther.* 1998;78:754-765.
33. McGill S. Low back exercises: prescription for the healthy back and when recovering from injury. In: *Resource Manual for Guidelines for Exercise Testing and Prescription.* 7th ed. Indianapolis: American College of Sports Medicine; 2005.
34. McGill SM. The biomechanics of low back injury: implications on current practice in industry and the clinic. *J Biomech.* 1997;30:465-475.
35. Nutter P. Aerobic exercise in the treatment and prevention of low back pain. *Occup Med.* 1988;3:137-145.
36. Adams MA, Dolan P. Recent advances in lumbar spinal mechanics and their clinical significance. *Clin Biomech (Bristol, Avon).* 1995;10:3-19.
37. Potvin J, Norman R: Can fatigue compromise lifting safety? In: *Proceedings of the Second North American Congress on Biomechanics*, Chicago, August 24-28, 1992, pp 513-514.
38. Frost H, Lamb SE, Doll HA, et al. Randomised controlled trial of physiotherapy compared with advice for low back pain. *BMJ.* 2004;329:708.
39. Haus BM, Micheli LJ. Back pain in the pediatric and adolescent athlete. *Clin Sports Med.* 2012;31:423-440.
40. Young WK, d'Hemecourt PA. Back pain in adolescent athletes. *Phys Sportsmed.* 2011;39:80-89.
41. King HA. Back pain in children. *Pediatr Clin North Am.* 1984;31:1083-1095.
42. Bhatia NN, Chow G, Timon SJ, Watts HG. Diagnostic modalities for the evaluation of pediatric back pain. *J Pediatr Orthop.* 2008;28:230-233.
43. Loud KJ, Micheli LJ. Common athletic injuries in adolescent girls. *Curr Opin Pediatr.* 2001;13:317-322.
44. Stoev I, Powers AK, Puglisi JA, Munro R, Leonard JR. Sacroiliac joint pain in pediatric population. *J Neurosurg Pediatr.* 2012;9:602-607.
45. Nachemson AL. Advances in low-back pain. *Clin Orthop Relat Res.* 1985;201:266-278.
46. Andersson G. The epidemiology of spinal disorders. In: Frymoyer J, Weinstein J, Ducker T, et al., eds. *The Adult Spine: Principles and Practice.* Philadelphia: Lippincott-Raven; 1991:107-146.
47. Szpalski M, Gunzburg R, Balague F, et al. A 2-year prospective longitudinal study on low back pain in primary school children. *Eur Spine J.* 2002;11:459-464.
48. Adams MA, Dolan P, Hutton WC, et al. Diurnal changes in spinal mechanics and their clinical significance. *J Bone Joint Surg Br.* 1990;72:266-270.
49. Snook SH, Webster BS, McGorry RW, et al. The reduction of chronic nonspecific low back pain through the control of early morning lumbar flexion: a randomized controlled trial. *Spine.* 1998;23:2601-2607.
50. Cyron BM, Hutton WC. The fatigue strength of the lumbar neural arch in spondylolysis. *J Bone Joint Surg Br.* 1978;60:234-238.
51. Herman MJ, Pizzutillo PD, Cavalier R. Spondylolysis and spondylolisthesis in the child and adolescent athlete. *Orthop Clin North Am.* 2003;34:461-467.
52. Jackson DW, Wiltse LL, Cirincoine RJ. Spondylolysis in the female gymnast. *Clin Orthop Relat Res.* 1976;117:68-73.
53. Soler T, Calderon C. The prevalence of spondylolysis in the Spanish elite athlete. *Am J Sports Med.* 2000;28:57-62.
54. El-Rassi G, Takemitsu M, Glutting J, et al. Clinical outcome and return to athletics after nonoperative treatment of spondylolysis in children. Presented at Scoliosis Research Society, Buenos Aires, 2004.
55. Bono CM. Low-back pain in athletes. *J Bone Joint Surg Am.* 2004;86:382-396.
56. Logroscino G, Mazza O, Aulisa G, et al. Spondylolysis and spondylolisthesis in the pediatric and adolescent population. *Childs Nerv Syst.* 2001;17:644-655.
57. Beck NA, Miller MS, Baldwin K, et al. Do oblique views add value in the diagnosis of spondylosis in adolescents? *J Bone Joint Surg.* 2013;95:e65(1-7).
58. Rush JK, Astur N, Scott S, et al. Use of magnetic resonance imaging in the evaluation of spondylolysis. *J Pediatr Orthop.* 2015;35:271-275.
59. Leono A, Cianfoni A, Cerase A, et al. Lumbar spondylolysis: a review. *Skeletal Radiol.* 2011;40(6):683-700.

60. Alkhawaldeh K, Ghuweri AA, Kawar J, Jaafreh A. Back pain in children and diagnostic value of MDP bone scintigraphy. *Acta Inform Med.* 2014;22:297-301.
61. Cavalier R, Herman MJ, Cheung EV, et al. Spondylolysis and spondylolisthesis in children and adolescents: I. Diagnosis, natural history, and nonsurgical management. *J Am Acad Orthop Surg.* 2006;14:417-424.
62. McNeely ML, Torrance G, Magee DJ. A systematic review of physiotherapy for spondylolysis and spondylolisthesis. *Man Ther.* 2003;8:80-91.
63. O'Sullivan PB, Phyty GD, Twomey LT, et al. Evaluation of specific stabilizing exercise in the treatment of chronic low back pain with radiologic diagnosis of spondylolysis or spondylolisthesis. *Spine.* 1997;22:2959-2967.
64. Salminen JJ, Erkintalo MO, Pentti J, et al. Recurrent low back pain and early disc degeneration in the young. *Spine.* 1999;24:1316-1321.
65. Vrable A, Sherman AL. Elite male adolescent gymnast who achieved union of a persistent bilateral pars defect. *Am J Phys Med Rehabil.* 2009;88(2):156-160.
66. Sairyo K, Sakai T, Yasui N, Dezama A. Conservative treatment for pediatric lumbar spondylolysis to achieve bone healing using a hard brace: what type and how long? *J Neurosurg Spine.* 2012;16:610-614.
67. Standaert CJ, Herring SA. Spondylolysis: a critical review. *Br J Sports Med.* 2000;34:415-422.
68. Dubousset J. Treatment of spondylolysis and spondylolisthesis in children and adolescents. *Clin Orthop Relat Res.* 1997;337:77-85.
69. Cheung EV, Herman MJ, Cavalier R, et al. Spondylolysis and spondylolisthesis in children and adolescents: II. Surgical management. *J Am Acad Orthop Surg.* 2006;14:488-498.
70. Chen JF, Lee ST. A physiological method for the repair of young adult simple isthmic lumbar spondylolysis. *Chang Gung Med J.* 2000;23:92-98.
71. Alton TB, Patel AM, Lee MJ, Chapman JR. Pediatric cervical spine spondylolysis and American football. *Spine J.* 2014;14:e1-e5.
72. Labelle H, Roussouly P, Berthonnaud E, et al. Spondylolisthesis, pelvic incidence, and spinopelvic balance: a correlation study. *Spine.* 2004;29:2049-2054.
73. Curylo LJ, Edwards C, DeWald RW. Radiographic markers in spondyloptosis: implications for spondylolisthesis progression. *Spine.* 2002;27:2021-2025.
74. Berk RH. [Lumbar spine injuries in pediatric and adolescent athletes]. *Acta Orthop Traumatol Turc.* 2004;38(suppl 1):S58-S63.
75. Wimberly RL, Lauerman WC. Spondylolisthesis in the athlete. *Clin Sports Med.* 2002;21:133-145.
76. Teitz CC, Cook DM. Rehabilitation of neck and low back injuries. *Clin Sports Med.* 1985;4:455-476.
77. Burkus JK, Lonstein JE, Winter RB, et al. Long-term evaluation of adolescents treated operatively for spondylolisthesis: a comparison of in situ arthrodesis only with in situ arthrodesis and reduction followed by immobilization in a cast. *J Bone Joint Surg Am.* 1992;74:693-704.
78. Lonstein JE. Spondylolisthesis in children: cause, natural history, and management. *Spine.* 1999;24:2640-2648.
79. Zindrick MR, Wiltse LL, Doornik A, et al. Analysis of the morphometric characteristics of the thoracic and lumbar pedicles. *Spine.* 1987;12:160-166.
80. Sorensen K. *Scheuermann's Juvenile Kyphosis: Clinical Appearances, Radiography, Aetiology and Prognosis.* Copenhagen: Mundsgaard; 1964.
81. Commandre F, Gagnerie G, Zakarian M. The child, the spine and sports. *J Sports Med Phys Fitness.* 1988;28:11-19.
82. Goldstein J, Berger P, Windier G. Spine injuries in gymnasts and swimmers: an epidemiologic investigation. *Am J Sports Med.* 1991;19:463-468.
83. Hellstrom M, Jacobsson B, Sward L. Radiologic abnormalities of the thoraco-lumbar spine in athletes. *Acta Radiol.* 1990;31:127-132.
84. Matheson G, Clement D, McKenzie D. Stress fractures in athletes: a study of 320 cases. *Am J Sports Med.* 1987;15:46-58.
85. Micheli L. Low back pain in the adolescent: differential diagnosis. *Am J Sports Med.* 1979;7:362-364.
86. Ohlen G, Wredmark T, Spangfort E. Spinal sagittal configuration and mobility related to low-back pain in the female gymnast. *Spine.* 1989;14:847-850.
87. Sward L, Hellstrom M, Jacobsson B. Back pain and radiologic changes in the thoraco-lumbar spine of athletes. *Spine.* 1990;15:124-129.
88. Sward L, Hellstrom M, Jacobsson B. Disc degeneration and associated abnormalities of the spine in elite gymnasts: a magnetic resonance imaging study. *Spine.* 1991;16:437-443.
89. Sward L, Hellstrom M, Jacobsson B. Vertebral ring apophysis injury in athletes: is the etiology different in the thoracic and lumbar spine? *Am J Sports Med.* 1993;21:841-845.
90. Tall R, DeVault W. Spinal injury in sport: epidemiologic considerations. *Clin Orthop Relat Res.* 1993;12:441-448.
91. Tsai L, Wredmark T. Spinal posture, sagittal mobility, and subjective rating of back problems in former female elite gymnasts. *Spine.* 1993;18:872-875.
92. Greene T, Hensinger R, Hunter L. Back pain and vertebral changes simulating Scheuermann's disease. *J Pediatr Orthop.* 1985;5:1-7.
93. Sward L, Eriksson B, Peterson L. Anthropometric characteristics, passive hip flexion, and spinal mobility in relation to back pain in athletes. *Spine.* 1990;15:376-382.
94. Schmorl G. Zur Kenntnis der Wirbelkorperepiphyse und der an ihr vorkommenden Verletzungen. *Arch Klin Chir.* 1928;153:35-45.
95. Siffert R. Classification of the osteochondroses. *Clin Orthop Relat Res.* 1981;158:10-18.
96. Heithoff KB, Gundry CR, Burton CV, et al. Juvenile discogenic disease. *Spine.* 1994;19:335-340.
97. Dimar JR 2nd, Glassman SD, Carreon LY. Juvenile degenerative disc disease: a report of 76 cases identified by magnetic resonance imaging. *Spine J.* 2007;7:332-337.
98. Durham SR, Sun PP, Sutton LN. Surgically treated lumbar disc disease in the pediatric population: an outcome study. *J Neurosurg.* 2000;92:1-6.
99. Epstein JA, Epstein NE, Marc J, et al. Lumbar intervertebral disk herniation in teenage children: recognition and management of associated anomalies. *Spine.* 1984;9:427-432.
100. Ishihara H, Matsui H, Hirano N, et al. Lumbar intervertebral disc herniation in children less than 16 years of age: long-term follow-up study of surgically managed cases. *Spine.* 1997;22:2044-2049.
101. Martinez-Lage JF, Poza M, Arcas P. Avulsed lumbar vertebral rim plate in an adolescent: trauma or malformation? *Childs Nerv Syst.* 1998;14:131-134.

102. Parisini P, Di Silvestre M, Greggi T, et al. Lumbar disc excision in children and adolescents. *Spine.* 2001;26:1997-2000.
103. Ikata T, Morita T, Katoh S, et al. Lesions of the lumbar posterior end plate in children and adolescents: an MRI study. *J Bone Joint Surg Br.* 1995;77:951-955.
104. Sassmannshausen G, Smith BG. Back pain in the young athlete. *Clin Sports Med.* 2002;21:121-132.
105. DeLuca PF, Mason DE, Weiand R, et al. Excision of herniated nucleus pulposus in children and adolescents. *J Pediatr Orthop.* 1994;14:318-322.
106. Shillito J Jr. Pediatric lumbar disc surgery: 20 patients under 15 years of age. *Surg Neurol.* 1996;46:14-18.
107. Ginsburg GM, Bassett GS. Back pain in children and adolescents: evaluation and differential diagnosis. *J Am Acad Orthop Surg.* 1997;5:67-78.
108. Gibson J, Waddell G. Surgery for degenerative lumbar spondylosis. *Cochrane Database Syst Rev.* 2005;(2):CD001352.
109. Hassard GH, Carmack WL, Dixon J, et al. Rehabilitation: a team approach to total patient care. The rehabilitation team. *J Pract Nurs.* 1978;28:22-25.
110. Lavelle WF, Bianco A, Mason R, Betz R, Albanese S. Pediatric disk herniation. *J Am Acad Orthop Surg.* 2011;19:649-656.
111. Papagelopoulos PJ, Shaughnessy WJ, Ebersold MJ, et al. Long-term outcome of lumbar discectomy in children and adolescents sixteen years of age or younger. *J Bone Joint Surg Am.* 1998;80:689-698.
112. Slotkin JR, Mislow JMK, Day AL, Proctor MR. Pediatric disk disease. *Neurosurg Clin N Am.* 2007;18:659-667.
113. Dang L, Liu Z. A review of current treatment for lumbar disc herniation in children and adolescents. *Eur Spine J.* 2010;19:205-224.
114. Beggs I, Addison J. Posterior vertebral rim fractures. *Br J Radiol.* 1998;71:567-572.
115. Skobowytsh-Okolot B. "Posterior apophysis" in L.IV—the cause of neuroradicular disturbance. *Acta Orthop Scand.* 1962;32:341-351.
116. Banerian KG, Wang AM, Samberg LC, et al. Association of vertebral end plate fracture with pediatric lumbar intervertebral disk herniation: value of CT and MR imaging. *Radiology.* 1990;177:763-765.
117. Dietemann JL, Runge M, Badoz A, et al. Radiology of posterior lumbar apophyseal ring fractures: report of 13 cases. *Neuroradiology.* 1988;30:337-344.
118. Dang L, Liu Z. A review of current treatment for lumbar disc herniation in children and adolescents. *Eur Spine J.* 2010;19:205-224.
119. Keller RH. Traumatic displacement of the cartilaginous vertebral rim: a sign of intervertebral disc prolapse. *Radiology.* 1974;110:21-24.
120. Lippit A. Fracture of the vertebral body end plate and disk protrusion causing subarachnoid block in an adolescent. *Clin Orthop Relat Res.* 1974;11:112-115.
121. Miyagi R, Sairyo K, Sakai T, et al. Persistent tight hamstrings following conservative treatment for apophyseal ring fracture in adolescent athletes: critical appraisal. *J Med Invest.* 2014;61:446-451.
122. Wu X, Ma W, Du H. A review of current treatment of lumbar posterior ring apophysis fracture with lumbar disc herniation. *Eur Spine J.* 2013;22:475-488.
123. Rihn JA, Anderson DT, Lamb K, et al. Cervical spine injuries in American football. *Sports Med.* 2009;39:697-708.
124. Proctor MR, Cantu RC. Head and neck injuries in young athletes. *Clin Sports Med.* 2000;19:693-715.
125. Kleiner D, Almquist J, Bailes J, et al. *Prehospital Care of the Spine-Injured Athlete: A Document from the Inter-Association Task Force for Appropriate Care of the Spine-Injured Athlete.* Dallas: National Athletic Trainers Association; 2001.
126. Cantu RC, Mueller FO. Catastrophic spine injuries in football (1977-1989). *J Spinal Disord.* 1990;3:227-231.
127. Cantu RC, Mueller FO. Catastrophic football injuries: 1977-1998. *Neurosurgery.* 2000;47:673-675.
128. Cantu RC, Mueller FO. Catastrophic spine injuries in American football, 1977-2001. *Neurosurgery.* 2003;53: 358-362.
129. Cantu RC, Mueller FO. Brain injury-related fatalities in American football, 1945-1999. *Neurosurgery.* 2003;52: 846-852.
130. Mueller FO, Cantu RC. Catastrophic injuries and fatalities in high school and college sports, fall 1982-spring 1988. *Med Sci Sports Exerc.* 1990;22:737-741.
131. Mueller FO, Cantu RC. The annual survey of catastrophic football injuries: 1977-1988. *Exerc Sport Sci Rev.* 1991;19:261-312.
132. Paulus S, Kennedy DJ. Return to play consideration for cervical spine injuries in athletes. *Phys Med Rehabil Clin N Am.* 2014;25:723-733.
133. Dailey A, Harrop JS, France JC. High-energy contact sports and cervical spine neuropraxia injuries. *Spine.* 2010;35:S193-S201.
134. Kepler CK, Vaccaro AR. Injuries and abnormalities of the cervical spine and return to play criteria. *Clin Sports Med.* 2012;31:499-508.
135. Meyer SA, Schulte KR, Callaghan JJ, et al. Cervical spinal stenosis and stingers in collegiate football players. *Am J Sports Med.* 1994;22:158-166.
136. Albright JP, McAuley E, Martin RK, et al. Head and neck injuries in college football: an eight-year analysis. *Am J Sports Med.* 1985;13:147-152.
137. Albright JP, VanGilder J, el Khoury GY, et al. Head and neck injuries in sports. In: Scott WN, Nisonson B, Nicholas JA, eds. *Principles of Sports Medicine.* Baltimore: Williams & Wilkins; 1984:40-86.
138. Bergfeld JA, Hershman E, Wilbourn A. Brachial plexus injury in sports: a five year follow-up. *Orthop Trans.* 1988;12:743-744.
139. Clancy WG Jr, Brand RL, Bergfield JA. Upper trunk brachial plexus injuries in contact sports. *Am J Sports Med.* 1977;5:209-216.
140. Funk FF, Wells RE. Injuries of the cervical spine in football. *Clin Orthop Relat Res.* 1975;109:50-58.
141. Rockett FX. Observations on the "burner": traumatic cervical radiculopathy. *Clin Orthop Relat Res.* 1982;164:18-19.
142. Speer KP, Bassett FH 3rd. The prolonged burner syndrome. *Am J Sports Med.* 1990;18:591-594.
143. Watkins RG. Neck injuries in football players. *Clin Sports Med.* 1986;5:215-246.
144. Quan D, Bird SJ. Nerve conduction studies and electromyography in the evaluation of peripheral nerve injuries. *Univ Pa Orthop J.* 1999;12:45-51.
145. Seddon HJ. Three types of nerve injuries. *Brain.* 1943;66:237.
146. Sunderland SA. A classification of peripheral nerve injuries producing loss of function. *Brain.* 1951;74:491-516.
147. Eismont FJ, Clifford S, Goldberg M, et al. Cervical sagittal spinal canal size in spine injury. *Spine.* 1984;9:663-666.

148. Castro FP Jr, Ricciardi J, Brunet ME, et al. Stingers, the Torg ratio, and the cervical spine. *Am J Sports Med.* 1997;25:603-608.
149. Torg JS, Pavlov H, Genuario SE, et al. Neurapraxia of the cervical spinal cord with transient quadriplegia. *J Bone Joint Surg Am.* 1986;68:1354-1370.
150. Pavlov H, Torg JS, Robie B, et al. Cervical spinal stenosis: determination with vertebral body ratio method. *Radiology.* 1987;164:771-775.
151. Kahanov L, Eberman L, Games K, Wasik M. Diagnosis, treatment and rehabilitation of stress fractures in the lower extremity in runners. *Open Access J Sports Med.* 2015;6:87-95.
152. Longhino V, Bonora C, Sansone V. The management of sacral stress fractures: current concepts. *Clin Cases Miner Bone Metab.* 2011;8:19-23.
153. Kivel CG, d'Hemecourt CA, Micheli LJ. Treatment of iliac crest apophysitis in the young athlete with bone stimulation: report of 2 cases. *Clin J Sport Med.* 2011;21:144-147.
154. Young S, Safran M. Greater trochanter apophysitis in the adolescent athlete. *Clin J sport Med.* 2015;25:e57-e58.
155. Clancy WG Jr, Foltz AS. Iliac apophysitis and stress fractures in adolescent runners. *Am J Sports Med.* 1976;4:214-218.
156. Doral MN, Aydog ST, Tetik O, et al. Multiple osteochondroses and avulsion fracture of anterior superior iliac spine in a soccer player. *Br J Sports Med.* 2005;39:e16.
157. Pointinger H, Munk P, Poeschl GP. Avulsion fracture of the anterior superior iliac spine following apophysitis. *Br J Sports Med.* 2003;37:361-362.
158. Dormans JP, Moroz L. Infection and tumors of the spine in children. *J Bone Joint Surg Am.* 2007;89(suppl 1):79-97.

CHAPTER 34 Congenital Anomalies of the Cervical Spine

Robert F. Murphy
Daniel J. Hedequist
Michael P. Glotzbecker

Introduction

Congenital anomalies of the cervical spine are an infrequent occurrence; physicians who manage children with these anomalies must be involved in the total care of the patient. Other anomalies are frequently present, including vascular, cardiac, renal, and musculoskeletal manifestations. An accurate diagnosis may be delayed because radiographic evaluation of pediatric patients can be difficult, and these anomalies frequently do not manifest until the patient is older.

This chapter is concerned with the evaluation and treatment of congenital anomalies of the pediatric cervical spine. Special consideration will be given to the role of radiographs and advanced imaging in making an accurate diagnosis, as well as surgical stabilization techniques.

Modern Cervical Instrumentation in Children

In the past, the only internal stabilization option available to surgeons treating children with cervical spine disorders was wiring techniques. These wires were traditionally sublaminar and were found to have acceptable rates of fusion and complications for a variety of cervical spine disorders. With advances in technology, screw options are now available for every segment of the cervical spine. Coupled with rigid rod connections, modern segmental screw instrumentation now affords surgeons a powerful and reliable tool to safely stabilize most pediatric cervical spine anomalies. These advanced constructs offer improved options for treating complex deformities associated with poor bone quality. A thorough understanding of the bony, neurologic, and vascular anatomy is paramount to successful implementation of these techniques.

Occipital Plating

Previous fixation options to the occiput included wiring techniques, such as loop-rod constructs. Modern techniques include the placement of occipital screws (most commonly through a plating system), which are then secured to a rod construct. Recent biomechanical data have demonstrated that occipital screws are superior to loop-rod wiring techniques in all planes of motion.[1] Placement of these screws is most commonly at the external occipital protuberance, and computed tomography (CT) scan–based studies have confirmed this as the thickest area of bone available for fixation with the ability to accept unicortical screws at acceptable pullout strength.[2–4] Studies specifically in children aged 2 to 6 years have confirmed this as the optimal location for screw placement[5] (Fig. 34.1). In a recent review of 70 children treated with occipital plating connected to cervical screws with rods, rates of fusion were high and complications rates were acceptable.[6]

C1 Screws

In congenital anomalies, sublaminar wiring of C1 in children is not always feasible, as the posterior arch of the atlas is not always completely formed. Furthermore, many procedures about the cervical spine require concomitant decompression of C1, which eliminates the ability to obtain wire fixation. Lateral mass screws can be safely placed in patients as young as 2 years old[5,7,8] (Fig. 34.2). CT studies of C1 in children have provided excellent information on the bony anatomy, including appropriate starting point and screw placement trajectory.

Salient principles of techniques for placement of C1 screws in children include a thorough understanding of the relationship of the vertebral artery to the bone (usually obtained by preoperative CT scan). In children, the location of the vertebral artery is usually closer than the traditional 1.5 cm from the midline, as described in adults,[9] and extra care should be assumed in the setting of congenital anomalies. In order to improve exposure of the starting point, some surgeons sacrifice the root of C2[10]; however, we have not consistently found this to be necessary. Hemostasis and control of the venous plexus found in this area are critical in the safe placement of C1 screws.

C1 lateral mass screw placement is successful in a variety of pediatric pathologies, including atlantoaxial instability, with low rates of complications, resulting in predictable fusion.[6,11,12]

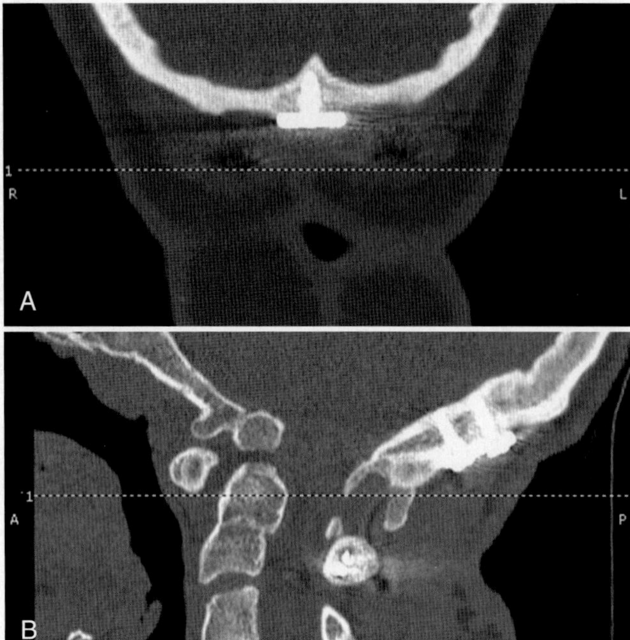

FIG. 34.1 (A) Coronal and (B) sagittal reformatted computed tomographic images showing that the external occipital protuberance is the thickest area of bone available for occipital screw purchase. If concerns of venous sinus penetration are present, unicortical screws may be used with little decrease to the biomechanical strength of the construct.

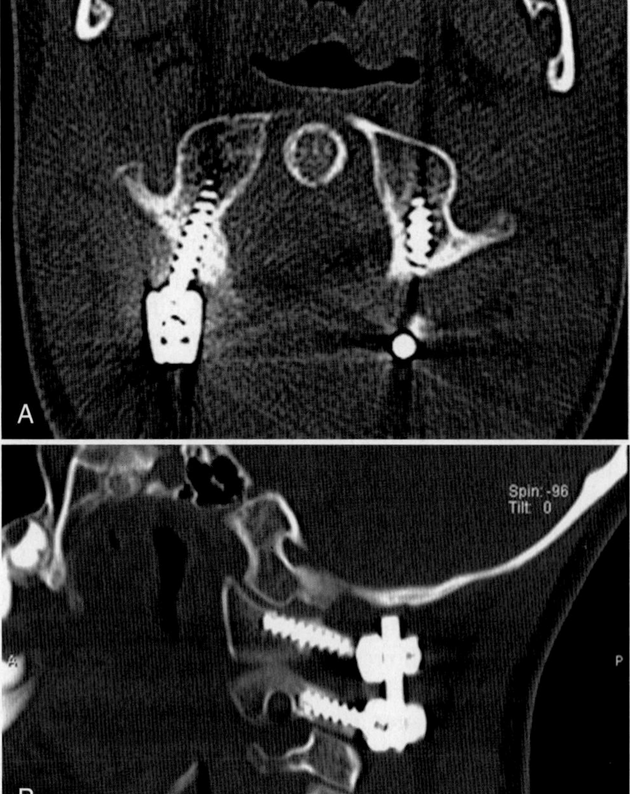

FIG. 34.2 (A) Axial and (B) sagittal reformatted computed tomographic images demonstrating appropriate placement of C1 lateral mass screws.

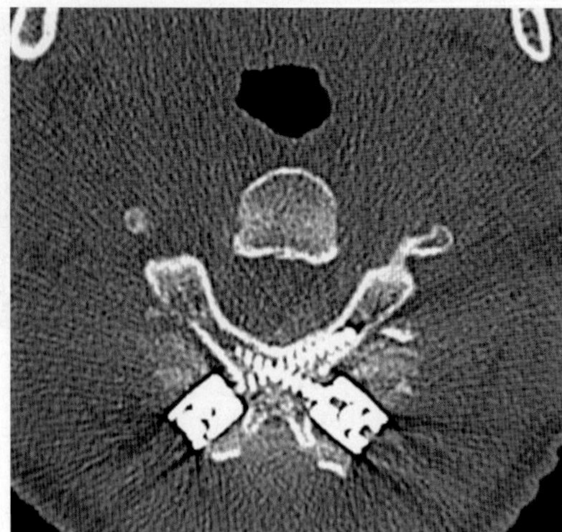

FIG. 34.3 Axial computed tomographic image demonstrating crossed laminar screws at C2.

C2 Screws

C2 is an important segment in pediatric cervical spine fusion constructs, as it can serve as the base of an occipitocervical construct, or the top of a lower cervical construct. Many screw options exist in C2, including laminar screws and pars/pedicle/isthmus screws. With limited space available for the cord at this segment, screw options are an attractive alternative to sublaminar wiring. As in the case of C1, adequate knowledge of the course of the vertebral artery is mandatory for successful implantation.[13]

The spinous process of C2 is the landmark for the entry point for translaminar screws, which are effective for construct rigidity.[14] Clinically, laminar screws are safe and efficacious.[14,15] Canal breach has not been reported in children[11,13] (Fig. 34.3).

Regarding the C2 pars/isthmus/pedicle, there is variability in the terminology. Technically, two separate screw paths exist, but the pars and pedicle are commonly intertwined in a shared mass of bone. Most frequently, surgeons select the course and tract of the screw based on maximum available bony purchase, as well as the location of the vertebral artery and C1–C2 articulation.

Rigid screw fixation, either through pars/pedicle or translaminar screws, is possible in almost all patients. This method serves as an excellent and reliable fixation point in pediatric deformity surgery without injury to the vertebral artery or malposition of screws in the vast majority of patients.[6,11,13]

C1–C2 Transarticular Screws

C1–C2 transarticular screws are a powerful, but challenging, fixation technique. The challenges of screw placement are threefold: dissection of the C2 isthmus must be adequate, dissection of the C1–C2 joint must be complete, and an understanding of the course of the vertebral artery in relation to C1 and C2 must be thorough. Common vertebral artery anomalies that preclude C1–C2 screws include high-riding vessels next to a small isthmus or medially deviated vessels blocking the optimal trajectory. The most common problematic vertebral

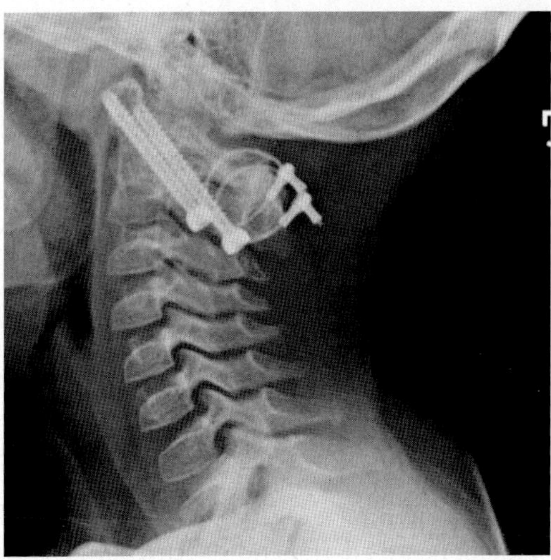

FIG. 34.4 Transarticular C1–C2 screws. Note posterior cables securing bone graft. This construct is powerful and stable if the surgeon is aware of the challenges associated with screw placement.

artery course in relation to C2 is a medial deviation.[13] To complicate matters in pediatric patients, few children younger than age 6 years have anatomy suitable for transarticular screws given either the size of the C2 isthmus or the course of the vertebral artery.[5] However, clinical studies have shown that, even in younger patients, screws may be safely placed if the preoperative imaging demonstrates anatomy that allows for safe screw placement[16,17] (Fig. 34.4). Some authors have found success in children younger than age 4 years, as long as safe anatomy on CT scan can be confirmed.[17,18] In cases of severe bony anomalies or aberrant vertebral artery courses, placement of a unilateral C1–C2 transarticular screw is a biomechanically reasonable consideration.[17]

Subaxial Lateral Mass Screws

Several studies have demonstrated that the use of lateral mass screws in children is safe and effective, as long as preoperative planning principles are maintained.[19,20] We use lateral mass screws for a variety of pediatric conditions. Postoperative CT has shown complete screw containment in all cases and there have been no vertebral artery injuries or postoperative nerve deficits.[19,20] (Fig. 34.5) Although subaxial lateral mass screws can be safely placed in children as young as 4 years, the indications are rare. We do not use cervical pedicle screws in pediatric patients given the cadaveric anatomic studies showing the size of the pedicle is not adequate for safe screw placement in the majority of patients.[21]

Halo

The halo orthosis is a powerful tool with a variety of uses in pediatric cervical spine pathology. In patients who present with substantial and significant deformity, the halo can be used to obtain an effective reduction prior to definitive surgical stabilization. Common principles in application of halo rings to pediatric patients include a greater number of pins

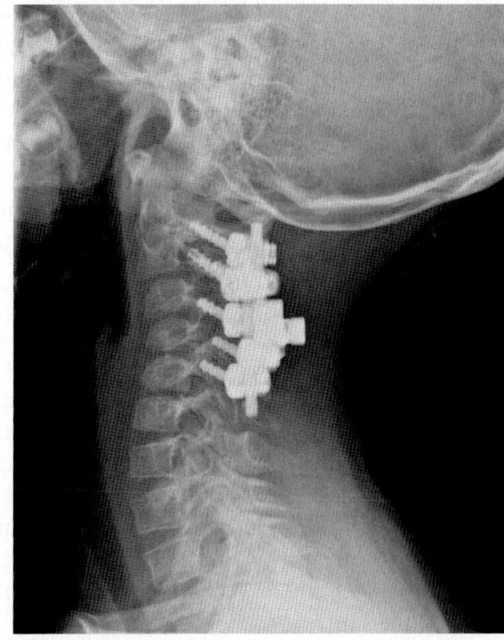

FIG. 34.5 Lateral mass screw placement for cervical instability.

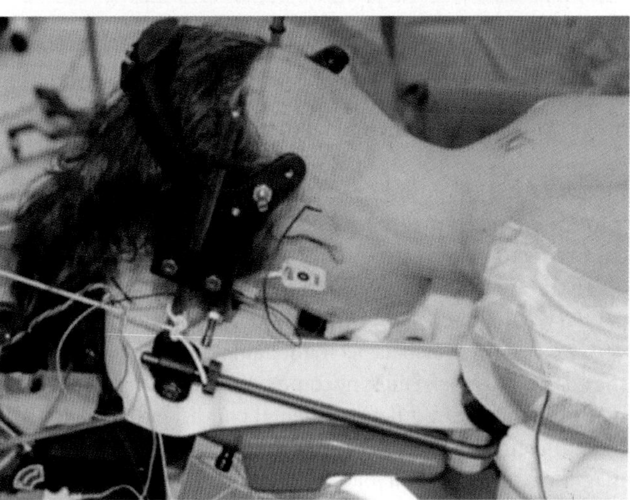

FIG. 34.6 A halo vest orthosis applied intraoperatively can maintain reduction and protect the eyes and face.

than traditionally utilized in adult patients, and less torque per pin. Care should be taken to avoid the supraorbital and supratrochlear nerve. The halo should be applied just superior to the equator of the head.[22]

Application and use of a halo vest orthosis preoperatively can aid the surgeon in maintaining reduction and protecting the patient during surgery. We commonly apply a halo vest orthosis once the patient has undergone general anesthesia. Once a reduction is obtained, the halo vest is secured. The patient is then turned into the prone position and the posterior leaf of the vest is removed. The reduction is reliably maintained for surgery, and pressure is removed from the face and eyes during the procedure (Fig. 34.6). Given the poor bone quality and pseudarthrosis rates in many pediatric cervical conditions, postoperative use of the halo vest provides additional security to the instrumented spine.

Halo vest orthoses are not benign devices; surgeons must use them judiciously. In a large series of patients, complications occurred in over half of patients. Neurologic changes are not rare when utilizing halo traction for reduction, and pin site infections are frequent.[23] This has led some authors to recommend pinless halo systems, which have been found to be safe in a variety of disorders.[24,25] Halo utilization in toddlers should be used with caution, as these children are prone to falls, which may destabilize the halo vest construct.[26]

Navigation

Improvements in image acquisition and computer-based planning software have afforded surgeons the ability to preoperatively plan and skillfully execute surgery using navigation technology. The feasibility and effectiveness of this technology has already been well explored in the thoracic and lumbar spines in pediatric patients.[27–30] New research is emerging on the utilization of this technology and its applications in pediatric cervical spine surgery.[31]

Specific Cervical Spine Conditions

Basilar Invagination

Basilar invagination (or impression) is a deformity of the base of the skull at the foramen magnum. The relationship between the base of the skull and upper cervical spine is altered, and the tip of the odontoid becomes more cephalad, protruding into the foramen magnum. This deformity may encroach on the brain stem, increasing the risk of neurologic damage.

There are two types of basilar impression. The first is a primary congenital abnormality often associated with other vertebral defects, such as occipitoatlantal fusion, hypoplasia of the atlas, or Klippel-Feil syndrome.[32] Secondary basilar invagination is an acquired developmental condition usually attributed to recurrent microfractures in the region of the foramen magnum from the axial load from the skull, which precipitates softening, flattening, and infolding of the posterior skull base. It is a potential sequela of osteogenesis imperfecta, neurofibromatosis, and other osteochondrodysplasias.[33–35]

Clinical Features

Patients with basilar invagination frequently have a deformity of the skull or neck, and may present with torticollis.[36,37] The symptoms (or lack thereof) are difficult to explain,[36,38] but are generally due to encroachment of the neural structures (particularly the medulla oblongata) at the level of the foramen magnum. The neurologic sequelae are determined by the degree of cranial migration of the dens. In addition to the direct compression of the ventral brain stem, the dens creates a fulcrum for traction on the cervical cord. Cerebellar dysfunction may arise from direct compression or reflect secondary herniation from the posterior fossa.

Basilar invagination is frequently associated with other neurologic conditions, such as Arnold-Chiari malformation[36] and syringomyelia[39–41]; therefore, the clinical picture may be unclear. Patients with pure basilar impression mainly complain of motor and sensory disturbances, such as weakness and paresthesia of the limbs within more severe cases of alteration of gait. In contrast, symptomatic patients with pure Chiari malformation are more likely to complain of cerebellar and vestibular disturbances (gait alteration, dizziness, and nystagmus). However, many patients will present with a combination of these symptoms, as these conditions commonly simultaneously coexist. In both conditions, there may be impingement of the lower cranial nerves as they emerge from the medulla oblongata. There may be pain in the nape of the neck from compression of the greater occipital nerve. Headache may also occur from blockage of the aqueduct of Sylvius, causing increased intracranial pressure.[36,42] Upon physical examination, many of these patients will have findings indicative of cord compression (myelopathy) or upper motor neuron dysfunction, such as a wide-based gait, decreased motor strength, and increased reflexes.

There is a high incidence of vertebral artery anomalies in basilar invagination.[43] The vessels may be compressed passing through the crowded foramen magnum, causing symptoms suggestive of vertebral artery insufficiency, such as dizziness, seizures, and syncope.[36,43,44] Compromise of vertebral arteries in the foramen magnum may lead to degeneration of the spinal cord and medulla, which may be an explanation for the frequent association with syringomyelia or syringobulbia.[45]

Many patients do not develop symptoms until the second or third decade of life[36] due to gradually increasing instability from ligamentous laxity caused by aging. These individuals often develop premature cervical osteoarthritis, and arteriosclerotic changes in the vertebral arteries may make these vessels more susceptible to minor constrictions.

Imaging

Basilar invagination is difficult to assess radiographically. Many measurement schemes have been proposed, such as the Chamberlain,[46] McGregor,[42] and McRae lines on the lateral radiograph (Fig. 34.7) and the Fischgold-Metzger line in the anteroposterior projection. The Chamberlain line[42,46] (a line drawn from the dorsal marginal hard palate to the posterior lip of the foramen magnum) is seldom used because the posterior lip of the foramen magnum (opisthion) is difficult to define on a standard radiograph and is often itself invaginated. The McGregor[42] line (a line drawn from the upper surface of the posterior edge of the hard palate to the most caudal point of the occipital curve of the skull) is easier to identify (Fig. 34.8). The position of the tip of the odontoid is measured in relation to this baseline, and any distance greater than 4.5 mm above the McGregor line is considered abnormal. The McRae line defines the opening of the foramen magnum and is an accurate guide in the clinical assessment of patients with basilar impression because if the tip of the odontoid lies below the opening of the foramen magnum, the patient is likely to be asymptomatic. A criticism of the lateral lines (McGregor and Chamberlain) is that the hard palate is not actually a part of the skull and may be distorted by an abnormal facial configuration or a highly arched palate, independent of a craniovertebral anomaly.[47]

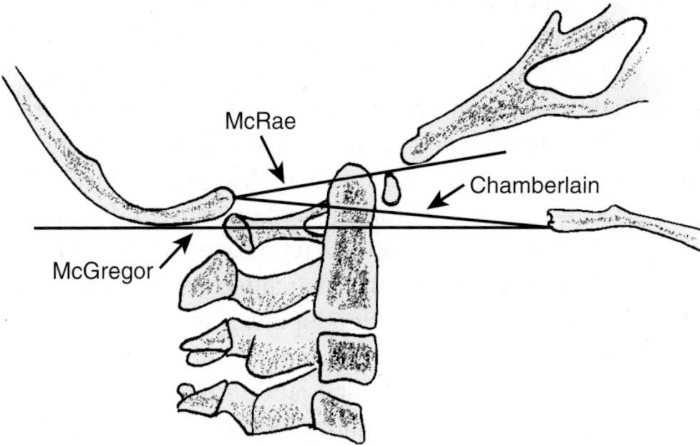

FIG. 34.7 Three lines used to determine basilar impressions. The Chamberlain line (1939) is drawn from the posterior lip of the foramen magnum (opisthion) to the dorsal margin of the hard palate. The McGregor line (1948) is drawn from the upper surface of the posterior edge of the hard palate to the most caudal point of the occipital curve of the skull. The McRae line (1953) defines the opening of the foramen magnum. The McGregor line is the best method for screening because the bony landmark can be clearly defined at all ages on routine lateral radiograph.

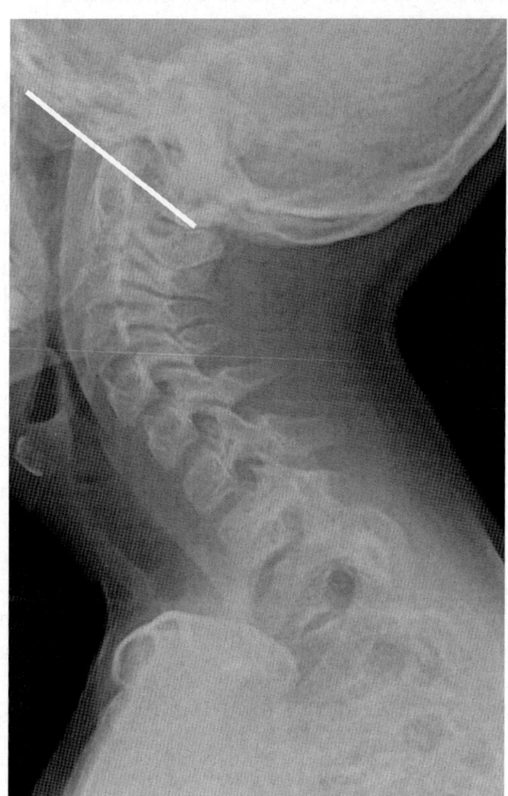

FIG. 34.8 A 12-year-old male presented with a history of unusual gait. Routine lateral radiograph suggested that the odontoid was displaced proximally into the opening of the foramen magnum. The McGregor line (*white*) has been drawn from the most caudal portion of the occiput to the hard palate. The tip of the odontoid is more than 4.5 mm above this line, indicating a basilar impression.

Since the advent of CT and magnetic resonance imaging (MRI), the diagnosis of basilar invagination can be made directly rather than based on radiographic lines.[48] MRI also allows direct assessment of neural compression and identifies the presence of associated pathologic processes, such as cord signal change, Chiari malformation, hydrocephalus, syringomyelia, or cerebellar herniation[35] (Fig. 34.9).

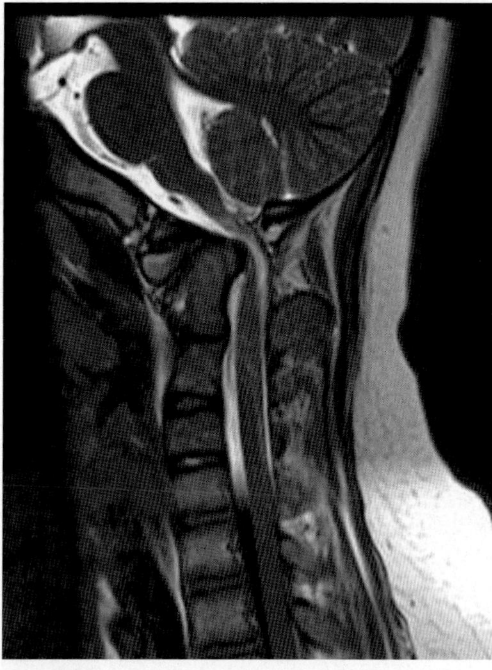

FIG. 34.9 Sagittal magnetic resonance image of basilar invagination shows cord signal change.

Treatment

Treatment of basilar invagination depends on the cause of the symptoms and is dictated by the severity of ventral neural compression and reducibility of the deformity. Absolute indications include symptomatic patients with documented impingement with spinal cord signal changes. Relative indications include progressive deformity or significant deformity with cord impingement in asymptomatic patients. Hydrocephalus from aqueductal stenosis, if present, must be addressed first with ventricular shunting before any other surgical interventions.[35]

In symptomatic patients, the cervical spine should initially be realigned using halo traction, which will also help decompress the neural elements. However, careful radiographic evaluation of the occipitocervical junction should precede use of traction,[49] as children with occipitocervical anomalies may be at increased risk of vertebral artery injury.

After application of halo traction, radiographs and MRI may be used to determine the adequacy of reduction and neural decompression. Patients who respond to closed reduction should be treated with posterior decompression via suboccipital craniectomy and upper cervical laminectomy, followed by occipitocervical arthrodesis to maintain stability and promote fusion.[35,37,50,51] The dura should be opened to look at any tight posterior dural bands.[36] In rare cases in which brain stem compression is not relieved by traction, circumferential anterior and posterior decompression, with resection of compressive elements, is recommended, followed by posterior fusion.[35,52–55] Anterior decompression can be performed through an open transoropharyngeal approach[56] or through an endoscopic approach.[57]

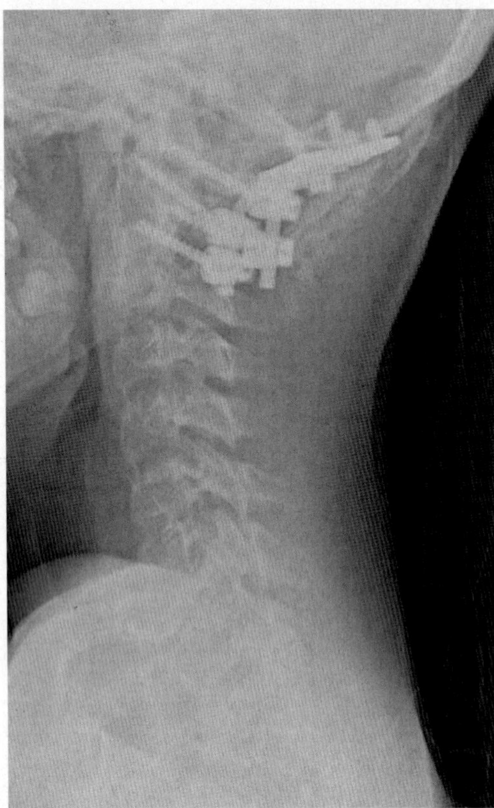

FIG. 34.10 A 10-year-old male with basilar invagination following posterior decompression and occiput to C2 instrumented spinal fusion. This is the same patient shown in Fig. 34.8; note the improved relationship of the odontoid to the foramen magnum.

Modern segmental fusion fixation constructs include occipital and cervical screws connected by a rod.[58] Occipitocervical arthrodesis from occiput–C2 can be performed with or without instrumentation at C1[6] (Fig. 34.10). In cases in which primary basilar invagination is diagnosed without neural injury, in situ stabilization without decompression may be beneficial to prevent further progression or neurologic compromise.

Posterior fossa decompression alone for symptomatic secondary basilar invagination typically provides only transient relief of symptoms and is not recommended, as recurrent neurologic deterioration inevitably occurs months to years later. This is because secondary basilar invagination tends to progress even after occipitocervical fusion with infolding of the skull base around the fusion mass and progressive forward bending.[34] Prolonged bracing with an orthotic device and lifelong surveillance may be necessary to halt further recurrence or symptomatic progression.[35,59] Bisphosphonates have shown some promise in being able to delay skull base malformations in some children with osteogenesis imperfecta, but routine surveillance is still required.[60] Some patients with secondary basilar invagination may benefit from surgical stabilization.

Occipitoatlantal Instability

Occipitoatlantal instability is rarely due to a congenital anomaly and is more often caused by trauma. In the past, most patients did not survive this injury; improved resuscitative measures have resulted in more patients surviving this condition. In both traumatic and congenital cases, the clinical and neurologic manifestations are due to trauma near the brain stem, and include motor weakness, pain, vertigo, and vomiting.[61] The most common anomalies of the upper cervical spine associated with this condition include Down syndrome and Klippel-Feil syndrome.[62] Patients who have Down syndrome fail to develop the normal curved architecture in the occipital condyle, resulting in the development of occipitoatlantal instability[63] (Fig. 34.11).

In cases of both congenital and traumatic atlantooccipital instability, surgical stabilization is recommended with arthrodesis from the occiput to C2.[64] Authors have reported successful outcomes using a variety of stabilization techniques.[65] In cases of trauma, neurologic sequelae are common. Any further deterioration should alert the clinician to the possibility of hydrocephalus.[66]

Occipitoatlantal Fusion (Occipitalization, Occipitocervical Synostosis)

Occipitoatlantal fusion is characterized by a partial or complete union between the base of the occiput and C1 (the atlas; Fig. 34.12). It ranges from a fibrous band connecting one or both of the occipital condyles to the atlas to complete osseous union.[67] Both upper and lower cervical anomalies may be associated with this condition, including occipital condyle hypoplasia, basilar impression, or Klippel-Feil syndrome. The incidence of occipitocervical malformations is around 2 per 1000 children, with a male predominance of 80%.[62,68,69]

Clinical Features

Patients with occipitoatlantal fusion have a short neck with limited cervical motion.[70,71] Associated spinal deformities, such as kyphosis and scoliosis, are frequent. Neurologic symptoms do not manifest during childhood, but develop in the third or fourth decades[69] in a slow, unrelenting manner.[72] It is unclear why neurologic problems develop so late and progress so slowly, but they are likely due to the degree of actual or relative basilar impression and the position of the odontoid. When the odontoid lies below the foramen magnum, the patient is usually asymptomatic,[73] but with fusion of the atlas to the occipital condyles, the odontoid may project far into the foramen magnum, producing brain stem pressure[70] (Fig. 34.13).

In this condition, the backward-projecting odontoid compresses the brain stem, causing upper motor neuron findings (spasticity, hyperreflexia, and muscle weakness) and cranial nerve involvement (diplopia, tinnitus, dysphagia, and auditory disturbances). The relative basilar invagination may cause vascular disturbances from vertebral artery involvement and irritation of the greater occipital nerve. Clinical manifestations include syncope, seizures, vertigo, and unsteady gait; dull, aching pain in the posterior occiput; and neck tenderness noted in the area of the posterior scalp. Rarely, acute

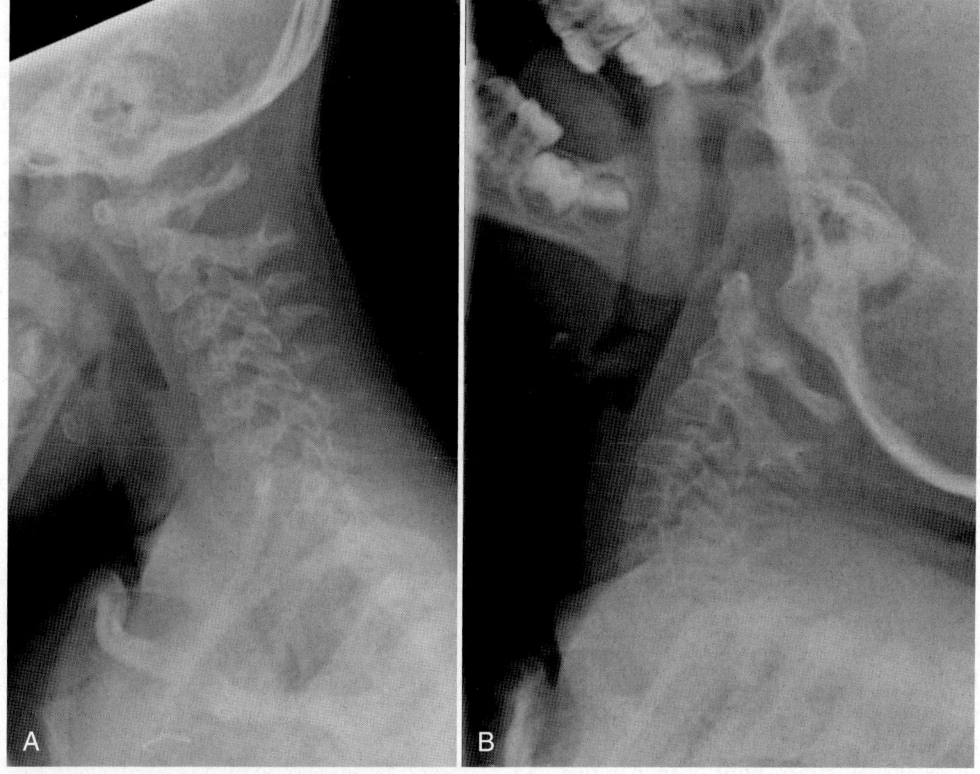

FIG. 34.11 (A) Flexion and (B) extension lateral radiographs in a patient with Down syndrome. Note the flattened occipital condyles and translation relative to the atlas. More attention is now being paid to craniocervical instability in Down syndrome.

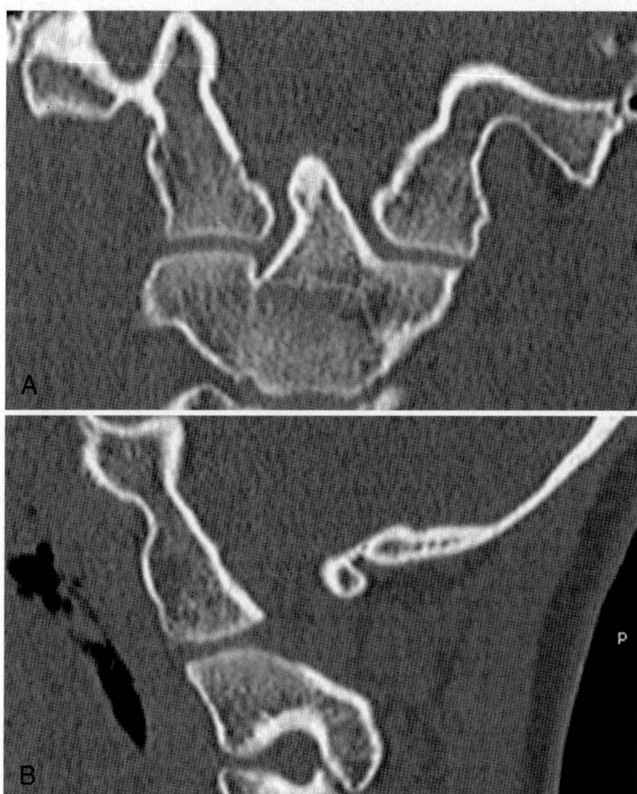

FIG. 34.12 (A) Coronal and (B) sagittal reformatted computed tomography scan images demonstrating complete fusion of the atlas to the occiput bilaterally.

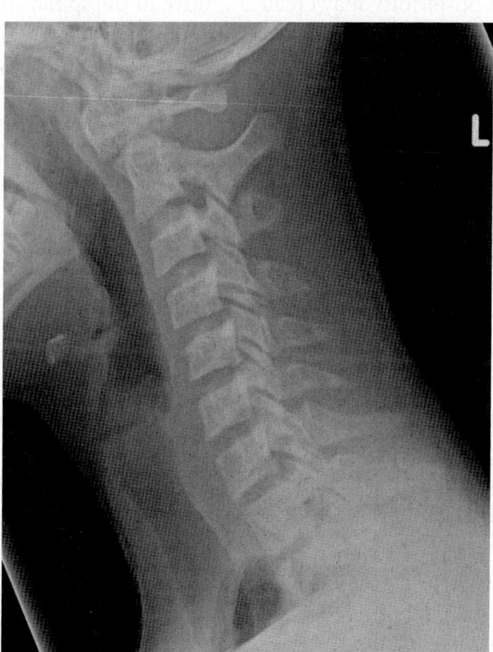

FIG. 34.13 Lateral radiograph demonstrating fusion C1 to the occiput. Note the relative basilar invagination, resulting in neurologic symptoms in this patient.

respiratory failure secondary to hypoventilation and sleep apnea may occur.[39]

Imaging

In children with occipitoatlantal fusion, radiographs are difficult to interpret, and advanced imaging, such as CT or MRI, may be necessary.[74,75] The condition may range from a bony or fibrous band to total fusion of the atlas into the occipital bone (see Fig. 34.12). Gholve et al.[69] proposed a morphologic classification of this anomaly: zone 1, a fused anterior arch; zone 2, fused lateral masses; zone 3, a fused posterior arch; and a combination of fused zones. Most commonly, the anterior arch of the atlas is fused to the occiput, with a hypoplastic posterior arch. Posterior fusion is not usually evident because this portion of the ring may only consist of a short bony fringe on the edge of the foramen magnum. Although innocuous in appearance, this fringe is frequently directed downward and inward and can compromise the spinal canal.

There is frequently an associated congenital fusion of C2–C3.[73] This results in greater demands being placed on the atlantoaxial articulation, particularly in flexion and extension,[71] resulting in atlantoaxial instability in 50% of patients.[76] Obtaining flexion-extension stress films is imperative. As mentioned earlier, with fusion of the atlas to the occiput, there is a relative loss of height of the atlas, allowing the odontoid to project upward into the foramen magnum and creating a basilar impression (see Fig. 34.13). Finally, a constricting band of dura posteriorly may create a groove in the spinal cord and may be the primary cause of symptoms. The band cannot be visualized on routine radiographs; therefore, MRI should be part of the evaluation.

Treatment

Management of this uncommon problem carries a high risk of morbidity and mortality.[70,77] In patients with persistent complaints of head and neck pain, initial nonoperative methods—such as antiinflammatories, rest, and cervical collars—may be initially attempted. With an unstable atlantoaxial complex and neurologic deficits, we recommend posterior decompression and posterior occipital cervical stabilization and fusion with rigid segmental instrumentation from the occiput to C2.[58] Further stability can be obtained by using a halo fixator in the postoperative period.[78] If reduction is possible and there are no neurologic signs, surgical intervention carries an improved prognosis.[70]

With irreducible ventral compression, transoral resection of the odontoid may be considered,[79] but may risk destabilizing the entire upper cervical spine.[80] We do not recommend isolated cervical laminectomy without instrumentation, as this may increase C1–C2 instability or lead to the late development of a cervical kyphosis, particularly if the laminectomy involves several levels.[81] We also strongly caution against operative reduction (rather than preoperative halo traction), which can result in death.

Anomalies of Ring of C1

In normal development, ossification of the atlas proceeds from paired centers, one for each of the lateral masses, then progresses posteriorly into the neural arches, which are fully ossified at birth except for a gap of 5 to 9 mm posteriorly that closes by the fourth year.[75] The anterior arch of the atlas ossifies from a single center, which appears during the first year of life and fuses to the remainder of the atlas by the third year.[68,75,82] The most common anomalies of C1 are a persistent bifid anterior (Fig. 34.14) and posterior (Fig. 34.15) arch, or a hemiatlas (absence of a C1 facet).

There is about a 3% incidence of failure of closure of either the anterior or posterior arch of the atlas beyond age 4 years.[83] This anomaly can be observed in several conditions, such as skeletal dysplasias, Goldenhar syndrome, Down syndrome, and Conradi syndrome.[51]

Anomalies of the posterior arch can be characterized as median clefts or hypoplasia. A classification scheme for congenital defects of the posterior arch of C1 has been proposed (Fig. 34.16). More than 90% of patients are asymptomatic with a type A median cleft variant, which is incidentally identified

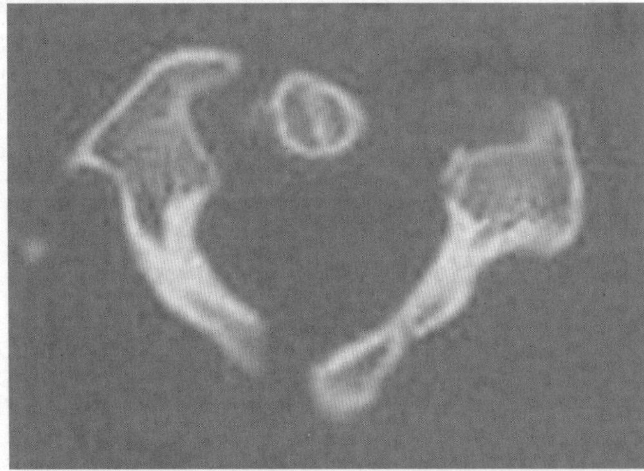

FIG. 34.14 Axial computed tomography scan demonstrating incomplete, or bifid, anterior arch.

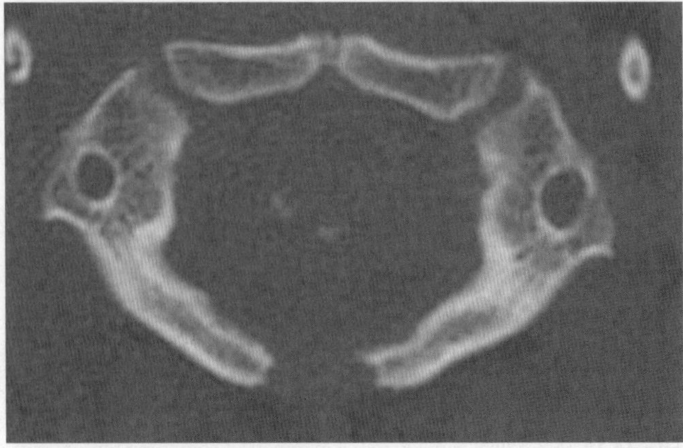

FIG. 34.15 Axial computed tomography scan demonstrating incomplete, or bifid, posterior arch.

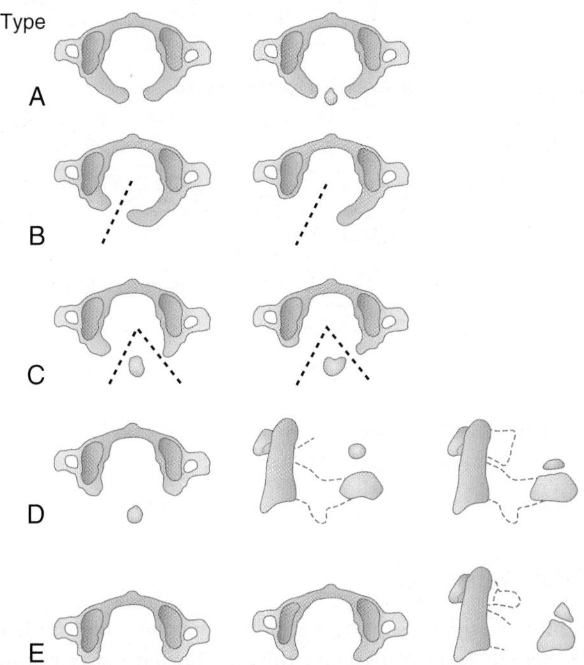

FIG. 34.16 Classification system for posterior C1 ring anomalies. *Type A* is small midline failure of fusion. *Type B* defects are unilateral clefts of variable size, ranging from small gap to complete absence of hemiarch. *Type C* indicates bilateral defects with preservation of most of the dorsal arch. *Type D* is complete absence of posterior arch with a retained, midline tubercle. *Type E* is a complete posterior arch and tubercle deficiency. (Modified from Currarino G, Rollins N, Diehl JT. Congenital defects of the posterior arch of the atlas. *Spine.* 2000;47:267–271.)

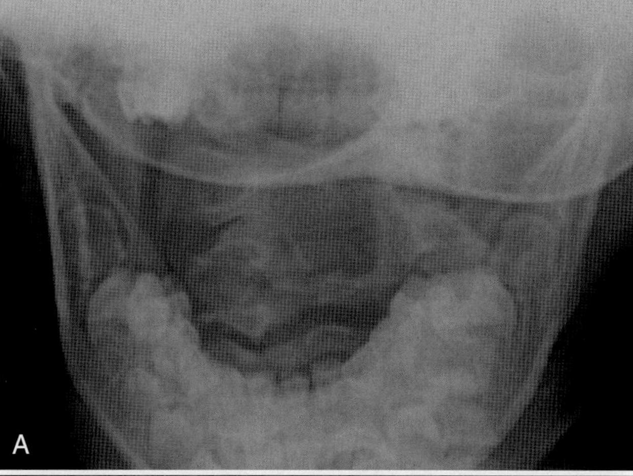

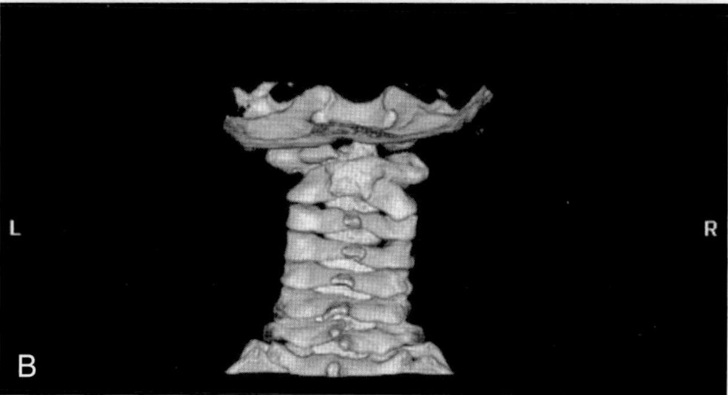

FIG. 34.17 Absence of C1 facet in a 5-year-old child with severe, progressive torticollis. (A) Open-mouth odontoid view shows absence of right C1. (B) Computed tomography scan with three-dimensional reconstructions viewed posteriorly shows absence of right C1. Note how the occipital condyle articulates with C2.

on radiographic studies.[83] Types C and D are accompanied by a free-floating posterior tubercle. These patients may experience neck pain and neurologic symptoms before discovery of the anomaly. The free posterior tubercle has been shown to move with neck extension, and in some cases may migrate anteriorly and traumatize the spinal cord with neck extension. Rarely, hypoplasia of the posterior arch occurs and has been associated with myelopathy.[84]

Dubousset[85] recognized the problem of the hemiatlas of C1, or absence of the facet of C1, which can lead to severe and progressive torticollis in young children (Fig. 34.17). Initially, the deformity is flexible but becomes more severe and eventually fixed as the child ages. CT is necessary to identify this deformity. It can accompany Klippel-Feil syndrome with anomalies of the lower cervical spine as well, and there is an increased incidence of anomalies of the vertebral vessels in these children. Clinicians should utilize arteriographic evaluation before the use of traction or surgical intervention. If the patient is passively correctable, a single posterior fusion, occiput to C2, is recommended.

Atlantoaxial Instability

Atlantoaxial instability can vary from subtle instability to frank fixed C1–C2 dislocation. It is commonly associated with syndromes or other systematic disorders. Specifically in patients with Down syndrome, generalized ligamentous laxity and flat facets predispose to hypermobility and pathologic motion at the craniovertebral and atlantoaxial articulations.[86,87] Up to 40% of these patients have radiologically detectable atlantoaxial instability,[88] although it is symptomatic in only 1% to 2% of cases.[89] Patients with congenital scoliosis, skeletal dysplasia, osteogenesis imperfecta, juvenile rheumatoid arthritis, and neurofibromatosis also can have significant atlantoaxial instability, which may be unrecognized. Other anomalies, such as os odontoideum, can manifest as atlantoaxial instability (see "Anomalies of the Odontoid" later in this chapter).[90]

The significance of anomalies at the atlantoaxial joint are related to the stability of the articulation between the atlas (C1) and the axis (C2), as this is the most mobile section of the vertebral column and consequently has the least stability. Normally, 90 degrees of rotatory motion exists in the cervical spine, and 50% occurs in the C1–C2 joint. Lateral slide is also a component of the rotatory motion. Limited flexion (5 degrees) and extension (10 degrees) are permitted.[91] The freedom of motion is primarily due to the lack of bony constraints, as the odontoid is the only bony buttress to prevent hyperextension. The integrity of the soft tissues (ligaments and capsular structures) provides the majority of stability at this articulation. Therefore, the atlantoaxial joint is extremely mobile but structurally weak. Furthermore, it is located between two relatively fixed points, the atlanto-occipital and C2–C3 joints, which puts C1–C2 at further risk.

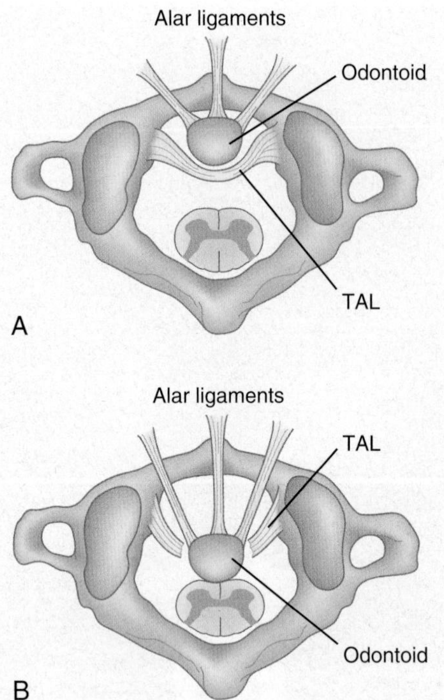

FIG. 34.18 Atlantoaxial joint as viewed from above. (A) Normal. (B) Disruption of transverse atlantal ligament (TAL): Odontoid occupies safe zone of Steel. Intact alar ligaments (second line of defense) prevent spinal cord compression.

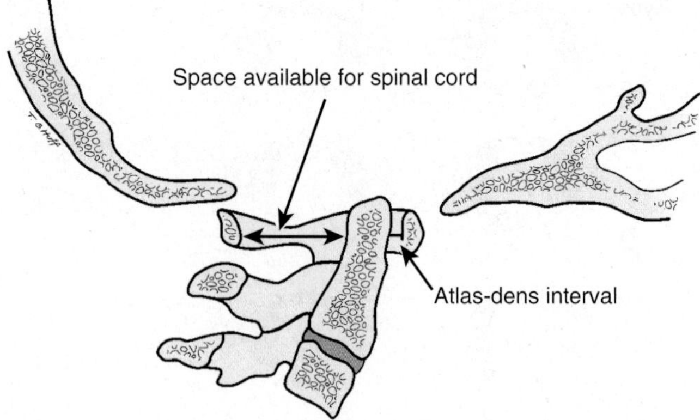

FIG. 34.19 Atlantoaxial joint showing the normal atlas-dens interval (ADI), normal space available for spinal cord (SAC), distance between posterior aspect of the odontoid, and the nearest posterior structure.

The primary ligamentous stabilizer is the transverse atlantal ligament. The alar ligaments form the second line of defense and act as a checkrein after disruption or laxity of the transverse atlantal ligament (Fig. 34.18). Although the alar ligaments appear thick and strong, they stretch with relative ease and permit significant displacement. This secondary stability plays an important role in patients with chronic atlantoaxial instability.

When evaluating this area, Steel defined the "rule of thirds": The area of the vertebral canal at C1 can be divided into one-third odontoid, one-third spinal cord, and one-third "space," which represents a safe zone in which displacement can occur without neurologic impingement and is roughly equivalent to the transverse diameter of the odontoid (usually 1 cm)[92] (see Fig. 34.12). In chronic atlantoaxial instability, the alar ligaments have failed and there is no longer a margin of safety. The patient has exceeded the "safe zone" of Steel and enters the area of impending spinal cord compression. The end result is narrowing of the spinal canal and impingement on the neural elements.[76]

Laxity of the transverse atlantal ligament is common in patients with Down syndrome, with a reported incidence of 15% found in all age groups.[89,93] These patients seem to have rupture or attenuation of the transverse atlantal ligament with encroachment of the safe zone of Steel, but at least initially they are protected by the checkrein action of the alar ligaments from spinal cord compression. In other words, many patients have excessive motion, but relatively few are symptomatic, and most cases are discovered only by radiologic survey.[94,95] MRI can be helpful in assessing the integrity of the transverse atlantal ligament.[96]

Clinical Presentation

In children, the presenting symptoms may be quite subtle and nonspecific. In most patients, the only presenting symptom is generalized weakness, manifested as lack of physical endurance, a history of frequent falling, or the child's asking to be carried.

As patients age, the central nervous system itself becomes less tolerant of intermittent compression, and its ability to recover is diminished. Even with hypermobility at this articulation, it is unusual for patients to become symptomatic before their third decade. When patients do become symptomatic, trauma is immediately suspected, but is often not the case. More likely, the degenerative changes of aging cause the lower cervical articulations to become more rigid. This gradual restriction of caudal motion places an increased demand on the ligaments and capsular structures of the atlantoaxial articulation, and instability develops.

With compression from the odontoid on the spinal cord, the symptoms and signs of upper motor neuron compression are commonly found.[70] If the primary area of impingement is posterior (from the foramen magnum, a dural band, or posterior ring of C1), symptoms are attributed to the posterior columns, with alterations in vibratory responses and proprioception. If there is also an associated cerebellar herniation, nystagmus, ataxia, and incoordination may be observed. Symptoms attributed to vertebral artery compression may occur.

Imaging

The atlas-dens interval (ADI) is the space seen on the lateral radiograph between the anterior aspect of the dens and the posterior aspect of the anterior ring of the atlas (Fig. 34.19). In children, the ADI should be no greater than 4 mm in flexion.[91] In children with ligamentous laxity (such as Down syndrome), instability is present with an ADI of more than 5 mm. Symptoms occur with instability greater than 7 to 10 mm. The ADI does not exceed 3 mm in adults if the transverse ligament is intact.[97]

However, in cases of congenital anomalies, ligamentous laxity, or chronic instability, the ADI is of limited value. In this

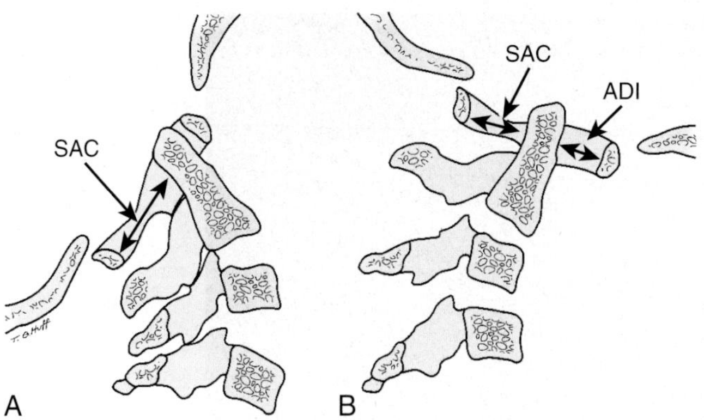

FIG. 34.20 Atlantoaxial instability. (A) Extension: forward sliding of the atlas with increased atlas-dens interval (ADI) and decreased space available for spinal cord (SAC). (B) Flexion: the ADI and SAC return to normal as the intact odontoid provides bony block to subluxation in hyperextension.

situation, attention should be directed to the amount of space available for the spinal cord (SAC). Determining the SAC is accomplished by measuring the distance from the posterior aspect of the odontoid or axis to the nearest posterior structure (foramen magnum or posterior ring of the atlas)[98] (Fig. 34.20). In adults, spinal cord compression does not occur if the SAC is 18 mm or more. While cord compression is possible between 15 and 17 mm, it frequently occurs if SAC is 14 mm or less.

Data on normal variations in sagittal and transverse diameter of the cervical spine have been collected for infants and children. As might be expected, these measurements generally are smaller than in adults and follow a predictable growth curve. Clinical significance is determined via comparison of the absolute diameter with the known norms for that vertebral level and age, and comparison of successive vertebral levels within the same individual. Comparisons between levels in the same patient is more sensitive in determining an abnormality. Jauregui et al.[33] found that Steel's rule of thirds generally applied throughout all of growth, and relative stenosis was defined at 13 mm in children.

Lateral flexion-extension views should be conducted voluntarily by the patient, and no effort should be made by the clinician to assist the patient. Although motion may be limited in certain cases, especially in the setting of pain or noncompliant children/poor effort, avoidance of precipitating a neurologic defect is paramount. Patients who present with a neurologic deficit usually exhibit significant instability (Fig. 34.21).

In patients with multiple anomalies or abnormal bone (such as Morquio syndrome or spondyloepiphyseal dysplasia), the usual radiographic views are not always reliable in confirming the presence or absence of an odontoid.[99] In these situations, dynamic CT scan with reconstruction views is helpful.[74,100] Although much attention has been paid to anterior translation of C1 on C2, extension views should not be ignored, as some patients have significant posterior subluxation.[101]

Dynamic MRI provides direct visualization of the neurologic structures and sites of bony impingement not appreciated on radiography.[74,96] While difficult to perform and time consuming, it is a reliable tool to diagnose instability.[102] MRI can evaluate the integrity of the transverse atlantal ligament, as well as other anomalies, such as the Chiari malformation and syringomyelia. Because excessive motion may lead to compression of the vertebral arteries,[75] arteriography is helpful in evaluating patients who exhibit symptoms of transient brain stem ischemia.[103,104]

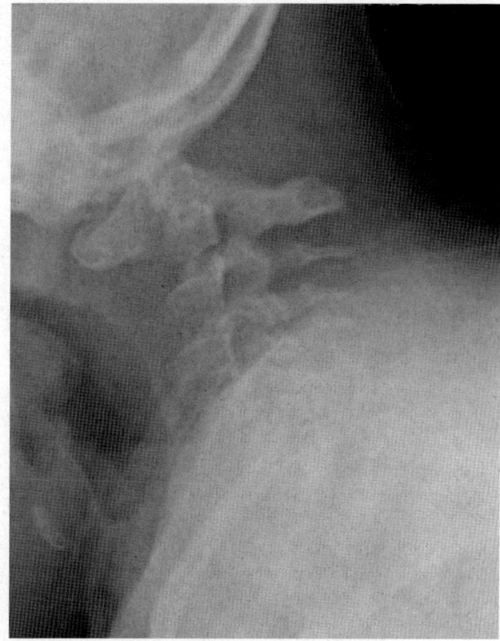

FIG. 34.21 Significant atlantoaxial instability in a patient with neurologic findings.

Current recommendations for radiographic screening for atlantoaxial instability in children with Down syndrome include lateral flexion-extension radiographs taken around age 3 years, and, if these are normal, the child may participate in activities but avoid contact sports.[93,105] Asymptomatic children with evidence of instability on radiographs should undergo MRI to determine if any neural compromise is present (or impending)[106] (Fig. 34.22). The Special Olympics requires repeat radiographs as evidence of ADI of less than 4.5 mm prior to participation in high-risk sports.[89,107,108]

Treatment

Nonoperative care plays a limited role in treatment of symptomatic atlantoaxial instability and is reserved for patients with no symptoms or neurologic findings. Fortunately, many patients remain asymptomatic throughout their life and need only be monitored periodically. Any new-onset pain or abnormalities in motor function should precipitate a thorough workup. In asymptomatic patients, there is currently no agreed upon indication for prophylactic fusion of C1 to C2; however, in cases of progressive instability and/or limited SAC, prophylactic fusion can be considered.

Effective treatment generally can be provided only if the exact cause of symptoms has been determined. Before surgical intervention, reduction of the atlantoaxial articulation should be achieved by either positioning or traction.[55,58,109] The patient

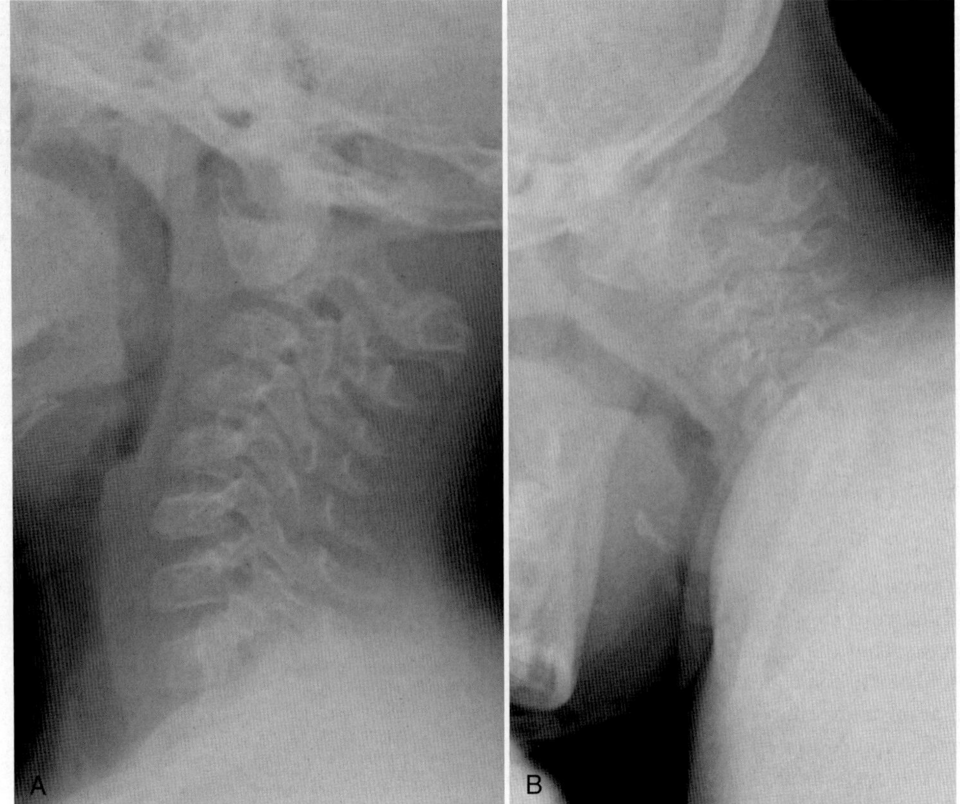

FIG. 34.22 A 5-year-old boy with Down syndrome atlantoaxial instability. (A) Neutral position. (B) In flexion, the atlas-dens interval is substantially increased.

should be maintained in the reduced position preoperatively and monitored for improvement in symptoms and neurologic status.

Prior to modern segmental screw and rod–based instrumentation, results of operative fusion, especially in Down syndrome patients, were disappointing.[110–112] With the advent of rigid internal fixation, such as C1 lateral mass to C2 screws, C1–C2 transarticular screws, and transoral decompression with posterior plating, rates of fusion have increased substantially[113–115] (Fig. 34.23). The improved rigidity afforded by modern segmental spinal instrumentation has substantially reduced the need for postoperative halo immobilization.[116,117] Choice of surgical procedure for stabilization must be individualized based on clinical presentation and surgeon expertise.[58]

Occult respiratory dysfunction in patients with atlantoaxial instability is important to recognize.[118] Many patients have an unrecognized decrease in vital capacity and chronic alveolar hypoventilation as a result of the neurologic injury to the brain stem. Periods of apnea and respiratory distress during surgery or in the immediate postoperative period have frequently resulted in death or have required prolonged respiratory support.[119]

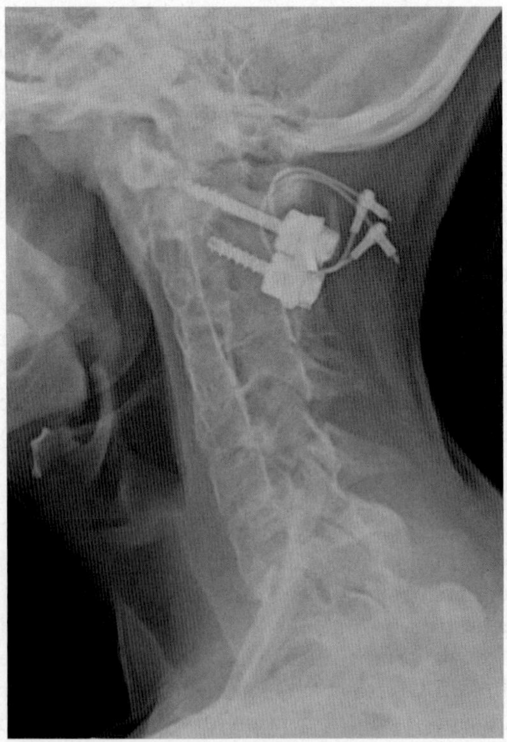

FIG. 34.23 Postoperative lateral radiograph of a Down syndrome patient with significant atlantoaxial instability who underwent C1–C2 fusion with C1 lateral mass and C2 pars screws. Note cables securing the iliac crest bone graft.

Anomalies of Odontoid (Dens)

Congenital anomalies of the odontoid occur on a spectrum, ranging from aplasia (complete absence) to hypoplasia (partial

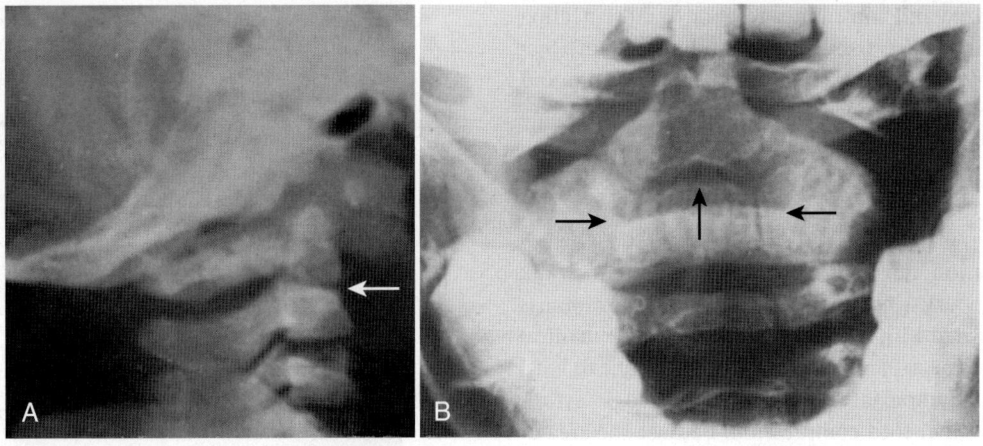

FIG. 34.24 (A) Radiograph of a 6-month-old infant. The odontoid is normally formed and recognizable on routine radiographs at birth, but is separated from the body of the axis by a broad cartilaginous band (*arrow*), similar in appearance to an epiphyseal plate. It represents the vestigial disc space and is referred to as *neurocentral synchondrosis*. (B) Neurocentral synchondrosis is not at anatomic base of the dens, at the level of the superior articular facets of the axis. This open-mouth view shows that the embryologic base of the odontoid is below the articular facets and contributes a substantial portion to the body of the axis. This radiolucent line is present in nearly all children at age 3 years and in 50% by age 4 years; it is absent in most individuals by age 5 years.

absence) to os odontoideum (an anomaly in which a partially or fully formed dens is in bony discontinuity with the body of the axis). Depending on the severity, potential neurologic sequelae may result from an unstable atlantoaxial complex.[120] The frequency of these anomalies is unknown. They are probably more common than typically appreciated, as they are often incidental findings. In the past, malformations of the dens were infrequently reported and considered rare[121–123]; however, improved imaging and awareness have led to an increase in diagnosis.

Ossification of the apex and body of the odontoid proceeds separately. The body is derived from the first cervical sclerotome and is the center of the first cervical vertebra. This center becomes separated from the atlas to fuse with the axis. The apex is derived from the mesenchyme of the most caudal occipital sclerotome.[124]

The body of the dens begins to ossify from two centers between the first and fifth prenatal months. These centers become a single mass by the time of birth.[82] At birth, the apex of the odontoid has not ossified, is V-shaped, and is known as a *dens bicornis*. A separate ossification center within the *dens bicornis* is known as an *ossiculum terminale*, which appears at age 3 years and fuses with the rest of the dens by age 12 years. An ossiculum terminale has been found in a quarter of normal children age 5 to 11 years.

However, an ossiculum terminale may never appear or may occasionally fail to fuse with the dens. In this case, it is considered an *ossiculum terminale persistens*, which is occasionally discernible as either a cyst or an area of increased density. These developmental anomalies are usually firmly bound to the main body of the dens by cartilage. They are of little clinical significance and seldom the source of instability,[125] but reports exist of serious neurologic sequelae.[126]

At birth, the dens is separated from the body of the axis by a cartilaginous band, or neurocentral synchondrosis, that represents the epiphyseal growth plate. It does not cross at the level of the superior articular facets, but lies well caudal to this level within the body of the axis (Fig. 34.24). It is present in almost all children by age 3 years and in 50% of children by age 4 years, but it is absent in most by age 6 years.[127] It rarely persists into adolescence and adult life.

The blood supply to the odontoid is from two sources.[128] The vertebral arteries provide anterior and posterior ascending arteries that originate at C3 and pass ventral and dorsal to the body of the axis and the odontoid. They anastomose in an arcade by the alar ligaments. These arteries supply small penetrating branches to the body of the axis and the odontoid. Lateral to the apex of the odontoid, the anterior ascending arteries and apical arcade receive anastomotic derivatives from the carotids by way of the base of the skull and the alar ligaments. This arrangement of the blood supply is necessary because of the embryologic development and anatomic function of the odontoid. The transient neurocentral synchondrosis between the odontoid and the axis prevents the development of any significant vascular channels between the two structures.[129] The body of the odontoid is surrounded entirely by synovial joint cavities; its fixed position relative to the rotation of the atlas precludes vascularization by direct branches from the vertebral arteries at the C1 segmental level.[124]

Theories on the etiology for os odontoideum are twofold. The first proposes a congenital theory, or failure of fusion of the dens to the body.[130,131] This is supported by a familial form[132] and os odontoideum in identical twins with no history of trauma.[133]

More likely, a traumatic etiology attributes an unrecognized fracture in the region of the base of the odontoid as the cause of os odontoideum.[101,123,134,135] After fracture of the odontoid, contracture of the alar ligaments exerts a distraction force that pulls the fragment away from the base and closer to their origin at the occiput. The delicate blood supply to the odontoid is easily traumatized and contributes to poor fracture healing or callus formation. Several cases of "os odontoideum" that developed several years after trauma when a normal odontoid was initially present have been reported.[134,136] Infection is a rare cause of dens abnormalities as well.[137]

Clinical Features

Clinical presentation can vary from no symptoms to frank myelopathy secondary to cord compression.[138] Minor trauma is commonly associated with the onset of symptoms. Mechanical symptoms, such as neck pain or headache, may be due to local irritation of the atlantoaxial articulation. Neurologic symptoms are due to spinal cord compression. Because the area of the spinal cord impingement is below the foramen magnum, these patients seldom have cranial nerve symptoms.[139]

If clinical manifestations are limited to mechanical symptoms without neurologic involvement, the prognosis is excellent.[101,139,140] Patients who exhibit only transient weakness of the extremities and paresthesias after minor trauma usually have complete return of function. More concerning are patients in whom there is an insidious onset and slowly progressive neurologic impairment, as they have a greater potential for permanent deficit.[101] Weakness and ataxia are the most common complaints, but sensory loss spasticity, increased deep tendon reflexes, clonus, loss of proprioception, and sphincter disturbances have been described.[98] In few patients, vertebral artery compression at the foramen magnum may lead to symptoms and signs of cerebral and brain stem ischemia, such as seizures, mental deterioration, syncope, vertigo, and visual disturbances.[141]

Radiographic Features

At birth, the normal odontoid can be visualized in the lateral view with an epiphyseal plate. A mistaken impression of hypoplasia may be given by a lateral extension radiograph because the anterior arch of the atlas may slide upward and protrude beyond the ossified tip of the dens, especially in very young patients.[142]

Agenesis or hypoplasia of the odontoid is an extremely rare anomaly that is best seen in the open-mouth view. The diagnostic feature is the absence of the basilar portion of the odontoid, which normally is well below the level of the superior articular facets of the axis. Hypoplasia manifests as a short, stubby peg of odontoid projecting just above the lateral facet articulations (Fig. 34.25). CT scan is necessary to confirm whether an os odontoideum is present in addition to the hypoplasia.

In the os odontoideum, there is a jointlike articulation between the odontoid and the body of the axis that appears radiologically as a wide radiolucent gap (Fig. 34.26). In children younger than 5 years, this gap may be confused with the normal neurocentral synchondrosis. The radiologic appearance of os odontoideum may be similar to a traumatic nonunion, and often they cannot be differentiated.[121] The location of lucency is usually the key to making the diagnosis. In the os odontoideum, the gap is above the level of the superior facets and is wide with a smooth edge. In traumatic nonunion, the gap between the fragments is characteristically narrow and irregular and frequently extends into the body of the axis below the level of the superior facets of the axis.

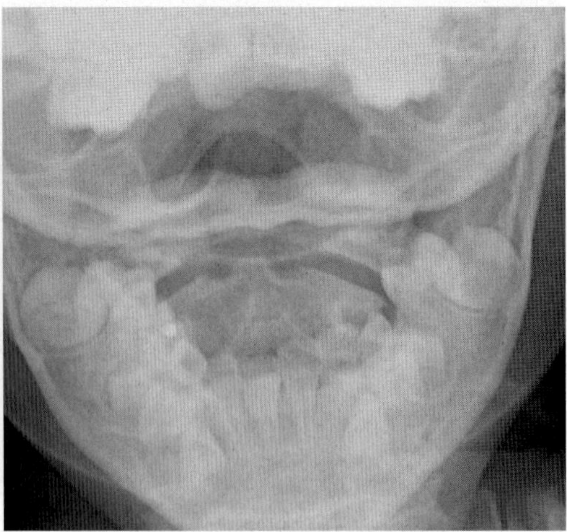

FIG. 34.25 Hypoplasia of the odontoid.

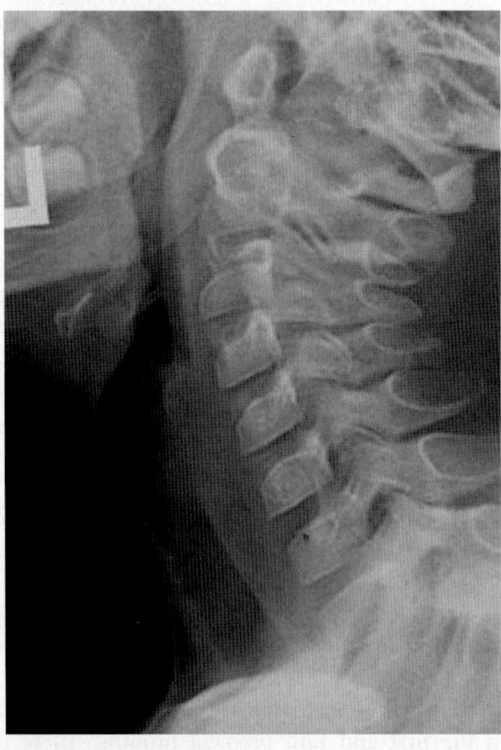

FIG. 34.26 Lateral radiograph of the cervical spine demonstrating wide lucency between the body of the dens and the os odontoideum.

Recommended radiographic views are open-mouth and lateral flexion-extension views. The free ossicle of the os odontoideum usually appears fixed to the anterior arch of the atlas and moves with it in flexion and extension (Fig. 34.27).[98,143] Since the os odontoideum moves with the ring of C1, measurements of its relationship to C1 are of little value. Instability can reduce the SAC but not the ADI.[91] Diminished space available for the cord with neck extension (SAC) significantly correlates with higher risk for myelopathy.[138] While the instability may be in any direction,[98,101] most commonly, the anterior

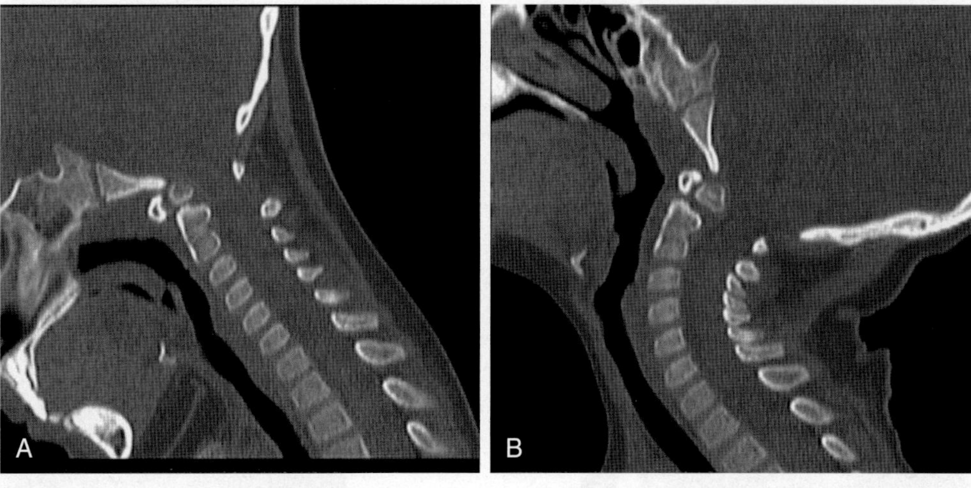

FIG. 34.27 Sagittal reformatted images from computed tomography scan demonstrating (A) dynamic flexion and (B) extension. Note posterior translation of the os odontoideum on the extension image.

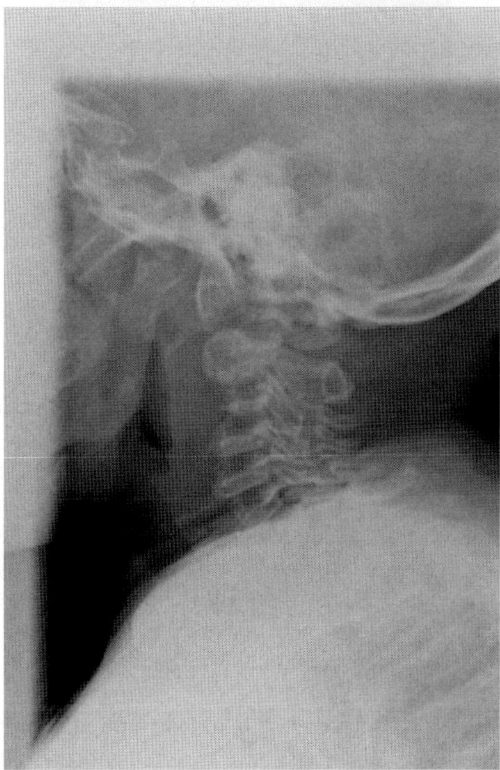

FIG. 34.28 Lateral radiograph of the cervical spine of a patient with Morquio syndrome; note the difficulty in identifying correct anatomy and potential pathology.

portion of the atlas is usually hypertrophied, and the posterior portion of the ring may be hypoplastic or absent.[144]

In patients with multiple cervical anomalies or those with abnormal bone (such as Morquio syndrome [Fig. 34.28] or skeletal dysplasia), the traditional radiographic views are not always reliable in confirming the presence or absence of an odontoid, as the odontoid may be present but dysplastic, or blend with the surrounding abnormal bone. In these situations, good results have been obtained by using CT scans to ascertain the character of the atlantoaxial articulation.

CT reconstructions are indicated when routine views are unsatisfactory in showing the anomaly. Lateral flexion-extension stress views should be conducted voluntarily by patients, particularly patients with a neurologic deficit. The degree of anteroposterior displacement of the atlas on the axis should be documented (see Fig. 34.20). CT scan can also help to define the anatomy of the craniocervical junction, including the completeness of the atlas ring and the position of the transverse foramina at C1 and C2.[145]

MRI is helpful for evaluating the SAC. MRI studies have shown a direct correlation between cord signal abnormality and the degree of myelopathy measured clinically.[146] Dynamic MRI[147] allows direct visualization of motion of the os odontoideum, atlas, and axis as well as surrounding motion throughout the full range of motion (ROM) of the cervical spine (Fig. 34.29). Open MRI configurations allow analysis of the cervical spine in the physiologic upright position, which may assist in identifying subtle pathology that is not apparent in the nonphysiologic supine position.

Treatment

Patients with congenital anomalies of the odontoid are at increased risk of neurologic injury, as a trivial insult superimposed on an already weakened and compromised structure may be catastrophic. The natural history is variable, and no predictive factors are apparent.[98] While strict indications for surgical stabilization are not apparent, we recommend considering surgery for persistent pain, myelopathy, or frank radiographic instability, as evidenced by instability of 10 mm or more in flexion and extension. Neural decompression must address bony or soft tissue impingement of the spinal cord.

Nonoperative treatment is possible in patients with os odontoideum who have no neurologic deficits or evidence of instability on radiographs. Patients with inflammatory symptoms or even transient myelopathies can expect recovery.[139,148] Cervical traction or immobilization may be helpful in such circumstances.

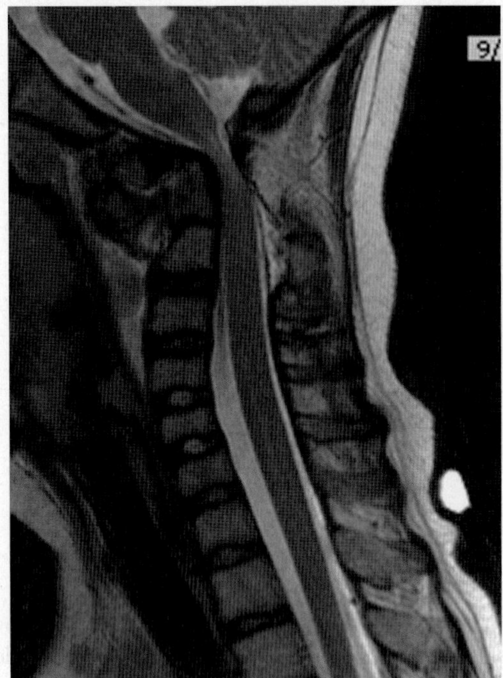

FIG. 34.29 Sagittal magnetic resonance image of the cervical spine showing cord compression in a patient with os odontoideum.

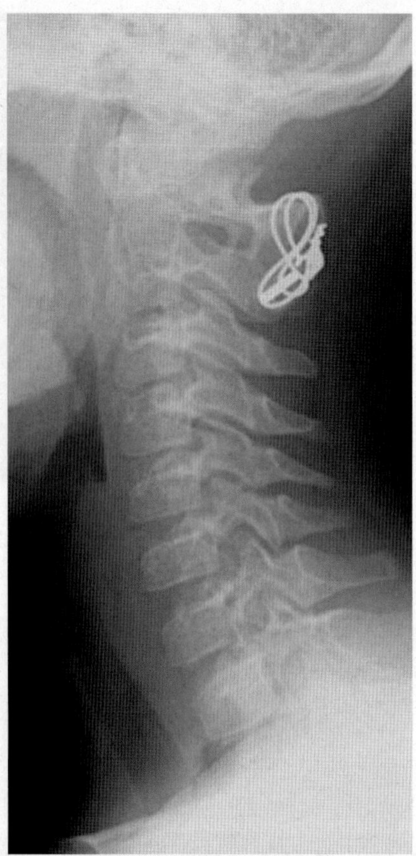

FIG. 34.30 Posterior cervical arthrodesis from C1–C2 with a wiring technique used to treat a symptomatic patient with os odontoideum.

Considerable controversy exists over the role of prophylactic stabilization in asymptomatic patients with instability. Surgical treatment is not required for every patient in whom an os odontoideum is identified. Patients who have no neurologic symptoms or instability at C1–C2 can be managed with periodic observation. The lack of C1–C2 instability at initial diagnosis does not guarantee that instability will not develop in these patients, however, or that they are not at higher risk for spinal cord injury with trauma.[149] For this reason, longitudinal follow-up with flexion-extension radiographs of these patients is recommended. Klimo and colleagues[98] recommended surgical stabilization for all patients with os odontoideum. The safety of stability and the ability to lead a normal active life may outweigh the possible complications of surgery or the catastrophic dangers of instability. Especially in the pediatric age group, it may be difficult or impossible to limit activity, even in the presence of instability.

When treating symptomatic patients, initial reduction of the atlantoaxial articulation must be accomplished prior to surgery, usually by skull-based halo-gravity traction.[150] Ideally, the patient should be maintained in the reduced position several days before surgery to allow recovery of neurologic function.[139]

Decompression of the neural elements by any offending lesion must be undertaken; the choice of approach depends on the site of compression and the comfort level of the surgeon. Both anterior and posterior decompression strategies can be undertaken with good results. Following any method of decompression, the suggested method of stabilization is posterior cervical arthrodesis and instrumentation of C1–C2. As discussed earlier, wiring techniques with iliac crest bone graft and halo immobilization have been reported with favorable results (Fig. 34.30).[151–155] However, concerns with neurologic injury[151] and incomplete posterior C1 arch formation[112] have made C1 lateral mass screws coupled with C2 screws a safe and reliable option.[8,11,156] In a small or poorly developed spinous process of C2, a threaded Kirschner wire (K-wire) through the spinous process can be helpful in improving the stability of the wiring technique.[157] In a patient with a marginally functioning neurologic status, it may be wiser to perform an occiput-to-C2 arthrodesis and plan to maintain immobilization with a halo vest in extension.

In patients who have a highly mobile but reducible C1–C2 articulation, several authors have reported good results using transarticular screws (see Fig. 34.4).[16,153,155,158,159] Atlantoaxial transarticular screws have been shown to be feasible in pediatric patients; the superior biomechanical stability may eliminate the need for prolonged postoperative halo vest immobilization.[16,160] As discussed earlier, a thorough understanding of the bony and vascular anatomy is paramount prior to attempting an instrumentation around C2.[13,88] When fusion is needed to subaxial levels, lateral mass screws at C3 and below can be used with good results.[11,155,161,162]

With transarticular fixation of C1–C2, the lamina of C1 can be removed without extending the fusion to the occiput. Although this technique is generally reliable and safe, in patients with spinal cord compression, fixed dislocations, or congenital ligamentous laxity, particularly in patients with Down syndrome, extra caution should be employed,[112] and a postoperative halo-vest orthosis should be considered. Smith and colleagues[163] reported significant problems with C1–C2 stabilization, particularly in patients who are very unstable or have myelopathy. Patients with failed fusions or irreducible dislocations were at high risk for perioperative neurologic complications.

Patients in whom the C1–C2 dislocation is unreducible pose a difficult management problem. Manipulative reduction during surgery is discouraged because it has proved extremely hazardous and may result in respiratory distress, apnea, or death. For patients with no neurologic deficit, a simple in situ posterior fusion is the least hazardous procedure. If neurologic findings are present, posterior decompression by laminectomy has been associated with increased morbidity and mortality[139] and may potentiate C1–C2 instability if performed in isolation. An occiput-to-C2 arthrodesis is recommended in these situations.[164] If reduction of the C1–C2 dislocation is considered necessary or if the clinical situation precludes posterior stabilization, an anterior or lateral retropharyngeal approach can be considered.[165]

Klippel-Feil Syndrome

In 1912, Klippel and Feil[166] published the first report of their eponymous syndrome. They presented a patient with shortening of the neck, a low posterior hairline, and severe restriction of neck motion. After the patient died, postmortem examination revealed complete fusion of the cervical vertebrae. Currently, the term *Klippel-Feil syndrome* (KFS) refers to patients with any congenital fusion of the cervical vertebrae, whether it involves two segments or the entire cervical spine (Fig. 34.31).

The embryologic etiology of KFS likely stems from failure of normal segmentation of the cervical somites during the third to eighth weeks of life. Between 20 and 30 days' gestational age, the paraxial mesoderm undergoes segmentation into spherical, discrete somites. As somites mature, they subdivide into sclerotomes, myotomes, and dermatomes. The sclerotomes, precursors of the adult vertebral bodies, undergo resegmentation such that the caudal section of one somite fuses with the cephalad segment of the adjacent one to form a vertebral body[167] (Fig. 34.32).

The precise reasons behind this failure of segmentation are yet to be elucidated, as only a few patients have inherited this condition.[168,169] Pedigree analysis and molecular studies have defined specific genetic abnormalities that may account for these anomalies. The gene *SGM1* has been identified as the first human Klippel-Feil locus (*SGM1*) in a large affected family. Experimental animal models have identified genes in segmentation and somitogenesis pathways, such as in the HOX, PAX, and Notch signaling pathways.[124]

As these embryologic abnormalities occur early in development, the pathology may not be limited to the cervical spine. Patients with KFS commonly have other defects in the genitourinary,[170,171] nervous,[172] cardiopulmonary,[173,174] and auditory systems.[175,176] Actually, many of these other abnormalities are more detrimental to the patient's general well-being than the cervical fusions. Because the incidence of related congenital

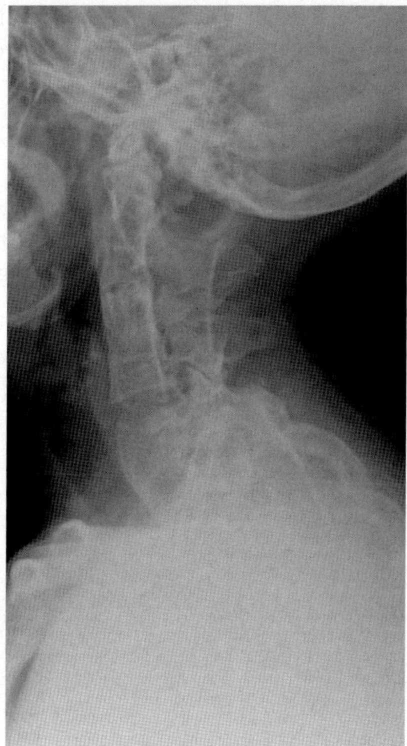

FIG. 34.31 Lateral cervical radiograph of a patient with Klippel-Feil syndrome. Note the multiple congenital cervical fusions.

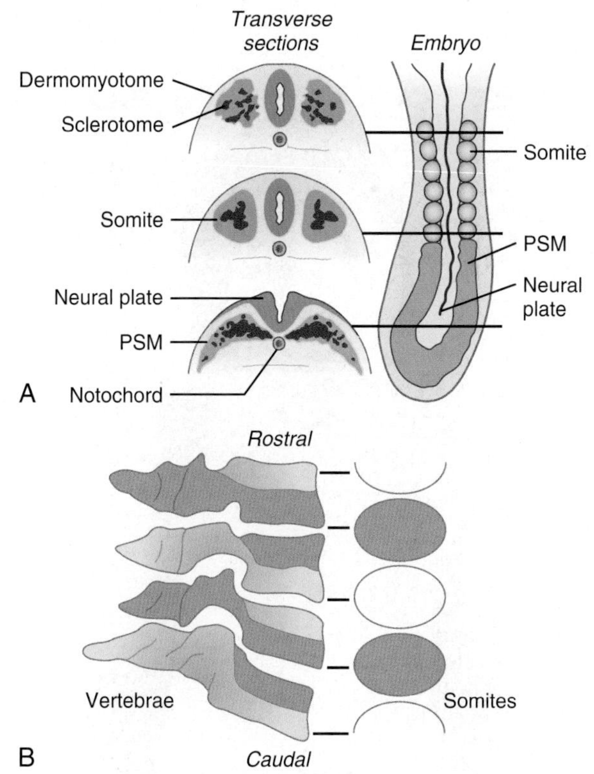

FIG. 34.32 (A) Embryologic differentiation of the mesoderm into pairs of somites on either side of the spinal cord. Somites divide further to form the ventral sclerotome and dorsal dermomyotome. (B) Cells from the rostral and caudal half of adjacent somites fuse to form future vertebral bodies and arches. Defects in this process have been theorized in Klippel-Feil syndrome. PSM, paraspinal muscles. (Modified from Tracy MR, Dormans JP, Kusumi K. Klippel-Feil syndrome. *Clin Orthop* 2004;424:183–190.)

SECTION IV

anomalies is fairly high, all patients with KFS should have the aforementioned organ systems thoroughly investigated[171] (Box 34.1).

Clinical Features

The classic description of KFS is a triad of low posterior hairline, short neck, and limitation of neck motion. However, fewer than half of patients have all three signs (Fig. 34.33).[171]

BOX 34.1 Abnormalities Associated With Klippel-Feil Syndrome

Common

Scoliosis: 60%
Renal abnormalities: 35%
Sprengel deformity: 30%
Deafness: 30%
Synkinesis: 20%
Congenital heart disease: 14%

Less Common

Ptosis
Duane contracture
Lateral rectus palsy
Facial nerve palsy
Syndactyly
Hypoplastic thumb
Upper extremity hypoplasia
Neurenteric cyst

Clinically, the most consistent finding is limitation of neck motion, which is directly related to the degree of cervical spine involvement. Generally, flexion-extension is better preserved than rotation or lateral bending. If fewer than three vertebrae are fused or if only the lower cervical segments are fused, the patient generally has no detectable limitation.[177] In addition, many patients with marked cervical involvement are able to compensate with hypermobility at the unfused joints and to maintain a deceptively good range of motion. Some patients may have 90 degrees of flexion-extension, only occurring at a single open interspace. Rarely, patients have fixed hyperextension of the neck; this is usually associated with iniencephaly (absence of the posterior cervical laminae and an enlarged foramen magnum[178]; Fig. 34.34).

Shortening of the neck is a rare finding, and a low posterior hairline is uncommon. Other head and neck manifestations—such as facial asymmetry, torticollis, or neck webbing—occur in fewer than 20% of patients.[171,177] In KFS, concomitant Sprengel deformity occurs in up to 35% of cases, either unilaterally or bilaterally[171,179] (Fig. 34.35). Since the scapula develops from mesodermal tissue high in the neck, it is thought to be due to the same interruption in the normal embryologic development pathway of the cervical somites.[177]

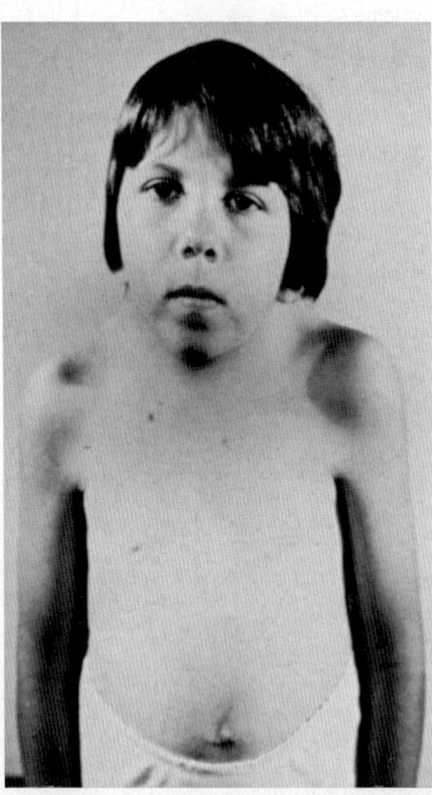

FIG. 34.33 A 9-year-old child with Klippel-Feil syndrome. Note short neck with tendency toward webbing, mild torticollis, and asymmetry of eye level. The patient clinically has marked restriction of neck motion, impaired hearing, and mirror motions (synkinesia) of upper extremities.

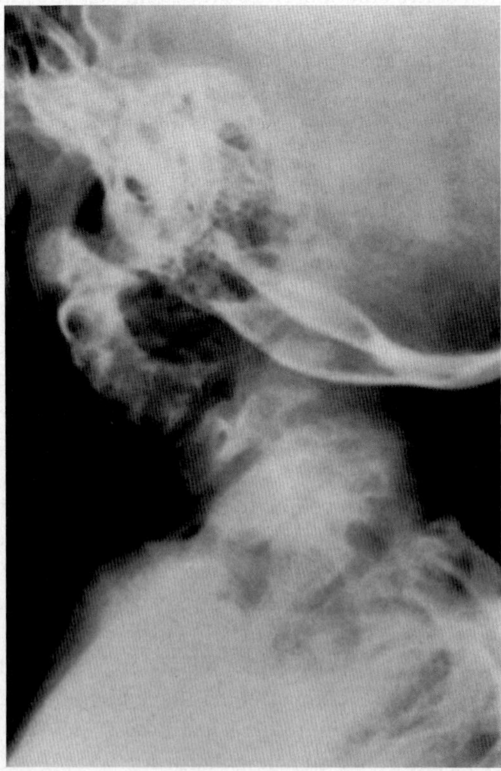

FIG. 34.34 A 12-year-old girl presented with Klippel-Feil syndrome and iniencephaly—enlarged foramen magnum and absent posterior laminae. Note fixed hyperextension and long segment of cervical fusion (C2–C6) and abnormal occipitocervical articulation. This pattern could be viewed as a more elaborate variation of the C2–C3 pattern of McRae. Flexion-extension and rotational forces are concentrated in the area of the abnormal occipitocervical junction. These patients may be at risk of developing instability with aging.

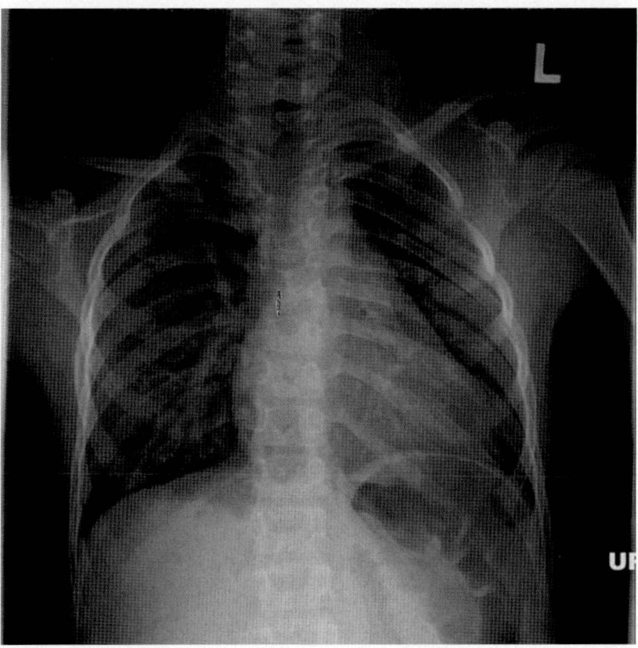

FIG. 34.35 A patient with concomitant Klippel-Feil syndrome and Sprengel deformity of the left scapula.

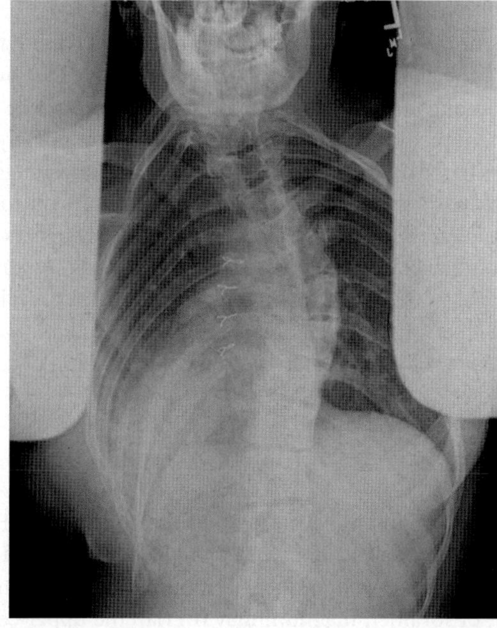

FIG. 34.36 Scoliosis below cervical deformity in a patient with Klippel-Feil syndrome. Note the previous Sprengel deformity correction.

Many patients are asymptomatic, but if they develop symptoms, they are generally localized to the head, neck, and upper extremities. The symptoms result from direct irritation or impingement of the cervical nerve roots, with radicular symptoms in the upper extremities.[45] Most patients who develop symptoms are in the second or third decade of life. Sources of the symptoms are either mechanical in nature due to inflammation of a cervical articulation, or neurologic in nature, owing to root irritation or spinal cord compression. Most symptoms originate at the open segments, where the remaining free articulations are hypermobile,[180] which can lead to instability or early arthritis. There may be constriction and narrowing of the nerve root at the foramen from osteophytic spurring.[181]

If joint instability is progressive or if there is appropriate trauma, myelopathy may occur, ranging from mild spasticity, hyperreflexia, and muscular weakness to sudden complete quadriplegia after minor trauma.[182,183] Syncope and neurologic compromise may be associated with mechanical compromise of the vertebral arteries secondary to hypermobility, with ischemic episodes.[184]

Associated Conditions

Scoliosis

Scoliosis is the most frequent anomaly found in association with KFS.[185,186] Up to 60% of patients have a significant degree of scoliosis, most of whom require treatment and should be followed through the growth years. Two types of scoliosis can be identified: congenital scoliosis, owing to vertebral anomalies and differential growth patterns (Fig. 34.36), and compensatory scoliosis, below the area of vertebral involvement. Congenital scoliosis is more frequent[171]; in fact, up to 5% of patients with congenital scoliosis have been found to have concomitant KFS.[187]

Radiographic examinations should include posteroanterior and lateral views of the spine to assess both coronal and sagittal plane deformities. If recognized early, many spinal deformities can be successfully managed with standard orthoses. Progressive curves are more likely associated with children who have extensive fusions,[186] and frequently occur in the normal-appearing vertebrae below the primary curve. Documented progression demands appropriate treatment to prevent serious additional deformity. Thoracic scoliosis may seriously compromise pulmonary function.[173] At present, many of these patients require posterior spinal stabilization.

Renal, Cardiac, Auditory Abnormalities

More than one-third of children with KFS can be expected to have a significant urinary tract anomaly, which is often asymptomatic. Ultrasonography is a noninvasive way to screen adequately for the anomalies associated with this syndrome.[188] Abnormalities include unilateral absence of a kidney, a double collecting system, renal ectopia, horseshoe kidney, and hydronephrosis from ureteropelvic obstruction. KFS is also associated with congenital heart disease (4.2–14%). The most common lesion reported has been an interventricular septal defect occurring alone or in combination with other defects, such as patent ductus arteriosus and abnormal position of the heart and aorta. The association of hearing impairment and deafness in KFS (>30%) is seldom mentioned in orthopaedic reports. There is no characteristic audiologic anomaly, and all types of hearing loss (conductive, sensorineural, and mixed) have been described. These patients should undergo a complete audiometric evaluation when defects are discovered.[130–136]

Mirror Motions (Synkinesis)

Mirror motion, or synkinesis, is involuntary paired movements of the hands in which the patient is unable to move one hand without similar reciprocal motion of the opposite hand. This phenomenon appears to occur in approximately 20% of patients with KFS[171]; thus, some authors have suggested that synkinesis should be included as part of the syndrome.[172] The etiology of synkinesis is unknown, but it appears to be a separate neurologic defect not caused by cervical vertebral fusions.[189] Autopsy specimens suggest that the clinical findings are due to inadequate or incomplete decussation of the pyramidal tracts in conjunction with a dysraphic cervical spinal cord.

Imaging

Adequate radiographic evaluation of the child with KFS can be difficult, especially if involvement is severe. Fixed bony deformities can prevent proper positioning, and the mandible, occiput, or foramen magnum may overlap the upper cervical vertebrae. Flexion-extension radiographs or CT scans may be necessary to provide information to assess stability.[181] With MRI, the relationship between the bony elements and neurologic structures (both the spinal cord and cervical nerve roots) can be assessed directly to show any potential sites of neural compression.[190,191]

The radiographic hallmark of KFS is fusion of any cervical vertebrae, whether a simple synostosis of two bodies (congenital block vertebrae; Fig. 34.37) or massive fusion of the entire cervical spine[166] (see Fig. 34.31). Other anomalies may be present, including flattening and widening of the involved vertebral bodies or an increase in the space available for the spinal cord.[192,193] Absent disc spaces or hypoplasia of the disc space can often be seen (Fig. 34.38). In a young child, narrowing of the cervical disc space cannot always be appreciated because the ossification of the vertebral body is incomplete, and the unossified endplates may give the false impression of a normal disc space. With continued growth, the ossification of the vertebral bodies is completed, however, and the fusion becomes obvious.[193]

Hemivertebrae are common (Fig. 34.39) occurring in up to 74% of patients. The incidence increases with the number of segments fused. Fusion of posterior elements usually parallels fusion of the vertebral bodies. In a young child, particular attention should be paid to the laminae because fusion posteriorly is often more apparent earlier.[171]

Knowledge of the normal variations in cervical spine mobility, particularly in children, is important in evaluating patients with KFS.[194] Pseudosubluxation of C2 on C3 with flexion can be observed in 45% of normal children younger than 8 years of age (Fig. 34.40).[127] Marked angulation at a single interspace during flexion, rather than a uniform arc of vertebral motion, can be observed in normal children (16%) and may be misinterpreted as vertebral fusion below. Advanced imaging with CT scan can aid surgeons in understanding bony abnormalities and also serve as an aid for preoperative planning.[195]

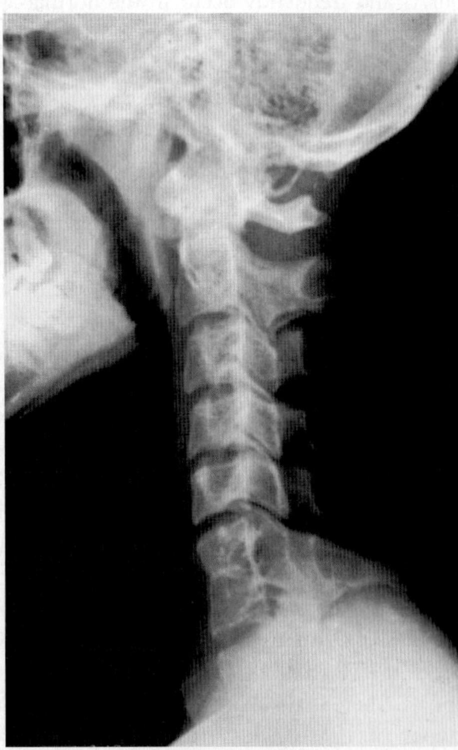

FIG. 34.37. Congenital block vertebrae at C6–C7. Symptoms are directly related to the number and level of involved vertebrae; this represents the most benign form of Klippel-Feil syndrome.

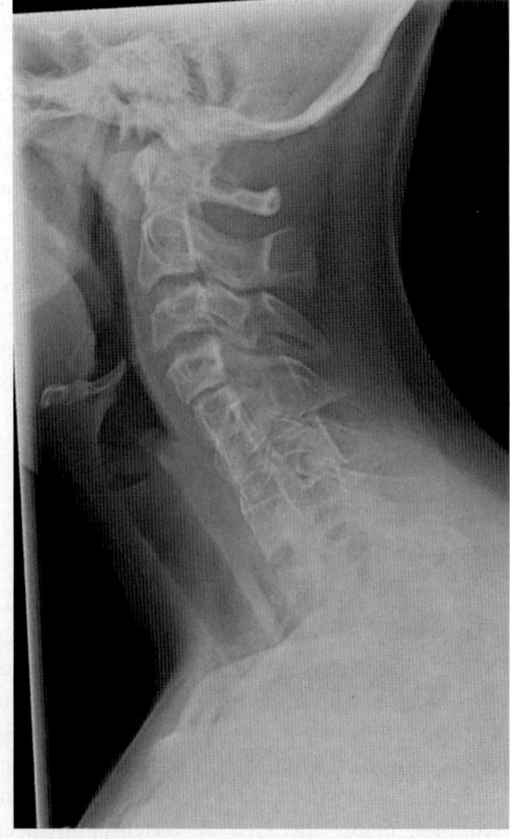

FIG. 34.38 Absent disc spaces in a patient with Klippel-Feil syndrome.

In KFS, the diameter of the spinal canal is usually normal. Narrowing occurs in adult life and is due to degenerative changes or hypermobility.[191,196,197] Enlargement of the canal is uncommon and may indicate conditions such as syringomyelia, hydromyelia, or Arnold-Chiari malformation. The intervertebral foramina are usually smooth in contour, but are frequently smaller than normal and oval rather than circular (Fig. 34.41). Posterior spina bifida is common (45%), but anterior spina bifida is rare. Rarely, there is complete absence of the posterior elements. This condition is usually accompanied by enlargement of the foramen magnum and fixed hyperextension of the neck, referred to as iniencephaly[178] (see Fig. 34.34).

Any KFS anomaly may extend into the thoracic spine. An anomaly of the thoracic spine on a routine chest radiograph may be the first clue to an unrecognized cervical synostosis. With a high thoracic congenital scoliosis, the radiographic evaluation should routinely include lateral views of the cervical spine.

Patterns of Cervical Motion

There are three patterns of cervical motion in KFS, described by Pizzutillo et al.[180]

FIG. 34.39 Cervical hemivertebra in Klippel-Feil syndrome.

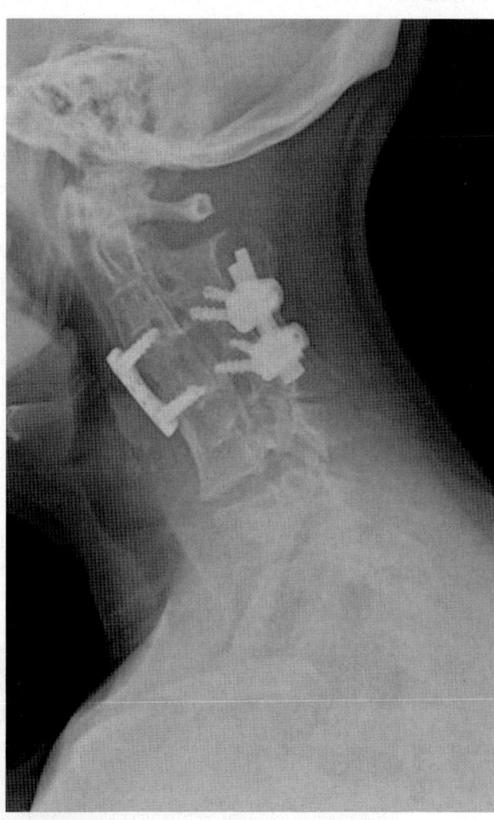

FIG. 34.41 Enlarged neural foramina in Klippel-Feil syndrome.

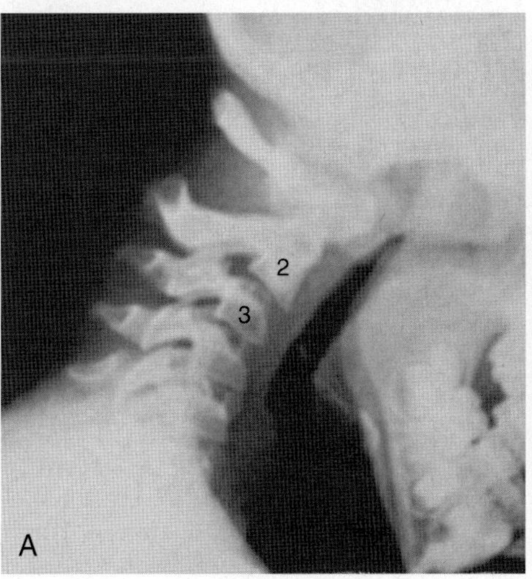

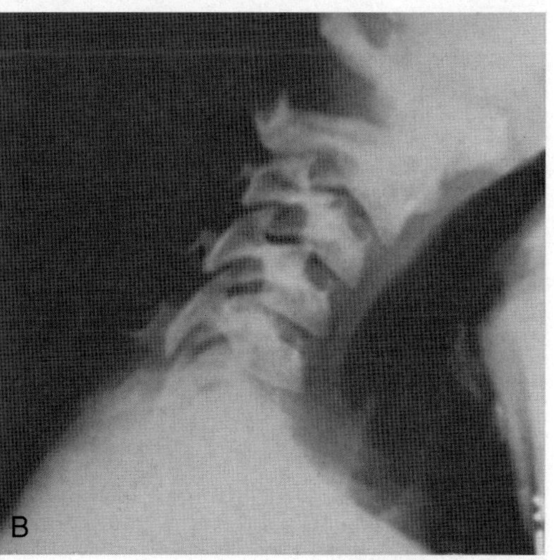

FIG. 34.40 (A) Pseudosubluxation of C2 on C3 in a child at age 5 years. (B) At age 10 years, flexion view of the cervical spine shows normal motion without pseudosubluxation. This normal variation can be found in more than half of children younger than 8 years.

Type 1 is fusion of C2 and C3 with occipitalization of the atlas. Flexion-extension is concentrated in the area of C1 and C2, and the odontoid can become hypermobile, narrowing the spinal canal and compromising the spinal cord and brain stem.

Type 2 is a long fusion with an abnormal occipitocervical junction. The center of flexion-extension and rotation is concentrated in the area of the abnormal odontoid or poorly developed ring of C1, which cannot withstand the wear and tear of aging.[197-199] It is important to differentiate this pattern from the pattern in a patient with a long fusion and a normal C1–C2 articulation (Fig. 34.42), which is usually compatible with a normal life expectancy.

Type 3 is a single open interspace between two fused segments (Fig. 34.43). As the cervical spine motion is concentrated at the single open articulation, this hypermobility may lead to frank instability or degenerative osteoarthritis.[180,200] This pattern can be easily recognized because the cervical spine appears to angle or hinge at the open segment.

Similarly, Samartzis et al.[198] studied cervical fusion patterns in patients with KFS. Their classification system encompassed three types: type I, single fusion; type II, multiple, noncontiguous fusions; and type III, multiple, contiguous fusions. Type I is associated with axial neck symptoms; types II and III were associated with radiculopathy and myelopathy.

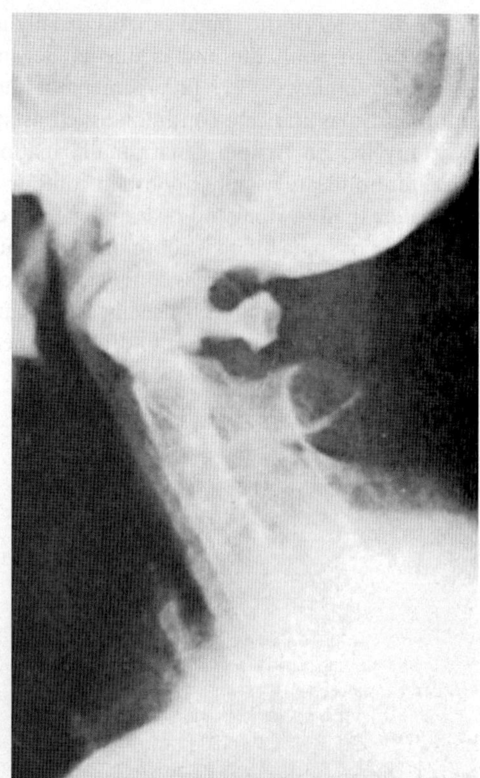

FIG. 34.42 Radiograph of a 45-year-old man with Klippel-Feil syndrome. The patient has complete fusion of C2–C7. Flexion-extension occurs only at atlantoaxial articulation. There are no symptoms referable to the neck despite two previous serious falls. This pattern seems to be relatively safe because a normal occipitocervical junction serves as protection from late instability.

Treatment

A patient with KFS with minimal involvement can be expected to lead a normal active life with no or only minor restrictions

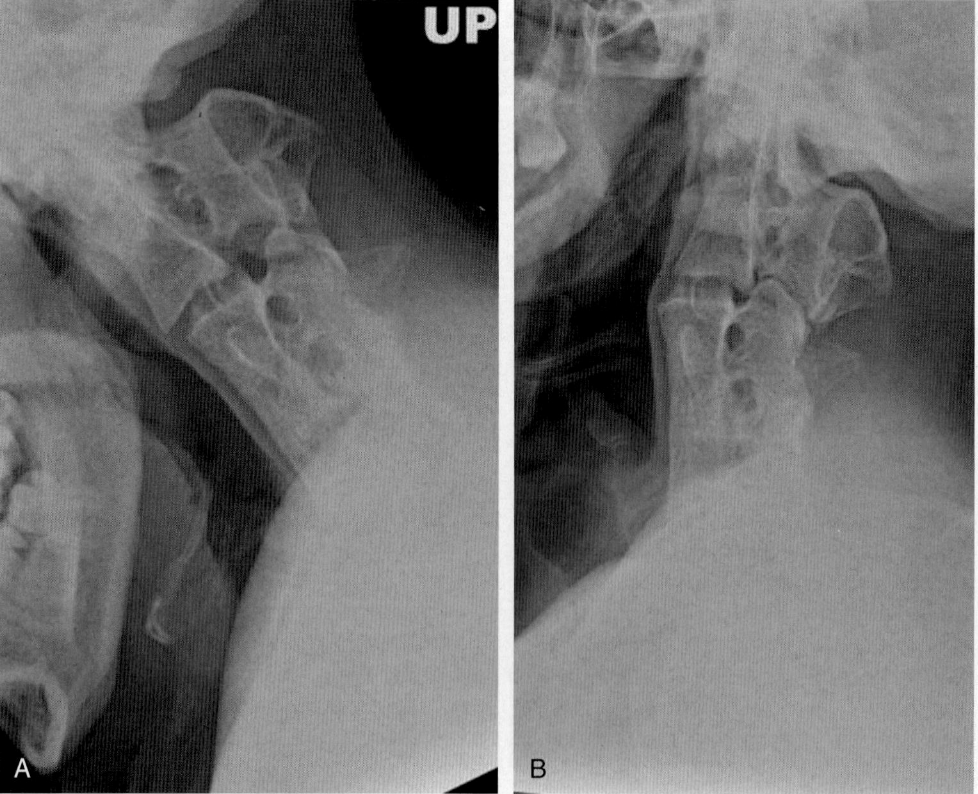

FIG. 34.43 (A) Flexion and (B) extension lateral radiographs show a single open interspace in Klippel-Feil syndrome.

or symptoms. In fact, the actual treatment of KFS is confined mostly to the area of associated conditions. Even patients with severe cervical involvement can have a good prognosis if early and appropriate treatment is instituted, especially regarding associated scoliosis and renal abnormalities.

Treatment options center on prophylaxis, mechanical treatment, and cosmetic treatment. Regarding prophylaxis, patients with long segments of cervical fusion or high-risk patterns of cervical spinal motion should avoid activities that might risk the cervical spine. In these patients, the mobile articulations are under greater mechanical demands and are less capable of protecting them against traumatic insults. Additionally, although neurologic compromise or death after minor trauma has been reported in patients with KFS,[182] the role of prophylactic surgical stabilization in asymptomatic patients has not yet been defined. There is no satisfactory definition of when the risk of instability warrants further reduction of neck motion.

For symptomatic patients with mechanical symptoms, conservative treatment measures are reasonable and may include antiinflammatories or a cervical collar. Symptoms that suggest neurologic compromise require consideration and thorough physical examination and radiologic evaluation. The area of neural compression must be determined before surgical intervention. Attempts should be made preoperatively to obtain reduction of the spinal column in advance of surgical stabilization. Also, the anesthesiologist may need to plan for airway management and be prepared for difficult intubation.[201]

Treatment of the cosmetic aspects of this deformity has found limited success. Occasionally, children's abnormal neck posture may be improved with bracing. Bracing requires long-term application, however, and excellent patient cooperation. Correction of the bony deformity by direct means, such as wedge osteotomy or hemivertebrae excision, has been done on a limited basis. Ruf et al.[202] reported hemivertebrae resection for correction of head tilt. Occasionally, carefully selected patients who have cervical congenital scoliosis may obtain some correction and improvement of appearance by use of the halo vest combined with posterior cervical fusion. Bonola[203] described a method of rib resection to attain apparent increase in neck length and motion. This procedure is an extensive surgical experience, however, and is a great risk to the patient. No subsequent reports have appeared in the literature.

Soft tissue procedures, Z-plasty, and muscle resection may achieve cosmetic improvement in properly selected patients. These procedures can restore a more natural contour to the shoulders and neck and an apparent increase in neck length. Neck motion is generally not increased, and the scars may be extensive, particularly in a patient with a large skin web. If an omovertebral bone is present or an abnormal connection to the clavicle,[204] its removal may permit an increase in neck and shoulder motion. The risk of brachial plexus injury from traction is higher in patients with KFS because there are likely to be anomalous origins of the cervical nerve roots in these patients.

Congenital Muscular Torticollis

Congenital muscular torticollis is a common condition caused by contracture of the sternocleidomastoid (SCM) muscle, usually discovered in the first 6 to 8 weeks of life. The head is tilted toward the involved side and the chin rotated toward the contralateral shoulder (Fig. 34.44). A palpable mass may be, but usually is not, detected within the first 4 weeks of life (Fig. 34.45).[205] It is a nontender, mobile enlargement beneath the skin, attached to or located within the body of the SCM. Ultrasonography may be helpful in assessing the mass.[206] After 4 to 6 months of age, the mass is usually absent, and the contracture of the SCM muscle and head posture are the only clinical findings (Fig. 34.46).

With progression of the condition, deformities of the face and skull can result.[207] Flattening of the face and skull (termed *plagiocephaly*) on the side of the contracted SCM muscle is due to the position of the child when sleeping. In the past, many children slept prone,[208] and the face remodeled to conform to the bed. The "Safe to Sleep" movement (formerly known as "Back to Sleep") has substantially decreased the percentage of children who sleep in the prone position.[209] In children who sleep supine, reverse modeling of the contralateral aspect of the skull is evident.

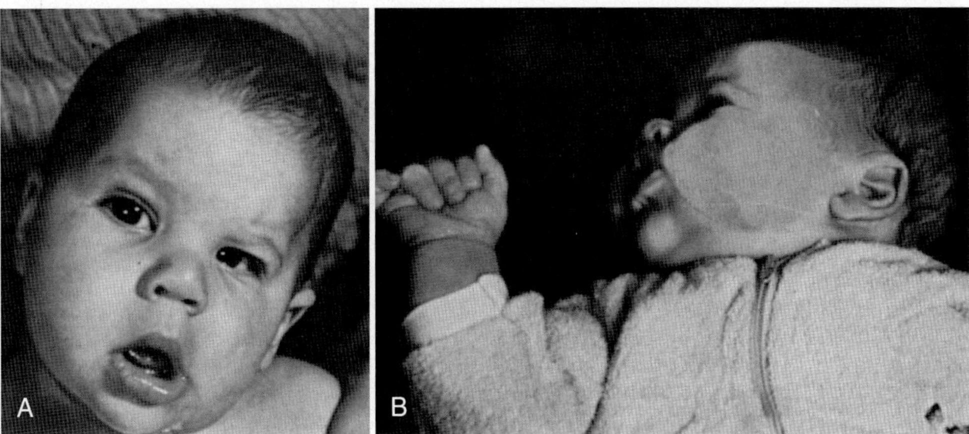

FIG. 34.44 A 6-month-old infant presented with right-sided congenital muscular torticollis. Note rotation of the skull and asymmetry and flattening of the face on the side of the contracted sternocleidomastoid.

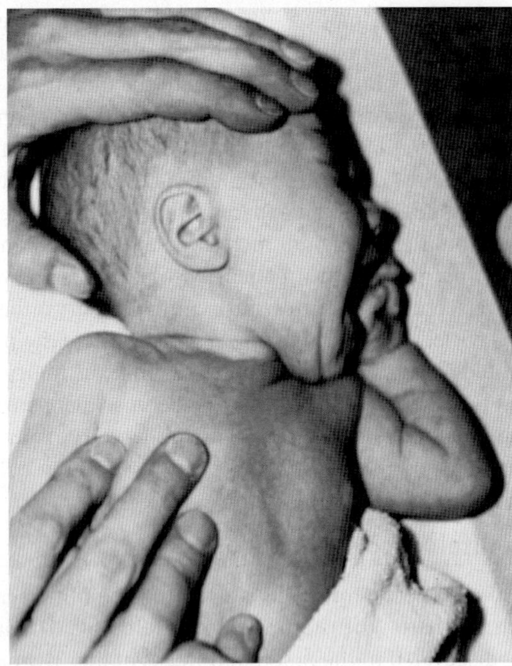

FIG. 34.45 A 6-week-old infant presented with swelling in the region of the sternocleidomastoid. The mass is usually soft, nontender, and mobile beneath the skin, but is attached to the muscle.

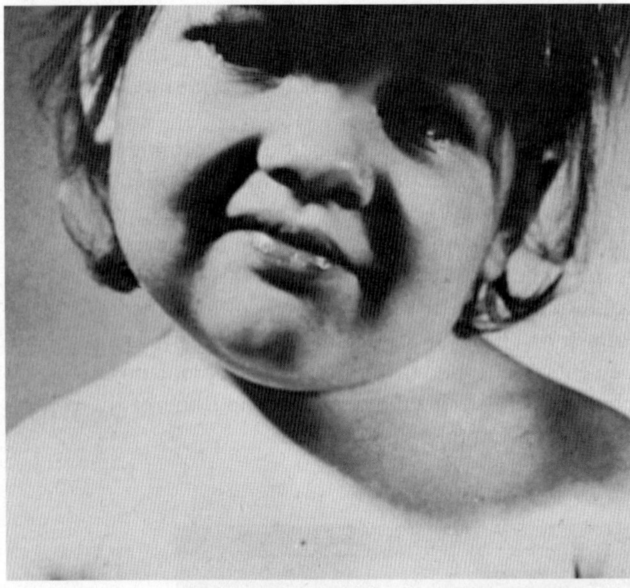

FIG. 34.46 This 18-month-old child had torticollis that was resistant to stretching exercises and required surgical release.

Clinical Presentation

Currently, the etiology of congenital muscular torticollis is thought to be due to compression of the SCM during delivery.[210] While most commonly unilateral, bilateral torticollis has been reported.[211] Although commonly associated with breech or difficult deliveries, it may occur after otherwise normal deliveries or in cesarean sections.[205]

In MRI studies of infants with congenital muscular torticollis, Davids et al.[210] found signal changes in the SCM muscle similar to changes observed in the forearm and leg after compartment syndrome. In cadaveric dissections, the fascia covers the entire SCM, strongly suggesting that congenital muscular torticollis represents a compartment syndrome. Experimental work with dogs suggests that the lesion is due to occlusion of the venous outflow of the SCM muscle. As in the sequelae of compartment syndrome in other locations of the body, the occlusion results in edema, degeneration of muscle fibers, and eventual fibrosis of the muscle body.

The clinical deformity is related to the ratio of fibrosis to remaining functional muscle.[207] With sufficient normal muscle, the SCM stretches with growth, and the child will not likely develop the torticollis posture. If fibrosis predominates, there is very little elastic potential, and deformity ensues. With time, the fibrosis of the sternal head may entrap and compromise the branch of the accessory nerve to the clavicular head of the muscle, leading to a late increase in the deformity due to progressive denervation.[212]

Congenital muscular torticollis is associated with uterine crowding, or "packaging syndrome," due to restriction of infant movement in the tight maternal space. In many children, the lesion is on the right side,[210,213] and up to 20% of children will have concomitant developmental dysplasia of the hip.[214,215] In one series, all patients with concomitant hip disease required treatment for their dysplasia. Some authors recommend screening hip ultrasounds for all patients with congenital muscular torticollis.[216]

Differential Diagnosis

Head and neck postural deformities are a common complaint in children. While congenital muscular torticollis is the most common cause of wry neck posture in infants and young children, the differential diagnosis is diverse, and many other problems may lead to this unusual posture (Tables 34.1 and 34.2), including bony deformities, soft tissue lesions, inflammatory conditions, and neurologic conditions.

In fact, coexisting bony anomalies are common in the setting of congenital muscular torticollis. In 20 cases of muscular torticollis, Gyorgyi[217] found congenital cervical fusions, asymmetrical facet joints, basilar impression, atlantoaxial dislocation, assimilation of the atlas, and deformities of the odontoid process. Occipitocervical malformations, basilar invagination, KFS, and asymmetrical development of the occipital condyles may manifest as torticollis.[36,68,171]

The posture of the head and neck, as well as the stiffness of the deformity, may provide clues as to the etiology. In the presence of both head tilt and rotatory deformity, the pathology is more likely at C1–C2, whereas head tilt alone indicates a more generalized problem in the cervical spine. Rigid deformity, especially without contracture of the SCM muscle, points to a bony anomaly of the cervical spine (particularly C1–C2) as a cause of torticollis.

Soft tissue problems are less frequent and may include excessive skin webs (pterygium colli), which maintain the neck posture. SCM muscle tumors, cystic hygroma, branchial cleft cyst, and thyroid teratoma are rare but possible. Inflammatory conditions include cervical lymphadenitis or retropharyngeal

TABLE 34.1 Differential Diagnosis of Torticollis

Congenital	Acquired
Occipitocervical anomalies	Neurogenic
Basilar impressions	Spinal cord tumors
Atlantooccipital fusion	Cerebellar tumors (posterior fossa)
Odontoid anomalies	Syringomyelia
Hemiatlas	Ocular dysfunction
Pterygium colli (skin web)	Bulbar palsies
Congenital muscular torticollis	Traumatic (particularly C1–C2)
Klippel-Feil syndrome	Subluxations Dislocations Fractures Inflammatory Cervical adenitis Spontaneous hyperemic atlantoaxial rotatory subluxation Tuberculosis Typhoid Rheumatoid arthritis Acute calcification of disc Miscellaneous Sandifer syndrome (hiatal hernia with esophageal reflux)

TABLE 34.2 Torticollis Caused by Bony Anomalies

Congenital Anomalies of Craniocervical Junction	Acquired Anomalies of Craniocervical Junction
Klippel-Feil syndrome	Traumatic
Atlantooccipital synostosis (unilateral)	Subluxations
Odontoid anomalies	Dislocations
Aplasia	Fractures
Hypoplasia	Inflammatory
Os odontoideum	Rheumatoid arthritis
Occipital vertebra	Idiopathic
Asymmetry of occipital condyles (hypoplasia)	Atlantoaxial rotatory displacement Subluxation Fixation

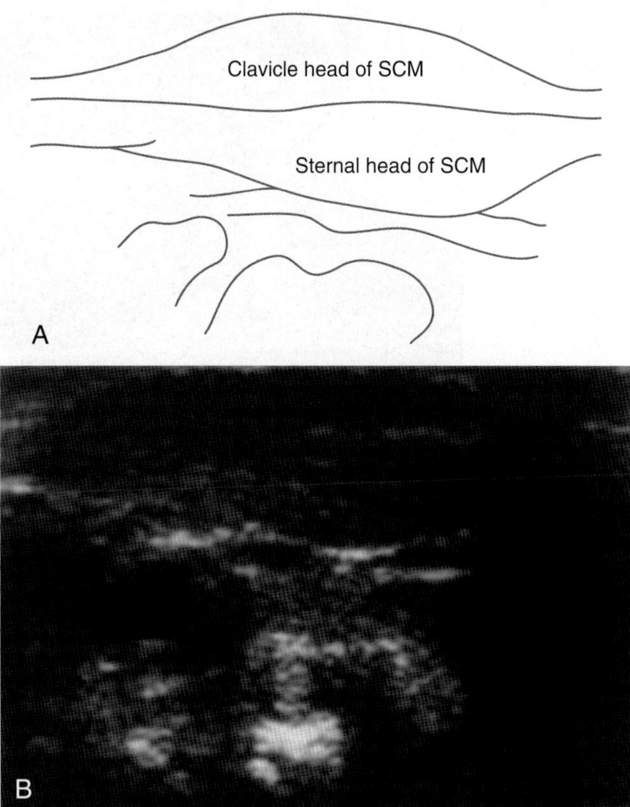

FIG. 34.47 (A) Abnormal appearance of sternocleidomastoid (SCM) in congenital muscular torticollis. (B) Ultrasonography shows homogeneous, hyperechoic mass on the SCM. (Modified from Tien YC, Su JY, Lin GT, et al. Ultrasonographic study of the coexistence of muscular torticollis and dysplasia of the hip. *J Pediatr Orthop* 2001;21:343–347.)

abscess.[218] Polyarticular juvenile rheumatoid arthritis may involve the cervical spine, and torticollis may be the only clinical sign. Following pharyngitis, spontaneous atlantoaxial rotatory subluxation may occur,[219,220] resulting in torticollis.

Traumatic causes should be considered also, as torticollis commonly follows injury to the C1–C2 articulation. Children with conditions with known C1–C2 instability (Morquio syndrome, spondyloepiphyseal dysplasia, and Down syndrome) should be evaluated thoroughly. Intermittent torticollis can occur, as in the case of a seizurelike disorder termed *benign paroxysmal torticollis of infancy*. Similarly, Sandifer syndrome, involving gastroesophageal reflux with sudden posturing of the trunk and neck, is a known etiology of torticollis in children with cerebral palsy.[221] Neurologic disorders, particularly space-occupying lesions of the central nervous system, are often accompanied by torticollis. Other neurologic causes include dystonia musculorum deformans and disorders of hearing and vision that can result in head tilt.[222]

In the setting of acute-onset torticollis, atlantoaxial rotatory subluxation must be part of the differential diagnosis. Early treatment is paramount, as acute treatment for this condition can often be nonoperative. Chronic or missed rotatory subluxation often will require more aggressive treatment.

Imaging

While the diagnosis of congenital muscular torticollis is most commonly made on clinical grounds, sometimes imaging modalities are needed for confirmation. Ultrasonography is now considered the most sensitive test for confirming the diagnosis of congenital muscular torticollis. A homogeneous, hyperechoic mass within the SCM muscle is diagnostic of congenital muscular torticollis.[223] Ultrasound has proven to be a very sensitive and specific modality in making the diagnosis[224] (Fig. 34.47).

Children with torticollis who fail to improve with routine conservative treatment should be evaluated with radiography to exclude an osseous abnormality or fracture. However, adequate radiographic interpretation (especially at the occipitocervical junction) may be difficult because of the abnormal head position. It is helpful to remember that the atlas moves with the occiput: a radiograph directed 90 degrees to the

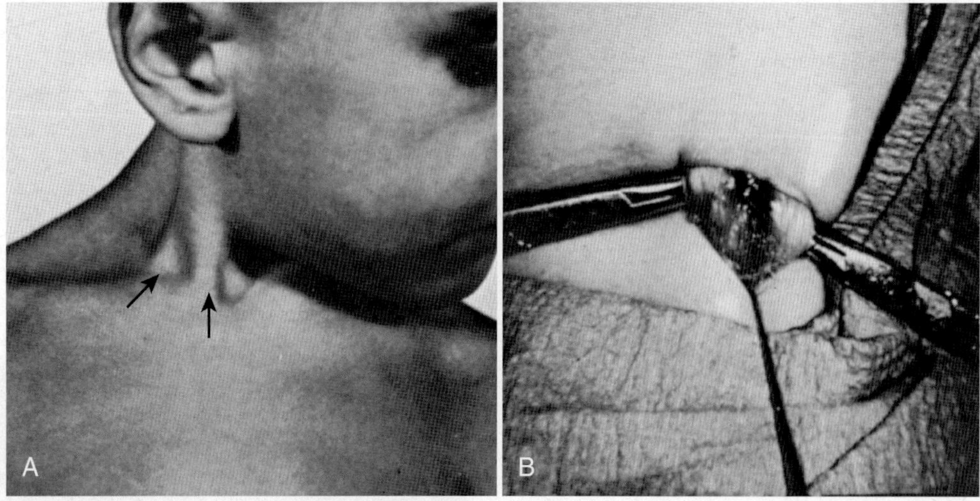

FIG. 34.48 (A) Clinical appearance of a 6-year-old child with congenital muscular torticollis. Note appearance of two heads of sternocleidomastoid (*arrows*). (B) Operative exposure of the same patient shows complete replacement with fibrous tissue of the two heads of the sternocleidomastoid..

lateral skull usually results in a satisfactory view of the occipitocervical junction. Flexion-extension films may also be necessary to reveal cervical instability.

CT scans may be beneficial, especially in the cases of discerning torticollis from atlantoaxial instability, or C1–C2 rotatory subluxation. This is because plain radiographs cannot differentiate the position of C1 and C2 during subluxation from that in a normal child whose head is rotated, as the images are identical. Using dynamic CT scans by rotating the head to the right and left, the clinician can determine the position of the facets.[220]

Nonoperative Treatment

Excellent results can be obtained with conservative measures in most patients,[205,213,225] which includes physical therapy and stretching exercises. Controlled manual stretching is safe and effective in greater than 95% of patients with congenital muscular torticollis when seen before the age of 1 year.[226] The most important prognostic factors for success are minimal rotational deficit, age less than 1 year, and absence of a palpable tight band or tumor in the affected SCM muscle.

Standard maneuvers include stretching the SCM muscle by positioning of the ear opposite the contracted muscle to the shoulder and touching the chin to the shoulder on the affected side.[227] Utilization of a physical therapist in performing exercises may be more beneficial than teaching parents on their own.[228] When adequate stretching has been obtained in the neutral position, these maneuvers are repeated with the head hyperextended to achieve maximal stretching. When plagiocephaly is present, the use of a sleeping helmet may reduce the deformity.

Surgery

There are no clear indications for surgery. In situations with persistent significant deformity persisting beyond 1 year of age with an obviously tight SCM, release of the muscle can be considered. In patients without functional deficit, indications for treatment are not clear. Early aggressive treatment of acute torticollis is important, as progression to chronic rotatory subluxation becomes a more significant problem requiring more aggressive treatment. Established facial asymmetry and motion limitations usually preclude a good result[225]; asymmetry of the skull and face improves as long as adequate growth potential remains after the deforming pull of the SCM is removed.[207] Although it has been traditionally thought that age greater than 1 year precluded good results, good cosmetic results can be obtained in children 5 to 7 years of age (Fig. 34.48).[229] Even patients older than 8 years can benefit from unipolar or bipolar release of the SCM and postoperative physical therapy.[230] Even if neglected, delayed release of the SCM has been found to be successful in improving both neck ROM and head and facial deformities.[231]

Surgery consists of resection of a portion of the distal SCM muscle. At least a 1-cm segment should be removed to guard against recurrence of the deformity. A transverse incision is made low in the neck to coincide with a normal skin fold.[232] The two heads of the SCM are identified, and both are sectioned. The investing fascia around the SCM must also be released.[205] Rotation of the chin and head at this point generally reveals the adequacy of the surgery, and palpation of the neck shows any extraneous tight bands that could lead to partial recurrence of incomplete correction. In an older child, an accessory incision (bipolar) is often required to section the muscle at its origin on the mastoid process. The whole muscle should not be excised because this may lead to reverse torticollis or asymmetry in the contour of the neck.[213] It is important not to place the incision near or very near the clavicle because scars in this area tend to spread and are cosmetically unacceptable.

The postoperative regimen includes passive stretching exercises of the SCM muscle, which should begin as soon as the patient can tolerate them. Occasionally, head traction at night is helpful, particularly in an older child. Bracing or cast correction may be necessary if the deformity has been of long duration or if the torticollis posture has become a habit for the child. In the right cohort of patients, results of surgery are uniformly good, with a low incidence of complications or recurrence. Slight restriction of the neck motion and anomalous reattachment can occur but are generally unnoticed by the patient, and recurrence is rare. Residual fascial bands may be an etiology for persistent neck posturing. The most common postoperative complaint is disfiguring scarring.[213,232]

Acknowledgment

We are deeply indebted to Dr. R. Hensinger, author of prior versions of this chapter. Much of the current work was built upon his previous efforts.

REFERENCES

1. Steinmetz MP, Mroz TE, Benzel EC. Craniovertebral junction: biomechanical considerations. *Neurosurgery*. 2010;66(3 suppl):7-12.
2. Ebraheim NA, Lu J, Biyani A, Brown JA, Yeasting RA. An anatomic study of the thickness of the occipital bone. Implications for occipitocervical instrumentation. *Spine*. 1996;21(15):1725-1729.
3. Haher TR, Yeung AW, Caruso SA, et al. Occipital screw pullout strength. A biomechanical investigation of occipital morphology. *Spine*. 1999;24(1):5-9.
4. Zipnick RI, Merola AA, Gorup J, et al. Occipital morphology: an anatomic guide to internal fixation. *Spine*. 1996;21(15):1719-1724.
5. Geck MJ, Truumees E, Hawthorne D, et al. Feasibility of rigid upper cervical instrumentation in children: tomographic analysis of children aged 2-6. *J Spinal Disord Tech*. 2014;27(3):E110-E117.
6. Hankinson TC, Avellino AM, Harter D, et al. Equivalence of fusion rates after rigid internal fixation of the occiput to C-2 with or without C-1 instrumentation. *J Neurosurg Pediatr*. 2010;5(4):380-384.
7. Chamoun RB, Whitehead WE, Curry DJ, Luerssen TG, Jea A. Computed tomography morphometric analysis for C-1 lateral mass screw placement in children. Clinical article. *J Neurosurg Pediatr*. 2009;3(1):20-23.
8. Harms J, Melcher RP. Posterior C1-C2 fusion with polyaxial screw and rod fixation. *Spine*. 2001;26(22):2467-2471.
9. Goldstein RY, Sunde CD, Assaad P, et al. Location of the vertebral artery at C1 in children: how far out laterally can one safely dissect? *J Bone Joint Surg Am*. 2014;96(18):1552-1556.
10. Patel AJ, Gressot LV, Boatey J, et al. Routine sectioning of the C2 nerve root and ganglion for C1 lateral mass screw placement in children: surgical and functional outcomes. *Childs Nerv Syst*. 2013;29(1):93-97.
11. Haque A, Price AV, Sklar FH, et al. Screw fixation of the upper cervical spine in the pediatric population. *J Neurosurg Pediatr*. 2009;3(6):529-533.
12. Desai R, Stevenson CB, Crawford AH, Durrani AA, Mangano FT. C-1 lateral mass screw fixation in children with atlantoaxial instability: case series and technical report. *J Spinal Disord Tech* 2010;23(7):474-479.
13. Hedequist D, Proctor M. Screw fixation to C2 in children: a case series and technical report. *J Pediatr Orthop*. 2009;29(1):21-25.
14. Lehman RA Jr, Dmitriev AE, Helgeson MD, et al. Salvage of C2 pedicle and pars screws using the intralaminar technique: a biomechanical analysis. *Spine*. 2008;33(9):960-965.
15. Chern JJ, Chamoun RB, Whitehead WE, et al. Computed tomography morphometric analysis for axial and subaxial translaminar screw placement in the pediatric cervical spine. *J Neurosurg Pediatr*. 2009;3(2):121-128.
16. Brockmeyer D, Apfelbaum R, Tippets R, Walker M, Carey L. Pediatric cervical spine instrumentation using screw fixation. *Pediatr Neurosurg*. 1995;22(3):147-157.
17. Brockmeyer DL, York JE, Apfelbaum RI. Anatomical suitability of C1-2 transarticular screw placement in pediatric patients. *J Neurosurg*. 2000;92(1 suppl):7-11.
18. Gluf WM, Brockmeyer DL. Atlantoaxial transarticular screw fixation: a review of surgical indications, fusion rate, complications, and lessons learned in 67 pediatric patients. *J Neurosurg Spine*. 2005;2(2):164-169.
19. Hedequist D, Hresko T, Proctor M. Modern cervical spine instrumentation in children. *Spine*. 2008;33(4):379-383.
20. Hedequist D, Proctor M, Hresko T. Lateral mass screw fixation in children. *J Child Orthop*. 2010;4(3):197-201.
21. Vara CS, Thompson GH. A cadaveric examination of pediatric cervical pedicle morphology. *Spine*. 2006;31(10): 1107-1112.
22. Bono CM. The halo fixator. *J Am Acad Orthop Surg*. 2007;15(12):728-737.
23. Limpaphayom N, Skaggs DL, McComb G, Krieger M, Tolo VT. Complications of halo use in children. *Spine*. 2009;34(8):779-784.
24. Skaggs DL, Lerman LD, Albrektson J, et al. Use of a noninvasive halo in children. *Spine*. 2008;33(15):1650-1654.
25. Bakhshi H, Kushare I, Banskota B, Nelson C, Dormans JP. Pinless halo in the pediatric population: indications and complications. *J Pediatr Orthop*. 2015;35(4): 374-378.
26. Caird MS, Hensinger RN, Weiss N, Farley FA. Complications and problems in halo treatment of toddlers: limited ambulation is recommended. *J Pediatr Orthop*. 2006;26(6):750-752.
27. Larson AN, Polly DW Jr, Guidera KJ, et al. The accuracy of navigation and 3D image-guided placement for the placement of pedicle screws in congenital spine deformity. *J Pediatr Orthop*. 2012;32(6):e23-e29.
28. Larson AN, Santos ER, Polly DW Jr, et al. Pediatric pedicle screw placement using intraoperative computed tomography and 3-dimensional image-guided navigation. *Spine*. 2012;37(3):E188-E194.
29. Luo TD, Polly DW Jr, Ledonio C, Wetjen NM, Larson AN. Accuracy of pedicle screw placement in children ≤10 years using navigation and intraoperative CT. *J Spinal Disord Tech* 2014.
30. Tormenti MJ, Kostov DB, Gardner PA, et al. Intraoperative computed tomography image-guided navigation for posterior thoracolumbar spinal instrumentation in spinal deformity surgery. *Neurosurg Focus*. 2010;28(3):E11.
31. Kovanda TJ, Ansari SF, Qaiser R, Fulkerson DH. Feasibility of CT-based intraoperative 3D stereotactic image-guided navigation in the upper cervical spine of children 10 years of age or younger: initial experience. *J Neurosurg Pediatr*. 2015;1-9.
32. Gosain AK, McCarthy JG, Pinto RS. Cervicovertebral anomalies and basilar impression in Goldenhar syndrome. *Plast Reconstr Surg*. 1994;93(3):498-506.

33. Jauregui N, Lincoln T, Mubarak S, Garfin S. Surgically related upper cervical spine canal anatomy in children. *Spine.* 1993;18(14):1939-1944.
34. Menezes AH, Vogel TW. Specific entities affecting the craniocervical region: syndromes affecting the craniocervical junction. *Childs Nerv Syst.* 2008;24(10):1155-1163.
35. Sawin PD, Menezes AH. Basilar invagination in osteogenesis imperfecta and related osteochondrodysplasias: medical and surgical management. *J Neurosurg.* 1997;86(6):950-960.
36. Caetano de Barros M, Farias W, Ataide L, Lins S. Basilar impression and Arnold-Chiari malformation. A study of 66 cases. *J Neurol Neurosurg Psychiatry.* 1968;31(6):596-605.
37. Goel A, Bhatjiwale M, Desai K. Basilar invagination: a study based on 190 surgically treated patients. *J Neurosurg.* 1998;88(6):962-968.
38. Samartzis D, Kalluri P, Herman J, Lubicky JP, Shen FH. Superior odontoid migration in the Klippel-Feil patient. *Eur Spine J.* 2007;16(9):1489-1497.
39. Bassi P, Corona C, Contri P, et al. Congenital basilar impression: correlated neurological syndromes. *Eur Neurol.* 1992;32(4):238-243.
40. Kohno K, Sakaki S, Nakamura H, et al. Foramen magnum decompression for syringomyelia associated with basilar impression and Chiari I malformation—report of three cases. *Neurol Med Chir (Tokyo).* 1991;31(11):715-719.
41. da Silva JA. Basilar impression and Arnold-Chiari malformation. Surgical findings in 209 cases. *Neurochirurgia (Stuttg).* 1992;35(6):189-195.
42. McGregor M. The significance of certain measurements of the skull in the diagnosis of basilar impression. *Br J Radiol.* 1948;21(244):171-181.
43. Bernini FP, Elefante R, Smaltino F, Tedeschi G. Angiographic study on the vertebral artery in cases of deformities of the occipitocervical joint. *Am J Roentgenol Radium Ther Nucl Med.* 1969;107(3):526-529.
44. Dickinson LD, Tuite GF, Colon GP, Papadopoulos SM. Vertebral artery dissection related to basilar impression: case report. *Neurosurgery.* 1995;36(4):835-838.
45. Michie I, Clark M. Neurological syndromes associated with cervical and craniocervical anomalies. *Arch Neurol.* 1968;18(3):241-247.
46. Chamberlain WE. Basilar impression (platybasia): a bizarre developmental anomaly of the occipital bone and upper cervical spine with striking and misleading neurologic manifestations. *Yale J Biol Med.* 1939;11(5):487-496.
47. Wellborn CC, Sturm PF, Hatch RS, Bomze SR, Jablonski K. Intraobserver reproducibility and interobserver reliability of cervical spine measurements. *J Pediatr Orthop.* 2000;20(1):66-70.
48. Cronin CG, Lohan DG, Mhuircheartigh JN, et al. MRI evaluation and measurement of the normal odontoid peg position. *Clin Radiol.* 2007;62(9):897-903.
49. Barker R, Fareedi S, Thompson D, Saunders D. The use of CT angiography in the preoperative planning of cervical spine surgery in children. *Childs Nerv Syst.* 2009;25(8):955-959.
50. Klimo P Jr, Rao G, Brockmeyer D. Congenital anomalies of the cervical spine. *Neurosurg Clin N Am.* 2007;18(3):463-478.
51. Menezes AH. Craniocervical developmental anatomy and its implications. *Childs Nerv Syst.* 2008;24(10):1109-1122.
52. Menezes AH, VanGilder JC. Transoral-transpharyngeal approach to the anterior craniocervical junction. Ten-year experience with 72 patients. *J Neurosurg.* 1988;69(6): 895-903.
53. Collignon FP, Cohen-Gadol AA, Krauss WE. Circumferential decompression of the foramen magnum for the treatment of syringomyelia associated with basilar invagination. *Neurosurg Rev.* 2004;27(3):168-172.
54. Zileli M, Cagli S. Combined anterior and posterior approach for managing basilar invagination associated with type I Chiari malformation. *J Spinal Disord Tech* 2002;15(4):284-289.
55. Kumar R, Kalra SK, Mahapatra AK. A clinical scoring system for neurological assessment of high cervical myelopathy: measurements in pediatric patients with congenital atlantoaxial dislocations. *Neurosurgery.* 2007;61(5):987-993.
56. Menezes AH. Surgical approaches: postoperative care and complications "transoral-transpalatopharyngeal approach to the craniocervical junction". *Childs Nerv Syst.* 2008;24(10):1187-1193.
57. McGirt MJ, Attenello FJ, Sciubba DM, Gokaslan ZL, Wolinsky JP. Endoscopic transcervical odontoidectomy for pediatric basilar invagination and cranial settling. Report of 4 cases. *J Neurosurg Pediatr.* 2008;1(4):337-342.
58. Ahmed R, Traynelis VC, Menezes AH. Fusions at the craniovertebral junction. *Childs Nerv Syst.* 2008;24(10):1209-1224.
59. Menezes AH. Specific entities affecting the craniocervical region: osteogenesis imperfecta and related osteochondrodysplasias: medical and surgical management of basilar impression. *Childs Nerv Syst.* 2008;24(10):1169-1172.
60. Arponen H, Vuorimies I, Haukka J, et al. Cranial base pathology in pediatric osteogenesis imperfecta patients treated with bisphosphonates. *J Neurosurg Pediatr.* 2015;15(3):313-320.
61. Georgopoulos G, Pizzutillo PD, Lee MS. Occipito-atlantal instability in children. A report of five cases and review of the literature. *J Bone Joint Surg Am.* 1987;69(3):429-436.
62. Yin YH, Wang P, Yu XG. Klippel-Feil syndrome associated with congenital atlantooccipital dislocation and absent C1 posterior arch. *Spine J.* 2015;15(6):1503-1505.
63. Browd SR, McIntyre JS, Brockmeyer D. Failed age-dependent maturation of the occipital condyle in patients with congenital occipitoatlantal instability and Down syndrome: a preliminary analysis. *J Neurosurg Pediatr.* 2008;2(5):359-364.
64. Hosalkar HS, Cain EL, Horn D, et al. Traumatic atlanto-occipital dislocation in children. *J Bone Joint Surg Am.* 2005;87(11):2480-2488.
65. Rahimi SY, Stevens EA, Yeh DJ, et al. Treatment of atlantoaxial instability in pediatric patients. *Neurosurg Focus.* 2003;15(6):ECP1.
66. Astur N, Klimo P Jr, Sawyer JR, et al. Traumatic atlanto-occipital dislocation in children: evaluation, treatment, and outcomes. *J Bone Joint Surg Am.* 2013;95(24):e194(1-8).
67. Chandraraj S, Briggs CA. Failure of somite differentiation at the cranio-vertebral region as a cause of occipitalization of the atlas. *Spine.* 1992;17(10):1249-1251.
68. Torklus DV, Gehle W. *The Upper Cervical Spine: Regional Anatomy, Pathology and Traumatology: A Systematic Radiological Atlas and Textbook.* London: Butterworth; 1972.
69. Gholve PA, Hosalkar HS, Ricchetti ET, et al. Occipitalization of the atlas in children. Morphologic classification, associations, and clinical relevance. *J Bone Joint Surg Am.* 2007;89(3):571-578.
70. Bharucha EP, Dastur HM. Craniovertebral anomalies (a report on 40 cases). *Brain.* 1964;87:469-480.
71. McRae DL, Barnum AS. Occipitalization of the atlas. *Am J Roentgenol Radium Ther Nucl Med.* 1953;70(1):23-46.

72. Hadley LA. *The Spine: Anatomico-Radiographic Studies: Development and the Cervical Region*. Springfield, IL: Thomas; 1956.
73. McRae DL. Bony abnormalities in the region of the foramen magnum: correlation of the anatomic and neurologic findings. *Acta Radiol*. 1953;40(2-3):335-354.
74. Gupta V, Khandelwal N, Mathuria SN, et al. Dynamic magnetic resonance imaging evaluation of craniovertebral junction abnormalities. *J Comput Assist Tomogr*. 2007;31(3):354-359.
75. Smoker WR, Khanna G. Imaging the craniocervical junction. *Childs Nerv Syst*. 2008;24(10):1123-1145.
76. Hosalkar HS, Sankar WN, Wills BP, et al. Congenital osseous anomalies of the upper cervical spine. *J Bone Joint Surg Am*. 2008;90(2):337-348.
77. Nicholson JT, Sherk HH. Anomalies of the occipitocervical articulation. *J Bone Joint Surg Am*. 1968;50(2):295-304.
78. Letts M, Slutsky D. Occipitocervical arthrodesis in children. *J Bone Joint Surg Am*. 1990;72(8):1166-1170.
79. Di Lorenzo N. Craniocervical junction malformation treated by transoral approach. A survey of 25 cases with emphasis on postoperative instability and outcome. *Acta Neurochir (Wien)*. 1992;118(3-4):112-116.
80. Dickman CA, Locantro J, Fessler RG. The influence of transoral odontoid resection on stability of the craniovertebral junction. *J Neurosurg*. 1992;77(4):525-530.
81. Aronson DD, Kahn RH, Canady A, Bollinger RO, Towbin R. Instability of the cervical spine after decompression in patients who have Arnold-Chiari malformation. *J Bone Joint Surg Am*. 1991;73(6):898-906.
82. Bailey DK. The normal cervical spine in infants and children. *Radiology*. 1952;59(5):712-719.
83. Senoglu M, Safavi-Abbasi S, Theodore N, et al. The frequency and clinical significance of congenital defects of the posterior and anterior arch of the atlas. *J Neurosurg Spine*. 2007;7(4):399-402.
84. Musha Y, Mizutani K. Cervical myelopathy accompanied with hypoplasia of the posterior arch of the atlas: case report. *J Spinal Disord Tech* 2009;22(3):228-232.
85. Dubousset J. Torticollis in children caused by congenital anomalies of the atlas. *J Bone Joint Surg Am*. 1986;68(2):178-188.
86. Spitzer R, Rabinowitch JY, Wybar KC. A study of the abnormalities of the skull, teeth and lenses in mongolism. *Can Med Assoc J*. 1961;84(11):567-572.
87. Brockmeyer D. Down syndrome and craniovertebral instability. Topic review and treatment recommendations. *Pediatr Neurosurg*. 1999;31(2):71-77.
88. Reilly CW, Choit RL. Transarticular screws in the management of C1-C2 instability in children. *J Pediatr Orthop*. 2006;26(5):582-588.
89. Pueschel SM, Scola FH. Atlantoaxial instability in individuals with Down syndrome: epidemiologic, radiographic, and clinical studies. *Pediatrics*. 1987;80(4):555-560.
90. Semine AA, Ertel AN, Goldberg MJ, Bull MJ. Cervical-spine instability in children with Down syndrome (trisomy 21). *J Bone Joint Surg Am*. 1978;60(5):649-652.
91. Locke GR, Gardner JI, Van Epps EF. Atlas-dens interval (ADI) in children: a survey based on 200 normal cervical spines. *Am J Roentgenol Radium Ther Nucl Med*. 1966;97(1):135-140.
92. Steel HH. Anatomical and mechanical considerations of the atlanto-axial articulations. *J Bone Joint Surg Am*. 1968; 50:1481.
93. Burke SW, French HG, Roberts JM, et al. Chronic atlanto-axial instability in Down syndrome. *J Bone Joint Surg Am*. 1985;67(9):1356-1360.
94. Davidson RG. Atlantoaxial instability in individuals with Down syndrome: a fresh look at the evidence. *Pediatrics*. 1988;81(6):857-865.
95. Elliott S, Morton RE, Whitelaw RA. Atlantoaxial instability and abnormalities of the odontoid in Down's syndrome. *Arch Dis Child*. 1988;63(12):1484-1489.
96. Dickman CA, Mamourian A, Sonntag VK, Drayer BP. Magnetic resonance imaging of the transverse atlantal ligament for the evaluation of atlantoaxial instability. *J Neurosurg*. 1991;75(2):221-227.
97. Fielding JW, Cochran G, Lawsing JF 3rd, Hohl M. Tears of the transverse ligament of the atlas. A clinical and biomechanical study. *J Bone Joint Surg Am*. 1974;56(8):1683-1691.
98. Klimo P Jr, Kan P, Rao G, Apfelbaum R, Brockmeyer D. Os odontoideum: presentation, diagnosis, and treatment in a series of 78 patients. *J Neurosurg Spine*. 2008;9(4):332-342.
99. Perovic MN, Kopits SE, Thompson RC. Radiological evaluation of the spinal cord in congenital atlanto-axial dislocation. *Radiology*. 1973;109(3):713-716.
100. Roach JW, Duncan D, Wenger DR, Maravilla A, Maravilla K. Atlanto-axial instability and spinal cord compression in children—diagnosis by computerized tomography. *J Bone Joint Surg Am*. 1984;66(5):708-714.
101. Fielding JW, Hensinger RN, Hawkins RJ. Os odontoideum. *J Bone Joint Surg Am*. 1980;62(3):376-383.
102. Weng MS, Haynes RJ. Flexion and extension cervical MRI in a pediatric population. *J Pediatr Orthop*. 1996;16(3):359-363.
103. Bhatnagar M, Sponseller PD, Carroll CT, Tolo VT. Pediatric atlantoaxial instability presenting as cerebral and cerebellar infarcts. *J Pediatr Orthop*. 1991;11(1):103-107.
104. Miyata I, Imaoka T, Masaoka T, Nishiura T, Ishimitsu H. Pediatric cerebellar infarction caused by atlantoaxial subluxation: case report. *Neurol Med Chir (Tokyo)*. 1994;34(4):241-245.
105. Ferguson RL, Putney ME, Allen BL Jr. Comparison of neurologic deficits with atlanto-dens intervals in patients with Down syndrome. *J Spinal Disord*. 1997;10(3):246-252.
106. Hankinson TC, Anderson RC. Craniovertebral junction abnormalities in Down syndrome. *Neurosurgery*. 2010;66(3 suppl):32-38.
107. Pueschel SM, Scola FH, Pezzullo JC. A longitudinal study of atlanto-dens relationships in asymptomatic individuals with Down syndrome. *Pediatrics*. 1992;89(6 Pt 2):1194-1198.
108. American Academy of Pediatrics. Committee on Sports Medicine. Atlantoaxial instability in Down syndrome. *Pediatrics*. 1984;74(1):152-154.
109. Fielding JW, Hawkins RJ, Ratzan SA. Spine fusion for atlanto-axial instability. *J Bone Joint Surg Am*. 1976;58(3):400-407.
110. Doyle JS, Lauerman WC, Wood KB, Krause DR. Complications and long-term outcome of upper cervical spine arthrodesis in patients with Down syndrome. *Spine*. 1996;21(10):1223-1231.
111. Segal LS, Drummond DS, Zanotti RM, Ecker ML, Mubarak SJ. Complications of posterior arthrodesis of the cervical spine in patients who have Down syndrome. *J Bone Joint Surg Am*. 1991;73(10):1547-1554.
112. Smith MD, Phillips WA, Hensinger RN. Fusion of the upper cervical spine in children and adolescents. An analysis of 17 patients. *Spine*. 1991;16(7):695-701.

113. Taggard DA, Menezes AH, Ryken TC. Treatment of Down syndrome-associated craniovertebral junction abnormalities. *J Neurosurg.* 2000;93(2 suppl):205-213.
114. Menezes AH, Ryken TC. Craniovertebral abnormalities in Down's syndrome. *Pediatr Neurosurg.* 1992;18(1):24-33.
115. Anderson RC, Ragel BT, Mocco J, Bohman LE, Brockmeyer DL. Selection of a rigid internal fixation construct for stabilization at the craniovertebral junction in pediatric patients. *J Neurosurg.* 2007;107(1 suppl):36-42.
116. Nader-Sepahi A, Casey AT, Hayward R, Crockard HA, Thompson D. Symptomatic atlantoaxial instability in Down syndrome. *J Neurosurg.* 2005;103(3 suppl):231-237.
117. Menezes AH. Specific entities affecting the craniocervical region: Down's syndrome. *Childs Nerv Syst.* 2008;24(10):1165-1168.
118. Krieger AJ, Rosomoff HL, Kuperman AS, Zingesser LH. Occult respiratory dysfunction in a craniovertebral anomaly. *J Neurosurg.* 1969;31(1):15-20.
119. Reddy KR, Rao GS, Devi BI, Prasad PV, Ramesh VJ. Pulmonary function after surgery for congenital atlantoaxial dislocation: a comparison with surgery for compressive cervical myelopathy and craniotomy. *J Neurosurg Anesthesiol.* 2009;21(3):196-201.
120. Hensinger RN. Osseous anomalies of the craniovertebral junction. *Spine.* 1986;11(4):323-333.
121. Wollin DG. The os odontoideum. Separate odontoid process. *J Bone Joint Surg Am.* 1963;45:1459-1471.
122. Gwinn JL, Smith JL. Acquired and congenital absence of the odontoid process. *Am J Roentgenol Radium Ther Nucl Med.* 1962;88:424-431.
123. Stevens JM, Chong WK, Barber C, Kendall BE, Crockard HA. A new appraisal of abnormalities of the odontoid process associated with atlanto-axial subluxation and neurological disability. *Brain.* 1994;117(Pt 1):133-148.
124. Herkowitz HN, Rothman RH, Simeone FA. *Rothman-Simeone, the Spine.* 5th ed. Philadelphia: Elsevier; 2006.
125. Evarts CM, Lonsdale D. Ossiculum terminale: an anomaly of the odontoid process. Report of a case of atlantoaxial dislocation with cord compression. *Cleve Clin Q.* 1970;37(1):73-76.
126. Swoboda B, Hirschfelder H, Hohmann D. Atlantoaxial instability in a 7-year-old boy associated with traumatic disrupture of the ossiculum terminale (apical odontoid epiphysis). *Eur Spine J.* 1995;4(4):248-251.
127. Cattell HS, Filtzer DL. Pseudosubluxation and other normal variations in the cervical spine in children. A study of one hundred and sixty children. *J Bone Joint Surg Am.* 1965;47(7):1295-1309.
128. Schiff DC, Parke WW. The arterial supply of the odontoid process. *J Bone Joint Surg Am.* 1973;55(7):1450-1456.
129. Parke WW. The vascular relations of the upper cervical vertebrae. *Orthop Clin North Am.* 1978;9(4):879-889.
130. Currarino G. Segmentation defect in the midodontoid process and its possible relationship to the congenital type of os odontoideum. *Pediatr Radiol.* 2002;32(1):34-40.
131. Flemming C, Hodson CJ. Os odontoideum; a congenital abnormality of the axis; case report. *J Bone Joint Surg Br.* 1955;37-B(4):622-623.
132. Morgan MK, Onofrio BM, Bender CE. Familial os odontoideum. Case report. *J Neurosurg.* 1989;70(4):636-639.
133. Kirlew KA, Hathout GM, Reiter SD, Gold RH. Os odontoideum in identical twins: perspectives on etiology. *Skeletal Radiol.* 1993;22(7):525-527.
134. Fielding JW, Griffin PP. Os odontoideum: an acquired lesion. *J Bone Joint Surg Am.* 1974;56(1):187-190.
135. Hawkins RJ, Fielding JW, Thompson WJ. Os odontoideum: congenital or acquired. A case report. *J Bone Joint Surg Am.* 1976;58(3):413-414.
136. Freiberger RH, Wilson PD Jr, Nicholas JA. Acquired absence of the odontoid process: a case report. *J Bone Joint Surg Am.* 1965;47:1231-1236.
137. Ahlback S, Collert S. Destruction of the odontoid process due to atlanto-axial pyogenic spondylitis. *Acta Radiol Diagn (Stockh).* 1970;10(5):394-400.
138. Watanabe M, Toyama Y, Fujimura Y. Atlantoaxial instability in os odontoideum with myelopathy. *Spine.* 1996;21(12):1435-1439.
139. Minderhoud JM, Braakman R, Penning L. Os odontoideum, clinical, radiological and therapeutic aspects. *J Neurol Sci.* 1969;8(3):521-544.
140. McKeever FM. Atlanto-axoid instability. *Surg Clin North Am.* 1968;48(6):1375-1390.
141. Ford FR. Syncope, vertigo and disturbances of vision resulting from intermittent obstruction of the vertebral arteries due to defect in the odontoid process and excessive mobility of the second cervical vertebra. *Bull Johns Hopkins Hosp.* 1952;91(3):168-173.
142. Elliott S. The odontoid process in children: is it hypoplastic? *Clin Radiol.* 1988;39(4):391-393.
143. Sankar WN, Wills BP, Dormans JP, Drummond DS. Os odontoideum revisited: the case for a multifactorial etiology. *Spine.* 2006;31(9):979-984.
144. Holt RG, Helms CA, Munk PL, Gillespy T 3rd. Hypertrophy of C-1 anterior arch: useful sign to distinguish os odontoideum from acute dens fracture. *Radiology.* 1989;173(1):207-209.
145. Fagan AB, Askin GN, Earwaker JW. The jigsaw sign. A reliable indicator of congenital aetiology in os odontoideum. *Eur Spine J.* 2004;13(4):295-300.
146. Yamashita Y, Takahashi M, Sakamoto Y, Kojima R. Atlantoaxial subluxation. Radiography and magnetic resonance imaging correlated to myelopathy. *Acta Radiol.* 1989;30(2):135-140.
147. Hughes TB Jr, Richman JD, Rothfus WE. Diagnosis of os odontoideum using kinematic magnetic resonance imaging. A case report. *Spine.* 1999;24(7):715-718.
148. Rowland LP, Shapiro JH, Jacobson HG. Neurological syndromes associated with congenital absence of the odontoid process. *AMA Arch Neurol Psychiatry.* 1958;80(3):286-291.
149. Clements WD, Mezue W, Mathew B. Os odontoideum: congenital or acquired? That's not the question. *Injury.* 1995;26(9):640-642.
150. Dai LY, Yuan W, Ni B, et al. Surgical treatment of nonunited fractures of the odontoid process, with special reference to occipitocervical fusion for unreducible atlantoaxial subluxation or instability. *Eur Spine J.* 2000;9(2):118-122.
151. Levy ML, McComb JG. C1-C2 fusion in children with atlantoaxial instability and spinal cord compression: technical note. *Neurosurgery.* 1996;38(1):211-215.
152. Huang CI, Chen IH. Atlantoaxial arthrodesis using Halifax interlaminar clamps reinforced by halo vest immobilization: a long-term follow-up experience. *Neurosurgery.* 1996;38(6):1153-1156.
153. Coyne TJ, Fehlings MG, Wallace MC, Bernstein M, Tator CH. C1-C2 posterior cervical fusion: long-term evaluation of results and efficacy. *Neurosurgery.* 1995;37(4):688-692.

154. Dickman CA, Crawford NR, Paramore CG. Biomechanical characteristics of C1-2 cable fixations. *J Neurosurg.* 1996;85(2):316-322.
155. Menendez JA, Wright NM. Techniques of posterior C1-C2 stabilization. *Neurosurgery.* 2007;60(1 Suppl 1):S103-S111.
156. Goel A, Desai KI, Muzumdar DP. Atlantoaxial fixation using plate and screw method: a report of 160 treated patients. *Neurosurgery.* 2002;51(6):1351-1356.
157. Mah JY, Thometz J, Emans J, Millis M, Hall JE. Threaded K-wire spinous process fixation of the axis for modified Gallie fusion in children and adolescents. *J Pediatr Orthop.* 1989;9(6):675-679.
158. Dickman CA, Sonntag VK. Posterior C1-C2 transarticular screw fixation for atlantoaxial arthrodesis. *Neurosurgery.* 1998;43(2):275-280.
159. Farey ID, Nadkarni S, Smith N. Modified Gallie technique versus transarticular screw fixation in C1-C2 fusion. *Clin Orthop Relat Res.* 1999;359:126-135.
160. Grob D, Crisco JJ 3rd, Panjabi MM, Wang P, Dvorak J. Biomechanical evaluation of four different posterior atlantoaxial fixation techniques. *Spine.* 1992;17(5):480-490.
161. Bambakidis NC, Feiz-Erfan I, Horn EM, et al. Biomechanical comparison of occipitoatlantal screw fixation techniques. *J Neurosurg Spine.* 2008;8(2):143-152.
162. Chamoun RB, Relyea KM, Johnson KK, et al. Use of axial and subaxial translaminar screw fixation in the management of upper cervical spinal instability in a series of 7 children. *Neurosurgery.* 2009;64(4):734-739.
163. Smith MD, Phillips WA, Hensinger RN. Complications of fusion to the upper cervical spine. *Spine.* 1991;16(7):702-705.
164. Dyck P. Os odontoideum in children: neurological manifestations and surgical management. *Neurosurgery.* 1978;2(2):93-99.
165. Whitesides TE Jr, McDonald AP. Lateral retropharyngeal approach to the upper cervical spine. *Orthop Clin North Am.* 1978;9(4):1115-1127.
166. Klippel M, Feil A. Un cas d'absence des vertèbres cervicales avec cage thoracique remontant jusqu'a la base du crane. *Nouv Icon Salpet.* 1912;25:223.
167. Tracy MR, Dormans JP, Kusumi K. Klippel-Feil syndrome: clinical features and current understanding of etiology. *Clin Orthop Relat Res.* 2004;424:183-190.
168. Clarke RA, Kearsley JH, Walsh DA. Patterned expression in familial Klippel-Feil syndrome. *Teratology.* 1996;53(3):152-157.
169. Clarke RA, Singh S, McKenzie H, Kearsley JH, Yip MY. Familial Klippel-Feil syndrome and paracentric inversion inv(8)(q22.2q23.3). *Am J Hum Genet.* 1995;57(6):1364-1370.
170. Ramsey J, Bliznak J. Klippel-Feil syndrome with renal agenesis and other anomalies. *Am J Roentgenol Radium Ther Nucl Med.* 1971;113(3):460-463.
171. Hensinger RN, Lang JE, MacEwen GD. Klippel-Feil syndrome; a constellation of associated anomalies. *J Bone Joint Surg Am.* 1974;56(6):1246-1253.
172. Baird PA, Robinson GC, Buckler WS. Klippel-Feil syndrome. A study of mirror movement detected by electromyography. *Am J Dis Child.* 1967;113(5):546-551.
173. Baga N, Chusid EL, Miller A. Pulmonary disability in the Klippel-Feil syndrome. A study of two siblings. *Clin Orthop Relat Res.* 1969;67:105-110.
174. Morrison SG, Perry LW, Scott LP 3rd. Congenital brevicollis (Klippel-Feil syndreom) and cardiovascular anomalies. *Am J Dis Child.* 1968;115(5):614-620.
175. Palant DI, Carter BL. Klippel-Feil syndrome and deafness. A study with polytomography. *Am J Dis Child.* 1972;123(3):218-221.
176. Stark EW, Borton TE. Hearing loss and the Klippel-Feil syndrome. *Am J Dis Child.* 1972;123(3):233-235.
177. Gray SW, Romaine CB, Skandalakis JE. Congenital fusion of the cervical vertebrae. *Surg Gynecol Obstet.* 1964;118: 373-385.
178. Sherk HH, Shut L, Chung S. Iniencephalic deformity of the cervical spine with Klippel-Feil anomalies and congenital elevation of the scapula; report of three cases. *J Bone Joint Surg Am.* 1974;56(6):1254-1259.
179. Samartzis D, Herman J, Lubicky JP, Shen FH. Sprengel's deformity in Klippel-Feil syndrome. *Spine.* 2007;32(18):E512-E516.
180. Pizzutillo PD, Woods M, Nicholson L, MacEwen GD. Risk factors in Klippel-Feil syndrome. *Spine.* 1994;19(18):2110-2116.
181. Ulmer JL, Elster AD, Ginsberg LE, Williams DW 3rd. Klippel-Feil syndrome: CT and MR of acquired and congenital abnormalities of cervical spine and cord. *J Comput Assist Tomogr.* 1993;17(2):215-224.
182. Shoul MI, Ritvo M. Clinical and roentgenological manifestations of the Klippel-Feil syndrome (congenital fusion of the cervical vertebrae, brevicollis); report of eight additional cases and review of the literature. *Am J Roentgenol Radium Ther Nucl Med.* 1952;68(3):369-385.
183. Illingworth RS. Attacks of unconsciousness in association with fused cervical vertebrae. *Arch Dis Child.* 1956;31(155):8-11.
184. Born CT, Petrik M, Freed M, DeLong WG Jr. Cerebrovascular accident complicating Klippel-Feil syndrome. A case report. *J Bone Joint Surg Am.* 1988;70(9):1412-1415.
185. Theiss SM, Smith MD, Winter RB. The long-term follow-up of patients with Klippel-Feil syndrome and congenital scoliosis. *Spine.* 1997;22(11):1219-1222.
186. Thomsen MN, Schneider U, Weber M, Johannisson R, Niethard FU. Scoliosis and congenital anomalies associated with Klippel-Feil syndrome types I-III. *Spine.* 1997;22(4):396-401.
187. Xue X, Shen J, Zhang J, et al. Klippel-Feil syndrome in congenital scoliosis. *Spine.* 2014;39(23):E1353-E1358.
188. Drvaric DM, Ruderman RJ, Conrad RW, et al. Congenital scoliosis and urinary tract abnormalities: are intravenous pyelograms necessary? *J Pediatr Orthop.* 1987;7(4): 441-443.
189. Gunderson CH, Solitare GB. Mirror movements in patients with the Klippel-Feil syndrome. Neuropathologic observations. *Arch Neurol.* 1968;18(6):675-679.
190. Guille JT, Miller A, Bowen JR, Forlin E, Caro PA. The natural history of Klippel-Feil syndrome: clinical, roentgenographic, and magnetic resonance imaging findings at adulthood. *J Pediatr Orthop.* 1995;15(5):617-626.
191. Ritterbusch JF, McGinty LD, Spar J, Orrison WW. Magnetic resonance imaging for stenosis and subluxation in Klippel-Feil syndrome. *Spine.* 1991;16(10 suppl): S539-S541.
192. Nguyen VD, Tyrrel R. Klippel-Feil syndrome: patterns of bony fusion and wasp-waist sign. *Skeletal Radiol.* 1993;22(7):519-523.
193. Samartzis D, Kalluri P, Herman J, Lubicky JP, Shen FH. The extent of fusion within the congenital Klippel-Feil segment. *Spine.* 2008;33(15):1637-1642.

194. Sullivan CR, Bruwer AJ, Harris LE. Hypermobility of the cervical spine in children; a pitfall in the diagnosis of cervical dislocation. *Am J Surg*. 1958;95(4):636-640.
195. Hedequist D, Emans J. Congenital scoliosis: a review and update. *J Pediatr Orthop*. 2007;27(1):106-116.
196. Hall JE, Simmons ED, Danylchuk K, Barnes PD. Instability of the cervical spine and neurological involvement in Klippel-Feil syndrome. A case report. *J Bone Joint Surg Am*. 1990;72(3):460-462.
197. Baba H, Maezawa Y, Furusawa N, et al. The cervical spine in the Klippel-Feil syndrome. A report of 57 cases. *Int Orthop*. 1995;19(4):204-208.
198. Samartzis D, Kalluri P, Herman J, Lubicky JP, Shen FH. The role of congenitally fused cervical segments upon the space available for the cord and associated symptoms in Klippel-Feil patients. *Spine*. 2008;33(13):1442-1450.
199. Shen FH, Samartzis D, Herman J, Lubicky JP. Radiographic assessment of segmental motion at the atlantoaxial junction in the Klippel-Feil patient. *Spine*. 2006;31(2):171-177.
200. Hensinger RN. Congenital anomalies of the cervical spine. *Clin Orthop Relat Res*. 1991;264:16-38.
201. Stallmer ML, Vanaharam V, Mashour GA. Congenital cervical spine fusion and airway management: a case series of Klippel-Feil syndrome. *J Clin Anesth*. 2008;20(6):447-451.
202. Ruf M, Jensen R, Harms J. Hemivertebra resection in the cervical spine. *Spine*. 2005;30(4):380-385.
203. Bonola A. Surgical treatment of the Klippel-Feil syndrome. *J Bone Joint Surg Br*. 1956;38-B(2):440-449.
204. Mooney JF 3rd, White DR, Glazier S. Previously unreported structure associated with Sprengel deformity. *J Pediatr Orthop*. 2009;29(1):26-28.
205. Ling CM, Low YS. Sternomastoid tumor and muscular torticollis. *Clin Orthop Relat Res*. 1972;86:144-150.
206. Chan YL, Cheng JC, Metreweli C. Ultrasonography of congenital muscular torticollis. *Pediatr Radiol*. 1992;22(5):356-360.
207. Coventry MB, Harris LE. Congenital muscular torticollis in infancy; some observations regarding treatment. *J Bone Joint Surg Am*. 1959;41-A(5):815-822.
208. Brackbill Y, Douthitt TC, West H. Psychophysiologic effects in the neonate of prone versus supine placement. *J Pediatr*. 1973;82(1):82-84.
209. Safe to Sleep Public Education Campaign. National Institute of Child Health and Human Development. https://www.nichd.nih.gov/sts/Pages/default.aspx.
210. Davids JR, Wenger DR, Mubarak SJ. Congenital muscular torticollis: sequela of intrauterine or perinatal compartment syndrome. *J Pediatr Orthop*. 1993;13(2):141-147.
211. Babu MK, Lee P, Mahadev A, Lee EH. Congenital bilateral sternocleidomastoid contracture: a case report. *J Pediatr Orthop B*. 2009;18(3):145-147.
212. Sarnat HB, Morrissy RT. Idiopathic torticollis: sternocleidomastoid myopathy and accessory neuropathy. *Muscle Nerve*. 1981;4(5):374-380.
213. Macdonald D. Sternomastoid tumour and muscular torticollis. *J Bone Joint Surg Br*. 1969;51(3):432-443.
214. Hummer CD, MacEwen GD. The coexistence of torticollis and congenital dysplasia of the hip. *J Bone Joint Surg Am*. 1972;54(6):1255-1256.
215. von Heideken J, Green DW, Burke SW, et al. The relationship between developmental dysplasia of the hip and congenital muscular torticollis. *J Pediatr Orthop*. 2006;26(6): 805-808.
216. Joiner ER, Andras LM, Skaggs DL. Screening for hip dysplasia in congenital muscular torticollis: is physical exam enough? *J Child Orthop*. 2014;8(2):115-119.
217. Gyorgyi G. [Morphological changes of the occipito-cervical region associated with torticollis]. *J Radiol Electrol Med Nucl*. 1964;45:797-802.
218. Bredenkamp JK, Maceri DR. Inflammatory torticollis in children. *Arch Otolaryngol Head Neck Surg*. 1990;116(3):310-313.
219. Fielding JW, Hawkins RJ. Atlanto-axial rotatory fixation (fixed rotatory subluxation of the atlanto-axial joint). *J Bone Joint Surg Am*. 1977;59(1):37-44.
220. Phillips WA, Hensinger RN. The management of rotatory atlanto-axial subluxation in children. *J Bone Joint Surg Am*. 1989;71(5):664-668.
221. Deskin RW. Sandifer syndrome: a cause of torticollis in infancy. *Int J Pediatr Otorhinolaryngol*. 1995;32(2):183-185.
222. Williams CR, O'Flynn E, Clarke NM, Morris RJ. Torticollis secondary to ocular pathology. *J Bone Joint Surg Br*. 1996;78(4):620-624.
223. Tien YC, Su JY, Lin GT, Lin SY. Ultrasonographic study of the coexistence of muscular torticollis and dysplasia of the hip. *J Pediatr Orthop*. 2001;21(3):343-347.
224. Wang L, Zhang L, Tang Y, Qiu L. The value of high-frequency and color Doppler ultrasonography in diagnosing congenital muscular torticollis. *BMC Musculoskelet Disord*. 2012; 13:209.
225. Canale ST, Griffin DW, Hubbard CN. Congenital muscular torticollis. A long-term follow-up. *J Bone Joint Surg Am*. 1982;64(6):810-816.
226. Cheng JC, Wong MW, Tang SP, et al. Clinical determinants of the outcome of manual stretching in the treatment of congenital muscular torticollis in infants. A prospective study of eight hundred and twenty-one cases. *J Bone Joint Surg Am*. 2001;83-A(5):679-687.
227. Oledzka M, Kaplan SL. Commentary on "adapting to higher demands: using innovative methods to treat infants presenting with torticollis and plagiocephaly". *Pediatr Phys Ther*. 2014;26(3):346.
228. Ohman A, Nilsson S, Beckung E. Stretching treatment for infants with congenital muscular torticollis: physiotherapist or parents? A randomized pilot study. *PM R*. 2010;2(12):1073-1079.
229. de Chalain TM, Katz A. Idiopathic muscular torticollis in children: the Cape Town experience. *Br J Plast Surg*. 1992;45(4):297-301.
230. Shim JS, Noh KC, Park SJ. Treatment of congenital muscular torticollis in patients older than 8 years. *J Pediatr Orthop*. 2004;24(6):683-688.
231. Kim HJ, Ahn HS, Yim SY. Effectiveness of surgical treatment for neglected congenital muscular torticollis: a systematic review and meta-analysis. *Plast Reconstr Surg*. 2015;136(1):67e-77e.
232. Staheli LT. Muscular torticollis: late results of operative treatment. *Surgery*. 1971;69(3):469-473.

CHAPTER 35 Congenital Anomalies of the Spinal Cord

Muhammad M. Abd-El-Barr
Kevin T. Huang
R. Michael Scott
Mark R. Proctor

Introduction

Congenital anomalies of the dorsal midline structures—including neural tissue, muscle, skin, and bones—fall into the broad category referred to as *neural tube defects* (NTDs). When referring to NTDs, there are several different types. They range from common entities that are not clinically important to major anomalies that have significant implications throughout the nervous system. *Spinal dysraphism* refers to a group of anomalies involving the bony or nervous components of the spine and, more specifically, the failure of fusion of these midline structures. *Spina bifida* refers to bony posterior structures that do not completely fuse in the midline. Although uncomplicated, bony spina bifida is a common asymptomatic radiographic finding. When it is associated with complex anomalies of the nerve roots, dura, and even organs outside the nervous system (such as those within the genitourinary or gastrointestinal systems), it can be a source of major disability. The embryologic defects related to spinal dysrhaphism can occur either due to failure of primary neurulation and closure of the neural tube, which should occur in the third or fourth fetal week of life, or later failures of secondary neurulation. The incidence of spinal dysraphism is estimated to be 0.05 to 0.25 per 1000 live births.[1]

Spinal dysraphism has been recognized since the earliest of times and in all cultures. The most severe of these defects can result in permanent disability to patients, depriving them of "those qualities held in high esteem by our society—independence, physical powers and intelligence."[2] Aristotle (384–322 BCE) recommended infanticide for these children, leading to an ongoing debate about the diagnosis and management of these difficult defects, including the current trend toward antenatal treatment.

Spinal dysraphism is divided into two main categories: (1) *Spina bifida aperta* is characterized by herniation of the spinal cord and nerves through a defect in the skin, apparent at birth and/or on prenatal imaging. *Myelomeningocele* (MMC) is the most common of these defects. (2) *Spina bifida occulta* involves less obvious defects, as the neural structures are covered by full-thickness skin. Although each can be associated with significant spinal cord pathology, the associated anomalies of the nervous system are far greater when the lesion is associated with a loss of spinal fluid (see discussion of "unified theory" in the myelomeningocele section later in the chapter). Management of spinal dysraphism involves three main stages: (1) accurate diagnosis; (2) surgical intervention, if warranted; and (3) postoperative care, which often includes lifelong management of neurologic deficits that can worsen over time. This chapter reviews the major types of congenital anomalies of the spinal cord, including the exciting but controversial subject of prenatal diagnosis and surgical intervention for open MMC defects.

Embryology

Many of these congenital anomalies are associated with presumed problems in embryogenesis; a review of relevant embryogenesis will be helpful for the practitioner to understand these anomalies.

The development of the spine occurs between the second and sixth week of gestation and progresses in the following stages: gastrulation, primary neurulation, secondary neurulation, and retrogressive differentiation. Gastrulation (day 16) occurs when the mesoblast (future mesoderm) converts the bilaminar embryonic disc to a trilaminar structure. By 18 days of development, all three germ layers are present. The neural groove, which is a longitudinal depression, is destined to be the brain and spinal cord.

Neurulation (beginning at day 22) is the process by which the neural groove deepens to become a hollow neural tube, and includes two phases. The rostral opening closes first in humans (day 24), while the caudal opening closes at 28 days of gestation. Primary neurulation is completed by the fourth week of gestation. Errors in this phase lead to open neural tube defects, such as MMC or encephalocele, when affecting the brain.

Secondary neurulation refers to the canalization of secondary tubules and the formation of a secondary neural tube caudal to the lower lumbar levels. This secondary neural tube will fuse with the primary neural tube. Errors during this process of secondary neurulation can lead to a terminal MMC or lipomyelomeningocele. The caudal cell mass, which is responsible for secondary neurulation, is also responsible for the formation of other organ systems, and accounts for the frequent association of anomalies of the distal spinal cord with those of the anorectal or genitourinary system.

At approximately 45 days of gestation, the caudal end of the neural tube (i.e., immature spinal cord) extends to the coccygeal spinal level. At this point, retrogressive differentiation is partly responsible for the cranial ascent of the neural tube as compared to the bony structures, although the differential growth of the spinal cord and spine is the major reason that, in a majority of adults, the conus medullaris corresponds to the level of the L1–L2 disc.[3]

Spina Bifida Aperta

The term *spina bifida* was first proposed by Nicolaas Tulp, a Dutch physician and surgeon who was pictured in Rembrandt's famous painting "Anatomy Lesson" for his description of MMC in 1651.[4] Originally, it was used to describe a duplication of the spinous process, but is currently still used for any malformation of the lumbar spine.[5]

Myelomeningocele

Embryology

MMC is the most common significant birth defect affecting the spine. It is characterized by herniation of a malformed spinal cord and its related meninges through a defect in the bony spinal canal and skin. MMC refers to herniation of the meninges through such a defect, without associated spinal cord tissue.

MMC most likely occurs when the posterior neuropore fails to close during primary neurulation, or if it reopens due to distention of the central canal by cerebrospinal fluid (CSF). This spinal abnormality is only one of the constitutive abnormalities seen in this disorder, which can also include Chiari II malformation, hydrocephalus, and multiple brain abnormalities, including partial agenesis of the corpus callosum, thalamic adhesions, and gyral malformations.

McLone and Naidich attempted to explain this constellation of findings with their "unified theory."[6] This theory hypothesizes that the open spinal defect and associated drainage of CSF leads to a loss of backpressure within the developing ventricular system of the brain, causing the collapse of the rhomboencephalic vesicle, which results in a small posterior fossa. This resultant small posterior fossa in effect forces the growing cerebellum and hindbrain to herniate downward into the cervical spinal canal, which is the hallmark finding of the Chiari II malformation. This downward herniation causes an obstruction of the fourth ventricle outlet, which causes hydrocephalus in the fetus or, in the newborn after closing the MMC, eliminates the spinal defect as a CSF drainage pathway.

Epidemiology

The incidence of MMC ranges from less than 1 case per 1000 live births to almost 9 cases per 1000 live births.[7] It is unclear what accounts for this regional variability. Ethnicity also appears to be involved in the epidemiology, with Hispanics having a higher rate of neural tube defects compared with African Americans and Asians in the United States, even after taking into account other factors.[8,9]

In the 1970s, it was noted that the red cell folate levels of women of lower socioeconomic status in the United Kingdom were lower than those of higher socioeconomic status, and that these women had a higher rate of pregnancies complicated by neural tube defects.[10] A double-blind randomized trial commissioned by the Medical Research Council Vitamin Study Group (UK) showed that periconceptional folic acid supplementation (4 mg/day in mothers with a previous history of NTDs) was associated with a substantial risk reduction of 72%.[11] The result of this study was the impetus of the US Centers for Disease Control and Prevention (CDC) recommending 4 mg/day folic acid supplementation for those mothers with a high risk of MMC due to a previously affected pregnancy.[12] A randomized study of more than 4000 low-risk Hungarian women found a statistically significant reduction of NTDs with folic acid supplementation (800 mg/day). This led to the further recommendation by the CDC that all women of reproductive age should take 400 mg folic acid daily in addition to consuming a folate-rich diet.[13]

Prenatal Diagnosis

Historically, the rates of prenatal diagnosis of MMC were relatively low, but this has changed in recent years, especially in developed countries. Serum screening of α-fetoprotein and acetylcholinesterase and the use of ultrasound yield current detection rates close to 80%.[14]

Ultrasound can be particularly effective in diagnosing MMC; as a result, rates of detection have increased dramatically over the last 2 decades. Both direct and indirect signs of MMC and other neural tube defects can be seen on ultrasonography. These indirect signs include the "lemon sign" (frontal bossing), the "banana sign" (deformation of the cerebellum), and obliteration of the cisterna magna (Fig. 35.1).[1] The diagnosis can be made as early as the tenth week of gestation in some cases, but the majority of cases are diagnosed between weeks 18 and 24.[15]

There is evidence, including sequential imaging studies, to suggest that the neurologic deficits in MMC may be progressive, with movement in the lower limbs decreasing with gestational age, and worsening of the hydrocephalus and hindbrain herniation.[16] Conversely, animal models of spina bifida showed preserved neurologic function and improved hindbrain herniation when there was prenatal coverage of the spinal defect.[17] This suggested that many of the final phenotypes of MMC may be due to a "two-hit" process, in which the spinal defect may initiate lower limb dysfunction, but the continued egress of CSF through the defect may cause some of the hindbrain defects, and further damage may

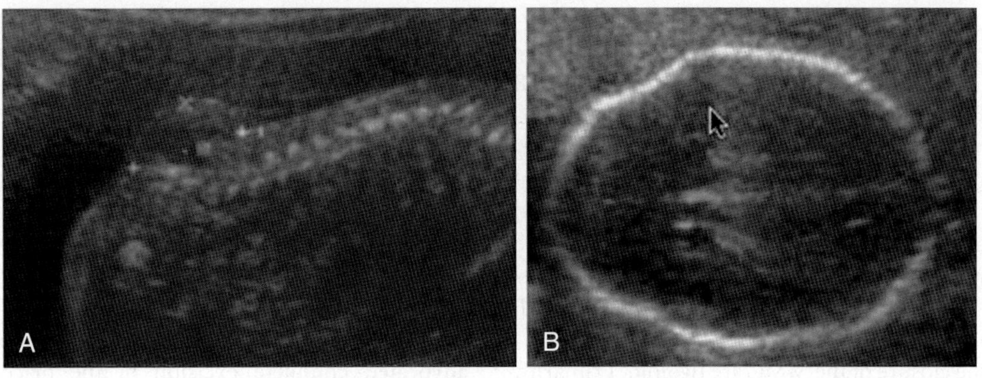

FIG. 35.1 Ultrasound findings of myelomeningocele. (A) Two-dimensional ultrasound showing fluid collection posterior to the spine, representing a myelomeningocele. (B) Frontal narrowing, or the banana sign. (From Zerah M, Kulkarni AV. Spinal cord malformations. *Handb Clin Neurol.* 2013;112:975-991.)

ensure exposure of the neural elements to the intrauterine environment.[18]

As can be imagined, once the diagnosis has been made, the parents and health care team are faced with an ethical dilemma. Termination of pregnancy is one option that is often pursued, with rates of termination around 20% in the United States and around 80% in Europe.[19] However, many countries have made termination of pregnancies illegal, even in the face of the most severe malformations. In addition, other families would not consider this a viable choice if it were permissible. Therefore, regardless of the choice made by the parents, a spina bifida center should include a multidisciplinary team consisting of neurosurgeons, orthopedists, neonatologists, urologists, and social workers.

TABLE 35.1 Segmental Innervation of Lower Extremity Muscles

Hip flexion	L1–L3
Hip adduction	L2–L4
Knee extension	L2–L4
Ankle inversion	L4
Toe extension	L5–S1
Hip abduction	L5–S1
Hip extension	L5–S1
Knee flexion	L5–S2
Ankle plantar flexion	S1–S2

From Sharrard WJ. The segmental innervation of the lower limb muscles in man. *Ann R Coll Surg Engl.* 1964;35:106–122.

Initial Management

A detailed physical examination is necessary when assessing an infant with an MMC. The physical examination evaluates the general well-being of the infant and the deficits associated with the MMC, and seeks to find associated anomalies. The physical examination should include an assessment of the actual MMC defect, with an eye toward surgical closure, and a complete neurologic examination with an emphasis on attempting to localize the functional level of the MMC. An assessment of any orthopedic deformity and urologic function is also important. It is critical to assess the patient clinically and radiographically for concomitant findings of hydrocephalus, as many of these infants will require treatment for the condition by either placement of a shunt or endoscopy. This can be assessed by head circumference, bulging of the fontanelle, and splaying of the cranial bones at the sutures. Hindbrain dysfunction or the concomitant finding of a Chiari II malformation can be suggested by the findings of stridor or apnea.

The condition of the MMC will determine the rapidity of surgical intervention. One should not rupture the sac if it is not ruptured, although this is uncommon. If the sac has ruptured, the neural placode should be readily visible and prophylactic antibiotics should be started. The lesion should be kept moist with a nonadherent dressing.

The neurologic examination should include cranial nerve examination, as Chiari II malformations can present with lower cranial nerve dysfunction, such as stridor from vocal cord paralysis or swallowing difficulty. Eye motion abnormalities and nystagmus are also common. Examination of the lower extremities is of paramount importance, as it allows one to assess the functional level of the MMC. Particular attention should be paid to the position of the legs at rest, as well as fixed contractures and wasting of particular muscles, as they suggest paralysis of the nerves innervating these muscles. One should also pay attention to the lowest level of reactivity to painful stimuli. Table 35.1 lists the segmental innervation of the lower extremities and can be used to assign a functional level to the defect.[20]

In addition to the neurologic assessment, a general orthopedic assessment of the lower extremities is also important, as many of these patients have clubfeet (equinovarus defects) and/or dislocated hips. Spine radiographs can be used to assess the associated scoliosis, although this can usually be done later. If a major gibbus is seen clinically, then the radiographs should be taken before closure of the MMC, as resection of the gibbus might be necessary.[21,22] Many patients with MMC have associated urologic problems; as such, clean intermittent catheterization should be initiated immediately to avoid urinary tract infections.

Postnatal Surgery for MMC Closure

Closure of the MMC defect should occur within 24 to 48 hours after birth to decrease the risk of meningitis and ventriculitis. It is important to note to the parents that the procedure is lifesaving and can prevent deterioration of function, but it does not improve neurologic function. If there is no evidence of hydrocephalus, then closure of the MMC can be done as an isolated procedure. If significant hydrocephalus is present, closure of the MMC should be accompanied by CSF diversion (discussed later).

The goals of the closure of the MMC are twofold. Primarily, it is to seal the spine and spinal cord and guard against the entry of bacteria. Second, it is to preserve neurologic function and to prevent tethering of the spinal cord, although it must be stressed that the rate of retethering is very high.

Surgically, the infant is put in the prone position after intubation under general anesthesia with gentle gel rolls so that the abdomen is free and to minimize epidural bleeding. An elliptical incision is made outside the normal skin and the zona epithelioserosa, which is a thin, pearly layer that surrounds the placode. It is important to excise this tissue, as leaving it may lead to the development of epidermoid inclusion cysts. For most MMC defects, the defect is oriented in the superior/posterior axis, making a vertical closure easier, but there are times when a horizontal closure may be easier[23] (Fig. 35.2).

Next, radial excision of the skin surrounding the placode is done, with care not to damage the placode. For MMCs with complete lack of distal neurologic function, some authors have advocated complete excision of the placode, which may prevent future tethering. However, most surgeons endeavor to preserve the placode. In fact, it may be beneficial to reconstruct the placode into a tubular form so that it fits into the dural sac and is less likely to tether.

Once this is done, the surgeon attempts to free the dura from the underlying fascia. The two edges of dura are then approximated and sewn together in a water-tight fashion.

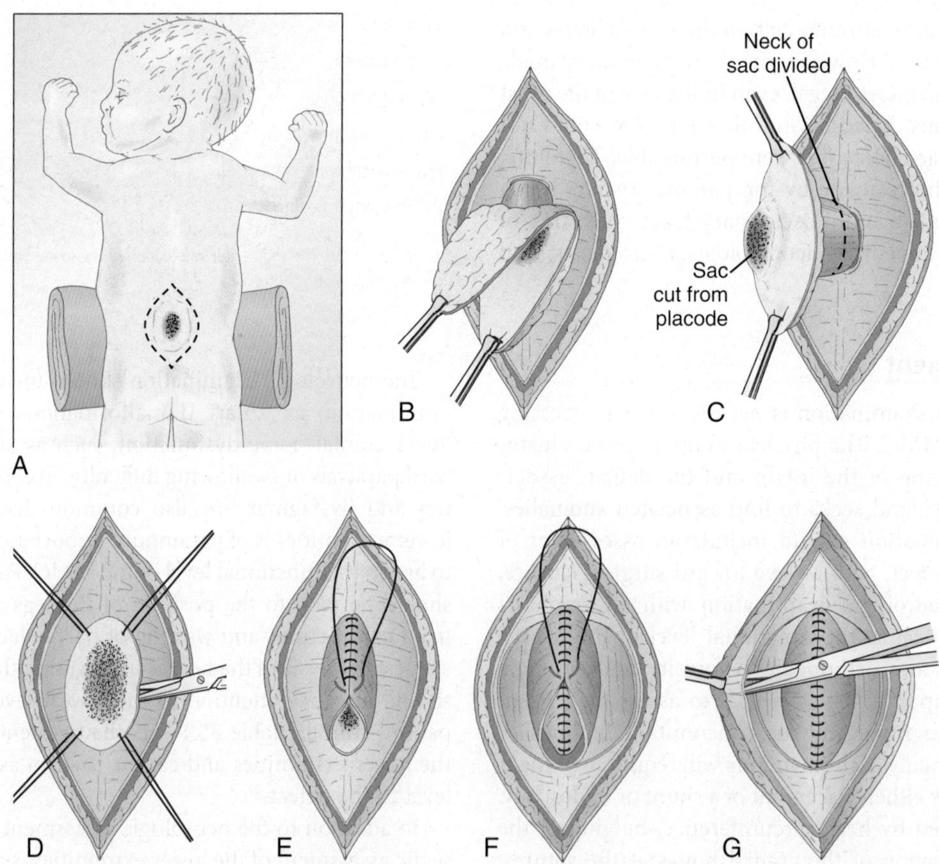

FIG. 35.2 Myelomeningocele closure. Technique for closure of myelomeningocele (see text). (A) The infant is placed in the prone position with towel rolls under the hips. An elliptic incision is outlined just outside the zona epithelioserosa, which may be oriented on the vertical or horizontal axis. (B) The incision is to the level of the lumbodorsal fascia. The apices of the island of skin within the incision are grasped with clamps, and the skin is undermined medially until the dural sac is seen to funnel through the fascial defect. (C) The dural sac is first incised at its base. The skin is excised from the placode and discarded, allowing the placode to fall into the spinal canal. (D) The everted dura is undermined and reflected medially to envelop the placode. The placode itself may be folded medially and sewn into a tube at this point. (E) The dural layer is closed with nonabsorbable suture, using a running stitch. (F) The fascia is incised to the muscle, undermined, and reflected medially to create second layer of closure. G, Skin is undermined using blunt techniques to permit closure.

Because the dura is often weak and the closure tenuous, it is a good idea to close the fascia in a separate layer. This is done by radially releasing the fascia from the overlying muscle and bringing the two edges of fascia together, over the closed dura. Next, to close the skin, undermining using blunt dissection is often necessary around to the abdomen. A two-layer closure is preferred, with interrupted nonabsorbable suture for large defects.

Larger defects require more complicated closure techniques; a close collaboration with plastic and reconstructive surgery is an important adjunct. The goal of closure is to minimize tension between individual tissue planes and to maximize tissue healing. One method to ensure this is to use an S-shaped skin opening, allowing for the use of local rotational flaps.[24] Rhomboid flaps and latissimus dorsi flaps can be used. We have also described using (1) local fascial turnover flaps with or without paraspinous muscle flaps for deep coverage of the dural repair followed by (2) linear, midline skin closure with good results[25] (Figs. 35.3 and 35.4).

Postoperatively, infants should be placed prone to avoid pressure on the incision. It is important to use a barrier dressing to avoid soiling with urine or stool. To monitor for the potential for hydrocephalus, daily head circumferences are measured and weekly head ultrasounds are obtained. It is important to have both orthopedic and urologic consultations to plan appropriate timing for repair of other associated anomalies and establish baseline urologic function. Routine catheterization is also important.

In Utero Closure

The first prenatal MMC repair was done in 1997. Early results suggested that this prenatal surgery had improved outcome for the infant in terms of decreased rates of hindbrain herniation, but also showed an increase in maternal risk, namely, the risk of preterm labor and uterine dehiscence.[26] These promising results were the impetus for the management of the Myelomeningocele Study (MOMS), which was a randomized trial at three tertiary centers that compared prenatal MMC closure to traditional postnatal closure.[18]

For this trial, the uterus was exposed via a low transverse laparotomy incision and exteriorized. The fetus and placenta were then located by ultrasound and hysterotomy. The MMC was closed in a standardized manner under magnification, generally using an allograft as a patch.

The primary outcome was the need for CSF shunting at 12 months. The prenatal group had a statistically significant lower rate compared with infants randomized to postnatal

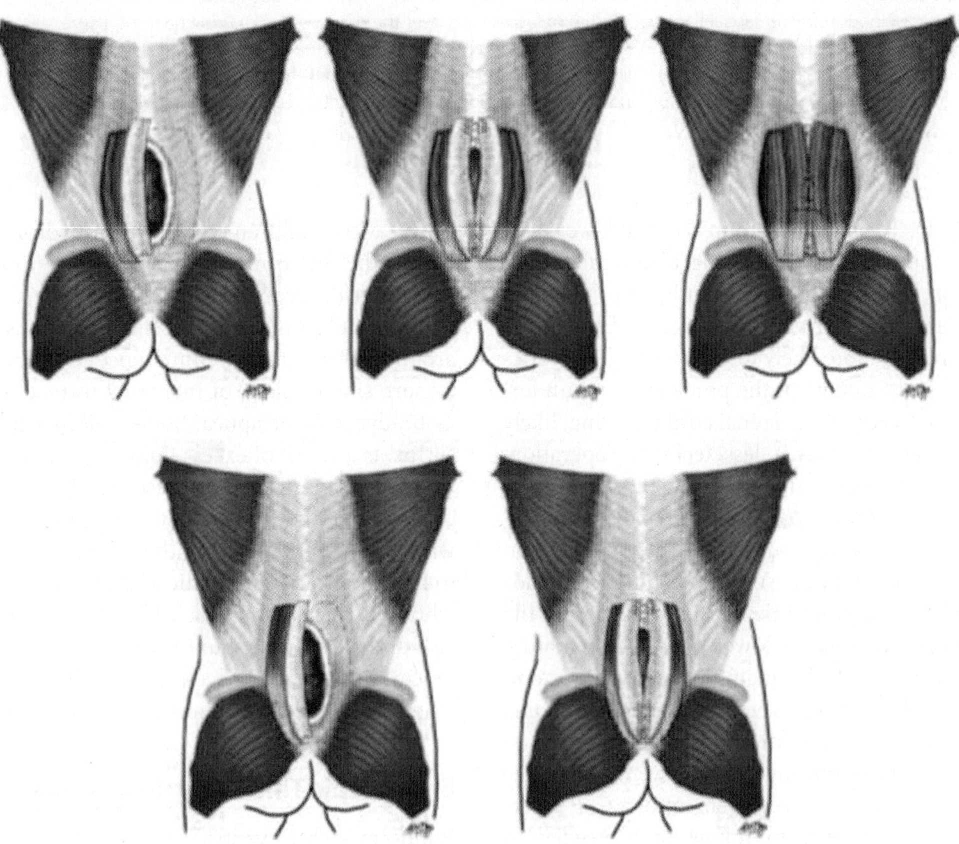

FIG. 35.3 Extradural myelomeningocele reconstruction. *Top,* Paraspinal muscle fascia is incised laterally and elevated medially over the underlying muscle. After the turnover fascial flaps are sutured together in the midline, the paraspinous muscles are then advanced medially. *Bottom,* If the majority of the defect is caudal to the paraspinous musculature, the paraspinous muscle fascia is turned over in continuity with the gluteal muscle fascia without additional muscle coverage. (From Patel KB, Taghinia AH, Proctor MR, Warf BC, Greene AK. Extradural myelomeningocele reconstruction using local turnover fascial flaps and midline linear skin closure. *J Plast Reconstr Aesthet Surg.* 2012;65[11]:1569-572.)

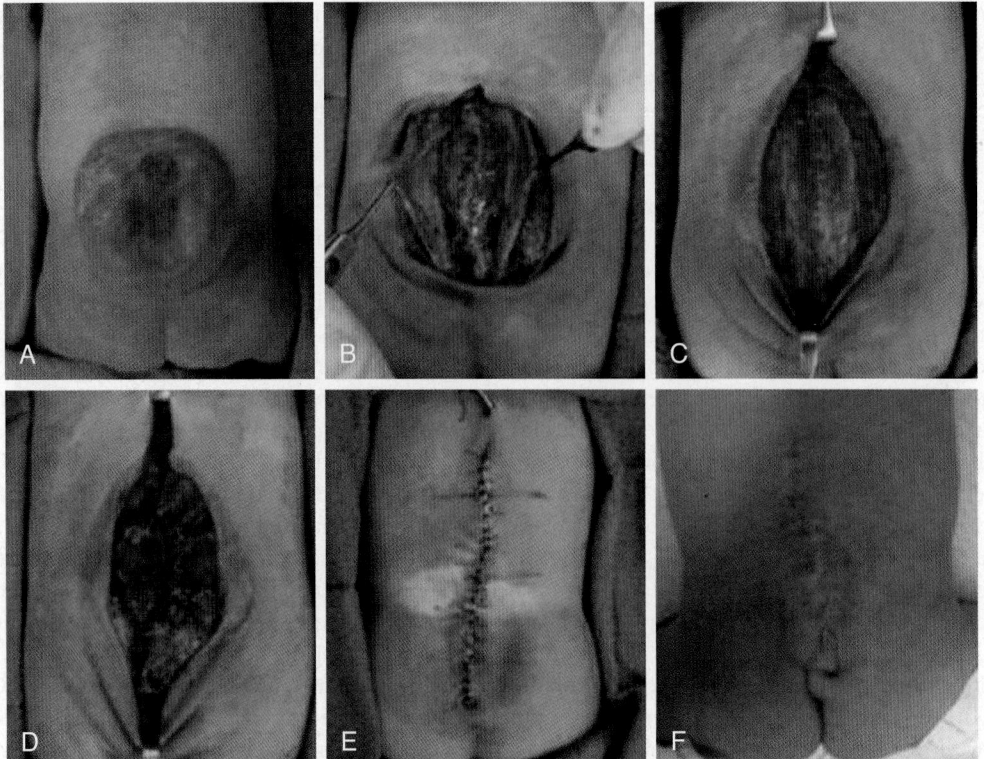

FIG. 35.4 (A) Two-day-old male with an 8.5 × 8.0 cm lumbosacral myelomeningocele. (B) Elevation of paraspinous turnover fascial flaps. (C) Closure of fascial flaps over the dural repair. (D) Additional soft tissue coverage using bilateral paraspinous muscle advancement flaps. (E) Widely undermined skin flaps advanced medially for midline linear closure. (F) Healed incision 4 months postoperatively. (From Patel KB, Taghinia AH, Proctor MR, Warf BC, Greene AK. Extradural myelomeningocele reconstruction using local turnover fascial flaps and midline linear skin closure. *J Plast Reconstr Aesthet Surg.* 2012;65[11]:1569-1572.)

closure (68% to 98%). The prenatal group also had lower rates of hindbrain herniation, brain stem kinking, abnormal fourth-ventricular location, and syringomyelia. Although the ability to walk is dependent on the level of the lesion, infants in the prenatal group were also more likely to walk without orthotics or devices. Interestingly, infants in the prenatal group underwent more delayed procedures for spinal cord tethering, likely because the initial closure was a less technical operation, aimed more at sealing the defect than releasing the spinal cord. Furthermore, the rates of maternal and pregnancy complications were higher with prenatal surgery. A later publication suggested that modification of the surgical technique, including not using a trochar and minimizing the separation of the amniotic membrane, resulted in lower rates of premature rupture of membranes and chorioamnion separation, and most infants were able to be delivered at a later gestational age.[27] A recent phase I study of an endoscopic approach to prenatal closure appears promising.[28] Larger ventricular size may be a prognostic sign for the requirement of a CSF diversion procedure.[29] More long-term follow-up is needed to ensure that these results hold up.

Ventriculoperitoneal Shunts

It is estimated that close to 80% of MMC patients will develop hydrocephalus, with 5% to 10% requiring CSF diversion at birth.[1] Most children who develop hydrocephalus will do so within the first 6 months of life. Interestingly, some patients develop hydrocephalus after MMC repair, as the egress of CSF from the defect is sealed off. The indications for CSF diversion are increasing head circumference, CSF leak from the MMC closure site, or signs of increased intracranial pressure, such as bradycardia or apnea. Some children may also develop a syrinx as a result of excess fluid buildup. If a CSF diversion is thought to be needed at the time of MMC repair, it can be done under the same anesthetic.[30] In a study comparing a wait-and-see approach for the placement of a ventriculoperitoneal shunt and automatic placement of the shunt, patients who had their shunts placed later had a significantly higher risk of developing a shunt infection.[31] However, by waiting to be certain that it is necessary, it is likely that some patients who would have been shunted can avoid this procedure.

Endoscopic Third Ventriculostomy

Endoscopic third ventriculostomy (ETV) is a procedure that was first proposed by W. Jason Mixter, founding chairman of neurosurgery at Massachusetts General Hospital, in 1923.[32] He used a urethroscope to puncture a hole in the floor of the third ventricle of a patient with noncommunicating hydrocephalus. Mixter's instrumentation and visualization were poor and cumbersome and did not have much appeal to his colleagues. As technology improved, specifically the development of charged-couple devices, which convert optical data to electrical impulses, better visualization, magnification, and lighting could be delivered to an endoscope and the size of the endoscopes could be reduced.[33] Recently, there has been a resurgence in interest in treating many types of hydrocephalus using ETV with and without choroid plexus cauterization (CPC), which is reducing the need for patients to have an implanted device (shunt). This can be of great value to patients if the efficacy and longevity of the ETV procedures are borne out over time, as implanted shunts are at permanent risk of mechanical failure, infection, and other complications. Interestingly, the efficacy of ETV with and without CPC was established, out of necessity, in Africa, where there was less access to implanted shunts and where it is often very difficult for these children to receive shunt revision surgery if the shunt fails.[34] This modality is now being introduced to first-world countries with widely accessible modern shunts, a rare transfer of medical innovation from less-developed to more-developed countries. In a large series of over 100 patients, Warf and Campbell showed that using ETV and CPC as a primary treatment of hydrocephalus in patients with MMC was successful in 76% of patients, with a predicted lifetime success rate of 76% if reopening of a closed ETV was performed.[34] Importantly, close to 10% of patients could not undergo ETV and CPC, most commonly due to postinflammatory distortion of intraventricular anatomy. Preliminary evidence in North American studies supports these results.[35] A recent meta-analysis of ETV of approximately 500 patients, 53% of whom presented with MMC, revealed a success rate of 55%.[36] Due to the high morbidity of shunt failures and infection in MMC, it may be reasonable to attempt an ETV with CPC in patients requiring CSF diversion; thus, we are likely to see reductions in the number of shunted patients in the future. There are caveats in that, for some patients, the intraventricular anatomy may not be ideal for the ETV procedures. When failures of ETV do occur, they are commonly within 6 months of treatment,[34,37] a time when the skull bones remain open. This means that, although some infants might be converted to an implanted shunt, ETV failure should not lead to increased intracranial pressure and a poor outcome, as the baby will generally present with a more benign acceleration of head growth. To date, there have been no studies looking at ETV for hydrocephalus that occurs after prenatal treatment of MMC.

Surgical Complications

Latex Allergy

There has been an observation of a definite increase in allergy to latex, as found in surgical gloves and urinary catheters, in patients with spinal dysraphism.[38] Health care providers must be vigilant in this regard, as the allergy is type I, an immediate immunoglobulin E (IgE) reaction that can result in anaphylaxis and death. This sensitization is thought to arise from repeated exposure to latex products, although there is evidence that patients with spinal dysraphism have higher levels of total and latex-specific IgE compared with normal patients.[39] For this reason, all surgical procedures on spina bifida patients are recommended to be done in a latex-free environment. At most pediatric centers, this latex-free precaution is established immediately, before any evidence of allergy is present, to prevent this reaction.

Late Deterioration

Although MMC is a congenital birth defect and most of the neurologic sequelae are present at birth, there is risk for progressive loss of function from several causes. Signs of worsening in a patient should be investigated, as early treatment affords the best outcome. Reasons for neurologic deterioration in an MMC patient include hydrocephalus, Chiari malformation, hydromyelia, tethered cord, and progressive spinal deformity. Many of these conditions can coexist; thus, it might not be easy to determine the exact reason for neurologic deterioration in an MMC patient. Therefore, it is generally best to consider a top-down approach.

Hydrocephalus can be the source of dysfunction for many reasons, including the primary effects of the progressive ventricle size, and the secondary effects this can have on the Chiari II malformation and the hydromyelia. Therefore, workup for MMC patients who present with neurologic deterioration should start with a brain scan. If this shows worsening ventriculomegaly, the treatment might be obvious. If the ventricles are not enlarging, paradoxically, the hydrocephalus can still cause worsening Chiari or syrinx symptoms; thus, the spine should be imaged. If the symptoms appear to be Chiari related (i.e., cranial nerve dysfunction) or syrinx related (i.e., upper extremity weakness) the treatment might still be for hydrocephalus, which will often improve these other conditions. If the findings are purely in the lower extremities or bowel/bladder, the tethered cord might be the source, in which case the treatment is directed there. The presence of findings is not always a mandate for surgery; rather, these findings should be placed in context to previous imaging and clinical presentation of the patient. It is therefore important that these patients are followed longitudinally by a highly specialized multidisciplinary clinic, including neurosurgeons, orthopedic surgeons, urologists, pediatricians, and physical therapists.

Shunt Malfunction/Increased Intracranial Pressure

Any neurologic deterioration in a patient with MMC should invoke a thorough investigation for increased intracranial pressure. If a shunt is present, it can malfunction, and even the ETV can fail. This is often confusing to first-line responders, who may not think of the possibility of hydrocephalus since no shunt is present. Studies have shown sudden death from hydrocephalus in patients treated with ETV alone.[40,41] It is important to note that many MMC patients have baseline ventriculomegaly, or "arrested" hydrocephalus. There is some evidence that some of these patients may benefit from an insertion of a new shunt or shunt revision,[42] which is a decision made carefully by the neurosurgeon. Eye examinations can be vitally important in looking for papilledema in these patients, and occasionally direct monitoring of intracranial pressure is needed. For patients who have undergone ETV, reopening of the ETV site has been shown to be effective, even if it is performed later.[43]

Tethered Cord

Tethered cord syndrome (TCS), in which the spinal cord is attached to the surrounding tissues and limited in its movements, can cause neural structures to stretch and lead to multiple neurologic, urologic, and orthopedic defects. It is important to note that by radiographic criteria, such as a low-lying conus or attachment of the spinal cord to overlying tissue, all MMC patients will have the picture of a "tethered cord," but it is only approximately 20% to 30% that will have symptomatic TCS.[44,45] Interestingly, fetal repair does not seem to change the incidence of this phenomenon, as 30% of patients that underwent a fetal repair subsequently presented with TCS, with 63% of these patients having a cutaneously derived intradural inclusion cyst. In fact, it may paradoxically increase this risk because the prenatal closure, despite its overall complexity, is a less technically exacting operation regarding the spinal cord.

Signs and symptoms of TCS are more likely to appear early in life, when growth is rapid. We often see spikes of presentation between 4 to 6 and 12 to 14 years of age, which coincide with growth spurts. Symptoms can include back and leg pain, urinary incontinence, gait abnormalities, progressive foot deformities, and kyphoscoliosis. In children whose function is already compromised, such as with gait abnormalities from low-lying lesions, loss of more function can significantly alter quality of life; thus, early diagnosis and treatment are essential.[46]

Surgery to detether a tethered cord is similar to that for a lipomyelomeningocele. It is important to identify the most cephalad normal lamina above the spina bifida defect. This most cephalad lamina is removed, and the underlying normal spinal cord is identified. Working in a caudal fashion, the dorsal and lateral attachments are detached using sharp dissection. This should continue until the cord is noted to fall into anterior spinal canal. There is some evidence that using electrophysiology—namely, electromyography (EMG)—and compound muscle action potentials can be helpful in making these dissections safer and perhaps decrease the rates of subsequent tethering.[47]

Although the aim of surgery is to halt neurologic deterioration, there is some evidence that detethering operations may actually improve neurologic function, including gait and motor difficulties and urinary incontinence.[48,49] It is for this reason that early detection and surgery are important.

Chiari Malformations

Chiari malformations refer to abnormalities of the hindbrain originally described by the Austrian pathologist Hans Christian in the early 1890s.[50] There are four main types described, but the most relevant to the topic of spinal dysraphism is the Chiari type II (CMII) malformation. CMII is almost always (>95%) associated with myelomeningocele or, rarely, other forms of spinal dysraphism.[51,52] In this malformation, there is downward displacement of the cerebellar vermis and brain stem through the foramen magnum (Fig. 35.5). Hydrocephalus is also present about 90% of the time.

Infants with CMII requiring treatment are in a fairly severe category and can present with inspiratory stridor due to vocal cord paralysis, bradycardia, or apnea.[53,54] Older children will

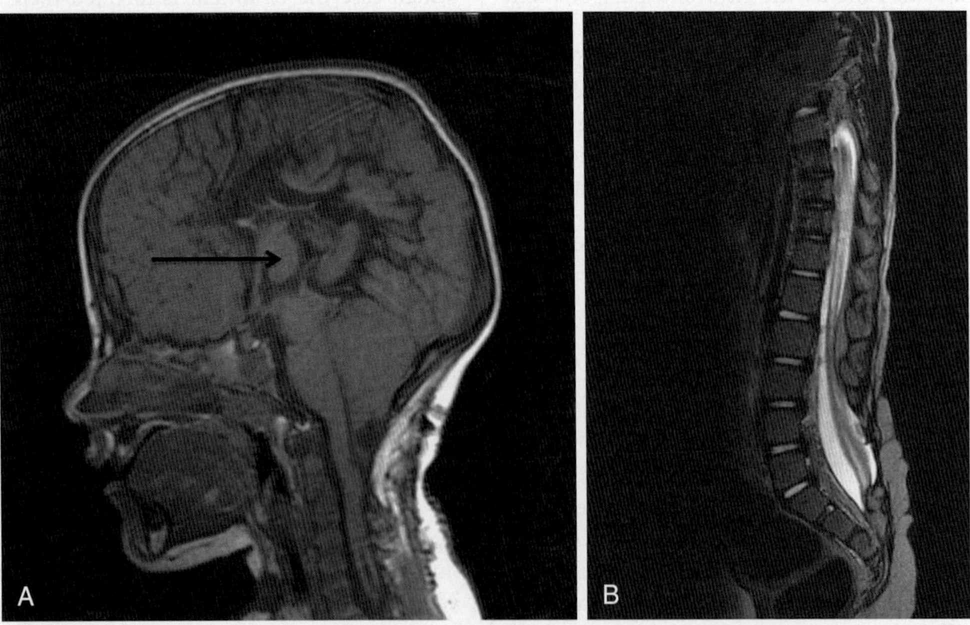

FIG. 35.5 Magnetic resonance imaging findings of Chiari II malformation. (A) Sagittal T1-weighted MRI reveals many of the associated findings in Chiari II malformations, including lack of corpus callosum, large massa intermedia (*arrow*), descent of the cerebellar tonsils, as well as descent of the brain stem. (B) Sagittal T2-weighted MRI reveals low-lying conus and myelomeningocele.

generally present with more mild symptoms, including lower cranial nerve palsies, ataxia, and tussive headaches.

The indications for surgical intervention for CMII lesions in myelomeningoceles are difficult, as many of these patients will have the radiographic findings of Chiari II but not require treatment. Generally, if patients present with these symptoms, treatment of the hydrocephalus can be effective in treating these Chiari symptoms, presumably by reducing the pressure from above that is putting downward pressure on the brain. However, some children do require Chiari decompression if the hydrocephalus treatment was not effective in relieving the symptoms.

The goal of surgery for Chiari malformations is to equilibrate CSF pressure dynamics between the intracranial and intraspinal subarachnoid spaces. This involves a posterior fossa decompression through a suboccipital craniotomy. Some centers do only bony decompression, while others advocate for at least a partial duraplasty, which involves thinning of the dura. The third option involves opening the dura at the craniocervical junction. A meta-analysis suggests that patients who undergo duraplasty have higher levels of symptom control and syrinx resolution, but also higher rates of CSF-related complications, such as CSF leaks or the development of a pseudomeningocele.[55]

Hydromyelia

Hydromyelia, or the abnormal widening of the central canal of the spinal cord due to the presence of CSF, is recognized with increasing frequency in association with MMC. The true incidence of hydromyelia in MMC patients may be close to 70%.[44] Some have posited that the presence of hydromyelia may be due to persistent hydrocephalus that transmits increased CSF pressure down the central canal.[56] Others have hypothesized that the hydromyelia is due to a transmission of a systolic pressure wave in the intracranial compartment to the cerebellar tonsils, which, in turn, is transmitted to the central canal.[57,58] This is why treatment of the hydrocephalus can be effective for treating the hydromyelia.

Whereas classic syringomyelia usually presents with dissociated sensory loss (presumably due to damage to the decussating anterior white commissure), hydromyelia associated with spina bifida can present with preserved sensation, but progressive bladder dysfunction and quadriparesis. Scoliosis also might be related to hydromyelia, but it can also be related to primary bone abnormalities, or spinal tethering.[59]

Spina Bifida Occulta

Spina bifida occulta represents the other major subcategory of spinal dysraphism. As opposed to spina bifida aperta, spina bifida occulta is a condition in which there is a congenital defect in the dorsal elements of the spinal canal, but the overlying skin is left intact, and the diagnosis is often not detected at birth. This is a distinct condition that may be associated with TCS and the risk for deterioration over time, which has different implications for both prognosis and treatment.

Embryology

In contrast to MMC, spina bifida occulta arises from defects at a later point in embryologic development. At 27 days of gestation, the neural tube has completely closed, finishing the process of primary neurulation.[60,61] This closure is the result of complex interactions between numerous intercellular signaling factors. By definition, this closure occurs successfully in all spina bifida occulta patients. The neural tube then separates from the overlying ectoderm in a process thought to be highly dependent on *cadherin* expression.[62,63] Following neural tube closure, canalization occurs from days 27 to 48. During this process, cells from the primitive streak distal to the caudal neuropore form a caudal cell mass, which, in turn, form vacuoles that go on to become the conus medullaris, cauda equina, and filum terminale.[64] These eventually fuse with the distal neuropore, forming the distal spinal cord.

The formation of the bony and muscular distal spinal elements occurs simultaneously. By the end of primary neurulation, paired mesoderm-derived somites have given rise to paired sclerotomes, flanking either side of the notochord ventral to the neural tube.[65] These sclerotomes migrate medially, meeting one another in the midline to eventually form the basis of the bony vertebral column. Sclerotomal cells then subsequently migrate dorsally to envelop the neural tube, forming the dorsal vertebral arch structures. The overlying back musculature and deep dermal tissues are simultaneously derived from the remaining somite cells left over after the sclerotomal cells have separated.

In spina bifida occulta, any number of these subsequent embryologic steps may be disrupted, leading to occult dysraphism. For example, failure of proper separation of elements during neural canalization can lead to either a fatty or fibrofatty filum terminale. Similarly, failure in the migration or fusion of dorsal sclerotomal cells may lead to malformation of the bony and muscular elements of the dorsal spine. Though these malformations may not become obvious or symptomatic until much later in development, many can be clearly traced to anomalies during early gestation.

Epidemiology

The true prevalence of occult spinal dysraphism is currently unclear, as many mild anomalies, such as a fibrofatty filum terminale, have an uncertain natural history.[66] As many of these abnormalities are detected either incidentally or as part of the workup of an overlying suspicious cutaneous sign, it is unclear how many of these anomalies become symptomatic, and, in turn, how many cases remain undiagnosed in the pediatric and adult populations. As a corollary, the measured incidence of occult spinal dysraphism has grown over time as imaging technology has become more widely available and awareness of screening for cutaneous manifestations has increased.

Estimates for lipomyelomeningocele and lipomeningocele have ranged from 0.3 to 1.6 per 10,000 live births with a higher incidence in Hispanic populations and a lower incidence in black populations.[67,68] The estimated prevalence of isolated filum terminale abnormalities are significantly higher. Cadaveric studies have yielded a presence of 4% to 6% for filum terminale lipomas.[69] Imaging prevalence studies have reported a slightly lower incidence: 0.2% to 4.0%.[70–72] Reports of the incidence of congenital dermal sinus tracts are somewhat more varied. Earlier studies, based on clinical examination of children, report a significantly higher incidence (1–4%) compared with later studies that supplement clinical investigation with imaging technology (~0.04%).[73–76] This is not surprising, as the vast majority of patients with suspicious cutaneous stigmata, even in prescreened populations, will not have underlying evidence of spinal dysraphism.[77] Other congenital malformations, such as spinal neurenteric cysts, diastematomyelia, and sacral agenesis, are rarer still, with data limited to case reports or small case series.

Of note, as opposed to the case of MMC, there have not been demonstrated associations of occult spinal dysraphism with folic acid deficiency. This has been most carefully studied in the specific case of lipomyelomeningocele. Repeated efforts have failed to find any reduced incidence of lipomyelomeningocele with dietary folic acid supplementation.[68,78] These data reinforce the idea that occult spinal dysraphism represents a pathologic entity distinct from MMC, with roots in developmental errors that occur after the complete neural tube closure.

Clinical Presentation

Occult spinal dysraphism should be suspected when there is the presence of suspicious cutaneous stigmata, syndromic or midline congenital malformations associated with spinal dysraphism, or symptoms suggestive of lower spinal cord pathology.

In terms of cutaneous stigmata, common suspicious lesions include the presence of a midline or paraspinal mass, a capillary hemangioma (port wine stain), a distinct lumbrosacral tuft of hair, a polypoid lesion or caudal appendage, hyper- or hypopigmented nodules or macules, an atretic meningocele, a sacral dimple, a sinus tract, or a significantly deviated gluteal cleft.[79,80] (Fig. 35.6). Due to the wide variety of possible manifestations, the incidence of some form of cutaneous stigmata is high, but only a fraction of those children have radiologic evidence of underlying spinal dysraphism on further investigation. There are reports that as many as 5% of all neonates bear some form of cutaneous stigmata, the most common of which is a sacral dimple, but only 7% of those bearing the stigmata go on to have signs of dysraphism on radiologic studies.[81] Nevertheless, due to the serious potential consequences of leaving an underlying malformation unrecognized, most children with suspicious cutaneous lesions should typically undergo further investigation.

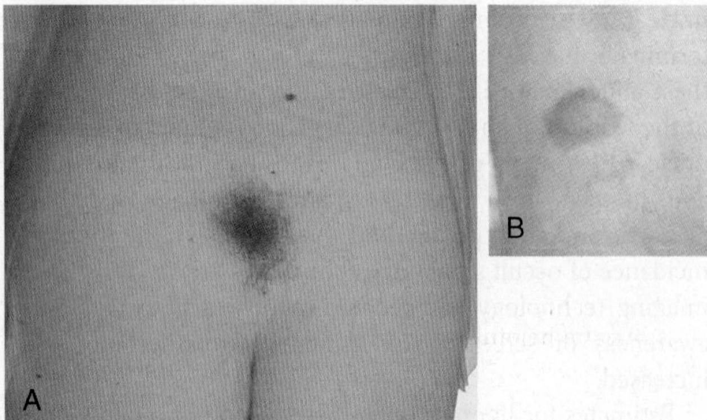

FIG. 35.6 Cutaneous stigmata of occult spinal dysraphism. (A) Hypertrichosis in a young woman, indicating underlying tethered cord. (B) Lumbosacral hemangioma.

Several congenital syndromes and associations are also known to be associated with occult spinal malformations; their presence typically warrants screening for spinal dysraphism. One of the more common is VACTERL, an association of co-occurrences involving the following, which comprise the acronym: vertebral anomalies, anal atresia, cardiac defects, tracheoesophageal fistula, esophageal atresia, renal and radial anomalies, and possibly limb defects. Though not linked through a common pathogenic pathway, these anomalies are known to be associated with one another. Tethered cord is a common occurrence in children with any type of anal and/or sacral anomaly, due to the common embryology of the caudal cell bud, VACTERL included. An estimated 8% to 45% of children with anorectal malformations have associated pathologic spinal abnormalities.[82–85] Other known syndromic associations include SACRAL syndrome (spinal dysraphism, anogenital, cutaneous, renal, and urologic anomalies) and the more recently coined PELVIS syndrome (perineal hemangioma, external genitalia malformations, lipomyelomeningocele, vesicorenal abnormalities, imperforate anus, and skin tag).[86,87] It should be noted that in all of these, there is a common thread of association between anorectal abnormalities and underlying spinal abnormalities.

Finally, if neither cutaneous manifestations nor nearby congenital abnormalities are present, progressive symptoms localized to the lower spinal cord and cauda equina should also raise suspicion for possible occult dysraphism. These symptoms include progressive lower extremity weakness, urinary incontinence and/or retention, bowel incontinence, high-arched feet, leg asymmetry, and/or scoliosis. It is important to recognize that these deficits may be present at birth, but more commonly present in a delayed fashion. As such, a detailed history and physical are, as always, critical to making a diagnosis. Lower extremity weakness may be particularly challenging, as younger children may be limited in their ability to give a clear history and/or participate in bedside examination. Thus, other associated signs—such as progressive inward toeing of the feet, refusal to walk or stand independently, or increased long-tract signs on examination—should also raise concern for underlying spinal cord issues. This suspicion should be particularly heightened in children who achieve a given developmental level and then experience unexplained regression.

Investigation

When an underlying occult spinal congenital malformation is suspected, the next step in workup is typically radiologic

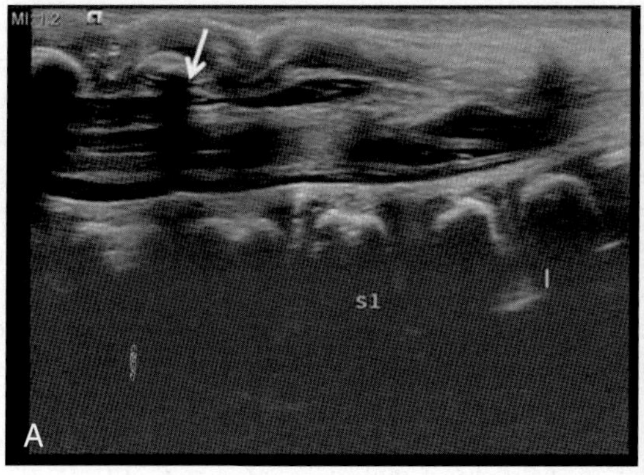

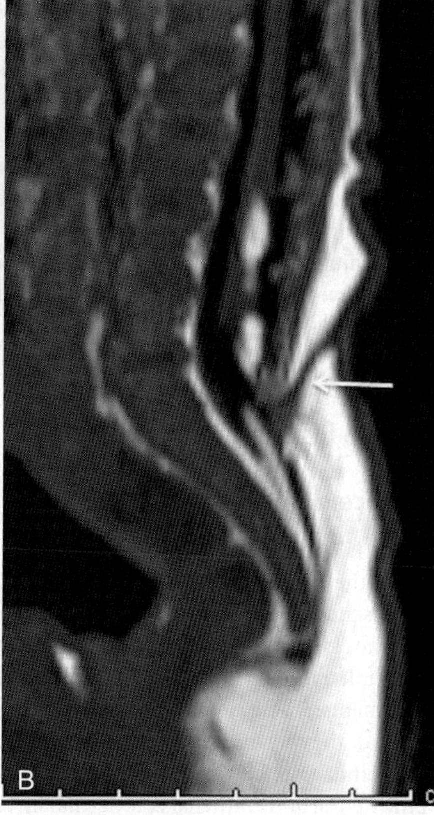

FIG. 35.7 Ultrasound findings of occult dysraphism. (A) Midsagittal ultrasound shows dermal sinus tract (*arrow*). (B) Midsagittal magnetic resonance image reveals dermal sinus tract in better resolution (*arrow*).

investigation. This can take the form of either a focused ultrasonography or magnetic resonance imaging (MRI), each with their distinct advantages and disadvantages.

Ultrasound studies are quick, cost effective, and generally give a good impression of the underlying structural composition of underlying structures if done before the ossification of the bones excludes effective imaging. Structures are contrasted based on their echogenicity; as such, bone, spinal fluid, and the spinal cord are well differentiated from one another. In addition, gross structural abnormalities, such as the presence of an MMC, a low-lying conus, or large lipoma, can also be examined, and even subtler details, such as a thickened filum terminale, can be identified[88] (Fig. 35.7). Moreover, this information can be obtained with some degree of motion tolerance, avoiding the need to sedate a child to obtain the study. Finally, cine views actually can show movement of the spinal cord, which can be limited in tethering conditions.

Ultrasonography has its limitations, however. Obtaining an adequate study can be dependent much more on technician experience and skill than in other imaging modalities. Furthermore, shadow effects created by highly echogenic structures, such as bone, can obscure the view of underlying structures; thus, these studies are only effective up to 3 to 4 months of age. Perhaps most important, tissues of similar echogenic properties are often poorly contrasted, leading to inadequate resolution of soft tissue structures. As such, while ultrasound is often an excellent initial study to evaluate the spine, and is useful for screening purposes, MRI studies may be needed to make a final diagnosis. In our practice, if the clinical suspicion is low to moderate and a high-quality ultrasound performed by an experienced radiologist is normal, no further workup is pursued.

MRI has the advantage of excellent soft tissue contrast, therefore being able to easily discern fat, fluid, fibrous, and neuronal content from one another. As such, it serves as the basis for the diagnosis of most forms of spinal dysraphism, both as a means to better characterize the suspected anomaly, and to help evaluate for any other associated lesions or changes to normal anatomy.[61] The main disadvantage of MRI in the pediatric population is the need to remain near motionless while images are being captured. For many children younger than 6 to 7 years of age, this requires sedation, rarely even general anesthesia, and all of the associated risks that these bring. As such, while MRI is often necessary for treatment planning and to confirm the final diagnosis in occult spinal dysraphism, it should only be pursued once clinical suspicion is high enough to justify the potential risks.

In addition to radiologic examination, other adjuvant tests may be helpful to determine if TCS exists. Urodynamic studies are a very objective way of determining any degree of urologic impairment, and whether it is neurogenic in origin. Patients whose primary complaint is urologic, such as enuresis or failure to potty train, often can have a broad differential diagnosis for their issues. A collection of urodynamic tests, including cystometry, uroflowmetry, abdominal leak point pressure, urethral pressure profile, stress testing, and post-void residual volume determination, can often help isolate the extent and nature of urologic complaints. Patients with spina bifida have been known to exhibit detrusor hyperreflexia and dyssynergia, detrusor hypocompliance, impaired bladder sensation, and absence of a bulbocavernosus reflex.[89,90] Moreover, urodynamic studies can not only help in the diagnosis of a patient's urologic complaints, but are also valuable to track any decrease in function over time or potential improvement with surgical correction.[90–95]

Specific Spina Bifida Occulta

Lipomyelomeningocele

Lipomyelomeningocele is one of the most common forms of occult spinal bifida. As the name implies, a lipomyelomeningocele refers to the presence of a subcutaneous lumbrosacral lipoma that is contiguous with the neural and meningeal elements that have extended through a congenital defect in the dorsal bony spinal elements. These neural elements are often not well formed; instead, they form a neural placode, similar to that found in spina bifida aperta.[96] This arises from premature disjunction of the neural and epithelial ectodermal layers. When this step occurs before the neural tube is completely closed, mesenchymal elements insert themselves into the closing neural placode, eventually becoming a mass of fat that prevents complete neural tube closure.[97]

As previously mentioned, lipomyelomeningocele is among the most common of spina bifida occulta lesions, although this might be because it is easily diagnosed on physical examination and does not actually represent a higher prevelance.[67,68] Unlike some other forms of occult deformities, the fatty mass is typically visible at birth; thus, the diagnosis often can be made before neurologic sequelae arise.[64]

Since most children with the defect will go on to present with gradually worsening neurologic deficits, surgical correction is advisable in most cases.[98] Timing can be somewhat controversial; however, some authors advocate correction early in life before symptoms develop, while others recommend delaying treatment until signs of deficit present. Since the risks of surgery are not trivial, and not all children will progress to have a neurologic deficit with this lesion, it is certainly justifiable to delay surgery until deficits are apparent. Treatment involves the resection of the lipoma and release of any tethered neural elements, with the ultimate goal of preventing any traction on the spinal cord as the child grows. Since the lipoma is intimately related to the neural placode, residual fat almost always must be left in place in order to minimize any deficits to the patient. Moreover, since there is a dural defect as well, repair involves either primary dural closure or a duraplasty, depending on the size of the defect (Fig. 35.8). Due to the complex nature of the lesion and the need to leave fatty elements on the neural placode, the rate of symptomatic retethering is high, with as many as 20% of patients presenting with retethering issues in a 10-year period.[99]

Filum Terminale Syndrome

Filum terminale syndrome refers to the scenario of progressive TCS in the setting of a thickened filum terminale. The pathogenesis is thought to arise from either excessive fibrous tissue in the filum or a filum lipoma, causing reduced inelasticity. As the bony spine grows and elongates, this inelastic filum is thought to "tether" the spinal cord, causing chronic traction, tension, and eventual ischemia-related oxidative stress on the lower spinal cord.[100] Classic radiologic evidence involves the presence of an abnormally thick (>2 mm) or fat-containing filum and a low-lying conus medularis, frequently defined as below the mid-vertebral level of L2.[72,101] However, it has become clear that the conus can be in a normal position even in symptomatic patients. Treatment typically involves a microsurgical exploration with sectioning of the filum, and often the procedure can be done with minimal to no bony removal (Fig. 35.9). It is important to stimulate the thickened filum to ensure that there are no important motor roots involved. Timing for treatment is somewhat controversial, with some authors arguing for early intervention while others advocate observation until the development of symptoms.[97,102] Risks of surgery are quite low.

Occult filum terminale syndrome, defined as the presence of symptoms of tethered cord in the setting of normal radiologic findings, has recently been a topic of ongoing interest. Surgical intervention in patients without radiographic abnormalities is a notion that has been met with significant controversy, and requires very thoughtful consideration and careful patient selection. However, case series–level data of tethered cord release have reported an 87% rate of improvement in urologic dysfunction in such patients.[103] Patients who appear to have more classic sequelae of TCS, such as presence of multiple concurrent orthopedic, urologic, neurologic, and/or cutaneous sequelae, as well as those with documented urodynamic dysfunction, tend to have higher success rates with detethering.[104,105]

Sacral Agenesis and Caudal Regression

Congenital absence of any part of the sacrum is, by definition, indicative of sacral agenesis. When combined with other congenital malformations of the caudal spine, lower limbs, urogenital system, and anus/rectum, it is known as caudal regression syndrome. In one particular subform, there is complete agenesis of the lower half of the sacrum associated with an anterior presacral mass and anorectal stenosis, in a hereditary, autosomal dominant condition known as the Currarino syndrome (also known as Currarino triad).[106,107] Sacral agenesis has multifactorial origins, with known strong associations with maternal diabetes.[108]

When detected, treatment of sacral agenesis is often conservative. Sacral anomalies often require no treatment, and surgical intervention is required only in cases of symptomatic spinal tethering or when the presacral mass is symptomatic (Fig. 35.10).[109] It is important to recognize that when the distal spine fails to form, often the distal spinal cord fails to form. Therefore, the neurologic deficit is not from tethering, but

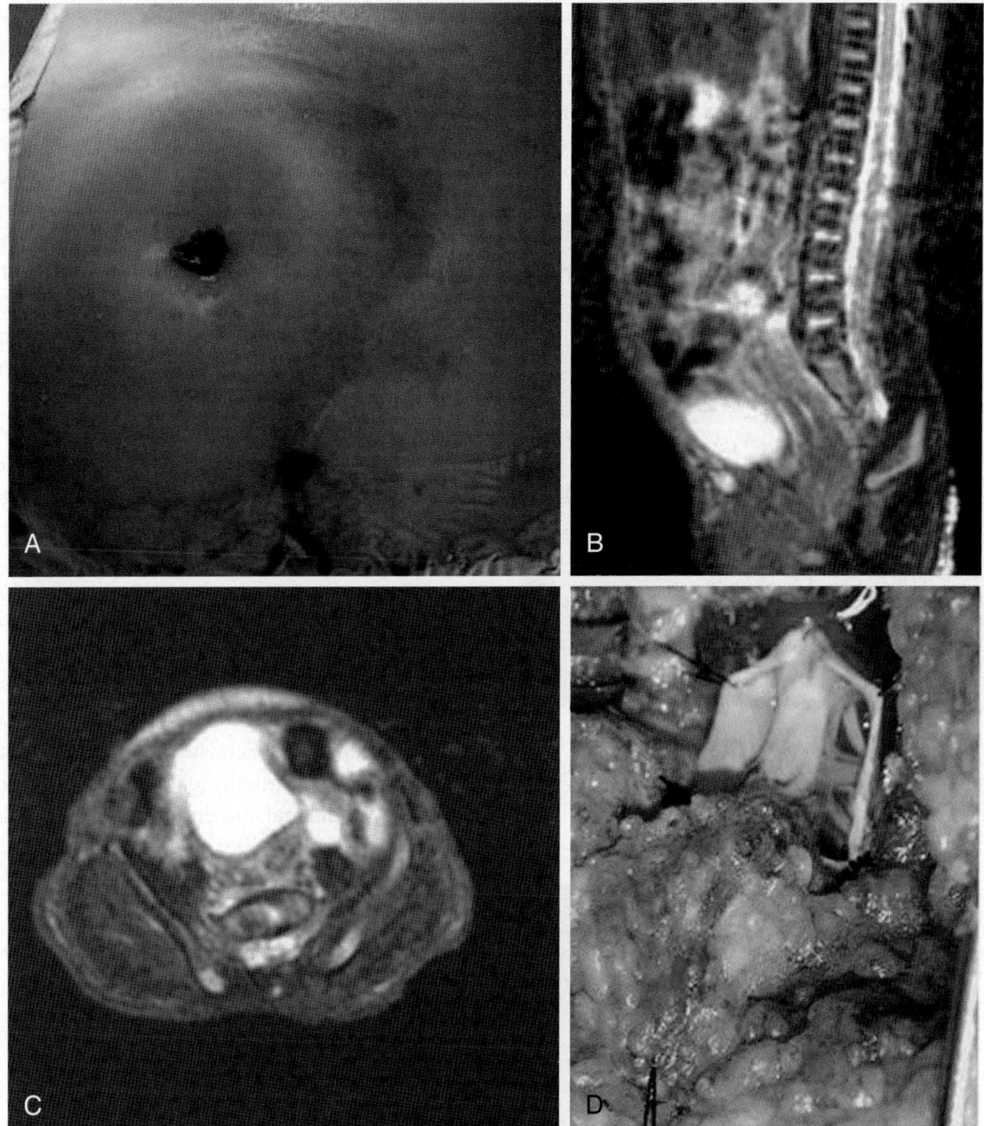

FIG. 35.8 Lipomeningocele. (A) The patient was noted to have a large mass in the back with an associated dimple at birth. (B) Sagittal fat-saturated T2-weighted magnetic resonance image showed evidence of low-lying conus. (C) Axial images showed evidence of fat past the conus. (D) At 6 months of age, after the dura was opened, a dorsal lipoma was found. A YAG laser was used to debulk the mass. Seven years later, the patient presented with symptoms of tethered cord and had to be detethered.

actually from absence of normal neural elements that cannot be fixed. Symptomatic dural stenosis can also be a feature in rare cases, with decompressive duraplasty being a necessary part of the repair.[110]

Congenital Dermal Sinus

Congenital dermal sinuses are abnormal tracts that communicate the overlying skin and the underlying intraspinal contents. As discussed previously, these are thought to arise from a focal failure of ectodermal separation.[75] The majority arise in the lumbrosacral region, though abnormal sinus tracts can develop all along the dorsal neuraaxis.[75] Though typically diagnosed based on observation of the tract on examination of the patient's skin, these lesions can also present with intraspinal infections, intradural dermoid or epidermoid cysts, focal neurologic deficits, and/or pain.[75,111,112] When encountered, surgical correction with intradural exploration and obliteration of the sinus tract is advised. This should be performed rapidly, as the complication of infection can turn a simple problem into a very complex one (Fig. 35.11).

Split Cord Anomalies

Congenital sagittal splitting of the spinal cord, known as split spinal cord malformation (SSCM) as well as diastematomyelia, are uncommon lesions with unclear embryologic origins. Two different subtypes exist, with SSCM type I lesions characterized as two hemicords with separate dural and arachnoid coverings separated by a bony cartilaginous septum, and SSCM type II lesions defined as those with a single dural and arachnoid sheath and fibrous septum dividing the two hemicords.[113,114] (Fig. 35.12). Though the exact pathogenesis has yet to be determined, it is hypothesized that the condition arises from an accessory neurenteric canal that splits the neural plate. This canal may allow for the connection of endodermal and ectodermal elements, which can later be populated by mesenchymal cells that go on to form the dividing septum.[114,115]

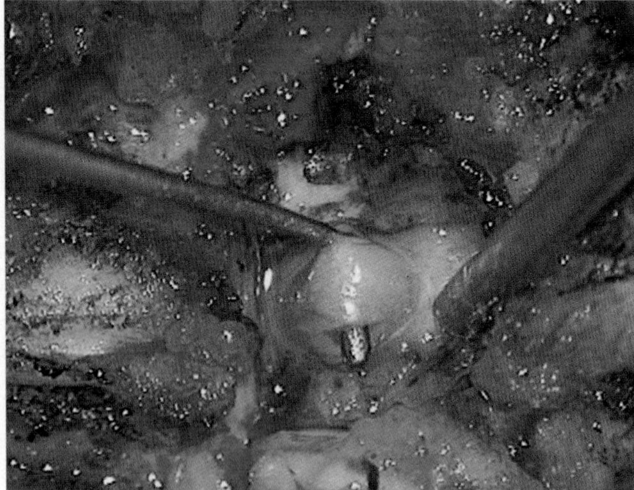

FIG. 35.9 Intraoperative findings in filum terminale syndrome. In this syndrome, a thickened filum terminale is found (elevated by a nerve hook). This is sectioned sharply after stimulating and ensuring that there are no involved motor roots.

Data on the natural history and treatment of these lesions are more limited, given their rarity. However, when encountered, prophylactic surgical treatment is generally considered, given the observation that children who present at older ages tend to have more significant deficits.[116] Surgical correction typically involves laminectomy, surgical removal of the intervening septum, and possibly reconstructive duraplasty, depending on the type of split cord abnormality. The association with other tethering lesions is very high; efforts should be made at the time of surgery to release concurrent tethering elements, such as fibrous bands, paramedian dorsal roots, and/or a thickened filum terminale.[117] Removal of the intervening septum before detethering is recommended if present because of the hypothetical risk of neurologic injury to the detethered cord if it recoils onto the septum.

Neurenteric Cyst

Neurenteric cysts are abnormalities that arise from focal persistence of parts of the neurenteric canal, which temporarily connects the amniotic sac and the yolk sac during the third week of gestation. Persistence of this canal can split the notochord and eventually lead to either abnormal attachments between ectodermal and endodermal elements, or a persistent

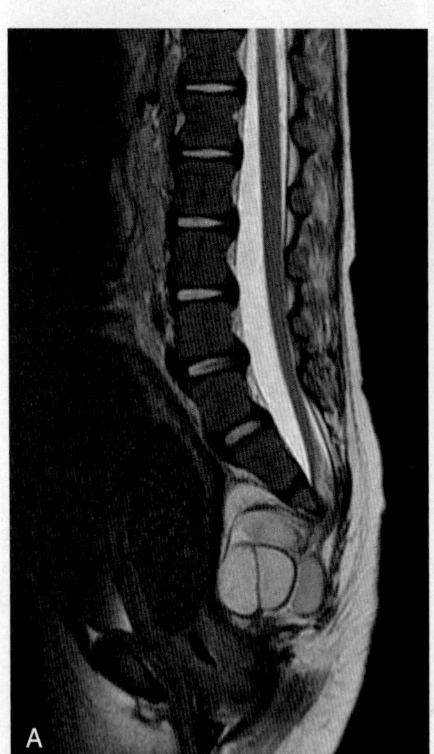

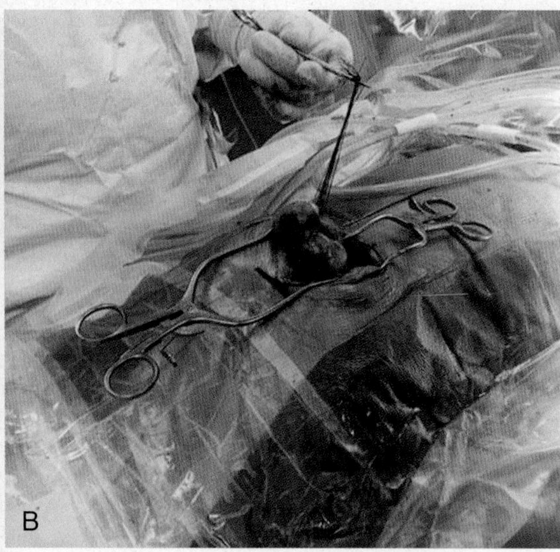

FIG. 35.10 Currarino syndrome in a 3-year-old female with chromosome 7 deletion with global developmental delay and microcephaly. She was found to have a sacral dimple. (A) T2-weighted sagittal magnetic resonance image showed a complex spinal dysraphism with a low conus ending in the sacral region attached to an intradural lipomatous mass, which was connected ventrally to a large presacral mass suggestive of a sacrococcygeal teratoma. The patient had chronic constipation. She was able to stand but not ambulate. Urodynamic studies were unremarkable. The patient underwent detethering of the conus and resection of the intradural fatty mass, which was found to contain hair and sebaceous material. (B) This mass was resected and disconnected from the ventral presacral mass. This mass was removed en bloc.

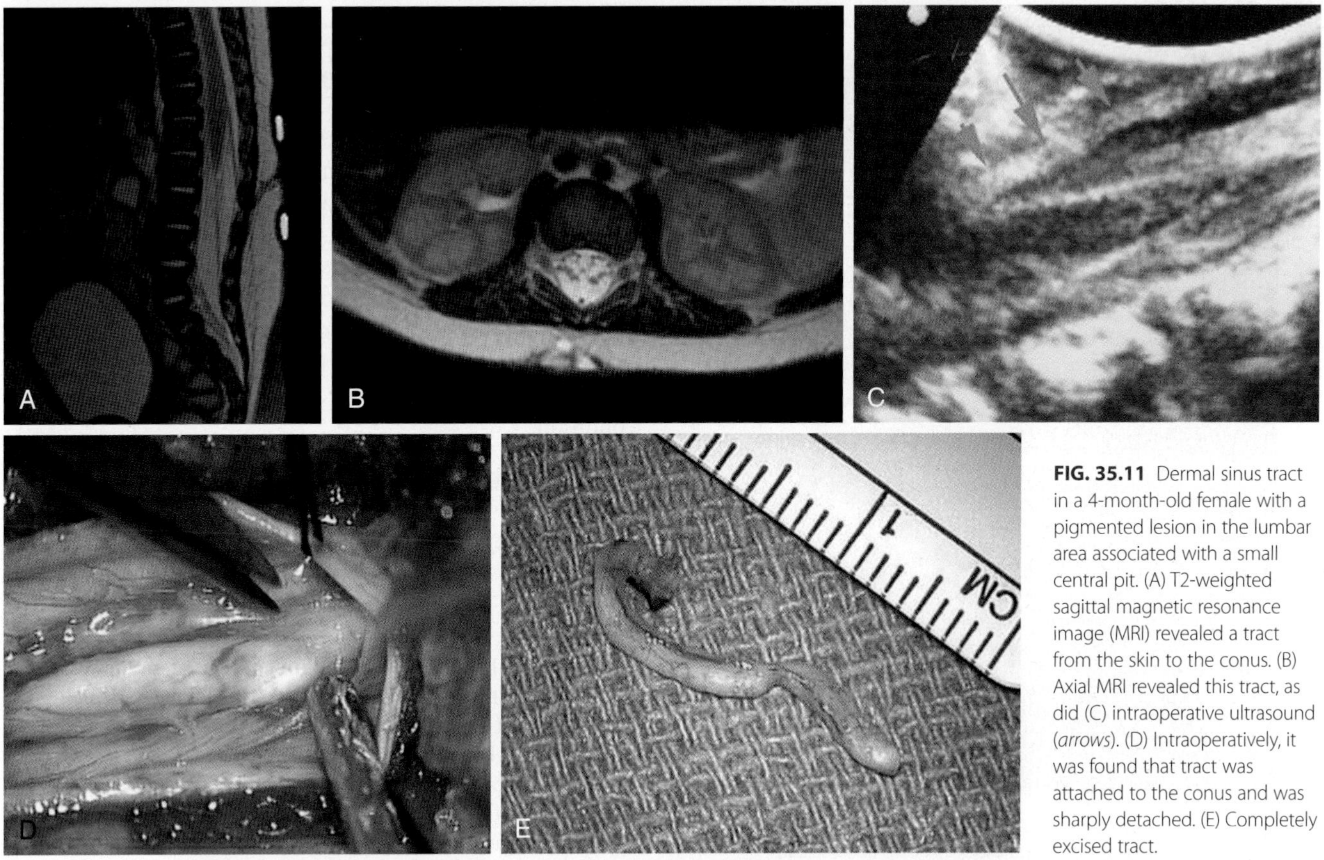

FIG. 35.11 Dermal sinus tract in a 4-month-old female with a pigmented lesion in the lumbar area associated with a small central pit. (A) T2-weighted sagittal magnetic resonance image (MRI) revealed a tract from the skin to the conus. (B) Axial MRI revealed this tract, as did (C) intraoperative ultrasound (*arrows*). (D) Intraoperatively, it was found that tract was attached to the conus and was sharply detached. (E) Completely excised tract.

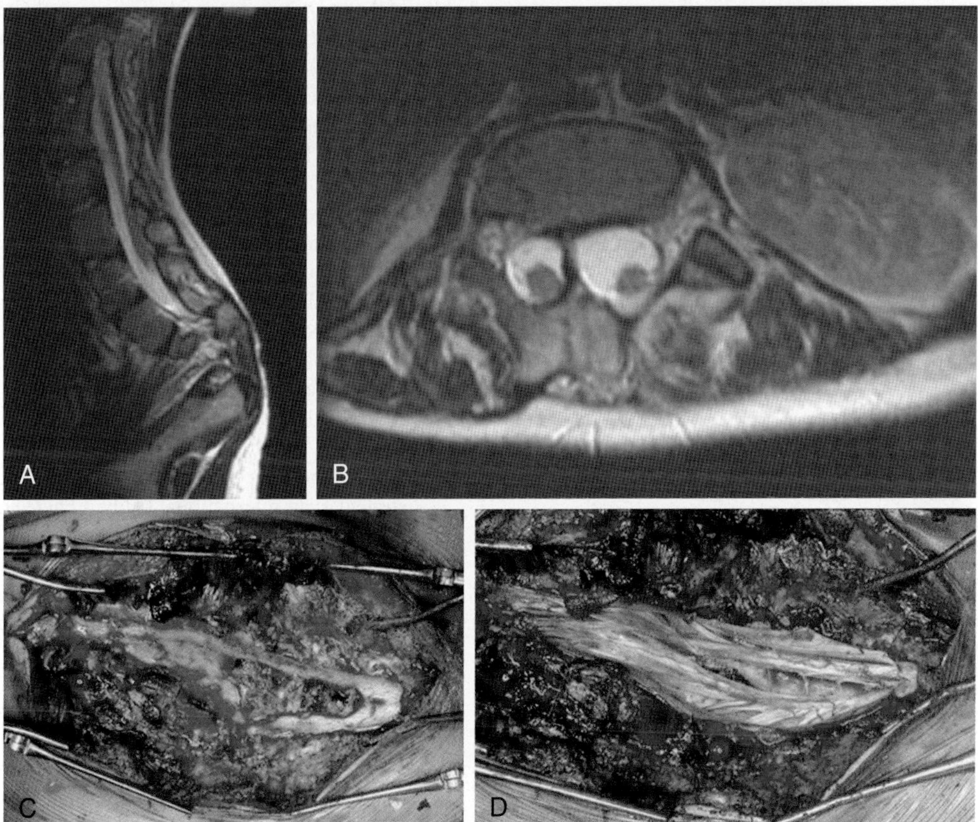

FIG. 35.12 Split cord syndrome in an 11-year-old girl with progressive scoliosis. She had severe distal lower extremity weakness, more marked on the left side than the right, with atrophy of both calves, more dramatic on the left, and weakness of both feet, more dramatic on the left. The patient also had a probable dermal sinus tract near the tip of the coccyx associated with a hair that entered the dermal sinus tract. (A) T2-weighted sagittal magnetic resonance imaging (MRI) revealed low conus, and (B) T2-weighted axial MRI revealed the presence of two dural tubes separated by a thick intervening bone. This separation appeared to extend into the thoracic spine. (C) Intraoperatively, a thick bony septum was found to separate the two dural tubes. (D) This was drilled off. The dura was closed primarily in the cephalad and rostral directions, but an allograft had to be placed where the bone was most prominent.

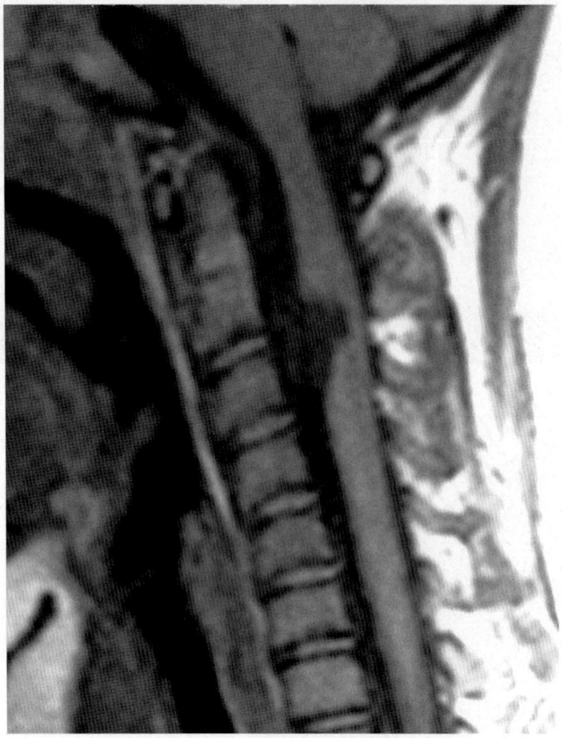

FIG. 35.13 Magnetic resonance imaging of cervical spine shows anteriorly placed neurenteric cyst compressing the spinal cord and causing myelopathy.

ventral cyst that goes on to be known as a neurenteric cyst[118] (Fig. 35.13). Neurenteric cysts are rare, with only case report and case series data available, but they have been known to occur throughout the neural axis.[119] The available data suggest that the natural history of these cysts is characterized by recurrent ruptures, gradual enlargement, and progressive motor weakness. As such, surgical excision is recommended.[120] Extramedullary lesions can often be excised completely, but intramedullary lesions may lack a clear cyst wall; thus, subtotal resection may be the best achievable result in certain cases.[120]

Conclusion

Spinal dysraphism represents a wide spectrum of abnormalities that may affect the spinal cord, and should be considered when assessing a spine patient—especially when they are "unknowns," such as onset scoliosis or lower extremity deformity. The spectrum of types of abnormality and complicated presentations makes these challenging diagnoses. The best treatment, with respect to both timing and type of intervention, is not always evident. The clinician must understand surgical and medical nuances of treatment, and these patients need long-term follow-up due to the risk of recurrence, as well as a strong support system due to the associated dysfunction of the bowel/bladder, lower extremity, and urogenital systems. Associated brain anomalies are often present as well. A multidisciplinary team—including a neurosurgeon, orthopedic surgeon, urologist, and specialized primary care physician—is necessary to ensure that the best care is delivered.

More work on uncovering genetic and environmental factors for the development of these defects will hopefully lead to measures to decrease their incidence. Prenatal surgery might offer hope as an alternate treatment option for spina bifida aperta, though it is clear that there are increased risks to the mother and more long-term follow-up is needed. ETV is reducing the need for shunts to treat hydrocephalus in these individuals, which is an exciting new development. Most important, as more of these children enter adulthood, for a disease that previously had a significantly reduced life expectancy, adult practitioners need to be more familiar with the condition.

REFERENCES

1. Zerah M, Kulkarni AV. Spinal cord malformations. *Handb Clin Neurol.* 2013;112:975-991.
2. French B. Midline fusion defects and defects in formation. In: Youmans J, ed. *Neurological Surgery.* 3rd ed. Philadelphia: WB Saunders; 1990:1081-1235.
3. Barson AJ. The vertebral level of termination of the spinal cord during normal and abnormal development. *J Anat.* 1970;106(Pt 3):489-497.
4. Rickham PP. Nicolaas Tulp and spina bifida. *Clin Pediatr (Phila).* 1963;2:40-42.
5. Afonso ND, Catala M. [Neurosurgical embryology. Part 7: development of the spinal cord, the spine and the posterior fossa]. *Neurochirurgie.* 2003;49(5):503-510.
6. McLone DG, Knepper PA. The cause of Chiari II malformation: a unified theory. *Pediatr Neurosci.* 1989;15(1):1-12.
7. Prevalence of neural tube defects in 20 regions of Europe and the impact of prenatal diagnosis, 1980-1986. EUROCAT Working Group. *J Epidemiol Community Health.* 1991;45(1):52-58.
8. Canfield MA, Annegers JF, Brender JD, Cooper SP, Greenberg F. Hispanic origin and neural tube defects in Houston/Harris County, Texas. II. Risk factors. *Am J Epidemiol.* 1996;143(1):12-24.
9. Canfield MA, Annegers JF, Brender JD, Cooper SP, Greenberg F. Hispanic origin and neural tube defects in Houston/Harris County, Texas. I. Descriptive epidemiology. *Am J Epidemiol.* 1996;143(1):1-11.
10. Rosano A, Smithells D, Cacciani L, et al. Time trends in neural tube defects prevalence in relation to preventive strategies: an international study. *J Epidemiol Community Health.* 1999;53(10):630-635.
11. Laurence KM, James N, Miller MH, Tennant GB, Campbell H. Double-blind randomised controlled trial of folate treatment before conception to prevent recurrence of neural-tube defects. *Br Med J (Clin Res Ed).* 1981;282(6275):1509-1511.
12. Pitkin RM. Folate and neural tube defects. *Am J Clin Nutr.* 2007;85(1):285S-288S.
13. Czeizel AE, Dudas I. Prevention of the first occurrence of neural-tube defects by periconceptional vitamin supplementation. *N Engl J Med.* 1992;327(26): 1832-1835.
14. Babcook CJ. Ultrasound evaluation of prenatal and neonatal spina bifida. *Neurosurg Clin N Am.* 1995;6(2):203-218.
15. Ghi T, Pilu G, Falco P, et al. Prenatal diagnosis of open and closed spina bifida. *Ultrasound Obstet Gynecol.* 2006;28(7):899-903.

16. Sival DA, Begeer JH, Staal-Schreinemachers AL, et al. Perinatal motor behaviour and neurological outcome in spina bifida aperta. *Early Hum Dev.* 1997;50(1):27-37.
17. Meuli M, Meuli-Simmen C, Yingling CD, et al. Creation of myelomeningocele in utero: a model of functional damage from spinal cord exposure in fetal sheep. *J Pediatr Surg.* 1995;30(7):1028-1032.
18. Adzick NS, Thom EA, Spong CY, et al. A randomized trial of prenatal versus postnatal repair of myelomeningocele. *N Engl J Med.* 2011;364(11):993-1004.
19. Koszutski T, Kawalski H, Kudela G, et al. Babies with myelomeningocele in Poland: parents' attitudes on fetal surgery versus termination of pregnancy. *Childs Nerv Syst.* 2009;25(2):207-210.
20. Sharrard WJ. The segmental innervation of the lower limb muscles in man. *Ann R Coll Surg Engl.* 1964;35:106-122.
21. Samagh SP, Cheng I, Elzik M, Kondrashov DG, Rinsky LA. Kyphectomy in the treatment of patients with myelomeningocele. *Spine J.* 2011;11(3):e5-e11.
22. Kaplan SC, Eksi MS, Bayri Y, Toktas ZO, Konya D. Kyphectomy and pedicular screw fixation with posterior-only approach in pediatric patients with myelomeningocele. *Pediatr Neurosurg.* 2015;50(3):133-144.
23. Bauman JASD, Welch WC, Sutton LN. Congenital anomalies of the spinal cord. In: Herkowitz HNGS, Eismont FJ, Bell GR, Balderston RA, eds. *Rothman-Simeone: The Spine.* Philadelphia: Elsevier; 2011.
24. Lien SC, Maher CO, Garton HJ, et al. Local and regional flap closure in myelomeningocele repair: a 15-year review. *Childs Nerv Syst.* 2010;26(8):1091-1095.
25. Patel KB, Taghinia AH, Proctor MR, Warf BC, Greene AK. Extradural myelomeningocele reconstruction using local turnover fascial flaps and midline linear skin closure. *J Plast Reconstr Aesthet Surg.* 2012;65(11):1569-1572.
26. Sutton LN, Adzick NS, Bilaniuk LT, et al. Improvement in hindbrain herniation demonstrated by serial fetal magnetic resonance imaging following fetal surgery for myelomeningocele. *JAMA.* 1999;282(19):1826-1831.
27. Bennett KA, Carroll MA, Shannon CN, et al. Reducing perinatal complications and preterm delivery for patients undergoing in utero closure of fetal myelomeningocele: further modifications to the multidisciplinary surgical technique. *J Neurosurg Pediatr.* 2014;14(1):108-114.
28. Pedreira DA, Zanon N, Nishikuni K, et al. Endoscopic surgery for the antenatal treatment of myelomeningocele: the CECAM trial. *Am J Obstet Gynecol.* 2016;214(1):111.e1-111.e11.
29. Tulipan N, Wellons JC 3rd, Thom EA, et al. Prenatal surgery for myelomeningocele and the need for cerebrospinal fluid shunt placement. *J Neurosurg Pediatr.* 2015;16(6):613-620.
30. Miller PD, Pollack IF, Pang D, Albright AL. Comparison of simultaneous versus delayed ventriculoperitoneal shunt insertion in children undergoing myelomeningocele repair. *J Child Neurol.* 1996;11(5):370-372.
31. Clemmensen D, Rasmussen MM, Mosdal C. A retrospective study of infections after primary VP shunt placement in the newborn with myelomeningocele without prophylactic antibiotics. *Childs Nerv Syst.* 2010;26(11):1517-1521.
32. Mixter WJ. Ventriculoscopy and puncture of floor of third ventricle. *Boston Med Surg J.* 1923;188:277-278.
33. Abd-El-Barr MM, Cohen AR. The origin and evolution of neuroendoscopy. *Childs Nerv Syst.* 2013;29(5):727-737.
34. Warf BC, Campbell JW. Combined endoscopic third ventriculostomy and choroid plexus cauterization as primary treatment of hydrocephalus for infants with myelomeningocele: long-term results of a prospective intent-to-treat study in 115 East African infants. *J Neurosurg Pediatr.* 2008;2(5):310-316.
35. Stone SS, Warf BC. Combined endoscopic third ventriculostomy and choroid plexus cauterization as primary treatment for infant hydrocephalus: a prospective North American series. *J Neurosurg Pediatr.* 2014;14(5):439-446.
36. Zandian A, Haffner M, Johnson J, et al. Endoscopic third ventriculostomy with/without choroid plexus cauterization for hydrocephalus due to hemorrhage, infection, Dandy-Walker malformation, and neural tube defect: a meta-analysis. *Childs Nerv Syst.* 2014;30(4):571-578.
37. Perez da Rosa S, Millward CP, Chiappa V, et al. Endoscopic third ventriculostomy in children with myelomeningocele: a case series. *Pediatr Neurosurg.* 2015;50(3):113-118.
38. Ellsworth PI, Merguerian PA, Klein RB, Rozycki AA. Evaluation and risk factors of latex allergy in spina bifida patients: is it preventable? *J Urol.* 1993;150(2 Pt 2):691-693.
39. Boettcher M, Goettler S, Eschenburg G, et al. Prenatal latex sensitization in patients with spina bifida: a pilot study. *J Neurosurg Pediatr.* 2014;13(3):291-294.
40. Bouras T, Sgouros S. Complications of endoscopic third ventriculostomy. *World Neurosurg.* 2013;79(suppl 2):S22 e9-S22 e12.
41. Javadpour M, May P, Mallucci C. Sudden death secondary to delayed closure of endoscopic third ventriculostomy. *Br J Neurosurg.* 2003;17(3):266-269.
42. Mataro M, Poca MA, Sahuquillo J, et al. Cognitive changes after cerebrospinal fluid shunting in young adults with spina bifida and assumed arrested hydrocephalus. *J Neurol Neurosurg Psychiatry.* 2000;68(5):615-621.
43. Marano PJ, Stone SS, Mugamba J, et al. Reopening of an obstructed third ventriculostomy: long-term success and factors affecting outcome in 215 infants. *J Neurosurg Pediatr.* 2015;15(4):399-405.
44. Talamonti G, D'Aliberti G, Collice M. Myelomeningocele: long-term neurosurgical treatment and follow-up in 202 patients. *J Neurosurg.* 2007;107(suppl 5):368-386.
45. Phuong LK, Schoeberl KA, Raffel C. Natural history of tethered cord in patients with meningomyelocele. *Neurosurgery.* 2002;50(5):989-993.
46. George TM, Fagan LH. Adult tethered cord syndrome in patients with postrepair myelomeningocele: an evidence-based outcome study. *J Neurosurg.* 2005;102(suppl 2):150-156.
47. Pouratian N, Elias WJ, Jane JA Jr, Phillips LH 2nd, Jane JA Sr. Electrophysiologically guided untethering of secondary tethered spinal cord syndrome. *Neurosurg Focus.* 2010;29(1):E3.
48. Reigel DH, Tchernoukha K, Bazmi B, Kortyna R, Rotenstein D. Change in spinal curvature following release of tethered spinal cord associated with spina bifida. *Pediatr Neurosurg.* 1994;20(1):30-42.
49. Heinz ER, Rosenbaum AE, Scarff TB, Reigel DH, Drayer BP. Tethered spinal cord following meningomyelocele repair. *Radiology.* 1979;131(1):153-160.
50. Abd-El-Barr MM, Strong CI, Groff MW. Chiari malformations: diagnosis, treatments and failures. *J Neurosurg Sci.* 2014;58(4):215-221.
51. Citton V, Toldo I, Balao L, et al. Chiari 2 without spinal dysraphism: does it blow a hole in the pathogenesis? *J Child Neurol.* 2012;27(4):536-539.

52. Fischer EG, Welch K, Shillito J Jr. Syringomyelia following lumboureteral shunting for communicating hydrocephalus. Report of three cases. *J Neurosurg.* 1977;47(1):96-100.
53. Bell WO, Charney EB, Bruce DA, Sutton LN, Schut L. Symptomatic Arnold-Chiari malformation: review of experience with 22 cases. *J Neurosurg.* 1987;66(6):812-816.
54. Patel DM, Rocque BG, Hopson B, et al. Sleep-disordered breathing in patients with myelomeningocele. *J Neurosurg Pediatr.* 2015;16(1):30-35.
55. Rocque BG, George TM, Kestle J, Iskandar BJ. Treatment practices for Chiari malformation type I with syringomyelia: results of a survey of the American Society of Pediatric Neurosurgeons. *J Neurosurg Pediatr.* 2011;8(5):430-437.
56. Hall PV, Campbell RL, Kalsbeck JE. Meningomyelocele and progressive hydromyelia. Progressive paresis in myelodysplasia. *J Neurosurg.* 1975;43(4):457-463.
57. Heiss JD, Snyder K, Peterson MM, et al. Pathophysiology of primary spinal syringomyelia. *J Neurosurg Spine.* 2012;17(5):367-380.
58. Oldfield EH, Muraszko K, Shawker TH, Patronas NJ. Pathophysiology of syringomyelia associated with Chiari I malformation of the cerebellar tonsils. Implications for diagnosis and treatment. *J Neurosurg.* 1994;80(1):3-15.
59. Dias MS. Neurosurgical causes of scoliosis in patients with myelomeningocele: an evidence-based literature review. *J Neurosurg.* 2005;103(suppl 1):24-35.
60. Anderson FM. Occult spinal dysraphism: a series of 73 cases. *Pediatrics.* 1975;55(6):826-835.
61. Lew SM, Kothbauer KF. Tethered cord syndrome: an updated review. *Pediatr Neurosurg.* 2007;43(3):236-248.
62. Detrick RJ, Dickey D, Kintner CR. The effects of N-cadherin misexpression on morphogenesis in *Xenopus* embryos. *Neuron.* 1990;4(4):493-506.
63. Fujimori T, Miyatani S, Takeichi M. Ectopic expression of N-cadherin perturbs histogenesis in *Xenopus* embryos. *Development.* 1990;110(1):97-104.
64. Hertzler DA 2nd, DePowell JJ, Stevenson CB, Mangano FT. Tethered cord syndrome: a review of the literature from embryology to adult presentation. *Neurosurg Focus.* 2010;29(1):E1.
65. Fleming A, Keynes RJ, Tannahill D. The role of the notochord in vertebral column formation. *J Anat.* 2001;199(Pt 1-2):177-180.
66. Drake JM. Occult tethered cord syndrome: not an indication for surgery. *J Neurosurg.* 2006;104(suppl 5):305-308.
67. Agopian AJ, Canfield MA, Olney RS, et al. Spina bifida subtypes and sub-phenotypes by maternal race/ethnicity in the National Birth Defects Prevention Study. *Am J Med Genet A.* 2012;158A(1):109-115.
68. McNeely PD, Howes WJ. Ineffectiveness of dietary folic acid supplementation on the incidence of lipomyelomeningocele: pathogenetic implications. *J Neurosurg.* 2004;100(2 suppl Pediatrics):98-100.
69. Emery JL, Lendon RG. Lipomas of the cauda equina and other fatty tumours related to neurospinal dysraphism. *Dev Med Child Neurol Suppl.* 1969;20:62-70.
70. Al-Omari MH, Eloqayli HM, Qudseih HM, Al-Shinag MK. Isolated lipoma of filum terminale in adults: MRI findings and clinical correlation. *J Med Imaging Radiat Oncol.* 2011;55(3):286-290.
71. Brown E, Matthes JC, Bazan C 3rd, Jinkins JR. Prevalence of incidental intraspinal lipoma of the lumbosacral spine as determined by MRI. *Spine.* 1994;19(7):833-836.
72. Uchino A, Mori T, Ohno M. Thickened fatty filum terminale: MR imaging. *Neuroradiology.* 1991;33(4):331-333.
73. Myrianthopoulos NC, Chung CS. Congenital malformations in singletons: epidemiologic survey. Report from the Collaborative Perinatal project. *Birth Defects Orig Artic Ser.* 1974;10(11):1-58.
74. Powell KR, Cherry JD, Hougen TJ, Blinderman EE, Dunn MC. A prospective search for congenital dermal abnormalities of the craniospinal axis. *J Pediatr.* 1975;87(5):744-750.
75. Ackerman LL, Menezes AH. Spinal congenital dermal sinuses: a 30-year experience. *Pediatrics.* 2003;112(3 Pt 1):641-647.
76. Kaufman BA. Neural tube defects. *Pediatr Clin North Am.* 2004;51(2):389-419.
77. Henriques JG, Pianetti G, Henriques KS, Costa P, Gusmao S. Minor skin lesions as markers of occult spinal dysraphisms: prospective study. *Surg Neurol.* 2005;63(suppl 1):S8-S12.
78. De Wals P, Van Allen MI, Lowry RB, et al. Impact of folic acid food fortification on the birth prevalence of lipomyelomeningocele in Canada. *Birth defects Res A.* 2008;82(2):106-109.
79. Kumar Sarin Y. Cutaneous stigmata of occult spinal dysraphism. *J Neonatal Surg.* 2013;2(1):15.
80. Davis DA, Cohen PR, George RE. Cutaneous stigmata of occult spinal dysraphism. *J Am Acad Dermatol.* 1994;31(5 Pt 2):892-896.
81. Kriss VM, Desai NS. Occult spinal dysraphism in neonates: assessment of high-risk cutaneous stigmata on sonography. *AJR Am J Roentgenol.* 1998;171(6):1687-1692.
82. Muthukumar N, Subramaniam B, Gnanaseelan T, Rathinam R, Thiruthavadoss A. Tethered cord syndrome in children with anorectal malformations. *J Neurosurg.* 2000;92(4):626-630.
83. Heij HA, Nievelstein RA, de Zwart I, et al. Abnormal anatomy of the lumbosacral region imaged by magnetic resonance in children with anorectal malformations. *Arch Dis Child.* 1996;74(5):441-444.
84. Davidoff AM, Thompson CV, Grimm JM, et al. Occult spinal dysraphism in patients with anal agenesis. *J Pediatr Surg.* 1991;26(8):1001-1005.
85. Long FR, Hunter JV, Mahboubi S, Kalmus A, Templeton JM Jr. Tethered cord and associated vertebral anomalies in children and infants with imperforate anus: evaluation with MR imaging and plain radiography. *Radiology.* 1996;200(2):377-382.
86. Stockman A, Boralevi F, Taieb A, Leaute-Labreze C. SACRAL syndrome: spinal dysraphism, anogenital, cutaneous, renal and urologic anomalies, associated with an angioma of lumbosacral localization. *Dermatology.* 2007;214(1):40-45.
87. Girard C, Bigorre M, Guillot B, Bessis D. PELVIS Syndrome. *Arch Dermatol.* 2006;142(7):884-888.
88. Scheible W, James HE, Leopold GR, Hilton SV. Occult spinal dysraphism in infants: screening with high-resolution real-time ultrasound. *Radiology.* 1983;146(3):743-746.
89. Sakakibara R, Hattori T, Uchiyama T, Kamura K, Yamanishi T. Uroneurological assessment of spina bifida cystica and occulta. *Neurourol Urodyn.* 2003;22(4):328-334.
90. Fone PD, Vapnek JM, Litwiller SE, et al. Urodynamic findings in the tethered spinal cord syndrome: does surgical release improve bladder function? *J Urol.* 1997;157(2):604-609.
91. Kondo A, Kato K, Kanai S, Sakakibara T. Bladder dysfunction secondary to tethered cord syndrome in adults: is it curable? *J Urol.* 1986;135(2):313-316.

92. Hellstrom WJ, Edwards MS, Kogan BA. Urological aspects of the tethered cord syndrome. *J Urol.* 1986;135(2):317-320.
93. De Gennaro M, Lais A, Fariello G, et al. Early diagnosis and treatment of spinal dysraphism to prevent urinary incontinence. *Eur Urol.* 1991;20(2):140-145.
94. Zoller G, Schoner W, Ringert RH. Pre- and postoperative urodynamic findings in children with tethered spinal cord syndrome. *Eur Urol.* 1991;19(2):139-141.
95. Meyrat BJ, Tercier S, Lutz N, et al. Introduction of a urodynamic score to detect pre- and postoperative neurological deficits in children with a primary tethered cord. *Childs Nerv Syst.* 2003;19(10-11):716-721.
96. Tortori-Donati P, Rossi A, Biancheri R, Cama A. Magnetic resonance imaging of spinal dysraphism. *Top Magn Reson Imaging.* 2001;12(6):375-409.
97. Warder DE. Tethered cord syndrome and occult spinal dysraphism. *Neurosurg Focus.* 2001;10(1):e1.
98. Kanev PM, Bierbrauer KS. Reflections on the natural history of lipomyelomeningocele. *Pediatr Neurosurg.* 1995;22(3):137-140.
99. Samuels R, McGirt MJ, Attenello FJ, et al. Incidence of symptomatic retethering after surgical management of pediatric tethered cord syndrome with or without duraplasty. *Childs Nerv Syst.* 2009;25(9):1085-1089.
100. Yamada S, Won DJ, Pezeshkpour G, et al. Pathophysiology of tethered cord syndrome and similar complex disorders. *Neurosurg Focus.* 2007;23(2):E6.
101. Raghavan N, Barkovich AJ, Edwards M, Norman D. MR imaging in the tethered spinal cord syndrome. *AJR Am J Roentgenol.* 1989;152(4):843-852.
102. Cornette L, Verpoorten C, Lagae L, et al. Tethered cord syndrome in occult spinal dysraphism: timing and outcome of surgical release. *Neurology.* 1998;50(6):1761-1765.
103. Selden NR. Occult tethered cord syndrome: the case for surgery. *J Neurosurg.* 2006;104(suppl 5):302-304.
104. Selcuki M, Coskun K. Management of tight filum terminale syndrome with special emphasis on normal level conus medullaris (NLCM). *Surg Neurol.* 1998;50(4):318-322, discussion 22.
105. Fabiano AJ, Khan MF, Rozzelle CJ, Li V. Preoperative predictors for improvement after surgical untethering in occult tight filum terminale syndrome. *Pediatr Neurosurg.* 2009;45(4):256-261.
106. Currarino G, Coln D, Votteler T. Triad of anorectal, sacral, and presacral anomalies. *AJR Am J Roentgenol.* 1981;137(2):395-398.
107. Lynch SA, Wang Y, Strachan T, Burn J, Lindsay S. Autosomal dominant sacral agenesis: Currarino syndrome. *J Med Genet.* 2000;37(8):561-566.
108. Passarge E, Lenz W. Syndrome of caudal regression in infants of diabetic mothers: observations of further cases. *Pediatrics.* 1966;37(4):672-675.
109. Muthukumar N. Surgical treatment of nonprogressive neurological deficits in children with sacral agenesis. *Neurosurgery.* 1996;38(6):1133-1137.
110. Pang D. Sacral agenesis and caudal spinal cord malformations. *Neurosurgery.* 1993;32(5):755-778.
111. Elton S, Oakes WJ. Dermal sinus tracts of the spine. *Neurosurg Focus.* 2001;10(1):e4.
112. Morandi X, Mercier P, Fournier HD, Brassier G. Dermal sinus and intramedullary spinal cord abscess. Report of two cases and review of the literature. *Childs Nerv Syst.* 1999;15(4):202-206.
113. Jankowitz BT, Albright AL. Cutaneous manifestations of split cord malformations. Report of three cases. *J Neurosurg.* 2007;107(suppl 3):240-243.
114. Pang D, Dias MS. Ahab-Barmada M. Split cord malformation: Part I: A unified theory of embryogenesis for double spinal cord malformations. *Neurosurgery.* 1992;31(3):451-480.
115. Rilliet B, Schowing J, Berney J. Pathogenesis of diastematomyelia: can a surgical model in the chick embryo give some clues about the human malformation? *Childs Nerv Syst.* 1992;8(6):310-316.
116. Ersahin Y. Split cord malformation types I and II: a personal series of 131 patients. *Childs Nerv Syst.* 2013;29(9):1515-1526.
117. Proctor MR, Bauer SB, Scott RM. The effect of surgery for split spinal cord malformation on neurologic and urologic function. *Pediatr Neurosurg.* 2000;32(1):13-19.
118. Brooks BS, Duvall ER, el Gammal T, et al. Neuroimaging features of neurenteric cysts: analysis of nine cases and review of the literature. *AJNR Am J Neuroradiol.* 1993;14(3):735-746.
119. Mann KS, Khosla VK, Gulati DR, Malik AK. Spinal neurenteric cyst. Association with vertebral anomalies, diastematomyelia, dorsal fistula, and lipoma. *Surg Neurol.* 1984;21(4):358-362.
120. Lippman CR, Arginteanu M, Purohit D, Naidich TP, Camins MB. Intramedullary neurenteric cysts of the spine. Case report and review of the literature. *J Neurosurg.* 2001;94(suppl 2):305-309.

SECTION V

CERVICAL DEGENERATIVE DISORDERS

CHAPTER 36 Cervical Spinal Disorders Associated With Skeletal Dysplasias and Metabolic Diseases

Bruce V. Darden II
Christopher O'Boynick
Jose Manuel Casamitjana

The sheer number of skeletal dysplasias and metabolic diseases associated with spinal disorders makes the topic quite daunting. This number is constantly growing and the boundaries are being redefined as modern medicine works to understand these complex entities. The limited literature on these topics does little to cover their wide gamut of pathologies. Notwithstanding the rarity of their presentation, it is vital that practitioners have a grasp on some of the key features of these diseases to accurately diagnose and select an appropriate treatment plan. Examination of these individuals with an awareness of the more commonplace cervical abnormalities is the safest option.

Skeletal Dysplasias and Metabolic Diseases

Skeletal dysplasias are typically identified at birth secondary to physical findings, family history, and imaging studies. The archetypal physical findings are body length and body proportions. Workup is indicated for any infant born to average-sized parents with a height below the fifth percentile and is also warranted if the child should ever move below the fifth percentile as he or she grows. These dysplasias typically come in one of two forms. The first is short limbs with a relatively normal trunk; the other is a short trunk with relatively normal limbs. It is important, but beyond the scope of this chapter, to identify the site of limb shortening. This can be in the proximal or distal aspect of the limb. Radiographs can be helpful to identify the affected region, whether it be the metaphysis or the epiphysis.

Mucopolysaccharidoses (MPS) are a group of several syndromes resulting from an abnormal metabolism of mucopolysaccharides. Many of these conditions are associated with short stature, thoracolumbar kyphosis, and cervical spine abnormalities. Diagnosis typically requires serum and urine markers. Accuracy of diagnosis is paramount, as there is significant variability in prognosis and treatment options between the syndromes.

Patient Evaluation

As with any pediatric condition, examination can be difficult, but it is paramount to a successful diagnosis. A meticulous history from the parent—including activity level, milestones, and bowel and bladder dysfunction—is very important. Children afflicted with these conditions rarely complain of pain.

A complete neurologic examination must be performed. Serial evaluations can be helpful to gauge progression of any condition. Distracting conditions related to the underlying disease, such as lower extremity deformities, can make examination more difficult and must be taken into account.

Imaging

Plain radiographs of the cervical spine are recommended as part of any evaluation. These should include sitting or standing anteroposterior and lateral views. Radiographs allow evaluation of the osseous structures of the cervical spine. Some of these conditions result in delayed ossification of the cervical elements and limit the usefulness of radiographs. Table 36.1 outlines imaging techniques and the abnormalities best visualized with each technique.

Flexion-extension lateral films focused on the occipitocervical junction are very useful for diagnosing instability (Fig. 36.1). Communication with the patient, family, and radiology staff about the goals of this procedure is necessary to obtain quality images. These images allow a measurement of key parameters related to upper cervical instability and upper cervical stenosis. It is important to know the normal values of cervical radiographic parameters when assessing patients with cervical deformities. These measurements include the anterior atlantodens interval (AADI) and the space available for the cord (SAC). The AADI measures the distance from the dens to the posterior border of the anterior arch of the atlas, and should be less than 5 mm in a normal child during flexion.[1] The SAC is a measurement of the distance from the

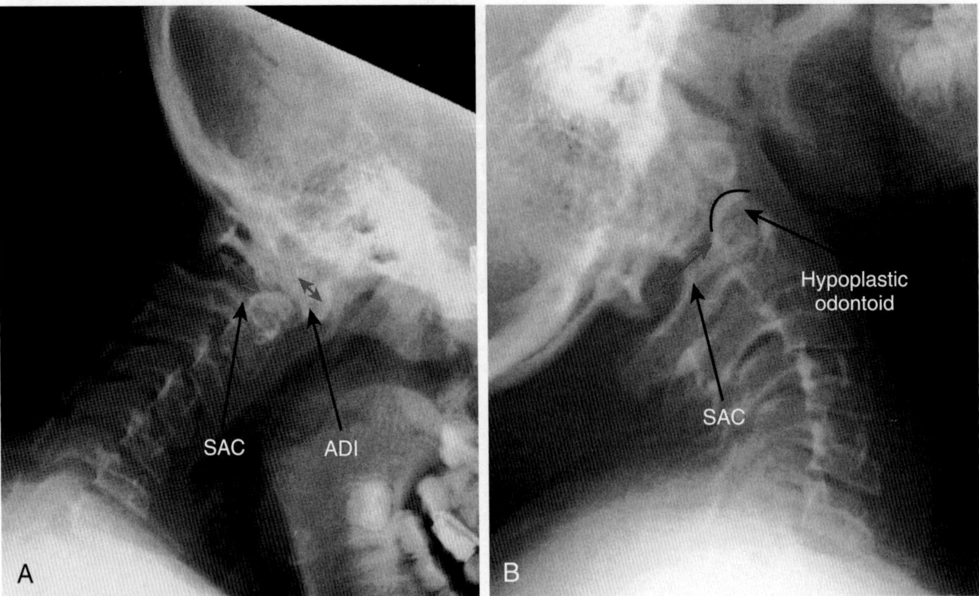

FIG. 36.1 (A) Extension and (B) flexion films focused on the occipitocervical junction can be very helpful in diagnosing instability. These images of a child with spondyloepiphyseal dysplasia congenita demonstrate instability in extension with the front of C1 riding over the hypoplastic odontoid. ADI, atlantodens interval; SAC, space available for the cord.

TABLE 36.1 Imaging Modalities

Imaging Modality	Abnormalities Best Visualized
Radiographs	Odontoid hypoplasia Os odontoideum Basilar invagination Fixed translational deformity Stenosis Upper cervical instability Platyspondyly
Computed tomography	Odontoid hypoplasia Os odontoideum Basilar invagination Fixed translational deformity Stenosis Upper cervical instability Platyspondyly Fine detail of bony anatomy Preoperative planning
Magnetic resonance imaging	Stenosis (dynamic and fixed) Cord compression Intrinsic cord abnormalities Cerebrospinal fluid flow dynamics Cerebral blood flow dynamics

dens to the anterior edge of the posterior ring of the atlas; the range of normal values can be found in Table 36.2.[2] An increasing AADI or a decreasing SAC can be indicative of instability and/or stenosis.

Computed tomography (CT) allows a more detailed examination of the bony anatomy, and is particularly useful in assessing the upper cervical spine. The quality of the images and the ability to create three-dimensional reconstructions based on CT data can be helpful tools for preoperative planning (Fig. 36.2). CT scans expose the pediatric patient to a

TABLE 36.2 Upper Cervical Spine Radiographic Parameters

Radiographic Parameters	Normal Values
Anterior atlantodens interval	Adult normal: <3.5 mm in flexion Child normal: <4.5 mm in flexion Abnormal: >5 mm
Space available for the cord at C2	Infant: 13 mm 3–6 y: 18 mm 7–10 y: 19 mm 11–14 y: 19.4 mm

significant amount of radiation, however, and thus should be used sparingly and only when absolutely necessary.

Magnetic resonance imaging (MRI) is another very useful tool for evaluating the cervical spine in patients with cervical deformity. MR images take more time to acquire than CT images and often require sedation to obtain satisfactory images. MRI is a very sensitive tool for detecting stenosis, cord compression, cord signal changes, and other cord abnormalities (Fig. 36.3). With the advent of flow-sensitive MRI techniques and magnetic resonance angiography (MRA) protocols, a complete picture of cerebrospinal fluid (CSF) dynamics and cerebral blood flow can also be assessed.

As with lateral C-spine radiographs, flexion-extension MRI can be performed to identify dynamic cord compression versus a fixed stenosis. Positioning is critical in these patients. A forced flexion position in a sedated child with undiagnosed atlantoaxial instability can have dire consequences. The child should be placed on a bolster, allowing the neck to fall into a neutral or extended position. The flexion position should be avoided until confirmation of a patent spinal canal.

Ultrasound has a limited role early in development and can be used to evaluate the spine and spinal cord in patients up to 6 months of age.[3,4]

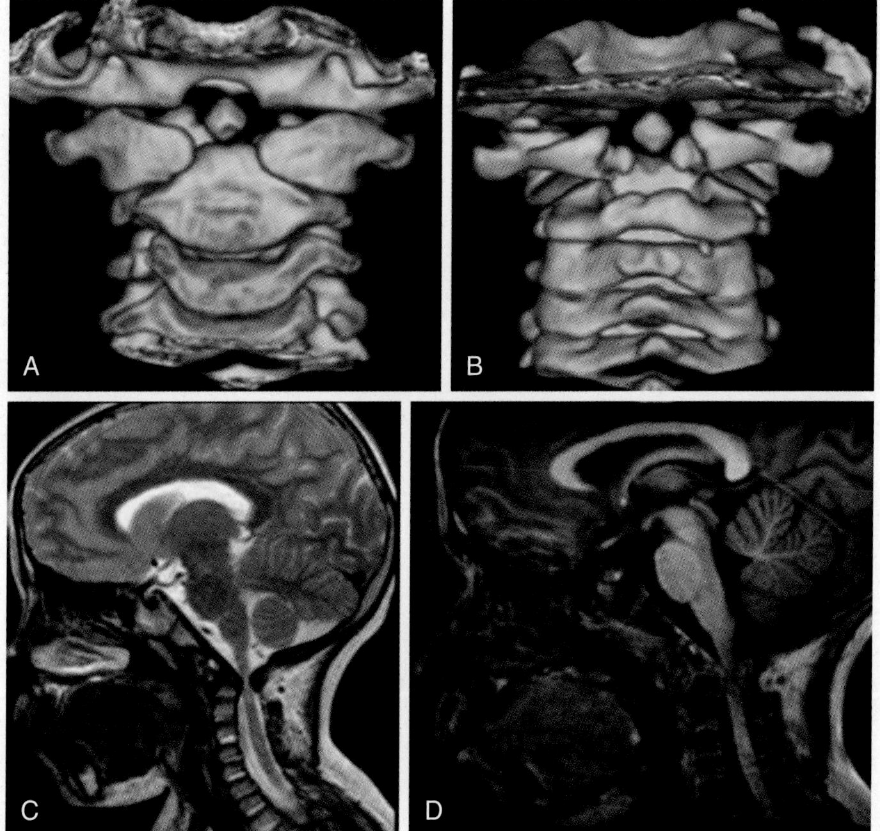

FIG. 36.2 (A–B) Three dimensional reconstructions of the upper cervical spine can aid in visualization of the complex deformities associated with these conditions and are helpful for preoperative planning. Computed tomography allows visualization of an os odontoideum in a child with Morquio syndrome. (C–D) Magnetic resonance imaging demonstrates the hypertrophied ventral soft tissue associated with Morquio syndrome that leads to craniocervical stenosis.

Treatment

These complex patients require a multidisciplinary approach. They are best served at high-volume centers with the training and facilities necessary to accommodate them. This would include a pediatric anesthesia team practiced in the intubation, positioning, and anesthetic requirements unique to these patients and procedures. Postoperatively, they will require care in the pediatric intensive care unit (ICU) and will need a treatment team familiar with the features of these conditions.

Children with skeletal dysplasias and metabolic syndromes typically fall into one of four categories when it comes to management. These include observation, observation with restrictions, relative indications for surgery, and absolute indications for surgery. The following section highlights the general principles of treatment. Specific treatment options are discussed later in the chapter as they apply to each condition.

Patients with skeletal dysplasia without evidence of neurocompromise or instability can be followed serially with observation. At a minimum, neurologic examination and cervical radiographs should be completed at each visit. Any change in neurologic examination would warrant an MRI.

A subset of patients will have radiographic evidence of mild, nonprogressive instability. These patients are best managed with a restriction from high-risk activities that would put their upper cervical spine at risk. Sports such as football, diving, and gymnastics should be included on this list. Communication about the risk associated with their condition is necessary when limiting activities.

A normal neurologic examination with radiographic evidence of significant stable kyphosis, with an AADI of 5 to 8 mm, or decreased SAC on MRI demonstrates relative indications for surgical intervention.

Absolute indications are reserved for patients with neurologic compromise, cord lesions, AADI greater than 8 mm, progressive kyphosis, and/or a dynamic instability resulting in severe reduction of the SAC.

The surgical procedure of choice is dependent on the underlying disease and surgical lesion. Treatment options include decompression, fusion, and decompression with fusion. Decompression should be reserved for patients with stenosis but without instability in a neutral or lordotic cervical spine. The concern with decompression alone is postlaminectomy kyphosis. Fusion alone is performed in patients demonstrating a dynamic instability that results in neurologic compromise without a fixed stenosis.[5–7] Decompression and fusion should be used to treat stenosis and instability and should also be used in those conditions associated with a postlaminectomy kyphosis.[8,9] Ventral procedures, including corpectomies and

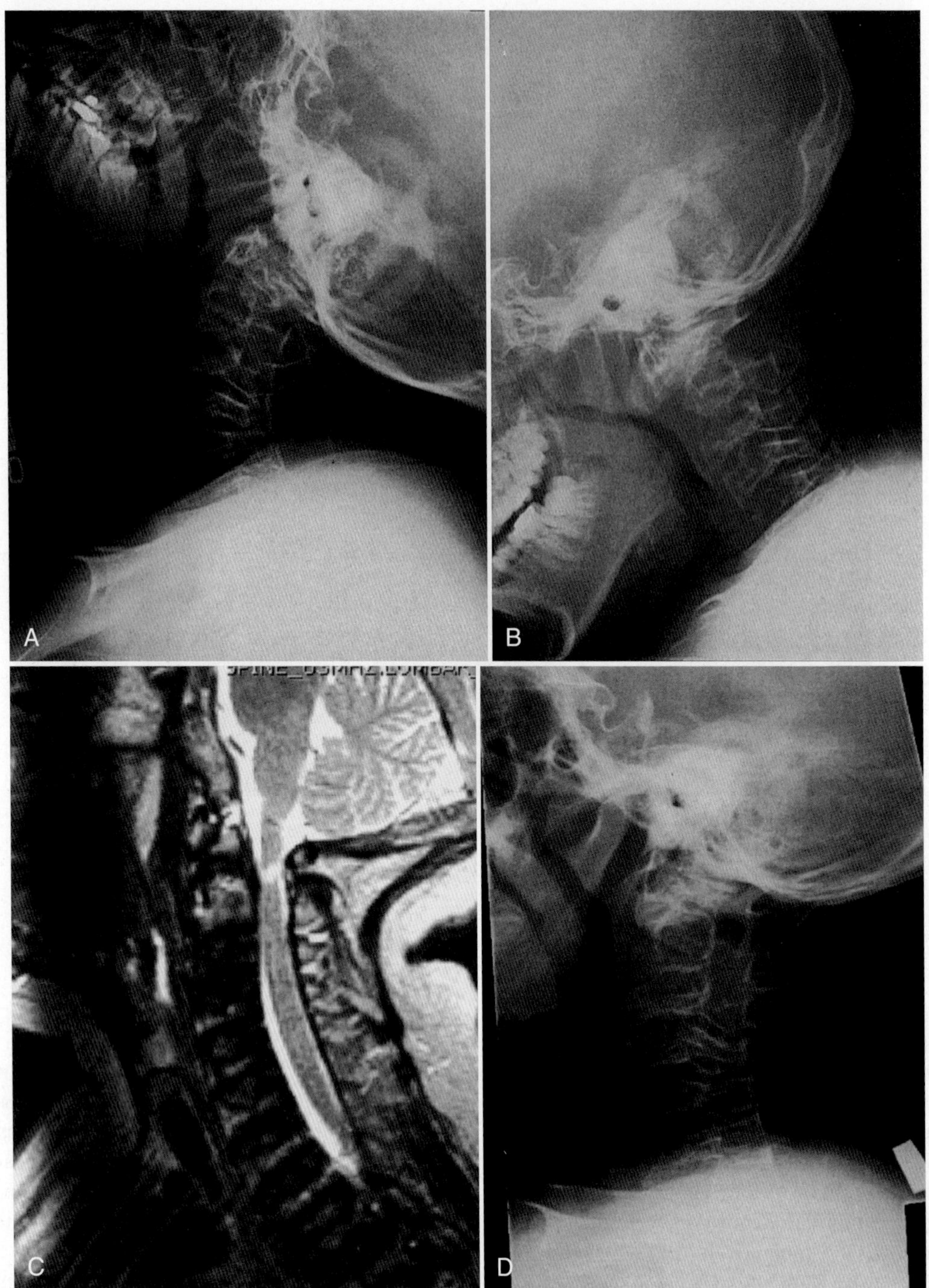

FIG. 36.3 (A–B) Flexion and extension radiographs demonstrating hypermobility at the C1–C2 joint. (C) Magnetic resonance imaging revealing signal changes within the cord secondary to compression. (D) Radiograph of the upper cervical spine after a noninstrumented occiput to C2 fusion.

strut grafting, should be reserved for conditions that result in a progressive kyphosis.[10]

Specific techniques of arthrodesis are beyond the scope of this chapter and have been previously described by multiple authors.[6,11,12] Close adherence to their described techniques should result in favorable outcomes. These procedures can be performed with or without internal fixation; the dysplastic anatomy is often the deciding factor regarding its implementation.[13,14] Preoperative CT scans with reconstructions and intraoperative navigation systems are excellent tools to aid in successfully instrumenting a deformed spine.[15]

In the setting of these procedures, diligent communication about the indications, anticipated outcomes, and possible complications is very important.

Postoperative immobilization is usually achieved by a halo or a brace. This will depend on the age and size of the child being treated. At a minimum, the halo should be MRI compatible. Pediatric patients require six to eight pins and have a lower torque allowance due to cranial size, skull thickness, and incomplete ossification. Regardless of the device, immobilization is maintained until radiographic evidence of solid fusion mass is identified.

Complications

Postoperative complications can be divided into early and delayed categories. Early complications include respiratory difficulty, wound drainage, and neurologic injury. Delayed complications include pseudarthrosis, infection, juxtafusional breakdown, and complications related to halo traction.

Respiratory difficulty is often multifactorial. These patients often have underlying lung and/or chest wall abnormalities that prevent normal lung function. Halo cast application and prolonged intubation superimposed on these preexisting conditions can lead to complications. Supportive ventilation techniques can be employed. As with all surgical patients, aggressive pulmonary toilet and rapid mobilization still remain the best options to prevent these complications.

Durotomy rates are increased in some forms of skeletal dysplasia. Shunting and duraplasty techniques at the time of index procedure can help to reduce this complication. CSF leaks can lead to wound compromise and breakdown.[12,16]

Neurologic injury typically results from a direct trauma to the spinal cord. In patients with preoperative neurologic compromise, the cord is already in a traumatized state and may be prone to added insult. In achondroplasia, it is recommended that no instruments be placed into the spinal canal secondary to the already reduced canal size. Neurologic injury can occur with or without instrumentation being placed in the spinal canal.[12,17] Somatosensory and motor evoked potentials should be considered in all cases to help reduce positional and instrument-related neurologic injury.[18]

Successful fusion has been linked to the use of autograft bone, meticulous surgical technique, and the use of internal fixation.[5,6,11,12] Numerous studies have outlined increased pseudarthrosis rates when allograft bone was utilized.[19,20] C1–C2 fusion rates were doubled with use of the transarticular screw technique over the sublaminar wiring technique in a study by Farey et al.[15]

Skeletal Dysplasias

Achondroplasia

Achondroplasia is by far the most common skeletal dysplasia routinely evaluated in the spine surgeon's office. This genetic defect of fibroblast growth factor receptor 3 function results in highly specific characteristics that make it recognizable at birth. These findings include rhizomelic extremities along with frontal bossing and nasal bridge depression. Head-to-body ratio can also be larger in patients with achondroplasia. Infants with this condition typically present with hypotonia in the trunk and extremities.

Stenosis of the craniocervical joint and upper cervical spine is present in nearly 60% of individuals.[21] However, all patients with achondroplasia have some component of foramen magnum stenosis. CT-based measurements have demonstrated a foramen magnum size three deviations below the mean in more than 90% of patients.[16] It is smaller than normal in all age-matched controls and has no association with head circumference.[22] This compression has two etiologies. The first is direct impingement of the spinal cord on the posterior rim of the foramen; the second is due to an invagination process of the foramen into the ring of C1.[23] Hecht et al.[22] reports that nearly one-third of these patients demonstrate symptoms of spinal cord compression, including sleep apnea, hypotonia, and quadriparesis. These factors all contribute to an increased risk of death in the first year of life.[24] Infants affected with this condition require careful neurologic examination, sleep laboratory studies, CT, and MRI evaluations during infancy. In addition to these tests, somatosensory evoked potentials have demonstrated excellent efficacy in diagnosing cervical myelopathy.[25,26]

Despite the plethora of diagnostic modalities, there still remains no consensus on patient selection or timing for operative intervention. Wang et al.[23] did correlate measurements of the foramen magnum with those who required decompression. The cross-sectional area of 239 mm^2 was found to be half that of normal controls.[23] Nelson et al.[25] found that cervicomedullary decompression was successful in reducing sleep apnea and improving sleep study results in affected patients. The abnormal CSF dynamics associated with achondroplasia result in a high rate of CSF leaks postoperatively and often benefit from the use of external ventricular drainage systems at the time of decompression.[16,27] Cervicomedullary decompression has been used successfully to treat a number of symptoms secondary to upper cervical stenosis; some authors go as far as to suggest that asymptomatic individuals with signal changes within the cord should also be treated.[28,29] Wassman et al.[30] prefer nonoperative management with continued sleep apnea monitoring while awaiting the natural enlargement of the foramen as the child matures.

Cervical stenosis in the subaxial cervical spine can also occur in patients with achondroplasia. While congenitally stenotic, subaxial cervical stenosis typically does not present until adulthood and is the result of the typical degenerative processes associated with normal individuals.[26,31] If symptoms of pain and/or weakness are present and are recalcitrant to nonoperative modalities, cervical decompression is the treatment of choice.[32,33] This can be done with laminectomy or laminoplasty per surgeon preference, along with selective foraminotomies, as indicated by imaging. Fusion is typically not necessary.

Cervical instability is relatively common in most skeletal dysplasias but is very rare in achondroplasia.[34,35]

Pseudoachondroplasia

Pseudoachondroplasia is a short-limbed form of dwarfism resulting from a defect in the cartilage oligomeric matrix protein. This results in a similar disruption to body proportions akin to that of achondroplasia, but that is where the similarities end.

Pseudoachondroplasia is associated with a generalized ligamentous laxity that results in atlantoaxial instability that increases with age.[36] It can also result from an os odontoideum and to a lesser extent odontoid hyperplasia or any combination of these factors.[5,36] Regardless of the cause, patients with this condition require lateral flexion and extension radiographs

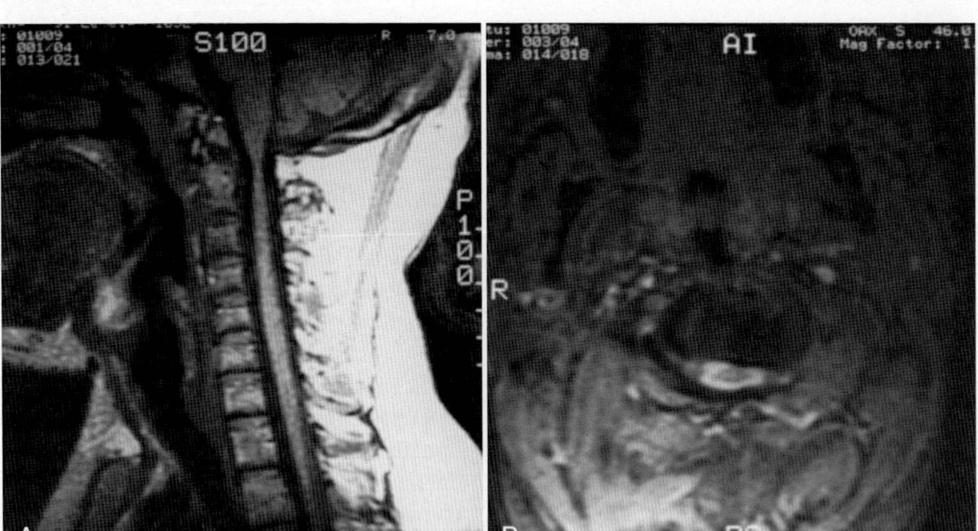

FIG. 36.4 (A) Sagittal and (B) axial magnetic resonance images of a patient with pseudoachondroplasia demonstrating marked stenosis at C1–C2. Note that the subaxial cervical spine demonstrates a normal spinal canal diameter without congenital stenosis.

prior to undergoing any procedure requiring intubation. Any instability that results in neurologic symptoms requires surgical fixation.

While achondroplasia results in severe congenital spinal stenosis, pseudoachondroplasia patients have a normal spinal canal diameter and relatively normal-sized bony anatomy; thus they can tolerate standard instrumentation (Fig. 36.4).

Spondyloepiphyseal Dysplasia

Spondyloepiphyseal dysplasia comes in two forms. The tarda type has a minimal effect on the cervical spine and is not discussed here. The congenital type is strongly associated with atlantoaxial instability secondary to ligamentous laxity, odontoid hypoplasia, or os odontoideum.[5,37–39] This condition results from a defect in type II collagen. Diagnosis is based on imaging findings of delayed ossification centers in the setting of a shortened trunk.[40]

Atlantoaxial instability presents in up to 50% of children with this condition.[41,42] Diagnosis can be made as early as in the first year of life and is usually associated with delayed motor milestones. This instability can occur in flexion or extension. Radiographic diagnosis can be difficult due to the delayed ossification of the posterior elements in this condition as well as the generalized flexibility of the juvenile cervical spine. Flexion-extension sagittal MRI is useful in this situation to quantify the amount of motion at this segment and to identify any stenosis or signal change within the cord. A patient with a normal MRI and less than 5 mm of translation on lateral C-spine films can be treated conservatively. If more than 5 mm of translation is visible on radiographs or there is evidence of spinal cord compression or cord signal change, then fusion without decompression is indicated. Decompression is reserved for patients with severe stenosis and myelopathy.[43]

The decision on the number of fusion levels is up to the discretion of the treating surgeon and may depend on the amount of ossification posteriorly in addition to the direction of instability. Fixation can be performed with or without halo application (Fig. 36.5). It is recommended that evoked potentials be monitored during the initial positioning as well as during the procedure. Ain et al.[44] demonstrated a better than 90% fusion rate with a similar rate of neurologic improvement in patients with atlantoaxial instability in the setting of skeletal dysplasia.

Kniest Dysplasia

Kniest dysplasia is another condition resulting from a defect in type II collagen production. From a cervical spine standpoint, this condition is very similar to spondyloepiphyseal dysplasia and results in atlantoaxial and occipitoatlantal instability.[44–47] Again, serial radiographs and sagittal flexion-extension MRIs can be used to determine any need for stabilization. The indications for surgical fixation are similar to those for spondyloepiphyseal dysplasia.

Metaphyseal Chondrodysplasia

The McKusick type, or cartilage-hair dysplasia, results in ligamentous laxity and atlantoaxial instability.[48,49] This condition has multiple physical abnormalities and is often associated with immunodeficiency.[48,49]

Metatropic Dysplasia

This condition arises from an uncoupling of endochondral and perichondral growth and results in short stature and dumbbell-shaped long bones.[50] Similar to most of the other dysplasias, atlantoaxial subluxation is a concern secondary to odontoid hypoplasia.[51] This condition has been associated with rotatory subluxation following failed fusion as well as C2–C3 instability due to anatomic abnormalities of the C2 lateral mass.[6] Leet et al.[52] has associated this condition with cervical spinal stenosis and identified patients

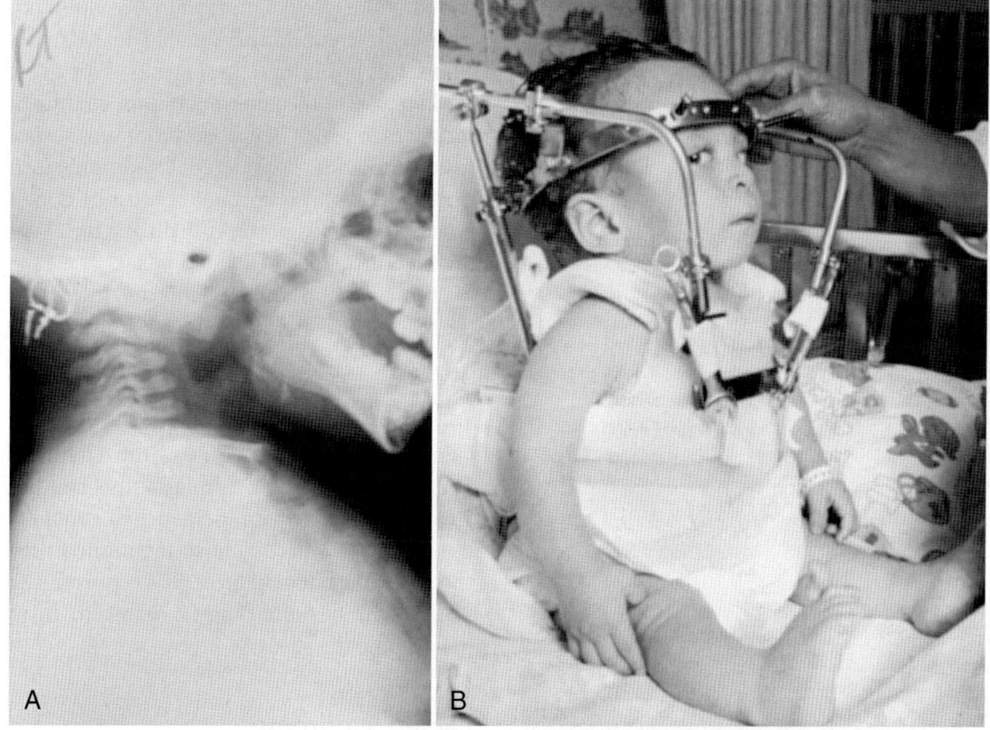

FIG. 36.5 (A) Radiograph of occipitoaxial wiring of an 18-month-old child with instability secondary to spondyloepiphyseal dysplasia. (B) Halo bracing can be used preoperatively, intraoperatively, and postoperatively to aid in reduction and to maintain stability when attempting fusion.

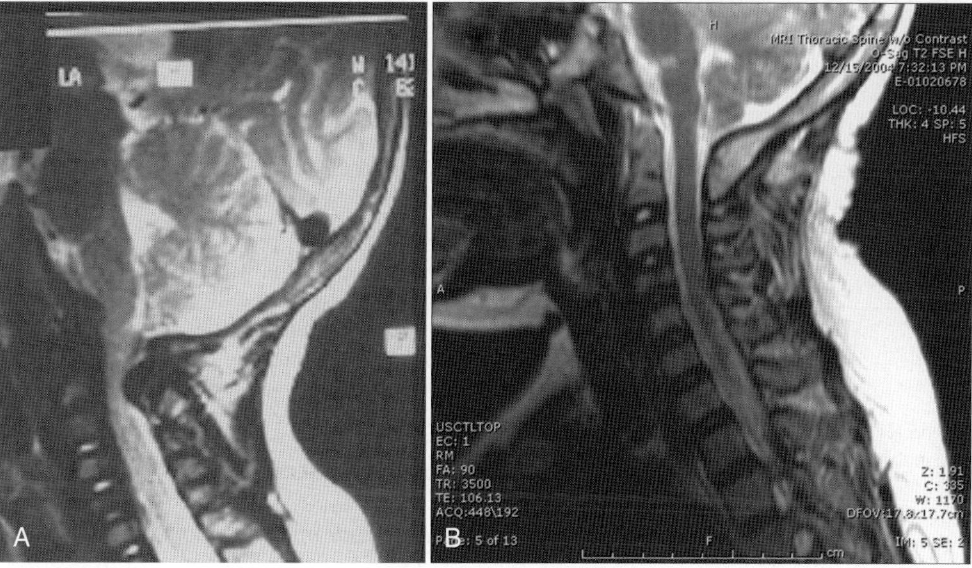

FIG. 36.6 (A) Preoperative and (B) postoperative images of a child with chondrodysplasia punctata treated with C1 laminectomy with occipitocervical fusion for cord compression. Postoperative magnetic resonance image shows a patent craniocervical junction without cord signal changes.

who may need decompression along with atlantoaxial fusion procedures.

Chondrodysplasia Punctata

This condition is characterized by short limbs, ichthyosis, and flat facial features. It has been associated with cervical cord compression from atlantoaxial instability (Fig. 36.6) as well as congenital cervical stenosis.[53] These patients can have subaxial kyphosis along with subluxation in the cervical spine, requiring radiographic and MRI evaluation.[54–57] Due to the dysplastic nature of the vertebral bodies and their association with kyphosis, a 360-degree fusion is recommended.[58]

Diastrophic Dysplasia

Diastrophic dysplasia arises from a defect in diastrophic dysplasia sulfate transportase. This condition has several key features associated with its diagnosis, including "hitchhikers thumb," "cauliflower ear," micromelia, and short stature.

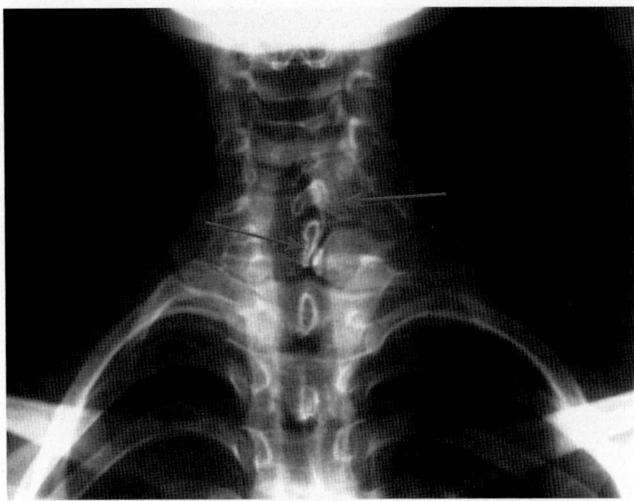

FIG. 36.7 Anteroposterior radiograph of the cervical spine demonstrating multilevel spina bifida common to diastrophic dysplasia.

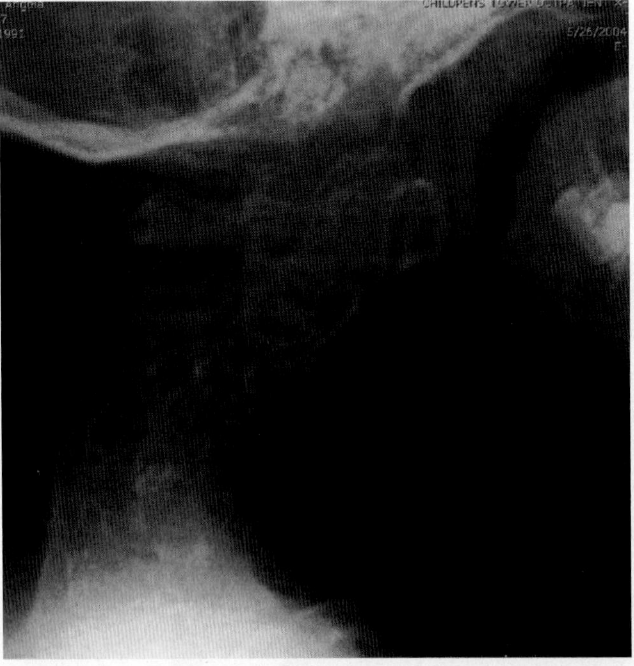

FIG. 36.8 Progressive cervical kyphosis typically requires 360-degree fusion procedures, as illustrated in this radiograph of a child with diastrophic dysplasia.

These patients all demonstrate spina bifida of the cervical spine (Fig. 36.7).[59,60] Upper cervical instability and upper cervical stenosis is not as common in diastrophic dysplasia as it is in some of the previously mentioned conditions, but it has been reported.[61,62] Perhaps the hallmark cervical abnormality associated with this condition is midcervical kyphosis (Fig. 36.8).[63,64] This may result from a combination of vertebral body wedging, ligamentous laxity, and the aforementioned cervical spina bifida.[10,60,65] This condition tends to resolve as the patients age.[59,65] In some cases, the kyphosis does not resolve and fusion becomes necessary. Kyphosis of greater than 60 degrees at initial evaluation has been linked to progression and can ultimately result in dire consequences.[59,65] Postmortem examinations of the spinal cord demonstrate changes in the anterior columns consistent with anterior cord compression. Kyphotic progression without neurologic compromise can be treated with posterior fusion alone. This posterior tethering allows for a gradual correction of the kyphosis as the anterior column continues to grow. In those instances in which neurocompromise is suspected, a 360-degree fusion should be considered. Decompression must occur anteriorly and kyphosis correction must be done carefully. Caution must also be used posteriorly during the exposure secondary to the high incidence of spina bifida.

These patients also develop cervical spondylosis as early as the second decade of life, which requires long-term follow-up.[61]

Camptomelic Dysplasia

Camptomelic dysplasia arises from a defect on the *SOX9* gene. Similar to diastrophic dysplasia, this condition results in cervical kyphosis, with an incidence of about 40%.[66–68] Treatment options are similar to those mentioned previously. However, the deformity and neurologic compromise in these patients often do not respond as favorably to fusion as they do in diastrophic dysplasia.[66–68]

Larsen Syndrome

This is a rare genetic condition of variable inheritance resulting from a mutation in the *filamin B* gene. This disrupts the normal skeletal development. Patients with Larsen syndrome often develop a progressive cervical kyphosis and should be managed similarly to patients with diastrophic dysplasia.[69]

22q11.2 Deletion Syndrome

This microdeletion has been linked to numerous syndromes, including velocardiofacial syndrome, DiGeorge syndrome, and conotruncal face anomaly syndrome. This syndrome is associated with multilevel hypermobility in addition to several bony abnormalities of the upper and subaxial cervical spine. All of these abnormalities can lead to significant instability and cervical stenosis.[69] Surgical treatment is specific to each individual and dependent on the deformities present.

Mucopolysaccharidoses

Hurler Syndrome: Mucopolysaccharidosis Type 1

This condition is associated with atlantoaxial instability and is typically a result of odontoid dysplasia.[70,71] Myelopathy can develop in these patients secondary to abnormal soft tissue formation on the tip of the dens. With the advent of bone marrow transplantation and enzyme replacement, there have been documented cases of resorption of this mass and resolution of symptoms.[72,73] These masses resolved slowly over the course of nearly 9 years.[73]

Hunter Syndrome: Mucopolysaccharidosis Type 2

Hunter syndrome is a lysosomal storage disease secondary to a defect in iduronate-2-sulfatase. The mucopolysaccharide is deposited posterior to the dens and can result in spinal stenosis.[74] Cervicomedullary decompression, along with laminectomy down to the subaxial cervical spine, is the recommended treatment for this condition.[75]

Morquio Syndrome: Mucopolysaccharidosis Type 4

Morquio syndrome comes in two varieties depending on the genetic defect and the resultant mucopolysaccharide that ultimately accumulates. This condition is perhaps the most severe of the metabolic syndromes as it relates to the craniocervical junction. Odontoid hypoplasia results in atlantoaxial instability, while ventral extradural soft tissues continue to hypertrophy and ultimately narrow the craniocervical junction.[76–78] This instability in the setting of severe stenosis has been linked to progressive myelopathy, quadriplegia, and sudden death.[79] The amount of hypertrophied tissue appears to correlate more with neurologic symptoms than does the odontoid dysplasia or direction of subluxation. As previously mentioned, workup typically includes flexion-extension radiographs and a flexion-extension MRI (Fig. 36.9). Criteria for fusion are similar to those mentioned for skeletal dysplasia, and fusion is recommended secondary to the high incidence of neurologic injury and poor recovery of myelopathic patients.[17,79] The hypertrophic craniocervical tissues tend to resolve after fusion, but direct anterior decompression can be performed transorally for significant compression (Fig. 36.10).[80,81]

Summary

The topic of cervical spine abnormalities associated with skeletal dysplasias and metabolic disease can be daunting.

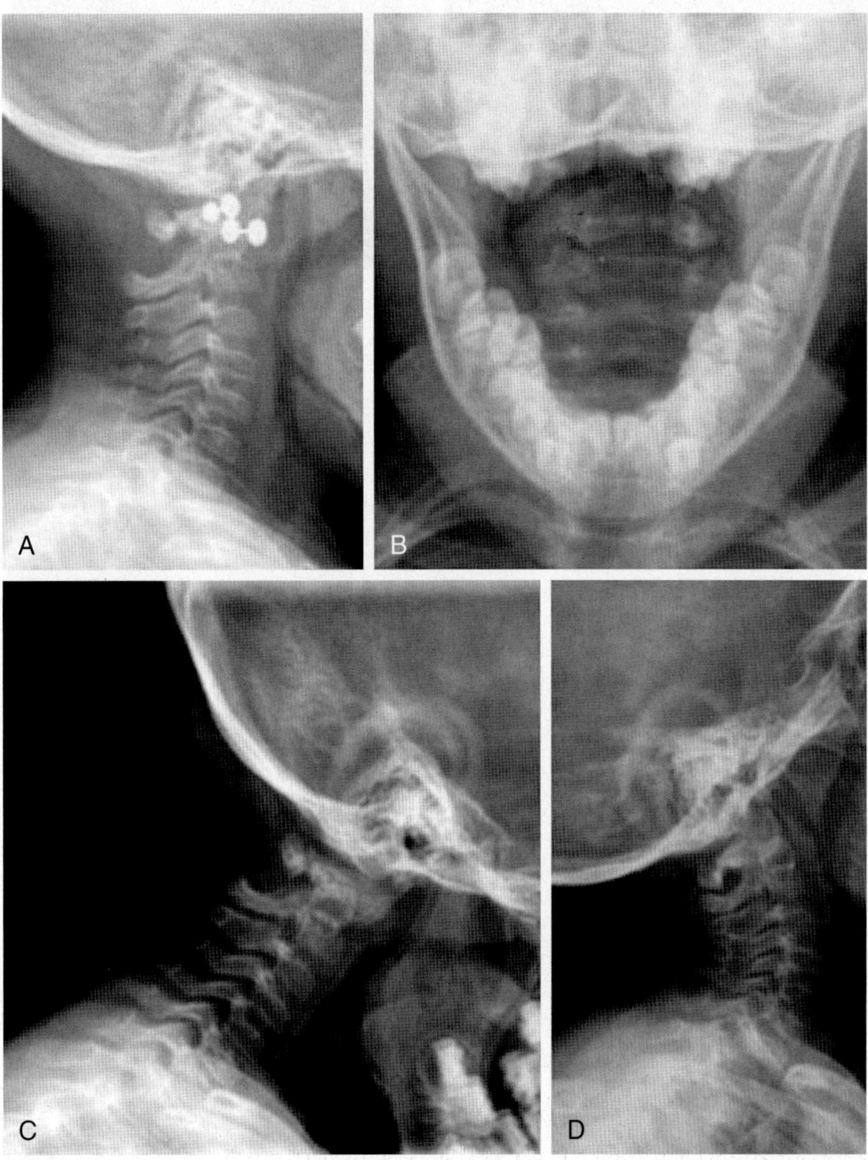

FIG. 36.9 (A–D) Plain radiographs of a child with Morquio syndrome. (B) The open-mouth view demonstrates hypoplasia of the odontoid. (C) Flexion and (D) extension views reveal a flexion instability with greater than 5 mm of motion. This is most easily visualized based on the relationship of the posterior ring of C1 to that of C2.

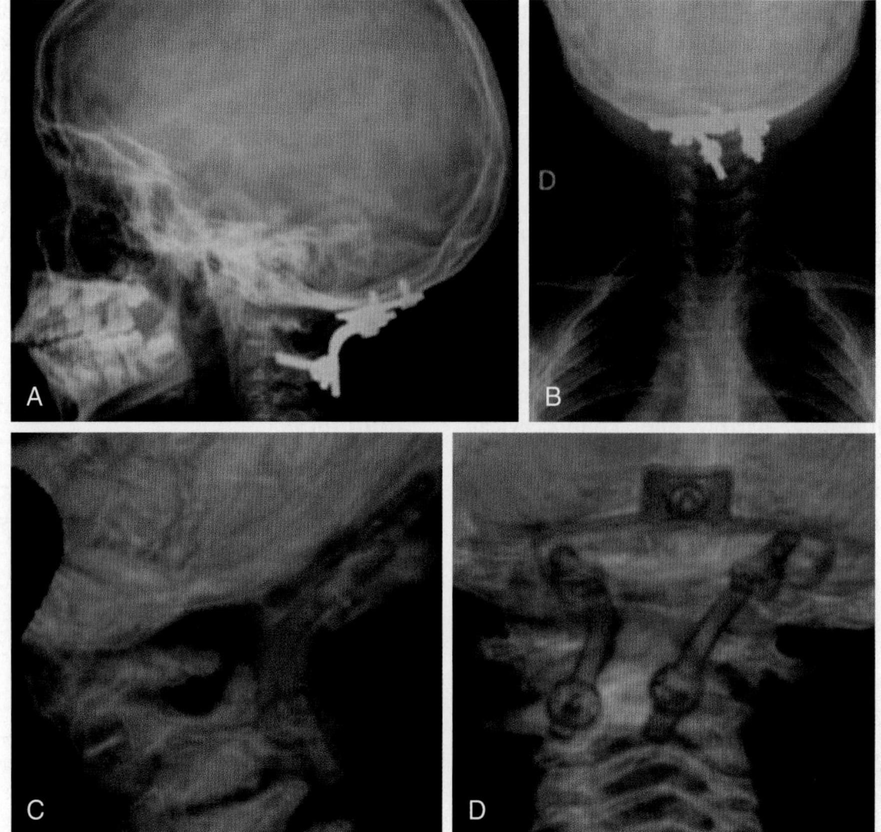

FIG. 36.10 Postoperative images of a child with Morquio syndrome following occiput to C2 fusion for a flexion instability.

TABLE 36.3 Skeletal Dysplasias and Cervical Spine Disorders

Skeletal Dysplasia	Cervical Pathology	Cause
Achondroplasia	Craniocervical stenosis Subaxial stenosis	Foramen magnum stenosis Basilar invagination Developmental
Pseudoachondroplasia	Atlantoaxial instability Subaxial cervical stenosis	Ligamentous laxity Os odontoideum Developmental
Spondyloepiphyseal dysplasia	Atlantoaxial instability	Odontoid hypoplasia Os odontoideum Ligamentous laxity
Spondylometaphyseal dysplasia	Atlantoaxial instability	Odontoid hypoplasia Ligamentous laxity
Kniest dysplasia	Atlantoaxial or occipitoatlantal instability	Ligamentous laxity
Metaphyseal chondrodysplasia	Atlantoaxial instability	Ligamentous laxity
Metatropic dysplasia	Atlantoaxial instability	Odontoid hypoplasia C2 lateral mass defect
Chondrodysplasia punctata	Atlantoaxial instability Subaxial stenosis Vertebral body hypoplasia	Os odontoideum
Diastrophic dysplasia	Progressive cervical kyphosis Atlantoaxial instability	Vertebral body hypoplasia Cervical spina bifida Hypotonia Odontoid dysmorphism

TABLE 36.3 Skeletal Dysplasias and Cervical Spine Disorders—Cont'd

Skeletal Dysplasia	Cervical Pathology	Cause
Camptomelic dysplasia	Kyphosis	Vertebral body malformation Spondylolisthesis Hypotonia
Hurler syndrome	Atlantoaxial instability Stenosis	Odontoid dysplasia Abnormal soft tissue about the dens
Hunter syndrome	Cervical stenosis	Thickening of the dura posterior to the dens
Morquio syndrome	Atlantoaxial instability Stenosis	Odontoid hypoplasia Ventral soft tissue hypertrophy
Larsen syndrome	Progressive cervical kyphosis	Vertebral body deformity
22q11.2 deletion syndrome	Cervical instability Congenital stenosis	Dysmorphic dens Incomplete C1 ring C2–C3 autofusion Decreased vertebral body width

Modified from Mackenzie WG, Shah SA, Takemitsu M. The cervical spine and skeletal dysplasia. In: Benzel EC, et al, eds. *The Cervical Spine*, ed 5. Philadelphia: Lippincott Williams & Wilkins; 2012:408–428.

While advances are made every day in diagnosis and medical management, surgical treatment of these patients evolving pathology remains the only option. Early recognition and accurate diagnosis of the underlying condition is vital. Table 36.3 serves as a quick reference guide for the syndromes discussed and their associated abnormalities.[82] A knowledge of the typical manifestations associated with each syndrome and an understanding of their workup will help to quickly and safely treat these patients.

KEY REFERENCES

1. Ain MC, Chaichana KL, Schkrohowsky JG. Retrospective study of cervical arthrodesis in patients with various types of skeletal dysplasia. *Spine (Phila Pa)*. 2006;31:E169-E174.
2. Remes V, Marttinen E, Poussa M, et al. Cervical kyphosis in diastrophic dysplasia. *Spine*. 1999;24:1990-1995.
3. McKay SD, Al-Omari A, Tomlinson LA, et al. Review of cervical spine anomalies in genetic syndromes. *Spine*. 2012;37:E269-E277.
4. Rodgers WB, Coran DL, Emans JB, et al. Occipitocervical fusions in children. Retrospective analysis and technical considerations. *Clin Orthop Relat Res*. 1999;359:125-133.
5. Farey ID, Nadkarni S, Smith N. Modified Gallie technique versus transarticular screw fixation in C1-C2 fusion. *Clin Orthop Relat Res*. 1999;359:126-135.

REFERENCES

1. Naik DR. Cervical spinal canal in normal infants. *Clin Radiol.* 1970;21:323-326.
2. Markuske H. Sagittal diameter measurements of the bony cervical spinal canal in children. *Pediatr Radiol.* 1977;6:129-131.
3. Cramer BC, Jequier S, O'Gorman AM. Sonography of the neonatal craniocervical junction. *Am J Roentgenol.* 1986;147:133-139.
4. Harlow CL, Drose JA. A special technique for cervical spine sonography. Illustrated by a patient with meningoencephalocele, Dandy-Walker variant, and syringomyelia. *J Ultrasound Med.* 1992;11:502-506.
5. Svensson O, Aaro S. Cervical instability in skeletal dysplasia. Report of 6 surgically fused cases. *Acta Orthop Scand.* 1988;59:66-70.
6. Koop SE, Winter RB, Lonstein JE. The surgical treatment of instability of the upper part of the cervical spine in children and adolescents. *J Bone Joint Surg Am.* 1984;66:403-411.
7. Ledoux MS, Naftalis RC, Aronin PA. Stabilization of the cervical spine in spondyloepiphyseal dysplasia congenita. *Neurosurgery*. 1991;28:580-583.
8. Lonstein JE. Post-laminectomy kyphosis. *Clin Orthop Relat Res.* 1977;128:93-100.
9. Mclaughlin MR, Wahlig JB, Pollack IF. Incidence of post-laminectomy kyphosis after Chiari decompression. *Spine.* 1997;22:613-617.
10. Forese LL, Berdon WE, Harcke HT, et al. Severe mid-cervical kyphosis with cord compression in Larsen's syndrome and diastrophic dysplasia: unrelated syndromes with similar radiographic findings and neurosurgical implications. *Pediatr Radiol.* 1995;25:136-139.
11. Dormans JP, Drummond DS, Sutton LN, et al. Occipitocervical arthrodesis in children. A new technique and analysis of results. *J Bone Joint Surg Am.* 1995;77:1234-1240.
12. Rodgers WB, Coran DL, Emans JB, et al. Occipitocervical fusions in children. Retrospective analysis and technical considerations. *Clin Orthop Relat Res.* 1999;364:125-133.
13. Brockmeyer D, Apfelbaum R, Tippets R, et al. Pediatric cervical spine instrumentation using screw fixation. *Pediatr Neurosurg.* 1995;22:147-157.
14. Meyer B, Vieweg U, Rao JG, et al. Surgery for upper cervical spine instabilities in children. *Acta Neurochir (Wien).* 2001;143:759-765.
15. Farey ID, Nadkarni S, Smith N. Modified Gallie technique versus transarticular screw fixation in C1-C2 fusion. *Clin Orthop Relat Res.* 1999;359:126-135.
16. Arynapur J, Hurko O, Francomano C, et al. Craniocervical decompression for cervicomedullary compression in pediatric patients with achondroplasia. *J Neurosurg.* 1990;73:375-382.
17. Ransford AO, Crockard HA, Stevens JM, et al. Occipito-atlanto-axial fusion in Morquio-Brailsford syndrome. A ten-year experience. *J Bone Joint Surg Br.* 1996;78:307-313.
18. Ofiram E, Lonstein JE, Skinner S, et al. "The disappearing evoked potentials"; a special problem of positioning patients with skeletal dysplasia: case report. *Spine.* 2006;31:E464-E470.
19. Shah SA, Taliwal RT, Mason DE, et al. *The treatment of cervical instability in children with skeletal dysplasia.* Proceedings of

the annual meeting of the Cervical Spine Research Society, 1999.

20. Stabler CL, Eismont FJ, Brown MD, et al. Failure of the posterior cervical fusions using cadaveric bone graft in children. *J Bone Joint Surg Am.* 1985;67:371-375.
21. Reid CS, Pyeritz RE, Kopits SE, et al. Cervicomedullary cord compression in young children with achondroplasia: value of comprehensive neurologic and respiratory evaluation. *Basic Life Sci.* 1988;48:199-206.
22. Hecht JT, Nelson FW, Butler IJ, et al. Computerized tomography of the foramen magnum: achondroplastic values compared to normal standards. *Am J Med Genet.* 1985;20:355-360.
23. Wang H, Rosenbaum AE, Reid CS, et al. Pediatric patients with achondroplasia: CT evaluation of the craniocervical junction. *Radiology.* 1987;164:515-519.
24. Pauli RM, Scott CI, Wassman ER Jr, et al. Apnea and sudden unexpected death in infants with achondroplasia. *J Pediatr.* 1984;104:342-348.
25. Nelson FW, Hecht JT, Horton WA, et al. Neurological basis of respiratory complications in achondroplasia. *Ann Neurol.* 1988;24:89-93.
26. Li L, Muller-Forell W, Oberman B, et al. Subcortical somatosensory evoked potentials after median nerve and posterior tibial nerve stimulation in high cervical cord compression of achondroplasia. *Brain Dev.* 2008;30:499-503.
27. Carson B, Winfield J, Wang H, et al. Surgical management of cervicomedullary compression in achondroplastic patients. In: Nicoletto B, Kopits SE, Ascani E, et al., eds. *Human Achondroplasia: A Multidisciplinary Approach.* New York: Plenum Press; 1988:207-214.
28. Ryken TC, Menzes AH. Cervicomedullary compression in achondroplasia. *J Neurosurg.* 1994;81:43-48.
29. Benglis DM, Sandberg DI. Acute neurological deficit after minor trauma in an infant with achondroplasia and cervicomedullary compression: case report and review of the literature. *J Neurosurg.* 2007;107(suppl 2):152-155.
30. Wassman ER Jr, Rimoin DL. Cervicomedullary compression with achondroplasia [letter]. *J Pediatr.* 1988;113:411.
31. Frigon VA, Castro FP, Whitecloud TS, et al. Isolated subaxial cervical spine stenosis in achondroplasia. *Curr Surg.* 2000;57:354-356.
32. Morgan DF, Young RF. Spinal neurological complications of achondroplasia: results of surgical treatment. *J Neurosurg.* 1980;52:463-472.
33. Pyeritz RE, Sack GH, Udvarhelyi GB. Cervical and lumbar laminectomy for spinal stenosis in achondroplasia. *Johns Hopkins Med J.* 1980;146:203-206.
34. Gulati DR, Rout D. Atlantoaxial dislocation with quadriparesis in achondroplasia [case report]. *J Neurosurg.* 1974;40:394-396.
35. Hammerschlag W, Ziv I, Wald U, et al. Cervical instability in an achondroplastic infant. *J Pedatr Orthop.* 1988;8:481-484.
36. Shetty GM, Song HR, Unnikrishnan R. Upper cervical spine instability in pseudoachondroplasia. *J Pediatr Orthop.* 2007;27:782-787.
37. Spranger JW, Langer LO Jr. Spondyloepiphyseal dysplasia congenital. *Radiology.* 1970;94:313-322.
38. Wynne-Davies R, Hall C. Two clinical variants of spondyloepiphyseal dysplasia congenital. *J Bone Joint Surg Br.* 1982;64:435-441.
39. Redl G. Massive pyramidal tract signs after endotracheal intubation: a case report of spondyloepiphyseal dysplasia congenital. *Anesthesiology.* 1998;89:1262-1264.
40. Spranger J, Wiedemann HR. Dysplasia spondyloepiphysaria congenital. *Helv Paediatr Acta.* 1966;21:598-611.
41. Walker BA, Scott CI, Hall JG, et al. Diastrophic dwarfism. *Medicine (Baltimore).* 1972;51:41-59.
42. Takeda E, Hashimoto T, Tayama M, et al. Diagnosis of atlanto-axial subluxation in Morquio's syndrome and spondyloepiphyseal dysplasia congenita. *Acta Paeditr Jpn.* 1991;33:633-638.
43. Miyoshi K, Nakamura K, Haga N, et al. Surgical treatment for atlantoaxial subluxation with myelopathy in spondyloepiphyseal dysplasia congenital. *Spine (Phila Pa).* 2004;31:E488-E491.
44. Ain MC, Chaichana KL, Schkrohowsky JG. Retrospective study of cervical arthrodesis in patients with various types of skeletal dysplasia. *Spine (Phila Pa).* 2006;31:E169-E174.
45. Merrill KD, Schmidt TL. Occipitoatlantal instability in a child with Kniest syndrome. *J Pediatr Orthop.* 1989;9:338-340.
46. Bethem D, Winter RB, Lutter L, et al. Spinal disorders of dwarfism. Review of the literature and report of eighty cases. *J Bone Joint Surg Am.* 1981;63:1412-1425.
47. Rimoin DL, Siggers DC, Lachman RS, et al. Metatropic dwarfism, the Kniest syndrome and pseudoachondroplastic dysplasias. *Clin Orthop Relat Res.* 1976;114:70-82.
48. Herring JA. Skeletal dysplasia. In: Herring JA, ed. *Tachdjian's Pediatric Orthopaedics.* 3rd ed. Philadelphia: W.B. Saunders; 2002.
49. Lachman RS. The cervical spine in skeletal dysplasias and associated disorders. *Pediatr Radiol.* 1997;27:402-408.
50. Boden SD, Kaplan FS, Fallon MD, et al. Meatropic dwarfism: uncoupling of endochondral and perichondral growth. *J Bone Joint Surg Am.* 1987;69:174-184.
51. Shohat M, Lachman R, Rimoin DL. Odontoid hypoplasia with vertebral cervical subluxation and ventriculomegaly in metatropic dysplasia. *J Pediatr.* 1989;114:239-243.
52. Leet AL, Sampath JS, Scott CI Jr, et al. Cervical spinal stenosis in metatropic dysplasia. *J Pediatr Orthop.* 2006;26:347-352.
53. Afshani E, Girdany BR. Atlanto-axial dislocation in chondrodyplasia punctata: report of the findings in two brothers. *Radiology.* 1972;102:399-401.
54. Khanna AJ, Braverman NE, Valle D, et al. Cervical stenosis secondary to rhizomelic chondrodysplasia punctata. *Am J Med Genet.* 2001;12:593-600.
55. Goddman P, Dominguez R. Cervicothoracic myelopathy in Conradi-Hunermann disease: MRI diagnosis. *Magn Reson Imaging.* 1990;8:647-650.
56. Violas P, Fraisse B, Chapuis M, et al. Cervical spine stenosis in chondrodysplasia punctata. *J Pediatr Orthop B.* 2007;16:443-445.
57. Garnier A, Dauger S, Eurin D, et al. Brachytelephalangic chondrodysplasia punctata with severe spinal cord compression: report of four new cases. *Eur J Pediatr.* 2007;166:127-131.
58. Wells TR, Landing BH, Bostwick FH. Studies of vertebral coronal cleft in rhizomelic chondrodysplasia punctata. *Pediatr Pathol.* 1992;12:593-600.
59. Bethem D, Winter RB, Lutter L. Disorders of the spine in diastrophic dwarfism: a discussion of nine patients and review the literature. *J Bone Joint Surg Am.* 1980;62:529-536.
60. Herring JA. The spinal disorder in diastrophic dwarfism. *J Bone Joint Surg Am.* 1978;60:177-182.
61. Remes V, Tervahartiala P, Poussa M, et al. Cervical spine in diastrophic dysplasia: an MRI analysis. *J Pediatr Orthop.* 2000;20:48-53.

62. Richards BS. Atlanto-axial instability in diastrophic dysplasia. A case report. *J Bone Joint Surg Am.* 1991;732:614-616.
63. Hensinger RN. Kyphosis secondary to skeletal dysplasias and metabolic disease. *Clin Orthop Relat Res.* 1977;128: 113-128.
64. Kopits SE. Orthopaedic complications of dwarfism. *Clin Orthop Relat Res.* 1976;114:153-179.
65. Remes V, Marttinen E, Poussa M, et al. Cervical kyphosis in diastrophic dysplasia. *Spine.* 1999;24:1990-1995.
66. Lekovic GP, Rekate HL, Dickman CA, et al. Congenital cervical instability in a patient with camptomelic dysplasia. *Childs Nerve Syst.* 2006;22:1212-1214.
67. Coscia MF, Bassett GS, Bowen JR, et al. Spinal abnormalities in camptomelic dysplasia. *J Pediatr Orthop.* 1989;9:6-14.
68. Ray S, Bowen JR. Orthopaedic problems associated with survival in camptomelic dysplasia. *Clin Orthop Relat Res.* 1984;185:77-82.
69. McKay SD, Al-Omari A, Tomlinson LA, et al. Review of cervical spine anomalies in genetic syndromes. *Spine.* 2012;37:E269-E277.
70. Thomas SL, Childress MH, Quinton B. Hypoplasia of the odontoid with atlanto-axial subluxation in Hurler's syndrome. *Pediatr Radiol.* 1985;15:353-354.
71. Brill CB, Rose JS, Godmilow L, et al. Spastic quadraparesis due to C1-C2 subluxation in Hurler syndrome. *J Pediatr.* 1978;92:441-443.
72. Tandon V, Williamson JB, Cowie RA, et al. Spinal problems in mucopolysaccharidosis I (Hurler syndrome). *J Bone Joint Surg Br.* 1996;78:938-944.
73. Hite SH, Peters C, Krivit W. Correction of odontoid dysplasia following bone-marrow transplantation and engraftment (in Hurler syndrome MPS1H). *Pediatr Radiol.* 2000;30: 464-470.
74. Parsons VJ, Hughes DG, Wraith JE. Magnetic resonance imaging of the brain, neck, and cervical spine in mild Hunter's syndrome (mucopolysaccharidosis type II). *Clin Radiol.* 1996;51:719-723.
75. O'Brien DP, Cowie RA, Wraith JE. Cervical decompression in mild mucopolysaccharidosis type II (Hunter syndrome). *Childs Nerv Syst.* 1997;13:87-90.
76. Blaw ME, Langer LO. Spinal cord compression in Morquio-Brailsford's disease. *J Pediatr.* 1969;74:595-600.
77. Beighton P, Craig J. Atlantoaxial subluxation in the Morquio syndrome. Report of a case. *J Bone Joint Surg Br.* 1973;55:478-481.
78. Taccone A, Tortori Donati P, Marzoli A, et al. Mucopolysaccharidosis: thickening of the dura mater at the craniocervical junction and other CT/MRI findings. *Pediatr Radiol.* 1993;23:349-352.
79. Lipson SJ. Dysplasia of the odontoid process in Morquio's syndrome causing quadriparesis. *J Bone Joint Surg Am.* 1977;59:340-344.
80. Ashraf J, Crockard HA, Ransford AO, et al. Transoral decompression and posterior stabilization in Morquio's disease. *Arch Dis Child.* 1991;66:1318-1321.
81. Stevens JM, Kendall BE, Crockhard HA, et al. The odontoid process in Morquio-Brailsford's disease. The effects of occipitocervical fusion. *J Bone Joint Surg Br.* 1991;73:851-858.
82. Mackenzie WG, Shah SA, Takemitsu M. The cervical spine and skeletal dysplasia. In: Benzel EC, et al., eds. *The Cervical Spine.* 5th ed. Philadelphia: Lippincott, Williams, & Wilkins; 2012:408-428.

37 CHAPTER Pathophysiology, Natural History, and Clinical Syndromes of Cervical Disc Disease

Sreeharsha V. Nandyala
A. Jay Khanna
Hamid Hassanzadeh

Cervical disc disease refers to a cascade of degenerative changes that results in spondylosis, which is the most common disorder in the aging adult cervical spine.[1] Spondylosis is often clinically benign and is ubiquitous within the population.[2,3] Radiographic evidence of cervical spondylosis is purported to be present in 25% of adults younger than 40 years of age, 50% of adults older than 40 years, and 85% of adults older than 60 years.[3,4] By age 65 years, 95% of individuals have radiographic findings suggestive of cervical spondylosis.[1]

The etiology of cervical spondylosis and stenosis can be classified into static and dynamic factors.[5,6] Static factors include congenital spinal stenosis, herniation of disc material, osteophytosis, and ligamentous hypertrophy and infolding (Fig. 37.1).[7] Conversely, the dynamic factors are characterized by motion aberrations (translation and angulation) that act on the spinal column during movement.[5] The combined effect of both the static and dynamic factors can decrease the sagittal diameter of the spinal canal and potentiate central and neuroforaminal compression.[8,9]

A multitude of biochemical and biomechanical abnormalities are associated with disc desiccation. Alterations—including a relative increase in the ratio of keratin sulfate to chondroitin sulfate, dehydration, and the loss of protein and mucopolysaccharides—have been described.[10,11] These changes decrease the viscoelasticity of the intervertebral disc, thereby promoting fibrosis and loss of disc height. The disc height loss occurs at a relatively greater magnitude in the ventral portion of the disc and results in a diminution of the normal cervical lordosis.[12] This facilitates the elongation of the ventral moment arm and causes ventral vertebral body compression and, eventually, kyphosis of the cervical spine.[12] In addition, the loss of disc height will cause hypertrophy and infolding of the ligamentum flavum and the facet joint capsule, further diminishing the dimensions of the spinal canal and the neuroforamina.

The greater loading forces that act on the ventral aspect of the cervical spine owing to disc height loss are transmitted to the uncovertebral and facet joints. In addition to promoting joint hypertrophy, the greater loads facilitate osteophyte formation at these joints and at the bare edges of the vertebral bodies. Furthermore, the shear biomechanical forces will separate Sharpey fibers and the peripheral fibers of the anulus fibrosus from the edges of the vertebral body, which can enable the nucleus pulposus to protrude or herniate into the spinal canal or the neuroforamen.[5] Additionally, the posterior longitudinal ligament will proceed to buckle when subjected to the greater loading forces. The C5–C6 interspace is the most commonly involved level, followed by the C6–C7 level and then the C4–C5 level.[4]

The conglomerate effect of cervical spondylosis can manifest as three distinct clinical syndromes: axial neck pain, cervical radiculopathy, and cervical spondylotic myelopathy. Axial neck pain denotes pain along the cervical spinal column and is related to facet arthrosis and the paraspinal musculoligamentous structures.[13] Cervical radiculopathy designates dermatomal findings in the arm that are characterized by sensory and/or motor disturbances owing to nerve root compression. Last, cervical spondylotic myelopathy is typically insidious and is associated with the hallmark long-tract signs. This chapter will elucidate the pathophysiology, natural history, and clinical findings associated with axial neck pain, cervical radiculopathy, and cervical spondylotic myelopathy.

Axial Neck Pain

Pathophysiology

Axial neck pain is defined as pain emanating from the region of the neck bounded superiorly by the superior nuchal line, laterally by the neck margins, and inferiorly by an imaginary transverse line through the T1 spinous process.[14,15] Anterior neck pain stems from strain of the sternocleidomastoid, the strap muscles, and their attachments. Posterior neck pain is thought to result from poor posture, faulty ergonomics, or muscle fatigue.[16] Frequently, subaxial neck pain can be associated with a postural adaptation relating to pain at the shoulder, craniovertebral junction, or at the temporomandibular joint.[16]

The pathophysiology of axial neck pain remains elusive and is subject to considerable scrutiny. However, numerous theories have been suggested. Disc desiccation is associated with inflammation, changes in disc innervation, and biomechanical hypermobility.[17,18] The plexus of the sinuvertebral nerve

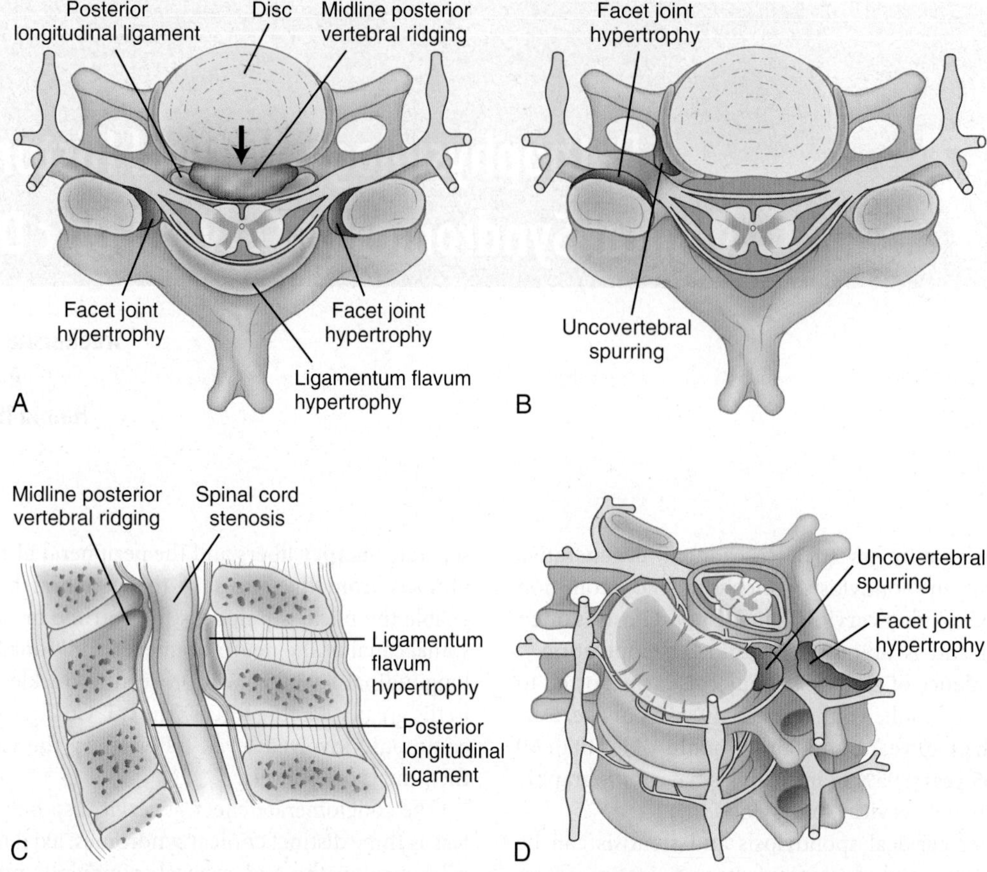

FIG. 37.1 Structural elements that can contribute to cervical spinal stenosis. (A, C) Central stenosis and (B, D) foraminal stenosis are shown. (Modified from Zebala LP, Buchowski JM, Daftary AR, O'Brien JR, Carrino JA, Khanna AJ. The cervical spine. In: Khanna AJ, ed. *MRI Essentials for the Spine Specialist*. New York: Thieme; 2014:111–154.)

innervates the dorsal portion of the cervical disc while the plexus of the cervical sympathetic trunk innervates the ventral portion.[19] With disc inflammation, biochemical mediators—including prostaglandin E_2, bradykinin, histamine, serotonin, and potassium—can sensitize the nociceptors present in these nerves.[17] In addition, elevated tissue levels of tumor necrosis factor-α (TNF-α) have downstream effects that can also sensitize nociceptors and stimulate cytokine production by promoting the formation of the nerve growth factor/TrkA receptor complex.[17,20] Recent studies have demonstrated the expression of the TrkA receptor in the mast cells of degenerative intervertebral discs and in chondrocytes.[20,21] These inflammatory mediators can also facilitate the degradation of the disc matrix, which can enhance hypermobility. Notably, the interleukin-1 (IL-1) and TNF-α–induced cascades—such as the mitogen-activated protein kinase, nuclear factor kappa B (NF-κB), and prostaglandin signal transduction pathways—have been implicated.[22] These inflammatory changes and biomechanical hypermobility are thought to contribute to the development of discogenic axial neck pain.

Some evidence suggests that the degeneration of the posterior facets can also contribute to axial neck pain. The facet joints from C3–C4 to C8–T1 receive innervation from the medial branches of the cervical dorsal rami above and below each joint, whereas the third occipital nerve innervates the C2–C3 facet joints.[16,19] The biomechanical hypermobility and greater loading forces that result from cervical spondylosis can increase motion about the posterior facets and generate pain.[23] Several studies have demonstrated that controlled diagnostic blocks of the cervical facet joints can relieve axial neck pain.[14,23-28] However, these studies are marred by mixed results.

Degenerative arthritis of the suboccipital spine can manifest as headache and can radiate caudally or to the back of the ear. In addition, suboccipital headaches can result from the irritation of the greater occipital nerve, which stems from the posterior rami of C2, C3, and C4.[16,29] Furthermore, the sinuvertebral nerves from C2–C3 can also contribute to suboccipital headache and neck pain, as they innervate the atlantoaxial ligament, tectorial membrane, and the dura mater of the upper cervical cord and posterior cranial fossa.[16,19]

Epidemiology and Natural History

Axial neck pain does not seem to carry a gender predisposition and is thought to be more prevalent in individuals with a history of injury, headaches, low back pain, or multiple medical comorbidities.[30] Some evidence suggests that nearly 66% of adults have experienced neck pain during their lifetime, 5% of whom are disabled by it.[31] Axial neck pain is often associated with injury to the cervical musculoligamentous complex and typically resolves within 6 weeks of onset with conservative treatment alone. However, chronic neck pain persists in 10% to 34% of adults.[32–34] Furthermore, of those with chronic neck pain, 50% will also report suboccipital headaches.

Few studies have characterized the natural history of axial neck pain. In general, nonoperative treatment is often the mainstay in the majority of patients with axial neck pain. Judicious utilization of analgesics, antiinflammatories, and physical therapy is warranted and has been demonstrated to relieve neck pain in 70% to 80% of cases.[35] DePalma et al. reported that 29% of patients had complete relief of neck symptoms, while 49% demonstrated improvement following 3 months of conservative treatment.[36] Similarly, Rothman and Rashbaum reported on the 5-year outcomes of patients with "predominantly" axial neck pain who were treated conservatively.[37] The authors demonstrated that 23% of patients remained disabled. In addition, there was no difference in outcomes between the operative and nonoperative cohorts at the 5-year follow-up period. As such, nonoperative management is advocated for nonneurogenic axial neck pain.[37]

Clinical Syndromes of Axial Neck Pain

Patients with axial neck pain from cervical degenerative disc disease will often report symptoms that have persisted for longer than 12 weeks. The pain is typically along the posterior neck and trapezius muscles with occasional radiation toward the head or into the periscapular region.[16] Localized pain suggests muscle sprain or a soft tissue injury.

Axial neck pain is worsened with flexion, which increases the loading forces on the discs. In addition, axial compression may also exacerbate the pain.[33,38] Prior to designating cervical spondylosis as the causative factor, signs and symptoms suggestive of a neoplastic or infectious process must be evaluated, including inquiry into nighttime pain, weight loss, or fevers and chills. Often, axial neck pain is encountered concomitantly with radicular or myelopathic symptoms, which warrants a full neurologic examination. Severe neck pain may overshadow radicular symptoms in the arm.[38] As such, provocative maneuvers that provide compression on the nerve roots, including the Spurling and L'Hermitte signs, should be elicited.

The determination of the point of maximal discomfort can also be of diagnostic value. Anterior neck pain stemming from muscular strain of the sternocleidomastoid or the strap muscles can be elicited by rotation of the neck to the contralateral side. Posterior neck pain that worsens with head extension and rotation is suggestive of discogenic pain. In addition, limited head rotation to one side is associated with dysfunction of the ipsilateral atlantoaxial articulation.[16] Pain with axial loading of the neck can be suggestive of facet-mediated pain.

Often, patients with shoulder and rotator cuff disease may present with neck pain. In addition, the patient may develop postural adaptations in the neck that result in overuse of the normal tissue, which may exacerbate the neck pain. Rotator cuff disease can be evaluated with the Neer and Hawkins tests for impingement as well as with abduction testing. The resolution of symptoms following a joint injection into the subacromial space may also aid in the diagnosis of rotator cuff pathology.[38]

Care must be taken to determine if C4 radiculopathy is the source of neck pain, as the C4 dermatome includes the proximal trapezial and posterior scapular regions.[13,38] Unilateral neck or scapular pain should raise suspicion of C4 radiculopathy.[38] To further investigate for potential radiculopathy, the patient should be asked about paresthesias within the C4 dermatome.[38]

In addition to organic musculoskeletal processes in the neck and shoulder, pathologic referred pain from the viscera can also elicit neck pain. Furthermore, inflammatory arthritis must be assessed with particular inquiry regarding morning stiffness, rigidity, or polyarticular symptoms.

Cervical Radiculopathy

Pathophysiology

Cervical radiculopathy is characterized by pain, loss of strength and/or sensation, or diminished reflexes in the upper extremity that follows a predictable dermatomal pattern. Radicular findings result from compression of the cervical nerve roots at a location between their origins from the spinal canal to their egress from the neural foramen.[16] Cervical spondylosis—characterized by the loss of disc height and disc herniation, infolding of the facet joint capsule and the ligamentum flavum, and osteophytosis—results in foraminal stenosis. In addition, osteophytes may compress the vascular supply to the nerve root, thereby causing spasm of the radicular arteries.[16] Furthermore, venous outflow may also be compromised, resulting in edema of the nerve roots.[39]

An inflammatory component is believed to be associated with radicular pain generated from nerve root compression.[40] Initially, neural compression results in edema that can eventually lead to fibrosis. This may lower the pain threshold of the nerve root.[40] Furthermore, the inflammation is perpetuated by the neuropeptides and other chemical mediators released by the compressed sensory nerve and by the desiccated disc material.[41] Some evidence suggests an increased concentration of neurogenic chemical mediators of pain, including substance P, in the dorsal root ganglion after 1 to 4 weeks of symptom onset.[41]

Biomechanical hypermobility may also contribute to dynamic compression of the nerve roots, thereby resulting in radicular symptoms when the patient moves the neck. Flexion of the cervical spine lengthens the neural foramen up to 31%, while extension shortens the foramina up to 22%.[42] Ipsilateral rotation narrows the foramen, while contralateral rotation widens it. With extension, the ligamentum flavum can become redundant and will taper the foraminal space. Flexion or extension can translate or angulate the vertebrae and can stretch the nerve root, resulting in radicular symptoms.[16] This dynamic compression can explain why some affected patients may not have radicular symptoms with the neck in a neutral static position.

SECTION V

The importance of nerve root tensioning is demonstrated by the relief of radicular findings with shoulder abduction, which is characterized by resting the hand on top of the head.[16,43] Some evidence suggests that shoulder abduction will decrease nerve root tension and can also lift the dorsal root ganglion cephalad, which distances it from the compressive lesion.[43] In addition, venous blood flow is also facilitated with shoulder abduction with the decompression of the epidural veins.

Epidemiology and Natural History

Incidence of cervical radiculopathy peaks in the sixth decade of life and has a point prevalence of 3.5 per 1000 persons.[44,45] Radiculopathy can be acute, subacute, or chronic.[45] Patients younger than 55 years of age often present with radiculopathy secondary to herniated disc material; older individuals often have osteophytosis causing the neuroforaminal stenosis.[46]

The natural history of radiculopathy has not been clearly elucidated, as treatment is typically provided to the patient. Favorable outcomes are often reported with nonoperative management. Radhakrishnan et al. demonstrated that 90% of patients with cervical radiculopathy remained asymptomatic or minimally affected at 5.9 years of follow-up.[44] As with axial neck pain, nonoperative management is primarily advocated. Nearly half of the patients with cervical radiculopathy report symptom resolution within 6 weeks of onset with nonoperative treatment.[46]

Clinical Syndromes of Cervical Radiculopathy

Radicular symptoms follow a predictable dermatomal distribution in the upper extremity. In addition to sensory and motor dysfunction, patients may report tingling and burning sensations across the affected dermatome.[16] It must be noted, however, that due to potential redundancies in neural innervation, clinical findings may overlap dermatomes. As such, a careful physical examination must be performed to delineate compressed nerve roots and to identify any potential neural redundancies.

Arm and neck pain that is associated with cervical radiculopathy is frequently unilateral. Patients may present with a head positional preference to the contralateral side of the arm pain.[16] The pain is exacerbated with extension and lateral rotation of the head to the side of the pain, termed the Spurling maneuver. This technique minimizes the dimensions of the foraminal space and specifically stresses the foraminal structures, including the nerve root and the vasculature. The Spurling maneuver enables the physician to distinguish cervical radiculopathy from other causes of neck and arm pain, including peripheral nerve compression.[16]

C3 radiculopathy results from pathology at the C2–C3 neuroforamina. C2–C3 has the largest foramen and contains the smallest cervical nerve root.[47] As such, C3 radiculopathy is relatively uncommon. Clinical symptoms that are associated with C3 nerve root compression include headache and sensory disturbance over the upper neck and occiput. No clear myotome has been identified for the C3 nerve root. As such, patients with C3 radiculopathy present similar to those with axial neck pain.[16,46]

The C4 nerve roots exit through the C3–C4 neuroforamina. Similar to C3 radiculopathy, pure C4 nerve root compression is unusual.[46] However, it must be noted that C4 radiculopathy can cause axial neck and shoulder pain.[48] It is associated with sensory disturbances in the lower neck extending to the trapezius region and to the anterior chest. In addition, because the C3–C5 nerve roots innervate the diaphragm via the phrenic nerve, patients with C4 radiculopathy may manifest paradoxical respiration, as evidenced with fluoroscopic evaluation.[49,50] The "sniff test" is performed under fluoroscopy and is characterized by rapid, repeated inspiration, which results in unilateral diaphragmatic paralysis in patients with C4 radiculopathy.[16,49,50]

C5 radiculopathy stems from compression of the C5 nerve root in the C4–C5 neuroforamen (Fig. 37.2).[51] It is characterized by pain that radiates from the neck, over the shoulder, and to the proximal lateral arm. Deltoid weakness often manifests and patients have difficulties with shoulder abduction. Often, patients report weakness with hair brushing or during dressing. In addition, the pectoralis, biceps, or the brachioradialis reflex can be diminished. Sensory deficit is localized to the lateral aspect of the arm, below the shoulder.[52] C5 radiculopathy must be distinguished from primary shoulder joint and rotator cuff dysfunction.[16,46]

C6 nerve root compression within the C5–C6 disc interspace will result in C6 radiculopathy, which is characterized by pain radiating from the base of the neck to the lateral aspect of the elbow and into the radial forearm and radial two digits[52] (Fig. 37.3).[51] This C5–C6 level pathology is the most common radiculopathy because the greatest amount of cervical spondylotic degeneration occurs at this disc interspace.[53,54] The increase in degenerative disease is due to greater angular mobility at this level, a higher mechanical load, and a smaller baseline canal diameter. A majority of flexion and extension of the subaxial spine occurs at segment C5–C6 in the anatomically normal cervical spine, causing this intervertebral level to be more subject to wear-and-tear forces. Additionally, C5–C6 also carries a large mechanical load in the normal cervical spine, also increasing risk of stenosis and degeneration.[55-57] Patients will present with weakness of the biceps muscle along with the extensor carpi radialis, which is solely innervated by the C6 nerve root. In addition, C6 radiculopathy is associated with diminished biceps and brachioradialis reflexes. The sensory changes are similar to that of carpel tunnel syndrome.[16,46]

C7 radiculopathy is associated with cervical spondylosis at the C6–C7 disc interspace (Fig. 37.4).[51] The C7 nerve root supplies the triceps muscle. Patients will present with weakness with arm extension about the elbow joint. In addition, it is associated with diminished triceps reflex. Of note, C7 radiculopathy may occur concurrently with Horner syndrome owing to sympathetic dysfunction, although some studies have suggested that this can be a variable finding.[52,58] Sensory dysfunction can be isolated to the middle and index finger, while pain can radiate from the interscapular area, through the midarm,

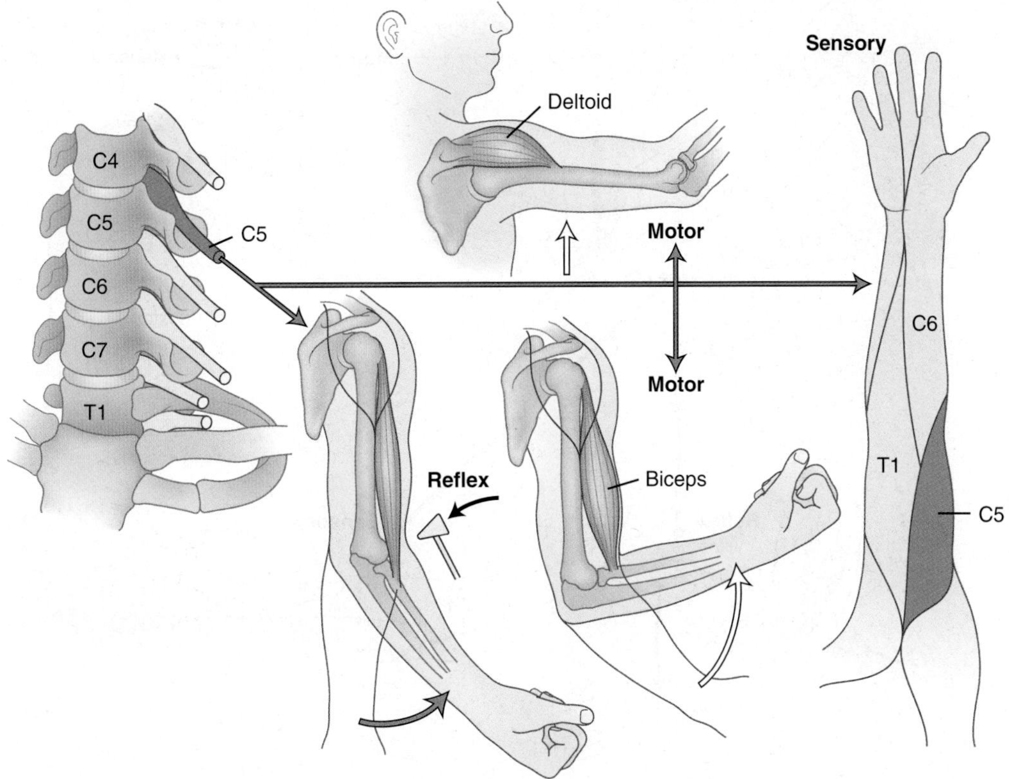

FIG. 37.2 C5 nerve root anatomy, dermatome, and myotome. (Modified from Paterno JM, Silverberg CM, Khanna AJ, Singla AK. Common clinical and correlative pain generators of the cervical and lumbosacral spine. In: Khanna AJ, ed. *MRI Essentials for the Spine Specialist*. New York: Thieme; 2014:45–67.)

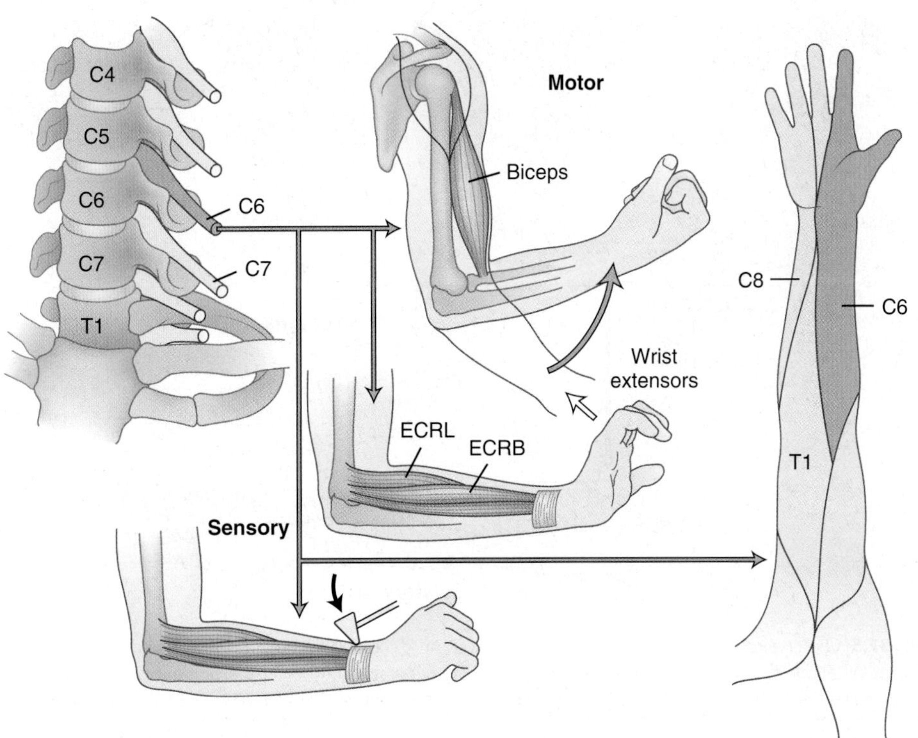

FIG. 37.3 C6 nerve root anatomy, dermatome, and myotome. ECRL, extensor carpi radialis longus; ERCB, extensor carpi radialis brevis. (Modified from Paterno JM, Silverberg CM, Khanna AJ, Singla AK. Common clinical and correlative pain generators of the cervical and lumbosacral spine. In: Khanna AJ, ed. *MRI Essentials for the Spine Specialist*. New York: Thieme; 2014:45–67.)

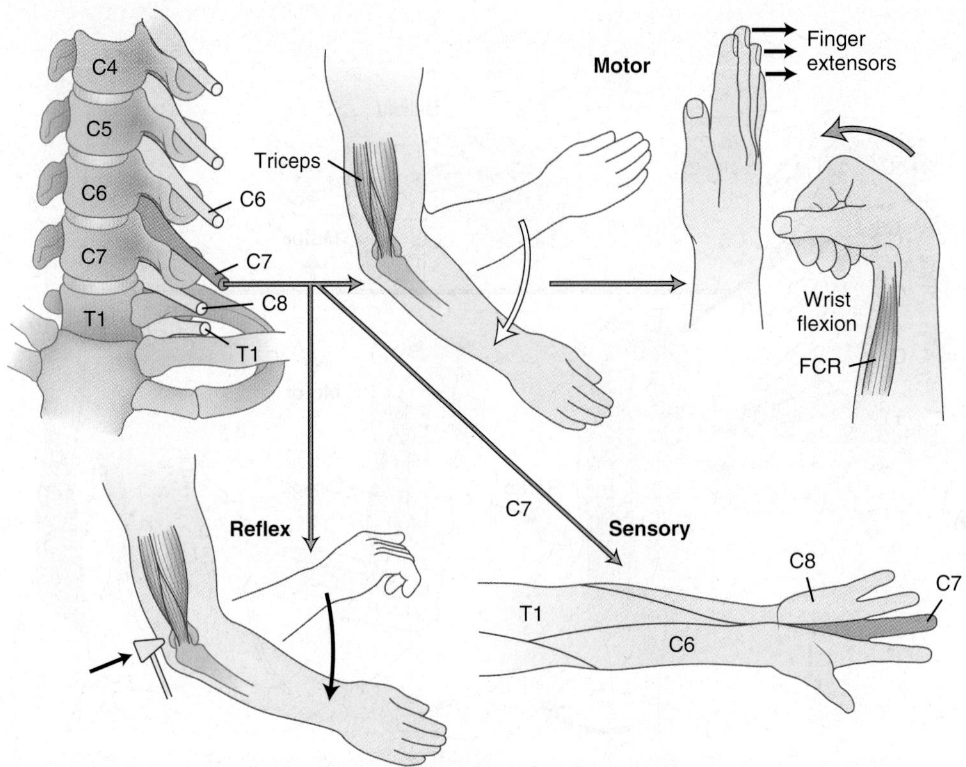

FIG. 37.4 C7 nerve root anatomy, dermatome, and myotome. FCR, flexor carpi radialis. (Modified from Paterno JM, Silverberg CM, Khanna AJ, Singla AK. Common clinical and correlative pain generators of the cervical and lumbosacral spine. In: Khanna AJ, ed. *MRI Essentials for the Spine Specialist.* New York: Thieme; 2014:45–67.)

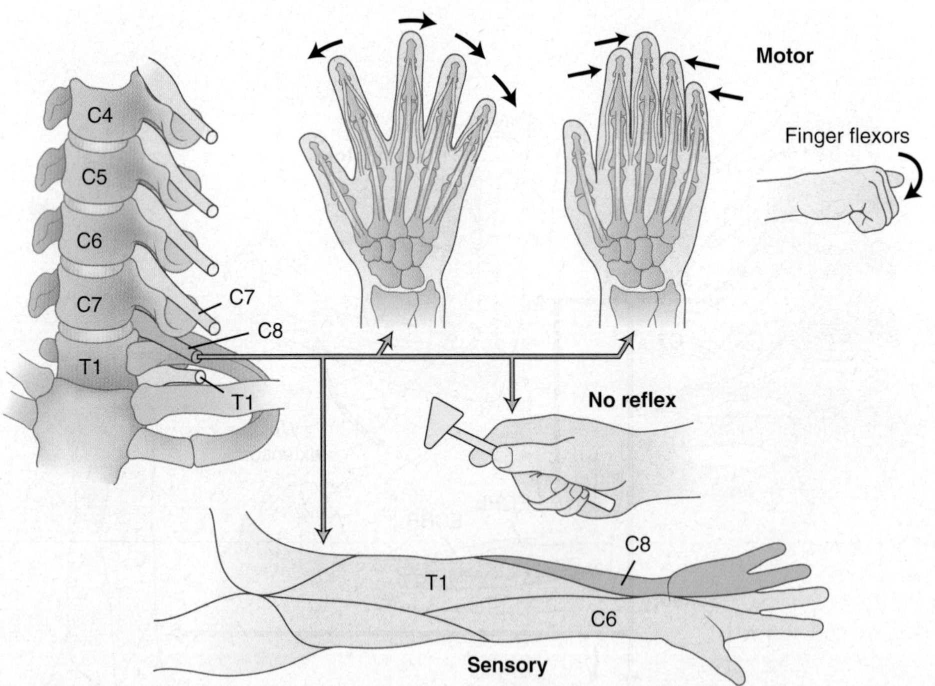

FIG. 37.5 C8 nerve root anatomy, dermatome, and myotome. (Modified from Paterno JM, Silverberg CM, Khanna AJ, Singla AK. Common clinical and correlative pain generators of the cervical and lumbosacral spine. In: Khanna AJ, ed. *MRI Essentials for the Spine Specialist.* New York: Thieme; 2014:45–67.)

and down the middle three fingers. In addition, chronic breast pain has been reported with C7 radiculopathy.[16,46,59]

Last, C8 radiculopathy is characterized by pathologic changes at the C7–C8 disc interspace (Fig. 37.5).[51] The C8 nerve root innervates the intrinsic hand muscles and finger flexors. The "benediction sign" is often present in patients with C8 radiculopathy and is characterized as weakness with extension of the fourth and fifth digits. Similar to C7 radiculopathy, sympathetic dysfunction may be present and can present with Horner syndrome.[52,58] Sensory changes can be localized to

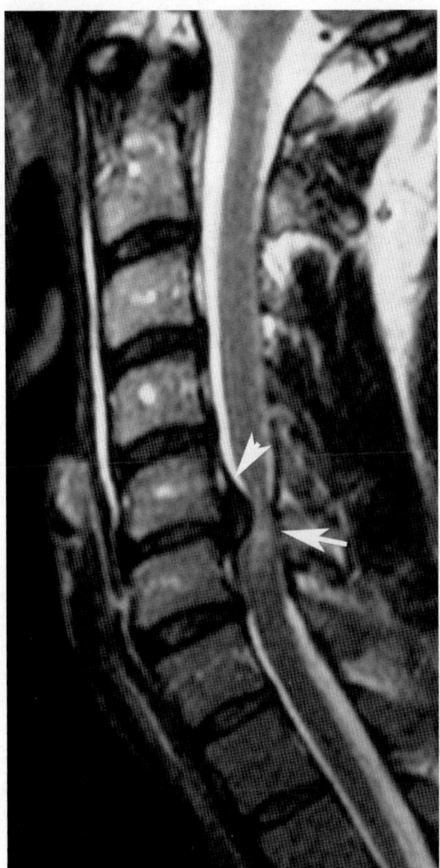

FIG. 37.6 Sagittal T2-weighted magnetic resonance image depicts C5–C6 disc herniation resulting in increased cord signal intensity (*arrow*) and elevation of the posterior longitudinal ligament (*arrowhead*). (From Zebala LP, Buchowski JM, Daftary AR, O'Brien JR, Carrino JA, Khanna AJ. The cervical spine. In: Khanna AJ, ed. *MRI Essentials for the Spine Specialist*. New York: Thieme; 2014:111–154.)

the medial aspect of the arm and forearm, and the ulnar two fingers. The patient can present with weakness of the wrist extensors, flexors, and intrinsics with the exception of the extensor carpi radialis and flexor carpi radialis. C8 radiculopathy can be distinguished from ulnar nerve entrapment as ulnar nerve pathology spares all of the short thenar muscles except the adductor pollicis.[16,45]

Cervical Myelopathy

Pathophysiology

Myelopathy is defined as the presence of long-tract signs secondary to mechanical compression of the afferent or efferent nerve tracts of the spinal cord.[46,60] Compression of the spinal cord is the result of both static (such as degenerative stenosis and disc protrusion) and dynamic (such as instability due to trauma) risk factors (Fig. 37.6).[7]

The normal anteroposterior diameter of the cervical spine is 17 to 18 mm in adults; the cervical cord itself measures 10 mm in diameter from anterior to posterior.[61–63] Congenital cervical stenosis is defined as a spinal canal that measures less than 13 mm.[61,62] While congenital stenosis may not be clinically symptomatic by itself, it is associated with a lower threshold for the magnitude of degenerative spondylotic changes that are required to compress the spinal cord to cause myelopathy.[16] In addition, the shape of the spinal cord in degenerative settings has been correlated with the development of cervical myelopathy.[63] If the cross-sectional area of the cord is reduced by the critical amount of 30% and the remaining transverse area is less than 60 mm^2, signs and symptoms of cervical cord compression can manifest.[63] Furthermore, a lower anteroposterior compression ratio of less than 0.4 correlates histologically with severe cord injury.[64–66] The Pavlov ratio, which is the anteroposterior diameter of the spinal canal divided by the anteroposterior diameter of the vertebral body at the same location, indicates developmental cervical narrowing if the value is less than 0.8.[16,64,65]

Dynamic factors are also correlated with the development of cervical myelopathy. Hyperextension of the neck is associated with buckling of the ligamentum flavum ventrally into the canal.[16] In addition, during extension, a retrolisthesed vertebral body can squeeze the cord between the inferoposterior edge of the vertebral body and the superior edge of the lamina caudal to it. Similarly, anterolisthesis during flexion can also compress the spinal cord.[16] Breig et al. demonstrated that the spinal cord thickens and shortens with extension, which potentiates compression from the redundant ligamentum flavum or the lamina[67] (Fig. 37.7). With flexion, the pressure within the cord can increase if a compressive lesion is pressing against the cord.[16]

Mechanical compression and ischemia can be concomitant in the development of cervical myelopathy. Breig et al. demonstrated that flow through the anterior spinal artery and the radicular arteries can diminish when the vessels are tented over a disc or vertebral body.[67] In particular, the transverse intramedullary arterioles are considered most vulnerable to vascular compression and they perfuse the gray matter and the adjacent lateral columns.[68] However, the blood flow through the posterior spinal arteries remains unaffected.[16]

Chronic cervical myelopathy is associated with demyelination and irreversible neurologic deficit likely due to ischemic death (apoptosis) of the oligodendrocytes (Fig. 37.8).[7] This cell lineage is the most susceptible to ischemic injury.[69,70]

Natural History

Cervical myelopathy develops in a small proportion of patients with spondylosis and is often encountered beyond the fifth decade.[71,72] Some evidence suggests that myelopathy is more common in men and in those with labor-intense occupations.[71,72] The development of cervical myelopathy is often insidious in its early stages. By the time a patient presents with overt clinical signs and symptoms, surgical management is often warranted. Numerous studies have demonstrated that cervical myelopathy is associated with a progressive deterioration of motor and sensory function, with 95% of patients who report gradual intervening periods of disease progression and stability.[73]

Some studies have demonstrated that the progression of cervical myelopathy is highly variable, with many patients

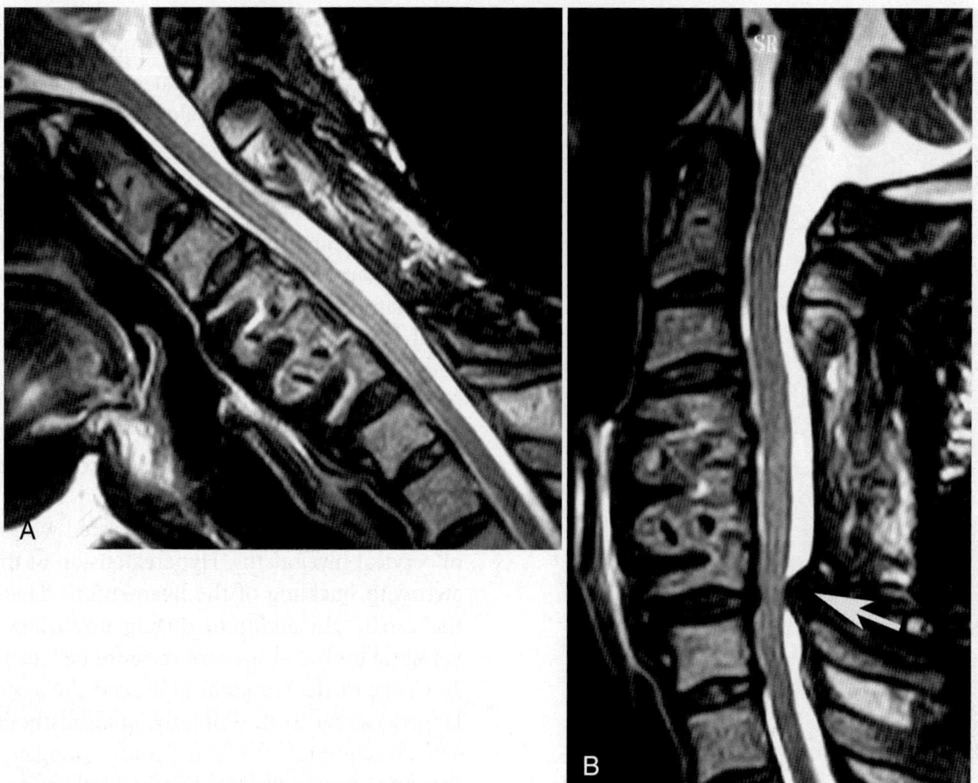

FIG. 37.7 Sagittal T2-weighted magnetic resonance images in a patient with previous C4–C6 anterior cervical discectomy and fusion with allograft and plate and prior multilevel laminectomy. (A) Flexion image demonstrating no stenosis. (B) Extension image of C6–C7 stenosis due to ligamentum flavum impingement (*arrow*) and continued disc bulge. (From Zebala LP, Buchowski JM, Daftary AR, O'Brien JR, Carrino JA, Khanna AJ. The cervical spine. In: Khanna AJ, ed. *MRI Essentials for the Spine Specialist*. New York: Thieme; 2014:111–154.)

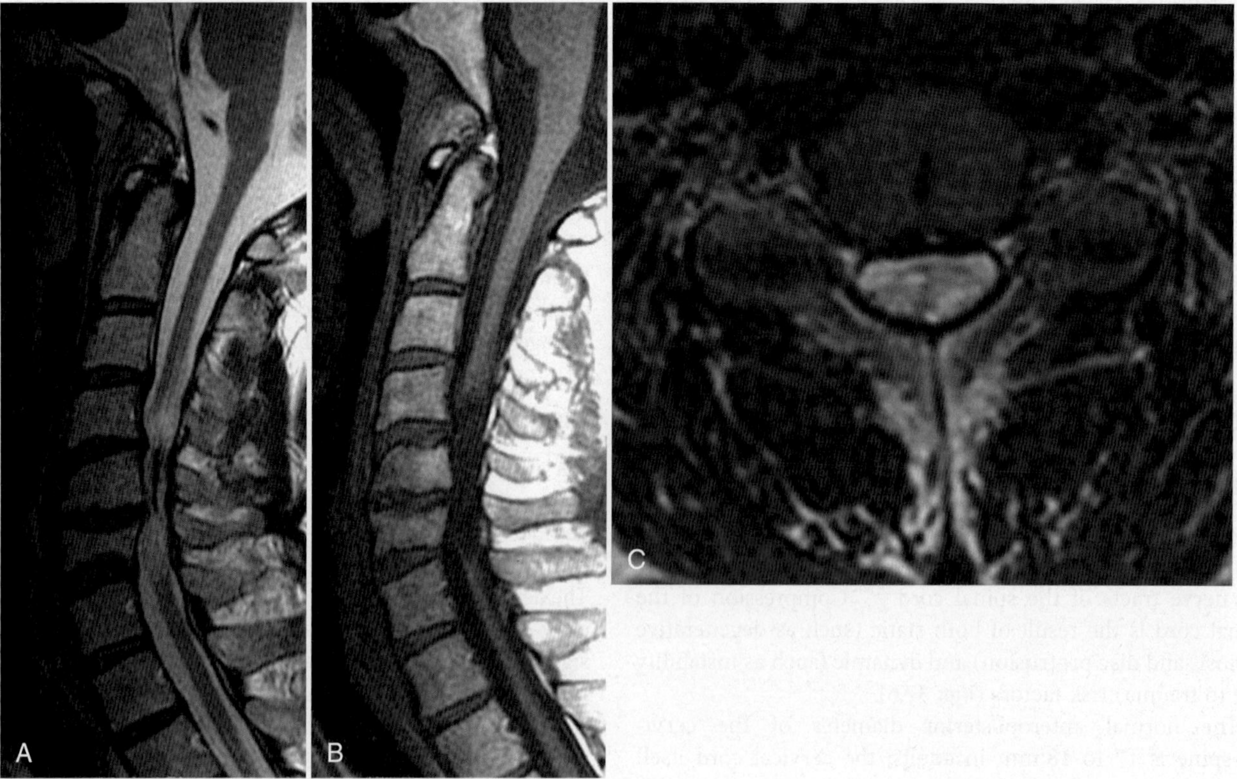

FIG. 37.8 Spinal cord atrophy as a result of persistent central canal stenosis. (A) Sagittal T2-weighted image showing C4–C6 stenosis and C5 spinal cord atrophy with surrounding edema. (B) Sagittal T1-weighted image demonstrates low cord signal intensity from C4–C5 to C6–C7. (C) Axial T2-weighted image at C4–C5 shows spinal cord atrophy. (From Zebala LP, Buchowski JM, Daftary AR, O'Brien JR, Carrino JA, Khanna AJ. The cervical spine. In: Khanna AJ, ed: *MRI Essentials for the Spine Specialist*. New York: Thieme, 2014: 111–154.)

who report a relatively benign form of the disease.[73–75] Epstein et al. reported that 38% of patients remained stable and 26% of patients deteriorated, with older patients most likely to experience worsening of symptoms.[74] However, the majority of patients who present with neurologic dysfunction do not have spontaneous improvement.[73]

Clinical Syndromes of Cervical Myelopathy

The anatomic site of compression dictates the clinical findings seen with cervical myelopathy. Sensory symptoms are related to three distinct sites of compression on the cervical cord: (1) the spinothalamic tract, which affects contralateral pain and temperature; (2) posterior columns, which involves ipsilateral position and vibration sense disturbances, leading to gait disturbances; and (3) dorsal root compression, which facilitates dermatomal findings.[16] At the level of the cervical lesions, lower motor neuron findings predominate and are characterized by hyporeflexia and weakness in the upper extremities. Conversely, caudal to the level of the cervical cord lesion, upper motor neuron signs are present, with hyperreflexia and spasticity in the lower extremities.

Patients can often present with difficulties with fine motor movements in the hands, characterized by difficulty with handwriting or typing.[76] This becomes progressively worse with gross motor dysfunction, characterized by gait abnormalities and falls. Gait may become spastic and patients may report weakness and wasting of the lower extremities. Severe chronic myelopathy can result in loss of proprioception, broad-based gait, and, eventually, quadriplegia.[16,77] Nurick et al. proposed a disability grading system based on these gait abnormalities[75] (Table 37.1).

Various physical examination findings are associated with cervical myelopathy. Often, patients can present with hyperreflexia of the deep tendon reflexes, changes in muscle tone or clonus, and the presence of long-tract signs, including the Babinski sign in the lower extremities and/or the Hoffman sign in the upper extremities.

In the upper extremity, the Hoffman sign (stimulation of the extensor tendon of the third digit with forcible flexion and sudden release of the distal phalanx, which prompts the thumb to flex and adduct along with concurrent flexion of the index finger) is often appreciated.[46,78,79] In addition, the inverted radial reflex is elicited by stimulating the distal brachioradialis tendon with gentle percussion, which yields hyperdynamic finger flexion.[80] The inverted radial reflex is associated with cord compression at C6.[16] Furthermore, poor ability to grip and release is often indicative of myelopathy in the hand.[81] Superficial reflexes, including the abdominal or cremasteric reflexes, are also compromised with cervical myelopathy.

In the lower extremity, the Babinski sign is elicited by rubbing the lateral aspect of the plantar surface of the foot from the heel to the metatarsal pads with a blunt object, which prompts the great toe to dorsiflex and the other toes to fan out if an upper motor neuron lesion is present.[46] It should be noted that numerous variations of the Babinski sign can be present in the patient, including the Oppenheim sign (apply heavy pressure with the thumb and index finger over the tibia and stroke down to the ankle), Gordon sign (apply pressure on the calf muscles), Schaefer sign (apply pressure on the calcaneal tendon), Bing sign (stimulate the great toe with a pin prick), Chaddock sign (stimulate the lateral foot with a blunt object), and the Gonda and Allen signs (provide forceful downward stretching of the distal phalanx of the second or fourth toe).[46,82] Any of these variations can be present in the patient.

Sensory deficits must also be evaluated in patients with cervical myelopathy. Crandall et al. reported on the various clinical findings associated with afferent nerve tract compression in patients with myelopathy.[53] Neck pain was present in 50% of patients, radicular pain in 38%, Lhermitte sign (shocklike sensation that radiates down the spine following flexion of the neck) in 27%, and sphincter tone changes in 44%.[53] In addition to these findings, changes in pain, temperature, proprioception, and dermatomal sensation may be present.

Signs and symptoms in the hands can often characterize the primary reason for why the patient seeks medical attention. Ono et al.[81] demonstrated two signs that are specific to "myelopathy hand": the finger-escapee sign (patient tries to extend digits fully with the palm facing down and the ulnar two or three digits drift into abduction and flexion after 30 seconds) and the grip and release test (suboptimal performance in the ability to open and close the fist rapidly).[16,81] Patients may also report diffuse numbness in the hands, which must be distinguished from carpal tunnel syndrome and peripheral neuropathy. In addition, wasting of the intrinsic hand muscles is often present.[16]

Myelopathy can often be accompanied by radicular findings in some patients. Myeloradiculopathy is associated with spinal stenosis with concurrent compression of the neuroforaminal contents. This can be reproduced with the Spurling maneuver, as described earlier.[46,53] Myeloradiculopathy produces lower motor neuron signs at the level of the cervical cord lesion and upper motor neuron signs caudal to the level of compression. In addition, Edwards et al. demonstrated that 13% of patients with spondylotic myelopathy present with both cervical and lumbar involvement.[83] These patients present with both upper and lower motor neuron findings in the lower extremities, which often complicates the clinical picture.

TABLE 37.1 Cervical Spondylosis Disability Grade

Grade	Signs
0	Signs or symptoms of root involvement without spinal cord disease
1	Signs of spinal cord disease without gait difficulty
2	Slight difficulty in gait that does not prevent full-time employment
3	Difficulty in walking that prevents full-time employment or housework but does not require assistance
4	Able to walk only with assistance or with aid of a frame
5	Chairbound or bedridden

Modified from Nurick S. The pathogenesis of the spinal cord disorder associated with cervical spondylosis. *Brain*. 1972;95:87-100.

Summary

Cervical disc disease describes a series of degenerative changes that can result in clinically significant radiculopathy and/or myelopathy. Numerous static and dynamic biomechanical and physiologic forces contribute to cervical spine degeneration. It becomes incumbent upon the spine surgeon to recognize clinical signs and symptoms consistent with clinically significant radiculopathy and/or myelopathy, as cervical spondylosis is ubiquitous among the aging general population.

REFERENCES

1. Garfin SR. Cervical degenerative disorders: etiology, presentation, and imaging studies. *Instr Course Lect.* 2000;49:335-338.
2. Boden SD, McCowin PR, Davis DO, et al. Abnormal magnetic-resonance scans of the cervical spine in asymptomatic subjects. A prospective investigation. *J Bone Joint Surg Am.* 1990;72:1178-1184.
3. Lehto IJ, Tertti MO, Komu ME, et al. Age-related MRI changes at 0.1 T in cervical discs in asymptomatic subjects. *Neuroradiology.* 1994;36:49-53.
4. Matsumoto M, Fujimura Y, Suzuki N, et al. MRI of cervical intervertebral discs in asymptomatic subjects. *J Bone Joint Surg Br.* 1998;80:19-24.
5. Morishita Y, Falakassa J, Naito M, et al. The kinematic relationships of the upper cervical spine. *Spine.* 2009;34:2642-2645.
6. Mullin JSD, Benzel E. Overview of cervical spondylosis pathophysiology and biomechanics. *World Spinal Column J.* 2011;2:89-97.
7. Zebala LP, Buchowski JM, Daftary AR, et al. The cervical spine. In: Khanna AJ, ed. *MRI Essentials for the Spine Specialist.* New York: Thieme; 2014:111-154.
8. Roh JS, Teng AL, Yoo JU, et al. Degenerative disorders of the lumbar and cervical spine. *Orthop Clin North Am.* 2005;36:255-262.
9. Shedid D, Benzel EC. Cervical spondylosis anatomy: pathophysiology and biomechanics. *Neurosurgery.* 2007;60:S7-S13.
10. Lipson SJ, Muir H. 1980 Volvo award in basic science. Proteoglycans in experimental intervertebral disc degeneration. *Spine.* 1981;6:194-210.
11. Pearce RH, Grimmer BJ, Adams ME. Degeneration and the chemical composition of the human lumbar intervertebral disc. *J Orthop Res.* 1987;5:198-205.
12. Benzel EC. *Biomechanics of Spine Stabilization.* New York: Thieme/AANS; 2015.
13. Connell MD, Wiesel SW. Natural history and pathogenesis of cervical disk disease. *Orthop Clin North Am.* 1992;23:369-380.
14. Bogduk N. The anatomy and pathophysiology of neck pain. *Phys Med Rehabil Clin N Am.* 2011;22:367-382.
15. Merskey HBN, ed. *Classification of Chronic Pain. Descriptions of Chronic Pain Syndromes and Definition of Pain Terms.* 2nd ed. Seattle, WA: IASP Press; 1994:103-111.
16. Rao R. Neck pain, cervical radiculopathy, and cervical myelopathy: pathophysiology, natural history, and clinical evaluation. *J Bone Joint Surg Am.* 2002;84-A:1872-1881.
17. Lotz JC, Ulrich JA. Innervation, inflammation, and hypermobility may characterize pathologic disc degeneration: review of animal model data. *J Bone Joint Surg Am.* 2006;88(suppl 2):76-82.
18. Galbusera F, van Rijsbergen M, Ito K, et al. Ageing and degenerative changes of the intervertebral disc and their impact on spinal flexibility. *Eur Spine J.* 2014;23(suppl 3):S324-S332.
19. Bogduk N, Windsor M, Inglis A. The innervation of the cervical intervertebral discs. *Spine.* 1988;13:2-8.
20. Freemont AJ, Watkins A, Le Maitre C, et al. Nerve growth factor expression and innervation of the painful intervertebral disc. *J Pathol.* 2002;197:286-292.
21. Freemont AJ, Jeziorska M, Hoyland JA, et al. Mast cells in the pathogenesis of chronic back pain: a hypothesis. *J Pathol.* 2002;197:281-285.
22. Shalom-Barak T, Quach J, Lotz M. Interleukin-17-induced gene expression in articular chondrocytes is associated with activation of mitogen-activated protein kinases and NF-kappaB. *J Biol Chem.* 1998;273:27467-27473.
23. Cooper G, Bailey B, Bogduk N. Cervical zygapophysial joint pain maps. *Pain Med.* 2007;8:344-353.
24. Aprill C, Bogduk N. The prevalence of cervical zygapophyseal joint pain. A first approximation. *Spine.* 1992;17:744-747.
25. Barnsley L, Lord SM, Wallis BJ, et al. The prevalence of chronic cervical zygapophysial joint pain after whiplash. *Spine.* 1995;20:20-25.
26. Bogduk N, Marsland A. The cervical zygapophysial joints as a source of neck pain. *Spine.* 1988;13:610-617.
27. Lord SM, Barnsley L, Wallis BJ, et al. Chronic cervical zygapophysial joint pain after whiplash. A placebo-controlled prevalence study. *Spine.* 1996;21:1737-1744.
28. Speldewinde GC, Bashford GM, Davidson IR. Diagnostic cervical zygapophyseal joint blocks for chronic cervical pain. *Med J Aust.* 2001;174:174-176.
29. Persson LC, Carlsson JY, Anderberg L. Headache in patients with cervical radiculopathy: a prospective study with selective nerve root blocks in 275 patients. *Eur Spine J.* 2007;16:953-959.
30. Cote P, Cassidy JD, Carroll L. The factors associated with neck pain and its related disability in the Saskatchewan population. *Spine.* 2000;25:1109-1117.
31. Cote P, Cassidy JD, Carroll L. The Saskatchewan Health and Back Pain Survey. The prevalence of neck pain and related disability in Saskatchewan adults. *Spine.* 1998;23:1689-1698.
32. Bovim G, Schrader H, Sand T. Neck pain in the general population. *Spine.* 1994;19:1307-1309.
33. Dvorak J. Epidemiology, physical examination, and neurodiagnostics. *Spine.* 1998;23:2663-2673.
34. Makela M, Heliovaara M, Sievers K, et al. Prevalence, determinants, and consequences of chronic neck pain in Finland. *Am J Epidemiol.* 1991;134:1356-1367.
35. Benzel EC. *The Cervical Spine.* 5th ed. Philadelphia: Lippincott Williams & Wilkins; 2012.
36. DePalma AF, Subin DK. Study of the cervical syndrome. *Clin Orthop Relat Res.* 1965;38:135-142.
37. Rothman RH, Rashbaum RF. Pathogenesis of signs and symptoms of cervical disc degeneration. *Instr Course Lect.* 1978;27:203-215.
38. Ahn NU, Ahn UM, Ipsen B, et al. Mechanical neck pain and cervicogenic headache. *Neurosurgery.* 2007;60:S21-S27.
39. Manifold SG, McCann PD. Cervical radiculitis and shoulder disorders. *Clin Orthop Relat Res.* 1999;368:105-113.
40. Cooper RG, Freemont AJ, Hoyland JA, et al. Herniated intervertebral disc-associated periradicular fibrosis and vascular abnormalities occur without inflammatory cell infiltration. *Spine.* 1995;20:591-598.

41. Cornefjord M, Olmarker K, Farley DB, et al. Neuropeptide changes in compressed spinal nerve roots. *Spine*. 1995;20:670-673.
42. Muhle C, Resnick D, Ahn JM, et al. In vivo changes in the neuroforaminal size at flexion-extension and axial rotation of the cervical spine in healthy persons examined using kinematic magnetic resonance imaging. *Spine*. 2001;26:E287-E293.
43. Davidson RI, Dunn EJ, Metzmaker JN. The shoulder abduction test in the diagnosis of radicular pain in cervical extradural compressive monoradiculopathies. *Spine*. 1981;6:441-446.
44. Radhakrishnan K, Litchy WJ, O'Fallon WM, et al. Epidemiology of cervical radiculopathy. A population-based study from Rochester, Minnesota, 1976 through 1990. *Brain*. 1994;117(Pt 2):325-335.
45. Salemi G, Savettieri G, Meneghini F, et al. Prevalence of cervical spondylotic radiculopathy: a door-to-door survey in a Sicilian municipality. *Acta Neurol Scand*. 1996;93:184-188.
46. Harrop JS, Hanna A, Silva MT, et al. Neurological manifestations of cervical spondylosis: an overview of signs, symptoms, and pathophysiology. *Neurosurgery*. 2007;60:S14-S20.
47. Payne EE, Spillane JD. The cervical spine; an anatomico-pathological study of 70 specimens (using a special technique) with particular reference to the problem of cervical spondylosis. *Brain*. 1957;80:571-596.
48. Jenis LG, An HS. Neck pain secondary to radiculopathy of the fourth cervical root: an analysis of 12 surgically treated patients. *J Spinal Disord*. 2000;13:345-349.
49. Buszek MC, Szymke TE, Honet JC, et al. Hemidiaphragmatic paralysis: an unusual complication of cervical spondylosis. *Arch Phys Med Rehabil*. 1983;64:601-603.
50. Cloward RB. Diaphragm paralysis from cervical disc lesions. *Br J Neurosurg*. 1988;2:395-399.
51. Paterno JM, Silverberg CM, Khanna AJ, Singla AK. Common clinical and correlative pain generators of the cervical and lumbosacral spine. In: Khanna AJ, ed. *MRI Essentials for the Spine Specialist*. New York: Thieme; 2014:45-67.
52. Murphey F, Simmons JC, Brunson B. Surgical treatment of laterally ruptured cervical disc. Review of 648 cases, 1939 to 1972. *J Neurosurg*. 1973;38:679-683.
53. Crandall PH, Batzdorf U. Cervical spondylotic myelopathy. *J Neurosurg*. 1966;25:57-66.
54. Penning L. Normal movements of the cervical spine. *AJR Am J Roentgenol*. 1978;130:317-326.
55. Lee MJ, Cassinelli EH, Riew KD. Prevalence of cervical spine stenosis. *J Bone Joint Surg Am*. 2007;89(2):376-380.
56. Morishita Y, Naito M, Hymanson H, et al. The relationship between the cervical spinal canal diameter and the pathological changes in the cervical spine. *Eur Spine J*. 2009;18(6):877-883.
57. Komura S, Miyamoto K, Hosoe H, Iinuma N, Shimizu K. Lower incidence of adjacent segment degeneration after anterior cervical fusion found with those fusing C5-6 and C6-7 than those leaving C5-6 or C6-7 as an adjacent level. *J Spinal Disord Tech*. 2012;25(1):23-29.
58. Harrop JS, Silva MT, Sharan AD, et al. Cervicothoracic radiculopathy treated using posterior cervical foraminotomy/discectomy. *J Neurosurg*. 2003;98:131-136.
59. LaBan MM, Meerschaert JR, Taylor RS. Breast pain: a symptom of cervical radiculopathy. *Arch Phys Med Rehabil*. 1979;60:315-317.
60. Kalsi-Ryan S, Karadimas SK, Fehlings MG. Cervical spondylotic myelopathy: the clinical phenomenon and the current pathobiology of an increasingly prevalent and devastating disorder. *Neuroscientist*. 2013;19:409-421.
61. Henderson CM, Hennessy RG, Shuey HM Jr, et al. Posterior-lateral foraminotomy as an exclusive operative technique for cervical radiculopathy: a review of 846 consecutively operated cases. *Neurosurgery*. 1983;13:504-512.
62. Rao RD, Gourab K, David KS. Operative treatment of cervical spondylotic myelopathy. *J Bone Joint Surg Am*. 2006;88:1619-1640.
63. Northover JR, Wild JB, Braybrooke J, et al. The epidemiology of cervical spondylotic myelopathy. *Skeletal Radiol*. 2012;41:1543-1546.
64. Bernhardt M, Hynes RA, Blume HW, et al. Cervical spondylotic myelopathy. *J Bone Joint Surg Am*. 1993;75:119-128.
65. Pavlov H, Torg JS, Robie B, et al. Cervical spinal stenosis: determination with vertebral body ratio method. *Radiology*. 1987;164:771-775.
66. Ono K, Ota H, Tada K, et al. Cervical myelopathy secondary to multiple spondylotic protrusions: a clinicopathologic study. *Spine*. 1977;2:109-125.
67. Breig A, Turnbull I, Hassler O. Effects of mechanical stresses on the spinal cord in cervical spondylosis. A study on fresh cadaver material. *J Neurosurg*. 1966;25:45-56.
68. Doppman JL. The mechanism of ischemia in anteroposterior compression of the spinal cord. *Invest Radiol*. 1975;10:543-551.
69. Baptiste DC, Fehlings MG. Pathophysiology of cervical myelopathy. *Spine J*. 2006;6:190S-197S.
70. Henderson FC, Geddes JF, Vaccaro AR, et al. Stretch-associated injury in cervical spondylotic myelopathy: new concept and review. *Neurosurgery*. 2005;56:1101-1113.
71. Asgari S. Cervical spondylotic myelopathy. In: Palmer JD, ed. *Neurosurgery '96: Manual of Neurosurgery*. New York: Churchill Livingstone; 1996:750-754.
72. Patten JP. *Neurological Differential Diagnosis*. London: Springer-Verlag; 1977.
73. Lees F, Turner JW. Natural history and prognosis of cervical spondylosis. *Br Med J*. 1963;2:1607-1610.
74. Epstein JA, Janin Y, Carras R, et al. A comparative study of the treatment of cervical spondylotic myeloradiculopathy. Experience with 50 cases treated by means of extensive laminectomy, foraminotomy, and excision of osteophytes during the past 10 years. *Acta Neurochir (Wien)*. 1982;61:89-104.
75. Nurick S. The pathogenesis of the spinal cord disorder associated with cervical spondylosis. *Brain*. 1972;95:87-100.
76. Emery SE. Cervical spondylotic myelopathy: diagnosis and treatment. *J Am Acad Orthop Surg*. 2001;9:376-388.
77. Spillane JD. Cervical spondylosis. *Lancet*. 1972;2:137.
78. Denno JJ, Meadows GR. Early diagnosis of cervical spondylotic myelopathy. A useful clinical sign. *Spine*. 1991;16:1353-1355.
79. Sung RD, Wang JC. Correlation between a positive Hoffmann's reflex and cervical pathology in asymptomatic individuals. *Spine*. 2001;26:67-70.
80. An HS. Cervical root entrapment. *Hand Clin*. 1996;12:719-730.
81. Ono K, Ebara S, Fuji T, et al. Myelopathy hand. New clinical signs of cervical cord damage. *J Bone Joint Surg Br*. 1987;69:215-219.
82. DeJong RN, Haerer AF. Case taking and the neurologic examination. In: Joynt RJ, ed. *Clinical Neurology*. Philadelphia: Lippincott; 1990:63-64.
83. Edwards WC, LaRocca SH. The developmental segmental sagittal diameter in combined cervical and lumbar spondylosis. *Spine*. 1985;10:42-49.

CHAPTER 38 Medical Myelopathies

Brandon L. Raudenbush
Olga Selioutski
Lawrence Samkoff
A. Jay Khanna
Addisu Mesfin

Medical myelopathies encompass a wide spectrum of conditions ranging from nutritional deficiencies to intrinsic spinal cord disorders and manifestations of systemic infections. Spine surgeons should maintain these conditions in their differential diagnosis for patients with myelopathy. Depending on the cause of the medical myelopathy, the spine surgeon should either manage it directly or refer it to appropriate providers.

Spinal Cord Anatomy

Longitudinal Orientation

The spinal cord starts at the foramen magnum and extends through the entire length of the vertebral canal in the embryonic phase. The spinal cord grows slower than the vertebral canal; in infancy, it extends to the L2 and L3, but may terminate anywhere between L1 and the second sacral (S2) vertebra.[1] In adults, the tip of the spinal cord (conus medullaris) ends at L1–L2.[2] The dissimilarity in growth between the cord and its canal leads to the lumbar nerve roots needing to descend within the subarachnoid space to reach the corresponding vertebral levels prior to exiting the spinal column, creating a group of roots called the cauda equina. The spinal cord has two enlargements (cervical and lumbar) at C3–T2 and L1–S3.[3] There are 31 segments in the spinal cord (8 cervical, 12 thoracic, 5 lumbar, 5 sacral, and 1 coccygeal).

Transverse Orientation

The spinal cord consists of white and gray matter strategically organized for rapid communication between peripheral structures and the brain. The structure has two identical semiovals separated by the deep ventral median fissure anteriorly and dorsal median sulcus posteriorly and joined only at the midline.[4]

The gray matter is an H-shaped, mirror-imaged structure, with each half subdivided into dorsal (containing sensory neurons) and ventral (containing lower motor neurons) horns and an intermediate column (containing autonomic neurons). The white matter is subdivided into anterior, lateral, and posterior columns containing either ascending or descending tracts. Three major tracts will be reviewed here.

Ascending Lateral Spinothalamic Tracts

The *ascending lateral spinothalamic tracts* relay pain, temperature, and crude touch sensation. The pain is transmitted to the dorsal root ganglia (DRG) neurons (first-order primary sensory neurons), which synapse ipsilaterally in the dorsal horn of the gray matter with the second-order neurons. The axons of the second-order neurons cross to the *contralateral side* via the anterior commissure two levels higher than the associated dermatome and ascend in the contralateral lateral column.

Ascending Dorsal Column–Medial Lemniscus Tracts

The *ascending dorsal column–medial lemniscus* tracts relay vibratory sensation, proprioception, and fine-touch discrimination. These sensory modalities are transmitted to the DRG neurons, axons of which enter the posterior columns forming fasciculi gracilis and cuneatus, remaining ipsilateral to the side of entry without crossing until the level of medulla, where they synapse with the second-order neurons. The axons of the second-order neurons decussate in the lower medulla and ascend as medial lemnisci to the level of the thalamus.[5] This pathway serves the basis for somatosensory-evoked potentials recording during intraoperative monitoring.

Descending Lateral Corticospinal (Pyramidal) Tracts

The fibers from the primary motor cortex descend via pyramidal tracts to synapse on the lower motor neurons of the anterior horns. The vast majority of these fibers decussate at the level of medulla (top of C1 level) prior to entering the lateral columns of the contralateral side.[6] This pathway serves as the basis for transcranial motor-evoked potentials recording during intraoperative monitoring.

Vascular Diseases of the Spinal Cord

Infarctions of the Spinal Cord

Arterial Spinal Cord Infarctions

Isolated spinal cord infarction is much less frequent than cerebral infarction, accounting for only 1% of all strokes.[7] Based on the pathogenesis, there are two main types of spinal cord ischemia: (1) mechanical disruption of the blood supply, resulting in anterior or posterior spinal artery infarcts, and (2) infarcts occurring after prolonged global hypotension or hypoperfusion, resulting in central and transverse infarcts.[8,9] Compromise of the spinal vascular supply results in a constellation of deficits specific to that vessel's territory.

Since the anterior spinal artery supplies the anterior two-thirds of the cord, its occlusion leads to abrupt flaccid paralysis (quadriplegia or paraplegia, depending on the level of ischemia) due to involvement of the bilateral descending corticospinal tracts, loss of superficial pain, and loss of temperature discrimination (bilateral ascending spinothalamic tracts) below the level of the vascular compromise, with preservation of vibration and position sense carried by the unaffected ascending posterior columns supplied by the posterior arteries. In addition, there is autonomic dysfunction with loss of sphincter control, bladder atonia, and paralytic ileus. Spasticity eventually ensues, with exaggerated deep tendon reflexes, positive Babinski responses, and ankle clonus.[9]

The occlusion of one of the posterior spinal arteries results in the infarction of the ipsilateral posterior third of the hemicord as well as alteration in specialized and complex discriminative sensory functions.[10]

In the context of surgical procedures, the most frequent mechanism of infarction is manipulation of the aorta or its branches. Nonsurgical etiologies include severe hypotension or hypovolemia from significant blood loss, aortic thrombosis, embolization, and aortic dissection, all resulting in global spinal hypoperfusion.[11]

Distinct from cerebral infarction, most (>80%) spinal infarcts are painful. Causes of ischemic spinal cord injury are listed in Box 38.1.

Spinal venous infarctions are rare, typically involving the thoracic cord and causing paraparesis and sensory disturbance of the lower extremities. Venous infarctions are subdivided into hemorrhagic or ischemic. Hemorrhagic and embolic venous infarctions have sudden onset and rapid progression and are painful. The clinical onset of a nonhemorrhagic infarction is protracted, with gradual evolution of the symptoms.[13]

Evaluation of Suspected Stroke of the Spinal Cord

Imaging

Computed tomography has little application to the diagnosis of spinal ischemia. It lacks the sensitivity, especially in the cervical region, to be adequate for reliable exclusion of ischemia, but may identify compressive causes of myelopathy (epidural hematoma, tumors). Spinal angiography (arteriography) is indicated occasionally, usually for diagnosis and treatment of a spinal arteriovenous malformation. Spinal magnetic resonance imaging (MRI) is a diagnostic test of choice for diagnosis of infarction.[14]

Treatment is guided by the underlying etiology. There are limited reports on use of recombinant tissue plasminogen activator in patients with spinal cord ischemia.[15] The goal is to improve spinal cord perfusion with permissive hypertension and maintenance of euvolemia, which may be supplemented by lumbar cerebrospinal fluid (CSF) draining to reduce intrathecal pressure and augment perfusion. Corticosteroids have no role in the treatment of spinal cord infarction unless noninfectious inflammation is established.[14]

The prognosis for functional recovery is guarded. Few patients improve; rarely (<10%), patients achieve a remarkable recovery of function, particularly of motor control and ability to walk. The short-term mortality rate is 20% to 25% over the first month following onset of symptoms. Overall life expectancy is diminished because of vascular, infectious, and other medical complications.

Spinal Cord Vascular Lesions

The vascular lesions are subdivided into neoplastic vascular lesions (hemangioblastoma, cavernous malformation), aneurysms, arteriovenous fistulas, and arteriovenous malformations (AVMs) (Box 38.2).[16]

BOX 38.1 Causes of Ischemic Spinal Cord Injury

Nonsurgical Vascular Pathology

Ischemic infarction due to arterial atherosclerosis/embolism
Ischemic infarction due to aortic dissection or thrombosis
Ischemic infarction due to fibrocartilaginous embolism[12]
Venous infarctions
Arteriovascular malformation (vascular steal)
Vasculitis
Decompression sickness
Vascular constriction (triptans, illicit substances)

Surgery Related

Hypoperfusion due to:

- Hypotension/cardiac arrest
- Hypovolemia (blood or volume loss)
- Clamping of the radicular feeding artery
- Clamping of the aorta

BOX 38.2 Classification of Vascular Malformations

Arteriovenous Malformations

Extradural-intradural
Intradural

- Intramedullary
- Conus

Arteriovenous Fistulas

Intradural
Extradural

Cavernous Hemangioma (Cavernomas)

Cavernomas are slow-growing, raspberry-shaped vascular malformations that become symptomatic in the case of bleeding or from direct cord compression. Symptoms depend on lesion location. Diagnosis is made with a characteristic spinal MRI appearance with evidence of blood degradation products at different stages. The lesions are well demarcated, with mixed signal intensity and popcorn appearance. The core is surrounded by a rim of low intensity that corresponds to hemosiderin. Hemosiderin-sensitive sequences (gradient echo or susceptibility-weighted imaging) are beneficial in the diagnosis of cavernous hemangiomas. Treatment of symptomatic patients requires surgical resection.[17]

Hemangioblastomas

These vascular lesions of the spinal cord can be sporadic or familial, as in case of von Hippel–Lindau syndrome. MRI is needed for diagnosis, and treatment entails surgical resection if the lesion is symptomatic.

Arteriovenous Malformations and Arteriovenous Fistulas

Spinal dural arteriovenous fistulas are the most common type of spinal cord vascular malformation.[18] These lesions are defined by abnormal connections between a radicular feeding artery and the coronal venous plexus of the spine without an intervening capillary bed. The actual fistula site is at the dural sleeve of the nerve root. The arterial blood flow is shunted directly into the venous plexus, leading to venous congestion, venous hypertension, and potential venous infarctions.[18] Clinical presentation is characterized by the insidious progression of weakness and sensory deficits in the lower extremities. MRI findings include presence of cord edema and dilated and tortuous perimedullary dural vessels. The gold standard for diagnosis is a catheter spinal angiography. Treatment is surgical disconnection or endovascular occlusion.[15]

Intramedullary (or glomus) AVMs are characterized by the presence of tightly compacted groups of arterial and venous vessels (nidus) inside the spinal cord. The AVM is supplied by multiple feeding arteries from the spinal arteries. This is a high-flow system shunting blood from the vital tissue and is often associated with aneurysms. The most common presentation is related to a hemorrhage, direct compression, or ischemia. Diagnosis is made by spinal MRI by demonstrating intramedullary flow voids and subsequent spinal catheter angiography.[15]

Inflammatory Spinal Cord Disorders

Transverse Myelitis

Transverse myelitis (TM) is an immune-mediated, inflammatory acute or subacute spinal cord disorder that causes a combination of motor, sensory, pain, and autonomic-sphincteric dysfunction that evolves over hours to days, but sometimes up to a few weeks. TM can be primary or idiopathic, or, more often, secondary to other systemic or neurologic disorders.[19] Although TM may result in complete disruption of all tracts across the spinal cord cross-section, more commonly there is variability in the severity of functional impairment. Thus, patients may present with variable degrees of sensory loss, weakness, neck or back pain, and bladder and bowel dysfunction. The pattern of weakness is usually level dependent, with quadriparesis with cervical cord TM and paraparesis with thoracolumbar TM; however, cervical cord disease often spares the upper extremities. Acutely, limbs may have flaccid weakness, with loss of deep tendon reflexes, although the presence of extensor plantar responses, urinary and bowel retention, and a protopathic (pain and temperature) sensory level localizes to the spinal cord. Some patients can present with a purely dorsal column syndrome, with loss of vibration and proprioception, resulting in a sensory ataxia. Patients with hemicord involvement may present with dissociated motor and sensory symptoms, ipsilateral weakness and loss of vibration and proprioception, and contralateral loss of ability to feel pain and temperature. This constellation of symptoms and signs is characteristic of Brown-Séquard syndrome, invariably localizing to the spinal cord. Pathology is usually 2 to 3 segments above the clinical sensory level but may be higher.[20]

The etiology of idiopathic TM is not established. It can occur following a nonspecific virus or vaccination.[19] TM secondary to a systemic or neurologic disorder is important to identify, as treatment of the underlying condition decreases the risk of relapse. Systemic diseases associated with TM include systemic lupus erythematosus (SLE), Sjögren syndrome, Behçet disease (BD), and sarcoidosis.[1,4] Both multiple sclerosis (MS) and neuromyelitis optica (NMO) very commonly present with TM and need to be considered in the differential diagnosis. These conditions are discussed later in this chapter.

MRI of the spine is the diagnostic test of choice in evaluating TM, often demonstrating a contrast-enhancing and expansile intrinsic cord lesion of variable length (Fig. 38.1).[2] It is important to note that clinical features of TM cannot be differentiated from spinal cord compression, necessitating emergent imaging to allow for expeditious surgery if necessary. Other diagnostic testing includes complete blood count, serum chemistries, rheumatologic screening (antinuclear antibody, anti-Ro/La antibodies), and serum angiotensin-converting enzyme. Lumbar puncture and brain MRI are helpful in the diagnosis of MS. Serum aquaporin-4 antibody is both highly specific and sensitive for NMO.[21]

The first line of treatment for idiopathic TM is pulse intravenous (IV) steroids, most often with methylprednisolone 1000 mg daily for 3 to 7 days, followed by a prednisone taper. Plasma exchange (5 to 6 treatments every other day) for steroid-refractory TM has demonstrated efficacy in patients with idiopathic TM, MS, and NMO, resulting in complete or near-complete recovery in the majority of patients.[19,22] Patients with TM secondary to another disorder will require long-term treatment for their underlying condition to prevent recurrence.

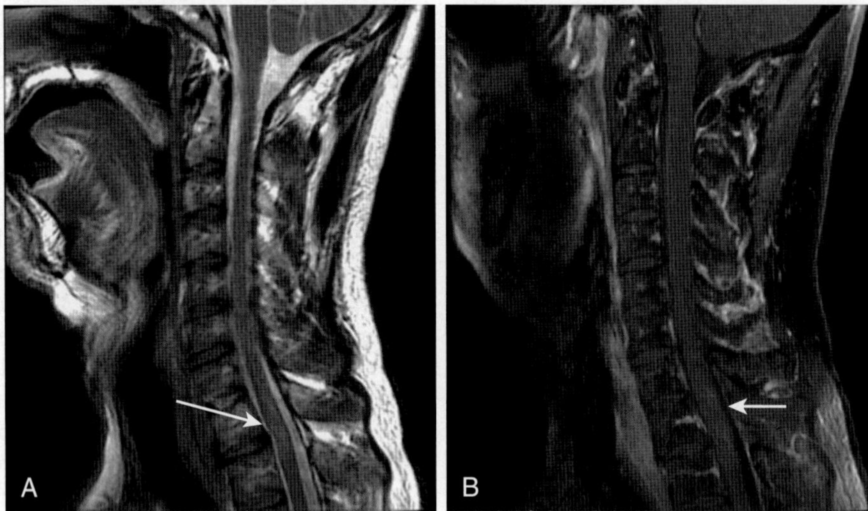

FIG. 38.1 (A) Sagittal T2-weighted magnetic resonance image (MRI) of a patient with neuromyelitis optica (NMO) demonstrating a longitudinally extensive transverse myelitis (*arrow*), increased signal change, and spinal cord expansion from C7 to T2. (B) Sagittal MRI with contrast enhancement of subacute longitudinally extensive transverse myelitis (*arrow*) in a patient with NMO.

Multiple Sclerosis

MS is a chronic immune-mediated disease of the central nervous system (CNS) that is a leading cause of neurologic disability in young adults. It is pathologically characterized by inflammation, demyelination (in both white and gray matter), and axonal degeneration. Although the etiology of MS is unknown, it is widely thought to be initiated by an aberrant immunologic response to an environmental agent in genetically predisposed individuals. While an infectious cause is suspected, no single virus or bacteria has been isolated. MS predominantly affects women by a 2:1 ratio and is more common in white individuals of Northern European descent and in those living in increasing latitudes away from the Equator. However, the disease tends to be more aggressive in those with African American ethnicity.

MS is classically described as a white matter disease disseminated in time and space. In 85% of patients, the disease presents with relapses and remissions (RRMS), with attacks of neurologic symptoms that resolve completely or nearly completely over weeks to months, followed by periods of clinical stability. Within 10 years, 50% of patients with RRMS will enter a secondary progressive phase (SPMS), with slowly accumulating disability, in large part due to myelopathy.[23,24] Approximately 15% of patients with MS present with progressive neurologic dysfunction at disease onset, usually due to myelopathy, classified as primary progressive MS (PPMS). A subset of patients with both SPMS and PPMS continue to have both clinical relapses and inflammatory radiologic disease and are categorized as having progressive MS with activity.

MS relapses are defined as new or worsening symptoms lasting at least 24 hours, not associated with a systemic illness, and separated by at least 30 days.[25] MS flares are associated with neurologic disability, functional impairment, and psychosocial disruption, all of which affect quality of life.[26] With increasing disease duration, patients tend to have less recovery from exacerbations, leading to accrual of disability. Clinical features of MS are varied and depend on regions of involvement. Most patients present with optic neuritis, brain stem–cerebellar syndrome, hemispheric disease, or spinal cord impairment.

Spinal cord disease in MS usually presents with upper motor deficits (facial-sparing hemiparesis, quadriparesis, paraparesis, with hyperreflexia, Babinski sign, and spasticity, due to corticospinal tract dysfunction); paresthesias and numbness of the limbs and trunk (often with a sensory level to pinprick due to spinothalamic involvement and/or proprioceptive and vibratory deficit, and Romberg sign due to posterior column dysfunction); Lhermitte phenomenon, a paroxysmal electrical sensation radiating from the neck down the midline spine and into all four limbs, triggered by neck flexion; and bladder and bowel dysfunction, including urinary urgency, urinary retention, urinary and fecal incontinence, and constipation. Optic neuritis is typically unilateral, with rapidly progressive monocular visual loss and pain with eye movement over several days, with an afferent pupillary defect on exam. Funduscopy is usually normal, since there is only retrobulbar optic nerve inflammation. Brain stem–cerebellar symptoms include diplopia with internuclear ophthalmoplegia or sixth nerve palsy, dysarthria, vertigo, facial numbness, unilateral trigeminal neuralgia or facial palsy, and truncal or limb ataxia. Hemispheric manifestations include contralateral hemiparesis, hemisensory loss, and cognitive impairment. In addition, many patients with MS complain of late-day fatigue, paroxysmal tonic limb spasms, and dysesthetic limb and trunk pain.

PPMS and SPMS most often present as an insidiously worsening myelopathy. Patients often complain of asymmetric leg weakness, eventually with involvement of the contralateral leg, and, later, the upper extremities. This is accompanied by neurogenic bladder and bowel, epicritic sensory loss, and limb spasticity. Less frequently, patients may develop progressive spastic hemiparesis or pancerebellar ataxia. Finally, cognitive dysfunction can affect from 40% to 70% of patients with MS, in both the relapsing and progressive stages of the disease, with impairment of short-term memory, attention and concentration, executive function, verbal fluency, and visuospatial processing, not uncommonly leading to a subcortical dementia. More rarely, PPMS may present as an isolated dementia.

The diagnosis of MS relies primarily on the clinical history and examination, with demonstration of events and neurologic signs disseminated in time and space.[25] The McDonald criteria for MS can be fulfilled without ancillary support on the basis of an appropriate history and neurologic exam, with the caveat that MS is the best explanation of the disorder. However, in the majority of individuals diagnostic testing is critical.

MRI is the most sensitive tool for both MS diagnosis and disease monitoring. The former is centered on demonstrating lesions that are both temporally and spatially disseminated. MS lesions are classically seen in the periventricular, juxtacortical (including the corpus callosum), and infratentorial regions and in the spinal cord. Brain lesions are typically ovoid in shape and configured perpendicularly to the ventricles. However, MS can also present with large, tumefactive hemispheric lesions, mimicking a mass. Spinal cord lesions are typically short segmented (one to two vertebral spaces) with a dorsal predilection. Both active and old lesions are hyperintense on T2 and fluid attenuation inversion recovery (FLAIR) sequences; gliotic lesions that correspond with axonal loss are hypointense on T1 sequences (Fig. 38.2). Active, inflammatory lesions are gadolinium enhancing, often with an open-ring configuration in the brain. The McDonald criteria define MRI dissemination in space (DIS) as 2 or more lesions in at least 2 of the periventricular, juxtacortical, infratentorial, or spinal cord regions. MRI dissemination in time can be established with either the presence of both asymptomatic gadolinium-enhancing and -nonenhancing lesions on a single scan or by the development of new T2/FLAIR or new gadolinium-enhancing lesions on sequential studies performed after the index study.[25]

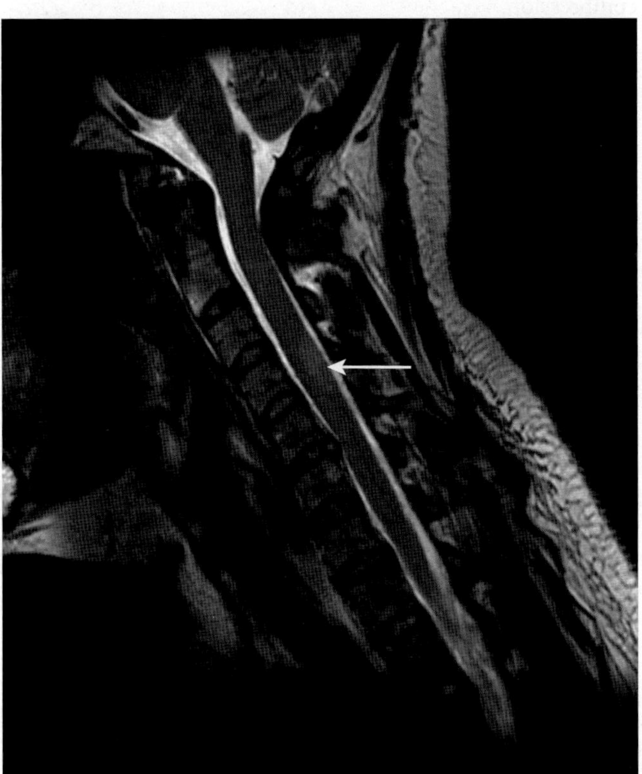

FIG. 38.2 Sagittal T2-weighted magnetic resonance image of a patient with multiple sclerosis and short-segment cervical myelitis at C4–C5 (*arrow*).

MRI is also useful in patients with PPMS whose history reveals a progressive neurologic impairment, usually referable to the spinal cord, that has evolved for at least 1 year. MRI criteria for DIS in PPMS relies on demonstration of two or more spinal cord lesions and at least one lesion in one of the aforementioned periventricular, juxtacortical, or infratentorial zones.[25]

CSF is often useful in confirming the diagnosis of MS when the clinical history and MRI findings are either nondiagnostic or atypical. The presence of CSF oligoclonal bands and/or elevated immunoglobulin (Ig) G index on isoelectric focusing is seen in more than 95% of patients with MS. Mild to moderate CSF lymphocytosis (≤50/μL) and protein elevation (≤100 mg/dL) may also be seen.

Because of the sensitivity of MRI, visual, brain stem auditory, and somatosensory evoked potentials are less commonly used in the diagnosis of MS. Of these, delayed latency of visual evoked responses are the most useful in establishing DIS in selected patients.

Differential diagnosis of MS is broad and includes systemic inflammatory disorders (sarcoidosis, vasculitis, connective tissue disease), CNS infection (Lyme disease, neurosyphilis, HIV related), neoplasm (CNS lymphoma, gliomatosis cerebri), nutritional deficiencies (B12, copper), and structural/compressive disorders (Chiari malformation, cervical spondylotic myelopathy). These diseases can usually be excluded by the clinical history, laboratory findings, and appropriate imaging.

Acute MS relapses are usually treated with short courses of steroids, most frequently with a 3- to 5-day course of high-dose IV methylprednisolone, followed by tapering prednisone for 2 weeks. Patients with severe neurologic deficits that are refractory to steroids may achieve enhanced recovery with plasma exchange.

The treatment of MS has been revolutionized with the development of disease-modifying therapies (DMT) in the early 1990s. There are now 11 Food and Drug Administration–approved injectable, parenteral, and oral agents for RRMS, including four formulations of interferon beta-1a or -1b, glatiramer acetate, mitoxantrone, natalizumab, fingolimod, teriflunomide, dimethyl fumarate, and alemtuzumab. However, the use of mitoxantrone has diminished due to complications of leukemia and cardiomyopathy.[27] Each of these DMTs have demonstrated efficacies in reducing annualized relapse rate and the development of new and contrast-enhancing lesions on brain MRI; the latter is an important component in monitoring patients on treatment.[28] Although there is no established therapy for PPMS, both rituximab and ocrelizumab, monoclonal antibodies that target CD20 B lymphocytes, have demonstrated efficacy in patients with PPMS with activity.[28–30] There are no approved medications for SPMS, although DMTs for RRMS are commonly used in patients with SPMS who have ongoing relapses.[27] The choice of therapy in a particular patient depends in large part on the severity of inflammatory disease activity, based both clinically and radiologically, with more potent but riskier agents (e.g., natalizumab, fingolimod, alemtuzumab) reserved for patients with aggressive disease.[31] Last, symptomatic treatment directed at MS-associated spasticity, neurogenic bladder and bowel, pain, fatigue, and mood dysfunction is an important facet of patient care.[31]

Neuromyelitis Optica

NMO is an autoimmune, relapsing disease of the CNS that is also characterized pathologically by inflammation and demyelination. NMO was historically portrayed as a monophasic illness related to MS that caused simultaneous optic neuritis and transverse myelitis, sparing the brain. However, with relatively recent advances in neuroimmunology, NMO is now known to be an autoantibody-mediated disorder that is usually distinguishable from MS, with uniquely characteristic involvement of not only the optic nerves and spinal cord, but also the cerebral hemispheres and brain stem. Unlike MS, relapses in NMO often cause severe neurologic disability that requires prompt evaluation and treatment. NMO affects women at a rate of 8:1, a higher ratio than MS. Its incidence in African Americans is also greater than that seen in MS.[32]

Optic nerve involvement in NMO may be unilateral or bilateral, resulting in severe visual loss, not infrequently associated with a long-segment optic neuritis on MRI. Spinal cord attacks are associated with severe quadriparesis or paraparesis, with associated spinothalamic and dorsal column deficits below the level of the lesion as well as urinary or bowel retention. MRI typically reveals a longitudinally extensive central intramedullary hyperintense lesion, spanning three or more vertebral levels, resulting in spinal cord expansion. Other less common manifestations of NMO include refractory hiccoughs or vomiting due to medullary disease, hypersomnolence and syndrome of inappropriate antidiuretic hormone with hypothalamic lesions, and encephalopathy with multifocal tumefactive subcortical inflammatory disease.[32]

Serum antibody to aquaporin-4 (also known as NMO-Ab), a CNS water channel that is expressed on foot processes on CNS astrocytes, is now established as pathogenic in NMO. The serum antibody is found in up to 85% of patients with a cell-based assay.[33] The presence of this antibody in patients presenting with syndromes associated with NMO is highly predictive of future relapse.[22,32]

NMO relapses are treated with high-dose IV steroids followed by a prolonged steroid taper, although plasma exchange is also frequently necessary to achieve satisfactory recovery. Long-term therapy with immunosuppressive agents is mandatory to prevent exacerbations. Although prednisone alone can be used, most clinicians use steroid-sparing agents, including azathioprine, mycophenolate, and rituximab, to reduce complications of chronic corticosteroids.[21] Novel monoclonal antibodies directed against downstream mechanisms of antibody-mediated, inflammatory cytotoxicity, including eculizumab and tocilizumab, are also under study for use in NMO.[34,35]

Myelopathy Due to Connective Tissue Conditions and Diseases

Rheumatoid Arthritis

There have been medical advancements over the last 20 years in the pharmacologic treatments for autoimmune diseases such as rheumatoid arthritis (RA). These treatments include the development of the biologic class of disease-modifying antirheumatic drugs (DMARDs), tissue necrosis factor-α (TNF-α) inhibitors, and traditional DMARDs such as methotrexate.[36] Due to the increased efficacy of these treatments, the true prevalence of cervical spine abnormalities in RA and other inflammatory arthropathies is not known.

RA most commonly affects the occiput–C1 articulation, a saddle joint, and the C1–C2 joint, a pivot joint. These are true synovial joints that RA and other inflammatory arthritides have a predilection to, including 65% of cases involving C1–C2 instability and 20% involving basilar invagination.[37–39] Radiographic findings include vertebral body and spinous process bony erosion and cystic changes, C2 pseudotumor and pannus formation, discitis, as well as ligamentous inflammation, laxity, and calcification.[38,39] RA can be a cause of spinal cord compression due to this degenerative cascade and resultant instability. Subaxial spine degeneration, especially after previous upper cervical spine fusion, should be followed clinically with dynamic radiographs and an MRI scan if upper motor neuron signs are present.[37,40,41] Further fusion and decompression surgery may be indicated depending on the patient's degree of cervical instability and spinal cord compression.

Systemic Lupus Erythematosus and Antiphospholipid Antibody Syndrome

SLE is a chronic and relapsing autoimmune connective tissue disease that affects multiple organ systems. SLE affects the skin, joints, kidneys, lungs, heart, blood, as well as the nervous system, primarily by activating the immune system with formation of immune complexes.[42] The CNS also can be affected by SLE. Patients can present with a headache or mild confusion all the way to seizure or frank myelopathy with or without optic neuritis.[43] There were 19 neuropsychiatric syndromes associated with SLE described by the American College of Rheumatology Research Committee in 1999.[44]

Patients with SLE myelopathy often have CSF abnormalities, including increased protein, pleocytosis, and decreased glucose. The term "longitudinal myelitis" has been given to the characteristic increased MRI signal seen on T2-weighted sequences over several continuous segments.[45]

Antiphospholipid antibody syndrome is characterized by a hypercoagulability and is associated with antiphospholipid antibodies. It is thought to be a possible variant of SLE. These antibodies include lupus anticoagulant, anticardiolipin, and antibodies against β_2-glycoprotein 1. As in SLE, there are wide ranges of neurologic disorders that can be associated with this condition, including myelopathy.

Therapies for these conditions include high-dose IV steroids for acute symptoms, IV immunoglobulin, cyclophosphamide, and plasmapheresis.[43,46]

Sjögren Disease

Sjögren disease is characterized by dry eyes (xerophthalmia), dry mouth (xerostomia), and a noninflammatory arthritis.[47] The disease is about 10 times more common in women than in men and can also have neurologic manifestations, including myelopathy, transverse myelitis, optic neuropathy, and necrotizing myelitis.[47–49] Treatment includes corticosteroids and, in some cases, plasma exchange.[47,49,50]

Behçet Disease

BD is a chronic inflammatory disorder of the blood vessels that can also involve inflammation of the parenchymal CNS (neuro-Behçet). The exact cause of this disease is unknown but thought to be autoimmune related.[51,52] Symptoms can include inflammation with sores or thrombosis in the mouth, eyes, skin, joints, digestive system, brain, and genital regions.

Neuro-Behçet affects approximately 5% to 49% of patients with this disease and can cause symptoms from confusion, psychosis, and mild weakness to complete paralysis.[51–56] Treatment includes high-dose IV steroids and/or TNF-α inhibitors such as infliximab and etanercept; adalimumab has shown variable results.[54,56]

Neurosarcoidosis

Sarcoidosis is a noncaseating granulomatous disease involving multiple organ systems and tissues. Its cause is believed to be autoimmune in nature, but the exact pathogenesis is not known.[57,58] The disease most commonly presents with bilateral hilar lymphadenopathy (>90%), pulmonary infiltrates, skin and eye lesions, and arthralgias. Granulomatous infiltrates can appear in any tissue, including the spine, and can cause arachnoiditis, cauda equina syndrome, intradural or extradural granulomas, and intramedullary spinal masses.

A small percentage of patients (5–10%) can develop CNS involvement, and a definitive diagnosis is difficult to obtain. The mean age of onset of neurologic symptoms is typically in the fourth decade of life.[59] Definitive diagnosis requires a biopsy that will demonstrate noncaseating epithelioid granulomas, and a biopsy sample of the spinal cord is not desirable. Biopsy of lung tissue is a less morbid procedure. MRI scan of the neural axis can be normal in some cases, but contrast-enhanced MRI may show a diffuse increased signal in parenchymal cord tissue or masses.[59–62]

Little is known about the natural history of patients with CNS involvement in sarcoidosis. Recovery over months or years occurs in 60% to 80% of patients with pulmonary disease, however. Treatment is similar to other autoimmune and connective tissue causes of myelopathy, and includes aggressive IV steroids, DMARDs, and TNF-α inhibitors.

Infectious Myelopathies

Several infections can lead to myelopathy in patients due to a variety of disease processes. Most commonly, a direct invasion of neural cells causing edema and permanent neurologic tissue scarring is the mechanism. There is a predilection for these processes to occur in the immunocompromised patients; however, it can occur in those in good health as well. A thorough history, physical examination, radiologic studies, and possibly invasive testing (e.g., CSF analysis) are necessary to make the diagnosis.

Viral Myelitis

Human Immunodeficiency Virus Infection

Human immunodeficiency virus (HIV) is the cause of acquired immunodeficiency syndrome (AIDS) in an estimated 30 million people worldwide.[63] HIV infection has been associated with immunodeficiency, neoplasia, and neurologic disease.[64] High rates of neurologic complications (up to 40–50%) have been reported.[65–67]

In patients with AIDS, vacuolar myelopathy (VM) is the most common spinal cord disease, found in up to 30% of patients prior to the antiretroviral therapy.[68] This most common form of myelopathy in HIV infection was first described by Petito and colleagues,[69] observing spinal cord degeneration. Autopsy revealed a high rate of spinal cord disease that was clinically not as prevalent and likely underrecognized.

Symptoms of VM can overlap with other myelopathies associated with HIV-1 infection; however, the pathologic appearance is distinct. There is a loss of myelin and spongy degeneration found on histologic examination, and the lateral and posterior columns are more affected. The microvacuolization of the white matter of the spinal cord resembles that of subacute combined degeneration. The vacuolization appears to result from intramyelin swelling, with axons being preserved, for the large part. Microglial nodules may be detected in the spinal cord gray matter.[69]

Symptoms of VM include a slowly progressive lower extremity weakness, lack of balance with gait instability and ataxia, dorsal column sensory changes in vibration and position, urinary frequency, urinary urgency, and erectile dysfunction. Spastic paraparesis is present, with weakness being greater than spasticity; prominent hyperreflexia and extensor plantar responses of the lower extremities are also usually present.

MRI findings in patients with AIDS-associated myelopathy can occur in up to 86% of patients. The most common finding is spinal cord atrophy followed by diffuse intrinsic cord signal abnormality.[70] Enhancement with gadolinium is not common. If the MRI of the spinal cord is lacking any findings, CSF can be examined for infection of other pathogens or for the presence of HIV.

Vacuolar myelopathy is a diagnosis of exclusion, as other opportunistic infections and conditions in HIV can be the cause of myelopathy in AIDS patients.

Human T-Cell Lymphotropic Virus Type 1

The human T-cell lymphotropic virus type 1 (HTLV-1) was the first oncogenic human retrovirus to be discovered in 1980.[71] It has since been implicated as the cause of cancer (adult T-cell leukemia/lymphoma) and several other spectrum inflammatory diseases.[72,73] It is believed to infect around 10 to 20 million people worldwide, and the clinical course is usually progressive without remission.[71–75] Infection can occur through a variety of methods, including mother to child, sexual activities, through the sharing of needles and syringes, and by the transfusion of infected blood products in countries that do not screen for HTLV-1 infection.[73,75,76]

The myelopathy that can develop in those infected with HTLV-1 is referred to as *tropical spastic paraparesis* or *HTLV-1 associated myelopathy* (TSP/HAM). It is characterized by chronic involvement of the pyramidal tracts, mainly at the thoracic level, causing lower extremity spasticity and weakness, urinary disturbances, pain, paresthesias, and sensory disturbances.[71,76,77] In a recent longitudinal cohort study by Tanajura and colleagues,[78] the development of neurologic signs and symptoms of HTLV-1 infection occurred in up to 30% of patients. The most common subjective findings were hand and feet numbness, nocturia, and urinary urgency. Lower extremity hyperreflexia and weakness with a positive Babinski sign were the most common objective findings.[78]

Infection of HTLV-1 shares a similar route of transmission as HIV, and dual infection is common.[79] The incidence of myelopathy among patients coinfected with both HIV and HTLV-1 is likely higher, especially in areas where HTLV-1 infection is endemic.[80] Treatment outcomes for TSP/HAM are disappointing; thus it remains as symptomatic therapy only.

Herpesviruses

Varicella-zoster virus (VZV) is a human neurotropic double-stranded DNA alpha-herpesvirus. VZV is the cause of chickenpox (varicella); after active infection, it remains latent for decades in the dorsal root and autonomic ganglia of the autonomic nervous system. As individuals age or become immunocompromised, a decrease in the VZV-specific cell-mediated immunity can occur, resulting in VZV reactivation, causing severely painful and blistering dermatomal eruptions called shingles (herpes zoster).[81–84]

Myelopathy associated with VZV can present as soon as days or weeks after acute varicella, and can present without the typical vesicular eruption and rash associated with herpes zoster.[82,85] Symptoms include a monophasic spastic paraparesis, with or without sensory features, and with or without sphincter problems.[81,82,85] The myelopathy can be insidious, progressive, and sometimes even fatal in immunocompromised patients, such as those with AIDS.[85] MRI can reveal serpiginous enhancing lesions and, in cases of VZV vasculopathy, can cause spinal cord infarcts seen on diffusion-weighted MRI.[85,86]

Diagnosis of VZV myelopathy can be confirmed with CSF analysis for virology. In myelopathy patients, the CSF usually contains a mild mononuclear pleocytosis with normal or slightly elevated protein. The CSF should be analyzed for DNA by polymerase chain reaction and for anti-VZV IgG and IgM.[81] Treatment for VZV myelopathy includes urgent IV acyclovir (10–15 mg/kg three times daily for 14 days) and possibly steroids, especially in those with VZV vasculopathy.[82,87,88]

Myelopathies Resulting From Bacterial Diseases

Syphilis

Sexually transmitted infections (STIs) take a huge toll on patients and society, both medically and economically. There are 20 million new STIs estimated to occur yearly in the United States, with direct and indirect medical costs estimated to exceed $16 billion.[89] Syphilis is an STI that accounts for 20% of these infections and occurs due to an infection by the bacterium *Treponema pallidum*.[89] In 2013, primary and secondary syphilis infection in the United States was estimated to occur in 5.3 cases per 100,000, more than double the lowest-ever rate of 2.1 in the year 2000.[90] The highest rates were found in men who have sex with men, with men accounting for more than 90% of syphilis cases in 2013.[89–91]

The *primary stage* of syphilis infection is marked by a single sore, or chancre, that occurs at the site where the bacterium entered the body. The chancre is firm, round, small, and painless. The time between infection and the first symptom can range from 10 to 90 days, and the chancre lasts 3 to 6 weeks before healing without treatment.[91] If no antibiotic treatment is sought, the infection progresses to the secondary stage.

The *secondary stage* of syphilis infection is characterized by a skin rash or rashes, typically nonpruritic in nature, and rough red to reddish brown spots located on the palms and the bottoms of the feet. Without antibiotic treatment, individuals will progress to tertiary or latent syphilis after the primary and secondary symptoms disappear. *Tertiary syphilis* can occur 10 to 20 years after the infection was acquired and affects up to 15% of those that were not treated at the primary or secondary stages.[91]

Invasion of the CNS by the *Treponema pallidum* bacterium usually occurs within 1 year of the primary infection. Headache and meningismus symptoms can be seen during the secondary syphilis stage, with up to 2% of patients having acute meningitis. Patients that are not treated with penicillin can develop neurosyphilis.

Tabes Dorsalis and Syphilitic Meningomyelitis

The spinal cord can be heavily affected by syphilis. Prior to the discovery of antibiotics, syphilis was believed to be the most common cause of spinal cord disease.[67,92] Tabes dorsalis is the prototypic spinal cord disease associated with syphilis and can be divided into three phases: the *preataxic phase*, the *ataxic phase*, and the *terminal* or *paralytic phase*. Currently, tabes dorsalis is thought to account for only 5% of neurosyphilis cases, but it is still a diagnostic and treatment dilemma in the developing world.[93,94] Testing for neurosyphilis includes algorithms for those with and those without HIV infection and may not catch all cases of chronic syphilis.[95,96] Tests include CSF VDRL (Venereal Disease Research Laboratory), CSF FTA-ABS (fluorescent treponemal antibody absorbed), CSF TPPA (*Treponema pallidum* particle agglutination assay), CSF T pallidum PCR (polymerase chain reaction), and CSF INNO-LIA (line blot immunoassay).[96]

Pathology of the spinal cord reveals overall atrophy in the posterior columns and spinal roots, with dorsal column demyelination of the fasciculus gracilis, root entry zone, and Lissauer tract. There is also thickening of the medium and small blood vessel walls. MRI findings include spinal cord atrophy and intramedullary hyperintensities, similar to findings seen in subacute combined degeneration; however, they can be normal in some cases.[94,97]

The *preataxic phase,* or period of "lightning pain," is the first phase occurring 10 to 15 years after primary infection and can last as long as 3 years. The majority of patients present with severe and lancinating pain. Other findings include a loss of muscle stretch reflexes, sensory losses, Romberg sign, and Argyll Robertson pupils (intact visual acuity but decreased pupillary light reflex and irregular pupils). Pain sensation is disturbed, with a delay in pain perception of approximately 15 seconds and an aftersensation lasting 30 seconds. Superficial pain sensation may be normal, but deep pain sensation is typically abnormal. Loss of deep pain sensation is reported with the application of pressure to the ulnar nerve (Biernacki sign), the Achilles tendon (Abadie sign), and the testicle (Pitres sign). Neuropathic pain is difficult to treat but can be attempted with gabapentin or other neuromodulatory agents.[98]

The *ataxic phase* is characterized by severe ataxia in the legs and has a variable duration of 2 to 10 years. Patients continue to lose deep pain sensation as well as proprioception and vibratory sense, which leads to a slapping and uncoordinated gait. These neurologic losses can lead to neuropathic joints and arthritic changes in the ankles, knees, hips, and spine.[99–102]

The final phase is known as the *terminal* or *paralytic phase.* The average duration of this final phase is between 2 and 10 years and is characterized by cachexia and paralysis, with severe constipation and urinary incontinence being prominent as well. Fatality is typically related to urosepsis or sepsis from decubitus ulcers.

Syphilitic meningomyelitis is seen most commonly in male patients between 25 and 40 years old and within 6 years of primary infection.[103,104] A slow and gradual leg weakness is noted and has similar symptoms as those with myelopathy due to cervical spondylosis. Muscle stretch reflexes are exaggerated with positive Babinski signs but muscle bulk is preserved. Autonomic dysfunction with urinary frequency, hesitancy, and impotence are common. On pathologic exam, the meninges are thickened and inflamed, with symmetrical involvement of the lateral columns. Granulomatous invasion with inflammation and vascular changes are noted in the medium and small vessels.

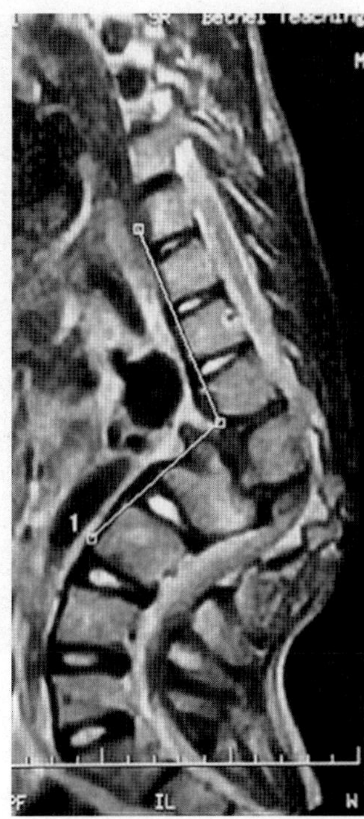

FIG. 38.3 Sagittal T2-weighted magnetic resonance image demonstrating a kyphotic deformity at the thoracolumbar junction arising from granulomatous disease (Pott disease).

Tuberculosis

Tuberculosis (TB) is caused by *Mycobacterium tuberculosis* and is a common source of neurologic complications in less-developed parts of the world. Skeletal manifestation of tuberculosis most commonly affects the spinal column in nearly 50% of cases.[105] Myelopathy occurring from spinal tuberculosis (Pott disease) is typically a compressive myelopathy due to a collapsing anterior spinal column from spinal instability as well as compression on the spinal cord from granulation tissue (Fig. 38.3).

Neurologic symptoms are present in more than 90% of patients with spinal TB and include sensory deficits, pain, paraplegia, and incontinence.[106] Thoracic spine involvement is most common (57%), followed by the cervical spine (29%).[106] The mainstay of treatment is medical, with long-term antibiotic therapy for at least 1 year, although 6 months may be adequate in some clinical situations.[107,108] Surgery has been noted to improve both pain and neurologic function in patients with progressive neurologic symptoms, but its usefulness is still debated.[109,110] Long-term sequelae and adverse outcomes can still be noted in those treated surgically, including chronic pain, deformity, and permanent neurologic injury.[105,106,109,110]

Spinal Epidural Abscesses

Spinal epidural abscesses (SEAs) are potentially devastating infections that can have a high mortality rate (Fig. 38.4). There are few high-quality studies to guide treatment of this potentially devastating condition.[111–113] Despite advances in early detection, diagnosis, and treatment, mortality rates can still

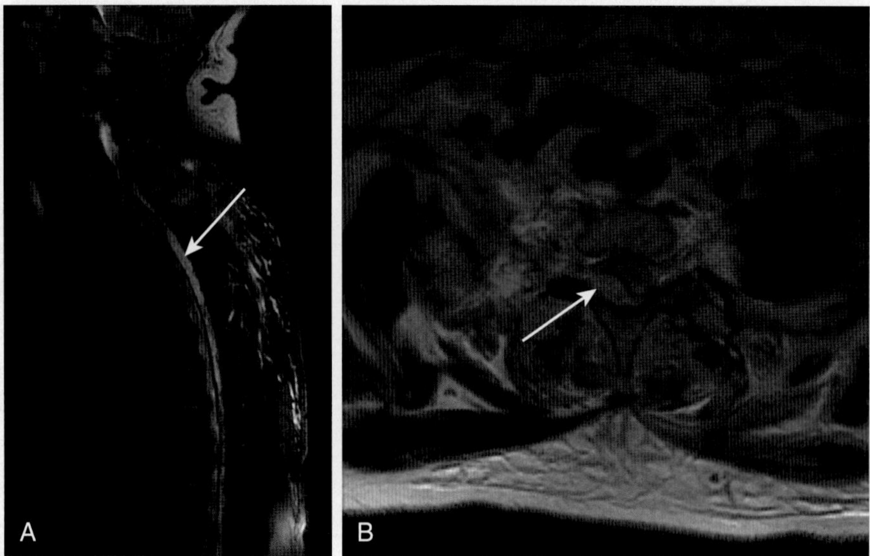

FIG. 38.4 (A) Sagittal T2-weighted short tau inversion recovery magnetic resonance image (MRI) of a patient with cervicothoracic epidural abscess compressing the spinal cord (*arrow*). (B) Axial T2-weighted MRI of the thoracic spine from the same patient demonstrating right-sided epidural spinal cord compression with cord deviation to the left (*arrow*).

approach 20%, and failure of medical treatment alone is as high as 75% to 99%.[111,113–115]

The incidence of SEAs is thought to be approximately 1.8 per 100,000 persons per year, with *Staphylococcus aureus* as the most common organism.[116] Several risk factors have been associated with SEAs, including HIV infection, IV drug use, diabetes mellitus, obesity, prior spinal surgery, advanced age, alcoholism, and liver disease.[108,111–115,117,118] Upper cervical epidural abscess, although rare, is associated with high rates of mortality and permanent neurologic deficits.[119]

In a recent database study by Schoenfeld et al., advanced age and liver disease were found to increase in-hospital mortality significantly; diabetes and chronic lung disease were the most frequently encountered comorbidity.[118] In the same study, hospital charges averaged nearly $160,000, with a range of $4000 to $3.3 million in charges. In addition to recalcitrant back pain, neurologic symptoms are present in a large portion of this population, with permanent paralysis as a known complication.

Practitioners should have a high index of suspicion for infection in patients presenting with back pain, subjective fevers, and weakness.[120] Other findings can include an increased white blood cell count, elevated C-reactive protein, and elevated erythrocyte sedimentation rate. Patients with multiple medical comorbidities and chronic immunosuppression may not have as prominent features compared with immunocompetent patients.

Noncontiguous SEAs have been reported by Ju et al., with risks being a delay in diagnosis (>7 days), a concomitant area of infection outside of the spine, and an erythrocyte sedimentation rate of greater than 95 mm/h.[112] Vertebral osteomyelitis is a common associated finding seen in approximately 86% of SEA cases.[108] In a recent retrospective review of electronic medical records in 355 patients over an 18-year period, Kim et al. determined patient characteristics that were prone to medical treatment failure. Factors associated with medical treatment failure included infection caused by methicillin-resistant *Staphylococcus aureus* (MRSA), patients older than 65 years, those with diabetes, and patients with major neurologic deficits.[115] Current treatment recommendations remain controversial, but there is a push for early surgical debridement in addition to long-term antibiotic treatment.

Nutritional Myelopathies

Vitamin B12 Deficiency

Vitamin B12 (cobalamin) deficiency is the most common nutritional cause of myelopathy.[121] Vitamin B12 is absorbed in the gastrointestinal tract via the intrinsic factor. Gastric parietal cells make intrinsic factor. Autoimmune-associated loss of parietal cells leads to lack of production of intrinsic factor. This is called pernicious anemia, and is the most common cause of vitamin B12 deficiency.[121] Myelopathy occurs in the setting of vitamin B12 deficiency because it is responsible for the myelination and maintenance of the CNS. Other causes of vitamin B12 deficiency include a history of gastric bypass surgery, a strict vegan diet, and nitrous oxide abuse.[122,123] Since vitamin B12 is found in meat and dairy, a vegan diet leads to inadequate intake. Nitrous oxide is a recreational inhaled drug that causes depletion of vitamin B12.

Clinically, patients will present with myelopathic signs and paresthesias of the upper and/or lower extremities. MRI of the spine in the setting of vitamin B12 deficiency will have a pathognomonic sign called the "inverted V sign" (Fig. 38.5).[124]

Lab work to determine serum vitamin B12 levels is the first step in evaluating for vitamin B12 deficiency.[121] If a low serum level is reported, additional testing of serum methylmalonic

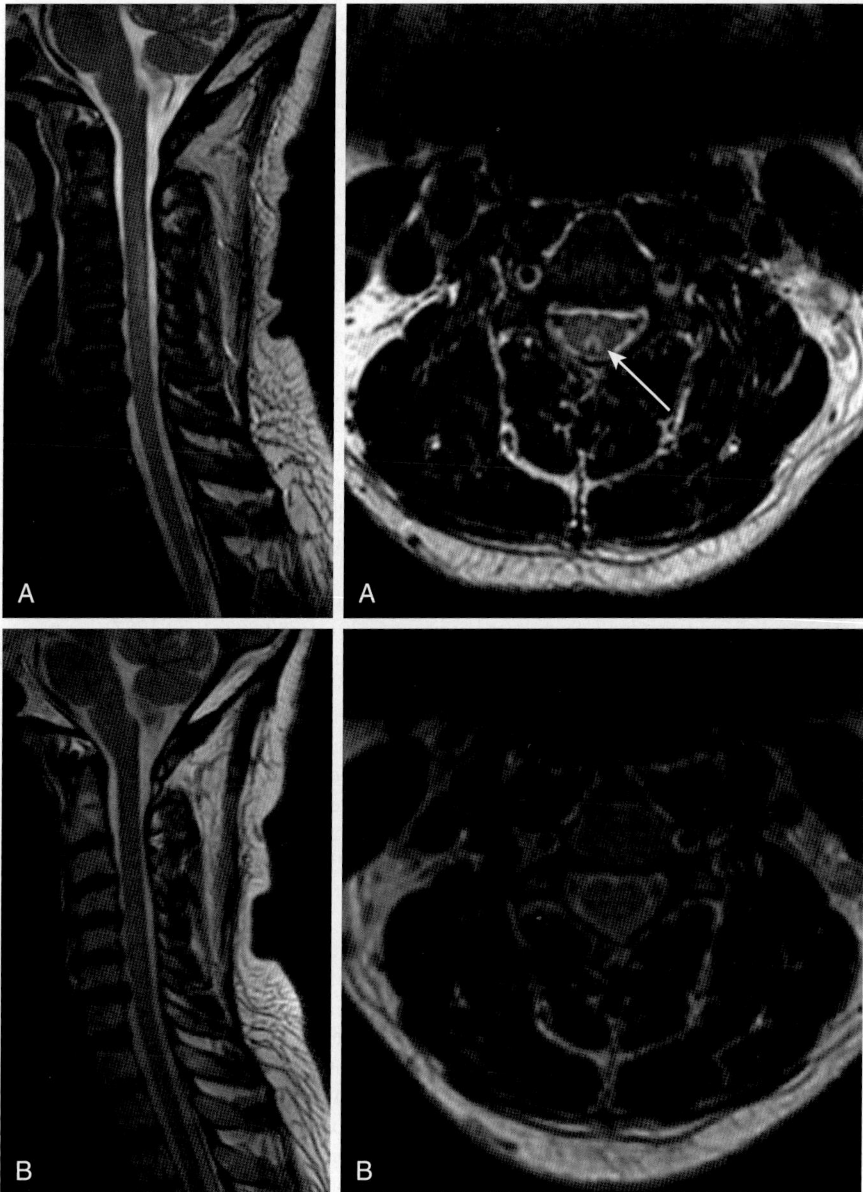

FIG. 38.5 (A) Sagittal and axial T2-weighted magnetic resonance imaging (MRI) of the cervical spine in patient with vitamin B12 deficiency. Note the "inverted V sign" on the axial MRI (*arrow*). (B) Sagittal and axial T2-weighted MRIs taken 6 months after the initiation of vitamin B12 injections demonstrating resolution of the nverted V sign.

acid and total homocysteine should be performed. In the presence of vitamin B12 deficiency, the serum level of these two proteins is highly elevated. If there are no dietary or other risk factors for vitamin B12 deficiency, then testing for pernicious anemia is recommended. Anti-intrinsic factor antibody and/or antiparietal cell antibody can be tested; a positive result is usually diagnostic of pernicious anemia.

Treatment of vitamin B12 deficiency consists of vitamin B12 injections (cyanocobalamin). Injections may consist of 1000 μg several times a week for up to 2 weeks, followed by monthly injections and clinical evaluation for resolution of symptoms alongside laboratory testing.[121] There are also options for oral vitamin B12 treatment. If the inverted V sign was present on spinal MRI on repeat imaging following vitamin B12 treatment, the sign will no longer be present. Pernicious anemia often requires lifelong treatment.

Copper Deficiency

Copper deficiency is a less common form of myelopathy and clinically presents in a manner similar to vitamin B12 deficiency.[125,126] Copper is important in the function of key enzymes, and deficiency can affect the CNS. Risk factors for inadequate gastrointestinal copper absorption and subsequent deficiency include gastric bypass surgery, increased zinc intake, and malabsorption syndromes. Diagnosis is via serum copper and ceruloplasmin levels and treatment is with supplementation of oral copper and elimination of risk factors if possible.

REFERENCES

1. Içten N, Memedova E, Süllü Y. Vertebral level of the ending of the spinal cord and its relationship to the length of the vertebral column in northern Turkish neonates. *Surg Radiol Anat*. 1995;17(4):315-318.
2. Brazis P, Masdeu J, Biller J. *Localization in Clinical Neurology*. 4th ed. Philadelphia: Lippincott Williams & Wilkins; 2001:101.
3. Patten J. *Neurological Differential Diagnosis*. 2nd ed. Springer; 1995:213.
4. Duane E. *Haines' Neuroanatomy. An Atlas of Structures, Section and Systems*. 4th ed. Williams and Wilkins; 1995:78.
5. Brazis P, Masdeu J, Biller J. *Localization in Clinical Neurology*. 4th ed. Philadelphia: Lippincott Williams & Wilkins; 2001:103.
6. Patten J. *Neurological Differential Diagnosis*. 2nd ed. Springer; 1995:214.
7. Sandson TA, Friedman JH. Spinal cord infarction: report of 8 cases and review of the literature. *Medicine (Baltimore)*. 1989;68:282-292.
8. Novy J, Carruzzo A, Maeder P, Bogousslavsky B. Spinal cord ischemia: clinical and imaging patterns, pathogenesis and outcomes in 27 patients. *Arch Neurol*. 2006;63:1113-1120.
9. Cheshire WP, Santos CC, Massey EW, Howard JF Jr. Spinal cord infarction: etiology and outcome. *Neurology*. 1996;47:321-330.
10. Davidoff RA. The dorsal columns. *Neurology*. 1989;39:1377-1385.
11. Robertson CE, Brown RD Jr, Wijdicks EF, Rabinstein AA. Recovery after spinal cord infarcts: long-term outcome in 115 patients. *Neurology*. 2012;78(2):114-121.
12. Tosi L, Rigoli G, Beltramello A. Fibrocartilaginous embolism of the spinal cord: a clinical and pathogenetic reconsideration. *J Neurol Neurosurg Psychiatry*. 1996;60:55-60.
13. Niino M, Isu T, Tashiro K. Nonhemorrhagic venous infarction of the spinal cord without spinal vascular malformation. *J Neurol*. 1999;246:852-854.
14. Rabinstein AA. Vascular myelopathies. *Continuum (Minneap Minn)*. 2015;21(1):67-83.
15. Restrepo L, Guttin J. Acute spinal cord ischemia during aortography treated with intravenous thrombolytic therapy. *Tex Heart Inst J*. 2006;33(1):74-77.
16. Spetzler RF, Detwiler PW, Riina HA, Porter RW. Modified classification of spinal cord vascular lesions. *J Neurosurg*. 2002;96:145-156.
17. Gonzalez LF, Spetzler RF. Treatment of spinal vascular malformations. *Clin Neurosurg*. 2005;52:192-201.
18. Fugate JE, Lanzino G, Rabinstein AA. Clinical presentation and prognostic factors of spinal dural arteriovenous fistulas: an overview. *Neurosurg Focus*. 2012;32(5):E17.
19. Greenberg BM, Frohman EM. Immune-mediated myelopathies. *Continuum (Minneap Minn)*. 2015;21:121-131.
20. Beh SC, Greenberg BM, Frohman T, Frohman EM. Transverse myelitis. *Neurol Clin*. 2013;31(1):79-138.
21. Tobin WO, Weinshenker BG, Lucchinetti CF. Longitudinally extensive transverse myelitis. *Curr Opin Neurol*. 2014;27(3):279-289.
22. Scott TF, Frohman EM, De Seze J, et al. Evidence-based guideline: clinical evaluation and treatment of transverse myelitis: report of the Therapeutics and Technology Assessment Subcommittee of the American Academy of Neurology. *Neurology*. 2011;77(24):2128-2134.
23. Weinshenker BG. The natural history of multiple sclerosis. *Neurol Clin*. 1995;13(1):119-146.
24. Kantarci OH, Weinshenker BG. Natural history of multiple sclerosis. *Neurol Clin*. 2005;23(1):17-38.
25. Polman CH, Reingold SC, Banwell B, et al. Diagnostic criteria for multiple sclerosis: 2010 revisions to the McDonald criteria. *Ann Neurol*. 2011;69(2):292-302.
26. Vollmer T. The natural history of relapses in multiple sclerosis. *J Neurol Sci*. 2007;256(suppl 1):S5-S13.
27. Torkildsen O, Myhr KM, Bo L. Disease-modifying treatments for multiple sclerosis: a review of approved medications. *Eur J Neurol*. 2016;23(suppl 1):18-27.
28. Wingerchuk DM, Carter JL. Multiple sclerosis: current and emerging disease-modifying therapies and treatment strategies. *Mayo Clin Proc*. 2014;89(2):225-240.
29. Castillo-Trivino T, Braithwaite D, Bacchetti P, Waubant E. Rituximab in relapsing and progressive forms of multiple sclerosis: a systematic review. *PLoS One*. 2013;8(7):e66308.
30. Kappos L, Li D, Calabresi PA, et al. Ocrelizumab in relapsing-remitting multiple sclerosis: a phase 2, randomised, placebo-controlled, multicentre trial. *Lancet*. 2011;378(9805):1779-1787.
31. Samkoff LM, Goodman AD. Symptomatic management in multiple sclerosis. *Neurol Clin*. 2011;29(2):449-463.
32. Wingerchuk DM, Banwell B, Bennett JL, et al. International consensus diagnostic criteria for neuromyelitis optica spectrum disorders. *Neurology*. 2015;85(2):177-189.
33. Melamed E, Levy M, Waters PJ, et al. Update on biomarkers in neuromyelitis optica. *Neurol Neuroimmunol Neuroinflamm*. 2015;2(4):e134.
34. Pittock SJ, Lennon VA, McKeon A, et al. Eculizumab in AQP4-IgG-positive relapsing neuromyelitis optica spectrum disorders: an open-label pilot study. *Lancet Neurol*. 2013;12(6):554-562.
35. Araki M, Matsuoka T, Miyamoto K, et al. Efficacy of the anti-IL-6 receptor antibody tocilizumab in neuromyelitis optica: a pilot study. *Neurology*. 2014;82(15):1302-1306.
36. Buckley F, Finckh A, Huizinga TW, Dejonckheere F, Jansen JP. Comparative efficacy of novel DMARDs as monotherapy and in combination with methotrexate in rheumatoid arthritis patients with inadequate response to conventional DMARDs: a network meta-analysis. *J Manag Care Spec Pharm*. 2015;21(5):409-423.
37. Kim HJ, Nemani VM, Riew KD, Brasington R. Cervical spine disease in rheumatoid arthritis: incidence, manifestations, and therapy. *Curr Rheumatol Rep*. 2015;17(2):9-014-0486-8.
38. Joaquim AF, Ghizoni E, Tedeschi H, Appenzeller S, Riew KD. Radiological evaluation of cervical spine involvement in rheumatoid arthritis. *Neurosurg Focus*. 2015;38(4):E4.
39. Quarta L, Corrado A, Melillo N, et al. Cervical myelopathy caused by periodontoid synovial pannus in a patient with psoriatic arthritis: a case report. *Clin Rheumatol*. 2007;26(8):1380-1382.
40. Clarke MJ, Cohen-Gadol AA, Ebersold MJ, Cabanela ME. Long-term incidence of subaxial cervical spine instability following cervical arthrodesis surgery in patients with rheumatoid arthritis. *Surg Neurol*. 2006;66(2):136-140.
41. Narvaez J, Narvaez JA, Serrallonga M, et al. Subaxial cervical spine involvement in symptomatic rheumatoid arthritis patients: comparison with cervical spondylosis. *Semin Arthritis Rheum*. 2015;45(1):9-17.
42. Merrill JT, Buyon JP, Utset T. A 2014 update on the management of patients with systemic lupus erythematosus. *Semin Arthritis Rheum*. 2014;44(2):e1-e2.

43. Hamming L, van der Meulen R, Vergouwen A, Siegert C. Myelopathy in systemic lupus erythematosus: a case report and a review of the literature. *Neth J Med*. 2015;73(6):290-292.
44. Yu C, Gershwin ME, Chang C. Diagnostic criteria for systemic lupus erythematosus: a critical review. *J Autoimmun*. 2014;48-49:10-13.
45. Tellez-Zenteno JF, Remes-Troche JM, Negrete-Pulido RO, Davila-Maldonado L. Longitudinal myelitis associated with systemic lupus erythematosus: clinical features and magnetic resonance imaging of six cases. *Lupus*. 2001;10(12):851-856.
46. Kovacs B, Lafferty TL, Brent LH, DeHoratius RJ. Transverse myelopathy in systemic lupus erythematosus: an analysis of 14 cases and review of the literature. *Ann Rheum Dis*. 2000;59(2):120-124.
47. de Paiva CS, Rocha EM. Sjogren syndrome: what and where are we looking for? *Curr Opin Ophthalmol*. 2015;26(6):517-525.
48. Thongpooswan S, Chapagain B, Bandagi S. A rare case of neuromyelitis optica spectrum disorder in patient with Sjogren's syndrome. *Case Rep Rheumatol*. 2014;2014:158165.
49. Manabe Y, Sasaki C, Warita H, et al. Sjogren's syndrome with acute transverse myelopathy as the initial manifestation. *J Neurol Sci*. 2000;176(2):158-161.
50. Rutan G, Martinez AJ, Fieshko JT, Van Thiel DH. Primary biliary cirrhosis, Sjogren's syndrome, and transverse myelitis. *Gastroenterology*. 1986;90(1):206-210.
51. Messina MJ, Rodegher M, Scotti R, Martinelli V. Treatment of myelitis in Behcet's disease with rituximab. *BMJ Case Rep*. 2014;May 30.
52. Noel N, Drier A, Wechsler B, et al. Neurological manifestations of Behcet's disease. *Rev Med Interne*. 2014;35(2):112-120.
53. Houman MH, Bellakhal S, Ben Salem T, et al. Characteristics of neurological manifestations of Behcet's disease: a retrospective monocentric study in Tunisia. *Clin Neurol Neurosurg*. 2013;115(10):2015-2018.
54. Kuroda R, Suzuki J, Muramatsu M, et al. Efficacy of infliximab in neuro-Behcet's disease presenting with isolated longitudinally extensive transverse myelitis. *J Neurol*. 2013;260(12):3167-3170.
55. Zhao B, He L, Lai XH. A case of neuro-Behcet's disease presenting with lumbar spinal cord involvement. *Spinal Cord*. 2010;48(2):172-173.
56. Coulter I, Huda S, Baborie A, Jacob A. Longitudinally extensive transverse myelitis as the sole presentation of neuro-Behcet's disease responding to infliximab. *J Spinal Cord Med*. 2012;35(2):122-124.
57. Kobak S. Sarcoidosis: a rheumatologist's perspective. *Ther Adv Musculoskelet Dis*. 2015;7(5):196-205.
58. Liu D, Birnbaum AD. Update on sarcoidosis. *Curr Opin Ophthalmol*. 2015;26(6):512-516.
59. Junger SS, Stern BJ, Levine SR, Sipos E, Marti-Masso JF. Intramedullary spinal sarcoidosis: clinical and magnetic resonance imaging characteristics. *Neurology*. 1993;43(2):333-337.
60. Endo T, Koike J, Kusama Y, Katsuta Y, Hayakawa H. Spinal cord sarcoidosis. *Neurology*. 1993;43(5):1059-1060.
61. Kameyama T, Ando T, Saito Y, Takahashi A, Yamada H. Spinal cord sarcoidosis—diagnostic value of Gd-enhanced MRI. *Rinsho Shinkeigaku*. 1992;32(6):631-636.
62. Morita H, Hayashi R, Tako K, Tsukada N, Yanagisawa N. Spinal cord sarcoidosis: MRI findings in response to treatment. *Eur Neurol*. 1992;32(3):126-129.
63. Hallett TB, Zaba B, Stover J, et al. Embracing different approaches to estimating HIV incidence, prevalence and mortality. *AIDS*. 2014;28(suppl 4):S523-S532.
64. Singer EJ, Valdes-Sueiras M, Commins D, Levine A. Neurologic presentations of AIDS. *Neurol Clin*. 2010;28(1):253-275.
65. Snider WD, Simpson DM, Nielsen S, et al. Neurological complications of acquired immune deficiency syndrome: analysis of 50 patients. *Ann Neurol*. 1983;14(4):403-418.
66. Levy RM, Bredesen DE, Rosenblum ML. Neurological manifestations of the acquired immunodeficiency syndrome (AIDS): experience at UCSF and review of the literature. *J Neurosurg*. 1985;62(4):475-495.
67. Berger JR, Moskowitz L, Fischl M, Kelley RE. Neurologic disease as the presenting manifestation of acquired immunodeficiency syndrome. *South Med J*. 1987;80(6):683-686.
68. Petito CK. Review of central nervous system pathology in human immunodeficiency virus infection. *Ann Neurol*. 1988;23(suppl):S54-S57.
69. Petito CK, Navia BA, Cho ES, et al. Vacuolar myelopathy pathologically resembling subacute combined degeneration in patients with the acquired immunodeficiency syndrome. *N Engl J Med*. 1985;312(14):874-879.
70. Chong J, Di Rocco A, Tagliati M, et al. MR findings in AIDS-associated myelopathy. *AJNR Am J Neuroradiol*. 1999;20(8):1412-1416.
71. Gessain A, Mahieux R. Tropical spastic paraparesis and HTLV-1 associated myelopathy: clinical, epidemiological, virological and therapeutic aspects. *Rev Neurol (Paris)*. 2012;168(3):257-269.
72. Proietti FA, Carneiro-Proietti AB, Catalan-Soares BC, Murphy EL. Global epidemiology of HTLV-I infection and associated diseases. *Oncogene*. 2005;24(39):6058-6068.
73. Verdonck K, Gonzalez E, Van Dooren S, et al. Human T-lymphotropic virus 1: recent knowledge about an ancient infection. *Lancet Infect Dis*. 2007;7(4):266-281.
74. Araujo AQ. Update on neurological manifestations of HTLV-1 infection. *Curr Infect Dis Rep*. 2015;17(2).
75. Carpentier A, Barez PY, Hamaidia M, et al. Modes of human T cell leukemia virus type 1 transmission, replication and persistence. *Viruses*. 2015;7(7):3603-3624.
76. Manns A, Hisada M, La Grenade L, Human T. lymphotropic virus type I infection. *Lancet*. 1999;353(9168):1951-1958.
77. Dias GA, Yoshikawa GT, Koyama RV, et al. Neurological manifestations in individuals with HTLV-1-associated myelopathy/tropical spastic paraparesis in the Amazon. *Spinal Cord*. 2016;54(2):154-157.
78. Tanajura D, Castro N, Oliveira P, et al. Neurological manifestations in human T-cell lymphotropic virus type 1 (HTLV-1)-infected individuals without HTLV-1-associated myelopathy/tropical spastic paraparesis: a longitudinal cohort study. *Clin Infect Dis*. 2015;61(1):49-56.
79. Casseb J, Posada-Vergara MP, Montanheiro P, et al. T CD4+ cells count among patients co-infected with human immunodeficiency virus type 1 (HIV-1) and human T-cell leukemia virus type 1 (HTLV-1): high prevalence of tropical spastic paraparesis/HTLV-1-associated myelopathy (TSP/HAM). *Rev Inst Med Trop Sao Paulo*. 2007;49(4):231-233.
80. Casseb J, de Oliveira AC, Vergara MP, et al. Presence of tropical spastic paraparesis/human T-cell lymphotropic virus type 1-associated myelopathy (TSP/HAM)-like among HIV-1-infected patients. *J Med Virol*. 2008;80(3):392-398.

81. Nagel MA, Gilden D. Complications of varicella zoster virus reactivation. *Curr Treat Options Neurol.* 2013;15(4): 439-453.
82. Nagel MA, Gilden D. Neurological complications of varicella zoster virus reactivation. *Curr Opin Neurol.* 2014;27(3):356-360.
83. Cohrs RJ, Gilden DH, Mahalingam R. Varicella zoster virus latency, neurological disease and experimental models: an update. *Front Biosci.* 2004;9:751-762.
84. Gilden D, Nagel MA, Cohrs RJ, Mahalingam R. The variegate neurological manifestations of varicella zoster virus infection. *Curr Neurol Neurosci Rep.* 2013;13(9):374-013-0374-z.
85. Gilden DH, Beinlich BR, Rubinstien EM, et al. Varicella-zoster virus myelitis: an expanding spectrum. *Neurology.* 1994;44(10):1818-1823.
86. Orme HT, Smith AG, Nagel MA, et al. VZV spinal cord infarction identified by diffusion-weighted MRI (DWI). *Neurology.* 2007;69(4):398-400.
87. Ben-Amor S, Lammouchi T, Benslamia L, Benammou S. Post varicella zoster virus myelitis in immunocompetent patients. *Neurosciences (Riyadh).* 2011;16(2):156-158.
88. de Silva SM, Mark AS, Gilden DH, et al. Zoster myelitis: improvement with antiviral therapy in two cases. *Neurology.* 1996;47(4):929-931.
89. Centers for Disease Control and Prevention: *Fact Sheet: Incidence, Prevalence, and Cost Associated with Sexually Transmitted Infections in the United States.* Available at http://www.cdc.gov/std/stats/sti-estimates-fact-sheet-feb-2013.pdf.
90. Patton ME, Su JR, Nelson R, Weinstock H, Centers for Disease Control and Prevention. Primary and secondary syphilis: United States, 2005-2013. *MMWR Morb Mortal Wkly Rep.* 2014;63(18):402-406.
91. Centers for Disease Control and Prevention. *Fact Sheet: Syphilis and MSM (Men Who Have Sex with Men).* Available at http://www.cdc.gov/std/syphilis/STDFact-MSM-Syphilis.htm.
92. Berger JR. Neurosyphilis and the spinal cord: then and now. *J Nerv Ment Dis.* 2011;199(12):912-913.
93. Sethi S, Das A, Kakkar N, et al. Neurosyphilis in a tertiary care hospital in north India. *Indian J Med Res.* 2005;122(3):249-253.
94. Zhang YQ, Huang M, Jia XY, Zou YF, Chen D. A clinical study of new cases of parenchymal neurosyphilis: has tabes dorsalis disappeared or been missed? *J Neuropsychiatry Clin Neurosci.* 2015;27(1):e17-e21.
95. Gatchel J, Legesse B, Tayeb S, Murray E, Price B. Neurosyphilis in psychiatric practice: a case-based discussion of clinical evaluation and diagnosis. *Gen Hosp Psychiatry.* 2015;37(5):459-463.
96. Wong T, Fonseca K, Chernesky MA, et al. Canadian Public Health Laboratory Network laboratory guidelines for the diagnosis of neurosyphilis in Canada. *Can J Infect Dis Med Microbiol.* 2015;26(supplA):18A-22A.
97. Pandey S. Magnetic resonance imaging of the spinal cord in a man with tabes dorsalis. *J Spinal Cord Med.* 2011;34(6):609-611.
98. Oshita K, Saeki N, Niinai H, Hamada H, Kawamoto M. Successful treatment of tabetic lightning pain and visceral crisis with gabapentin. *J Anesth.* 2011;25(6):952.
99. Liu JT, Li XF, Xu KL, et al. Bilateral total knee arthroplasty for Charcot knees associated with tabes dorsalis. *Pain Physician.* 2014;17(6):E796-E799.
100. Lakjiri S, Mernissi FZ. Tabetic arthropathy revealing neurosyphilis: a new observation. *Pan Afr Med J.* 2014;18:198.
101. Samia M, Ezzahra AF, Khadija B, et al. Bilateral neuro-arthropathy of the ankle as a sequela of undiagnosed tabes dorsalis. *Joint Bone Spine.* 2013;80(6):664.
102. Moreau S, Lonjon G, Jameson R, Judet T, Garreau de Loubresse C. Do all Charcot spines require surgery? *Orthop Traumatol Surg Res.* 2014;100(7):779-784.
103. Fisher M, Poser CM. Syphilitic meningomyelitis. A case report. *Arch Neurol.* 1977;34(12):785.
104. Strom T, Schneck SA. Syphilitic meningomyelitis. *Neurology.* 1991;41(2 Pt 1):325-326.
105. Trecarichi EM, Di Meco E, Mazzotta V, Fantoni M. Tuberculous spondylodiscitis: epidemiology, clinical features, treatment, and outcome. *Eur Rev Med Pharmacol Sci.* 2012;16(suppl 2):58-72.
106. Chandra SP, Singh A, Goyal N, et al. Analysis of changing paradigms of management in 179 patients with spinal tuberculosis over a 12-year period and proposal of a new management algorithm. *World Neurosurg.* 2013;80(1-2):190-203.
107. Agarwal A, Kant KS, Kumar A, Shaharyar A. One-year multidrug treatment for tuberculosis of the cervical spine in children. *J Orthop Surg (Hong Kong).* 2015;23(2): 168-173.
108. Boody BS, Jenkins TJ, Maslak J, Hsu WK, Patel AA. Vertebral osteomyelitis and spinal epidural abscess: an evidence-based review. *J Spinal Disord Tech.* 2015;28(6): E316-E327.
109. Batirel A, Erdem H, Sengoz G, et al. The course of spinal tuberculosis (Pott disease): results of the multinational, multicentre Backbone-2 study. *Clin Microbiol Infect.* 2015;21(11):1008.
110. Qu JT, Jiang YQ, Xu GH, et al. Clinical characteristics and neurologic recovery of patients with cervical spinal tuberculosis: should conservative treatment be preferred? A retrospective follow-up study of 115 cases. *World Neurosurg.* 2015;83(5):700-707.
111. Schoenfeld AJ, Hayward RA. Predictive modeling for epidural abscess: what we can, can't, and should do about it. *Spine J.* 2015;15(1):102-104.
112. Ju KL, Kim SD, Melikian R, Bono CM, Harris MB. Predicting patients with concurrent noncontiguous spinal epidural abscess lesions. *Spine J.* 2015;15(1):95-101.
113. Reihsaus E, Waldbaur H, Seeling W. Spinal epidural abscess: a meta-analysis of 915 patients. *Neurosurg Rev.* 2000;23(4):175-204.
114. Alton TB, Patel AR, Bransford RJ, et al. Is there a difference in neurologic outcome in medical versus early operative management of cervical epidural abscesses? *Spine J.* 2015;15(1):10-17.
115. Kim SD, Melikian R, Ju KL, et al. Independent predictors of failure of nonoperative management of spinal epidural abscesses. *Spine J.* 2014;14(8):1673-1679.
116. Zimmerer SM, Conen A, Muller AA, et al. Spinal epidural abscess: aetiology, predisponent factors and clinical outcomes in a 4-year prospective study. *Eur Spine J.* 2011;20(12): 2228-2234.
117. Ghobrial GM, Viereck MJ, Margiotta PJ, et al. Surgical management in 40 consecutive patients with cervical spinal epidural abscesses: shifting toward circumferential treatment. *Spine.* 2015;40(17):E949-E953.
118. Schoenfeld AJ, Wahlquist TC. Mortality, complication risk, and total charges after the treatment of epidural abscess. *Spine J.* 2015;15(2):249-255.

119. Al-Hourani K, Al-Aref R, Mesfin A. Upper cervical epidural abscess in clinical practice: diagnosis and management. *Global Spine*. 2016;6(4):383-393.
120. Patel AR, Alton TB, Bransford RJ, et al. Spinal epidural abscesses: risk factors, medical versus surgical management, a retrospective review of 128 cases. *Spine J*. 2014;14(2): 326-330.
121. Stabler SP. Clinical practice. Vitamin B12 deficiency. *N Engl J Med*. 2013;368(2):149-160.
122. Ghobrial GM, Dalyai R, Flanders AE, Harrop J. Nitrous oxide myelopathy posing as spinal cord injury. *J Neurosurg Spine*. 2012;16(5):489-491.
123. Moore CE, Sherman V. Effectiveness of B vitamin supplementation following bariatric surgery: rapid increases of serum vitamin B12. *Obes Surg*. 2015; 25(4):694-699.
124. Sun HY, Lee JW, Park KS, Wi JY, Kang HS. Spine MR imaging features of subacute combined degeneration patients. *Eur Spine J*. 2014;23(5):1052-1058.
125. Jaiser SR, Winston GP. Copper deficiency myelopathy. *J Neurol*. 2010;257(6):869-881.
126. Plantone D, Primiano G, Renna R, et al. Copper deficiency myelopathy: a report of two cases. *J Spinal Cord Med*. 2015;38(4):559-562.

39

CHAPTER

Nonoperative Management of Disc and Degenerative Disorders

SECTION V

Daniel Park
Jad G. Khalil
Michael P. Planalp

Introduction

Axial neck pain is a significant and highly prevalent cause of disability. Cross-sectional, population-based surveys have demonstrated that acute and chronic neck pain permeates the population at large.[1-3] In population registries from Norway, and later corroborated in Finland,[3] Bovim and colleagues[1] showed an overall prevalence of neck pain of 34.4%, with 13.8% of these individuals reporting chronic neck pain of greater than 6 months' duration. In their evaluation of 1131 patients, Cote and colleagues[2] found that 54% of subjects had experienced significant neck pain, 5% of which was reported as highly disabling. In the acute setting, the majority of neck pain can be thought of as resulting from soft tissue sprains and muscle strain. Chronic pain, on the other hand, is more likely to be caused by a degenerative etiology.

Degeneration, or spondylosis, of the cervical spine is a descriptor applied to a wide range of cervical disorders. Pain etiology can be discogenic, radiculopathic, and myelopathic in nature, all of which usually originate with degenerative changes of the cervical disc space. Degeneration of the healthy disc can lead to subsequent bulge or herniation, leading to impingement of the neural structures adjacent to the disc. In addition to neuropathic pain, disc degeneration can lead to loss of the normal cervical alignment and collapse into kyphosis due to loss of disc height. This degenerative cascade can also lead to instability of the cervical motion segments and compensatory osteophytosis, providing another vehicle for compressive potential. Posterior neural impingement can also occur through hypertrophy of the facet joints and ligamenta flava.

These conditions can happen independently or together and may lead to axial neck pain, causing patients to seek medical attention for relief of neck pain, arm pain, weakness, or numbness. Many of these problems are self-limited; for this reason, the vast majority of patients are successfully treated nonoperatively, using a combination of established methods. Surgery is typically reserved for patients with myelopathy or severe, progressive weakness. This chapter will discuss the various nonoperative modalities focusing on the degenerative causes, particularly axial neck pain and cervical radiculopathy. We will not address the impact of myelopathy due to the surgical nature of this disorder.

General Treatment Approach

Once the diagnosis is made, a discussion must take place between the physician and patient regarding the direction of treatment. Initial treatment decisions are based upon the disease course. Fortunately, the natural history of nonmyelopathic spondylotic cervical disorders is statistically favorable. In their long-term study of 205 patients with axial neck pain, Gore et al. showed 79% improved with nonoperative care.[4] In this study, only one-third of patients reported persistent moderate to severe pain, with initial symptom severity and specific injury being the only predictors of refractory disease.

With regard to radiculopathy, results of conservative management are similar. In their 1965 study, DePalma and Subin[5] found that 75% to 90% of patients will have symptomatic improvement of radicular pain with nonoperative therapy. These data are corroborated in the classic study by Lees and Turner,[6] who found the natural history of cervical radiculopathy to be generally favorable, with only 25% of patients having persistent or worsening symptoms and no patients with radiculopathy progressing to myelopathy. It is important to note the distinction in treating cervical myelopathy, which is generally considered a surgical disorder because of the progressive nature of disease.[7] Surgery has been shown to improve prognosis in myelopathy, with better functional and neurologic outcomes versus nonoperative care.[8]

In the clinical setting, it is difficult to predict which patients suffering from axial neck pain or radiculopathy are likely to improve and which are likely to fail nonoperative measures. Because of this and because research has shown that an overwhelming proportion of patients are likely to improve with conservative management alone, nonoperative treatment is the initial approach of choice for patients with axial neck pain or radiculopathy. Surgery is reserved for patients with neurologic deficits, progressive dysfunction, or failure to improve after an appropriate course of nonoperative treatment. The definition of what constitutes an appropriate course of nonoperative treatment (in terms of duration and actual regimen) has not been standardized, however.

The rationale for initially avoiding surgery is clear, but it is more difficult to identify if nonoperative measures can actually improve the natural history. No controlled trials have compared the various nonoperative regimens (e.g., physical therapy modalities, traction, medications, manipulation, and immobilization) versus the natural history (i.e., no treatment at all). Several studies have looked at various treatment regimens and algorithms but are limited by lack of sufficient control groups to definitively compare outcomes to natural history. As a baseline, the nonoperative progression consisting of immobilization, ice, rest, nonsteroidal antiinflammatory drugs (NSAIDs), traction, postural education and strengthening, oral steroid tapers, acupuncture, and transcutaneous electrical nerve stimulation can be used. This regimen was analyzed by Lees and Turner[6] and resulted in 77% of patients having good to excellent results. Based on comparison with previously published surgical series, the authors suggested that their nonoperative outcomes were comparable to surgical outcomes and superior to the natural history of cervical radiculopathy. This interpretation is limited, however, by the absence of true controls in the surgical or natural history categories, as previously mentioned.

There are also no studies adequately assessing outcomes of surgical versus nonsurgical treatment. Saal et al. studied a group of patients divided into surgical and nonsurgical arms and concluded there were more favorable outcomes in the nonsurgical group.[9] However, valid conclusions are difficult to make from this study due to more disease severity at initial presentation in the surgical group. This study and others[4–6,9,10] have shown correlation between higher disease severity at initial presentation and failure of nonsurgical treatment; these patients may be better suited to operative intervention. There remains an unknown dividing line between patients who could benefit from conservative management and those who should be offered immediate surgery at the outset to avoid delays in delivering the ultimately needed treatment.

Regardless of whether surgical or nonsurgical treatment is selected, there are certain modifiable risks of which every patient should be made aware. Smoking is a well-documented risk factor for neck pain[11–13] and has been shown to advance degeneration of the intervertebral disc and connective tissues. Occupations requiring excessive cervical motion and overhead work may accelerate the process of disc degeneration, as can vibration caused by heavy equipment.[11,13–15] Lifestyle and occupation changes may be a necessary first step in the treatment process to prevent and alleviate symptoms.

Mechanical Treatment Modalities

From cited literature, the natural history of cervical spondylosis trends toward resolution. Therefore, the immediate goals of the physician are to control the patient's pain, minimize the disruption of the patient's life and work, and educate the patient about the problem and prognosis.

When tailoring treatment for each patient, the initial approach should be directed at pain control and the restoration of movement. Pain is usually the first complaint; patients will frequently limit their activities or even immobilize themselves in order to prevent pain exacerbation. Immobility can quickly lead to deconditioning, leading to further decreases in activity, further deconditioning, and chronic pain. It is therefore crucial to encourage participation in physical therapy to regain strength and retrain proper alignment. Table 39.1 summarizes available nonoperative treatments for cervical degenerative disorders.

Immobilization

Activity can often lead to pain exacerbation, causing a patient to decrease participation. A short course of cervical spine immobilization can be used initially to decrease local inflammation of painful joints and soft tissues around nerve roots. Immobilization may also diminish muscle spasm, and the warmth provided by wearing the collar may be therapeutic.[16] While the use of collars has theoretical benefits, there is no evidence to suggest their efficacy. Their use has neither limited the duration or severity of radiculopathy[17] nor decreased the degree or duration of neck pain after whiplash injury.[18]

Since their use has not been statistically delineated, we believe that the use of collars should be reserved to the short term, not to exceed 2 weeks. Prolonged immobilization should be avoided to prevent deconditioning and atrophy of the cervical musculature. Nighttime collar wear may be helpful by maintaining proper cervical alignment during the entire night and protecting the discs from abnormal loads associated with poor posture while the patient is not in control.

Temperature Therapy

As mentioned, heat from a cervical collar has been shown to provide subjective therapeutic benefits, but cold therapy can also relieve discomfort due to pain and spasm. In the acute period, inflammatory changes may be exacerbated by external heat sources and should be avoided in favor of cryotherapy. After the acute pain period has started to wane and motion has started to return, heat may see added benefit. These measures can generally be tried by the patient at home and do not require the attention of a physician unless they are used directly to facilitate an active rehabilitation program.

Passive Modalities

Massage, ultrasound, and iontophoresis all have failed to be of proven long-term efficacy.[19] Other passive modalities that require no effort on the part of the patient may also be of limited value because the patient is not an active participant in his or her own recovery.

Traction

In the literature, traction has not proven to show any long-term benefit.[20–23] However, patient reports suggest it continues to be a

TABLE 39.1 Nonoperative Modalities for Treatment of Cervical Disc and Degenerative Disorders

Modality	Pros	Cons
Cervical collars	Immobilization may decrease inflammation and muscle spasm.	Muscle atrophy from prolonged use.
Ice or heat	Ice may relieve acute pain and spasm; heat beneficial when regaining motion.	Heat may exacerbate pain in acute period.
Traction	With neck in flexion, may relieve foraminal compression.	Avoid in myelopathic patients; if neck extended, may worsen compression of narrowed foramen.
NSAIDs	Safe, cost-effective method to decrease inflammation.	Gastrointestinal side effects, cardiovascular risks with COX-2 inhibitors.
Narcotics	Rapid pain relief in acute period.	Constipation, sedation, depression, and potential for abuse.
Corticosteroids	May decrease radicular pain acutely.	Avascular necrosis, increased blood glucose, unproven long-term benefits.
Muscle relaxants	Acute relief of muscle spasms.	Sedation, fatigue, abuse potential, limits participation in rehabilitation.
Exercise and physical therapy	Well tolerated, aerobic conditioning.	No long-term pain benefits shown, forceful passive range of motion may lead to further injury and increased pain.
Cervical manipulation	Some anecdotal reports of relief.	No objective evidence of improvement in pain; rare potential complications, including myelopathy, spinal cord injury, vascular injury.
Cervical steroid injections	Antiinflammatory effect, interruption of nociceptive input/sympathetic blockade, mechanical disruption of adhesions.	Rare complications include dural puncture, meningitis, epidural abscess, intraocular hemorrhage, epidural hematoma, adrenocortical suppression, paralysis.

COX-2, cyclooxygenase-2; NSAIDs, nonsteroidal antiinflammatory drugs.

home therapy and is said to provide intermittent symptom relief for patients with axial neck pain or radiculopathy. The presence of myelopathy is a contraindication to traction, as it can put the spinal cord under stretch and cause further damage. If traction is to be employed at home, care should be taken to explain the need for a flexion-type moment to expand the available space for the nervous structures. Extension can increase the stenosis in an already compromised neural foramen.

Pharmacotherapy

The following medications are among the most frequently used drugs to combat cervical disc disease.[24]

Nonsteroidal Antiinflammatory Drugs

NSAIDs are the most common intervention prescribed for nonmalignant chronic pain in the United States[25] and they should be considered first-line pharmacotherapy for the patient who presents with cervical spondylosis and radiculopathy. In a retrospective review of patients with neck pain and other disorders from 2000 to 2014, Wong[26] found evidence to suggest that NSAID use is more effective than placebo, despite finding no increased benefit in treating low back pain. The mechanism of action aims to decrease prostaglandin synthesis, thereby decreasing the inflammatory response. It also has analgesic properties.

There are many drugs currently on the market that are over the counter and possess safe side effect profiles, but there are risks associated with long-term use, including liver, cardiac, kidney, and gastrointestinal problems. The low cost and relative effectiveness of these drugs make them an ideal first-line agent. Most over-the-counter NSAIDs inhibit cyclooxygenase-1 (COX-1) and COX-2. There are now a range of selective COX-2 inhibitors that avoid the side effects associated with inhibiting the COX-1 enzyme, including gastrointestinal problems and platelet dysfunction. However, selective COX-2 inhibitors have not proven to be any more effective than their nonselective relatives in controlled trials of osteoarthritis.[27–29] Selective inhibitors are also associated with higher cost and potential cardiovascular complications.[30]

Oral Corticosteroids

Much like NSAIDs, corticosteroids are utilized for their antiinflammatory properties. Unlike NSAIDs, however, corticosteroids possess no analgesic properties. Used systemically, corticosteroids are often administered to patients with acute neck or arm pain.[24] Oral tapers are most commonly used with good anecdotal results but little clinical data. Theoretically, their antiinflammatory properties should decrease any swelling surrounding impinged nerve roots, and may diminish radicular pain. It is thought they are more effective at treating radicular arm pain than axial pain, but no long-term benefit in altering the natural history has been shown. The side effect profile can include immunocompromise, metabolic derangement, and avascular necrosis of the femoral and humeral head. Because of these rare but significant complications, corticosteroids should be used judiciously. They may be contraindicated in patients with severe diabetes because of effects on blood glucose, and patients being administered steroids need to be counseled appropriately.

Opioids

Opioid analgesics should be used with care in the patient with axial neck pain. There is a role for their use in the acute setting of pain exacerbation, but due to their addictive and tolerance-building properties they should not be used by the spine surgeon to manage chronic neck pain. Opioids are best reserved for the acute setting as breakthrough treatment to supplement NSAIDs or in patients who cannot tolerate NSAIDs. Once an acute exacerbation of pain is controlled, weaning should immediately commence.

Opioid medications are one of the most studied drug classes, and their side effects are well established. Constipation, sedation, depressant qualities, abuse potential, and the tendency to develop tolerance all limit their effective use. As patients develop more tolerance to their current opioid level, the dosage will need to increase in order to continue effectiveness. Extended-release opioids provide a more even blood level for longer periods, but the use of these medications should be judicious. In practice, the spine surgeon should work closely with a pain management specialist to manage patients requiring such regimens. A multidisciplinary pain program should also include a psychological evaluation and emotional support, while seeking to decrease the patient's pain level and teaching the patient to deal with unresolved pain.

Neuropathic Pain

Amitriptyline is an antidepressant commonly used for patients with cervical disc disease.[24] Its benefit is multifactorial in that it is able to treat depression, sleeplessness, and pain, all of which can be associated with chronic neck pain. While the mechanism is currently not fully understood, amitriptyline has shown some analgesic benefit in a placebo-controlled trial of lower back pain and lumbar radiculopathy.[31] There is currently no replicative study in the cervical spine, but extrapolation may be possible.

Gabapentin is an anticonvulsant medication frequently used to treat radicular pain. While the mechanism has not been fully described, it is an analog of the γ-aminobutyric acid (GABA) neurotransmitter and is currently Food and Drug Administration (FDA) approved to treat neuropathic pain. Robertson et al. found gabapentin to have greater efficacy in pain reduction compared to placebo in patients with neuropathic pain due to sciatica.[32] Reported side effects were minimal and included dizziness, somnolence, chest pain, dry mouth, constipation, headache, and peripheral edema.

Both gabapentin and amitriptyline have a time lag of several weeks before they show therapeutic benefit. There are clear uses elsewhere in the body, but limited research related to the cervical spine to clearly identify their role in treatment.

Muscle Relaxants

Muscular spasm can be a significant component associated with degenerative cervical disease, and antispasmodic medications are commonly prescribed. Similar to opioids, muscle relaxants tend to cause sedation and fatigue, and they are increasingly being recognized for their abuse potential. Their depressive effect may be more pronounced when administered simultaneously with opioids. Muscle relaxants should only be used as short-term treatment because they may impair the patient's ability to participate in rehabilitation.

Exercise and Physical Therapy

Over the long-term course of disease, there is inadequate data to show if physical therapy can alter the natural history of cervical radiculopathy.[33,34] Several short-term studies have shown good results, however, when compared to surgical groups. Enqquist et al.[35] conducted a prospective randomized trial looking at patients with cervical radiculopathy treated with anterior cervical decompression and fusion with physiotherapy compared to physiotherapy alone. The surgical group resulted in more rapid pain improvement in the first postoperative year, but by the conclusion of the study at 2-year follow-up, the differences between groups decreased. Peolsson et al.[36] found similar results while evaluating physical function after 2-year follow up. The conclusion from these studies is that a structured physiotherapy program should be tried on all patients and those who fail should be counseled regarding surgery.

In the acute pain period, patients may have difficulty participating in aggressive therapy regimens. A graduated program of physical therapy is commonly prescribed for these patients, starting with initial passive modalities and progressing to active modalities in order to regain strength lost during any immobilization. There has not been any proven benefit from passive modalities in the long term,[37] but they are well tolerated short term when patients are too symptomatic to participate in an active therapy regimen. Eventually, when the acute pain resolves, a program of isometric exercises is started allowing strengthening without potentially painful cervical motion. This program can help regain strength lost due to intentional or unintentional immobilization, and also teach proper posture and biomechanics to prevent further harm. Concern does exist that isometric contraction of the cervical musculature can cause increased intervertebral disc loading force, exacerbating pain, but often the benefit outweighs this theoretical disadvantage. In general, passive modalities pose greater risk than active exercises and should be limited in their use. At the extremes of motion, patients are not able to protect themselves and forcible motion can result in worsening pain and loss of motion.

After the initial passive and isometric phase, active range of motion and resistance exercises are typically added as tolerated by the patient. An expanded program addressing weaknesses of the entire body, but focusing on the neck and shoulder girdle,[34] may be instituted to improve biomechanics and posture. For a patient with cervical disc disease, special attention should be given to the scapular stabilization muscles, including the trapezius, deltoids, latissimus dorsi, and rhomboids. Aerobic conditioning may also be helpful in relieving symptoms but is ideally limited to low-impact activities, such as walking, cycling, swimming, and use of elliptical trainers.

Once the patient has gained familiarity with the exercises, the program will shift from recovery to prevention in a long-term home exercise regimen. This will include simple exercises that can be performed easily on a daily basis with inexpensive equipment found at home.

Manipulation

There are no quality data to suggest clinical effectiveness of manipulative therapy on the cervical spine[38] and its efficacy for the treatment of cervical radiculopathy has not been established.[39–42] Further, although there are many theories, the mechanisms of action for manipulation are poorly understood.[43] There is some evidence that cervical manipulation can provide some short-term relief from cervicogenic headaches and neck pain[39] but no data to suggest long-term effectiveness.

There are, however, several rare and potentially catastrophic complications of cervical manipulation, including radiculopathy, myelopathy, spinal cord injury, and vascular injury.[41] The complication rate is admittedly small, at 5 to 10 per 10 million manipulations.[39] Thomas[44] showed the risk of carotid artery dissection and vertebral artery dissection with manipulative therapy to be less than the risk in the general population. Nevertheless, in the absence of objective evidence showing any proven benefit and given the known risks (albeit low probability), cervical manipulation is not routinely recommended for patients with cervical radiculopathy and should be strongly avoided in patients with known myelopathy.

As with all therapeutic interventions, the patient should be made aware of any potential complications associated with intervention. If manipulation is employed, the clinician should be able to identify patients at risk for injury and be able to recognize any suspicious symptoms. Absolute contraindications for spinal manipulation include vertebral fracture or dislocation, infection, malignancy, spondylolisthesis, myelopathy, vertebral hypermobility, Marfan and Ehlers-Danlos syndromes, osteoporosis, spondyloarthropathies, severe diabetes mellitus, anticoagulation therapy, and objective signs of spinal nerve root compromise.[38] A radiographic screen for cervical instability should be performed prior to manipulative therapy.

Injections

According to current literature, steroid injections into the cervical spine can be expected to yield 50% to 80% good to excellent results in patients with cervical radiculopathy. However, unlike the lumbar spine, there is a paucity of studies to adequately evaluate the true efficacy of cervical injections. With current research, it is unclear how to compare with either the natural history of radiculopathy or surgical management. A possible reason for the lack of data for cervical injections is the increased risk of performing them relative to lumbar injections. Nonetheless, the theoretical benefits are the same, and since disease pathophysiology of disc degeneration and radiculopathy is similar in the lumbar and cervical spine, benefit should likewise be found in the cervical spine. The effects of steroids are multifactorial: an antiinflammatory effect, with inhibition of prostaglandin synthesis; interruption of nociceptive input from somatic nerves; a direct membrane-stabilizing effect; blockade of neuropeptide synthesis; sympathetic blockade; the mechanical effect of the injectant breaking up epidural adhesions; and blockade of C fiber activity in the dorsal root ganglion.

Epidural Injections

Injections of steroid into the epidural space are a mainstay of management for lumbar degenerative disease. In the cervical spine, however, there is little well-designed literature to adequately judge clinical effectiveness. In their prospective analysis of 42 patients, Stav et al.[45] injected methylprednisolone into either the epidural space or the posterior cervical musculature. There was a statistically significant difference in outcomes at 1 week, with the epidural group reporting 76% good to excellent results using the visual analog scale versus 36% in the musculature group. The difference in groups continued to the 1-year follow-up (68% good to excellent results for epidural injections vs. 12% for muscle injections).

In a retrospective analysis, Cicala and colleagues[46] found 56% to 80% good to excellent results at 6 months after C7–T1 epidural steroid injections; but their patient population was mostly a multitude of neck pain instead of radiculopathy. They also had no control group, making it virtually impossible to find a difference between the injection group and the natural history of disease in these patients. A separate investigation by Rowlingson and Kirschenbaum[47] looked at 25 patients with a clinical diagnosis of radiculopathy. Their analysis showed 64% good to excellent results at 15 months after C6–C7 or C7–T1 epidural steroid injections—but, again, without a control group. Finally, Ferrante and colleagues[48] reviewed 100 patient charts in search of predictors of good outcomes with cervical epidural steroid injection. Age greater than 50 years with radicular pain had better outcomes at 13.5 months unless radiculopathy was due to disc herniation.

Selective Nerve Root Blocks

A variant of epidural steroid injections, selective nerve root blocks instead bathe a specific nerve root in steroid injectant. These injections can be considered more localized, as they can direct a higher concentration of steroid solely at the inciting nerve rather than the entire cord. From a safety standpoint, they also decrease the risk of direct cord injury, as they are targeting a root instead. Retrospectively, Slipman and colleagues[49] found 60% good to excellent results at 21 months after injection. Vallee and colleagues[50] found 50% good to excellent results at 12 months in their prospective evaluation.

Complications and Efficacy

Like surgery, cervical injection therapies are an invasive measure and there are well-documented complications that can result, including infection (1–2%), neurologic deterioration, intravascular injections (7.9–11.6%), cerebrospinal fluid fistulas (0.4–6%), persistent positional headaches (28%), arachnoiditis (6–16%), hydrocephalus, air embolism, urinary retention, allergic reactions, stroke, blindness, hematomas, seizures, and death.[51]

There is insufficient literature to date to definitively establish a long-term benefit of cervical injections when compared to the natural history of disease. Successful treatment by injections is often defined by transient pain relief, but it is difficult to differentiate between treatment success and the normal self-limited course of disease. Recent evidence has suggested there may be little long-term difference between injection of steroid versus saline.[52,53] In addition, multiple studies have followed patients over 1- to 2-year intervals after treatment with epidural methylprednisolone and determined the treatment did not result in functional benefit or decrease the need for eventual surgery.[54,55] Epstein[51] concluded in a 2013 review that although cervical injections may offer transient pain relief in this patient population, the plethora of risks outweighs the benefits. In practice, the risks of injection should not be taken lightly; thus, a discussion of the risks and benefits needs to take place with the patient.

If injection therapy is pursued, there are several strategies to help minimize the incidence of complications. Utilizing an interlaminar approach at C6–C7 or C7–T1 can be safer, because the epidural space is typically larger there. Epidural injections should also be avoided at the level of a large herniated disc, where the cord may be displaced more posteriorly into the epidural space and preclude safe needle entry. If a dural puncture does occur during the procedure, the injection should be aborted because of a conduit that now connects the spinal and epidural spaces. There is potential neurotoxicity with certain injection preparations (e.g., Depo-Medrol formulation of methylprednisolone acetate, which contains ethylene glycol, a substance associated with arachnoiditis). Finally, injection can be performed with only light sedation so that the patient can report pain and neuropathic symptoms during the procedure. Selective root blocks are theoretically safer than epidural injections, although both have relatively few reported complications.

Diagnostic Injections

Theoretically, if injection of local anesthetic with or without steroid gets rid of a patient's pain, this finding can confirm the anatomic location of the patient's symptoms. The targeted use of selective root blocks should therefore provide confirmatory diagnostic information for preoperative planning. Unfortunately, there is only limited evidence suggesting validity of this notion. Sasso et al.[56] found they could accurately identify radiculopathy by performing selective nerve root injections. They looked at 101 patients in which MRI findings were equivocal, multilevel, or do not agree with the patient's symptoms and found that a negative diagnostic injection was superior in predicting the absence of an offending lesion.

Biotechnology and Future Treatment Strategies

Over the last 20 years, the largest area of progress has been with regard to disc biology and potential targets of pharmaceutical therapy. But while we have seen a veritable explosion of literature, there is still a relative paucity of data to begin implementing these theoretical treatments into clinical practice.

Many inflammatory cytokines and growth factors have been shown to be relevant to the biology of intervertebral disc degeneration, including interleukin (IL)1-β, IL-6, IL-8, transforming growth factor β, bone morphogenetic protein 7/osteogenic protein 1, bone morphogenetic protein 2, prostaglandin E_2, nitric oxide, platelet-derived growth factor, and insulin growth factor 1. These molecules will be the targets of future research. By increasing the action of anabolic factors and decreasing the action of catabolic factors, we can achieve a net healing vector to the intervertebral disc space. How we deliver the message will come in several forms.

Medications

Antiinflammatory medications are designed to decrease production or action of some of these molecules. Several NSAIDs can inhibit the prostaglandin family, but research into the specific roles of these other proinflammatory molecules is in its relative infancy and directed medications acting on growth factors are yet to be trialed.

Direct Injection

Whether a single growth factor is injected or a combination of many, the goal will be to change the balance of catabolism to anabolism. Goni and collegues[57] ran a pilot study comparing the epidural perineural injection of methylprednisolone against autologous conditioned serum. Autologous conditioned serum is known to have high quantities of IL-1 receptor antagonist, and since IL-1 is thought to play a part in pain generation of radiculopathy, they hypothesized that injection of a local antagonist might reduce the symptoms of cervical radiculopathy. Their trial was small, with only 40 randomized patients, but showed similar effectiveness to epidural perineural injection of steroid, while effecting longer symptom relief.

Platelet-rich plasma is another preparation containing many growth factors in a high concentration after it is spun down from a patient's blood. Currently, it is used to stimulate wound healing, and is being evaluated in other areas of orthopaedics as well to stimulate cell proliferation and prostaglandin and collagen synthesis.[58] A limitation to direct injection of growth factors is the relatively short-term effectiveness of the drug. Degradation and diffusion can limit the therapeutic effect. Also, given that the intervertebral disc is the largest avascular tissue in the body, results of local injection may be short-lived without a method of increased nutrient delivery.[59]

Gene Therapy

As the disc tissue degenerates, growth factors may need to be present for an extended exposure to net a positive effect. Direct injection may last in the short term of weeks to months, but definitive change may need a constant replenishment of growth factors to the desired tissue. In this application, gene therapy can be used to transfer the genetic material to encode and produce a protein into a target cell that can then be implanted or injected in the local disc environment. There are already several ongoing human studies that are trying to replicate previous data built with animal models.[60,61]

Cell-Based Therapies

Growth factors work at the level of the microenvironment, stimulating their effect on individual cells. With significant degeneration, the entire disc macroenvironment can be altered. The tissue architecture is such that nutrient supply is diminished, and a positive feedback loop exists whereby degeneration leads to more degeneration. Cell-based therapies aim to resupply cells and extracellular matrix to the disc space. At the time of this publication, there are several stem cell–based studies currently ongoing.[62,63] Cellular senescence is thought to play a pivotal role in age-related degenerative changes of the intervertebral disc.[64,65] In the lumbar spine, several studies looking at reimplantation of disc tissue have been done, leading to excitement regarding the future prospects of cellular therapy. Multipotent stem cells[66-68] and platelet-rich plasma[69] are gaining research support in other areas of orthopaedics, and now are an active area of research for regenerating cellularity and engendering repair within the degenerated nucleus pulposus. Human studies are still needed to better clarify usefulness of treatments like these.

Summary

The natural history of cervical disc and degenerative disorders is statistically a favorable one. For this reason, nonoperative treatment is the initial recommendation for patients without neurologic deficit. While there is no standardized algorithm by which clinicians may progress, several modalities have shown short-term benefit in reducing pain. However, due to a lack of quality literature, none of the commonly used nonoperative therapies has been proven to alter the long-term course of disease. In a retrospective literature review of conservative treatment of radiculopathy and myelopathy between 1953 and 2013, Alentado and colleagues[70] found limited evidence supporting an optimal period of nonsurgical management prior to operative intervention. Their analysis of outcomes and cost-effectiveness supported operative intervention between 4 and 8 weeks of symptom onset, but evidence-based conclusions could not be made, and further research must be done. Similarly, there are no high-level studies comparing operative to nonoperative treatment, but there are smaller studies that have shown benefit to surgical intervention for radicular and myelopathic symptoms within 3 months of symptom onset. Alvin[71] reviewed all published economic data through January 2014 evaluating cost-effectiveness of surgical interventions for degenerative cervical diseases. There is currently no consensus as to the cost-effectiveness of nonoperative versus operative intervention for mild cervical myelopathy and radiculopathy; further research is needed to elucidate the optimal treatment algorithm. Until such studies are available, empirical and anecdotal evidence must be used.

In the absence of proven benefit, treatments should be used only if they are associated with a reasonably low level of risk. A program of gradual, progressive nonoperative treatment seems most reasonable, adding therapies in a stepwise fashion as failure of symptoms to resolve dictates. Short-term bracing and rest, NSAIDs, oral corticosteroid taper, short-term narcotics, physical therapy, and corticosteroid injections can be used judiciously by the treating physician. In patients with myelopathy, progressive or severe neurologic dysfunction, or failure to improve despite time and nonoperative treatment, surgical management should be discussed.

KEY REFERENCES

1. Lees F, Turner JWA. Natural history and prognosis of cervical spondylosis. *BMJ*. 1963;2:1607-1610.
   In this classic study, the natural history of cervical radiculopathy was shown to be generally favorable.
2. Gore D, Sepic S, Gardner G, et al. Neck pain: a long term follow-up of 205 patients. *Spine*. 1987;12:1-5.
   In this study of 205 patients with axial neck pain and an average follow-up of 15.5 years, 79% noted improvement with nonoperative care, 43% reported a pain-free state, and 32% continued to complain of moderate to severe persistent pain. The severity of the symptoms at initial presentation and a history of a specific injury were suggestive of long-term persistent symptoms.
3. Dillin W, Uppal GS. Analysis of medications used in the treatment of cervical disc degeneration. *Orthop Clin North Am*. 1992;23:421-433.
   This article presents an analysis of commonly used medications for the treatment of cervical disc disease.
4. Tan JC, Nordin M. Role of physical therapy in the treatment of cervical disk disease. *Orthop Clin North Am*. 1992;23:435-449.
   This study highlights the role of physical therapy and suggests that it is best for patients to be involved in a whole-body exercise program, with special attention to the shoulder girdle and neck musculature.
5. Sasso RC, Macadaeg K, Nordmann D, et al. Selective nerve root injections can predict surgical outcome for lumbar and cervical radiculopathy: comparison to magnetic resonance imaging. *J Spinal Disord Tech*. 2005;18:471-478.
   This analysis of 101 patients found that a diagnostic selective nerve root injection could safely and accurately discern the presence or absence of cervical radiculopathy. The investigators noted that in cases in which MRI findings are equivocal, multilevel, or do not agree with the patient's symptoms, the result of a negative diagnostic injection becomes superior in predicting the absence of an offending lesion.
6. Kepler CK, Anderson DG, Tannoury C, et al. Intervertebral disk degeneration and emerging biologic treatments. *J Am Acad Orthop Surg*. 2011;19:543-553.
   This article reviews the current state of future biologic treatments for spine degenerative disorders.

REFERENCES

1. Bovim G, Schrader H, Sand T. Neck pain in the general population. *Spine*. 1994;19:1307-1309.
2. Cote P, Cassidy J, Carroll L. The factors associated with neck pain and its related disability in the Saskatchewan population. *Spine*. 2000;25:1109-1117.
3. Makela M, Heliovara M, Sievers K, et al. Prevalence, determinants and consequences of chronic neck pain in Finland. *Am J Epidemiol*. 1991;134:1356-1367.

4. Gore D, Sepic S, Gardner G, et al. Neck pain: a long term follow-up of 205 patients. *Spine*. 1987;12:1-5.
5. DePalma AF, Subin DK. Study of the cervical syndrome. *Clin Orthop Relat Res*. 1965;38:135-142.
6. Lees F, Turner JWA. Natural history and prognosis of cervical spondylosis. *BMJ*. 1963;2:1607-1610.
7. Nurick S. The natural history and the results of surgical treatment of the spinal cord disorder associated with cervical spondylosis. *Brain*. 1972;95:101-108.
8. Sampath P, Bendebba M, Davis JD, et al. Outcome of patients treated for cervical myelopathy: a prospective, multi-center study with independent clinical review. *Spine*. 2000;25: 670-676.
9. Saal JS, Saal JA, Yurth EF. Nonoperative management of herniated cervical intervertebral disc with radiculopathy. *Spine*. 1996;21:1877-1883.
10. Heckmann JG, Lang CJ, Zobelein I, et al. Herniated cervical intervertebral discs with radiculopathy: an outcome study of conservatively or surgically treated patients. *J Spinal Disord*. 1999;12:396-401.
11. Frymoyer JL, Pope M, Constanza ML, et al. Epidemiologic studies of low back pain. *Spine*. 1980;5:419-423.
12. Holmes S, Nachemson A. Nutrition of the intervertebral disc: acute effects of cigarette smoking: an experimental animal study. *Int J Microcirc Clin Exp*. 1985;3:406.
13. Kelsey J, Githens P, O'Connor T, et al. Acute prolapsed lumbar intervertebral disc: an epidemiologic study with special reference to driving automobiles and cigarette smoking. *Spine*. 1984;9:608-613.
14. Anderson G. Epidemiologic aspects of low back pain in industry. *Spine*. 1981;6:53-60.
15. Kelsey J, Githens P, White A, et al. An epidemiologic study of lifting and twisting on the job and risk for acute prolapsed lumbar intervertebral disc. *J Orthop Res*. 1984;2:61-66.
16. Kurz LT. Cervical disc disease: nonoperative treatment. In: Herkowitz HN, Rothman RH, Simeone FA, eds. *Rothman-Simeone The Spine*. 4th ed. Philadelphia: WB Saunders; 1999:496.
17. Naylor JR, Mulley GP. Surgical collars: a survey of their prescription and use. *Br J Rheumatol*. 1991;30:282-284.
18. Gennis P, Miller L, Gallagher EJ, et al. The effect of soft cervical collars on persistent neck pain in patients with whiplash injury. *Acad Emerg Med*. 1996;3:568-573.
19. Philadelphia Panel evidence-based clinical practice guidelines on selected rehabilitation interventions for neck pain. *Phys Ther*. 2001;18:1701-1717.
20. Pain in the neck and arm: a multicentre trial of the effects of physiotherapy, arranged by the British Association of Physical Medicine. *BMJ*. 1966;5482:253-258.
21. Moeti P, Marchetti G. Clinical outcome from mechanical intermittent cervical traction for the treatment of cervical radiculopathy: a case series. *J Orthop Sports Phys Ther*. 2001; 31:207-213.
22. Moeti P, Marchetti G. Erratum: clinical outcome from mechanical intermittent cervical traction for the treatment of cervical radiculopathy: a case series. *J Orthop Sports Phys Ther*. 2001;31:538.
23. Swezey RL, Swezey AM, Warner K. Efficacy of home cervical traction therapy. *Am J Phys Med Rehabil*. 1999;78:30-32.
24. Dillin W, Uppal GS. Analysis of medications used in the treatment of cervical disc degeneration. *Orthop Clin North Am*. 1992;23:421-433.
25. Rasu RS, Vouthy K, Crowl AN, et al. Cost of pain medication to treat adult patients with nonmalignant chronic pain in the United States. *J Manag Care Pharm*. 2014;20(9):921-928.
26. Wong JJ, Cote P, Ameis A, et al. Are non-steroidal anti-inflammatory drugs effective for the management of neck pain and associated disorders, whiplash-associated disorders, or non-specific low back pain? A systematic review of systematic reviews by the Ontario Protocol for Traffic Injury Management (OPTIMa) Collaboration. *Eur Spine J*. 2016;25(1):34-61.
27. Bensen WG. Antiinflammatory and analgesic efficacy of COX-2 specific inhibition: from investigational trials to clinical experience. *J Rheumatol Suppl*. 2000;60:17-24.
28. Bensen WG, Zhao SZ, Burke TA, et al. Upper gastrointestinal tolerability of celecoxib, a COX-2 specific inhibitor, compared to naproxen and placebo. *J Rheumatol*. 2000;27:1876-1883.
29. Day R, Morrison B, Luza A, et al. A randomized trial of the efficacy and tolerability of the COX-2 inhibitor rofecoxib vs ibuprofen in patients with osteoarthritis. Rofecoxib/Ibuprofen Comparator Study Group. *Arch Intern Med*. 2000;160: 1781-1787.
30. Graham DJ, Campen D, Hui R, et al. Risk of acute myocardial infarction and sudden cardiac death in patients treated with cyclo-oxygenase 2 selective and non-selective non-steroidal anti-inflammatory drugs: nested case-control study. *Lancet*. 2005;365:475-481.
31. Atkinson JH, Slater MA, Williams RA, et al. A placebo-controlled randomized clinical trial of nortriptyline for chronic low back pain. *Pain*. 1998;76:287-296.
32. Robertson K, Marshman LA, Plummer D. Pregabalin and gabapentin for treatment of sciatica. *J Clin Neurosci*. 2016; 26:1-7.
33. Levine MJ, Albert TJ, Smith MD. Cervical radiculopathy: diagnosis and nonoperative management. *J Am Acad Orthop Surg*. 1996;4:305-316.
34. Tan JC, Nordin M. Role of physical therapy in the treatment of cervical disk disease. *Orthop Clin North Am*. 1992;23:435-449.
35. Enqquist M, Lofgren H, Oberg B, et al. Surgery versus nonsurgical treatment of cervical radiculopathy: a prospective, randomized study comparing surgery plus physiotherapy with physiotherapy alone with a 2-year follow-up. *Spine*. 2013;38(20):1715-1722.
36. Peolsson A, Soderlund A, Enqquist M, et al. Physical function outcome in cervical radiculopathy patients after physiotherapy alone compared with anterior surgery followed by physiotherapy: a prospective randomized study with a 2-year follow-up. *Spine*. 2013;38(4):300-307.
37. Santiesteban AJ. The role of physical agents in the treatment of spine pain. *Clin Orthop Relat Res*. 1983;24-30.
38. LaBan MM, Taylor RS. Manipulation: an objective analysis of the literature. *Orthop Clin North Am*. 1992;23:451-459.
39. Haldeman S, Kohlbeck FJ, McGregor M. Unpredictability of cerebrovascular ischemia associated with cervical spine manipulation therapy: a review of sixty-four cases after cervical spine manipulation. *Spine*. 2002;27:49-55.
40. Stevinson C, Honan W, Cooke B, et al. Neurological complications of cervical spine manipulation. *J R Soc Med*. 2001;94:107-110.
41. Schellhas KP, Latchaw RE, Wendling LR, et al. Vertebrobasilar injuries following cervical manipulation. *JAMA*. 1980;244:1450-1453.
42. Wei X, Wang S, Li J, et al. Complementary and alternative medicine for the management of cervical radiculopathy:

an overview of systematic reviews. *Evid Based Complement Alternat Med*. 2015;2015:793649.
43. Pickar JG. Neurophysiological effects of spinal manipulation. *Spine J*. 2002;2:357-371.
44. Thomas LC. Cervical arterial dissection: an overview and implications for manipulative therapy practice. *Man Ther*. 2016;21:2-9.
45. Stav A, Ovadia L, Sternberg A, et al. Cervical epidural steroid injection for cervicobrachialgia. *Acta Anaesthesiol Scand*. 1993;37:562-566.
46. Cicala RS, Thoni K, Angel JJ. Long-term results of cervical epidural steroid injections. *Clin J Pain*. 1989;5:143-145.
47. Rowlingson JC, Kirschenbaum LP. Epidural analgesic techniques in the management of cervical pain. *Anesth Analg*. 1986;65:938-942.
48. Ferrante FM, Wilson SP, Iacobo C, et al. Clinical classification as a predictor of therapeutic outcome after cervical epidural steroid injection. *Spine*. 1993;18:730-736.
49. Slipman CW, Lipetz JS, Plastaras CT, et al. Therapeutic zygapophyseal joint injections for headaches emanating from the C2-3 joint. *Am J Phys Med Rehabil*. 2001;80:182-188.
50. Vallee JN, Feydy A, Carlier RY, et al. Chronic cervical radiculopathy: lateral-approach periradicular corticosteroid injection. *Radiology*. 2001;218:886-892.
51. Epstein NE. The risks of epidural and transforaminal steroid injections in the spine: commentary and a comprehensive review of the literature. *Surg Neurol Int*. 2013;4(2):S74-S93.
52. Valat JP, Giraudeau B, Rozenberg S, et al. Epidural corticosteroid injections for sciatica: a randomized, double blind controlled clinical trial. *Ann Rheum Dis*. 2003;62(7):639-643.
53. Anderberg L, Annertz M, Persson L, et al. Transforaminal steroid injections for the treatment of cervical radiculopathy: a prospective and randomized study. *Eur Spine J*. 2007;16(3):321-328.
54. Carette S, Leclair R, Marcoux S, et al. Epidural corticosteroid injections for sciatica due to herniated nucleus pulposus. *N Engl J Med*. 1997;336(23):1634-1640.
55. Arden NK, Price C, Reading I, et al. A multicentre randomized controlled trial of epidural corticosteroid injections for sciatica: the WEST study. *Rheumatology (Oxford)*. 2005;44(11):1399-1406.
56. Sasso RC, Macadaeg K, Nordmann D, et al. Selective nerve root injections can predict surgical outcome for lumbar and cervical radiculopathy: comparison to magnetic resonance imaging. *J Spinal Disord Tech*. 2005;18:471-478.
57. Goni VG, Jhala SS, Gopinathan NR, et al. Efficacy of epidural perineural injection of autologous conditioned serum in unilateral cervical radiculopathy. *Spine*. 2015;40:E915-E921.
58. Akeda K, An HS, Pichika R, et al. Platelet-rich plasma (PRP) stimulates the extracellular matrix metabolism of porcine nucleus pulposus and annulus fibrosus cells cultured in alginate beads. *Spine*. 2006;31:959-966.
59. Park DK, Ellman MB, Singh K, An HS. The future: disc regeneration and other technologies. In: Bridwell K, Kulko T, eds. *The Textbook of Spinal Surgery*. 3rd ed. 2011.
60. Moon SH, Gilbertson LG, Nishida K, et al. Human intervertebral disc cells are genetically modifiable by adenovirus-mediated gene transfer: implications for clinical management of intervertebral disc disorders. *Spine*. 2000;25:2573-2579.
61. Moon SH, Nishida K, Gilbertson L, et al.: *Responsiveness of human intervertebral disc cells to adenovirus-mediated TGF-β1 cDNA transfer in 2D and 3D culture system: comparison with exogenous TGF-β1 treatment*. In Proceedings of the International Society for the Study of the Lumbar Spine. Adelaide, Australia, 2000.
62. Henriksson HB, Svanvik T, Jonsson M, et al. Transplantation of human mesenchymal stems cells into intervertebral discs in a xenogeneic porcine model. *Spine*. 2009;34:141-148.
63. Orozco L, Soler R, Morera C, et al. Intervertebral disc repair by autologous mesenchymal bone marrow cells: a pilot study. *Transplantation*. 2011;92:822-828.
64. Kepler CK, Anderson DG, Tannoury C, et al. Intervertebral disk degeneration and emerging biologic treatments. *J Am Acad Orthop Surg*. 2011;19:543-553.
65. Le Maitre CL, Freemont AJ, Hoyland JA. Accelerated cellular senescence in degenerate intervertebral discs: a possible role in the pathogenesis of intervertebral disc degeneration. *Arthritis Res Ther*. 2007;9(3):R45.
66. Risbud MV, Albert TJ, Guttapalli A, et al. Differentiation of mesenchymal stem cells towards a nucleus pulposus-like phenotype in vitro: implications for cell-based transplantation therapy. *Spine*. 2004;29(23):2627-2632.
67. Zhang YG, Guo X, Xu P, et al. Bone mesenchymal stem cells transplanted into rabbit intervertebral discs can increase proteoglycans. *Clin Orthop Relat Res*. 2005;430:219-226.
68. Sakai D, Mochida J, Iwashina T, et al. Regenerative effects of transplanting mesenchymal stem cells embedded in atelocollagen to the degenerated intervertebral disc. *Biomaterials*. 2006;27(3):335-345.
69. Nagae M, Ikeda T, Mikami Y, et al. Intervertebral disc regeneration using platelet-rich plasma and biodegradable gelatin hydrogel microspheres. *Tissue Eng*. 2007;13(1): 147-158.
70. Alentado VJ, Lubelski D, Steinmetz MP, et al. Optimal duration of conservative management prior to surgery for cervical and lumbar radiculopathy: a literature review. *Global Spine J*. 2014;4:279-286.
71. Alvin MD, Qureshi S, Klineberg E, et al. Cervical degenerative disease: systematic review of economic analyses. *Spine*. 2014;39(22 suppl 1):S53-S64.

40 CHAPTER Surgical Management of Axial Neck Pain

Raj Rao
Satyajit Marawar

Axial neck pain refers to posterior neck pain without radicular symptoms in upper extremities. The patient's description of the neck pain can vary and is frequently poorly defined. The pain may be dominant on one side or bilateral, and may be associated with headaches or neck stiffness. The pain is often associated with referral to the trapezius muscles, shoulder blades, or interscapular region.

Most people experience neck pain at some point in their lifetime. A 2010 study on the global burden of disease estimates that 332 million people are afflicted with neck pain worldwide. Among all musculoskeletal conditions, neck pain is the second highest contributor to years lived with disability (33.6 million years lived with disability), ranking only behind low back pain, the leading cause of musculoskeletal disability worldwide.[1] The United States Bone and Joint Initiative task force on neck pain reported a 12-month prevalence of neck pain ranging as high as 30% to 50%, although the prevalence of activity-limiting pain was between 1.7% and 11.5 %.[2] Neck pain also impacts the workforce, with 11% to 14% of workers reporting neck pain that limited activity in the past year.[3] A study of work absenteeism in a cohort of claimants at the Ontario Workplace Safety and Insurance Board showed that an estimated 11.3% of claimants who lost time from work listed neck pain as the reason.[4] Prevalence of neck pain increases with older age, peaking in middle years and declining in later years of life.[3]

Only a small proportion of subjects with neck pain are disabled enough to seek medical attention, and only a fraction of the population with chronic neck pain will ever see a surgeon. The role of surgical fusion has traditionally been limited in the treatment of patients with only axial neck pain. At the same time, the number of surgical procedures done for cervical degenerative pathology in general has been exponentially increasing in the last 2 decades. Marawar et al.[5] analyzed data collected in the National Hospital Discharge Survey from 1990 to 2004 and reported that from 2000 to 2004, a total of 451,166 anterior cervical discectomy and fusion (ACDF) surgeries were performed in United States. The authors found an overall 8-fold increase in the total number of ACDFs performed over the three 5-year time periods between 1990 and 2004. The greatest proportion (49%) of surgeries was in the group of patients aged 46 to 64 years. Over the same time period, utilization rates for ACDF dramatically increased (28-fold) in the group of patients aged 65 years and older. Interestingly, the number of ACDFs done in patients younger than 45 years also rose significantly, from 27,278 from 1990 to 1994 to 151,407 from 2000 to 2004.[5] The reasons behind this enormous increase in the number of ACDFs performed are likely multifactorial. Aging of the population, a greater access to diagnostic imaging, patient demand for pain relief, and an increased number of fellowship-trained spine surgeons may all play a role.

The proportion of procedures that were carried out for axial neck pain, as opposed to neurologic findings, is not clear from the databases mentioned earlier. There are, however, other outcome studies that shed some light on the prevalence of surgery for the subgroup of patients with axial neck pain. Palit et al. noted that 38 (22%) out of 175 ACDF procedures done in their medical group from 1989 to 1994 were for patients with nonradicular neck pain.[6] Eck et al., while comparing outcome of ACDF in patients with and without radicular symptoms, reported that 41 (21%) of 202 patients who underwent ACDF by two surgeons had axial neck pain alone.[7] On the other hand, Lied et al. from Norway reported that 20 (5.1%) of 390 patients who underwent ACDF for cervical disc degeneration had neck pain only without radicular or myelopathic symptoms.[8] Reasonable conclusions from these datasets are that (1) global variations exist in the utilization of surgery to treat axial neck pain, and (2) with the large increases in the overall number of ACDF procedures being done in the United States, there is likely a proportional increase in the utilization of surgery to treat patients with purely axial neck pain. It is therefore critical to continually evaluate the available evidence to define the role of surgery in treating axial neck pain.

Etiology and Pathophysiology of Axial Neck Pain

Smith and Robinson described "cervical disc syndrome" in patients with cervical disc degeneration as a constellation of symptoms that included chronic pain in the posterior part of the neck, shoulder, occiput, and arm; paresthesias in the arm; limitation of movement of the neck; and roentgenographic evidence of cervical disc degeneration.[9] Although the clinical approach to neck pain has focused on the degenerated cervical disc as the primary pain generator, neck pain is most certainly multifactorial in nature. The cervical motion segment is a five-joint complex comprised of a disc, and paired uncovertebral joints anteriorly, and paired facet joints posteriorly. Stabilizing soft tissue structures include the ligamentum nuchae, which attaches to the spinous processes in the midline and surrounding musculature, including the trapezius and deeper paraspinal muscles (semispinalis capitis, splenius capitis, longissimus and interspinalis). All of these structures could potentially play a role in pain generation.

Disc degeneration is thought to begin with loss of proteoglycans and consequent desiccation of the disc nucleus. This results in changes in the mechanical properties of the disc, with increasing stresses on the outer anulus and the facet joint. This can cause annular disruption, resulting in increased motion and abnormal stresses at the facet and uncovertebral joints, even under physiologic loading conditions. Eventually, the collective result of these changes can cause central canal and foraminal narrowing, with impingement of the neurologic structures.

Although the anatomic process of degeneration is reasonably well defined, the correlation of axial neck pain to the degenerative process is poorly understood. The sinuvertebral nerve, a branch of the dorsal ramus that supplies the posterior anulus, can get irritated by an annular tear and lead to neck pain.[10] Chemonociceptors and altered stresses at the facet joint capsule can contribute to neck pain. Myofascial trigger points are also commonly found in patients with neck pain. Han et al. reported that the incidence of myofascial pain syndrome with associated trigger points varied between 30% and 85% in people presenting to pain clinics with persistent pain in the head, neck, shoulders, or low back.[11]

There is little evidence in the literature to support disc degeneration as a primary etiology of neck pain. Multiple studies have found cervical disc degeneration on MRI scans in asymptomatic volunteers.[12–17] Further, disc degeneration seen on MRI in asymptomatic subjects is often accompanied by other common degenerative findings, such as disc bulging,[12,16] annular tears, narrowing of the disc space, and foraminal stenosis.[12–14] The Bone and Joint Decade 2000–2010 Task Force on Neck Pain and its Associated Disorders in fact concluded that there was no evidence to suggest that common degenerative changes seen on imaging studies were strongly correlated with neck pain symptoms.[12–14]

The role of prior soft tissue trauma in causation of neck pain is even more controversial. Whiplash-associated disorders (WAD) is a term assigned to the symptom complex that patients present with after a rear-end mechanism vehicular collision. Neck pain and headaches are the major symptoms. A Quebec task force on whiplash injury reported that WAD is almost always self-limited and rarely results in permanent harm.[18] On the other hand, Freeman and colleagues[19] reviewed the literature refuting the role of whiplash syndrome and determined: "There is no epidemiologic or scientific basis in the literature for the following statement: whiplash injuries do not lead to chronic pain, rear impact collisions that do not result in vehicle damage are unlikely to cause injury, and whiplash trauma is biomechanically comparable to common movements of daily living." Macnab[20] reported that 45% of the patients with whiplash injuries had continued symptoms 2 years after a court settlement action. He suggested that, in his experience, "10% to 20% are left with discomfort of sufficient severity to interfere with their ability to do work or enjoy themselves in leisure hours." Sterner et al.[21] reported on a prospective study of 356 patients with a whiplash trauma to the cervical spine. Of the patients, 32% reported persisting disability at 1-year follow-up. Pretraumatic neck pain, low educational level, and female gender were found to be significantly associated with poor prognosis. The Bone and Joint Decade 2000–2010 Task Force on Neck Pain and its Associated Disorders found that eliminating insurance payments for pain and suffering was associated with a lower incidence of whiplash-associated disorder injury claims. They did not find any evidence in the literature of a demonstrable ligamentous injury on MRI in patients with whiplash-associated disorders.[22]

Natural History and Prognosis Factors for Neck Pain

Knowledge of natural history provides perspective on the patient's history of pain, and sets patient expectations on the course of their pain. It also helps study if the interventions provided have altered the course of neck pain and associated disability in a particular patient. Understanding the natural history of neck pain can also identify modifiable and non-modifiable risk factors that affect prognosis. This can help the physician determine which individuals have a higher risk of persistent or worsening disability.

Cote et al.[23] reported on incidence and course of neck pain by studying a cohort of 1100 randomly selected adults and following up on them at 6 months and 1 year. They found that annual incidence of neck pain was 14.6%. On follow-up of adults with neck pain, 36.6 % had complete resolution of neck pain and another 32.7% reported improvement, while 37.3% reported persistent neck pain and 9.9% reported worsening of their symptoms. In general, in the population with neck pain, most subjects did not have complete resolution of neck pain. A quarter of the people who reported neck pain improvement at interim follow-up complained of recurrence of pain on final follow-up. The authors found that women were more likely to develop neck pain and have persistent pain on follow-up as compared with men. In another cohort of 7669 adults from the general population, neck pain was reported by 17.7%.[24] At 1-year follow-up of people with neck pain at baseline, 48% reported neck pain lasting for more than 1 day in the previous month. Baseline characteristics that predicted persistent neck pain were age between 45 and 59 years (odds ratio [OR], 3.4), being off work at the time of the baseline survey (OR, 1.6), comorbid low back pain (OR, 1.6), and cycling as a regular activity (OR, 2.4).[24] Vos et al.[25] followed 187 patients who presented with acute neck pain to a general practice for 1 year. Of the 138 that provided follow-up data, 76% had fully or partially recovered, although 47% reported some persistent symptoms. Almost half the patients who were on sick leave at baseline returned to work in 7 days. Interestingly, they found that the highest association with recovery was the advice of the general practitioner "to wait and see" (OR, 6.7), while a referral to physical therapy or to a medical specialist showed the highest association (OR, 2.8) with a prolonged sick leave.

In a study from Sweden, Pernold et al.[26] reported on a follow-up of 439 patients seeking care for neck and shoulder disorders. The highest improvements in pain and disability, both in men and in women, were seen after 3 months. After that, improvements were minor. At 5 years, 22% of the men and 15% of the women from the initial group had no neck pain, while 75% of the men and 59% of the women had reported some decrease in neck pain intensity. Van Eard et al.[27] describe the course of lost time claims involving neck pain in workers compensated by the Ontario Workplace Safety and Insurance Board (WSIB). They reported that, although most workers who had a lost work claim for neck pain at baseline did not have a second claim for neck pain in the following 2 years, 14.1% of the initial claimants had repeated claims for lost work due to neck pain. Overall, in a segment of the population that has neck pain, recurrence and persistence is frequent. These individuals usually seek a surgical opinion.

Clinical Evaluation of the Patient With Neck Pain

Patients with long-standing neck pain have typically tried a variety of conservative treatment modalities prior to being seen by a surgeon. The chronicity and severity of their disability, associated with failure of multiple prior treatment modalities, leads to frustration and overall disenchantment with medical modalities. It is important that a solid patient-physician relationship is established, as this will play an important role in surgical decision making. A thorough history and physical examination is the first step in that direction.

Axial neck pain is typically along the posterior musculature of the cervical spine, occasionally radiating to the trapezius, shoulder blade, or interscapular areas. Radiation of pain along the trapezius, particularly if unilateral and accompanied by tingling, may suggest C4 radiculopathy. Neck pain and suboccipital headaches radiating to the retroauricular region has been noted in patients with high cervical (C3, C4) radiculopathy.[28,29] Even when neck pain is dominant, care should be taken to rule out neurologic symptoms or findings of cervical radiculopathy and myelopathy.

Some patients with instability will report feeling occasional "clunks" as they move their neck through a range of motion. Worsening of neck pain with flexion or pain exacerbated by whole body vibration during driving may indicate a discogenic source of pain. In patients with axial neck pain, the physician needs to be vigilant to detect any red flags that may suggest serious underlying pathology (Table 40.1).[30]

Obtaining a social history can play an important role in determining treatment options. Exaggeration of pain, history of litigation, clinical depression, drug-seeking behavior, and

TABLE 40.1 Red Flags in the Patient With Axial Neck Pain

Red Flag	Potential Source of Pain
Minor trauma leading to fracture	Pathologic fracture from osteoporosis or spinal metastasis
A history of malignancy with unexplained weight loss and constitutional symptoms	Spinal metastasis; pathologic fracture
A history of ankylosing spondylitis or inflammatory bowel disease	Inflammatory arthropathy affecting the spine, unsuspected trauma, epidural hematoma
Fever in patients with immunosuppressed status or history of recent urinary tract, dental, or skin infections	Osteomyelitis, discitis, epidural abscess

lack of even temporary pain relief with any treatment modalities previously tried will have an adverse impact on prognosis following surgery. Such patients should have a formal psychosocial evaluation and should be referred to a multidisciplinary pain program.

The visual analog scale SF-36 and the Neck Disability Index questionnaire can help understand the patient's current perceived disability and are used to monitor changes in symptoms and disability over time. Pain diagrams and patient expectations may impact the patient's prognosis after surgery.[31] A nonorganic pain diagram as opposed to one suggesting an anatomic source of pain (Fig. 40.1), when associated with drug-seeking behavior or litigation, can increase the risk of a poor outcome after surgical fusion.[32] Together, these surveys can help the surgeon and the patient choose appropriate and effective treatment.

On physical examination, specific areas of tenderness, range of motion of the cervical spine, and any worsening of radicular symptoms on provocation should be noted. The Spurling test has been reported to have low to moderate sensitivity and high specificity for detecting nerve root impingement.[33,34] A detailed neurologic examination is necessary to rule out radiculopathy or myelopathy.

In patients with purely axial neck pain, an exaggerated pain response to light touch can be an indication of a nonorganic basis of pain. Waddell described signs of nonorganic pain in the lumbar spine,[35] which can be similarly utilized in patients with cervical symptoms.[36] Nondermatomal numbness, cogwheel or jerking motion on strength testing, and inconsistencies when certain tests are repeated are signs of nonorganic origin of pain. Although nonorganic signs may not be necessarily associated with secondary gain, they have been correlated with a poor outcome after surgical management.[37] In these patients, a multidisciplinary pain clinic referral should be sought.

Imaging Studies

Radiographs

In the absence of any red flags, plain radiographs are obtained for the patient who continues to have axial neck pain despite 6 weeks of conservative treatment. Anteroposterior, lateral,

PAIN DIAGRAM

Name: JOHN DOE Date: 00/00/0000

Please use the symbols below to show the area, upon the body outlines, in which you are experiencing pain.

Ache-A
Burning-B
Numbness-N
Pins and Needles-P
Stabbing-S
Other-O

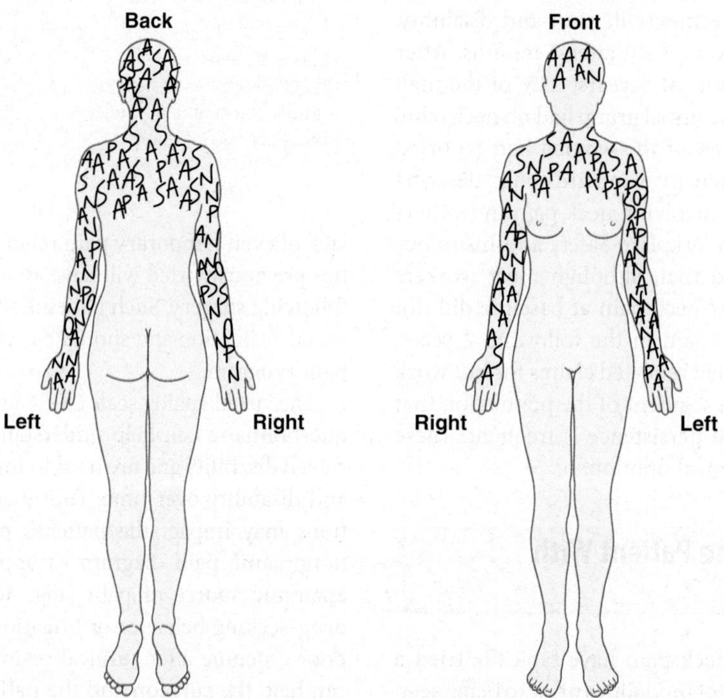

The line below represents the intensity of the pain you are experiwncing. Please make an "X" at the postion on the scale which indicates how much pain you are feeling ***at this time***.

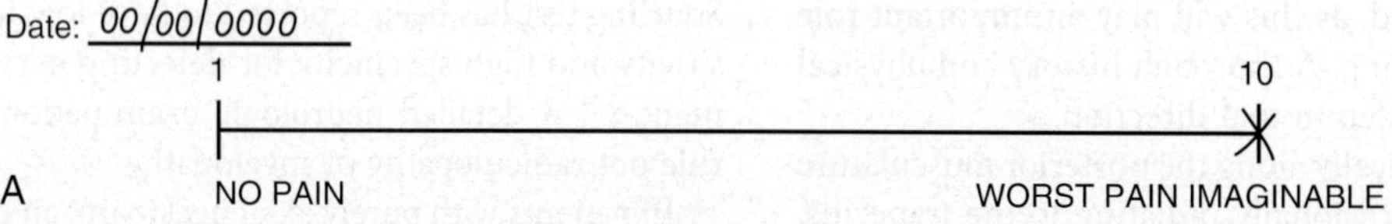

FIG. 40.1 Pain diagram suggestive of (A) nonorganic pathology compared with the pain diagram suggestive of (B) organic pathology presenting as axial neck pain.

and flexion-extension views are obtained. Overall alignment and any evidence of instability are noted. Degenerative changes—such as loss of disc height, endplate sclerosis, and bone spurs—are ubiquitous in the population and will generally be present in the patient with axial neck pain as well. The clinical significance of these radiographic changes and their correlation with neck pain and disability is debatable. Peterson et al. reported that there was no difference in reported pain and disability levels between those with and those without evidence of cervical spine degeneration on plain radiographs.[38] Gore et al. also reported that degenerative changes are common in plain radiographs in asymptomatic people.[39] They later reported on a radiographic and clinical follow-up of a group of 159 previously asymptomatic people at 10 years from their first evaluation. There was an increase in degenerative changes with increasing age. Neck pain was reported by 15% of the previously asymptomatic subjects. In this study, presence of degenerative changes at C6–C7 was a statistically significant predictor of pain.[40] Other serious and destructive pathologies, such as metastatic tumors or discitis-osteomyelitis, can be detected on plain radiographs if advanced enough. Such findings should lead to prompt referral for advanced imaging studies.

Advanced Imaging Studies

In the absence of red flags in patients with predominant axial neck pain, advanced imaging studies should be obtained if the patient has persistent disability despite 4 to 6 months of conservative management. Magnetic resonance imaging (MRI) shows degenerated and narrowed discs, vacuum disc phenomenon, annular tears, or disc bulges. However, such changes are

PAIN DIAGRAM

Name: JANE DOE Date: 00/00/0000

Please use the symbols below to show the area, upon the body outlines, in which you are experiencing pain.

Ache-A
Burning-B
Numbness-N
Pins and Needles-P
Stabbing-S
Other-O

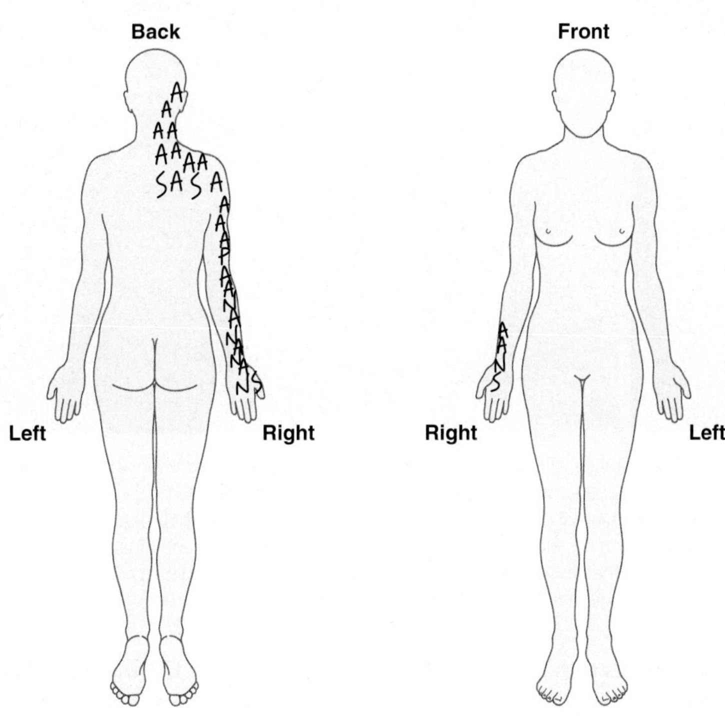

The line below represents the intensity of the pain you are experiwncing. Please make an "X" at the postion on the scale which indicates how much pain you are feeling ***at this time***.

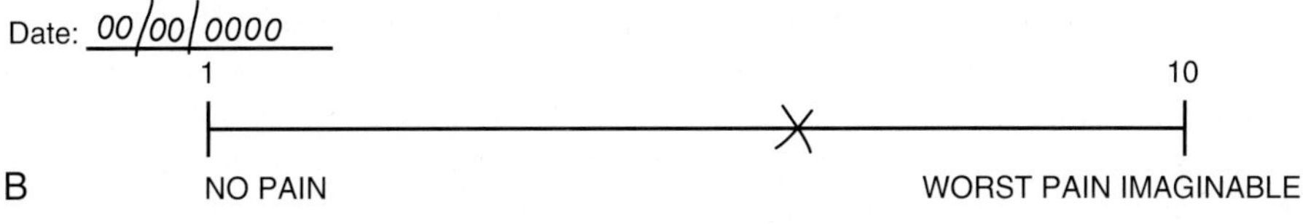

FIG. 40.1, cont'd

also frequently seen in asymptomatic patients,[12–17] and the utility of these findings in determining a clear pain generator is limited. CT scans are done in patients with a contraindication for MRI. CT scans provide more details about bony anatomy, especially in patients with trauma, tumor, or infection. As is the case with MRI, utility of the CT scan in determining the pain generator in patients with axial neck pain is limited.

Cervical Discography

The need to more definitively identify a disc that may be a pain generator led to cervical discography. Cervical discography was described in 1957 by Smith and Nichols,[41] and in 1958 by Cloward.[42] Using image-guided techniques, the cervical disc is cannulated and contrast material injected into the disc (Fig. 40.2). Abnormal morphology of the disc as well as concordant pain provocation by the injection are both considered diagnostic of pain-generating disc levels. Despite its frequent use in prior decades, the procedure is now generally regarded with caution due to risks from its invasive nature and the operator-dependent nature of the technique and interpretation.

Yin et al.[43] carried out a retrospective review of patients with neck pain who underwent diagnostic blocks and provocative discography to determine the causes of neck pain. Among the 46% of the patients who completed all investigations, the prevalence of zygapophyseal joint pain was 55%, discogenic pain was 16%, and lateral atlantoaxial joint pain was 9%. Bogduk and Aprill[44] reported on the causes of neck pain in 56 patients with posttraumatic neck pain. They reported that only 20% of the patients had exclusively discogenic pain with positive discograms.

A high false-positive rate is a major argument against cervical discography. Schellhas et al.[45] compared responses to discography

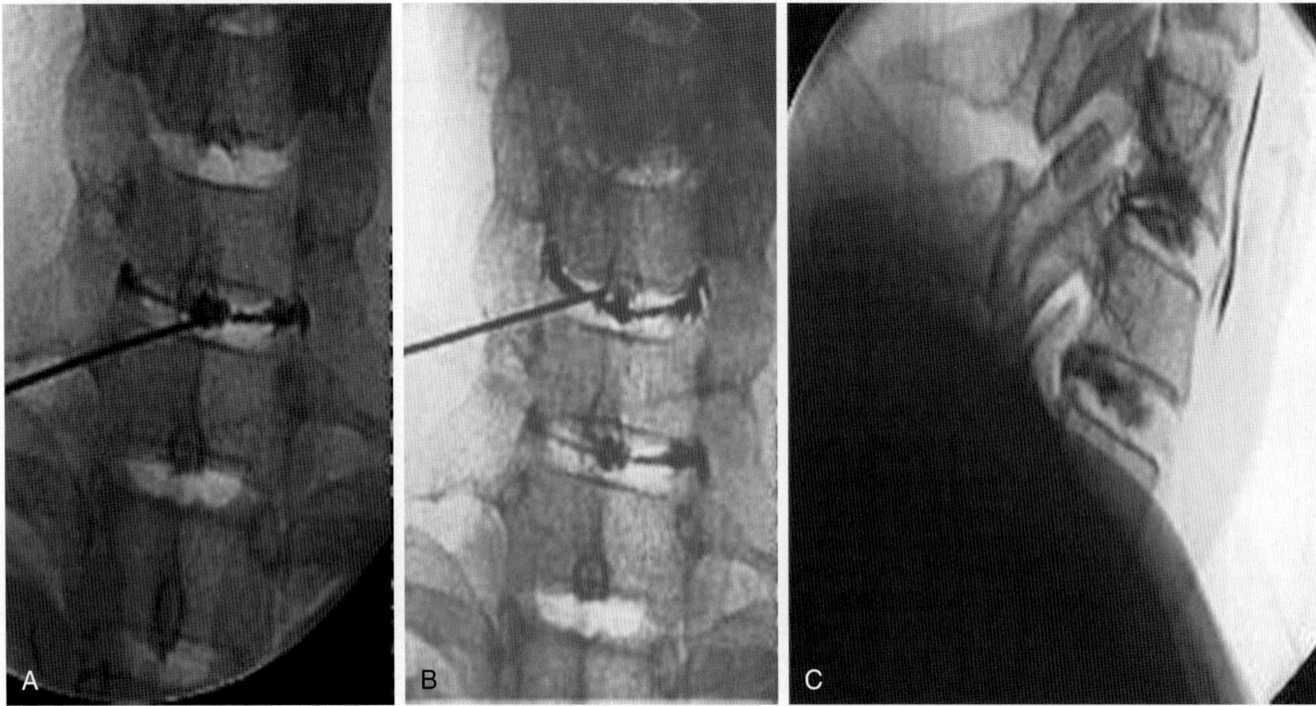

FIG. 40.2 (A) Anteroposterior (AP) view after discogram at the C6–C7 level demonstrates extravasation of contrast beyond the lateral disc margin. (B) AP view after discogram at the C5–C6 level, which was injected as the control, showing the normal distribution of the contrast that remains within the disc margins. (C) Lateral view after the discogram in (A) and (B) showing that the contrast remains predominantly in the center of the disc at the C5–C6 level, whereas it leaks beyond the posterior margin of the disc at C6–C7 level. (Courtesy Dr. A. Gangi, Dr. Sveta Trikha, Neuroradiology, Syracuse VA Medical Center, and www.openradiology.org.)

in asymptomatic volunteers and patients with neck pain. They reported that asymptomatic subjects had a painful response to disc injection, usually a 4 to 5 on a scale of 0 to 10. Although the patient group reported greater mean pain responses with disc injection compared with the asymptomatic group ($P < .0001$), production of pain on discography in both symptomatic and asymptomatic groups underlines the risk of false-positive responses on discography. However, it is difficult to determine the exact false-positive rate of discography, as a positive discogram, by definition, has to elicit concordant pain, which is not possible in asymptomatic subjects.

There is lack of standardization in terms of number of levels to be injected during a cervical discogram, with recommendations ranging from injecting all cervical levels[46] to injecting at least one level below and one level above the suspected level based on imaging studies.[6,47] There is lack of consensus on pain threshold level and on what constitutes a positive response on discogram. Schellhas et al.[45] recommend that the patient must rate the intensity of produced pain as 7 or greater on a 10-point numeric scale for it to be considered positive on discogram. Singh et al.[46] suggest that the discogram is positive when the patient reports pain that closely resembles symptomatic pain in intensity and location. Zheng et al.[48] consider moderate to severe reproduction of the patient's typical pain as the determinant for a symptomatic disc.

Nordin et al.[30] reviewed the literature available on cervical discography and did not find any scientifically admissible phase III or phase IV studies that tested the validity of discography as demonstrating primary discogenic pain in the cervical spine. On the other hand, Onyewu et al. concluded that there was level II-2 strength of evidence for diagnostic accuracy of cervical discography. This recommendation should be taken lightly, as they also point out in this review that there was a paucity of literature with widespread discrepancies in methodology of cervical discography and outcome measurement. They found only five studies in the post-MRI era reporting surgical outcome based on cervical discography,[6,48–51] of which there was only one study that had employed controlled provocation discography, with two adjacent discs being injected as controls.[6] Additionally, there are concerns about the effects of annular puncture of control discs during a discogram. Carragee et al.[52] reported accelerated disc degeneration and an increased incidence of disc herniation after lumbar discography as compared to matched controls at 10-year follow-up after discography. Although these results were reported after lumbar discography, it is possible that, in the longer term, annular puncture during cervical discography can lead to accelerated degeneration, even if a small-gauge needle is used with low pressurization. For the surgeon considering surgery in a patient with axial neck pain, discography remains a controversial choice.

Surgery for Axial Neck Pain

Determination of fusion levels in the patient with axial neck pain requires deliberate evaluation of all available clinical and radiographic information. Improved surgical outcomes will be obtained if multiple clinical and radiographic findings all point to the same disc as the source of pain. This clinical algorithm should include (1) clinical judgment on the need for surgery, given the patient's reported pain and disability; (2) clinical assessment of secondary gain or other potential nonstructural issues that may be contributing to the patient's pain level and will result in a diminished surgical outcome; (3) assessment of current or historical clinical findings that may point to a specific level, such as unilateral tingling over the trapezius muscle may suggest ipsilateral C4 nerve root irritation; (4) radiographs that show degenerative changes prominently at a single level with relatively normal adjacent levels; (5) lateral radiographs or flexion-extension radiographs that show translation at a specific level suggestive of instability; (6) MRI showing marked disc space narrowing at a single level, or marked endplate changes at the level; and (7) discography with clearly concordant pain at the same disc. In patients with axial neck pain considering surgery, determination of surgical levels is largely surgeon dependent, will remain controversial, and needs careful and deliberate decision making.

The surgical treatment for axial neck pain is anterior cervical discectomy and fusion at the presumed painful disc level. The removal of the degenerated discs theoretically eliminates the pain generator and also stabilizes the uncovertebral joints and facet joints, thereby reducing their role. Using a Smith-Robinson approach,[9] all disc material is removed and endplates cleaned of all cartilaginous material while preserving the bony endplate. A few small perforations through the endplate using a high-speed burr or a curette facilitate fusion across the disc space. Under gentle distraction, an interbody spacer is inserted. Anterior cervical plating provides immediate stability and allows early mobilization, diminishing the need for postoperative external immobilization. In multilevel fusions, use of an anterior cervical plate reduces pseudarthrosis rates[53–55] and graft-related complications.[53,56] Instrumentation also maintains overall lordosis better and significantly improves segmental lordosis compared with unplated constructs.[57] The length of the plate chosen should allow at least 5 mm between the ends of the plate and adjacent disc levels. Segmental screw fixation is carried out for multilevel fusions.

Several options are available in choosing the interbody spacer and bone graft for anterior cervical fusion. Structural iliac crest bone graft is still considered the gold standard for success of fusion, but is increasingly viewed as an unacceptable option due to the morbidity and pain at the harvest site.[58,59] Earlier reports showed high pseudarthrosis rates with allograft use for ACDF compared with iliac crest autograft, especially for multilevel fusions and in smokers.[60,61] Recent reports, however, show fusion rates and clinical outcome comparable to that of autograft when using allograft spacers with rigid plate fixation, even in multilevel fusions.[62–64] Today, polyetheretherketone (PEEK) interbody spacers filled with allograft and/or demineralized bone matrix are being increasingly used. Fusion rates for PEEK interbody spacers with anterior cervical plating have not been evaluated in prospective studies. In retrospective studies, fusion rates with PEEK spacers have been found to be comparable to that of tricortical iliac crest autograft.[65] In our experience, both tricortical allograft spacers and PEEK spacers filled with bone graft extenders are reasonable alternatives to iliac crest autograft in one- or two-level anterior cervical fusion procedures (Fig. 40.3).

Cervical disc arthroplasty offers a motion-sparing treatment modality for cervical disc pathology with the potential advantage of avoiding increased stresses at the adjoining discs and reduction in the risk of adjacent-segment disease. In patients with cervical radiculopathy, short-term and midterm data comparing cervical disc arthroplasty and ACDF have shown comparable results.[66–71] Some recent studies of cervical disc arthroplasty have included patients with neck or arm pain but have not reported outcome data separately for the subset of patients with predominant axial neck pain.[70,71] The complex multifactorial etiology of neck pain, the difficulty in identifying a pain generator in this subset of patients, and the absence of outcome data on benefits from a motion-sparing device in these patients suggest that disc arthroplasty should not be recommended for these patients.

Axial Neck Pain Secondary to Pseudarthrosis From Prior Surgery

Despite a reduction in the incidence following the use of cervical plating, pseudarthrosis following anterior cervical fusion surgery is reported to occur with an incidence of 10% to 40% in multilevel anterior fusion procedures.[54–56] Pseudarthrosis rates after posterior cervical laminectomy and fusion have been reported to range from 1% to 38%.[72–75] A pseudarthrosis associated with a stable fibrous union can be asymptomatic, but a small proportion of patients with pseudarthrosis present with neck pain due to instability.[76,77] Interbody graft collapse associated with nonunion can result in foraminal stenosis as well as recurrent axial neck pain and radiculopathy. Failure of hardware and progressive deformity can contribute to the symptomatology. CT is the imaging modality of choice to diagnose a nonunion and assess the status of the interbody graft and the hardware.

The treatment approach in patients with symptomatic anterior pseudarthrosis remains a matter of debate. Both anterior revision fusion and posterior stabilization have been reported as effective approaches[78–81]; however, there are no randomized controlled trials comparing the outcomes of these approaches for treating cervical pseudarthrosis. While the anterior procedure allows access to the site of nonunion and lets the surgeon address hardware failure, graft collapse or dislodgment, recurrent foraminal stenosis, and kyphosis, it requires dissecting through the surgical scar with potentially increased risks of iatrogenic injury to neurovascular structures, the esophagus, and the trachea, as well as increased incidence of postoperative dysphagia.[82] On the other hand, posterior fusion surgery involves larger intraoperative blood loss, longer hospital stay, and a higher complication rate compared with anterior revisions.[83] McAnany et al.[84] carried out a meta-analysis of clinical outcomes following treatment of symptomatic cervical pseudarthrosis with either anterior revision surgery or posterior fusion. While the fusion rate was significantly higher in the posterior group as compared to anterior revision (97.1% vs. 86.4%; $P = .028$), clinical outcome

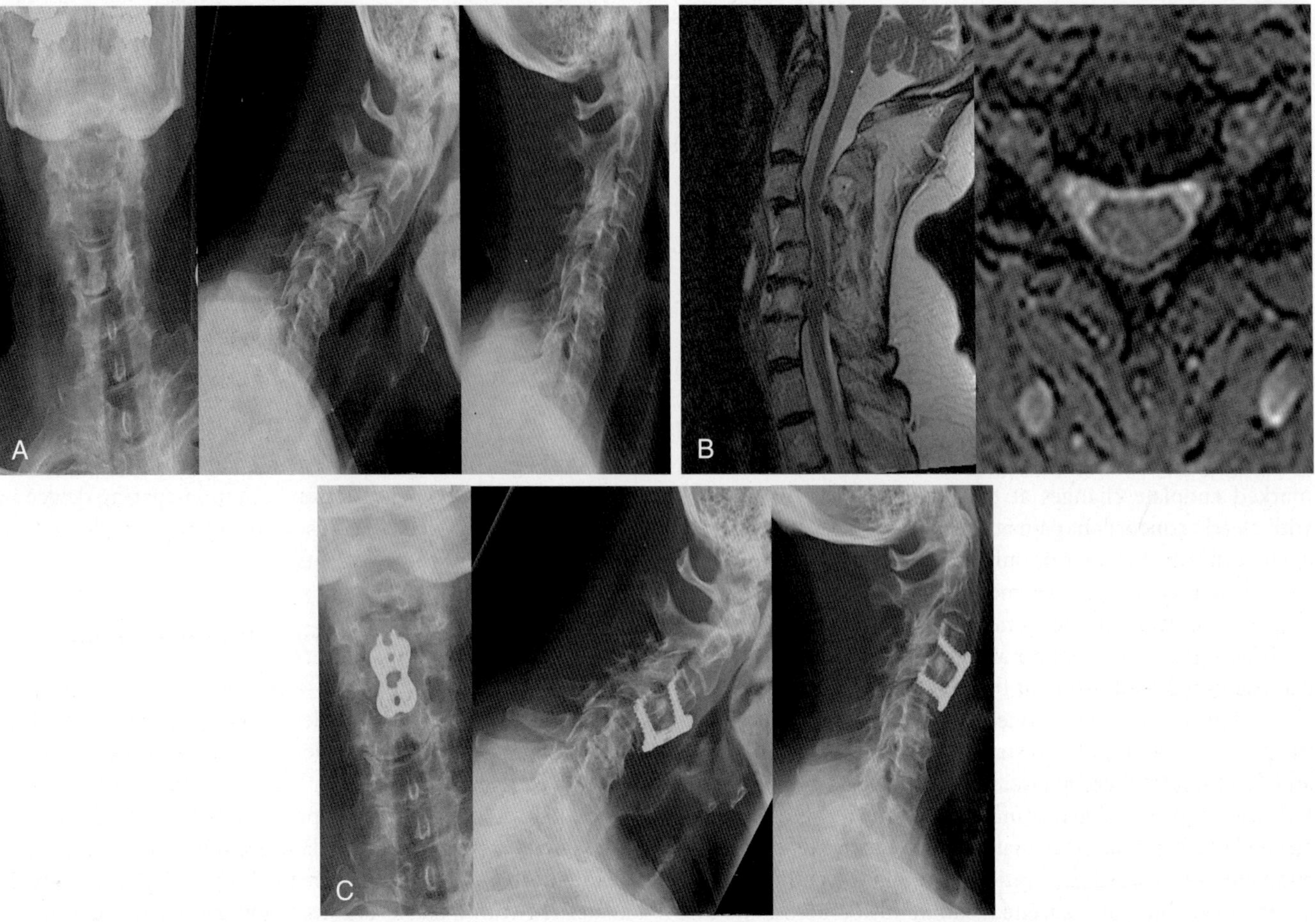

FIG. 40.3 A 70-year-old woman with chronic, intractable axial neck pain in the posterior cervical musculature and no evidence of cervical radiculopathy or myelopathy. (A) Preoperative radiographs and (B) sagittal and axial weighted T2-weighted magnetic resonance images show degenerative changes at multiple levels throughout the cervical spine, with spondylolisthesis at the C3–C4 level. (C) Postoperative radiographs 2 years following anterior fusion at the C3–C4 level with allograft bone and an anterior plate. The patient had complete resolution of her symptoms and return to active function.

was similar. They suggested that this divergence could be due to the higher complication rate and postoperative neck pain associated with posterior fusion.

Outcome After Surgery for Axial Neck Pain

The earliest reports of anterior cervical fusion procedures include axial neck pain as an indication for surgery. In their 1958 article describing the surgical technique for anterior cervical discectomy and fusion, Smith and Robinson reported that three of the 14 patients in the study had disc degeneration alone without nerve root irritation.[9] Yet, surgical intervention for patients who present with axial neck pain alone has always generated controversy. In 1978, Rothman and Rashbaum[85] reported that 23% of the patients with significant cervical degenerative symptoms remained partially or totally disabled after conservative management at 5-year follow-up. However, little functional difference was noted in patients who underwent surgery for dominant neck pain. DePalma et al.[86] reported that 78% of 255 patients treated conservatively for "cervical syndrome" obtained either complete or partial relief, with 22% of patients having poor results. They reported on the results of 58 patients who underwent an anterior fusion procedure after failure of 6 months of conservative management. The outcome was rated as excellent in 74%, improved in 15%, and poor in 11%. They concluded that anterior surgery has "improved to excellent" outcome in this group of patients, with better results than posterior fusion.

Variations of the ACDF procedure have been reported by several authors. Kambin et al.[87] reported on anterior cervical discectomy and fusion using a vertical self-locking T graft. In the group of 50 patients who had neck pain without neurologic findings, "excellent" results were reported in 37, "good" in 10, and "satisfactory" in 3. Brodke and Zdeblick[88] reported on using Caspar pins for intervertebral distraction and a reversed iliac crest graft in 51 patients. Neck pain was the primary symptom in nine of the 51 patients. Outcome was reported as excellent in 36, very good in 11, good in 3, and poor in 1 of the 51 patients. Outcome in patients with neck pain as the primary symptom was not reported separately.

Kikuchi et al.[89] reported on the outcome of surgical fusion in a mixed group of 41 patients with predominant axial neck pain alone as well as 97 patients who had neck pain and radicular symptoms. Diagnostic discography was performed in all patients on four adjacent discs. The discogram was considered positive on production of concordant pain. One year from surgery, 80% of all patients were reported to be either totally free of symptoms or had discomfort that did not interfere with their work or social life. The outcome in patients with only neck pain was not reported separately. Zheng et al.[48] attempted to correlate discography findings with MRI findings in 55 patients undergoing ACDF for axial neck pain. The authors considered 79 of 161 levels to be discogram positive. At a minimum follow-up of 2 years, successful fusion was achieved in 95% of the patients, and an overall satisfactory result was achieved in 76%. Abnormal MRI morphology was found in 100 of the 161 levels that underwent discography. Of the 79 levels that were discogram positive, MRI was abnormal at 58 levels. Based on these findings, they determined that MRI had a false-positive rate of 51% and a false-negative rate of 27%.

A frequently cited study in support of surgery for axial neck pain is a retrospective review of 38 patients by Palit et al.,[6] published in 1999. Cervical discography, MRI, and CT scans were used to determine the levels at which fusion was carried out. Discography was carried out at the disc that was suspected of being the pain generator based on the imaging studies and at least two adjacent levels as controls. Anterior cervical discectomy and fusion was carried out using tricortical iliac crest allograft. All patients completed a numeric rating scale (NRS) to measure pain and the Oswestry Disability Index (ODI) to measure function. After an average follow-up period of 53 months after surgery (range, 24–87 months), the mean NRS for neck pain reduced from 8.3 to 4.1 ($P < .001$). The ODI score improved from 57.5 to 38.9 ($P < .001$). Although the results of the study are generally supportive of surgery for neck pain, there are certain methodologic problems that should be pointed out. The author elaborates that patients with 75% or more neck pain and 25% or less arm pain were considered eligible for inclusion in this study. Thus, it seems that this group included patients with some radicular symptoms. They also excluded some patients based on psychological evaluation. However, the number of patients excluded on this basis was not reported. Although they reported obtaining radiographs at 1 and 3 months after surgery, outcome parameters were reported only for the final follow-up, which was performed by telephone at a widely variable period from surgery (24 to 87 months). At final follow-up, 30 of 38 patients (79%) reported that they were satisfied with surgery and 8 patients (21%) reported that they were not satisfied. However, while 20 patients were not working before surgery because of neck pain, 15 were still not working at final follow-up.

Garvey et al.[90] conducted a retrospective review on 87 patients who had undergone an anterior cervical discectomy and fusion for dominant mechanical neck pain, defined as neck pain greater than arm pain. At a mean follow-up period of 4.4 ± 1.5 years, this group of patients completed outcome questionnaires that included a visual analog pain score, a modified ODI, and a modified Roland Morris disability index. The authors reported that 82% of the patients reported their outcome to be good, very good, or excellent. The average visual analog score reduced from 8.4 ± 1.7 before surgery to 3.8 ± 2.8 ($P < .01$) after surgery. The ODI improved from 58.8 ± 19.8 before surgery to 30.7 ± 21.4 at final follow-up ($P < .01$), while the Roland Morris disability score improved from 15.8 ± 6.4 before surgery to 7.6 ± 6.5 at final follow-up ($P < .01$). Although this retrospective study reports an overall positive outcome after surgery for axial neck pain, the indications for surgery appear to be heterogeneous. The authors report that 66 of 87 patients who underwent surgery had preoperative discography, but 31 of 66 (46%) had nonclassic findings on discography with pain greater than 4 or 5 out of 10 at adjacent segments. The role of routine imaging studies in determining indication for surgery is not clarified. The authors point out that, despite improvement in pain and self-rated disability scores, global patient satisfaction after surgery showed a mixed distribution and did not seem to correlate well with improvements in pain scores and disability ratings.

A small number of reviews of available literature on surgery for axial neck pain have been reported. In a report on best evidence synthesis for utility of surgical interventions for neck pain, as part of the Bone and Joint Decade 2000–2010 Task Force on Back Pain and its Associated Disorders, Carragee et al.[91] reported that they found no well-designed randomized controlled trials of open surgery for treatment of neck pain alone in patients with common degenerative changes on imaging in the absence of radiculopathy, myelopathy, or serious pathology, such as tumors or infection. They did not find any evidence in the available literature that showed a better outcome after surgery for neck pain that could be attributed to surgery and not to the natural history of neck pain in patients with degenerative pathology. They concluded that there was no evidence in the literature to support use of anterior cervical discectomy and fusion, or disc arthroplasty in patients with neck pain without radiculopathy or serious structural pathology.

Riew et al.[92] conducted a systematic review of articles published up to 2010 to examine the clinical outcome in patients who underwent ACDF for axial neck pain without radicular or myelopathic symptoms. They did not identify any comparative studies. The authors reported three case series that met the criterion to be included in their review.[6,7,90] They reported that all studies showed a mean improvement of pain of 50% at approximately 4-year follow-up with patients' satisfaction rates ranging from 56% to 79%. They concluded that there is low evidence in the literature that patients with axial neck pain without radicular or myelopathic symptoms will receive some improvement in pain and function following an ACDF. Additionally, there is no evidence to clarify whether the benefit from surgery is better than no treatment or other conservative treatment modalities.

Summary

Neck pain is a widely prevalent, though frequently self-limiting, condition. Some individuals develop persistent and disabling neck pain, refractory to conservative treatment. The etiology of neck pain is multifactorial, and degenerated discs may be the primary pain generator in only a minority of cases; identification of a pain generator is frequently difficult. Discography has been frequently used in the past in an attempt to identify the pain-generating disc level. The procedure is currently more controversial due to a lack of standard methodology, variation in outcome measurement, limited evidence to its utility in improving surgical outcome, and the potential for annular injury to uninvolved discs. Currently available review of literature points to a lack of reliable and controlled studies that show improved outcome with surgery for axial neck pain as compared to nonsurgical modalities or nonintervention. Commonly cited case series supporting surgery for axial neck pain suffer from methodological flaws, lack of control groups, and the absence of long-term outcome data. Further long-term studies may help us better understand the utility of surgical intervention in patients with axial neck pain.

KEY REFERENCES

1. Carragee EJ, Hurwitz EL, Cheng I, et al. Treatment of neck pain: injections and surgical interventions: results of the Bone and Joint Decade 2000-2010 Task Force on Neck Pain and its Associated Disorders. *Spine.* 2008;33(4 suppl):S153-S169.
2. Garvey TA, Transfeldt EE, Malcolm JR, Kos P. Outcome of anterior cervical discectomy and fusion as perceived by patients treated for dominant axial-mechanical cervical spine pain. *Spine.* 2002;27(17):1887-1894.
3. Marawar S, Girardi FP, Sama AA, et al. National trends in anterior cervical fusion procedures. *Spine.* 2010;35(15):1454-1459.
4. Palit M, Mark S, Jerome G, et al. Anterior discectomy and fusion for the management of neck pain. *Spine.* 1999;24(21):2224.
5. Riew KD, Ecker E, Dettori JR. Anterior cervical discectomy and fusion for the management of axial neck pain in the absence of radiculopathy or myelopathy. *Evid Based Spine Care J.* 2010;1(3):45-50.

REFERENCES

1. Vos T, Flaxman AD, Naghavi M, et al. Years lived with disability (YLDs) for 1160 sequelae of 289 diseases and injuries 1990-2010: a systematic analysis for the global burden of disease study 2010. *Lancet.* 2012;380(9859):2163-2196.
2. Hogg-Johnson S, van der Velde G, Carroll LJ, et al. The burden and determinants of neck pain in the general population: results of the Bone and Joint Decade 2000-2010 Task Force on Neck Pain and its Associated Disorders. *Spine.* 2008;33(4 suppl):S39-S51.
3. Cote P, van der Velde G, Cassidy JD, et al. The burden and determinants of neck pain in workers: results of the Bone and Joint Decade 2000-2010 Task Force on Neck Pain and its Associated Disorders. *Spine.* 2008;33(4 suppl):S60-S74.
4. Cote P, Kristman V, Vidmar M, et al. The prevalence and incidence of work absenteeism involving neck pain: a cohort of Ontario lost-time claimants. *Spine.* 2008;33(4 suppl):S192-S198.
5. Marawar S, Girardi FP, Sama AA, et al. National trends in anterior cervical fusion procedures. *Spine.* 2010;35(15):1454-1459.
6. Palit M, Mark S, Jerome G, et al. Anterior discectomy and fusion for the management of neck pain. *Spine.* 1999;24(21):2224.
7. Eck JC, Humphreys SC, Hodges SD, Levi P. A comparison of outcomes of anterior cervical discectomy and fusion in patients with and without radicular symptoms. *J Surg Orthop Adv.* 2006;15(1):24-26.
8. Lied B, Roenning PA, Sundseth J, Helseth E. Anterior cervical discectomy with fusion in patients with cervical disc degeneration: a prospective outcome study of 258 patients (181 fused with autologous bone graft and 77 fused with a PEEK cage). *BMC Surg.* 2010;21(10):10.
9. Smith GW, Robinson RA. The treatment of certain cervical-spine disorders by anterior removal of the intervertebral disc and interbody fusion. *J Bone Joint Surg Am.* 1958;40-A(3):607-624.
10. Bogduk N, Windsor M, Inglis A. The innervation of the cervical intervertebral discs. *Spine.* 1988;13(1):2-8.
11. Han SC, Harrison P. Myofascial pain syndrome and trigger-point management. *Reg Anesth.* 1997;22(1):89-101.
12. Boden SD, McCowin PR, Davis DO, et al. Abnormal magnetic-resonance scans of the cervical spine in asymptomatic subjects. A prospective investigation. *J Bone Joint Surg Am.* 1990;72(8):1178-1184.
13. Ernst CW, Stadnik TW, Peeters E, Breucq C, Osteaux MJ. Prevalence of annular tears and disc herniations on MR images of the cervical spine in symptom free volunteers. *Eur J Radiol.* 2005;55(3):409-414.
14. Matsumoto M, Fujimura Y, Suzuki N, et al. MRI of cervical intervertebral discs in asymptomatic subjects. *J Bone Joint Surg Br.* 1998;80-B(1):19-24.
15. Matsumoto M, Okada E, Ichihara D, et al. Age-related changes of thoracic and cervical intervertebral discs in asymptomatic subjects. *Spine.* 2010;35(14):1359-1364.
16. Nakashima H, Yukawa Y, Suda K, et al. Abnormal findings on magnetic resonance images of the cervical spines in 1211 asymptomatic subjects. *Spine.* 2015;40(6):392-398.
17. Okada E, Matsumoto M, Fujiwara H, Toyama Y. Disc degeneration of cervical spine on MRI in patients with lumbar disc herniation: comparison study with asymptomatic volunteers. *Eur Spine J.* 2011;20(4):585-591.
18. Spitzer WO, Skovron ML, Salmi LR, et al. Scientific monograph of the Quebec task force on whiplash-associated disorders: redefining "whiplash" and its management. *Spine.* 1995;20(8 suppl):1S-73S.
19. Freeman MD, Croft AC, Rossignol AM, Weaver DS, Reiser M. A review and methodologic critique of the literature refuting whiplash syndrome. *Spine.* 1999;24(1):86-96.
20. Macnab I. Acceleration injuries of the cervical spine. *J Bone Joint Surg Am.* 1964;46:1797-1799.
21. Sterner Y, Toolanen G, Gerdle B, Hildingsson C. The incidence of whiplash trauma and the effects of different factors on recovery. *J Spinal Disord Tech.* 2003;16(2):195-199.
22. Carroll LJ, Holm LWD, Hogg Johnson S, et al. Course and prognostic factors for neck pain in whiplash-associated disorders (WAD): results of the Bone and Joint Decade 2000-2010 Task Force on Neck Pain and its Associated Disorders. *Spine.* 2008;33(4 suppl):S83-S92.
23. Cote P, Cassidy DJ, Carroll LJ, Kristman V. The annual incidence and course of neck pain in the general population: a population-based cohort study. *Pain.* 2004;112(3):267-273.
24. Hill J, Lewis M, Papageorgiou AC, Dziedzic K, Croft P. Predicting persistent neck pain: a 1-year follow-up of a population cohort. *Spine.* 2004;29(15):1648-1654.
25. Vos CJ, Verhagen AP, Passchier J, Koes BW. Clinical course and prognostic factors in acute neck pain: an inception cohort study in general practice. *Pain Med.* 2008;9(5): 572-580.
26. Pernold G, Mortimer M, Wiktorin C, et al. Neck/shoulder disorders in a general population. Natural course and influence of physical exercise: a 5-year follow-up. *Spine.* 2005;30(13):E363-E368.

27. Van Eerd D, Cote P, Kristman V, et al. The course of work absenteeism involving neck pain: a cohort study of Ontario lost-time claimants. *Spine*. 2011;36(12):977-982.
28. Jenis LG, An HS. Neck pain secondary to radiculopathy of the fourth cervical root: an analysis of 12 surgically treated patients. *J Spinal Disord*. 2000;13(4):345-349.
29. Park MS, Kelly MP, Min W, Rahman RK, Riew KD. Surgical treatment of C3 and C4 cervical radiculopathies. *Spine*. 2013;38(2):112-118.
30. Nordin M, Carragee EJ, Hogg Johnson S, et al. Assessment of neck pain and its associated disorders: results of the Bone and Joint Decade 2000-2010 Task Force on Neck Pain and its Associated Disorders. *Spine*. 2008;33(4 suppl):S101-S122.
31. Carr FA, Healy KM, Villavicencio AT, et al. Effect on clinical outcomes of patient pain expectancies and preoperative mental component summary scores from the 36-item short form health survey following anterior cervical discectomy and fusion. *J Neurosurg Spine*. 2011;15(5):486-490.
32. Anderson PA, Subach BR, Riew KD. Predictors of outcome after anterior cervical discectomy and fusion: a multivariate analysis. *Spine*. 2009;34(2):161-166.
33. Rubinstein SM, Pool JJ, van Tulder MW, Riphagen II, de Vet HC. A systematic review of the diagnostic accuracy of provocative tests of the neck for diagnosing cervical radiculopathy. *Eur Spine J*. 2007;16(3):307-319.
34. Wainner RS, et al. Reliability and diagnostic accuracy of the clinical examination and patient self-report measures for cervical radiculopathy. *Spine*. 2003;28(1):52-62.
35. Waddell G, McCulloch JA, Kummel E, Venner RM. Nonorganic physical signs in low-back pain. *Spine*. 1980;5(2):117-125.
36. Sobel JB, Sollenberger P, Robinson R, Polatin PB, Gatchel RJ. Cervical nonorganic signs: a new clinical tool to assess abnormal illness behavior in neck pain patients: a pilot study. *Arch Phys Med Rehabil*. 2000;81(2):170-175.
37. Fishbain DA, et al. A structured evidence-based review on the meaning of nonorganic physical signs: Waddell signs. *Pain Med*. 2003;4(2):141-181.
38. Peterson C, et al. A cross-sectional study correlating degeneration of the cervical spine with disability and pain in United Kingdom patients. *Spine*. 2003;28(2):129-133.
39. Gore DR, Sepic SB, Gardner GM. Roentgenographic findings of the cervical spine in asymptomatic people. *Spine*. 1986;11(6):521-524.
40. Gore DR. Roentgenographic findings in the cervical spine in asymptomatic persons: a ten-year follow-up. *Spine*. 2001;26(22):2463-2466.
41. Smith GW, Nichols P Jr. The technic of cervical discography. *Radiology*. 1957;68(5):718-720.
42. Cloward RB. Cervical diskography: technique, indications and use in diagnosis of ruptured cervical disks. *Am J Roentgenol Radium Ther Nucl Med*. 1958;79(4):563-574.
43. Yin W, Bogduk NDS. The nature of neck pain in a private pain clinic in the United States. *Pain Med*. 2008;9(2):196-203.
44. Bogduk N, Aprill C. On the nature of neck pain, discography and cervical zygapophysial joint blocks. *Pain*. 1993;54(2):213-217.
45. Schellhas KP, Smith MD, Gundry CR, Pollei SR. Cervical discogenic pain. prospective correlation of magnetic resonance imaging and discography in asymptomatic subjects and pain sufferers. *Spine*. 1996;21(3):300-311.
46. Singh V. The role of cervical discography in interventional pain management. *Pain Physician*. 2004;7(2):249-255.
47. Onyewu O, Manchikanti L, Falco FJ, et al. An update of the appraisal of the accuracy and utility of cervical discography in chronic neck pain. *Pain Physician*. 2012;15(6):E777-E806.
48. Zheng Y, Liew SM, Simmons ED. Value of magnetic resonance imaging and discography in determining the level of cervical discectomy and fusion. *Spine*. 2004;29(19):2140-2145.
49. Connor PM, Darden BV 2nd. Cervical discography complications and clinical efficacy. *Spine*. 1993;15(18):2035-2038.
50. Motimaya A, Arici M, George D, Ramsby G. Diagnostic value of cervical discography in the management of cervical discogenic pain. *Conn Med*. 2000;64(7):395-398.
51. Siebenrock KA, Aebi M. Cervical discography in discogenic pain syndrome and its predictive value for cervical fusion. *Arch Orthop Trauma Surg*. 1994;113(4):199-203.
52. Carragee EJ, Don A, Hurwitz EL, et al. Does discography cause accelerated progression of degeneration changes in the lumbar disc: a ten-year matched cohort study. *Spine*. 2009;34(21):2338-2345.
53. Wang JC, McDonough PW, Endow KK, Delamarter RB. Increased fusion rates with cervical plating for two-level anterior cervical discectomy and fusion. *Spine*. 2000;25(1):41-45.
54. Wang JC, McDonough PW, Kanim LEA, Endow KK, Delamarter RB. Increased fusion rates with cervical plating for three-level anterior cervical discectomy and fusion. *Spine*. 2001;26(6):643-646.
55. Bolesta MJ, Rechtine GR 2nd, Chrin AM. One- and two-level anterior cervical discectomy and fusion: the effect of plate fixation. *Spine J*. 2002;2(3):197-203.
56. Kaiser MG, Haid RW Jr, Subach BR, Barnes B, Rodts GE Jr. Anterior cervical plating enhances arthrodesis after discectomy and fusion with cortical allograft. *Neurosurgery*. 2002;50(2):229-236.
57. Troyanovich SJ, Stroink AR, Kattner KA, Dornan WA, Gubina I. Does anterior plating maintain cervical lordosis versus conventional fusion techniques? A retrospective analysis of patients receiving single-level fusions. *J Spinal Disord Tech*. 2002;15(1):69-74.
58. Silber JS, Anderson DG, Daffner SD, et al. Donor site morbidity after anterior iliac crest bone harvest for single-level anterior cervical discectomy and fusion. *Spine*. 2003;28(2):134-139.
59. Malloy KM, Hilibrand AS. Autograft versus allograft in degenerative cervical disease. *Clin Orthop Relat Res*. 2002;(394):27-38.
60. An HS, Simpson JM, Glover JM, Stephany J. Comparison between allograft plus demineralized bone matrix versus autograft in anterior cervical fusion. A prospective multicenter study. *Spine*. 1995;20(20):2211-2216.
61. Zdeblick TA, Ducker TB. The use of freeze-dried allograft bone for anterior cervical fusions. *Spine*. 1991;16(7):726-729.
62. Yue WM, Brodner W, Highland TR. Long-term results after anterior cervical discectomy and fusion with allograft and plating: a 5- to 11-year radiologic and clinical follow-up study. *Spine*. 2005;30(19):2138-2144.
63. Miller LE, Block JE. Safety and effectiveness of bone allografts in anterior cervical discectomy and fusion surgery. *Spine*. 2011;36(24):2045-2050.
64. Samartzis D, Shen FH, Matthews DK, et al. Comparison of allograft to autograft in multilevel anterior cervical discectomy and fusion with rigid plate fixation. *Spine J*. 2003;3(6):451-459.
65. Vanek P, Bradac O, DeLacy P, et al. Comparison of 3 fusion techniques in the treatment of the degenerative cervical

spine disease. Is stand-alone autograft really the "gold standard?" Prospective study with 2-year follow-up. *Spine*. 2012;37(19):1645-1651.

66. Burkus JK, Traynelis VC, Haid RW Jr, Mummaneni PV. Clinical and radiographic analysis of an artificial cervical disc: 7-year follow-up from the PRESTIGE prospective randomized controlled clinical trial. *J Neurosurg Spine*. 2014;21(4):516-528.
67. Coric D, Nunley PD, Guyer RD, et al. Prospective, randomized, multicenter study of cervical arthroplasty: 269 patients from the kineflex|C artificial disc investigational device exemption study with a minimum 2-year follow-up. *J Neurosurg Spine*. 2011;15(4):348-358.
68. Davis RJ, Kim KD, Hisey MS, et al. Cervical total disc replacement with the Mobi-C cervical artificial disc compared with anterior discectomy and fusion for treatment of 2-level symptomatic degenerative disc disease: a prospective, randomized, controlled multicenter clinical trial. *J Neurosurg Spine*. 2013;19(5):532-545.
69. Gornet MF, Burkus JK, Shaffrey ME, et al. Cervical disc arthroplasty with PRESTIGE LP disc versus anterior cervical discectomy and fusion: a prospective, multicenter investigational device exemption study. *J Neurosurg Spine*. 2015;Jul(31):1-16.
70. Hisey MS, Bae HW, Davis R, et al. Multi-center, prospective, randomized, controlled investigational device exemption clinical trial comparing Mobi-cervical artificial disc to anterior discectomy and fusion in the treatment of symptomatic degenerative disc disease in the cervical spine. *Int J Spine Surg*. 2014;1:8.
71. Vaccaro A, Beutler W, Peppelman W, et al. Clinical outcomes with selectively constrained SECURE-C cervical disc arthroplasty: two-year results from a prospective, randomized, controlled, multicenter investigational device exemption study. *Spine*. 2013;38(26):2227.
72. Heller JG, Edwards CC 2nd, Murakami H, Rodts GE. Laminoplasty versus laminectomy and fusion for multilevel cervical myelopathy: an independent matched cohort analysis. *Spine*. 2001;26(12):1330-1336.
73. Highsmith JM, Dhall SS, Haid RW Jr, Rodts GE Jr, Mummaneni PV. Treatment of cervical stenotic myelopathy: a cost and outcome comparison of laminoplasty versus laminectomy and lateral mass fusion. *J Neurosurg Spine*. 2011;14(5):619-625.
74. Woods BI, Hohl J, Lee J, Donaldson W 3rd, Kang J. Laminoplasty versus laminectomy and fusion for multilevel cervical spondylotic myelopathy. *Clin Orthop Relat Res*. 2011;469(3):688-695.
75. Yoon ST, Hashimoto RE, Raich A, et al. Outcomes after laminoplasty compared with laminectomy and fusion in patients with cervical myelopathy: a systematic review. *Spine*. 2013;38(22 suppl 1):S183-S194.
76. Newman M. The outcome of pseudarthrosis after cervical anterior fusion. *Spine*. 1993;18(16):2380-2382.
77. Phillips FM, Carlson G, Emery SE, Bohlman HH. Anterior cervical pseudarthrosis: natural history and treatment. *Spine*. 1997;22(14):1585-1589.
78. Kuhns CA, Geck MJ, Wang JC, Delamarter RBM. An outcomes analysis of the treatment of cervical pseudarthrosis with posterior fusion. *Spine*. 2005;30(21):2424-2429.
79. Liu H, Ploumis A, Schwender JD, Garvey TA. Posterior cervical lateral mass screw fixation and fusion to treat pseudarthrosis of anterior cervical fusion. *J Spinal Disord Tech*. 2012;25(3):138-141.
80. Tribus CB, Corteen DP, Zdeblick TA. The efficacy of anterior cervical plating in the management of symptomatic pseudoarthrosis of the cervical spine. *Spine*. 1999;24(9):860-864.
81. Zdeblick TA, Hughes SS, Riew KD, Bohlman HH. Failed anterior cervical discectomy and arthrodesis: analysis and treatment of thirty-five patients. *J Bone Joint Surg Am*. 1997;79-A(4):523-532.
82. Coric D, Branch CL Jr, Jenkins JD. Revision of anterior cervical pseudoarthrosis with anterior allograft fusion and plating. *J Neurosurg*. 1997;86(6):969-974.
83. Carreon L, Glassman SD, Campbell MJ. Treatment of anterior cervical pseudoarthrosis: posterior fusion versus anterior revision. *Spine J*. 2006;6(2):154-156.
84. McAnany SJ, Baird EO, Overley SC, et al. A meta-analysis of the clinical and fusion results following treatment of symptomatic cervical pseudarthrosis. *Global Spine J*. 2015;5(2):148-155.
85. Rothman R, Rashbaum R. Pathogenesis of signs and symptoms of cervical disc degeneration. *Instr Course Lect*. 1978;27:203-215.
86. DePalma AF, et al. Study of the cervical syndrome. *Clin Orthop Relat Res*. 1965;38:135-142.
87. Kambin P. Anterior cervical fusion using vertical self-locking T-graft. *Clin Orthop Relat Res*. 1980;153:132-137.
88. Brodke DS, Zdeblick T. Modified Smith-Robinson procedure for anterior cervical discectomy and fusion. *Spine*. 1992;17(10 suppl):S427-S430.
89. Kikuchi S, Macnab I, Moreau P. Localisation of the level of symptomatic cervical disc degeneration. *J Bone Joint Surg Br*. 1981;63-B(2):272-277.
90. Garvey TA, Transfeldt EE, Malcolm JR, Kos P. Outcome of anterior cervical discectomy and fusion as perceived by patients treated for dominant axial-mechanical cervical spine pain. *Spine*. 2002;27(17):1887-1894.
91. Carragee EJ, Hurwitz EL, Cheng I, et al. Treatment of neck pain: injections and surgical interventions: results of the Bone and Joint Decade 2000-2010 Task Force on Neck Pain and its Associated Disorders. *Spine*. 2008;33(4 suppl):S153-S169.
92. Riew KD, Ecker E, Dettori JR. Anterior cervical discectomy and fusion for the management of axial neck pain in the absence of radiculopathy or myelopathy. *Evid Based Spine Care J*. 2010;1(3):45-50.

41 CHAPTER Cervical Radiculopathy: Surgical Management

Sheeraz A. Qureshi
Steven J. McAnany
Dante Leven

Introduction

Cervical radiculopathy was first described in the early 20th century and recognized as a common type of nerve root impingement.[1] Stookey first reported on the presentation of symptoms, which resulted from a cervical disc causing compression of cervical nerve roots in 1928. Originally, the disc pathology was thought to be a type of chondroma, though later histologic studies proved that these findings were incorrect. The underlying degenerative process was then thought to be inflammatory or infectious, thus the condition was given the name *spondylitis*. Brain et al.[2] later recognized the compressive effect of cervical disc herniations causing nerve root compression and subsequent radicular burning pain in a series of 10 patients. Several recent studies have shown that cervical radiculopathy can be a debilitating condition with a significant impact on quality of life.[3–7] The presentation commonly occurs in the setting of degenerative cervical pathology, most commonly spondylosis, which complicates the diagnostic workup and management options.[4,7]

Studies have shown that about 10% of individuals have radiographic signs of cervical spondylosis by 25 years old and about 95% have these findings by 65 years old.[2,5] The annual incidence of cervical radiculopathy has a rate of 107 per 100,000 in men and 64 per 100,000 in women in the United States.[8] The growing number of elderly people will increase the prevalence of cervical radiculopathy over the next few decades. The demands on spine surgeons to provide efficacious and financially sound treatment options begins with a comprehensive understanding of this condition.

Pathophysiology

Cervical radiculopathy is a condition that results from nerve root compression in the cervical spine, causing various upper extremity symptoms, which include impaired sensation, parasthesias, weakness, and burning pain.[4,7,9] This can lead to impaired ability to function, work, and perform normal daily activities.

The mechanism of nerve root impingement is most commonly from one of two causes: (1) osteophyte formation or (2) disc herniation posterolaterally, typically in the neural foramen. Spondylosis, trauma, tumors, deformity, or spinal instability can also cause radiculopathy.[10,11] However, most commonly (75% of cases), a combination of degenerative changes and disc space narrowing leads to osteophyte formation and facet joint spondylosis, which encroach on the exiting nerve root. In cases of severe disc herniations causing radiculopathy, usually some degree of underlying spondylosis is contributory.[1,5]

This progressive degenerative process often begins with the cervical discs (nucleus pulposus and anulus fibrosus) losing water, proteoglycans, and nutritional support with aging, which subsequently leads to a decrease in viscoelasticity and inability to properly distribute weight and transfer load. Disc material may then bulge posteriorly (worsened by flexed postures of the neck) into the spinal canal or exiting neural foramen. The surrounding structures experience an increase in loading, which causes excess force through the uncovertebral, intervertebral, and zygaphophyseal joints. Similar to other osteoarthritic processes, osteophyte formation develops as a reactive process and an attempt to increase the stability of these joints, which have developed excessive motion.

The ligamentum flavum, anterior longitudinal ligament, and posterior longitudinal ligament (PLL) undergo hypertrophy during the degenerative process and some degree of buckling and stiffening as disc height is lost.[10] As the process progresses in severity and time, these changes produce prolonged compression and ischemic changes within the nerve roots and spinal cord. Typically, radiculopathy develops prior to the onset of myelopathic changes.

Both myelopathy and radiculopathy have been described based on dynamic and static mechanisms. During motion (dynamic), the nerve roots can be compressed by osteophytes, disc herniations, or hypertrophied ligaments. For example, with the Spurling maneuver (flexion and ipsilateral rotation and lateral bending), the posterolateral uncovertebral osteophytes encroach on the exiting nerve root, producing radicular symptoms. Over time, chronic compression (static) on the nerve roots can produce radicular symptoms and pain from ischemia and neuroinflammation, which may respond differently once the compressive force is removed with a discectomy or foraminotomy. With this prolonged compression, demyelination, scarring, atrophy, interneuronal loss, and degeneration of the spinal tracts may eventually develop, which can also alter the postoperative course.[7,10,11]

The prolonged dynamic or static compression on the nerve roots increases the permeability of the endothelial cells lining the blood vessels along the blood-brain barrier and decreases the total number of endothelial cells.[9] This allows for entry of inflammatory cells and toxins into the spinal parenchyma. The combination of neuroinflammation and toxins can worsen the compression and hypoxic environment, which worsens the underlying pain and radicular symptoms. Chemical mediators released from the disc tissue and sensory neurons perpetuate the inflammatory response, and chronic edema may increase the sensitivity of the nerve roots to pain. The dorsal root ganglion has also been implicated in the development of radiculopathy, as these cell bodies produce chemical mediators and the surrounding membrane is more permeable than other regions of the nerve root.

Though less common with radiculopathy, spinal deformity may contribute to this cascade of events. The degenerative process often results in segmental or global cervical kyphosis and the nerve roots and spinal cord are driven anteriorly, which tensions these structures, exacerbating the inflammatory and compressive pathologies. The C5–C7 spinal levels are responsible for the greatest amount of motion and force distribution in the subaxial spine and are most commonly involved in cervical radiculopathy. The apex of the cervical lordosis is found at C5, and loss of the normal cervical curvature in the sagittal or coronal plane places excessive stress on adjacent spinal levels. If the underlying process is left untreated, the degenerative changes commonly proceed cephalad and caudally.

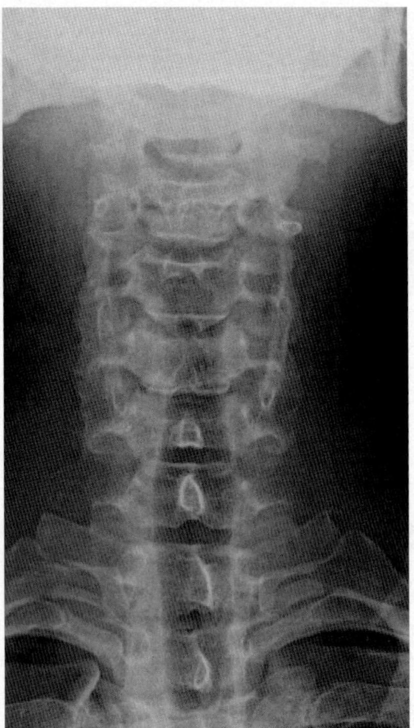

FIG. 41.1 Anteroposterior radiograph of the cervical spine demonstrating normal alignment with no significant uncovertebral arthrosis.

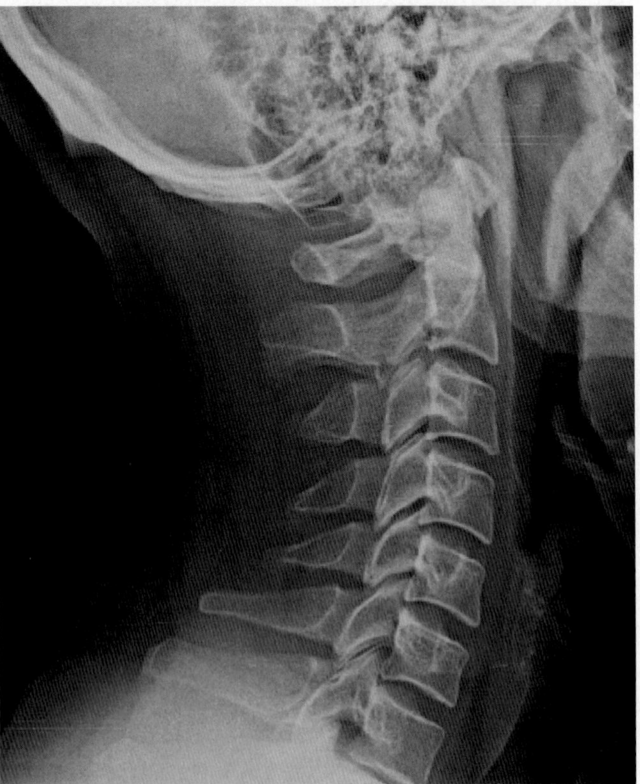

FIG. 41.2 Lateral cervical radiograph demonstrating preserved cervical lordosis, and no evidence of central stenosis or cervical spondylosis.

Radiographic Evaluation

Patients presenting with an acute episode of cervical radiculopathy do not require immediate imaging in the setting of a normal neurologic examination. If the patient continues to be symptomatic after 6 weeks of appropriate conservative management, plain cervical radiographs consisting of an anteroposterior and lateral radiograph can be obtained (Fig. 41.1). The lateral radiograph is particularly helpful in determining the space available for the cord in the anteroposterior diameter (Fig. 41.2).

Flexion and extension radiographs should be considered to rule out segmental instability (Fig. 41.3). Oblique cervical radiographs can also be helpful, as they can identify areas of foraminal stenosis that may be correlated with the clinical symptoms of the patient. Overall, the series of plain radiographs is useful for identifying areas of foraminal stenosis, the presence of significant osteophytes/spondylosis, and the presence of spinal instability.

Magnetic resonance imaging (MRI) remains the gold standard for the diagnosis of cervical radiculopathy. Wilson et al.[12] were among the first groups to correlate MRI findings of nerve root compression with intraoperative findings. MRI offers several advantages, including excellent visualization of the neural elements and soft tissues, the ability to directly identify soft disc herniations, and no radiation exposure for the patient (Fig. 41.4). Park at al.[13] recently evaluated the diagnostic utility of oblique MRI images for improving the

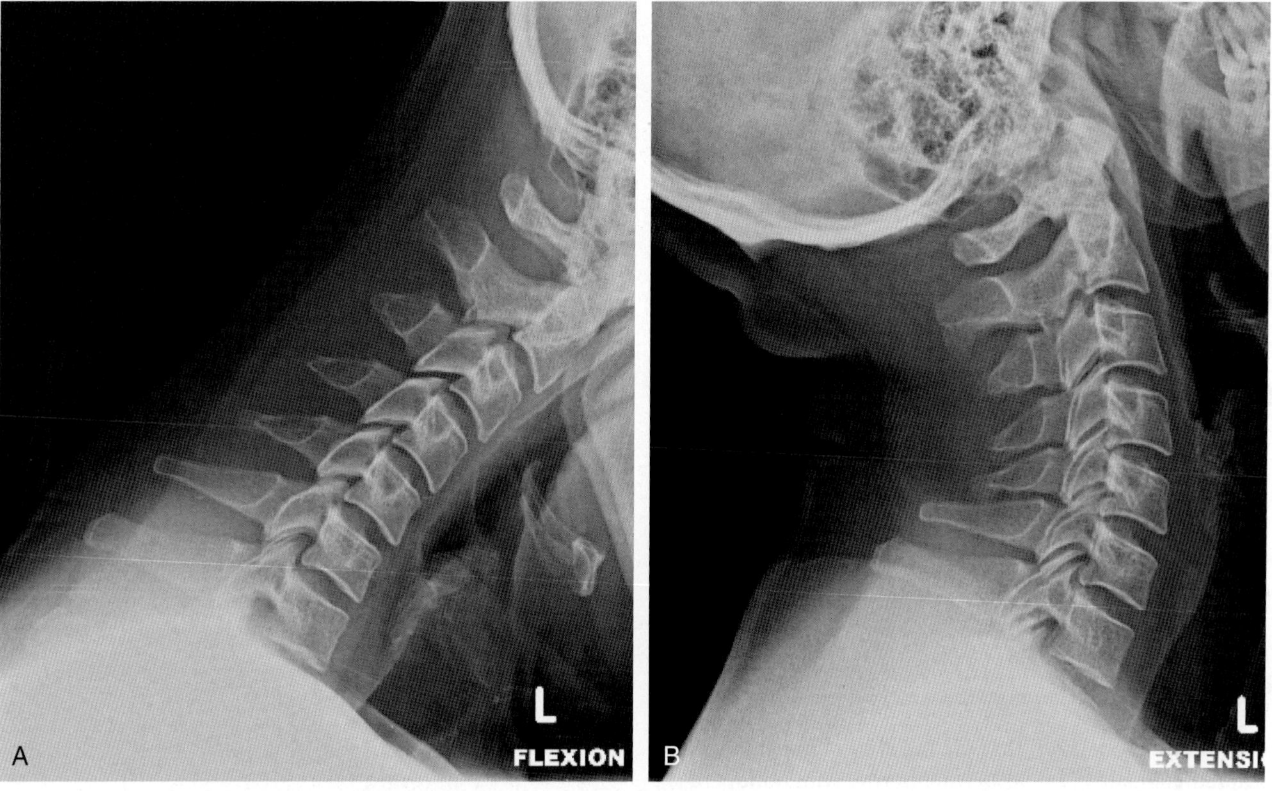

FIG. 41.3 (A) Flexion and (B) extension lateral cervical radiographs with no evidence of segmental instability.

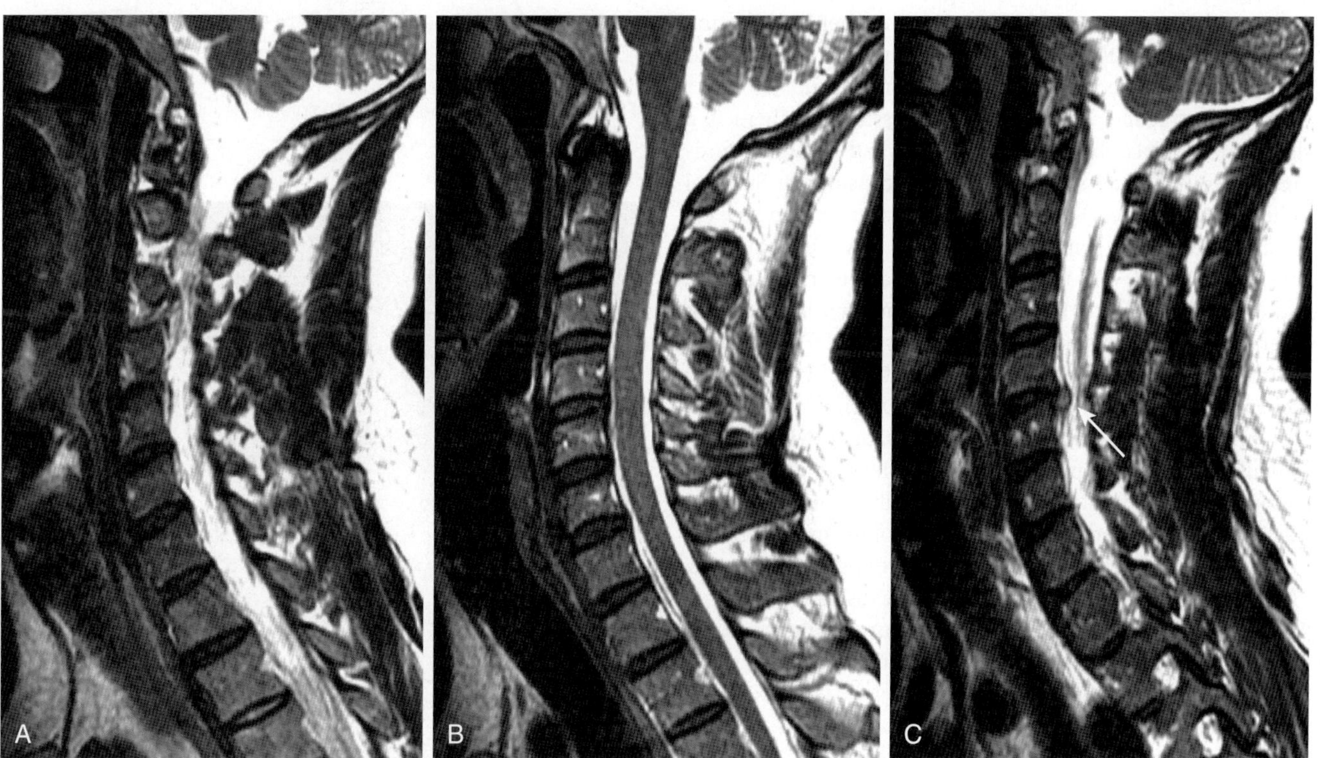

FIG. 41.4 (A–C) Sagittal and parasagittal T2-weighted cervical magnetic resonance images demonstrating a right C4–C5 disc herniation with root compression *(arrow)*.

diagnostic accuracy in foraminal stenosis. The authors concluded that oblique MRI views of the cervical spine significantly reduce the degree of intraobserver and interobserver variabilities and increase observer confidence in the assessment of foraminal stenosis.

Computed tomography (CT) myelography remains a useful tool in the diagnosis of cervical radiculopathy, particularly in patients who have had previous instrumentation in the cervical spine. Myelography can also be used in patients who have a contraindication to receiving an MRI.

Surgical Indications

The surgical indications for the treatment of cervical radiculopathy include (1) persistent radicular symptoms that have not improved with an appropriate trial of conservative care, (2) a neurologic deficit that is progressive, and/or (3) a neurologic deficit that is associated with significant radicular pain.

Surgical Treatment

Several studies have shown that the majority of patients with cervical radiculopathy (75–90%) will improve with nonoperative treatment.[8,14] However, other studies have shown that more than 55% of patients presenting with cervical radiculopathy have little or no improvement in symptoms.[15] Regardless, with patients presenting without significant motor weakness, a reasonable course of conservative treatment—including nonsteroidal antiinflammatory drugs, physical therapy, and epidural steroid injections—should be considered.

If nonoperative treatment is unsuccessful and there is a clear concordance between symptoms and imaging findings, several surgical strategies may be considered. Surgical indications include (1) progressive cervical radiculopathy, (2) persistent radicular symptoms after 4 to 8 weeks of nonoperative treatment, (3) instability with radicular symptoms, and (4) motor deficits. Posterior foraminotomy/laminotomy, anterior cervical discectomy and fusion (ACDF), and disc arthroplasty are all surgical options that should be considered after a careful review of the risks and potential benefits of each procedure. In a randomized trial of patients with cervical radiculopathy, Peolsson et al.[16] placed patients in one of three cohorts: ACDF, physical therapy, or collar immobilization. They found improved pain scores at 4 months in the surgical group, but no difference in the three groups at 12 months. However, the surgery group had favorable disability ratings at 12 months. These findings may support surgical intervention, though only following the completion of a structured physical therapy program.

Anterior Approach

The anterior approach was first described in the 1960s by Robinson and Smith, and later modified by several surgeons to include a formal discectomy, foraminotomy, and corpectomy (when necessary).[17–19]

The anteromedial approach is the most common approach utilized for anterior procedures. The patient is placed supine, with the neck in neutral or slight extension and a towel roll, intravenous bag or blood pressure cuff placed behind the neck or scapular region to enhance access. Fig. 41.5 demonstrates the typical anatomic landmarks that can be used for localization.

For surgery on lower cervical levels (C6–C7), the shoulders are carefully taped down (tensioned caudally) to improve radiographic access. Gardner-Wells tongs may be used to help position the head and provide slight traction during the approach.

A transverse or oblique incision is utilized in line with the skin creases for optimal cosmesis (Fig. 41.6). For multilevel

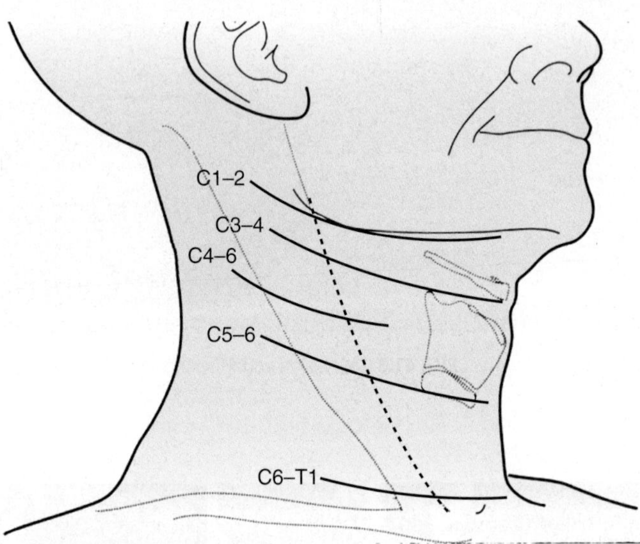

FIG. 41.5 Superficial landmarks are helpful in identifying the correct level for skin incision.

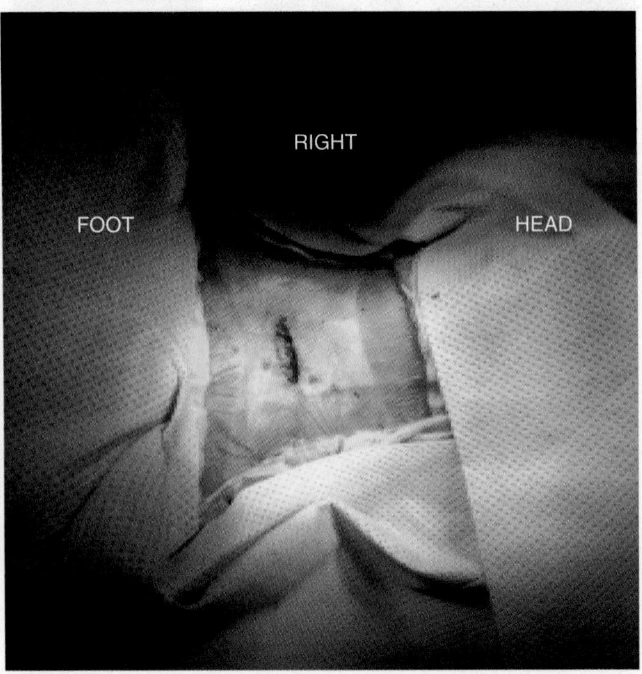

FIG. 41.6 Intraoperative image with a typical Smith-Robinson anterior cervical type approach.

procedures, an oblique incision is more commonly used in line with the medial edge of the sternocleidomastoid. For primary procedures, the left- or right-sided approach may be utilized; no studies have shown a consistent advantage of either approach. The side of surgical approach is dictated by surgeon preference, though the concerns regarding the recurrent laryngeal nerve support a left-sided approach, as the course of this nerve is more consistent within the carotid sheath. However, the thoracic duct may potentially be injured from the left side with access to more caudal cervical levels.

The superficial fascia is often encountered overlying the platysma, which runs from the midline of the mandible vertically to the medial border of the sternocleidomastoid. The muscle is sectioned transversely, perpendicular to the muscle fibers, which allows visualization of the deep cervical fascia. Depending on the number of spinal levels being addressed, the platysma may be undermined in a cephalad and caudal direction to mobilize the soft tissue window. Careful palpation is utilized to identify the carotid sheath and identify the plane between the sternocleidomastoid laterally and the trachea and esophagus medially. A combination of blunt and sharp dissection is used to continue through the deep cervical fascia, which is encountered in layers. Palpation of osteophytes can help identify the midline of the anterior cervical spine. The pretracheal and prevertebral fascia are released with an elevator or electrocautery to expose the anterior vertebral body and intervertebral disc. The longus colli are encountered and also released laterally to the lateral border of the vertebral body. Once the disc space is clearly identified, a bent 18-gauge needle is placed into the disc space to confirm the spinal level with a lateral radiograph.

Typically, the disc is incised with a long No. 15 blade scalpel and the anterior anulus is removed with a straight pituitary (Fig. 41.7A). The disc is then removed with curettes and Kerrison rongeurs in a systematic manner, proceeding posteriorly with awareness of the uncovertebral joints laterally and the posterior depth within the disc space (Fig. 41.7B). A high-speed burr is used to prepare the endplates of the caudal and cephalad levels until punctate bleeding is encountered.

Overall, this is a muscle-sparing approach with little muscle dissection and minimal postoperative pain. The advantages include low infection rates, low wound complications, and less pain, which may improve the rate of postoperative recovery and minimize the use of postoperative narcotics.[9]

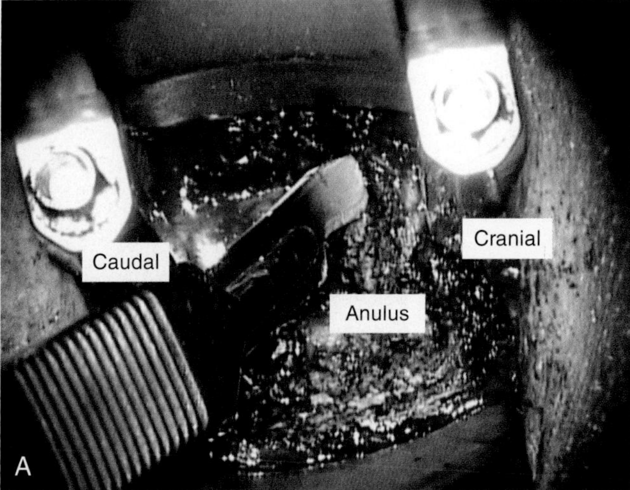

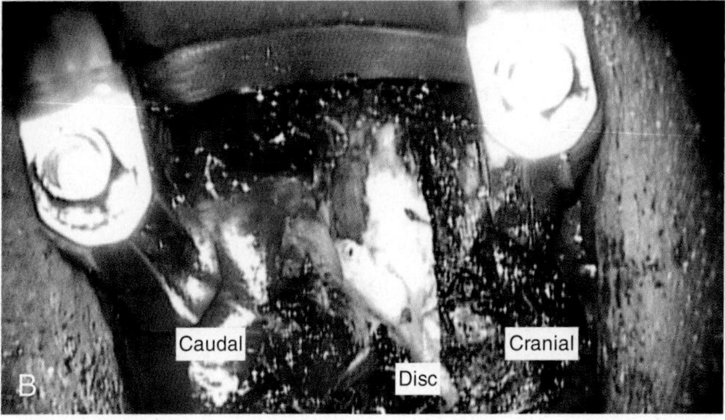

FIG. 41.7 Intraoperative images showing (A) incision of the anulus and (B) removal of the disc material.

Anterior Cervical Discectomy and Fusion

ACDF allows access to the majority of compressive pathologies (intervertebral discs, ventral osteophytes, foraminal compression, and ossification of the posterior longitudinal ligament) and is a good option for most single- and two-level pathologies (Fig. 41.8). The efficacy of ACDF for relief of arm pain and neurologic deficits and successful patient-reported outcomes has been extensively reported.[19–23] Additional benefits of ACDF include the restoration of cervical lordosis, decompression in the presence of kyphotic deformities, and the indirect decompression that is also provided by placement of the spacer or bone graft within the disc space. Axial neck pain from underlying spondylosis or disc degeneration can also be addressed with ACDF, although the results may be inferior compared to relief of radicular pain.

Overall complication rates with anterior procedures are often higher than with posterior procedures, which include pseudarthrosis, adjacent-segment degeneration (ASD), plate- and graft-related complications, and approach-related complications.[23–28] Important variables include patient factors, number of spinal levels, and use of plating or ventral fixation. Recent literature has shown comparable complication rates between anterior and posterior procedures, with higher complication rates in combined anterior-posterior procedures. Zhu et al. compared anterior (n = 245) and posterior (n = 285) procedures; the reoperation rate was significantly higher in the anterior group (21/245, 8.57% vs. 1/285, 0.3%; $P < .001$). Of the 21 who underwent reoperation, 13 of 21 (62%) were for pseudarthrosis, 7 of 21 (33.3%) for adjacent deterioration, and 1 of 21 (4.8%) for loosening of implant. In the posterior group, only 1 (0.3%) required reoperation for radiculopathy due to a new herniation, which is consistent with other studies.[29] However, postoperative neurologic function and outcomes were more favorable in the anterior group ($P < 0.05$).

In several well-designed investigations, anterior plating has been shown to improve fusion rates compared with stand-alone grafts and cages.[30–32] Newer-design stand-alone spacers with anterior fixation need further long-term studies

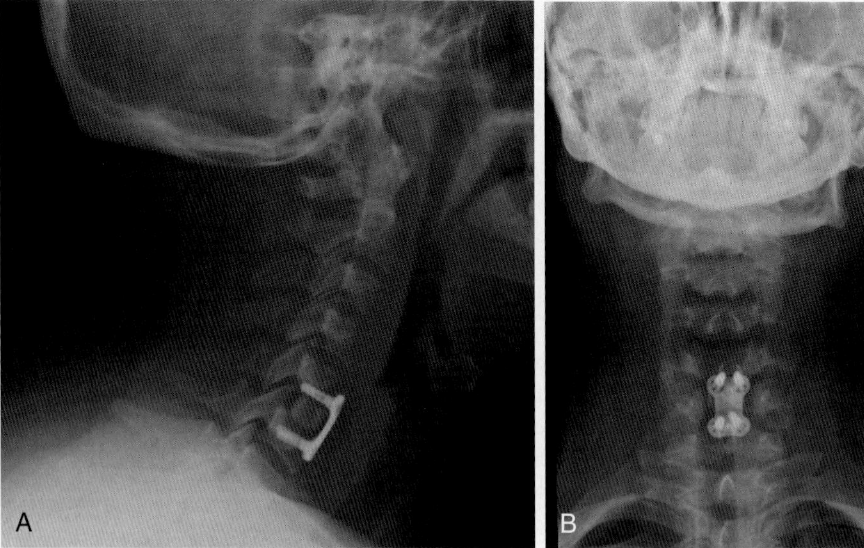

FIG. 41.8 (A) Lateral and (B) anteroposterior cervical radiographs in a patient after anterior cervical discectomy and fusion at C5–C6.

to analyze patient outcomes, complications, and fusion rates. Fusion rates of 96% and 91% for one- and two-level ACDF with anterior plate fixation compared with 90% and 72% without anterior fixation ($P < .05$) were shown in a retrospective review of 540 patients.[13] In a meta-analysis of 2682 patients, Fraser et al.[31] assessed fusion rates in ACDF and anterior cervical corpectomy and fusion (ACCF) procedures with and without plate fixation. Plate fixation improved fusion rates for all one-, two-, and three-level ACDFs ($P <.0001$, .0001, and .05, respectively). They also concluded that for three-level procedures, corpectomy with plate placement was associated with slightly higher fusion rates than discectomy without plate placement (82.5% vs. 96.2%; $P < .05$).

ASD is a common complication following ACDF with an incidence of 2.9% per year.[35,36] Lee et al.[33] showed that patients undergoing posterior arthrodesis were 7.5 times more likely to undergo reoperation due to ASD than patients undergoing posterior decompression only, and three times more likely to undergo reoperation due to ASD than patients undergoing anterior arthrodesis.

In a large recent study of approach-related complications in patients undergoing ACDF, the overall incidence of dysphagia, hoarseness, and unilateral vocal cord paralysis was 12.3%, 4.9%, and 1.4%, respectively.[34] Dysphagia and hoarseness are common postoperative complications that require close monitoring, though typically resolve by 6 months.

Multilevel Pathology

Cervical radiculopathy commonly involves one spinal level, though with prolonged degenerative changes, several levels may become involved. Bolesta et al. found high pseudarthrosis rates in a review of patients undergoing three- and four-level ACDFs with iliac crest autograft and locking plates.[35] Pseudarthrosis was found in 53% (8/16) of patients, though less than half (3/8) had enough pain to warrant a revision procedure. The authors concluded that, though plating may improve fusion rates for ACDFs, three- and four-level fusions appear to have unacceptably high failure rates.

The choice of interbody implant remains an area of controversy and interest. Historically, iliac crest autograft has been the gold standard, with fusion rates approaching 100% in some series. However, harvesting of iliac crest autograft is not without complications. These include chronic graft site harvest pain, infection, hematoma formation, and pelvic bone fracture. Allograft bone, while it eliminates the possibility of graft harvest complications, may have a slower time to union compared with autograft. Additionally, the overall fusion rate for a single-level ACDF may be lower than what is seen with autograft. Additional interbody options after ACDF include polyetheretherketone as well as titanium cages. Both have shown fusion rates comparable to allograft.

Cervical Arthroplasty

Cervical disc arthroplasty (CDA) is an option for patients with cervical radiculopathy that provides decompression without a fusion, and good midterm patient-reported outcomes have been reported[36–40] (Fig. 41.9). The surgical approach is essentially the same as for ACDF; thus, approach-related complications are reportedly similar, though some have reported longer operative times and more blood loss with cervical arthroplasty.[41] This motion-sparing procedure may minimize the complications of ASD, plate and screw complications, plate and soft tissue irritation, and nonunion. Additionally, ACDF may lead to higher rates of surrounding joint arthropathy and disc degeneration as a compensatory mechanism to the fusion, though some studies support that this is a natural development in the patient with underlying spondylosis and degenerative changes.[42] For example, the ASD rate of 2.9% per year has been reported regardless of the index procedure (ACDF, CDA, posterior foraminotomy),[33,43,44] and several studies

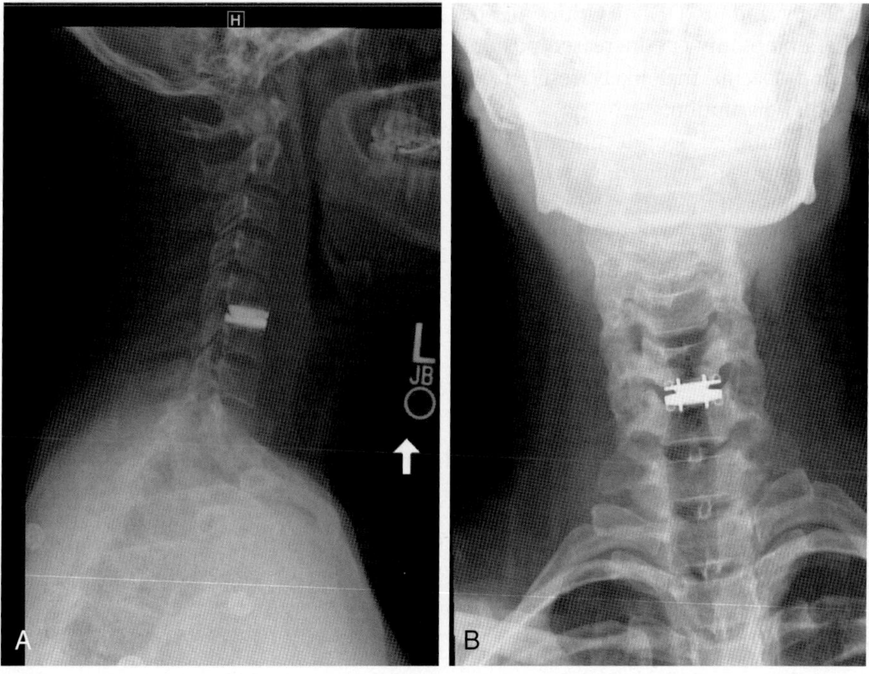

FIG. 41.9 (A) Lateral and (B) anteroposterior cervical radiographs in a patient who underwent a C5–C6 cervical disc arthroplasty.

comparing arthrodesis with motion-sparing procedures have shown comparable rates of ASD.[27,42] There are limited studies analyzing the development of long-term changes in patients following CDA compared with ACDF.

As some patients with ASD are asymptomatic, describing this complication based on whether surgery was indicated may be a more relevant factor. Lee et al.[33] conducted a study of 1358 patients undergoing ACDF, laminoplasty, foraminotomy, CDA, posterior or combined anterior and posterior arthrodesis. The rate of ASD that required a reoperation (ASD that occurred at a level cephalad or caudal to the index procedure that did not respond to conservative treatment, which was consistent with the patients' symptoms and imaging) was compared between the groups. The positive predictors were female sex, smoking, and posterior or combined anterior and posterior fusion ($P < .05$). Patients undergoing ACDF, CDA, or posterior decompression had similar rates of ASD. These findings support that the development of ASD may be more related to the natural progression of the underlying pathology than the type of procedure.

In a meta-analysis by Gao et al.[41] comparing ACDF and CDA, neurologic outcomes and neck and arm pain scores were more favorable in the arthroplasty cohort, while the neck disability index (NDI) was similar between the two groups. The underlying etiology of these findings could not be determined; however, the ACDF group had a higher rate of requiring a secondary surgical procedure (odds ratio [OR], 0.52; $P = .01$).

Sasso et al[39] reported promising 4-year results in a study comparing CDA with ACDF. Statistically significant outcomes favoring the CDA cohort were found for Short Form-36 scores and arm pain while NDI, range of motion and adverse events were similar between the two groups. Another investigation reported on 7-year follow-up of patients treated with CDA or ACDF. Patients in the CDA cohort were found to have lower rates of subsequent procedures for ASD and lower reoperation rates. NDI and neurologic improvement were also favorable in the CDA group.[45] As more long-term studies come to fruition, the mid- and long-term complications and patient-reported outcomes associated with CDA will be better understood and the optimal treatment options can be more clearly discussed during patient counseling.

Posterior Cervical Foraminotomy

A number of surgical techniques have been employed for the treatment of cervical radiculopathy. Surgeons have at their disposal a number of evolving technologies, including the use of minimally invasive surgery (MIS), to treat the pathology. The decision to treat cervical radiculopathy from an anterior- or posterior-based approach or through an open or MIS approach is determined by both the surgeon's comfort with the particular technique and, highly important, the location of the pathology.

The use of a posterior-based approach for the treatment of cervical radiculopathy was first described over 65 years ago by Mixter.[46] Frykholm[47] and Scoville[48] further popularized the posterior cervical foraminotomy technique. In the 1980s, the technique underwent advancement and refinement with the development of the keyhole laminoforaminotomy, as popularized by Fager,[49] Epstein,[50] and Casotto.[51] In small case series, a clinical success rate approaching 90% was found with this new technique. More recently, success rates approaching 95% have been reported using the open technique.[52] Furthermore, recent studies have shown no difference in clinical outcomes or surgical complication rates when comparing posterior cervical laminoforaminotomy and ACDF.[53,54] Critics of the open posterior cervical foraminotomy cite increased postoperative axial neck pain and spasms that likely result from increased muscle damage and disruption.

As an alternative to the traditional open technique, minimally invasive posterior cervical foraminotomy techniques have been developed. Proponents of the MIS technique cite a shorter hospital stay, less blood loss, faster recovery time, and equivalent or better clinical outcomes.[55–57] Furthermore, by eliminating the subperiosteal dissection of muscle, the MIS techniques result in less acute muscle injury and denervation, which may improve long-term cervical biomechanics when compared with the open technique.

Indications for Posterior Cervical Foraminotomy

Posterior cervical foraminotomy via an open or MIS approach is indicated for patients with cervical radiculopathy resulting from compression of the nerve root within the neural foramen as a result of an osteophyte, spondylosis, or a lateral disc herniation. Patients should have received appropriate conservative management for a minimum of 6 weeks prior to being indicated for surgery. Furthermore, the patient's pattern of radiculopathy should correlate with findings on advanced imaging, including CT, MRI, or a CT myelogram. Absolute contraindications for posterior cervical foraminotomy include local segmental kyphosis or instability, evidence of spinal cord compression or myelopathy, or symptomatology not referable to findings on the imaging studies.

Open Technique

The open posterior cervical laminoforaminotomy is performed with the patient in the prone position. Mayfield three-pin tongs may be applied to secure the head to the table. The head of the patient is placed into gentle flexion to decrease the cervical lordosis, which facilitates visualization of the superior facet of the caudal vertebral segment. The bed is then positioned in the reverse Trendelenburg position, with the knees flexed to less than 90 degrees, which helps to reduce epidural venous bleeding. Surgical tape may be used to lower the shoulders to facilitate imaging of the lower cervical levels as well as to flatten any possible skin creases. A lateral cervical radiograph using a metallic marker or needle is used to determine the appropriate operative level.

A midline skin incision is made centered over the spinous process of the intended level. For a single-level foraminotomy, the length of the skin incision should be approximately 2 cm. The skin incision is carried down to the fascia of the nuchal ligament, which is divided in the midline to expose the spinous processes. A metal clamp can then be attached to the spinous process, and a lateral cervical radiograph is used to again confirm the correct operative level. Dissection is then continued in a subperiosteal fashion, elevating the paravertebral muscles from the lamina. The dissection is carried laterally to the facet joint with careful attention paid to not violate the facet capsule. Once the inferior articular process (IAP) of the cephalad vertebra is identified, a high-speed burr is used to remove the medial third of the IAP and the inferior portion of the superior lamina. A Kerrison rongeur (1 or 2 mm) is used to enlarge the space until the ligamentum flavum is identified. Once this is removed, the exiting nerve is able to be identified within the foramen. Additional bone can be removed until a nerve probe can be easily placed within the neuroforamen.

If there is a discrete disc herniation, the nerve root can be gently retracted superiorly to expose the extruded disc fragments or the distended PLL. A discectomy can be performed by sharply incising the PLL overlying the herniated fragments. Once all of the visible fragments are removed, irrigation of the disc space and the use of reverse angle curettes and upgoing pituitaries can remove any additional fragments that are not readily visualized.

After completing the decompression, the wound is copiously irrigated with antibiotic saline. The fascia is then reapproximated, and the wound is closed in layers.

Minimally Invasive Technique

Following the induction of anesthesia, the bed is positioned so that the operative side is away from the anesthesia equipment. The patient is then placed in a sitting or semirecumbent position utilizing a Mayfield three-point head fixation. Similar to the positioning utilized in the open technique, the patient's head is placed into gentle flexion. The bed is placed in the reverse Trendelenburg position, with knee flexion.

The target level is initially localized by placing a spinal needle lateral to the neck and checked fluoroscopically. A longitudinal 1.5- to 1.8-cm incision is made 1.5 cm lateral to the midline on the operative side. The ideal trajectory is to angle slightly cephalad from the skin to the lamina. A Kirschner wire (K-wire) is then introduced through the skin incision and advanced to the inferomedial edge of the rostral lateral mass at the operative level. A lateral fluoroscopic image is obtained to confirm the level. It is important at this step to fully release the deep cervical fascia with a pair of scissors, as this can restrict the passage of the tube dilators. Once this is done, serial dilators are passed to create the appropriately sized working portal.

Once confirmed to be on the lamina, the first dilator is passed over the wire to the bone, and the wire is removed (Fig. 41.10). Once the final dilator is in place, the operative tube is positioned caudally over the lamina with fluoroscopic confirmation until centered over the target disc space before anchoring to the table-mounted arm (Fig. 41.11).

The remaining muscle overlying the bone is removed with a pituitary rongeur. At this point, the microendoscope is brought in to use from the cephalad side for visualization. The medial facet and lateral lamina can usually be visualized at this point. Any remaining soft tissue obstructing the view is either removed or cauterized to shrink out of the way. The laminoforaminotomy is then initiated using a high-speed drill, removing the outer cortical layer and cancellous bone of the lamina as well as the medial aspect of the facet. Once a small opening is made through the deep cortical bone over the lateral canal, a Kerrison rongeur is used to complete the

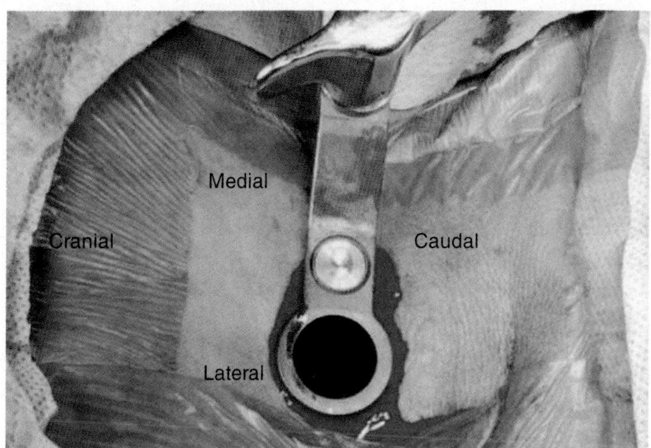

FIG. 41.10 Intraoperative image demonstrating the tube placement during a minimally invasive posterior cervical foraminotomy.

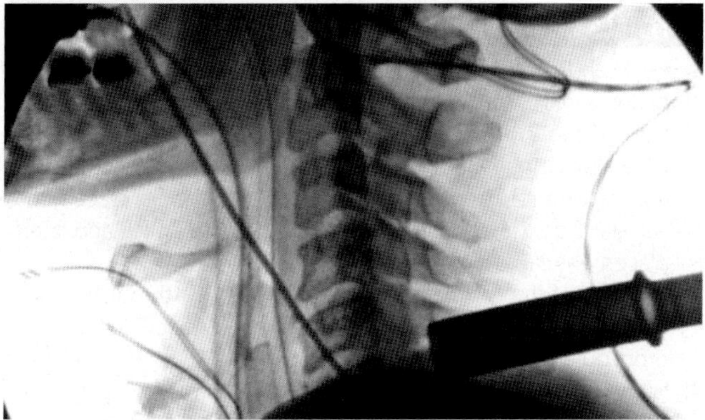

FIG. 41.11 Intraoperative lateral cervical radiograph showing the tube placement overlying the C5–C6 lateral mass.

foraminotomy. Identifying the medial and cephalad margins of the pedicle is useful for medial/lateral orientation. The foraminotomy is extended laterally until the lateral margin of the pedicle begins to fall away. At this point, only a third to a half of the medial facet has been removed and should not impact stability. A small laminotomy in the caudal lamina is useful to visualize the lateral margin of the thecal sac. A nerve hook can be introduced to retract the nerve root superiorly to allow access to the disc space. Loose disc fragments can be mobilized into the axilla, where they can be removed with a micropituitary rongeur. Similar to the open procedure, contained fragments may require an incision of the PLL and the use of reverse-angle curettes and downgoing pituitaries to facilitate removal of the disc herniation.

Once hemostasis is obtained with electrocautery or hemostatic foam, the wound is carefully irrigated. The operative cylinder is removed and the wound closed in a standard layered fashion.

Surgical Outcomes

The posterior cervical foraminotomy is a safe, highly efficacious procedure that provides significant symptom relief to those patients with foraminal-based compression of the nerve root resulting in radiculopathy. The traditional open, midline-based approach has been refined over several decades. In recent years, MIS-based techniques have been developed as an alternative to the standard open procedure. Proponents of the open technique cite the familiarity of the posterior approach to the cervical spine, avoidance of the steep learning curve associated with MIS techniques, and avoidance of the complications associated with MIS techniques, including misplacement of the percutaneous K-wire and medial/lateral migration of the tubular retractor, causing spinal cord/nerve root injury. Advocates of the MIS approach cite shorter hospital stays, less blood loss, and a quicker return to function.

Many small case series have reported on the results of either the open or MIS technique. Kang et al.[58] performed a retrospective review of 135 patients who underwent a posterior cervical foraminotomy, with 117 also receiving a discectomy. Clinical success was determined by excellent or good outcomes as defined by Odom criteria. Overall, 106 of 117 (90.6%) patients were deemed to have a successful outcome. Additionally, neck and radicular visual analog scale (VAS) scores improved by 2.1 and 3.2 points, respectively. Witzmann et al.[59] reported similar findings following an open posterior cervical foraminotomy, with a clinical success rate of 90%. Ruetten et al.[54] performed a randomized controlled trial of endoscopic foraminotomy versus ACDF. Clinical success was achieved in 96.6% of the foraminotomy patients. Another retrospective review of 100 patients undergoing a microendoscopic posterior cervical foraminotomy found that at an average follow-up of 14.8 months, 97% of patients were deemed to have achieved a clinical success.[55]

There are a limited number of studies directly comparing the results of open versus MIS posterior cervical foraminotomy. Winder et al.[60] found significant differences favoring the MIS cohort with respect to decreased intraoperative blood loss, postoperative analgesic use, and length of hospital stay. However, there were no differences in operative time or operative complications. The authors also noted that the results did not take into account the associated learning curve of the individual surgeons, which could have an impact on the observed complication rates. It is important to consider the learning curve when mastering any sort of novel technique. In one study, blood loss, operative time, and complications were all higher during the initial learning curve.[56] The authors noted an initial durotomy rate of 9%, which fell to less than 1% as experience increased. Lee et al.[61] found that surgeons reach the end of their initial learning curve after 30 cases with the MIS transforaminal lumbar interbody fusion technique.

In the only prospective, randomized clinical trial comparing open and MIS posterior cervical foraminotomy techniques, Kim et al.[62] performed an open procedure in 19 patients and a tubular retractor–assisted MIS technique in 22 patients. The length of incision, duration of hospital stay, and amount of postoperative narcotic use all favored the MIS group. However, there were no significant differences found in radicular pain at any time point. At 2-year follow-up, clinical success was achieved in 16 of 19 (84.2) of the open cohort and 19 of 22 (86.4%) of the MIS cohort.

A recent systematic review by Clark et al.[63] compared open and MIS foraminotomy results. The authors were able to identify 19 studies that met inclusion criteria. Summative results indicated that patients undergoing MIS foraminotomy had lower blood loss, a shorter operative time, less analgesic utilization, and a shorter hospital stay. McAnany et al.[64] in a meta-analysis comparing the open and MIS techniques found an overall clinical success rate as defined by Odom or Prolo criteria of 92.7% in the open group and 94.9% in the MIS group, which did not achieve statistical significance.

The anterior approach to the cervical spine, as pioneered by Smith and Robinson[18] and Cloward,[17] has largely remained the gold standard for the treatment of cervical radiculopathy. However, the posterior cervical foraminotomy has been shown over the last 4 decades to be a highly efficacious procedure with excellent clinical outcomes. Advantages of the posterior approach when compared to the anterior approach include improved access to posterolateral disc herniations, decreased risk of iatrogenic kyphosis, no risk for graft subsidence, and no risk for pseudarthrosis.[52,65] Furthermore, the risk of adjacent-segment disease remains a clinical concern following an ACDF.[66] After an ACDF, biomechanics studies have demonstrated that an arthrodesis affects the mechanical properties of the adjacent discs, resulting in hypermobility and increased internal stress responses.[42,67,68] A purported advantage of posterior cervical laminoforaminotomy is the motion preservation that can potentially prevent ASD. However, in a recent study by Skovrlj et al.,[69] the authors found a rate of ASD of 0.9% per year, which is similar to recent rates found in the literature following ACDF. Similarly, Lubelski et al.[70] found no difference in the reoperation rates between ACDF and posterior cervical foraminotomy at 2 years. A recent cost analysis comparing ACDF and posterior cervical foraminotomy found that ACDF is 89% more expensive and in the context of equivalent outcomes may not be the ideal surgical strategy.[71]

Summary

Cervical radiculopathy remains one of the most common complaints treated by spine surgeons. While most patients can be effectively managed with conservative care, surgical treatment of cervical radiculopathy is associated with good clinical outcomes and resolution of symptoms. The pathology associated with cervical radiculopathy can be effectively managed with either an anterior- or posterior-based approach. From an anterior-based approach, ACDF and CDA have been shown to have equivalent outcomes. Posteriorly, foraminal-based compression of the nerve can be treated with an open or MIS laminoforaminotomy. There are no differences in clinical outcomes when choosing between open and MIS-based approaches.

PEARLS

1. Flexion-extension radiographs should be obtained prior to considering a posterior-based laminoforaminotomy, as this procedure can worsen any preexisting segmental instability.
2. Oblique cervical radiographs and/or MRI can be utilized to more accurately assess foraminal-based pathology and can be used to correlate with clinical symptomatology.
3. During anterior-based procedures, taping of the shoulders can often facilitate radiographic visualization of lower cervical levels.
4. Palpation of bony landmarks, including the thyroid cartilage (C4–C5), cricoid cartilage (C6), and the carotid tubercle (C6), can be useful when planning the incision for anterior-based procedures.
5. When preparing the endplates during cervical disc arthroplasty, it is important to remove all of the disc material or the implant may shift position.
6. The lateral fluoroscopic radiograph is critical when implanting a cervical disc arthroplasty, as splaying of the facet joints may indicate that the implant is too large and a gap between the implant and the endplate indicates that the implant is undersized.
7. In a revision anterior procedure, the surgeon should consider an otolaryngology evaluation to assess the status of the vocal cords and function of the recurrent laryngeal nerve.

PITFALLS

1. Cervical disc arthroplasty should not be considered in those patients with significant facet joint degeneration or severe cervical spondylosis.
2. When localizing with the Steinmann pin in MIS foraminotomies, it is important to accurately place the pin, as medial placement can damage the spinal cord in the interlaminar space and lateral placement can damage the exiting nerve root.
3. Violation of the endplates during cervical disc arthroplasty can result in implant subsidence and the need for a revision procedure.
4. When performing a posterior cervical foraminotomy, care should be taken to avoid removal of greater than 50% of the facet joint, as this may result in segmental instability.

REFERENCES

1. Brain WR, Knight GC, Bull JW. Discussion of rupture of the intervertebral disc in the cervical region. *Proc R Soc Med.* 1948;41(8):509-516.
2. Garfin SR. Cervical degenerative disorders: etiology, presentation, and imaging studies. *Instr Course Lect.* 2000;49:335-338.
3. Baptiste DC, Fehlings MG. Pathophysiology of cervical myelopathy. *Spine J.* 2006;6(6 suppl):190S-197S.
4. Rhee JM, Yoon T, Riew KD. Cervical radiculopathy. *J Am Acad Orthop Surg.* 2007;15(8):486-494.
5. Shedid D, Benzel EC. Cervical spondylosis anatomy: pathophysiology and biomechanics. *Neurosurgery.* 2007;60(1 Suppl 1):S7-S13.
6. Caridi JM, Pumberger M, Hughes AP. Cervical radiculopathy: a review. *HSS J.* 2011;7(3):265-272.
7. Tetreault L, Goldstein CL, Arnold P, et al. Degenerative cervical myelopathy: a spectrum of related disorders affecting the aging spine. *Neurosurgery.* 2015;77(suppl 4):S51-S67.
8. Radhakrishnan K, Litchy WJ, O'Fallon WM, Kurland LT. Epidemiology of cervical radiculopathy. A population-based study from Rochester, Minnesota, 1976 through 1990. *Brain.* 1994;117(Pt 2):325-335.
9. Rao RD, Gourab K, David KS. Operative treatment of cervical spondylotic myelopathy. *J Bone Joint Surg Am.* 2006;88(7):1619-1640.
10. Cooper RG, Freemont AJ, Hoyland JA, et al. Herniated intervertebral disc-associated periradicular fibrosis and

vascular abnormalities occur without inflammatory cell infiltration. *Spine*. 1995;20(5):591-598.
11. Kalsi-Ryan S, Karadimas SK, Fehlings MG. Cervical spondylotic myelopathy: the clinical phenomenon and the current pathobiology of an increasingly prevalent and devastating disorder. *Neuroscientist*. 2013;19(4):409-421.
12. Wilson DW, Pezzuti RT, Place JN. Magnetic resonance imaging in the preoperative evaluation of cervical radiculopathy. *Neurosurgery*. 1991;28(2):175-179.
13. Park MS, Moon SH, Lee HM, et al. Diagnostic value of oblique magnetic resonance images for evaluating cervical foraminal stenosis. *Spine J*. 2015;15(4):607-611.
14. Sampath P, Bendebba M, Davis JD, Ducker T. Outcome in patients with cervical radiculopathy. Prospective, multicenter study with independent clinical review. *Spine*. 1999;24(6):591-597.
15. Lees F, Turner JW. Natural history and prognosis of cervical spondylosis. *Br Med J*. 1963;2(5373):1607-1610.
16. Peolsson A, Soderlund A, Engquist M, et al. Physical function outcome in cervical radiculopathy patients after physiotherapy alone compared with anterior surgery followed by physiotherapy: a prospective randomized study with a 2-year follow-up. *Spine*. 2013;38(4):300-307.
17. Cloward RB. The anterior approach for removal of ruptured cervical disks. *J Neurosurg*. 1958;15(6):602-617.
18. Smith GW, Robinson RA. The treatment of certain cervical-spine disorders by anterior removal of the intervertebral disc and interbody fusion. *J Bone Joint Surg Am*. 1958;40-A(3):607-624.
19. Klein GR, Vaccaro AR, Albert TJ. Health outcome assessment before and after anterior cervical discectomy and fusion for radiculopathy: a prospective analysis. *Spine*. 2000;25(7):801-803.
20. Cloward RB. Cervical diskography; technique, indications and use in diagnosis of ruptured cervical disks. *Am J Roentgenol Radium Ther Nucl Med*. 1958;79(4):563-574.
21. Bohlman HH, Emery SE, Goodfellow DB, Jones PK. Robinson anterior cervical discectomy and arthrodesis for cervical radiculopathy. Long-term follow-up of one hundred and twenty-two patients. *J Bone Joint Surg Am*. 1993;75(9):1298-1307.
22. Bohlman HH. Cervical spondylosis and myelopathy. *Instr Course Lect*. 1995;44:81-97.
23. Zhu B, Xu Y, Liu X, Liu Z, Dang G. Anterior approach versus posterior approach for the treatment of multilevel cervical spondylotic myelopathy: a systemic review and meta-analysis. *Eur Spine J*. 2013;22(7):1583-1593.
24. Heller JG, Silcox DH 3rd, Sutterlin CE 3rd. Complications of posterior cervical plating. *Spine*. 1995;20(22):2442-2448.
25. Lowery GL, Swank ML, McDonough RF. Surgical revision for failed anterior cervical fusions. Articular pillar plating or anterior revision? *Spine*. 1995;20(22):2436-2441.
26. Sevki K, Mehmet T, Ufuk T, et al. Results of surgical treatment for degenerative cervical myelopathy: anterior cervical corpectomy and stabilization. *Spine*. 2004;29(22):2493-2500.
27. Buchowski JM, Liu G, Bunmaprasert T, Rose PS, Riew KD. Anterior cervical fusion assessment: surgical exploration versus radiographic evaluation. *Spine*. 2008;33(11):1185-1191.
28. Yoon ST, Raich A, Hashimoto RE, et al. Predictive factors affecting outcome after cervical laminoplasty. *Spine*. 2013;38(22 suppl 1):S232-S252.
29. Liu X, Wang H, Zhou Z, Jin A. Anterior decompression and fusion versus posterior laminoplasty for multilevel cervical compressive myelopathy. *Orthopedics*. 2014;37(2):e117-e122.
30. Bolesta MJ, Rechtine GR 2nd, Chrin AM. One- and two-level anterior cervical discectomy and fusion: the effect of plate fixation. *Spine J*. 2002;2(3):197-203.
31. Fraser JF, Hartl R. Anterior approaches to fusion of the cervical spine: a metaanalysis of fusion rates. *J Neurosurg Spine*. 2007;6(4):298-303.
32. Wright IP, Eisenstein SM. Anterior cervical discectomy and fusion without instrumentation. *Spine*. 2007;32(7):772-774.
33. Lee JC, Lee SH, Peters C, Riew KD. Risk-factor analysis of adjacent-segment pathology requiring surgery following anterior, posterior, fusion, and nonfusion cervical spine operations: survivorship analysis of 1358 patients. *J Bone Joint Surg Am*. 2014;96(21):1761-1767.
34. Baron EM, Soliman AM, Gaughan JP, Simpson L, Young WF. Dysphagia, hoarseness, and unilateral true vocal fold motion impairment following anterior cervical diskectomy and fusion. *Ann Otol Rhinol Laryngol*. 2003;112(11):921-926.
35. Bolesta MJ, Rechtine GR 2nd, Chrin AM. Three- and four-level anterior cervical discectomy and fusion with plate fixation: a prospective study. *Spine*. 2000;25(16):2040-2044.
36. Murrey D, Janssen M, Delamarter R, et al. Results of the prospective, randomized, controlled multicenter Food and Drug Administration investigational device exemption study of the ProDisc-C total disc replacement versus anterior discectomy and fusion for the treatment of 1-level symptomatic cervical disc disease. *Spine J*. 2009;9(4):275-286.
37. Burkus JK, Haid RW, Traynelis VC, Mummaneni PV. Long-term clinical and radiographic outcomes of cervical disc replacement with the Prestige disc: results from a prospective randomized controlled clinical trial. *J Neurosurg Spine*. 2010;13(3):308-318.
38. Coric D, Nunley PD, Guyer RD, et al. Prospective, randomized, multicenter study of cervical arthroplasty: 269 patients from the Kineflex|C artificial disc investigational device exemption study with a minimum 2-year follow-up: clinical article. *J Neurosurg Spine*. 2011;15(4):348-358.
39. Sasso RC, Anderson PA, Riew KD, Heller JG. Results of cervical arthroplasty compared with anterior discectomy and fusion: four-year clinical outcomes in a prospective, randomized controlled trial. *Orthopedics*. 2011;34(11):889.
40. Harrod CC, Hilibrand AS, Fischer DJ, Skelly AC. Adjacent segment pathology following cervical motion-sparing procedures or devices compared with fusion surgery: a systematic review. *Spine*. 2012;37(22 suppl):S96-S112.
41. Gao Y, Liu M, Li T, et al. A meta-analysis comparing the results of cervical disc arthroplasty with anterior cervical discectomy and fusion (ACDF) for the treatment of symptomatic cervical disc disease. *J Bone Joint Surg Am*. 2013;95(6):555-561.
42. Eck JC, Humphreys SC, Lim TH, et al. Biomechanical study on the effect of cervical spine fusion on adjacent-level intradiscal pressure and segmental motion. *Spine*. 2002;27(22):2431-2434.
43. Lunsford LD, Bissonette DJ, Jannetta PJ, Sheptak PE, Zorub DS. Anterior surgery for cervical disc disease. Part 1: treatment of lateral cervical disc herniation in 253 cases. *J Neurosurg*. 1980;53(1):1-11.
44. Henderson CM, Hennessy RG, Shuey HM Jr, Shackelford EG. Posterior-lateral foraminotomy as an exclusive operative technique for cervical radiculopathy: a review of 846 consecutively operated cases. *Neurosurgery*. 1983;13(5):504-512.

45. Burkus JK, Traynelis VC, Haid RW Jr, Mummaneni PV. Clinical and radiographic analysis of an artificial cervical disc: 7-year follow-up from the Prestige prospective randomized controlled clinical trial: clinical article. *J Neurosurg Spine.* 2014;21(4):516-528.
46. Mixter WJ. Rupture of the intervertebral disk; a short history of this evolution as a syndrome of importance to the surgeon. *J Am Med Assoc.* 1949;140(3):278-282.
47. Frykholm R. Lower cervical nerve roots and their investments. *Acta Chir Scand.* 1951;101(6):457-471.
48. Scoville WB, Whitcomb BB, McLaurin R. The cervical ruptured disc; report of 115 operative cases. *Trans Am Neurol Assoc.* 1951;56:222-224.
49. Fager CA. Posterolateral approach to ruptured median and paramedian cervical disk. *Surg Neurol.* 1983;20(6):443-452.
50. Epstein JA, Janin Y, Carras R, Lavine LS. A comparative study of the treatment of cervical spondylotic myeloradiculopathy. Experience with 50 cases treated by means of extensive laminectomy, foraminotomy, and excision of osteophytes during the past 10 years. *Acta Neurochir (Wien).* 1982;61(1-3):89-104.
51. Casotto A, Buoncristiani P. Posterior approach in cervical spondylotic myeloradiculopathy. *Acta Neurochir (Wien).* 1981;57(3-4):275-285.
52. Jagannathan J, Shaffrey CI, Oskouian RJ, et al. Radiographic and clinical outcomes following single-level anterior cervical discectomy and allograft fusion without plate placement or cervical collar. *J Neurosurg Spine.* 2008;8(5):420-428.
53. Wirth FP, Dowd GC, Sanders HF, Wirth C. Cervical discectomy. A prospective analysis of three operative techniques. *Surg Neurol.* 2000;53(4):340-346.
54. Ruetten S, Komp M, Merk H, Godolias G. Full-endoscopic cervical posterior foraminotomy for the operation of lateral disc herniations using 5.9-mm endoscopes: a prospective, randomized, controlled study. *Spine.* 2008;33(9):940-948.
55. Adamson TE. Microendoscopic posterior cervical laminoforaminotomy for unilateral radiculopathy: results of a new technique in 100 cases. *J Neurosurg.* 2001;95(1 suppl):51-57.
56. Fessler RG, Khoo LT. Minimally invasive cervical microendoscopic foraminotomy: an initial clinical experience. *Neurosurgery.* 2002;51(5 suppl):S37-S45.
57. Coric D, Adamson T. Minimally invasive cervical microendoscopic laminoforaminotomy. *Neurosurg Focus.* 2008;25(2):E2.
58. Kang MS, Choi KC, Lee CD, et al. Effective cervical decompression by the posterior cervical foraminotomy without discectomy. *J Spinal Disord Tech.* 2014;27(5):271-276.
59. Witzmann A, Hejazi N, Krasznai L. Posterior cervical foraminotomy. A follow-up study of 67 surgically treated patients with compressive radiculopathy. *Neurosurg Rev.* 2000;23(4):213-217.
60. Winder MJ, Thomas KC. Minimally invasive versus open approach for cervical laminoforaminotomy. *Can J Neurol Sci.* 2011;38(2):262-267.
61. Lee KH, Yue WM, Yeo W, Soeharno H, Tan SB. Clinical and radiological outcomes of open versus minimally invasive transforaminal lumbar interbody fusion. *Eur Spine J.* 2012;21(11):2265-2270.
62. Kim KT, Kim YB. Comparison between open procedure and tubular retractor assisted procedure for cervical radiculopathy: results of a randomized controlled study. *J Korean Med Sci.* 2009;24(4):649-653.
63. Clark JG, Abdullah KG, Steinmetz MP, Benzel EC, Mroz TE. Minimally invasive versus open cervical foraminotomy: a systematic review. *Global Spine J.* 2011;1(1):9-14.
64. McAnany SJ, Kim JS, Overley SC, et al. A meta-analysis of cervical foraminotomy: open versus minimally-invasive techniques. *Spine J.* 2015;15(5):849-856.
65. Samartzis D, Shen FH, Lyon C, et al. Does rigid instrumentation increase the fusion rate in one-level anterior cervical discectomy and fusion? *Spine J.* 2004;4(6):636-643.
66. Hilibrand AS, Carlson GD, Palumbo MA, Jones PK, Bohlman HH. Radiculopathy and myelopathy at segments adjacent to the site of a previous anterior cervical arthrodesis. *J Bone Joint Surg Am.* 1999;81(4):519-528.
67. Maiman DJ, Kumaresan S, Yoganandan N, Pintar FA. Biomechanical effect of anterior cervical spine fusion on adjacent segments. *Biomed Mater Eng.* 1999;9(1):27-38.
68. Lopez-Espina CG, Amirouche F, Havalad V. Multilevel cervical fusion and its effect on disc degeneration and osteophyte formation. *Spine.* 2006;31(9):972-978.
69. Skovrlj B, Gologorsky Y, Haque R, Fessler RG, Qureshi SA. Complications, outcomes, and need for fusion after minimally invasive posterior cervical foraminotomy and microdiscectomy. *Spine J.* 2014;14(10):2405-2411.
70. Lubelski D, Healy AT, Silverstein MP, et al. Reoperation rates after anterior cervical discectomy and fusion versus posterior cervical foraminotomy: a propensity-matched analysis. *Spine J.* 2015;15(6):1277-1283.
71. Mansfield HE, Canar WJ, Gerard CS, O'Toole JE. Single-level anterior cervical discectomy and fusion versus minimally invasive posterior cervical foraminotomy for patients with cervical radiculopathy: a cost analysis. *Neurosurg Focus.* 2014;37(5):E9.

42 CHAPTER Management of Cervical Myelopathy: Surgical Treatment

Brett D. Rosenthal
Barrett S. Boody
Wellington K. Hsu
Alpesh A. Patel

Introduction

Cervical myelopathy is a condition of chronic progressive atraumatic spinal cord compression that, over time, may cause a decline in physical function and quality of life. Cervical spondylotic myelopathy (CSM) is the most common form of spinal cord dysfunction in the world and is more common in men than women.[1] In a separate disease process, Asian individuals are at increased risk of cervical myelopathy due to the increased prevalence of ossification of the posterior longitudinal ligament (OPLL) in this population.[1,2] The natural history of CSM results in progressive neurologic deterioration that is frequently recalcitrant to nonoperative measures. Surgical management, on the other hand, can often successfully halt, and potentially reverse, patients' neurologic decline. Thus, operative management is the standard of care for patients with moderate to severe myelopathy. The choice of which operative procedure to perform is a complex issue that must be determined based on the patient's individual symptoms, radiographic findings, and risk profile.

Pathophysiology

Cervical myelopathy is a syndrome of clinical findings caused by spinal cord compression secondary to narrowing of the spinal canal, which can be attributed to developmental stenosis, degenerative spondylosis, and/or OPLL. Furthermore, congenitally stenotic cervical spines with a canal diameter of less than 13 mm are associated with increased risk of pathologic changes in cervical intervertebral discs, which may further accelerate the development of cervical myelopathy.[3] Degenerative changes of intervertebral discs are commonly the first changes seen in the development of cervical stenosis. Subsequent alterations in cervical spine biomechanics result in hypertrophy of the ligamentum flavum and facet joint laxity.[4] With aging, osteophyte formation, vertebral subluxation, facet osteoarthritis, and uncovertebral joint thickening may also occur and further contribute to cervical cord compression.[5] Although degenerative changes in the cervical spine are commonly seen with advanced age, the association with myelopathic symptoms is unclear. One study found that among 200 asymptomatic individuals aged 60 to 65 years, radiographic signs of degeneration were found in 95% of men and 70% of women.[6] The clinical signs and symptoms of myelopathy have multiple hypothesized etiologies aside from the direct compression of nervous tissue, including (1) vascular disruption, (2) blood–spinal cord barrier disruption, (3) neuroinflammation, and (4) hypoxia-induced apoptosis of neurons and oligodendrocytes.[4]

Natural History

Early literature by Lees and Turner depicted myelopathy as a disease largely characterized by long periods of stable disability punctuated by intermittent exacerbations.[7] Nurick's retrospective review of the disease's natural history also identified prolonged static periods throughout conservative management of the disease process.[8] It has been hypothesized that these exacerbations may be triggered by minor traumas. While this has been supported by the literature in the setting of patients with OPLL,[9] a recent systematic review found insufficient evidence to support or refute this claim in patients with either asymptomatic spondylotic cord compression or myelopathy in the absence of OPLL.[10]

Symptomatic patients are commonly recommended for surgical management of cervical myelopathy because of the risk of progression; however, nonoperative care may be reasonable in those with mild manifestations. In a systematic review of the literature performed by Rhee et al. in 2013, a strong recommendation was made against routinely prescribing nonoperative treatment as the primary modality for patients with moderate to severe myelopathy given the naturally progressive history of this disease.[10] The same review cautioned that frequent monitoring should be performed

TABLE 42.1 Ranawat Classification

Class	Exam Findings
I	Pain, no neurologic deficits
II	Subjective weakness, hyperreflexia, dysesthesias
IIIA	Objective weakness, long tract signs, ambulatory
IIIB	Objective weakness, long tract signs, nonambulatory

to identify subtle neurologic deterioration in patients who are treated nonoperatively with mild myelopathy. Patients undergoing conservative management should be counseled on the prevalence of disease progression and the importance of the longitudinal follow-up for subtle progression of CSM symptomatology. Neurologic decline in conservatively managed patients with CSM occurs in 20% to 62% of patients at 3- to 6-year follow-up.[4,11–13] Likewise, with 6.5 years of follow-up, one retrospective comparative study identified a failure of nonoperative treatment with conversion to operative management rate of 37%.[12]

Classification

A major limitation of current research is the dearth of an ideal classification/grading system for cervical myelopathy. Historically, the Nurick classification system classified patients with cervical spondylotic myelopathy on the basis of symptoms and lower extremity functional status.[14] Criticisms of this classification system include the lack of assessment of upper extremity dysfunction and difficulty with use in elderly. The Ranawat classification improves upon the Nurick scale by emphasizing both subjective complaints and objective findings,[15] but it is limited by having only three classification groups (Table 42.1). The Japanese Orthopaedic Association (JOA) scoring system measures function as a continuous variable, allowing it to identify and classify subtle deterioration and/or improvement (Table 42.2). The JOA assessment tool contains a 24-item self-administered questionnaire that was devised based on statistical analysis of an initial, much larger survey.[16] The final score system has six subscores based on the patient's following functions: upper extremity motor, lower extremity motor, upper extremity sensory, truncal sensory, lower extremity sensory, and bladder. Test-retest reliability has been shown to be acceptable when comparing patients' responses at 4 weeks apart with no changes in symptoms.[17]

History and Physical Examination

Patients with cervical spondylotic myelopathy have been shown to have severely impaired quality of life in comparison to the general population, as measured by the Medical Outcomes Study Short Form Health Survey (SF-36).[18] Specifically, the most notable declines in health-related quality of life were noted in the role-physical, role-emotional, and social function subscales of the SF-36 survey.

TABLE 42.2 Japanese Orthopaedic Association Myelopathy Scoring System

Neurologic Status	Score
Lower Limb Motor Dysfunction	
Unable to walk	0
Able to walk on flat floor with walking aid	1
Able to walk up and down stairs with handrail	2
Lack of stability and smooth reciprocation of gait	3
No dysfunction	4
Lower Limb Sensory Deficit	
Severe sensory loss or pain	0
Mild sensory deficit	1
No deficit	2
Trunk Sensory Deficit	
Severe sensory loss or pain	0
Mild sensory deficit	1
No deficit	2
Sphincter Dysfunction	
Unable to void	0
Marked difficulty in micturition	1
Minor difficulty in micturition	2
No dysfunction	3

Cervical myelopathy can display a variety of upper and lower extremity symptoms and signs due to the location of neurologic compression. It is important to obtain an in-depth history in order to identify the patient's overall level of disability as well as that likely attributable to CSM. Patients with cervical myelopathy may complain of loss of upper extremity dexterity, gait imbalance, and/or nonspecific weakness. Bowel and bladder symptoms are less commonly the primary complaint.[19] An understanding of the duration of symptoms, severity of disability, and course of disease progression aids clinical decision making. Clinical presentations often include a combination of radicular (lower motor neuron) and long tract (upper motor neuron) signs. Most commonly, lower motor neuron signs, such as radicular pain and weakness, will be present at the presumed clinically significant level of cervical stenosis with upper motor neuron signs, such as hyperreflexia and spastic gait, at the levels discussed later.[19]

Certain upper motor neuron reflexes can frequently be elicited in myelopathic patients. To elicit a Hoffman reflex, the examiner flicks the terminal phalanx of the middle or ring finger. A positive test is signified by the reflexive flexion of the terminal phalanx of the thumb and index finger. To elicit an inverted brachioradialis test, the examiner strikes the brachioradialis tendon with a reflex hammer. A positive test is present when there exists a diminished brachioradialis reflex alongside a reflexive contraction of the finger flexors. In the lower extremity, a Babinski sign may indicate upper motor neuron compression, resulting in damage to the corticospinal tract. To perform this test, a blunt, pointed instrument is stroked in a curved trajectory along the lateral aspect of the sole of the foot from the heel toward the toes. A positive test result is indicated by an extension of the hallux.

Although each patient is different, cervical spondylotic myelopathy often involves compression of the lateral corticospinal tracts, which are responsible for voluntary skeletal muscle control, and the spinocerebellar tracts (anterior and posterior), which convey proprioceptive information to the cerebellum.[20] Together, these deficits are responsible for the wide-based spastic gait with clumsy upper extremity function that is classic to cervical myelopathy. Additional commonly involved spinal cord regions are the spinothalamic tracts, which are responsible for contralateral pain and temperature sensation, the posterior columns, which are responsible for ipsilateral position and vibration sense, and the dorsal nerve root, which is responsible for dermatomal sensation.[19]

Concomitant spinal pathologies may further complicate the clinical picture and surgical planning. Patients with OPLL, ankylosing spondylitis, and diffuse idiopathic skeletal hyperostosis require special consideration when formulating preoperative plans.

Tandem stenosis should be considered as a possible contributing factor to the patient's reported symptoms. One cadaveric study identified the presence of stenosis in one region of the spine (cervical or lumbar) as positively predicting stenosis of the other 15.3% to 32.4% of the time.[21] This may be partly explained by the positive association between congenital stenosis of the lumbar and cervical spines.[22] Clinically speaking, a patient's presentation may be an amalgam of signs from each disease process, and disability from lumbar stenosis should be considered. If the surgeon deems the lumbar stenosis to be clinically relevant, surgical planning for these patients may include consideration of single-stage versus two-stage decompression. One retrospective cohort study did not identify a significant difference between single- and two-stage decompression with respect to JOA or Oswestry Disability Index scores.[23]

A comprehensive understanding of all prior treatments received, including surgical procedures, assists with further treatment recommendations and preoperative planning. An account of the patient's comorbidities should be taken into consideration to determine the patient's suitability for surgical procedures. Given the progressive natural history of the disease process, timely medical optimization of comorbidities, when possible, is preferred in patients at increased perioperative risk.

Imaging

Preoperative imaging is essential for confirming the presence of cervical stenosis and preoperative planning. Every patient undergoing a workup for CSM should have upright cervical spine radiographs, including flexion/extension views. The clinician should note degeneration of uncovertebral and facet joints, subluxation, the presence of osteophytes, narrowing of disc spaces, or decreased sagittal diameter of the spinal canal.

On the lateral radiographs, the Pavlov ratio, which is the ratio of the canal diameter (measured from the posterior aspect of the vertebral body to the corresponding spinolaminar line) to the vertebral body width (measured anterior to posterior), should be determined. If the ratio is less than 0.8, congenital narrowing of the spinal canal is present, which greatly increases the patient's risk of symptomatic stenosis and cord compression.[24] The Pavlov ratio has been found to have excellent correlation to narrowing identified on computed tomography (CT) and magnetic resonance imaging (MRI; Fig. 42.1).[25] Based on a lateral radiograph, a canal diameter of 12 mm or less will often indicate cord compression, whether or not the patient is symptomatic, because the spinal cord diameter is approximately 10 mm in the midcervical spine and soft tissues are not accounted for on plain films. The surgeon should also note the presence of any radiographic evidence of OPLL, although CT is the most diagnostically accurate method of identifying this abnormality, especially if it is segmental or localized.[26] CT provides additional information regarding the extent of OPLL and/or osteophytes. CT myelography, although invasive, may be useful in patients who cannot have an MRI or have a substantial artifact secondary to local hardware.

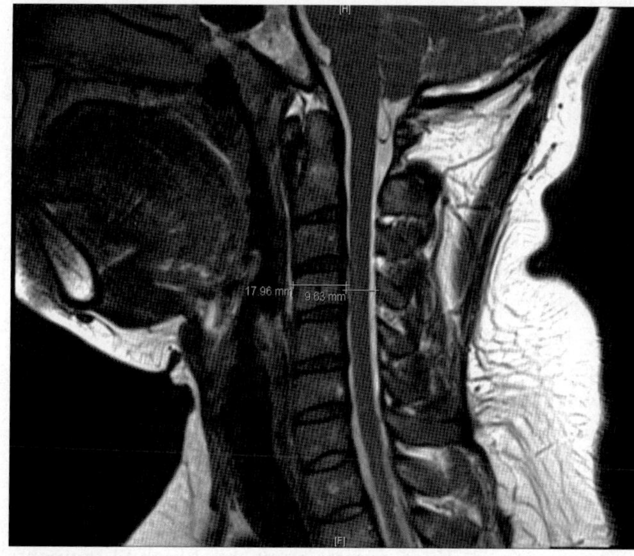

FIG. 42.1 T2-weighted midsagittal magnetic resonance imaging (MRI) slice from a 26-year-old woman with congenital stenosis of the cervical spine. Although Pavlov's ratio is traditionally measured on a lateral radiograph, this MRI slice demonstrates a ratio of 0.53 and highlights the limited space available for the spinal cord.

Sagittal plane alignment should also be assessed on the upright lateral radiographs. Sagittal plane malalignment can contribute to neurologic decline by increasing tension, increasing pressure, and flattening/deforming the spinal cord.[27] Additionally, small feeder blood vessels to the cord can be compromised as deformity ensues, further compromising the patient's neurologic status.[28] With progressive kyphosis, the cord is increasingly tensioned and draped across the anterior vertebral body osteophytes and/or disc herniations, which may necessitate anterior decompression. Flexion-extension views are used to identify the presence of any angular or translational instability that may be present. Hypermobility, or "compensatory subluxation," of segments one or two levels away from stiff segments is not uncommon, and may contribute to cord compression. The sagittal plane alignment is significant in preoperative planning because the neurologic compression from cervical stenosis with kyphosis may not be completely addressed with posterior spinal procedures.

MRI is a crucial imaging modality in the setting of neurologic deficits. It is an essential part of the preoperative workup for a patient whose presentation is concerning for CSM. The MRI is integral to confirming the diagnosis and providing prognostic information with regard to surgical intervention. A systematic review by Tetreault et al. in 2013 identified 3 important negative predictors of neurologic recovery after surgery.[29] First, high signal intensity (SI) changes on T2-weighted images (T2WI) in combination with low SI changes on T1-weighted images (T1WI) correlated with a poorer JOA recovery rate[30,31] and poorer motor symptom (e.g., weakness, spasticity, wasting, and so on) recovery.[32] Second, a high ratio of T2 SI between compressed and noncompressed (C7–T1) segments also was repeatedly associated with a poorer JOA recovery rate.[33,34] Third, greater numbers of high SI segments on T2WI had a negative association with JOA recovery[35] and Neurosurgical Cervical Spine Scale (NCSS) recovery.[36] These findings should not deter surgical intervention when it is indicated; they should simply be used to guide expectations during preoperative discussions with the patient.

Goals of Management

The overlying goals of management for cervical myelopathy are cord decompression, stabilization, preservation and improvement of cord vascularity, and restoration of normal sagittal alignment. As discussed previously, nonoperative management for patients with significant and/or progressive symptoms should not be routinely recommended.[10] Law et al. identified several poor prognostic factors for conservative treatment and put them forward as absolute surgical indications. They recommended surgery for the following: progression of signs or symptoms, duration of symptoms greater than 6 months, compression ratio (cord sagittal diameter/transverse diameter) 0.4 or less, or transverse area of the cord less than 40 mm^2.[37] More recently, a consensus statement recommended surgical intervention once a diagnosis of CSM was made.[38] Regardless, timeliness of intervention is critical as patients with milder myelopathy and those with symptom duration less than 6 months have improved outcomes after surgery.[39]

Contraindications for surgical management of CSM are based on the patient's inability to tolerate the physiologic stresses of surgery. As always, patient-specific risk factors should be identified preoperatively and discussed openly with the patient. Increased surgical mortality has been associated with patients who have heart failure (odds ratio [OR], 4.59; 95% confidence interval [CI], 3.62–5.82), pulmonary circulatory disorders (OR, 11.29; 95% CI, 8.24–15.47), and pathologic weight loss (OR, 5.43; 95% CI, 4.07–7.26) preoperatively.[40] Tetreault, Karpova, and Fehlings reviewed the literature and, by metaanalysis, identified age as the most powerful predictor of perioperative morbidity and worse neurologic recovery.[41] Similarly, a recent clinical prediction model that was internally and externally validated (on different subject populations) identified the following as the most significant predictors of surgical outcome: preoperative severity of myelopathy, age, smoking status, and presence of impaired gait.[42] While most of these are nonmodifiable risk factors, smoking cessation should be encouraged for all patients.

Surgical Approach Considerations

Many factors must be considered when determining the procedure needed to adequately achieve the aforementioned goals of management. The sagittal alignment, source of compression, number of segments involved, presence of axial neck pain, shape of pathoanatomy, and/or history of prior surgeries must all be taken into account when planning. The first decision point is whether an anterior, posterior, or combined approach is necessary to manage the patient's pathology. Each approach has its own merits and unique risks.

Posterior approaches should be considered for surgical management of multilevel (more than three) cervical stenosis, OPLL, congenital stenosis, and posterior compression. The posterior approaches provide direct and/or indirect decompression of the spinal cord. Direct decompression may occur in cases of compressive posterior element pathology (e.g., ossification of the yellow ligament or infolding of ligamentum flavum). Indirect decompression, more frequently the goal of posterior procedures, allows the spinal cord and thecal sac to drift posteriorly away from anterior sources of compression, but is most successful in the absence of kyphosis. Kyphotic alignment is often regarded to be an absolute contraindication to posterior approaches in isolation.[43] The two primary procedures performed with a posterior approach are (1) laminectomy with or without posterior spinal fusion and (2) laminoplasty. Both are useful when treating a patient with more than three levels of pathology because, in this situation, the posterior techniques have less additive morbidity.[44–47]

Laminectomy without fusion places the spine at risk for postlaminectomy kyphosis with delayed neurologic deterioration.[48–55] The incidence of postlaminectomy kyphosis ranges from 6% to 47% in adults and nearly 100% in children.[56] While most patients have neurologic recovery in the short term regardless of their sagittal alignment, delayed neurologic deterioration has been documented in 10% to 39% of patients who have cervical laminectomy without fusion.[56] The review of the literature by McAllister et al.[56] identified two predictors of success for laminectomy without fusion: preoperative lordosis greater than 10 degrees and absence of instability on flexion-extension views. These authors still reserved isolated laminectomies only for elderly patients with multiple comorbidities who had these predictors for success because posterior spinal instrumentation and arthrodesis by means of lateral mass fixation is a relatively safe, expedient, and successful procedure. Postlaminectomy kyphosis has multiple hypothesized etiologies. Some believe that it is due to disruption of the posterior tension band with load redistribution; others attribute it to iatrogenic destabilization from aggressive facet resection. Regardless, arthrodesis is indicated in the vast majority of patients. An additional benefit of arthrodesis, in addition to the avoidance of instability and sagittal malalignment, is the possibility of alleviating pain generators responsible for axial neck pain.

Laminoplasty evolved as a technique to minimize stripping of the posterior elements, maintain the posterior tension band, and maintain the patient's range of cervical motion. While many variants of the technique have been described, they all aim to expand the spinal canal by opening the posterior arch without removing it. Laminoplasty should not be performed in the setting of instability because a fusion procedure is required to avoid iatrogenic sagittal malalignment. The decision to perform a laminoplasty or a laminectomy with fusion is a complex issue that depends upon the presence of axial neck pain, surgeon preference, and desire to maintain cervical motion.

Anterior approaches allow for direct decompression of anterior compressive structures. In the presence of kyphosis, anterior approaches are preferred. Cord compression at only the level of the discs (retrodiscal) can be successfully managed with an anterior cervical discectomy and fusion (ACDF). If the pathology extends above or below the disc space (retrovertebral), anterior cervical corpectomy and fusion (ACCF) should be considered because the surgeon cannot safely address this pathology through the exposure afforded by discectomy alone. Extensive, multilevel anterior pathology can be seen with OPLL as well as spondylosis. Due to the limitations of exposure and technical challenges with multilevel fixation and fusion, a combined approach is recommended when addressing pathology at greater than three levels requiring anterior decompression.

One review of prospectively collected data identified a higher postoperative wound infection rate in patients undergoing a posterior approach but no difference in overall complication rates, C5 palsies, or dysphagia.[57] Luo et al.[58] conducted a systematic review and meta-analysis of the literature pertaining to multilevel CSM management, identifying anterior approaches as having significantly better postoperative JOA scores. Recovery rates, however, were no different between anterior and posterior approaches. The anterior approach had higher blood loss, operation times, and complication rates but a shorter length of stay than posterior approaches. However, given the heterogeneity of patients and disease processes included in the metaanalysis, these generalizations may not be completely accurate reflections of approach-related morbidity, especially since the analysis did not control for number of levels, extent of disease, and procedures performed. Without a clear consensus of superiority, most reviews of the literature conclude that, given equivalent effectiveness of anterior and posterior approaches, an individualized approach based on the patient's specific pathology should be taken.[37,59,60]

Anterior Procedures for the Cervical Spine

Anterior procedures can address spinal cord compression secondary to uncovertebral osteophytes, spondylotic bars, and disc osteophyte complexes. Anterior procedures also have the benefit of being able to restore sagittal malalignment much more than posterior techniques. In the setting of significant axial neck pain with spondylotic changes of the intervertebral discs, anterior fusion procedures are preferred over posterior approaches. While stand-alone anterior procedures are successful when treating one or two levels of appropriate pathology, controversy exists over whether a three-level procedure is best handled anteriorly or posteriorly.[37,61] As the number of surgically treated levels increases to greater than three, anterior procedures commonly need to be supplemented with posterior procedures to provide the necessary stability for fusion.

Anterior Approach to the Cervical Spine

Both ACDF and ACCF procedures can be performed with the anterior approach to the cervical spine, the Smith-Robinson approach, which provides access from C2 to T1, spanning the majority of cervical spondylotic pathology. The course of the vertebral arteries should be reviewed on all available imaging preoperatively to note any aberrancies. Prior to the induction of general anesthesia and intubation, the degree of neck extension that the patient can tolerate is important to determine; fiber-optic intubation may be necessary.[62]

The patient is positioned supine with neutral head rotation. The use of a foam donut to prevent pressure sores of the occiput is encouraged. A bump at the level of the shoulders allows for additional extension of the cervical spine, improving access to the anterior elements. For low cervical pathology, the shoulders may be taped down to allow for easier radiographs.

The incision can be made transversely when treating one or two levels of pathology in order to provide a more cosmetic scar. Alternatively, a longitudinal incision provides access to three or more levels at the expense of scar cosmesis. Surface landmarks help guide the level of the incision: C2 at the level of the angle of the mandible, C3 at the level of the hyoid, C4–C5 at the level of the thyroid cartilage, and C6 at the level of both the carotid tubercle and the cricoid cartilage (Fig. 42.2). Preoperative and intraoperative radiographs should also be used to determine the level of the incision.

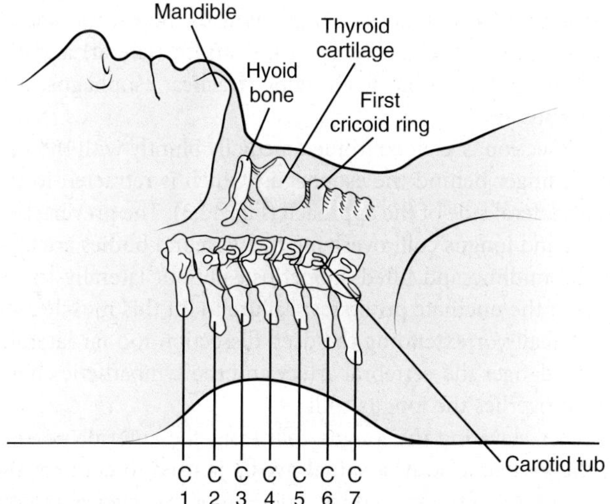

FIG. 42.2 Palpable landmarks and their relationship to the cervical spine. (From Hoppenfeld S. *Physical Examination of the Spine and Extremities.* Norwalk, CT: Appleton & Lange; 1976:110.)

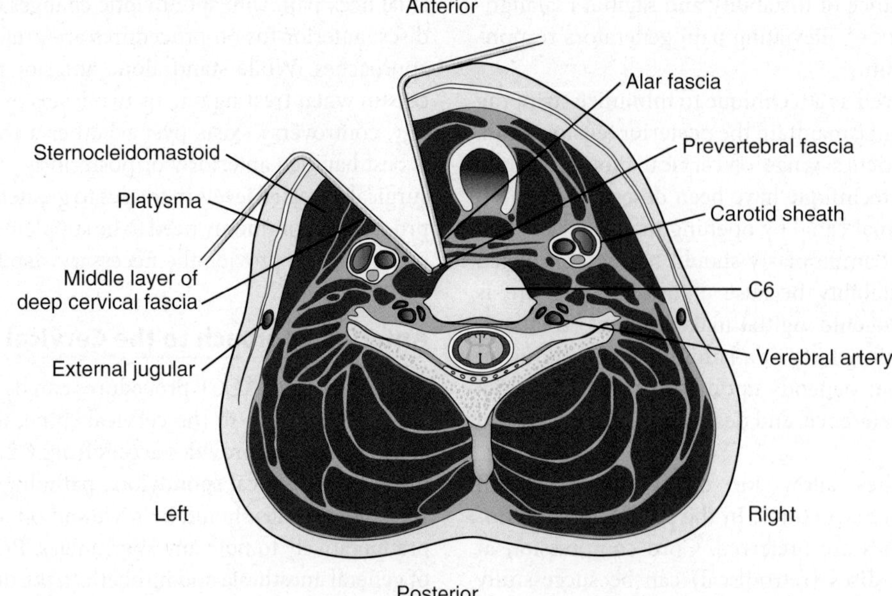

FIG. 42.3 Plane of surgical dissection during the anterior approach to the cervical spine. The carotid sheath is lateral to the plane of dissection, and the esophagus is medial to it. (From Silber JS, Albert TS. Anterior and anterolateral, mid and lower cervical spine approaches: transverse and longitudinal [C3 to C7]. In Herkowitz HN, editor. *The Cervical Spine Surgery Atlas*, ed 2. Philadelphia: Lippincott Williams & Wilkins; 2004:91.)

After the incision is made with a scalpel, electrocautery can be used to dissect down through the subcutaneous fat to the level of the platysma, which is subsequently divided in line with the incision using electrocautery. Care must be taken during this stage to avoid injury to the external jugular vein or other superficial veins that may be crossing the operative field; ligation may be necessary if the veins cannot be adequately mobilized.[62]

With the platysma retracted, the anterior border of the sternocleidomastoid is identifiable. The dissection is continued through the deep cervical (investing) fascia just medial to the sternocleidomastoid (SCM). The SCM can subsequently be retracted laterally; the carotid pulse is then palpated. The pretracheal fascia that is contiguous with the carotid sheath can be split in a plane between the sheath (lateral) and the medial structures that it envelops (trachea, esophagus, and strap muscles).

Dissection is then continued medially bluntly with the surgeon's finger behind the esophagus, which is retracted to the contralateral side of the approach (Fig. 42.3). The prevertebral fascia and longus colli overlying the vertebral bodies are split in the midline and lifted subperiosteally out laterally to the level of the uncinate processes. Failure to lift this muscle subperiosteally or extending the deep dissection too far laterally will endanger the vertebral artery and the sympathetic chain, which overlies the longus colli.

After elevating the longus colli from the anterior portion of the vertebral body, a spinal needle is used to confirm the correct level of the procedure. Wide, smooth-edged retractors are preferred in the coronal plane to avoid damage to the adjacent structures. Sharp retractors can cause inadvertent injury to the esophagus medially or carotid sheath laterally. Narrow retractors can inadvertently damage the vertebral artery by slipping between the transverse processes.[63]

Complications and Risks of the Anterior Approach to the Cervical Spine

Certain risks are associated with the Smith-Robinson approach, regardless of the spinal procedure performed. Esophageal perforation is a devastating complication that may occur secondary to improper retractor placement or inadvertent injury with a sharp instrument or the burr. The incidence is estimated as 0.2% to 0.4%.[64,65] A general or thoracic surgery consultation should be made intraoperatively if there is any concern for potential esophageal perforation.

Vertebral artery injury is a rare, but significant, potential complication of anterior cervical spine surgery. Failure to identify aberrancy in the vertebral artery course preoperatively can increase the risk of inadvertent injury. Excessively wide corpectomies can increase the risk of vertebral artery injury, as can off-center or oblique corpectomies. A retrospective review of 1976 cases reported an incidence of iatrogenic vertebral artery injury as 0.3%.[66] In the setting of vertebral artery injury, temporary hemostasis can be achieved via tamponade, and a vascular surgery consultation should be made. Intraoperative angiography should be performed prior to considering ligation as a definitive method of attaining hemostasis. Repairs should be performed if possible.

Dural tears are also a possibility during anterior cervical spine procedures. One large series identified an overall CSF leak rate of 1% with no significant difference between anterior or posterior approaches.[67] Patients with OPLL were 13.74 (95% CI, 4.53–41.61) times more likely to have a cerebrospinal fluid (CSF) leak than patients without OPLL.[67] The treating physician should be prepared to place a lumbar CSF drain in the presence of a substantial dural tear that cannot be closed with a watertight primary repair.

Radiculopathies have also been attributed to anterior cervical spine procedures. The incidence is most frequently reported as 2% to 4%.[68–70] Most often, C5 is the level involved. Previous studies have found that higher rates of radiculopathy are present as the number of levels fused increases.[70] While the etiology of this is not entirely elucidated, some theorize that the more obtuse angle that the C5 nerve root attaches to the cord and/or increased posterior drift at this level may be responsible for its increased susceptibility to injury.

The recurrent laryngeal nerve is also at risk of injury with this approach. Traditionally, it was believed that the surgery should be approached from the left side preferentially due to the increased risk of aberrancy of the right recurrent laryngeal nerve, but recent studies demonstrate no appreciable difference in injury rates.[71,72] Our preferred technique is to approach from the side contralateral from radicular symptoms (if any) such that a foraminotomy can be performed intraoperatively with greater ease. If there are no radicular symptoms preoperatively, the approach should be from the side the surgeon finds most comfortable. In revision surgery, preoperative evaluation should include direct laryngoscopy prior to approaching from the contralateral side of previous surgeries. Any prior injuries to the recurrent laryngeal nerve need to be identified before a contralateral approach is attempted to prevent bilateral recurrent laryngeal nerve injury, a devastating complication that could compromise the patient's airway. In the setting of unilateral vocal cord dysfunction, procedures should be approached from the dysfunctional side.

Dysphagia is also a frequent complication of anterior approaches to the cervical spine. Most often, it is transient. The reported incidence of dysphagia after an anterior cervical approach is highly variable, from 3% to 67%.[73,74] The reason for such variability of reported incidences is unclear, but is likely due to the variation in methods of measurement, surgical technique used, definition of dysphagia, and reporting consistency. One series has demonstrated 80% underreporting of dysphagia by surgeons in comparison to patient surveys.[75] Evidence has suggested that increased retraction pressures,[76] scar tissue,[77] osteophytes,[77] vagus nerve dysfunction,[77] and soft tissue swelling[73] may all be contributing factors. Although many series have conflicting data, various risk factors have also been implicated, including preoperative swallowing difficulties, increased age,[47,78] increased duration of pain prior to intervention,[79] gender,[47] bone morphogenetic protein use,[47] smoking,[80] and number of levels.[73]

Dysphonia, like dysphagia, is a frequent complication of anterior cervical spine surgery. The reported prevalence ranges from 1% to 51%.[81,82] Similar to dysphagia, one series identified greater than 85% underreporting by spine surgeons compared with patient surveys.[75] Dysphonia is one potential manifestation of a recurrent laryngeal nerve palsy. More severe injuries may present with other symptoms, such as postoperative airway obstruction, persistent cough, or aspiration. The mechanism of injury is most often a stretch-induced neurapraxia.[83] Risk factors of developing postoperative dysphonia include more extensive dissection, aggressive retraction,[84] longer cuff inflation time,[85] and elevated endotracheal tube pressures.[85]

Depending on the level of dissection, various other structures are at risk as well. The superior thyroid vessels typically cross the operative field around C3–C4, and the inferior thyroid vessels usually cross around C6–C7. These should be preserved if possible but may require ligation without any substantial deficit incurred to the patient. The omohyoid is also crossing the operative field obliquely at approximately the level of C6; it may be divided if needed to extend the exposure in the rostral-caudal direction.

Access to C2–C3 may be limited in the Smith-Robinson approach by the mandible, thus should be assessed with a lateral radiograph preoperatively. To further facilitate access to C2–C3, nasotracheal intubation should be considered so that the mandible can be fully closed. With the rostral extents of this approach, there is an increased risk of injury to the hypoglossal nerve, hypopharynx, and the hypoglossal and mandibular branches of the facial nerve.[86]

Access to the cervicothoracic junction is also limited in the Smith-Robinson approach without the use of special techniques to increase exposure, which include detaching the SCM from its insertion, sectioning strap muscles, and mobilizing the clavicle and manubrium. This approach is outside the scope of this current chapter.

Anterior Cervical Discectomy and Fusion

Procedure

Preoperative planning for an ACDF must include considerations of the graft or implant to be used. Historically, an autologous tricortical iliac crest bone graft has been used for grafting, but our current preferred approach is to use a cage device to avoid donor site morbidity. Shriver et al. reviewed the literature and found that fusion occurs in 99.1% of autograft cases compared with 95.2% of allograft cases.[87]

After exposure and confirmation of the appropriate level, Caspar posts are placed into the vertebral bodies above and below the disc to be excised, providing distraction at the level of the disc. These will assist with visualization of the posterior aspect of the disc space once the discectomy is underway. The Caspar pins should be placed in the midline to avoid screw path issues from the subsequent plating procedure. Alternatively, an intervertebral spreader can be used once the discectomy has been initiated. Anterior vertebral body osteophytes should be removed, which will (1) improve visualization within the disc space, (2) facilitate placement of the implant at an appropriate depth, and (3) minimize plate prominence.

A rectangular annulotomy is performed with a No. 15 scalpel blade on a long handle. A pituitary rongeur can then be used to excise the majority of the disc material. A straight curette can be used to further remove disc material and begin the resection of the cartilage from the endplates. The lateral extent of the resection should be made to the level of the uncinate process. The use of a Kerrison rongeur may facilitate resection of disc material at the edges of the uncinate processes. Resection farther laterally can risk injury to the vertebral artery. Decortication of the endplate can subsequently be continued with a burr. Care should be taken to not decorticate deeper than the subchondral bone to reduce the risk of graft/implant subsidence. Uncovertebral osteophytes must be resected to fully decompress the foramina. If the posterior aspect of the anulus is intact, a curette may be used to create a vertical rent in the anulus to provide subsequent access for a Kerrison rongeur.

If a foraminotomy is necessary, the PLL should be left intact until it is completed because it plays a protective role. The medial posterior uncinate process can be thinned with a burr. The surgeon should keep in mind the location of the vertebral arteries as determined from preoperative imaging to avoid inadvertent arterial injury. The microscope (if used) should be angled into the wound toward the foramen to be decompressed. Decompression of the contralateral side can subsequently be performed with a Kerrison rongeur and curette. When probing with a nerve hook to assess the adequacy of the foraminotomy, one must remember that the nerve exits at an approximately 45-degree angle ventrolaterally; thus, the nerve hook should glide along the posterior surface of the uncinate to avoid inadvertent injury. A blush of blood from the neural foramen often signifies an adequate decompression. The PLL can be excised with a Kerrison rongeur after the foraminotomy is completed. After the disc material has been resected, the endplates have been decorticated, and the PLL has been excised, a nerve hook should be used to identify any further sources of compression. Attention should be paid to the cranial and caudal aspects of the disc space to identify posterior osteophytes behind the adjacent vertebra.

Trial sizers should be used next to identify the appropriate size for the final graft/implant. Sequential sizers are inserted until there is a snug fit within the disc space. Typically, the graft/implant should measure 2 to 3 mm greater than what is measured on a lateral preoperative film. After the height of the trial is determined, the depth should also be assessed with a depth gauge. The appropriately sized graft or implant can be inserted using a tamp and mallet. The graft should be countersunk approximately 2 mm relative to the anterior cortex of the adjacent vertebral bodies. Excessive countersinking should be avoided to prevent spinal canal intrusion. After the graft has been positioned, anterior plating to the adjacent vertebral bodies is commonly performed. The plate should be the shortest length possible to span the fusion site, and screws should be angled away from the graft to improve screw length. Minimizing plate contact with the adjacent motion segments is thought to decrease adjacent-segment ossification. Final implant and plate positioning should be confirmed on intraoperative radiographs or fluoroscopy.

A layered closure, with or without a drain, is performed. The drain is pulled on postoperative day 1, barring excessive drainage. Postoperatively, patients typically do not need further immobilization if anterior plating is performed, but a soft collar may be provided for additional comfort. No postoperative rehabilitation is required. Postoperative diet must account for the higher incidence of dysphagia, and often slowly advancing from mechanical soft to general diets is appropriate. Full activity is often resumed by 3 months.

Fig. 42.4 depicts a case example of a patient treated with ACDF for cervical myelopathy. This patient had previously had a C5–C6 and C6–C7 ACDF. Adjacent-segment degeneration of C3–C4 and C4–C5 subsequently occurred, resulting in recurrence of myelopathy. Given the presence of predominantly anterior pathology and segmental kyphosis, ACDF of C3–C4 and C4–C5 was our preferred treatment. The patient was sent to an ear, nose, and throat specialist for preoperative evaluation of vocal cord function for the reasons discussed previously.

Outcomes, Complications, and Other Considerations

ACDFs have highly reproducible outcomes. Fusion rates have improved over time, whether it has been due to surgical technique or advancements in anterior cervical plating. Fusion rates vary based on the number of levels addressed. Single-, two-, and three-level ACDFs have fusion rates of 97.1%, 95.9%, and 89.8%, respectively, when anterior plating is used.[88] Fusion rates prior to routine use of anterior cervical plating were substantially lower.[89,90] Long-term outcomes demonstrate maintained improvements in JOA scores and a change in the disease course of cervical myelopathy.[91]

Pseudarthrosis rates are lower among patients whose fusion used autograft bone instead of allograft (0.9% vs. 4.8%, respectively).[87] Many of the patients who do develop a pseudarthrosis after ACDF remain asymptomatic. An additional risk of arthrodesis from an anterior approach is the risk of accelerated spondylosis of a vertebral segment adjacent to the level of the procedure. The incidence of symptomatic adjacent-segment disease (ASD) is 2.9% per year, with 26% symptomatic at 10-year postoperative follow-up.[92] One retrospective cohort study identified an overall revision rate after single-level ACDF (for all diagnoses) of 15%, with a mean follow-up of 31 months. ASD and pseudarthrosis were the most common reasons for revision, accounting for 47.5% and 45.5% of cases, respectively.[93]

Substantial controversy exists as to whether a hard cervical collar is needed for two-level or greater level fusion procedures. The literature has not shown any benefit for the use of a collar for single-level ACDFs. One survey of treating physicians identified 70% of spine surgeons reporting the use of a cervical collar (the majority rigid) for two-level ACDF procedures.[94] We prefer, however, to not use a cervical collar for two-level ACDFs given the increased risk of neck disability in the perioperative period, increased neck stiffness, and lack of proven benefit.[95]

Anterior Cervical Corpectomy and Fusion

Procedure

ACCFs require more extensive preoperative planning than ACDFs, including considerations for graft donor site and obtaining appropriately sized grafts. For single-level, and sometimes two-level, corpectomies, autologous iliac crest

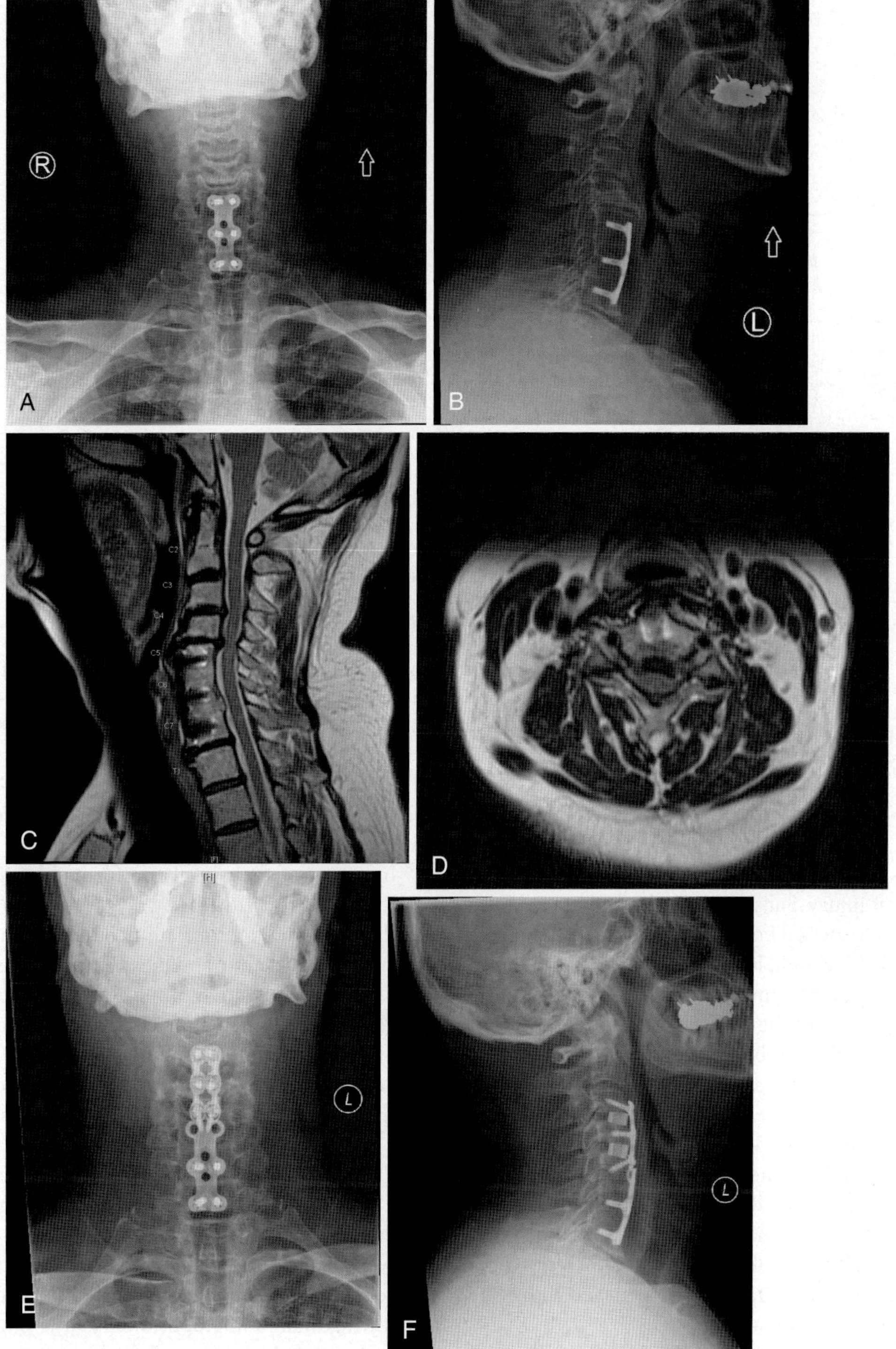

FIG. 42.4 Patient treated with anterior cervical discectomy and fusion for cervical myelopathy. (A) Preoperative anteroposterior radiograph. (B) Preoperative lateral radiograph. (C) Preoperative T2-weighted midsagittal magnetic resonance imaging (MRI) slice. (D) Preoperative T2-weighted axial MRI slice. (E) Postoperative anteroposterior radiograph. (F) Postoperative lateral radiograph.

graft can be considered, while autograft or allograft fibula is often used in larger reconstructions. A cage or spacer is an alternative to structural allograft/autograft that avoids donor-site morbidity and is easy to use.

After exposure and confirmation of the appropriate level, Caspar posts are placed into the vertebral bodies above and below the levels to be excised to provide distraction. Discectomies are performed at the levels cranial and caudad to the planned resection. Osteophytes are removed to improve visualization of the uncovertebral joints, which are used to center the resection. The ventral aspects of the vertebral bodies are debulked with a Leksell rongeur (Fig. 42.5). A 5-mm

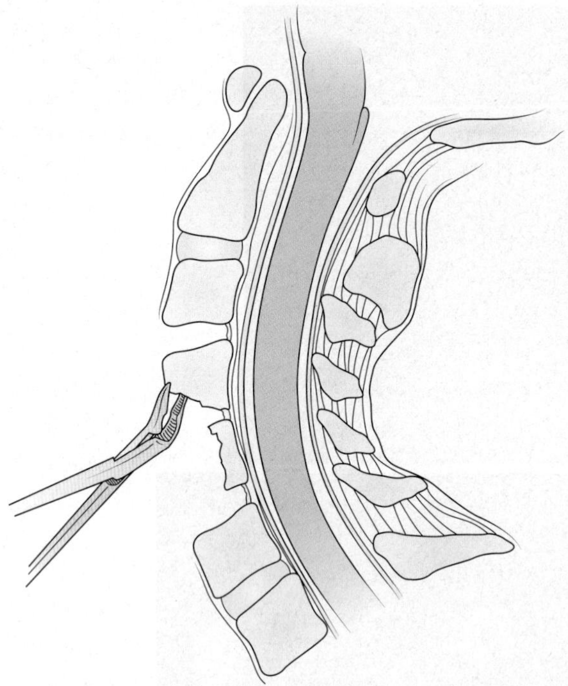

FIG. 42.5 After discectomies are completed, the anterior two-thirds of the vertebral bodies to be removed can be safely excised with a rongeur. (From Whitecloud TS. Multilevel cervical vertebrectomy and stabilization using cortical bone. In: Sherk H, Dunn EJ, Eismont FJ, et al, eds. *The Cervical Spine: An Atlas of Surgical Procedures.* Philadelphia: JB Lippincott; 1994:202.)

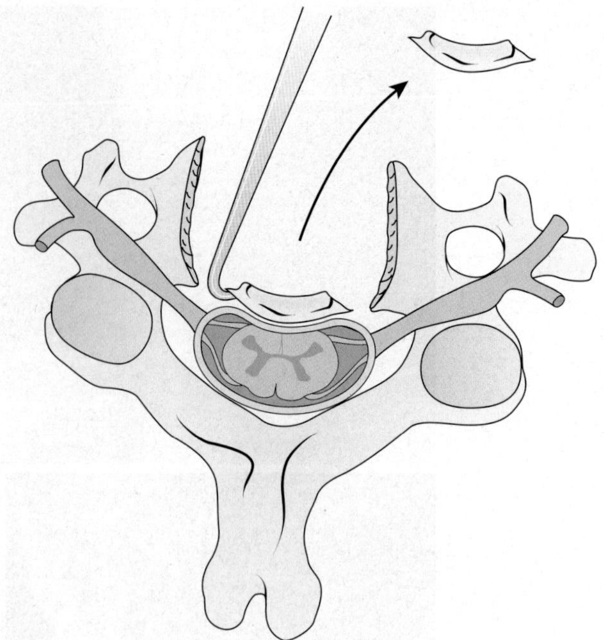

FIG. 42.6 A small angled curette can be used to excise the thinned posterior cortex of the vertebral body. Force must be directed anteriorly to avoid inadvertent damage to the dura and spinal cord. (Modified from Smith MD. Cervical spondylosis. In: Bridwell KH, DeWald RL, eds. *The Textbook of Spinal Surgery*, ed 2. Philadelphia: Lippincott-Raven; 1997:1411.)

midline trough is developed to minimize the risk of the burr causing inadvertent injury. Subsequently, the high-speed burr is used to resect the vertebral bodies in line with the uncovertebral joints. The width should be approximately 15 to 18 mm such that a graft can be accommodated. The burr should be used to debulk a majority of the vertebral body down to a thin posterior cortex, which can be subsequently excised with small angled curettes pulling away from the PLL and dura (Fig. 42.6). The PLL can then be excised with a small Kerrison rongeur. In the setting of OPLL, this may not be possible because the PLL may be adherent to the dura; aggressive attempts at resection can cause dural tear or, rarely, neurologic injury.[96] In cases of OPLL, a small bone island, decompressed and separated from all four borders but still adherent to the PLL, can be left behind. Hemostasis can be achieved with bone wax and thrombin-soaked sponges.

Regardless of whichever graft is selected, the endplates must be prepared to appropriately dock the graft and provide a good bed for subsequent fusion. A high-speed burr is used to remove the cartilage from the endplates, exposing punctate bleeding subchondral bone, which facilitates fusion. After the endplates are prepared, they are measured with a ruler or 18-gauge wire. The depth of the defect should also be measured before harvesting or selecting the graft/cage to use.

Iliac crest bone graft may be used due to its simplicity of harvesting, subcutaneous location, and autogenous source with robust osteogenic, osteoinductive, and osteoconductive properties. Tricortical grafts should be harvested with an oscillating saw. The anterior surface of the iliac crest graft may be best used to recreate the posterior vertebral body wall.[63] Alternatively, fibular graft or cage implants may be used.

Insertion of the graft is performed by increasing cervical traction to distract the bony defect further (~30 lb). The graft is placed in the appropriate position by means of a Kocher clamp and bone tamp, and the traction is subsequently released (Fig. 42.7). The position of the graft should be confirmed fluoroscopically, monitoring for any displacement or subsidence. The appropriate positioning is for the graft to be centered on the cephalad and caudad endplate subchondral bone. The graft's stability can be tested by using an instrument to gently pull on it.

Plating may be performed to increase construct stability. The plate size should adequately span the region of the corpectomy. Fixation is obtained via purchase into the vertebral body cephalad and caudad to the corpectomy. After plate placement, its position should be confirmed fluoroscopically. Following final radiographs, hemostasis should be confirmed, and a layered closure is performed.

Postoperatively, patients may have supplemental immobilization with a semirigid orthosis for 6 to 10 weeks based on the final construct's stability, as determined intraoperatively. Until fusion is completed, cervical spine twisting/bending and overhead lifting should be avoided.[63]

Fig. 42.8 depicts a case example of a patient who underwent a corpectomy for cervical myelopathy. The anterior source of spinal cord compression led to the decision to perform an anterior decompressive procedure. Given the retrovertebral (as opposed to retrodiscal) pathology at C5, an ACDF was not optimal for that level because it would inadequately decompress the spinal canal. For these reasons, our preferred

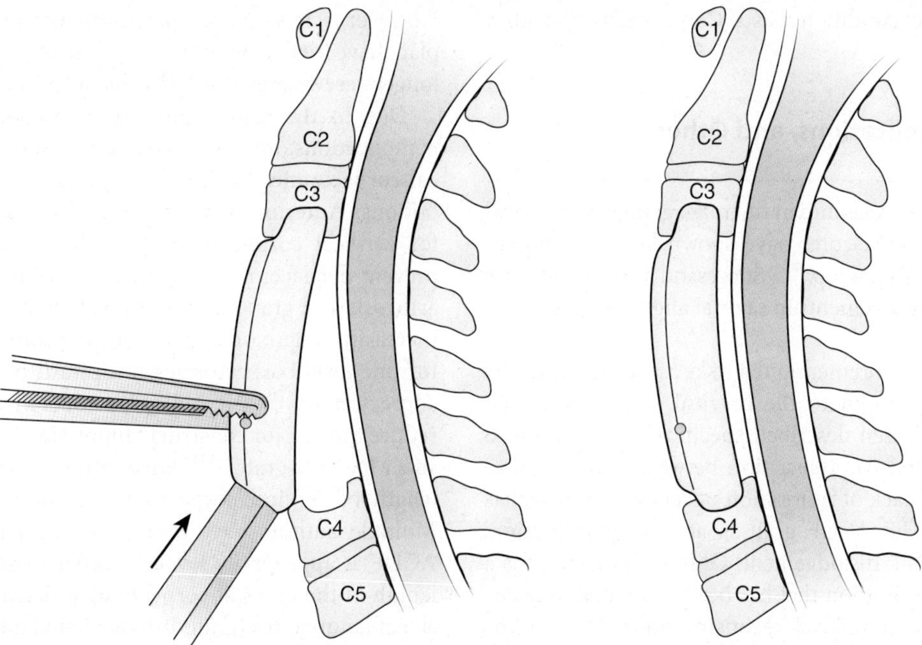

FIG. 42.7 The graft is seated into the cranial end of the corpectomy defect. Traction is subsequently applied to the patient's head. The distal end of the graft is seated with a tamp. A Kocher clamp is used to prevent graft displacement during this process. (Modified from Smith MD. Cervical spondylosis. In: Bridwell KH, DeWald RL, eds. *The Textbook of Spinal Surgery*, ed 2. Philadelphia: Lippincott-Raven; 1997:1411.)

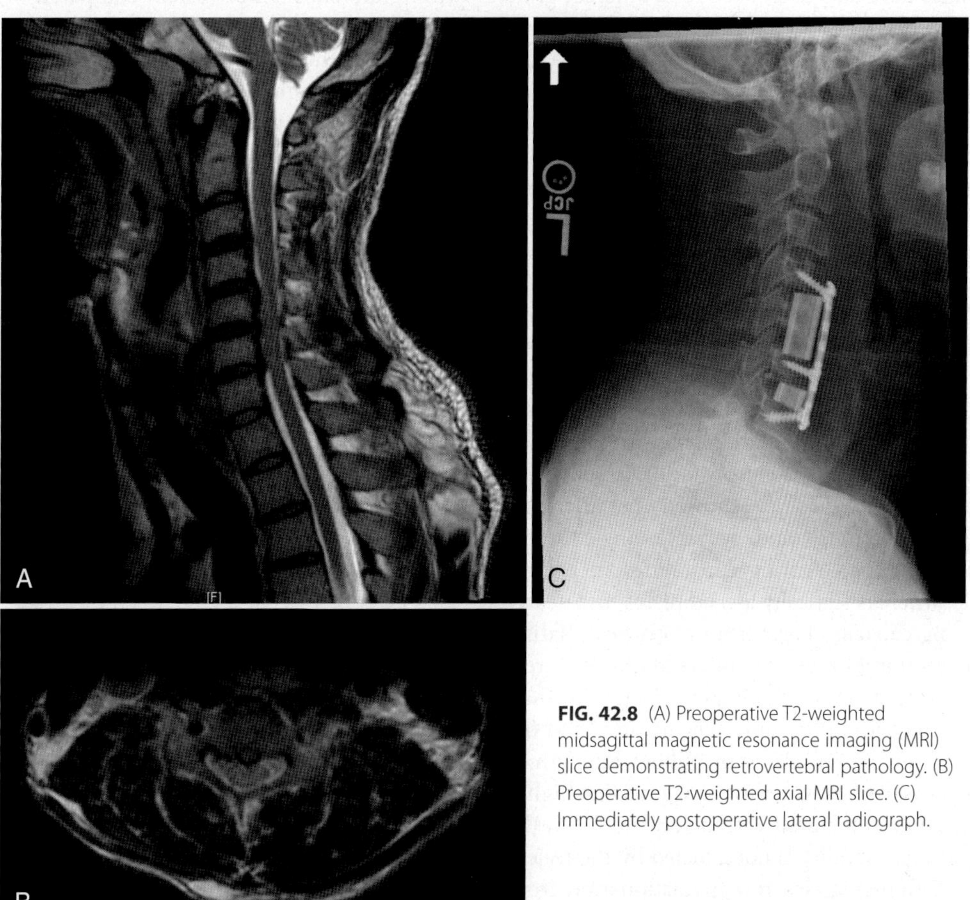

FIG. 42.8 (A) Preoperative T2-weighted midsagittal magnetic resonance imaging (MRI) slice demonstrating retrovertebral pathology. (B) Preoperative T2-weighted axial MRI slice. (C) Immediately postoperative lateral radiograph.

management of this condition was a C5 corpectomy with a C6–C7 ACDF.

Outcomes, Complications, and Other Considerations

ACCF is an effective procedure in the management of cervical myelopathy. Mean JOA scores have shown lasting improvement at long-term follow-up.[97,98] Successful fusion rates are 92% to 96%.[97–99] Improvements in sagittal alignment have also been long-standing.

In addition to the aforementioned risks associated with the Smith-Robinson approach to the cervical spine, additional complications have been described specifically in relation to the ACCF procedure. An association between postoperative axial neck pain and lack of restoration of cervical lordosis has been identified.[98] The ACCF graft is at risk of migration, subsidence, and frank dislodgement. Graft dislodgement is a well-described complication that has been estimated to occur in 4.9% to 29% of multilevel reconstructions.[100–104] In the setting of these complications, neurologic injury and the need for revision surgery may arise. Attempts to minimize the incidence of these complications have been made with anterior plating techniques that gain fixation at the cephalad and caudad vertebral bodies adjacent to the graft. Unfortunately, these have been associated with hardware failure and pseudarthrosis rates of up to 40%, which are partially attributed to the plate inadvertently distracting across the intended fusion site.[103] Buttress plates have also been used to counteract graft displacement, but success was also limited, and complications were occasionally devastating.[103] To provide additional stabilization and minimize the risk of graft dislodgement, posterior stabilization should be considered in addition to ACCF for larger reconstructions.

Successful fusion of multilevel cervical corpectomies requires an understanding of optimal cervical plate and screw placement, as the anterior cervical plates used for multilevel cervical corpectomies are vulnerable biomechanically. Singh and colleagues[105] reviewed multilevel cervical corpectomies (two or more levels), noting significant increases of approximately 30% greater motion in flexion-extension, lateral bending, and axial rotation for stand-alone anterior fixation compared with anterior fixation augmented with posterior lateral mass fixation and stand-alone posterior lateral mass fixation. Brodke and colleagues[106,107] showed that dynamic plates, including translational and variable angle screw constructs, retain their load sharing capabilities in a graft subsidence model, whereas statically locked plates lose nearly 70% of load sharing capacity. Furthermore, cervical plating techniques for corpectomies requires understanding of screw biomechanics. Locking screws exhibit greater rigidity than nonlocking screws for both initial and cyclic loading, and the length of screws positively correlates to pullout strength.[108] Finite element analysis of screw trajectory suggests that higher stresses are imparted onto the graft with divergence from the endplates, yet rotational stability is not affected by the trajectory of the screw. With increased screw angulation away from the endplate, the construct becomes more load sharing.[109] However, screws placed perpendicular to the vertebral endplate have higher pullout strength than angled screws, despite longer screw length with divergent trajectories.[110]

Due to the significant risk of pseudarthrosis and graft complications, interest in developing stable fixation for cervical corpectomies has produced a variety of instrumentation options. Anterior cervical plating provides buttress support for cervical corpectomies to stabilize the graft as well as prevent displacement and excessive settling. Risks for pseudarthrosis and graft complications increase exponentially with increasing length of corpectomy procedures, ranging from 7% for one-level corpectomies to upward of 75% for multilevel corpectomies.[111–113] Avoiding postoperative hyperlordosis can reduce the risk for construct failure, since extension can excessively load the graft.[113,114] Furthermore, use of ACDF to reduce length of cervical corpectomy can decrease failure rates.[113] Multiple authors have found that hybrid techniques using ACDF at appropriate levels in order to shorten the required length of the cervical corpectomy procedure can reduce construct failure rates (graft dislodgement and construct revision) seen with long cervical corpectomy procedures.[115,116] Various modifications for anterior cervical plating have been designed to improve fusion rate and minimize complications. Dynamic plating with variable angle screws in nonslotted plate designs may allow a degree of toggling to provide translation with graft subsidence while avoiding uncontrolled graft settling.[117] Similarly, translational plating allows for telescoping of the plate to provide continued fixation and improved graft loading with graft subsidence when compared with conventional locked plating.[118] However, excessive settling with these dynamic plating options can lead to implant failure, kyphosis, and construct failure.

Despite our understanding of optimal cervical plate and screw biomechanics, the data on clinical outcomes for ACCF plating techniques are sparse. Early experience with hybrid plating (use of variable angled screws at inferior margin of plate) has produced successful fusion and clinical results for one-level anterior cervical corpectomies.[119] Additionally, data on translational plating for corpectomies are largely limited to ACDF studies. Despite conceptual improvements over existing technology, similar rates of fusion have been reported with use of static, dynamic, and translational plating for two-level ACDF.[120–122] While dynamic plate designs with variable screw angle and translational designs to maintain load sharing with graft subsidence still may be conceptually useful in ACCF clinical scenarios, there are limited clinical data to support this.

Anterior Cervical Discectomy and Fusion Versus Anterior Cervical Corpectomy and Fusion

ACDF and ACCF are both successful techniques in the management of anterior compression sources in cervical myelopathy, especially in the setting of kyphosis when posterior approaches should not be done in isolation. A recent meta-analysis compared the two procedures. Operative times, fusion rates, postoperative JOA scores, JOA recovery rates, and visual analog scale pain scores were not significantly different between the two techniques. Blood loss was greater and complications were more frequent in ACCF compared with ACDF.[123] One systematic review identified graft dislodgement as having a significantly higher incidence in ACCF procedures than ACDF (4.9% vs. 1.7%).[104] Review of the literature suggests that the greater the number of levels involved, the higher the risk of nonunion for both procedures. One systematic review identified a nonunion rate of 18.4% for two-level ACDFs (compared with 5.1% for single-level ACCF) and 37.3% for three-level ACDFs (compared with 15.2% for two-level ACCFs).[104] Although the data available are limited by low numbers, multiple metaanalyses agree that ACDFs provide better restoration of cervical lordosis postoperatively compared with ACCF when treating multilevel CSM.[124,125]

Posterior Procedures for the Cervical Spine

Posterior approaches to the cervical spine have the benefit of familiarity of the surgical approach. Additionally, the easily expansile nature of the approach allows for straightforward management of multilevel spinal pathology, including OPLL and congenital cervical stenosis. Irreducible kyphosis is a contraindication to posterior procedures done in isolation because their success is contingent on posterior drift of the spinal cord (Fig. 42.9).

Posterior Approach to the Cervical Spine

As with the anterior approach, an assessment of the patient's asymptomatic cervical range of motion (ROM) should be assessed preoperatively to determine whether a fiber-optic intubation is necessary. Awake intubation may be considered for severely myelopathic patients.[126]

The patient is placed prone with slight neck flexion to open the posterior elements and facilitate access. Mayfield clamps or Gardner-Wells tongs may be used for additional stabilization of the cervical spine. Bony prominences and peripheral nerves must be padded to prevent pressure ulcerations and neurapraxias, respectively. The abdomen should be allowed to hang freely, and a slight reverse Trendelenburg position should be used, which both reduce epidural venous congestion as well as intraoperative bleeding. The patient's shoulders should be pulled and taped caudad to allow for easier radiographic assessment intraoperatively. Before prepping and draping, radiographs should be taken, and the appropriate level of surgery should be identified with a radiopaque marker to help guide the position of the incision.[126]

A midline posterior incision is made centered around the level(s) of interest. Sharp dissection is performed down through the midline. The dissection should attempt to remain within the relatively avascular region of the median raphe of the ligamentum nuchae because it will minimize blood loss that would otherwise obscure visualization. Once the spinous processes are reached, the interspinous musculature is elevated off of the laminae bilaterally in a subperiosteal fashion. A Cobb elevator is helpful for both the dissection and retraction. As the dissection continues laterally, care must be taken not to disturb the facet joint capsules unless arthrodesis is planned.[126] The interspinous ligaments at the cephalad and caudad ends of the planned construct should be spared. Additionally, the C2 and C7 spinous processes should be left intact because they serve as an attachment site of the nuchal

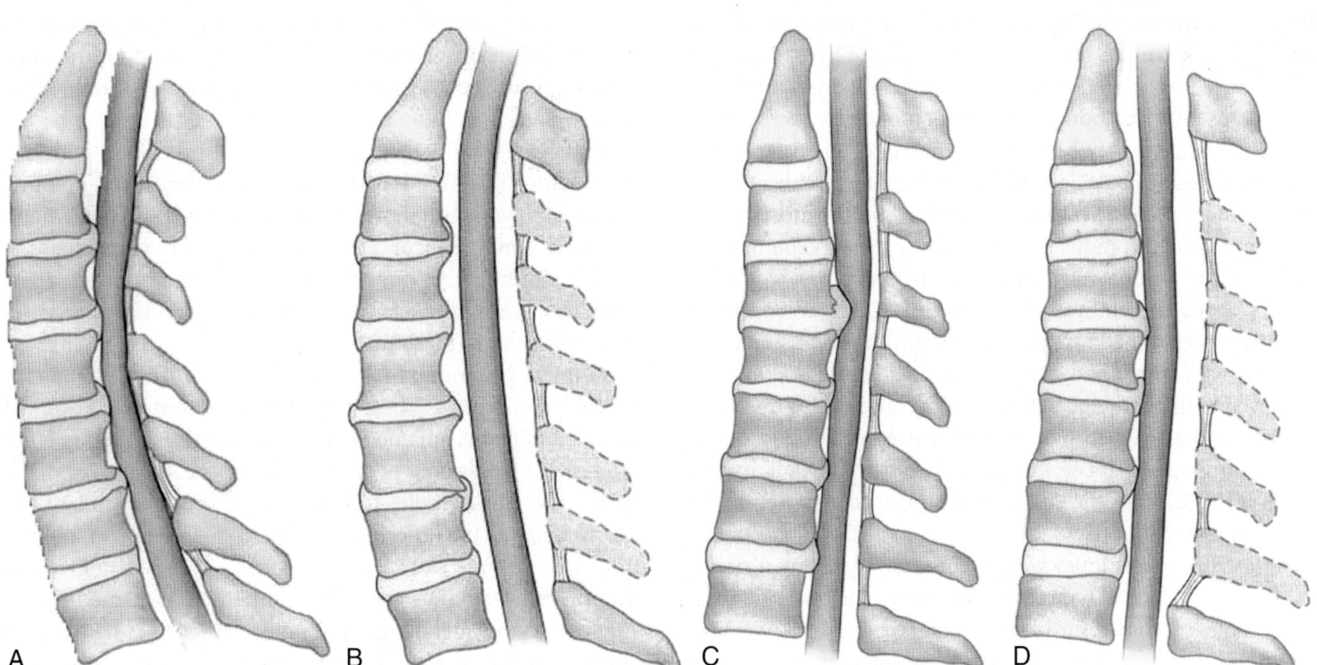

FIG. 42.9 Effect of cervical sagittal alignment on the success of posterior cervical decompressive procedures. (A) Multilevel cord compression in the setting of lordotic cervical alignment. (B) Dorsal drift of the spinal cord away from impinging structures after multilevel laminoplasty. (C) Multilevel cord compression in the setting of kyphotic cervical alignment. (D) Persistent spinal cord impingement after laminoplasty.

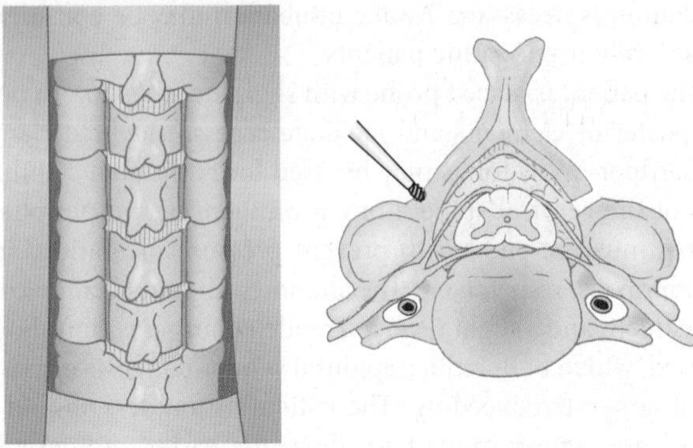

FIG. 42.10 Bilateral laminotomies are made with a high-speed burr at the lamina-facet junction. (From Komotar RJ, Mocco J, Kaiser MG. Surgical management of cervical myelopathy: indications and techniques for laminectomy and fusion. *Spine J.* 2006;6:258S.)

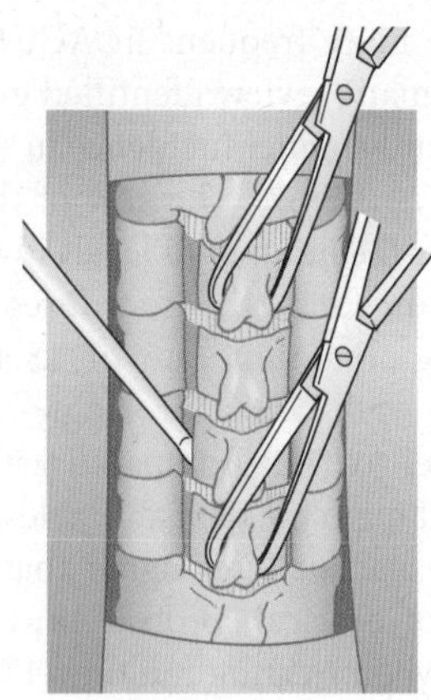

FIG. 42.11 Towel clamps on the most cranial and caudal spinous processes are used to carefully lift the laminae and ligamentum flavum en bloc. (From Komotar RJ, Mocco J, Kaiser MG. Surgical management of cervical myelopathy: indications and techniques for laminectomy and fusion. *Spine J.* 2006;6:259S.)

ligaments and may result in increased risk of postoperative kyphotic deformity and axial pain if disrupted.[127,128] If needed, dome laminectomies can be performed at these levels with minimal disruption to the attachment points.

Laminectomy and Fusion

Procedure

The levels of dissection should be confirmed radiographically with a radiopaque object (e.g., Kocher clamp on the spinous process). The extents of the planned construct should be demarcated with a Leksell rongeur by removing a fragment of the spinous processes. Subsequently, the lamina-facet junction should be identified bilaterally. A high-speed burr may then be used to initiate the lamina trough. An attempt should be made to remove the laminae en bloc (Fig. 42.10). After the burr is used to create a trough through the outer cortex and cancellous layers of bone, either a diamond burr or a 1-mm Kerrison rongeur may be used to remove the far cortex. This trough is performed bilaterally, allowing full mobilization of the laminae en bloc. Towel clamps placed on the most cranial and most caudal spinous processes allow the surgeon to carefully lift the laminae and ligamentum flavum en bloc (Fig. 42.11). Prior to removal of the laminae, the surgeon must carefully assess for adhesions between the bone or ligamentum flavum with the dura. Any adhesions present should be removed with an angled curette prior to attempting elevation of the laminae. An en bloc resection is considered less time consuming and is a safe technique because it avoids instrument intrusion into the central canal prior to completing the decompression.[129]

If any foraminotomies were preoperatively deemed necessary due to radicular symptoms, they may now be performed. Alternatively, some surgeons prefer to perform keyhole foraminotomies prior to the en bloc laminectomy to use the lamina as a protective barrier during drilling.[129] The surgeon should orient himself or herself to the margins of the foramen and assess the degree of compression with a nerve hook. The high-speed burr can then be used to resect the medial half of the facet articulation until a thin shell of bone remains. A Kerrison rongeur should be used to carefully remove the bone just dorsal to the nerve root. No more than 50% of the facet should be resected at a single level, or iatrogenic instability may occur.[130] The nerve hook can be used once again to confirm the adequacy of the decompression.

Instrumented fusion via a screw and rod–based construct is our preferred method of fixation. Lateral mass fixation can be achieved successfully at C3 to C6. Pedicle screw fixation is possible at C2 and C7 due to the pedicle size and relatively safe location from adjacent vasculature. Traditionally, it was believed that a hybrid construct of lateral mass screws and pedicle screws at C7 would be biomechanically superior; however, this may not be the case.[131] Regardless, we recommend fixation distal to the cervicothoracic junction in most multilevel cases even though rod contouring may prove more challenging.

Entry sites for pedicle screws should be drilled with the burr before decompression is performed because anatomic landmarks will be more recognizable. Screw placement, however, should occur after decompression such that the pedicle can be palpated with a nerve hook to improve accuracy. The hemostatic agent can be packed into the entry sites until it is time to place the screws.

Many techniques have been described for the placement of lateral mass screws. These techniques evolved as a result of insufficient pedicle diameter and excessive risk to the vertebral arteries for traditional pedicle screws in the subaxial cervical spine. The Roy-Camille technique uses the midpoint of the lateral mass as the entry point with 10-degree lateral angulation and 0-degree rostrocaudal angulation. The Jeanneret and Magerl technique has an entry point 1 to 2 mm medial and superior to the lateral mass midpoint with a 15- to 25-degree lateral angulation and 30-degree rostral angulation. Advantages of this technique include a decreased risk of facet violation and improved pullout strength[132,133]; no differences in morbidity between the two techniques were identified.[132] Both techniques were designed to have the screw miss the vertebral artery laterally. The Roy-Camille trajectory aims the screw to miss the exiting nerve inferiorly; the Magerl technique misses the exiting nerve superiorly. The Anderson et al.[127] technique is a modification of the Magerl technique, with a starting point 1 mm medial to the midpoint of the lateral mass, with 20-degree lateral angulation and 30-degree rostral angulation. For simplicity's sake, one can approximate these angles by leaning the drill on the next caudal spinous process. If adequate lateral angulation cannot be achieved due to impingement on the spinous process, it may be removed with a rongeur. Unicortical lateral mass screw placement is recommended by drilling in 2-mm increments until the ventral cortex is reached. There appears to be no obvious biomechanical advantage to bicortical screw placement, but there are risks (vascular and neurologic) to such a procedure.[134]

Pedicle screw fixation can be achieved at C2 and C7, which in some studies has been shown to have superior biomechanics over lateral mass fixation. Preoperatively, pedicle diameters should be measured based on the available imaging. While hybrid constructs have not shown improved biomechanics, the ability to place a pedicle screw at these levels should be a part of any surgeon's armamentarium. C2 "pedicle screws" are actually placed through the pars interarticularis. The screw entry point is in the superior medial quadrant of the lateral mass, 3 mm lateral to the medial edge of the isthmus, and in line with the superior margin of the C2 lamina. The trajectory is 15 to 25 degrees medially and 20 to 30 degrees cranially.

Preoperative imaging should be reviewed carefully prior to placement of C7 pedicle screws. Approximately 0.6% to 0.8% of patients have a vertebral artery present within the C7 transverse foramen.[135,136] C7 pedicle screws have a trajectory parallel to the C7 endplate and 20 degrees medial.

A well-prepared fusion bed is crucial to achieve bony fusion. A high-speed burr is used to decorticate the proximal and dorsal aspects of the facet joints to be fused. The facet capsule and the cartilaginous endplate should also be removed. We prefer the use of autograft bone from the laminectomies to maximize fusion potential, although allograft or synthetic materials may be used to supplement the fusion.

With unclear benefits, but minimal risk, many surgeons add 1 g of vancomycin powder overlying the paraspinal musculature to minimize the risk of surgical site infection.[137,138] A layered closure over a drain is then performed. A watertight closure is critical.

Fig. 42.12 demonstrates a case example of a laminectomy with fusion and instrumentation performed for cervical myelopathy. The patient's multilevel pathology as well as cervical scoliosis made a C2–T1 laminectomy with fusion our preferred treatment because it allowed for decompression and stabilization.

Outcomes, Complications, and Other Considerations

Anderson et al.[48] performed a systematic review in which it was determined that laminectomy with fusion resulted in neurologic improvement consistently in 70% to 95% of patients. The neurologic recovery rate was typically around 50% of the JOA score deficit.

Concomitant posterolateral arthrodesis is routinely recommended with cervical laminectomy; otherwise, postlaminectomy kyphosis may occur. The incidence of postlaminectomy kyphosis ranges from 6% to 47% in adults who have cervical laminectomies in isolation.[56] Fusion rates using lateral mass screw fixation in large series have been reported as over 97%.[139]

Emerging evidence suggests that the width of the C5 laminectomy performed, as well as the degree of spinal cord posterior drift, are associated with the incidence of postoperative C5 nerve palsy.[140] It is unclear currently if strategies to reduce the width of this laminectomy will reduce the rate of postoperative C5 palsies.

Cervical Laminoplasty

Many varieties of cervical laminoplasty have been described, most of which are derivatives of Hirabayashi's "open-door" or Kurokawa's "French door" procedures. Our preferred technique, the "open-door" laminoplasty, is described later. Both of these techniques evolved with the intention of avoiding the devastating postlaminectomy kyphosis while maintaining ROM and providing safe, predictable neurologic recovery. These procedures relatively spare the posterior column, allowing it to retain its load-bearing abilities. As such, it is rare to have postoperative instability secondary to laminoplasty procedures. Most laminoplasty innovations have come out of Japan due to the high rates of OPLL and congenital cervical stenosis within the native population requiring multilevel reconstructions. Traditional teaching on the matter is that laminoplasty does not reliably provide relief for axial neck pain; thus, arthrodesis should be considered if that is the patient's primary complaint, although some attribute postoperative axial neck pain after laminoplasty to overly protective immobilization used in historic protocols. A recent meta-analysis does not identify differences in axial pain between laminoplasty and laminectomy with fusion[141]; thus, this may not be an appropriate consideration during preoperative planning.

Open-Door Laminoplasty Procedure

Open-door laminoplasty requires the creation of two osteotomy troughs, one complete and one incomplete, which will be used as the hinge to open the posterior elements. After exposure is completed and the appropriate levels are determined, the lamina–lateral mass junction is identified bilaterally and can be marked with a marking pen. Arthrosis may obscure these landmarks; thus, preoperative imaging should be reviewed for additional guidance. A high-speed burr is used to create the troughs at the bilateral lamina–lateral mass junctions, which usually have a subtle inflection point to guide the surgeon intraoperatively. The trough should not be greater than 4 mm in depth; trough depth greater than this should clue the surgeon to an excessively lateral trough, which could result in vertebral artery injury.

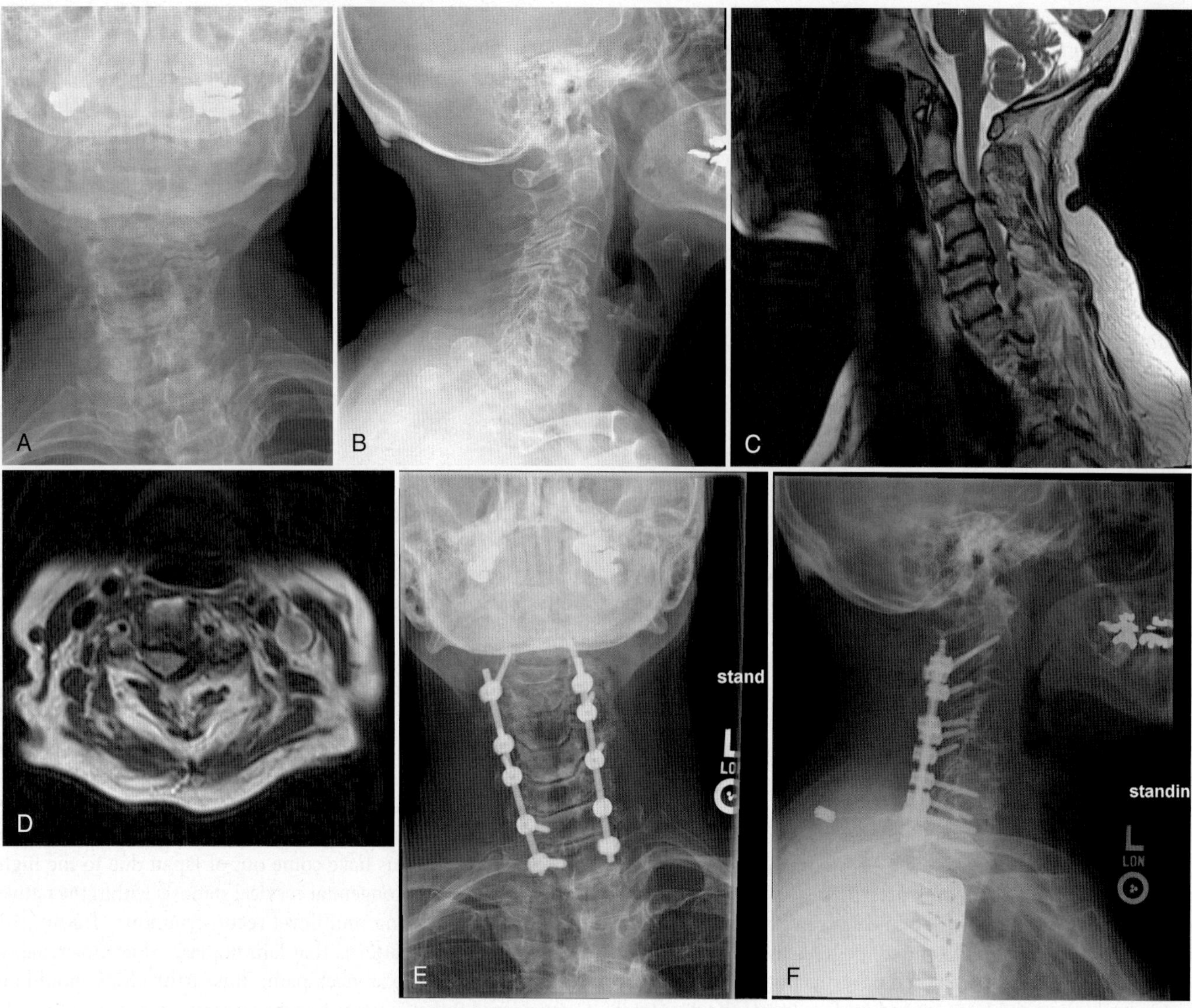

FIG. 42.12 (A) Preoperative anteroposterior radiograph of the cervical spine. (B) Preoperative lateral radiograph of the cervical spine. (C) Preoperative midsagittal magnetic resonance imaging (MRI) slice of the cervical spine. (D) Preoperative axial MRI slice of the cervical spine. (E) Immediately postoperative anteroposterior radiograph of the cervical spine. (F) Immediately postoperative lateral radiograph of the cervical spine.

Our preferred method is to perform the complete osteotomy first, starting at the inferior aspect of each lamina. Once the osteotomy has reached the appropriate depth, the ligamentum flavum will be visible. The remainder of the osteotomy to the superior half of each lamina can be completed with a diamond-tipped burr or a Kerrison rongeur. On the contralateral side, the hinge/incomplete osteotomy is performed at the same inflection point between the lamina and lateral mass. The dorsal cortical bone and cancellous bone are removed with a burr until a thin unicortical hinge remains. Excessive removal of bone should be avoided because it may result in a weak hinge.

The spinous processes of each level can subsequently be used to lever away from the complete osteotomy and toward the hinge osteotomy (Fig. 42.13). The surgeon must be extremely careful to avoid the devastating complication of having the posterior elements spring back and cause spinal cord injury. We recommend placing a thumb on the spinous process and curette within the complete osteotomy site while performing this levering maneuver. After levering, open the posterior elements; the spinal canal area is enlarged. Any fibrous adhesions between the dura and the undersurface of the lamina can be divided with scissors.[142]

Historically, suture fixation was used to keep the laminoplasty door open.[142] Alternatively, bone graft could be wedged into the defect. Our preferred approach, however, is the use of a laminoplasty plate to maintain the integrity of the door and avoid the "spring-back" complication (Fig. 42.14). Laminoplasty plates typically involve the placement of screw fixation into both the lamina and the lateral mass to rigidly fix the space between the two structures.

Fig. 42.15 demonstrates a case example of a laminoplasty with plating performed for cervical myelopathy. Given the multilevel pathology, stability on plain radiographs, as well as autofusions of C4–C5 and C5–C6, preventing ACDF, our preferred technique for management was a C3–C6 laminoplasty with laminectomy and foraminal decompression of C7.

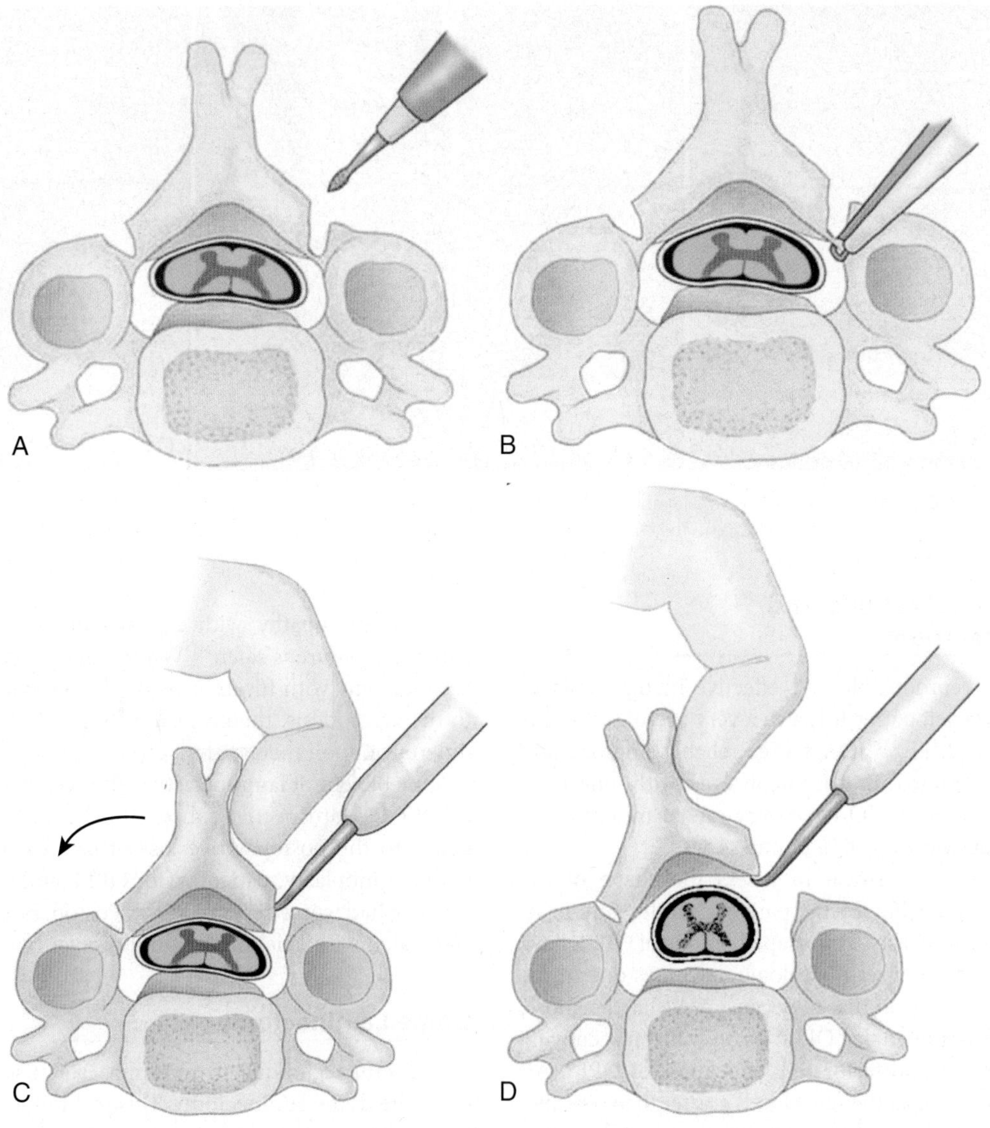

FIG. 42.13 Open-door laminoplasty technique. (A) Unicortical gutters at the lamina-facet junction are created with the high-speed burr. (B) A curette or micro-Kerrison rongeur is used to breach the ventral cortex on the side to be opened. (C–D) With the concomitant use of a finger and an instrument, the posterior arch is expanded by pushing, elevating toward the hinge side.

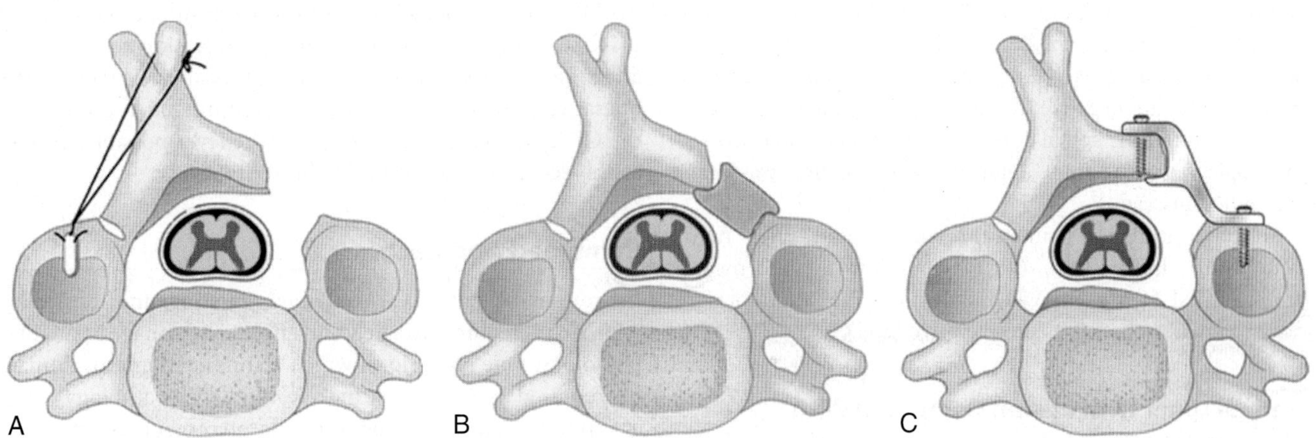

FIG. 42.14 Various methods to stabilize an open-door laminoplasty. (A) Lateral mass suture anchor tethering. (B) Strut grafting to prop open the expanded spinal canal. (C) Intrasegment fixation with a plate and screw system.

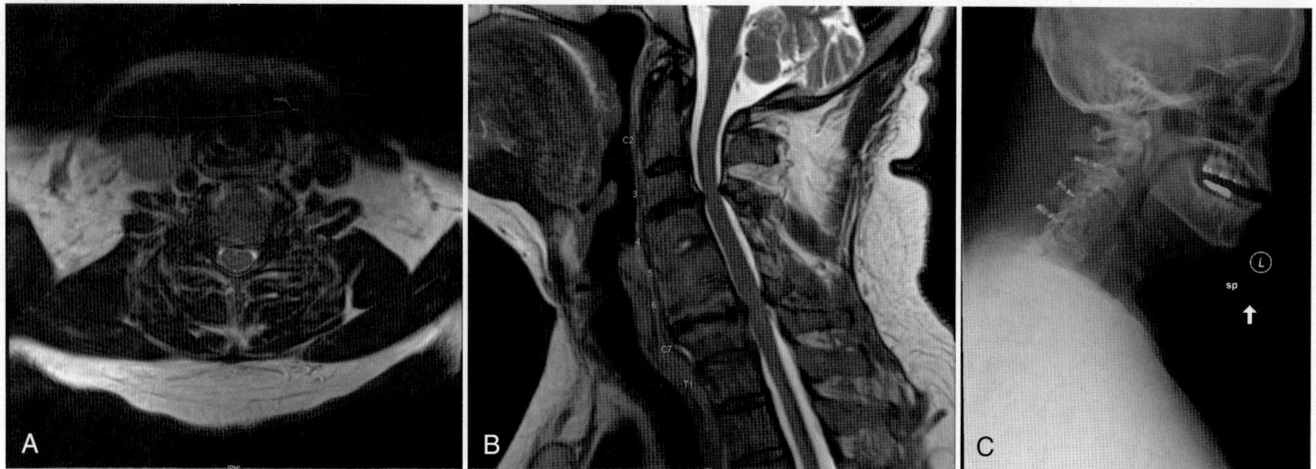

FIG. 42.15 (A) Preoperative axial magnetic resonance imaging (MRI) slice of a stenotic cervical level. (B) Preoperative sagittal MRI slice of the cervical spine. (C) Postoperative lateral radiograph of the cervical spine.

Outcomes, Complications, and Other Considerations

Laminoplasty is reproducible and effective in the management of cervical myelopathy. It is also a very useful technique in the setting of OPLL.[143] JOA scores reliably improve and demonstrate maintained improvement, even with long-term follow-up.[144,145] The mean JOA recovery rate at minimum of 10-year follow-up was over 55% in one series.[144]

Preoperatively, it is critical to assess the shape of the pathoanatomy responsible for the patient's myelopathy prior to performing laminoplasty. Hill-shaped lesions of OPLL have been associated with poorer neurologic outcomes due to the focal anterior compression that they cause.[146,147] Furthermore, Iwasaki et al.[147] determined that OPLL lesions with an occupying ratio (maximal anteroposterior [AP] thickness of OPLL/AP diameter of spinal canal at the same level) greater than 60% had poor or fair neurologic outcomes. An anterior procedure may be required to fully decompress the cord in these situations.

Similarly, Fujiyoshi et al.[148] described a radiographic marker known as the K-line, which can preoperatively predict the neurologic recovery of patients with OPLL undergoing laminoplasty. The K-line is a straight line that connects the midpoints of the spinal canal at C2 and C7 on a lateral radiograph. If the OPLL lesions lie entirely anterior to the K-line, they are referred to as K-line positive; otherwise, they are considered K-line negative. K-line-negative patients had less posterior shift of the spinal cord after laminoplasty and worse neurologic recovery; thus, anterior decompression was recommended instead.[148]

Although no fusion is intended, laminar autofusions may occur, which limit ROM. At 10-year follow-up, the mean cervical ROM of patients who had undergone laminoplasty was 25% to 47% that of its preoperative level.[144,149]

Laminectomy With Fusion Compared With Laminoplasty

A recent meta-analysis concluded that laminoplasty and laminectomy with fusion are similarly effective in the treatment of cervical myelopathy with insufficient evidence to identify which procedure is safer.[141] While some surgeons believe that laminectomy with fusion provides better axial pain relief due to the arthrodesis, there was low evidence demonstrating no difference upon metaanalysis.[141]

One benefit of laminoplasty is the retention of some cervical ROM. A prospective cohort study identified a time dependence to the postoperative loss of cervical ROM associated with laminoplasty; patients with OPLL and autofusion of the laminae had worse cervical ROM. Postoperative ROM was not associated with axial neck pain, however.[150]

Dome Laminectomy

One useful technique to minimize soft tissue dissection at C7 is the dome laminectomy. This technique has evolved as a means of preventing the detachment of the cervical extensor muscles, which heavily attach to C7. The technique involves creating a dome-shaped resection of the superior lamina of C7 and, in doing so, sparing the C7 spinous process. Proponents of this technique believe that it reduces the incidence of postoperative axial neck pain.[151] In a recent systematic review of the literature by Riew et al.,[152] it was determined that there is conflicting evidence as to whether preservation of muscular attachments to C7 (and C2) reduces axial neck pain postoperatively. Regardless, the authors recommended preserving the C7 (and C2) spinous processes whenever possible as long as the decompression is not compromised.

Combined Approaches

In certain scenarios, a combined anterior and posterior approach is required to safely and effectively manage a patient's pathology. One scenario in which a combined approach may be required is in the setting of multilevel pathology with a kyphotic deformity. The kyphotic alignment can be corrected anteriorly, and decompression can subsequently be performed posteriorly. Alternatively, a combined approach may be needed in the setting of multilevel pathology with a focal anterior source of compression. For instance, a patient with diffuse OPLL, but a hill-shaped thickening at a particular level, would likely require a combined approach for management. A patient with multilevel pathology addressed with an ACCF may require posterior arthrodesis for added construct stability as well. As mentioned previously, no single approach is optimal for all patients. An individualized treatment plan must be designed based on the patient's sagittal alignment, source of compression, number of levels involved, presence of axial neck pain, shape of pathoanatomy, and/or history of prior surgeries.

Conclusion

Cervical spondylotic myelopathy is the most common cause of spinal cord dysfunction in the world.[1] The condition is characterized by a generally progressive neurologic decline, which fails to respond to nonoperative measures and, once symptomatic, often benefits from operative management. Anterior and posterior spine surgical procedures can effectively halt or slow the neurologic decline associated with CSM. With a careful history, physical, and review of available imaging, an individualized treatment plan can be constructed to safely and appropriately care for a patient with cervical myelopathy.

KEY REFERENCES

1. Anderson PA, et al. Laminectomy and fusion for the treatment of cervical degenerative myelopathy. *J Neurosurg Spine.* 2009;11:150-156.
2. Fraser JF, Härtl R. Anterior approaches to fusion of the cervical spine: a metaanalysis of fusion rates. *J Neurosurg Spine.* 2007;6:298-303.
3. Hilibrand AS, Carlson GD, Palumbo MA, Jones PK, Bohlman HH. Radiculopathy and myelopathy at segments adjacent to the site of a previous anterior cervical arthrodesis. *J Bone Joint Surg Am.* 1999;81:519-528.
4. Jiang S-D, Jiang L-S, Dai L-Y. Anterior cervical discectomy and fusion versus anterior cervical corpectomy and fusion for multilevel cervical spondylosis: a systematic review. *Arch Orthop Trauma Surg.* 2012;132:155-161.
5. Kawaguchi Y, et al. Minimum 10-year followup after en bloc cervical laminoplasty. *Clin Orthop.* 2003;129-139.
6. Kimura I, Shingu H, Nasu Y. Long-term follow-up of cervical spondylotic myelopathy treated by canal-expansive laminoplasty. *J Bone Joint Surg Br.* 1995;77:956-961.
7. Lees F, Turner JWA. Natural history and prognosis of cervical spondylosis. *Br Med J.* 1963;2:1607-1610.
8. Matsumoto M, Chiba K, Toyama Y. Surgical treatment of ossification of the posterior longitudinal ligament and its outcomes: posterior surgery by laminoplasty. *Spine.* 2012;37:E303-E308.
9. Wen Z-Q, Du J-Y, Ling Z-H, Xu H-D, Lin X-J. Anterior cervical discectomy and fusion versus anterior cervical corpectomy and fusion in the treatment of multilevel cervical spondylotic myelopathy: systematic review and a meta-analysis. *Ther Clin Risk Manag.* 2015;11:161-170.

REFERENCES

1. Kalsi-Ryan S, Karadimas SK, Fehlings MG. Cervical spondylotic myelopathy: the clinical phenomenon and the current pathobiology of an increasingly prevalent and devastating disorder. *Neurosci. Rev. J. Bringing Neurobiol. Neurol. Psychiatry.* 2013;19:409-421.
2. Fujimori T, et al. Ossification of the posterior longitudinal ligament of the cervical spine in 3161 patients: a CT-based study. *Spine.* 2015;40:E394-E403.
3. Morishita Y, et al. The relationship between the cervical spinal canal diameter and the pathological changes in the cervical spine. *Eur Spine J.* 2009;18:877-883.
4. Karadimas SK, Erwin WM, Ely CG, Dettori JR, Fehlings MG. Pathophysiology and natural history of cervical spondylotic myelopathy. *Spine.* 2013;38:S21-S36.
5. Tracy JA, Bartleson JD. Cervical spondylotic myelopathy. *Neurologist.* 2010;16:176-187.
6. Gore DR, Sepic SB, Gardner GM. Roentgenographic findings of the cervical spine in asymptomatic people. *Spine.* 1986;11:521-524.
7. Lees F, Turner J. Natural history and prognosis of cervical spondylosis. *Br Med J.* 1963;2:1607-1610.
8. Nurick S. The natural history and the results of surgical treatment of the spinal cord disorder associated with cervical spondylosis. *Brain.* 1972;95:101-108.
9. Katoh S, Ikata T, Hirai N, Okada Y, Nakauchi K. Influence of minor trauma to the neck on the neurological outcome in patients with ossification of the posterior longitudinal ligament (OPLL) of the cervical spine. *Paraplegia.* 1995;33:330-333.
10. Rhee JM, et al. Nonoperative management of cervical myelopathy: a systematic review. *Spine.* 2013;38:S55-S67.
11. Sumi M, et al. Prospective cohort study of mild cervical spondylotic myelopathy without surgical treatment. *J Neurosurg Spine.* 2012;16:8-14.
12. Yoshimatsu H, et al. Conservative treatment for cervical spondylotic myelopathy. Prediction of treatment effects by multivariate analysis. *Spine J.* 2001;1:269-273.
13. Shimomura T, et al. Prognostic factors for deterioration of patients with cervical spondylotic myelopathy after nonsurgical treatment. *Spine.* 2007;32:2474-2479.
14. Nurick S. The pathogenesis of the spinal cord disorder associated with cervical spondylosis. *Brain J. Neurol.* 1972;95:87-100.
15. Ranawat CS, et al. Cervical spine fusion in rheumatoid arthritis. *J Bone Jt. Surg Am.* 1979;61:1003-1010.
16. Fukui M, et al. An outcome measure for patients with cervical myelopathy: Japanese Orthopaedic Association Cervical Myelopathy Evaluation Questionnaire (JOACMEQ): part 1. *J Orthop Sci.* 2007;12:227-240.
17. Fukui M, et al. Japanese Orthopaedic Association Cervical Myelopathy Evaluation Questionnaire: part 3. Determination of reliability. *J Orthop Sci.* 2007;12:321-326.
18. Zhang Y, Zhou F, Sun Y. Assessment of health-related quality of life using the SF-36 in Chinese cervical spondylotic myelopathy patients after surgery and its consistency with neurological function assessment: a cohort study. *Health Qual Life Outcomes.* 2015;13:39.
19. Clark CR. Cervical spondylotic myelopathy: history and physical findings. *Spine.* 1988;13:847-849.
20. Singh A, et al. A summary of assessment tools for patients suffering from cervical spondylotic myelopathy: a systematic review on validity, reliability and responsiveness. *Eur Spine J.* 2015;24(suppl 2):209-228.
21. Lee MJ, Garcia R, Cassinelli EH, Furey C, Riew KD. Tandem stenosis: a cadaveric study in osseous morphology. *Spine J.* 2008;8:1003-1006.

22. Bajwa NS, Toy JO, Young EY, Ahn NU. Is congenital bony stenosis of the cervical spine associated with lumbar spine stenosis? An anatomical study of 1072 human cadaveric specimens. *J Neurosurg Spine*. 2012;17:24-29.
23. Eskander MS, et al. Is there a difference between simultaneous or staged decompressions for combined cervical and lumbar stenosis? *J Spinal Disord Tech*. 2011;24:409-413.
24. Pavlov H, Torg JS, Robie B, Jahre C. Cervical spinal stenosis: determination with vertebral body ratio method. *Radiology*. 1987;164:771-775.
25. Suk K-S, et al. Reevaluation of the Pavlov ratio in patients with cervical myelopathy. *Clin. Orthop. Surg*. 2009;1:6-10.
26. Kang MS, Lee JW, Zhang HY, Cho YE, Park YM. Diagnosis of cervical OPLL in lateral radiograph and MRI: is it reliable? *Korean J. Spine*. 2012;9:205.
27. Ames CP, et al. Cervical radiographical alignment: comprehensive assessment techniques and potential importance in cervical myelopathy. *Spine*. 2013;38:S149-S160.
28. Shimizu K, et al. Spinal kyphosis causes demyelination and neuronal loss in the spinal cord: a new model of kyphotic deformity using juvenile Japanese small game fowls. *Spine*. 2005;30:2388-2392.
29. Tetreault LA, et al. Systematic review of magnetic resonance imaging characteristics that affect treatment decision making and predict clinical outcome in patients with cervical spondylotic myelopathy. *Spine*. 2013;38:S89-S110.
30. Kim H-J, et al. Diabetes and smoking as prognostic factors after cervical laminoplasty. *J Bone Joint Surg Br*. 2008;90:1468-1472.
31. Zhang L, et al. Preoperative evaluation of the cervical spondylotic myelopathy with flexion-extension magnetic resonance imaging: about a prospective study of fifty patients. *Spine*. 2011;36:E1134-E1139.
32. Suri A, Chabbra RPS, Mehta VS, Gaikwad S, Pandey RM. Effect of intramedullary signal changes on the surgical outcome of patients with cervical spondylotic myelopathy. *Spine J*. 2003;3:33-45.
33. Zhang Y-Z, et al. Magnetic resonance T2 image signal intensity ratio and clinical manifestation predict prognosis after surgical intervention for cervical spondylotic myelopathy. *Spine*. 2010;35:E396-E399.
34. Wang L-F, et al. Using the T2-weighted magnetic resonance imaging signal intensity ratio and clinical manifestations to assess the prognosis of patients with cervical ossification of the posterior longitudinal ligament. *J Neurosurg Spine*. 2010;13:319-323.
35. Wada E, Yonenobu K, Suzuki S, Kanazawa A, Ochi T. Can intramedullary signal change on magnetic resonance imaging predict surgical outcome in cervical spondylotic myelopathy? *Spine*. 1999;24:455-461.
36. Park Y-S, et al. Predictors of outcome of surgery for cervical compressive myelopathy: retrospective analysis and prospective study. *Neurol Med Chir (Tokyo)*. 2006;46:231-238.
37. Law MD, Bernhardt M, White AA. Cervical spondylotic myelopathy: a review of surgical indications and decision making. *Yale J Biol Med*. 1993;66:165-177.
38. Fehlings MG, et al. Symptomatic progression of cervical myelopathy and the role of nonsurgical management: a consensus statement. *Spine*. 2013;38:S19-S20.
39. Lesoin F, Bouasakao N, Clarisse J, Rousseaux M. Jomin, M. Results of surgical treatment of radiculomyelopathy caused by cervical arthrosis based on 1000 operations. *Surg Neurol*. 1985;23:350-355.
40. David Kaye I, et al. Predictors of morbidity and mortality among patients with cervical spondylotic myelopathy treated surgically. *Eur Spine J*. 2015;doi:10.1007/s00586-015-4010-2.
41. Tetreault LA, Karpova A, Fehlings MG. Predictors of outcome in patients with degenerative cervical spondylotic myelopathy undergoing surgical treatment: results of a systematic review. *Eur Spine J*. 2015;24(suppl 2):236-251.
42. Tetreault LA, et al. A clinical prediction model to assess surgical outcome in patients with cervical spondylotic myelopathy: internal and external validations using the prospective multicenter AOSpine North American and international datasets of 743 patients. *Spine J. Off. J. North Am. Spine Soc*. 2015;15:388-397.
43. Epstein JA. The surgical management of cervical spinal stenosis, spondylosis, and myeloradiculopathy by means of the posterior approach. *Spine*. 1988;13:864-869.
44. O'Neill KR, Neuman B, Peters C, Riew KD. Risk factors for postoperative retropharyngeal hematoma after anterior cervical spine surgery. *Spine*. 2014;39:E246-E252.
45. Marquez-Lara A, Nandyala SV, Fineberg SJ, Singh K. Incidence, outcomes, and mortality of reintubation after anterior cervical fusion. *Spine*. 2014;39:134-139.
46. Veeravagu A, Cole T, Jiang B, Ratliff JK. Revision rates and complication incidence in single- and multilevel anterior cervical discectomy and fusion procedures: an administrative database study. *Spine J*. 2014;14:1125-1131.
47. Singh K, Marquez-Lara A, Nandyala SV, Patel AA, Fineberg SJ. Incidence and risk factors for dysphagia after anterior cervical fusion. *Spine*. 2013;38:1820-1825.
48. Anderson PA, et al. Laminectomy and fusion for the treatment of cervical degenerative myelopathy. *J Neurosurg Spine*. 2009;11:150-156.
49. Herkowitz HN. A comparison of anterior cervical fusion, cervical laminectomy, and cervical laminoplasty for the surgical management of multiple level spondylotic radiculopathy. *Spine*. 1988;13:774-780.
50. Kaptain GJ, Simmons NE, Replogle RE, Pobereskin L. Incidence and outcome of kyphotic deformity following laminectomy for cervical spondylotic myelopathy. *J Neurosurg*. 2000;93:199-204.
51. Kato Y, Iwasaki M, Fuji T, Yonenobu K, Ochi T. Long-term follow-up results of laminectomy for cervical myelopathy caused by ossification of the posterior longitudinal ligament. *J Neurosurg*. 1998;89:217-223.
52. Ryken TC, et al. Cervical laminectomy for the treatment of cervical degenerative myelopathy. *J Neurosurg Spine*. 2009;11:142-149.
53. Ebersold MJ, Pare MC, Quast LM. Surgical treatment for cervical spondylitic myelopathy. *J Neurosurg*. 1995;82:745-751.
54. Arnold H, Feldmann U, Missler U. Chronic spondylogenic cervical myelopathy. A critical evaluation of surgical treatment after early and long-term follow-up. *Neurosurg Rev*. 1993;16:105-109.
55. Snow RB, Weiner H. Cervical laminectomy and foraminotomy as surgical treatment of cervical spondylosis: a follow-up study with analysis of failures. *J Spinal Disord*. 1993;6:245-250.
56. McAllister BD, Rebholz BJ, Wang JC. Is posterior fusion necessary with laminectomy in the cervical spine? *Surg. Neurol. Int*. 2012;3:S225-S231.

57. Fehlings MG, et al. Perioperative and delayed complications associated with the surgical treatment of cervical spondylotic myelopathy based on 302 patients from the AOSpine North America Cervical Spondylotic Myelopathy Study. *J Neurosurg Spine*. 2012;16:425-432.
58. Luo J, et al. Comparison of anterior approach versus posterior approach for the treatment of multilevel cervical spondylotic myelopathy. *Eur Spine J*. 2015;24:1621-1630.
59. Kiely PD, Quinn JC, Du JY, Lebl DR. Posterior surgical treatment of cervical spondylotic myelopathy: review article. *HSS J. Musculoskelet. J. Hosp. Spec. Surg*. 2015;11:36-42.
60. Lawrence BD, et al. Anterior versus posterior approach for treatment of cervical spondylotic myelopathy: a systematic review. *Spine*. 2013;38:S173-S182.
61. Yonenobu K, et al. Choice of surgical treatment for multisegmental cervical spondylotic myelopathy. *Spine*. 1985;10:710-716.
62. Heflin J, Rhee JM. Anterior cervical approaches. In: Wiesel SW, ed. *Operative Techniques in Orthopaedic Surgery*. Philadelphia: Lippincott Williams & Wilkins; 2011:4507-4515.
63. Spiker WR, Brodke DS. Cervical vertebrectomy and plating. In: Zdeblick TA, Albert TJ, eds. *Master Techniques in Orthopaedic Surgery: The Spine*. 3rd ed. Philadelphia: Lippincott Williams & Wilkins; 2013.
64. Orlando ER, Caroli E, Ferrante L. Management of the cervical esophagus and hypofarinx perforations complicating anterior cervical spine surgery. *Spine*. 2003;28:E290-E295.
65. Bertalanffy H, Eggert HR. Complications of anterior cervical discectomy without fusion in 450 consecutive patients. *Acta Neurochir (Wien)*. 1989;99:41-50.
66. Burke JP, Gerszten PC, Welch WC. Iatrogenic vertebral artery injury during anterior cervical spine surgery. *Spine J*. 2005;5:508-514.
67. Hannallah D, Lee J, Khan M, Donaldson WF, Kang JD. Cerebrospinal fluid leaks following cervical spine surgery. *J Bone Joint Surg Am*. 2008;90:1101-1105.
68. Saunders RL. On the pathogenesis of the radiculopathy complicating multilevel corpectomy. *Neurosurgery*. 1995;37:408-412.
69. Ikenaga M, Shikata J, Tanaka C. Radiculopathy of C-5 after anterior decompression for cervical myelopathy. *J Neurosurg Spine*. 2005;3:210-217.
70. Wada E, et al. Subtotal corpectomy versus laminoplasty for multilevel cervical spondylotic myelopathy: a long-term follow-up study over 10 years. *Spine*. 2001;26:1443-1447; discussion 1448.
71. Kilburg C, Sullivan HG, Mathiason MA. Effect of approach side during anterior cervical discectomy and fusion on the incidence of recurrent laryngeal nerve injury. *J Neurosurg Spine*. 2006;4:273-277.
72. Beutler WJ, Sweeney CA, Connolly PJ. Recurrent laryngeal nerve injury with anterior cervical spine surgery risk with laterality of surgical approach. *Spine*. 2001;26:1337-1342.
73. Frempong-Boadu A, et al. Swallowing and speech dysfunction in patients undergoing anterior cervical discectomy and fusion: a prospective, objective preoperative and postoperative assessment. *J Spinal Disord Tech*. 2002;15:362-368.
74. Robinson RA, Walker AE, Ferlic DC, Wiecking DK. The results of anterior interbody fusion of the cervical spine. *J. Bone Jt. Surg*. 1962;44:1569-1587.
75. Edwards CC, et al. Accurate identification of adverse outcomes after cervical spine surgery. *J Bone Joint Surg Am*. 2004;86-A:251-256.
76. Tortolani PJ, et al. A comparison of retraction pressure during anterior cervical plate surgery and cervical disc replacement: a cadaveric study. *J Spinal Disord Tech*. 2006;19:312-317.
77. Winslow CP, Meyers AD. Otolaryngologic complications of the anterior approach to the cervical spine. *Am J Otolaryngol*. 1999;20:16-27.
78. Smith-Hammond CA, et al. Prospective analysis of incidence and risk factors of dysphagia in spine surgery patients: comparison of anterior cervical, posterior cervical, and lumbar procedures. *Spine*. 2004;29:1441-1446.
79. Riley LH, Skolasky RL, Albert TJ, Vaccaro AR, Heller JG. Dysphagia after anterior cervical decompression and fusion: prevalence and risk factors from a longitudinal cohort study. *Spine*. 2005;30:2564-2569.
80. Olsson EC, Jobson M, Lim MR. Risk factors for persistent dysphagia after anterior cervical spine surgery. *Orthopedics*. 2015;38:e319-e323.
81. Winslow CP, Winslow TJ, Wax MK. Dysphonia and dysphagia following the anterior approach to the cervical spine. *Arch Otolaryngol Head Neck Surg*. 2001;127:51-55.
82. Grisoli F, et al. Anterior discectomy without fusion for treatment of cervical lateral soft disc extrusion: a follow-up of 120 cases. *Neurosurgery*. 1989;24:853-859.
83. Netterville JL, Koriwchak MJ, Winkle M, Courey MS, Ossoff RH. Vocal fold paralysis following the anterior approach to the cervical spine. *Ann Otol Rhinol Laryngol*. 1996;105:85-91.
84. Apfelbaum RI, Kriskovich MD, Haller JR. On the incidence, cause, and prevention of recurrent laryngeal nerve palsies during anterior cervical spine surgery. *Spine*. 2000;25:2906-2912.
85. Jellish WS, Jensen RL, Anderson DE, Shea JF. Intraoperative electromyographic assessment of recurrent laryngeal nerve stress and pharyngeal injury during anterior cervical spine surgery with Caspar instrumentation. *J Neurosurg*. 1999;91:170-174.
86. Haller JM, Iwanik M, Shen FH. Clinically relevant anatomy of high anterior cervical approach. *Spine*. 2011;36:2116-2121.
87. Shriver MF, et al. Pseudoarthrosis rates in anterior cervical discectomy and fusion: a meta-analysis. *Spine J*. 2015;15:2016-2027.
88. Fraser JF, Härtl R. Anterior approaches to fusion of the cervical spine: a metaanalysis of fusion rates. *J Neurosurg Spine*. 2007;6:298-303.
89. Bolesta MJ, Rechtine GR, Chrin AM. One- and two-level anterior cervical discectomy and fusion: the effect of plate fixation. *Spine J*. 2002;2:197-203.
90. Mobbs RJ, Rao P, Chandran NK. Anterior cervical discectomy and fusion: analysis of surgical outcome with and without plating. *J Clin Neurosci*. 2007;14:639-642.
91. Li J, et al. Anterior surgical options for the treatment of cervical spondylotic myelopathy in a long-term follow-up study. *Arch Orthop Trauma Surg*. 2013;133:745-751.
92. Hilibrand AS, Carlson GD, Palumbo MA, Jones PK, Bohlman HH. Radiculopathy and myelopathy at segments adjacent to the site of a previous anterior cervical arthrodesis. *J Bone Joint Surg Am*. 1999;81:519-528.
93. van Eck CF, Regan C, Donaldson WF, Kang JD, Lee JY. The revision rate and occurrence of adjacent segment disease after anterior cervical discectomy and fusion: a study of 672 consecutive patients. *Spine*. 2014;39:2143-2147.
94. Bible JE, et al. Postoperative bracing after spine surgery for degenerative conditions: a questionnaire study. *Spine J*. 2009;9:309-316.

95. Baird EO, Rhee JM, Dodwad S-NM, Patel AA. Do you need to use a collar after a 2-level instrumented ACDF? *J Spinal Disord Tech*. 2015;28:199-201.
96. Smith MD, Bolesta MJ, Leventhal M, Bohlman HH. Postoperative cerebrospinal-fluid fistula associated with erosion of the dura. Findings after anterior resection of ossification of the posterior longitudinal ligament in the cervical spine. *J Bone Joint Surg Am*. 1992;74:270-277.
97. Gao R, et al. Long term results of anterior corpectomy and fusion for cervical spondylotic myelopathy. *PLoS One*. 2012;7:e34811.
98. Andaluz N, Zuccarello M, Kuntz C. Long-term follow-up of cervical radiographic sagittal spinal alignment after 1- and 2-level cervical corpectomy for the treatment of spondylosis of the subaxial cervical spine causing radiculomyelopathy or myelopathy: a retrospective study. *J Neurosurg Spine*. 2012;16:2-7.
99. Uribe JS, Sangala JR, Duckworth EAM, Vale FL. Comparison between anterior cervical discectomy fusion and cervical corpectomy fusion using titanium cages for reconstruction: analysis of outcome and long-term follow-up. *Eur Spine J*. 2009;18:654-662.
100. Bernard TN, Whitecloud TS. Cervical spondylotic myelopathy and myeloradiculopathy. Anterior decompression and stabilization with autogenous fibula strut graft. *Clin Orthop*. 1987;221:149-160.
101. Fernyhough JC, White JI, LaRocca H. Fusion rates in multilevel cervical spondylosis comparing allograft fibula with autograft fibula in 126 patients. *Spine*. 1991;16: S561-S564.
102. Zeidman SM, Ducker TB, Raycroft J. Trends and complications in cervical spine surgery: 1989-1993. *J Spinal Disord*. 1997;10:523-526.
103. Riew KD, Sethi NS, Devney J, Goette K, Choi K. Complications of buttress plate stabilization of cervical corpectomy. *Spine*. 1999;24:2404-2410.
104. Jiang S-D, Jiang L-S, Dai L-Y. Anterior cervical discectomy and fusion versus anterior cervical corpectomy and fusion for multilevel cervical spondylosis: a systematic review. *Arch Orthop Trauma Surg*. 2012;132:155-161.
105. Singh K, et al. Biomechanical comparison of cervical spine reconstructive techniques after a multilevel corpectomy of the cervical spine. *Spine*. 2003;28:2352-2358.
106. Brodke DS, et al. Dynamic cervical plates: biomechanical evaluation of load sharing and stiffness. *Spine*. 2001;26:1324-1329.
107. Brodke DS, Klimo P, Bachus KN, Braun JT, Dailey AT. Anterior cervical fixation: analysis of load-sharing and stability with use of static and dynamic plates. *J Bone Joint Surg Am*. 2006;88:1566-1573.
108. Spivak JM, Chen D, Kummer FJ. The effect of locking fixation screws on the stability of anterior cervical plating. *Spine*. 1999;24:334-338.
109. Hussain M, et al. Screw angulation affects bone-screw stresses and bone graft load sharing in anterior cervical corpectomy fusion with a rigid screw-plate construct: a finite element model study. *Spine J*. 2009;9:1016-1023.
110. Dipaola CP, Jacobson JA, Awad H, Conrad BP, Rechtine GR. Screw orientation and plate type (variable- vs. fixed-angle) effect strength of fixation for in vitro biomechanical testing of the Synthes CSLP. *Spine J*. 2008;8:717-722.
111. Vaccaro AR, et al. Early failure of long segment anterior cervical plate fixation. *J Spinal Disord*. 1998;11:410-415.
112. Daubs MD. Early failures following cervical corpectomy reconstruction with titanium mesh cages and anterior plating. *Spine*. 2005;30:1402-1406.
113. Okawa A, et al. Risk factors for early reconstruction failure of multilevel cervical corpectomy with dynamic plate fixation. *Spine*. 2011;36:E582-E587.
114. DiAngelo DJ, Foley KT, Vossel KA, Rampersaud YR, Jansen TH. Anterior cervical plating reverses load transfer through multilevel strut-grafts. *Spine*. 2000;25:783-795.
115. Odate S, Shikata J, Kimura H, Soeda T. Hybrid decompression and fixation technique versus plated three-vertebra corpectomy for four-segment cervical myelopathy: analysis of 81 cases with a minimum 2-year follow-up. *J Spinal Disord Tech*. 2013. Available at: http://journals.lww.com/jspinaldisorders/Abstract/publishahead/Hybrid_Decompression_and_Fixation_Technique_Versus.99549.aspx.
116. Wei-bing X, et al. Reconstructive techniques study after anterior decompression of multilevel cervical spondylotic myelopathy. *J Spinal Disord Tech*. 2009;22:511-515.
117. Rhee JM, Park J-B, Yang J-Y, Riew DK. Indications and techniques for anterior cervical plating. *Neurol India*. 2005;53:433-439.
118. Rapoff AJ, Conrad BP, Johnson WM, Cordista A, Rechtine GR. Load sharing in Premier and Zephir anterior cervical plates. *Spine*. 2003;28:2648-2650.
119. Epstein NE. The management of one-level anterior cervical corpectomy with fusion using Atlantis hybrid plates: preliminary experience. *J Spinal Disord*. 2000;13: 324-328.
120. Ragab AA, Hodges FS, Hill CP, McGuire RA, Tucci M. Dynamic anterior cervical plating for multi-level spondylosis: does it help? *Evid Based Spine Care J*. 2010; 1:41-46.
121. Saphier PS, Arginteanu MS, Moore FM, Steinberger AA, Camins MB. Stress-shielding compared with load-sharing anterior cervical plate fixation: a clinical and radiographic prospective analysis of 50 patients. *J Neurosurg Spine*. 2007;6:391-397.
122. Barnes B, Haid RW, Rodts GE, Subach BR, Kaiser M. Early results using the Atlantis anterior cervical plate system. *Neurosurg Focus*. 2002;12:E13.
123. Wen Z-Q, Du J-Y, Ling Z-H, Xu H-D, Lin X-J. Anterior cervical discectomy and fusion versus anterior cervical corpectomy and fusion in the treatment of multilevel cervical spondylotic myelopathy: systematic review and a meta-analysis. *Ther Clin Risk Manag*. 2015;11:161-170.
124. Huang Z-Y, et al. Comparison of two anterior fusion methods in two-level cervical spondylosis myelopathy: a meta-analysis. *BMJ Open*. 2014;4:e004581.
125. Xiao S-W, Jiang H, Yang L-J, Xiao Z-M. Anterior cervical discectomy versus corpectomy for multilevel cervical spondylotic myelopathy: a meta-analysis. *Eur Spine J*. 2015;24:31-39.
126. Rao R, Marawar SV. Posterior cervical approaches. In: Wiesel SW, ed. *Operative Techniques in Orthopaedic Surgery*. Philadelphia: Lippincott Williams & Wilkins; 2011.
127. Anderson PA, Finn MA. Laminectomy and posterior fusion. In: Zdeblick TA, Albert TJ, eds. *Master Techniques in Orthopaedic Surgery: The Spine*. 3rd ed. Philadelphia: Lippincott Williams & Wilkins; 2013.
128. Zhang P, et al. Preserving the C7 spinous process in laminectomy combined with lateral mass screw to prevent axial symptom. *J Orthop Sci*. 2011;16:492-497.

129. Komotar RJ, Mocco J, Kaiser MG. Surgical management of cervical myelopathy: indications and techniques for laminectomy and fusion. *Spine J*. 2006;6: 252S-267S.
130. Zdeblick TA, et al. Cervical stability after foraminotomy. A biomechanical in vitro analysis. *J Bone Joint Surg Am*. 1992;74:22-27.
131. Regan CM, Emmanuel S, Hornik C, Weinhold P, Lim MR. Lateral mass versus hybrid construct for cervical laminectomy and fusion. *Orthopedics*. 2013;36:e484-e488.
132. Heller JG, Carlson GD, Abitbol JJ, Garfin SR. Anatomic comparison of the Roy-Camille and Magerl techniques for screw placement in the lower cervical spine. *Spine*. 1991;16:S552-S557.
133. Montesano PX, Jauch E, Jonsson H. Anatomic and biomechanical study of posterior cervical spine plate arthrodesis: an evaluation of two different techniques of screw placement. *J Spinal Disord*. 1992;5:301-305.
134. Seybold EA, et al. Characteristics of unicortical and bicortical lateral mass screws in the cervical spine. *Spine*. 1999;24:2397-2403.
135. Wakao N, et al. Variance of cervical vertebral artery measured by CT angiography and its influence on C7 pedicle anatomy. *Spine*. 2014;39:228-232.
136. Takeuchi M, et al. Prevalence of C7 level anomalies at the C7 level: an important landmark for cervical nerve ultrasonography. *Acta Radiol*. 2015;doi:10.117 7/0284185115579078.
137. Hall WA. Vancomycin powder in spine surgery: still a work in progress. *World Neurosurg*. 2015;83:1051-1052.
138. Kang DG, Holekamp TF, Wagner SC, Lehman RA. Intrasite vancomycin powder for the prevention of surgical site infection in spine surgery: a systematic literature review. *Spine J*. 2015;15:762-770.
139. Katonis P, et al. Lateral mass screw complications: analysis of 1662 screws. *J Spinal Disord Tech*. 2011;24:415-420.
140. Radcliff KE, et al. Cervical laminectomy width and spinal cord drift are risk factors for postoperative C5 palsy. *J Spinal Disord Tech*. 2014;27:86-92.
141. Yoon ST, et al. Outcomes after laminoplasty compared with laminectomy and fusion in patients with cervical myelopathy: a systematic review. *Spine*. 2013;38:S183-S194.
142. Hirabayashi K, et al. Expansive open-door laminoplasty for cervical spinal stenotic myelopathy. *Spine*. 1983;8:693-699.
143. Matsumoto M, Chiba K, Toyama Y. Surgical treatment of ossification of the posterior longitudinal ligament and its outcomes: posterior surgery by laminoplasty. *Spine*. 2012;37:E303-E308.
144. Kawaguchi Y, et al. Minimum 10-year followup after en bloc cervical laminoplasty. *Clin Orthop*. 2003;411:129-139.
145. Kimura I, Shingu H, Nasu Y. Long-term follow-up of cervical spondylotic myelopathy treated by canal-expansive laminoplasty. *J Bone Joint Surg Br*. 1995;77:956-961.
146. Yoon ST, et al. Predictive factors affecting outcome after cervical laminoplasty. *Spine*. 2013;38:S232-S252.
147. Iwasaki M, et al. Surgical strategy for cervical myelopathy due to ossification of the posterior longitudinal ligament. Part 1: clinical results and limitations of laminoplasty. *Spine*. 2007;32:647-653.
148. Fujiyoshi T, et al. A new concept for making decisions regarding the surgical approach for cervical ossification of the posterior longitudinal ligament: the K-line. *Spine*. 2008;33:E990-E993.
149. Motosuneya T, Maruyama T, Yamada H, Tsuzuki N, Sakai H. Long-term results of tension-band laminoplasty for cervical stenotic myelopathy: a ten-year follow-up. *J Bone Joint Surg Br*. 2011;93:68-72.
150. Hyun S-J, Riew KD, Rhim S-C. Range of motion loss after cervical laminoplasty: a prospective study with minimum 5-year follow-up data. *Spine J*. 2013;13:384-390.
151. Sakaura H, et al. Preservation of muscles attached to the C2 and C7 spinous processes rather than subaxial deep extensors reduces adverse effects after cervical laminoplasty. *Spine*. 2010;35:E782-E786.
152. Riew KD, Raich AL, Dettori JR, Heller JG. Neck pain following cervical laminoplasty: does preservation of the C2 muscle attachments and/or C7 matter? *Evid Based Spine Care J*. 2013;4:42-53.

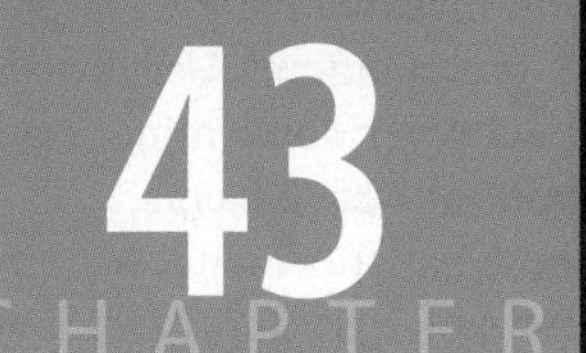

Ossification of the Posterior Longitudinal Ligament

Bhavuk Garg
Alok Sharan

Ossification of the posterior longitudinal ligament (OPLL) is a common cause of cervical myelopathy. Nearly 25% of patients with cervical myelopathy have been estimated to have OPLL.[1] The highest prevalence of OPLL is seen in the Japanese population, with a reported range of 1.9% to 4.3% in patients older than 30 years.[2] In the United States, the reported prevalence is around 0.1% to 0.7%.[2] The usual age of onset of OPLL is 50 years and is found twice as often in males as compared to females.[3]

Although most common in the cervical spine, it is also found less commonly in the thoracic and lumbar spine. Approximately 70% of cases occur in the cervical spine, followed by 15% in thoracic and 15% in the upper lumbar spine from L1 to L3.[3] Park et al.[3a] reported a 33.8% occurrence of thoracic OPLL in patients with cervical OPLL and recommended that the whole spine should be screened in patients with cervical OPLL.

Key[4] published the first report of OPLL causing compressive myelopathy in 1838 in Guy's Hospital Report and Oppenheimer[5] published a report in 1942. Numasawa[6] reported the first case of compressive myelopathy in the Japanese population due to OPLL based on autopsy findings in 1960.

Etiology

OPLL is a multifactorial disease with both genetic and environmental factors playing a role. Broadly, OPLL can be divided into two types: primary, or idiopathic, and secondary, or syndromic. The majority of OPLL cases are idiopathic. Secondary OPLL has been described with hypophosphatemic rickets, osteomalacia, and various endocrine disorders, such as hypoparathyroidism, acromegaly, and gigantism.[7]

Genetic Factors

Many genomic, linkage, and association studies have shown a strong genetic predisposition for OPLL.[7] Matsunaga et al. reported a high prevalence of identical human leukocyte antigen haplotypes in families of 24 patients.[8] Karasugi et al. reported linkages on 1p, 2p, 7q, 16q, and 20p in a genome-wide linkage study of 410 Japanese individuals.[9] A number of candidate genes/loci, including nucleotide pyrophosphatase/phosphodiesterase ENNP1, transforming growth factor-β1, estrogen receptor, interleukin-1β, vitamin D receptor, bone morphogenetic proteins (BMP) 2 and 9, runt-related transcription factor 2, toll-like receptor 5, and interleukin-15 receptor subunit alpha have been studied and reported to enhance susceptibility to OPLL.[7] Candidate gene approach has also linked collagen genes *COL11A2* and *COL6A1* genes with OPLL.[6,10] Kawaguchi et al.[11] reported that transforming growth factor-β1 polymorphism is related to the extent of ossification in OPLL rather than in its pathogenesis.

Environmental Factors

Various environmental factors have also been linked to the pathogenesis of OPLL. Mechanical stresses on the head have been postulated as a cause leading to hyperexpression of several bone-forming proteins, such as BMP and osteopontin, leading to ossification of several ligaments, including OPLL.[12] There is a high prevalence of type 2 diabetes and glucose intolerance in patients with OPLL.[13,14] Increasing age, obesity, and a vitamin A–rich diet have also been linked with OPLL.[12,14,15] Various musculoskeletal disorders, including ankylosing spondylitis, diffuse idiopathic skeletal hyperostosis, and other spondyloarthropathies have also been associated with OPLL.[16–19] Matsunaga et al.[20] reported a 20% incidence of OPLL in schizophrenia patients.

Various other environmental factors, such as the excessive consumption of pickles, hypertension, family history of myocardial infarction, high body mass index at age 40, long working hours, and working the night shift have also been reported as risk factors for OPLL. On the other hand, frequent intake of chicken or soy products and good sleeping habits have been shown to reduce the risk of OPLL.[3,16]

BMP is also believed to play an important role in OPLL. BMP-2 induces differentiation of ligament cells and leads to ossification by enchondral ossification.[21,22] Li et al.[23] reported that elevated insulin levels lead to an increased expression of insulin receptors, proliferation of spinal ligament cells, and induction of osteogenic differentiation through the PI3-K/Akt pathway in rats. This may explain the high association of

OPLL in type 2 diabetes. Some studies have also correlated high serum levels of activin with OPLL.[22]

Pathology

Ossification of the posterior longitudinal ligament occurs due to both enchondral and intramembranous ossification, resulting in the formation of ectopic lamellar bone; however, enchondral ossification plays the major role.[24] McAfee et al.[25] extensively reported the histopathology of OPLL, which is composed of lamellar bone with mature haversian canals. Ishida and Kawai reported that cells from nonossified areas in patients with OPLL have a high alkaline phosphatase activity and a high response to calcitonin and calcitriol.[26] Epstein et al.[1] reported that ossification of the PLL starts with vascular fibrosis, leading to calcification, cartilage proliferation, and then ossification.

Classification

The Japanese Investigation Committee on the Ossification of the Spinal Ligaments classified OPLL into four subtypes depending on its extent[3,27]:

Continuous: OPLL extends over several contiguous vertebrae.
Segmental: OPLL is seen behind several vertebrae, but there is interruption at the disc level.
Mixed: Combination of continuous and segmental type.
Others: OPLL is confined to the disc space only.

In terms of distribution, the segmental type is the most common (39%), followed by mixed (29%), continuous (27%), and focal (5%).[3,28] Some authors have also classified OPLL into the plateau type and hill type depending on its sagittal morphology. The plateau type is common in the segmental and continuous variety, whereas the hill type is common in the focal type.

Natural History

OPLL is a disease most commonly seen in individuals after the fifth decade of life. Chiba et al[29] and Hori et al[30,31] studied the progression of OPLL and found that the rate of progression was maximal for continuous and mixed types. They also found that C3 involvement was an important predictor of progression, with frequent progression seen at the C2–C4 level. Matsunaga et al[32] studied 450 patients with OPLL for at least 10 years and reported that only 17% of patients without myelopathy at the initial visit developed myelopathy; thus, they recommended that prophylactic decompression is not always required.

Clinical Features

Most of the patients with OPLL are asymptomatic and are diagnosed when imaging is done for other reasons or for nonspecific symptoms. As discussed earlier, OPLL is most common in the cervical region, followed by the thoracic and lumbar regions. Patients with OPLL in the cervical and thoracic regions usually present with myelopathy, whereas in the lumbar region stenosis is the presentation.[3] Usually, these symptoms are gradual in onset; however, some minor trauma may lead to an acute presentation in these patients.

On physical examination, these patients may reveal upper motor neuron signs, such as a Hoffman sign, finger escape sign, inability to perform the grasp and release test after 10 seconds, inverted brachioradialis reflex, and Babinski sign. These patients may also exhibit gait abnormalities. Axial tenderness is usually absent, except in patients with a history of trauma. Patients with lumbar spine involvement may show signs of canal stenosis, including sensory abnormalities in lower limbs.

Risk Factors for Myelopathy

Many static and dynamic risk factors[3,32,33] have been identified for the development or progression of myelopathy in patients with OPLL. These may include:

- More than 60% canal involvement by OPLL
- Laterally deviated OPLL
- Progression of OPLL
- Type of OPLL, with segmental type having the greatest risk
- Increased cervical range of motion

Imaging

Improvement in imaging techniques, including computed tomography (CT) and magnetic resonance imaging (MRI), has led to a better understanding of OPLL. However, plain radiographs still remain useful and are the simplest screening tool for OPLL.

Plain Radiographs

Plain radiographs can diagnose OPLL in a majority of cases. A longitudinal ossified strip along the posterior border of the vertebrae on lateral radiographs is a distinctive finding. Radiographs may also show the presence of other associated diseases, such as diffuse idiopathic skeletal hyperostosis or ankylosing spondylitis. It is not uncommon to see findings of cervical spondylotic myelopathy in the form of degenerated collapsed disc spaces; however, the disc space is usually preserved in the OPLL involved area. Dynamic radiographs can be useful if there is any doubt regarding instability or if the surgeon is planning to add instrumentation.

Lateral radiographs can also be used for calculation of canal occupancy by OPLL. Fujiyoshi et al.[34] presented the concept of a K line to help in choosing the optimal approach for OPLL. This K line extends from the midpoint of the spinal canal at C2 to the midpoint of the spinal canal at C7. He defined two groups: K line positive and K line negative. In K line positive patients, the OPLL lies ventral to the K line; in K line negative patients, it extends dorsal to it. Their series found

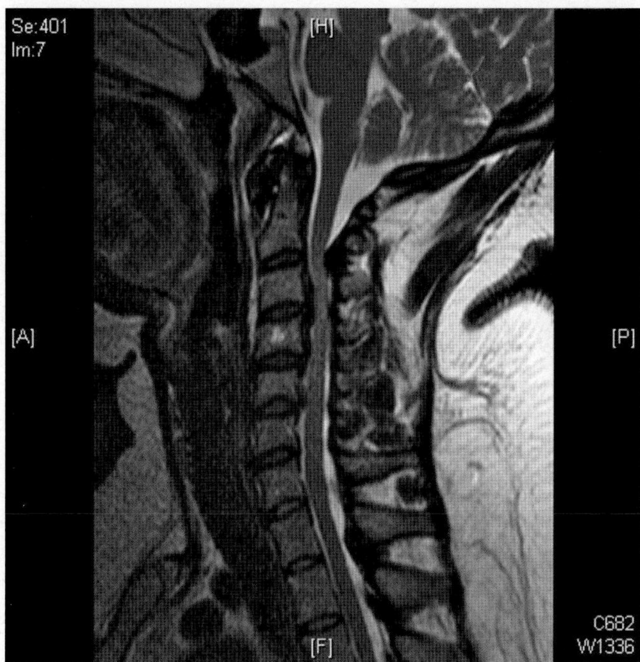

FIG. 43.1 This 35-year-old female presented with neck and midback pain, along with increasing gait disturbance and difficulty with fine hand coordination. Sagittal T2-weighted magnetic resonance imaging demonstrates stenosis due to ossification of the posterior longitudinal ligament and C3–C4 and C4–C5.

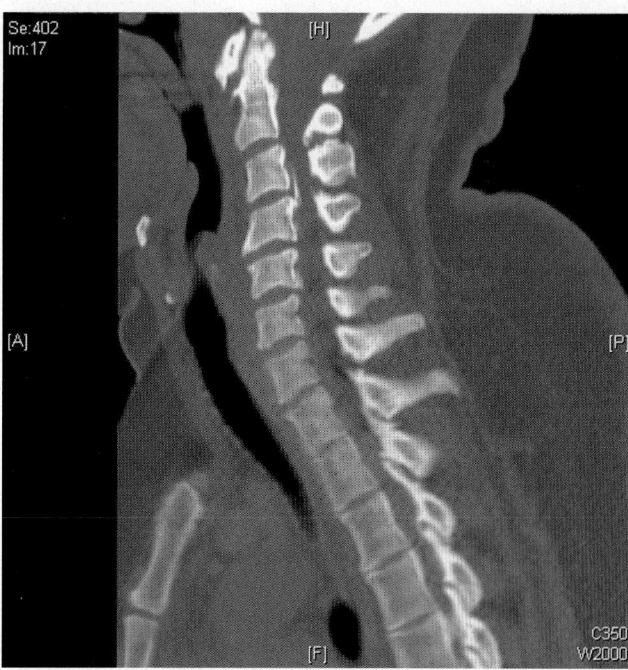

FIG. 43.2 Sagittal computed tomographic scan demonstrating ossification of the posterior longitudinal ligament at the C3–C4 level.

that posterior decompression was effective only in the K line positive group; the spinal cord had very little potential for shifting following posterior decompression in the K line negative group. Recently, the same K line has been described on MRI instead of radiographs.

Computed Tomography

CT has emerged as an invaluable modality to assess the type and extent of OPLL.[3,35] Axial CT scan best demonstrates the OPLL with an ossified mass extending from the posterior margin of the vertebrae into the cervical canal. It is also necessary to image the whole spine due to a very high association of thoracic and thoracolumbar OPLL, along with ossification of the ligamentum flavum (Figs. 43.1 through 43.5).[36] A sagittal section best shows the extent of OPLL, helping in classification. CT myelography can show the extent of cord compression and is particularly useful in patients for whom MRI is contraindicated.

A single- or double-layer sign[35] has been described for possible penetrance of the dural sac by OPLL on bony window CT cuts. A single-layer sign is defined as the presence of a single hyperdense ossified tissue behind the vertebral window, while double-layer is defined as two hyperdense ossified masses separated by a central hypodense linear rim produced by a hypertrophied, but nonossified, remnant of the PLL. The double-layer sign is more pathognomonic of dural involvement. Dural penetrance creates a surgical challenge, as removal of the mass will lead to a dural defect and cerebrospinal fluid leak in the postoperative period. A canal occupancy of more than 60% with OPLL has also been linked to a high incidence of dural penetrance. The anterior approach is not favorable in such cases and should be planned with careful consideration of this possibility. Dural ossification is more common in thoracic OPLL. Min et al.[36a] reported an 80% dural ossification rate in thoracic OPLL.

Magnetic Resonance Imaging

MRI has emerged as an essential modality to evaluate spinal cord status in OPLL. However, it may not reveal much information about OPLL itself. Classic OPLL is hypointense both on T1- and T2-weighted images. A T2-weighted image can show the presence of edema, gliosis, or myelomalacia.[3] Presence of intramedullary high signal intensity on T2-weighted MRI images has also been linked to poor surgical outcome following surgery.

Matsuyama and colleagues[36b] classified OPLL based on the MRI cross-sectional appearance of the spinal canal shape at the level of maximum compression. He classified the spinal canal as triangular, boomerang, and teardrop types. He found that neurologic outcome was worst for the triangular and best for the teardrop type, while the boomerang type had moderately good prognoses.

Treatment for OPLL Involving the Cervical Spine

Conservative Treatment

Conservative treatment is warranted when patients present with minimal or no symptoms. Treatment may consist of

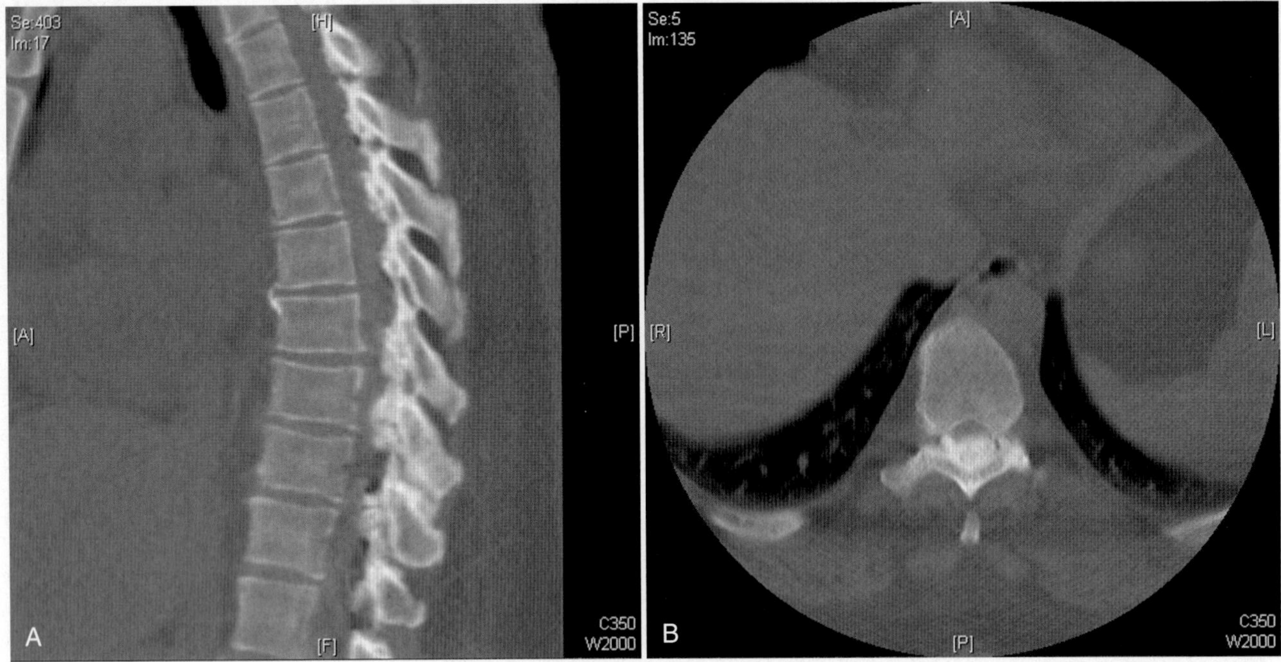

FIG. 43.3 (A) Sagittal and (B) axial computed tomographic scans of the thoracic spine demonstrating the presence of severe concomitant ossification of the ligamentum flavum.

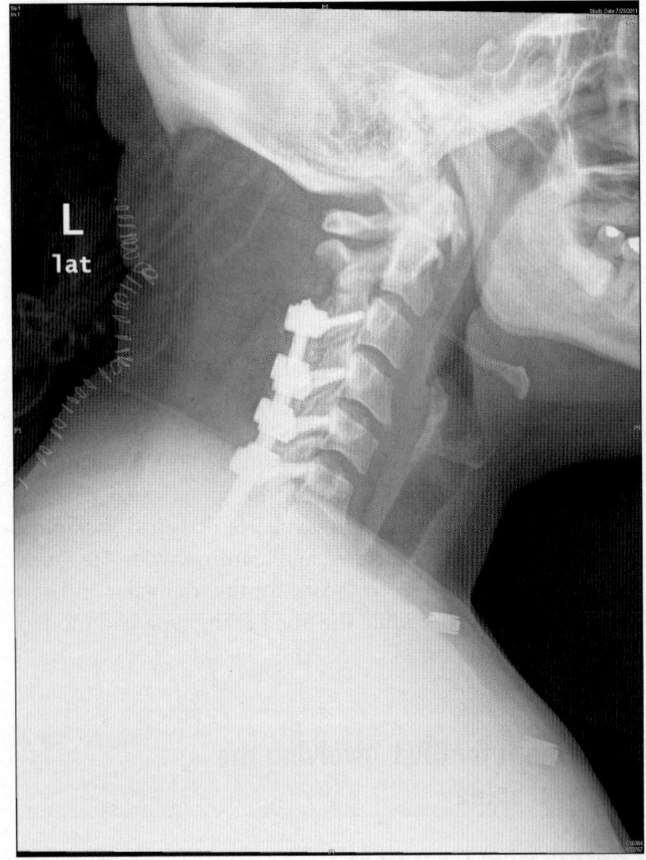

FIG. 43.4 Postoperative sagittal computed tomographic scan of the cervical spine demonstrating decompression and instrumentation through a posterior approach.

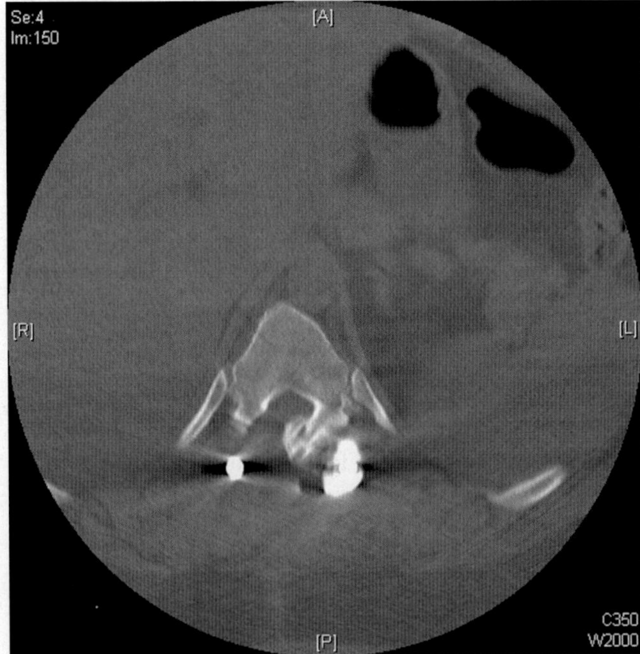

FIG. 43.5 Postoperative axial computed tomographic scan of the thoracic spine demonstrating decompression of the thoracic segment.

observation, use of cervical orthotic devices, traction, and the use of nonsteroidal antiinflammatory drugs. Recently, famotidine has been found to suppress progression of OPLL in mice and thus may be a useful drug in the future.[37]

Surgical Treatment

The surgical treatment of OPLL can be divided into anterior or posterior surgeries depending on the approach. The anterior approach usually directly targets the ossified mass and its removal; posterior approaches involve standard techniques of decompression, as used for cervical spondylotic myelopathy, such as laminectomy, laminectomy with fusion, or laminoplasty. Intraoperative neuromonitoring should be strongly considered for these surgeries.

Anterior Approaches

The usual indication for an anterior approach is a localized or segmental type involving fewer than three levels, between C2 and T1 without the presence of congenital stenosis. The other factors favoring an anterior approach are the presence of local kyphosis and a higher than 60% canal occupancy ratio. The anterior approach usually involves corpectomy and the excision of the ossified mass, followed by fusion.[3] Other options are skip corpectomy, oblique corpectomy, open-window corpectomy, and anterior decompression through a transvertebral approach.

Complications associated with the anterior approach involve graft extrusion, pseudarthrosis, hardware failure, and dural tear with cerebrospinal fluid leak. The risk of dural tears following anterior surgery for OPLL has been quoted as 4.3% to 32% in various series.[38] Some surgeons prefer to use the "floating dura" technique, in which they leave just the thin shell of ossification as an island to the dura.[39]

Posterior Approaches

The posterior approach is usually reserved for patients with more than three-level involvement, age greater than 65 years, and cervical lordosis.[3] Posterior options include laminectomy with or without instrumentation and laminoplasty. Although laminectomy is a straightforward surgery with a low complication rate, the risks of late complications include spinal instability, postlaminectomy kyphosis, and OPLL progression. The addition of posterior instrumentation prevents postlaminectomy kyphosis, but it is ineffective in the presence of preoperative severe kyphosis and large OPLL. There are two main techniques for laminoplasty: open-door and double-door techniques. While useful for certain cases, both types of laminoplasty are ineffective in the presence of preoperative severe kyphosis and large OPLL.[21]

Outcome of Surgical Treatment

The anterior approach in patients with OPLL is relatively difficult. However, the surgical results are much better (as high as 92%), with fewer complications compared to posterior approaches (67% for laminoplasty, 42% for laminectomy).[3,32,40–42] Tani et al[41] reported a 58% success rate with anterior surgery as compared to 13% with laminoplasty. He also reported significant neurologic deficit in 5 patients following laminoplasty. OPLL has been shown to progress even after laminoplasty, and the frequency is reported to be very high (70%), leading to late-onset neurologic decline. Symptomatic neurologic deficit is relatively rare, however.[3,42,43] Iwasaki et al. reported 16% late neurologic deficit following laminoplasty.[43] Recently, Katsumi et al. reported that the addition of posterior instrumentation following laminoplasty reduces the progression of OPLL.[44]

Factors Associated With Poor Surgical Outcome

Several risk factors have been identified that are associated with poor surgical outcome following surgery of OPLL[3,40,45–48]:

- Advanced age
- Malalignment of the cervical spine
- Greater than 60% canal occupancy by OPLL
- OPLL segmental type having the greatest risk
- Preoperative neurologic status
- Dural penetrance
- Intramedullary high signal intensity on T2-weighted MRI images
- Diabetes mellitus[49]

Treatment for OPLL Involving Thoracic Spine

Outcome of thoracic OPLL has been linked to preoperative duration of symptoms as well as severity of OPLL. Results of surgical treatment of OPLL in the thoracic spine are poorer compared to the cervical spine. Several factors[3] have been implicated for this poor outcome:

- Natural kyphosis of the thoracic spine prevents posterior translation of the spinal cord after laminectomy, thus limiting its effectiveness.
- Poor vascularity of the spinal cord at the site of compression.
- Presence of the rib cage limits the anterior approach.

Posterior approaches alone are usually not effective for thoracic OPLL. However, in a multicentric study, Matsumoto[50] reported that laminoplasty is a useful and safe technique for OPLL involving the upper nonkyphotic thoracic spine from T1 to T4. Tokuhashi et al[51] studied the critical kyphotic angle and found that if kyphosis at the decompression site is more than 23 degrees, posterior decompression alone is not effective. The anterior approach for OPLL removal is technically demanding and carries a poor prognosis.[21]

Tomita et al.[52] described a circumferential decompression technique in 1990 for removal of OPLL, which was modified in 2001 by including dekyphosing stabilization.[53] This is a two-stage operation that initially consists of performing a wide posterior laminectomy. The inner part of the facets and pedicles are then drilled down lateral to the dura. Lateral gutters are made in the vertebral body. Doing so allows the posterior release of any adhered OPLL laterally. In their original paper, these authors describe placing the patient in a lateral decubitus position for the second stage. A corpectomy is then completed of the affected level. This exposes the adhered OPLL, which allows the surgeon to perform a microscope-assisted removal of the OPLL. A strut allograft is then subsequently placed into the corpectomy defect. Yang et al.[54] reported that the posterolateral approach is a safe and effective technique for treating thoracic OPLL. In view of current surgical advances, anterior decompression can be done by an anterior, lateral, or posterior approach. Recently, Liu et al.[55] reported that circumferential decompression via the posterior approach is an effective surgical technique for thoracic spinal stenosis caused by multilevel OPLL of the thoracic spine. They also emphasized that complete resection of the OPLL gives better results compared with the floating technique.

Summary

Ossification of the posterior longitudinal ligament can present in a variety of different forms. A small percentage of patients who present with OPLL do not develop any symptoms. Unfortunately, the majority of patients do develop myelopathic symptoms that progress to require intervention. Nonoperative treatment in these patients tends not to alleviate their symptoms; surgery is therefore indicated in the majority of these patients. Due to adhesions of the OPLL on the dura, careful consideration must be taken of the approach that is used because of the high complication rate typically seen. Depending on the region of the spine, anterior, posterior, and combined approaches with or without instrumentation have been described, all with mixed success rates. Spine surgeons should be aware of the various complication rates seen in patients with OPLL before undertaking treatment of these patients.

REFERENCES

1. Epstein N. Ossification of the cervical posterior longitudinal ligament: a review. *Neurosurg Focus.* 2002;13:2ECP1.
2. Kim TJ, Bae KW, Uhm WS, et al. Prevalence of ossification of the posterior longitudinal ligament of the cervical spine. *Joint Bone Spine.* 2008;75(4):471-474.
3. Kalb S, Martirosyan NL, Perez-Orribo L, Kalani MY, Theodore N. Analysis of demographics, risk factors, clinical presentation, and surgical treatment modalities for the ossified posterior longitudinal ligament. *Neurosurg Focus.* 2011;30(3):E11.

3a. Park JY, Chin DK, Kim KS, Cho YE. Thoracic ligament ossification in patients with cervical ossification of the posterior longitudinal ligaments: tandem ossification in the cervical and thoracic spine. *Spine.* 2008;33:E407-E410.

4. Key GA. On paraplegia depending on the ligament of the spine. *Guys Hosp Rep.* 1838;3:17-34.
5. Oppenheimer A. Calcification and ossification of vertebral ligaments (spondylitis ossificans ligamentosa): roentgen study of pathogenesis and clinical significance. *Radiology.* 1942;38:160-173.
6. Numasawa T, Koga H, Ueyama K, et al. Human retinoic X receptor beta: complete genomic sequence and mutation search for ossification of posterior longitudinal ligament of the spine. *J Bone Miner Res.* 1999;14:500-508.
7. Ikegawa S. Genetics of ossification of the posterior longitudinal ligament of the spine: a mini review. *J Bone Metab.* 2014;21(2):127-132.
8. Matsunaga S, Yamaguchi M, Hayashi K, et al. Genetic analysis of ossification of the posterior longitudinal ligament. *Spine.* 1999;24:937-939.
9. Karasugi T, Nakajima M, Ikari K, et al. A genome-wide sib-pair linkage analysis of ossification of the posterior longitudinal ligament of the spine. *J Bone Miner Metab.* 2013;31:136-143.
10. Tanaka T, Ikari K, Furushima K, et al. Genomewide linkage and linkage disequilibrium analyses identify COL6A1, on chromosome 21, as the locus for ossification of the posterior longitudinal ligament of the spine. *Am J Hum Genet.* 2003;73:812-822.
11. Kawaguchi Y, Furushima K, Sugimori K, Inoue I, Kimura T. Association between polymorphism of the transforming growth factor-beta1 gene with the radiologic characteristic and ossification of the posterior longitudinal ligament. *Spine.* 2003;28:1424-1426.
12. Taguchi T. Etiology and pathogenesis. In: Yonenobu K, Nakamura K, Toyama Y, eds. *Ossification of the Posterior Longitudinal Ligament.* 2nd ed. Tokyo: Springer; 2006:33-35.
13. Kobashi G, Washio M, Okamoto K, et al. High body mass index after age 20 and diabetes mellitus are independent risk factors for ossification of the posterior longitudinal ligament of the spine in Japanese subjects: a case-control study in multiple hospitals. *Spine.* 2004;29:1006-1010.
14. Shingyouchi Y, Nagahama A, Niida M. Ligamentous ossification of the cervical spine in the late middle-aged Japanese men: its relation to body mass index and glucose metabolism. *Spine.* 1996;21:2474-2478.
15. Wu JC, Liu L, Chen YC, et al. Ossification of the posterior longitudinal ligament in the cervical spine: an 11-year comprehensive national epidemiology study. *Neurosurg Focus.* 2011;30:E5.
16. Choi BW, Song KJ, Chang H. Ossification of the posterior longitudinal ligament: a review of literature. *Asian Spine J.* 2011;5(4):267-276.
17. Ehara S, Shimamura T, Nakamura R, Yamazaki K. Paravertebral ligamentous ossification: DISH, OPLL and OLF. *Eur J Radiol.* 1998;27:196-205.
18. Kim TJ, Kim TH, Jun JB, Joo KB, Uhm WS. Prevalence of ossification of posterior longitudinal ligament in patients with ankylosing spondylitis. *J Rheumatol.* 2007;34(12):2460-2462.
19. Ramos-Remus C, Russell AS, Gomez-Vargas A, et al. Ossification of the posterior longitudinal ligament in three geographically and genetically different populations of ankylosing spondylitis and other spondyloarthropathies. *Ann Rheum Dis.* 1998;57:429-433.
20. Matsunaga S, Koga H, Kawabata N, et al. Ossification of the posterior longitudinal ligament in dizygotic twins with schizophrenia: a case report. *Mod Rheumatol.* 2008;18:277-280.
21. Saetia K, Cho D, Lee S, Kim DH, Kim SD. Ossification of the posterior longitudinal ligament: a review. *Neurosurg Focus.* 2011;30(3):E1.
22. Yonemori K, Imamura T, Ishidou Y, et al. Bone morphogenetic protein receptors and activin receptors are highly expressed in ossified ligament tissues of patients with ossification of the posterior longitudinal ligament. *Am J Pathol.* 1997;150:1335-1347.
23. Li H, Liu D, Zhao CQ, Jiang LS, Dai LY. Insulin potentiate the proliferation and bone morphogenetic protein-2-induced osteogenic differentiation of rat spinal ligament cells via extracellular signal-regulated kinase and phosphatidylinositol 3-kinase. *Spine.* 2008;33:2394-2402.
24. Frymoyer J. *Orthopaedic Knowledge Update 4.* Rosemont, IL: American Academy of Orthopaedic Surgeons; 1993:296.

25. McAfee PC, Regan JJ, Bohlman HH. Cervical cord compression from ossification of the posterior longitudinal ligament in non-Orientals. *J Bone Joint Surg Br*. 1987;69:569-575.
26. Ishida Y, Kawai S. Effects of bone-seeking hormones on DNA synthesis, cyclic AMP level, and alkaline phosphatase activity in cultured cells from human posterior longitudinal ligament of the spine. *J Bone Miner Res*. 1993;8:1291-1300.
27. Tsuyama N. Ossification of the posterior longitudinal ligament of the spine. *Clin Orthop Relat Res*. 1984;184:71-84.
28. Epstein N. Diagnosis and surgical management of cervical ossification of the posterior longitudinal ligament. *Spine J*. 2002;2:436-449.
29. Chiba K, Yamamoto I, Hirabayashi H, et al. Multicenter study investigating the postoperative progression of ossification of the posterior longitudinal ligament in the cervical spine: a new computer-assisted measurement. *J Neurosurg Spine*. 2005;3:17-23.
30. Hori T, Kawaguchi Y, Kimura T. How does the ossification area of the posterior longitudinal ligament progress after cervical laminoplasty? *Spine*. 2006;31:2807-2812.
31. Hori T, Kawaguchi Y, Kimura T. How does the ossification area of the posterior longitudinal ligament thicken following cervical laminoplasty? *Spine*. 2007;32:E551-E556.
32. Matsunaga S, Sakou T, Taketomi E, Komiya S. Clinical course of patients with ossification of the posterior longitudinal ligament: a minimum 10-year cohort study. *J Neurosurg*. 2004;100(3 supplSpine):245-248.
33. Mochizuki M, Aiba A, Hashimoto M, Fujiyoshi T, Yamazaki M. Cervical myelopathy in patients with ossification of the posterior longitudinal ligament. Clinical article. *J Neurosurg Spine*. 2009;10:122-128.
34. Fujiyoshi T, Yamazaki M, Kawabe J, et al. A new concept for making decisions regarding the surgical approach for cervical ossification of the posterior longitudinal ligament: the K-line. *Spine*. 2008;33:E990-E993.
35. Hida K, Iwasaki Y, Koyanagi I, Abe H. Bone window computed tomography for detection of dural defect associated with cervical ossified posterior longitudinal ligament. *Neurol Med Chir (Tokyo)*. 1997;37:173-176.
36. Shepard NA, Shenoy K, Cho W, Sharan AD. Extensive ossification of the ligamentum flavum treated with triple stage decompression: a case report. *Spine J*. 2015;15(4):e9-e14.
36a. Min JH, Jang JS, Lee SH. Significance of the double- and single-layer signs in the ossification of the posterior longitudinal ligament of the thoracic spine. *Neurosurgery*. 2007;61:118-122.
36b. Matsuyama Y, Kawakami N, Yanase M, et al. Cervical myelopathy due to OPLL: clinical evaluation by MRI and intraoperative spinal sonography. *J Spinal Disord Tech*. 2004;17:401-404.
37. Maeda Y, Yamamoto K, Yamakawa A, et al. The H2 blocker famotidine suppresses progression of ossification of the posterior longitudinal ligament in a mouse model. *RMD Open*. 2015;1(1):e000068.
38. Mazur M, Jost GF, Schmidt MH, Bisson EF. Management of cerebrospinal fluid leaks after anterior decompression for ossification of the posterior longitudinal ligament: a review of the literature. *Neurosurg Focus*. 2011;30(3):E13.
39. Sugrue PA, McClendon J Jr, Halpin RJ, et al. Surgical management of cervical ossification of the posterior longitudinal ligament: natural history and the role of surgical decompression and stabilization. *Neurosurg Focus*. 2011;30(3):E3.
40. Iwasaki M, Okuda S, Miyauchi A, et al. Surgical strategy for cervical myelopathy due to ossification of the posterior longitudinal ligament. Part 1: clinical results and limitations of Laminoplasty. *Spine*. 2007;32:647-653.
41. Tani T, Ushida T, Ishida K, et al. Relative safety of anterior microsurgical decompression versus laminoplasty for cervical myelopathy with a massive ossified posterior longitudinal ligament. *Spine*. 2002;27:2491-2498.
42. Kato Y, Iwasaki M, Fuji T, Yonenobu K, Ochi T. Long-term follow-up results of laminectomy for cervical myelopathy caused by ossification of the posterior longitudinal ligament. *J Neurosurg*. 1998;89:217-223.
43. Iwasaki M, Kawaguchi Y, Kimura T, Yonenobu K. Long-term results of expansive laminoplasty for ossification of the posterior longitudinal ligament of the cervical spine: more than 10 years follow up. *J Neurosurg*. 2002;96(2 suppl):180-189.
44. Katsumi K, Izumi T, Ito T, et al. Posterior instrumented fusion suppresses the progression of ossification of the posterior longitudinal ligament: a comparison of laminoplasty with and without instrumented fusion by three-dimensional analysis. *Eur Spine J*. 2015;25(5):1634-1640.
45. Koyanagi I, Iwasaki Y, Hida K, Imamura H, Abe H. Magnetic resonance imaging findings in ossification of the posterior longitudinal ligament of the cervical spine. *J Neurosurg*. 1998;88:247-254.
46. Masaki Y, Yamazaki M, Okawa A, et al. An analysis of factors causing poor surgical outcome in patients with cervical myelopathy due to ossification of the posterior longitudinal ligament: anterior decompression with spinal fusion versus laminoplasty. *J Spinal Disord Tech*. 2007;20:7-13.
47. Yagi M, Ninomiya K, Kihara M, Horiuchi Y. Long-term surgical outcome and risk factors in patients with cervical myelopathy and a change in signal intensity of intramedullary spinal cord on magnetic resonance imaging. *J Neurosurg Spine*. 2010;12:59-65.
48. Kim B, Yoon do H, Shin HC, et al. Surgical outcome and prognostic factors of anterior decompression and fusion for cervical compressive myelopathy due to ossification of the posterior longitudinal ligament. *Spine J*. 2015;15(5):875-884.
49. Choi JH, Shin JJ, Kim TH, et al. Does intramedullary signal intensity on MRI affect the surgical outcomes of patients with ossification of posterior longitudinal ligament? *J Korean Neurosurg Soc*. 2014;56(2):121-129.
50. Matsumoto M, Chiba K, Toyama Y, et al. Surgical results and related factors for ossification of posterior longitudinal ligament of the thoracic spine: a multi-institutional retrospective study. *Spine*. 2008;33:1034-1041.
51. Tokuhashi Y, Matsuzaki H, Oda H, Uei H. Effectiveness of posterior decompression for patients with ossification of the posterior longitudinal ligament in the thoracic spine: usefulness of the ossification-kyphosis angle on MRI. *Spine*. 2006;31:E26-E30.
52. Tomita K, Kawahara N, Baba H, Kikuchi Y, Nishimura H. Circumspinal decompression for thoracic myelopathy due to combined ossification of the posterior longitudinal ligament and ligamentum flavum. *Spine*. 1990;15:1114-1120.
53. Kawahara N, Tomita K. Circumspinal decompression for thoracic myelopathy due to combined ossification of the posterior longitudinal ligament and yellow ligament. *J Jpn Spine Res Soc*. 2001;12:450-456.
54. Yang C, Bi Z, Fu C, Zhang Z. A modified decompression surgery for thoracic myelopathy caused by ossification of posterior longitudinal ligament: a case report and literature review. *Spine*. 2010;35:E609-E613.
55. Liu X, Zhu B, Liu X, Liu Z, Dang G. Circumferential decompression via the posterior approach for the surgical treatment of multilevel thoracic ossification of the posterior longitudinal ligaments: a single institution comparative study. *Chin Med J*. 2014;127(19):3371-3377.

44 CHAPTER Cervical Disc Replacement

Abhishek Kannan
Wellington K. Hsu
Rick C. Sasso

Background

The cervical spine consists of seven vertebrae that comprise the axial skeleton of the neck. The five vertebral bodies of the *subaxial cervical spine,* C3 to C7, have unique structural characteristics that affect normal physiology and pathophysiology and directly influence considerations of surgical management. The vertebral bodies, the axial load-bearing elements of the vertebral column, are mobile segments joined by cartilaginous intervertebral discs. A single intervertebral disc is composed of a central nucleus pulposus with a surrounding anulus fibrosus (composed of highly elastic mucoprotein gel and collagen fibers, respectively). The vertebral column is the central axis of the human body, serving roles in biomechanical function through muscular attachment and motion. The spine also serves a neuroprotective role, as it houses the spinal cord and exiting spinal nerve roots.

Disc degeneration is a disease state marked by progressive wear and tear on the intervertebral discs, which contributes to changes such as mild to more severe spondylosis and spinal stenosis. Disc degeneration can compress or stretch nerve roots, resulting in myelopathy, radiculopathy, and repeated trauma to the spinal cord. Historically, surgical management of patients with symptomatic degenerative disc disease (DDD) included removal of pathologic disc material and fusion of the interspace.

Since its introduction in the 1950s by Robinson and Smith,[1] anterior cervical discectomy and fusion (ACDF) has been widely used to treat spondylotic radiculopathy and myelopathy while demonstrating long-term clinical success.[2,3] ACDF has become one standard of care for treating cervical disc disease in symptomatic patients, as it achieves neural decompression and segmental stabilization. ACDF consists of neurologic decompression by discectomy followed by the use of intervertebral graft to maintain disc height and instrumentation (plating) to improve the rate of fusion. Anterior cervical plates may span the rostral to caudal vertebral bodies included in discectomies and have thereby made postoperative immobilization less critical. Furthermore, plating has been shown to decrease pseudarthrosis rates for multilevel fusions[4] while maintaining sagittal balance through segments within the construct.[5]

ACDF, however, can pose a number of limitations, including loss of cervical range of motion (ROM), dysphagia, pseudarthrosis, autograft harvest site pain, and increased segmental motion leading to adjacent disease.[6–11] Adjacent segment degeneration remains a major concern and is a direct result of altered biomechanics of the cervical spine. Arthrodesis at any given level can lead to increased load bearing at levels above and below the construct, accelerating the degenerative process. The radiographic demonstration of these changes is called *adjacent segment degeneration*, while consequent clinical symptomatology in the form of myelopathy or radiculopathy is diagnosed as *adjacent segment disease*. Goffin et al. report the radiographic incidence of adjacent segment degeneration to be as high as 92% after anterior cervical interbody fusion.[3]

Clinical studies have demonstrated the postoperative occurrence of adjacent segment disease, including Hilibrand et al., who reported an annualized incidence of 2.9% per year in 374 patients after ACDF.[12] In the 10 years following ACDF, they estimated 25% of patients undergoing cervical fusion will develop radiographic degeneration of adjacent spinal segments, of which two-thirds would go on to require additional surgery. In a retrospective clinical study of 888 patients undergoing ACDF, Xu et al.[13] identified 108 patients who developed adjacent segment disease necessitating a reoperation. Of the 108 who underwent a revision procedure, 27 developed recurrent disease requiring a third cervical fusion. This study demonstrates that patients who underwent a second cervical fusion developed adjacent segment disease at both higher and faster rates, which were statistically significant. Notably, patients who were revised via an anterior approach had a higher chance of recurring disease versus patients who underwent a posterior procedure. Bydon et al. reported that patients are more likely to develop disease above the index level of fusion as compared to below, even for patients undergoing a revision procedure, and predicted a rate of adjacent segment disease development of 31% at 10 years.[14]

Biomechanical analyses have also demonstrated that vertebral levels adjacent to the index level ACDF have demonstrated increased intradiscal pressures and ROM during both flexion and extension.[9,15] Clinical prevalence of adjacent segment disease coupled with in vitro biomechanical findings suggest that ACDF accelerates degeneration of intervertebral discs, resulting in altered physiologic biomechanics and the resultant pathogenesis of adjacent segment disease.

Cervical pseudarthrosis is another well-established complication of ACDF, described as failure of solid arthrodesis at 12 months. Pseudarthrosis rates following ACDF have been reported in the range of 3% to 20% for single-level fusions and 21% to 46% for two- and three- level fusions, respectively.[16,17] Factors that impact fusion rates include number of levels involved, surgical technique, patient comorbidities, and choice of graft.

In an effort to improve on fusion rates after ACDF, an extensive body of literature has emerged investigating various choices of bone graft. Historically, iliac crest bone graft (ICBG) was considered the gold standard for use in ACDF, utilizing the anterior crest as a donor site. However, a significant drawback of this option is the involved donor site morbidity, manifesting as persistent pain, numbness, and ambulatory impairment.[18] ICBG harvest has also been associated with superficial infection, wound complications, sensory abnormalities, hematomas, and tissue herniation through donor site, with reported complication rates of 10% to 39%.[19,20]

While the use of allograft avoids the donor site morbidity and associated risks of ICBG, there have been reports of disease transmission and bioincompatibility.[21] Although advances have been made in cadaveric tissue screening and processing, interest in bone graft substitutes continues to grow, with emerging in vitro and in vivo studies investigating the use of demineralized bone matrix, ceramic-based bone grafts, and nanofiber-based collagen scaffolds.[22,23]

Recombinant human bone morphogenetic protein-2 (rhBMP2) was first approved by the US Food and Drug Administration (FDA) for use in an anterior lumbar interbody cage in 2002. It was initially received as a novel bone graft substitute to ICBG, demonstrating fusion rates as high as 98%[24] with shorter length of surgery and shorter hospital stays.[25] However, multiple studies have demonstrated potential adverse effects in the cervical spine, including postoperative prevertebral swelling, hematoma formation, and heterotopic ossification.[26–28] The increasing prevalence of off-label use coupled with controversial indications for clinical use of rhBMP-2 have led to significant criticism of its application in both academic and clinical settings.[29,30] These considerations make a strong case for fusion alternatives in the treatment of DDD of the cervical spine.

There is a growing body of literature surrounding the use of total intervertebral disc arthroplasty (TDA) as an alternative to traditional fusion in restoring mobility and function at the involved spinal segments. Proposed advantages of TDA include maintenance of cervical ROM, restoration of cervical disc height and spinal alignment, as well as avoidance of pseudarthrosis, adjacent segment degeneration, and adjacent segment disease. The procedure also avoids the potential surgical morbidity of autograft harvest while avoiding complications associated with postoperative immobilization.

History of Disc Arthroplasty and Device Design

Arthroplasty aims to provide a stable, biomechanically efficient construct that is safe for patient use and reduces symptomatology associated with disc disease. The unique anatomic characteristics of the cervical spine necessitate specific considerations regarding TDA device design that may not be applicable in other major joint replacements. Bone stock in the cervical spine is limited, resulting in less flexibility when making bony cuts to accommodate an implant prosthesis. In contrast to knee and hip joints, the intervertebral disc plays a major role in spinal stability by maintaining balance of the anterior and middle columns. TDA candidates are typically younger than patients receiving lower extremity joint replacements; a longer expected lifespan (between 30 and 50 years longer) entails an estimated 100 million flexion cycles for a given implant. This raises concern for device bearing and wear characteristics as well as articular constraint. Given the proximity of the implant to the spinal cord and critical structures of the anterior neck, wear debris and the potential ensuing inflammatory reaction are major topics under investigation. Local and systemic responses to debris may be evaluated in the context of biocompatibility, neurologic response, tissue response, and toxicity. Extremes of motion may lead to abnormal wear, contributing to debris formation. Therefore, static and dynamic characterization of a given device should involve compression-shear testing using the maximum theoretical ROM in one or more directions.[31]

The earliest application of TDA in humans was in the late 1980s by Cummins et al. in the United Kingdom.[31a] This group developed a metal-on-metal ball-and-socket device for implant in the cervical spine. Over the past 2 decades, the original artificial disc has been further developed to incorporate newer materials and methods of fixation in the cervical vertebral bodies. The Prestige ST (stainless steel; Medtronic), a direct descendant of the original Bristol-Cummins device, is made of stainless steel and was approved by the FDA for human use in 2007 (Figs. 44.1 and 44.2). The Prestige low-profile (LP) (Medtronic), the fifth iteration of the original Bristol-Cummins device, was also recently approved for use in the US market. Other FDA-approved devices include ProDisc-C Total Disc Replacement (DePuy Synthes) (Figs. 44.3 and 44.4), Bryan Cervical Disc (Medtronic) (Figs. 44.5 through 44.7), Mobi-C Cervical Disc (Zimmer Biomet), and SECURE-C Cervical Artificial Disc (Globus Medical Inc.).

A more recent addition to the metal-on-metal category of arthroplasty devices includes the Kineflex-C disc (SpinalMotion) for which the FDA investigational device exemption (IDE) trial has been completed. A summary of the design characteristics of each of these devices is presented in Table 44.1. The seventh FDA-approved cervical disc arthroplasty device is the PCM disc (NuVasive).

The Cervical Spine Study Group classifies TDA devices as nonarticulating, uniarticulating, and biarticulating. The device may be modular (with replaceable components) or nonmodular (with nonreplaceable components).[32] Disc prostheses can also be classified as unconstrained, semiconstrained, and

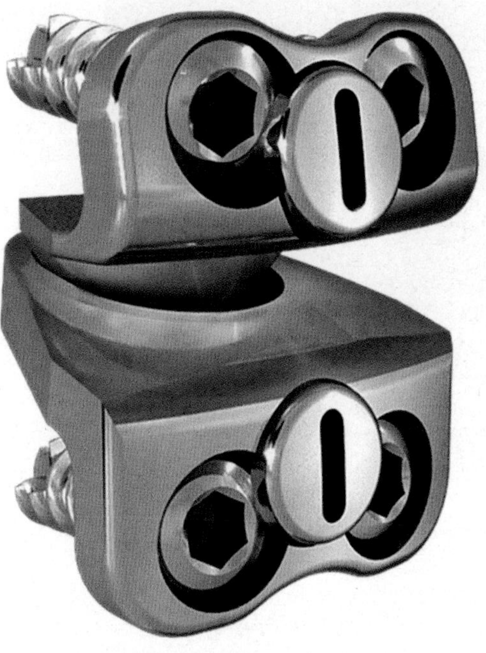

FIG. 44.1 The Prestige ST Cervical Disc prosthesis is currently approved by the Food and Drug Administration for use in the United States. This stainless steel uniarticulating device attains primary fixation to the vertebral bodies via use of locked screws. (Courtesy Medtronic, Minneapolis, MN.)

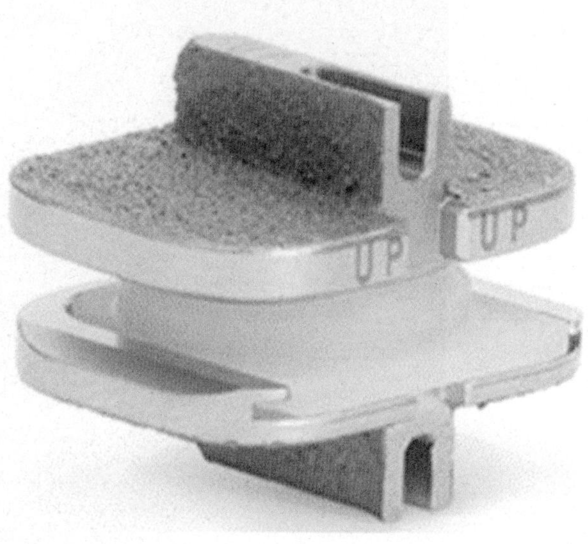

FIG. 44.3 Ex vivo image of the ProDisc-C. This device is approved by the Food and Drug Administration in the United States for cervical arthroplasty and obtains initial fixation via a central keel. Bone ingrowth is promoted via the surface alterations of the superior and inferior endplates of this device. (Courtesy DePuy Synthes Spine, Raynham, MA.)

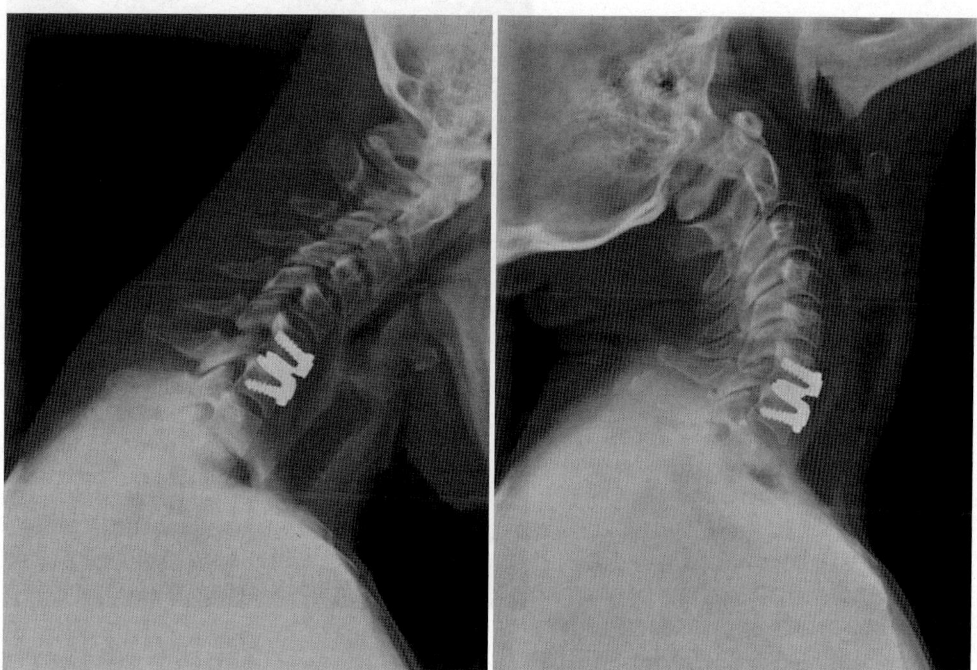

FIG. 44.2 Prestige ST Cervical Disc prosthesis in C5–C6 arthroplasty. Lateral flexion and extension radiographs show motion through the arthroplasty device in this postoperative patient. (Courtesy Medtronic, Minneapolis, MN.)

constrained, depending on the degrees of freedom allowed by a specific design. The ball-and-socket motif, consisting of a gliding interface between two rigid components, is shared by all three designs.[33] Devices considered constrained in certain planes restrict motion to less than that seen physiologically. Semiconstrained designs allow motion similar to that seen physiologically. Devices are considered unconstrained if there is no mechanical stop to motion relying on soft tissues and the inherent compression across the disc space to provide the primary restraint to extremes of motion.[34]

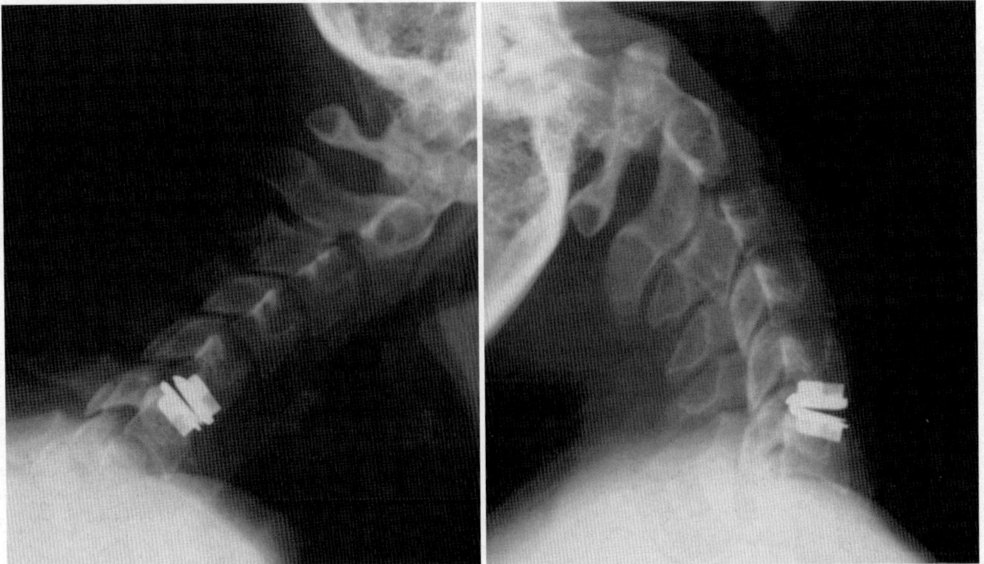

FIG. 44.4 ProDisc-C is visualized on lateral flexion-extension radiographs. The device retains motion at the index surgical level in this patient successfully treated with arthroplasty at C5–C6. (Courtesy DePuy Synthes Spine, Raynham, MA.)

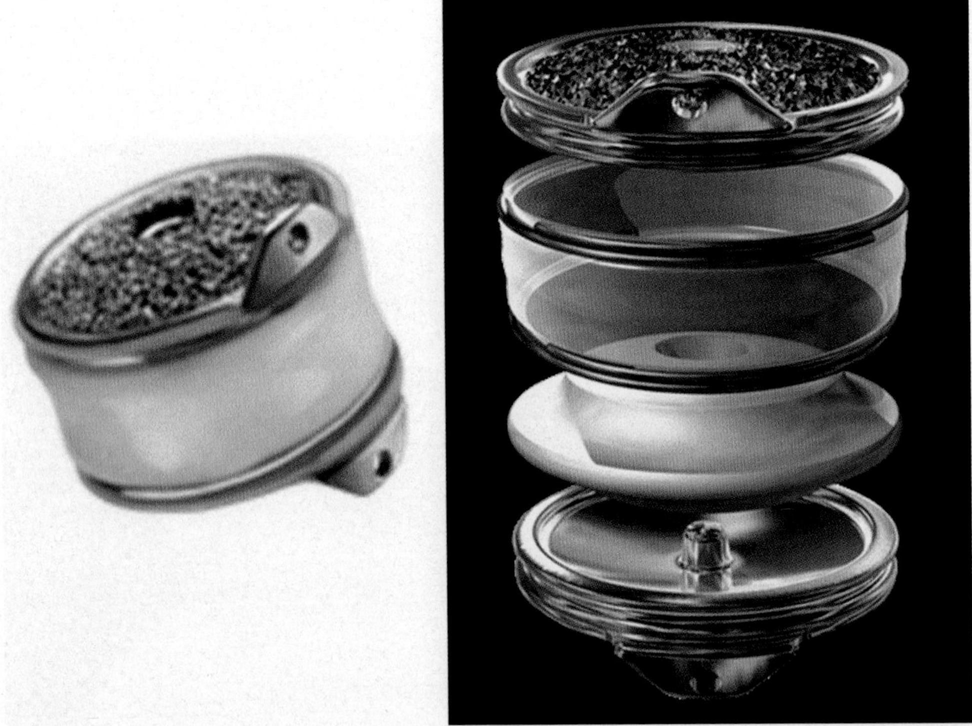

FIG. 44.5 Bryan Cervical Disc prosthesis is shown ex vivo and in unassembled form. The endplates of this device are unique in their design and promote ingrowth of bone into the metallic surface. (Courtesy Medtronic, Minneapolis, MN.)

Indications for Use, Contraindications, and Complications

The FDA-approved indication for cervical disc arthroplasty is single- and double-level cervical DDD causing radiculopathy and/or myelopathy in patients of adult age.[35] Exhaustion of conservative management options for single-level spondylosis should precede the discussion of operative management. Additional indications for TDA include soft- or hard-disc herniation or foraminal osteophytes causing radiculopathy, and soft-disc herniation causing myelopathy.[36] There is concern that motion preservation may not create an environment for maximum neurologic recovery in patients with

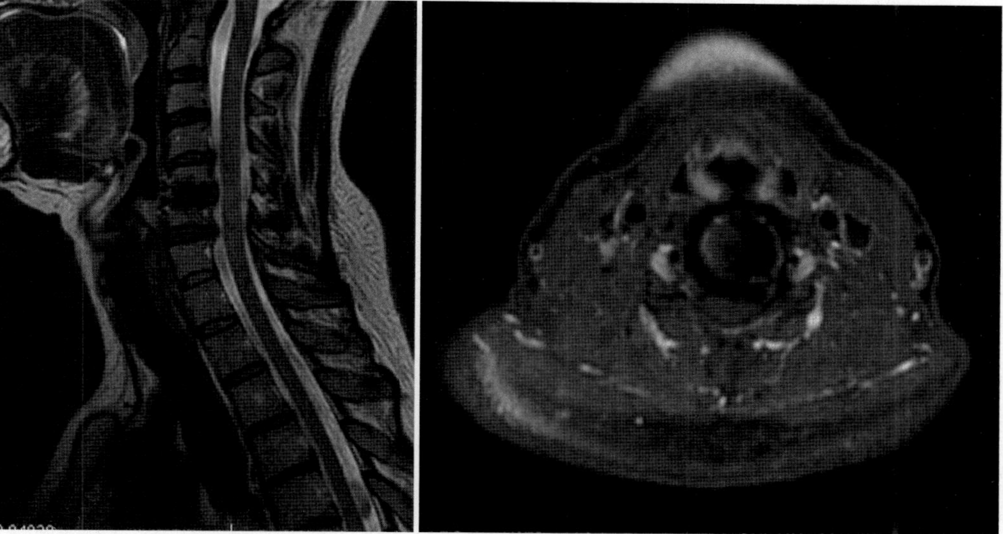

FIG. 44.6 Bryan Cervical Disc prosthesis is visualized on postoperative magnetic resonance imaging (MRI). Titanium alloy devices such as the Bryan device may have less MRI artifact than similar devices constructed with cobalt-chromium or stainless steel. These images show the imaging characteristics of this device at index and adjacent surgical levels. (Courtesy Rick Sasso, Indianapolis, IN.)

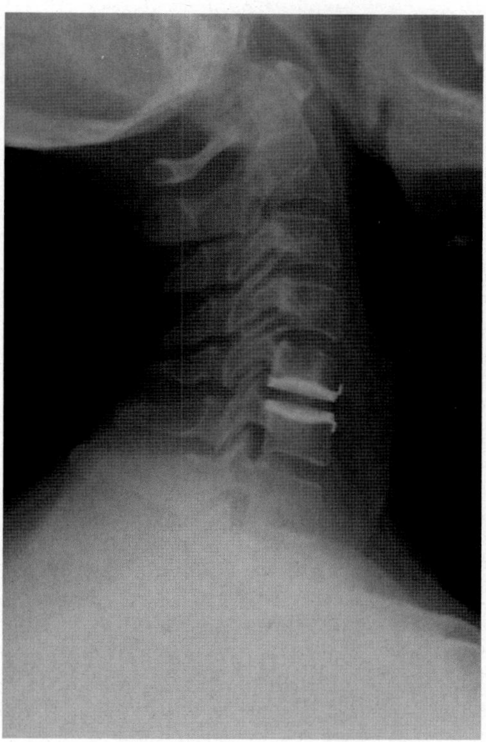

FIG. 44.7 Upright lateral view of a patient who underwent successful cervical arthroplasty at C5–C6 with a Bryan Cervical Disc prosthesis. (Courtesy Medtronic, Minneapolis, MN.)

cervical myelopathy. However, Riew et al. have shown that in patients with single-level disease, clinical improvement measured via Nurick grade, neck disability index, 36-Item Short Form Health Survey (SF-36) scores, and visual analog scale (VAS) was similar between patients treated with fusion and those treated with arthroplasty.[37] Thus, for cervical myelopathy not caused by retrovertebral compression secondary to ligamentum flavum hypertrophy, ossification of the posterior longitudinal ligament, or congenital stenosis, a cervical disc prosthesis accompanied by a meticulous decompression would be a reasonable treatment option.[38]

Complications and adverse events associated with cervical disc arthroplasty involve both surgical approach and device-related issues. General postoperative complications include infection, newly occurring neurologic deficits, implant migration, intervertebral subluxation, vascular injury, dural injury, cerebrospinal fluid leak, and epidural abscess formation.

Heterotopic ossification (HO) in the region of the arthroplasty device is a unique complication reported after TDA. The proposed mechanism of HO involves differentiation of mesenchymal cells originating from bone or muscle to osteoblasts, which are able to spread into the vasculature of surrounding soft tissue. The osteogenic agents released from tissues attached to bone are a result of local intraoperative injury.[39] HO tends to develop relatively early postoperatively following cervical disc arthroplasty, and may be seen in as high as 34% of patients at 4 years and in 38% of patients at 6 years.[40] Early postoperative use of nonsteroidal antiinflammatory drugs is reported to decrease the incidence and severity of HO, similar to its effect in HO prevention after total hip replacement. Delayed hypersensitivity reactions also pose a threat after TDA, in which critical structures, primarily the spinal cord, are at risk of exposure to implant materials and wear debris.

Contraindications for cervical disc arthroplasty include active or prior infection, severe osteoporosis, severe facet arthrosis, ankylosis, congenital cervical stenosis, and segmental cervical instability (>3.5 mm of translation or >11 degrees of kyphosis). Additionally, as intact posterior elements are essential to prosthesis stability, prior laminectomy or excessive facet removal are contraindications to disc arthroplasty. The current approval status of cervical disc arthroplasty devices can be found in Table 44.2.

TABLE 44.1 Design Characteristics of Past and Present Cervical Arthroplasty Devices

Device	Design	Modular	Articulating Method	Implant Composition	Bearing Surface	Primary Fixation	Secondary Fixation	Manufacturer
Bristol/ Cummins	Ball and socket	No	Uniarticulating	316L stainless steel	316L on 316L	Vertebral body screws	Vertebral body screws	None; technology by Medtronic
Bryan	Biarticulating contained bearing	No	Biarticulating	Titanium, central polymer	Titanium alloy on polymer	Milled vertebral endplates	Endplate ingrowth	Medtronic
CerviCore	Ellipsoid saucer	No	Uniarticulating	Cobalt-chromium	Cobalt-chromium on cobalt-chromium	Ridged rails	Endplate ongrowth to titanium spray	Stryker, IDE status revoked
DISCOVER	Spherical bearing between superior titanium endplate and UHMWPE core	No	Uniarticulating	Titanium and UHMWPE	Titanium on UHMWPE	Teeth on superior and inferior endplates	Endplate ongrowth	DePuy Synthes, IDE in progress
Frenchay/ Prestige I[a]		No	Uniarticulating	316L stainless steel	316L on 316L	Locked vertebral body screws, posterior endplate lip	Locked vertebral body screws, posterior endplate lip	None; technology by Medtronic
Kineflex-C	Modular three-piece bearing system with two endplates and mobile metallic core	Yes	Biarticulating	CCM	CCM modular core between two CCM endplates	Vertical keel and ridged endplate surface	Endplate ongrowth	SpinalMotion
Mobi-C	Superior endplate with ball and socket motion; inferior endplate with sliding constraint	Yes	Biarticulating	Titanium	Titanium on polyethylene modular core	Lateral self-retaining teeth	Endplate ongrowth	Zimmer Biomet
Prestige II[a]	Ellipsoid saucer	No	Uniarticulating	316L stainless steel	316L on 316L	Locked vertebral body screws	Locked vertebral body screws	None; technology by Medtronic
Prestige LP	Ellipsoid saucer	No	Uniarticulating	Titanium/ ceramic composite	Titanium/ ceramic composite	Dual rails	Endplate ongrowth	Medtronic
Prestige ST	Ellipsoid saucer	No	Uniarticulating	316L stainless steel	316L on 316L	Locked vertebral body screws	Locked vertebral body screws	Medtronic
Prestige STLP[a]	Ellipsoid saucer	No	Uniarticulating	316L stainless steel	316L on 316L	Dual rails	Endplate ongrowth	None; technology by Medtronic
ProDisc-C	Ball and socket	No	Uniarticulating	Cobalt-chromium, UHMWPE	Cobalt-chromium on UHMWPE	Central keel	Endplate ongrowth	DePuy Synthes
PCM	Upper endplate translation on fixed UHMWPE	No	Uniarticulating	Cobalt-chromium, UHMWPE	Cobalt-chromium on UHMWPE	Ridged metallic endplates	Endplate ongrowth	NuVasive
SECURE-C	Metal on polyethylene		Biarticulating	Cobalt-chromium, UHMWPE	Cobalt-chromium on UHMWPE	Ridged central keel	Endplate ongrowth	Globus Medical

CCM, cobalt-chrome-molybdenum; IDE, investigational device exemption; UHMWPE, ultrahigh-molecular-weight polyethylene.
[a]Devices not currently in production, current/known clinical use, or IDE investigation at the time of this writing.

Preoperative Imaging

Preoperative imaging for TDA should include anteroposterior (AP) and lateral radiographs of the cervical spine (including neutral, flexion, and extension views) and bilateral oblique views. Care must be taken to ensure visibility of potential short neck, high shoulders, and the C6–C7 level on lateral radiograph. The surgeon should assess preexisting spondylosis, making note of anterior or posterior osteophytes and ligament ossification. It is important to ensure proper disc height and motion in operation segments, as both are prerequisites for

TABLE 44.2 Current Status of Cervical Arthroplasty Devices in the United States

Device	Manufacturer	U.S. FDA Status
Prestige ST	Medtronic Sofamor Danek	Approved
Prestige LP	Medtronic Sofamor Danek	Approved
ProDisc-C	Synthes Spine	Approved
Bryan disc	Medtronic Sofamor Danek	Approved
Mobi-C disc	LDS Spine	Approved
SECURE-C	Globus Medical	Approved
PCM disc	NuVasive	Approved
Kineflex-C disc	SpinalMotion	IDE clinical trial complete

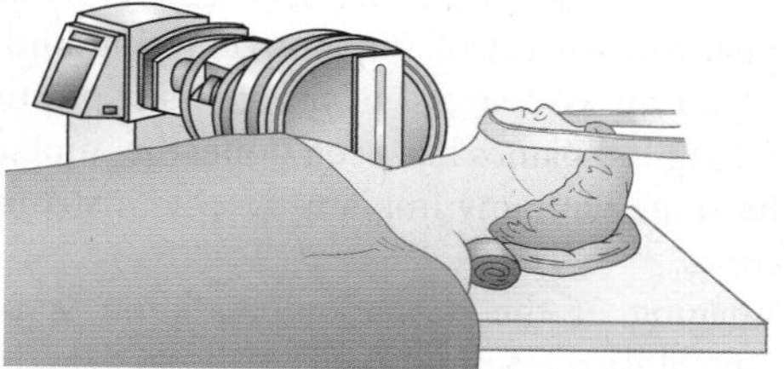

FIG. 44.8 Positioning for cervical arthroplasty is as crucial to the technique as any portion of the procedure. Correct positioning of a patient maintains physiologic lordosis without creating hyperlordosis in the cervical spine, and may be facilitated through use of a towel roll placed under the cervical spine. Techniques have moved away from traction through the spine (as shown in this illustration). Preoperative and intraoperative use of fluoroscopy allows for confirmation of patient positioning and device alignment. (Courtesy Rick Sasso, Indianapolis, IN.)

successful arthroplasty. Computed tomography (CT) and/or magnetic resonance imaging (MRI) are also essential to observe surrounding anatomy and potential pathology.

Technique of Implantation

Intraoperatively, patient position is even more critical than that of a fusion procedure. A "physiologic" or slightly lordotic cervical spine position is preferred.[41] Assessment prior to incision via fluoroscopy (C-arm) is crucial to patient positioning, as well as the implant insertion and fixation portions of these procedures. It is important to keep the head, neck, and shoulders in a stable and neutral position throughout this surgical procedure. A small towel roll may be placed under the neck to assist with appropriate positioning of the neck and shoulders, and to keep a physiologic lordosis without creating a hyperlordosis (Fig. 44.8). This positioning technique differs from the typical placement of a roll under the shoulders or thoracic spine, which could place the cervical spine in hyperlordosis. The head can be placed on a doughnut-type pillow or a folded towel to keep it from rolling during the procedure. Careful positioning of the shoulders with a taping technique can also allow for less motion during this procedure, but must be carefully weighed against the risk of traction to the shoulders.

A standard right- or left-sided Smith-Robinson approach may proceed, with appropriate localization and exposure of the index surgical level being the intent of this exposure. It is crucial to obtain a surgical exposure that facilitates identification of the center of the index disc and vertebral bodies for later placement of the arthroplasty device. Disc arthroplasty implantation is performed only after adequate decompression of the affected cervical level. At the surgeon's discretion for treatment of the index neurologic complaint, this may involve a complete discectomy from ventral to dorsal that also allows for placement of a device of appropriate width and adequate decompression, symmetrical resection of uncovertebral osteophytes and spurs, resection of all or part of the posterior longitudinal ligament, and any resection of central spondylotic osteophytes associated with DDD. A thorough and complete decompression is even more critical in a TDA procedure compared to an ACDF because of the incidence of recurrent radiculopathy from persistent foraminal stenosis. Meticulous hemostasis is recommended throughout this procedure to diminish blood loss and minimize the risk of heterotopic ossification. It may become clear at any point during the neurologic decompression, endplate preparation, or device trialing process that arthroplasty is contraindicated. Should this occur, the surgeon must adjust the surgical plan intraoperatively and proceed with a fusion-based alternative.

After neurologic decompression, assessment for placement of an appropriately sized disc and planning for proper orientation of the implant are crucial to successful arthroplasty. To this end, it should be the surgeon's goal to place an appropriately sized implant (depth, width, and height) in the prepared space.[42] Device-specific tools may aid in this assessment. Before any intervention that prepares the endplates, it is important to ensure the exact sagittal position of the vertebrae with lateral fluoroscopic imaging. AP views are important to place the spinous processes at the target disc level between the pedicles to ensure perfect alignment and centering in the coronal plane. Sizing of a cervical arthroplasty device may be determined with a combination of preoperative templates and preoperative radiographic studies, including CT. The use of intraoperative trials and fluoroscopic imaging allows for additional assessment of proper device sizing and placement in the coronal and sagittal planes.

Endplates are prepared in a manner consistent with the device to be implanted. This preparation may include milling of the endplate (as in the Bryan device) or creation of a bony trough to accommodate an endplate keel (as in the ProDisc-C device). Preservation of subchondral bone is otherwise crucial to the prevention of implant subsidence. Instrumentation specific to each arthroplasty device may be of great assistance in endplate preparation and may include special endplate distracters, keel preparation mills, rasps, and endplate mills. After the endplate preparation has been completed, it is appropriate to reassess the centering of the preparation and recheck the neurologic decompression.

Insertion of the artificial disc device may proceed, and is implant specific. Common to all devices is the principle of implantation to an appropriate depth based on implant design, with a repeat assessment of implant centering and endplate coverage. After an assessment of the implant position in the coronal and sagittal planes has been done, the implant may be fixed to the spine with any implant-specific instrumentation, such as screws.

Final imaging of the device implantation is performed before wound closure. Hemostasis is rechecked, and the surgical wound is closed in a standard fashion. Postoperative immobilization is not required. Upright flexion-extension radiographs may be obtained before discharge from the hospital and serve as a comparison to postdischarge radiographs for the purposes of follow-up.

Postoperative Imaging

The current generation of disc arthroplasty devices retains metallic components in either the endplate or bearing mechanism, making radiation-based imaging the preferred modality for postoperative evaluation. Plain radiography, including flexion and extension views of the cervical spine, is a mainstay in the postoperative period, and is useful for observing device placement, identifying potential displacement or dislodgement of device components, and assessing maintenance of motion. Special attention should be paid to device fixation at the endplate-device interface, and sagittal balance of the entire cervical spine (C2–C7) must be assessed.

MRI has been proposed as an alternative modality for follow-up imaging, allowing for postoperative assessment of the spinal canal, neural foramina, and neurologic status at the index and adjacent levels. When evaluating the amount of metal artifact on MRI with spinal implants, Wang et al. found that titanium-based devices produced significantly less artifact as compared to stainless steel and other alloys.[43] Sekhon et al.[44] used a scoring system to analyze surgeon interpretation of randomized postoperative MRI and found that the titanium-based devices (Bryan and Prestige LP) scored significantly higher than chromium-cobalt-molybdenum (Cr-Co-Mb) devices (ProDisc-C and PCM). These findings suggest that titanium-based devices produced less artifact while the Cr-Co-containing devices obscured the index and adjacent levels.

Although the MRI characteristics of all devices on the market (including those utilizing 316 stainless steel and/or Cr-Co-Mb) have not been studied, device composition may play a role in surgeon preference with regard to follow-up imaging. Initial MRI studies and the resulting image obscurity caused by such devices may affect future material choices and design strategies for cervical disc prostheses in the future.

As postoperative use of MRI may not be optimal secondary to artifacts generated by instrumentation, CT myelogram is a viable option to visualize the neural canal and offers superior visualization of neurologic and motions segments. CT imaging may also be used to identify complications, including implant malpositioning, subsidence, failure, or fracture.[45] A disadvantage of CT is high-dose radiation exposure to the patient.

Clinical Studies

The primary rationale for cervical disc arthroplasty in the treatment of DDD and symptomatic spondylosis is motion preservation, as well as reduction of adjacent-segment degeneration and consequent adjacent-level disease. The evidence-based literature is rapidly evolving as both short- and mid-term results become available.

Prestige Disc

The Prestige ST artificial disc is a ball-and-trough design made of stainless steel and contains iron, carbon, chromium, nickel, and molybdenum. The device design includes two-screw fixation to each adjacent vertebral body with thin anterior flanges. The 2-year and 5-year results of the Prestige ST FDA IDE clinical trials were published in 2007 and 2010.[35,46] Mummaneni et al.[35] published the 2-year results of a prospective, randomized, multicenter study comparing single-level cervical disc arthroplasty with the Prestige ST to single-level ACDF in the treatment of cervical DDD and radiculopathy. At 24-month follow-up, the arthroplasty group demonstrated a statistically significant higher rate of neurologic success, lower rate of secondary surgeries, and a lower rate of adjacent segment reoperations (1.1% in the arthroplasty group vs. 3.4% in the ACDF group; $P < .05$). The arthroplasty group also demonstrated earlier return to work compared to the ACDF group (45 vs. 61 days, respectively).[47]

In 2010, Burkus et al.[46] published the 5-year results of the aforementioned FDA IDE clinical trial, which showed significant improvements in the Neck Disability Index (NDI), SF-36 scores, and Neck and Arm Pain Numerical Rating Scale scores in both the arthroplasty and ACDF groups. Segmental motion was preserved at the index level at 3 years (mean, 7.3 degrees) and 5 years (mean, 6.5 degrees) postoperatively. Notably, reoperation rates differed significantly between treatment groups, with 0% of the arthroplasty group requiring revision surgery (defined as any procedure that adjusted or modified the original implant configuration) compared to 1.9% of the ACDF group undergoing revision procedure ($P = .028$).

The Prestige LP is a titanium and ceramic composite disc with rails that provide friction against migration and a plasma spray coating on the superior and inferior surfaces to promote bony ingrowth from vertebral endplates.[32] In 2015, in a prospective, multicenter investigational device exemption study, Gornet et al.[48] collected Prestige LP data from 20 investigational sites and compared the data with the control ACDF patients in the initial Prestige ST FDA IDE study.[35] Clinical outcomes data included NDI, SF-36, Neck and Arm Pain scale, work status, ROM, disc height, adverse events, additional procedures, and neurologic status. Clinical and radiographic evaluations were completed preoperatively, intraoperatively, and postoperatively up to 24 months. Significant improvements were achieved with respect to NDI, neck/arm pain, SF-36, and neurologic status in both the Prestige LP and ACDF groups by 1.5 months and were sustained at 24 months postoperatively. Mean angular motion with the Prestige LP device was maintained at 12 months (7.9 degrees) and 24 months (7.5 degrees). Neurologic success at 24 months was 93.5% in the investigational group and 83.5% in the control group. The authors of the study supported Prestige LP superiority on overall success and as a safe and efficacious alternative to ACDF for cervical DDD with radiculopathy and/or myelopathy. In mid-2014, Medtronic announced FDA approval to market the Prestige LP Cervical Disc System for the treatment of single-level cervical disc disease (radiculopathy and/or myelopathy).

ProDisc-C

The FDA IDE trial for ProDisc-C was a prospective, randomized, controlled multicenter trial that studied patients with single-level symptomatic cervical disc disease between C3–C7 who were unresponsive to 6 weeks of conservative treatment, with a total of 209 patients enrolled: 106 underwent ACDF, and 103 underwent TDA with ProDisc-C. Both groups showed significant improvement from baseline, but there was no statistical significance in the improvement between groups at 24 months. Device success, defined as lack of revision surgeries at the index level, was 98.1% in the ProDisc-C group and 91.5% in the ACDF group; this difference was statistically significant ($P < .05$). Overall success was 68.3% in the ACDF group compared to 72.3% in the ProDisc-C group, demonstrating noninferiority of the ProDisc-C cervical disc arthroplasty.

Zigler et al.[49] reported the 5-year interim results for the ProDisc-C IDE study, which demonstrated that ProDisc-C patients had statistically significantly reduced neck pain intensity and frequency when compared to the ACDF-treated group. There were no reports of device failures or implant migration 5 years postoperatively, and ProDisc-C patients had a lower rate of reoperation compared with ACDF patients (2.9% vs. 11.3%, respectively), which was also statistically significant.

Kelly et al.[50] compared adjacent segment motion in patients following TDA with ProDisc-C and those treated with ACDF. Nearly complete elimination of motion was observed at the index level in patients who underwent ACDF, while a small but statistically significant increase in ROM (1.01 degrees) was observed in the TDA group. This study demonstrated no significant difference in adjacent-segment ROM between the two groups. Long-term clinical follow-up is necessary to determine whether differences in adjacent-segment motion may ultimately affect the prevalence of adjacent-segment disease in those treated with ProDisc-C arthroplasty or ACDF.

Bryan Disc

Heller et al.[51] conducted a prospective, randomized, multicenter study as part of the 2009 FDA IDE trial investigating the safety and efficacy of TDA using the Bryan Cervical Disc. The investigational group included 242 patients treated with arthroplasty; the control group included 221 patients who underwent single-level ACDF. Patients completed clinical and radiographic follow-up at regular intervals for 24 months. Pain and function were assessed using NDI and SF-36 scores, as well as numerical rating scales for neck and arm pain. While both groups showed improvement compared to preoperative scores, the investigational group demonstrated significantly favorable results in several outcomes, including NDI, neck pain, and return to work. Arm pain scores, SF-36 physical and mental components, and rates of neurologic success, while significantly reduced in both treatment groups compared with preoperative levels, did not show significant differences between groups. At 24 months postoperatively, overall success was achieved in 82.6% of the TDA group and 72.7% of the ACDF group, which was statistically significant.[51]

Sasso et al.[52] reported 48-month follow-up to the pivotal FDA clinical trial, including 319 subjects (181 arthroplasty, 138 fusion). While at every time point the two groups were significantly improved from their respective preoperative state with regard to the NDI, the arthroplasty group was significantly superior when compared to the arthrodesis group. At every time point postoperatively, the percentage of the arthroplasty group with reduction of greater than 15 points in NDI scores was significantly higher than that of the fusion group, with NDI success achieved in 90.6% of the TDA cohort and 79.0% of the ACDF cohort. Neurologic success rates at 48 months were similar to those observed at the 24-month time point, and difference in mean rates between the two groups was not statistically significant. Mean cervical spine motion in the single-level TDA group increased from 6.5 degrees at baseline to 8.08 degrees at 24 months and 8.5 degrees at 48 months; this increase was significant at all time points after 3 months. Ryu et al.[53] completed an in vivo prospective study of patients treated with single-level BRYAN disc arthroplasty investigating whether artificial disc replacement could maintain physiologic kinematics at the index and adjacent levels, concluding that there is minimal change in the device kinematic behavior at early follow-up and that kinematics of the BRYAN Disc are predictable and durable at 5 years postoperatively.

Mobi-C

The Mobi-C cervical disc prosthesis remains the only FDA-approved prosthesis for two-level cervical disc arthroplasty.[54] Twenty-three patients were included in a retrospective study on single-level TDA that showed statistically significant improvements in VAS arm and neck pain scores at 6-month follow-up. All patients were able to return to work within 1 month postoperatively, and there were no complications observed. Cervical mobility was preserved at the index and adjacent levels at 6-month follow-up. Park et al. retrospectively studied a cohort of 53 patients who underwent operative treatment (21 treated with single-level TDA and 32 treated with ACDF) for cervical disc herniations.[55] This study demonstrated statistically significant improvements in return to work and shorter mean hospital stays in the TDA patients. While there were no postoperative complications in the group treated with the Mobi-C prosthesis, there were five instances of cage subsidence in the fusion group.

In a prospective study analyzing sagittal balance in 40 patients after TDA, Guérin et al. demonstrated maintenance

SECTION V

of ROM, cervical lordosis, and sagittal alignment 2 years postoperatively.[56] This study also showed statistically significant improvements in NDI, VAS, and SF-36 scores for patients who underwent TDA with Mobi-C. Beaurain et al. reported the intermediate results of an ongoing multicenter prospective study of 76 patients treated with Mobi-C TDA.[57] The study showed improvements in NDI, VAS arm and neck pain indices, and SF-36 scores, all of which were statistically significant. Through radiologic evaluation, the authors demonstrated preservation of segmental motion, with flexion-extension ROM of treated levels averaging 9.9 degrees preoperatively and 9 degrees at 2 years postoperatively.

In regard to two-level TDA, Davis et al. published the results of a prospective, randomized, FDA IDE trial that compared Mobi-C TDA to ACDF for two-level contiguous cervical DDD with 2-year follow-up.[58] Of 330 patients enrolled in the study, 225 (68%) were treated with two-level TDA while 105 (32%) underwent ACDF. Both groups demonstrated statistically significant improvements in NDI and VAS arm and neck pain scores when compared to preoperative values. The TDA group experienced significantly greater improvement in the NDI score when compared to the fusion group. The ACDF group also demonstrated a higher reoperation rate (11.4% vs. 3.1% reoperation after TDA).

While one-level Mobi-C TDA is noninferior, but not superior, to one-level ACDF, and two-level Mobi-C TDA may be superior to two-level ACDF, long-term studies are necessary to evaluate outcomes and to elucidate complications associated with the device. Critics would also argue that substantial evidence beyond the findings of studies with significant conflict of interest is still lacking.[59]

Future Direction

Several of the aforementioned studies published in the last decade, regardless of arthroplasty device, have attempted to demonstrate that cervical TDA reduces the incidence of adjacent-segment degeneration in the cervical spine. However, there is a growing segment of the current literature critical of the data comparing TDA to ACDF with regard to the incidence of adjacent-segment disease (ASD) postoperatively. Points of contention include short follow-up period, cohort size, disproportionate numbers of subjects among treatment groups, and parameters used for assessing the incidence of ASD.

Nunley et al. studied 173 patients among the FDA IDE trials for four separate disc replacement devices, with the primary objective of identifying the incidence of and factors influencing ASD after TDA.[60] Patients included in the analysis demonstrated one- and/or two-level symptomatic cervical DDD, had failed at least 6 months of active conservative management, and completed at least 4 years' follow-up. This study identified a 3.1% annual incidence of symptomatic ASD after cervical TDA, regardless of patient's age, sex, smoking habits, and implant device. Meanwhile, patients participating in the control arm treated with ACDF had a 2.8% annual incidence of ASD—a difference that was not statistically significant.

In addition to a lower incidence of ASD, the proposed benefits of TDA include better function (per NDI, pain assessment, SF-36, and neurologic status) and a lower incidence of reoperation. Yin et al. performed a meta-analysis of functional scores, reoperation rates, and major complications following TDA, identifying 2227 patients from 10 randomized controlled trials.[61] Fewer major surgical complications (including implant wear, migration, dislodgement and subsidence, graft donor site morbidity, and graft extrusion) occurred in TDA patients than in fusion patients; this difference was statistically significant. While segmental motion at the index level was retained in the setting of TDA, motion at adjacent levels was not greater than that of the fusion group. Furthermore, there was not a statistically significant difference in reoperation rates at adjacent levels after TDA or fusion at 4 to 5 years' mean follow-up. Verma et al. described similar results in a meta-analysis of 6 prospective studies, including IDE and non-IDE trials with at least 2 years' follow-up.[62] In a sample size of 1586 patients (777 ACDF, 809 TDA) and 70% follow-up, there was no detectable difference in reoperation rates between groups.

While the FDA IDE trials remain a primary source of truly randomized, collected, and validated data, independently funded, blinded, long-term follow-up prospective studies are necessary to further compare the effects that motion-preserving devices and fusion methods have on adjacent spinal levels. The fact that osteopenia and concurrent lumbar DDD significantly increase the risk of ASD has been established in the literature. However, the theoretical assumption that motion-sparing TDA may significantly reduce the incidence of future ASD when compared to ACDF requires further corroboration.

Biomechanics

The goals of TDA with respect to biomechanical parameters are as follows: restoration of physiologic kinematics and mobility while avoiding spinal instability; protection of biologic structures including adjacent discs, facet joints, and ligaments from overloading; restoration of correct spinal alignment; and device stability and response to wear debris.[33] The most studied parameter concerning spinal kinematics after TDA is ROM, that is, the rotation from one extreme to the other of the physiologic range of rotation of a specific motion. The majority of ex vivo studies that quantify motion alternations after TDA find a general preservation of motion at the index level, with ROMs nearly similar to physiologic values regardless of prosthesis design.[6,63–65]

Normal cervical spine motion exhibits AP translation during flexion and extension. The cervical spine motion segments are complex joints, each consisting of three compartments: the disc and two facets. Disc prosthesis design must consider the three compartments as well as the multiple ligamentous structures of the cervical spine.

Biomechanical studies suggest that the semiconstrained design (ball-in-trough) of the PRESTIGE cervical disc provides for normal kinematics in all ROMs. However, DiAngelo et al. reported that a constrained design (ball-in-socket), such as that of the ProDisc-C prosthesis, failed to reproduce normal motion in extension.[63] The ball-in-socket design does not reproduce the natural AP translation seen in the normal motion of the facet joint. The complexity of the cervical spine requires a "balance" of all the significant structures, including facets and ligaments.

The most significant effect of this change in balance is in extension. When the spine goes into flexion, the facets "unshingle" and reduce their involvement in constraining the motion of the functional spine unit. When the spine goes into extension, the facets "shingle" and become more involved in constraining the motion. With a constrained facet joint and a constrained disc joint, one would expect to see binding or limited motion (also known as *kinematic conflict*), as one joint works against the other. This binding would give rise to decreased motion or increased stress on the system.

Balancing the kinematics in the functional spine unit is crucial. A constrained disc replacement may be unable to provide the normal kinematics of the cervical spine. AP translation is anatomic and must be allowed to restore normal motion. The Prestige Cervical Disc was shown to maintain normal kinematics through all ROMs. Similar results would be expected from the Bryan Cervical Disc system because it is also semiconstrained and allows for AP translation in flexion and extension.

Sasso and colleagues[66] studied the kinematics of cervical motion from patients enrolled in a prospective, randomized, multicenter clinical trial. Radiographic data, including flexion, extension, and neutral lateral radiographs, were obtained preoperatively and at regular postoperative intervals up to 24 months. All patients had received either a single-level anterior cervical plate (Atlantis anterior cervical plate, n = 221) or a single-level artificial cervical disc (Bryan Cervical Disc prosthesis, n = 242) at C3 to C7. Cervical vertebral bodies were tracked to calculate the functional spinal unit motion parameters. Parameters measured included flexion-extension ROM and translation. These data were recorded at the index surgical level and, if visible, at the functional spinal units cranial and caudal to it.

More motion was retained in the disc replacement group than the plated group at the index level, a statistically significant finding. At 24 months, the arthroplasty group retained an average of 7.95 degrees (average, 6.43 degrees preoperatively). In the control ACDF cohort, the average ROM in the fusion group was 1.11 degrees at the 3-month follow-up and gradually decreased to 0.87 degrees at 24 months (average, 8.39 degrees preoperatively). In the Bryan cohort, index-level functional spinal unit translation averaged 0.36 mm at 24 months, a data point that was statistically unchanged from the first postoperative measurement of translation at 3 months. No investigational devices showed radiographic evidence of subsidence at 24 months, and no HO was observed in the BRYAN cohort.

Angular ROM at adjacent levels cranial and caudal to the index surgical functional spinal unit was measured and was not statistically different between the two cohorts preoperatively. At 24 months, these differences were unchanged in both groups (statistically similar). There was no consistent correlation between angular ROM at adjacent or index levels and standard outcome measures of success in the investigational group. These data were not analyzed in the control. This study showed that the Bryan disc maintains mobility at the level of the prosthesis over 24 months. No conclusions with regard to the adjacent segments could be statistically reached at this early follow-up interval.

In an in vitro biomechanical analysis, Gandhi et al.[67] found that after single-level arthroplasty, the motion at implanted levels increased in all directions. The Prestige LP disc demonstrated increased motion by 26% in flexion-extension, 33% in lateral bending, and 6% in axial rotation. TDA with the Bryan disc demonstrated an increase of 25% in flexion-extension, 8% in lateral bending, and 1% in axial rotation.[67]

SECTION V

PEARLS

1. Disc arthroplasty is the most favorable intervention when degenerative conditions of the anterior cervical spine are largely limited to pathology of the disc with a sparing of degeneration of the facet joints.
2. During the procedure, the surgeon should intermittently relax retraction to allow recovery of surrounding soft tissues. This has been suggested to decrease the duration and severity of postoperative dysphagia.
3. Care should be taken to size the disc prosthesis appropriately.[68] A prosthesis should be selected that optimally covers the vertebral body endplates on AP and lateral fluoroscopic views. Implant-specific sizing and alignment guides should be used judiciously.
4. Proper orientation of the implant is crucial to a successful outcome.[68] The AP fluoroscopic view should be oriented so that the spinous process is equidistant between the pedicles of the cranial and caudal vertebral bodies. The surgeon should ensure that the midline is well marked after it has been determined fluoroscopically and should be careful not to stray from the midline during implant preparation. The surgeon should ensure that the implant is directly in the center of the disc space on the AP view. Implant-specific instrumentation should be employed for the purposes of endplate preparation and distraction.

PITFALLS

1. Lack of meticulous hemostasis has been implicated as a factor in HO.
2. Care should be taken not to overdistract the posterior facets during implantation of the device.

KEY POINTS

1. Cervical disc arthroplasty is proposed as a safe, effective alternative to ACDF in patients with symptomatic cervical radiculopathy or myelopathy related to cervical DDD.
2. Cervical arthroplasty is designed to preserve motion and avoid some of the limitations and morbidity of cervical fusion, such as pseudarthrosis, bone graft harvest and allograft issues, anterior cervical plating, and cervical immobilization.
3. In addition to the primary goal of relief of symptoms from cervical DDD, the technique of cervical arthroplasty has been theorized to provide an advantageous biomechanical environment that may counter the adjacent-segment degeneration that has been observed in patients treated with ACDF.

4. At 24 months, arthroplasty seems to compare favorably with traditional ACDF in prospective randomized multicenter trials examining the outcomes of devices including the Bryan, Prestige ST, and ProDisc-C devices.
5. Intermediate-term and long-term follow-up are crucial to the assessment of devices used in this technique because the short-term data may not be an appropriate representation of the primary and secondary outcomes for motion-sparing technologies.

KEY REFERENCES

1. Mummaneni PV, Burkus JK, Haid RW, et al. Clinical and radiographic analysis of cervical disc arthroplasty compared with allograft fusion: a randomized controlled clinical trial. *J Neurosurg Spine*. 2007;6:198-209.
2. Heller JG, Sasso RC, Papadopoulos SM, et al. Comparison of BRYAN cervical disc arthroplasty with anterior cervical decompression and fusion: clinical and radiographic results of a randomized, controlled, clinical trial. *Spine*. 2009;34:101-107.
3. Hilibrand AS, Carlson GD, Palumbo MA, et al. Radiculopathy and myelopathy at segments adjacent to the site of a previous anterior cervical arthrodesis. *J Bone Joint Surg*. 1999;81A:519-528.
4. Bohlman HH, Emery SE, Goodfellow DB, et al. Robinson anterior cervical discectomy and arthrodesis for cervical radiculopathy. Long-term follow-up of one hundred and twenty-two patients. *J Bone Joint Surg*. 1993;75A:1298-1307.
5. Goffin J, Geusens E, Vantomme N, et al. Long-term follow-up after interbody fusion of the cervical spine. *J Spinal Disord Tech*. 2004;17:79-85.

REFERENCES

1. Robinson RA. Fusions of the cervical spine. *J Bone Joint Surg Am*. 1959;41:1-6.
2. Bohlman HH, Emery SE, Goodfellow DB, et al. Robinson anterior cervical discectomy and arthrodesis for cervical radiculopathy. Long-term follow-up of one hundred and twenty-two patients. *J Bone Joint Surg*. 1993;75A:1298-1307.
3. Goffin J, Geusens E, Vantomme N, et al. Long-term follow-up after interbody fusion of the cervical spine. *J Spinal Disord Tech*. 2004;17:79-85.
4. Wang JC, McDonough PW, Endow KK, et al. Increased fusion rates with cervical plating for two-level anterior cervical discectomy and fusion. *Spine*. 2000;25:41-45.
5. Yoon DH. Cervical disk arthroplasty techniques. In: Kim DH, ed. *Surgical Anatomy & Techniques to the Spine*. 2nd ed. Philadelphia: Elsevier; 2013:187-195.
6. Dmitriev AE, Cunningham BW, Hu N, et al. Adjacent level intradiscal pressure and segmental kinematics following a cervical total disc arthroplasty: an in vitro human cadaveric model. *Spine*. 2005;30:1165-1172.
7. Phillips FM, Carlson G, Emery SE, et al. Anterior cervical pseudarthrosis. Natural history and treatment. *Spine*. 1997;22:1585-1589.
8. Katsuura A, Hukuda S, Saruhashi Y, et al. Kyphotic malalignment after anterior cervical fusion is one of the factors promoting the degenerative process in adjacent intervertebral levels. *Eur Spine J*. 2001;10:320-324.
9. Eck JC, Humphreys SC, Lim TH, et al. Biomechanical study on the effect of cervical spine fusion on adjacent-level intradiscal pressure and segmental motion. *Spine*. 2002;27:2431-2434.
10. Silber JS, Anderson DG, Daffner SD, et al. Donor site morbidity after anterior iliac crest bone harvest for single-level anterior cervical discectomy and fusion. *Spine*. 2003;28:134-139.
11. Riley LH 3rd, Skolasky RL, Albert TJ, et al. Dysphagia after anterior cervical decompression and fusion: prevalence and risk factors from a longitudinal cohort study. *Spine*. 2005;30:2564-2569.
12. Hilibrand AS, Carlson GD, Palumbo MA, et al. Radiculopathy and myelopathy at segments adjacent to the site of a previous anterior cervical arthrodesis. *J Bone Joint Surg*. 1999;81A:519-528.
13. Xu R, Bydon M, Macki M, et al. Adjacent segment disease after anterior cervical discectomy and fusion: clinical outcomes after first repeat surgery versus second repeat surgery. *Spine*. 2014;39:120-126.
14. Bydon M, Xu R, Macki M, et al. Adjacent segment disease after anterior cervical discectomy and fusion in a large series. *Neurosurgery*. 2014;74:139-146.
15. Park DH, Ramakrishnan P, Cho TH, et al. Effect of lower two-level anterior cervical fusion on the superior adjacent level. *J Neurosurg Spine*. 2007;7:336-340.
16. Mutoh N, Shinomiya K, Furuya K, et al. Pseudarthrosis and delayed union after anterior cervical fusion. *Int Orthop*. 1993;17:286-289.
17. Simmons EH. Anterior cervical discectomy and fusion. *Proc R Soc Med*. 1970;63:897-898.
18. Samartzis D, Shen FH, Goldberg EJ, et al. Is autograft the gold standard in achieving radiographic fusion in one-level anterior cervical discectomy and fusion with rigid anterior plate fixation? *Spine*. 2005;30:1756-1761.
19. Robertson PA, Wray AC. Natural history of posterior iliac crest bone graft donation for spinal surgery: a prospective analysis of morbidity. *Spine*. 2001;26:1473-1476.
20. Behairy YM, Al-Sebai W. A modified technique for harvesting full-thickness iliac crest bone graft. *Spine*. 2001;26:695-697.
21. Transmission of HIV through bone transplantation: case report and public health recommendations. *MMWR Morb Mortal Wkly Rep*. 1988;37:597-599.
22. Hsu EL, Ghodasra JH, Ashtekar A, et al. A comparative evaluation of factors influencing osteoinductivity among scaffolds designed for bone regeneration. *Tissue Eng Part A*. 2013;19:1764-1772.
23. Hsu WK, Polavarapu M, Riaz R, et al. Nanocomposite therapy as a more efficacious and less inflammatory alternative to bone morphogenetic protein-2 in a rodent arthrodesis model. *J Orthop Res*. 2011;29:1812-1819.
24. Burkus JK, Sandhu HS, Gornet MF, et al. Use of rhBMP-2 in combination with structural cortical allografts: clinical and radiographic outcomes in anterior lumbar spinal surgery. *J Bone Joint Surg*. 2005;87A:1205-1212.
25. Mulconrey DS, Bridwell KH, Flynn J, et al. Bone morphogenetic protein (RhBMP-2) as a substitute for iliac crest bone graft in multilevel adult spinal deformity surgery: minimum two-year evaluation of fusion. *Spine*. 2008;33:2153-2159.
26. Carragee EJ, Hurwitz EL, Weiner BK. A critical review of recombinant human bone morphogenetic protein-2 trials in spinal surgery: emerging safety concerns and lessons learned. *Spine J*. 2011;11:471-491.
27. Smucker JD, Rhee JM, Singh K, et al. Increased swelling complications associated with off-label usage of rhBMP-2 in the anterior cervical spine. *Spine*. 2006;31:2813-2819.
28. Vaidya R, Carp J, Sethi A, et al. Complications of anterior cervical discectomy and fusion using recombinant human bone morphogenetic protein-2. *Eur Spine J*. 2007;16:1257-1265.

29. Hsu WK. Recombinant human bone morphogenetic protein-2 in spine surgery. *J Bone Joint Surg Rev*. 2014;2.
30. Kannan A, Dodwad SN, Hsu WK. Biologics in spine arthrodesis. *J Spinal Disord Tech*. 2015;28:163-170.
31. Center for Devices and Radiological Health. *Guidance for Industry and FDA Staff: Preparation and Review of Investigational Device Exemption Applications (IDEs) for Total Artificial Discs*. Rockville, MD: 2008:1-28.
31a. Cummins BH, Robertson JT, Gill SS. Surgical experience with an implanted artificial cervical joint. *J Neurosurg*. 1998;88:943-948.
32. Mummaneni PV, Robinson JC, Haid RW Jr. Cervical arthroplasty with the PRESTIGE LP cervical disc. *Neurosurgery*. 2007;60:310-314.
33. Galbusera F, Bellini CM, Brayda-Bruno M, et al. Biomechanical studies on cervical total disc arthroplasty: a literature review. *Clin Biomech (Bristol, Avon)*. 2008;23:1095-1104.
34. Jaramillo-de la Torre JJ, Grauer JN, Yue JJ. Update on cervical disc arthroplasty: where are we and where are we going? *Curr Rev Musculoskelet Med*. 2008;1:124-130.
35. Mummaneni PV, Burkus JK, Haid RW, et al. Clinical and radiographic analysis of cervical disc arthroplasty compared with allograft fusion: a randomized controlled clinical trial. *J Neurosurg Spine*. 2007;6:198-209.
36. Hashmi SZ, Hsu WK. Cervical disc arthroplasty. *Contemp Spine Surg*. 2014;15:1-8.
37. Riew KD, Buchowski JM, Sasso R, et al. Cervical disc arthroplasty compared with arthrodesis for the treatment of myelopathy. *J Bone Joint Surg Am*. 2008;90A:2354-2364.
38. Hsu WK. The rationale for cervical disc arthroplasty. *Tech Orthop*. 2010;25:84-87.
39. van Loon J, Goffin J. Unanticipated outcomes after cervical disk arthroplasty. *Semin Spine Surg*. 2012;24:20-24.
40. Walraevens J, Demaerel P, Suetens P, et al. Longitudinal prospective long-term radiographic follow-up after treatment of single-level cervical disk disease with the Bryan Cervical Disc. *Neurosurgery*. 2010;67:679-687.
41. Anderson PA, Sasso RC, Rouleau JP, et al. The Bryan Cervical Disc: wear properties and early clinical results. *Spine J*. 2004;4:S303-S309.
42. Wigfield CC, Gill SS, Nelson RJ, et al. The new Frenchay artificial cervical joint: results from a two-year pilot study. *Spine*. 2002;27:2446-2452.
43. Wang JC, Yu WD, Sandhu HS, et al. A comparison of magnetic resonance and computed tomographic image quality after the implantation of tantalum and titanium spinal instrumentation. *Spine*. 1998;23:1684-1688.
44. Sekhon LH, Duggal N, Lynch JJ, et al. Magnetic resonance imaging clarity of the Bryan, Prodisc-C, Prestige LP, and PCM cervical arthroplasty devices. *Spine*. 2007;32:673-680.
45. Robinson Y, Sanden B. Spine imaging after lumbar disc replacement: pitfalls and current recommendations. *Patient Saf Surg*. 2009;3:15.
46. Burkus JK, Haid RW, Traynelis VC, et al. Long-term clinical and radiographic outcomes of cervical disc replacement with the Prestige disc: results from a prospective randomized controlled clinical trial. *J Neurosurg Spine*. 2010;13:308-318.
47. Wu J-C, Meyer SA, Gandhoke G, et al. PRESTIGE cervical arthroplasty: past, present, and future. *Semin Spine Surg*. 2012;24:14-19.
48. Gornet MF, Burkus JK, Shaffrey ME, et al. Cervical disc arthroplasty with PRESTIGE LP disc versus anterior cervical discectomy and fusion: a prospective, multicenter investigational device exemption study. *J Neurosurg Spine*. 2015;1-16.
49. Zigler JE, Delamarter R, Murrey D, et al. ProDisc-C and anterior cervical discectomy and fusion as surgical treatment for single-level cervical symptomatic degenerative disc disease: five-year results of a Food and Drug Administration study. *Spine*. 2013;38:203-209.
50. Kelly MP, Mok JM, Frisch RF, et al. Adjacent segment motion after anterior cervical discectomy and fusion versus Prodisc-C cervical total disk arthroplasty: analysis from a randomized, controlled trial. *Spine*. 2011;36:1171-1179.
51. Heller JG, Sasso RC, Papadopoulos SM, et al. Comparison of BRYAN cervical disc arthroplasty with anterior cervical decompression and fusion: clinical and radiographic results of a randomized, controlled, clinical trial. *Spine*. 2009;34:101-107.
52. Sasso RC, Anderson PA, Riew KD, et al. Results of cervical arthroplasty compared with anterior discectomy and fusion: four-year clinical outcomes in a prospective, randomized controlled trial. *J Bone Joint Surg*. 2011;93A:1684-1692.
53. Ryu WHA, Kowalczyk I, Duggal N. Long-term kinematic analysis of cervical spine after single-level implantation of Bryan cervical disc prosthesis. *Spine J*. 2013;13:628-634.
54. Kim SH, Shin HC, Shin DA, et al. Early clinical experience with the Mobi-C disc prosthesis. *Yonsei Med J*. 2007;48:457-464.
55. Park JH, Roh KH, Cho JY, et al. Comparative analysis of cervical arthroplasty using Mobi-C and anterior cervical discectomy and fusion using the Solis Cage. *J Korean Neurosurg Soc*. 2008;44:217-221.
56. Guerin P, Obeid I, Gille O, et al. Sagittal alignment after single cervical disc arthroplasty. *J Spinal Disord Tech*. 2012;25:10-16.
57. Beaurain J, Bernard P, Dufour T, et al. Intermediate clinical and radiological results of cervical TDR (Mobi-C) with up to 2 years of follow-up. *Eur Spine J*. 2009;18:841-850.
58. Davis RJ, Kim KD, Hisey MS, et al. Cervical total disc replacement with the Mobi-C cervical artificial disc compared with anterior discectomy and fusion for treatment of 2-level symptomatic degenerative disc disease: a prospective, randomized, controlled multicenter clinical trial. *J Neurosurg Spine*. 2013;19:532-545.
59. Alvin MD, Abbott EE, Lubelski D, et al. Cervical arthroplasty: a critical review of the literature. *Spine J*. 2014;14:2231-2245.
60. Nunley PD, Jawahar A, Cavanaugh DA, et al. Symptomatic adjacent segment disease after cervical total disc replacement: re-examining the clinical and radiological evidence with established criteria. *Spine J*. 2013;13:5-12.
61. Yin S, Yu X, Zhou S, et al. Is cervical disc arthroplasty superior to fusion for treatment of symptomatic cervical disc disease? A meta-analysis. *Clin Orthop Relat Res*. 2013;471:1904-1919.
62. Verma K, Gandhi SD, Maltenfort M, et al. Rate of adjacent segment disease in cervical disc arthroplasty versus single-level fusion: meta-analysis of prospective studies. *Spine*. 2013;38:2253-2257.
63. DiAngelo DJ, Foley KT, Morrow BR, et al. In vitro biomechanics of cervical disc arthroplasty with the ProDisc-C total disc implant. *Neurosurg Focus*. 2004;17:E7.
64. Puttlitz CM, Rousseau MA, Xu Z, et al. Intervertebral disc replacement maintains cervical spine kinetics. *Spine*. 2004;29:2809-2814.
65. Rabin D, Pickett GE, Bisnaire L, et al. The kinematics of anterior cervical discectomy and fusion versus artificial cervical disc: a pilot study. *Neurosurgery*. 2007;61:100-104.

SECTION V

66. Sasso RC, Best NM, Metcalf NH, et al. Motion analysis of bryan cervical disc arthroplasty versus anterior discectomy and fusion: results from a prospective, randomized, multicenter, clinical trial. *J Spinal Disord Tech*. 2008;21: 393-399.
67. Gandhi AA, Kode S, DeVries NA, et al. Biomechanical analysis of cervical disc replacement and fusion using single level, two level and hybrid constructs. *Spine*. 2015.
68. Anderson PA, Sasso RC, Riew KD. Update on cervical artificial disk replacement. *Instr Course Lect*. 2007;56:237-245.

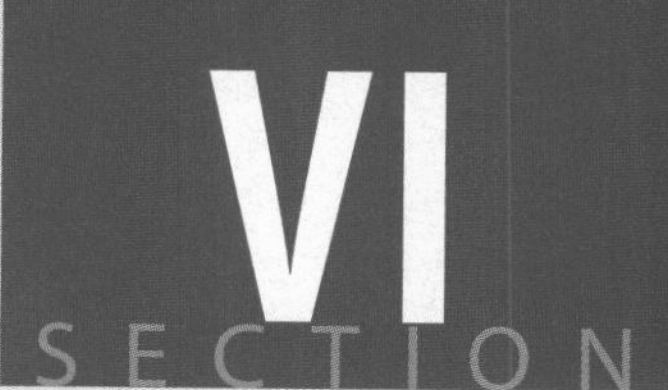

SECTION VI

THORACIC AND LUMBAR DISC DISEASE

SECTION VI

45 CHAPTER Thoracic Disc Disease

Bradford L. Currier
Jason C. Eck
Frank J. Eismont
Barth A. Green

Thoracic disc herniation is an uncommon disease. Diagnosis is often difficult owing to myriad presenting symptoms. Advances in diagnostic methods, specifically magnetic resonance imaging (MRI), have led to earlier diagnosis of both symptomatic and asymptomatic disc herniation. The natural history of thoracic disc herniation is unclear because improved diagnostic methods identify an increasing prevalence of asymptomatic thoracic herniated discs. The vast majority of thoracic disc herniations remain asymptomatic and are treated nonoperatively. However, surgery generally is regarded as the treatment of choice for a symptomatic herniated thoracic disc with myelopathy to prevent the sequelae of spinal cord compression. The prognosis associated with surgical decompression has improved dramatically with selection of surgical approach and the advent of techniques for disc excision without cord manipulation.

Historical Background

In 1838, Key[1] wrote the first report of a thoracic herniated disc causing spinal cord compression. Middleton and Teacher[2] reported the second case 73 years later. The first reported surgical treatment of a thoracic herniated disc was in 1922 by Adson, who performed a laminectomy and disc removal.[3] In their classic 1934 monograph on ruptured intervertebral discs, Mixter and Barr[4] described four cases of thoracic disc herniation; two of three patients treated surgically via laminectomy were rendered paraplegic, emphasizing the challenge in the management of the disease. In the ensuing years, many reports helped define the disease and document that treatment by laminectomy was unpredictable and very risky.[3,5–16]

The costotransversectomy approach was introduced by Menard[17] in 1900. Capener[18] later modified the procedure for use in the treatment of Pott disease. At Alexander's suggestion, Hulme[19] was the first to use this approach in the management of a herniated thoracic disc. Hulme reported his experience with six patients treated by costotransversectomy and showed that it was a safer, more effective approach than laminectomy. In a later literature review of 49 surgical cases using costotransversectomy, Arce and Dohrmann[20] noted that 82% of patients improved, the condition was unchanged in 14% of patients, and only 4% of patients experienced worsening of their condition.

Hodgson and Stock[21] popularized the anterior approach to the spine for the treatment of Pott disease. In 1958, Crafoord and colleagues[22] reported the first transthoracic procedure on the spine for a herniated disc. They performed a *fenestration,* or windowing, of the disc without any attempt at disc removal or cord decompression. The one patient described in their article did well. Simultaneous reports by Perot and Munro[23] and Ransohoff and colleagues[24] in 1969 established transthoracic spinal cord decompression as a viable alternative to costotransversectomy. The posterolateral approach to the thoracic disc space was described by Carson and colleagues[25] in 1971 and was modified by Patterson and Arbit[26] in 1978.

All the surgical approaches have undergone minor modifications, including the application of microsurgical techniques.[27–29] Developments in the use of video-assisted thoracoscopic surgery (VATS) have provided an additional option in surgical treatment of a symptomatic thoracic herniated disc.[30–33] Each technique has advantages and disadvantages, and all but laminectomy are currently acceptable.

The diagnostic use of MRI has had a profound influence on the treatment of thoracic disc herniation.[34–42] At most centers, MRI has replaced myelography as the standard for the diagnosis of this condition. Because MRI is rapid, noninvasive, and increasingly available, its use is likely to decrease delay in diagnosis and lead to earlier treatment and perhaps improved prognosis. A new challenge is likely to be avoiding overdiagnosis and unnecessary operations on asymptomatic lesions.[41,43]

Epidemiology

The true incidence of thoracic herniated discs is unknown; many cases go unrecognized, or patients are asymptomatic. Most patients are in the fourth through sixth decades of life (Fig. 45.1).[3,6,44,45] In a review of 288 cases reported in the literature, Arce and Dohrmann[44] noted a slight male preponderance (1.5 : 1), although most series show an approximately even sex

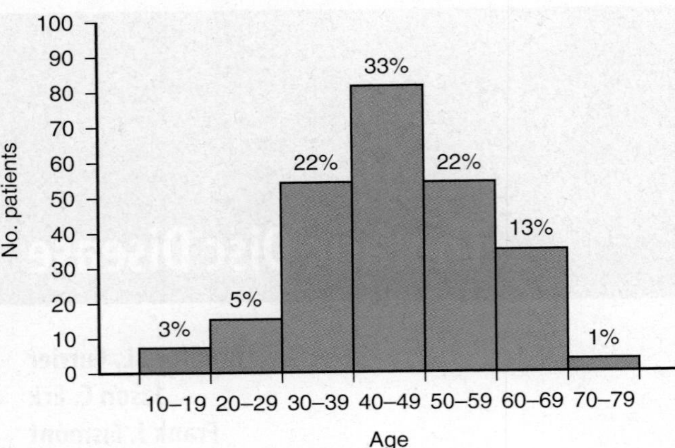

FIG. 45.1 Distribution of 280 cases of thoracic disc herniation according to age. (From Arce CA, Dohrmann GJ. Herniated thoracic disks. *Neurol Clin.* 1985;3:383–392.)

distribution.[5,11,46,47] Cases have been reported in patients ranging in age from 11 to 75 years.[25,48,49]

Historically, only 0.15% to 4% of all symptomatic protrusions of an intervertebral disc are in the thoracic spine.[3,5,6,12,44,50–52] Surgically, thoracic disc excision accounts for 0.2% to 1.8% of all operations performed on symptomatic herniated discs.[5,29,39,44,53–56] In 1950, Love and Kiefer[47] reported on 17 cases seen over 26 years. Logue[12] reported a thoracic herniated disc in 11 of 250 discectomies (4%). Otani and colleagues[51] later reported symptomatic thoracic disc herniation in 15 of 857 discectomies (1.8%) over a 15-year period. In a cadaveric study, Haley and Perry[57] showed that 11% of unselected autopsies revealed protruded thoracic discs; 2 of 99 specimens in their series had discs protruding 4 to 7 mm into the canal. The prevalence of herniated thoracic discs with an associated neurologic deficit has been estimated to be 1 per 1 million population.[25,42,47,52,58]

Improvements in imaging techniques have resulted in an increased detection of thoracic abnormalities and, concurrently, of herniated thoracic discs. Ryan and colleagues[59] reviewed 270 patients undergoing computed tomography (CT) of the thorax for suspected malignancy and found four (1.5%) who had asymptomatic calcified herniated thoracic discs. In a retrospective review of combined CT and myelography in 360 patients, Awwad and colleagues[60] found 54 herniations of a thoracic disc in 40 patients (11%) who were asymptomatic. In their study, 88% of the asymptomatic thoracic discs showed some deformity of the spinal cord; there was no single feature or combination of features clearly separating asymptomatic from symptomatic thoracic herniated discs.

The advent of MRI and its inherent sensitivity has increased further the reported incidence of thoracic disc herniations. Williams and colleagues[41] retrospectively reviewed 48 patients who underwent MRI for oncologic evaluation and reported a thoracic herniated disc in seven (15%). Ross and colleagues[39] diagnosed 20 cases (16 confirmed) by MRI in a 2-year period compared with the initial report of Love and Kiefer[47] in 1949 of 17 cases seen over a 26-year period. Wood and colleagues[42] reported that 66 of 90 asymptomatic individuals (73%) had positive anatomic findings at one or more thoracic levels. Findings included herniation of a disc in 33 subjects (37%), bulging of a disc in 48 (53%), an annular tear in 52 (58%), and deformation of the spinal cord in 26 (29%). These investigators reported no association between age and the prevalence of disc herniation. Compared with the MRI findings of 18 patients treated operatively for thoracic disc herniations in their study, the overall prevalence of these findings in the group that had thoracic pain was not significantly different from the asymptomatic population.

Williams and colleagues[41] suggested that thoracic disc herniation may be common enough to be considered a normal variant on MRI. More recently, Niemelainen and colleagues[61] reported that degenerative thoracic MRI changes were less common than previously reported. In a cross-sectional study of men 35 to 70 years old from the Finnish Twin Cohort study, only 9.2% of subjects had posterior disc bulging. Anterior disc bulging was much more common, found in 45.2%. The presence of anterior disc bulging was positively correlated with age ($r = 0.15$ to 0.23, $P < .005$). Moderate to severe disc height narrowing ranged from 5.4% to 9.5% by level in the thoracic spine.

Etiology

Most authors favor degenerative processes as the major cause of thoracic disc herniation.[3,20,57] This theory is supported by the higher incidence of herniation in the thoracolumbar spine, where greater degenerative changes occur.[34,40,62] In a review of MRI findings and their relationship to thoracic and lumbar disc degeneration in a cohort of 232 subjects, Videman and colleagues[40] noted that moderate and severe osteophytes were most common at the T11–T12 level (20.7% of subjects); upper endplate irregularities were most common at levels T8–T12, typically in the middle of the endplates in the thoracolumbar spine compared with more peripheral endplate changes in the lumbar spine. These results were later supported by Niemelainen and colleagues,[61] who reported moderate to severe disc height narrowing in 21.4% of subjects.

The role of trauma as a cause of herniated thoracic discs is controversial. A history of trauma can be elicited in 14% to 63% of patients.[35,45] The mean prevalence in 10 random series was 34%. In some patients, the causal relationship is undeniable; in others, trauma may have been an aggravating factor or purely coincidental. The degree of reported trauma responsible for herniation ranges from minor twisting strains and chiropractic manipulation to major falls or motor vehicle accidents.[63]

Several authors[35,54,64] have suggested an association between Scheuermann disease and herniated thoracic discs. The primary pathogenic process of the disease or secondary disc degeneration may be the factors promoting herniation. Wood and colleagues[42] noted that endplate changes consistent with Scheuermann disease were more prevalent in their symptomatic patient group than in the asymptomatic population.

Pathogenesis

The pathogenesis of neurologic compromise secondary to herniated thoracic discs is believed to be a combination of direct neural compression and vascular insufficiency.[2,3,6,12,26] Middleton and Teacher[2] suggested this in a case reported in 1911. Severe back pain developed while this patient was lifting a heavy object. Approximately 20 hours later, he felt a sudden severe pain shoot from his chest to his feet and he became almost completely paraplegic. The patient died 16 days later of urosepsis. The autopsy revealed a herniated thoracic disc opposite a section of cord that was compressed, degenerated, and hemorrhagic. A thrombosed vessel was found in the section of cord showing the most hemorrhage.

Several anatomic features make the thoracic cord vulnerable to manipulation and trauma.[26] The thoracic spinal canal is small, and most of its available space is occupied by the cord. The blood supply to the cord is tenuous in this region, especially in the "critical zone" of T4–T9.[65] In addition, thoracic disc protrusions are more common centrally than laterally, are often calcified, and may adhere to or penetrate the dura.[3,12,16,20,23,66,67]

The theory of direct compression causing neural compromise is supported by the report by Logue[12] of a patient who died after a 14-month course of progressive paraplegia. The autopsy showed extreme distortion of the cord, but the anterior spinal artery and vein were patent and showed no evidence of damage. Kahn[68] suggested that, in addition to direct anterior compression by the herniated disc, the dentate ligaments may resist posterior displacement of the cord, leading to traction and distortion of neural structures.

Vascular insufficiency has been the explanation for unusual cases, such as cases with transitory paresis and instances in which the segmental level of involvement was higher than expected from the location of the herniated disc.[3,6] Significant neural deficits may be caused by herniations that appear too small to cause significant compression. This theory also helps explain patients who show no improvement after complete decompression and patients who had an abrupt onset of paraplegia in the presence of a chronic calcified disc. The theory is supported by patients in whom the disc herniation has been shown to cause anterior spinal artery thrombosis.[12]

Doppman and Girton[69] performed an angiographic study on animals on the effect of laminectomy in the presence of acute anterior epidural masses. They found that when decompression restored normal arteriovenous hemodynamics, the animals were neurologically intact despite significant cord distortion. When either the artery or the vein remained obstructed, however, the animals remained paraplegic.

Clinical Presentation

There is extreme variation in the clinical presentation of patients who have a herniated thoracic disc. This variation explains why no clear-cut syndrome has been identified. The signs and symptoms may depend on the location of herniation in the sagittal plane and transverse plane. Additional factors may include size of the lesion, duration of compression, degree of vascular compromise, size of the bony canal, and health of the spinal cord.

In symptomatic cases, the condition is dynamic and can progress.[9] Tovi and Strang[16] outlined the usual chronologic progression, which begins with thoracic pain followed by sensory disturbances, weakness, and finally bowel and bladder dysfunction. Arce and Dohrmann[20] confirmed this pattern in their review of the literature: of 179 patients who described their initial symptoms, 57% described pain, 24% described sensory disturbance, 17% described motor weakness, and 2% described bladder dysfunction (Table 45.1). By the time of presentation, 90% of the patients had signs and symptoms of cord compression, 61% had motor and sensory complaints, and 30% had bowel or bladder dysfunction (Table 45.2). The duration of symptoms before presentation ranged from hours to 16 years in one series.[3] In a report of 55 patients initially treated conservatively, Brown and colleagues[70] reported anterior bandlike chest pain as the most common early symptom in 67% of patients; lower extremity complaints were present in 20% of patients and ranged from paresthesia (4%) to frank muscle weakness (16%). Additional symptoms included intrascapular pain (8%) and epigastric pain (4%).

Thoracic pain can be midline, unilateral, or bilateral, depending on the location of the herniation. In some cases, there may be no pain. Coughing and sneezing may aggravate pain, as with herniated discs in the cervical and lumbar regions. With herniation of the T1 disc, the pain may be in the neck and upper extremity, and simulate a cervical disc problem, causing upper extremity numbness, intrinsic muscle weakness, and Horner syndrome.[5,26,71]

When the herniation is in the midthoracic spine, radiation of pain into the chest or abdomen can simulate cardiac or abdominal disease, clouding an already complex clinical

TABLE 45.1 Initial Symptoms of Protruded Thoracic Disc

Symptom	No. Patients (%)
Pain	102 (57)
Sensory	42 (24)
Motor	31 (17)
Bladder	4 (2)

From Arce CA, Dohrmann GJ. Herniated thoracic disks. *Neurol Clin.* 1985;3:383–392.

TABLE 45.2 Presenting Features of Thoracic Disc Herniation

Feature	No. Patients (%)
Motor and sensory signs and symptoms	131 (61)
Brown-Séquard syndrome	18 (9)
Sensory signs and symptoms only	33 (15)
Motor signs and symptoms only	13 (6)
Radicular pain only	20 (9)
Bladder or sphincter features	65 (30)

From Arce CA, Dohrmann GJ. Herniated thoracic disks. *Neurol Clin.* 1985;3:383–392.

picture. In the four cases reported by Epstein,[7] one patient underwent an unnecessary thoracotomy for excision of a pericardial cyst, hysterectomy and salpingo-oophorectomy were performed in another patient, and a third patient almost underwent an abdominal exploration for endometriosis before the true cause of her symptoms was identified. Pain from a lower thoracic disc herniation may radiate to the groin or flank and simulate ureteral calculi or renal disease.[62,72,73] Abdominal wall paresis and abdominal hernia have also been presenting signs for thoracic disc herniations.[74,75] Herniated discs at the lowest thoracic levels can impinge on the cauda equina and on the distal spinal cord, causing lower extremity pain or weakness and mimic a herniated lumbar disc.[76,77] On physical examination, flexion of the neck may induce back or root pain with lesions below the midthoracic level.[25] A thorough neurologic examination is mandatory; the examiner should pay close attention to long tract signs and other evidence of myelopathy. Cases of unexplained abdominal pain or lower extremity complaints with normal abdominal and lumbar imaging should be evaluated for the possibility of thoracic disc herniation.[78,79]

Some investigators believe that the occurrence of pronounced sensory changes with relatively minor motor deficits is highly suggestive of a herniated thoracic disc.[25,80] Sensory disturbances, motor weakness, sphincter dysfunction, and gait abnormalities should direct the examiner's attention to the nervous system as the source of the problem.

Level and Classification of Herniation

Three-fourths of cases occur between T8 and L1; the peak is at T11–T12, where 26% to 50% of herniations occur (Fig. 45.2).[20,40] Herniations are uncommon in the upper thoracic spine.[20,26,71] Haley and Perry[57] found a similar distribution in their cadaveric study of 99 spines and theorized that the increased incidence in the thoracolumbar area is due to the greater degree of motion in this region. The reason that the incidence at T11–T12 is greater than that at T12–L1 (9%) may be the facet orientation. Malmivaara and colleagues[81] believed that the coronally oriented facets in the upper thoracolumbar region have less torsional resistance than the sagittally oriented facets at T12–L1; thus, the T11–T12 disc is exposed to greater stress and has a high likelihood of degeneration.

Herniated thoracic discs can be classified by location or by symptoms. Most authors describe the location of the herniation as central, centrolateral, or lateral, and roughly 70% of the cases are either central or centrolateral.[20,60] In a comparison of characteristics on CT myelography of asymptomatic and symptomatic herniated thoracic discs, Awwad and colleagues[60] reported that 90% of herniations were central or parasagittal versus lateral in asymptomatic patients, whereas 80% were central or parasagittal in symptomatic patients. No identifiable radiographic features could reliably classify a herniated thoracic disc as symptomatic or asymptomatic. Abbott and Retter[5] classified cases by symptoms and reported that lateral protrusions cause root compression, and that patients have radicular

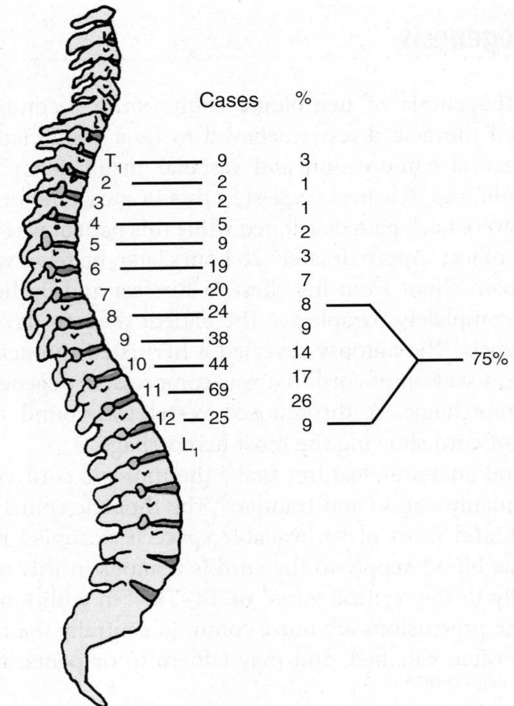

FIG. 45.2 Levels of thoracic disc protrusion in 280 cases. (From Arce CA, Dohrmann GJ. Herniated thoracic disks. *Neurol Clin.* 1985;3:383–392.)

pain and minimal or no signs of cord compression. Patients with central disc herniation in the upper and middle thoracic spine can have signs of myelopathy caused by spinal cord compression. Protrusions at T11 and T12 compress the conus medullaris and cauda equina, and may cause pain referred to the lower limbs and sphincter disturbance.

Few cases of intradural herniation of thoracic discs have been reported, suggesting that the incidence is low.[3,8,16,26,82–86] Love and Schorn[3] reported a series of 61 cases in which seven (11%) showed disc erosion through the anterior dura. In a review of the literature, Epstein and colleagues[83] noted that 5% of all intradural disc herniations were found in the thoracic spine. Similar to the cervical spine, the low incidence was attributed to the lack of significant dural adhesions of the thoracic dura to the posterior longitudinal ligament and anulus fibrosus. Patients with intradural thoracic disc herniations tended to present with a higher incidence of Brown-Séquard syndromes and paraplegia.[44] In most cases, the presence of an intradural thoracic disc herniation is not identified preoperatively. CT myelography seems to have a higher sensitivity to detect this than MRI even with the addition of gadolinium.[82]

The exact incidence of multilevel herniations is unknown.[5,14,35,87] Arseni and Nash[6] reviewed the literature in 1960 and found multiple herniations in only 4 of 106 cases reported. A report by Bohlman and Zdeblick[35] suggested, however, that the incidence may be much higher than previously recognized. Of their 19 patients, three (16%) had herniations at two levels. The sensitivity of MRI may be partially responsible for this increased frequency.[37,39] Ross and colleagues[39] reported that three of 13 patients (23%) whose herniation was diagnosed by MRI had multilevel involvement; Wood and colleagues[42] reported multiple disc herniations in 39% of asymptomatic volunteers that were diagnosed by MRI. These rates are similar to the findings in the autopsy study by Haley and Perry,[57] in which two of seven patients had more than one protruded disc.

Van Landingham[64] suggested an association between Scheuermann disease and multilevel herniation. Wood and colleagues[42] noted that endplate changes consistent with Scheuermann disease were more prevalent in the group with thoracic pain and disc herniation than in the asymptomatic population. Conversely, Lesoin and colleagues[54] reported six cases of single-level herniations only in patients with Scheuermann disease, suggesting a lack of significant association with multiple herniations.

Natural History

There are few long-term reports of untreated adults with herniated thoracic discs. In 1992, Brown and colleagues[70] reported a 2-year follow-up on 55 patients found to have thoracic disc herniation on MRI and concurrent pain; 11 (20%) initially had lower extremity complaints. Initial treatment in 54 patients included bed rest; nonsteroidal antiinflammatory drugs; and controlled physical therapy involving hyperextension strengthening, postural training, and body mechanics education. Ultimately, 15 patients (27%) underwent operation. Of the remaining 40 patients treated nonoperatively, 31 (78%) returned to their prior level of activity. Nine of the 11 patients presenting with lower extremity complaints of pain or weakness underwent operation; 55% of herniated discs in the operative group were at or below T9. In contrast, 48% of the discs in the nonoperative group were at T6–T9.

In patients with lower extremity complaints, the natural history of the disorder is typically one of progression, and nearly all patients eventually undergo operation for progressive neurologic deficit or unremitting pain.[3,11] The most characteristic chronologic progression of symptoms is pain followed by sensory disturbance, weakness, and bowel and bladder dysfunction.[16] The course can be extremely variable, however, and it is unknown whether neurologic signs or symptoms ever would have developed in patients operated on for pain alone. Some patients might have improved spontaneously if not subjected to surgical treatment. Haro and colleagues[88] reported on two patients with acute onset of symptomatic thoracic disc herniation with signs of myelopathy that resolved without surgery. Both patients had lower extremity signs of myelopathy, but neither developed bowel or bladder dysfunction or progressive motor weakness. Treatment with steroids and prostaglandin E_1 led to resolution of symptoms and resorption of thoracic disc herniation on follow-up MRI scans.

Arseni and Nash[6] described two general patterns for the time course of symptoms. The first, which occurs in younger patients with a history of trauma, is backache that can be followed by a rapidly evolving myelopathy. In the second pattern, which typically occurs in patients past middle age who have degenerative disc disease without any significant trauma, signs and symptoms of cord compression develop slowly and progressively. Tovi and Strang[16] found that when the first symptom to develop was unilateral, the course tended to be one of slow progression with periods of stabilization and occasional slight remission. Rapid, irreversible progression generally was noted in cases with a bilateral onset.

Calcification of the disc in children is considered to be a painful but self-limited process, with eventual resolution of the pain and resorption of the calcified deposit. It generally occurs in the cervical spine. About half of cases are preceded by a history of trauma (30%) or upper respiratory tract infection.[89,90] The natural history of herniated calcified thoracic discs in children was reviewed by Nicolau and colleagues.[91] The course was similar to cases without herniation; the patients improved spontaneously as the calcified fragment resorbed. The progression is not always benign, however. Two cases in children have been reported in which myelopathy developed from cord compression and required operation.[13,67]

Disc calcification in adults differs from that in children. The thoracolumbar spine is the most frequent site of calcification, and the condition is generally asymptomatic unless herniation of the disc occurs.[89] The deposits may accelerate degeneration by interfering in the biomechanics and nutrition of the disc.[89,92] Disc calcification is found on routine radiographs in 4% to 6% of patients without disc herniation compared with up to 70% of patients with disc prolapse.[12,89] The natural history of disc herniation in adults has not been conclusively shown to be altered by disc calcification.

Differential Diagnosis

Love and Schorn[3] reported that before myelography the correct diagnosis was made in 13 of 61 patients and was considered in the differential diagnosis in only 7 others; even after myelography, the correct diagnosis was made preoperatively in only 56% of patients. With greater awareness of the diagnosis and improved imaging techniques now available, the correct diagnosis should be made before operation in almost all cases.

The differential diagnosis of back pain includes spinal tumors, infection, ankylosing spondylitis, fracture, intercostal neuralgia, herpes zoster, and cervical and lumbar herniated discs. Diseases of the thoracic and abdominal viscera may have a similar presentation. Neurosis is another possibility. The differential diagnosis of myelopathy includes demyelinating and degenerative processes of the central nervous system (CNS), such as multiple sclerosis and amyotrophic lateral sclerosis.[93,94] Intraspinal tumors, brain tumors, and cerebrovascular accidents also should be considered.[20,63]

In patients who have a neurologic deficit and radiographic evidence of Scheuermann disease, the differential diagnosis includes an extradural cyst or compression from an angular kyphosis.[54,95] In the series by Lesoin and colleagues,[54] the mean age of the patients who had a herniated thoracic disc in association with Scheuermann disease was 44 years, similar to the population without Scheuermann disease. This is in contrast to a mean age of 17 years in three patients in whom neurologic compromise developed secondary to bony cord compression at the apex of the kyphosis.[95]

Diagnostic Evaluation

Spine Radiographs

Plain radiographs of the spine generally are diagnostic only if they show disc calcification. The calcified disc is not always the one that is herniated, but the association at least suggests the diagnosis.[3,96] A calcified disc in the canal is pathognomonic of disc herniation.[12,27,28,96] Baker and colleagues[96] identified two radiographic patterns of calcification (Fig. 45.3). One consisted of extensive calcification posteriorly in the interspace and bulging into the canal. The other pattern, which is subtle and often overlooked initially, is a small nidus just posterior to the narrowed interspace. Studies[35,59] of adult lumbar discs have shown that the deposits may be calcium pyrophosphate dihydrate or calcium hydroxyapatite. The clinical significance of the different radiographic patterns or chemical compositions has not been determined.

The proposed association between Scheuermann disease and herniated thoracic discs has been discussed previously. A patient found to have kyphosis with vertebral body wedging and endplate irregularity in association with back pain or a neurologic deficit should undergo other studies to eliminate the possibility of a herniated disc. Other radiographic findings, such as narrowing and hypertrophic changes, are nonspecific and are not helpful in the diagnosis.[3,12,96]

Myelography

The thoracic spine is difficult to image by myelography because of the thoracic kyphosis and superimposition of mediastinal structures. Myelography alone is diagnostic in only 56% of cases and has a false-negative rate of 8%.[3] A complete block is found in 10% to 15% of cases.[16,96] Myelography is performed by injecting water-soluble contrast agent in the lumbosacral canal, removing the spinal needle, and placing the patient supine so that the contrast agent pools in the dependent thoracic kyphosis.[36] Anteroposterior and lateral films are essential. A herniated disc appears as a central filling defect at the level of the disc space (Fig. 45.4). Central protrusions produce discrete oval or round filling defects. In large protrusions, a complete block occurs with a blunt, convex leading edge.[12,96] Lateral discs produce triangular or semicircular indentations with displacement of the cord to the opposite side (Fig. 45.5).[96] Evaluation of cerebrospinal fluid (CSF) at the time of myelography is nonspecific.[9] The protein content is increased in less than 50% of patients and helps only to focus attention on the central nervous system. It generally is in the range of 50 to 100 mg/dL but may be greater than 400 mg/dL.[53] Currently, myelography is most helpful in localizing lesions to allow directed CT and in preparation for operation.[35,97]

Computed Tomography

Enhanced CT after myelography with a water-soluble contrast agent is an extremely valuable technique, which has been the diagnostic standard (Fig. 45.6).[35,36,39,44,50,60] When combined with standard myelography, CT not only improves sensitivity and accuracy, but also detects intradural penetration of the disc.[44,83]

CT alone may be helpful when the disc is calcified (Fig. 45.7), but it is not as sensitive as CT with intrathecal injection of a contrast agent.[65] The criterion for diagnosis of a herniated disc by CT is a focal extension of the disc beyond the posterior aspect of the vertebral body with spinal cord compression or displacement.[39]

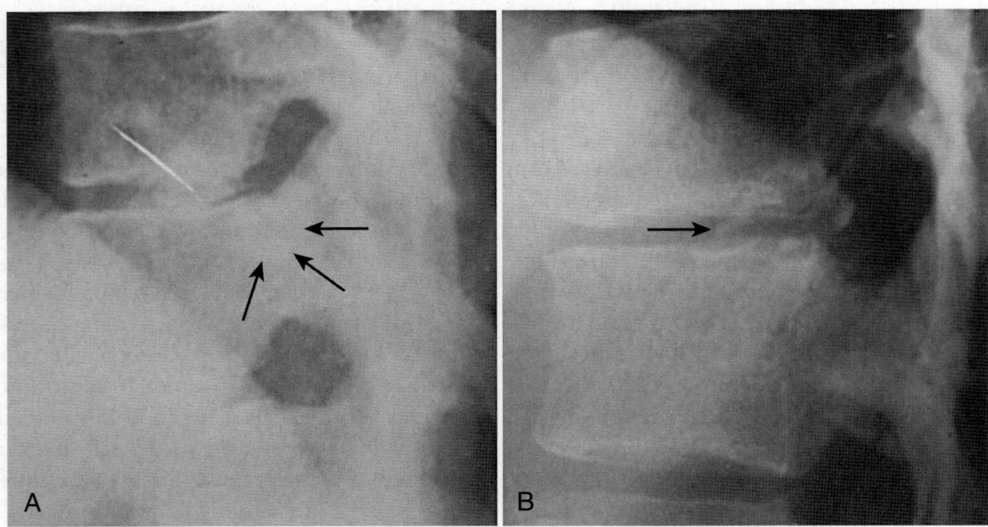

FIG. 45.3 Plain radiographs can be used to diagnose herniated discs only when calcification is seen within the spinal canal. (A) Large calcified disc within canal (*arrows*) is nearly obscured by overlying ribs (see Figs. 45.7 and 45.8, respectively for computed tomographic and magnetic resonance images from the same patient). (B) Tiny nidus of calcium is visible in the canal posterior to the narrowed 11th interspace (*arrow*).

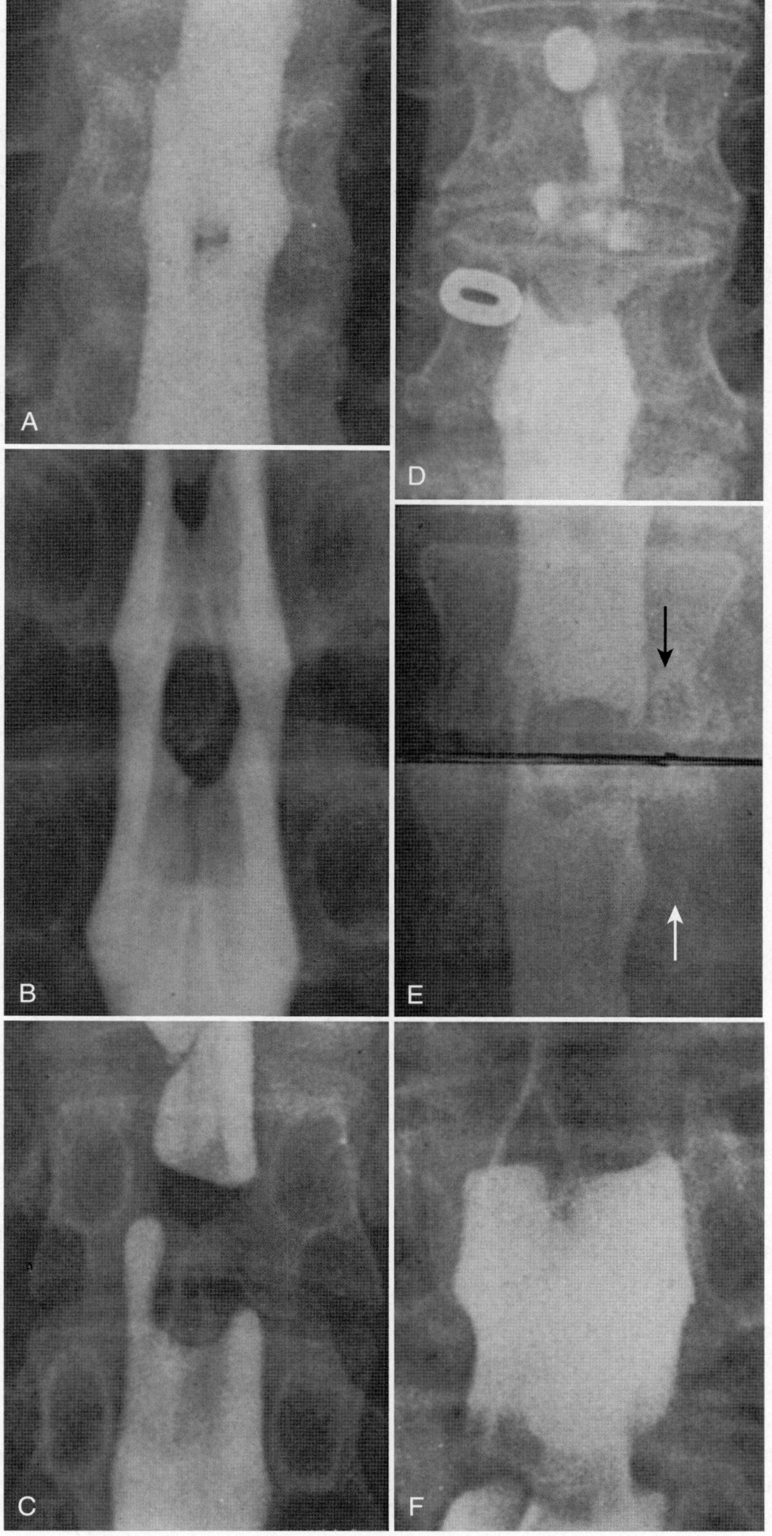

FIG. 45.4 Oval filling defects in the opaque column of an iophendylate (Pantopaque) myelogram resulting from central protruded thoracic discs. Note the midline position of the spinal cord in all cases. (A) Tiny protrusion visible at the T9 interspace. (B) Small protrusion at T12. (C) Moderately large, slightly obstructing protrusion at T12. (D) Large, severely obstructing protrusion at T12. (E) Upper margin was outlined only when oil flowed caudad (*arrows*). (F) Completely obstructing protrusion at T12. Note the blunt, convex leading edge of column. (From Baker HL Jr, Love JG, Uihlein A. Roentgenologic features of protruded thoracic intervertebral disks. *Radiology.* 1965;84:1059–1065.)

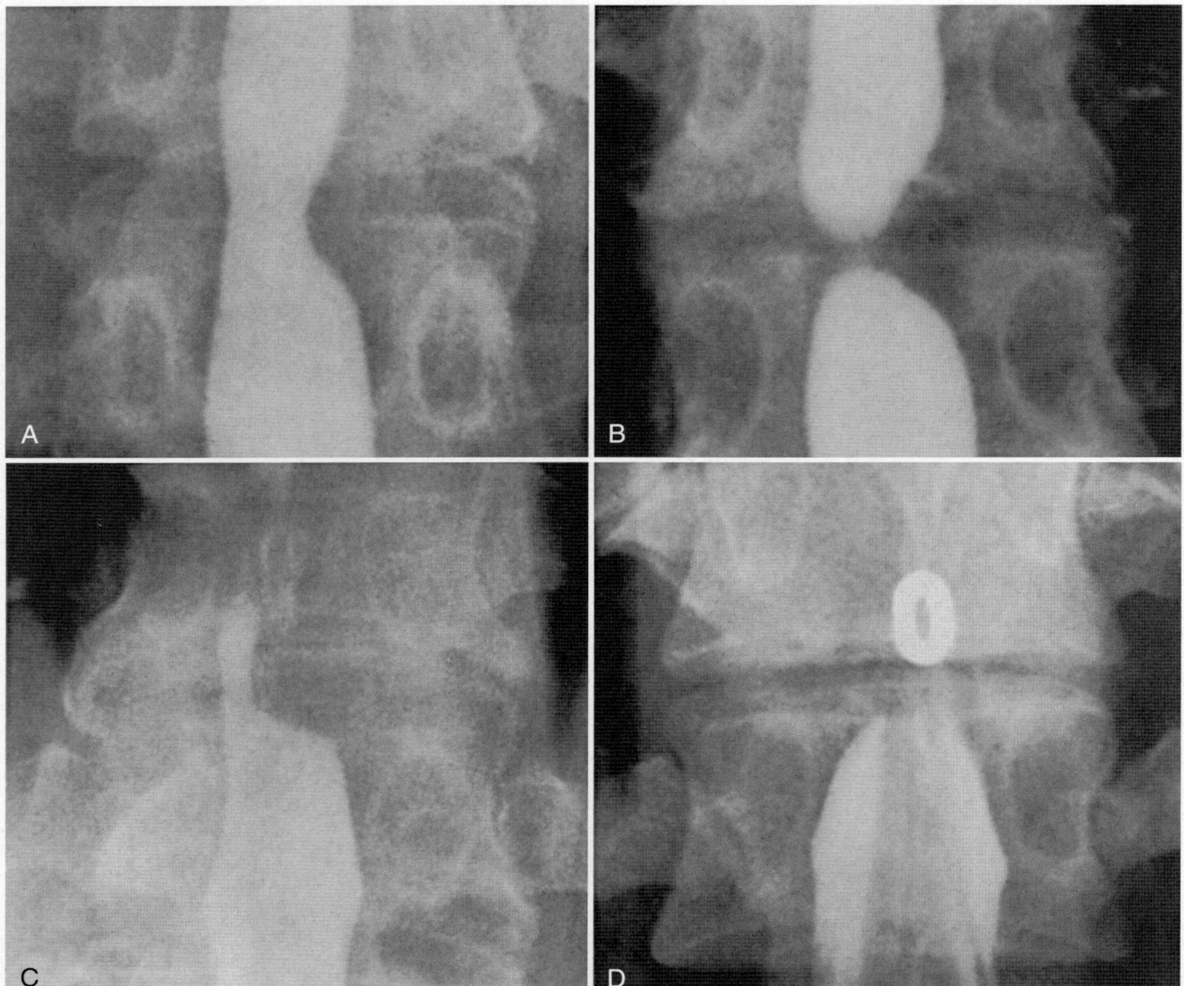

FIG. 45.5 Filling defects in the opaque column of an iophendylate (Pantopaque) myelogram resulting from a lateral protruded thoracic disc. Note the lateral displacement of the spinal cord in several cases. (A) Small lateral protrusion at T11. (B) Moderately large, slightly obstructing protrusion at T10. (C) Large obstructing protrusion at T9. (D) Completely obstructing protrusion at T10. Note the pointing of the column and deviation of the spinal cord to the left. (From Baker HL Jr, Love JG, Uihlein A. Roentgenologic features of protruded thoracic intervertebral disks. *Radiology.* 1965;84:1059–1065.)

Magnetic Resonance Imaging

MRI has revolutionized the diagnostic evaluation of thoracic disc disease. Most centers rely on MRI almost exclusively, but others still perform myelography and CT when operative treatment is being considered.[35–37] MRI is a rapid, noninvasive outpatient procedure that does not use ionizing radiation and causes no morbidity. It is a sensitive and specific technique that makes it easy to obtain sagittal sections of the entire thoracic spine.[36,37,39] Findings on MRI are similar to findings of myelography and CT, but it is necessary to use information from sagittal T1-weighted and T2-weighted and axial T1-weighted images to achieve similar sensitivity (Fig. 45.8).[39]

MRI is a highly technical procedure; the expertise of the radiologist and the design of the scanner determine the accuracy of the test to a great degree. There are pitfalls of MRI, such as partial volume averaging (owing to the relatively large section thickness), the CSF flow void sign (regions of low signal intensity within the fluid owing to its pulsatile motion), signal dropout from calcified discs, chemical shift artifacts from marrow fat, and mismapped signal from cardiac motion.[36,39,98] Addition of gadolinium as a contrast agent has been reported to help in differentiating between thoracic disc herniations and small meningiomas; herniated disc material does not enhance, whereas spinal meningiomas show a very early, homogeneous, and intense uptake of contrast agent.[38]

Despite improved imaging and increased sensitivity, findings of thoracic disc herniation on MRI must be interpreted with caution and closely correlated with clinical findings. Several reports noted significant disc protrusion and spinal cord deformation in 30% of asymptomatic individuals.[42,60] In their large MRI series, Wood and colleagues[42] noted that the overall prevalence of thoracic disc herniation in the group with thoracic pain was not significantly different from the asymptomatic population.

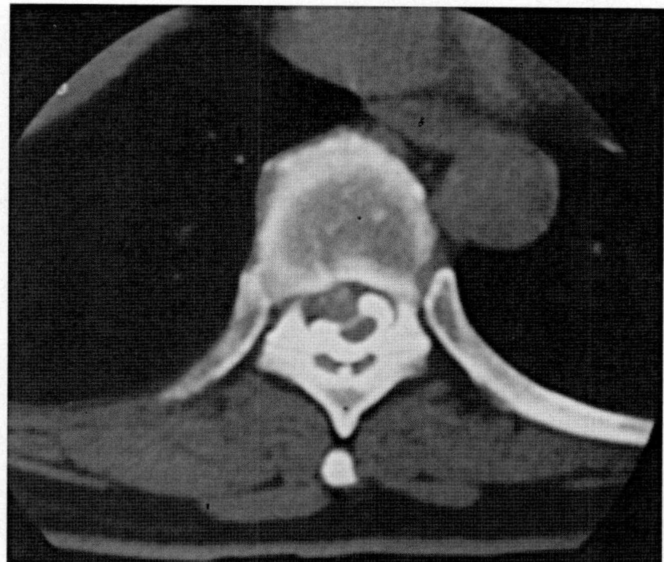

FIG. 45.6 Postmyelography computed tomographic scan showing a large, right centrolateral herniated disc at T8–T9.

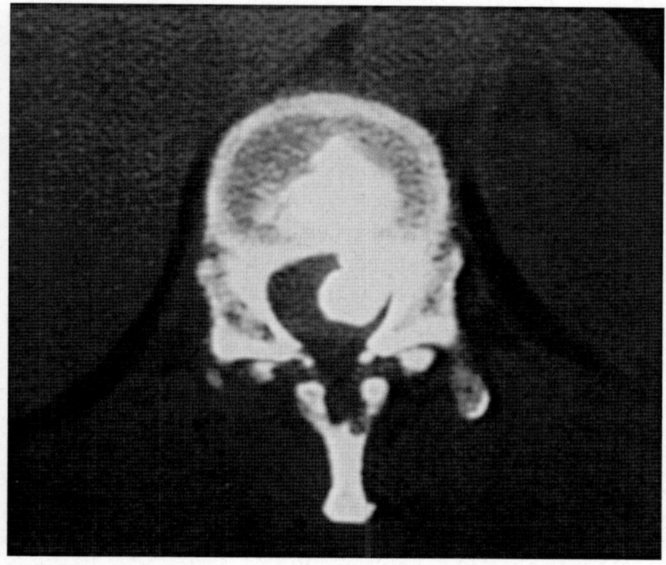

FIG. 45.7 Computed tomographic scan showing calcification of a centrolateral herniated thoracic disc.

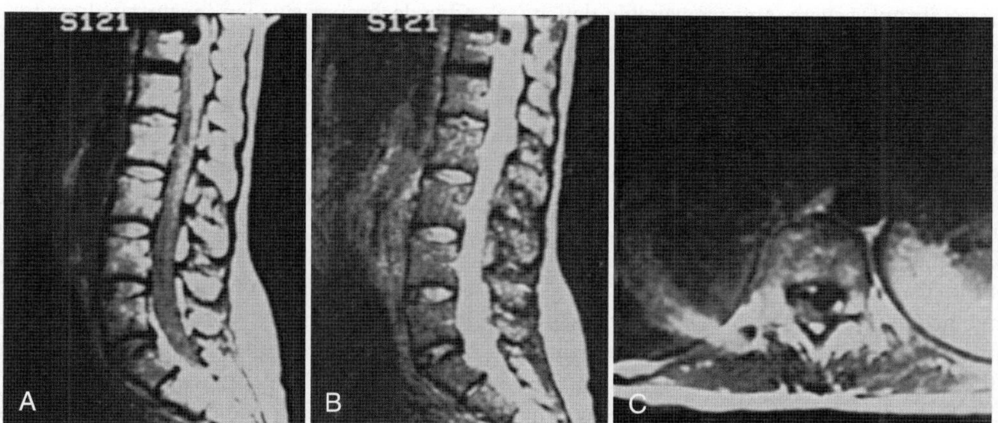

FIG. 45.8 Magnetic resonance image of the same patient in Fig. 45.7 showing a large, calcified, herniated thoracic disc at T11–T12. (A) T1-weighted sagittal image. (B) T2-weighted sagittal image. (C) T1-weighted axial image.

Discography

The general sensitivity but lack of specificity of thoracic MRI in diagnosing painful thoracic disc disease sometimes may require the supplemental use of provocative discography to identify a specific thoracic disc pain source. In a retrospective review, Schellhas and colleagues[99] showed thoracic discography as a safe and reliable technique.

In a controlled prospective study, Wood and colleagues[100] compared MRI and discography in asymptomatic and symptomatic individuals. In asymptomatic volunteers, the mean pain response with discography was 2.4 out of 10. On discography, 27 of 40 discs were abnormal, with endplate irregularities, annular tears, or herniations. Ten discs read as initially normal on MRI showed annular pathology on discography. In symptomatic patients with chronic thoracic pain, the pain response with discography was 6.3 out of 10. Of the 49 discs studied in this group, 55% had a concordant pain response, 39% had a discordant pain response, and 6% had no pain. On MRI, 21 of 49 discs appeared normal; however, on discography, only 10 were judged as normal. The only correlative pathology seemed to be Scheuermann endplate pathology, as seen on MRI, and Schmorl nodes as seen on discography.

In a systematic review of the literature, Buenaventura and colleagues[101] reported there is limited evidence to support the role of discography for the diagnosis of chronic thoracic discogenic pain. Given the general prevalence of degenerative thoracic disc pathology in asymptomatic individuals, discography apparently should be reserved for individuals with interdiscal pathology on MRI and thoracic axial pain unresponsive to an appropriate duration of nonsurgical treatment. Additionally, results from discography can be highly variable based on the examiner. Consideration should be given to the possibility of needle penetration by discography and deleterious effects from the contrast agent leading to progressive degenerative changes as reported clinically in the lumbar spine as well as in vitro studies.[102,103]

Treatment

The majority of thoracic disc herniations remain asymptomatic and are even considered a normal incidental finding. In these cases, observation is the treatment of choice. Indications for surgery include (1) progressive myelopathy, (2) lower extremity weakness or paralysis, (3) bowel or bladder dysfunction, and (4) radicular pain refractory to conservative measures. Brown and colleagues[70] reported that 77% of patients with radicular pain as the primary presentation improved after a course of physical therapy. In cases of radicular presentation only, some authors believe that if the protrusion is far lateral with nerve root compression only, the situation is not urgent, and the decision to operate should be based on the degree of pain.[7] Conversely, there have been reports of lateral lesions causing severe neurologic deficits from compression of a major medullary feeder vessel.[55] Small herniations also should be respected because abrupt, severe, and irreversible deficits can occur. Some investigators have concluded that there is no relationship between the size of the herniation and the gravity of the clinical picture.[11,27]

In cases of myelopathy and lower extremity involvement, most authors recommend early decompression. In cases of late treatment, favorable results are still possible despite significant delays and the presence of major neurologic deficits.[35] A less aggressive approach may be taken in children because the natural history of the disorder seems to be different.[91]

The surgical management of this disorder has evolved in recent years. Laminectomy with disc excision was the benchmark approach 30 years ago, but has been abandoned because of the risk of neurologic deterioration (Fig. 45.9). After the introduction of alternative techniques of decompression, Ravichandran and Frankel[104] noted a significant decrease in admission to spinal cord injury centers of patients with paralysis after treatment of herniated thoracic discs. In a review of 135 cases, Arce and Dohrmann[20] found that after laminectomy 58% of the patients were improved, 10% were unchanged, 28% were worse, and 4% had died. There is also evidence that patients who do not improve or who are made worse by laminectomy are less likely to be helped by later anterior decompression.[93] The best results are achieved in patients who have lateral lesions above T11, who have minimal neurologic deficits, who have a soft disc, and who are operated on early after the onset of symptoms.[3,7,16,23,84,105,106]

Patients with myelopathy caused by ossification of the posterior longitudinal ligament have worse rates of recovery.[105] Although laminectomy is still occasionally advocated for lateral lesions, most authors think that the procedure is contraindicated.[28,107] Singounas and Karvounis[108] described good results in patients treated by decompressive laminectomy alone without attempted disc removal. Several studies[8,12] described disastrous results with this technique, however. Studies in animals found consistent neurologic deterioration after decompressive laminectomy alone for anterior epidural masses.[69,109]

Costotransversectomy is an effective technique for managing herniated thoracic discs (Fig. 45.10).[10,45,110] Disc excision is performed through a paramedian incision with the patient prone[10] or in a modified lateral decubitus position.[110] The paraspinal muscles are either retracted medially or split transversely.[10,45] The posterior portion of each rib on the side of the herniated disc is excised, and the pleura is mobilized and reflected anterolaterally. The transverse processes and remaining head and neck of each excised rib are removed. The intervertebral foramen is located by tracing the intercostal nerve medially. The foramen is enlarged by partial removal of the corresponding pedicles, and the dural sac is exposed. A

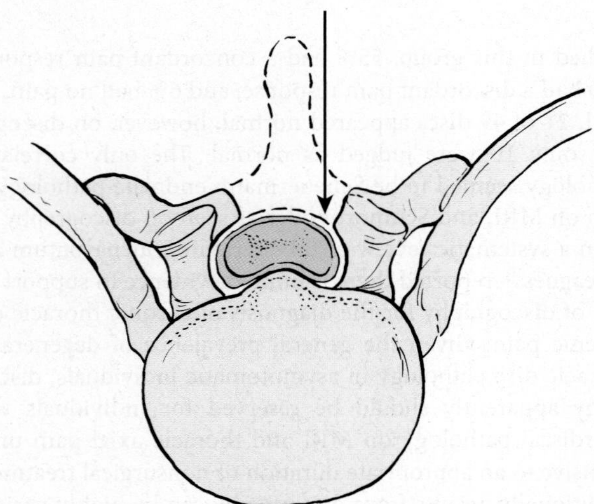

FIG. 45.9 Attempted decompression by laminectomy would require manipulation of the cord and a high risk of neurologic deterioration.

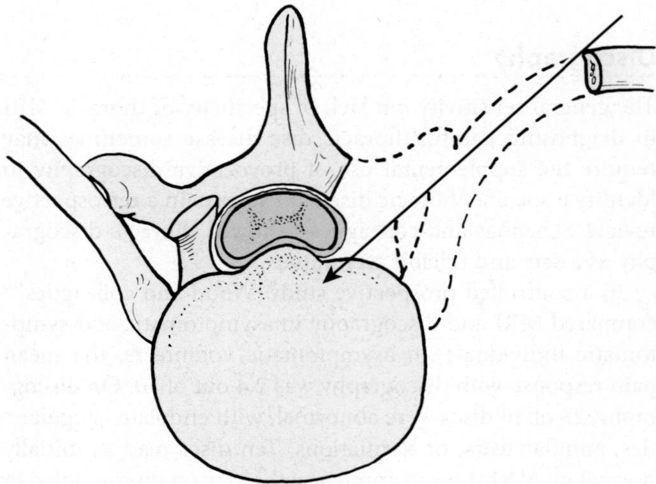

FIG. 45.10 Decompression by costotransversectomy is possible without manipulation of the cord.

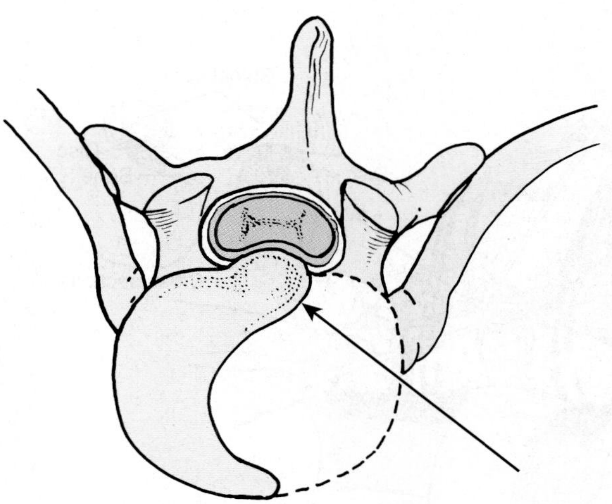

FIG. 45.11 Transthoracic decompression allows the most direct approach to the lesion without manipulation of the cord.

cavity is created in the posterior aspect of the bodies and disc, allowing gentle removal of disc fragments through the defect without manipulation of the spinal cord.[10,45,111,112]

Transthoracic spinal cord decompression has been shown to be a viable alternative to costotransversectomy (Fig. 45.11).[23,24] Advantages include a more direct approach to the lesion and better visualization, facilitating excision of central herniations and herniations with intradural penetration. Disadvantages of the procedure include the potential complications associated with a thoracotomy.

Although many complications have been described after thoracotomy for other disorders, few have been reported after discectomy.[20,23,24,35,46,93,113,114] The results of transthoracic decompression are similar to results of costotransversectomy. In 53 cases collected from the literature, 52 patients improved, and 1 was unchanged. Bohlman and Zdeblick[35] reported the outcome in 19 patients treated by costotransversectomy or transthoracic decompression. The two poor outcomes in their series were in cases treated by costotransversectomy. They concluded that the transthoracic approach with its superior exposure was the preferred procedure. Lubelski and collegues compared results of the lateral extracavitary versus costotransversectomy approaches to the thoracic spine and found similar rates of complications, but slightly increased rates of blood loss and hospital stay with the more invasive extracavitary approach.[115]

Some authors[23,24,49,84,116] recommended preoperative angiography to determine the location of the artery of Adamkiewicz and other major medullary feeder vessels. If such a vessel is found at the level of the disc herniation, the spine could be approached from the opposite side. Alternatively, by carefully avoiding dissection in the neural foramina, this problem can be obviated without the need for an arteriogram. There is generally abundant collateral circulation in the region of the neural foramina that provides blood flow to the cord even with ligation of the artery of Adamkiewicz.[65,117,118] We routinely ligate the segmental vessels adjacent to the herniated disc midway between the foramina and the aorta, and have not observed any untoward effects (Fig. 45.12).[93]

The patient is placed in the lateral decubitus position. A lateral prolapse is best approached from the ipsilateral side; a midline herniation may be approached from either side. In the upper or middle thoracic spine, the right side has the advantage of avoiding the great vessels and the heart. There also is statistically less risk to the artery of Adamkiewicz because this vessel is on the left in approximately 80% of patients.[65] When the herniation is in the lower thoracic spine, a left thoracotomy is preferred because it is easier to mobilize the aorta than the vena cava, and the liver does not crowd the field.[23,35]

The level of rib resection is chosen to give the most direct access to the affected disc (see Fig. 45.12A). A horizontal line drawn on a chest radiograph from the disc space to the chest wall intersects the rib that should be resected. This is generally one to two ribs above the affected disc in the middle and lower thoracic spine.[84] In the upper thoracic spine, the exposure is limited by the scapula; it is generally necessary to excise the fifth or sixth rib, then work craniad.

The recommended extent of bone and disc removal varies from a relatively small trough in the posterior aspect of the disc to complete discectomy with partial corpectomy of the adjacent bodies (see Fig. 45.12B).[23,28,35,84,93] We believe that the latter approach is safer because it provides the greatest degree of visualization and allows complete discectomy without disturbing the foraminal vessels. In either case, great care is taken to perform the decompression without any manipulation or pressure to the spinal cord.

Fusion is indicated when stability is compromised by the decompression and in cases associated with Scheuermann disease.[45] When only a small amount of bone and disc is excised, fusion generally is not recommended.[23,28,35,84] Conversely, with complete discectomy, fusion is mandatory (see Fig. 45.12C). In addition to providing stability, fusion may limit local pain secondary to motion of the degenerated segment. Recurrence of thoracic disc herniation has not been reported, but complete discectomy and fusion theoretically is the best way to prevent this complication. At the conclusion of the procedure, a chest tube is placed and attached to waterseal suction. If fusion has been performed, a thoracolumbosacral orthosis brace should be used.

Otani and colleagues[49] described a modification of the transthoracic procedure in which the pleura is dissected away from the chest wall after rib excision. This modification allows the approach to be entirely extrapleural. Their results were similar to results in other series of transthoracic decompressions. The advantage of the technique is the avoidance of a chest tube postoperatively. Claims of a lower incidence of pulmonary complications may be more theoretical than real because few such complications have been reported, but the reduction in pain caused by the chest tube is a definite advantage.

A posterolateral approach was described by Carson and colleagues[25] in 1971 (Fig. 45.13). They performed a complete laminectomy of the vertebrae adjacent to the herniated disc combined with a medial facetectomy and excision of the transverse process. A T-shaped incision through the erector

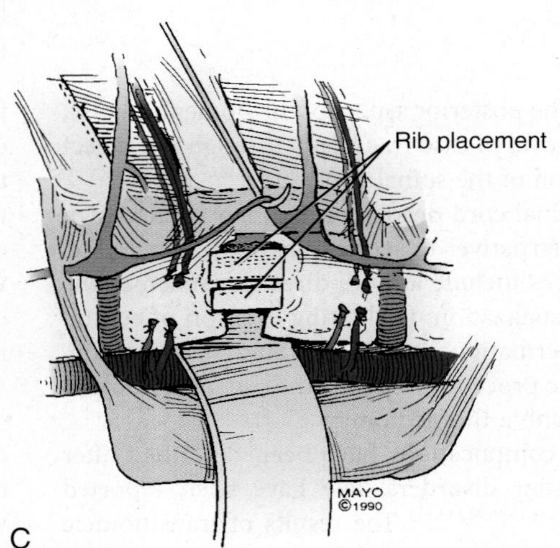

FIG. 45.12 (A) Exposure provided by the transthoracic approach. The great vessels are mobilized by ligation of the segmental vessels midway between the aorta and neural foramina. A malleable retractor may be placed for protection of the great vessels. (B) Complete discectomy and partial corpectomy of adjacent vertebral bodies provides excellent visualization and allows complete decompression without disturbance of collateral vessels within the neural foramina. (C) Fusion is indicated when stability is compromised by decompression. (Courtesy the Mayo Foundation.)

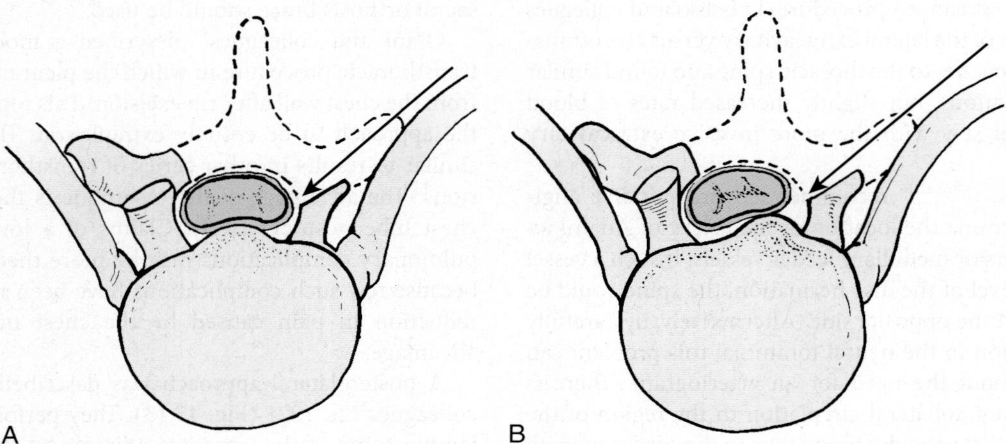

FIG. 45.13 Posterolateral decompression. (A) Removal of central herniation would require some manipulation of the cord. (B) Lateral herniations may be approached by this technique without manipulation of the cord.

muscle of the spine allowed an oblique approach to the anterior epidural space. Patterson and Arbit[26] modified the approach in 1978 to include the removal of the facet and pedicle of the vertebra caudal to the protruded disc through a straight midline incision. The central portion of the disc is removed by creating a cavity. The protruded material is excised by reduction of disc and bone into the cavity before removal. After anterior decompression, a complete laminectomy can be performed. Le Roux and colleagues[53] reported the results of the transpedicular approach and use of the operative microscope in 20 patients; all patients symptomatically improved postoperatively, 40% became asymptomatic, and no complications were noted.

Lesoin and colleagues[27] reported good results with a slightly more extensive exposure in which the transverse process, articular facets, and portions of the adjacent pedicles are removed. The extent of bone removal requires that a fusion be performed; these authors recommended unilateral Harrington rod instrumentation. Spinal deformity has been reported to occur after posterolateral decompression without fusion.[15] In the 45 cases in the literature, 40 patients noted improvement (89%), the condition was unchanged in 3 patients, and it was worse in 1 patient; 1 patient died.[30] Some authors claim that intradural disc herniation can be dealt with much more easily with this approach than with any other; however, approaching anterior dural erosion by this technique requires some degree of manipulation of the cord.[99]

Zhuang and collegues[119] reported on a posterior transfacet approach to thoracic disc herniations. A complete laminectomy was performed, and bilateral facet joints were removed. The disc was exposed and removed bilaterally through the intervertebral foramen. The anterior thecal sac was released posterior to the longitudinal ligament and anulus with a down-biting curette. The superior and inferior portions of the vertebral bodies were then removed as needed with an L-shaped osteotome to allow access to central calcified thoracic discs. This remaining portion of the disc could then be safely removed with down-biting curettes. This technique was performed on 27 patients with excellent recovery in 12 patients, good in 6, fair in 5, and unchanged in 1. No patients were worse postoperatively.

Other, less common approaches have also been described for upper thoracic disc herniations. Ulivieri and colleagues[120] described a transmanubrial osteomuscular-sparing approach for T1–T2 disc herniations. A transvertebral herniotomy has also been reported for a T2–T3 lesion.[121]

Video-Assisted Thoracoscopic Surgery

The continuing evolution of VATS has provided experienced surgeons an alternative approach for thoracic disc herniation decompression. The VATS technique was first described by Mack and colleagues[122] in 1993 for the drainage of thoracic paravertebral abscess. In 1994, Horowitz and colleagues[123] reported the clinical application of VATS for the treatment of thoracic disc herniation. Subsequently, several authors reported larger clinical series documenting the outcome of VATS-treated thoracic disc herniation.[1,19,30–32,56,124–126]

Reported advantages of VATS include reduced perioperative morbidity from minimal surgical dissection and avoidance of rib resection or spreading, enhanced visualization for the operating surgeons and support team, reduced postoperative pain with improved ventilatory excursion, shorter hospitalization and rehabilitation, and consequent decreased overall medical costs.[1,26] Disadvantages of VATS include the required coordination of two operative surgeons, an acquired technical skill set with a steep learning curve, specialized thoracoscopic instrumentation, and the required deflation of the ipsilateral lung for the procedure to be successful.

Indications for VATS application for thoracic disc herniation are similar to the indications for the anterior thoracic approach. The procedure can be performed in patients ranging in age from pediatric to geriatric. The minimally invasive nature of the VATS approach and consequent reduced postoperative pain and inspiratory splinting make this approach applicable in patients less able to tolerate the physiologic effects of open thoracotomy, such as patients with chronic obstructive pulmonary disease or interstitial fibrosis. Patients with contraindications for VATS include patients intolerant of single-lung ventilation and patients with severe or acute respiratory insufficiency, high airway pressures with positive-pressure ventilation, and pleural scarring. Relative contraindications include previous tube thoracostomy or previous thoracotomy. For technical details of the VATS technique, see Chapter 25.

In addition to numerous case reports, several authors have reported on large series of thoracic disc herniation treated by VATS.[30,32,56,124,125] In 1998, Regan and colleagues[32] reported their preliminary experience in 29 patients. Mean operative time was 175 minutes. The surgical complication rate was 14%, primarily from intercostal neuralgia and atelectasis. At 1-year follow-up, 76% of patients related satisfactory results; 24% of patients reported dissatisfaction or no change.

In a further extension of their series, Anand and Regan[30] reported outcomes on 100 consecutive cases with minimal 2-year follow-up. In 100 patients, 117 discs were excised; 40 patients underwent fusion: 27 with autologous rib strut and 13 with a threaded interbody fusion cage. Mean operative time was 173 minutes, mean blood loss was 259 mL, and average length of stay was 4 days. The surgical complication rate was 21%; 75% of the complications were pulmonary related (pleural effusion, pneumothorax, atelectasis, and pneumonia). Intercostal neuralgia occurred in six patients (6%) early in the series and declined subsequent to use of soft flexible intercostal trocars. One patient incurred a 2500-mL blood loss; open conversion to thoracotomy was done in one patient. Five patients underwent reoperation: four for secondary fusion secondary to discogram-positive intractable axial pain and one for pseudarthrosis with a threaded interbody fusion device that was removed and replaced with a rib graft strut.

At final follow-up, 88 patients were available for evaluation. Of the 68 who responded to the patient satisfaction survey, 18% rated their procedure satisfaction as excellent, 54% as good, 16% as fair, and 12% as poor. Oswestry scores improved with 36% of patients with preoperative scores greater than 50 and 23% of patients with preoperative scores less than 50.

Patient satisfaction was greatest in patients with preoperative findings of myelopathy or lower extremity radicular pain or both and least in patients with pure thoracic radicular pain as the preoperative presentation.

Kim and colleagues[124] reported on the use of VATS in 20 consecutive patients with various thoracic pathologies. These investigators found VATS to be an effective minimally invasive technique, but with a steep learning curve.

McAfee and colleagues[56] reported on the incidence of VATS complications in a series of 78 consecutive patients, 41 of whom underwent VATS for thoracic discectomy. Six patients showed a transient postoperative intercostal neuralgia; the incidence diminished with subsequent use of soft trocars. Atelectasis or effusion resulting in a prolonged hospital stay was seen in five patients. Blood loss greater than 2500 mL occurred in two patients. Penetration of the right hemidiaphragm occurred in one case, with mild parenchymal laceration to the liver repaired thoracoscopically without postoperative sequelae. Intraoperative conversion to open thoracotomy was required in one patient secondary to scarring from a previous costotransversectomy.

Hur and collegues[126] used VATS combined with an O-arm CT-based navigation system for treatment of 10 patients with thoracic disc herniation. They reported the addition of 29.4 minutes for the use of the image guidance system, but reported no complications in their series. Additional reported advantages of combining VATS with computer guidance were improved visualization of the operative field, improved surgical planning, optimization of the surgical approach involving the establishment of correct drilling trajectory, and safe decompression of the spinal cord.

Methodologic review of VATS emphasizes the necessity of initial portal placement at the midaxillary sixth or seventh intercostal space to avoid injury to vital organs. The recommended use of soft trocar portals and a meticulous technique emphasizing the constant visualization of all instrumentation tips was believed to be cardinal in the reduction of VATS-associated complications. Gille and colleagues[125] reported on the results of VATS in 18 cases of hard thoracic disc herniation. In 11 of the patients, there was no definitive plane between the calcified disc and the dura. Seven patients developed a dural tear with a high risk of CSF fistula. Four of these seven patients required revision surgery.

Minimally Invasive Techniques

There have been several more recent reports of using minimally invasive techniques for the surgical treatment of thoracic disc herniations.[127–131] In a cadaveric and initial clinical study, Lidar and colleagues[129] reported the minimally invasive technique to be safe and effective. These investigators used a series of sequentially larger tubular dilators inserted on the lateral border of the rib head to allow visualization of the space between the costotransverse joint and caudal border of the costovertebral joint (Fig. 45.14). The joints are disarticulated, and the rib is freed and cut 2 cm distal to the costotransverse joint. The neurovascular bundle is identified and gently retracted. The transverse process is removed. The working tube is inserted deeper and medially. The pedicle is removed, starting at the foramen, allowing access to the disc.

The feasibility of this technique was first verified using four cadaveric specimens. Following that, Lidar and colleagues[129] used the technique on 10 patients with myelopathy secondary to thoracic disc herniation. The mean operative time was 171 minutes (range, 150 to 220 minutes), mean blood loss was 215 mL (range, 60 to 350 mL), and all patients had a one-night hospital stay and returned to work within 4 weeks. There were no documented operative or postoperative complications.

Smith and collegues[131] reported on a series of 16 patients with thoracic disc herniation treated with a minimally

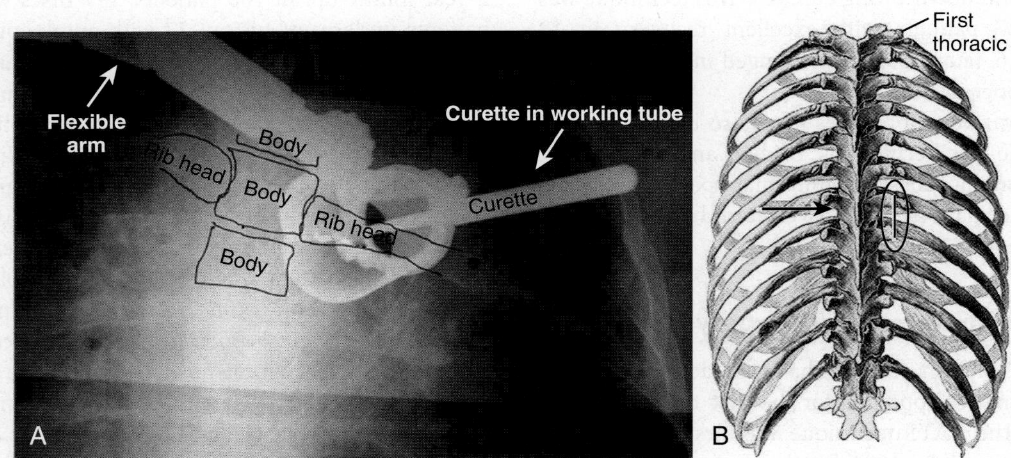

FIG. 45.14 (A) Intraoperative radiograph detailing minimally invasive approach through a dilated tube with a curette placed on the inferior border of the rib head. (B) Schematic drawing showing the working area of the tube. The *arrow* shows the desired discectomy level. The *oval* shows the working tube placement. The *vertical line* inside the oval shows the skin incision. (From Lidar Z, Lifshutz J, Bhattacharjee S, et al. Minimally invasive, extracavitary approach for thoracic disc herniation: technical report and preliminary results. *Spine J.* 2006;6:157–163.)

invasive thoracic microendoscopic discectomy technique. The approach was performed with a tunular retractor system placed through a muscle dilating technique and visualization through an endoscope. No complications were reported, with a mean operative time of 153 minutes per level and hospital stay of 21 hours. Reported outcomes were excellent or good in 13 (81%), fair in 1 (6%), and poor in 2 (13%). The two poor outcomes were related to neurologic diagnoses, not to the surgical approach or procedure.

Summary

Symptomatic herniated thoracic discs are uncommon lesions that usually affect middle-aged adults. Diagnosis is difficult owing to myriad symptoms, and there is no clear-cut clinical syndrome. The natural history is unclear; improved diagnostic techniques have identified an increasing prevalence of asymptomatic herniated thoracic discs. The natural history of symptomatic patients generally is progression, often starting with pain followed sequentially by sensory, motor, gait, and sphincter disturbances. Many patients complain of pain only; others present with painless myelopathy.

Most herniations occur in the lower thoracic region; central protrusions are more frequent than lateral protrusions. Multiple herniations and intradural penetration are uncommon. In most cases, the cause is a degenerative process, but a history of trauma can be elicited in approximately one-third of cases; an association with Scheuermann disease has been suggested by several authors. The pathogenesis of neurologic compromise in thoracic disc herniation is believed to be a combination of direct neural compression and vascular insufficiency. The differential diagnosis is long and requires careful consideration. Radiologic evaluation is essential for the diagnosis, but plain films are helpful only if disc calcification is present. Myelography, CT, and MRI are considered standard diagnostic tools, although no specific imaging features can reliably classify a herniated disc as symptomatic or asymptomatic.

Laminectomy is no longer indicated for treatment of thoracic disc herniation because of a high risk of neurologic deterioration and the fact that it may compromise the results of later anterior decompression. Discectomy may be performed by various surgical approaches: costotransversectomy, transthoracic, posterolateral, or video-assisted. The most rational way to manage the problem may be to select the approach best suited to the disease that is present and to the surgeon's experience. Posterolateral techniques are ideal for lateral lesions and may be the best choice for herniated discs with coexistent stenosis.[132] The transthoracic approach permits the best visualization for central lesions. Upper thoracic lesions are more difficult to approach through the chest and may be managed best by costotransversectomy. Depending on the experience of the surgeon, video-assisted approaches can provide an alternative with reportedly less surgical morbidity. Newer minimally invasive approaches are also being developed that may offer less pain and quicker recovery.

The prognosis of patients who have herniated thoracic discs treated surgically is favorable, and early operative intervention is advised in cases of myelopathy or refractory radicular pain. The techniques are exacting, however, and still carry a significant risk of neurologic deterioration.

PEARLS

1. Of asymptomatic adults, 73% have positive anatomic findings, including 37% with disc herniation and 29% with spinal cord deformation.
2. Disc calcification can be seen in 70% of patients with thoracic disc prolapse.
3. For symptomatic central thoracic disc herniation, the transthoracic approach is probably the safest.

PITFALLS

1. Surgical treatment of thoracic disc herniation by laminectomy has a 28% chance of worsening symptoms.
2. Blood supply to the spinal cord is tenuous in the thoracic spine, especially from T4 to T9, and ligation of blood vessels within the neural foramina should be avoided whenever possible because this may cause paralysis.

KEY POINTS

1. The true incidence of thoracic herniated discs is unknown; many cases are unrecognized, or patients are asymptomatic.
2. Surgically, thoracic disc excision accounts for 0.2% to 1.8% of all operations performed on symptomatic herniated discs.
3. The pathogenesis of neurologic compromise secondary to herniated thoracic discs is believed to be a combination of direct neural compression and vascular insufficiency.
4. A thorough neurologic examination is mandatory; the examiner should pay close attention to long tract signs and other evidence of myelopathy.
5. Indications for surgery include progressive myelopathy, lower extremity weakness or paralysis, bowel or bladder dysfunction, and radicular pain refractory to conservative measures.
6. The recommended extent of bone and disc removal varies from a relatively small trough in the posterior aspect of the disc to complete discectomy with partial corpectomy of adjacent bodies.
7. Reported advantages of VATS include reduced perioperative morbidity from minimal surgical dissection and avoidance of rib resection or spreading, enhanced visualization for the operating surgeons and support team, reduced postoperative pain with improved ventilatory excursion, shorter hospitalization and rehabilitation, and consequent decreased overall medical costs.
8. The prognosis of patients who have herniated thoracic discs treated surgically is favorable, and early operative intervention is advised in cases of myelopathy or refractory radicular pain.

KEY REFERENCES

1. Anand N, Regan JJ. Video-assisted thoracoscopic surgery for thoracic disc disease. *Spine*. 2002;27:871-879.
   The authors describe the technique and clinical outcome of video-assisted thoracic disc decompression.
2. Arce CA, Dohrmann G. Herniated thoracic disks. *Neurol Clin*. 1985;3:383-392.
   This review of the literature details the clinical presentation and progression of thoracic disc herniation.
3. Bohlman HH, Zdeblick TA. Anterior excision of herniated thoracic discs. *J Bone Joint Surg Am*. 1988;70:1038-1047.
   This article describes the technique of transthoracic disc decompression and clinical outcomes.

SECTION VI

4. Brown CW, Deffer PA, Akmakjian J, et al. The natural history of thoracic disc herniation. *Spine*. 1992;17:S97-S102.
The clinical method and the outcome of nonoperative thoracic disc herniation treatment are presented.
5. Currier BL, Eismont FJ, Green BA. Transthoracic disc excision and fusion for thoracic herniated discs. *Spine*. 1994;3:323-328.
This article is a summary of the early experience of the authors of this chapter using the transthoracic approach for treating patients with symptomatic thoracic herniated discs.
6. Wood KB, Garvey TA, Gundry C, et al. Magnetic resonance imaging of the thoracic spine. *J Bone Joint Surg Am*. 1995;77:1631-1638.
A clinical review is provided of MRI-detected thoracic disc herniation in an asymptomatic patient population.

REFERENCES

1. Key CA. On paraplegia: depending on disease of the ligaments of the spine. *Guys Hosp Rep*. 1838;3:17-24.
2. Middleton GS, Teacher JH. Injury of the spinal cord due to rupture of an intervertebral disc during muscular effort. *Glasgow Med J*. 1911;76:1.
3. Love JG, Schorn VG. Thoracic disk protrusions. *JAMA*. 1965;191:627-631.
4. Mixter WJ, Barr JS. Rupture of the intervertebral disc with involvement of the spinal canal. *N Engl J Med*. 1934;211:210-218.
5. Abbott KH, Retter RH. Protrusions of thoracic intervertebral disc. *Neurology*. 1956;6:1-10.
6. Arseni C, Nash F. Thoracic intervertebral disc protrusion: a clinical study. *J Neurosurg*. 1960;17:418-430.
7. Epstein JA. The syndrome of herniation of the lower thoracic intervertebral discs with nerve root and spinal cord compression: a presentation of four cases with a review of the literature, methods of diagnosis, and treatment. *J Neurosurg*. 1954;11:525-538.
8. Fisher RG. Protrusions of thoracic disc: the factor of herniation through the dura mater. *J Neurosurg*. 1965;22:591-593.
9. Hawk WA. Spinal compression caused by enchondrosis of the intervertebral fibrocartilage with a review of the recent literature. *Brain*. 1936;59:204-224.
10. Huang T, Hsu RW, Sum C, et al. Complications in thoracoscopic spinal surgery: a study of 90 consecutive patients. *Surg Endosc*. 1999;19:346-350.
11. Kite WC Jr, Whitfield RD, Campbell E. The thoracic herniated intervertebral disc syndrome. *J Neurosurg*. 1957;14:61-67.
12. Logue V. Thoracic intervertebral disc prolapse with spinal cord compression. *J Neurol Neurosurg Psychiatry*. 1952;15:227-241.
13. Peck FC Jr. A calcified thoracic intervertebral disk with herniation and spinal cord compression in a child: case report. *J Neurosurg*. 1957;14:105-109.
14. Svien HJ, Karavitis AL. Multiple protrusions of intervertebral disks in the upper thoracic region: report of case. *Mayo Clin Proc*. 1954;29:375-378.
15. Terry AF, McSweeney T, Jones HWF. Paraplegia as a sequela to dorsal disc prolapse. *Paraplegia*. 1981;19:111-117.
16. Tovi D, Strang RR. Thoracic intervertebral disk protrusions. *Acta Chir Scand Suppl*. 1960;267:6.
17. Menard V. *Etude Pratique sur le Mal de Pott*. Paris: Masson; 1900.
18. Capener N. The evolution of lateral rachiotomy. *J Bone Joint Surg Br*. 1954;36:173-179.
19. Hulme A. The surgical approach to thoracic intervertebral disc protrusions. *J Neurol Neurosurg Psychiatry*. 1960;23:133-137.
20. Arce CA, Dohrmann G. Herniated thoracic disks. *Neurol Clin*. 1985;3:383-392.
21. Hodgson AR, Stock FE. Anterior spinal fusion: a preliminary communication on the radical treatment of Pott's disease and Pott's paraplegia. *Br J Surg*. 1956;44:266-275.
22. Crafoord C, Hiertonn T, Lindblom K, et al. Spinal cord compression caused by a protruded thoracic disc: report of a case treated with anterolateral fenestration of the disc. *Acta Orthop Scand*. 1958;28:103-107.
23. Perot PH Jr, Munro DD. Transthoracic removal of midline thoracic disc protrusions causing spinal cord compression. *J Neurosurg*. 1969;31:452-458.
24. Ransohoff J, Spencer F, Siew F, et al. Case reports and technical notes on transthoracic removal of thoracic disc: report of three cases. *J Neurosurg*. 1969;31:459-461.
25. Carson J, Gumpert J, Jefferson A. Diagnosis and treatment of thoracic intervertebral disc protrusions. *J Neurol Neurosurg Psychiatry*. 1971;34:67-68.
26. Patterson RH Jr, Arbit E. A surgical approach through the pedicle to protruded thoracic discs. *J Neurosurg*. 1978;48:768-772.
27. Lesoin F, Rousseaux M, Autricque A, et al. Thoracic disc herniations: evolution in the approach and indications. *Acta Neurochir (Wien)*. 1986;80:30-34.
28. Safdari H, Baker RL. Microsurgical anatomy and related techniques to an anterolateral transthoracic approach to thoracic disc herniations. *Surg Neurol*. 1985;23:589-593.
29. Signorini G, Baldini M, Vivenza C, et al. Surgical treatment of thoracic disc protrusion. *Acta Neurochir (Wien)*. 1979;49:245-254.
30. Anand N, Regan JJ. Video-assisted thoracoscopic surgery for thoracic disc disease: classification and outcome study of 100 consecutive cases with a 2-year minimum follow-up period. *Spine*. 2002;27:871-879.
31. Regan JJ, Mack MJ, Picetti GD. A technical report on video-assisted thoracoscopy in thoracic spine surgery: preliminary description. *Spine*. 1995;20:831-837.
32. Regan JJ, Ben-Yishay A, Mack MJ. Video-assisted thoracoscopic excision of herniated thoracic disc: description of technique and preliminary experience in the first 29 cases. *J Spinal Disord*. 1998;11:183-191.
33. Rosenthal D, Rosenthal R, de Simone A. Removal of a protruded thoracic disc using microsurgical endoscopy: a new technique. *Spine*. 1994;19:1087-1091.
34. Blumenkopf B. Thoracic intervertebral disc herniations: diagnostic value of magnetic resonance imaging. *Neurosurgery*. 1988;23:36-40.
35. Bohlman HH, Zdeblick TA. Anterior excision of herniated thoracic discs. *J Bone Joint Surg Am*. 1988;70:1038-1047.
36. Chambers AA. Thoracic disk herniation. *Semin Roentgenol*. 1988;23:111-117.
37. Francavilla TL, Powers A, Dina T, et al. MR imaging of thoracic disk herniations. *J Comput Assist Tomogr*. 1987;11:1062-1065.
38. Parizel PM, Rodesch G, Baleriaux D, et al. Gd-enhanced MR in thoracic disc herniations. *Neuroradiology*. 1989;31:75-79.
39. Ross JS, Perez-Reyes N, Masaryk TJ, et al. Thoracic disc herniation: MR imaging. *Radiology*. 1987;165:511-515.
40. Videman T, Battie MC, Gill K, et al. Magnetic resonance imaging findings and their relationships in the thoracic and

lumbar spine: insights into the etiopathogenesis of spinal degeneration. *Spine*. 1995;20:928-935.
41. Williams MP, Cherryman GR, Husband JE. Significance of thoracic disc herniations demonstrated by MR imaging. *J Comput Tomogr*. 1989;13:212-214.
42. Wood KB, Garvey TA, Gundry C, et al. Magnetic resonance imaging of the thoracic spine. *J Bone Joint Surg Am*. 1995;77: 1631-1638.
43. Williams MP, Cherryman GR. Thoracic disc herniation: MR imaging [letter]. *Radiology*. 1988;167:874-875.
44. Arce CA, Dohrmann G. Thoracic disc herniation: improved diagnosis with computed tomographic scanning and a review of the literature. *Surg Neurol*. 1985;23:356-361.
45. Benson MKD, Byrnes DP. The clinical syndromes and surgical treatment of thoracic intervertebral disc prolapse. *J Bone Joint Surg Br*. 1975;57:471-477.
46. Albrand OW, Corkill G. Thoracic disc herniation: treatment and prognosis. *Spine*. 1979;4:41-46.
47. Love JG, Kiefer EJ. Root pain and paraplegia due to protrusions of thoracic intervertebral disks. *J Neurosurg*. 1950;7:62-69.
48. Brennan M, Perrin JCS, Canady A, et al. Paraparesis in a child with a herniated thoracic disc. *Arch Phys Med Rehabil*. 1987;68:806-808.
49. Otani KI, Yoshida M, Fujii E, et al. Thoracic disc herniation: surgical treatment in 23 patients. *Spine*. 1988;13:1262-1267.
50. Alvarez O, Roque CT, Pampati M. Multilevel thoracic disk herniations: CT and MR studies. *J Comput Assist Tomogr*. 1988;12:649-652.
51. Otani K, Manxoku S, Shibaski K, et al. The surgical treatment of thoracic and thoracolumbar disc lesions using the anterior approach. *Spine*. 1977;2:266-275.
52. Russell T. Thoracic intervertebral disc protrusion: experience of 67 cases and a review of the literature. *Br J Neurosurg*. 1989;3:153-160.
53. Le Roux PD, Haglund MM, Harris AB. Thoracic disc disease: experience with the transpedicular approach in twenty consecutive patients. *Neurosurgery*. 1993;33: 58-66.
54. Lesoin F, Leys D, Rousseaux M, et al. Thoracic disk herniation and Scheuermann's disease. *Eur Neurol*. 1987;26:145-152.
55. Mansour H, Hammoud F, Vlahovitch B. Brown-Séquard syndrome caused by foramen and calcified disk herniation responsible for direct compression of Adamkiewicz's artery. *Neurochirurgie*. 1987;33:478-481.
56. McAfee PC, Regan JR, Zdeblick T, et al. The incidence of complications in endoscopic anterior thoracolumbar spinal reconstructive surgery: a prospective multicenter study comprising the first 100 cases. *Spine*. 1995;20:1624-1632.
57. Haley JC, Perry JH. Protrusion of intervertebral discs: study of their distribution, characteristics and effects on the nervous system. *Am J Surg*. 1950;80:394-404.
58. Ridenour TR, Haddad SF, Hitchon PW, et al. Herniated thoracic disks: treatment and outcome. *J Spinal Disord*. 1993;6:218-224.
59. Ryan RW, Lally JF, Kozic Z. Asymptomatic calcified herniated thoracic disks: CT recognition. *AJNR Am J Neuroradiol*. 1988;9:363-366.
60. Awwad EE, Martin DS, Smith KR Jr, et al. Asymptomatic versus symptomatic herniated thoracic discs: their frequency and characteristics as detected by computed tomography after myelography. *Neurosurgery*. 1991;28:180-186.
61. Niemelainen R, Battie MC, Gill K, et al. The prevalence and characteristics of thoracic magnetic resonance imaging findings in men. *Spine*. 2008;33:2552-2559.
62. Tahmouresie A. Herniated thoracic intervertebral disc: an unusual presentation: case report. *Neurosurgery*. 1980;7: 623-625.
63. Landreneau RJ, Hazelrigg SR, Mack MJ, et al. Post-operative pain-related morbidity: video-assisted thoracic surgery versus thoracotomy. *Ann Thorac Surg*. 1993;56:1285-1289.
64. Van Landingham JH. Herniation of thoracic intervertebral discs with spinal cord compression in kyphosis dorsalis juvenilis (Scheuermann's disease). Case report. *J Neurosurg*. 1954;11:327-329.
65. Dommisse GF. The blood supply of the spinal cord: a critical vascular zone in spinal surgery. *J Bone Joint Surg Br*. 1974;56:225-235.
66. Hochman MS, Pena C, Ramirez R. Calcified herniated thoracic disc diagnosed by computerized tomography. *J Neurosurg*. 1980;52:722-723.
67. Maccartee CC Jr, Griffin PP, Byrd EB. Ruptured calcified thoracic disc in a child. *J Bone Joint Surg Am*. 1972;54: 1271-1274.
68. Kahn EA. The role of the dentate ligaments in spinal cord compression and the syndrome of lateral sclerosis. *J Neurosurg*. 1944;4:191-199.
69. Doppman JL, Girton M. Angiographic study of the effect of laminectomy in the presence of acute anterior epidural masses. *J Neurosurg*. 1976;45:195-202.
70. Brown CW, Deffer PA, Akmakjian J, et al. The natural history of thoracic disc herniation. *Spine*. 1992;17(suppl 6):S97-S102.
71. Gelch MM. Herniated thoracic disc at T1-2 level associated with Horner's syndrome. *J Neurosurg*. 1978;48:128-130.
72. Fransen P, Collignon F, Van Den Heule B. Foraminal disc herniation Th9-Th10 mimicking abdominal pain. *Acta Orthop Belg*. 2008;74:881-884.
73. Ozturk C, Tezer M, Sirvanci M, et al. Far lateral thoracic disc herniation presenting with flank pain. *Spine J*. 2006;6:201-203.
74. LaBan MM, Gorin G. A thoracic disc herniation presenting as an abdominal hernia. *Am J Phys Med Rehabil*. 2007;86:601.
75. Stetkarova I, Chrobok J, Ehler E, et al. Segmental abdominal wall paresis caused by lateral low thoracic disc herniation. *Spine*. 2007;32:E635-E639.
76. Deitch K, Chudnofsky C, Young M. T2-3 thoracic disc herniation with myelopathy. *J Emerg Med*. 2009;36:138-140.
77. Papapostolou A, Tsivgoulis G, Papadopoulou M, et al. Bilateral drop foot due to thoracic disc herniation. *Eur J Neurol*. 2007;14:E5.
78. Cho HL, Lee SH, Kim JS. Thoracic disk herniation manifesting as sciatica-like pain. *Neurol Med Chir (Tokyo)*. 2011;51:67-71.
79. Lara FJP, Berges AF, Quesada JQ, et al. Thoracic disk herniation, a not infrequent cause of chronic abdominal pain. *Int Surg*. 2012;97:27-33.
80. Kuhlendahl H. Der Thorakale Bandscheibenprolaps als extramedullarer Spinaltumor und in seinen Beziehungen zu internen Organsyndromen. *Arztl Wochenschr*. 1951;6:154-157.
81. Malmivaara A, Videman T, Kuosma E, et al. Facet joint orientation, facet and costovertebral joint osteoarthrosis, disc degeneration, vertebral body osteophytosis, and Schmorl's nodes in the thoracolumbar junctional region of cadaveric spines. *Spine*. 1987;12:458-463.
82. Almond LM, Hamid NA, Wasserberg J. Thoracic intradural disc herniation. *Br J Neurosurg*. 2007;21:32-34.

83. Epstein NE, Syrquin MS, Epstein JA, et al. Intradural disc herniations in the cervical, thoracic, and lumbar spine: report of three cases and review of the literature. *J Spinal Disord.* 1990;3:396-403.
84. Fidler MW, Goedhard ZD. Excision of prolapse of thoracic intervertebral disc: a transthoracic technique. *J Bone Joint Surg Br.* 1984;66:518-522.
85. Isla A, Roda JM, Benscome J, et al. Intradural herniated dorsal disc: case report and review of the literature. *Neurosurgery.* 1988;22:737-738.
86. Jefferson A. The treatment of thoracic intervertebral disc protrusion. *Clin Neurol Neurosurg.* 1975;78:1.
87. Chin LS, Black KL, Hoff JT. Multiple thoracic disc herniations. Case report. *J Neurosurg.* 1987;66:290-292.
88. Haro H, Domoto T, Maekawa S, et al. Resorption of thoracic disc herniation: report of 2 cases. *J Neurosurg Spine.* 2008;8:300-304.
89. Bullough PG, Boachie-Adjei O. *Atlas of Spinal Diseases.* Philadelphia: JB Lippincott; 1988.
90. Sonnabend DH, Taylor TKF, Chapman GK. Intervertebral disc calcification syndromes in children. *J Bone Joint Surg Br.* 1982;64:25-31.
91. Nicolau A, Diard F, Darrigade JM, et al. Posterior herniation of a calcified disc in children: a report of two cases. *J Radiol.* 1985;66:683-688.
92. Weinberger A, Myers AR. Intervertebral disk calcification in adults: a review. *Semin Arthritis Rheum.* 1978;8:69-75.
93. Currier BL, Eismont FJ, Green BA. Transthoracic disc excision and fusion for thoracic herniated discs. *Spine.* 1994;3:323-328.
94. Roosen N, Dietrich U, Nicola N, et al. Case report: MR imaging of calcified herniated thoracic disk. *J Comput Assist Tomogr.* 1987;11:733-735.
95. Ryan MD, Taylor TKF. Acute spinal cord compression in Scheuermann's disease. *J Bone Joint Surg Br.* 1982;64:409-412.
96. Baker HL Jr, Love JG, Uihlein A. Roentgenologic features of protruded thoracic intervertebral disks. *Radiology.* 1965;84:1059-1065.
97. Alberico A, Sahni KS, Hall JA Jr, et al. High thoracic disc herniation. *Neurosurgery.* 1986;19:449-451.
98. Enzmann DR, Griffin C, Rubin JB. Potential false-negative MR images of the thoracic spine in disk disease with switching of phase and frequency encoding gradients. *Radiology.* 1987;165:635-637.
99. Schellhas KP, Pollei SR, Dorwart RH. Thoracic discography: a safe and reliable technique. *Spine.* 1994;19:2103-2109.
100. Wood KB, Schellhas KP, Garvey TA, et al. Thoracic discography in healthy individuals: a controlled prospective study of magnetic resonance imaging and discography in asymptomatic and symptomatic individuals. *Spine.* 1999;24:1548-1555.
101. Buenaventura RM, Shah RV, Patel V, et al. Systematic review of discography as a diagnostic test for spinal pain: an update. *Pain Physician.* 2007;20:147-164.
102. Gruber HE, Rhyne AL 3rd, Hansen KJ, et al. Deleterious effects of discography radiocontrast solution on human annulus cell in vitro: changes in cell viability, proliferation, and apoptosis in exposed cells. *Spine J.* 2012;12(4):329-335.
103. Carragee EJ, Don AS, Hurwitz EL, et al. Does discography cause accelerated progression of degeneration changes in the lumbar disc: a ten-year matched cohort study. *Spine.* 2009;34(21):2338-2345.
104. Ravichandran G, Frankel HL. Paraplegia due to intervertebral disc lesions: a review of 57 operated cases. *Paraplegia.* 1981;19:133-139.
105. Aizawa T, Sato T, Sasaki H, et al. Results of surgical treatment for thoracic myelopathy: minimum 2-year follow-up study in 132 patients. *J Neurosurg Spine.* 2007;7:13-20.
106. Yi S, Kim H, Shin HC, et al. Outcome of surgery for a symptomatic herniated thoracic disc in relation to preoperative characteristics of the disc. *Acta Neurochir (Wien).* 2007;149:1139-1145.
107. Fessler RG, Sturgill M. Review: Complications of surgery for thoracic disc disease. *Surg Neurol.* 1998;49:609-618.
108. Singounas EG, Karvounis PC. Thoracic disc protrusion (analysis of 8 cases). *Acta Neurochir (Wien).* 1977;39:251-258.
109. Bennett MH, McCallum J. Experimental decompression of the spinal cord. *Surg Neurol.* 1977;8:63-67.
110. Simpson JM, Silveri CP, Simeone FA, et al. Thoracic disc herniation: re-evaluation of the posterior approach using a modified costotransversectomy. *Spine.* 1993;13:1872-1877.
111. Chesterman PJ. Spastic paraplegia caused by sequestrated thoracic intervertebral disc. *Proc R Soc Med.* 1964;57:87-88.
112. Garrido E. Modified costotransversectomy: a surgical approach to ventrally placed lesions in the thoracic spinal canal. *Surg Neurol.* 1980;13:109-113.
113. Hulme A. The surgical approach to thoracic intervertebral disc protrusions. *J Neurol Neurosurg Psychiatry.* 1960;23:133-137.
114. Amini A, Apfelbaum RI, Schmidt MH. Chylorrhea: a rare complication of thoracoscopic discectomy of the thoracolumbar junction. *J Neurosurg Spine.* 2007;6:563-566.
115. Lubelski D, Abdullah KG, Mroz TE, et al. Lateral extracavitary vs. costotransversectomy approaches to the thoracic spine: reflections on lessons learned. *Neurosurgery.* 2012;71(6):1096-1102.
116. Maiman DJ, Larson SJ, Luck E, et al. Lateral extracavitary approach to the spine for thoracic disc herniations: report of 23 cases. *Neurosurgery.* 1984;14:178-182.
117. DiChiro G, Fried LC, Doppman JL. Experimental spinal cord angiography. *Br J Radiol.* 1970;43:19-20.
118. Lazorthes G, Gouzae A, Zadeh JO, et al. Arterial vascularization of the spinal cord: recent studies of the anastomotic substitution pathways. *J Neurosurg.* 1971;35:253-262.
119. Zhuang QS, Lun DX, Xu ZW, Dai WH, Liu DY. Surgical treatment for central calcified thoracic disk herniation: a novel L-shaped osteotomy. *Orthopedics.* 2015;38(9):e794-e798.
120. Ulivieri S, Oliveri G, Petrini C, et al. Transmanubrial osteomuscular sparing approach for T1-T2 thoracic disc herniation. *Minerva Chir.* 2008;63:421-423.
121. Kawahara N, Demura S, Marukami H, et al. Transvertebral herniotomy for T2/3 disc herniation—a case report. *J Spinal Disord Tech.* 2009;22:62-66.
122. Mack MJ, Regan JJ, Bobechko WP, et al. Present role of thoracoscopy for diseases of the spine. *Ann Thorac Surg.* 1993;56:736-738.
123. Horowitz MB, Moossy JJ, Julian T, et al. Thoracic discectomy using video assisted thoracoscopy. *Spine.* 1994;19:1082-1086.
124. Kim SJ, Sohn MJ, Ryoo JY, et al. Clinical analysis of video-assisted thoracoscopic spinal surgery in the thoracic or thoracolumbar spinal pathologies. *J Korean Neurosurg Soc.* 2007;42:293-299.

125. Gille O, Soderlund C, Razafimahandri HJC, et al. Analysis of hard thoracic herniated discs: review of 18 cases operated by thoracoscopy. *Eur Spine J*. 2006;15:537-542.
126. Hur JW, Kim JS, Cho DY, et al. Video-assisted thoracoscopic surgery under O-arm navigation system guidance for the treatment of thoracic disk herniations: surgical techniques and early clinical results. *J Neurol Surg A Cent Eur Neurosurg*. 2014;75(6):415-421.
127. Bartels RH, Peul WC. Mini-thoracotomy or thoracoscopic treatment for medially located thoracic herniated disc? *Spine*. 2007;32:E581-E584.
128. Chi JH, Dhall SS, Kanter AS, et al. The mini-open transpedicular thoracic discectomy: surgical technique and assessment. *Neurosurg Focus*. 2008;25:E5.
129. Lidar Z, Lifshutz J, Bhattacharjee S, et al. Minimally invasive, extracavitary approach for thoracic disc herniation: technical report and preliminary results. *Spine J*. 2006;6:157-163.
130. Sheikh H, Samartzis D, Perez-Cruet MJ. Techniques for the operative management of thoracic disc herniation: minimally invasive thoracic microdiscectomy. *Orthop Clin North Am*. 2007;38:351-361.
131. Smith JS, Eichholz KM, Shafizadeh S, et al. Minimally invasive thoracic microendoscopic diskectomy: surgical technique and case series. *World Neurosurg*. 2013;80(3-4): 421-427.
132. Ungersbock K, Perneczky A, Korn A. Thoracic vertebrostenosis combined with thoracic disc herniation: case report and review of the literature. *Spine*. 1987;12:612-615.

CHAPTER 46

Lumbar Disc Disease

Makarand V. Risbud
Gunnar B.J. Andersson

Introduction

The location of the anatomic pain generator in patients with low back pain is often difficult to discern. Pain can originate from several anatomic structures within the spine, making it difficult for both the patient and physician to localize. The intervertebral disc (IVD) is a widely accepted source of chronic low back pain (LBP). A study reviewing magnetic resonance images (MRIs) of patients with persistent LBP showed disc degeneration in 87% of participants.[1] Additionally, patients with severely degenerate discs are 3.2 times more likely to have LBP.[2] Despite this robust link between disc degeneration and back pain, degeneration is a normal consequence of aging that does not routinely cause discomfort, even with a corresponding reduction in biomechanical function.[3,4] However, there is still much work to be done to identify the underlying pathology that distinguishes painful degenerate disc disease from nonpainful age-related changes.

Common subgroups of LBP of IVD origin include lumbar disc herniation, internal disc disruption, and degenerative disc disease. Lumbar disc herniation causes an acute onset of pain, while degenerative disc disease is linked to chronic LBP. Degenerative disc disease also contributes to the pathogenesis of secondary spinal disorders such as spinal stenosis and degenerative spondylolisthesis. Improved understanding of the pathophysiology of IVD disorders has led to a resurgence of enthusiasm in the development of new pharmacobiologics and treatment techniques for this common disorder. New advances in physical therapy and operative technologies, such as IVD replacement and minimally invasive surgical techniques, are challenging traditional methods of treatment.

This chapter discusses the anatomy, pathophysiology, diagnosis, and treatment of primary disc disorders, namely internal disc disruption (IDD) and degenerative disc disease (DDD). Disorders arising secondarily from the IVD are beyond the scope of this chapter.

Natural History

Sixty to eighty percent of the adult population can be expected to experience LBP at some point during their lifetime. The annual incidence of back pain in the adult population is 15%, and its point prevalence is about 30%.[5] By the age of 30 years almost half the population will have experienced a substantive episode of LBP.[6] Fortunately, the vast majority of symptoms are short lived; it is generally believed that 80% to 90% of patients with episodes of LBP will recover within 6 weeks of onset regardless of the type of treatment.[7]

Even though resolution of symptoms is the common and expected outcome, there is also a high recurrence rate. Croft et al.[8] reported that although 90% of subjects stopped pursuing treatment for their symptoms within 3 months, most still had substantial LBP and related disability. In addition, only 25% of the patients who sought consultation for LBP had fully recovered within12 months. In a survey of the British general population, 38% of adults reported a significant episode of LBP within a 1-year period, of which one-third had experienced symptoms for longer than 4 weeks.[9] Inability to return to work within 3 months of symptom onset is a poor prognostic indicator. Only 20% of patients still disabled after 1 year will return to work, and only 2% return after 2 years.[10]

The clinical onset and course of LBP may be prolonged for many patients and may best be represented as a continuum of back-related disability and distress.[11] A significant number of patients presenting with acute LBP have a prior history of chronic back pain.[12] The strongest predictive factor for a new episode of LBP is a previous episode.[13,14]

The natural history of DDD is largely unknown. Smith et al.[15] reported on the outcome of 25 discogram-positive patients treated nonoperatively and found that 68% of patients improved by the 3-year minimum follow-up. Although 60% of the patients were involved with worker's compensation and 32% were being treated for psychiatric diagnoses, this study suggests that at least two-thirds of those with discogenic pain improve with conservative therapy. The retrospective study design and small sample size limit the conclusions, and since only patients with significant symptoms typically undergo discography, the natural history of untreated, less-severe cases of symptomatic DDD is likely to result in more improvement than the cited study.

In their classic description, Kirkaldy-Willis et al.[16] classified the degenerative process into three distinct phases: dysfunction, instability, and stabilization. In the first phase the disc loses its normal function as the degenerative process begins. This is followed by a period of relative instability as degeneration progresses with intermittent episodes of pain. During the instability phase abnormal motion can occasionally be seen on flexion-extension radiographs; however, the spinal segments during this phase of degeneration more often show no demonstrable radiographic instability. The final phase—stabilization—results when the spinal segment has reached a new equilibrium because of loss of height and compression of disc tissue; at this point the patient typically no longer has episodes of back pain. A problem with this theory is that patients who meet either the radiographic diagnostic criteria of DDD—loss of height, osteophytes, or even olisthesis—or show the MRI signs of disc degeneration—signal changes when compared with adjacent levels—can be completely symptom free. Waris et al.,[17] in a study with 17 years of follow-up MRIs, showed that young patients with DDD did show radiographic evidence of progression, but it was not significantly associated with LBP or a higher rate of surgery.

Relevant Anatomy

The major functional role of the IVD is mechanical; it supports the compressive load of the torso while allowing for polyaxial flexion, extension, and torsion. Although the movement capable of a single spinal motion segment is quite limited, the range of motion supported by the 24 presacral motion segments of the spine in its entirety is remarkable. Found between two rigid vertebral bodies, the disc allows this movement while simultaneously supporting compressive loads. The discs themselves are complex organs comprising central proteoglycan-rich nucleus pulposus surrounded circumferentially by fibrocartilaginous anulus fibrosus. The nucleus pulposus is bound caudally and cephalically by the cartilage end plates of the contiguous vertebrae. Major characteristics of these tissue components of the disc are highlighted below.

Nucleus Pulposus

The central nucleus pulposus is derived from the embryonic notochord, and notochordal cells remain in the tissue after birth and into adult life. During development, the nucleus is highly cellular; after birth and an initial period of cell growth, the number of cells declines. In the adult, the cell density is very low.[18] The histology of the nucleus pulposus cells is unique and complex; large cells are arranged mainly in clusters separated by an abundant extracellular matrix. Among the large notochordal cells, much smaller cells, possibly derived from the notochordal sheath, can also be seen.[19] The large cells appear to have numerous vacuoles, which have prompted some to describe them as "physaliphorus."[20] Transition electron microscopic analysis showed that the nucleus pulposus contained cell clusters embedded in a proteoglycan-collagen matrix. The cells exhibit a well-defined Golgi system, an extensive endoplasmic reticulum, and a complex vesicular system filled with beaded structures. Neither necrotic nor apoptotic cells are evident. Although a defining characteristic of the cells is the presence of numerous cytoplasmic processes, a remarkable finding is that the cells contain few, if any, mitochondria. Moreover, since the nucleus pulposus has no blood supply, the oxygen tension within the disc is very low. These limitations have prompted one study group to note that nucleus pulposus cells "tune" their metabolism to the available oxygen supply.[21] In this case, nucleus pulposus cells rely to a large extent on the glycolytic pathway to generate metabolic energy.[22]

With respect to the extracellular matrix, nucleus pulposus cells secrete aggrecan as well as collagen II and, to a very small extent, collagen I. The matrix also contains collagen IX and XI, and collagen X has also been reported to be present during degeneration. Because of the presence of hydrophilic aggrecan, the disc exhibits a high osmotic pressure. The high water content of a healthy nucleus pulposus, as evidenced by the intense bright signal on T2-weighted MRI, is responsible for supporting compressive loads.

Anulus Fibrosus

Compressive deformation of the nucleus pulposus is limited circumferentially by the anulus fibrosus, which experiences the compressive loads of the torso as hoop stress. Since the anulus fibrosus experiences tensile stress as opposed to compression, its anatomy and biochemical composition are distinct from the nucleus pulposus. The anulus is not a homogeneous tissue; it is divided into an inner region and an outer, or peripheral, fibrous zone.[23] The outer anulus fibrosus is composed of very well-defined collagen I fibers that bundle to form long parallel concentric lamellae. Marchand and Ahmed[24] showed that the number of fiber bundles varies from 20 to 62. The thickness of lamellae varies both circumferentially and radially. Age, location, and vertebral type also influence lamellar architecture. The central anulus fibers insert into the end plate cartilage, whereas those at the periphery anchor to the vertebral bone.

The inner anulus fibrosus represents approximately 50% of the total radial thickness. Many consider the inner anulus a transition zone because it differs substantially from the outer region. Compared with the outer anulus fibrosus, where the cells are elongated and fusiform aligned with the long axis of the fibrils, the cells of the inner anulus are spherical in shape and more closely resemble chondrocytes. These cells are few in number with short processes. A further difference between the inner and outer anulus is their chemical composition. The inner anulus contains collagen I and II as well as versican. Although aggrecan is present in both regions of the anulus, decorin and biglycan are found mainly in the outer anulus. The other protein of significance is elastin, which accounts for 2% of the dry tissue weight and aids the anulus in its role of withstanding cyclic tensile forces.

End Plate Cartilage

The third component of the disc is end plate cartilage, which is located at the junction of the vertebral body and the disc. This thin layer of hyaline-like cartilage is most thick in the newborn and thins with age. It serves as an interface between the soft nucleus pulposus and the dense bone of the vertebrae as well as a biomechanical barrier that prevents the disc from applying pressure directly to the bone. In addition, the end plate cartilage plays a role in maintaining nucleus pulposus cell viability and controlling biosynthetic activities.[18,25] In the adult human, the width of the end plate is up to 1 mm. It contains chondrocytes embedded in an aggrecan-rich and collagen II extracellular matrix. Although the cells do not undergo terminal differentiation, collagen X may be present in the central region of the end plate, perhaps in relationship to focal areas of endochondral bone formation. The end plate transitions into bone through a region of calcified cartilage. Work in rabbit and rat models suggests that end plate chondrocytes may contribute a cell fraction that makes up some of the nucleus pulposus and the anulus fibrosus in normal development and during injury.[26,27] However, cell lineage studies are required before a definitive contribution of such a homeostatic mechanism is understood. The presence of the cartilage layer provides the motion segment with its jointlike characteristics.

In his review on the end plate, Moore[28] noted that vascular channels penetrate the cartilage during development, but at maturity the vessels become narrow or even obliterated. It is likely that this change impacts the nutrient supply to both the cartilage and the disc. Nachemson et al.[29] showed that, at the tissue periphery, the cartilage is much less permeable to low-molecular-weight dyes. Supporting this, Crock and Yoshizawa[30] showed that the central region of the end plate, where there is a high concentration of channels, is freely permeable to small molecules. Clinically, it is not uncommon to note that the central region undergoes sclerosis or mineralization with alterations in the mechanical properties of the cartilage. When this occurs, nucleus pulposus tissue can be forced through the end plate into the underlying bone of the vertebrae. This phenomenon is referred to as Schmorl's nodes, which Schmorl himself considered to be linked to degenerative changes at the cartilage-bone interface.

Defining the IVD Niche: Molecular Characters

One overriding aspect of disc cell biology is that nucleus pulposus and cells residing in the inner anulus are removed from the blood supply. Blood vessels originating in the vertebral body traverse the superficial region of the end plates, but none of these vessels infiltrates the nucleus pulposus. Gruber and colleagues[31] showed that the anulus is avascular except for small capillary beds in the dorsal and ventral surfaces, and this vasculature never enters the nucleus pulposus.[32,33] The lack of penetrating vasculature suggests that the disc is a low-oxygen environment. Studies have confirmed that this logic holds true in vivo. Experimental measurements done in canine discs[34] as well as modeling studies by Bartels et al.[35] indicate that the pO_2 within the disc is indeed low. Thus, it is now widely recognized that the nucleus pulposus cells reside in a hypoxic niche.[36]

However, this raises an important question: How do cells survive in this unique niche? Due to pioneering studies by Semenza and others, it is now evident that the key molecule regulating energy metabolism and survival activity under hypoxia is hypoxia-inducible factor 1 (HIF-1),[37] a member of the basic helix-loop-helix (bHLH)–PER-ARNT-SIM family of proteins. HIF-1 is composed of a constitutively expressed β-subunit and a regulatory α-subunit. The α-subunit is stable under hypoxia but is rapidly degraded in normoxia.[38] Transactivation of HIF-1 target genes involves dimerization of the two subunits and binding to an enhancer, the hypoxia-response element in target genes. HIF-1 serves as a key transcription factor that regulates the expression of glycolytic enzymes, and enzymes that control the activity of the tricarboxylic acid cycle and oxidative phosphorylation.[37,39,40] Additional target genes include those that contribute to apoptosis, autophagy, and matrix synthesis pathways.[41-43] Details of these relationships are shown schematically in Fig. 46.1. Other isoforms of HIF exist, the most important being HIF-2α. Recent evidence suggests that HIF-1α and HIF-2α are not redundant, and that the relative importance of each of the homologues, in response to hypoxia, varies among different cell types.[44] In addition to these genes, the Sox family of transcription factors that are essential for the development and function of the nucleus pulposus are hypoxia and HIF sensitive.[45-48] However, the relationship between Sox proteins and HIF in the hypoxic niche of the IVD is not yet clearly demonstrated. The influence of HIF on cell function is vast, warranting further

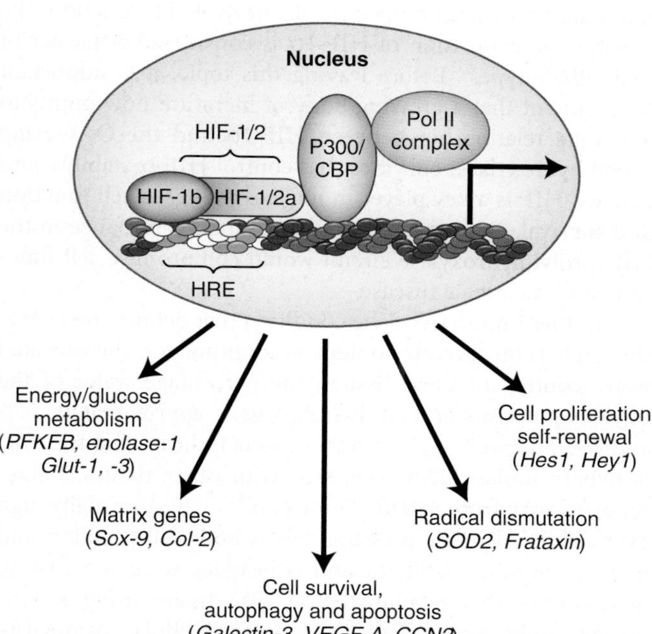

FIG. 46.1 Functional activity of hypoxia-inducible factor (HIF) target genes. Critical functions include energy metabolism, angiogenesis, cell survival, autophagy and apoptosis, matrix synthesis, proliferation, self-renewal and differentiation, radical dismutation, and pH regulation. Many of these functions are critical for survival and functioning of the nucleus pulposus cells in the avascular niche of the intervertebral disk. Hypoxia/HIF-sensitive proteins that are identified in the nucleus pulposus cells are shown in parentheses. (Modified from Risbud MV, Schipani E, Shapiro IM, et al. Hypoxic regulation of nucleus pulposus cell survival: from niche to notch. *Am J Pathol.* 2010;176[4]:1577–1583.)

study, but it is evident that this protein is responsible for nucleus pulposus survival in the hypoxic disc.

A number of reports showed that there is a robust HIF response by nucleus pulposus cells. The response is evident across species; more importantly, HIF-1α activity is unresponsive to the oxemic state of the tissue.[22,36,49] Accordingly, when compared with most other tissues, there are important underlying differences in the HIF status and reactivity of disc cells. HIF-1α expression and activity is always "on." This unique response suggests that stabilization of HIF-1α in nucleus pulposus cells ensures that transcriptional activity is a major governor of their function. The second HIF homologue, HIF-2α, is robustly expressed by nucleus pulposus cells. Like HIF-1α, steady-state protein levels are similar in both hypoxia and normoxia, suggesting that it is stabilized as well.[50] Recent work by Merceron and colleagues[51] has unequivocally demonstrated that HIF-1 is indispensable for nucleus pulposus cell survival in vivo. Conditional deletion of HIF-1α in mouse notochord by FoxA2-driven Cre recombinase results in massive apoptotic cell death in the nucleus pulposus at birth, likely due to energetic failure by decreased glycolysis. Eventually the nucleus pulposus is replaced with a fibrocartilaginous tissue with inferior biomechanical properties. Interestingly, lineage-tracing studies clearly showed the notochordal lineage of the nucleus pulposus cells, and their replacement with nonnotochordal cells, likely migrate into the tissue from the inner anulus or end plate cartilage (Fig. 46.2). Thus, because of the necessity of HIF-1α in maintaining nucleus pulposus cell survival and function, the constitutive expression of HIF-1α is considered a marker of their phenotype.[52] Before leaving this topic, it is important to comment that a growing body of literature now points to a unique relationship between HIF-1α and the O_2-sensing prolyl hydroxylase, enzymes that control HIF-α stability and activity. HIF is a key player in nucleus pulposus cell function and survival. Consequently it is likely that disturbance in the HIF–prolyl hydroxylase circuit would compromise cell function and exacerbate disease.

Another important niche condition that defines the IVD is the high proteoglycan content accounting for the elevated water content in these tissues; the percentage water of the nucleus pulposus and anulus fibrosus is approximately 77% and 70%, respectively.[53] Several reports indicate that the IVD is hyperosmolar when compared with other tissues. Values reported vary from 430 to 496 mOsm.[54,55] This unusually high extracellular osmotic pressure affects both cell function and matrix synthesis. Ishihara and colleagues were the first to demonstrate this relationship in disc tissue using bovine nucleus pulposus explants.[54] How extracellular osmolarity regulates the expression levels of specific matrix molecules has received intense study in recent years. In human nucleus pulposus and anulus cells, expression levels of aggrecan and collagen II were increased in cells under hyperosmotic conditions (500 mOsm), whereas collagen I expression was downregulated.[56] Similarly, in bovine nucleus pulposus cells, an increase in medium osmolarity from 300 to 500 mOsm increased aggrecan expression and decreased levels of matrix metalloproteinase (MMP)-3 mRNA.[57] To relate osmolarity to

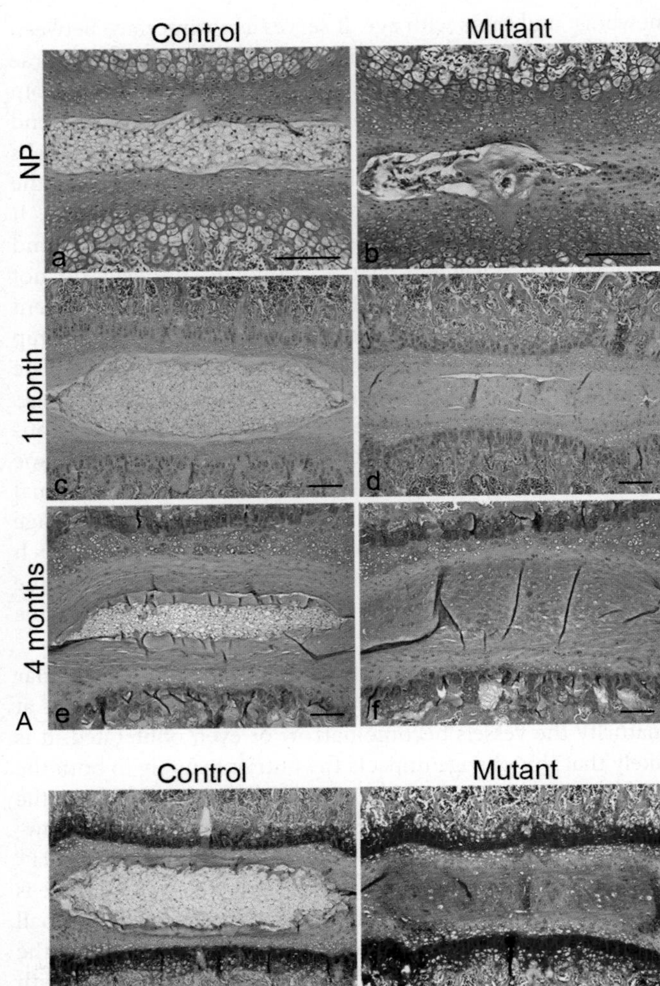

FIG. 46.2 Progressive disappearance of the nucleus pulposus (NP) postnatally in mice with conditional deletion of HIF-1α in NP. (A) Hematoxylin and eosin staining of newborn *(a,b)* and at 1 month *(c,d)* and 4 months *(e,f)*. Results are shown for control ($Foxa2^{Cre}$;HIF-$1\alpha^{f/+}$) and mutant ($Foxa2^{Cre}$;HIF-$1\alpha^{f/f}$) mice. Bar = 50 μm. (B) Safranin O staining of NP at 1 month *(a,b)* in control (HIF-$1\alpha^{f/f}$) and mutant ($Foxa2^{Cre}$;HIF-$1\alpha^{f/f}$) mice. Bar = 100 μm. (Modified from Merceron C, Mangiavini L, Robling A, et al. Loss of HIF-1α in the notochord results in cell death and complete disappearance of the nucleus pulposus. *PLoS One.* 2014;9:e110768.)

loading, rabbit discs were cultured under hyperosmotic conditions (485 mOsm 8 h/day); although loading did not influence proteoglycan content or disc cell viability, after 28 days in culture the raised osmotic pressure prevented aberrant overexpression of collagen I and appeared to influence aggrecan expression.[58]

Loading of the hydrostatically pressurized IVD results in minute-to-minute fluctuations in extracellular osmolarity.[59,60] From this perspective, it is not surprising that tonicity enhancer binding protein (TonEBP), the only known mammalian transcription factor responsive to changes in osmolarity, is robustly expressed in both nucleus pulposus and anulus fibrosus tissues.[61] Importantly, decreased expression of TonEBP correlated to increased evidence of cell death, suggesting that this protein is necessary for nucleus pulposus cell viability in the hypertonic milieu of the disc. Later studies showed that TonEBP controls expression of critical matrix-related targets as well as the water channel AQP2.[62,63] Analogous to the importance of HIF for the survival of the disc due to its hypoxic niche, TonEBP may prove to play a central role in disc survival in the hypertonic stress. For detailed discussion of osmosensing in intervertebral disc see recent review by Johnson et al.[64]

In addition to the above niche conditions, the IVD is also largely aneural, with innervation in a healthy disc limited to the peripheral fibers of the anulus. The sinuvertebral nerve innervates the disc, posterolateral ligament, ventral dura, posterior anulus, and blood vessels. It is composed of a sensory branch from the ventral root and a sympathetic branch from the gray rami communicans near the distal pole of the dorsal root ganglion. The sinuvertebral nerve is believed to have three segmental levels of overlap, which makes it difficult to localize pain originating in the disc, dura, and posterolateral ligament. Nakamura et al.[65] treated 33 patients with a selective L2 nerve root block and showed good relief of back pain. These authors hypothesized that the main afferent pathways of pain from lower lumbar IVDs in patients with discogenic back pain are sympathetic in nature and are mediated through the L2 nerve root via the sinuvertebral nerve; this hypothesis has yet to be validated, however.

Changes in Disc Structure With Aging and Degeneration

Changes that almost universally occur in the IVD with aging include reduction in disc volume, shape, and content. Alterations in gene expression and transcription factors may be responsible for cell senescence within the disc. These senescent cells lose biochemical and synthetic capabilities, which ultimately diminishes the ability of the disc to recover from deformation and renders the matrix more vulnerable to progressive fatigue failure. The nucleus pulposus gradually becomes less hydrated, and by the third decade of life there is usually already a significant decline in the number of viable cells and a loss of proteoglycans.

The early degenerative process affects the nucleus pulposus and the end plate more than the anulus fibrosus. Both anabolic and catabolic processes are upregulated during the early stages of degeneration; however, anabolic repair processes fail to keep up with the catabolic processes and matrix degeneration ensues over time. As the process progresses, the inner layers of the anulus and the nucleus pulposus gradually become indistinguishable and change into a stiff desiccated fibrocartilaginous material.

The number of arterioles supplying the peripheral disc diminishes significantly as remaining blood vessels are obliterated by calcification of the cartilaginous end plates. Loss of end plate vascularity and porosity leads to a reduction in the influx of nutrients and efflux of waste products. Lactate levels rise locally within the hypovascular disc secondary to increased production and decreased removal. Cell apoptosis occurs as a result of decreased tissue pH,[66] and the biosynthetic reparative capability of the disc is thus further impaired.

Thinning and microfracture of the end plate alter its diffusion properties. This may allow rapid outflow of fluid through the cartilage end plate upon loading, thereby rendering the hydrostatic pressure mechanisms involved in load transference less effective and uniform. Focal elevations in shear stresses at the disc level may further adversely affect the disc structure and result in anular damage. Over time cracks develop between and through the anular lamellae. Eventually communicating channels may develop between the peripheral layers of the anulus and the nucleus, and disc material can then herniate through these fissures. The weakened anulus can develop a full-thickness defect and allow near-complete herniation of the nucleus pulposus, particularly when the disc is loaded in flexion and torsion.

The degenerative process resulting from matrix changes and internal structural disruption sets the stage for abnormal motion at the degenerated segment. Changes in disc structure alter the loading response and alignment of the spinal column. These changes can influence the facet joints, ligaments, and paraspinal muscles, which may also become pain generators. However, pain does not always correlate with morphologic changes in the disc and mechanical compression.[67] MacNab[68] described traction osteophytes around the vertebrae originating 2 mm from the anterior end plate at the site of attachment of the outermost anular fibers. These osteophytes were thought to be signs of abnormal biomechanics caused by traction at the insertion of the anular fibers into the vertebral bodies. Subsequent studies found these osteophytes to be inconsistently present.

Thus multiple factors lead to disc degeneration, including insufficient nutritional supply, reduction in the amount of viable cells, degradative enzymatic activity, and cell senescence and apoptosis. Alteration in loading patterns between the end plate and disc leads to anular damage and the potential for herniation. Perturbation of the disc also leads to degeneration and pain in other segmental structures such as the facet joints, ligaments, and paraspinal muscles. The initiating event(s) leading to the onset of degeneration remains unknown.

Associated Factors

Various risk factors have been implicated in the pathogenesis of lumbar disc degeneration. Hangai et al.,[69] in a recent review of factors associated with IVD degeneration in the elderly, cited increased age, high body mass index, occupational lifting, sporting activities, and factors associated with atherosclerosis as risk factors. Multiple studies have demonstrated genetic contributions to degenerative LBP.[70] Battié et al.[71] estimated the familial contribution to IVD degeneration to be between 34% and 61%. Cigarette smoking has also been implicated and appears to have an adverse vasoconstrictive and atherosclerotic effect on the nutrition of the IVD.[72,73] Interestingly. effects of cigarette smoking on disc degeneration seem to be gender specific, with males, but not females, being prone to smoking-induced pathology.[74,75] Type of occupation has also been demonstrated to have an adverse effect on lumbar spinal segment degeneration, increasing the risk of symptomatic DDD. Studies have implicated occupations that require repetitive lifting or pulling, prolonged sitting[76] (such as motor vehicle driving[77]), and whole-body vibration.[78]

Arun et al.[79] used serial postcontrast MRI to study the effect of prolonged mechanical load on diffusion into the IVD. These authors reported that 4.5 hours at a load corresponding to 50% body weight significantly retarded the diffusion of small solutes into the center of the IVD, and 3 hours in an unloaded recovery phase were required to return the diffusion rate to that seen in the unloaded disc. Prolonged mechanical load can therefore cause a disruption of diffusion that may accelerate disc degeneration; however, this hypothesis is yet to be confirmed clinically.

The genetic predisposition to lumbar DDD and lifetime exposures were studied in a classic monozygotic twin study by Battié et al.[71] They reviewed 115 male identical twin pairs for exposures to common risk factors such as occupation, recreational activities, driving, and smoking. Disc degeneration was determined by MRI and clinical evaluation. In the upper lumbar spine only 7% of the variability was explained by occupation, 16% by age, and 77% by familial aggregation. In the lower lumbar spine recreational physical loading explained 2% of variability, age explained 9%, and familial aggregation explained 43%. The authors concluded that primarily genetic and other unexplained factors result in DDD, whereas commonly implicated environmental factors have only modest effects. In a 5-year follow-up study of the same twin population, the authors reaffirmed that genetics have a dominant role in the progression of DDD, whereas occupational lifting and leisure activity had only modest effects.[80] The important role of genetic factors has been corroborated in other twin studies[81,82] but appears to be less of an explaining factor for back pain in older populations.[83]

Several gene loci have been determined to be associated with increased risk for DDD. Type IX collagen was one of the first gene loci identified with some aberrant alleles imparting a 3- or 4-fold increase in relative risk.[84-86] More recent publications also implicate collagen type XI, interleukin-1, aggrecan, the vitamin D receptor, MMP-3, and corticotropin-like immediate lobe peptide as candidate genes.[87] In a meta-analysis of 4600 subjects using disc space narrowing and osteophyte growth as a continuous trait, Williams et al.[88] identified four signal nucleotide polymorphisms with a *P* value $< 5 \times 10^{-8}$. Among these identified signal nucleotide polymorphisms was a polymorphism in the intron of the Parkinson protein 2, E3 ubiquitin protein ligase (PARK2) gene on chromosome 6 (rs926849) significantly associated with lumbar disc degeneration, a subset of the patients also exhibited differential methylation at one CpG island in the PARK2 promoter, providing additional evidence indicating the importance of this gene to DDD. Another study looking at 4043 DDD patients and 28,599 controls identified carbohydrate sulfotransferase 3 (CHST3) as a susceptibility gene for disc degeneration based on enhanced microRNA binding. CHST3 catalyzes proteoglycan sulfation.[89] The discovery of these genetic risk factors has yet to inform new useful diagnostic and treatment modalities, but they offer novel unbiased insight into the pathophysiology of disc degeneration.

Pathophysiology

Internal Disc Disruption

Henry Crock coined the term "internal disc disruption" in 1970 and defined it as a painful increase in biologic activity of the IVD after injury with normal radiographic, computerized tomographic, and myelographic examinations but an abnormal discogram.[67] IDD as a cause of discogenic back pain remains controversial. The advent of MRI has dramatically improved the suspect presence of this entity; IDD presents as a dark disc with relatively preserved height and contour. Pain in IDD is believed to be caused by mechanical and chemical stimulation of nociceptors within the anulus or on the surface layers of the anulus and the overlying ligamentous tissue. The hallmark of IDD is the absence of disc herniation, prolapsed disc material, segmental instability, or other radiographic abnormality.[67,90] Nerve root irritation, radicular pain, and neurologic deficits are also absent. Radiographic changes associated with DDD—such as significant disc space narrowing, end plate osteophyte formation, end plate sclerosis, and gas formation within the disc space—are not seen in IDD.[91] MRI (dark disc), and positive discography (concordant pain in the abnormal level, not at normal adjacent levels) are required to make the diagnosis of IDD. Because of the poor sensitivity and specificity of discography, there are many disbelievers of the existence of IDD as a clinical entity. It is important to note that there is a growing consensus spearheaded by Carragee that discography may accelerate disc degeneration, loss of disc height, and overall progression of pathology and symptoms.[92] Advanced imaging technologies offer a noninvasive way to measure degeneration in intact discs. T1ρ MRI imaging can discriminate painful from nonpainful discs, and T1ρ values strongly correlate with in vivo opening pressure measurements obtained by discography.[93]

Degenerative Disc Disease

The relationship between DDD and LBP is not well understood. Two potential sources that have been implicated as contributors to discogenic pain are sensitization of nerve endings by release of chemical mediators and neurovascular ingrowth into the degenerated disc. The precise pathophysiologic mechanism for chemically mediated induction of hyperalgesia within the disc has yet to be fully elucidated. Radial anular tears provide a route for nuclear material and noxious chemicals to leak from the disc and contact the dural sac and nerve roots; some studies have shown that autologous nucleus pulposus alone has the capacity to produce a robust inflammatory response. The presence of nerve endings in the disc is a controversial topic; abundance of neurovascular ingrowth into the degenerate disc has been less substantiated by recent studies.[94] Some of the important features of the degenerating disc are described below.

Defining Features of the Degenerating Disc

Both nucleus pulposus and anulus fibrous cells are able to secrete a variety of inflammatory cytokines in response to various noxious stimuli and altered mechanics. During the degenerative process, disc cells secrete elevated levels of tumor necrosis factor-α (TNF-α), interleukin-1β (IL-1β), IL-6, and IL-17. These cytokines stimulate the production of additional cytokines, induce matrix catabolism, alter cell protein synthesis, and affect the biophysical properties of nucleus pulposus cells. Matrix destruction is mediated by cytokine-induced expression of MMP and a disintegrin and metalloproteinase with thrombospondin motifs (ADAMTS).[95] This system amounts to a positive feedback loop in which disc degeneration stimulates cytokine production, which in turn stimulates more disc degeneration and cytokine production.

IL-1β and TNF-α are the two most widely studied cytokines in the pathogenesis of disc degeneration. IL-1β is synthesized in an inactive pro-IL-1β form and activated by caspase-1 before secretion. IL-1β binds to IL-1β receptor that acts through the myeloid differentiation primary response gene 88 (MYD88) to induce expression of matrix-degrading enzymes.[52,96] Expression of both IL-1β and its receptor increases in correspondence to the severity of disc disease. Not only does IL-1β signaling induce matrix catabolism by inducing matrix-degrading enzymes, signaling also interferes with aggrecan and collagen II synthesis.[97] TNF-α, on the other hand, is synthesized as a type II transmembrane cytokine. TNF-α-converting enzyme cleaves the membrane-bound portion to generate secreted TNF-α. Nuclear factor-κB light chain enhancer of activated B cells and mitogen-activated protein kinase pathways are the two primary downstream targets of TNF-α signaling in disc cells (see Fig. 46.1).[52] Importantly, in addition to transcriptional induction of several catabolic mediators, TNF-α promotes ADAMTS-5 processing and activation by elevating cell surface levels of syndecan-4, a heparan sulfate proteoglycan.[98] A recent study has also shown the critical contribution of syndecan-4 in controlling TNF-α–mediated transcriptional induction of MMP-3.[99] In addition to their well-described catabolic functions, higher levels of inflammatory cytokines TNF-α and IL-6 have been shown to cause cell death in dorsal root ganglion neurons.[100] Moreover, IL-6 and IL-8 are correlated with painful degenerate discs.[101] Both IL-1β and TNF-α also upregulate nerve growth factor, with IL-1β also inducing the expression of brain-derived neurotrophic factor and substance P.[102-104] Thus, not only could these neurotrophic factors cause pain by dorsal root ganglion sensitization and through retrograde signaling, but substance P has been shown to upregulate synthesis of inflammatory cytokines (IL-6, IL-8, and TNF-α), further exacerbating to progression of disc degeneration.[105] Although it is evident that inflammatory phenotype characterizes degenerate discs, little is known about how the inflammation is initiated and sustained to give rise to chronic LBP.

Subclinical Bacterial Infection of the Spinal Motion Segment as a Possible Initiator of Low Back Pain

There is growing interest and controversy in the notion that subclinical anaerobic bacterial infection could play a role in symptomatic disc degeneration. This subclinical infection is in contrast to LBP from overt discitis, in which 80% of patients present with elevations in erythrocyte sedimentation rate and 50% present with a fever.[106,107] Changes in end plate radiologic appearance may lead to clues to identifying patients who have bacteria-mediated LBP. Modic et al.[108] used MRI to detect changes in vertebral bone marrow associated with DDD. Type 1 changes were described as decreased signal intensity on T1-weighted images with increased signal intensity on T2-weighted images; type 2 changes were described as increased signal intensity on T1-weighted images with slightly increased intensity on T2-weighted images. Fat appears bright and increases the signal intensity on T1-weighted images, whereas water increases signal intensity on T2-weighted images. Consequently, painful type 1 changes are associated with edema in the vertebral bodies. More recently, Jensen et al.[109] showed that these same Modic type 1 changes are strongly correlated with LBP. Albert et al.[110] proposed that anaerobic bacteria, predominantly *Propionibacterium acnes,* might be responsible for radiologic changes associated with LBP. The discs in their study infected with anerobic bacteria were significantly more likely to have Modic type 1 changes than discs infected with aerobic bacteria or discs with no detectable infection.[110] (Of note, whenever bacterial culture is taken from a surgical sample, there is a chance of environmental contamination, which could have affected these authors' results.) However, they found a difference between the aerobic and anaerobic bacteria groups. Simple environmental contamination would not likely favor anaerobic bacteria over the more commonly aerobic skin flora. Moreover, other studies have also found anaerobic bacteria in nucleus material, thus adding strength to the notion that the hypoxic conditions in the inner anulus and nucleus pulposus may be preferable for survival and colonization of anerobic microorganisms.[111,112]

The hypothesis that subclinical bacterial infection can cause LBP is further supported by the ability of antibiotic treatment to resolve back pain in patients with Modic type 1 changes. In a double-blind, randomized, controlled clinical trial, Albert et al.[113] found that a 100-day course of amoxicillin-clavulanate resulted in significant improvement in both disability and pain of patients with LBP. This is one of the most strikingly successful experimental treatments for LBP to date; however, along with the possible shortcomings of their earlier study, there are possible confounding effects of amoxicillin-clavulanate. There is some evidence suggesting that clavulanate has antiinflammatory action in the treatment of ulcerative colitis and analgesic properties during morphine withdrawal in mice, which could lead to a misinterpretation of this clinical study.[114,115] It is important to note that treating back pain with long-term antibiotics also raises global health concerns by exacerbating the

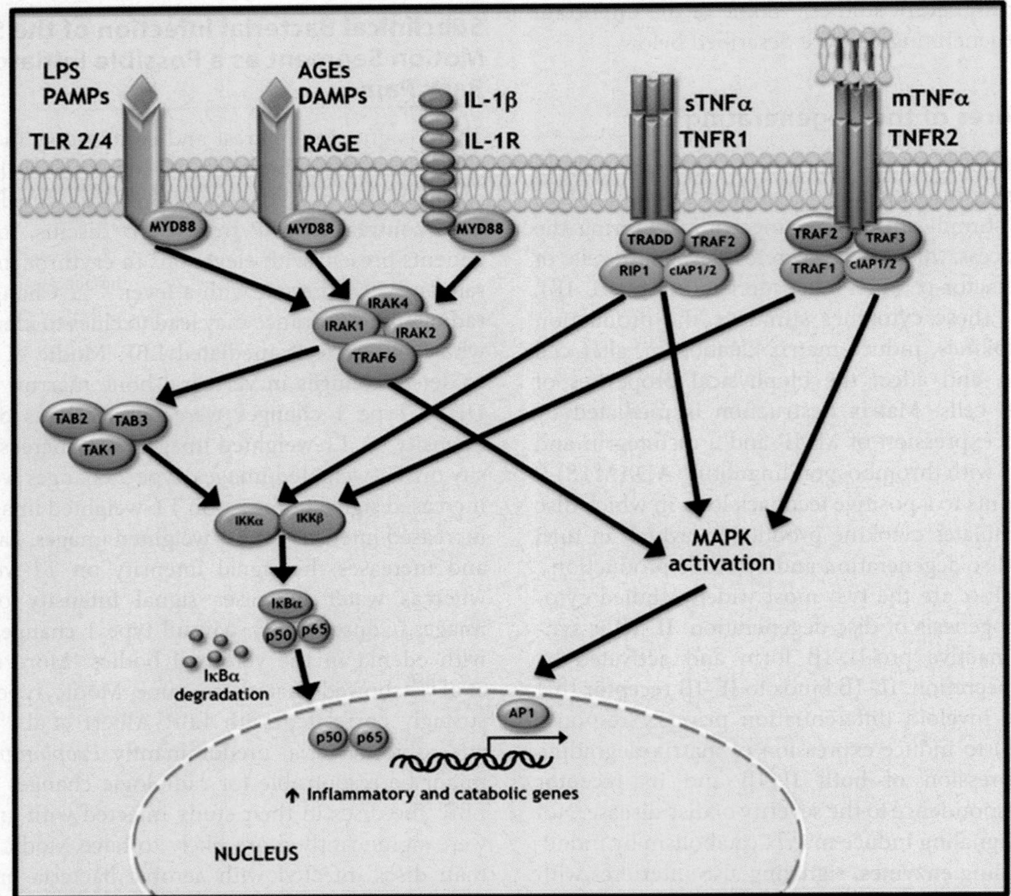

FIG. 46.3 Signaling pathways driving inflammation. Toll-like receptor (TLR), RAGE, and interleukin-1 (IL-1) all initiate their inflammatory effects through MYD88 with subsequent recruitment of members of the IRAK family that activate TRAF6. Tumor necrosis factor-α can stimulate the cell in both its soluble and membrane bound form by activating TNFR1 and TNFR2, respectively. TNFR1 ligand binding results in a conformational change leading to the recruitment of TRADD, RIP1, TRAF2, and CIAP1/2. Ligand binding to TNFR2 results in the recruitment of similar downstream factors. All five of these receptor pathways converge on nuclear factor (NF)-κB and mitogen-activated protein kinase (MAPK) activation to induce their inflammatory and catabolic effects. AGEs, advanced glycation end products; DAMP, damage-associated molecular patterns; LPS, lipopolysaccharide; PAMPs, pathogen-associated molecular patterns. (Reproduced from Gorth DJ, Shapiro IM, Risbud MV. Discovery of the drivers of inflammation induced chronic low back pain: from bacteria to diabetes. *Discov Med.* 2015;20[110]:177–184.)

already serious problem of antibiotic resistance.[116] Despite these limitations, subclinical bacterial infection is a promising new theory of LBP. Additional investigation into the underlying mechanisms linking anaerobic bacterial infection to LBP could enhance our collective understanding of the disease and identify treatments directly targeting the pathways contributing to painful disc degeneration.

Damage-Associated Molecular Patterns as Mediators of Chronic Inflammation and Low Back Pain

Some endogenous molecules and their atypical cleavage products have the ability to stimulate sterile inflammation in the disc. This family of molecules, collectively called damage-associated molecular patterns (DAMPs), include fragments of commonly found extracellular matrix molecules such as hyaluronan and fibronectin as well as high-mobility group protein B1 (HMGB1), a protein involved in chromatin assembly. Hyaluronic acid fragments (12–24 mer) have been reported to enhance the production of IL-1β, IL-6, IL-8, and matrix-degrading enzymes MMP-1, MMP-3, and MMP-13. These effects are mediated by Toll-like receptor-2 (TLR2) signaling and can be inhibited by high-molecular-weight hyaluronan.[117] The TLR2 signaling cascade activated by hyaluronan fragments is the same MyD88-IRAK-TRAF6–dependent cascade activated by both lipopolysaccharide and CpG sequence DNA binding (Fig. 46.3).[118,119] It is interesting to note that by binding TLR2 instead of TLR4 or CD44, hyaluronan fragments stimulate nucleus pulposus cells in a manner that more closely resembles macrophages than chondrocytes, hinting at the unique nature and origin of these cells.[120-122]

HMGB1 is another DAMP that is receiving attention in the disc field. HMGB1 is both passively released from necrotic cells and secreted by monocytes. It likely exerts its inflammatory function by binding to TLR2/4 as well as RAGE receptors.[122,123] It is important to note that redox status of HMGB1 is shown to play an important role in the biologic outcomes it produces.[124] Delivery of anti-HMGB1 reduces pain and TNF expression after application of nucleus pulposus tissue to DRG in a rat model.[125] Fibronectin fragments are another possible inflammatory mediator in disc degeneration. Fibronectin fragments are absent in infant human IVDs, but increase in concentration with aging and severity of disc degeneration.[126] Delivery of a 30-kDa fibronectin fragment into rabbit lumbar discs induced a degenerative phenotype similar to spontaneous human disc degeneration; it caused a significant decrease in disc height and proteoglycan synthesis.[127] These effects could be due to increased MMP-9 and MMP-13 expression along with decreased collagen II and aggrecan expression observed in vitro after stimulation with fibronectin fragments.[128] In contrast to signaling through RAGE and TLR, fibronectin fragments exert their catabolic effects through integrin $\alpha_5\beta_1$.[129] The enhanced catabolism caused by fibronectin fragments could also be a result of their outcompeting CCN2 for $\alpha_5\beta_1$ binding. CCN2 causes context-dependent effects in the disc, promoting aggrecan expression and inhibiting the catabolic effects of IL-1β when bound to $\alpha_5\beta_1$ and, conversely, possibly through HSPGs, promoting catabolism.[130] Thus, atypical matrix cleavage products may interfere with disc homeostasis, pushing the homeostatic balance more toward catabolism.

Systemic Metabolic Syndrome as a Driver of Disc Inflammation and Low Back Pain

Obesity and diabetes are two epidemics in Western society that increase the risk of developing painful disc degeneration. Beyond the greater forces that the spinal motion segments of an obese individual experiences, diabetes creates a niche environment that can drive disc degeneration. Advanced glycation end products (AGEs) associated with diabetes can accelerate disc degeneration by inducing catabolism and promoting inflammation. Although diabetes and obesity are linked, recent research has attempted to isolate the effects of diabetes from the effects of obesity by comparing both obese Sprague-Dawley rats to diabetic obese UCD-T2DM rats while using lean rats as an additional control. The diabetic rats alone had an elevated AGE concentration, which was associated with diminished glycosaminoglycan and water content of discs. These compositional changes resulted in an experimentally consistent decrease in disc mechanics.[131] In a separate study, Tsai and colleagues showed that treatment with AGEs of both rat and human nucleus pulposus cells caused a dose-dependent increase in MMP-2, extracellular signal-related kinases (ERK) activity, and elevation in advanced AGE-specific receptor (RAGE) mRNA expression, which all could lead to enhanced NF-κB activation.[132] Inhibiting RAGE-induced disc degeneration offers an accessible possible therapeutic target; both the antiinflammatory pentosan-polysulfate and AGE inhibitor pyridoxamine are already Food and Drug Administration (FDA) approved compounds and have been shown to reduce the deleterious effects of streptozotocin-induced diabetes on disc health in mice.[133] Independent of the aberrant reactions caused by hyperglycemia leading to AGE production, elevated blood glucose concentration, common to diabetes, has been shown to inhibit nucleus pulposus cell proliferation in vitro, which could further alter cellular homeostasis in the disc.[134] Although in vitro data and in vivo studies suggest that diabetes contributes to disc degeneration, the clinical data have not been as conclusive. A study evaluating nine pairs of monozygotic twins discordant for insulin-dependent diabetes mellitus did not show increased incidence of disc degeneration in the diabetic twin.[134a] A larger study focusing on non–insulin-dependent diabetes showed no increase in diabetic patient disc disease when controlled for body mass index.[134b] Taken together these studies suggest that diabetes, obesity, and their mechanical and metabolic consequences may compromise disc health and promote degeneration.

Effect of Disc Degeneration on Nerves

Degradative changes can occur within nerve roots exposed to nuclear material even in the absence of mechanical compression.[90,135-137] Weinstein et al.[138] investigated the reproduction of pain on discography and concluded that various neurochemical changes within the disc are expressed by sensitized anular nociceptors. These nociceptors are terminal nerve endings of sensory neurons that selectively respond to painful stimuli by the release of substance P.[139] These chemicals are leaked into the epidural space and transported into the axons of the exiting nerve roots. Within the nerve root they alter the excitability of type C nerve fibers and initiate the production of inflammatory agents such as prostaglandins as well as inflammatory cytokines, which results in radicular pain.[68,140,141]

In addition to material from the nucleus pulposus many other substances in the degenerated disc have been implicated in pain generation. The role of nitric acid and phospholipase A_2 in irritation of nerve roots has been well documented.[140,142-145] Phospholipase A_2 has been implicated in multiple aspects: direct activation of nociceptors, nerve injury from degradation of cell membrane phospholipids, and nerve injury from inflammatory mediators created from the arachidonic acid cascade (i.e., prostaglandins and leukotrienes).[146-148] Burke et al.[149] reported on the elevation of inflammatory mediators within the disc such as IL-6, IL-8, and prostaglandin E_2. Other studies have demonstrated the presence of inflammatory cytokines in the facet joints,[150] suggesting facet involvement of a pain generator via a biochemical mechanism as well. Ohtori et al.[151] reported on ingrowth of nerve tissue immunoreactive for TNF and neuronal marker protein gene peptide 9.5 (PGP) in 18 surgically harvested vertebral end plates of patients with Modic type 1 and 2 changes who had undergone surgery. Their findings suggest that axon ingrowth into the vertebral end plate in association with Modic changes was induced by TNF and may be related to pain generation.

Neurovascular proliferation within and around degenerated disc elements has been proposed as another mechanism of pain generation. Normal IVDs have sparse innervation and vascularity that is solely distributed within the outer lamellae (3 mm) of the anulus fibrosus,[152,153] whereas degenerated discs have significant neurovascular ingrowth within the inner anulus and nucleus pulposus,[154] although this observation remains a subject of controversy with the field. Immunoreactive staining and acetylcholinesterase studies have demonstrated penetration of nerve fibers within the inner third of the anulus in association with neovascularized granulation tissue.[142,152] Peng et al.[155] recently reported on a histological study of 19 IVDs harvested from surgery compared with normal control discs. The distinctive histologic characteristic of painful discs was a zone of richly innervated vascular granulation tissue extending from the outer anulus to the nucleus along the edges of fissures. Proliferation of vascular channels and sensory nerve endings rich in the calcitonin gene-related peptide (CGRP) has also been observed in the end plate region and vertebral body adjacent to the degenerated disc. These findings suggest a role for the vertebral end plate and body as additional pain generators in DDD.[156]

Other recent studies suggest that the sensory nerve supply within the IVD is similar to visceral innervation patterns,[157] with CGRP immunoreactive fibers that pass through the sympathetic trunks.[158] This visceral pattern of innervation is potentially susceptible to central sensitization, which may further complicate chronic LBP with psychosomatic overtones.[159] Psychosocial and chronic non–back pain syndromes have been implicated in recent publications as having a significant effect in patients with LBP.[160-164]

Clinical Picture

Internal Disc Disruption

The diagnosis of IDD is not readily apparent on a routine clinical workup. The patient is typically a younger individual between the ages of 20 and 50 years, with recurrent or persistent back pain. There may be a history of antecedent trauma or a forceful provocative event such as heavy lifting, or unexpected flexion or compression force on the lumbar spine, but more often the pain is gradual in onset with no associated event or date.

The pain is characterized as a deep, dull ache in the lower lumbar region, exacerbated by rotation, flexion, and side-bending movements and partially relieved by rest. Sitting intolerance may be a primary complaint, and pain is often relieved in a lateral recumbent position. Occasionally there is a complaint of pain in the buttock or posterior thigh, but there is a conspicuous lack of radiculopathic symptoms. In the rare instances of associated leg pain it is usually a late finding and pain does not follow any dermatomal pattern. O'Neill et al.,[165] in a study involving intradiscal electrothermal annuloplasty in 25 patients, showed that stimulation of the IVD may result in low back and referred leg pain in patients presenting with symptoms of IDD. The distal distribution of pain was found to depend on the intensity of stimulation, and occasional pain extending below the knee was produced.

Physical examination of these patients reveals decreased range of motion of the back and tenderness of the paraspinal musculature but is otherwise normal. The straight-leg raise test may reproduce back pain but not leg pain. LBP may also be reproduced at 20 to 30 degrees of flexion when rising from a flexed position. The sensorimotor examination is unremarkable, and deep tendon reflexes are normal and symmetric.

Degenerative Disc Disease

Patients with DDD typically present with a history of persistent LBP over the lumbosacral spine, sacroiliac joints, and radiating into the buttocks and posterior thighs. Symptoms are often exacerbated with sitting and prolonged walking; signs of neurologic claudication in the legs are not seen unless associated with concomitant lumbar stenosis. Radicular symptoms are rarely seen in the early stages of the disease. In end-stage DDD significant disc collapse may result in foraminal stenosis and late-onset radicular symptoms.

The physical examination is typically unremarkable except for point tenderness over the lumbar spine in the midline and over the sacroiliac joints. Range of motion of the lumbar spine may be reduced, most specifically in flexion. Extreme flexion usually causes significant discomfort as well as returning to upright from a flexed position. Extension is usually the least painful maneuver and may actually relieve pain. The straight-leg raise test may elicit some posterior thigh pain, which is often described as a stretching or pulling sensation, but there is no true radicular pain distal to the knee unless there is coexisting foraminal stenosis. The sensorimotor examination is usually unremarkable, and deep tendon reflexes are normal and symmetric.

Diagnostic Imaging

Plain Radiography

Plain radiographs are the recommended initial imaging modality for patients with LBP. Classic comparative and cost benefit studies have been performed to determine when and what radiographs to obtain.[166,167] In 1982 Liang et al.[168] published a comparison study between performing radiographs on all patients versus only on patients whose pain did not improve within 8 weeks of presentation. They found that risks and costs did not justify obtaining radiographs on initial presentation. Scavone et al.[169] reviewed the radiographs of 782 patients and found that spot lateral and oblique films only added diagnostic information in 2% of patients. They recommended that a spine series in patients with LBP should consist only of anteroposterior and lateral films. In general, flexion-extension and oblique views are only necessary in patients suspected of having instability or a pars fracture. The presence of so-called red flags increase the chances of diagnostic radiographic findings and may prompt the physician to obtain early radiographic studies (Box 46.1).[170]

Typical radiographic findings for patients with DDD include narrowing of the disc space (loss of height), end plate

BOX 46.1 Practice Guidelines: Red Flags

Anteroposterior and lateral radiographs are generally not useful in the acute setting but may be warranted with the following:

- Unrelenting night pain or pain at rest (increased incidence of clinically significant pathology)
- History or suspicion of cancer (rule out metastatic disease)
- Fever above 38°C (100.4°F) for >48 hours
- Osteoporosis
- Other systemic diseases
- Neuromotor or sensory deficit
- Chronic oral steroid administration
- Immunosuppression
- Serious accident or injury (fall from heights, blunt trauma, motor vehicle accident), not including twisting or lifting injury unless other risk factors are present (e.g., history of osteoporosis)
- Clinical suspicion of ankylosing spondylitis

Other conditions that may warrant anteroposterior or lateral radiographs:

- Age >50 years (increased risk of malignancy, compression fracture)
- Failure to respond to 4 to 6 weeks of conservative therapy
- Drug or alcohol abuse (increased incidence of osteomyelitis, trauma, fracture)

Oblique radiographs are not recommended; they add only minimal information in a small percentage of cases and more than double the exposure to radiation.

From Institute for Clinical Systems Improvement (ICSI). *Adult low back pain.* Bloomington, MN: ICSI; 2008.

sclerosis, and the presence of osteophytes. These are, however, late changes occurring when the degeneration is advanced. Degenerative spondylolisthesis and scoliosis may occur as degeneration progresses. Advanced stages of disc degeneration may demonstrate vacuum phenomenon within the discs, a finding that represents nitrogen collection within voids in the disc.

The radiographs in patients with IDD typically show well-preserved height in the IVD and are normal in appearance other than occasional benign spinal alignment changes. Nonstructural scoliosis and loss of lumbar lordosis may safely be observed in patients with sciatic list and paraspinal spasm.

Computed Tomography

Computed tomography (CT) is an excellent method to assess osseous pathology, but it is generally not the imaging modality of choice for either IDD or DDD because they are primarily soft tissue disorders. Injecting contrast material into the vertebral canal (CT myelography) significantly improves the accuracy of the CT scan for demonstrating pathology within the canal such as masses or stenosis; although they are not a primary feature of DDD, they frequently occur secondarily. CT myelography is the diagnostic imaging study of choice in patients with significant scoliosis or those who are unable to undergo MRI examination due to implanted metal, aneurysm clips, pacemaker, obesity, or claustrophobia.

CT scanning has largely been replaced by MRI scanning because the disc is not adequately imaged, and CT exposes the patient to radiation. As is discussed later, CT is also used in combination with discography.

Magnetic Resonance Imaging

T1- and T2-weighted MRI is used in standard protocols. A semiquantitative method is often used to classify degenerative grades. The 5-scale grading system by Pfirrman combines structural changes with distinction of nucleus and anulus, signal intensity, and height of the disc. Quantitative MRI techniques such as relaxation times and T1ρ have the potential to biochemically assess disc tissue but are currently rarely used in clinical practice. Diffusion of water protons and contrast agents are other quantitative methods primarily used in research. MRI spectroscopy is challenging in vivo but may in the future provide important information about the source of pain.

MRI is the best imaging modality for visualization and evaluation of the neuronal and discal elements and is the most valuable adjunctive diagnostic tool in assessing disc pathology. The IVDs are a highly unlikely cause of pain if the patient's MRI is completely normal and all discs are well hydrated. General MRI findings indicative of DDD include loss of water, loss of disc height, disc bulges, and signal or morphologic irregularity within the nucleus pulposus and end plates. In addition, MRIs are often examined for three specific types of findings: a high-intensity zone (HIZ) in the posterior anulus, dark disc with or without loss of height, and end plate signal changes.

The MRI finding of an HIZ was originally described by Aprill and Bogduk[171] in 1992 and is believed to represent an anular tear (see Fig. 46.1). Postmortem studies have demonstrated three types of tears that can occur in the anulus: concentric, transverse, and radial.[172,173] A concentric tear is a crescentic or oval cavity created by a disruption in the short transverse fibers interconnecting the anular lamellae and is usually not visible on MRI. These concentric tears are occasionally referred to as *delamination*. A transverse tear represents a rupture of the Sharpey's fibers near their attachments to the ring apophysis at the disc periphery; these tears are typically thought to be clinically insignificant. A radial tear extending from the nucleus pulposus to the outermost surface of the posterior anulus is manifest on MRI as an HIZ.[174] The HIZ is visualized on T2-weighted spin-echo images as high-intensity signal located within the anulus fibrosus that is clearly distinguishable from the nucleus pulposus.

Decreased signal within the IVD on T2-weighted images with relative preservation of disc height is a relatively common finding in asymptomatic individuals. Such a disc appearance is frequently referred to as *dark disc disease*; however, whether these discs constitute a potential pain generator is unclear. In the absence of any psychometric abnormalities, an isolated dark disc in a patient with no other identifiable causes of back pain is considered by many clinicians to be a source of back pain even though the evidence is weak to absent.

End plate changes (see Fig. 46.2) that occur with disc degeneration have been well described by Modic.[175] Stage 1 change represents edema and is characterized by decreased signal on T1-weighted images and bright signal on T2-weighted images within the end plate. In stage 2, fatty degeneration in the bone adjacent to the end plates is represented by bright signal on T1-weighted images and intermediate signal on T2-weighted images. Lastly, stage 3 changes correspond with advanced degenerative changes and end plate sclerosis and are characterized on MRI by decreased signal intensity on both T1- and T2-weighted images.

When interpreting MRI findings, the clinician must be careful to consider the high prevalence of clinically false-positive findings. Abnormal disc findings on MRI are often found in clinically asymptomatic individuals. Boden et al.[176] showed that approximately 30% of asymptomatic individuals have a major finding on lumbar MRIs. In patients older than 60 years those abnormal findings are almost universally present irrespective of symptoms. Jensen et al.[177] reported on 98 asymptomatic patients aged 20 to 80 years and found that 52% overall had disc bulge in at least one level on MRI. Stadnik et al.[178] showed an unusually high rate of disc bulge (81%) and anular tears (56%) on MRI in their 30 asymptomatic volunteers.

Abnormal MRI findings in asymptomatic patients are not indicators of future problems. Borenstein et al.[179] reported on 50 of the 67 patients from the Boden study at a 7-year follow-up interval and found that incidental MRI findings were not predictive of the development or duration of LBP. Jarvik et al.[180] studied 148 veterans who had been asymptomatic of LBP for at least 4 months. They found an incidence of moderate to severe desiccation in at least one disc in 83%, disc bulge in 64%, and loss of disc height in 58%. In a 3-year follow-up of the same cohort, the investigators found no association between the development of new back pain and incidental MRI findings such as Modic changes, disc degeneration, anular tears, or facet degeneration. The single greatest risk factor for developing LBP in the 3-year interval was depression.[160]

Jarvik et al.[181] also published a report on the use of early MRI in the primary care setting. A total of 380 patients with LBP were randomized to receive either initial spine imaging via rapid MRI or plain radiography. These authors reported that substituting rapid MRI for radiographic studies in the primary care setting offered little additional benefit to patients in terms of secondary outcomes measures at 1 year and had the potential to increase the cost of care by $320 per patient (in 2002 dollars). Carragee et al.[182] performed a prospective study of 200 asymptomatic patients to determine the rate at which new episodes of LBP are associated with changes on MRI. On follow-up MRI in 51 patients who had an episode of LBP, 84% had no new finding. The most common new findings were disc signal loss (dark disc), progressive facet arthrosis, and increased end plate changes. New findings were not more common in patients developing back pain after minor trauma. The conclusion was that new findings on MRI within 12 weeks of onset of a serious episode of LBP were unlikely to represent any significant structural change and preexisted the onset.

In consideration of the high prevalence of false-positive MRI findings, the clinician does well to remember that the MRI does not stand alone in the evaluation of spinal pathology. Together with the patient's history, physical findings, and plain radiographs, selective use of MRI can provide valuable information on the source of a patient's lumbar complaints.

Contrast-Enhanced Magnetic Resonance Imaging

The use of intravenous gadolinium diethylenetriaminepentaacetic acid (DTPA) contrast with MRI in the setting of discogenic pain has also been explored. The addition of gadolinium to a lumbar MRI is known to be useful for differentiating scar tissue from recurrent disc herniation, as the latter fails to enhance while the vascular scar tissue will take up the contrast. It appears unlikely that gadolinium-enhanced MRI helps determine if a degenerative disc is painful. Lappalainen et al.,[183] in an animal study of surgically created anular tears, showed that gadolinium-enhanced MRI did not detect all tears; specifically the peripheral, small tears were not visualized. Yoshida et al.[184] investigated the relationship between T2-weighted gadolinium-DTPA–enhanced MRI and a positive pain response with discography of 56 lumbar discs in 23 patients with chronic LBP. The sensitivity, specificity, positive predictive value, and negative predictive value of the unenhanced T2-weighted images in detecting the symptomatic disc were 94%, 71%, 59%, and 97%, respectively. With enhancement the corresponding values were 71%, 75%, 56%, and 86%, respectively.

High-Intensity Zone

The presence of an HIZ indicates the presence of an anular fissure. Aprill and Bogduk[185] correlated the finding of an HIZ with CT discography and found an 86% positive predictive value for a positive discogram; however, the predictive value and clinical significance of the HIZ on MRI has more recently been brought into question. The results vary among publications. Multiple authors have found a positive correlation between the finding of an HIZ and concordant pain on discography similar to the findings of Aprill and Bogduk,[186-189] whereas others have documented the correlation but found unacceptably low sensitivity.[190,191]

Kang et al.,[192] in a study of 62 patients aged 17 to 68 years, found that only an HIZ in association with disc protrusion correlated with concordant pain on discography. The specificity was 98% and positive predictive value was 87%; however, the sensitivity was low at 46%. An HIZ in association with either a normal or bulging disc on MRI was not found to be associated with a positive discogram. Ricketson et al.,[193] in a 30-patient study, found no correlation between the presence of an HIZ on MRI and a concordant pain response on discography; however, they did note that an HIZ was never visualized in a disc found to be morphologically normal on discography. Further studies[144,187,194-196] attempting to correlate positive HIZ findings on MRI and painful discography suggest that, although lumbar IVDs with posterior combined anular tears are likely to produce pain, the validity of these signs for predicting discogenic lumbar pain is limited.

Although the prevalence is unknown, an HIZ is frequently seen in asymptomatic individuals.[139] Carragee et al.[162] reported the presence of an HIZ in 59% of their symptomatic patient population and in 24% of asymptomatic individuals. In the asymptomatic group, 69% of the discs with an HIZ were positive on discography, whereas 10% of the discs without an HIZ were positive. The authors also reported that 50% of the discs with an HIZ were positive on discography in patients with normal psychometric testing compared with 100% positive discography results in patients with abnormal psychometric testing and chronic pain. They concluded that the presence of an HIZ does not reliably indicate the presence of symptomatic IDD due to the high prevalence of the HIZ in asymptomatic people.

In 2004 Mitra et al.[197] followed 56 LBP patients with the finding of an HIZ longitudinally for 6 to 72 months with MRI. Changes in the HIZ on follow-up MRI—either an increase in intensity or spontaneous resolution—were not correlated to changes in Visual Analog Scale (VAS) score, Oswestry Disability Index (ODI), or symptoms, which again calls into question the clinical significance of the HIZ. Although the finding of an HIZ on MRI has been found in some studies to have good specificity and positive predictive value for concordant pain generation on discography, it has low sensitivity, high false-positive rates, and therefore questionable clinical significance.

Dark Disc

It is quite clear that the majority of patients with a dark disc are asymptomatic. Dark disc is, however, clearly the sign of a degenerative process. Milette et al.[198] found that loss of disc height or abnormal signal intensity were highly predictive of symptomatic tears extending beyond the anulus. Horton and Daftari[199] reported a positive discogram in 50% of patients with dark discs without evidence of an anular tear. An isolated dark disc with concordant pain on provocative discography is often considered to be pathologic in the absence of other potential sources of pain and in the absence of confounding psychosocial issues; however, as discussed previously, this evidence is weak.

Modic End Plate Changes

The various stages of Modic change are thought to be specifically linked with phases of the degenerative disc process. Toyone et al.[200] evaluated the MRIs of 74 patients with Modic changes and found that type 1 changes tended to be associated with complaint of LBP and correlated to segmental hypermobility. Other investigators have also described Modic 1 changes as specifically associated with LBP.[201,202] In a recent large retrospective review by Thompson et al.,[203] Modic changes in 736 patients were correlated to provocative discogram. The authors found that Modic type 1 changes had a high positive predictive value (0.81) for a positive discogram. Modic type 2 had a lower positive predictive value (0.64), and the predictive value of Modic type 3 was not statistically significant.

In the original Modic et al.[175] description of vertebral body marrow changes, conversion between signal characteristics from type 1 to type 2 was described in five of six patients over the course of 14 months to 3 years. Mitra et al.[204] performed a prospective evaluation of 48 patients with Modic type 1 changes. At 12-month to 3-year follow-up, 37% were found to have progressed to Modic type 2, 15% partially progressed, and 40% had no change in type but more extensive Modic 1 changes. Type 1 changes are believed by many to represent an unstable, dynamic phase of the degenerative process and tend to either convert to a type 2 pattern or become more pervasive. Modic type 2 changes are thought to be stable and less associated with painful episodes, but there have been reports of type 2 converting back to type 1.[205] Kuisma et al.[206] reported the prevelance of Modic changes in 60 patients treated nonoperatively for sciatica to be 23%. In a longitudinal follow-up of the same patients at 3 years, 14% were noted to have changed type. Those levels that did not convert to type 2 were found to have more extensive type 1 changes. Development of a Modic change at previously unaffected levels was found in 6%.

Many authors have explored the correlation between Modic changes on MRI with positive concordant pain on discography. Sandhu et al.[207] found that while both were relatively specific for discogenic pain, there was no significant correlation between them. Braithwaite et al.[208] found that Modic changes did not predict a positive response on discography; they concluded that Modic changes may represent a specific but relatively insensitive sign of discogenic LBP. Kokkonen et al.[209] observed that contrast injection during discography reflected pain of discogenic origin well, whereas the pain associated with end plate damage was usually not demonstrated by CT discography. The authors found a stronger association between end plate degeneration and disc degeneration than between end plate degeneration and anular tears, which may explain why Modic changes have been found to be less sensitive for discogenic pain than discography.

Conversely, other studies have found better correlation between back pain and Modic changes than the correlation between back pain and discography. Carragee et al.[161] reported on 100 prospectively followed patients recruited from a study population of asymptomatic persons at high risk for developing disabling back pain. Of all the incidental diagnostic findings, only moderate or severe Modic changes of the vertebral end plates were found to be weakly associated with subsequent development of a disabling episode of back pain. Other structural MRI findings as well as concordant pain with discography correlated only weakly with previous back pain episodes and had no association with future disability or medical consultations for back pain. Interestingly, psychosocial, neurophysiologic (chronic nonlumbar pain), and occupational factors strongly predicted future disabling episodes and consultations for back pain.

Schenk et al.,[210] in a cross-sectional study of 109 women from two groups (nursing or administrative professions), found that Modic changes and nerve root compromise were the only MRI findings that were statistically significant predictors of LBP. Disc degeneration, disc herniation, HIZs, and facet arthritis were found in both groups but were not significant risk factors for LBP.

Similar findings were reported in a study by Kjaer et al.,[211] in which LBP was correlated to MRI findings in a random selection of 412 Danish subjects. Although Modic changes occurred in less than 25% of subjects (16% Modic type 1 and 7% Modic type 2), this finding had the strongest correlation with complaints of back pain. When the subjects were evaluated clinically, the authors found that patients with both radiographic evidence of DDD and Modic changes had the best clinical evidence of disc disease. Clinical findings in patients with radiographic evidence of disc degeneration without Modic changes were not significantly different from the baseline population. The authors concluded that a Modic change was a critical finding in relation to history of LBP and clinical findings.[212] In a follow-up study of the same Danish population, Modic changes correlated with type of occupation, history of smoking, and overweight body habitus. The odds ratio for heavy labor combined with smoking was 4.9 for the presence of Modic changes on MRI.[213]

A recent meta-analysis review of Modic changes by Jensen et al.[214] found that the median prevalence of Modic changes from all studies was 43% in patients with nonspecific LBP. Seven of 10 studies reported a positive association between LBP and Modic changes with odds ratios between 2.0 and 19.9.

Axially and Vertically Loaded Magnetic Resonance Imaging

Axially loaded MRIs have been used to evaluate patients afflicted with lumbar spinal diseases. The idea is to better reproduce the anatomy of the disc under physiologic load. The utility of axially loaded MRI has been primarily studied in the spinal stenosis and spondylolisthesis patient populations.[215-218] Danielson and Willén[219] observed a significant decrease in dural cross-sectional area between a psoas-relaxed position and axial compression in extension in 56% of asymptomatic individuals. The decrease was most pronounced at L4–L5 and greater in older individuals. Saifuddin et al.[220] postulated that lumbar spine MRI with axial loading may increase the sensitivity for the detection of HIZs; however, this hypothesis remains untested.Vertical MRI has also been introduced to represent a loaded spine situation, but no evidence suggests a role in pure DDD.

Discography

Discography is another diagnostic modality for the evaluation of the integrity of the lumbar disc. There is significant controversy surrounding its usefulness. Some investigators consider discography to be the single most important tool in the diagnosis of IDD,[138,221] but recent outcome studies[222] and a practice guideline by the American Pain Society[223] have recommended against the use of provocative discography in the diagnosis of discogenic back pain.

Discography is the only widely available physiologic modality used to determine if a specific disc is a pain generator. Although several attempts have been made to explain the pathogenesis of pain provocation during discography, the precise pathomechanism is not well understood. There are four components to the evaluation of a discogram: (1) the pressure and volume of fluid injected into the disc, (2) the morphology of the disc being injected, (3) the subjective pain response at the level of interest, and (4) the pain response when adjacent control levels are injected.[224,225] The subjective pain response to low-pressure provocation is believed to be the most important determinant of disc derangement; reproduction of the patient's symptoms upon injection of the diseased level is essential to a positive test. A normal disc nucleus can accept 1.0 to 1.5 mL of contrast media. If 2.0 mL or more of contrast is easily introduced, some degree of disc degeneration is assumed with contrast leakage from the nucleus. The use of postdiscography CT increases the sensitivity for the diagnosis of radial tears of the anulus[226]; however, because of low specificity and sensitivity, postdiscography CT is not as helpful in the diagnosis of IDD. Most authors feel that to be diagnostic the pain should be concordant on low-pressure injection and a normal control disc should be pain free.

Despite being used since 1948, discography remains controversial. In the 1960s, Holt et al.[221] and Massie et al.[227] reported on the high false-positive rate of lumbar discography, which was found to be as high as 26% by Holt. Walsh et al.[228] later published a rigorous study on the reliability of lumbar discography. Ten normal volunteers were compared with seven symptomatic patients. Although 17% of the normal discs were found to be morphologically abnormal, there were no positive pain responses. They concluded that with modern techniques the false-positive rate of lumbar discography is not as high as reported by Holt. Derby et al.[229] found similar results in a more recent study of 90 LBP patients and 16 controls. Morphologically, the prevalence of grade III anular tears was 58% among the asymptomatic control population. Presumably asymptomatic discs in symptomatic individuals on pressure-controlled discography demonstrated pain levels and responses similar to the control group, whereas patients with true-positive discography demonstrated pain characteristics concordant with their usual symptoms. The authors concluded that pressure-controlled discography can differentiate between asymptomatic discs and morphologically abnormal discs.

Carragee et al.[163] studied the false-positive rate of low-pressure discography in a comparison of 69 volunteers with no significant LBP and 52 patients undergoing discography in consideration for treatment of discogenic pain. Low-pressure discography was positive in at least one level in 27% of the LBP patients and in 25% of the controls. The false-positive rate of discography was 25% and correlated with psychosocial factors and history of chronic pain of a non–lumbar spine origin. In another publication from Carragee's group,[164] psychosocial factors and chronic nonlumbar pain, such as cervical pain and somatization disorder, also correlated with positive discography in patients asymptomatic for LBP. The authors concluded that false-positive rates can be low with strict application of the Walsh protocol[228] in patients who do not have positive psychometric issues or other chronic pain syndromes.

In contrast to reports of high false-positive rates, two recent meta-analyses of low-pressure discography reported strong evidence to support the role of discography in identifying patients with discogenic pain.[230,231] Combined data from all studies demonstrated an overall false-positive rate of 9.3% per patient and 6.0% per disc. False-positive rates among asymptomatic patients was 3.0% per patient and 2.1% per disc. Chronic pain was not found to be a confounder, and strength of evidence was reported as level 2 in support of the diagnostic accuracy of discography.

Finding a gold standard to which discography results can be compared remains a problem. Few studies have compared the use of discography and outcomes after surgical fusion, which is perhaps the best measure for the validity of discography. Colhoun et al.,[232] in a study of 137 patients, reported 89% favorable outcomes in patients with positive concordant pain on discography versus 52% favorable outcomes among those who had no painful response. Madan et al.[233] had different findings; 81% of 41 patients who underwent fusion based on MRI findings had satisfactory outcomes versus 76% of 32 patients who had surgery based on discography. Perhaps the most rigorous study to date was published by Carragee et al.[234] Success of surgical fusion was compared in 32 patients with single-level positive discogram and a matched cohort of 34 patients with single-level spondylolisthesis. Seventy-two percent of the spondylolisthesis patients met the highly effective success criteria for surgery versus only 27% of patients with discogenic pain. Minimal acceptable success criteria were 91% and 43%, respectively. The authors calculated a best-case positive predictive value for discography of 50% to 60% and concluded that provocative discography was not highly predictive of single-level discogenic back pain.

In an attempt to improve on the poor reliability of discography, interest has turned to functional anesthetic discograms, also called discoblocks. This is a modification of discography in which a local anesthetic, usually bupivacaine, is infused with the contrast agent into the disc to enhance the diagnostic capability of the procedure. Relief of pain after discoblock is considered diagnostic for discogenic pain. A recent randomized controlled study comparing standard provocative discogram to discoblock in diagnosing discogenic LBP was published by Ohtori et al.[235] Anterior lumbar interbody fusion procedures were performed in 15 patients who were diagnosed with discogenic pain by discography and 15 patients diagnosed by discoblock. Outcome measures (ODI, VAS, and Japanese Orthopedic Association score) at 3 years' follow-up showed statistically significantly better results in the group diagnosed by discoblock.

Regardless of the details of how discography is performed, some authors have posed the question of potential ill effects resulting from perforating the lumbar disc. Carragee et al.[222] recently published a report on the effect of lumbar discography in precipitating accelerated degeneration in a matched cohort study. Ten-year follow-up demonstrated that discs that had been punctured had a greater progression of disc degeneration (35% vs. 14% in the control group). There were 55 new disc herniations in the discography group versus 22 in the control group. The authors concluded that despite utilizing modern discography techniques with small-gauge needles, there is still an increased risk of disc degeneration, disc herniation, changes in disc and end plate signal, and loss of disc height when discography is performed.

Although discography has the potential for diagnosing disc derangement, its reliance on the patient's subjective pain response can also be problematic when secondary gain may be an issue. Psychosocial factors and chronic nonlumbar pain have also been shown to alter the diagnostic capabilities of the procedure. Finally, consideration of the consistent reports of the high false-positive rates, as well as new findings of accelerated degeneration in discs that undergo discography, make it difficult to recommend the procedure for the diagnosis of discogenic back pain. Indeed, the validity of lumbar discography is very much in doubt, which is underscored by a recent practice recommendation published by the American Pain Society. The society's current recommendation is that provocative lumbar discography should not be used for making the diagnosis of a discogenic source of pain in the setting of nonradicular LBP.[223] The value of using discography to assess the levels to be operated on in patients with multilevel disc degeneration has not been adequately established scientifically.

Treatment

Once a clinician has gathered all the data from the history and physical examination along with appropriate diagnostic studies, decisions must be made regarding treatment. All available information should be used in formulating a treatment plan to ensure a successful outcome. Sole reliance on individual clinical findings or imaging studies drastically lowers the success rate because the incidence of disc abnormality in asymptomatic patients approaches 30% to 40% and increases with advancing age.

In 2009, the American Pain Society published five practice guidelines regarding the management of chronic nonradicular back pain based on the best available evidence for the various diagnostic and treatment modalities available. Those recommendations are summarized in Box 46.2.[223] These treatment modalities, along with others not mentioned in the treatment recommendations, are discussed in detail along with brief summaries of the current supporting and opposing literature.

Nonoperative Treatment

Nonoperative treatment of lumbar disc disorders has been extensively discussed in the literature.[236,237] Physical therapy, pharmcology, and spinal manipulations have all been supported by mutliple studies of reasonable quality, but it is difficult to fully evaluate most of these studies because of a generalized lack of randomized control design, blind observers, compliance measures, and cointerventions. Additionally, very little of the literature on these nonoperative treatments is specific for the diagnosis of IDD or DDD, but rather is generalized to chronic and acute LBP, which may have multiple etiologies.

BOX 46.2 American Pain Society Recommendations Regarding Management of Chronic Nonradicular Low Back Pain

Recommendation 1

- Strong recommendation against use of provocative discography as a procedure for diagnosing discogenic low back pain (moderate-quality evidence).
- Insufficient evidence to evaluate validity of diagnostic selective nerve root block, facet joint block, medial branch block, or sacroiliac joint block as diagnostic procedures.

Recommendation 2

- In patients who do not respond to usual, noninterdisciplinary interventions, clinicians should consider intensive interdisciplinary rehabilitation with a cognitive/behavioral emphasis (high-quality evidence).
- Clinicians should counsel patients about interdisciplinary rehabilitation as an initial treatment option.

Recommendation 3

- Facet joint corticosteroid injection, prolotherapy, and intradiscal corticosteroid injection are not recommended (moderate-quality evidence).
- Insufficient evidence to adequately evaluate benefits of local injections, botulinum toxin injection, epidural steroid injection, intradiscal electrothermal therapy, therapeutic medial branch block, radiofrequency denervation, sacroiliac joint steroid injection, or intrathecal therapy with opioids or other medications.

Recommendation 4

- Clinicians should discuss risks and benefits of surgery including a specific discussion about intensive interdisciplinary rehabilitation as a similarly effective option, the small to moderate average benefit of surgery over noninterdisciplinary nonsurgical therapy, and the fact that the majority of patients who undergo surgery do not experience an optimal outcome (moderate-quality evidence).

Recommendation 5

- Insufficient evidence to adequately evaluate long-term benefits and harms of vertebral disc replacement.

From Chou R, et al. Interventional therapies, surgery, and interdisciplinary rehabilitation for low back pain: an evidence-based clinical practice guideline from the American Pain Society. *Spine.* 2009;34:1066–1077.

Bed Rest and Advice to Stay Active

The use of bed rest and its duration has long been debated in the literature. Treatment schedules ranging from 2 days to 6 weeks have been described.[238-240] The currently accepted recommendation[170] is limited bed rest for a maximum of 2 days in patients with acute severe pain because longer durations of bed rest may be detrimental to the patient's general health while offering no benefit to the back pain. Even a short period of bed rest may not be beneficial. Allen et al.[241] published a review of studies of bed rest as treatment for 15 different conditions and found that for patients with acute LBP there was significant worsening of outcome measures. A Cochrane Review of bed rest for treatment of acute LBP reported high-quality evidence that advice to rest in bed is less effective than advice to stay active.[242] Progressive return to activity and the initiation of a formal physical therapy or home exercise program are recommended after any initial short period of rest.

Verbunt et al.[243] explored reasons why patients sometimes use prolonged bed rest in the setting of acute episodes of LBP. Among the study population of 282 patients, 33% reported using bed rest, and 8% remained in bed for longer than 4 days. Behavioral factors, catastrophizing, and fear of injury were associated with use of prolonged bed rest. History of back pain and pain intensity was not associated with patient use of prolonged bed rest. Additionally, patients who used prolonged bed rest in the early phase of acute LBP were more disabled after 1 year.

Patient education and advice to stay active is now the favored recommendation. A Cochrane Review[244] of patient education and advice to stay active demonstrated strong evidence that individual instructional sessions of 2.5 hours are more effective in returning patients to work than no intervention; however, in the setting of chronic back pain, patient education was less effective than more intensive interventions. Education sessions of shorter duration or written information was no more effective than no intervention. Another meta-analysis[245] of 39 randomized controlled studies evaluated whether advice to stay active alone was as effective as advice in combination with other interventions such as "back school" or specific exercise routines. Advice as an adjunct to a specific exercise program was the most common form of treatment in the reviewed studies and was best supported for chronic LBP. Outcomes among acute LBP patients were generally poor, but advice to stay active alone was found to be the best recommendation.

Brox et al.[246] published a systematic review of brief education in the clinical setting involving examination, information, reassurance, and advice to stay active. The authors found strong evidence that brief education was more effective for return to work but was no more effective than usual care for reduction of pain. There was limited evidence that exercise was more effective than dissemination of a back book or an educational internet session.

Orthotics

Another common conservative management technique involves the use of lumbar supports. Calmels et al.,[247] based on the results of a randomized clinical trial, recommended the limited use of a lumbar belt to improve functional status and pain and reduce medication use. Oleske et al.[248] performed a randomized clinical trial of back supports and patient education in work-related back pain. The authors found no effect on patient self-report of recovery or lost work time between brace use and controls, but back supports were found to have value in preventing recurrence of work-related back pain. A Cochrane systematic review[249] of brace treatment for LBP failed to find sufficient evidence to support the use of lumbar supports to treat LBP. Moderate evidence was found that braces are no more effective than no treatment or physical training in preventing episodes of back pain.

Shoe insoles have been recommended in the past for both treatment and prevention of nonspecific LBP. The most recent Cochrane systematic review[250] of six randomized control trials reported strong evidence that use of insoles does not prevent episodes of LBP. Limited evidence was found that insoles alleviated LBP, but no conclusions or recommendations were made for use in the treatment of patients with LBP.

Physical Therapy

A large number of physical therapy modalities and routines have been described in the literature. They include land-based and aquatic programs, specific protocols and exercise routines, and group treatment programs—so-called *back schools*. Adjunctive modalities include ultrasound, iontophoresis, transcutaneous electrical nerve stimulation, and heat and cold therapy. Exercise programs commonly use aerobic exercise, stretching, flexion and extension routines, core conditioning, and back stabilization protocols. The goal is to improve core strength, flexibility of the trunk and hip muscles, and conditioning. Patients often respond differently to physical therapy so treatment programs must be tailored to the individual. Periods of activity modification may be necessary. Patients should also be educated on proper body biomechanics, lifestyle, and healthy living habits such as weight control, proper nutrition, stress relaxation, and cessation of smoking.

Several published randomized controlled trials have supported different therapy routines or programs. Although a comprehensive review of all the various programs is not in the scope of this chapter, some critical updates in recent years are worthy of discussion. Recent prospective randomized trials comparing physical therapy to fusion have emphasized the importance of a multidisciplinary approach with cognitive therapy, fear-avoidance counseling, and intensive exercise programs.[251-253] A recent systematic review[246] found moderate evidence that fear-avoidance training emphasizing exposure is more effective than graded activity increase for improvement of pain, disability, and fear avoidance.

Intensive interdisciplinary rehabilitation with emphasis on cognitive and behavioral intervention is one of the treatment recommendations by the American Pain Society.[223] Interdisciplinary rehabilitation was defined as an integrated intervention with rehabilitation and a psychological and/or social or occupational component. Noninterdisciplinary or "traditional" physical therapy is also efficacious in this patient population, but no one specific program, method, or technique is significantly better than another. A recent study of 3094 patients treated with physical therapy for back pain concluded that the treatment is safe but did not reach minimally effective clinical level.[254]

Back schools are another commonly discussed therapy modality, and there is some indication that low-intensity back schools may have some efficacy. Heymans et al.,[255] in a randomized controlled trial, found that low-intensity back school patients experienced fewer sick leave days (68 days) than usual care patients (75 days) and those who attended high-intensity back school (85 days). Functional status and kinesiophobia were improved at 3 months, but there was no difference in pain intensity and perception of recovery among the groups. In another randomized controlled trial, however, Kaapa et al.[256] found no significant benefit of back school compared with physical therapy combined with cognitive therapy at 6-month, 1-year, and 2-year follow-up.

A 2004 systematic Cochrane Review[257] concluded there was moderate evidence suggesting that back schools in an occupational setting reduce pain and improve function and return-to-work status compared with other forms of therapy such as exercises, manipulation, myofascial therapy, advice, placebo, and waiting list controls. Brox et al.[246] published a separate systematic review of back schools and found moderate evidence that back schools were no better than waiting lists, no intervention, placebo, or general exercises for reduction of pain.

A European economic evaluation of a randomized controlled study[258] of intensive group therapy found no significant cost difference between intensive group therapy and standard physiotherapy. There was also no difference in clinical effect between the groups at 1 year follow-up.[259] To date there are no economic studies of group therapy back schools in the United States. Although low-intensity back school and programs in a work setting may have a benefit versus other forms of nonoperative treatment, most of the current literature demonstrates that back schools offer little benefit over standard physiotherapy and cognitive therapy.

Adjunctive Modalities

Another treatment option for LBP includes adjunctive physical therapy modalities such as transcutaneous electrical nerve stimulation (TENS), electrical muscle stimulation, ultrasound, and iontophoresis. Poitras and Brosseau[260] published a review of randomized controlled data on the use of TENS and found that it may be useful for immediate short-term pain reduction but has little impact on patient perception of disability or long-term pain control. A 2008 Cochrane Review of TENS versus placebo[261] concluded there is currently not enough evidence to support the routine use of TENS for the management of chronic LBP.[262] There is even less literature available on the use of iontophoresis and ultrasound in the setting of discogenic back pain. The few randomized controlled trials that exist focus on ultrasound in conjunction with other physical therapy regimens. The efficacy of these modalities as well as heat and cold treatments in isolation has not been determined.

Manual Therapy and Complementary/Alternative Medicine Therapies

Several studies have reported beneficial effects of chiropractic treatment for acute nonspecific LBP.[263-265] The role of chiropractic manipulations for the treatment of IDD or DDD of the lumbar spine has not been studied. Chiropractic manipulation is generally not considered effective in the treatment of chronic back pain resulting from disorders of the IVDs.[266] A Cochrane Review[267] reported there was no evidence that spinal manipulative therapy was superior to general practioner care, analgesics, physical therapy, exercises, or back school in the treatment of both acute and chronic LBP.

Eisenberg et al.[268] published a randomized trial of usual care therapy (nonsteroidal antiinflammatory drugs [NSAIDs], educational and activity modification) versus the addition of the patient's choice of alternative therapy—chiropracty, acupuncture, or therapeutic massage—in the treatment of acute LBP. Outcomes using the Roland-Morris scale and subjective assessment of symptoms demonstrated no statistically significant improvement in patients who underwent alternative therapies. The study did, however, demonstrate an increase in patient satisfaction with alternative therapy.

Hurwitz et al.[269] had similar findings in a randomized prospective study of 681 patients with chronic LBP comparing chiropractic care to medical treatment with 18 months of follow-up. Although less than 20% of the patients experienced overall relief of pain and differences in outcome measures were not clinically significant, patients in the chiropractic group were more likely to perceive that their symptoms had improved.

Andersson et al.[270] compared osteopathic manual therapy to usual care in patients with a 3- to 6-month history of back pain and found that the overall results were similar, but the manual therapy group required fewer medications.

Other alternative medical therapies such as acupuncture, prolotherapy, and massage have also been evaluated. A Cochrane Review of acupuncture[271] showed superiority to placebo sham therapy and also a short-term benefit that did not extend beyond first follow-up when acupuncture was used in conjunction with other conventional therapies. However, a more recent systematic review by Ammendolia et al.[272] questioned inconclusive evidence of the success of acupuncture versus sham acupuncture and called for further randomized trials to rule out the possibility of a placebo effect.

Prolotherapy is a technique that attempts to regenerate ligamentous and tendinous structures of the spine via injections of various irritant solutions. The treatment is usually performed in conjunction with spinal manipulation. There is no consensus on method, type of solution injected, or frequency of sessions. Most practitioners use various combinations of saline, dextrose, glycerin, phenol, and lidocaine. Reports of the efficacy of prolotherapy are conflicted among many randomized trials and systematic reviews.[273-275] No evidence has been reported for the efficacy of prolotherapy without cointerventions such as spinal manipulation or exercise.

The efficacy of complementary and alternative modalities for the treatment of chronic LBP remains in question. The benefit of spinal manipulative therapy is also controversial but may improve patient satisfaction with care and perception of symptoms.

Pharmacotherapy

Judicious use of narcotic pain medications, oral steroids, and NSAIDs in patients with severe, acute back pain can provide good pain relief. The majority of patients with painful degenerative discs can be treated adequately on an outpatient basis. NSAIDs and acetaminophen are common over-the-counter medications used to treat back pain. A Cochrane Review[276] included 65 studies on NSAID use in LBP. NSAIDs were found to be superior to placebo but had significantly more side effects. There is no documented difference between type of NSAID, including cyclooxygenase-2 inhibitors. Acetaminophen has an effect similar to NSAIDs, but it has less risk of associated side effects when taken as directed and generally should be tried before NSAIDs. A Cochrane group concluded that NSAIDs are effective for short-term treatment of acute and chronic LBP, but the size of the effect is small.

Opioid formulations are also commonly used to treat back pain, but considering their widespread use there is a surprising paucity of high-quality randomized controlled data available on their efficacy. A Cochrane meta-analysis[277] of opioid use found only four studies, three of which focused on the use of tramadol. Pooled data found that tramadol, an atypical opioid, was more effective than placebo for pain relief and showed a slight improvement in functional scores. The only randomized controlled study of classic opioids[278] was a comparison to naproxen. Opioids were found to be more effective for pain relief but were not more effective for improving function than naproxen. The Cochrane authors concluded that the benefits of opioids for the treatment of chronic LBP are questionable, and further well-designed randomized controlled studies need to be performed. Two systematic reviews[279,280] of opioid use in the setting of chronic LBP have concluded there is evidence to support the efficacy of opioids for short-term relief of pain only. There is little evidence for long-term opioid use, which is fraught with an incidence of aberrant consumptive behavior approaching 25%.

Opioid pain medication use has many problems, ranging from minor side effects such as constipation and nausea to severe complications including respiratory depression, altered mental status, and insidious issues with tolerance and addiction. Another concern is the combination of opioids and acetaminophen in commonly prescribed formulations.[281] Hepatotoxicity and death from acetaminophen overdose is rare when the dose is less than 7.5 to 10 g in an 8-hour period,[282] but concern arises when patients inadvertently take larger doses in the setting of prescription drug abuse. An FDA advisory committee[283] recommended the addition of a boxed warning on the risk of acetaminophen overdose and also suggested elimination of combination opioid-acetaminophen formulations. Opioid pain medications should be given for only a few days in the setting of severe acute back pain. Opioid prescriptions for patients with chronic back pain are not recommended.

Oral tapering courses of steroids have been found to decrease symptoms of LBP in patients with radiculopathy from disc herniations.[175,284] In patients with axial LBP, steroids are not recommended.[285] Steroids can cause gastrointestinal bleeding; simultaneous use of gastrointestinal protective agents with oral steroids can reduce the risk of this complication.

Muscle relaxants are another class of medication routinely used in the treatment of muscle spasm associated with LBP. Their use should also be limited to very short courses due to their addictive potential. A Cochrane Review[286] of muscle relaxants for the treatment of back pain included 30 trials evaluating the use of benzodiazepines, nonbenzodiazepines, and antispasmotic muscle relaxants. Strong evidence for the efficacy of muscle relaxants over placebo was reported for short-term pain relief in the setting of acute back pain. No difference between the various drugs and classes was discerned. More trials to determine the efficacy of muscle relaxants compared with other analgesics and NSAIDs were recommended.

The last class of medications commonly prescribed in the setting of back pain are antidepressants. Their use may be particularly beneficial in patients presenting with chronic LBP in association with altered mental status, depression, anhedonia, sleep disturbances, agitation, and anorexia. Clinical studies[287-289] supporting the use of tricyclic antidepressants (TCAs) have shown an improvement in mood and sleep patterns. Low doses of TCAs also affect membrane potentials of peripheral nerves, which may be a mechanism by which they produce pain reduction. A 2003 review[290] of antidepressants in the treatment of chronic LBP found TCAs have a moderate effect on pain reduction in patients with no history of depression but reported conflicting evidence for improvement in functional outcomes. Physicians prescribing TCAs should be aware of potentially serious side effects involving orthostatic hypotension and cardiovascular perturbations. Selective serotonin reuptake inhibitors, another common class of antidepressants, failed to show efficacy in the treatment of chronic LBP and should be reserved for emotional or psychiatric disturbances related to back pain, not as a primary treatment for symptoms of back pain.[291]

Keller et al.[292] published a recent meta-analysis of nonsurgical management options for LBP. The authors reported that behavioral therapy, exercise therapy, and NSAIDs had the largest effect of those modalities studied. Machado et al.[293] published a separate large meta-analysis of placebo-controlled randomized trials of various forms of nonoperative treatment for nonspecific LBP. Small improvements in pain were found in patients treated with traction, physical therapy, antidepressants, and NSAIDs; moderate improvements were reported in patients treated with opioid analgesics, muscle relaxants, facet injections, and nerve blocks.

Nonsurgical Interventional Therapies

Nonsurgical treatment alternatives range from short-term temporizing measures, such as epidural injections, to procedures designed to be definitive treatments, such as intradiscal electrothermal therapy (IDET).

Epidural Spinal Injection

The advantage of epidural injections over oral steroids is the ability to achieve higher concentrations of steroid at the suspected site of pain while minimizing systemic effects. Epidural steroids typically work well when administered in the setting of radicular pain and not well in the setting of axial pain. Patients with foraminal stenosis secondary to loss of disc height may benefit from selective nerve root blocks either as a diagnostic or a therapeutic tool. Many clinicians recommend epidural steroid injections as second-line therapy in the treatment of lumbar disc disorders. Epidural steroids are commonly administered by three different routes: caudal, interlaminar, and transforaminal. The transforaminal approach is generally considered best because it achieves a better anterior epidural distribution. Complications from injection exist but are uncommon.[294,295]

Reports on the efficacy of epidural injections in the literature are contradictory. Manchikanti et al.[296] published preliminary results of a randomized trial of serial caudal epidural injections in patients with discogenic pain without disc herniation or radiculitis. The authors reported greater than 50% pain relief in 72% to 81% of patients and 40% reduction in ODI scores in 81% of patients. They concluded that caudal epidural injections with or without steroid are effective in treating discogenic back pain in more than 70% of patients. Two other observational studies[297,298] by the same authors had similar findings for the beneficial effects of caudal epidural injections in the specific setting of discogenic LBP.

Buttermann[299] studied patients with DDD and back pain of greater than 1 year duration who were candidates for fusion. There was initial success of treatment in greater than 50% of patients, but the success rate declined to between 23% and 29% by 1- to 2-year follow-up. The study had a high dropout rate, with more than two-thirds of the patients seeking another invasive treatment within 2 years. The authors concluded that patients with DDD but without spinal stenosis may experience a short-term benefit from epidural injections, with only one-fourth to one-third experiencing long-term improvement in pain and function. Other earlier studies of both caudal and transforaminal approaches have reported similar good short-term results, with up to 59% of patients having greater than 50% improvement in symptoms and function at a 1-year interval.[297,300]

A systematic review[301] criticized the literature on epidural injections for a lack of careful control of route of administration and patient diagnosis. In one evaluation of the pooled data, the only evidence found to support epidural injections was for short-term symptom relief in nonspecific LBP. No well-designed randomized trials were found specific to discogenic back pain. A 2008 Cochrane Review[302] of injection therapy for LBP failed to find sufficient evidence to make a recommendation. A systematic review by Chou et al.,[303] as part of the American Pain Society practice recommendations, found fair evidence that epidural steroid injection is moderately effective for short-term pain relief; however, the literature supporting its use in nonradicular LBP is sparse and has not shown significant benefit. No specific recommendation for the use of epidural steroid injections or the route of administration was made by the pain society.

Intradiscal Injection

Direct intradiscal injection, usually with a steroid solution, is another intervention that has been described in the literature for IDD. The desired effect is suppression of an inflammatory process within the disc, which is thought to be the cause of the discogenic pain. Intradiscal steroid injections were reported in an early case series by Feffer,[304] in which 47% of patients reportedly had remission of discogenic symptoms. Similar results were found by Wilkinson and Schuman.[305] Fayad et al.[306] reported short-term improvement in VAS score at a 1-month follow-up with intradiscal steroid injection in patients with Modic types 1 and 1 to 2 changes on MRI, but there was no long-term benefit. The only two major prospective randomized trials[307,308] of intradiscal steroid injection have failed to find a statistically significant benefit versus placebo in the treatment of discogenic back pain. Other authors have attempted intradiscal injection of various other substances, including solutions of chondroitin and dextrose,[309] hypertonic dextrose,[310] methylene blue,[311] and oxygen-ozone gas mixtures.[312,313] Although these studies report promising results, they have yet to be proven efficacious by rigorous randomized controlled trials.

Thermal Annuloplasty

Intradiscal electrothermal therapy (IDET) involves percutaneous insertion of a thermally controlled catheter into the IVD, usually the posterior anulus, and heating the tissue to a specific temperature (90°C) for a prescribed period of time (e.g., 20 minutes).

The proposed mechanism of action for these procedures is twofold: (1) elimination of nociceptive pain fibers and aberrant painful responses to the disrupted disc, and (2) collagen rearrangement in the anulus with resultant spinal segment stabilization. The biologic effects are not well understood and there is a lack of clear consensus regarding the effects on neuronal deafferentiation, collagen modulation, and spinal stability. Freeman et al.[314] studied the effect of nociceptor destruction via IDET on experimentally created anular tears in a sheep model. The authors failed to find any difference in the amount of neoinnervation in the anulus between specimens that underwent IDET and those that did not, which calls into question the theory of deafferentiation of the anulus. Whether collagen rearrangement with resultant shrinkage and stabilization of the discal element is a viable mechanism for IDET also remains in question.[315,316] Cadaveric studies of the effect of IDET on anular collagen have been performed by Kleinstueck et al.,[316] which showed a 10% to 16.7% reduction in tissue volume immediately adjacent to the electrode.

To destroy nociceptors in the anulus fibrosus temperatures must be raised to a minimum of 42°C to 45°C.[317,318] It is not possible to generate sufficient temperatures in the anulus with a radiofrequency probe placed in the center of the disc, as demonstrated by Houpt et al.[319] Temperature changes at distances further than 11 mm were insufficient to raise the tissue temperature of the outer anulus to the 42°C needed for neuronal ablation. Ashley et al.[320] compared temperature distribution in the disc between a radiofrequency needle and a navigable Spinecath. Using this method, they were able to deliver thermal energy to the anulus more effectively and achieved sufficient temperatures to cause denervation. Karasek and Bogduk[321] have recommended inserting the IDET electrode so as to remain within 5 mm of the outer surface of the anulus. Placement of the probe in the interlamellar plane rather than inside the innermost layer of the anulus allows for sufficient heat generation to destroy the nociceptors in the outer layers of the anulus.

Complications secondary to any of the thermal annulopasty procedures are rare. There has been one reported case of postoperative cauda equina syndrome caused by inadvertent placement of the catheter in the spinal canal,[322] and a few reports of broken catheters with no resultant adverse effect. There have been no reports of infection, bleeding, or other equipment- or technique-related complications.

Early uncontrolled clinical trials of IDET were promising, with improvement in 50% to 70% of patients,[137,321,323,324] but randomized controlled trials have produced conflicting results. Freeman et al.[325] found no significant improvement in outcome measures compared with sham surgery at 6-month follow-up. The opposite findings were reported by Pauza et al.[326] in patients with discographically diagnosed LBP of greater than 6 months' duration. The authors found that 40% of their patients who underwent IDET experienced at least 50% relief of pain, whereas a significant portion of the control group experienced symptom progression. They concluded that the IDET procedure is an effective intervention for a selective patient population and reported a needed-to-treat number of five to achieve 75% relief of pain. Barendse et al.[327] reported on a trial of intradiscal radiofrequency thermocoagulation in patients with chronic discogenic back pain. An 8-week follow-up assessment showed no difference from sham surgery in VAS score, global perceived effect, and ODI outcome measures.

Andersson et al.[328] published a systematic review of IDET versus spinal fusion in patients with disc degeneration and disruption. Similar median percentage improvement was noted between the two interventions for pain severity and quality-of-life outcomes. Fusion demonstrated better functional improvement but had a higher rate of complications. The authors concluded that IDET offers similar symptom relief with less risk of complications compared with fusion. Derby et al.,[329] in a systematic review, concluded that IDET is generally safer and cheaper than more invasive surgical techniques despite the fact that the best evidence available demonstrates only modest improvement in pain relief and functional outcomes.

Other systematic reviews of IDET have been more critical. Helm et al.[330] reported level 2 evidence in support of IDET in the setting of discogenic back pain based on two of the above randomized trials and a number of observational studies. Two observational studies were found by the authors in support of radiofrequency intradiscal thermocoagulation for level 3 evidence. Evidence in support of biacuplasty was lacking and was assigned as level 3 evidence. Freeman[331] published a systematic review of the literature that criticized generally poor outcomes even among studies in support of IDET. The author concluded that evidence for the efficacy of IDET is weak and has not passed the standard of scientific proof.

In summary of all nonoperative interventional therapies, Chou et al.[303] published a systematic review as part of the American Pain Society practice recommendations published in 2009. The authors reported fair evidence that epidural steroid injections are effective for short-term relief of pain. Good evidence was reported that prolotherapy, facet injection, intradiscal steroid, and intradiscal radiofrequency thermocoagulation are not effective. For IDET, no conclusions were made due to the fact that available randomized controlled trials are conflicting. IDET may best be indicated for less functionally impaired patients with well-maintained disc heights and discogenic pain from anular tears.[329]

Surgical Treatment

Once all conservative measures have been exhausted or if symptom nature warrants, surgical intervention may be required. The most common surgical treatment used for recalcitrant discogenic back pain and DDD is arthrodesis (fusion). Lumbar disc arthroplasty is another method approved by the FDA but is not currently in widespread use. Other motion-preserving options being investigated include dynamic stabilization of the motion segment and biologic disc repair.

Chou et al.[332] published a systematic review of surgical treatment for nonradicular LBP as part of the American Pain Society's practice recommendations. The authors found fair evidence that surgical fusion is no better than intensive rehabilitation with a cognitive behavioral emphasis. Surgically treated patients were noted as performing poorly, with less than 50% obtaining optimal outcome with fusion. The benefits of instrumented fusion compared with noninstrumented fusion were not clear. Fair evidence was found that arthroplasty performs as well as fusion for single-level DDD, but long-term outcome data were lacking.

The American Pain Society[223] practice recommendations, published in 2009, encourage clinicians to offer intensive interdisciplinary rehabilitation as an option with outcomes similar to surgery in the setting of nonradicular LBP. The report states that the majority of patients with nonradicular pain who undergo surgery do not experience an optimal outcome, which was defined by the pain society as (1) minimal or no pain, (2) discontinuation of or only occasional use of pain medications, and (3) return to high-level function. The society also suggested that there is insufficient evidence at this time to support disc arthroplasty for patients with nonradicular LBP. Other treatment guidelines also take a cautious view on spinal fusion for DDD, yet in some patients the symptoms are so severe that the chance for a good result makes surgical management attractive, especially when nonoperative treatment has failed.

Spinal Fusion

Surgical treatment for unremitting discogenic back pain has traditionally been spinal fusion. Most clinicians find that it is acceptable to perform spinal fusion for DDD in patients who have not responded to conservative care. The role of spinal fusion in the management of IDD is more controversial.[333]

Three high-quality randomized controlled studies have evaluated spinal fusion compared with nonoperative treatment in the setting of chronic LBP and DDD. Fritzell et al.[334] published a randomized controlled multicenter study of severe chronic LBP comparing fusion of the lower lumbar spine with nonsurgical therapy. The study involved a total of 222 operative and 72 nonoperative patients between the ages of 25 and 65 years with chronic LBP of at least 2 years' duration and radiologic evidence of disc degeneration at L4–L5, L5–S1, or both. The nonsurgical group received physical therapy, patient education, and alternative pain control modalities, such as TENS units, acupuncture, and injections. Results at 2-year follow-up were found to be significantly better in the fusion group, with back pain reduced by 33% compared with 7% in the nonsurgical group. Pain improvement was most significant during the first 6 months postoperatively but then gradually deteriorated thereafter. Disability according to ODI was reduced by 25% compared with 6% among nonsurgical patients, and 63% of surgical patients rated themselves as "much better" or "better" compared with 29% of nonsurgical patients. The "net back to work rate" was 36% in the surgical group and 13% in the nonsurgical group. The early complication rate in the surgical group was 17%. The authors concluded that surgical treatment of severe chronic LBP provides improved results compared with nonoperative treatment in carefully selected patients.

Brox et al.[251] published another randomized trial comparing outcomes of lumbar instrumented fusion versus cognitive intervention and exercise in 64 patients with chronic LBP and DDD. The critical component of this study was the addition of cognitive therapy to an intensive rehabilitation program. The mean change in ODI for the surgical fusion group was from 41 preoperatively to 26 at 1-year follow-up; mean change for the rehab group was from 42 to 30. The authors reported no significant difference in back pain, use of analgesics, emotional distress, and life satisfaction between the groups. Return-to-work rate at 1 year was 22% in the surgical group and 33% in the rehab group. The rehab group experienced greater improvement in fear-avoidance beliefs and fingertip-to-floor distance, while the surgical group had greater improvement in associated symptoms of leg pain. The overall success rate for surgical intervention was rated at 70% and 76% for nonoperative cognitive therapy. The authors concluded that there were near-equivalent outcomes between the groups, which was offset by an 18% complication rate among the surgical group.

The last major randomized clinical trial of surgery versus nonoperative therapy was published by Fairbank et al.[253] The MRC Spine Stabilization Trial was a randomized controlled trial comparing surgical treatment and intensive rehabilitation in 349 patients with chronic LBP. Similar to the Brox study, the intensive physical therapy program in the MRC trial also incorporated principles of cognitive behavioral therapy. At 1-year follow-up the mean ODI scores decreased from 46.5 to 34.0 in the surgical group and from 44.8 to 36.1 in the rehabilitation group. No significant differences were found between the groups in the shuttle walking test and Short Form-36 outcomes. The authors concluded that although the surgical group enjoyed a small—but statistically significant—benefit in one of the primary outcome measures (ODI), this was contradicted by the additional cost and potential risk of complication associated with surgery.

In a separate publication on the MRC trial, Rivero-Arias et al.[335] performed a cost analysis at 2-year follow-up. The cost per patient over the study time frame in the surgical group was estimated to be £7830 ($12,450), versus £4526 ($7200) in the rehabilitation group. There was no significant difference in mean quality-adjusted life-years between the groups. The authors concluded that surgical treatment was not a cost-effective use of health care funds compared with therapy, although the authors pointed out that ultimate costs could vary depending on the number of patients in either group that require subsequent intervention after the 2-year follow-up period.

Meta-analyses of surgical versus nonoperative treatment have paralleled the findings of Brox et al.[251] and the MRC trials.[253] Ibrahim et al.[336] pooled the data from these three randomized trials and found that a modest improvement in mean ODI scores among surgical patients should not be used as justification for routine operative treatment in light of a 16% early complication rate. Mirza et al.,[337] in a separate systematic review, concluded that surgical outcomes are equivalent to a structured rehabilitation program with cognitive behavioral therapy.

Phillips et al.[338] performed a systematic review of fusion in the treatment of DDD. They concluded that comparing surgery to nonoperative treatment obviates the fact that the treatments generally are performed in sequence, with surgery occurring when nonoperative treatment has failed. They further concluded that lumbar spine fusions result in meaningful improvements in pain and function.

Fusion Technologies

Over the years there has been a change from posterolateral and anterior stand-alone fusions to circumferential fusions. In recent years lateral fusion techniques have grown in popularity, as have minimally invasive fusion techiques. There is little question that minimally invasive approaches will grow in use; in fact, all procedures today are done with less-invasive techniques than in the past.

The use of new materials in implants and osteobiologics are discussed elsewhere in this text. Iliac crest bone grafts are today rarely used in the United States.

Adjacent-Segment Degeneration

A serious adverse effect of fusion surgery is adjacent-segment pathology. Sometimes it is an imaging finding without clinical importance, but sometimes it results in pain and may result in an extension of the fusion.[339,340]

As a consequence motion-preservation techniques have developed such as disc replacements and posterior motion preservation systems. These techniques are discussed in other chapters of this text.

Biologic Treatment of Degenerative Disc Disease

Over the past few decades research into biologic repair of disc degeneration has grown substantially. Molecular therapy, gene therapy, and stem cell disc regeneration are all viable alternatives but are not yet at the stage where they can be used clinically with predictable success.[341-343] Tissue engineering approaches are challenged by the complexity and stresses of the IVD.[344] Biologic repair will undoubtedly succeed at some time in the future but is not an immediate solution.

Summary

Lumbar disc disease is a common problem that affects many people at various ages in the form of IDD and DDD. Detailed history and physical examination are vital components in harmony with imaging modalities to make an accurate diagnosis. Recent practice guidelines have reaffirmed that the first line of treatment for those who have LBP of a discogenic source, with or without radicular symptoms, is conservative therapy. New emphasis has been placed on multidisciplinary therapy incorporating cognitive and behavioral treatment. Intradiscal therapy remains controversial, and many patients who undergo this procedure may eventually require arthrodesis. Surgical fusion, in all the various forms, is an appropriate option for patients who do not improve with appropriate nonoperative therapy. Preliminary studies of lumbar total disc replacement report equivalence to arthrodesis for the management of this patient population. Development of new motion-preserving techniques will likely change the treatment approach, as will emerging biologic techniques.

KEY POINTS

1. Detailed history and physical examination in conjunction with radiographic and MRI findings such as loss of disc height, disc signal changes, HIZs, and Modic changes are the best means available for diagnosing IDD and DDD.
2. Routine use of lumbar discography is not recommended for diagnosing a discogenic LBP.
3. Recent practice guidelines have reaffirmed that the first line of treatment for patients with LBP of a discogenic source, with or without radicular symptoms, is conservative therapy, and new emphasis has been placed on multidisciplinary therapy incorporating cognitive and behavioral treatment.
4. IDET remains controversial, and many patients who undergo this procedure still require arthrodesis. Other forms of less-invasive therapy, such as prolotherapy and intradiscal corticosteroid injections, are not recommended in this patient population.
5. Surgical fusion is an appropriate option for patients who do not improve with exhaustive nonoperative therapy.
6. No one method for achieving segmental fusion has clearly been shown to be better than another.
7. Preliminary studies of lumbar total disc replacement report equivalence to arthrodesis for the surgical management of this patient population, but there is still insufficient evidence to evaluate the long-term benefits and complications.

KEY REFERENCES

1. Aprill C, Bogduk N. High-intensity zone: a diagnostic sign of painful lumbar disc on magnetic resonance imaging. *Br J Radiol.* 1992;65(773):361-369.
   This study focuses on HIZ as a diagnostic sign of an anular tear.

2. Boden S, McCowin P, Davis D, et al. Abnormal magnetic-resonance scans of the lumbar spine in asymptomatic subjects: a prospective investigation. *J Bone Joint Surg Am*. 1990;72(3):403-408.
Abnormal MRI of the lumbar spine often reveals abnormalities in asymptomatic subjects, as illustrated by this article.
3. Brox J. Randomized clinical trial of lumbar instrumented fusion and cognitive intervention and exercises in patients with chronic low back pain and disc degeneration. *Spine*. 2003;28:1913-1921.
This article reports the outcomes of a randomized controlled trial of operative versus cognitive therapy and intensive exercise for the treatment of chronic low back pain and shows near-equivalent outcomes between the groups.
4. Carragee E. A gold standard evaluation of the "discogenic pain" diagnosis as determined by provocative discography. *Spine*. 2006;31:2115-2123.
This article calculates a best possible positive predictive value of lumbar discography in diagnosing discogenic back pain based on success of fusion in patients with positive discography versus a cohort of spondylolisthesis patients treated surgically.
5. Carragee E, Paragioudakis S, Khurana S. Lumbar high-intensity zone and discography in subjects without low back problems. *Spine*. 2000;25(23):2987-2992.
This article points out the low predictive value of lumbar HIZ and discography.
6. Chou R, Baisden J, Carragee EJ, et al. Surgery for low back pain: a review of the evidence for an American Pain Society Clinical Practice Guideline. *Spine*. 2009;34(10):1094-1109.
This meta-analysis reviews the best available evidence for surgical treatment of patients with low back pain as part of the American Pain Society's current practice guidelines.
7. Chou R, Loeser JD, Owens DK, et al. American Pain Society Low Back Pain Guideline Panel. Interventional therapies, surgery, and interdisciplinary rehabilitation for low back pain: an evidence-based clinical practice guideline from the American Pain Society. *Spine*. 2009;34(10):1066-1077.
This article reports the American Pain Society's current practice recommendations for the treatment of chronic low back pain.
8. Crock H. Internal disc disruption: a challenge to disc prolapse fifty years on. *Spine*. 1986;11(6):650-653.
The concept of IDD was elaborated in this article.
9. Fairbank J. Randomised controlled trial to compare surgical stabilisation of the lumbar spine with an intensive rehabilitation programme for patients with chronic low back pain: the MRC spine stabilisation trial. *BMJ*. 2005;330:1233.
This large randomized controlled trial compared operative and interdisciplinary physical therapy programs in the treatment of chronic low back pain. A small benefit was shown for the surgically treated group but with a significant increase in cost and complications.
10. Fritzell P, et al. Lumbar fusion versus nonsurgical treatment for chronic low back pain: a multicenter randomized controlled trial from the Swedish Lumbar Spine Study Group. *Spine*. 2001;26(23):2521-2532.
This multicenter, randomized controlled trial comparing lumbar fusion and nonsurgical treatment for chronic back pain showed superiority for the fusion alternative.
11. Modic M, Steinberg P, Ross J, et al. Degenerative disc disease: assessment of changes in vertebral body marrow with MR imaging. *Radiology*. 1988;166(1 Pt 1):193-199.
The changes observed in vertebrae adjacent to the degenerative disc are described and classified.

REFERENCES

1. Arnbak B, Jensen TS, Egund N, et al. Prevalence of degenerative and spondyloarthritis-related magnetic resonance imaging findings in the spine and sacroiliac joints in patients with persistent low back pain. *Eur Radiol*. 2016;26(4):1191-1203.
2. Livshits G, Popham M, Malkin I, et al. Lumbar disc degeneration and genetic factors are the main risk factors for low back pain in women: the UK Twin Spine Study. *Ann Rheum Dis*. 2011;70(10):1740-1745. doi:10.1136/ard.2010.137836.
3. Cheung KM, Karppinen J, Chan D, et al. Prevalence and pattern of lumbar magnetic resonance imaging changes in a population study of one thousand forty-three individuals. *Spine*. 2009;34(9):934-940.
4. Dreischarf M, Albiol L, Rohlmann A, et al. Age-related loss of lumbar spinal lordosis and mobility–a study of 323 asymptomatic volunteers. *PLoS One*. 2014;9(12):e116186.
5. Andersson G. Epidemiological features of chronic low-back pain. *Lancet*. 1999;354:581-585.
6. Papageorgiou AC, Croft PR, Ferry S, Jayson MI, Silman AJ. Estimating the prevalence of low back pain in the general population. Evidence from the South Manchester Back Pain Survey. *Spine*. 1995;20:1889-1894.
7. Waddell G. A new clinical model for the treatment of low-back pain. *Spine*. 1987;12:632-644.
8. Croft PR, Macfarlane GJ, Papageorgiou AC, Thomas E, Silman AJ. Outcome of low back pain in general practice: a prospective study. *BMJ*. 1998;316:1356-1359.
9. Walsh K, Cruddas M, Coggon D. Low back pain in eight areas of Britain. *J Epidemiol Community Health*. 1992;46:227-230.
10. Andersson GB, Svensson HO, Odén A. The intensity of work recovery in low back pain. *Spine*. 1983;8:880-884.
11. Wahlgren DR, Atkinson JH, Epping-Jordan JE, et al. One-year follow-up of first onset low back pain. *Pain*. 1997;73:213-221.
12. Carey TS, Garrett JM, Jackman AM. Beyond the good prognosis. Examination of an inception cohort of patients with chronic low back pain. *Spine*. 2000;25:115-120.
13. Roland MO, Morrell DC, Morris RW. Can general practitioners predict the outcome of episodes of back pain? *Br Med J (Clin Res Ed)*. 1983;286:523-525.
14. Papageorgiou AC, Croft PR, Thomas E, et al. Influence of previous pain experience on the episode incidence of low back pain: results from the South Manchester Back Pain Study. *Pain*. 1996;66:181-185.
15. Smith SE, Darden BV, Rhyne AL, Wood KE. Outcome of unoperated discogram-positive low back pain. *Spine*. 1995;20:1997-2000.
16. Kirkaldy-Willis WH, Farfan HF. Instability of the lumbar spine. *Clin Orthop Relat Res*. 1982;165:110-123.
17. Waris E, et al. Disc degeneration in low back pain: a 17-year follow-up study using magnetic resonance imaging. *Spine*. 2007;32:681-684.
18. Dahia CL, Mahoney EJ, Durrani AA, Wylie C. Intercellular signaling pathways active during intervertebral disc growth, differentiation, and aging. *Spine*. 2009;34:456-462.
19. Risbud MV, Shapiro IM. Notochordal cells in the adult intervertebral disc: new perspective on an old question. *Crit Rev Eukaryot Gene Expr*. 2011;21(1):29-41.
20. Gan JC, Ducheyne P, Vresilovic EJ, Swaim W, Shapiro IM. Intervertebral disc tissue engineering I: characterization of the nucleus pulposus. *Clin Orthop Relat Res*. 2003;411:305-314.

21. Risbud MV, Schipani E, Shapiro IM. Hypoxic regulation of nucleus pulposus cell survival: from niche to notch. *Am J Pathol.* 2010;176(4):1577-1583.
22. Agrawal A, Guttapalli A, Narayan S, et al. Normoxic stabilization of HIF-1alpha drives glycolytic metabolism and regulates aggrecan gene expression in nucleus pulposus cells of the rat intervertebral disk. *Am J Physiol Cell Physiol.* 2007;293:C621-C631.
23. Souter WA, Taylor TK. Sulphated acid mucopolysaccharide metabolism in the rabbit intervertebral disc. *J Bone Joint Surg Br.* 1970;52:371-384.
24. Marchand F, Ahmed AM. Investigation of the laminate structure of lumbar disc anulus fibrosus. *Spine.* 1990;15:402-410.
25. Arana CJ, Diamandis EP, Kandel RA. Cartilage tissue enhances proteoglycan retention by nucleus pulposus cells in vitro. *Arthritis Rheum.* 2010;62(11):3395-3403.
26. Kim KW, Lim TH, Kim JG, et al. The origin of chondrocytes in the nucleus pulposus and histologic findings associated with the transition of a notochordal nucleus pulposus to a fibrocartilaginous nucleus pulposus in intact rabbit intervertebral discs. *Spine.* 2003;28(10):982-990.
27. Kim KW, Ha KY, Park JB, et al. Expressions of membrane-type I matrix metalloproteinase, Ki-67 protein, and type II collagen by chondrocytes migrating from cartilage endplate into nucleus pulposus in rat intervertebral discs: a cartilage endplate-fracture model using an intervertebral disc organ culture. *Spine.* 2005;30(12):1373-1378.
28. Moore RJ. The vertebral end-plate: what do we know? *Eur Spine J.* 2000;9:92-96.
29. Nachemson A, Lewin T, Maroudas A, Freeman MA. In vitro diffusion of dye through the end-plates and the annulus fibrosus of human lumbar inter-vertebral discs. *Acta Orthop Scand.* 1970;41:589-607.
30. Crock HV, Yoshizawa H. The blood supply of the lumbar vertebral column. *Clin Orthop Relat Res.* 1976;115:6-21.
31. Gruber HE, Ashraf N, Kilburn J, et al. Vertebral endplate architecture and vascularization: application of micro-computerized tomography, a vascular tracer, and immunocytochemistry in analyses of disc degeneration in the aging sand rat. *Spine.* 2005;30:2593-2600.
32. Hassler O. The human intervertebral disc: A micro-angiographical study on its vascular supply at various ages. *Acta Orthop Scand.* 1969;40:765-772.
33. Rudert M, Tillmann B. Lymph and blood supply of the human intervertebral disc: cadaver study of correlations to discitis. *Acta Orthop Scand.* 1993;64:37-40.
34. Ejeskär A, Holm S. Oxygen tension measurements in the intervertebral disc. A methodological and experimental study. *Ups J Med Sci.* 1979;84(1):83-93.
35. Bartels EM, Fairbank JC, Winlove CP, Urban JP. Oxygen and lactate concentrations measured in vivo in the intervertebral discs of patients with scoliosis and back pain. *Spine.* 1998; 23:1-7.
36. Rajpurohit R, Risbud MV, Ducheyne P, Vresilovic EJ, Shapiro IM. Phenotypic characteristics of the nucleus pulposus: expression of hypoxia inducing factor-1, glucose transporter-1 and MMP-2. *Cell Tissue Res.* 2002;308:401-407.
37. Semenza GL, Roth PH, Fang HM, Wang GL. Transcriptional regulation of genes encoding glycolytic enzymes by hypoxia-inducible factor 1. *J Biol Chem.* 1994;269:23757-23763.
38. Wang GL, Jiang BH, Rue EA, Semenza GL. Hypoxia-inducible factor 1 is a basic-helix-loop-helix-PAS heterodimer regulated by cellular O2 tension. *Proc Natl Acad Sci USA.* 1995;92:5510-5514.
39. Papandreou I, Cairns RA, Fontana L, Lim AL, Denko NC. HIF-1 mediates adaptation to hypoxia by actively downregulating mitochondrial oxygen consumption. *Cell Metab.* 2006;3:187-197.
40. Fukuda R, Zhang H, Kim JW, et al. HIF-1 regulates cytochrome oxidase subunits to optimize efficiency of respiration in hypoxic cells. *Cell.* 2007;129:111-122.
41. Schipani E, Ryan HE, Didrickson S, et al. Hypoxia in cartilage: HIF-1 alpha is essential for chondrocyte growth arrest and survival. *Genes Dev.* 2001;15:2865-2876.
42. Zhang H, Bosch-Marce M, Shimoda LA, et al. Mitochondrial autophagy is an HIF-1–dependent adaptive metabolic response to hypoxia. *J Biol Chem.* 2008;283:10892-10903.
43. Hofbauer KH, Gess B, Lohaus C, et al. Oxygen tension regulates the expression of a group of procollagen hydroxylases. *Eur J Biochem.* 2003;270:4515-4522.
44. Sowter HM, Raval RR, Moore JW, Ratcliffe PJ, Harris AL. Predominant role of hypoxia-inducible transcription factor (Hif)-1 alpha versus Hif-2 alpha in regulation of the transcriptional response to hypoxia. *Cancer Res.* 2003;63:6130-6134.
45. Smits P, Lefebvre V. Sox5 and Sox6 are required for notochord extracellular matrix sheath formation, notochord cell survival and development of the nucleus pulposus of intervertebral discs. *Development.* 2003;130:1135-1148.
46. Lafont JE, Talma S, Murphy CL. Hypoxia-inducible factor 2alpha is essential for hypoxic induction of the human articular chondrocyte phenotype. *Arthritis Rheum.* 2007;56:3297-3306.
47. Khan WS, Adesida AB, Hardingham TE. Hypoxic conditions increase hypoxia-inducible transcription factor 2alpha and enhance chondrogenesis in stem cells from the infrapatellar fat pad of osteoarthritis patients. *Arthritis Res Ther.* 2007;9:R55.
48. Kanichai M, Ferguson D, Prendergast PJ, Campbell VA. Hypoxia promotes chondrogenesis in rat mesenchymal stem cells: a role for AKT and hypoxia-inducible factor (HIF)-1alpha. *J Cell Physiol.* 2008;216:708-715.
49. Risbud MV, Guttapalli A, Stokes DG, et al. Nucleus pulposus cells express HIF-1alpha under normoxic culture conditions: a metabolic adaptation to the intervertebral disc microenvironment. *J Cell Biochem.* 2006;98:152-159.
50. Agrawal A, Gajghate S, Smith H, et al. Cited2 modulates hypoxia-inducible factor-dependent expression of vascular endothelial growth factor in nucleus pulposus cells of the rat intervertebral disc. *Arthritis Rheum.* 2008;58:3798-3808.
51. Merceron C, Mangiavini L, Robling A, et al. Loss of HIF-1α in the notochord results in cell death and complete disappearance of the nucleus pulposus. *PLoS One.* 2014;9:e110768.
52. Risbud MV, Shapiro IM. Role of cytokines in intervertebral disc degeneration: pain and disc content. *Nat Rev Rheumatol.* 2014;10:44-56.
53. Roberts S, Urban JPG. Intervertebral discs. In: Riihimäki H, Viikari-Juntura E, eds. *Encyclopedia of Occupational Health and Safety.* Geneva: International Labor Organization; 2011.
54. Ishihara H, Warensjo K, Roberts S, Urban JP. Proteoglycan synthesis in the intervertebral disk nucleus: the role of extracellular osmolality. *Am J Physiol.* 1997;272:C1499-C1506.
55. Van Dijk B, Potier E, Ito K. Culturing bovine nucleus pulposus explants by balancing medium osmolarity. *Tissue Eng C Methods.* 2011;17:1089-1096.

56. Wuertz K, Urban JPG, Klasen J, et al. Influence of extracellular osmolarity and mechanical stimulation on gene expression of intervertebral disc cells. *J Orthop Res.* 2007;25:1513-1522.
57. Neidlinger-Wilke C, Mietsch A, Rinkler C, et al. Interactions of environmental conditions and mechanical loads have influence on matrix turnover by nucleus pulposus cells. *J Orthop Res.* 2012;30:112-121.
58. Haschtmann D, Stoyanov JV, Ferguson SJ. Influence of diurnal hyperosmotic loading on the metabolism and matrix gene expression of a whole-organ intervertebral disc model. *J Orthop Res.* 2006;24:1957-1966.
59. Urban JP. The chondrocyte: a cell under pressure. *Br J Rheumatol.* 1994;33:901-908.
60. Roberts N, Hogg D, Whitehouse GH, Dangerfield P. Quantitative analysis of diurnal variation in volume and water content of lumbar intervertebral discs. *Clin Anat.* 1998;11:1-8.
61. Tsai TT, Danielson KG, Guttapalli A, et al. TonEBP/OREBP is a regulator of nucleus pulposus cell function and survival in the intervertebral disc. *J Biol Chem.* 2006;281:25416-25424.
62. Hiyama A, Gogate SS, Gajghate S, et al. BMP-2 and TGF-beta stimulate expression of beta1,3-glucuronosyl transferase 1 (GlcAT-1) in nucleus pulposus cells through AP1, TonEBP, and Sp1: role of MAPKs. *J Bone Miner Res.* 2010;25:1179-1190.
63. Gajghate S, Hiyama A, Shah M, et al. Osmolarity and intracellular calcium regulate aquaporin2 expression through TonEBP in nucleus pulposus cells of the intervertebral disc. *J Bone Miner Res.* 2009;24:992-1001.
64. Johnson ZI, Shapiro IM, Risbud MV. Extracellular osmolarity regulates matrix homeostasis in the intervertebral disc and articular cartilage: evolving role of TonEBP. *Matrix Biol.* 2014;40:10-16.
65. Nakamura SI, et al. The afferent pathways of discogenic low-back pain. Evaluation of L2 spinal nerve infiltration. *J Bone Joint Surg Br.* 1996;78:606-612.
66. Buckwalter JA. Aging and degeneration of the human intervertebral disc. *Spine.* 1995;20:1307-1314.
67. Crock HV. Internal disc disruption. A challenge to disc prolapse fifty years on. *Spine.* 1986;11:650-653.
68. Macnab I. The traction spur. An indicator of segmental instability. *J Bone Joint Surg Am.* 1971;53:663-670.
69. Hangai M, Kaneoka K, Kuno S, et al. Factors associated with lumbar intervertebral disc degeneration in the elderly. *Spine J.* 2008;8:732-740.
70. Kalichman L, Hunter DJ. The genetics of intervertebral disc degeneration. Familial predisposition and heritability estimation. *Joint Bone Spine.* 2008;75:383-387.
71. Battié MC, Videman T, Gibbons LE, et al. 1995 Volvo Award in clinical sciences. Determinants of lumbar disc degeneration. A study relating lifetime exposures and magnetic resonance imaging findings in identical twins. *Spine.* 1995;20:2601-2612.
72. An HS, Silveri CP, Simpson JM, et al. Comparison of smoking habits between patients with surgically confirmed herniated lumbar and cervical disc disease and controls. *J Spinal Disord.* 1994;7:369-373.
73. Kauppila LI. Atherosclerosis and disc degeneration/low-back pain—a systematic review. *Eur J Vasc Endovasc Surg.* 2009;37:661-670.
74. Hassett G, Hart DJ, Manek NJ, Doyle DV, Spector TD. Risk factors for progression of lumbar spine disc degeneration: the Chingford Study. *Arthritis Rheum.* 2003;48(11):3112-3117.
75. Takatalo J, Karppinen J, Taimela S, et al. Body mass index is associated with lumbar disc degeneration in young Finnish males: subsample of Northern Finland birth cohort study 1986. *BMC Musculoskelet Disord.* 2013;14:87.
76. Lis AM, Black KM, Korn H, Nordin M. Association between sitting and occupational LBP. *Eur Spine J.* 2007;16:283-298.
77. Kelsey JL, Hardy RJ. Driving of motor vehicles as a risk factor for acute herniated lumbar intervertebral disc. *Am J Epidemiol.* 1975;102:63-73.
78. Wilder DG. The biomechanics of vibration and low back pain. *Am J Ind Med.* 1993;23:577-588.
79. Arun R, Freeman BJ, Scammell BE, et al. What influence does sustained mechanical load have on diffusion in the human intervertebral disc? an in vivo study using serial postcontrast magnetic resonance imaging. *Spine.* 2009;34:2324-2337.
80. Videman T, Battié MC, Ripatti S, et al. Determinants of the progression in lumbar degeneration: a 5-year follow-up study of adult male monozygotic twins. *Spine.* 2006;31:671-678.
81. MacGregor AJ, Andrew T, Sambrook PN, Spector TD. Structural, psychological, and genetic influences on low back and neck pain: a study of adult female twins. *Arthritis Rheum.* 2004;51:160-167.
82. Hestbaek L, Iachine IA, Leboeuf-Yde C, Kyvik KO, Manniche C. Heredity of low back pain in a young population: a classical twin study. *Twin Res.* 2004;7:16-26.
83. Hartvigsen J, Christensen K, Frederiksen H, Petersen HC. Genetic and environmental contributions to back pain in old age: a study of 2,108 Danish twins aged 70 and older. *Spine.* 2004;29:897-901.
84. Paassilta P, Lohiniva J, Göring HH, et al. Identification of a novel common genetic risk factor for lumbar disc disease. *JAMA.* 2001;285:1843-1849.
85. Jim JJ, Noponen-Hietala N, Cheung KM, et al. The TRP2 allele of COL9A2 is an age-dependent risk factor for the development and severity of intervertebral disc degeneration. *Spine.* 2005;30:2735-2742.
86. Solovieva S, Lohiniva J, Leino-Arjas P, et al. Intervertebral disc degeneration in relation to the COL9A3 and the IL-1ss gene polymorphisms. *Eur Spine J.* 2006;15: 613-619.
87. Kalichman L, Hunter DJ. The genetics of intervertebral disc degeneration. Associated genes. *Joint Bone Spine.* 2008;75:388-396.
88. Williams FM, Bansal AT, van Meurs JB, et al. Novel genetic variants associated with lumbar disc degeneration in northern Europeans: a meta-analysis of 4600 subjects. *Ann Rheum Dis.* 2013;72(7):1141-1148.
89. Song YQ, Karasugi T, Cheung KM, et al. Lumbar disc degeneration is linked to a carbohydrate sulfotransferase 3 variant. *J Clin Invest.* 2013;123(11):4909-4917.
90. Crock HV. A reappraisal of intervertebral disc lesions. *Med J Aust.* 1970;1:983-989.
91. Haughton VM. MR imaging of the spine. *Radiology.* 1988;166:297-301.
92. Cuellar JM, Stauff MP, Herzog RJ, et al. Does provocative discography cause clinically important injury to the lumbar intervertebral disc? A 10-year matched cohort study. *Spine J.* 2016;16(3):273-280.
93. Borthakur A, Maurer PM, Fenty M, et al. T1ρ magnetic resonance imaging and discography pressure as novel biomarkers for disc degeneration and low back pain. *Spine.* 2011;36(25):2190-2196.

94. Binch AL, Cole AA, Breakwell LM, et al. Nerves are more abundant than blood vessels in the degenerate human intervertebral disc. *Arthritis Res Ther*. 2015;17:370.
95. Maidhof R, Jacobsen T, Papatheodorou A, Chahine NO. Inflammation induces irreversible biophysical changes in isolated nucleus pulposus cells. *PLoS One*. 2014;9:1-11.
96. Ellman MB, Kim J-S, An HS, et al. Toll-like receptor adaptor signaling molecule MyD88 on intervertebral disk homeostasis: in vitro, ex vivo studies. *Gene*. 2012;505:283-290.
97. Le Maitre CL, Freemont AJ, Hoyland JA. The role of interleukin-1 in the pathogenesis of human intervertebral disc degeneration. *Arthritis Res Ther*. 2005;7:R732-R745.
98. Wang J, Markova D, Anderson DG, et al. TNF-α and IL-1β promote a disintegrin-like and metalloprotease with thrombospondin type I motif-5-mediated aggrecan degradation through syndecan-4 in intervertebral disc. *J Biol Chem*. 2011;286:39738-39749.
99. Wang X, Wang H, Yang H, et al. Tumor necrosis factor-α- and interleukin-1β-dependent matrix metalloproteinase-3 expression in nucleus pulposus cells requires cooperative signaling via syndecan 4 and mitogen-activated protein kinase-nuclear factor κB axis: implications in inflammatory disease. *Am J Pathol*. 2014;184:1-13.
100. Murata Y, Rydevik B, Nannmark U, et al. Local application of interleukin-6 to the dorsal root ganglion induces tumor necrosis factor-α in the dorsal root ganglion and results in apoptosis of the dorsal root ganglion cells. *Spine (Phila Pa)*. 2011;36:926-932.
101. Burke JG, Watson RWG, McCormack D, et al. Intervertebral discs which cause low back pain secrete high levels of proinflammatory mediators. *J Bone Joint Surg Br*. 2002;84: 196-201.
102. Abe Y, Akeda K, An HS, et al. Proinflammatory cytokines stimulate the expression of nerve growth factor by human intervertebral disc cells. *Spine (Phila Pa)*. 2007;32: 635-642.
103. García-Cosamalón J, del Valle ME, Calavia MG, et al. Intervertebral disc, sensory nerves and neurotrophins: who is who in discogenic pain? *J Anat*. 2010;217:1-15.
104. Purmessur D, Freemont AJ, Hoyland JA. Expression and regulation of neurotrophins in the nondegenerate and degenerate human intervertebral disc. *Arthritis Res Ther*. 2008;10:R99.
105. Kepler CK, Markova DZ, Hilibrand AS, et al. Substance P stimulates production of inflammatory cytokines in human disc cells. *Spine J*. 2012;12:S109.
106. Carragee EJ, Kim D, van der Vlugt T, Vittum D. The clinical use of erythrocyte sedimentation rate in pyogenic vertebral osteomyelitis. *Spine (Phila Pa)*. 1997;18:2089-2093.
107. Sapico FL, Montgomerie JZ. Pyogenic vertebral osteomyelitis: report of nine cases and review of the literature. *Rev Infect Dis*. 1979;1:754-776.
108. Modic MT, Steinberg PM, Ross JS, Masaryk TJ, Carter JR. Degenerative disk disease: assessment of changes in vertebral body marrow with MR imaging. *Radiology*. 1988;166: 193-199.
109. Jensen TS, Karppinen J, Sorensen JS, Niinimäki J, Leboeuf-Yde C. Vertebral endplate signal changes (Modic change): A systematic literature review of prevalence and association with non-specific low back pain. *Eur Spine*. 2008;17:1407-1422.
110. Albert HB, Lambert P, Rollason J, et al. Does nuclear tissue infected with bacteria following disc herniations lead to Modic changes in the adjacent vertebrae? *Eur Spine J*. 2013;22:690-696.
111. Agarwal VJ, Golish R, Kondrashov D, Alamin TF. Results of bacterial culture from surgically excised intervertebral disc in 52 patients undergoing primary lumbar microdiscectomy at a single level. *Spine J*. 2010;10:S45-S46.
112. Fritzell P, Bergström T, Welinder-Olsson C. Detection of bacterial DNA in painful degenerated spinal discs in patients without signs of clinical infection. *Eur Spine J*. 2004;13:702-706.
113. Albert HB, Sorensen JS, Christensen BS, Manniche C. Antibiotic treatment in patients with chronic low back pain and vertebral bone edema (Modic type 1 changes): a double-blind randomized clinical controlled trial of efficacy. *Eur Spine J*. 2013;22:697-707.
114. Casellas F, Borruel N, Papo M, et al. Antiinflammatory effects of enterically coated amoxicillin-clavulanic acid in active ulcerative colitis. *Inflamm Bowel Dis*. 1998;4:1-5.
115. Hajhashemi V, Dehdashti K. Antinociceptive effect of clavulanic acid and its preventive activity against development of morphine tolerance and dependence in animal models. *Res Pharm Sci*. 2014;9:315-321.
116. Roca I, Akova M, Baquero F, et al. The global threat of antimicrobial resistance: Science for intervention. *New Microbes New Infect*. 2015;6:22-29.
117. Quero L, Klawitter M, Schmaus A, et al. Hyaluronic acid fragments enhance the inflammatory and catabolic response in human intervertebral disc cells through modulation of toll-like receptor 2 signalling pathways. *Arthritis Res Ther*. 2013;15:R94.
118. Kawagoe T, Sato S, Matsushita K, et al. Sequential control of Toll-like receptor-dependent responses by IRAK1 and IRAK2. *Nat Immunol*. 2008;9:684-691.
119. Scheibner KA, Lutz MA, Boodoo S, et al. Hyaluronan fragments act as an endogenous danger signal by engaging TLR2. *J Immunol*. 2006;177:1272-1281.
120. Campo GM, Avenoso A, D'Ascola A, et al. Hyaluronan differently modulates TLR-4 and the inflammatory response in mouse chondrocytes. *Biofactors*. 2012;38:69-76.
121. Campo GM, Avenoso A, Campo S, et al. Small hyaluronan oligosaccharides induce inflammation by engaging both toll-like-4 and CD44 receptors in human chondrocytes. *Biochem Pharmacol*. 2010;80:480-490.
122. Scaffidi P, Misteli T, Bianchi ME. Release of chromatin protein HMGB1 by necrotic cells triggers inflammation. *Nature*. 2002;418:191-195.
123. Voll RE, Urbonaviciute V, Herrmann M, Kalden JR. High mobility group box 1 in the pathogenesis of inflammatory and autoimmune diseases. *Isr Med Assoc J*. 2008;10:26-28.
124. Tang D, Kang R, Cheh CW, et al. HMGB1 release and redox regulates autophagy and apoptosis in cancer cells. *Oncogene*. 2010;29(38):5299-5310.
125. Otoshi K, Kikuchi S, Kato K, Sekiguchi M, Konno S. Anti-HMGB1 neutralization antibody improves pain-related behavior induced by application of autologous nucleus pulposus onto nerve roots in rats. *Spine (Phila Pa)*. 2011;36:E692-E698.
126. Ruel N, Markova DZ, Adams SL, et al. Fibronectin fragments and the cleaving enzyme ADAM-8 in the degenerative human intervertebral disc. *Spine (Phila Pa)*. 2014;39:1274-1279.
127. Liu H-F, Zhang H, Qiao G-X, et al. A novel rabbit disc degeneration model induced by fibronectin fragment. *Joint Bone Spine*. 2013;80:301-306.

128. Anderson DG, Li X, Balian GA. Fibronectin fragment alters the metabolism by rabbit intervertebral disc cells in vitro. *Spine (Phila Pa)*. 2005;30:1242-1246.
129. Xia M, Zhu Y. Fibronectin fragment activation of ERK increasing integrin α5 and β1 subunit expression to degenerate nucleus pulposus cells. *J Orthop Res*. 2011;29: 556-561.
130. Tran CM, Schoepflin ZR, Markova DZ, et al. CCN2 suppresses catabolic effects of interleukin-1β through α5β1 and αVβ3 integrins in nucleus pulposus cells: implications in intervertebral disc degeneration. *J Biol Chem*. 2014;289:7374-7387.
131. Fields AJ, Berg-Johansen B, Metz LN, et al. Alterations in intervertebral disc composition, matrix homeostasis and biomechanical behavior in the UCD-T2DM rat model of type 2 diabetes. *J Orthop Res*. 2015;33:738-746.
132. Tsai T-T, Ho NY-J, Lin Y-T, et al. Advanced glycation end products in degenerative nucleus pulposus with diabetes. *J Orthop Res*. 2014;32:238-244.
133. Illien-Junger S, Grosjean F, Laudier DM, et al. Combined anti-inflammatory and anti-AGE drug treatments have a protective effect on intervertebral discs in mice with diabetes. *PLoS One*. 2013;8:e64302.
134. Johnson WEB, Stephan S, Roberts S. The influence of serum, glucose and oxygen on intervertebral disc cell growth in vitro: implications for degenerative disc disease. *Arthritis Res Ther*. 2008;10:R46.
134a. Videman T, Battie MC, Gibbons LE, et al. Disc degeneration and bone density in monozygotic twins discordant for insulin-dependent diabetes mellitus. *J Orthop Res*. 2000;18(5):768-772.
134b. Fabiane SM, Ward KJ, Iatridis JC, et al. Does type 2 diabetes mellitus promote intervertebral disc degeneration? *Eur Spine J*. 2016;25(9):2716-2720.
135. Deyo RA, et al. Outcome measures for low back pain research. A proposal for standardized use. *Spine*. 1998;23:2003-2013.
136. Spruit M, Jacobs WC. Pain and function after intradiscal electrothermal treatment (IDET) for symptomatic lumbar disc degeneration. *Eur Spine J*. 2002;11:589-593.
137. Derby R, Eek B, Chen Y. Intradiscal electrothermal annuloplasty (IDET): a novel approach for treating chronic discogenic back pain. *Neuromodulation*. 2000;3(2):82-88.
138. Weinstein J, Claverie W, Gibson S. The pain of discography. *Spine*. 1988;13:1344-1348.
139. Weinstein J. Neurogenic and nonneurogenic pain and inflammatory mediators. *Orthop Clin North Am*. 1991;22:235-246.
140. Kawakami M, et al. Possible mechanism of painful radiculopathy in lumbar disc herniation. *Clin Orthop Relat Res*. 1998;351:241-251.
141. Byröd G, et al. A rapid transport route between the epidural space and the intraneural capillaries of the nerve roots. *Spine*. 1995;20:138-143.
142. Freemont AJ, et al. Nerve ingrowth into diseased intervertebral disc in chronic back pain. *Lancet*. 1997;350:178-181.
143. Evans W, Jobe W, Seibert C. A cross-sectional prevalence study of lumbar disc degeneration in a working population. *Spine*. 1989;14:60-64.
144. Gibson MJ, et al. Magnetic resonance imaging and discography in the diagnosis of disc degeneration. A comparative study of 50 discs. *J Bone Joint Surg Br*. 1986;68:369-373.
145. Saal JS, et al. High levels of inflammatory phospholipase A2 activity in lumbar disc herniations. *Spine*. 1990;15:674-678.
146. Nygaard OP, Mellgren SI, Osterud B. The inflammatory properties of contained and noncontained lumbar disc herniation. *Spine*. 1997;22:2484-2488.
147. O'Donnell JL, O'Donnell AL. Prostaglandin E2 content in herniated lumbar disc disease. *Spine*. 1996;21:1653-1655.
148. Franson RC, Saal JS, Saal JA. Human disc phospholipase A2 is inflammatory. *Spine*. 1992;17(suppl 6):S129-S132.
149. Burke JG, Watson RW, McCormack D, et al. Intervertebral discs which cause low back pain secrete high levels of proinflammatory mediators. *J Bone Joint Surg Br*. 2002;84:196-201.
150. Igarashi A, Kikuchi S, Konno S, Olmarker K. Inflammatory cytokines released from the facet joint tissue in degenerative lumbar spinal disorders. *Spine*. 2004;29:2091-2095.
151. Ohtori S, et al. Tumor necrosis factor-immunoreactive cells and PGP 9.5-immunoreactive nerve fibers in vertebral endplates of patients with discogenic low back pain and Modic type 1 or type 2 changes on MRI. *Spine*. 2006;31:1026-1031.
152. Ashton IK, et al. Substance P in intervertebral discs. Binding sites on vascular endothelium of the human annulus fibrosus. *Acta Orthop Scand*. 1994;65:635-639.
153. Palmgren T, et al. An immunohistochemical study of nerve structures in the anulus fibrosus of human normal lumbar intervertebral discs. *Spine*. 1999;24:2075-2079.
154. Coppes MH, et al. Innervation of "painful" lumbar discs. *Spine*. 1997;22:2342-2349.
155. Peng B, et al. The pathogenesis of discogenic low back pain. *J Bone Joint Surg Br*. 2005;87:62-67.
156. Brown MF, et al. Sensory and sympathetic innervation of the vertebral endplate in patients with degenerative disc disease. *J Bone Joint Surg Br*. 1997;79:147-153.
157. Takebayashi T, et al. Sympathetic afferent units from lumbar intervertebral discs. *J Bone Joint Surg Br*. 2006;88:554-557.
158. Aoki Y, et al. Innervation of the lumbar intervertebral disc by nerve growth factor-dependent neurons related to inflammatory pain. *Spine*. 2004;29:1077-1081.
159. Edgar MA. The nerve supply of the lumbar intervertebral disc. *J Bone Joint Surg Br*. 2007;89:1135-1139.
160. Jarvik JG, et al. Three-year incidence of low back pain in an initially asymptomatic cohort: clinical and imaging risk factors. *Spine*. 2005;30:1541-1548.
161. Carragee EJ, et al. Discographic, MRI and psychosocial determinants of low back pain disability and remission: a prospective study in subjects with benign persistent back pain. *Spine J*. 2005;5:24-35.
162. Carragee EJ, Paragioudakis SJ, Khurana S. 2000 Volvo Award winner in clinical studies: Lumbar high-intensity zone and discography in subjects without low back problems. *Spine*. 2000;25:2987-2992.
163. Carragee EJ, Alamin TF, Carragee JM. Low-pressure positive discography in subjects asymptomatic of significant low back pain illness. *Spine*. 2006;31:505-509.
164. Carragee EJ, et al. The rates of false-positive lumbar discography in select patients without low back symptoms. *Spine*. 2000;25:1373-1380.
165. O'Neill CW, et al. Disc stimulation and patterns of referred pain. *Spine*. 2002;27:2776-2781.

166. Deyo RA, Diehl AK. Lumbar spine films in primary care: current use and effects of selective ordering criteria. *J Gen Intern Med*. 1986;1:20-25.
167. Torgerson WR, Dotter WE. Comparative roentgenographic study of the asymptomatic and symptomatic lumbar spine. *J Bone Joint Surg Am*. 1976;58:850-853.
168. Liang M, Komaroff AL. Roentgenograms in primary care patients with acute low back pain: a cost-effectiveness analysis. *Arch Intern Med*. 1982;142:1108-1112.
169. Scavone JG, Latshaw RF, Weidner WA. Anteroposterior and lateral radiographs: an adequate lumbar spine examination. *AJR Am J Roentgenol*. 1981;136:715-717.
170. Institute for Clinical Systems Improvement. *Adult low back pain*; 2008. Institute for Clinical Systems Improvement. Bloomington, MN.
171. Aprill C, Bogduk N. High-intensity zone: a diagnostic sign of painful lumbar disc on magnetic resonance imaging. *Br J Radiol*. 1992;65:361-369.
172. Yu SW, et al. Tears of the anulus fibrosus: correlation between MR and pathologic findings in cadavers. *AJNR Am J Neuroradiol*. 1988;9:367-370.
173. Osti OL, Vernon-Roberts B, Moore R, Fraser RD. Annular tears and disc degeneration in the lumbar spine. A post-mortem study of 135 discs. *J Bone Joint Surg Br*. 1992;74:678-682.
174. Morgan S, Saifuddin A. MRI of the lumbar intervertebral disc. *Clin Radiol*. 1999;54:703-723.
175. Modic MT, et al. Degenerative disc disease: assessment of changes in vertebral body marrow with MR imaging. *Radiology*. 1988;166:193-199.
176. Boden SD, et al. Abnormal magnetic-resonance scans of the lumbar spine in asymptomatic subjects. A prospective investigation. *J Bone Joint Surg Am*. 1990;72:403-408.
177. Jensen MC, et al. Magnetic resonance imaging of the lumbar spine in people without back pain. *N Engl J Med*. 1994;331:69-73.
178. Stadnik TW, et al. Annular tears and disc herniation: prevalence and contrast enhancement on MR images in the absence of low back pain or sciatica. *Radiology*. 1998;206:49-55.
179. Borenstein DG, et al. The value of magnetic resonance imaging of the lumbar spine to predict low-back pain in asymptomatic subjects : a seven-year follow-up study. *J Bone Joint Surg Am*. 2001;83-A:1306-1311.
180. Jarvik JJ, et al. The Longitudinal Assessment of Imaging and Disability of the Back (LAIDBack) study: baseline data. *Spine*. 2001;26:1158-1166.
181. Jarvik JG, et al. Rapid magnetic resonance imaging vs radiographs for patients with low back pain: a randomized controlled trial. *JAMA*. 2003;289:2810-2818.
182. Carragee E, et al. Are first-time episodes of serious LBP associated with new MRI findings? *Spine J*. 2006;6:624-635.
183. Lappalainen AK, et al. The diagnostic value of contrast-enhanced magnetic resonance imaging in the detection of experimentally induced anular tears in sheep. *Spine*. 2002;27:2806-2810.
184. Yoshida H, et al. Diagnosis of symptomatic disc by magnetic resonance imaging: T2-weighted and gadolinium-DTPA-enhanced T1-weighted magnetic resonance imaging. *J Spinal Disord Tech*. 2002;15:193-198.
185. Aprill C, Bogduk N. High-intensity zone: a diagnostic sign of painful lumbar disc on magnetic resonance imaging. *Br J Radiol*. 1992;65:361-369.
186. Lim CH, et al. Discogenic lumbar pain: association with MRI imaging and CT discography. *Eur J Radiol*. 2005;54:431-437.
187. Lam KS, Carlin D, Mulholland RC. Lumbar disc high-intensity zone: the value and significance of provocative discography in the determination of the discogenic pain source. *Eur Spine J*. 2000;9:36-41.
188. Schellhas KP, et al. Lumbar disc high-intensity zone. Correlation of magnetic resonance imaging and discography. *Spine*. 1996;21:79-86.
189. Peng B, et al. The pathogenesis and clinical significance of a high-intensity zone (HIZ) of lumbar intervertebral disc on MR imaging in the patient with discogenic low back pain. *Eur Spine J*. 2006;15:583-587.
190. Lei D, et al. Painful disc lesion: can modern biplanar magnetic resonance imaging replace discography? *J Spinal Disord Tech*. 2008;21:430-435.
191. Saifuddin A, et al. The value of lumbar spine magnetic resonance imaging in the demonstration of anular tears. *Spine*. 1998;23:453-457.
192. Kang CH, et al. Can magnetic resonance imaging accurately predict concordant pain provocation during provocative disc injection? *Skeletal Radiol*. 2009;38:877-885.
193. Ricketson R, Simmons JW, Hauser BO. The prolapsed intervertebral disc. The high-intensity zone with discography correlation. *Spine*. 1996;21:2758-2762.
194. Schneiderman G, et al. Magnetic resonance imaging in the diagnosis of disc degeneration: correlation with discography. *Spine*. 1987;12:276-281.
195. Ito M, et al. Predictive signs of discogenic lumbar pain on magnetic resonance imaging with discography correlation. *Spine*. 1998;23:1252-1258.
196. Simmons JW, et al. Awake discography. A comparison study with magnetic resonance imaging. *Spine*. 1991;16(suppl 6): S216-S221.
197. Mitra D, Cassar-Pullicino VN, McCall IW. Longitudinal study of high intensity zones on MR of lumbar intervertebral discs. *Clin Radiol*. 2004;59:1002-1008.
198. Milette P, et al. Differentiating lumbar disc protrusions, disc bulges, and discs with normal contour but abnormal signal intensity: magnetic resonance imaging with discographic correlations. *Spine*. 1999;24:44-53.
199. Horton WC, Daftari TK. Which disc as visualized by magnetic resonance imaging is actually a source of pain? A correlation between magnetic resonance imaging and discography. *Spine*. 1992;17(suppl 6):S167-S171.
200. Toyone T, et al. Vertebral bone-marrow changes in degenerative lumbar disc disease. An MRI study of 74 patients with low back pain. *J Bone Joint Surg Br*. 1994;76:757-764.
201. Kuisma M, et al. Modic changes in endplates of lumbar vertebral bodies: prevalence and association with low back and sciatic pain among middle-aged male workers. *Spine*. 2007;32:1116-1122.
202. Albert HB, Manniche C. Modic changes following lumbar disc herniation. *Eur Spine J*. 2007;16:977-982.
203. Thompson KJ, et al. Modic changes on MR images as studied with provocative discography: clinical relevance—a retrospective study of 2457 discs. *Radiology*. 2009;250:849-855.
204. Mitra D, Cassar-Pullicino VN, McCall IW. Longitudinal study of vertebral type-1 end-plate changes on MR of the lumbar spine. *Eur Radiol*. 2004;14:1574-1581.
205. Marshman LA, et al. Reverse transformation of Modic type 2 changes to Modic type 1 changes during sustained chronic

low-back pain severity. Report of two cases and review of the literature. *J Neurosurg Spine*. 2007;6:152-155.

206. Kuisma M, et al. A three-year follow-up of lumbar spine endplate (Modic) changes. *Spine*. 2006;31:1714-1718.
207. Sandhu HS, et al. Association between findings of provocative discography and vertebral endplate signal changes as seen on MRI. *J Spinal Disord*. 2000;13:438-443.
208. Braithwaite I, et al. Vertebral end-plate (Modic) changes on lumbar spine MRI: correlation with pain reproduction at lumbar discography. *Eur Spine J*. 1998;7:363-368.
209. Kokkonen SM, et al. Endplate degeneration observed on magnetic resonance imaging of the lumbar spine: correlation with pain provocation and disc changes observed on computed tomography discography. *Spine*. 2002;27:2274-2278.
210. Schenk P, et al. Magnetic resonance imaging of the lumbar spine: findings in female subjects from administrative and nursing professions. *Spine*. 2006;31:2701-2706.
211. Kjaer P, et al. Magnetic resonance imaging and low back pain in adults: a diagnostic imaging study of 40-year-old men and women. *Spine*. 2005;30:1173-1180.
212. Kjaer P, Korsholm L, Bendix T, Sorensen JS, Leboeuf-Yde C. Modic changes and their associations with clinical findings. *Eur Spine J*. 2006;15:1312-1319.
213. Leboeuf-Yde C, et al. Self-reported hard physical work combined with heavy smoking or overweight may result in so-called Modic changes. *BMC Musculoskelet Disord*. 2008;9:5.
214. Jensen TS, et al. Vertebral endplate signal changes (Modic change): a systematic literature review of prevalence and association with non-specific low back pain. *Eur Spine J*. 2008;17:1407-1422.
215. Huang KY, et al. Factors affecting disability and physical function in degenerative lumbar spondylolisthesis of L4-5: evaluation with axially loaded MRI. *Eur Spine J*. 2009;18:1851-1857.
216. Hansson T, et al. The narrowing of the lumbar spinal canal during loaded MRI: the effects of the disc and ligamentum flavum. *Eur Spine J*. 2009;18:679-686.
217. Jayakumar P, et al. Dynamic degenerative lumbar spondylolisthesis: diagnosis with axial loaded magnetic resonance imaging. *Spine*. 2006;31:E298-E301.
218. Hiwatashi A, et al. Axial loading during MR imaging can influence treatment decision for symptomatic spinal stenosis. *AJNR Am J Neuroradiol*. 2004;25:170-174.
219. Danielson B, Willén J. Axially loaded magnetic resonance image of the lumbar spine in asymptomatic individuals. *Spine*. 2001;26:2601-2606.
220. Saifuddin A, McSweeney E, Lehovsky J. Development of lumbar high intensity zone on axial loaded magnetic resonance imaging. *Spine*. 2003;28:E449-E451.
221. Holt EP Jr. The question of lumbar discography. *J Bone Joint Surg Am*. 1968;50:720-726.
222. Carragee EJ, et al. Does discography cause accelerated progression of degeneration changes in the lumbar disc: a ten-year matched cohort study. *Spine*. 2009;34(21):2338-2345.
223. Chou R, et al. Interventional therapies, surgery, and interdisciplinary rehabilitation for low back pain: an evidence-based clinical practice guideline from the American Pain Society. *Spine*. 2009;34:1066-1077.
224. Aprill C. Diagnostic Disc Injection. In: Frymoyer J, ed. *The Adult Spine: Principles and Practice*. New York: Raven Press; 1991.
225. Guyer RD, Ohnmeiss DD. Lumbar discography. Position statement from the North American Spine Society Diagnostic and Therapeutic Committee. *Spine*. 1995;20:2048-2059.
226. Bernard TN Jr. Lumbar discography followed by computed tomography. Refining the diagnosis of low-back pain. *Spine*. 1990;15:690-707.
227. Massie W. A critical evaluation of discography: scientific exhibit. *J Bone Joint Surg Am*. 1967;49:1243-1244.
228. Walsh TR, et al. Lumbar discography in normal subjects. A controlled, prospective study. *J Bone Joint Surg Am*. 1990;72:1081-1088.
229. Derby R, et al. Comparison of discographic findings in asymptomatic subject discs and the negative discs of chronic LBP patients: can discography distinguish asymptomatic discs among morphologically abnormal discs? *Spine J*. 2005;5:389-394.
230. Buenaventura RM, et al. Systematic review of discography as a diagnostic test for spinal pain: an update. *Pain Physician*. 2007;10:147-164.
231. Wolfer LR, et al. Systematic review of lumbar provocation discography in asymptomatic subjects with a meta-analysis of false-positive rates. *Pain Physician*. 2008;11:513-538.
232. Colhoun E, et al. Provocation discography as a guide to planning operations on the spine. *J Bone Joint Surg Br*. 1988;70:267-271.
233. Madan S, et al. Does provocative discography screening of discogenic back pain improve surgical outcome? *J Spinal Disord Tech*. 2002;15:245-251.
234. Carragee EJ, et al. A gold standard evaluation of the "discogenic pain" diagnosis as determined by provocative discography. *Spine*. 2006;31:2115-2123.
235. Ohtori S, et al. Results of surgery for discogenic low back pain: a randomized study using discography versus discoblock for diagnosis. *Spine*. 2009;34:1345-1348.
236. Deyo RA. Conservative therapy for low back pain. Distinguishing useful from useless therapy. *JAMA*. 1983;250:1057-1062.
237. Moss IL, An HS, Shen FH, et al. The nonsurgical treatment of back pain. In: Shapiro IM, Risbud MV, eds. *The Intervertebral Disc*. New York: Springer-Verlag; 2014:247-259.
238. Deyo RA, Diehl AK, Rosenthal M. How many days of bed rest for acute low back pain? A randomized clinical trial. *N Engl J Med*. 1986;315:1064-1070.
239. Quinet RJ, Hadler NM. Diagnosis and treatment of backache. *Semin Arthritis Rheum*. 1979;8:261-287.
240. Rowe ML. Low back pain in industry. A position paper. *J Occup Med*. 1969;11:161-169.
241. Allen C, Glasziou P, Del Mar C. Bed rest: a potentially harmful treatment needing more careful evaluation. *Lancet*. 1999;354:1229-1233.
242. Hagen KB, et al. Bed rest for acute low-back pain and sciatica. *Cochrane Database Syst Rev*. 2004;(8):CD001254.
243. Verbunt JA, et al. A new episode of low back pain: who relies on bed rest? *Eur J Pain*. 2008;12:508-516.
244. Engers A, et al. Individual patient education for low back pain. *Cochrane Database Syst Rev*. 2008;(1):CD004057.
245. Liddle SD, Gracey JH, Baxter GD. Advice for the management of low back pain: a systematic review of randomised controlled trials. *Man Ther*. 2007;12:310-327.
246. Brox JI, et al. Evidence-informed management of chronic low back pain with back schools, brief education, and fear-avoidance training. *Spine J*. 2008;8:28-39.

247. Calmels P, et al. Effectiveness of a lumbar belt in subacute low back pain: an open, multicentric, and randomized clinical study. *Spine*. 2009;34:215-220.
248. Oleske DM, et al. Are back supports plus education more effective than education alone in promoting recovery from low back pain? Results from a randomized clinical trial. *Spine*. 2007;32:2050-2057.
249. van Duijvenbode IC, et al. Lumbar supports for prevention and treatment of low back pain. *Cochrane Database Syst Rev*. 2008;(2):CD001823.
250. Sahar T, et al. Insoles for prevention and treatment of back pain. *Cochrane Database Syst Rev*. 2007;(4):CD005275.
251. Brox JI, et al. Randomized clinical trial of lumbar instrumented fusion and cognitive intervention and exercises in patients with chronic low back pain and disc degeneration. *Spine*. 2003;28:1913-1921.
252. Keller A, et al. Trunk muscle strength, cross-sectional area, and density in patients with chronic low back pain randomized to lumbar fusion or cognitive intervention and exercises. *Spine*. 2004;29:3-8.
253. Fairbank J, Frost H, Wilson-MacDonald J, et al. Randomised controlled trial to compare surgical stabilisation of the lumbar spine with an intensive rehabilitation programme for patients with chronic low back pain: the MRC spine stabilisation trial. *BMJ*. 2005;330:1233.
254. Eleswarapu AS, et al. How effective is physical therapy for common low back pain diagnosis. *Spine*. 2016;41(16): 1325-1329.
255. Heymans MW, et al. The effectiveness of high-intensity versus low-intensity back schools in an occupational setting: a pragmatic randomized controlled trial. *Spine*. 2006;31:1075-1082.
256. Kääpä EH, et al. Multidisciplinary group rehabilitation versus individual physiotherapy for chronic nonspecific low back pain: a randomized trial. *Spine*. 2006;31:371-376.
257. Heymans MW, van Tulder MW, Esmail R, Bombardier C, Koes BW. Back schools for non-specific low-back pain. *Cochrane Database Syst Rev*. 2004;(4):CD000261.
258. van der Roer N, et al. Economic evaluation of an intensive group training protocol compared with usual care physiotherapy in patients with chronic low back pain. *Spine*. 2008;33:445-451.
259. van der Roer N, et al. Intensive group training protocol versus guideline physiotherapy for patients with chronic low back pain: a randomised controlled trial. *Eur Spine J*. 2008;17:1193-1200.
260. Poitras S, Brosseau L. Evidence-informed management of chronic low back pain with transcutaneous electrical nerve stimulation, interferential current, electrical muscle stimulation, ultrasound, and thermotherapy. *Spine J*. 2008;8:226-233.
261. Khadilkar A, et al. Transcutaneous electrical nerve stimulation (TENS) versus placebo for chronic low-back pain. *Cochrane Database Syst Rev*. 2008;(4):CD003008.
262. van Middlekoop M, Rubinstein SM, Kuipers T, et al. A systemic review on the effectiveness of physical and rehabilitation interventions for chronic non-specific low back pain. *Eur Spine J*. 2011;20(1):19-39.
263. Hoiriis KT, et al. A randomized clinical trial comparing chiropractic adjustments to muscle relaxants for subacute low back pain. *J Manipulative Physiol Ther*. 2004;27:388-398.
264. Haas M, Groupp E, Kraemer DF. Dose-response for chiropractic care of chronic low back pain. *Spine J*. 2004;4: 574-583.
265. McMorland G, Suter E. Chiropractic management of mechanical neck and low-back pain: a retrospective, outcome-based analysis. *J Manipulative Physiol Ther*. 2000;23:307-311.
266. Ernst E, Canter PH. A systematic review of systematic reviews of spinal manipulation. *J R Soc Med*. 2006;99:192-196.
267. Assendelft WJ, et al. Spinal manipulative therapy for low back pain. *Cochrane Database Syst Rev*. 2004;(1):CD000447.
268. Eisenberg DM, et al. Addition of choice of complementary therapies to usual care for acute low back pain: a randomized controlled trial. *Spine*. 2007;32:151-158.
269. Hurwitz EL, et al. A randomized trial of chiropractic and medical care for patients with low back pain: eighteen-month follow-up outcomes from the UCLA low back pain study. *Spine*. 2006;31(6):611-621.
270. Andersson GBJ, Lucente T, Davos AM, et al. A comparison of osteopathic spinal manipulation therapy and usual care for patients with subchronic low back pain. *N Engl J Med*. 1999;341:1126-1431.
271. Furlan AD, et al. Acupuncture and dry-needling for low back pain. *Cochrane Database Syst Rev*. 2005;(1):CD001351.
272. Ammendolia C, et al. Evidence-informed management of chronic low back pain with needle acupuncture. *Spine J*. 2008;8:160-172.
273. Yelland MJ, et al. Prolotherapy injections, saline injections, and exercises for chronic low-back pain: a randomized trial. *Spine*. 2004;29:9-16.
274. Dagenais S, et al. Evidence-informed management of chronic low back pain with prolotherapy. *Spine J*. 2008;8:203-212.
275. Rabago D, et al. A systematic review of prolotherapy for chronic musculoskeletal pain. *Clin J Sport Med*. 2005;15:376-380.
276. Roelofs PD, et al. Non-steroidal anti-inflammatory drugs for low back pain. *Cochrane Database Syst Rev*. 2008;(1):CD000396.
277. Deshpande A, et al. Opioids for chronic low-back pain. *Cochrane Database Syst Rev*. 2007;(3):CD004959.
278. Jamison RN, et al. Opioid therapy for chronic noncancer back pain. A randomized prospective study. *Spine*. 1998;23:2591-2600.
279. Martell BA, et al. Systematic review: opioid treatment for chronic back pain: prevalence, efficacy, and association with addiction. *Ann Intern Med*. 2007;146:116-127.
280. Schofferman J, Mazanec D. Evidence-informed management of chronic low back pain with opioid analgesics. *Spine J*. 2008;8:185-194.
281. Armstrong TA, Rohal GM. Potential danger from too much acetaminophen in opiate agonist combination products. *Am J Health Syst Pharm*. 1999;56:1774-1775.
282. *Physicians Desk Reference*. 63rd ed. Montvale, NJ: Thomson PDR; 2009.
283. Krenzelok EP. The FDA Acetaminophen Advisory Committee Meeting: what is the future of acetaminophen in the United States? The perspective of a committee member. *Clin Toxicol*. 2009;47:784-789.
284. Vamvanij V, et al. Surgical treatment of internal disc disruption: an outcome study of four fusion techniques. *J Spinal Disord*. 1998;11:375-382.
285. Chou R, Huffneu Lit. Medications for acute and chronic low back pain: a review of evidence for an American Pain Society clinical practice guideline. *Ann Intern Med*. 2007;147(7):492-504.

286. van Tulder MW, et al. Muscle relaxants for non-specific low back pain. *Cochrane Database Syst Rev*. 2003;(2):CD004252.
287. Alcoff J, et al. Controlled trial of imipramine for chronic low back pain. *J Fam Pract*. 1982;14:841-846.
288. Pheasant H, et al. Amitriptyline and chronic low-back pain. A randomized double-blind crossover study. *Spine*. 1983;8:552-557.
289. Ward NG. Tricyclic antidepressants for chronic low-back pain. Mechanisms of action and predictors of response. *Spine*. 1986;11:661-665.
290. Staiger TO, et al. Systematic review of antidepressants in the treatment of chronic low back pain. *Spine*. 2003;28:250-255.
291. Chang V, Gonzalez P, Akuthota V. Evidence-informed management of chronic low back pain with adjunctive analgesics. *Spine J*. 2008;8:21-27.
292. Keller A, et al. Effect sizes of non-surgical treatments of non-specific low-back pain. *Eur Spine J*. 2007;16:1776-1788.
293. Machado LA, et al. Analgesic effects of treatments for non-specific low back pain: a meta-analysis of placebo-controlled randomized trials. *Rheumatology*. 2009;48:520-527.
294. Delaney TJ, et al. Epidural steroid effects on nerves and meninges. *Anesth Analg*. 1980;59:610-614.
295. Fairbank JC, et al. Apophyseal injection of local anesthetic as a diagnostic aid in primary low-back pain syndromes. *Spine*. 1981;6:598-605.
296. Manchikanti L, et al. Preliminary results of a randomized, equivalence trial of fluoroscopic caudal epidural injections in managing chronic low back pain. Part 1: discogenic pain without disc herniation or radiculitis. *Pain Physician*. 2008;11:785-800.
297. Manchikanti L, et al. Effectiveness of caudal epidural injections in discogram positive and negative chronic low back pain. *Pain Physician*. 2002;5:18-29.
298. Manchikanti L, et al. Caudal epidural injections with sarapin or steroids in chronic low back pain. *Pain Physician*. 2001;4:322-335.
299. Buttermann GR. The effect of spinal steroid injections for degenerative disc disease. *Spine J*. 2004;4:495-505.
300. Rosenberg SK, et al. Effectiveness of transforaminal epidural steroid injections in low back pain: a one year experience. *Pain Physician*. 2002;5:266-270.
301. DePalma MJ, Slipman CW. Evidence-informed management of chronic low back pain with epidural steroid injections. *Spine J*. 2008;8:45-55.
302. Staal JB, et al. Injection therapy for subacute and chronic low-back pain. *Cochrane Database Syst Rev*. 2008;(3):CD001824.
303. Chou R, et al. Nonsurgical interventional therapies for low back pain: a review of the evidence for an American Pain Society clinical practice guideline. *Spine*. 2009;34:1078-1093.
304. Feffer HL. Therapeutic intradiscal hydrocortisone. A long-term study. *Clin Orthop Relat Res*. 1969;67:100-104.
305. Wilkinson HA, Schuman N. Intradiscal corticosteroids in the treatment of lumbar and cervical disc problems. *Spine*. 1980;5:385-389.
306. Fayad F, et al. Relation of inflammatory Modic changes to intradiscal steroid injection outcome in chronic low back pain. *Eur Spine J*. 2007;16:925-931.
307. Simmons JW, et al. Intradiscal steroids. A prospective double-blind clinical trial. *Spine*. 1992;17(suppl 6):S172-S175.
308. Khot A, et al. The use of intradiscal steroid therapy for lumbar spinal discogenic pain: a randomized controlled trial. *Spine*. 2004;29:833-836.
309. Klein RG, et al. Biochemical injection treatment for discogenic low back pain: a pilot study. *Spine J*. 2003;3:220-226.
310. Miller MR, Mathews RS, Reeves KD. Treatment of painful advanced internal lumbar disc derangement with intradiscal injection of hypertonic dextrose. *Pain Physician*. 2006;9:115-121.
311. Peng B, et al. Intradiscal methylene blue injection for the treatment of chronic discogenic low back pain. *Eur Spine J*. 2007;16:33-38.
312. Gallucci M, et al. Sciatica: treatment with intradiscal and intraforaminal injections of steroid and oxygen-ozone versus steroid only. *Radiology*. 2007;242:907-913.
313. Muto M, et al. Low back pain and sciatica: treatment with intradiscal-intraforaminal O(2)-O (3) injection. Our experience. *Radiol Med*. 2008;113:695-706.
314. Freeman BJ, et al. Does intradiscal electrothermal therapy denervate and repair experimentally induced posterolateral annular tears in an animal model? *Spine*. 2003;28:2602-2608.
315. Shah RV, et al. Intradiscal electrothermal therapy: a preliminary histologic study. *Arch Phys Med Rehabil*. 2001;82:1230-1237.
316. Kleinstueck FS, et al. Acute biomechanical and histological effects of intradiscal electrothermal therapy on human lumbar discs. *Spine*. 2001;26:2198-2207.
317. Strohbeln JW. Temperature distributions from interstitial RF electrode hyperthermia systems: theoretical predictions. *Int J Radiat Oncol Biol Phys*. 1983;9:1655-1667.
318. Troussier B, et al. Percutaneous intradiscal radio-frequency thermocoagulation. A cadaveric study. *Spine*. 1995;20:1713-1718.
319. Houpt JC, Conner ES, McFarland EW. Experimental study of temperature distributions and thermal transport during radiofrequency current therapy of the intervertebral disc. *Spine*. 1996;21:1808-1812.
320. Ashley J, Gharpuray V, Saal J. Temperature distribution in the intervertebral disc: a comparison of intranuclear radiofrequency needle to a novel heating catheter. Proceedings of the 1999 Bioengineering Conference. 1999;42:77.
321. Karasek M, Bogduk N. Twelve-month follow-up of a controlled trial of intradiscal thermal anuloplasty for back pain due to internal disc disruption. *Spine*. 2000;25:2601-2607.
322. Hsia AW, Isaac K, Katz JS. Cauda equina syndrome from intradiscal electrothermal therapy. *Neurology*. 2000;55:320.
323. Bogduk N, Karasek M. Two-year follow-up of a controlled trial of intradiscal electrothermal anuloplasty for chronic low back pain resulting from internal disc disruption. *Spine J*. 2002;2:343-350.
324. Saal JA, Saal JS. Intradiscal electrothermal treatment for chronic discogenic low back pain: prospective outcome study with a minimum 2-year follow-up. *Spine*. 2002;27:966-973.
325. Freeman BJ, et al. A randomized, double-blind, controlled trial: intradiscal electrothermal therapy versus placebo for the treatment of chronic discogenic low back pain. *Spine*. 2005;30:2369-2377.
326. Pauza KJ, et al. A randomized, placebo-controlled trial of intradiscal electrothermal therapy for the treatment of discogenic low back pain. *Spine J*. 2004;4:27-35.

327. Barendse GA, et al. Randomized controlled trial of percutaneous intradiscal radiofrequency thermocoagulation for chronic discogenic back pain: lack of effect from a 90-second 70 C lesion. *Spine*. 2001;26:287-292.
328. Andersson GB, Mekhail NA, Block JE. Treatment of intractable discogenic low back pain. A systematic review of spinal fusion and intradiscal electrothermal therapy (IDET). *Pain Physician*. 2006;9:237-248.
329. Derby R, et al. Evidence-informed management of chronic low back pain with intradiscal electrothermal therapy. *Spine J*. 2008;8:80-95.
330. Helm S, et al. Systematic review of the effectiveness of thermal annular procedures in treating discogenic low back pain. *Pain Physician*. 2009;12:207-232.
331. Freeman BJ. IDET: a critical appraisal of the evidence. *Eur Spine J*. 2006;15(suppl 3):S448-S457.
332. Chou R, et al. Surgery for low back pain: a review of the evidence for an American Pain Society Clinical Practice Guideline. *Spine*. 2009;34:1094-1109.
333. Deyo RA, Nachemson A, Mirza SK. Spinal-fusion surgery—the case for restraint. *N Engl J Med*. 2004;350:722-726.
334. Fritzell P, et al. Lumbar fusion versus nonsurgical treatment for chronic low back pain: a multicenter randomized controlled trial from the Swedish Lumbar Spine Study Group. *Spine*. 2001;26:2521-2532.
335. Rivero-Arias O, et al. Surgical stabilisation of the spine compared with a programme of intensive rehabilitation for the management of patients with chronic low back pain: cost utility analysis based on a randomised controlled trial. *BMJ*. 2005;330:1239.
336. Ibrahim T, Tleyjeh IM, Gabbar O. Surgical versus non-surgical treatment of chronic low back pain: a meta-analysis of randomised trials. *Int Orthop*. 2008;32:107-113.
337. Mirza SK, Deyo RA. Systematic review of randomized trials comparing lumbar fusion surgery to nonoperative care for treatment of chronic back pain. *Spine*. 2007;32:816-823.
338. Phillips FM, Slosar PJ, Youssef JA, Andersson G. Papatheofaris F. Lumbar spine fusion for chronic low back pain due to degenerative disc disease. *Spine*. 2013;38(7):409-422.
339. Anderson PA, Andersson GBJ, Arnold PM, et al. Terminology. *Spine*. 2012;37(22s):58-59.
340. Lund T, Oxland TR. Adjacent level disc disease – is it really fusion disease? *Orthop Clinic North Am*. 2011;42:529-541.
341. Bae WC, Masuda K. Emerging technologies for molecular therapy for intervertebral disc degeneration. *Ortrhop Clin North Am*. 2011;42:585-601.
342. Woods BL, Vo N, Sowa G, Kang JD. Gene therapy for intervertebral disc degeneration. *Orthop Clin North Am*. 2011;42:563-574.
343. Sakai D. Stem cell regeneration of the intervertebral disc. *Orthop Clin North Am*. 2011;42:555-562.
344. Leung VYL, Tam V, Chan D, Chen BP, Cheung KMC. Tissue engineering for intervertebral disc degeneration. *Orthop Clin North Am*. 2011;42:575-583.

SECTION VI

CHAPTER 47 Lumbar Disc Herniations

Amandeep Bhalla
Christopher M. Bono
Andrew J. Schoenfeld
Steven R. Garfin

Lumbar disc herniations are a common manifestation of degenerative disease.[1-3] They tend to occur early within the degenerative cascade, representing the tensile failure of the anulus to contain the gel-like nuclear portion of the disc. With improvements in advanced imaging techniques, lumbar disc herniations have been increasingly recognized in symptomatic and asymptomatic individuals.[4]

Treatment decision making for patients with herniated discs can be challenging. Nonoperative treatment can be effective in most cases.[5–9] Other authors have indicated that surgery leads to superior results, especially in short-term pain relief.[1,7–10] Several authors have highlighted the influence of fragment location and pattern, as well as social and psychological factors on outcomes.[7–9,11–13] The exact natural history and complex interaction of biologic, psychosocial, ergonomic, and cultural variables have not been well established.

In the best-case scenario, the clinician can radiologically identify a single culprit disc that positively correlates with clinical findings. In patients who do not respond to nonoperative management, disagreement remains concerning the optimal period of observation, timing of surgery, method of excision, and type of postoperative rehabilitation. In less evident cases, one or more minor disc bulges may be identified that are difficult to attribute to the patient's signs and symptoms. The use of diagnostic injections can be helpful in localizing symptomatic regions. Empiricism and reliance primarily on intuition may lead to inferior results. Strict agreement between a patient's signs, symptoms, and correlative diagnostic tests needs to exist when predicating treatment recommendations.

To address these questions, the wealth of classic and contemporary contributions made to the understanding of lumbar disc herniations has been reviewed. This chapter synthesizes the information and organizes it to help clinicians' understanding and recommendations of management of this seemingly simple, but realistically challenging, problem.

Pathoanatomy

Effective evaluation is based on an intimate understanding of the relationship of the lumbar intervertebral disc to its surrounding structures. The disc is the anterior border of the spinal canal at the facet joint level. It is covered by the thin posterior longitudinal ligament, which is concentrated in the midline, from which small bands extend laterally to cover the inferior aspect of the disc (Fig. 47.1). This configuration leaves the superior part of the posterolateral disc bare, and is thought to contribute to the fact that posterolateral (or paracentral) herniations are the most frequent location for herniations to occur. Cumulative degenerative changes occur in this region of the disc from concentration of torsional, axial loading, and flexion-induced biomechanical strains.

The spinal cord ends at approximately the L1 level in adults to form the conus medullaris. The cauda equina is located within the lumbar spinal canal. It contains the lumbar and sacral nerve roots bathed in cerebrospinal fluid contained—or encapsulated—by the pia, arachnoid, and dural membranes (meninges). Nerve roots branch from the cauda equina one level above their exiting foramen (Fig. 47.2). The L5 nerve root leaves the cauda equina approximately at the level of the L4 vertebral body. It descends inferolaterally to pass anterior to the L4–L5 facet joint and posterior to the L4–L5 disc. Intimately associated with the inferomedial aspect of the L5 pedicle, the root turns lateral to enter the L5–S1 intervertebral (neural) foramen just proximal to the L5–S1 disc. Within the foramen, sensory cell bodies form the dorsal root ganglion. The root, now called a *postganglionic spinal nerve,* exits the neural foramen, where it is in close proximity to the lateral aspect of the L5–S1 disc. Fibrous bands (called *Hoffman ligaments*) often tether the nerve to the disc in this region.[14,15] After a short extraspinal course, the nerve divides into a ventral and dorsal primary ramus.

The location of the disc herniation determines which root is primarily affected. The spinal canal can be divided into longitudinal zones (Fig. 47.3). The *central zone* is delineated by the lateral borders of the cauda equina. The *lateral recess* is between the lateral border of the cauda equina and the medial border of the pedicle. Although the term *lateral recess* is frequently used to describe stenosis from bony encroachment (*lateral recess stenosis*), it sufficiently describes the location of *paracentral, posterolateral,* or *juxtacentral* herniations. Within the lateral recess, fragments medial to the nerve root,

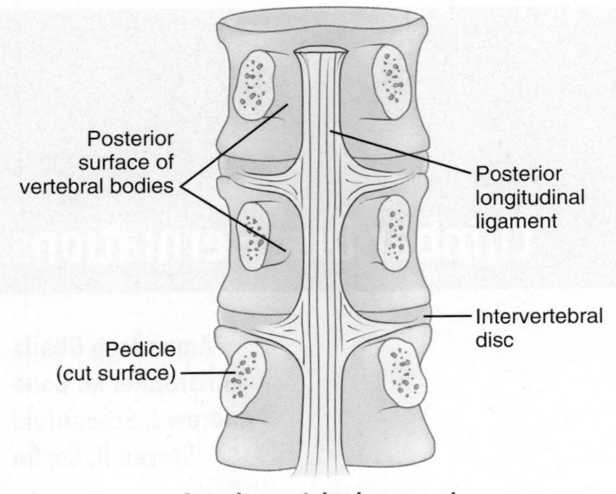

FIG. 47.1 The posterior longitudinal ligament incompletely covers the posterior portion of the disc. Specifically, the superolateral aspect of the disc remains uncovered, which may help explain why disc herniations are most common in this region.

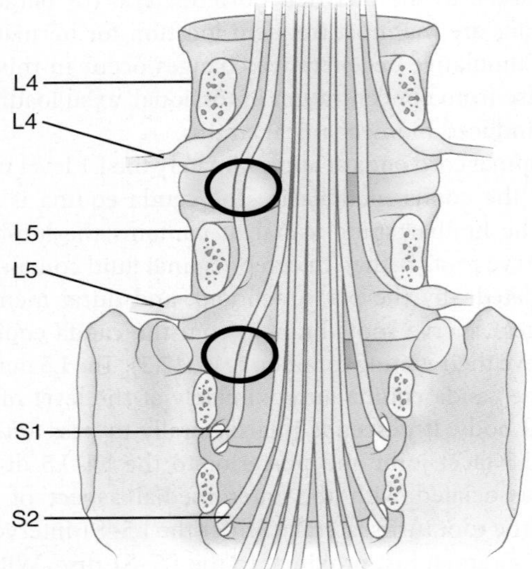

FIG. 47.2 Lumbar nerve root branches exit the dural sac one vertebral level above their respective foramen. Paracentral disc herniations tend to affect the traversing nerve root as it crosses the intervertebral disc.

interposed between it and the cauda equina, are called *axillary* herniations (Fig. 47.4). The *foraminal* zone is between the medial and lateral borders of the pedicle. Herniations beyond the lateral border of the pedicle are within the far-lateral or *extraforaminal* zone. Herniations in the foraminal or extraforaminal zones usually affect the exiting nerve.

Fragments can displace cranially or caudally. Axillary herniations have a tendency to migrate distally, lying inferior to the disc space. Superior migration of the fragment can position it behind the adjacent cranial vertebral body. Locating the fragment preoperatively is crucial to successful operative excision.

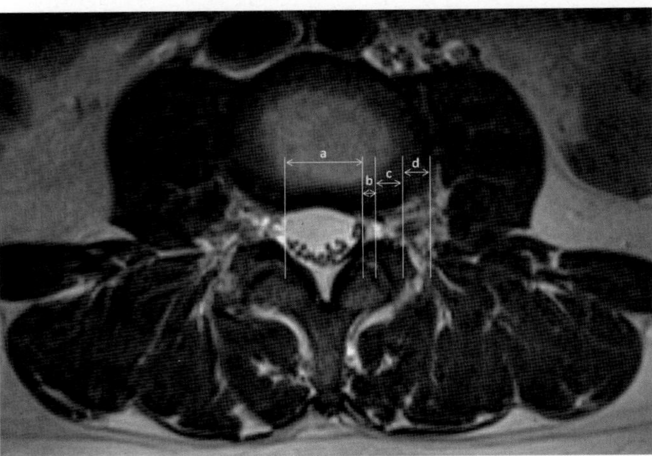

FIG. 47.3 Considered in cross-section, the spinal canal can be divided into anatomic zones to describe better the location of lumbar disc herniations. *The central zone* (*a*) is within the borders of the cauda equina dural sac. The *lateral recess* (*b*), which paracentral disc herniations can compromise, is bordered by the lateral aspect of the dural sac and the medial aspect of the pedicle and neural foramen. In this zone, the nerve root descends within the spinal canal toward its respective foramen. The *foraminal zone* (*c*) is the space between adjacent ipsilateral pedicles. The *extraforaminal zone* (*d*) is the space lateral to the pedicles. Disc herniations in this region, commonly referred to as *far lateral,* affect the exiting nerve root.

Pathophysiology

Disc Degeneration and Herniation

Disc herniation is one stage of the lumbar degenerative cascade. It is considered one of the earlier stages, following internal disc disruption. Herniation occurs through a tear in the anulus fibrosus. The anulus is the thick outer layer that normally withstands tensile forces transferred from the compressed nucleus pulposus (Fig. 47.5).[16,17] Force transfer works only if the nucleus-anulus-endplate complex acts as a closed-volume system.[18] Normally, compression across the disc space leads to increased pressure within the nucleus. The soft nucleus deforms and flattens, pushing against the annular fibers, which then generates tensile hoop stresses. The circumferential fibers are placed under tension, dissipating stresses and containing the anulus.

With disruption of the anulus, the soft nucleus can be pushed through (i.e., herniated) if placed under sufficient pressure. The nucleus must be fluid, or "dynamic," enough to permit herniation to occur. Discs in younger individuals that have a well-hydrated nucleus are more likely to herniate. Older patients with desiccated discs are less prone to herniation. The ejected portion is typically a fibrocartilaginous fragment.[19] In some cases, a piece of anulus or endplate fibrocartilage can be associated with it. In juveniles, an apparent herniation may represent a Salter type II fracture of the vertebral ring apophysis with its attached anulus.

When a portion of the nucleus is ejected, disc mechanics are altered. Frei and colleagues[17] showed that nucleotomy alters the loading pattern across the disc space, with the anulus sustaining higher compression forces than normal.

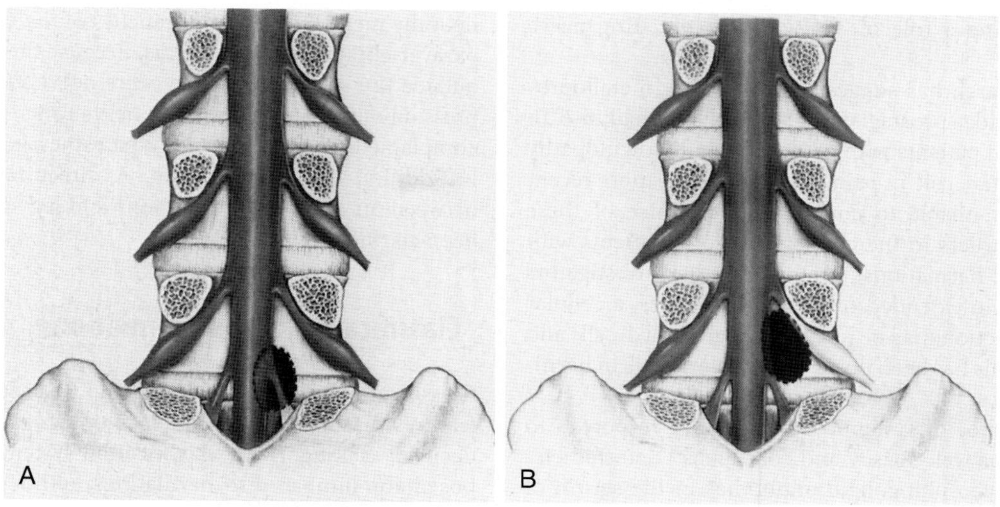

FIG. 47.4 (A) Most commonly, paracentral disc herniations compress the traversing (descending) nerve root along its lateral aspect. (B) In some cases, the disc fragment can be interposed between the nerve root and lateral border of the cauda equina sac. These are known as *axillary disc herniations*.

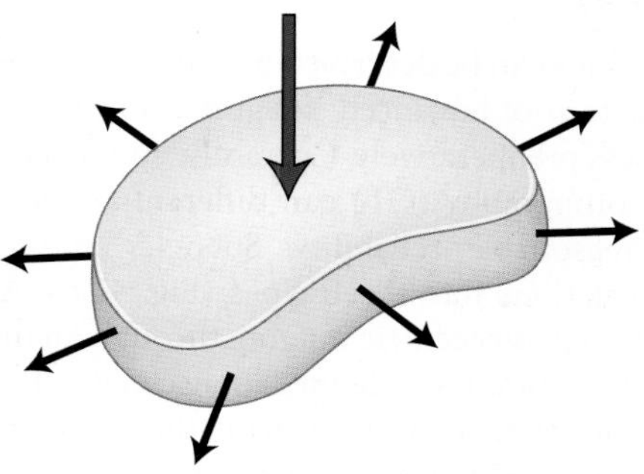

FIG. 47.5 The thick, outer anulus normally withstands tensile forces transferred from a compressed nucleus pulposus. This force transfer works, however, only if the nucleus-anulus-endplate acts as a closed-volume system. An annular defect disrupts this closed-volume system and can allow a portion of the nucleus to escape (or herniate).

This situation can lead to increases in endplate pressures along the periphery where the anulus attaches to the bone. Chondro-osseous metaplastic changes such as osteophytes or sclerosis in these regions are a response to long-standing abnormal loading patterns.

The exact inciting event leading to disc herniation is unknown. Some authors believe that an acute traumatic episode leads to displacement of the disc, although this is most likely related to force imparted onto a previously degenerated disc, which has developed a focal annular weakness. Acute sciatica from a disc herniation is often associated with a prodromal history of back pain.

Postural variations can influence intradiscal pressures. The highest pressures have been recorded in patients with the torso forward flexed with weight in hand. In an elegant biomechanical study, Wilder and colleagues[16] found that combined lateral bend, flexion, and axial rotation with 15 minutes of exposure to vibration can lead to tears extending from the nucleus across the anulus. This finding may have significance for occupations with exposure to long periods of vibratory stimuli, such as truck drivers and machine workers.

Disc Herniation and Sciatica

The most classic symptom of a herniated disc is radicular pain in the lower extremity following a dermatomal distribution. Focal neurologic deficits attributable to the same nerve root are sometimes present and lend further diagnostic accuracy. The relationship between disc herniation and sciatica is incompletely understood, however.

In animals and humans, pure compression of a noninflamed nerve produces sensory and motor changes without pain, whereas pain is elicited with manipulation of inflamed nerves.[20] These findings suggest that herniated discs large enough to cause mechanical compression of a nerve root may produce focal deficits, but that associated sciatic-type pain is produced only if the nerve root is concurrently irritated or inflamed. Inflammation may be produced by prolonged neuroischemia of the microvasculature of the nerve root from mechanical compression or by nonmechanical, possibly biochemical, factors. This phenomenon helps explain why some patients with small bulges or protrusions contacting inflamed nerves have pain that does not seem to be consistent with the "small" degree of neural compression. Additionally, these patients frequently do not have demonstrable sensory or motor deficit.

Neurochemical factors also have a role in the production of sciatic pain. This role may be related to initiation of an immune response locally or systemically, or both. Spiliopoulou and colleagues[21] examined immunoglobulin G (IgG) and IgM levels in discs excised from patients with sciatica and controls. Although IgG levels were equivalent, elevated levels of IgM were found in discs from sciatica patients but not in controls, suggesting a local and humoral antigenic inflammatory reaction as a contributor to pain. Other investigators have shown the role of cytokines in the mediation of root pain. Olmarker and Rydevik[22] studied the effects of selective inhibition of tumor necrosis factor-α (TNF-α) in a herniated disc model in pigs. They found preservation of nerve conduction velocity and decreased nerve root injury in treated animals versus controls, suggesting a role of TNF-α in potentiating nerve dysfunction.

Similarly, research has suggested that matrix metalloproteinase, nitric oxide, prostaglandin E_2, and interleukin-6 in discs excised from patients with herniation and radiculopathy may have a causative role in pain production.[23] A more recent investigation was unable to confirm the presence of these inflammatory markers in the epidural space of patients with symptomatic disc herniations, however.[24] Other investigators have shown that in extruded or sequestered discs, a cellular inflammatory reaction may be locally mediated via T cells and macrophages[25]; this has been postulated to play a role in herniated disc regression.[26]

There is evidence of systemic inflammatory responses to disc herniations as well. Brisby and colleagues[27] detected elevated levels of glycosphingolipid antibodies in the serum of patients with sciatica and disc herniation compared with healthy volunteers. Elevations were equivalent to those found in patients with autoimmune neurologic disorders, such as Guillain-Barré syndrome. Brisby and colleagues[27] suggested that a systemic autoimmune response to disc tissue may result in damage, or alteration, of nerve tissue. After age 12 years, the endplate apophyseal vessels close, which may facilitate an amnestic antigenic response to exposure to extruded nucleus pulposus tissue. These findings are helpful in considering patients who have severe sciatic pain with minimal mechanical compression and patients who seem to have persistent symptoms despite surgical decompression.

Disc Herniation and Back Pain

Most patients with symptomatic disc herniations present with leg and back pain (Table 47.1). The mechanism of degenerative back pain remains elusive, although many authors have suggested mechanisms. Accepting that herniation is a stage within the continuum of lumbar degeneration, discogenic pain generators may be a factor. Innervation of the posterior anulus by branches of the sinuvertebral nerve have been well documented and are a suggested pathway of nociceptive pain transmission from disc degeneration. An annular tear and nuclear herniation could result in similar pain transmission.

The concept of *vertebrogenic pain* has also been suggested. Jinkins and colleagues[28] studied the contribution of anterior disc herniations to back pain. They believed that the pain was neurally mediated through branches of the ventral ramus and paravertebral autonomic plexus. Because the herniations were outside the spinal canal, they were not associated with compression of the cauda equina or nerve roots, but most patients complained of lower extremity paresthesias, mostly bilateral, in addition to low back pain. A direct causal relationship between anterior disc herniations and leg symptoms has not been clarified.

TABLE 47.1 Prevalence of Back Pain and Sciatica in Adults

Characteristic	Prevalence (%)
Any low back pain	60–80
Any low back pain persisting at least 2 wk	14
Low back pain persisting at least 2 wk at a given time (point prevalence)	7
Back pain with features of sciatica lasting at least 2 wk	1.6
Lumbar spine surgery	1–2

From Deyo RA, Loeser J, Bigos S. Herniated lumbar intervertebral disc. *Ann Intern Med.* 1990;112:598–603.

Classification of Disc Herniations

Classification of any disorder should be based on identifiable features that have some influence on prognosis or treatment decision making. Many classification systems have been proposed for lumbar disc herniations, although none are all-inclusive or ideal.[29,30] It is more appropriate to consider them as tools to describe the herniation.

Morphology

Disc herniations can be described by their morphology. Before the introduction of advanced imaging, morphology was difficult to assess preoperatively. Currently, and to a lesser extent, computed tomography (CT) can differentiate disc morphology with reasonable reliability. Spengler and colleagues[13] divided herniations into three types (Fig. 47.6). A *protruded* disc was defined as eccentric bulging through an intact anulus fibrosus. An *extrusion* was defined as disc material that crosses the anulus but is in continuity with the remaining nucleus within the disc space. A *sequestered* disc represents a herniation that is not continuous with the disc space; this is the typical "free fragment."

Other authors have classified discs as either contained or uncontained.[31] *Contained* disc herniations are subligamentous. It is presumed that they have not passed beyond the limits of the posterior longitudinal ligament or the outer layer of the anulus. *Uncontained* disc herniations have crossed this boundary. Advocates of this system describe contained and uncontained extrusions, with the former remaining beneath the outer layers of the anulus.[31]

Location

Herniations can be described topographically according to anatomic location (see Fig. 47.3). The herniation can be located within the central zone, lateral recess, foraminal, or extraforaminal regions. Herniations can also exhibit cranial or caudal migration in relation to the disc space.

Timing

Lumbar disc herniations can be organized according to the time from initial symptom onset. These may be arbitrarily divided as acute or chronic. Acute herniations are present for less than 3 to 6 months, whereas chronic discs cause symptoms for a longer time. Breakdown according to this time frame is based on our sense of what is a reasonable cutoff point. Because

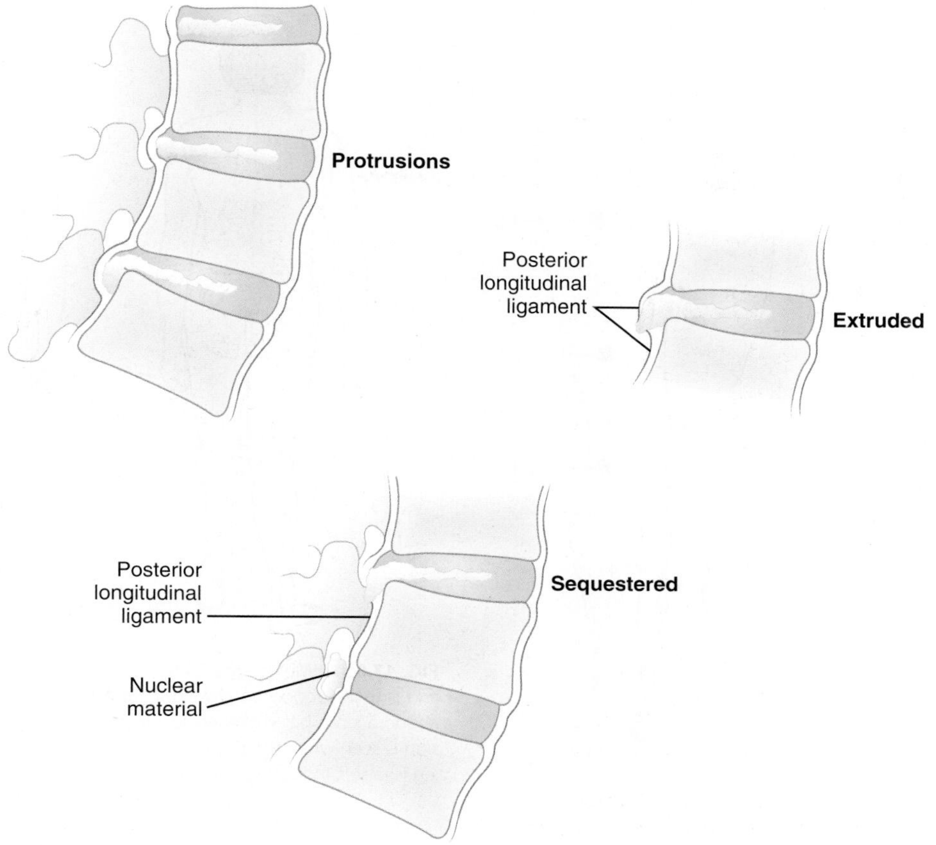

FIG. 47.6 Classification of disc herniations as described by Spengler and colleagues.[13] *Disc protrusion* is defined as a bulging, displaced nucleus that has not extended beyond the limits of the anulus fibrosus. *Extrusion* extends beyond the anulus fibrosus but is still in continuity, at least partially, with the parent disc. *Sequestered* disc herniation implies that a fragment has broken free (i.e., free fragment) and is no longer in continuity with the parent disc. In some cases, in which disc herniation lies immediately behind the vertebral body, it is difficult to tell from which disc the herniated fragment originated.

the results of disc excision seem to be influenced by the timing of surgery, this categorization is important. From a survey of the literature, it seems that the results of disc excision are compromised if delayed more than 2 to 16 months from symptom onset.[12,32–34]

History and Symptoms

Many patients describe a prodromal history of long-standing mild to moderate back pain. Although trauma is not the only component leading to a disc herniation, some patients describe a specific incident attributable to the onset of leg and back pain. This incident may be a fall, a twist, or lifting of a heavy item. Specific postures can lead to exponential increases in intradiscal pressure, which can predispose to disc injury.[18] Exposure to vibrational energy combined with sustained lateral flexion and rotation may also predispose to herniation.[16] The exact history of the incident and the presence of preexistent back or leg pain must be explored; this is particularly important in work-related injuries.

Pain is the most common complaint. Axial back pain is typically present, although some patients do not have this complaint. Radicular pain is more typical and often the more "treatable" of the complaints. The pattern of lower extremity radiation depends on the level of the herniation. Lower lumbar or lumbosacral disc herniations can lead to the classic symptoms of pain radiating below the knee. Often pain extends into the foot and can follow a dermatomal distribution. S1 radicular pain may radiate to the back of the calf or the lateral aspect or sole of the foot. L5 radicular pain can lead to symptoms on the dorsum of the foot (Fig. 47.7). Radiculopathy from involvement of the upper lumbar roots can lead to more proximal symptoms. L2 and L3 radiculopathy can produce anterior or medial thigh and groin pain. Groin pain may also be indicative of L1 pathology. Radicular pain can be difficult to discern and is often not "classic." Many patients do not exhibit pain in a specific dermatomal distribution, or the radiation does not extend along the entire leg. It may radiate only into the hip region or just the foot or any portion of the leg.

The character of radicular pain can be sharp, dull, burning, or dysesthetic. It can be exacerbated by coughing, bending, or lifting. A relieving maneuver may be lying supine with the knees and hips flexed, particularly with lower lumbar herniations. In contrast to patients with lumbar stenosis, patients

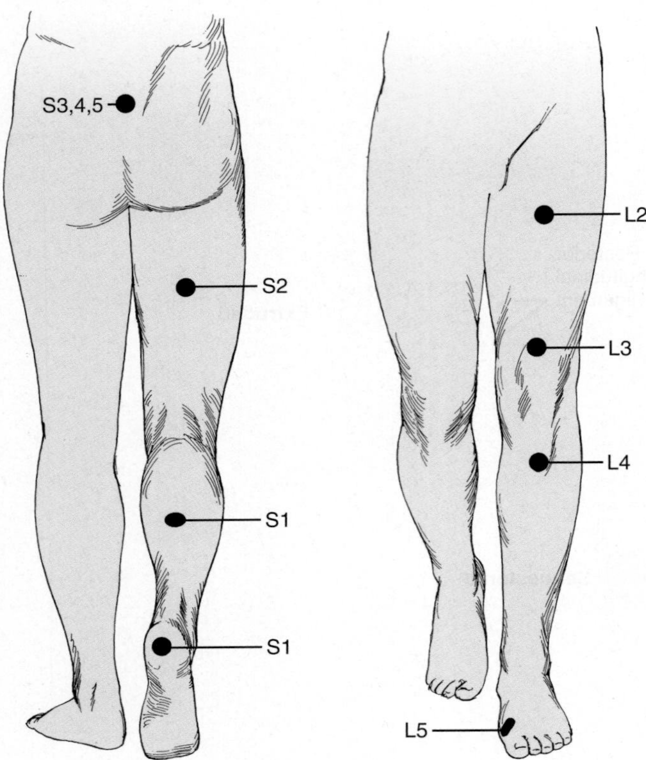

FIG. 47.7 The location of the pain can help localize the nerve root involved. Pain may radiate to small, isolated areas along the course of the dermatome.

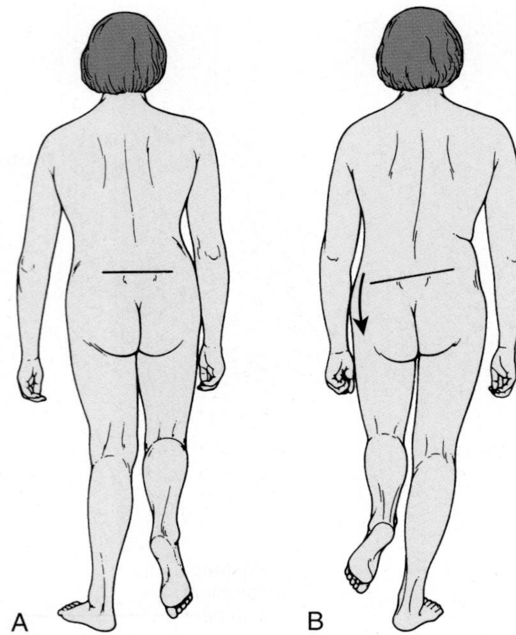

FIG. 47.8 (A) With normal L5 nerve root function, hip abductors are strong and able to support body weight. (B) With L5 nerve root compression, hip abductors can be weakened, leading to positive Trendelenburg sign. This sign is seen when the iliac crest (pelvis) tilts down onto the side where the leg is raised, indicating contralateral hip abductor (L5) weakness.

with disc herniations more typically complain of constant pain that is not exacerbated by ambulation. Buttock pain is also common and can be referred or radicular in nature. Patients may interpret this as back pain, but the pathoanatomic significance of pain in this area is different than true axial pain. Pain is one component of radiculopathic complaints. Nerve compression can lead to motor and sensory deficits. Weakness may be reported as a slapping gait, footdrop, knee buckling, or imbalance when walking.

It is important to ask questions pertaining to bowel and bladder function. The examiner should inquire about urgency and frequency and fecal and urinary incontinence. Questions must be direct because most patients report constipation, which is often related to narcotic usage or inactivity, as a change in bowel habits. Acute bowel or bladder symptoms can be the sign of a cauda equina syndrome, which should mandate urgent surgical decompression.

The influence of social and psychological factors on the outcomes of disc surgery has been well documented. It is highly recommended to obtain a social and at least cursory psychiatric history. Prescription use of antidepressants is an important clue, although depression is often undiagnosed and untreated at the time of initial presentation. Other personality factors—such as chronic headaches, hysteria, hypochondriasis, nervous disorders, and impulsivity—can also be influential.[13,35] Work history, pending litigation, and type of work should be obtained. A history of smoking is an independent risk factor for low back pain and a risk factor for a poor result after back surgery.[35,36]

Physical Examination

Inspection

Inspection is the first step in the physical examination. As the patient walks into the examining room, gait should be observed. A sciatic list may be present, usually manifested as the patient leaning away from the side of leg pain. This sciatic list is thought to be associated with a paracentral herniation lateral to the nerve root. Axillary herniations may cause a list toward the side of herniation. The list is an attempt to relieve neuromeningeal tension by drawing the nerve root away from the herniated fragment. Another feature of gait that should be noted is a wide-based gait, indicative of lumbar or more cranial canal stenosis. A footdrop or foot slapping gait may occur with L4 or L5 paresis. A Trendelenburg gait can suggest hip abductor weakness (Fig. 47.8), which may be a clue to L5 nerve root compression because the gluteus medius is most often an L5 dominant muscle.

Alignment of the spine should be noted. There can be loss of normal lumbar lordosis from muscular spasm. Hip flexion can relieve pain, leading some patients to lean forward or be reluctant to place the affected foot flat on the floor. In some cases, a nonstructural "sciatic scoliosis" can be noted on radiographs or examination of the back.

Palpation and Percussion

Examination should include a systematic examination of the back. The spinous processes are palpated individually and in stepwise fashion. Tenderness to palpation of one or two levels is more consistent with bony pathology than tenderness at multiple levels. In some cases, pressure on the spinous processes can reproduce sciatic symptoms. Continuing caudally, the lumbosacral junction and the sacral prominences and sacroiliac joint area can be palpated and percussed. Inflammation in these regions can manifest with sciatica, feigning disc herniation.

The musculature is examined next. The paraspinal muscles should be palpated. Spasm can be noted in addition to tenderness; this may be present as a "ball" of contracted muscle in one region. These findings are nonspecific and are of minimal diagnostic value. Muscular atrophy can be a sign of long-standing neural compression and is more likely isolated to one motor group. Generalized, symmetric muscle atrophy can suggest a more systemic neurologic disorder, such as a demyelinating disease.

Neurologic Examination

A neurologic examination is required in all patients with suspected herniated discs. Sensation of light touch is tested along dermatomes from L1 to S1. Standard dermatomal charts can be helpful, but there is variability among individuals; thus, this is highly subjective. In testing the upper lumbar roots, there is often a significant amount of overlap. The most discrete levels of testing are for L4, L5, and S1 nerve roots.[37] These nerve roots are the most often affected by lumbar disc herniations. L4 sensory function is tested at the medial ankle; L5, at the first webspace between the great and second toes; and S1, at the lateral aspect of the sole of the foot. Sensation is difficult to "grade." It is more useful to document sensation as normal, diminished, or absent. Sensory function should be compared with the contralateral side because this may help detect differences. The examiner should be wary of the presence of a glove-and-stocking distribution sensory loss, which can indicate a peripheral neuropathy—such as that associated with diabetes, or functional overlay—as it is not anatomic.

The motor examination should proceed in a routine manner. In the lower extremity, it is better to test movements rather than specific muscles. S1 motor function is assessed by testing plantarflexion, whereas L5 is tested by toe dorsiflexion, particularly the great toe (extensor hallucis longus), and hip abduction. L4 involvement most often affects ankle dorsiflexion (anterior tibialis), although quadriceps function can be compromised. There is a significant amount of overlap of upper lumbar motor innervation. Knee extension can be considered L3 function (although L2 and L4 contribute); hip flexion, an assessment of L1–L2 function; and hip adduction, an assessment of L2 function. Motor function is graded as 0 to 5, with 5 being full strength against active resistance (Table 47.2). In particular, S1 function should be assessed by asking the patient to toe raise repeatedly or toe-walk. Because of the enormous strength of the gastrocnemius complex, even a weakened muscle can overcome the examiner's hand. Toe-walking can show smaller differences, however, from side to side by using the weight of the patient's body as the resistance. Repetitive toe raising may help detect smaller differences.

TABLE 47.2 Motor Strength Grading System by Physical Examination

Grade	Definition
0	No visible muscle contraction
1	Visible muscle contraction; no joint movement
2	Can move joint, but not overcome gravity
3	Able to overcome gravity, but cannot overcome any examiner resistance
4	Able to overcome some, but not full, examiner resistance
5	Full strength; able to resist full examiner force

Deep tendon reflexes are tested at the patella and Achilles tendons. The patellar tendon reflex may be diminished or absent with L3 or L4 involvement, whereas the Achilles tendon reflex is affected primarily by S1. There is no specific reflex that reliably reflects L5 function. Reflexes are tested bilaterally and can be graded. Symmetrically decreased reflexes are not helpful in isolating a lesion. Generally, reflexes are anticipated to be decreased in response to nerve root compression from a herniated disc. Increased reflexes (hyperreflexia), especially if bilaterally symmetric, can indicate spinal cord compression at the thoracic or cervical level.

Specific Tests

The straight-leg raise (SLR) test is an extremely useful provocative test in examining patients with a herniated disc (Fig. 47.9). The classic test is performed with the patient in the supine position. The heel of a relaxed leg is cupped by the examiner's hand and elevated slowly. The knee is kept in extension while the hip is flexed. The test is considered positive if sciatic pain is reproduced between 35 and 70 degrees of elevation. Studies have determined that in the first 35 degrees of elevation, the slack in the nerves is taken up, and at 35 degrees or more, tension is placed on the nerves. More than 70 degrees of elevation causes no further stretch of the nerve roots. The SLR test is best for eliciting L4, L5, or S1 radiculopathy. It is not useful for upper lumbar roots, for which a femoral stretch test should be used. A positive SLR test is indicative of nerve root compression in 90% of cases.[38] It does not implicate a herniated disc as the source of compression, however, because foraminal encroachment or other mass lesions can lead to a positive SLR test as well.

The SLR test should always be performed bilaterally. If raising the contralateral leg reproduces symptoms in the ipsilateral side, this is highly suggestive for a herniated disc. It should be considered strong evidence of the diagnosis and is more specific for a free disc fragment. The Lasègue maneuver is a modification of the SLR test. The leg is raised until radiating symptoms are produced. Then, the foot of the ipsilateral leg is maximally dorsiflexed. By increasing the tension along

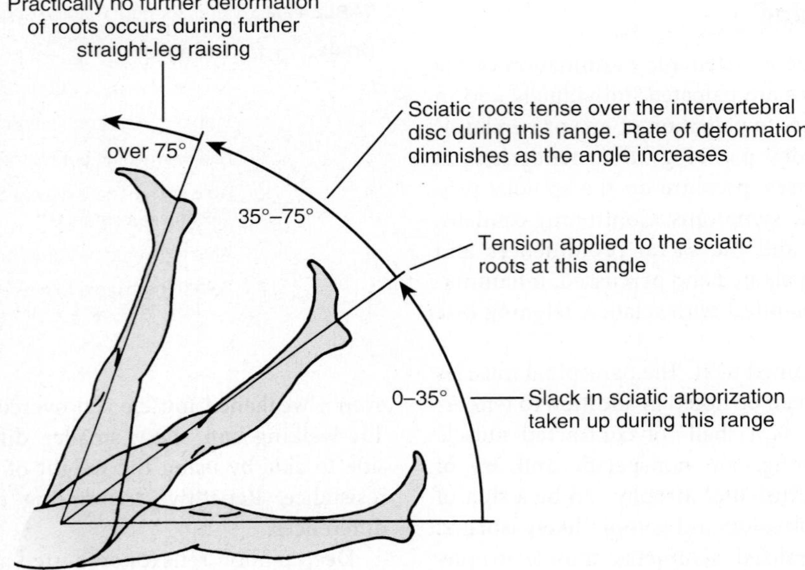

FIG. 47.9 Supine straight-leg raise test.

the sciatic nerve and lower lumbar nerve roots, dorsiflexion exacerbates pain and is considered a positive examination.

An important variant of the supine SLR test is the seated SLR test. When a patient is initially examined, the patient is usually seated at the side of the examining table with the knees and hips flexed at about 90 degrees. In this position, the heel is cupped, and the leg is extended at the knee. With a herniated fragment causing nerve root tension, the patient reflexively extends at the hip and leans back to relieve the ensuing sciatic pain. If the patient is comfortable with the seated SLR test but has a positive supine SLR test, symptom magnification must be considered because these findings are pathoanatomically contradictory.

The so-called slump test is a variant of the Lasègue test and SLR test. This test is performed in the seated position; the patient is asked to flex the thoracic and lumbar spine while fully flexing the neck. Next, the SLR test is performed while the foot is dorsiflexed on the same side, as denoted by the Lasègue test. The combination of these maneuvers adds cephalad gliding of the spinal cord to the examination, whereas the SLR test and Lasègue test by themselves produce only caudal tension on the nerve roots. A more recent study found that the slump test was more sensitive than the SLR test in patients with lumbar disc herniations, whereas the SLR test was more specific.[39]

Another tension sign is the bowstring test. Starting with a typical SLR test, the leg is raised until symptoms are produced. The leg is flexed at the knee, and the tibial and peroneal nerves (distal aspect of the sciatic nerve) are placed on tension by palpation in the popliteal space. Reproduction of pain is considered a positive sign of root tension.

The femoral stretch test is performed in the prone position. The leg is flexed at the knee while pulling the hip into extension. Reproduction of anterior thigh pain is indicative of upper lumbar root pathology.

Differential Diagnosis

The differential diagnosis should be narrowed based on history, physical examination, and selected imaging tests. Radicular pain can be caused by numerous compressive disorders, such as spinal stenosis, abscess, tumor, or vascular disease. Intrinsic nerve problems, such as nerve tumors or multiple sclerosis, can produce similar symptoms. Peripheral neuropathies, such as tarsal tunnel syndrome, meralgia paresthetica, and obturator or piriformis syndrome, can also lead to similar sciatic-type pain.

Diagnostic Imaging

We use a simple imaging algorithm for patients with suspected lumbar herniated discs. If the patient presents acutely, within the first 2 weeks of the incident, the examination is typically masked by a large amount of spasm, back pain, and generalized tenderness. If the mechanism of injury involved substantial trauma, plain radiographs are obtained. For low-energy injury, radiographs can be delayed until the follow-up examination at 6 weeks. Numerous patients will have recovered substantially by 6 weeks, obviating the need for further workup. For patients whose pain has not improved or perhaps has worsened, plain radiographs are obtained. Advanced imaging is reserved for patients in whom pain is persistent, the diagnosis is unclear, or surgical treatment is planned. "Red flags" in a patient's history that should prompt early MRI include constitutional symptoms (i.e., fever, chills, and sweats), a history of malignancy, osteoporosis, progressive neurologic deficits, or bowel and bladder incontinence.

Plain Radiographs

Plain radiographs cannot show a herniated disc. They can show changes that are suggestive of a herniated disc, however. As stated previously, a scoliotic list can be present on radiographs. This list may be convex or concave to the ipsilateral side and is not specific for a level.

Other findings that can be noted on plain films are changes consistent with disc degeneration, including osteophytes; disc space narrowing; or subtle changes in translation, facet hypertrophy, or changes in sagittal alignment. Most commonly, plain films are negative, especially in younger patients with an acute herniation. Plain films are important in ruling out obvious underlying problems, such as lytic lesions, tumors, infections, inflammatory spinal disorders, or instabilities (e.g., spondylolisthesis).

High-quality anteroposterior (AP) and lateral radiographs are prerequisites to planning operative interventions such as discectomy. It is crucial to recognize if there is an anomalous number of lumbar vertebrae, such as spines with a "lumbarized" first sacral segment (i.e., six lumbar vertebrae), because this can influence intraoperative identification of the correct disc level. Plain films can help detect other congenital anomalies, such as spina bifida occulta defects, which can influence surgical exposure and dissection.

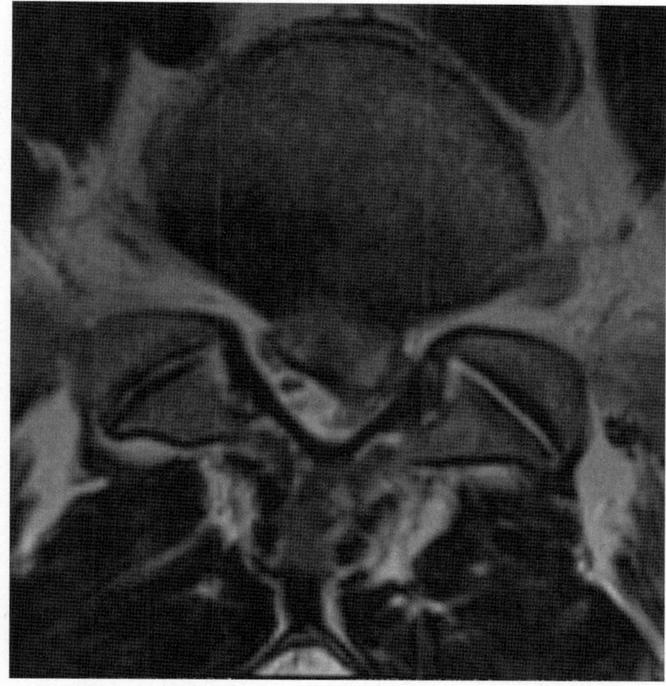

FIG. 47.10 T2-weighted magnetic resonance image has myelogram-like appearance, in which cerebrospinal fluid within dural sac is bright. This makes compression from disc herniations readily visible, as can be visualized in this case of a large extruded paracentral disc herniation.

Magnetic Resonance Imaging

MRI is the most popular modality for advanced imaging of lumbar disc herniations. MRI is superior to CT in delineating soft tissues. The disc and fragments that may have herniated from it are readily visualized. Free fragments (sequestered) can be differentiated from extruded disc herniations (Fig. 47.10), and a symmetric bulge can be differentiated from a contained protrusion. The neural elements themselves are well visualized. Neural encroachment can be detected within the spinal canal, the foramina, or extraforaminally. MRI is also useful in differentiating disc herniations from tumors, vascular anomalies, or bony compression.

Numerous features of a herniated disc can be noted on MRI. The size and type of disc herniation can be reliably determined using MRI, which may have prognostic significance.[11,40,41] Carragee and Kim[11] correlated outcomes with herniated fragment size and its effect on canal area. Larger discs (>6 mm) were more likely to have a positive SLR test or femoral stretch test (Wasserman sign). In the operative group, larger discs were predictive of a better outcome. The fair and poor outcomes in operative patients were in patients with small discs (<6 mm).

Attempts to correlate MRI findings with clinical symptoms have been made. In 33 patients in whom disc herniation was diagnosed clinically and 5 control patients with low back pain alone, Kikkawa and colleagues[42] performed three-dimensional MRI using a fast low-angle shot with gadolinium enhancement. Dorsal root ganglion enhancement was found to be nonspecific, occurring in controls and sciatica patients. Enhancement of the root proper was detected, however, in 11 of 30 symptomatic patients, with patients having a statistical tendency for more severe motor involvement. There was no significant association of diffuse versus local enhancement with the positivity of the SLR test or sensory changes. Central compression of the cauda equina did not lead to enhancement in any cases. Although these results are modest, they suggest a future use of gadolinium-enhanced MRI as a noninvasive method of determining the microvascular response to compression of neural structures.

Komori and colleagues[41] studied the significance of enhancement around the herniated fragment itself. Patients with radiculopathy underwent initial and follow-up gadolinium-enhanced MRI to correlate clinical improvement with the degree of enhancement. Patients with marked decrease in size of the herniation showed good clinical resolution. This resolution was most significant in the "migrating"-type discs, which were closest to sequestered discs according to the authors' description. Decrease in fragment size was associated with a gradual increase in the area of enhancement in 17 of 22 sequestered disc herniations, all of which had improvement of radicular pain. Five cases of sequestered discs without enhancement or size decrease had a poor clinical result. Enhancement was less marked in extruded versus sequestered herniations; however, herniations that did show enhancement had a significantly better clinical course. From these data, Komori and colleagues[41] recommended this test as a prognostic tool in guiding the treatment of patients with extruded or sequestered herniated discs.

Of more recent interest is the influence of posture on the MRI appearance of discs and their relationship to the neural structures. Because images are traditionally acquired in the supine position, the spine is not axially loaded as it is during everyday activities. Weishaupt and colleagues[43] performed positional MRI in patients with low back or leg pain for 6 weeks that was not responding to conservative treatment. Images were obtained in the usual supine position and with a seated flexed and extended posture. Changes in foraminal size and neural compression occurred with flexion and extension. Changes in foraminal size correlated with increased pain scores. These findings are probably most significant for low-grade herniations (i.e., bulges or protrusions) in which there is still a fixed-volume system within the disc space provided by an intact outer annular layer. Similar findings have been shown using dynamic functional plain myelography.[44]

Magnetic Resonance Imaging in the Postoperative Spine

Not all patients respond well to surgical discectomy. Failures may be related to numerous factors, including psychosocial disturbance, recurrence, infection, wrong-level surgery, poor surgical indications, and improper operative technique. Residual or recurrent back and leg complaints often prompt practitioners to seek postoperative imaging. Plain radiographs can show overall alignment, with flexion-extension views useful in detecting instability, spondylolisthesis, or disc space collapse, which is a frequent occurrence after discectomy in adult patients. Contrast-enhanced CT is best to show if there is associated bone or soft tissue impingement of the space available for the neural elements.

As the modality of choice for imaging the neural structures, MRI is frequently obtained. Because of edema, hematoma, and formation of surgical scar, MRI is best delayed until 6 months after surgery,[45] if symptoms allow. The main challenge is differentiating scar from new-onset disc. On standard T1-weighted sequences, this differentiation can be difficult. In the early days of MRI, T2-weighted images were not as useful because of longer scan times with inadequate magnet strength.[46]

The superiority of MRI over CT to distinguish scar from disc has evolved with the introduction of gadolinium contrast agent; this is based on T1-weighted sequences and has been shown by many researchers. Opinions have been changing regarding this test as the gold standard. A herniated disc fragment may eventually enhance if enough time passes before it is imaged. This enhancement can lead to recurrent or residual disc fragments being interpreted as extradural fibrosis or scar. Enhancement of scar should occur within 15 minutes of injection.

Evidence suggests that sophisticated T2 image analysis might supplant the need for gadolinium-enhanced MRI. Barrera and colleagues[47] compared different imaging sequences with and without gadolinium contrast agent. These investigators documented 100% sensitivity for detecting scar for T2-weighted turbo-spin echo (TSE) and fluid-attenuated inversion recovery (FLAIR) sequences compared with T1-weighted images with gadolinium. Specificity was 94% and 92% for TSE T2 and FLAIR images. Barrera and colleagues[47] concluded that standard TSE T2 images acquired using a rapid sequence are extremely sensitive and specific in distinguishing disc from scar in most cases, and that the use of gadolinium contrast agent should be reserved for the rare situation in which that distinction cannot be made. These recommendations are supported by others.[46]

Grane and Lindqvist[45] studied the role of gadolinium enhancement of the nerve roots after discectomy. These investigators found intradural (within the cauda equina) nerve root enhancement in 59% of patients with recurrent clinical symptoms. Recurrent symptoms occurred, however, in 84% of patients with focal (extradural, after the nerve root has exited the cauda equina) enhancement and 86% of patients with nerve root thickening. Enhancement occurred in patients with and without evidence of nerve root displacement by scar or disc. This finding indicates that although symptoms may correlate with MRI enhancement, it is not associated with a compressive mass lesion.

In an early report on the use of MRI without gadolinium, Bundschuh and colleagues[48] studied 20 patients after failed disc surgery who had a strong likelihood of undergoing further surgery. In 14 patients, CT with contrast agent was also performed. The authors found that free fragments of disc had a mildly increased signal on T1 images compared with scar, whereas scar and disc were similarly hyperintense on T2 images. Overall, Bundschuh and colleagues[48] believed that MRI was at least comparable to CT with contrast agent in differentiating scar from disc, confirmed by intraoperative findings.

In general, patients requesting repeat imaging after a first episode of acute sciatica should be informed about the difficulty of MRI interpretation with respect to symptomatology. In a recent randomized clinical trial by Barzouhi et al., which compared surgery and prolonged nonoperative care for sciatica from lumbar disc herniation did not distinguish between patients with a favorable outcome and those with an unfavorable outcome.[49] Importantly, patients enrolled had an acute diagnosis of sciatica with a dermatomal pattern of pain distribution corresponding to the identified nerve root on MRI, and the character of the herniations were classified. Repeat MRI images at 1 year showed herniated discs in 35% of patients with favorable outcomes and in 33% of patients with unfavorable outcomes.

Myelography

Plain myelography previously was the imaging modality of choice in detecting herniated discs. It involves injection of intrathecal contrast material to outline the boundaries of the subarachnoid space and silhouette the enclosed neural elements. It is invasive and cannot show compression beyond the confines of the subarachnoid space. Extradural compression caused by a foraminal or extraforaminal disc can be missed. Advantages of myelography are that it is a dynamic test because images can be made with the patient standing.[44] Myelography should be reserved for cases in which noninvasive imaging, such as CT or MRI, are nondiagnostic, equivocal, or contraindicated. Currently, myelography is rarely used for the routine workup of herniated discs. When used, it is usually followed by a CT scan.

Computed Tomography

Before the advent of MRI, CT was the imaging modality of choice for evaluation of herniated discs. Using bone and soft tissue imaging techniques, herniations can be detected in various regions independent of the dural cavity. It has been shown to be 93% accurate in predicting surgical findings at discectomy. CT can also be performed with intrathecal contrast injection (CT myelography). We currently use this test for patients in whom MRI is contraindicated or cannot be obtained.

Some disc herniations can contain gas (Knuttson phenomenon), noted on CT images. Mortensen and colleagues[50] reported four such cases that responded well to surgical discectomy. It is unknown if the gas forms before or after herniation. The clinical significance of the gas is not well understood. Ford and colleagues[51] determined that intradiscal gas is composed predominantly of nitrogen.

Natural History

The key to enhancing one's skills as an intelligent diagnostician and patient advisor is understanding the available knowledge related to the natural history of degenerative lumbar disc disease. The exact natural history of lumbar disc herniations is variable and incompletely understood. A few well-performed natural history investigations are available. Some studies are of patients treated by various nonoperative methods. Others represent the nonoperative arm of operative versus nonoperative comparison studies.

In a widely quoted retrospective study, Saal and Saal[5] found a 90% good or excellent outcome in patients treated nonoperatively for a lumbar disc herniation diagnosed by clinical examination and CT. Inclusion criteria were strict, including patients with SLR test positive at 60 degrees or less, leg pain greater than back pain, and electromyographic evidence of radiculopathy. Of patients, 92% returned to work. Nonoperative treatment consisted of aggressive physical therapy and back school education. A possible confounding factor is that many patients were referred for a second opinion regarding surgical versus nonsurgical treatment because they were anxious to avoid surgery. This may have introduced preselection bias error because the authors of the study were not surgeons. Concern has been raised about eventual fibrosis formation with nonoperative treatment of herniated discs. In a follow-up MRI study,[6] the same investigators documented no increased risk for perineural fibrosis or adhesions with nonsurgical management.

Other authors have reported more modest results. In the nonoperative arm of Weber's[10] classic randomized study, the long-term outcome of lumbar disc herniations was observed in 49 patients. Inclusion criteria were clinical signs and symptoms of L5 or S1 radiculopathy in addition to myelographic evidence of nerve root compression. Treatment included full-time bed rest for 1 week followed by partial bed rest the second week and back school instruction as an inpatient. At 1 year, 33% had good results, 49% had a fair result, and 18% had a poor result. At 4 years, good results were reported in 51%, fair results were reported in 39%, and poor or bad results were reported in 10%. Because the tiered system is slightly different than that used by Saal and Saal,[5] a direct comparison of the studies is difficult. If Weber's good and fair results are equated to Saal's excellent and good results, an 89% success rate achieved in the former at 4 years may be considered comparable to the latter's 90% success. Many of Saal and Saal's patients ultimately dropped out of the study and underwent surgical discectomy; thus, their 90% success rate might represent an overestimation.

In another nonoperative arm of a comparative study, 10-year follow-up results from the prospective Maine Lumbar Spine Study showed 61% improvement in the predominant symptom, 40% resolution of low back symptoms, and 56% satisfaction rate.[7] Work and disability status were comparable between operative and nonoperative groups in this investigation. Similar findings were reported for the observational cohort of the Spine Patient Outcomes Research Trial (SPORT).[8]

In a subgroup analysis of SPORT data, obese patients, defined as having a body mass index (BMI) greater than or equal to 30 kg/m^2, were found to have less clinical benefit from both operative and nonoperative treatment. More important, the benefit of surgery over nonoperative treatment was not affected by BMI.[52] McGuire et al. found a greater surgical treatment effect for highly obese patients primarily due to the poor outcomes of nonoperative management.[53] Rihn et al., in an analysis of the as-treated SPORT data, found that duration of symptoms affected outcomes following the treatment of lumbar disc herniation.[54] For patients with symptoms present for more than 6 months prior to seeking treatment, outcomes of nonoperative treatment were statistically significantly worse than those with symptom duration less than 6 months.

Methods of Nonoperative Treatment

Physiotherapy

Bed rest should be limited to no more than 2 to 3 days.[55] Greater periods of inactivity can potentiate prolonged disability and continued or augmented pain. Exercise therapy and physical rehabilitation should be included in the nonoperative care of herniated discs. Treatment goals are to restore strength, flexibility, and function that were lost secondary to pain, splinting, and spasm. Postural education to avoid activities that can increase intradiscal pressure or neuromeningeal tension, or both, should be provided.

Various regimens have been advocated, with none clearly superior. In our practice, physical therapy prescription usually includes torso stabilization training; paraspinal muscle stretching and strengthening; and a focus on gluteal, hamstrings, and abdominal exercises. These muscles are important in the static and dynamic stabilization of the spinal column. Some authors suggest concentration on flexion or extension maneuvers. In our experience, it is difficult, however, to predict if one or both of these movements would aggravate pain or help. Provisions for either flexion or extension concentration, at times combined with lateral shifts, are best left to the therapist's assessment because the therapist can actively assess what is provoking pain. Concomitant facet arthritis, painful disc degeneration, and muscular pain can influence pain patterns and aggravating movements.

Adjunctive modalities can aid in relieving some associated symptoms. These modalities include ultrasound treatment, electrical stimulation, and massage. These may be helpful in short-term, symptomatic relief of back pain. Traction is also commonly prescribed. It theoretically may diminish intradiscal pressure, increase foraminal dimensions, and possibly relieve radicular pain secondary to herniated discs.[56] The role of chiropractic manipulation is controversial. Although some patients believe that manipulations have "reversed" the herniation, there is no evidence to support the ability of chiropractic manipulation to alter the normal or pathologic morphology of the disc.[57]

Pharmacologic Treatment

Medications can be useful in decreasing disc-related symptoms. Because a local or systemic inflammatory reaction may participate in pain generation, antiinflammatory agents are believed to be beneficial. Nonsteroidal antiinflammatory drugs (NSAIDs) are first-line agents. Numerous choices are currently available, including cyclooxygenase-2 inhibitors. In prescribing NSAIDs, several important issues must be considered. The medications can have side effects. A history of gastrointestinal bleeding or peptic ulcers can be a contraindication to NSAID use. Although this risk is reduced with cyclooxygenase-2 agents, it is not nil, and the patient should be warned of the possibility. Additionally with NSAIDs, other systems, such as the kidneys and liver, may be detrimentally affected.

In the acute setting, back and radicular pain can be severe. Short-term narcotic use, such as a single dose of a morphine-derivative analgesic, can be useful. Narcotics should not be prescribed or administered in an extended manner; they should preferably be limited to a 2- to 3-day course. Also in the acute setting, a tapering dosage regimen of oral steroids can be helpful in decreasing inflammation-generated pain from nerve root irritation. In a randomized, double-blind, placebo-controlled trial of patients with acute sciatica due to herniated disc, Goldberg et al. demonstrated that a 15-day tapered dose of oral prednisone, compared with placebo, resulted in statistically significant, though modest, functional improvement without improvement in pain.[58]

So-called muscle relaxants are frequently prescribed. Although the drug class name implies a direct muscular effect, these medications have more significant sedative effects. Medications such as diazepam and methocarbamol should be used sparingly. Truly antispasmodic medications such as baclofen or cyclobenzaprine can have a more direct effect on muscle spasms.

Selective transforaminal steroid injections can produce symptomatic relief in many patients. In our treatment protocol, injections are offered to patients who have failed noninvasive measures but either are not interested in or are not good candidates for discectomy. In patients with more than one level of herniation, selective nerve root injection can be useful in determining the symptomatic level. That said, similar efficacy in pain relief between fluoroscopically guided epidural steroid injection and local anesthetic injection has been demonstrated in a recent double-blind, randomized controlled study.[59]

In a prospective series touted as a natural history study, Bush and colleagues[60] reported the results of 159 patients with CT-confirmed disc herniations treated with epidural steroid injections. Although 91% avoided surgery, this underscores a glaring problem of so-called natural history studies in that an interventional treatment was used. Although its exact biochemical effects are still being elucidated, steroid injections may be effective in "avoiding" surgery. In an analysis of SPORT data, Radcliff et al. noted that a higher percentage of patients randomized to surgery who subsequently received an epidural steroid injection switched to the nonsurgical treatment group (41%) compared to patients randomized to have surgery who did not have an epidural steroid injection (12%).[61] The authors concluded that this is confounded by the higher baseline desire to avoid surgery in the group of patients who received epidural steroid injections.

With TNF-α being considered a significant contributor to radicular symptoms associated with lumbar disc herniation,[62] recent attention has been paid to delivering anti-TNF-α medications into the epidural space. Freeman et al conducted a multicenter, randomized, double-blind, placebo-controlled phase IIa clinical trial to examine the efficacy of etanercept, a TNF-α inhibitor, injected transforaminally to treat symptomatic disc herniation.[63] Compared to placebo, etanercept was found safe and effective in providing significant therapeutic relief for patients with sciatica. When compared to epidural dexamthasone injection, etanercept has shown similar clinical efficacy in back and leg pain reduction, with no significant difference between the two medications.[64] There has also been recent interest in the use of transforaminal epidural clonidine injections, for its potential to dual action as an antiinflammatory and analgesic,[65] though this remains controversial.

In a well-designed retrospective study, Wang and colleagues[66] studied 69 patients who failed nonoperative (or, more accurately, noninvasive) care and had requested surgery as treatment. Instead, each patient was advised to undergo one or more transforaminal steroid injections at the affected root level. Of patients, 77% had clinical resolution and had not undergone surgery at an average follow-up of 1.5 years. In agreement with other studies, clinical success was not related to disc size, percentage canal compromise, or degree of motor weakness. From these findings, selective nerve root steroid injections seem to produce at least short-term relief of radicular symptoms from a herniated disc.

Operative Versus Nonoperative Treatment

The results of operative and nonoperative treatment for symptomatic herniated discs have been compared in numerous studies. The Maine Lumbar Spine Study group published

1-year and 5-year results of an ongoing comparison of surgically and nonsurgically treated patients.[1,67] More than 500 patients were included in the prospective observational study without stringent clinical or radiographic criteria except for disc-related sciatica treated with at least 2 weeks of nonoperative care within 2 months of onset. The decision to undergo surgery was determined on an individual basis and was not randomized. At 1-year follow-up, surgically treated patients were less symptomatic than patients in the nonoperative group, despite the former being *more* symptomatic at initial presentation. Relief of back or leg pain was reported by 71% of operated patients compared with 43% of the nonoperative group. High satisfaction levels and improved quality of life were documented for the operative group. For the workers' compensation group, there was no difference in time to return to work between operative and nonoperative groups. A criticism of the study is a substantial attrition rate, with 24% of patients unavailable for final follow-up.

In the 5-year outcome report, 70% of surgical patients reported back or leg pain improvement, whereas 56% of nonoperatively treated patients reported improvement.[1] As with the 1-year results, a similar percentage of patients were receiving workers' compensation benefits in both groups with no difference in return to work at final follow-up. Reoperations were performed in 20% of the operative patients; 16% of patients initially treated nonsurgically went on to operation. The authors noted that the benefits of surgery versus nonoperative treatment were greatest in the early part of the study, within the first 2 years, and that at final follow-up these advantages were less apparent.

Most recently, the Maine Lumbar Spine Study Group published their 10-year follow-up results.[7] Of the eligible patients initially enrolled, data were available for 85% of patients treated surgically and 82% of patients treated nonoperatively. A significantly larger percentage of surgical patients reported relief of low back and leg pain than patients treated nonoperatively. Similarly, surgical patients exhibited better function and satisfaction compared with nonoperative patients. Nonetheless, improvement in dominant symptoms was reported for both treatment groups. Work and disability status were similar for both groups.

The 2006 SPORT investigation was designed to be a rigorous, randomized, prospective, controlled study.[8,9,68] In its execution, there was a high rate of crossover between operative and nonoperative groups and a substantial portion of patients not willing to be randomized, resulting in a large observational group. The randomized and observational arms of the investigation reported improvement in bodily pain, physical function, and Oswestry Disability Index (ODI) scores regardless of intervention. In the randomized arm of the study, between-group differences favored surgical intervention, but these differences did not reach statistical significance in an intention-to-treat analysis. With the difficulties encountered with nonadherence to assigned treatments (i.e., crossover), the intention-to-treat analysis may not be reflective of the true outcomes. In an as-treated analysis, surgical treatment showed statistically superior results compared with nonoperative treatment. Similar results were found in the observational arm of SPORT. These results have proven to be durable, as there has been little to no degradation of outcomes in either the nonoperative group or the operative group in 8-year follow-up reports.[69] With the analysis adjusted for the treatment received, operated patients still maintained clinically significant greater improvement in all primary outcomes compared to the nonoperative group, as was reported at earlier follow-up time points.

The classic work by Weber[10] reported similar results to these findings. As briefly discussed in the prior section on natural history, Weber[10] compared surgery versus nonoperative care in a randomized, prospective study. There were three study groups: one group "required surgery"; another showed no indications for surgery; and the third was the "undecided" group, in which it was unclear if surgery would be beneficial. Only the third group was randomly assigned to surgical or nonsurgical treatment.

At 1 year, good results were reported in 33% of the nonoperative group versus 66% in the surgical group; at 4 years, 51% versus 66%; and at 10 years, 55% versus 57%. These findings show that operative and nonoperative treatment outcomes seem to converge with time, being nearly the same at 10 years, and that the benefits of surgery are early. The 5- and 10-year results from the Maine study are similar, although the larger numbers of the Maine study achieved statistical significance. Both studies are flawed by patient selection bias. Weber randomly assigned only patients in the "unclear" group, whereas the Maine group had no specific criteria and included patients per individual physician investigators' usual practice.

Alaranta and colleagues[70] also prospectively compared operated versus nonoperated patients. In contrast to other similar studies, the nonoperative group was subdivided into cases with and without myelographic evidence of nerve root compression, whereas all operated patients had a positive myelogram. At 1-year follow-up, 91% of operated and 82% of nonoperatively treated patients with positive myelograms had improved pain levels. Only 51% of nonoperatively treated patients with negative myelograms had improvement. These data suggest that a distinctly worse natural history exists for patients with sciatica and no evidence of root compression. Although not specified by the investigators, this group probably represents sciatica from an extraspinal or non–disc-related origin. In a companion study published by the same authors, they further identified this group as having a high incidence of generalized pain (e.g., concomitant occipital headaches), more physically strenuous jobs, and lower pain thresholds.[71] This study could possibly point to a preponderance of psychosocial and behavioral factors involved in the perpetuation of the symptom complex.

Operative Treatment

Indications

An absolute indication for lumbar discectomy is a progressive neurologic deficit. In this circumstance, operative intervention may be considered conservative care, provided that no medical contraindications exist. Progressive neurologic deficit is most commonly associated with a cauda equina syndrome and is discussed in more detail later. The relative indications for discectomy vary among surgeons and patients. Discectomy, in its many shapes and forms, can produce symptomatic relief in appropriately selected patients. It is the surgeon's obligation to identify the patients in whom the anticipated benefits outweigh the attendant risks of surgery.

A prerequisite is radiologic identification of compressive pathology that is concordant with the patient's physical signs and symptoms. A patient with a large left L4–L5 level who presents with leg pain that radiates to the dorsum of the foot, weakness of toe dorsiflexion, decreased sensation in the first dorsal webspace, and a distinctly positive ipsilateral and contralateral SLR is an ideal candidate after failure of appropriate nonoperative treatment. In this "ideal" situation, the clinical and radiologic findings point toward compression of the L5 nerve root. To idealize the presentation further, the patient has a strong desire to return to work; is not involved in litigation, disability, or workers' compensation issues; and does not have any psychological issues. Important questions remain unanswered even in such cases, however, including optimal surgical timing, the method of disc excision, and the postoperative rehabilitation protocol.

Only a few patients match such textbook descriptions. Most patients lack one or more of the supportive diagnostic clues, making it more difficult to support the decision to operate. This situation does not represent a contraindication to surgery, however, because many published series show approximately 85% success rates in patient groups with lesser percentages of objective motor and sensory findings.[3,38,67,72–79] The slim chance of back pain relief in relation to leg pain with discectomy that surgeons obligatorily confess to their patients is also probably an underestimation because most series document at least modest improvements in back pain. It is incumbent on clinicians to discuss the advantages, disadvantages, risks, alternatives, and estimated expected outcomes with patients.

Available Techniques

A vast array of techniques exist for surgical treatment of herniated discs.[80–85] Standard open discectomy is the most common surgical approach.[72,77,86,87] It involves careful incision planning, laminotomy or partial laminectomy to provide adequate visualization of the pathology, gentle retraction of the neural elements, and direct excision of the herniation. As an adjunct to open discectomy, some surgeons advocate the use of a microscope for better visualization and minimizing incision size.[31,79,83,88,89] The purported advantage of the microscope is the ability for the surgeon and the assistant to visualize the operative field equally through a smaller surgical wound.

Alternatives to interlaminar techniques have been developed for excision of foraminal and extraforaminal lateral disc herniations, which involve exposures between the transverse processes and lateral to the pars interarticularis.[14,89] Although some surgeons have advocated the addition of fusion,[76,90] this practice is unpopular.[81] Advocates hold that fusion decreases the chance for reherniation; however, only a complete discectomy with interbody reconstruction can eliminate this risk. Long-term effects such as an adjacent-segment degeneration and the additional morbidity and complication rates are potential disadvantages.[76,81,90,91]

With increased interest in smaller incisions and minimally invasive surgery, various percutaneous methods of treatment have been developed. Some methods entail placement of a cutting device intradiscally to decompress the disc space to retract the herniated fragment.[92–95] Other methods involve percutaneous techniques of directly visualizing the neural elements and disc using an endoscope.[80,96] Chemical digestion of the disc (i.e., chemonucleolysis) had enjoyed popularity in the past. However, enzyme-related complications and results inferior to open discectomy limited continued popularity in the United States.[92,97,98]

Repair of the anulus fibrosus following lumbar discectomy is an emerging technology, with various techniques and devices introduced in recent years. There remains a paucity of published studies concerning the clinical outcomes of newer devices, though data are forthcoming. In one published prospective randomized trial, an annular repair technique did not show statistically significant benefit in patient symptoms, but did reduce the need for subsequent surgery.[99]

Open Simple Discectomy

Timing

Disagreement exists regarding the optimal timing for surgery. The question is how long should nonoperative care be continued (without improvement) before the outcomes of surgery are detrimentally affected? Stated another way, in patients who are not responding to nonoperative measures, when should surgery be performed? In evaluating the currently available surgical results, this interval may be 2 to 16 months. The clear exception to delaying surgery is a patient who is experiencing a progressive neurologic deficit or cauda equina syndrome.

Rotheorl and colleagues[33] stratified operatively treated patients according to time from presentation to surgery. Patients with symptom duration of more than 2 months had a statistically significantly worse outcome than patients operated on within 2 months. There was no difference if surgery was performed within 1 or 2 months. Likewise, Hurme and Alaranta[12] found the best results in patients operated on within 2 months of the onset of disabling sciatica. Nygaard and colleagues[32] reported worse results in patients with leg pain for 8 months or more; Jansson and colleagues[36] found similar results in their analysis of the Swedish registry data, which included greater than 27,000 patients. Sorensen and colleagues[34] found that symptom duration greater than 16 months was predictive of poor results, but this was highly influenced by patient personality and social factors. The disparity between these findings is difficult to explain. Randomized prospective data comparing early versus late surgery are lacking. In our practice, surgery is performed within 6 months from symptom onset if nonoperative care has failed. The important message is that there is not an urgency to perform surgery. Nerve roots, as compared with the spinal cord, are fairly resilient.

Other factors can influence the time to surgery. Ito and colleagues[40] found that patients with uncontained herniations had surgery much earlier than patients with contained herniations. Specifically, 56% of patients with uncontained herniations and 21% of patients with contained herniations had surgery within 1 month. This finding was not correlated to outcomes but was influenced more by the severity of symptoms. Early surgery does not seem to affect the rate of neurologic recovery; objective improvements in motor and sensory deficits do not seem to correlate with symptomatic relief and overall success rates.[100]

Technique

General endotracheal anesthesia is induced. Alternatively, spinal anesthesia can be used. The patient is carefully logrolled into the prone position. An Andrews frame can be attached to a regular operating table to facilitate the prone kneeling position. Special spine frames, such as the sling attachment for the Jackson (OSI) table (Mizuho OSI, Union City, CA), can be used. These frames allow hip flexion to produce some flexion of the lumbar spine, which widens the interlaminar space (Fig. 47.11). The kneeling position also allows the abdomen to hang free, which helps indirectly to reduce the epidural venous pressure and reduce intraoperative blood loss. One set of hip pads is placed just distal to the anterior superior iliac crest. Adequate padding protects against lateral femoral cutaneous nerve injury. The thighs are allowed to flex at the hip, with the knees resting within the sling. The sling should be positioned low enough to allow adequate hip and knee flexion and is padded with gel pads and pillows. A pad is placed between the knees and medial malleoli to prevent pressure necrosis. The transverse chest pad is placed just above the xiphoid process.

With either table, the arms are placed in the 90-90 position with the cubital tunnels protected. The advantages of the Jackson table include that it allows a one-step turn to the prone position (avoiding the second step of pulling the patient's buttocks to the posterior pads with the Andrews frame) and its complete radiolucency. The disadvantage is that the table cannot be rotated away from the surgeon to allow better visualization by the assistant. With the patient secure, the superior aspects of the crests are palpated and marked; this usually corresponds to the level of the L4–L5 disc space or the L3–L4 interspinous process interval. The midline spinous processes are marked, and the interspinous regions are counted from the sacrum up. The target interspinous space can be indicated with a marker or scratched in the skin using a sterile 25-gauge needle after alcohol skin preparation. If the patient is unusually large and landmarks cannot be palpated, a radiograph can be taken to determine the level of skin incision before preparation. The lumbar region is then prepared and draped. A 3- to 5-cm midline skin incision is made, and can be extended if necessary in obese patients.

The subcutaneous tissue is dissected down to the level of the lumbar fascia. The spinous processes are palpated in the midline. The deep lumbar fascia is incised, on the side of the herniation, adjacent to the spinous process. The fascial incision spans the spinous processes of the adjacent segments. An intraoperative lateral radiograph should be obtained at this time to confirm the correct level. A marker, either a Kocher clamp or a spinal needle, can be placed along the interspinous ligaments. On the radiograph, the marker should point toward the operative disc space. It should angle superiorly in line with the interspinous process space.

The paraspinal muscles are subperiosteally elevated from the lateral aspect of the spinous processes using electrocautery. It is usually necessary to expose only the superior and inferior aspects of the adjacent segments. At the junction of the spinous process and lamina, blunt dissection is performed laterally along the interlaminar space using a large Cobb elevator. Care is taken to expose, but not violate, the facet joint.

A Taylor retractor is positioned to maintain exposure of the interlaminar space. The tip of the retractor is inserted lateral to the facet joint, and the instrument is levered laterally. A roller-gauze is looped underneath the surgeon's foot and tied to the handle of the Taylor retractor. Appropriate foot leverage maintains its position. Alternatively, numerous small retraction systems can be used. Meticulous hemostasis is achieved with a bipolar electrocautery. Extraneous posterior muscle and soft tissues that impair vision should be removed using a large curette and rongeur. The interspinous ligaments should not be disrupted.

A medium-sized curette is used to detach the ligamentum flavum from the inferior aspect of the superior lamina (Fig. 47.12). Because the ligamentum inserts along the anterior aspect of the lamina, the curette needs to be introduced at an angle with the spoon facing cephalad. The instrument is worked from side to side to release all layers of the ligamentum. In some cases, it is difficult to release the ligamentum flavum completely without removing a portion of the inferior

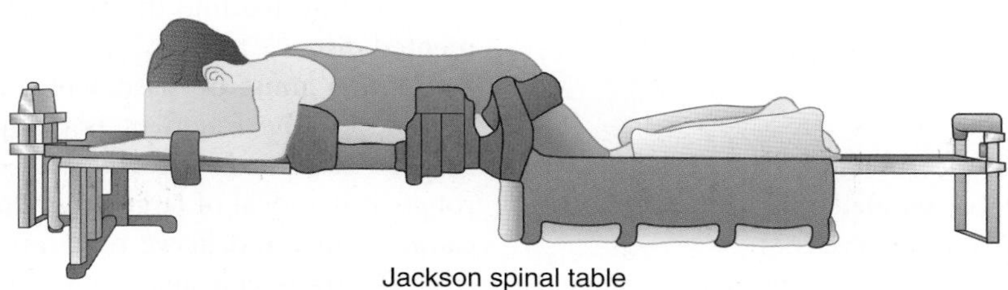

FIG. 47.11 The Jackson (OSI) table can be used to place the patient into a kneeling position, increasing interlaminar lumbar space while allowing the abdomen to hang free.

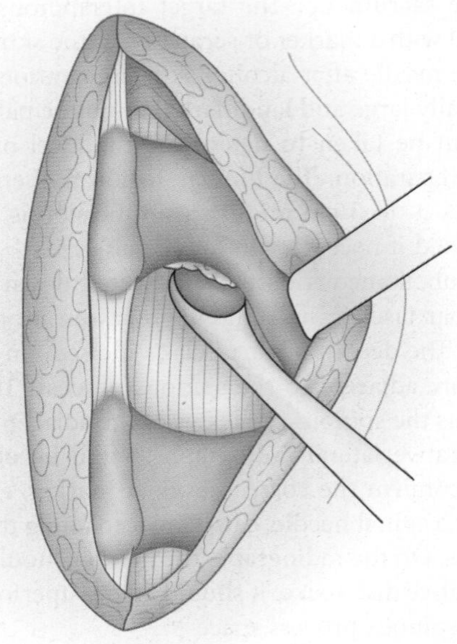

FIG. 47.12 The ligamentum is released from the inferior aspect of the superior lamina. The cup of the curette should face away from the dural sac to avoid inadvertent injury or tear.

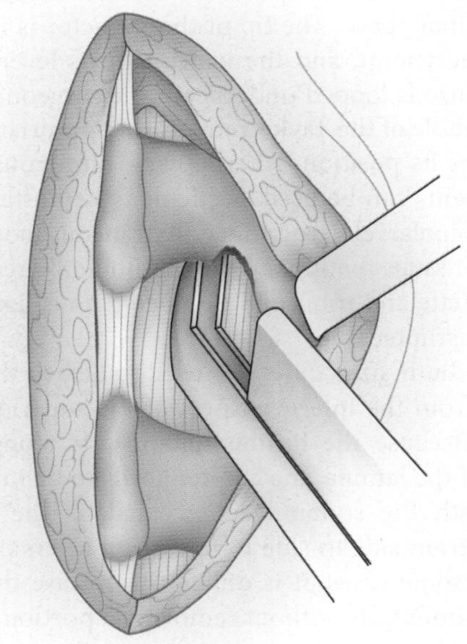

FIG. 47.13 In some cases, particularly above the L5–S1 level, a small portion of lamina must be removed to release the ligamentum flavum fully.

hemilamina (Fig. 47.13). Bone resection can be kept to a minimum but should not be avoided if it jeopardizes the exposure of the cauda equina and nerve root.

After the ligamentum is released superiorly, an angled probe, such as a Woodson elevator, can be inserted just deep to the ligamentum flavum (the yellow ligament). The Woodson elevator is positioned along the periphery near the bone. A long-handle No. 15 blade scalpel is carefully used to incise the flavum directly on top of the Woodson elevator, which protects the dural sac deep to it, which may often be displaced posteriorly by a large herniated disc. The blade should not be inserted deep to the ligament or the elevator. If concerns exist, the ligamentum flavum should be incised layer by layer with consecutive passes of the blade until the Woodson elevator pops through; this is continued along the periphery of the interlaminar window. Optionally, the medial aspect of the ligamentum flavum can be left attached, and the ligamentum can be flapped open. At the completion of the discectomy, the flap can be replaced to act as a barrier against epidural adhesions.

With the ligamentum retracted or removed, epidural fat is visualized. In some cases, the fat layer has thinned from a displaced or inflamed nerve root. If present, the epidural fat is swept away from the dura with a Penfield No. 4 elevator. The focus of this maneuver is to identify the lateral aspect of the exiting nerve root and cauda equina. Epidural vessels are coagulated using irrigating bipolar cautery, as necessary.

A medial facetectomy often must be performed to visualize the nerve root adequately. A 3-mm or 4-mm Kerrison rongeur can be used in a back-hand manner to resect the medial aspect of the facet joint. Excessive resection should be avoided because the integrity of the facet and pars interarticularis is crucial to maintaining stability. It is wise to protect the underlying dura by pointing the Kerrison rongeur in the direction of the exiting nerve root. The endpoint of resection is adequate visualization of the shoulder of the descending nerve root adjacent to the medial border of the pedicle.

Before discectomy, a blunt-tipped probe is passed along the root and out the foramen to assess the amount of space available. Using a Penfield No. 4 elevator, the nerve root is mobilized medially. This mobilization can be facilitated using the bipolar cautery to lyse adhesions between the dura and the posterior disc. Retracting the nerve root medially shows the posterior anulus or the herniated fragment, or both. A nerve root retractor is used to maintain retraction (Fig. 47.14).

The disc fragment may be extirpated using the Penfield elevator to ensure that it is free of dural adhesions. With clear visualization of the fragment and its distinction from the neural elements, a pituitary rongeur can be used to explant it. If the fragment is extruded or sequestered, one can often identify a tear in the posterolateral or central anulus. If the herniation is subligamentous, a No. 15 blade scalpel can be used to create a small annulotomy to gain access to the herniated nuclear material. A pituitary rongeur can be carefully inserted into the annular defect to remove the fragmented disc.

Caution must be used when removing an axillary disc herniation. The fragment is easily visualized, tempting the surgeon to proceed directly with excision with the pituitary rongeur. Removal of large fragments that extend deep to the cauda equina and nerve root can lead to excessive bleeding from the transverse anastomoses of the epidural veins in the axillary region. It is preferable to retract the root medially and remove the fragment from a lateral approach, if possible.

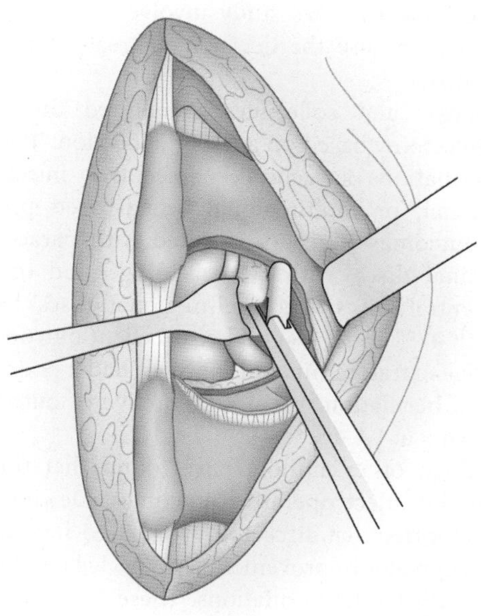

FIG. 47.14 A nerve root retractor is used to retract gently the descending nerve root and cauda equina toward the midline to visualize the disc space and herniation.

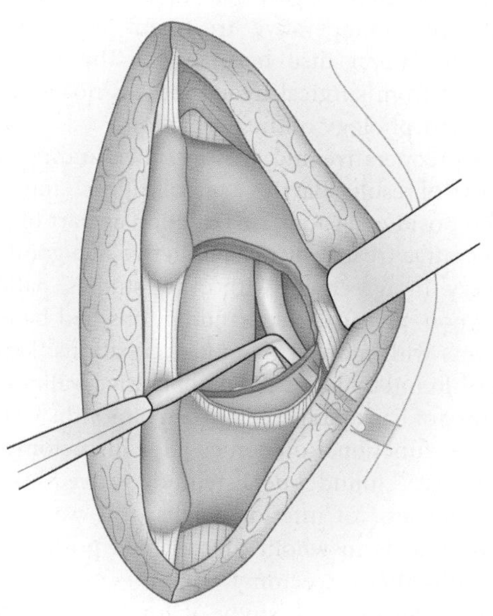

FIG. 47.15 After the herniated fragment has been removed, the spinal canal should be systematically inspected for any remaining fragments. A Woodson elevator is used to ensure that the neural foramen and nerve root are free. If the root is not completely free, additional fragments or compression may be present.

The mobility of the nerve root is assessed using a Penfield No. 4 or Woodson elevator (Fig. 47.15). After discectomy, the nerve root should be freely mobile and under no tension or compression. If it is not, additional pathology should be suspected. Using a Woodson elevator, the epidural space must be systematically inspected in a clockwise fashion, checking the canal ventral to the thecal sac and the patency of the foramen. A concomitant lateral recess or foraminal stenosis from bony encroachment is decompressed with Kerrison rongeurs. Finally, the disc space is irrigated with normal saline to dislodge any remaining loose fragments.

If the ligamentum flavum was spared, it can be loosely replaced. A fat graft placed over the dura does not improve clinical results but does facilitate reexploration and theoretically prevents adhesions from inhibiting normal neuromeningeal motion.[101,102] The wound is copiously irrigated. Adequate epidural hemostasis is ensured before closure. In most cases, a drain is not needed. All retractors are removed, and the deep lumbar fascia is approximated with interrupted No. 1 absorbable suture. The subcutaneous layer is closed in two layers, and the skin is approximated with a subcuticular stitch or staples. The wound is cleaned, and a sterile dressing is applied.

Postoperative Care and Rehabilitation

After an uncomplicated simple open discectomy, the patient is discharged on postoperative day 1 or 2. Outpatient discectomy can be performed on selected patients with appropriate presurgical planning and postdischarge discussion.[86] The level of activity in the first week after surgery usually is limited by incisional pain. If leg symptoms were predominant preoperatively, the patient typically reports immediate relief.

The activity level recommended after surgery varies among surgeons. Concerns are that aggressive movements and loads can predispose to reherniation or excessive scarring. This concern leads many surgeons to limit lifting and bending after discectomy for about 3 to 4 weeks. Although this is probably the predominant practice, there is little literature to support such extended periods of protected activity.

Unrestricted activity protocols have shown success rates comparable to other series. Carragee and colleagues[87] conducted an uncontrolled, prospective trial of 152 patients who were allowed full activity after lumbar discectomy. Approximately one-third of patients returned to work in 1 week, with most (97%) returning to work within 8 weeks. Recurrent sciatica occurred in 17 patients and was considered possible reherniation (11%). Nine of these patients experienced improvement, and eight underwent repeat surgery. This rate is similar to reherniation rates previously reported, which have ranged from 0% to 13%. Carragee and colleagues[87] concluded that an unrestricted activity protocol does not negatively affect results after discectomy.

Other studies have focused on possible advantages to an early rehabilitation protocol after discectomy. Kjellby-Wendt and Styf[103] performed a prospective, randomized, controlled study comparing an early active versus traditional training program. The focus of early activity was to reduce lumbar edema and maintain mobility of the neural elements through motion and trunk-strengthening exercises. A pain-coping program was included in the early active group that was not included in the traditional group. There was greater range of motion and decreased pain at 12 weeks in the early group.

At 1-year follow-up, both groups were equivalent. Patient satisfaction was ultimately greater in the early active group (88%) versus the control group (67%), although this was not statistically significant. In critique of the study, it was unclear why the difference in subjective outcome was not accompanied by sustained objective benefits. Inclusion of the pain-coping program in the study group, which would have minimal influence on range of motion, may have positively influenced patients' perception of their residual impairment. In support of the findings by Carragee and colleagues,[87] there was no difference in reherniation rates between the two groups.

Gencay-Can and colleagues performed a clinical trial comparing patients undergoing lumbar discectomy treated with a supervised aerobic exercise program starting 1 month after surgery in addition to home exercises with patients performing home exercises alone.[104] While there was no significant advantage in visual analog scale (VAS) back and leg pain, there was significantly better functional improvement in the aerobic exercise group as measured by the Roland Morris Disability Index. As one may expect, the functional recovery did not carry forward once the exercise program was discontinued.

Alaranta and colleagues[105] performed a randomized trial comparing an "immediate" versus "normal" rehabilitation program. Physical activities, such as sports and games, were encouraged in the immediate activity group; psychological and social counseling were also provided. Details of the normal rehabilitation protocol were not provided. At 1-year follow-up, there were no differences in subjective outcomes, postoperative impairments, or return-to-work statistics. These results further indicate that early activity programs do not seem to be harmful but offer only minimal, if any, long-term benefits. Our decision to initiate early return to unrestricted activity is made on an individual basis.

Outcomes

The outcomes of surgical discectomy are reliable when one adheres to strict preoperative selection criteria. Factors that can influence these outcomes, such as location of the herniation, preoperative psychological status, surgeon experience, and work status, have been extensively analyzed.

Carragee and Kim[11] correlated operative outcomes with herniated fragment size and its effect on the canal area. Using axial MRI, these authors recorded several parameters, including disc area, canal area, AP disc length, and AP canal length. Patients with larger discs (>6 mm) were more likely to have positive SLR or femoral stretch tests. Comparing patients with operative and nonoperative treatment, the former had larger AP disc lengths and larger ratios of disc to canal area. In the operative group, larger discs were predictive of a better outcome. In the nonoperative group, symptom duration less than 6 months before presentation, no litigation, and younger age were predictive of a better outcome. All of the fair and poor outcomes in operative patients were in patients with small discs (<6 mm). Summarizing these findings, it seems that larger discs respond to surgery better than small discs and that disc size is less predictive of outcomes in the nonoperative group. A criticism of this study involves the existence of a selection bias because the decision to treat operatively was nonrandomized.

Knop-Jergas and colleagues[106] analyzed the results of lumbar discectomy based on anatomic location. They characterized herniations as central, paracentral, intraforaminal, extraforaminal, or multiregional broad-based protrusions. The best outcomes were documented with paracentral and intraforaminal discs, with 80% yielding good or excellent results. Central discs and multiregional discs had worse results, with 47% and 54% good or excellent outcomes. There was only one extraforaminal disc, which had a poor outcome. The level of herniation was not predictive of outcome, with 59% occurring at L4–L5.

In contrast, other authors have found that the level of herniation can affect operative outcomes. Dewing and colleagues[107] reported that discectomy for L5–S1 herniations had significantly greater improvements in VAS leg and ODI scores compared with L4–L5 herniations. These authors also found that patients with sequestered disc fragments had significantly better outcomes than patients with contained disc herniations. In a post-hoc analysis of SPORT trial data, Pearson and colleagues[68] examined the influence of disc herniation location (central or lateral) and morphology (protrusion, extrusion, or sequestration) on the results of operative and nonoperative treatment. Their data suggest that the advantages of surgical treatment over nonoperative treatment were greatest for patients with lateral disc herniations. The magnitude of improvement from surgical treatment was not related to the location or morphology of the herniation.

Various preoperative and postoperative findings may also be predictive of results. Barrios and colleagues[73] found that the use of (and positive response to) traction as part of preoperative conservative treatment was predictive of a good outcome with surgery. In agreement with other studies, patients with sedentary, non–physically demanding jobs had better results than patients with more strenuous occupations. Jansson and colleagues[36] found that reduced preoperative walking distance and a history of back pain greater than 6 months were predictors of lower functional outcomes after discectomy. Jonsson and Stromqvist[108] found a persistently positive SLR test to be a reliable indicator of inferior results; this was particularly evident in patients in whom the test was positive for more than 4 months after discectomy.

As part of an ongoing study of lumbar discectomy, the Maine group published an investigation comparing operative rates and outcomes between high versus low rate of surgery regions within the state.[109] The data suggest that, in the high-rate region, the results were inferior compared with the low-rate region. These calculations were based on the rate of surgery per capita (population). The investigators concluded that this difference was most significantly related to the surgical indications used by the individual physicians and that, in the higher-rate areas, the indications may have been less stringent. This might have been true, but an additional factor was not highlighted, which we calculated from the data. In the high-rate region, there were more surgeries done per capita, but the number of operations done per physician was lower, averaging 11 surgeries per surgeon. In the low-rate region, surgeons averaged 26 operations each, although the overall rate of surgery was lower per capita. This factor directly supports previous analyses of the results of total joint arthroplasty, which indicate better results in high-volume hospitals because of concentrated experience. From these data, discectomy is optimally performed by an experienced, high-volume surgeon who employs strict indications.

Psychological and social factors have been shown by many investigators to influence profoundly the surgical results of lumbar discectomy.[34,74] Sorensen and colleagues[34] found that preoperative psychological assessment was 86% predictive of surgical results after discectomy. Cashion and Lynch[74] found that patients with a good outcome were more self-confident individuals, were only mildly depressed, and were generally optimistic about the outcome of surgery. Slover and colleagues[35] found that a history of chronic headaches, smoking, depression, and self-rated poor health were associated with poor outcomes after discectomy. Jansson and colleagues[36] found that smoking was the most significant risk factor in patients who failed to improve after surgery. Olson et al. found that patients with higher education level demonstrated significantly greater improvement with nonoperative treatment, while surgical outcomes were not affected.[110]

With increased attention on the use of opioid analgesics in the United States, Radcliff et al. examined whether the use of these agents had an effect on outcomes for patients with lumbar disc herniation.[111] While patients who were treated with opioids had significantly worse baseline pain and quality of life, at 4-year follow-up, there was no long-term difference in outcome associated with opioid medication use. They also found that opioid use was not associated with surgical avoidance.

Spengler and colleagues[13] calculated preoperative assessment scores for 84 patients before discectomy and correlated these with outcomes. The four components of the score were neurologic signs, clinical tension signs, psychological factors, and imaging evidence of neural compression. Imaging studies were most predictive of operative findings but not of outcome. The best predictor of outcome was the psychological score. This was based on the Minnesota Multiphasic Personality Inventory.

Hurme and Alaranta[12] prospectively studied 220 patients after discectomy, analyzing preoperative and perioperative factors. Optimistic patients had better results. Patients who preoperatively decided not to return to work had poorer outcomes. Patients who perceived their jobs to be physically strenuous had inferior results. The most predictive factors of a poor outcome were the decision not to return to work, marital status (divorced or widowed), age older than 40 years, a protracted period of sciatic pain, and multiple nonspecific somatic complaints. Predictors of good results were a high preoperative pain index, higher education level, overall satisfaction with life, and the perception that the patient's job was of light or suitable duty. Patients with a highly positive SLR test and younger patients with large disc herniations tended to have better results. This study highlights the importance of psychological, social, and objective physical factors in predicting the outcome of lumbar disc excision.

Dvorak and colleagues[112] retrospectively applied a set of "accepted" operative indications—including radicular pain, positive SLR, contralateral SLR, dermatomal hypesthesia, motor deficit, and diminished deep tendon reflexes—to a series of patients who underwent discectomy. Of the patients, 65% fulfilled these criteria, and 35% did not. The long-term outcomes were not significantly different between these two groups. Patients who returned to work postoperatively were on disability compensation less than 2 months before surgery, whereas patients who did *not* return to work were on disability compensation an average of 4 months before surgery. Indications based on objective physical findings alone do not ensure a satisfactory outcome. The preoperative period of disability is a significant factor.

Some proponents of microscopically assisted discectomy purport that results are superior compared with standard techniques. In a published review of the literature by one of the strongest advocates of microdiscectomy, McCulloch[88] concluded that the available data are insufficient to show its superiority. He noted that successful results have ranged from 80% to 96%, regardless of the technique used, and highlighted the importance of patient selection as the more important determinant of outcome. Series of microsurgical discectomy report comparable rates of complications, such as dural tear and recurrent herniations.[113,114] In a report with 5-year follow-up, long-term outcomes for minimally invasive techniques are comparable to those reported using standard techniques.[115] It is important to note that radiation exposure to the surgical team and the patient can be 10 to 20 times greater with the use of minimally invasive techniques.[116]

There is disagreement regarding the efficacy of simple fragment excision (the so-called Williams sequestrectomy[117]) versus more extensive nucleus curettage. In a retrospective study of 200 patients, Faulhauer and Manicke[77] showed a lower reherniation rate with fragment excision alone. This comparison was inherently flawed. The standard discectomy group, by definition, had herniations that were in continuity with the disc space and could be characterized as subligamentous (contained). The fragment excision group obligatorily had displaced fragments that were not contained within the disc space. The most useful information perhaps is that when an extruded or sequestered (uncontained) fragment is found, acceptable results with a low herniation rate can be expected with fragment excision alone. Although aggressive methods of removal of further nuclear material may not be warranted, meticulous examination of all quadrants of the epidural space surrounding the nerve root and cauda equina should be performed in each case to avoid missing disc fragments.

Balderston and colleagues[72] compared 40 patients who underwent simple fragment excision in one center with 40 patients who underwent excision and curettage in another center. The reherniation rate was not significantly different: 12.5% in the former group and 11.6% in the latter group. There was also no difference in the rate of disc space narrowing between the two groups. The only difference was a higher rate of postoperative back pain in the curettage group at a minimum 2-year follow-up. In distinction to Faulhauer and Manicke's work,[77] the types of disc herniation were not different between the two groups.

Carragee and colleagues[118] reported the results of a prospective, controlled study comparing subtotal versus limited discectomy. In the latter group, only the extruded disc material and loose fragments present in the disc space were removed. In the former, a more aggressive disc space curettage and debridement was performed in addition to removal of the extruded fragments. Early findings suggested a shorter convalescence in the limited discectomy group but decreased VAS and ODI scores in the subtotal group. These differences were not statistically significant at 2-year follow-up. Although the reherniation rate in the limited group was 18% compared with 9% in the subtotal group, this difference was not significant with the numbers available. Type II (beta) error cannot be excluded, however, because a significant difference may have been detected with greater patient numbers. The clinical significance of a 9% difference in reherniation rate may outweigh the lack of statistical significance.

Complications

Numerous complications can occur with lumbar discectomy, albeit at acceptably low rates. Recurrence rates range from 0% to 18%. In addition to differences in surgical technique and other factors, this broad range may reflect differences in the definition of recurrence. In some series, *recurrence* is defined as recurrent sciatica, whereas in others use of the term is limited to patients who required reoperation. The strictest definition is a true reherniation at the level and side previously operated, which ultimately leads to a frequency of 2% to 5%.

Wound infections have been reported in 0% to 3% of cases.[12,72,77,84,86,117] These may be superficial or deep. Superficial infections may be managed with local wound care and antibiotics. Deep infections should be surgically debrided and irrigated. Epidural abscess is rare, with reported rates of 0.3%, and should be managed with surgical evacuation.[119] The microscope has been considered a possible source of contamination because of the exposed unsterile optics that are in close proximity over the wound.[88,120] Infection rates are comparable, however, to cases performed without the microscope.

Pyogenic discitis may occur after discectomy 2.3% of the time.[12,119] Early detection is crucial in avoiding extensive bone involvement. Intravenous antibiotic therapy is usually successful, with rare cases requiring surgical debridement. MRI findings, including increased bone edema near the endplates and loss of disc space height, are difficult to discern from typical degenerative Modic-type changes. Laboratory evidence, such as elevated erythrocyte sedimentation rates and C-reactive protein levels, is important in confirming the diagnosis.

Vascular injuries are exceedingly rare. Injury to anterior vessels from perforation of the disc space have been documented in a few case reports.[121,122] Arteriovenous fistula has also been documented.[123,124] The most important component of managing these complications is prompt recognition and aggressive treatment, including vascular repair. Excessive epidural bleeding is uncommon, although one series documented blood loss of more than 300 mL in 4% of cases.[12]

Incidental durotomy occurs 0% to 4% of the time.[8,72,84,113,125] It has been associated with a poor outcome in some series. At an average of 10 years after surgery, Saxler and colleagues[125] reported a lower rate of symptom resolution and a greater rate of chronic pain and headaches in patients who sustained an incidental durotomy. This study did not discern between primary and revision cases, which may have been a potential confounder. The potential for long-term clinical sequelae after incidental durotomy during discectomy is most likely influenced by the size of the tear, the ability to repair it, and the coexistence of neurologic injury.

Instability is quite rare after discectomy. Preservation of the facet joints is helpful in avoiding this sequela, although in our experience, a large percentage of the facet joint can be resected unilaterally without adverse effect. Some authors have indicated that instability can occur 30% of the time. This percentage is highly dependent on the definition of instability. Padua and colleagues[126] found radiographic evidence of instability, detected by flexion-extension films, in 20% of patients who underwent discectomy. Only 6% seemed to be symptomatic, however. In contrast, Faulhauer and Manicke[77] defined instability by clinical findings, such as apprehension with flexion or extension, instead of radiographic measurements. These authors reported rates of 16% and 30% with two different operative techniques; 3% had severe enough symptoms to warrant a brace, and only one patient eventually went on to fusion. Kotilainen and Valtonen[119] found that the presence of clinical apprehension postoperatively was predictive of a poor result after surgery. These data highlight the importance of documenting preoperative radiographic and clinical instability so that the effects of the discectomy itself can be better assessed in the postoperative period.[127] Biomechanically, simple discectomy is not a destabilizing procedure if performed properly.

Recurrent Disc Herniations

The distinguishing histologic feature of recurrent disc herniation is the presence of large collagen bundles associated with a fibrillar framework.[128] Granulation tissue found in recurrences is not present in primary disc herniations. This fact indicates that the pathophysiology of recurrent disc herniations may be different than in primary cases.

Depending on the definition, recurrent disc herniations can occur in 18% of cases. Clinical presentation is usually of recurrent sciatic leg pain. Jonsson and Stromqvist[129] attempted to determine the relative frequency of clinical signs and symptoms after discectomy to differentiate better perineural fibrosis from true recurrent herniation. Pain reproduced by cough and a positive SLR were more frequent with recurrent disc herniations. These findings were also present in many patients with fibrosis alone, however; thus, imaging modalities are crucial to the diagnosis. As discussed previously, MRI is best delayed for at least 6 months after surgery.

Recurrences can occur at the same level, same side, opposite side, or entirely different level. To be considered a recurrence, there must have been a pain-free (or relief) time period after the index surgery. A nonoperative treatment regimen, including a period of observation, physical therapy, medications, and other modalities, should be used in the initial treatment of recurrent disc herniations unless progressive neurologic deterioration occurs.

Important questions arise after the decision to proceed with surgery is made. The main focus of current investigations is whether or not comparable or inferior results can be expected after discectomy for a recurrent disc herniation. Some authors have documented inferior results after repeat surgery,[130] although most failures were reported in patients operated on without imaging evidence of neural compression.

Suk and colleagues[131] retrospectively examined their results in a highly select group of patients. Recurrence was defined as a reherniation at the same level (ipsilateral or contralateral) after a pain-free interval of 6 months or more. These authors used gadolinium-enhanced MRI to confirm the diagnosis. They found that the second surgery was significantly longer and that recurrent disc herniations were typically larger. Clinical success was documented in 71.1% of cases, which was comparable to their results after primary discectomy (79.3%). In a similar study, Cinotti and colleagues[132] examined their results with same-level contralateral reherniations only. At 2-year follow-up, surgery for recurrences resulted in satisfactory outcomes in 88% of cases and in 90% of primary discectomies. The only difference noted was more back pain in the reherniation group at 6 months, although this difference was not noted at 2 years.

Cinotti and colleagues[133] also studied a group of patients with ipsilateral lumbar disc reherniation and compared these patients with patients after primary surgery as a control group. Satisfactory results were reported in 85% of patients with ipsilateral lumbar disc reherniation and 88% of control patients. Noted differences were a higher degree of disc degeneration in the recurrence group. Although epidural fibrosis was abundant in the study group, its presence or amount did not adversely influence outcome. There was no difference in the psychological profiles of recurrent versus primary discectomy groups. In a similar study, Papadopoulos and colleagues[134] reported 85% improvement after discectomy for reherniations compared with 80% improvement for primary herniations at an average of 53.6 months follow-up. Herron[135] reported 69% good and 24% fair results after laminectomy and discectomy for recurrences at the same and other levels.

Most authors do not recommend fusion after a first-time recurrent disc herniation.[135,136] After any lumbar surgery involving facetectomy and bone resection, preoperative and intraoperative assessment of stability is a major determinant of the decision to fuse. Although investigational evidence is lacking, we consider fusion after a second reherniation at the same level.

Discectomy in Children

The role of trauma in causing disc herniations in children is believed to be more significant than in adults.[3,137,138] Children are unlikely to have disc degeneration or the antecedent period of back pain before herniation. Clinical signs and symptoms are similar to adults but are much more acute in onset. The clinical and imaging evaluation is similar to adults.

The literature of discectomy in children reveals prolonged length of follow-up. Initial results are excellent, but results tend to deteriorate with time. At 1-year follow-up, Papagenlopoulos and colleagues[139] reported 93% good or excellent results. At final follow-up, ranging from 12 to 45 years, 92% were good or excellent; however, there was a 28% reoperation rate. Parisini and colleagues[140] documented 95% success at short-term follow-up, whereas at long-term follow-up (average, 12.4 years), good or excellent outcomes were documented in 87% of cases. These investigators found a 10% reoperation rate at 10 years. DeOrio and Bianco[141] showed 96% good or excellent results at initial follow-up, trending down to 74% at final examination. Numerous other series document similar results.[3,137,142]

Fusion has been reported in a small percentage of pediatric patients. Well-defined selection criteria are lacking, however. The influence of congenital anomalies has been considered previously. There does not seem to be a correlation between any one anomaly and disc herniation. It is important to recognize anomalies, such as spina bifida, during routine preoperative planning to avoid iatrogenic neurologic injury.

Discectomy in Elderly Patients

Lumbar disc herniations are much less common in elderly patients. The nucleus desiccates with age and is less likely to herniate. Underlying stenosis and bony overgrowth is a more common problem. Regardless, herniations can still occur, with or without the presence of stenosis. The results of discectomy in this population are comparable to younger patients, assuming the correct diagnosis is made.

Maistrelli and colleagues[143] reported results of discectomy in 32 patients older than 60 years. Clinical findings were similar, with 81% of patients having root tension signs such as a positive SLR. At an average follow-up of 50 months, good or excellent results were found in 87% of cases. None of the patients had evidence of neurogenic claudication, which is an important distinguishing feature when making the diagnosis of a disc herniation versus stenosis. Jonsson and Stromqvist[144] also found disc surgery to be gratifying in patients older than 70 years, with good results documented at 2-year follow-up.

Foraminal and Extraforaminal (Far-Lateral) Herniations

So-called far-lateral disc herniations require special consideration. Surgical excision is more easily accomplished through

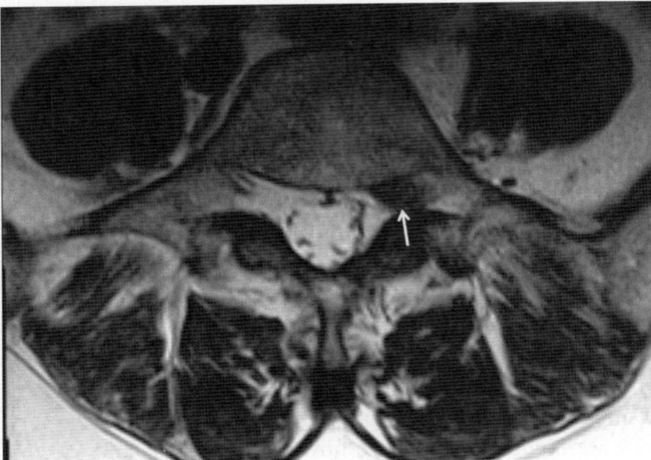

FIG. 47.16 Magnetic resonance imaging can readily show foraminal disc herniations that may otherwise be missed by computed tomographic or plain myelograms because neural compression is extradural.

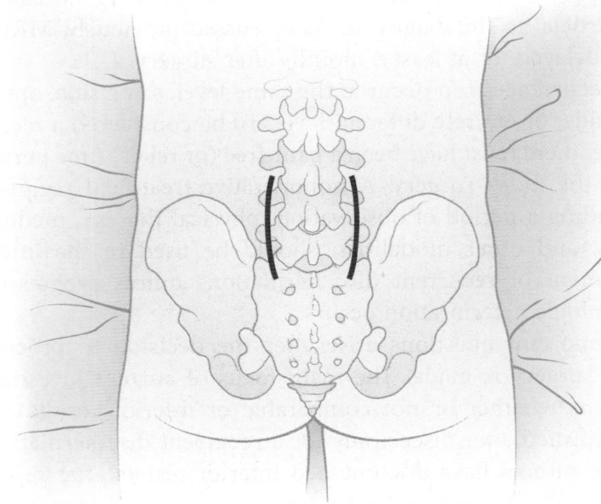

FIG. 47.17 The Wiltse muscle-splitting approach, using a paramedian incision, can be used to access the intertransverse process region.

modified operative techniques. Foraminal and extraforaminal disc herniations are more common in older patients. Symptoms are more likely to be isolated to one particular nerve root. In contrast to paracentral discs, they lead to compression of the exiting nerve root rather than the descending root. Diagnosis is best by MRI or CT (Fig. 47.16). Because the compression is usually extradural, myelography does not show a filling defect.

Different techniques have been advocated for the foraminal or extraforaminal herniation. Compression of the nerve root occurs outside of the spinal canal, making visualization of the herniation challenging through a standard laminotomy or laminectomy performed from within the canal. Garrido and Connaughton[145] advocated a unilateral facetectomy. Bone is removed along the entire path of the nerve root from its exit from the cauda equina out and through the foramen; this necessitates complete removal of the facet on the side of exposure. Although symptom relief was not well documented, painful radiographic instability was detected in only 1 of 35 (3%) cases. This patient had pain relief after fusion.

Donaldson and colleagues[146] advocated a less destabilizing procedure. They considered identification of the nerve within the intertransverse process "blind." As a solution, they performed a partial hemilaminectomy at the level above the disc at the point where the root exited the cauda equina. They followed it laterally beneath the bone of the remaining pars interarticularis. By placing a probe over the root and advancing it laterally, they were able to identify the root and facilitate its dissection between the transverse processes before discectomy was performed through this interval. They reported good or excellent pain relief in 72% of patients. No cases of instability were reported.

Melvill and Baxter[14] used the intertransverse approach for discectomy in 40 patients with extraforaminal herniations. They performed this using standard midline dissection that was extended subperiosteally out and over the facets to expose the transverse processes. This is in contrast to the classic description of the Wiltse paraspinal muscle–splitting approach. Complete resolution of leg pain was reported in 85% of cases. Melvill and Baxter[14] noted a fibrous band that was present tethering the nerve root to the lateral aspect of the disc in an associated cadaveric study.

In an investigation with midterm follow-up, satisfactory results were reported using the Wiltse paraspinal muscle–splitting approach for so-called lateral disc herniations.[147] Satisfaction was reported by 85% of patients, with 60% of patients reporting complete resolution of pain. At 5 years' follow-up, 20% of patients had developed some degree of instability, half of whom ultimately underwent fusion. Assuming uniformity of the definition of instability and indications for fusion in these cases, this finding is supportive of the hypothesis by McCulloch and Transfelt[31] that lateral disc herniations were a precursor to the development of degenerative spondylolisthesis.

A thorough knowledge of the anatomy in this region is imperative to performing an effective discectomy without undue bleeding or injury to the nerve root.[89] We prefer to excise foraminal or extraforaminal discs through a true Wiltse paraspinal muscle–splitting approach to the intertransverse interval. It is easiest through a paramedian incision (Fig. 47.17). Identification of the correct level of incision is crucial in minimizing the length of the incision.

Cauda Equina Syndrome

Cauda equina syndrome (CES) most commonly occurs from a herniated lumbar disc. It is more common with central herniation (27% of central herniations), although it can occur with paracentral or lateral herniations as well.[148,149] It is more frequent in men in their fourth decade. The odds of developing CES are significantly higher in overweight and obese individuals.[150] An L4–L5 disc is the usual cause.[148] CES should be considered a true surgical urgency because neurologic results are affected by the time to decompression. The clinical

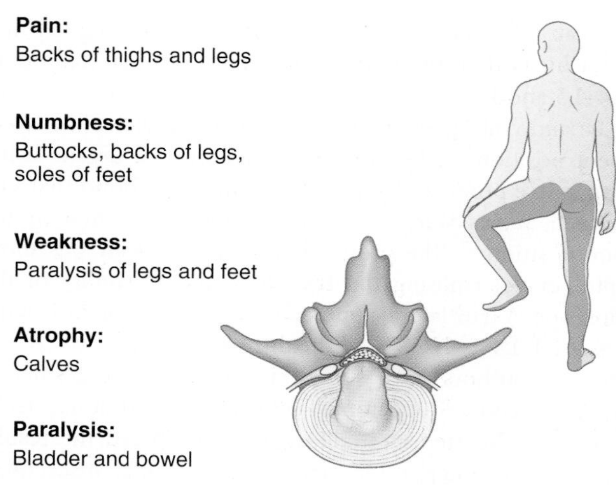

FIG. 47.18 Cauda equina syndrome is characterized by saddle anesthesia, motor weakness, and loss of bowel and bladder control.

diagnosis of CES relies on many components, including perineal sensory deficit (so-called saddle anesthesia), bowel or bladder incontinence, new-onset lower extremity sensory deficit, and a new or progressive motor deficit (Fig. 47.18). In addition to a meticulous physical examination, evaluation of CES should include measurement of a bladder postvoid residual. Normally, the postvoid residual should be less than 50 to 100 mL. The postvoid residual is often abnormal preoperatively and can be an important parameter to follow postoperatively.[151]

Decompression and discectomy can be via a laminotomy or through a formal laminectomy. Proponents of laminectomy believe that this provides superior visualization of the dura and avoids excessive traction.[152–154] Adequate exposure is particularly relevant for removal of central disc herniations.

The effect of timing of surgery on outcomes continues to be debated. Although a number of studies have reported that surgical decompression within 48 hours of the onset of symptoms is a safe time point within which to perform surgery, more recent systematic reviews have concluded that there is no strong support for the often-cited 24- or 48-hour thresholds nor that the earlier the decompression, the better the outcomes.[151,154–156]

DeLong et al., in a metaanalysis of a number of observational cohort series, found a statistically significant relative risk for timing of surgery greater than 24 hours.[157] These authors remarked that higher-quality scientific study is difficult to obtain on this subject since equipoise is lacking, making a prospective randomized study difficult to execute. In analyzing the effect of early surgical decompression on urinary function, it is important to differentiate patients who have incomplete cauda equina syndrome (CES), characterized as "altered urinary sensation, loss of desire to void, poor urinary stream, and the need to strain in order to micturate" from CES with retention, characterized as "painless urinary retention and overflow incontinence, when the bladder is no longer under executive control," the former of which was found to have a better prognosis.[158] In one study, decompressive surgery within 24 hours of onset of autonomic symptoms in CES reduces bladder dysfunction at initial follow-up, while no statistically significant difference was observed in CES with retention regarding timing of operation.[159]

Strength may continue to improve for 1 year after surgery.[154] Although the postvoid residual usually decreases to less than 110 mL by 6 weeks, bladder function may continue to improve for 16 months.[149] Early surgery does not seem to substantially affect the resolution of postoperative pain compared with delayed intervention.[160] In a systematic review of the literature reporting dysfunction of micturition, defecation, and/or sexual dysfunction following CES secondary to herniated disc, Korse and colleagues reported considerable continued impairment. At a minimum of 17 months follow-up, 42.5% of patients reported micturition dysfunction, 49.6% reported defecation dysfunction, and 44% reported sexual dysfunction.[161] Above all, preoperative neurologic status seems to be the greatest predictor of recovery.[162] This is evident in that many patients are found to have residual neurologic deficits despite timely and effective surgical intervention.[160]

Alternatives to Standard Discectomy

Endoscopic Discectomy

The use of the endoscope to perform lumbar discectomy has enthusiastic proponents. Improvements in equipment have made the technique more user-friendly and facile. Still, endoscopic discectomy remains a technically demanding procedure, and the results depend heavily on surgeon experience.[163] It is beneficial to have prior training in minimally invasive spine surgery.[164] Although it is not yet a replacement for standard discectomy techniques, more recent series have shown the ability to achieve comparable results in some surgeons' hands.[80,165,166]

Purported advantages of endoscopic lumbar discectomy include less intraoperative blood loss and smaller surgical wounds. A study by Pan and colleagues did not show a significant difference in patient-reported pain when comparing endoscopic and traditional open discectomy, though postoperative inflammatory markers such as interleukin-6 and C-reactive protein were reduced in the endoscopic group.[167] DeAntoni and colleagues[96] reported results of translaminar epidural endoscopic discectomy in 190 patients. Using a lateral decubitus position, the technique uses a small paramedian incision for introduction of the instruments. Dilators are used to strip the muscles subperiosteally from the adjacent lamina as far lateral as the facet joint. The arthroscope (endoscope) is inserted through a 6-mm working cannula. An additional lateral paraspinal incision is made for an outflow cannula. A shaver is used to remove bone within the interlaminar window until the attachments of the ligamentum flavum can be visualized. The ligamentum flavum is elevated using a Penfield dissector and removed with a Kerrison rongeur, similar to a standard open approach. A root retractor pulls the nerve root and dura medially, allowing access to the disc space. The anulus is incised, and the herniation is removed. The endoscope can be inserted into the disc space to look for any additional loose fragments (so-called discoscopy). Good or

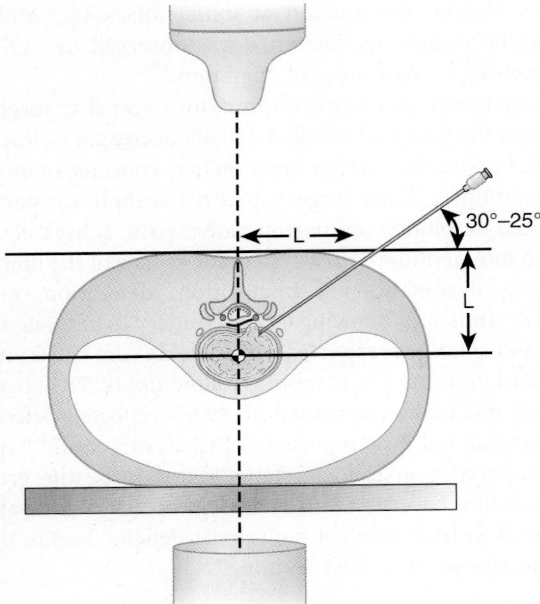

FIG. 47.19 The transforaminal endoscopic approach for disc excision. (From Yeung AT, Tsou PM. Posterolateral endoscopic excision for lumbar disc herniation. *Spine (Phila Pa 1976).* 2002;27:722–731.)

excellent results were documented in 92% of cases with a minimum 2-year follow-up. There was only one dural laceration that did not need repair, there was no instability, and there were no neurologic injuries.

Yeung and Tsou[80] reported results of 307 endoscopically assisted transforaminal discectomies. The patient is positioned supine on a radiolucent table. Local anesthesia with light sedation is used. In this technique, intraoperative fluoroscopy is crucial. A standard discogram is performed first, injecting blue dye into the disc space to help identify the herniated tissue. Along the same path, a series of dilators and ultimately a single working cannula is inserted percutaneously through the intervertebral foramen (Fig. 47.19). One cannula is used for inflow, outflow, and instrument insertion. The cannula has a shielded tip that allows aggressive discectomy with the use of graspers and shavers while retracting the exiting nerve root. As stated, this is performed through the intervertebral foramen. The nerve root can be visualized by rotating the cannula, allowing assessment of its integrity and mobility. Satisfactory results were reported in 89.3% of patients. Six patients (2%) had lower extremity dysesthesia that lasted longer than 6 weeks, two had thrombophlebitis, two had discitis, and one had a dural tear that did not require repair. Yoshimoto and colleagues demonstrated transforaminal microendoscopic decompression to be effective for treating far-lateral disc herniations.[168]

This technique has been shown to be safe and effective for recurrent disc herniations as well.[166] In a prospective evaluation of 262 consecutive cases of reherniation treated by an endoscopically assisted transforaminal technique, Hoogland and colleagues[166] reported an 85% success rate and 3.8% complication rate at 2-year follow-up. Kim and colleagues reported that percutaneous endoscopic interlaminar discectomy can be successful for reherniation by avoiding the iliac crest, which can be prohibitive with transforaminal techniques at L4–L5 and L5–S1.[169]

Lee and colleagues prospectively studied the influence of patient position on the location of abdominal organs using preoperative prone and supine CT scans, and found that safe approach angles were significantly more horizontal in the prone position.[170] The prone abdominal CT scan was more helpful in determining the trajectory and feasibility of the endoscope. A true lateral approach was possible for 75% of the discs at L3–L4 and 76.7% of the discs at L4–L5.

Several authors have sought to compare the results of microendoscopic discectomy with more traditional techniques.[171–173] Ruetten and colleagues[173] compared the results of endoscopic interlaminar and transforaminal discectomy with microsurgical discectomy. They showed no clinically significant differences between the endoscopic and microsurgical groups and identical reherniation rates (6.2% for each).[173] Analogous findings have been reported with comparisons of endoscopic and standard open discectomy.[171,172] However, Teli et al. reported higher rates of dural tears and recurrent herniation in endoscopic surgery compared to traditional techniques, with similar patient-reported outcomes at 2 years.[174] Garg et al., in a prospective randomized study, reported shorter hospital stay and earlier return to work in the microendoscopic group compared to the open discectomy group.[174a] In a systematic review of randomized controlled studies comparing microendoscopic technique with open discectomy or microdiscectomy, Smith and colleagues found that patient-reported outcome measures were similar with all three techniques.[175]

In a recent retrospective review of over 10,000 patients who had undergone percutaneous endoscopic lumbar discectomy, Choi and colleagues sought to find common causes of surgical failure, defined as a case requiring reoperation within 6 weeks.[176] They found that 4.3% of cases were failures, and over half of these were due to incomplete removal of herniated disc, of which inappropriate positioning of the working channel was the cause in 33.6% of cases. Exiting root injury is another complication of endoscopic surgery. Choi et al. analyzed the radiologic risk factors for exiting root injury by retrospectively reviewing the preoperative MRIs of patients undergoing endoscopic discectomy who experienced this complication.[177] They determined that if the distance between the exiting nerve root and the superior articular process of the caudal level is inadequate to accept the diameter of the working cannula without compressing the nerve root, an alternative technique, such as microdiscectomy or open discectomy, should be employed.

Percutaneous Automated Discectomy

Because of the evolution of percutaneous techniques of discectomy, there is considerable "overlap" in the names of different procedures. Although endoscopic discectomy can be considered percutaneous, it is not what is typically considered *percutaneous automated discectomy*. This term refers specifically to a procedure introduced in the early 1980s.

Using a posterolateral approach, a tissue-removing device is introduced into the disc space in a similar path as the needle of a discogram; this is guided by intraoperative fluoroscopy. Earlier techniques used a direct lateral approach that led to (or raised concern of) viscous perforation in some patients. The instrument is used to remove nucleus material in small increments. This removal theoretically can decrease intradiscal pressure. There is no direct visualization of the nerve roots, dura, or disc material. Neurologic decompression cannot be assessed with this technique.

Results of automated discectomy are inferior to standard open discectomy. Shapiro[93] showed only partial improvement of leg pain in 57% of patients undergoing this procedure. More disappointing was that only 5% had complete sciatica relief. All patients had disc bulges or protrusions, with none having free fragments. These results are less positive than the results documented with open discectomy.

In contrast, Hoppenfeld[94] reported more successful results, with relief of sciatica and sensory deficit in 86% of patients. He determined, however, that patients with sequestered discs do not reliably respond well to the procedure. Kotilainen and Valtonen[95] treated 41 patients with small protrusions or prolapses (bulges) with percutaneous automated discectomy. Sciatica had completely resolved in 78% of patients. From these data, it can be inferred that automated discectomy can be reasonably effective in patients with small disc bulges or protrusions that are in direct continuity with the remaining nucleus. Only in this select group of patients is there the possibility of relieving the neural compression. The procedure should not be used in patients with sequestered or extruded fragments (uncontained herniations) or most patients with disc herniations.

Chemonucleolysis

Chemonucleolysis involves the chemical digestion of nucleus material via injection of an agent, such as chymopapain, into the intervertebral disc. Ideally, the agent not only decompresses the central aspect of the disc space (producing a similar effect as percutaneous automated discectomy), but also might directly attack the herniated fragment. The clinical success of the procedure has not been supportive.

Chemonucleolysis has been rigorously examined in numerous clinical investigations. In a randomized prospective trial comparing chemonucleolysis and standard discectomy, Muralikuttan and colleagues[98] concluded that it leads to inferior results. There was a high rate of conversion to open surgery in the chemonucleolysis group because of continued, unrelieved symptoms. Crawshaw and colleagues[178] found extremely high failure rates—47% to 52%—after chemonucleolysis compared with 11% with open surgery. van Alphen and colleagues[82] documented increased radicular pain after chemonucleolysis in 22% of patients treated. Salvage discectomy after failed chemonucleolysis leads to worse results than primary surgery.[82,98,178] In addition to these poor results, neurologic complications, such as transverse myelitis associated with the use of chymopapain, have all but eliminated the procedure from continued use in the United States.

PEARLS

1. Most lumbar disc herniations respond well to conservative treatment within the first 3 months from the onset of symptoms.
2. In patients who fail conservative treatment, surgery consistently showed better outcomes than continued nonoperative care.
3. The type and size of disc herniations and psychosocial factors are the primary determinants of outcomes after discectomy.
4. Although minimally invasive techniques, such as endoscopic and percutaneous laser discectomy, can be effective in experienced hands, it is unclear whether they would ever replace the gold standard operation of open discectomy (with or without the use of a microscope).

PITFALLS

1. Patients with extraforaminal (far lateral) and central disc herniations should be advised that surgical outcomes may be inferior compared with outcomes for more common and typical paracentral herniations.
2. Patients should be informed that a lumbar discectomy is primarily indicated for leg pain. Back pain, numbness, and weakness are less reliably alleviated after surgery.
3. Recurrent disc herniations, which can occur in 18% of patients, remain problematic and may be more prevalent in patients who have large annular defects after discectomy.
4. Although simple discectomy for a recurrent disc herniation can yield outcomes equivalent to the index procedure, the addition of fusion may be considered after a second recurrence.

KEY POINTS

1. Patients should be carefully counseled preoperatively on the risk and benefits of surgery so that they may make a well-informed decision according to their specific functional demands and expectations.
2. Positioning a patient in a flexed or kneeling position can help open the interlaminar window to allow easier entry into the spinal canal.
3. Regardless of the technique of discectomy, a successful operation is contingent on adequate exposure that enables careful and minimally traumatic identification of the cauda equina, descending nerve root, and exiting nerve root before retraction to retrieve the herniated fragments.
4. During discectomy, the amount and location of the disc herniation should be commensurate with that shown on preoperative MRI.
5. The spinal canal and disc space should be thoroughly inspected before closure to avoid retained disc fragments.

KEY REFERENCES

1. Atlas SJ, Keller RB, Wu YA, et al. Long-term outcomes of surgical and nonsurgical management of sciatica secondary to a lumbar disc herniation: 10 year results from the Maine Lumbar Spine Study. *Spine*. 2005;30:927-935.
   This article details the 10-year follow-up results from the Maine lumbar spine study that prospectively evaluated patients with operative and nonoperative treatment for lumbar disc herniations. In this nonrandomized study, surgical treatment produced better results than nonoperative treatment, and the benefits were maximally appreciated at the 2-year mark.
2. Weinstein JN, Lurie JD, Tosteson TD, et al. Surgical vs nonoperative treatment for lumbar disk herniation: the Spine

Patient Outcomes Research Trial (SPORT) observational cohort. *JAMA*. 2006;296:2451-2459.
This article outlines the results of the nonrandomized patients in the SPORT trial for lumbar disk herniations. In this analysis, surgery resulted in better outcomes than nonoperative treatment.

3. Weinstein JN, Tosteson TD, Lurie JD, et al. Surgical vs nonoperative treatment for lumbar disk herniation: the Spine Patient Outcomes Research Trial (SPORT): a randomized trial. *JAMA*. 2006;296:2441-2450.
In this article, intention-to-treat analysis showed no statistical differences between surgery and nonoperative treatment of lumbar disc herniations. This trial has been widely criticized for its high crossover rate between groups, however.

4. Weber H. Lumbar disc herniation: a controlled, prospective study with ten years of observations. *Spine*. 1983;8:131-140.
This classic study was a randomized controlled trial of operative versus nonoperative treatment for lumbar disc herniations. It showed statistically better results with surgery at 1-year and 4-year follow-up but no difference at 10-year follow-up.

5. Carragee EJ, Kim D. A prospective analysis of magnetic resonance imaging findings in patients with sciatica and lumbar disc herniation: correlation of outcomes with disc fragment and canal morphology. *Spine*. 1997;22:1650-1660.
This article correlates the size of a disc herniation (at least 6 mm anteroposterior dimension) with better outcomes after surgery.

REFERENCES

1. Atlas SJ, Keller RB, Chang Y, et al. Surgical and nonsurgical management of sciatic secondary to a lumbar disc herniation: five-year outcomes from the Maine Lumbar Spine Study. *Spine*. 2001;26:1179-1187.
2. DePalma AF, Rothman RH. Surgery of the lumbar spine. *Clin Orthop Relat Res*. 1969;63:162-170.
3. Fisher RG, Saunders RL. Lumbar disc protrusion in children. *J Neurosurg*. 1981;54:480.
4. Boden SD, Davis DO, Dina TS, et al. Abnormal magnetic resonance scans of the lumbar spine in asymptomatic subjects: a prospective investigation. *J Bone Joint Surg Am*. 1990;72:403-408.
5. Saal JA, Saal JS. Nonoperative treatment of herniated lumbar intervertebral disc with radiculopathy: an outcome study. *Spine*. 1989;14:431-437.
6. Saal JA, Saal JS, Herzog RJ. The natural history of lumbar intervertebral disc extrusions treated nonoperatively. *Spine*. 1990;15:683-686.
7. Atlas SJ, Keller RB, Wu YA, et al. Long-term outcomes of surgical and nonsurgical management of sciatica secondary to a lumbar disc herniation: 10 year results from the Maine Lumbar Spine Study. *Spine*. 2005;30:927-935.
8. Weinstein JN, Lurie JD, Tosteson TD, et al. Surgical vs nonoperative treatment for lumbar disk herniation: the Spine Patient Outcomes Research Trial (SPORT) observational cohort. *JAMA*. 2006;296:2451-2459.
9. Weinstein JN, Tosteson TD, Lurie JD, et al. Surgical vs nonoperative treatment for lumbar disk herniation: the Spine Patient Outcomes Research Trial (SPORT): a randomized trial. *JAMA*. 2006;296:2441-2450.
10. Weber H. Lumbar disc herniation: a controlled, prospective study with ten years of observations. *Spine*. 1983;8:131-140.
11. Carragee EJ, Kim D. A prospective analysis of magnetic resonance imaging findings in patients with sciatica and lumbar disc herniation: correlation of outcomes with disc fragment and canal morphology. *Spine*. 1997;22:1650-1660.
12. Hurme M, Alaranta H. Factors predicting the results of surgery for lumbar intervertebral disc herniation. *Spine*. 1987;12:933-938.
13. Spengler DM, Ouellette EA, Battie M, et al. Elective discectomy for herniation of a lumbar disc: additional experience with an objective method. *J Bone Joint Surg Am*. 1990;72:320-327.
14. Melvill RL, Baxter BL. The intertransverse approach to extraforaminal disc protrusion in the lumbar spine. *Spine*. 1994;19:2707-2714.
15. Grimes PF, Massie JB, Garfin SR. Anatomic and biomechanical analysis of the lower lumbar foraminal ligaments. *Spine*. 2000;25:2009-2014.
16. Wilder DG, Pope MH, Frymoyer JW. The biomechanics of lumbar disc herniation and the effect of overload and instability. *J Spinal Disord*. 1988;1:16-32.
17. Frei H, Oxland TR, Rathonyi GC, et al. The effect of nucleotomy on lumbar spine mechanics in compression and shear loading. *Spine*. 2001;26:2080-2089.
18. White A, Panjabi M. *Clinical Biomechanics of the Spine*. 2nd ed. Philadelphia: Lippincott-Raven; 1990.
19. Repanti M, Korovessis PG, Stamatakis MV, et al. Evolution of disc degeneration in lumbar spine: a comparative histological study between herniated and postmortem retrieved disc specimens. *J Spinal Disord*. 1998;11:41-45.
20. Smyth MJ, Wright VJ. Sciatica and the intervertebral disc: an experimental study. *J Bone Joint Surg Am*. 1958;40:1401.
21. Spiliopoulou I, Korovessis P, Konstantinou D, et al. IgG and IgM concentration in the prolapsed human intervertebral disc and sciatica etiology. *Spine*. 1994;19:1320-1323.
22. Olmarker K, Rydevik B. Selective inhibition of tumor necrosis factor-alpha prevents nucleus pulposus-induced thrombus formation, intraneural edema, and reduction of nerve conduction velocity: possible implications for future pharmacologic treatment strategies of sciatica. *Spine*. 2001;26:863-869.
23. Kang JD, Stefanovic-Racic M, McIntyre LA, et al. Toward a biochemical understanding of human intervertebral disc degeneration and herniation: contributions of nitric oxide, interleukins, prostaglandin E2, and matrix metalloproteinases. *Spine*. 1997;22:1065-1073.
24. Scuderi GJ, Brusovanik GV, Anderson DG, et al. Cytokine assay of the epidural space lavage in patients with lumbar intervertebral disk herniation and radiculopathy. *J Spinal Disord Tech*. 2006;19:266-269.
25. Arai Y, Yasuma T, Shitoto K, et al. Immunohistochemical study of intervertebral disc herniation of lumbar spine. *J Orthop Sci*. 2000;5:229-231.
26. Hatano E, Fujita T, Ueda Y, et al. Expression of ADAMTS-4 (aggrecanase-1) and possible involvement in regression of lumbar disc herniation. *Spine*. 2006;31:1426-1432.
27. Brisby H, Balague F, Schafer D, et al. Glycosphingolipid antibodies in serum in patients with sciatica. *Spine*. 2002;27:380-386.
28. Jinkins JR, Whittemore AR, Bradley WG. The anatomic basis of vertebrogenic pain and the autonomic syndrome associated with lumbar disc extrusion. *AJR Am J Roentgenol*. 1989;152:1277-1289.
29. Fardon DF, Milette PC. Nomenclature and classification of lumbar disc pathology. Recommendations of the combined task forces of the North American Spine Society, American Society of Spine Radiology, and American Society of Neuroradiology. *Spine*. 2001;26:E93-E113.

30. Fardon DF. Nomenclature and classification of lumbar disc pathology. *Spine*. 2001;26:461-462.
31. McCulloch JA, Transfelt EE. *Macnab's Backache*. Baltimore: Williams & Wilkins; 1997.
32. Nygaard OP, Kloster R, Solberg T. Duration of leg pain as a predictor of outcome after surgery for lumbar disc herniation: a prospective cohort study with 1-year follow up. *J Neurosurg*. 2000;92:131-134.
33. Rothoerl RD, Woertgen C, Brawanski A. When should conservative treatment for lumbar disc herniation be ceased and surgery considered? *Neurosurg Rev*. 2002;25:162-165.
34. Sorensen LV, Mors O, Skovlund O. A prospective study of the importance of psychological and social factors for the outcome after surgery in patients with slipped lumbar disk operated upon for the first time. *Acta Neurochir (Wien)*. 1987; 88:119-125.
35. Slover J, Abdu WA, Hanscom B, et al. The impact of comorbidities on the change in Short-Form 36 and Oswestry scores following lumbar spine surgery. *Spine*. 2006;31: 1974-1980.
36. Jansson KA, Nemeth G, Granath F, et al. Health-related quality of life in patients before and after surgery for a herniated lumbar disc. *J Bone Joint Surg Br*. 2005;87:959-964.
37. Weise MD, Garfin SR, Gelberman RH, et al. Lower-extremity sensibility testing in patients with herniated lumbar intervertebral discs. *J Bone Joint Surg Am*. 1985;67:1219-1224.
38. Kosteljanetz M, Espersen JO, Halaburt H, et al. Predictive value of clinical and surgical findings in patients with lumbago-sciatica: a prospective study (part I). *Acta Neurochir (Wien)*. 1984;73:67-76.
39. Majlesi J, Togay H, Unalan H, et al. The sensitivity and specificity of the slump and the straight leg raising tests in patients with lumbar disc herniation. *J Clin Rheumatol*. 2008;14:87-91.
40. Ito T, Takano Y, Yuasa N. Types of lumbar herniated disc and clinical course. *Spine*. 2001;26:648-651.
41. Komori H, Okawa A, Haro H, et al. Contrast-enhanced magnetic resonance imaging conservative management of lumbar disc herniation. *Spine*. 1998;23:67-73.
42. Kikkawa I, Sugimoto H, Saita K, et al. The role of Gd enhanced three dimensional MRI fast low-angle shot (FLASH) in the evaluation of symptomatic lumbosacral nerve roots. *J Orthop Sci*. 2001;6:101-109.
43. Weishaupt D, Schmid MR, Zanetti M, et al. Positional MR imaging of the lumbar spine: does it demonstrate nerve root compromise not visible at conventional MR imaging. *Radiology*. 2000;215:247-253.
44. Botwin KP, Skene G, Tourres-Ramos FM, et al. Role of weightbearing flexion and extension myelography in evaluating the intervertebral disc. *Am J Phys Med Rehabil*. 2001;80:289-295.
45. Grane P, Lindqvist M. Evaluation of the postoperative lumbar spine with MR imaging: the role of contrast enhancement and thickening in nerve roots. *Acta Radiol*. 1997;38:1035-1042.
46. Heithoff KB. *Recurrent disc herniation and gadolinium*. SpineLine Sept/Oct:23-26, 2002.
47. Barrera MC, Alustiza JM, Gervas C, et al. Postoperative lumbar spine: comparative study of TSE T2 and turbo FLAIR sequences vs contrast-enhanced SE T1. *Clin Radiol*. 2001;56:133-137.
48. Bundschuh CV, Modic MT, Ross JR, et al. Epidural fibrosis and recurrent disc herniation in the lumbar spine: MR imaging assessment. *AJR Am J Roentgenol*. 1988;150:923-932.
49. el Barzouhi A, Vleggeert-Lankamp CL, Lycklama a Nijeholt GJ, et al. Magnetic resonance imaging in follow-up assessment of sciatica. *N Engl J Med*. 2013;368(11):999-1007.
50. Mortensen WW, Thorne TP, Donaldson WF. Symptomatic gas-containing disc herniation: report of four cases. *Spine*. 1991;16:190-192.
51. Ford LT, Gilula LA, Murphy WA, et al. Analysis of gas in vacuum lumbar disc. *AJR Am J Roentgenol*. 1977;128: 1056-1057.
52. Rihn JA, Kurd M, Hilibrand AS, et al. The influence of obesity on the outcome of treatment of lumbar disc herniation: analysis of the Spine Patient Outcomes Research Trial (SPORT). *J Bone Joint Surg Am*. 2013;95(1):1-8.
53. McGuire KJ, Khaleel MA, Rihn JA, et al. The effect of high obesity on outcomes of treatment for lumbar spinal conditions: subgroup analysis of the spine patient outcomes research trial. *Spine*. 2014;39(23):1975-1980.
54. Rihn JA, Hilibrand AS, Radcliff K, et al. Duration of symptoms resulting from lumbar disc herniation: effect on treatment outcomes: analysis of the Spine Patient Outcomes Research Trial (SPORT). *J Bone Joint Surg Am*. 2011;93(20):1906-1914.
55. Deyo RA, Diehl AK, Rosenthal M. How many days of bedrest for acute low back pain? A randomized clinical trial. *N Engl J Med*. 1986;315:1064-1070.
56. Krause M, Reshauge KM, Dessen M, et al. Lumbar spine traction: evaluation of effects and recommended application for treatment. *Man Ther*. 2000;5:72-81.
57. Polkinghorn BS, Colloca CJ. Treatment of symptomatic lumbar disc herniation using activator methods chiropractic technique. *J Manipulative Physiol Ther*. 1998;21:187-196.
58. Goldberg H, Firtch W, Tyburski M, et al. Oral steroids for acute radiculopathy due to a herniated lumbar disk: a randomized clinical trial. *JAMA*. 2015;313(19):1915-1923.
59. Manchikanti L, Singh V, Cash KA, et al. Effect of fluoroscopically guided caudal epidural steroid or local anesthetic injections in the treatment of lumbar disc herniation and radiculitis: a randomized, controlled, double blind trial with a two-year follow-up. *Pain Physician*. 2012;15(4):273-286.
60. Bush K, Cowan N, Katz DE, et al. The natural history of sciatica associated with disc pathology: a prospective study with clinical and independent radiographic follow-up. *Spine*. 1992;17:1205-1212.
61. Radcliff K, Hilibrand A, Lurie JD, et al. The impact of epidural steroid injections on the outcomes of patients treated for lumbar disc herniation: a subgroup analysis of the SPORT trial. *J Bone Joint Surg Am*. 2012;94(15):1353-1358.
62. Hou SX, Tang JG, Chen HS, Chen J. Chronic inflammation and compression of the dorsal root contribute to sciatica induced by the intervertebral disc herniation in rats. *Pain*. 2003;105(1-2):255-264.
63. Freeman BJ, Ludbrook GL, Hall S, et al. Randomized, double-blind, placebo-controlled, trial of transforaminal epidural etanercept for the treatment of symptomatic lumbar disc herniation. *Spine*. 2013;38(23):1986-1994.
64. Ohtori S, Miyagi M, Eguchi Y, et al. Epidural administration of spinal nerves with the tumor necrosis factor-alpha inhibitor, etanercept, compared with dexamethasone for treatment of sciatica in patients with lumbar spinal stenosis: a prospective randomized study. *Spine*. 2012;37(6):439-444.
65. Burgher AH, Hoelzer BC, Schroeder DR, Wilson GA, Huntoon MA. Transforaminal epidural clonidine versus

corticosteroid for acute lumbosacral radiculopathy due to intervertebral disc herniation. *Spine*. 2011;36(5):E293-E300.

66. Wang JC, Lin E, Brodke DS, et al. Epidural injections for the treatment of symptomatic lumbar herniated discs. *J Spinal Disord*. 2002;15:269-272.
67. Atlas SJ, Deyo RA, Keller RB, et al. The Maine Lumbar Spine Study, Part II: 1-year outcomes of surgical and nonsurgical management of sciatica. *Spine*. 1996;21:1777-1786.
68. Pearson AM, Blood EA, Frymoyer JW, et al. SPORT lumbar intervertebral disk herniation and back pain: does treatment, location, or morphology matter? *Spine*. 2008;33:428-435.
69. Lurie JD, Tosteson TD, Tosteson AN, et al. Surgical versus nonoperative treatment for lumbar disc herniation: eight-year results for the spine patient outcomes research trial. *Spine*. 2014;39(1):3-16.
70. Alaranta H, Hurme M, Einola S, et al. A prospective study of patients with sciatica: a comparison between conservatively treated patients and patients who have undergone operation. Part II: results after one year follow-up. *Spine*. 1990;15:1345-1349.
71. Hurme M, Alaranta H, Einola S, et al. A prospective study of patients with sciatica: a comparison between conservatively treated patients and patients who have undergone operation. Part I: patient characteristics and differences between groups. *Spine*. 1990;15:1340-1344.
72. Balderston RA, Gilyeard GG, Jones AA, et al. The treatment of lumbar disc herniation: simple fragment excision versus disc space curettage. *J Spinal Disord*. 1991;4:22-25.
73. Barrios C, Ahmed M, Arrotegui JI, et al. Clinical factors predicting outcome after surgery for herniated lumbar disc: an epidemiological multivariate analysis. *J Spinal Disord*. 1990;3:205-209.
74. Cashion EL, Lynch WJ. Personality factors and results of lumbar disc surgery. *Neurosurgery*. 1979;4:141-145.
75. Daneyemez M, Sali A, Kahraman S, et al. Outcome analyses in 1072 surgically treated lumbar disc herniations. *Minim Invasive Neurosurg*. 1999;42:63-68.
76. Eie N. Comparison of the results in patients operated for ruptured lumbar discs with and without spinal fusion. *Acta Neurochir (Wien)*. 1978;41:107-113.
77. Faulhauer K, Manicke C. Fragment excision versus conventional disc removal in the microsurgical treatment of herniated lumbar disc. *Acta Neurochir (Wien)*. 1995;133:107-111.
78. Jonsson B, Stromqvist B. Motor affliction of the L5 nerve root in lumbar nerve root compression syndromes. *Spine*. 1995;20:2012-2015.
79. Kulali A, von Wild K. Microsurgical management of the lumbar intervertebral disc-disease. *Neurosurg Rev*. 1995;18:183-188.
80. Yeung AT, Tsou PM. Posterolateral endoscopic excision for lumbar disc herniation. *Spine*. 2002;27:722-731.
81. White AH, von Rogov P, Zucherman J, et al. Lumbar laminectomy for herniated disc: a prospective controlled comparison with internal fixation fusion. *Spine*. 1987;12:305-307.
82. van Alphen HA, Braakman R, Berfelo MW, et al. Chemonucleolysis or discectomy? Results of a randomized multicentre trial in patients with a herniated lumbar intervertebral disc (a preliminary report). *Acta Neurochir Suppl (Wien)*. 1988;43:35-38.
83. Tullberg T, Isacson J, Weidenhielm L. Does microscopic removal of lumbar disc herniation lead to better results than the standard procedure? Results of a one-year randomized study. *Spine*. 1993;18:24-27.
84. Soldner F, Hoelper BM, Wallenfang T, et al. The translaminar approach to canalicular and craniodorsolateral lumbar disc herniations. *Acta Neurochir (Wien)*. 2002;144:315-320.
85. Pointillart V, Broc G, Senegas J. A novel paraspinal surgical approach for lumbar lateral extraforaminal root entrapment. *Eur Spine J*. 1997;6:102-105.
86. An HS, Simpson JM, Stein R. Outpatient laminotomy and discectomy. *J Spinal Disord*. 1999;12:19-26.
87. Carragee EJ, Han MY, Yang B, et al. Activity restrictions after posterior lumbar discectomy: a prospective study of outcomes in 152 cases with no postoperative restrictions. *Spine*. 1999;24:2346-2351.
88. McCulloch JA. Focus issue on lumbar disc herniation: macro- and microdiscectomy. *Spine*. 1996;21:45S-56S.
89. Reulen HJ, Muller A, Ebeling U. Microsurgical anatomy of the lateral approach to extraforaminal lumbar disc herniations. *Neurosurgery*. 1996;39:345-350.
90. Eie N, Solgaard T, Kleppe H. The knee-elbow position in lumbar disc surgery: a review of complications. *Spine*. 1983;8:897-900.
91. Miyamoto K. Long-term follow-up results of anterior discectomy and interbody fusion for lumbar disc herniation. *J Jpn Orthop Assoc*. 1991;65:1179-1190.
92. Revel M, Payan C, Vallee C, et al. Automated percutaneous lumbar discectomy versus chemonucleolysis in the treatment of sciatica: a randomized multicenter trial. *Spine*. 1993;18:1-7.
93. Shapiro S. Long-term followup of 57 patients undergoing automated percutaneous discectomy. *J Neurosurg*. 1995;83:31-33.
94. Hoppenfeld S. Percutaneous removal of herniated lumbar discs: 50 cases with ten-year follow-up periods. *Clin Orthop Relat Res*. 1989;238:92-97.
95. Kotilainen E, Valtonen S. Long-term outcome of patients who underwent percutaneous nucleotomy for lumbar disc herniation: results after a mean follow-up of 5 years. *Acta Neurochir (Wien)*. 1998;140:108-113.
96. DeAntoni DJ, Claro ML, Poehling GG, et al. Translaminar lumbar epidural endoscopy: technique and clinical results. *J South Orthop Assoc*. 1998;7:61-62.
97. Fraser RD. Chymopapain for the treatment of intervertebral disc herniation: the final report of a double-blind study. *Spine*. 1984;9:815-818.
98. Muralikuttan KP, Hamilton A, Kernohan WG, et al. A prospective randomized trial of chemonucleolysis and conventional disc surgery in single level lumbar disc herniation. *Spine*. 1992;17:381-387.
99. Bailey A, Araghi A, Blumenthal S, Huffmon GV. Prospective, multicenter, randomized, controlled study of anular repair in lumbar discectomy: two-year follow-up. *Spine*. 2013;38(14):1161-1169.
100. Weber H. The effect of delayed disc surgery on muscular paresis. *Acta Orthop Scand*. 1975;46:631-642.
101. MacKay MA, Fischgrund JS, Herkowitz HN, et al. The effect of interposition membrane on the outcome of lumbar laminectomy and discectomy. *Spine*. 1995;20:1793-1796.
102. Bernsmann K, Kramer J, Ziozios I, et al. Lumbar micro disc surgery with and without autologous fat graft: a prospective randomized trial evaluated with reference to clinical and social factors. *Arch Orthop Trauma Surg*. 2001;121:476-480.

103. Kjellby-Wendt G, Styf J. Early active training after lumbar discectomy: a prospective, randomized, and controlled study. *Spine*. 1998;23:2345-2351.
104. Gencay-Can A, Gunendi Z, Suleyman Can S, Sepici V, Ceviker N. The effects of early aerobic exercise after single-level lumbar microdiscectomy: a prospective, controlled trial. *Eur J Phys Rehabil Med*. 2010;46(4):489-496.
105. Alaranta H, Hurme M, Einola S, et al. Rehabilitation after surgery for lumbar disc herniation: results of a randomized clinical trial. *Int J Rehabil Res*. 1986;9:247-257.
106. Knop-Jergas BM, Zucherman JF, Hsu KY, et al. Anatomic position of a herniated nucleus pulposus predicts the outcome of lumbar discectomy. *J Spinal Disord*. 1996;9:246-250.
107. Dewing CB, Provencher MT, Rifenburgh RH, et al. The outcomes of lumbar microdiscectomy in a young, active population: correlation by herniation type and level. *Spine*. 2008;33:33-38.
108. Jonsson B, Stromqvist B. Significance of a persistent positive straight leg raising test after lumbar disc surgery. *J Neurosurg*. 1999;91:50-53.
109. Keller RB, Atlas SJ, Soule DN, et al. Relationship between rates and outcomes of operative treatment for lumbar disc herniation and spinal stenosis. *J Bone Joint Surg Am*. 1999;81:752-762.
110. Olson PR, Lurie JD, Frymoyer J, et al. Lumbar disc herniation in the Spine Patient Outcomes Research Trial: does educational attainment impact outcome? *Spine*. 2011;36(26):2324-2332.
111. Radcliff K, Freedman M, Hilibrand A, et al. Does opioid pain medication use affect the outcome of patients with lumbar disc herniation? *Spine*. 2013;38(14):E849-E860.
112. Dvorak J, Gauchat MH, Valach L. The outcome of surgery for lumbar disc herniation, I: a 4-17 years follow-up with emphasis on somatic aspects. *Spine*. 1988;13:1418-1422.
113. Kotilainen E, Valtonene S, Carlson CA. Microsurgical treatment of lumbar disc herniation: follow-up of 237 patients. *Acta Neurochir (Wien)*. 1993;120:143-149.
114. Goffin J. Microdiscectomy for lumbar disc herniations. *Clin Neurol Neurosurg*. 1994;96:130-134.
115. Casal-Moro R, Castro-Menendez M, Hernandez-Blanco M, et al. Long-term outcome after microendoscopic diskectomy for lumbar disk herniation: a prospective clinical study with a 5-year follow-up. *Neurosurgery*. 2011;68(6):1568-1575.
116. Mariscalco MW, Yamashita T, Steinmetz MP, et al. Radiation exposure to the surgeon during open lumbar microdiscectomy and minimally invasive microdiscectomy: a prospective, controlled trial. *Spine*. 2011;36(3):255-260.
117. Wenger M, Mariani L, Kalbarczyk A, et al. Long-term outcome of 104 patients after lumbar sequestrectomy according to Williams. *Neurosurgery*. 2001;49:329-334.
118. Carragee EJ, Spinnickie AO, Alamin TF, et al. A prospective controlled study of limited versus subtotal posterior discectomy: short-term outcomes in patients with herniated lumbar intervertebral discs and large posterior anular defect. *Spine*. 2006;31:653-657.
119. Kotilainen E, Valtonen S. Clinical instability of the lumbar spine after microdiscectomy. *Acta Neurochir (Wien)*. 1993;125:120-126.
120. Tronnier V, Schneider R, Kunz U, et al. Postoperative spondylodiscitis: results of a prospective study about the aetiology of spondylodiscitis after operation for lumbar disc herniation. *Acta Neurochir (Wien)*. 1992;117:149-152.
121. Sande E, Myhre HO, Witsoe E, et al. Vascular complications of lumbar disc surgery (case report). *Eur J Surg*. 1991;157:141-143.
122. Ewah B, Calder I. Intraoperative death during lumbar discectomy. *Br J Anaesth*. 1991;66:712-723.
123. Christensen C, Bank A. Arteriovenous fistula complicating lumbar disc surgery (case report). *Eur J Surg*. 1991;157:145-147.
124. Farouk M, Murie JA. Postlaminectomy arteriovenous fistula formation: a continuing problem. *J R Coll Surg Edinb*. 1991;36:130-131.
125. Saxler G, Kramer J, Barden B, et al. The long-term clinical sequelae of incidental durotomy in lumbar disc surgery. *Spine*. 2005;30:2298-2302.
126. Padua R, Padua S, Romanini E, et al. Ten to 15 year outcome of surgery for lumbar disc herniation: radiographic instability and clinical findings. *Eur Spine J*. 1999;8:70-74.
127. Kotilainen E. Long-term outcome of patients suffering from clinical instability after microsurgical treatment of lumbar disc herniation. *Acta Neurochir (Wien)*. 1998;140:120-125.
128. Laus M, Bertoni F, Bacchini P, et al. Recurrent lumbar disc herniation: what recurs? (A morphological study of recurrent disc herniation). *Chir Organi Mov*. 1993;78:147-154.
129. Jonsson B, Stromqvist B. Clinical characteristics of recurrent sciatica after lumbar discectomy. *Spine*. 1996;21:500-505.
130. Vik A, Zwart JA, Hullberg G, et al. Eight year outcome after surgery for lumbar disc herniation: a comparison of reoperated and nonreoperated patients. *Acta Neurochir (Wien)*. 2001;143:607-610.
131. Suk KS, Lee HM, Moon SH, et al. Lumbosacral scoliotic list by lumbar disc herniation. *Spine*. 2001;26:667-671.
132. Cinotti G, Gumina S, Giannicola G, et al. Contralateral recurrent lumbar disc herniation: results of discectomy compared with those in primary herniation. *Spine*. 1999;24:800-806.
133. Cinotti G, Roysam GS, Eisenstein SM, et al. Ipsilateral recurrent lumbar disc herniation: a prospective, controlled study. *J Bone Joint Surg Br*. 1998;80:825-832.
134. Papadopoulos EC, Girardi FP, Sandhu HS, et al. Outcome of revision discectomies following recurrent lumbar disc herniation. *Spine*. 2006;31:1473-1476.
135. Herron L. Recurrent lumbar disc herniation: results of repeat laminectomy and discectomy. *J Spinal Disord*. 1994;7:161-166.
136. Stambough JL. Recurrent same-level, ipsilateral lumbar disc herniation. *Orthop Rev*. 1994;23:810-816.
137. Kurihara A, Kataoka O. Lumbar disc herniation in children and adolescents: a review of 70 operated cases and their minimum 5-year follow-up studies. *Spine*. 1980;5:443-451.
138. Garrido E. Lumbar disc herniation in the pediatric patient. *Neurosurg Clin N Am*. 1993;4:149-152.
139. Papagenlopoulos PJ, Shaughnessy WJ, Ebersold MJ, et al. Long-term outcome of lumbar discectomy in children and adolescents sixteen years of age or younger. *J Bone Joint Surg Am*. 1998;80:689-698.
140. Parisini P, DiSilvestre M, Greggi T, et al. Lumbar disc excision in children and adolescents. *Spine*. 2001;26:1997-2000.
141. DeOrio JK, Bianco AJ. Lumbar disc excision in children and adolescents. *J Bone Joint Surg Am*. 1982;64:991-996.
142. Shillito J. Pediatric lumbar disc surgery: 20 patients under 15 years of age. *Surg Neurol*. 1996;46:14-18.
143. Maistrelli GL, Vaughan PA, Evans DC, et al. Lumbar disc herniation in the elderly. *Spine*. 1987;12:63-66.

144. Jonsson B, Stromqvist B. Lumbar spine surgery in the elderly: complications and surgical results. *Spine*. 1994;19: 1431-1435.
145. Garrido E, Connaughton PN. Unilateral facetectomy approach for lateral lumbar disc herniation. *J Neurosurg*. 1991;74: 754-756.
146. Donaldson WF, Star MJ, Thorne RP. Surgical treatment for the lateral herniated lumbar disc. *Spine*. 1993;18:1263-1267.
147. Weiner BK, Dabbah M. Lateral lumbar disc herniations treated with a paraspinal approach: an independent assessment of longer-term outcomes. *J Spinal Disord Tech*. 2005;18:519-521.
148. Walker JL, Schulak D, Murtagh R. Midline disk herniations of the lumbar spine. *South Med J*. 1993;86:13-17.
149. Tay ECK, Chacha PB. Midline prolapse of a lumbar intervertebral disc with compression of the cauda equina. *J Bone Joint Surg Br*. 1979;61:43-46.
150. Venkatesan M, Uzoigwe CE, Perianayagam G, Braybrooke JR, Newey ML. Is cauda equina syndrome linked with obesity? *J Bone Joint Surg Br*. 2012;94(11):1551-1556.
151. Nielsen B, de Nully M, Schmidt K, et al. A urodynamic study of cauda equina syndrome due to lumbar disc herniation. *Urol Int*. 1980;35:167-170.
152. Kostuik JP, Harrington I, Alexander D, et al. Cauda equina syndrome and lumbar disc herniation. *J Bone Joint Surg Am*. 1986;68:386-391.
153. Choudry AR, Taylor JC. Cauda equina syndrome in lumbar disc disease. *Acta Orthop Scand*. 1980;51:493-499.
154. Shapiro S. Cauda equina syndrome secondary to lumbar disc herniation. *Neurosurgery*. 1993;32:743-747.
155. Chau AM, Xu LL, Pelzer NR, Gragnaniello C. Timing of surgical intervention in cauda equina syndrome: a systematic critical review. *World Neurosurg*. 2014;81(3-4):640-650.
156. Ahn UM, Ahn NU, Buchowski JM, et al. Cauda equina syndrome secondary to lumbar disc herniation. *Spine*. 2000;25:1515-1522.
157. DeLong WB, Polissar N, Neradilek B. Timing of surgery in cauda equina syndrome with urinary retention: meta-analysis of observational studies. *J Neurosurg Spine*. 2008;8(4):305-320.
158. Gleave JR, Macfarlane R. Cauda equina syndrome: what is the relationship between timing of surgery and outcome? *Br J Neurosurg*. 2002;16(4):325-328.
159. Srikandarajah N, Boissaud-Cooke MA, Clark S, Wilby MJ. Does early surgical decompression in cauda equina syndrome improve bladder outcome? *Spine*. 2015;40(8):580-583.
160. McCarthy MJ, Aylott CE, Grevitt MP, et al. Cauda equina syndrome: factors affecting long-term functional and sphincteric outcome. *Spine*. 2007;32:207-216.
161. Korse NS, Jacobs WC, Elzevier HW, Vleggeert-Lankamp CL. Complaints of micturition, defecation and sexual function in cauda equina syndrome due to lumbar disk herniation: a systematic review. *Eur Spine J*. 2013;22(5):1019-1029.
162. Chang HS, Nakagawa H, Mizuno J. Lumbar herniated disc presenting with cauda equina syndrome. *Surg Neurol*. 2002;53: 100-105.
163. Yeung AT, Yeung CA. Minimally invasive techniques for the management of lumbar disc herniation. *Orthop Clin North Am*. 2007;38:363-372.
164. Wang H, Huang B, Li C, et al. Learning curve for percutaneous endoscopic lumbar discectomy depending on the surgeon's training level of minimally invasive spine surgery. *Clin Neurol Neurosurg*. 2013;115(10):1987-1991.
165. Sencer A, Yorukoglu AG, Akcakaya MO, et al. Fully endoscopic interlaminar and transforaminal lumbar discectomy: short-term clinical results of 163 surgically treated patients. *World Neurosurg*. 2014;82(5):884-890.
166. Hoogland T, van den Brekel-Dijstra K, Schubert M, et al. Endoscopic transforaminal discectomy for recurrent lumbar disc herniation: a prospective, cohort evaluation of 262 consecutive cases. *Spine*. 2008;33:973-978.
167. Pan L, Zhang P, Yin Q. Comparison of tissue damages caused by endoscopic lumbar discectomy and traditional lumbar discectomy: a randomised controlled trial. *Int J Surg*. 2014;12(5):534-537.
168. Yoshimoto M, Iwase T, Takebayashi T, Ida K, Yamashita T. Microendoscopic discectomy for far lateral lumbar disk herniation: less surgical invasiveness and minimum 2-year follow-up results. *J Spinal Disord Tech*. 2014;27(1):E1-E7.
169. Kim CH, Chung CK, Sohn S, Lee S, Park SB. The surgical outcome and the surgical strategy of percutaneous endoscopic discectomy for recurrent disk herniation. *J Spinal Disord Tech*. 2014;27(8):415-422.
170. Lee DH, Kim NH, Park JB, et al. CT scan assessment of the pathway of the true lateral approach for transforaminal endoscopic lumbar discectomy: is It possible? *J Bone Joint Surg Br*. 2011;93(10):1395-1399.
171. Wu X, Zhuang S, Mao Z, et al. Microendoscopic discectomy for lumbar disc herniation: surgical technique and outcome in 873 consecutive cases. *Spine*. 2006;31:2689-2694.
172. Righesso O, Falavigna A, Avanzi O. Comparison of open discectomy with microendoscopic discectomy in lumbar disc herniations: results of a randomized controlled trial. *Neurosurgery*. 2007;61:545-549.
173. Ruetten S, Komp M, Merk H, et al. Full-endoscopic interlaminar and transforaminal lumbar discectomy versus conventional microsurgical technique: a prospective, randomized, controlled study. *Spine*. 2008;33:931-939.
174. Teli M, Lovi A, Brayda-Bruno M, et al. Higher risk of dural tears and recurrent herniation with lumbar micro-endoscopic discectomy. *Eur Spine J*. 2010;19(3):443-450.
174a. Garg B, Nagraja UB, Jayaswal A. Microendoscopic versus open discectomy for lumbar disc herniation: a prospective, randomized study. *J Orthop Surg (Hong Kong)*. 2011;19(1): 30-34.
175. Smith N, Masters J, Jensen C, Khan A, Sprowson A. Systematic review of microendoscopic discectomy for lumbar disc herniation. *Eur Spine J*. 2013;22(11):2458-2465.
176. Choi KC, Lee JH, Kim JS, et al. Unsuccessful percutaneous endoscopic lumbar discectomy: a single-center experience of 10,228 cases. *Neurosurgery*. 2015;76(4):372-380.
177. Choi I, Ahn JO, So WS, et al. Exiting root injury in transforaminal endoscopic discectomy: preoperative image considerations for safety. *Eur Spine J*. 2013;22(11):2481-2487.
178. Crawshaw C, Frazer AM, Merriam WF, et al. A comparison of surgery and chemonucleolysis in the treatment of sciatica: a prospective randomized trial. *Spine*. 1984;9:195-198.

CHAPTER 48

Annular Repair

Gregory Lopez
Gunnar B.J. Andersson

Introduction

The anulus fibrosus is an important part of the intervertebral disc. Like the other disc components, the anulus undergoes changes with aging and with degeneration.[1,2] The degenerative process leads to a weakening of the anulus; delamination, fissures, and cracks result. Occasionally, the nucleus pulposus can herniate into those cracks and actually through the entire annular wall, causing pain due to both local inflammatory response and nerve root ischemia. Also, as part of surgical procedures to address contained disc herniations, iatrogenic holes in various shapes and locations are made into the anulus.

In recent years, there has been increasing interest in strengthening the annular structure, which is important to regain the normal function of the disc.[3] There is also interest in repairing degenerative and iatrogenic cracks, tears, and holes in the anulus to prevent recurrence of disc herniations, and to slow the degenerative process following discectomy. The purpose of this chapter is to review some of these strategies and put them in the context of successful treatment of different types of painful spinal conditions. The focus will be on the lumbar discs.

Anulus Fibrosus

The anulus fibrosus is a laminate structure surrounding the central nucleus pulposus and inserting into the endplates and vertebral body. It consists primarily of water, collagen, proteoglycans, and noncollagenous proteins. The laminates are organized in layers, mainly composed of type I collagen fibers, which alternate in angles with respect to the transverse plane. Between the layers are so-called interlaminar spaces containing proteoglycans (aggrecan, versican) and other link elements.[4] In the center, the fibers insert into the cartilaginous endplates; in the periphery, they bypass the endplates and insert into the bone, called Sharpey's fibers. The inner and outer parts of the anulus are different in that, in the inner part, the layers are less well organized and more widely spaced. The proportion of type I collagen increases from the inner anulus to the outer anulus; type II collagen is more common in the inner than outer anulus. Small proteoglycans (decorin and biglycan) are found primarily in the outer anulus, while elastin is present throughout. Elastin constitutes 1.7% to 2.0% of the dry weight of the anulus. In the outer anulus, elastin is present within the lamella running parallel to the collagen and in the same direction.[5] In the inner anulus, elastin is also organized within the lamellae. Fiber networks bind adjacent lamellae together, preventing them from separation.[6,7] Table 48.1 compares the outer and inner anulus.

The cell density in the anulus pulposus is about twice that of the nucleus pulposus.[8] In the outer anulus, the cells are fusiform shaped and align with the collagen fibers alternating with each lamella. These cells produce mainly type I collagen. In the inner anulus, the cells are more similar to those of the nucleus pulposus. They are chrondrocyte-like and produce mainly type II collagen.

The mechanical exposures of the different parts of the anulus are initially different. The inner anulus is primarily subjected to the hydrostatic pressures of the nucleus pulposus; the outer anulus is more under compression or tension, depending on the direction of movement. As are other connective tissue structures, the anulus is anisotropic and adapted to the principal directions of load.

Effect of Aging on the Anulus Fibrosus

A variety of chemical and structural changes occur with aging. These changes appear to occur first in the inner anulus, which loses a large part of its proteoglycan and water and gradually assumes a more nucleus-like structure.[2]

Both the overall proteoglycan and collagen concentrations decrease with aging, probably reflecting a decrease in cellular biochemical activity. Among smaller nonaggregating proteoglycans, decorin levels decrease with aging in the outer anulus, while biglycan and fibromodulin levels increase. In the inner anulus, decorin levels have been found to increase with aging. The mechanical properties are altered with aging as well. Peak compressive stresses are increased by 160%, and the width of the anulus is thickened by 80%.[9]

TABLE 48.1 Characteristics of the Outer Versus the Inner Anulus

	Outer Anulus	Inner Anulus
Collagen	40–60% dry weight	25–40% dry weight
Type collagen	Type I mainly	Type II mainly
Proteoglycan	5–8% dry weight	11–20% dry weight
Cells	Fusion from	Chondrocyte-like

Healing of the Anulus

Early studies in dogs showed comparatively poor healing when larger defects were created in the annular wall.[10] Smith and Walmsley[11] reported that after an incision, the outer anulus healed by fibrous tissue ingrowth from the sides and that there was also a gradual healing of the inner anulus over a 1-year period. Long-term collagen fibers gradually invaded the nuclear tissue, some of which remained in the annular incisions. Fazzalari et al.,[12] in an ovine model, introduced needle punctures and concentric tears, and tested the specimen mechanically up to 18 months. Significant changes occurred in disc biomechanics in both cases, and remained significant over time. The annular lamellae thickened and the adjacent vertebral body bone volume fraction increased. While this model is not a herniation model, it shows the poor healing of concentric tears and their effect on disc biomechanics. There is limited information on annular repair in humans after discectomy. Current information suggests a limited healing potential after annulotomy. This increases the risk of reherniation. Reoperation rates for recurrent herniations ranging from 3% to up to 27% have been reported.[13–16] The frequency of reoperations appears to be related to the size of the annular defect.

Biologic Repair

At least four types of annular repair are discussed in the literature: collagen modification, cell therapy, gene therapy, and tissue-engineered scaffolds. Gene and cell therapies are unlikely to repair existing cracks, tears, and incisions unless combined with scaffolds. Also, current gene delivery systems use virus-mediated gene transfer to enhance matrix deposition within the disc[17,18]; however, infection is always a risk with viral delivery systems.

A number of studies have been published in which scaffolds have been populated with cells, with various success rates reported. Most of these studies have been performed in vitro, but a few animal studies have been reported. Gene and growth factor therapies can repair annular needle punctures in the early stages. Most anulus fibrosus scaffolds use collagen type II, despite type I being more abundant in the outer layers of the anulus. Saad et al. demonstrated a higher production of extracellular matrix with type II collagen.[19] Many growth factors appear to have a stronger effect on proteoglycan than collagen. Zhang et al.[20] reported that collagen synthesis was enhanced by bone morphogenetic protein 13 (BMP-13) and Sox9.

Bron et al.[3] list a number of requirements for anulus fibrosus scaffolds. The scaffolds should:

- Fix and/or repair the anulus fibrosus gap to contain the nucleus pulposus (or its replacement).
- Allow fixation to surrounding structures.
- Allow anulus fibrosus cells (or stem cells) to survive and secrete extracellular matrix.
- Have the characteristic anisotropic behavior to maintain/restore the mechanical properties of a spinal motion segment.
- Not irritate or adhere to the perineurium.

To date, no single approach has met all these requirements, but several scaffolds hold promise.[21–24]

Surgical Repair

A few alternatives have been developed to address the closure of an annular defect caused by a discectomy. In an in vitro study, a laboratory simulation of intradiscal pressures of the lumbar spine was conducted to compare nonrepaired versus repaired annular defects. Bartlett and colleagues concluded that repair of the anulus may be beneficial to retaining disc material and preventing reherniation.[25] Synthetic materials are advantageous as well, as the materials are predictably reproduced. Wang et al.[26] put gelfoam, platinum core, bone cement, and tissue glue into an 18-gauge needle defect. Gelfoam appeared to have the best result. The size of the defect in this model is so small, however, that it is difficult to extrapolate this model to a discectomy. Sutures have been used in a sheep model.[27] The healing effect was not statistically significant.

More recently, sutures with anchors (Xclose) have been introduced (Anulex Technologies, Inc.; Fig. 48.1). A retrospective case series presented in 2009 at a society meeting compared 133 microdiscectomy cases without anulus repair to 59 with anulus repair. There were 16 reoperations within 12 months in the nonrepair group (12.9%) compared to four in the annular repair group (6.8%).[28] More recently, Bailey et al. reported their results using the Xclose from a prospective, multicenter, single-blind, randomized, controlled clinical trial of individuals who were candidates for a one- or two-level discectomy with persistent leg pain.[29] Although visual analog scale leg and back pain, Oswestry Disability Index, and Short Form-12 outcomes improved, there was no statistically significant difference between the groups at any of the follow-up points. Symptomatic reherniation rates also did not statistically differ at any of the follow-up points. To what degree sutures can be used when larger defects exist remains unknown. It is also not clear how well they reverse the biomechanical changes caused by the defect.

Barricaid is another commercially available implant that anchors into the vertebral body and supports a woven mesh barrier inserted into the defect (Intrinsic Therapeutics Inc.; Fig. 48.2). In a multicenter prospective cohort study, recurrent herniation, disc height loss, and pain scores were monitored, with 2-year follow-up. Thirty patients underwent implantation of the device, while 46 had no implant placement. Although not statistically significant, at 2 years no patient with

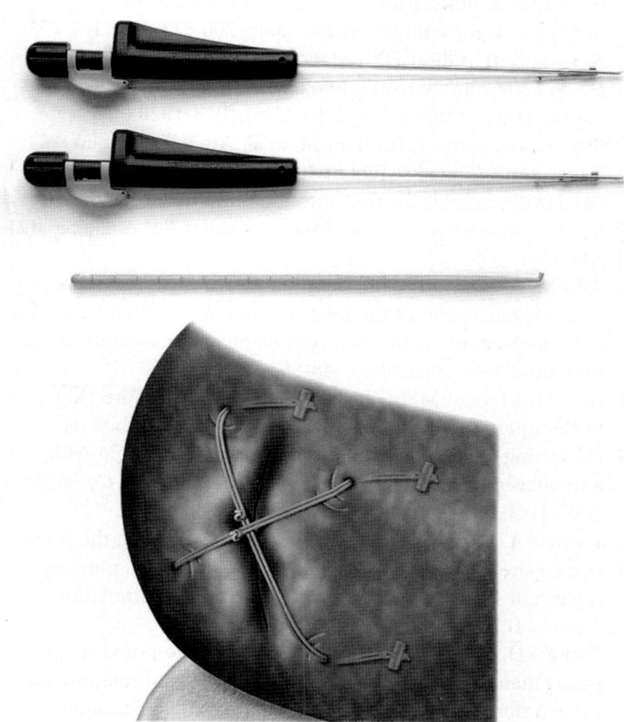

FIG. 48.1 Xclose implant. (Courtesy Anulex Technologies, Inc., Eden Prairie, MN.)

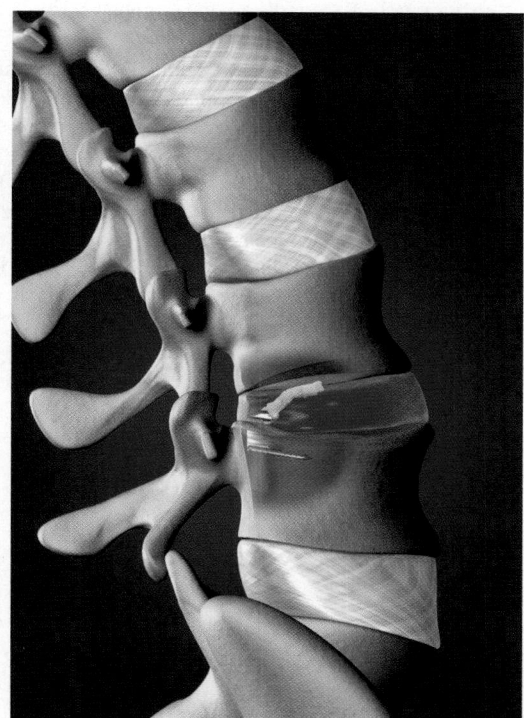

FIG. 48.2 Barricaid implant. (Courtesy Intrinsic Therapeutics, Inc., Woburn, MA.)

an implanted device had a symptomatic recurrent disc herniation, while there were three in the control group. Significant scores were achieved with the implanted device cohort as they reported less leg pain, back pain, and disability at 1 year postoperatively.

Other implants are in various stages of development and likely to be presented at meetings in the near future.

Summary

Annular repair is an exciting developing technology to address the age- and degeneration-related changes of the anulus, as well as annular tears occurring from disc herniations or in the treatment of herniations. We can expect clinical data in the next several years, but it may take a decade or more to determine how effective annular strengthening is in retarding the development of degenerative and age-related changes.

KEY REFERENCES

1. Osti OL, Vernon-Roberts B, Moore R, Fraser RD. Annular tears and disc degeneration in the lumbar spine. A post-mortem study of 135 discs. *J Bone Joint Surg Br.* 1992;74(5):678-682.
   This is a classic study of anatomic findings of the anulus fibrosus of humans.
2. Bron JL, Heider MN, Meisel H-J, Van Royen BJ, Smit TH. Repair, regenerative and supportive therapies of the annulus fibrosus: achievements and challenges. *Eur Spine J.* 2009;18:301-313.
   This is a review article on repair of the anulus fibrosus.
3. Carragee EJ, Han MY, Suen PW, Kim D. Clinical outcomes after lumbar discectomy for sciatica: the effects of fragment type and anular competence. *J Bone Joint Surg Am.* 2007;85(1):102-108.
   This article describes the risk of reherniation in relation to the type of herniation and the size of the annular defect.
4. Hartman L, Griffith SL, Melone B, Melone D. *Surgical Outcome of Lumbar Microdiscectomy With Emphasis on Annular Repair Techniques.* New Orleans, LA: American Meeting of the Congress of Neurological Surgeons; 2009.
   This study of a mechanical repair technique shows promising results.

REFERENCES

1. Osti OL, Vernon-Roberts B, Moore R, Fraser RD. Annular tears and disc degeneration in the lumbar spine. A post-mortem study of 135 discs. *J Bone Joint Surg Br.* 1992;74(5):678-682.
2. Singh K, Masuda K, Thonar EJ-M, An HS, Cs-Szabo G. Age-related changes in the extracellular matrix of mucleus pulposus and annulus fibrosus of human intervertebral disc. *Spine.* 2008;34:10-16.
3. Bron JL, Heider MN, Meisel H-J, Van Royen BJ, Smit TH. Repair, regenerative and supportive therapies of the annulus fibrosus: achievements and challenges. *Eur Spine J.* 2009;18: 301-313.
4. Pezowicz CA, Robertson PA, Broom ND. The structural basis of interlamellar cohesion in the intervertebral disc well. *J Anat.* 2006;208(3):317-330.
5. Smith LJ, Byers S, Costi JJ, Fazzalari NL. Elastic fibers enhance the mechanical integrity of the human lumbar annulus fibrosus in rha radial direction. *Ann Biomed Eng.* 2008;36(2):214-223.
6. Yu J, Tirlapur U, Fairbank J, et al. Microfibrils, elastin fibres and collagen fibres in the human intervertebral disc and bovine tail disc. *J Anat.* 2007;210(4):460-471.
7. Melrose J, Smith SM, Appleyard RC, et al. Aggrecan, vernican and type VI collagen are components of annular translamellar cross bridges in the intervertebral disc. *Eur Spine J.* 2008;17: 314-324.

8. Roughley PJ. Biology of intervertebral disc aging and degeneration: involvement of the extracellular matrix. *Spine.* 2004;29(23):2691-2699.
9. Adams MA, McNally DS, Dolan P. Stress' distributions inside intervertebral discs. The effects of age and degeneration. *J Bone Joint Surg Br.* 1996;78:965-972.
10. Key JA, Ford LT. Experimental intervertebral-disc lesions. *J Bone Joint Surg Am.* 1948;30:621-630.
11. Smith JW, Walmsley R. Experimental incision of the intervertebral disc. *J Bone Joint Surg Br.* 1951;33-B(4):612-625.
12. Fazzalari NL, Costi JJ, Hearn TC, et al. Mechanical and pathologic consequences of induced concentric anular tears in an ovine model. *Spine.* 2001;26(23):2572-2581.
13. Carragee EJ, Han MY, Suen PW, Kim D. Clinical outcomes after lumbar discectomy for sciatica: the effects of fragment type and anular competence. *J Bone Joint Surg Am.* 2007;85(1): 102-108.
14. Ebeling U, Kalbarcyk H, Reulen HJ. Microsurgical re-operation following lumbar disc surgery: timing, surgical findings, and outcome in 92 patients. *J Neurosurg.* 1989;70:397-404.
15. Ambrossi GLG, MCGirt MJ, Sciobba DA, et al. Recurrent lumbar disc herniation after single level discectomy: Incidence and health care cost analysis. *Neurosurgery.* 2009;65:574-578.
16. Watters WC, McGirt MJ. An evidence-based review of the literature on the consequences of conservative versus aggressive discectomy for the treatment of primary disc herniation with radiculopathy. *Spine J.* 2009;9:240-257.
17. Liang H, Ma SY, Feng G, Shen FH, Joshua LX. Therapeutic effects of adenovirus-mediated growth and differentiation factor-5 in a mice disc degeneration model induced by annulus needle puncture. *Spine J.* 2010;10:32-41.
18. Yoon ST, Park JS, Kim KS, et al. ISSLS prize winner: LMP-1 upregulates intervertebral disc cell production of proteoglycans and BMPs in vitro and in vivo. *Spine.* 2004;29:2603-2611.
19. Saad L, Spector M. Effects of collagen type on the behavior of adult canine annulus fibrosus cells in collagen-glycosaminoglycan scaffolds. *J Biomed Mater Res A.* 2004;71:233-241.
20. Zhang Y, Anderson DB, Phillips FM, et al. Comparative effects of bone morphogenetic proteins and Sox9 overexpression on matrix accumulation by bovine annulus fibrosus cells: implications for annular repair. *Spine.* 2007;32(23):2515-2520.
21. Nerurkar NL, Elliott DM, Mauck RL. Mechanics of oriented electrospun nanofibrous scaffolds for annulus fibrosus tissue engineering. *J Orthop Res.* 2007;25(8):1018-1028.
22. Sato M, Asazuma T, Ishihara M, et al. An atelocollagen honeycomb-shaped scaffold with a membrane seal (ACHMS-scaffold) for the culture of annulus fibrosus cells from an intervertebral disc. *J Biomed Mater Res A.* 2003;64(2): 248-256.
23. Sato M, Asazuma T, Ishihara M, et al. An experimental study of the regeneration of the intervertebral disc with an allograft of cultured annulus fibrosus cells using a tissue-engineering method. *Spine.* 2003;28(6):548-553.
24. Sato M, Kikuchi M, Ishihara M, et al. Tissue engineering of the intervertebral disc with cultured annulus fibrosus cells using atelocollagen honeycomb-shaped scaffold with a membrane seal (ACHMS scaffold). *Med Bio Eng Comput.* 2003;41(3):365-371.
25. Bartlett A, Wales L, Houfburg R, et al. Optimizing the effectiveness of a mechanical suture-based anulus fibrosus repair construct in an acute failure laboratory simulation. *J Spinal Disord Tech.* 2013;26(7):393-399.
26. Wang YH, Kuo TF, Wang JL. The implantation of non-cell-based materials to prevent the recurrent disc herniation: an in vivo porcine model using quantitative discomanometry examination. *Eur Spine J.* 2007;16(7):1021-1027.
27. Ahlgren BD, Lui W, Herkowitz HN, Panjabi MM, Guiboux JP. Effect of annular repair on the healing strength of the intervertebral disc: a sheep model. *Spine.* 2000;25(17): 2165-2170.
28. Hartman L, Griffith SL, Melone B, Melone D. *Surgical Outcome of Lumbar Microdiscectomy With Emphasis on Annular Repair Techniques.* New Orleans, LA: American Meeting of the Congress of Neurological Surgeons; 2009.
29. Bailey A, Araghi A, Blumenthal S, Huffmon GV, Anular Repair Clinical Study Group. Prospective, multicenter, randomized, controlled study of anular repair in lumbar discectomy: two-year follow-up. *Spine (Phila Pa 1976).* 2013;38(14):1161-1169. Erratum. *Spine.* 2013;38(17):1527.

Lumbar Disc Degeneration: Anterior Lumbar Interbody Fusion, Degeneration, and Disc Replacement

Robert Johnson
Richard D. Guyer

Low back pain has long been noted to be one of the most disabling conditions in the United States and the Western world. Disability from back pain has been reported to cost approximately $100 billion annually.[1] Lumbar disc degeneration is often divided into three basic categories: internal disc derangement, degenerative disc disease (DDD), and motion segment instability. Internal disc derangement[2] encompasses annular tears and dark disc disease. DDD describes isolated disc resorption and spondylosis. Motion segment instability involves listhesis and scoliotic changes. This description of lumbar disc degeneration, although oversimplified, encompasses a dynamic process with overlapping findings at individual and adjacent levels. DDD, although controversial in its exact role in patients with back pain, has been shown to be a pain source generator.[3,4] Removal of the pain generator, the intervertebral disc, is a viable and logical approach for selected patients.

Determining the ideal candidate for surgical management of DDD can be more challenging than performing the procedure itself because of the unclear relationship between patient symptoms, diagnostic studies, and surgical outcomes. The patient should have not responded to conservative management—including oral medication, lifestyle modification, active rehabilitation, and injections—before surgical intervention for a minimum of 6 months. To maximize the predictive value of lumbar interbody fusion or disc replacement for the treatment of lumbar disc degeneration, the patient's history should be consistent with mechanical back pain, and radiographic studies should show degeneration at discrete levels. While a good history, physical examination, and diagnostic radiographs—including standing flexion and extension views along with MRI—will allow diagnosis of discogenic pain, discography is useful in those equivocal cases and should reproduce concordant pain and show abnormal disc morphology (Fig. 49.1). Patients with a significant behavioral component to their pain should be considered poor surgical candidates. Preoperative psychological screening can be helpful in the evaluation of those patients.[5]

Anterior lumbar interbody fusion (ALIF) and total disc replacement (TDR), as options for treating DDD, have had a tumultuous history with increasing and decreasing interest and success over the years. ALIF as a procedure favors load transmission through the anterior column, recreates lordosis, restores disc height, and tensions lateral and posterior annular or ligamentous fibers (Fig. 49.2).[6] TDR likewise removes the diseased disc, indirectly decompresses posterior structures, and replaces the diseased disc with an artificial one while preserving aspects of normal biomechanical function. Direct anterior exposure allows complete removal of disc material, increasing the fusion rate,[7] and prepares the disc space while avoiding trauma to the posterior musculature, making it an attractive option for the treatment of DDD. In the United States, most approaches to the anterior spine are performed by general/vascular surgeons, though, depending on training, some US spine surgeons do their own.

Anterior Lumbar Surgical Approach

Relative contraindications to anterior lumbar approaches include advanced atherosclerosis of the major vessels and obesity. Some consideration should be given to patients who have previously undergone prior abdominal surgery or have inflammatory diseases because these conditions create significant scarring that may increase the risk or preclude one from successful surgery. Both the retroperitoneal and transperitoneal approaches may be used in these patients, but extra care and consideration should be taken into account. Transperitoneal approaches have been associated with higher rates of retrograde ejaculation in comparison to retroperitoneal with elevation of the hypogastric plexus. Given the decrease in the rate of peritoneal scarring and retrograde ejaculation with retroperitoneal approaches, it has become the preferred approach by many surgeons. Therefore, the retroperitoneal approach will be the primary approach covered in this chapter.

The retroperitoneal approach can proceed from various incisions, including vertical midline, paramedian, oblique, and transverse. Extensive lateral incisions should be avoided because this may denervate the medially situated rectus muscle. The incision needs to take into account the spinal level and number of lumbar levels to be exposed. An infraumbilical transverse or vertical incision can accommodate most approaches to the L4–L5 and L5–S1 disc levels, whereas a more obliquely or vertically oriented incision is favored for

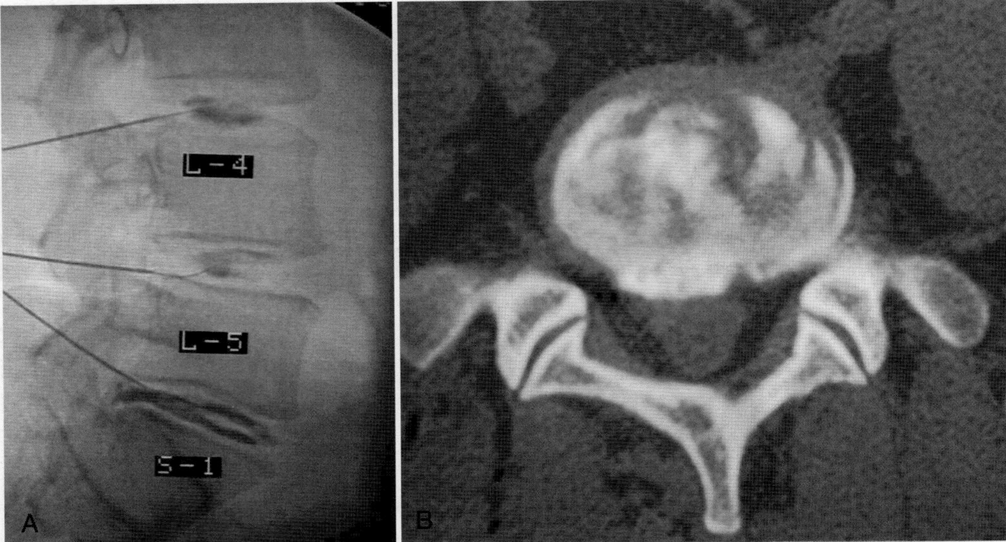

FIG. 49.1 (A) Lateral fluoroscopic image after discography with dye leaking into periphery of an abnormal L5–S1 disc. (B) Axial computed tomographic scan after discography shows abnormal disc morphology and dye extrusion into the peripheral anulus.

access to disc levels above L4 (Figs. 49.3 and 49.4). This incision allows for access to the L2–L3 disc level and possibly the L1–L2 disc level in patients with a favorable body habitus.

In most nonobese patients, palpation by an experienced access surgeon can be used to locate the sacral prominence to identify the L5–S1 disc space. An approach to the L4–L5 level should be directed at approximately the level of the anterior superior iliac spine, although fluoroscopic confirmation should be used if there is any question. All of the landmarks can be confirmed by fluoroscopic guidance. Fluoroscopy is especially important in patients who have distorted spine anatomy, who have had prior spine surgery, or are obese.

The incision is made and cautery is used to deepen the incision to the level of the anterior rectus sheath fascia. The fascia is incised; superior and inferior fascial flaps are then raised at the linea alba. Care should be taken in patients who have had previous Pfannenstiel incisions because they may have unrecognized midline incisional hernias. The mobilization of the fascial flaps provides for less tethering of the deeper tissues and rectus muscle. The left rectus muscle is bluntly mobilized to a lateral position, taking care to identify the inferior epigastric vessels and small perforators. By dissecting deep to these vessels, they can be preserved; however, they can be clipped and divided if necessary.

Inspection and gentle finger dissection can be used to identify the inferior edge of the posterior rectus sheath. This provides the landmark to begin blunt separation of the peritoneal cavity laterally to start the exposure into the retroperitoneal space (Figs. 49.5 and 49.6). The left ureter easily rolls up as part of this maneuver. The landmark to feel is the bulge of the psoas muscle and the pulse of the common iliac artery. A common mistake is to persist in aggressive dissection lateral to the psoas muscle thinking that the planes may be adhesed.

When the peritoneum has started to roll medially and the iliac artery has been palpated, the next landmark to be palpated should be the L5–S1 disc level. The L5–S1 disc space can be mobilized with the use of Kittner dissectors. The middle sacral vessels can be mobilized and divided between ligatures or small clips. Occasionally, anomalous venous drainage may be present across the sacral spine. This may include a single vessel as a bridging iliac vein to a confluent venous plexus across the region. The iliolumbar vein typically branches off posterior to the common iliac vein at the L5 vertebral level, and is an important consideration for exposure for the L4–L5 disc space above. Most of the time, it may be identified within 2 cm of the L4–L5 disc space. In a small percentage of patients, it may not be present. The common iliac artery can be easily visualized lateral to the vein and is usually bifurcating into the internal and external iliac arteries at the L5–S1 level. Blunt dissection generally can be used to expose the entire face of the L5–S1 disc level without significant need for major vascular mobilization (Fig. 49.7). Care should be taken during the mobilization to elevate the superior hypogastric plexus with the peritoneum, helping to avoid nerve injury and retrograde ejaculation in males. This plexus typically feels like a fibrous band within the peritoneal fat, and typically elevates with the peritoneal packet.

The L4–L5 disc level is generally the most difficult level to provide full access to for the spine surgeon. It is often at this level where the bifurcation commences, and can be difficult to mobilize. It is also important to look for vascular calcifications because calcification increases the potential risk for complications with an exposure at the L4–L5 level. After the retroperitoneum has been exposed, a plain film can be obtained to confirm the disc level. Gentle blunt dissection can be used to mobilize the left common iliac artery. This dissection should be continued distally well onto the external iliac artery to minimize potential trauma to the artery. Generally, the vascular structures should be mobilized as paired structures. If it is a high bifurcation, a thorough mobilization of the left common

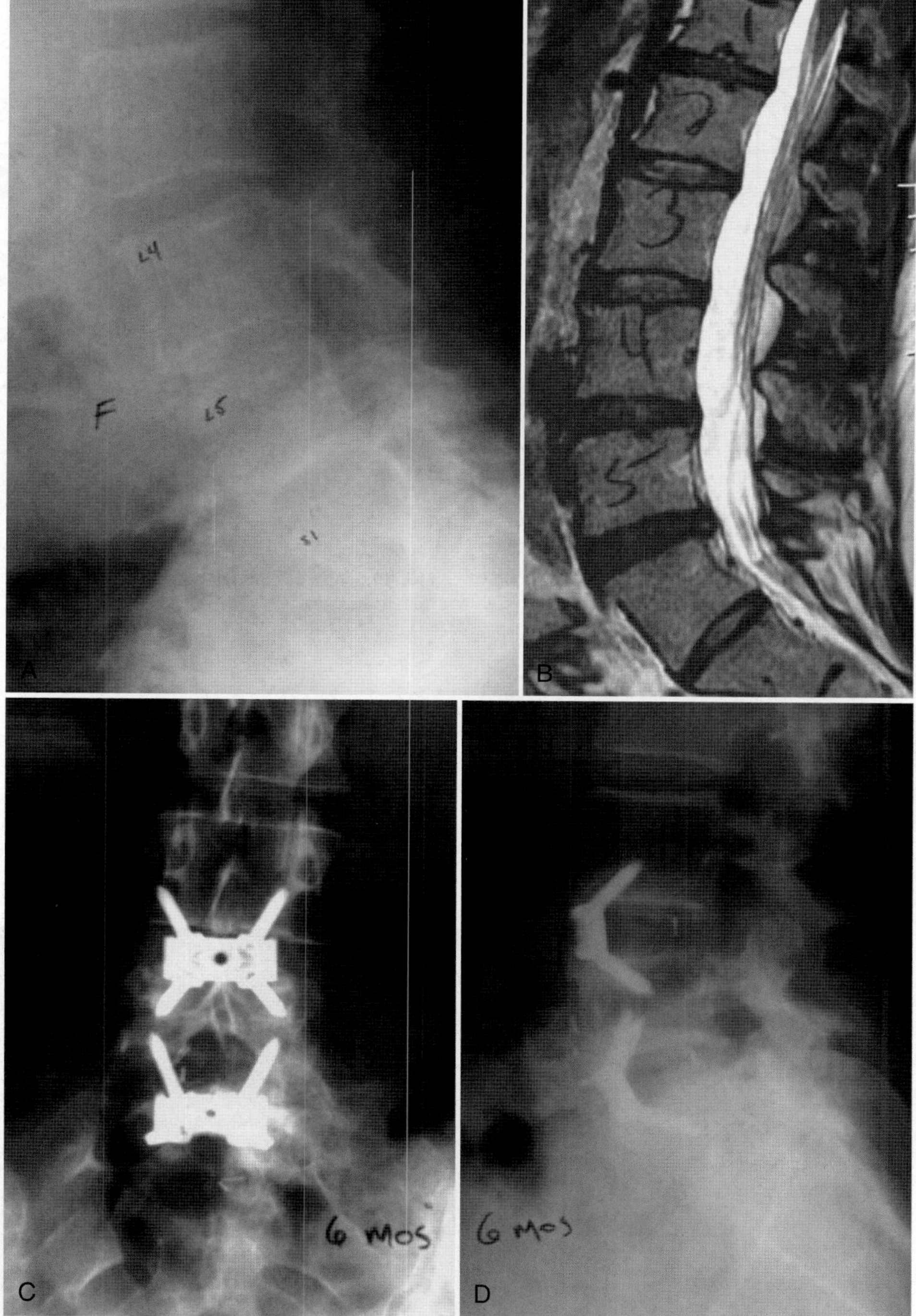

FIG. 49.2 (A) Preoperative plain radiograph and (B) T2-weighted sagittal magnetic resonance image showing two-level degenerative disc disease and 6-month postoperative plain (C) anteroposterior and (D) lateral radiographs. Note significant disc space and foraminal restoration using an anterior interbody spacer.

iliac artery and vein may allow them to be retracted laterally. Gentle Kittner dissection shows the iliolumbar vein as it branches off the posterolateral aspect of the common iliac vein, inferior to the L4–L5 disc. If it is not identified within approximately 15 to 20 mm of the disc space, it may not impede the exposure and, if not under tension, may be left intact.

Additional mobilization of the segmental vessels immediately adjacent and superior to the L4–L5 region is sometimes necessary (Fig. 49.8). Pulse oximetry, though optional, can be helpful when mobilizing vascular structures. Before retraction or mobilization, the oxygen saturation and waveform of a left lower extremity pulse oximeter should be evaluated. When retraction has been applied, if the saturation diminishes to

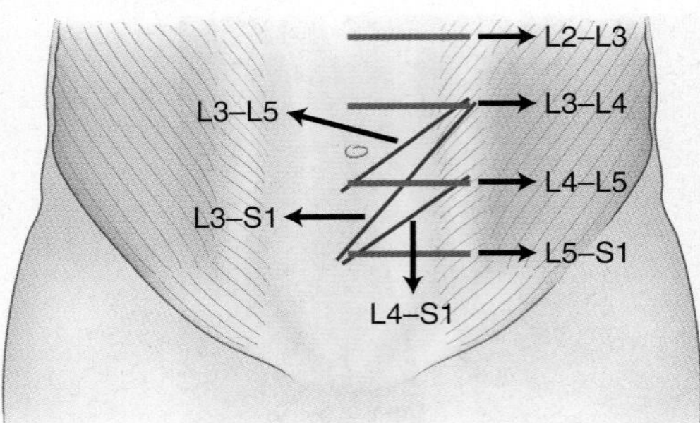

FIG. 49.3 Approximate level of incision.

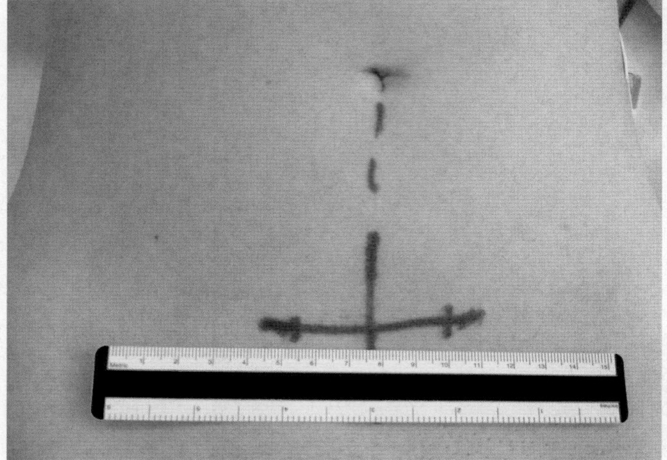

FIG. 49.4 Skin marking for the L5–S1 approach.

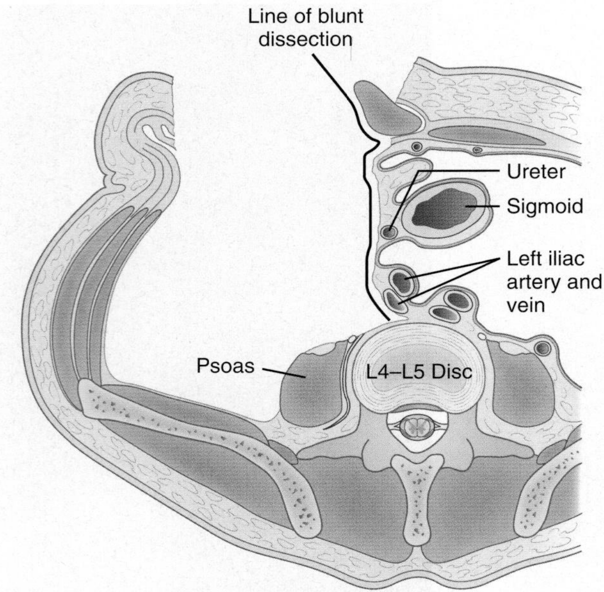

FIG. 49.6 Approach to retroperitoneum with the peritoneal packet mobilized medially.

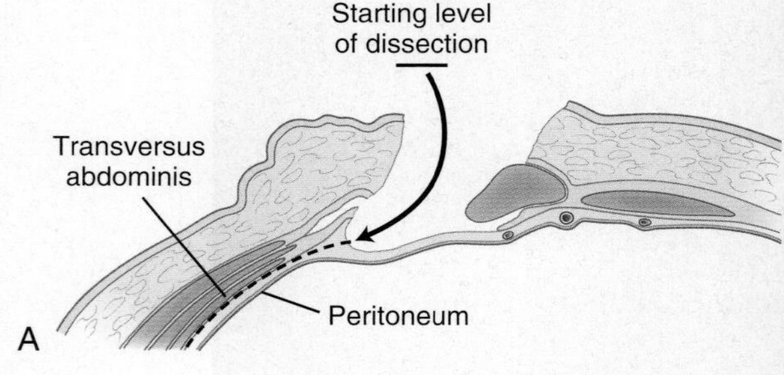

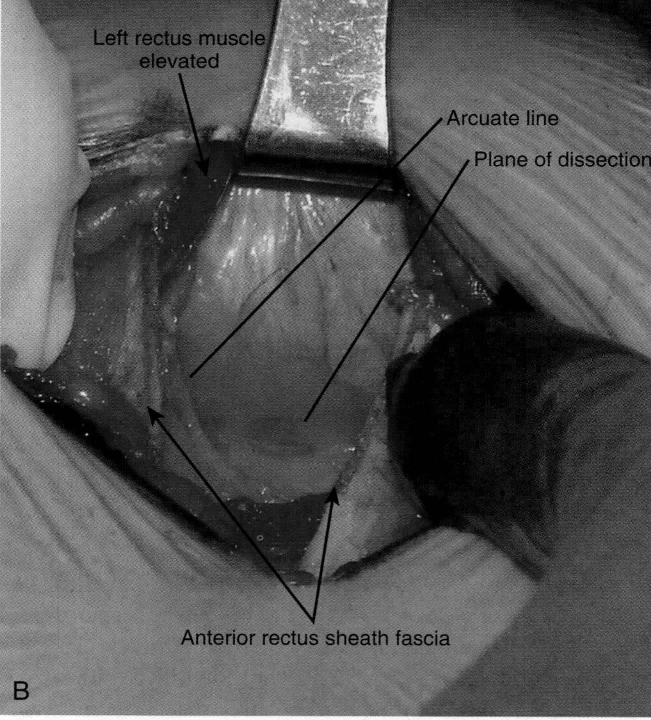

FIG. 49.5 (A) Initial retroperitoneal approach. (B) Initial approach with the peritoneum separated from the posterior rectus fascia.

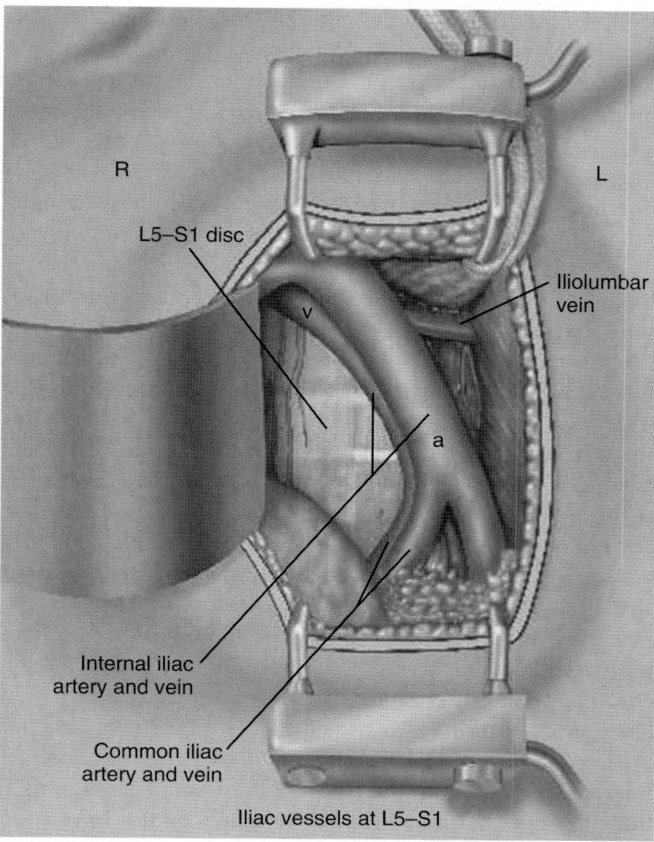

FIG. 49.7 Exposure of L5–S1 disc. a, artery; L, left; R, right; v, vein.

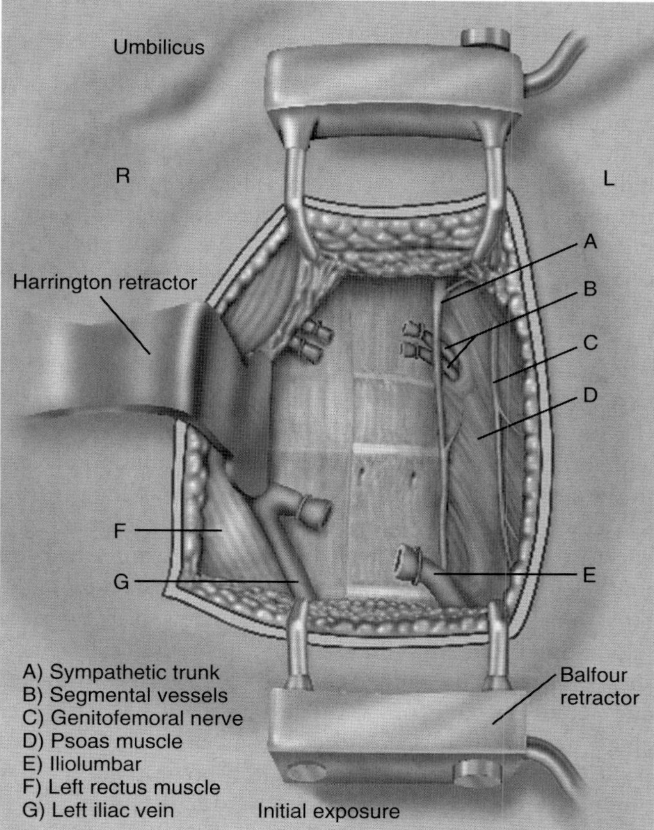

FIG. 49.8 Exposure of L4–L5 disc. L, left; R, right.

zero, the surgeon has approximately 45 to 50 minutes before the retraction should be released to allow for resumption of unimpeded blood flow. The waveform should normalize over a brief period before replacement of the retractors. This can be repeated with periodic release of the retractors every 30 minutes or so after that. If there is not a return to baseline over a few minutes, vascular examination with ultrasound should be performed.

Indications for Interbody Fusions

Choosing to proceed with operative intervention on the spine should be a joint decision reached by the patient and the physician. Prospective patients should have tried and failed nonoperative management, and the clinical and radiographic picture should correlate to maximize results and patient satisfaction. ALIF can be chosen to aid patients with (1) DDD and the spectrum of clinical and radiographic changes noted under this umbrella term; (2) pain after prior posterior surgery, such as laminectomy, in which significant epidural scar may complicate a revision surgery; and (3) significant low back pain with two or more recurrent herniated discs.

Axial back pain caused by the degenerative process of the disc and spine as a whole is currently the main indication for ALIF. By correctly identifying discogenic pain via radiographs, magnetic resonance imaging (MRI), and provocative discography, one can remove the pathologic disc and stabilize the segment with an interbody graft (see Figs. 49.1 and 49.2). Using an ALIF procedure, patients with associated radicular leg pain secondary to foraminal narrowing can be indirectly decompressed by restoring the foraminal height, elongating redundant posterior and lateral anulus (if not removed), and realigning overlapping incongruent facet joints and more directly decompressed by removing compressive nuclear material.[8,9] Patients with a herniated nucleus pulposus can undergo direct decompression and discectomy via an anterior exposure. Interbody implants placed through an anterior approach can be used alone or in conjunction with posterior fusion techniques for cases requiring a more robust fusion construct.

Interbody Implants and Graft Material

The race between temporary mechanical support and biology has been run since the origins of orthopaedic care. In the spine, the goal of any interbody device is to provide anterior column mechanical support while a bony fusion develops. A single question remains to be answered: How rigid does a construct need to be to provide early stability without negatively affecting the spine when fusion is present? Creating an unnecessarily stiff construct may lead to stress shielding,[10] additional surgery, and implantation of costly implants; however, too little stiffness leads to biomechanical failure or pseudarthrosis. Pilliar and colleagues[11] showed that small micro-motion of 28 µm does not affect bone ingrowth into porous-surfaced implants and large micro-motion greater

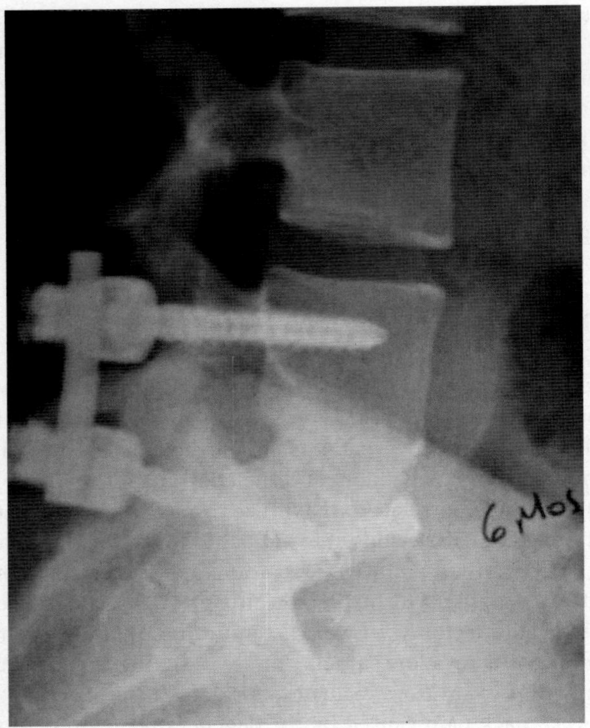

FIG. 49.9 Six-month follow-up lateral radiograph of graft using femoral ring allograft and bone morphogenetic protein, with posterior bilateral pedicle screws showing bone bridging and solid fusion.

than 150 μm can produce a fibrous interface. Nevertheless, the current consensus seems to be that adequate stabilization must greatly increase the stiffness above the native segment.

Femoral ring allograft (FRA), a frequently used method, obviates the need for cortical autograft and provides a strut with significant compressive strength,[12,13] incorporates with host bone, and provides a medium easier than metal to evaluate graft incorporation (Fig. 49.9). Previously, allograft rings were fashioned by surgeons on back operating room tables, but now can be commercially obtained. To augment fusion, allograft or autograft cancellous bone can be placed in the center of the cortical ring. FRA as a stand-alone intervertebral spacer has been shown to have a high rate of pseudarthrosis and subsidence.[14,15] Anterior or posterior augmentation has been recommended.

Transforaminal lumbar interbody fusion and posterior lumbar interbody fusion have allowed surgeons to place interbody grafts from posterior approaches, providing anterior column support and negating anterior exposures. Posterior-based surgery has been shown, however, to have increased operative time, patient morbidity, and complications compared with anterior-based surgery.[16,17] Also, patient anatomy and the degree of pathology can make achieving an adequate discectomy and ideal graft size and position and placement a challenge. These factors have contributed to less restoration of disc height, less than complete fusion bed preparation, and less mechanical stability at the time of implantation than with ALIF.

Previously, stand-alone anterior interbody grafts were fraught with reported complications, such as migration, subsidence, and pseudarthrosis. As interbody graft technology has progressed, there has been renewed interest, however, in stand-alone anterior interbody fusion, single-approach procedures. Biomechanical studies have reported that stand-alone anterior interbody grafts without fixation are weakest in shear strength, rotation, and extension.[18] The addition of a blocking screw or plate for FRA and synthetic spacers such as polyetheretherketone (PEEK) has minimized the occurrence of anterior migration. Currently available in PEEK, metal carbon fiber, and machined allograft and other various materials and combinations, interbody synthetic grafts have been optimized compared with their predecessors. Cage design from cylindric to a box shape has led to better matching of the endplate geometry and has been shown to decrease motion at the intervertebral segment.[19] Grant and colleagues,[20] performing a human cadaveric biomechanical investigation, showed that lumbar endplate density and thickness increased toward the periphery, with the strongest being posterolateral just in front of the pedicles.

Larger, more robust, locking and nonlocking plates have been used to augment a stand-alone interbody graft; although effective, these plates require increased exposure and have a large anterior profile. To negate the exposure necessary for plating and minimize soft tissue and vessel irritation, anterior interbody synthetic products with incorporated plates or fixation through the graft into the vertebral bodies have been developed. By increasing their stand-alone biomechanical strength to minimize extension and shear forces, one hopes that these products may negate the need for a robust anterior plating and posterior surgery.

Many studies have shown the stability-enhancing effect of integrated anterior instrumentation and a biomechanical argument for stand-alone ALIF (Figs. 49.9 and 49.10). Kuzhupilly and colleagues[21] looked at stand-alone FRA versus industrial FRA with integrated crossed cancellous screws into the adjacent vertebral bodies. They found significant improvement in extension stability only. Le Huec and colleagues[22] tested a lateral entry–placed cage with plate augmentation and found a significant increase in stiffness in all loading directions. No statistical significance was noted whether or not the plate was attached to the cage.

Schleicher and colleagues[23] compared the SYNFIX LR (DePuy Synthes) and the STALIF (Centinel Spine), two stand-alone ALIF cages, and found a statistically significant increase in stiffness over the native in vitro segment, with the SYNFIX LR, a locking four-screw implant, showing a higher stabilizing effect in lateral bending than the STALIF. Flexion-extension finite element analysis revealed that the cage bears most of the force in flexion, and the screws and the screw–plate interface take most of the stress in extension. Cain and colleagues[24] showed the SYNFIX LR had equal stiffness versus 270-degree and 360-degree constructs. The test device showed a higher ability to withstand axial torque compared with standard pedicle screw instrumentation. At the present time, a few products have US Food and Drug Administration (FDA) approval for stand-alone interbody use, with many more devices seeking approval.

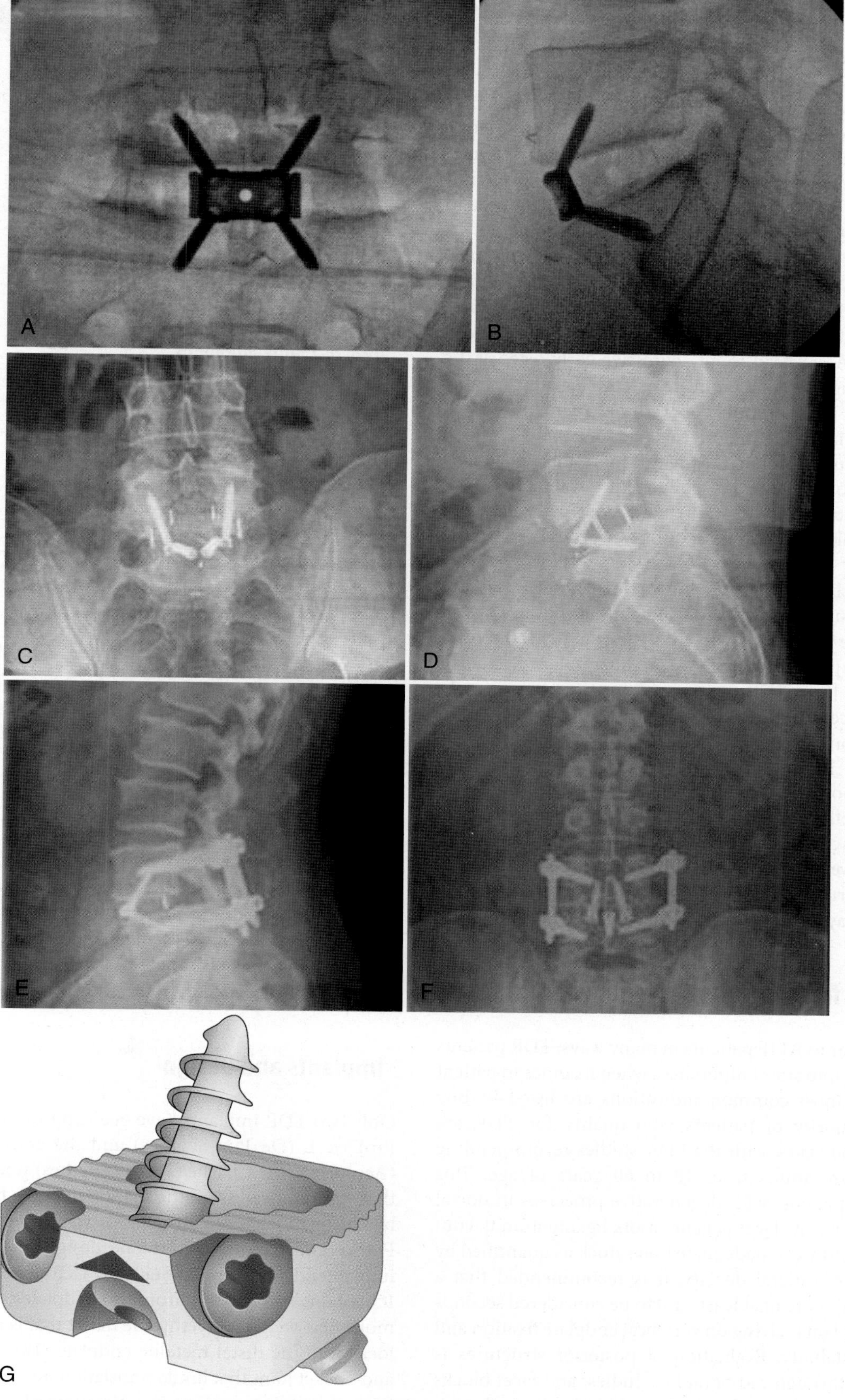

FIG. 49.10 (A) Anteroposterior and (B) lateral radiographs of the lumbar spine demonstrating a standalone L5–S1 interbody fusion cage (Arcadius L, Aesculap). (C) Anteroposterior and (D) lateral radiographs of MIDLINE II (Centinel Spine) cage utilized in a 360-degree fusion construct. (E) Lateral and (F) anteroposterior radiographs of MIDLINE II (Centinel Spine) cage in a 360-degree fusion construct. (G) Depiction of MIDLINE II. (G, Courtesy Centinel Spine, West Chester, PA.)

Most current implants allow the incorporation of graft material to augment the fusion process. Historically, the gold standard has been autogenous morcellized bone graft; however, to minimize patient morbidity, allograft and biologic materials have been developed. Multiple studies have evaluated allograft efficacy in fusion patients as extenders and stand-alone with good results.[25] The addition of the recombinant human bone morphogenetic protein (rhBMP-2) Infuse Bone Graft (Medtronic) has been shown to promote osteoinduction and to stimulate early incorporation of grafts (see Fig. 49.9).[26,27] Burkus and colleagues[27] reported 100% fusion rate with stand-alone interbody fusion using threaded cylinder allograft dowels with rhBMP compared with autograft. Pradhan and colleagues[28] showed, however, that the use of rhBMP-2 with stand-alone FRA can lead to an aggressive early osteoclastic response, causing graft and endplate osteolysis with potential subsidence risk. These authors believed that augmenting with intersegmental instrumentation can support the FRA with bone morphogenetic protein during this mechanically vulnerable time. Although bone morphogenetic protein has been shown to enhance fusions, it still remains controversial due to its perceived link to increased rates of cancer and retrograde ejaculation.[29]

Now the technology is moving to incorporate titanium porous-coated surfaces to allow better initial interference fit and to promote bone ingrowth into the cage (MIDLINE II [Centinel Spine], Arcadius^{XP} L [Aesculap Implant Systems], Lucent Ti-Bond [Spinal Elements]), making the cages not only function as spacers and carriers of the graft, but as part of the fusion mass. Some of these new cages are prior PEEK cages that have been impregnated with porous titanium at their contact with bony endplates, while others are completely made out of metal alloy. Some even go further by incorporating new manufacturing procedures, such as three-dimensional printing, to give increased surface area for bone ingrowth (ALIF Spine Truss System [4WEB Medical]). These newer cage designs may also be classified as bioactive implants.

BOX 49.1 Common Indications and Contraindications for Lumbar Total Disc Arthroplasty

Indications

- Age 18 to 60 y
- Symptomatic degenerative disc disease L3–L4 to L5–S1 with or without confirmatory discography
- Failure of nonoperative therapy for at least 6 mo
- No significant facet disease
- Bone density dual-energy x-ray absorptiometry T-score >–1.0
- No previous retroperitoneal approach
- No significant arterial calcification
- Spondylolisthesis or pars defects
- Recurrent disc herniation contiguous with disc space with significant low back pain in a patient with no other contraindication who would be considered to be a fusion candidate

Absolute Contraindications

- Poor bone quality (e.g., osteoporosis, osteopenia, metabolic bone disease, tumor)
- Severe facet degeneration
- Spondylolisthesis and spondylolysis
- Circumferential stenosis
- Scoliotic deformity >11 degrees
- Current or past trauma to involved vertebrae
- Morbid obesity
- Infection
- Autoimmune disorder

Relative Contraindications

- Age older than 60 y
- Psychosocial disorder
- Multiple degenerative disc disease levels
- Obesity
- Previous lumbar surgery if facet joint compromised

Indications for Total Disc Replacement

Although similar to ALIF patients in many ways, TDR patients have some very important differences when it comes to patient selection. The most common indications are listed in Box 49.1.[30] The majority of patients who qualify for TDR are younger than 60 years, with the FDA studies recommending skeletally mature adults from 18 to 60 years of age. This excludes most patients with degenerative processes in dorsal spinal structures (e.g., facet degeneration, ligamentum flavum hypertrophy) and with inadequate bone stock as quantified by evaluating bone mineral density. It is recommended that a patient have a T-score of at least –1.0 to be considered secondary to TDR implants relying on vertebral endplate fixation and ingrowth for stability. Evaluation of posterior structures is typically done through radiographic studies, and facet blocks may be used to diagnose facet-mediated pain. Even though ventral insertion of a TDR may offer some indirect decompression, circumferential stenosis is best treated by direct decompression of neural elements through a dorsal approach with fusion, if needed. Studies have shown that the disc space preparation necessary for insertion of a TDR can increase rotational instability of the spine. The currently available semiconstrained disc replacements do not fully restore this stability.[31] Therefore, TDR in a spine with preexisting rotational instability (Cobb angle >11 degrees) might be expected to result in higher failure rates, thus is not recommended.

Implants and Design

Only two TDR implants have been approved by the FDA, the ProDisc L (De Puy Synthes) and the activL Artificial Disc (Aesculap). The Charité (DePuy Synthes) was a previous TDR that was removed from the market due to a business decision by the manufacturer. ProDisc L was developed in 1990 in France and has undergone one design revision. It was first implanted in the United States in October 2001 (Fig. 49.11). It contains two cobalt-chromium endplates, with a ultrahigh-molecular-weight polyethylene insert that is monoconvex and locks into the distal metallic endplate. This results in a ball-and-socket joint that limits translation but allows rotation and limited bending, making it a constrained device in terms of translation. A central keel on the endplates and plasma-sprayed titanium coating allow for bony fixation and ingrowth.

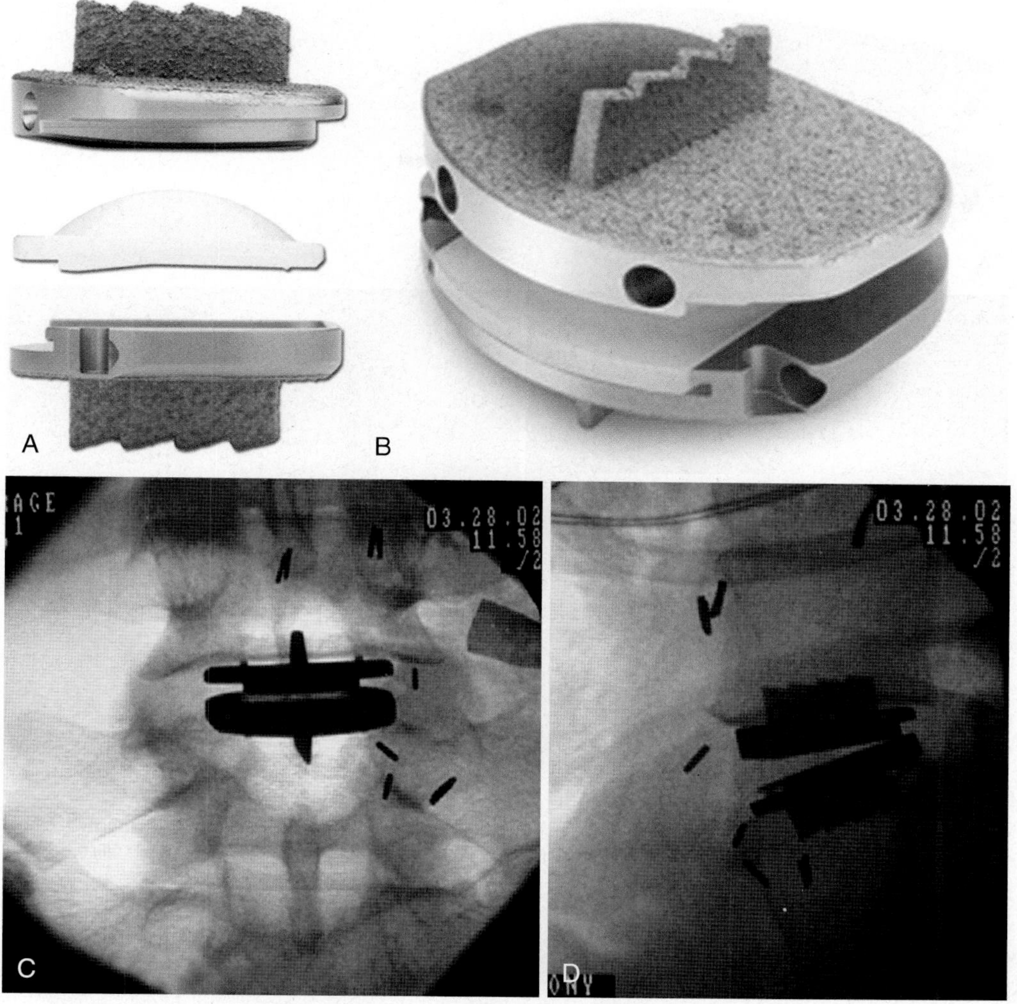

FIG. 49.11 ProDisc L lumbar disc replacement. (A) Three components. (B) Implant with ultrahigh-molecular-weight polyethylene component attached to caudal endplate, nested with cephalad endplate as it rests in vivo. (C) Anteroposterior and (D) lateral radiographs of device in vivo. (A and B, Courtesy DePuy Synthes, West Chester, PA.)

It is important when discussing disc replacements and their ability to maintain spinal motion to classify them in terms of degrees of freedom and constraint. There is controversy regarding the level of constraint in these implants. Most are classified as semiconstrained due to partial loss of degrees of freedom. The ball-and-socket articulation of the ProDisc L classifies it as being semiconstrained (see Fig. 49.11).

The activL was first released in June 2015 in the US market (Fig. 49.12). It is classified as a mobile bearing implant secondary to its translational abilities along with its traditional ball-and-socket attributes. The activL allows for continued rotation and bending motion, but also allows anterior to posterior translation. It also has a titanium coating (Plasmapore), making it a bioactive implant similar to the ProDisc L. The activL comes in a spike-and-keel version, but only the spike design is FDA approved in the United States. It does offer a wider range of implant sizes and angles, along with a sacral-specific design, than the ProDisc L. At this time, other designs have been approved for use in Europe with similar designs and features, but they have yet to be approved in the United States (Table 49.1). Many discs have undergone the investigational device exemption (IDE) trials, but have never been approved secondary to various reasons, including implant design (metal on metal), product safety, patient issues, and the extensive financial burden of the approval process.

Numerous studies have demonstrated the effectiveness of lumbar TDR. There are multiple FDA IDE trials with 2-year and 5-year follow-up and one with 10 years in a subset of patients.[32–40] There are multiple studies from Europe with over 10 years of follow-up.[34,41–43] There are three FDA IDE randomized control trials comparing TDR to fusion (ProDisc L, Charité, Maverick [Medtronic]) that consistently found TDR to have similar or superior outcomes compared with fusion.[35,36,44] The other 5-year study was an FDA IDE trial comparing two TDRs (Kineflex [SpinalMotion] vs. Charité) with good results in both groups.[45] Two studies have had a

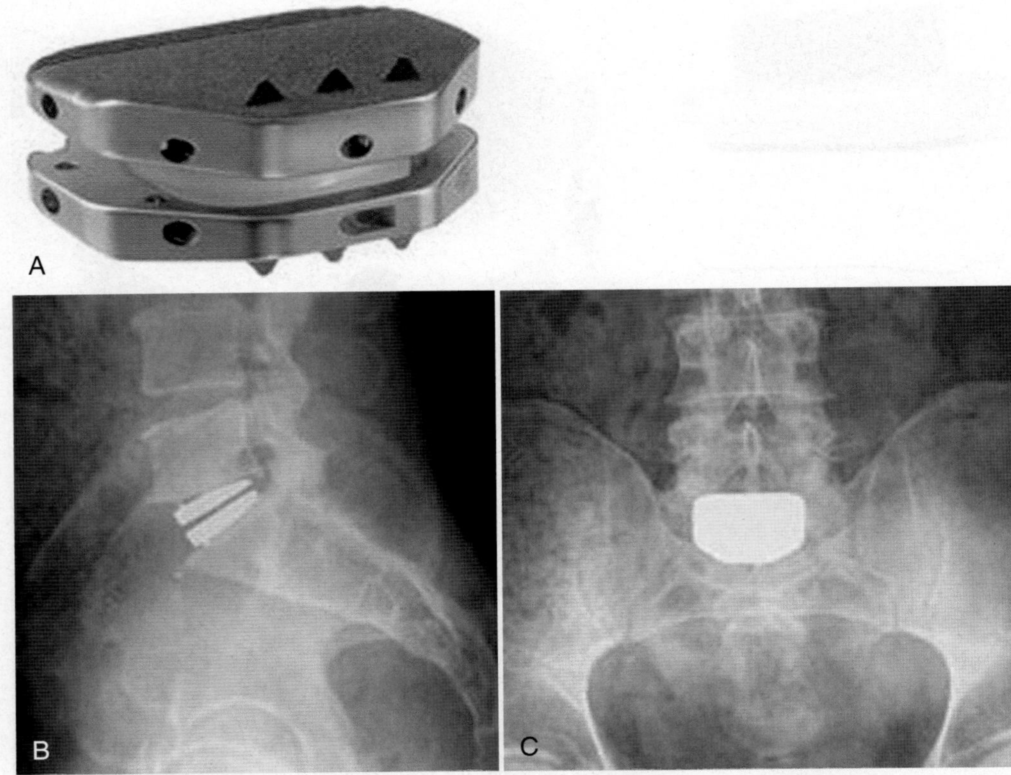

FIG 49.12 (A) Three components of the activL disc replacement: superior and inferior endplates with the ultrahigh-molecular-weight polyethylene component sliding into the inferior plate. (B) Anteroposterior view of an L5–S1 activL disc implanted. (C) Lateral radiograph of the activL disc implanted. (A, Courtesy Aesculap, Center Valley, PA.)

TABLE 49.1 Current Lumbar Total Disc Replacement Designs

Implant	Manufacturer	Key Features	Approved Use
Charité	DePuy Synthes	Two metal endplates with biconvex mobile with unconstrained motion and UHMWPE insert	Single-level lumbar disc replacement (discontinued 9/2011)
ProDisc L	DePuy Synthes	Two metal endplates with fixed uniconvex UHMWPE insert, ball-and-socket articulation with fixed center of rotation and constrained motion	Single-level lumbar disc replacement
Maverick	Medtronic	Two metal endplates with metal-on-metal articulation ball-and-socket type with constrained motion	Withdrawn due to patent issues
FlexiCore	Stryker Spine	Two metal endplates with metal-on-metal articulation ball-and-socket type with constrained motion	Withdrawn by Stryker
Kineflex	SpinalMotion	Two metal endplates with metal-on-metal articulation and semiconstrained motion	Withdrawn by sponsor
activL	Aesculap	Two metal endplates with UHMWPE insert with constrained motion	Single-level lumbar disc replacement
Freedom	Axiomed	Two titanium bead–coated endplates with rails for short-term fixation, notched endcap for device positioning with viscoelastic polymer core	FDA IDE study data collection is ongoing
M6 L	Spinal Kinetics	Two metal plates with UHMWPE artificial anulus and artificial polymer nucleus and viscoelastic motion	Not yet studied in the United States, but used in Europe
Mobidisc	Zimmer Biomet	Two metal endplates with self-centered UHMWPE creating an unconstrained motion	Being implanted in Europe

FDA, Food and Drug Administration; IDE, investigational device exemption; UHMWPE, ultrahigh-molecular-weight polyethylene.

2-year follow-up comparing TDR to fusion (ProDisc L two-level IDE, FlexiCore [Stryker]) with TDR outcomes similar or superior to fusion.[33,39]

Specifically, the ProDisc L two-level study enrolled 237 patients with 2-year follow-up that resulted in significantly less operative time, blood loss, and hospital stay compared with fusion.[33] The TDR group demonstrated preservation of range of motion (ROM) with greater improvements in visual analog scale (VAS) and Short Form-36) scores as well as patient satisfaction. In regard to two-level surgery, results of

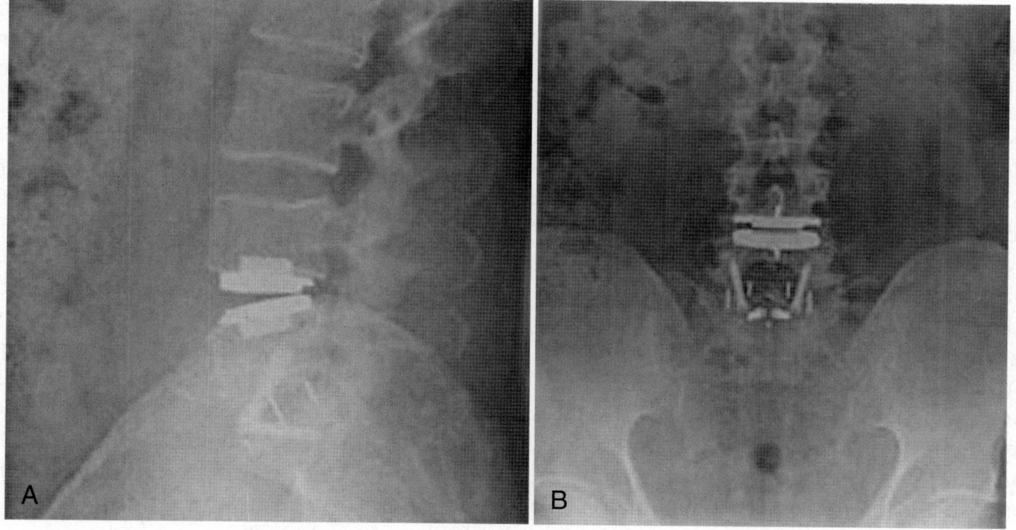

FIG. 49.13 Anteoposterior (A) and (B) lateral radiographs of a hybrid implantation with a ProDisc L and Arcadius L stand-alone interbody fusion device in a patient with two-level disc pathology with differing stages of degeneration.

10-year follow-up have been reported in a relatively small sample of patients from one site participating in the FDA trial.[41] They found that patient satisfaction was 92%, with 85% clinical success. The significant improvement in Oswestry Disability Index (ODI) scores were maintained during the long-term follow-up. Overall, there was a trend of similar or superior outcomes in the studies done in the United States comparing TDR to fusion and comparing different TDRs done for one- and two-level DDD.

Multiple studies from Europe have had a 5- to 10-year follow-up. In a 5-year study from Siepe et al., with a more than 90% follow-up rate, the satisfaction rate was 86.3% and there was a 2.2% adjacent-segment reoperation rate.[46] They also found that a one-level TDR had statistically better results on some measures compared with a two-level TDR, including a lower complication rate (11.9% vs. 17.6%), lower VAS and ODI scores, and higher satisfaction. Another long-term study was by Lemaire et al., with a minimum 10-year follow up with the Charité.[32] More than 90% of patients returned to work, and good/excellent outcomes and maintenance of ROM were found in over 95% of patients. Other studies with more than a 10-year follow-up replicated the results. Regarding other implants, there is a study from Lovi et al. with 51 patients from two centers in Europe using the Maverick at a single level.[34] They reported that back pain was improved in 84% of patients. There were no significant changes in adjacent discs and facet joints based on MRI at 10-year follow-up. Overall, studies in Europe had longer follow-up and replicated the results from the United States.

One of the major potential clinical benefits of lumbar TDR is reducing the occurrence of adjacent-level degeneration. Biomechanically, fusion increases intradiscal pressure, facet loading, and hypermobility above and beyond natural history. Risk factors for adjacent-level disease are pedicle screws, facet joint violation, sagittal malalignment, and fusion length. There is evidence showing significant difference in adjacent-level disease comparing TDR versus fusion (9.2% vs. 28.6%, respectively).[35] In the same study, among patients with normal adjacent levels preoperatively, significantly more TDR patients had no changes in these levels at 5 years postoperatively (90.8%) compared to fusion (71.4%). Adjacent segments were reoperated in 1.9% of patients who underwent TDR and in 4% of fusion patients.

A *hybrid construct* refers to the use of a lumbar disc replacement adjacent to a fusion. The TDR may be performed along with fusion of an adjacent level, or it may be performed adjacent to a previously fused level (Fig. 49.13). Both of these clinical scenarios are considered off-label use for the prostheses currently available for use in the United States based on the inclusion and exclusion criteria from the FDA IDE trials. The theoretical advantages of preventing adjacent-segment disease may have more utility when used in hybrid constructs. The advantages would be increased in longer fusions, which have a higher incidence of adjacent-segment disease.[47–50] Aunoble and colleagues[51] implanted hybrid constructs in 42 patients and followed them prospectively. At 2 years, ODI decreased by 53%. However, no prospective randomized level 1 data or long-term prospective data exist to support the regular use of these hybrid constructs.

Despite the overwhelming amount of scientific data supporting TDR in the lumbar spine, there still is a lack of approval by insurance companies for its use, with many of the major insurance carriers claiming TDR is still experimental or that it is a more costly procedure. However, when compared to fusion, as previously mentioned, it shows higher patient satisfaction outcomes and is more cost-effective than ALIF and anteroposterior procedures.[52–56] Along with almost no catastrophic failures or high revision rates, the TDR revision burden fell within range of hip and knee replacement, which are generally considered successful and cost-effective procedures.[52–56]

Postoperative Management

Postoperative management is quite similar for ALIF and TDR. Patient-controlled analgesia is instituted for pain control and weaned as bowel function and oral tolerance allow. The patient is mobilized the day of surgery, starting with chair transfers and assisted ambulation. A liquid diet is started after surgery and progressed as tolerated. Hospital stay is typically 1 to 3 days, based on patient type and surgery performed. Bracing is variable, dependent on stability of fixation, and is surgeon specific, ranging from an abdominal binder for comfort and incision healing to a rigid orthosis. The addition of instrumentation, bone morphogenetic proteins, and similar substances may obviate the need for rigid bracing in fusion patients. Activity should include limited bending and twisting motions, and lifting initially should be limited to 10 pounds or less. TDR patients are explicitly counseled to refrain from extension of the spine during the immediate postoperative period. Return to activities of daily living is progressively allowed and encouraged. Return to work and sports depends on the patient and surgeon, based on the patient's requirements, status of fusion, and fixation method. In general, TDR patients are released for all activities at 3 months.

Evaluation of fusion progression can be difficult in the presence of an interbody graft. Evaluation of fusions that is 100% reliable is available only with histologic examination, which is rarely possible or done. Radiolucent and nonferromagnetic implants, such as carbon fiber and polymer synthetics, have been developed to allow better visualization of surrounding bone and soft tissues on plain radiographs, MRI, and computed tomography (CT). Cizek and Boyd[57] evaluated cadaveric implant models radiographically and found neither CT nor radiographic interpretation reliable. Evidence of a fusion can be evaluated by the following radiographic features: (1) no motion on flexion-extension films (≤5 degrees has been accepted as fused in the literature and by the FDA); (2) anterior or posterior bridging bone across the disc space, called the *sentinel sign*[58]; (3) bridging trabecular bone across the intervertebral space and endplates; and (4) the absence of "a windshield wiping halo," or lucency around instrumentation, indicating implant motion.

In disc replacement patients, fixation of the implant is equally difficult. Once soft tissues are healed, fixation of the implant to the endplates is best judged on plain film radiographic images demonstrating good endplate–implant interface apposition and secondary bony integration, which usually occurs by 3 months. As with fusion and other implants, radiolucency of the bone-implant interface is indicative of motion and loosening.

Complications

The incidence of complications in anterior spinal surgery is often difficult to assess because of the different types of procedures, surgeons performing them, implants used, and experience of the operative team. Poor outcome is the number one surgical complication, and poor patient selection is often to blame; one must be vigilant in diagnostic workup and adhere to surgeries that address the patient's pain generators.

Vascular injury to the common iliac vessels with L5–S1 exposure is most commonly seen upon exposure for both TDR and ALIF patients. Clear identification of the disc space before discectomy must be obtained and maintained during the operation. In particular, the common iliac vein, being compressible and dorsal to the artery, can be mistaken for soft tissue during the approach. The iliolumbar vein, also called the *ascending lumbar vein,* is at risk during approaches to the L4–L5 interspace, and should be controlled as dictated by the amount of exposure necessary. Some surgeons believe that ligation of this vessel should be obtained in 100% of exposures to minimize the risk of tearing during retraction. Arterial thrombosis from aggressive retraction or injury, or both, has also been reported.[59,60]

Retrograde ejaculation as a result of hypogastric plexus injury has been reported to range from 0.4%[61] to 8%.[62] In one of the largest single ALIF trials to date, Kuslich and colleagues[63] reported a 4% rate in 591 patients. Loguidice and colleagues[64] in 58 patients and Brau[65] in 686 exposures each noted only one case of retrograde ejaculation. The preaortic (prevertebral) sympathetic plexus runs along the anterolateral edge of the vertebral bodies, adjacent to the psoas, then traverses over the aortic bifurcation and common iliac vessels forming the hypogastric plexus. Blunt dissection to mobilize the more cephalad prevertebral plexus before the hypogastric plexus can aid the exposure. Aggressive electrocautery should be minimized during the approach in this area and during the disc space preparation. Male patients should be counseled on this potential adverse event and advised that there also is a chance of spontaneous recovery. Most patients, even if retrograde ejaculation occurs, are still able to achieve sexual satisfaction, but may still have difficulty fathering a child. If the patient is concerned, he can predonate and store sperm, or some urologists recommend recovery of the sperm in affected individuals.

Injury to the alimentary tract can be minimized by packing the peritoneum behind self-retaining retractors. Postoperative ileus occurs and can be effectively managed with restricted oral intake, proper fluid hydration, and gastric suction, as indicated. Damage to the bladder and ureter, rare in primary cases, can be minimized by routine use of a Foley catheter and, in revision cases, with proper identification and the placement of preoperative ureteral stents.

Fusion implant-related complications, such as graft subsidence, malposition, extrusion, and pseudarthrosis, as alluded to previously in this chapter, can be minimized with careful patient selection, careful implant selection, and meticulous discectomy to optimize the fusion bed without disrupting the structural integrity of the subchondral bony endplates. The proper height graft should be selected to restore "normal" disc height, avoiding overdistraction.

Complications in TDR surgery can be divided into previously mentioned approach-related, device-related, and patient-related complications.[66] Device-related complications include implant subsidence, migration or extrusion, malposition, and material wear or reaction. Subsidence is by far the most common issue, seen in up to 9% of TDRs in older studies and from 0% to 3% of patients in more recent trials.[30,36,67] Subsidence has also been observed in up to 67% of patients with failed TDR outcomess.[68] Of note, no clear clinical effect of subsidence on outcomes has yet been demonstrated. This complication may be minimized by excluding patients with poor bone quality and seating the largest implants on the more cortical peripheral edges of the vertebral endplates. The risk of device migration or extrusion depends significantly on implant design, placement, and sizing. A TDR inserted in the midline—which can be fixed to bone with spikes or keels, promotes bony ingrowth to the endplates, and is sized to provide good soft tissue tension—would have a very low chance of migrating. In earlier studies, the rates of migration were up to 7%,[68] but with improved designs and surgical experience, more recent studies have shown rates of 0% to 2.4%.[36,42] There have been several reports of confirmed adverse reactions to particulate wear debris. There are also controversies surrounding metal-on-metal implants, mostly due to the concerns existing about the release of metal ions into the bloodstream.[69] Most device-related complications are iatrogenic and can be minimized with proper patient selection, operative technique, and implant sizing and position. Malpositioning is the main reason for significant wear in these implants.

Patient-related complications include adjacent-level disc degeneration, same-level facet degeneration, and heterotopic ossification. Successful motion preservation is the main mechanical goal of lumbar TDR. This has been well documented.[37,70] Adjacent-segment degeneration seen after arthrodesis is thought to be related to increased stress at adjacent segments due to transfer of extra motion and loads from the fused segment. Currently, there is only one long-term study that definitively shows that motion preservation using TDR avoids accelerated adjacent-segment degeneration in a 5-year follow-up.[35] Intermediate-term data by Huang et al. using the PRODISC show that ROM of at least 5 degrees is needed for improved clinical outcomes and reduction in degeneration of adjacent discs.[71]

The presence of degenerative disease in the facet joints is a contraindication to lumbar TDR. Early disease in the facets may be missed during initial screening, and patients may continue to experience pain after surgery from persistent motion in these degenerated posterior structures. In a study assessing 175 patients complaining of persistent pain after PRODISC II implantation, facet joints were confirmed as a source of pain by fluoroscopically guided blocks in 12.6% of patients, mostly at the index level (84%).[43] Van Ooij et al. reported facet joint arthrosis in 42% of patients with persistent pain after Charité TDR.[68] All 29 patients with failed TDRs in a study by Rosen et al. had evidence of facet distraction or compression on CT.[57] Facet distraction was also associated with radiculopathy, likely from capsular stretch.

TDR design may also affect the manner in which the facets are loaded. In the normal lumbar spine, facets are loaded with ventral shear forces. Implants with a fixed center of rotation, such as the ProDisc, absorb anteroposterior shear forces, thus creating greater stress within the implant and at the implant–bone interface, while sparing the facets. The fixed center of rotation creates a greater arc of motion to compensate for the lack of translation. This changes the kinematics of a facet joint, causing greater stresses at the extremes of flexion and extension.[72]

Heterotopic ossification, limiting TDR's ROM, is of some concern. Although it was observed often with earlier implant designs, studies with modern TDRs show significantly lower rates. In addition, Tortolani et al. reviewed data from the Charité IDE study and evaluated the clinical significance of heterotopic ossification.[73] Of 276 patients, 12 (4.3%) had radiographic evidence of new bone formation. All of these patients had ROMs and clinical outcomes similar to the rest of the study population.

The complication rates with TDR surgeries are relatively low. Nevertheless, strategies for revision have been developed. If additional surgery is necessary, either an anterior or a posterior approach is used. Repeat ventral surgery carries a significantly higher risk of intraoperative complications. In the Charité IDE study, the incidence of vessel injury during reoperation was significantly greater than that with the index operation (16.7% vs. 3.6%), mostly because of scarring to the vertebral column.[74] Other structures at risk due to scarring and distorted anatomy are the ureters and the lumbosacral trunk. These complications may be minimized with use of preoperative angiography and the intraoperative placement of intravascular balloons and ureteral stents.

An alternative revision procedure involves posterior fusion with rigid instrumentation. This strategy avoids the area of previous surgery and solves problems of instability. Cunningham et al. performed an in vitro biomechanical analysis of such a construct. They found that augmentation of an anteriorly placed TDR with posteriorly placed pedicle screws provided stability similar to that of the combination of anterior cage and posterior pedicle screws (circumferential fusion construct).[75] If TDR components must be removed because of dislodgement or malposition, however, the posterior approach is inadequate. Alternative approaches, such as transperitoneal, contralateral retroperitoneal, and transpsoas (for levels L4–L5 and above), have been described.[76–78] A prophylactic strategy involves placing an antiadhesive barrier over the vertebral column after TDR implantation to prevent scarring after a primary anterior approach. Various liquid and solid products are available and have been shown to be effective in adhesion prevention with abdominal and pelvic surgery.[79]

Acknowledgment

We thank Karl Lelkes, MD, and Ernesto Lopez, MD, for their contributions to this chapter.

PEARLS AND PITFALLS: ALIF

1. Careful patient selection is the key to successful surgery and maximization of outcomes.
2. Meticulous disc space preparation that avoids endplate violation is important for proper fit of the implant.

3. Selection of an implant depends on the disc space anatomy to allow the best fit and contact with endplates.
4. An implant of the proper height should be selected to restore "normal" disc height, avoiding overdistraction.

PEARLS: TDR

1. Level 1 scientific evidence for the efficacy of lumbar TDR exists for one- and two-level DDD, although US FDA approval is currently only for single-level use.
2. Preoperative CT scans should be considered in all lumbar TDR patients to assess for facet arthrosis and to ensure that there is no preoperative unrecognized spondylolysis.
3. DEXA scans should be obtained preoperatively in patients older than 50 years or if there are other clinical risk factors for osteoporosis because osteopenia (T-score of ≤−1.0) is a contraindication to lumbar disc replacement.
4. Care should be taken to preserve the bony endplates. Endplate insufficiency is an indication to convert to fusion.
5. Radiographic confirmation of the midline in the coronal plane (on anteroposterior fluoroscopic view) is imperative before final disc space preparation and implant insertion.

PITFALLS: TDR

1. Failure to identify the patient's pain generator adequately may lead to a higher clinical failure rate than published series.
2. Extremely easy mobilization and distraction of a collapsed disc space may point to unrecognized defects in the pars interarticularis.
3. Failure to mobilize the motion segment adequately before implant insertion or attempts to stuff the disc space with the tallest TDR implant would result in limited postoperative ROM.
4. Implant insertion with inadequate anterior exposure may result in device positioning unacceptably off the midline.
5. For revision anterior surgery for device removal, the surgeon should consider an alternative approach to the disc space from the original approach.

KEY POINTS: ALIF

1. Knowledge of the retroperitoneal anatomy is essential.
2. Both TDR and ALIF are safe and effective procedures in the hands of experienced spine surgeons.
3. Patient selection is key to a successful outcome.
4. A wide variety of graft materials and constructs are available with varying degrees of stability that may or may not necessitate posterior fixation.
5. Complications can be kept to a minimum with careful surgical technique.

KEY POINTS: TDR

1. The US FDA IDE clinical trials for the various devices provide level 1 prospective randomized data showing clinical success for fusion and TDR for properly selected patients with chronic back pain secondary to disc degeneration.
2. Despite the noninferiority design of the clinical trials, the published data seem to indicate that a well-implanted, functional disc replacement can result in a better clinical outcome than a fused segment.
3. Revision and removal of the current lumbar TDR devices remain quite technically challenging.
4. Long-term results are also needed to see if current motion preservation designs are effective in preventing adjacent-segment degeneration seen with lumbar fusions.

KEY REFERENCES

1. Burkus JK, Gornet MF, Dickman CA, et al. Anterior lumbar interbody fusion using rhBMP-2 with tapered interbody cages. *J Spinal Disord Tech*. 2002;15:337-349.
   This article provides strong evidence in favor of the use of bone morphogenetic protein as an alternative to harvesting iliac crest autograft for patients undergoing ALIF.
2. Brau S. Mini-open approach to the spine for anterior lumbar interbody fusion: description of the procedure, results and complications. *Spine*. 2002;2:216-223.
   This article presents a single surgeon's experience with 686 cases illustrating a very low complication rate associated with a mini-open approach to the anterior spine.
3. Cain CM, Schleicher P, Gerlach R, et al. A new stand-alone anterior lumbar interbody fusion device: biomechanical comparison with established fixation techniques. *Spine*. 2005;30:2631-2636.
   This article provides early in vitro biomechanical evidence for stand-alone ALIF using an integrated interbody device with screw fixation. The future success of these devices remains to be seen; however, they are an attractive option to decrease patient morbidity associated with posterior-based surgery.
4. Schofferman J, Slosar P, Reynolds J, et al. A prospective randomized comparison of 270 degrees fusions to 360 degrees fusions (circumferential fusions). *Spine*. 2001;26:E207-E212.
   The authors of this article challenge the need for posterolateral fusion in the setting of ALIF with anterior column support and pedicle screw fixation. They illustrate equal clinical outcomes and fusion rates with decreased cost, blood loss, and operative time.
5. Stauffer RN, Coventry MB. Anterior interbody lumbar spine fusion: analysis of Mayo Clinic series. *J Bone Joint Surg Am*. 1972;54:756-768.
   Early proponents of ALIF described the procedure as an alternative for patients who had previously undergone posterior decompressive surgery with persistent symptoms. Current proponents continue to praise the avoidance of revision canal surgery while providing anterior column support, restoration of disc height and lordosis, and indirect decompression of the neural elements.
6. Blumenthal S, McAfee PC, Guyer RD, et al. A prospective, randomized, multicenter Food and Drug Administration investigational device exemptions study of lumbar total disk replacement with the CHARITÉ™ artificial disc versus lumbar fusion. Part I: evaluation of clinical outcomes. *Spine*. 2005;30:1565-1575.
7. Cunningham BW. Basic scientific considerations in total disc arthroplasty. *Spine J*. 2004;4(suppl 6):219S-230S.
8. Zigler JE, Glenn J, Delamarter RB. Five-year adjacent-level degenerative changes in patients with single-level disease treated using lumbar total disc replacement with ProDisc-L versus circumferential fusion. *J Neurosurg Spine*. 2012;17:504-511.
9. Huang RC, Girardi FP, Cammisa FP Jr, et al. Correlation between range of motion and outcome after lumbar total disc replacement: 8.6-year follow-up. *Spine*. 2005;30:1407-1411.
10. Zigler J, Delamarter R, Spivak JM, et al. Results of the prospective, randomized, multicenter Food and Drug Administration investigational device exemption study of the ProDisc-L total disc replacement versus circumferential fusion for the treatment of 1-level degenerative disc disease. *Spine*. 2007;32:1155-1162.
    This article presents the data for the Prodisc-L pivotal FDA IDE study, finding one-level Prodisc-L noninferior to anteroposterior fusion for ODI and VAS pain improvement and significantly better than fusion for neurologic recovery, SF-36 improvement, and VAS

patient satisfaction at 2 years postoperatively, with an average maintenance of 7.7 degrees of flexion-extension motion.

11. Guyer RD, McAfee PC, Banco RJ, et al. Prospective, randomized, multicenter Food and Drug Administration investigational device exemption study of lumbar total disc replacement with the Charité artificial disc versus lumbar fusion: five-year follow-up. *Spine J*. 2009;9:374-386.
This article presents the 5-year follow-up data for the Charité pivotal FDA IDE study, which found maintenance of the 24-month result showing noninferiority of a one-level Charité TDR to ALIF with Bagby and Kuslich cages and iliac autograft at 5 years after the procedure.

REFERENCES

1. Katz JN. Lumbar disc disorders and low-back pain: socioeconomic factors and consequences. *J Bone Joint Surg Am*. 2006;88(suppl 2):21-24.
2. Crock HV. A reappraisal of intervertebral disc lesions. *Med J Aust*. 1970;16:983-989.
3. Freemont AJ, Peacock TE, Gourille P, et al. Nerve ingrowth into diseased intervertebral disc in chronic back pain. *Lancet*. 1997;350:178-181.
4. Weinstein J, Claverie W, Gibson S. The pain of discography. *Spine*. 1988;13:1344-1348.
5. Block AR, Ohnmeiss DD, Guyer RD, et al. The use of presurgical psychological screening to predict the outcome of spine surgery. *Spine J*. 2001;1:274-282.
6. Evans JH. Biomechanics of lumbar fusion. *Clin Orthop Relat Res*. 1985;193:38-46.
7. McAfee PC, Lee GA, Fedder IL, et al. Anterior BAK instrumentation and fusion: complete versus partial discectomy. *Clin Orthop Relat Res*. 2002;394:55-63.
8. Chen D, Fay LA, Lok J, et al. Increasing neuroforaminal volume by anterior interbody distraction in degenerative lumbar spine. *Spine*. 1995;20:74-79.
9. Sandu HS, Turner S, Kabo JM, et al. Distractive properties of a threaded interbody fusion device: an in vivo model. *Spine*. 1996;21:1201-1210.
10. Craven TG, Carson WL, Asher MA, et al. The effects of implant stiffness on the bypassed bone mineral density and facet fusion stiffness of the canine spine. *Spine*. 1994;19:1664-1673.
11. Pilliar RM, Lee JM, Maniatopoulous C. Observations on the effect of movement on bone ingrowth into porous-surfaced implants. *Clin Orthop Relat Res*. 1986;208:108-113.
12. Janssen ME, Nguyen C, Beckham R, et al. Biologic cages. *Eur Spine J*. 2000;9(suppl 1):S102-S109.
13. Summers BN, Eisenstein SN. Donor site pain from the ilium: a complication of lumbar spine fusion. *J Bone Joint Surg Br*. 1989;71:677-680.
14. Flynn JC, Hogue MA. Anterior fusion of the lumbar spine: end-result study with long-term follow-up. *J Bone Joint Surg Am*. 1979;61:1143-1150.
15. Kumar A, Kozak JA, Doherty BJ, et al. Interspace distraction and graft subsidence after anterior lumbar fusion with femoral strut allograft. *Spine*. 1993;18:2393-2400.
16. Fritzell P, Hagg O, Wessberg P, et al. Chronic low back pain and fusion: a comparison of three surgical techniques: a prospective multicenter randomized study from the Swedish Lumbar Spine Study Group. *Spine*. 2002;27:1131-1141.
17. Scaduto AA, Gamradt SC, Yu WD, et al. Perioperative complications of threaded cylindrical lumbar interbody fusion devices: anterior versus posterior approach. *J Spinal Disord Tech*. 2003;16:502-507.
18. Pizen T, Matthis D, Steudel WI. The effect of posterior instrumentation following PLIF with BAK cages is most pronounced in weak bone. *Acta Neurochir (Wien)*. 2002;144:121-128.
19. Tsantrizos A, Andreou A, Aebi M, et al. Biomechanical stability of five stand-alone anterior lumbar interbody fusion constructs. *Eur Spine J*. 2000;9:14-22.
20. Grant JP, Oxland TR, Dvorak MF. Mapping the structural properties of the lumbosacral vertebral endplates. *Spine*. 2001;26:889-896.
21. Kuzhupilly RR, Lieberman IH, McLain RF, et al. In vitro stability of FRA spacers with integrated crossed screws for anterior lumbar interbody fusion. *Spine*. 2002;27(9):923-928.
22. Le Huec J, Liu M, Skalli W, et al. Lumbar lateral interbody cage with plate augmentation: in vitro biomechanical analysis. *Eur Spine J*. 2002;11:130-136.
23. Schleicher P, Gerlach R, Schar B, et al. Biomechanical comparison of two different concepts for stand alone anterior lumbar interbody fusion. *Eur Spine J*. 2008;17:1757-1765.
24. Cain CM, Schleicher P, Gerlach R, et al. A new stand-alone anterior lumbar interbody fusion device: biomechanical comparison with established fixation techniques. *Spine*. 2005;30:2631-2636.
25. Hashimoto T, Shigenobu K, Kanayama M, et al. Clinical results of single-level posterior lumbar interbody fusion using the Brantigan I/F carbon cage filled with a mixture of local morselized bone and bioactive ceramic granules. *Spine*. 2002;27:258-262.
26. Boden SD, Zdeblick TA, Sandhu HS, et al. The use of rhBMP-2 in interbody fusion cages: definitive evidence of osteoinduction in humans: a preliminary report. *Spine*. 2000;25:376-381.
27. Burkus JK, Gornet MF, Dickman CA, et al. Anterior lumbar interbody fusion using rhBMP-2 with tapered interbody cages. *J Spinal Disord Tech*. 2002;15:337-349.
28. Pradhan BB, Bae HW, Kropf MA, et al. Kyphoplasty reduction of osteoporotic vertebral compression fractures: correction of local kyphosis versus overall sagittal alignment. *Spine*. 2006;31:435-441.
29. Dyrda L. *The future of spinal fusion: where BMP stands today & tomorrow. Becker's Spine Review*. 2014 Feb 12. Available at: http://www.beckersspine.com/spine/item/19610-the-future-of-spinal-fusion-where-bmp-stands-today-tomorrow.html.
30. Patel VV, Estes S, Lindley EM, et al. Lumbar spinal fusion versus anterior lumbar disc replacement: the financial implications. *J Spinal Disord Tech*. 2008;21:473-476.
31. McAfee PC, Cunningham BW, Hayes V, et al. Biomechanical analysis of rotational motions after disc arthroplasty: implications for patients with adult deformities. *Spine*. 2006;31:S152-S160.
32. Lemaire JP, Carrier H, Sariali el-H, et al. Clinical and radiological outcomes with the Charite artificial disc: a 10-year minimum follow-up. *J Spinal Disord Tech*. 2005;18:353-359.
33. Delamarter R, Zigler JE, Balderston RA, et al. Prospective, randomized, multicenter Food and Drug Administration Investigational Device Exemption study of the ProDisc-l total disc replacement compared with circumferential arthrodesis for the treatment of two-level lumbar degenerative disc disease: results at twenty-four months. *J Bone Joint Surg Am*. 2011;93:1-11.
34. Lovi A, Brayda-Bruno M, Hugues D, et al. *10 years follow up with Maverick total disc arthroplasty: clinical and radiological*

results. Miami, FL: International Society for the Advancement of Spine Surgery; 2014.
35. Zigler JE, Glenn J, Delamarter RB. Five-year adjacent-level degenerative changes in patients with single-level disease treated using lumbar total disc replacement with ProDisc-L versus circumferential fusion. *J Neurosurg Spine*. 2012;17: 504-511.
36. Guyer RD, Pettine K, Roh JS, et al. Comparison of 2 lumbar total disc replacements: results of a prospective, randomized, controlled multicenter Food and Drug Administration trial with 24-month follow-up. *Spine*. 2014;39:925-931.
37. Guyer RD, McAfee PC, Banco RJ, et al. Prospective, randomized, multicenter Food and Drug Administration Investigational Device Exemption study of lumbar total disc replacement with the CHARITE artificial disc versus lumbar fusion: five-year follow-up. *Spine J*. 2009;9:374-386.
38. Bertagnoli R, Yue JJ, Nanieva R, et al. Lumbar total disc arthroplasty in patients older than 60 years of age: a prospective study of the ProDisc prosthesis with 2-year minimum follow-up period. *J Neurosurg Spine*. 2006;4:85-90.
39. Sasso RC, Foulk DM, Hahn M. Prospective, randomized trial of metal-on-metal artificial lumbar disc replacement: initial results for treatment of discogenic pain. *Spine*. 2008;33: 123-131.
40. Thierry D. Long-term results of one-level lumbar arthroplasty: minimun 10-year follow-up of the CHARITE artificial disc in 106 patients. *Spine*. 2007;32:661-666.
41. Balderston JR, Gertz ZM, McIntosh T, et al. Long-term outcomes of 2-level total disc replacement using ProDisc-L: nine- to 10-year follow-up. *Spine*. 2014;39:906-910.
42. Tropiano P, Huang RC, Girardi FP, et al. Lumbar total disc replacement. Seven to eleven-year follow-up. *J Bone Joint Surg Am*. 2005;87:490-496.
43. Siepe CJ, Korge A, Grochulla F, et al. Analysis of post-operative pain patterns following total lumbar disc replacement: results from fluoroscopically guided spine infiltrations. *Eur Spine J*. 2008;17:44-56.
44. Blumenthal S, McAfee PC, Guyer RD, et al. A prospective, randomized, multicenter Food and Drug Administration investigational device exemptions study of lumbar total disk replacement with the CHARITÉ™ artificial disc versus lumbar fusion. Part I: evaluation of clinical outcomes. *Spine*. 1565–1575;30:2005.
45. Guyer RD, Pettine K, Coric D, et al. *Five-year follow-up of a prospective, randomized FDA IDE trial comparing two lumbar total disc replacements: clinical outcome and serum ion level analysis for a metal-on-metal device*. Scottsdale, AZ: International Society for the Study of the Lumbar Spine; 2013.
46. Siepe CJ, Heider F, Wiechert K, et al. Mid- to long-term results of total lumbar disc replacement: a prospective analysis with 5- to 10-year follow-up. *Spine J*. 2014;14:1417-1431.
47. Gillet P. The fate of the adjacent motion segments after lumbar fusion. *J Spinal Disord Tech*. 2003;16:338-345.
48. Hilibrand AS, Robbins M. Adjacent segment degeneration and adjacent segment disease: the consequences of spinal fusion? *Spine J*. 2004;4(6 suppl):190S-194S.
49. Park P, Garton HJ, Gala VC, et al. Adjacent segment disease after lumbar or lumbosacral fusion: review of the literature. *Spine*. 1938-1944;29:2004.
50. Throckmorton TW, Hilibrand AS, Mencio GA, et al. The impact of adjacent level disc degeneration on health status outcomes following lumbar fusion. *Spine*. 2003;28:2546-2550.
51. Aunoble S, Meyrat R, Al Sawad Y, et al. Hybrid construct for two levels disc disease in lumbar spine. *Eur Spine J*. 2010;19: 290-296.
52. Levin DA, Bendo JA, Quirno M, et al. Comparative charge analysis of one- and two-level lumbar total disc arthroplasty versus circumferential lumbar fusion. *Spine*. 2007;32: 2905-2909.
53. Guyer RD, Tromanhauser SG, Regan JJ. An economic model of one-level lumbar arthroplasty versus fusion. *Spine J*. 2007;7: 558-562.
54. Kurtz SM, Lau E, Ianuzzi A, et al. National revision burden for lumbar total disc replacement in the United States: epidemiologic and economic perspectives. *Spine*. 2010;35:690-696.
55. Johnsen LG, Hellum C, Storheim K, et al. Cost-effectiveness of total disc replacement versus multidisciplinary rehabilitation in patients with chronic low back pain: a Norwegian multicenter RCT. *Spine*. 2014;39:23-32.
56. Fritzell P, Berg S, Borgstrom F, et al. Cost effectiveness of disc prosthesis versus lumbar fusion in patients with chronic low back pain: randomized controlled trial with 2-year follow-up. *Eur Spine J*. 2011;20:1001-1011.
57. Cizek GR, Boyd LM. Imaging pitfalls of interbody spinal implants. *Spine*. 2000;25:2633-2636.
58. McAfee PC. Interbody fusion cages in reconstructive operations on the spine. *J Bone Joint Surg Am*. 1999;81: 859-880.
59. Rajaraman V, Vingan R, Roth P, et al. Visceral and vascular complications resulting from anterior lumbar interbody fusion. *J Neurosurg*. 1999;91(1 suppl):60-64.
60. Hackenberg L, Liljenqvist U, Halm H, et al. Occlusion of the left common iliac artery and consecutive thromboembolism of the left popliteal artery following anterior lumbar interbody fusion. *J Spinal Disord*. 2001;14:365-368.
61. Flynn JC, Price CT. Sexual complications of anterior fusion of the lumbar spine. *Spine*. 1984;9:489-492.
62. Christensen FB, Bunger CE. Retrograde ejaculation after retroperitoneal lower lumbar interbody fusion. *Int Orthop*. 1997;21:176-180.
63. Kuslich SD, Ulstrom CL, Griffith SL, et al. The Bagby and Kuslich method of lumbar interbody fusion: history, techniques, and 2-year follow-up results of a United States prospective, multicenter trial. *Spine*. 1998;23:1267-1278.
64. Loguidice VA, Johnson RG, Guyer RD, et al. Anterior lumbar interbody fusion. *Spine*. 1988;13:366-369.
65. Brau S. Mini-open approach to the spine for anterior lumbar interbody fusion: description of the procedure, results and complications. *Spine*. 2002;2:216-223.
66. Bertagnoli R, Zigler J, Karg A, et al. Complications and strategies for revision surgery in total disc replacement. *Orthop Clin North Am*. 2005;36:389-395.
67. Cinotti G, David T, Postacchini F. Results of disc prosthesis after a minimum follow-up period of 2 years. *Spine*. 1996;21: 995-1000.
68. van Ooij A, Oner FC, Verbout AJ. Complications of artificial disc replacement: a report of 27 patients with the SB Charite disc. *J Spinal Disord Tech*. 2003;16:369-383.
69. Cunningham BW. Basic scientific considerations in total disc arthroplasty. *Spine J*. 2004;4(suppl 6):219S-230S.
70. Zigler J, Delamarter R, Spivak JM, et al. Results of the prospective, randomized, multicenter Food and Drug Administration investigational device exemption study of the ProDisc-L total disc replacement versus circumferential fusion

for the treatment of 1-level degenerative disc disease. *Spine*. 2007;32:1155-1162.

71. Huang RC, Girardi FP, Cammisa FP Jr, et al. Correlation between range of motion and outcome after lumbar total disc replacement: 8.6-year follow-up. *Spine*. 2005;30:1407-1411.
72. Huang RC, Wright TM, Panjabi MM, et al. Biomechanics of nonfusion implants. *Orthop Clin North Am*. 2005;36:271-280.
73. Tortolani PJ, Cunningham BW, Eng M, et al. Prevalence of heterotopic ossification following total disc replacement. A prospective, randomized study of two hundred and seventy-six patients. *J Bone Joint Surg Am*. 2007;89:82-88.
74. McAfee PC, Geisler FH, Saiedy SS, et al. Revisability of the CHARITE artificial disc replacement: analysis of 688 patients enrolled in the U.S. IDE study of the CHARITE artificial disc. *Spine*. 2006;31:1217-1226.
75. Cunningham BW, Hu N, Beatson HJ, et al. Revision strategies for single- and two-level total disc arthroplasty procedures: a biomechanical perspective. *Spine J*. 2009;9:735-743.
76. Pimenta L, Diaz RC, Guerrero LG. Charite lumbar artificial disc retrieval: use of a lateral minimally invasive technique. Technical note. *J Neurosurg Spine*. 2006;5:556-561.
77. Wagner WH, Regan JJ, Leary SP, et al. Access strategies for revision or explantation of the Charite lumbar artificial disc replacement. *J Vasc Surg*. 2006;44:1266-1272.
78. Pimenta L, Oliveira L, Schaffa T, et al. Lumbar total disc replacement from an extreme lateral approach: clinical experience with a minimum of 2 years' follow-up. *J Neurosurg Spine*. 2011;14:38-45.
79. Patel AA, Brodke DS, Pimenta L, et al. Revision strategies in lumbar total disc arthroplasty. *Spine*. 2008;33:1276-1283.

SECTION VI

50 CHAPTER Posterior Lumbar Interbody Fusion

William J. Molinari III
Nathan H. Lebwohl

Introduction

The technique of posterior lumbar interbody fusion (PLIF) has become an important part of the modern spine surgeon's armamentarium. This was not always so; for nearly half a century after the introduction of this technique, it was performed routinely by only a handful of surgeons. Most surgeons condemned the technique as unnecessary, technically difficult, or even dangerous.[1,2] Controversy persists regarding the safety of PLIF compared with other approaches to the intervertebral space and regarding the benefit that PLIF adds to the outcome of surgical treatment for various spinal pathologies.

PLIF is an operation in which the disc space is exposed from a posterior approach, similar to that used in a discectomy, and a fusion is performed by directly grafting the intervertebral space. Classically, PLIF is performed via bilateral exposure of the disc space, with some retraction of the dura to expose the disc. When PLIF was first described, before the era of spinal instrumentation, advocates of the operation argued that it prevented collapse of the disc space after discectomy and maintained the height of the neural foramen, keeping the root free of bony compression. These advocates also believed that placing bone graft directly in the disc space would more likely result in healing of the fusion because the bone would be subject to compressive forces. Critics argued that the operation required excessive epidural dissection and nerve root retraction with a high risk of dural tear, epidural fibrosis, nerve root injury, and chronic arachnoiditis, and that graft displacement could lead to late neurologic compromise.

Historical Perspective

Attempts to identify the first surgeon to perform an interbody fusion from a posterior approach are muddled by several reports appearing in the published literature beginning in 1944,[3–5] but no one disputes that credit for initially developing the techniques and key principles of the operation as it is practiced today belongs to Cloward,[6] who emphasized the importance of a wide exposure of the spinal canal to minimize nerve root injuries, the use of structural graft to prevent intervertebral collapse, and the complete removal of nuclear material from the disc space and replacement with bone to promote fusion. Cloward was widely criticized for his operation, probably as much because he advocated that it be included as part of the routine surgical treatment for all lumbar disc herniations as for the frequency of poor outcomes and complications when it was attempted by other surgeons. A few surgeons embraced Cloward's operation, and several large surgical series were published in the literature reporting good outcomes and high fusion rates.[7–10] Widespread interest in and acceptance of PLIF as a valuable technique did not occur, however, until the introduction of pedicle screw instrumentation.

With the early generation of pedicle instrumentation, screw fracture was a common occurrence. Fracture especially occurred if a dramatic change in spinal alignment was achieved, such as in the reduction of a high-grade spondylolisthesis. Even without large changes in alignment, screw fracture occurred commonly in overweight patients or when the disc space was distracted.[11] In those cases, the mechanical loads that the instrumentation was subjected to exceeded the fatigue properties of the screws. Surgeons, in particular Steffee and Sitkowski,[12] recognized that a structural graft placed in the disc space would divert some of the load, decreasing the forces on the posterior instrumentation, and reduce the frequency of instrumentation failure. Steffee and Sitkowski[12] reported their experiences with reduction of high-grade spondylolisthesis. In each of the first three patients treated with pedicle screws, the instrumentation failed, and alignment was lost. In the next 11 patients, an interbody graft was placed. All of these patients developed solid fusions with no loss of alignment. With PLIF, the load-sharing anterior column support could be added to protect the pedicle screws without the need for a separate anterior incision (Fig. 50.1).

Simultaneous with the benefit of PLIF on reducing failures of the new instrumentation, pedicle instrumentation had a beneficial effect on the outcome of PLIF surgery. For the first time, rigid fixation was available that could effectively stabilize the lumbar spine after laminectomy. This fixation virtually eliminated the complication of graft displacement

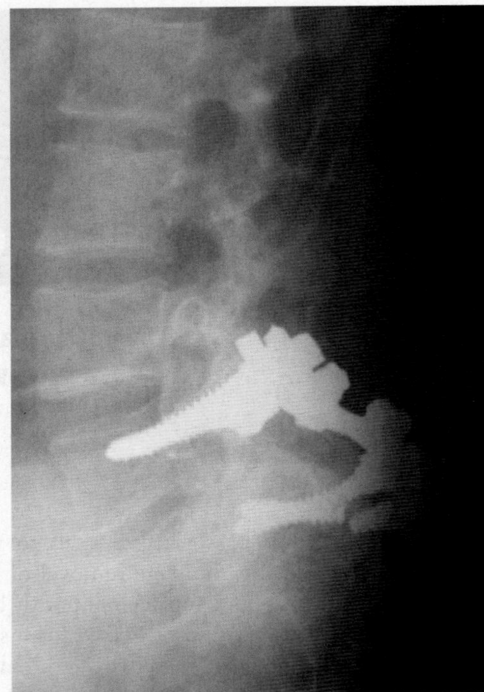

FIG. 50.1 Screw fracture and loss of alignment is a common complication after reduction of spondylolisthesis if anterior column support is not added.

that had previously been associated with PLIF in some surgeons' hands.

The addition of instrumentation also improved the fusion rate of PLIF. Many of the previously held objections to PLIF surgery were no longer applicable when PLIF was combined with pedicle instrumentation.

Another development that favored the adoption of PLIF was the invention of the interbody fusion cage by Brantigan and the titanium mesh cage by Harms. Their designs eliminated the need to harvest a structural graft from the iliac crest, which was a major source of morbidity previously associated with the PLIF procedure. The cage provided the structure,[13] and the osteogenic potential for fusion came from cancellous bone packed into the cage, which could be obtained from the iliac crest more easily than a structural graft, with less injury to the patient. Before the invention of the cages, it was possible to avoid the morbidity associated with graft harvest by using allograft bone, as advocated by Cloward.[14,15] Concerns about availability, disease transmission, healing potential, delayed healing, and wide variation in the structural integrity of available grafts all contributed to the limited enthusiasm for the use of allograft bone for interbody fusion.[16,17] The availability of cages overcame another common objection to the PLIF operation.

The availability of pedicle screw instrumentation and intervertebral cages contributed to progressively greater acceptance of the operation first pioneered by Cloward. Better alignment and higher fusion rates are routinely achieved using these devices. The training of surgeons and marketing of these devices by their manufacturers have also contributed to wider adoption of PLIF in surgical practice. Not all of these devices have proven to be successful, however. Cylindrical threaded fusion cages enjoyed brief popularity as PLIF devices that did not require supplementary fixation, but mediocre results and high complication rates associated with their use resulted in their virtual disappearance as a posterior spinal implant.[18] The clinical experience with threaded implants and the study of the relevant biomechanics have helped surgeons understand the PLIF operation better, however, and develop the operation that is currently performed. Although more recent advances, such as the development of the transforaminal and direct lateral approaches to the disc space, have decreased the frequency with which PLIF is performed, PLIF remains an important and powerful tool for spinal surgeons.

Indications for Interbody Fusion

Some surgeons believe that an interbody fusion is indicated whenever a lumbar fusion is done. They argue that the intervertebral space is biologically and mechanically superior for fusion compared with the intertransverse plane because of the larger surface area of the highly vascular bony endplate and because the interbody bone graft is subject to compressive forces. In addition, they criticize the large amount of muscle damage that occurs from exposure of the spine for posterolateral fusion. Despite these theoretical advantages, it is difficult to show clinical superiority of interbody fusions over posterolateral fusions for most lumbar degenerative conditions, and most published studies comparing the techniques reveal similar outcomes regardless of what fusion technique is used.[19–22] There are, however, certain circumstances when interbody fusion offers definite advantages. Adding an interbody fusion to a posterolateral fusion increases the rate of achieving successful arthrodesis. This is especially true when a long fusion extends to the sacrum, which is historically associated with a high risk of lumbosacral pseudarthrosis.[23]

Some authors have argued that interbody fusion should be combined with posterolateral fusion in other patients at high risk for failed fusion, such as smokers.[24] Witham et al. reviewed 103 patients that were either treated with a posterolateral arthrodesis alone or a posterolateral arthrodesis with PLIF or transforaminal lumbar interbody fusion (TLIF) for degenerative or isthmic spondylolisthesis. They found that a posterolateral fusion combined with an interbody fusion correlated with a greater amount of correction as well as a decreased need for reoperation related to pseudarthrosis, progression of listhesis, instrumentation failure, and adjacent-segment disease. They argue that adding an interbody fusion to the index procedure is most worthwhile to decrease the need for reoperation, which is more than seven times likely in the posterolateral fusion–only group.[25] In patients with pseudarthrosis after failed posterolateral fusion, an interbody fusion is a good salvage operation, allowing the fusion to occur in a well-vascularized bony bed rather than attempting fusion again in the scarred devascularized posterolateral space.[26] Interbody fusion offers a particular advantage in the treatment of scoliosis and kyphosis or flatback deformities. The destabilizing effect of disc space preparation facilitates rotational correction, and distraction of the intervertebral space allows correction of segmental kyphosis and asymmetrical tilt of the vertebrae. In patients with isthmic spondylolisthesis who undergo deformity reduction, it has been well shown that an interbody graft offers a biomechanical advantage, which protects instrumentation by load sharing, helping to maintain the alignment achieved at surgery. Also, the L5 transverse process is often hypoplastic in these patients; thus, the increased bone surface area of the vertebral endplate offers a vastly larger area to which bone can fuse.

Most series evaluating the role of interbody fusion in isthmic spondylolisthesis show substantial clinical and radiographic benefit.[27,28] Finally, the most common indication for interbody fusion, but probably the most controversial, is ablation of the disc space in patients with discogenic pain.[29,30] Many advocates for surgical treatment of this entity argue that only interbody fusion can completely remove motion of the painful disc and that complete removal of nuclear material is necessary to eliminate the anatomic source of pain.

Regardless of the indication, interbody fusion can be performed from anterior and posterior approaches. The relative advantages of these approaches are influenced by many factors, and it is essential that the spinal surgeon be well trained in various approaches so that the most appropriate one can be chosen for each unique clinical situation. Specific advantages of the posterior approach include the ability to simultaneously decompress the spinal canal directly and stabilize the spine more effectively with instrumentation. Although safe techniques of anterior fixation have become available more recently, if multilevel instrumentation is needed, posterior approaches are preferred. In patients with spinal deformity, bilateral facet resection allows more effective destabilization of the motion segment, allowing greater corrections than can be obtained by anterior disc removal alone, again favoring a posterior approach to the intervertebral disc. Posterior approaches avoid manipulation of the great vessels, of special concern in patients with atherosclerosis or a history of venous thrombosis. Also, posterior approaches avoid injury to the hypogastric plexus, which can result in retrograde ejaculation and sterility; thus, they are generally preferred in young men.

When there has been extensive posterior surgery and scarring, anterior approaches to the disc space avoid the increased risks of dural tear and nerve root injury associated with reoperation on the spinal canal. If a conjoined root is identified on preoperative imaging, the risk of root injury is also higher, and an anterior approach is preferred. A wider exposure of the disc space can also be achieved anteriorly, theoretically allowing better preparation of the endplates and more complete packing of the interspace with bone graft. Some surgeons prefer the anterior approach in patients at high risk for pseudarthrosis. An anterior approach may also be preferred when trying to increase lordosis. Dividing the anterior longitudinal ligament may allow for greater anterior distraction and more lordosis. Despite this theoretical advantage, in our experience, anterior approaches are more effective than posterior approaches in achieving lordosis only when the facet joints are highly mobile or have first been resected through a posterior approach.

Biomechanics of Interbody Fusion

An appreciation of the mechanical properties of the spine after interbody fusion is essential to understanding the benefits and pitfalls of this operation. It seems intuitively obvious that placing a solid block in the disc space would prevent flexion of the vertebral motion segment. This is what occurs—whether the graft is placed from an anterior or posterior approach. This fact has important implications for protection of posterior instrumentation. Interbody grafts significantly decrease the strain in posterior spinal implants when they are subjected to compression or flexion loads, which are the common modes of failure of these constructs in clinical practice. Various authors have shown that placing intervertebral cages decreases forces and strain in posterior implants by 56% to 80%,[29,30] and the clinical benefit of establishing anterior load sharing to prevent implant and construct failure is well established (Fig. 50.2).[31]

Increasing stability when the spine is subject to flexion loading does not mean that the spine is more stable when subject to forces in every direction. After interbody graft placement, the motion segment is more unstable in certain directions. The pattern of instability is determined to a great extent by the direction from which the graft is placed and represents the destabilizing effect of the surgical approach[32] and the preparation of the disc space. Grafts placed from an anterior approach result in increased motion when force is applied in extension; this likely represents the effect of dividing the anterior longitudinal ligament. Grafts placed from a posterior approach result in increased axial rotation of the motion segment owing to the resection of the posterior facet complexes necessary to avoid excessive dural retraction.[33–37] The design of the cage—vertical, box, or threaded, and whether or not the cage engages the endplates—does not seem to matter with regard to the patterns of instability created by intervertebral placement. Only the structures sacrificed during the approach to the disc are important in determining instability of the final construct (Fig. 50.3).[38,39]

Most surgeons make the assumption that a PLIF procedure is a stabilizing operation. The biomechanical data show that this is not entirely true. Understanding that placing an interbody graft or cage can lead to destabilization of the motion segment in certain directions is important for understanding why interbody fusion done without supplementary fixation has a high failure rate, especially when done from a posterior approach. Proponents of threaded fusion cages, which were designed to be used without supplementary fixation, argued that distraction of the disc space would stabilize the motion segment through ligamentotaxis. This argument is true. Increasing the size of the cage used to distract the disc space results in greater stabilization of the motion segment on mechanical testing.[40] After cyclic loading, some subsidence is inevitable, however, and biomechanical tests done after cyclic loading of threaded cage constructs reveal decreased stability in all directions.[41]

The destabilizing effects of interbody fusion are overcome by adding pedicle screw instrumentation; this is true whether

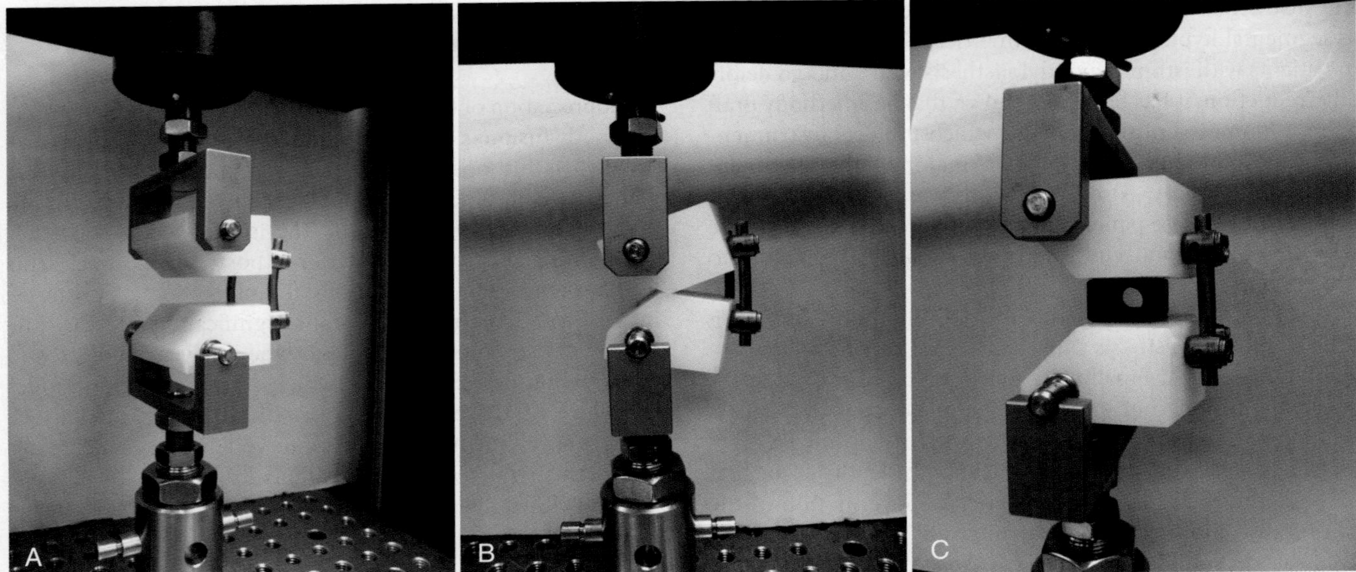

FIG. 50.2 Reduction in strain on posterior implants when a cage is placed in the intervertebral disc space. This model of a spinal motion segment with pedicle screw fixation has no anterior column support. (A) Alignment with no load applied. (B) Loss of alignment with only 700 N of load, the physiologic equivalent of standing in place. (C) Protective effect of an implant placed in the disc space. (Courtesy Hassan Serhan, PhD.)

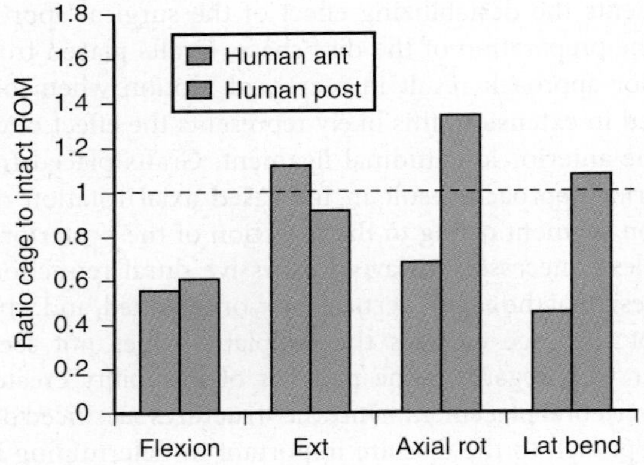

FIG. 50.3 Summation of five biomechanical studies of stability after anterior (ant) cage placement in human cadaver models, and three studies of posterior (post) cage placement. The data for each direction of testing is presented as the ratio of range of motion (ROM) after interbody cage placement compared with the motion of the unoperated segment. A ratio of 1.0 implies the same motion as the intact specimen. Note that placement from an anterior approach stiffens the spine in flexion, axial rotation (rot), and lateral bending (Lat bend), while placement from a posterior approach only stiffens the spine in extension (Ext). When testing axial rotation, placing a cage from a posterior approach creates more motion than the unoperated spine. (Modified from Oxland TR, Lund T. Biomechanics of stand-alone cages and cages in combination with posterior fixation: a literature review. *Eur Spine J.* 2000;9:S95–S101.)

the fusion is done from an anterior or posterior approach. These biomechanical data correlate well with the substantially greater clinical reliability of achieving an arthrodesis when interbody fusion is done with supplementary pedicle fixation compared with the variable results reported with stand-alone interbody fusion procedures.

Although cage design characteristics do not seem to have a significant effect on segmental motion, these characteristics do influence the risk of subsidence, the healing of bone within the cage, and the alignment achieved. In addition, endplate preparation and vertebral bone density have important effects on the extent of subsidence.

Cage Characteristics

The optimal cage material is unknown. Cloward[42] advocated the use of ethylene oxide sterilized allograft bone. Brantigan and colleagues[16] tested 18 tricortical iliac specimens obtained from bone banks and determined that 3 were not strong enough to sustain anticipated loads without collapse.

Current allograft products available for intervertebral use are made primarily of cortical bone and have adequate compressive strength. In designing his cage, Brantigan chose carbon fiber–reinforced polymer because of its strength and because its modulus of elasticity is similar to that of cortical bone.[13] In the United States, other materials commonly used in commercially available cages are polyetheretherketone, a nonreinforced polymer, and titanium, which has a modulus of elasticity significantly greater than that of cortical bone. The stiffness of the cage is determined not only by the mechanical properties of the material but also by the shape and design characteristics of the cage. The ideal stiffness and its role in limiting subsidence or enhancing fusion are unknown. Finite-element data have suggested that stiffer cages are more likely to subside,[43] but animal data have not supported this hypothesis,[44] and clinical reports have not convincingly shown that metal cages are more likely to subside than cages made of polymer (Fig. 50.4).

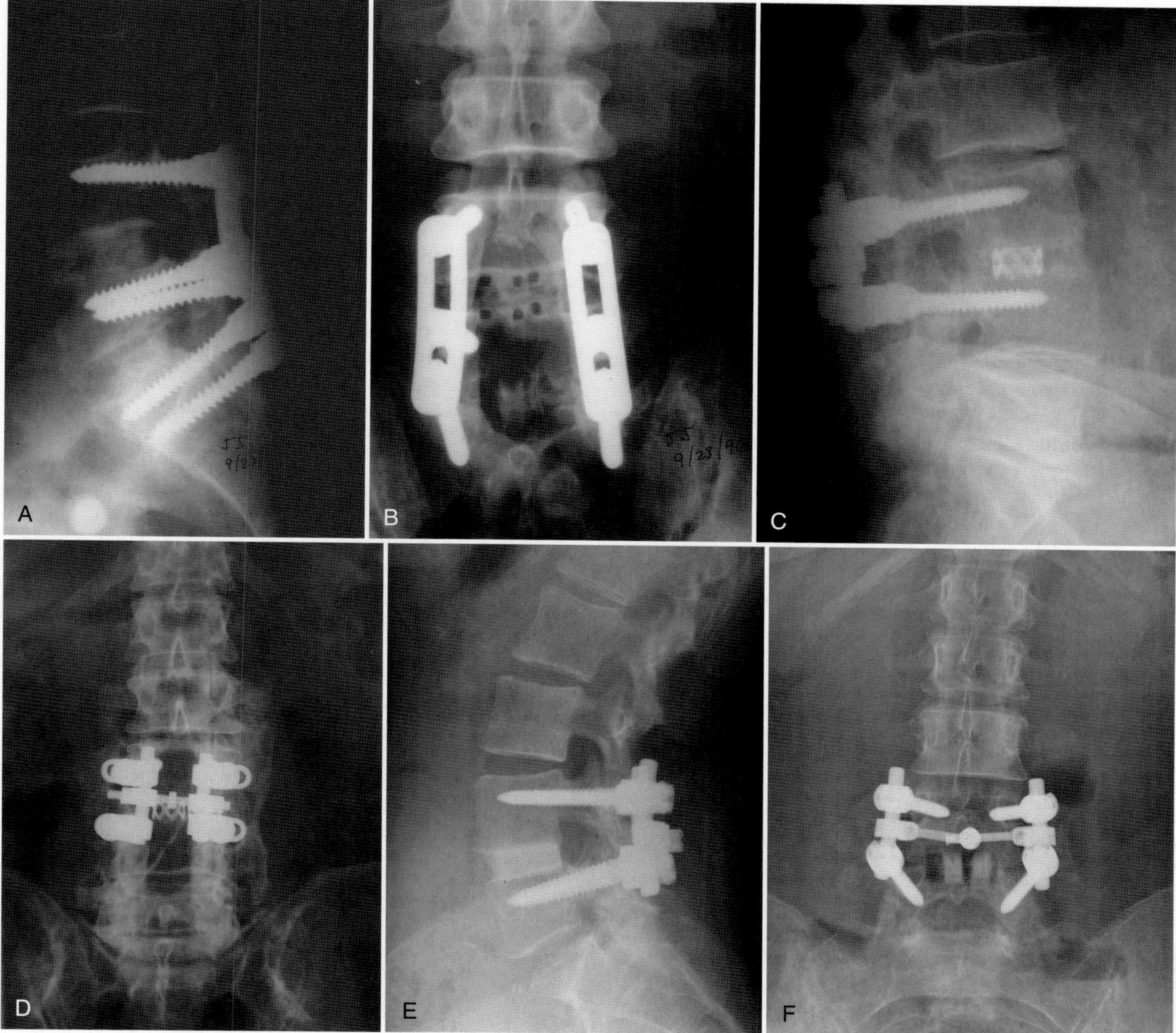

FIG. 50.4 Anteroposterior (AP) and lateral radiographs of successful interbody fusions with (A–B) carbon fiber–reinforced polymer cages, (C–D) titanium mesh cages, and (E–F) allograft wedge spacers. Incorporation of bone graft and replacement by new bone is most easily visualized with the polymer cages because they are radiolucent. The outline of the polymer can be seen on the AP view as four radiolucent squares at the periphery of the implant. With titanium mesh cages, healed bone graft is visualized in front and behind the implants, but assessment of the graft within the cage is difficult with standard radiographs. When nonunion occurs with allograft implants, a radiolucency is usually seen adjacent to the allograft. (A–B, Courtesy John Brantigan, MD.)

Kanayama and colleagues[45] studied the effect of cage design on stress shielding of the graft inside the cage. They determined that it was the pore size, not the stiffness of the material, that determined the load experienced by the graft. The total pore size was not important; rather, it was the size of the largest contiguous opening that determined how much force was transferred to the graft. It was implied that minimizing stress shielding is important to promote fusion, but no data were presented to support that presumption. One clinical study consistent with this hypothesis compared narrow and standard carbon fiber–reinforced polymer cages. The pore opening in the narrow cage was 36% smaller than the pore opening in the standard cage. There was a small but statistically significant reduction in fusion rate, 91.1% compared with 98.9%, but the conclusions have limitations because of methodologic flaws.[46] A larger pore size seems desirable as long as the design of the cage provides adequate structural support for the endplate.

Trabecular metal, another material often used for interbody fusion, offers a porous tantalum surface for fusions. This differs from the standard cage design in which there is space in the center of the cage to fill with additional graft material. Tantalum has a modulus of elasticity similar to cancellous bone and a friction coefficient substantially higher than autograft, allograft, or other common implantable materials. Van de Kelft and Van Goethem[47] have shown that these trabecular metal spacers do provide an adequate environment for interbody fusions when used in a stand-alone fashion or reinforced with pedicle screw fixation. They reported a 94% and 97% fusion rate, respectively, when comparing stand-alone trabecular spacers versus trabecular spacers with pedicle screw fixation in single-level interbody fusions. Subsidence rates were acceptably low in both groups.

Implant design also influences the alignment achieved. An increasingly large body of evidence shows that maintaining or restoring lumbar lordosis is an important surgical goal and that lordosis correlates with the outcome of surgery.[48] Early cage designs were rectangular and tended to force the vertebral endplates into parallel alignment. It is possible to achieve lordosis with rectangular cages, either by resecting bone posteriorly or by compressing the posterior disc space and causing the posterior portion of the cage to subside.[49] A disadvantage of this approach is that it results in loss of posterior disc space height, which can lead to foraminal narrowing. A better solution is to use a cage that is tapered to achieve lordosis.[50–52] It is commonly said that anterior distraction is necessary to achieve lordosis, but distraction of the disc space with an implant that is not tapered flattens the spine. Placing large cages to achieve lordosis is a mistake. They require more root retraction to place, which is more likely to result in nerve injury. A better solution is to use a tapered device and not to strive for maximal anterior height restoration (Fig. 50.5).

Subsidence

In addition to achieving fusion, avoiding subsidence to maintain alignment is an important goal of interbody fusion surgery. In mechanical testing, endplate failure has a linear correlation with decreased bone density,[53] and severe osteoporosis is considered to be a relative contraindication to interbody fusion because of the risk of endplate collapse. Severe osteoporosis, according to Oh et al., is defined as a T-score less than −3.0 on bone mineral density scanning.[54] This study group found subsidence of cages 3 mm or greater more prevalent in their severely osteoporotic study population compared to those patients with higher T-scores. Although the incidence of subsidence was greater, they did not correlate this finding with a negative impact on clinical outcomes.[54] The strength of the endplate is not uniform, and the central portion, where most surgeons place their grafts, is the weakest. Mapping studies have shown that the posterolateral portion of the endplate is most resistant to compression.[55,56] Placing the cage or graft in the area where the bone is strongest makes biomechanical sense,[57] but may not be consistent with the goals of an individual surgical case. If it is necessary to increase lordosis, better results are achieved by anterior placement. Putting the graft in the posterolateral position might be stronger, but would block compression of the posterior disc space and limit lordosis. This is especially true with rectangular cage designs or vertical titanium mesh cages.

Cage designs that optimize contact with the strongest portions of the endplate are desirable, and include cloverleaf designs and large round cages, both of which have peripheral endplate contact.[58] Practical use of large round cages is limited to anterior surgery because of the excessive dural retraction

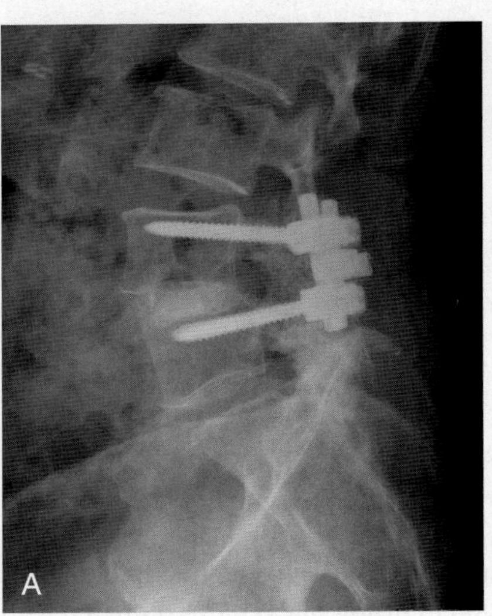

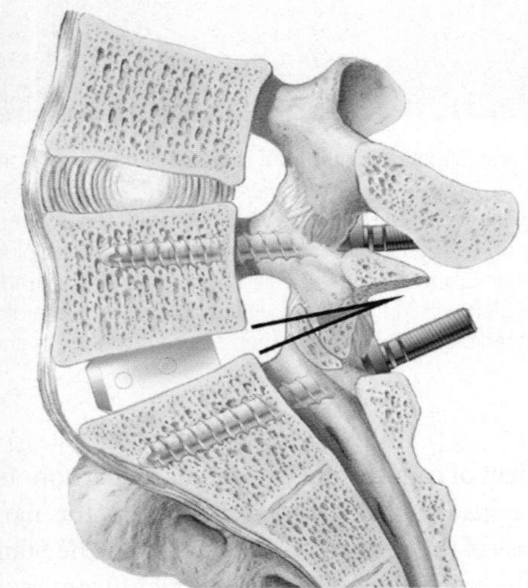

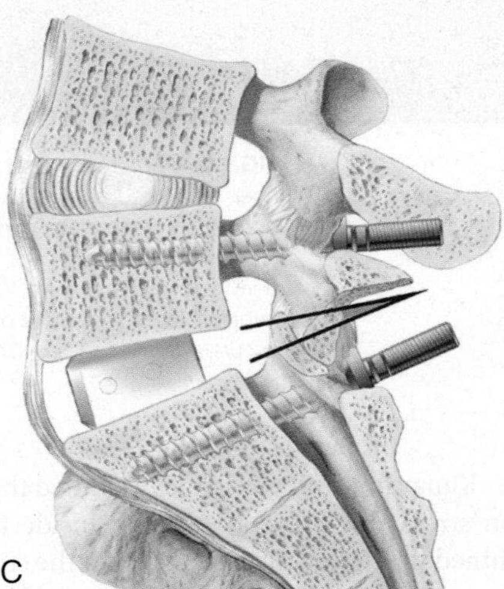

FIG. 50.5 Using a tapered cage or spacer is the best way to achieve lordosis. Facet resection is sometimes needed to allow the back of the disc space to narrow adequately. An advantage of allograft bone is the ease with which it can be sculpted intraoperatively to achieve the desired shape. (A) In this case, more lordosis was achieved than would be typically possible using commercially prepared devices by using a burr to increase the taper of the graft. (B–C) Using larger grafts and distracting the disc space more does not increase lordosis; it only increases the amount of dural retraction needed and increases the difficulty of the surgery. (B–C, Courtesy Depuy Synthes Spine, West Chester, PA.)

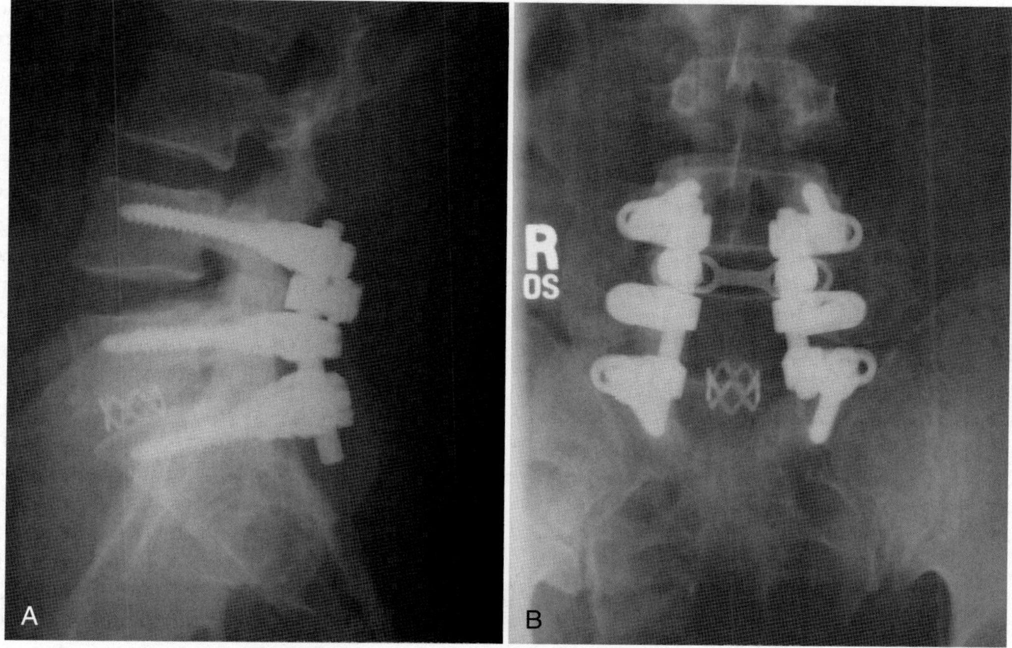

FIG. 50.6 Obvious subsidence of the cage into the inferior endplate of L5. Technical factors that may have predisposed to subsidence include the use of a single small cage placed centrally. Endcaps were not used, which would have increased the surface area of metal supporting the endplate. Inadequate grafting of the interspace around the cage may also have been a factor, suggested by the absence of bone in the disc space. Fortunately, a solid posterolateral fusion was achieved.

that would be necessary to place such an implant. Lordotic cages placed laterally also achieve near-optimal endplate contact. The surface area of the endplate that needs to be in contact with the graft is unknown, but is commonly stated to be 30%. This percentage is based on a study of thoracic vertebrae subjected to a physiologic load of 600 N. Failure of the endplate occurred in 80% of specimens subjected to that load when the grafts were 25% or less of the endplate surface area. When the grafts exceeded 30% of the endplate surface, 88% of the specimens remained intact (Fig. 50.6).[59]

Preservation of the endplate is important to maintain the structural integrity of the vertebra. Oxland and colleagues[60] removed slightly less than 1 mm of cortical endplate with a power burr to expose trabecular bone; this resulted in a 33% reduction in compressive resistance of the vertebra. If the endplate is decorticated where it is not in contact with the cage, the strength of the remaining endplate is preserved.[61] Consequently, it is recommended that the endplates be carefully preserved during preparation of the disc space wherever they are in contact with the implant, but that areas of the endplate that are not load bearing can be decorticated to increase contact of graft placed outside the cage with trabecular bone.

Our Preferred Technique

Our experience with PLIF dates back to 1994; the method of interbody fusion described here has been used without modification since 1999. Early results were reported in 2000 with an interbody fusion rate of 92%.[62] It is our practice always to perform a posterolateral fusion simultaneously with the PLIF to ensure the highest chance of achieving an arthrodesis. The technique for PLIF evolved from that described by Steffee and Biscup (personal communication, October 1994) for insertion of trapezoidal "ramps" made of carbon fiber–reinforced polymer. Their method was to insert the ramps sideways and rotate them into their final position, minimizing the amount of root retraction needed and simplifying placement of a lordotic graft.

We prefer to use a commercially prepared trapezoidal allograft wedge for two reasons. First is that its size and shape can be easily customized intraoperatively with a power burr to match the individual patient's anatomy. The second is that, in contrast to titanium and polymer cages, this structural device has the potential to incorporate in the fusion. Although the graft is placed primarily as a spacer and it is the autologous bone placed around the graft that is relied on to achieve arthrodesis, incorporation of the allograft generally occurs, resulting in a more robust fusion. There is no potential for polymer or metal to incorporate and contribute to the fusion; thus, a smaller area of the endplate is available to participate in healing when using devices made of those materials. Ceramic blocks have been used in Asia because of the potential for bone ingrowth, but there is no experience with that material in the United States, and it does not share the ability to be easily sculpted intraoperatively. Currently, several manufacturers produce allograft implants of this design.

The technique described here for preparation of the intervertebral space is applicable to any intervertebral cage or graft,

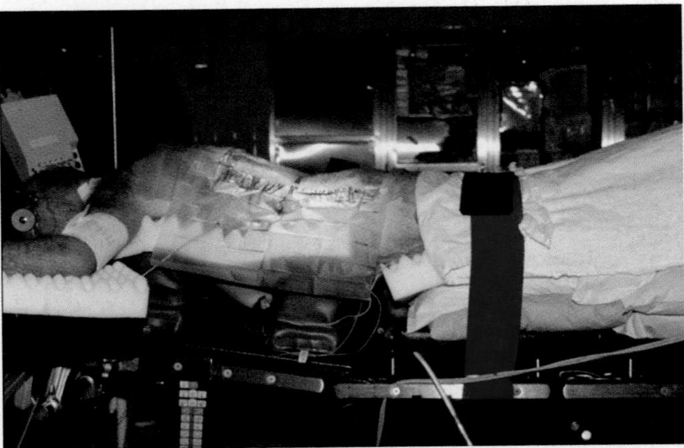

FIG. 50.7 The patient is positioned in hyperextension, with pillows under the thighs and the head of the bed elevated to help achieve maximum lordosis. The abdomen hangs free to allow unimpeded venous return. Electromyelographic monitoring is used to help prevent nerve injury due to excessive traction.

and the principles outlined help prevent neural injury and other complications that have been associated with this operation. The procedure begins with proper positioning, which is essential to achieve a good outcome. The patient is positioned in hyperextension to help create lumbar lordosis. The abdomen should hang free for unimpeded venous return; this decompresses the epidural venous plexus and helps reduce bleeding. A radiolucent positioning frame is useful so that intraoperative fluoroscopic images can be obtained to confirm correct placement of screws and grafts (Fig. 50.7). Pedicle screws should be placed before beginning the interbody fusion. PLIF destabilizes the motion segment and should not be done unless adequate pedicle fixation can be achieved.

A wide laminectomy and resection of the medial portion of the facet joints is essential to minimize retraction of the dura and nerve roots. The wide exposure helps avoid traction injury to the lumbar roots, which can cause neuropathic pain and weakness. Generally, the exposure of the disc space should extend lateral to the medial border of the pedicle below. Adequate exposure may require sacrifice of the facet joints, especially in the upper lumbar spine. This sacrifice is of little consequence because stability is restored by pedicle screw fixation. The facets should always be excised when correcting deformity because this helps loosen the spine and facilitates correction. The superior edge of the upper lamina should be preserved to maintain the posterior ligamentous attachments to the vertebra above the fusion.

An abundant epidural plexus is usually encountered at the lateral border of the spinal canal. Bipolar electrocautery and packing with cottonoid patties can prevent the excessive bleeding that sometimes accompanies interbody fusion procedures. A paste made from absorbable gelatin foam powder and saline is very helpful in controlling bleeding. The venous plexus should be sharply divided to facilitate mobilization of the nerve roots and dura. A nerve root retractor is used to protect the dura, and a rectangular opening is cut in the anulus with a scalpel. When extending the annular opening laterally, care is taken to protect the exiting nerve root. This is easily done by sweeping any soft tissue toward the root with a No. 1 Penfield elevator and leaving the elevator in place to protect the root while working laterally.

The anulus is opened bilaterally, and the disc space is distracted with intervertebral spreaders. These are bars of increasing width with rounded edges. They are inserted into the disc space horizontally and rotated 90 degrees, distracting the disc space. If the disc space is initially very narrow, it is sometimes helpful to use a smaller instrument first, such as a No. 4 Penfield elevator, to identify the path. It is important not to use force in order to avoid inadvertent penetration into the vertebral body. Lateral fluoroscopy can be helpful to confirm that the starting tools are correctly placed in the interspace. The disc is gradually distracted, working from side to side with increasingly large spreaders until resistance is met. The interspace should not be overdistracted, or the endplates may collapse. It is not necessary to maximize distraction to achieve lordosis, and decompression of the nerve roots should be accomplished by aggressive foraminotomy, not aggressive distraction. Placing a maximally tapered graft is the best way to increase lordosis. Trying to place a tall graft has many negative effects. It increases the amount of dural retraction necessary, it increases the volume of bone graft needed to fill the interspace, and it increases the distance over which the fusion must occur (Fig. 50.8).

After distracting the space to a comfortable working distance, usually 11 or 12 mm, one of the spreaders is removed, and a four-sided Collis curette 1 or 2 mm smaller than the largest spreader used is inserted horizontally, then rotated clockwise and counterclockwise to separate the cartilage from the bony endplate. This step is repeated at various depths and angles to clean as much of the endplate as possible. These curettes can be very aggressive, and it is important to be careful not to cut into the endplate. A Kerrison rongeur is used to resect loosened anulus flush with the vertebral endplates; this allows better visualization of the disc space so that a more complete discectomy can be done.

The discectomy is completed with standard curettes and pituitary rongeurs. A reverse curette is very effective in removing any remaining cartilage from the endplates. It is helpful to mark the curettes so that they are not inserted past a depth of 30 mm. In most cases, the anterior anulus prevents protrusion anterior to the vertebra, but the anulus is sometimes deficient, especially in patients with spondylolisthesis. Thus, it is important to avoid anterior protrusion of the instruments and visceral injury. After cleaning the interspace, the intervertebral spreader is reinserted, usually one size larger than was possible before removing the disc and cartilaginous endplate. Next, the opposite side of the disc is prepared in the same fashion.

It now is obvious that the interspace has been grossly destabilized. If a rotational deformity is present, it can be corrected by rotating the bilateral intervertebral spreaders simultaneously and "walking" the displaced vertebra into alignment. If no rotational deformity is present, the spreaders should be turned in opposite directions so that a rotational deformity is not induced. A graft is chosen to fit into the

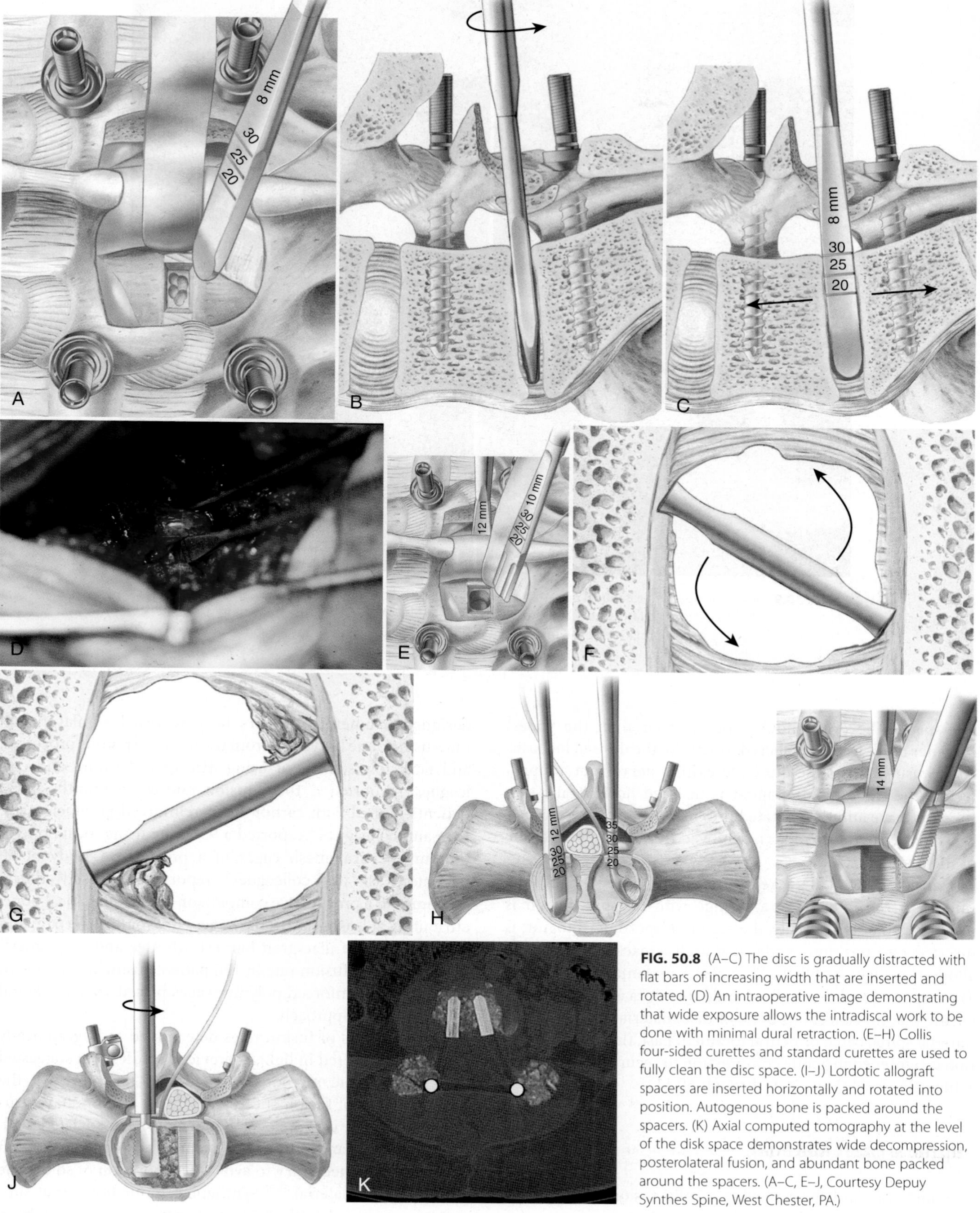

FIG. 50.8 (A–C) The disc is gradually distracted with flat bars of increasing width that are inserted and rotated. (D) An intraoperative image demonstrating that wide exposure allows the intradiscal work to be done with minimal dural retraction. (E–H) Collis four-sided curettes and standard curettes are used to fully clean the disc space. (I–J) Lordotic allograft spacers are inserted horizontally and rotated into position. Autogenous bone is packed around the spacers. (K) Axial computed tomography at the level of the disk space demonstrates wide decompression, posterolateral fusion, and abundant bone packed around the spacers. (A–C, E–J, Courtesy Depuy Synthes Spine, West Chester, PA.)

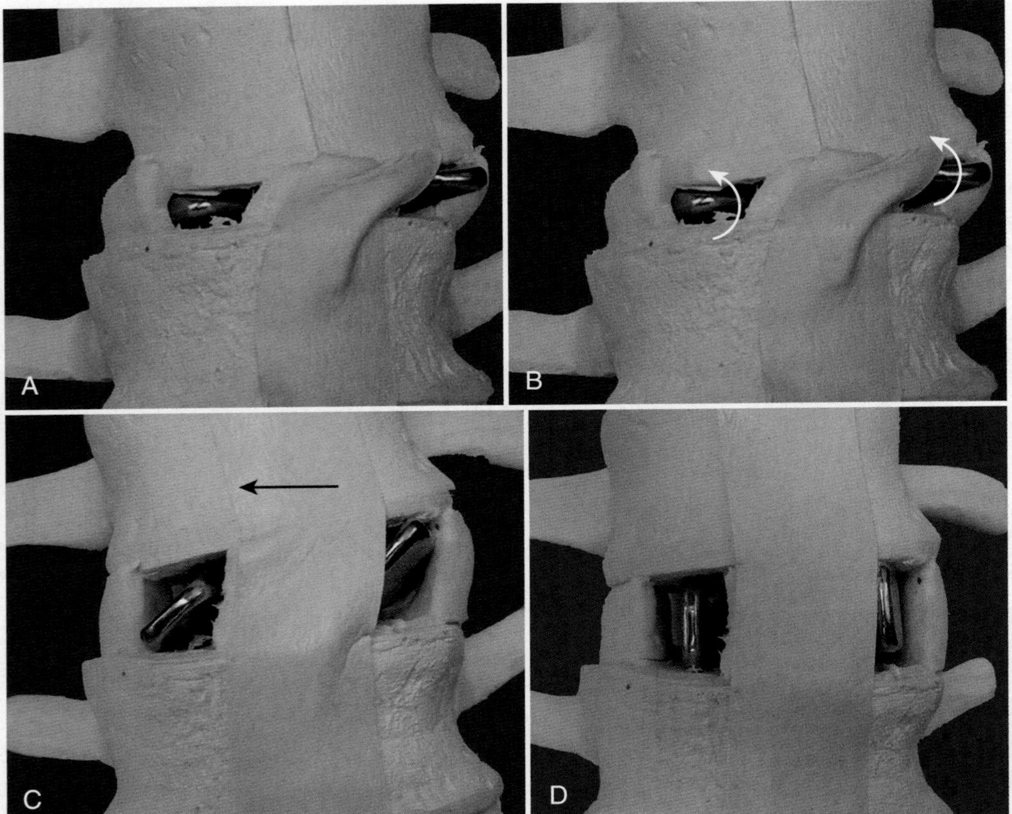

FIG. 50.9 Lateral listhesis and rotational deformity can be corrected efficiently with posterior lumbar interbody fusion. The spine is destabilized by bilateral facet excision and complete discectomy. The distraction paddles can now be used to translate the vertebra laterally, correcting axial rotation, lateral listhesis, and asymmetric disc space collapse.

interspace. The graft should not be taller than the widest spreader used. It can be tapered to achieve the desired lordosis. After ensuring that the dura and exiting nerve root are protected, the trapezoidal allograft is inserted horizontally into the disc space and then rotated into its final lordotic position. The intervertebral spreader is removed from the opposite side of the disc space.

Cancellous graft is packed from the opposite side into the middle of the interspace; a syringe with the end cut off is useful for this step. Finally, the second trapezoidal allograft is inserted into position. Additional graft is packed around the allograft wedges to fill the disc space maximally with bone. The foramina and the midline under the dura are inspected to ensure that no cancellous bone or disc material was displaced into the spinal canal or neural foramen. Last, the instrumentation is tightened in gentle compression to secure the grafts and achieve lordosis (Figs. 50.9 through 50.11).

Optimal Graft Material

The gold standard for achieving a solid fusion is cancellous autograft bone, regardless of which cage device or intervertebral spacer is chosen. Brantigan[63] reported a 97.7% fusion rate when using autologous cancellous graft in the cage that he designed. Numerous authors have reported similar fusion rates using bone harvested from the lamina, spinous processes, and facet joints, without using iliac graft.[64] Miura and colleagues[65] reported a 100% fusion rate at 12 months in 32 patients treated with carbon fiber–reinforced polymer cages. Kim and colleagues[66] reported a 95% rate using local bone in titanium vertical mesh cages in a prospective study of 50 patients. Kasis and colleagues[67] reported improved clinical outcomes in a prospective comparison when using local bone, attributing at least some of the benefit to avoiding the pain and complications of iliac graft harvest. McAfee and colleagues[68] reported a 98% fusion rate in 120 patients using local bone in carbon fiber–reinforced polymer cages placed via a unilateral transforaminal approach.

These reports of fusion rates determined radiographically must be interpreted in light of previous studies that suggested that radiographic methods have limited reliability for the determination of fusion success.[69,70] Other authors have cautioned that the use of local bone may be associated with pseudarthrosis, and if local bone is used, careful preparation and cleaning is necessary to avoid incorporation of soft tissue with the graft material.[63,71] Synthetic ceramic bone graft substitutes combined with iliac crest aspirate have also been reported to be highly effective for achieving interbody fusion,[72] but experience is limited.

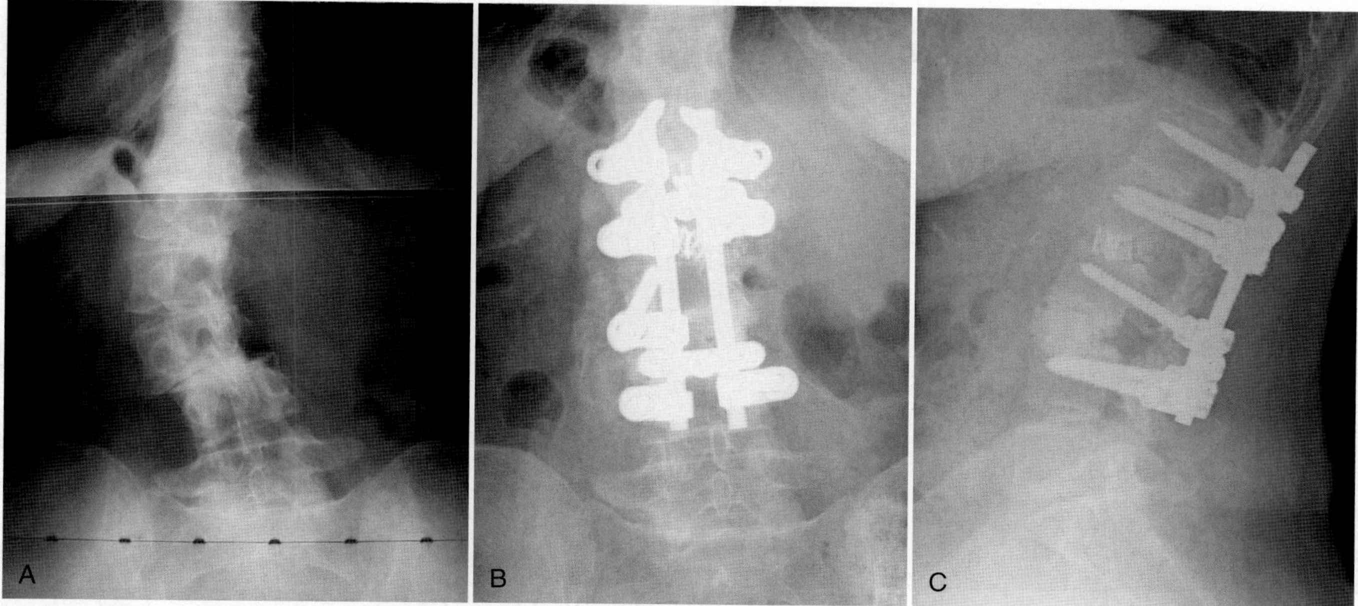

FIG. 50.10 Acute rotational deformity causing degenerative scoliosis is corrected by posterior lumbar interbody fusion. Note that the deformity at L4–L5 was flexible and resolved spontaneously with correction of the structural deformity at L3–L4.

More recently, there has been a surge of enthusiasm for the use of bone morphogenetic protein to achieve spinal fusion.[73] Recombinant human bone morphogenetic protein (rhBMP-2) was shown to be highly effective in achieving spinal fusion when used inside a titanium-threaded cage placed anteriorly in the intervertebral space. In a 2-year prospective randomized trial of 279 patients, fusion was achieved in 94.5% of patients compared with 88.7% in the control group in whom iliac autograft was used.[74] Although not approved by the US Food and Drug Administration (FDA) for posterior use, many surgeons have extrapolated the outcomes documented in the anterior clinical trial to posterior intervertebral applications. Review of the published data on outcomes of posterior interbody use of this material reveals conflicting results. Although some authors report universal fusion with few complications,[75] others have reported a worrisome list of unexpected outcomes.

A clinical trial of rhBMP-2 used in posterior threaded fusion cages was stopped by the FDA because of a high rate of new bone formation (28 of 34 patients) in the spinal canal or neuroforamina, although the authors of the study were enthusiastic about the fusion results and believed that there was no clinical significance to the new bone formation.[76] Radiculopathy and neurologic deficit associated with ectopic bone have been reported by other authors,[77,78] and radiculitis has been reported with the use of rhBMP-2 even when no ectopic bone has formed. The use of a barrier between rhBMP-2 and the neural elements has been reported to eliminate this complication.[79,80] Osteolysis and endplate resorption resulting in subsidence and cage migration have also been reported as a complication of using rhBMP-2. Reports regarding the clinical significance of these radiographic findings vary significantly, and many surgeons continue to advocate for the use of rhBMP-2 in posterior interbody applications.[81-84] Optimal dosing and methods of application of this recombinant protein are unclear at this time. Although fusion rates seem to be high with the use of rhBMP-2, questions remain regarding safety, superiority, and cost effectiveness.

Posterior Lumbar Interbody Fusion Versus Transforaminal Lumbar Interbody Fusion

Although Cloward, Stefee, Branch, and others emphasized the importance of a wide exposure to minimize dural retraction and nerve root injuries during PLIF, other authors described a more medial approach, which was often associated with a high incidence of nerve root injuries. This association was especially true before the advent of posterior instrumentation, when it was often recommended that the facet joints be preserved to avoid destabilizing the motion segment.[85] Dural and root injuries were particularly prevalent when threaded fusion cages were used posteriorly because of the emphasis on using large devices to achieve stability through annular distraction.[86] Because the cylinders were designed to cut into the endplates, the diameter needed was sometimes 50% greater than the height of the interspace achieved.[39] Even when using smaller devices, rates of neurologic complications of 17% were reported.[87]

In 1997, Harms and colleagues[88] reported a technique for performing a posterior interbody fusion through a more lateral approach than previously described.[89] These investigators advocated a unilateral approach to the disc space through the neural foramen by removing the facet joint. This approach allowed access to the disc space through the triangular "safe zone" between the exiting nerve root and the lateral dural

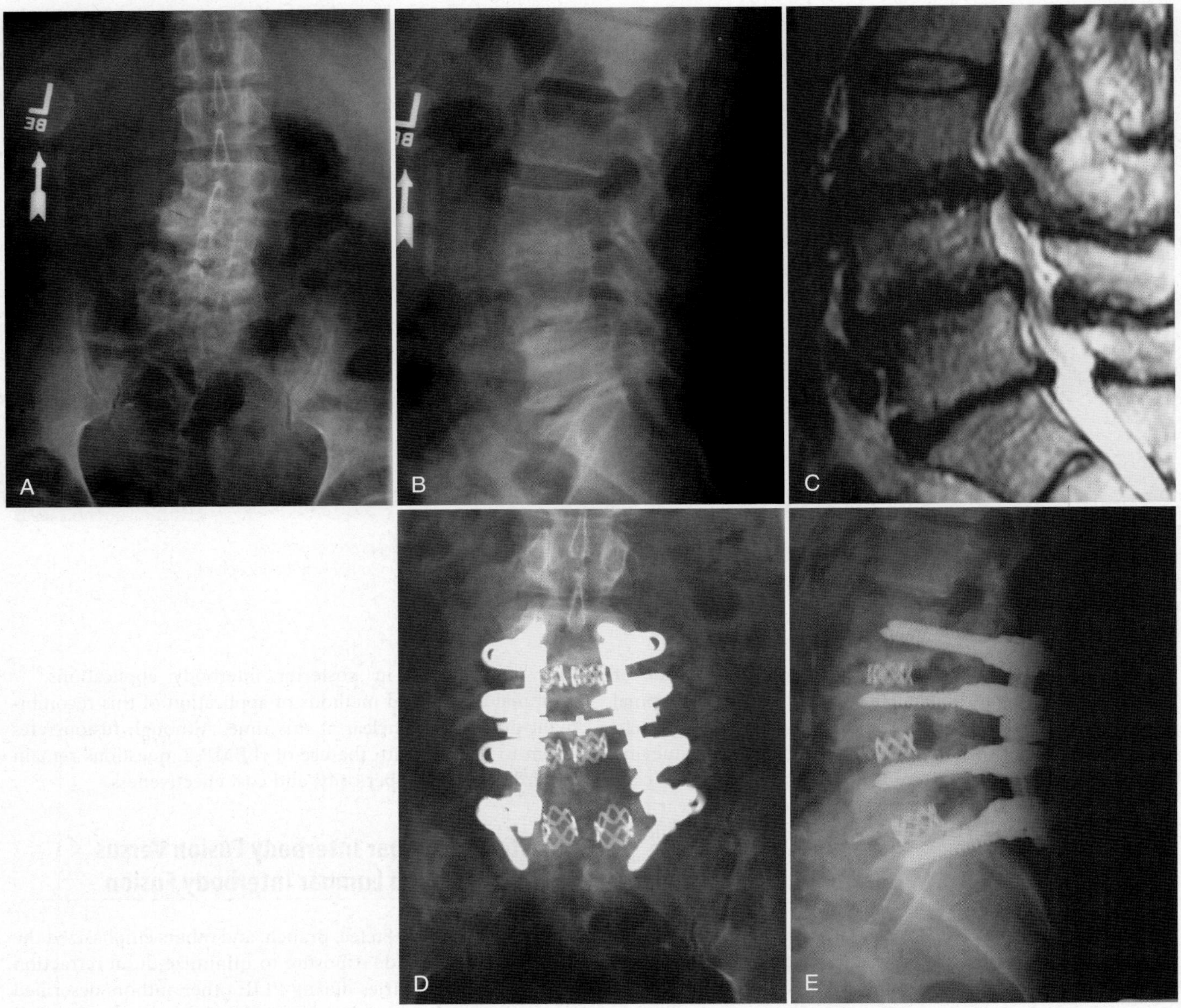

FIG. 50.11 In this patient, severe degenerative disease of the lumbar spine has resulted in spinal stenosis, degenerative spondylolisthesis, and asymmetric disc space collapse. Because a posterior decompression is needed to treat the patient's stenosis and pseudoclaudication, posterior lumbar interbody fusion is the most efficient way to simultaneously correct the patient's deformity and achieve fusion.

edge.[90] In this way, an interbody fusion could be performed with minimal or no retraction of the dura. The transforaminal technique has been enthusiastically adopted by many surgeons; a number of studies have shown a reduction of nerve root injuries when comparing PLIF and TLIF in their hands.[91,92] The increased incidence of iatrogenic nerve root injuries, reported by some authors, during a PLIF versus a TLIF may be due to the technical aspects of the PLIF technique, which requires a more complete exposure of the thecal sac as well as dural retraction. Surgeons who favor the TLIF also report decreased blood loss, operative time, dural tears, and need for reoperation. Although these differences are quoted in the literature, this has not been our experience.[91-93]

One theoretical disadvantage of the TLIF technique is that, because only a unilateral approach to the disc space is done, it is impossible to remove the disc material completely. Javernick and colleagues[94] showed that, on average, 31% more disc material could be removed when a bilateral approach was done. This finding leads to concern that the fusion rate might not be satisfactory with a unilateral approach. McAfee and colleagues[95] showed that, for anterior interbody fusions, 100% of patients who underwent complete discectomies achieved a solid arthrodesis, whereas only 86% of patients with incomplete discectomies achieved solid fusion. In an animal model, the inclusion of disc material with autologous bone in cages led to a significant impairment of fusion.[96] Despite these concerns, although no prospective randomized comparison has been done, the unilateral approach to the disc space seems to result in adequate fusion rates.

In our experience, the unilateral transforaminal approach is useful when extensive postoperative scar makes mobilization of the dura or exposure of one side of the disc difficult. When trying to correct deformity, the greater laxity of the motion segment achieved by a bilateral approach makes PLIF the preferred technique, however. The technique of PLIF described in this chapter involves extensive or complete facet resection, eliminating any differences in risk of nerve root or dural injury between PLIF and TLIF.

Outcome and Complications of Posterior Lumbar Interbody Fusion

The outcome of PLIF surgery depends on many factors. Probably the most important, as with any operation on the lumbar spine, is proper patient selection. Lumbar fusion done for the wrong reasons or on the wrong patient uniformly yields bad results. Review of the published outcomes of PLIF surgery makes it clear that PLIF is a technically demanding procedure. Variations in technique, care, and skill have significant influence on the rate of fusion and the frequency with which complications occur.

In large series, fusion rates greater than 95% have routinely been reported with PLIF, regardless of whether carbon fiber–reinforced cages, polymer cages, vertical titanium mesh cages, allograft bone spacers, or stand-alone cylindrical threaded cages have been used.[19,96–99] In contrast, only 77% of the patients reported by Rivet and colleagues[100] achieved solid arthrodesis, despite the use of cancellous iliac graft and supplementary pedicle fixation. Fuji and colleagues[101] reported a nonunion rate of 72% in their series of threaded cages placed posteriorly without supplementary fixation. It is unclear whether poor technique or other factors are responsible for the poor fusion results reported in those series.

Probably the most devastating complication that can occur with PLIF procedures is a nerve root injury.[102] The reported incidence of this complication varies widely, suggesting that surgical technique is an important factor affecting the frequency with which this complication occurs. Hosono and colleagues, in their review of 240 patients operated on by four surgeons, correlated complication rates with the experience of the surgeon.[87] In that series, 41 patients had some kind of nerve injury, mostly transient. In Brantigan's series,[63] despite previous failed discectomy and the associated epidural scar in 83% of his patients, postoperative radiculitis was reported in only 2 of 100 patients, and one patient experienced a footdrop.

In the larger series of carbon fiber–reinforced polymer cages submitted to the FDA in which 221 patients were operated on by 15 surgeons, 3 cases of reflex sympathetic dystrophy and 3 cases of motor deficit, 1 of which was permanent, were reported.[97] Davne and Myers[103] reported only a 0.4% rate of traction root injury in their series of 384 PLIF procedures.

Krishna and colleagues[104] reported postoperative neuralgia in 7.1% of their patients, but they were able to reduce the incidence of this complication by half by modifying their technique and removing the superior facet to widen the exposure. Barnes and colleagues[86] reported a 13.6% incidence of permanent nerve root injury when using threaded fusion cages but no nerve root injury when using much smaller allograft wedges. These results reinforce the principle that wide exposure, careful technique, and avoiding oversized grafts can minimize the risk of neurologic injury in PLIF.

Graft displacement and loosening is another complication that was associated with PLIF when the technique was first described. This is a rare complication, however, with the addition of posterior pedicle screw stabilization. Subsidence of the implants can occur with PLIF. Most authors have not carefully documented this phenomenon. Factors predisposing to subsidence include inadequate graft technique and sizing, and endplate injury during preparation. Patient factors such as weight and osteoporosis are likely important.[105] Implant type may be a factor, but convincing evidence of this has not been presented.[106,107] Pedicle screws alone do not prevent subsidence after PLIF.[108]

Vertebral compression fractures at the adjacent proximal or distal level to the interbody fusion have also been reported. Osteopenia/osteoporosis, short segment fusions, female gender, and age older than 65 years were cited to increase the risk of compression fractures at the nonfused vertebrae after interbody fusion.[109]

Other complications of PLIF are similar to the complications encountered in all lumbar spine surgery. Epidural hematoma, wound infections, and other non–implant-related complications seem to occur with similar frequency in PLIF as in other reconstructive operations on the lumbar spine.

Summary

PLIF is a technically demanding operation that has an important role in the modern management of lumbar spine problems. Careful surgical technique emphasizing wide exposure and avoiding oversized implants can lead to excellent results with a low rate of complications and high fusion rates. Many different types of implants and grafts are available, without a clear-cut advantage of one type of device over another. Excellent results have been reported with most commercially available cages and grafts. PLIF is a useful way to provide anterior column support without the need for an anterior incision. PLIF is especially helpful to avoid failure of posterior instrumentation in patients who have undergone realignment of high-grade spondylolisthesis and to prevent distal instrumentation failure in long fusions to the sacrum.[110]

Although PLIF with supplementary fixation creates a very stiff motion segment, the PLIF operation by itself destabilizes the motion segment. This destabilization is useful for correcting spinal deformity but makes the addition of posterior fixation, such as pedicle screw fixation, important to ensure successful healing of the fusion. In the treatment of degenerative conditions of the lumbar spine and back pain, PLIF offers some theoretical advantages over traditional posterolateral fusion techniques. Clinical studies generally have failed to show superiority of PLIF convincingly over other techniques, however. In clinical situations involving degenerative conditions of the lumbar spine and back pain, the role of PLIF as part of the surgical treatment of the patient has more to do with the experience of the surgeon than with any other factor.

REFERENCES

1. White AH. Editorial commentary. In: White AH, Rothman RH, Ray CD, eds. *Lumbar Spine Surgery Techniques and Complications*. St Louis: CV Mosby; 1987:294-295.
2. Verlooy J, Smedt KD, Selosse P. Failure of a Modi ED posterior lumbar interbody fusion technique to produce adequate pain relief in isthmic spondylolytic grade 1 spondylolisthesis patients. *Spine*. 1993;18:1491-1495.
3. Briggs H, Milligan PR. Chip fusion of the low back following exploration of the spinal canal. *J Bone Joint Surg Am*. 1944;26:125-130.
4. Ovens JM, Williams HG. Intervertebral spine fusion with removal of herniated intervertebral disk. *Am J Surg*. 1945;70:24-26.
5. Jaslow IA. Intercorporeal bone graft in spinal fusion after disc removal. *Surg Gynecol Obstet*. 1946;82:215.
6. Cloward RB. The treatment of ruptured intervertebral discs by vertebral body fusion: indications, operative technique, after care. *J Neurosurg*. 1953;10:154-168.
7. Collis JS. Total disc replacement: a modified posterior lumbar interbody fusion: report of 750 cases. *Clin Orthop Relat Res*. 1985;193:64-67.
8. Ma GW. Posterior lumbar interbody fusion with specialized instruments. *Clin Orthop Relat Res*. 1985;193:57-63.
9. Lin PM, Cautilli RA, Joyce MF. Posterior lumbar interbody fusion. *Clin Orthop Relat Res*. 1983;180:154-168.
10. Hutter CG. Posterior lumbar interbody fusion, a 25 year study. *Clin Orthop Relat Res*. 1983;179:86-96.
11. Cohen DS. *Etiology of broken pedicle screw instrumentation in the treatment of spondylolisthesis*. Proceedings of the North American Spine Society 11th Annual Conference, Vancouver, 1996, pp 168-169.
12. Steffee AD, Sitkowski DJ. Posterior lumbar interbody fusion and plates. *Clin Orthop Relat Res*. 1988;227:99-102.
13. Brantigan JW, Steffee AD, Geiger JM. A carbon fiber implant to aid interbody lumbar fusion: mechanical testing. *Spine*. 1991;16(6 suppl):S277-S282.
14. Cloward RB. Gas-sterilized cadaver bone grafts for spinal fusion operations: a simplified bone bank. *Spine*. 1980;5:4-10.
15. Cloward RB. Posterior lumbar fusion updated. *Clin Orthop Relat Res*. 1985;193:16-19.
16. Brantigan JW, Cunningham BW, Warden K, et al. Compression strength of donor bone for posterior lumbar interbody fusion. *Spine*. 1993;18:1213-1221.
17. Brantigan JW. Pseudarthrosis rate after allograft posterior lumbar interbody fusion with pedicle screw and plate fixation. *Spine*. 1994;19:1271-1279.
18. Barnes B, Rodts GE, Haid R, et al. Allograft implants for posterior lumbar interbody fusion: results comparing cylindrical dowels and impacted wedges. *Neurosurgery*. 2002;51:1191-1198.
19. Kim KT, Lee SH, Lee YH, et al. Clinical outcomes of 3 fusion methods through the posterior approach in the lumbar spine. *Spine*. 2006;31:1351-1357.
20. Fritzell P, Hägg O, Wessberg P, et al. Chronic low back pain and fusion: a comparison of three surgical techniques: a prospective multicenter randomized study from the Swedish Lumbar Spine Study Group. *Spine*. 2002;27:1131-1141.
21. Jacobs WC, Vreeling A, DeKleuver M. Fusion for low-grade adult isthmic spondylolisthesis: a systematic review of the literature. *Eur Spine J*. 2006;15:391-402.
22. Abdu W, Lurie J, Spratt K, et al. Degenerative spondylolisthesis: does fusion method influence outcome? Four-year results of the Spine Patient Outcomes Research Trial (SPORT). *Spine*. 2009;34(21):2351-2360.
23. Byrd JA 3rd, Scoles PV, Winter RB, et al. Adult idiopathic scoliosis treated by anterior and posterior spinal fusion. *J Bone Joint Surg Am*. 1987;69:843-850.
24. DiPaola CP, Molinari RW. Posterior lumbar interbody fusion. *J Am Acad Orthop Surg*. 2008;16:130-139.
25. Macki M, Bydon M. Posterolateral fusion with interbody for lumbar spondylolisthesis is associated with less repeat surgery than posterolateral fusion alone. *Clin Neurol Neurosurg*. 2015;138:117-123.
26. Cohen DB, Chotivichit A, Fujita T, et al. Pseudarthrosis repair: autogenous iliac crest versus femoral ring allograft. *Clin Orthop Relat Res*. 2000;371:46-55.
27. Molinari RW, Bridwell KH, Lenke LG, et al. Anterior column support in surgery for high-grade, isthmic spondylolisthesis. *Clin Orthop Relat Res*. 2002;394:109-120.
28. Suk SI, Lee CK, Kim WJ, et al. Adding posterior lumbar interbody fusion to pedicle screw fixation and posterolateral fusion after decompression in spondylolytic spondylolisthesis. *Spine*. 1997;22:210-219.
29. Barrick WT, Schofferman JA, Reynolds JB, et al. Anterior lumbar fusion improves discogenic pain at levels of prior posterolateral fusion. *Spine*. 2000;25:853-857.
30. Nachemson A, Zdeblick TA, O'Brien JP. Lumbar disc disease with discogenic pain: what surgical treatment is most effective? *Spine*. 1996;21:1835-1838.
31. McCormack T, Karaikovic E, Gaines RW. The load sharing classification of spine fractures. *Spine*. 1994;19:1741-1744.
32. Oxland TR, Lund T. Biomechanics of stand-alone cages and cages in combination with posterior fixation: a literature review. *Eur Spine J*. 2000;9:S95-S101.
33. Tencer AF, Hampton D, Eddy S. Biomechanical properties of threaded inserts for lumbar interbody spinal fusion. *Spine*. 1995;20:2408-2414.
34. Voor MJ, Mehta S, Wang M, et al. Biomechanical evaluation of posterior and anterior lumbar interbody fusion techniques. *J Spinal Disord*. 1998;11:328-334.
35. Dimar JR, Beck DJ, Glassman SD, et al. Posterior lumbar interbody cages do not augment segmental biomechanical stability. *Am J Orthop*. 2001;8:636-639.
36. Brodke DS, Dick JC, Kunz DN, et al. Posterior lumbar interbody fusion: a biomechanical comparison, including a new threaded cage. *Spine*. 1997;22:26-31.
37. Pitzen T, Geisler FH, Matthis D, et al. Motion of threaded cages in posterior lumbar interbody fusion. *Eur Spine J*. 2000;9:571-576.
38. Lund T, Oxland TR, Jost B, et al. Interbody cage stabilization in the lumbar spine: biomechanical evaluation of cage design, posterior instrumentation and bone density. *J Bone Joint Surg Br*. 1998;80:351-359.
39. Tsantrizos A, Baramki HG, Zeidman S, et al. Segmental stability and compressive strength of posterior lumbar interbody fusion implants. *Spine*. 2000;25:1899-1907.

40. Goh JC, Wong HK, Thambyah A, et al. Influence of PLIF cage size on lumbar spine stability. *Spine*. 2000;25:35-39.
41. Kettler A, Wilke HJ, Dietl R, et al. Stabilizing effect of posterior lumbar interbody fusion cages before and after cyclic loading. *J Neurosurg*. 2000;92(1 suppl):87-92.
42. Cloward RB. Gas sterilized cadaver bone grafts for spinal fusion operations. A simplified bone bank. *Spine*. 1980;5:4.
43. Vadapalli S, Sairyo K, Goel VK, et al. Biomechanical rationale for using polyetheretherketone (PEEK) spacers for lumbar interbody fusion: a finite element study. *Spine*. 2006;31: E992-E998.
44. van Dijk M, Smit TH, Sugihara S, et al. The effect of cage stiffness on the rate of lumbar interbody fusion: an in vivo model using poly(l-lactic acid) and titanium cages. *Spine*. 2002;27:682-688.
45. Kanayama M, Cunningham BW, Haggerty CJ, et al. In vitro biomechanical investigation of the stability and stress-shielding effect of lumbar interbody fusion devices. *Neurosurgery*. 2000;93(2 suppl):259-265.
46. Fogel GR, Toohey JS, Neidre A, et al. Outcomes of posterior lumbar interbody fusion with the 9-mm width lumbar I/F cage and the variable screw placement system. *J Surg Orthop Adv*. 2009;18:77-82.
47. Van de Kelft E, Van Goethem J. Trabecular metal spacers as standalone or with pedicle screw augmentation, in posterior lumbar interbody fusion: a prospective, randomized controlled trial. *Eur Spine J*. 2015;24:2597-2606.
48. Glassman SD, Bridwell K, Dimar JR, et al. The impact of positive sagittal balance in adult spinal deformity. *Spine*. 2005;30:2024-2029.
49. Groth AT, Kuklo TR, Klemme WR, et al. Comparison of sagittal contour and posterior disc height following interbody fusion: threaded cylindrical cages versus structural allograft versus vertical cages. *J Spinal Disord Tech*. 2005;18: 332-336.
50. Sears W. Posterior lumbar interbody fusion for lytic spondylolisthesis: restoration of sagittal balance using insert-and-rotate interbody spacers. *Spine J*. 2005;5:161-169.
51. Gödde S, Fritsch E, Dienst M, et al. Influence of cage geometry on sagittal alignment in instrumented posterior lumbar interbody fusion. *Spine*. 2003;28:1693-1699.
52. Brantigan JW, Neidre A. Achievement of normal sagittal plane alignment using a wedged carbon fiber reinforced polymer fusion cage in treatment of spondylolisthesis. *Spine J*. 2003;3:186-196.
53. Jost B, Cripton PA, Lund T, et al. Compressive strength of interbody cages in the lumbar spine: the effect of cage shape, posterior instrumentation and bone density. *Eur Spine J*. 1998;7:132-141.
54. Oh KW, Lee JH, et al. The correlation between cage subsidence, bone mineral density, and clinical results in posterior lumbar interbody fusion. *Clin Spine Surg*. 2016. Epub ahead of print.
55. Grant JP, Oxland TR, Dvorak MF. Mapping the structural properties of the lumbosacral vertebral endplates. *Spine*. 2001;26:889-896.
56. Lowe TG, Hashim S, Wilson LA, et al. A biomechanical study of regional endplate strength and cage morphology as it relates to structural interbody support. *Spine*. 2004;29: 2389-2394.
57. Labrom RD, Tan JS, Reilly CW, et al. The effect of interbody cage positioning on lumbosacral vertebral endplate failure in compression. *Spine*. 2005;30:E556-E561.
58. Tan JS, Bailey CS, Dvorak MF, et al. Interbody device shape and size are important to strengthen the vertebra-implant interface. *Spine*. 2005;30:638-644.
59. Closkey RF, Parsons JR, Lee CK, et al. Mechanics of interbody spinal fusion: analysis of critical bone graft area. *Spine*. 1993; 18:1011-1015.
60. Oxland TR, Grant JP, Dvorak MF, et al. Effects of endplate removal on the structural properties of the lower lumbar vertebral bodies. *Spine*. 2003;28:771-777.
61. Steffen T, Tsantrizos A, Aebi M. Effect of implant design and endplate preparation on the compressive strength of interbody fusion constructs. *Spine*. 2000;25:1077-1084.
62. Lebwohl NH, Green BA, Buck BE. *Technique indications complications, and outcomes of allograft PLIF*. In Proceedings of the Scoliosis Research Society 35th Annual Meeting, Cairns, Australia, 2000, Exhibit #66.
63. Brantigan JW. A prospective study of 100 consecutive cases. In: Brantigan JW, Lauryssen C, eds. *Intervertebral Fusion Using Carbon Fiber Reinforced Polymer Implants*. St Louis: Quality Medical Publishing; 2006:231-248.
64. Arai Y, Takahashi M, Kurosawa H, et al. Comparative study of iliac bone graft and carbon cage with local bone graft in posterior lumbar interbody fusion. *J Orthop Surg*. 2002;10: 1-7.
65. Miura Y, Imagama S, Yoda M, et al. Is local bone viable as a source of bone graft in posterior lumbar interbody fusion? *Spine*. 2003;28:2386-2389.
66. Kim KT, Lee SH, Lee YH, et al. Clinical outcomes of 3 fusion methods through the posterior approach in the lumbar spine. *Spine*. 2006;31:1351-1357.
67. Kasis AG, Marshman LA, Krishna M, et al. Significantly improved outcomes with a less invasive posterior lumbar interbody fusion incorporating total facetectomy. *Spine*. 2009; 34:572-577.
68. McAfee PC, DeVine JG, Chaput CD, et al. The indications for interbody fusion cages in the treatment of spondylolisthesis: analysis of 120 cases. *Spine*. 2005;30(6 suppl):S60-S65.
69. Blumenthal SL, Gill K. Can lumbar spine radiographs accurately determine fusion in postoperative patients? Correlation of routine radiographs with a second surgical look at lumbar fusions. *Spine*. 1993;18:1186-1189.
70. Brodsky AE, Kovalsky ES, Khalil MA. Correlation of radiologic assessment of lumbar spine fusions with surgical exploration. *Spine*. 1991;16(6 suppl):S261-S265.
71. Togawa D, Bauer TW, Lieberman IH, et al. Lumbar intervertebral body fusion cages: histological evaluation of clinically failed cages retrieved from humans. *J Bone Joint Surg Am*. 2004;86:70-79.
72. Peterson M, Weinman C, Lewis M. The use of ultraporous a-tricalcium phosphate supplementing local autograft in lumbar interbody fusion surgery. *Spine J*. 2005;5(suppl):S171.
73. Rihn JA, Gates C, Glassman SD, et al. The use of bone morphogenetic protein in lumbar spine surgery. *J Bone Joint Surg Am*. 2008;90:2014-2025.
74. Burkus JK, Gornet MF, Dickman CA, et al. Anterior lumbar interbody fusion using rhBMP-2 with tapered interbody cages. *J Spinal Disord Tech*. 2002;15:337-349.
75. Geibel PT, Boyd DL, Slabisak V. The use of recombinant human bone morphogenic protein in posterior interbody fusions of the lumbar spine: a clinical series. *J Spinal Disord Tech*. 2009;22:315-320.
76. Haid RW Jr, Branch CL Jr, Alexander JT, et al. Posterior lumbar interbody fusion using recombinant human bone

morphogenetic protein type 2 with cylindrical interbody cages. *Spine J*. 2004;4:527-538.
77. Wong DA, Kumar A, Jatana S, et al. Neurologic impairment from ectopic bone in the lumbar canal: a potential complication of off-label PLIF/TLIF use of bone morphogenetic protein-2 (BMP-2). *Spine J*. 2008;8: 1011-1018.
78. Chen NF, Smith ZA, Stiner E, et al. Symptomatic ectopic bone formation after off-label use of recombinant human bone morphogenetic protein-2 in transforaminal lumbar interbody fusion. *J Neurosurg Spine*. 2010;12:40-46.
79. Rihn JA, Patel R, Makda J, et al. Complications associated with single-level transforaminal lumbar interbody fusion. *Spine J*. 2009;9:623-629.
80. Villavicencio AT, Burneikiene S, Nelson EL, et al. Safety of transforaminal lumbar interbody fusion and intervertebral recombinant human bone morphogenetic protein-2. *J Neurosurg Spine*. 2005;3:436-443.
81. Smoljanovic T, Bojanic I, Delimar D. Adverse effects of posterior lumbar interbody fusion using rhBMP-2. *Eur Spine J*. 2009;18:920-923.
82. Vaidya R, Sethi A, Bartol S, et al. Complications in the use of rhBMP-2 in PEEK cages for interbody spinal fusions. *J Spinal Disord Tech*. 2008;21:557-562.
83. Rihn JA, Makda J, Hong J, et al. The use of RhBMP-2 in single-level transforaminal lumbar interbody fusion: a clinical and radiographic analysis. *Eur Spine J*. 2009;18:1629-1636.
84. Meisel HJ, Schnöring M, Hohaus C, et al. Posterior lumbar interbody fusion using rhBMP-2. *Eur Spine J*. 2008;17: 1735-1744.
85. Lin PM. Posterior lumbar interbody fusion technique: complications and pitfalls. *Clin Orthop Relat Res*. 1985;193: 90-102.
86. Barnes B, Rodts GE Jr, Haid RW Jr, et al. Allogra implants for posterior lumbar interbody fusion: results comparing cylindrical dowels and impacted wedges. *Neurosurgery*. 2002;51:1191-1198.
87. Hosono N, Namekata M, Makino T, et al. Perioperative complications of primary posterior lumbar interbody fusion for nonisthmic spondylolisthesis: analysis of risk factors. *J Neurosurg Spine*. 2008;9:403-407.
88. Harms J, Jeszenszky D, Stoltze D, et al. True spondylolisthesis reduction and monosegmental fusion in spondylolisthesis. In: Bridwell KH, Dewald RL, eds. *Textbook of Spine Surgery*. 2nd ed. Philadelphia: Lippincott-Raven; 1997:1337-1347.
89. Harms JG, Jeszenszky D. Die posteriore, lumbale, interkorporelle fusion in unilateraler transforaminaler technik. *Oper Orthop Traumatol*. 1998;10:90-102.
90. Kambin P. Arthroscopic microdiskectomy. *Mt Sinai J Med*. 1991;58:159-164.
91. Humphreys SC, Hodges SD, Patwardhan AG, et al. Comparison of posterior and transforaminal approaches to lumbar interbody fusion. *Spine*. 2001;26:567-571.
92. Cole CD, McCall TD, Schmidt MH, et al. Comparison of low back fusion techniques: transforaminal lumbar interbody fusion (TLIF) or posterior lumbar interbody fusion (PLIF) approaches. *Curr Rev Musculoskelet Med*. 2009;2: 118-126.
93. Liu J, Deng H, et al. A comparative study of perioperative complications between transforaminal versus posterior lumbar interbody fusion in degenerative lumbar spondylolisthesis. *Eur Spine J*. 2015;doi:10.1007/s00586-015-4086-8.
94. Javernick MA, Kuklo TR, Polly DW Jr. Transforaminal lumbar interbody fusion: unilateral versus bilateral disk removal—an in vivo study. *Am J Orthop*. 2003;32:344-348.
95. McAfee PC, Lee GA, Fedder IL, et al. Anterior BAK instrumentation and fusion: complete versus partial discectomy. *Clin Orthop Relat Res*. 2002;394:55-63.
96. Li H, Zou X, Laursen M, et al. The influence of intervertebral disc tissue on anterior spinal interbody fusion: an experimental study on pigs. *Eur Spine J*. 2002;11:476-481.
97. Brantigan JW, Steffee AD, Lewis ML, et al. Lumbar interbody fusion using the Brantigan I/F cage for posterior lumbar interbody fusion and the variable pedicle screw placement system: two-year results from a Food and Drug Administration investigational device exemption clinical trial. *Spine*. 2000;25:1437-1446.
98. Arnold PM, Robbins S, Paullus W, et al. Clinical outcomes of lumbar degenerative disc disease treated with posterior lumbar interbody fusion allograft spacer: a prospective, multicenter trial with 2-year follow-up. *Am J Orthop*. 2009;38: E115-E122.
99. Kuslich SD, Danielson G, Dowdel JD, et al. Four-year follow-up results of lumbar spine arthrodesis using the Bagby and Kuslich lumbar fusion cage. *Spine*. 2000;25:2656-2662.
100. Rivet DJ, Jeck D, Brennan J, et al. Clinical outcomes and complications associated with pedicle screw fixation-augmented lumbar interbody fusion. *J Neurosurg Spine*. 2004;1:261-266.
101. Fuji T, Oda T, Kato Y, et al. Posterior lumbar interbody fusion using titanium cylindrical threaded cages: is optimal interbody fusion possible without other instrumentation? *J Orthop Sci*. 2003;8:142-147.
102. Wetzel FT, LaRocca H. The failed posterior lumbar interbody fusion. *Spine*. 1991;16:839-845.
103. Davne SH, Myers DL. Complications of lumbar spinal fusion with transpedicular instrumentation. *Spine*. 1992;17(6 suppl): S184-S189.
104. Krishna M, Pollock RD, Bhatia C. Incidence, etiology, classification, and management of neuralgia after posterior lumbar interbody fusion surgery in 226 patients. *Spine J*. 2008;8:374-379.
105. Okuda S, Oda T, Miyauchi A, et al. Surgical outcomes of posterior lumbar interbody fusion in elderly patients. *J Bone Joint Surg Am*. 2006;88:2714-2720.
106. Abbushi A, Cabraja M, Thomale UW, et al. The influence of cage positioning and cage type on cage migration and fusion rates in patients with monosegmental posterior lumbar interbody fusion and posterior fixation. *Eur Spine J*. 2009;18:1621-1628.
107. Tokuhashi Y, Ajiro Y, Umezawa N. Subsidence of metal interbody cage after posterior lumbar interbody fusion with pedicle screw fixation. *Orthopedics*. 2009;32:259.
108. Brantigan JW. Pseudarthrosis rate after allograft posterior lumbar interbody fusion with pedicle screw and plate fixation. *Spine*. 2004;19:1271-1279.
109. Li YC, Yang SC, et al. Impact of lumbar instrumented circumferential fusion on the development of adjacent vertebral compression fracture. *Bone Joint J*. 2015;97-B(10): 1411-1416.
110. Lee JY, Milne EL, Shufflebarger HL, et al. *Anterior column support in long segment kyphosis constructs*. In Proceedings of the Scoliosis Research Society 32nd Annual Meeting, St. Louis, 1997, Paper #50.

CHAPTER 51 Posterolateral and Lateral Corpectomies

Raghav Badrinath
T. Barrett Sullivan
Steven R. Garfin
R. Todd Allen

Posterolateral and lateral approaches to disc disease in the thoracic spine developed as a consequence of poor outcomes after traditional posterior laminectomies, generally due to the approach morbidity and inadequacy of ventral decompression achieved by these procedures in surgical management of central and paramedian herniated discs. Posterolateral approaches to the thoracic spine are varied and include costotransversectomy, transforaminal, transpedicular, transfacet pedicle sparing, and transverse arthropediculectomy. Variations among these approaches largely hinge on the amount of bone resected to achieve decompression. These may be seen as in a continuum with the lateral approaches, namely the lateral rhachotomy, the lateral extracavitary approach, and the lateral parascapular extrapleural approach. Improved exposure offered by these approaches facilitates better decompression of centrally located, larger, or highly calcified disc herniations, among many other pathologies. However, these techniques come at a cost of being technically demanding and require significant soft tissue manipulation and dissection.

In the lumbar spine, posterolateral corpectomy and arthrodesis is a fairly common procedure performed for pathologies such as spinal deformity, degenerative disease, trauma, tumor and infection. In many patients corpectomy can serve as a workhorse for more complex disorders requiring effective interbody fusion, and use of a less-invasive lateral approach to perform lateral corpectomy and arthrodesis is increasingly common and used for more complex disorders of the spine. Interest in the procedure has exponentially increased after its introduction.

Although the focus of this section is thoracic and lumbar disc disease, posterolateral and lateral approaches to corpectomy are among the most versatile of approaches for vertebral body resections and have been adapted for use in spinal deformity and scoliosis, thoracic and thoracolumbar vertebral body trauma, vertebral neoplasm, and vertebral osteomyelitis.

Posterolateral and Lateral Corpectomy in the Thoracic Spine

Historical Perspective

Spinal cord decompression for thoracic disc herniation traditionally involved simple laminectomies. Adson performed the first laminectomy and decompression for thoracic disc herniation in 1922.[1] Mixter and Barr reported on laminectomies for 19 disc herniations in 1934, of which 4 were in the thoracic spine.[2] Two of these patients developed transverse myelopathy postoperatively, and another recurrence of symptoms was noted shortly thereafter. Similar results were noted by multiple other series, with significant morbidity and mortality associated with the procedure.[3-8] Perot and Munro in 1969 reviewed 91 cases of thoracic disc herniations treated with dorsal laminectomy and noted persistence of symptoms or paralysis in 40 of these patients.[9] Importantly, they were able to demonstrate improved outcomes with lateral disc herniations compared with centrally located protrusions.

Costotransversectomy was introduced by Menard in 1895, as with many approaches to the spine, for the treatment of Pott disease.[10,11] Variations were developed by Seddon (1935) and Capener (1954).[12,13] Hulme (1960) is believed to have been the first to perform the procedure for thoracic disc herniation, although his technique was a modification of the original and involved a more extensive transverse arthropediculectomy.[5] The lateral extracavitary approach (LECA) was originally developed by Alexander[14] and a modified version by Capener[15] in the treatment of tuberculous spondylitis. The procedure was later introduced by Larson[16] in 1976, allowing for wide exposure using a fully extrapleural approach, which gave surgeons the ability to span the thorax and abdomen without taking down the diaphragm.[17,18] Several authors have subsequently, and in recent decades, used modified versions of the procedure to access and treat all types of anterior spinal pathology while allowing for the placement of posterior instrumentation. Patterson and Arbit[19] described the transpedicular approach in 1978, which involved removal of the entire pedicle and facet, affording a more direct exposure of ventral disc space. This approach offers the advantage of not placing radicular vessels at risk but still provides reasonable access to central and calcified discs.

The development of these approaches was driven out of goals to improve the management of degenerative disease and disc pathology via decreased morbidity with improved decompression and *partial* corpectomy. These techniques, however, have been modernized to facilitate greater degrees of corpectomy and even vertebrectomy in the management of more diverse pathologies, including vertebral body fractures, neoplasms, vertebral osteomyelitis, and spinal deformity (e.g. kyphosis, kyphoscoliosis) to generate greater sagittal and coronal plane corrections.

Indications and Choice of Approach

Absolute indications for surgical management of thoracic disc disease, and cord compression from a variety of pathologies, remain poorly defined. The natural history of the disease is not well captured, and thus is relatively unknown, and symptoms do not always correlate with the extent of disease noted on imaging.[20-23] In general, patients with severe, intractable radicular pain, progressive myelopathy, lower extremity weakness, or bowel and bladder dysfunction with evidence of cord compression on magnetic resonance imaging are considered to be good candidates for surgical treatment, not uncommonly requiring partial corpectomy for decompression. Indications for more extensive corpectomy or vertebrectomy via posterolateral and lateral approaches are outlined in separate sections, but this chapter is focused on cord compression, progressive neurologic deficits, or spinal column instability resulting from degenerative, deformity, traumatic, infectious, or neoplastic processes leading to destruction of the vertebral body that causes anterior column instability or direct cord compression via mass effect.

Surgeon opinion regarding choice of approach is also inconsistent. Each approach carries with it unique benefits and risks. Choice of approach requires careful evaluation of patient-specific pathology and overall medical status as well as a consideration of surgeon experience with a particular technique. In all cases, the most important goal during treatment is to minimize manipulation of a damaged/compressed spinal cord while ensuring complete decompression and stabilization. Transpedicular and pedicle-sparing transfacet approaches are often cited as technically simpler than other approaches, allowing for minimal bone removal and decreased operative time.[21,22,24,25] Costotransversectomy requires more extensive soft tissue dissection and rib removal and comes with increased risk of blood loss.[24,26,27] There also exists the potential for vascular compromise due to poor visualization of the radicular vessels, especially when operating between T7 and L2 due to possible disruption of the artery of Adamkiewicz.[28,29] The extrapleural nature of these approaches usually eliminates the need for a chest tube. Posterior and posterolateral approaches, particularly when made via a central midline incision, also allow for posterior instrumentation without the need for an additional incision.

Transpedicular and pedicle-sparing approaches are suited for more laterally located pathologies or in the treatment patients with multiple medical comorbidities, who require less anesthesia and historically a more expedient procedure.[19,25,30] Densely calcified discs or centrally located pathologies have been suggested to be better managed with a more direct transthoracic or thoracoscopic approach.[9,31] However, some authors continue to prefer a costotransversectomy approach with an interbody fusion after removal of more ventral disc, then impacting the calcified compressive disc away from the dural sac and spine. Lateral and costotransversectomy approaches tend to offer advantages in exposure with paramedian pathology or lateral disc herniations with calcification,[21,25,32-34] although it has been suggested that a direct lateral approach can achieve decompressions in a variety of ventral pathologies. As mentioned, vascular compromise must be guarded against in these approaches, and some recommend routine angiography in cases where the planned procedure places multiple radicular vessels at risk.[10,24,35] New modifications of and indications for these approaches continue to be described.[21,36] Beyond thoracic disc herniations, many of these techniques have been used extensively for neoplasm, trauma, deformity, and infection with good results.[33,37-41] The extent of corpectomy varies with the burden of disease. Vertebrectomy is more commonly indicated in cases of extensive vertebral osteomyelitis, fracture, or neoplasm but also facilitates improved decompression or deformity correction in kyphosis/kyphoscoliosis. These approaches often require anterior interbody fusion devices and posterior instrumentation and arthrodesis depending on the amount of bone removed and subsequent instability.

Surgical Technique

Posterolateral Approaches

In posterior/posterolateral approaches, the patient is prone or in a modified prone/laterally tilted position. The approach side is based on the laterality of the pathology, and a right-sided approach is often preferred in central pathology to avoid the descending aorta. Special consideration must also be given to the artery of Adamkiewicz with left-sided approaches in the lower thoracic spine.[5,42,43] Care must be taken intraoperatively to accurately identify and mark the correct surgical level, and intraoperative fluoroscopic images should be compared with preoperative radiographs to account for vertebral level anomalies.[22,24] With a costotransversectomy, the incision is typically midline and vertical rather than curving out over the rib. Dissection is carried through the fascia, and subperiosteal dissection proceeds for optimal spine exposure. The costotransverse articulation is an important landmark. It approaches medially and ends just at and above the pedicle, to articulate with the vertebral body and disc space, crossing along the undersurface of the transverse process. The trapezius and nondissected erector spinae muscles are further exposed and dissection proceeds through the rib periosteum as laterally as needed prior to rib removal. The intercostal neurovascular bundle is identified on the rib undersurface and separated from the rib, and the rib is then cut and disarticulated from the vertebral body. A periosteal tissue plane can protect the pleura during dissection. The pleura is mobilized (preferably behind a subperiosteal tissue plane of the vertebra) and reflected anterolaterally, protected with malleable retractors and moistened sponges. The intercostal nerve can be followed medially to identify the intervertebral foramen. Visualization is improved several ways, including laminectomy and by partial removal of the pedicles, and the dural sac is exposed. Having achieved visualization of the neural elements and remaining bony landmarks, the surgeon can subsequently proceed with partial or near complete corpectomy without manipulation of the dura. If circumferential decompression is desired, bilateral costotransversectomy can be performed.[27,43] When this is performed, a temporary rod should be placed contralateral to the side of decompression to maintain spinal stability, optimize complete decompression, and reduce risk of iatrogenic injury to the spinal cord.[27] An interbody cage can be placed posterolaterally to fill either the discectomy or corpectomy defect. For larger defects, the spinal root often may need to be tied and resection, allowing greater exposure for placement of larger interbody devices, such as titanium mesh cages, expandable cages, or structural bony grafts (e.g., femoral and humeral allografts).

The transpedicle and transfacet approaches use a posterior midline incision. Paraspinal musculature is reflected from the spinous processes and laminae via subperiosteal dissection, facilitating access to the posterior aspect of the spinal for facet and/or pedicle removal and subsequent partial discectomy or corpectomy. In the case of central pathology, bilateral facetectomies may be performed for improved access.[19,31,44,45] Once again a central cavity allows for anterior decompression. Posterior instrumentation can be accomplished from the same incision, and excised bone can be used if an arthrodesis is desired in addition to the decompression.

Lateral Approaches

LECA has historically used a curvilinear incision extending from the midline to approximately 7 to 12 cm lateral at its apex (e.g., "hockey stick" incision). A thick cutaneous flap down to the thoracodorsal fascia is mobilized and retracted. A vertical incision is made in the latissimus dorsi parallel to its fibers at the lateral extent of the incision down to the ribs, and is mobilized. This mobile mass of latissimus and paraspinal musculature can be mobilized medially for rib resection and laterally for access to the central pathology. The rib at the inferior level of the pathology is isolated from the neurovascular bundle and intercostal muscles, cut laterally, and disarticulated.[16,46-48] A LECA can, in practicality, be performed via a midline incision if extensile enough. The key difference between the costotransversectomy and the LECA is not only the central midline versus a more hockey stick–like incision in LECA, but also in the amount of rib resection, with the LECA generally resecting greater than 6 cm of rib. At this point, the ipsilateral facet complex, transverse process, and laminae can be resected for exposure of the dural sac and posterior spine. A partial or complete corpectomy and complete decompression can then be accomplished. As with posterolateral approaches, interbody fusion and posterior instrumentation and arthrodesis can be accomplished with the same incision.

With upper thoracic disc herniations (T1–T4), additional challenges are encountered, including a narrowed thoracic cage, accentuated kyphosis, greater proximity to the brachial plexus and mediastinal structures, and scapular bone and surrounding musculature.[49] A proximal approach, or lateral parascapular extrapleural approach, involves a curvilinear midline incision around the scapula. The trapezius and rhomboids are transected, mobilized, and reflected as a myocutaneous flap, allowing the scapula to retract laterally. At this point, the paraspinal musculature can be elevated subperiosteally off the spinous processes and dissection proceeds as for the LECA.

The direct lateral thoracic approach for the thoracic spine is a modification of a standard thoracotomy; the direct lateral lumbar spine approach is detailed later in this chapter. During the direct lateral thoracic approach, the patient is placed in the lateral decubitus position (typically with sticky rolls), with the torso, pelvis, and legs secured. We prefer not to "break" the table or bend open the disc space for thoracic discs. However, during the approach to the thoracolumbar spine, gently opening this space can be beneficial to pull the ribs proximally and with little morbidity or concern for plexus injuries. Obtaining an anteroposterior (AP) fluoroscopy image, followed by an orthogonal view directly lateral (perpendicular to the floor and parallel to the disc space endplates), centered at the disc space of interest to minimize parallax, is crucial to decrease the risk of surgical injury during discectomy and corpectomy, as well as during cage and instrumentation placement. The table should be adjusted to provide true AP and lateral images when the C-arm is horizontal and vertical, respectively. Once identified, disc spaces of interest are marked on the lateral skin parallel to the ribs, then sterile prep and drape is performed. Entry into the thoracic cavity can then be performed via partial rib resection or in between ribs for single-level disc access. We prefer a partial rib resection to decrease the risk of postoperative radiculitis or rib pain due to retractor pressure at the rib undersurface. Care should be taken to avoid the neurovascular bundle that lies on the inferior surface of each rib. An oblique incision is made and the rib dissected through the periosteum. Depending on the segments of interest and size of the incision, multiple ribs can be exposed. The rib is dissected circumferentially with the direct undersurface protecting the pleura from being breached, and the rib is cut at the desired interval. Recall that one can work in between ribs if single-level disc pathology is approached. Once the portion of the rib is cut and removed, dissection ensues around the posterior wall in a preferably retropleural tissue plane on the undersurface of the thoracic cage. This proceeds to the disc of interest via blunt dissection, often following a rib head to the disc space, prior to localization. Discectomy ensues after ensuring the retractor blades are centered around the desired area in the lateral and then AP planes. Alternatively, the index finger can be used to enter the pleural space and digitally displace the lung and pleural structures anteriorly. Posteriorly introducing the inner dilator behind this and onto the disc, at the junction of the rib head and vertebral body, can be performed. The lung does not need to be deflated. Some authors prefer variations of this approach, which typically requires a chest tube. If the surgeon remains in a plane mostly behind the parietal pleura, and discectomy/corpectomy performed, a malleable tube or red rubber catheter can be placed during closure and removed prior to sealing the cavity without chest tube placement. Once the dilator is positioned (preferably in the posterior third of the disc) and lateral fluoroscopic imaging is performed, an inner wire and serial dilation ensues until the retractor is docked in the appropriate trajectory (e.g., parallel to the disc space) and stabilized via the retractor arm to the bed. For corpectomy, thorough discectomies can be performed above and below the vertebra of interest, followed by expansion of the retractor over the vertebral body, using the prior discectomies, proximal pedicle, and posterior vertebral body as a guide to placement. Once placed and expanded to the appropriate size, orthogonal lateral and AP fluoroscopic imaging should be obtained, followed by corpectomy and thorough canal decompression. A key anatomic structure to identify is the pedicle, in reference to its relationship to the posterior vertebral body, rib, and disc. Several interbody options can be used to span the corpectomy site, and instrumentation can be applied via the same approach.

Outcomes

Disc Herniation

In general, outcomes are comparable between the posterolateral, lateral and transthoracic approaches when used for disc herniation. However, studies do not specifically identify the extent of corpectomy performed in addition to the disc excision and decompression. Mulier et al reviewed 331 cases of thoracic disc herniation and noted improved outcomes in 93% of patients treated with the transthoracic approach, 87% of patients treated with posterolateral approaches, and 80% of patients treated with lateral approaches.[21] Worse outcomes were noted with the presence and degree of preoperative paresis, absence of radiculopathy, duration of symptoms, and a history of previous surgery. Outcome does not appear to be related to level of herniation, multiplicity, or the presence of calcification or intradural penetration. Fessler et al, in their meta-analysis comparing approaches to thoracic disc herniation, noted a 10% morbidity rate with the transthoracic and LECA approaches.[26] They noted lower morbidity rates with costotransversectomy (2%) and transpedicular approaches (1%), although relatively few patients underwent these procedures in their analysis. Although the transthoracic approach appears to cause the most reliable symptom relief, it poses a greater risk. McCormick et al performed a meta-analysis of complications after various approaches between 1934 and 1998.[24] They noted a 13.4% rate of complications with the transthoracic approach compared with 5.4% with costotransversectomy, 2.8% with LECA, and 4.6% with the transfacet pedicle-sparing approach. They noted no complications associated with the transpedicle approach in their review. However, postoperative infections, pneumonia, and cerebrospinal fluid leak were specifically excluded from their analysis due to a relative lack of data in the literature.[24] Common complications noted were neurologic compromise, misidentification of the surgical level, postoperative instability, cerebrospinal fluid leak, pulmonary complications, surgical infection, intercostal neuralgia and general surgical complications such as deep venous thrombosis and pulmonary embolus.

A more recent review by Lubelski et al compared thoracotomy, costotransversectomy, and LECA, analyzing 774 cases in the literature between 1991 and 2011.[27,32] The thoracotomy approach had the highest rate of complications (39%), reoperations (3.5%), and death (1.5%) among the three approaches. LECA had a complication rate of 17%, with the need for a thoracostomy tube (9.6%) and wound infections (5.7%) being the most common complications. Costotransversectomy had a 15% complication rate. Wound infection (3.7%) and deep vein thrombosis/pulmonary embolism (DVT/PE) (3.7%) were the most common complications. Reoperation rate (1.3% with LECA vs. 1.2% with costotransversectomy) and mortality rate (0.6% for LECA vs. 1.2% with costotransversectomy) were similar between the two approaches. Average operating time with LECA was 544 minutes, and average estimated blood loss was 3.3 L. With costotransversectomy, average operating time was 405 minutes, average estimated blood loss was 2.0 L, and average postoperative length of hospital stay was 6.7 days.

Results of operative management of traumatic, neoplastic, infectious, or degenerative deformity pathologies with corpectomy or vertebrectomy in the thoracic spine are addressed in their respective chapters in this text.

Posterolateral and Lateral Corpectomy in the Lumbar Spine

Historical Perspective

Spinal fusion surgery was first introduced by Hibbs and Albee in 1911 for the treatment of Pott disease.[50,51] Following Chandler's description of lumbar fusion for low back pain, corpectomy and arthrodesis gained in popularity as surgeons recognized that disc excision alone did not alleviate symptoms of discogenic back pain.[2,52] Watkins later introduced the technique of posterolateral fusion with the aim of reducing high rates of pseudarthrosis encountered in posterior fusion surgery.[53] Partial corpectomy with interbody fusion was subsequently proposed by Cloward[54] in 1953, and this technique quickly gained favor as a means by which to increase fusion and graft compression surface area.[55] Although reports of poor outcomes in arthrodesis in the 1970s led the technique to briefly fall out of favor, focus on the technique was reinvigorated by development of the pedicle screw, fusion cages, and modern biologics seen in the 1990s.[56-59]

More recently, interest in reducing postoperative hospitalization time and operative morbidity through minimizing exposure and soft tissue trauma has been a driving force in the development of minimally invasive techniques for spinal decompression and fusion. Although approaches for percutaneous posterior instrumentation are relatively straightforward, addressing the anterior aspect of the spinal column through minimally invasive methods is limited by the abdominal and thoracic viscera in the lumbar and thoracic regions of the spine. Historically, approaches to the anterior aspect of the spinal column required violation of the peritoneum or pleura, frequently necessitating the involvement of access surgeons. As minimally invasive techniques evolved with the development and implementation of laparoscopic and thoracoscopic instrumentation, limitations in postoperative visceral complications, a steep learning curve, and access surgeon support persisted. It was, at least in part, in the interest of developing an extracavitary approach to the anterior aspect of the spinal column via tissue planes not requiring violation of the pleura or peritoneum that the lateral transpsoas approach was developed.

Initially reported as an endoscopic retroperitoneal technique in 2001, the direct lateral approach was quickly adapted into an open, minimally invasive, psoas-splitting technique.[60] Developed for treatment of degenerative disc disease, indications for the approach grew to predominantly mirror those for anterior and posterior approaches to spinal fusion: unstable degenerative disc disease, degenerative spondylolisthesis, degenerative scoliosis, disc herniation, and even trauma, infection, or neoplastic processes.[60-64] As with other posterolateral approaches, the transpsoas approach (or direct lateral in the thoracolumbar or thoracic spines) can be combined with partial corpectomy or vertebrectomy to facilitate desired deformity correction, decompression, or preparation for interposition constructs.

Indications

Absolute indications stem from preservation of neurologic function due to severe retrovertebral compression and/or spinal instability, with many contributing diagnoses such as trauma, tumor, deformity, infection/spondylodiscitis, and advanced degenerative disease. Precise indications for posterolateral and lateral corpectomies in cases of degenerative disc disease are ill defined, yet roughly 51% of lumbar spinal fusion surgery is performed for a diagnosis of degenerative disc disease.[58,65-68] As expected in cases of chronic low back pain associated with degenerative disease, initial nonoperative measures including rest, activity modification, physical therapy, antiinflammatory medications, and often epidural steroid or other injections focused on the pathology.[70-79] As with many cases of lumbar degenerative disease, symptoms nonresponsive to aggressive nonoperative management are indications for surgery, with clear priority given to progressive neurologic deficits, saddle anesthesia, or bowel and bladder dysfunction. Although specific indications for partial corpectomy or vertebrectomy and fusion in the setting of trauma, neoplasm, infection, or degenerative deformity are discussed in their respective chapters, intervention in each of these conditions is recommended in the presence of progressive neurologic deficits or spinal column instability.

Technique

Posterolateral

After induction of anesthesia and intubation, the patient is placed in a prone position typically on a Jackson table. Care is taken to pad all prominences and fluoroscopy is utilized to identify appropriate spinal levels. Posterolateral extracavitary corpectomy is typically performed through a posterior midline approach. Open approaches, even in fairly good bone, typically require 2 levels of instrumented stabilization above and below the corpectomy site, though 3 levels should be considered with larger deformity corrections and/or poor bone quality. Once incision is made, subperiosteal dissection proceeds to expose spinal lamina, pars and facets, then spinous processes are removed and laminectomy is performed using a high-speed burr and Kerrison punches/rongeurs. Transverse processes, pars and facets are decorticated to stimulate fusion. This allows access to the pedicles and lateral vertebral body, and pedicle resection and corpectomy may be performed using the curettes and pituitary rongeur if desired.[69] Autograft or allograft graft material is placed over the decorticated areas. Fusion may be augmented with various osteoconductive or osteoinductive materials. Stabilization may be enhanced by the addition of posterior pedicle screws from the same approach.

Lateral Transpsoas Approach (Extreme or Direct Lateral Approach)

This procedure was first reported in the literature by Ozgur et al in 2006.[60] The following procedural description is based on their work, with slight modification. After induction of anesthesia, the patient is typically placed in the left side up, right side down lateral decubitus position using anterior and posterior sticky rolls, with an axillary roll in place. Tape is used to secure the patient to the bed, at the torso and between the ilium and greater trochanter. The break in the table is placed just above the greater trochanter, and the table is often gently flexed to pull the iliac wing caudal and the ribs proximally. We strongly prefer, however, to use angled instruments rather than break or bend the table. When required, it is broken *as little as possible* and only if access to the spine needs to be improved or optimized. Attempts should be made to minimize table break so that little, if any, significant stretching the lumbar plexus or psoas occurs. Mild forward flexion of the patient may assist to distract the posterior elements and may increase working room between the iliac wing and the twelfth rib. Intraoperative fluoroscopy is then used, first obtaining a perfect AP image with spinous process splitting the pedicles symmetrically, then obtaining a later image in which the caudal vertebral body has a flat endplate and the pedicles overlap. Once fluoroscopic confirmation is achieved by using orthogonal views that the patient is in the true 90-degree lateral orientation, discs of interest are marked on the lateral abdominal wall using a radiopaque marker, and sterile prep and drape is performed. A 1.5- to 2-cm posterolateral incision can be made overlying the border between the abdominal obliques and the erector spinae as an access portal to the retroperitoneal space via a Kocher clamp and then blunt finger dissection. The posterolateral incision also allows for gentle retraction of the peritoneum during passage of dilators through the lateral approach.

After gaining access to the retroperitoneal space the surgeon's finger can be used to gently lift the peritoneum anteriorly in a sweeping fashion, thereby facilitating palpation down to the psoas muscle and transverse process. After separating these tissue planes the surgeon's finger can then be redirected superficially to directly under the lateral approach marking, further facilitating anterior retraction of the peritoneum from the abdominal wall. A surgical blade is then used to make a skin incision overlying the direct lateral mark, and an initial dilator (with attached free-run electromyographic neuromonitoring) is then passed through this incision and the surgeon's index finger, passed into the retroperitoneal space via the posterolateral incision, is used to gently guide the soft tissue dilator to the psoas muscle with care taken to protect the peritoneum by lifting it anteriorly during passage. Once the dilator has reached the psoas muscle, it is used to split the psoas fibers at the middle to anterior third of the muscle to reduce risk to more posteriorly located nerve roots and the lumbar plexus. Neurologic monitoring cannot be overemphasized as a means to reduce risk of injury to the lumbar plexus and roots during this process. After the initial dilator has reached the disc space, intraoperative lateral fluoroscopy is used to confirm appropriate positioning. Once confirmed, an inner wire is placed into the disc space. After confirmation, sequential dilators are used until a retractor can be inserted over the final dilator and secured to a retractor arm. Gentle, controlled distraction can then be used to generate the desired exposure. At this point, we prefer to confirm neural elements are out of the field using a neuromonitoring probe in all quadrants of the disc space and retractor bed. Once lateral and AP fluoroscopy is used to verify appropriate retractor positioning, the surgeon proceeds with discectomy. Care should be taken of all opposite-side structures, particularly if the annulus is released via a cobb or other method. Our preference for lateral corpectomy is to perform discectomy at the proximal disc space, identify the pedicle and posterior body wall, and then perform caudal interbody space discectomy. Once caudal discectomy is performed, the posterior vertebral wall and pedicle are identified once again, and the retractor is opened to access the vertebral body for corpectomy. At the onset, a lateral fluoroscopic image is crucial to ensure one is not overlying the canal and that the retractor is in an optimal position. Once confirmed, and the pedicle and posterior vertebral body are identified, the segmental artery is transected using a bipolar and/or clips and a bovie. We then proceed with corpectomy, or vertebrectomy and subsequent interposition construct insertion.[70] In addition to placement of static or expandable interbody devices of titanium, polyetheretherketone, or bone, one can consider lateral fixation options such as a plate or screw-rod constructs, the latter being our preference when required. After completion of instrumentation, copious irrigation, and optimization of hemostasis, the retractor is slowly removed with direct visualization used to confirm closure of the psoas and ensure excellent hemostasis. Incision sites are then closed in a layered fashion and dressed with sterile dressings.

Outcomes

In general, and as may be expected, outcome studies specifically analyzing corpectomy for degenerative disease are not readily available. The following data help to define some of the roles for which the LECA and minimally invasive direct lateral approach have been used in a variety of pathologies.

Lateral Extracavitary Approach

The versatility of the LECA allows for its use for a wide range of spinal pathologies, including tumor, trauma, and infection in addition to disc disease. However, good-quality, larger scale studies specifically evaluating approach as the variable are difficult to come by.

Resnick et al performed a retrospective review of 33 patients with thoracic and thoracolumbar fractures treated by LECA in an effort to outline complications from the approach.[33] Patients were overwhelmingly male (91%), with a mean age of 32.5 years. Fractures were largely at the thoracolumbar junction. Mean blood loss was 3.1 L, and mean operative time was 7.74 hours. Complications were observed in 55% of patients. The most common complication (33%) was a hemothorax or pleural effusion requiring chest tube placement. Pneumonia occurred in 21% of patients, and wound complications were observed in 12% of patients. Other complications included incisional hernias, sepsis, gastrointestinal bleeding secondary to anticoagulation, and implant malposition. There were no cases of neurologic worsening or death. Arnold and colleagues reviewed 33 patients undergoing LECA for nontuberculous thoracic and lumbar osteomyelitis.[71] Of these, 22 patients with extensive disease required fusion. Graft material used included the rib in the thoracic spine and iliac crest in the lumbar spine. They noted good neurologic recovery after the procedure. Three of seven paraplegic patients improved, with one patient regaining ambulation. All 11 patients with mild weakness became neurologically intact, and 10 of 11 patients with severe preoperative weakness achieved good functional recovery. Although details on specific complications were not provided, the authors reported on two reoperations, and no deaths. McCormick et al. studied 12 patients with dumbbell or paraspinal tumors treated with LECA.[72] They noted gross total removal of tumor, confirmed by computed tomography or magnetic resonance imaging, in 10 patients. At mean follow-up of 34 months, nine patients showed no evidence of residual tumor. There were two deaths from systemic tumor dissemination and recurrence in one patient. The study notes no significant perioperative complications, although two patients did require chest tube placement for pleural entry. Lubelski et al compared LECA to costotransversectomy performed for any indication, including disc herniation, trauma, osteomyelitis, scoliosis, and kyphosis.[32] Overall, 54 patients were included in the study, 19 of whom underwent LECA. The average age was 53.7 years, and 74% were male. Mean blood loss was 2.1 L, and average length of stay was 17.2 days.

Complications were noted in 68% of patients. Approximately half of these were classified as intraoperative complications. The common intraoperative complications included need for transfusion, need for a thoracostomy, and DVT/PE. The most common postoperative complications were pleural effusion, infection, and reoperation. Of note, complications were not found to be different between the two approaches studied. Similarly, Graham et al. looked at 29 patients with significant medical comorbidities and anterior spinal cord compression secondary to a variety of diagnoses who underwent LECA.[73] The average age was 53 years, and the population was 34% male. They noted death secondary to pneumonia in one patient, and two patients had postoperative infections. Overall, they concluded that LECA offered a useful one-stage treatment in medically complex patients for whom a two-stage procedure may not be preferable.

Summarizing these and other studies, Foreman et al. performed a meta-analysis of the literature examining the use of LECA for any indication.[48] They included 11 studies covering 278 patients in addition to their own series of 65 patients. They noted improved neurologic outcomes in 75% of patients and improved pain outcomes in 85%. Thirty-two percent of patients were noted to have at least one complication.

Costotransversectomy

Costotransversectomy has perhaps been most studied in its application to address tumors in the thoracolumbar spine. Sciubba and colleagues noted the utility of the surgery in addressing spinal cord compression secondary to metastatic lesions, effectively improving neurologic outcomes.[74] One of the earlier studies, by Cybulski et al., reported on performing corpectomy and decompression in 15 patients with metastatic tumors of the thoracic spine, 10 of whom also underwent posterior instrumentation.[75] They noted neurologic improvement in 75% of patients and, importantly, no neurologic deterioration. More recently, Chong and colleagues retrospectively analyzed 105 patients undergoing single-stage posterior decompression with or without corpectomy for thoracic vertebral metastases.[76] Twenty percent of patients noted an improvement in Frankel grade, and 10 of 21 Frankel grade C patients became ambulatory. Pain improvement was especially pronounced in patients with anterior column reconstruction and more than four fixation levels. Wiggins and colleagues performed a retrospective review of their prospective database and compared outcomes of 29 patients undergoing costotransversectomy with 18 patients undergoing anterior procedures for neoplasms.[77] They found a complication rate of 38% in the costotransversectomy group and noted that it was similar between the two groups. However, they did note two cases of neurologic deterioration and one death in the costotransversectomy group compared with none in the anterior group. Lu et al. similarly compared outcomes after thoracolumbar corpectomy with the transpedicular approach in 34 patients with the anterior approach in 46 patients, noting similar rates of complications, blood loss, and operative time between groups.[78] Good results have been noted using the approach for large intradural ventral neoplastic lesions, as noted in the series by Ito et al.[79] and Kim et al.[80] Thorat and colleagues reported on their series of 11 patients with dumbbell tumors of the thoracic spine treated with single-stage corpectomy using the costotransversectomy approach.[81] They noted the ability to obtain total excision in 10 of the 11 patients. No significant neurologic worsening was noted postoperatively, and two patients required thoracostomy tube placement. Similar results were also noted by Ando et al. in their series of 16 patients undergoing a modified costotransversectomy for thoracic dumbbell tumors.[82]

Besides applications in tumor, the approach is fairly versatile and also allows for more extensive decompression, circumferential arthrodesis, and multilevel corpectomies for any indication.[83-86] In their meta-analysis, Lubelski et al. looked at 13 papers in the literature that detailed a costotransversectomy approach for a variety of spinal disorders.[27] They noted an overall complication rate of 15%, with wound infection (3.7%) and DVT/PE (3.7%) being the most common complications. They also noted a mortality rate of 1.2% and a reoperation rate of 4.3%.

Lateral/Posterolateral/Posterior Minimally Invasive Surgical Thoracic and Lumbar Corpectomy

Increasing familiarity of lateral access anatomy, instrumentation, and implants has led to advanced applications of lateral surgery for all types of spine disorders. Kim et al[87] were among the first to describe minimally invasive posterolateral corpectomy in a combined cadaver and case series, including two burst fractures, one plasmacytoma, and one metastatic lesion. In their clinical cases a mean 79.2% of corpectomy procedures were facilitated via the approach, with all patients achieving satisfactory neural decompression, though they did report difficulty with contralateral decompression. Average estimated blood loss was 495 mL, with a mean operating room time of 5.8 hours. In 2010, Smith et al.[88] treated 52 patients with unstable thoracic or lumbar burst fractures with mini-open lateral corpectomy. All patients received supplemental fixation with anterolateral plating or transpedicular fixation, and titanium cages were used in 35% of patients. Average operative time was 128 minutes, estimated blood loss was 300 mL, and the complication rate was 13.5%. No patients had neurologic deterioration, and postoperative American Spinal Injury Association (ASIA) score significantly improved. Khan et al.[89] reported on the use of a minimally invasive extreme lateral approach to the thoracolumbar spine for corpectomy and reconstruction in 25 patients with varying pathology, which included tumor, infection, and fracture. Thirteen patients underwent anterior-only fixation, and the remaining 12 had a staged posterior procedure. Mean operative time was 188.5 minutes, and average blood loss was 423 mL. Although mean follow-up was only 5.1 months, these authors observed no implant failures or wound complications at final follow-up, and patients reported a 62% decrease in visual analog scale score. Gandhoke and colleagues[90] used a minimally invasive extreme lateral approach to treat thoracolumbar burst fractures in two patients with incomplete spinal cord injury. Estimated blood loss was less than 500 mL in both patients, with an operating room time of 4 hours in one case and 4.5 hours in the second case. Both patients were neurologically intact without pain at roughly 1 year follow-up, and both patients had maintained their restored lordosis.

In addition to direct lateral approaches, posterolateral and posterior transpedicular modifications using less-invasive retractors and paramedian incisions have been used for vertebral corpectomy. Deutsch et al.[91] reported their results of a minimally invasive transpedicular corpectomy without instrumentation in eight patients with metastatic disease. Operations were planned as palliative procedures, but the authors reported a 75% decompression of the canal with a unilateral approach. They also described an average blood loss of 227 mL and mean operating room time of 2.2 hours, a marked improvement over traditionally reported operative times and estimated blood loss. Sixty-three percent (63%) of patients had a postoperative improvement of at least one Nurick grade.[91] Smith and colleagues[92] reported the results of a cadaveric feasibility study for a minimally invasive LECA for corpectomy. They performed the procedure in three human cadavers and achieved a circumferential volume decompression of 48% and mean vertebral body resection of 72%. Average anterior height expansion was 47 mm and posterior height expansion was 61 mm. No dural or pleural tears were encountered, and of 24 screws placed there was only one lateral breach. In the three clinic cases (a T11 burst fracture, a T7 plasmacytoma, and a T4–T5 tuberculosis lesion), estimated blood loss was 517 mL and average operating room time was 4.75 hours. Patients were all determined to have excellent outcomes, and the authors concluded that the procedure was safe and associated with reduced blood loss and minimal morbidity. Chou and Lu performed a case series analysis consisting of minimally invasive transpedicular corpectomy and cage reconstruction in eight patients compared with a similar cohort treated with an open procedure. They reported similar findings.[93,94] In a comparative study, Lau and Lou[95] compared mini-open versus open posterior thoracic corpectomy with cage reconstruction in oncology patients with metastatic disease. Twenty-one patients underwent mini-open surgery and 28 patients had open surgery, with mean operative times similar at approximately 4 hours. In the mini-open group, however, significantly reduced blood loss and shorter length of hospital stay were observed. No differences were found in complication rate, revision rate, or postoperative ASIA change. There was a nonsignificant trend toward reduced infection rate in the mini-open technique.[95]

Summary

From the time of tuberculous pathology, deformity, and disc disease, successful treatment of this and more advanced pathologies has been made possible by the versatility of extracavitary, costotransversectomy, and now lateral approaches to the spine. Although several reports allow conclusions to be drawn regarding exceptional surgical utility, high-level outcome studies remain elusive. Future investigation will likely require prospective, multicenter study designs to determine how truly impactful these approaches are toward removing offending pathology and improving patient quality of life.

REFERENCES

1. Adson AW, Ott WO. Results of the removal of tumors of the spinal cord. *Arch Neurol Psychiatry*. 1922;8(5):520-537.
2. Mixter WJ, Barr JS. Rupture of the intervertebral disc with involvement of the spinal canal. *NEJM*. 1934;211(5):210-215.
3. Arce C, Dohrmann G. Herniated thoracic disks. *Neurol Clin*. 1985;3(2):383-392.
4. Hawk WA. Spinal compression caused by ecchondrosis of the intervertebral fibrocartilage: with a review of the recent literature. *Brain*. 1936;59(2):204-224.
5. Hulme A. The surgical approach to thoracic intervertebral disc protrusions. *J Neurol Neurosurg Psychiatry*. 1960;23(2): 133-137.
6. Kite WC Jr, Whitfield RD, Campbell E. The thoracic herniated intervertebral disc syndrome. *J Neurosurg*. 1957;14(1):61-67.
7. Logue V. Thoracic intervertebral disc prolapse with spinal cord compression. *J Neurol Neurosurg Psychiatry*. 1952;15(4):227-241.
8. Love JG, Kiefer EJ. Root Pain and Paraplegia Due to Protrusions of Thoracic Intervertebral Disks. *J Neurosurg*. 1950;7(1):62-69.
9. Perot PL Jr, Munro DD. Transthoracic removal of midline thoracic disc protrusions causing spinal cord compression. *J Neurosurg*. 1969;31(4):452-458.
10. Burke TG, Caputy AJ. Treatment of thoracic disc herniation: evolution toward the minimally invasive thoracoscopic technique. *Neurosurg Focus*. 2000;9(4):1-7.
11. Menard V. Traitement de la paraplegie du mal de Pott par le drainage lateral: costotransversectomie. *Rev Orthop Paris*. 1895;6:134-146.
12. Capner N. The evolution of lateral rachiotomy. *J Bone Joint Surg Br B*. 1954;36:173-179.
13. Seddon H. Pott's paraplegia: prognosis and treatment. *Br J Surg*. 1935;22(88):769-799.
14. Alexander G. Neurological complications of spinal tuberculosis. *Proc R Soc Med*. 1946;39(730):1945-1946.
15. Capener N. The evolution of lateral rhachotomy. *Bone Joint J*. 1954;36(2):173-179.
16. Larson SJ, et al. Lateral extracavitary approach to traumatic lesions of the thoracic and lumbar spine. *J Neurosurg*. 1976; 45(6):628-637.
17. Maiman DJ, et al. Lateral extracavitary approach to the spine for thoracic disc herniation: report of 23 cases. *Neurosurgery*. 1984;14(2):178-182.
18. Sekhar LN, Jannetta PJ. Thoracic disc herniation: operative approaches and results. *Neurosurgery*. 1983;12(3):303-305.
19. Patterson RH Jr, Arbit E. A surgical approach through the pedicle to protruded thoracic discs. *J Neurosurg*. 1978;48(5):768-772.
20. Brown CW, et al. The natural history of thoracic disc herniation. *Spine*. 1992;17(6):S97-S102.
21. Mulier S, Debois V. Thoracic disc herniations: transthoracic, lateral, or posterolateral approach? A review. *Surg Neurol*. 1998;49(6):599-608.
22. Yoshihara H. Surgical treatment for thoracic disc herniation: an update. *Spine*. 2014;39(6):E406-E412.
23. Arce CA, Dohrmann GJ. Thoracic disc herniation: improved diagnosis with computed tomographic scanning and a review of the literature. *Surg Neurol*. 1985;23(4):356-361.

24. McCormick WE, Will SF, Benzel EC. Surgery for thoracic disc disease. Complication avoidance: overview and management. *Neurosurg Focus*. 2000;9(4):1-6.
25. Stillerman CB, et al. Experience in the surgical management of 82 symptomatic herniated thoracic discs and review of the literature. *J Neurosurg*. 1998;88(4):623-633.
26. Fessler RG, Sturgill M. Review: complications of surgery for thoracic disc disease. *Surg Neurol*. 1998;49(6): 609-618.
27. Lubelski D, et al. Lateral extracavitary, costotransversectomy, and transthoracic thoracotomy approaches to the thoracic spine: review of techniques and complications. *Clin Spine Surg*. 2013;26(4):222-232.
28. Dommisse G. The blood supply of the spinal cord. *Bone Joint J*. 1974;56(2):225-235.
29. Mansour H, Hammoud F, Vlahovitch B. [Brown-Sequard syndrome caused by foramen and calcified disk herniation, responsible for direct compression of Adamkiewicz's artery]. *Neurochirurgie*. 1986;33(6):478-481.
30. Le Roux PD, Haglund MM, Harris AB. Thoracic disc disease: experience with the transpedicular approach in twenty consecutive patients. *Neurosurgery*. 1993;33(1):58-66.
31. Carson J, Gumpert J, Jefferson A. Diagnosis and treatment of thoracic intervertebral disc protrusions. *J Am Acad Orthop Surg*. 1971;34(1):68-77.
32. Lubelski D, et al. Lateral extracavitary vs costotransversectomy approaches to the thoracic spine: reflections on lessons learned. *Neurosurgery*. 2012;71(6):1096-1102.
33. Resnick DK, Benzel EC. Lateral extracavitary approach for thoracic and thoracolumbar spine trauma: operative complications. *Neurosurgery*. 1998;43(4):796-802.
34. Yi S, et al. Outcome of surgery for a symptomatic herniated thoracic disc in relation to preoperative characteristics of the disc. *Acta Neurochir (Wien)*. 2007;149(11):1139-1145.
35. Benson M, Byrnes D. The clinical syndromes and surgical treatment of thoracic intervertebral disc prolapse. *J Bone Joint Surg Br*. 1975;57(4):471-477.
36. Yamasaki R, et al. Surgical outcomes of posterior thoracic interbody fusion for thoracic disc herniations. *Eur Spine J*. 2013;22(11):2496-2503.
37. Lesoin F, et al. Thoracic disk herniation and Scheuermann's disease. *Eur Neurol*. 1987;26(3):145-152.
38. Lesoin F, et al. Thoracic disc herniations: evolution in the approach and indications. *Acta Neurochir (Wien)*. 1986; 80(1-2):30-34.
39. Rath SA, et al. Neurosurgical management of thoracic and lumbar vertebral osteomyelitis and discitis in adults: a review of 43 consecutive surgically treated patients. *Neurosurgery*. 1996;38(5):926-933.
40. Shaw B, Mansfield FL, Borges L. One-stage posterolateral decompression and stabilization for primary and metastatic vertebral tumors in the thoracic and lumbar spine. *J Neurosurg*. 1989;70(3):405-410.
41. Van Landingham JH. Herniation of thoracic intervertebral discs with spinal cord compression in kyphosis dorsalis juvenilis (Scheuermann's disease): case report. *J Neurosurg*. 1954;11(3):327-329.
42. Garrido E. Modified costotransversectomy: a surgical approach to ventrally placed lesions in the thoracic spinal canal. *Surg Neurol*. 1980;13(2):109.
43. Simpson JM, et al. Thoracic disc herniation: re-evaluation of the posterior approach using a modified costotransversectomy. *Spine*. 1993;18(13):1872-1877.
44. Bransford R, et al. Early experience treating thoracic disc herniations using a modified transfacet pedicle-sparing decompression and fusion. *J Neurosurg Spine*. 2010;12(2): 221-231.
45. Stillerman CB, et al. The transfacet pedicle-sparing approach for thoracic disc removal: cadaveric morphometric analysis and preliminary clinical experience. *J Neurosurg*. 1995;83(6):971-976.
46. Delfini R, et al. Surgical treatment of thoracic disc herniation: a reappraisal of Larson's lateral extracavitary approach. *Surg Neurol*. 1996;45(6):517-522.
47. Wolfla CE, Maiman DJ. Lateral extracavitary approach. *Tech Neurosurg*. 2003;8(2):93-100.
48. Foreman PM, et al. The lateral extracavitary approach to the thoracolumbar spine: a case series and systematic review. *J Neurosurg Spine*. 2016;24(4):570-579.
49. Fessler RG, et al. Lateral parascapular extrapleural approach to the upper thoracic spine. *J Neurosurg*. 1991;75(3): 349-355.
50. Albee FH. Transplantation of a portion of the tibia into the spine for Pott's disease: a preliminary report. *J Am Med Assoc*. 1911;57(11):885-886.
51. Hibbs RA. THE CLASSIC: An Operation for progressive spinal deformities: a preliminary report of three cases from the service of the orthopaedic hospital. *Clin Orthop Relat Res*. 2007;460:17-20.
52. Barr JS. Ruptured intervertebral disc and sciatic pain. *J Bone Joint Surg Am*. 1947;29(2):429-437.
53. Watkins MB. Posterolateral fusion of the lumbar and lumbosacral spine. *J Bone Joint Surg Am*. 1953;35(4): 1014-1018.
54. Cloward RB. The treatment of ruptured lumbar intervertebral discs by vertebral body fusion: I. Indications, operative technique, after care. *J Neurosurg*. 1953;10(2):154-168.
55. Barrick WT, et al. Anterior lumbar fusion improves discogenic pain at levels of prior posterolateral fusion. *Spine*. 2000;25(7):853-857.
56. Bono CM, Lee CK. Critical analysis of trends in fusion for degenerative disc disease over the past 20 years: influence of technique on fusion rate and clinical outcome. *Spine*. 2004; 29(4):455-463.
57. Deyo RA, et al. United States trends in lumbar fusion surgery for degenerative conditions. *Spine*. 2005;30(12):1441-1445.
58. Deyo RA, Mirza SK. Spinal-fusion surgery: the case for restraint. *N Engl J Med*. 2004;350(7):722.
59. Glassman SD, et al. Posterolateral lumbar spine fusion with INFUSE bone graft. *Spine J*. 2007;7(1):44-49.
60. Ozgur BM, et al. Extreme Lateral Interbody Fusion (XLIF): a novel surgical technique for anterior lumbar interbody fusion. *Spine J*. 2006;6(4):435-443.
61. Berjano P, Lamartina C. Far lateral approaches (XLIF) in adult scoliosis. *Eur Spine J*. 2013;22(2):242-253.
62. Phillips FM, et al. Adult degenerative scoliosis treated with XLIF: clinical and radiographical results of a prospective multicenter study with 24-month follow-up. *Spine*. 2013; 38(21):1853-1861.
63. Formica M, et al. Extreme lateral approach to the spine in degenerative and post traumatic lumbar diseases: selection process, results and complications. *Eur Spine J*. 2014;23(6): 684-692.
64. Alimi M, et al. Extreme lateral interbody fusion for unilateral symptomatic vertical foraminal stenosis. *Eur Spine J*. 2015; 24(3):346-352.

65. Herkowitz HN, Sidhu KS. Lumbar spine fusion in the treatment of degenerative conditions: current indications and recommendations. *J Am Acad Orthop Surg*. 1995;3(3):123-135.
66. Lee CK, Langrana NA. A review of spinal fusion for degenerative disc disease: need for alternative treatment approach of disc arthroplasty? *Spine J*. 2004;4(6):S173-S176.
67. Resnick DK, et al. Guidelines for the performance of fusion procedures for degenerative disease of the lumbar spine. Part 7: intractable low-back pain without stenosis or spondylolisthesis. *J Neurosurg Spine*. 2005;2(6):670-672.
68. Vamvanij V, et al. Surgical treatment of internal disc disruption: an outcome study of four fusion techniques. *Clin Spine Surg*. 1998;11(5):375-382.
69. Street J, et al. Single-stage posterolateral vertebrectomy for the management of metastatic disease of the thoracic and lumbar spine: a prospective study of an evolving surgical technique. *Clin Spine Surg*. 2007;20(7):509-520.
70. Sun J-C, et al. Surgical incision and approach in thoracolumbar extreme lateral interbody fusion surgery: an anatomic study of the diaphragmatic attachments. *Spine*. 2016;41(4):E186-E190.
71. Arnold PM, et al. Surgical management of nontuberculous thoracic and lumbar vertebral osteomyelitis: report of 33 cases. *Surg Neurol*. 1997;47(6):551-561.
72. McCormick PC. Surgical management of dumbbell and paraspinal tumors of the thoracic and lumbar spine. *Neurosurgery*. 1996;38(1):67-75.
73. Graham AW, Mac Millan M, Fessler RG. Lateral extracavitary approach to the thoracic and thoracolumbar spine. *Orthopedics*. 1997;20(7):605-610.
74. Sciubba DM, et al. Diagnosis and management of metastatic spine disease: a review. *J Neurosurg Spine*. 2010;13(1):94-108.
75. Cybulski GR, Stone JL, Opesanmi O. Spinal cord decompression via a modified costotransversectomy approach combined with posterior instrumentation for management of metastatic neoplasms of the thoracic spine. *Surg Neurol*. 1991;35(4):280-285.
76. Chong S, et al. Single-stage posterior decompression and stabilization for metastasis of the thoracic spine: prognostic factors for functional outcome and patients' survival. *Spine J*. 2012;12(12):1083-1092.
77. Wiggins GC, et al. Perioperative complications with costotransversectomy and anterior approaches to thoracic and thoracolumbar tumors. *Neurosurg Focus*. 2001;11(6):1-9.
78. Lu DC, et al. The transpedicular approach compared with the anterior approach: an analysis of 80 thoracolumbar corpectomies. *J Neurosurg Spine*. 2010;12(6):583-591.
79. Ito K, et al. Surgery for ventral intradural thoracic spinal tumors with a posterolateral transpedicular approach. *Acta Neurochir (Wien)*. 2016;158(8):1563-1569.
80. Kim CH, Chung CK. Surgical outcome of a posterior approach for large ventral intradural extramedullary spinal cord tumors. *Spine*. 2011;36(8):E531-E537.
81. Thorat JD, et al. Single-stage posterior midline approach for dumbbell tumors of the thoracic spine, with intraoperative CT guidance. *Surg Neurol Int*. 2011;2.
82. Ando K, et al. Removal of thoracic dumbbell tumors through a single-stage posterior approach: its usefulness and limitations. *J Orthop Sci*. 2013;18(3):380-387.
83. Snell BE, Nasr FF, Wolfla CE. Single-stage thoracolumbar vertebrectomy with circumferential reconstruction and arthrodesis: surgical technique and results in 15 patients. *Neurosurgery*. 2006;58(4):263-269.
84. Chandra SP, et al. Extended costotransversectomy to achieve circumferential fusion for pathologies causing thoracic instability. *Spine J*. 2014;14(9):2094-2101.
85. Lau D, et al. Perioperative characteristics, complications, and outcomes of single-level versus multilevel thoracic corpectomies via modified costotransversectomy approach. *Spine*. 2013;38(6):523-530.
86. Hofstetter CP, et al. Posterior approach for thoracolumbar corpectomies with expandable cage placement and circumferential arthrodesis: a multicenter case series of 67 patients. *J Neurosurg Spine*. 2011;14(3):388-397.
87. Kim D-H, et al. Minimally invasive posterolateral thoracic corpectomy: cadaveric feasibility study and report of four clinical cases. *Neurosurgery*. 2009;64(4):746-753.
88. Smith WD, et al. Minimally invasive surgery for traumatic spinal pathologies: a mini-open, lateral approach in the thoracic and lumbar spine. *Spine*. 2010;35(26S):S338-S346.
89. Khan SN, et al. Minimally invasive thoracolumbar corpectomy and reconstruction. *Orthopedics*. 2012;35(1):e74-e79.
90. Gandhoke GS, et al. Technical nuances of the minimally invasive extreme lateral approach to treat thoracolumbar burst fractures. *Eur Spine J*. 2015;24(3):353-360.
91. Deutsch H, Boco T, Lobel J. Minimally invasive transpedicular vertebrectomy for metastatic disease to the thoracic spine. *Clin Spine Surg*. 2008;21(2):101-105.
92. Smith ZA, et al. Minimally invasive lateral extracavitary corpectomy: cadaveric evaluation model and report of 3 clinical cases: Laboratory investigation. *J Neurosurg Spine*. 2012;16(5):463-470.
93. Chou D, Lu DC. Mini-open transpedicular corpectomies with expandable cage reconstruction: technical note. *J Neurosurg Spine*. 2011;14(1):71-77.
94. Lall RR, et al. Minimally invasive thoracic corpectomy: surgical strategies for malignancy, trauma, and complex spinal pathologies. *Minim Invasive Surg*. 2012;2012:213791.
95. Lau D, Chou D. Posterior thoracic corpectomy with cage reconstruction for metastatic spinal tumors: comparing the mini-open approach to the open approach. *J Neurosurg Spine*. 2015;23(2):217-227.

SECTION VI

CHAPTER 52 Dynamic Stabilization: What's Current and What's the Potential

Dilip K. Sengupta

Dynamic stabilization in the treatment of activity-related mechanical low back pain was introduced nearly three decades ago (Graf ligament in 1989[1] and Dynesys in 1994[2]).

The need for dynamic stabilization originated from the limitations of spinal fusion, which may not always result in successful clinical outcome,[3,4] and may lead to accelerated degeneration of the adjacent segments.[5,6] Nearly every possible flexible design of dynamic stabilization devices has been introduced for clinical application without proper biomechanical evaluation or design rationale. During the turn of the 21st century, the use of dynamic stabilization devices gained momentum, but the enthusiasm has declined recently, as the mechanical failure of the devices and failure of clinical success were increasingly recognized. Dynamic stabilization is broadly classified into pedicle screw–based posterior dynamic stabilization (PDS) devices and interspinous/interlaminar distraction (IPD) devices.

Understanding Spinal Instability

When abnormal increased motion—in particular, translation—is present on flexion-extension radiographs, especially in the setting of spondylolisthesis, fusion is accepted as a reasonable option.[7] By this standard, however, relatively few patients with low back pain have clear subjective or objective evidence of instability. Biomechanical and radiologic studies using open magnetic resonance imaging in flexion and extension have shown that segmental motion either does not change significantly with lumbar disc degeneration,[8–10] or may decrease, except during early stages of disc degeneration.[11]

Panjabi redefined spinal instability as an abnormal-quality motion, often accompanied by an increased neutral zone (NZ) motion caused by ligament laxity, even when range of motion (ROM) is diminished.[12] Panjabi uses the analogy of a marble rolling in a soup bowl (Fig. 52.1).

Mulholland and Sengupta[13] hypothesize that spinal instability does not mean "increased motion" as commonly misunderstood,[14,15] but it indicates abnormal load distribution across the vertebral endplate. The normal disc is isotropic; it consists of a homogeneous gel of collagen and proteoglycan, and behaves like a fluid-filled bag that allows distribution of load uniformly across the vertebral endplates.[13] Disc degeneration alters the isotropic properties of the disc. The disc becomes nonhomogeneous, with areas of fragmented and condensed collagen, cartilage fragments, fluid, and gas.[16] The nucleus becomes depressurized and an increasingly larger load is transmitted through the anulus, which leads to splitting and inward folding of the anulus.[17] Load transmission over the endplates, therefore, becomes uneven.[18,19] Focal loading of the endplate cartilage and subchondral bony trabeculae can occur with certain positions, leading to a sharp increase in back pain, analogous to a stone in the shoe, a concept proposed by Mulholland and Sengupta.[13] This explains the clinical sign of *instability catch* in mechanical back pain. Mulholland's hypothesis of abnormal loading as the primary cause of mechanical back pain was supported by a close association of abnormal disc pressure profiles to positive discography with pain provocation.[20] This was established by a pressure profilometry study by McNally and Adams.[21]

There is no real conflict between Panjabi's abnormal motion theory and Mulholland's abnormal load distribution theory of spinal instability. These two factors may be interrelated. An abnormal motion may cause abnormal load distribution, which, in turn, may cause pain. On the other hand, it may be anticipated that, if an abnormal motion does not cause abnormal load distribution, it may not be associated with pain production, and explains why many dark discs do not hurt.

Biomechanical Goals of a Posterior Dynamic Stabilization Device

Survival of a PDS device against fatigue failure in the long term and its clinical success depend on how closely its design adheres to the biomechanical goals.

Motion Preservation

The primary goal of dynamic stabilization is to preserve as much normal motion as possible and limit any abnormal motion. Since clinical instability occurs mostly during the

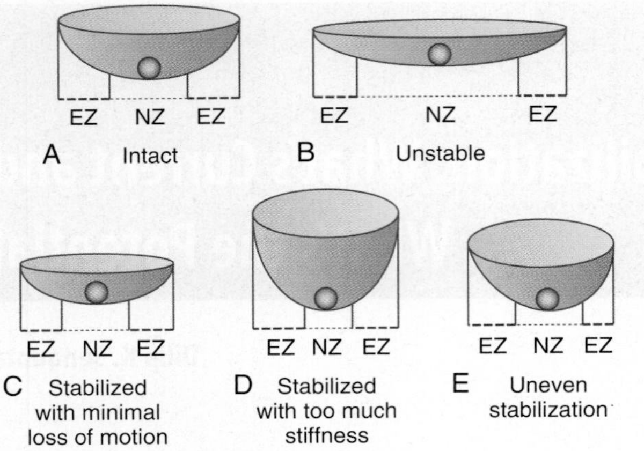

FIG. 52.1 Panjabi's analogy of a marble in a soup bowl, explaining the relationship between spinal instability and change in range of motion. (A) In an intact spine, the marble can move with little resistance across the neutral zone (NZ) but faces increasing resistance toward the elastic zone (EZ). (B) With an unstable motion segment the bowl is flat, allowing the marble to move to and fro with little resistance; that is, increased NZ with no increase in EZ. (C) A stabilized segment has a smaller cup that reduces primarily the NZ, with minimal reduction of EZ movement. (D) A stabilized segment, but with too much loss of motion, which is undesirable. (E) Uneven stabilization, which has different stiffness in two directions, which is again undesirable. (Modified from Sengupta DK. Use of posterior motion-sparing instrumentation and interspinous devices for the treatment of degenerative disorders of the lumbar spine. In: Shen FH, Shaffrey CL, eds. *Arthritis and Arthroplasty: The Spine*. Philadelphia: Elsevier; 2010:349–356.)

NZ motion secondary to ligament laxity, the key to stabilization should be restriction of the NZ while preserving the elastic zone (EZ) motion as much as possible. All PDS systems, regardless of their mechanism of action, can reduce NZ motion, which explains their short-term clinical success. In postlaminectomy instability, the ROMs may be increased with abnormal translation and the goal of the PDS device should be to restore a normal range and quality of motion. Normally, it is unlikely that a dynamic stabilization device will increase the ROM of a degenerated segment unless it induces a favorable biologic reaction to the facet joint and disc, such as restoring the height of a collapsed disc by offloading these structures.

Load Transmission

The mechanism of pain relief with dynamic stabilization may be unloading the disc and the facet joints by load sharing, thereby preventing abnormal load distribution and high spot loading.[13] How much load should be shared by the device is not clear, but it should alleviate any elevated intradiscal pressure.

Resistance to Fatigue Failure

The most important challenge for dynamic stabilization devices is to survive against fatigue failure despite allowing continued motion. The key to survival against fatigue of a PDS device, which is structurally weaker than a fusion rod, is appropriate quality and quantity of motion restriction and load sharing so that the device is never exposed to an abnormal load.

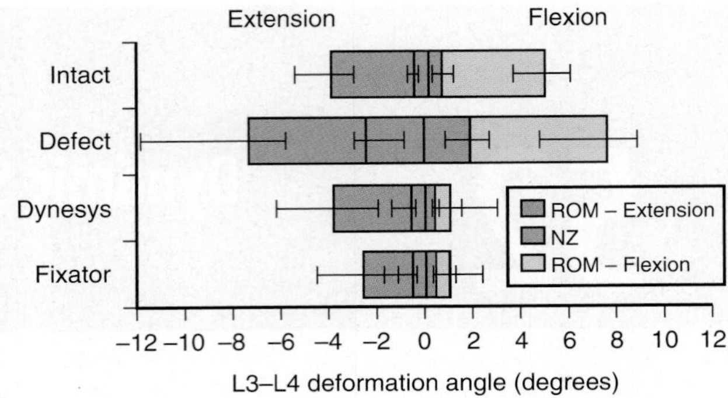

FIG. 52.2 Dynesys restricts flexion too much, equivalent to rigid fixation, but permits near-normal extension in the cadaver spine. NZ, neutral zone. (Modified from Schmoelz W, et al. Dynamic stabilization of the lumbar spine and its effects on adjacent segments: an in vitro experiment. *J Spinal Disord Tech*. 2003;16[4]:418–423.)

There are two important biomechanical principles to ensure that the device or the device-bone junction is not exposed to a failure load. Motion restriction should be uniform throughout the ROM. Should the device cause too much restriction at any phase of motion—for example, Dynesys controlling flexion smoothly, but acting as an extension block—the device may be exposed to unusually high stress in extension repeatedly and may fail eventually (Fig. 52.2). The second biomechanical principle is that load-sharing should be uniform throughout the ROM. If the device may unload the disc too much in one phase of motion, often in extension, the device has to bear an unusually high load during that motion and becomes likely to fail (Fig. 52.3).

The fatigue property of a fusion device is normally tested in an ASTM standard spine model consisting of two plastic cubes as vertebral bodies, but there is nothing available to represent anatomic structures such as the disc or the facet joints. Dynamic stabilization devices are expected to share load with the disc and facet joints. Therefore, unfortunately, the fatigue property of a dynamic stabilization device cannot be tested directly in a spine model. A crude estimation of the fatigue load that a PDS device may encounter can be assessed indirectly by studying the changes in the kinetic and kinematic properties of the motion segment before and after application of the PDS device. These may include the instantaneous axis of rotation (IAR), intradiscal pressure changes, and pedicle-to-pedicle distance excursion before and after application of the device in a cadaver spine or model.

Normally, the disc pressure increases both in flexion and extension and is lowest in neutral position. A PDS device should ideally permit the rise in disc pressure in both flexion and extension but to a smaller magnitude due to load sharing (see Fig. 52.3). If the disc pressure does not rise at all, particularly in extension, it may indicate that the device is acting like a total load-bearing structure during extension rather than as a load-sharing structure in extension. Similarly, a mismatch in the location of the IAR of the device and the motion segment is a predictor of the device encountering a higher load and being more likely to undergo fatigue failure.

A normal pedicle-to-pedicle excursion during flexion-extension may be as large as 6 to 9 mm, less in lateral bending,

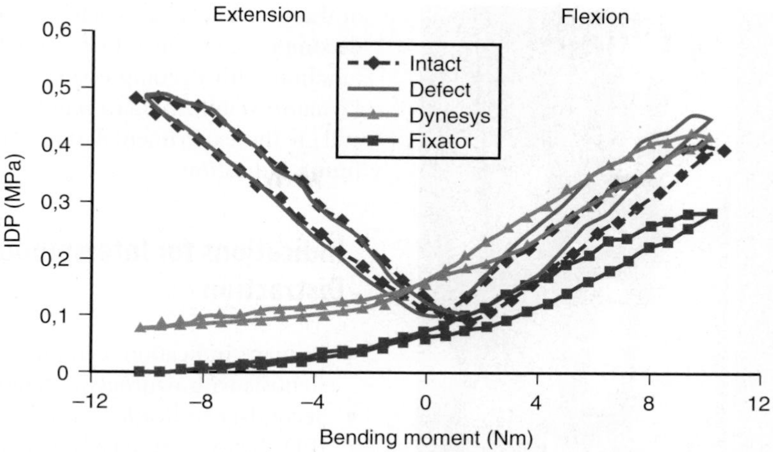

FIG. 52.3 Intradiscal pressure (IDP) changes with flexion-extension motion. Normally, the pressure at the center of the disc rises both in flexion and extension. Stabilization with Dynesys restores disc pressure in flexion to normal but unloads the disc completely and behaves like a total load-bearing structure, without sharing any load with the disc. (From Schmoelz W, Huber JF, Nydegger T, Claes L, Wilke HJ. Influence of a dynamic stabilisation system on load bearing of a bridged disc: an in vitro study of intradiscal pressure. *Eur Spine J.* 2006;15[8]:1276–1285.)

and minimal in rotation (Fig. 52.4). The device should permit a normal pedicle-to-pedicle distance excursion to permit normal ROM and ensure that the device does not act as a motion stopper in any direction or phase of motion. Unfortunately, only a few dynamic stabilization devices can accommodate such a large degree of flexibility.

Nonmetallic devices may deform, soften, and creep to adapt to the kinematics of the motion segment and survive fatigue better at the cost of reduced efficacy over time. Is creep and softening of a nonmetallic device a disadvantage? One may argue that dynamic stabilization may stimulate a favorable biologic response to repair the motion segment, and its subsequent creep or softening is truly an advantage, when its function is over. Conversely, metallic spring devices may retain their mechanical property over a long period but are more subject to fatigue failure should there be any mismatch in kinematics. It is important to note that fatigue failure of a nonmetallic device may not be recognized radiologically unless there is screw loosening or breakage, but failure of a metallic device cannot hide!

The following are design rationales for PDS devices:

1. Motion preservation with uniform effect throughout ROM
2. Load sharing uniformly throughout ROM
3. Minimum conflict with the IAR, intradiscal pressure, and pedicle-to-pedicle distance excursion of the motion segment

Other design-related factors are as follows:

1. Safe and easy salvage—conversion to fusion in case of failure
2. Ease of implantation—top-loading screws
3. Compatibility with minimally invasive procedures
4. Restoration of normal sagittal alignment, for example, lordosis
5. Biomaterial—metallic versus nonmetallic
6. Easy salvage procedure to address failure of the device, such as conversion to fusion with a rod (Fig. 52.5).

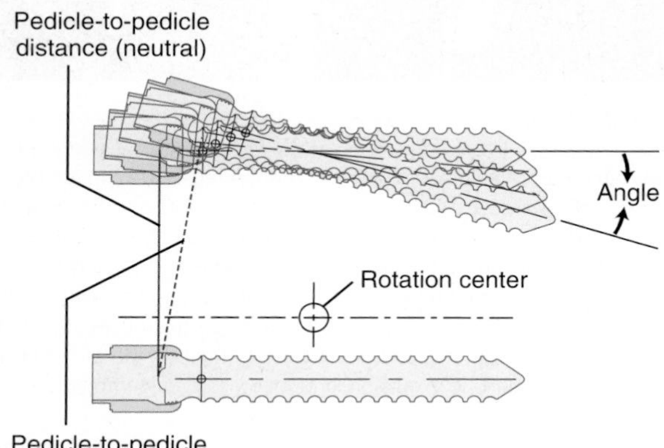

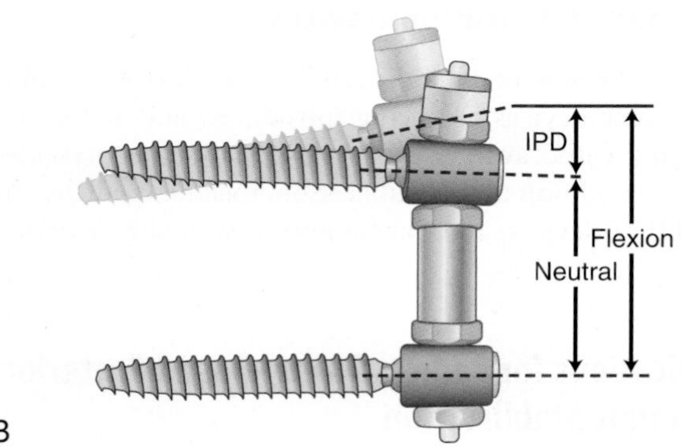

FIG. 52.4 (A) The pedicle-to-pedicle distance from flexion to extension may be as large as 8 to 9 mm to preserve normal motion. (B) Dynamic stabilization (e.g., Transition; Globus Medical) may need to permit an excursion of the pedicle screw heads by the same magnitude. IPD, interspinous/interlaminar distraction. (From Sengupta DK. Use of posterior motion-sparing instrumentation and interspinous devices for the treatment of degenerative disorders of the lumbar spine. In: Shen FH, Shaffrey CL, eds. *Arthritis and Arthroplasty: The Spine*. Philadelphia: Elsevier; 2010:349–356.)

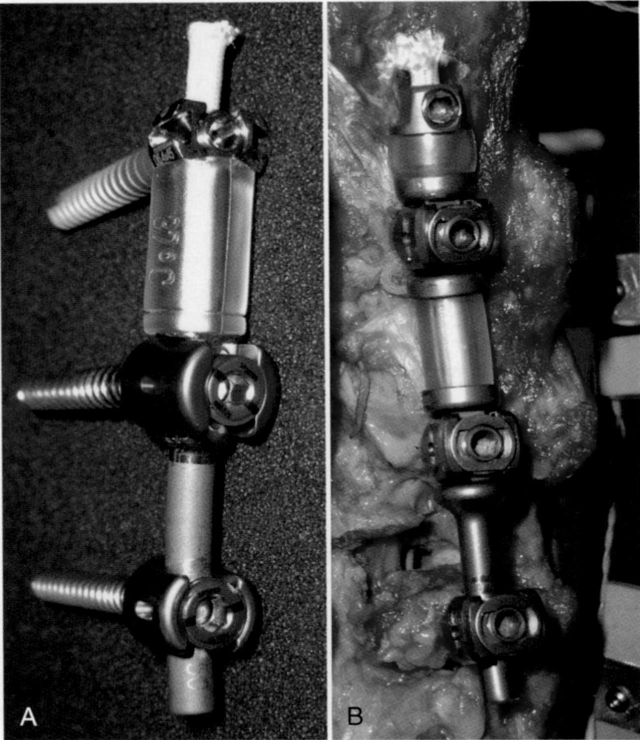

FIG. 52.5 Design rationale between second- versus third-generation posterior dynamic stabilization devices. (A) Dynesys uses a side-loading screw, which is not suitable for rod insertion. A recent design adaptation, Dynesys DTO, makes it suitable for use in conjunction with fusion at an adjacent segment and requires three different types of screws. It needs in situ assembly and tensioning. (B) Transition has been designed to accommodate implantation in isolation and in conjunction with adjacent-segment fusion using the same pedicle screw design. It uses top-loading screws for all the segments, lordosis is built in, the bumper at the end offers larger pedicle-to-pedicle excursion, and it comes preassembled or can be assembled on the back table.

Dynamic Stabilization Devices

The classification of dynamic stabilization devices is a moving target; new devices are being introduced and some devices are being withdrawn. A broad classification, as presented in the earlier edition of this publication, includes pedicle-screw–based PDS devices, and interspinous distraction devices (Box 52.1).

Indications for Pedicle Screw–Based Posterior Dynamic Stabilization

The primary indication of dynamic stabilization is treatment of mechanical back pain due to spinal instability. Radicular pain or claudication pain can be adequately treated by decompression alone; the role of additional dynamic stabilization here is only to prevent instability and back pain. Application of a dynamic stabilization device with concomitant decompression to address radicular or claudication leg pain may not be accepted as evidence in support of their efficacy to relieve back pain. Such efficacy can only be established by application of the device to treat mechanical back pain in the absence of decompression. Once that is established, application in conjunction with decompression procedures could be justified. Dynamic stabilization to supplement total disc replacement is still in the experimental stage and may be considered as a future indication.

Indications for Interspinous Process Distraction

- Primary indication: central spinal canal and/or foraminal stenosis with neurogenic claudication
- Secondary indication: Axial mechanical back pain

IPD devices are ideally suited for indirect, less invasive decompression of the spinal canal or the foramen causing claudication pain. Direct decompression by conventional laminectomy may achieve a more definitive and longer-lasting relief of symptoms. Intuitively, interspinous distraction may produce less postoperative morbidity. Its use may only be justified in elderly patients with multiple comorbidities. Osteoporosis and scoliosis may be relative contraindications for IPD because of high incidence of device failure. Proponents and enthusiasts of interspinous distraction sometimes recommend its use in the treatment of axial back pain. This is a questionable indication. IPD devices can reduce the laxity of the motion segment and secondarily reduce the unstable motion in the NZ. This action may also address mechanical back pain to some extent. Currently, a sound rationale, justification, or evidence in favor of such indication is lacking.

Clinical Experience With Dynamic Stabilization

Pedicle Screw–Based Posterior Dynamic Stabilization Devices

One of the earliest dynamic stabilization devices is the *Graf ligament*, described by Henry Graf in 1992.[1] This is the first-generation PDS device, and forms the basis of many other devices introduced subsequently. The mechanism of action or the design rationale has never been published in the English literature. The monograph from the inventor in French describes that the device locks the facet joints to reduce painful motions.

The Graf ligament consists of braided polypropylene bands that span between flanges at the titanium pedicle screw heads under tension, locking the facet joints. The surgical procedure is simple and, unlike fusion, it avoids exposure of the transverse processes or the need to harvest bone graft. Unfortunately, as a result of compression applied to the screws, there is a high incidence of radicular symptoms secondary to either disc herniation or foraminal narrowing.[22,23] Increased facet loading may lead to back pain.

The clinical outcome during short-term follow-up (up to 2 years) is reported to be as good as with conventional fusion.[23] However, the long-term outcome with Graf ligament stabilization has conflicting reports in the literature. Gardner[24] and Markwalder and Wenger[25] reported reasonably good results with

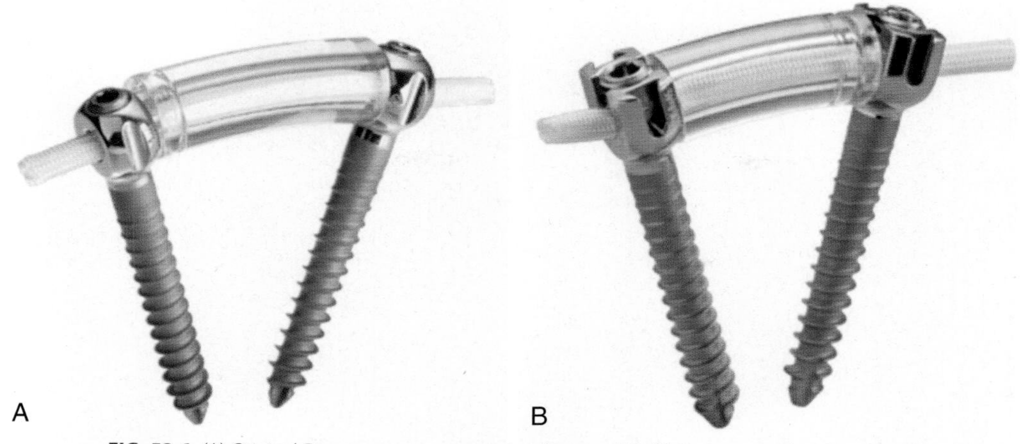

FIG. 52.6 (A) Original Dynesys, now presented as Dynesys LIS. (B) Dynesys top-loading device.

BOX 52.1 Classification of Dynamic Stabilization Devices

Pedicle Screw–Based Posterior Dynamic Stabilization (PDS) Devices

Nonmetallic Devices

Dynesys LIS and Dynesys top-loading system (Zimmer-Biomet)
Transition (Globus Medical)

Metallic Devices

DSS-II Dynamic Stabilization System (Abbott Spine)
BioFlex (Bio-Spine
Stabilimax NZ (Applied Spine Technologies)
Cosmic Posterior Dynamic System (Ulrich GmbH)

Hybrid Devices (Metallic Component With Plastic Bumper)

CD Horizon Agile (Medtronic Sofamor Danek)
Dynesys DTO system (Zimmer-Biomet)
NFlex (Synthes GmbH)
Transition (Globus Medical)

Interspinous Distraction (IPD) Devices

Rigid Devices With Free Flexion

X-Stop interspinous process decompression device (Medtronic Sofamor Danek)
Flexus (Globus Medical)
Superion (VertiFlex)

Rigid Devices With Restricted Flexion

Wallis system (Zimmer-Biomet)
Interspinous Locker (NHS)

Flexible Devices

Nonmetallic: DIAM (Medtronic Sofamor Danek)
Metallic: Coflex (Paradigm Spine)

Indications for IPD Devices

Primary: spinal stenosis with neurogenic claudication
Secondary: axial-mechanical back pain

the Graf ligament even at 5- to 10-year follow-up. On the other hand, from a retrospective case control study, Hadlow et al[22] reported that the Graf ligament produces a worse outcome at 1 year and a significantly higher revision rate at 2 years compared to the fusion group. The Graf ligament is still used in a few centers in both Europe and Asia, but its use has declined.[24,26]

Dynesys Dynamic Stabilization System

The most extensively used pedicle screw–based PDS system to date is Dynesys (Zimmer-Biomet).[2,27] This was introduced in Europe as a true dynamic stabilization device, to be used without fusion. In 2004, Dynesys was introduced in the US market as a fusion device under 510(k) US Food and Drug Administration (FDA) approval.

The design incorporates a plastic cylinder (Sulene-polycarbonate urethane) around the cord to apply a distraction force unloading the facet joints, which is thought to be the cause of back pain with the Graf ligament. This is a design improvement over the Graf ligament and may be considered as a second-generation PDS device (Fig. 52.6). A review of the literature provides the best resource for understanding the mechanism of PDS systems in general.

The design rationale or the mechanism of action of Dynesys has never been presented in the English literature. The current designs of Dynesys are the original lateral side-loading system, Dynesys LIS, and an alternative Dynesys top-loading system. In biomechanical testing on a cadaver spine, the Dynesys device is shown to reduce range of flexion more than extension,[28] (see Fig. 52.2), apparently because the device holds the segment in close to full flexion. The extension is produced by an abnormal distraction of the disc space, with the plastic cylinder acting like a fulcrum. This is evidenced by an abnormal negative disc pressure during extension.[29] Conversely, in vivo, Dynesys limits extension more than flexion,[30] as expected, because the device acts like an extension stop. In flexion, Dynesys acts as an ideal load-sharing device. However, in extension, Dynesys acts as an extension stop, and becomes totally load-bearing, allowing no load transmission through the disc[29] (see Fig. 52.3). Because of uneven restriction of motion and uneven load-sharing properties, Dynesys may be subjected to high stress at the pedicle screws.[31] This may explain why screw loosening and breakage had been so rare with the Graf ligament but fairly common with Dynesys, as high as 17% in some clinical series[27,32] (Fig. 52.7).

The clinical outcome with Dynesys used as a dynamic stabilization device, as reported by the inventor group in Europe, was comparable to spinal fusion but without the need

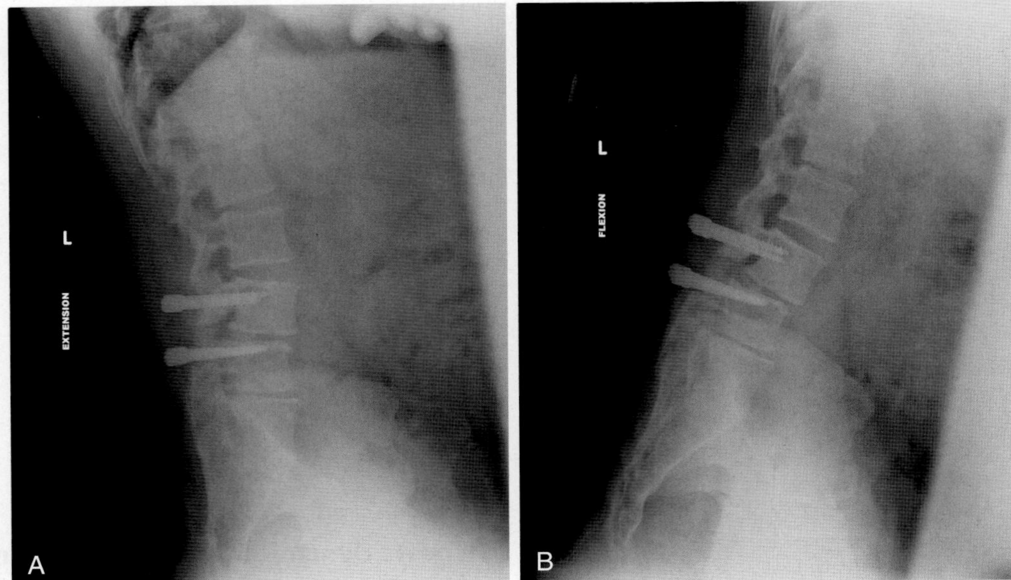

FIG. 52.7 Dynesys LIS stabilization at L4–L5 segment in (A) extension and (B) flexion. The segment is held in the flexed position and does not permit extension of the index segment. The screws are loose in both L4 and L5.

for fusion.[2] Over 60% of their cases had spinal stenosis and Dynesys was used in conjunction with decompression. This made it difficult to evaluate whether the good outcome was secondary to Dynesys or decompression. Subsequent studies by Grob et al.[27] found that stand-alone Dynesys produced a good outcome in only 39% of cases compared to 69% when combined with decompression. A similar experience was reported by other independent researchers.[33]

Most clinical outcome studies with Dynesys were reported from outside of the United States. Dynesys was introduced in the United States as a fusion device. The initial clinical outcome reported from the United States involved Dynesys as a fusion device, used with posterolateral bone graft.[34]

Dynesys has been used in the United States since 2004, when it was approved by the FDA for stabilization of spinal segments as an adjunct to fusion.[35] In 2009, an FDA-controlled investigations device exemption (IDE) clinical trial was completed for use of Dynesys as a stand-alone PDS device. The Orthopaedic and Rehabilitation Devices Panel of the FDA released an Executive Summary available on their website.[36]

The objective of this FDA IDE study was to assess the safety and efficacy of the Dynesys system for patients requiring one-level or contiguous two-level posterior spinal stabilization of the lumbar and/or sacral spine following decompression for degenerative back and leg pain. The outcome with the Dynesys system was compared to a posterolateral spinal fusion procedure using autogenous bone graft with a rigid posterior instrumentation (Silhouette Spinal Fixation System).

The IDE study database was initially closed on September 20, 2007, but was reopened for additional data entry on November 6, 2008, in order to respond to deficiencies pointed out by the FDA. It was closed again on March 13, 2009. The original study design was approved for 399 patients at 30 sites (266 Dynesys, 133 Silhouette). The final study design involved a total of 367 patients, randomized in 2:1 ratio (253 Dynesys, 114 Silhouette) at 26 sites. A total of 28 patients were nonrandomized and are referred to as the Dynesys training cohort.

The inclusion criteria emphasized predominant leg pain, with a leg pain visual analog scale (VAS) score greater than 4 out of 10. Patients with predominant axial mechanical back pain and back pain more than leg pain were excluded. A total of 74.6% of Dynesys patients and 70% of Silhouette patients have reached the 24-month primary endpoint, but only 57.3% and 56%, respectively, completed data entry within the protocol-defined study window. The study reported 52.1% overall clinical success rate in Dynesys patients compared with 40.4% in Silhouette patients. The overall clinical success rates drop to 47.0% for Dynesys and 37.5% for Silhouette if only patients in the protocol-defined windows are considered.

The Dynesys and Silhouette patients experienced differential results depending on primary indication, instability versus stenosis, and one versus two levels. For instability, Dynesys patients performed notably better; 64.6% achieved success criteria with Dynesys as opposed to 41.5% with Silhouette. However, for central canal stenosis, the outcome was reversed, with Silhouette patients (54.5%) performing better than Dynesys patients (37.3%) in achieving success criteria. Single-level disease had better outcome compared to two-level disease in both the groups.

The FDA panel pointed out several deficiencies in this study. The study was not blinded, which may have led to reporting bias among patients and investigators, potentially in favor of the investigational treatment. The study design was noninferiority in nature, and the follow-up rate in both the groups was very low. At the end, the FDA did not approve Dynesys for use as a nonfusion device.

The failure of Dynesys as a stand-alone nonfusion stabilization device by the FDA resulted in a sharp decline of its use in the United States. Most of the recent clinical outcome studies are reported from Europe and Asia.[37–43]

Hoppe et al.,[37] in a review of 39 cases treated with Dynesys for monosegmental (L4–L5) instability with a mean 7-year follow-up, reported high success rates (>85% of patients) in long-term, low adjacent-segment disease (ASD). They concluded that Dynesys stabilization is a possible alternative to other stabilization devices. Zhang et al.[43] from China reported a review of 46 cases treated with the Dynesys system compared to 50 cases with posterior lumbar interbody fusion (PLIF) with a greater than 4-year follow-up. The authors concluded that both Dynesys and PLIF can improve the clinical outcomes for lumbar degenerative disease. Compared to PLIF, Dynesys stabilization partially preserves the ROM of the stabilized segments, limits hypermobility in the upper adjacent segment, and may prevent the occurrence of ASD. Conversely, St. Pierre et al.[41] reviewed their 52 cases treated with the Dynesys system in Canada with 5-year follow-up and concluded that Dynesys was associated with a high rate of ASD over long-term follow-up, despite maintaining a low fusion rate. Prior ASD was the strongest predictor of progressive ASD. In a recent meta-analysis, Lee et al.[39] reported that spinal fusion still remains the method of choice for advanced degeneration and gross instability; however, spinal degenerative disease with or without grade 1 spondylolisthesis, particularly in patients who require a quicker recovery, will likely constitute the main indication for PDS using the Dynesys system.

The Transition Stabilization System (Globus Medical) evolved from Dynesys, addressing several limitations in implant design. This system uses a regular top-loading pedicle screw, actively creates lordosis, and permits increased pedicle-to-pedicle distance excursion, and is preassembled. It may therefore be considered as a third-generation PDS device. It consists of a cylindrical polycarbonate urethane spacer around a polyethylene tetraphthalate (PET) cord similar to Dynesys. The system comes preassembled or can be assembled in the back table and does not require in situ tensioning. It is implanted between regular, top-loading pedicle screws, making insertion and conversion to fusion as a salvage procedure simple (see Fig. 52.5B). It incorporates a soft bumper at the end, which allows adequate pedicle-to-pedicle excursion in flexion-extension (see Fig. 52.5B). The length of the spacer defines the unloading of the facet joint. The capability of creating an active lordosis is built into the metal spools that connect the soft section of the device to the pedicle screws. Lordosis ensures unloading of the disc. These two important mechanical properties permit uniform motion restriction in all directions and uniform load sharing throughout the ROM, which is important to increase resistance to fatigue. Although this device has made several design improvements compared to Dynesys, its advantages remain to be established. The device has only been approved by the FDA under 510(k) as a fusion device, but no clinical outcome has been reported yet. The failure rate of the device in terms of screw loosening or breakage are found to be not superior compared to Dynesys (Fig. 52.8).

The DSS-II dynamic stabilization system[44] was developed by the author and is one of the earliest titanium metallic springs used for dynamic stabilization. Its predecessor, the

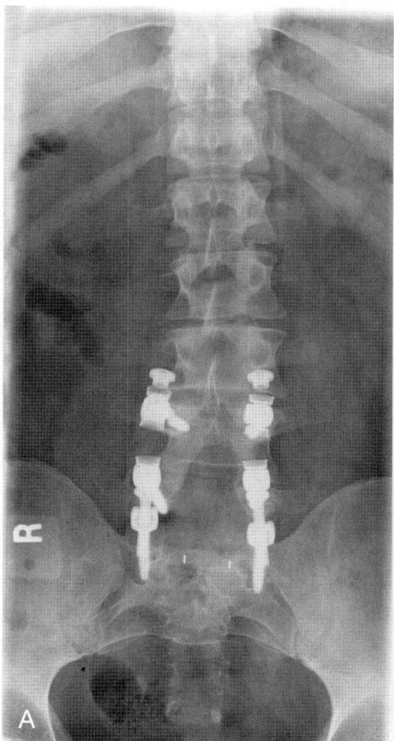

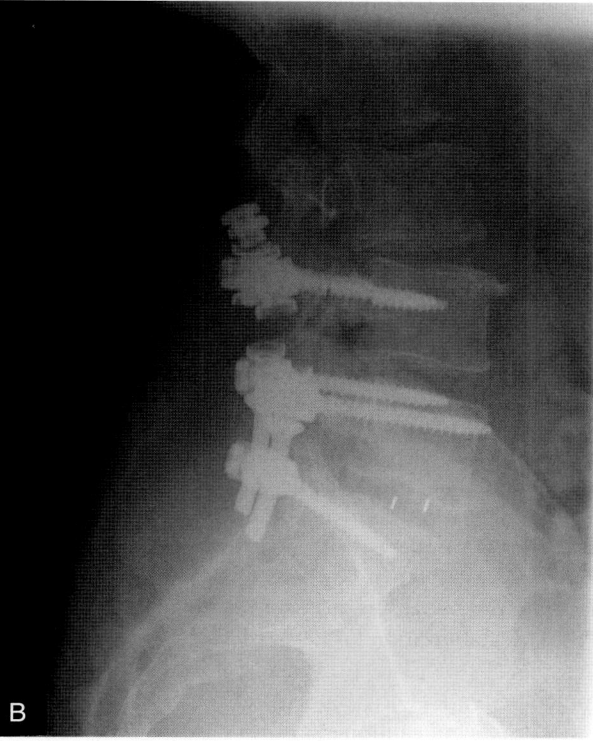

FIG. 52.8 Transition system used for rigid fusion at the L5–S1 segment (S1 is lumbarized) and dynamic stabilization at L4–L5. Note screw breakage at L4 at 18-month follow-up.

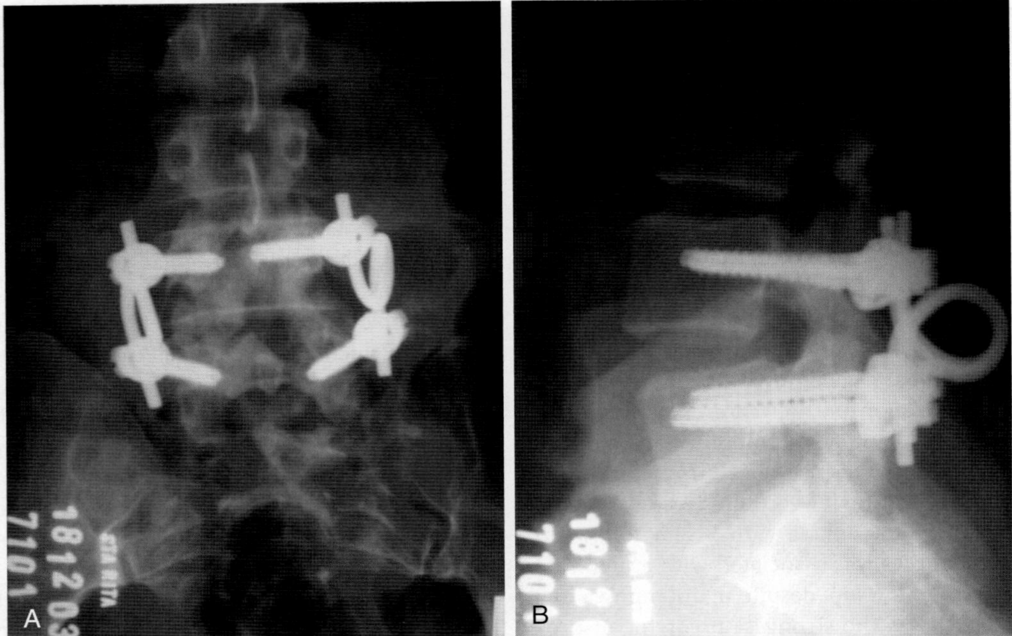

FIG. 52.9 DSS-II system for stabilization of L4–L5 motion segment: (A) anteroposterior and (B) lateral radiographs.

DSS-I, was a C-shaped titanium spring which, on biomechanical testing, showed uneven restriction to extension and excessive unloading of the disc in extension, indicating possibility of fatigue failure. It was therefore never used clinically. The second-generation DSS-II is an α-shaped titanium spring implanted between the pedicle screws. This design improvement produces active lordosis and permits adequate pedicle-to-pedicle excursion and physiologic translation of the IAR of the motion segment. The system allows uniform motion restriction and uniform load sharing throughout the ROM, the two essential biomechanical characteristics for survival of the implant against fatigue failure. The device has never been introduced for general use, but a pilot clinical trial in a small group of patients (n = 19) was completed in Sao Paulo, Brazil for patients with mechanical back pain without needing decompression (Fig. 52.9). The clinical outcome was encouraging, but, more important, no implant failure was observed in 2 to 3 years of follow-up.[44]

The BioFlex (Bio-Spine Corporation),[45] a coil spring made of nitinol 4 mm in diameter for increased flexibility, has been used extensively in Seoul, Korea. This device has been used most commonly in conjunction with interbody cages to achieve fusion, although it has also been used alone as a nonfusion device.[46] Recently, a titanium version of the device has been approved by the FDA under 510(k) as a fusion device, but no clinical use in the United States has been reported yet. In a retrospective study, Yang et al.[47] reported a review of 28 cases treated with BioFlex stabilization for L4–L5 degenerative spondylolisthesis, with 82% of cases experiencing good or excellent clinical outcome. Park et al.[48] reported encouraging clinical outcomes in 27 cases but cautioned against hardware-related complications that they encountered in five cases at 1-year follow-up (Fig. 52.10).

Stabilimax NZ (Applied Spine Technologies),[49] a dual-core spring device developed by Panjabi, is designed to apply soft resistance against both compression and distraction. The design rationale is to limit the NZ motion but leave the elastic zone unaffected. Currently, the device is undergoing an FDA-controlled IDE trial to assess whether it is at least as safe and effective as fusion in patients receiving decompression surgery for the treatment of clinically symptomatic spinal stenosis at one or two contiguous vertebral levels from L1–S1.[49,50]

The Cosmic Posterior Dynamic System (Ulrich GmbH)[51] has a unique design that incorporates a rigid rod connected to the pedicle screws with a hinged screw head, which is expected to permit motion. No biomechanical data are available in the peer-reviewed literature. There are some clinical reports of its use in journals that are not peer reviewed.[52] In a retrospective study, Yang et al.[47] reported a review of 23 cases treated with Cosmic stabilization for L4–L5 degenerative spondylolisthesis, with 78% of cases experiencing good or excellent clinical outcome. Kaner et al.[53] reported only one case with screw loosening, but no screw breakage, at 2- to 5-year follow-up in a review of 30 cases treated with Cosmic stabilization following decompression.

The AccuFlex (Globus Medical) titanium rod has a spiral cut to make the rod flexible and can be inserted between regular pedicle screws. This device has been used clinically for fusion[54] but not for nonfusion dynamic stabilization as yet. This metallic device offers some flexibility but does not permit any significant pedicle-to-pedicle excursion.

Hybrid devices incorporate a metallic rod connected to a flexible segment, with a nonmetallic bumper to allow shock absorption as well as some degree of pedicle-to-pedicle excursion. The primary clinical indication is to address

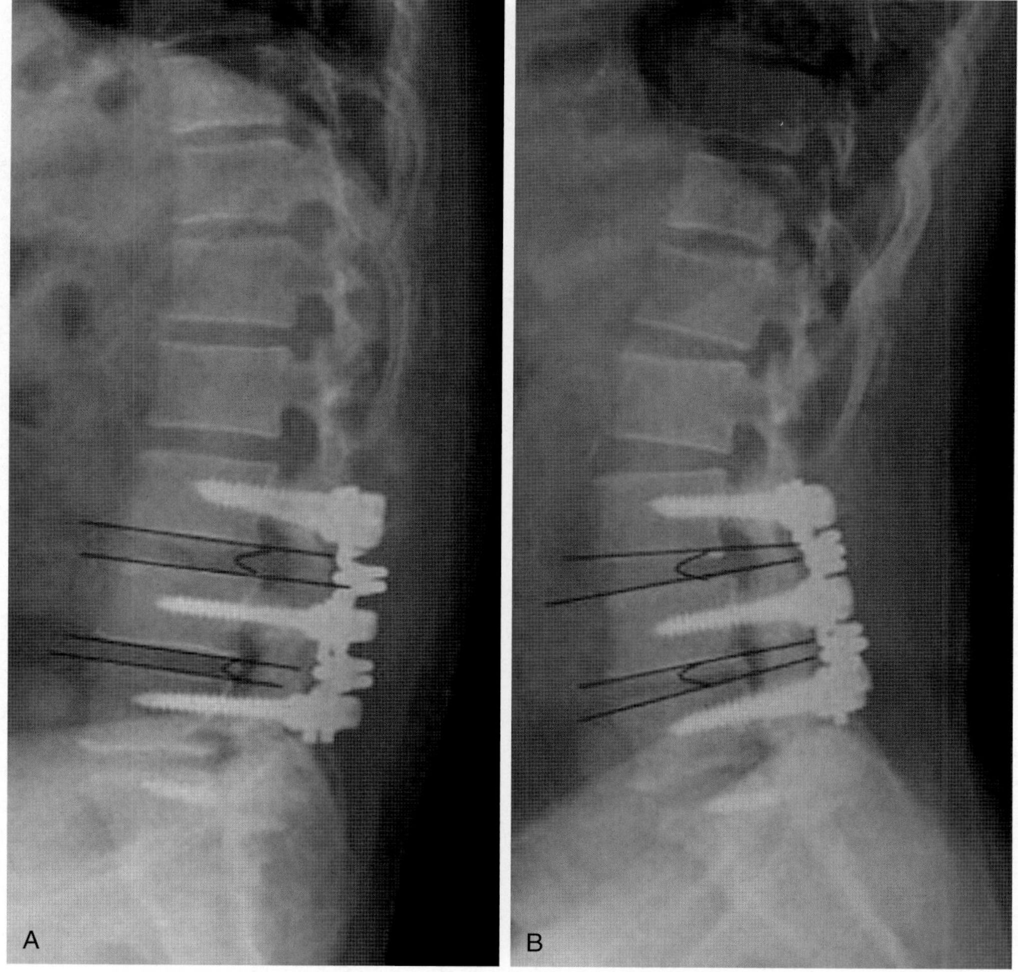

FIG. 52.10 BioFlex system for stabilization of L3–L4 and L4–L5 segments in (A) flexion and (B) extension.

advanced degenerated segments with rigid fusion and address moderately degenerated adjacent segments by stabilizing with a flexible device without fusion in order to prevent progression of degeneration. The Transition system described earlier is an example that can be used as a dynamic stabilization system only as well as a rigid to flexible hybrid system.

The CD Horizon Agile (Medtronic Sofamor Danek) system incorporates a soft cylindrical bumper at the end of a fusion rod, held by a metallic cable in its center, similar to the fabric cord as used in the Dynesys system described earlier. Following initial clinical use, the device was recalled by the company for reported fatigue failure of the cable.

The Dynesys Transition Optima (DTO) implant (Zimmer-Biomet) is a modification of the original Dynesys system that combines a hybrid rigid to dynamic stabilization. This transition system allows for arthrodesis of critically unstable vertebrae in combination with the dynamic stabilization of adjacent moderately degenerated segments. In a recent study, Lee et al.[55] reported their small experience using this hybrid system in 15 cases. They reported better outcome and greater preservation of posterior disc height with the use of the hybrid system compared to rigid fusion (see Fig. 52.5).

NFlex (Synthes GmbH) has a similar design, in which a 6.0-mm titanium fusion rod is connected to a flexible end made of 3.25-mm titanium core and a polycarbonate urethane sleeve. The sleeve allows soft resistance to both flexion and extension, permitting the essential pedicle-to-pedicle excursion. Although the device may permit compression and elongation, its ability to permit anteroposterior translation remains a concern. The device has been used clinically since the fall of 2006.[56] In 2012, Coe et al.[57] reported 2-year outcomes in 65 of 72 cases treated in five centers. They concluded that the NFlex system was effective in improving pain and functional scores at 2 years and may be considered an effective alternative to rigid fusion with appropriate patient selection (Fig. 52.11).

Interspinous Distraction Devices

One of the earliest and most frequently used IPDs was the X-Stop device (Medtronic). This titanium spacer can be inserted with a minimally invasive approach under local anesthesia; therefore, elderly patients with medical comorbidities are considered ideal candidates. Biomechanical studies in

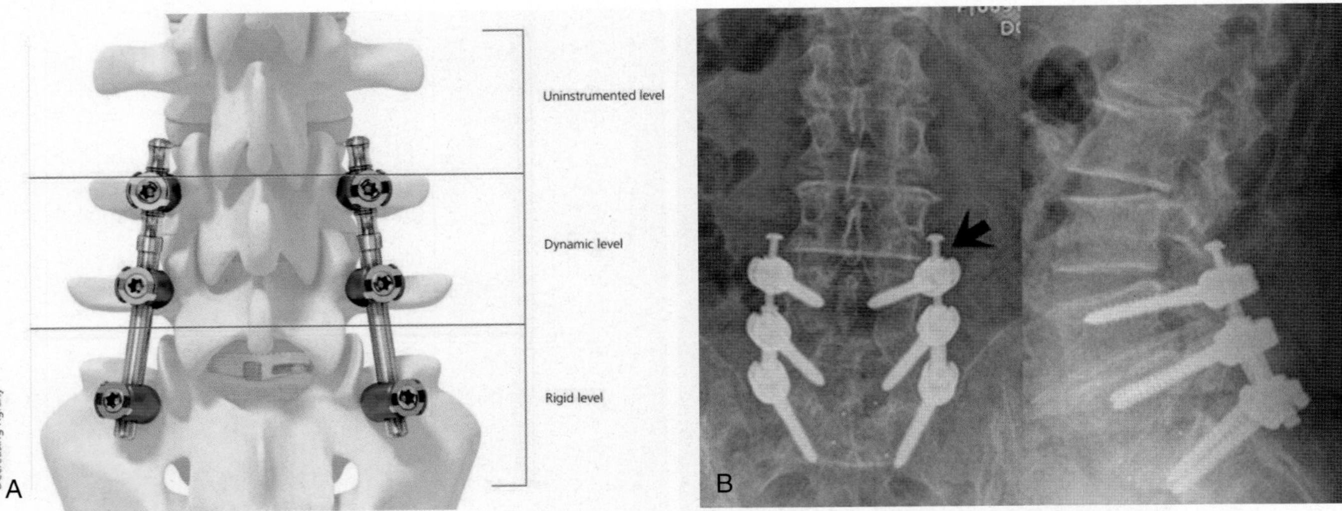

FIG. 52.11 (A) NFlex system schematic indicating the rigid and dynamic levels. (B) Clinical application at the L4–L5 and L5–S1 segments.

cadaver spines have demonstrated that X-Stop significantly decreases posterior intradiscal pressure[58,59] and reduces facet pressures; it decreases the contact area at the facets as well.[60] An in vivo study with MRI scan also demonstrated that X-Stop increases the spinal canal and foramen diameter during extension.[61] This device holds the spine into a position of flexion, a position of relief from claudication pain. Because it is not tied with Dacron ligament to the adjacent spinous process, it can permit further flexion.

In a prospective randomized, multicenter study on 191 patients with neurogenic intermittent claudication, the efficacy of X-Stop was compared to nonoperative treatment.[62] At 2-year follow-up, the X-Stop group had improved symptom severity, physical function, and patient satisfaction scores at all of the time points compared to the nonoperative group. The reoperation rate was 6% at 2 years for the X-Stop group, which is comparable to the reoperation rate for lumbar decompression procedures. There were some limitations to this study, including a lack of blinding and loss to follow-up. But the major limitation of the study was failure to compare the efficacy of X-Stop to a conventional surgical treatment for spinal stenosis, that is, decompressive laminectomy. The device received FDA approval for use in one- or two-level stenosis in patients over 50 years with significant neurogenic claudication with or without back pain after failed conservative treatment for at least 6 months.

The main complication of this device is dislodgement of the spacer with or without breakage of the spinous process. This is because the device is not flexible and does not permit extension movement of the spine. In a randomized control trial, Anderson et al.[63] reported that the X-Stop device was more effective than nonoperative treatment in the management of neurogenic claudication secondary to degenerative lumbar spondylolisthesis. However, in another study, Verhoof et al.[64] reported failure of X-Stop in seven of 15 (58%) consecutive cases within 2 years when the device was used for degenerative spondylolisthesis. A similar experience was reported by other authors as well.[65]

The Superion device (Vertiflex) is another metallic device similar to X-Stop, but with a smaller profile, and can be inserted through a minimally invasive approach without disrupting the interspinous ligament. This device is also metallic and not flexible, permitting flexion but no extension. Patel et al.[66] reported 3-year clinical outcomes of a randomized, controlled FDA IDE trial of Superion (190 cases) compared to a control group with X-Stop (201 cases) for the treatment of moderate degenerative lumbar spinal stenosis. They reported better outcomes with Superion, achieving a success rate of 80% for each of the individual components of the primary endpoint (Fig. 52.12).

The Wallis device (Zimmer Spine) is an example of a rigid nonmetallic polyetheretherketone spacer, retained between the spinous processes by a Dacron tape, which prevents its accidental dislodgement.[67] This device holds the spine into flexion and stops extension. In addition, the holding ligaments also restrict further flexion. As a result, its manufacturers and inventors have recommended its use for indications beyond spinal stenosis, for example, mechanical back pain with early disc degeneration.[68,69]

An FDA IDE trial is currently comparing the Wallis system to total disc replacement for the treatment of mild to moderate degenerative disc disease of the lumbar spine at the L4–L5 level.[70] An updated report of this trial is not available, but a prospective randomized controlled trial to assess the efficacy of the Wallis system has been reported from Europe.[71] Sixty patients with an average age of 58 years (range, 34–81 years) with spinal stenosis were randomly assigned to two groups with an equal number of patients: decompression alone or decompression with Wallis implant. The Wallis group had better improvement of symptoms, but it was not statistically significant. Korovessis et al[72] reported a prospective controlled study, designed to investigate if the implantation of Wallis implant cephalad to short segment instrumented fusion in 25 cases, and a control group without; they found that the adjacent segments with Wallis implant stabilization resisted degeneration more than in the control group. Floman et al[68]

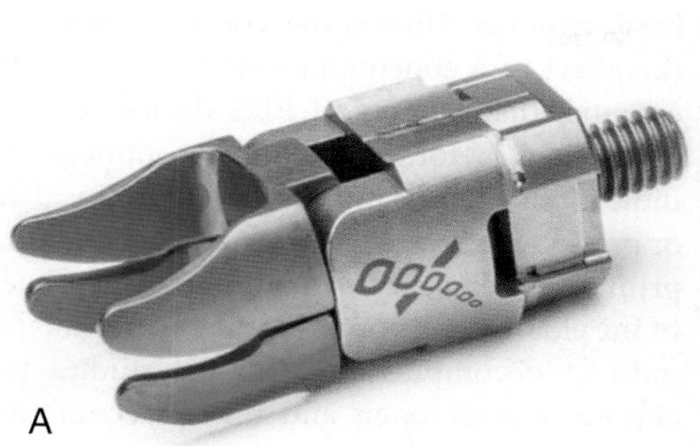

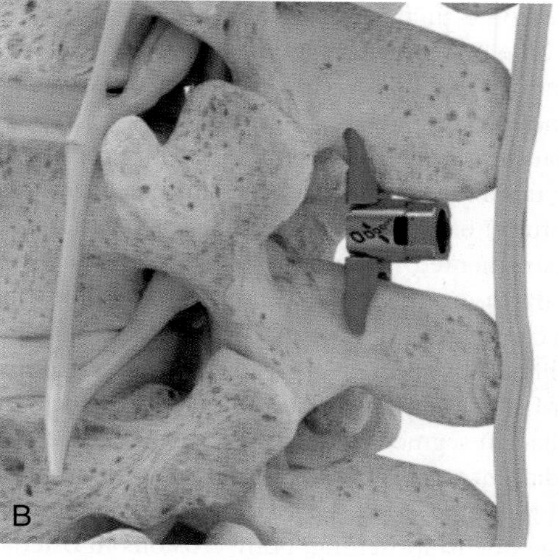

FIG. 52.12 Superion system (A) collapsed and (B) expanded after insertion between the spinous processes.

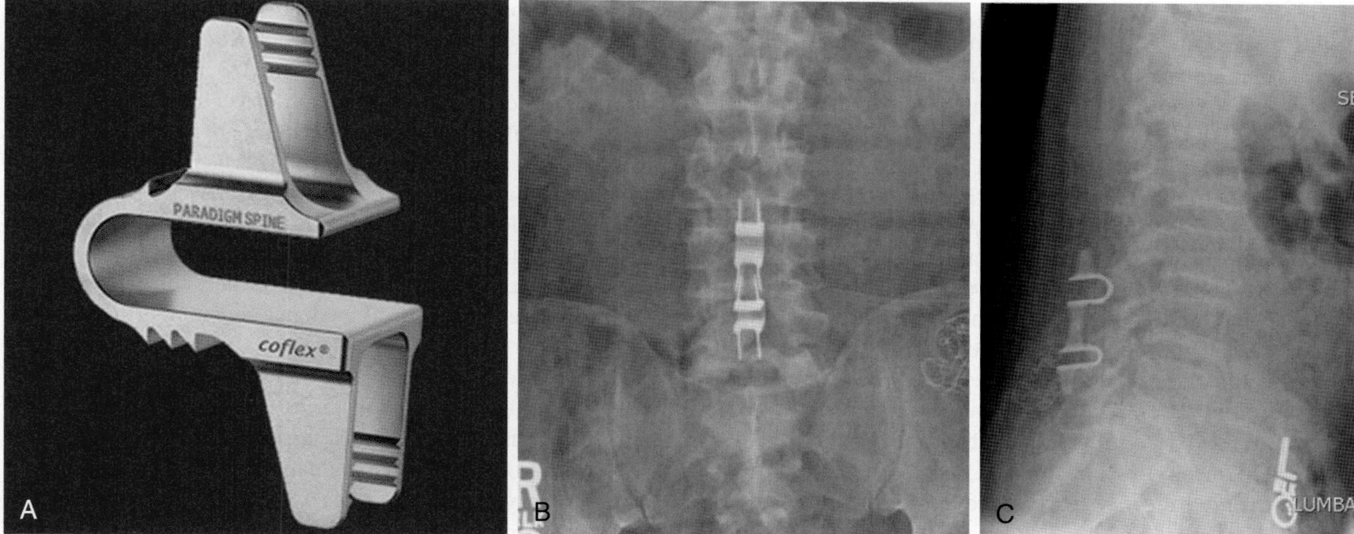

FIG. 52.13 The Coflex system. Clinical application to L4–L5 and L5–S1 segments in (A) anteroposterior and (B) lateral radiographs.

reported failure of the Wallis interspinous implant to lower the incidence of recurrent lumbar disc herniation in patients undergoing primary disc excision.

The DIAM system (Medtronic Sofamor Danek) is an H-shaped, polyester-covered, silicone bumper that is placed between the spinous processes with a suture to hold it in place. The device has been used in Europe for a few years. A recent clinical study failed to establish efficacy of DIAM in improving back pain when compared to decompression alone.[73] An FDA-regulated clinical trial for DIAM was initiated in late 2006 for patients with lumbar spinal stenosis. The FDA also granted another IDE trial to study DIAM in patients with low back pain caused by degenerative disc disease.[74] In February of 2016, the Orthopaedic and Rehabilitation Devices Panel of the FDA Medical Devices Advisory Committee presented its report on the DIAM Spine Stabilization Trial.[75] This was a prospective, randomized, controlled pivotal clinical trial, with nonoperative control, randomized at a 2 : 1 ratio, no blinding, and the primary endpoint to be determined at the 12-month time point. Inclusion criteria were degenerative disc disease, in the 18 to 70 years age group, with Oswestry Disability Index score greater than 30 and visual analog scale (VAS) score for back pain greater than or equal to 8 out of 10. Study success was defined as superiority in the treatment group at 12 months. The DIAM subjects reported better outcomes (64%) as compared to the control group (24.5%) in the primary and secondary effectiveness assessments. Spinous process erosions and spinous process fractures were observed in DIAM subjects throughout the course of this clinical trial. Despite significantly superior clinical outcome in the DIAM group, the panel suggested a postapproval study to provide long-term safety and effectiveness data with the device with 5-year follow-up.

The Coflex device (Paradigm Spine), is a U-shaped titanium device, retained in place by clamping its wings around the adjacent spinous processes (Fig. 52.13). In contrast to other IPD devices, it allows both flexion and extension and does not act as an extension stop. Biomechanical studies report that it restores normal flexion-extension in a destabilized spine rather than holding the spine in flexion.[76] Kong et al. reported a comparable outcome at 1-year follow-up with Coflex versus PLIF for degenerative back pain.[77] However, the Coflex group had preserved motion and the PLIF group had an adverse effect on the adjacent segment. Bae et al.[78] recently reported the 3-year follow-up of the prospective randomized controlled trial (FDA IDE study) of Coflex interlaminar stabilization (n = 196) versus instrumented fusion (n = 94) in patients with lumbar stenosis. Both groups showed improvement, but the percentage with a clinically significant improvement (≥15) in the Oswestry Disability Index seemed larger for the Coflex group. In addition, ROM was maintained with the Coflex device in the index and adjacent segment compared to increased ROM in the superior adjacent segment in the fusion group. Five-year follow-up data of the same study showed a similar outcome.[79]

Device slippage due to loosening, bony erosions in osteoporotic bones, and/or progression of instability are the main concerns with the Coflex device.[80] Because of the smaller size of the S1 spinous process, there is a concern of failure of the Coflex device at the L5–S1 level. However, in a retrospective study, Xu et al.[81] reported a consecutive series of 33 patients with degenerative lumbar spinal stenosis or lumbar disc herniation at the L5–S1 level, stabilized successfully with Coflex, and observed no significant implant failure.

Many other spinous process distraction devices are being developed or are beginning an FDA trial. A comprehensive review is beyond the scope of this chapter. A systematic review comparing four different commonly used IPD devices (DIAM, Wallis, Coflex, and X-Stop) was reported by Lee et al.[82] Out of a total of 286 articles, 20 were included in the final assessment. Two assessors independently extracted data. The authors found that the complication rate of combined interspinous dynamic stabilization and decompression treatment (32.3%) was greater than that of decompression alone (6.5%), but no complication that significantly affected treatment results was found. Interspinous dynamic stabilization produced slightly better clinical outcomes than conservative treatments for spinal stenosis. No significant difference in treatment outcomes was found in the studies that compared interspinous dynamic stabilization with decompression or fusion alone. The authors concluded that clinical outcomes with the IPD devices were similar to those of conventional techniques and that no additional clinical advantage could be attributed to interspinous dynamic stabilization. However, few studies have been conducted on the long-term efficacy of interspinous dynamic stabilization.

Summary

PDS evolved from failure of fusion to address mechanical back pain due to spinal instability. IPD devices have been primarily introduced to treat spinal stenosis with claudication or radicular pain by indirect decompression. Spinal instability is poorly defined, but the current understanding is abnormal quality of motion, leading to uneven load transmission. This occurs mostly during NZ motion. The biomechanical goals of PDS devices are to preserve motion as much as possible but prevent any abnormal motion and to unload the disc and facet joints by load sharing. The biggest challenge for PDS devices is to survive fatigue failure despite allowing continued motion. The key to this survival is uniform load sharing and uniform restriction of motion throughout ROM. Unfortunately, many PDS devices have been introduced without any biomechanical basis, and their clinical success was confounded by combining the effect of a concomitant decompression for leg pain. It is essential that efficacy of PDS devices to treat back pain be established before they are recommended for secondary indications, such as preventing instability after decompression or preventing adjacent-segment degeneration. IPD devices are primarily indicated for treatment of neurogenic claudication in the elderly with comorbidities by minimal intervention and indirect decompression. Clinical studies to establish their efficacy against open and direct decompression is lacking. Their recommendation in the treatment of mechanical back pain does not have any scientific basis. Product development and marketing is expensive; therefore, most clinical trials are aimed at establishing clinical success rather than a proper scientific evaluation of their clinical efficacy. Most of the new PDS devices are introduced in the US market with FDA approval under 510(k) as a fusion device. The clinical use for dynamic stabilization without an attempt of fusion has become an off-label use in the United States. This has led to the concept of soft fusion, which indicates intertransverse fusion only, using a PDS device. Expectation is that resultant fusion would be less stiff than conventional fusion with rigid instrumentation and therefore less likely to produce adjacent-segment disease. There is no clinical evidence to support this concept yet. Dynamic stabilization has raised a great deal of enthusiasm, theoretical promises, and many expectations. Like any new technology, these procedures are apt to breed clinical failures. The need for detailed consideration of design rationale and proper clinical evaluation without confounding factors to prove safety and efficacy cannot be overemphasized. Fusion remains the method of choice for advanced disc/facet degeneration and gross instability. However, disc degeneration in multiple segments—particularly in young patients with concerns about adjacent-segment disease following fusion—will likely constitute the main indication for PDS. Future applications of dynamic stabilization may include salvage of failed disc prosthesis or nuclear replacement. In the future, PDS may be considered to provide temporary mechanical support for any pharmacologic treatment aiming for repair or regeneration of the intervertebral disc.

PEARLS

1. Clinical instability causing mechanical back pain may be defined as abnormal quality of motion leading to uneven load distribution in the motion segment.
2. The goals of PDS are motion preservation and to prevent abnormal motion in the NZ.
3. The mechanism of pain relief by PDS is load sharing with the disc and the facet joints.
4. The goal of interspinous distraction is indirect decompression for the spinal stenosis, with minimal intervention.
5. The primary indication for PDS is activity-related mechanical back pain.

6. The secondary indications for PDS are prevention of instability, prevention of iatrogenic instability after decompression, and stabilization of the adjacent motion segment.
7. The primary indication for IPD is spinal stenosis with claudication.
8. The secondary indication for IPD is mechanical back pain.
9. Contraindications for dynamic stabilization are osteoporosis, advanced disc degeneration with complete collapse of disc height, scoliosis, and spondylolisthesis greater than grade 1.

PITFALLS

1. The biggest challenge for dynamic stabilization devices is survival against fatigue, despite allowing continued motion.
2. Avoid too much distraction and kyphosis with a PDS device, which increases the poor outcome and device failure.
3. Avoid using any dynamic stabilization device in the presence of osteoporosis to prevent implant loosening.
4. For advanced disc degeneration, fusion remains the gold standard of surgical treatment.

KEY REFERENCES

1. Mulholland RC, Sengupta DK. Rationale, principles and experimental evaluation of the concept of soft stabilization. *Eur Spine J.* 2002;11(suppl 2):S198-S205.
   In this landmark review article, Mulholland and Sengupta describe the concept of instability as a function of abnormal load distribution as opposed to abnormal motion. They also describe the "stone in the shoe concept" and the rationale of design and mechanism of action of various dynamic stabilization devices.
2. Panjabi MM. Clinical spinal instability and low back pain. *J Electromyogr Kinesiol.* 2003;13:371-379.
   Panjabi presents his understanding of clinical instability causing low back pain as a function of abnormal motion during the neutral zone.
3. Bono CM, Kadaba M, Vaccaro AR. Posterior pedicle fixation based dynamic stabilization devices for the treatment of degenerative diseases of the lumbar spine. *J Spinal Disord Tech.* 2009;22:376-383.
   This literature review reports clinical results of using pedicle-based PDS systems and facet replacement devices in the lumbar spine.
4. Stoll TM, Dubois G, Schwarzenbach O. The dynamic neutralization system for the spine: a multi-center study of a novel non-fusion system. *Eur Spine J.* 2002;11(suppl 2):S170-S178.
   This was the first report of clinical outcome of the Dynesys PDS system from its inventor Dubois.
5. Zucherman JF, Hsu KY, Hartjen CA, et al. A multicenter, prospective, randomized trial evaluating the X STOP interspinous process decompression system for the treatment of neurogenic intermittent claudication: two-year follow-up results. *Spine (Phila Pa 1976).* 2005;30:1351-1358.
   This was the first report of a randomized, controlled, prospective multicenter trial comparing the outcomes of neurogenic claudication patients treated with the X-Stop with patients treated nonoperatively.

REFERENCES

1. Sengupta DK, Herkowitz HN. Pedicle screw-based posterior dynamic stabilization: literature review. *Adv Orthop.* 2012;2012:424268.
2. Stoll TM, Dubois G, Schwarzenbach O. The dynamic neutralization system for the spine: a multi-center study of a novel non-fusion system. *Eur Spine J.* 2002;11(suppl 2): S170-S178.
3. Bono CM, Lee CK. Critical analysis of trends in fusion for degenerative disc disease over the past 20 years: influence of technique on fusion rate and clinical outcome. *Spine.* 2004;29(4):455-463.
4. Gibson JN, Waddell G. Surgery for degenerative lumbar spondylosis. *Cochrane Database Syst Rev.* 2005;(2):CD001352.
5. Cheh G, et al. Adjacent segment disease followinglumbar/thoracolumbar fusion with pedicle screw instrumentation: a minimum 5-year follow-up. *Spine.* 2007;32(20):2253-2257.
6. Panjabi MM. Hybrid multidirectional test method to evaluate spinal adjacent-level effects. *Clin Biomech (Bristol, Avon).* 2007;22(3):257-265.
7. Sengupta DK, Herkowitz HN. Degenerative spondylolisthesis: review of current trends and controversies. *Spine.* 2005;30(6 suppl):S71-S81.
8. Okawa A, et al. Dynamic motion study of the whole lumbar spine by videofluoroscopy. *Spine.* 1998;23(16):1743-1749.
9. Murata M, Morio Y, Kuranobu K. Lumbar disc degeneration and segmental instability: a comparison of magnetic resonance images and plain radiographs of patients with low back pain. *Arch Orthop Trauma Surg.* 1994;113(6):297-301.
10. Paajanen H, Tertti M. Association of incipient disc degeneration and instability in spondylolisthesis. A magnetic resonance and flexion-extension radiographic study of 20-year-old low back pain patients. *Arch Orthop Trauma Surg.* 1991;111(1):16-19.
11. Fujiwara A, et al. The relationship between disc degeneration, facet joint osteoarthritis, and stability of the degenerative lumbar spine. *J Spinal Disord.* 2000;13(5):444-450.
12. Panjabi MM. Clinical spinal instability and low back pain. *J Electromyogr Kinesiol.* 2003;13(4):371-379.
13. Mulholland RC, Sengupta DK. Rationale, principles and experimental evaluation of the concept of soft stabilization. *Eur Spine J.* 2002;11(suppl 2):S198-S205.
14. Frymoyer JW, Krag MH. Spinal stability and instability: definitions, classification, and general principles of management. In: Dunsker SB, et al., eds. *The Unstable Spine.* New York: Grune & Stratton; 1986.
15. Pope MH, Panjabi M. Biomechanical definitions of spinal instability. *Spine.* 1985;10(3):255-256.
16. Moore RJ, et al. The origin and fate of herniated lumbar intervertebral disc tissue. *Spine.* 1996;21(18):2149-2155.
17. McNally DS. The objectives for the mechanical evaluation of spinal instrumentation have changed. *Eur Spine J.* 2002; 11(suppl 2):S179-S185.
18. Keller TS, et al. Regional variations in the compressive properties of lumbar vertebral trabeculae. Effects of disc degeneration. *Spine.* 1989;14(9):1012-1019.
19. Simpson EK, et al. Intervertebral disc disorganization is related to trabecular bone architecture in the lumbar spine. *J Bone Miner Res.* 2001;16(4):681-687.
20. McNally DS, et al. In vivo stress measurement can predict pain on discography. *Spine.* 1996;21(22):2580-2587.
21. McNally DS, Adams MA. Internal intervertebral disc mechanics as revealed by stress profilometry. *Spine.* 1992; 17(1):66-73.
22. Hadlow SV, et al. The Graf ligamentoplasty procedure. Comparison with posterolateral fusion in the management of low back pain. *Spine.* 1998;23(10):1172-1179.
23. Grevitt MP, et al. The Graf stabilisation system: early results in 50 patients. *Eur Spine J.* 1995;4(3):169-175.

24. Gardner A, Pande KC. Graf ligamentoplasty: a 7-year follow-up. *Eur Spine J*. 2002;11(suppl 2):S157-S163.
25. Markwalder TM, Wenger M. Dynamic stabilization of lumbar motion segments by use of Graf's ligaments: results with an average follow-up of 7.4 years in 39 highly selected, consecutive patients. *Acta Neurochir (Wien)*. 2003;145(3): 209-214.
26. Kanayama M, et al. A minimum 10-year follow-up of posterior dynamic stabilization using Graf artificial ligament. *Spine*. 2007;32(18):1992-1996.
27. Grob D, et al. Clinical experience with the Dynesys semirigid fixation system for the lumbar spine: surgical and patient-oriented outcome in 50 cases after an average of 2 years. *Spine*. 2005;30(3):324-331.
28. Schmoelz W, et al. Dynamic stabilization of the lumbar spine and its effects on adjacent segments: an in vitro experiment. *J Spinal Disord Tech*. 2003;16(4):418-423.
29. Schmoelz W, et al. Influence of a dynamic stabilisation system on load bearing of a bridged disc: an in vitro study of intradiscal pressure. *Eur Spine J*. 2006;15(8):1276-1285.
30. Beastall J, et al. The Dynesys lumbar spinal stabilization system: a preliminary report on positional magnetic resonance imaging findings. *Spine*. 2007;32(6):685-690.
31. Meyers K, et al. The use of instrumented pedicle screws to evaluate load sharing in posterior dynamic stabilization systems. *Spine J*. 2007.
32. Sapkas GS, et al. Stabilization of the lumbar spine using the dynamic neutralization system. *Orthopedics*. 2007;30(10): 859-865.
33. Wurgler-Hauri CC, et al. Dynamic neutralization of the lumbar spine after microsurgical decompression in acquired lumbar spinal stenosis and segmental instability. *Spine*. 2008; 33(3):E66-E72.
34. Anand N, Baron EM. Role of dynesys as pedicle-based nonfusion stabilization for degenerative disc disorders. *Adv Orthop*. 2012;2012:218385.
35. Welch WC, et al. Clinical outcomes of the Dynesys dynamic neutralization system: 1-year preliminary results. *Neurosurg Focus*. 2007;22(1):E8.
36. FDA Orthopedic and Rehabilitation Devices Panel. *FDA Executive Summary for Zimmer Spine's Dynesys Spinal System*. Available at www.fda.gov/downloads/advisorycommittees/committeesmeetingmaterials/medicaldevices/medicaldevicesadvisorycommittee/orthopaedicandrehabilitationdevicespanel/ucm188734.pdf. Last accessed 2009.
37. Hoppe S, et al. Long-term outcome after monosegmental l4/5 stabilization for degenerative spondylolisthesis with the Dynesys device. *Clin Spine Surg*. 2016;29(2):72-77.
38. Hsieh CT, et al. Clinical experiences of dynamic stabilizers: Dynesys and Dynesys top loading system for lumbar spine degenerative disease. *Kaohsiung J Med Sci*. 2016;32(4): 207-215.
39. Lee CH, et al. Dynamic stabilization using the Dynesys system versus posterior lumbar interbody fusion for the treatment of degenerative lumbar spinal disease: a clinical and radiological outcomes-based meta-analysis. *Neurosurg Focus*. 2016;40(1):E7.
40. Pham MH, et al. Complications associated with the Dynesys dynamic stabilization system: a comprehensive review of the literature. *Neurosurg Focus*. 2016;40(1):E2.
41. St Pierre GH, et al. Nonfusion does not prevent adjacent segment disease: dynesys long-term outcomes with minimum five-year follow-up. *Spine*. 2016;41(3):265-273.
42. Wang Q, et al. Short-term effects of a dynamic neutralization system (Dynesys) for multi-segmental lumbar disc herniation. *Eur Spine J*. 2016;25(5):1409-1416.
43. Zhang Y, et al. Comparison of the Dynesys dynamic stabilization system and posterior lumbar interbody fusion for lumbar degenerative disease. *PLoS One*. 2016;11(1): e0148071.
44. Sengupta DK. Dynamic stabilization system. In: Yue JJ, McAfee PC, An HS, eds. *Motion Preservation Surgery of the Spine: Advanced Techniques and Controversies*. Philadelphia: Elsevier; 2008:472-475.
45. Kim YS, Moon BJ. Bioflex spring rod pedicle screw system. In: Kim DH, Fessler RG, eds. *Dynamic Reconstruction of the Spine*. New York.: Thieme; 2006:340-346.
46. Kim YS, et al. Nitinol spring rod dynamic stabilization system and Nitinol memory loops in surgical treatment for lumbar disc disorders: short-term follow up. *Neurosurg Focus*. 2007;22(1):E10.
47. Yang JS, et al. Dynamic radiographic results of different semi-rigid fusion devices for degenerative lumbar spondylolisthesis: "dynamic rod" vs. "dynamic screw head". *Turk Neurosurg*. 2016;26(2):268-273.
48. Park H, et al. Change of lumbar motion after multi-level posterior dynamic stabilization with Bioflex system: 1 year follow up. *J Korean Neurosurg Soc*. 2009;46(4): 285-291.
49. Yue JJ, et al. Clinical application of the Panjabi neutral zone hypothesis: the Stabilimax NZ posterior lumbar dynamic stabilization system. *Neurosurg Focus*. 2007;22(1):E12.
50. Yue JJ, Malcolmon G, Timm JP. The Stabilimax NZ posterior lumbar dynamic stabilization system. In: Yue JJ, McAfee PC, An HS, eds. *Motion Preservation Surgery of the Spine: Advanced Techniques and Controversies*. Philadelphia: Elsevier; 2008:476-482.
51. Karabekir HS, Sedat C, Mehmet Z. Clinical outcomes Of Cosmic dynamic neutralization system: preliminary results of 1-year. *The Internet Journal of Minimally Invasive Spinal Technology*. 2008;2(3).
52. von Strempel A, et al. Stabilisation of the degenerated lumbar spine in the nonfusion technique with Cosmic posterior dynamic system. *World Spine J*. 2006;1(1):40-47.
53. Kaner T, et al. Clinical outcomes of degenerative lumbar spinal stenosis treated with lumbar decompression and the Cosmic "semi-rigid" posterior system. *SAS J*. 2010;4(4):99-106.
54. Mandigo CE, Sampath P, Kaiser MG. Posterior dynamic stabilization of the lumbar spine: pedicle based stabilization with the AccuFlex rod system. *Neurosurg Focus*. 2007;22(1):E9.
55. Lee SE, Jahng TA, Kim HJ. Hybrid surgery combined with dynamic stabilization system and fusion for the multilevel degenerative disease of the lumbosacral spine. *Int J Spine Surg*. 2015;9:45.
56. Wallach CJ, Teng AL, Wang JC. NFlex. In: Yue JJ, McAfee PC, An HS, eds. *Motion Preservation Surgery of the Spine: Advanced Techniques and Controversies*. Philadelphia: Elsevier; 2008:505-510.
57. Coe JD, et al. NFlex dynamic stabilization system: two-year clinical outcomes of multi-center study. *J Korean Neurosurg Soc*. 2012;51(6):343-349.
58. Lindsey DP, et al. The effects of an interspinous implant on the kinematics of the instrumented and adjacent levels in the lumbar spine. *Spine*. 2003;28(19):2192-2197.
59. Swanson KE, et al. The effects of an interspinous implant on intervertebral disc pressures. *Spine*. 2003;28(1):26-32.

60. Wiseman CM, et al. The effect of an interspinous process implant on facet loading during extension. *Spine*. 2005;30(8): 903-907.
61. Richards JC, et al. The treatment mechanism of an interspinous process implant for lumbar neurogenic intermittent claudication. *Spine*. 2005;30(7):744-749.
62. Zucherman JF, et al. A multicenter, prospective, randomized trial evaluating the X-STOP interspinous process decompression system for the treatment of neurogenic intermittent claudication: two-year follow-up results. *Spine*. 2005;30(12):1351-1358.
63. Anderson PA, Tribus CB, Kitchel SH. Treatment of neurogenic claudication by interspinous decompression: application of the X-STOP device in patients with lumbar degenerative spondylolisthesis. *J Neurosurg Spine*. 2006;4(6):463-471.
64. Verhoof OJ, et al. High failure rate of the interspinous distraction device (X-STOP) for the treatment of lumbar spinal stenosis caused by degenerative spondylolisthesis. *Eur Spine J*. 2008;17(2):188-192.
65. Huddleston P. X-STOP resulted in a higher reoperation rate than minimally invasive decompression, but both decreased symptoms of neurogenic intermittent claudication in patients with lumbar spinal stenosis. *J Bone Joint Surg Am*. 2015;97(22):1889.
66. Patel VV, et al. Superion InterSpinous Spacer for treatment of moderate degenerative lumbar spinal stenosis: durable three-year results of a randomized controlled trial. *J Pain Res*. 2015;8:657-662.
67. Senegas J. Mechanical supplementation by non-rigid fixation in degenerative intervertebral lumbar segments: the Wallis system. *Eur Spine J*. 2002;11(suppl 2):S164-S169.
68. Floman Y, et al. Failure of the Wallis interspinous implant to lower the incidence of recurrent lumbar disc herniations in patients undergoing primary disc excision. *J Spinal Disord Tech*. 2007;20(5):337-341.
69. Senegas J, et al. Long-term actuarial survivorship analysis of an interspinous stabilization system. *Eur Spine J*. 2007;16(8): 1279-1287.
70. Christie SD, Song JK, Fessler RG. Dynamic interspinous process technology. *Spine*. 2005;30(16 suppl):S73-S78.
71. Marsh GD, Mahir S, Leyte A. A prospective randomised controlled trial to assess the efficacy of dynamic stabilisation of the lumbar spine with the Wallis ligament. *Eur Spine J*. 2014;23(10):2156-2160.
72. Korovessis P, et al. Does Wallis implant reduce adjacent segment degeneration above lumbosacral instrumented fusion? *Eur Spine J*. 2009;18(6):830-840.
73. Kim KA, et al. Dynamic intraspinous spacer technology for posterior stabilization: case-control study on the safety, sagittal angulation, and pain outcome at 1-year follow-up evaluation. *Neurosurg Focus*. 2007;22(1):E7.
74. Food and Drug Administration. *DIAM Spinal Stabilization System vs. Decompression, Formerly vs. Posterolateral Fusion*. Available at: https://clinicaltrials.gov/ct2/show/NCT00627497.
75. Food and Drug Administration. *DIAM Spinal Stabilization System (P140007)*. Available at: https://www.fda.gov/downloads/AdvisoryCommittees/CommitteesMeetingMaterials/MedicalDevices/MedicalDevicesAdvisoryCommittee/OrthopaedicandRehabilitationDevicesPanel/UCM486692.pdf..
76. Tsai KJ, et al. A biomechanical evaluation of an interspinous device (Coflex) used to stabilize the lumbar spine. *J Surg Orthop Adv*. 2006;15(3):167-172.
77. Kong DS, Kim ES, Eoh W. One-year outcome evaluation after interspinous implantation for degenerative spinal stenosis with segmental instability. *J Korean Med Sci*. 2007;22(2): 330-335.
78. Bae HW, et al. Three-year follow-up of the prospective, randomized, controlled trial of Coflex interlaminar stabilization vs instrumented fusion in patients with lumbar stenosis. *Neurosurgery*. 2016;79(2):169-181.
79. Musacchio MJ, et al. Evaluation of decompression and interlaminar stabilization compared with decompression and fusion for the treatment of lumbar spinal stenosis: 5-year follow-up of a prospective, randomized, controlled trial. *Int J Spine Surg*. 2016;10:6.
80. Park SC, et al. Minimum 2-year follow-up result of degenerative spinal stenosis treated with interspinous U (Coflex). *J Korean Neurosurg Soc*. 2009;46(4):292-299.
81. Xu C, et al. Application of the Coflex interlaminar stabilization in patients with L5/S1 degenerative diseases: minimum 4-year follow-up. *Am J Ther*. 2016;23(6):e1813-e1818.
82. Lee SH, et al. A systematic review of interspinous dynamic stabilization. *Clin Orthop Surg*. 2015;7(3):323-329.

Index

Page numbers followed by "*f*" indicate figures, "*t*" indicate tables, and "*b*" indicate boxes.

B

C

F

G

J

K

N

O

P

Q

R

S

W

Rothman-Simeone and Herkowitz's

The Spine

Rothman-Simeone and Herkowitz's

The Spine

SEVENTH EDITION

Steven R. Garfin, MD
Distinguished Professor and Chair
Department of Orthopaedic Surgery
University of California, San Diego
San Diego, California

Frank J. Eismont, MD
Leonard M. Miller Professor and Chairman
Department of Orthopaedic Surgery
University of Miami Miller School of Medicine
Miami, Florida

Gordon R. Bell, MD
Emeritus Staff
Former Director, Center for Spine Health
Cleveland Clinic
Cleveland, Ohio

Jeffrey S. Fischgrund, MD
Harry N. Herkowitz Professor and Chairman
Department of Orthopaedic Surgery
Beaumont Health
Royal Oak, Michigan

Christopher M. Bono, MD
Chief, Orthopaedic Spine Service
Department of Orthopaedic Surgery
Associate Professor of Orthopaedic Surgery
Harvard Medical School
Brigham and Women's Hospital
Boston, Massachusetts

ELSEVIER

ELSEVIER

1600 John F. Kennedy Blvd.
Ste 1800
Philadelphia, PA 19103-2899

ROTHMAN-SIMEONE AND HERKOWITZ'S THE SPINE,
SEVENTH EDITION

ISBN: 978-0-323-39397-3

Senior Content Strategist: Kristine Jones
Senior Content Development Specialist: Joanie Milnes
Publishing Services Manager: Patricia Tannian
Senior Project Manager: Carrie Stetz
Design Direction: Maggie Reid

Printed in China

Last digit is the print number: 9 8 7 6 5 4 3 2 1

This edition is dedicated to our esteemed colleague and close friend, Harry N. Herkowitz, MD, who passed away, too early, in June 2013. In a humble attempt to honor him and his legacy, we list Harry's name along with our mentors, thus changing the title of this book to *Rothman-Simeone and Herkowitz's The Spine*. Harry abruptly and unintentionally left the editorship of this great work, of which he truly was the lead and driving force for the first six editions. We present this seventh edition proudly and with the hope that our departed friend would approve. To fill the void left by this one man, we have added two new editors whom Harry respected immensely.

Harry was a luminary in spine. Orthopedic surgeons and neurosurgeons worldwide have benefited from his extensive and significant contributions to the field. Harry worked incredibly hard and accomplished much during his career, rising to the presidency of multiple organizations. He was an excellent and exceptionally active surgeon. He was a surgeon's surgeon, as we say, who was respected as a superb educator, a leader among leaders, and a shining example of a clinical researcher. Harry emphasized and fostered patient-oriented care long before it was in vogue. His manner of practice and teaching epitomized evidence-based medicine, once again before it became a defined process. With an intrinsic drive, he continued to search for excellence. His accomplishments, for a single person, were extraordinary.

Unlike most of us, Harry did not begin his career in a university setting with its attendant peer pressure to publish and produce; his was an internal force. Ultimately he surpassed his original goals. "Don't worry, I will get it done," was a consoling and affirming phrase he used often. And after he uttered those words, we didn't worry, and he would always get it done. Today, it would be unusual to get through a round of fellowship candidate interviews without hearing the word "privademics," and it is to this type of practice that many of our young colleagues aspire. Harry, under the guidance of our mentor Richard Rothman, MD, PhD, blazed a trail into this heretofore unknown hybrid world brilliantly and selflessly, setting aside his and his group's personal finances and time.

In so many ways and in so many settings, Harry changed the lives of patients, colleagues, and trainees. He rewarded those who lived up to his expectations with a lifetime of honor and friendship. He changed the course of contemporary spine surgery through his research and his leadership of numerous professional organizations, not the least of which was the American Board of Orthopaedic Surgery.

Harry was cordial to everyone, tough when needed, and extremely loyal to his friends. His professional and personal life was about giving and sharing with others what he had learned along the way (much of which was from Richard Rothman). Those of us who knew him well saw his softer side. Besides being a great, loyal, and true friend, he was, most importantly, a devoted family man. He adored his wife, Jan, and children, Seth (and wife Lauren) and Rachel (and husband Michael). Sadly, he never met his granddaughter.

We all strive to move forward, improving on the past when possible and appropriate. But the spine world, and the friends Harry left behind, are not the same without him. He bound contemporary orthopedic and spine communities together.

Thank you to Harry's mentors, and family, who shared this giant with us.

Contributors

Muhammad M. Abd-El-Barr, MD, PhD
Resident Neurosurgeon
Harvard Medical School
Brigham and Women's Hospital
Boston Children's Hospital
Boston, Massachusetts

Steven S. Agabegi, MD
Assistant Professor
Department of Orthopaedic Surgery and Sports Medicine
Division of Spine Surgery
University of Cincinnati College of Medicine
Cincinnati, Ohio

Todd J. Albert, MD
Surgeon in Chief and Medical Director
Korein-Wilson Professor of Orthopaedic Surgery
Hospital for Special Surgery
Weill Cornell Medical College
New York, New York

Ilyas S. Aleem, MD, MSc, FRCSC
Assistant Professor, Spine Surgery
Departments of Orthopaedic Surgery and Neurosurgery
University of Michigan
Ann Arbor, Michigan

R. Todd Allen, MD, PhD
Assistant Clinical Professor
Spine Fellowship Program Director
Department of Orthopaedic Surgery
University of California, San Diego
San Diego, California

Howard S. An, MD
The Morton International Endowed Chair
Professor of Orthopaedic Surgery
Director of Spine Surgery and Spine Fellowship Program
Department of Orthopaedic Surgery
Rush University Medical Center
Chicago, Illinois

Dheera Ananthakrishnan, MD, MSE
Assistant Professor
Department of Orthopaedic Surgery
Emory University
Atlanta, Georgia

D. Greg Anderson, MD
Professor
Departments of Orthopaedic and Neurological Surgery
Rothman Institute, Thomas Jefferson University
Philadelphia, Pennsylvania

Paul A. Anderson, MD
Professor
Orthopedic Surgery and Rehabilitation
University of Wisconsin
Madison, Wisconsin

Gunnar B.J. Andersson, MD, PhD
Professor and Chairman Emeritus
Department of Orthopedic Surgery
Rush University Medical Center
Chicago, Illinois

M. Saeid Asadollahi
Graduate Research Assistant
Engineering Center for Orthopaedic Research Excellence (E-CORE)
Department of Bioengineering
College of Engineering
University of Toledo
Toledo, Ohio

John Attenello, MD
Orthopaedic Surgery Resident
Division of Orthopaedic Surgery
University of Hawaii
Honolulu, Hawaii

Raghav Badrinath, MD
Resident
Department of Orthopedic Surgery
University of California, San Diego
San Diego, California

Michele C. Battié, PhD
Professor
Faculty of Rehabilitation Medicine
University of Alberta
Edmonton, Alberta, Canada

Jennifer J. Beck, MD
Assistant Professor
Orthopedic Surgery
Orthopedic Institute for Children/UCLA
Los Angeles, California

Gordon R. Bell, MD
Emeritus Staff
Former Director, Center for Spine Health
Cleveland Clinic
Cleveland, Ohio

Carlo Bellabarba, MD
Professor
Orthopaedic and Neurological Surgery
University of Washington;
Chief, Orthopaedics and Sports Medicine
Harborview Medical Center
Seattle, Washington

David M. Benglis Jr, MD
Atlanta Brain and Spine Care
Atlanta, Georgia

Amandeep Bhalla, MD
Spine Surgery Fellow
Department of Orthopaedic Surgery
Harvard Medical School
Boston, Massachusetts

Mohit Bhandari, MD, PhD, FRCSC
Professor and Academic Head
Canada Research Chair in Evidence-Based Orthopaedics
Division of Orthopaedic Surgery
McMaster University
Hamilton, Ontario, Canada

Nitin N. Bhatia, MD
Vice Chairman
Chief, Spine Service
Residency Program Director
Department of Orthopaedic Surgery
University of California, Irvine
Orange, California

Jesse E. Bible, MD, MHS
Assistant Professor
Department of Orthopaedics
Penn State Milton S. Hershey Medical Center
Hershey, Pennsylvania

Christopher M. Bono, MD
Chief, Orthopaedic Spine Service
Department of Orthopaedic Surgery
Brigham and Women's Hospital;
Associate Professor of Orthopaedic Surgery
Harvard Medical School
Boston, Massachusetts

Barrett S. Boody, MD
Resident Physician
Department of Orthopaedic Surgery
Northwestern University
Chicago, Illinois

David G. Borenstein, MD
Clinical Professor of Medicine
Division of Rheumatology
Department of Medicine
George Washington University Medical Center;
Partner, Arthritis and Rheumatism Associates
Washington, DC

Richard J. Bransford, MD
Professor
Orthopaedic and Neurological Surgery
University of Washington
Harborview Medical Center
Seattle, Washington

Zorica Buser, PhD
Senior Research Associate
Department of Orthopaedic Surgery
Keck School of Medicine
University of Southern California
Hoffman Medical Research Center
Los Angeles, California

Eugene Carragee, MD
Professor
Department of Orthopedics
Stanford University School of Medicine
Stanford, California

Jose Manuel Casamitjana, MD
Senior Consultant
Orthopaedic Surgeon
Cervical Spine Pathology
Orthopaedic and Trauma Hospital
Barcelona, Spain

Samuel H. Cass, BS
MD Candidate
University of Miami Miller School of Medicine
Miami, Florida

Saad B. Chaudhary, MD, MBA
Assistant Professor
Minimally Invasive and Complex Spine Surgery
Department of Orthopaedic Surgery
Icahn School of Medicine at Mount Sinai
New York, New York

Jeffrey L. Chen, MD, MHS
Assistant Clinical Professor
Department of Anesthesiology
Center for Pain Medicine
University of California San Diego
La Jolla, California

Boyle C. Cheng, PhD
Director of Research
Neuroscience Institute
Allegheny Health Network
Pittsburgh, Pennsylvania

Daniel Cher, MD
Vice President of Clinical Affairs
SI-BONE, Inc.
San Jose, California

Jason Pui Yin Cheung, MBBS, MMedSc
Clinical Assistant Professor
Department of Orthopaedics and Traumatology
University of Hong Kong
Pokfulam, Hong Kong

Kenneth M.C. Cheung, MBBS(UK), MD(HK)
Jessie Ho Professor in Spine Surgery
Chair Professor and Head
Department of Orthopaedics and Traumatology
University of Hong Kong
Pokfulam, Hong Kong

Matthew R. Cohn, MD
Department of Orthopedic Surgery
Rush University Medical Center
Chicago, Illinois

Daniel Cook, BS
Laboratory Manager, Spine and Biomechanics Laboratory
Neuroscience Institute
Allegheny Health Network
Pittsburgh, Pennsylvania

Edward C. Covington, MD
Medical Consulting and Education
Emeritus Staff
Neurologic Institute
Cleveland Clinic
Cleveland, Ohio

Alvin H. Crawford, MD
Professor Emeritus
Orthopaedic Surgery
University of Cincinnati, College of Medicine;
Founding Director, Crawford Spine Center
Cincinnati Children's Hospital;
Orthopaedic Surgery
Christ Hospital
Westchester Community Hospital
Cincinnati, Ohio

Shari Cui, MD
Assistant Professor, Spine Surgery
Department of Orthopaedic Surgery
West Virginia University
Morgantown, West Virginia

Bradford L. Currier, MD
Professor of Orthopedics
Mayo Clinic College of Medicine;
Director, Spinal Fellowship Program
Mayo Clinic College of Medicine
Rochester, Minnesota

Scott D. Daffner, MD
Associate Professor
Department of Orthopaedics
West Virginia University School of Medicine
Morgantown, West Virginia

Kevin L. Dalal, MD
Assistant Professor
Department of Physical Medicine and Rehabilitation
University of Miami Miller School of Medicine
Miami, Florida

Bruce V. Darden II, MD
Fellowship Director
Orthocarolina Spine Center
Charlotte, North Carolina

Sara Davin, PsyD, MPH
Staff Psychologist
Chronic Pain Rehabilitation Section
Center for Neurological Restoration
Cleveland Clinic
Cleveland, Ohio

Scott Delp, PhD
James H. Clark Professor
Departments of Bioengineering, Mechanical Engineering, and Orthopaedic Surgery
Schools of Engineering and Medicine
Stanford University
Stanford, California

Richard Derby, MD
Medical Director
Spinal Diagnostics and Treatment Center
Daly City, California

Peter B. Derman, MD
Orthopedic Surgery Resident
Hospital for Special Surgery
New York, New York

Clinton J. Devin, MD
Associate Professor of Orthopaedic Surgery and Neurosurgery
Vanderbilt University Medical Center
Nashville, Tennessee

Elizabeth A. Dugan, PhD
Postdoctoral Associate
Miami Project to Cure Paralysis
University of Miami Miller School of Medicine
Miami, Florida

Alexandra Miller Dunham, MD
Resident
Orthopaedic Surgery
Johns Hopkins University School of Medicine
Baltimore, Maryland

Richard W. Easton, MD
Assistant Professor
Department of Orthopaedic Surgery
Oakland University William Beaumont School of Medicine
Rochester Hills, Michigan;
Section Head
Orthopaedic and Spine Surgery
Beaumont Hospital
Troy, Michigan

Jason C. Eck, DO, MS
Spine Surgeon
Center for Sports Medicine and Orthopaedics
Chattanooga, Tennessee

Frank J. Eismont
Leonard M. Miller Professor and Chairman
Department of Orthopaedic Surgery
University of Miami Miller School of Medicine
Miami, Florida

Todd M. Emch, MD
Staff
Division of Neuroradiology
Imaging Institute
Cleveland Clinic
Cleveland, Ohio

Sanford E. Emery, MD, MBA
Professor and Chairman
Department of Orthopaedics
West Virginia University
Morgantown, West Virginia

Yashar Eshraghi, MD
Assistant Clinical Professor
Department of Anesthesiology and Perioperative Care
School of Medicine
University of California, Irvine
Irvine, California

Saif Aldeen Farhan, MD
Research Spine Fellow
Department of Orthopaedic Surgery
University of California, Irvine
Irivine, California

Timothy J. Furnish, MD
Associate Clinical Professor of Anesthesiology
Center for Pain Medicine
Pain Fellowship Program Director
University of California, San Diego Medical Center
San Diego, California

Shyam Gajavelli, PhD
Associate Scientist
Department of Neurosurgery
Miami Project to Cure Paralysis
University of Miami Miller School of Medicine
Miami, Florida

Steven R. Garfin, MD
Distinguished Professor and Chair
Department of Orthopaedic Surgery
University of California, San Diego
San Diego, California

Bhavuk Garg, MD
Associate Professor
Department of Orthopaedics
All India Institute of Medical Sciences
New Delhi, India

Matthew F. Gary, MD
Assistant Professor of Neurosurgery and Orthopaedic Surgery
Emory Spine Center
Emory University School of Medicine
Atlanta, Georgia

Joseph P. Gjolaj, MD
Assistant Professor
Orthopaedic Surgery
University of Miami Miller School of Medicine;
Orthopaedic Spine Surgeon
Orthopaedic Surgery
Jackson Memorial Hospital
Miami, Florida

Paul Glazer, MD
Spine Specialists of Boston
Chestnut Hill, Massachusetts

Michael P. Glotzbecker, MD
Assistant Professor
Department of Orthopaedic Surgery
Boston Children's Hospital
Boston, Massachusetts

Vijay K. Goel, PhD
Distinguished University Professor
Endowed Chair and McMaster-Gardner Professor of Orthopaedic Bioengineering
Co-Director, Engineering Center for Orthopaedic Research Excellence (E-CORE)
Departments of Bioengineering and Orthopaedic Surgery
Colleges of Engineering and Medicine
University of Toledo
Toledo, Ohio

Jonathan N. Grauer, MD
Associate Professor
Department of Orthopaedics and Rehabilitation
Yale University School of Medicine
New Haven, Connecticut

Barth A. Green, MD
Professor of Neurological Surgery
University of Miami Miller School of Medicine
Miami, Florida

Ajay Gupta, MD
Head, Pediatric Epilepsy
Director, Tuberous Sclerosis Program
Associate Professor, Cleveland Clinic Lerner College of Medicine
Cleveland Clinic Foundation
Cleveland, Ohio

Richard D. Guyer, MD
Past President
Director, Spine Fellowship
Texas Back Institute
Plano, Texas;
Clinical Associate Professor
Department of Orthopaedic Surgery
University of Texas Southwestern School of Medicine
Dallas, Texas

Aldric Hama, PhD
Study Director
Hamamatsu Pharma Research
Hamamatsu, Japan

Hamid Hassanzadeh, MD
Assistant Professor
Department of Orthopaedic Surgery
University of Virginia
Charlottesville, Virginia

Spencer Hauser, MD
Fellow, Orthopaedic Surgery
Duke University School of Medicine
Durham, North Carolina

Robert F. Heary, MD
Professor of Neurosurgery
Rutgers New Jersey Medical School
Director, Spine Center of New Jersey
Newark, New Jersey

Daniel J. Hedequist, MD
Associate Professor
Department of Orthopaedic Surgery
Boston Children's Hospital
Boston, Massachusetts

Stanley A. Herring, MD
Clinical Professor
Rehabilitation Medicine, Orthopaedics and Sports Medicine and Neurological Surgery
University of Washington;
Director, UW Medicine Sports Health and Safety System
Co-Medical Director, UW Medicine Sports Concussion Program
Harborview Medical Center and Seattle Children's Hospital
Seattle, Washington

Kenneth A. Hood, DO
Assistant Clinical Professor, Spine Surgery
Department of Orthopaedic Surgery
University of Arizona
Tucson, Arizona

Wellington K. Hsu, MD
Clifford C. Raisbeck Distinguished Professor of Orthopaedic Surgery
Director of Research
Department of Orthopaedic Surgery
Northwestern University Feinberg School of Medicine
Chicago, Illinois

Serena S. Hu, MD
Professor and Vice Chair
Chief, Spine Service
Department of Orthopedic Surgery
Stanford University
Stanford, California

Xiaobang Hu, PhD
Research Director
Scoliosis and Spine Tumor Center
Texas Back Institute
Texas Health Presbyterian Hospital
Plano, Texas

Kevin T. Huang, MD
Department of Neurosurgery
Boston Children's Hospital
Harvard Medical School
Boston, Massachusetts

Andre M. Jakoi, MD
Department of Orthopedic Surgery
Spine Division
University of Southern California
Los Angeles, California

Pawel P. Jankowski, MD
Chief Resident
Department of Neurosurgery
University of California, San Diego
San Diego, California

Andrew Jea, MHA, FACS, FAAP
Pediatric Neurosurgeon
Goodman Campbell Brain and Spine;
Professor and Chief
Section of Pediatric Neurosurgery
Department of Neurological Surgery
Indiana University School of Medicine
Indianapolis, Indiana

Walter J. Jermakowicz, MD, PhD
Resident
Department of Neurological Surgery
University of Miami Miller School of Medicine
Miami, Florida

Xavier F. Jimenez, MD
Medical Director
Chronic Pain Rehabilitation Program
Chronic Pain Rehabilitation Section
Cleveland Clinic
Cleveland, Ohio

Jeremiah N. Johnson, MD
Assistant Professor
Department of Neurosurgery
Baylor College of Medicine
Houston, Texas

Robert Johnson, DO
Orthopaedic Spine Surgeon
Idaho Back Institute
Blackfoot, Idaho

James D. Kang, MD
Thornhill Family Professor of Orthopaedic Surgery
Harvard Medical School;
Chairman, Department of Orthopaedic Surgery
Brigham and Women's Hospital
Boston, Massachusetts

Abhishek Kannan, MD
Resident Physician
Department of Orthopaedic Surgery
Northwestern University Feinberg School of Medicine
Chicago, Illinois

Jaakko Kaprio, MD, PhD
Academy Professor
Director, Institute for Molecular Medicine Finland (FIMM)
Nordic EMBL Partnership for Molecular Medicine
University of Helsinki
Helsinki, Finland

Lori A. Karol, MD
Assistant Chief of Staff
Orthopaedic Surgery
Texas Scottish Rite Hospital for Children;
Professor
Orthopaedic Surgery
University of Texas-Southwestern
Dallas, Texas

Jad G. Khalil, MD
Attending Spine Surgeon
William Beaumont Hospital
Royal Oak, Michigan

Safdar N. Khan, MD
Benjamin R. and Helen Slack Wiltberger Endowed Chair in Orthopaedic Spine Surgery
Associate Professor and Chief, Division of Spine Surgery
Department of Orthopaedic Surgery
Associate Professor, Department of Integrated Systems Engineering
Clinical Co-Director, Spine Research Institute
Ohio State University Wexner Medical Center
Columbus, Ohio;
Director, The Spine Program at Wooster Hospital
Wooster, Ohio

A. Jay Khanna, MD, MBA
Vice Chair and Professor
Department of Orthopaedic Surgery
Johns Hopkins University
Baltimore, Maryland

Shinichi Kikuchi, MD, PhD
Orthopedic Department
Fukushima Medical University
Fukushima, Japan

Choll W. Kim, MD, PhD
Director, Advanced Spine and Joint Institute
University of California, San Diego;
Spine Institute of San Diego
Center for Minimally Invasive Spine Surgery at Alvarado Hospital
San Diego, California

David H. Kim, MD
Associate Clinical Professor
Orthopaedic Surgery
Tufts University School of Medicine;
Director of Medical Education
Department of Orthopaedic Surgery
New England Baptist Hospital
Boston, Massachusetts

Theodore D. Koreckij, MD
Dickson-Diveley Midwest Orthopaedic Clinic;
Clinical Assistant Professor
Orthopaedic Surgery
University of Missouri-Kansas City;
Kansas City Orthopaedic Institute
Leawood, Kansas

Tyler Kreitz, MD
Department of Orthopaedic Surgery
Thomas Jefferson University
Philadelphia, Pennsylvania

Jonathan D. Krystal, MD
Clinical Instructor
Orthopedic Surgery
Thomas Jefferson University Hospital;
Spine Fellow
Spine Surgery
Rothman Institute
Philadelphia, Pennsylvania

Mark F. Kurd, MD
Assistant Professor
Department of Orthopaedic Surgery
Thomas Jefferson University
Rothman Institute
Philadelphia, Pennsylvania

Swamy Kurra, MBBS
Research Fellow
SUNY Upstate Medical University
Syracuse, New York

Kenny Kwan, BMBCh(Oxon)
Clinical Assistant Professor
Department of Orthopaedics and Traumatology
Li Ka Shing Faculty of Medicine
University of Hong Kong
Pokfulam, Hong Kong

Brian Kwon, MD
Assistant Clinical Professor
Orthopedic Surgery
Tufts University School of Medicine;
Department of Orthopaedic Surgery
New England Baptist Hospital
Boston, Massachusetts

Lauren LaMont, MD
Orthopedic Surgeon
Department of Pediatric Orthopedics
Cook Children's Hospital
Fort Worth, Texas

Joseph M. Lane, MD
Professor of Orthopaedic Surgery
Orthopaedic Surgery
Chief, Metabolic Bone Disease Service
Hospital for Special Surgery
New York, New York

William F. Lavelle, MD
Associate Professor
Departments of Orthopaedic Surgery and Pediatrics
SUNY Upstate Medical University
Syracuse, New York

Darren R. Lebl, MD
Spine and Scoliosis Surgery
Hospital for Special Surgery
New York, New York

Nathan H. Lebwohl, MD
Chief of Spinal Deformity Surgery
Department of Orthopaedics
University of Miami Miller School of Medicine
Miami, Florida

Joon Yung Lee, MD
Associate Professor, Department of Orthopedic Surgery
Medical Director, Ferguson Laboratory
Associate Program Director, Orthopedic Residency
University of Pittsburgh Medical Center
Pittsburgh, Pennsylvania

Scott I. Lee, MD
Orthopedic Spine Surgeon
Adventist Health
White Memorial Medical Center
Los Angeles, California;
Glendale Adventist Medical Center
Glendale, California

Yu-Po Lee, MD
Clinical Professor
Department of Orthopaedic Surgery
University of California, Irvine
Irvine, California

Ronald A. Lehman Jr, MD
Professor of Orthopaedic Surgery
Chief, Degenerative, MIS, and Robotic Spine Surgery
Director, Athletics Spine Center
Director, Spine Research
Co-Director, Adult and Pediatric Spine Fellowship
Advanced Pediatric and Adult Deformity Service
The Spine Hospital
New York–Presbyterian/The Allen Hospital
New York, New York

Lawrence G. Lenke, MD
Professor and Chief of Spinal Surgery
Chief of Spinal Deformity Surgery
Department of Orthopedic Surgery
Columbia University College of Physicians and Surgeons;
Surgeon-in-Chief
The Spine Hospital
New York–Presbyterian/The Allen Hospital
New York, New York

Dante Leven, MD
Total Orthopedics and Sports Medicine
Associate Professor
Nassau University Medical Center
East Meadow, New York

Allan D. Levi, MD, PhD
Chair, Department of Neurological Surgery
Professor of Neurological Surgery, Orthopedics, and Rehabilitation Medicine
University of Miami Miller School of Medicine
Chief of Neurosurgery
Jackson Memorial Hospital
Miami, Florida

Richard L. Lieber, PhD
Senior Vice President and Chief Scientific Officer
Rehabilitation Institute of Chicago;
Professor of Physiology and Biomedical Engineering
Northwestern University
Chicago, Illinois

Isador H. Lieberman, MD
Director
Scoliosis and Spine Tumor Center
Texas Back Institute
Texas Health Presbyterian Hospital
Plano, Texas

Richard A. Lindtner, MD, PhD
Trauma Surgeon
Department of Trauma Surgery and Sports Medicine
Medical University of Innsbruck
Innsbruck, Austria

Gregory Lopez, MD
Assistant Professor of Spine Surgery
Rush University
Chicago, Illinois

J. Diego Lozano, MD
Interventional Neuroradiologist
Providence Little Company of Mary Medical Center
Mechanical Thrombectomy-Ready Advanced Primary Stroke Center
Torrance, California

Prasath Mageswaran, PhD
Research Associate
Spine Research Institute
Ohio State University
Columbus, Ohio

Kamran Majid, MD
Physician
Orthopedic Spine Surgery
Kaiser Permanente
Oakland, California

Antonios Mammis, MD
Assistant Professor, Neurological Surgery and Anesthesiology
Director, Center for Neuromodulation
Director, Functional and Restorative Neurosurgery
Senator, Rutgers University
Rutgers New Jersey Medical School
Newark, New Jersey

Satyajit Marawar, MD
Orthopedic Spine Surgeon
Veterans Affairs Medical Center
Syracuse, New York

William S. Marras, PhD, CPE
Honda Chair Professor
Integrated Systems Engineering/Spine Research Institute
Ohio State University
Columbus, Ohio

Eric A.K. Mayer, MD
Associate Director, Clinical Transformation
Cleveland Clinic Center for Spine Health
Cleveland, Ohio

Tom G. Mayer, MD
Harvard College
Columbia College of Physicians and Surgeons
New York, New York

Daniel Mazanec, MD
Physician Emeritus
Cleveland Clinic
Cleveland, Ohio;
Chief Medical Officer
Dorsata
Arlington, Virginia

Steven J. McAnany, MD
Spine Surgery
Assistant Professor of Orthopaedic Surgery
Washington University Orthopaedics
St. Louis, Missouri

Paul C. McCormick, MD, MPH
Herbert and Linda Gallen Professor of Neurological Surgery
Director
Spine Hospital at the Neurological Institute of New York;
Attending Physician
New York–Presbyterian/Columbia University Medical Center
New York, New York

Zachary McCormick, MD
Assistant Professor of Physical Medicine and Rehabilitation
Department of Orthopaedics
University of California, San Francisco
San Francisco, California

Nagy A. Mekhail, MD, PhD
Carl Wasmuth Professor and Chair
Director, Evidence-Based Pain Management and Research
Cleveland Clinic
Cleveland, Ohio

Ehud Mendel, MD
President Elect, Ohio State Neurosurgical Society
Justine Skestos Endowed Chair
Professor of Neurosurgery, Oncology, Orthopedics, and Systems Engineering
Vice Chair Clinical/Academic Affairs
Clinical Director, OSU Spine Research Institute
Director, Spine Program, Complex/Oncological Fellowship Program
Ohio State University Wexner Medical Center
James Cancer Hospital
Columbus, Ohio

Addisu Mesfin, MD
Associate Professor
Orthopaedic Surgery
University of Rochester
Rochester, New York

Umesh Metkar, MD
Orthopaedic Spine Surgeon
Spine Center at Beth Israel Deaconess Medical Center
Boston, Massachusetts

Lyle J. Micheli, MD
Director
Division of Sports Medicine
O'Donnell Family Professor of Orthopaedics and Sports Medicine
Boston Children's Hospital
Boston, Massachusetts

Megan Mignemi, MD
Assistant Professor of Orthopedics and Rehabilitation
Division of Pediatric Orthopedics
Monroe Carell Jr. Children's Hospital at Vanderbilt
Nashville, Tennessee

Andrew Z. Mo, MD
Orthopaedic Surgery
Lenox Hill Hospital
New York, New York

William J. Molinari III, MD
Orthopedic Surgeon
Residency Program Site Director
Department of Orthopedics
Malcolm Randall VA Medical Center;
Spine Surgeon
Assistant Residency Program Director
Department of Orthopedics
University of Florida
Gainesville, Florida

David M. Montgomery, MD
Associate Professor
Department of Orthopaedic Surgery
Oakland University/William Beaumont School of Medicine
Royal Oak, Michigan

Thomas Mroz, MD
Director, Center for Spine Health
Director, Clinical Research
Center for Spine Health
Departments of Orthopaedic and Neurological Surgery
Cleveland Clinic
Cleveland, Ohio

Scott J. Mubarak, MD
Surgeon in Chief
Emeritus Chair, Division of Pediatric Orthopedics
Rady Children's Hospital;
Clinical Professor
Department of Orthopedics
University of California, San Diego Medical Center
San Diego, California

Charles N. Munyon, MD
Director of Functional and Restorative Neurosurgery
Assistant Professor of Neurosurgery
Lewis Katz School of Medicine at Temple University
Philadelphia, Pennsylvania

Robert F. Murphy, MD
Assistant Professor
Department of Orthopaedics
Medical University of South Carolina
Charleston, South Carolina

George F. Muschler, MD
Vice Chair, Orthopaedic and Rheumatologic Institute
Cleveland Clinic Foundation
Cleveland, Ohio

Robert R. Myers, PhD
Professor of Anesthesiology and Pathology
University of California, San Diego School of Medicine
San Diego, California

Dileep R. Nair, MD
Section Head of Adult Epilepsy
Epilepsy Center
Cleveland Clinic
Cleveland, Ohio

Sreeharsha V. Nandyala, MD
Orthopaedic Surgery Resident
Massachusetts General Hospital
Harvard Medical School
Boston, Massachusetts

Raj Nangunoori, MD
Department of Neurosurgery
Allegheny Health Network
Pittsburgh, Pennsylvania

Randy Neblett, MA, LPC, BCB
Psychology Department Coordinator and Biofeedback Coordinator
Productive Rehabilitation Institute of Dallas for Ergonomics (PRIDE);
Research Coordinator
PRIDE Research Foundation
Dallas, Texas

David Nelles, MD
Orthopedic Spine Surgery
Muir Orthopedic Surgeons
Walnut Creek, California

Peter O. Newton, MD
Chief
Department of Pediatric Orthopedics
Rady Children's Hospital;
Clinical Professor
Orthopaedic Surgery
University of California, San Diego
San Diego, California

Christopher O'Boynick, MD
Physician
Premier Care Orthopedics and Sports Medicine
St. Louis, Missouri

Joseph R. O'Brien, MD, MPH
Washington Spine and Scoliosis Clinic
Medical Director, Minimally Invasive Spine Surgery
Virginia Hospital Center
Mayo Clinic Care Network
Arlington, Virginia

Kjell Olmarker, MD, PhD
Musculoskeletal Research
Department of Medical Chemistry and Cell Biology
Institute of Biomedicine
Sahlgrenska Academy
University of Gothenburg
Gothenburg, Sweden

Adam S. Olsen, MD
Resident Physician
Department of Orthopaedic Surgery
University of Pittsburgh Medical Center
Pittsburgh, Pennsylvania

John E. O'Toole, MD
Professor
Department of Neurosurgery
Rush University Medical Center
Chicago, Illinois

Sohrab Pahlavan, MD
Spine Surgery Fellow
Department of Orthopaedic Surgery
University of Miami/Jackson Memorial Hospital
Miami, Florida

Daniel Park, MD
Assistant Professor
Department of Orthopedics
William Beaumont Hospital
Royal Oak, Michigan

Alpesh A. Patel, MD
Professor of Orthopaedic Surgery
Director, Orthopaedic Spine Surgery
Co-director, Northwest Spine Center
Northwestern University Feinberg School of Medicine
Chicago, Illinois

Chetan K. Patel, MD
Medical Director
Spine Health Institute
Florida Hospital Medical Group
Altemonte Springs, Florida

Neil N. Patel, MD
Orthopedic Spine Surgeon
Spine Team Texas
Southlake, Texas

Adam M. Pearson, MD
Assistant Professor
Orthopaedic Surgery
Geisel School of Medicine at Dartmouth
Hanover, New Hampshire

Martin H. Pham, MD
Resident Physician
Department of Neurosurgery
University of Southern California
Los Angeles, California

Frank M. Phillips, MD
Professor
Department of Orthopaedic Surgery
Rush University Medical Center;
Co-Director, Spine Fellowship
Rush University Medical Center
Chicago, Illinois

Christine Piper, MD
Resident Physician
Department of Orthopaedic Surgery
George Washington University
Washington, DC

Nicolas S. Piuzzi, MD
Orthopaedic Regenerative Medicine and Cellular Therapy Clinical Scholar
Department of Orthopaedic Surgery and Biomedical Engineering
Cleveland Clinic
Cleveland, Ohio

Michael P. Planalp, MD
Orthopaedic Surgery Resident
William Beaumont Hospital
Royal Oak, Michigan

Peter B. Polatin, MD, MPH
Consultant Physician
Production Rehabilitation Institute of Dallas for Ergonomics;
Senior Faculty
Harvard Program in Refugee Trauma
Boston, Massachusetts

Sina Pourtaheri, MD
Assistant Professor
Department of Orthopaedic Surgery
University of California, San Diego
San Diego, California;
Assistant Professor
Department of Orthopaedic Surgery
University of California, Los Angeles
Los Angeles, California

Mark R. Proctor, MD
Associate Professor of Neurosurgery
Harvard Medical School
Boston Children's Hospital
Boston, Massachusetts

Andrew J. Pugely, MD
Assistant Professor of Spine Surgery
Department of Orthopaedic Surgery
University of Iowa
Iowa City, Iowa

Ajit S. Puri, MD
Associate Professor of Radiology, Neurology, and Neurosurgery
Division of Neuroimaging and Intervention
University of Massachusetts Medical School
Worcester, Massachusetts

Varun Puvanesarajah, MD
Department of Orthopaedic Surgery
Johns Hopkins University
Baltimore, Maryland

Sheeraz A. Qureshi, MD, MBA
Associate Professor, Orthopaedic Surgery
Minimally Invasive Spine Surgery
Hospital for Special Surgery
Weill Cornell Medical College
New York, New York

Dipak B. Ramkumar, MD
Resident in Orthopaedic Surgery
Instructor in Anatomy
Department of Orthopaedic Surgery
Dartmouth-Hitchcock Medical Center
Geisel School of Medicine at Dartmouth
Lebanon, New Hampshire

Raj Rao, MD
Professor of Orthopaedic Surgery and Neurosurgery
Chairman, Department of Orthopaedic Surgery
George Washington University
Washington, DC

Alexandre Rasouli, MD
Spinal Surgeon
Center of Excellence
Cedars-Sinai Medical Center
Los Angeles, California

Brandon L. Raudenbush, MD
Fellow
Orthopaedic Surgery
University of Rochester
Rochester, New York

W. Carlton Reckling, MD, MBA
Chief Medical Officer and Vice President of Medical Affairs
SI-BONE, Inc.
San Jose, California

K. Daniel Riew, MD
Professor of Orthopaedic Surgery
Columbia University;
Chief, Cervical Spine Surgery and Co-Director, Spine Division
Co-Director, Columbia University Spine Fellowship
Department of Orthopaedic Surgery
The Spine Hospital
New York–Presbyterian/The Allen Hospital
New York, New York

Jeffrey Rihn, MD
Associate Professor
Department of Orthopedic Surgery
Rothman Institute
Thomas Jefferson University Hospital
Philadelphia, Pennsylvania

Makarand V. Risbud, PhD
James J. Maguire Jr. Professor of Spine Research
Director of Spine Research Program
Department of Orthopaedic Surgery
Professor and Co-Director, Cell Biology and Regenerative Medicine PhD Program
Thomas Jefferson University
Philadelphia, Pennsylvania

Brett D. Rosenthal, MD
Senior Housestaff Physician
Department of Orthopaedic Surgery
Northwestern University
Chicago, Illinois

Jeffrey S. Ross, MD
Neuroradiology Division
Department of Radiology
Senior Associate Consultant
Mayo Clinic Arizona;
Professor of Radiology
Mayo Clinic College of Medicine
Phoenix, Arizona

Glenn Russo, MD, MS
Department of Orthopaedics and Rehabilitation
Yale University School of Medicine
New Haven, Connecticut

Björn Rydevik, MD, PhD
Department of Orthopaedics
University of Gothenburg
Gothenburg, Sweden

Jacqueline Sagen, PhD
Professor of Neurosurgery
Miami Project to Cure Paralysis
University of Miami Miller School of Medicine
Miami, Florida

Comron Saifi, MD
Assistant Professor of Orthopaedic Surgery and Neurosurgery
Director of Clinical Spine Research
University of Pennsylvania
Philadelphia, Pennsylvania

Rajiv Saigal, MD, PhD
Assistant Professor of Surgery
Department of Surgery
University of Washington
Seattle, Washington

Lawrence Samkoff, MD
Associate Professor of Neurology
Attending Neurologist
Neuroimmunology Unit
Department of Neurology
University of Rochester Medical Center
Rochester, New York

Rick C. Sasso, MD
Professor
Chief of Spine Surgery
Department of Orthopaedic Surgery
Indiana University School of Medicine
Carmel, Indiana

Michael Saulino, MD, PhD
Physiatrist
MossRehab
Elkins Park, Pennsylvania;
Assistant Professor
Rehabilitation Medicine
Jefferson Medical College
Philadelphia, Pennsylvania

Judith Scheman, PhD
Director, Behavioral Medicine
Digestive Disease and Surgery Institute
Cleveland Clinic
Cleveland, Ohio

Andrew J. Schoenfeld, MD, MSc
Assistant Professor
Department of Orthopaedic Surgery
Brigham and Women's Hospital
Harvard Medical School
Boston, Massachusetts

Gregory D. Schroeder, MD
Rothman Institute
Thomas Jefferson University
Philadelphia, Pennsylvania

Alexandra Schwartz, MD
Clinical Professor
Orthopaedic Surgery
University of California, San Diego
San Diego, California

James D. Schwender, MD
Staff Surgeon
Twin Cities Spine Center
Minneapolis, Minnesota

R. Michael Scott, MD
Fellows Family Chair in Pediatric Neurosurgery
Neurosurgeon-in-Chief, Emeritus
Boston Children's Hospital;
Professor of Neurosurgery
Harvard Medical School
Boston, Massachusetts

Olga Selioutski, DO
Assistant Professor
Strong Epilepsy Center
Department of Neurosurgery
University of Rochester
Rochester, New York

Dilip K. Sengupta, MD, DrMed
Director
Center for Scoliosis and Advanced Spine Surgery
Dallas, Texas

Eiman Shafa, MD
Fellow in Spine Surgery
Twin Cities Spine Center
Minneapolis, Minnesota

Ashish H. Shah, MD
Jackson Memorial Hospital
University of Miami
Miami, Florida

Neel Shah, MD
Department of Orthopedic Surgery
New England Baptist Hospital
Boston, Massachusetts

Suken A. Shah, MD
Division Chief, Spine and Scoliosis Center
Department of Orthopaedics
Nemours/Alfred I. duPont Hospital for Children
Wilmington, Delaware;
Associate Professor of Orthopaedic Surgery and Pediatrics
Department of Orthopaedic Surgery
Sidney Kimmel Medical College of Thomas Jefferson University
Philadelphia, Pennsylvania

Alok Sharan, MD, MHCDS
Co-Director, WESTMED Spine Center
Yonkers, New York;
Assistant Professor
Albert Einstein College of Medicine
New York, New York;
Distinguished Visiting Research Fellow
Center for Complex Systems and Enterprises
Stevens Institute of Technology
Hoboken, New Jersey

Andrew L. Sherman, MD, MS
Professor and Vice Chair
Department of Physical Medicine and Rehabilitation
University of Miami Miller School of Medicine
Miami, Florida

Adam L. Shimer, MD
Associate Professor
Orthopedic Surgery
University of Virginia
Charlottesville, Virginia

Shyam Shridharani, MD
Section Chief, Spine Surgery
Department of Orthopaedic Surgery
University of Arizona
Tucson, Arizona

J. Alex Sielatycki
Department of Orthopaedics
Vanderbilt University
Nashville, Tennessee

Krzysztof B. Siemionow, MD, PhD
Chief of Spine Surgery
Department of Orthopedic Surgery
University of Illinois
Chicago, Illinois

Fernando E. Silva, MD
Southeast Texas Spine Center
CHRISTUS Southeast Texas St. Elizabeth Hospital
Beaumont, Texas

Andrew K. Simpson, MD
Spine Surgeon
Texas Back Institute
Dallas, Texas

J. David Sinclair, MD
Medical Director, Paradigm Outcomes
Walnut Creek, California;
Independent Consultant for the Management of Chronic Pain
Seattle, Washington

Evan J. Smith, MD
Resident Physician
Department of Orthopaedic Surgery
George Washington University
Washington, DC

Gwendolyn Sowa, MD, PhD
Professor and Chair, Department of Physical Medicine and Rehabilitation
Co-Director, Ferguson Laboratory for Orthopaedic and Spine Research
Pittsburgh, Pennsylvania

Paul D. Sponseller, MD, MBA
Professor and Head
Pediatric Orthopaedics
Johns Hopkins Bloomberg Children's Center
Baltimore, Maryland

Kevin Spratt, MD
Dartmouth-Hitchcock Medical Center
Lebanon, New Hampshire;
Geisel School of Medicine at Dartmouth
Hanover, New Hampshire

Christopher J. Standaert, MD
Clinical Professor
Department of Rehabilitation Medicine
University of Washington
Seattle, Washington

Michael Stauff, MD
Assistant Professor
Department of Orthopedics and Physical Rehabilitation
University of Massachusetts Medical School
Worcester, Massachusetts

T. Barrett Sullivan, MD
Resident Physician
Department of Orthopedic Surgery
University of California, San Diego
San Diego, California

Ryan A. Tauzell, PT, MA, CMDT
Physical Therapist
Choice Physical Therapy and Wellness
Christiansburg, Virginia

Jinny Tavee, MD
Neuromuscular Fellowship Program Director
Associate Professor
Cleveland Clinic Lerner College of Medicine
Cleveland, Ohio

Bobby K.-B. Tay, MD
Professor
Orthopaedic Surgery
UCSF Medical Center
San Francisco, California

Dinesh P. Thawrani, MD
Assistant Professor
Department of Orthopedic Surgery
University of Cincinnati College of Medicine;
Attending Physician
Orthopaedic Surgery
Cincinnati VA Medical Center
Cincinnati, Ohio

Clifford B. Tribus, MD
Professor
Department of Orthopedic Surgery and Rehabilitative Medicine
University of Wisconsin-Madison
Madison, Wisconsin

Eeric Truumees, MD
Professor of Surgery and Perioperative Care
Dell Medical School
University of Texas;
Chief Executive Officer
Seton Brain and Spine Institute
Austin, Texas

Alexander R. Vaccaro, MD, PhD, MBA
Richard H. Rothman Professor and Chairman
Department of Orthopaedic Surgery
Professor of Neurosurgery
Co-Director, Delaware Valley Spinal Cord Injury Center
Co-Chief of Spine Surgery
Sidney Kimmel Medical Center at Thomas Jefferson University
President, Rothman Institute
Philadelphia, Pennsylvania

Steve Vanni, DO
University of Miami
Miami, Florida

Arya G. Varthi, MD
Spine Surgery Fellow
Rush University Medical Center
Chicago, Illinois

Anita Vasavada, PhD
Associate Professor
Voiland School of Chemical Engineering and Bioengineering
Department of Integrative Physiology and Neuroscience
Washington State University
Pullman, Washington

Michael J. Vives, MD
Associate Professor and Chief of Spine Surgery
Department of Orthopedics
Rutgers University–New Jersey Medical School
Newark, New Jersey

Nam Vo, PhD
Associate Professor
Co-Director, Ferguson Laboratory for Spine Research
Department of Orthopaedic Surgery
Department of Pathology
McGowan Institute for Regenerative Medicine
Stimulating Pittsburgh in Geroscience (SPRIG)
Pittsburgh, Pennsylvania

Ajay K. Wakhloo, MD, PhD, FAHA
Professor of Radiology, Neurology, and Neurosurgery
Division of Neuroimaging and Intervention
University of Massachusetts Medical School
Worcester, Massachusetts

Mark S. Wallace, MD
Professor of Clinical Anesthesiology
Department of Anesthesiology
Division of Pain Medicine
University of California, San Diego
San Diego, California

Emily Walsh, BA
Research Intern
Neuroscience Institute
Allegheny Health Network
Pittsburgh, Pennsylvania

Jeffrey C. Wang, MD
Chief, Orthopaedic Spine Service
Professor of Orthopaedic Surgery and Neurosurgery
Co-Director, USC Spine Center
Los Angeles, California

Samuel R. Ward, PT, PhD
Professor of Radiology, Orthopaedic Surgery, and Bioengineering
University of California, San Diego
San Diego, California

Matthew L. Webb, MD
Resident Physician
Department of Orthopaedic Surgery
Hospital of the University of Pennsylvania
Philadelphia, Pennsylvania

James N. Weinstein, MD
Dartmouth-Hitchcock Health
Dartmouth Institute for Health Policy and Clinical Practice
Lebanon, New Hampshire;
Geisel School of Medicine at Dartmouth
Hanover, New Hampshire

Dennis R. Wenger, MD
Director of Orthopedic Training Program
Rady Children's Hospital
Clinical Professor of Orthopedic Surgery (volunteer)
University of California, San Diego
San Diego, California

F. Todd Wetzel, AB, MD
Professor and Vice Chair
Department of Orthopaedic Surgery and Sports Medicine
Professor
Department of Neurosurgery
Temple University School of Medicine
Philadelphia, Pennsylvania

Peter G. Whang, MD, FACS
Associate Professor
Orthopaedics and Rehabilitation
Yale University School of Medicine
New Haven, Connecticut

Seth K. Williams, MD
Assistant Professor
Department of Orthopedics and Rehabilitation
University of Wisconsin School of Medicine and Public Health
Madison, Wisconsin

Lee Wolfer, MD
Medical Director
Bay Area Integrative Orthopedics
San Francisco, California

Kuan Wen Wu, MD
Department of Orthopaedic Surgery
National Taiwan University Hospital
Taipan, Taiwan

Burt Yaszay, MD
Associate Clinical Professor
Rady Children's Hospital
University of California, San Diego
San Diego, California

Anthony T. Yeung, MD
Associate, Desert Institute for Spine Care
Voluntary Professor, University of New Mexico School of Medicine
Albuquerque, New Mexico

Christopher A. Yeung, MD
President
Desert Institute for Spine Care
Phoenix, Arizona

Terri A. Zachos, MD, PhD, DVM
Diplomate, American College of Veterinary Surgeons
Clinical Research Fellow in Orthopaedic Traumatology
Department of Orthopaedic Surgery
Geisinger Health Systems
Geisinger Commonwealth School of Medicine
Danville, Pennsylvania

Jie Zheng, MD
Department of Neurosurgery
Allegheny Health Network
Pittsburgh, Pennsylvania

Jack E. Zigler, MD
Medical Director
Texas Back Institute
Plano, Texas

Vinko Zlomislic, MD
Assistant Clinical Professor
Department of Orthopaedic Surgery
University of California, San Diego
San Diego, California

Preface

As can be seen from the Dedication and Acknowledgment pages, the Editorial Board for this seventh edition of *The Spine* has undergone some changes. With the passing of Harry N. Herkowitz, MD, and the fact this may be the last edition for some of the remaining long-term editors, two new editors—Christopher N. Bono, MD, and Jeffrey S. Fischgrund, MD—have stepped in, and up, to help us create this new edition of *Rothman-Simeone and Herkowitz's The Spine*. We hope readers will find this edition—as well as future editions—as important and useful as previous ones.

This edition of *The Spine* comes 7 years after the sixth edition. We have strived to continue the original concepts of Richard H. Rothman, MD, PhD, and Frederick A. Simeone, MD, which was to correlate basic science, knowledge of the natural history, and clinical course of spinal disorders with current treatments based on established scientific principles and evidence-based literature. This edition, as in those of the past, provides a comprehensive look at spinal disorders affecting adults and children. It is directed at clinicians of all levels and specialties who treat spinal conditions and who need and appreciate our underlying principles, which ultimately lead to enhanced quality of care for patients.

Since this may be the last edition for some of the editors, we feel it is important to briefly describe the background for this seventh edition of *The Spine*. In our Preface to the sixth edition, we highlighted each of the previous editions by choosing important wording from the Prefaces. We have followed the same pattern here so that new readers, as well as long-term ones, can put this edition in historical perspective.

The forerunner to *The Spine* was *The Intervertebral Disc* by Drs. Rothman and DePalma. In their preface written in 1970, the authors wrote: "The role of the intervertebral disc in the production of neck and back pain, with or without radiation into one of the extremities, has been the subject of much investigation for many decades…The disc has been attacked from every conceivable angle, the most important of which is its biochemical nature and its response to physiologic aging and trauma. In spite of the exhaustive studies recorded in the literature, it is alarming to find how little of this knowledge has been acquired by those concerned with neck and back disorders…We are sure that much that is recorded in this book is still very controversial. Yet, we believe that our approach to this complex problem will be helpful and rewarding to others." This comprehensive monograph on the disc totaled 373 pages. It crystallized concepts of the disc for spine physicians of the day and served as the forerunner of many books to follow.

In the Preface to the first edition, Rothman and Simeone stated, "*The Spine* had as its genesis a strong feeling on the part of its editors that a need existed for a comprehensive textbook to include all aspects of diagnosis and treatment of spinal disease. Our goals were to lower the traditional disciplinary barriers and biases and to present a uniform guideline to problem solving in this area…This book has been designed to include all facets of disease related to the spine, whether orthopedic, neurosurgical, or medical in nature… An attempt has been made to achieve completeness without exhaustive and burdensome details. The contributing authors have not merely recorded the possibilities in diagnosis and treatment of spinal disorders, but have relied on their personal experience to offer concrete recommendations." The first edition of *The Spine*, following the dictates of the editors, covered the full range of knowledge of spinal disorders known at the time and became an essential component of the libraries of all medical personnel who dealt with spinal disorders. The authors, one a neurosurgeon (F.A.S.) and one an orthopedic surgeon (R.H.R.), combined their efforts to teach the world not only diseases of the spine, but also the importance of working together in an attempt to understand and treat the disease processes. Their spinal fellowship, as well as personal fellowship, was based on this multidisciplinary yet regimented approach to the spine and has been the model that we have sought to achieve in our own clinical and teaching environments.

The Preface to the second edition of *The Spine* stated, "Advancements in medicine generally follow broader scientific and even social trends. The treatment of spine diseases is no exception. Consequently, increments of new information have been added to the general body of knowledge in spotty, but predictable, areas. These new developments constitute the raison d'être for this second edition. The dramatic progress in radiologic imaging stands out as the most useful innovation [at that time, computed tomography]. Each contributor has demonstrated his commitment to summarizing the most recent information in a manner useful to students and clinicians alike, and for this the editors are proud and appreciative."

The Preface to the third edition included the following: "The current edition has new editorial leadership. Those of us involved in the direction of this project have tried to follow the model previously established by Drs. Rothman and Simeone in finding the best authors for each chapter. We, hopefully, have emphasized, as in the past editions, the importance of understanding the basic science in a concise manner, which leads to the ability to make appropriate decisions and manage patients with simple or complex spinal problems. We have attempted to update each section, have eliminated those areas that are not current, and have separated some components of the basic science from the clinical to aid readers in locating pertinent information in the ever-increasing body of knowledge related to the spine."

The Editorial Board for the fourth edition of *Rothman-Simeone The Spine* carried over from the third edition. "It provided expanded information on magnetic resonance imaging and laparoscopic and endoscopic surgery. It contained a comprehensive discussion of disc degeneration and its treatment. This edition also introduces a chapter on outcomes research and its importance to our assessment of functional outcome in addition to the more traditional measurements of success, including radiographic parameters."

The fifth edition of *The Spine* added much new information, along with significant updates in content and references. This edition introduced Key Points, which were four or five important concepts and facts contained at the end of many of the clinical chapters. A Key References section was added for each chapter that highlighted the most significant references. Chapters new to the fifth edition included surgical management of osteopenic fractures, disc and nuclear replacement, management of flat back deformity, use of transforaminal lumbar interbody fusion, and use of bone graft extenders and bone morphogenetic protein in the lumbar spine. Other new chapters included thoracoscopic surgery and its clinical applications and intraoperative monitoring, including motor-evoked potentials. A new chapter on genetic application and its exciting role for future treatments of degenerative disease was included in the basic science section. Minimally invasive posterior approaches to the lumbar spine were also introduced in that edition.

The sixth continued under the same Editorial Board as the fifth edition. The editors were charged with ensuring that the chapters within their sections contained the latest evidence-based information whenever available. New chapters included those devoted to arthroplasty for cervical and lumbar degenerative disorders. In addition, revision strategies for failed disc replacements highlighted the potential difficulties in dealing with this complex surgical problem. The sixth edition also significantly expanded the discussion of minimally invasive techniques with six chapters devoted to the rationale for minimally invasive surgery and the surgical techniques, results, and complications. A chapter devoted to soft stabilization for lumbar fixation was also added. Also new to that edition were a chapter devoted to anulus repair and a chapter devoted to the basic science of spinal cord injury. As had been done in previous editions, chapter updates were incorporated throughout the book whenever appropriate.

This, the seventh edition of *The Spine*, includes many of the chapters and authors from the sixth edition. However, all have been updated to include what is new in the basic and clinical sciences related to the topic, with relevant references and updates on clinical outcomes where warranted. In essence, as in all other editions, these chapters epitomize the newer academic catchphrase of "clinical translational research."

We have also expanded international authorship, including adding new contributors. The genetics chapters have been enhanced with both basic and clinically relevant information. Even more content on minimally invasive surgery has been added, with updates on outcomes, approaches, and techniques. We have eliminated some topics (e.g., facet replacement) that have fallen out of favor and/or use. We have added discussion on the sacroiliac joint, since that is one of the newest areas in spine care. We have updated the current status on motion-sparing techniques, including disc replacement with now longer-term follow-up and experiential updates in complications and their treatment. Although this is specifically important to disc replacement, it is the crux of change in most preexisting chapters.

The current Editorial Board remains committed to the broad-based appeal of this book. The authors include basic scientists, neuroradiologists, neurologists, physiatrists, and rheumatologists, along with orthopedic surgeons and neurosurgeons. In addition, this book remains unique in providing comprehensive sections on pediatric disorders and adult disease. Its comprehensive content ranges from degenerative disease to deformity to trauma and tumor. Afflictions of the spinal cord, along with detailed discussions of complications and their management, contribute to this book's broad appeal.

We feel this edition of *The Spine* continues to be the primary reference resource for all physicians and other clinicians with an interest in spinal disorders and treatments.

Steven R. Garfin
Frank J. Eismont
Gordon R. Bell
Jeffrey S. Fischgrund
Christopher M. Bono

Acknowledgment

In the past six editions, the editors have always dedicated this book to our mentors Drs. Rothman and Simeone, our families, and our associates, who have given us the time, support, love, and energy to pursue our careers as well as to coordinate, write, and edit this tome, which in fact was a dedication of love toward Drs. Rothman and Simeone. All of this is still true today. This edition, however, represents our feelings toward Harry N. Herkowitz, MD, our deceased lead editor and organizer, colleague, and close, close friend (see Dedication). The senior editors would like to thank and acknowledge our new "junior" editors, Christopher M. Bono, MD, and Jeffrey S. Fischgrund, MD, who have accepted this responsibility for now and the future—carrying on the spine care educational lineage provided by Drs. Rothman, Simeone, and Herkowitz. They stepped in as if they had been with us since the first edition. In addition, the full editorial team would like to thank all of the authors and contributors, some who have done this many times before and accepted our request to submit an updated chapter because it was dedicated to Harry, as well as the new contributors, who did the same thing. It is a monumental effort on everyone's part. We truly appreciate all of them and their hard work. We also thank the readers and the publishers, who have made this one of, if not the, longest-lasting and most-read complete texts on spine care in the world.

Contents

VOLUME 1

Section I
BASIC SCIENCE

Section II
DIAGNOSIS

Section III
SURGICAL ANATOMY AND APPROACHES

Section IV
PEDIATRICS

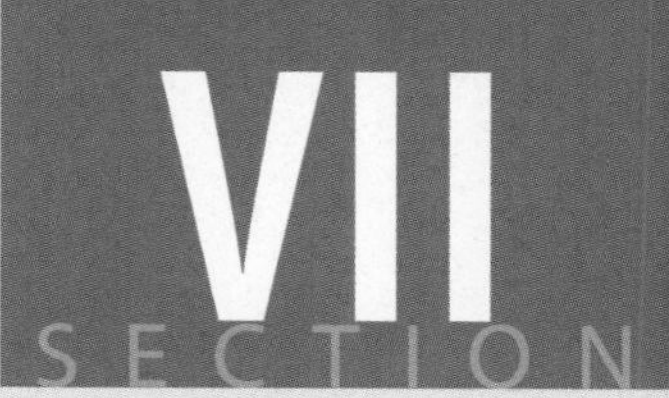

SECTION VII MINIMALLY INVASIVE SURGERY

SECTION VII

53 CHAPTER Rationale of Minimally Invasive Spine Surgery

Choll W. Kim
Steven R. Garfin

Introduction

The goal of minimally invasive spine (MIS) surgery is to accomplish the intended goals of treatment, whether they be decompression, fusion, and/or realignment. The key concepts that guide MIS approaches are to (1) decrease muscle crush injuries during retraction; (2) avoid detachment of tendons to the posterior bony elements, especially the multifidus attachments to the spinous process and superior articular processes; (3) maintain the integrity of the dorsolumbar fascia; (4) limit bony resection; (5) utilize known neurovascular planes; and (6) decrease the size of the surgical corridor to coincide with the area of the surgical target site. Recent advances in instrumentation, combined with refinement of surgical techniques, have allowed treatment of an ever increasing number of spinal disorders.

Anatomy of the Posterior Paraspinal Muscles

The posterior lumbar paraspinal muscles are part of a larger biomechanical system that includes the abdominal muscles and their fibrous attachment to the spine through the dorsolumbar fascia. This network of muscles is responsible for generating movements of the spine while maintaining its stability.[1,2] In addition to maintaining spinal posture in its neutral position, the paraspinal muscles guard the spine from excessive bending that would otherwise endanger the integrity of the intervertebral discs and ligaments.[3] Panjabi et al. have proposed that the paraspinal muscles apply minimal resistance inside the neutral zone, but increase their stiffness exponentially once the range of motion falls outside this neutral zone.[4,5] This dynamic stabilizing system is controlled by an interconnected chain of mechanoreceptors imbedded in the muscle fascicles, disc anulus, and spinal ligaments.[6] Functional electromyelography (EMG) studies reveal that spinal stability is achieved by the simultaneous contraction of several agonist-antagonist muscles.[3,7,8] Architectural studies suggest that the individual paraspinal muscles may have different primary roles as either movers or stabilizers of the spinal column.[9] The anatomic position of the intermuscular planes vary from level to level and may affect the proper location of the incisions.[10,11] In general, the intermuscular plane at the L1–L2 level is closer to the midline than at the L5–S1. Placement of the paramedian incisions should take into consideration this finding along with other characteristics unique to the individual patient, including the depth of the surgical target site from the skin and the trajectory of the pedicles in cases in which the same incision will be used for pedicle screw insertion.

Multifidus Muscle

The posterior paraspinal muscles are composed of two muscle groups: the deep paramedian transversospinalis muscle group, which includes the multifidus, interspinales, intertransversarii and short rotators, and the more superficial and lateral erector spinae muscles, which include the longissimus and iliocostalis (Fig. 53.1). These muscles run along the thoracolumbar spine and attach caudally to the sacrum, sacroiliac joint, and iliac wing. The multifidus is the most medial of the major posterior paraspinal muscles and is the largest muscle that spans the lumbosacral junction. It is believed to be the major posterior stabilizing muscle of the spine.[3,9,12] Compared to other paraspinal muscles, the multifidus muscle is short and stout. It has a large physiologic cross-sectional area (PCSA) but short fiber lengths. This unique architectural anatomy is designed to create large forces over relatively short distances (Fig. 53.2A).[9] Furthermore, the multifidus sarcomere length is positioned on the ascending portion of the length-tension curve (Fig. 53.2B). When our posture changes from standing erect to bending forward, the multifidus is able to produce more force as the spine flexes forward. This serves to protect the spine at its most vulnerable position. Not only is the multifidus muscle designed for maximal active force generation during spinal flexion and extension maneuvers, passive stability is created through increased stiffness of the extracellular matrix surrounding the multifidus muscle at the muscle bundle level.[13]

The multifidus is the only muscle that is attached to both posterior parts of the L5 and S1 vertebrae and is, therefore, the sole posterior stabilizer that both originates and inserts to this segment. The morphology of the lumbar multifidus is complex.[14] Unlike the other paraspinal muscles that have specific origins and insertions, the multifidus muscle is formed by five separate bands, each having its own origin and several different insertion sites. Each band consists of several fascicles arising from the tip of the spinous process and the lateral surface of the vertebral lamina. Caudally, the different fascicles diverge to separate attachments into the mammillary processes of the caudal vertebrae 2 to 5 levels below their origin and downward through each vertebra to the sacrum. For example, fibers from the L1 band insert into the mammillary processes of the L3, L4, and L5 vertebrae; to the dorsal part of S1; and to the posterior superior iliac spine. Biomechanical analyses, based on the multifidus muscle anatomy, show that it produces posterior sagittal rotation of the vertebra, which opposes a counter-rotation generated by the abdominal muscles. The multifidus can further increase lumbar spine stability through a "bowstring" mechanism in which the muscle, positioned posterior to the lumbar lordosis, produces compressive forces on the vertebrae interposed between its attachments.[15]

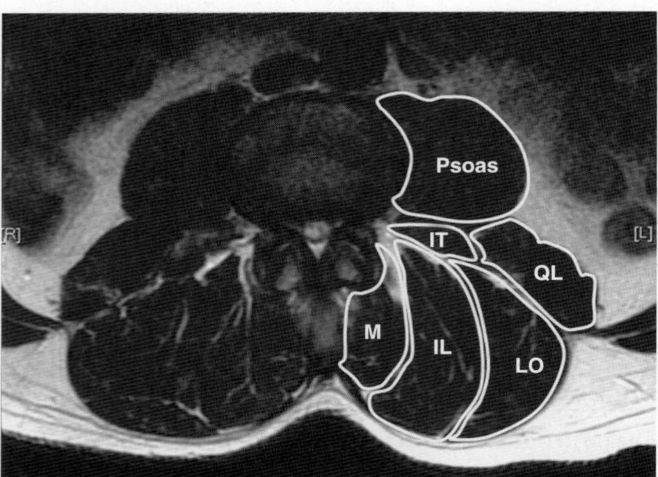

FIG. 53.1 Magnetic resonance cross-sectional image through the L4–L5 disk space showing the multifidus (M), iliocostalis (IL), longissimus (LO), quadratus lumborum (QL), intertransversarii (IT), and psoas muscles.

Erector Spinae Muscles

The erector spinae muscles are composed of the longissimus, iliocostalis, and spinalis (in the thoracic area).[14,16] In the lumbar spine, the longissimus is positioned medially and arises from the transverse and accessory processes; it inserts caudally into the ventral surface of the posterior superior iliac spine. The laterally positioned iliocostalis arises from the tip of the transverse processes and the adjacent middle layer of the thoracolumbar fascia; it inserts into the ventral edge of the iliac crest caudally.[17] Unilateral contraction of the lumbar erector spinae laterally flexes the vertebral column; bilateral contraction produces extension and posterior rotation of the vertebrae in the sagittal plane. In addition to their role as the major extensor muscles of the trunk, the iliocostalis and longissimus also exert large compressive loads as well as lateral and posterior shear forces at the L4 and L5 segments. While these forces increase the stiffness and stability of the normal vertebral column, the shearing forces may also exacerbate instability and deformity in a malaligned spine.[18] In contrast to the multifidus muscle, microarchitectural studies reveal that these muscles are designed as long muscle fascicles with relatively small PCSA. This anatomic morphology suggests that they serve to move the trunk to extension, lateral bending, and rotation. With this type of design, they are less likely to act as primary stabilizers of the vertebral column.[19]

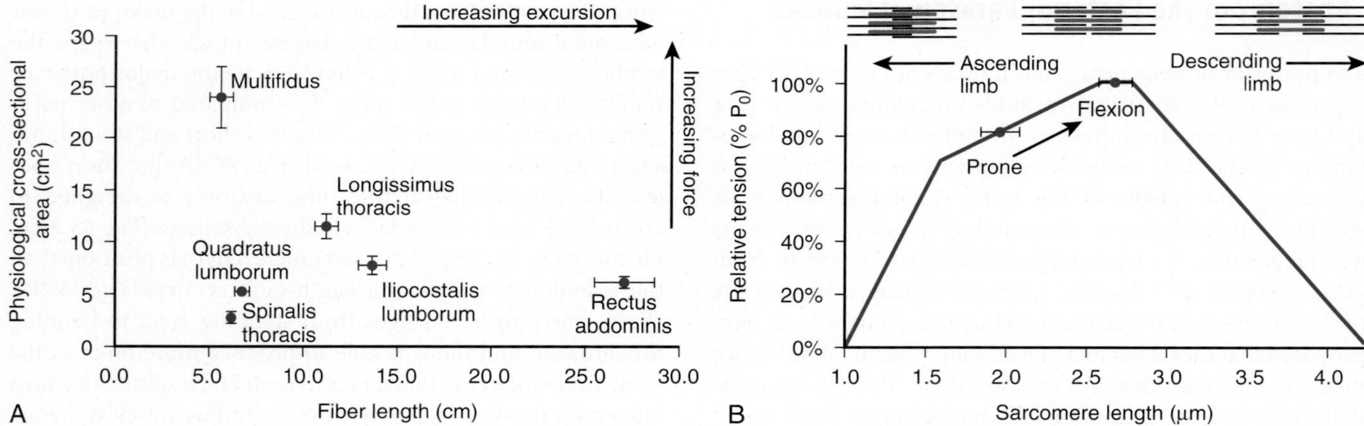

FIG. 53.2 (A) Scatter plot of physiologic cross-sectional area (PCSA) versus fiber length. Since PCSA is proportional to muscle force and fiber length is proportional to muscle excursion, this type of plot illustrates the functional design of a muscle. These data illustrate that the multifidus has the largest force-generating capacity in the lumbar spine and is designed for stability. (B) Sarcomere length operating range of the multifidus plotted on the human skeletal muscle sarcomere length-tension curve (*black line*). These data demonstrate that the multifidus muscle operates on the ascending limb of the length-tension curve and becomes intrinsically stronger as the spine is flexed (*arrow*). Schematic sarcomeres are shown on the ascending and descending limb to scale based on the quantification of actin and myosin filament lengths. (From Ward SR, Kim CW, Eng CM, et al. Architectural analysis and intraoperative measurements demonstrate the unique design of the multifidus muscle for lumbar spine stability. *J Bone Joint Surg Am.* 2009;91:176-185.)

Interspinales, Intertransversarii, and Short Rotator Muscles

The interspinales, intertransversarii, and short rotator muscles are short, flat muscles that lie dorsal to the intertransverse ligament (see Fig. 53.1). The intertransversarii and interspinales run along the intertransverse and the interspinous ligaments of each segment. The short rotators originate from the posterior-superior edge of the lower vertebra and attach to the lateral side of the upper vertebral lamina. Because of their small PCSA, they are not able to generate the forces needed for movement or stability of the spinal column. More likely, they act as proprioceptive sensors, rather than force-generating structures.[20]

Innervation of the Posterior Paraspinal Muscles

The innervation of all of the posterior paraspinal muscles is derived from the dorsal rami. The iliocostalis is innervated by the lateral branch, while the lumbar fibers of the longissimus receive innervation from the intermediate branch. The multifidus is innervated by the medial branch of the dorsal rami (Fig. 53.3). The medial branch curves around the root of the superior articular process and passes between the mammillary and accessory processes to the vertebral lamina, where it branches to supply the multifidus muscle, the intertransversarii and interspinales muscles, and the zygapophyseal joints.[21]

During its extramuscular course, the medial branch is strongly attached to the vertebral body in two locations. The first attachment is to the periosteum lateral to the zygapophyseal joints by fibers of the intertransverse ligament. The mammilloaccessory ligament provides the second attachment in the lumbar spine. This strong ligament covers the medial branch and is often calcified.[22] These attachments to the vertebra are of clinical importance, as they expose the medial branch to possible damage during a midline posterior surgical approach.[23]

Direct damage to the nerve is also possible during insertion of pedicle screws.[13] Insertion of a pedicle screw in the area of the mammillary process can injure the medial branch arising from the cephalad-level nerve root, causing denervation injury and consequent atrophy to the multifidus fascicles that arise from the adjacent cephalad level.[24–26] For instance, pedicle screws placed at L2 may damage the L1 nerve, which denervates the multifidus bands that originate at L1 and insert into the vertebrae caudally. Moreover, the monosegmental innervation of the multifidus makes it particularly susceptible to atrophy, as it lacks a collateral nerve supply from adjacent muscle segments.[14] It is intriguing to consider that dysfunction of this muscle could contribute to adjacent-level disc degeneration.

Fiber Type Characteristics of the Paraspinal Muscles

Fiber type analysis can provide important information about the use pattern of a muscle.[27,28] There are two major fiber types in skeletal muscles: type I, also known as a "slow twitch," and type II, or "fast twitch." The type I fibers possess low adenosine triphosphatase (ATPase) activity, prolonged twitch duration (hence, "slow twitch"), and a low maximal velocity. In addition, type I fibers contain higher mitochondrial content and greater oxidative enzyme complements than type II fibers. Type II fibers are characterized by higher ATPase activities and correspondingly shorter isometric twitch durations. With this design, they are better suited to support the regeneration of adenosine triphosphate through anaerobic mechanisms. Type II fibers can be further subdivided into type IIa and IIx fibers. Type IIx fibers are generally more extreme in each of these respects than the type IIa fibers.[28–30]

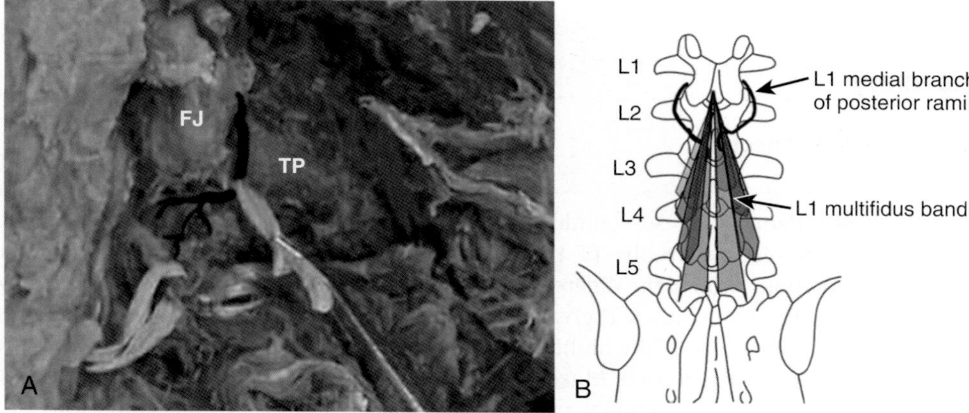

FIG. 53.3 (A) Anatomic specimen showing the spatial relationship of the medial branch of the posterior rami (MBPR) nerve (*highlighted in black and retracted with a rubber vessel loop*), the facet joint (FJ), and transverse process (TP). (B) Path of the L1 medial branch of posterior rami nerve to the L1 multifidus muscle. The L1 MBPR traverses the L2 transverse process and rises posteriorly to innervate the multifidus muscle that originates from the L1 spinous process. The L1 multifidus then separates into four bands that insert into the lamina and superior articular processes of the L3, L4, L5, and S1. (From Regev GJ, Lee YP, Taylor WR, Garfin SR, Kim CW. Nerve injury to the posterior rami medial branch during the insertion of pedicle screws: comparison of mini-open versus percutaneous pedicle screw insertion techniques. *Spine (Phila Pa 1976)*. 2009;34:1239-1242.)

One of the most striking features of the lumbar paraspinal muscles is the predominance of type I muscle fibers compared with other skeletal muscles. Polgar and Johnson studied the distribution of fiber types in 36 human muscles.[31] A significantly larger type I to type II fiber ratio was observed in the multifidus, longissimus, and iliocostalis muscles compared to muscles of the extremities. The predominance of type I fibers and selective type II atrophy has been found in other studies that analyzed fiber type distribution and size in normal paraspinal muscles. It is presumed that, along with the adaptation to their stabilizing tonic work characteristics, the phenomenon of type II atrophy can be explained by the sedentary modern lifestyle that deprives these muscles of stimulation from exercise.[32] The relatively larger size of type II fibers in professional athletes further supports this assumption.[33,34]

The morphology of fiber type distribution between the different paraspinal muscles and in different areas inside the muscle is well known. Jorgensen et al. reported a higher proportion of type I fibers in the longissimus than in the multifidus or iliocostalis muscles.[35] Furthermore, the multifidus muscle is composed of a relatively high percentage of type I fibers, consistent with a postural function. The psoas muscle, on the other hand, is composed of a higher percentage of type II fibers, such as in the appendicular muscles.[36] Mannion et al. showed that, in women, the mean size of the type I fiber is significantly greater than that of either the type IIA or the type IIx, while men have relatively larger-sized type II fibers.[37] In the older population, a loss of muscle mass leads to a decrease in both fiber type sizes with slightly more effect in type II fibers.[38–40] The most profound changes in fiber size and fiber type distribution occur in patients with degenerative conditions of the spine.[29] Compared with the control, the muscle of low back pain patients had a significantly higher proportion of type IIx fibers than type I fibers. They proposed that the relatively low proportion of type I fibers in patients with low back pain render them less resistant to fatigue and more susceptible to injury.

Paraspinal Muscle Injury

Characteristics of Paraspinal Muscles in the Postsurgical Spine

Spine surgery inherently causes damage to surrounding muscles.[41] This injury can be followed by atrophy of the muscles and subsequent loss of function. Among the different surgical approaches to the spine, injury to the muscle is greatest when using the midline posterior approach.[42] The multifidus muscle is most injured when using this approach. Muscle atrophy coincides with decreased muscle cross-sectional area (CSA), which, in turn, correlates with decreased force production capacity of the muscle.[41,43–49]

Muscle biopsies obtained from patients undergoing revision spinal surgery exhibit an array of pathologic features that include selective type II fiber atrophy, widespread fiber type grouping (a sign of reinnervation), and "moth eaten" appearance of muscle fibers.[40] Although these pathologic changes can occasionally be found in biopsies from normal individuals, the pathologic changes are more prevalent after surgery.[50] Atrophy of the paraspinal muscles can readily be seen in postsurgical back patients.[51] Reductions in the CSA of the paraspinal muscles are greatest following a midline approach for a posterolateral fusion.[42,47,52] Using electromyography, paraspinal muscle function adjacent to instrumented fusions was significantly diminished after traditional midline open transforaminal lumbar interbody fusion (TLIF).[53] In contrast, electromyography evidence of muscle function was well maintained after minimally invasive transforaminal lumbar interbody fusion (MIS TLIF).[53]

Mechanism of Paraspinal Muscle Injury During Surgery

The factors responsible for muscle injury during surgery have been well studied in both animals and humans. Muscle damage can be caused by several different mechanisms. Direct injury to the muscle is caused by dissection and stripping of tendinous attachments from the posterior elements of the spine. Additionally, extensive use of electrocautery causes localized thermal injury and necrosis to the tissues. The most significant factor responsible for muscle injury is likely the use of forceful self-retaining retractors. Kawaguchi and co-workers quantified the factors responsible for muscle necrosis following a standard open midline posterior approach.[54–56] They proposed that injury is induced by a crush mechanism similar to that caused by a pneumatic tourniquet during surgery of the limbs. During the application of self-retaining retractors, elevated pressures lead to decreased intramuscular perfusion.[57–60] The severity of the muscle injury is closely correlated to the degree of intramuscular pressure and length of retraction time. A pressure-time parameter can be calculated by multiplying the intramuscular pressure and the length of time of the surgery. A high pressure-time product was shown to be tightly correlated to muscle necrosis. They concluded that muscle damage can be reduced by intermittent release of the retractors during prolonged surgery combined with a relatively longer incision that allows reduced retraction pressures.

Denervation is yet another mechanism that leads to muscle degeneration and atrophy following surgery. Muscle denervation can occur in a discrete location along the supplying nerve or can be located in several points along the nerve and the neuromuscular junction. As previously described, nerve supply to the multifidus is especially vulnerable to injury because of its monosegmental innervation pattern.[14] Muscle denervation is also possible through damage to the neuromuscular junction following long muscle retraction and necrosis. Shorter retraction time or an intermittent release of muscle retraction has been shown to significantly decrease degeneration and denervation of the muscles.[59] Gejo et al. examined the relationship between retraction time and postoperative damage to the paraspinal muscle by measuring postoperation signal intensity of the multifidus muscle using T2-weighted MRI.[61] Long retraction time during surgery was found to correlate with high signal intensity in the multifidus muscle even at 6 months after surgery. They proposed that these findings reflect chronic denervation of the muscle caused by damage to the neuromuscular synapses.

Correlation of Muscle Injury With Clinical Outcomes

There appears to be a correlation between muscle damage and long-term postoperative pain. Sihvonen et al. found signs of severe denervation of the multifidus muscle in patients with failed back syndrome.[62] Muscle biopsies showed signs of advanced chronic denervation consisting of group atrophy, marked fibrosis, and fatty infiltration. Moreover, fiber type grouping, a histologic sign of reinnervation, was rare. They hypothesized that the denervation injury resulted from direct damage to the medial branch of the posterior rami during muscle retraction associated with the posterior midline approach. The lack of reinnervation was thought to result from the absence of intersegmental nerve supply to the multifidus. Signs of severe denervation of the paraspinal muscles correlate with poor outcome of postsurgical patients. They also showed that poor clinical outcomes are associated with abnormal EMG patterns 2 to 5 years after surgery.

Changes in multifidus CSA and T2 signal intensity vary significantly depending on the surgical approach. There is significantly less atrophy after MIS TLIF compared with open TLIF. These changes are correlated with improved pain scores, disability, and creatine kinase levels.[63] Changes in the paraspinal atrophy were significant in the multifidus muscle but not in the longissimus muscle between open TLIF and MIS TLIF groups.[64] Other parameters of surgical success seem to favor a minimally invasive approach.

The integrity of the paraspinal muscles may have an effect on fusion rates.[65] Patients with less atrophy of the paraspinal muscle group had higher rates of solid fusion than patients with more significant paraspinal atrophy.[65] The most clinically obvious and pronounced benefit of minimally invasive posterior techniques over the conventional midline open approaches is the decreased postoperative infections. The Scoliosis Research Society Morbidity and Mortality studies show a nearly 5-fold decrease in rates of deep surgical site infections when a TLIF is performed using MIS techniques. This has been shown in several other studies, with a wide range of significant differences.[66] In a more direct comparison of open TLIF versus MIS TLIF, Ee et al. showed that the relative risk of deep surgical site infections.[67]

Preservation of Muscle Function and Integrity

MIS surgery techniques strive to minimize muscle injury during surgery. By minimizing the use of self-retaining retractors, intramuscular retraction pressure is reduced, leading to less crush injury. Furthermore, focusing the surgical corridor directly over the surgical target site allows for less muscle stripping that may otherwise disrupt its tendinous attachments or damage their neurovascular supply. Kim et al. compared trunk muscle strength between patients treated with open posterior instrumentation versus percutaneous instrumentation.[68] Tests were performed isometrically at multiple flexion positions. Patients undergoing percutaneous instrumentation displayed over 50% improvement in extension strength, while patients undergoing traditional midline open surgery had no significant improvement in lumbar extension strength. Extension strength correlated with preservation of multifidus CSA as measured on MRI. In a similar study, Stevens et al. assessed the postsurgical appearance of the multifidus muscle using a high-definition MRI sequence.[69] In patients treated via an open posterior TLIF technique, marked intermuscular and intramuscular edema was observed on postsurgical MRI at 6 months after surgery. In contrast, patients in the MIS TLIF group had a normal appearance on MRI following surgery.

Hyun et al. retrospectively assessed a group of patients who underwent unilateral TLIF with ipsilateral instrumented posterior spinal fusion via an open technique.[45] Contralateral instrumented posterior spinal fusion was performed at the same level employing a paramedian, intermuscular (Wiltse) minimally invasive approach. Postoperatively, there was a significant decrease in the CSA of the multifidus on the side of the open approach while no reduction in the multifidus CSA on the contralateral side was observed.

Decreases in tissue trauma not only have local effects but alter overall systemic physiology. Kim et al. studied circulating markers of tissue injury in patients undergoing open versus MIS fusions.[69,70] Markers of skeletal muscle injury (creatinine kinase, aldolase), proinflammatory cytokines (interleukin 6 [IL-6], IL-8), and antiinflammatory cytokines (IL-10, IL-1 receptor antagonist) were analyzed with enzyme-linked immunosorbent assay techniques. Twofold to sevenfold increases in all markers were observed in the open surgery group. The greatest difference between the groups occurred on the first postoperative day. Most markers returned to baseline in 3 days for the MIS group, whereas the open surgery group required 7 days. IL-6 and IL-8 are known cytokines that participate in various systemic inflammatory reactions.[71–73] It is possible that such elevations in inflammatory cytokines have direct effects beyond the surgical site. As such, persistently elevated levels of proinflammatory cytokines have been associated with organ failure in postsurgical patients.[74]

Preservation of the Bone-Ligament Complex

It is well accepted that excessive facet resection leads to altered motion and spinal instability.[75–78] Furthermore, a laminectomy leads to loss of the midline supraspinous/interspinous ligament complex, which can contribute to flexion instability.[79,80] In cases in which significant bony resection is required, or when there is an underlying relative instability (such as in spondylolisthesis), concomitant fusion is often recommended following a decompressive laminectomy.[79–82] Efforts to limit such potentially destabilizing surgery have been pursued via unilateral laminotomies in which the spinous processes and corresponding tendinous attachments of the multifidus muscle and the supraspinous/interspinous ligaments are preserved (Fig. 53.4). When this technique is combined with minimally invasive tubular retractors, bilateral decompression

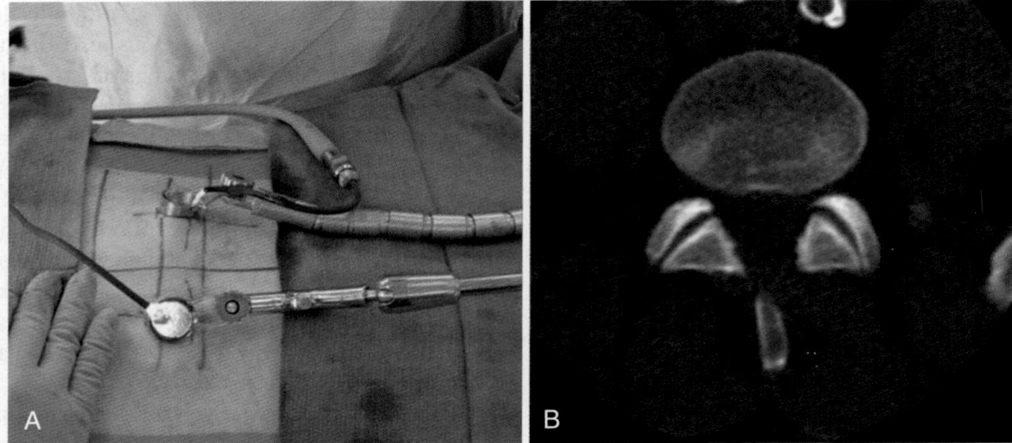

FIG. 53.4 (A) A minimally invasive decompression procedure for the treatment of L4–L5 spinal stenosis. The strategy is to use a bilateral paramedian approach that spares the tendinous attachment of the multifidus muscle at the spinous process. (B) Postoperative computed tomographic scan demonstrating good decompression of the spinal canal without noticeable damage to the posterior paraspinal muscles. Decompression of the left lateral recess via the right paramedian approach (and vice versa) allows minimal facet resection during decompression of the lateral recess.

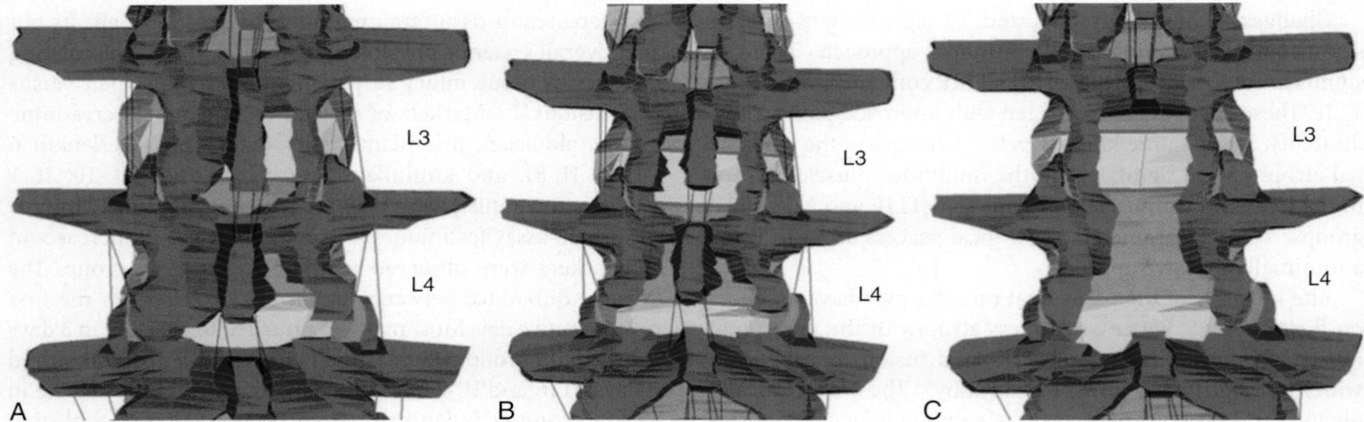

FIG. 53.5 Posterior view illustrating three different decompression methods tested by finite element analysis: (A) minimally invasive unilateral laminotomies; (B) midline interlaminar decompression, which retains the spinous process but sacrifices the interspinous/supraspinous ligaments; and (C) midline open laminectomies with resection of the spinous processes. (From Bresnahan L, Ogden AT, Natarajan RN, Fessler RG. A biomechanical evaluation of graded posterior element removal for treatment of lumbar stenosis: comparison of a minimally invasive approach with two standard laminectomy techniques. *Spine (Phila Pa 1976)*. 2009;34:17-23.)

for stenosis can be achieved with good clinical results.[83–85] The long-term outcome of such MIS procedures and their effect on spinal stability have yet to be shown clinically. However, biomechanical studies suggest that such MIS techniques have significant effects on spinal stability.

Biomechanical and finite element analyses have been used to assess the consequences of various lumbar decompressive procedures on spinal motion.[86,87] Bresnahan et al. compared three decompressive techniques to treat two-level spinal stenosis: open laminectomies versus interlaminar midline decompression (which retains the spinous process but sacrifices the interspinous/supraspinous ligaments) versus MIS unilateral laminotomies (Fig. 53.5).[87] These studies show that open laminectomy produces marked increases in flexion, extension, and axial rotation. For flexion-extension, there is a greater than twofold increase in motion, which leads to increased stress on the anulus. No changes in flexion were noted when the interlaminar or MIS models were studied. Axial rotation increased by 2.5-fold in the open and interlaminar groups but only 1.3-fold in the MIS group. Similar findings have been shown in biomechanical studies in human lumbar cadaveric specimens.[86] These findings lend further support to the concept that MIS techniques have relevant effects on spinal motion and stability.

Summary

Preservation of normal spinal motion and stability constitutes the best means for ensuring improved long-term outcomes following the surgical treatment of spinal disorders. In the living organism, stability and motion are controlled by active and passive means. The lumbar spine is surrounded by powerful muscles that actively control movement and confer dynamic stability. Concurrently, the ligaments, bones, cartilage, and discs provide for passive stability. Emerging MIS surgery techniques seek to minimize surgical damage and thereby preserve normal function. The rationale of this approach relies on limiting the surgical corridor to the minimum necessary to safely expose the surgical target site. This minimizes the destruction of anatomic structures necessary for normal function, namely, the relevant osseoligamentous, neurovascular, and musculotendinous anatomy. In addition, the traditional use of larger self-retaining retractors, which can induce crush injuries to adjacent tissues, have been supplanted by table mounted, tubular-type retractors that minimize pressure on muscles, vessels, and nerves. Continued development of minimally invasive techniques remains a vital effort in the advancement of spinal surgery.

KEY REFERENCES

1. Gejo R, Matsui H, Kawaguchi Y, Ishihara H, Tsuji H. Serial changes in trunk muscle performance after posterior lumbar surgery. *Spine*. 1999;24:1023-1028.
   In this clinical study of patients undergoing posterior lumbar surgery, back muscle injury was directly related to muscle retraction time.
2. Kim DY, Lee SH, Chung SK, Lee HY. Comparison of multifidus muscle atrophy and trunk extension muscle strength: percutaneous versus open pedicle screw fixation. *Spine*. 2005;30:123-129.
   The use of percutaneous pedicle screw insertion techniques, compared to traditional midline open approaches, leads to less muscle injury and allows for greater recovery of muscle function.
3. Kim KT, Lee SH, Suk KS, Bae SC. The quantitative analysis of tissue injury markers after mini-open lumbar fusion. *Spine*. 2006;31:712-716.
   In patients undergoing posterior lumbar surgery, the use of minimally invasive techniques leads to lower levels of proinflammatory cytokines detected in the bloodstream.
4. MacIntosh JE, Bogduk N. The morphology of the lumbar erector spinae. *Spine*. 1987;12:658-668.
   This classic study has formed the basis of our general understanding of the posterior lumbar muscle anatomy.
5. Ward SR, Kim CW, Eng CM, et al. Architectural analysis and intraoperative measurements demonstrate the unique design of the multifidus muscle for lumbar spine stability. *J Bone Joint Surg Am*. 2009;91:176-185.
   This study shows the multifidus is designed to exert high forces over short distances, suggesting it plays a key role in spinal stability.

REFERENCES

1. Brown SH, McGill SM. Muscle force-stiffness characteristics influence joint stability: a spine example. *Clin Biomech (Bristol, Avon)*. 2005;20:917-922.
2. Brown SH, Potvin JR. Constraining spine stability levels in an optimization model leads to the prediction of trunk muscle cocontraction and improved spine compression force estimates. *J Biomech*. 2005;38:745-754.
3. Cholewicki J, Panjabi MM, Khachatryan A. Stabilizing function of trunk flexor-extensor muscles around a neutral spine posture. *Spine*. 1997;22:2207-2212.
4. Panjabi MM. The stabilizing system of the spine. Part I. Function, dysfunction, adaptation, and enhancement. *J Spinal Disord*. 1992;5:383-389.
5. Panjabi MM. The stabilizing system of the spine. Part II. Neutral zone and instability hypothesis. *J Spinal Disord*. 1992;5:390-396.
6. Panjabi MM, White AA 3rd. Basic biomechanics of the spine. *Neurosurgery*. 1980;7:76-93.
7. McGill SM. Electromyographic activity of the abdominal and low back musculature during the generation of isometric and dynamic axial trunk torque: implications for lumbar mechanics. *J Orthop Res*. 1991;9:91-103.
8. Cholewicki J, McGill SM, Norman RW. Lumbar spine loads during the lifting of extremely heavy weights. *Med Sci Sports Exerc*. 1991;23:1179-1186.
9. Ward SR, Kim CW, Eng CM, et al. Architectural analysis and intraoperative measurements demonstrate the unique design of the multifidus muscle for lumbar spine stability. *J Bone Joint Surg Am*. 2009;91:176-185.
10. Deng X, Zhu Y, Wang S, et al. CT and MRI determination of intermuscular space within lumbar paraspinal muscles at different intervertebral disc levels. *PLoS ONE*. 2015;10:e0140315.
11. Li H, Yang L, Chen J, et al. Magnetic resonance imaging-based anatomical study of the multifidus-longissimus cleavage planes in the lumbar spine. *Am J Transl Res*. 2016;8:109-116.
12. Donisch EW, Basmajian JV. Electromyography of deep back muscles in man. *Am J Anat*. 1972;133:25-36.
13. Ward SR, Tomiya A, Regev GJ, et al. Passive mechanical properties of the lumbar multifidus muscle support its role as a stabilizer. *J Biomech*. 2009;42:1384-1389.
14. MacIntosh JE, Bogduk N. The morphology of the lumbar erector spinae. *Spine*. 1987;12:658-668.
15. Bogduk N, Macintosh JE, Pearcy MJ. A universal model of the lumbar back muscles in the upright position. *Spine*. 1992;17:897-913.
16. Macintosh JE, Bogduk N. The attachments of the lumbar erector spinae. *Spine*. 1991;16:783-792.
17. Bustami FM. A new description of the lumbar erector spinae muscle in man. *J Anat*. 1986;144:81-91.
18. Bogduk N. A reappraisal of the anatomy of the human lumbar erector spinae. *J Anat*. 1980;131:525-540.
19. Delp SL, Suryanarayanan S, Murray WM, Uhlir J, Triolo RJ. Architecture of the rectus abdominis, quadratus lumborum, and erector spinae. *J Biomech*. 2001;34:371-375.
20. Bogduk N. The innervation of the lumbar spine. *Spine*. 1983;8:286-293.
21. Bogduk N, Long DM. The anatomy of the so-called "articular nerves" and their relationship to facet denervation in the treatment of low-back pain. *J Neurosurg*. 1979;51:172-177.
22. Bogduk N, Tynan W, Wilson AS. The nerve supply to the human lumbar intervertebral discs. *J Anat*. 1981;132:39-56.
23. Boelderl A, Daniaux H, Kathrein A, Maurer H. Danger of damaging the medial branches of the posterior rami of spinal nerves during a dorsomedian approach to the spine. *Clin Anat*. 2002;15:77-81.
24. Bogduk N. Lumbar lateral branch neuralgia: a complication of rhizolysis. *Med J Aust*. 1981;1:242-243.

25. Bogduk N, Lambert GA, Duckworth JW. The anatomy and physiology of the vertebral nerve in relation to cervical migraine. *Cephalalgia*. 1981;1:11-24.
26. Bogduk N. The lumbar mamillo–accessory ligament. Its anatomical and neurosurgical significance. *Spine*. 1981;6:162-167.
27. Kirschbaum BJ, Schneider S, Izumo S, et al. Rapid and reversible changes in myosin heavy chain expression in response to increased neuromuscular activity of rat fast-twitch muscle. *FEBS Lett*. 1990;268:75-78.
28. Edgerton VR, Roy RR. Regulation of skeletal muscle fiber size, shape and function. *J Biomech*. 1991;24(suppl 1):123-133.
29. Mannion AF, Kaser L, Weber E, et al. Influence of age and duration of symptoms on fibre type distribution and size of the back muscles in chronic low back pain patients. *Eur Spine J*. 2000;9:273-281.
30. Mannion AF. Fibre type characteristics and function of the human paraspinal muscles: normal values and changes in association with low back pain. *J Electromyogr Kinesiol*. 1999;9:363-377.
31. Johnson MA, Sideri G, Weightman D, Appleton D. A comparison of fibre size, fibre type constitution and spatial fibre type distribution in normal human muscle and in muscle from cases of spinal muscular atrophy and from other neuromuscular disorders. *J Neurol Sci*. 1973;20:345-361.
32. Crossman K, Mahon M, Watson PJ, Oldham JA, Cooper RG. Chronic low back pain-associated paraspinal muscle dysfunction is not the result of a constitutionally determined "adverse" fiber-type composition. *Spine*. 2004;29:628-634.
33. Puustjarvi K, Tammi M, Reinikainen M, Helminen HJ, Paljarvi L. Running training alters fiber type composition in spinal muscles. *Eur Spine J*. 1994;3:17-21.
34. Short KR, Vittone JL, Bigelow ML, et al. Changes in myosin heavy chain mRNA and protein expression in human skeletal muscle with age and endurance exercise training. *J Appl Physiol*. 2005;99:95-102.
35. Jorgensen K, Nicholaisen T, Kato M. Muscle fiber distribution, capillary density, and enzymatic activities in the lumbar paravertebral muscles of young men. Significance for isometric endurance. *Spine*. 1993;18:1439-1450.
36. Regev GJ, Kim CW, Thacker BE, et al. Regional myosin heavy chain distribution in selected paraspinal muscles. *Spine*. 2010;35:1265-1270.
37. Mannion AF, Weber BR, Dvorak J, Grob D, Muntener M. Fibre type characteristics of the lumbar paraspinal muscles in normal healthy subjects and in patients with low back pain. *J Orthop Res*. 1997;15:881-887.
38. Rantanten J, Rissanen A, Kalimo H. Lumbar muscle fiber size and type distribution in normal subjects. *Eur Spine J*. 1994;3:331-335.
39. Zhu XZ, Parnianpour M, Nordin M, Kahanovitz N. Histochemistry and morphology of erector spinae muscle in lumbar disc herniation. *Spine*. 1989;14:391-397.
40. Mattila M, Hurme M, Alaranta H, et al. The multifidus muscle in patients with lumbar disc herniation. A histochemical and morphometric analysis of intraoperative biopsies. *Spine*. 1986;11:732-738.
41. Gejo R, Matsui H, Kawaguchi Y, Ishihara H, Tsuji H. Serial changes in trunk muscle performance after posterior lumbar surgery. *Spine*. 1999;24:1023-1028.
42. Gille O, Jolivet E, Dousset V, et al. Erector spinae muscle changes on magnetic resonance imaging following lumbar surgery through a posterior approach. *Spine*. 2007;32:1236-1241.
43. Datta G, Gnanalingham KK, Peterson D, et al. Back pain and disability after lumbar laminectomy: is there a relationship to muscle retraction? *Neurosurgery*. 2004;54:1413-1420.
44. Granata C, Cervellati S, Ballestrazzi A, Corbascio M, Merlini L. Spine surgery in spinal muscular atrophy: long-term results. *Neuromuscul Disord*. 1993;3:207-215.
45. Hyun SJ, Kim YB, Kim YS, et al. Postoperative changes in paraspinal muscle volume: comparison between paramedian interfascial and midline approaches for lumbar fusion. *J Korean Med Sci*. 2007;22:646-651.
46. Mayer TG, Vanharanta H, Gatchel RJ, et al. Comparison of CT scan muscle measurements and isokinetic trunk strength in postoperative patients. *Spine*. 1989;14:33-36.
47. Motosuneya T, Asazuma T, Tsuji T, et al. Postoperative change of the cross-sectional area of back musculature after 5 surgical procedures as assessed by magnetic resonance imaging. *J Spinal Disord Tech*. 2006;19:318-322.
48. Kawaguchi Y, Matsui H, Gejo R, Tsuji H. Preventive measures of back muscle injury after posterior lumbar spine surgery in rats. *Spine*. 1998;23:2282-2287.
49. Rantanen J, Hurme M, Falck B, et al. The lumbar multifidus muscle five years after surgery for a lumbar intervertebral disc herniation. *Spine*. 1993;18:568-574.
50. Weber BR, Grob D, Dvorak J, Muntener M. Posterior surgical approach to the lumbar spine and its effect on the multifidus muscle. *Spine*. 1997;22:1765-1772.
51. Mayer TG, Vanharanta H, Gatchel RJ, et al. Comparison of CT scan muscle measurements and isokinetic trunk strength in postoperative patients. *Spine*. 1989;14:33-36.
52. Suwa H, Hanakita J, Ohshita N, et al. Postoperative changes in paraspinal muscle thickness after various lumbar back surgery procedures. *Neurol Med Chir (Tokyo)*. 2000;40: 151-154.
53. Cawley DT, Alexander M, Morris S. Multifidus innervation and muscle assessment post-spinal surgery. *Eur Spine J*. 2014;23:320-327.
54. Kawaguchi Y, Matsui H, Tsuji H. Back muscle injury after posterior lumbar spine surgery. Part 1: histologic and histochemical analyses in rats. *Spine*. 1994;19:2590-2597.
55. Kawaguchi Y, Matsui H, Tsuji H. Back muscle injury after posterior lumbar spine surgery. Part 2: histologic and histochemical analyses in humans. *Spine*. 1994;19:2598-2602.
56. Kawaguchi Y, Matsui H, Tsuji H. Back muscle injury after posterior lumbar spine surgery. A histologic and enzymatic analysis. *Spine*. 1996;21:941-944.
57. Styf J, Korner L, Suurkula M. Intramuscular pressure and muscle blood flow during exercise in chronic compartment syndrome. *J Bone Joint Surg Br*. 1987;69:301-305.
58. Styf J, Lysell E. Chronic compartment syndrome in the erector spinae muscle. *Spine*. 1987;12:680-682.
59. Styf JR, Willen J. The effects of external compression by three different retractors on pressure in the erector spine muscles during and after posterior lumbar spine surgery in humans. *Spine*. 1998;23:354-358.
60. Taylor H, McGregor AH, Medhi-Zadeh S, et al. The impact of self-retaining retractors on the paraspinal muscles during posterior spinal surgery. *Spine*. 2002;27:2758-2762.
61. Gejo R, Kawaguchi Y, Kondoh T, et al. Magnetic resonance imaging and histologic evidence of postoperative back muscle injury in rats. *Spine*. 2000;25:941-946.

62. Sihvonen T, Herno A, Paljarvi L, et al. Local denervation atrophy of paraspinal muscles in postoperative failed back syndrome. *Spine*. 1993;18:575-581.
63. Fan S, Hu Z, Zhao F, et al. Multifidus muscle changes and clinical effects of one-level posterior lumbar interbody fusion: minimally invasive procedure versus conventional open approach. *Eur Spine J*. 2010;19:316-324.
64. Putzier M, Hartwig T, Hoff EK, Streitparth F, Strube P. Minimally invasive TLIF leads to increased muscle sparing of the multifidus muscle but not the longissimus muscle compared with conventional PLIF—a prospective randomized clinical trial. *Spine J*. 2016;16:811-819.
65. Choi MK, Kim SB, Park BJ, Park CK, Kim SM. Do trunk muscles affect the lumbar interbody fusion rate?: correlation of trunk muscle cross sectional area and fusion rates after posterior lumbar interbody fusion using stand-alone cage. *J Korean Neurosurg Soc*. 2016;59:276-281.
66. McAfee PC, Garfin SR, Rodgers WB, et al. An attempt at clinically defining and assessing minimally invasive surgery compared with traditional "open" spinal surgery. *SAS J*. 2011;5:125-130.
67. Ee WW, Lau WL, Yeo W, Von Bing Y, Yue WM. Does minimally invasive surgery have a lower risk of surgical site infections compared with open spinal surgery? *Clin Orthop Relat Res*. 2014;472:1718-1724.
68. Kim SB, Jeon TS, Heo YM, et al. Radiographic results of single level transforaminal lumbar interbody fusion in degenerative lumbar spine disease: focusing on changes of segmental lordosis in fusion segment. *Clin Orthop Surg*. 2009;1:207-213.
69. Stevens KJ, Spenciner DB, Griffiths KL, et al. Comparison of minimally invasive and conventional open posterolateral lumbar fusion using magnetic resonance imaging and retraction pressure studies. *J Spinal Disord Tech*. 2006;19: 77-86.
70. Kim KT, Lee SH, Suk KS, Bae SC. The quantitative analysis of tissue injury markers after mini-open lumbar fusion. *Spine*. 2006;31:712-716.
71. Igonin AA, Armstrong VW, Shipkova M, et al. Circulating cytokines as markers of systemic inflammatory response in severe community-acquired pneumonia. *Clin Biochem*. 2004;37:204-209.
72. Baggiolini M, Dahinden CA. CC chemokines in allergic inflammation. *Immunol Today*. 1994;15:127-133.
73. Baggiolini M, Dewald B, Moser B. Interleukin-8 and related chemotactic cytokines–CXC and CC chemokines. *Adv Immunol*. 1994;55:97-179.
74. Ogawa M. Acute pancreatitis and cytokines: "second attack" by septic complication leads to organ failure. *Pancreas*. 1998;16:312-315.
75. Zander T, Rohlmann A, Klockner C, Bergmann G. Influence of graded facetectomy and laminectomy on spinal biomechanics. *Eur Spine J*. 2003;12:427-434.
76. Natarajan RN, Andersson GB, Patwardhan AG, Andriacchi TP. Study on effect of graded facetectomy on change in lumbar motion segment torsional flexibility using three-dimensional continuum contact representation for facet joints. *J Biomech Eng*. 1999;121:215-221.
77. Lee KK, Teo EC, Qiu TX, Yang K. Effect of facetectomy on lumbar spinal stability under sagittal plane loadings. *Spine*. 2004;29:1624-1631.
78. Abumi K, Panjabi MM, Kramer KM, et al. Biomechanical evaluation of lumbar spinal stability after graded facetectomies. *Spine*. 1990;15:1142-1147.
79. Tuite GF, Doran SE, Stern JD, et al. Outcome after laminectomy for lumbar spinal stenosis. Part II: radiographic changes and clinical correlations. *J Neurosurg*. 1994;81:707-715.
80. Tuite GF, Stern JD, Doran SE, et al. Outcome after laminectomy for lumbar spinal stenosis. Part I: clinical correlations. *J Neurosurg*. 1994;81:699-706.
81. Fischgrund JS, Mackay M, Herkowitz HN, et al. 1997 Volvo Award winner in clinical studies. Degenerative lumbar spondylolisthesis with spinal stenosis: a prospective, randomized study comparing decompressive laminectomy and arthrodesis with and without spinal instrumentation. *Spine*. 1997;22:2807-2812.
82. Herkowitz HN, Kurz LT. Degenerative lumbar spondylolisthesis with spinal stenosis. A prospective study comparing decompression with decompression and intertransverse process arthrodesis. *J Bone Joint Surg Am*. 1991;73:802-808.
83. Palmer S, Turner R, Palmer R. Bilateral decompression of lumbar spinal stenosis involving a unilateral approach with microscope and tubular retractor system. *J Neurosurg*. 2002;97:213-217.
84. Guiot BH, Khoo LT, Fessler RG. A minimally invasive technique for decompression of the lumbar spine. *Spine*. 2002;27:432-438.
85. Shin MH, Kim JS, Ryu KS, Hur JW. Bilateral decompression via microscopic tubular crossing laminotomy (MTCL) for lumbar spinal stenosis: technique and early surgical result. *Neurol Med Chir (Tokyo)*. 2015;55:570-577.
86. Smith ZA, Vastardis GA, Carandang G, et al. Biomechanical effects of a unilateral approach to minimally invasive lumbar decompression. *PLoS One*. 2014;9:e92611.
87. Bresnahan L, Ogden AT, Natarajan RN, Fessler RG. A biomechanical evaluation of graded posterior element removal for treatment of lumbar stenosis: comparison of a minimally invasive approach with two standard laminectomy techniques. *Spine*. 2009;34:17-23.

CHAPTER 54 Minimally Invasive Posterior Approaches to the Spine

Choll W. Kim

The term *minimally invasive spine* (MIS) *surgery* describes a variety of surgical techniques that employ key concepts in spinal surgery. The guiding principles of MIS are to (1) decrease muscle crush injuries during retraction, (2) avoid injury of osseotendinous attachments important for spinal stability, (3) maintain the integrity of the dorsolumbar fascia, (4) limit bony resection, (5) avoid injury to the neurovascular supply of muscle compartments by using known anatomic planes, and (6) decrease the size of the surgical corridor to coincide with the area of the surgical target site. These principles can be used in a variety of settings. In the lumbar spine, the most significant application of these principles has been for posterior approaches to the lumbar spine.

Surgical Anatomy of the Posterior Paraspinal Muscles

The posterior lumbar paraspinal muscles are responsible for maintaining spinal posture in its neutral position. Furthermore, the paraspinal muscles guard the spine from excessive bending that would otherwise endanger the integrity of the intervertebral discs, facet joints, and ligaments.[1] It is the body's dynamic stabilizing system that prevents pain and injury to the spinal column due to repetitive loads during the course of daily activities. The posterior paraspinal muscles are composed of several muscle groups that run along the thoracolumbar spine and attach caudally to the sacrum, sacroiliac joint, and iliac wing.

Posterior spine surgery using midline approaches inherently causes damage to surrounding muscles.[2,3] Muscle injury leads to long-term muscle atrophy, which, in turn, leads to decreased force production capacity of the muscle.[2,4–12] The multifidus muscle is most severely injured when using this approach for several reasons. First, its medial location inherently requires that it be displaced most during retraction. This predisposes the muscle to greater retraction pressures and makes it more vulnerable to disruption of its neurovascular supply.[2,7] Of equal importance, the midline posterior approach inevitably leads to disruption of the multifidus tendon attachment to the spinous process and the integrity of the dorsolumbar fascia.

Key Concepts for Minimally Invasive Spine Retraction Systems

A key advance in minimally invasive surgery came from Perez-Cruet and colleagues[13] with the development of the tubular retractor. A cylindrical retractor allows the surgical corridor to be opened via serial dilation using sequentially larger concentric tubes. This decreases the need for muscle stripping during the exposure. Furthermore, a tubular retractor maximizes the surface contact area, which, in turn, minimizes the pressure per unit area. Another key concept in MIS is use of a retractor holder mounted to the table instead of using a "self-retaining" mechanism. In a self-retaining retractor system, constant pressure on the tissues must be exerted to hold the retractor in place. Studies show that the maximum intermuscular pressure around a tubular retractor decreases by 50% within 3 seconds.[14] Thereafter, the pressure is undetectable. With self-retaining retractors, the pressure remains unchanged.

Minimally Invasive Spine Surgical Corridor

The guiding principles of MIS posterior lumbar surgery are to avoid injury to the multifidus tendon attachment to the spinous process and to maintain dorsolumbar fascia integrity. This is accomplished by using paramedian approaches rather than midline approaches. Decompression, microdiscectomy, interbody fusion, posterolateral fusion, and pedicle screw instrumentation can be accomplished through this surgical corridor. Emerging techniques for advanced reconstruction—including posterior corpectomies and strut fusion for burst fractures, tumors, and infections—are also possible.

Posterior Lumbar Approaches

Tubular Microdiscectomy

The treatment of herniated discs via MIS tubular microdiscectomy is the most common technique currently used in the United States. This system, developed by Foley and Smith, consists of a series of concentric dilators and thin-walled

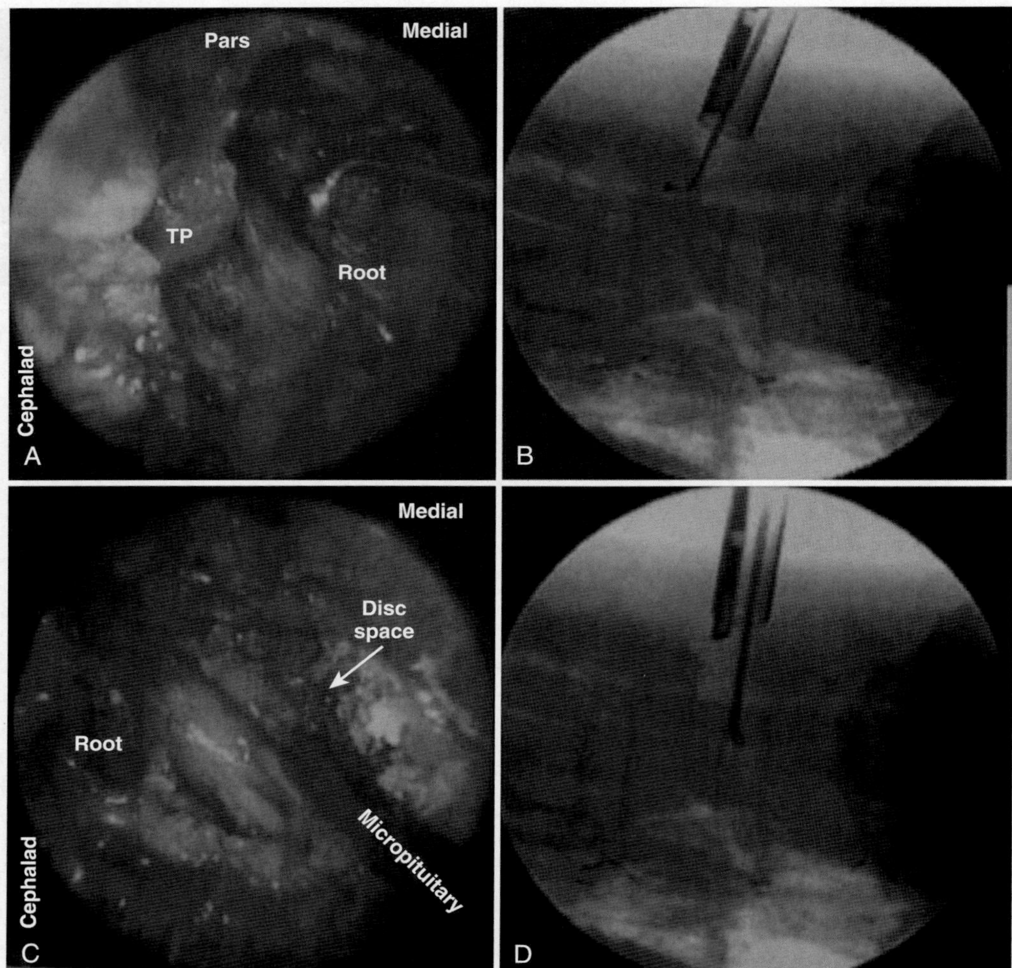

FIG. 54.1 Intraoperative and fluoroscopic images of the tubular microdiscectomy technique. (A, C) Intraoperative image and (B, D) corresponding to the lateral fluoroscopic image of the surgical target site showing the lateral pars and inferomedial transverse process (TP) after removal with a fine Kerrison rongeur. This maneuver allows for palpation of the pedicle and assists identification of the exiting nerve root adjacent to the ball-tip probe.

tubular retractors of variable length. The use of the tubular retractor rather than blades allows the retractor itself to be thin walled (0.9 mm). The tube circumferentially defines a surgical corridor through the erector spinae muscles. The appropriate depth of retractor prevents the muscle from intruding into the field of view. The retractor allows for the appropriately sized working channel to permit spinal decompression. The typical retractor size is approximately 18 mm for microdiscectomy (Fig. 54.1). Surgery is typically performed using an operating microscope. Several randomized controlled trials have been performed to compare traditional open microdiscectomy with minimally invasive tubular microdiscectomy.[15–17] These studies all show that tubular microdiscectomy is safe and efficacious compared with well-established traditional techniques. However, clinically significant superiority was not shown, likely reflecting the difficulty in demonstrating differences between the two already successful procedures. In a meta-analysis of 6 trials comprising 837 patients, clinical improvements in pain and function were similar in both the minimally invasive and traditional open groups, but there were higher risks of incidental durotomies and reoperations for recurrent disc herniations.[17a]

Lumbar Decompression

An important goal of minimally invasive posterior surgery is maintaining the tendinous attachment of the multifidus to the spinous process. During a traditional laminectomy, the spinous process is removed and the multifidus muscle is retracted laterally. Upon wound closure, the multifidus origin can no longer be repaired to the spinous process. The midline approach affords a symmetrical view of the posterior elements, which allows for safe resection of the lamina, ligamentum flavum, and medial facets. The symmetrical view allows the surgeon to readily identify and orient the surgical corridor. However, a thorough decompression can be achieved without need for removal of the spinous process. In a technique originally described by Weiner and colleagues,[18] the spinal canal can be approached through a unilateral portal via a hemilaminectomy technique. Decompression of the central canal and

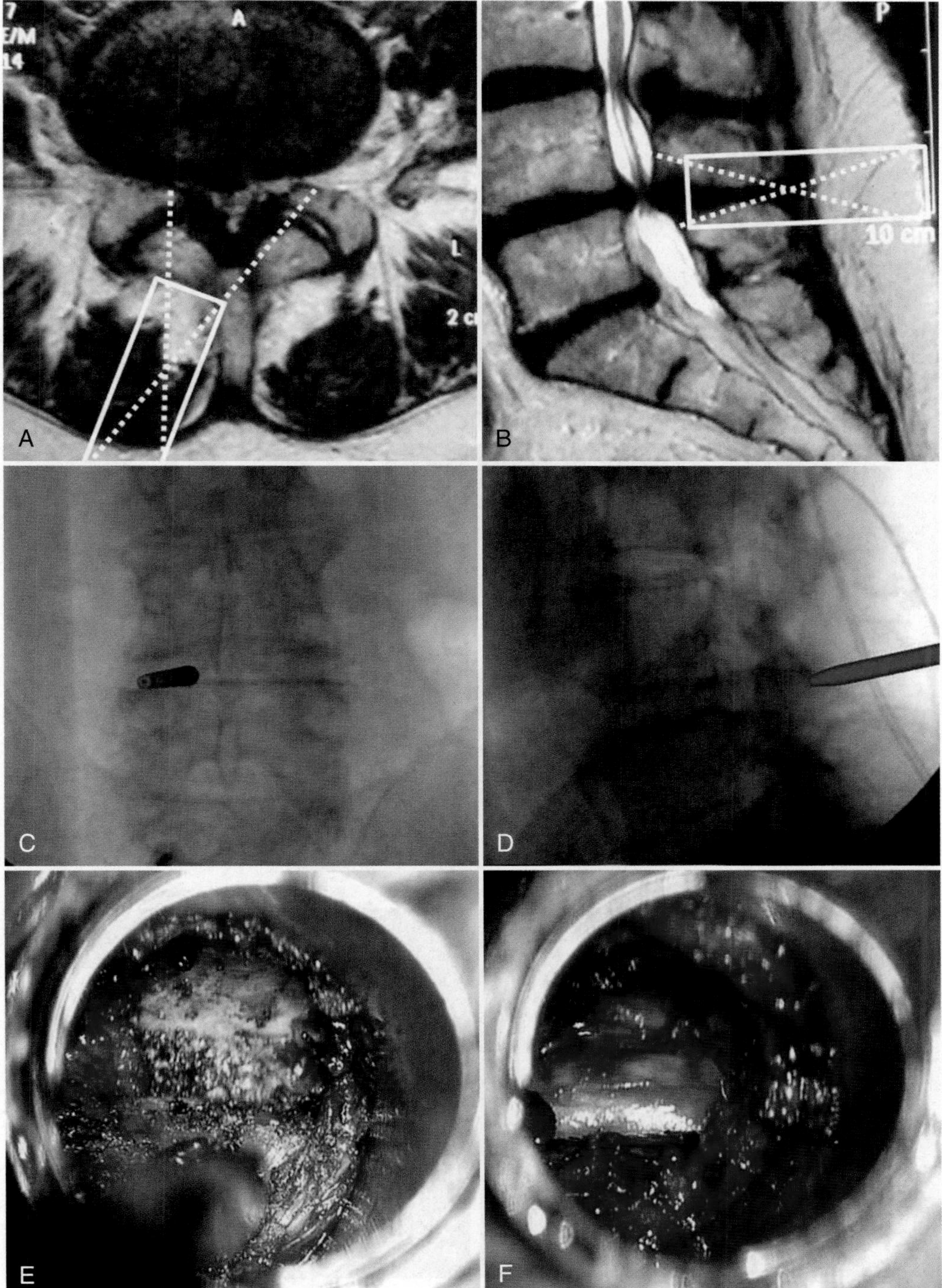

FIG. 54.2 Magnetic resonance (A) axial and (B) sagittal images in a patient with spinal stenosis. Intraoperative fluoroscopic navigation (C) anteroposterior and (D) lateral images showing insertion of the initial dilator. The surgical corridor is overlaid with the tubular retractor in *solid white* and surgical target sites in *dashed lines*. (E–F) Intraoperative photomicrographs of the surgical target site. (E) Initial bony exposure of the base of the spinous process and facet joint line; top is medial. (F) Visualization of the dural tube to the contralateral side using a unilateral approach.

contralateral recess can be achieved by angling the tubular retractor dorsally to view the undersurface of the spinous process and contralateral lamina (Fig. 54.2). The dural tube can be gently pushed down and the ligamentum flavum and contralateral superior articular process resected to achieve a bilateral decompression.

The efficacy and safety of minimally invasive posterior lumbar decompression have been assessed in multiple studies.[18–24] In a review by Asgarzadie and Khoo,[25] this technique provides long-term symptomatic relief equivalent to traditional open surgery but with significant reductions in operative blood loss, postoperative pain, hospital stay, and

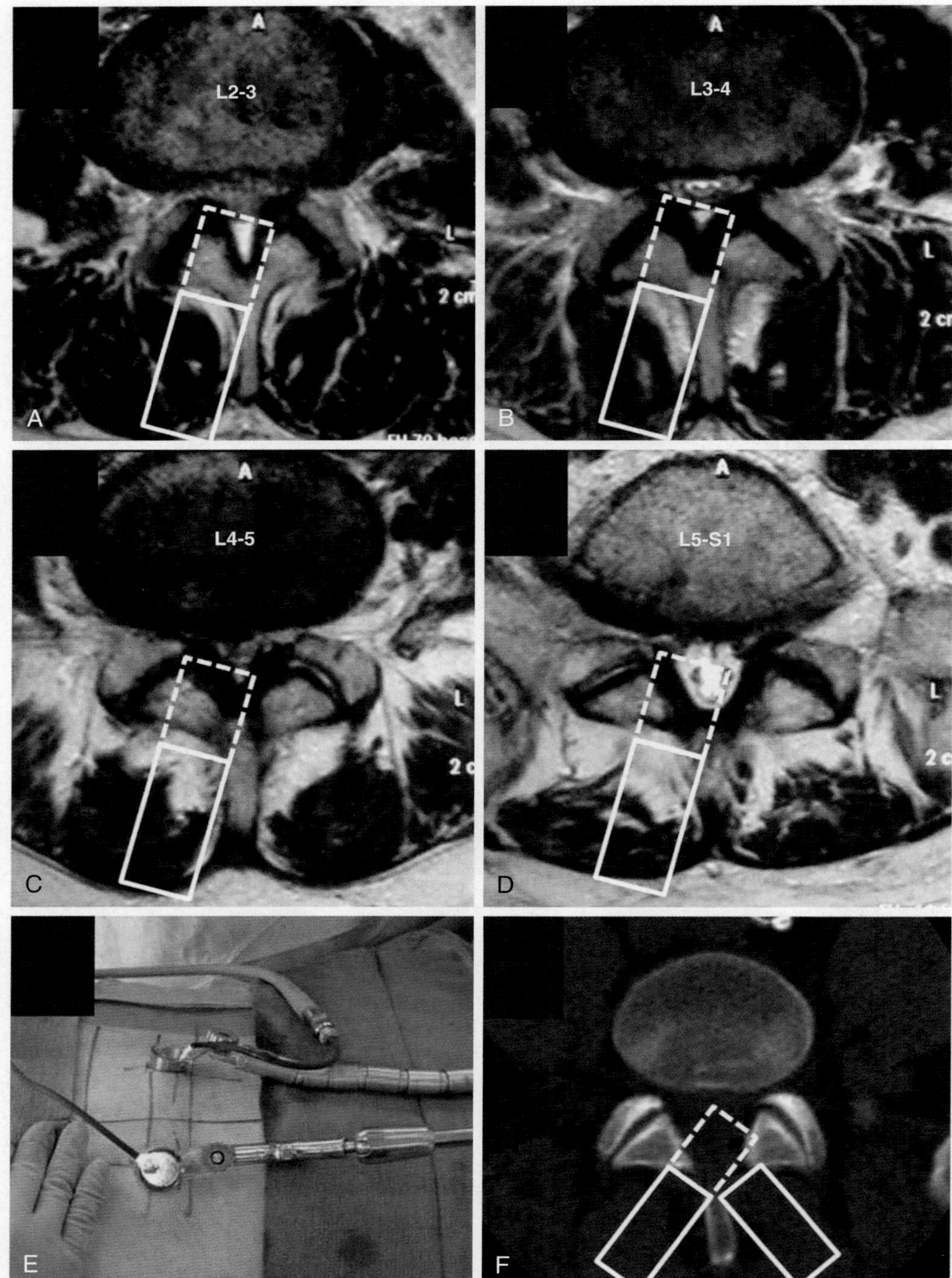

FIG. 54.3 Magnetic resonance cross-sectional image through disc space of (A) L2–L3, (B) L3–L4, (C) L4–L5, and (D) L5–S1. The outline of the tubular retractor is overlaid on each image. Note the proximity of the ipsilateral facet joint at the higher lumbar levels. At L3–L4 and above, care must be exercised to avoid inadvertent injury to the ipsilateral facet joint. (E) A bilateral approach can be used to decompress the lateral recess from the contralateral sides (F).

narcotic usage. The effect of the MIS learning curve remains a significant concern, as increased complication rates are seen during the initial series of patients.[26] Despite the learning curve, the overall complication rates remain low, even in patients who are elderly or medically frail.[27–29]

It is important to consider the anatomic variation of the lower lumbar spine with the upper lumbar spine with this particular technique. At L3 and above, the lamina between the spinous process and facet joint can be narrow (Fig. 54.3). With a unilateral approach, it may be difficult to reach the ipsilateral recess without excessively removing the ipsilateral inferior articular process. An option is to use a bilateral crossover technique to reach the right lateral recess from a left-sided hemilaminectomy and vice versa.[2] Anatomically, the lateral

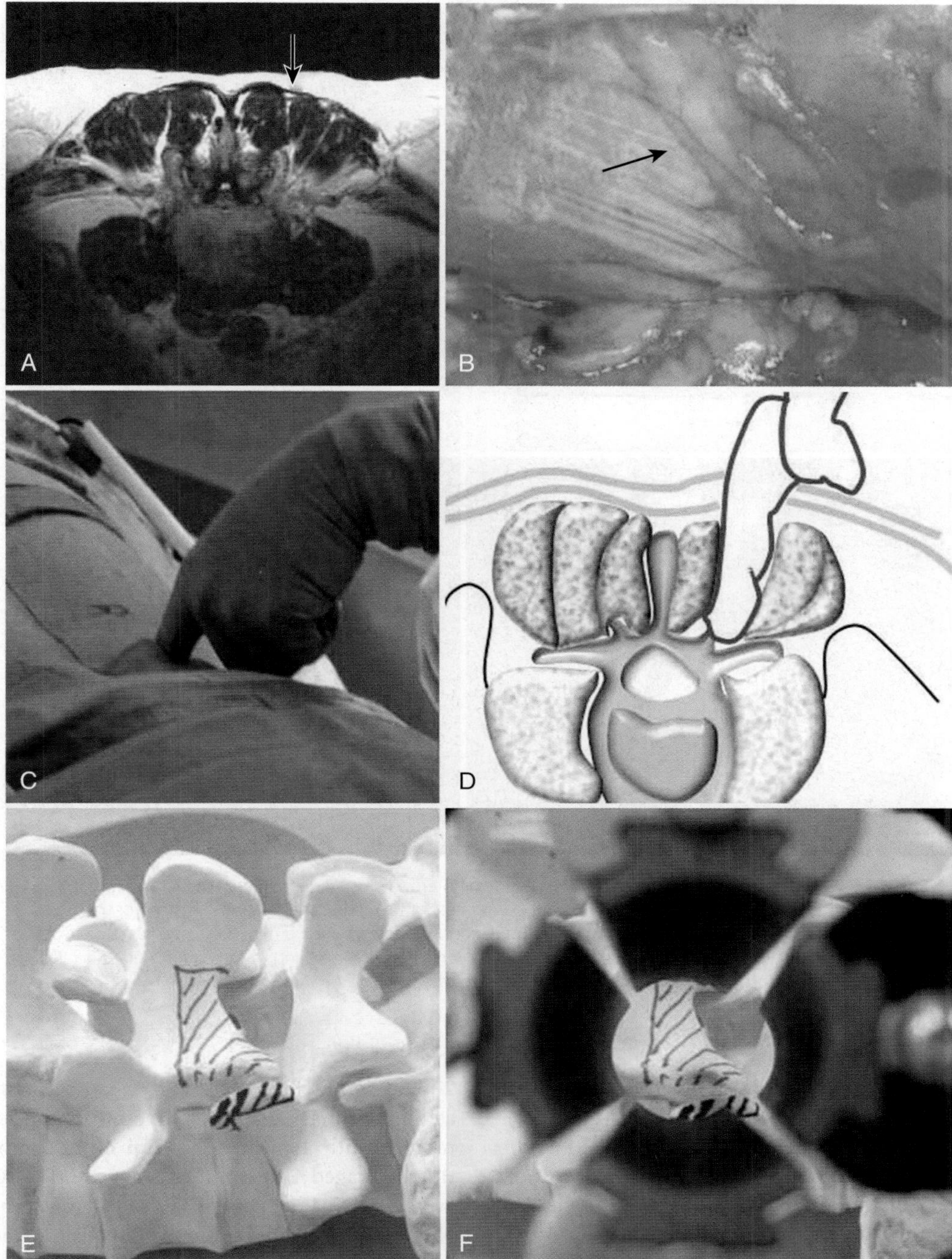

FIG. 54.4 Minimally invasive spine transforaminal lumbar interbody fusion surgical corridor is shown. (A) Magnetic resonance cross-sectional image through the L4–L5 disc space showing the neurovascular plane between the multifidus and longissimus muscles (*arrow*). (B) Intraoperative photomicrograph showing the lateral aspect of the multifidus muscle and the neurovascular bundle (*arrow*). (C) Intraoperative image and (D) corresponding illustration showing the technique of manual blunt dissection to the surgical target site. (E) Image of a spine model with the surgical target site noted (*red and black lines*). (F) View of the surgical target site through a minimally invasive retractor.

recess is more accessible through a contralateral approach when using the unilateral approach. In a preliminary study of four patients and seven levels of decompression, the total operating time was 32 minutes per level and the estimated blood loss was 75 mL. The average postoperative stay was 1.2 days. All patients had resolution of neurogenic claudication and there were no complications.[30]

Posterior Lumbar Interbody Fusion

An extension of the minimally invasive hemilaminectomy technique is transforaminal lumbar interbody fusion (MIS TLIF). The unilateral approach is used to perform the analogous decompression and is combined with a complete facetectomy. The surgical corridor is in the neurovascular plane between the multifidus and longissimus muscles (Fig. 54.4). A

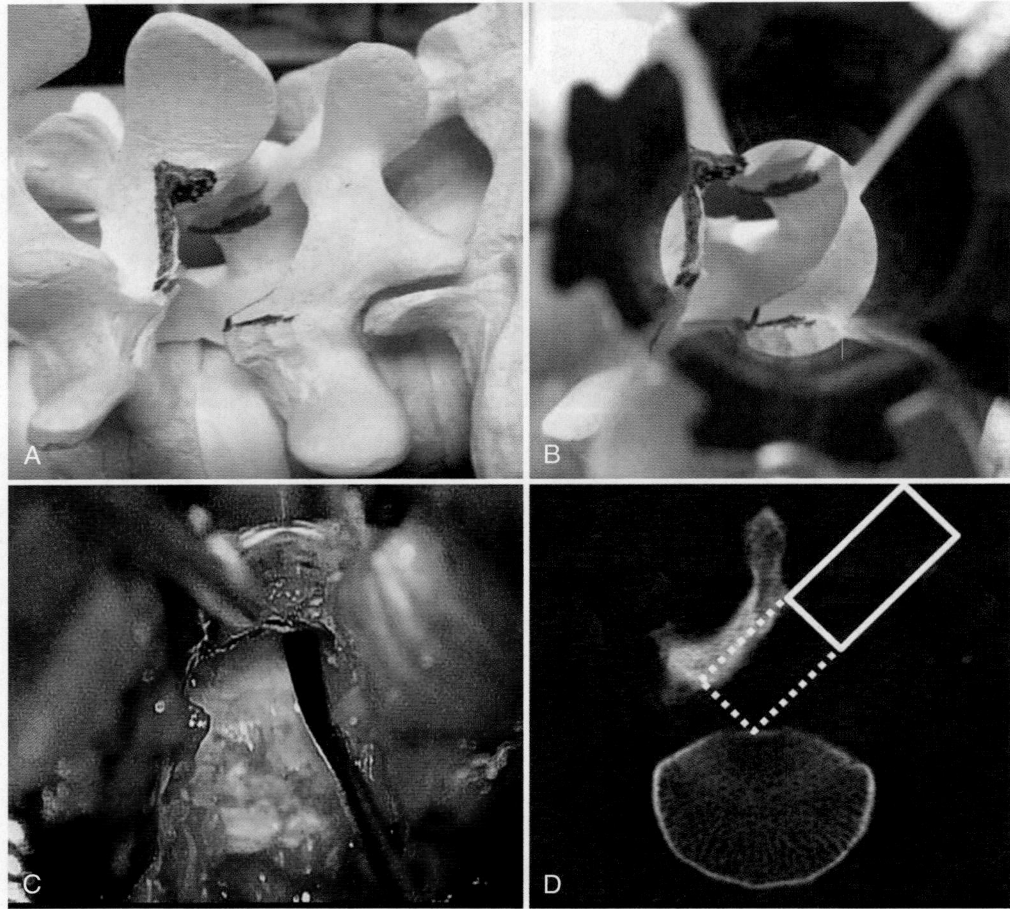

FIG. 54.5 Minimally invasive spine transforaminal lumbar interbody fusion decompression is shown. (A) Image of a spine model with removal of the inferior articular process of the cephalad level and overhang of the superior articular process of the caudad level. (B) Corresponding view through a minimally invasive retractor. (C) Intraoperative photomicrograph of the dural tube with a Penfield probe reaching to the contralateral side. (D) Postoperative computed tomographic scan with overlay of the surgical corridor.

complete facetectomy allows for decompression of the spinal canal from the ipsilateral to the contralateral side (Fig. 54.5). Access to the disc space is through a window bordered medially by the dural tube, proximally by the exiting nerve root, and distally by the pedicle and superior endplate of the caudad vertebra, thus forming within the Kambin triangle (Fig. 54.6). Angled curettes are used to perform a subtotal discectomy from a unilateral approach. If necessary, an osteotome is used to remove the overhanging rim of the posterior vertebral endplate during discectomy. Fusion is performed using interbody spacers that can be placed anteriorly for maximum lordosis correction. A second cage may be inserted by using the smooth trials to push the first cages to the far side of the disc space. Dual cage constructs may be desirable when there is significant osteoporosis or at L5–S1 in a multilevel fusion.

The clinical safety and efficacy of this technique has been well established. Schwender and colleagues[31] reported on 49 patients who underwent MIS TLIF through a paramedian, muscle-sparing approach using an expandable tubular retractor system. Of these patients, 26 patients had degenerative disc disease with herniated nucleus pulposus, 22 had spondylolisthesis, and 1 had a Chance-type fracture as their primary diagnosis. The minimum follow-up was 18 months with a mean follow-up of 22.6 months. Operative time averaged 240 minutes (range, 110–310 minutes), and average estimated blood loss was 140 mL (range, 50–450 mL). No patients required a blood transfusion, and there were no intraoperative complications. Length of hospital stay was 1.9 days on average (range, 1–4 days). All 45 patients who had preoperative radicular symptoms had resolution of their symptoms. All patients with mechanical low back pain had postoperative improvement of their pain. Four complications were noted postoperatively (two from malpositioned screws, one from graft dislodgement causing new radiculopathy, and the last from radiculopathy caused by contralateral neuroforaminal stenosis). Visual Analog Scale pain scores improved from 7.2 to 2.1, and Oswestry Disability Index scores improved from 46% to 14% at last follow-up.

Numerous studies have since confirmed the safety and efficacy of this technique.[32–40] These studies show that MIS TLIF can achieve results comparable with traditional open techniques but with less postoperative pain, decreased blood

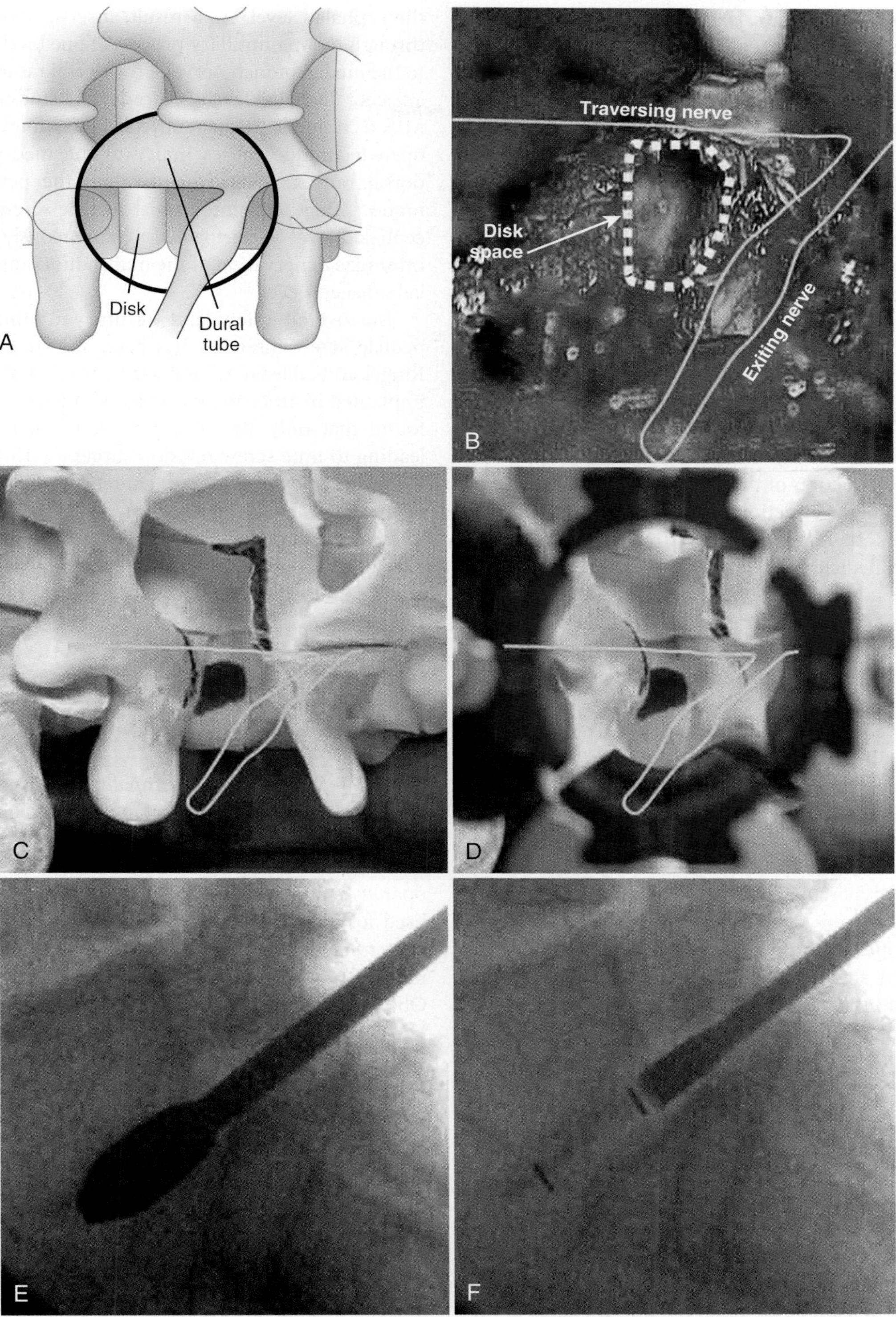

FIG. 54.6 Minimally invasive spine transforaminal lumbar interbody fusion discectomy is shown. (A) Illustration and (B) corresponding photomicrograph of the surgical target site after facetectomy to expose the Kambin triangle, which is bounded medially by the dural tube, proximally by the exiting nerve root, and distally by the pedicle and superior endplate of the caudad vertebra. (C) Image of a spine model after facetectomy. The Kambin triangle is in red. (D) Corresponding view through a minimally invasive retractor. (E) Intraoperative image during discectomy showing a paddle distractor and sizer and (F) during cage insertion.

loss, and shorter hospital stays, particularly when compared with anteroposterior circumferential fusion.[41] Another significant advantage of MIS is the marked decrease in rates of surgical site infections. Several studies show several-fold decreases in deep infection rates with MIS posterior lumbar fusions.[41a-41d] Shorter hospital stay, faster return to work, and decreased rates of reoperations due to infections lead to decreased overall cost of care.[41d-41h] The long-term benefits of minimally invasive fusion techniques have yet to be elucidated. It is intriguing to consider that preservation of the osseomusculotendinous complex may provide dynamic stability to the adjacent segments and provide some degree of protection from adjacent-segment disease.[41i,41j]

Percutaneous Pedicle Screw Instrumentation

Insertion of pedicle screws through a midline approach requires massive retraction of the multifidus muscle, subjecting the muscle to high retraction pressures and disruption of its osseotendinous attachments and neurovascular supply. The rationale for MIS pedicle screw insertion lies in the preservation of multifidus muscle function. Pedicle screw insertion can be performed percutaneously or via a paramedian mini-open technique. With the percutaneous technique, the pedicle is entered using a Jamshidi-type trocar needle under fluoroscopic control (Fig. 54.7). Once the needles are within the pedicle, the stylets are removed and guidewires inserted. The guidewire is then used to direct cannulated taps and screws into the pedicle (Fig. 54.8). Sequential soft tissue dilators are used to create a path for the tap and screw. The outermost dilator can be used as a protective sleeve during pedicle tapping. A cannulated pedicle screw is then placed over the guidewire. Rods are inserted percutaneously to minimize soft tissue trauma.

In the mini-open technique, a longitudinal, paramedian incision is placed slightly lateral to the lateral edge of the pedicles. Dissection is performed through the intermuscular plane between the multifidus and longissimus muscles. A tubular retractor system is subsequently deployed after tissue dilation is performed. The pars interarticularis and the mammillary processes of the cephalad and caudal levels are exposed with gentle electrocautery. A high-speed burr to create a starting point and pedicle probes are used to enter the pedicle. Cannulated or noncannulated pedicle screws can be used with this technique. The exposure allows for decortication of the pars, facet joint, and transverse processes for bone grafting and fusion. A standard rod and end caps can then be placed.

The mini-open technique offers several advantages over the percutaneous method. It allows for direct visualization of the anatomy and the choice of using either cannulated or noncannulated pedicle screw systems. The mini-open technique also allows for greater access for bone grafting posteriorly. On the other hand, the mini-open technique threatens the medial branch of the dorsal rami, which extends downward to the transverse process of the caudal level, where it passes between the mammillary and accessory processes. It then curves posteriorly, where it branches to supply the multifidus muscle, the intertransverse muscles and ligaments, and the facet joint of the cephalad level. As a result, insertion of a pedicle screw through the mammillary process at one level can cause injury to the medial branch nerve of the dorsal rami that supplies the adjacent cephalad level. In a cadaveric study comparing these MIS techniques, Regev and colleagues found that the mini-open technique causes injury to the medial branch of the dorsal rami more frequently than the percutaneous technique.[42] They recommend that pedicle screw insertion at the cephalad level be performed percutaneously if one desires to minimize denervation of the multifidus complex at the cephalad adjacent level.

The overall safety and accuracy of minimally invasive pedicle screw insertion has been shown in several studies. Ringel and colleagues[43] assessed a total of 488 pedicle screws implanted in 103 patients via a percutaneous technique. They found that only 3% of screws were rated as unacceptable, leading to nine screw revision surgeries. These results mirror a growing body of evidence that reflects the safety and efficacy of minimally invasive posterior spinal instrumentation.[31,44,45] These results are comparable with pedicle screws inserted via a traditional open approach. In a meta-analysis of 130 studies and 37,337 pedicle screws placed, the overall screw accuracy was 91.3%.[46]

Limitations and Drawbacks

Radiation Exposure

Several techniques for minimally invasive posterior screw insertion exist, but the percutaneous pedicle screw technique is the least tissue disruptive and is currently adapted for single or multilevel fusions. Its use, however, depends on intraoperative fluoroscopy. In the past, fluoroscopy was mainly used for lateral fluoroscopic pedicle screw guidance in open surgery. However, multiplanar fluoroscopic techniques are necessary for minimally invasive spinal instrumentation. Obtaining multiple views in several planes increases accuracy but increases operating times. The operative time for two screws on the same vertebra level reaches 10 minutes or longer using advanced fluoroscopic techniques, whereas lateral-only fluoroscopic methods require less than 5 minutes per level.[47–49] With increased insertion times associated with advanced fluoroscopic guidance, the cumulative exposure to radiation increased concomitantly.

Studies have shown that fluoroscopically guided pedicle screw placement exposes surgeons to 10 to 12 times the dose of radiation required when compared with nonspinal musculoskeletal procedures.[50] Despite these concerns, the convenience of the C-arm, combined with a high degree of accuracy, has made intraoperative fluoroscopy an increasingly necessary part of advanced spinal surgery. The addition of navigation technology is a promising means of decreasing radiation exposure to the surgical team. Kim and colleagues[51] showed that the use of navigation-assisted fluoroscopy for MIS TLIF markedly decreases direct exposure to radiation. In addition to reducing radiation exposure, navigation eliminates the need for cumbersome protective lead gear and clears the surgical field by removing the C-arm during surgery.

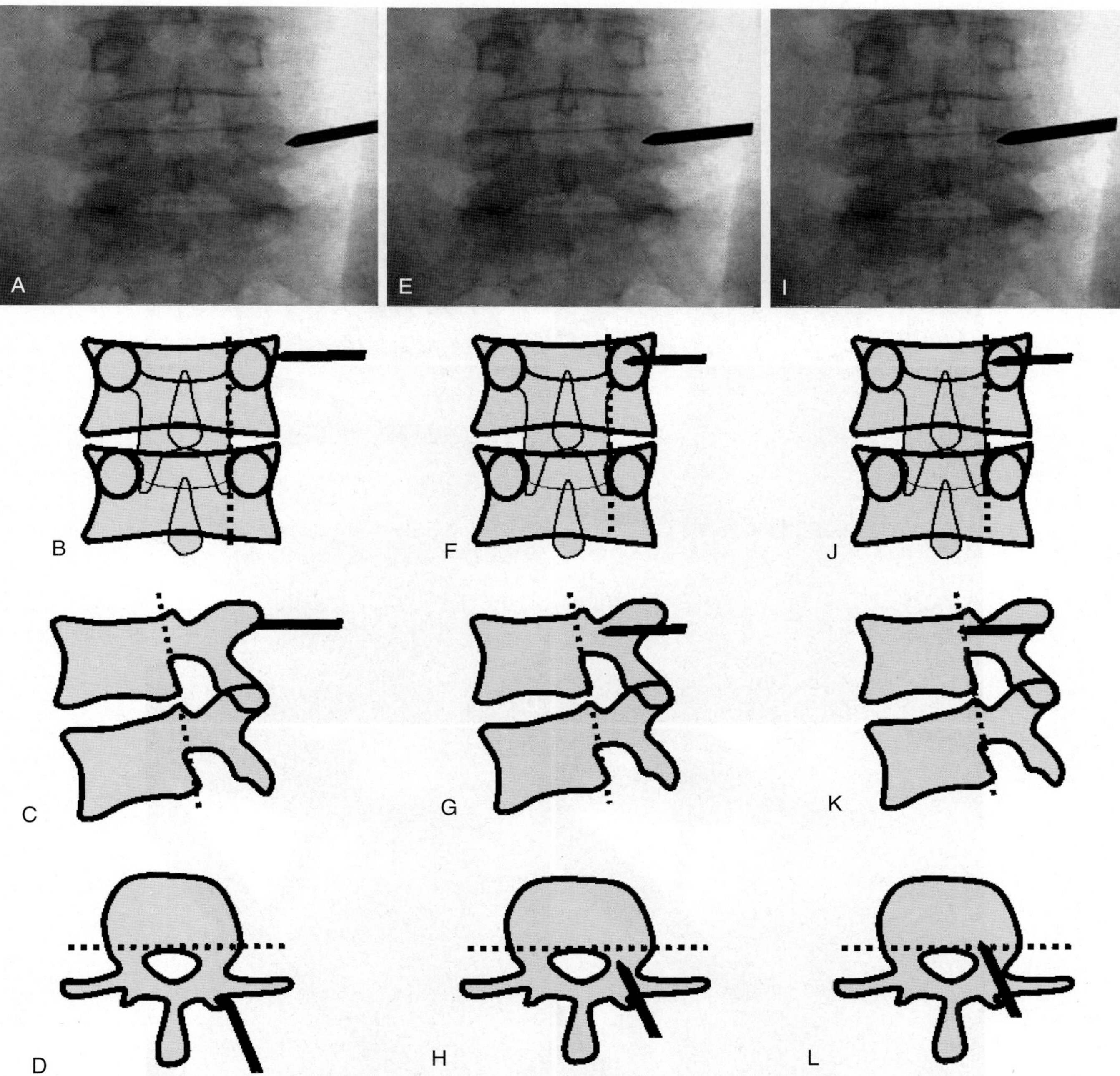

FIG. 54.7 Percutaneous pedicle screw insertion requires scrupulous intraoperative imaging. (A, E, I) The trocar needle is inserted using a perfect en face anteroposterior image of the pedicle. The endplates should be flat and the top of the pedicle is in line with the superior endplate. The needle is inserted from a lateral to medial direction until the tip reaches the medial border of the pedicle (I and J). The C-arm is then brought under the table for a lateral view (B, F, J). If the needle is correctly inserted into the pedicle, the tip should be past the posterior vertebral body line (K and L). (A–D) Initial position of the needle in the anteroposterior, lateral, and axial planes, respectively. (E–H) Needle halfway across the pedicle. (I–L) Needle at the medial border of the pedicle. Once past the posterior vertebral body line, the needle can be inserted another 5 mm in preparation for insertion of the guidewire.

Learning Curve for Minimally Invasive Spinal Surgery

The barriers to widespread adoption of minimally invasive techniques appear to be related to technical difficulties of the procedures and a lack of adequate training opportunities. In a survey of spinal surgeons, Webb and colleagues[52] showed that most surgeons perceive MIS to be efficacious and want to perform more MIS procedures. However, most have not pursued MIS surgery because of concerns with technical difficulties of the procedure and a lack of adequate training opportunities. The technical difficulty of the procedure, combined with inadequate training, is evident in initial studies of MIS surgery. Nowitzke evaluated the learning curve for tubular decompression and

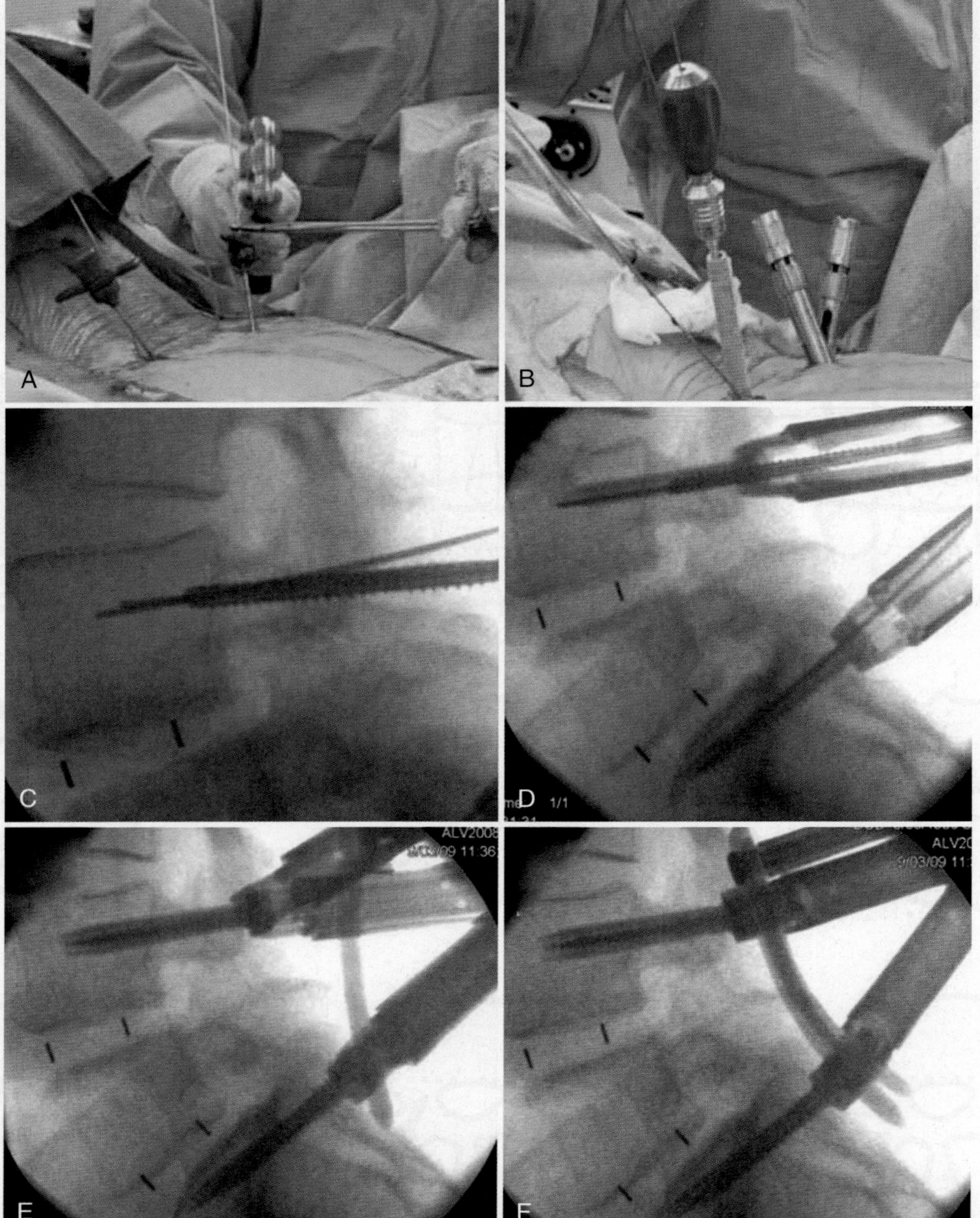

FIG. 54.8 Percutaneous pedicle screw insertion uses guidewires to guide the taps and screws through the pedicle and into the vertebral body in a reliable manner. (A) Once the Jamshidi needle is safely passed through the pedicle and into the vertebral body, the inner stylet is removed and the guidewire inserted. (B) The cannula is then removed and soft tissues opened with serial dilators. (C) The tap is then passed over the guidewire and into the dilator sleeves, which is monitored on a lateral fluoroscopic image. It is critical to maintain control of the guidewire to avoid inadvertent advancement into the abdominal cavity. (D) After tapping, cannulated pedicle screws with extension sleeves are inserted over the guidewire. Again, a lateral image is used to monitor the guidewire and to insert the tulips to a consistent depth. (E) Once all the screws are in place, a contoured rod is inserted under the dorsolumbar fascia and through the rod sleeves. (F) The rod sleeves are then used to reduce the rod to the tulips and insert the locking caps.

noted that 3 of the first 7 but none of the subsequent 28 cases required conversion to open surgery.[53] Villavicencio and colleagues[41] noted a higher rate of overall perioperative complications, Dhall and colleagues[54] found a higher rate of instrumentation complications, and Peng and colleagues[55] noted longer operative times when comparing MIS TLIF versus open TLIF. However, it is important to note that a better understanding of the learning curve may decrease the complication rates associated with initial adoption of MIS techniques.[56]

Summary

The posterior spine is dynamically stabilized by a diverse group of muscles that lie in close proximity to the vertebral column. These muscles possess a single tendon origin at the spine process and multiple tendon insertion sites distally along the superior articular processes. Each of these muscles possesses unique anatomic and structural characteristics that reflect their primary role. The multifidus muscles are made up of short and powerful fibers that enable them to produce large forces over short distances, making them a powerful stabilizer. Traditional posterior midline open approaches disrupt the function of these muscles through tendon detachment, devascularization, and crush injury. Currently, minimally invasive techniques use surgical approaches in which these events are minimized. Paramedian incisions avoid detachment of the multifidus tendon origin. Table-mounted, tubular retractors minimize retraction pressure. Specialized surgical instruments and implants accommodate narrow surgical corridors. The short-term results of these techniques are well demonstrated in multiple studies. The long-term effects of minimally invasive posterior spinal surgery are not yet known, but it is anticipated that maintaining muscle function will have effects on future events such as adjacent-level degeneration and level of function.

PEARLS

1. Ensure adequate preparation and training for all MIS procedures by performing the entire procedure, skin to skin, on a cadaveric specimen.
2. Use intraoperative imaging to precisely position the retractor directly in line with the intended surgical corridor.
3. Avoid the temptation to excessively open the retractor because this leads to additional muscle creep that further obscures the surgical target site.
4. Use instruments specifically designed for MIS procedures that are properly angled and bayoneted for use down a long, narrow surgical corridor.
5. Consider the use of expandable tubular retractors that contain a gap between the blades to allow increased angulation of instruments.

PITFALLS

1. MIS procedures are reliant on fluoroscopic imaging, which can lead to excessive radiation exposure to the surgical team. Proper protective wear should include not only a lead gown but also a thyroid shield and protective eyewear. Strong consideration should be given to use of protective gloves.
2. Unintentional durotomies more often occur in patients with severe stenosis and facet cysts. Meticulous release of the tissue adherent to the dural tube before use of the Kerrison rongeur decreases this risk.
3. Insertion of an interbody cage during MIS TLIF procedures endangers the exiting nerve root. Care should be taken to maintain the pars interarticularis, which serves to protect the nerve during cage insertion. Similarly, the dural tube should be adequately released and decompressed to allow the traversing nerve root to move out of the path of the cage during insertion.

SECTION VII

KEY POINTS

1. The posterior paraspinal musculature, particularly the multifidus muscle, provides a critical dynamic stabilizing function.
2. Prevention of multifidus muscle injury is the main concept in minimally invasive posterior lumbar surgery.
3. Multifidus muscle injury can occur by detachment of the tendon origin at the spinous process.
4. Table-mounted, tubular retractors minimize muscle crush injury by maximizing the surface area of the retractor and avoiding the prolonged elevated retraction pressures associated with self-retaining retractors.
5. Minimally invasive posterior lumbar techniques remain technically demanding, leading to higher complication rates and longer operative times during the early period of the learning curve.
6. A difficult learning curve demands that surgeons have sufficient preclinical training and that education is obtained before the application of MIS surgery in clinical practice.
7. Meticulous use of fluoroscopic imaging is required to prevent instrumentation-related complications.

KEY REFERENCES

1. Stevens KJ, Spenciner DB, Griffiths KL, et al. Comparison of minimally invasive and conventional open posterolateral lumbar fusion using magnetic resonance imaging and retraction pressure studies. *J Spinal Disord Tech*. 2006;19:77-86.
   Cadaveric studies of muscle compartment pressures combined with a clinical study using specialized postoperative MR imaging show that minimally invasive tubular retractors minimize retraction pressure and subsequent muscle injury during minimally invasive posterior lumbar approaches.
2. Foley KT, Gupta SK. Percutaneous pedicle screw fixation of the lumbar spine: preliminary clinical results. *J Neurosurg*. 2002;97:7-12.
   The fundamental basis for percutaneous pedicle screw insertion and percutaneous rod delivery using screw extension sleeves is described.
3. Schwender JD, Holly LT, Rouben DP, et al. Minimally invasive transforaminal lumbar interbody fusion (TLIF): technical feasibility and initial results. *J Spinal Disord Tech*. 2005;18(suppl):S1-S6.
   The most commonly used and accepted technique for minimally invasive transforaminal lumbar interbody fusion is described, along with the results that have been commonly found in subsequent studies.
4. Peng CW, Yue WM, Poh SY, et al. Clinical and radiological outcomes of minimally invasive versus open transforaminal lumbar interbody fusion. *Spine*. 2009;34:1385-1389.
   This prospective study of 29 MIS TLIF and 29 open TLIF patients with at least 2-year follow-up shows that the MIS technique is associated with less blood loss, shorter hospital stay, and lower narcotic needs but has similar clinical results in terms of fusion rates, pain relief, and quality-of-life scores.

5. Parker SL, Adogwa O, Witham TF, et al. Post-operative infection after minimally invasive versus open transforaminal lumbar interbody fusion (TLIF): literature review and cost analysis. *Minim Invasive Neurosurg.* 2011;54:33-37.
This is a systematic review showing a greater than 6-fold decrease in postoperative infection rates after MIS vs. open TLIF (0.6% vs. 4.0%, respectively).

REFERENCES

1. Cholewicki J, Panjabi MM, Khachatryan A. Stabilizing function of trunk flexor-extensor muscles around a neutral spine posture. *Spine.* 1997;22:2207-2212.
2. Gejo R, Kawaguchi Y, Kondoh T, et al. Magnetic resonance imaging and histologic evidence of postoperative back muscle injury in rats. *Spine.* 2000;25:941-946.
3. Gille O, Jolivet E, Dousset V, et al. Erector spinae muscle changes on magnetic resonance imaging following lumbar surgery through a posterior approach. *Spine.* 2007;32:1236-1241.
4. Datta G, Gnanalingham KK, Peterson D, et al. Back pain and disability after lumbar laminectomy: is there a relationship to muscle retraction? *Neurosurgery.* 2004;54:1413-1420.
5. Gejo R, Matsui H, Kawaguchi Y, et al. Serial changes in trunk muscle performance after posterior lumbar surgery. *Spine.* 1999;24:1023-1028.
6. Hyun SJ, Kim YB, Kim YS, et al. Postoperative changes in paraspinal muscle volume: comparison between paramedian interfascial and midline approaches for lumbar fusion. *J Korean Med Sci.* 2007;22:646-651.
7. Kawaguchi Y, Matsui H, Gejo R, et al. Preventive measures of back muscle injury after posterior lumbar spine surgery in rats. *Spine.* 1998;23:2282-2287.
8. Mayer TG, Vanharanta H, Gatchel RJ, et al. Comparison of CT scan muscle measurements and isokinetic trunk strength in postoperative patients. *Spine.* 1989;14:33-36.
9. Motosuneya T, Asazuma T, Tsuji T, et al. Postoperative change of the cross-sectional area of back musculature after 5 surgical procedures as assessed by magnetic resonance imaging. *J Spinal Disord Tech.* 2006;19:318-322.
10. Rantanen J, Hurme M, Falck B, et al. The lumbar multifidus muscle five years after surgery for a lumbar intervertebral disc herniation. *Spine.* 1993;18:568-574.
11. Granata KP, Marras WS. An EMG-assisted model of loads on the lumbar spine during asymmetric trunk extensions. *J Biomech.* 1993;26:1429-1438.
12. Marras WS, Davis KG, et al. Trunk muscle activities during asymmetric twisting motions. *J Electromyogr Kinesiol.* 1998;8:247-256.
13. Perez-Cruet MJ, Foley KT, Isaacs RE, et al. Microendoscopic lumbar discectomy: technical note. *Neurosurgery.* 2002;51:S129-S136.
14. Stevens KJ, Spenciner DB, Griffiths KL, et al. Comparison of minimally invasive and conventional open posterolateral lumbar fusion using magnetic resonance imaging and retraction pressure studies. *J Spinal Disord Tech.* 2006;19:77-86.
15. Arts MP, Brand R, van den Akker ME, et al. Tubular diskectomy vs conventional microdiskectomy for sciatica: a randomized controlled trial. *JAMA.* 2009;302:149-158.
16. Ryang YM, Oertel MF, Mayfrank L, et al. Standard open microdiscectomy versus minimal access trocar microdiscectomy: results of a prospective randomized study. *Neurosurgery.* 2008;62:174-181.
17. Righesso O, Falavigna A, Avanzi O. Comparison of open discectomy with microendoscopic discectomy in lumbar disc herniations: results of a randomized controlled trial. *Neurosurgery.* 2007;61:545-549.

17a. Dasenbrock HH, Juraschek SP, Schultz LR, et al. The efficacy of minimally invasive discectomy compared with open discectomy: a meta-analysis of prospective randomized controlled trials. *J Neurosurg Spine.* 2012;16:452-462.

18. Weiner BK, Walker M, Brower RS, et al. Microdecompression for lumbar spinal canal stenosis. *Spine.* 1999;24:2268-2272.
19. Palmer S, Turner R, Palmer R. Bilateral decompressive surgery in lumbar spinal stenosis associated with spondylolisthesis: unilateral approach and use of a microscope and tubular retractor system. *Neurosurg Focus.* 2002;13:E4.
20. Palmer S, Turner R, Palmer R. Bilateral decompression of lumbar spinal stenosis involving a unilateral approach with microscope and tubular retractor system. *J Neurosurg.* 2002;97:213-217.
21. Costa F, Sassi M, Cardia A, et al. Degenerative lumbar spinal stenosis: analysis of results in a series of 374 patients treated with unilateral laminotomy for bilateral microdecompression. *J Neurosurg Spine.* 2007;7:579-586.
22. Iwatsuki K, Yoshimine T, Aoki M. Bilateral interlaminar fenestration and unroofing for the decompression of nerve roots by using a unilateral approach in lumbar canal stenosis. *Surg Neurol.* 2007;68:487-492.
23. Khoo LT, Fessler RG. Microendoscopic decompressive laminotomy for the treatment of lumbar stenosis. *Neurosurgery.* 2002;51:S146-S154.
24. Rahman M, Summers LE, Richter B, et al. Comparison of techniques for decompressive lumbar laminectomy: the minimally invasive versus the "classic" open approach. *Minim Invasive Neurosurg.* 2008;51:100-105.
25. Asgarzadie F, Khoo LT. Minimally invasive operative management for lumbar spinal stenosis: overview of early and long-term outcomes. *Orthop Clin North Am.* 2007;38:387-399.
26. Ikuta K, Tono O, Tanaka T, et al. Surgical complications of microendoscopic procedures for lumbar spinal stenosis. *Minim Invasive Neurosurg.* 2007;50:145-149.
27. Podichetty VK, Spears J, Isaacs RE, et al. Complications associated with minimally invasive decompression for lumbar spinal stenosis. *J Spinal Disord Tech.* 2006;19:161-166.
28. Rosen DS, O'Toole JE, Eichholz KM, et al. Minimally invasive lumbar spinal decompression in the elderly: outcomes of 50 patients aged 75 years and older. *Neurosurgery.* 2007;60:503-509.
29. Sasaki M, Abekura M, Morris S, et al. Microscopic bilateral decompression through unilateral laminotomy for lumbar canal stenosis in patients undergoing hemodialysis. *J Neurosurg Spine.* 2006;5:494-499.
30. Regev G, Taylor W, Garfin SR, et al.: *The Use of Concurrent Bilateral Minimally Invasive Approach for Central and Neuroforaminal Spinal Decompression.* Poster Presentation at 2008 Annual Meeting of the Society for Minimally Invasive Spine Surgery, San Diego, 2008.
31. Schwender JD, Holly LT, Rouben DP, et al. Minimally invasive transforaminal lumbar interbody fusion (TLIF): technical feasibility and initial results. *J Spinal Disord Tech.* 2005;18(suppl):S1-S6.
32. Anand N, Hamilton JF, Perri B, et al. Cantilever TLIF with structural allograft and RhBMP2 for correction and maintenance of segmental sagittal lordosis: long-term clinical, radiographic, and functional outcome. *Spine.* 2006;31:E748-E753.

33. Deutsch H, Musacchio MJ Jr. Minimally invasive transforaminal lumbar interbody fusion with unilateral pedicle screw fixation. *Neurosurg Focus*. 2006;20:E10.
34. Isaacs RE, Podichetty VK, Santiago P, et al. Minimally invasive microendoscopy-assisted transforaminal lumbar interbody fusion with instrumentation. *J Neurosurg Spine*. 2005;3:98-105.
35. Joseph V, Rampersaud YR. Heterotopic bone formation with the use of rhBMP2 in posterior minimal access interbody fusion: a CT analysis. *Spine*. 2007;32:2885-2890.
36. Park Y, Ha JW. Comparison of one-level posterior lumbar interbody fusion performed with a minimally invasive approach or a traditional open approach. *Spine*. 2007;32: 537-543.
37. Salerni AA. A minimally invasive approach for posterior lumbar interbody fusion. *Neurosurg Focus*. 2002;13:e6.
38. Selznick LA, Shamji MF, Isaacs RE. Minimally invasive interbody fusion for revision lumbar surgery: technical feasibility and safety. *J Spinal Disord Tech*. 2009;22:207-213.
39. Sethi A, Lee S, Vaidya R. Transforaminal lumbar interbody fusion using unilateral pedicle screws and a translaminar screw. *Eur Spine J*. 2009;18:430-434.
40. Shen FH, Samartzis D, Khanna AJ, Anderson DG. Minimally invasive techniques for lumbar interbody fusions. *Orthop Clin North Am*. 2007;38:373-386.
41. Villavicencio AT, Burneikiene S, Bulsara KR, et al. Perioperative complications in transforaminal lumbar interbody fusion versus anterior-posterior reconstruction for lumbar disc degeneration and instability. *J Spinal Disord Tech*. 2006;19:92-97.
41a. Wong AP, Smith ZA, Nixon AT, et al. Intraoperative and perioperative complications in minimally invasive transforaminal lumbar interbody fusion: a review of 513 patients. *J Neurosurg Spine*. 2015;22:487-495.
41b. McAfee PC, Garfin SR, Rodgers WB, et al. An attempt at clinically defining and assessing minimally invasive surgery compared with traditional "open" spinal surgery. *SAS J*. 2011;5:125-130.
41c. Smith JS, Shaffrey CI, Sansur CA, et al. Rates of infection after spine surgery based on 108,419 procedures. *Spine*. 2011;36:556-563.
41d. Parker SL, Adogwa O, Witham TF, et al. Post-operative infection after minimally invasive versus open transforaminal lumbar interbody fusion (TLIF): literature review and cost analysis. *Minim Invasive Neurosurg*. 2011;54:33-37.
41e. Pelton MA, Phillips FM, Singh K. A comparison of perioperative costs and outcomes in patients with and without workers' compensation claims treated with minimally invasive or open transforaminal lumbar interbody fusion. *Spine*. 2012;37:1914-1919.
41f. McGirt MJ, Parker SL, Lerner J, et al. Comparative analysis of perioperative surgical site infection after minimally invasive versus open posterior/transforaminal lumbar interbody fusion: analysis of hospital billing and discharge data from 5170 patients. *J Neurosurg Spine*. 2011;14:771-778.
41g. Adogwa O, Parker SL, Bydon A, Cheng J, McGirt MJ. Comparative effectiveness of minimally invasive versus open transforaminal lumbar interbody fusion: 2-year assessment of narcotic use, return to work, disability, and quality of life. *J Spinal Disord Tech*. 2011;24:479-484.
41h. Wang MY, Lerner J, Lesko J, McGirt MJ. Acute hospital costs after minimally invasive versus open lumbar interbody fusion: data from a US national database with 6106 patients. *J Spinal Disord Tech*. 2012;25:324-328.
41i. Yee TJ, Terman SW, La Marca F, Park P. Comparison of adjacent segment disease after minimally invasive or open transforaminal lumbar interbody fusion. *J Clin Neurosci*. 2014;21:1796-1801.
41j. Radcliff KE, Kepler CK, Maaieh M, et al. What is the rate of lumbar adjacent segment disease after percutaneous versus open fusion? *Orthop Surg*. 2014;6:118-120.
42. Regev GJ, Lee YP, Taylor WR, et al. Nerve injury to the posterior rami medial branch during the insertion of pedicle screws: comparison of mini-open versus percutaneous pedicle screw insertion techniques. *Spine*. 2009;34:1239-1242.
43. Ringel F, Stoffel M, Stuer C, et al. Minimally invasive transmuscular pedicle screw fixation of the thoracic and lumbar spine. *Neurosurgery*. 2006;59:ONS361-ONS366.
44. Foley KT, Gupta SK. Percutaneous pedicle screw fixation of the lumbar spine: preliminary clinical results. *J Neurosurg*. 2002;97:7-12.
45. Eck JC, Hodges S, Humphreys SC. Minimally invasive lumbar spinal fusion. *J Am Acad Orthop Surg*. 2007;15:321-329.
46. Kosmopoulos V, Schizas C. Pedicle screw placement accuracy: a meta-analysis. *Spine*. 2007;32:E111-E1120.
47. Merloz P, Troccaz J, Vouaillat H, et al. Fluoroscopy-based navigation system in spine surgery. *Proc Inst Mech Eng H*. 2007;221:813-820.
48. Assaker R, Cinquin P, Cotten A, et al. Image-guided endoscopic spine surgery: Part I. A feasibility study. *Spine*. 2001;26:1705-1710.
49. Assaker R, Reyns N, Pertruzon B, et al. Image-guided endoscopic spine surgery: Part II: clinical applications. *Spine*. 2001;26:1711-1718.
50. Rampersaud YR, Foley KT, Shen AC, et al. Radiation exposure to the spine surgeon during fluoroscopically assisted pedicle screw insertion. *Spine*. 2000;25:2637-2645.
51. Kim CW, Lee YP, Taylor W, et al. Use of navigation-assisted fluoroscopy to decrease radiation exposure during minimally invasive spine surgery. *Spine J*. 2008;8:584-590.
52. Webb J, Gottschalk L, Lee YP, et al. Surgeon perceptions of minimally invasive spine surgery. *SAS J*. 2008;2:62-66.
53. Nowitzke AM. Assessment of the learning curve for lumbar microendoscopic discectomy. *Neurosurgery*. 2005;56: 755-762.
54. Dhall SS, Wang MY, Mummaneni PV. Clinical and radiographic comparison of mini-open transforaminal lumbar interbody fusion with open transforaminal lumbar interbody fusion in 42 patients with long-term follow-up. *J Neurosurg Spine*. 2008;9:560-565.
55. Peng CW, Yue WM, Poh SY, et al. Clinical and radiological outcomes of minimally invasive versus open transforaminal lumbar interbody fusion. *Spine*. 2009;34:1385-1389.
56. Sclafani JA, Kim CW. Complications associated with the initial learning curve of minimally invasive spine surgery: a systematic review. *Clin Orthop Relat Res*. 2014;472:1711-1717.

55 CHAPTER Minimally Invasive Posterior Lumbar Instrumentation

Eiman Shafa
James D. Schwender

Overview

Various surgical fields have been revolutionized by expansion of minimally invasive techniques in the recent past. In spine surgery, minimally invasive surgical (MIS) techniques have evolved to safely allow access to the spine with less collateral damage compared to traditional open surgical approaches. The basic principles and treatment goals are unchanged. The most basic tenet of minimally invasive spine surgery is to perform the same surgery as has traditionally been done open but with less approach-related morbidity and equal or better outcomes. MIS techniques have demonstrated less blood loss, decreased postoperative pain and narcotic demand, shorter hospital stays, earlier mobilization and return to work, lower disability index at 2 years postoperatively, and lower infection rates as compared with open surgical techniques.[1–5,6] However, adoption of minimally invasive lumbar surgery techniques is associated with a prolonged learning curve, initially longer operative times, and higher initial rate of complications.[7] Nonetheless, with increasing popularization of MIS techniques and incorporation in surgical training programs, these practices are progressively utilized successfully in patient care.

The concept of percutaneous spinal fixation was first introduced by Magerl in 1982 for management of thoracolumbar trauma.[8] To decrease the related high risk of pin tract infection and screw loosening, in 1995, Matthews and Long described a technique for percutaneous transpedicular screw fixation connected by a subcutaneous plate.[9] This was both poorly tolerated by the patient due to prominent instrumentation and associated with a high nonunion rate. Today, a variety of different instrumentation systems may be used in posterior-based minimally invasive lumbar spine surgery. These primarily include traditional pedicle screws, percutaneous pedicle screws, facet screws, and cortical screws. Each type of instrumentation has been shown to be safely and effectively used in minimally invasive surgery.

Indications and Contraindications

The indications for minimally invasive posterior spinal instrumentation are similar to traditional open surgery. Minimally invasive posterior spinal fusion with instrumentation has been used safely and effectively to treat instability associated with spondylolisthesis, degenerative disc disease, large or recurrent disc herniations, postlaminectomy instability, degenerative scoliosis, and trauma. Minimally invasive fusion with instrumentation can be performed safely in the revision setting and is often advantageous, as it allows the surgeon to access the spine through a native surgical corridor free of scar tissue.

A number of high-quality studies have shown the harmful effect of open exposure related to muscle detachment, ligamentous disruption, denervation, adjacent facet joint disruption, and prolonged muscle retraction. In all, these events can lead to increased risk of local instability and adjacent-level disease, requiring further surgery. Kim et al.[10] compared open versus percutaneous posterior pedicle screw fixation and found significantly greater cross-sectional area of the multifidus muscle and greater trunk extension strength in the percutaneous posterior fixation cohort. Kim et al.[11] compared conventional open versus mini-open posterior spinal fusion and instrumentation. They reported increased postoperative serum levels of proinflammatory cytokines interleukin (IL)-6 and IL-8 as well as increased serum creatinine kinase and aldolase in cohort undergoing open procedure. Hu et al.[12] have shown the accuracy of postoperative MRI in evaluating multifidus injury and atrophy.

Though there are no absolute contraindications to minimally invasive posterior spinal instrumentation, relative contraindications include high-grade spondylolisthesis (grade 3 or 4) and previous posterior fixation requiring an open approach for removal or extension of instrumentation.

Obesity poses an interesting case for minimally invasive surgical techniques. Obesity (body mass index [BMI] >30) remains a national epidemic, with a prevalence of 35.7% in the United States.[13] Complication rates as high as 36% to 50% have been reported for obese patients undergoing lumbar fusion.[14] Although obesity certainly makes minimally invasive surgery more challenging, it can be done safely and effectively in this population. In obese patients, we have found it helpful to measure the distance from the dorsal aspect of the facet at the level of the intended procedure on the preoperative magnetic resonance imaging (MRI) to help determine the length of retractor needed (Fig. 55.1). This measurement is often a lower

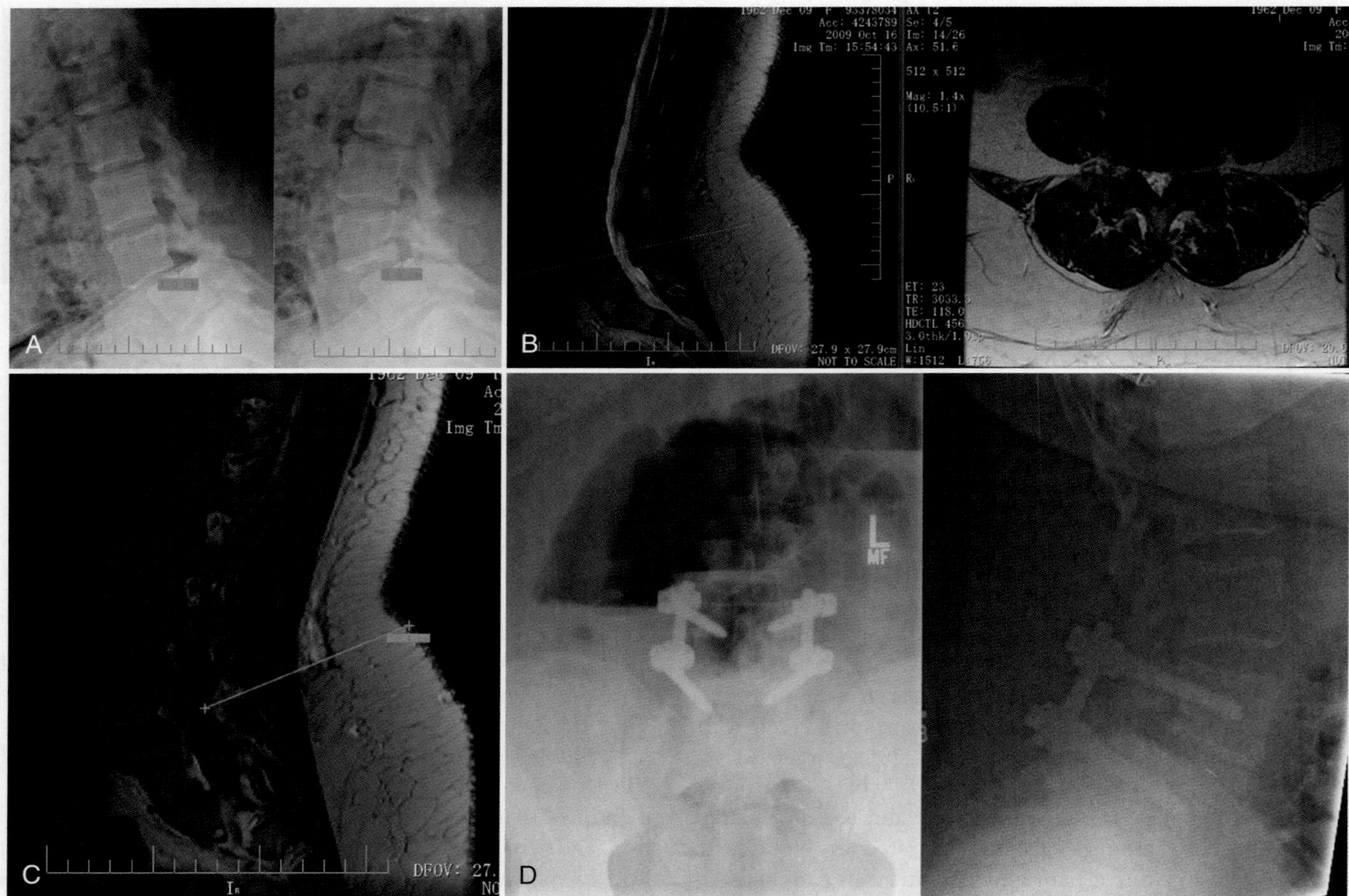

FIG. 55.1 Degenerative spondylolisthesis with body mass index (BMI) >40. A 43-year-old woman (BMI = 41) presented with neurogenic claudication. (A) Flexion-extension radiographs show unstable degenerative spondylolisthesis. (B) Magnetic resonance imaging (MRI) shows bilateral subarticular stenosis and facet arthropathy. (C) The expected length of tubular retractor is measured from the skin edge to the facet joint on axial and sagittal MRI. (D) Postoperative radiographs after minimally invasive transforaminal lumbar interbody fusion, posterior spinal fusion, and decompression at L4–L5. Visual analog scale score: preoperative = 10, postoperative = 1.

estimate, as the patient is lying supine during MRI yet positioned prone for surgery. The surgeon should consider the technical challenges of performing MIS procedures that become progressively demanding as the working depth increases. This is particularly true for fusion surgery. During a surgeon's initial experience with minimally invasive lumbar fusion surgery, patients with an expected retractor length greater than 80 mm are a relative contraindication, particularly early in the learning stages. However, with experience, obesity becomes a relative indication for minimally invasive fusion and instrumentation rather than a contraindication, as tubular retractors and percutaneous techniques drastically minimize surgical exposure in obese patients where adipose tissue and the deep (often thick) musculature make traditional open techniques difficult. Our personal experience has found that pedicle screws often can be placed more easily through a minimally invasive Wiltse-type approach as compared with midline approaches because there is much less muscle, fat, and soft tissue retraction necessary to obtain the correct screw trajectory.

Minimally invasive lumbar surgery in obese patients also creates less postoperative dead space, which may lead to lower infection rates. O'Toole and colleagues[15] reviewed surgical site infections in MIS decompressions, discectomy, and fusion cases. A total of 1338 cases were included for the review. Three postoperative surgical site infections were identified. Two patients developed superficial cellulitis after minimally invasive fusions and one patient developed discitis after a microendoscopic discectomy. The reported surgical site infection rate for simple decompressive procedures was 0.1% and 0.74% for fusion with internal fixation. The overall infection rate for the entire cohort was 0.22%. The reported infection rate for minimally invasive fusion compares favorably with open fusion infection rates. Importantly, there were no cases of postoperative deep wound infection in O'Toole and colleagues' cohort. The one patient with discitis developed symptoms 1 month after developing a lower extremity cellulitis. The disc space biopsy grew the same organism as the cellulitis. No patient in their series required reoperation for a deep wound infection. In contrast, Picada and colleagues[16] reported a 3.2%

deep wound infection after reviewing 817 patients who underwent an open lumbosacral fusion.

Technical Outcomes of Transpedicular Lumbar Instrumentation

The goal of lumbar instrumentation is to provide stability required to improve the rate of spinal fusion. Pedicle screws engage all three anatomic columns of the vertebra as defined by Denis.[17] This biomechanical advantage allows the need for fewer instrumented levels, early postoperative mobilization, and obviates the need for casting or rigid orthoses.

Lonstein et al. reviewed their experience with pedicle screw instrumentation over a 10-year period.[18] Of the 4790 pedicle screws reviewed, 94.9% were placed fully within the pedicle and vertebral body. Only 0.2% were associated with nerve root irritation due to improper screw placement. Overall, they concluded that with attention to technical details of the operative technique, there were few complications with use of pedicle screws. In a more recent review, Parker et al.[19] revisited pedicle screw placement accuracy. In a review of 6816 consecutively placed pedicle screws, they found a 0.9% rate of pedicle breach. These findings suggest pedicle screw placement to be a safe procedure with low rates of complications due to misplacement, which can certainly still occur even with experience and routine use.

Traditional ("Mini-Open") Pedicle Screws

Minimally invasive fusions use the surgical corridor as described by Wiltse[20] between the multifidus and longissimus paraspinal muscles (Fig. 55.2). This trajectory is ideal for pedicle screw placement as well as decompression and disc space preparation if required for fusion. Anatomic localization can be done using standard fluoroscopy and a radiographic marker placed on the skin.

After the appropriate trajectory is localized with fluoroscopy, sequential dilators are passed through the fascia and docked onto the facet joint. A tubular retractor (typically 20 or 22 mm) is then docked and secured over the dilators. The use of an expandable retractor allows the blades to expand cephalad or caudad, creating a corridor for pedicle screw placement (Fig. 55.3). Soft tissue is cleared to expose the standard pedicle screw entry points (Fig. 55.4). Screws can be placed using a variety of methods—including freehand, under C-arm guidance, or using navigation—depending on surgeon preference. In addition, both posted- and tulip-style screws can be used if working through the tubular retractor systems that are available.

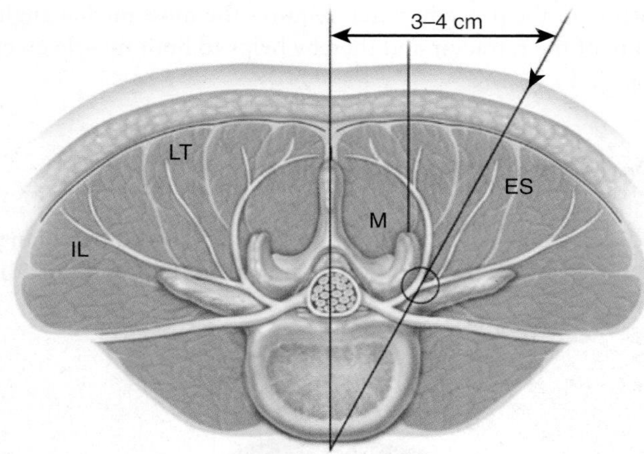

FIG. 55.2 Wiltse approach. ES, erector spinae; IL, iliocostalis lumborum; LT, longissimus; M, multifidus.

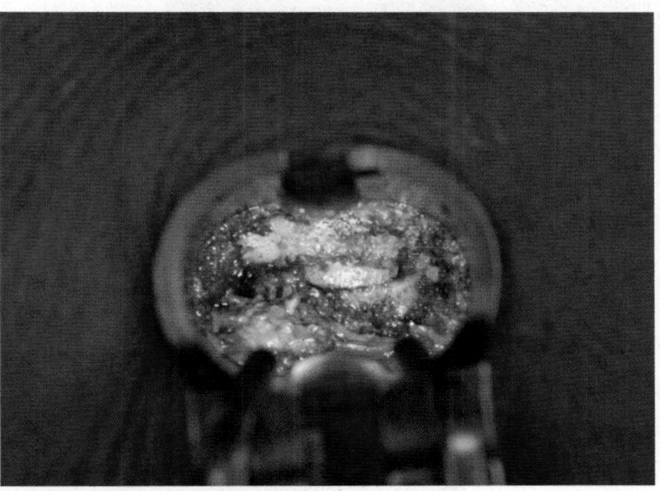

FIG. 55.3 Tubular retractor docked on desired facet and expanded.

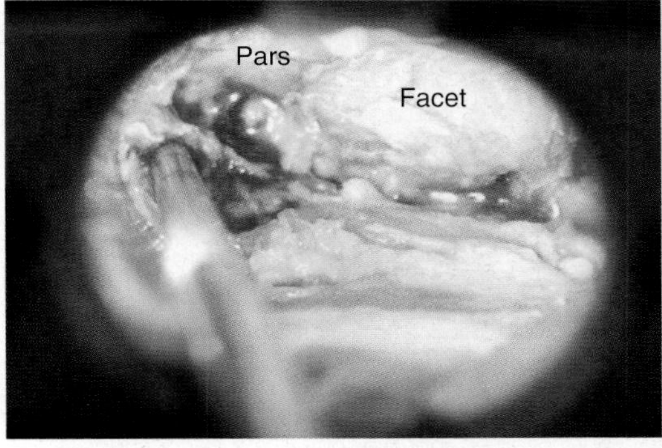

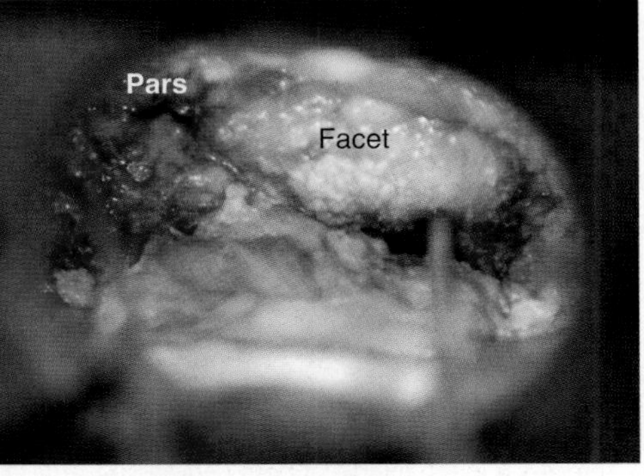

FIG. 55.4 Pedicle screw entry sites visualized through a tubular retractor.

Surgeon preference dictates the sequence of steps when planning for minimally invasive fusion. Early on in a surgeon's experience, it may be easiest to place the pedicle screw tracts first, before the decompression or facetectomy. This will preserve "normal" anatomy to help orient the surgeon to the anatomic starting points. However, our experience has shown that it is more efficient to perform the decompression and interbody spacer placement before screw tract preparation if required. This minimizes the surgical exposure during the portion of the procedure that requires the most medial angulation of the retractor and thereby helps to limit muscle creep (Fig. 55.5).

Percutaneous Pedicle Screws

Pedicle screws can be safely and effectively placed percutaneously to avoid the additional dissection required for the placement of traditional pedicle screws. Percutaneous pedicle screw placement has the advantage of less muscle injury and less potential damage to the medial branch nerve (innervation of the multifidus), and it can be used effectively over long segment fusions.[10,21] The placement of percutaneous pedicle screws can require more operative time and more radiation exposure for accurate placement.

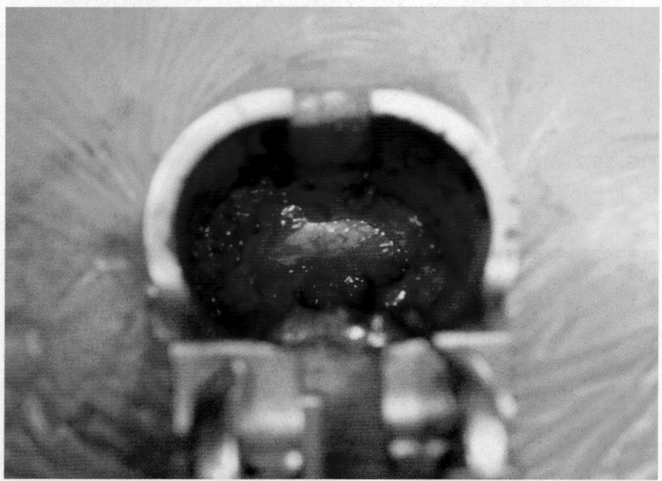

FIG. 55.5 Visualization of dura and transforaminal lumbar interbody fusion discectomy through a tubular retractor.

Technique of Percutaneous Pedicle Screw Placement

We prefer to place percutaneous pedicle screws using fluoroscopy as it is readily available, though navigation technology is becoming more widely accessible. The orientation of the C-arm beam is of critical importance. The anteroposterior (AP) images must be true AP images of each pedicle for which the surgeon is planning screw placement (Fig. 55.6). The spinous process should be in the midline of the vertebral body, equally spaced between both pedicles. The superior and inferior endplates should be parallel, and the pedicles should be appropriately located at the caudal end of the ascending articular process. On the lateral view, the superior endplate should appear as one line and the pedicles should overlap and thus appear as one. True AP and lateral radiographs are of critical importance because a small variance can produce a large degree of error.

The pedicle of interest is localized using the AP fluoroscopic image. The skin is incised just lateral to the lateral pedicle border. The thoracolumbar dorsal fascia and muscle fascia are incised in line with the skin incision. A Jamshidi trocar is used to cannulate the pedicle. The ideal starting point is at the 10 and 2 o'clock positions on the left and right pedicles, respectively. The Jamshidi trocar is slowly advanced a few millimeters to gain purchase in bone. A lateral fluoroscopic image is obtained and should confirm that the trocar is placed within the center of the pedicle. Under AP fluoroscopic imaging, the trocar is advanced approximately 20 mm. The tip should

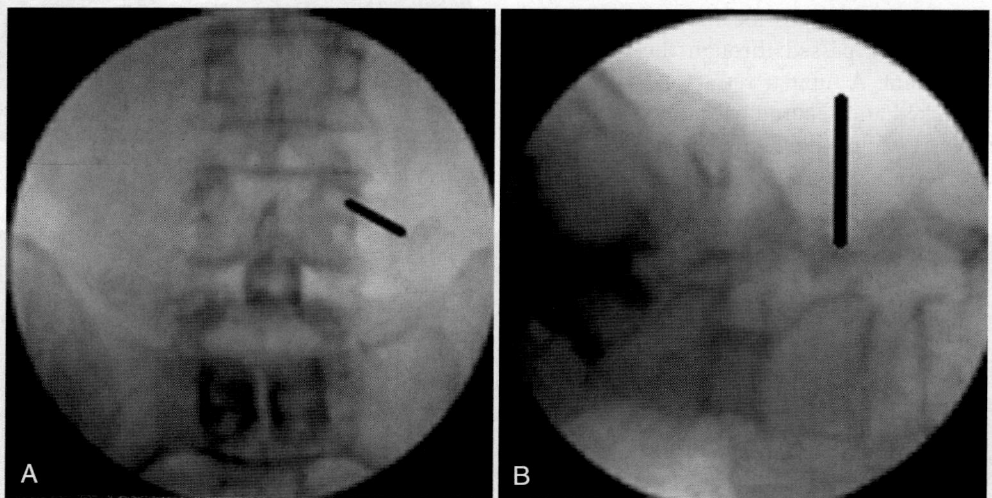

FIG. 55.6 Fluoroscopic imaging for percutaneous pedicle screw placement. (A) "True AP": pedicles are located just below the ascending articular process, and the superior endplate is parallel to the x-ray beam. The spinous process is in the middle of both pedicles. (B) "True lateral": both pedicles appear as one. The superior endplate is parallel to the x-ray beam.

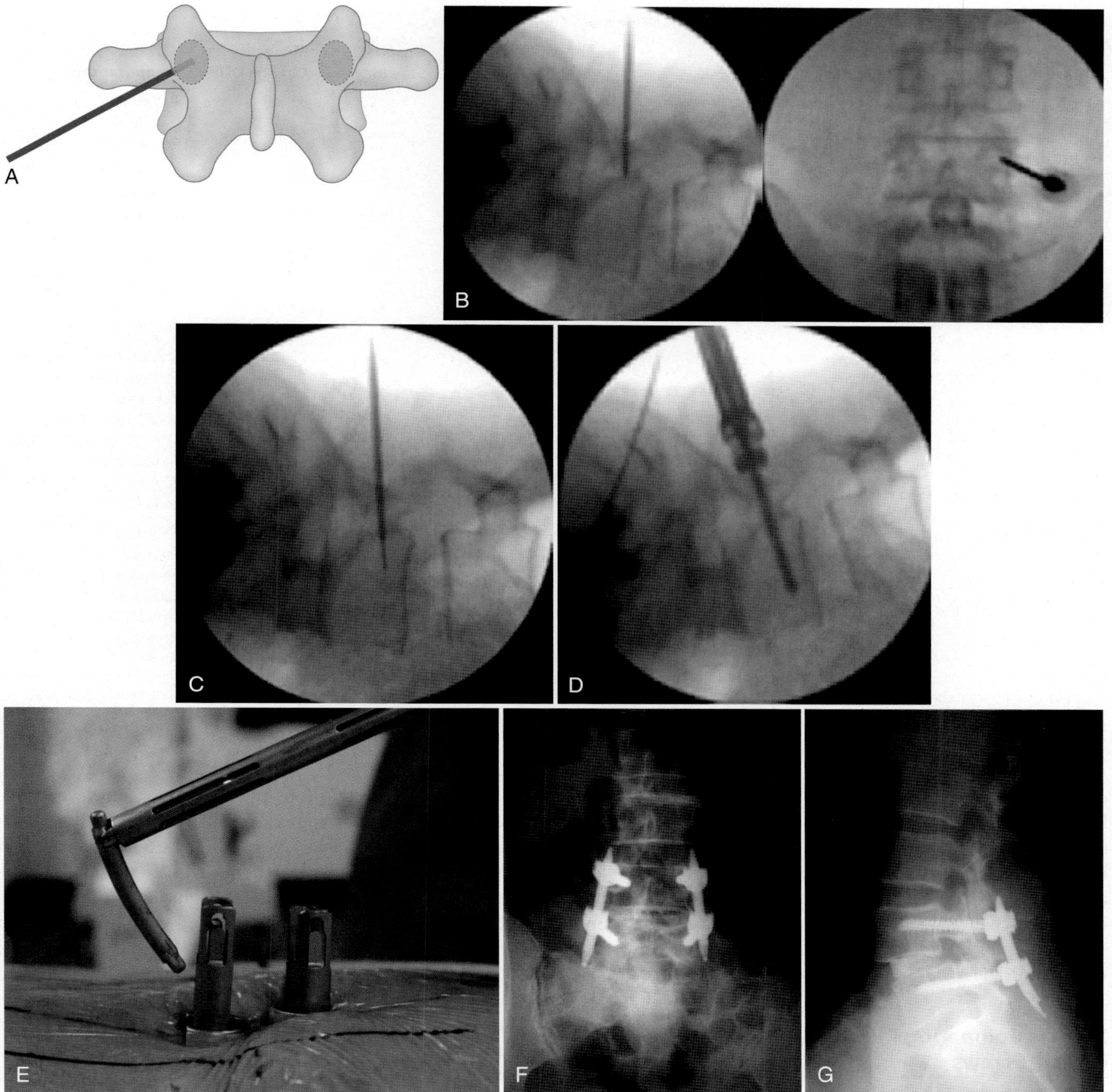

FIG. 55.7 Pedicle cannulation. (A) The ideal anteroposterior starting point. (B) The Jamshidi trocar has been advanced until it sits within the center of the pedicle. A lateral view is obtained. If the Jamshidi tip is at the neurocentral junction, then it may be safely advanced under lateral fluoroscopy. (C) Once the trocar is placed past the neurocentral junction in a satisfactory position, the guidewire may be inserted and advanced into the cancellous bone. (D) Screw holes are tapped, and screws are passed over the guidewires. Intermittent fluoroscopy is recommended to identify potential guidewire migration. (E) The appropriately sized rod is passed. Use direct visualization and palpation to avoid trapping muscle beneath the rod, which can lead to severe postoperative pain. (F–G) Final images.

remain lateral to the medial border of the pedicle. A lateral image is obtained and should show the tip of the trocar at or past the neurocentral junction. If so, the trocar can be safely advanced to its desired depth. If the tip of the trocar is at or medial to the medial border of the pedicle on the AP view and has not yet passed the neurocentral junction on the lateral, the pedicle screw tract has breached the medial border of the pedicle (Fig. 55.7).

After appropriate placement of the Jamshidi trocar is confirmed radiographically on orthogonal views, a guidewire is passed. These steps are repeated at each pedicle. The Kirschner wires (K-wires) are secured out of the field, and the

TABLE 55.1 Minimally Invasive Surgery Transforaminal Lumbar Interbody Fusion (TLIF) Results

Study	Procedure	Diagnosis	EBL (mL)	OR Time (min)	Hospital Stay (days)	Mean Change ODI	Complications
Schwender et al.[5] (2005)	MIS TLIF–PS (n = 49)	DDD + HNP, spondylolisthesis	<140	240	1.9	32	Technical: 4 Pseudo: 0 Revisions: 4
Park and Ha[2] (2007)	MIS PLIF–PS (n = 32)	Spondylolisthesis, large HNP	433	192	5.3	NR	Technical: 2 Revisions: 4
	Open PLIF (n = 29)		738	149	10.8	NR	Technical: 0 Revisions: 2
Schizas et al.[4] (2009)	MIS TLIF–PS (n =18)	DDD, spondylolisthesis	456	NR	6.1	22	Technical: 2 Pseudo: 3
	Open TLIF (n = 18)		961		8.2	27	Technical: 2 Pseudo: 0
Peng et al.[3] (2009)	MIS TLIF–PS (n = 29)	Spondylolisthesis, DDD	150	216	4	29	Complication rate: 6.9% Technical: NR Revisions: 0 Solid fusion: 80%[a]
	Open TLIF (n = 29)		681	171	6.7	30	Complication rate: 13.8% Technical: NR Revisions: 0 Solid fusion: 87%[a]
Dhall et al.[1] (2008)	MIS TLIF–MO (n = 21)	Spondylolisthesis, DDD	194	199	3	NR	Technical: 2 Pseudo: 1 Revisions: 3
	Open TLIF (n = 21)		505	237	5.5		Technical: 2 Pseudo: 0 Revisions: 1

DDD, degenerative disc disease; EBL, estimated blood loss; HNP, herniated nucleus pulposus; MIS TLIF–MO, minimally invasive transforaminal lumbar interbody fusion with screws placed by a mini-open technique; MIS TLIF–PS, minimally invasive transforaminal lumbar interbody fusion with percutaneous pedicle screws; NR, not reported in the study; ODI, Oswestry Disability Index; OR, operating room; PLIF, posterior lumbar interbody fusion; pseudo, pseudoarthrosis.

[a]Not statistically significant.

decompressive and interbody work are performed. A cannulated pedicle screw is then placed over each K-wire and the appropriately sized rod is passed. It is critical to continue lateral C-arm visualization to ensure that the K-wire is not advanced anteriorly during this process. When first performing this procedure, we encourage the liberal use of fluoroscopy. With experience, radiographic exposure and operative time will diminish.

Studies Comparing Mini-Open and Percutaneous Pedicle Screws

The decision regarding which minimally invasive instrumentation technique to use is largely surgeon dependent. Regev and colleagues[21] compared mini-open pedicle screw placement with percutaneous pedicle screw insertion in cadavers. After screw placement, the authors dissected out the medial branch nerve, which originates from the dorsal rami of each spinal nerve and innervates the multifidus muscle. In this study, percutaneous pedicle screw placement better preserved the segmental innervation of the multifidus, with only 20% of cases causing disruption of this innervation compared with 84% medial branch nerve transection using the mini-open pedicle screw insertion technique. The clinical significance of this difference is unknown.

To date, no clinical studies have directly compared the use of traditional pedicle screws placed through a tubular retractor (mini-open) to percutaneous pedicle screws. However, multiple studies have reported perioperative data regarding percutaneous versus open screw insertion (Table 55.1). Schizas and colleagues[4] reported their experience with 18 minimally invasive transforaminal lumbar interbody fusions (TLIFs) using percutaneous pedicle screw fixation and compared this with 18 open TLIFs. The percutaneous pedicle screw patients used 2.7 cGy/cm^2 of radiation as compared with 1.8 cGy/cm^2 in the open TLIF group. The minimally invasive TLIF operative time averaged 4.3 hours in the last third of their experience. Their estimated blood loss was 456 mL. Peng and colleagues[3] also reviewed the results of minimally invasive TLIFs. They used an average 105 seconds of fluoroscopy, estimated blood loss (EBL) of 150 mL, and operative time of 216 minutes. Neither of these studies reported any technical complications with minimally invasive TLIFs performed by percutaneous screws. Foley's[22] initial experience was similar, with an average operative time of 290 minutes and EBL of 25 mL. He reported one technical complication of a loose locking plug that required revision. Dhall and colleagues[1] compared minimally invasive TLIFs with traditional pedicle screws with open TLIFs. Their average EBL was 194 mL, and their average operating room time was 199 minutes. There were two technical complications in the minimally invasive group with one misplaced pedicle screw and one case of interbody cage migration. The open group also had one misplaced screw. Schwender and colleagues[5] reported on their initial experience with minimally invasive TLIFs and percutaneous screw insertion. Their average operative time was 240 minutes and EBL of 140 mL. In this series there were two misplaced screws and interbody cage dislodgement. Park and Ha[2] compared 32 minimally invasive posterior lumbar interbody fusions (PLIFs) with 29 open PLIFs. All minimally invasive cases were stabilized with percutaneous screws. The average operating room time was longer for the minimally invasive cases compared with open cases, 191 minutes and 150 minutes, respectively. The average EBL in the minimally invasive cases was 432 mL compared with 737 mL. There were two technical complications, one screw malposition and one interbody cage migration, reported in the minimally invasive group and none in the open group. These differences were not statistically significant.

In 2005, Kim and colleagues[10] compared longitudinal changes in multifidus cross-sectional area and trunk extension strength in both open and percutaneous pedicle screw constructs. The T2 cross-sectional area of the multifidus muscle was recorded on preoperative and postoperative MRIs. Trunk extension strength was measured using a MedX lumbar extension machine. Multifidus cross-sectional area decreased from 1140 to 800 mm^2 in open pedicle screw constructs as compared with percutaneous pedicle screw constructs in which multifidus area decreased from 1320 to 1270 mm^2. Trunk extension strength increased in both open and percutaneous pedicle screw constructs, but the improvements in strength were only statistically significant in the percutaneous pedicle screw cohort.

Overall, there are not enough comparative data to make any evidence-based decisions between the use of traditional pedicle screws through tubular retractors and percutaneous pedicle screws. More clinical data are necessary.

Consideration for Radiation Exposure

As discussed, minimally invasive spine surgery, particularly percutaneous techniques for which no exposed anatomy is available for guidance, requires greater use of fluoroscopy. The clear concern with the use of fluoroscopy is exposure to ionizing radiation to the surgeon, the operative room staff, and the patient. Rampersaud et al.[23] performed a cadaveric study to determine occupational radiation exposure during lumbar fluoroscopy. They noted 10 to 12 times greater radiation exposure to the surgeon during thoracolumbar pedicle screw placement than other, nonspinal musculoskeletal procedures that use fluoroscopy. Exposure was greatest to the torso and hand when the surgeon was positioned ipsilateral to the beam source and increased with cadavers with larger dorsal body surface. Kim and colleagues[24] performed a two-phased cadaveric and prospective clinical review comparing navigation-assisted fluoroscopy and standard fluoroscopy use in minimally invasive TLIFs. In the cadaveric study, they noted a longer setup time for navigation (9.7 minutes) compared with fluoroscopy (4.8 minutes). The mean fluoroscopic time was 42 seconds in the fluoroscopy group and 29 seconds in the navigation group. The average radiation exposure to the surgeon was undetectable in the navigation group and was 12.4 mrem in the fluoroscopic group. Clinically, minimally invasive TLIFs with navigation used 57 seconds of fluoroscopy and minimally invasive TLIFs with fluoroscopy used 147 seconds. They found that total fluoroscopy time was statistically greater with standard fluoroscopy and that radiation exposure to the surgeon was undetectable with the navigation-assisted technique. Kim and colleagues reported no cases of screw malposition in either group and blood loss, operating time, and hospital stay were similar in both groups.[25] In a 2014 prospective randomized study, Villard et al.[26] showed that the use of intraoperative three-dimensional, fluoroscopy-based navigation reduced surgeon exposure to ionizing radiation almost 10-fold compared to the freehand, nonnavigated technique; radiation exposure to the patient was decreased in the navigated group but did not reach statistical significance. Bindal et al. prospectively recorded radiation exposure in 24 consecutive minimally invasive TLIF procedures.[27] The mean fluoroscopy time was 1.69 minutes (101 seconds). The mean exposure was 76 mrem at the surgeon's dominant hand, 27 mrem under a lead apron, and 32 mrem at an unprotected thyroid level. The mean exposure to the patient's skin was between 59 mrem and 78 mrem depending on the orientation to the x-ray beam. According to Bindal and colleagues,[27] the radiation exposure to both surgeon and patient was relatively low. They extrapolated that it would take 194 cases to exceed the acceptable torso radiation limits. The radiation levels that they observed also compared favorably with other fluoroscopic procedures, such as percutaneous coronary interventions. Nonetheless, all surgeons should be judicious with the use of intraoperative radiation. Computer-assisted navigation has been proposed as one means to reduce the need for fluoroscopy.

Fluoroscopic Versus Navigation-Assisted Spinal Instrumentation

Fluoroscopically guided percutaneous posterior lumbar instrumentation is considered an accurate and safe procedure.[28,29] However, the AP and lateral images are limited in assessing the screw in the axial plane that best demonstrates the position of the intended screw in relation to the neural elements.

Navigation-assisted pedicle screw placement is gaining popularity around the United States and worldwide. These techniques are designed to improve intraoperative orientation and hence the accuracy and precision of instrumentation. Additionally, navigated procedures significantly reduce or eliminate radiation exposure. This technology pairs preoperative or intraoperatively obtained imaging of the spine to corresponding intraoperative anatomy. Currently, four types of navigation guidance are available: fluoroscopic navigation, intraoperative isocentric fluoroscopic navigation, preoperative computed tomography (CT), and intraoperative CT. To achieve the goal of providing real-time three-dimensional guidance, algorithms establish a spatial relationship between image data and surgical anatomy. There are three distinct ways to achieve this: "surface matching," paired point registration, and automated registration. The specifics of navigation technology are beyond the scope of this chapter. Data suggest that navigation can be used safely for percutaneous pedicle screw placement and there is evidence that its use improves accuracy rate. However, caution is warranted when known identifiable landmarks are not visualized and great care must be taken to avoid dislodgement of the positioning arrays, which can cause the navigation to err.

Waschke et al.[30] reviewed their experience with CT navigation and fluoroscopically guided 4500 pedicle screw placements. They did find a statistically significant improvement in accuracy when utilizing CT navigation and 3D reconstruction and intraoperative CT control of the screw position. This difference was most pronounced in the thoracic spine. Gelalis and colleagues[31] performed a systematic review of prospective in vivo studies comparing freehand, fluoroscopy-guided, and navigation techniques; 26 studies and 6617 screws were included in their analysis. They concluded that all techniques were considered safe; however, navigation did exhibit the greatest accuracy and increased safety. The percentage of pedicle screws fully confined within bony anatomy ranged from 69% to 94% in the freehand group, 28% to 85% in the fluoroscopy-guided group, 81% to 92% for the fluoroscopy-based navigation group, and 89% to 100% in the CT-based navigation group.

Intraoperative Electrophysiological Monitoring

Calcancie and colleagues first described intraoperative electromyographic monitoring as a nonimaging modality for assessment of pedicle screw placement.[32] This can be used in conjunction with techniques described earlier or independently. Dermal or subdermal needle electrodes are placed in given muscles of the lower extremities and a monopolar probe is used by the surgeon to touch the exposed pedicle screw head, delivering progressively increased current intensities. Recordings from distal electrodes identify motor function of individual nerve roots. The pedicle wall provides an anatomic barrier without breach of the bony wall. A stimulation threshold of 10 to 20 mA strongly suggests that the screw does not breach the medial pedicle wall. An elicited action potential with a current intensity of 8 mA or less should prompt inspection and repositioning of the screw. A stimulation threshold above 15 mA is associated with a 98% likelihood for accurate screw placement when postoperative CT scan was obtained.[33] Raynor et al. retrospectively analyzed their experience with 4857 pedicle screws using evoked electromyography in addition to intraoperative imaging and direct palpation of the pedicle border and found improved accuracy of screw placement.[34]

PEARLS AND PITFALLS

1. When working through a tubular retractor, remember to move the retractor to see what you want to see and to allow you to position instrumentation in the direction you want to direct it. Do not let the retractor dictate what you see and do.
2. When first placing screws through a tubular retractor, expose the pars and the medial portion of the transverse process well.
3. Pedicle screw tracks may be easier to prepare before performing the decompression and facetectomy when more bony landmarks are present.
4. When placing percutaneous screws, fluoroscopic images must be "perfect" AP and lateral views. Otherwise, percutaneous screw placement may be aberrant.
5. Start simple. Surgeons should build confidence and skill beginning with less technically demanding procedures and anatomy.

KEY POINTS

1. Minimally invasive pedicle screw instrumentation is associated with less blood loss and shorter hospital stays but longer initial operative times.
2. Minimally invasive instrumentation has a lower infection rate than open instrumentation.
3. Obesity is an initial contraindication to minimally invasive instrumentation and fusion, but as a surgeon gains experience, obesity is a relative indication.
4. Technical complications have been comparable in minimally invasive instrumentation and open instrumentation.

KEY REFERENCES

1. Dhall S, Wang M, Mummaneni P. Clinical and radiographic comparison of mini-open transforaminal lumbar interbody fusion with open transforaminal lumbar interbody fusion in 42 patients with long term follow-up. *J Neurosurg Spine.* 2008;9:560-564.
   Retrospective review demonstrating less blood loss and shorter hospital stays, but possibly higher technical complications in 21 patients who underwent a mini-open TLIF compared with 21 patients who underwent a traditional open TLIF.
2. Park P, Upadhyaya H, Garton H, et al. The impact of minimally invasive spine surgery on perioperative complications in overweight or obese patients. *Neurosurgery.* 2008;62:693-699.
   The authors found similar perioperative complication rates in patients with a BMI greater than 25 kg/m² compared with patients with a BMI less than 25 kg/m² who underwent minimally invasive spine procedures.
3. Peng C, Yue W, Poh S, et al. Clinical and radiological outcomes of minimally invasive versus open transforaminal lumbar interbody fusion. *Spine.* 2009;34:1385-1389.
   MIS TLIFs were found to have less blood loss, less postoperative pain, shorter hospital stays, and equivalent 2-year clinical results compared with traditional open TLIFs.
4. O'Toole J, Eichholz K, Fessler R. Surgical infection rates after minimally invasive spinal surgery. *J Neurosurg Spine.* 2009;11:471-476.
   The authors report a 0.22% surgical site infection rate after reviewing 1338 minimally invasive surgical procedures.
5. Kim D, Lee S, Chung S, et al. Comparison of multifidus muscle atrophy and trunk extension muscle strength. Percutaneous versus open pedicle screw fixation. *Spine.* 2005;30:123-129.
   Multifidus muscle cross-sectional area and trunk extension muscle strength were compared in patients undergoing open and percutaneous pedicle screw fixation.

REFERENCES

1. Dhall SS, Wang MY, Mummaneni PV. Clinical and radiographic comparison of mini-open transforaminal lumbar interbody fusion with open transforaminal lumbar interbody

fusion in 42 patients with long-term follow-up. *J Neurosurg Spine*. 2008;9:560-565.

2. Park Y, Ha JW. Comparison of one-level posterior lumbar interbody fusion performed with a minimally invasive approach or a traditional open approach. *Spine*. 2007;32:537-543.
3. Peng CW, Yue WM, Poh SY, et al. Clinical and radiological outcomes of minimally invasive versus open transforaminal lumbar interbody fusion. *Spine*. 2009;34:1385-1389.
4. Schizas C, Tzinieris N, Tsiridis E, et al. Minimally invasive versus open transforaminal lumbar interbody fusion: evaluating initial experience. *Int Orthop*. 2009;33:1683-1688.
5. Schwender JD, Holly LT, Rouben DP, et al. Minimally invasive transforaminal lumbar interbody fusion (TLIF): technical feasibility and initial results. *J Spinal Disord Tech*. 2005;18 (suppl 1):S1-S6.
6. Goldstein CL, et al. Perioperative outcomes and adverse events of minimally invasive versus open posterior lumbar fusion: meta-analysis and systematic review. *J Neurosurg Spine*. 2016;24:416-427.
7. Silva PS, et al. Learning curve and complications of minimally invasive transforaminal lumbar interbody fusion. *Neurosurg Focus*. 2013;35(2):E7.
8. Magerl F. External skeletal fixation of the lower thoracic and lumbar spine. In: Uhthoff H, Stahl E, eds. *Current Concepts of External Fixation of Fractures*. New York: Springer-Verlag; 1982:353-366.
9. Matthews H, Long B. Endoscopy assisted percutaneous anterior interbody fusion with subcutaneous suprafascial internal fixation: evolution of technique and surgical considerations. *Orthopaedics*. 1995;3:496-500.
10. Kim DY, Lee SH, Chung SK, et al. Comparison of multifidus muscle atrophy and trunk extension muscle strength: percutaneous versus open pedicle screw fixation. *Spine*. 2005;30:123-129.
11. Kim KT, Lee SH, Suk KS, et al. The quantitative analysis of tissue injury markers after mini-open lumbar fusion. *Spine*. 2006;31:712-716.
12. Hu ZJ, et al. Accuracy of magnetic resonance imaging signal intensity ratio measurements in the evaluation of multifidus muscle injury and atrophy relative to that of histological examinations. *Spine*. 2014;39(10):E623-E629.
13. Ogden CL, Carroll MD, Fryar CD, Flegal KM. Prevalence of obesity among adults and youth: United States, 2011-2014. *NCHS Data Brief*. 2015;219:1-8.
14. Rosen DS, Ferguson SD, Ogden AT, et al. Obesity and self-reported outcome after minimally invasive lumbar spinal fusion surgery. *Neurosurgery*. 2008;63:956-960.
15. O'Toole JE, Eichholz KM, Fessler RG. Surgical site infection rates after minimally invasive spinal surgery. *J Neurosurg Spine*. 2009;11:471-476.
16. Picada R, Winter RB, Lonstein JE, et al. Postoperative deep wound infection in adults after posterior lumbosacral spine fusion with instrumentation: incidence and management. *J Spinal Disord*. 2000;13:42-45.
17. Denis F. The three column spine and its significance in the classification of acute thoracolumbar spinal injuries. *Spine*. 1983;8(8):817-831.
18. Lonstein JE. Complications associated with pedicle screws. *J Bone Joint Surg Am*. 1999;81(11):1519-1528.
19. Parker SL, McGirt MJ, Farber SH, et al. Accuracy of free-hand pedicle screws in the thoracic and lumbar spine: analysis of 6816 consecutive screws. *Neurosurgery*. 2011;68: 170-178.
20. Wiltse LL, Bateman JG, Hutchinson RH, et al. The paraspinal sacrospinalis-splitting approach to the lumbar spine. *J Bone Joint Surg Am*. 1968;50:919-926.
21. Regev GJ, Lee YP, Taylor WR, et al. Nerve injury to the posterior rami medial branch during the insertion of pedicle screws: comparison of mini-open versus percutaneous pedicle screw insertion techniques. *Spine*. 2009;34:1239-1242.
22. Foley KT, Holly LT, Schwender JD. Minimally invasive lumbar fusion. *Spine*. 2003;28:S26-S35.
23. Rampersaud YR, Foley KT, Shen AC, et al. Radiation exposure to the spine surgeon during fluoroscopically assisted pedicle screw insertion. *Spine*. 2000;25(20):2637-2645.
24. Kim CW, Lee YP, Taylor W, et al. Use of navigation-assisted fluoroscopy to decrease radiation exposure during minimally invasive spine surgery. *Spine J*. 2008;8:584-590.
25. Kim CW, Lee YP, Taylor W, et al. Use of navigation-assisted fluoroscopy to decreased exposure during minimally invasive spine surgery. *Spine J*. 2008;8(4):584-590.
26. Villard J, Ryang YM, Demetriades AK, et al. Radiation exposure to the surgeon and the patient during posterior lumbar spinal instrumentation. *Spine*. 2014;39(13): 1004-1009.
27. Bindal RK, Glaze S, Ognoskie M, et al. Surgeon and patient radiation exposure in minimally invasive transforaminal lumbar interbody fusion. *J Neurosurg Spine*. 2008;9: 570-573.
28. Hansen-Algenstaedt N, et al. Accuracy and safety of fluoroscopic guided percutaneous pedicle screws in thoracic and lumbosacral spine: a review of 2000 screws. *Spine*. 2015;40(17):E954-E963.
29. Koktekir E, et al. Accuracy of fluoroscopically-assisted pedicle screw placement: analysis of 1,218 screws in 198 patients. *Spine J*. 2014;14:1702-1708.
30. Waschke A, et al. CT-navigation versus fluoroscopy-guided placement of pedicle screws at the thoracolumbar spine: single center experience of 4,500 screws. *Eur Spine J*. 2013;22: 654-660.
31. Gelalis ID, et al. Accuracy of pedicle screw placement: a systematic review of prospective in vivo studies comparing free hand, fluoroscopy guidance and navigation techniques. *Eur Spine J*. 2012;21:247-255.
32. Calcancie B, Lebwohl N, Madsen P, et al. Intraoperative evoked EMG monitoring in an animal model: a new technique for evaluating pedicle screw placement. *Spine*. 1992;17:1229-1235.
33. Glassman SD, Dimar JD, Puno RM, et al. A prospective analysis of intraoperative electromyographic monitoring of pedicle screw placement with computed tomographic scan confirmation. *Spine*. 1995;20:1375-1379.
34. Raynor BL, Lenke LG, Bridwell KH, et al. Correlation between low triggered electromyographic thresholds and lumbar pedicle screw malposition: analysis of 4857 screws. *Spine*. 2007;32:2673-2678.

CHAPTER 56

Minimally Invasive Posterior Lumbar Fusion Techniques

SECTION VII

D. Greg Anderson
Jonathan D. Krystal

Introduction

Lumbar spinal fusion has long been used in the treatment of a wide variety of spinal pathologies causing spinal instability and pain. Various spinal fusion techniques are the subject of ongoing clinical investigations, with the goal of improving surgical technique, graft biomaterials, and implant designs in order to achieve a stable symptom-free spinal column with the least chance of patient morbidity.

Surgical morbidity after spinal fusion remains significant, despite multiple advances in technique and implant design. The standard open paraspinal approach involves extensive stripping of the paraspinal musculature, which has been shown to lead to denervation and atrophy.[1,2] Additionally, the large dissection may be associated with prolonged recovery and in-hospital complications.[3–7]

The development of less invasive surgical techniques has allowed surgeons to accomplish their treatment goals without utilizing the traditional open dissection. This approach may lead to lower surgical blood loss, lower transfusion rates, and shorter hospital stays for similar outcomes.[8–13] Additional benefits have been shown in regard to total cost and utility, with decreasing perioperative costs and less utilization of hospital resources and operative time.[14–16]

Minimally invasive spinal surgery (MIS) is a rapidly evolving field that is supported by a number of technological innovations. These include the operative microscope, C-arm fluoroscopy, tubular retractor systems, cannulated pedicle screws, and, for some, image guidance systems. The basic hand instruments used during a minimally invasive spinal procedure are similar to those used during a traditional spinal case, but are often longer and bayoneted to improve visualization through a tubular retraction system. A high-speed burr or drill, with a long and thin shaft, is useful in decorticating or thinning the bony elements of the spine. To be successful with MIS, a surgeon must be familiar with the microscopic anatomy of the spine. The surgeon must gain the skills necessary to work safely and efficiently despite a limited field of view and must become facile with the use of MIS equipment. Numerous surgeons have evaluated the learning curve needed to become proficient with minimally invasive techniques. With increasing experience, operative time, blood loss, and outcomes improve.[17,18] Care should be taken when first introducing MIS lumbar fusion techniques, as the overall complication rate has been shown to be significantly higher during a surgeon's first 20 to 30 cases.[19] The learning process is best accomplished in a slow, stepwise fashion, mastering basic skills with simple cases before attempting to approach the more challenging spinal pathologies in an MIS fashion. This chapter will provide an overview to the field of MIS as it applies to lumbar fusion techniques for common conditions of the lumbar spine.

Principles of Minimally Invasive Spinal Surgery

Whether using traditional open approaches or a minimally invasive technique, the goal is to treat and correct the underlying spinal pathology. MIS has the additional goal of doing this while minimizing damage to the paraspinal muscle envelope. As with any spinal surgery, careful analysis of preoperative imaging and patient symptomatology are important to correctly localize the pathology and devise an effective treatment plan. Localizing fluoroscopy is used to localize the pathologic levels and plan the skin incision to offer the most direct access to the necessary structures. It is important to note that the paraspinal musculature should not be cut or resected, but rather should be split inline with the muscle fibers using serial tubular dilators (Fig. 56.1). Exposure should be limited only to those areas of the spine that are necessary for the procedure, and electrocautery should be limited.

There are two distinct paraspinal muscle compartments that need to be considered when planning the surgical approach. Overlying the midline spinal structures is the multifidus compartment. This midline compartment contains the large multifidus muscle, which surrounds the spinous process, lamina, and facet joints. The multifidus is innervated by the medial branches of the dorsal rami and receives its vasculature from the segmental vessels, which course along the base of the transverse process and enter the lateral margin of the muscle in the region of the pars interarticularis. Overlying the transverse processes is the lateral compartment (Fig. 56.2). Within the lateral compartment, the erector spinae muscle group lies with its longitudinally oriented fibers. The starting point for lumbar pedicle screws lies within the lateral

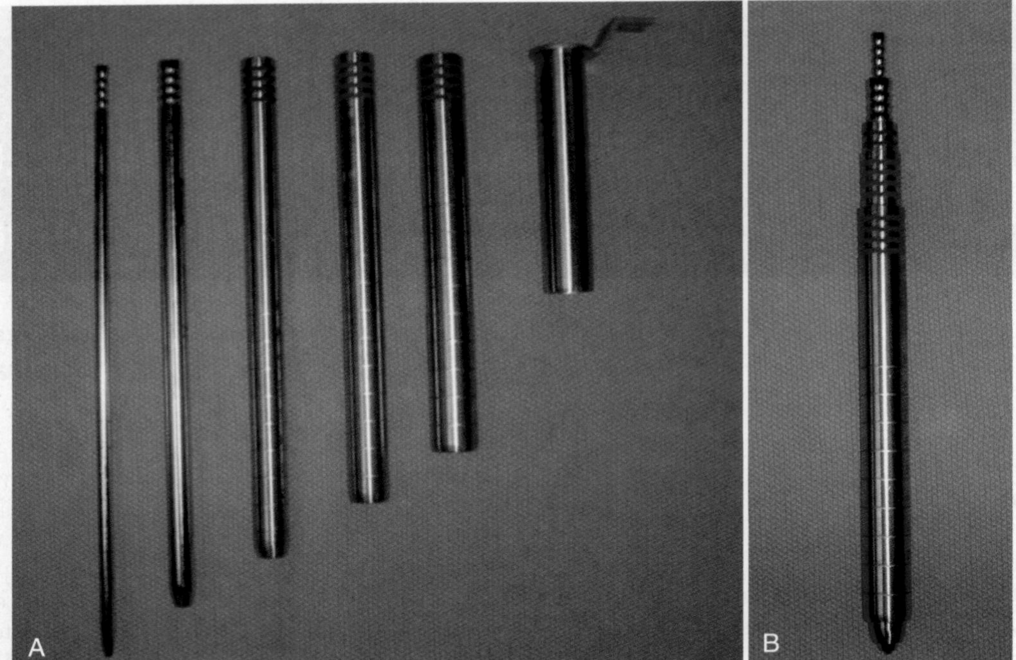

FIG. 56.1 (A) Individual and (B) assembled serial tubular dilators are used to gain access to the spine through muscle splitting rather than cutting through the paraspinal muscles.

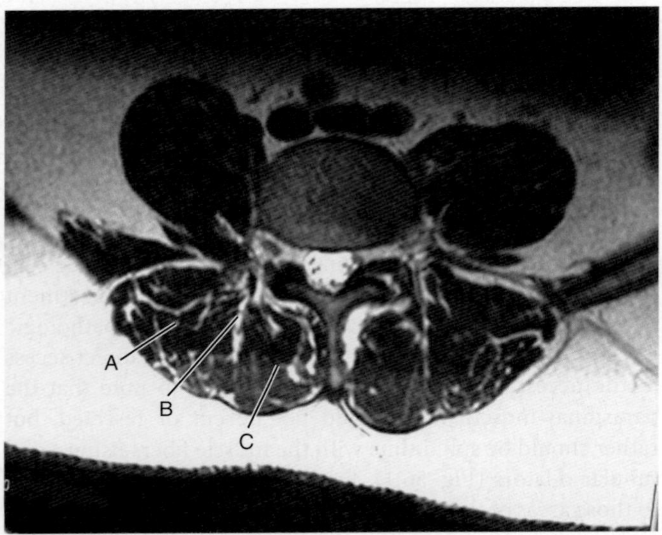

FIG. 56.2 Deep paraspinal muscle compartment: The multifidus muscle *(C)* overlies the midline, and the lateral compartment *(A, B)* contains the longissimus and iliocostalis muscles, overlying the transverse processes.

compartment, as do the transverse processes, which provide a fusion surface for a posterolateral onlay fusion.

Many procedures will require access to both compartments. In the multifidus compartment, the midline structures will be accessible, and the lateral compartment will need to be utilized for the placement of pedicle screws and posterolateral fusion. Operating in a paraspinal compartment requires a fascial incision over each individual compartment. The underlying muscle should be split or dilated in order to reach the desired structure below. Care should be taken not to divide the fascial barrier between compartments, which can disrupt the blood supply to the multifidus muscle. Separate fascial incisions should be made to access the two compartments separately; however, a well-placed single skin incision can be made to access both regions.

Both the surgeon and patient must understand the benefits and limitations of MIS compared with other options, including open surgery. The surgeon and patient should discuss the goal of surgery and treatment of the underlying spinal pathology, and it should be made clear to the patient that the approach is a secondary issue. Surgical consent should always include the possibility that the less invasive procedure may have to be aborted in favor of an open procedure if the pathology proves too difficult to treat though an MIS approach.

Surgical Setup for a Posterior Fusion Procedure

Setup and Imaging

Following placement of surgical monitoring equipment and the induction of general anesthesia, the patient should be positioned prone on a radiolucent spinal frame (Fig. 56.3). The abdomen should be free of compression and free access to the lumbar region for fluoroscopy should be confirmed. The preoperative imaging studies should be available in the room, with the operative plan clearly marked. The surgeon should ensure the availability of the proper implants and instruments prior to commencing with the operative procedure.

After a sterile skin preparation and draping, the C-arm mobile fluoroscopy unit is used to demarcate the location of bony landmarks, which are drawn on the skin. A critical step is to ensure that the skin incisions are localized in an optimal position to allow access to the underlying spinal pathology. In some cases, it may be useful to introduce a spinal needle along the proposed trajectory of the surgical incision and check the position of the needle on both anteroposterior (AP) and lateral fluoroscopic views to ensure that an optimal path to the pathology is achieved.

Care should be taken in positioning and planning for C-arm use in order to minimize intraoperative radiation exposure. On average, a surgeon performing an MIS procedure is likely to receive about 10 to 20 times the radiation exposure compared with an open technique. Additionally, operating on patients with a body mass index greater than 35 kg/m^2 has been shown to significantly increase the radiation exposure to the patient, physician, and nursing staff.[20,21] While the clinical significance of this increased exposure is unclear, planning and judicious use of fluoroscopy to limit radiation exposure is recommended.

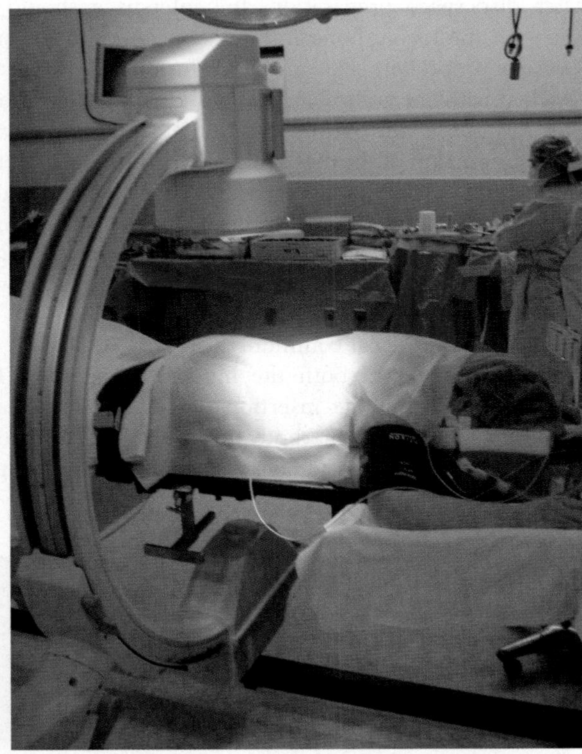

FIG. 56.3 The patient is positioned prone on a radiolucent spinal frame.

Surgical Incisions and Approach

The number and length of skin incisions should correspond to the surgical plan, which must be more thoroughly planned compared to a traditional open surgery. A single skin incision may be used during different phases of the surgical procedure to reach different areas of the spine. For instance, one incision may initially be used to decompress the neural elements in the multifidus compartment. Subsequently, the same skin incision may be used to perform a posterolateral fusion and place pedicle screw instrumentation in the lateral compartment. Although a single skin incision is used, separate fascial incisions should be used to reach each individual compartment.

When working through perimedian incisions, two distinct fascial layers will be encountered. The superficial layer corresponds to the thoracodorsal fascia, while the deeper layer is a thin fascia that overlies the muscle of the compartment. Both fascial incisions should be a little longer than the corresponding skin incision to allow the subsequently placed tubular retractors to be maneuvered and angulated freely as needed to reach the various areas of the spine necessary to perform the operation. The muscles of the compartment can be split with the surgeon's digit or with an instrument such as a Cobb elevator. It is often helpful to palpate bony landmarks, such as the facet joint or transverse processes, to assist with placement of the initial instruments through the skin and muscle portal to the vertebral column.

When operating through a tubular retractor, the smallest dilator is then docked at the appropriate bony site and serial dilation is used to expand the operative corridor. Care should be taken when bringing each subsequent dilator into contact with the bony vertebra. The correct length of the tubular retractor can then be selected, inserted, and secured using an operating table–mounted retractor holder. Once the tubular retractor is in place, the position of the retractor should be verified using fluoroscopy (Fig. 56.4).

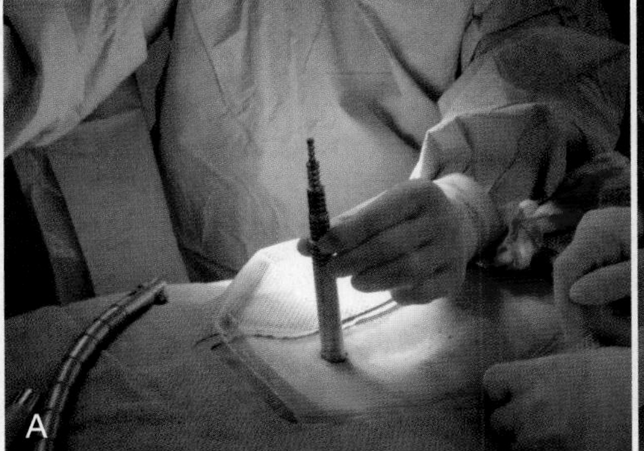

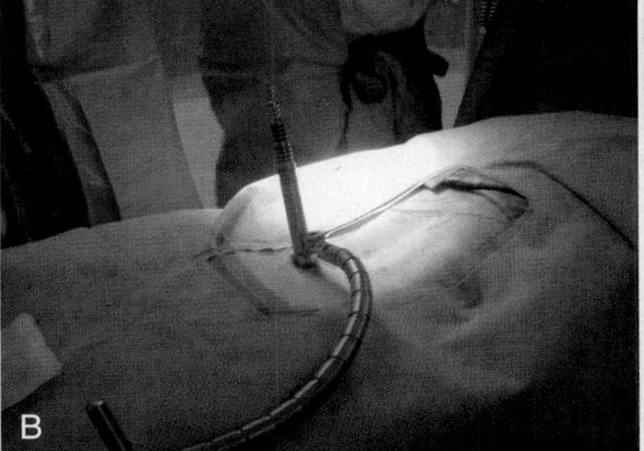

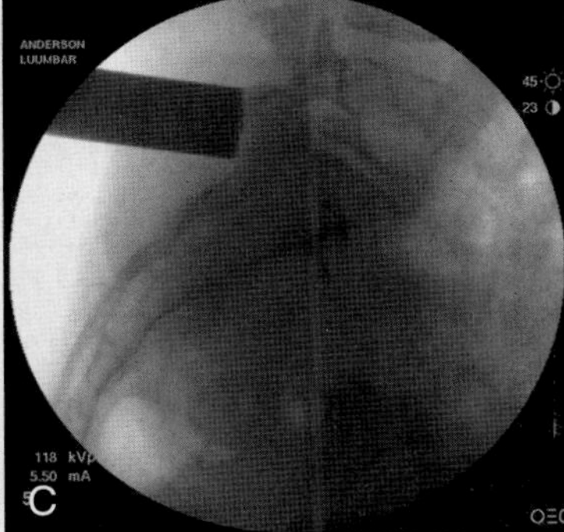

FIG. 56.4 (A) Following insertion of the tubular dilator system, (B) the tubular retractor is secured in place using an operating table–mounted rigid retractor holder. (C) Fluoroscopy is used to verify correct positioning of the tubular retractor.

Spinal Decompression

The topic of spinal decompression is substantial and exceeds the goals of this chapter; however, a few points deserve mention. Our preference is to perform the decompression first when performing both a decompression and fusion of the lumbar spine. This allows the surgeon to obtain local autologous bone from the decompression site that may be used for the spine fusion and exposes important bony landmarks, such as the pedicle, that will be useful in subsequent stages of the procedure. The decompression will be done by entering and traversing the multifidus compartment. Thus, it is useful to perform a facet fusion during this phase of the procedure before exiting the multifidus compartment.

Posterior Interbody and Transforaminal Interbody Fusion

When performing a posterior lumbar interbody fusion (PLIF) or transforaminal lumbar interbody fusion (TLIF) via a minimally invasive approach, it is important to align the tubular retractor collinear with the disc space on the lateral view (see Fig. 56.5). When performing a TLIF procedure, the tubular retractor must be aligned with enough lateral to medial angulation to allow the surgeon to reach the contralateral side of the disc space for preparation of an adequate fusion bed (Fig. 56.6). During the exposure, an adequate amount of facet joint must be removed to minimize retraction of the neural elements and provide working access to the disc space.[22]

The detrimental effects of overretraction of the neural elements with the PLIF procedure have been well documented in the literature.[23] Facet removals for a PLIF or TLIF can be achieved with either osteotomes or a high-speed burr. It is helpful to skeletonize the upper and medial portions of the caudal pedicle (e.g., L5 pedicle for an L4–L5 TLIF) to gain adequate access to the disc space and allow safe retraction/protection of the dural/neural elements.

Once the disc space has been adequately exposed, the posterolateral anulus is incised with a scalpel and the posterior margin of the disc is removed. The posterior "lip" of the vertebral body should be resected so that the opening is flush with the most concaved portions of the disc space. Disc material and cartilaginous endplate are thoroughly debrided from the interbody space using curettes, shavers, and/or pituitary rongeurs until the interspace is clean, leaving intact only bony endplates to support the interbody cage. If the disc space is collapsed, the endplates should be dilated to restore the foraminal height and improve the sagittal contour of the spine.

After disc space preparation, the interspace should be packed with autologous bone graft or an adequate fusion substrate. An appropriately sized interbody fusion cage is selected and packed with the graft material before impacting the cage into the disc space. The optimal position of the cage is toward the anterior portion of the disc space.[24,25] This produces better reconstruction of the sagittal contour of the spine and allows ample bone graft material to be packed around and behind the cage. With correct placement of interbody fusion cages, similar improvements in sagittal contour have been seen with both MIS and open surgery.[26]

Instrumentation, most commonly with pedicle screws, is a standard component of both the modern PLIF and TLIF procedures. Following the insertion of pedicle screws and rods, compression of the interbody construct is performed to restore the lumbar lordosis and ensure compressive loading of the interbody grafts.

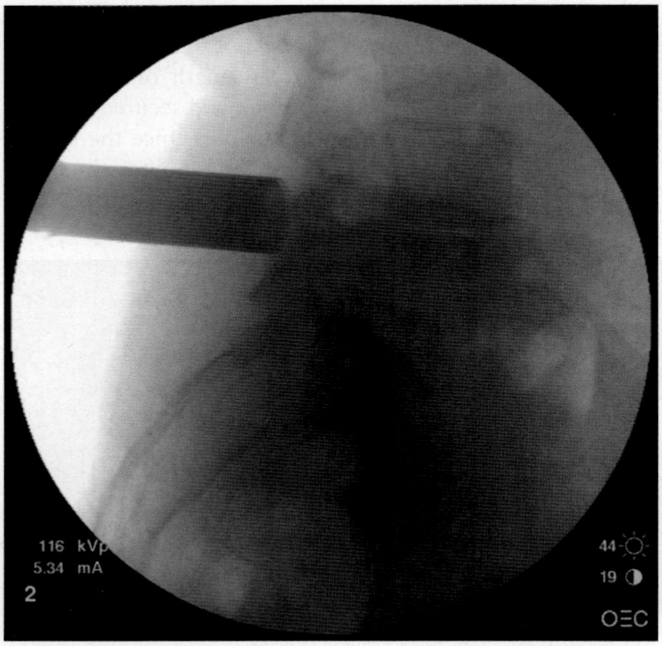

FIG. 56.5 Lateral fluoroscopic view shows the tubular retractor positioned in a proper alignment (i.e., collinear with the disc space).

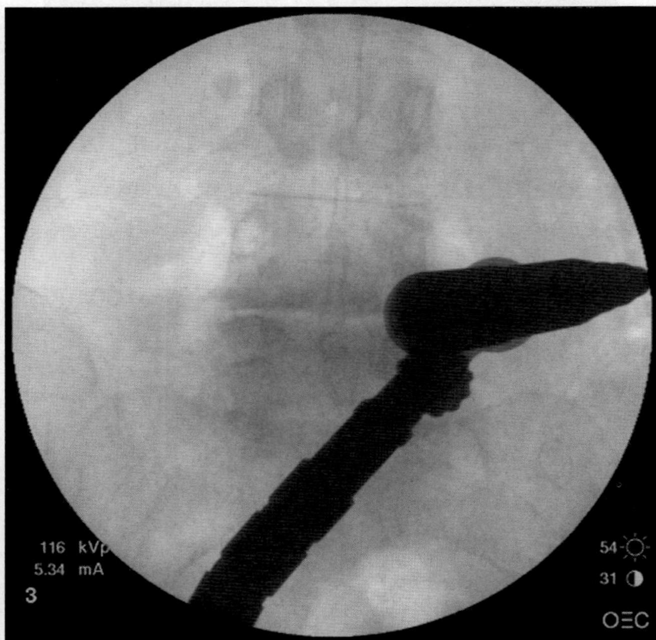

FIG. 56.6 Angulation of the tubular retractor system allows access to the contralateral side of the disc space and therefore preparation of the fusion bed.

Posterolateral Fusion (Intertransverse Onlay Fusion)

From the traditional midline approach, access to the intertransverse region for onlay fusion requires complete stripping of the paraspinal muscles to the tips of the transverse processes, an act that causes destruction of the multifidus muscle and significant postoperative scarring.[2] Using the paraspinal muscle–splitting approach (Wiltse approach), exposure of the intertransverse region is simple to achieve without major muscle stripping. This provides direct access to the intertransverse region for fusion.

The skin incision for a paraspinal approach with intertransverse fusion is made at least 3.5 to 4 cm lateral to the midline. The fascia is divided in line with the skin incision and the paraspinal muscles are split in line with their fibers to expose the transverse processes. For fusion purposes, the entire transverse process at both levels should be exposed. Either a tubular retractor (preferably an expandable tubular retractor) or side-to-side retractor (e.g., McCullough retractor) can be utilized to visualize the intertransverse interval. We prefer to use an expandable tubular retractor, which allows both transverse processes to be simultaneously exposed (Fig. 56.7).

Once the intertransverse region has been exposed, the soft tissues are meticulously cleaned away from the transverse processes and intertransverse membrane. The transverse processes are decorticated using a high-speed burr. Then, the interval is packed with autologous bone graft or a suitable graft material. Care should be taken when withdrawing the retractors in order not to displace the graft materials from the fusion bed.

Facet Fusion

Fusion of the facet joints is a useful adjunct to interbody or intertransverse fusion, but has not been well accepted as stand-alone fusion due to the relatively small surface area of the facet joints. However, the facet joint offers a number of theoretical advantages as a fusion site, including the ease of access to the joint, the small gap across which the fusion must heal, and the compression of the fusion site that is achieved during normal upright posture of the patient. In addition, a facet fusion is a quick, simple, and low-morbidity procedure.

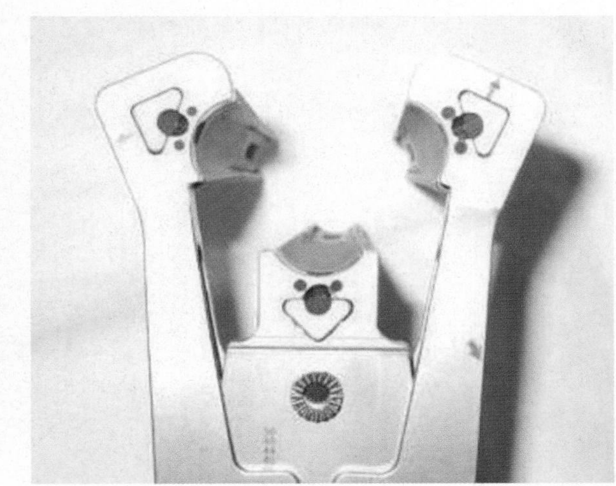

FIG. 56.7 Use of an expandable tubular retractor allows simultaneous exposure of both transverse processes.

To perform a facet fusion, the retractor should be docked on the facet that resides in the lateral portion of the multifidus compartment. If decompression of the spinal canal is required, facet fusion can easily be performed during the exposure through the multifidus compartment. Once the facet is exposed, the capsule is removed with electrocautery, and the articular surfaces of the inferior and superior articular processes are identified. A high-speed burr is used to decorticate the facet joint along its entire length, and the joint space is packed with fragments of autologous bone or a suitable bone substitute. In some cases, osteophytic bone material may overlie the true facet joint, which should be removed to expose the native joint surfaces. The surgeon should be cognizant of the normal anatomy of the facet joint, with the superior articular process lying lateral and deep to the inferior articular process. The specific topography of the facet joint can also be defined preoperatively by analyzing imaging studies, either magnetic resonance imaging (MRI) or computed tomography (CT).

Pedicle Screw Instrumentation

Pedicle screw instrumentation has emerged as the most common form of internal fixation used for thoracolumbar arthrodesis. Pedicle screws offer numerous advantages compared with hooks or wires, which are less rigid. Pedicle screws can be used when posterior spinal elements are deficient due to prior surgery and provide rigid segmental immobilization, minimizing the need for postoperative brace immobilization. Because of the three-column support provided by the transpedicular fixation, these implants are effectively used in various complex spinal pathologies, including deformities, where corrective forces must be employed.[27]

With the advent of cannulated pedicle screw systems, these implants can be placed through the same skin incisions used for the decompression or fusion portions of the spinal operation. Our preference is to place instrumentation as the final stage of surgery so that the bulk of the implants will not physically interfere with other stages of the operation.

Some surgeons prefer to use noncannulated pedicle screws, placed with direct visualization of the spinal anatomy, using an expandable tubular retractor system. This approach is best used for short procedures (one or two levels), in the lower lumbar spine, where the natural spinal lordosis brings the trajectory of the pedicles into close proximity. In such a situation, it is not difficult to place pedicle screws at adjacent levels using a small, paramedian incision and appropriate expandable retractor system. Placement of pedicle screws in an MIS fashion offers significant advantages compared to traditional pedicle screw instrumentation, which requires full exposure of the spine and major paraspinal muscle stripping.

Cannulated Pedicle Screw Insertion

The first step in placing cannulated pedicle screws involves obtaining a true AP image of each vertebra to be instrumented (Fig. 56.8). Because of the natural sagittal contour of the spine, the C-arm must be angulated to the specific sagittal profile of each individual vertebra in order to obtain the true AP view. It is helpful to have the radiology technician mark the exact angle of the C-arm where the true AP image can be obtained to facilitate rapid return to the proper image (Fig. 56.9). A properly aligned AP C-arm image will demonstrate the superior vertebral endplate as a single, dense line and the pedicles will be localized just below the upper endplate. Correct rotation of the vertebra is ensured when the spinous process shadow is centered between the pedicles. The true AP view is most useful when cannulating the pedicle during pedicle screw insertion.

True lateral fluoroscopic images are also used during pedicle screw instrumentation, particularly during assembly of the construct. The true lateral image will demonstrate the superior endplate as a single, dense line (Fig. 56.10). The pedicles will be superimposed. The posterior cortex of the vertebral body should also appear to be a single radiopaque line, confirming that no rotation of the vertebra is present. The true lateral view is useful during pedicle tapping, placement of pedicle screws, and assembly of the construct. In cases in which scoliosis is present, the C-arm may need to be angled ("wig-wagged") to obtain a true lateral view of each individual vertebra.

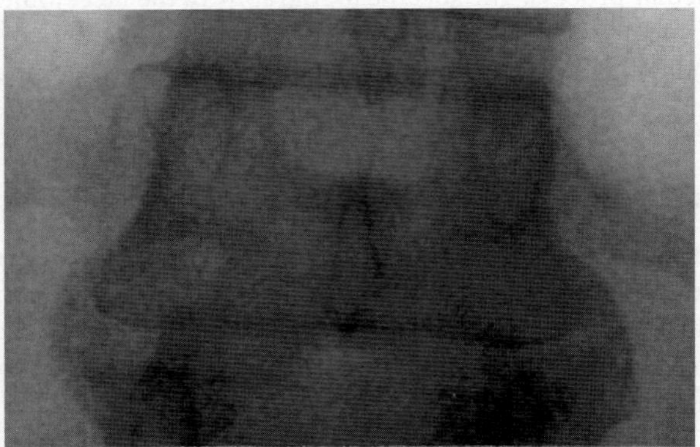

FIG. 56.8 True anteroposterior imaging of each vertebra to be instrumented is crucial for safe pedicle screw placement.

When performing percutaneous instrumentation, obtaining properly aligned C-arm images is, by far, the most important step in the procedure. Thus, it cannot be overemphasized that good images should be obtained prior to attempting to implant percutaneous pedicle screws. If adequate C-arm images cannot be obtained due to severe osteopenia, obesity, intraabdominal contrast or any other reason, placement of percutaneous pedicle screw implants should not be attempted.

After obtaining a true AP fluoroscopic image of a given level, a Kirschner wire (K-wire) should be aligned over the skin of the back so that it appears to bisect the pedicles (Fig. 56.11). Next, a horizontal line is drawn along the skin using the K-wire (Fig. 56.12). This step should be repeated using a true AP image for each of the vertebrae in the construct. Vertical lines are then drawn (using a K-wire placed over the skin of the back) along the lateral pedicle shadow (Fig. 56.13). Skin incisions for percutaneous pedicle screw insertion should be placed about 1 cm lateral to the vertical line (Fig. 56.14).

Once the skin and fascia have been divided, the surgeon can digitally palpate the transverse process of the vertebra whose pedicles are to be cannulated. A Jamshidi needle is then placed at the base of the transverse process (at the junction of the transverse process and superior articular process) and a true AP image is obtained (Fig. 56.15). The goal is to position the tip of the needle directly over the lateral margin of the pedicle shadow (at the 3 and 9 o'clock positions) on the true AP view (Fig. 56.16). The tip of the needle should be adjusted until it lies directly at the lateral border of the pedicle. The

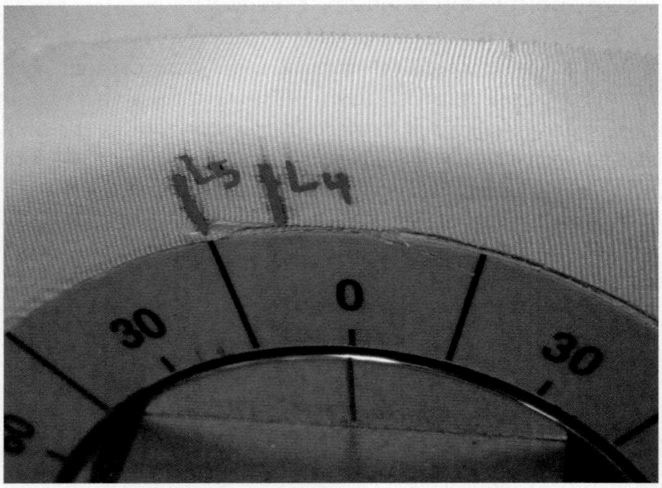

FIG. 56.9 Marking of the exact C-arm angle where the true anteroposterior image can be obtained helps the radiology technician and assists rapid return to the proper image.

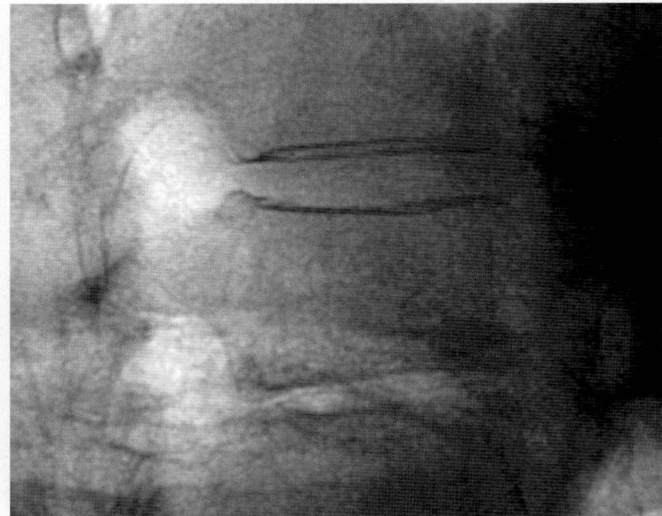

FIG. 56.10 True lateral images are also necessary for proper pedicle screw instrumentation.

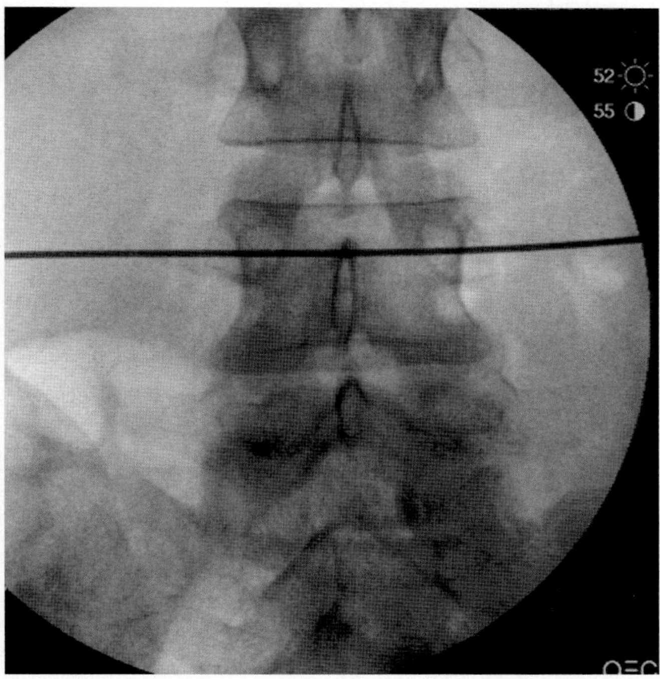

FIG. 56.11 Marking the skin (horizontally): With fluoroscopic assistance, a K-wire is placed horizontally over the skin of the back, bisecting the pedicles of the level to be addressed.

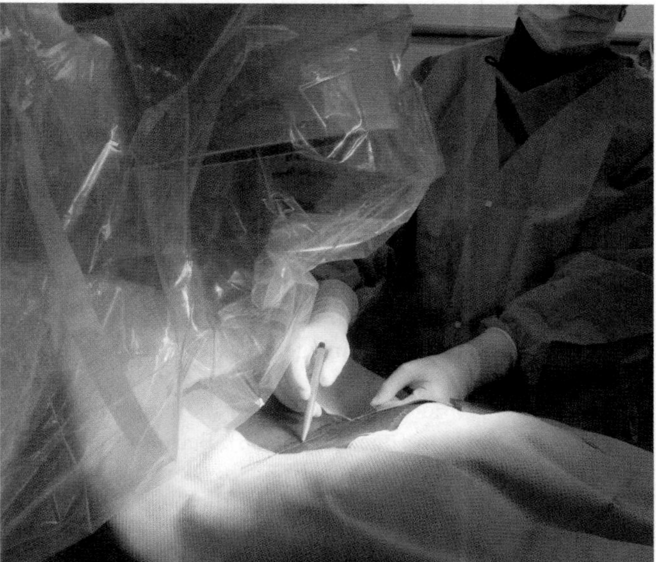

FIG. 56.12 The skin is marked using the K-wire to draw a horizontal line.

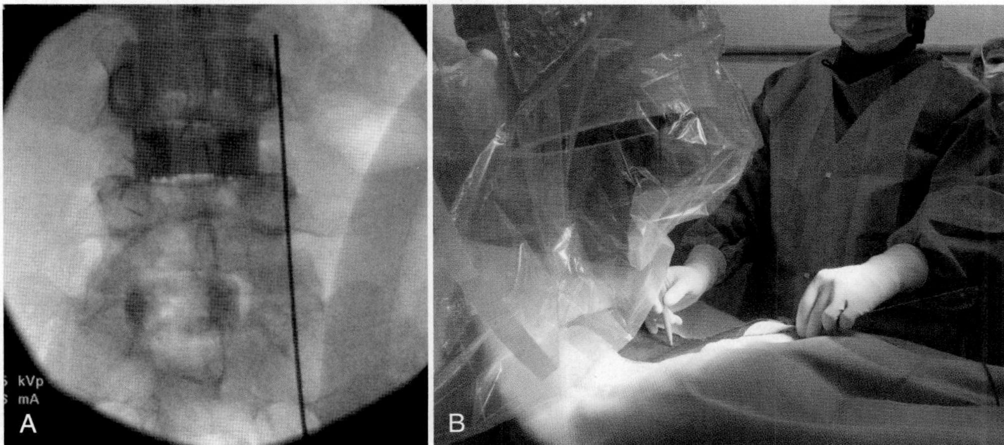

FIG. 56.13 (A) Marking the skin (vertically). Under fluoroscopy, the K-wire is vertically placed over the skin of the back and positioned along the lateral pedicle shadow. (B) The skin is then marked using the K-wire as a reference to draw a vertical line.

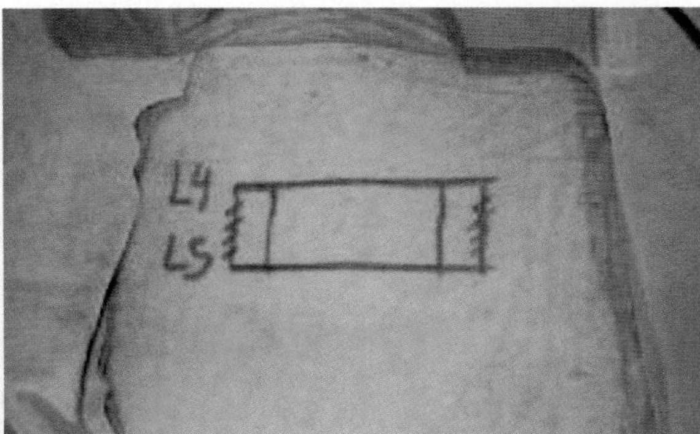

FIG. 56.14 Skin incisions, for percutaneous pedicle screw instrumentation, are placed 1 cm lateral to the marked vertical lines.

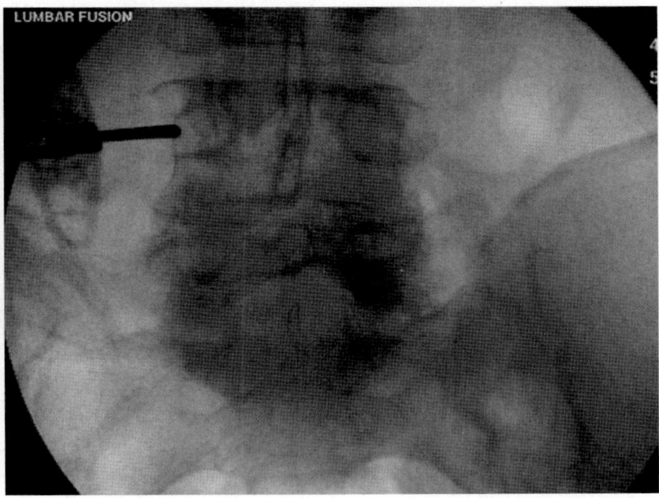

FIG. 56.15 The Jamshidi needle is placed, with fluoroscopic assistance, at the base of the transverse process.

needle shaft is then aligned parallel to the endplate (or transverse process) on the AP image, which ensures a needle trajectory parallel to the central axis of the pedicle (Fig. 56.17). The shaft of the needle should also be held with a lateral to medial trajectory of approximately 10 to 15 degrees, depending on the level to approximate the normal divergence of the pedicles anatomically. Then, the needle is tapped gently a few times to seat the needle tip into the bone and ensure that slippage of the needle tip does not occur as the needle is driven through the pedicle. A final true AP image is checked to be sure that the needle is properly positioned and aligned.

Next, a line is drawn on the shaft of the Jamshidi needle, 20 mm above the skin edge (Fig. 56.18). Because the average length of the pedicle is 20 mm from the starting point, this line is used to determine the depth of the needle tip as it is driven through the pedicle. With the Jamshidi needle properly aligned, the needle is tapped with a mallet to drive the needle through the bone of the central pedicle. When this line on the needle shaft reaches the skin edge, the needle tip has traversed the pedicle isthmus and is at approximately the depth of the base of the pedicle. At this point, another true AP fluoroscopic image is obtained to ensure that the needle tip lies well within the pedicle shadow, no more than three-fourths of the distance (from lateral to medial) across the pedicle (Fig. 56.19). This true AP image should be critically analyzed—if the needle tip

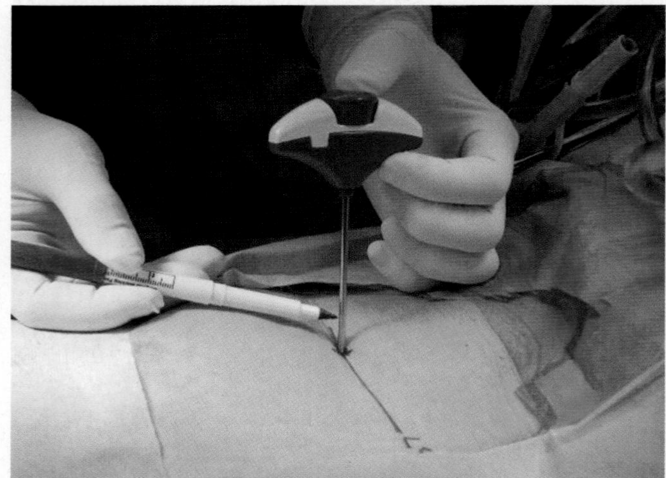

FIG. 56.18 The Jamshidi needle is marked 20 mm above the skin edge, an estimate of the depth of the pedicle.

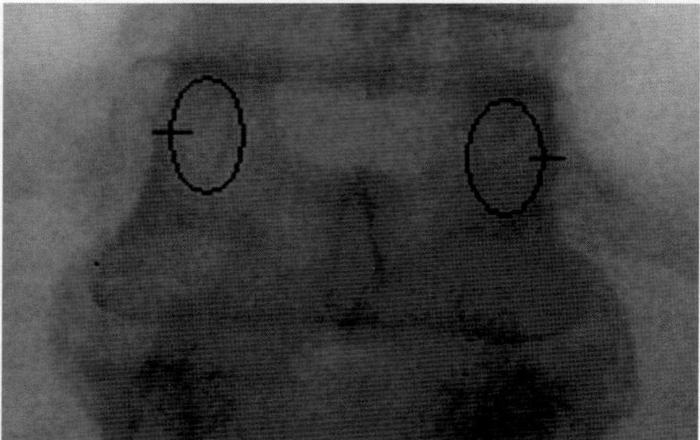

FIG. 56.16 True anteroposterior view illustrates the recommended positioning of the needle tip over the lateral margin of the pedicle shadow at the 3 and 9 o'clock positions.

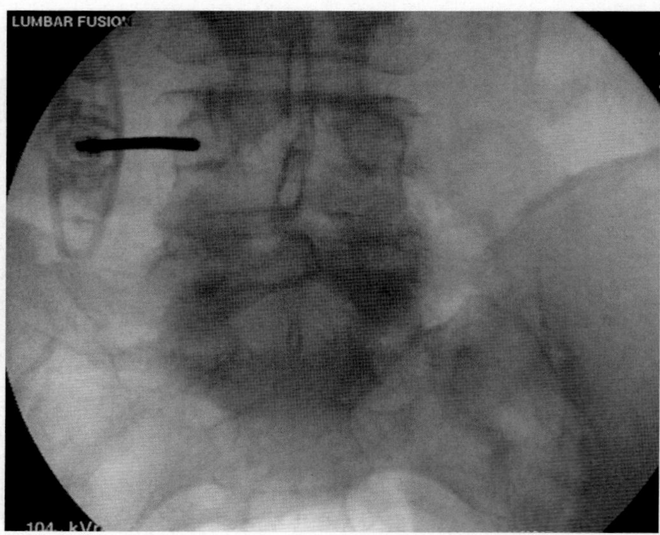

FIG. 56.19 On true anteroposterior fluoroscopy, the needle tip should be located within the pedicle shadow, no more than three-fourths of the distance across the pedicle.

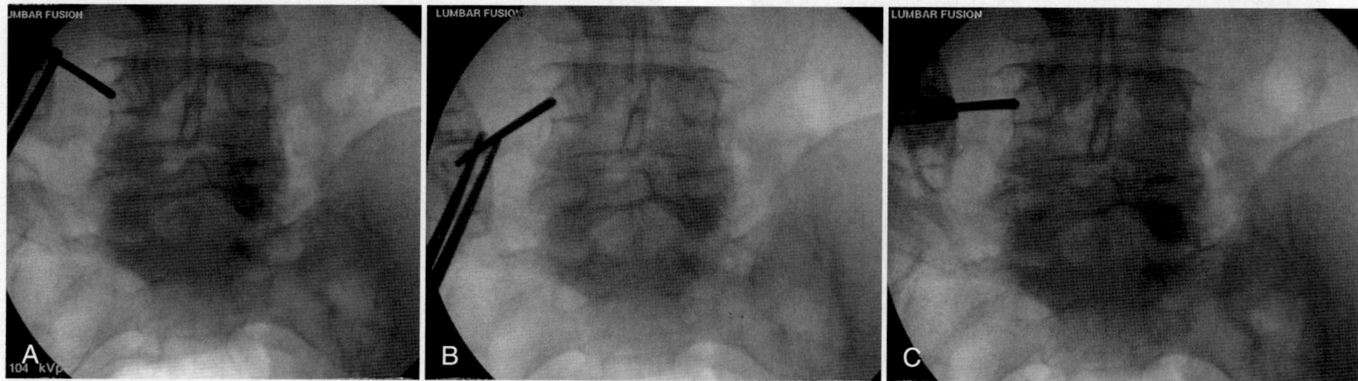

FIG. 56.17 Fluoroscopy is valuable in localizing the needle tip at the (A–B) lateral border of the pedicle and (C) the needle shaft parallel to the endplate.

is in proper position, then it is deemed acceptable for pedicle screw insertion.

Subsequently, the Jamshidi needle is driven 5 to 10 mm deeper into the vertebral body and a guidewire is inserted through the Jamshidi needle into the cancellous bone of the vertebral body. The surgeon should feel "crunchy" cancellous bone at the base of the needle and will generally be able to insert the guidewire 10 to 15 mm beyond the needle tip into the vertebral body with manual pressure. If the bone is too hard for manual insertion, a Kocher clamp can be placed on the guidewire 10 mm above the top of the Jamshidi needle and tapped with a mallet to achieve the positioning of the guidewire into the vertebral body. The same procedure is repeated for all the pedicles in the surgical construct. Our preference is to cannulate all pedicles in the construct using AP fluoroscopy before adjusting the C-arm into the lateral position.

Once all of the pedicles in the construct have been cannulated and guidewires have been placed, the C-arm is adjusted to obtain true lateral images of the spine (Fig. 56.20). The position of the guidewires on the lateral fluoroscopic view is verified prior to proceeding with pedicle preparation. Pedicle preparation and pedicle screw placement are then carried starting from one end of the construct in an "assembly line" fashion. Each pedicle is tapped using a cannulated tap. We prefer to stimulate the tap using stimulus-evoked electromyelography (EMG) to ensure that no low-voltage activity is present that might indicate a breach of the pedicle. Then, cannulated pedicle screws are placed over the guidewires at each level and threaded into the pedicles. The pedicle screws are adjusted in height as needed to maintain polyaxial motion of the screw crowns and to achieve a smooth contour of the screws at adjacent levels (necessary for rod seating). It is also our preference to stimulate each pedicle screw, after insertion with stimulus-evoked EMG, using an insulated port over the screws (Fig. 56.21).

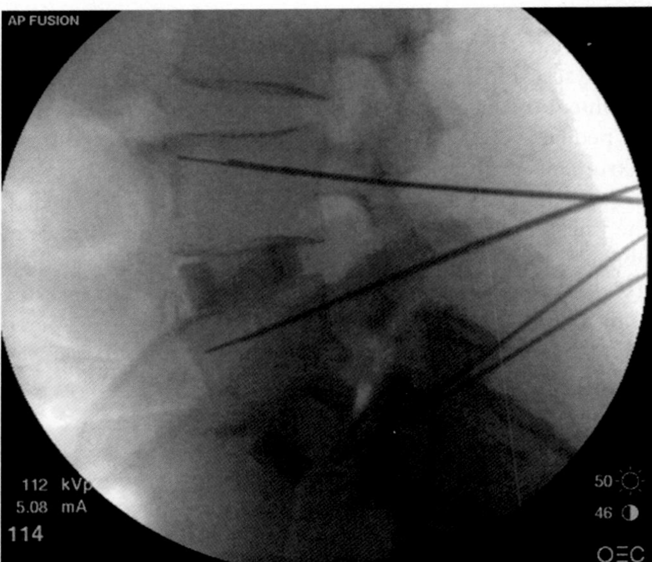

FIG. 56.20 True lateral fluoroscopic image showing the guidewires properly placed within the pedicles.

Once the screws are positioned, the proper rod length is measured and rods are inserted through the screw extensions and into the screw crowns. The details of rod insertion differ slightly between different manufacturers of cannulated screw systems. The surgeon should be familiar with the details of the specific system selected. After the rods are placed, screw caps are inserted into each screw to capture the rod. Compression or distraction of the construct can be performed as needed, followed by final tightening of the construct. At the conclusion of the procedure, AP and lateral imaging of the entire construct should be obtained (Fig. 56.22).

Technical Tips

A few technical points are worth mentioning. First, the advancement of the Jamshidi needle across the pedicle should proceed smoothly with light to moderate taps of the mallet. If the surgeon encounters very hard bone, it generally indicates that the needle tip is displaced medially into the facet joint (the needle tip is striking the hard cortical surface of the superior articular facet). In this instance, the surgeon should withdraw the needle tip and begin with a slightly more lateral starting point to prevent the needle tip from slipping into the facet joint. Another useful tip is to consider the en face view if the AP view fails to clearly show the outline of the pedicle. This is most commonly a concern at the L5 level. To obtain an en face view, start with a true AP view and then angulate the C-arm 10 to 15 degrees in the axial plane to line up the beam with the pedicle axis (Fig. 56.23). Using the en face view, the center of the pedicle should be targeted, keeping the shaft of the needle in line with the C-arm beam. Another useful tip is to consider making minor adjustments to a cannulated pedicle screw trajectory. In such a case, the pedicle can be tapped (with a cannulated tap) to the base of the pedicle. Then, leaving the tap in place, the guidewire can be withdrawn into the tap, allowing the trajectory of the tap to be adjusted as desired with the assistance of fluoroscopy. Once the new trajectory is achieved, the guidewire is reinserted into the vertebral body

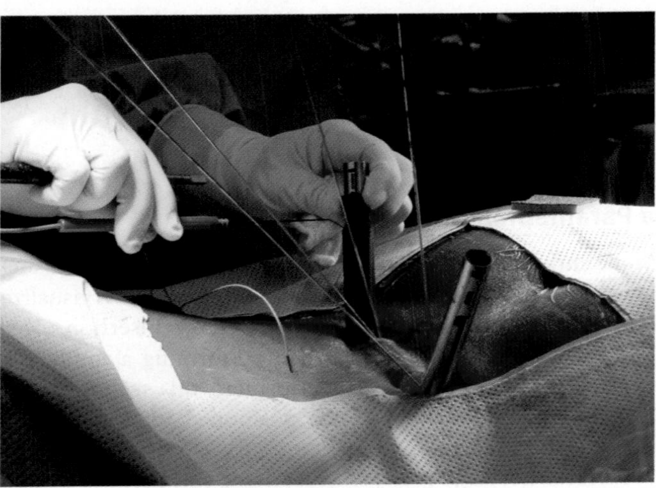

FIG. 56.21 Following their insertion, pedicle screws are tested with stimulus-evoked electromyography using an insulated port.

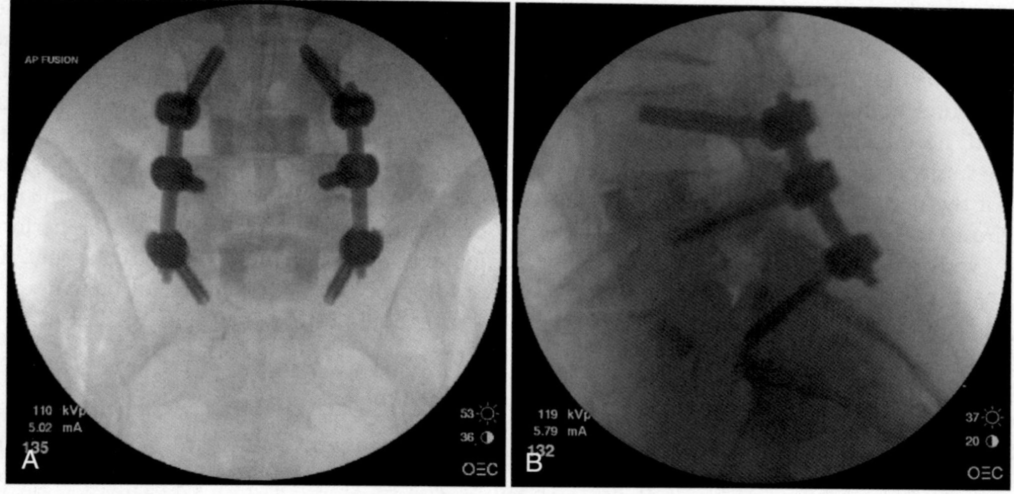

FIG. 56.22 (A) Anteroposterior and (B) lateral fluoroscopic views of the construct at the conclusion of the procedure.

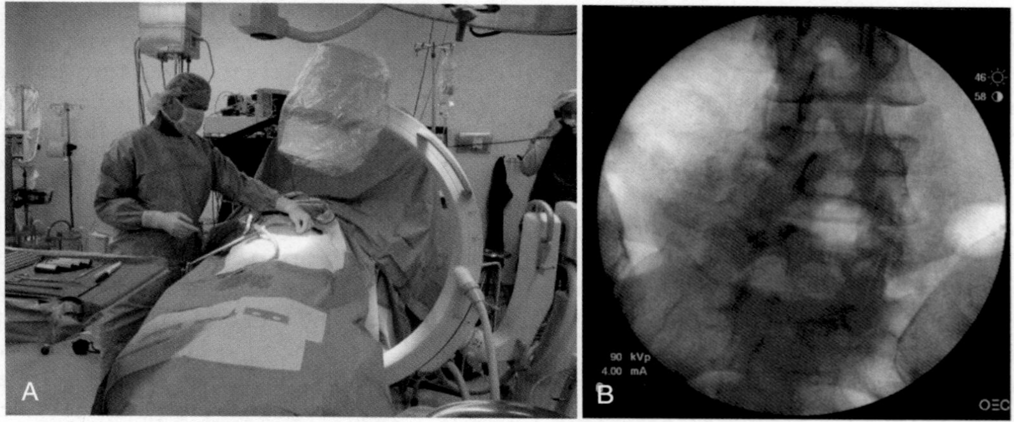

FIG. 56.23 (A) En face view obtained through angulating the C-arm 10 to 15 degrees in the axial plane to (B) line up the beam with the pedicle axis.

along the new trajectory. Finally, stimulus-evoked EMG testing of the taps and screws has proven to be a useful adjuvant to the placement of percutaneous pedicle screws. Any low-voltage activity (<8 mV) should alert the surgeon to the need to pursue additional measures to ensure correct placement of the implant.

Direct Pedicle Screw Insertion via a Paramedian Approach

Some surgeons prefer direct insertion of pedicle screws, using an expandable tubular retractor system to directly visualize the anatomic landmarks for pedicle screw insertion. This approach is especially useful when performing a minimally invasive TLIF procedure. In performing this technique, an expandable tubular retractor is positioned to visualize the junction between the base of the transverse process and the superior articular process. Any overlying soft tissue is cleared away using electrocautery to expose the bony landmarks. A starting hole for the pedicle screw insertion is then made using the normal anatomic landmarks as with traditional open pedicle screw insertion. C-arm fluoroscopy can be utilized to document the location of the starting point and trajectory for the pedicle cannulation. A "gear shift" or similar type blunt instrument is inserted into the starting hole and passed through the pedicle, using fluoroscopic guidance as needed. The walls of the pedicle are palpated to ensure the absence of a breach. Next, the site is tapped and the walls of the pedicle are again palpated for integrity. Pedicle screws are inserted using a technique analogous to open pedicle screw placement. Electrical testing of the screw can be used if desired, followed by the introduction of a rod and caps.

Facet Screw Instrumentation

Although pedicle screws are the workhorse for most spinal fixation strategies, facet screws offer certain advantages in selected cases. Facet screws are quick and relatively easy to place. They are generally less expensive compared with pedicle screw implants and yet offer comparable initial stiffness for

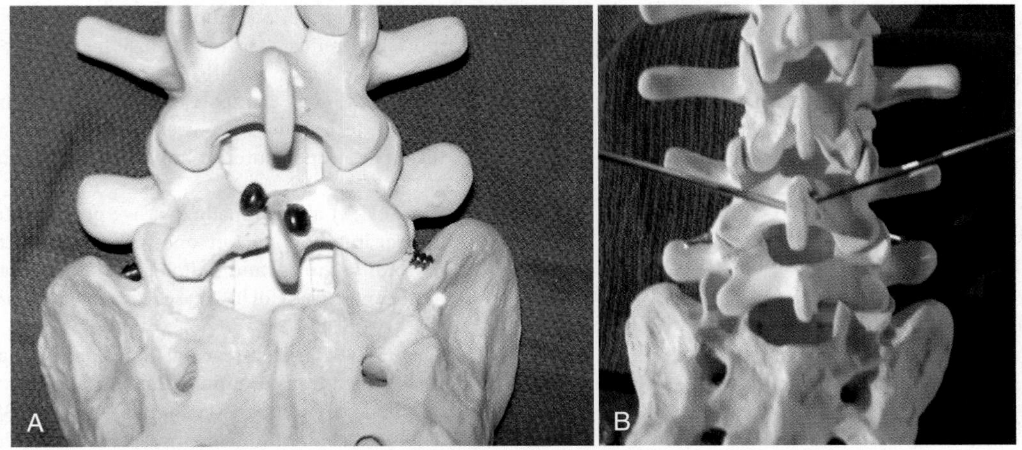

FIG. 56.24 Facet screw instrumentation. (A) The screw path begins at the base of the spinous process on one side and then (B) advances across the contralateral lamina and facet joint.

short constructs.[28] In certain clinical situations, such as following anterior lumbar interbody fusion, facet screw instrumentation has been shown to produce favorable clinical results.[29,30] Additionally, recent studies have suggested similar results with lower costs for patients undergoing minimally invasive TLIF surgery who have unilateral pedicle screws and contralateral facet screws compared to traditional bilateral pedicle screw fixation.[31]

Magerl et al. described a technique using large fragment (4.5-mm) cortical bone screws to perform a translaminar fixation of the facet joint.[32] The screw path begins at the base of the spinous process on one side and is then advanced across the contralateral lamina and facet joint (Fig. 56.24). Two screws are placed to immobilize the facet joints bilaterally using a mini-open or percutaneous technique.[33,34]

To insert translaminar facet screws, using the mini-open technique, a midline incision is performed and the spinous processes, bilateral laminae, and facet joints are exposed. The facet joint capsules may be removed and the joint decorticated and packed with bone graft to promote local fusion following instrumentation. When placing translaminar facet screws, pilot holes are made on each side of the spinous process in line with the anticipated screw trajectories. The pilot holes should be slightly staggered to prevent the two screws from contacting one another as they cross through the base of the spinous process.

Next, the trajectory for each screw is defined, using fluoroscopy if desired. Some surgeons prefer to make a small laminotomy and palpate the medial wall of the pedicle as a landmark and to ensure direct visualization of the dura while drilling the screw trajectory. Additionally, decompressions of the lateral recess using fenestration can be performed if necessary.

Next, a line connecting the mid-facet (or medial border of the pedicle) and the pilot hole is marked on the skin. This trajectory can be extended superiorly and laterally to the midline incision. A small, percutaneous incision is made along this line, about 10 to 12 cm from the midline such that the drill trajectory will be in line with the contralateral lamina.

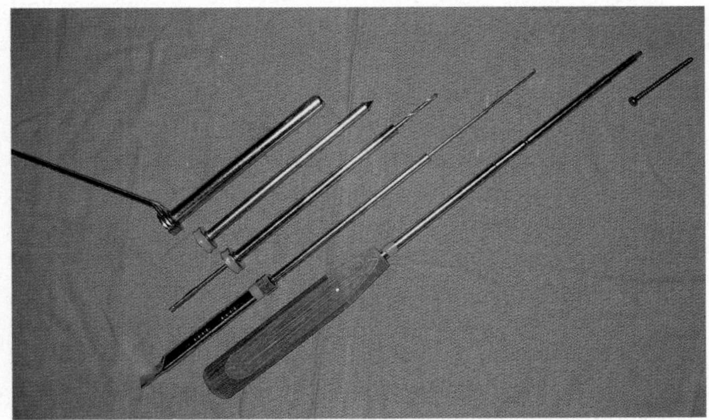

FIG. 56.25 Various instruments (e.g., drill guides, depth gauge, screws) are used during percutaneous facet screw placement.

A drill guide is inserted into the percutaneous incision and advanced into the midline exposure (Fig. 56.25). The drill is inserted and seated into the pilot hole at the base of the spinous process. The drill is adjusted as necessary so that it will traverse the lamina and then the facet joint. As the drill is advanced, the surgeon should feel uniform resistance until the facet joint has been breached. A momentary change in resistance may be noted as the facet joint space is traversed, but the cortical bone of the superior articular process will then be encountered. After drilling, the length of the screw path is measured. Then, a 4.5-mm, fully threaded cortical screw is placed to secure the position of the facet joint. A similar percutaneous technique has been described, relying only on fluoroscopic images to ensure adequate placement of the translaminar facet screw implants.[30]

Patient Selection

Patient selection remains the most crucial outcome variable for any spinal procedure. The same selection criteria that have been shown to produce success in traditional spinal surgery apply to patient selection for an MIS approach. In addition, patients being considered for an MIS approach have some additional selection criteria that should be considered.[35]

In the early learning curve of an individual surgeon, only simple cases should be considered for an MIS approach. Experience can be gained working with MIS equipment, such as tubular retractors and microscopes, by performing straightforward cases (e.g., microdiscectomy). As a surgeon gains experience with minimally invasive spinal procedures, progressively more complex cases may be tackled in a minimally invasive fashion. Other aspects should be considered as well, including the size of the patient (obese patients will be more difficult), severity of the pathologies, and history of any prior spinal surgery.

Summary

It appears likely that MIS will become an increasingly important component of the spinal surgical armamentarium in the future. With the advances in MIS techniques, spinal fusions and instrumentations are now being achieved with less morbidity and faster recovery compared to traditional open surgical approaches. However, surgical expertise in MIS can be reached only by ascending a learning curve. Thus, surgeons interested in this innovative field must be willing to spend the time and effort necessary to become proficient in MIS techniques.

In skilled hands, the benefits of MIS procedures appear to outweigh the risks. Additional long-term outcome data are still needed to define the efficacy of these approaches compared to traditional open spinal fusion approaches. However, early data suggest that surgeons willing to spend the time and energy necessary to gain proficiency in MIS can expect to be rewarded through the benefits provided to their surgical patient population, especially with regard to reduced blood loss and a shorter recovery period.

REFERENCES

1. Gille O, et al. Erector spinae muscle changes on magnetic resonance imaging following lumbar surgery through a posterior approach. *Spine*. 2007;32:1236-1241.
2. Motosuneya T, et al. Postoperative change of the cross-sectional area of back musculature after 5 surgical procedures as assessed by magnetic resonance imaging. *J Spinal Disord Tech*. 2006;19:318-322.
3. Fritzell P, Hägg O, Nordwall A. Complications in lumbar fusion surgery for chronic low back pain: comparison of three surgical techniques used in a prospective randomized study. A report from the Swedish Lumbar Spine Study Group. *Eur Spine J*. 2003;12:178-189.
4. Katz JN. Lumbar spinal fusion. Surgical rates, costs, and complications. *Spine*. 1995;20:78S-83S.
5. Malter AD, McNeney B, Loeser JD, Deyo RA. 5-year reoperation rates after different types of lumbar spine surgery. *Spine*. 1998;23:814-820.
6. Stauffer RN, Coventry MB. Posterolateral lumbar-spine fusion. *J Bone Joint Surg Am*. 1972;54:1195-1204.
7. Pumberger M, et al. National in-hospital morbidity and mortality trends after lumbar fusion surgery between 1998 and 2008. *J Bone Joint Surg Br*. 2012;94-B:359-364.
8. Kepler CK, et al. Comparison of open and minimally invasive techniques for posterior lumbar instrumentation and fusion after open anterior lumbar interbody fusion. *Spine J*. 2013;13:489-497.
9. Giorgi H, et al. Minimally invasive posterior transforaminal lumbar interbody fusion: one-year postoperative morbidity, clinical and radiological results of a prospective multicenter study of 182 cases. *Orthop Traumatol Surg Res*. 2015;101:S241-S245.
10. Seng CM, et al. Five-year outcomes of minimally invasive versus open transforaminal lumbar interbody fusion: a matched-pair comparison study. *Spine*. 2013;38:2049-2055.
11. Patel AA, et al. Minimally invasive versus open lumbar fusion: a comparison of blood loss, surgical complications, and hospital course. *Iowa Orthop J*. 2015;35:130-134.
12. Foley KT, Holly LT, Schwender JD. Minimally invasive lumbar fusion. *Spine*. 2003;28:S26-S35.
13. Benglis DM, Elhammady MS, Levi AD, Vanni S. Minimally invasive anterolateral approaches for the treatment of back pain and adult degenerative deformity. *Neurosurgery*. 2008;63:191-196.
14. Vertuani S, et al. A Cost-effectiveness analysis of minimally invasive versus open surgery techniques for lumbar spinal fusion in Italy and the United Kingdom. *Value Health*. 2015;18:810-816.
15. Singh K, et al. A perioperative cost analysis comparing single-level minimally invasive and open transforaminal lumbar interbody fusion. *Spine J*. 2014;14:1694-1701.
16. Rampersaud YR, Gray R, Lewis SJ, Massicotte EM, Fehlings MG. Cost-utility analysis of posterior minimally invasive fusion compared with conventional open fusion for lumbar spondylolisthesis. *SAS J*. 2011;5:29-35.
17. Lee JC, Jang H-D, Shin B-J. Learning curve and clinical outcomes of minimally invasive transforaminal lumbar interbody fusion: our experience in 86 consecutive cases. *Spine*. 2012;37:1548-1557.
18. Ahn J, et al. Minimally invasive lumbar decompression—the surgical learning curve. *Spine J*. 2016;16:909-916. doi:10.1016/j.spinee.2015.07.455.
19. Sclafani JA, Kim CW. Complications associated with the initial learning curve of minimally invasive spine surgery: a systematic review. *Clin Orthop*. 2014;472:1711-1717.
20. Kukreja S, Haydel J, Nanda A, Sin AH. Impact of body habitus on fluoroscopic radiation emission during minimally invasive spine surgery. *J Neurosurg Spine*. 2015;22:211-218.
21. Ropper AE, Chi JH. Maximal radiation exposure during minimally invasive spine surgery? *Neurosurgery*. 2011;68:N23-N24.
22. Kasis AG, Marshman LAG, Krishna M, Bhatia CK. Significantly improved outcomes with a less invasive posterior lumbar interbody fusion incorporating total facetectomy. *Spine*. 2009;34:572-577.
23. Krishna M, Pollock RD, Bhatia C. Incidence, etiology, classification, and management of neuralgia after posterior lumbar interbody fusion surgery in 226 patients. *Spine J*. 2008;8:374-379.
24. Kwon BK, et al. Radiographic analysis of transforaminal lumbar interbody fusion for the treatment of adult isthmic spondylolisthesis. *J Spinal Disord Tech*. 2003;16:469-476.

25. Quigley KJ, Alander DH, Bledsoe JG. An in vitro biomechanical investigation: variable positioning of Leopard carbon fiber interbody cages. *J Spinal Disord Tech*. 2008;21:442-447.
26. Oh CH, et al. Slip reduction rate between minimal invasive and conventional unilateral transforaminal interbody fusion in patients with low-grade isthmic spondylolisthesis. *Korean J Spine*. 2013;10:232-236.
27. Liljenqvist U, Lepsien U, Hackenberg L, Niemeyer T, Halm H. Comparative analysis of pedicle screw and hook instrumentation in posterior correction and fusion of idiopathic thoracic scoliosis. *Eur Spine J*. 2002;11:336-343.
28. Ferrara LA, et al. A biomechanical comparison of facet screw fixation and pedicle screw fixation: effects of short-term and long-term repetitive cycling. *Spine*. 2003;28:1226-1234.
29. Volkman T, Horton WC, Hutton WC. Transfacet screws with lumbar interbody reconstruction: biomechanical study of motion segment stiffness. *J Spinal Disord*. 1996;9:425-432.
30. Shim CS, et al. Fluoroscopically assisted percutaneous translaminar facet screw fixation following anterior lumbar interbody fusion: technical report. *Spine*. 2005;30:838-843.
31. Awad BI, et al. Bilateral pedicle screw fixation versus unilateral pedicle and contralateral facet screws for minimally invasive transforaminal lumbar interbody fusion: clinical outcomes and cost analysis. *Global Spine J*. 2013;3:225-230.
32. Benini A, Magerl F. Selective decompression and translaminar articular facet screw fixation for lumbar canal stenosis and disc protrusion. *Br J Neurosurg*. 1993;7:413-418.
33. Montesano PX, Magerl F, Jacobs RR, Jackson RP, Rauschning W. Translaminar facet joint screws. *Orthopedics*. 1988;11:1393-1397.
34. Hailong Y, Wei L, Zhensheng M, Hongxun S. Computer analysis of the safety of using three different pedicular screw insertion points in the lumbar spine in the Chinese population. *Eur Spine J*. 2007;16:619-623.
35. German JW, Adamo MA, Hoppenot RG, Blossom JH, Nagle HA. Perioperative results following lumbar discectomy: comparison of minimally invasive discectomy and standard microdiscectomy. *Neurosurg Focus*. 2008;25:E20.

57 CHAPTER Posterolateral Endoscopic Lumbar Discectomy

Christopher A. Yeung
Anthony T. Yeung

Posterolateral endoscopic lumbar surgery is a less invasive surgical procedure to address lumbar pathology in the disc and bony foramen. Like any surgical procedure, it is based on visual identification and exposure of the target pathology and adequate surgical tools to address the offending pathology. Modern endoscopic technology allows for discectomy and decompression of the traversing and exiting nerve roots from a percutaneous posterolateral/transforaminal approach under continuous direct visualization. This is safe and equally efficacious to microscopic discectomy in properly selected patients.[1–4] Recent advances also allow for bony decompression of foraminal stenosis.[5,6]

Advances in the ability to perform endoscopic discectomy have paralleled other specialties, yet endoscopic spinal surgery has not met with the same peer recognition as the other fields. This is due in part to the high success rate and relative low morbidity of the current gold standard, posterior microscopic lumbar discectomy. However, this approach still requires a 1-inch midline incision, muscle and ligament stripping, prolonged muscle retraction, partial facet and lamina resection, and both nerve root and dura retraction. This can weaken the muscular lumbar stabilizers, create instability and facet arthrosis, cause traction neurapraxia, promote epidural scarring, and make revision surgery more difficult.

Another barrier for more widespread adoption was the relative paucity of peer-reviewed literature, and critics noted that only a few authors were contributing to this body of literature. Recently, there have been many more published results of posterolateral endoscopic discectomy from around the world; the preponderance of evidence supports its efficacy.

Numerous other nonvisualized, percutaneous techniques often get categorized and confused with posterolateral endoscopic lumbar discectomy. These include automated percutaneous lumbar discectomy, percutaneous laser discectomy, and percutaneous discectomy with the Dekompressor or Arthrocare wand (Coblation). These are all fluoroscopically guided, nonvisualized procedures that access the disc via the same posterolateral approach as endoscopic lumbar surgery. The underlying principle of these procedures is that, through central nucleus removal or ablation, intradiscal pressure can be substantially lowered. This was based on the work of Hirsh and his postulated relationship between intradiscal pressure, disc herniation, and low back pain.[7] He hypothesized that lowering this pressure in an injured disc could be efficacious in the relief of sciatica. Multiple studies described decreases in intradiscal pressures of 50% or greater.[8–10]

The results of these types of indirect decompressive procedures have been similar, with initial favorable reports. However, subsequent studies have shown varying degrees of success. The inability to consistently see the decompressed nerve or the targeted pathoanatomy has limited the use of these nonvisualized decompressive procedures.[11–14] It is unfortunate that these interventional procedures and their results are mistaken for posterolateral endoscopic discectomy surgery.

History

The basis for percutaneous lumbar disc procedures came from accepted posterolateral percutaneous biopsy techniques of the lumbar vertebrae. These procedures were initially performed with the use of a Craig needle to perform a posterolateral biopsy for neoplastic conditions.[15,16]

Minimally invasive surgery for lumbar disc herniation was first independently reported by Kambin and colleagues[17] and Hijikata[18] in 1975. A posterolateral approach was used to position a small cannula in the foraminal zone of the disc bordered by the traversing nerve dorsally, the exiting nerve ventrally, and the endplate of the inferior vertebra caudally. Mechanical instruments were used to remove disc tissue. The early efforts were limited to a nonvisualized central discectomy to achieve an indirect decompression of the nerve roots.[17–19] The goal was to decompress nerve roots secondary to lumbar disc herniation by the inside-out technique of central and posterior nuclectomy and fragmentectomy.

The addition of an endoscope to help with the decompression developed in stages. Initially, an arthroscope was used to inspect the disc and anulus intermittently through the cannula while the mechanical nuclectomy was done under fluoroscopic guidance. The introduction of a biportal approach allowed for direct visualization of instruments introduced through a cannula inserted into the disc from the opposite posterolateral portal. The later development of an operating spine scope with a working channel for instruments allowed for surgical removal of disc material and visualization of foraminal anatomy under direct visualization via a uniportal approach.

Kambin performed the first true endoscopic lumbar procedures. The arthroscope was at first used intermittently through the working cannula. At certain stages of the procedure, such as perforating the disc in the triangular working zone, the arthroscope would be placed in the cannula. The nonworking-channel scope was used for identification of the anulus and periannular structures. The basis was to see that the nerve was not in the way before advancing the cannula. Once the cannula was safely within the disc, the nucleotome, an arthroscopic shaver, and pituitary rongeurs were passed through the cannula to perform mechanical disc removal. The majority of the procedure was only fluoroscopically visualized.[17] Kambin reported an 88% success rate in his first 100 patients.[20,21]

The early endoscopic procedures were limited by the absence of a working-channel arthroscope. This led Kambin to the development of a biportal technique in which the scope was inserted on one side and the working cannula on the opposite side. Kambin's indications for a biportal approach included large subligamentous herniations, extraligamentous herniations, and arthroscopic interbody fusion.[22] In later studies, Kambin reports results from both uniportal and biportal procedures together. Overall results ranged from 85% to 92% satisfactory results at a minimum 2-year follow-up. There was no differentiation made between the results of uniportal versus biportal approaches.[23–25]

Kambin's first prototype of the working-channel scope was not fully developed and was not successfully marketed. The problems with the initial scope included fragility, limited degree of angulation for the working instruments, and the inability to establish sufficient inflow or outflow for adequate visualization.[26] Yeung developed the first working-channel endoscope to become widely available. The scope was developed in 1997 and was approved for use by the US Food and Drug Administration in March 1998. The Yeung Endoscopic Spine Surgery system (Richard Wolf Surgical Instruments) modified the scope by adding multichannel integrated irrigation, specialized beveled cannulas, a two-hole obturator, and newly designed discectomy tools that allowed for constant real-time visualization with a uniportal technique[27] (Fig. 57.1).

Another major change, which allowed for advancement in the field of endoscopic spinal surgery, was Yeung and Mathews' emphasis on placement of the cannula closer to the epidural space and the base of the targeted disc herniation leading to the so-called targeted technique. They promoted routine visualization of the epidural space and greater access to the traversing nerve root.[28] This enabled surgeons to target extruded herniations in addition to contained herniations. Previous percutaneous modalities all focused on entry through Kambin's triangle and working within the center of the disc with the cannula anchored inside the anulus. The cannula was advanced past the anulus and remained intradiscal for the procedure.

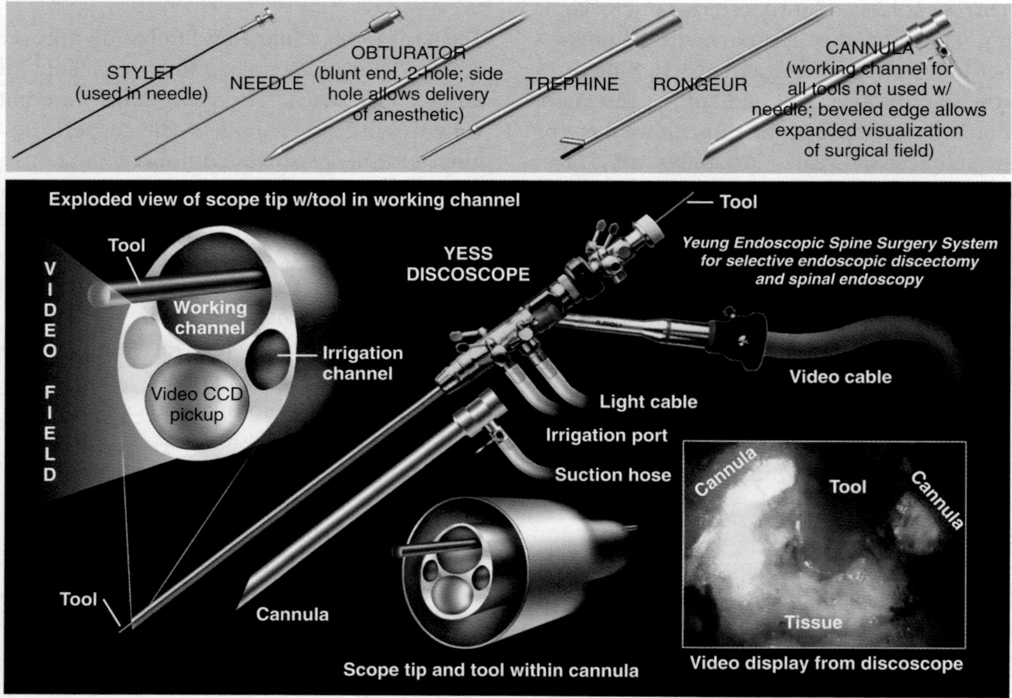

FIG. 57.1 The Yeung Endoscopic Spine Surgery system. (Courtesy Richard Wolf Surgical Instruments, Vernon Hills, IL.)

The development of a working-channel scope and use of the transforaminal approach using beveled and slotted cannulas enhanced endoscopic lumbar surgery. Using this approach, surgeons could operate under full visualization throughout most of the procedure and follow the neural structures into the epidural space. The specialized cannulas provide greater access to pathology and help protect and retract sensitive anatomy, such as the exiting nerve and dorsal root ganglion. The working channel also allows the passage of high-speed burrs for bone removal and direct foraminal enlargement and decompression of foraminal stenosis (foraminoplasty). This facet decompression also allows the surgeon to access the midline of the disc and the epidural space. Thus, it is feasible to treat the full spectrum of disc herniations with advanced endoscopic instrumentation and techniques that can either target the extruded fragment directly or with a combination of the inside-out technique.[29]

Improvements in surgical equipment and technique have evolved gradually since 1975. A systematic fluoroscopically guided approach method introduced by Yeung and reported by Tsou[30–32] outlined a consistent and safe technique for entry into all lumbar posterior disc spaces, including the L5–S1 level. This specific technique has been termed selective endoscopic discectomy but can be classified under the more general descriptive term of posterolateral endoscopic lumbar discectomy (PELD) that other authors describe. In the past 15 years, the important major equipment improvements have included various-sized high-resolution rod lens operating endoscopes with variable-sized working channels, more variety of beveled and slotted cannulas, flexible shavers and pituitary forceps, a bipolar flexible high-frequency/low-temperature radiofrequency electrode, multidirectional holmium yttrium-aluminum-garnet (YAG) lasers, and high-speed diamond burrs and motorized shavers to decompress the foramen.[29] These refinements have enhanced the capabilities of foraminal endoscopic discectomy to deliver surgical results similar to the results obtainable by traditional transcanal approaches for treating common lumbar disc herniations.[1–4]

Recent development of expandable and cannulated interbody fusion devices has allowed truly minimally invasive interbody fusion procedures to become feasible. The RISE IntraLIF (Globus Medical) expandable interbody device can fit down an 8.5-mm access cannula after endoscopic discectomy and endplate preparation. The OptiMesh (Spineology) expandable polyetheretherketone mesh cage is another example. Early studies are just starting to get reported.[33]

Anatomy

Posterolateral endoscopic lumbar surgery is performed through what has been named the *triangular working zone*, or *Kambin's triangle* (Fig. 57.2). This triangular zone is defined as a safe zone in the posterolateral anulus between the exiting and traversing nerve roots. The exiting nerve root forms the anterior border of the triangular zone as it exits under the cephalad pedicle. The superior endplate of the caudal vertebral body forms the inferior border and the articular process and superior articulating facet of the caudal vertebra form the posterior border. The working zone is bordered medially by the traversing nerve root and dura. From cadaveric measurements, it was determined that cannulas ranging from 4 to 10 mm could be safely used in the triangular working zone.[22,34–37] A thorough understanding of the three-dimensional anatomy is necessary to understand and perform posterior percutaneous lumbar surgery.

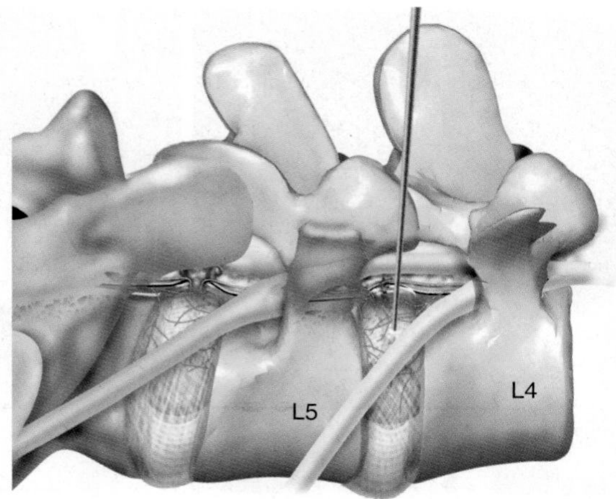

FIG. 57.2 Triangular working zone at L4–L5 (Kambin triangle). This is the access point for posterolateral disc access. The exiting nerve root is the hypotenuse of the triangle, the superior endplate of the caudal vertebral body/sacrum is the base (width), and the traversing nerve root/dura is the height of the triangle.

Indications and Contraindications

Current indications for the use of an endoscopic posterolateral approach to the lumbar spine include foraminal and far-lateral disc herniations, contained central and paracentral disc herniations, small nonsequestered extruded disc herniations, recurrent herniations, symptomatic annular tears, synovial cysts, biopsy and debridement of discitis, decompression of foraminal stenosis with or without spondylolisthesis, visualized total nuclectomy (before nucleus replacement), and visualized discectomy with endplate preparation before interbody fusion.

Perhaps the ideal lesions for posterolateral selective endoscopic discectomy are the foraminal and extraforaminal disc herniations. The cannula inserts directly at the herniation site, and the exiting nerve is routinely visualized and protected (Fig. 57.3). This approach requires less manipulation of the exiting nerve root than the paramedian posterior approach.

Any herniation contiguous with the disc space not sequestered and migrated is amenable to endoscopic disc excision if the bony anatomy permits an unobstructed approach. A targeted technique can be utilized or the inside-out technique, in which the herniation is grasped from its base within the disc, pulled back into the working intradiscal cavity, and removed via the cannula. The size and types of herniations chosen by the surgeon for endoscopic excision will depend on the skill and experience of the surgeon. Certainly, all contained disc

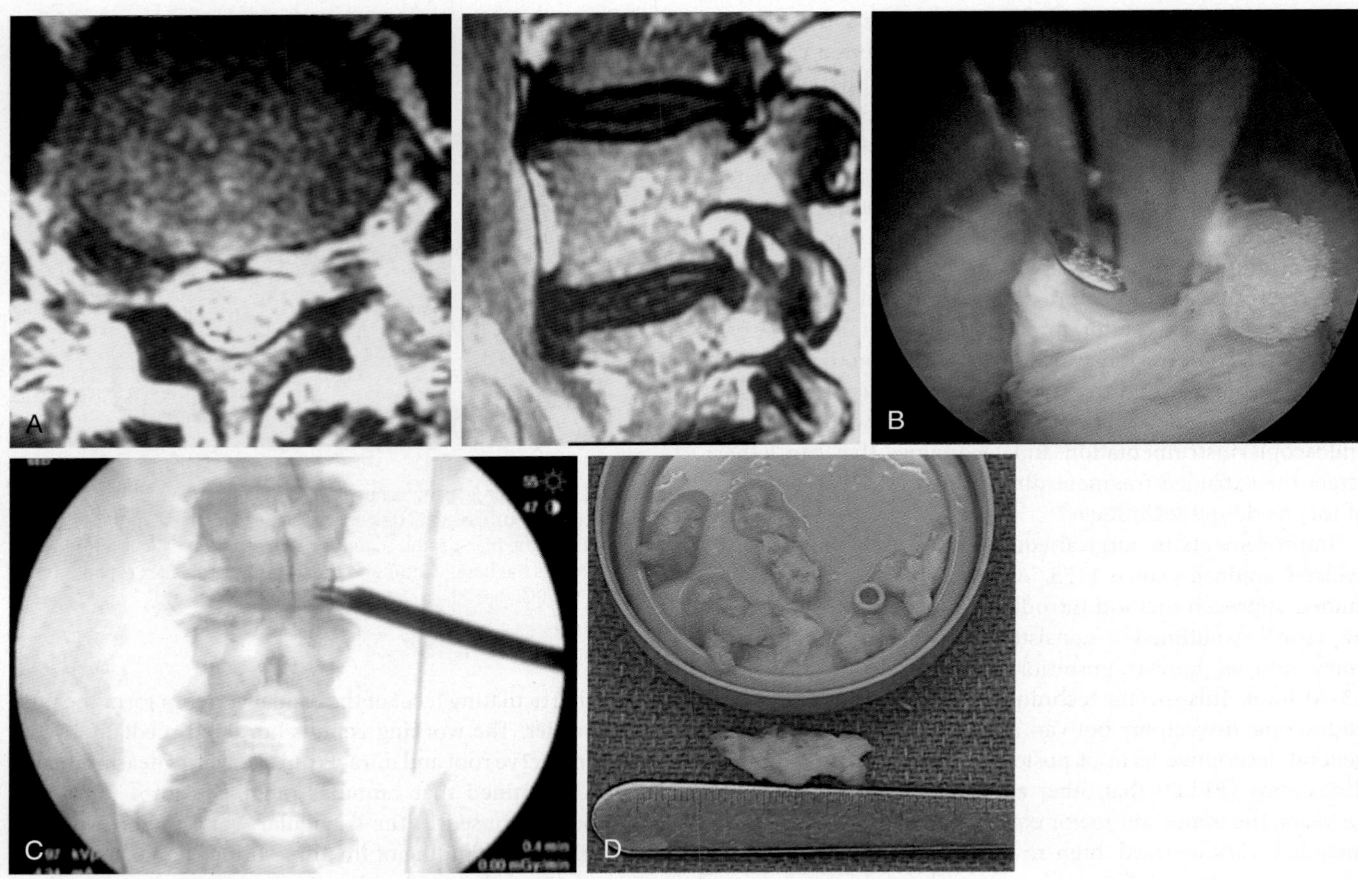

FIG. 57.3 Treatment of a foraminal herniated disc. (A) Magnetic resonance image of an extruded right L3–L4 foraminal herniation with some cephalad migration. (B) Fluoroscopic anteroposterior image shows the pituitary forceps positioned to grab the herniation in the epidural space in the axilla of the exiting nerve root. The forceps are within the working channel of the scope and the herniation is removed under direct endoscopic visualization. (C) Endoscopic picture of the extruded herniation abutting the axilla of the exiting right L3 nerve root. (D) The large extruded fragment that was removed. Note the red, white, and blue stained portions of the fragment. The red portion is the part that was extruded and has some inflammatory tissue, the white portion is the part trapped within the anulus, and the blue part is the intradiscal portion that is stained by the injected indigo carmine dye.

herniations are appropriate for endoscopic decompression. With experience, extruded herniations can be routinely addressed. This approach is especially attractive for recurrent herniations after a traditional posterior approach because the surgeon can avoid the scar tissue from the previous surgery.

Extruded herniations with limited cephalad/caudal migration can be removed with the outside-in technique. If the herniation is sequestered and a free fragment, then posterolateral endoscopic discectomy is relatively contraindicated.

Radiofrequency energy can be applied to the annular tears under direct visualization to contract the collagen and ablate ingrown granulation tissue, neoangiogenesis, and sensitized nociceptors.[38] Frequently, interpositional nuclear tissue is seen within the fibers of the annular tear, preventing the tear from healing. This tissue can then be removed to allow the tear to heal.

Endoscopic foraminoplasty can be readily achieved with bone trephines/rasps, the side-firing holmium-YAG laser, and endoscopic high-speed drills.[5,6] The roof of the foramen is formed by the undersurface of the superior articular facet. This is easily visualized and accessed via the endoscope, and the previously mentioned tools are used to remove bone and enlarge the foraminal opening. Synovial cysts can sometimes be visualized and removed as well, depending on their location.

In cases of discitis, the posterolateral endoscopic approach will provide a robust biopsy for culture diagnosis, and the infected/necrotic disc tissue can be thoroughly debrided to reduce the bacterial load and accelerate healing and potential in situ fusion.[39] This approach also limits the spread of the infection since no approach-related dead space is created.

Contraindications include any pathology not accessible from the posterolateral endoscopic approach. This may include some extruded sequestered disc herniations, extruded migrated disc herniations (migrated extent greater than the measured height of the posterior marginal disc space on T2 sagittal magnetic resonance imaging [MRI]), larger herniations occupying greater than 50% of the spinal canal,[4] moderate to severe central canal stenosis, and hard calcified herniations. These contraindications are considered relative contraindications dependent on the surgeon's technical experience and comfort level. More experienced endoscopic surgeons can gain greater access to pathology using advanced techniques for bone removal of osteophytes, stenosis, and the posterolateral corner of the vertebral body before addressing the pathology. Other relative contraindications include inadequate support staff or equipment to successfully perform procedure and uncooperative patients.

Posterolateral Endoscopic Lumbar Discectomy

Different styles of posterolateral endoscopic discectomy have been described in the literature. The inside-out technique initially positions the cannula within the disc near the base of the herniation as a safe starting point. The cannula is gradually backed out and the surgeon works toward the base of the herniation and epidural space to directly remove the herniated fragment in addition to some of the underlying unstable nucleus. The outside-in technique positions the cannula immediately in the epidural space where the herniated fragment is. The fragment is removed and the surgeon only minimally enters the disc space or does not enter it at all, thus performing more of a fragmentectomy. This is especially useful for extruded migrated disc herniations. The targeted technique is a blend of these two techniques, in which the initial cannula placement is at the site of the herniation. The herniated fragment is removed and the surgeon enters the disc space to then remove any loose unstable nucleus. All of these techniques are effective; the main difference is simply the starting point of the cannula position in relation to the disc. After that initial starting point, the surgery progresses to attempt removal of the offending disc herniation completely by using the same instruments.

The different types and locations of herniations also dictate the location of the skin incision (skin window). The approach trajectory gets shallower if you start farther away from the midline. Foraminal herniations are more easily removed with a more steep approach trajectory into the disc, about 45 to 55 degrees. It is better to have a shallower 20- to 40-degree approach trajectory for paracentral herniations in order to fully access them. Central or large paracentral herniations may utilize an extreme lateral approach with a 0- to 20-degree approach trajectory, but care must be taken to avoid breaching the retroperitoneal or peritoneal space.

Most surgeons operate with the patient placed in a prone position, but some prefer the patient to be in a lateral decubitus position. It is more ergonomic to operate with the patient prone, which is our preferred position.

The basic inside-out technique for a typical paracentral herniation is described in detail next.

Step-by-Step Operative Technique

Patient Positioning

The patient is prone on a hyperkyphotic frame with a radiolucent table. The endoscope is on one side and the fluoroscopic unit is on the opposite side of the patient.

Anesthesia

Although some experienced international endoscopic surgeons prefer general anesthesia, we recommend mild sedation and local anesthesia so that the patient is awake and responsive throughout the procedure. The patient can then provide real-time feedback in case of nerve irritation from instrument pressure or retraction, adding a layer of safety and allowing the surgeon to adjust the instruments accordingly. We use midazolam (Versed) and fentanyl for sedation and recommend against using general anesthetics like propofol, which can produce temporary total analgesia, eliminating the patient's responsiveness to any nerve stimuli. The skin, needle tract, and anulus are anesthetized with 0.5% lidocaine. This allows anesthesia without motor block of the nerve roots.

Needle Placement

Optimal needle placement is the most crucial step of the procedure and is based on the type of pathology being addressed.[30] The skin window (needle insertion site) is determined using this protocol. This will typically be about 12 to 15 cm lateral to the midline aligned parallel to the disc inclination (Fig. 57.4). The starting point can be adjusted based on the location of the targeted herniation. You would start closer to the midline for foraminal/extraforaminal herniations and more lateral for central herniations.

Once the starting point is determined, the skin window and subcutaneous tissue are infiltrated with 0.5% lidocaine. A 6-inch, 18-gauge needle is then inserted from the skin window at the desired trajectory, typically at a 30-degree angle to the floor (coronal plane) and passed anteromedially toward the anatomic disc center. Infiltrating the needle tract with 0.5% lidocaine as you advance the needle will anesthetize the tissue tract, avoiding pain when the dilator is passed later in the procedure.

In order to avoid puncturing the dura with a trajectory that is too shallow, we advance the needle with the C-arm in the posteroanterior view and never advance the needle tip medial to the medial border of the pedicle without checking a lateral view first. The C-arm lateral projection should confirm the needle tip's correct annular location at the annular window (annular entry point). In the posteroanterior view, the needle tip should be at the disc between the pedicles. In the lateral view, the correct needle tip position should be just touching the posterior anulus surface. These two views of the C-arm confirm that the needle tip has engaged the safe zone, the center of the foraminal annular window.

While monitoring the posteroanterior view, advance the needle tip through the anulus to the midline (anatomic disc center). Then, check the lateral view. If the needle tip is in the center of the disc on the lateral view, you have a central needle placement, which is good for a central nucleotomy and foraminal herniations. Ideally the needle tip will be in the posterior third of the disc, indicating posterior needle placement if you are attempting to access paracentral herniations.

SECTION VII

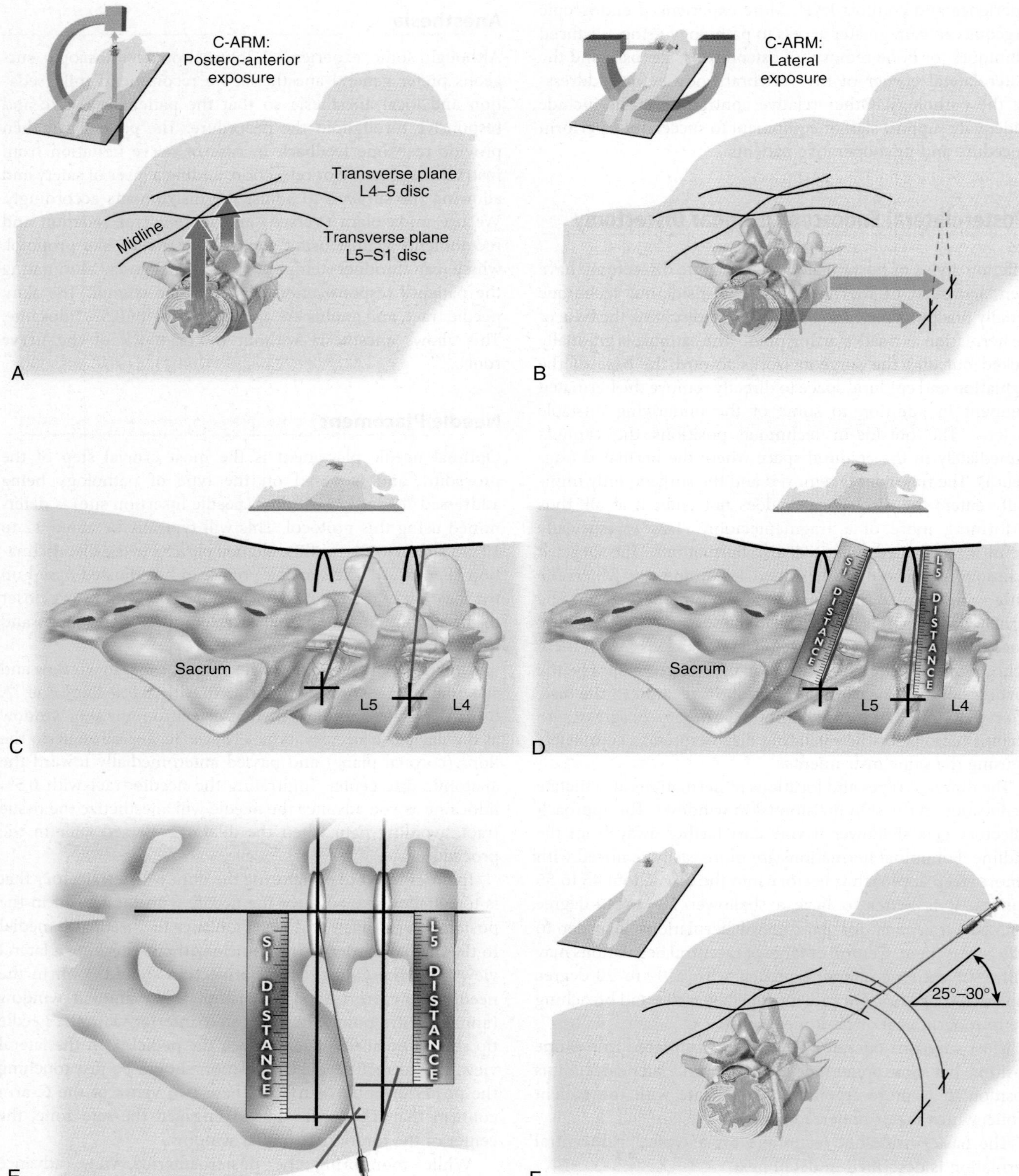

FIG. 57.4 Protocol for optimal needle placement. (A) Posteroanterior (PA) fluoroscopic view enables topographic location of the midline and the transverse disc plane. The intersection of these lines is the PA anatomic disc center. (B) Lateral fluoroscopic view enables topographic location of the disc inclination plane. (C) The inclination plane of each target disc is drawn on the skin from the lateral disc center. (D) The distance from the lateral disc center to the posterior skin plane is measured along the inclination plane. (E–F) This same distance is measured from the midline along the transverse disc plane for each target disc. At the end of this measure, a line parallel to the midline is drawn to intersect the disc inclination line. This is the skin entry point or skin window for the needle.

Evocative Chromodiscography

Perform confirmatory contrast discography at this time. Historically, the following contrast mixture was used: 9 mL of Isovue 300 (iopamidol injection) with 1 mL of indigo carmine dye. This combination of contrast ratio gives readily visible radiopacity on the discography images and intraoperative light blue chromatization of pathologic nucleus and annular fissures, which help guide the targeted fragmentectomy. Indigo carmine was recently discontinued; substitution with methylene blue dye is now used.

Instrument Placement

Insert a guidewire through the 18-gauge needle channel. Advance the guidewire tip, 1 to 2 cm deep into the anulus; then, remove the needle. Slide the bluntly tapered tissue-dilating obturator over the guidewire until the tip of the obturator is firmly engaged in the annular window. An eccentric parallel channel in the obturator allows for four-quadrant annular infiltration using small incremental volumes of 0.5% lidocaine in each quadrant, enough to anesthetize the anulus but not the nerves. If the patient has some radicular nerve pain while placing the needle in one of these quadrants, the surgeon is alerted to the nerve's close proximity to the obturator. Hold the obturator firmly against the annular window surface and remove the guidewire.

The next step is the through-and-through fenestration of the annular window by advancing the bluntly tapered obturator with a mallet. Annular fenestration is the most painful step of the entire procedure. Advise the anesthesiologist to heighten the sedation level just before annular fenestration. Advance the obturator tip deep into the anulus and confirm on the C-arm views. Now, slide the beveled access cannula over the obturator toward the disc. Advance the cannula until the beveled tip is deep in the annular window, with the beveled opening facing dorsally. Remove the obturator and insert the endoscope to get a view of the disc nucleus and anulus (Fig. 57.5). If the targeting has been ideal and the cannula is within the base of the herniation, the surgeon will be looking right at the herniated disc material that requires removal. The subsequent steps depend on the goal of the procedure and pathology being addressed. The basic endoscopic method to excise a noncontained paramedian extruded lumbar herniated disc via a uniportal technique is described here. Different steps are used for other pathology and are beyond the scope of this chapter.

Performing the Discectomy

Oftentimes, there are some annular fibers at the base of the herniation that need to be resected in order to remove the herniation easily. In this situation, enlarge the annulotomy medially to the base of the herniation with cutting forceps. The side-firing holmium-YAG laser can also be used to enlarge and widen the annulotomy. This is performed to release the annular fibers at the herniation site that may pinch off or prevent the extruded portion of the herniation from being

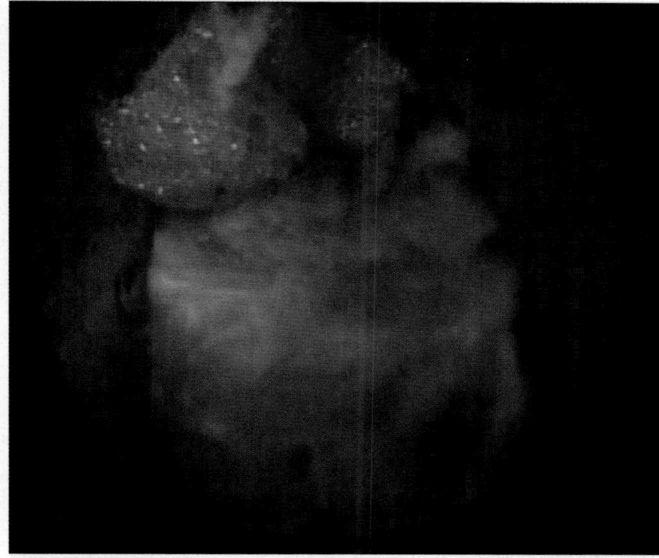

FIG. 57.5 Uniportal endoscopy for paracentral herniation. The cannula is positioned near the base of the herniation. The epidural fat can be seen at the top of the image. The extruded herniation is stained blue with indigo carmine dye and is seen here extruding through the thinned-out annular fibers seen coursing horizontally in this image. At this point, the annular fibers are cut to enlarge the annulotomy with the cutting forceps and the side-firing laser to allow the apex of the herniation to be pulled back into the disc and out the cannula with pituitary rongeurs.

extracted. Directly under the herniation apex, a large amount of blue-stained nucleus is usually present, likened to the submerged portion of an iceberg. The nucleus here represents a migrated and unstable nucleus. The endoscopic rongeurs are used to extract the blue-stained nucleus pulposus under direct visualization. The larger straight and hinged rongeurs are used directly through the cannula after the endoscope is removed. Fluoroscopy and surgeon feel guide this step. By grabbing the base of the herniated fragment, one can usually extract the extruded portion of the herniation. Initial medialization and widening of the annulotomy reduce the prospect of breaking off the herniated nucleus and retaining the apex of the herniation in the spinal canal. The traversing nerve root is readily visualized after removal of the extruded herniation (Fig. 57.6).

Next, perform a minimal bulk decompression by using a straight and flexible suction-irrigation shaver. This step requires shaver head C-arm localization before power is activated to avoid nerve/dura injury and anterior annular penetration. The cavity thus created is called the *working cavity*. The debulking removes the loose, unstable nucleus material to prevent future reherniation.

Inspect the working cavity. If a noncontained extruded disc fragment is still present by finding blue-stained nucleus material posteriorly, then these fragments are teased into the working cavity with the endoscopic rongeurs, curved nerve hooks, and the flexible radiofrequency trigger-flex bipolar probe (Elliquence) and removed. Creation of the working cavity allows the herniated disc tissue to follow the path of least resistance into the cavity. The flexible radiofrequency bipolar probe is used to contract and thicken the annular

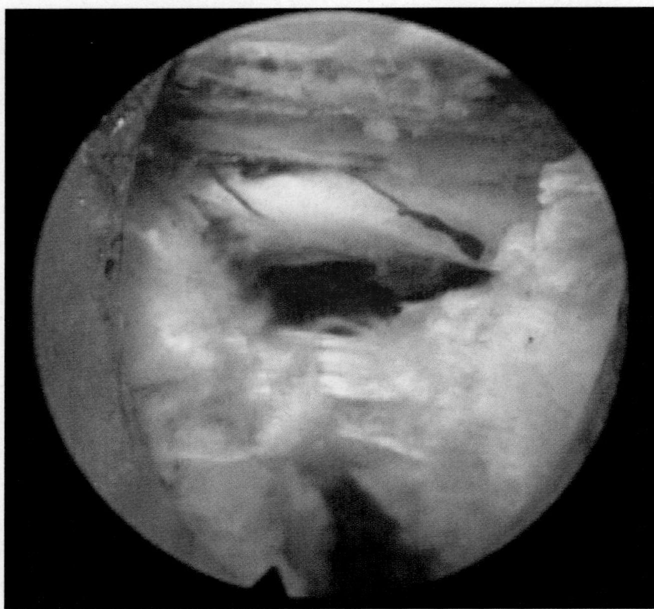

FIG. 57.6 Inspection of the freed traversing nerve root. After successful removal of an extruded paracentral herniation, the traversing nerve root is visualized, confirming complete decompression of the nerve. This is routine in extruded herniations. If the herniation is a contained herniation, the surgeon would visualize the undersurface of the thinned-out posterior annular fibers rather than the traversing nerve root because the herniation did not extrude past the posterior anulus.

collagen at the herniation site. It is also used for hemostasis throughout the case.

The vast majority of herniations can be treated via the uniportal technique. Sometimes for large central herniations and herniations at L5–S1, the disc needs to be approached from both sides, a biportal technique. This allows the use of larger articulating instruments that fit through the contralateral 7-mm access cannula and can reach more posteriorly to extract the herniated fragment under direct endoscopic vision.

Clinical Outcomes

Yeung has reported his initial results using the Yeung Endoscopic Spine Surgery system in his first 307 patients with disc herniations who were candidates for open microdiscectomy.[31] The study included intracanal and extracanal herniations. Recurrent herniations and patients with previous surgery at the same level were not excluded. Results were reported with 1-year follow-up. Overall patient satisfaction was found to be 91%. The same percentage of patients said that they would undergo the procedure again if faced with the same diagnosis. The overall complication rate was 3.5%.[31] Tsou and Yeung separated out a subgroup of 219 patients with noncontained herniations and reported results at 1 year. Patient satisfaction was 91%.[32] These initial results demonstrated that endoscopic surgery could provide equivalent results to reported results of open microdiscectomy, even with noncontained herniations.

There are three prospective randomized studies comparing traditional microdiscectomy and percutaneous endoscopic discectomy. Hermantin et al.[1] performed a prospective randomized study with 30 patients in each group. The mean duration of follow-up was 31 months. Patient satisfaction was 93% in the open surgical group and 97% in the endoscopic group. The endoscopic group had shorter duration of narcotic use and shorter time out of work compared with the open discectomy group. Mayer and Brock[2] performed a randomized prospective study in 1993 with 20 patients in each group. They chose return to previous occupation as the measurement of success. This study showed a significant difference in this outcome measure. In the percutaneous group, 95% of patients returned to their previous profession, whereas only 72% of the microdiscectomy group returned to a previous profession. In 2008, Ruetten et al.[3] compared traditional microdiscectomy with full endoscopic discectomy via either the transforaminal or interlaminar route. There were 178 patients (87 microdiscectomy and 91 endoscopic) with 2-year follow-up. The microdiscectomy group had a 79% success rate and the full endoscopic group had an 85% success rate with no leg pain at all. It is noteworthy that all three of these prospective randomized studies showed a trend toward better outcomes with the endoscopic procedure, but statistically they were comparable.

Kambin et al.[40] reported an 82% success rate for the treatment of lateral recess stenosis and foraminal herniations using an oval cannula with two portals and the transforaminal approach. Even though they were working next to the exiting nerve root, they reported no neurovascular complications in their series. Successful posterolateral endoscopic treatment of foraminal and extraforaminal herniations has been described by many authors. Lew et al. reported an 85% success rate in 47 patients,[41] Choi et al. reported a 92% success rate in 41 patients,[42] Jang et al. reported an 85% success rate in 35 patients,[43] and Sasani et al. reported an 89% success rate in 66 patients.[44]

Yue et al.[45] described excellent results treating single-level, multifocal subarticular and paracentral and/or far-lateral lumbar disc herniations with a single-incision posterolateral endoscopic surgery in 15 patients with 15.3-month follow up. These herniations typically require both a posterior intracanal and extraforaminal surgical approach to alleviate compression of both exiting and traversing nerve roots. Total facetectomy and transforaminal lumbar interbody fusion is also often performed for this type of complex herniation.

Knight and Goswami[6] have reported on the use of the endoscope in foraminal decompressions for isthmic spondylolisthesis. In 79% of patients, a good or excellent outcome was obtained with an average follow-up of 34 months. Of the initial group, only two went on to have spinal fusion. Madhavan et al.[46] also described a case report using posterolateral endoscopic foraminal decompression to avoid fusion in a 31-year-old patient with isthmic spondylolisthesis. The patient was asymptomatic with 2-year follow-up.

Ahn and colleagues[47] reported an 81% success rate with PELD in 43 patients with recurrent disc herniations after a posterior microdiscectomy. Hoogland et al. also had good success (85%) using endoscopic transforaminal discectomy for recurrent herniations in 262 consecutive cases from 1994 to 2002.[48] Of the 262 patients, 194 had a previous posterior microdiscectomy and 68 had a prior endoscopic discectomy. Both studies pointed out the advantage of avoiding the posterior scar tissue. Ruetten et al. also reported a prospective randomized study of 87 patients treated endoscopically after a recurrent herniation, with 79% reporting no leg pain and 16% with occasional leg pain.[49]

The ability to effectively remove pathology using endoscopic surgery has been validated by postprocedure imaging studies. Casey and colleagues[50] looked at a group of patients who had immediate postoperative computed tomography scans. The imaging studies demonstrated that 88.9% of patients undergoing biportal endoscopy had significant reduction in the amount of neural compromise. The results of uniportal, extraforaminal, and foraminal herniations showed only mild to moderate change in canal diameter. They concluded that arthroscopic discectomy had a high rate of canal clearance and removal of disc fragments.[50]

Lee and colleagues[4] reported on a matched cohort comparing radiographic changes 3 years postsurgery in PELD versus posterior microdiscectomy. They revealed less degenerative progression in the PELD group, with loss of disc height and foraminal height being statistically significant. Clinical success rates were 96% in the PELD group and 93% in the microdiscectomy group. The authors conclude that PELD is a less invasive procedure that causes less approach-related damage and less damage to the targeted disc.

Complications and Avoidance

The risks of serious complications or injury are low. The usual risks of infection, nerve injury, dural tears, bleeding, and scar tissue formation are present, as with any surgery. Because the transforaminal endoscopic approach passes adjacent to the exiting spinal nerve root and dorsal root ganglion, there is potential for nerve irritation (dysesthesia) or overt nerve damage. Dysesthesia occurrence is 5% to 15% and is almost always transient.[31,32] This rate of occurrence is similar to dysesthesia rates in posterior open discectomy. However, in the latter situation, because the dysesthesia affects the retracted traversing nerve root that was already the source of radiculopathy, the transient persistent or increased postoperative dysesthesia is generally not considered a complication after posterior discectomy. Both situations are transient the vast majority of the time. Routine injection of 80 mg of methylprednisolone acetate (Depo-Medrol) steroid medication in the foramen at the conclusion of the endoscopic discectomy has reduced the rates of dysesthesia significantly.

Avoidance of complications is enhanced by the ability to clearly visualize normal anatomy and pathoanatomy, the use of local anesthesia and conscious sedation rather than general or spinal anesthesia, and the use of a standardized needle placement protocol. The procedure is usually accomplished with the patient remaining comfortable during its entirety and should be done without the patient feeling severe pain except when expected, such as during evocative discography, annular fenestration, or when instruments are manipulated past the exiting nerve. Local anesthesia using 0.5% lidocaine allows generous use of this dilute anesthetic for pain control and still allows the patient to feel pain when the nerve root is manipulated. Thus, the awake and aware patient serves as the best indicator to avoid any nerve irritation/damage. Dural tears can be treated with a visualized blood patch or a hemostatic matrix such as Floseal (Baxter Healthcare) and observation because there is no dead space for cerebrospinal fluid collection or drainage.

Future Considerations

Perhaps the best future indication for the use of this technique and approach is in the realm of motion preservation (nucleus augmentation/replacement). A partial nuclectomy tract can be created and filled with one or more expandable hydrogel sticks to augment the degenerated nucleus. Alternatively, a complete endoscopic nuclectomy can be performed followed by insertion of a polymer to completely fill the nuclear cavity, redistribute the load across the disc space, and protect the anulus. Early companies focused on nucleus replacement completed pilot studies, but did not complete an IDE study. Interest in this technology has recently been rekindled.

Radical endoscopic discectomy with burring of the endplates and subsequent delivery of an interbody prosthesis with bone graft or bone morphogenetic protein can yield a truly minimally invasive interbody fusion, and early results of this technique are just starting to get reported. Transforaminal anatomy will limit the size of implant that can be delivered; this problem can be overcome by using expandable interbody or graft containment devices.

Future advances in the use of biomaterials and biologics may allow endoscopic annular reinforcement, tissue repair, tissue regeneration, anterior column stabilization by disc arthroplasty, and other alternatives to fusion for pain reduction. The future of spine surgery will most likely involve a mix of endoscopic and traditional open procedures. Studies comparing open and endoscopic procedures will have to be performed to determine which conditions will be best treated by minimally invasive procedures.

PEARLS

1. Initial proper placement of a needle or guide pin is critical to the entire procedure. Take the time to have best possible needle placement in both anteroposterior and lateral projections.
2. Use the inside-out technique when first adopting spinal endoscopy. Start the endoscopy by first entering the disc and then address the pathology accordingly. This is a safe starting point to avoid getting disoriented to your cannula position. Once you are within the disc, the herniation is between you and the affected nerve; this is advantageous because it protects the nerve from iatrogenic injury.
3. Fluoroscopy should be used to confirm location if there is any uncertainty about anatomy or location during endoscopy.
4. It is helpful to use the specially designed cannulas with a Penfield-like extension to retract and protect the exiting nerve when working in the foramen.

5. The patient is awake; thus, use this to your advantage! If significant leg pain is experienced, stop and reevaluate the patient; ask the patient about the distribution of the pain and reassess the position using fluoroscopy to prevent complications.
6. When bleeding is encountered, advance the scope back into the disc and slowly pull back the scope, cauterizing the bleeders when seen at the edge of the cannula.

PITFALLS

1. Make sure that the MRI and plain radiographs are numbered the same (i.e., look out for patients with transitional or six lumbar vertebrae).
2. Always visualize the action portion of your endoscopic tools to avoid dura or nerve injury. You want to clearly see the tissue you are grasping with the pituitary forceps, ablating with the bipolar radiofrequency probe, and firing the laser at.
3. It is recommended that the patient be *awake and alert* until the endoscope is within the disc space to avoid nerve injury. Avoiding excessive sedation before this point in the procedure is crucial, especially during needle insertion and dilator and cannula passage. We recommend against the use of a general anesthetic such as propofol.

KEY POINTS

1. PELD is a directly visualized surgical procedure and is not to be confused with the many nonvisualized percutaneous discectomy procedures for indirect disc decompression.
2. The surgeon can visually confirm that the traversing nerve root is adequately decompressed when removing an extruded paracentral herniation.
3. The literature shows that PELD is at least as safe and effective as traditional open posterior discectomy.

KEY REFERENCES

1. Hermantin FU, Peters T, Quartararo L, et al. A prospective randomized study comparing the results of open discectomy with those of video-assisted arthroscopic microdiscectomy. *J Bone Joint Surg*. 1999;81-A:958-965.
   The authors showed comparable success rates between open discectomy and arthroscopic microdiscectomy (posterolateral endoscopic discectomy), but the latter group had less narcotic use and shorter time off work.
2. Ahn Y, Lee SH, Park WM, et al. Percutaneous endoscopic lumbar discectomy for recurrent disc herniation: surgical technique, outcome, and prognostic factors of 43 consecutive cases. *Spine*. 2004;29:326-332.
   The authors were able to avoid the posterior scar tissue in patients with recurrent herniations after a posterior discectomy and achieve an 81% success rate by using the posterolateral endoscopic approach.
3. Yeung AT, Tsou PM. Posterolateral endoscopic excision for lumbar disc herniation: surgical technique, outcome and complications in 307 consecutive cases. *Spine*. 2002;27:722-731.
   Results of more than 300 patients with 2-year follow-up using the endoscopic technique and working channel scope. Excellent description of authors' technique and outcomes rated using patient satisfaction.
4. Ruetten S, Komp M, Merk H, et al. Full-endoscopic interlaminar and transforaminal lumbar discectomy versus conventional microsurgical technique: a prospective, randomized, controlled study. *Spine*. 2008;33:930-939.
   This large prospective, randomized study directly compared standard microdiscectomy to both posterolateral and posterior interlaminar endoscopic techniques.
5. Lee SH, Kang B, Ahn Y, et al. Operative failure of percutaneous endoscopic lumbar discectomy: a radiologic analysis of 55 cases. *Spine*. 2006;31:E285-E290.
   The authors identify high-grade canal compromise (>50%) and high-grade migration as herniation characteristics that predispose for a higher failure rate with posterolateral endoscopic lumbar discectomy.

REFERENCES

1. Hermantin FU, Peters T, Quartararo L, et al. A prospective randomized study comparing the results of open discectomy with those of video-assisted arthroscopic microdiscectomy. *J Bone Joint Surg*. 1999;81-A:958-965.
2. Mayer HM, Brock M. Percutaneous endoscopic discectomy: surgical technique and preliminary results compared to microsurgical discectomy. *J Neurosurg*. 1993;78:216-225.
3. Ruetten S, Komp M, Merk H, et al. Full-endoscopic interlaminar and transforaminal lumbar discectomy versus conventional microsurgical technique: a prospective, randomized, controlled study. *Spine*. 2008;33:930-939.
4. Lee SH, Chung SE, Ahn Y, et al. Comparative radiologic evaluation of percutaneous endoscopic lumbar discectomy and open microdiscectomy: a matched cohort analysis. *Mt Sinai J Med*. 2006;73:795-801.
5. Knight MTN, Goswami AKD. Endoscopic laser foraminoplasty. In: Savitz MH, Chiu JC, Yeung AT, eds. *The Practice of Minimally Invasive Spinal Technique*. Richmond, VA: AAMISMS Education; 2000:337-340.
6. Knight M, Goswami A. Management of isthmic spondylolisthesis with posterolateral endoscopic foraminal decompression. *Spine*. 2003;28:573-581.
7. Hirsh C, Ingelmark B, Miller M. The anatomic basis for low back pain. *Acta Orthop Scand*. 1963;33:1-17.
8. Choy DS, Altman P. Fall of intradiscal pressure with laser ablation. *J Clin Laser Med Surg*. 1995;13:149-151.
9. Prodoehl JA, Lane GJ, Black J, et al. The effects of lasers on intervertebral disc pressures. *Spine*. 1993;7:17-21.
10. Nerubay J, Caspi I, Levinkopf M, et al. Percutaneous laser nucleolysis of the intervertebral lumbar disc. *Clin Orthop*. 1997;337:42-44.
11. Chatterjee S, Foy PM, Findlay GF. Report of a controlled clinical trial comparing automated percutaneous lumbar discectomy and microdiscectomy in the treatment of contained lumbar disc herniation. *Spine*. 1995;20:734738.
12. Grevitt MP, McLaren A, Shakelford IM, et al. Automated percutaneous lumbar discectomy—an outcome study. *J Bone Joint Surg Br*. 1995;77-B:626-629.
13. Ramberg N, Sahlstrand T. Early and long-term follow-up after automated percutaneous lumbar discectomy. *J Spinal Disord*. 2001;14:511-517.
14. Choy DS, Asher PW, Ran HS, et al. Percutaneous laser decompression: a new therapeutic modality. *Spine*. 1992;17:949-956.
15. Valls J, Ottolenghi CE, Schajowicz F. Aspiration biopsy in diagnosis of lesions of vertebral bodies. *JAMA*. 1948;136:376-382.
16. Craig FS. Vertebral-body biopsy. *J Bone Joint Surg Am*. 1956;38A:93-102.
17. Kambin P, Gellman H. Percutaneous lateral discectomy of the lumbar spine. *Clin Orthop*. 1983;174:127-132.

18. Hijikata S, Yamagishi N, Nakayama T, et al. Percutaneous discectomy: a new treatment method for lumbar disc herniation. *J Toden Hosp.* 1975;5:5-13.
19. Onik GM, Helms C, Hoaglund F, et al. Successful percutaneous lumbar discectomy using a new aspiration probe: a case report. *Am J Radiol.* 1985;6:290-293.
20. Kambin P, Schaffer JL. Percutaneous posterolateral discectomy and decompression with a 6.9 mm cannula. *J Bone Joint Surg Am.* 1991;73-A:822-831.
21. Kambin P. Arthroscopic microdiscectomy. *Arthroscopy.* 1992;8: 287-295.
22. Kambin P, McCullen G, Parke W, et al. Minimally invasive arthroscopic spinal surgery. *Instr Course Lect.* 1997;46:1443-1461.
23. Kambin P, O'Brien E, Zhou L, et al. Arthroscopic microdiscectomy and selective fragmentectomy. *Clin Orthop.* 1998;347:150-167.
24. Kambin P, Savitz MH. Arthroscopic microdiscectomy: an alternative to open disc surgery. *Mt Sinai J Med.* 2000;67: 283-287.
25. Kambin P, Zhou L. Arthroscopic discectomy of the lumbar spine. *Clin Orthop.* 1997;337:49-57.
26. Kambin P, Zhou L. History and current status of percutaneous arthroscopic disc surgery. *Spine.* 1996;21:57S-61S.
27. Yeung AT. The evolution of percutaneous spinal endoscopy and discectomy: state of the art. *Mt Sinai J Med.* 2000;67:327-332.
28. Mathews HH. Transforaminal endoscopic microdiscectomy. *Neurosurg Clin N Am.* 1996;7:59-63.
29. Yeung AT, Yeung CA. In vivo endoscopic visualization of patho-anatomy in painful degenerative conditions of the lumbar spine. *Surg Technol Int.* 2006;XV:243-256.
30. Yeung AT, Yeung CA. Posterolateral selective endoscopic discectomy: the YESS Technique. In: Kim D, Fessler R, Regan J, eds. *Endoscopic Spine Surgery and Instrumentation: Percutaneous Procedures.* New York: Thieme; 2004:201-211.
31. Yeung AT, Tsou PM. Posterolateral endoscopic excision for lumbar disc herniation: surgical technique, outcome and complications in 307 consecutive cases. *Spine.* 2002;27:722-731.
32. Tsou PM, Yeung AT. Transforaminal endoscopic decompression for radiculopathy secondary to intracanal noncontained lumbar disc herniations: outcome and technique. *Spine J.* 2002;2:41-48.
33. Wang MY, Grossman J. Endoscopic minimally invasive transforaminal interbody fusion without general anesthesia: initial clinical experience with 1-year follow-up. *Neurosurg Focus.* 2016;40(2):E13.
34. Kambin P, Bradger MD. Percutaneous posterolateral discectomy: anatomy and mechanism. *Clin Orthop.* 1987; 223:145-154.
35. Kambin P. *Arthroscopic Microdiscectomy: Minimal Intervention in Spinal Surgery.* Baltimore: Urban and Schwarzenberg; 1991.
36. Mirkovic SR, Schwartz DG, Glazier KD. Anatomic considerations in lumbar posterolateral percutaneous procedures. *Spine.* 1995;20:1965-1971.
37. Hardenbrook M, Lombardo S, Wilson MC, Telfeian AE. The anatomic rationale for transforaminal endoscopic interbody fusion: a cadaveric analysis. *Neurosurg Focus.* 2016;40(2):E12.
38. Tsou PM, Yeung CA, Yeung AT. Posterolateral transforaminal selective endoscopic discectomy and thermal annuloplasty for chronic lumbar discogenic pain: a minimal access visualized intradiscal surgical procedure. *Spine J.* 2004;4:564-573.
39. Ito M, Abumi K, Kotani Y, et al. Clinical outcome of posterolateral endoscopic surgery for pyogenic spondylodiscitis: results of 15 patients with serious comorbid conditions. *Spine.* 2007;32:200-206.
40. Kambin P, Casey K, O'Brien E, et al. Transforaminal arthroscopic decompression of the lateral recess stenosis. *J Neurosurg.* 1996;84:462-467.
41. Lew SM, Mehalic TF, Fagone KL. Transforaminal percutaneous endoscopic discectomy in the treatment of far-lateral and foraminal lumbar disc herniation. *J Neurosurg.* 2001;94:216-220.
42. Choi G, Lee SH, Bhanot A, et al. Percutaneous endoscopic discectomy for extraforaminal lumbar disc herniations. *Spine.* 2007;32:93-99.
43. Jang JS, An SH, Lee SH. Transforaminal percutaneous endoscopic discectomy in the Treatment of foraminal and extraforaminal lumbar disc herniations. *J Spinal Discord Tech.* 2006;19:338-343.
44. Sasani M, Oktenoglu T, Canbulat N, et al. Percutaneous endoscopic discectomy for far lateral lumbar disc herniations: prospective study and outcome of 66 patients. *Minim Invasive Neurosurg.* 2007;50:91-97.
45. Yue JJ, Scott DL, Han X, Yacob A. The surgical treatment of single level multi-focal subarticular and paracentral and/ or far-lateral lumbar disc herniations: the single incision full endoscopic approach. *Int J Spine Surg.* 2014 Dec 1;8.
46. Madhavan K, Chieng LO, Hofstetter CP, Wang MY. Transforaminal endoscopic discectomy to relieve sciatica and delay fusion in a 31-year-old man with pars defects and low-grade spondylolisthesis. *Neurosurg Focus.* 2016;40(2):E4.
47. Ahn Y, Lee SH, Park WM, et al. Percutaneous endoscopic lumbar discectomy for recurrent disc herniation: surgical technique, outcome, and prognostic factors of 43 consecutive cases. *Spine.* 2004;29:326-332.
48. Hoogland T, van den Brekel-Dijkstra K, Schubert M, et al. Endoscopic transforaminal discectomy for recurrent lumbar disc herniation: a prospective, cohort evaluation of 262 consecutive cases. *Spine.* 2008;33:973-978.
49. Ruetten S, Komp M, Merk H, Godolias G. Recurrent lumbar disc herniation after conventional discectomy: a prospective, randomized study comparing full-endoscopic interlaminar and transforaminal versus microsurgical revision. *J Spinal Disord Tech.* 2009;22(2):122-129.
50. Casey KF, Chang MK, O'Brien ED, et al. Arthroscopic microdiscectomy: comparison of preoperative and postoperative imaging studies. *Arthroscopy.* 1997;13: 438-445.

CHAPTER 58 Interspinous Process Decompressive Devices

Clifford B. Tribus

Introduction

The interspinous process space has become a target for spinal implants to address degenerative conditions of the lumbar spine. The interspinous process decompression (IPD) devices employ a range of insertion techniques and materials but share the common goal of distraction to be maintained between the adjacent spinous processes to incur a clinical result. The variety of materials employed include titanium, polyetheretherketone, Silastic compounds, and allograft. Many of the implants are devised to be static in nature, while some employ dynamic techniques.[1,2] The clinical use of the Interspinous process space has continued to evolve. The indications have become less refined and the data mixed; leaving clinicians and payors less guidelines to follow.

The X-Stop (Medtronic International) is a titanium implant that was the first US Food and Drug Administration (FDA)-approved IPD device marketed in the United States, having been cleared by the FDA in November 2005 through an investigational device exemption (IDE) study. The indication for its use is spinal stenosis leading to neurogenic claudication. Medtronic recently chose to discontinue the marketing and sales of X-Stop. Coflex (Paradigm Spine LLC) received premarket approval in October of 2012 and Superion (VertiFlex Inc.) received premarket approval in May of 2015, both for similar indications.[3]

Many other IPD devices are marketed outside of the United States, including the following: Aperius (Medtronic), DIAM (Medtronic/Sofamor Danek), Wallis (Zimmer Spine), Viking (Sintea), Ellipse (Sintea), BacJac (Pioneer), ExtendSure (Nuvasiv), Promise, Rocker (Biomech), Helifix (Alphatec Spine), Biolig (Cousin Biotech), In-Space (Synthes), InSWing (Orthofix), I-MAXX (Maxx Spine), Flexus (GlobusMedical), and Spinos (Privelop).

Biomechanical studies of IPD devices have demonstrated the implants' ability to change forces in the disc and facet joints. These findings have led to diagnoses potentially helped by this technology, yet to be cleared by the FDA, as indications to include discogenic back pain, facet arthropathy, disc herniation, degenerative disc disease, and instability, including degenerative spondylolisthesis. Clinical studies differentiating these indications and guidance for utilization are lacking.

IPD devices all share characteristics that are relatively unique among spinal implants of the lumbar spine. They can be implanted with a modest degree of destruction to the local anatomy. Several do not require exposure of the neural elements, they are at least partially motion preserving, and they are relatively reversible. These features coalesce to an implant with a very favorable risk profile. It is up to randomized controlled studies to prove the efficacy, indications, and ultimately role in the armamentarium available to the spine surgeon in the care of the spinal patient.

The interspinous process space has also been exploited by a similar family of devices that were FDA approved as supplemental fusion devices: Affix (Nuvasiv), Aileron (LifeSpine), Aspen (Lanx), Axle (X-Spine), BacFuse (Pioneer Surgical), BridgePoint (Alphatec Spine), Inspan (SpineFrontier Inc.), PrimaLOK (OsteoMed), Octave (Life Spine), Spire (Medtronic/Sofamor Danek), SP-Fix (Globus), and Stabilink (Southern Spine). These devices have expanded the use of the interspinous spinal device but have a different surgical goal, which is fusion.

Design Rationale

Early criticisms of interspinous process decompression devices stem from the apparent kyphosing nature of the implant. It is indeed counterintuitive to apply posterior distraction to the lumbar spine. Yet, one need only look at the clinical presentation of a patient with lumbar spinal stenosis to appreciate the design rationale. A patient with lumbar stenosis typically walks with a forward stooped gate. Additionally, patients with spinal stenosis obtain symptom relief upon sitting down. The common feature in both of these postures is the relative flexion of the lumbar spine or avoidance of extension. Human beings are unable to segmentally kyphose their lumbar spine. Muscle insertions allow global motions of flexion and extension. However, spinal stenosis is often a focal phenomenon presenting with its worst clinical level at one or two lumbar segments. Therefore, the rationale of the device is to implant the interspinous process decompression device at the one or two levels where the stenosis is most severe. The implant then segmentally kyphoses the lumbar spine at the level of most severe stenosis and allows the rest of the lumbar spine to fall into its natural posture of extension, having relieved the local stenosis.

An additional concept in the treatment of patients with lumbar spinal stenosis is how much nerve compression is clinically significant. While several studies have tried to elucidate this measurement, it appears to be an elusive number. Any clinician who has been involved in the care of the stenosis patient can appreciate the fact that for every octogenarian who presents with new-onset stenotic symptoms who has a spinal canal that is extraordinarily narrow, there is another patient who presents with similar symptoms in their 50s with magnetic resonance imaging (MRI) findings that are not nearly as impressive. With this variation in mind, it can be appreciated that spinal stenosis is a threshold disease. That is to say, the degree of tightness that elicits symptoms in any particular patient may in part be somewhat unique for that patient. Therefore, by extension, a device that can create additional room for the neural elements may only need to create enough room to get that patient to the other side of the threshold for symptoms. As surgeons, we may be a bit uncomfortable with this rationale, preferring to directly decompress the neural elements in their entirety and confirm this by direct visualization. This may represent overtreatment, however.

If we accept the concept of focal spinal stenosis causing symptoms at a particular threshold, then it must be shown that interspinous process decompressive devices can enact an effect on the canal diameter with acceptably minimal alterations to spine biomechanics. The majority of the current literature on this topic relates to the X-Stop interspinous process device. Whether this data can be extrapolated to other products in this category is up to the reader's discretion; however, these studies are presented as a design rationale for IPD devices.

The first reasonable question to pose in evaluating the design rationale of an IPD device is what is its net effect, on implantation, on the dimensions of the spinal canal. Richards et al.[4] attempted to address this question in studying eight cadaver specimens from L2–L5 that underwent MRI preimplantation and postimplantation of an X-Stop device at the L3–L4 level. Canal and foraminal dimensions were measured. The specimens were positioned and parameters measured in both 15 degrees of flexion and 15 degrees of extension. In extension, the canal area was increased by 18% when compared to the noninstrumented spine. Similarly, the subarticular diameter was increased by 50%, the canal diameter by 10%, the foraminal area by 25%, and the foraminal width by 41%.[4] In a subsequent in vivo study, Siddiqui et al.[5,6] presented results on 12 patients with 17 instrumented levels in which positional MRIs were obtained presurgery and postsurgery in the sitting flexed, sitting extended, and sitting neutral postures, as well as standing positions. The area for the dural sac increased from 77.8 to 93.4 mm at 6 months after surgery in the standing position. There was a similar increase in the foramina. It is important to note that no change in overall lumbar lordosis was observed.

These studies demonstrate the passive decompression obtained in placing an interspinous process decompression device. The question remains as to whether this degree of passive decompression is enough to be clinically relevant.

The other area of study as it relates to implantation of the interspinous process decompression device is the net effect on the kinematics and load sharing within the lumbar spine at both the instrumented level and the adjacent levels.[7] Swanson et al.[8] presented data on eight human cadaveric lumbar spines in which they tested intradiscal pressure preimplantation and postimplantation. The spines were positioned in flexion, neutral, and extension with intradiscal pressure transducers placed in the anterior and posterior aspect of the nucleus pulposus. The implants were placed at L3–L4 and the measurements of intradiscal pressure taken at L2–L3, L3–L4, and L4–L5. The device proved to be load sharing in both the extension and neutral positions. At L3–L4, which was the instrumented level, the authors measured a 63% decrease in pressure at the posterior anulus and a 41% decrease in pressure in the nucleus pulposus in extension. In the neutral position, the decrease in pressure was 38% in the posterior anulus and 20% in the nucleus pulposus. The adjacent levels did not show any significant change in intradiscal pressure.

Wiseman et al.[9] presented a similar study as it relates to facet loading. Pressure film was placed in the facets at the instrumented level, which was L3–L4, as well as the facets at L2–L3 and L4-L5. The film could then be measured for contact area, mean force, mean pressure, and peak pressure. At the implanted level, the contact area decreased by 47%, mean force decreased by 68%, mean pressure decreased by 39%, and peak pressure decreased by 55%. No changes of facet pressure were seen at adjacent levels. These mechanical studies provide the basis for the assumption that interspinous process decompression devices may be helpful in the clinical treatment of patients suffering from facet arthropathy or discogenic or degenerative disc–induced back pain. Yet, these are only biomechanical studies; the efficacy of IPD devices has not been shown clinically in these conditions.

The effect of the X-Stop IPD device on spinal kinematics was further measured by Lindsey et al.[10] Seven cadaveric specimens from L2–L5 were loaded in flexion, extension, axial rotation, and lateral bending to 7.5 Nm. There was a superimposed axial load of 700 N applied. Rigid markers were placed in each vertebral body as well as the supporting frame to measure the relative motion. Measurements were taken both preimplantation and postimplantation of an L3–L4 IPD device. There was no change in range of motion as measured in axial rotation or lateral bending. The intervertebral angle was changed by 1.9 degrees. An average of 7.6 degrees of extension at L3–L4 was reduced to 3.1 degrees after implantation of the device. Notably, the adjacent levels were not affected in flexion or extension with a device in place.

Two studies are presented to assess the question of kyphosis of the lumbar spine. Siddiqui et al., as referenced earlier, studied 12 patients with 17 implanted levels.[5-7] Comparing his postoperative to preoperative MRIs, the mean intervertebral angle changed less than 1 degree in extension. The overall mean lumbar lordosis changed 8 degrees in extension. Therefore, the change in overall lumbar lordosis was not statistically significant.[5-7] The mean intervertebral angle and mean lumbar lordosis were also measured in the pivotal study trial for FDA submission. This included 41 patients with data available preoperatively and postoperatively. In the 23 patients receiving a single-level implant, the mean lumbar lordosis changed 0.1 degree in extension. In 18 patients who underwent double-level implants, the mean lumbar lordosis changed 1.2 degrees in extension.[11]

Surgical Technique

Surgical technique is variable depending on the implant used and surgeon preference. Placement of an IPD device may be performed in the outpatient setting. While the patient may be positioned prone, my preferred technique is to position the patient lateral, under general anesthesia, with the hips and knees flexed and taped in this position. The lumbar spine is forced into relative flexion to facilitate placement of the implant. The various devices are placed either as a primary decompression device or as a stabilization device after a direct surgical decompression. Fluoroscopy is used. Of note, the spinous processes may often be difficult to visualize, while the disc spaces are generally better delineated. The surgeon should watch for distraction of the appropriate disc space to confirm the surgical level. For the majority of the IPD devices, the implant should be positioned as far anterior as possible. Placement is planned and confirmed fluoroscopically.

Clinical Results

The X-Stop device was approved in 2005. Over the last decade, clinical studies have been reported comparing various interspinous devices to more traditional approaches. The data are evolving, as is the role for interspinous decompressive devices. The surgeon needs to be exacting in review of the literature. As alluded to earlier in this discussion, many of the IPD devices are placed with a simultaneous traditional open decompression (Wallis, Coflex) while others do not require direct neural decompression (X-Stop, Superion), relying on local distraction to provide a passive decompression. The implication is that the former are stabilization devices, with device efficacy difficult to distinguish from direct neural decompression versus lower surgical risk in the devices that obviate the need for direct decompression, though they do not permit the surgeon direct visualization of the neural elements. This latter technique may be viewed as an advantage because of decreased surgical risk or as a disadvantage because of the inability to visualize the neural elements. Clinical results of these latter devices, however, are easier to interpret.

Zucherman et al.[11] reported in 2005 on 191 age-matched patients enrolled in a prospective, randomized, multicenter study comparing X-Stop to controls. The 91 control patients consisted primarily of patients undergoing epidural steroid treatment. The 100 patients selected for the X-Stop had one (76 patients) or two (24 patients) implants placed. The levels instrumented were predominantly L3–L4 and L4–L5. Both study groups required symptoms to be refractory to 6 months of nonoperative care. The degree of stenosis could not exceed 50% of the normal canal diameter. All patients had to be older than 50 years, able to walk at least 50 feet, and obtain symptom relief with sitting. Outcomes were measured by the Zurich Claudication Questionnaire, Short-Form 36 questionnaire, and radiographic measurements. Results favored the instrumented group by showing statistically significant pain reduction and increase in physical function, which was obtained by 6 weeks' follow-up and maintained for the 2-year study period. Complications included incisional pain, hematoma, wound swelling, wound dehiscence, implant dislodgement, implant malposition, spinous process fracture, coronary ischemia, and respiratory distress.

Spinous process fracture warrants specific mention, as clinical outcomes are not always failures. The tip of the spinous process may fracture on insertion; yet, if the implant can still be positioned anterior to the fracture in a stable position, the outcome may still be good. If the fracture obviates stable intraoperative placement or the implant posteriorly displaces in the postoperative period, results may suffer but surprisingly not always or even routinely.

Anderson et al.[12] restudied a subgroup of 75 patients in the initial cohort who carried the additional diagnosis of grade 1 degenerative spondylolisthesis. This subgroup of patients similarly followed the index group by showing statistically significant pain reduction and increase in physical function obtained by 6 weeks' follow-up and maintained for the 2-year study period. Additionally, there was no increase in the degree of spondylolisthesis in the study group.

In a study with 13 years' follow-up, Senegas et al.[13] reported on 107 patients completing health questionnaires who were initially scheduled for decompression and fusion for canal stenosis, herniated nucleus pulposus, or both. They underwent decompression and stabilization with the Wallis device. Twenty patients had undergone revision fusion during the study period, while 80% of the patients reported good clinical results.

Verhoof et al.[14] reported on 12 patients treated with the X-Stop device for spinal stenosis in the setting of degenerative spondylolisthesis. The authors also showed no progression of the deformity. Four of their initial patients showed no improvement in symptoms, while eight patients showed complete resolution of their symptoms. Three of this latter group eventually developed recurrent symptoms for a failure rate of 58%.

Kondrashov et al.[15] presented further results of a subgroup of the initial cohort with 4 years' follow-up. A total of 77% of patients had experienced at least a 15-point improvement in their Oswestry Disability Index, which was maintained at the 4-year postoperative follow-up.

More recently, Stromqvist[16] presented 100 patients randomized in a prospective controlled study comparing 50 patients treated with the X-Stop and 50 patients undergoing traditional decompressive surgery. Both groups enjoyed significant clinical improvement as measured by the Zurich Claudication Questionnaire (ZCQ), the Visual Analog Scale and the Short-Form 36 questionnaire, which could not be distinguished at any time period to 2 years postoperatively. However, the X-Stop group had a 26% reoperation rate, while the decompressive group had a 6% reoperation rate.

The Superion IPD device recently obtained FDA approval. The FDA-IDE pivotal trial data were presented by Patel et al.[17] A total of 391 patients were randomized between the X-Stop and Superion. Noninferiority was demonstrated. With the ZCQ being the primary outcomes instrument, leg pain clinical success was 76% and 77% with Superion and X-Stop, respectively, at 2 years. Back pain clinical success was 67% and 68%, respectively. Patients' self-ratings of their treatment were "satisfied" or "somewhat satisfied" in 86% for the Superion group and 89% of the X-Stop group at 2 years. A total of 83% of the Superion group and 84% of the X-Stop reported that they would undergo the same treatment again. Reoperation rates were 23% for the Superion group and 19% the X-Stop group, primarily for inadequate pain relief or return of symptoms.[17]

In 2011, Wooter et al.[18] reported a meta-analysis on the effectiveness of IPD surgery in claudicant patients. Eleven studies were analyzed with combined databases on ZCQ questionnaires favoring IPD treatment over nonoperative care. The authors warned of "relatively soft" data and high costs.

Moojen[19] then reported in 2013 on a randomized controlled trial of IPD devices versus conventional decompressive surgery. At 1 year, there was no difference in ZCQ disability, yet the reoperation rate of 29% in the IPD group was substantially higher than the conventional decompression group (6%).

Then, 1 year later, the same research group reported on the cost-effectiveness of the IPD devices utilizing quality-adjusted life years and societal costs, concluding that IPD devices are highly unlikely to be cost-effective in the surgical treatment of lumbar spinal stenosis compared to conventional decompression.[20]

In a more favorable review, Gazzeri et al.[21] reported on a multicenter study of 1108 patients who underwent placement of one or two IPD devices in the lumbar spine for stenosis. A total of 8 different implants were represented with a variety of clinical indications. At 2 years' follow-up, 76.2% were very satisfied with their clinical result, 12.5% were somewhat satisfied, and 11.2% were not satisfied. The reoperation rate was 9.6%, with a mean follow-up of 44.8 months. Chief reasons for reoperation were implant dislocation (20 cases), no improvement (18 cases), spinous process fracture, overdistraction (27 cases), and/or recurrent symptoms after initial improvement (42 cases).

Summary

The interspinous process space is an appealing surgical target. The exposure is minimally destructive; therefore, the risk profile is relatively low. Broad clinical outcomes data from the various devices are evolving. Additionally, clinical outcomes data comparing interspinous process devices to more traditional surgical approaches are also lacking. The challenging subgroup of stenosis patients with concomitant degenerative spondylolisthesis or degenerative scoliosis needs to be vetted. These patients may benefit from IPD devices, as their insertion does not destabilize the spine and they perhaps offer a fusion alternative. Yet, while recent studies have shown clinical outcomes using IPD devices to be comparable to traditional decompressive surgery, surgeons sometimes are reluctant to use them because of higher cost and higher revision rates. Outcome studies for specific diagnoses and surgeon opinion, as well as reimbursement, will ultimately define their relative role in the armamentarium of surgical procedures utilized in the care of the stenosis patient.

PEARLS

1. Mark the planned incision with the patient upright.
2. Position the patient in maximum flexion.
3. Use disc space as a reference for confirming the surgical level.

PITFALLS

1. Avoid violating the supraspinous ligament (X-Stop).
2. Avoid overdistraction.
3. Assure anterior placement of the implant.

KEY POINTS

1. IPD devices are motion-preserving devices utilized in the treatment of spinal stenosis and neurogenic claudication.
2. Clinical results for IPD devices are less predictable than traditional surgical approaches but they have a favorable risk profile, especially when compared to decompression and fusion cases.

KEY REFERENCES

1. Siddiqui M, Nicol M, Karadimas E, Smith F, Wardlaw D. The positional magnetic resonance imaging changes in the lumbar spine following insertion of a novel interspinous process distraction device. *Spine*. 2005;30(23):2677-2682.
   In 12 patients with 17 distracted levels, the area of the dural sac at these levels increased from 77.8 to 93.4 mm after surgery in the standing position (P =.006), with increase in the exit foramina, but no change in lumbar posture.
2. Lindsey DP, Swanson KE, Fuchs P, et al. The effects of an interspinous implant on the kinematics of the instrumented and adjacent levels in the lumbar spine. *Spine*. 2003;28(19):2192-2197.
   The flexion-extension range of motion was significantly reduced at the instrumented level. Axial rotation and lateral bending ranges of motion were not affected at the instrumented level. The range of motion in flexion-extension, axial rotation, and lateral bending at the adjacent segments was not significantly affected by the implant.
3. Zucherman JF, Hsu KY, Hartjen CA, et al. A multicenter, prospective, randomized trial evaluating the X STOP interspinous process decompression system for the treatment of neurogenic intermittent claudication: two-year follow-up results. *Spine*. 2005;30(12):1351-1358.
   At every follow-up visit, X-Stop patients had significantly better outcomes in each domain of the Zurich Claudication Questionnaire. At 2 years, the X-Stop patients improved by 45.4% over the mean baseline symptom severity score compared with 7.4% in the control group; the mean improvement in the Physical Function domain was 44.3% in the X-Stop group and –0.4% in the control group. In the X-Stop group, 73.1% of patients were satisfied with their treatment compared with 35.9% of control patients.

REFERENCES

1. Bono CM, Vaccaro AR. Interspinous process devices in the lumbar spine. *J Spinal Disord Tech*. 2007;20(3):255-261.
2. Wilke HJ, Drumm J, Häussler K, et al. Biomechanical effect of different interspinous implants on flexibility and intradiscal pressure. *Eur Spine J*. 2008;17(8):1049-1056.

3. US Food and Drug Administration. Premarket approval: Coflex and Superion. Available at https://www.accessdata.fda.gov/scripts/cdrh/cfdocs/cfPMA/pma.cfm?id=P110008 and https://www.accessdata.fda.gov/scripts/cdrh/cfdocs/cfPMA/pma.cfm?id=P140004.
4. Richards JC, Majumdar S, Lindsey DP, Beaupré GS, Yerby SA. The treatment mechanism of an interspinous process implant for lumbar neurogenic intermittent claudication. *Spine*. 2005;30(7):744-749.
5. Siddiqui M, Karadimas E, Nicol M, Smith FW, Wardlaw D. Influence of X Stop on neural foramina and spinal canal area in spinal stenosis. *Spine*. 2006;31(25):2958-2962.
6. Siddiqui M, Nicol M, Karadimas E, Smith F, Wardlaw D. The positional magnetic resonance imaging changes in the lumbar spine following insertion of a novel interspinous process distraction device. *Spine*. 2005;30(23):2677-2682.
7. Siddiqui M, Karadimas E, Nicol M, Smith FW, Wardlaw D. Effects of X-STOP device on sagittal lumbar spine kinematics in spinal stenosis. *J Spinal Disord Tech*. 2006;19(5):328-333.
8. Swanson KE, Lindsey DP, Hsu KY, Zucherman JF, Yerby SA. The effects of an interspinous implant on intervertebral disc pressures. *Spine*. 2003;28(1):26-32.
9. Wiseman CM, Lindsey DP, Fredrick AD, Yerby SA. The effect of an interspinous process implant on facet loading during extension. *Spine*. 2005;30(8):903-907.
10. Lindsey DP, Swanson KE, Fuchs P, et al. The effects of an interspinous implant on the kinematics of the instrumented and adjacent levels in the lumbar spine. *Spine*. 2003;28(19):2192-2197.
11. Zucherman JF, Hsu KY, Hartjen CA, et al. A multicenter, prospective, randomized trial evaluating the X STOP interspinous process decompression system for the treatment of neurogenic intermittent claudication: two-year follow-up results. *Spine*. 2005;30(12):1351-1358.
12. Anderson PA, Tribus CB, Kitchel SH. Treatment of neurogenic claudication by interspinous decompression: application of the X STOP device in patients with lumbar degenerative spondylolisthesis. *J Neurosurg Spine*. 2006;4(6):463-471.
13. Senegas J, Vital JM, Pointillart V, Mangione P. Clinical evaluation of a lumbar interspinous dynamic stabilization device (the Wallis system) with a 13-year mean follow-up. *Neurosurg Rev*. 2009;32(3):335-341, discussion 341-342.
14. Verhoof OJ, Bron JL, Wapstra FH, van Royen BJ. High failure rate of the interspinous distraction device (X-Stop) for the treatment of lumbar spinal stenosis caused by degenerative spondylolisthesis. *Eur Spine J*. 2008;17(2):188-192.
15. Kondrashov DG, Hannibal M, Hsu KY, Zucherman JF. Interspinous process decompression with the X-STOP device for lumbar spinal stenosis: a 4-year follow-up study. *J Spinal Disord Tech*. 2006;19(5):323-327.
16. Strömqvist BH, Berg S, Gerdhem P, et al. X-stop versus decompressive surgery for lumbar neurogenic intermittent claudication: randomized controlled trial with 2-year follow-up. *Spine*. 2013;38(17):1436-1442.
17. Patel VV, Whang PG, Haley TR, et al. Superion interspinous process spacer for intermittent neurogenic claudication secondary to moderate lumbar spinal stenosis: two-year results from a randomized controlled FDA-IDE pivotal trial. *Spine*. 2015;40(5):275-282.
18. Moojen WA, Arts MP, Bartels RHMA, Jacobs WCH, Peul WC. Effectiveness of interspinous implant surgery in patients with intermittent neurogenic claudication: a systematic review and meta-analysis. *Eur Spine J*. 2011;20:1596-1606.
19. Moojen WA, Arts MP, Jacobs WC, et al. Interspinous process device versus standard conventional surgical decompression for lumbar spinal stenosis: randomized controlled trial. *BMJ*. 2013;347:f6415.
20. van den Akker-van Marle ME, Moojen WA, Arts MP, et al., for the Leiden-The Hague Spine Intervention Prognostic Study Group (SIPS). Interspinous process devices versus standard conventional surgical decompression for lumbar spinal stenosis: cost-utility analysis. *Spine J*. 2014;16(6):702-710.
21. Gazzeri R, Galarza M, Neroni M, et al. Failure rates and complications of interspinous process decompression devices: a European multicenter study. *Neurosurg Focus*. 2015;39(4):E14.

CHAPTER 59 Minimally Invasive Cervical Spine Techniques

Scott I. Lee
Vinko Zlomislic

Introduction

Minimally invasive surgical techniques have gained increasing popularity, particularly for lumbar spine applications. While there is no strict definition of a minimally invasive technique, the proposed hallmarks include smaller incisions, muscle-splitting rather than muscle stripping, limiting soft tissue damage, and variable soft tissue retraction for visualization. Lumbar spine applications include tubular retractors for decompression and interbody fusions and percutaneous methods for posterior instrumentation.[1] Such techniques propose to reduce approach-related soft tissue injury associated with traditional open procedures. Subperiosteal muscle dissection and soft tissue retraction time and pressure have been shown to induce muscle edema and subsequent muscle necrosis.[2] This undoubtedly has an effect on a patient's pain, analgesic requirement, and functional recovery. Proponents of minimally invasive techniques point to early, albeit growing, evidence that these techniques result in less postoperative pain, decreased hospital length of stay, decreased blood loss, fewer surgical site infections, and a quicker return to function.[3]

Traditional open cervical spine techniques are well established with good clinical outcomes and relatively low complication rates. This brings into question whether there is even a role for minimally invasive techniques in the cervical spine. Approach-related morbidity in the cervical spine, while low, still leaves room for improvement. For example, the incidence of dysphagia following cervical surgery has been quoted to be as high as 71%.[4] While postoperative dysphagia is likely multifactorial in nature, retraction time and pressure have been proposed as contributing factors.[4,5] Furthermore, posterior cervical approaches are well known to cause significant postoperative pain and higher analgesic requirements due to muscle stripping and injury.[6] Furthermore, disruption of the posterior musculature and bony-ligamentous posterior tension band have been linked to instability and progressive kyphotic deformity.[7] In an analysis of Medicare trends, the adjusted rates of cervical spine fusions rose 206% from 1992 to 2005.[8] This increase in cervical spine surgery is partially related to a growing elderly population and resultant increase in cervical degenerative pathology amenable to surgical intervention. If minimally invasive techniques can reduce approach-related morbidity and subsequently improve patient recovery and outcomes, there certainly is a growing patient population that may benefit from these techniques.

This chapter describes approaches and applications of minimally invasive techniques for the cervical spine while highlighting existing evidence for their role in modern spine surgery.

Anterior Cervical Minimally Invasive Applications

Anterior cervical discectomy and fusion (ACDF) has long been the standard operation for cervical disc herniations that cause spinal cord and/or symptomatic root compression. While clinical outcomes are often excellent, ACDF still has its issues. Implant-related irritation, loss of segmental motion leading to adjacent-segment disease, pseudarthrosis, and the direct cost of surgical implants are just some of the issues with ACDF.[9,10] These issues have led to the development of minimally invasive anterior cervical techniques that may limit some of the downsides associated with ACDF while maximizing the benefits of anterior-based approaches (e.g., direct access to disc herniation for neural decompression, avoidance of paraspinal muscle dissection and associated patient discomfort). The following techniques will be highlighted: endoscopic anterior discectomy and cervical microendoscopic discectomy and fusion (CMEDF).

Endoscopic Anterior Discectomy

Indications and Contraindications

Endoscopic anterior discectomy (EAD) has been described for the treatment of unilateral cervical disc herniations and/or spondylotic osteophytes causing symptomatic unilateral radiculopathy. EAD does not require fusion and is a motion-sparing operation, as it avoids a complete discectomy, only targets symptomatic areas of unilateral foraminal stenosis, and does not disrupt the posterior bony/ligamentous tension band. Contraindications to this technique include cervical myelopathy or severe cervical spinal stenosis, large disc herniations (particularly central, requiring near-complete discectomy), bilateral radiculopathy, preexisting cervical instability or fracture, calcified disc herniations, axial neck pain, and significant anterior cervical soft tissue scarring (e.g., prior surgery, radiation, tracheostomy).

Clinical Evaluation

History should focus on the location and quality of unilateral radicular complaints while simultaneously ruling out other potential etiologies for pain. Patients should complete a recommended course of conservative management (e.g., activity modification, physical therapy, medication, injections) prior to consideration for surgical intervention. A thorough neurologic examination should also ensure that there are no signs of myelopathy. Imaging evaluation should include radiographs (anteroposterior, lateral, flexion-extension) to ensure no cervical fracture or instability. Noncontrast magnetic resonance imaging (MRI) is essential to visualize the location and size of disc herniation, location and size of uncovertebral osteophytes, caliber of the spinal canal, presence or absence of myelomalacia, as well as any aberrant vertebral artery anatomy. A noncontrast computed tomography (CT) scan can also help further delineate bony anatomy.

Surgical Technique

The patient is positioned supine under general anesthesia. The arms are positioned at the side. A towel roll can be placed between the scapulae to aid cervical extension with or without use of Mayfield clamps. The cervical vertebrae and discs are palpated in the interval between the esophagus/trachea and sternocleidomastoid on the side of symptomatic nerve root compression. Skin markings and use of anteroposterior and lateral fluoroscopy can help aid localization toward the indicated disc level. A 5-mm skin incision is made to allow blunt dissection down to the platysma. A small transverse incision is made in the platysma to allow eventual passage of an initial blunt, thin dilator. With use of an index finger, bluntly sweep subplatysmal structures away through finger dissection. Care should be taken to palpate the trachea, larynx, carotid artery, and the desired cervical disc. Insert the initial blunt dilator to open the prevertebral fascia and sequentially dilate up. Fluoroscopy should confirm docking on the appropriate disc space in anteroposterior and lateral planes. The following represents the transuncal approach described by Jho in 1996[11] and Saringer and colleagues in 2003.[12] The longus colli is retracted to expose the disc space and lower vertebrae. The endoscope is then inserted (Figs. 59.1 and 59.2). While maintaining visualization and continuous irrigation with 0.9% saline, a 2-mm, high-speed burr is used to remove a thin cortical portion of the uncinate process. Maintain a thin lateral wall, as this will help to protect the vertebral artery, as well as a thin dorsal edge to protect the exiting nerve root. Alternating use of curettes

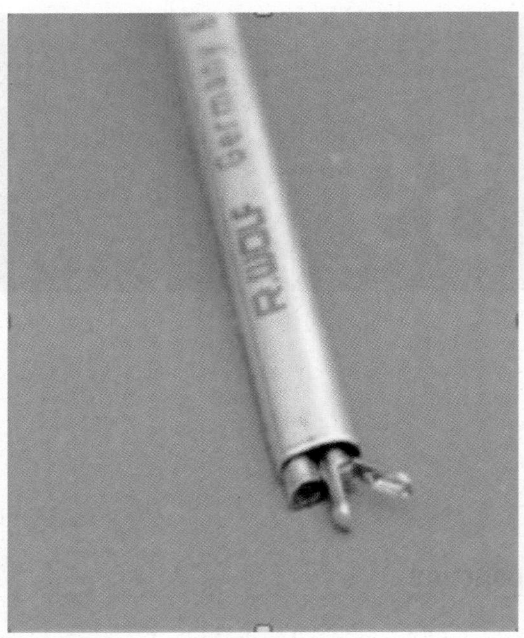

FIG. 59.1 Example of endoscopic anterior cervical discectomy instrumentation, consisting of an optic in an oval sheath with adjacent inserted rongeur.

and a Kerrison rongeur under endoscopic visualization will allow safe removal of disc material until visualization of the posterior longitudinal ligament. Care is taken to remove all herniated disc material using microsurgical instruments under endoscopic visualization. Complete the foraminotomy while ensuring protection of the exiting nerve root. Bipolar electrocautery and Gelfoam can help achieve hemostasis. The endoscope and outer sheaths are removed under direct visualization. The wound is closed in standard fashion without a drain. A soft collar can be used for the first 2 weeks to allow wound healing, after which the brace can be worn for comfort.

Clinical Outcomes and Published Studies

Published clinical studies have shown encouraging results. Saringer et al. reported a series of 16 patients treated with EAD and reported overall good results with 87.6% satisfaction rate, reduction in neck disability index score, and 96% reduction in visual analog scale score for radicular pain.[12] Ruetten et al. designed a prospective randomized controlled trial comparing ACDF versus EAD.[13] The study reports no intraoperative complications, no significant difference in incidence of postoperative dysphagia, and significantly reduced operative time favoring EAD (32 minutes versus 62 minutes). Over the 2-year follow-up, clinical outcomes were noted to be "good" with similar low rates of revision surgery for persistent radicular arm pain (7.4% in the EAD group revised to ACDF, 6.1% in ACDF group revised with posterior laminoforaminotomy). Radiographic examination revealed no spontaneous fusion or adjacent-segment degeneration. However, 25% of the EAD patients developed degeneration

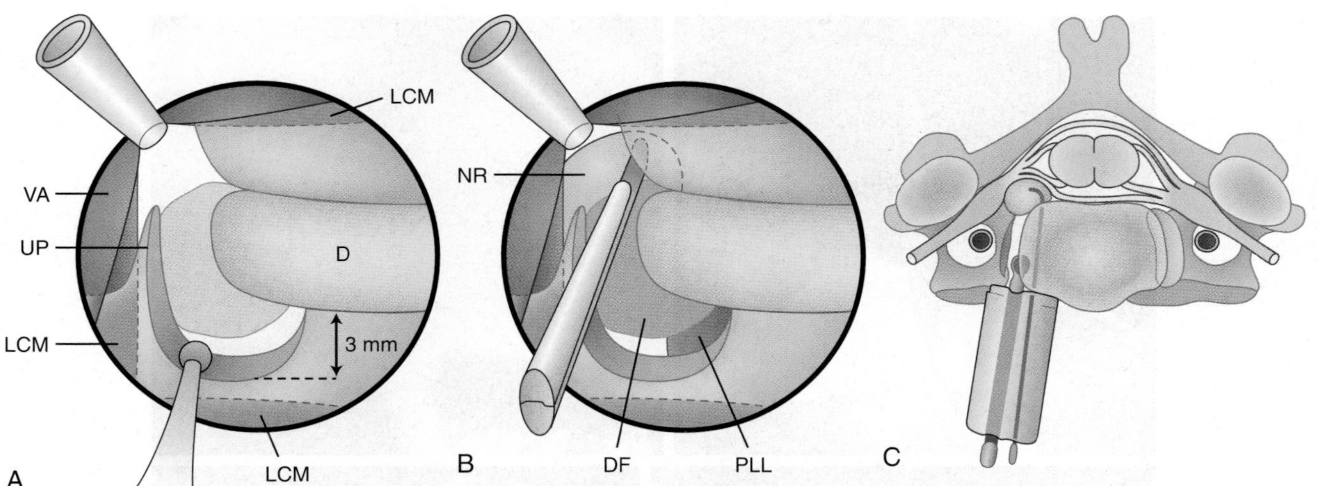

FIG. 59.2 Endoscopic anterior cervical discectomy technique for cervical disc herniation. (A) The medial edge of the longus colli muscle (LCM) is exposed in standard fashion, allowing visualization of the uncinate process (UP) and lateral edge of the intervertebral disc (D). The UP is drilled, leaving a thin edge as a landmark and to protect the adjacent vertebral artery (VA). (B) Fibrous annular disc material between the tip of the UP and caudal endplate is removed, allowing exposure of the underlying disc fragment (DF), nerve root (NR), and a portion of the posterior longitudinal ligament (PLL). (C) Maintaining constant visualization, a 1- or 2-mm Kerrison rongeur is used to remove disc fragments as well as the dorsolateral disc osteophyte complex from the nerve root.

of the operative disc level. In a retrospective study, Yang et al. examined 97 patients who had undergone a modified EAD.[14] The study reports 81% excellent results over an average of 4-year follow-up with no reported complications or cervical instability.

In these limited studies, the technique appears to be safe with good clinical outcomes and relief of radicular complaints on par with ACDF. However, one cannot ignore the strict indications for this technique as well as the potential for accelerated disc degeneration at the operative level, as observed by Ruetten et al.[13] The 25% incidence of disc degeneration in the 2-year study far exceeds the quoted rates of symptomatic disc degeneration (1.6–4.2% per year) following arthrodesis in the cervical spine.[10] EAD is a technique that appears to have clinical value but requires further clinical studies to ascertain its true benefit and complication rate.

Cervical Microendoscopic Discectomy and Fusion

Indications and Contraindications

CMEDF is indicated for symptomatic cervical spinal cord and/or nerve root compression from herniated disc material, osteophytes, spondylosis, congenital canal stenosis, and dynamic instability. CMEDF utilizes a similar approach as EAD. However, in contrast to EAD, the addition of a complete discectomy and placement of an interbody device for fusion opens up the indications to include patients with cervical myelopathy, large central disc herniations, bilateral radiculopathy, preexisting cervical instability or fracture, and axial neck pain. Contraindications include significant anterior cervical soft tissue scarring (e.g., prior surgery, radiation, tracheostomy), aberrant anatomy, retrovertebral stenosis, and multiple levels of symptomatic neurologic compression.

Clinical Evaluation

History should focus on the location and quality of unilateral radicular complaints while simultaneously ruling out other potential etiologies for pain. Patients should complete a recommended course of conservative management (e.g., activity modification, physical therapy, medication, injections) prior to consideration for surgical intervention unless the patient exhibits symptoms and signs of myelopathy. A thorough neurologic history and examination should be performed, with particular emphasis placed on motor strength, sensory function, balance, reflexes, and bowel/bladder function. Imaging evaluation should include radiographs (anteroposterior, lateral, flexion-extension) to ensure no cervical fracture or instability. Noncontrast MRI is essential to visualize the location and size of disc herniation, location, and size of uncovertebral osteophytes, caliber of the spinal canal, presence or absence of myelomalacia, and any aberrant vertebral artery anatomy. Noncontrast CT scan can also help further delineate bony anatomy.

Surgical Technique

Surgical setup and general concepts are very similar to that described for EAD (see earlier section). This section highlights key differences between EAD and CMEDF. A 2-cm transverse incision over the appropriate disc level affords sufficient exposure with eventual aid of the tubular retractor. Incise the

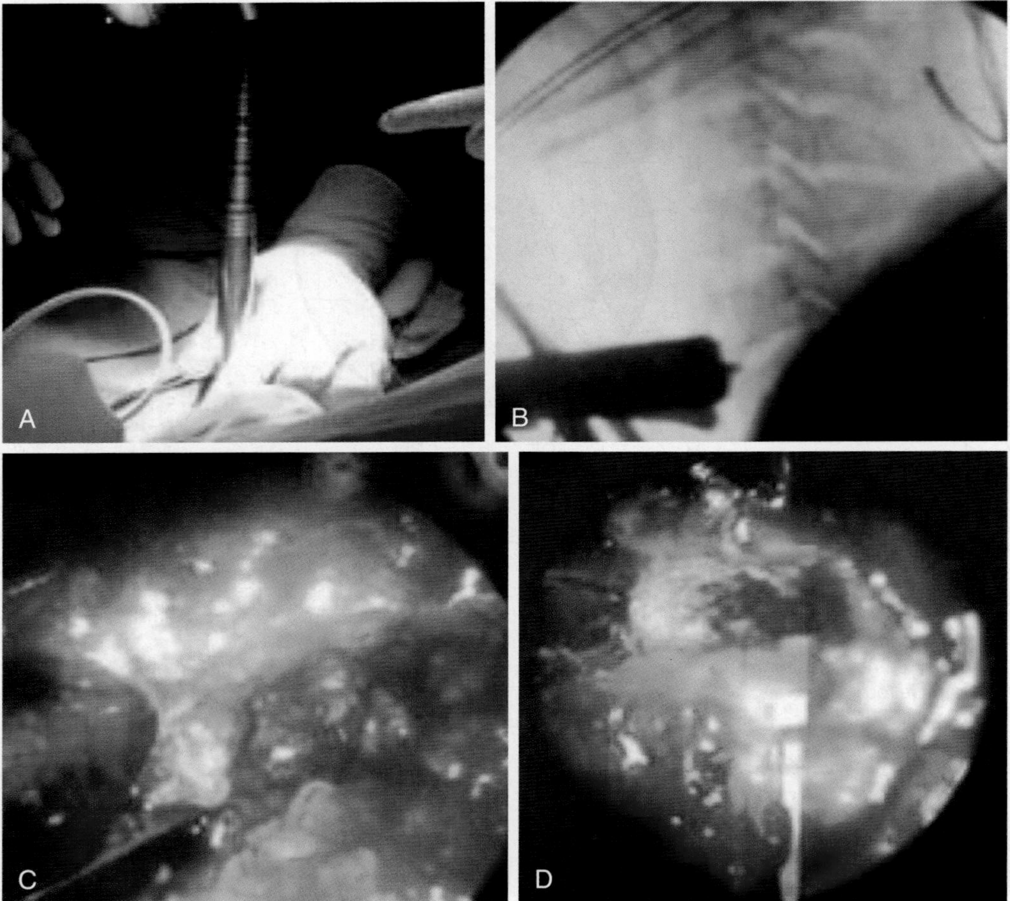

FIG. 59.3 Intraoperative endoscopic views. (A) Sequential placement of endoscopic dilators between strap muscles and esophagus medially and carotid sheath laterally. (B) Fluoroscopic imaging to confirm appropriate retractor positioning and level. (C) Begin discectomy with removal of anterior osteophytes immediately adjacent to the disc space. (D) Endoscopic view upon completion of discectomy with placement of graft.

platysma and bluntly dissect through subplatysmal structures to localize the trachea, esophagus, carotid sheath, and desired disc space. Endoscopic dilators are sequentially placed under fluoroscopic guidance. The final dilator is replaced with a tubular retractor that is secured to the operating table (Fig. 59.3). Subtle adjustments in angulation, tension, and placement of the retractor, as well as use of a mobile window, can help aid visualization of the appropriate disc space(s) while limiting soft tissue tension. After obtaining fluoroscopic images confirming that the retractor is docked at the correct disc level, remove the dilators and begin endoscopic discectomy (see Fig. 59.3). All steps for discectomy, endplate preparation, and interbody graft placement are similar to a standard open procedure. Manual cervical traction or sequential dilation of the disc space with osteotomes can help aid discectomy and interbody graft placement (Fig. 59.4). Published studies of this technique have not used an anterior cervical plate.[1,15,16] After obtaining appropriate hemostasis, the wound is closed in standard fashion without a drain. The patient is placed in a hard cervical collar for 4 to 8 weeks.

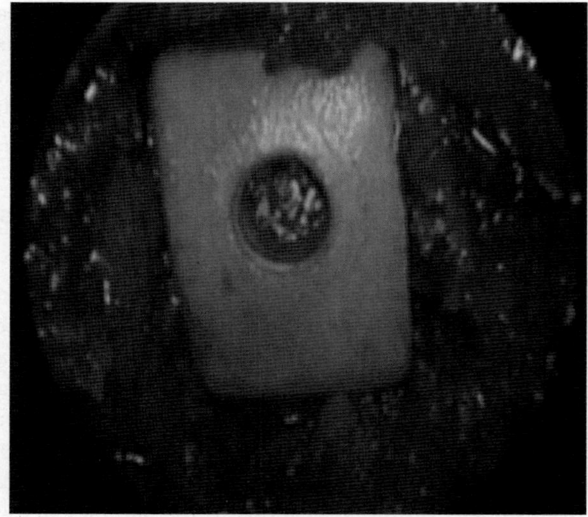

FIG. 59.4 Endoscopic image after graft placement.

Clinical Outcomes and Published Studies

In 2008, Tan et al. reported their short-term results of CMEDF in 36 patients: no intraoperative complications, no dysphagia, and significant improvement in Japanese Orthopaedic Association and visual analog scale scores over a mean 38-month follow-up.[15] While there was one postoperative hematoma, the study noted overall good clinical results and improved cosmesis. Yao et al. reported 5-year follow-up results of 67 patients who underwent CMEDF with carbon fiber interbody graft augmented with iliac crest bone graft.[1] In keeping with other studies, the technique was associated with good to excellent clinical results, with minimal blood loss, no intraoperative complications, and no persistent dysphagia. Furthermore, 91.1% of patients achieved radiographic fusion by 6 months. There was a 6% incidence of cage subsidence and the remaining patients either achieved radiographic fusion after 6 months or were noted to have asymptomatic pseudarthrosis. Only one patient required adjacent-segment ACDF for symptomatic disc herniation at 6 years postoperatively. Soliman reported results of a blinded randomized controlled trial comparing ACDF to CMEDF.[16] Both techniques were without anterior cervical plating and resulted in 91% good to excellent results in both groups. The study noted a significant reduction in average length of hospital stay (47 hours for ACDF, 26 hours for CMEDF), decreased self-reported rates of dysphagia, and decreased analgesic requirement favoring the CMEDF group. At 1 year, all patients had achieved fusion except for one asymptomatic pseudarthrosis in the CMEDF group.

CMEDF appears to be a viable option, with clinical and radiographic results in published studies that match those of ACDF. The purported benefits of cosmesis, reduced hospital stay, reduced pain, and reduced dysphagia are encouraging and require additional study to ascertain if these are true benefits over traditional ACDF.

Posterior Cervical Minimally Invasive Applications

Posterior-based techniques are attractive, as they can address neurologic compression while avoiding anterior structures (e.g., trachea, esophagus, vertebral artery, recurrent laryngeal nerve) and potentially preserving cervical motion. Posterior cervical laminoforaminotomy, first described by Spurling and Scoville[17] in 1944, has been shown to produce favorable results in treating cervical radiculopathy.[18] However, approach-related morbidity can make open posterior techniques less attractive due to considerable muscle injury, pain and spasms, and potential instability and progressive sagittal deformity due to disruption of the posterior tension band.[7,19] Preoperative sagittal alignment and the amount of operative muscular dissection and bony resection increase the risk of developing postoperative cervical kyphosis.[7,20] Concerns regarding postoperative kyphosis may prompt the addition of posterior instrumented fusion or a reconsideration of performing an anterior-based procedure. Supplementation with posterior instrumentation increases operative time, blood loss, potential risks to the patient, and pain and rehabilitation. Minimally invasive posterior cervical techniques may prove advantageous by limiting the extent of muscle dissection and minimizing the risk of postoperative instability. The following techniques will be highlighted: minimally invasive cervical laminoforaminotomy, minimally invasive posterior cervical discectomy, and minimally invasive lateral mass fixation.

Minimally Invasive Cervical Laminoforaminotomy

Indications and Contraindications

Minimally invasive cervical laminoforaminotomy is indicated for the treatment of cervical radiculopathy resulting from soft lateral disc herniation and/or foraminal stenosis. It can be performed for single- or multilevel disease and can be an effective treatment for patients with recurrent radicular symptoms following ACDF. Cases of bilateral same-level radiculopathy and/or foraminal stenosis from uncinate spurs may achieve better neurologic decompression from an anterior-based approach. Central disc herniations are not amenable to this technique due to the unsafe spinal cord retraction that would be required to access the disc space and herniated material. Other contraindications to minimally invasive cervical laminoforaminotomy include patients with cervical kyphosis, fracture or instability, axial neck pain, and severe central or retrovertebral stenosis with or without myelomalacia. Patients with these characteristics are likely better candidates for an anterior-based approach.

Clinical Evaluation

A thorough history and physical examination will localize the involved cervical nerve root(s) while also screening for cervical myelopathy. The patient should also be screened for axial neck pain and other sources of arm/shoulder pain. Radiographic examination should include anteroposterior, lateral, and flexion-extension views to evaluate for fracture and instability. A noncontrast MRI is essential to localize compressive pathology and evaluate the health of the cervical spine. The MRI should also be studied for any aberrant vertebral artery anatomy. A noncontrast CT scan can be helpful to further delineate bony anatomy but is not absolutely necessary for most cases. Prior to surgical intervention, the patient should undergo appropriate conservative treatment measures consisting of activity modification, medications, physical therapy, and injections.

Surgical Technique

After induction with general endotracheal anesthesia, the patient is placed in the prone position. The head can either be secured with use of Mayfield clamps or can be positioned on a well-padded headrest. Take care to ensure that there is no pressure on bony prominences or the eyes and that the

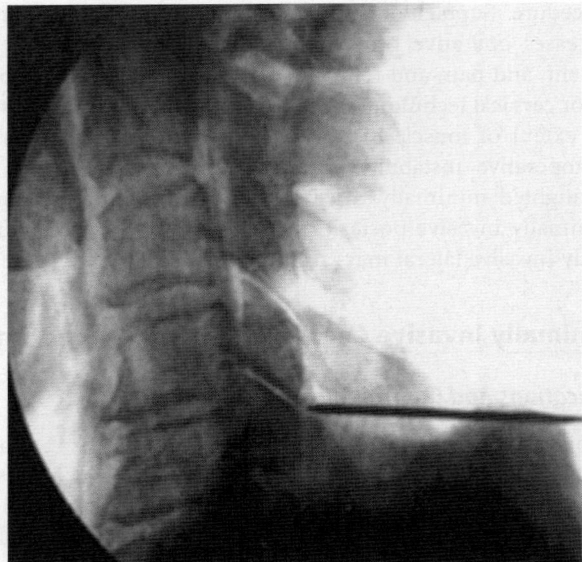

FIG. 59.5 A K-wire is advanced through posterior cervical musculature under fluoroscopic guidance and docked at the inferomedial edge of the cephalad lateral mass of the desired level.

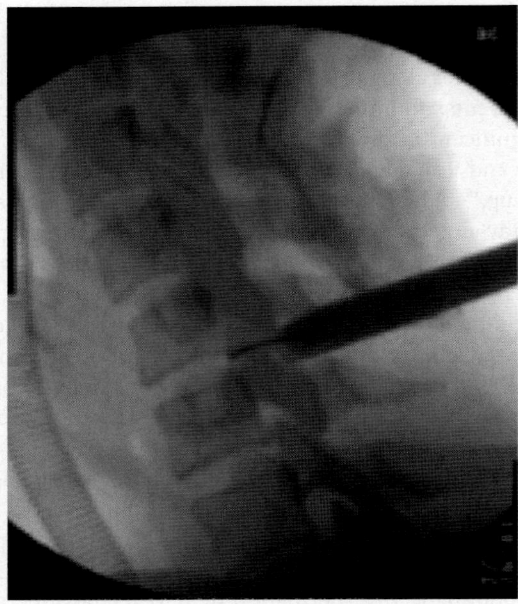

FIG. 59.6 Intraoperative fluoroscopic image demonstrating positioning of working retractor with a Penfield elevator positioned on the dorsal anulus following safe removal of a herniated disc ventral to the nerve root.

endotracheal tube is secure. Slight flexion through the cervical spine and a military chin tuck can aid exposure.

With aid of posteroanterior fluoroscopic images, mark the skin in line with the location and orientation of the lateral masses and facet joints of the side of the proposed operation. Under lateral fluoroscopic views, mark the skin over the desired cervical segment(s), taking into account the trajectory of the lateral masses and laminae. The skin markings and subsequent incision will be 5 to 15 mm off of midline ipsilateral to and at the target level. If planning to decompress multiple levels, the incision can be made midway between the two desired levels. After making a stab incision, bluntly dissect through subcutaneous tissue. Using lateral fluoroscopic guidance, slowly advance a Kirschner wire (K-wire) through posterior musculature and dock at the inferomedial edge of the desired lateral mass (Fig. 59.5). Extend the stab incision approximately 1 cm cephalad and caudad to the K-wire. Dissect through the cervical fascia with monopolar electrocautery. Place the tubular dilators over the K-wire to serially dilate down to the desired cervical level. After confirming the correct level with a lateral fluoroscopic image, secure the tubular retractor to the table.

Alternatively, the procedure can be performed through a midline posterior incision centered over the spinous process(es) of the desired level(s). Incise through the underlying fascia 4 to 6 mm off of the midline. For bilateral procedures, make two separate fascial incisions to each side of the midline. Use finger dissection to bluntly dissect the paraspinal musculature until palpation of the facet joint. Introduce the smallest dilator and confirm the level with a lateral fluoroscopic image. After serially dilating, secure the tubular retractor to the table.

Decompression can be performed under loupe magnification, microscope magnification, or with use of an endoscope. Bipolar electrocautery can help remove any residual soft tissue overlying the desired lateral mass and facet. The ligamentum flavum is detached from the inferior edge of the lamina with use of a straight curette. Identify the medial edge of the facet as it joins into the lamina. This will help avoid over-resection of the facet articulation that could lead to iatrogenic instability and degeneration. Use Kerrison rongeurs and/or a high-speed burr to begin the laminotomy. Removal of the dorsolateral portion of the lamina as well as the medial border of the inferior articular facet will allow visualization of the exiting nerve root. Angled curettes can help dissect a safe tissue plane out laterally into the foramen. Bipolar electrocautery can help aid dissection, particularly of any overlying venous plexus. Straight or angled Kerrison rongeurs can complete the decompression of the foramen and exiting nerve root. When a Woodson elevator can be freely passed over the nerve root to the lateral pedicle border, the nerve root has been adequately decompressed in the foramen. Ensure that the nerve root has no additional ventral compression on imaging and with direct palpation ventral to the nerve with a Woodson elevator or small, angled curette (Fig. 59.6). If there is herniated disc material, the nerve root can be gently retracted medially to allow visualization of the disc space. If visualization is limited by bony anatomy, use a high-speed burr or Kerrison rongeurs to resect additional lamina and the superomedial pedicle to allow safe removal of herniated disc material with use of curettes and pituitary rongeurs. If there are additional levels for decompression, the tubular retractor can be angled and translated utilizing a mobile window for visualization. After manipulation of the retractor, be sure to confirm the level with a lateral fluoroscopic image. After irrigation and appropriate hemostasis, the incision is closed in standard fashion without a drain. A soft collar can be used for the first 1 to 2 weeks to allow wound healing, following which it can be discontinued.

Clinical Outcomes and Published Studies

Fessler et al. first reported their initial clinical experience in treating 25 patients with minimally invasive cervical laminoforaminotomy in 2002.[21] Clinical outcomes were equivalent to open posterior laminoforaminotomy with the added benefits of decreased blood loss, shorter postoperative stays (20 vs. 68 hours) and reduced narcotic requirements. These initial short-term benefits have been confirmed by multiple other studies including a randomized controlled trial comparing open posterior laminoforaminotomy versus tubular retractor assisted cervical laminoforaminotomy and discectomy.[6] In a recent systematic review, Clark et al.[22] reported 19 studies comparing minimally invasive cervical laminoforaminotomy to open posterior decompression for cervical radiculopathy. Across these studies, the minimally invasive procedure was found to have decreased blood loss (52.8 vs. 173.5 mL), a shorter surgical time (58 vs. 108 minutes), less inpatient analgesic use (2.5 vs. 27.6 Eq), and a shorter hospital stay (1.0 vs. 3.2 days). Symptom relief following minimally invasive cervical laminoforaminotomy across the literature is between 87% and 97%.[18] The advantages of the minimally invasive approach appear to be long-lasting. Lawton et al. reported on the long-term outcomes of minimally invasive cervical laminoforaminotomy with up to 6-year follow-up data showing persistence of patient satisfaction, low neck disability index scores, and low visual analog scale for both neck and arm.[23]

Currently, ACDF remains the most-common operation for cervical radiculopathy. However, minimally invasive cervical laminoforaminotomy compares favorably to ACDF. Ruetten et al.[13] reported a prospective randomized trial comparing 175 patients randomly assigned to ACDF versus full-endoscopic posterior cervical laminoforaminotomy. In 2-year follow-up, clinical results were similar in both groups with 87.4% of patients reporting complete relief of arm pain and 9.2% with occasional arm pain. The minimally invasive group had a 3.4% recurrence rate which was similar to the ACDF group and comparable to other published data.

Minimally invasive posterior cervical laminoforamintomy appears to be clinically efficacious when used for the correct indications. However, it is still a posterior-based approach. As such, concerns remain for the development of neck pain, instability, and adjacent-segment degeneration due to potential iatrogenic violation of the bony and ligamentous posterior tension band without an adjunct instrumented fusion for support. In a retrospective review of 303 patients following posterior cervical laminoforaminotomy, Clarke et al. found the annual rate of developing same-segment or adjacent-segment pathology to be 0.7%.[24] This is similar to published data in regard to ACDF; the risk of developing clinically significant adjacent-segment pathology following ACDF is 1.6% to 4.2% per year.[10] In regard to neck pain, Steinberg et al. found no difference in the postoperative neck pain visual analog scale or neck disability index scores of patients undergoing minimally invasive cervical laminoforaminotomy and ACDF.[25] Such data suggest that the minimally invasive approach helps preserve the posterior tension band, preventing the need for secondary fusion. However, if there is clinically significant neck pain, instability, and/or recurrent radicular symptoms following minimally invasive cervical laminoforaminotomy, ACDF is a potential treatment option. Skovrlj et al.[18] examined a prospective cohort of 70 patients following minimally invasive cervical laminoforaminotomy; 7.1% of patients required ACDF at a mean of 55 months from the index procedure either at the index level or adjacent level for symptomatic disc pathology. This incidence of revision following minimally invasive cervical laminoforaminotomy is lower than quoted rates for revision following ACDF. A meta-analysis of class I US Food and Drug Administration trials for ACDF reported a 9.8% reoperation rate due to pseudarthrosis, adjacent-level disease, and recurrent radicular symptoms following ACDF.[26]

Multiple studies describe an initial learning period with this technique. Complication rates are low, with studies citing rates from 1.1% to 9% and include durotomy and radicular injury secondary to root manipulation.[21,23,27,28] Minimally invasive cervical laminoforaminotomy is an evolving surgical technique with good clinical outcomes. Given that much of the concerns with open, posterior-based approaches is centered on soft tissue disruption, this is an ideal clinical scenario to apply this minimally invasive technique.

Minimally Invasive Lateral Mass Fixation

Indications and Contraindications

Lateral mass screws can be placed using minimally invasive techniques in most clinical scenarios that require posterior cervical instrumented fusion. It can be combined with minimally invasive cervical laminoforaminotomy and discectomy if neurologic decompression is required. It is also an excellent option when decompression is not necessary and the patient requires only supplemental fixation and stability (e.g., prior multilevel anterior corpectomy). This technique is contraindicated in patients with lateral mass fracture, small or absent lateral mass, or abnormal vertebral artery anatomy.

Surgical Technique

After induction with general endotracheal anesthesia, the patient is placed in the prone position. The head can either be secured with use of Mayfield clamps or can be positioned on a well-padded headrest. Take care to ensure that there is no pressure on bony prominences or the eyes and that the endotracheal tube is secure. Slight flexion through the cervical spine and a military chin tuck can aid exposure.

The procedure is performed through a midline posterior incision centered over the spinous process(es) of the desired level(s). Fluoroscopy can help localize the incision. Incise through the underlying fascia 4 to 6 mm off of the midline bilaterally. Use finger dissection to bluntly dissect the paraspinal musculature until palpation of the facet joint. Take care not to dissect past the lateral border of the lateral mass, as this is unnecessary muscle dissection that can lead to significant bleeding. Introduce the smallest dilator and confirm the level with a lateral fluoroscopic image. The dilators should be placed

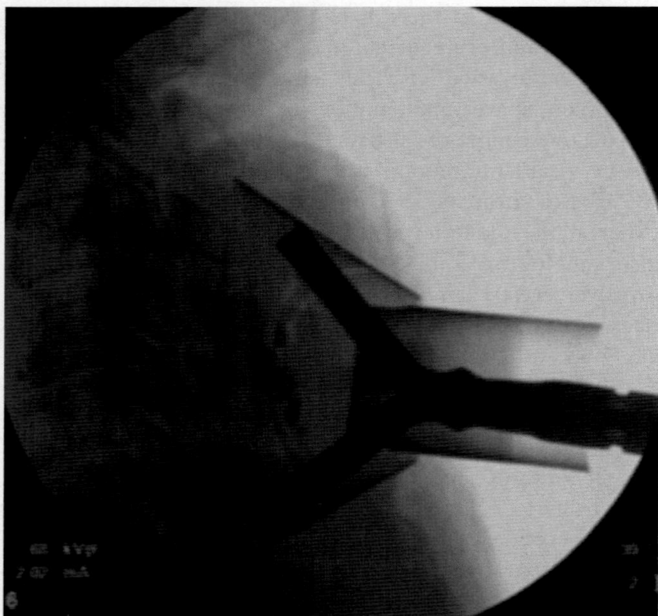

FIG. 59.7 Intraoperative fluoroscopic image demonstrating expansion of a deployed rivet retractor to allow deep exposure over multiple levels. It is necessary to use fluoroscopy during expansion to ensure that retraction remains seated over the intended surgical levels.

with a 15-degree cephalad angulation to help facilitate proper trajectory for screw placement. After serially dilating, secure the tubular retractor to the table, ensuring proper trajectory. Obtain a lateral fluoroscopic image to confirm docking at the desired level. A sliding rivet retractor can also help with visualization of multiple levels (Fig. 59.7). Use bipolar electrocautery and pituitary rongeurs to clear off the lateral mass to enable complete visualization of the medial, lateral, cephalad, and caudad borders (Fig. 59.8). Take care not to violate the facet articulations of segments not included in the fusion construct.

Placement of lateral mass instrumentation is in standard fashion as open techniques. Preoperative templating on MRI and CT scan is invaluable in determining drill/screw length and trajectory. Use a drill with a preset drill depth (8–14 mm) to avoid blowing out the lateral mass and subsequently risking injury to neurovascular structures. The starting point is in the center of the lateral mass relative to the cephalad-caudad borders and 1 mm medial to the center of the lateral mass relative to the medial-lateral borders. The drill should be angled approximately 15 to 20 degrees cephalad to match the trajectory of the lateral mass. It should also be angled 25 to 30 degrees lateral to avoid injury to the superior facet articulation, exiting nerve root, and the vertebral artery. The drill hole is then checked with a ball-tip feeler to ensure no cortical wall breech. Trajectory and length can also be checked on lateral fluoroscopic imaging. The hole is then tapped prior to placement of a 3.5-mm polyaxial screw. For each additional level, the retractor should be translated to ensure appropriate visualization of bony anatomy. Confirm on lateral fluoroscopic image that the retractor is well seated on the posterior aspect of the desired lateral mass and the trajectory has not changed. Once lateral mass screws are secured, the exposed posterior cortical surfaces and facet articulations are decorticated with a high-speed burr. Local bone autograft, iliac crest bone autograft, and allograft can be packed onto the decorticated surfaces prior to placement of an appropriately lordosed rod. After the rod is secured into place, the tubular retractor is slowly removed while maintaining visualization to ensure appropriate hemostasis. The wound is closed in standard fashion without a drain. The patient is then placed in a hard cervical collar.

Clinical Outcomes and Published Studies

Lateral mass screw fixation has been shown to be safe and effective in promoting stability and fusion in large patient studies.[29,30] While there are very few clinical studies examining the minimally invasive technique, the available data indicate that the technique enables safe placement of instrumentation while minimizing violation of the posterior musculature and ligaments.[31] In a retrospective analysis, Wang et al. noted no intraoperative complications, bony fusion in all cases, and no aberrant screw placement, as confirmed by CT scan.[31] The study did note that two patients had to be converted to an open procedure, as fluoroscopic imaging was inadequate at the lower cervical levels due to patient anatomy. Wang et al. also limited the minimally invasive technique to two-level fusions. Mikhael et al. demonstrated minimally invasive lateral mass fixation in C3–C7 constructs.[32]

Conclusions

Minimally invasive techniques are continually evolving in spine surgery. The application of these techniques to the cervical spine has lagged behind the techniques in use for the lumbar spine. However, there is certainly a role for these techniques in both anterior and posterior cervical applications. Studies have shown that these techniques are safe and demonstrate similar or superior clinical efficacy compared to traditional open techniques, with the added benefit of significantly reducing approach-related soft tissue morbidity. This has a profound impact on postoperative pain and recovery; as such, these minimally invasive techniques represent an attractive surgical option. Certainly, these techniques are still relatively new and require additional study before widespread application. It is important to use these techniques for the proper indications and not lose sight of the traditional open procedures. Like any new technique, there is an associated learning curve. Having a strong foundation with the open procedures can help avoid complications, solve intraoperative issues, and reinforce anatomy. Minimally invasive techniques require appropriate visualization (via direct visualization, endoscope, microscope, and fluoroscopy) in order to safely operate through a smaller window. As these techniques are refined, the surgical indications may expand. Regardless, further clinical study will be essential to improve these techniques.

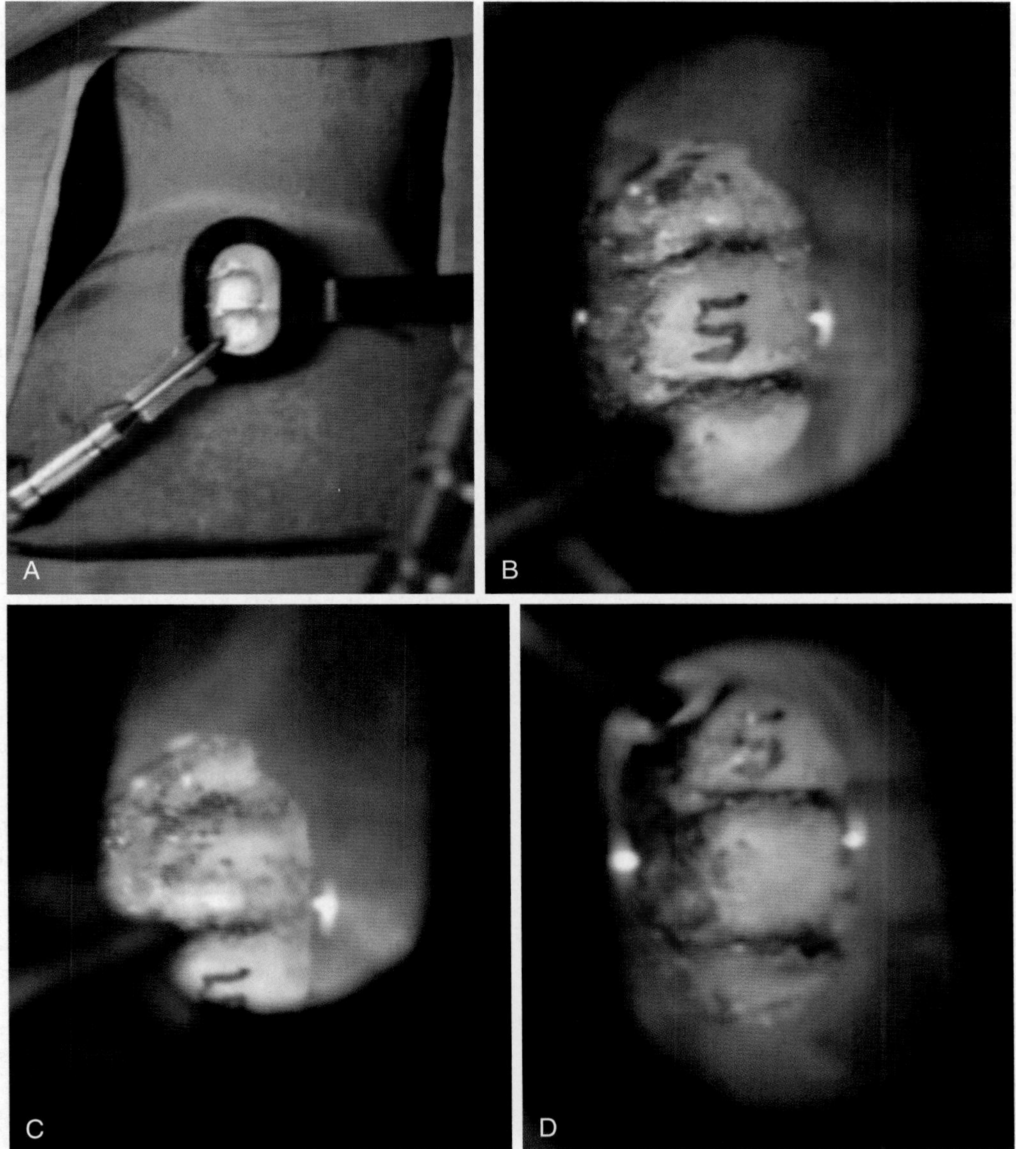

FIG. 59.8 (A) Intraoperative image showing final retractor setup with attachment to flexible mounting system. (B) This allows for complete exposure of the lateral mass, with visualization of the medial and lateral facet joint. Repositioning and angulation of the retractor allows for easy access to the (C) cephalad and (D) caudad levels if necessary.

KEY REFERENCES

1. Yao N, Wang C, Wang W, Wang L. Full-endoscopic technique for anterior cervical discectomy and interbody fusion: 5-year follow-up results of 67 cases. *Eur Spine J*. 2011;20(6):899-904.
2. Jho HD. Microsurgical anterior cervical foraminotomy for radiculopathy: a new approach to cervical disc herniation. *J Neurosurg*. 1996;84(2):155-160.
3. Saringer WF, Reddy B, Nöbauer-Huhmann I, et al. Endoscopic anterior cervical foraminotomy for unilateral radiculopathy: anatomical morphometric analysis and preliminary clinical experience. *J Neurosurg*. 2003;98(2 suppl):171-180.
4. Tan J, Zheng Y, Gong L, et al. Anterior cervical discectomy and interbody fusion by endoscopic approach: a preliminary report. *J Neurosurg Spine*. 2008;8(1):17-21.
5. Fessler RG, Khoo LT. Minimally invasive cervical microendoscopic foraminotomy: an initial clinical experience. *Neurosurgery*. 2002;51(5 suppl):S37-S45.
6. Clark JG, Abdullah KG, Steinmetz MP, Benzel EC, Mroz TE. Minimally invasive versus open cervical foraminotomy: a systematic review. *Global Spine J*. 2011;1(1):9-14.
7. Wang MY, Levi AD. Minimally invasive lateral mass screw fixation in the cervical spine: initial clinical experience with long-term follow-up. *Neurosurgery*. 2006;58(5):907-912.

REFERENCES

1. Yao N, Wang C, Wang W, Wang L. Full-endoscopic technique for anterior cervical discectomy and interbody fusion: 5-year follow-up results of 67 cases. *Eur Spine J*. 2011;20(6):899-904.

2. Kawaguchi Y, Matsui H, Tsuji H. Back muscle injury after posterior lumbar spine surgery. A histologic and enzymatic analysis. *Spine*. 1996;21(8):941-944.
3. Lubelski D, Mihalovich KE, Skelly AC, et al. Is minimal access spine surgery more cost-effective than conventional spine surgery? *Spine*. 2014;39(22 suppl 1):S65-S74.
4. Cho SK, Lu Y, Lee DH. Dysphagia following anterior cervical spinal surgery: a systematic review. *Bone Joint J*. 2013;95-B(7):868-873.
5. Joaquim AF, Murar J, Savage JW, Patel AA. Dysphagia after anterior cervical spine surgery: a systematic review of potential preventative measures. *Spine J*. 2014;14(9):2246-2260.
6. Kim KT, Kim YB. Comparison between open procedure and tubular retractor assisted procedure for cervical radiculopathy: results of a randomized controlled study. *J Korean Med Sci*. 2009;24(4):649-653.
7. Kaptain GJ, Simmons NE, Replogle RE, Pobereskin L. Incidence and outcome of kyphotic deformity following laminectomy for cervical spondylotic myelopathy. *J Neurosurg*. 2000;93(2 suppl):199-204.
8. Wang MC, Kreuter W, Wolfla CE, Maiman DJ, Deyo RA. Trends and variations in cervical spine surgery in the United States: medicare beneficiaries, 1992 to 2005. *Spine*. 2009;34(9):955-961.
9. Mansfield HE, Canar WJ, Gerard CS, O'toole JE. Single-level anterior cervical discectomy and fusion versus minimally invasive posterior cervical foraminotomy for patients with cervical radiculopathy: a cost analysis. *Neurosurg Focus*. 2014;37(5):E9.
10. Lawrence BD, Hilibrand AS, Brodt ED, Dettori JR, Brodke DS. Predicting the risk of adjacent segment pathology in the cervical spine: a systematic review. *Spine*. 2012;37(22 suppl): S52-S64.
11. Jho HD. Microsurgical anterior cervical foraminotomy for radiculopathy: a new approach to cervical disc herniation. *J Neurosurg*. 1996;84(2):155-160.
12. Saringer WF, Reddy B, Nöbauer-Huhmann I, et al. Endoscopic anterior cervical foraminotomy for unilateral radiculopathy: anatomical morphometric analysis and preliminary clinical experience. *J Neurosurg*. 2003;98(2 suppl):171-180.
13. Ruetten S, Komp M, Merk H, Godolias G. Full-endoscopic anterior decompression versus conventional anterior decompression and fusion in cervical disc herniations. *Int Orthop*. 2009;33(6):1677-1682.
14. Yang B, Xie J, Yin B, et al. Treatment of cervical disc herniation through percutaneous minimally invasive techniques. *Eur Spine J*. 2014;23(2):382-388.
15. Tan J, Zheng Y, Gong L, et al. Anterior cervical discectomy and interbody fusion by endoscopic approach: a preliminary report. *J Neurosurg Spine*. 2008;8(1):17-21.
16. Soliman HM. Cervical microendoscopic discectomy and fusion: does it affect the postoperative course and the complication rate? A blinded randomized controlled trial. *Spine*. 2013;38(24):2064-2070.
17. Spurling RG, Scoville WB. Lateral rupture of the cervical intervertebral disc: a common cause of shoulder and arm pain. *Surg Gynecol Obstet*. 1944;78:350-358.
18. Skovrlj B, Gologorsky Y, Haque R, Fessler RG, Qureshi SA. Complications, outcomes, and need for fusion after minimally invasive posterior cervical foraminotomy and microdiscectomy. *Spine J*. 2014;14(10):2405-2411.
19. Hosono N, Yonenobu K, Ono K. Neck and shoulder pain after laminoplasty. A noticeable complication. *Spine*. 1996;21(17):1969-1973.
20. Albert TJ, Vacarro A. Postlaminectomy kyphosis. *Spine*. 1998;23(24):2738-2745.
21. Fessler RG, Khoo LT. Minimally invasive cervical microendoscopic foraminotomy: an initial clinical experience. *Neurosurgery*. 2002;51(5 suppl):S37-S45.
22. Clark JG, Abdullah KG, Steinmetz MP, Benzel EC, Mroz TE. Minimally invasive versus open cervical foraminotomy: a systematic review. *Global Spine J*. 2011;1(1):9-14.
23. Lawton CD, Smith ZA, Lam SK, et al. Clinical outcomes of microendoscopic foraminotomy and decompression in the cervical spine. *World Neurosurg*. 2014;81(2):422-427.
24. Clarke MJ, Ecker RD, Krauss WE, McClelland RL, Dekutoski MB. Same-segment and adjacent-segment disease following posterior cervical foraminotomy. *J Neurosurg Spine*. 2007; 6(1):5-9.
25. Steinberg JA, German JW. The effect of minimally invasive posterior cervical approaches versus open anterior approaches on neck pain and disability. *Int J Spine Surg*. 2012;6:55-61.
26. Pettine KA, Eiserman L. *Meta-analysis of class I results of anterior cervical decompression and fusion with allograft and plating*. Abstract presented at the annual meeting of American Academy of Orthopaedic Surgeons, February 7, 2012, San Francisco, CA.
27. McAnany SJ, Kim JS, Overley SC, et al. A meta-analysis of cervical foraminotomy: open versus minimally-invasive techniques. *Spine J*. 2015;15(5):849-856.
28. Wang TY, Lubelski D, Abdullah KG, et al. Rates of anterior cervical discectomy and fusion after initial posterior cervical foraminotomy. *Spine J*. 2015;15(5):971-976.
29. Katonis P, Papadakis SA, Galanakos S, et al. Lateral mass screw complications: analysis of 1662 screws. *J Spinal Disord Tech*. 2011;24(7):415-420.
30. Sekhon LH. Posterior cervical lateral mass screw fixation: analysis of 1026 consecutive screws in 143 patients. *J Spinal Disord Tech*. 2005;18(4):297-303.
31. Wang MY, Levi AD. Minimally invasive lateral mass screw fixation in the cervical spine: initial clinical experience with long-term follow-up. *Neurosurgery*. 2006;58(5):907-912.
32. Mikhael MM, Celestre PC, Wolf CF, Mroz TE, Wang JC. Minimally invasive cervical spine foraminotomy and lateral mass screw placement. *Spine*. 2012;37(5):E318-E322.

CHAPTER

60 Future Directions in Minimally Invasive Spinal Surgery

SECTION VII

Xiaobang Hu
Isador H. Lieberman

The use of minimally invasive spinal surgery (MIS) is a philosophy focused on targeting the offending pathology while minimizing the collateral tissue damage. MIS is not any single specific device, technique, or use of an implant. The principal goal of MIS is to reduce approach-related soft tissue injury and complications while reducing postoperative pain, blood loss, and recovery time, still achieving the same or even better clinical outcomes as compared with traditional open surgery.[1,2] Over the past 2 decades, advances in tissue retractors, intraoperative navigation, specialized minimally invasive instruments, and visualization through microscopy and endoscopy have revolutionized the field of MIS. Over the same time span, continuing advances in diagnostic capabilities and biologic therapeutics have evolved that will no doubt merge with MIS techniques to further advance treatment options and minimize the need for traditional invasive surgical procedures. This chapter explores several exciting areas in MIS and discusses possible future directions.

Minimally Invasive Approaches to the Spine: Understanding the Anatomy and Designing Retractors

The first report of using a tubular retractor system (METRx, Medtronic) to treat symptomatic herniated discs was described by Foley and Smith in 1997.[3] The pioneering MIS approach that they described demonstrated that microdiscectomy, a routine spine procedure, can be performed using a novel retractor system and an attachable endoscope, allowing for visualization of the pathology with minimal tissue trauma and virtually no obstruction for the passage of instruments through a defined working channel.[4] Several prospective, randomized studies confirmed that minimally invasive tubular microdiscectomy is as safe and effective as traditional open microdiscectomy.[5–7] The patients who underwent a tubular microdiscectomy had lesser operative time and intraoperative blood loss, lower complication rates, a shorter duration of postoperative disability, and less narcotic usage.[6,7] Today, treatment of herniated discs via minimally invasive tubular microdiscectomy is one of the most commonly performed MIS techniques in the United States.[8] In recent years, working through a defined corridor or channel has evolved to be used for various spinal disorders, including decompression for lumbar stenosis and epidural compression due to metastatic or primary tumors of the spine.[9–12]

Over the last 10 years, by virtue of the experience gained with tubular microdiscectomy, surgeons implemented various design modifications to the tubular retractor, which have now allowed spine surgeons to perform spinal fusions through far less invasive approaches, including direct lateral transpsoas and posterolateral transforaminal approaches. The current technique of minimally invasive transforaminal lumbar interbody fusion (MI-TLIF) for the treatment of low-grade spondylolisthesis, recurrent disc herniation, degenerative disc disease, postlaminectomy instability, and spinal trauma has become a popular approach for interbody fusion. Recent studies have shown that MI-TLIF is associated with reduced blood loss, decreased complication rates, and shorter hospital length of stay. Meanwhile, the rates of fusion and operative time are similar between MI-TLIF and open TLIF.[13,14] Some authors suggest that this technique will be the gold standard to evaluate emerging techniques for the treatment of spondylolisthesis and degenerative disc disease in the future.[4] Newly designed implants, such as deployable cages, along with biologic materials to provide osteoinductive, osteoconductive, and osteogenic potential, will facilitate the evolution of spinal fusion from an inpatient procedure to a day surgery procedure.

The future of tubular spine surgery techniques lies in the surgeon's ability to understand the anatomy, to place the tube, and provide a corridor to the offending pathology in the least invasive and shortest distance from skin to target. This will be accomplished with either guidance technology, such as robotics or navigation, or with mechanically manipulated technology, such as flexible endoscopy.

Percutaneous Pedicle Screw Placement, Image Guidance and Robotics

Traditional open spinal fusion procedures require extensive tissue dissection to expose the entry points and provide adequate lateral to medial orientation for optimal pedicle screw trajectory. This extensive dissection leads to muscular denervation, facet capsule disruption, proximal facet joint damage, and weakening of ligamentous structures, which could lead to prolonged postoperative pain and morbidity.[15] These disadvantages have led to the increasingly popular minimally invasive percutaneous pedicle screw fixation technique, especially in the lumbar spine. The traditional midline incision and extensive paraspinal muscle dissection is largely eliminated with minimally invasive percutaneous pedicle screw fixation. Traditionally, percutaneous pedicle screw placement is performed with the use of C-arm fluoroscopy.[16,17] However, accurate percutaneous pedicle screw placement is often challenging because subtle anatomic variations and altered screw trajectories that are identifiable with open approaches may not be easily identified with fluoroscopic MIS approaches due to poor image quality or image parallax, which distorts the anatomy. In addition, the surgeon cannot rely on bony palpable and visual landmarks,which they typically use to guide placement.[18]

In the past decade, various intraoperative image-assisted line-of-sight navigation systems and robotic guidance systems have been developed with the aim of increasing the accuracy of percutaneous pedicle screw placement. The most commonly used image-assisted navigation systems use two-dimensional (2D) fluoroscopy, or cone-beam computed tomography (CT), or three-dimensional (3D) CT image acquisition to register and reference the spine in 3D space.[19,20] At present, the only US Food and Drug Administration (FDA)–approved robotic guidance system is a bone-mounted hexapod miniature robot consisting of a cylindrical device composed of two endplates and six pistons that maneuver the endplates over six degrees of freedom.[21] This system relies on 2D fluoroscopy image acquisition, which is matched to a preoperative CT scan for registration and referencing. Multiple recent studies have shown that percutaneous pedicle screw placement using image-assisted navigation or robotic guidance are both safe and effective, and provided improved overall accuracy compared with conventional fluoroscopic techniques.[21–24] However, image-assisted navigation and robotic-guided surgery should be considered as an adjunct to a surgeon's thorough knowledge of spinal anatomy and should not be used as a substitute for it.[25] These technologies could be technically demanding and the learning curve can be treacherous. The future success of these technologies will depend on the ease of use and increased efficiency that they can provide. Meanwhile, further studies are needed to better assess the cost effectiveness of these technologies and their contribution to patient outcomes. Remember that both image-assisted navigation and robotic guidance will not make a bad surgeon good. Both, however, do make a good surgeon more efficient and precise.

Motion Preservation Techniques

Discectomy and fusion has been considered the gold standard for the treatment of symptomatic degenerative discs. However, a commonly recognized adverse outcome of spinal fusion is the development of adjacent-level deterioration above or below the fused segments. The nonfused segments adjacent to the fusion are subject to concentrated stresses and strains depending on the level within the spine and the sagittal balance after the fusion.[26–28] In the past decade, significant progress has been made in the field of motion preservation techniques. The primary goal of these techniques is to closely replicate normal or near-normal biomechanics of the motion segment in an effort to restore patient mobility and minimize the development of clinically significant adjacent-segment disc disease.[29]

Currently, the most commonly performed motion-preserving surgery is total disc replacement (TDR). Most TDR devices today require an anterior approach, which, over time and with experience, has become far less invasive. The use of a focused retroperitoneal approach has minimized much of the morbidity associated with the traditional thoracoabdominal or transperitoneal approaches.

The clinical effectiveness of lumbar TDR has long been a source of debate. There is still currently much skepticism and limited acceptance of lumbar TDR in the United States, although several recent reports suggest that, at long-term follow-up, lumbar TDR is superior for the treatment of symptomatic lumbar degenerative discs compared with fusion.[30,31]

Contrasting cervical TDR with lumbar TDR, the safety and efficacy of cervical TDR have been more easily established with a series of prospective, randomized clinical trials with intermediate and long-term follow-up.[32–35] Currently, cervical TDR is considered to be a viable alternative to anterior cervical discectomy and fusion in select patients with symptomatic one- and two-level cervical radiculopathy or myelopathy.[32]

Despite the previously described advances, the question as to whether TDR can reduce the incidence of adjacent-segment disc degeneration remains unclear. Solid long-term data will be needed before the role of TDR can be fully appraised.

The enthusiasm for motion preservation has also led to the development of several devices, particularly in the lumbar spine, such as interspinous spacers, dynamic stabilization screws and rods, and total facet replacement products. Currently, there is a lack of studies regarding the long-term effectiveness of these devices, and many of the specific devices originally conceived and used are no longer clinically available or failed to prove their effectiveness in clinical trials.[29]

The field of spine motion preservation surgery is constantly evolving, and we are likely to see many new devices in the near future. There is no doubt that second to sagittal alignment, the restoration of native disc function, including axial load-bearing properties, will be important in the advancement of minimally invasive disc replacement technologies.

Spinal Radiosurgery for the Treatment of Metastatic Spine Diseases

Metastatic spine tumors may occur in up to 30% of all cancer patients at some point in their disease course.[36] Spinal cord compression and myelopathy could occur in 25% to 50% of these patients.[37] The treatment goals for metastatic spine tumors include an improvement in the patient's quality of life, relief of tumor-mediated or biomechanically mediated pain, and preservation or restoration of neurologic function. The most common treatments for metastatic spine tumors are palliative in nature and consist of radiation therapy, systemic chemotherapy, surgery, or some combination of these depending on the histology and behavior of the malignancy.

Recent advances in radiation oncology have ushered in the era of spinal stereotactic radiosurgery (SRS), which has had a profound impact on patient outcomes and function. The use of SRS has demonstrated improved local tumor control compared to conventional external beam radiation.[38] In the spine, SRS allows for the delivery of a high dose of radiation to the tumor site while minimizing the amount delivered to the healthy neighboring tissues. Total radiation doses ranging from 8 to 30 Gy can be safely given as a single fraction or even in multiple fractions with SRS.[39] Tumors that have typically been considered radioresistant, such as renal cell carcinoma, are now becoming target sites of treatment with SRS.[40]

SRS can be applied as isolated treatment or after spine surgery for the treatment of metastatic spine diseases. The development of newer technologies has allowed spine surgeons to perform minimally invasive surgical decompression, which removes only the compressive component of a tumor. This will allow an appropriate separation between the tumor and the spinal cord so that a high dose of radiation can be delivered with minimal risk of radiation-induced spinal cord myelopathy. SRS can be applied as soon as 2 weeks after the surgery to achieve durable local tumor control without the concern of skin damage and delayed healing.[40] Various studies have shown that the majority of patients treated with SRS reported effective palliation of pain and improvement of progressive neurologic symptoms.[38,41–43] SRS will likely become an essential tool in the multimodality treatment for spine tumors in the near future.

The addition of percutaneous vertebral augmentation, vertebroplasty and kyphoplasty, along with SRS, have also changed the surgical paradigm for treating spinal tumors. Vertebral augmentation provides structural stability, while SRS provides tumor burden control.[44] Current efforts are now exploring the addition of radiotherapeutics and chemotherapeutics in the cement substrate to provide even more local tumor control.[45,46]

Spinal Biologics

Ongoing research and development of biologic materials for the treatment of spinal disorders is one of the most exciting areas in this field. Various bone graft extenders, such as demineralized bone matrices and calcium phosphate salts, as well as substitutes, such as bone morphogenetic proteins (BMPs), have been used by spine surgeons to enhance fusion rates and avoid the morbidity of harvesting iliac crest bone graft.[47] However, as with all new technologies, the long-term problems may not be readily recognized. This, in turn, has led to controversies regarding the use of BMPs in spine surgeries. Recently, a systematic data analysis was not able to find convincing data to warrant recombinant human BMP-2 (rhBMP-2) use over iliac crest bone graft.[48,49] It has been suggested that rhBMP-2 should be reserved for patients whose risk of failed spine surgery outweighs the risks of rhBMP-2 (theoretical risks of retrograde ejaculation, heterotrophic bone formation, or induction of malignancy), as rhBMP-2 still remains one of the most powerful commercially available osteogenic agents.[50] Polymethylmethacrylate has been an effective filler material for the treatment of vertebral compression fractures, but development of alternate materials with improved biomechanical and biologic properties, good radiopacity and handling for vertebroplasty and kyphoplasty is also underway.[51–53]

Significant progress in the fields of tissue engineering, regenerative medicine, and harvesting and propagation of stem cells has fueled many in the spine field to start using these technologies with the aim of treating and reversing disc degeneration. Biologic therapies can be protein based or cell based.[54] Protein-based therapy involves administration of biologic factors into the disc to delay degeneration, stop inflammation, or enhance matrix synthesis using various proteins, such as osteogenic protein-1, growth factors, interleukin-1 receptor antagonists, and platelet-rich plasma.[55–59] The goal of cell-based therapy is to either replace necrotic or apoptotic cells or minimize cell death. Various cell sources, such as autologous chondrocytes, disc cells, and mesenchymal stem cells, have been considered for cell replacement for treating symptomatic degenerative discs. However, the science is still not fully supportive of these treatment options.[60–62] Many technical challenges associated with biologic treatments and their application still exist, and their use is still far from clinical practice.[54] Further knowledge about the molecular mechanisms of disc degeneration and a more thorough understanding of various biomolecules, as well as a better understanding of the degenerative environment of the host disc space, will allow the future development of multidisciplinary approaches for the treatment of symptomatic disc degeneration.

Summary

The field of MIS will continue to evolve. The continued development and incorporation of MIS techniques into the field of spine surgery has the potential of greatly benefiting all those afflicted with spinal pathology. In the meantime, more vigorous, prospective, long-term clinical studies, coupled with surgeons' and scientists' insatiable imaginations, will be needed to critically evaluate these new techniques and technologies.

REFERENCES

1. O'Toole JE, Eichholz KM, Fessler RG. Minimally invasive spine surgery. *Neurosurg Clin N Am*. 2006;17:ix-x.
2. Smith ZA, Fessler RG. Minimally invasive spine surgery. *Neurosurg Clin N Am*. 2014;25:xiii.
3. Foley KT, Smith MM. Microendoscopic discectomy. *Tech Neurosurg*. 1997;3:301-307.
4. Kazemi N, Crew LK, Tredway TL. The future of spine surgery: new horizons in the treatment of spinal disorders. *Surg Neurol Int*. 2013;4:S15-S21.
5. Arts MP, Brand R, van den Akker ME, et al. Tubular diskectomy vs conventional microdiskectomy for the treatment of lumbar disk herniation: 2-year results of a double-blind randomized controlled trial. *Neurosurgery*. 2011;69:135-144.

SECTION VII

6. Hermantin FU, Peters T, Quartararo L, et al. A prospective, randomized study comparing the results of open discectomy with those of video-assisted arthroscopic microdiscectomy. *J Bone Joint Surg Am*. 1999;81:958-965.
7. Ryang YM, Oertel MF, Mayfrank L, et al. Standard open microdiscectomy versus minimal access trocar microdiscectomy: results of a prospective randomized study. *Neurosurgery*. 2008;62:174-181.
8. Kim CW, Siemionow K, Anderson DG, et al. The current state of minimally invasive spine surgery. *J Bone Joint Surg Am*. 2011;93:582-596.
9. Alimi M, Hofstetter CP, Pyo SY, et al. Minimally invasive laminectomy for lumbar spinal stenosis in patients with and without preoperative spondylolisthesis: clinical outcome and reoperation rates. *J Neurosurg*. 2015;22:339-352.
10. Hudak EM, Perry MW. Outpatient minimally invasive spine surgery using endoscopy for the treatment of lumbar spinal stenosis among obese patients. *J Orthop*. 2015;12:156-159.
11. Haji FA, Cenic A, Crevier L, et al. Minimally invasive approach for the resection of spinal neoplasm. *Spine*. 2011;36:E1018-E1026.
12. Nzokou A, Weil AG, Shedid D. Minimally invasive removal of thoracic and lumbar spinal tumors using a nonexpandable tubular retractor. *J Neurosurg*. 2013;19:708-715.
13. Khan NR, Clark AJ, Lee SL, et al. Surgical outcomes for minimally invasive vs open transforaminal lumbar interbody fusion: an updated systematic review and meta-analysis. *Neurosurgery*. 2015;77(6):847-874.
14. Wong AP, Smith ZA, Stadler JA 3rd, et al. Minimally invasive transforaminal lumbar interbody fusion (MI-TLIF): surgical technique, long-term 4-year prospective outcomes, and complications compared with an open TLIF cohort. *Neurosurg Clin N Am*. 2014;25:279-304.
15. Skovrlj B, Gilligan J, Cutler HS, et al. Minimally invasive procedures on the lumbar spine. *World J Clin Cases*. 2015;3:1-9.
16. Lowery GL, Kulkarni SS. Posterior percutaneous spine instrumentation. *Eur Spine J*. 2000;9(suppl 1):S126-S130.
17. Powers CJ, Podichetty VK, Isaacs RE. Placement of percutaneous pedicle screws without imaging guidance. *Neurosurg Focus*. 2006;20:E3.
18. Bourgeois AC, Faulkner AR, Bradley YC, et al. Improved accuracy of minimally invasive transpedicular screw placement in the lumbar spine with 3-dimensional stereotactic image guidance: a comparative meta-analysis. *J Spinal Disord Tech*. 2015;28:324-329.
19. Gebhard F, Weidner A, Liener UC, et al. Navigation at the spine. *Injury*. 2004;35(suppl 1):S-A35-45.
20. Sembrano JN, Yson SC, Santos ERG, et al. Percutaneous pedicle screws. In: Phillips FM, Lieberman IH, Polly DW Jr, eds. *Minimally Invasive Spine Surgery: Surgical Techniques and Disease Management*. New York: Springer; 2014:129-139.
21. Hu X, Lieberman IH. Robotic-assisted spine surgery. In: Phillips FM, Lieberman IH, Polly DW Jr, eds. *Minimally Invasive Spine Surgery: Surgical Techniques and Disease Management*. New York: Springer; 2014:61-66.
22. Mason A, Paulsen R, Babuska JM, et al. The accuracy of pedicle screw placement using intraoperative image guidance systems. *J Neurosurg*. 2014;20:196-203.
23. Shin BJ, James AR, Njoku IU, et al. Pedicle screw navigation: a systematic review and meta-analysis of perforation risk for computer-navigated versus freehand insertion. *J Neurosurg*. 2012;17:113-122.
24. Shweikeh F, Amadio JP, Arnell M, et al. Robotics and the spine: a review of current and ongoing applications. *Neurosurg Focus*. 2014;36:E10.
25. Rahmathulla G, Nottmeier EW, Pirris SM, et al. Intraoperative image-guided spinal navigation: technical pitfalls and their avoidance. *Neurosurg Focus*. 2014;36:E3.
26. Carrier CS, Bono CM, Lebl DR. Evidence-based analysis of adjacent segment degeneration and disease after ACDF: a systematic review. *Spine J*. 2013;13:1370-1378.
27. Helgeson MD, Bevevino AJ, Hilibrand AS. Update on the evidence for adjacent segment degeneration and disease. *Spine J*. 2013;13:342-351.
28. Lee JC, Choi SW. Adjacent segment pathology after lumbar spinal fusion. *Asian Spine J*. 2015;9:807-817.
29. Murtagh R, Castellvi AE. Motion preservation surgery in the spine. *Neuroimaging Clin N Am*. 2014;24:287-294.
30. Nie H, Chen G, Wang X, et al. Comparison of total disc replacement with lumbar fusion: a meta-analysis of randomized controlled trials. *J Coll Physicians Surg Pak*. 2015;25:60-67.
31. Siepe CJ, Heider F, Wiechert K, et al. Mid- to long-term results of total lumbar disc replacement: a prospective analysis with 5- to 10-year follow-up. *Spine J*. 2014;14:1417-1431.
32. Coric D. ISASS policy statement: cervical artificial disc. *Int J Spine Surg*. 2014;8.
33. Davis RJ, Nunley PD, Kim KD, et al. Two-level total disc replacement with Mobi-C cervical artificial disc versus anterior discectomy and fusion: a prospective, randomized, controlled multicenter clinical trial with 4-year follow-up results. *J Neurosurg*. 2015;22:15-25.
34. Zhang HX, Shao YD, Chen Y, et al. A prospective, randomised, controlled multicentre study comparing cervical disc replacement with anterior cervical decompression and fusion. *Int Orthop*. 2014;38:2533-2541.
35. Hyun Oh C, Hwan Yoon S. Past, present, and future of cervical arthroplasty. *Keio J Med*. 2015;62:47-52.
36. Wong DA, Fornasier VL, MacNab I. Spinal metastases: the obvious, the occult, and the impostors. *Spine*. 1990;15:1-4.
37. Rades D, Abrahm JL. The role of radiotherapy for metastatic epidural spinal cord compression. *Nat Rev Clin Oncol*. 2010;7:590-598.
38. Ryu S, Yoon H, Stessin A, et al. Contemporary treatment with radiosurgery for spine metastasis and spinal cord compression in 2015. *Radiat Oncol J*. 2015;33:1-11.
39. Joaquim AF, Ghizoni E, Tedeschi H, et al. Stereotactic radiosurgery for spinal metastases: a literature review. *Einstein (Sao Paulo)*. 2013;11:247-255.
40. Sharan AD, Szulc A, Krystal J, et al. The integration of radiosurgery for the treatment of patients with metastatic spine diseases. *J Am Acad Orthop Surg*. 2014;22:447-454.
41. Bate BG, Khan NR, Kimball BY, et al. Stereotactic radiosurgery for spinal metastases with or without separation surgery. *J Neurosurg*. 2015;22:409-415.
42. Bishop AJ, Tao R, Rebueno NC, et al. Outcomes for spine stereotactic body radiation therapy and an analysis of predictors of local recurrence. *Int J Radiat Oncol Biol Phys*. 2015;92:1016-1026.
43. Harel R, Emch T, Chao S, et al. Quantitative evaluation of local control and wound healing following surgery and stereotactic spine radiosurgery (SRS) for spine tumors. *World Neurosurg*. 2016;87:48-54.
44. Papanastassiou ID, Filis AK, Gerochristou MA, et al. Controversial issues in kyphoplasty and vertebroplasty in malignant vertebral fractures. *Cancer Control*. 2014;21:151-157.

45. Kaneko TS, Sehgal V, Skinner HB, et al. Radioactive bone cement for the treatment of spinal metastases: a dosimetric analysis of simulated clinical scenarios. *Phys Med Biol.* 2012;57:4387-4401.
46. Handal JA, Schulz JF, Pahys JM, et al. Evaluation of elution and mechanical properties of two injectable chemotherapeutic bone cements. *Chemotherapy.* 2011;57:268-274.
47. Kaiser MG, Groff MW, Watters WC 3rd, et al. Guideline update for the performance of fusion procedures for degenerative disease of the lumbar spine. Part 16: bone graft extenders and substitutes as an adjunct for lumbar fusion. *J Neurosurg.* 2014;21:106-132.
48. Fu R, Selph S, McDonagh M, et al. Effectiveness and harms of recombinant human bone morphogenetic protein-2 in spine fusion: a systematic review and meta-analysis. *Ann Intern Med.* 2013;158:890-902.
49. Simmonds MC, Brown JV, Heirs MK, et al. Safety and effectiveness of recombinant human bone morphogenetic protein-2 for spinal fusion: a meta-analysis of individual-participant data. *Ann Intern Med.* 2013;158:877-889.
50. Tannoury CA, An HS. Complications with the use of bone morphogenetic protein 2 (BMP-2) in spine surgery. *Spine J.* 2014;14:552-559.
51. Aghyarian S, Hu X, Lieberman IH, et al. Two novel high performing composite PMMA-CaP cements for vertebroplasty: an ex vivo animal study. *J Mech Behav Biomed Mater.* 2015;50:290-298.
52. Holub O, Lopez A, Borse V, et al. Biomechanics of low-modulus and standard acrylic bone cements in simulated vertebroplasty: a human ex vivo study. *J Biomech.* 2015;48:3258-3266.
53. Lieberman IH, Togawa D. Kayanja MM. Vertebroplasty and kyphoplasty: filler materials. *Spine J.* 2005;5:305S-316S.
54. Vasiliadis ES, Pneumaticos SG, Evangelopoulos DS, et al. Biologic treatment of mild and moderate intervertebral disc degeneration. *Mol Med.* 2014;20:400-409.
55. Feng C, Liu H, Yang Y, et al. Growth and differentiation factor-5 contributes to the structural and functional maintenance of the intervertebral disc. *Cell Physiol Biochem.* 2015;35:1-16.
56. Formica M, Cavagnaro L, Formica C, et al. What is the preclinical evidence on platelet rich plasma and intervertebral disc degeneration? *Eur Spine J.* 2015;24:2377-2386.
57. Gorth DJ, Mauck RL, Chiaro JA, et al. IL-1ra delivered from poly(lactic-co-glycolic acid) microspheres attenuates IL-1beta-mediated degradation of nucleus pulposus in vitro. *Arthritis Res Ther.* 2012;14:R179.
58. Ren S, Liu Y, Ma J, et al. Treatment of rabbit intervertebral disc degeneration with co-transfection by adeno-associated virus-mediated SOX9 and osteogenic protein-1 double genes in vivo. *Int J Mol Med.* 2013;32:1063-1068.
59. Wang Z, Hutton WC, Yoon ST. Bone morphogenetic protein-7 antagonizes tumor necrosis factor-alpha-induced activation of nuclear factor kappaB and up-regulation of the ADAMTS, leading to decreased degradation of disc matrix macromolecules aggrecan and collagen II. *Spine J.* 2014;14:505-512.
60. Wang Z, Perez-Terzic CM, Smith J, et al. Efficacy of intervertebral disc regeneration with stem cells—a systematic review and meta-analysis of animal controlled trials. *Gene.* 2015;564:1-8.
61. Oehme D, Goldschlager T, Rosenfeld JV, et al. The role of stem cell therapies in degenerative lumbar spine disease: a review. *Neurosurg Rev.* 2015;38:429-445.
62. Richardson SM, Kalamegam G, Pushparaj PN, et al. Mesenchymal stem cells in regenerative medicine: focus on articular cartilage and intervertebral disc regeneration. *Methods.* 2016;99:69-80.

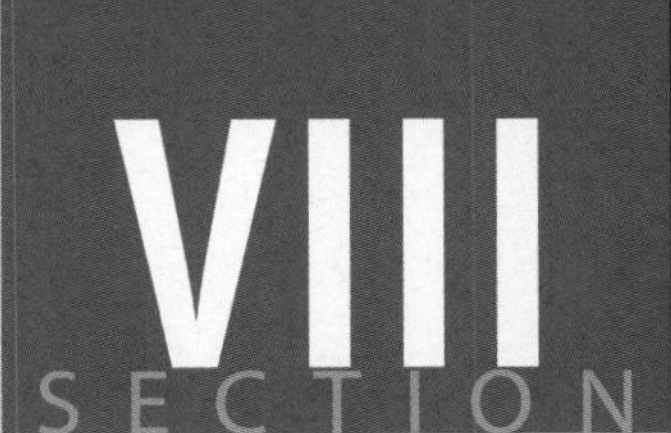
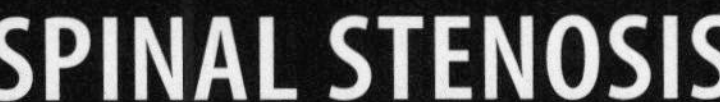

SECTION VIII
SPINAL STENOSIS

CHAPTER 61 Spinal Stenosis: Pathophysiology, Clinical Diagnosis, and Differential Diagnosis

Chetan K. Patel
Eeric Truumees

Spinal stenosis is one of the most common conditions in the elderly. It is defined as a narrowing of the spinal canal. The term *stenosis* is derived from the Greek word for narrow, which is *stenos*. The first description of this condition is attributed to Antoine Portal in 1803. Verbiest[1–10] is credited with coining the term *spinal stenosis* and the associated narrowing of the spinal canal as its potential cause. Kirkaldy-Willis[11–15] subsequently described the degenerative cascade in the lumbar spine as the cause for the altered anatomy and pathophysiology in spinal stenosis.

The term *spinal stenosis* refers to an anatomic diagnosis that increases with age and can occur in asymptomatic individuals.[16,17] The exact reason for why some with this condition have debilitating symptoms while others have no symptoms is not well understood. These differences in presentation may be related to the different abilities of individuals to compensate for the anatomic changes that have occurred. When symptoms do present, they usually occur on the basis of the location of neural compression. Patients with central canal stenosis typically present with neurogenic claudication, whereas those with lateral recess and foraminal stenosis present with radicular pain. Patients with significant symptoms that do not respond to conservative treatment often elect surgical treatment. In fact, in adults older than age 65, spinal stenosis is the most common reason to undergo lumbar spine surgery.[18,19]

Anatomy

In order to understand how spinal stenosis causes symptoms, we must first have a good understanding of the normal anatomy of the lumbar spine. The spinal canal's anterior border is formed by the vertebral body, the disc, and the posterior longitudinal ligament. The lateral border is formed by the pedicles, the lateral ligamentum flavum, and the neural foramen. The posterior border is formed by the facet joints, lamina, and ligamentum flavum. The shape of the spinal canal may be circular, oval, or trefoil (Fig. 61.1). The circular and oval canal shapes provide the most space for the neural elements centrally and in the lateral recess. The trefoil canal has the smallest cross-sectional area.[20] It is present in 15% of individuals and predisposes these individuals to lateral recess stenosis.

Disc

Disc degeneration is believed to be the first step in degeneration of the spine. At birth, the nucleus pulposus and the anulus occupy roughly 50% of the disc area. The nucleus is gelatinous and there is a discrete boundary between the nucleus and the anulus. Over time, the collagen content increases and the demarcation between the nucleus and the anulus becomes less distinct. Other structures within the disc also change with aging. The chondroitin sulfate concentration decreases, and the ratio of keratin sulfate to chondroitin sulfate increases. Because keratin sulfate has less hydrophilic potential, the disc dehydrates over time.

Hydration of the disc also changes due to an alteration in the type of collagen within the disc over time. The anulus contains 60% type II and 40% type I collagen, whereas the disc contains mainly type II collagen. Type I collagen is associated with decreased water content compared with type II collagen. Thus, as the type I collagen content increases with age, hydration of the disc decreases. The normal nucleus pulposus typically consists of 85% water, whereas the anulus consists of 78% water. With degeneration of the disc, the water content drops to roughly 70%. A desiccated disc has a decreased ability to handle mechanical load.

The Kirkaldy-Willis[21] theory explains how these changes progress over time. This theory is based on viewing the spine as a tripod, with the disc and the two facet joints making up the three legs. This analogy makes it easier to understand how alteration in one joint can alter the others. The initial stage in the degenerative cascade is circumferential tearing of the anulus, which progresses to radial tears. This, along with the biochemical changes in the disc described previously, lead to further degeneration of the disc and disc height loss. Altered disc structure and disc height loss lead to bulging of the disc and the posterior longitudinal ligament. This causes narrowing of the spinal canal and potential neural impingement. The lost disc height also leads to buckling of the ligamentum flavum and settling of the facet joints. The facet joints

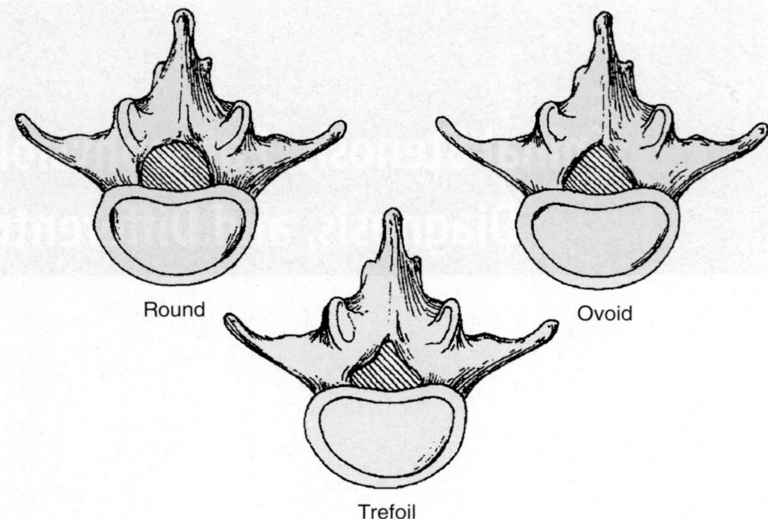

FIG. 61.1 The three typical shapes of the spinal canal. Trefoil canals have the smallest cross-sectional area. (From Hilibrand AS, Rand N. Degenerative lumbar stenosis: diagnosis and management. *J Am Assoc Orthop Surg.* 1999;7:239–248.)

subsequently deteriorate and form osteophytes, which further narrows the spinal canal. The ligamentum flavum also hypertrophies over time. The altered structure, motion, and biomechanics then lead to additional disc deterioration, which propagates the cycle of degeneration.

Facet Joints

The lumbar facet joints are encapsulated structures that have a uniform cartilaginous surface to produce a smooth gliding motion. The superior articular process is concave and its articular surface faces medially and dorsally. The inferior articular process is convex and its articular surface faces laterally and ventrally. Lumbar facet joints are oriented 90 degrees in the sagittal plane and 45 degrees anterior in the coronal plane. Studies show that more sagittally oriented facet joints are associated with a degenerative spondylolisthesis. The two facet joints are usually symmetrical with respect to their joint angles at each level. Facet tropism refers to an asymmetry between the facet joints and has been theorized to lead to degeneration.

As the disc degenerates and narrows, the facet joints settle and increased stress is placed across the facet joint. This leads to facet joint degeneration, hypertrophy, and osteophyte formation. These osteophytes can cause impingement of the thecal sac within the spinal canal or the nerve root in the neural foramen.

Intervertebral Foramen

The anterior boundary of the intervertebral foramen is made up of the posterior wall of the vertebral body and the disc. The posterior boundary is made up of the lateral aspect of the facet joint and the ligamentum flavum. Superior and inferior boundaries are formed by the pedicles of the vertebral bodies corresponding to that segment. The foramen is typically larger than the ganglion and the nerve that it contains. The additional space is occupied by fat and loose areolar tissue that can accommodate for changes in size of the foramen with motion. With degeneration, hypertrophy of the facets can cause posterior compression of the neural elements (Fig. 61.2). Anterior compression of the neural elements usually arises from endplate osteophytes or foraminal disc herniations. Decrease in disc height with degeneration can cause a decrease in the foraminal height and neural compression. This type of vertical or up-down foraminal stenosis is important to recognize because a posterior decompression alone may not significantly improve the vertical compression and may result in persistent symptoms after surgery.

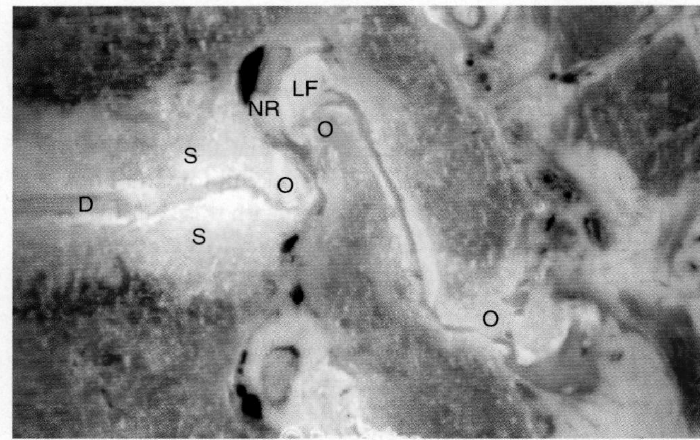

FIG. 61.2 Sagittal cross-section demonstrating disc desiccation (D), endplate sclerosis (S), osteophyte formation (O), hypertrophy and buckling of the ligamentum flavum (LF), and nerve root (NR) compromise within the foramen. (From Gallego J, Schnuerer AP, Manuel C. *Basic Anatomy and Pathology of the Spine*. Memphis, TN: Medtronic Sofamor Danek; 2001. Photograph by Wolfgang Rauschning, MD, PhD.)

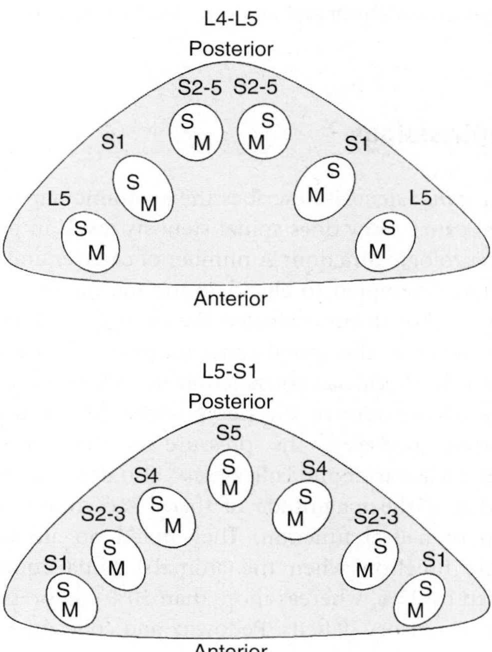

FIG. 61.3 Neural organization within the thecal sac at the L4–L5 and L5–S1 disc levels. M, motor components; S, sensory components. (From Garfin SR, Herkowitz HN, Mirkovic S. Spinal stenosis: instructional course lecture. *J Bone Joint Surg Am.* 1999;81:572–586.)

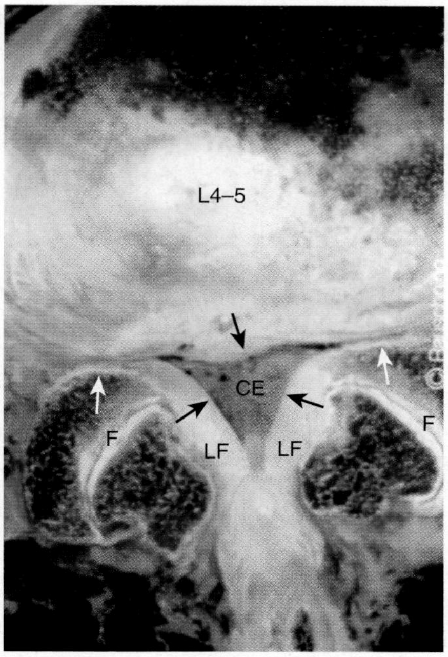

FIG. 61.4 Axial cross-section view at the L4–L5 disc level showing advanced degenerative changes. Cauda equina (CE) compression is caused by hypertrophic facets (F) and ligamentum flavum (LF) disc protrusion. (From Gallego J, Schnuerer AP, Manuel C. *Basic Anatomy and Pathology of the Spine*. Memphis, TN: Medtronic Sofamor Danek; 2001. Photograph by Wolfgang Rauschning, MD, PhD.)

Cauda Equina

The thecal sac lies in the spinal canal and gives rise to nerve roots at each segment. The nerve root initially courses along the medial aspect of the pedicle and then progresses laterally, inferior to the pedicle in the neural foramen. The nerve roots within the cauda equina are arranged in a predictable pattern within the thecal sac (Fig. 61.3). Cross-section of the thecal sac demonstrates the most caudal roots to be present in a central and posterior position. The more cephalad roots are located sequentially, and are more lateral and anterior. At each level, the motor fibers of a root are anterior and medial to the larger sensory component. Dorsal root ganglia exist at every level and can be intraspinal or intraforaminal. A variety of clinical presentations arise on the basis of the anatomic location of neural compression.

Classification

Stenosis can be anatomically classified as central, lateral recess, and foraminal on the basis of the location of neural compression. With aging, central canal stenosis occurs as degenerative changes progress. As the axial height of the disc and facet joints decreases, the disc bulges into the spinal canal. The central canal is further narrowed by posterior impingement from enlarged facets and the hypertrophied ligamentum flavum (Fig. 61.4). Hypertrophy of the soft tissues is responsible for 40% of spinal stenosis.[22] With extension, the hypertrophied ligamentum buckles centrally into the canal and worsens the central stenosis. This explains why patients with stenosis typically report worsening of their symptoms in extension.

Lateral recess stenosis typically results from posterior disc protrusion in combination with some superior articular facet hypertrophy. Lateral recess stenosis can present with lumbar radiculopathy; incidence of lateral recess stenosis ranges from 8% to 11%.[23–25] These patients present with pain or neurologic symptoms in a dermatomal distribution on the basis of the nerve that is compressed in the lateral recess.

Foraminal stenosis causes compression of the exiting nerve root and ganglion and leads to lumbar radiculopathy. Foraminal stenosis occurs most commonly in the lower lumbar spine, with the fifth lumbar nerve root being the most commonly involved. Foraminal stenosis can occur from loss of disc height, vertebral endplate osteophytes, facet osteophytes, spondylolisthesis, and disc herniations. Like central canal stenosis, foraminal stenosis is worse in extension; thus, exacerbating and alleviating factors for symptoms from foraminal compression are similar to those from central canal stenosis.[26]

Spinal stenosis can also be classified on the basis of the etiology, which can be congenital, acquired, or both. Congenital stenosis is present as a normal variant in the population and is a feature of certain conditions, such as dwarfism. In these conditions, patients have short pedicles that are closer together than in the normal lumbar spine.[6] In congenital stenosis, few degenerative changes are required to cause neural compression

BOX 61.1 Classification of Spinal Stenosis

I. Congenital/Developmental

A. Idiopathic
B. Achondroplastic
C. Osteopetrosis

II. Acquired

A. Degenerative
   1. Central
   2. Lateral recess
   3. Foraminal
B. Iatrogenic
   1. Postlaminectomy
   2. Adjacent to fusion
   3. Malposition of hardware in the canal
   4. Postprocedure epidural hematoma
C. Miscellaneous disorders
   1. Acromegaly
   2. Paget disease
   3. Fluorosis
   4. Ankylosing spondylitis
D. Traumatic

III. Combined

Any combination of congenital/developmental or acquired stenosis

and symptoms. As one would expect, congenital stenosis becomes symptomatic much earlier in life and patients usually become symptomatic in the fourth decade. Acquired stenosis can be caused by trauma, neoplasms, and infection, along with other causes listed in Box 61.1.

Deformity and Instability

The static changes discussed thus far can be worsened by dynamic factors such as segmental instability. Instability typically arises from degenerative changes and can be in the form of translational or rotational abnormality. Translational abnormality is found most commonly in women as a degenerative anterolisthesis of L4 on L5.[27] The attachment of the iliolumbar ligaments to the L5 level may act as a restraining force and cause more relative motion at L4–L5. The more sagittally oriented facet joints between the fourth and fifth lumbar vertebrae can be an additional predisposing factor for instability at this level.[28] Because the lamina and the spinous process typically project inferior to the vertebral body, the amount of room available between the inferior aspect of the L4 lamina and the posterior superior aspect of L5 is substantially decreased. This anterior translation of the L4 posterior elements, along with hypertrophy of the facets and ligamentum flavum, leads to central and lateral recess stenosis. Foraminal stenosis can also occur in this setting, with collapse of the disc space, disc herniation, endplate osteophytes, or facet hypertrophy. With scoliosis, lateral subluxation and rotational instability can cause altered biomechanics that accelerate further degeneration. The altered anatomy can also directly cause narrowing of the central canal, lateral recess, and foraminal regions. Degenerative changes superimposed on abnormal anatomy lead to stenosis in these patients.

Pathophysiology

The term *spinal stenosis* describes the anatomic narrowing of the spinal canal. How does spinal stenosis result in pain and altered neurologic function? A number of cadaver and animal studies have attempted to elucidate the mechanism of these symptoms. Schonstorm evaluated the changes in nerve pressure that occur as the spinal canal narrows.[29] In his human cadaver study, thecal sac constriction of 45% or more led to an increased pressure in the nerve roots. As the degree of compression increased, the pressure in the nerve roots increased. Delamarter and colleagues[30] also demonstrated the importance of the magnitude of thecal sac compression in alteration of neural function. They noted no alteration in neurologic function when the animal's cauda equina was constricted by 25%, whereas more than 50% compression led to motor or sensory deficits. Pedowitz and colleagues[31] demonstrated that the duration of compression was also an important factor in neural dysfunction.

Rydevik and colleagues[32–37] demonstrated another effect of compression of the thecal sac. They noted that once pressure of more than 50 mm Hg was achieved, capillary restriction and electrophysiologic alteration occurred in the nerve roots. Even at pressures as low as 5 to 10 mm Hg, venous congestion of the intraneural microcirculation occurred. Solute transport decreased 45% across nerve root segments with the low pressure of 10 mm Hg. This suggests that low-grade sustained compression of the nerve roots could lead to vascular impairment and potential detrimental changes in the function of the nerve roots. In addition to neural compression and altered nutrition, inflammatory chemical mediators have also been shown to be a cause of pain.[38–43]

The presence of stenosis increases with aging; however, it often does not produce any symptoms. What causes pain in some individuals with mild spinal stenosis and no symptoms in others with severe stenosis? The experimental evidence reviewed earlier suggests that each individual may have an innate ability to compensate for the accumulating pathologic changes. Because the magnitude an individual can compensate for is different for different people, two individuals with the same amount of stenosis may not exhibit the same symptoms. The rate at which these changes are occurring also appears to be important. Individuals may become symptomatic with a lower magnitude of compression if it occurs rapidly. This explains how a patient with stenosis can become symptomatic with an acute mild disc herniation.

Natural History

Patients with congenital stenosis typically become symptomatic earlier in life. Due to congenital narrowing of the canal in these patients, significant stenosis is present at multiple levels even with little degenerative change.[44] Patients with degenerative stenosis present later in life (during their 60s) and have far more advanced degeneration in their spine. Females are more commonly affected with stenosis, with the L4–L5 level being the most common segment involved.[45]

Recent studies have also shed light on the prevalence and likelihood of developing symptoms from spinal stenosis. A portion of the Framingham Heart Study participants were prospectively enrolled in a study evaluating lumbar symptoms and computed tomography (CT) findings of the lumbar spinal canal.[46] In the group of 191 study participants with the mean age of 52.6 years, the prevalence of lumbar stenosis was 23.6%. The prevalence of lumbar stenosis increased with age, as expected, and led to a threefold higher risk of having symptoms. Will the patients without any symptoms continue to remain asymptomatic? A separate retrospective study of asymptomatic lumbar stenosis attempted to answer this question. A group of 41 patients with cervical myelopathy who had asymptomatic lumbar stenosis and a mean age of 69 years were followed.[47] At a mean of 5 years after the diagnosis, 23% developed symptoms, suggesting that patients with known asymptomatic stenosis should be informed of symptoms that could develop.

Multiple studies have looked at the short-term and long-term results of nonoperative treatment of patients with symptomatic lumbar stenosis.[48–55] These studies show that a significant number of patients respond favorably to nonoperative treatment. Some patients, however, do not improve and some even worsen. Johnsson and colleagues reviewed the results of 32 patients who declined to have surgery at a 4-year follow-up period.[56] They noted that 70% of patients were unchanged, while 15% were the same and 15% worsened.

Recently, prospective studies have reported short-term and long-term results of nonoperative and operative treatment. The prospective observational Maine Lumbar Spine Study reported 8- to 10-year follow-up results on 97 patients.[57] They noted that a large number of patients (39%) that had initially elected nonsurgical treatment subsequently elected to undergo surgery. Of the patients who continued nonoperative treatment, most had stable symptoms. Miyamoto and colleagues reported prospective results of nonsurgical treatment in 120 patients.[58] Of these patients, 16% required surgical treatment during the follow-up period of 5 years. Of the nonsurgically treated patients, 53% reported no hindrance during the activities of daily living. No sudden neurologic deterioration was reported. Roughly 23% of patients had worsened but did not elect to undergo surgical intervention.

The Finnish Lumbar Spinal Research Group reported the results of a randomized controlled trial in 2007.[59] They randomized 94 patients with mild to moderate stenosis into either the surgical group or nonoperative group. At the 2-year follow-up, patients in both groups noted improvement of symptoms; however, the outcome of patients undergoing surgical treatment was significantly better. The most recent prospective study to evaluate patients with lumbar stenosis is the Spine Patient Outcomes Research Trial (SPORT).[60–62] This study reported prospective outcomes of 634 patients at 2-, 4- and 8-year follow-up. Patients undergoing surgical treatment had better outcomes than those who underwent nonsurgical treatment in the as-treated analysis at each of the time points. Pain, function, satisfaction, and self-rated progress were all better in those that underwent surgery. Patients in the nonsurgical treatment group showed small improvements in most outcome measures. It should be noted that no disastrous neurologic deterioration was noted with nonoperative treatment.

The original and recent updated North American Spine Society evidence-based guidelines for diagnosis and treatment of lumbar stenosis provide some tangible conclusions from these studies.[63,64] They state that in one-third to one-half of patients with mild to moderate stenosis, the natural history is favorable. Unfortunately, predicting which patients with stenosis will worsen over time is impossible. In some studies, symptomatic patients with severe stenosis did poorly over time, but overall there is not sufficient evidence to draw any conclusions. What is known is that rapid or catastrophic deterioration is rare in patients with spinal stenosis. Knowing this can be helpful in guiding treatment and evaluating these patients. When a patient with spinal stenosis has rapidly worsening neurologic status, other causes of neurologic dysfunction should be investigated.

Clinical Presentation

Patients with lumbar spinal stenosis most commonly present with leg pain.[22] This leg pain presents as either neurogenic claudication or radicular leg pain. Patients with neurogenic claudication report a feeling of pain, heaviness, numbness, cramping, burning, or weakness. The symptoms typically start from the back or the buttocks and bilaterally radiate down below the knees. One lower extremity may be worse than the other; however, both legs are typically involved. Symptoms usually do not follow a dermatomal pattern and are usually related to activities. These abnormal sensations are typically worse with extension of the lumbar spine during walking or standing for a prolonged time. Some report worsening weakness if they keep walking. They may note ankle dorsiflexion weakness that is typically described as feet slapping or even falling as they attempt to keep walking. Walking downhill is more challenging for these patients as the lumbar spine is extended while going downhill. Most describe a set distance they can walk before the symptoms become disabling. As the stenosis worsens, this distance typically decreases, further disrupting the daily life and function of these patients. Relief of symptoms typically comes from flexing the lumbar spine by leaning forward, sitting, or lying down. As discussed earlier, the degree of stenosis decreases as the lumbar spine is flexed and patients naturally learn to position themselves in a posture that minimizes discomfort and maximizes function. Keeping this in mind, it is easy to understand why these patients typically lean forward on a grocery cart and have an easier time riding a bike, walking uphill, or driving while sitting in a car.

In contrast to neurogenic claudication arising from compression of the thecal sac, radicular pain arises from compression of a particular nerve root in the lateral recess or the neural foramen. Unlike claudication, radicular leg pain is described by the patients in a specific dermatomal pattern corresponding to the compressed nerve root. The most common presentation of this is L5 radiculopathy from lateral recess stenosis causing compression of the L5 nerve root. In addition to numbness in the L5 distribution, weakness can be seen in the extensor hallucis longus and tibialis anterior muscle groups.

Low back pain is also a common complaint in patients with stenosis. Although most patients note the radiation of this pain into their legs, some present without leg pain or note radiation of the pain only into their buttocks. Exacerbating and alleviating factors for claudicatory low back pain are similar to those for the leg pain. Spondylotic change with or without spondylolisthesis is a common finding in this patient population and often the cause for low back pain. Patients with symptoms in both the low back and leg have a greater disability than those who have symptoms only in one location.[65]

Severe neurologic symptoms, such as bowel and bladder incontinence or profound weakness, are uncommon in patients with stenosis. Urinary dysfunction is a common complaint in this elderly population and can be present in 50% to 80% of patients.[66,67] Because various causes of urinary dysfunction (such as preexisting stress incontinence, urinary tract infections, and prostatic hypertrophy) are common in this population, a careful history can help exclude these nonspinal causes. The factors more commonly noted in patients with neurogenic bladder dysfunction are perianal sensory disturbance, longer duration of symptoms, and higher mean residual volumes on urodynamic studies.[68]

In addition to obtaining a history specific to the patient's pain and neurologic symptoms, it is important to obtain a comprehensive medical history. A patient's report of preexisting peripheral arterial occlusive disease, hip arthritis, multiple sclerosis, or neuropathy would substantially alter what symptoms are attributed to the stenosis. Similarly, obtaining an overall picture of the medical comorbidities and physiologic condition will also shed light on the ability of the patient to safely undergo any invasive procedures. Knowing the patient's other medical conditions can also help identify patients who may be at risk for inferior outcomes. Cardiovascular comorbidities, depression, and disorders influencing walking ability have all been noted to be preoperative predictors of poor postoperative outcomes.[69]

Physical Examination

A good physical examination of patients with lumbar spinal stenosis should start with observation. Often, these patients will be sitting flexed forward on a chair in the examination room. While standing and ambulating, stenosis patients still often flex their trunk forward to decrease their symptoms. This may also be noticed when checking their range of motion as a decrease in the active lumbar extension. Reproduction of the patient's usual symptoms by prolonged lumbar extension can also be helpful in confirming the diagnosis. Neurologic examination is often normal in spite of long-standing debilitating symptoms. Lateral recess stenosis is more commonly responsible for neurologic changes.[70] When motor weakness or sensory deficit is present, it is most often in the L5 distribution. A frequent neurologic finding is an asymmetrical deep tendon reflex at the patellar or Achilles tendon. A symmetrical decrease in the reflexes is more indicative of age-related changes. Nerve root tension signs are usually not present.[71] Changes in neurologic examination may become more obvious after stressing the patient's neurologic system. This can be accomplished by asking the patient to walk until he or she experiences significant symptoms. Reexamination at this point may reveal changes in motor, sensory, or reflex examination that were not detected before the stress.

It is useful to review physical examination findings found in some studies to get a better idea of their frequency. Amundsen and colleagues[72] prospectively evaluated the clinical and radiographic features of 100 patients with symptomatic spinal stenosis. They reported a motor weakness in 23% and sensory deficit in 51%. In the 2007 randomized controlled trial of 94 stenosis patients from the Finnish Lumbar Spinal Research Group,[59] 22% of patients had an L5 motor weakness and 19% had a sensory deficit. The straight-leg raise test was positive in 3% of the patients. In the recent SPORT study, asymmetrical reflexes were noted in 26%, motor weakness was noted in 28%, and sensory deficit was noted in 29%.[60-62]

An important part of the physical examination is identifying other common causes of similar symptoms. The neurologic examination should focus on eliciting signs that would suggest other neurologic causes of the patient's symptoms. Hyperreflexia, clonus, and upgoing toes, along with other upper motor neuron findings, can suggest the presence of myelopathy from cord compression. Sensory disturbance in a stocking distribution suggests the presence of neuropathy. A general musculoskeletal examination must include assessing the irritability and limitation of motion in the hips to rule out hip pathology. Palpation of the greater trochanter and iliotibial band can help detect pathology in these easily treated structures. Diminished peripheral pulses along with diminished skin hair are important clues that the symptoms may be coming from vascular claudication.

Diagnostic Studies

Radiography

The diagnostic testing of patients with spinal stenosis often starts with plain radiographs. In addition to the anteroposterior and lateral radiographs, flexion and extension lateral views should be obtained. Most patients suspected of having stenosis are elderly and thus likely demonstrate a variety of spondylotic changes on radiographs. Particular attention should be paid to diagnosing scoliosis and spondylolisthesis in addition to any dynamic instability that can be detected on the flexion–extension views. If scoliosis is noted, long-cassette scoliosis films would be helpful in evaluating the full extent of the deformity in both the coronal and sagittal planes. Narrowing of the neural foramen and inferred narrowing of the spinal canal from the location and extent of degenerated structures

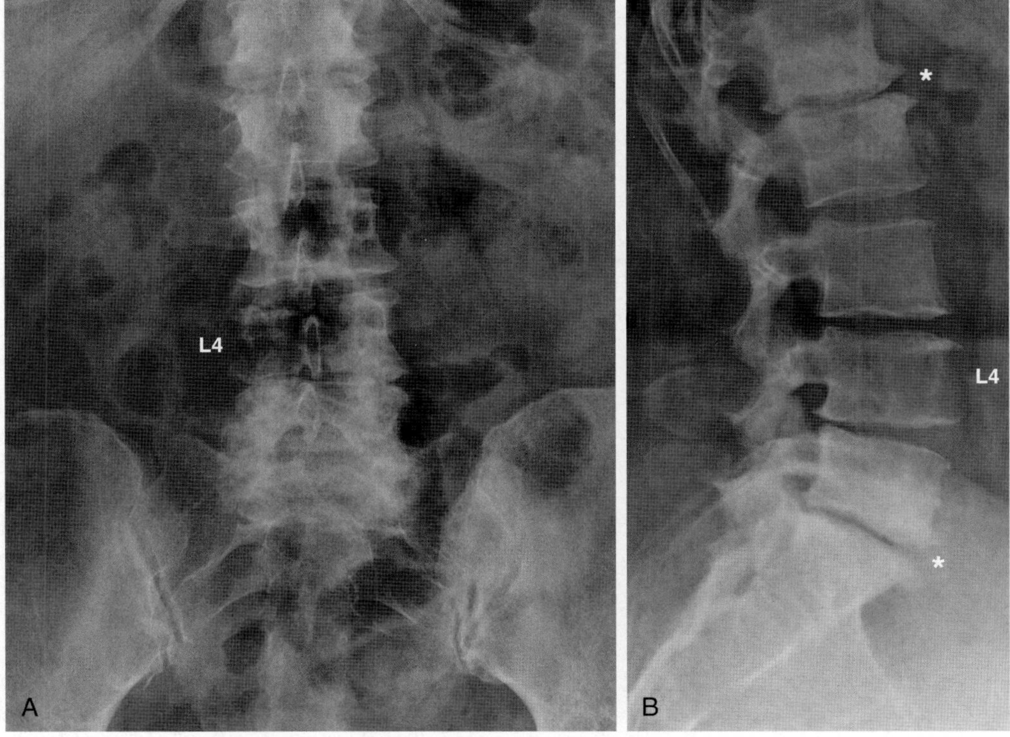

FIG. 61.5 (A) Anteroposterior (AP) and (B) lateral radiographs of a patient with progressively worsening right lumbar radiculopathy. *Asterisk* denotes the degenerative changes in the form of disc height collapse, endplate sclerosis, and osteophytes. On the AP radiograph, the right side of the superior and lateral walls of the vertebral body are indistinct, with collapse of the height of L4 on the right compared with the left. On the lateral radiograph, radiolucency is present in the L4 body along with an indistinct anterior wall. After additional workup, this patient was diagnosed with multiple myeloma in the L4 vertebral body.

should be evaluated. Ossification of ligamentous structures, ankylosis of the spine, erosion of the disc space, or any abnormal appearance of the bony structures should be assessed (Fig. 61.5). It should be kept in mind that even severe degenerative changes can be seen in asymptomatic patients.[73]

Computed Tomography With and Without Myelography

Prior to the common availability of magnetic resonance imaging (MRI), a CT scan was the study of choice for visualizing pathologic anatomy in the axial plane. Because a significant portion of the stenosis comes from soft tissue pathology, visualization of the soft tissues is the top priority in axial imaging. A CT scan is a poor modality for detailed analysis of the soft tissue pathology (Fig. 61.6). A metaanalysis demonstrated that the sensitivity of a CT scan in detecting spinal stenosis ranges from 70% to 100%.[74]

Diagnostic utility of the CT scan can be improved by combining it with myelography.[75,76] The dye injected in the cerebrospinal fluid during a myelogram provides good contrast between the thecal sac and the surrounding soft tissue and bony pathology. Preoperative complete contrast block on a CT-myelogram has been correlated with an improved surgical outcome.[77] The invasiveness of the myelogram and the radiation associated with the CT are the two biggest drawbacks of this diagnostic modality. Given these limitations, patients who

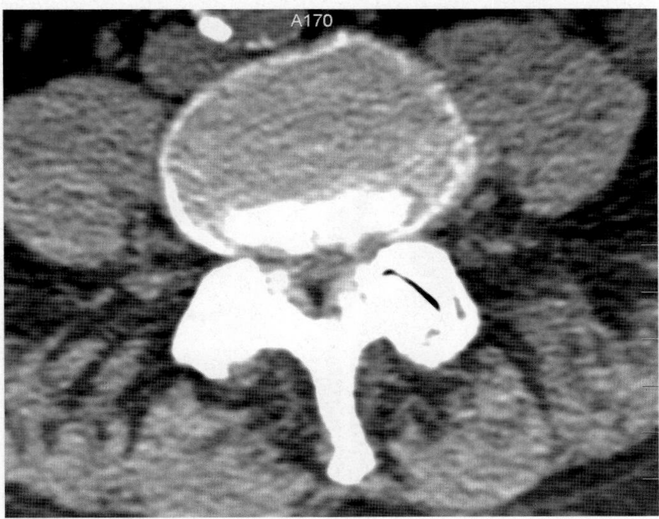

FIG. 61.6 Soft tissue window of a computed tomography scan through the L4–L5 level demonstrating stenosis. Note the facet and ligamentum hypertrophy are better seen on the magnetic resonance imaging of this patient in Figs. 61.9 and 61.10.

are unable to have an MRI, who have scoliosis, or who have previous spinal instrumentation are the most likely to undergo this study (Figs. 61.7 and 61.8). In cases in which MRI findings are unclear, a CT or a CT-myelogram should be considered to gain further information about the pathology.

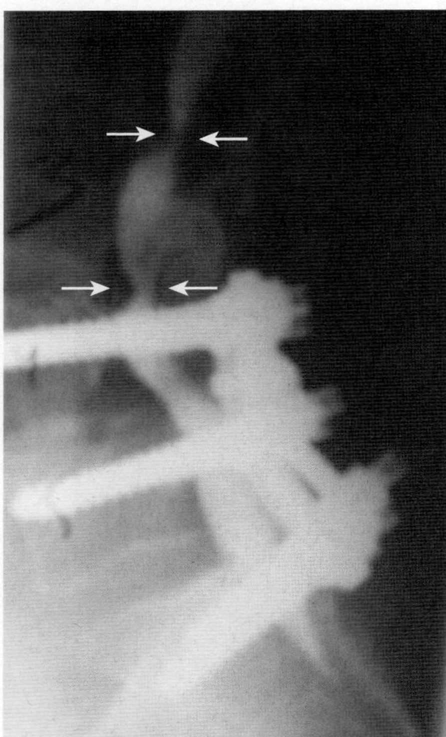

FIG. 61.7 Myelogram of a patient with neurogenic claudication who had a history of a previous lumbar instrumented fusion. The *arrows* identify the two levels of adjacent-level stenosis.

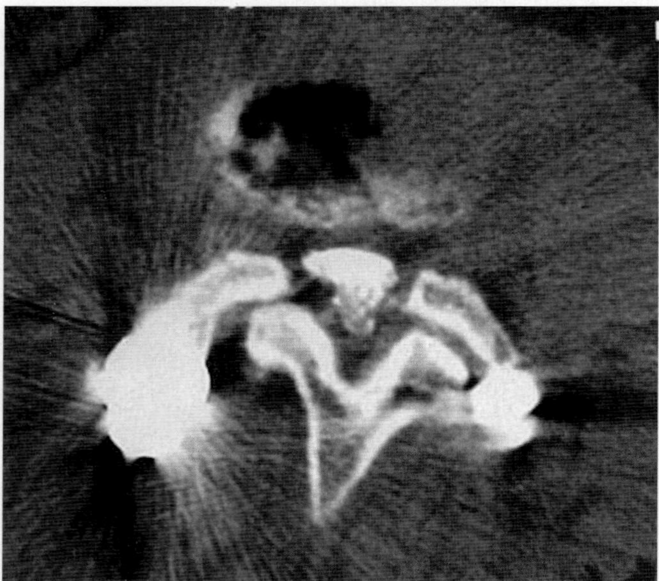

FIG. 61.8 Postmyelogram computed tomography through the adjacent-level stenosis of the patient in Fig. 61.7.

Magnetic Resonance Imaging

MRI is the diagnostic modality of choice in patients with suspected lumbar spinal stenosis. It is noninvasive and provides images in axial, coronal, and sagittal planes. MRI offers details of both the bony and soft tissue anatomy. It provides improved visualization of the soft tissue elements of the spine (Figs. 61.9 and 61.10). The degree of compression of the neural elements and the offending pathology are both easily visualized. The central canal, lateral recess, and neural foramen can all be visualized along with the degree of stenosis that is present in each of these regions. Facet arthropathy, ligamentum hypertrophy, disc bulges or herniations, and other compressive pathology, such as synovial cysts, are easily identified on MRI (Fig. 61.11). Foraminal stenosis is best visualized on T1-weighted sagittal images in which the nerve root and dorsal root ganglion are contrasted with the surrounding fat.

Overall, the diagnostic accuracy of MRI is similar to that of the CT-myelogram and does not have the drawbacks of ionizing radiation and contrast injection in the cerebrospinal fluid.[78–81] The reliability of MRI interpretation has also been investigated, and there appears to be significant inter-reader variability in assessing some anatomic locations.[82–85] The measurement of thecal sac area, as well as the ratings of the degree of central and foraminal stenosis, show good reliability.[86] The reading of the degree of lateral recess stenosis, on the other hand, shows significant variability. Although some have noted correlation between the degree of stenosis and outcomes of treatment, others have not been able to identify any such relationship.[87–90] The nerve root sedimentation sign describes the typical sedimentation of lumbar nerve roots in the dorsal part of the thecal sac due to gravity. The absence of this sedimentation is considered a positive sign of lumbar stenosis.[91]

It has been theorized that supine MRIs may understate the degree of stenosis because the patients may not be in the position of the worst compression during the study. Attempts have been made to demonstrate pathology in MRI scans that is obvious only under dynamic conditions.[92-96] A typical supine static MRI that demonstrates fluid-filled facets on T2-weighted axial images may indicate instability and would require careful scrutiny of flexion–extension radiographs.[97] Alternatively, MRIs in flexion, extension, axial loading, and upright positions can be performed. Investigation of this approach, however, has not provided any conclusive evidence regarding its utility. It is unclear what the results of invasive treatment will be for those patients whose stenosis can only be detected under dynamic conditions. What the existing studies do point out is that the static images on the current MRIs should be supplemented with the dynamic information available from clinical presentation as well as flexion and extension radiographs. One study noted that supine MRIs performed with the lumbar spine extended (by having the hips and knees extended) demonstrated more thecal sac compression than the images obtained in the flexed position.[98] This suggests that position of the lower extremities during the MRI should be ascertained as a routine part of the patient's history.

Electromyography, Nerve Conduction Studies, and Somatosensory Evoked Potentials

Electromyography (EMG), nerve conduction studies (NCSs), and somatosensory evoked potentials (SSEPs) are not part of the routine workup of patients with spinal stenosis. EMG

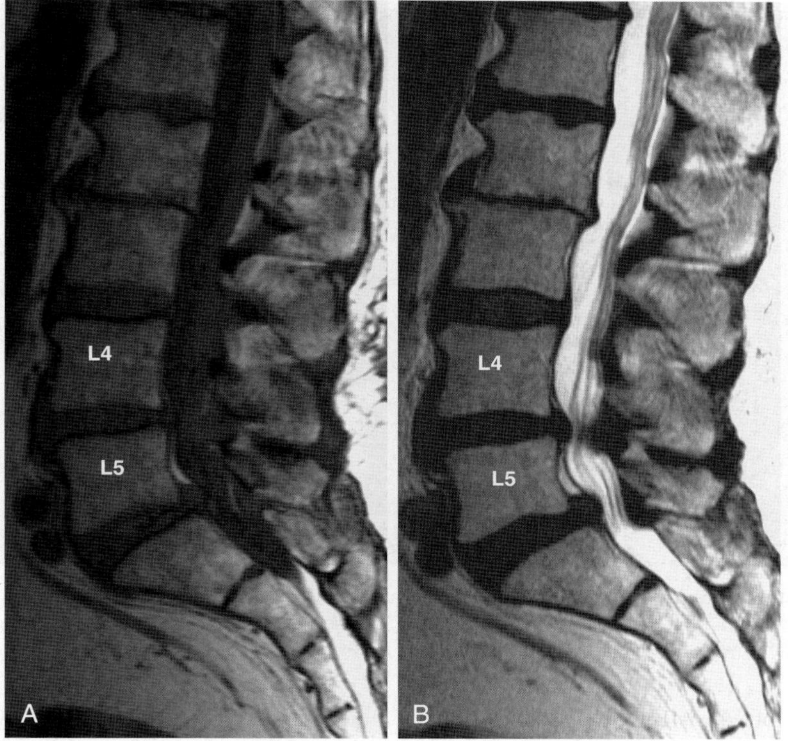

FIG. 61.9 (A) T1-weighted and (B) T2-weighted sagittal MRI of the patient in Fig. 61.6 with L4–L5 and L5–S1 stenosis. Note the disc bulges and ligamentum hypertrophy at the L4–L5 and L5–S1 levels.

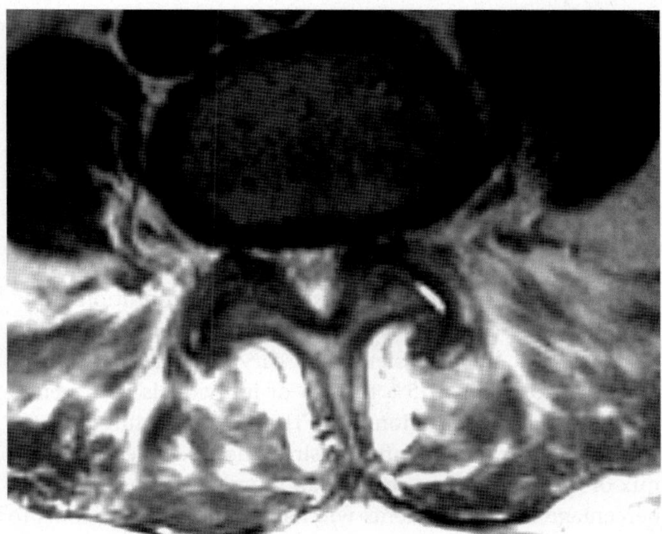

FIG. 61.10 Axial T2-weighted magnetic resonance imaging of the patient in Fig. 61.6 through the L4–L5 level demonstrating facet and ligamentum hypertrophy along with a disc bulge causing stenosis. Note increased T2 signal in the facet joint corresponding to the instability that this patient had on flexion-extension radiographs at the L4–L5 level.

identifies the effect of nerve function through recording the electrical activity of muscle at rest and with stimulation. EMG identifies lower motor neuron dysfunction and does not evaluate any sensory dysfunction. Electromyographic changes have been documented in up to 80% of patients with spinal stenosis.[90,99–102] EMG can be useful in differentiating chronic changes from active ongoing denervation. However, it should be kept in mind that there is a significant incidence of false-negative electromyograms in patients with spinal stenosis. This can be attributed to the fact that EMG does not measure sensory dysfunction and thus does not catch the more common abnormality in patients with neurogenic claudication. EMG also does not help differentiate symptomatic from asymptomatic patients.

NCSs measure the speed with which impulses travel down an axon. NCSs are useful in differentiating changes that are occurring from neuropathy versus radiculopathy. SSEPs measure the electrical transmission of sensory stimulation starting from the peripheral nerves and going through the spinal cord and brain. A lesion in the peripheral nerve will prolong the latency response, whereas lesions of the root and cord will cause changes in the waveform. An SSEP is more sensitive and specific compared with an EMG, although there continue to be false-negatives and false-positives.[103–105]

Differential Diagnosis

Neurogenic claudication is the hallmark of spinal stenosis. Patients describe a variety of abnormal sensations that radiate down their legs with ambulation. Symptoms are typically relieved by forward flexion of the lumbar spine and are worse with extension. Sudden onset or severe motor weakness and bowel and bladder dysfunction in these patients should prompt evaluation of other etiologies of these symptoms, such as cord compression. In spite of various attempts to create

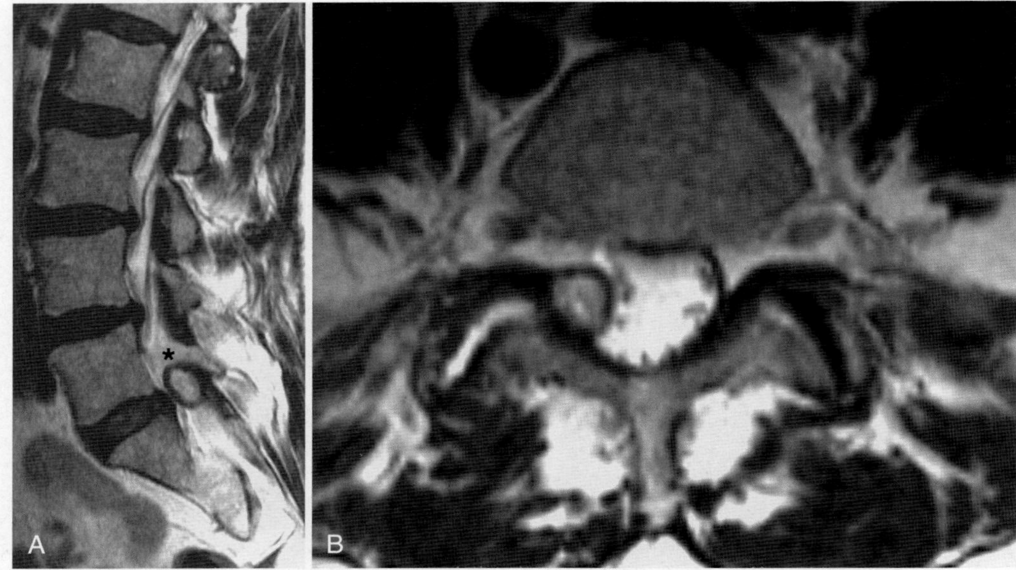

FIG. 61.11 T2-weighted (A) sagittal and (B) axial magnetic resonance imaging of a patient with a right L5–S1 synovial cyst causing a right lumbar radiculopathy. *Asterisk* denotes the synovial cyst on the sagittal view. In the axial view, the cyst is noted to arise from the right facet joint and causes neural compression.

a single validated method of consistently diagnosing spinal stenosis, no single test or algorithm is available to accurately diagnose all patients with symptomatic spinal stenosis.[63,106–108]

The differential diagnosis of spinal stenosis includes vascular claudication, lumbar spondylosis, lower extremity arthritis, cord compression, neurologic disorders, peripheral neuropathy, infection, tumors, and lumbosacral plexus lesions. Symptoms from neurogenic claudication start proximally and progress distally, whereas symptoms from vascular claudication start distally and progress proximally. Vascular claudication causes symptoms with a constant level of exertion regardless of the position of the lumbar spine. Thus, leaning forward on a grocery cart or going uphill does not allow these patients to walk longer. Similarly, patients with vascular claudication continue to be limited on a bike, while the patients with neurogenic claudication have better endurance on a bike. On physical examination, painless full extension of the lumbar spine; shiny, hairless legs; and weak peripheral pulses are all hallmarks of vascular claudication. If clinical suspicion of vascular claudication exists, then a peripheral pulse examination is not sufficient to diagnose peripheral arterial occlusive disease. Ankle brachial index and toe brachial index tests should be obtained. In a recent prospective study of 201 patients with lumbar stenosis, peripheral arterial disease was also present in 26% of patients, with a significant number of these cases only diagnosed using a combination of ankle brachial index and toe brachial index tests.[109]

Lumbar spondylosis typically causes pain in the low back without significant pain or abnormal sensation in the legs. Peripheral neuropathy typically causes burning pain and paresthesias that are unrelated to activity. A history of diabetes, vitamin deficiencies, alcoholism, chemotherapy, drug abuse, and exposure to toxins should be elicited in these patients. Physical examination in neuropathy patients will typically demonstrate hypoesthesia or dysesthesia in a glove-and-stocking distribution. Ankle reflexes will often be absent bilaterally. NCSs are helpful in establishing a diagnosis in these patients.

A history of isolated joint pain with ambulation will help identify patients with lower extremity arthritis. Hip arthritis typically presents with groin pain radiating into the anterior thigh but can also be a cause of buttock pain. Physical examination demonstrating hip irritability and limitation in internal rotation suggests that hip pathology is symptomatic. A thorough history and physical examination can thus help eliminate the majority of common conditions that mimic lumbar spinal stenosis. Presence of constitutional symptoms and intense nighttime pain suggest a possible infection or malignancy. These symptoms should trigger an MRI and laboratory studies, which would help eliminate these more rare conditions.

Finally, the coexistence of more than one condition must be considered. Tandem stenosis of cervical and lumbar spine is known to occur in 5% to 25% of individuals with neural compression in one region.[110–113] The clinical picture in these patients can be quite confusing since they will present with a mix of symptoms from cervical and lumbar stenosis. A small percentage of these patients will have sufficient symptoms to require surgical treatment of both conditions.[47] Thus, every patient diagnosed with lumbar stenosis should be carefully evaluated for cervical stenosis and any signs or symptoms of myelopathy.[112]

Summary

Lumbar spinal stenosis is a common finding in the elderly. With the aging population in the United States, the number of patients with spinal stenosis seeking treatment will dramatically increase over the next decade. Because pathologic changes can be present in asymptomatic patients, abnormalities found on imaging modalities are not a good method of diagnosing symptomatic spinal stenosis. Findings from a thorough history and physical examination should be correlated with corresponding pathologic abnormalities on MRI or a CT-myelogram. This is especially important if any invasive treatment will be recommended. Plain radiographs complement the other imaging modalities to create a full clinical picture that includes the detection of any dynamic instability. EMG, NCSs, and SSEPs are typically not helpful in confirming the diagnosis of stenosis. Despite our long history of treating patients with spinal stenosis, there is no single diagnostic test that can help identify patients with symptomatic spinal stenosis.

PEARLS

1. In patients with mild to moderate lumbar spinal stenosis, rapid or catastrophic neurologic deterioration is rare.
2. MRI is the noninvasive study of choice in patients suspected of having spinal stenosis.
3. Imaging studies should be correlated with specific findings on history and physical examination that would be expected on the basis of the specific neural elements that are compressed.
4. No single diagnostic test can confirm the presence of symptomatic spinal stenosis.

PITFALLS

1. Abnormal imaging is not a reliable method of diagnosing symptomatic lumbar spinal stenosis. The incidence of clinically silent lumbar degenerative disease is high.
2. A small but significant number of patients with lumbar stenosis will also have cervical myelopathy.
3. Lumbar stenosis and peripheral arterial occlusive disease often coexist. A peripheral pulse examination alone is not sufficient to exclude peripheral arterial occlusive disease in patients suspected of having vascular claudication.
4. Electrodiagnostic studies are not typically helpful in the diagnosis of spinal stenosis.
5. Most patients with spinal stenosis have a normal neurologic examination.
6. In evaluating patients with stenosis, do not forget to examine the hip joints and lower extremity vascularity.

KEY POINTS

1. Lumbar disc degeneration is a nearly universal finding in the aging population.
2. Degeneration alone does not imply a pathologic entity. A disease may be said to exist relative to the symptoms with which the patient presents.
3. In the absence of pathognomonic findings, the diagnosis of spinal stenosis rests on a Venn diagram approach in which historical elements overlap with physical examination and imaging findings.
4. Once symptomatic, most patients will continue to have symptoms on at least an intermittent basis.
5. Lumbar stenosis does not progress rapidly and catastrophic neurologic deterioration is rare. Therefore, a trial of nonoperative management is indicated in most cases.
6. Patients with symptomatic stenosis may present with one or more of a combination of axial pain, radiculopathy, and neurogenic claudication. Each of these is associated with different historical and examination findings.
7. Patients with lumbar stenosis often have other coexisting pathologies—such as hip or knee arthritis, vascular claudication, and cervical myelopathy—that may confuse the clinical picture.
8. Every patient with lumbar stenosis should be screened for cervical myelopathy.

KEY REFERENCES

1. Lurie JD, Tosteson TD, Tosteson A, et al. Long term outcomes of lumbar spinal stenosis: eight-year results of the Spine Patient Outcomes Research Trial (SPORT). *Spine*. 2015;40:63-76.
   Eight-year outcomes of a large prospective study evaluating nonsurgical and surgical treatment of lumbar spinal stenosis.
2. Kreiner DS, Shaffer WO, Baisden JL, et al. An evidence-based clinical guideline for the diagnosis and treatment of degenerative lumbar spinal stenosis (update). *Spine J*. 2013; 13:734-743.
   Evidence-based guidelines produced by North American Spine Society regarding diagnosis and treatment of patients with lumbar spinal stenosis.
3. Atlas SJ, Keller RB, Wu YA, et al. Long-term outcomes of surgical and nonsurgical management of lumbar spinal stenosis: 8 to 10 year results from the Maine Lumbar Spine Study. *Spine*. 2005; 30:936-943.
   A prospective observational cohort study evaluating outcomes of surgical and nonsurgical treatment after 8 to 10 years.
4. Kirkaldy-Willis WH, Wedge JH, Yong-Hing K, et al. Pathology and pathogenesis of lumbar spondylosis and stenosis. *Spine*. 1978;3:319-328.
   A classic article describing the pathogenesis of lumbar stenosis.
5. Verbiest H. A radicular syndrome from developmental narrowing of the lumbar vertebral canal. *J Bone Joint Surg Br*. 1954;36: 230-237.
   A historical perspective on diagnosis and treatment of lumbar spinal stenosis.

REFERENCES

1. Verbiest H. A radicular syndrome from developmental narrowing of the lumbar vertebral canal. *J Bone Joint Surg Br*. 1954;36:230-237.
2. Verbiest H. Further experiences on pathologic influence of a developmental stenosis of the lumbar vertebral canal. *J Bone Joint Surg Br*. 1956;38:576-583.
3. Verbiest H. Spondylolisthesis: the value of radicular signs and symptoms. *J Int Coll Surg*. 1963;39:461-481.
4. Verbiest H. Unilateral lumbo-sacral radicular symptoms due to sequestrated disc material in the spinal canal. *Cesk Neurol*. 1968;31:93-101.
5. Verbiest H. Neurogenic intermittent claudication in cases with absolute and relative stenosis of the lumbar vertebral canal (ASLC and RSLC), in cases with narrow lumbar intervertebral foramina, and in cases with both entities. *Clin Neurosurg*. 1973;20:204-214.
6. Verbiest H. Pathomorphic aspects of developmental lumbar stenosis. *Orthop Clin North Am*. 1975;6:177-196.
7. Verbiest H. Results of surgical treatment of idiopathic developmental stenosis of the lumbar vertebral canal. *J Bone Joint Surg Br*. 1977;59:181-188.
8. Verbiest H. The treatment of lumbar spondyloptosis or impending lumbar spondyloptosis accompanied by neurologic deficit and/or neurogenic intermittent claudication. *Spine*. 1979;4:68-77.
9. Verbiest H. Stenosis of the lumbar vertebral canal and sciatica. *Neurosurg Rev*. 1980;3:75-89.

10. Verbiest H. Developmental stenosis of the bony lumbar vertebral canal. *Acta Orthop Belg*. 1987;53:373-387.
11. Kirkaldy-Willis WH, Paine KWE, Cauchoix J, et al. Lumbar spinal stenosis. *Clin Orthop*. 1974;99:30-50.
12. Kirkaldy-Willis WH, Wedge JH, Yong-Hing K, et al. Pathology and pathogenesis of lumbar spondylosis and stenosis. *Spine*. 1978;3:319-328.
13. Kirkaldy-Willis WH. Lumbar spinal nerve entrapment. *Clin Orthop*. 1982;169:171-178.
14. Kirkaldy-Willis WH. The relationship of structural pathology to the nerve root. *Spine*. 1984;9:49.
15. Kirkaldy-Willis WH. Presidential symposium on instability of the lumbar spine. *Spine*. 1985;10:254-291.
16. Boden SD, Davis DO, Dina TS, et al. Abnormal magnetic-imaging scans of the lumbar spine in asymptomatic subjects: a prospective investigation. *J Bone Joint Surg Am*. 1990; 72:403-408.
17. Jensen MC, Brant-Zawadzki MN, Obuchowski N, et al. Magnetic resonance imaging of the lumbar spine in people without back pain. *N Engl J Med*. 1994;331:69-73.
18. Deyo RA, Ciol MA, Cherkin DC, et al. Lumbar spinal fusion: a cohort study of complications, reoperations, and resource use in the Medicare population. *Spine*. 1993;18: 1463-1470.
19. Deyo RA, Gray DT, Kreuter W, et al. United States trends in lumbar fusion surgery for degenerative conditions. *Spine*. 2005;30:1441-1445.
20. Hillabrand AS, Rand N. Degenerative lumbar stenosis: diagnosis and management. *J Am Acad Orthop Surg*. 1999;7:239-248.
21. Yong-Hing K, Kirkaldy-Willis WH. The pathophysiology of disc degeneration of the lumbar spine. *Orthop Clin North Am*. 1983;14(3):59-64.
22. Arbit E, Pannullo S. Lumbar stenosis: a clinical review. *Clin Orthop Relat Res*. 2001;384:137-143.
23. Vanderlinden R. Subarticular entrapment of the dorsal root ganglion as a cause of sciatic pain. *Spine*. 1984;9:19-22.
24. Kunogi J, Hasue M. Diagnosis, operative treatment of intraforaminal, extraforaminal nerve root compression. *Spine*. 1991;16:1312-1330.
25. Porter R, Hibbert C, Evans C. The natural history of root entrapment syndrome. *Spine*. 1984;9:418-421.
26. Morishita Y, Hida S, Naito M, et al. Measurement of the local pressure in the intervertebral foramen and the electrophysiologic values of the spinal nerve roots in the vertebral foramen. *Spine*. 2006;31:3076-3080.
27. Rosenburg NJ. Degenerative spondylolisthesis: predisposing factors. *J Bone Joint Surg Am*. 1975;67:240-246.
28. Spivak JM. Degenerative lumbar spinal stenosis: current concepts review. *J Bone Joint Surg Am*. 1998;80:1053-1066.
29. Schonstorm N, Bolender NF, Spengler DM, et al. Pressure changes within the cauda equine following constriction of the dural sac. An in vitro experimental study. *Spine*. 1984;9: 604-607.
30. Delamarter RB, Bohlmann HH, Dodge LD, et al. Experimental lumbar spinal stenosis: analysis of the cortical evoked potentials, microvasculature, and histopathology. *J Bone Joint Surg Am*. 1990;72:110-120.
31. Pedowitz R, Garfin S, Massie J, et al. Effects of magnitude and duration of compression on spinal nerve root conduction. *Spine*. 1992;17:194-199.
32. Rydevick B, Lundborg G. Permeability of intraneural microvessels and perineurium following acute, graded experimental nerve compression. *Scand J Plast Reconstr Surg*. 1977;11:179-187.
33. Rydevick B, Lundborg G, Bagge U. Effects of graded compression on intraneural blood flow. An in vivo study on rabbit tibial nerve. *J Hand Surg Am*. 1981;6:3-12.
34. Rydevick B, Nordborg G. Changes in nerve function and nerve fiber structure induced by acute, graded compression. *J Neurol Neurosurg Psychiatry*. 1981;43:1070-1082.
35. Rydevick B, Brown M, Lundborg G. Pathoanatomy and pathophysiology of nerve root compression. *Spine*. 1984;9: 7-15.
36. Rydevick B, Holm S, Brown MD, et al. Diffusion from the cerebrospinal fluid as a nutritional pathway for spinal nerve roots. *Acta Physiol Scand*. 1990;138:247-248.
37. Rydevick B, Pedowitz RA, Hargens AR, et al. Effects of acute, graded compression on spinal nerve root function and structure. An experimental study of the pig cauda equina. *Spine*. 1991;16:487-493.
38. Kang JD, Georgescu HI, Larkin L, et al. Herniated lumbar intervertebral discs spontaneously produce matrix metalloproteinases, nitric oxide, interleukin-6, and prostaglandin E2. *Spine*. 1996;21:271-277.
39. O'Donnel JL, O'Donnel AL. Prostaglandin E2 content in herniated lumbar disc disease. *Spine*. 1996;21:1653-1656.
40. Olemarker K, Nordborg C, Larsson K, et al. Ultrastructural changes in spinal nerve roots induced by autologous nucleus pulposus. *Spine*. 1996;21:411-414.
41. Muramoto T, Atsuta Y, Iwahara T, et al. The action of prostaglandin E2 and triamcinolone acetonide on the firing activity of lumbar nerve roots. *Orthopedics*. 1997;21:172-175.
42. Hashizume H, Kawakami M, Nishi H, et al. Histochemical demonstration of nitric oxide in herniated lumbar discs: a clinical and animal model study. *Spine*. 1997;22:1080-1084.
43. Yabuki S, Kikuchi S, Olemarker K, et al. Acute effects of nucleus pulposus on blood flow and endoneurial fluid pressure in rat dorsal root ganglia. *Spine*. 1998;23:2517-2523.
44. Singh K, Samartzis D, Vacarro AR, et al. Congenital lumbar spinal stenosis: a prospective, control-matched, cohort radiographic analysis. *Spine J*. 2005;5:615-622.
45. Hall S, Bartleson JD, Onofrio BM, et al. Lumbar spinal stenosis: clinical features, diagnostic procedures, and results of surgical treatment in 68 patients. *Ann Intern Med*. 1985;103:271-275.
46. Kalichman L, Cole R, Kim DH, et al. Spinal stenosis prevalence and association with symptoms: the Framingham study. *Spine J*. 2009;9:545-550.
47. Tsutsumimoto T, Shimogata M, Yui M, et al. The natural history of asymptomatic lumbar canal stenosis in patients undergoing surgery for cervical myelopathy. *J Bone Joint Surg Br*. 2012;94-B:378-384.
48. Jones RA, Thomson JL. The narrow lumbar canal: a clinical and radiological review. *J Bone Joint Surg Br*. 1968;50:595-605.
49. Tile M, McNeil SR, Zarins RK, et al. Spinal stenosis: results of treatment. *Clin Orthop*. 1976;115:104-108.
50. Blau JN, Logue V. The natural history of intermittent claudication of the cauda equina: a long term follow-up study. *Brain*. 1978;101:211-222.
51. Rosomoff HL, Rosomoff RS. Nonsurgical aggressive treatment of lumbar spinal stenosis. *Spine*. 1987;1:383.
52. Postacchini F, Cinotti G, Gumina S, Perugia D. Long-term results of surgery in lumbar stenosis: 8-year review of 64 patients. *Acta Orthop Scand Suppl*. 1993;251:78-80.

53. Herno A, Airaksinen O, Saari T, Luukkonen M. Lumbar spinal stenosis: a matched-pair study of operated and non-operated patients. *Br J Neurosurg*. 1996;10: 461-465.
54. Benoist M. The natural history of lumbar degenerative spinal stenosis. *Joint Bone Spine*. 2002;69:450-457.
55. Atlas SJ, Keller RB, Robson D, et al. Surgical and nonsurgical management of lumbar spinal stenosis. *Spine*. 2000;25: 556-562.
56. Johnsson KE, Rosen I, Uden A. The natural course of lumbar spinal stenosis. *Clin Orthop Relat Res*. 1992;279:82-86.
57. Atlas SJ, Keller RB, Wu YA, et al. Long-term outcomes of surgical and nonsurgical management of lumbar spinal stenosis: 8 to 10 year results from the Maine Lumbar Spine Study. *Spine*. 2005;30:936-943.
58. Miyamoto H, Sumi M, Uno K, et al. Clinical outcome of nonoperative treatment for lumbar spinal stenosis, and predictive factors relating to prognosis, in a 5-year minimum follow-up. *J Spinal Disord Tech*. 2008;21:563-568.
59. Malmivaara A, Slatis P, Heliovaara M, et al. Surgical or non-operative treatment of lumbar spinal stenosis? *Spine*. 2007;32:1-8.
60. Weinstein JN, Tosteson TD, Lurie JD, et al. Surgical versus nonsurgical therapy for lumbar spinal stenosis. *N Engl J Med*. 2008;358:794-810.
61. Weinstein JN, Tosteson TD, Lurie JD, et al. Surgical versus non-operative treatment for lumbar spinal stenosis: four-year results of the Spine Patient Outcomes Research Trial (SPORT). *Spine*. 2010;35:1329-1338.
62. Lurie JD, Tosteson TD, Tosteson A, et al. Long term outcomes of lumbar spinal stenosis: eight-year results of the Spine Patient Outcomes Research Trial (SPORT). *Spine*. 2015;40:63-76.
63. Waters WC, Baisden J, Gilbert TJ, et al. Degenerative lumbar spinal stenosis: an evidence based clinical guideline for the diagnosis and treatment of degenerative lumbar spinal stenosis. *Spine J*. 2008;8:305-310.
64. Kreiner DS, Shaffer WO, Baisden JL, et al. An evidence-based clinical guideline for the diagnosis and treatment of degenerative lumbar spinal stenosis (update). *Spine J*. 2013; 13:734-743.
65. Lin S-I, Lin R-M, Huang L-W. Disability in patients with degenerative lumbar spinal stenosis. *Arch Phys Med Rehabil*. 2006;87:1250-1256.
66. Hellstrom PA, Tammela TL, Niinimaki TJ. Voiding dysfunction and urodynamic findings in patients with lumbar spinal stenosis and the effect of decompressive laminectomy. *Scand J Urol Nephrol*. 1995;29:167-171.
67. Johnsson KE. Lumbar spinal stenosis: a retrospective study of 163 cases in southern Sweden. *Acta Orthop Scand*. 1995;66:403-405.
68. Kawaguchi Y, Kanamori M, Ishihara H, et al. Clinical symptoms and surgical outcome in lumbar spinal stenosis patients with neuropathic bladder. *J Spinal Disord*. 2001;14:404-410.
69. Aalto TJ, Malmivaara A, Kovacs F, et al. Preoperative predictors of postoperative clinical outcome in lumbar spinal stenosis. *Spine*. 2006;31:E648-E663.
70. Ciric I, Mikhael M, Tarkington J, et al. The lateral recess syndrome. *J Neurosurg*. 1980;53:433-443.
71. Rainville J, Lopez E. Comparison of radicular symptoms caused by lumbar disc herniation and lumbar spinal stenosis in the elderly. *Spine*. 2013;38:1282-1287.
72. Amundsen T, Weber H, Lilleas F, et al. Lumbar spinal stenosis: clinical and radiologic features. *Spine*. 1995;20: 1178-1186.
73. Frymoyer JW, Newberg A, Pope MH, et al. Spine radiographs in patients with low-back pain: an epidemiological study in men. *J Bone Joint Surg Am*. 1984;66:1048-1055.
74. Kent DL, Haynor DR, Larson EB. Diagnosis of lumbar spinal stenosis in adults: a meta-analysis of the accuracy of CT, MR, and myelography. *AJR Am J Roentgenol*. 1992;158: 1135-1144.
75. Herkowitz HN, Garfin SR, Bell GR, et al. The use of computed tomography in evaluating non-visualized vertebral levels caudad to a complete block on a lumbar myelogram: a review of 32 cases. *J Bone Joint Surg Am*. 1987;69:218-224.
76. Bell GR, Rothman RH, Booth RE, et al. A study of computer assisted tomography: II. Comparison of metrizamide myelography and computed tomography in the diagnosis of herniated lumbar disc and spinal stenosis. *Spine*. 1984;9:552-556.
77. Herno A, Airaksinen O, Saari T, et al. The predictive value of preoperative myelography in lumbar spinal stenosis. *Spine*. 1994;19:1335-1338.
78. Modic MT, Masaryk T, Boumphrey F, et al. Lumbar herniated disk disease and canal stenosis: prospective evaluation by surface coil MR, CT, and myelography. *AJR Am J Roentgenol*. 1986;147:757-765.
79. Schnebel B, Kingston S, Watkins R, et al. Comparison of MRI to contrast CT in diagnosis of spinal stenosis. *Spine*. 1989;14:332-337.
80. Postacchini F, Amatruda A, Morace GB, et al. Magnetic resonance imaging in the diagnosis of lumbar spinal canal stenosis. *Ital J Orthop Traumatol*. 1991;17:327-337.
81. Bischoff RJ, Rodriguez RP, Gupta K, et al. A comparison of computed tomography-myelography, magnetic resonance imaging, and myelography in the diagnosis of herniated nucleus pulposus and spinal stenosis. *J Spinal Disord*. 1993;6:289-295.
82. Hamanishi C, Matukura N, Fujita M, et al. Cross-sectional area of the stenotic lumbar dural tube measured from the transverse views of magnetic resonance imaging. *J Spinal Disord*. 1994;7:388-393.
83. Speciale AC, Pietrobon R, Urban CW, et al. Observer variability in assessing lumbar spinal stenosis severity on magnetic resonance imaging and its relation to cross-sectional spinal canal area. *Spine*. 2002;27:1082-1086.
84. Weiner BK, Patel NM, Walker MA. Outcomes of decompression for lumbar spinal canal stenosis based upon pre-operative radiographic severity. *J Orthop Surg*. 2007;2:3.
85. Song K, Jang E, Jung H, et al. Observer variability in the evaluation of multiple lumbar stenosis by routing MR-myelography and MRI. *J Spinal Disord Tech*. 2008;21:569-574.
86. Lurie JD, Tosteson AN, Tosteson TD, et al. Reliability of readings of magnetic resonance imaging features of lumbar spinal stenosis. *Spine*. 2008;33:1605-1610.
87. Uden A, Johnsson KE, Johnsson K, et al. Myelography in the elderly and the diagnosis of spinal stenosis. *Spine*. 1985;10:171-174.
88. Ogikubo O, Forsberg L, Hansson T. The relationship between the cross-sectional area of the cauda equine and the pre-operative symptoms in central lumbar spinal stenosis. *Spine*. 2007;13:1423-1428.

89. Geisser ME, Haig AJ, Tong HC, et al. Spinal canal size and clinical symptoms among persons diagnosed with lumbar spinal stenosis. *Clin J Pain*. 2007;23:780-785.
90. Haig AJ, Geisser ME, Tong HC, et al. Electromyography and magnetic resonance imaging to predict lumbar stenosis, low back pain, and no back symptoms. *J Bone Joint Surg*. 2007;89:358-366.
91. Barz T, Melloh M, Staub LP, et al. Nerve root sedimentation sign: evaluation of a new radiologic sign in lumbar spinal stenosis. *Spine*. 2010;35:892-897.
92. Schmid MR, Strucki G, Duewell S, et al. Changes in cross-sectional measurements of the spinal canal and intervertebral foramina as a function of body position: in vivo studies on an open-configuration MR system. *AJR Am J Roentgenol*. 1999;172:1095.
93. Zamani AA, Moriarty T, Hsu L, et al. Functional MRI of the lumbar spine in erect position in a superconducting open-configuration MR system: preliminary results. *J Magn Reson Imaging*. 1998;8:1329-1333.
94. Vitzthum HE, Konig A, Seifert V. Dynamic examination of the lumbar spine by using vertical, open magnetic resonance imaging. *J Neurosurg*. 2000;93:58-64.
95. Weishaupt D, Schmid MR, Zanetti M, et al. Positional MR imaging of the lumbar spine: does it demonstrate nerve root compromise not visible at conventional MR imaging? *Radiology*. 2000;215:247-253.
96. Willen J, Wessberg PJ, Danielsson B. Surgical results in hidden lumbar spinal stenosis detected by axial loaded computed tomography and magnetic resonance imaging. *Spine*. 2008;33:E109-E115.
97. Schinnerer KA, Katz LD, Grauer JN. MR findings of exaggerated fluid in facet joints predicts instability. *J Spinal Disord Tech*. 2008;21:468-472.
98. Madsen R, Jensen TS, Ope M, et al. The effect of body position and axial load on spinal canal morphology. *Spine*. 2008;33:61-67.
99. Jacobsen RE. Lumbar stenosis: an electromyographic evaluation. *Clin Orthop*. 1976;115:68-72.
100. Spengler DM. Degenerative stenosis of the lumbar spine. *J Bone Joint Surg Am*. 1987;69:305-308.
101. Johnsson KE, Rosen I, Uden A. Neurophysiologic investigation of patients with spinal stenosis. *Spine*. 1987;12:483-487.
102. Chiodod A, Haig AJ, Yamakawa KSJ, et al. Magnetic resonance imaging vs electrodiagnostic root compromise in lumbar spinal stenosis. *Am J Phys Med Rehabil*. 2008;87:789-797.
103. Dvonch V, Scoff T, Bunch WH, et al. Dermatomal somatosensory evoked potentials: their use in lumbar radiculopathy. *Spine*. 1984;9:291-293.
104. Keim HA, Hajdu M, Gonzales EG, et al. Somatosensory evoked potentials as an aid in diagnosis and intraoperative management of spinal stenosis. *Spine*. 1985;10:338-388.
105. Kondo M, Matsuda H, Kureya S, et al. Electrophysiological studies of intermittent claudication in lumbar stenosis. *Spine*. 1989;14:862-866.
106. Tenhula J, Lenke LJ, Bridwell KH, et al. Prospective functional evaluation of the surgical treatment of neurogenic claudication in patients with lumbar spinal stenosis. *J Spinal Disord*. 2000;13:276-282.
107. Graff ID, Park A, Bierma-Zeinstra S, et al. Diagnosis of lumbar spinal stenosis: a systematic review of the accuracy of the diagnostic tests. *Spine*. 2006;31:1168-1176.
108. Konno S, Hayashino Y, Fukuhara S, et al. Development of a clinical diagnosis support tool to identify patients with lumbar spinal stenosis. *Eur Spine J*. 2007;16:1951-1957.
109. Imagama S, Matsuyama Y, Sakai Y, et al. An arterial pulse examination is not sufficient for diagnosis of peripheral arterial disease in lumbar spinal canal stenosis. *Spine*. 2011;36:1204-1210.
110. Dagi TF, Tarkington MA, Leech JJ. Tandem lumbar and cervical spinal stenosis. Natural history, prognostic indices, and results after surgical decompression. *J Neurosurg*. 1987;66:842-849.
111. LaBan MM, Green ML. Concurrent (tandem) cervical and lumbar spinal stenosis: a 10-yr review of 54 hospitalized patients. *Am J Phys Med Rehabil*. 2004;83:187-190.
112. Park MS, Moon S, Kim T, et al. Asymptomatic stenosis in the cervical and thoracic spines of patients with symptomatic lumbar stenosis. *Global Spine J*. 2015;5:366-371.
113. Adamova B, Bednarik J, Andrasinova T, et al. Does lumbar spinal stenosis increase the risk of spondylotic cervical spinal cord compression? *Eur Spine J*. 2015;24:2946-2953.

CHAPTER 62 Nonoperative Management of Lumbar Spinal Stenosis

Daniel Mazanec

Lumbar spinal stenosis (LSS) is best defined as a clinical syndrome of buttock or lower extremity pain, with or without low back pain, resulting from diminished space for neurovascular elements in the spinal canal.[1] A clinical definition is preferred because imaging findings do not correlate with symptoms. Approximately 20% of asymptomatic individuals older than 60 years have stenosis on magnetic resonance imaging (MRI).[2] Anteroposterior spinal canal diameter is not predictive of symptoms or prognosis.[3] Since its description as a distinct clinical entity in the early 1950s, LSS has been increasingly identified as a common clinical problem in older adults and now represents the most common diagnosis requiring spinal surgery in patients older than 65 years.[4]

Clinical Aspects

The classic symptom of LSS is pseudoclaudication—leg pain, paresthesias, and/or weakness provoked by walking or standing and relieved with forward flexion (i.e., sitting or squatting), noted in more than 90% of patients.[5] Though axial lumbar pain may be present, most patients with LSS report greater lower extremity discomfort than spinal pain. Physical examination in patients with LSS may be unremarkable, with a minority of patients demonstrating provocation of leg symptoms with spinal extension or an abnormal Romberg test. Findings such as diminished patellar or Achilles reflexes, focal muscle weakness, or positive nerve tension signs are noted in only a minority of patients.

The physical examination is crucial, however, in identifying common alternative causes of back and leg pain in this population, including osteoarthritis of the hip, peripheral arterial disease, and greater trochanteric pain syndrome. These conditions may produce symptoms that superficially mimic the pseudoclaudication of LSS. In addition, older patients with LSS may have coexisting hip or vascular disease (i.e., the "hip-spine syndrome").

Natural History of Lumbar Spinal Stenosis

Understanding the natural history of untreated spinal stenosis is crucial to making any recommendation for treatment, medical or surgical. Unfortunately, surprisingly little information about the course of untreated LSS is available. Johnson[6] reported the course of 32 patients with myelographically confirmed stenosis and radicular or claudication pain followed for a mean of almost 4 years without any medical/interventional or surgical treatment. Pain, as assessed by visual analog scores, was unchanged in 70% at final follow-up, improved in 15%, and worse in 15%, suggesting a benign course in most patients. Functionally, walking capacity at 4 years was unchanged from baseline. In these untreated patients, no severe or catastrophic neurologic deterioration occurred.

Several studies have compared surgical and nonsurgical treatment in patients with LSS, but none has included an untreated control group. As a result, they do not provide further insight into the natural history of untreated LSS. However, the results do suggest that approximately 50% of patients with mild to moderate LSS who were managed without surgery have a favorable course. Malmivaara[7] reported a prospective randomized controlled trial comparing surgical treatment (undercutting laminectomy) with medical management (physical therapy) in 94 patients with symptomatic LSS severe enough to warrant treatment. Both groups demonstrated improvement at their 2-year follow-up. Clinically significant improvement in the Oswestry Disability Index (ODI) was noted in 55% of surgical patients and 42% of nonoperative patients. No difference in walking ability was detected. Weinstein reported a prospective randomized trial with an observational cohort comparing surgical and nonsurgical treatment in patients with LSS who were believed to be surgical candidates.[8] Though surgical patients demonstrated superior improvement at 2 years, nonoperatively treated patients demonstrated improvements as well, in the ODI and bodily pain and physical function indices of the Short-Form 36 questionnaire. The Maine Lumbar Spine Study reported the results of a prospective cohort trial comparing medical and surgical treatment of 148 patients with LSS, some followed for up to 10 years.[9,10] Patients were treated in community-based orthopedic and neurosurgery practices in Maine. Medical treatment was not specified by the study, but most frequently included physical therapy (modalities and exercises), manipulation, analgesics, and epidural injections. After 4 years, 70% of the surgically treated patients and 52% of the medically treated patients reported improvement in their dominant symptom. After 8 to 10 years, a similar percentage of surgical and medically treated patients available for evaluation reported improvement in their predominant symptom (54% vs. 42%). Both groups reported comparable satisfaction with their current status (55% and 49%). In a cohort of 68 patients with LSS with moderate symptoms who were treated medically, Amundsen reported about 70% of persons had good outcomes at 10 years.[11] Medical treatment included a 1-month stay in a rehabilitation unit with bracing. Outcomes in conservatively managed patients who ultimately required surgery did not differ from patients who were selected for initial surgical treatment (i.e., delay in surgery did not adversely affect results). Finally, Delitto et al. reported the results of a randomized study in 169 patients with stenosis who had been consented for surgery and then randomized to surgical decompression or a 6-week structured physical therapy program with 2-year follow up.[12] Intention-to-treat analysis demonstrated no difference in physical function; however, 57% of patients randomized to physical therapy crossed over to surgery. Successful outcomes of treatment were found in 61% of surgical patients, 55% of crossover patients, and 52% of physical therapy patients.

These studies suggest that, although surgical results are generally superior in the short term (1–4 years), a significant proportion of patients do well with nonoperative care for as long as 10 years without catastrophic neurologic deterioration. In most trials, the decision for early surgery was based on severity of symptoms rather than anatomic factors such as spinal canal dimensions, which are not predictive of symptoms, much less need for urgent surgical intervention. The study by Delitto et al.[12] suggests that crossover patients who tried physical therapy (mean, 7.8 visits) had comparable success to patients who had earlier surgery. This would suggest that delaying surgery for several weeks does not adversely impact outcome. In patients with moderate or less severe symptoms, on the basis of these data, a trial of conservative management is certainly reasonable. None of these trials included an untreated control group, however, making attribution of success to a specific treatment impossible.

Nonoperative Management

Whether medical and interventional treatments improve the outcome of patients with spinal stenosis compared with the generally favorable natural history of the disease remains uncertain. A recent Cochrane review of nonoperative treatment for LSS with neurogenic claudication including 21 trials (1851 participants) concluded that "moderate and high-quality evidence for nonoperative treatment is lacking and thus prohibits recommendations for guiding clinical practice."[13] Another systematic review of the literature found no direct comparisons of active treatment to an untreated control group.[1] Medical treatment is therefore based primarily on clinical experience and training guided by limited clinical outcome data. In most patients, a combination of physical therapy, medications, and spinal injections are considered with the objectives of relieving pain and functionally improving walking and standing time.

Drug Therapy

Though widely used, the efficacy of analgesics and nonsteroidal antiinflammatory drugs (NSAIDs) has not been investigated in patients with lumbar stenosis. In the absence of studies demonstrating that NSAIDs are superior to simple analgesics, the risk of NSAID toxicity becomes the determining factor in therapeutic decision making. For osteoarthritis, on the basis of cost and toxicity associated with NSAIDs, the American College of Rheumatology and the European League Against Rheumatism have both recommended acetaminophen as initial therapy.[14] However, a recent study comparing acetaminophen to placebo in acute back pain found no difference in outcome.[15] In addition, a systematic review and metaanalysis of acetaminophen for spinal pain also concluded that the drug is ineffective.[16] Typically, patients with LSS are older and more likely to have common comorbidities, including hypertension, cardiovascular disease, and diabetes, that increase the risk of NSAID-induced cardiovascular, renal, and gastrointestinal toxicity.[17–19] Extrapolating from these guidelines, pure analgesics—including opioids—would be the agents of first choice in patients with LSS. The fact that inflammation is not believed to play a central role in the pathogenesis of LSS lends further rationale for the choice of a pure analgesic in this high-risk population. However, even therapy with opioid analgesics often fails to produce significant functional improvement, as assessed by increased walking or standing tolerance. The adverse effects of long-term opioid therapy, including cognitive impairment and sedation, are of particular concern in older stenosis patients at increased risk of falls.[20]

Gabapentin is an anticonvulsant and analgesic agent that has been found in multiple trials to be effective in the treatment of various neuropathic pain syndromes, including diabetic neuropathy and postherpetic neuralgia.[21] Two small trials of gabapentin suggest possible efficacy in patients with LSS. Yaksi et al. reported a randomized trial of 57 patients comparing standard treatment (physical therapy, NSAIDs) with standard treatment plus gabapentin. Gabapentin resulted in significantly increased walking distance, as well as improved pain scores and recovery of sensory deficits.[22] A more recent 4-week prospective cohort study using an extended-release form of gabapentin reported significant improvement in sleep and pain.[23] Careful attention to common adverse effects of gabapentin, particularly sedation and dizziness, is crucial in treating patients with LSS. Other drugs used to treat neuropathic pain syndromes—including pregabalin, tricyclic antidepressants, and duloxetine—have not been studied in LSS. Because of potential cardiovascular toxicity, tricyclics should be used with caution in this population.

Physical Therapy

Though nonoperative treatment of spinal stenosis typically includes physical therapy, a recent systematic review of physical therapy interventions for degenerative LSS found that evidence was scarce and insufficient to identify which physical therapy treatment is best.[24] The authors found no evidence that addition of physical therapy modalities (ultrasound, transcutaneous electrical nerve stimulation, heat packs) to exercise had any impact on outcome. Exercise was superior to no exercise but specific exercise programs have not been well studied. Traditional empirically based exercise programs in patients with stenosis have focused on the goals of decreasing lumbar lordosis and extension forces on the spine while improving abdominal "core" strength. Commonly, flexion-based lumbar stabilization exercises are recommended. This approach should include identification and treatment of hip flexion contractures, which may result in increased lumbar lordosis. Many patients with LSS are deconditioned as a result of symptom-limited walking and age-related comorbidities. Options for low-impact, aerobic training include stationary cycling, elliptical trainers, or aquatic exercise programs. Recent trials comparing structured physical therapy approaches in younger (mean age, 58 years) LSS patients demonstrated comparable improvement in walking tolerance, pain, and ODI scores with body weight–supported treadmill walking and cycling as the cardiovascular/aerobic component of a therapy program.[25,26] Other potential benefits of active aerobic exercise include improvement in depression, assistance with weight control, and opportunities for increased socialization (group exercise programs). Physical therapy programs must be tailored to individual circumstances to optimize compliance, particularly in older, frailer patients.

A lightweight lumbar corset that maintains a slight degree of lumbar flexion may offer some patients modest benefit. Prateepavanich and colleagues[27] noted improved treadmill walking distance and decreased pain in 21 patients with neurogenic claudication who were provided a lumbosacral corset.

Epidural Corticosteroid Injection

Epidural steroid injection (ESI) for spinal stenosis is directed at treatment of the presumed inflammatory reaction and edema present at the stenotic segment. Fluoroscopic guidance is strongly recommended for caudal, interlaminar, or transforaminal injection to ensure accurate needle placement. Renfrew et al.[28] demonstrated that nonfluoroscopically assisted injections were actually in the epidural space in only 62% of procedures performed by experienced physicians.

Whether ESI results in significant long-term improvement in patients with LSS is uncertain. A recent subgroup analysis of the Spine Patient Outcomes Research Trial (SPORT) found that ESIs were associated with less improvement at 4 years among all patients, whether treated nonoperatively or surgically.[29] Ng and colleagues[30] found no difference in pain or walking distance at 12-week follow-up between patients with LSS who received a single transforaminal, fluoroscopically guided ESI. A randomized trial comparing epidural steroid injections with epidural injections of lidocaine only in 400 patients with spinal stenosis found no difference in functional outcomes at 6 weeks.[31]

However, several case series using a multiple injection regimen in patients with LSS suggest that from one-third to two-thirds of patients may experience long-term improvement extending to almost 2 years. In a multiple-injection protocol, after an initial injection, an additional injection is performed only when severe symptoms recur. Botwin and colleagues[32] reported a prospective series of 34 patients with LSS treated with a multiple-injection protocol of transforaminal lumbar epidural steroid injections and followed for 12 months. Of the patients, 75% had at least a 50% improvement in pain scores, and 64% noted improvement in walking tolerance. The average number of injections per patient was 1.9. Hoogmartens and colleagues[33] reported that 32% of patients with severe pseudoclaudication defined by a walking distance of less than 100 m treated with multiple caudal injections reported good to excellent improvement in symptoms at an average follow-up of 23 months. In a more recent retrospective study of 140 patients with LSS treated with either fluoroscopically guided transforaminal or caudal ESI, Delport and colleagues reported that 32% of patients experienced pain relief at their 2-month follow-up after an average of 2.23 injections.[34] Of the patients, 53% reported improvement in their functional abilities.

Before an epidural injection, anticoagulants and antiplatelet agents, including NSAIDs and clopidogrel, are usually discontinued for approximately 1 week. In anticoagulated patients with severe comorbid cardiovascular disease with LSS who are not surgical candidates, this may be contraindicated, eliminating this nonoperative option. A relatively common adverse effect, transient headache, is seen in up to one-quarter of patients treated with epidural steroids.[35] More serious complications—including epidural abscess, meningitis, and spinal hematomas—are rare.[36]

Lumbar Spinal Stenosis: Evidence-Informed Approach to Management

Evidence-informed treatment of symptomatic lumbar stenosis rests on at least three principles derived from the recent clinical studies reviewed earlier:

1. Severity of symptoms rather than spinal canal dimensions should dictate aggressiveness of treatment because the correlation between spinal anatomy and symptoms is poor.
2. Surgical treatment offers patients with severe pain and functional impairment more rapid short-term improvement.
3. Because up to 70% of patients with LSS have a favorable untreated or medically treated long-term outcome and catastrophic neurologic deterioration is rare, most patients should be offered a trial of medical treatment.

For most individuals, an informed choice of initial medical or surgical treatment is influenced by severity of pain, functional status, comorbid medical conditions, and personal preference.

Choice of medical treatments is also influenced by severity of symptoms. A reasonable, evidence-informed approach in most patients begins with the least invasive options—physical therapy and gabapentin. Because of frailty or severe comorbid medical conditions, however, some persons may be unable to engage in even limited exercise programs. In such patients, a trial of bracing may be appropriate. For some severely limited nonsurgical patients, a rolling walker significantly improves walking distance and balance. Patients with a significant component of back pain in addition to pseudoclaudication may benefit from an analgesic. A trial of an epidural injection is reasonable in patients without contraindications whose leg pain has not responded to simpler meabat di sures. If the response to a single injection is significant and somewhat durable, a multiple-injection approach over time may be effective in some patients.

PEARLS

1. LSS is a clinical diagnosis. Most patients with radiographic stenosis do not exhibit symptoms of pseudoclaudication.
2. Most patients (70%) with LSS do well with nonoperative care without catastrophic neurologic decline.
3. Gabapentin may be superior to pure analgesics in treating the neuropathic pain of LSS.
4. Episodic epidural steroid injections may provide longer-term relief of pain with improved function in some patients with LSS.

PITFALLS

1. Imaging findings of LSS are found in up to 20% of persons without the clinical syndrome.
2. NSAIDs have not been shown superior to pure analgesics in LSS and pose a greater risk of adverse effects in this older population.
3. Frail, elderly LSS patients with severe comorbid medical conditions may be unable to engage in even limited trials of exercise-oriented physical therapy.

KEY POINTS

1. LSS is a clinical diagnosis. Radiographic stenosis is common in asymptomatic persons.
2. Though the diagnosis of LSS is based primarily on the history of neurogenic claudication, the physical examination is crucial in identifying alternative diagnoses that may mimic LSS, including hip disease and peripheral arterial disease.
3. The long-term (10-year) outcome of patients with LSS treated medically compares favorably with surgically treated patients.
4. For most patients with LSS, appropriate initial medical treatment includes physical therapy and gabapentin or a pure analgesic.
5. For most patients, an informed choice of initial medical or surgical treatment is influenced by severity of pain, functional status, comorbid medical conditions, and personal preference.

KEY REFERENCES

1. Watters WC, Baisden J, Gilbert TJ, et al. Degenerative lumbar spinal stenosis: an evidence-based clinical guideline for the diagnosis and treatment of degenerative lumbar spinal stenosis. *Spine J*. 2008;8:305-310.
   This current evidence-based review addresses key clinical questions regarding diagnosis and treatment of lumbar spinal stenosis.
2. Gazzi Macedo L, Hum A, Kuleba L, et al. Physical therapy interventions for degenerative lumbar spinal stenosis: a systematic review. *Phys Ther*. 2013;93:1646-1660.
   This is a comprehensive, current review of physical therapy options in patients with lumbar stenosis.
3. Delitto A, Piva SR, Moore CG, et al. Surgery versus nonsurgical treatment of lumbar spinal stenosis. A randomized trial. *Ann Intern Med*. 2015;162:465-473.
   This study compares surgical treatment with a well-conceived, consistent physical therapy approach.
4. Yaksi A, Ozgonenel B. The efficacy of gabapentin therapy in patients with lumbar canal stenosis. *Spine*. 2007;32:939-942.
   This is a rare study demonstrating efficacy of a pharmacologic therapy in patients with LSS.
5. Botwin KP, Gruber RD, Bouchlas CG, et al. Fluoroscopically guided lumbar transforaminal epidural steroid injections in degenerative lumbar stenosis. An outcome study. *Am J Phys Med Rehabil*. 2002;81:898-905.
   This small prospective study demonstrated benefit in the majority of patients treated with a multiple-injection protocol.

REFERENCES

1. Watters WC, Baisden J, Gilbert TJ, et al. Degenerative lumbar spinal stenosis: an evidence-based clinical guideline for the diagnosis and treatment of degenerative spinal stenosis. *Spine J*. 2008;8:305-310.
2. Boden SD, Davis DO, Dina TS, et al. Abnormal magnetic-resonance scans of the lumbar spine in asymptomatic subjects. A prospective investigation. *J Bone Joint Surg Am*. 1990;72A:403-408.
3. Geisser ME, Haig AJ, Tong HC, et al. Spinal canal size and clinical symptoms among persons diagnosed with lumbar spinal stenosis. *Clin J Pain*. 2007;23:780-785.
4. Chad DA. Lumbar spinal stenosis. *Neurol Clin*. 2007;25:407-418.
5. Katz JN, Dalgas M, Stucki G, et al. Degenerative lumbar spinal stenosis: diagnostic value of the history and physical examination. *Arthritis Rheum*. 1995;38:1236-1241.
6. Johnson EK, Rosen I, Uden A. The natural course of lumbar spinal stenosis. *Clin Orthop Relat Res*. 1992;279:82-86.
7. Malmivaara A, Slatis P, Heliovaara M, et al. Surgical or nonoperative treatment for lumbar spinal stenosis? A randomized controlled trial. *Spine*. 2007;32:1-8.
8. Weinstein JN, Tosteson TD, Lurie JD, et al. Surgical versus nonsurgical therapy for lumbar spinal stenosis. *N Engl J Med*. 2008;358:794-810.
9. Atlas SJ, Keller RB, Wu YA, et al. Long-term outcomes of surgical and nonsurgical management of lumbar spinal stenosis: 8 to 10 year results from the Maine Lumbar Spine Study. *Spine*. 2005;30:936-943.
10. Atlas SJ, Keller RB, Robson D, et al. Surgical and nonsurgical management of lumbar spinal stenosis. Four-year outcomes from the Maine Lumbar Spine Study. *Spine*. 2000;25:556-562.
11. Amundsen T, Weber H, Nordal HJ, et al. Lumbar spinal stenosis: conservative or surgical management? A prospective 10 year study. *Spine*. 2000;25:1424-1436.
12. Delitto A, Piva SR, Moore CG, et al. Surgery versus nonsurgical treatment of lumbar spinal stenosis. A randomized trial. *Ann Intern Med*. 2015;162:465-473.
13. Ammendolia C, Sturber KJ, Rok E, et al. Nonoperative treatment for lumbar spinal stenosis with neurogenic claudication. *Cochrane Database Syst Rev*. 2013;(8):CD010712.
14. American College of Rheumatology Ad Hoc Group on the Use of Selective and Nonselective Nonsteroidal Antiinflammatory Drugs. Recommendations for use of selective and nonselective nonsteroidal antiinflammatory drugs: an American College of Rheumatology White Paper. *Arthritis Rheum*. 2008;59:1058-1073.
15. Williams CM, Maher CG, Latimer J, et al. Efficacy of paracetamol for acute low-back pain: a double-blind, randomized controlled trial. *Lancet*. 2014;384:1586-1596.
16. Machado GC, Maher CG, Ferreira PH, et al. Efficacy and safety of paracetamol for spinal pain and osteoarthritis: systematic

review and meta-analysis of randomized placebo controlled trials. *BMJ*. 2015;350h:1225.
17. Gutthann SP, Garcia Rodriguez LA, Railford DS. Individual nonsteroidal anti-inflammatory drugs and other risk factors for upper gastrointestinal bleeding and perforation. *Epidemiology*. 1997;8:18-24.
18. Griffin MR, Yared RA, Ray WA. Nonsteroidal anti-inflammatory drugs and acute renal failure in elderly persons. *Am J Epidemiol*. 2000;151:488-496.
19. Bennett JS, Daugherty A, Herrington D, et al. The use of nonsteroidal anti-inflammatory drugs (NSAIDs): a science advisory from the American Heart Association. *Circulation*. 2005;111:1713-1716.
20. Schofferman J, Mazanec D. Evidence-informed management of chronic low back pain with opioid analgesics. *Spine J*. 2008;8:185-194.
21. Wong MC, Chung JW, Wong TK. Effects of treatments for symptoms of painful diabetic neuropathy: systematic review. *BMJ*. 2007;335:87.
22. Yaksi A, Ozgonenel L, Ozgonenel B. The efficacy of gabapentin therapy in patients with lumbar canal stenosis. *Spine*. 2007;32:939-942.
23. Kaye AD, Rivera Bueno F, Katalenich B, et al. The effects of gastroretentive gabapentin (Gralise) on spinal stenosis patients with radicular pain. *Pain Physician*. 2014;17:169-178.
24. Gazzi Macedo L, Hum A, Kuleba L, et al. Physical therapy interventions for degenerative lumbar spinal stenosis: a systematic review. *Phys Ther*. 2013;93:1646-1660.
25. Whitman JM, Flynn TW, Childs JD, et al. A comparison between two physical therapy treatment programs for patients with lumbar spinal stenosis. A randomized clinical trial. *Spine*. 2006;31:2541-2549.
26. Pua Y, Cong-Cong C, Kian-Chong L. Treadmill walking with body weight support is no more effective than cycling when added to an exercise program for lumbar spinal stenosis: a randomized controlled trial. *Aust J Physiother*. 2007;53:83-89.
27. Prateepavanich P, Thanapipatsiri S, Santisatisakul P, et al. The effectiveness of lumbosacral corset in symptomatic degenerative lumbar spinal stenosis. *J Med Assoc Thai*. 2001;84:572-576.
28. Renfrew DL, Moore TE, Kathol MH, et al. Correct placement of epidural steroid injections: fluoroscopic guidance and contrast administration. *AJNR Am J Neuroradiol*. 1991;12:1003-1007.
29. Radcliff K, Kepler C, Hilibrand A, et al. Epidural steroid injections are associated with less improvement in patients with lumbar spinal stenosis. *Spine*. 2013;38:279-291.
30. Ng L, Chaudhary N, Sell P. The efficacy of corticosteroids in periradicular infiltration for chronic radicular pain: a randomized, double-blind, controlled trial. *Spine*. 2005;30:857-862.
31. Friedly JL, Comstock BA, Turner JA, et al. A randomized trial of epidural glucocorticoid injections for spinal stenosis. *N Engl J Med*. 2014;371:11-21.
32. Botwin KP, Gruber RD, Bouchlas CG, et al. Fluoroscopically guided lumbar transforaminal epidural steroid injections in degenerative lumbar stenosis. An outcome study. *Am J Phys Med Rehabil*. 2002;81:898-905.
33. Hoogmartens M, Morelle P. Epidural injection in the treatment of spinal stenosis. *Acta Orthop Belg*. 1987;53:409-411.
34. Delport EG, Cucuzzella AR, Marley JK, et al. Treatment of lumbar spinal stenosis with epidural steroid injections: a retrospective outcome study. *Arch Phys Med Rehabil*. 2004;85:479-484.
35. Carette S, Leclaire R, Marcoux S, et al. Epidural corticosteroid injections for sciatica due to herniated nucleus pulposus. *N Engl J Med*. 1997;336:1634-1640.
36. Armon C, Argoff CE, Samuels J, Backonja MM. Assessment: use of epidural steroid injections to treat radicular lumbosacral pain. *Neurology*. 2007;68:723-729.

SECTION VIII

CHAPTER 63

Surgical Management of Lumbar Spinal Stenosis

Peter B. Derman
Jeffrey Rihn
Todd J. Albert

Indications for Surgery

Spinal stenosis is the most common reason for lumbar spine surgery in adults older than 65 years of age.[1] Lumbar stenosis occurs secondary to spondylotic changes at the facet joints and uncinate processes, spondylolisthesis, ligamentum flavum buckling or hypertrophy, disc herniations or bulging, and/or a congenitally narrow canal. Pathologic changes affect the central vertebral canal, lateral recess, and neural foramina (Fig. 63.1). Spondylotic lateral recess stenosis typically emanates from the superior articular process of the caudal vertebra. This compresses the traversing nerve root, leading to neurogenic claudication (e.g., overgrowth of the superior articular process of L5 produces stenosis at the L4–L5 level, which compresses the L5 nerve root; Fig. 63.2). Spinal stenosis does not necessarily worsen over time, and a substantial proportion of patients remain unchanged or even improved with nonoperative treatment.[2]

Proper patient selection is critical to achieving a good outcome with spinal stenosis surgery. Ultimately, patient desire combined with failure of conservative treatment (physical therapy, activity modification, medication, and steroid injections) drive the decision for operative treatment. The ideal patient has symptoms of neurogenic claudication, which include pain, numbness, and paresthesias in the posterolateral legs and thighs associated with prolonged walking or with activities that cause back extension (e.g., standing). Neurogenic claudication may also manifest as cramping or fatigue in the lower extremities. Activities such as sitting, leaning forward on a walker or shopping cart, and riding a bicycle typically alleviate the symptoms. It is important to rule out vascular claudication as a source of lower extremity symptoms.

Deen and colleagues[3] performed a review of patients with early failure after lumbar laminectomy and found that the most common presentation prior to the index procedure was an absence of classic symptoms of neurogenic claudication coupled with a lack of severe stenosis on imaging studies. Other authors have reported that surgical outcomes are significantly better in patients who preoperatively exhibited greater disability, predominant leg pain over low back pain, neuroforaminal stenosis, or a neurologic deficit; not lifting at work and not smoking have also been associated with better outcomes.[4–6] Selective nerve root blocks are good prognostic indicators of surgical outcome. Patients who obtain more than 50% relief of leg pain for at least 1 week after an injection tend to have greater relief of leg pain after surgery.[7] Additionally, those with long-standing symptoms (>12 months) are less likely to have a positive surgical outcome and are more likely to undergo reoperation.[7,8]

Surgical decompression can be performed on an elective basis unless the patient has a rapidly progressing neurologic deficit or bowel/bladder dysfunction, both of which are rare presentations of spinal stenosis. Before surgical intervention, we routinely obtain standing anteroposterior, lateral, and flexion-extension radiographs, as well as magnetic resonance imaging (MRI) or computed tomography (CT) myelogram. It is important to recognize that instability is a dynamic process that is most evident on flexion-extension radiographs and may not necessarily be apparent on static supine imaging. Although numerous surgical techniques have been described to treat lumbar stenosis, there currently is insufficient evidence to determine which is most effective.[9,10] Surgical options include decompressive laminectomy with or without fusion, laminotomy, minimally invasive decompression, and placement of an interspinous process device.

Laminectomy

Laminectomy has been the gold standard for the surgical treatment of central, lateral recess, and foraminal stenosis in the absence of instability.[10] After induction of anesthesia, the patient is positioned face down on an operating table. Surgeons can choose from several different positions (e.g., prone and kneeling) and support devices, each with its own set of advantages and disadvantages.[11,12] The Andrews frame, for instance, places the patient in a kneeling position, which has been shown to decrease vena caval and central venous pressures, leading to a reduction in blood loss when compared with a Cloward surgical saddle.[13,14] In addition, flexion of the hips reduces normal lumbar lordosis and widens the interlaminar space, making it easier to access the spinal canal. Use of a Wilson frame also allows for reduction of lumbar lordosis

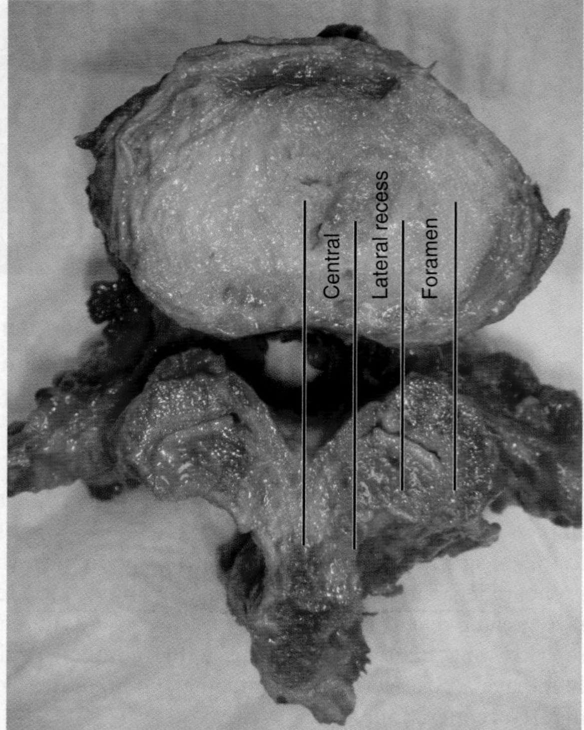

FIG. 63.1 Lumbar stenosis is anatomically categorized into compression within the central canal, lateral recess (subarticular), and neural foramina.

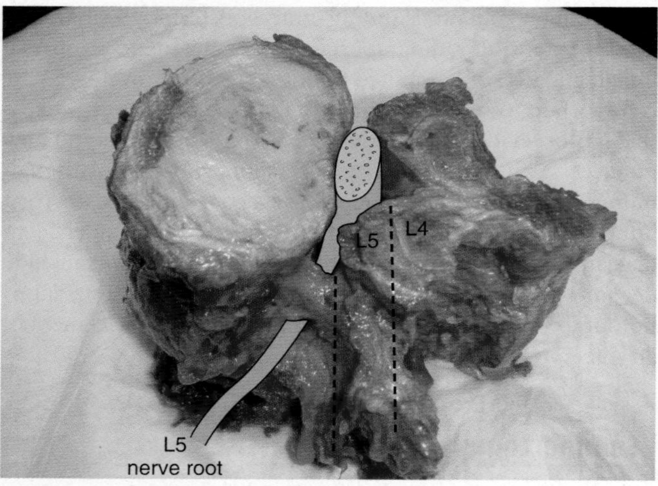

FIG. 63.2 Stenosis at the lateral recess leads to compression of the traversing nerve root by the superior articular process of the caudal vertebra (e.g., spondylosis at the L4–L5 level leads to compression of the L5 nerve root as it traverses the lateral recess before exiting the foramen).

during decompression, although not to the same degree as the Andrews frame. It is important to note that placing a patient in a kneeling position can lead the surgeon to underestimate the true degree of stenosis when compared to the lordotic position obtained on a flat Jackson table. Also, when performing a fusion in addition to a decompression on a lordosis-reducing frame, care must be taken to avoid the tendency to fuse the lumbar spine in a hypolordotic position. The Wilson frame can be used in the fully cranked position for the laminectomy and then uncranked for the final fusion to prevent arthrodesis in a nonlordotic position. Given the ease of use and more accurate portrayal of native lordosis, we prefer to use a flat Jackson table with bolsters as long as the patient can be supported with the abdomen hanging free. We believe that flexion of the knees with the use of pillows under the shins is also important because it has the potential to reduce tension on the sciatic nerve.

We routinely use ×2.5 or ×3.5 loupe magnification and an operating headlight. The relationship of the iliac crests to the lower lumbar levels on preoperative radiographs should be carefully examined to help guide placement of the incision. Using a scalpel, a standard midline skin incision is made over the desired levels. The incision should be long enough to allow for exposure of the pedicles of the cephalad and caudal levels to be decompressed. For example, an L3 to L5 pedicle-to-pedicle decompression requires enough exposure such that the inferior aspect of the L3 pedicle and the superior aspect of the L5 pedicle can be easily palpated at the end of the decompression. Dissection is carried down to the thoracolumbar fascia using electrocautery. The fascia should be clearly exposed approximately 1 cm off of midline with a Cobb elevator to ensure a distinct layer for fascial closure at the conclusion of the case. The spinous processes are easily palpated and can be used to fine-tune the fascial incision for exposure of the appropriate levels. Electrocautery is then used to dissect just lateral to the spinous processes, taking care to preserve the supraspinous and interspinous ligaments.

At this point, a Kocher clamp is placed on the cephalad aspect of one of the spinous processes so that the clamp is in line with the pedicle of interest. Alternatively, a Woodson elevator can be placed in the interlaminar space to mark the appropriate surgical level. An intraoperative radiograph that includes the Kocher clamp or Woodson elevator and the sacrum is then taken in order to confirm. This step is critical because, despite the potentially disastrous repercussions of wrong-level surgery, 50% of spine surgeons report performing at least one such case over the course of their careers, and 71% of the wrong-level cases occur in the lumbar spine.[15]

Once the correct levels are identified, subperiosteal dissection of the paraspinal muscles is carried laterally with a combination of a Cobb elevator and electrocautery, allowing for exposure of the spinous processes and lamina. During the dissection, the midlateral pars (MLP) must be clearly identified so that it can be used later as a landmark for bony resection (Fig. 63.3). As the dissection is carried out laterally, care should be taken to preserve the facet joint capsules, which lie superficial to the level of the lamina and MLP. It has been demonstrated in cadaveric models that excision of the capsule and cartilage of the facets results in increased motion in both the sagittal and axial planes, potentially leading to clinical instability.[16] For an isolated laminectomy, dissection should be carried out as far laterally as the lateral aspect of the facet capsule. Hemostasis with bipolar electrocautery is critical for visualization, particularly around the facet joint, where bleeding may occur from medial and lateral parafacetal arteries.[17] If a posterolateral fusion is planned, the dissection needs to extend laterally to the transverse processes, taking

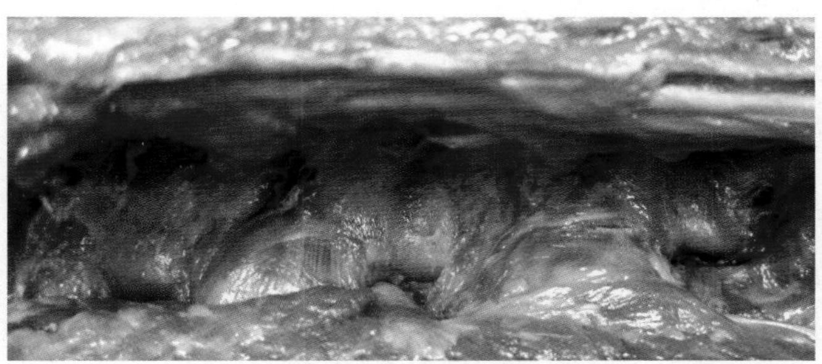

FIG. 63.3 Exposure for a laminectomy must include clear delineation of the midlateral pars at each level, as this landmark provides a guideline for the degree of final bony resection. Dissection should be taken out to the lateral aspect of the facet, taking care to preserve the facet capsule.

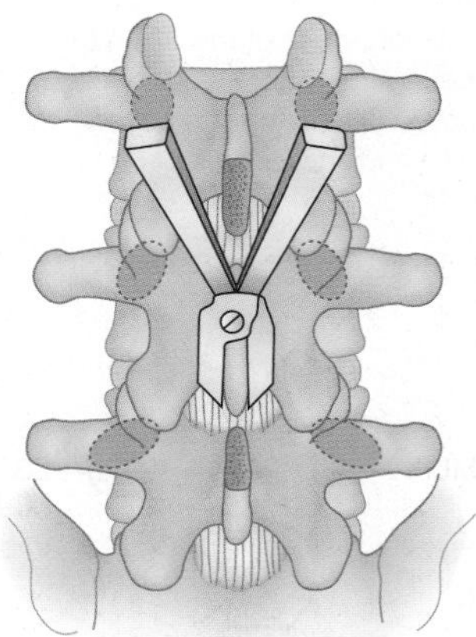

FIG. 63.4 Decompression begins by delineating the extent of bony resection with a rongeur. For an L3–L5 decompression, this includes the inferior half of the L3 spinous process and the superior half of the L5 spinous process (*shaded area*). A Horsley bone cutter is used to remove the intervening spinous processes down to the level of the spinous process/lamina junction.

care to maintain the integrity of the intertransverse membrane between each level.

The cephalad and caudal limits of the laminectomy are delineated with a Leksell rongeur. The inferior half of the spinous process at the cranial aspect of the decompression and the superior half of the spinous process of the most caudal aspect of the decompression are removed. Performing a laminectomy between these bounds is typically sufficient to permit palpation of the pedicles of the cephalad and caudal levels to be decompressed. A Horsley bone cutter is used to remove the intervening spinous processes (Fig. 63.4). These are resected down to the spinous process/laminar junction. The rongeur is then used to thin the lamina. Any bleeding from cancellous bone should be controlled with bone wax.

The decompression should begin centrally because the central zone is typically the least stenotic. The laminae of the lower spine have a much greater proportion of their anterior surface covered by the deep layer of the ligamentum flavum (Fig. 63.5).[18,19] A curette is used to dissect the underlying ligamentum flavum from the inferior aspect of the lamina (Fig. 63.6). A Kerrison punch is then used to remove bone from the inferior aspect of the lamina, using the ligamentum flavum as a protective layer. The decompression is carried cephalad until

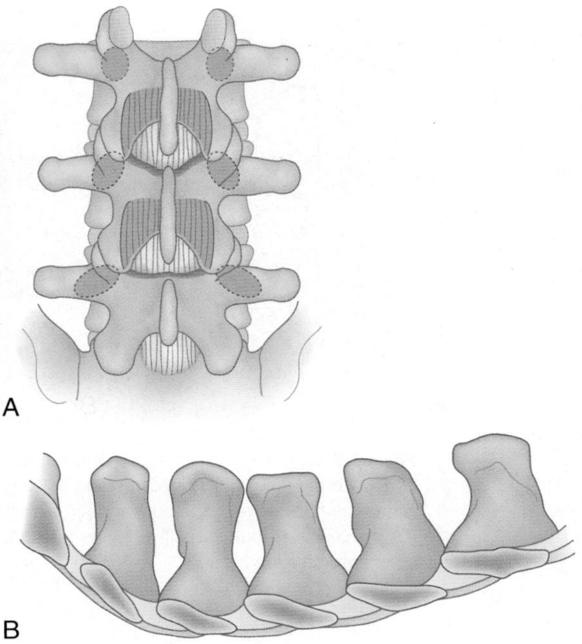

FIG. 63.5 (A) In general, the ligamentum flavum originates from halfway up the lamina of the cephalad level and inserts onto the superior aspect of the caudal lamina. (B) From the sagittal view, the laminae of the lower spine have a much greater proportion of their anterior surface covered by the deep layer of the ligamentum flavum. (From Olszewski AD, Yaszemski MJ, White AA III. The anatomy of the human lumbar ligamentum flavum. New observations and their surgical importance. *Spine.* 1996;21:2307–2312.)

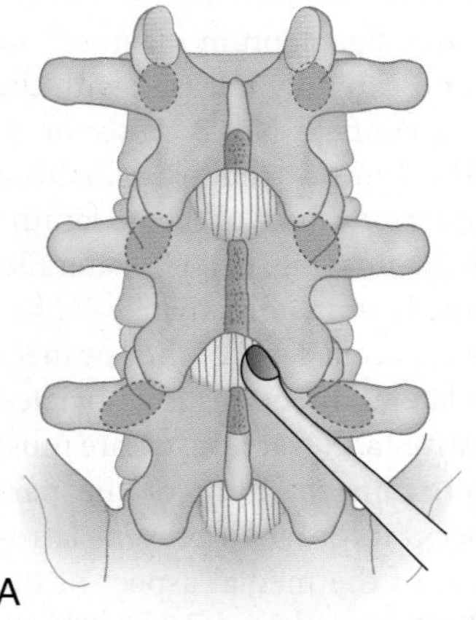

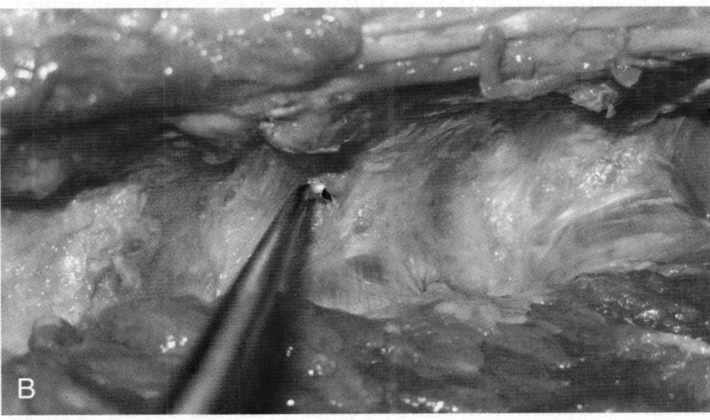

FIG. 63.6 A curette is used to dissect the underlying ligamentum flavum from the inferior aspect of the lamina.

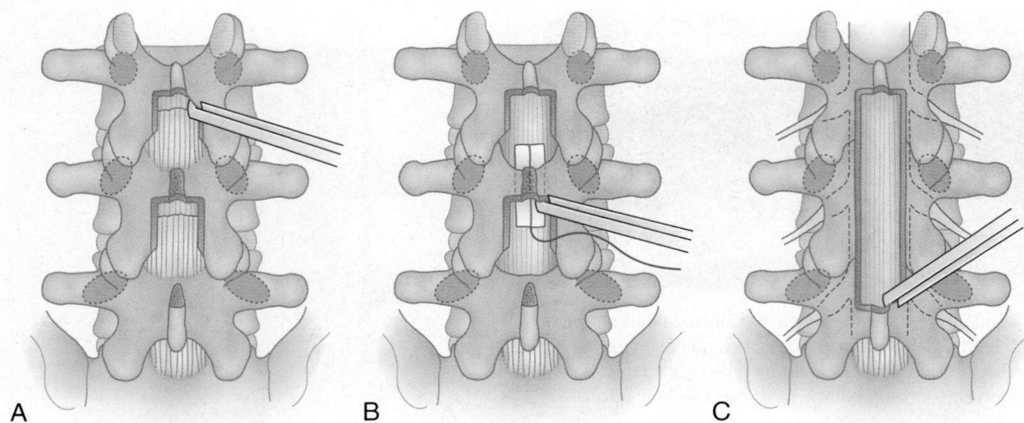

FIG. 63.7 (A) In an L3 to L5 decompression, we recommend beginning at the inferior aspect of the L4 lamina and, once the dura is identified, moving on to removing the inferior aspect of the L3 lamina. (B) A cottonoid is then placed between the dura and remaining L4 laminar bridge, which is removed with a Kerrison punch. (C) The central trough is finalized by removing the superior aspect of the L5 lamina and any residual ligamentum flavum.

the ligamentum flavum ends and epidural fat or dura is encountered. In our experience, this typically occurs at the level of the inferior aspect of the pedicle of the lamina being removed. In an L3 to L5 decompression, we recommend beginning at the inferior aspect of the L4 lamina and, once the dura is identified, moving on to removing the inferior aspect of the L3 lamina (Fig. 63.7A). A cottonoid is then placed between the dura and remaining L4 laminar bridge, which is removed with a Kerrison punch (Fig. 63.7B). Fibrous connections between the dura and the ligamentum flavum[20] or laminae[21] should be identified and carefully released with the use of a Woodson elevator or a Penfield No. 3 dissector to avoid inadvertent durotomy. The central trough is finalized with complete removal of the superior aspect of the L5 lamina and any remaining ligamentum flavum (Fig. 63.7C). Laterally, resection of more than 25% of the lamina immediately cephalad to the inferior articular process at the level of the laminectomy (measured in a medial to lateral direction) is associated with increased risk of postoperative facet fracture.[22] Care must also be taken to preserve approximately 1 cm of the pars interarticularis during this process in order to prevent iatrogenic pars fracture. The location of the medial aspect of the pedicle with respect to the MLP varies with each lumbar level. Su and colleagues[23] described the percentage of pedicle medial and lateral to the MLP and found that less pars remains when the decompression is carried out to the medial aspect of the pedicle in the more cephalad levels (Fig. 63.8). Particular caution should be taken at levels cephalad to L4 to not take too much of the lamina, leaving a narrow pars susceptible to fracture. As such, with a decompression from L2 to S1, the laminectomy should appear to be trapezoidal with a narrower laminectomy trough in the more cephalad levels and a wider trough in the more caudal levels.

The next step involves decompression of the lateral recesses. The most common technical error resulting in early failure after lumbar laminectomy is inadequate neural decompression[3]; thus, careful attention to the lateral recesses is critical.

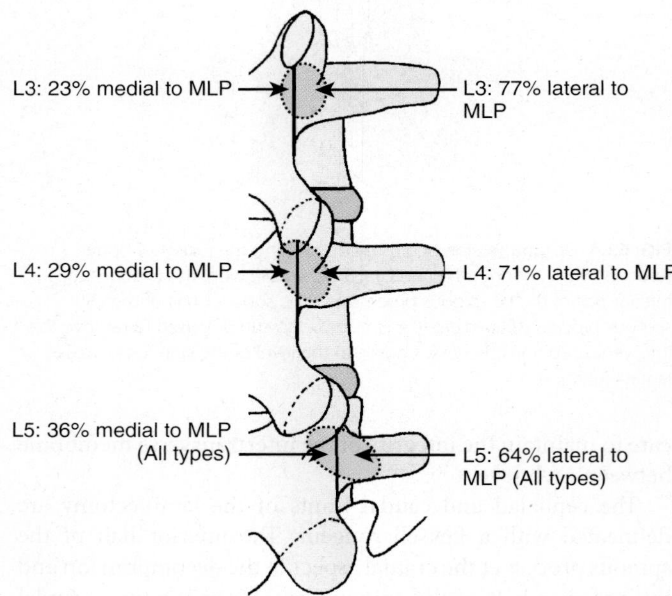

FIG. 63.8 At more cephalad levels, there is less distance between the medial pedicle to the midlateral pars (MLP). Particular caution should be taken at levels cephalad to L4 to not take too much of the lamina, leaving a narrow pars susceptible to fracture. As such, with a decompression from L2 to S1, the laminectomy should appear to be trapezoidal with a narrower laminectomy trough in the more cephalad levels and a wider trough in the more caudal levels. (From Su BW, Kim PD, Cha TD, et al. An anatomical study of the mid-lateral pars relative to the pedicle footprint in the lower lumbar spine. *Spine [Phila Pa 1976]*. 2009;34:1355–1362.)

A high-speed burr may be used cautiously to thin the lamina and delineate the area of bony resection. The surgeon must be particularly careful at the cephalad aspect of the lamina, where the cortical bone is thin and not protected by the ligamentum flavum. Lateral recess decompression is performed with a Kerrison punch (Fig. 63.9). Depending on the surgeon's experience, the medial aspect of the inferior facet can be removed

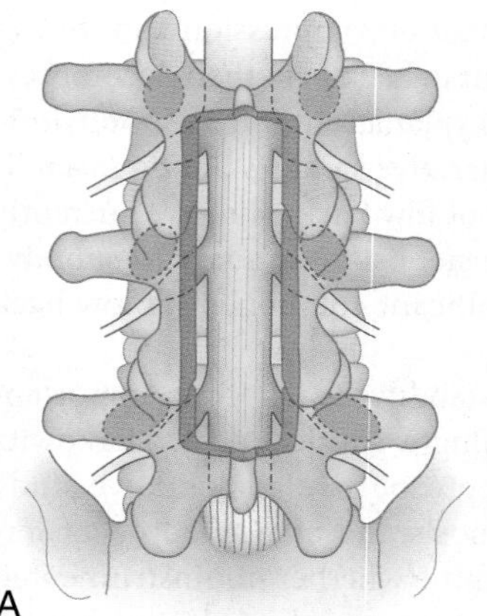

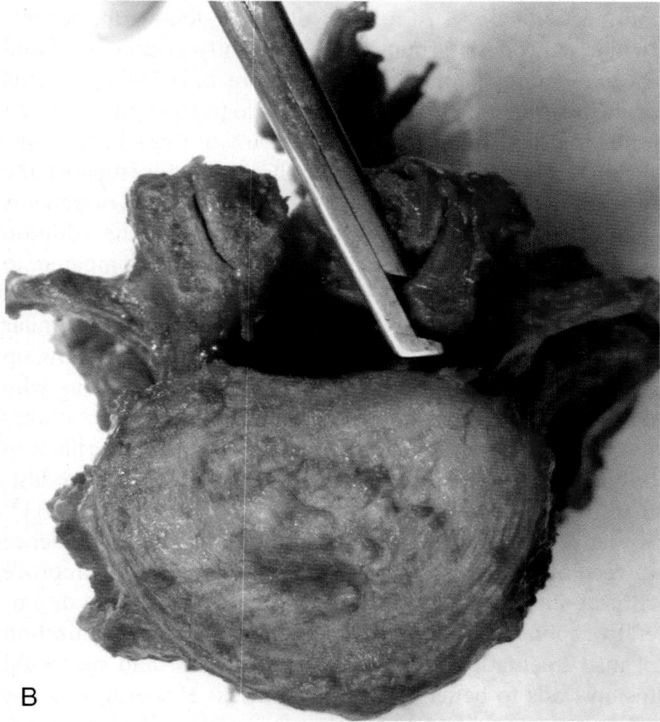

FIG. 63.9 (A) Lateral recess decompression is performed with a Kerrison punch and should preserve at least 50% of the facet joint (*axial view*). (B) Final decompression after undercutting the lateral recess.

using an osteotome, exposing the underlying superior facet. Undercutting the superior facet using a Kerrison punch assists in bone removal while preserving the facet joint and the pars interarticularis. Because of the angle of approach, this maneuver should be performed from the opposite side of the operating table to ensure complete visualization of the dura during the decompression. Decompression should progress laterally until the medial wall of the pedicle is easily palpated with a Woodson or angled dural elevator. Cadaveric studies have shown that decompression with even partial medial facetectomy results in measurable increases in segmental range of motion and decreases in stiffness.[24] In addition, postlaminectomy CT scans reveal that, on average, patients suffering from postoperative facet fracture had significantly more of the articular surface resected than those without fractures.[22] As such, we ensure that at least 50% of each facet joint is preserved to minimize postoperative instability. In the cranial-caudal dimension, the pedicles of the superior and inferior segments should be palpable. Decompression of the lateral recess often leads to bleeding from the epidural venous plexus. Hemostasis is obtained with the use of bipolar electrocautery and hemostatic agents, such as an absorbable gelatin sponge and cross-linked gelatin granules with topical human thrombin.

The last stage of the decompression involves foraminotomies at each level. Each nerve root should be traced as it passes underneath the pedicle and into the foramen. Any compressing bone or soft tissue is removed with a Kerrison punch placed dorsal and parallel to the root as it exits the foramen. In the presence of exit-zone stenosis, bony spurs from the dorsal and lateral aspect of the superior facet should be resected. As in lateral recess decompression, this should be performed from the contralateral side to prevent iatrogenic durotomy of the nerve root sleeve. A Woodson elevator or Murphy probe is used to assess the decompression by passing it into the foramen dorsal to the nerve root; a 4-mm ball tip probe should pass without difficulty.[25] The nerve root can also be assessed for mobility by gently retracting the dural sac and nerve root medially into the canal with a Penfield No. 4 dissector. The nerve should demonstrate 1 cm of medial displacement if adequately decompressed.[25] At the end of the decompression, any sharp spikes of bone should be smoothed with a curette or a Kerrison punch to prevent them from lacerating the dura. Finally, each level should be examined for an extruded herniated disc fragment, which should then be removed in a routine manner. We do not recommend a discectomy for well-contained discs. Before closure, hemostasis is once again obtained, and the wound is irrigated. We routinely place a 15-Fr fully fluted Blake drain in the deep wound. The fascia is closed with interrupted figure-of-eight No. 1 absorbable sutures. The subcutaneous tissue is closed with buried 2-0 absorbable sutures, and the skin is closed with a nonlocked running 3-0 nylon suture or 3-0 absorbable subcuticular suture.

Outcomes of Laminectomy

The evidence to support surgical decompression for the treatment of patients with symptomatic lumbar stenosis has been mounting, with evidence-based guidelines now finding sufficient data to recommend operative intervention for moderate to severe lumbar stenosis when nonoperative modalities have failed.[26] The largest and most well-known study addressing this subject, the Spine Patient Outcomes Research Trial (SPORT), was a multicenter randomized controlled trial with a concurrent observational cohort that evaluated the surgical treatment of conditions associated with low back and leg pain, including lumbar stenosis.[27] In 2008, the 2-year outcomes of the SPORT study evaluating laminectomy versus conservative treatment for lumbar stenosis were reported.[28] All patients who had a history of at least 12 weeks of symptomatic lumbar stenosis without spondylolisthesis were considered surgical candidates. A total of 289 patients were enrolled in the randomized cohort, and 365 patients were enrolled in the observational cohort. By 2-year follow-up, however, 43% of those who were randomly assigned to receive nonsurgical care underwent surgery (compared to 67% of the patients randomly assigned to the operative group). Despite the high incidence of crossover, intention-to-treat analysis revealed a significant treatment effect favoring surgery on the Short-Form 36 General Health Survey (SF-36) scale for bodily pain. However, there were no significant differences in scores on the SF-36 scale for physical function or on the modified Oswestry Disability Index (ODI). The as-treated analysis, which included the randomized and observational cohorts, showed a significant advantage for surgery compared with nonoperative treatment by 3 months for the ODI and both SF-36 components. These changes remained significant for all subsequent time points in the 2-year duration of the study. At 2-year follow-up, on the basis of the as-treated analysis, 63% of patients treated surgically rated themselves as having major improvement with their condition versus 29% of the group treated nonoperatively.[28]

The long-term outcomes of the SPORT study were published in 2015.[29] At 8-year follow-up, no significant differences remained between randomized cohorts in intent-to-treat analysis. By this point, however, 52% of those randomized to nonoperative care had undergone surgery, which began to approach the 70% of patients in the operative group who actually underwent surgery. As-treated analysis of the randomized group showed that the benefit of surgery diminished over time and was not significant after 5 years. However, the significantly better early outcomes (SF-36 bodily pain and physical function, ODI) associated with surgery in the observational group were maintained out to 8 years. These results suggest that laminectomy for symptomatic degenerative spinal stenosis provides significant improvements in function, pain, and disability, but that these effects likely diminish to some degree over the long term. From a financial standpoint, comparative effectiveness analysis of the SPORT data shows that, even over a 4-year horizon, laminectomy for spinal stenosis produces good value compared to nonoperative care with a cost per quality-adjusted life year (QALY) gained of $59,400 in 2004 dollars[30] (approximately $74,400 in 2015 dollars).

Arthrodesis After Laminectomy

Some authors have recommended that arthrodesis be performed when stenosis is associated with spondylosis and substantial low back pain or with instability.[31,32] Grob and colleagues[33] randomized 45 patients with lumbar spinal stenosis (LSS) without instability to receive decompression with and without arthrodesis. Instability was defined as greater than 5 mm of motion between segments in the sagittal plane or greater than 5 mm of lateral offset in the coronal plane. All patients had significant clinical improvement compared with preoperative values at an average of 28-month follow-up with no significant differences between fusion and nonfusion groups. These results suggest that, in the absence of instability, decompression with care taken to not destabilize the spine does not necessitate an arthrodesis. However, authors of a more recent retrospective review of 50 elderly patients with LSS without instability found that decompression with fusion resulted in greater improvement in back pain than decompression alone.[34] The most likely explanation is that spondylotic changes in patients with degenerative stenosis but no instability contribute to a component of low back pain. We currently do not fuse patients who have stenosis secondary to spondylosis unless they exhibit a significant component of low back pain.

As mentioned earlier, instability is another important factor to consider when creating a surgical plan. Herkowitz and colleagues[35] performed a prospective comparative study of 50 patients with spinal stenosis and associated degenerative spondylolisthesis to determine whether noninstrumented arthrodesis produced better outcomes than decompressive laminectomy alone. At a mean of 3-year follow-up, patients in the arthrodesis group had significantly greater back and lower extremity pain relief. Furthermore, only 28% of patients in the fusion group experienced slip progression after surgery, while the slip distance increased in 96% of those in the nonfusion group. Fischgrund and colleagues[36] investigated the effects of instrumentation in a randomized study of patients with spondylolisthesis and stenosis. Although the addition of instrumentation increased the fusion rate compared to noninstrumented arthrodesis (82% vs. 45%) in the 67 patients available for 2-year follow-up, clinical outcomes were similar between the groups.[36] However, longer-term follow-up (average, 7 years, 8 months) of the cohort of patients who underwent noninstrumented fusion from these two studies revealed that clinical outcomes were significantly more likely to be good or excellent in patients who achieved solid arthrodesis than in those with a pseudarthosis (86% vs. 56%, $P = .01$).[37] Evidence-based guidelines have not found sufficient evidence to recommend the addition of instrumentation to improve clinical outcomes in patients with spinal stenosis and degenerative spondylolisthesis[32] despite the findings that utilization of instrumentation increases rates of fusion[36] and successful fusion leads to better clinical outcomes.[37] However, it is our current practice to perform arthrodesis with pedicular fixation along with decompressive laminectomy if there is associated instability at the involved motion segments (>5 mm), degenerative scoliosis (curve progression or >30 degrees), revision decompression at the same level, or resection of greater than 50% of the facet joints.[17]

The cost per QALY gained with surgical treatment of spinal stenosis with degenerative spondylolisthesis has been calculated for patients in the SPORT study at $64,300 in 2004 dollars over a 4-year postoperative time frame[30] (or approximately $80,500 in 2015 dollars). This figure is about 8% higher than that reported for isolated spinal stenosis.[30] The fact that patients without spondylolisthesis tended to undergo decompression alone while those with stenosis and spondylolisthesis typically underwent fusion as well (which carries a higher upfront surgical cost) likely contributed to this difference. The value of surgical treatment of spinal stenosis with degenerative spondylolisthesis may improve with longer-term follow-up, assuming that the observed improvements in quality of measures are lasting and that the need for additional treatment and revision surgery is minimal.

Laminotomy

In patients with primarily lateral recess stenosis, laminotomy (or laminoforaminotomy) is an alternative to laminectomy. Laminotomy involves performing a decompression through a microdiscectomy-like approach to target the stenotic levels either unilaterally or bilaterally. Only the caudal aspect of the superior lamina and the cephalad portion of the inferior lamina at the stenotic level are resected, leaving the spinous process and interspinous and supraspinous ligaments intact.[10] This is performed via a unilateral approach for unilateral pathology, while bilateral stenosis can be addressed either via bilateral approaches or through a unilateral approach for bilateral decompression (Fig. 63.10).[10] Advocates argue that leaving the midline structures intact decreases the chance of iatrogenic instability and back pain.[38,39] Others believe that little additional stability is gained by performing multiple laminotomies compared to a facet-sparing laminectomy because the majority of stability is provided by the intervertebral disc and the facet–joint capsule complex.[38]

Gurelik and colleagues[40] performed a randomized trial comparing unilateral laminotomy for bilateral decompression to laminectomy for the treatment of lumbar stenosis in 52 patients split evenly between groups. Average follow-up was 9.1 months. While maximal walking distance and ODI scores improved in both groups, the authors observed no statistically significant difference between the groups in the magnitude of these effects. They did find that laminectomy resulted in a significantly larger increase in dural sac area than laminotomy. Postoperative instability occurred in five of the laminectomy patients and none of the laminotomy patients; however, unilateral total facetectomy was performed in 27% of patients in the laminectomy group and none of those in the laminotomy cohort.

Thomé and colleagues[41] compared bilateral laminotomy, unilateral laminotomy for bilateral decompression, and conventional laminectomy for lumbar stenosis. Forty patients were randomized to each group, and the mean follow up was 15.5 months. Bilateral laminotomy resulted in a significantly lower complication rate than laminectomy (5.0% vs. 22.5%, $P < .05$) but did not differ significantly from unilateral laminotomy (17.5%). Dural tear was the most common complication in all groups. While all three techniques produced highly significant symptomatic and functional improvement (e.g., visual analog [VAS], SF-36, walking distance, patient satisfaction scores), bilateral laminotomy demonstrated the best overall outcomes, with unilateral laminotomy and laminectomy providing similar results.

Celik and colleagues[42] conducted a randomized trial comparing bilateral laminotomy to conventional laminectomy. Each group had 40 patients, and average follow-up was 5 years. Postoperative CT and MRI demonstrated adequate decompressions in both groups. The laminectomy groups suffered from significantly more perioperative complications and postoperative instability, and there was a nonsignificant trend toward superior walking distance, pain control, and disability scores in the laminotomy group.

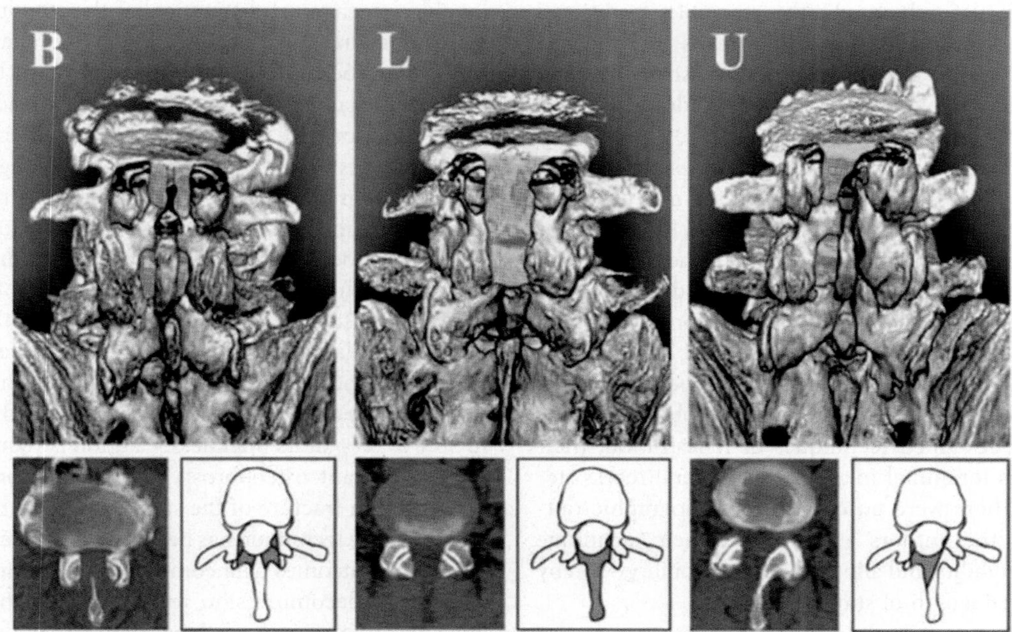

FIG. 63.10 *Top,* Postoperative three-dimensional reconstructions of lumbar computed tomographic (CT) scans following bilateral laminotomy (*B*), laminectomy (*L*), and unilateral laminotomy for bilateral decompression (*U*). In each technique, different osseous windows are created to access the spinal canal (*yellow*). *Bottom,* Axial postoperative CT scans and corresponding illustrations demonstrating the surgical corridors (*gray*). (From Thomé C, Zevgaridis D, Leheta O, et al. Outcome after less-invasive decompression of lumbar spinal stenosis: a randomized comparison of unilateral laminotomy, bilateral laminotomy, and laminectomy. *J Neurosurg Spine.* 2005;3[2]:129–141.)

In similar study performed by Fu and colleagues,[43] 152 patients were evenly randomized between bilateral laminotomy and conventional laminectomy. Functional outcomes were evaluated at approximately 40 months postoperatively. A total of 89% of the patients in the laminotomy group and 63% of the patients in the laminectomy group had good to excellent results, suggesting that a laminotomy can lead to good long-term results with few complications.

These studies and several others were synthesized in a 2015 Cochrane review, which was able to draw a limited number of conclusions based on the existing data.[10] The authors concluded that bilateral laminotomy resulted in better perceived recovery at final follow-up than laminectomy. Unilateral laminotomy for bilateral decompression and bilateral laminectomy led to lower rates of iatrogenic instability than conventional laminectomy (although the rates were low in all groups). There was a clinically small but statistically significant difference in the severity of postoperative low back pain favoring bilateral laminotomy over laminectomy. However, there was insufficient evidence to show a difference in complications, procedure length, length of hospital stay, or postoperative walking distance between techniques. It is our recommendation that a less invasive unilateral or bilateral laminoforaminotomy is a reasonable option in one- or two-level lateral recess stenosis without significant central stenosis.

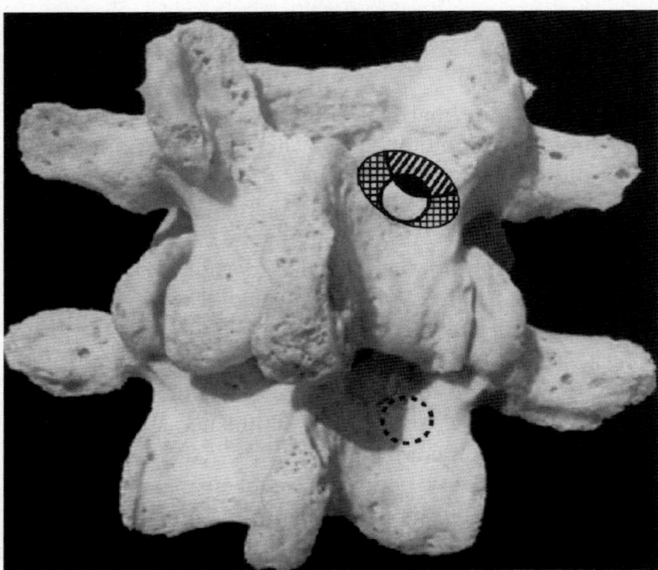

FIG. 63.11 Fenestration technique. A view of the lower lumbar spine showing the position of the laminal fenestration in relation to the superior articular facet. The *dotted circle* is the laminal fenestration. *Solid shading* is the portion of the pedicle drilled away through the hole. *Diagonal lines* represent the part of the pedicle undercut through the hole. *Hatched lines* represent the amount of laminal undercutting through the hole. (From Shenouda EF, Gill SS. Laminal fenestration for the treatment of lumbar nerve root foraminal stenosis. *Br J Neurosurg.* 2002;16:494–496.)

Fenestration

The use of fenestration to treat stenosis has been described in multiple reports but with notable variability in surgical techniques, many of which closely resemble traditional laminotomy.[44–49] While the nomenclature is nonspecific, these procedures aim to preserve the midline structures and minimize soft tissue and bony resection while addressing sites of neurologic compression.

Shenouda and Gill[46] described a unique fenestration technique that involves decompression through a 5-mm drill hole in the pars interarticularis immediately below the superior facet. The hole exposes the inferior aspect of the pedicle and the nerve root in the foramen. Using a 2-mm diamond drill bit through an operating microscope, the inferior aspect of the superior pedicle is drilled away, and the dorsal aspect of the nerve root is decompressed by undercutting the lamina and hypertrophied facet (Fig. 63.11). The authors note that, unlike other previously described techniques of fenestration, their method addresses foraminal in addition to lateral recess stenosis. Although there were no clinical or radiographic outcomes reported, the authors suggest that their technique preserves spinal stability and allows for early mobility, thereby shortening hospital length of stay.[46]

Laminoplasty

Distraction laminoplasty and expansive lumbar laminoplasty are two alternatives to standard laminectomy. Distraction laminoplasty is a technique for decompression of central and lateral recess stenosis with minimal bony resection. This method, formally described by O'Leary and colleagues,[50] involves mechanical distraction of the stenotic interspace to facilitate spinal canal access. Similar to a standard laminectomy, the procedure begins with removal of the inferior half of the cephalad vertebra's spinous process and lamina as well as the superior edge of the caudal vertebra. Distraction is then applied across the spinous processes of the segments, opening the interlaminar working space by mobilizing the cephalad lamina proximally and the caudad lamina distally (Fig. 63.12). The motion occurs through the facet joints and disc, and the increase in interlaminar space (typically 1 cm) allows for improved visualization. After removal of the ligamentum flavum, the lateral recesses are decompressed by removing 10% to 20% of the facet joint in a tapered fashion. The undersurface of the cephalad lamina is then thinned from inside out to 30% to 50% of its thickness. Caution is required in patients with significant osteoporosis in whom vigorous distraction may result in fracture of the spinous process or laminar edge. Although the technique has been well described, there is a lack of clinical outcomes data comparing distraction laminoplasty with other decompression techniques. In the setting of an open decompression, we have found that use of a laminar spreader between the spinous processes tenses the dura, making neural decompression easier and decreasing the chance of dural violation.

Expansive lumbar laminoplasty is a technique developed by Tsuji and colleagues[51] that aims to provide osteoplastic enlargement of the spinal canal while retaining spinal stability in the treatment of spinal stenosis. The technique is analogous to cervical laminoplasty, and involves opening one side of the lamina by using the contralateral side as a hinge (Fig. 63.13). Bone grafts from excised spinous processes are placed in the opened laminae and fixed with braided wire or nylon suture. The original developers of the technique reported the outcomes of 54 patients undergoing expansive lumbar laminoplasty with an average follow-up of 5.5 years.[52] Average intraoperative blood loss was higher and operative time longer than that typical of standard laminectomy. At final follow-up, the average Japanese Orthopaedic Association (JOA) score had improved significantly compared to preoperative baselines. Patients aged 56 years or older had significantly less improvement than those aged 55 years or younger. Nine patients had worsening of their JOA scores, seven of whom developed lesions at adjacent levels. Five patients developed new spondylolisthesis at an adjacent level. Interlaminar fusion was observed in 43% of patients, and range of motion was reduced to 58% of the preoperative range in those who avoided interlaminar fusion. The authors concluded that these results were "satisfactory" and suggested that the best indications for the procedure were young and active patients with isolated central spinal stenosis.

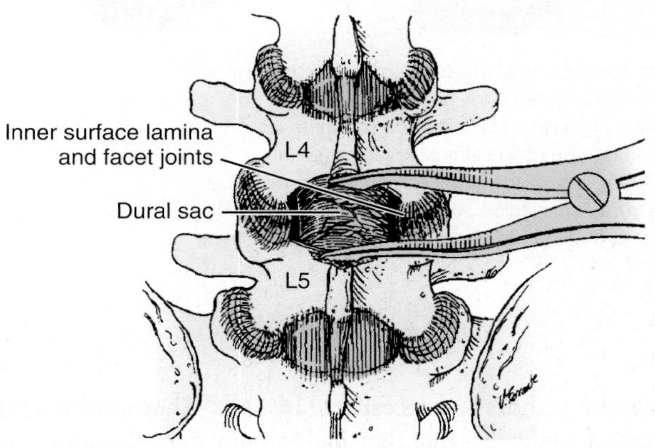

FIG. 63.12 Distraction laminoplasty. Distraction is applied across the spinous processes of the segments. This expands the interlaminar working space by mobilizing the cephalad lamina proximally and the caudal lamina distally. The lamina is then undercut to address the stenosis. (From O'Leary PF, McCance SE. Distraction laminoplasty for decompression of lumbar spinal stenosis. *Clin Orthop Relat Res.* 2001;384:26-34.)

Sangwan and colleagues[53] performed a review of 25 patients who underwent expansive lumbar laminoplasty with follow-up ranging from 3 to 5 years. Patients experienced an average enlargement in anteroposterior spinal canal diameter of 124% (as measured on CT scan), and 22 had good or excellent results. However, because of the inability of this operation to fully address lateral recess stenosis, mediocre clinical outcomes, and the high interlaminar fusion rate, we do not currently employ this procedure for the treatment of lumbar stenosis.

Microendoscopic Decompressive Laminotomy

Many authors have advocated the concept of minimally invasive decompression, which involves decompression of the neural elements through a smaller skin incision with preservation of soft tissue and bony anatomy. Although procedures such as laminotomy and fenestration are considered less

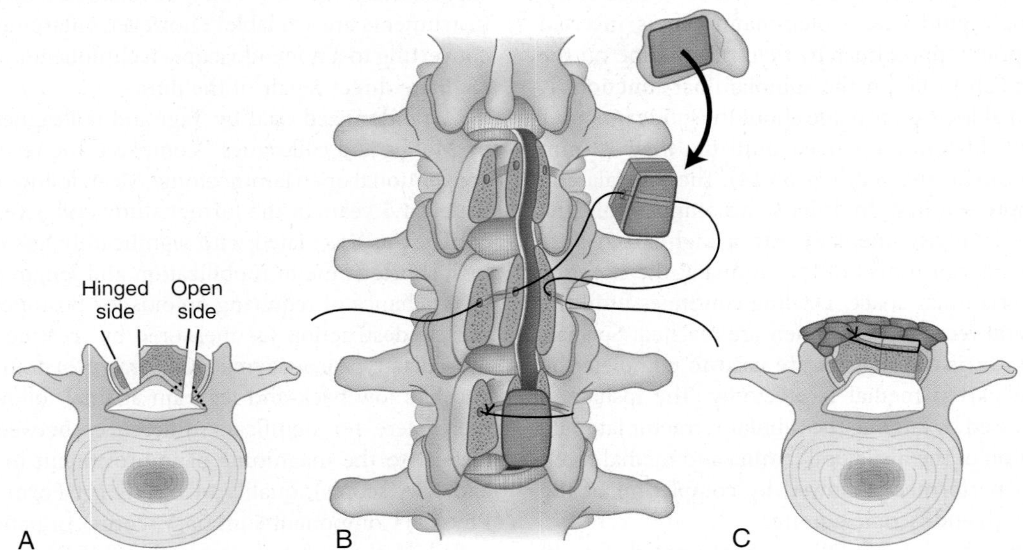

FIG. 63.13 Expansive lumbar laminoplasty technique. (A) After the spinous process is removed, a high-speed burr is used to make a groove in either side of the lamina. One groove extends completely through the lamina, while the other is incomplete. (B) The lamina is hinged open through the site of the incomplete groove and held open with autograft from the excised spinous processes. These are secured with a wire or suture. (C) This increases the cross-sectional area of the spinal canal. Additional bone graft is packed dorsally over the osteotomy sites. (From Kawaguchi Y, Kanamori M, Ishihara H, et al. Clinical and radiographic results of expansive lumbar laminoplasty in patients with spinal stenosis. *J Bone Joint Surg Am.* 2005;87[Suppl 1, Pt 2]:292–299.)

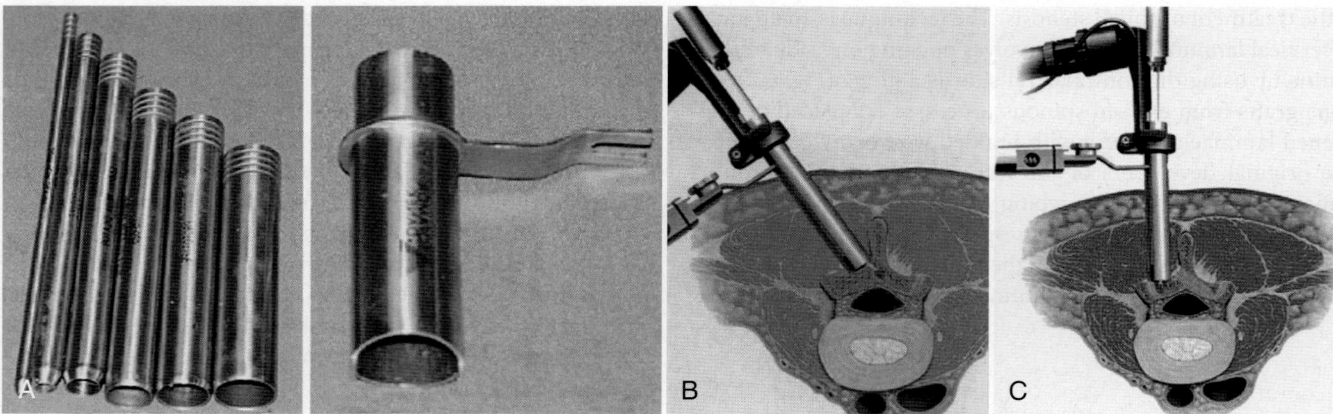

FIG. 63.14 Bilateral decompression through a unilateral microscopic decompressive laminotomy approach. (A) METRx sequential soft tissue dilators and 18-mm working channel with retractor. (B) Medial angulation of the retractor tube ensures optimal visualization of the spinolaminar junction and facilitates a proper trajectory for drilling of the anterior aspect of the lamina. Drilling continues until the contralateral lateral recess and foramen are reached. (C) The tubular retractor is then angled laterally toward the ipsilateral lamina–medial facet junction, and decompression is performed on this side as well. (From Asgarzadie F, Khoo LT. Minimally invasive operative management for lumbar spinal stenosis: overview of early and long-term outcomes. *Orthop Clin North Am* 2007;38:387–399.)

invasive than conventional laminectomy, the term "minimally invasive" has been tied to microendoscopic decompression by surgeons, patients, and industry. Microendoscopic decompressive laminotomy (MEDL) was first investigated in a 2002 cadaveric study that used postdecompression CT scans to demonstrate that endoscopic techniques could be used to achieve equivalent bony resection compared to open decompression.[54] Asgarzadie and Khoo[55] described a surgical technique for bilateral decompression through a unilateral MEDL approach using the METRx system (Medtronic). Under fluoroscopic guidance, a Steinmann pin is inserted from a starting point approximately 3 cm off midline on the side of the approach to lie on the spinolaminar junction. A 2.5-cm longitudinal incision is made about the guide pin, over which a series of dilators are passed until the final 18-mm tubular retractor can be inserted (Fig. 63.14). The contralateral lamina is decompressed first. In order to accomplish this, the tubular retractor is angled medially and a high-speed burr used to drill the anterior aspect of the lamina at the superior aspect of the interlaminar space. Drilling continues until the contralateral lateral recess and foramen are reached. Specialized endoscopic Kerrison rongeurs are used to complete the laminotomy and partial medial facetectomy. The ipsilateral side is then addressed by angling the tubular retractor laterally toward the junction of the ipsilateral lamina and medial facet. Drilling is again performed, followed by completion of the decompression with endoscopic curettes.

Four-year outcomes of MEDL were presented for 48 patients with lumbar central and/or lateral recess stenosis but no instability or deformity.[55] Of the patients, 80% had an increase in walking endurance, and 88% of patients reported an improvement in symptoms. There were no cases of neurologic injury or subsequent instability requiring fusion. The rate of dural violations (4%) was notably less than that reported by the same authors 5 years earlier (16%).[55,56] They attributed this decrease to the fact that they had initially been decompressing the ipsilateral side first, which they believe increased the risk of dural tears because unprotected dura was exposed while subsequently drilling the contralateral side.[55] For procedures in which a cerebrospinal fluid leak was encountered, direct repair was difficult secondary to the small surgical working field. The authors used fibrin glue or fat and muscle grafts to tamponade small leaks rather than attempt direct repair. They suggest that large leaks could be repaired if special endoscopic instruments are available[55]; however, enlarging the incision or converting to a nonendoscopic technique may be necessary to facilitate direct repair of the dura.

A randomized trial by Yagi and colleagues[57] and another by Mobbs and colleagues[58] compared the results of MEDL to conventional open laminectomy. Mean follow-up was approximately 1.5 years in the former study and 3 years in the latter. MEDL was associated with significantly less operative blood loss, shorter time to mobilization and length of hospital stay, lower chance of requiring opioids for postoperative pain, less muscle destruction (as measured by creatine phosphokinase muscular-type isoenzyme levels drawn 24 hours after surgery), and less low back and leg pain at final follow-up. However, there were no significant differences between groups with respect to the magnitude of improvement in function (ODI and JOA scores), quality of life (Short-Form 12 Mental and Physical Component Summary scores), or patient satisfaction.

While these data suggest that MEDL produces comparable outcomes to open laminectomy, potentially with less perioperative morbidity, there is a learning curve for all new techniques, and it is essential to become closely familiar with the endoscopic system and anatomy by performing the procedure in cadaveric specimens before attempting it in a clinical setting.

Interspinous Process Devices

Interspinous process (ISP) devices distract the spinous processes. This causes relative kyphosis of the instrumented segment, which stretches the infolded ligamentum flavum to achieve indirect canal decompression. Additionally, longitudinal distraction between two vertebrae increases the neuroforaminal dimensions, resulting in indirect decompression of the exiting nerve roots. Richards and colleagues[59] used MRI to quantify the spinal canal and neural foramina dimensions of cadaveric lumbar spines before and after placement of an ISP device. During extension, the implant increased the canal area by 18% and the foraminal area by 25%.[59] Clinically, positional MRIs performed on patients before and 6 months after implantation of an ISP device demonstrated that, in extension, the left and right foramina increased by 34.2% and 25.4%, respectively; the dural sac area increased by 20% in standing and 16.3% in neutral.[60]

There are two categories of ISP spacers: static and dynamic. Static devices are available in a variety of different noncompressible materials that maintain a constant amount of distraction between spinous processes.[61] For instance, the X-STOP device (Medtronic) is composed of an oblong central core that is stabilized by two lateral wings (Fig. 63.15). It is inserted as two components that are fixed to each other to straddle the interspinous region (Fig. 63.16). The device is composed of titanium so that it is compatible with postoperative MRI. Because static implants have a tendency to fit tighter when the lumbar spine is positioned in extension than flexion, some static devices include features intended to supplement fixation.[61] The Wallis ISP device (Zimmer Biomet), for example, has polyester bands that encircle the spinous processes on either end of the device to more broadly distribute the distraction forces during flexion. Alternatively, dynamic ISP devices, which compress during extension and expand during flexion, have been developed.[61] These include the Coflex device (Paradigm Spine), an axially compressible U-shaped titanium component, and the DIAM (Device for Intervertebral Assisted Motion; Medtronic), which is composed of silicone and polyester and acts as a rubbery spacer between the spinous processes.

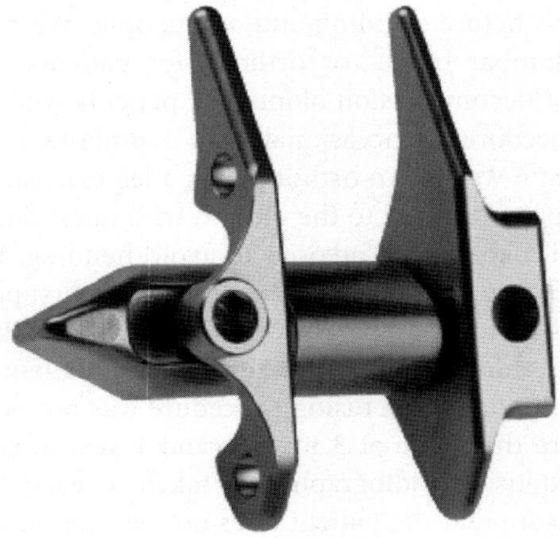

FIG. 63.15 The X-STOP device is a titanium spacer composed of an oblong central core stabilized by two lateral wings that straddle the interspinous region. (From Bono CM, Vaccaro AR. Interspinous process devices in the lumbar spine. *J Spinal Disord Tech.* 2007;20:255–261.)

ISP spacers are not recommended for use in patients with low bone mineral density. These individuals may not have sufficiently strong bone stock to support these devices and may suffer intraoperative or postoperative fractures.[61–64] Talwar and colleagues[65] performed a cadaveric biomechanical study utilizing the X-STOP spacer and found that the lateral force necessary to place the device averaged 66 N (range, 11–150 N), and the lateral force necessary to fracture the spinous process averaged 317 N (range, 95–786 N). While these means were statistically significantly different, there was some overlap in the ranges such that the greatest insertion force was sufficient to break the weakest spinous process. Furthermore, there was a significant positive correlation between bone mineral density and failure force. Idler and colleagues[66] attempted to address this issue by developing a technique for augmenting the spinous processes of osteoporotic patients with polymethylmethacrylate (PMMA) in order to decrease the risk of ISP device-related fracture. After injecting osteoporotic cadaveric spinous processes with PMMA and placing an ISP spacer, the mean failure load of the PMMA-treated specimens was significantly higher than that of the nonaugmented group.[66]

Wu and colleagues[67] performed a meta-analysis to determine the effectiveness of ISP spacers versus traditional decompression for LSS. They included two randomized controlled trials and three nonrandomized prospective studies with a total of 204 ISP device and 217 traditional decompression patients in their analysis. The authors found that there were no significant differences in 12- to 24-month results between the groups with respect to low back or leg pain, ODI scores, Roland Disability Questionnaire scores, or complication rates. However, traditional decompressive surgery was associated with a significantly lower reoperation rate than ISP device implantation (relative risk, 3.34; 95% confidence interval, 1.77–6.31; $P < .001$). Because ISP devices can be inserted through minimally invasive, percutaneous approaches or via open surgery, the authors performed subgroup analyses to independently compare each of these approaches to traditional decompression. They again found similar clinical outcomes but significant reoperation rates with ISP spacers.

Hong and colleagues[68] performed their own meta-analysis, and identified 21 publications with a total of 3155 ISP device and 50,983 open decompression patients for analysis. Follow-up ranged from 6 to 54 months, but was 1 year or longer in 90% of the trials. Investigators determined that there was no significant difference in ODI scores, improvement rates, or VAS scores for back or leg pain between ISP device and open decompressive surgery groups. ISP spacer use led to a significantly faster operative time, less perioperative blood loss, lower postoperative complication rate (1.7% vs. 2.1%; $P = .02$), and shorter hospital length of stay. However, the ISP spacer group also had a significantly higher reoperation rate (16.2% vs. 8.7%; $P < .001$). As a result, the authors concluded that ISP spacers may be a viable alternative in the treatment of lumbar

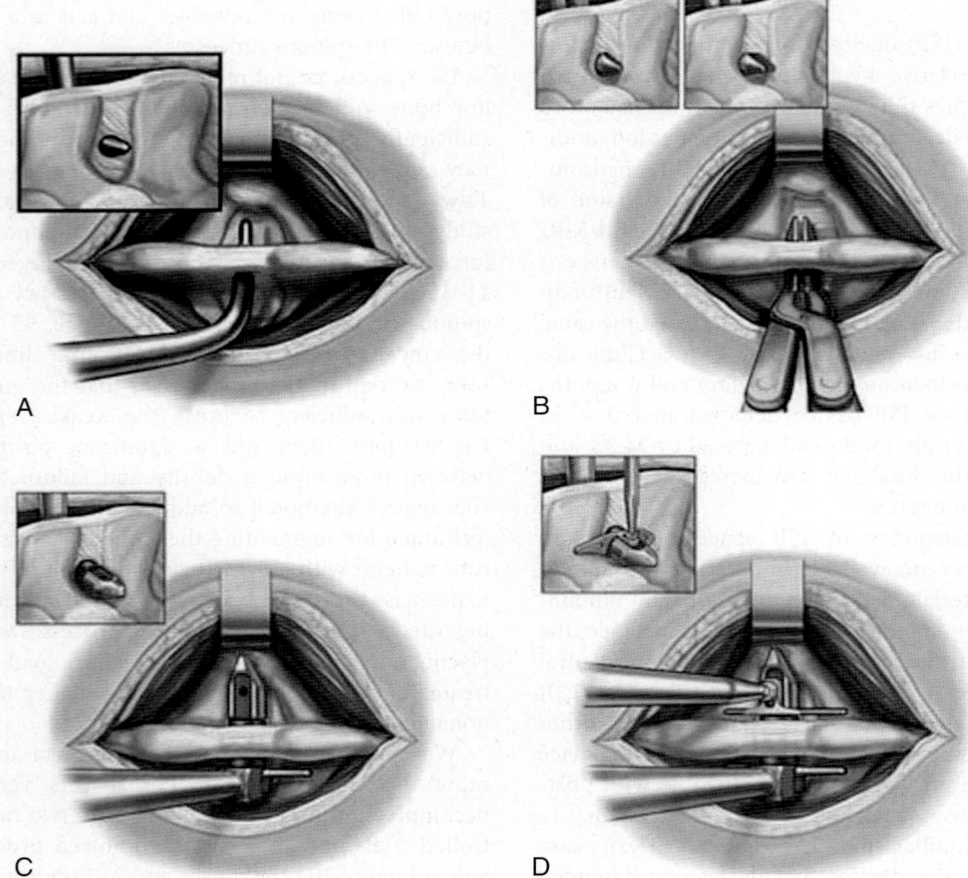

FIG. 63.16 X-STOP interspinous process device insertion. (A) The curved dilator is inserted into the anterior margin of the interspinous space. (B) The sizing distractor is inserted to determine the implant size. (C) The X-STOP is inserted into the interspinous space. (D) The adjustable wing is fastened to the implant. (From Zucherman JF, Hsu KY, Hartjen CA, et al. A prospective randomized multi-center study for the treatment of lumbar spinal stenosis with the X-STOP interspinous implant: 1-year results. *Eur Spine J.* 2004;13:22–31.)

stenosis but that open decompressive surgery remains the gold standard.

Because of the lack of sufficient long-term follow-up in a large cohort of patients, we still perform a laminotomy or laminectomy when there is stenosis in the absence of instability. Our primary indication for use of an ISP device is for patients with mild to moderate intermittent neurologic claudication with grade 1 degenerative spondylolisthesis who cannot tolerate a decompression and fusion procedure. We do not recommend use of an interspinous device for greater than a grade 1 spondylolisthesis. When considering utilizing the procedure, it is essential that the patient's symptoms of neurogenic claudication are alleviated within 5 minutes of sitting because spinal unit distraction is the mechanism by which the device functions.

Postoperative Care

All patients are encouraged to get out of bed with physical therapy and ambulate as soon as possible. Even in the setting of a short-segment fusion, patients are given a long-acting local anesthetic and mobilized the day of surgery. In the event of a dural tear, however, the patient is placed on bed rest for 1 to 2 days before standing and ambulating. We rarely prescribe a lumbar binder or orthotic for patients who have undergone decompression alone. For patients who receive a fusion procedure, we occasionally use a lumbosacral orthotic for the first 6 weeks. An orthotic with a leg extension is used for those patients fused to the sacrum with questionable bone quality. All patients are advised to avoid bending, lifting, or twisting for 6 to 12 weeks postoperatively. The first postoperative visit is typically at 2 to 3 weeks, at which time the wound is assessed, radiographs are taken, and outpatient physical therapy is initiated. If a fusion procedure was not performed, patients are then seen at 3 months and 1 year after surgery. Flexion-extension radiographs are taken at each follow-up visit to ensure that the patient does not develop instability at the decompressed level. If a fusion procedure was performed, patients are seen more frequently: at 6 weeks, 3 months, 6 months, 1 year, and annually up to year 5 postoperatively. This long-term follow-up is required to ensure that fusion is obtained and that there are no hardware-related complications. Radiographic evidence of a posterolateral fusion is typically evident at 6 months to 1 year with complete arthrodesis expected at 2 years. Absence of bridging bone at 2 years and symptoms suggestive of a pseudarthrosis should prompt a CT to better assess the fusion mass.

Complications

Complications of lumbar decompressive surgery include dural tear, nerve root injury, infection, vascular complications, epidural hematoma, nonunion or hardware failure following fusion, instability, bony regrowth, and adjacent-segment degeneration.

Dural tears are a well-known complication of lumbar stenosis surgery, with rates in the literature ranging from 1.8%[69] to 17.4%.[70] Khan and colleagues[71] performed a large retrospective series of 3183 consecutive degenerative lumbar spine operations (decompression and/or fusion) and identified a dural tear rate of 7.6% during primary cases and 15.9% for revision procedures. Incidental durotomies are most commonly created while the surgeon is using the Kerrison punch.[72] It is our protocol to perform a closure of all dural tears at the time of durotomy. Primary repair is performed with 6-0 Gortex suture followed by placement of a spinal sealant system such as DuraSeal (Covidien) and/or Duragen (Integra LifeSciences). All repairs are tested with a Valsalva maneuver. Closed-suction wound drainage does not appear to aggravate the leak and can be used safely in the presence of a dural repair.[73] Patients are given ceftriaxone for meningitis prophylaxis, placed on bed rest for 24 to 48 hours, and then slowly permitted to ambulate. Primary watertight closure of the dura has been shown to produce good results without long-term deleterious effects or increased rates of postoperative infection, neural damage, or arachnoiditis.[73] However, others have reported inferior 10-year outcomes with significantly greater chance of headaches and lower Tegner scores for general activities of daily living in patients whose surgeries were complicated by dural tear.[74] After primary closure, a small fraction of patients may require a secondary procedure for a persistent spinal fluid leak; this represented 1.8% of the patients in the Khan et al. series described earlier.[71] In this scenario, a promptly performed direct repair or a fascia lata graft typically leads to good results.[71,75]

The vascular complications of posterior lumbar surgery include deep vein thrombosis (DVT), pulmonary embolism (PE), postoperative hematoma, and catastrophic vascular events. Although major vascular injury during lumbar decompression is rare, it is important to recognize this complication in the operating room or in the early postoperative period because the best prognosis for recovery occurs with immediate treatment within 24 to 48 hours.[76] Unexplained hypotension is highly suggestive of a vascular catastrophe, and is an indication for arteriography in the stable patient and laparotomy in the unstable patient. Patients with preexisting vascular disease are predisposed to such injuries.[76]

DVT is a more common vascular complication, with rates of 5% after lumbar laminectomy and 3.1% after lumbar fusion procedures reported in a systematic review by Glotzbecker and colleagues.[77] No instances of PE were reported in these patients. The authors recommended the use of compression stockings and pneumatic sequential compression devices as a primary method of prophylaxis, as this was associated with a lower overall rate of DVT. There was insufficient evidence to support the use of pharmacologic prophylaxis or DVT screening in patients undergoing routine elective spinal surgery.[77] However, others suggest that mechanical prophylaxis for thromboembolism may not be sufficiently protective for patients undergoing combined anterior/posterior spine surgery.[78] This ambiguity manifests as wide variability in spinal surgeons' estimation of DVT rates as well as in their choice and timing of thromboembolic prophylaxis.[79] We currently feel that the relatively low risk of postoperative DVT and PE, when weighed against the potentially disastrous effect of epidural hematoma, does not justify the use of pharmacologic DVT prophylaxis with lumbar decompression surgery. We routinely use sequential compression stockings and early ambulation in patients undergoing elective posterior spinal surgery.

Infection rates after surgery for lumbar stenosis were investigated by Deyo and colleagues[80] using the Veterans Affairs National Surgical Quality Improvement Program database. In the 12,154 decompression and/or fusion procedures identified, the 30-day rate of superficial wound infection, deep wound infection, and wound disruption were 1.9%, 1.2%, and 0.3%, respectively. Higher American Society of Anesthesiologists class and fusion procedures (as opposed to decompression alone) were associated with significantly elevated rates of these wound complications. Infection rates in other large series for lumbar spine surgery have ranged from 2%[48] to 4.4%.[81] Fang and colleagues[81] observed that the majority of infections occurred during the early postoperative period (<3 months). Age older than 60 years, smoking, diabetes, previous surgical infection, increased body mass index, and alcohol abuse were statistically significant preoperative risk factors.[81] Instrumented fusion has also been reported as a risk factor for infection.[82]

It is critical to diagnose infections early in the postoperative period. Measuring C-reactive protein (CRP) levels has been shown to be a useful adjunct to physical examination findings. Mok and colleagues[83] examined perioperative trends in CRP and erythrocyte sedimentation rate in 149 patients who underwent spine surgery. Postoperative infection complicated 20 (13%) of these cases. In patients with an uncomplicated postoperative course, CRP peaked 2.7 days after surgery, then showed an exponential decrease with a half-life of 2.6 days.[83] A second rise or a failure to decrease as expected had a sensitivity, specificity, positive predictive value, and negative predictive value of 82%, 48%, 41%, and 86%, respectively, for infectious complications. Erythrocyte sedimentation rate was a less predictable and responsive measure.[83] Once diagnosed, postoperative wound infections should be aggressively managed with operative irrigation and debridement and a minimum of 6 weeks of culture-guided intravenous antibiotics.[84] Loose bone graft should be removed, but intact hardware should be maintained unless the infection cannot be controlled otherwise.[84] Repeat irrigation and debridement may be indicated 48 to 72 hours postoperatively in the presence of extensive muscular necrosis, an immunocompromised host, or multiorganism infection.[84] In instrumented cases, antibiotics will ideally postpone the need for hardware removal until a fusion mass has formed.[84] This approach has led to good clinical results[82] with similar functional outcome scores at a mean follow-up of 62 months when compared with a cohort of noninfected patients.[85]

Prophylactic antibiotics significantly reduce the risk of postoperative spinal wound infections[86]; they should be administered prior to incision, then postoperatively for up to 24 hours.[84] However, prolonged antibiotic treatment has been shown to prolong the duration of hospitalization, inhibit normalization of body temperature, and elevate CRP levels.[87] We routinely administer perioperative antibiotics immediately before surgery and for 24 hours thereafter.

Meningitis is a rare complication of spinal surgery, with a documented incidence of 0.18% in a series of 2180 spinal operations.[88] Patients typically present with fever, headache, photophobia, and neck stiffness within 6 to 14 days after surgery.[88] Good outcomes can be expected with prompt diagnosis and treatment.[88]

Although spondylotic spinal stenosis is typically a condition of older patients with greater comorbidities, several studies have demonstrated that decompression and/or fusion in elderly patients is relatively safe with an acceptable rate of morbidity when compared with younger patients.[89–93] Benz and colleagues[89] found that preoperative medical comorbidities did not predict early postoperative complications in patients older than 70 years who underwent spinal decompression. The total complication rate was 40%, and serious complications potentially affecting quality of life occurred in 12% of patients. The early mortality rate was 1.4%.[89] Ragab and colleagues[90] found an overall morbidity rate of 20% in a group of patients aged 70 to 101 years with spinal stenosis who underwent decompressive surgery. Because their results were comparable to those reported in younger populations, they concluded that advanced age does not increase the morbidity associated with lumbar decompression.[90] Reindl and colleagues[91] compared complications of elective spinal decompression with those of total hip arthroplasty in patients aged 65 to 80 years and found that these surgeries resulted in a similar number of life-threatening complications (approximately 20%).[91] However, it should be noted that there were twice as many minor complications in the spinal decompression group.[91] An analysis of patients at least 80 years of age with lumbar stenosis and degenerative spondylolisthesis from the SPORT trial found that operative treatment produced significant benefit over nonoperative treatment.[93] Furthermore, this older population experienced no significant increases in complication or mortality rates after surgery compared with younger patients. Finally, Glassman and colleagues[92] studied the 2-year outcomes of single-level decompression and posterolateral arthrodesis with iliac crest bone graft for single-level degenerative disc disease in patients older and younger than 65 years. Older patients actually experienced significantly greater relief of leg pain with similar improvements in ODI scores, back pain, and SF-36 scores at final follow-up. However, there were significantly more serious postoperative adverse events in the older patient group (38% vs. 17%; $P = .003$), including significantly more cardiac events, respiratory events, and infections.[92]

Despite adequate decompression, substantial back and leg symptoms develop in up to 10% to 15% of patients who have undergone an adequate lumbar decompression.[94] Early studies suggested that osseous regrowth after decompression may be the cause of symptomatic recurrence and decreased patient satisfaction.[95,96] Chen and colleagues[96] followed 48 patients treated for lumbar stenosis for an average of 4.5 years after posterior decompression. Plain radiographs were used to quantify the amount of bone regrowth at the original laminectomy site. Of the patients, 44% were observed to have more than 40% regrowth of the lamina, and spinal instability was found to accelerate this process. Patients with moderate and marked osseous regrowth exhibited statistically significantly poorer clinical outcomes than those with no significant and mild regrowth. However, more recent studies have contradicted these findings. Guigui and colleagues[97] evaluated 23 patients for an average of 8 years following laminectomy using both plain radiographs and CT. They found that radiographs significantly overestimated bone regrowth compared with CT scans. Using axial imaging, they determined that mean regrowth at final follow-up was only 7.7%, with no patients exhibiting greater than 20% regrowth. Furthermore, no association between osseous regrowth and clinical outcome was identified. Similarly, Dohzono and colleagues[98] found relatively low degrees of bone regrowth on CT scan with no correlation between regrowth and clinical outcomes after microscopic bilateral decompression via a unilateral approach in a group of 85 patients. The authors postulated that the minimally invasive technique allowed for greater preservation of the facet joints, which led to less iatrogenic instability and therefore a relatively small amount of osseous regrowth. In light of this conflicting evidence, it seems reasonable to take precautions to avoid destabilization of the spine, as bone regrowth may result in neural compression and recurrent symptoms.

Adjacent-segment pathology is one of the main clinical issues encountered after lumbar fusion.[99] In a systematic review containing 27 studies, the incidence of radiographic evidence of adjacent-level degeneration ranged from 8% to 100%, but only 0% to 27.5% of patients were symptomatic.[100] The wide range of estimates may be due to varying definitions, measurement methodologies, and follow-up periods in each study. Nonetheless, the results suggest that degeneration is commonly observed on radiographs but is only clinically symptomatic in a subset of these patients. Ghiselli and colleagues[101] reported on 215 patients who underwent posterior lumbar arthrodesis with mean follow-up of 6.7 years. Over the course of the study, 27% of the patients had evidence of degeneration at adjacent levels and elected to undergo additional surgery. The rate of surgery to address adjacent segments was predicted to be 16.5% at 5 years and 36.1% at 10 years following the index procedure. However, Radcliff and colleagues,[8] in a subgroup analysis of the SPORT study, demonstrated that the addition of fusion (with or without instrumentation) in the surgical treatment of spinal stenosis without instability did not result in increased reoperation rates at the index or adjacent levels when compared to decompression alone over a 4-year period. This refutes the classical hypothesis that lumbar fusion results in elevated rates of adjacent-segment disease.

PEARLS AND PITFALLS

1. The surgical exposure should clearly identify the midlateral pars and facet capsule to prevent overresection of bone, which can lead to iatrogenic pars interarticularis fractures.
2. Laminectomy should begin centrally, starting from the caudal portion of the lamina where the ligamentum flavum protects the dura, followed by decompression of the lateral recesses.
3. Distraction laminoplasty using a laminar spreader between spinous processes at the level of interest allows for improved visualization of the spinal canal during decompression, with minimal resection of the posterior osseous elements.
4. Decompression of the lateral recess and foramen should be performed from the contralateral side to avoid iatrogenic durotomy.

KEY POINTS

1. Ideal surgical candidates have symptoms of neurogenic claudication in a distribution that correlates with radiographic findings of spinal stenosis.
2. Open decompressive laminectomy is the gold standard for treatment of stable lumbar stenosis.
3. Fusion should be performed in conjunction with decompressive laminectomy in the presence of instability at the involved motion segment (>5 mm), degenerative scoliosis (curve progression or >30 degrees), prior decompression at the same level, or the need to resect greater than 50% of the facet joints.
4. The SPORT study, the largest level 1 prospective randomized study to evaluate the surgical treatment of conditions associated with low back and leg pain, demonstrated the efficacy of operative treatment over nonoperative treatment for spinal stenosis.
5. Candidates for interspinous process devices should have neurogenic claudication completely relieved with sitting and no greater than a grade 1 spondylolisthesis.

KEY REFERENCES

1. Fry RW, Alamin TF, Voronov LI, et al. Compressive preload reduces segmental flexion instability after progressive destabilization of the lumbar spine. *Spine*. 2014;39(2): E74-E81.
   This cadaveric study showed that decompression with even partial medial facetectomy results in measurable increases in segmental range of motion and decreases in stiffness.
2. Weinstein JN, Tosteson TD, Lurie JD, et al. Surgical versus nonsurgical therapy for lumbar spinal stenosis. *N Engl J Med*. 2008;358:794-810.
   The 2-year outcomes of the SPORT study, a large multicenter randomized controlled trial with a concurrent observational cohort evaluating laminectomy versus conservative treatment for lumbar stenosis, were reported in 2008. All patients who had a history of at least 12 weeks of symptomatic lumbar stenosis without spondylolisthesis were considered surgical candidates. A total of 289 patients were enrolled in the randomized cohort, and 365 patients were enrolled in the observational cohort. By 2-year follow-up, however, 43% of those who were randomly assigned to receive nonsurgical care underwent surgery (compared to 67% of the patients randomly assigned to the operative group). Despite the high incidence of crossover, the intention-to-treat analysis revealed a significant treatment effect favoring surgery on the SF-36 scale for bodily pain. However, there were no significant differences in scores on the SF-36 scale for physical function or on the modified ODI. The as-treated analysis, which included the randomized and observational cohorts, showed a significant advantage for surgery compared with nonoperative treatment by 3 months for the ODI and both SF-36 components. These changes remained significant for all subsequent time points in the 2-year duration of the study. At 2-year follow-up, on the basis of the as-treated analysis, 63% of patients treated surgically rated themselves as having major improvement with their condition versus 29% of the group treated nonoperatively.
3. Lurie JD, Tosteson TD, Tosteson A, et al. Long-term outcomes of lumbar spinal stenosis: eight-year results of the Spine Patient Outcomes Research Trial (SPORT). *Spine*. 2015;40(2):63-76.
   The long-term outcomes of the SPORT study were published in 2015. At 8-year follow-up, no significant differences remained between randomized cohorts in intent-to-treat analysis. By this point, however, 52% of those randomized to nonoperative care had undergone surgery, which began to approach the 70% of patients in the operative group who actually underwent surgery. As-treated analysis of the randomized group showed that the benefit of surgery diminished over time and was not significant after 5 years. However, the significantly better early outcomes (SF-36 bodily pain and physical function, ODI) associated with surgery in the observational group were stably maintained out to 8 years. These results suggest that laminectomy for symptomatic degenerative spinal stenosis provides significant improvements in function, pain, and disability but that these effects likely diminish to some degree over the long term.
4. Grob DT, Humke T, Dvorak J. Degenerative lumbar spinal stenosis. Decompression with and without arthrodesis. *J Bone Joint Surg Am*. 1995;77:1036-1041.
   The authors randomized 45 patients with lumbar spinal stenosis without instability to receive decompression with and without arthrodesis. Instability was defined as greater than 5 mm of motion between segments in the sagittal plane or greater than 5 mm of lateral offset in the coronal plane. All patients had significant clinical improvement compared with preoperative values at an average of 28-month follow-up with no significant differences regardless of whether or not a fusion was performed. These results suggest that, in the absence of instability, decompression with care taken to not destabilize the spine does not necessitate an arthrodesis.
5. Herkowitz HN, Kurz LT. Degenerative lumbar spondylolisthesis with spinal stenosis. A prospective study comparing decompression with decompression and intertransverse process arthrodesis. *J Bone Joint Surg Am*. 1991;73:802-808.
   This study randomized 50 patients with spinal stenosis and associated degenerative spondylolisthesis to determine whether noninstrumented arthrodesis produced better outcomes than decompressive laminectomy alone. At a mean of 3-year follow-up, patients in the arthrodesis group had significantly greater back and lower extremity pain relief. Furthermore, only 28% of patients in the fusion group experienced slip progression after surgery, while the slip distance increased in 96% of those in the nonfusion group.
6. Fischgrund JS, Mackay M, Herkowitz HN, et al. Degenerative lumbar spondylolisthesis with spinal stenosis: a prospective, randomized study comparing decompressive laminectomy

and arthrodesis with and without spinal instrumentation. *Spine*. 1997;22:2807-2812.
This study investigated the effects of instrumentation in a randomized trial of patients with spondylolisthesis and stenosis. Although the addition of instrumentation increased the fusion rate compared to noninstrumented arthrodesis (82% vs. 45%) in the 67 patients available for 2-year follow-up, clinical outcomes were similar between the groups (P <.435).

7. Kornblum MB, Fischgrund JS, Herkowitz HN, et al. Degenerative lumbar spondylolisthesis with spinal stenosis: a prospective long-term study comparing fusion and pseudarthrosis. *Spine*. 2004;29:726-733.
A longer-term follow-up (average 7 years, 8 months) of the cohort of patients who underwent uninstrumented fusion from the above two studies revealed that clinical outcomes were significantly more likely to be good or excellent in patients who achieved solid arthrodesis than in those with a pseudarthosis (86% vs. 56%, P = .01).

8. Overdevest GM, Jacobs W, Vleggeert-Lankamp C, et al. Effectiveness of posterior decompression techniques compared with conventional laminectomy for lumbar stenosis. *Cochrane Database Syst Rev*. 2015;(3):CD010036.
A 2015 Cochrane review compared posterior decompression techniques for lumbar stenosis. The authors concluded that bilateral laminotomy resulted in better perceived recovery at final follow-up than laminectomy. Unilateral laminotomy for bilateral decompression and bilateral laminotomy led to lower rates of iatrogenic instability than conventional laminectomy (although the rates were low in all groups). There was a clinically small but statistically significant difference in the severity of postoperative low back pain favoring bilateral laminotomy over laminectomy. However, there was insufficient evidence to show a difference in complications, procedure length, length of hospital stay, or postoperative walking distance between techniques.

9. Hong P, Liu Y, Li H. Comparison of the efficacy and safety between interspinous process distraction device and open decompression surgery in treating lumbar spinal stenosis: a meta-analysis. *J Invest Surg*. 2015;28(1):40-49.
A meta-analysis comparing the outcomes of ISP spacers versus open decompression for lumbar stenosis. The authors identified 21 publications with a total of 3155 ISP device and 50,983 open decompression patients for analysis. Follow up ranged from 6 to 54 months, but was 1 year or longer in 90% of the trials. Investigators determined that there was no significant difference in ODI score, improvement rate, or VAS scores for back or leg pain between ISP device and open decompressive surgery groups. ISP spacer use led to a significantly faster operative time, less perioperative blood loss, lower postoperative complication rate (1.7% vs 2.1%, P =.02), and shorter hospital length of stay. However, the ISP spacer group also had a significantly higher reoperation rate (16.2% vs 8.7%, P <.001). As a result, the authors concluded that ISP spacers may be a viable alternative in the treatment of lumbar stenosis but that open decompressive surgery remains the gold standard.

10. Wang JC, Bohlman HH, Riew KD. Dural tears secondary to operations on the lumbar spine. Management and results after a two-year-minimum follow-up of eighty-eight patients. *J Bone Joint Surg Am*. 1998;80:1728-1732.
A total of 641 patients who underwent lumbar decompression (14% of whom had a dural tear) were reviewed. The article describes primary repair of the tear followed by bed rest. Closed-suction wound drainage did not appear to aggravate the leak and can be used safely in the presence of a dural repair. Primary watertight closure of the dura produced good results without long-term deleterious effects or increased rates of postoperative infection, neural damage, or arachnoiditis.

11. Pearson A1, Lurie J, Tosteson T, et al. Who should have surgery for spinal stenosis? Treatment effect predictors in SPORT. *Spine*. 2012;37(21):1791-1802.
An analysis of SPORT study data demonstrated that surgical outcomes for spinal stenosis are significantly better in patients who preoperatively exhibited greater disability, predominant leg pain over low back pain, neuroforaminal stenosis, or a neurologic deficit; not lifting at work and not smoking were associated with better outcomes.

REFERENCES

1. Deyo RA, Gray DT, Kreuter W, et al. United States trends in lumbar fusion surgery for degenerative conditions. *Spine*. 2005;30:1441-1445.
2. Benoist M. The natural history of lumbar degenerative spinal stenosis. *Joint Bone Spine*. 2002;69:450-457.
3. Deen HG Jr, Zimmerman RS, Lyons MK, et al. Analysis of early failures after lumbar decompressive laminectomy for spinal stenosis. *Mayo Clin Proc*. 1995;70:33-36.
4. Atlas SJ, Deyo RA, Keller RB, et al. The Maine Lumbar Spine Study, Part III. 1-year outcomes of surgical and nonsurgical management of lumbar spinal stenosis. *Spine*. 1996;21:1787-1794.
5. Atlas SJ, Keller RB, Robson D, et al. Surgical and nonsurgical management of lumbar spinal stenosis: four-year outcomes from the Maine Lumbar Spine Study. *Spine*. 2000;25:556-562.
6. Pearson A, Lurie J, Tosteson T, et al. Who should have surgery for spinal stenosis? Treatment effect predictors in SPORT. *Spine*. 2012;37(21):1791-1802.
7. Derby R, Kine G, Saal JA, et al. Response to steroid and duration of radicular pain as predictors of surgical outcome. *Spine*. 1992;17:S176-S183.
8. Radcliff K, Curry P, Hilibrand A, et al. Risk for adjacent segment and same segment reoperation after surgery for lumbar stenosis: a subgroup analysis of the Spine Patient Outcomes Research Trial (SPORT). *Spine*. 2013;38(7):531-539.
9. Gibson JN, Waddell G. Surgery for degenerative lumbar spondylosis: updated Cochrane Review. *Spine*. 2005;30:2312-2320.
10. Overdevest GM, Jacobs W, Vleggeert-Lankamp C, et al. Effectiveness of posterior decompression techniques compared with conventional laminectomy for lumbar stenosis. *Cochrane Database Syst Rev*. 2015;(3):CD010036.
11. Schonauer C, Bocchetti A, Barbagallo G, Albanese V, Moraci A. Positioning on surgical table. *Eur Spine J*. 2004;13(suppl 1):S50-S55.
12. Shriver MF, Zeer V, Alentado VJ, et al. Lumbar spine surgery positioning complications: a systematic review. *Neurosurg Focus*. 2015;39(4):E16.
13. DiStefano VJ, Klein KS, Nixon JE, et al. Intra-operative analysis of the effects of position and body habitus on surgery of the low back. A preliminary report. *Clin Orthop Relat Res*. 1974;99:51-56.
14. McNulty SE, Weiss J, Azad SS, et al. The effect of the prone position on venous pressure and blood loss during lumbar laminectomy. *J Clin Anesth*. 1992;4:220-225.
15. Mody MG, Nourbakhsh A, Stahl DL, et al. The prevalence of wrong level surgery among spine surgeons. *Spine*. 2008;33:194-198.
16. Boden SD, Martin C, Rudolph R, et al. Increase of motion between lumbar vertebrae after excision of the capsule and

cartilage of the facets. A cadaver study. *J Bone Joint Surg Am.* 1994;76:1847-1853.

17. Yuan PS, Booth RE Jr, Albert TJ. Nonsurgical and surgical management of lumbar spinal stenosis. *Instr Course Lect.* 2005;54:303-312.
18. Olszewski AD, Yaszemski MJ, White AA 3rd. The anatomy of the human lumbar ligamentum flavum. New observations and their surgical importance. *Spine.* 1996;21:2307-2312.
19. Chau AM, Pelzer NR, Hampton J, et al. Lateral extent and ventral laminar attachments of the lumbar ligamentum flavum: cadaveric study. *Spine J.* 2014;14(10):2467-2471.
20. Connor MJ, Nawaz S, Prasad V, et al. The posterior epidural ligaments: a cadaveric and histological investigation in the lumbar region. *ISRN Anat.* 2013;2013:424058.
21. Kimmell KT, Dayoub H, Shakir H, Sincoff EH. Spinal dural attachments to the vertebral column: an anatomic report and review of the literature. *Surg Neurol Int.* 2011;2:97.
22. Rosen C, Rothman S, Zigler J, et al. Lumbar facet fracture as a possible source of pain after lumbar laminectomy. *Spine.* 1991;16:S234-S238.
23. Su BW, Kim PD, Cha TD, et al. An anatomical study of the mid-lateral pars relative to the pedicle footprint in the lower lumbar spine. *Spine.* 2009;34:1355-1362.
24. Fry RW, Alamin TF, Voronov LI, et al. Compressive preload reduces segmental flexion instability after progressive destabilization of the lumbar spine. *Spine.* 2014;39(2):E74-E81.
25. Truummees E, Herkowitz H. Lumbar spinal stenosis: treatment options. *AAOS Instr Course Lect.* 2003;107-115.
26. Kreiner DS, Shaffer WO, Baisden JL, et al., North American Spine Society. An evidence-based clinical guideline for the diagnosis and treatment of degenerative lumbar spinal stenosis (update). *Spine J.* 2013;13(7):734-743.
27. Birkmeyer NJ, Weinstein JN, Tosteson AN, et al. Design of the Spine Patient Outcomes Research Trial (SPORT). *Spine.* 2002;27:1361-1372.
28. Weinstein JN, Tosteson TD, Lurie JD, et al. Surgical versus nonsurgical therapy for lumbar spinal stenosis. *N Engl J Med.* 2008;358:794-810.
29. Lurie JD, Tosteson TD, Tosteson A, et al. Long-term outcomes of lumbar spinal stenosis: eight-year results of the Spine Patient Outcomes Research Trial (SPORT). *Spine.* 2015;40(2):63-76.
30. Tosteson AN, Tosteson TD, Lurie JD, et al. Comparative effectiveness evidence from the Spine Patient Outcomes Research Trial surgical versus nonoperative care for spinal stenosis, degenerative spondylolisthesis, and intervertebral disc herniation. *Spine.* 2011;36(24):2061-2068.
31. Nasca RJ. Rationale for spinal fusion in lumbar spinal stenosis. *Spine.* 1989;14:451-454.
32. Watters WC 3rd, Bono CM, Gilbert TJ, et al., North American Spine Society. An evidence-based clinical guideline for the diagnosis and treatment of degenerative lumbar spondylolisthesis. *Spine J.* 2009;9(7):609-614.
33. Grob D, Humke T, Dvorak J. Degenerative lumbar spinal stenosis. Decompression with and without arthrodesis. *J Bone Joint Surg Am.* 1995;77:1036-1041.
34. Lee CH, Hyun SJ, Kim KJ, Jahng TA, Kim HJ. Decompression only versus fusion surgery for lumbar stenosis in elderly patients over 75 years old: which is reasonable? *Neurol Med Chir (Tokyo).* 2013;53(12):870-874.
35. Herkowitz HN, Kurz LT. Degenerative lumbar spondylolisthesis with spinal stenosis. A prospective study comparing decompression with decompression and intertransverse process arthrodesis. *J Bone Joint Surg Am.* 1991;73:802-808.
36. Fischgrund JS, Mackay M, Herkowitz HN, et al. Degenerative lumbar spondylolisthesis with spinal stenosis: a prospective, randomized study comparing decompressive laminectomy and arthrodesis with and without spinal instrumentation. *Spine.* 1997;22:2807-2812.
37. Kornblum MB, Fischgrund JS, Herkowitz HN, et al. Degenerative lumbar spondylolisthesis with spinal stenosis: a prospective long-term study comparing fusion and pseudarthrosis. *Spine.* 2004;29:726-733.
38. Benz RJ, Garfin SR. Current techniques of decompression of the lumbar spine. *Clin Orthop Relat Res.* 2001;384:75-81.
39. Bresnahan L, Ogden AT, Natarajan RN, Fessler RG. A biomechanical evaluation of graded posterior element removal for treatment of lumbar stenosis: comparison of a minimally invasive approach with two standard laminectomy techniques. *Spine.* 2009;34(1):17-23.
40. Gurelik M, Bozkina C, Kars Z, et al. Unilateral laminotomy for decompression of lumbar stenosis is effective and safe: a prospective randomized comparative study. *J Neurol Sci.* 2012;29(4):744-753.
41. Thomé C, Zevgaridis D, Leheta O, et al. Outcome after less-invasive decompression of lumbar spinal stenosis: a randomized comparison of unilateral laminotomy, bilateral laminotomy, and laminectomy. *J Neurosurg Spine.* 2005;3(2):129-141.
42. Celik SE, Celik S, Göksu K, Kara A, Ince I. Microdecompressive laminotomy with a 5-year follow-up period for severe lumbar spinal stenosis. *J Spinal Disord Tech.* 2010;23(4):229-235.
43. Fu YS, Zeng BF, Xu JG. Long-term outcomes of two different decompressive techniques for lumbar spinal stenosis. *Spine.* 2008;33(5):514-518.
44. Aryanpur J, Ducker T. Multilevel lumbar laminotomies: an alternative to laminectomy in the treatment of lumbar stenosis. *Neurosurgery.* 1990;26:429-432.
45. Mackay DC, Wheelwright EF. Unilateral fenestration in the treatment of lumbar spinal stenosis. *Br J Neurosurg.* 1998;12:556-558.
46. Shenouda EF, Gill SS. Laminal fenestration for the treatment of lumbar nerve root foraminal stenosis. *Br J Neurosurg.* 2002;16:494-496.
47. Young S, Veerapen R. O'Laoire SA: Relief of lumbar canal stenosis using multilevel subarticular fenestrations as an alternative to wide laminectomy: preliminary report. *Neurosurgery.* 1988;23:628-633.
48. Aizawa T, Ozawa H, Kusakabe T, et al. Reoperation rates after fenestration for lumbar spinal canal stenosis: a 20-year period survival function method analysis. *Eur Spine J.* 2015;24(2):381-387.
49. Morimoto D, Isu T, Kim K, et al. Microsurgical medial fenestration with an ultrasonic bone curette for lumbar foraminal stenosis. *J Nippon Med Sch.* 2012;79(5):327-334.
50. O'Leary PF, McCance SE. Distraction laminoplasty for decompression of lumbar spinal stenosis. *Clin Orthop Relat Res.* 2001;384:26-34.
51. Tsuji H, Itoh T, Sekido H, et al. Expansive laminoplasty for lumbar spinal stenosis. *Int Orthop.* 1990;14:309-314.
52. Kawaguchi Y, Kanamori M, Ishihara H, et al. Clinical and radiographic results of expansive lumbar laminoplasty in patients with spinal stenosis. *J Bone Joint Surg Am.* 2004;86-A:1698-1703.

53. Sangwan SS, Kundu ZS, Walecha P, et al. Degenerative lumbar spinal stenosis—results of expansive laminoplasty. *Int Orthop*. 2008;32(6):805-808.
54. Guiot BH, Khoo LT, Fessler RG. A minimally invasive technique for decompression of the lumbar spine. *Spine*. 2002;27:432-438.
55. Asgarzadie F, Khoo LT. Minimally invasive operative management for lumbar spinal stenosis: overview of early and long-term outcomes. *Orthop Clin North Am*. 2007;38:387-399.
56. Khoo LT, Fessler RG. Microendoscopic decompressive laminotomy for the treatment of lumbar stenosis. *Neurosurgery*. 2002;51:S146-S154.
57. Yagi M, Okada E, Ninomiya K, Kihara M. Postoperative outcome after modified unilateral-approach microendoscopic midline decompression for degenerative spinal stenosis. *J Neurosurg Spine*. 2009;10(4):293-299.
58. Mobbs RJ, Li J, Sivabalan P, Raley D, Rao PJ. Outcomes after decompressive laminectomy for lumbar spinal stenosis: comparison between minimally invasive unilateral laminectomy for bilateral decompression and open laminectomy. *J Neurosurg Spine*. 2014;21(2):179-186.
59. Richards JC, Majumdar S, Lindsey DP, et al. The treatment mechanism of an interspinous process implant for lumbar neurogenic intermittent claudication. *Spine*. 2005;30:744-749.
60. Siddiqui M, Nicol M, Karadimas E, et al. The positional magnetic resonance imaging changes in the lumbar spine following insertion of a novel interspinous process distraction device. *Spine*. 2005;30:2677-2682.
61. Bono CM, Vaccaro AR. Interspinous process devices in the lumbar spine. *J Spinal Disord Tech*. 2007;20:255-261.
62. Zucherman JF, Hsu KY, Hartjen CA, et al. A prospective randomized multi-center study for the treatment of lumbar spinal stenosis with the X STOP interspinous implant: 1-year results. *Eur Spine J*. 2004;13:22-31.
63. Davis RJ, Errico TJ, Bae H, Auerbach JD. Decompression and Coflex interlaminar stabilization compared with decompression and instrumented spinal fusion for spinal stenosis and low-grade degenerative spondylolisthesis: two-year results from the prospective, randomized, multicenter, Food and Drug Administration Investigational Device Exemption trial. *Spine*. 2013;38(18):1529-1539.
64. Gazzeri R, Galarza M, Alfieri A. Controversies about interspinous process devices in the treatment of degenerative lumbar spine diseases: past, present, and future. *Biomed Res Int*. 2014;2014:975052.
65. Talwar V, Lindsey DP, Fredrick A, et al. Insertion loads of the X STOP interspinous process distraction system designed to treat neurogenic intermittent claudication. *Eur Spine J*. 2006;15(6):908-912.
66. Idler C, Zucherman JF, Yerby S, et al. A novel technique of intra-spinous process injection of PMMA to augment the strength of an inter-spinous process device such as the X STOP. *Spine*. 2008;33:452-456.
67. Wu AM, Zhou Y, Li QL, et al. Interspinous spacer versus traditional decompressive surgery for lumbar spinal stenosis: a systematic review and meta-analysis. *PLoS One*. 2014;9(5):e97142.
68. Hong P, Liu Y, Li H. Comparison of the efficacy and safety between interspinous process distraction device and open decompression surgery in treating lumbar spinal stenosis: a meta analysis. *J Invest Surg*. 2015;28(1):40-49.
69. Wang JC, Bohlman HH, Riew DK. Dural tears secondary to operations on the lumbar spine: management and results after a two-year-minimum follow-up of eighty-eight patients. *J Bone Joint Surg Am*. 1998;80:1728-1732.
70. Stolke D, Sollmann W, Seifert V. Intra- and postoperative complications in lumbar disc surgery. *Spine*. 1989;14:56-59.
71. Khan MH, Rihn J, Steele G, et al. Postoperative management protocol for incidental dural tears during degenerative lumbar spine surgery: a review of 3,183 consecutive degenerative lumbar cases. *Spine*. 2006;31:2609-2613.
72. Sin AH, Caldito G, Smith D, et al. Predictive factors for dural tear and cerebrospinal fluid leakage in patients undergoing lumbar surgery. *J Neurosurg Spine*. 2006;5:224-227.
73. Wang JC, Bohlman HH, Riew KD. Dural tears secondary to operations on the lumbar spine. Management and results after a two-year-minimum follow-up of eighty-eight patients. *J Bone Joint Surg Am*. 1998;80:1728-1732.
74. Saxler G, Krämer J, Barden B, et al. The long-term clinical sequelae of incidental durotomy in lumbar disc surgery. *Spine*. 2005;30(20):2298-2302.
75. Eismont FJ, Wiesel SW, Rothman RH. Treatment of dural tears associated with spinal surgery. *J Bone Joint Surg Am*. 1981;63:1132-1136.
76. Smith DW, Lawrence BD. Vascular complications of lumbar decompression laminectomy and foraminotomy. A unique case and review of the literature. *Spine*. 1991;16:387-390.
77. Glotzbecker MP, Bono CM, Wood KB, et al. Thromboembolic disease in spinal surgery: a systematic review. *Spine*. 2009;34:291-303.
78. Dearborn JT, Hu SS, Tribus CB, et al. Thromboembolic complications after major thoracolumbar spine surgery. *Spine*. 1999;24:1471-1476.
79. Glotzbecker MP, Bono CM, Harris MB, et al. Surgeon practices regarding postoperative thromboembolic prophylaxis after high-risk spinal surgery. *Spine*. 2008;33:2915-2921.
80. Deyo RA, Hickam D, Duckart JP, Piedra M. Complications after surgery for lumbar stenosis in a veteran population. *Spine*. 2013;38(19):1695-1702.
81. Fang A, Hu SS, Endres N, et al. Risk factors for infection after spinal surgery. *Spine*. 2005;30:1460-1465.
82. Weinstein MA, McCabe JP, Cammisa FP Jr. Postoperative spinal wound infection: a review of 2,391 consecutive index procedures. *J Spinal Disord*. 2000;13:422-426.
83. Mok JM, Pekmezci M, Piper SL, et al. Use of C-reactive protein after spinal surgery: comparison with erythrocyte sedimentation rate as predictor of early postoperative infectious complications. *Spine*. 2008;33:415-421.
84. Sasso RC, Garrido BJ. Postoperative spinal wound infections. *J Am Acad Orthop Surg*. 2008;16(6):330-337.
85. Mok JM, Guillaume TJ, Talu U, et al. Clinical outcome of deep wound infection after instrumented posterior spinal fusion: a matched cohort analysis. *Spine*. 2009;34:578-583.
86. Barker FG II. Efficacy of prophylactic antibiotic therapy in spinal surgery: a meta-analysis. *Neurosurgery*. 2002;51:391-400.
87. Ohtori S, Inoue G, Koshi T, et al. Long-term intravenous administration of antibiotics for lumbar spinal surgery prolongs the duration of hospital stay and time to normalize body temperature after surgery. *Spine*. 2008;33:2935-2937.
88. Twyman RS, Robertson P, Thomas MG. Meningitis complicating spinal surgery. *Spine*. 1996;21:763-765.
89. Benz RJ, Ibrahim ZG, Afshar P, et al. Predicting complications in elderly patients undergoing lumbar decompression. *Clin Orthop Relat Res*. 2001;384:116-121.

90. Ragab AA, Fye MA, Bohlman HH. Surgery of the lumbar spine for spinal stenosis in 118 patients 70 years of age or older. *Spine*. 2003;28:348-353.
91. Reindl R, Steffen T, Cohen L, et al. Elective lumbar spinal decompression in the elderly: is it a high-risk operation? *Can J Surg*. 2003;46:43-46.
92. Glassman SD, Polly DW, Bono CM, et al. Outcome of lumbar arthrodesis in patients sixty-five years of age or older. *J Bone Joint Surg Am*. 2009;91:783-790.
93. Rihn JA, Hilibrand AS, Zhao W, et al. Effectiveness of surgery for lumbar stenosis and degenerative spondylolisthesis in the octogenarian population: analysis of the Spine Patient Outcomes Research Trial (SPORT) data. *J Bone Joint Surg Am*. 2015;97(3):177-185.
94. Diwan AD, Parvartaneni H, Cammisa F. Failed degenerative lumbar spine surgery. *Orthop Clin North Am*. 2003;34:309-324.
95. Postacchini F, Cinotti G. Bone regrowth after surgical decompression for lumbar spinal stenosis. *J Bone Joint Surg Br*. 1992;74:862-869.
96. Chen Q, Baba H, Kamitani K, et al. Postoperative bone re-growth in lumbar spinal stenosis. A multivariate analysis of 48 patients. *Spine*. 1995;19:2144-2149.
97. Guigui P, Barre E, Benoist M, Deburge A. Radiologic and computed tomography image evaluation of bone regrowth after wide surgical decompression for lumbar stenosis. *Spine*. 1999;24(3):281-288.
98. Dohzono S, Matsumura A, Terai H, et al. Radiographic evaluation of postoperative bone regrowth after microscopic bilateral decompression via a unilateral approach for degenerative lumbar spondylolisthesis. *J Neurosurg Spine*. 2013;18(5):472-478.
99. Lee JC, Choi SW. Adjacent segment pathology after lumbar spinal fusion. *Asian Spine J*. 2015;9(5):807-817.
100. Harrop JS, Youssef JA, Maltenfort M, et al. Lumbar adjacent segment degeneration and disease after arthrodesis and total disc arthroplasty. *Spine*. 2008;33:1701-1707.
101. Ghiselli G, Wang JC, Bhatia NN, et al. Adjacent segment degeneration in the lumbar spine. *J Bone Joint Surg Am*. 2004;86-A:1497-1503.

CHAPTER 64 Degenerative Spondylolisthesis

Andrew Z. Mo
Gordon R. Bell
Darren R. Lebl

Degenerative spondylolisthesis (DS) was first described in 1930 by Junghanns, who coined the term *pseudospondylolisthesis* to describe the presence of forward slippage of a vertebral body in the presence of an intact neural arch.[1] The clinical and pathologic features of this entity were further defined by Macnab, who described the condition as "spondylolisthesis with an intact neural arch."[2] The term *degenerative spondylolisthesis* was originally used by Newman and Stone[3] and is the terminology most commonly used to describe the anterior slippage of one vertebral body on another in the presence of an intact neural arch. More recently, an etiology-based classification has been proposed that distinguishes between the pathologic processes that may cause spondylolisthesis.[4] Under this classification, two broad types of spondylolisthesis have been defined: *developmental* and *acquired.* DS, as described initially by Macnab and subsequently by Newman and Stone, is a subtype of the *acquired* form subsequently described by Marchetti and Bartolozzi.[4,5] In that classification, DS may be either primary or secondary. *Primary degenerative spondylolisthesis* is typically seen in middle-aged women and usually presents with clinical spinal stenosis. *Secondary degenerative spondylolisthesis* occurs as a result of a predisposing factor, such as adjacent-segment degeneration and slip above a preexisting fusion.

Epidemiology and Biomechanics

DS is a condition of older people and rarely affects those younger than 40 years of age. It most commonly involves the L4–L5 level, although other levels may be affected. It much less commonly involves the L5–S1 level, in contrast to isthmic spondylolisthesis, which most commonly occurs at L5–S1. Factors that have been reported to predispose to anterolisthesis at the lumbosacral junction include an L5 vertebral body that is less deeply seated within the pelvis, a more slender L5 transverse process, and increased sacral inclination, all of which are more common in women than men.[6]

DS is approximately four to five times more common in females than in males and is more common in black females than in white females.[7] The female preponderance is thought to be due to greater ligamentous laxity and hormonal effects.[8–10] A significantly increased expression of estrogen receptors has been found in facet joints of postmenopausal women having severe facet arthritis associated with DS compared with those with spinal stenosis only. It was not clear whether the higher expression of estrogen receptors aggravated the degenerative facet changes or was a causative factor for DS.[9]

In an epidemiologic survey of 4151 patients, the Copenhagen Osteoarthritis Study found that the incidence of DS was 2.7% in males and 8.4% in females.[11] The only factors associated with an increased risk of DS in women were elevated body mass index, increased age, and increased angle of lordosis. In men, only increased age was associated with a higher risk of DS. There was no association between DS and age at menopause, smoking, or occupational lifting exposure.

It is likely that the development of DS is multifactorial and dependent on anatomic factors, such as intervertebral disc pathology, ligament laxity, posterior facet joint arthrosis, the amount of lumbar lordosis, hormonal factors, and prior pregnancy. Genetic factors are also a likely contributor to the development of spinal stenosis with DS in some patients. One study demonstrated that a type IX collagen gene polymorphism that introduced a tryptophan residue into the protein's triple helix predisposed its carriers to development of spinal stenosis with DS.[12] Results from another study linked estrogen receptor alpha gene polymorphisms to the prevalence of DS.[13]

A cadaveric model investigating the relative contributions of disc integrity and the anterior and posterior longitudinal ligaments in the development of low-grade anterolisthesis found that integrity of the disc was more important than ligamentous factors, although disruption of both was necessary to produce significant destabilization.[14] The effect of facet joint orientation has also been reported to be a potential factor in the development of DS. Specifically, more sagittally oriented L4–L5 facet joints have been implicated as a cause of DS.[15–17] In one study, individuals in whom both L4–L5 facet joint angles were sagittally oriented more than 45 degrees were 25 times more likely to have DS than those with less than 45 degrees of facet angulation.[14] Whether the sagittal orientation is developmental or acquired is unclear and is a matter of debate. One study reported that sagittal orientation is a result of facet joint remodeling associated with arthrosis rather than the cause of anterior subluxation.[17] In another study, it was found that destabilization of both the facet complex and disc was required to achieve anterior listhesis consistent with DS.[18]

A retrospective, age- and sex-matched, case-control radiographic study of middle-aged women found that decreased anterior disc height and increased lumbar index (lumbar index = posterior vertebral body height/anterior vertebral body height) were two independent predictors of DS.[19]

Natural History

The natural history of DS, like many other spinal conditions, is not well characterized.[20] A meta-analysis of the literature on DS between 1970 and 1993 found that only 25 of the 152 studies reviewed, representing 889 patients, satisfied their inclusion criteria.[21] Only three of these studies, encompassing 278 patients, described the natural history of DS.[22,23] Overall, 90 of these 278 patients (32%) achieved satisfactory results without treatment. A study by Matsunaga and colleagues[24] represented the best of the three studies and was the only true natural history study. In that study, 40 patients who received no treatment were followed from 5 to 14 years (mean, 8.25 years). Only 4 of 40 patients (10%) showed clinical deterioration over the course of the study and all were in the group of 28 patients who exhibited no slip progression over the follow-up period. Progressive slip was noted in 12 patients (30%), although none of the 12 patients exhibited clinical deterioration. The majority of the patients in this study showed slight improvement in their clinical symptoms over time. In general, no correlation was noted between slip progression and clinical deterioration. No slip progression was noted in patients with intervertebral disc narrowing, spur formation, subcartilaginous sclerosis, or ligamentous ossification, suggesting that these anatomic factors were protective against further slip and represented a mechanism of spinal restabilization. The lack of correlation between slip progression and progression of symptoms has also been reported by other authors.[20,25,26] The generally favorable prognosis of DS was confirmed by a North American Spine Society work group consensus statement that summarized evidence-based clinical guidelines on the diagnosis and treatment of DS.[20] Although it did not distinguish between natural history and conservative care, that committee reported that most patients without neurologic signs or symptoms did well without surgery.

Clinical Features

The clinical features of DS are the same as those of spinal stenosis. DS, like spinal stenosis, may be either asymptomatic or may produce low back and/or leg pain. Back pain with DS is typically mechanical and may be aggravated by back extension or by arising from a bent posture. It is to be distinguished from discogenic back pain, which is typically provoked by flexion or sitting. Only a small percentage of patients with DS may experience low back pain. A report that investigated a small cohort of patients from the Framingham Heart Study concluded that there did not appear to be an association between low back pain and DS as diagnosed by computed tomography.[27]

TABLE 64.1 Characteristics of Vascular vs. Neurogenic Claudication

Evaluation	Vascular	Neurogenic
Walking distance	Fixed	Variable
Palliative factors	Standing	Sitting/bending
Provocative factors	Walking	Walking/standing
Walking uphill	Painful	Painless
Bicycle test	Positive (painful)	Negative (painless)
Pulses	Absent	Present
Skin	Loss of hair/shiny	Normal
Weakness	Rarely	Occasionally
Back pain	Occasionally	Commonly
Back motion	Normal	Limited
Pain character	Cramping/distal to proximal	Numbness/aching/ proximal to distal
Atrophy	Uncommon	Occasionally

Leg pain may be either radicular or referred in a characteristic pattern of neurogenic claudication. *Neurogenic claudication,* also known as *pseudoclaudication,* is a clinical condition consisting of leg pain associated with walking.[28] Neurogenic claudication must be distinguished from vascular claudication, which has slightly different clinical features, a different etiology, and completely different treatment (Table 64.1). Neurogenic claudication is defined as lower extremity pain, paresthesias, or weakness associated with walking or standing.[29,30] Pain is the predominant symptom, being present in up to 94% of patients with spinal stenosis, with numbness (63%) and weakness (43%) being less common.[29,30] Bilateral involvement is common. Patients with neurogenic claudication may present with either unilateral radicular pain or with diffuse, nondermatomal symptoms beginning in the buttocks and extending a variable distance into the legs. Radicular pain is typically dermatomal in distribution and is often unilateral. It is the presenting type of symptom in 6% to 13% of symptomatic patients with stenosis.[30] It is often seen with lateral recess stenosis, foraminal stenosis, or concomitant disc herniation. The clinical effects of spinal canal narrowing are magnified by the presence of a degenerative slip that further narrows the spinal canal.

Typical neurogenic claudication is less dermatomal in character than is radicular pain. It is frequently bilateral and may have a radicular component to it. Symptoms are typically produced by standing or walking and are relieved by sitting or bending forward (see Table 64.1). Patients may preferentially assume a stooped-over posture when walking or standing to ameliorate symptoms ("shopping cart sign"). Other leg symptoms, such as weakness or numbness, may also occur in association with standing or walking. Night pain is an uncommon feature of spinal stenosis, although it has been described in patients with lateral stenosis (lateral recess stenosis or foraminal stenosis). Unusual symptoms of spinal stenosis, such as priapism associated with intermittent claudication during walking, have also been reported.

The relationship of symptoms to posture can be explained on the basis of variation in canal size with posture.[31,32] Cadaveric studies have demonstrated that spinal canal cross-sectional area, midsagittal diameter, subarticular sagittal diameter, and foraminal size are significantly reduced in extension and are increased with flexion.[31] Similarly, neural compression is greater in extension than in flexion. An association between posture and epidural pressure measurements has also been demonstrated. In vivo studies relating posture to epidural pressure measurements have shown that epidural pressures at the level of stenosis were higher in standing compared with lying and sitting, and were increased with extension and decreased with flexion.[31]

Neurogenic claudication should be distinguished from vascular claudication because their causes and treatments are different (see Table 64.1). Although both conditions may present as leg pain associated with walking, only patients with neurogenic claudication typically have leg pain with standing. Leg pain associated with neurogenic claudication is highly position dependent, whereas vascular claudication is unaffected by back flexion or extension. Leg pain with cycling in a sitting position is common with vascular claudication but not with neurogenic claudication.[33] Patients with vascular claudication will typically have more leg pain produced by walking uphill than downhill, whereas patients with a neurogenic claudication will typically have less pain walking uphill owing to the slightly flexed posture of the lumbar spine that results in neuroforaminal widening and reduced neural compression. Patients with neurogenic claudication may actually have increased leg pain when walking down an incline owing to associated lumbar lordosis and consequent neuroforaminal narrowing.

The radicular pattern of spinal stenosis with DS most commonly involves the L5 nerve root, which is usually compressed within the lateral recess. This radicular pain is typically located in the posterolateral thigh, extending into the lateral calf and occasionally into the dorsum of the foot. The presence of a degenerative slip also narrows the L4–L5 neural foramen and can therefore result in L4 radicular pain from foraminal compression of the L4 nerve root. Pain in an L4 distribution is characteristically located in the anterior thigh to the knee and along the anterior shin. It can occasionally be confused with pain from a hip etiology; thus, careful attention must be given to the possibility of hip pathology as a cause for anterior thigh pain.

Radiographic Diagnosis

The diagnosis of DS is a radiographic diagnosis that is made on the lateral lumbar radiograph (Fig. 64.1). Although the slippage (anterolisthesis) may also be evident on a supine lateral radiograph, it is important that the lateral radiograph be performed in the standing position because there can be a dynamic component to the slip, causing it to reduce in the supine position and appear normal.[34] One recent study investigated asymmetric facet hypertrophy at C3–C4 and C4–C5, finding an association with lumbar degenerative spondylolisthesis on upright lateral films even in the absence of anterolisthesis on supine magnetic resonance imaging (MRI).[35] It is not unusual for a patient to present with a normally aligned supine MRI study as the only radiographic study. Unless standing lumbar radiographs are obtained, however, the presence of a degenerative slip could be missed. In a recent study, 22% of L4–L5 degenerative slips, as documented by standing lateral flexion–extension radiographs, were not detectable on supine MRI.[36] Other dynamic radiographic views, such as sitting or standing flexion–extension views and distraction–compression radiography, may also be considered.

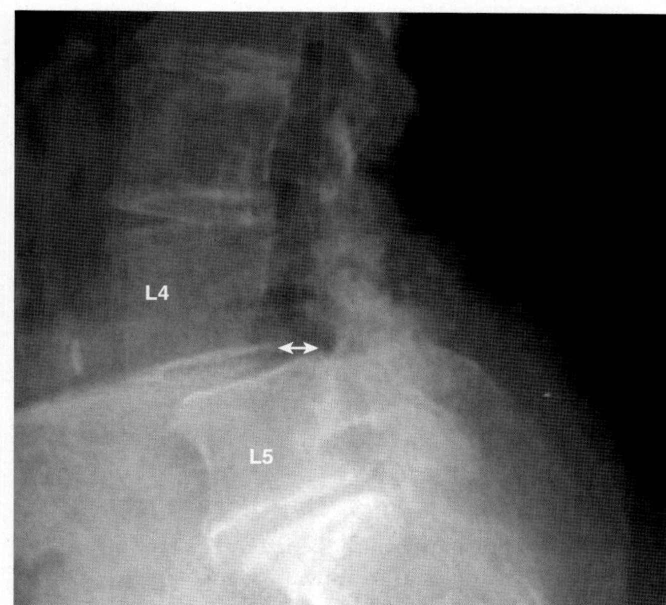

FIG. 64.1 Standing lateral lumbar radiograph showing the anterior slippage (*arrow*) of L4 on L5.

MRI may show an increased signal within a facet joint at the level of the slip.[36–38] Large facet effusions greater than 1.5 mm were found to be highly predictive of L4–L5 DS, even in the absence of a measurable slip on the supine MRI.[36] Therefore, a patient who presents with only an MRI should be suspected of having a DS if a large facet effusion is detected, in which case standing lumbar radiographs should be obtained. Alternatively, the slip can be documented by upright or axial loaded MRI.[37,39]

Although the actual measurement of translation is generally straightforward, the distinction between what is normal dynamic translation and abnormal segmental motion (instability) is not.[40,41] There is no consensus as to what constitutes clinically significant radiographic instability of the lumbar spine, nor even what is considered to be the normal range of translation between motion segments.[40,41] As with routine radiographs, there exists a spectrum of normal translation that can exist in the absence of symptoms.[40,41] One study showed that more than 90% of asymptomatic volunteers exhibited between 1 mm and 3 mm of translation on flexion-extension lateral lumbar radiographs and that a dynamic change of greater than 4 mm was therefore considered abnormal.[40]

It is important not to base the decision for type of surgery on the MRI or myelography/CT findings without obtaining a preoperative standing lateral lumbar radiograph. Failure to identify a listhesis preoperatively could result in performing the incorrect procedure, namely, isolated decompression rather than decompression and fusion. Furthermore, without preoperative standing lateral radiographs, it cannot be determined if the presence of postoperative spondylolisthesis in a patient with poor pain relief after surgery was the result of destabilization from the surgery or if it was a preexisting condition.

Treatment

As mentioned previously, both the natural history of DS and, until recently, its optimal treatment are incompletely understood. The well-publicized Spine Patient Outcomes Research Trial (SPORT) was a prospective evaluation of the 2-year[42] and 4-year[20,43] outcomes of 607 patients with DS. Half of the patients were enrolled in a randomized cohort and half in an observational cohort. Preenrollment nonoperative care was not specified, and the type of surgery or nonoperative treatment during the study period was left to the discretion of the treating physicians. This study was hampered by a significant crossover and nonadherence to treatment between the two groups, leading to both an *as-treated* and an *intent-to-treat* analysis of the data. When both the randomized and observational cohorts were combined, the as-treated analysis revealed that the surgically treated patients had significantly better outcomes for both pain and function at 2-year and 4-year follow-ups. This study did not allow comparison of types of treatments; thus, it did not answer the question of which surgical treatments provided better outcomes.

That same SPORT trial examined radiographic predictors of outcome in both surgically and nonoperatively treated patients.[44] Radiographic features examined included degree of slip (grade I vs. grade II), disc height (<5 mm vs. >5 mm), and mobility (stable vs. hypermobile). As noted previously, surgically treated patients had better outcomes than nonsurgically treated patients across all three radiographic parameters examined. For nonoperative patients, those with a grade I slip did better than those with a grade II slip, and those with a hypermobile slip did better than those with a stable slip.

In a long-term follow-up of patients with DS, progressive slip was noted in 34% of the 145 nonsurgically managed patients who were observed for a minimum of 10 years.[45] This study was not a true natural history study because it included patients who had various nonsurgical interventions. Seventy-five percent of the patients were neurologically normal at the beginning of the study and the majority (76%) remained so at final follow-up. Of the 34% who had neurologic symptoms, 83% experienced neurologic deterioration and had a poor outcome. There was no correlation between slip progression and clinical symptoms. This study suggested that conservative (nonsurgical) treatment in neurologically normal patients can result in a satisfactory clinical outcome at an average of 10 years' follow-up in the majority of patients.

Decompression Without Fusion

A review of Medicare patients undergoing surgery for stenosis, with or without spondylolisthesis, from 2002 to 2007 found that only 21% of patients undergoing surgery for stenosis with spondylolisthesis in 2007 had simple decompression surgery compared with 79% having some form of decompression with fusion.[46] Although the trend in type of surgical procedure performed over this 6-year period was not examined for patients with stenosis associated with DS, the study noted that for patients with stenosis the trend was one of increasing complexity of surgical procedure. The rate of *complex* fusion, defined as fusion involving more than two levels or a 360-degree fusion, increased 15-fold from 2002 to 2007. It is likely that a similar increase in the rate of complex surgery occurred for patients with stenosis associated with DS.

One reason for considering decompression without fusion in select patient populations is that it is less invasive than fusion and reduces the morbidity and mortality associated with spinal fusion in elderly patients.[46–50] In the retrospective review of Medicare claims for patients undergoing surgery for spinal stenosis between 2002 and 2007, patients having a complex fusion had greater morbidity, more life-threatening complications, greater likelihood of rehospitalization within 30 days of surgery, and higher costs compared with patients having decompression alone or decompression with *simple* fusion (defined as one- or two-level fusion through a single surgical approach).[46] In a recent retrospective review of Medicare claims from 2005 to 2009, 1-year readmission rates after spinal stenosis decompression surgery with and without fusion were found to be 9.7% and 7.2%, respectively.[51]

A meta-analysis of the literature on DS between 1970 and 1993 found only 11 papers, encompassing 216 patients, reporting outcome measures after decompression without fusion that met their inclusion criteria (Table 64.2).[21] One of these studies was retrospective and nonrandomized[22]; two were prospective and randomized[52,53]; and the remaining eight were retrospective, nonrandomized, and uncontrolled. Overall, 69% of patients in this meta-analysis reported a satisfactory outcome with decompression alone, with 31% having an unsatisfactory result.

One report that supported decompression without fusion for DS reviewed an elderly (average age, 67 years) population

TABLE 64.2 Results of Decompression Without Fusion for Degenerative Spondylolisthesis: Meta-Analysis of Literature, 1970–1993 (11 Articles)

Total No. of Patients	Satisfactory	Unsatisfactory	Progressive Slip
216	140 (69%)[a]	75 (31%)[a]	67 (31%)[b]

From Mardjetko SM, Connolly PJ, Shott S. Degenerative lumbar spondylolisthesis: a meta-analysis of literature, 1970–1993. *Spine.* 1994;19(20 Suppl):2556S–2565S.
[a]Weighted pooled proportion.
[b]Reported in only 9 of 11 articles.

of 290 patients, 250 of whom had a one-level slip and 40 of whom had a two-level slip.[54] The data from that study were self-reported by the surgeons and were retrospective. The decompressive procedures included laminectomy in 249 patients and fenestration procedures in 41 patients. Fenestration procedures typically involved bilateral laminotomy with partial medial facetectomy and foraminotomy. Only patients with a "stable" slip having less than 4-mm translation and less than 10 to 12 degrees of angulation on dynamic lateral radiographs were included. At an average follow-up of 10 years (range, 1 to 27 years), 69% of patients reported an excellent outcome, 13% good outcome, 12% fair outcome, and 6% poor outcome. These authors concluded that 82% excellent/good outcomes was acceptable in this elderly population, in whom fusion is associated with higher morbidity and mortality.

Similar results were reported in a retrospective review of 49 elderly patients (mean age, 68.7 years) with symptomatic degenerative lumbar spondylolisthesis, without evidence of hypermobility on flexion–extension radiographs and who underwent decompression without fusion.[55] At a mean follow-up of 3.73 years, 73.5% of the patients reported excellent or good results, although 10% underwent revision surgery with an instrumented fusion. The study concluded that limited decompression alone can be helpful in a select group of elderly patients without hypermobility.

Bilateral decompression through a unilateral approach has also been described in patients with spinal stenosis, both with and without DS. A retrospective study using that technique compared patients with and without spondylolisthesis and showed similar functional outcomes between the two groups at 2 years.[56] Although there was a statistically significant increase in the percentage slip postoperatively in the patients with spondylolisthesis, it did not appear to produce an adverse functional outcome. Nevertheless, the presence of an increased slip at 2 years is a cause for concern and caution.

One prospective study assigned a group of 67 patients with spinal stenosis to either laminectomy or multilevel laminotomy and included a small subgroup of patients with DS.[57] Nine of the patients assigned to the laminotomy group crossed over to the laminectomy group, which caused some difficulty in interpreting the results. However, no patient who underwent multilevel laminotomy developed instability as a result of the surgery, compared with three patients who developed instability following laminectomy. These authors recommended multilevel laminotomies for patients with developmental stenosis, mild to moderate degenerative stenosis, or DS. Bilateral laminectomy was recommended for patients with severe degenerative stenosis or marked DS.

Another study prospectively evaluated 54 consecutive patients who underwent decompression without fusion for spinal stenosis.[58] In the small subgroup of 15 patients who had concomitant DS, 87% (13 of 15 patients) showed no change in the amount of preoperative slip. Overall, 88% of the 54 patients reported a good/excellent clinical outcome; the results were comparable between patients with and without DS. The study concluded that degenerative spinal stenosis, including patients with DS, can be decompressed effectively without the need for fusion.

Noninstrumented Posterolateral Fusion

Although the beneficial role of fusion in the surgical treatment of spinal stenosis associated with DS is less controversial than the role of fusion in the treatment of other degenerative back conditions, incontrovertible evidence supporting fusion is sparse. An attempted meta-analysis of literature reported between 1970 and 1993 found only six studies meeting the inclusion criteria that reported results of decompression with noninstrumented fusion for DS.[21] In that review, 90% of patients having decompression with noninstrumented fusion reported a satisfactory clinical outcome and 86% achieved a solid arthrodesis, although the fusion rate varied from 90% to 100% (Table 64.3).[59] Patients undergoing decompression with noninstrumented fusion achieved a statistically significantly better clinical outcome than those treated with decompression alone (90% vs. 69%, respectively).

Many studies on the surgical treatment of DS report unfavorable outcomes after decompression without fusion. One early small study by two groups of surgeons from two different institutions included two populations of patients with spinal stenosis and DS: one group underwent decompression alone and the other had decompression and fusion.[22] In the patients undergoing decompression alone, 5 of 11 (45%) were rated as having a good (satisfactory) outcome and 6 of 11 (55%) as having a fair/poor (unsatisfactory) outcome. In contrast, 5 of 8 patients (63%) undergoing decompression with in situ posterolateral fusion achieved a satisfactory outcome. This study suggested that patients did better when their decompression was accompanied by noninstrumented fusion.

Several studies have supported the position that patients undergoing fusion with decompression for DS do clinically better than those undergoing decompression alone.[22,53,60] It is difficult to gain a clear understanding of this issue from a review of existing literature, however, because well-done studies reporting surgical outcome after surgery for DS are uncommon.

Although most studies report no correlation between clinical outcome and the amount of slip progression, one study suggested that poor outcome was associated with slip progression.[52] That study was a prospective randomized study that included a subgroup of 11 patients undergoing decompression and noninstrumented fusion for DS. Of the 10 patients available for follow-up, only 3 (30%) reported improved functional outcome and 7 had an increase in their preoperative

TABLE 64.3 Results of Decompression With Noninstrumented Fusion: Meta-Analysis of Literature, 1970–1993 (Six Articles)

Total No. of Patients	Satisfactory Clinical Outcome	Unsatisfactory Clinical Outcome	Fusion
74 (clinical outcome)	90%[a,b]	10%[a,b]	86%[a]
84 (fusion outcome)			

From Mardjetko SM, Connolly PJ, Shott S. Degenerative lumbar spondylolisthesis: A meta-analysis of literature, 1970–1993. *Spine*. 1994;19(20 Suppl):2556S–2565S.
[a]Weighted pooled proportion.
[b]Data from 5 of 6 articles reported.

TABLE 64.4 Prospective, Randomized Comparison of Decompression vs. Decompression and Noninstrumented Spinal Fusion for Degenerative Spondylolisthesis

Outcome	Arthrodesis ($n = 25$)	No Arthrodesis ($n = 25$)
Excellent	11 (44%)	2 (8%)
Good	13 (52%)	9 (36%)
Fair	1 (4%)	12 (48%)
Poor	0 (0%)	2 (8%)
Mean increase in slip (preoperative to postoperative)	0.5 mm	2.6 mm ($P = .002$)

From Herkowitz HN, Kurz LT. Degenerative lumbar spondylolisthesis with spinal stenosis: a prospective study comparing decompression with decompression and intertransverse process arthrodesis. *J Bone Joint Surg Am.* 1991;73:802–808.

spondylolisthesis, suggesting that slip progression was associated with poor clinical outcome.

A landmark prospective randomized study comparing decompression alone with decompression and noninstrumented posterolateral spinal fusion in the treatment of L3–L4 and L4–L5 DS with spinal stenosis reported superior results when concomitant fusion was performed with the decompression.[53] A satisfactory outcome was more than twice as common in the fused group compared with the unfused group (96% vs. 44%, respectively). Furthermore, the percentage of excellent results was significantly and dramatically greater in the fused group (44% excellent) than in the unfused group (8% excellent; $P < .0001$) (Table 64.4). This study concluded that the results of surgical decompression with in situ arthrodesis were superior to those of decompression alone in the treatment of spinal stenosis associated with L3–L4 or L4–L5 DS. Outcome was influenced by neither the age nor sex of the patient nor the preoperative height of the disc space. These authors concluded that the decision for concomitant arthrodesis should be based purely on the presence or absence of a preoperative slip rather than on other preoperative factors, such as the age or sex of the patient, disc height, or intraoperative factors (e.g., amount of bone resected during the decompression). This study showed that the results of decompression with an *attempted* arthrodesis produced superior results to decompression alone, even if the fusion was unsuccessful (pseudarthrosis). Although, postoperatively, there was a significant ($P = .002$) increase in the slip in patients not receiving an arthrodesis compared with those undergoing fusion, 36% of the arthrodesis group were also noted to have a pseudarthrosis, although all had an excellent or good result.

A long-term review of 96 patients undergoing decompressive surgery for spinal stenosis followed for at least 5 years included a subset of patients with associated DS.[61] Although this subgroup was not fully analyzed separately and the study itself was retrospective, nonrandomized, and uncontrolled, some important trends were noted. Twenty-six patients (27%) of the entire group were considered failures: 16 because of recurrent neural symptoms and 10 because of low back pain. The incidence of DS was significantly greater in the surgical failure group (12 of 26 patients [46%]) than in the surgical successes (16 of 64 [25%]). These authors concluded that, because of the higher incidence of recurrent symptoms in patients with preexisting DS, all patients with an associated slip should be fused.

TABLE 64.5 Relationship Between Outcome and Fusion in Patients With Degenerative Spondylolisthesis

	No. of Patients	Excellent	Good	Fair	Poor
Fusion	10	3	5	2	0
No fusion	6	0	2	1	3

From Postacchini F, Cinotti G. Bone regrowth after surgical decompression for lumbar spinal stenosis. *J Bone Joint Surg Br.* 1992;74:862–869.

One well-recognized cause of long-term failure of decompression for spinal stenosis is subsequent bone regrowth causing recurrent neural compression. One study reported the relationship between bone regrowth, occurring an average of 8.6 years after surgical decompression for spinal stenosis, and long-term outcome.[59] Of the 40 patients in the study, 16 had preoperative DS, 10 of whom had concomitant arthrodesis. Although all 16 patients with preexisting DS showed some bone regrowth, the degree of regrowth was less severe in the 10 patients undergoing arthrodesis than in the 6 patients who were not fused (Table 64.5). Furthermore, the proportion of satisfactory results was significantly higher in patients who had spinal fusion. Although this study was retrospective and not randomized, it suggested that arthrodesis stabilized the spine, resulting in less bone regrowth causing recurrent stenosis, and produced superior long-term results.

One problem associated with noninstrumented in situ fusion is the difficulty, if not inability, to restore normal lumbar lordosis. This is particularly true with a multilevel noninstrumented fusion, which can produce a flatback deformity, although it can occur even with a single-level noninstrumented fusion. It has been demonstrated that an L4–L5 in situ fusion that produces kyphosis or hypolordosis results in increased motion at the adjacent L3–L4 level.[62] Such hypermobility may be one factor in adjacent-level degeneration after fusion.

An important issue with the use of spinal instrumentation in the elderly patient is its potential biomechanical effect on adjacent unfused levels. There is concern and evidence that the rigidity produced by a solid fusion, particularly with instrumentation, may cause significant stresses at adjacent levels above or below the fusion, with the potential for adjacent-level failure (Fig. 64.2). Such failure may be manifested by symptomatic or asymptomatic degeneration or by adjacent-level vertebral compression fracture or stress fracture because of the osteoporotic nature of the bone. The use of instrumentation may also produce direct injury to the superior facet by either capsular disruption or articular facet damage. These are arguments against pedicle screw fixation in the elderly patient with osteoporosis. Therefore, the use of less rigid instrumentation or no instrumentation may be preferable to rigid instrumentation because of theoretically reduced stresses on adjacent levels by the presence of a less

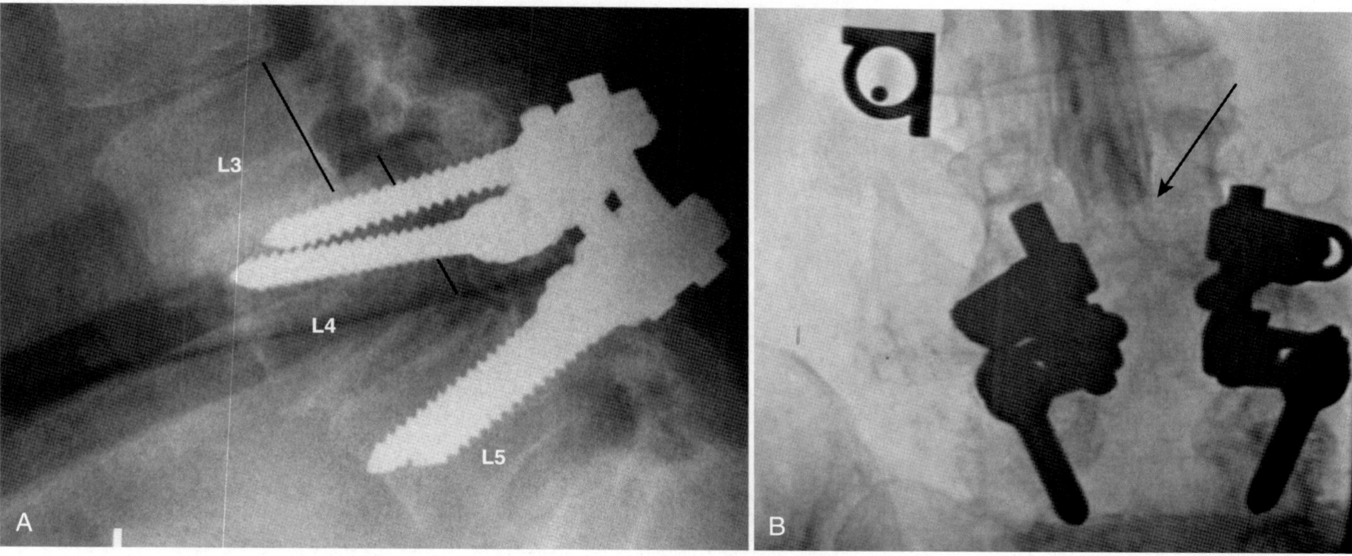

FIG. 64.2 (A) Standing lateral lumbar radiograph showing 7-year follow-up of L4–L5 instrumented fusion for L4–L5 degenerative spondylolisthesis. Note the adjacent-level degeneration at L3–L4, characterized by disc space collapse and L3–L4 slip (posterior aspect of L3 and L4 vertebral bodies marked by line). (B) Anteroposterior lumbar myelogram of the same patient as shown in (A), showing complete block of dye (*arrow*) at the level of the L3–L4 slip.

rigid fusion or even a stable pseudarthrosis, or by less risk to the superior facet joint by a pedicle screw.

A common clinical and radiographic scenario in older patients is the presence of symptomatic multiple-level spinal stenosis and a single-level (usually L4–L5) DS. Some of the possible permutations of treatment options include multilevel decompression of all stenotic levels without fusion, multilevel decompression with instrumented fusion of all decompressed levels, multilevel decompression with instrumented fusion at the listhetic level only, multilevel decompression with noninstrumented L4–L5 fusion only, and multilevel decompression and noninstrumented fusion of all decompressed levels. A multilevel decompression without any fusion is certainly a reasonable option in some elderly patients, particularly those with multiple comorbidities, even though the literature generally supports concomitant fusion. A multilevel instrumented fusion is a significant operative procedure in many older patients and may not be warranted because of the magnitude of the surgery. A one-level instrumented fusion with a multilevel decompression runs the risk of creating a stiff instrumented segment, which can result in transmission of significant forces to the adjacent decompressed segments, thereby rendering them potentially unstable and increasing the risk of developing a slip at another level. Multilevel noninstrumented fusion carries a high probability of pseudarthrosis at one or more levels and runs the risk of producing iatrogenic flatback deformity. Thus, it is reasonable to decompress all symptomatic stenotic levels and to perform a noninstrumented fusion at only the spondylolisthetic level. Even if this results in a stable pseudarthrosis rather than a solid arthrodesis, this may be sufficient to minimize the risk of slip progression and is less likely to transmit significant forces to adjacent decompressed levels, therefore creating less risk of adjacent-level failure.

Posterior Instrumented Fusion

The long-term clinical outcome of surgical decompression with instrumented spinal fusion for DS, particularly when compared with the outcome of decompression with noninstrumented fusion, is not completely known. A comprehensive search of the English literature on lumbar or lumbosacral fusion from 1979 to 2000[63] identified only two prospective and randomized studies that were limited to DS.[53,64] Although that study identified a nonsignificant trend toward greater use of instrumentation technology for lumbar fusion, generally, the clinical benefit of that pattern was unclear.

A Cochrane review of lumbar surgery found that there was limited evidence that fusion produced a better outcome or resulted in less slip progression than decompression alone. Although there was strong evidence that the use of adjunct instrumentation produced a higher fusion rate than noninstrumented fusion with decompression, a superior outcome was not demonstrated.[65]

A randomized controlled trial comparing surgery with nonsurgical treatment for spinal stenosis found that patients undergoing fusion with decompression had less pain and better functional outcomes at 2-year follow-up than patients undergoing decompression alone.[66] This was also true for a smaller subset of patients with DS who underwent instrumented fusion. Although the number of patients undergoing instrumented fusion was too small to permit extensive analysis, these authors felt that instrumented fusion should be considered for stenosis associated with DS.

A prospective nonrandomized study of patients with grade I DS compared decompression alone with decompression with instrumented fusion with 1-year follow-up.[67] The study demonstrated statistically significant functional improvement in the fusion group compared with the decompression group

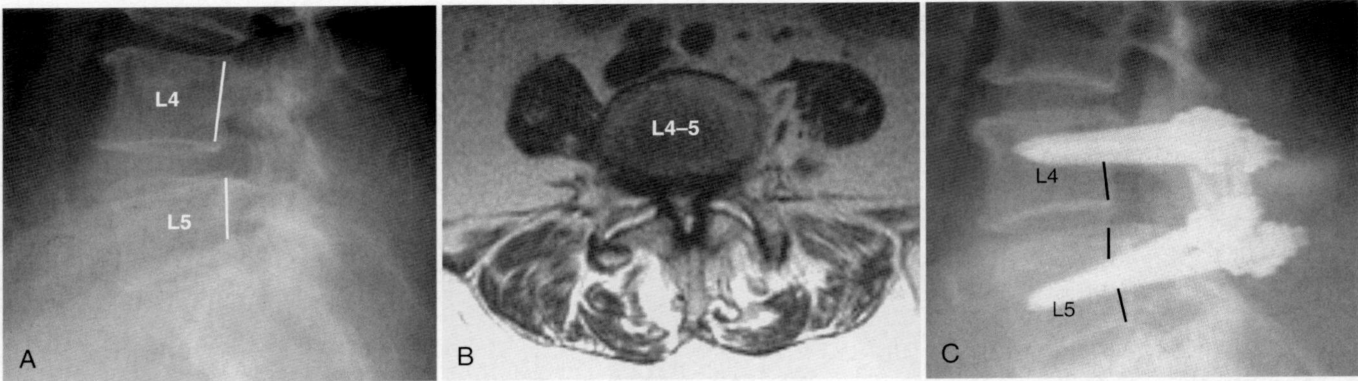

FIG. 64.3 (A) Preoperative standing lateral lumbar radiograph showing a small L4–L5 degenerative spondylolisthesis. The posterior borders of the L4 and L5 vertebral bodies are outlined (*white lines*). (B) Axial magnetic resonance imaging showing severe canal narrowing at the L4–L5 level. (C) Postoperative standing lateral lumbar radiograph showing the reduction of the L4–L5 spondylolisthesis. The posterior borders of the L4 and L5 vertebral bodies are outlined (*black lines*).

by Oswestry Disability Index and Short Form-36 (SF-36). The type of surgery was at the discretion of the treating surgeon and was done at two institutions by two surgeons. The nonrandom nature of the study and its restriction to patients with grade I slips only limited the generalization of the conclusions.

Most studies looking at fusion with instrumentation in the treatment of DS involve concomitant decompression (Fig. 64.3). One study, however, investigated the role of instrumented fusion with slip reduction and minimal decompression for DS.[68] The decompression involved only bilateral foraminotomies to safely visualize and mobilize the exiting nerve root. At a mean month follow-up of 33 months, 82% of patients with leg pain and 75% of those with back pain showed relief. The degree of anterolisthesis was reduced by 90% at follow-up. These authors concluded that the clinical, functional, and radiographic outcomes produced results comparable with the published outcomes of in situ fusion after formal laminectomy and that formal laminectomy may not always be necessary in the treatment of degenerative lumbar spinal stenosis with spondylolisthesis.

Although there is little argument that segmental instrumentation produces a more solid arthrodesis than noninstrumented fusion, there are conflicting data relating a solid arthrodesis to better clinical outcome. The multicenter historical cohort study of spinal fusion using pedicle screw fixation involved a retrospective review of 2684 patients with DS.[69] Solid radiographic fusion was noted in 89% of patients undergoing pedicle screw fixation compared with 70% of those without instrumentation. The clinical outcome was also better in the group of patients undergoing instrumented fusion. This report, however, was a retrospective historical review rather than a prospective randomized study; the validity of its conclusions is therefore limited.

A prospective randomized study followed 124 patients for 1 year after either instrumented or noninstrumented fusion for various diagnoses, including DS.[60] Two types of spinal instrumentation were employed: a rigid system and a semirigid system. Outcome was based primarily on radiographic fusion rate. The overall fusion rate was 65% for the noninstrumented group, 77% for the semirigid fixation group, and 95% for the rigid fixation group. For the subgroup of patients with DS, fusion was achieved in 65% of the noninstrumented patients, 50% of the semirigid fixation group, and 86% of the rigid fixation group. A trend of better clinical outcomes with increasing rigidity of fixation was also observed: 71% of the noninstrumented group, 89% of the semirigid group, and 95% of the rigid group reported excellent or good results.

A retrospective review of 30 patients undergoing decompression and instrumented fusion for DS reported both radiographic outcomes by fusion rate and functional outcomes by patient questionnaire and the SF-36 survey.[70] Both fusion rate and patient satisfaction were 93%. However, 13 patients (43%) had complications, including dural tears (3 patients), excessive blood loss (2 patients), pseudarthrosis (2 patients), pulmonary embolus (1 patient), deep infection (1 patient), urinary tract infections (3 patients), and unstable angina (1 patient). Patients with complications were found to have poorer outcomes. The study concluded that patients treated with decompression and fusion for DS had improved patient-reported functional outcomes but a significant risk of complications.

Some studies have concluded that the addition of spinal instrumentation to a fusion did not necessarily improve outcome. A randomized prospective study of patients undergoing posterolateral lumbar fusion, with and without pedicle screw instrumentation, for a variety of conditions concluded that the addition of instrumentation did not produce a significant incremental clinical benefit to that obtained from noninstrumented fusion, although there was a slight but nonsignificant trend toward higher fusion rate in the instrumented fusion group.[71] Overall, there was no statistical difference in patient-reported outcomes between the two groups. Although there was a slight nonsignificant trend toward an increased radiographic fusion rate in the group with instrumentation, this did not correlate with increased patient-reported improvement. For the entire group, the results did not show a

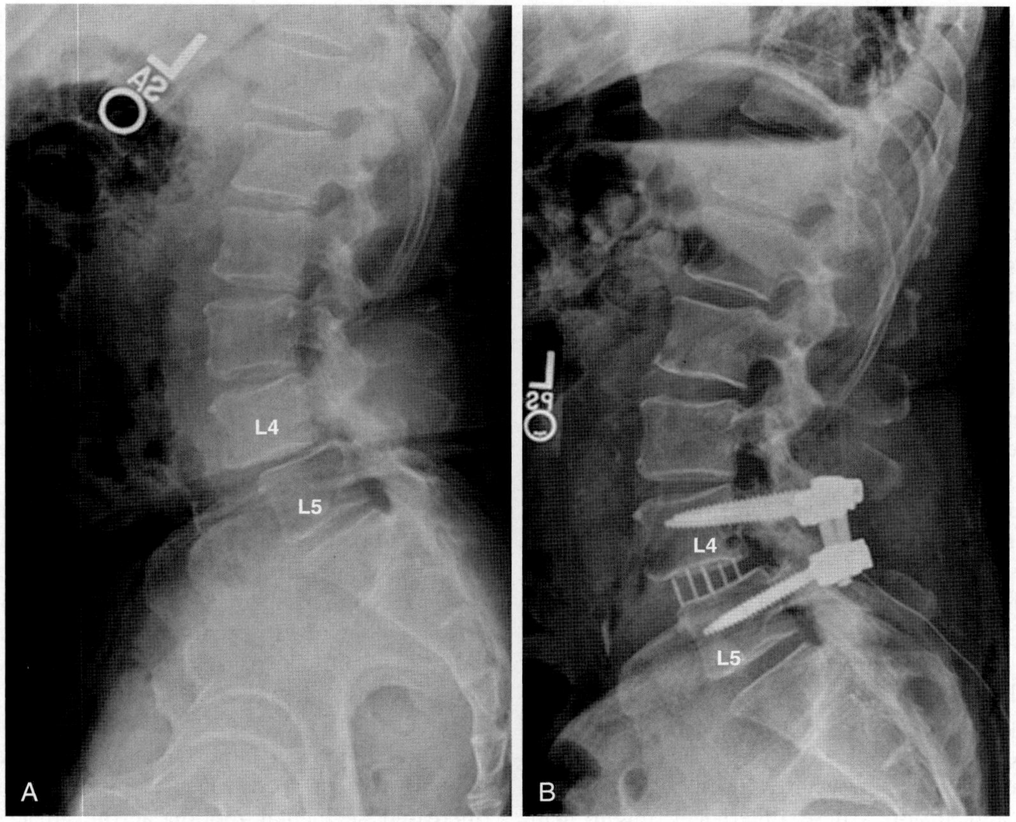

FIG. 64.4 (A) Preoperative standing lateral lumbar radiograph showing L4–L5 degenerative spondylolisthesis. (B) Postoperative standing lateral lumbar radiograph after extreme lateral interbody fusion showing the reduction of the L4–L5 spondylolisthesis. Visible are pedicle screw constructs and interbody cage, depicting stabilization and fusion of the L4–L5 level.

clinical benefit from the addition of instrumentation in elective lumbar fusions. For a small subgroup of 10 patients who had DS, 5 underwent instrumented fusion and 5 underwent noninstrumented in situ fusion. Four of the five patients with DS undergoing instrumented fusion achieved an excellent/good outcome, compared with two of five of those undergoing noninstrumented fusion. For this small subgroup of patients with DS, the clinical outcome appeared to be better than that of the overall population studied, although this subgroup was too small to achieve statistical significance.

A prospective randomized study of 68 patients with spinal stenosis and DS compared decompression and arthrodesis without instrumentation to decompression with segmental transpedicular instrumentation.[64] At an average of 2 years' follow-up, successful fusion was significantly more common in the instrumented group than in the noninstrumented group (83% vs. 45%, respectively), although there was no significant improvement in clinical outcome between the two groups (76% vs. 85% excellent/good outcomes, respectively). These authors concluded that the presence of successful fusion did not predict or influence short-term clinical outcome at 2 years.

In a long-term follow-up of 58 patients previously reported and prospectively randomized to decompression with noninstrumented fusion,[53,64] 47 were available for review at an average of 7 years, 8 months postoperatively (range, 5 to 14 years).[72] Excellent and good clinical outcomes were reported in 86% of patients achieving a solid arthrodesis but in only 56% of those patients having a pseudarthrosis. Patients with a solid fusion had significantly less back pain and better function than those with a pseudarthrosis. This study demonstrated a clear benefit of a solid arthrodesis on clinical outcome for patients undergoing decompression for spinal stenosis with DS. The short-term improvement in outcome noted at 2 years' follow-up in Herkowitz and Kurz's[53] and Fischgrund and colleagues'[64] initial studies deteriorated at final follow-up in patients who did not achieve a solid arthrodesis. The finding of better clinical outcome associated with solid fusion was also confirmed in another retrospective comparison of patients having a solid noninstrumented arthrodesis compared with patients with a pseudarthrosis.[73]

A 7-year follow-up of 47 patients treated with decompression and noninstrumented fusion found that long-term outcome was better in patients having a solid arthrodesis compared with those with a pseudarthrosis.[72] These authors inferred that the use of adjunct instrumentation might produce better long-term clinical outcomes than fusion without instrumentation. However, they did not compare the long-term clinical outcomes of the noninstrumented but solidly fused patients from their initial study with instrumented patients from their subsequent study; thus, a definitive conclusion on the value of instrumentation on clinical outcome could not be made.[64,74] Therefore, the issue of whether the addition of spinal instrumentation confers long-term clinical outcome that is superior to, worse than, or the same as that of a solid noninstrumented arthrodesis has not been answered by this or any other study.[75–77]

Most recently, Ghogawala et al. published 4-year results of a prospective randomized controlled trial that compared laminectomy alone to laminectomy and instrumented posterolateral fusion in 66 patients with degenerative spondylolisthesis and stenosis.[78] They found greater improvements in SF-36 scores with fusion than laminectomy alone. In contrast, Oswestry Disability Index scores were not significantly different between treatment groups. The most striking difference between treatments was the reoperation rate, which was 14% in the fusion group and 34% in the laminectomy-alone group. Most reoperations following fusion were for adjacent-level disease; most in the decompression-alone group were for recurrent stenosis. Published in the same issue, Försth et al. reported no difference in a subgroup of patients with degenerative spondylolisthesis and stenosis who were treated with decompression alone versus decompression and fusion.[79] Methodologically, these two studies differed in that the former controlled all aspects of the surgical technique and the indications for surgery were determined by a physician panel. In the latter, there were a variety of surgical techniques, both for decompression and fusion. These differences might help explain the disparate findings between the two studies.

Posterior Fusion With Anterior Column Support

Some authors have recommended the use of concomitant posterior fusion with anterior column support in the surgical management of some types of spondylolisthesis. Most commonly, anterior column support is provided by either a posterior lumbar interbody fusion (PLIF) or a transforaminal lumbar interbody fusion (TLIF), although anterior lumbar interbody fusion has also been used. Recent advances have allowed for lateral lumbar interbody fusion, in particular, minimally invasive lumbar interbody fusion (so-called extreme lateral interbody fusion [XLIF] and direct lateral interbody fusion) and minimally invasive TLIF (MIS TLIF) (Fig. 64.4). Minimally invasive surgical techniques such as XLIF and MIS TLIF allow for a smaller surgical site with similar, if not decreased, surgical complications and decreased surgical recovery times compared to traditional open approaches. A retrospective review comparing PLIF and MIS TLIF found that patients undergoing PLIF experienced higher operative blood loss, higher volume of blood transfusion, and increased complications compared to those who underwent TLIF, although hospital length of stay was comparable.[80] In a recent prospective multicenter study, Sembrano et al. found similar clinical outcomes at 2-year follow-up when comparing XLIF to MIS TLIF, in particular, back and leg pain relief when compared to baseline (73% and 64%, respectively).[81] Anterior column support has been more commonly recommended for isthmic spondylolisthesis, although its use for DS has also been advocated.[82–85] As with posterior instrumented fusion, generally, convincing data comparing posterior fusion with anterior column augmentation with other types of fusion do not exist. Furthermore, there is no evidence to suggest that the biomechanics and potential mechanism of failure for isthmic spondylolisthesis are the same as those for DS.

Purported advantages of interbody fusion with PLIF, TLIF, or XLIF compared with posterior instrumented fusion without an interbody fusion include greater likelihood of fusion, better indirect foraminal decompression, better reduction of the spondylolisthesis, and better lordosis.[81,82,85] In a one-level spondylolisthesis, however, it is not clear whether a slight improvement in slip reduction or lordosis produces a better clinical outcome. Nor is it known whether the potential for a slight incremental improvement in sagittal alignment or an increase in lordosis is worth the risk of potential nerve root injury as a result of interbody fusion.

Options for interbody fusion devices include metallic cages, carbon fiber cages, polyetheretherketone cages, or bone. A study comparing combined anterior and posterior lumbar reconstruction using anterior cages to posterior pedicle screw fixation alone investigated the biomechanical effects of interbody cages on construct stiffness, pedicle screw strain, and adjacent-level changes.[86] This study found that for spinal instability with preserved anterior load sharing, pedicle screw fixation alone was biomechanically adequate and recommended that interbody cages not be used because they further increased segmental motion at the adjacent level. Where anterior column support was deficient, however, posterior stabilization with pedicle screws alone provided inadequate stability and resulted in a high level of implant strain. Under such circumstances, the addition of an interbody cage significantly increased the construct stiffness and decreased hardware strain, although it resulted in increased motion at the adjacent segment. Similar adverse effects on the adjacent level were demonstrated in another biomechanical study that showed that rigid fusion using posterior pedicle screw fixation and an interbody cage produced higher loads at the superior adjacent level than posterior instrumented fusion without an interbody cage because of the increased stiffness of the fixed segments using the cage.[87]

In the absence of a head-to-head, prospective, randomized controlled study comparing the clinical outcome of instrumented to noninstrumented fusion for DS, it is difficult to know which treatment is better. In the absence of such data, the decision for treatment will inevitably be based largely on complications and cost.

From a societal perspective, fusion, particularly instrumented fusion, adds significantly to the incremental costs of treating spinal stenosis with DS. Kuntz and colleagues looked at the 10-year costs, quality-adjusted life-years (QALY), and incremental cost-effectiveness ratios (reported as dollars per quality-adjusted year of life gained) for patients undergoing decompressive surgery, with or without spinal fusion, for spinal stenosis with DS.[88] Laminectomy with noninstrumented fusion was found to cost $56,500 per QALY versus laminectomy without fusion. The cost-effectiveness ratio of instrumented fusion, compared with noninstrumented fusion, was $3,112,800 per QALY. A cost-effectiveness ratio of $82,400 per

QALY was calculated if the proportion of patients experiencing symptom relief after instrumented fusion was 90% as compared with 80% for patients with noninstrumented fusion. The study concluded that the cost-effectiveness of laminectomy with noninstrumented fusion compared favorably with other surgical interventions, such as lumbar discectomy for treatment of herniated lumbar disc or coronary artery bypass grafting for triple-vessel coronary artery disease. The cost-effectiveness, however, depended greatly on the true effectiveness of the surgery to alleviate symptoms and also on how patients valued the quality-of-life effect of relieving severe stenosis symptoms. Instrumented fusion was expensive compared with the incremental gain in health outcome. The study further concluded that better data on the effectiveness of this and other alternative procedures were necessary to justify their incremental cost.

The SPORT looked at the cost-effectiveness of spine surgery at 2-year follow-up.[89] This study evaluated the 61% of patients with DS who had surgery. Of these surgical patients, 93% had fusion, most (78%) with instrumentation. The study found that surgery significantly improved quality of life compared with nonoperative treatment, with an average cost of $115,000 per QALY gained. These authors concluded that surgery was not highly cost-effective compared with other elective orthopaedic surgeries over the 2-year follow-up period but did compare favorably with many other health interventions. Whether or not surgery for DS is cost-effective in the long run depends on long-term benefits and the ongoing costs associated with fusion surgery (e.g., the potential for future revision surgery).

The cost-effectiveness of fusion was also examined in a Swedish study that compared a group of patients who were randomized to one of four treatment groups for chronic low back pain: noninstrumented posterolateral fusion, instrumented posterolateral fusion, instrumented posterolateral fusion with interbody fusion, and a nonsurgical control group.[90] This study did not specifically examine patients with spinal stenosis and DS but concluded that the cost of treatment of chronic low back pain at 2-year follow-up was significantly higher if fusion was performed. Although the treatment effect of all surgical groups was found to be better than the control (nonoperative) group, the added (incremental) cost per QALY for fusion compared with nonoperative care ranged from $52,000 to $157,000 in the United States, depending on the magnitude of the assumed average annual QALY.

A recent study that reviewed major medical complications and charges associated with surgery for spinal stenosis in Medicare patients from 2002 to 2007 found that adjusted mean hospital charges for *complex* fusion procedures, defined as fusion involving more than two levels or a 360-degree (interbody) fusion, cost $80,888 compared with $23,724 for decompression alone.[46]

Besides the added cost of instrumented fusion, other adverse effects of fusion have been noted. It has been demonstrated that lumbar fusion is associated with greater morbidity than decompression alone.[47,48,50] In addition, a greater potential for complications exists with instrumentation than without it. A retrospective 6.5-year follow-up (range, 5–10.75 years) of 36 patients undergoing instrumented fusion for DS reported a patient satisfaction rate of 83%.[91] Although there were no neurologic deficits, pseudarthroses, recurrent stenosis at the fused segment, or progression of deformity at the fused level, five patients had symptomatic adjacent-level degeneration (transition syndrome) and an additional seven patients had asymptomatic radiographic transition syndromes. These authors concluded that although the rate of major complications (2%), implant failures (2%), and symptomatic pseudarthroses (0%) was low, radiographic degeneration at levels adjacent to the fused levels (transition syndrome) was common.

Alternative Surgical Strategies

Indirect spinal canal and foraminal decompression via interspinous process distraction has been proposed as an alternative to decompression for spinal stenosis with DS.[92] A randomized controlled study of 42 patients with spinal stenosis associated with DS was compared with 33 control patients treated nonoperatively.[92] The study found that the use of an interspinous process distraction device produced a better functional outcome than nonoperative management in patients with neurogenic claudication associated with degenerative spondylolisthesis. The question of whether or not that device was as good as, worse, or better than traditional decompression or decompression and fusion was not addressed by this study.

A contrary view of interspinous process distraction was reported in a study of 12 consecutive patients with DS and DS treated by interspinous process distraction and followed for a mean of 30 months.[93] That study reported a high failure rate: although two-thirds of patients had complete relief of their preoperative symptoms, one-third had no relief and 58% underwent surgical decompression and fusion within 24 months of their index procedure.

Significant reduction in total sagittal range of motion has been reported with one interspinous process distraction device that used both a mechanical blocking component and a tension band.[93] The tension band resulted in a significant additional restriction in total motion, including flexion, compared with the device without the tension band (43% reduction in motion compared with 16% reduction).

The use of motion-sparing technology has been advocated by some authors as an effective alternative to fusion that can reduce the potential for adjacent-level degeneration.[56,94–96] One prospective, minimum 4-year follow-up study of 26 consecutive patients with DS reported significantly improved pain and walking distance without progression of the spondylolisthesis.[56,95] Three patients demonstrated radiographic screw loosening and one patient had screw breakage. Nearly half of the patients showed some degeneration at adjacent levels. Comparable clinical outcome using the same device was reported in a prospective randomized, multicenter U.S. Food and Drug Administration investigational device exemption trial with a 1-year follow-up.[96] Early results from that study showed significant improvement in both back and leg pain, as well as function, but the study cautioned that further follow-up was necessary.

Summary of Treatment Options

Currently, there does not appear to be a clear consensus as to the optimal way to treat patients with symptomatic DS. Some studies suggest that patients undergoing surgery do better when decompression is accompanied by fusion. It is less clear, however, whether fusion should be augmented with instrumentation. Although a fusion is more robust and solid with instrumentation than without it, the incremental benefits of instrumentation on clinical outcome are less clear. It seems reasonable that in the presence of clear evidence of instability on flexion–extension radiographs, the immediate stability provided by instrumentation warrants the additional time, expense, and potential morbidity associated with its use. This is especially appropriate for young active patients with good bone stock. On the other hand, the indication for the use of hardware in a patient with a collapsed disc space, no motion at the spondylolisthetic level, or the presence of osteoporotic bone is less clear. A 2005 focus issue in *Spine* on lumbosacral fusion contained a combined position statement by *Spine* and the Scoliosis Research Society. It noted a positive long-term correlation between fusion and improved clinical outcome. It also noted a clear association between the use of instrumentation and higher fusion rates. Accordingly, the use of spinal instrumentation was recommended for spinal stenosis associated with DS. The position statement concluded by stating that the effectiveness of other posterior or anterior techniques (e.g., interbody fusion techniques) has yet to be established.[97]

Summary

The optimal surgical treatment of spinal stenosis, particularly when associated with DS, is still somewhat controversial. Such controversy involves the method and extent of decompression, the role of fusion, and the use of spinal instrumentation. Although spinal stenosis is a diffuse degenerative condition with many segmental levels often showing evidence of radiographic stenosis, decompression of *every* level showing *any* degree of radiographic stenosis is clearly not always warranted. Obviously, all symptomatic levels should be decompressed. There is no clear consensus, however, on whether to decompress asymptomatic levels; this decision depends on many factors. Because restenosis at a previously decompressed level or the development of symptomatic stenosis at a previously asymptomatic and unoperated stenotic level is a common reason for failure of surgery for spinal stenosis, it is generally more prudent to decompress any stenotic level suspected of being potentially symptomatic than not to. When diffuse degenerative changes produce unilateral symptoms with multilevel stenosis, particularly in an elderly patient, decompression by multilevel unilateral hemilaminectomies is a good therapeutic option. If symptoms are bilateral and the stenosis is diffuse and multilevel, multiple bilateral laminotomies, rather than multiple complete laminectomies, can be considered. Multilevel decompression with bilateral laminectomies carries the risk of developing instability and therefore mandates consideration of fusion to ameliorate this risk.

Because fusion is associated with higher morbidity in the elderly population, it is prudent to consider a less extensive surgical decompression that could obviate the need for fusion in these patients. Such an approach reduces the need for concomitant fusion by preserving the uninvolved laminae and ligamentous structures, thereby minimizing the risk of developing late instability. The arguments against such limited decompression are the risk of performing an inadequate decompression, the potential for recurrence of stenosis, and technical challenges associated with a unilateral approach. Unilateral (foraminal) neural decompression without sacrificing the facet joint is difficult in the presence of an intact spinous process because the spinous process inhibits the ability to angle instruments enough to adequately decompress the neural foramen. This can be obviated to some degree by the use of angled rongeurs, although foraminal decompression is still difficult with intact midline structures.

As noted previously, many studies suggest that patients with spinal stenosis and DS have better clinical outcomes when decompression is accompanied by arthrodesis. The issue of whether to augment the fusion with segmental (pedicle) instrumentation is not yet completely resolved. In a *younger, healthy, and active patient* with focal spinal stenosis associated with DS, particularly if associated with well-maintained disc height, fusion of the listhetic level is recommended, usually with segmental fixation, because of the risk of developing subsequent instability. For an *older patient* with combined stenosis and DS, fusion is also generally warranted, particularly if the patient is active and generally healthy. The issue of whether to instrument the fusion, however, is not completely resolved. Although most studies show the beneficial effect of instrumentation on fusion rate, its relationship to improved short-term clinical outcome is not completely known. Because long-term clinical outcome is improved by the presence of a solid fusion and because the use of instrumentation has been shown to increase the likelihood of achieving a solid fusion, instrumentation is generally recommended. In *elderly low-demand patients with multiple comorbidities,* the decision to fuse must be balanced against the increased morbidity associated with arthrodesis. Arthrodesis may not be a therapeutic imperative in the elderly low-demand patient with a listhetic level associated with decreased disc height, spur formation, subchondral sclerosis, or ligament ossification because these degenerative changes may provide enough stability to the listhetic level to minimize the risk of slip progression. Under such conditions, consideration of hemilaminectomies or unilateral or bilateral laminotomies to preserve uninvolved stabilizing structures is warranted.

Decompression and fusion with pedicle fixation are indicated and recommended as a means to promote stability at the level of the slip for active, healthy, physiologically young patients with spinal stenosis associated with DS. Decompression and instrumented fusion is also generally recommended for older, healthy, active patients with a relatively well-maintained disc height at the listhetic level. Elderly and inactive patients can be managed by decompression with either instrumented or noninstrumented fusion. Elderly low-demand patients with multiple comorbidities and significant degenerative changes that reduce the likelihood of slip progression are usually best managed by limited decompression without fusion or decompression with noninstrumented fusion.

PEARLS AND PITFALLS

1. Degenerative spondylolisthesis (DS), also known as spondylolisthesis with an intact neural arch, is an acquired condition that rarely presents before the age of 50 years.
2. DS most commonly affects the L4–L5 level, although other levels may be affected; it rarely affects the L5–S1 level, in contrast to isthmic spondylolisthesis, which most commonly affects L5–S1.
3. It is important to always get a standing anteroposterior and lateral lumbar radiograph of any patient suspected of having a DS because supine radiographs may fail to detect the slip.
4. DS may be asymptomatic or may present with low back pain and neurogenic claudication.
5. In general, the surgical treatment of DS is decompressive laminectomy and fusion.
6. Long-term surgical outcome appears better with a solid arthrodesis than with a pseudarthrosis. It has been shown that posterior instrumented fusion produces a more solid arthrodesis than noninstrumented fusion. Therefore, the durability of surgery may be more reliable with instrumented fusion than with noninstrumented fusion.
7. The role of fusion in the elderly patient with DS must be balanced against the potential morbidity of fusion surgery. Decompression without fusion may be the better option in selected elderly patients with significant medical comorbidities and limited activity.

KEY REFERENCES

1. Macnab I. Spondylolisthesis with an intact neural arch: the so-called pseudo-spondylolisthesis. *J Bone Joint Surg Br.* 1950;32:325-333.
   This classic article by Ian Macnab describes the etiology, clinical findings, and treatment of degenerative spondylolisthesis.
2. Newman P, Stone K. The etiology of spondylolisthesis. *J Bone Joint Surg Br.* 1963;45:39-59.
   Another classic article that describes the etiology, biomechanics, and mechanism of slipping in spondylolisthesis. It is the most commonly used classification of spondylolisthesis.
3. Herkowitz H, Kurz L. Degenerative lumbar spondylolisthesis with spinal stenosis: a prospective study comparing decompression with decompression and intertransverse process arthrodesis. *J Bone Joint Surg Am.* 1991;73:802-808.
   This classic, prospective, randomized, controlled study showed that decompression and noninstrumented fusion was superior to decompression alone in the treatment of degenerative spondylolisthesis.
4. Fischgrund J, Mackay M, Herkowitz H, et al. Degenerative lumbar spondylolisthesis with spinal stenosis: a prospective, randomized study comparing decompressive laminectomy and arthrodesis with and without spinal instrumentation. *Spine.* 1997;22:2807-2812.
   This prospective, randomized study compared posterior pedicle screw fixation with noninstrumented posterolateral fusion and found that the fusion rate at 2 years was better in the instrumented group than in the noninstrumented group, although the clinical outcome was similar in both.
5. Kornblum MB, Fischgrund JS, Herkowitz HN, et al. Degenerative lumbar spondylolisthesis with spinal stenosis: a prospective long-term study comparing fusion and pseudarthrosis. *Spine.* 2004;29:726-733.
   This long-term follow-up of patients undergoing posterolateral fusion and decompression for degenerative spondylolisthesis found that patients with a solid arthrodesis had a superior clinical outcome to those with a pseudarthrosis.
6. Mardjetko S, Connolly P, Shott S. Degenerative lumbar spondylolisthesis: a meta-analysis of literature, 1970-1993. *Spine.* 1994;19(20 suppl):2256S-2265S.
   This is a review of 24 years of literature on degenerative spondylolisthesis. The results of this analysis support the conclusions reached by Herkowitz and his group: patients do better with decompression in conjunction with fusion, and instrumentation enhances the fusion rate.
7. Ghogawala Z, Dziura J, Butler WE, et al. Laminectomy plus fusion versus laminectomy alone for lumbar spondylolisthesis. *N Engl J Med.* 2016;374:1424-1434.
   This prospective, randomized controlled study compared laminectomy alone to laminectomy and instrumented posterolateral fusion in 66 patients with degenerative spondylolisthesis and stenosis. The most striking difference between treatments was the reoperation rate, which was 14% in the fusion group and 34% in the laminectomy alone group.
8. Försth P, Ólafsson G, Carlsson T, et al. A randomized, controlled trial of fusion surgery for lumbar spinal stenosis. *N Engl J Med.* 2016;374:1413-1423.
   Another prospective, randomized controlled study, reporting no difference between decompression alone versus decompression and fusion in patients with degenerative spondylolisthesis and stenosis.

REFERENCES

1. Junghanns H. Spondylolisthesen ohne Spalt in Zwischengelenkstueck. *Arch Orthop Unfallchir.* 1930;29:118-127.
2. Macnab I. Spondylolisthesis with an intact neural arch: the so-called pseudo-spondylolisthesis. *J Bone Joint Surg Br.* 1950;32:325-333.
3. Newman P, Stone K. The etiology of spondylolisthesis. *J Bone Joint Surg Br.* 1963;45:39-59.
4. Marchetti PG, Bartolozzi P. Spondylolisthesis: classification of spondylolisthesis as a guideline for treatment. In: Bridwell R, Dewald R, eds. *The Textbook of Spinal Surgery.* 2nd ed. Philadelphia: Lippincott Williams & Wilkins; 1997:1211-1254.
5. Hammerberg KW. New concepts on the pathogenesis and classification of spondylolisthesis. *Spine.* 2005;30(suppl):S4-S11.
6. Hosoe H, Ohmori K. Degenerative lumbosacral spondylolisthesis: possible factors which predispose the fifth lumbar vertebra to slip. *J Bone Joint Surg Br.* 2008;90:356-359.
7. Rosenberg N. Degenerative spondylolisthesis: surgical treatment. *Clin Orthop Relat Res.* 1976;117:112-120.
8. Bird HA, Eastmond CJ, Hudson A, Wright V. Is generalized joint laxity a factor in spondylolisthesis? *Scand J Rheumatol.* 1980;9:203-205.
9. Ha Kee-Yong, Chang Cheong-Ho, Kim Ki-Won, et al. Expression of estrogen receptor of the facet joints in degenerative spondylolisthesis. *Spine.* 2005;30:562-566.
10. Sanderson PL, Fraser RD. The influence of pregnancy on the development of degenerative spondylolisthesis. *J Bone Joint Surg Br.* 1996;78:951-954.
11. Jacobsen S, Sonne-Holm S, Rovsing H, et al. Degenerative lumbar spondylolisthesis: an epidemiological perspective: the Copenhagen Osteoarthritis Study. *Spine.* 2007;32:120-125.

12. Matsui Y, Mirza SK, Wu JJ, et al. The association of lumbar spondylolisthesis with collagen IX tryptophan alleles. *J Bone Joint Surg Br*. 2004;86:1021-1026.
13. Lee JS, Suh KT, Kim JI, Lim JH, Goh TS. Association of estrogen receptor gene polymorphism in patients with degenerative lumbar spondylolisthesis. *J Korean Neurosurg Soc*. 2011;50:415-419.
14. Crawford NR, Cagli S, Sonntag VK, et al. Biomechanics of grade 1 degenerative spondylolisthesis: I. In vitro model. *J Neurosurg Spine*. 2001;94:51-60.
15. Boden SD, Riew KD, Yamaguchi K, et al. Orientation of the lumbar facet joints: association with degenerative disc disease. *J Bone Joint Surg Am*. 1996;78:403-411.
16. Grobler LJ, Robertson PA, Novotny JE, Pope MH. Etiology of spondylolisthesis: assessment of the role played by lumbar facet joint morphology. *Spine*. 1993;18:80-91.
17. Love TW, Fagan AB, Fraser RD. Degenerative spondylolisthesis: developmental or acquired? *J Bone Joint Surg Br*. 1999;81:670-674.
18. Melnyk AD, Kingwell SP, Zhu Q, et al. An in vitro model of degenerative lumbar spondylolisthesis. *Spine*. 2013;38:E870-E877.
19. Chen I-Ru, Wei Ta-Sen. Disc height and lumbar index as independent predictors of degenerative spondylolisthesis in middle-aged women with low back pain. *Spine*. 2009;34:1402-1409.
20. Watters WC, Bono CM, Gilbert TJ, et al. An evidence-based clinical guideline for the diagnosis and treatment of degenerative lumbar spondylolisthesis. *Spine J*. 2009;9:609-614.
21. Mardjetko S, Connolly P, Shott S. Degenerative lumbar spondylolisthesis: a meta-analysis of literature, 1970-1993. *Spine*. 1994;19(20 suppl):2256S-2265S.
22. Feffer H, Weisel S, Cuckler JM, Rothman RH. Degenerative spondylolisthesis: to fuse or not to fuse. *Spine*. 1985;10:286-289.
23. Saal JA, Saal JA, Parthasarathy R. *The Natural History of Lumbar Spinal Stenosis. The Results of Non-operative Treatment*. Presented at 10th annual meeting of the North American Spine Society (NASS). Washington, DC, 1995.
24. Matsunaga S, Sakou T, Morizono Y, et al. Natural history of degenerative spondylolisthesis: pathogenesis and natural course of the slippage. *Spine*. 1990;15:1204-1210.
25. Cinotti G, Postacchini F, Fassari F, et al. Predisposing factors in degenerative spondylolisthesis: a radiographic and CT study. *Int Orthop*. 1997;21:337-342.
26. Grob D, Humke T, Dvorak J. Degenerative lumbar spinal stenosis decompression with and without arthrodesis. *J Bone Joint Surg Am*. 1995;77:1036-1041.
27. Kalichman L, Kim DH, Li L, et al. Spondylolysis and spondylolisthesis: prevalence and association with low back pain in the adult community-based population. *Spine*. 2009;34:199-205.
28. Verbiest H. A radicular syndrome from developmental narrowing of the lumbar vertebral canal. *J Bone Joint Surg Br*. 1954;36:230-237.
29. Katz JN, Dalgas M, Stucki G, et al. Degenerative lumbar spinal stenosis: diagnostic value of the history and physical examination. *Arthritis Rheum*. 1995;38:1236-1241.
30. Katz J, Lipson S, Larson M, et al. The outcome of decompressive laminectomy for degenerative lumbar stenosis. *J Bone Joint Surg Am*. 1991;73:809-816.
31. Inufusa A, An HS, Lim TH. Anatomic changes of the spinal canal and intervertebral foramen associated with flexion-extension movement. *Spine*. 1996;21:2412-2420.
32. Yoshida M, Shima K, Taniguchi Y. Hypertrophied ligamentum flavum in lumbar spinal canal stenosis: pathogenesis and morphologic and immunohistochemical observation. *Spine*. 1992;17:1353-1360.
33. Dyck P, Doyle JB Jr. "Bicycle test" of van Gelderen in diagnosis of intermittent cauda equina compression syndrome: case report. *J Neurosurg*. 1977;46:667-670.
34. Bendo JA, Ong B. Importance of correlating static and dynamic imaging studies in diagnosing degenerative lumbar spondylolisthesis. *Am J Orthop*. 2001;30:247-250.
35. Chaput C, Allred J, Pandorf J, et al. The significance of facet joint cross-sectional area on magnetic resonance imaging in relationship to cervical degenerative spondylolisthesis. *Spine J*. 2013;13(8):856-861.
36. Chaput C, Padon D, Rush J, et al. The significance of increased fluid signal on magnetic resonance imaging in lumbar facets in relationship to degenerative spondylolisthesis. *Spine*. 2007;32:1883-1887.
37. Ben-Galim P, Reitman CA. The distended facet sign: an indicator of position-dependent spinal stenosis and degenerative spondylolisthesis. *Spine J*. 2007;7:245-248.
38. Schinnerer K, Katz L, Grauer J. MR findings of exaggerated fluid in facet joints predicts instability. *J Spinal Disord Tech*. 2008;21(7):468-472.
39. Jayakumar P, Nnadi C, Saifuddin A, et al. Dynamic degenerative lumbar spondylolisthesis: diagnosis with axial loaded magnetic resonance imaging. *Spine (Phila Pa 1976)*. 2006;31:E298-E301.
40. Boden SD, Wiesel SW. Lumbosacral segmental motion in normal individuals: have we been measuring instability properly? *Spine*. 1990;5:571-576.
41. Hayes MA, Howard TC, Gruel CR, et al. Roentgenographic evaluation of lumbar spine flexion-extension in asymptomatic individuals. *Spine*. 1989;14:327-331.
42. Weinstein JN, Lurie JD, Tosteson TD, et al. Surgical versus nonsurgical treatment for lumbar degenerative spondylolisthesis. *N Engl J Med*. 2007;356:2257-2270.
43. Weinstein JN, Lurie JD, Tosteson TD, et al. Surgical compared with nonoperative treatment for lumbar degenerative spondylolisthesis. *J Bone Joint Surg Am*. 2009;91-A:1295-1304.
44. Pearson AM, Lurie JD, Blood EA, et al. Spine Patient Outcomes Research Trial. radiographic predictors of clinical outcomes after operative or nonoperative treatment of degenerative spondylolisthesis. *Spine*. 2008;33:2759-2766.
45. Matsunaga S, Ijiri K, Hayashi K. Nonsurgically managed patients with degenerative spondylolisthesis: a 10- to 18-year follow-up study. *J Neurosurg*. 2000;93(2 suppl):194-198.
46. Deyo RA, Mirza SK, Martin BI, et al. Trends, major medical complications, and charges associated with surgery for lumbar spinal stenosis in older adults. *JAMA*. 2010;303:1259-1265.
47. Deyo R, Cherkin D, Loeser J, et al. Morbidity and mortality in association with operations on the lumbar spine. *J Bone Joint Surg Am*. 1992;74:536-543.
48. Deyo R, Ciol M, Cherkin D, et al. Lumbar spinal fusion: a cohort study of complications, reoperations, and resource use in the Medicare population. *Spine*. 1993;18:1463-1470.
49. Oldridge N, Yuan Z, Stoll J, Rimm A. Lumbar spine surgery and mortality among Medicare beneficiaries, 1986. *Am J Public Health*. 1994;84:1292-1298.
50. Turner JA, Ersek M, Herron L, et al. Patient outcomes after lumbar spinal fusions. *JAMA*. 1992;268:907-911.
51. Modhia U, Takemoto S, Braid-Forbes MJ, et al. Readmission rates after decompression surgery in patients with lumbar

spinal stenosis among Medicare beneficiaries. *Spine*. 2013;38(7):591-596.

52. Bridwell K, Sedgewick TA, O'Brien MF, et al. The role of fusion and instrumentation in the treatment of degenerative spondylolisthesis with spinal stenosis. *J Spinal Disord*. 1993;6:461-472.
53. Herkowitz H, Kurz L. Degenerative lumbar spondylolisthesis with spinal stenosis: a prospective study comparing decompression with decompression and intertransverse process arthrodesis. *J Bone Joint Surg Am*. 1991;73:802-808.
54. Epstein N, Epstein J. Decompression in the surgical management of degenerative spondylolisthesis: advantages of a conservative approach in 290 patients. *J Spinal Disord*. 1998;11:116-122.
55. Kristof RA, Aliashkevich AF, Schuster M, et al. Degenerative lumbar spondylolisthesis-induced radicular compression: nonfusion-related decompression in selected patients without hypermobility on flexion-extension radiographs. *J Neurosurg*. 2002;97(3 suppl):S281-S286.
56. Sasai K, Umeda M, Maruyama T, et al. Microsurgical bilateral decompression via a unilateral approach for lumbar spinal canal stenosis including degenerative spondylolisthesis. *J Neurosurg Spine*. 2008;9:554-559.
57. Postacchini F, Cinotti G, Perugia D, et al. The surgical treatment of central lumbar stenosis: multiple laminotomy compared with total laminectomy. *J Bone Joint Surg Br*. 1993;75:386-392.
58. Kleeman TJ, Hiscoe AC, Berg EE. Patient outcomes after minimally destabilizing lumbar stenosis decompression: the "port-hole" technique. *Spine*. 2000;25:865-870.
59. Postacchini F, Cinotti G. Bone regrowth after surgical decompression for lumbar spinal stenosis. *J Bone Joint Surg Br*. 1992;74:862-869.
60. Zdeblick T. A prospective, randomized study of lumbar fusion: preliminary results. *Spine*. 1993;18:983-991.
61. Caputy A, Luessenhop A. Long-term evaluation of decompressive surgery for degenerative lumbar stenosis. *J Neurosurg*. 1992;77:669-676.
62. Akamaru T, Kawahara N, Tim Yoon S, et al. Adjacent segment motion after a simulated lumbar fusion in different sagittal alignments: a biomechanical analysis. *Spine*. 2003;28:1560-1566.
63. Bono CM, Lee CK. Critical analysis of trends in fusion for degenerative disc disease over the past 20 years: influence of techniques on fusion rate and clinical outcome. *Spine*. 2004;29:455-463.
64. Fischgrund J, Mackay M, Herkowitz H, et al. Degenerative lumbar spondylolisthesis with spinal stenosis: a prospective, randomized study comparing decompressive laminectomy and arthrodesis with and without spinal instrumentation. *Spine*. 1997;22:2807-2812.
65. Gibson JN, Grant IC, Waddell G. The Cochrane review of surgery for lumbar disc prolapse and degenerative lumbar spondylosis. *Spine*. 1999;24:1820-1832.
66. Malmivaara A, Slätis P, Heliövaara M, et al. Surgical or nonoperative treatment for lumbar spinal stenosis? A randomized controlled trial. *Spine*. 2007;32:1-8.
67. Ghogawala Z, Benzel EC, Amin-Hanjani S, et al. Prospective outcomes evaluation after decompression with or without instrumented fusion for lumbar stenosis and degenerative Grade I spondylolisthesis. *J Neurosurg Spine*. 2004;1:267-272.
68. Bednar DA. Surgical management of lumbar degenerative spinal stenosis with spondylolisthesis via posterior reduction with minimal laminectomy. *J Spinal Disord Tech*. 2002;15:105-109.
69. Yuan HA, Garfin SR, Dickman CA, et al. A historical cohort study of pedicle screw fixation in thoracic lumbar, and sacral spinal fusions. *Spine*. 1994;19(20 suppl):2279-2296.
70. Nork SE, Serena SH, Workman KL, et al. Patient outcomes after decompression and instrumented posterior spinal fusion for degenerative spondylolisthesis. *Spine*. 1999;24:561-569.
71. France JC, Yaszemski MJ, Lauerman WC, et al. A randomized prospective study of posterolateral lumbar fusion outcomes with and without pedicle screw instrumentation. *Spine*. 1999;24:553-560.
72. Kornblum MB, Fischgrund JS, Herkowitz HN, et al. Degenerative lumbar spondylolisthesis with spinal stenosis: a prospective long-term study comparing fusion and pseudarthrosis. *Spine*. 2004;29:726-733.
73. Tsutsumimoto T, Shimogata M, Yoshimura Y, et al. Union versus nonunion after posterolateral lumbar fusion: a comparison of long-term surgical outcomes in patients with degenerative lumbar spondylolisthesis. *Eur Spine J*. 2008;17:1107-1112.
74. Katz JN. Point of view. *Spine*. 2004;29:733-734.
75. Fischgrund JS. The argument for instrumented posterolateral fusion for patients with spinal stenosis and degenerative spondylolisthesis [editorial]. *Spine*. 2004;29:173-174.
76. McLain RF. Instrumented fusion for degenerative spondylolisthesis: is it necessary [editorial]? *Spine*. 2004; 29:170.
77. Phillips FM. The argument for noninstrumented posterolateral fusion for patients with spinal stenosis and degenerative spondylolisthesis [editorial]. *Spine*. 2004;29:170-172.
78. Ghogawala Z, Dziura J, Butler WE, et al. Laminectomy plus fusion versus laminectomy alone for lumbar spondylolisthesis. *N Engl J Med*. 2016;374:1424-1434.
79. Försth P, Ólafsson G, Carlsson T, et al. A randomized, controlled trial of fusion surgery for lumbar spinal stenosis. *N Engl J Med*. 2016;374:1413-1423.
80. Patel AA, Zfass-Mendez M, Lebwohl NH, et al. Minimally invasive versus open lumbar fusion: a comparison of blood loss, surgical complications, and hospital course. *Iowa Orthop J*. 2015;35:130-134.
81. Sembrano J, Tohmeh A, Isaacs R. Two-year comparative outcomes of MIS lateral and MIS transforaminal interbody fusion in the treatment of degenerative spondylolisthesis. Part I: clinical findings. *Spine*. 2016;41(suppl 8):S123-S132.
82. Jagannathan J, Sansur C, Oskouian R Jr, et al. Radiographic restoration of lumbar alignment after transforaminal lumbar interbody fusion. *Neurosurgery*. 2009;64:955-963.
83. Park P, Foley KT. Minimally invasive transforaminal lumbar interbody fusion with reduction of spondylolisthesis: technique and outcomes after a minimum of 2 years' follow-up. *Neurosurg Focus*. 2008;25:E16.
84. Xu H, Tang H, Li Z. Surgical treatment of adult degenerative spondylolisthesis by instrumented transforaminal lumbar interbody fusion in the Han nationality. *J Neurosurg Spine*. 2009;10:496-499.
85. McAfee PC, DeVine JG, Chaput CD, et al. The indications for interbody fusion cages in the treatment of spondylolisthesis: analysis of 120 cases. *Spine*. 2005;30(suppl):S60-S65.
86. Oda I, Abumi K, Yu BS, et al. Types of spinal instability that require interbody support in posterior lumbar reconstruction: an in vitro biomechanical investigation. *Spine*. 2003;28:1573-1580.

87. Sudo H, Oda I, Abumi K, et al. In vitro biomechanical effects of reconstruction on adjacent motion segment: comparison of aligned/kyphotic posterolateral fusion with aligned posterior lumbar interbody fusion/posterolateral fusion. *J Neurosurg*. 2003;99(2 suppl):221-228.
88. Kuntz KM, Snider RK, Weinstein JN, et al. Cost-effectiveness of fusion with and without instrumentation for patients with degenerative spondylolisthesis and spinal stenosis. *Spine*. 2000;25:1132-1139.
89. Tosteson AN, Lurie JD, Tosteson TD, et al. Surgical treatment of spinal stenosis with and without degenerative spondylolisthesis: cost-effectiveness after 2 years. *Ann Intern Med*. 2008;149:845-853.
90. Fritzell P, Hägg O, Jonsson D, Nordwall A. Cost-effectiveness of lumbar fusion and nonsurgical treatment for chronic low back pain in the Swedish Lumbar Spine Study: a multicenter, randomized controlled trial from the Swedish lumbar spine study group. *Spine*. 2004;29:421-434.
91. Booth KC, Bridwell KH, Eisenberg BA, et al. Minimum 5-year results of degenerative spondylolisthesis treated with decompression and instrumented posterior fusion. *Spine*. 1999;24:1721-1727.
92. Anderson P, Tribus C, Kitchel S. Treatment of neurogenic claudication by interspinous decompression: application of the X STOP device in patients with lumbar degenerative spondylolisthesis. *J Neurosurg Spine*. 2006;4:463-471.
93. Verhoof O, Bron J, Wapstra F, et al. High failure rate of the interspinous distraction device (X-Stop) for the treatment of lumbar spinal stenosis caused by degenerative spondylolisthesis. *Eur Spine J*. 2008;17:188-192.
94. Kanayama M, Hashimoto T, Shigenobu K, et al. Non-fusion surgery for degenerative spondylolisthesis using artificial ligament stabilization: surgical indication and clinical results. *Spine*. 2005;30:588-592.
95. Schaeren S, Broger I, Jeanneret B. Minimum four-year follow-up of spinal stenosis with degenerative spondylolisthesis treated with decompression and dynamic stabilization. *Spine*. 2008;33:E636-E642.
96. Welch W, Cheng B, Awad T, et al. Clinical outcomes of the Dynesys dynamic neutralization system: 1-year preliminary results. *Neurosurg Focus*. 2007;22:E8.
97. Mardjetko S, Albert T, Andersson G, et al. Spine/SRS Spondylolisthesis Summary Statement. *Spine*. 2005;30(6 suppl):S3.

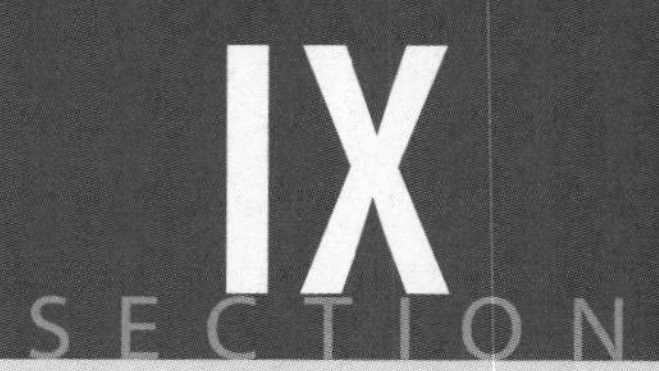

SPINAL FUSION AND INSTRUMENTATION

CHAPTER 65 Techniques and Complications of Bone Graft Harvesting

SECTION IX

Kenny Kwan
Kenneth M.C. Cheung

Solid spinal fusion requires bone healing, similar to the process of fracture healing, through a combination of intramembranous and enchondral ossification. Spinal fusion in a rabbit model is comprised of three distinct phases: early inflammatory phase (weeks 1–3), the middle reparative phase (weeks 4–5), and the late remodeling phase (weeks 6+).[1]

Local bone graft from spinous processes and laminae can be effective in lumbar fusion, either as standalone graft or as graft extender in combination with nonlocal autogenous graft. One study has shown that the mean volume of local bone graft harvested can be approximately 25 mL.[2] A retrospective comparative study showed that for single-level fusion in degenerative lumbar cases, the fusion rate was similar between local bone and iliac crest graft. However, in multilevel fusion, defined as two or more levels, the fusion rate was significantly lower in the local bone group.[3] However, in children undergoing surgery for adolescent idiopathic scoliosis, fusion rate is not greatly influenced by the type of bone graft used.[4,5]

Iliac crest bone graft (ICBG) is still considered the gold standard for spinal fusion by many surgeons today. It is readily available, has inherent fusion-developing properties (i.e., osteogenic potential, osteoinductivity, and osteoconductivity), is biocompatible, and can provide structural support. Harvested bone contains osteoblasts, bony matrix, and factors such as bone morphogenetic proteins, and transforming growth factor-β. The cancellous bone from ICBG contains readily available channels for vascularization[6,7] and important growth factors that facilitate each of the three phases of fusion.

Apart from local bone and ICBG, other sources of autologous bone graft in spine surgery include the rib and both vascularized and nonvascularised fibula.

Surgical Anatomy and Techniques

Anterior Iliac Crest

The ilium was introduced by Abbott in 1942 as a bone graft reserve,[8] and since then the iliac crest and outer table of the ilium have been used as a source of cancellous or corticocancellous bone grafting. Corticocancellous graft can be harvested from the anterior iliac crest. It can be bicortical or tricortical bone graft for use in anterior cervical arthrodesis after discectomy or corpectomy. This is the preferred site for anterior spinal surgery due to easier access without the need to turn the patient prone.

The patient is placed in the supine position. A roll or sandbag is placed underneath the gluteal area of the side from which bone graft will be harvested. This elevates and internally rotates the iliac crest, making it more readily accessible. This area is prepped and draped separately from the main wound. It is our practice to prep this area in all cases of anterior cervical spine surgery in the event that autogenous bone graft is needed.

The surgical incision is made parallel to the iliac crest, beginning at least 2 cm posterior and lateral to the anterior superior iliac spine (ASIS), at the iliac tubercle (Fig. 65.1A). This incision can reduce the amount of fibrous scar healing by preserving the skin around the ASIS.[9] The skin is pulled superiorly so the incision is not directly on the crest itself. This maneuver can reduce discomfort from having a scar directly over a bony prominence. The iliac tubercle marks the anterior portion of the ilium and is the area containing the largest amount of corticocancellous bone. An incision here will avoid a variant course of the lateral femoral cutaneous nerve (LFCN). The LFCN most commonly exits the pelvis about 2 cm medial to the ASIS and passes beneath the inguinal ligament and sartorius muscle, both of which attach to the ASIS. The most superficial and dangerous variant course (in about 4% of cases) occurs when the LFCN exits through the abdominal wall, approximately 2 cm posterior to the ASIS, and crosses the iliac crest.[10] An incision at least 2 cm lateral to the ASIS should avoid the LFCN.

After incising the skin, the incision is continued through the subcutaneous fat and deep fascia onto the periosteum (Fig. 65.1B). The deep fascia can be incised in the manner of a flap, such that after closure it can act as "tent" to cover up the defect. The next step depends on whether cancellous bone or corticocancellous bone graft is required. If only cancellous bone is required, a trapdoor method is used to elevate the cortex of the iliac crest, which can subsequently be "closed" after the cancellous bone is harvested to maintain the contour of the iliac crest. An osteotome is used to make horizontal cut over the crest and at the outer periosteal table, while the inner table is kept intact by the periosteum and fascial attachments of

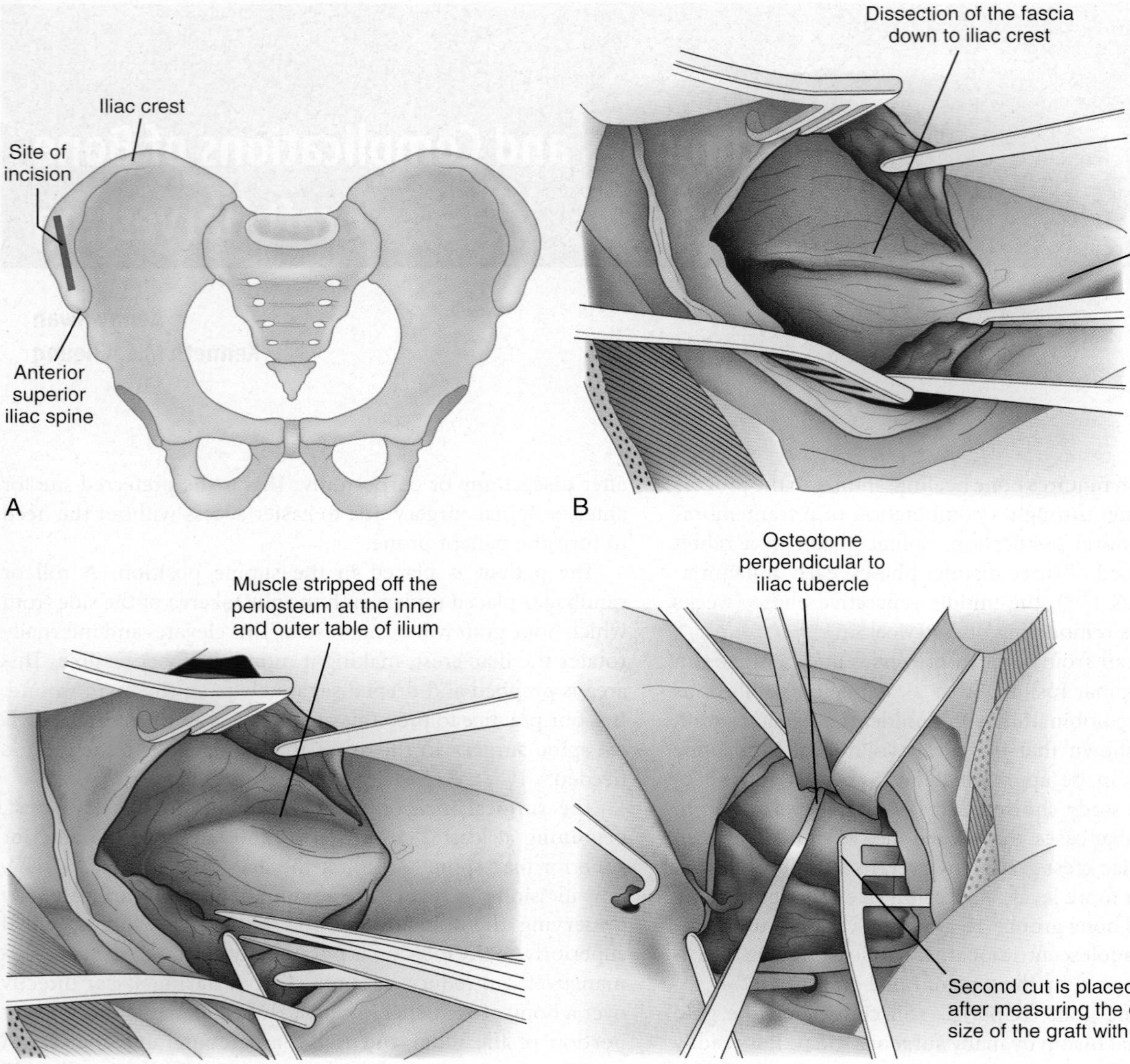

Iliac crest
Site of incision
Anterior superior iliac spine

A

Dissection of the fascia down to iliac crest
ASIS

B

Muscle stripped off the periosteum at the inner and outer table of ilium

C

Osteotome perpendicular to iliac tubercle
Second cut is placed here after measuring the desired size of the graft with caliper

D

2 parallel perpendicular cuts made and further cut at the base of the iliac crest to obtain tricortical graft

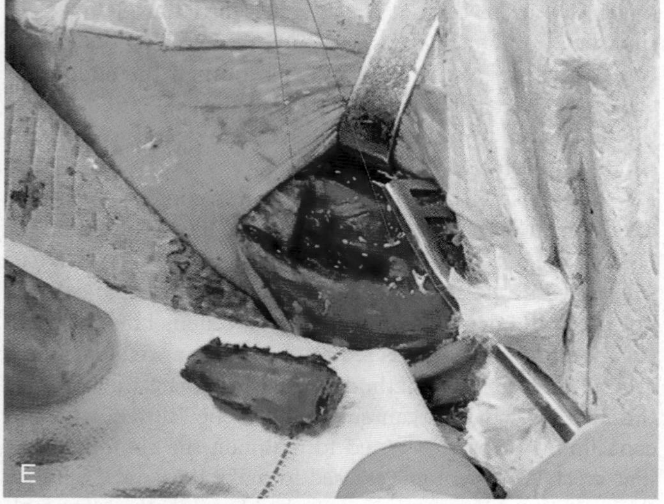

FIG. 65.1 (A) Incision is made 2 cm posterolateral to the anterior superior iliac spine over the iliac crest. This decreases the risk of fracture, and the incision is not made directly over the bone defect. (B) Incision is continued over the skin, subcutaneous tissues, and a deep fascia flap. (C) The deep fascia and muscles are stripped from the periosteum so the surfaces of the iliac crest are exposed. (D) An osteotome or oscillating saw can be used to make a cut perpendicular to the iliac tubercle. A spare saw blade can be left in place to guide a second parallel cut of the predetermined-size bone graft. The graft cut is completed with an osteotome at the base of the bone. (E) A tricortical bone graft of the desirable size is harvested.

iliacus and the abdominal wall muscles. This serves as a hinge for the cortex to "open" like a trapdoor, and cancellous bone can be harvested with a curette. The periosteum and fascia can be approximated subsequently and the cortex of the crest will heal in its original position.

For harvesting tricortical cancellous graft, subperiosteal stripping of the muscles off the inner and outer table either using cauterization or a periosteal elevator and sponge packing provides adequate exposure (Fig. 65.1C). The length and depth of the required graft are measured with a caliper. The harvest site must be at least 2 fingerbreadths posterior to the ASIS to reduce the likelihood of a stress fracture from the downward pull of the sartorius and rectus femoris. A complete block of the ilium can be removed with an oscillating saw or osteotome to make two cuts perpendicular to the surface of the iliac tubercle (Fig. 65.1D) and is completed with an osteotome at the base of the crest (Fig. 65.1E). To obtain cuts parallel to each other, a spare saw blade can be placed in the first cut to act as a guide for the second cut. Hemostasis with bone wax and gel foam can be applied to the defect, and the fascia is repaired. We do not routinely use a drain at the harvest site.

Posterior Iliac Crest

The superior and posterior margin of this bone graft donor site is the posterior iliac crest, with the inferior margin being the greater sciatic notch. The anterior margin is the anterior limit of the superior limb of the sacroiliac joint, although this remains unseen during the bone graft harvest.

This site of harvest is typically used in posterior spinal surgery since the patient is already placed in the prone position. The posterior superior iliac spine (PSIS) and the subcutaneous part of the iliac crest are readily palpable. Either an oblique incision centered over the PSIS in line with the crest (Fig. 65.2A) or a longitudinal incision can be used. An anatomic study using cadavers and dry ilium specimens showed that the average distance from the superior cluneal nerve laterally to the PSIS medially was 68.8 mm.[11] The incision therefore should be placed well within this distance to avoid injury to this nerve and formation of painful neuromas. Alternatively, if the patient is undergoing lumbosacral spinal surgery, the incision can be extended distally and the posterior iliac crest can be accessed via the midline fascial splitting technique.

The midline fascial splitting approach was described by Hutchinson and Dall.[12] After incising the dorsal lumbar fascia and releasing the fascial insertion from the spinous process, the two posterior planes of the fascia (i.e., the fascial extension of the latissimus dorsi and the fascia of the erector spinae muscles) are separated. Both fascial layers attach to the iliac crest, so the surgeon is led directly to the border of the iliac crest. Electrocautery is used to cut directly down onto the crest to release the insertion of the fascia of the gluteus maximus. The gluteus can be elevated from the crest subperiosteally with a Cobb elevator (Fig. 65.2B–C).

Xu et al.[11] proposed that the largest and thickest area of the posterior iliac crest was bound by the superior extension of the posterior border of the superior limb of the articular surface anteriorly, and a line extending from the PSIS to the apex of the sacroiliac joint and oriented perpendicular to the posterior margin of the superior limb inferiorly. The average anterior limit was 34 mm lateral to the PSIS, with an average maximum thickness of 17.1 mm.

An osteotome is used to make an initial cut parallel to the superior aspect of the iliac crest. Then longitudinal cuts are made to the outer cortical table and completed with a gouge at the inferior limit to obtain cortical strips of bone graft (Fig. 65.2D). Afterward, the exposed underlying cancellous bone can be removed by careful stripping using the gouge without breaching the inner table (Fig. 65.2E). Both cortical and cancellous bone grafts can be obtained and used as needed (Fig. 65.2F). When both the outer cortical table and the cancellous bone beneath it are harvested, significantly more bone can be obtained than when just the cancellous bone is taken from between the inner and outer cortices (average 36 g vs. 25.7 g).[13] Before closure, hemostasis should be achieved with bone wax and gel foam. The wound is thoroughly irrigated before closing the incision in layers. We do not routinely use a suction drain at the harvest site because there is evidence suggesting that suction drainage does not improve patient outcomes.[14-16]

Rib

During anterior thoracic or thoracoabdominal approaches to the spine, a piece of rib may be excised to facilitate access to the thoracic cavity. The rib can be saved and trimmed to the appropriate size for the graft.

The incision should be centered over the appropriate rib, and skin, subcutaneous tissue, and the intercostal muscles are incised down to the rib. The periosteum is stripped with a periosteal elevator, taking care not to inadvertently incise the parietal pleura during this stage (Fig. 65.3). The costochondral junction can be cut medially with a rib cutter, as close to the angle of the rib as possible. The rib can then be wrapped with a piece of wet gauze until the graft is needed. The rib should be cleared of soft tissue to ensure good bony fusion and cut to the appropriate size.

Fibula

Autogenous fibula graft is rarely used these days because other sites for harvesting or allograft bone are usually available. The relatively high morbidity of autogenous fibular harvest precludes its routine use because it may affect ambulation. Nevertheless, the fibula can be used as a strut graft for anterior reconstruction after multilevel corpectomies in the cervical and thoracic spine.

A direct lateral incision is made parallel to the posterior border of fibula, at the middle third of the fibula, and carried directly down to the bone. The superficial peroneal nerve and surrounding soft tissues should be protected. Subperiosteal elevation of the peronei, extensor digitorum longus, tibialis posterior, flexor hallucis longus, and soleus from the bone is performed (Fig. 65.4). Once stripped of the muscles, a suitable length of bone can be harvested with an oscillating saw.

The syndesmosis of the ankle joint is 10 cm proximal to the joint, so harvesting should extend no more distally than 10 cm

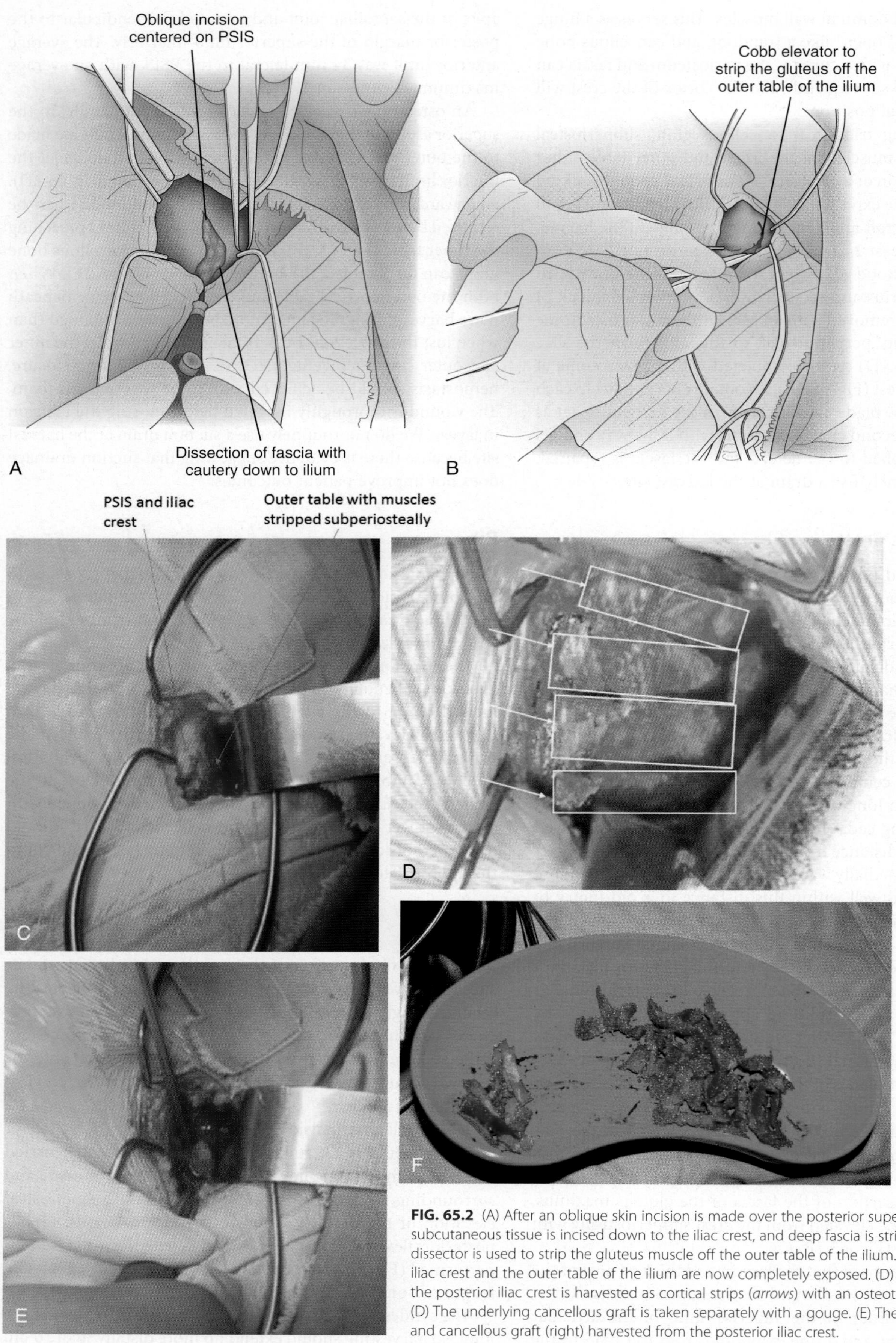

FIG. 65.2 (A) After an oblique skin incision is made over the posterior superior iliac crest, subcutaneous tissue is incised down to the iliac crest, and deep fascia is stripped. (B) A Cobb dissector is used to strip the gluteus muscle off the outer table of the ilium. (C) The top of the iliac crest and the outer table of the ilium are now completely exposed. (D) The outer cortex of the posterior iliac crest is harvested as cortical strips (*arrows*) with an osteotome and gouge. (D) The underlying cancellous graft is taken separately with a gouge. (E) The cortical strips (left) and cancellous graft (right) harvested from the posterior iliac crest.

above the ankle joint, or else there is a risk of ankle joint instability. Proximally, the common peroneal nerve courses over the neck of the fibula within the substance of the peroneus longus muscle, then divides into the deep and superficial branches. Hence the ideal harvest site lies at the junction of the distal third and middle third of the fibula.

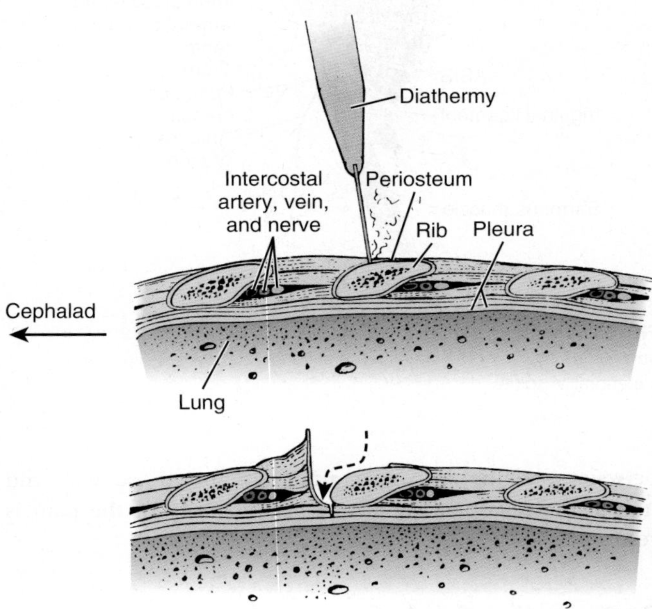

FIG. 65.3 The pleura is entered superior to the rib to avoid damage to the intercostal neurovascular bundle, which courses along the rib's posteroinferior border.

Complications of Bone Graft Harvesting

General

Hematoma

Arterial injury is uncommon during bone graft harvesting. Harvesting bone grafts from the inner table of the anterior ilium can damage the arterial anastomoses formed by the lumbar artery, iliolumbar artery, and deep circumflex iliac artery that supplies iliacus. In posterior bone grafting, the superior gluteal artery can be injured (see below).

After the bone graft is harvested, adequate hemostasis must be obtained with bone wax applied over the cancellous bone surfaces and other sites of bleeding and filled with gel foam. If adequate hemostasis is achieved intraoperatively, a suction drain is optional.

Infection

Donor site infection is uncommon and no more likely than in other orthopedic procedures. The principles of treatment are identical to any other surgical site infections.

Anterior Iliac Crest

Complications include pain, infection, cosmetic deformity, peritoneal perforation, and herniation of abdominal contents through the defect in the ilium. Stress fracture of the anterior ilium has also been reported.

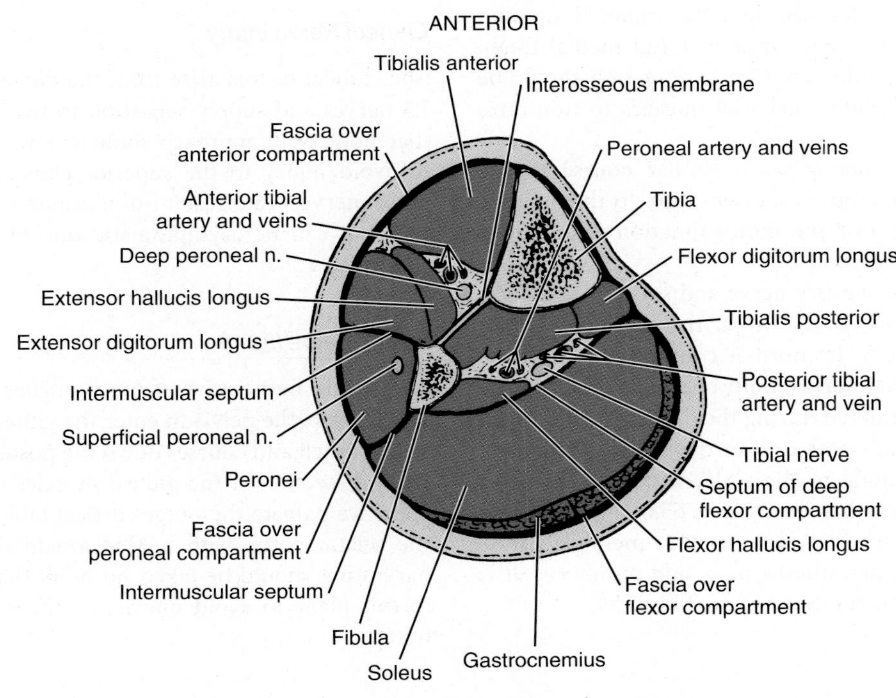

FIG. 65.4 Axial view of the lower leg depicting the fibro-osseus compartments as well as the neurovascular structures.

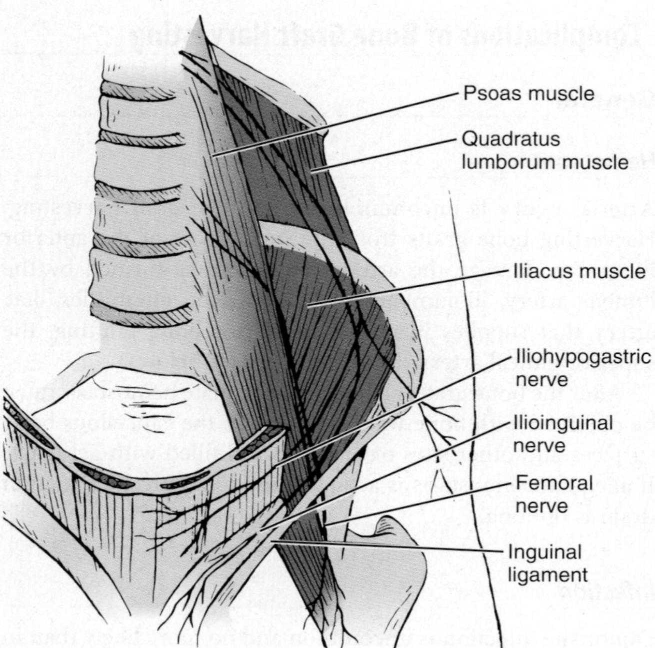

FIG. 65.5 Anteroposterior view of the abdomen and pelvis showing the normal course of the ilioinguinal, iliohypogastric, and femoral nerves.

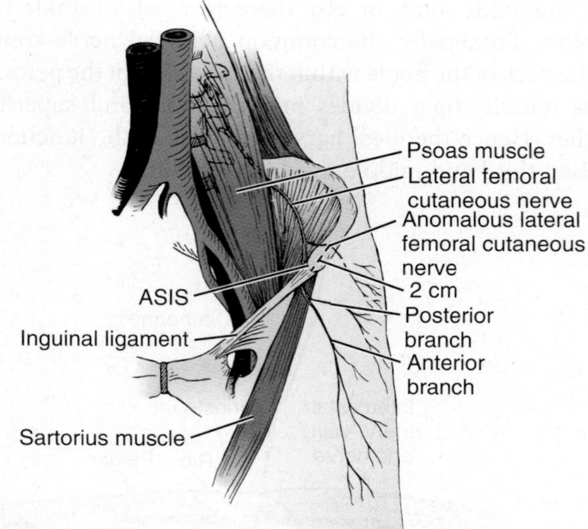

FIG. 65.6 Anteroposterior view of the pelvis depicting the normal and anomalous course of the lateral femoral cutaneous nerve. ASIS, anterior superior iliac spine.

Nerve Injuries

Nerve injuries are uncommon, but the ilioinguinal, iliohypogastric, and lateral femoral cutaneous nerves can be injured during anterior bone graft harvesting (Fig. 65.5).

The ilioinguinal nerve is a branch of L1. It traverses the internal oblique and transversus abdominis, passes under the external oblique, and enters the inguinal canal. It supplies sensation to parts of the penis, proximal and medial thigh, scrotum, and adjacent abdomen. Gentle retraction should be applied to iliacus and abdominal wall muscles to minimize injury to this nerve.

The iliohypogastric nerve has a similar course to the ilioinguinal nerve and supplies the sensation to the anterior two-thirds of the iliac crest and motor function of the lower portion of the abdominal wall.

The LFCN is a pure sensory nerve and supplies sensation to the anterolateral aspect of the thigh. The nerve passes into the thigh near the ASIS. Its normal course is beneath the inguinal ligament and sartorius, both of which attach to the ASIS, and is not encountered during the dissection. However, in 10% of cases the nerve crosses over the anterior iliac crest approximately 2 cm lateral to the ASIS, making it liable to damage during bone graft harvesting (Fig. 65.6). LFCN neurapraxia due to retraction will present itself as meralgia paresthetica, manifesting as paresthesia, pain, and numbness. It is usually self-limiting and resolves within 3 months.

Pain

The incidence of persistent donor site pain from anterior iliac crest harvesting ranges between 2% and 40%. Nonetheless, no differences have been found in health-related outcomes between patients who had autograft and those who did not; at 6 weeks postoperatively, the majority of the pain is resolved.[17]

Posterior Iliac Crest

Pain, cluneal nerve injury, infection, stress fracture, sacroiliac joint injury, alterations in gait (i.e., gluteal gait), vascular injury, and ureteral injury have been reported.

Cluneal Nerve Injury

The cluneal nerves arise from the dorsal rami of L1, L2, and L3 nerves and supply sensation to the buttocks. A posterior iliac bone graft approach should be within 8 cm of the PSIS to avoid injury to the superior cluneal nerves. Damage to these nerves can result in numbness and painful neuromas but can be asymptomatic due to cross-innervation in this area.

Sciatic Nerve Injury

The sciatic nerve arises from branches of the sacral plexus L4–S3, exits the pelvis to enter the gluteal region through the sciatic notch and courses down the posterior thigh (Fig. 65.7). After dissection of the gluteal muscles off the posterior iliac crest, we palpate the outer cortical table of the ilium toward the sciatic notch with a MacDonald dissector. Subsequent harvesting should be taken no more than 1 cm in proximity to this plane to avoid injuries to the contents of the sciatic notch.

Superior Gluteal Artery Injury

Injury of the superior gluteal vessels can cause a false aneurysm, arteriovenous fistula, and hemorrhage. The superior

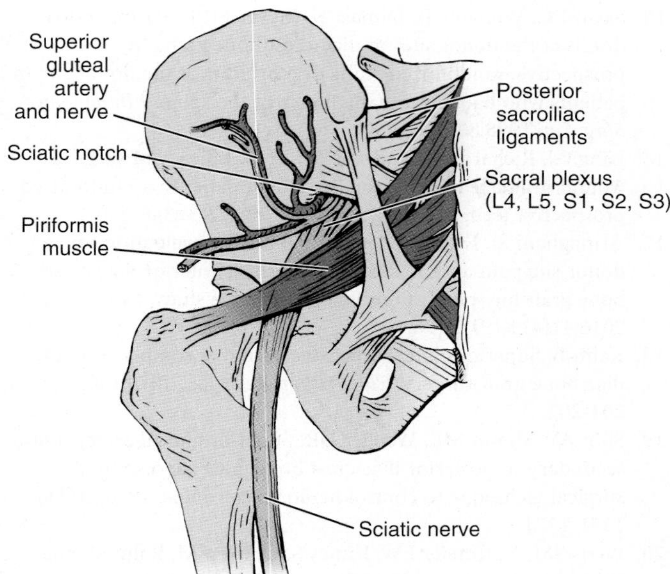

FIG. 65.7 Posteroanterior view of the pelvis showing the neurovascular structures in the sciatic notch.

gluteal vessels leave the pelvis through the superior portion of the greater sciatic notch, staying against the bone. The average distance between the PSIS and the superior gluteal vessels was 62.4 mm from anatomic studies of dry specimens.

Management of superior gluteal artery injury includes direct pressure, enlargement of the upper margin of the sciatic notch to allow better access to bleeding vessels, immediate supine positioning to allow approach to the vessels anteriorly, angiographic-controlled embolization,[18] and subperiosteal elevation of the gluteus maximus to identify the vessel at the superior border of piriformis.[19]

Pain

A retrospective study found that most patients who had ICBG were unable to identify which side the iliac crest had been harvested.[20] Another study found that in patients who did not have any ICBG harvesting, 51% had tenderness over the iliac crest, and patients who had ICBG harvesting had an equal likelihood of having pain over the unharvested ilium as the harvested one.[21] Other studies have also found that patients may not be able to differentiate between donor site pain and residual low back pain.[22] These studies put in perspective the general gluteal pain experienced by patients after posterior lumbar fusion and dispute the common belief of the severity and frequency of donor site pain.

Nonetheless, some studies have shown significant rates of persistent pain and morbidity from iliac bone graft harvest.[23] One prospective observational cohort study found that at 12 months postoperatively, 15.5% of patients reported more severe pain from the harvest site than from the primary operative site, and 29.1% reported numbness. Reported effects have included functional limitation due to harvest site pain, including difficulty in walking (15.1%) and problems with employment (5.2%), recreation (12.9%), household chores (14.1%), sexual activity (7.6%), and irritation from clothing (5.9%).[24]

Fracture

Iliac crest fractures have been reported after ICBG harvesting.[25,26] Risk factors include age, osteoporosis, and comorbidities.

The best way to reduce the risk of structurally weakening the posterior crest is to maintain its continuity and enter the bone below the crest on the outer table. Graft sites that cross the anterior plane of the sacroiliac joint are subjected to tensile and shear forces that may exceed the strength of the remaining bone. Hence, pelvic integrity is least compromised if the area of harvest is limited to the iliac bone posterior to the posterior coronal plane of the sacroiliac joint to avoid pelvic ring fracture.

Kurz and colleagues[14] recommend that long splitting of the iliac tables should be avoided to prevent undue stress concentrating on the remaining ilium.

Fibula

The incidence of complications after fibula bone graft harvesting ranges from 40% to 57.7%. The most common short-term complication is pain at the donor site for up to 3 months postoperatively. Infection either in the form of cellulitis or deep wound infection has also been reported. Long-term complications include incisional pain lasting more than 3 months postoperatively, injury to the superficial peroneal nerve causing paresthesia and neuroma, infection, tibial stress fractures, and ankle instability. Other complications that have been reported include delayed wound healing, contracture of the flexor hallucis longus, and weakness of toe flexor and extensor muscles due to disruption of the interosseous membrane.

Rib

Each intercostal neurovascular bundle is located in the groove on the posteroinferior edge of the rib. Subperiosteal dissection of the rib should avoid damage to these structures. Intercostal analgesia near the costovertebral junction before wound closure can decrease postoperative pain.

KEY REFERENCES

1. Sandhu HS, Grewal HS, Parvataneni H. Bone grafting for spinal fusion. *Orthop Clin North Am*. 1999;30(4):685-698.
2. Xu R, Ebraheim NA, Yeasting RA, Jackson WT. Anatomic considerations for posterior iliac bone harvesting. *Spine*. 1996; 21(9):1017-1020.
3. Kurz LT, Garfin SR, Booth RE Jr. Harvesting autogenous iliac bone grafts. A review of complications and techniques. *Spine*. 1989;14(12):1324-1331.
4. Howard JM, Glassman SD, Carreon LY. Posterior iliac crest pain after posterolateral fusion with or without iliac crest graft harvest. *Spine J*. 2011;11(6):534-537.
5. Banwart JC, Asher MA, Hassanein RS. Iliac crest bone graft harvest donor site morbidity. A statistical evaluation. *Spine*. 1995;20(9):1055-1060.

REFERENCES

1. Boden SD, Schimandle JH, Hutton WC, Chen MI. The use of an osteoinductive growth factor for lumbar spinal fusion. Part I: biology of spinal fusion. *Spine*. 1995;20(24):2626-2632.
2. Carragee EJ, Comer GC, Smith MW. Local bone graft harvesting and volumes in posterolateral lumbar fusion: a technical report. *Spine J*. 2011;11(6):540-544.
3. Sengupta DK, Truumees E, Patel CK, et al. Outcome of local bone versus autogenous iliac crest bone graft in the instrumented posterolateral fusion of the lumbar spine. *Spine*. 2006;31(9):985-991.
4. Price CT, Connolly JF, Carantzas AC, Ilyas I. Comparison of bone grafts for posterior spinal fusion in adolescent idiopathic scoliosis. *Spine*. 2003;28(8):793-798.
5. Theologis AA, Tabaraee E, Lin T, Lubicky J, Diab M. Spinal Deformity Study Group. Type of bone graft or substitute does not affect outcome of spine fusion with instrumentation for adolescent idiopathic scoliosis. *Spine*. 2015;40(17):1345-1351.
6. Sandhu HS, Grewal HS, Parvataneni H. Bone grafting for spinal fusion. *Orthop Clin North Am*. 1999;30(4):685-698.
7. Rihn JA, Gates C, Glassman SD, et al. The use of bone morphogenetic protein in lumbar spine surgery. *Instr Course Lect*. 2009;58:677-688.
8. Abbott LC. The use of iliac bone in the treatment of ununited fractures. *AAOS Instructional Course Lectures*. 1944;13-22.
9. Hwang K, Nam YS, Kim DJ, Han SH, Hwang SH. Could skin retraction incision minimize nerve injury over the iliac crest? *J Craniofac Surg*. 2007;18(6):1447-1450.
10. Aszmann OC, Dellon ES, Dellon AL. Anatomical course of the lateral femoral cutaneous nerve and its susceptibility to compression and injury. *Plast Reconstr Surg*. 1997;100(3):600-604.
11. Xu R, Ebraheim NA, Yeasting RA, Jackson WT. Anatomic considerations for posterior iliac bone harvesting. *Spine*. 1996; 21(9):1017-1020.
12. Hutchinson MR, Dall BE. Midline fascial splitting approach to the iliac crest for bone graft. A new approach. *Spine*. 1994;19(1):62-66.
13. Mirovsky Y, Neuwirth MG. Comparison between the outer table and intracortical methods of obtaining autogenous bone graft from the iliac crest. *Spine*. 2000;25(13):1722-1725.
14. Kurz LT, Garfin SR, Booth RE Jr. Harvesting autogenous iliac bone grafts. A review of complications and techniques. *Spine*. 1989;14(12):1324-1331.
15. Sasso RC, Williams JI, Dimasi N, Meyer PR Jr. Postoperative drains at the donor sites of iliac-crest bone grafts. A prospective, randomized study of morbidity at the donor site in patients who had a traumatic injury of the spine. *J Bone Joint Surg Am*. 1998;80(5):631-635.
16. Lang GJ, Richardson M, Bosse MJ, et al. Efficacy of surgical wound drainage in orthopaedic trauma patients: a randomized prospective trial. *J Orthop Trauma*. 1998;12(5):348-350.
17. Armaghani SJ, Even JL, Zern EK, et al. The evaluation of donor site pain after harvest of tricortical anterior iliac crest bone graft for spinal surgery: a prospective study. *Spine*. 2016;41(4):E191-E196.
18. Kahn B. Superior gluteal artery laceration, a complication of iliac bone graft surgery. *Clin Orthop Relat Res*. 1979;140: 204-207.
19. Shin AY, Moran ME, Wenger DR. Superior gluteal artery injury secondary to posterior iliac crest bone graft harvesting. A surgical technique to control hemorrhage. *Spine*. 1996;21(11): 1371-1374.
20. Pirris SM, Nottmeier EW, Kimes S, O'Brien M, Rahmathulla G. A retrospective study of iliac crest bone grafting techniques with allograft reconstruction: do patients even know which iliac crest was harvested? *J Neurosurg Spine*. 2014;21(4):595-600.
21. Howard JM, Glassman SD, Carreon LY. Posterior iliac crest pain after posterolateral fusion with or without iliac crest graft harvest. *Spine J*. 2011;11(6):534-537.
22. Delawi D, Dhert WJ, Castelein RM, Verbout AJ, Oner FC. The incidence of donor site pain after bone graft harvesting from the posterior iliac crest may be overestimated: a study on spine fracture patients. *Spine*. 2007;32(17):1865-1868.
23. Fernyhough JC, Schimandle JJ, Weigel MC, Edwards CC, Levine AM. Chronic donor site pain complicating bone graft harvesting from the posterior iliac crest for spinal fusion. *Spine*. 1992;17(12):1474-1480.
24. Kim DH, Rhim R, Li L, et al. Prospective study of iliac crest bone graft harvest site pain and morbidity. *Spine J*. 2009;9(11): 886-892.
25. Hu RW, Bohlman HH. Fracture at the iliac bone graft harvest site after fusion of the spine. *Clin Orthop Relat Res*. 1994;309: 208-213.
26. Banwart JC, Asher MA, Hassanein RS. Iliac crest bone graft harvest donor site morbidity. A statistical evaluation. *Spine*. 1995;20(9):1055-1060.

CHAPTER 66 Principles of Bone Fusion

Terri A. Zachos
Nicolas S. Piuzzi
Thomas Mroz
Krzysztof B. Siemionow
George F. Muschler

Spinal fusion may be defined as a bony union between two or more vertebral bodies. Spinal fusion was first reported in 1911 for treatment of Pott disease. The mechanical stability provided by fusion was intended to inhibit progressive deformity and the spread of the tuberculous infection.[1] Surgery to accomplish spinal fusion has now been extended to treat a variety of spinal conditions, including scoliosis, kyphosis, fracture, dislocation, spondylolisthesis, and intervertebral disc disease.

Much has changed since the pioneering efforts of Albee[1] and Hibbs[2] in the early part of the twentieth century. Specialized techniques and surgical approaches have been developed for internal fixation and fusion of every part of the spine. Additionally, there have been significant advances in diagnostic techniques, intraoperative image guidance, intraoperative monitoring, minimally invasive surgical approaches, and bone graft materials. These advances have allowed for the aggressive correction of many severe spinal deformities with relative safety and predictability. Furthermore, the biologic principles on which these procedures are based have become better understood and used.

All fusion surgery involves preparation of bony surfaces at the site of the intended fusion. This usually involves the removal of soft tissues and decortication of bony surfaces. The stimulus for the bone healing response, commonly referred to as the "bone graft," may be autologous or homologous bone (i.e., allograft bone) or one of an increasing number of synthetic materials or bioactive substances. As the graft is incorporated, bone tissue is formed by osteogenic cells. Union is accomplished when the newly synthesized bone matrix becomes mineralized and remodels with mature bone, having sufficient strength to bear physiologic loads without injury, thus becoming mechanically contiguous with the local host bone. Failure of bone formation, union, or effective remodeling results in pseudarthrosis. The incidence of pseudarthrosis ranges from 5% to 34% in large adult series.[3–11] A recent review of revision spine fusion procedures found that 23.6% were performed for pseudarthrosis.[10,11]

The fundamental requirements for a successful spinal fusion are (1) availability of an adequate population of osteogenic cells; (2) the presence of an osteoconductive matrix within the region where new bone tissue is desired, osteoinductive signals within the graft site; (3) an adequate local blood supply to support a bone healing response; and (4) a local mechanical environment suitable for bone formation. The following is a discussion of these fundamental concepts and principles, with a review of the orthopaedic and neurosurgical literature regarding the bone grafting materials that are currently used or under evaluation in clinical spine fusion.

Biology of Fusion Sites

Bone growth between vertebrae in a spinal fusion, as in all bone healing, is a cellular process, and unless cells are added to the fusion site, the tissues at the site are the only source of viable cells. Conventional *autogenous* bone grafts add osteogenic cells; however, it has long been recognized that only a small fraction of these cells survive.[12–17] Consequently, preparation of the fusion site and handling of the tissue bed are of paramount importance for a successful arthrodesis. The components of the tissue bed that contribute most to the healing process are the local population of osteogenic stem cells and progenitor cells, local vascular tissues, the cells contributing to the inflammatory response, and the formation of a stable clot within the void spaces of the graft site. Bone, fat, and muscle have all been shown to contain osteogenic stem cells and progenitors that can contribute to new bone formation.[18–26] These basic elements of the graft bed may be affected by local or systemic disease. However, the quality of these elements within the graft site is largely determined by surgical technique.

To preserve the local blood supply, the surgeon must attempt to minimize trauma to the host tissue bed imposed by the trauma of retraction, cautery, and/or desiccation. Any avascular, nonviable, or heavily traumatized tissues should be removed. The importance of the local blood supply cannot be overstated. The blood supply serves as (1) a source of oxygen and other nutrients to the healing tissue as well as control of local pH; (2) a vehicle for endocrine stimulation; (3) a conduit for recruitment of inflammatory cells, which both produce paracrine factors, which may mediate the early proliferation of osteoblastic progenitor cells, and serve to reduce the potential for infection; (4) a source of endothelial cells that produce paracrine factors, which may enhance osteoblastic differentiation[27,28]; and (5) a potential source of osteoblastic progenitors in the form of the vascular pericyte[29,30] or circulating osteogenic cells.[31,32]

The effect of the postoperative hematoma on the success of fusion has been debated. It has been suggested that spinal fusion wounds should not be drained because the fibrin-rich local hematoma may provide an osteoconductive scaffold or matrix, which may assist some of the initial phases of bone healing. Additionally, the trapped platelets in the hematoma release platelet-derived growth factor (PDGF), epidermal growth factor (EGF), basic fibroblast growth factor (bFGF or FGF-2), vascular endothelial growth factors (VEGFs), transforming growth factor beta (TGF-β), and other growth factors that play a critical role during the repair process (discussed later).[33–35] On the other hand, the presence of a large hematoma may displace some of the vascular tissue surrounding the graft site away from the graft, slowing the vascularization of the graft site. It may also increase the chance for displacement of the graft and the potential for nonunion or bone formation outside the intended site.

The inflammatory response in the wound site and the grafted bed represents a critical event in the healing process. This response will involve the removal of necrotic tissue debris, lysis of the local fibrin clot, the establishment and reestablishment of a vascular supply to the graft and host tissue, and synthesis of an early matrix rich in hyaluronic acid.[14,36–42] After the surgical procedure, polymorphonuclear cells, lymphocytes, monocytes, and macrophages migrate to the fusion site and perform their various functions. Among these, and possibly the most important in terms of affecting vascular endothelial cells and osteoblastic progenitors in the graft site, is the local production of paracrine signals: cytokines, kinins, and prostaglandins. These messages act as chemotactic signals and growth factors, affecting the proliferation, migration, differentiation, and activity of a variety of cells, as well as modulation of local blood flow, vascular permeability, and angiogenic response of local endothelial cells. In this way, the inflammatory response establishes the local environment in which the early events of the bone healing response occur. It is not surprising, therefore, that agents that inhibit the inflammatory response have been shown to alter or inhibit bone healing.[43–48] While the use of nonsteroidal antiinflammatory drugs (NSAIDs) has been associated with impaired healing in patients undergoing spinal fusion,[48] a more recent meta-analysis of clinical trials did not support the hypothesis that use of NSAIDs increases the risk of nonunion.[49] NSAIDs reduce inflammation by inhibiting cyclooxygenases (COX). The *COX-2* isoform specifically induces osteogenesis via the anabolic effect of prostaglandin E_2 and the subsequent upregulation of *Runx2*, a transcription factor that is necessary for osteoblastogenesis.[50] These findings have led to the recommendation that clinicians weigh the theoretical risks of impaired bone healing against the potential for pain benefit of NSAID therapy.[42,51]

In addition to the influence of the local blood supply and the inflammatory response, the host bone surface itself is known to have a profound effect on the healing process in spinal fusions. When properly prepared by the surgeon, local bone will serve as a reservoir of osteogenic cells and osteoinductive signals. It also provides an osteoconductive surface for graft incorporation and serves as part of the local blood supply to the graft site. As such, the goal of surgical preparation of local bone is to minimize cellular and mechanical damage to the host bone, while maximizing the availability of osteoprogenitor cells and the osteoconductive and osteoinductive properties of this surface. This is generally achieved by subperiosteal dissection with or without decortication or roughening of the underlying bone to expose vascular osteonal or endosteal bone spaces. Decortication can be achieved with manual tools such as a rongeur or osteotome. Alternatively, a power burr may be used, provided that caution is exercised to prevent thermal necrosis of the bone owing to the heat of friction at the site by using continuous irrigation and limiting periods of contact between the burr and bone at any one site.[52] The surface area of cancellous bone exposed during decortication is another factor thought to affect the success of a spinal fusion. Increasing the available surface area also increases the number of osteogenic cells at the fusion site, which should have a positive effect on the amount of bone formed and the rate of graft incorporation. Additionally, increasing the area of contact between the osteogenic host bone and the graft material should lead to an increase in the osteoconductive surface area available and potentially lead to greater mechanical strength of the subsequent bony union. This may account for the greater success of allografts in anterior fusions[53] as compared with posterior fusions, which generally rely on a smaller area of decorticated bone per fusion segment. Similarly, this may also contribute to the lower fusion rates seen in myelomeningocele,[54,55] in which the laminae are not available as a surface for fusion. In theory, any exposure of the local bone surface, osteonal spaces, or marrow spaces that does not excessively weaken the mechanical strength of local bone should increase the number of osteoblastic progenitors with access to the graft site.[56,57]

Bone Graft Biology and Materials

Bone grafting is performed to accelerate, augment, or substitute for the normal regenerative capacity of bone. There is no single ideal or optimal graft. The functional demands and the biologic assets and deficiencies of each graft site vary with the clinical setting. As a result, the surgeon must rely on both past experience and clinical judgment and must be familiar with the new and expanding knowledge base of bone healing biology and clinical grafting materials.

All bone-grafting strategies involve either the transplantation or targeting of osteoblastic stem cells or progenitor cells. Bone grafts have been described as having osteogenic, osteoinductive, and osteoconductive properties. Grafts may also contribute to mechanical stability and vascularity at the graft site.[58-60] Detailed reviews of the principles underlying these practical clinical concepts have been published.[15,59-63]

The osteogenic property of a graft is derived from viable stem and progenitor cells that may be transplanted as part of the graft under conditions in which they can survive and contribute directly to new bone formation. Osteoinductive activity refers to the capacity of some stimuli, usually peptide growth factors, to stimulate cellular events that transform an uncommitted cell into a cell that becomes activated and committed to new bone formation. The prototype for osteoinductive factors is the family of bone morphogenetic proteins (BMPs), particularly BMPs 2, 4, 6, 7, and 9, which appear to be the most osteoinductive. However, other matrix-bound and soluble growth factors also contribute to this process, such as TGF-β, insulin-like growth factors I and II (IGF-I and IGF-II), and bFGF. These factors may also be delivered as autocrine and paracrine factors that are released from or secreted by local or transplanted stem cells and progenitor cells, platelets, or other cells associated with the local inflammatory response.

In contrast to osteoinduction, osteoconduction is the result of the structural and surface features of a graft matrix. Osteoconductivity refers to the capacity of a graft matrix to enhance the attachment, migration, proliferation, and differentiation of osteoblastic stem cells and progenitors as well as other cells that contribute to the bone healing response. As a result, osteoconduction promotes the distribution of a bone healing response of the graft. The osteoconductivity of a matrix is a function of its macrostructure or architecture, the size and connection between pores on the material, and its surface chemistry and surface texture. In the case of degradable materials, the degradation properties of the material are also critical, specifically the degradation rate, the chemical species that are released by degradation, and their rate of clearance from the site.[15,64,65]

Cell attachment and migration is mediated by the presence of cell adhesion molecules and other proteins in or bound to the surface of a matrix. These matrix ligands can also have a profound effect on the survival and retention of cells within the graft site and on their differentiation. Examples of biomolecules that may serve as adhesion molecules are collagens, fibronectin, osteonectin, laminin, vitronectin, hyaluronan, bone sialoprotein, heparin, and various proteoglycans. Binding domains similar to those provided by these molecules can also be provided by smaller peptides of 7 to 30 amino acids, a strategy that is being exploited in many current development efforts. The extracellular matrix of an allograft is a prototype for an osteoconductive scaffold, which assists the distribution of a bone healing process throughout a graft site.

The following section reviews the specific functional elements and clinical outcomes of each of the major spinal fusion grafting options.

Autogenous Cancellous Bone

Autologous cancellous bone has traditionally been considered to be the gold standard of graft materials. Autograft has maintained a track record as the most reliable and effective graft material, particularly in the challenging clinical setting of spinal fusion.[66-69] This finding is reinforced by the recognition that an autogenous cancellous graft provides all three areas of functionality: osteogenic bone and marrow cells; an osteoconductive matrix of collagen, mineral, and matrix proteins; and a spectrum of osteoinductive proteins provided within the transplanted matrix of cells. However, the limitations and disadvantages of autogenous cancellous bone have become increasingly evident in recent years as more effective and less morbid grafting options have become available.

The principal disadvantage of autogenous cancellous bone graft relates to the process of graft harvest. Autograft harvest adds operative time, pain, and blood loss. It also carries an increased risk of infection, cutaneous nerve damage, and even local fracture. Autograft harvest leaves the patient with permanent scars and a risk of long-term pain at the graft site.[70-73] Increased blood loss attributable to the graft harvest results in an increased potential exposure to blood products along with all the associated costs and risks of transfusion. The incidence of major complications associated with the harvest of iliac crest bone graft (ICBG) was, in earlier studies, reported to be 5% to 10%.[74-76] A subsequent prospective study of 170 patients undergoing spinal fusion with autologous ICBG found that 24% reported numbness at the graft harvest site 3.5 years postoperatively, and 19% reported that the pain at their graft harvest sites impaired their ability to perform routine chores.[77] However, there is marked variability in techniques to retrieve bone (e.g., cortical window for cancellous, tricortical for structural) in the reported incidence and severity of pain as well as other major and minor complications associated with harvest of ICBG.[70,76-91] Less invasive bone graft harvest methods may decrease the incidence of complications and pain.[78,92] While randomized controlled trials (RCTs) have shown no differences in clinical outcome measures between patients undergoing lumbar fusion with ICBG and those receiving bone graft substitutes without ICBG,[78,85,93,94] these studies specifically investigated and reported the incidence of bone graft pain in the ICBG groups and not in the groups receiving bone graft substitutes. ICBG donor site pain may be overestimated, however, since patients undergoing lumbar spine fusion have difficulty distinguishing between residual back pain and donor site pain.[78,92,95]

A second disadvantage of autograft is that, in addition to its cost and morbidity, the amount of autogenous bone is limited and may be insufficient in many settings, particularly in children undergoing arthrodesis over multiple segments. Autogenous bone also has a biologic limitation as a cellular graft. Although cancellous bone from the pelvis is the most abundant source of osteoblastic stem cells and progenitors, these cells represent only about 1 in 20,000 cells in normal bone marrow. ICBG is packed with many other cells that do not necessarily contribute to bone healing. When autogenous cancellous bone is harvested, its diverse mixture of highly metabolic cells is dissociated from its blood supply and is then implanted under conditions in which each cell must compete with all of the other cells in bone and marrow for the limited amount of oxygen and other nutrients that are available to diffuse into the graft site. The metabolic demand within the graft site far exceeds the capacity for nutrient diffusion. This results in profound hypoxia as one moves more than 1 to 2 mm into the graft, and few deeply placed cells survive. This fact was recognized by Burwell from histologic assessment in the 1960s and can now be defined in more quantitative terms on the basis of chemical engineering principles,[16,96] Necrosis within the graft places an additional burden on the site. Necrotic debris must be removed before new bone formation can occur. In addition, cell debris and the cytokines that are released by dying cells escalate the local inflammatory response, bringing in additional cells that further increase local metabolic demand.

Autologous Cortical Bone

Cortical bone grafts are less biologically active than cancellous grafts as a result of several factors. Cortical bone contains fewer osteoblastic stem cells and progenitors than trabecular bone. Furthermore, the cells that are present are less likely to survive because a larger fraction of cells are located within osteons, which are buried in the matrix, where diffusion is insufficient to provide adequate nutrients to support viability. The absence of nonosteogenic marrow cells and endothelial cells further limits the biologic potential of a cortical graft. In addition, in contrast to trabecular bone, cortical grafts have a much lower available surface area per unit volume. This reduces the potential surface for new bone formation (and therefore osteoconductive potential) and may also reduce the bioavailability of osteoinductive factors buried in the matrix. The marked reduction in porosity of cortical bone also represents a barrier to vascular ingrowth and bony remodeling, both of which are critical to bone healing and the development of optimal mechanical strength.

The only advantage of cortical bone versus cancellous bone and other graft materials is its superior mechanical strength and the availability of cortical segments of sufficient size to fill virtually any skeletal defect. The ability to provide immediate mechanical strength at the time of implantation is a critical advantage in many situations, particularly in anterior interbody fusions. However, the mechanical strength of a cortical graft is not constant over time. Allograft bone is remodeled by the process of creeping substitution, resulting in increased porosity and progressive loss of strength during the first 12 to 24 months after implantation before remodeling and new bone formation reconstitutes the mechanical properties of the grafted segment.[58,97–101] This is associated with increased risk of graft failure and collapse during the first 24 months after implantation.

Combined grafts consisting of intact cortical and cancellous bone from the iliac crest are common and readily available graft materials with good mechanical properties and biologic properties of incorporation. The mechanical strength of these grafts is variable, however. Grafts from the anterior crest exhibit greater mechanical compressive strength than grafts from the posterior crest.[60,102]

Vascularized Autologous Grafts

Vascularized grafts are used extensively in many centers for musculoskeletal reconstructive procedures. High rates of vascular patency can be achieved by experienced microsurgeons. Many studies have shown clear advantages to using vascularized grafts in a number of settings.[103–109] In anterior spinal fusions, donor vessels are available to support the vascularized graft. Suitable grafts with good mechanical strength are available from the anterior iliac crest, posterior iliac crest,[110] fibula,[107,111] or rib.[112] An iliac graft pedicle flap on quadratus lumborum has also been described.[113] In intrathoracic procedures, a vascularized rib graft may be mobilized on its intercostal pedicle, with limited additional morbidity and in much less time than a free vascularized graft.[114,115] However, a rib graft provides less mechanical strength when compared with the iliac crest or fibula[116] and therefore must be mechanically supplemented by additional cortical bone or internal fixation.

Although routine use of vascular grafts is limited by concerns regarding their increased operative time, technical difficulty, and added morbidity, the improved incorporation of these grafts may make them highly desirable in some settings in which incorporation of avascular grafts may be compromised, such as in areas of radiation-induced fibrosis, dense scar, or previous infection.[107] The ability of vascular grafts to withstand higher levels of irradiation than nonvascularized grafts has markedly increased the use of vascularized grafts in the treatment of bone tumors.[104,107,117–119]

Autologous Bone Marrow

Bone marrow is a valuable and easily accessible source of osteogenic cells that is probably underused in contemporary clinical practice. The osteogenic potential of transplanted bone marrow was first documented in 1869 by Goujon[120] and later in 1889 by Senn.[121] Studies by Burwell in the 1960s concluded that the formation of new bone following autografting resulted from the differentiation of osteogenic precursor cells contained within the marrow in addition to osteoblasts on the surface of the graft material itself.[16] Burwell postulated that, following transplantation, these reticular cells free themselves from the sinusoidal walls to become primitive migratory cells. They then differentiate into osteogenic cells when they are exposed to osteoinductive substances released from the necrotic portion of the graft[122] or perhaps from osteoinductive materials contained within or secreted by the marrow itself.

Many studies have demonstrated the ability of marrow cells to form bone intramuscularly,[123,124] subcutaneously,[125] interperitoneally,[126–128] in the anterior chamber of eye,[129] and orthotopically. Using a suspension of marrow cells in diffusion chambers, Friedenstein showed that hematopoietic cells die following transplantation, whereas fibroblasts and other stromal elements are more resistant to hypoxia and may proliferate close to the surface of the graft to produce immature bone, suggesting the presence of an undifferentiated precursor cell in postnatal marrow.[125,128,130,131] It has been well established that the osteogenic cells that contribute to this response are not derived from one homogeneous population of cells but rather appear to come from two or more compartments of stem cells or progenitor cells that are upstream from the osteoblastic population in bone.[63,125,132,133] A more mature preosteoblastic

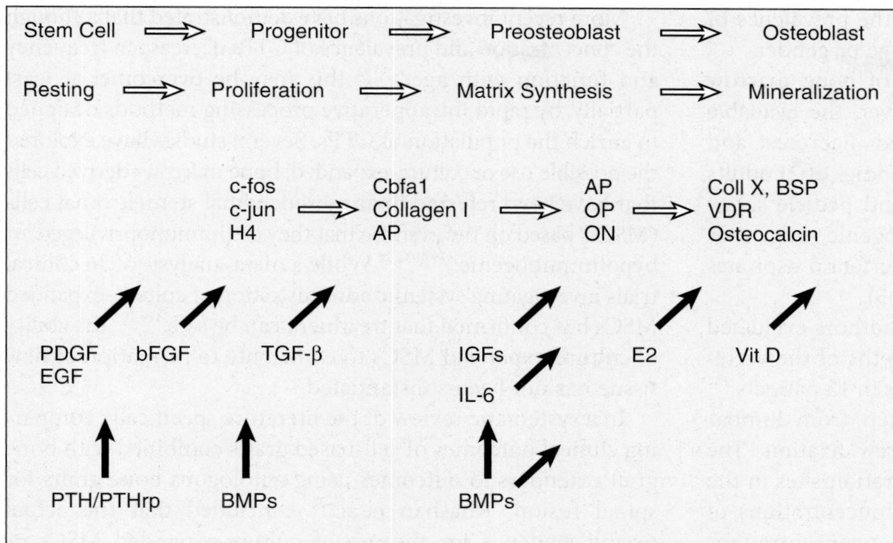

FIG. 66.1 The osteoblastic pathway. This figure illustrates the stages of osteoblastic differentiation, the predominant activity of the differentiation cell at each stage, some of the characteristic genes expressed at each stage, and the approximate site of principal action for some of the principal osteotropic growth factors and hormones. AP, alkaline phosphatase; bFGF, basic fibroblast growth factor; BMPs, bone morphogenetic protein family members; BSP, bone sialoprotein; E2, estradiol; EGF, epithelial growth factor; H4, H4 histone; IGFs, insulin-like growth factors I and II; IL-6, interleukin-6; ON, osteonectin; OP, osteopontin; PDGF, platelet-derived growth factor; TGF-β, transforming growth factor-beta; VDR, vitamin D receptor; Vit D, vitamin D_3.

cell appears to be localizable to the marrow space adjacent to trabecular surfaces or osteonal bone. One or more populations of less mature and potentially multipotent cells appear to be present in the more liquid phase of bone marrow space, possibly including cells associated with perivascular tissue of vascular sinusoids or other marrow vessels. Overall, one can estimate that, on average, 60% to 70% of osteogenic stem and progenitor cells are from the trabecular surface population.[134]

Osteoblastic differentiation proceeds in a series of steps, which can be conceptually divided into phases.[135,136] An initial proliferative phase is characterized by expression of H4 histone, c-*fos,* and c-*jun.* A matrix synthesis phase is characterized by a reduction in proliferation and upregulation of gene products for type I collagen, osteopontin, osteonectin, and alkaline phosphatase. Finally, a matrix mineralization phase culminates in an osteoblastic phenotype characterized by expression of osteocalcin, bone sialoprotein, and responsiveness to 1,25-dihydroxyvitamin D and parathyroid hormone. A conceptual summary of the large body of literature related to osteoblastic differentiation is presented in Fig. 66.1.[63,137]

The value of bone marrow as a bone graft, used alone or as a component in a composite bone graft material, has been supported by numerous studies in rats and rabbits.[122,125,128–130,138–145] Lane et al.[146] demonstrated the efficacy of autogenous bone marrow grafting in a 5-mm rat femoral defect and showed that the efficacy of bone marrow grafts were dependent on transplantation of viable cells. Yasko et al.[147] also showed that bone marrow enhanced the performance of an effective synthetic BMP-2 material in rats, a finding consistent with prior materials.[143] However, in contrast to clinical practice, almost all of these studies in rodents have used bone marrow obtained by open harvesting of bone and/or irrigation of bone explants rather than by aspiration.

Increasing evaluation of bone marrow grafting has been carried out in larger nonrodent models. Johnson et al.[148] found canine bone marrow much less osteogenic than rabbit marrow when transplanted in diffusion chambers. Using a canine tibial model, Tiedeman et al.[144] found that the percutaneous injection of marrow mixed with demineralized bone matrix powder produced overall results comparable with open cancellous grafting.

There have been series of reports showing that aspirated bone marrow can improve bone healing.[122,140,149–154] Connolly reported successful treatment of 18 of 20 nonunions treated with casting or intramedullary nails plus percutaneous marrow injection.[139]

Recognizing the potential biologic value in various clinical settings, many surgeons currently use bone marrow as an adjuvant to allograft bone. This practice is indicated primarily because the risk and morbidity of bone marrow aspiration from the iliac crest are low. The prospective trials needed to document the value or limitations of bone marrow grafting are only now being organized. These investigations are justified by a significant volume of clinical information regarding methods and cellular yield of bone marrow aspiration[155–157] and by a robust set of preclinical studies.[158–162]

The method of bone marrow aspiration has a significant effect on the concentration and prevalence of bone marrow–derived osteogenic cells. Muschler et al.,[156] in a cohort of normal subjects undergoing elective orthopaedic procedures, showed that a mean of approximately 2100 osteoblastic progenitors (colony-forming units or CFU-Os) could be harvested in a 2-mL aspirate of human bone marrow from the iliac crest and that the mean prevalence of CFU-Os among nucleated marrow cells was approximately 1 in 37,000 cells.

They further documented that the yield of CFU-Os harvested dropped rapidly as the volume of bone marrow aspirated was increased owing to dilution with peripheral blood. On the basis of these findings, they recommended that aspiration of marrow be limited to 2 mL from each aspiration site in order to maximize the concentration of CFU-Os in the marrow graft. Further studies have demonstrated that the yield of osteoblastic stem cells and progenitors tends to decrease with age and that the prevalence of these cells may decrease more rapidly in women than in men.[155,157,163–165] However, these data also show that there is marked variation from individual to individual in the cellularity of marrow and the prevalence of osteogenic cells that is not associated with age or gender.

The vertebral pedicle can be a source of bone marrow aspiration during spinal arthrodesis; however, the available volume is limited. McLain et al.[166] obtained iliac crest and transpedicular aspirates from the vertebral bodies of 21 adults undergoing posterior lumbar arthrodesis and pedicle screw instrumentation. The concentration of osteogenic progenitor cells was, on average, 71% higher in the vertebral aspirates than in the paired iliac crest samples ($P = .05$).

In a subsequent clinical study, the same authors evaluated sequential aspirations from the different depths of the vertebral body, along the same transpedicular axis in 13 patients.[167] Four aspirations of 2.0 mL each were taken from lumbar pedicles prior to placement of pedicle screw fixation. The authors found that the most superficial aspiration sites in the vertebral bodies had significantly greater concentrations of connective tissue progenitors (CTPs) and that concentrations decreased progressively and significantly with sequentially deeper aspirates.

Several authors have addressed the potential value of harvesting bone marrow by aspiration and then processing the cells that are collected to concentrate those that are most likely to be of value while eliminating cells that may not contribute to fusion or inhibit fusion. Connolly et al.[138] described concentration of marrow-derived cells using centrifugation techniques and showed that a three-fold to four-fold increase in the concentration of nucleated cells increased the amount of bone formation in a diffusion chamber in the rabbit. Several recent reports have described the results of clinical spine fusion procedures using bone marrow as a cell source and concentrating marrow-derived cells using a centrifuge (density separation).[168–171] Other methods have been described that allow rapid intraoperative concentration and selection of osteoblastic stem cells and progenitors from bone marrow using an appropriately designed implantable allograft matrix as an affinity column to select osteoblastic cells on the basis of attachment behavior (i.e., selective retention).[159,160,172,173] Both density separation and selective retention can be used to rapidly concentrate marrow-derived nucleated cells. However, selective retention has the theoretical advantage of concentrating osteogenic CTP-Os; while removing 50% to 80% of the other nucleated cells (non-CTPs) may improve the survival of transplanted cells and reduce local inflammation associated with necrotic cell debris.[172] A clinical cohort study using bone marrow concentration strategies to lumbar interbody fusion has also reported a fusion rate of 85%, comparable with historical autograft controls.[174] Use of bone marrow aspirate from the vertebral body, as accessed during spinal fusion procedures utilizing instrumentation, has been shown to augment fusion rates in the absence of donor site morbidity.[175–178]

Muschler et al.[15,62,63,179,180] have published four more detailed reviews of the biologic principles and practical strategies for harvest and use of stem cells and progenitor cells for bone healing applications. Use of genetically modified cells as a delivery system for gene products promoting bone fusion has been explored in several studies. This strategy is addressed in other chapters in this text.[181–191]

More recent investigations have demonstrated that although the concentration and prevalence of CTPs decrease in frequency and function with age,[179,192] this may be overcome, at least partially, by rapid intraoperative processing methods designed to enrich the population of CTPs. Several studies have explored the possible use of culture-expanded, bone marrow–derived cells that have been referred to as mesenchymal stem/stromal cells (MSCs) based on the premise that they are immunoprivileged, or hypoimmunogenic.[179,193,194] While a meta-analysis of 36 clinical trials investigating systemic administration of culture-expanded MSCs has confirmed that treatment can be safe,[179,195] the ability of culture-expanded MSCs to contribute to formation of new tissue has not been substantiated.

In a systematic review of the literature specifically comparing clinical outcomes of cell-based grafts combined with bone graft extenders to outcomes using autologous bone grafts for spinal fusion, Khashan et al.[196] concluded that the actual overall evidence for the use of culture-expanded MSCs or BMA combined with synthetic or allograft materials is insufficient to support their use as a substitute for iliac crest grafts. A paucity of high-quality, prospective, comparative controlled trials currently limit the use of these cell-based therapies in place of autograft or allograft bone for spinal fusion.[196] In another recent systematic review, Hsu et al.[197] concluded that there were no studies available providing data of sufficient quality to assess the cost-effectiveness of cell-based products and other synthetic carriers.

RIA (Reamer-Irrigator-Aspirator)

Recent studies have evaluated the potential for use of a reamer-irrigator-aspirator (RIA), a novel system for harvest of intramedullary reamings and fatty marrow contents from the intramedullary canal of the femur and tibia. There are clinical reports that RIA grafts have osteoconductive and angiogenic properties comparable to ICBGs.[198,199] If the intramedullary canal of the femur or tibia is readily available in the operative field, RIA provides a large volume of graft compared with ICBG harvest procedures.[200–202] However, the clinical utility for spine fusion is debated, as is the extra cost of the RIA device as compared to the ICBG. In addition, Henrich et al. found that culture-expanded MSCs from the femur harvested with the RIA had reduced expression of *BMP2* and *WNT* family genes, compared with MSCs obtained from the iliac crest by aspiration.[203] They also found trends toward increased methylation of the *RUNX2* gene, as well as decreased methylation of the *SMAD5* and *WNT3A* genes. Biologic potential of cells harvested by RIA may be altered by different mechanical stresses on the cells or by harvest of a mixture of fat and bone-derived CTPs. RIA harvests are prone to variation in the amount of cells harvested from patient to patient and due to differences in reamer diameter and the bone endosteal diameter.

Structural Bone Allografts and Cages

Use of allograft bone has been well characterized over the past 30 years.[204] There are four principal advantages of allografts.

First, they eliminate the morbidity associated with harvesting autologous bone. Second, and in contrast to autograft bone, the volume of available allograft is essentially unlimited. Third, because cortical allografts can be selected from any bone (not just the iliac crest or tibial hemicortex), they provide the surgeon with access to grafts that have mechanical strength and options for shaping that are superior to any autograft site. Fourth, allograft bone can be preprocessed into a wide range of specialized physical forms (e.g., blocks, threaded or non-threaded dowels, sized rings and wedges, chips, fibers, powder) prepared from cortical and/or cancellous bone. These preprocessed grafts provide the opportunity to customize and pre-certify the physical form and architectural properties (shape, size, mechanical strength, surface area, porosity) of a graft matrix to an individual site.

The method of sterilization and preparation of allograft tissue has a significant impact on osteoconductive, osteoinductive, and mechanical properties, as well as immunogenicity.[101,205–208] Donor cells and cell fragments are the most immunogenic material in allogeneic bone. Processing of allograft bone therefore includes steps that attempt to remove as many cells as possible from the graft. Immunogenicity is further reduced, although not eliminated, by freezing to −20° C.[209–217] Freeze-drying is even more effective at reducing the immunogenicity of allogeneic bone, but at the price of reducing mechanical strength by 50%.[211,218]

Using contemporary processing and storage techniques, clinical evidence of overt immunologic reaction against the graft is rare. Even so, histologic evidence of a low-grade inflammatory reaction can be found around essentially all allografts. This reaction probably slows the incorporation of many allografts and may contribute to the failure of some, as suggested by several canine studies that have documented improved biologic behavior in antigen-matched allografts.[206,207,218,219] Antigen matching is not currently considered practical in the clinical setting, however. The relatively high current success rates for allografts makes the large cost of antigen matching not feasible and is probably unwarranted in general practice.[220]

Sterility of frozen allografts is ensured through expedient postmortem harvesting using sterile surgical technique and careful monitoring using surface cultures and polymerase chain reaction screening for bacterial and viral genome fragments. The American Association of Tissue Banks (www.aatb.org) requires screening tests of all allografts as well as screening of patients' medical histories. Musculoskeletal allografts are tested for hepatitis B virus, hepatitis C virus, human T-lymphotrophic virus types I and II, and syphilis (*Treponema pallidum*).[221] It is difficult to determine exact risks of transmission, particularly in spinal surgery patients, who often have multiple comorbidities and may have had blood transfusions in addition to receiving tissue allografts. Differences in reporting and investigating these infections may also prevent precise determination of incidences of these events. Allograft transmission rates are estimated by risks of blood transmission of these viruses. The risk of transmission of hepatitis B virus in fresh-frozen allograft is estimated to be 1 in 63,000. Risk of transmission of hepatitis C virus is 1 in 1,000,000. The risk of transmission of HIV is between 1 in 1,000,000 and 1 in 1,600,000 for fresh-frozen allograft bone.[221–226]

A variety of secondary sterilization procedures have been designed and may be used, depending on the source of the allograft. Ethylene oxide sterilization was evaluated by Cornell,[227] who found a 70% decrease in bone induction by demineralized bone powder in rats. Other authors have reported variable changes in inductive capacity of ethylene oxide sterilized matrix.[228–231] Heating or autoclaving bone tissue is generally avoided due to their disruption of matrix proteins. Some processing techniques, such as high-dose irradiation, compromise both the biologic potential of bone matrix, reducing bone formation and union rates,[232,233] and also alter the mechanical properties of the graft.[234–242] For example, irradiation to 2.5 mrad or freeze-dried processing may reduce the torsional strength of the cortical allograft by as much as 50%.[218] Islam et al.[242] showed that, in contrast to the previously documented two- to threefold decreases in strength, Young's modulus, and ductility determined with monotonic tests, by their group and others,[237,238,243] gamma irradiation induces a more than 15-fold reduction in the high-cycle fatigue life of cortical bone at physiologically relevant stress levels.

Results from other clinical and experimental studies using allograft bone alone in spinal fusions have been mixed. Some investigators have found allograft to be significantly inferior to autogenous bone grafting when compared with other distinctive preparation methods,[53,55,235,244–256] whereas others find little or no difference between them.[53,114,256–270]

Angevine et al.[271] documented similar cost-effectiveness ratios between iliac crest autograft bone and allograft bone for single-level anterior cervical decompression and fusion (ACDF) for patients with cervical spondylosis.

Allograft bone appears to be particularly valuable in settings that require the graft to serve a significant mechanical function, such as struts or ring allografts for anterior lumbar interbody fusions (ALIF)[272–276] or as struts or bone–wire fixation constructs in the upper cervical spine.[277–286] In these settings, allografts have essentially replaced the use of autografts from rib, fibula, tricortical iliac crest, and tibial hemicortex grafts, which are all associated with significant donor site morbidity.

Several synthetic materials have expanded the options for structural support. These include interbody fusion cages comprised of titanium, carbon fiber–reinforced polymers, and polyetheretherketone (PEEK).[286–295] These materials provide the structural function that is necessary to maintain the height and stability of the interbody site. These cages and wedges lack some of the osteoconductive capacity of allograft bone. Furthermore, they lack the capacity of allograft bone to be biologically incorporated into the fusion mass and remodeled, remaining in the site essentially as a permanent foreign body. Metal cages create artifacts on magnetic resonance imaging and computed tomography, which makes radiographic assessment of fusion difficult. However, in comparison with allograft, synthetic materials offer the advantage of more consistent material properties, specifically strength and fracture resistance. Recent studies have begun to evaluate absorbable designs, such as polylactic acid–polyglycolic acid copolymers, as well as poly(L-lactide-coD,L-lactide). However, the current data regarding the latter and former is insufficient to support broad clinical use at this time.[295]

Regardless of material used for structural support, there is general consensus that in order to achieve optimal rates of spinal fusion, the environment within and around these structural allografts or cages should be further supplemented with other osteogenic, osteoconductive, and/or osteoinductive graft materials. Autogenous cancellous bone, bone marrow aspirate,[296] processed bone marrow–derived cells,[174] processed nonstructural allograft materials, and BMPs[3,297] are most commonly considered.

Demineralized Allograft Bone Matrix

Demineralization is one means by which the biologic activity of allograft bone can be modified. In settings in which mechanical properties are not critical to the graft application, demineralization may enhance the osteoinductive activity of the allograft matrix by making growth factors embedded in the matrix more available. Several preparations of demineralized bone matrix (DBM) are available; however, these materials may vary in biologic activity, as discussed later.

The history of demineralization as a means to enhance allograft performance is richly linked to many of the recent biologic insights into bone biology and bone healing. It was more than a century ago, in 1889, that Senn reported the repair of long bone and cranial defects in patients with chronic osteomyelitis using hydrochloric acid–treated decalcified heterologous bone implants.[121] Although his primary motive was to promote antisepsis within the bone cavities, Senn observed rapid substitution of the demineralized tissue with new bone formation invading from the perimeter of the defects. However, several of Senn's contemporaries obtained equivocal results and clinical efforts over the next 70 years were minimal.[277,298–300]

Reddi and Huggins[301,302] revived this concept when they reported on their observation that demineralized matrix induced bone formation in rats. Marshall Urist went on to demonstrate bone induction using a variety of demineralized matrix preparations in muscular pouches of rabbits, rats, mice, and guinea pigs.[303] Subsequently, matrix-induced heterotopic bone formation was documented at many soft tissue sites, including muscle, tendon, and fascia,[301,303–305] as well as in the thymus[125] and soft connective tissue of visceral organs.[306] Nathanson also observed the differentiation of neonatal embryonic skeletal tissue into cartilage when cultured on demineralized bone matrix substratum and suggested that the tissue transformation of bone induction was analogous to embryonic bone tissue differentiation.[307–309]

Reddi subsequently characterized the inductive phenomenon of bone matrix as a cascade of events parallel to those occurring in endochondral ossification and postulated that the process was the result of stimulation by a series of soluble matrix factors that potentiated events along the cascade.[310–312] In this paradigm, bioactive factors in bone matrix stimulate activation and migration of osteogenic stem cells and progenitor cells. Mitogenic factors promote cell proliferation. Angiogenic factors promote local revascularization, and osteoinductive factors promote osteoblastic differentiation. Subsequently, bone matrix has been shown to contain a rich variety of growth factors and other bioactive molecules in concentrations that are bioactive.[313,314]

Sato and Urist[315] showed that demineralized bone matrix was both inductive and was synergistic with bone marrow–derived cells in healing of rat femoral defects. They went on to provide a clinical outlet for these discoveries by developing a "chemosterilized, autolyzed, antigen-extracted allogeneic bone (AAA)," prepared using chloroform-methanol extraction, 0.6 N hydrochloric acid extraction of soluble proteins with partial demineralization, and neutral phosphate autodigestion.[316–319] This preparation appeared to reduce the immunogenicity of the allograft matrix without loss of inductive properties. Using this preparation, Urist and Dawson reported on 40 patients undergoing posterolateral lumbar spinal fusion with an 80% success rate and a pseudarthrosis rate of 12%.[320]

The value of a variety of DBM preparations (chips, fibers, powders) has subsequently been described in a number of settings by a series of authors. Glowacki et al.[321–323] were among the first to report successful repair of craniofacial defects. Tiedeman et al.[144] and Wilkins et al.[324] both reported clinical efficacy in long bone defects. Other reports have also shown efficacy for DBM in spine fusion models.[325,326] Some studies have reported a benefit of adding DBM to autograft or ceramic matrices in animal spine fusion models.[142,327–330] There is also recent evidence that some DBM preparations can be used as a substrate for selective attachment and concentration of bone marrow–derived osteogenic stem cells and progenitors.[174,331]

Because demineralized bone preparations do not have mechanical properties sufficient to resist external forces, they can easily be dislodged from a graft site. The use of these materials is therefore primarily restricted to grafting of contained defects or graft sites that are protected by rigid internal fixation or to settings in which demineralized matrix is combined with other allograft or synthetic materials that resist displacement or compression.

Of recent clinical concern is evidence that suggests that the biologic efficacy of commercially available preparations of DBM materials can vary significantly, depending on the method of processing, the individual batch of bone that is processed, or the donor of the bone that is used. This variation has raised questions about the possible value of implementing generalized standards for either in vitro or in vivo biologic assays for bone from each batch and donor in order to limit the potential for biologically deficient materials from compromising the performance of clinical grafting procedures. At present,[204,225,332] without evidence that failed graft procedures cluster around individual donors or batches of demineralized bone and that these failures can be predicted by any of the available assays, the clinical value and cost-effectiveness of biologic assays is uncertain. Regardless, some providers of demineralized bone have elected to implement some form of bioassay and use these data to exclude some bone from use and to make claims of superior or more reliable performance in the marketplace.

Deproteinated Heterologous Bone

In contrast to allograft bone, heterologous bone (xenograft) fails to induce osseous repair due to its high level of antigenicity. Partially deproteinated and partially defatted heterologous bone (Kiel bone or Oswestry bone) does exhibit greatly reduced antigenicity and therefore evokes a minimal immune response.[333] The denaturing process, however, also destroys osteoinductive matrix proteins. Accordingly, implantation of such materials in bone defects and muscular compartments has failed to generate bone formation.[150]

The impregnation of this material with cells capable of osteogenic activity, however, has been studied. Salama et al.[150] and Plenk et al.[334] demonstrated that deproteinated xenograft bone supplemented with autologous marrow assisted osteogenesis in both experimental animals and humans. In these experiments, deproteinated bone served as an osteoconductive scaffolding, providing a stable mechanical environment for revascularization and proliferation and differentiation of osteogenic cells. Salama and Weissman[151] reported satisfactory results in clinical attempts to use composite xenograft/autograft (Kiel bone/marrow) in a variety of bone defects. More recently, Rawlinson et al.[335] reported poor results using bovine-derived Cloward grafts. Due to the wide availability of more effective allograft matrix materials in the United States at similar costs, xenograft materials are not currently used.

Synthetic Bioactive Bone Graft Materials

Recent years have seen an explosion of new information about the cellular and molecular events involved in the bone healing response (see Fig. 66.1) and has increased the potential for clinical applications of growth factors with and without traditional bone grafts and bone graft substitutes. Purified human recombinant growth factors are becoming available. Many are active in multiple events in the bone healing process and are therefore candidates as potential therapeutic agents. In addition, developments in porous ceramic materials and bioerodible polymers of biologic and synthetic polymers enable the design of customized matrix materials that can be used both as osteoconductive scaffolds and as delivery systems for bioactive molecules. These converging events are now producing an army of first-generation and second-generation biosynthetic bone grafting materials. One of the prototype materials designed used in combination with bone marrow aspirate (BMA) is a matrix comprised of type I bovine collagen fiber coated with hydroxyapatite. Several studies compared BMA-collagen-ceramic composite to ICBG in transforaminal lumbar interbody fusion (TLIF), posterior lumbar interbody fusion (PLIF), and posterolateral spine fusion, finding similar outcomes but a lower radiographic fusion rate.[336–339] It is beyond the scope of this chapter to comprehensively review any one of these areas. Several recent reviews are available.[15,205,340–342] The following is intended as an overview of some of the ongoing developments in this area, specifically the application of growth factors, collagen matrices, and ceramics in synthetic bone grafting materials.

Bone Morphogenetic Proteins

A major advance occurred in 1978, when Urist et al.[343] reported the isolation of a hydrophobic, low-molecular-weight protein fraction from insoluble bone matrix gelatin that was responsible for osteoinductive activity.[344] Further characterization of this inductive factor, BMP, was made possible by quantitative extraction accomplished by differential precipitation in a buffer containing 4M guanidine hydrochloride.[345] Lovell and Dawson went on to report the success of a partly purified BMP preparation on polylactic acid strips in a canine segmental spinal fusion model.[346]

After an extensive search for the protein responsible for the inductive activity of bone matrix extract, Wozney et al.[347] identified and characterized three proteins isolated from a highly purified preparation from bovine bone in 1988, each capable of inducing bone formation in a rat subcutaneous bioassay. Human complementary DNA clones for each peptide were isolated and expressed as recombinant human proteins. Two of the encoded proteins were homologous and described as members of the TGF-β super gene family, whereas the third appeared to be a novel polypeptide (BMP-1). BMP-1 has turned out not to be a growth factor at all. Rather, this molecule has been characterized as a procollagen C-proteinase, which may have a biologic function in the activation of TGF-β–like molecules, including the BMPs.[348,349]

At least 17 BMPs have been identified, but only BMP-2, BMP-4, BMP-6, BMP-7, and BMP-9 have been documented to have significant osteogenic properties.[347,350–352] The BMP family are homologous proteins with molecular weight of 12 to 14 kD that are posttranscriptionally modified by glycosylation and are secreted as homodimers or heterodimers linked by one disulfide bond (≈30 kD).[347,353,354] In vivo, these proteins are secreted as soluble factors that have autocrine and paracrine effects. BMP-7 (OP-1) can also be found in systemic circulation and may also have effects on kidney function.[355,356] BMPs are present in bone matrix, both as homodimers and as heterodimers at a concentration of roughly 1 mg/kg of bone, where they are believed to play a role in bone remodeling and the coupling of osteoclastic and osteoblastic activity. BMP-3 is the most abundant BMP in demineralized bone, comprising as much as 65% of the BMP in bone matrix. However, BMP-3 is a negative regulator of bone formation, antagonizing the effects of BMP-2[357] and increasing levels of chondrogenic markers, such as aggrecan and type II collagen.[358] Daluiski et al. found that BMP-3 knockout mice have twice as much trabecular bone as controls.[359]

There are four subfamilies of BMP ligands based on their degree of sequence similarity and functions[360,361]: subfamily (I), containing BMP-2 and BMP-4; subfamily (II), containing BMP-5, BMP-6, BMP-7, BMP-8a, and BMP-8b; subfamily (III), containing BMP-9 and BMP-10; and subfamily (IV), containing BMP-3, BMP-3b, BMP-11, BMP-13, BMP-14, BMP-15, and BMP-16. BMP-3 (as stated earlier)[357–359] and BMP-13[361,362]

BMP-1	Procollagen C-proteinase		
BMP-2	BMP-2a		
BMP-3	Osteogenin		
BMP-4	BMP-2b		
BMP-5			
BMP-6	VgR1		
BMP-7	OP-1		
BMP-8	OP-2		
BMP-9		GDF-2	
BMP-10			
BMP-11		GDF-11	
BMP-12		GDF-7	CDMP-3
BMP-13		GDF-6	CDMP-2
BMP-14	MP53	GDF-5	CDMP-1
BMP-15		GDF-9	

FIG. 66.2 The bone morphogenetic protein (BMP) family of proteins. This figure lists the known members of the BMP family of proteins and some of the corresponding names that identify the same protein using other classification terminology. CDMP, cartilage-derived matrix protein; GDF, growth and differentiation factor.

have been shown to be inhibitory. Subfamily (IV) contains those BMPs that do not have osteogenic properties.

Fig. 66.2 summarizes these proteins along with synonyms or alternative names that are now, or have been, used for some of these molecules. There is RNA sequence homology within and between subgroups of the BMP protein family. Each of these proteins can interact with one or more of a family of cell surface receptors. Cells must express both type I and type II receptors (serine/threonine kinases) in order to be responsive to BMPs because a type I and type II receptor must interact in the presence of a BMP to mediate a cellular response. To date, three type I and three type II BMP receptors have been identified. BMPR-IA binds only BMPs. BMPR-IB binds BMPs and müllerian inhibitory substance. ALK-2 (also a type I receptor) binds BMPs and activin. BMPR-II binds only BMPs, and the activin type II receptors, ActR-IIA and ActR-IIB, bind both BMPs and activin.[363] In vitro, BMPs demonstrate dose-responsive modulation in responsive cells, both in primary osteogenic cells and in cell lines, in the range of 1 to 100 ng/mL, but each BMP demonstrates a unique and variable binding pattern for the individual receptors, as illustrated in Fig. 66.3. These genes are independently regulated in both space and time in embryonic development and in bone healing settings, but a great deal of functional redundancy and promiscuity between these proteins and receptors is present. Expression of specific inhibitors of BMP function (e.g., noggin, chordin, connective tissue growth factor, follistatin) also plays a role.[353,364–369]

Binding of BMP homodimers to type I and type II receptors can also be modulated by three families of co-receptors[361]: (1) betaglycan or type III TGF-β receptor[370] and Endoglin (aka CD105)[371]; (2) the EGF-CFC family (which includes Cripto)[372]; and (3) the glycosyl-phosphatidylinositol-linked family of repulsive guidance molecules (RGM),[373,374] which includes RGMa, TGMb or DRAGON, RGMc or hemojuvelin, and RGMd.[375] This complex system of activators, inhibitors, receptors, and modulators creates a rich field of potential therapeutic targets for purposed modulation. Spine fusion has been at the heart of both development and controversy in the rapidly

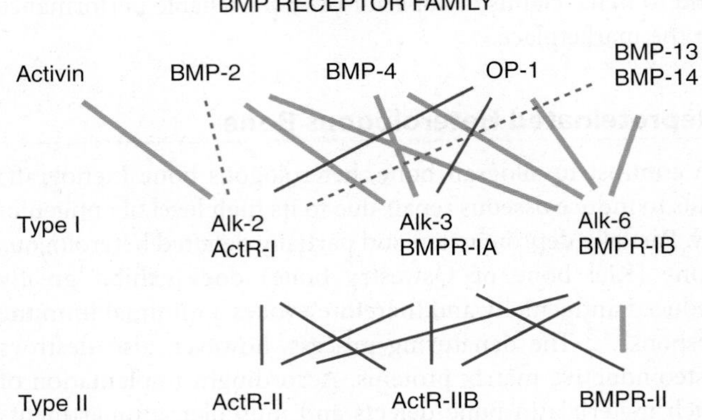

FIG. 66.3 The bone morphogenetic protein (BMP) receptor family. BMPs act on cells through interaction with a family of membrane-bound cell surface receptors. Cells must express one or more of the type I and the type II receptors in order to be responsive to BMPs. Some of the cross-reactivity between BMP-7, BMP-4, and another TGF-β superfamily member, Activin A, are illustrated. BMPs bind first to a type I receptor, including Alk-2, Alk-3, Alk-4, and Alk-6. The relative binding affinity of each BMP is reflected by the thickness of the connecting line. The BMP–type I receptor complex is then phosphorylated by a type II receptor protein to activate the signal transduction mechanism in the cell, which results in the BMP-induced response acting through the SMAD pathway.

evolving and promising field of targeted delivery of potent bioactive agents for tissue regeneration and repair.

Among the BMP homodimers that are most active in bone induction in vivo are BMP-2 (i.e., INFUSE), BMP-4, BMP-6, BMP-7 (i.e., osteogenic protein-1, or OP-1), and BMP-9. BMP-2 and BMP-7 have both been developed for clinical applications in bone grafting and skeletal reconstruction. BMP-13 (aka, GDF-6, CDMP-2) and BMP-14 (aka, GDF-5, CDMP-1) have been investigated.[358,361,376,377] BMP-14 (GDF-5) is present in varying levels in nucleus pulposus and anulus fibrosus of both normal and degenerative intervertebral disc tissue from patients with lumbar intervertebral disc disease, and it has been proposed that BMP-14 (GDF-5) may play an inhibitory role in progression of intervertebral disc disease.[378] At present, only BMP-2 has been approved by the US Food and Drug Administration (FDA) for use in spinal fusion. This approval is specifically limited to use in an absorbable collagen sponge (ACS) carrier (INFUSE Bone Graft, Medtronic) with a metallic lumbar tapered fusion device (INFUSE Bone Graft/LT-Cage Lumbar Tapered Fusion Device; Medtronic) in the setting of single-level ALIF from L2 to S1 for degenerative disc disease.[379] BMP-2 is also approved for use in open tibial shaft fractures stabilized with an intramedullary nail and treated within 14 days of initial injury.[380,381] BMP-7 (OP-1) received FDA approval under a humanitarian device exemption as an alternative to autograft in patients who have failed a previous spinal fusion surgery and are not able to provide their own bone or bone marrow for grafting because of a condition such as osteoporosis, diabetes, or smoking.[178] BMP-7–based products (OP-1 IMPLANT, OP-1 PUTTY, BioEZE, and BioVERSE) were removed from the US market in 2014.

A large number of animal studies have demonstrated the promise and relative safety for these proteins as powerful stimulants of a local bone-healing response in rodents, sheep, canines, and nonhuman primates, using various carrier matrices and a dosage range of 100 to 10,000 μg/mL.[354,383–411]

Several of the early prospective clinical trials strongly supported the value of BMPs (particularly BMP-2) in the setting of spinal fusion, reporting fusion rates that were comparable with autogenous cancellous bone between 80% and 99%.[412–421]

In a prospective, consecutive patient enrollment with a minimum 24-month follow-up, 30 patients underwent anterior interbody allografts alone and 45 patients underwent anterior interbody allograft filled with rhBMP-2. All cases had posterior pedicle screw instrumentation. A total of 165 surgical levels (62 allograft alone; 103 allograft + BMP) were included. In the allograft-rhBMP-2 group, fusion rates were 94%, 100%, and 100% at 6, 12, and 24 months, respectively, after surgery. In the allograft-only group, fusion rates were 66%, 84%, and 89%, respectively, at the same time intervals. Clinical outcomes were significantly improved in the rhBMP-2 group when compared with the allograft group at 6 months. There were no revisions in the rhBMP-2 group and four revision fusion surgeries (13%) in the allograft group.[422] In a randomized, controlled trial in patients older than 60 years, Glassman et al.[423] also found that rhBMP-2/ACS (INFUSE Bone Graft) is a viable ICBG replacement in older patients in terms of safety, clinical efficacy, and cost-effectiveness.

Taking advantage of the clinical availability of BMP-2, several investigators began evaluating the use of BMPs for expanded off-label indications. One of the first areas was anterior cervical spine surgery.[424–426] Anterior cervical discectomy and fusion performed with rhBMP-2 (0.9 mg BMP per level) allograft was found to be as effective as iliac bone graft in terms of patient outcomes and fusion rates. However, safety concerns were raised related to neck swelling in the BMP group.[425] Vaidya et al.[304] compared 22 patients treated with rhBMP-2 and PEEK cages with 24 patients in whom allograft spacers and DBM was used. Radiographic examination following surgery revealed endplate resorption in all patients in whom rhBMP-2 was used, followed by a period of new bone formation commencing at 6 weeks. In contrast, allograft patients showed a progressive fusion. Dysphagia was a common complication; it was significantly more frequent and more severe at 1 and 6 weeks in patients in whom rhBMP-2 was used. There was no significant difference in the clinical outcome of patients in the two groups at 2 years. The authors concluded that, despite good fusion rates, they abandoned using rhBMP-2 and PEEK cages for anterior cervical fusion, due to side effects, high cost, and the availability of a suitable alternative. Shields et al.[427] reviewed 151 patients who underwent either an anterior cervical discectomy and fusion (n = 138) or anterior cervical vertebrectomy and fusion (n = 13) augmented with high-dose BMP-2 and found a 23% complication rate attributable to BMP-2. The authors concluded that an inflammatory effect involving adjacent critical structures led to increased postoperative morbidity.[427] Smucker et al.[428] and Crawford et al.[429] also reported similar findings.

Although BMPs clearly provide valuable tools for use in stimulation of spinal fusion, the next set of challenges is to optimize their use in a broader range of applications. This includes defining those clinical settings in which the current formulation of BMPs does or does not provide optimally effective biologic effects. This includes identification of patient groups or settings in which clinical performance may be limited even for on-label applications (e.g., high-risk patients—diabetes, steroid use, tobacco use, pseudarthrosis). It also includes identification of potential value settings that are currently off label, such as posterolateral lumbar fusion and applications in the cervical spine. These must be assessed through prospective trials or carefully selected and documented clinical experience. Until data regarding the use of BMPs in these settings become available, surgeons must remain cautious to avoid overoptimism or wishful thinking that may result in the use of these products in settings in which their performance is still to be proven. The following discussion regarding published complications associated with the clinical use of BMPs brings to light the importance of this vigilance on the part of surgeons to avoid being "overwhelmed by their enthusiasm of using recombinant human bone morphogenetic protein type 2."[430,431]

Risks and Adverse Events Associated With Use of Bone Morphogenetic Proteins in Spine Fusion

The initial clinical studies using BMPs reported few and often no complications.[93,94,412–414,430–434] However, this was not always the case. Lewandrowski et al.[435] reported vertebral osteolysis with the use of rhBMP-2 in PLIF with 5 out of 68 patients developing osteolysis within 4 months of surgery. Violation of the endplate during decortication was thought to be a contributing factor. This often resolves spontaneously. Similar observations were made in the cervical spine by Vaidya et al.[424]

As clinical experience expanded and BMP-2 was used in many settings beyond anterior lumbar spinal fusion, awareness of risks and adverse effects became more evident. This assessment began by a review of the concerns raised by Poynton and Lane (also discussed earlier) in 2002,[403] warning that "Safety issues associated with the use of bone morphogenetic proteins in spine applications include the possibility of bony overgrowth, interaction with exposed dura, cancer risk, systemic toxicity, reproductive toxicity, immunogenicity, local toxicity, osteoclastic activation, and effects on distal organs."

Despite initial reports of excellent outcomes, data first became available in 2006 citing adverse event rates between 20% and 70%, leading to the issue of a Public Health Notification by the FDA in June 2008[379] regarding life-threatening complications associated with the use of rhBMP-2. Despite initial reports of no adverse events regarding the use of rhBMP-2 for spinal fusions,[93,94,412,434,436] in 2011, Carragee et al.[431] systematically reviewed the published data on rhBMP-2, comparing results of early industry-funded studies with FDA reports and later independent reviews of outcomes and clinical trial data. In this review, concern was expressed regarding an increased risk of malignancy with high doses—specifically with use of AMPLIFY, developed by Medtronic, which is reported to have a dose (concentration × graft volume) 33% higher than INFUSE Bone Graft). There was also strong level 1 evidence demonstrating morbidity equal to or greater than that in patients undergoing harvest of ICBG, specifically a two- to threefold increase in early back and leg pain (16–18% with INFUSE and 25–30% with AMPLIFY). The rate of wound complications was estimated to be two to five times the rate of those seen in patients not receiving rhBMP-2 (level 3 evidence). Carragee et al.[431] criticized the study design as having potentially biased clinical outcomes against the ICBG group, as the study protocols (1) limited the quantities of ICBG that could be used, (2) required discarding local bone graft, and (3) did not allow preparation of facets for arthrodesis, all changes from standard surgical procedures for PLIF.[431,437–439] In a more recent review of the literature, Walker et al.[297] concluded that rhBMP-2 might be useful in improving rates of radiographic arthrodesis in PLF, specifically in patients at high risk for pseudarthrosis, such as smokers.

Focusing on studies using rhBMP-2 for ALIF,[413,414,432,440,441] which previously had unreported complications, a later review on available FDA data and recent publications reported complications including osteolysis, subsidence, implant loosening, and migration at rates significantly greater than those in controls.[431] In addition, a statistical higher rate of retrograde ejaculation (RE) was seen in male patients (6–9%), two to four times greater than that in patients not receiving rhBMP-2. The rate of urogenital adverse events (described as mainly urinary retention) was twice that in controls (level 2 evidence). The rates of delayed infections in anterior and anteroposterior fusion procedures were significantly increased in patients receiving rhBMP-2, with the infection rate being as high as five times greater for delayed wound infections (level 2 evidence).[431]

In analysis that followed, Siemionow and Singh[442] advise caution in interpreting these findings, asserting that the current available evidence may be biased in favor of finding a correlation between rhBMP-2 and RE. However, they agreed with the prior assertion by Mroz et al.[443] that validated methods for preoperative and postoperative assessments of RE should be used in patients undergoing ALIF and that the lack of these standardized methods in the previous literature may have even contributed to previous underreporting.

Focusing on studies in which BMP-2 was used for PLIF despite initial reports of no adverse events, Carragee et al.[431] found that the morbidity in the patients receiving rhBMP-2 was the same as or greater than associated with harvest of ICBG (level 2 evidence). There was level 1 evidence of formation of ectopic bone into the spinal canal/foramen at a frequency six times that seen in patients not receiving rhBMP-2. In 50% to 70% of patients receiving rhBMP-2 for PLIF, complications included osteolysis, subsidence, implant migration, and/or loss of lordosis (level 1 and level 2 evidence). These problems usually do not resolve. Patients receiving rhBMP-2 for PLIF had poorer outcome scores: they were more dissatisfied with their surgery. The external validity of this finding was difficult to assess, as the RCT in question was discontinued prior to enrollment of a number of patients sufficient to provide statistical power to support further analysis of the data (level 2 evidence). Carragee et al.[431] criticized the use of ICBG as the source of autogenous bone in the PLIF trial. They asserted that prior to the publication of the industry-sponsored trial evaluating rhBMP-2 in PLIF,[430] the efficacy of local bone graft for PLIF had been established.[444] They argued that harvest of ICBG increased pain that would have been minimal or absent if local bone graft had been used alone or used to supplement the ICBG controls.[431] They proposed that the use of ICBG in controls may have unnecessarily handicapped the control group. More recent trials had confirmed the efficacy of local bone in single-level PLF,[445–447] and Carragee et al. emphasized that despite this handicap, no advantage was found for the use of rhBMP-2 in PLIF.[431] Haid et al.[430] later conceded, despite no discussion of adverse events in the initial reports, that the study was discontinued as a result of bony overgrowth into the spinal canal in patients receiving rhBMP-2.

Focusing on studies using rhBMP-2 in ACDF, despite initial reports of no device-related adverse events and claims of a 100% fusion rate with no significant morbidity in patients receiving rhBMP-2,[433,448] the Carragee et al.[431] review of later available FDA data and more recent publications revealed the following. There was increased perioperative mortality in the rhBMP-2 group (level 2 evidence). Perioperative wound complications, difficulty swallowing, and impaired vocalization were seen in rates 40% higher during the acute hospitalization in patients receiving rhBMP-2 (level 2 evidence). Patients in the rhBMP-2 group also experienced prolonged dysphagia requiring tube feeding even when a lower-dose formulation of rhBMP-2 was used (level 3 and level 4 evidence). Finally, endplate resorption, subsidence, and loss of alignment were seen in more than 50% of patients receiving rhBMP-2 for ACDF (level 3 evidence).

The findings of Carragee et al.[431] have been supported by more recent meta-analyses on the use of rhBMP-2 and rhBMP-7.[449,450] In addition to concerns regarding study design and the possible role of bias in reporting of the earlier industry-funded studies, Carragee et al.[431] drew attention to the importance of caution in large-scale clinical application of biologics that have known potential for safety concerns based on preclinical data, including intense inflammatory response and comprising neural elements.[403,410] These concerns, particularly regarding off-label use, were echoed by Epstein et al.[451]

In a prospective, randomized, controlled clinical and radiographic trial conducted in Belgium, Michielsen et al.[452] found no differences in clinical outcomes between use of rhBMP-2 and ICBG in patients undergoing single-level PLIF. Fusion was equally achieved between groups, but formation of trabecular bone was slower and interbody bone density was lower in the first year postoperatively in the rhBMP-2 group. The incidences of ectopic bone formation and osteolysis were high in the rhBMP-2 group. Because there was no evidence of ectopic bone formation, cystic formation, or osteolysis in the control group and because the ectopic bone extended posteriorly along the path of cage implantation, the authors concluded that these complications were directly related to use of rhBMP-2.

A cohort-controlled study confirmed previously published findings demonstrating a higher rate of RE in patients undergoing ALIF with rhBMP-2 at a single level (6.7%) when compared with control patients undergoing single-level (0%) and two-level (1.6%) ALIF without rhBMP-2.[453] Glassman et al.[454] reported that use of rhBMP-2 in posterolateral fusion does not adversely affect postoperative leg pain to a clinically significant level in patients with dural tears specifically. There were no differences in leg pain scores or in any other health-related quality-of-life outcome measure between the group with dural tears and the group with no dural tears. However, the number of patients with neurologic deficits preoperatively was too small to determine whether or not there was a differential rate of recovery of neurologic function. Mannion et al.[455] reported on the use of rhBMP-2 with autograft for minimally invasive lumbar interbody fusion (PLIF or TLIF) performed at either one or two levels in 30 patients (36 levels). Using their technique of placement of a low dose of rhBMP-2 (1.4 mg) and locally harvested bone graft, almost all patients (33 of 36 levels) had evidence of fusion within 7.1 months. Complications related to rhBMP-2 occurred in 5 of 30 patients and included vertebral body osteolysis with nonunion (3.3%), heterotopic ossification in the neural foramen (6.6%), and cyst formation (6.6%). One patient required revision surgery. Practicing in the United Kingdom and Australia, they emphasized the importance of two potential obstacles to widespread use of rhBMP-2 in publicly funded health care systems: cost and adverse effects. They cautioned that, given that high rates of interbody fusion can be achieved with minimally invasive techniques without rhBMP-2,[456] the added cost and potential morbidity associated with use of this product should limit its applications to cases in which preexisting risks of nonunion are considerable.

In a retrospective study of patients undergoing TLIF with rhBMP-2, Helgeson et al.[457] reported that the incidence of osteolysis was high: 54% at 3 to 6 months postoperatively. While this decreased to 41% at 1 to 2 years, 76% of cases of osteolysis did not resolve. While this affected neither the rate of fusion nor the final outcome (overall union rate of 83%), a bony void was still present at the time of ultimate fusion. The authors noted that this patient population (at a military hospital) was younger, on average (38.2 years), than patients in other published studies.

Despite the fact that early studies documented little to no morbidity to the nervous system,[401] the incidences of back and leg adverse events were noted by the FDA to be markedly higher in the early postoperative period in patients undergoing PLF with both the INFUSE and AMPLIFY (Medtronic) rhBMP-2 formulations.[458] Concerns regarding the effects of rhBMP-2 in the setting of spinal cord injury led to in vivo studies in a rat model of penetrating spinal cord injury, in which Dmitriev et al.[459] performed PLF with or without rhBMP-2 at varying intervals after injury. They found significant intraparenchymal inflammatory changes with use of rhBMP-2 at all time points. Further studies with this model confirmed the presence of intraparenchymal inflammation at both early and late time points.[460] An unexpected finding was the difference in the need for treatment for self-mutilation behavior, a response to neuropathic pain in rats,[461] in the rhBMP-2–treated group (56%) compared with controls (31%). The authors proposed that these histochemical and clinical findings in rats correlated with clinical reports on early postoperative radiculitis in patients undergoing single-level TLIF with rhBMP-2.[462] This relative time interval (10 days in rats) is believed to correlate to several months in human patients.[463] This finding appears to be supported by FDA clinical data documenting the effects of radiculitis in these patients persisting for approximately 3 months postoperatively. The authors concluded that the mechanism of this observed allodynia is potentially via BMP-2–mediated inflammation in and around the dorsal root ganglion and emphasize the importance of careful consideration of risks associated with off-label use of rhBMP-2.[465]

In a meta-analysis of RCTs evaluating clinical outcomes of use of BMP versus ICBG for lumbar fusion in patients with degenerative disc disease, Noshchenko et al.[466] found significant improvements in the Oswestry Disability Index (ODI) and 36-Item Short Form Health Survey (SF-36) scores as well as in back and leg pain in both groups at 24 months. The rate of patient satisfaction was approximately 80% in both groups. The only difference in patient-reported clinical outcome measures between the two groups was a significantly greater improvement in the SF-36 (physical scale) scores in the BMP groups. However, the authors reported that the difference was heterogeneous, raising concerns regarding low levels of evidence.[466–468]

Malham et al.[469] reported results of a prospective study of 131 consecutive patients undergoing ALIF with a PEEK cage filled with rhBMP-2 and a separate anterior titanium plate, performed by a single spine surgeon and a single vascular surgeon with goal of prospectively evaluating complication rates, particularly RE. Of note, this patient population is closest in age (mean age, 45.3 years; range, 23–70 years) to that of Helgeson et al.[457] (mean age, 38.2 years; range, 23–81 years). Malham et al.[469] reported lower complication rates than those in the literature for ALIF patients, reported to be as high as 40%. Their total perioperative complication rate was 10.1%, with minor complications in 13.0% and major complications in 6.1%. Perhaps most noteworthy was that only 1 of 67 male patients in this series experienced RE (1.5%). This is in contrast to previous studies with published rates of RE of 7.9%,[470] 3.4%,[471] and 7.2%,[453] which led to conclusions that use of rhBMP-2 in lumbosacral ALIF was associated with an increased risk of RE. The overall fusion rate in this study (for ALIF and hybrid patients receiving rhBMP-2) was 96.9%. Only 4 of 131 patients had not experienced fusion at 12 months postoperatively. This was the 12-month fusion rate (12.9%) reported by Burkus et al.[414]

In the largest reported series of adult patients receiving high-dose rhBMP-2 (≥40 mg), Mesfin et al.[472] reported short- and long-term results in 502 adult patients at a single institution. The average length of follow-up was 42 months (range, 14–92 months). The majority of this caseload was comprised of adult spinal deformity cases, noted for having high complication rates, ranging from 35.9% to 46%.[473–475] Further, 47% of their cases were revisions, known to have a documented higher risk of major complications.[474] The authors stated that one of the main reasons they elected to use rhBMP-2 was the potential for decreasing the high risk for pseudarthrosis in this challenging patient population. Compared with a published pseudarthrosis rate of 17%, cited in studies performed prior to the use of rhBMP-2, Mesfin et al.[476] reported a rate of 5%; 52% of their patients developing pseudarthrosis were patients undergoing revision procedures. In a patient population receiving an average dose of 115 mg of rhBMP-2 (range, 40–351 mg), with an average of 11.5 levels instrumented (range, 3–19 levels), these authors reported a lower prevalence of cancer in this patient group, when compared with the general population, and the dose of patients in this group who had cancer received a lower dose of rhBMP-2 than those in the noncancer group (although the dose was not significantly lower). At 1%, the rate of postoperative radiculopathy (in five patients, four undergoing TLIF) was also lower in this study than the rates of 5.4% to 11% reported in other studies evaluating rhBMP-2 in TLIF,[472,477,478] and the authors found no correlation between dose of rhBMP-2 and development of postoperative radiculopathy. These results challenge the findings in the literature regarding these complications and the associated discussions regarding potential for dose-related escalations in risk, particularly a study published at the same time by Carragee et al.[479] reporting on 463 patients with 86% follow-up at 2 years. In patients undergoing single-level instrumented posterolateral arthrodesis, at 2 years the incidence rate of cancer was 6.8-fold greater in the rhBMP-2 (40 mg) group in a compression-resistant matrix when compared with autogenous bone graft (control). In addition, fivefold more patients in the rhBMP-2/CRM group developed one or more cancers compared with the control group, also a statistically significant difference. The authors concluded that use of 40 mg of rhBMP-2/CRM was associated with an increased risk of new cancers.[479]

In a larger, population-based retrospective cohort study, Cooper et al.[480] compared the rate of new cancers in Medicare beneficiaries aged 67 years and older undergoing lumbar spinal fusion with rhBMP between 2003 and 2008 to patients who did not receive rhBMP. The authors identified 146,278 patients meeting these criteria. Mean duration of surveillance was 4.7 years. The authors used data from the Surveillance, Epidemiology, and End Results (SEER) Program[481] to determine whether the incidence of cancer was different from the general population. There was no association of administration of rhBMP with cancer incidence.

In response to concerns regarding the safety of INFUSE, Medtronic, Yale University, Oregon Health and Science University, the University of York in the United Kingdom, and Fu et al.,[482] via the Yale University Open Data Access (YODA) Project, conducted a meta-analysis of individual-patient data from 13 RCTs (12 sponsored by Medtronic and one by Norton Healthcare). The goals of this study were (1) to estimate the effectiveness and harm of rhBMP-2 in spinal fusion and (2) to assess reporting biases in published articles of industry-sponsored studies.[482] The authors found that the main sources of bias were lack of blinding of surgeons, patients, and outcome assessors. They concluded that there was no difference between the effectiveness of rhBMP-2 and ICBG when used in spinal fusion, specifically in ALIF and PLF. They found the evidence available insufficient to make conclusions regarding the effectiveness of rhBMP-2 compared with ICBG in other surgical approaches for spinal fusion.

In agreement with the findings (discussed earlier) by Carragee et al.,[431] Fu et al.[482] also concluded that use of rhBMP-2 in ACDF was associated with statistically significant increases in adverse events overall, wound complications, and dysphonia and dysphagia. They found that adverse events were common with the use of both rhBMP-2 and ICBG for lumbar fusion, with both on-label and off-label use. The authors stated that although this review did raise concerns regarding the possibility of increased risks of RE, urinary retention, and ectopic bone formation with rhBMP-2, the data on these events were sparse and "the quality of ascertainment was often poor," leading them to conclude that there was insufficient evidence regarding the risks of these complications in patients receiving rhBMP-2.

Fu et al.[482] also found that, consistent with previous findings, rhBMP-2 was associated with an increased risk for cancer through 24 months of follow-up but recommended caution in interpretation of this finding, as cancer cases were found to be heterogeneous and were underreported. They agreed with Carragee et al.[431] that publications of data reporting both on-label and off-label use of rhBMP-2 in journals favored the reporting of results favoring rhBMP-2 over ICBG and that adverse events of five trials were, in fact, underreported. They conceded that results were not previously made available to the public.

In another publication funded by the YODA Project, Simmonds et al.[484] evaluated individual-participant data in a meta-analysis of 11 Medtronic RCTs and one additional RCT comparing effectiveness of rhBMP-2 to ICBG. The authors concluded that rhBMP-2 improves rates of fusion compared with ICBG. However, they noted that inconsistency across trials was high. They also found that rhBMP-2 improves back pain and quality of life (based on ODI or SF-36 scores) between 6 and 24 months postoperatively, but that these improvements in pain were not clinically significant. They noted the limitation that patients were not blinded regarding treatment and, as such, may have been biased toward reporting better function and less pain if they were in the rhBMP-2 treatment group. This study also found increased pain in the immediate postoperative period in the rhBMP-2 group, but concluded that rhBMP-2 reduced pain in the longer term. This study reported an increase in the risk of cancer associated with rhBMP-2 administration, with this treatment group having almost twice the incidence of new cancer cases when compared with patients in the ICBG group, consistent with previously reported concerns regarding cancer risks.[485] However, they note that the overall absolute cancer risk in both groups is low and question whether this increased risk is genuine. This is not consistent with the increased risk of malignancy reported by the FDA with use of AMPLIFY, in which a 3.8% incidence of new malignancies was found when compared with 0.89% in controls. This difference was statistically significant, with the statistical analysis performed reporting a 90% to 95% probability that this association was genuine.[431,458] Regarding concerns about increases in formation of heterotopic bone, osteolysis, radiculitis, and RE,[485] Simmonds et al.[484]

advised that these findings should be interpreted with caution, as they were based on less extensive and less detailed clinical data than that in the YODA Project. Analysis of YODA studies found no difference in effectiveness (based on ODI/SF-36 scores, safety, or cancer risk between patients receiving the licensed INFUSE product and the unlicensed AMPLIFY preparation (which contained a higher concentration of rhBMP-2). However, the authors did concede that, overall, rhBMP-2 may lead to an increase in incidence of cancer and that this is a finding important for clinicians to discuss with patients when facilitating informed decision making. Regardless of the low published risks, Tannoury and An[486] advise that the observed increases in cancer incidence associated with use of rhBMP-2 should remain a critically important concern to clinicians based on longer-term reviews of the literature.[487]

Hustedt and Blizzard[178] subsequently expanded on the findings of the YODA studies, clarifying the rationale and logistics of the collaboration between Medtronic and Yale University. They summarized the findings resulting from all studies in the YODA Project as follows:

- There were no differences in fusion rates between rhBMP-2 and autograft ICBG.
- Both rhBMP-2 and ICBG are associated with similar rates of RE and neurologic complications when used in ALIF or PLF.
- There is clear evidence that use of rhBMP-2 leads to high complication rates in anterior cervical spine procedures and high rates of formation of ectopic bone in posterior lumbar interbody procedures.
- While there is a slight increase in the risk of cancer with use of rhBMP-2, the absolute risk remains very small and is therefore most likely clinically insignificant.

They also summarized the current recommendations for the use of rhBMP-2 based on the results of YODA analyses, as shown in Table 66.1.

TABLE 66.1 Recommendations for Use of rhBMP-2, per YODA[178,482,484] Analyses

Procedure	Recommendation
ALIF	There is no difference between rhBMP-2 and ICBG. However, ICBG requires an additional surgical site. When autograft bone is not available or harvest/use of autograft is not desired, rhBMP-2 is a reliable alternative to ICBG. RE and neurologic complications in patients treated with rhBMP-2 and ICBG were equal.
Anterior cervical fusion	The FDA has issued a warning stating that rhBMP-2 should not be used in the anterior cervical spine due to inflammation causing severe dysphagia and airway compromise.
PLF	There is no difference between rhBMP-2 and ICBG. However, ICBG harvest requires an additional surgical site. When autograft bone is not available or the harvest procedure is not desired, rhBMP-2 is a reliable alternative.
PLIF	Use of rhBMP-2 is associated with high rates of ectopic bone formation leading to neurologic compromise. ICBG is preferred.
TLIF	Use of rhBMP-2 is associated with seroma formation and neurologic compromise. Further evidence is needed. Judicious use of rhBMP-2 is advised based on reported complications.

ALIF, anterior lumbar interbody fusion; FDA, US Food and Drug Administration; ICBG, iliac crest bone graft; PLF, posterolateral fusion; PLIF, posterior lumbar interbody fusion; RE, retrograde ejaculation; rhBMP, recombinant human bone morphogenetic protein; TLIF, transforaminal lumbar interbody fusion; YODA, Yale University Open Data Access.

Cahill et al.[488] reviewed and summarized the findings of both YODA meta-analyses[482,484] and articles in the English language meeting their criteria of being published studies with at least 1 year of follow-up,[472,479] which included three large population-based studies.[480,489,490] With the addition of the population-based analyses, the advantages of the inclusion of massive data sets (MarketScan,[490] Medicare Beneficiary Data,[480] and PearlDiver[489] Medicare Data), the authors noted the clear advantages of larger sample sizes in risk assessment regarding postoperative carcinogenesis in patients receiving rhBMP-2 for spine fusion procedures. In combining these sources, Cahill et al.[488] concluded that the overall risk of cancer development is low and that there is no clear association between postoperative cancer formation and use of rhBMP-2 in spinal fusion.

In a meta-analysis of studies reporting on spinal fusion with rhBMP-2 in human patients, Vavken et al.[491] identified 26 studies with outcomes on a total of 184,324 patients (28,815 experimental patients and 155,509 controls) with a mean age of 51.1 ± 1.8 years. Using random-effects modeling to calculate pooled odds ratios (ORs), they found significantly higher risks of the following in patients receiving rhBMP-2 compared with ICBG: general complications (OR, 1.78), heterotopic ossification (OR, 5.57), RE (OR, 3.31), and cervical swelling (OR, 4.72). The pooled OR for new onset of tumor was slightly higher (OR, 1.35) for patients receiving rhBMP-2, but did not differ significantly between groups.

Favorable long-term outcomes of use of rhBMPs in spinal surgery were recently reported by Malham et al.[492] in a retrospective cohort study of patients in the state of Victoria, Australia. In 527 patients undergoing anterior, lateral, posterior, or posterolateral lumbar fusion performed by two spine surgeons between 2002 and 2012 with either rhBMP-2 (INFUSE) or rhBMP-7 (OP-1), with a mean follow-up period of 4.4 years (range, 1.8–11.5 years) and a mean age of 58.4 years (range, 21.3–93.0 years), fusion rates were similar (90.1% for rhBMP-2 and 91.9% for rhBMP-7). The success rate of interbody fusion was 93.5% at 12 months with no difference found between rhBMP-2 and rhBMP-7. The authors commented that they have not harvested ICBG since initiating the use of rhBMP in their practice in 2002. Reporting of cancer diagnoses in the state of Victoria, Australia to the Victorian Cancer Registry is mandated by law. The authors used this database to identify new cancers occurring during the duration of patient follow-up (2002–13) and compared this to the incidence of cancer in the population of Victoria. There was no significant difference in the incidence of cancer in their patient cohort when compared with age- and sex-specific rates for the population of Victoria. The authors noted that while their analysis criteria were more strict, these estimates of risk in their patient cohort are similar to those reported by Cooper and Kou.[480] They also cited that their findings differed from those of Fu et al.,[482] Simmonds et al.,[484] and Carragee et al.,[479] all of whom reported increased cancer risks in patients who underwent spinal surgery utilizing rhBMP-2.

Opportunities for Improving or Refining the Use of BMPs and Other Bioactive Molecules

The mechanism of action of BMPs provides many opportunities for further advancement and refinement, including modification of dose, formulation, delivery systems, changes in molecular structure, and means of optimizing the environment into which these agents are placed. One of the principal requirements for optimal BMP activity is the presence of a local population of target cells that are responsive to the protein (i.e., they express appropriate receptors). In order for a BMP to be optimally effective, these target cells must be both available and activated in sufficient numbers to produce the desired result. If an optimal number of responsive cells are not present within the tissue volume that is exposed to the protein, the biologic response will inevitably be reduced and the implantation of a BMP (or any agent) may be completely ineffective. Variation in the concentration or biologic potential of target cell populations in bone, bone marrow, periosteum, and other tissues (e.g., muscle, fat) may explain much of the apparent variation in the magnitude and type of response seen to BMPs and other growth factors from site to site and individual to individual.[156,157,493,494]

Preclinical evaluation of BMPs in a series of animal models from rats to rabbits to dogs to nonhuman primates demonstrated the need for delivery of dramatically high concentrations of BMP to graft sites in higher animals.[386] In fact, the formulation of BMP currently available delivers an amount of BMP that is roughly 50 times greater than the total amount of BMP that is present in an entire human skeleton. INFUSE delivers BMP-2 in solution at a concentration of 1.5 mg/mL to be combined with a collagen carrier, resulting in an implanted concentration of slightly less than 1 mg/mL. The reason for this escalation of dose has not been clearly established, though several factors are likely to contribute. Species-specific differences in dose response may exist at the target cell level, though this has not been a consistent finding in in vitro culture of primary osteogenic cells. However, individual species do demonstrate significant differences in the concentration and prevalence of responsive target cells in local tissues and consistently lower numbers in higher animals. The geometry involved in delivery of BMP to a sufficient volume of a responsive target population of cells in larger graft sites increases with the cube of the dimension, which also contributes. A huge dose may be necessary to provide a burst of BMP delivery that is sufficiently large that the BMP diffusing away from the graft site will penetrate into regional tissues to a sufficient depth at a sufficiently large concentration to activate enough stem cells and progenitors or the graft site becomes larger. Similarly, if the concentration and prevalence of target cells in regional tissues decrease, as they do in higher animals, activation of a similar number of cells will require even deeper tissue penetration. These factors likely contribute to the seemingly exponential increase in dose that is necessary in larger animals.[15] A second possible explanation for the massive dose relates to the issue of BMP retention at the graft site. A massive initial dose may also ensure that a sufficient, though perhaps small, quantity of BMP will remain at the site long enough to result in activation of target cells that may not enter the graft site until several days after implantation, with the associated inflammatory response or angiogenic response following the surgical trauma. These issues in BMP delivery and function in a graft site suggest a number of options that could be used to increase the exposure of BMP to an appropriate target population of cells, thereby improving its performance. Direct delivery or supplementation of the target cell population in the graft site is one option. Evidence is provided by a number of studies that addition of a target population (e.g., bone marrow–derived cells) to a site of BMP implantation will significantly improve bone healing.[147,493,494] Another possible method for enhancing the performance of BMPs is to refine the method and rate of BMP delivery into the graft site. The chemical surface of the matrix may influence the protein binding, its conformation, and stability. In some cases, BMP binding to matrix can actually enhance the biologic performance.[495–497] The four major categories of BMP carrier materials are natural polymers, such as collagen, hyaluronans, fibrin, chitosan, silk, alginate, and agarose; inorganic materials such as low- and high-temperature calcium orthophosphates (calcium phosphate cements and sintered ceramics) and calcium sulfate cements; poly(α-hydroxy acid) synthetic polymers such as polylactic acid, polyglycolide (PLG); and their copolymers (poly[D,L-lactide-co-glycolide]) (PLGA).[498] Furthermore, the carrier (collagen, ceramic, polymer) may have its own biologic effects associated with the release of ions or other degradation products.[15] Currently INFUSE uses an absorbable type I bovine collagen sponge (ACS) as the carrier, on which BMP-2 is reversibly absorbed. A recent study in canines suggested that if BMP-2 is implanted in an environment containing $CaPO_4$ ceramic, BMP-2 and BMP-2–associated bone formation will concentrate around the ceramic.[172] Other options include controlled release from degradable polymers, liposomes, collagen-hydroxyapatite microspheres, and potentially an osteogenic and antiadipogenic molecule known as Oxy133 (recently evaluated in rodent and rabbit models).[499–502] Tethering BMP or other bioactive agents to the surface of a substrate using covalent linkage or a matrix-specific binding peptide is also being explored.[503]

Yet another option for enhancing the performance of BMPs is to prolong the period of time that effective concentrations of the protein are present in the graft site. Residence time of bioactive protein in a graft site is a complex function of the rate of delivery (e.g., release or solubilization); the rate of consumption within the graft site (e.g., degradation, inactivation, binding to inhibitors); and the rate of clearance from the graft site (e.g., diffusion, convection). With the current BMP preparations, release kinetics is relatively rapid. BMP diffuses rapidly out of the immediate graft site and appears at low concentrations, in systemic circulation, where it is rapidly cleared. Fifty percent of the rhBMP-2 is cleared from the site in 48 hours and less than 1% is remaining at 2 weeks.[504] Approximately 50% is excreted in the urine.[494]

Longer residence time within the site is associated with improved efficacy at lower protein concentration.[505] Residence time is influenced by the affinity of the protein to the carrier.[506,507] Residence time can also be increased by modifying the BMP protein itself to reduce its solubility and therefore its rate of diffusion out of the implant.[508] Prolonged residence time within the graft site may have two effects. It may allow the initial gradient of protein concentration around the site to be maintained for a longer period, which may positively influence chemotactic effects that may be mediated by the protein and draw more activated progenitors and other cells into the defect. Prolonged residence may also serve to maintain a functional concentration of protein in the graft site for a longer time, providing the opportunity for additional stem cells and progenitors to migrate into the graft site where they may become activated.

Other Growth Factors

A large number of peptide growth factors and hormones are known to have important effects on the recruitment, proliferation, and differentiation of osteoblastic progenitors, which may have potential therapeutic importance.[509,510] EGF and PDGF are both capable of inducing colony formation by osteoblastic progenitors in vitro,[33] and local injection of PDGF has been shown to result in induction of new bone formation when applied close to a bone surface. A PDGF product has been introduced for use in ankle fusion but has no current indication or data related to spine fusion.[511,512] Basic fibroblast growth factor (FGF; also called bFGF or FGF-2) will also increase proliferation of human osteoblastic progenitors and reversibly inhibit the expression of alkaline phosphatase and matrix synthesis in addition to its known potent angiogenic effects. FGF has been evaluated in preclinical studies using a hyaluronic acid delivery system and has been shown to increase local bone formation and union rates.[513]

VEGFs are a family of proteins that function as dimers. They have a structure similar to PDGF and interact with transmembrane receptors Flt-1, Flk-1, and Flt-4 to activate a tyrosine kinase signaling cascade. VEGFs play several important roles in angiogenesis, osteoclast migration, and osteoblastic activity.[514,515] VEGFs do not induce bone directly but, in addition to angiogenic effects, VEGF delivery has been shown to upregulate BMP activity in fracture healing and distraction osteogensis.[516,517] When used in combination, VEGFs may enhance the performance of BMPs.[518,519]

Transforming growth factor beta (TGF-β) is another potent osteotropic factor. Of the five known isoforms of TGF-β, two—TGF-β1 and TGF-β2—are synthesized by bone cells. In fact, bone matrix deposited by osteoblasts is the largest source of TGF-β and is mostly present in a latent form that is released during bone remodeling.[520,521] TGF-β has effects on bone formation and remodeling. It will induce new bone formation, but only when implanted or injected in close proximity to bone, suggesting that its bone formation effects are mediated primarily by trabecular or periosteal cells, a different or more limited target cell population than the BMPs.[522] For example, Joyce et al.[523] showed that subperiosteal injection of TGF-β can produce a marked periosteal response resulting in rapid formation of a cartilage tissue mass and bone formation via endochondral ossification. IGF-I and IGF-II potentiate a mature osteoblastic phenotype in culture.[58,524,525] Both TGF-β and IGF-I have been shown to promote spine fusion in a sheep model.[526,527]

Collagen

The major components of organic matrix of bone are type I collagen (90% dry weight), a large number of noncollagenous matrix proteins, at least two proteoglycans (biglycan and decorin), and several minor collagens (mostly types III and X). These proteins contribute an osteoconductive substrate for cell attachment and migration and are necessary elements of new bone formation and mineralization. The precise contribution of each element of organic bone matrix is not known. Nor is it understood how the structural organization of the various components within the matrix influences the biologic function of these proteins, making the engineering of synthetic matrices that mimic specific functional relationships between these proteins difficult.

Type I collagen has been the focus of many efforts to develop optimal tissue engineering scaffolds. Most of the noncollagenous proteins in bone matrix can be solubilized using 4 M guanidine. However, the majority of type I collagen in bone matrix is heavily interconnected by covalent pyridinium cross-links. This makes native collagen I insoluble and virtually impossible to manipulate as a reagent to create new structures. In addition, demineralized extracted collagen matrix is only modestly effective as osteoconductive material, though it has been used effectively as a delivery vehicle for purified proteins and extracts of bone matrix.

In contrast, fibrillar collagen (uncross-linked collagen) is soluble and can be extracted from bone and skin. Fibrillar collagen can be engineered to produce a variety of matrices, such as gels, sponges, and filaments. These are often secondarily cross-linked to stabilize their structure using a variety of chemical methods. Again, few of these engineered collagen matrices are effective by themselves in strongly promoting bone formation. Some formulations have appeared to actually compromise the efficacy of autograft in a graft site.[162] However, in general, collagen matrices have been effective as delivery systems for bone marrow–derived cells[146] and for growth factors. Both BMP-2 and OP-1 used collagen I as their delivery vehicle when introduced. Interconnected porous meshes of purified bovine collagen (pore size ≈50 μm) with a coating of hydroxyapatite precipitated on its surface have also been specifically developed and marketed as a delivery system for bone marrow harvested by aspiration.[339,528]

Noncollagenous Matrix Proteins

Bone matrix contains many proteins other than collagens and growth factors.[155,313,529–531] These proteins may serve a role in organization of the collagenous matrix and other proteins into higher-ordered structures. They may provide attachment sites for cells or binding sites for growth factors. They may serve as regulators of mineralization, as in the case of bone and dentin phosphoproteins, bone sialoprotein, osteonectin, and osteocalcin.[532–534] They may also provide a source for release of locally active growth factors and other bioactive molecules during the process of matrix turnover and remodeling, as previously discussed.

Other than growth factors that are embedded in bone matrix, it is difficult to ascribe any one factor with exceptional function in the setting of bone grafting or a high potential for future clinical application. However, some may be relevant and deserve mention. For example, osteoblasts and osteoblastic cell lines appear to express integrins that bind selectively to both fibronectin and vitronectin[535–537] and possibly osteopontin, bone sialoprotein, and laminin. In addition, osteocalcin appears to be chemotactic for osteoclasts and monocytes,[538] critical elements of normal bone remodeling. Although these proteins are not likely to be exploited in terms of recombinant manufacturing processes used for BMPs, it is possible that these functions may be localized to specific functional domains of these proteins. This knowledge may be used to design specific low-molecular-weight surrogates that may be applied to tissue engineering constructs.

Ceramics

Calcium phosphate biomaterials fused at their crystal grain boundaries into polycrystalline ceramics by high-temperature sintering confer stability to these minerals and reduce bioresorbability.[539] A variety of ceramics are currently being evaluated, most of which are composed of either hydroxyapatite (HA) or tricalcium phosphate (TCP). Ceramics may be prepared as porous three-dimensional implants, dense block implants, granular particles (usually 0.5–3 mm in size), or thin surface coatings. Almost all calcium phosphate ceramics have a high degree of biocompatibility,[330,540] and some have already been extensively used in dentistry and maxillofacial surgery.[330,341,540–547]

The minimal macropore size in porous ceramics needed for effective ingrowth of bone is approximately 100 μm.[548,549] Most porous ceramics currently being manufactured contain interconnecting macropores ranging from 100 to 400 μm. The various calcium phosphate ceramics generally differ with regard to their bioresorbability characteristics. A number of investigators have reported that ceramic HA that does not exhibit bioresorption is essentially inert.[539,540,550,551] Conversely, there is unequivocal evidence that ceramic TCP undergoes biodegradation.[330,473,539,540,550]

Early studies of ceramics suggested that they may be capable of osteogenic stimulation.[552] In fact, one can often find new bone formation in an HA ceramic implant placed at heterotopic sites in the absence of other stimuli. This occurs only after several months and would not be likely to contribute to the early success of a bone graft. The role of ceramics, therefore, is primarily that of osteoconduction.[553] One possible mechanism for this apparent late osteoinductive property of HA ceramics is that an implanted HA implant will selectively bind proteins to its surface on the basis of their relative affinity to HA. This may result in the accumulation of some protein growth factors, such as BMPs, TGF-βs, and insulin-like binding protein-5, which have strong affinity to HA. Accumulation of these low-abundance proteins and their presentation on a stable surface may secondarily create a local growth factor environment on the ceramic surface that is capable of recruiting local osteoblastic progenitors and inducing bone formation. This affinity of many osteotropic growth factors for the highly charged surface of HA may also make HA ceramics an effective delivery system for growth factors as composite synthetic bone grafting materials are developed.[554]

The stability of a bone-ceramic interface and preparation of local bone are also important. Cameron et al.[555] demonstrated that ceramic implants placed against an unprepared bony cortex do not exhibit bone ingrowth and simply resorb over time. However, when placed subperiosteally and immobilized on a scarified cortex, bone ingrowth readily takes place. The sensitivity of these materials to micromotion likely results from magnification of the mechanical strain within the graft site at the interface between local tissues and the surface of a rigid ceramic block. Similar magnification of strain will occur in the regions of tissue between adjoining ceramic granules, inhibiting bone formation. As a result, the optimal settings for use of these materials may be limited to settings in which mechanical micromotion can be well controlled.

Another drawback of ceramic implants is that they are brittle and have low impact and fracture resistance.[556] Furthermore, the limited solubility and remodeling capacity of highly crystalline HA ceramics may retard late stages of bone healing and remodeling and may compromise late mechanical properties of the bone formed in a fusion site.[539,556] This concern has been reduced by the work of Ohgushi et al.,[557] which showed that ceramic combined with bone marrow exhibited greater biomechanical properties following implantation with marrow cells as a result of new bone formation in the implant. In addition, Muschler et al.[161,162,557] have performed a series of spinal fusion experiments evaluating composites of collagen and ceramic granules (60% hydroxyapatite, 40% TCP). Although these studies found that all composites tested had a significantly higher nonunion rate than autogenous cancellous bone graft, the mechanical properties of successful unions achieved with the collagen ceramic composites were comparable with the mechanical properties of unions resulting from autogenous bone graft, despite the presence of unresorbed granules in the fusion mass.

A modest volume of clinical literature is available related to ceramic materials in spine fusion. Several injectable ceramic preparations that crystallize at body temperature have also been described. Resorption rates vary significantly, from weeks to months. These may provide means for improving the initial mechanical fixation for acute fractures, though they do not seem well conceived for achieving long-term fixation. These injectable setting ceramics may also have potential utility in providing extended local delivery for bioactive proteins.[558] In a prospective, randomized study with 3-year follow-up, Dai et al.[559] compared beta-tricalcium phosphate versus autograft in patients undergoing single-level instrumented posterolateral fusion of lumbar spine with beta-tricalcium phosphate versus autograft. The authors reported similar clinical outcomes and fusion rates and suggested that beta-TCP as bone graft substitute may eliminate the need for bone graft harvesting from the ilium.[559] In a different prospective study, Chen et al.[560] placed autologous iliac crest bone graft in one posterolateral gutter; on the other side, an equal quantity of autogenous laminectomy bone supplemented with calcium sulfate was placed. In a prospective, matched, and controlled study, Acharya et al.[561] evaluated HA-bioactive glass ceramic composite as a stand-alone graft substitute for posterolateral fusion of lumbar spine by placing it in the left intertransverse bed. The autograft was placed in the right intertransverse bed. At the end of 1 year, excellent radiologic outcome was seen on the right side (autogenous graft) in all the cases, whereas 95% (21 of 22) of the cases had poor consolidation on the left side (HA composite). Epstein[562] found a 15% pseudarthrosis rate following multilevel laminectomy and one- to two-level noninstrumented posterolateral fusion using lamina autograft/β-TCP. Enriched bone-marrow–derived mesenchymal stem cells were combined with porous beta-tricalcium phosphate in 41 patients undergoing posterior spinal fusion.[563] After 34.5 months, 95.1% of cases had good spinal fusion results.

Nickoli et al.[564] reported an overall fusion rate for all ceramic products as a bone graft extender in the lumbar spine to be 86.4% and that ceramics used in combination with local autograft resulted in significantly higher fusion rates. Kaiser et al.[565] provided an evidence-based guideline for performance of fusion procedures for degenerative disease of the lumbar spine, using HA/calcium extenders. β-tricalcium phosphate (β-TCP)/local autograft can substitute for autologous ICBG for single-level instrumented posterolateral fusion (one level 2 study). HA with local bone autograft/bone marrow aspirate (BMA) can be a substitute for ICBG in instrumented posterolateral fusion (one level 2 study). Use of HA can be a bone graft extender when mixed with ICBG for instrumented posterolateral fusions (multiple level 5 studies). Use of calcium sulfate preparations mixed with local autograft can be a substitute for ICBG in instrumented posterolateral fusions (one level 4 study and several level 5 studies). Finally, there is insufficient evidence to recommend an HA-glass/BMA composite as a substitute for autograft for posterolateral fusion.

Systemic/Patient-Specific Factors Influencing Bone Healing in Spine Fusion

Many systemic factors have been shown to influence bone healing in the laboratory. Clinically, these factors are also likely to play an important role. A list of systemic factors and their relative effects on bone healing is shown in Table 66.2. Given the complexity of various factors in the clinical setting, it is difficult to demonstrate on a case-by-case basis or in a clinical series that each of these factors results in significant alterations of fracture healing or the success of spinal fusion procedures. Nevertheless, the surgeon should optimize each factor whenever possible.

Nutritional status has been shown to affect the clinical outcome of surgical procedures generally[566] and on bone healing specifically.[567] Identification of a nutritional deficit using anthropomorphic measurements, serum albumin levels, lymphocyte count, skin antigen testing, and nitrogen balance studies can be important in selected patients. Recent weight loss, anergy in skin testing, serum albumin levels less than 3.4 mg/dL, or a total lymphocyte count of less than 1500 are clinical red flags indicating the need for a careful nutritional evaluation and a possible need for nutritional support.[568] Lenke et al.[569] documented that patients undergoing multiple-level spinal fusion procedures may take 6 to 12 weeks to recover from the perioperative nutritional insult and suggested more aggressive nutritional assessment in these patients. Because most evidence suggests that the critical period in determining the success of a fusion attempt occurs in the first 3 to 7 days of healing, manipulation of systemic factors should be carefully controlled during this time period, especially the administration of radiation,[570] chemotherapeutic agents,[571] nonsteroidal antiinflammatory drugs,[43,44] and corticosteroids. Tobacco use, specifically nicotine, is a clinical factor that is both reversible and most strongly associated with negative results.[406,572–577]

TABLE 66.2 Systemic Factors Influencing Bone Healing

Positive Factors	Negative Factors
Insulin	Corticosteroids
Insulin-like growth factor and other somatomedins	Vitamin A intoxication
	Vitamin D deficiency
Testosterone	Vitamin D intoxication
Estrogen	Iron deficiency anemia
Growth hormone	Negative nitrogen balance
Thyroxine	Calcium deficiency
Parathyroid hormone	Nonsteroidal antiinflammatory drugs
Calcitonin	Adriamycin
Vitamin A	Methotrexate
Vitamin D	Rheumatoid arthritis
Anabolic steroids	Syndrome of inappropriate antidiuretic hormone
Vitamin C	
	Castration
	Tobacco
	Sepsis

Local Factors Influencing Bone Healing in Spine Fusion

Many local factors also influence bone healing; a partial list of these is shown in Table 66.3. In some cases, these factors are unavoidable. In other cases, rational methods can be employed to limit the negative effects. Osteoporosis is generally assumed to be an undesirable factor in fracture healing, but this is without direct clinical evidence. This is probably true but could relate to both mechanical and biologic factors. The quality of internal fixation is significantly affected by bone mass and is an important variable in the outcome of spinal fusions. Furthermore, it has been reported that the quality of local bone marrow and other regional tissues in terms of the concentration, prevalence, and biologic potential of local osteogenic stem cells and progenitors may be reduced in the elderly patient, particularly patients with low rates of bone

TABLE 66.3 Local Factors Influencing Bone Healing

Positive Factors	Negative Factors
Increased surface area (bone and viable local tissue)	Osteoporosis
Local stem cell sources (e.g., bone marrow, periosteum)	Radiation scar
Osteoconductive scaffold (e.g., fibrin clot or other matrix material)	Radiation
Mechanical stability	Denervation
Mechanical loading	Tumor
Factors promoting recruitment, activation, and proliferation of osteoblastic stem cells (e.g., platelet degranulation products including PDGF, EGF)	Marrow-packing disorder
Osteoinductive factors (e.g., BMPs)	Infection
Factors promoting angiogenesis (e.g., FGF, EGF, VEGF)	Local bone disease
Electrical stimulation	Mechanical motion
	Bone wax (other materials inducing foreign body reaction)

BMPs, bone morphogenetic proteins; EGF, epidermal growth factor; FGF, fibroblast growth factor; PDGF, platelet-derived growth factor; VEGF, vascular endothelial growth factor.

remodeling.[15,62,578,579] These age-related changes may or may not be directly related to the pathophysiology of osteoporosis but likely have a negative impact on the biology of the graft site for spinal arthrodesis. These effects may be partly reversed by strategies that allow concentration of osteogenic cells from bone marrow or other tissues. The use of antiresorptive agents that inhibit osteoclasts would theoretically reduce bone formation and remodeling. Antiresorption medications affect bone remodeling, which is a central part of graft incorporation and fusion. In a recent review, Lubelski et al. concluded that although there have been numerous animal studies, there is limited clinical evidence on the use of antiresorptive medication and spinal fusion. Further clinical data are needed to understand the relative advantages/disadvantages of antiresorptive compared to anabolic agents and the impact of administration of these medications before or after fusion surgery.[578]

The mechanical stability of the graft site is generally a factor that the surgeon can control. Solid internal fixation increases the chances of achieving a successful fusion. The anatomic site, patient's weight, patient's activity level, and use of external immobilization are additional variables. The generally higher union rates seen in patients with spinal muscular atrophy[580] and Duchenne muscular dystrophy[581,582] may be the result of decreased voluntary motion and improved local mechanics despite the presence of osteopenia.

Local tumor invasion can replace normal marrow and weaken bone, and it may directly invade the fusion site. These problems may be partly overcome by the use of special fixation techniques[583] and adjuvant radiation and chemotherapy depending on the individual tumor. Use of autologous bone or bone marrow is desirable, but harvest must be performed in a separate surgical field to prevent tumor seeding in the donor site.

Marrow-packing disorders, such as thalassemia major, may decrease the osteogenic potential of marrow by overgrowth of normal marrow cells, altering the marrow growth factor environment and/or crowding out osteogenic stem cells. Similarly, local bone disease, such as Paget disease or fibrous dysplasia, can replace the population of normal osteogenic cells with abnormal cells, preventing or eroding into a successful fusion mass.

Radiation is an adverse factor for bone healing, especially when administered perioperatively. This may be a function of its direct cytotoxic effects on proliferating cells or the intense vasculitis induced by radiation injury. Long after the acute phase, radiation-induced osteonecrosis and the dense hypovascular scar left in the radiation bed may leave a poor environment for fusion. In some cases, therefore, it may be advantageous to use free vascularized grafts and donor vessels outside the area of previous radiation to enhance the vascular supply of local tissues and the likelihood of a successful fusion. Emery et al.[584–586] have shown that the timing of radiation after a spine fusion procedure has a significant effect on outcome and that radiation has the least adverse effect if given at least 3 weeks after grafting. Radiation was best timed to be performed either preoperatively or in the late postoperative period, avoiding the early postoperative period when vascular invasion of the graft site and proliferating osteogenic progenitors would be most vulnerable. Settings of marrow replacement or regional scarring secondary to radiation or other causes are perhaps most likely to benefit from methods designed to supplement or replace the local population of osteogenic cells. However, their value is as yet unproven in clinical trials.

Ma et al.[587] reported on a series of 22 consecutive patients with giant cell tumor of the cervical spine. Of these, 18 received postoperative radiation therapy 4 to 6 weeks following either subtotal resection or en bloc resection with total spondylectomy, with reconstruction with titanium plate and titanium mesh with autogenous bone graft for anterior reconstruction and pedicle screw placement for posterior reconstruction. While the authors caution that radiation myelopathy and radiation-induced sarcoma remain legitimate clinical concerns in any patients undergoing radiation therapy of the spine, their patients in this series experienced neither of these complications (with a follow-up period ranging from 36 to 124 months).

Electrical stimulation has been shown to be of potential benefit in the treatment of nonunions,[588,589] failed arthrodeses,[590–592] and congenital pseudarthroses,[590] consistent with spinal fusions in animal models.[593–595] Nonetheless, firm conclusions about efficacy are difficult to establish because of inconsistencies in both determining a reliable, reproducible endpoint for fusion and in incorporating the effect of patient parameters.[596]

Several of these clinical studies have been small series, often without a randomized control population.[594,597–599] A recent double-blind clinical trial in 201 evaluable patients found a benefit of electrical stimulation following uninstrumented posterolateral lumbar fusions but only in women.[600] Another randomized trial in 179 patients with both instrumented and uninstrumented posterolateral fusions found a union score of 85% among treated patients compared with

65% in placebo controls.[601] Application of extracorporeal shock wave treatment to enhance spinal fusion is another promising technique.[602,603]

Future Considerations

Advances that have already been made in the strategies and graft materials available for spinal fusion in the past several years have not yet eliminated the need for harvest of cortical or cancellous bone autografts, sparing patients the significant morbidity and cost of these procedures and their complications.

The potential for further advancement in the area of spinal fusion and tissue repair and regeneration in the spine is tremendous. Advances in stem cell biology, biomaterials, manufacture and purification of growth factors and other biomolecules, and the delivery of these agents is proceeding rapidly. In addition, methods for clinical evaluation and surgical and anesthetic techniques will offer surgeons and patients ever increasing reliable options, safer methods, and potentially entirely new strategies for repair and regeneration of bone and other tissues in the spine.

The clinically effective preparations of purified recombinantly manufactured protein growth factors are available. However, the efficacy and risks of these agents vary significantly with dose, carrier, and anatomic site. Clinical trials to date demonstrate clinical efficacy only for the limited indication of interbody lumbar fusion instrumented using a cage and, even then, only in carefully selected patients. Prudence and caution are indicated until additional data become available demonstrating that these materials or future materials will be effective in other settings and in less selected populations to minimize the chance of exposing patients to potentially ineffective treatment without the benefit of systematic controls or means of generalizable analysis.

Optimizing the use of current and future grafting materials will increasingly require a detailed understanding of the cell biology, materials science, and engineering principles upon which tissue engineering strategies are based.[15,60,62,63,205,415,604] Central to this process is the recognition that stem cell and progenitor populations that are capable of proliferating and differentiating to form new tissues are the direct or indirect target cells for all implantable osteoconductive biomaterials, all bioactive or osteoinductive proteins, and all methods for biophysical physical intervention (i.e., mechanical or electrical stimulation).

Future strategies will use the rapidly evolving knowledge and capabilities of many converging fields. We will design more efficient, more effective, and less invasive methods for surgical exposure, manipulation, and mechanical control over spinal segments and tissues. We will define methods to characterize and optimize the stem cell and progenitor populations in our spinal fusion sites, especially in settings where these essential target cells may be deficient in number or biologic potential. This will include the harvest, concentration, selection, and transplantation of osteogenic stem and progenitor cells when needed. We will develop more efficient and more effective methods for delivery of bioactive factors to responsive target cells. Finally, advances in biomaterials will also allow us to design and provide a milieu in which the conditions necessary for the activation, migration, proliferation, differentiation, and survival of osteogenic cells (and other cells that are essential to the bone healing response) can be customized to the unique biologic situation presented by each clinical setting and each graft site.

KEY POINTS

1. Graft site preparation is of paramount importance in fusion procedures regardless of whether or not biologics are used. Care needs to be taken to ensure that all of the soft tissues have been removed and that the bone surfaces are decorticated.
2. Host factors—such as diabetes, immunosuppression, nutritional depletion, and tobacco—play an important role in bone fusion; effort should be made to optimize reversible factors before undergoing elective spinal procedures.
3. Knowledge of the cell biology of spinal fusion and the attributes and synergies of available materials for bone grafting as well as clinical literature is essential for optimal selection of surgical techniques and graft materials.
4. BMP-2 is a powerful and potentially effective agent in enhancing bone regeneration. However, use of BMP-2 must be balanced by increased awareness of potential adverse effects and cost.

KEY REFERENCES

1. McLain RF, Fleming JE, Boehm CA, et al. Aspiration of osteoprogenitor cells for augmenting spinal fusion: comparison of progenitor cell concentrations from the vertebral body and iliac crest. *J Bone Joint Surg Am*. 2005;87:2655-2661.
Aspirates were obtained from two depths within the vertebral body and were quantified relative to matched, bilateral aspirates from the iliac crest that were obtained from the same patient at the same time and served as a control. Aspirates of vertebral marrow demonstrated comparable or greater concentrations of progenitor cells compared with matched controls from the iliac crest. The authors concluded that the vertebral body is a suitable site for aspiration of bone marrow for graft augmentation during spinal arthrodesis.
2. Vaccaro AR, Whang PG, Patel T, et al. The safety and efficacy of OP-1 (rhBMP-7) as a replacement for iliac crest autograft for posterolateral lumbar arthrodesis: minimum 4-year follow-up of a pilot study. *Spine J*. 2008;8:457-465.
Thirty-six patients undergoing decompressive laminectomy and single-level uninstrumented fusion for degenerative spondylolisthesis and symptomatic spinal stenosis were randomized in a 2:1 fashion to receive either OP-1 Putty (24 patients) or autogenous iliac crest bone graft (12 patients). At the 48-month time point, complete radiographic and clinical data were available for 22 of 36 patients (16 OP-1 Putty and six autograft) and 25 of 36 patients (18 OP-1 Putty and seven autograft), respectively. Radiographic evidence of a solid arthrodesis was present in 11 of 16 OP-1 Putty patients (68.8%) and 3 of 6 autograft patients (50%). Clinically successful outcomes defined as at least a 20% improvement in preoperative Oswestry scores were experienced by 14 of 19 OP-1 Putty patients (73.7%) and 4 of 7 autograft patients (57.1%); these clinical findings were corroborated by similar increases in SF-36 scores. The respective overall success rates of the OP-1 Putty and autograft group were 62.5% and 33.3%. In this study, there were no incidents of local or systemic toxicity, ectopic bone production, or other adverse events directly related to the use of OP-1 Putty.

3. Shields LB, Rague GH, Glassman SD, et al. Adverse effects associated with high-dose recombinant human bone morphogenetic protein-2 use in anterior cervical spine fusion. *Spine.* 2006;31:542-547.
The authors reviewed 151 patients who underwent either anterior cervical discectomy and fusion (n = 138) or anterior cervical vertebrectomy and fusion (n = 13) augmented with high-dose INFUSE. They found a high morbidity rate with a total of 35 (23.2%) patients having complications that the authors thought were attributable to the use of high-dose INFUSE in the cervical spine. Fifteen patients were diagnosed with a hematoma, including 11 on postoperative day 4 or 5, eight of whom were surgically evacuated. Thirteen individuals had either a prolonged hospital stay (>48 hours) or hospital readmission because of swallowing/breathing difficulties or dramatic swelling without hematoma. The authors concluded that putative inflammatory effect that contributes to the effectiveness of INFUSE in inducing fusion may spread to adjacent critical structures and lead to increased postoperative morbidity.

4. Muschler GF, Nakamoto C, Griffith LG. Engineering principles of clinical cell-based tissue engineering. *J Bone Joint Surg Am.* 2004;86:1541-1558.
This review highlights the current state of cell-based tissue engineering and the central engineering principles and strategies involved in the design and use of cell-based tools and strategies, particularly the challenges of mass transport and the influence of cell biology on the design and development of biologic osteoconductive scaffold materials.

5. Burkus JK, Gornet MF, Dickman CA, et al. Anterior lumbar interbody fusion using rhBMP-2 with tapered interbody cages. *J Spinal Disord Tech.* 2002;15:337-349.
The authors presented results of a multicenter, prospective, randomized, nonblinded study of patients with degenerative lumbar disc disease undergoing interbody fusion using two tapered, threaded fusion cages. The investigational group (143 patients) received rhBMP-2 on an absorbable collagen sponge. A control group (136 patients) received autogenous iliac crest bone grafts. At 24 months the BMP-2 group's fusion rate was 94.5% and the control group's was 88.7%.

REFERENCES

1. Albee F. Transplantation of a portion of the tibia into the spine for Pott's disease. *JAMA.* 1911;57:885-886.
2. Hibbs R. A report of fifty-nine cases of scoliosis treated by the fusion operation. *J Bone Joint Surg Am.* 1924;6.
3. Boden S. Clinical Applications of BMPs for Spine Fusion. *Pittsburgh Bone Symp.* 2003;425-433.
4. DePalma A, Rothman R. The nature of pseudarthrosis. *Clin Orthop.* 1968;59:113-118.
5. Eie N, Solgaard T, Kleppe H. The knee-elbow position in lumbar disc surgery: a review of complications. *Spine.* 1983;8:897-900.
6. May VJ, Mauck W. Exploration of the spine for pseudarthrosis following spinal fusion in the treatment of scoliosis. *Clin Orthop.* 1967;53.
7. O'Beirne J, O'Neill D, Gallagher J, Williams D. Spinal fusion for back pain: a clinical and radiological review. *J Spinal Disord.* 1992;5.
8. Steinmann J, Herkowitz H. Pseudarthrosis of the spine. *Clin Orthop.* 1992;284:983-991.
9. Zdeblick T. A prospective, randomized study of lumbar fusion. Preliminary results. *Spine.* 1993;18:983-991.
10. Martin B, Mirza S, Comstock B, Gray D. Reoperation rates following lumbar spine surgery and the influence of spinal fusion procedures. *Spine.* 2007;32:382-3870.
11. Raizman N, O'Brien J, Poehling-Monaghan K, Yu W. Pseudarthrosis of the spine. *J Am Acad Orthop Surg.* 2009;17:494-503.
12. Bos GD, Goldberg VM, Gordon NH, et al. The long-term fate of fresh and frozen orthotopic bone allografts in genetically defined rats. *Clin Orthop Relat Res.* 1985;245-254.
13. Burwell R. The fate of bone grafts. In: Apley AG, ed. *Recent Advances in Orthopaedics.* Baltimore: William & Wilkins; 1969:115-207.
14. Urist M. Bone transplants and implants. In: Urist MR, ed. *Fundamental and Clinical Bone Physiology.* Philadelphia: Lippincott; 1980:131.
15. Muschler GF, Nakamoto C, Griffith LG. Engineering principles of clinical cell-based tissue engineering. *J Bone Joint Surg Am.* 2004;86:1541-1558.
16. Burwell R. Studies in the transplantation of bone. VII. The fresh composite homograft-autograft of cancellous bone; an analysis of factors leading to osteogenesis in marrow transplants and in marrow-containing bone grafts. *J Bone Joint Surg Br.* 1964;46:110-140.
17. Burwell R. Studies in the transplantation of bone. Treated composite homograft-autografts of cancellous bone: an analysis of inductive mechanisms in bone transplantation. *J Bone Joint Surg Br.* 1966;48:8.
18. Beresford J, Graves S, Smoothy C. Formation of mineralized nodules by bone derived cells in vitro: a model of bone formation? *Am J Med Genet.* 1993;45:163-178.
19. Bosch P, Musgrave DS, Lee JY, et al. Osteoprogenitor cells within skeletal muscle. *J Orthop Res.* 2000;18:933-944.
20. Halvorsen YC, Wilkison WO, Gimble JM. Adipose-derived stromal cells–their utility and potential in bone formation. *Int J Obes Relat Metab Disord.* 2000;24(suppl 4):S41-S44.
21. Katzburg S, Lieberherr M, Ornoy A, et al. Isolation and hormonal responsiveness of primary cultures of human bone-derived cells: gender and age differences. *Bone.* 1999; 25:667-673.
22. Lopez MJ, McIntosh KR, Spencer ND, et al. Accleration of spinal fusion using syngenic and allogenic adult adipose derived stem cells in a rat model. *J Orthop Res.* 2009;27:366-373.
23. Robey PG. Collagenase-treated trabecular bone fragments: a reproducible source of cells in the osteoblastic lineage. *Calcif Tissue Int.* 1995;56(suppl 1):S11-S12.
24. Sheyn D, Pelled G, Zilberman Y, et al. Nonvirally engineered porcine adipose tissue-derived stem cells: use in posterior spinal fusion. *Stem Cells.* 2008;26:1056-1064.
25. Zuk PA, Zhu M, Mizuno H, et al. Multilineage cells from human adipose tissue: implications for cell-based therapies. *Tissue Eng.* 2001;7:211-228.
26. Tuli R, Tuli S, Nandi S, et al. Characterization of multipotential mesenchymal progenitor cells derived from human trabecular bone. *Stem Cells.* 2003;21:681-693.
27. Villanueva JE, Nimni ME. Promotion of calvarial cell osteogenesis by endothelial cells. *J Bone Miner Res.* 1990;5:733-739.
28. Gittens RA, Olivares-Navarrete R, Schwartz Z, Boyan BD. Implant osseointegration and the role of microroughness and nanostructures: lessons for spine implants. *Acta Biomater.* 2014;10:3363-3371.
29. Brighton CT, Lorich DG, Kupcha R, et al. The pericyte as a possible osteoblast progenitor cell. *Clin Orthop Relat Res.* 1992;287-299.
30. Beamer B, Hettrich C, Lane J. Vascular endothelial growth factor: an essential component of angiogenesis and fracture healing. *HSS J.* 2010;6:85-94.

31. Zvaifler NJ, Marinova-Mutafchieva L, Adams G, et al. Mesenchymal precursor cells in the blood of normal individuals. *Arthritis Res*. 2000;2:477-488.
32. McDonald CA, Oehme D, Pham Y, et al. Evaluation of the safety and tolerability of a high-dose intravenous infusion of allogeneic mesenchymal precursor cells. *Cytotherapy*. 2015;17:1178-1187.
33. Gronthos S, Simmons PJ. The growth factor requirements of STRO-1-positive human bone marrow stromal precursors under serum-deprived conditions in vitro. *Blood*. 1995;85:929-940.
34. Tan HB, Giannoudis PV, Boxall SA, McGonagle D, Jones E. The systemic influence of platelet-derived growth factors on bone marrow mesenchymal stem cells in fracture patients. *BMC Med*. 2015;13:6.
35. Alvarez LM, Rivera JJ, Stockdale L, et al. Tethering of epidermal growth factor (EGF) to beta tricalcium phosphate (βTCP) via fusion to a high affinity, multimeric βTCP-binding peptide: effects on human multipotent stromal cells/connective tissue progenitors. *PLoS One*. 2015;10:e0129600.
36. *Orthopaedic Basic Science*. Rosemont, IL: American Academy of Orthopaedic Surgeons; 1999.
37. Cruess R. Healing of bone, tendon, and ligament. In: Rockwood CA Jr, Green DP, eds. *Fractures in Adults*. Vol 1. 2nd ed. Philadelphia: Lippincott; 1984:153.
38. Prolo D, Rodrigo J. Contemporary bone graft physiology and surgery. *Clin Orthop*. 1985;(200):322-342.
39. Simmons D. Fracture healing perspectives. *Clin Orthop Relat Res*. 1985;(200):100-113.
40. Dickson K, Katzman S, Paiement G. The importance of the blood supply in the healing of tibial fractures. *Contemp Orthop*. 1995;30:489-493.
41. Schmidt-Bleek K, Schell H, Kolar P, et al. Cellular composition of the initial fracture hematoma compared to a muscle hematoma: a study in sheep. *J Orthop Res*. 2009;27:1147-1151.
42. Shantz JS, Marcucio R, Kim HT, Miclau T. Bone and cartilage healing. In: Court-Brown C, Heckman JD, McKee M, et al., eds. *Rockwood and Green's Fractures in Adults*. Vol 1. 8th ed. Philadelphia: Lippincott; 2015.
43. Glassman SD, Rose SM, Dimar JR, et al. The effect of postoperative nonsteroidal anti-inflammatory drug administration on spinal fusion. *Spine*. 1998;23:834-838.
44. Keller JC, Trancik TM, Young FA, St Mary E. Effects of indomethacin on bone ingrowth. *J Orthop Res*. 1989;7:28-34.
45. Long J, Lewis S, Kuklo T, Zhu Y, Riew KD. The effect of cyclooxygenase-2 inhibitors on spinal fusion. *J Bone Joint Surg Am*. 2002;84A:1763-1768.
46. McLaren AC. Prophylaxis with indomethacin for heterotopic bone. After open reduction of fractures of the acetabulum. *J Bone Joint Surg Am*. 1990;72:245-247.
47. Nilsson OS, Bauer HC, Brosjö O, Törnkvist H. Influence of indomethacin on induced heterotopic bone formation in rats. Importance of length of treatment and of age. *Clin Orthop Relat Res*. 1986;239-245.
48. Riew KD, Long J, Rhee J, et al. Time-dependent inhibitory effects of indomethacin on spinal fusion. *J Bone Joint Surg Am*. 2003;85–A:632-634.
49. Dodwell ER, Latorre JG, Parisini E, et al. NSAID exposure and risk of nonunion: a meta-analysis of case-control and cohort studies. *Calcif Tissue Int*. 2010;87:193-202.
50. Zhang X, Schwarz EM, Young DA, et al. Cyclooxygenase-2 regulates mesenchymal cell differentiation into the osteoblast lineage and is critically involved in bone repair. *J Clin Invest*. 2002;109:1405-1415.
51. Pountos I, Georgouli T, Blokhuis TJ, Pape HC, Giannoudis PV. Pharmacological agents and impairment of fracture healing: what is the evidence? *Injury*. 2008;39:384-394.
52. Sucato DJ, Welch RD, Pierce B, et al. Thoracoscopic discectomy and fusion in an animal model: safe and effective when segmental blood vessels are spared. *Spine*. 2002;27:880-886.
53. Brown MD, Malinin TI, Davis PB. A roentgenographic evaluation of frozen allografts versus autografts in anterior cervical spine fusions. *Clin Orthop Relat Res*. 1976;231-236.
54. Allen BL, Ferguson RL. The operative treatment of myelomeningocele spinal deformity—1979. *Orthop Clin North Am*. 1979;10:845-862.
55. Curtis B. Orthopaedic management of muscular dystrophy. *Instr Course Lect*. 1970;19:78-89.
56. Lim TH, Kwon H, Jeon CH, et al. Effect of endplate conditions and bone mineral density on the compressive strength of the graft-endplate interface in anterior cervical spine fusion. *Spine*. 2001;26:951-956.
57. Hou Y, Luo Z. A study on the structural properties of the lumbar endplate: histological structure, the effect of bone density, and spinal level. *Spine*. 2009;34:E427-E433.
58. Muschler G, Lane J. Clinical applications in orthopaedic surgery. In: Habal MB, Reddi AH, eds. *Bone Grafts and Bone Substitutes*. Philadelphia: WB Saunders; 1992.
59. Egol KA, Nauth A, Lee M, et al. Bone grafting: sourcing, timing, strategies, and alternatives. *J Orthop Trauma*. 2015;29:S10-S14.
60. Pape HC, Evans A, Kobbe P. Autologous bone graft: properties and techniques. *J Orthop Trauma*. 2010;24 (suppl 1):S36-S40.
61. Lane JM. Spine fusion: principles of bone fusion. In: Herkowitz HN, Garfin SR, Balderston RA, et al., eds. *The Spine*. 4th ed. Philadelphia: WB Saunders; 1999:1573-1589.
62. Muschler GF, Midura RJ. Connective tissue progenitors: practical concepts for clinical applications. *Clin Orthop Relat Res*. 2002;66-80.
63. Muschler G, Midura R, Nakamoto C. Practical modeling concepts for connective tissue stem cell and progenitor compartment kinetics. *J Biomed Biotechnol*. 2003;2003(3):170-193.
64. Hak DJ. The use of osteoconductive bone graft substitutes in orthopaedic trauma. *J Am Acad Orthop Surg*. 2007;15:525-536.
65. Beuerlein MJS, McKee MD. Calcium sulfates: what is the evidence? *J Orthop Trauma*. 2010;24(suppl 1):S46-S51.
66. Heiple KG, Chase SW, Herndon CH. A comparative study of the healing process following different types of bone transplantation. *J Bone Joint Surg Am*. 1963;45:1593-1616.
67. Oikarinen J, Korhonen LK. The bone inductive capacity of various bone transplanting materials used for treatment of experimental bone defects. *Clin Orthop Relat Res*. 1979;208-215.
68. Tuli SM. Bridging of bone defects by massive bone grafts in tumorous conditions and in osteomyelitis. *Clin Orthop Relat Res*. 1972;87:60-73.
69. Wilson PD, Lance EM. Surgical reconstruction of the skeleton following segmental resection for bone tumors. *J Bone Joint Surg Am*. 1965;47:1629-1656.

70. Banwart JC, Asher MA, Hassanein RS. Iliac crest bone graft harvest donor site morbidity. A statistical evaluation. *Spine*. 1995;20:1055-1060.
71. Loeffler BJ, Kellam JF, Sims SH, Bosse MJ. Prospective observational study of donor-site morbidity following anterior iliac crest bone-grafting in orthopaedic trauma reconstruction patients. *J Bone Joint Surg Am*. 2012;94:1649-1654.
72. Robertson PA, Wray AC. Natural history of posterior iliac crest bone graft donation for spinal surgery: a prospective analysis of morbidity. *Spine*. 2001;26:1473-1476.
73. Younger EM, Chapman MW. Morbidity at bone graft donor sites. *J Orthop Trauma*. 1989;3:192-195.
74. Ackerman SJ, Mafilios MS, Polly DW. Economic evaluation of bone morphogenetic protein versus autogenous iliac crest bone graft in single-level anterior lumbar fusion: an evidence-based modeling approach. *Spine*. 2002;27:S94-S99.
75. Hu RW, Bohlman HH. Fracture at the iliac bone graft harvest site after fusion of the spine. *Clin Orthop Relat Res*. 1994;208-213.
76. Younger EM, Chapman MW. Morbidity at bone graft donor sites. *J Orthop Trauma*. 1989;3:192-195.
77. Schwartz CE, Martha JF, Kowalski P, et al. Prospective evaluation of chronic pain associated with posterior autologous iliac crest bone graft harvest and its effect on postoperative outcome. *Health Qual Life Outcomes*. 2009;7:49.
78. Howard J, Glassman S, Carreon L. Posterior iliac crest pain after posterolateral fusion with or without iliac crest graft harvest. *Spine J*. 2011;11:534-537.
79. Ahlmann E, Patzakis M, Roidis N, Shepherd L, Holtom P. Comparison of anterior and posterior iliac crest bone grafts in terms of harvest-site morbidity and functional outcomes. *J Bone Joint Surg Am*. 2002;84A:716-720.
80. Arrington ED, Smith WJ, Chambers HG, Bucknell AL, Davino NA. Complications of iliac crest bone graft harvesting. *Clin Orthop Relat Res*. 1996;300-309.
81. Castelein RM, Sauter AJ. Lumbar hernia in an iliac bone graft defect. A case report. *Acta Orthop Scand*. 1985;56:273-274.
82. Kurz LT, Garfin SR, Booth RE. Harvesting autogenous iliac bone grafts. A review of complications and techniques. *Spine*. 1989;14:1324-1331.
83. Shin AY, Moran ME, Wenger DR. Superior gluteal artery injury secondary to posterior iliac crest bone graft harvesting. A surgical technique to control hemorrhage. *Spine*. 1996;21:1371-1374.
84. Varga E, Hu R, Hearn TC, Woodside T, Yang JP. Biomechanical analysis of hemipelvic deformation after corticospongious bone graft harvest from the posterior iliac crest. *Spine*. 1996;21:1494-1499.
85. Dimar JR, Glassman SD, Burkus JK, et al. Two-year fusion and clinical outcomes in 224 patients treated with a single-level instrumented posterolateral fusion with iliac crest bone graft. *Spine J*. 2009;9:880-885.
86. Fernyhough JC, Schimandle JJ, Weigel MC, Edwards CC, Levine AM. Chronic donor site pain complicating bone graft harvesting from the posterior iliac crest for spinal fusion. *Spine*. 1992;17:1474-1480.
87. Heary RF, Schlenk RP, Sacchieri TA, Barone D, Brotea C. Persistent iliac crest donor site pain: independent outcome assessment. *Neurosurgery*. 2002;50:510-516.
88. Keller EE, Triplett WW. Iliac bone grafting: review of 160 consecutive cases. *J Oral Maxillofac Surg*. 1987;45:11-14.
89. Kim DH, Rhim R, Li L, et al. Prospective study of iliac crest bone graft harvest site pain and morbidity. *Spine J*. 2009;9:886-892.
90. Silber JS, Anderson DG, Daffner SD, et al. Donor site morbidity after anterior iliac crest bone harvest for single-level anterior cervical discectomy and fusion. *Spine*. 2003;28:134-139.
91. Summers BN, Eisenstein SM. Donor site pain from the ilium. A complication of lumbar spine fusion. *J Bone Joint Surg Br*. 1989;71B:677-680.
92. Hu S. Commentary: Iliac crest bone graft: are the complications overrated? *Spine*. 2011;11:538-539.
93. Dawson E, Bae HW, Burkus JK, Stambough JL, Glassman SD. Recombinant human bone morphogenetic protein-2 on an absorbable collagen sponge with an osteoconductive bulking agent in posterolateral arthrodesis with instrumentation. A prospective randomized trial. *J Bone Joint Surg Am*. 2009;91:1604-1613.
94. Dimar JR, Glassman SD, Burkus JK, et al. Clinical and radiographic analysis of an optimized rhBMP-2 formulation as an autograft replacement in posterolateral lumbar spine arthrodesis. *J Bone Joint Surg Am*. 2009;91:1377-1386.
95. Delawi D, Dhert WJA, Castelein RM, Verbout AJ, Oner FC. The incidence of donor site pain after bone graft harvesting from the posterior iliac crest may be overestimated: a study on spine fracture patients. *Spine*. 2007;32:1865-1868.
96. Heylman CM, Caralla TN, Boehm CA, Patterson TE, Muschler GF. Slowing the onset of hypoxia increases colony forming efficiency of connective tissue progenitor cells in vitro. *J Regen Med Tissue Eng*. 2013;26:2.
97. Burchardt H. The biology of bone graft repair. *Clin Orthop Relat Res*. 1983;28-42.
98. Enneking WF, Burchardt H, Puhl JJ, Piotrowski G. Physical and biological aspects of repair in dog cortical-bone transplants. *J Bone Joint Surg Am*. 1975;57:237-252.
99. Reikerås O, Reinholt FP, Zinöcker S, Shegarfi H, Rolstad B. Healing of long-term frozen orthotopic bone allografts is not affected by MHC differences between donor and recipient. *Clin Orthop Relat Res*. 2011;469:1479-1486.
100. Stevenson S, Li XQ, Martin B. The fate of cancellous and cortical bone after transplantation of fresh and frozen tissue-antigen-matched and mismatched osteochondral allografts in dogs. *J Bone Joint Surg Am*. 1991;73:1143-1156.
101. Beebe KS, Benevenia J, Tuy BE, et al. Effects of a new allograft processing procedure on graft healing in a canine model: a preliminary study. *Clin Orthop Relat Res*. 2009;467:273-280.
102. Takeda M. Experience in posterior lumbar interbody fusion: unicortical versus bicortical autologous grafts. *Clin Orthop Relat Res*. 1985;120-126.
103. Dell PC, Burchardt H, Glowczewskie FP. A roentgenographic, biomechanical, and histological evaluation of vascularized and non-vascularized segmental fibular canine autografts. *J Bone Joint Surg Am*. 1985;67:105-112.
104. Shaffer JW, Field GA, Goldberg VM, Davy DT. Fate of vascularized and nonvascularized autografts. *Clin Orthop Relat Res*. 1985;32-43.
105. Weiland AJ, Moore JR, Daniel RK. Vascularized bone autografts. Experience with 41 cases. *Clin Orthop Relat Res*. 1983;87-95.
106. Weiland AJ, Phillips TW, Randolph MA. Bone grafts: a radiologic, histologic, and biomechanical model comparing autografts, allografts, and free vascularized bone grafts. *Plast Reconstr Surg*. 1984;74:368-379.

107. Ackerman DB, Rose PS, Moran SL, et al. The results of vascularized-free fibular grafts in complex spinal reconstruction. *J Spinal Disord Tech.* 2011;24: 170-176.
108. Al-Jabri T, Mannan A, Giannoudis P. The use of the free vascularised bone graft for nonunion of the scaphoid: a systematic review. *J Orthop Surg Res.* 2014;9:21.
109. Allsopp BJ, Hunter-Smith DJ, Rozen WM. Vascularized versus nonvascularized bone grafts: what is the evidence? *Clin Orthop Relat Res.* 2016;474:1319-1327.
110. Hayashi A, Maruyama Y, Okajima Y, Motegi M. Vascularized iliac bone graft based on a pedicle of upper lumbar vessels for anterior fusion of the thoraco-lumbar spine. *Br J Plast Surg.* 1994;47:425-430.
111. Hubbard LF, Herndon JH, Buonanno AR. Free vascularized fibula transfer for stabilization of the thoracolumbar spine. A case report. *Spine.* 1985;10:891-893.
112. Lascombes P, Grosdidier G, Olry R, Thomas C. Anatomical basis of the anterior vertebral graft using a pediculated rib. *Surg Radiol Anat.* 1991;13:259-263.
113. Hartman JT, McCarron RF, Robertson WW. A pedicle bone grafting procedure for failed lumbosacral spinal fusion. *Clin Orthop Relat Res.* 1983;223-227.
114. McBride GG, Bradford DS. Vertebral body replacement with femoral neck allograft and vascularized rib strut graft. A technique for treating post-traumatic kyphosis with neurologic deficit. *Spine.* 1983;8:406-415.
115. Rose G, Owen R, Sanderson J. Transposition of rib with blood supply for the stabilization of a spinal kyphosis. *J Bone Joint Surg Br.* 1975;57–B:112.
116. Bradford DS. Anterior vascular pedicle bone grafting for the treatment of kyphosis. *Spine.* 1980;5:318-323.
117. Goldberg VM, Shaffer JW, Field G, Davy DT. Biology of vascularized bone grafts. *Orthop Clin North Am.* 1987;18:197-205.
118. Tonoli C, Bechara AHS, Rossanez R, Belangero WD, Livani B. Use of the vascularized iliac-crest flap in musculoskeletal lesions. *Biomed Res Int.* 2013;2013:237146.
119. Wright NM, Kaufman BA, Haughey BH, Lauryssen C. Complex cervical spine neoplastic disease: reconstruction after surgery by using a vascularized fibular strut graft. Case report. *J Neurosurg.* 1999;90:133-137.
120. Goujon E. Researches experimentals sur les propiete physiologiques de la moelle des os. *J l'Anatomie Physiol Norm Pathol l'Homme des Animaux.* 1869;6:399.
121. Senn S. On the healing of aseptic cavities by implantation of antiseptic decalcified bone. *Am J Med Sci.* 1889;98:219.
122. Burwell RG. The function of bone marrow in the incorporation of a bone graft. *Clin Orthop Relat Res.* 1985;125-141.
123. Nade S. Clinical implications of cell function in osteogenesis. A reappraisal of bone-graft surgery. *Ann R Coll Surg Engl.* 1979;61:189-194.
124. Nade S. Osteogenesis after bone and bone marrow transplantation. II. The initial cellular events following transplantation of decalcified allografts of cancellous bone. *Acta Orthop Scand.* 1977;48:572-579.
125. Friedenstein A. Determined and inducible osteogenic precursor cells. *Ciba Found Symp New Ser.* 1973;11:170-185.
126. Ashton BA, Allen TD, Howlett CR, et al. Formation of bone and cartilage by marrow stromal cells in diffusion chambers in vivo. *Clin Orthop Relat Res.* 1980;294-307.
127. Budenz RW, Bernard GW. Osteogenesis and leukopoiesis within diffusion-chamber implants of isolated bone marrow subpopulations. *Am J Anat.* 1980;159:455-474.
128. Friedenstein AJ, Chailakhyan RK, Latsinik NV, Panasyuk AF, Keiliss-Borok IV. Stromal cells responsible for transferring the microenvironment of the hemopoietic tissues. Cloning in vitro and retransplantation in vivo. *Transplantation.* 1974;17:331-340.
129. Pfeiffer C. Development of bone from transplanted marrow in mice. *Anat Rec.* 1948;102:225.
130. Friedenstein AJ. Precursor cells of mechanocytes. *Int Rev Cytol.* 1976;47:327-359.
131. Friedenstein AJ, Petrakova KV, Kurolesova AI, Frolova GP. Heterotopic of bone marrow. Analysis of precursor cells for osteogenic and hematopoietic tissues. *Transplantation.* 1968;6:230-247.
132. Owen M. The origin of bone cells in the postnatal organism. *Arthritis Rheum.* 1980;23:1073-1080.
133. Vaughan J. Osteogenesis and haematopoiesis. *Lancet.* 1981;2:133-136.
134. Patterson TE, Boehm C, Nakamoto C, et al. The efficiency of bone marrow aspiration for harvest of connective tissue progenitors from the human iliac crest. *J Bone Joint Surg Am.* 2017; in press.
135. Maniatopoulos C, Sodek J, Melcher AH. Bone formation in vitro by stromal cells obtained from bone marrow of young adult rats. *Cell Tissue Res.* 1988;254:317-330.
136. Lian JB, Stein GS. Concepts of osteoblast growth and differentiation: basis for modulation of bone cell development and tissue formation. *Crit Rev Oral Biol Med.* 1992;3:269-305.
137. Aubin J. Osteogenic cell differentiation. *Bone Eng.* 2000;19-30.
138. Connolly J, Guse R, Lippiello L, Dehne R. Development of an osteogenic bone-marrow preparation. *J Bone Joint Surg Am.* 1989;71:684-691.
139. Connolly JF, Guse R, Tiedeman J, Dehne R. Autologous marrow injection as a substitute for operative grafting of tibial nonunions. *Clin Orthop Relat Res.* 1991;259-270.
140. Healey JH, Zimmerman PA, McDonnell JM, Lane JM. Percutaneous bone marrow grafting of delayed union and nonunion in cancer patients. *Clin Orthop Relat Res.* 1990;280-285.
141. Paley D, Young MC, Wiley AM, Fornasier VL, Jackson RW. Percutaneous bone marrow grafting of fractures and bony defects. An experimental study in rabbits. *Clin Orthop Relat Res.* 1986;300-312.
142. Ragni P, Lindholm TS, Lindholm TC. Vertebral fusion dynamics in the thoracic and lumbar spine induced by allogenic demineralized bone matrix combined with autogenous bone marrow. An experimental study in rabbits. *Ital J Orthop Traumatol.* 1987;13:241-251.
143. Takagi K, Urist MR. The role of bone marrow in bone morphogenetic protein-induced repair of femoral massive diaphyseal defects. *Clin Orthop Relat Res.* 1982;224-231.
144. Tiedeman JJ, Connolly JF, Strates BS, Lippiello L. Treatment of nonunion by percutaneous injection of bone marrow and demineralized bone matrix. An experimental study in dogs. *Clin Orthop Relat Res.* 1991;294-302.
145. Tiedeman JJ, Huurman WW, Connolly JF, Strates BS. Healing of a large nonossifying fibroma after grafting with bone matrix and marrow. A case report. *Clin Orthop Relat Res.* 1991;302-305.

146. Lane J, Muschler G, Werntz J, et al. The use of composite bone graft materials in a segmental defect model in the rat. *J Orthop Trauma*. 1988;2:57-58.
147. Yasko AW, Lane JM, Fellinger EJ, et al. The healing of segmental bone defects, induced by recombinant human bone morphogenetic protein (rhBMP-2). A radiographic, histological, and biomechanical study in rats. *J Bone Joint Surg Am*. 1992;74:659-670.
148. Johnson KA, Howlett CR, Bellenger CR, Armati-Gulson P. Osteogenesis by canine and rabbit bone marrow in diffusion chambers. *Calcif Tissue Int*. 1988;42:113-118.
149. Garg NK, Gaur S, Sharma S. Percutaneous autogenous bone marrow grafting in 20 cases of ununited fracture. *Acta Orthop Scand*. 1993;64:671-672.
150. Salama R, Burwell RD, Dickson IR. Recombined grafts of bone and marrow. The beneficial effect upon osteogenesis of impregnating xenograft (heterograft) bone with autologous red marrow. *J Bone Joint Surg Br*. 1973;55:402-417.
151. Salama R, Weissman SL. The clinical use of combined xenografts of bone and autologous red marrow. A preliminary report. *J Bone Joint Surg Br*. 1978;60:111-115.
152. Fernandez-Bances I, Perez-Basterrechea M, Perez-Lopez S, et al. Repair of long-bone pseudoarthrosis with autologous bone marrow mononuclear cells combined with allogenic bone graft. *Cytotherapy*. 2013;15:571-577.
153. Hernigou P, Poignard A, Beaujean F, Rouard H. Percutaneous autologous bone-marrow grafting for nonunions. Influence of the number and concentration of progenitor cells. *J Bone Joint Surg Am*. 2005;87:1430-1437.
154. Hernigou P, Flouzat-Lachaniette C-H, Delambre J, et al. Osteonecrosis repair with bone marrow cell therapies: state of the clinical art. *Bone*. 2015;70:102-109.
155. Majors AK, Boehm CA, Nitto H, Midura RJ, Muschler GF. Characterization of human bone marrow stromal cells with respect to osteoblastic differentiation. *J Orthop Res*. 1997;15:546-557.
156. Muschler GF, Boehm C, Easley K. Aspiration to obtain osteoblast progenitor cells from human bone marrow: the influence of aspiration volume. *J Bone Joint Surg Am*. 1997;79:1699-1709.
157. Muschler GF, Nitto H, Boehm C, Easley K. Age- and gender-related changes in the cellularity of human bone marrow and the prevalence of osteoblastic progenitors. *J Orthop Res*. 2001;19:117-125.
158. Curylo LJ, Johnstone B, Petersilge CA, Janicki JA, Yoo JU. Augmentation of spinal arthrodesis with autologous bone marrow in a rabbit posterolateral spine fusion model. *Spine*. 1999;24:434-438.
159. Kadiyala S, Kraus K, Attawia M, Bruder S. *Rapid bone regeneration in femoral defects by an autologous osteoprogenitor cell concentrate prepared using an intraoperative selective cell retention technique (paper #0317)*. Presented at the 49th Annual Meeting of the Orthopaedic Research Society; 2003.
160. Kadiyala S, Kraus K, Attawia M, Bruder S. *Use of intra-operative selective cell retention technique to regenerate canine femoral segmental defects*. Presented at the 5th International Meeting of thhe Tissue Engineering Society; 2002.
161. Muschler GF, Huber B, Ullman T, et al. Evaluation of bone-grafting materials in a new canine segmental spinal fusion model. *J Orthop Res*. 1993;11:514-524.
162. Muschler GF, Negami S, Hyodo A, et al. Evaluation of collagen ceramic composite graft materials in a spinal fusion model. *Clin Orthop Relat Res*. 1996;250-260.
163. Erdmann J, Kögler C, Diel I, Ziegler R, Pfeilschifter J. Age-associated changes in the stimulatory effect of transforming growth factor beta on human osteogenic colony formation. *Mech Ageing Dev*. 1999;110:73-85.
164. Manolagas SC, Jilka RL. Bone marrow, cytokines, and bone remodeling. Emerging insights into the pathophysiology of osteoporosis. *N Engl J Med*. 1995;332:305-311.
165. Nishida S, Endo N, Yamagiwa H, Tanizawa T, Takahashi HE. Number of osteoprogenitor cells in human bone marrow markedly decreases after skeletal maturation. *J Bone Miner Metab*. 1999;17:171-177.
166. McLain R, Fleming J, Boehm C, Muschler G. Aspiration of osteoprogenitor cells for augmenting spinal fusion: comparison of progentior cell concentrations from the vertebral body and iliac crest. *J Bone Joint Surg Am*. 2005;87:2655-2661.
167. McLain R, Boehm C, Rufo-Smith C, Muschler G. Transpedicular aspiration of osteoprogenitor cells from the vertebral body: progenitor cell concentrations affected by serial aspiration. *Spine J*. 2009;9:995-1002.
168. Johnson RG. Bone marrow concentrate with allograft equivalent to autograft in lumbar fusions. *Spine*. 2014;39:695-700.
169. Khashan M, Inoue S, Berven SH. Cell based therapies as compared to autologous bone grafts for spinal arthrodesis. *Spine*. 2013;38:1885-1891.
170. Odri GA, Hami A, Pomero V, et al. Development of a per-operative procedure for concentrated bone marrow adjunction in postero-lateral lumbar fusion: radiological, biological and clinical assessment. *Eur Spine J*. 2012;21:2665-2672.
171. Vadalà G, Di Martino A, Tirindelli MC, Denaro L, Denaro V. Use of autologous bone marrow cells concentrate enriched with platelet-rich fibrin on corticocancellous bone allograft for posterolateral multilevel cervical fusion. *J Tissue Eng Regen Med*. 2008;2:515-520.
172. Luangphakdy V, Shinohara K, Pan H, et al. Evaluation of rhBMP-2/collagen/TCP-HA bone graft with and without bone marrow cells in the canine femoral multi defect model. *Eur Cell Mater*. 2015;29:57-68.
173. Muschler GF, Matsukura Y, Nitto H, et al. Selective retention of bone marrow-derived cells to enhance spinal fusion. *Clin Orthop Relat Res*. 2005;242-251.
174. Youssef J, Brodke D, Haynesworth S, et al. Selective cell retention technology in spinal fusion. *Spine J*. 2003;3:114S-115S.
175. Badrinath R, Bohl DD, Hustedt JW, Webb ML, Grauer JN. Only prolonged time from abstraction found to affect viable nucleated cell concentrations in vertebral body bone marrow aspirate. *Spine J*. 2014;14:990-995.
176. Hustedt JW, Jegede KA, Badrinath R, et al. Optimal aspiration volume of vertebral bone marrow for use in spinal fusion. *Spine J*. 2013;13:1217-1222.
177. Risbud MV, Shapiro IM, Guttapalli A, et al. Osteogenic potential of adult human stem cells of the lumbar vertebral body and the iliac crest. *Spine*. 2006;31:83-89.
178. Hustedt JW, Blizzard DJ. The controversy surrounding bone morphogenetic proteins in the spine: a review of current research. *Yale J Biol Med*. 2014;87:549-561.
179. Marcucio RS, Nauth A, Giannoudis PV, et al. Stem cell therapies in orthopaedic trauma. *J Orthop Trauma*. 2015;29:24-27.
180. Patterson TE, Kumagai K, Griffith L, Muschler GF. Cellular strategies for enhancement of fracture repair. *J Bone Joint Surg Am*. 2008;90(suppl 1):111-119.

181. Boden SD, Hair GA, Viggeswarapu M, Liu Y, Titus L. Gene therapy for spine fusion. *Clin Orthop Relat Res.* 2000;S225-S233.
182. Boden SD, Titus L, Hair G, et al. Lumbar spine fusion by local gene therapy with a cDNA encoding a novel osteoinductive protein (LMP-1). *Spine.* 1998;23:2486-2492.
183. Cui Q, Ming Xiao Z, Balian G, Wang GJ. Comparison of lumbar spine fusion using mixed and cloned marrow cells. *Spine.* 2001;26:2305-2310.
184. Kim H-S, Viggeswarapu M, Boden SD, et al. Overcoming the immune response to permit ex vivo gene therapy for spine fusion with human type 5 adenoviral delivery of the LIM mineralization protein-1 cDNA. *Spine.* 2003;28: 219-226.
185. Lieberman JR. Orthopaedic gene therapy. Fracture healing and other nongenetic problems of bone. *Clin Orthop Relat Res.* 2000;S156-S158.
186. Lieberman JR, Ghivizzani SC, Evans CH. Gene transfer approaches to the healing of bone and cartilage. *Mol Ther.* 2002;6:141-147.
187. Riew KD, Lou J, Wright NM, et al. Thoracoscopic intradiscal spine fusion using a minimally invasive gene-therapy technique. *J Bone Joint Surg Am.* 2003;85–A:866-871.
188. Wang JC, Kanim LEA, Yoo S, et al. Effect of regional gene therapy with bone morphogenetic protein-2-producing bone marrow cells on spinal fusion in rats. *J Bone Joint Surg Am.* 2003;85–A:905-911.
189. Zachos TA, Shields KM, Bertone AL. Gene-mediated osteogenic differentiation of stem cells by bone morphogenetic proteins-2 or -6. *J Orthop Res.* 2006;24:1279-1291.
190. Ishihara A, Zachos TA, Bartlett JS, Bertone AL. Evaluation of permissiveness and cytotoxic effects in equine chondrocytes, synovial cells, and stem cells in response to infection with adenovirus 5 vectors for gene delivery. *Am J Vet Res.* 2006;67:1145-1155.
191. Zachos T, Diggs A, Weisbrode S, Bartlett J, Bertone A. Mesenchymal stem cell-mediated gene delivery of bone morphogenetic protein-2 in an articular fracture model. *Mol Ther.* 2007;15:1543-1550.
192. Haynesworth S, Goldberg V, Caplan A. Diminution of the number of mesenchymal stem cells as a cause for skeletal aging. In: Buckwalter JA, Goldberg VM, Woo SL-Y, eds. *Musculoskeletal Soft Tissue Aging: Impact on Mobility (Symposium).* American Academy of Orthopaedic Surgeons; 1994:79-87.
193. Bartholomew A, Sturgeon C, Siatskas M, et al. Mesenchymal stem cells suppress lymphocyte proliferation in vitro and prolong skin graft survival in vivo. *Exp Hematol.* 2002;30:42-48.
194. Klyushnenkova E, Mosca JD, Zernetkina V, et al. T cell responses to allogeneic human mesenchymal stem cells: immunogenicity, tolerance, and suppression. *J Biomed Sci.* 2005;12:47-57.
195. Lalu MM, McIntyre L, Pugliese C, et al. Safety of cell therapy with mesenchymal stromal cells (SafeCell): a systematic review and meta-analysis of clinical trials. *PLoS One.* 2012;7:e47559.
196. Khashan M, Inoue S, Berven SH. Cell based therapies as compared to autologous bone grafts for spinal arthrodesis. *Spine.* 2013;38:1885-1891.
197. Hsu WK, Hashimoto RE, Berven SH, Nassr A. Biological substitutes/extenders for spinal arthrodesis: which agents are cost-effective? *Spine.* 2014;39:S86-S98.
198. Henrich D, Seebach C, Sterlepper E, et al. RIA reamings and hip aspirate: a comparative evaluation of osteoprogenitor and endothelial progenitor cells. *Injury.* 2010;41(suppl 2): S62-S68.
199. Schmidmaier G, Herrmann S, Green J, et al. Quantitative assessment of growth factors in reaming aspirate, iliac crest, and platelet preparation. *Bone.* 2006;39:1156-1163.
200. Stafford PR, Norris BL. Reamer-irrigator-aspirator bone graft and bi Masquelet technique for segmental bone defect nonunions: a review of 25 cases. *Injury.* 2010;41(suppl 2):S72-S77.
201. McCall TA, Brokaw DS, Jelen BA, et al. Treatment of large segmental bone defects with reamer-irrigator-aspirator bone graft: technique and case series. *Orthop Clin North Am.* 2010;41:63-73.
202. Belthur MV, Conway JD, Jindal G, Ranade A, Herzenberg JE. Bone graft harvest using a new intramedullary system. *Clin Orthop Relat Res.* 2008;466:2973-2980.
203. Henrich D, Nau C, Kraft S, et al. Effect of the harvest procedure and tissue site on the osteogenic function of and gene expression in human mesenchymal stem cells. *Int J Mol Med.* 2016;37(4):976-988.
204. Abjornson C, Lane J: *Bone allograft preparations: A critical review.* Presented at the Pittsburgh Bone Symposium, Aug 20-23, 2003.
205. Bauer TW, Muschler GF. Bone graft materials. An overview of the basic science. *Clin Orthop Relat Res.* 2000;10-27.
206. Stevenson S. The immune response to osteochondral allografts in dogs. *J Bone Joint Surg Am.* 1987;69:573-582.
207. Stevenson S, Hohn RB, Templeton JW. Effects of tissue antigen matching on the healing of fresh cancellous bone allografts in dogs. *Am J Vet Res.* 1983;44:201-206.
208. Tomford WW, Starkweather RJ, Goldman MH. A study of the clinical incidence of infection in the use of banked allograft bone. *J Bone Joint Surg Am.* 1981;63:244-248.
209. Bos GD, Goldberg VM, Zika JM, Heiple KG, Powell AE. Immune responses of rats to frozen bone allografts. *J Bone Joint Surg Am.* 1983;65:239-246.
210. Chalmers J. Transplantation immunity in bone homografting. *J Bone Joint Surg Br.* 1959;41B:160-179.
211. Friedlaender GE, Mankin HJ. Bone banking: current methods and suggested guidelines. *Instr Course Lect.* 1981;30:36-55.
212. Friedlaender GE, Strong DM, Sell KW. Studies on the antigenicity of bone. I. Freeze-dried and deep-frozen bone allografts in rabbits. *J Bone Joint Surg Am.* 1976;58: 854-858.
213. Friedlaender GE, Strong DM, Sell KW. Studies on the antigenicity of bone. II. Donor-specific anti-HLA antibodies in human recipients of freeze-dried allografts. *J Bone Joint Surg Am.* 1984;66:107-112.
214. Halloran PF, Lee EH, Ziv I, Langer F, Gross AE. Orthotopic bone transplantation in mice. II. Studies of the alloantibody response. *Transplantation.* 1979;27:420-426.
215. Langer F, Czitrom A, Pritzker KP, Gross AE. The immunogenicity of fresh and frozen allogeneic bone. *J Bone Joint Surg Am.* 1975;57:216-220.
216. Lee E, Langer F, Halloran P. The immunogenicity of osteochondral and massive allografts. *Trans Orthop Res Soc.* 1979;61.
217. Muscolo DL, Kawai S, Ray RD. Cellular and humoral immune response analysis of bone-allografted rats. *J Bone Joint Surg Am.* 1976;58:826-832.

218. Pelker RR, Friedlaender GE, Markham TC. Biomechanical properties of bone allografts. *Clin Orthop Relat Res.* 1983;54-57.
219. Bos GD, Goldberg VM, Powell AE, Heiple KG, Zika JM. The effect of histocompatibility matching on canine frozen bone allografts. *J Bone Joint Surg Am.* 1983;65:89-96.
220. Muscolo DL, Caletti E, Schajowicz F, Araujo ES, Makino A. Tissue-typing in human massive allografts of frozen bone. *J Bone Joint Surg Am.* 1987;69:583-595.
221. McAllister DR, Joyce MJ, Mann BJ, Vangsness CT. Allograft update: the current status of tissue regulation, procurement, processing, and sterilization. *Am J Sports Med.* 2007;35:2148-2158.
222. Friedlaender G. Appropriate screening for prevention of infection transmission by musculoskeletal allografts. *Instr Course Lect.* 2000;49:615-619.
223. Tomford WW. Transmission of disease through transplantation of musculoskeletal allografts. *J Bone Joint Surg Am.* 1995;77:1742-1754.
224. Mroz TE, Joyce MJ, Steinmetz MP, Lieberman IH, Wang JC. Musculoskeletal allograft risks and recalls in the United States. *J Am Acad Orthop Surg.* 2008;16:559-565.
225. Boyce T, Edwards J, Scarborough N. Allograft bone: The influence of processing on safety and performance. *Orthop Clin North Am.* 1999;30:571-581.
226. Mroz TE, Joyce MJ, Lieberman IH, et al. The use of allograft bone in spine surgery: is it safe? *Spine J.* 2009;9:303-308.
227. Cornell C, Lane J, Nottebaert M. The effect of ethylene oxide sterilization upon the bone inductive properties of demineralized bone matrix. *Orth Trans.* 1987;31:1.
228. Doherty MJ, Mollan RA, Wilson DJ. Effect of ethylene oxide sterilization on human demineralized bone. *Biomaterials.* 1993;14:994-998.
229. Ijiri S, Yamamuro T, Nakamura T, Kotani S, Notoya K. Effect of sterilization on bone morphogenetic protein. *J Orthop Res.* 1994;12:628-636.
230. Thorén K, Aspenberg P. Ethylene oxide sterilization impairs allograft incorporation in a conduction chamber. *Clin Orthop Relat Res.* 1995;259-264.
231. Prolo DJ, Oklund SK, Borer M. Efficacy and safety of ethylene oxide sterilization of allogeneic bone for human transplantation: a forty-year experience. *Cureus.* 2013;5:e121.
232. Dziedzic-Goclawska A, Ostrowski K, Stachowicz W, Michalik J, Grzesik W. Effect of radiation sterilization on the osteoinductive properties and the rate of remodeling of bone implants preserved by lyophilization and deep-freezing. *Clin Orthop Relat Res.* 1991;30-37.
233. Zhang Q, Cornu O, Delloye C. Ethylene oxide does not extinguish the osteoinductive capacity of demineralized bone. A reappraisal in rats. *Acta Orthop Scand.* 1997;68:104-108.
234. Akkus O, Rimnac CM. Fracture resistance of gamma radiation sterilized cortical bone allografts. *J Orthop Res.* 2001;19:927-934.
235. Cornu O, Banse X, Docquier PL, Luyckx S, Delloye C. Effect of freeze-drying and gamma irradiation on the mechanical properties of human cancellous bone. *J Orthop Res.* 2000;18:426-431.
236. Fideler BM, Vangsness CT, Lu B, Orlando C, Moore T. Gamma irradiation: effects on biomechanical properties of human bone-patellar tendon-bone allografts. *Am J Sports Med.* 1995;23:643-646.
237. Godette GA, Kopta JA, Egle DM. Biomechanical effects of gamma irradiation on fresh frozen allografts in vivo. *Orthopedics.* 1996;19:649-653.
238. Hamer AJ, Strachan JR, Black MM, et al. Biochemical properties of cortical allograft bone using a new method of bone strength measurement. A comparison of fresh, fresh-frozen and irradiated bone. *J Bone Joint Surg Br.* 1996;78:363-368.
239. Jinno T, Miric A, Feighan J, et al. The effects of processing and low dose irradiation on cortical bone grafts. *Clin Orthop Relat Res.* 2000;275-285.
240. Loty B, Courpied JP, Tomeno B, et al. Bone allografts sterilised by irradiation. Biological properties, procurement and results of 150 massive allografts. *Int Orthop.* 1990;14:237-242.
241. Sugimoto M, Takahashi S, Toguchida J, et al. Changes in bone after high-dose irradiation. Biomechanics and histomorphology. *J Bone Joint Surg Br.* 1991;73:492-497.
242. Islam A, Chapin K, Moore E, et al. Gamma radiation sterilization reduces the high-cycle fatigue life of allograft bone. *Clin Orthop Relat Res.* 2016;474:827-835.
243. Currey JD, Foreman J, Laketić I, et al. Effects of ionizing radiation on the mechanical properties of human bone. *J Orthop Res.* 1997;15:111-117.
244. Bowen JR, Angus PD, Huxster RR, MacEwen GD. Posterior spinal fusion without blood replacement in Jehovah's Witnesses. *Clin Orthop Relat Res.* 1985;284-288.
245. Brantigan JW. Pseudarthrosis rate after allograft posterior lumbar interbody fusion with pedicle screw and plate fixation. *Spine.* 1994;19:1271-1279.
246. Fernyhough JC, White JI, LaRocca H. Fusion rates in multilevel cervical spondylosis comparing allograft fibula with autograft fibula in 126 patients. *Spine.* 1991;16:S561-S564.
247. Jorgenson SS, Lowe TG, France J, Sabin J. A prospective analysis of autograft versus allograft in posterolateral lumbar fusion in the same patient. A minimum of 1-year follow-up in 144 patients. *Spine.* 1994;19:2048-2053.
248. Kozak JA, Heilman AE, O'Brien JP. Anterior lumbar fusion options. Technique and graft materials. *Clin Orthop Relat Res.* 1994;45-51.
249. Nugent PJ, Dawson EG. Intertransverse process lumbar arthrodesis with allogeneic fresh-frozen bone graft. *Clin Orthop Relat Res.* 1993;107-111.
250. Oikarinen J. Experimental spinal fusion with decalcified bone matrix and deep-frozen allogeneic bone in rabbits. *Clin Orthop Relat Res.* 1982;210-218.
251. Stabler CL, Eismont FJ, Brown MD, Green BA, Malinin TI. Failure of posterior cervical fusions using cadaveric bone graft in children. *J Bone Joint Surg Am.* 1985;67:371-375.
252. Tenholder MJ, Kneisl JS, Harrow ME, Peindl RD, Stanley KJ. Biomechanical effects of processing bulk allograft bone with negative-pressure washing. *Am J Orthop.* 2003;32:289-297.
253. Wetzel FT, Hoffman MA, Arcieri RR. Freeze-dried fibular allograft in anterior spinal surgery: cervical and lumbar applications. *Yale J Biol Med.* 1993;66:263-275.
254. Zdeblick TA, Cooke ME, Wilson D, Kunz DN, McCabe R. Anterior cervical discectomy, fusion, and plating. A comparative animal study. *Spine.* 1993;18:1974-1983.
255. Zdeblick TA, Ducker TB. The use of freeze-dried allograft bone for anterior cervical fusions. *Spine.* 1991;16:726-729.
256. Miller LE, Block JE. Safety and effectiveness of bone allografts in anterior cervical discectomy and fusion surgery. *Spine.* 2011;36:2045-2050.

257. Aurori BF, Weierman RJ, Lowell HA, Nadel CI, Parsons JR. Pseudarthrosis after spinal fusion for scoliosis. A comparison of autogeneic and allogeneic bone grafts. *Clin Orthop Relat Res*. 1985;153-158.
258. Bridwell KH, Lenke LG, McEnery KW, Baldus C, Blanke K. Anterior fresh frozen structural allografts in the thoracic and lumbar spine. Do they work if combined with posterior fusion and instrumentation in adult patients with kyphosis or anterior column defects? *Spine*. 1995;20:1410-1418.
259. Collis JS. Total disc replacement: a modified posterior lumbar interbody fusion. Report of 750 cases. *Clin Orthop Relat Res*. 1985;64-67.
260. Fabry G. Allograft versus autograft bone in idiopathic scoliosis surgery: a multivariate statistical analysis. *J Pediatr Orthop*. 1991;11:465-468.
261. Gepstein R, Nakamura K, Latta M. Posterior spinal fusion using preserved bone allografts. *Trans Orthop Res Soc*. 1986;73-76.
262. Grossman W, Peppelman WC, Baum JA, Kraus DR. The use of freeze-dried fibular allograft in anterior cervical fusion. *Spine*. 1992;17:565-569.
263. Malinin TI, Rosomoff HL, Sutton CH. Human cadaver femoral head homografts for anterior cervical spine fusions. *Surg Neurol*. 1977;7:249-251.
264. McCarthy RE, Peek RD, Morrissy RT, Hough AJ. Allograft bone in spinal fusion for paralytic scoliosis. *J Bone Joint Surg Am*. 1986;68:370-375.
265. Nasca RJ, Whelchel JD. Use of cryopreserved bone in spinal surgery. *Spine*. 1987;12:222-227.
266. Savolainen S, Usenius JP, Hernesniemi J. Iliac crest versus artificial bone grafts in 250 cervical fusions. *Acta Neurochir (Wien)*. 1994;129:54-57.
267. Schneider JR, Bright RW. Anterior cervical fusion using preserved bone allografts. *Transplant Proc*. 1976;8:73-76.
268. Tiedeman JJ, Garvin KL, Kile TA, Connolly JF. The role of a composite, demineralized bone matrix and bone marrow in the treatment of osseous defects. *Orthopedics*. 1995;18:1153-1158.
269. Whitehill R, Wilhelm CE, Moskal JT, Kramer SJ, Ruch WW. Posterior strut fusions to enhance immediate postoperative cervical stability. *Spine*. 1986;11:6-13.
270. Young WF, Rosenwasser RH. An early comparative analysis of the use of fibular allograft versus autologous iliac crest graft for interbody fusion after anterior cervical discectomy. *Spine*. 1993;18:1123-1124.
271. Angevine PD, Zivin JG, McCormick PC. Cost-effectiveness of single-level anterior cervical discectomy and fusion for cervical spondylosis. *Spine*. 2005;30:1989-1997.
272. Cohen DB, Chotivichit A, Fujita T, et al. Pseudarthrosis repair. Autogenous iliac crest versus femoral ring allograft. *Clin Orthop Relat Res*. 2000;46-55.
273. Janssen ME, Nguyen C, Beckham R, Larson A. Biological cages. *Eur Spine J*. 2000;9(suppl 1):S102-S109.
274. Kleinstueck FS, Hu SS, Bradford DS. Use of allograft femoral rings for spinal deformity in adults. *Clin Orthop Relat Res*. 2002;84-91.
275. Liljenqvist U, O'Brien JP, Renton P. Simultaneous combined anterior and posterior lumbar fusion with femoral cortical allograft. *Eur Spine J*. 1998;7:125-131.
276. Siff TE, Kamaric E, Noble PC, Esses SI. Femoral ring versus fibular strut allografts in anterior lumbar interbody arthrodesis. A biomechanical analysis. *Spine*. 1999;24:659-665.
277. Deaver J. Secondary bone implantation by a modification of Senn's method. *Med News*. 1889;55:714.
278. Kaiser MG, Haid RW, Subach BR, Barnes B, Rodts GE. Anterior cervical plating enhances arthrodesis after discectomy and fusion with cortical allograft. *Neurosurgery*. 2002;50:229-236.
279. Kummer FJ, Chen D, Spivak JM. Optimal selection and preparation of fresh frozen corticocancellous allografts for cervical interbody spinal fusion. *Spine*. 1998;23:2295-2298.
280. Löfgren H, Johansson V, Olsson T, Ryd L, Levander B. Rigid fusion after cloward operation for cervical disc disease using autograft, allograft, or xenograft: a randomized study with radiostereometric and clinical follow-up assessment. *Spine*. 2000;25:1908-1916.
281. Martin GJ, Haid RW, MacMillan M, Rodts GE, Berkman R. Anterior cervical discectomy with freeze-dried fibula allograft. Overview of 317 cases and literature review. *Spine*. 1999;24:852-858.
282. McKoy BE, Wingate JK, Poletti SC, et al. Fibular allograft after anterior cervical corpectomy: long term follow-up. *Iowa Orthop J*. 2002;22:42-46.
283. McLaughlin MR, Purighalla V, Pizzi FJ. Cost advantages of two-level anterior cervical fusion with rigid internal fixation for radiculopathy and degenerative disease. *Surg Neurol*. 1997;48:560-565.
284. Parthiban JKBC, Singhania BK, Ramani PS. A radiological evaluation of allografts (ethylene oxide sterilized cadaver bone) and autografts in anterior cervical fusion. *Neurol India*. 2002;50:17-22.
285. Shapiro S, Bindal R. Femoral ring allograft for anterior cervical interbody fusion: technical note. *Neurosurgery*. 2000;47:1457-1459.
286. Vaccaro AR, Cirello J. The use of allograft bone and cages in fractures of the cervical, thoracic, and lumbar spine. *Clin Orthop Relat Res*. 2002;19-26.
287. Chen L, Tang T, Yang H. Complications associated with posterior lumbar interbody fusion using Bagby and Kuslich method for treatment of spondylolisthesis. *Chin Med J*. 2003;116:99-103.
288. DeBerard MS, Colledge AL, Masters KS, Schleusener RL, Schlegel JD. Outcomes of posterolateral versus BAK titanium cage interbody lumbar fusion in injured workers: a retrospective cohort study. *J South Orthop Assoc*. 2002;11:157-166.
289. Hacker RJ, Cauthen JC, Gilbert TJ, Griffith SL. A prospective randomized multicenter clinical evaluation of an anterior cervical fusion cage. *Spine*. 2000;25:2646-2654.
290. McAfee PC, Fedder IL, Saiedy S, Shucosky EM, Cunningham BW. SB Charité disc replacement: report of 60 prospective randomized cases in a US center. *J Spinal Disord Tech*. 2003;16:424-433.
291. McAfee PC, Lee GA, Fedder IL, Cunningham BW. Anterior BAK instrumentation and fusion: complete versus partial discectomy. *Clin Orthop Relat Res*. 2002;55-63.
292. Merk H, Koch H, Liebau C, et al. [Implantation of a Harms titanium mesh cylinder for vertebral body replacement in spinal metastases]. *Z Orthop Ihre Grenzgeb*. 2000;138:169-173.
293. Togawa D, Bauer TW, Brantigan JW, Lowery GL. Bone graft incorporation in radiographically successful human intervertebral body fusion cages. *Spine*. 2001;26:2744-2750.

294. Togawa D, Bauer TW, Lieberman IH, Lowery GL, Takikawa S. Histology of tissues within retrieved human titanium mesh cages. *Spine*. 2003;28:246-253.
295. Chong E, Pelletier MH, Mobbs RJ, Walsh WR. The design evolution of interbody cages in anterior cervical discectomy and fusion: a systematic review. *BMC Musculoskelet Disord.* 2015;16:99.
296. Espersen JO, Buhl M, Eriksen EF, et al. Treatment of cervical disc disease using Cloward's technique. I. General results, effect of different operative methods and complications in 1,106 patients. *Acta Neurochir (Wien)*. 1984;70:97-114.
297. Walker B, Koerner J, Sankarayanaryanan S, Radcliff K. A consensus statement regarding the utilization of BMP in spine surgery. *Curr Rev Musculoskelet Med.* 2014;7:208-219.
298. Weir R. Antiseptic irrigation for synovitis of the bone: implantation of mucus membrane in traumatic structure of the urethra. Implantation of Bone. *Med News.* 1890;56:125.
299. Mackie W. Clinical observation of the healing of aseptic bone cavities by Senn's method of implantation of antiseptic decalcified bone. *Med News*. 1890;57:202.
300. Miller A. A case of bone grafting with decalcified bone chips. *Lancet.* 1890;618.
301. Reddi AH, Huggins C. Biochemical sequences in the transformation of normal fibroblasts in adolescent rats. *Proc Natl Acad Sci USA*. 1972;69:1601-1605.
302. Reddi AH. Bone matrix in the solid state: geometric influence on differentiation of fibroblasts. *Adv Biol Med Phys.* 1974;15:1-18.
303. Urist MR. Bone: formation by autoinduction. *Science.* 1965;150:893-899.
304. Vaidya R, Carp J, Sethi A, et al. Complications of anterior cervical discectomy and fusion using recombinant human bone morphogenetic protein-2. *Eur Spine J.* 2007;16:1257-1265.
305. Van de Putte KA, Urist MR. Osteogenesis in the interior of intramuscular implants of decalcified bone matrix. *Clin Orthop Relat Res.* 1986;43:257-270.
306. Chalmers J, Gray DH, Rush J. Observations on the induction of bone in soft tissues. *J Bone Joint Surg Br.* 1975;57:36-45.
307. Nathanson MA. Analysis of cartilage differentiation from skeletal muscle grown on bone matrix. III. Environmental regulation of glycosaminoglycan and proteoglycan synthesis. *Dev Biol.* 1983;96:46-62.
308. Nathanson MA, Hay ED. Analysis of cartilage differentiation from skeletal muscle grown on bone matrix. I. Ultrastructural aspects. *Dev Biol.* 1980;78:301-331.
309. Nathanson MA, Hay ED. Analysis of cartilage differentiation from skeletal muscle grown on bone matrix. II. Chondroitin sulfate synthesis and reaction to exogenous glycosaminoglycans. *Dev Biol.* 1980;78:332-351.
310. Reddi AH. Extracellular bone matrix dependent local induction of cartilage and bone. *J Rheumatol Suppl.* 1983;11:67-69.
311. Reddi AH. Cell biology and biochemistry of endochondral bone development. *Coll Relat Res.* 1981;1:209-226.
312. Muthukumaran N, Reddi AH. Bone matrix-induced local bone induction. *Clin Orthop Relat Res.* 1985;159-164.
313. Mohan S, Baylink DJ. Bone growth factors. *Clin Orthop Relat Res.* 1991;30-48.
314. Linkhart TA, Mohan S, Baylink DJ. Growth factors for bone growth and repair: IGF, TGF beta and BMP. *Bone.* 1996;19:1S-12S.
315. Sato K, Urist MR. Induced regeneration of calvaria by bone morphogenetic protein (BMP) in dogs. *Clin Orthop Relat Res.* 1985;301-311.
316. Van de Putte KA, Urist MR. Osteogenesis in the interior of intramuscular implants of decalcified bone matrix. *Clin Orthop Relat Res.* 1966;43:257-270.
317. Urist MR, Nakagawa M, Nakata N, Nogami H. Experimental myositis ossificans: cartilage and bone formation in muscle in response to a diffusible bone matrix-derived morphogen. *Arch Pathol Lab Med.* 1978;102:312-316.
318. Urist MR, Iwata H, Ceccotti PL, et al. Bone morphogenesis in implants of insoluble bone gelatin. *Proc Natl Acad Sci USA.* 1973;70:3511-3515.
319. Urist MR, Hay PH, Dubuc F, Buring K. Osteogenetic competence. *Clin Orthop Relat Res.* 1969;64:194-220.
320. Urist MR, Dawson E. Intertransverse process fusion with the aid of chemosterilized autolyzed antigen-extracted allogeneic (AAA) bone. *Clin Orthop Relat Res.* 1981;97-113.
321. Kaban LB, Mulliken JB, Glowacki J. Treatment of jaw defects with demineralized bone implants. *J Oral Maxillofac Surg.* 1982;40:623-626.
322. Glowacki J, Kaban LB, Murray JE, Folkman J, Mulliken JB. Application of the biological principle of induced osteogenesis for craniofacial defects. *Lancet.* 1981;1:959-962.
323. Glowacki J, Altobelli D, Mulliken JB. Fate of mineralized and demineralized osseous implants in cranial defects. *Calcif Tissue Int.* 1981;33:71-76.
324. Wilkins R, Stringer E. Demineralized bone powder use in grafting space-occupying lesions of bone. *Int Orthop.* 1994;2:71-78.
325. Morone MA, Boden SD. Experimental posterolateral lumbar spinal fusion with a demineralized bone matrix gel. *Spine.* 1998;23:159-167.
326. Martin GJ, Boden SD, Titus L, Scarborough NL. New formulations of demineralized bone matrix as a more effective graft alternative in experimental posterolateral lumbar spine arthrodesis. *Spine.* 1999;24:637-645.
327. Zerwekh JE, Kourosh S, Scheinberg R, et al. Fibrillar collagen-biphasic calcium phosphate composite as a bone graft substitute for spinal fusion. *J Orthop Res.* 1992;10:562-572.
328. Lindholm TS, Ragni P, Lindholm TC. Response of bone marrow stroma cells to demineralized cortical bone matrix in experimental spinal fusion in rabbits. *Clin Orthop Relat Res.* 1988;296-302.
329. Frenkel SR, Moskovich R, Spivak J, Zhang ZH, Prewett AB. Demineralized bone matrix. Enhancement of spinal fusion. *Spine.* 1993;18:1634-1639.
330. Flatley TJ, Lynch KL, Benson M. Tissue response to implants of calcium phosphate ceramic in the rabbit spine. *Clin Orthop Relat Res.* 1983;246-252.
331. Muschler GF, Nitto H, Matsukura Y, et al. Spine fusion using cell matrix composites enriched in bone marrow-derived cells. *Clin Orthop Relat Res.* 2003;102-118.
332. Chakkalakal DA, Strates BS, Garvin KL, et al. Demineralized bone matrix as a biological scaffold for bone repair. *Tissue Eng.* 2001;7:161-177.
333. Elves MW, Salama R. A study of the development of cytotoxic antibodies produced in recipients of xenografts (heterografts) of iliac bone. *J Bone Joint Surg Br.* 1974;56:331-339.
334. Plenk H, Hollmann K, Wilfert KH. Experimental bridging of osseous defects in rats by the implantation of Kiel bone

containing fresh autologous marrow. *J Bone Joint Surg Br.* 1972;54:735-743.
335. Rawlinson JN. Morbidity after anterior cervical decompression and fusion. The influence of the donor site on recovery, and the results of a trial of surgibone compared to autologous bone. *Acta Neurochir (Wien).* 1994;131:106-118.
336. Carter JD, Swearingen AB, Chaput CD, Rahm MD. Clinical and radiographic assessment of transforaminal lumbar interbody fusion using HEALOS collagen-hydroxyapatite sponge with autologous bone marrow aspirate. *Spine J.* 2009;9:434-438.
337. Kitchel SH. A preliminary comparative study of radiographic results using mineralized collagen and bone marrow aspirate versus autologous bone in the same patients undergoing posterior lumbar interbody fusion with instrumented posterolateral lumbar fusion. *Spine J.* 2006;6:405-411.
338. Neen D, Noyes D, Shaw M, et al. Healos and bone marrow aspirate used for lumbar spine fusion: a case controlled study comparing Healos with autograft. *Spine.* 2006;31:E636-E640.
339. Ploumis A, Albert TJ, Brown Z, Mehbod AA, Transfeldt EE. Healos graft carrier with bone marrow aspirate instead of allograft as adjunct to local autograft for posterolateral fusion in degenerative lumbar scoliosis: a minimum 2-year follow-up study. *J Neurosurg Spine.* 2010;13:211-215.
340. Alsaleh KAM, Tougas CA, Roffey DM, Wai EK. Osteoconductive bone graft extenders in posterolateral thoracolumbar spinal fusion: a systematic review. *Spine.* 2012;37:E993-E1000.
341. Costantino PD, Friedman CD. Synthetic bone graft substitutes. *Otolaryngol Clin North Am.* 1994;27:1037-1074.
342. Vacanti CA, Vacanti JP. Bone and cartilage reconstruction with tissue engineering approaches. *Otolaryngol Clin North Am.* 1994;27:263-276.
343. Urist MR, Mikulski A, Lietze A. Solubilized and insolubilized bone morphogenetic protein. *Proc Natl Acad Sci USA.* 1979;76:1828-1832.
344. Urist MR, Silverman BF, Büring K, Dubuc FL, Rosenberg JM. The bone induction principle. *Clin Orthop Relat Res.* 1967;53:243-283.
345. Urist MR, Lietze A, Mizutani H, et al. A bovine low molecular weight bone morphogenetic protein (BMP) fraction. *Clin Orthop Relat Res.* 1982;219-232.
346. Lovell TP, Dawson EG, Nilsson OS, Urist MR. Augmentation of spinal fusion with bone morphogenetic protein in dogs. *Clin Orthop Relat Res.* 1989;266-274.
347. Wozney JM, Rosen V, Celeste AJ, et al. Novel regulators of bone formation: molecular clones and activities. *Science.* 1988;242:1528-1534.
348. Kessler E, Takahara K, Biniaminov L, Brusel M, Greenspan DS. Bone morphogenetic protein-1: the type I procollagen C-proteinase. *Science.* 1996;271:360-362.
349. Reddi AH. BMP-1: resurrection as procollagen C-proteinase. *Science.* 1996;271:463.
350. Israel D, Nove J, Kerns K, Moutsatsos I, Kaufman R. Expression and characterization of bone morphogenetic protein-2 in Chinese hamster ovary cells. *Growth Factors.* 1992;7:139-150.
351. Wozney J, Rosen V. Bone morphogenetic protein and bone morphogenetic protein gene family in bone formation and repair. *Clin Orthop Relat Res.* 1998;346:26-37.
352. Even J, Eskander M, Kang J. Bone morphogenetic protein in spine surgery: current and future uses. *J Am Acad Orthop Surg.* 2012;20:547-552.
353. Rosen V, Wozney J. Bone morphogenetic protein. *Princ Bone Biol.* 2002;919-928.
354. Wozney JM. The bone morphogenetic protein family and osteogenesis. *Mol Reprod Dev.* 1992;32:160-167.
355. Hruska KA, Guo G, Wozniak M, et al. Osteogenic protein-1 prevents renal fibrogenesis associated with ureteral obstruction. *Am J Physiol Renal Physiol.* 2000;279:F130-F143.
356. Vukicevic S, Basic V, Rogic D, et al. Osteogenic protein-1 (bone morphogenetic protein-7) reduces severity of injury after ischemic acute renal failure in rat. *J Clin Invest.* 1998;102:202-214.
357. Bahamonde ME, Lyons KM. BMP3: to be or not to be a BMP. *J Bone Joint Surg Am.* 2001;83–A(suppl):S56-S62.
358. Cheng H, Jiang W, Phillips FM, et al. Osteogenic activity of the fourteen types of human bone morphogenetic proteins (BMPs). *J Bone Joint Surg Am.* 2003;85:1544-1552.
359. Daluiski A, Engstrand T, Bahamonde ME, et al. Bone morphogenetic protein-3 is a negative regulator of bone density. *Nat Genet.* 2001;27:84-88.
360. Lissenberg-Thunnissen SN, De Gorter DJJ, Sier CFM, Schipper IB. Use and efficacy of bone morphogenetic proteins in fracture healing. *Int Orthop.* 2011;35:1271-1280.
361. Sanchez-Duffhues G, Hiepen C, Knaus P, ten Dijke P. Bone morphogenetic protein signaling in bone homeostasis. *Bone.* 2015;80:43-59.
362. Shen B, Bhargav D, Wei A, et al. BMP-13 emerges as a potential inhibitor of bone formation. *Int J Biol Sci.* 2009;5:192-200.
363. Miyazono K. Bone morphogenetic protein receptors and actions. *Princ Bone Biol.* 2002;929-942.
364. Abreu JG, Ketpura NI, Reversade B, De Robertis EM. Connective-tissue growth factor (CTGF) modulates cell signalling by BMP and TGF-beta. *Nat Cell Biol.* 2002;4:599-604.
365. Bostrom MP, Saleh KJ, Einhorn TA. Osteoinductive growth factors in preclinical fracture and long bone defects models. *Orthop Clin North Am.* 1999;30:647-658.
366. Brunet LJ, McMahon JA, McMahon AP, Harland RM. Noggin, cartilage morphogenesis, and joint formation in the mammalian skeleton. *Science.* 1998;280:1455-1457.
367. Lieberman JR, Daluiski A, Einhorn TA. The role of growth factors in the repair of bone. Biology and clinical applications. *J Bone Joint Surg Am.* 2002;84A:1032-1044.
368. Merino R, Macias D, Gañan Y, et al. Expression and function of Gdf-5 during digit skeletogenesis in the embryonic chick leg bud. *Dev Biol.* 1999;206:33-45.
369. Tsumaki N, Nakase T, Miyaji T, et al. Bone morphogenetic protein signals are required for cartilage formation and differently regulate joint development during skeletogenesis. *J Bone Miner Res.* 2002;17:898-906.
370. Bilandzic M, Stenvers KL. Betaglycan: a multifunctional accessory. *Mol Cell Endocrinol.* 2011;339:180-189.
371. ten Dijke P, Goumans M-J, Pardali E. Endoglin in angiogenesis and vascular diseases. *Angiogenesis.* 2008;11:79-89.
372. Yeo C-Y, Whitman M. Nodal signals to smads through cripto-dependent and cripto-independent mechanisms. *Mol Cell.* 2001;7:949-957.
373. Babitt JL, Zhang Y, Samad TA, et al. Repulsive guidance molecule (RGMa), a DRAGON homologue, is a bone morphogenetic protein co-receptor. *J Biol Chem.* 2005;280:29820-29827.

374. Samad TA, Rebbapragada A, Bell E, et al. DRAGON, a bone morphogenetic protein co-receptor. *J Biol Chem.* 2005;280:14122-14129.
375. Corradini E, Babitt JL, Lin HY. The RGM/DRAGON family of BMP co-receptors. *Cytokine Growth Factor Rev.* 2009;20:389-398.
376. Kuniyasu H, Hirose Y, Ochi M, et al. Bone augmentation using rhGDF-5-collagen composite. *Clin Oral Implants Res.* 2003;14:490-499.
377. Settle SH, Rountree RB, Sinha A, et al. Multiple joint and skeletal patterning defects caused by single and double mutations in the mouse Gdf6 and Gdf5 genes. *Dev Biol.* 2003;254:116-130.
378. Li Y-F, Tang X-Z, Liang C-G, et al. Role of growth differentiation factor-5 and bone morphogenetic protein type II receptor in the development of lumbar intervertebral disc degeneration. *Int J Clin Exp Pathol.* 2015;8: 719-726.
379. Food and Drug Administration. *FDA Public Health Notification: Life-Threatening Complications Associated With Recombinant Human Bone Morphogenetic Protein in Cervical Spine Fusion.* Available at http://www.fda.gov/MedicalDevices/Safety/AlertsandNotices/PublicHealthNotifications/ucm062000.htm.
380. Alt V, Borgman B, Eicher A, et al. Effects of recombinant human bone morphogenetic protein-2 (rhBMP-2) in grade III open tibia fractures treated with unreamed nails: a clinical and health-economic analysis. *Injury.* 2015;46:2267-2272.
381. Wei S, Cai X, Huang J, et al. Recombinant human BMP-2 for the treatment of open tibial fractures. *Orthopedics.* 2012;35:e847-e854.
382. Deleted in review.
383. Boden SD, Martin GJ, Horton WC, Truss TL, Sandhu HS. Laparoscopic anterior spinal arthrodesis with rhBMP-2 in a titanium interbody threaded cage. *J Spinal Disord.* 1998;11:95-101.
384. Boden SD, Martin GJ, Morone M, et al. The use of coralline hydroxyapatite with bone marrow, autogenous bone graft, or osteoinductive bone protein extract for posterolateral lumbar spine fusion. *Spine.* 1999;24:320-327.
385. Boden SD, Martin GJ, Morone MA, Ugbo JL, Moskovitz PA. Posterolateral lumbar intertransverse process spine arthrodesis with recombinant human bone morphogenetic protein 2/hydroxyapatite-tricalcium phosphate after laminectomy in the nonhuman primate. *Spine.* 1999;24:1179-1185.
386. Boden SD, Moskovitz PA, Morone MA, Toribitake Y. Video-assisted lateral intertransverse process arthrodesis. Validation of a new minimally invasive lumbar spinal fusion technique in the rabbit and nonhuman primate (rhesus) models. *Spine.* 1996;21:2689-2697.
387. Boden SD, Schimandle JH, Hutton WC. The use of an osteoinductive growth factor for lumbar spinal fusion. Part II: study of dose, carrier, and species. *Spine.* 1995;20: 2633-2644.
388. Boden S, Schimandle J, Hutton W. *Evaluation of a bovine-derived osteoinductive bone protein in a non-human primate model of lumbar fusion.* Presented at the 48th Annual Meeting of the Orthopaedic Research Society; 1996.
389. Boden SD, Schimandle JH, Hutton WC. Lumbar intertransverse-process spinal arthrodesis with use of a bovine bone-derived osteoinductive protein. A preliminary report. *J Bone Joint Surg Am.* 1995;77:1404-1417.
390. Boden SD, Schimandle JH, Hutton WC, et al. In vivo evaluation of a resorbable osteoinductive composite as a graft substitute for lumbar spinal fusion. *J Spinal Disord.* 1997;10:1-11.
391. Cook SD. Preclinical and clinical evaluation of osteogenic protein-1 (BMP-7) in bony sites. *Orthopedics.* 1999;22:669-671.
392. Cunningham B, Kanayama M, Parker L, et al. *Osteogenic protein versus autologous fusion in the sheep thoracic spine.* A comparative endoscopic study using the BAK interbody fusion device. Presented at the 42nd Annual Meeting of the Orthopaedic Research Society; 1996.
393. Cunningham BW, Kanayama M, Parker LM, et al. Osteogenic protein versus autologous interbody arthrodesis in the sheep thoracic spine. A comparative endoscopic study using the Bagby and Kuslich interbody fusion device. *Spine.* 1999;24:509-518.
394. Damien CJ, Grob D, Boden SD, Benedict JJ. Purified bovine BMP extract and collagen for spine arthrodesis: preclinical safety and efficacy. *Spine.* 2002;27:S50-S58.
395. David S, Gruber H, Murakami T. *Lumbar spinal fusion using recombinant human bone morphogenetic protein (rhBMP-2) a randomized, blinded and controlled study.* Presented at the 42nd Annual Meeting of the Orthopaedic Research Society; 1996.
396. Grauer JN, Patel TC, Erulkar JS, et al. Evaluation of OP-1 as a graft substitute for intertransverse process lumbar fusion. *Spine.* 2001;26:127-133.
397. Holliger EH, Trawick RH, Boden SD, Hutton WC. Morphology of the lumbar intertransverse process fusion mass in the rabbit model: a comparison between two bone graft materials—rhBMP-2 and autograft. *J Spinal Disord.* 1996;9:125-128.
398. Magin MN, Delling G. Improved lumbar vertebral interbody fusion using rhOP-1: a comparison of autogenous bone graft, bovine hydroxylapatite (Bio-Oss), and BMP-7 (rhOP-1) in sheep. *Spine.* 2001;26:469-478.
399. Martin GJ, Boden SD, Titus L. Recombinant human bone morphogenetic protein-2 overcomes the inhibitory effect of ketorolac, a nonsteroidal anti-inflammatory drug (NSAID), on posterolateral lumbar intertransverse process spine fusion. *Spine.* 1999;24:2188-2193.
400. Martin GJ, Boden SD, Marone MA, Moskovitz PA. Posterolateral intertransverse process spinal arthrodesis with rhBMP-2 in a nonhuman primate: important lessons learned regarding dose, carrier, and safety. *J Spinal Disord.* 1999;12:179-186.
401. Meyer RA, Gruber HE, Howard BA, et al. Safety of recombinant human bone morphogenetic protein-2 after spinal laminectomy in the dog. *Spine.* 1999;24:747-754.
402. Paramore CG, Lauryssen C, Rauzzino MJ, et al. The safety of OP-1 for lumbar fusion with decompression—a canine study. *Neurosurgery.* 1999;44:1151-1155.
403. Poynton AR, Lane JM. Safety profile for the clinical use of bone morphogenetic proteins in the spine. *Spine.* 2002;27:S40-S48.
404. Sandu H, Kanim L, Kabo M, et al. *Effective doses of recombinant human bone morphogenetic protein-2 in experimental spinal fusion.* Presented at the 42nd Annual Meeting of the Orthopaedic Research Society; 1996.
405. Schimandle JH, Boden SD, Hutton WC. Experimental spinal fusion with recombinant human bone morphogenetic protein-2. *Spine.* 1995;20:1326-1337.

406. Silcox DH, Boden SD, Schimandle JH, et al. Reversing the inhibitory effect of nicotine on spinal fusion using an osteoinductive protein extract. *Spine*. 1998;23:291-296.
407. Suh DY, Boden SD, Louis-Ugbo J, et al. Delivery of recombinant human bone morphogenetic protein-2 using a compression-resistant matrix in posterolateral spine fusion in the rabbit and in the non-human primate. *Spine*. 2002;27:353-360.
408. Cook SD, Dalton JE, Tan EH, Whitecloud TS, Rueger DC. In vivo evaluation of recombinant human osteogenic protein (rhOP-1) implants as a bone graft substitute for spinal fusions. *Spine*. 1994;19:1655-1663.
409. Fu T-S, Chen W-J, Chen L-H, et al. Enhancement of posterolateral lumbar spine fusion using low-dose rhBMP-2 and cultured marrow stromal cells. *J Orthop Res*. 2009;27:380-384.
410. Muschler GF, Hyodo A, Manning T, Kambic H, Easley K. Evaluation of human bone morphogenetic protein 2 in a canine spinal fusion model. *Clin Orthop Relat Res*. 1994;229-240.
411. Valdes M, Moore DC, Palumbo M, et al. rhBMP-6 stimulated osteoprogenitor cells enhance posterolateral spinal fusion in the New Zealand white rabbit. *Spine J*. 2007;7:318-325.
412. Boden SD, Kang J, Sandhu H, Heller JG. Use of recombinant human bone morphogenetic protein-2 to achieve posterolateral lumbar spine fusion in humans: a prospective, randomized clinical pilot trial: 2002 Volvo Award in clinical studies. *Spine*. 2002;27:2662-2673.
413. Boden SD, Zdeblick TA, Sandhu HS, Heim SE. The use of rhBMP-2 in interbody fusion cages. Definitive evidence of osteoinduction in humans: a preliminary report. *Spine*. 2000;25:376-381.
414. Burkus JK, Gornet MF, Dickman CA, Zdeblick TA. Anterior lumbar interbody fusion using rhBMP-2 with tapered interbody cages. *J Spinal Disord Tech*. 2002;15:337-349.
415. Laursen M, Høy K, Hansen ES, et al. Recombinant bone morphogenetic protein-7 as an intracorporal bone growth stimulator in unstable thoracolumbar burst fractures in humans: preliminary results. *Eur Spine J*. 1999;8:485-490.
416. McKay B, Sandhu HS. Use of recombinant human bone morphogenetic protein-2 in spinal fusion applications. *Spine*. 2002;27:S66-S85.
417. Sandhu HS, Khan SN. Recombinant human bone morphogenetic protein-2: use in spinal fusion applications. *J Bone Joint Surg Am*. 2003;85A(suppl):89-95.
418. Vaccaro AR, Anderson DG, Toth CA. Recombinant human osteogenic protein-1 (bone morphogenetic protein-7) as an osteoinductive agent in spinal fusion. *Spine*. 2002;27:S59-S65.
419. Kanayama M, Hashimoto T, Shigenobu K, et al. A prospective randomized study of posterolateral lumbar fusion using osteogenic protein-1 (OP-1) versus local autograft with ceramic bone substitute: emphasis of surgical exploration and histologic assessment. *Spine*. 2006;31:1067-1074.
420. Singh K, Smucker JD, Gill S, Boden SD. Use of recombinant human bone morphogenetic protein-2 as an adjunct in posterolateral lumbar spine fusion: a prospective CT-scan analysis at one and two years. *J Spinal Disord Tech*. 2006;19:416-423.
421. Vaccaro AR, Whang PG, Patel T, et al. The safety and efficacy of OP-1 (rhBMP-7) as a replacement for iliac crest autograft for posterolateral lumbar arthrodesis: minimum 4-year follow-up of a pilot study. *Spine J*. 2008;8:457-465.
422. Slosar PJ, Josey R, Reynolds J. Accelerating lumbar fusions by combining rhBMP-2 with allograft bone: a prospective analysis of interbody fusion rates and clinical outcomes. *Spine J*. 2007;7:301-307.
423. Glassman SD, Carreon LY, Djurasovic M, et al. RhBMP-2 versus iliac crest bone graft for lumbar spine fusion: a randomized, controlled trial in patients over sixty years of age. *Spine*. 2008;33:2843-2849.
424. Vaidya R, Sethi A, Bartol S, et al. Complications in the use of rhBMP-2 in PEEK cages for interbody spinal fusions. *J Spinal Disord Tech*. 2008;21:557-562.
425. Buttermann GR. Prospective nonrandomized comparison of an allograft with bone morphogenic protein versus an iliac-crest autograft in anterior cervical discectomy and fusion. *Spine J*. 2008;8:426-435.
426. Tumialán LM, Pan J, Rodts GE, Mummaneni PV. The safety and efficacy of anterior cervical discectomy and fusion with polyetheretherketone spacer and recombinant human bone morphogenetic protein-2: a review of 200 patients. *J Neurosurg Spine*. 2008;8:529-535.
427. Shields LBE, Raque GH, Glassman SD, et al. Adverse effects associated with high-dose recombinant human bone morphogenetic protein-2 use in anterior cervical spine fusion. *Spine*. 2006;31:542-547.
428. Smucker JD, Rhee JM, Singh K, Yoon ST, Heller JG. Increased swelling complications associated with off-label usage of rhBMP-2 in the anterior cervical spine. *Spine*. 2006;31:2813-2819.
429. Crawford CH, Carreon LY, McGinnis MD, Campbell MJ, Glassman SD. Perioperative complications of recombinant human bone morphogenetic protein-2 on an absorbable collagen sponge versus iliac crest bone graft for posterior cervical arthrodesis. *Spine*. 2009;34:1390-1394.
430. Haid RW, Branch CL, Alexander JT, Burkus JK. Posterior lumbar interbody fusion using recombinant human bone morphogenetic protein type 2 with cylindrical interbody cages. *Spine J*. 2004;4:527-538.
431. Carragee EJ, Hurwitz EL, Weiner BK. A critical review of recombinant human bone morphogenetic protein-2 trials in spinal surgery: emerging safety concerns and lessons learned. *Spine J*. 2011;11:471-491.
432. Burkus JK, Transfeldt EE, Kitchel SH, Watkins RG, Balderston R. Clinical and radiographic outcomes of anterior lumbar interbody fusion using recombinant human bone morphogenetic protein-2. *Spine*. 2002;27:2396-2408.
433. Baskin DS, Ryan P, Sonntag V, Westmark R, Widmayer MA. A prospective, randomized, controlled cervical fusion study using recombinant human bone morphogenetic protein-2 with the CORNERSTONE-SR allograft ring and the ATLANTIS anterior cervical plate. *Spine*. 2003;28:1219-1224.
434. Dimar JR, Glassman SD, Burkus KJ, Carreon LY. Clinical outcomes and fusion success at 2 years of single-level instrumented posterolateral fusions with recombinant human bone morphogenetic protein-2/compression resistant matrix versus iliac crest bone graft. *Spine*. 2006;31:2534-2539.
435. Lewandrowski K-U, Nanson C, Calderon R. Vertebral osteolysis after posterior interbody lumbar fusion with recombinant human bone morphogenetic protein 2: a report of five cases. *Spine J*. 2007;7:609-614.
436. Glassman SD, Carreon L, Djurasovic M, et al. Posterolateral lumbar spine fusion with INFUSE bone graft. *Spine J*. 2007;7:44-49.

437. Ohtori S, Suzuki M, Koshi T, et al. Single-level instrumented posterolateral fusion of the lumbar spine with a local bone graft versus an iliac crest bone graft: a prospective, randomized study with a 2-year follow-up. *Eur Spine J.* 2011;20:635-639.
438. Inage K, Ohtori S, Koshi T, et al. One, two-, and three-level instrumented posterolateral fusion of the lumbar spine with a local bone graft: a prospective study with a 2-year follow-up. *Spine.* 2011;36:1392-1396.
439. Carragee EJ, Comer GC, Smith MW. Local bone graft harvesting and volumes in posterolateral lumbar fusion: a technical report. *Spine J.* 2011;11:540-544.
440. Burkus JK, Heim SE, Gornet MF, Zdeblick TA. Is INFUSE bone graft superior to autograft bone? An integrated analysis of clinical trials using the LT-CAGE lumbar tapered fusion device. *J Spinal Disord Tech.* 2003;16:113-122.
441. Burkus JK. Bone morphogenetic proteins in anterior lumbar interbody fusion: old techniques and new technologies. Invited submission from the Joint Section Meeting on Disorders of the Spine and Peripheral Nerves, March 2004. *J Neurosurg Spine.* 2004;1:254-260.
442. Siemionow K, Sundberg E, Tyrakowski M, Nandyala SV, Singh K. Point-counter-point debate: the association between recombinant human bone morphogenetic protein utilization and complications in spine surgery. *Curr Rev Musculoskelet Med.* 2014;7:200-207.
443. Mroz T, Abdullah K, Benzel E. Commentary: Retrograde ejaculation and the use of rhBMP-2 for anterior lumbar interbody fusion: what does the evidence say to surgeons and to patients? *Spine J.* 2012;12:891-893.
444. Branch C, Branch C. Posterior lumbar interbody fusion with the keystone graft: technique and results. *Surg Neurol.* 1987;27:449-454.
445. Miura Y, Imagama S, Yoda M, Mitsuguchi H, Kachi H. Is local bone viable as a source of bone graft in posterior lumbar interbody fusion? *Spine.* 2003;28:2386-2389.
446. Ito Z, Matsuyama Y, Sakai Y, et al. Bone union rate with autologous iliac bone versus local bone graft in posterior lumbar interbody fusion. *Spine.* 2010;35:E1101-E1105.
447. Kim D-H, Jeong S-T, Lee S-S. Posterior lumbar interbody fusion using a unilateral single cage and a local morselized bone graft in the degenerative lumbar spine. *Clin Orthop Surg.* 2009;1:214-221.
448. Boakye M, Mummaneni PV, Garrett M, Rodts G, Haid R. Anterior cervical discectomy and fusion involving a polyetheretherketone spacer and bone morphogenetic protein. *J Neurosurg Spine.* 2005;2:521-525.
449. Schenker M. Building better bone: the weaving of biologic and engineering strategies for managing bone loss. Bone graft and bone graft substitutes. *Progr Book, Annu Meet Orthop Res Soc.* 2016;34.
450. Vavken J, Vavken P, Mameghani A, Schaeren S. Union rate and complications in spine fusion with recombinant human bone morphogenetic protein-7: systematic review and meta-analysis. *Global Spine J.* 2016;6:124-132.
451. Epstein NE. Pros, cons, and costs of INFUSE in spinal surgery. *Surg Neurol Int.* 2011;2:10.
452. Michielsen J, Sys J, Rigaux A, Bertrand C. The effect of recombinant human bone. *J Bone Joint Surg Am.* 2013;873-880.
453. Carragee E, Mitsunaga K, Hurwitz E, Scuderi G. Retrograde ejaculation after anterior lumbar interbody fusion using rhBMP-2: a cohort controlled study. *Spine J.* 2011;11: 511-516.
454. Glassman S, Gum J, Crawford C, Shields C, Carreon L. Complications with recombinant human bone morphogenetic protein-2 in posterolateral spine fusion associated with a dural tear. *Spine J.* 2011;11:522-526.
455. Mannion R, Nowitzke A, Wood M. Promoting fusion in minimally invasive lumbar interbody stabilization with low-dose bone morphogenic protein-2—but what is the cost? *Spine J.* 2011;11:527533.
456. Joseph V, Rampersaud YR. Heterotopic bone formation with the use of rhBMP2 in posterior minimal access interbody fusion: a CT analysis. *Spine.* 2007;32:2885-2890.
457. Helgeson M, Lehman R, Patzkowski J, et al. Adjacent vertebral body osteolysis with bone morphogenetic protein use in transforaminal lumbar interbody fusion. *Spine J.* 2011;11:507-510.
458. Medtronic's AMPLIFY rhBMP-2 Matrix. *Food Drug Administration Executive Summary.* Available at https://www.fda.gov/AdvisoryCommittees/Calendar/ucm217433.htm.
459. Dmitriev AE, Farhang S, Lehman RA, Ling GSF, Symes AJ. Bone morphogenetic protein-2 used in spinal fusion with spinal cord injury penetrates intrathecally and elicits a functional signaling cascade. *Spine J.* 2010;10:16-25.
460. Dmitriev AAE, Lehman RRA, Symes AAJ. Bone morphogenetic protein-2 and spinal arthrodesis: the basic science perspective on protein interaction with the nervous system. *Spine J.* 2011;11:500-505.
461. Stuesse SL, Crisp T, McBurney DL, et al. Neuropathic pain in aged rats: behavioral responses and astrocytic activation. *Exp Brain Res.* 2001;137:219-227.
462. Rihn JA, Makda J, Hong J, et al. The use of RhBMP-2 in single-level transforaminal lumbar interbody fusion: a clinical and radiographic analysis. *Eur Spine J.* 2009;18:1629-1636.
463. Gordon T, Brushart TM, Amirjani N, Chan KM. The potential of electrical stimulation to promote functional recovery after peripheral nerve injury—comparisons between rats and humans. *Acta Neurochir Suppl.* 2007;100:3-11.
464. Deleted in review.
465. Dmitriev AE, Lehman RA, Symes AJ. Bone morphogenetic protein-2 and spinal arthrodesis: the basic science perspective on protein interaction with the nervous system. *Spine J.* 2011;11:500-505.
466. Noshchenko A, Hoffecker L, Lindley EM, et al. Perioperative and long-term clinical outcomes for bone morphogenetic protein versus iliac crest bone graft for lumbar fusion in degenerative disk disease: systematic review with meta-analysis. *J Spinal Disord Tech.* 2014;27:117-135.
467. Atkins D, Briss PA, Eccles M, et al. Systems for grading the quality of evidence and the strength of recommendations II: pilot study of a new system. *BMC Health Serv Res.* 2005;5:25.
468. Liberati A, Altman DG, Tetzlaff J, et al. The PRISMA statement for reporting systematic reviews and meta-analyses of studies that evaluate health care interventions: explanation and elaboration. *Ann Intern Med.* 2009;151:W65-W94.
469. Malham GM, Parker RM, Ellis NJ, et al. Anterior lumbar interbody fusion using recombinant human bone morphogenetic protein-2: a prospective study of complications. *J Neurosurg Spine.* 2014;21:851-860.
470. FDA: *Summary of Safety and Effectiveness Data for InFUSE Bone Graft for Spinal Fusion Procedures.* Available at https://www.accessdata.fda.gov/cdrh_docs/pdf/P000058b.pdf.

471. Burkus JK, Dryer RF, Peloza JH. Retrograde ejaculation following single-level anterior lumbar surgery with or without recombinant human bone morphogenetic protein-2 in 5 randomized controlled trials: clinical article. *J Neurosurg Spine*. 2013;18:112-121.
472. Mesfin A, Buchowski JM, Zebala LP, et al. High-dose rhBMP-2 for adults: major and minor complications. *J Bone Joint Surg Am*. 2013;95:1546.
473. Zimmerman RM, Mohamed AS, Skolasky RL, Robinson MD, Kebaish KM. Functional outcomes and complications after primary spinal surgery for scoliosis in adults aged forty years or older: a prospective study with minimum two-year follow-up. *Spine*. 2010;35:1861-1866.
474. Cho SK, Bridwell KH, Lenke LG, et al. Major complications in revision adult deformity surgery: risk factors and clinical outcomes with 2- to 7-year follow-up. *Spine*. 2012;37: 489-500.
475. Hassanzadeh H, Jain A, El Dafrawy MH, et al. Clinical results and functional outcomes of primary and revision spinal deformity surgery in adults. *J Bone Joint Surg Am*. 2013;95:1413-1419.
476. Mesfin A, Buchowski JM, Zebala LP, et al. High-dose rhBMP-2 for adults: major and minor complications: a study of 502 spine cases. *J Bone Joint Surg Am*. 2013;95(17):1546-1553.
477. Rihn JA, Currier BL, Phillips FM, Glassman SD, Albert TJ. Defining the value of spine care. *J Am Acad Orthop Surg*. 2013;21:419-426.
478. Mindea SA, Shih P, Song JK. Recombinant human bone morphogenetic protein-2-induced radiculitis in elective minimally invasive transforaminal lumbar interbody fusions: a series review. *Spine*. 2009;34:1480-1484.
479. Carragee EJ, Chu G, Rohatgi R, et al. Cancer risk after use of recombinant bone morphogenetic protein-2 for spinal arthrodesis. *J Bone Joint Surg Am*. 2013;95:1537-1545.
480. Cooper GS, Kou TD. Risk of cancer after lumbar fusion surgery with recombinant human bone morphogenic protein-2 (rh-BMP-2). *Spine*. 2013;38:1862-1868.
481. Howlander N, Noone A, Krapcho M, et al. *SEER Cancer Statistics Review, 1975-2009*. Bethesda, MD: National Cancer Institute; 2011.
482. Fu R, Selph S, McDonagh M, et al. Effectiveness and harms of recombinant human bone morphogenetic protein-2 in spine fusion: a systematic review and meta-analysis. *Ann Intern Med*. 2013;158:890-902.
483. Deleted in review.
484. Simmonds MC, Brown JVE, Heirs MK, et al. Review: safety and effectiveness of recombinant human bone morphogenetic protein-2 for spinal fusion. A meta-analysis of individual-participant data. *Ann Intern Med*. 2013;158:877-889.
485. Carragee EJ, Hurwitz EL, Weiner BK. A critical review of recombinant human bone morphogenetic protein-2 trials in spinal surgery: emerging safety concerns and lessons learned. *Spine J*. 2011;11:471-491.
486. Tannoury CA, An HS. Complications with the use of bone morphogenetic protein 2 (BMP-2) in spine surgery. *Spine J*. 2014;14:552-559.
487. Thawani JP, Wang AC, Than KD, et al. Bone morphogenetic proteins and cancer: review of the literature. *Neurosurgery*. 2010;66:233-246.
488. Cahill KS, McCormick PC, Levi AD. A comprehensive assessment of the risk of bone morphogenetic protein use in spinal fusion surgery and postoperative cancer diagnosis. *J Neurosurg Spine*. 2015;23:1-8.
489. Kelly MP, Savage JW, Bentzen SM, et al. Cancer risk from bone morphogenetic protein exposure in spinal arthrodesis. *J Bone Joint Surg Am*. 2014;96:1417-1422.
490. Lad SP, Bagley JH, Karikari IO, et al. Cancer after spinal fusion: the role of bone morphogenetic protein. *Neurosurgery*. 2013;73:440-449.
491. Vavken J, Mameghani A, Vavken P, Schaeren S. Complications and cancer rates in spine fusion with recombinant human bone morphogenetic protein-2 (rhBMP-2). *Eur Spine J*. 2016;25(12):3979-3989.
492. Malham GM, Giles GG, Milne RL, Blecher CM, Brazenor GA. Bone Morphogenetic Proteins in Spinal Surgery: What Is the Fusion Rate and Do They Cause Cancer? *Spine*. 2015;40:1737-1742.
493. Takigami H, Latson L, Togawa D, et al. *Bone formation following OP-1 implantation is improved by addition of autogenous bone marrow*. Presented at the American Society of Bone Mineral Research 25th Annual Meeting; 2003.
494. Takigami H, Kumagai K, Latson L, et al. Bone formation following OP-1 implantation is improved by addition of autogenous bone marrow cells in a canine femur defect model. *J Orthop Res*. 2007;25:1333-1342.
495. Arteaga-Solis E, Gayraud B, Lee SY, et al. Regulation of limb patterning by extracellular microfibrils. *J Cell Biol*. 2001;154:275-281.
496. Larraín J, Oelgeschläger M, Ketpura NI, et al. Proteolytic cleavage of Chordin as a switch for the dual activities of Twisted gastrulation in BMP signaling. *Development*. 2001;128:4439-4447.
497. Ohkawara B, Iemura S, ten Dijke P, Ueno N. Action range of BMP is defined by its N-terminal basic amino acid core. *Curr Biol*. 2002;12:205-209.
498. Issa JPM, Bentley MVLB, Iyomasa MM, Sebald W, De Albuquerque RF. Sustained release carriers used to delivery bone morphogenetic proteins in the bone healing process. *Anat Histol Embryol*. 2008;37:181-187.
499. Akamaru T, Suh D, Boden SD, et al. Simple carrier matrix modifications can enhance delivery of recombinant human bone morphogenetic protein-2 for posterolateral spine fusion. *Spine*. 2003;28:429-434.
500. Minamide A, Kawakami M, Hashizume H, Sakata R, Tamaki T. Evaluation of carriers of bone morphogenetic protein for spinal fusion. *Spine*. 2001;26:933-939.
501. Seeherman H, Wozney J, Li R. Bone morphogenetic protein delivery systems. *Spine*. 2002;27:S16-S23.
502. Scott TP, Phan KH, Tian H, et al. Comparison of a novel oxysterol molecule and rhBMP2 fusion rates in a rabbit posterolateral lumbar spine model. *Spine J*. 2015;15: 733-742.
503. Alvarez LM, Rivera JJ, Stockdale L, et al. Tethering of epidermal growth factor (EGF) to beta tricalcium phosphate (βTCP) via fusion to a high affinity, multimeric βTCP-binding peptide: effects on human multipotent stromal cells/connective tissue progenitors. *PLoS One*. 2015;10:e0129600.
504. Louis-Ugbo J, Kim H-S, Boden SD, et al. Retention of 125I-labeled recombinant human bone morphogenetic protein-2 by biphasic calcium phosphate or a composite sponge in a rabbit posterolateral spine arthrodesis model. *J Orthop Res*. 2002;20:1050-1059.

505. Uludag H, D'Augusta D, Golden J, et al. Implantation of recombinant human bone morphogenetic proteins with biomaterial carriers: a correlation between protein pharmacokinetics and osteoinduction in the rat ectopic model. *J Biomed Mater Res.* 2000;50:227-238.
506. Ruhe PQ, Hedberg EL, Padron NT, et al. rhBMP-2 release from injectable poly(DL-lactic-co-glycolic acid)/calcium-phosphate cement composites. *J Bone Joint Surg Am.* 2003;85A(suppl):75-81.
507. Seeherman H, Li R, Wozney J. A review of preclinical program development for evaluating injectable carriers for osteogenic factors. *J Bone Joint Surg Am.* 2003;85A(suppl):96-108.
508. Brekke JH, Toth JM. Principles of tissue engineering applied to programmable osteogenesis. *J Biomed Mater Res.* 1998;43:380-398.
509. Rosen V. *Growth factors involved in bone formation and repair.* Proceedings of the Pittsburgh Bone Symposium; 2003.
510. Zachos TA, Bertone AL. Growth factors and their potential therapeutic applications for healing of musculoskeletal and other connective tissues. *Am J Vet Res.* 2005;66:727-738.
511. Daniels TR, Younger ASE, Penner MJ, et al. Prospective randomized controlled trial of hindfoot and ankle fusions treated with rhPDGF-BB in combination with a β-TCP-collagen matrix. *Foot Ankle Int.* 2015;36:739-748.
512. DiGiovanni CW, Lin SS, Baumhauer JF, et al. Recombinant human platelet-derived growth factor-BB and beta-tricalcium phosphate (rhPDGF-BB/β-TCP): an alternative to autogenous bone graft. *J Bone Joint Surg Am.* 2013;95:1184-1192.
513. Radomsky ML, Aufdemorte TB, Swain LD, et al. Novel formulation of fibroblast growth factor-2 in a hyaluronan gel accelerates fracture healing in nonhuman primates. *J Orthop Res.* 1999;17:607-614.
514. Folkman J. Seminars in Medicine of the Beth Israel Hospital, Boston. Clinical applications of research on angiogenesis. *N Engl J Med.* 1995;333:1757-1763.
515. Zelzer E, McLean W, Ng Y-S, et al. Skeletal defects in VEGF(120/120) mice reveal multiple roles for VEGF in skeletogenesis. *Development.* 2002;129:1893-1904.
516. Bouletreau PJ, Warren SM, Spector JA, et al. Hypoxia and VEGF up-regulate BMP-2 mRNA and protein expression in microvascular endothelial cells: implications for fracture healing. *Plast Reconstr Surg.* 2002;109:2384-2397.
517. Eckardt H, Bundgaard KG, Christensen KS, et al. Effects of locally applied vascular endothelial growth factor (VEGF) and VEGF-inhibitor to the rabbit tibia during distraction osteogenesis. *J Orthop Res.* 2003;21:335-340.
518. Kempen DHR, Lu L, Heijink A, et al. Effect of local sequential VEGF and BMP-2 delivery on ectopic and orthotopic bone regeneration. *Biomaterials.* 2009;30:2816-2825.
519. Peng H, Wright V, Usas A, et al. Synergistic enhancement of bone formation and healing by stem cell-expressed VEGF and bone morphogenetic protein-4. *J Clin Invest.* 2002;110:751-759.
520. Bonewald LF, Mundy GR. Role of transforming growth factor beta in bone remodeling: a review. *Connect Tissue Res.* 1989;23:201-208.
521. Bonewald LF, Mundy GR. Role of transforming growth factor-beta in bone remodeling. *Clin Orthop Relat Res.* 1990;261-276.
522. Pfeilschifter J, Wolf O, Naumann A, et al. Chemotactic response of osteoblastlike cells to transforming growth factor beta. *J Bone Miner Res.* 1990;5:825-830.
523. Joyce ME, Roberts AB, Sporn MB, Bolander ME. Transforming growth factor-beta and the initiation of chondrogenesis and osteogenesis in the rat femur. *J Cell Biol.* 1990;110:2195-2207.
524. Baylink DJ, Finkelman RD, Mohan S. Growth factors to stimulate bone formation. *J Bone Miner Res.* 1993;8(suppl 2):S565-S572.
525. Canalis E. The hormonal and local regulation of bone formation. *Endocr Rev.* 1983;4:62-77.
526. Kandziora F, Pflugmacher R, Scholz M, et al. Dose-dependent effects of combined IGF-I and TGF-beta1 application in a sheep cervical spine fusion model. *Eur Spine J.* 2003;12:464-473.
527. Kandziora F, Schmidmaier G, Schollmeier G, et al. IGF-I and TGF-beta1 application by a poly-(D,L-lactide)-coated cage promotes intervertebral bone matrix formation in the sheep cervical spine. *Spine.* 2002;27:1710-1723.
528. Kunakornsawat S, Kirinpanu A, Piyaskulkaew C, Sathira-Angkura V. A comparative study of radiographic results using HEALOS collagen-hydroxyapatite sponge with bone marrow aspiration versus local bone graft in the same patients undergoing posterolateral lumbar fusion. *J Med Assoc Thai.* 2013;96:929-935.
529. Khan SN, Tomin E, Lane JM. Clinical applications of bone graft substitutes. *Orthop Clin North Am.* 2000;31:389-398.
530. Lane JM, Sandhu HS. Current approaches to experimental bone grafting. *Orthop Clin North Am.* 1987;18:213-225.
531. Palecek SP, Loftus JC, Ginsberg MH, Lauffenburger DA, Horwitz AF. Integrin-ligand binding properties govern cell migration speed through cell-substratum adhesiveness. *Nature.* 1997;385:537-540.
532. Termine J, Kleinman H, Whitson S. Osteonectin, a bone-specific protein linking mineral to collagen. *Cell.* 1981;26:99-105.
533. Nawrot C, Campbell D, Schroeder J. Dental phosphoprotein-induced formation of hydroxylapatite during in vitro synthesis of amorphous calcium phosphate. *Biochemistry.* 1976;15:3445-3449.
534. Stanford C, Jacobson P, Eanes E. Rapidly forming apatitic mineral in an osteoblastic cell line (UMR 106-01 BSP). *J Biol Chem.* 1995;270:9420-9428.
535. Hughes D, Salter D, Dedhar S. Integrin expression in human bone. *J Bone Miner Res.* 1993;8:527-533.
536. Saito T, Albelda S, Brighton C. Identification of integrin receptors on cultured human bone cells. *J Orthop Res.* 1994;12:384-394.
537. Weiss R, Reddi A. Role of fibronectin in collagenous matrix-induced mesenchymal cell proliferation and differentiation in vivo. *Exp Cell Res.* 1981;133:247-254.
538. Mundy G, Poser J. Chemotactic activity of the gamma-carboxyglutamic acid containing protein in bone. *Calcif Tissue Int.* 1983;35:164-168.
539. Jarcho M. Calcium phosphate ceramics as hard tissue prosthetics. *Clin Orthop.* 1981;259-278.
540. Jarcho M, Kay J, Gumaer K. Tissue, cellular and subcellular events at a bone-ceramic hydroxylapatite interface. *J Bioeng.* 1977;1:79-92.
541. Profeta AC, Huppa C. Bioactive-glass in oral and maxillofacial surgery. *Craniomaxillofac Trauma Reconstr.* 2016;9:1-14.
542. Denissen HW, de Groot K. Immediate dental root implants from synthetic dense calcium hydroxylapatite. *J Prosthet Dent.* 1979;42:551-556.

543. Costantino PD, Hiltzik D, Govindaraj S, Moche J. Bone healing and bone substitutes. *Facial Plast Surg.* 2002;18: 13-26.
544. Atkinson PJ, Roberts EW, Khudayer ZM. Porous ceramic materials as immediate root implants. *J Dent.* 1984;12:189-202.
545. Samavedi S, Whittington AR, Goldstein AS. Calcium phosphate ceramics in bone tissue engineering: a review of properties and their influence on cell behavior. *Acta Biomater.* 2013;9:8037-8045.
546. Montazerian M, Zanotto ED. Bioactive and inert dental glass-ceramics. *J Biomed Mater Res A.* 2017;105(2):619-639.
547. Glowacki J. Demineralized Bone and BMPs: Basic science and clinical utility. *J Oral Maxillofac Surg.* 2015;73:S126-S131.
548. Klawitter J, Hulbert S. Application of porous ceramics for the attachment of load bearing orthopaedic applications. *J Biomed Mater Res.* 1971;2:161.
549. Klawitter JJ, Weinstein AM. The status of porous materials to obtain direct skeletal attachment by tissue ingrowth. *Acta Orthop Belg.* 1974;40:755-765.
550. Hoogendoorn HA, Renooij W, Akkermans LM, Visser W, Wittebol P. Long-term study of large ceramic implants (porous hydroxyapatite) in dog femora. *Clin Orthop Relat Res.* 1984;281-288.
551. Ricci JL, Spivak JM, Alexander H, Blumenthal NC, Parsons JR. Hydroxyapatite ceramics and the nature of the bone-ceramic interface. *Bull Hosp Jt Dis Orthop Inst.* 1989;49:178-191.
552. Ragni P, Lindholm TS. Interaction of allogeneic demineralized bone matrix and porous hydroxyapatite bioceramics in lumbar interbody fusion in rabbits. *Clin Orthop Relat Res.* 1991;292-299.
553. Cornell CN, Lane JM. Current understanding of osteoconduction in bone regeneration. *Clin Orthop Relat Res.* 1998;S267-S273.
554. Takigami H, Kumagai K, Latson L, et al. Bone formation following OP-1 implantation is improved by addition of autogenous bone marrow cells in a canine femur defect model. *J Orthop Res.* 2007;25:1333-1342.
555. Cameron HU, Macnab I, Pilliar RM. Evaluation of biodegradable ceramic. *J Biomed Mater Res.* 1977;11: 179-186.
556. Bhaskar SN, Brady JM, Getter L, Grower MF, Driskell T. Biodegradable ceramic implants in bone. Electron and light microscopic analysis. *Oral Surg Oral Med Oral Pathol.* 1971;32:336-346.
557. Ohgushi H, Goldberg VM, Caplan AI. Heterotopic osteogenesis in porous ceramics induced by marrow cells. *J Orthop Res.* 1989;7:568-578.
558. Constantz BR, Ison IC, Fulmer MT, et al. Skeletal repair by in situ formation of the mineral phase of bone. *Science.* 1995;267:1796-1799.
559. Dai L-Y, Jiang L-S. Single-level instrumented posterolateral fusion of lumbar spine with beta-tricalcium phosphate versus autograft: a prospective, randomized study with 3-year follow-up. *Spine.* 2008;33:1299-1304.
560. Chen W-J, Tsai T-T, Chen L-H, et al. The fusion rate of calcium sulfate with local autograft bone compared with autologous iliac bone graft for instrumented short-segment spinal fusion. *Spine.* 2005;30:2293-2297.
561. Acharya NK, Kumar RJ, Varma HK, Menon VK. Hydroxyapatite-bioactive glass ceramic composite as stand-alone graft substitute for posterolateral fusion of lumbar spine: a prospective, matched, and controlled study. *J Spinal Disord Tech.* 2008;21:106-111.
562. Epstein NE. An analysis of noninstrumented posterolateral lumbar fusions performed in predominantly geriatric patients using lamina autograft and beta tricalcium phosphate. *Spine J.* 2008;8:882-887.
563. Gan Y, Dai K, Zhang P, et al. The clinical use of enriched bone marrow stem cells combined with porous beta-tricalcium phosphate in posterior spinal fusion. *Biomaterials.* 2008;29:3973-3982.
564. Nickoli MS, Hsu WK. Ceramic-based bone grafts as a bone grafts extender for lumbar spine arthrodesis: a systematic review. *Global Spine J.* 2014;4:211-216.
565. Kaiser MG, Groff MW, Watters WC, et al. Guideline update for the performance of fusion procedures for degenerative disease of the lumbar spine. Part 16: bone graft extenders and substitutes as an adjunct for lumbar fusion. *J Neurosurg Spine.* 2014;21:106-132.
566. Einhorn TA, Bonnarens F, Burstein AH. The contributions of dietary protein and mineral to the healing of experimental fractures. A biomechanical study. *J Bone Joint Surg Am.* 1986;68:1389-1395.
567. Dickhaut SC, DeLee JC, Page CP. Nutritional status: importance in predicting wound-healing after amputation. *J Bone Joint Surg Am.* 1984;66:71-75.
568. Jensen JE, Jensen TG, Smith TK, Johnston DA, Dudrick SJ. Nutrition in orthopaedic surgery. *J Bone Joint Surg Am.* 1982;64:1263-1272.
569. Lenke LG, Bridwell KH, Blanke K, Baldus C. Prospective analysis of nutritional status normalization after spinal reconstructive surgery. *Spine.* 1995;20:1359-1367.
570. Coventry MB, Scanlon PW. The use of radiation to discourage ectopic bone. A nine-year study in surgery about the hip. *J Bone Joint Surg Am.* 1981;63:201-208.
571. Nilsson OS, Bauer HC, Brostrom LA. Comparison of the effects of adriamycin and methotrexate on orthotopic and induced heterotopic bone in rats. *J Orthop Res.* 1990;8:199-204.
572. Wing KJ, Fisher CG, O'Connell JX, Wing PC. Stopping nicotine exposure before surgery. The effect on spinal fusion in a rabbit model. *Spine.* 2000;25:30-34.
573. Theiss SM, Boden SD, Hair G, et al. The effect of nicotine on gene expression during spine fusion. *Spine.* 2000;25:2588-2594.
574. Silcox DH, Daftari T, Boden SD, et al. The effect of nicotine on spinal fusion. *Spine.* 1995;20:1549-1553.
575. Patel TC, Erulkar JS, Grauer JN, et al. Osteogenic protein-1 overcomes the inhibitory effect of nicotine on posterolateral lumbar fusion. *Spine.* 2001;26:1656-1661.
576. Glassman SD, Anagnost SC, Parker A, et al. The effect of cigarette smoking and smoking cessation on spinal fusion. *Spine.* 2000;25:2608-2615.
577. Andersen T, Christensen FB, Laursen M, et al. Smoking as a predictor of negative outcome in lumbar spinal fusion. *Spine.* 2001;26:2623-2628.
578. Lubelski D, Choma TJ, Steinmetz MP, Harrop JS, Mroz TE. Perioperative medical management of spine surgery patients with osteoporosis. *Neurosurgery.* 2015;77(suppl 4):S92-S97.
579. Muschler GF, Nitto H, Boehm CA, Easley KA. Age- and gender-related changes in the cellularity of human bone marrow and the prevalence of osteoblastic progenitors. *J Orthop Res.* 2001;19:117-125.

580. Aprin H, Bowen JR, MacEwen GD, Hall JE. Spine fusion in patients with spinal muscular atrophy. *J Bone Joint Surg Am.* 1982;64:1179-1187.
581. Bunch W. Muscular dystrophy. *Spinal Deform Neurol Muscular Disord.* 1974;92-110.
582. Swank SM, Brown JC, Perry RE. Spinal fusion in Duchenne's muscular dystrophy. *Spine (Phila Pa 1976).* 1982;7:484-491.
583. Clark CR, Keggi KJ, Panjabi MM. Methylmethacrylate stabilization of the cervical spine. *J Bone Joint Surg Am.* 1984;66:40-46.
584. Bouchard JA, Koka A, Bensusan JS, Stevenson S, Emery SE. Effects of irradiation on posterior spinal fusions. A rabbit model. *Spine.* 1994;19:1836-1841.
585. Emery SE, Brazinski MS, Koka A, Bensusan JS, Stevenson S. The biological and biomechanical effects of irradiation on anterior spinal bone grafts in a canine model. *J Bone Joint Surg Am.* 1994;76:540-548.
586. Emery SE, Hughes SS, Junglas WA, Herrington SJ, Pathria MN. The fate of anterior vertebral bone grafts in patients irradiated for neoplasm. *Clin Orthop Relat Res.* 1994;207-212.
587. Junming M, Cheng Y, Dong C, et al. Giant cell tumor of the cervical spine: a series of 22 cases and outcomes. *Spine.* 2008;33:280-288.
588. Bassett CA, Mitchell SN, Gaston SR. Treatment of ununited tibial diaphyseal fractures with pulsing electromagnetic fields. *J Bone Joint Surg Am.* 1981;63:511-523.
589. Paterson D. Treatment of nonunion with a constant direct current: a totally implantable system. *Orthop Clin North Am.* 1984;15:47-59.
590. Bassett CA, Pilla AA, Pawluk RJ. A non-operative salvage of surgically-resistant pseudarthroses and non-unions by pulsing electromagnetic fields. A preliminary report. *Clin Orthop Relat Res.* 1977;128-143.
591. Bassett CA, Mitchell SN, Gaston SR. Pulsing electromagnetic field treatment in ununited fractures and failed arthrodeses. *JAMA.* 1982;247:623-628.
592. Bassett CA. The development and application of pulsed electromagnetic fields (PEMFs) for ununited fractures and arthrodeses. *Orthop Clin North Am.* 1984;15:61-87.
593. Toth JM, Seim HB, Schwardt JD, et al. Direct current electrical stimulation increases the fusion rate of spinal fusion cages. *Spine.* 2000;25:2580-2587.
594. Kahanovitz N, Arnoczky SP, Hulse D, Shires PK. The effect of postoperative electromagnetic pulsing on canine posterior spinal fusions. *Spine.* 1984;9:273-279.
595. MacEwan MR, Talcott MR, Moran DW, Leuthardt EC. Novel spinal instrumentation to enhance osteogenesis and fusion: a preliminary study. *J Neurosurg Spine.* 2016;1-10. doi:10.3171/2016.1.SPINE13979.
596. Hodges SD, Eck JC, Humphreys SC. Use of electrical bone stimulation in spinal fusion. *J Am Acad Orthop Surg.* 2003;11:81-88.
597. Kucharzyk DW. A controlled prospective outcome study of implantable electrical stimulation with spinal instrumentation in a high-risk spinal fusion population. *Spine.* 1999;24:465-468.
598. Nerubay J, Marganit B, Bubis JJ, Tadmor A, Katznelson A. Stimulation of bone formation by electrical current on spinal fusion. *Spine.* 1986;11:167-169.
599. Simmons JW. Treatment of failed posterior lumbar interbody fusion (PLIF) of the spine with pulsing electromagnetic fields. *Clin Orthop Relat Res.* 1985;127-132.
600. Linovitz RJ, Pathria M, Bernhardt M, et al. Combined magnetic fields accelerate and increase spine fusion: a double-blind, randomized, placebo controlled study. *Spine.* 2002;27:1383-1389.
601. Goodwin CB, Brighton CT, Guyer RD, et al. A double-blind study of capacitively coupled electrical stimulation as an adjunct to lumbar spinal fusions. *Spine.* 1999;24:1349-1356.
602. Lee T-C, Huang H-Y, Yang Y-L, et al. Application of extracorporeal shock wave treatment to enhance spinal fusion: a rabbit experiment. *Surg Neurol.* 2008;70:129-134.
603. Lee T-C, Wang C-J, Yang Y-L, et al. Bone morphogenetic protein-2 expression in spinal fusion masses enhanced by extracorporeal shock wave treatment: a rabbit experiment. *Acta Neurochir (Wien).* 2010;152:1779-1784.
604. Fleming JE, Cornell CN, Muschler GF. Bone cells and matrices in orthopedic tissue engineering. *Orthop Clin North Am.* 2000;31:357-374.

SECTION IX

CHAPTER 67 Bone Substitutes: Basic Science and Clinical Applications

Jeffrey C. Wang
Zorica Buser

Spine disorders are one of the most common medical problems worldwide, with low back and cervical pain being among the top contributors to high disability rates.[1] Choosing the right treatment is very challenging due to the complexity of degenerative changes, patient comorbidities, and psychosocial factors. Spinal fusion is a common treatment for various conditions, including deformity, trauma, and degenerative disc disease with instability. Nonetheless, significant rates of pseudarthrosis (up to 26%) have been reported in the literature.[2] Advances in surgical techniques and instrumentation, a variety of biologics, and better knowledge of fusion biology have increased fusion rates, but symptomatic pseudarthrosis still occurs in 10% to 15% of cases.[3–7] Nonunion may result in poor clinical outcomes and extensive medical expenditure. New bone formation is essential to arthrodesis of the spine and is heavily influenced by the local bone environment and grafting substitutes.

Successful grafting materials require three essential components: an osteogenic potential capable of directly providing mature osteoblasts and stem cells that will drive new bone formation, osteoinductive factors that are able to signal the osteoblastic differentiation of osteoprogenitor stem cells, and an osteoconductive scaffold that assists neovascularization and supports the ingrowth of bone. In addition to these properties, the ideal bone substitute should be without risks of disease transmission. Autologous bone grafts are the only grafting materials that possess all three properties; they can provide immediate and long-term mechanical stability, and are therefore considered the standard. Autogenous grafts can be divided into two groups: local bone (laminae, spinous processes, or facet joints) and extraspinal material (iliac crest bone graft [ICBG]). Local bone is a cortical bone graft in which cell migration is decreased due to small pore size. ICBG, on the other hand, is cancellous bone that provides a great environment for rapid new bone formation but lacks the ability to withstand compressive loading. Both grafting materials have similar fusion rates in single-level fusions; however, it has been shown that ICBG outperforms local autograft for multilevel fusions.[8] The main challenges with both grafting materials are bone quality, particularly in older patients, and the amount of autograft needed for long-segment fusions or revision surgeries. Furthermore, ICBG harvesting is associated with considerable donor site morbidity, increased operative time, and increased blood loss.[9] Up to 30% of all patients undergoing the harvesting of ICBG will experience significant postoperative pain or complications including infection, hematoma, nerve or vascular injury, fracture, persistent pain, abdominal herniation, or pelvic instability.[4,5,10–23] Some older studies report autologous bone graft harvest to be associated with major complications in 8.6% of patients and minor complications in 20.6%.[19] For these reasons, other grafting materials were developed to augment, expand, or substitute for autogenous bone grafts.

In order to avoid morbidity associated with harvesting autogenous graft and to optimize bone formation for fusion, several classes of bone substitutes have been developed. These include allografts, ceramics, demineralized bone matrices (DBMs), osteoinductive factors and bone marrow aspirates (BMAs), autogenous platelet concentrate, mesenchymal stem cells, and gene therapy (Table 67.1). Although bone substitutes do not provide the same osteogenic, osteoinductive, and osteoconductive properties as autografts, various grafting materials have demonstrated efficiency for bone formation in basic science and clinical studies. Furthermore, advances in the understanding of bone remodeling, the development of osteoinductive proteins and small molecules, and the synthesis of new osteoconductive carriers hold a promising future for biologic treatments of spinal conditions.

Allografts

Allografts are composed of cadaveric bone and have been employed traditionally as bone graft extenders. Allografts have good osteoconductive and minimal osteoinductive properties; however, they lack growth factors and osteogenic cells due to the processing that they undergo in order to decrease their antigenicity. Allograft bone may be applied to the graft bed in a crushed particulate form or can be formulated to create structural spacers. Cortical allografts offer substantial structural

TABLE 67.1 Properties of Bone Substitutes

Bone Graft Substitute	Osteogenic Cells	Osteoinductive Factors	Osteoconductive Matrix	Initial Biomechanical Strength	Donor Site Morbidity
Autogenous bone, cancellous	+++	++	+++	–	++
Autogenous bone, cortical	+	+	+	+++	++
Allograft, frozen	–	+	+	++	–
Allograft, lyophilization	–	+	+	+	–
Ceramics	–	–	+++	+	–
Demineralized bone matrix	–	++	+	–	–
Osteoinductive growth factors	–	+++	–	–	+
Unfractionated bone marrow	++	+	–	–	+
Mesenchymal stem cells	+++	–	–	–	+
Autologous platelet concentrate	–	++	–	–	–
Gene therapy, in vivo	–	+++	–	–	–
Gene therapy, ex vivo	++	+++	–	–	+

–, none; +, low; ++, medium; +++, high.

stability and are best suited for interbody arthrodesis but suffer from increased graft resorption and slow bone remodeling. Corticocancellous allografts initially impart little mechanical support to the fusion site but, because of its relatively large surface area, are integrated more rapidly than cortical bone.[24,25] Genetic incompatibility between donor and recipient has been found to be associated with increased resorption of the allograft and histologic evidence of rejection.[26]

After the harvest, allograft bone undergoes debridement of soft tissue, removal of bacteria and viruses, and antibiotic bath. Preservation is achieved through freezing or freeze-drying in order to decrease its antigenicity and permit storage for extended periods of time.[27] Frozen allografts may be stored for up to 1 year. Freeze-drying reduces immunogenicity even more than freezing, but on rehydration, these grafts may lose up to 50% of their mechanical strength.[28] Other sterilization techniques, such as ethylene oxide or irradiation, may compromise the material properties and osteoinductive capacity or leave toxic residues behind.

Disease transmission is one of the main concerns with allografts, particularly viral diseases, such as human immunodeficiency virus and hepatitis. Nevertheless, there have been only two documented cases of human immunodeficiency virus transmission from allograft bone, both of which involved unprocessed grafts.[29] The combination of rigorous donor screening and tissue processing has lowered the risk of infection to less than one per million transplants.[30] A retrospective review of US Food and Drug Administration (FDA) data from 1994 to July 2007 found that 96.5% of all recalled allografts were musculoskeletal. Most were recalled between 2006 and 2007 because of improper donor evaluation.[31] Other complications observed after the implantation of structural allografts include nonunion and fracture of the graft due to the slower rates of incorporation.[32,33]

Structural allografts have been used extensively for anterior cervical discectomy and fusion (ACDF). Studies evaluating patients undergoing single-level ACDF with either allograft or autogenous bone have demonstrated similar fusion rates.[34,35] Furthermore, Jagannathan and colleagues reported 94% fusion rates for single-level ACDF with freeze-dried cortical allograft without plate fixation or postoperative rigid cervical collar.[35a] For two-level ACDFs, several studies reported higher fusion and lower nonunion rates with autografts compared to allografts.[36,37] Advances in plate fixation have increased the fusion rates in both single-level and multilevel ACDFs. Samartzis et al. noted similar fusion rates between allografts (94.3%) and autografts (100%) in two- and three-level ACDFs.[38]

In the posterior lumbar spine, autogenous bone graft appears to be superior to allograft for promoting posterolateral arthrodesis. Jorgenson and colleagues[39] conducted a prospective analysis of autografts versus allografts in posterolateral lumbar fusion in the same patient and concluded that ethylene oxide–treated allograft is inferior to autograft and should not be used for posterior lumbar fusions. Another prospective study of adult posterolateral lumbar spinal fusion reported that autografts alone or combined with allograft resulted in solid fusion in 80% and 50% of the cases, respectively. Freeze-dried allograft produced no solid fusions, and frozen allograft led to partial fusion in only 40% of the cases.[40] While allografts alone were not able to achieve a sufficient fusion rate for posterior spinal fusion, they contributed to solid fusion as bone extenders in adolescent idiopathic scoliosis. Jones and colleagues conducted a retrospective review of long-segment spinal fusion with cancellous freeze-dried allograft in patients with pediatric idiopathic scoliosis. They reported a 92.7% fusion rate and an average of 3.4 degrees of loss of curve correction at 39 months' follow-up.[41] A multicenter retrospective study with 111 patients undergoing spinal fusion for adolescent idiopathic scoliosis reported a 2.7% pseudarthrosis rate and 5.9 degrees loss of correction when freeze-dried allograft and autograft were used together.[42]

Additional studies have reported excellent outcomes with the use of femoral ring allografts in the anterior lumbar spine, with freeze-dried allografts having higher risk of nonunion compared to frozen allograft.[43–45] In cases involving revision anterior lumbar fusions, one study found that the results obtained with tricortical allograft may be comparable with those obtained with autogenous bone graft taken from the iliac crest.[46] Overall, these studies suggest that allografts may be efficacious alone or as graft extenders in anterior cervical and lumbar fusions and in patients with scoliosis deformities.

Ceramics

Ceramics are osteoconductive bone substitutes without cells and growth factors.[47] The most commonly used ceramic scaffolds for spinal fusion are calcium sulfates, silicate-substituted calcium phosphate, calcium phosphates (hydroxyapatite [HA], β-tricalcium phosphate [β-TCP]), or a combination of these materials. Ceramics are favorable bone substitutes because they are biodegradable, nontoxic, nonimmunogenic, easy to sterilize, and available in virtually unlimited supply without donor site morbidity or infection risk. The bioresorbability of a ceramic is influenced by the shape, density, and chemical composition of the material. HA is a relatively inert substance that is retained in vivo for prolonged periods of time, whereas the more porous tricalcium phosphate typically biodegrades in about 6 weeks.[48] When loaded with a source of osteogenic cells, such as autogenous bone or bone marrow, ceramic scaffolds assist cellular adhesion, support vascular ingrowth, and promote new bone formation.[49] Disadvantages of ceramic structures are their brittle structure and reduced shear strength and resistance to fracture. Because they offer minimal mechanical stability in the immediate postoperative period, ceramics are commonly used in conjunction with rigid internal fixation and must be protected from loading forces until they are incorporated into the surrounding bone.

With rigid instrumentation, several studies have reported that ceramic scaffolds are efficient bone graft extenders when used with the local bone in posterolateral spinal fusion.[50–52] In a prospective single-center study, patients underwent posterior lumbar interbody fusion (PLIF) or posterior lumbar fusion (PLF) with laminectomized bone chips and HA or ICBG.[53] At 12 months, the fusion rates were 86.7% in the HA group and 88.9% in the autograft group, with the average fusion mass volume being greater in the HA/local graft group. In a prospective PLF study done by Korovessis et al.,[54] patients were divided into three groups based on the grafting material: ICBG bilaterally, ICBG on one side and HA plus BMA and local autograft on the other side, and HA plus BMA plus local bone bilaterally. Solid intertransverse and posterior fusion was observed only in the ICBG group, deeming HA inappropriate as a stand-alone grafting material. Similar results were reported by Thalgott and colleagues,[55–57] who retrospectively evaluated the efficacy of coralline HA as a bone replacement in anterior interbody fusion in both the cervical and lumbar spine. Yoshii et al.[57a] reported positive results for HA as bone extender in ACDF. HA and percutaneously harvested trephine chips led to similar fusion rates as ICBG, had lower blood loss, and no donor site complications or fragmentation of the HA graft.

On the other hand, successful results have been reported for the implantation of ceramic scaffolds for posterior spinal fusion in scoliosis cases, which require extensive bone graft.[58–60] Ransford and colleagues[59] conducted a prospective randomized study to evaluate the use of a synthetic porous ceramic as a bone graft substitute in posterior spinal fusion for idiopathic scoliosis; they concluded that porous ceramic is a safe and effective bone substitute. Lerner and coworkers reported similar results with the use of β-TCP as a local bone extender in the posterior correction of adult idiopathic scoliosis.[60] They reported loss of correction for the β-TCP group of 2.6 degrees compared to 4.2 degrees in the ICBG group. Furthermore, β-TCP was shown to be a good bone extender in posterior lumbar fusion, achieving 100% fusion rates, as with ICBG at a 3-year follow-up.[61]

Calcium sulfate is another synthetic graft substitute. It was initially used as filler for traumatic bone defects or as an antibiotic carrier. It has been linked to increased wound and infection rates, however.[62] Furthermore, Niu et al. reported low fusion rates in patients on the side treated with calcium sulfate and BMA (41%) compared to the side treated with ICBG (91%).[63] Silicate-substituted calcium phosphate (SiCaP) has been shown to contain some osteogenic properties in addition to osteoconduction. However, data on the success of SiCaP in fusion is inconclusive. In a randomized clinical trial, SiCaP led to 100% fusion rates in patients undergoing PLIF for degenerative disc disease. The authors also reported that patients with SiCaP showed reduced back pain at 6 weeks and better quality-of-life measurements at 6 months compared to a recombinant human bone morphogenetic protein 2 (rhBMP2) group.[64] On the other hand, Nandyala and colleagues reported poor outcomes with SiCaP in minimally invasive transforaminal lumbar interbody fusion (TLIF). They recorded lower fusion rates (65%) and higher pseudarthosis rates (35%) with SiCaP when compared to rhBMP2.[65]

Ceramic carriers may also function as effective vehicles for the delivery of osteoinductive growth factors.

Demineralized Bone Matrices

DBMs are derived from allograft bone by removing the mineralized component and antigenic markers, thereby reducing its immunogenicity. DBMs have osteoconductive and some osteoinductive properties. The osteoconductive matrix consists of type I collagen, glycoproteins, calcium sulfate, and debris. The osteoinductive properties of DBMs were first recognized by Urist[66] in 1965, when he reported that the introduction of decalcified bone brought about the formation of heterotopic bone in rodents. The bone morphogenetic proteins (BMPs) represent less than 0.1% of all bone proteins by weight,[67] but these growth factors are essential to the process of osteoinduction, initiating a cascade of cellular events leading to bone formation. Other growth factors include bone sialoprotein, osteopontin, transforming growth factor-β (TGF-β), and insulin-like growth factor-1.[68] With aging, the levels of BMPs decrease; however, TGF-β and insulin-like growth factor-1 levels are not affected and extend

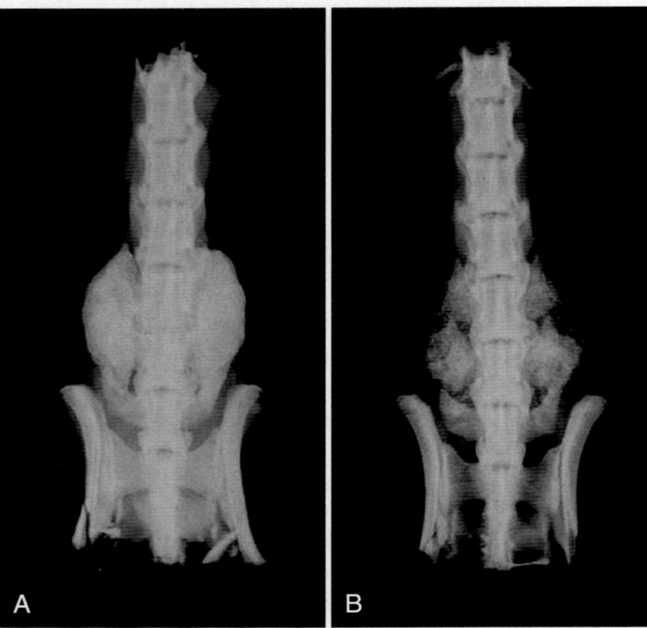

FIG. 67.1 Demineralized bone matrix (DBM) preparations possess variable osteoinductive activities. (A) Implantation of DBM induces an intertransverse spinal fusion in a rat model. (B) Implantation of another DBM does not result in a solid fusion, suggesting that there are significant differences in the osteoinductive potentials of commercially available DBM products.

osteoinduction via interaction with BMP proteins.[69] Commercially available DBMs have demonstrated marked variability in osteoinductive potential that may reflect differences in their BMP content in rat spinal fusion models (Fig. 67.1).[70–72]

Rabbit, dog, and nonhuman primate models of posterolateral spinal fusion have demonstrated good results with DBMs alone or in conjunction with autograft.[73–76] Clinical studies also support the efficacy of DBMs as bone graft extenders for posterolateral spinal fusion.[77,78] A composite consisting of DBM putty and aspirated bone marrow offers similar performance to autograft in posterolateral spinal fusion. A multicenter prospective study that compared the effectiveness of Grafton (Osteotech) DBM gel composite with iliac crest autograft in posterolateral spinal fusion demonstrated that Grafton DBM could extend a volume of autograft that was less than that normally required to achieve a solid spinal fusion.[79] DBM and bone marrow composite has been successful for posterior spinal fusion in scoliosis surgeries as well, and the fusion rates have been reported to be comparable with those of autograft.[80] One case series of anterior lumbar interbody fusions (ALIFs) with DBM composites consisting of titanium mesh cages, coralline HA, and DBM concluded that the DBM composite was effective for anterior interbody fusion of the lumbar spine when used as part of a rigidly instrumented circumferential fusion.[56] On the other hand, An and colleagues[81] prospectively compared the fusion rates of an allograft-DBM composite with autograft in anterior cervical fusion and concluded that the allograft-DBM construct resulted in a higher rate of graft collapse and pseudarthrosis than autograft alone. The low fusion rates reported in that study have prompted surgeons to look for an alternative in DBM delivery. Several studies conducted prospective evaluations of DBM with or without autograft packed into polyetherether ketone (PEEK) cages.[82,83] Park et al. observed 97% fusion rates in ACDF patients with DBM and local autograft packed in PEEK cages.[82] Moon and colleagues reported fusion in 77.8% of patients at a mean 25.5-months' follow-up in two-level ACDFs with PEEK cages packed with Grafton DBM without plate fixation. Regional alignment and cervical global alignment were improved postoperatively; however, 84% of the patients had some subsidence of the cages.[83]

In a direct comparison of multiple formulations of the same DBM, the putty and flexible sheet forms enhanced spinal fusion to a greater extent than a gel, most likely because the former are fiber-based preparations and exhibit improved handling characteristics over the gel form.[84] Apart from bone extenders, DBM was tested as a delivery vehicle for growth factors, cells, and antibiotics. In a rat PLF model, DBM with adenovirus carrying a *Nell-1* gene was implanted at L4–L5; at 6 weeks postoperatively, micro-CT demonstrated a 70% fusion rate.[85] High doses of Grafton DBM had a nephrotoxic effect in a rat model but not in human studies.[86]

Osteoinductive Growth Factors

Numerous growth factors capable of signaling cell-surface receptors and directing cellular activities are involved in the regeneration of bone tissue. In 1965, Urist[66] first observed that DBM possessed osteoinductive ability; subsequently, the osteoinductive BMPs were isolated and characterized. BMPs are members of the TGF-β superfamily. By binding to specific receptors present on the surface of the osteogenic progenitor, intracellular cascades that recapitulate endochondral ossification are activated. BMPs also stimulate mesenchymal stem cells to differentiate. Initially, BMPs were extracted from large amounts of bone: 10 kg of cortical bone yielded less than 20 g of osteoinductive protein.[87] In addition, these crude preparations contained a heterogeneous collection of growth factors, including several different types of BMPs, as well as other biologically inactive proteins.

With advantages in molecular biology, the genes encoding the BMP proteins were sequenced and subsequently cloned (recombinant DNA), allowing for the mass production of single BMPs, including BMP-2 and BMP-7 (also known as osteogenic protein-1 [OP-1]).[88] Because they are available in almost unlimited quantities, BMP-2 and BMP-7 have become the most widely used recombinant BMPs for animal studies and are the only BMPs currently being evaluated in human clinical trials. In contrast to purified extracts, recombinant growth factors are free of impurities and do not elicit a host immune response. Recombinant human BMPs (rhBMPs) are soluble factors that tend to diffuse away from the fusion site when used alone, resulting in attenuation of their osteoinductive capacity. For this reason, before implantation, these factors are combined with a carrier matrix that serves to restrict their movement, confine them to the location where they are needed, and allow them to release consistently over time. Current osteoinductive carriers used to deliver rhBMPs include autogenous bone graft, DBMs, collagen, ceramics, and polylactic acid.[88–100] Depending on the specific clinical application and the location into which the growth factors will be introduced, some carriers might be superior to others. Minamide et al. demonstrated in their rabbit lumbar fusion model that rhBMP-2 delivered onto bone cement coated with type I collagen had better fusion rates and more mature bone with higher tensile strength and stiffness than rhBMP-2 delivered onto a type I collagen sheet.[101] Multiple animal studies, many of which were performed in nonhuman primates, have established that the implantation of BMP-2 and BMP-7 in the posterior spine results in fusion rates equivalent to or superior to those obtained with autogenous bone graft. Furthermore, they may generate fusion masses with improved biomechanical properties that may obviate the need for decortication of the posterior elements, a procedure that is normally required to provide endogenous growth factors that are essential for successful posterolateral spine arthrodesis.[102] Boden and colleagues[103] conducted one of the first prospective randomized clinical pilot studies on the use of rhBMP-2 for posterolateral fusion in humans. In that study, the authors randomly divided the enrolled patients into three treatment groups, as follows: autograft with instrumentation, rhBMP-2/ceramic granules with instrumentation, and rhBMP-2/ceramic granules without instrumentation. They reported that the fusion rate of the rhBMP-2/ceramic granules without instrumentation group was 100%, which was superior to the autograft with instrumentation group (40%).[103] Following this pilot study, Dimar and colleagues[104] conducted a prospective randomized study comparing the use of ICBG to rhBMP-2 combined with a carrier (bovine collagen and tricalcium/HA) for single-level posterolateral fusions. Those authors reported that the rhBMP-2 group demonstrated increased fusion rates (91%) as compared with the autograft group (73%).[104] In another study, Boden and colleagues[105] described the human pilot trial of the use of rhBMP-2/collagen inside lumbar interbody spinal fusion cages. Although the number of patients enrolled in that study was small, they reported at the 2-year follow-up that fusion occurred more reliably in patients treated with rhBMP-2-filled cages than in controls treated with autogenous bone graft.[105] Burkus and colleagues also conducted a prospective study on the use of rhBMP-2/collagen sponge with allograft dowels or tapered cylindrical fusion devices in ALIF and concluded that the use of those rhBMP-2 composites showed promise in assisting anterior intervertebral spinal fusion.[106–108] Slosar and colleagues,[109] in a prospective study on ALIFs, compared patients treated with allografts, either with or without the addition of rhBMP-2, with posterior instrumentation and demonstrated excellent results with the use of rhBMP-2. These reports supported the use of rhBMP-2 for ALIF and contributed to approval by the FDA in 2002. Because of its high fusion rates in ALIF, rhBMP-2 use was extended "off-label" to PLIF, TLIF, and cervical fusion. An increase in the number of procedures with rhBMP-2 has generated a large body of literature on adverse events and complications. Resorption of an implanted graft before osteoinduction and interbody fusion occurs was associated with the rhBMP-2 use. McClellan and colleagues[110] retrospectively investigated cases with a TLIF with BMP and reported a high rate of bone resorption, thereby assuming that the osseous remodeling potential of rhBMP-2 may lead to bone resorption within the vertebral body. In another TLIF study, 7.4% of the patients who received rhBMP-2 developed vertebral osteolysis within 4 months postoperatively.[111] Pradhan and colleagues[112] reported that the pseudarthrosis rate among patients who received femoral ring allografts with rhBMP-2 was higher than that in patients who received femoral ring allografts with autogenous iliac bone. They concluded that this appeared to be caused by the aggressive resorptive phase of allograft incorporation, which occurs before the osteoinduction phase.[112] These results suggested that caution must be exercised in deciding between autograft and rhBMP-2 for anterior lumbar interbody fusion and that further clinical studies were warranted. In a canine lumbar spine fusion model, the placement of OP-1 (BMP-7) over a dural tear stimulated new bone formation in the subarachnoid space, resulting in mild spinal stenosis at the site of dural decompression.[113] Several other rhBMP-2 complications have been documented in the lumbar spine including heterotopic/ectopic bone formation, radiculitis, and wound infections.[114–117] In a minimally invasive TLIF and PLIF study, 21% of the patients with rhBMP-2 presented with heterotopic bone formation; however, they were not associated with any further adverse events.[116] The rate of radiculitis in patients undergoing minimally invasive TLIF with rhBMP-2 was 11% within the first few days postoperatively.[117] Vaccaro and coworkers reported wound infections in 4 out of 24 patients (16.7%) who had single-level uninstrumented fusion with OP-1.[118] A recent meta-analysis reported that the overall data on the benefits and harms of BMP are underreported and often industry biased, making their accuracy inconclusive.[119,120]

It appears that the osteoinductive activity of the BMPs may compensate for the inhibitory effects of nicotine and nonsteroidal antiinflammatory drugs, two agents implicated in hindering spinal fusion in humans.[121–124] As noted previously, recombinant growth factors have been used in conjunction with intervertebral fusion devices in an attempt to achieve arthrodesis of the anterior spinal column. Titanium cages or cortical allograft dowels loaded with rhBMPs proved to be more efficacious than similar devices carrying autogenous bone for stimulating interbody fusion in a number of different animal models, a finding that was consistent whether these composite grafts were implanted in the cervical, thoracic, or lumbar spine.[123–125] These encouraging results were corroborated by a prospective, randomized clinical trial in which patients with degenerative disc disease limited to a single level of the lumbar spine were treated with a threaded cylindrical cage filled with either rhBMP-2 protein or autograft.[126] After 24 months, all 11 patients who had received rhBMP-2 exhibited radiographic evidence of solid fusion, compared with only two of the three control patients who were implanted with interbody devices containing their own iliac crest bone. Patients in the rhBMP-2 group initially experienced a more rapid resolution of their original symptoms, although at 6 months both groups demonstrated similar levels of clinical improvement. In addition, no complications were reported with the use of rhBMP-2. These studies have confirmed that partially purified BMP extracts and recombinant growth factors are able to induce spinal fusion in animals and humans. In all of these studies, however, the concentration of BMP necessary to bring about adequate bone formation in this environment was several magnitudes of order greater than normal physiologic levels, an observation that raised potential safety concerns. Furthermore, a recent meta-analysis summarized rhBMP-2 concentrations for various spinal procedures, and found poor study quality and large discrepancies in BMP doses within each procedure.[127]

In contrast to anterior lumbar fusion, there are studies that caution against the use of high-dose rhBMP-2 for cervical anterior spinal fusion. Shields and colleagues[128] reported a retrospective review of patients who underwent anterior cervical fusion using high-dose rhBMP-2/collagen sponge. The authors reported that 23.2% of patients suffered complications, such as hematomas, dysphagia, and excessive edema. Vaidya and colleagues[129] also reported that complications were associated with anterior cervical spinal fusion using rhBMP-2, including dysphagia, which was shown to be significantly more frequent and more severe in patients in whom rhBMP-2 was used. As a consequence, in July 2009, the FDA issued a Public Health Notification citing serious adverse effects with use of BMP in the cervical spine. Several systematic reviews looked at rhBMP-2 complications in the cervical spine. Tannoury and colleagues reported that the most common complications were dysphagia and neck swelling, hematoma, vertebral edema, osteolysis, and wound infections.[114] In order to minimize the quantities of BMP required for a successful fusion and outcome, it will be important to establish the appropriate dose for each spinal application and develop efficient carrier systems to deliver these osteoinductive factors.

New adjuvant agents such as bone morphogenetic binding peptide (BBP), which may enhance the efficiency of BMP, are under investigation in animal and in vitro studies. BBP is a BMP-specific binding protein that was isolated on the basis of the early work of Urist. BBP binds rhBMP-2 with an intermediate affinity, which makes it an ideal "slow release" agent.[129] As such, BBP may reduce the time to fusion and more thoroughly control the distribution of bone healing in spinal fusion.

Autologous Platelet Concentrate

Platelet degranulation is part of the normal cascade of bone healing with release of several growth factors, such as platelet-derived growth factor and TGF-β. These growth factors promote chemotaxis and proliferation of mesenchymal stem cells and osteoblasts and enhance bone healing.[130,131] By concentrating these platelet factors as autologous growth factor (AGF) concentrate, one may enhance the formation of new bone in lumbar spinal fusion when used in combination with autografts.[132] In the autologous platelet gel systems currently in development, platelet-rich plasma is separated from a sample of the patient's blood and concentrated in a fibrinogen matrix. This fibrinogen preparation is combined with thrombin, forming a fibrin clot that can be administered with an osteoconductive scaffold or a source of osteogenic cells to form a composite bone graft. However, AGFs have several disadvantages: blood draw, platelet processing, and longer surgery time. Recently, several reports have addressed in detail the efficacy of AGF for spinal fusion.[133–136] Weiner and colleagues[134] retrospectively compared autograft alone with an autograft with AGF in posterolateral spinal fusion; the authors reported that the use of AGF resulted in inferior rates of fusion compared with those of autograft alone. Hee and colleagues[135] conducted a prospective study on AGF in instrumented TLIF and concluded that the use of AGF in TLIF procedures did not increase overall fusion rates, although it might promote a faster rate of fusion. Carreon and colleagues[136] retrospectively investigated the effectiveness of platelet gel in instrumented posterolateral fusion and reported that platelet gel failed to enhance the fusion rate when added to autograft. On the other hand, Jenis et al. reported similar fusion rates between ICBG (85%) and autograft supplemented with AGF (89%) in one- or two-level lumbar interbody fusion with posterior fixation.[137] In current systems, autologous platelet concentrate has not been conclusively shown to enhance fusion; thus, further investigation may be warranted.

Mesenchymal Stem Cells

Mesenchymal stem cells (MSCs) are self-renewing and pluripotent cells and have been identified in a variety of tissues, including bone marrow,[138] muscle,[139,140] periosteum,[141] and adipose tissue.[142] In a variety of animal models, bone marrow–derived MSCs have demonstrated an efficacy in spinal fusion. Minamide and colleagues[143] cultured MSCs derived from bone marrow and implanted these cells onto the posterolateral lumbar transverse process with an HA-granule carrier in a rabbit model; five of seven rabbits in the high-number cultured cell group were deemed to be fused using manual palpation. The authors demonstrated that these cells acted as a substitute for the autograft in spinal fusion.[140] Using a rhesus monkey model, Wang and colleagues[144] expanded autologous MSCs derived from bone marrow in culture, stimulated them with osteogenic supplements, and constructed calcium phosphate ceramic composites with MSCs. They demonstrated that autologous MSC composites could enhance bone regeneration and achieve osseous spinal fusion in an anterior interbody fusion model. Clinically, Gan and colleagues[145] used bone marrow–derived MSCs combined with porous β-TCP for posterior spinal fusion and reported 95.1% spinal fusion.

Unfractionated bone marrow (BMA) has osteoinductive (growth factors) and some osteogenic potential. The bone marrow of healthy adults contains only one MSC for every 50,000 nucleated cells; this population is even further diminished in older patients and those with metabolic diseases such as osteoporosis.[143–145] Moreover, as bone marrow is aspirated from the iliac crest, it undergoes extensive dilution with peripheral blood, further decreasing the concentration of MSCs. Amplification or concentration of BMA may improve the yield of osteogenic MSCs from bone marrow. BMA is always combined with a carrier (DBM or collagen I sponge) to supplement mechanical properties. Taghavi and colleagues retrospectively reviewed a cohort of patients undergoing instrumented revision PLF with at least 24 months' follow-up.[146] Patients were divided into three groups: autograft only, BMA and autograft, and rhBMP-2 on a collagen sponge. They found that all grafting options achieved solid single-level fusion (100%). However, the multilevel BMA group had only a 63.6% fusion rate, while the other two groups had 100%. Clinical outcomes in all three groups were similar at 2 years, leading to the conclusion that BMA is a viable option for single-level procedures. Another single-level PLF study showed good fusion rates with BMA and autogenous bone chips (85.7%) similar to ICBG alone (90.5%). However, the calcium sulfate and BMA group had only a 45.5% fusion rate compared to the control side that received ICBG (90.9% fusion).[63] In a systematic review, Khashan et al. reported several PLF studies comparing local bone graft to BMA with various carriers (ceramics, DBM, or collagen). All of them showed similar fusion rates between BMA and ICBG groups, but the overall level of evidence was weak.[147] At the same time, multiple studies have confirmed that the amplification of osteoprogenitor cells that occurs after the culture expansion of MSCs results in greater bone formation than the use of unfractionated bone marrow, which demonstrates a relative paucity of osteogenic cells.[148,149] The introduction of culture-expanded MSCs has also been shown to be superior to bone marrow for eliciting the repair of critical-sized skeletal defects in an animal model.[150] While MSCs can play an important role in replacing the autogenous bone graft for spinal fusion, there are significant limitations, such as in vitro expansion, potential contamination, and revision surgery.

Gene Therapy

Gene therapy involves the delivery of a vector with a specific DNA sequence, or gene, to target cells that subsequently express the therapeutic protein. Recombinant BMPs have been used successfully to stimulate fusion in several clinical trials.[103,105,151–156] The advantages of gene therapy are that it can provide longer release of osteogenic proteins at levels more closely resembling physiologic levels than the administration of a single large dose of recombinant proteins. Delivery vehicles include viral and nonviral vectors that can be delivered in vivo (nonspecific and can elicit host immune response) or ex vivo (transfection of isolated autologous cell). Nonviral vectors are easier to produce, they are more stable, less antigenic, and are theoretically safer than viral vectors. Common nonviral vectors include naked DNA, liposomes, or polyplexes (DNA embedded into lipids or polymers). Nevertheless, viral vectors are often favored over nonviral strategies because of their superior transduction efficiencies. Replication-deficient adenoviral vectors have been successful in animal experiments. Lu and colleagues[85] tested a new osteoinductive factor, Nell-1 (Nel-like molecule-1) with DBM carrier, for in vivo gene therapy in the posterior rat spinal fusion model and reported 70% fusion rates at 6 weeks. However, there are several drawbacks

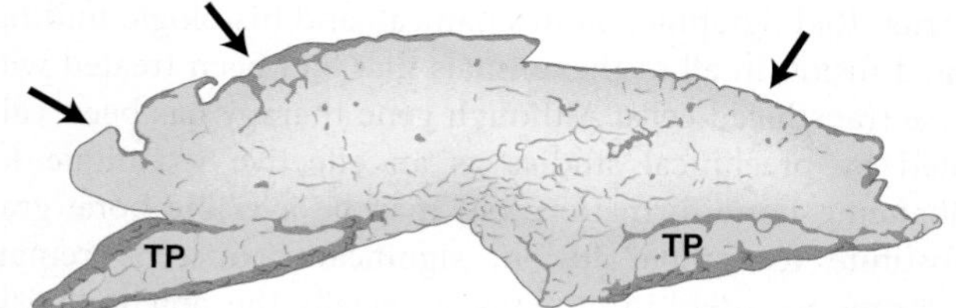

FIG. 67.2 Ex vivo gene therapy using rat bone marrow cells transduced with the bone morphogenic protein-2 gene successfully induces spinal fusion in rats. A sagittal section through the posterolateral spine demonstrates a solid fusion mass (*arrows*) spanning two adjoining transverse processes (TP).

with adenoviral vectors. Although these vectors transfect both dividing and nondividing cells, they cannot integrate into the host genome, thereby limiting protein production to several weeks.[157] Furthermore, adenoviral vectors generally retain their ability to synthesize adenoviral proteins, which stimulate the host immune response.[158,159] Recently, in order to compensate for the disadvantage of adenoviral vectors, various other viral vectors, such as adeno-associated viral vector and lentiviral vector, have been tested[160–162] and improvements have been implemented to ensure safety.[162–164]

Using cells, in particular stem cells, as a delivery vehicle in gene therapy could potentially hold a two-fold benefit for spine fusion by providing both osteogenic and osteoinductive characteristics. This bone grafting technique has been implemented in several animal models for spinal arthrodesis.[161,165–171] Wang and colleagues[168] employed ex vivo gene therapy to promote posterolateral spinal fusions in rats. Rat bone marrow cells transduced with the *BMP-2* gene were combined with a guanidine-extracted DBM and implanted in the posterolateral spine. Treatment with BMP-2-producing marrow cells generated solid fusion masses comparable with those resulting from the use of recombinant BMP-2 protein (Fig. 67.2). Even though high rates of fusion were observed, there are several safety concerns with use of viral vectors in humans. Furthermore, cells have to be isolated, expanded, and successfully transfected. Focusing on one or a combination of two BMPs is only capturing a certain stage of bone remodeling and might not provide long-term results. To overcome some of these obstacles, several studies looked at the markers of early bone pathway. Boden and colleagues[169] achieved single-level posterior fusions of the lumbar and thoracic spines in rats by supplying bone marrow cells with the gene encoding the LIM mineralization protein (LMP-1), a signaling protein that stimulates the expression of multiple osteoinductive growth factors. Consistent fusions were obtained in all of the animals receiving bone marrow cells containing the LMP-1 DNA sequence, whereas no bone formation was observed in those implanted with cells carrying an inactive copy of the gene. Another study on LIM-1 looked at the transfection dose response in vitro and the fusion rates in vivo using buffycoat cells derived from either bone marrow or peripheral blood.[170] After being infected for only 10 minutes with an adenoviral vector bearing the *LIM-1* gene, these cells were placed in the posterolateral spine in conjunction with an osteoconductive carrier. Radiographic, biomechanical, and histologic findings noted fusion in all of the animals that had been treated with these transduced cells. Although gene therapy has been validated by preclinical studies as an effective technique for enhancing bone formation and may be a viable bone graft substitute for spinal fusion, significant concerns remain regarding its safety in humans, especially the potential risks related to the use of viruses. Although these viruses are unable to replicate, it is still conceivable that they may regain the ability to propagate and trigger an uncontrollable infection. Some viruses insert randomly into the DNA of target cells, raising the possibility of malignant transformation. In addition, the cost-effectiveness of gene transfer methods has not been definitively established. These safety and economic issues may ultimately determine whether gene therapy is viewed as an acceptable alternative to autogenous bone graft for augmenting spinal fusion.

Conclusion

There is a wide array of bone substitutes for spinal fusion. Despite the existing literature on each of those graft substitutes, a strong level of clinical evidence is still absent. Most of the grafting materials do not require FDA approvals and thus lack preclinical research. At the same time, there are ample clinical studies on local autograft, bone morphogenetic proteins, and bone marrow aspirates. Unlike autogenous bone, which remains the gold standard because it contributes osteogenic cells, osteoinductive factors, and an osteoconductive matrix, none of the other individual bone substitutes provides all three components required for bone regeneration. As such, optimal use of bone substitutes may combine several techniques to construct a composite graft with an even greater capacity to enhance spinal arthrodesis. Understanding the biology and specificity of each bone substitute is critical for achieving successful spinal fusion. Expanding the number of clinical studies on each grafting substitute is warranted.

KEY POINTS

1. Bone substitutes can act as graft extenders (combined with autologous bone in order to reduce the amount of needed autograft), enhancers (combined with autograft to enhance fusion), or substitutes.
2. Autogenous bone graft, usually harvested from the iliac crest, is the only graft that possesses all components needed for bone formation: osteoconductive matrix, osteoinductive proteins, and osteogenic cells. The optimal bone substitute may be a composite of materials to share some of these properties.
3. Autogenous bone graft may be limited in quantity, and its harvest is associated with complications.
4. Potential forms of bone substitutes include allograft bone, DBM, ceramics, osteoinductive proteins, autologous platelet concentrate, mesenchymal stem cells, bone marrow aspirates, and gene delivery systems.
5. Each bone graft carries risks and benefits; the right choice strongly depends on the medical condition of the patient and the type of surgery.

KEY REFERENCES

1. Boden SD, Zdeblick TA, Sandhu HS, et al. The use of rhBMP-2 in interbody fusion cages. Definitive evidence of osteoinduction in humans: a preliminary report. *Spine*. 2000;25:376-381.
   A prospective human pilot trial of the use of rhBMP-2/collagen inside lumbar interbody spinal fusion cages showed at 2-year follow-up that fusion was observed to occur more reliably in patients treated with rhBMP-2-filled cages than in controls treated with autogenous bone graft.
2. Cammisa FP Jr, Lowery G, Garfin SR, et al. Two-year fusion rate equivalency between Grafton DBM gel and autograft in posterolateral spine fusion: a prospective controlled trial employing a side-by-side comparison in the same patient. *Spine*. 2004;29:660-666.
   In a multicenter prospective study that compared the effectiveness of a Grafton DBM gel composite with an iliac crest autograft in posterolateral spinal fusion, Grafton DBM could only extend an autograft that was smaller than is normally required to achieve a solid spinal fusion.
3. Muschik M, Ludwig R, Halbhubner S, et al. Beta-tricalcium phosphate as a bone substitute for dorsal spinal fusion in adolescent idiopathic scoliosis: preliminary results of a prospective clinical study. *Eur Spine J*. 2001;10(suppl 2):S178-S184.
   A prospective study on beta-tricalcium phosphate as a bone graft extender for posterior spinal fusion in scoliosis cases demonstrates that beta-tricalcium phosphates were a valuable alternative to allografts as a bone extender, even when large amounts of bone were necessary.
4. Khashan M, Inoue S, Berven SH. Cell based therapies as compared to autologous bone grafts for spinal arthrodesis. *Spine*. 2013;38(21):1885-1891.
   A systematic review of literature found that the current evidence on use of MSC or BMA as bone graft enhancers or substitutes in spine fusions was weak. After the exclusion and inclusion criteria only seven studies qualified for the analysis; however, their quality of evidence was low.
5. Hofstetter CP, Hofer AS, Levi AD. Exploratory meta-analysis on dose-related efficacy and morbidity of bone morphogenetic protein in spinal arthrodesis surgery. *J Neurosurg Spine*. 2016;24(3):457-475. [Epub 2015 Nov 27].
   A metaanalysis on currently available literature on BMP dosing concluded that there was a large discrepancy in the BMP dose for specific fusion procedures. For certain approaches the quality of evidence was weak, preventing any conclusions or recommendations on dosage.

REFERENCES

1. Global Burden of Disease Study 2013 Collaborators. Global, regional, and national incidence, prevalence, and years lived with disability for 301 acute and chronic diseases and injuries in 188 countries, 1990-2013: a systematic analysis for the Global Burden of Disease Study 2013. *Lancet*. 2015;386(9995):743-800.
2. Steinmann JC, Herkowitz HN. Pseudarthrosis of the spine. *Clin Orthop*. 1992;284:80-90.
3. Hamer AJ, Strachan JR, Black MM, et al. Biomechanical properties of cortical allograft bone using a new method of bone strength measurement: a comparison of fresh, fresh frozen, and irradiated bone. *J Bone Joint Surg Br*. 1996;78:363-368.

4. Silcox DH, Boden SD, Schimandle JH, et al. Reversing the inhibitory effect of nicotine on spinal fusion using an osteoinductive protein extract. *Spine*. 1998;23:291-296.
5. Alden TD, Pittman DD, Beres EJ, et al. Percutaneous spinal fusion using bone morphogenetic protein-2 gene therapy. *J Neurosurg*. 1999;90:109-114.
6. Chun DS, Baker KC, Hsu WK. Lumbar pseudarthrosis: a review of current diagnosis and treatment. *Neurosurg Focus*. 2015;39(4):E10.
7. Raizman NM, O'Brien JR, Poehling-Monaghan KL, Yu WD. Pseudarthrosis of the spine. *J Am Acad Orthop Surg*. 2009;17(8):494-503.
8. Sengupta DK, Truumees E, Patel CK, et al. Outcome of local bone versus autogenous iliac crest bone graft in the instrumented posterolateral fusion of the lumbar spine. *Spine*. 2006;31(9):985-991.
9. Gruskay JA, Basques BA, Bohl DD, Webb ML, Grauer JN. Short-term adverse events, length of stay, and readmission after iliac crest bone graft for spinal fusion. *Spine*. 2014;39(20):1718-1724.
10. Reid RL. Hernia through an iliac bone graft donor site. A case report. *J Bone Joint Surg Am*. 1968;50:757-760.
11. Cockin J. Autogenous bone graft complications and the donor site. *J Bone Joint Surg Br*. 1971;53:153.
12. Coventry MB, Tapper EM. Pelvic instability—a consequence of removing iliac crest for bone grafting. *J Bone Joint Surg Am*. 1972;54:83-101.
13. Challis JA, Lyttle JA, Stuart AE. Strangulated lumbar hernia and volvulus following removal of iliac crest bone graft. *Acta Orthop Scand*. 1975;46:230-233.
14. Escales F, DeWald RL. Combined traumatic arteriovenous fistula and urethral injury: a complication of bone grafting. *J Bone Joint Surg Am*. 1977;59:270-271.
15. Cowley SP, Anderson LD. Hernias through donor sites for iliac crest bone grafts. *J Bone Joint Surg Am*. 1983;65:1023-1025.
16. Kuhn DA, Moreland MS. Complications following iliac crest bone grafting. *Clin Orthop*. 1986;209:224-226.
17. Kurz LT, Garfin SR, Booth RE. Harvesting autogenous iliac bone grafts: a review of complications and techniques. *Spine*. 1989;14:1324-1331.
18. Summers BN, Eisenstein SM. Donor site pain from the ilium: a complication of lumbar spine fusion. *J Bone Joint Surg Br*. 1989;71:677-680.
19. Younger EM, Chapman MW. Morbidity at bone graft donor sites. *J Orthop Trauma*. 1989;3:192-194.
20. Catinella FP, Delaria GA, DeWald RL. False aneurysm of the superior gluteal artery—a complication of iliac crest bone grafting. *Spine*. 1990;15:1360-1362.
21. Fernyhough JC, Schimandle JJ, Weigel MC, et al. Chronic donor site pain complicating bone graft harvesting from the posterior iliac crest for spinal fusion. *Spine*. 1992;17:1474-1480.
22. Banwart JC, Asher MA, Hassanein RS. Iliac crest bone graft harvest donor site morbidity: a statistical evaluation. *Spine*. 1994;20:1055-1060.
23. Myeroff C, Archdeacon M. Autogenous bone graft: donor sites and techniques. *J Bone Joint Surg Am*. 2011;93(23):2227-2236.
24. Goulet JA, Senunas LE, DeSilva GL, et al. Autogenous iliac crest bone graft. Complications and functional assessment. *Clin Orthop*. 1997;339:76-81.
25. Stevenson S, Horowitz M. The response to bone allografts. *J Bone Joint Surg Am*. 1992;74:939-950.
26. Bauer TW, Muschler GF. Bone graft materials. An overview of the basic science. *Clin Orthop*. 2000;371:10-27.
27. Stevenson S, Emery SE, Goldberg VM. Factors affecting bone graft incorporation. *Clin Orthop*. 1996;324:66-74.
28. Hamer AJ, Strachan JR, Black MM, et al. Biomechanical properties of cortical allograft bone using a new method of bone strength measurement: a comparison of fresh, fresh frozen, and irradiated bone. *J Bone Joint Surg Br*. 1996;78:363-368.
29. Tomford WW. Transmission of disease through transplantation of musculoskeletal allografts. *J Bone Joint Surg Am*. 1995;77:1742-1754.
30. Asselmeier MA, Casperi RB, Bottenfeld S. A review of allograft processing and sterilization techniques and their role in transmission of the human immunodeficiency virus. *Am J Sports Med*. 1993;21:170-175.
31. Mroz TE, Joyce MJ, Lieberman IH, et al. The use of allograft bone in spine surgery: is it safe? *Spine J*. 2009;9(4):303-308.
32. Sim FH, Frassica FJ. Use of allografts following resection of tumors of the musculoskeletal system. *Instr Course Lect*. 1993;42:405-413.
33. Tsuang YH, Yang RS, Chen PQ, et al. Experimental allograft in spinal fusion in dogs. *Taiwan Yi Xue Hui Za Zhi*. 1989;88:989-994.
34. Cloward RB. The anterior approach for removal of ruptured cervical discs. *J Neurosurg*. 1958;15:602.
35. Brown MD, Malinin TI, Davis PB. A roentgenographic evaluation of frozen allografts versus autografts in anterior cervical spine fusions. *Clin Orthop*. 1976;119:231-236.
35a. Jagannathan J, Shaffrey CI, Oskouian RJ, et al. Radiographic and clinical outcomes following single-level anterior cervical discectomy and allograft fusion without plate placement or cervical collar. *J Neurosurg Spine*. 2008;8(5):420-428.
36. Young WF, Rossenwasser RH. An early comparative analysis of the use of fibular allograft versus autologous iliac crest graft for interbody fusion after anterior cervical discectomy. *Spine*. 1993;18:1123-1124.
37. Zdeblick TA, Ducker TB. The use of freeze-dried allograft bone for anterior cervical fusions. *Spine*. 1991;16:726-729.
38. Samartzis D, Shen FH, Matthews DK, et al. Comparison of allograft to autograft in multilevel anterior cervical discectomy and fusion with rigid plate fixation. *Spine J*. 2003;3(6):451-459.
39. Jorgenson SS, Lowe TG, France J, et al. A prospective analysis of autograft versus allograft in posterolateral lumbar fusion in the same patient. A minimum of 1-year follow-up in 144 patients. *Spine*. 1994;19:2048-2053.
40. An HS, Lynch K, Toth J. Prospective comparison of autograft vs. allograft for adult posterolateral lumbar spine fusion: differences among freeze-dried, frozen, and mixed grafts. *J Spinal Disord*. 1995;8(2):131-135.
41. Jones KC, Andrish J, Kuivila T, Gurd A. Radiographic outcomes using freeze-dried cancellous allograft bone for posterior spinal fusion in pediatric idiopathic scoliosis. *J Pediatr Orthop*. 2002;22(3):285-289.
42. Knapp DR Jr, Jones ET, Blanco JS, Flynn JC, Price CT. Allograft bone in spinal fusion for adolescent idiopathic scoliosis. *J Spinal Disord Tech*. 2005;18(suppl):S73-S76.
43. Kozak JA, Heilman AE, O'Brian JP. Anterior lumbar fusion options: techniques and graft materials. *Clin Orthop*. 1994;300:45-51.
44. Silcox DH. Laparoscopic bone dowel fusions of the lumbar spine. *Orthop Clin North Am*. 1998;29:655-663.

45. Thalgott JS, Fogarty ME, Giuffre JM, et al. A prospective, randomized, blinded, single-site study to evaluate the clinical and radiographic differences between frozen and freeze-dried allograft when used as part of a circumferential anterior lumbar interbody fusion procedure. *Spine*. 2009;34(12): 1251-1256.
46. Butterman GR, Glazer PA, Hu SS, Bradford DS. Revision of failed lumbar fusions. A comparison of anterior autograft and allograft. *Spine*. 1997;22:2748-2755.
47. Tay BK, Patel VV, Bradford DS. Calcium sulfate and calcium phosphate-based bone substitutes. Mimickry of the moneral phase of bone. *Orthop Clin North Am*. 1999;30:615-623.
48. Jarcho M. Calcium phosphate ceramics as hard tissue prosthetics. *Clin Orthop*. 1981;157:259-278.
49. Ohgushi H, Goldberg VM, Caplan AI. Heterotopic osteogenesis in porous ceramics induced by marrow cells. *J Orthop Res*. 1989;7:568-578.
50. Chen WJ, Tsai TT, Chen LH, et al. The fusion rate of calcium sulfate with local autograft bone compared with autologous iliac bone graft for instrumented short-segment spinal fusion. *Spine*. 2005;30:2293-2297.
51. Epstein NE. A preliminary study of the efficacy of beta tricalcium phosphate as a bone expander for instrumented posterolateral lumbar fusions. *J Spinal Disord Tech*. 2006;19:424-429.
52. Xie Y, Chopin D, Morin C, et al. Evaluation of the osteogenesis and biodegradation of porous biphasic ceramic in the human spine. *Biomaterials*. 2006;27:2761-2767.
53. Lee JH, Hwang CJ, Song BW, et al. A prospective consecutive study of instrumented posterolateral lumbar fusion using synthetic hydroxyapatite (Bongros-HA) as a bone graft extender. *J Biomed Mater Res A*. 2009;90(3):804-810.
54. Korovessis P, Koureas G, Zacharatos S, et al. Correlative radiological, self-assessment and clinical analysis of evolution in instrumented dorsal and lateral fusion for degenerative lumbar spine disease. Autograft versus coralline hydroxyapatite. *Eur Spine J*. 2005;14:630-638.
55. Thalgott JS, Fritts K, Giuffre JM, et al. Anterior interbody fusion of the cervical spine with coralline hydroxyapatite. *Spine*. 2001;24:1295-1299.
56. Thalgott JS, Giuffre JM, Klezl Z, et al. Anterior lumbar interbody fusion with titanium mesh cages, coralline hydroxyapatite, and demineralized bone matrix as part of a circumferential fusion. *Spine J*. 2002;2:63-69.
57. Thalgott JS, Klezl Z, Timlin M, et al. Anterior lumbar interbody fusion with processed sea coral (coralline hydroxyapatite) as part of a circumferential fusion. *Spine*. 2002;27:E518-E525.
57a. Yoshii T, Yuasa M, Sotome S, et al. Porous/dense composite hydroxyapatite for anterior cervical discectomy and fusion. *Spine*. 2013;38(10):833-840.
58. Passuti N, Daculsi G, Rogez JM, et al. Macroporous calcium phosphate ceramic performance in human spine fusion. *Clin Orthop Relat Res*. 1989;248:169-176.
59. Ransford AO, Morley T, Edgar MA, et al. Synthetic porous ceramic compared with autograft in scoliosis surgery. A prospective, randomized study of 341 patients. *J Bone Joint Surg Br*. 1998;80:13-18.
60. Lerner T, Bullmann V, Schulte TL, Schneider M, Liljenqvist U. A level-1 pilot study to evaluate of ultraporous beta-tricalcium phosphate as a graft extender in the posterior correction of adolescent idiopathic scoliosis. *Eur Spine J*. 2009;18(2):170-179.
61. Dai LY, Jiang LS. Single-level instrumented posterolateral fusion of lumbar spine with beta-tricalcium phosphate versus autograft: a prospective, randomized study with 3-year follow-up. *Spine*. 2008;33(12):1299-1304.
62. Ziran BH, Smith WR, Morgan SJ. Use of calcium-based demineralized bone matrix/allograft for nonunions and posttraumatic reconstruction of the appendicular skeleton: preliminary results and complications. *J Trauma*. 2007;63(6):1324-1328.
63. Niu CC, Tsai TT, Fu TS, et al. A comparison of posterolateral lumbar fusion comparing autograft, autogenous laminectomy bone with bone marrow aspirate, and calcium sulphate with bone marrow aspirate: a prospective randomized study. *Spine*. 2009;34(25):2715-2719.
64. Licina P, Coughlan M, Johnston E, Pearcy M. Comparison of silicate-substituted calcium phosphate (Actifuse) with recombinant human bone morphogenetic protein-2 (Infuse) in posterolateral instrumented lumbar fusion. *Global Spine J*. 2015;5(6):471-478.
65. Nandyala SV, Marquez-Lara A, Fineberg SJ, Pelton M, Singh K. Prospective, randomized, controlled trial of silicate-substituted calcium phosphate versus rhBMP-2 in a minimally invasive transforaminal lumbar interbody fusion. *Spine*. 2014;39(3):185-191.
66. Urist MR. Bone: formation by autoinduction. *Science*. 1965;150:893-899.
67. Sandhu HS, Grewal HS, Parvataneni H. Bone grafting for spinal fusion. *Orthop Clin North Am*. 1999;30:685-698.
68. Salih E, Wang J, Mah J, Fluckiger R. Natural variation in the extent of phosphorylation of bone phosphoproteins as a function of in vivo new bone formation induced by demineralized bone matrix in soft tissue and bony environments. *Biochem J*. 2002;364(Pt 2):465-474.
69. Blum B, Moseley J, Miller L, Richelsoph K, Haggard W. Measurement of bone morphogenetic proteins and other growth factors in demineralized bone matrix. *Orthopedics*. 2004;27(1 suppl):s161-s165.
70. Lee YP, Jo M, Luna M, et al. The efficacy of different commercially available demineralized bone matrix substances in an athymic rat model. *J Spinal Disord Tech*. 2005;18:439-444.
71. Peterson B, Whang PG, Iglesias R, et al. Osteoinductivity of commercially available demineralized bone matrix. Preparations in a spine fusion model. *J Bone Joint Surg Am*. 2004;86-A:2243-2250.
72. Wang JC, Alanay A, Mark D, et al. A comparison of commercially available demineralized bone matrix for spinal fusion. *Eur Spine J*. 2007;16:1233-1240.
73. Choi Y, Oldenburg FP, Sage L, et al. A bridging demineralized bone implant facilitates posterolateral lumbar fusion in New Zealand white rabbits. *Spine*. 2007;32:36-41.
74. Louis-Ugbo J, Murakami H, Kim HS, et al. Evidence of osteoinduction by Grafton demineralized bone matrix in nonhuman primate spinal fusion. *Spine*. 2004;29:360-366.
75. Yee AJ, Bae HW, Friess D, et al. Augmentation of rabbit posterolateral spondylodesis using a novel demineralized bone matrix-hyaluronan putty. *Spine*. 2003;28:2435-2440.
76. Frenkel SR, Moskovich R, Spivak J, et al. Demineralized bone matrix: enhancement of spinal fusion. *Spine*. 1993;18:1634-1639.
77. Girardi FP, Cammisa FP Jr. The effect of bone graft extenders to enhance the performance of iliac crest bone

grafts in instrumented lumbar spine fusion. *Orthopedics.* 2003;26:s545-s548.

78. Sassard WR, Eidman DK, Gray PM, et al. Augmenting local bone with Grafton demineralized bone matrix for posterolateral lumbar spine fusion: avoiding second site autologous bone harvest. *Orthopedics.* 2000;23:1059-1064.
79. Cammisa FP Jr, Lowery G, Garfin SR, et al. Two-year fusion rate equivalency between Grafton DBM gel and autograft in posterolateral spine fusion: a prospective controlled trial employing a side-by-side comparison in the same patient. *Spine.* 2004;29:660-666.
80. Vaccaro AR, Stubbs HA, Block JE. Demineralized bone matrix composite grafting for posterolateral spinal fusion. *Orthopedics.* 2007;30:567-570.
81. An HS, Simpson JM, Glover JM, et al. Comparison between allograft plus demineralized bone matrix versus autograft in anterior cervical fusion. A prospective multicenter study. *Spine.* 1995;20:2211-2216.
82. Park HW, Lee JK, Moon SJ, et al. The efficacy of the synthetic interbody cage and Grafton for anterior cervical fusion. *Spine.* 2009;34(17):E591e5.
83. Moon HJ, Kim JH, Kim JH, et al. The effects of anterior cervical discectomy and fusion with stand-alone cages at two contiguous levels on cervical alignment and outcomes. *Acta Neurochir (Wien).* 2011;153(3):559e65.
84. Martin GJ, Boden SD, Titus L, et al. New formulations of demineralized bone matrix as a more effective graft alternative in experimental posterolateral lumbar spine arthrodesis. *Spine.* 1999;24:637-645.
85. Lu SS, Zhang X, Soo C, et al. The osteoinductive properties of Nell-1 in a rat spinal fusion model. *Spine J.* 2007;7:50-60.
86. Bostrom MP, Yang X, Kennan M, et al. An unexpected outcome during testing of commercially available demineralized bone graft materials: how safe are the nonallograft components? *Spine.* 2001;26:1425-1428.
87. Wang EA, Rosen V, D'Alessandro JS, et al. Recombinant human bone morphogenetic protein induces bone formation. *Proc Natl Acad Sci USA.* 1990;87:2220-2224.
88. Boden SD, Schimandle JH, Hutton WC. 1995 Volvo award in basic sciences. The use of an osteoinductive growth factor for lumbar spinal fusion. Part II: study of dose, carrier, and species. *Spine.* 1995;20:2633-2644.
89. Silcox DH, Boden SD, Schimandle JH, et al. Reversing the inhibitory effect of nicotine on spinal fusion using an osteoinductive protein extract. *Spine.* 1998;23:291-296.
90. Martin GJ, Boden SD, Titus L. Recombinant human bone morphogenetic protein-2 overcomes the inhibitory effect of ketorolac, a nonsteroidal anti-inflammatory drug (NSAID), on posterolateral lumbar intertransverse spine fusion. *Spine.* 1999;24:2188-2193.
91. Cook SD, Dalton JE, Tan EH, et al. In vivo evaluation of recombinant human osteogenic protein (rhOP-1) implant as a bone graft substitute for spinal fusions. *Spine.* 1994;19:1655-1663.
92. Schimandle JH, Boden SD, Hutton WC. Experimental spinal fusion with recombinant human bone morphogenetic protein-2. *Spine.* 1995;20:1326-1337.
93. Boden SD, Moskovitz PA, Morone MA, et al. Video-assisted lateral intertransverse process arthrodesis. Validation of a new minimally invasive lumbar spinal fusion technique in the rabbit and nonhuman primate (rhesus) models. *Spine.* 1996;21:2689-2697.
94. Boden SD, Martin GJ, Morone M, et al. The use of coralline hydroxyapatite with bone marrow, autogenous bone graft, or osteoinductive bone protein extract for posterolateral lumbar spinal fusion. *Spine.* 1999;24:320-327.
95. Boden SD, Martin GJ, Morone M, et al. Posterolateral lumbar intertransverse process spine arthrodesis with recombinant human bone morphogenetic protein 2/hydroxyapatite-tricalcium phosphate after laminectomy in the nonhuman primate. *Spine.* 1999;24:1179-1185.
96. Lovell TP, Dawson EG, Nilsson OS, et al. Augmentation of spinal fusion with bone morphogenetic protein in dogs. *Clin Orthop.* 1989;243:266-274.
97. Muschler GF, Hyodo A, Manning T, et al. Evaluation of human bone morphogenetic protein 2 in a canine spinal fusion model. *Clin Orthop.* 1994;308:229-240.
98. Sandu HS, Kanim LE, Kabo JM, et al. Evaluation of rhBMP-2 with an OPLA carrier in a canine posterolateral (transverse process) spinal fusion model. *Spine.* 1995;20: 2669-2682.
99. Sandu HS, Kanim LE, Kabo JM, et al. Effective doses of recombinant human bone morphogenetic protein-2 in experimental spinal fusion. *Spine.* 1996;21:2115-2122.
100. Patel TC, Erulkar JS, Grauer JN, et al. Osteogenic protein-1 overcomes the inhibitory effect of nicotine on posterolateral lumbar fusion. *Spine.* 2001;26:1656-1661.
101. Minamide A, Kawakami M, Hashizume H, Sakata R, Tamaki T. Evaluation of carriers of bone morphogenetic protein for spinal fusion. *Spine.* 2001;26(8):933-939.
102. Peterson B, Whang PG, Iglesias R, et al. Osteoinductivity of commercially available demineralized bone matrix. Preparations in a spine fusion model. *J Bone Joint Surg Am.* 2004;86-A:2243-2250.
103. Boden SD, Kang J, Sandhu H, et al. Use of recombinant human bone morphogenetic protein-2 to achieve posterolateral lumbar spine fusion in humans: a prospective, randomized clinical pilot trial. *Spine.* 2002;27:2662-2673.
104. Dimar JR, Glassman SD, Burkus KJ, et al. Clinical outcomes and fusion success at 2 years of single-level instrumented posterolateral fusions with recombinant human bone morphogenetic protein-2/compression resistant matrix versus iliac crest bone graft. *Spine.* 2006;31:2534-2539.
105. Boden SD, Zdeblick TA, Sandhu HS, et al. The use of rhBMP-2 in interbody fusion cages. Definitive evidence of osteoinduction in humans: a preliminary report. *Spine.* 2000;25:376-381.
106. Burkus JK, Dorchak JD, Sanders DL. Radiographic assessment of interbody fusion using recombinant human bone morphogenetic protein type 2. *Spine.* 2003;28:372-377.
107. Burkus JK, Gornet MF, Dickman CA, et al. Anterior lumbar interbody fusion using rhBMP-2 with tapered interbody cages. *J Spinal Disord Tech.* 2002;15:337-349.
108. Burkus JK, Transfeldt EE, Kitchel SH, et al. Clinical and radiographic outcomes of anterior lumbar interbody fusion using recombinant human bone morphogenetic protein-2. *Spine.* 2002;27:2396-2408.
109. Slosar PJ, Josey R, Reynolds J. Accelerating lumbar fusions by combining rhBMP-2 with allograft bone: a prospective analysis of interbody fusion rates and clinical outcomes. *Spine J.* 2007;7:301-307.
110. McClellan JW, Mulconrey DS, Forbes RJ, et al. Vertebral bone resorption after transforaminal lumbar interbody fusion with bone morphogenetic protein (rhBMP-2). *J Spinal Disord Tech.* 2006;19:483-486.

111. Lewandrowski KU, Nanson C, Calderon R. Vertebral osteolysis after posterior interbody lumbar fusion with recombinant human bone morphogenetic protein 2: a report of five cases. *Spine J*. 2007;7(5):609-614.
112. Pradhan BB, Bae HW, Dawson EG, et al. Graft resorption with the use of bone morphogenetic protein: lessons from anterior lumbar interbody fusion using femoral ring allografts and recombinant human bone morphogenetic protein-2. *Spine*. 2006;31:E277-E284.
113. Sandhu HS, Toth JM, Diwan AD, et al. Histologic evaluation of the efficacy of rhBMP-2 compared with autograft bone in sheep spinal anterior interbody fusion. *Spine*. 2002;27:567-575.
114. Tannoury CA, An HS. Complications with the use of bone morphogenetic protein 2 (BMP-2) in spine surgery. *Spine J*. 2014;14(3):552-559.
115. Chrastil J, Low JB, Whang PG, Patel AA. Complications associated with the use of the recombinant human bone morphogenetic proteins for posterior interbody fusions of the lumbar spine. *Spine*. 2013;38(16):E1020-E1027.
116. Joseph V, Rampersaud YR. Heterotopic bone formation with the use of rhBMP2 in posterior minimal access interbody fusion: a CT analysis. *Spine*. 2007;32(25):2885-2890.
117. Mindea SA, Shih P, Song JK. Recombinant human bone morphogenetic protein-2-induced radiculitis in elective minimally invasive transforaminal lumbar interbody fusions: a series review. *Spine*. 2009;34(14):1480-1484.
118. Vaccaro AR, Whang PG, Patel T, et al. The safety and efficacy of OP-1 (rhBMP-7) as a replacement for iliac crest autograft for posterolateral lumbar arthrodesis: minimum 4-year follow-up of a pilot study. *Spine J*. 2008;8(3):457-465.
119. Fu R, Selph S, McDonagh M, et al. Effectiveness and harms of recombinant human bone morphogenetic protein-2 in spine fusion: a systematic review and meta-analysis. *Ann Intern Med*. 2013;158:890-902.
120. Simmonds MC, Brown JV, Heirs MK, et al. Safety and effectiveness of recombinant human bone morphogenetic protein-2 for spinal fusion: a meta-analysis of individual-participant data. *Ann Intern Med*. 2013;158:877-889.
121. Silcox DH, Boden SD, Schimandle JH, et al. Reversing the inhibitory effect of nicotine on spinal fusion using an osteoinductive protein extract. *Spine*. 1998;23:291-296.
122. Martin GJ, Boden SD, Titus L. Recombinant human bone morphogenetic protein-2 overcomes the inhibitory effect of ketorolac, a nonsteroidal anti-inflammatory drug (NSAID), on posterolateral lumbar intertransverse process spine fusion. *Spine*. 1999;24:2188-2193.
123. Zdeblick TA, Ghanayem AJ, Rapoff AJ, et al. Cervical interbody fusion cages. An animal model with and without bone morphogenetic protein. *Spine*. 1998;23:758-765.
124. Cunningham BW, Kanayama M, Parker LM, et al. Osteogenic protein versus autologous interbody arthrodesis in the sheep thoracic spine. A comparative endoscopic study using the Bagby and Kuslich interbody fusion device. *Spine*. 1999;24:509-518.
125. Boden SD, Nartin GJ, Horton WC, et al. Laparoscopic anterior spinal arthrodesis with rhBMP-2 in a titanium interbody threaded cage. *J Spinal Disord*. 1998;11:95-101.
126. Hecht BP, Fischgrund JS, Herkowitz HN, et al. The use of recombinant human bone morphogenetic protein 2 (rhBMP-2) to promote spinal fusion in a nonhuman primate anterior interbody fusion model. *Spine*. 1999;24:629-636.
127. Hofstetter CP, Hofer AS, Levi AD. Exploratory meta-analysis on dose-related efficacy and morbidity of bone morphogenetic protein in spinal arthrodesis surgery. *J Neurosurg Spine*. 2016;24(3):457-475.
128. Shields LB, Raque GH, Glassman SD, et al. Adverse effects associated with high-dose recombinant human bone morphogenetic protein-2 use in anterior cervical spine fusion. *Spine*. 2006;31:542-547.
129. Vaidya R, Carp J, Sethi A, et al. Complications of anterior cervical discectomy and fusion using recombinant human bone morphogenetic protein-2. *Eur Spine J*. 2007;16:1257-1265.
130. Alanay A, Chen C, Lee S, et al. The adjunctive effect of a binding peptide on bone morphogenetic protein enhanced bone healing in a rodent model of spinal fusion. *Spine*. 2008;33:1709-1713.
131. Guizzardi S, Di Silvestre M, Scandroglio R, et al. Implants of heterologous demineralized bone matrix for induction of posterior spinal fusion in rats. *Spine*. 1992;17:701-707.
132. Lindholm TS, Ragni P, Lindholm TC. Response of bone marrow stroma cells to demineralized cortical bone matrix in experimental spinal fusion in rabbits. *Clin Orthop*. 1988;230:296-302.
133. Lowery GL, Kulkarni S, Pennisi AE. Use of autologous growth factors in lumbar spinal fusion. *Bone*. 1999;25:47S-50S.
134. Weiner BK, Walker M. Efficacy of autologous growth factors in lumbar intertransverse fusions. *Spine*. 2003;28:1968-1970.
135. Hee HT, Majd ME, Holt RT, et al. Do autologous growth factors enhance transforaminal lumbar interbody fusion? *Eur Spine J*. 2003;12:400-407.
136. Carreon LY, Glassman SD, Anekstein Y, et al. Platelet gel (AGF) fails to increase fusion rates in instrumented posterolateral fusions. *Spine*. 2005;30:E243-E246.
137. Jenis LG, Banco RJ, Kwon B. A prospective study of Autologous Growth Factors (AGF) in lumbar interbody fusion. *Spine J*. 2006;6(1):14-20.
138. Caplan AI, Bruder SP. Mesenchymal stem cells: building blocks for molecular medicine in the 21st century. *Trends Mol Med*. 2001;7:259-264.
139. Jackson KA, Mi T, Goodell MA. Hematopoietic potential of stem cells isolated from murine skeletal muscle. *Proc Natl Acad Sci USA*. 1999;96:14482-14486.
140. Williams JT, Southerland SS, Souza J, et al. Cells isolated from adult human skeletal muscle capable of differentiating into multiple mesodermal phenotypes. *Am Surg*. 1999;65:22-26.
141. Nakahara H, Dennis JE, Bruder SP, et al. In vitro differentiation of bone and hypertrophic cartilage from periosteal-derived cells. *Exp Cell Res*. 1991;195:492-503.
142. Zuk PA, Zhu M, Mizuno H, et al. Multilineage cells from human adipose tissue: implications for cell-based therapies. *Tissue Eng*. 2001;7:211-228.
143. Minamide A, Yoshida M, Kawakami M, et al. The use of cultured bone marrow cells in type I collagen gel and porous hydroxyapatite for posterolateral lumbar spine fusion. *Spine*. 2005;30:1134-1138.
144. Wang T, Dang G, Guo Z, et al. Evaluation of autologous bone marrow mesenchymal stem cell-calcium phosphate ceramic composite for lumbar fusion in rhesus monkey interbody fusion model. *Tissue Eng*. 2005;11:1159-1167.
145. Gan Y, Dai K, Zhang P, et al. The clinical use of enriched bone marrow stem cells combined with porous beta-tricalcium

phosphate in posterior spinal fusion. *Biomaterials*. 2008;29:3973-3982.
146. Taghavi CE, Lee KB, Keorochana G, et al. Bone morphogenetic protein-2 and bone marrow aspirate with allograft as alternatives to autograft in instrumented revision posterolateral lumbar spinal fusion: a minimum two-year follow-up study. *Spine*. 2010;35(11):1144-1150.
147. Khashan M, Inoue S, Berven SH. Cell based therapies as compared to autologous bone grafts for spinal arthrodesis. *Spine*. 2013;38(21):1885-1891.
148. Muschler GF, Boehm C, Easley KA. Aspiration to obtain osteoblast progenitor cells from human bone marrow: the influence of aspiration volume. *J Bone Joint Surg Am*. 1997;79:1699-1709.
149. Kahn A, Gibbons R, Perkins S, et al. Age-related bone loss: a hypothesis and initial assessment in mice. *Clin Orthop*. 1995;313:69-75.
150. Kadiyala S, Jaiswal N, Bruder SP. Culture-expanded bone marrow derived mesenchymal stem cells can regenerate a critical-sized segmental bone defect. *Tissue Eng*. 1997;3:173-185.
151. Baskin DS, Ryan P, Sonntag V, et al. A prospective, randomized, controlled cervical fusion study using recombinant human bone morphogenetic protein-2 with the CORNERSTONE-SR allograft ring and the ATLANTIS anterior cervical plate. *Spine*. 2003;28:1219-1224.
152. Vaccaro AR, Whang PG, Patel T, et al. The safety and efficacy of OP-1 (rhBMP-7) as a replacement for iliac crest autograft for posterolateral lumbar arthrodesis: minimum 4-year follow-up of a pilot study. *Spine J*. 2007;8:457-465.
153. Vaccaro AR, Anderson DG, Patel T, et al. Comparison of OP-1 putty (rhBMP-7) to iliac crest autograft for posterolateral lumbar arthrodesis: a minimum 2-year follow-up pilot study. *Spine*. 2005;30:2709-2716.
154. Vaccaro AR, Patel T, Fischgrund J, et al. A pilot safety and efficacy study of OP-1 putty (rhBMP-7) as an adjunct to iliac crest autograft in posterolateral lumbar fusions. *Eur Spine J*. 2003;12:495-500.
155. Vaccaro AR, Patel T, Fischgrund J, et al. A 2-year follow-up pilot study evaluating the safety and efficacy of OP-1 putty (rhBMP-7) as an adjunct to iliac crest autograft in posterolateral lumbar fusions. *Eur Spine J*. 2005;14:623-629.
156. Vaccaro AR, Patel T, Fischgrund J, et al. A pilot study evaluating the safety and efficacy of OP-1 putty (rhBMP-7) as a replacement for iliac crest autograft in posterolateral lumbar arthrodesis for degenerative spondylolisthesis. *Spine*. 2004;29:1885-1892.
157. Feeley BT, Conduah AH, Sugiyama O, et al. In vivo molecular imaging of adenoviral versus lentiviral gene therapy in two bone formation models. *J Orthop Res*. 2006;24:1709-1721.
158. Mack CA, Song WR, Carpenter H, et al. Circumvention of anti-adenovirus neutralizing immunity by administration of an adenoviral vector of an alternate serotype. *Hum Gene Ther*. 1997;8:99-109.
159. Yang Y, Nunes FA, Berencsi K, et al. Cellular immunity to viral antigens limits E1-deleted adenoviruses for gene therapy. *Proc Natl Acad Sci USA*. 1994;91:4407-4411.
160. Chen Y, Luk KD, Cheung KM, et al. Gene therapy for new bone formation using adeno-associated viral bone morphogenetic protein-2 vectors. *Gene Ther*. 2003;10: 1345-1353.
161. Miyazaki M, Sugiyama O, Tow B, et al. The effects of lentiviral gene therapy with bone morphogenetic protein-2-producing bone marrow cells on spinal fusion in rats. *J Spinal Disord Tech*. 2008;21:372-379.
162. Sugiyama O, An DS, Kung SP, et al. Lentivirus-mediated gene transfer induces long-term transgene expression of BMP-2 in vitro and new bone formation in vivo. *Mol Ther*. 2005;11:390-398.
163. Stieger K, Le Meur G, Lasne F, et al. Long-term doxycycline-regulated transgene expression in the retina of nonhuman primates following subretinal injection of recombinant AAV vectors. *Mol Ther*. 2006;13:967-975.
164. Zufferey R, Dull T, Mandel RJ, et al. Self-inactivating lentivirus vector for safe and efficient in vivo gene delivery. *J Virol*. 1998;72:9873-9880.
165. Dumont RJ, Dayoub H, Li JZ, et al. Ex vivo bone morphogenetic protein-9 gene therapy using human mesenchymal stem cells induces spinal fusion in rodents. *Neurosurgery*. 2002;51:1239-1244.
166. Hidaka C, Goshi K, Rawlins B, et al. Enhancement of spine fusion using combined gene therapy and tissue engineering BMP-7-expressing bone marrow cells and allograft bone. *Spine*. 2003;28:2049-2057.
167. Peterson B, Iglesias R, Zhang J, et al. Genetically modified human derived bone marrow cells for posterolateral lumbar spine fusion in athymic rats: beyond conventional autologous bone grafting. *Spine*. 2005;30:283-289.
168. Wang JC, Kanim LE, Yoo S, et al. Effect of regional gene therapy with bone morphogenetic protein-2-producing bone marrow cells on spinal fusion in rats. *J Bone Joint Surg Am*. 2003;85-A:905-911.
169. Boden SD, Titus L, Hair G, et al. Lumbar spine fusion by local gene therapy with a cDNA encoding a novel osteoinductive protein (LMP-1). *Spine*. 1998;23:2486-2492.
170. Viggeswarapu M, Boden SD, Liu Y, et al. Adenoviral delivery of LIM mineralization protein-1 induces new-bone formation in vitro and in vivo. *J Bone Joint Surg Am*. 2001;83-A:364-376.
171. Helm GA, Alden TD, Beres EJ, et al. Use of bone morphogenetic protein-9 gene therapy to induce spinal arthrodesis in the rodent. *J Neurosurg*. 2000;92(2 suppl):191-196.

CHAPTER 68 Electrical Stimulation for Spinal Fusion

Ilyas S. Aleem
Paul Glazer
Mohit Bhandari

Achieving a consistently successful fusion continues to be a challenge in spinal surgery.[1] Approximately 25% to 81% of lumbar fusion procedures fail to solidly fuse[2] and may require further operative or nonoperative intervention. Numerous factors affect fusion rates, including patient age, smoking status, medical comorbidities, graft source, and levels of fusion.[3–5] Electrical stimulation is a limited-risk adjunctive therapy that has been advocated to promote spinal fusion. Three types of electrical stimulation are currently employed: direct current (DC), capacitive coupling (CC), and inductive coupling (IC). IC includes the mechanisms of pulsed electromagnetic fields (PEMFs) and combined magnetic fields (CMFs).[6–8] Clinical data have demonstrated an enhancement in bone healing rates with electrical stimulation even before the true mechanisms of action of these technologies were well understood. Recent evidence provides support for the use of electrical stimulation for decreasing pain and radiographic nonunion rates.[9] This chapter reviews the history of electrical stimulation, the types of electrical stimulation and their mechanism of action, and the quality of the evidence behind the use of electrical stimulators for bone healing.

History of Electrical Stimulation

The role of bone electrical potential is increasingly being recognized as an important component in bone healing.[10,11] The earliest use of electrical currents was in 1841, when Hartshorne reported its use on a patient with a tibial nonunion.[12] In 1850, Lente reported successful use of galvanic current in the treatment of patients with delayed union or nonunions.[13] In 1957, Fukada and Yasuda[14] subsequently developed the concept of piezoelectric fields on bone healing, suggesting that electrical potentials of bone are altered in response to compression and tension. The authors reported that the areas of bone under compression were electronegative and those under tension were electropositive. In 1974, Dwyer and Wickham advanced this concept to spinal fusion, first reporting the use of electrical stimulation as an adjunct to lumbar spinal fusion.[15] The mechanism of action of electrical stimulation therapy is not clearly understood but is generally thought to work by stimulating the calcium-calmodulin pathway secondary to the upregulation of bone morphogenetic proteins (BMPs), transforming growth factor-β, and other cytokines.[16–21]

Methods of Electrical Stimulation

Three types of electrical stimulation have received US Food and Drug Administration approval for treating spinal fusions. These technologies include DC electrical stimulation, CC stimulation, and IC stimulation, such as PEMFs and CMFs. DC stimulation requires implantation of the device at the surgical site, whereas IC and CC methods are used noninvasively.

Direct Current Electrical Stimulation

DC stimulation involves the surgical implantation of electrodes connected to a battery. The cathodes are in direct contact with the exposed fusion bed. The cathode's effective stimulation distance is 5 to 8 mm. The batteries deliver a constant DC for a total of 6 to 9 months. The surgical implantation of the device obviates the need for patient compliance. However, there are disadvantages to the placement of the device because the manufacturer recommends removing the battery in 6 to 9 months, which entails a second surgical procedure. Also, there is a rare but reported risk of seeding the battery from systemic infection.

Direct Current Stimulation: Mechanism of Action

DC stimulation enhances the production of a number of osteoinductive factors that are normal regulators of bone matrix formation. This mechanism of action was discovered using Boden's animal model of spinal fusion,[17] which uses a New Zealand White rabbit intertransverse process fusion model for spinal fusion using autogenous bone graft. The model involves a surgical procedure similar to that performed in humans and has a similar nonunion rate to that of autograft.[17] Morone and colleagues[22] studied this model further and showed that within the developing fusion mass, there is a distinct temporal and anatomic location for the production of BMPs and other factors that are necessary to achieve a solid fusion.

Fredericks and colleagues[23] used this animal model to study the effects of DC on the temporal expression of growth factors in the developing fusion mass. They demonstrated that there was an upregulation in the production of BMP-2, BMP-6, and BMP-7 relative to controls. In addition, the use of DC stimulation avoided the potential complications seen with the application of a single high dose of growth factor to achieve fusion. Complications of ectopic bone formation, bone resorption, or antibody formation against the single growth factor have been reported with the application of a single growth factor.[23]

The use of DC stimulation creates an electrochemical reaction at the cathode. This creates a faradic reaction, lower oxygen concentration, increased pH, and hydrogen peroxide production. Decreased oxygen concentration has been shown to increase the activity of osteoblasts. An increase in local pH decreases the activity of osteoclasts and enhances the activity of osteoblasts. Furthermore, the elevation in pH can stimulate the release of vascular endothelial growth factor (VEGF) from local macrophages. VEGF has been shown to be another factor involved in enhancing vascular ingrowth and stimulating bone formation.

Direct Current Stimulation: Clinical Application

The clinical use of DC current stimulation began as early as 1974 by Dwyer, who demonstrated clinical success in 11 out of 12 patients who received an implanted bone stimulator.[15,24] Kane reported the results of a multicenter trial involving 84 patients who had an implantable DC current stimulator.[25] This group was compared with a historical control group of 159 patients. The experimental group using the DC current stimulator had a higher percentage of patients who had previous surgery and nonunion. Despite this bias favoring the control group, there was a significant increase in successful fusion in the DC-stimulated group: 91% versus 83% in controls. In 1988, Kane published an additional study of "difficult" patients undergoing posterior spinal fusion.[25] These patients were deemed difficult because they (1) had one or more previous failed spinal fusions; (2) had grade II or worse spondylolisthesis; (3) required extensive bone grafting necessary for a multilevel fusion; or (4) had other risk factors, such as obesity. He found that there was a statistically significant improvement in fusion rate of 81% in the electrically stimulated group versus 54% in controls.

In 1994, Meril reported a 93% fusion rate in patients who had undergone anterior lumbar or posterior lumbar interbody fusion with DC current stimulation compared with a 75% fusion rate in the control group.[2] In 1996, Rogozinski published a study that analyzed the use of DC stimulation in patients undergoing posterior lumbar spinal fusion with pedicle screw instrumentation and autograft.[26] The electrical stimulation group had a 96% successful fusion rate as compared with 85% in the control group. The higher rate of fusion in the Rogozinski study as compared with that in the Kane study may be related to the use of spinal instrumentation.

Kucharzyk[27] reported the outcome of a controlled prospective study in a high-risk fusion population. The study involved two groups, each with 65 patients with similar diagnoses. All patients underwent posterolateral fusions with pedicle screw instrumentation and the use of autologous bone graft. They were divided into two groups: those with or without the use of DC electrical stimulation. The average follow-up was 3.8 years. That study reported a 95% successful fusion in the stimulated group versus 79% in the control group.[27]

In 1996, Tejano and colleagues[28] evaluated a series of patients undergoing posterolateral intertransverse process fusion and facet fusions, either as a primary procedure or as a pseudarthrosis repair. They reported a 91.5% fusion rate in the primary surgery group and an 80% fusion in the pseudarthrosis group.

Capacitive Coupling Electrical Stimulation

CC is a noninvasive electrical stimulation technology used to enhance spinal fusions. This device consists of electrodes placed directly on the skin, over the area of the spine undergoing fusion. The pair of external plates produce electric fields when an electric current is applied by the alternating-current signal generator. The device is worn continuously for 6 to 9 months. The success of this technology, however, depends heavily on patient compliance. Brighton first reported CC electrical stimulation to treat recalcitrant nonunions in 1985.[29]

Capacitive Coupling Stimulation: Mechanism of Action

CC perturbs bone cell membrane potentials, which then activate membrane proteins and affect healing. Osteopromotive factors are upregulated by CC electrical stimulation. Using Boden's rabbit model for posterolateral spinal fusions,[17] Fredericks and colleagues[23] found that the normal physiologic expression of the following growth factors is upregulated by CC stimulation: BMP-2, BMP-4, BMP-6, BMP-7, transforming growth factor-β, fibroblast growth factor 2, and VEGF.

Lorich and colleagues[30] studied the response of bone cells to CC. They found that CC stimulation involves transmembrane calcium translocation using voltage-gated calcium channels. This mechanism increased intracellular calcium concentration and calmodulin activation, which has been shown to enhance bone cell proliferation. Zhuang and colleagues[31] further documented that this enhancement of calcium and calmodulin also promotes the synthesis of transforming growth factor-β. Brighton and colleagues[32] studied the signal transduction in electrically stimulated bone cells using CC. These studies demonstrated a dose-response effect, showing increased cell proliferation with longer treatment times.[32]

Capacitive Coupling Stimulation: Clinical Application

Goodwin and colleagues[33] performed a multicenter, randomized double-blind study of CC stimulation. Patients underwent either anterior interbody or posterolateral lumbar fusions. Clinical and radiographic results were assessed, and CC stimulation had a higher success rate of 84.7% versus 64.9% for the control group, although the surgeries varied in terms of use of instrumentation and type of bone graft material.

Inductive Coupling Electrical Stimulation

IC stimulation includes the mechanism of PEMF and CMF. The PEMF device is a noninvasive technology consisting of external current-carrying coils, driven by a signal generator. The CMF device differs from that of the PEMF device in that it involves a time-varying magnetic field superimposed on a static magnetic field. Bone generates a biphasic electrical potential when stress is applied. These electrical potentials are thought to be the signal for bone degradation and formation. The biochemical pathway mediating the effects of CMF may involve an increase in osteoblast responsiveness to insulin-like growth factor II by modulating receptor availability.

The PEMF coils must be worn across the area of the spinal fusion for approximately 6 to 8 hours daily for 3 to 6 months. Many clinical trials have shown that PEMF devices may help heal nonunions.[34] As with CC stimulation, however, patient compliance is essential.

Pulsed Electromagnetic Fields: Mechanism of Action

The mechanism of action of the PEMF is not well understood and its effect on enhancement of spinal fusion is not as conclusive as with DC electrical stimulation. Several animal studies show no significant differences with PEMF-treated groups and controls. In rabbits, there was an increase in stiffness, area under the load displacement, and load to failure of the fusion mass in the stimulated group versus controls. There are no in vivo animal studies using CMF for spinal fusions.

Clinical Studies of Pulsed Electromagnetic Fields

In one study, 13 patients with documented pseudarthrosis following posterior lumbar interbody fusion procedures achieved fusion after being treated with PEMF. Lee reported a 67% success rate for treatment of posterior pseudarthrosis with PEMF.[35] Mooney[36] reported a randomized, sham-controlled double-blind trial of 195 patients comparing PEMF versus placebo using a brace containing PEMF to induce an electromagnetic field in patients undergoing interbody fusion. They reported a 92% fusion with PEMF compared with 65% fusion in controls.[36]

Electrical Stimulators: Quality of the Evidence

In 2013, Tian et al. conducted a meta-analysis looking at the efficacy of various types of electrical stimulation on spinal fusion.[37] A total of 21 articles with 1381 patients were evaluated. The pooled fusion rate for all studies was found to be 85% (95% confidence interval [CI], 79–90%). No statistical difference was found between the three electrical stimulation methods. Further, subgroup analysis suggested that various patient and surgical factors—such as age, sex, smoking status, surgery type, fusion levels, implant use, and graft type—did not significantly influence the fusion rate.[37] However, although the authors compared DC, CC, and IC, the specific question of stimulation versus no stimulation was not addressed. Furthermore, there were several major limitations of that study,[38] including combining randomized trials with observational studies, no adjudication of the confidence in the effect estimates, no exploration of heterogeneity, no risk of bias assessment, and no presentation of results in a clinically applicable format (number needed to treat or minimal clinically important difference). Park et al.[39] performed the most recent systematic review of electrical stimulation following lumbar spinal fusion procedures; a statistical meta-analysis, however, was not performed by the authors.

A number of factors limit the quality of the evidence in studies assessing adjuvants to bone healing. First, in keeping with other orthopaedic studies of fracture healing, the definition of radiographic union has proved troublesome and inconsistent.[40–42] Static anteroposterior and lateral radiographs or computed tomography scans are generally the most common method for assessing bony union. Although use of standardized checklists can improve agreement,[40,43] none of the trials described used these checklists. Multiple, independent blinded assessors would also increase the reliability of union assessment. Second, most studies reported only surrogate endpoints; similar to other studies on orthopaedic adjunct devices, larger effects are typically reported for surrogates compared with direct measures of function.[44] In addition, patient-reported outcomes are inconsistently utilized in fusion studies. Finally, certain disadvantages of electrical stimulation—such as cost, patient inconvenience, and self-limited local conditions (e.g., skin irritation or superficial hematoma)—were rarely assessed.[33,45] Given the potential benefit in preventing nonunion, however, it is unlikely that these disadvantages would be a significant deciding factor for patients or clinicians. An economic evaluation by Wu et al.[46] demonstrated that electrical stimulation for bone healing is a more cost-effective fracture nonunion treatment when compared to either ultrasound or no stimulation and that patients receiving electrical stimulation had lower total health care resource use and overall costs.

In order to address many of the methodological limitations of previous studies, a rigorous meta-analysis of sham-controlled randomized trials was recently reported.[9] The study involved 15 sham-controlled randomized clinical trials that included 1247 patients total. The authors identified all trials randomizing patients to electrical or sham stimulation for bone healing and included acute fractures, nonunion/delayed unions, osteotomy, and spinal fusions. The assumption that electrical stimulation has a similar effect on all bone healing was hypothesized based on the consistency of the biologic process across all bone healing[47–50] This hypothesis was then tested using the interaction test, which found no evidence to support a difference in treatment effect due to treatment indication. The authors found moderate-quality evidence supporting that electrical stimulation decreased pain ($P = .02$)

and radiographic nonunion rates by 35% (95% CI, 19–47%). A subgroup analysis assessing only spinal fusions found an even greater effect of electrical stimulation with a nonunion risk reduction of 38% (95% CI, 45–84%).[9]

Conclusions and Future Direction

The clinical benefits of electrical stimulation in spinal fusion surgery have been well recognized and evidence supporting the use of electrical stimulators for spinal fusion continues to grow. Numerous studies demonstrate a consistent enhancement of successful fusion with electrical stimulation. Recent studies further show that electrical stimulation not only decreases rates of nonunion, but also improves patient-reported outcomes, such as pain.[9]

Future large, rigorously designed trials using an intention-to-treat analysis with clear reporting of methodologic quality are warranted.[51] Furthermore, future investigation into the use of electrical stimulators in higher-risk populations—such as smokers, those undergoing multilevel procedures, or those with reoperations—may allow clinicians to determine who may benefit most from this intervention. Additionally, although union is a continuous process and there is no commonly accepted radiographic definition, a consistent and valid method for defining union should be considered in future trials.[52] Finally, high-quality randomized trials assessing patient-important outcomes, such as function, are warranted.[9]

KEY POINTS

1. Three types of electrical stimulation are described for spinal fusion: direct current, capacitive coupling, and inductive coupling.
2. The mechanism of action of electrical stimulation therapy is not clearly understood but is generally thought to work by stimulating the calcium-calmodulin pathway secondary to the upregulation of bone morphogenetic proteins, transforming growth factor-β, and other cytokines.
3. The clinical benefits of electrical stimulation in spinal fusion surgery have been well recognized and evidence supporting the use of electrical stimulators for spinal fusion continues to grow.

KEY REFERENCES

1. Kahanovitz N. Spine update. The use of adjunctive electrical stimulation to enhance the healing of spine fusions. *Spine.* 1996;21(21):2523-2525.
2. Fredericks DC, Smucker J, Petersen EB, et al. Effects of direct current electrical stimulation on gene expression of osteopromotive factors in a posterolateral spinal fusion model. *Spine.* 2007;32(2):174-181.

REFERENCES

1. Zdeblick TA. A prospective, randomized study of lumbar fusion. Preliminary results. *Spine.* 1993;18(8):983-991.
2. Meril AJ. Direct current stimulation of allograft in anterior and posterior lumbar interbody fusions. *Spine.* 1994;19(21):2393-2398.
3. Boden SD. The biology of posterolateral lumbar spinal fusion. *Orthop Clin North Am.* 1998;29(4):603-619.
4. Boden SD. Biology of lumbar spine fusion and use of bone graft substitutes: present, future, and next generation. *Tissue Eng.* 2000;6(4):383-399.
5. Boden SD. Overview of the biology of lumbar spine fusion and principles for selecting a bone graft substitute. *Spine.* 2002;27(16 suppl 1):S26-S31.
6. Bush JL, Vaccaro AR. Electrical stimulation in lumbar spinal fusion. *Orthopedics.* 2000;23(7):737-743.
7. Kahanovitz N. Spine update. The use of adjunctive electrical stimulation to enhance the healing of spine fusions. *Spine.* 1996;21(21):2523-2525.
8. Oishi M, Onesti ST. Electrical bone graft stimulation for spinal fusion: a review. *Neurosurgery.* 2000;47(5):1041-1055.
9. Aleem IA I, Evaniew N, Busse J, et al. *Efficacy of Electrical Stimulators for Bone Healing: A Meta-Analysis of Randomized Sham-Controlled Trials. American Academy of Orthopaedic Surgeons Annual Meeting*; 2016; Orlando, FL.
10. Cook JJ, Summers NJ, Cook EA. Healing in the new millennium: bone stimulators: an overview of where we've been and where we may be heading. *Clin Podiatr Med Surg.* 2015;32(1):45-59.
11. Zigman T, Davila S, Dobric I, et al. Intraoperative measurement of bone electrical potential: a piece in the puzzle of understanding fracture healing. *Injury.* 2013;44(suppl 3): S16-S19.
12. Hartshorne E. On the causes and treatment of pseudarthrosis and especially that form of it sometimes called supernumerary joint. *Am J Med.* 1841;1:121-156.
13. Lente R. Cases of ununited fracture treated by electricity. *NY State J Med.* 1850;5:317-319.
14. Fukada E, Yasuda I. On the piezoelectric effect of bone. *J Physiol Soc Jpn.* 1957;12:1158-1162.
15. Dwyer AF, Wickham GG. Direct current stimulation in spinal fusion. *Med J Aust.* 1974;1(3):73-75.
16. Aaron RK, Boyan BD, Ciombor DM, Schwartz Z, Simon BJ. Stimulation of growth factor synthesis by electric and electromagnetic fields. *Clin Orthop Relat Res.* 2004;419:30-37.
17. Boden SD, Schimandle JH, Hutton WC. An experimental lumbar intertransverse process spinal fusion model. Radiographic, histologic, and biomechanical healing characteristics. *Spine.* 1995;20(4):412-420.
18. Ciombor DM, Aaron RK. The role of electrical stimulation in bone repair. *Foot Ankle Clin.* 2005;10(4):579-593, vii.
19. France JC, Norman TL, Santrock RD, McGrath B, Simon BJ. The efficacy of direct current stimulation for lumbar intertransverse process fusions in an animal model. *Spine.* 2001;26(9): 1002-1008.
20. Heckman JD, Sarasohn-Kahn J. The economics of treating tibia fractures. The cost of delayed unions. *Bull Hosp Jt Dis.* 1997;56(1):63-72.
21. Haddad JB, Obolensky AG, Shinnick P. The biologic effects and the therapeutic mechanism of action of electric and electromagnetic field stimulation on bone and cartilage: new findings and a review of earlier work. *J Altern Complement Med.* 2007;13(5):485-490.
22. Morone MA, Boden SD, Hair G, et al. The Marshall R. Urist Young Investigator Award. Gene expression during autograft lumbar spine fusion and the effect of bone morphogenetic protein 2. *Clin Orthop Relat Res.* 1998;351:252-265.
23. Fredericks DC, Smucker J, Petersen EB, et al. Effects of direct current electrical stimulation on gene expression of osteopromotive factors in a posterolateral spinal fusion model. *Spine.* 2007;32(2):174-181.

24. Dwyer AF. The use of electrical current stimulation in spinal fusion. *Orthop Clin North Am*. 1975;6(1):265-273.
25. Kane WJ. Direct current electrical bone growth stimulation for spinal fusion. *Spine*. 1988;13(3):363-365.
26. Rogozinski A, Rogozinski C. Efficacy of implanted bone growth stimulation in instrumented lumbosacral spinal fusion. *Spine*. 1996;21(21):2479-2483.
27. Kucharzyk DW. A controlled prospective outcome study of implantable electrical stimulation with spinal instrumentation in a high-risk spinal fusion population. *Spine*. 1999;24(5):465-468.
28. Tejano NA, Puno R, Ignacio JM. The use of implantable direct current stimulation in multilevel spinal fusion without instrumentation. A prospective clinical and radiographic evaluation with long-term follow-up. *Spine*. 1996;21(16):1904-1908.
29. Brighton CT, Pollack SR. Treatment of recalcitrant non-union with a capacitively coupled electrical field. A preliminary report. *J Bone Joint Surg Am*. 1985;67(4):577-585.
30. Lorich DG, Brighton CT, Gupta R, et al. Biochemical pathway mediating the response of bone cells to capacitive coupling. *Clin Orthop Relat Res*. 1998;350:246-256.
31. Zhuang H, Wang W, Seldes RM, et al. Electrical stimulation induces the level of TGF-beta1 mRNA in osteoblastic cells by a mechanism involving calcium/calmodulin pathway. *Biochem Biophys Res Commun*. 1997;237(2):225-229.
32. Brighton CT, Wang W, Seldes R, Zhang G, Pollack SR. Signal transduction in electrically stimulated bone cells. *J Bone Joint Surg Am*. 2001;83-A(10):1514-1523.
33. Goodwin CB, Brighton CT, Guyer RD, et al. A double-blind study of capacitively coupled electrical stimulation as an adjunct to lumbar spinal fusions. *Spine*. 1999;24(13):1349-1356.
34. Bassett CA. The development and application of pulsed electromagnetic fields (PEMFs) for ununited fractures and arthrodeses. *Orthop Clin North Am*. 1984;15(1):61-87.
35. Lee K. *Clinical investigation of the spinal stem system, open trial phase: pseudarthrosis stratum*. Las Vegas, NV: American Academy of Orthopaedic Surgeons; 1989.
36. Mooney V. A randomized double-blind prospective study of the efficacy of pulsed electromagnetic fields for interbody lumbar fusions. *Spine*. 1990;15(7):708-712.
37. Tian NF, Wu YS, Zhang XL, et al. Efficacy of electrical stimulation for spinal fusion: a meta-analysis of fusion rate. *Spine J*. 2013;13(10):1238-1243.
38. Murad MH, Montori VM, Ioannidis JP, et al. How to read a systematic review and meta-analysis and apply the results to patient care: users' guides to the medical literature. *JAMA*. 2014;312(2):171-179.
39. Park P, Lau D, Brodt ED, Dettori JR. Electrical stimulation to enhance spinal fusion: a systematic review. *Evid Based Spine Care J*. 2014;5(2):87-94.
40. Kuurstra N, Vannabouathong C, Sprague S, Bhandari M. Guidelines for fracture healing assessments in clinical trials. Part II: electronic data capture and image management systems–Global Adjudicator system. *Injury*. 2011;42(3):317-320.
41. McKee MD. Displaced fractures of the clavicle: who should be fixed?: commentary on an article by Robinson CM, et al.: "Open reduction and plate fixation versus nonoperative treatment for displaced midshaft clavicular fractures. A multicenter, randomized, controlled trial". *J Bone Joint Surg Am*. 2013;95(17):e1291-e1292.
42. Bhandari M, Petrisor B, Schemitsch E. Outcome measurements in orthopedic. *Indian J Orthop*. 2007;41(1):32-36.
43. Bhandari M, Chiavaras M, Ayeni O, et al. Assessment of radiographic fracture healing in patients with operatively treated femoral neck fractures. *J Orthop Trauma*. 2013;27(9):e213-e219.
44. Busse JW, Kaur J, Mollon B, et al. Low intensity pulsed ultrasonography for fractures: systematic review of randomised controlled trials. *BMJ*. 2009;338:b351.
45. Andersen T, Christensen FB, Ernst C, et al. The effect of electrical stimulation on lumbar spinal fusion in older patients: a randomized, controlled, multi-center trial: part 1: functional outcome. *Spine*. 2009;34(21):2241-2247.
46. Wu NL, Lee YC, Segina D, et al. Economic burden of illness among US patients experiencing fracture nonunion. *Orthop Res Rev*. 2013;5:21-33.
47. Academy of Orthopedic Surgery. *Musculoskeletal Injuries Report: Incidence, Risk Factors and Prevention*; 2000. Rosemont, IL: American Academy of Orthopaedic Surgeons.
48. Khan SN, Cammisa FP Jr, Sandhu HS, et al. The biology of bone grafting. *J Am Acad Orthop Surg*. 2005;13(1):77-86.
49. Marsell R, Einhorn TA. The biology of fracture healing. *Injury*. 2011;42(6):551-555.
50. Day SO, Ostrum RF, Chao EYS, et al. *Orthopaedic Basic Science: Biology and Biomechanics of the Musculoskeletal System*. 2nd ed. Rosemont, IL: American Academy of Orthopaedic Surgeons; 2000.
51. Chan S, Bhandari M. The quality of reporting of orthopaedic randomized trials with use of a checklist for nonpharmacological therapies. *J Bone Joint Surg Am*. 2007;89(9):1970-1978.
52. Bhandari M, Fong K, Sprague S, Williams D, Petrisor B. Variability in the definition and perceived causes of delayed unions and nonunions: a cross-sectional, multinational survey of orthopaedic surgeons. *J Bone Joint Surg Am*. 2012;94(15):e1091-e1096.

CHAPTER 69 Cervical Instrumentation: Anterior and Posterior

Eeric Truumees

Introduction and Overview

In the late 1890s, B.E. Hadra of Galveston, Texas, stabilized a cervical fracture-dislocation in the first modern report of spine instrumentation.[1] Hadra later used this technique in Pott disease.[2] For the next hundred years, cervical instrumentation remained limited to various posterior wiring schemes, of which Rogers' technique was the most frequently used.[3] In the 1980s, wiring patterns began to include corticocancellous bone struts for added extension stiffness.[4] In the last 2 decades rigid, segmental fixation, including lateral mass and pedicle screws, has dominated.

Anterior instrumentation could not be considered until Smith and Robinson popularized the anteromedial approach.[5] Even then, the simple plating systems carried over from appendicular stabilization were fraught with loosening, back-out, and other devastating soft tissue consequences. Dedicated anterior cervical plating systems were first described in the 1970s. Bicortical purchase decreased screw back-out and instrumentation failure rates but added canal penetration and cord injury risk. In the 1980s, locking mechanisms enabled safe unicortical purchase while preventing screw migration.[6]

Cervical instrumentation continues to evolve with new disc replacement systems, dynamic and low-profile anterior plates, cervical cages, and resorbable implants. While promising, some of these newer technologies have been incorporated into clinical practice without evidence of added benefit. Since the last edition of this textbook, interest in resorbable implants has waxed and waned.

Before recommending an implant system, American surgeons must consider its Food and Drug Administration (FDA) status. Often a device will be cleared for some, but not all, of its common indications. The reasoning is usually obscure and bureaucratic and does not always reflect safety or efficacy. Read the device's package inserts and direct questions to the manufacturer's legal counsel or to the FDA (800-638-2041).

The FDA is not empowered to dictate patient care. Off-label use of cervical instrumentation may occur in two settings, each establishing different demands on the physician. The practice of medicine includes use of FDA-cleared, marketed devices for indications not listed on the FDA approved labeling. When the indication or intended patient population lies outside the device's labeling, surgeons may still legally use the device per their best judgment but must be able to support the decision with reliable scientific evidence. It is prudent, though not specifically required, to discuss the proposed implant's FDA status and rationale with the patient. No investigational device exemption (IDE) or institutional review board (IRB) review is needed in practice of medicine cases. The second off-label implant setting involves experimental or investigational devices. If the FDA has not cleared the device for market for any indication, clinical use requires an IDE. Even then, the implant may be used only in accordance to the approved protocol's plan of investigation. A separate, formal informed consent must be obtained from the patient. Physicians involved in the study may not share the device with other physicians.

Since the last edition of this text, placement of screws in the posterior elements of the cervical spine, including pedicle and lateral mass screws, has received FDA labeling for most common indications. That said, several implants, such as some expandable cages, remain off-label when used in the cervical spine.[7-9]

Cervical spine implants are used in wide-ranging indications, including trauma, tumor, deformity, infection, and degenerative disease. In each group, the goals are the same; implants can reduce deformity, provide stability, and share loads with host and graft tissues until healing occurs. Most of these devices aim to support the fusion process. Some laminoplasty plates, for example, are approved as "bone graft containment devices." Newer devices seek to improve on their predecessors by emphasizing previously ancillary goals: minimization of adjacent-segment degeneration, surgical morbidity, iatrogenic neurologic deficits, and unintended-level fusion. For example, interest in motion-preserving devices is increasing. This chapter is written to assist spine surgeons in rational selection of implants by discussing their evolution, biomechanics, indications, outcomes, and complications.

Relevant Anatomy for Spinal Instrumentation

For the purposes of reconstruction, the cervical spine is divided into three regions: the cervicocranium, mid-cervical spine, and cervicothoracic junction. Each region's unique anatomic and biomechanical considerations influence the instrumentation chosen.

The cervicocranium includes the skull base, atlas, and axis. The cervicocranial joints' size, shape, and location allow more motion than those in the subaxial spine and render arthrodesis particularly challenging.[10,11] The bony elements of the cervicocranium, beginning with the occiput, are unique. The clivus ends in the basion, the anterior border of the foramen magnum. The opisthion refers to its dorsal border. From the foramen magnum, the occipital squama curves 90 degrees cranially toward the inion (or external occipital protuberance [EOP]).

Embryologically, the C1 vertebral body is absorbed into the dens. The absence of a C1 vertebral body means there is no disc between the occiput and C1 or between C1 and C2. The posterior C1 arch forms two-thirds of the ring. There is no spinous process, but rather a posterior tubercle to which the rectus minor and suboccipital membrane attaches. Critically, the vertebral artery runs along a groove on the cranial surface of the posterior ring. More than 1.5 cm from the midline, the groove becomes very shallow. Exposure of the ring's superior aspect risks vertebral artery injury. C1 has a lateral mass on each side, but no pedicle or laminae. While the arches are thin, the lateral masses are heavy, thick structures, each with concave superior articulating surface.

The occiput–C1 articulation includes convex occipital condyles lateral to the foramen magnum articulating with the concave C1 lateral masses. Normal occipitocervical extension is limited to 21 degrees when the occiput abuts the C1 posterior arch.[12,13] More than 8 degrees of rotation between the occiput and C1 is pathologic. In children, the flatter occiput–C1 joints are less able to restrict motion, predisposing them to injury.[14]

Atlantoaxial motion occurs through two sets of two joints. First, the slightly convex inferior facets of the axis meet the slightly convex superior facets of the atlas. These joints are oriented in the horizontal plane and have no interlocking bone to prevent subluxation. They allow 43 degrees of rotation, nearly half of normal cervical rotation.[15] The second set of atlantoaxial joints arises from the cranial projection of the odontoid projecting into axis ring. The dens acts as the focal point of a network of ligaments providing resistance to translation, flexion, extension, and rotation. Dens resection leads to vertical and atlantoaxial instability.[16]

The axis, the largest and heaviest cervical vertebra, bears a large, bifid spinous process. The bony isthmus between the facets is often called the pedicle. Technically, this represents the C2 pars and is a large dense structure that projects medially at 30 degrees and superiorly at 20 degrees. The short, stout, nearly horizontal C2 pedicle lies between the C1–C2 facet and the vertebral body.

The lower cervicocranium (C2–C3) transitions into the more homogeneous subaxial patterns.[17,18] The C3–C6 vertebrae exhibit a uniform configuration but increase gradually in size. The vertebral bodies are roughly twice as wide as they are deep. Each contains a body, paired pedicles and articular masses, laminae, and a single, bifid spinous process. The transverse process projects laterally from the superolateral aspect of the body and anterior surface of the articular mass and contains the foramen transversarium. The transverse process ends in anterior and posterior tubercles. At C6, the prominent anterior (carotid) tubercle can be palpated for intraoperative localization.

Morphometric data from 100 CT studies revealed mean vertebral body widths of 24.6 and 23.0 mm wide in males and females, respectively.[19] The narrowest measured 17 and 14 mm, respectively. In the midsagittal plane, the average anteroposterior (AP) diameter was 18 mm in males (smallest, 13 mm) and 16 mm in females (smallest, 10 mm). A morphometric analysis of critical cervical pedicle dimensions recorded a wide range of values and only fair interobserver correlation.[20] Transverse angulation was constant at 40 degrees. Relative to the lateral mass axis, the C3 and C4 pedicles were oriented superiorly, whereas C6 and C7 were oriented inferiorly. The dorsal entry point of the pedicle on the lateral mass defined by transverse and sagittal offset had similar mean values with wide ranges and variable topography. Sufficient variation exists to preclude safe instrumentation with topographic landmarks alone. Ludwig and colleagues recommended laminoforaminotomy or image guidance to place these screws.[20]

Because bony element size varies considerably, preoperative planning with axial and sagittal images decreases the risk of screw placement. For example, verify that the C2 isthmus is large enough to accommodate a 3.5 mm screw. If bony element size is questionable on magnetic resonance imaging (MRI), a 2-mm computed tomographic (CT) slice limited to the levels of surgical interest should be obtained. Request that the CT gantry be reangled to parallel the endplate at each disc level. Clear preoperative measurements of the bony elements allow larger screws to be used. Otherwise, smaller screws with lower pullout and fatigue strength characteristics are used. Similarly, preoperative planning allows improved screw trajectory to incorporate better triangulation and subchondral bone purchase. Upper cervical anterior plating may benefit from coronal CT or MRI images above C3 because anatomic variation is considerable and makes this technique inadvisable in up to 20% of cases.[21]

The uncinate process projects cephalad from the inferior mid-cervical vertebral endplates. The immediately superior vertebral endplate receives the uncinate via a contiguous lateral indentation. Together, the process and indentation form the synovial uncovertebral joint (of Luschka). Biomechanically, the uncovertebral joints regulate extension and lateral bending. The posterior uncovertebral joint has a secondary role in torsional control.[22,23]

Posterior midline cervical approaches first encounter the spinous process. The bifid process may be taller on one side or the other. The surgeon must therefore pay critical attention to the midline. Deep in the subperiosteal plane, no sharp demarcation exists between the spinous process and the lamina. Spinous process wiring techniques therefore require great care to avoid inadvertent spinal canal entry. Working laterally, an inferior notch at the junction between the lateral mass and the lamina is typically encountered. At the medial boundary of the lateral mass, this notch serves as an excellent landmark both for lateral mass fixation and en bloc decompression procedures. The articular masses (or pillars) are dense, heavy, rhomboid structures formed by junction of the superior and inferior articular processes. Average facet inclination is 35 degrees from vertical.

Successful cervical instrumentation requires a detailed understanding of vascular anatomy. First, placement of occipital screws risks dural sinus injury. Venous sinus injury is especially likely with screw placement within 1 cm of the EOP.[24] The internal carotid artery (ICA) runs a mean 2.9 mm from the anterior C1 lateral mass and is therefore at risk with Magerl and Harms screw constructs.[25] ICA injury could lead to life-threatening hemorrhage and stroke, but only one clinical report has, as yet, emerged.[26] In this case, a 60-year-old man presented with an 8-month history of recurrent cerebral infarcts more than 3 years after atlantoaxial stabilization with transarticular screws. The screw tip impinged the ICA, leading to both high-grade arterial stenosis and a pseudoaneurysm. On the other hand, in a retrospective review of 50 random contrast CTs of the head and neck, the artery's course would place it at risk during C1 lateral mass screw placement in 58% of cases.[27] Medial screw angulation decreases risk.

Vertebral artery injury may occur with both anterior and posterior cervical procedures. Although clinically evident injuries are rare, catastrophic consequences include fistula, pseudoaneurysm, cerebral ischemia, and death.[28,29] Because the vertebral arteries are paired, injury to one rarely results in significant neurologic deficit. If intraoperative vertebral artery injury is suspected, do not attempt exposure or screw placement on the contralateral side. In anterior procedures, dissection lateral to the vertebral body puts the vertebral artery at risk.[29] On approach, carefully mark the midline. Previously, with both anterior and posterior vertebral artery injury, attempts were made to tie off the vessel. Posteriorly, the vertebral arteries are vulnerable to injury during insertion of Magerl and C2 pars and pedicle screws because the drill bit traverses the C2 body. Especially in rheumatoid patients, a high rate of erratic and variable arterial courses has been reported and may preclude safe screw placement in 20% of sides (Fig. 69.1)[28,30,31] Thus, with any significant cervical reconstruction procedure, preoperative investigation of the artery's course is mandatory.[32] Although recommendations today vary, the advent of endovascular repair has prompted many spine surgeons to request an intraoperative vascular surgery consultation. For many of these injuries, local bleeding is controlled and the patient is taken to the vascular suite for stent placement. Consider permanent occlusion or ligation only if the contralateral vertebral artery provides adequate collateral circulation.

Less frequently, a variable course of the posterior inferior cerebellar artery could pass through the skull into the upper cervical spine, where it is vulnerable to C1 lateral mass screw placement.[33]

Another major anatomic factor limiting safe cervical spine instrumentation is individual variation. In children, for example, standard implant sizes may be too large. Because their fusion potential is so high, onlay bone grafts alone are a good option in most children. However, in children with neuromuscular disorders or greater degrees of instability, rigid stabilization should be considered.[34]

In one study of 28 children with skeletal dysplasia, nonrigid implants with postoperative halo immobilization were compared with rigid implants. Nonunion was seen in nine of 14 nonrigid cases and one of 14 rigid cases. That said, two of the children in whom rigid implant placement was attempted had intraoperative vertebral artery injuries. No new neurologic deficits were seen in either group, however.[35]

Recent anatomic studies have suggested that, in children as young as 2 years, the occipital keel, C1 lateral mass, and C2 lamina offer adequate space for 3.5 mm screw placement in "almost all cases."[36] Transarticular screw placement was not considered safe in the majority of these younger patients. Successful use of C2 laminar screws in children was recently reported.[37] Caution is certainly advised for patients younger than 6 years.[38-40] Other implants modified for use in small children, including craniofacial miniplates, have been described.[40]

Body habitus also affects instrumentation choices. For example, obtaining a shallow trajectory for dens screw placement in barrel-chested patients is difficult. A preoperative CT

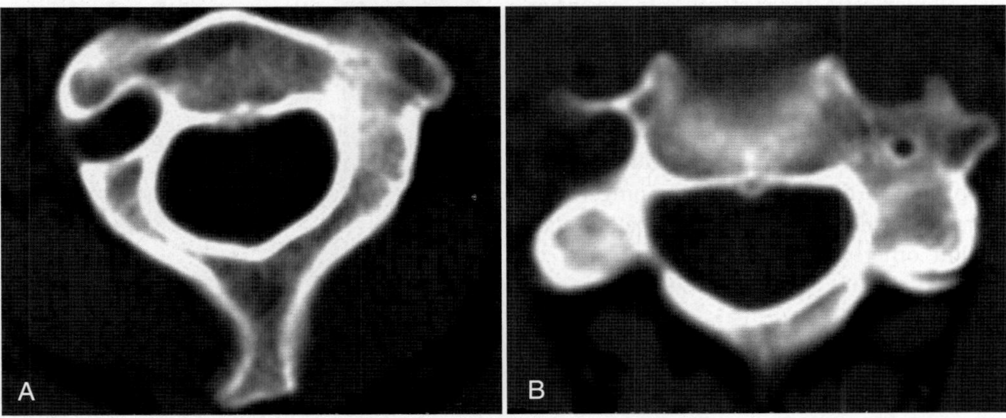

FIG. 69.1 Asymmetric course of right vertebral artery at (A) C2 and (B) C6. Risks of screw placement vary significantly from right to left sides.

topogram should be used to assess this option. Similarly, transarticular screw placement is more challenging in patients with marked thoracic kyphosis. If the topogram does not include enough of the patient's frame, check the screw's inclination angle by holding a guide wire alongside the neck and obtaining lateral fluoroscopic images. Adjusting the patient's position often allows the case to go forward. Failure to make these changes before incision adds significantly to the time, risk, and complexity of the procedure. Occasionally, coronal images are useful. Structures at risk include the vertebral artery and the hypoglossal nerve. Note the size and caudal extent of the jawline, which may limit anterior upper cervical instrumentation angulation options.

Significant interindividual variability also affects reconstruction options at the cervicothoracic junction. Typically, the Southwick and Robinson anteromedial exposure is difficult below T1–T2.[41] Even in cases in which the disc space can be safely reached, orthogonal screw placement is affected by the manubrium.[42] In Sharan's study of 106 consecutive MRIs, while T3 was often cranial to the sternal notch, a straight trajectory was limited to the T1–T2 disc space.[43] Transmanubrial or transsternal approaches increase exposure to T3 but are associated with significant morbidity.[44] Below T4, a formal thoracotomy is often required. In one study, the size of the thoracic outlet, as measured by the instrument manubrial thoracic distance, served as a key guide to the optimal anterior approach.[45] Still, marked interindividual variability of the cervicothoracic angle and the cranial extent (and cervical level) of the superior manubrium (i.e., short- and long-necked patients) greatly affects selection, ease, and safety of anterior approaches.[43,46]

Although cervical instrumentation relies on standard spinal approaches, a wider exposure than that for simple decompression or uninstrumented fusion procedures is often needed. Small incisions with tight fascial constraints may force suboptimal screw trajectories. Because rigid implants "lock in" segmental alignment, careful attention to positioning is mandatory.

Percutaneous placement of cervical instrumentation from both anterior and posterior approaches is being reported with increasing frequency in the literature.[47] For example, to protect the midline tension band, lateral mass screw constructs have been implanted via tubular retractor systems.[48] In posterior cervical reconstruction, smaller, midline open approaches may complement percutaneous screw delivery.

The fluoroscope should be set up so that AP and lateral images can be easily obtained. For technically challenging cases such as dens or Magerl screw fixation, simultaneous AP and lateral fluoroscopy may be helpful. Prior to draping, check the alignment fluoroscopically. While certain pathologies reduce better in flexion, others align with extension.

Fluoroscopy and Navigation for Cervical Spine Instrumentation

Safe instrumentation of the cervical spine requires avoidance of vascular and neurologic structures that are often not exposed for implant placement. Historically, intraoperative fluoroscopy has been used to confirm level localization, optimize spinal alignment, and assess screw trajectory. Fluoroscopy can be used in real time to guide entry point selection or after placement to confirm acceptable positioning. Some techniques, such as cervical disc arthroplasty, require a real-time approach to ensure proper implant centering and alignment. Other indications for continuous or pulsed live imaging include cervical vertebroplasty and debridement of distant structures (Fig. 69.2).[49,50]

At the occipitocervical and cervicothoracic junctions, overlying bony structures such as the jaw and shoulders frustrate fluoroscopy.[51] Other limitations of fluoroscopy include increased surgical time, possible sterile field contamination, and radiation exposure.[52] Delineation of which cases intraoperative fluoroscopy is "necessary" remains controversial.[53-55] In one study of 419 cervical pedicle screws, 17 were malpositioned.[53] Given the risks associated with malposition, the authors concluded that pedicle axis/en face views improved safety. Even with intraoperative imaging, malposition rates from 2.7% to 34% are reported.[54,56-58]

In another series, the accuracy of intraoperative AP fluoroscopy was compared with use of bony landmarks (the uncovertebral joints) when centering a cervical disc prosthesis.[59] Postoperative CT scan demonstrated acceptable accuracy with anatomic alignment alone. A variety of intraoperative guides to improve aim and placement have been devised but have gained only limited popularity.[60]

Overlapping anatomic structures, difficulty imaging the cervicothoracic junction, and the desire for intraoperative axial images have fostered increased interest in "three-dimensional" fluoroscopy.[51] The reconstructed axial images are not real CT slices, but intraoperative CT simulation was found to have 100% concordance with postoperative CT.[61] The bulk and radiation required limit the utility of these systems in real-time imaging applications. Typically, they are used at the end of the procedure to document appropriate implant

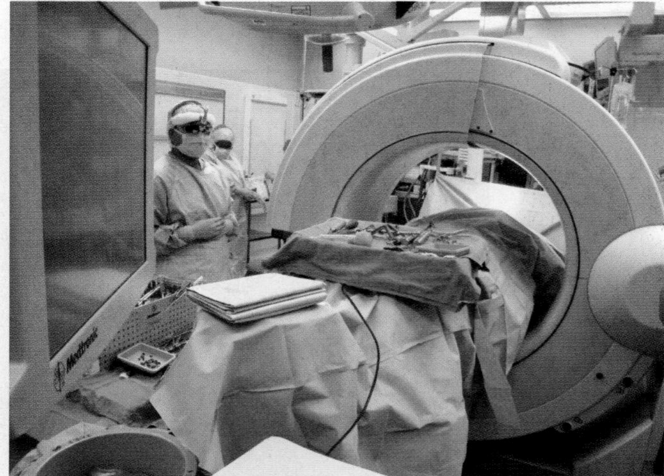

FIG. 69.2 Intraoperative image using O-Arm navigation (Medtronic) in a complex cervical reconstruction.

positioning or as part of a frameless stereotactic guidance system.[62] Although these systems continue to rapidly evolve, significant controversy remains as to their accuracy in cervical applications.[63,64] Ludwig and others found computer guidance more accurate than topographic landmarks or a laminoforaminotomy in accurate cervical pedicle screw placement.[20]

Beyond improving safety of screw insertion, computer-aided spinal navigation has fostered enthusiasm for smaller incisions and less soft tissue mobilization.[65]

Use of image guidance to place C2 pedicle screws in a minimally invasive manner was compared with standard open placement. Accuracy rates were similar but time and blood loss were lower in the minimally invasive group.[66] Another recent study of eight children with failed wiring for atlantoaxial instability underwent successful, rigid stabilization using CT navigation.[67] Most conclude that navigation improves, but does not eliminate, the risk of critical screw malpositioning. Computer guidance systems may be particularly helpful in patients with previous surgery, deformity, or destructive processes that obliterate landmarks.[68-70]

Limitations of computer navigation include displacement with drilling forces, cervical mobility requiring frequent reregistration, small structure size at the limits of device accuracy, and steep trajectories outside device pathways.[71] The surgeon must understand the principles of the tracking system to prevent misinterpretation of computer-generated information.[72] Navigation systems should only be used by experienced surgeons who can, if necessary, continue the procedure with conventional techniques.

Selecting the Biomechanically Correct Implant

The most common preventable cause of instrumentation failure arises from surgical judgment errors. Although modern implants are overengineered for their designated function, their success requires understanding of their biomechanical function.[73-75] Direct failure of the implant is most often due to improper selection or fatigue. The average spine cycles 3 million times per year.[76,77] If bone healing fails to occur, the implant will ultimately fail, either at its anchor points in the bone or in the material itself. The novelty and technical challenge of safe implant placement should not divert the surgeon's attention from meticulous preparation of the fusion bed and grafting technique. Occasionally, misplaced implants fail. However, careful surgical exposure and intraoperative radiographic confirmation reduces misplacement (Box 69.1). More typically, failure occurs when the surgeon fails to fully understand one of four things: (1) the forces to which the spine will be subjected, (2) the planes in which the spine is unstable, (3) how the implants are meant to counteract these forces, and (4) how instrumentation affects forces passing through structural grafts.

Unlike typical fracture healing, which passes through Hunter's stages of bone repair (inflammation, soft callus, hard callus, and remodeling), most modern cervical implants seek primary healing in which osteon cutting heads directly cross segmental gaps.[78,79] This approach requires near-anatomic alignment and rigid stabilization. Excessive strain or poor bone-to-bone contact stimulates fibrous tissue deposition and, ultimately, construct failure. The importance of restoration of proper spinal alignment in reducing stresses on the construct and graft has become increasingly clearer.[80]

BOX 69.1 Important Factors in Selection of Cervical Implants

Pathoanatomy: mechanism of injury and direction of instability
- Mode of failure (in trauma, direction and magnitude of injury vector)
- Direction of instability
- Degree of instability
- Compromised stabilizing structures:
  - Number of levels
  - Number of spinal columns per level
  - Bone vs. ligament (anticipated healing)

Host bone quality
Graft bone quality
Expected level of patient loading
Availability of postoperative immobilization
Surgeon familiarity with techniques
Availability of implants

No clear line divides the "stable" from the "unstable" spine. In serial sectioning studies, White and Panjabi concluded that more than 11 degrees of sagittal angulation and 3.5 mm of sagittal plane translation represented instability.[75] These values are most helpful in the acute trauma setting but are less meaningful with chronic destruction, such as with infection. In many cases cervical instrumentation is not meant to correct any innate spinal instability, but rather to reverse the iatrogenic instability associated with decompression. Because each structure contributes to normal stability and kinematics, minimizing disruption of intact structures during decompression is key.[82] For example, a two-level cervical anterior approach is less destabilizing than a one-level corpectomy.[83] Another classic example of iatrogenic spinal destabilization is postlaminectomy kyphosis.[84] The difficulty in treating this condition fostered interest in laminoplasty.

The surgeon must ask: what is unstable, which planes are affected, and how badly? In trauma, for example, identifying the primary plane or mode of failure is critical. For example, a transverse atlantal ligament rupture leads to flexion instability, whereas posteriorly displaced dens fractures are unstable in extension as well. Posterior C1–C2 wiring is mechanically more rational for transverse acetabular ligament rupture than for displaced dens fracture.

Account for patient-specific factors when planning cervical instrumentation. Children's excellent healing potential may require less rigid fixation.[85] On the other hand, even with excellent graft carpentry and implant placement, osteoporosis increases segmental motion and decreases construct pullout and fatigue strength.[86] Other physiologic factors, such as the challenged healing environments in diabetics and smokers and after chemotherapy and radiation, as well as in larger or poorly compliant patients, may require a more aggressive, rigid implant strategy.[87]

Increase the strength of any spinal construct with added fixation points, triangulated placement, or the goal of aiming for the dense subchondral bone of the vertebral endplate. Alternatively, extend postoperative immobilization.[88] For cervical bone screw placement, insertional torque, pullout strength, and bone mineral density are highly correlated.[89,90] Bone mineral density has a greater impact on pullout strength than bicortical purchase,[91] yet the relative merits of unicortical versus bicortical screw purchase continue to be debated.[92] In both anterior and posterior applications, bicortical screws exhibit significantly greater holding power in terms of both immediate pullout strength and fatigue resistance.[84,93-95] Yet even in the trauma setting, unicortical fixation maintains reduction and confers high fusion rates.[96] The advantages of bicortical purchase are magnified in osteoporosis, wide decompression, multilevel procedures, and when the available fixation points are limited.[89,97-99]

Adding polymethylmethacrylate (PMMA) to the screw tract significantly increases the screw's torque and pullout strength.[100,101] Bone loss may affect pedicle screws because they engage cortical bone rather than the lateral mass's cancellous bone, later and to a lesser degree.[63] Other physiologic factors, such as challenged healing environments after chemotherapy and radiation, may mitigate for more rigid fixation.

Once the surgeon has delineated the "personality" of the pathology, implant options should be considered. Ideally, the surgeon should be facile with a wide array of implants and techniques to tailor the treatment to the patient's needs. That is, having decided which issues the implant is meant to address, the surgeon should review the available options while noting each implant's limitations and risks. Implantation risks vary and decrease with experience. Each institution may offer a variety of tools, such as fluoroscopy, navigation systems, and intraoperative monitoring, that may improve safety.

Early attempts at surgical fixation were complicated by infection, devascularization, inadequate metallurgy, and metal allergy. Better antisepsis, soft tissue handling, and materials evolved. Then, a limited understanding of the bone biology and mechanics resulted in poorly conceived implants and techniques. Over time, biomechanical studies have improved implant design. Unfortunately, these studies underestimate the importance of soft tissue and muscular tension. Most biomechanical research is limited by its ex vivo nature. Cadaveric, animal, or plastic spines are tested in laboratory settings with various pure or complex loads, but these studies do not take into account the importance of muscle forces, tissue healing, or the possibility of gradual ligamentous relaxation (creep).[102,103]

The surgeon should seek to optimize the healing environment by limiting unnecessary exposure, denervation, and devascularization of the paraspinal muscles. Compromised extensor musculature allows collapse into kyphosis above or below the instrumentation.[48] Increasingly, surgeons are exploring midline sparing, less-invasive approaches to the placement of cervical implants, even in anatomically challenging regions such as the C2 pedicle.[104] Careful muscular repair may protect the construct.[105] In the posterior cervical spine, a multilayered closure, including the suboccipital triangle and ligamentum nuchae, improves balance and decreases eccentric implant loading.[48,106]

Biomechanical Principles and Functional Modes

Most cervical spine implants are made of stainless steel, pure titanium or, most commonly, titanium-aluminum-vanadium alloy. Steel implants usually have cobalt chrome and molybdenum to enhance corrosion resistance and have a modulus of elasticity 12 times that of normal bone. That means that steel is significantly stiffer than bone. Titanium alloys tend to have greater native biocompatibility and corrosion resistance. Furthermore, titanium has a modulus only six times greater than bone. Use of titanium alloys is increasing because of their high strength/weight ratio, enhanced ductility, and increased fatigue life.

The material's ultimate tensile strength refers to the area under its stress-strain curve up to the point where elastic deformation becomes plastic deformation. That is, ultimate tensile strength is the maximum stress a material can sustain without changing shape. This value is different for different materials and ranges from 50 MPa for trabecular bone to 650 MPa for titanium.[74] Ultimate tensile strength of a material may become altered during surgery. Compromise of the implant's integrity by repeatedly bending and unbending is common. Titanium is especially sensitive to notching. The implant's material properties are also affected by manufacturing elements such as drill holes, structural imperfections, and surface irregularities. Hardness is a surface characteristic referring to the material's ability to resist plastic deformation. Hardness can be enhanced with surface coating, but improper handling may destroy the surface coating and compromise implant hardness.

During the 1950s, Danis and Müller refined the principles of internal fixation.[107] Stable internal fixation fulfills the spine's local biomechanical demands without concomitant external immobilization. Fixation strategies can be subdivided by implant constraint. A constrained system's locking mechanism rigidly binds the individual components (e.g., the screw and plate). The surgeon should achieve maximum rigidity by segmental fixation of each vertebra to a constrained system. A nonconstrained construct is fixed only at the ends of a multilevel construct or includes nonrigid connections between the screws and longitudinal member.

Spinal implants function in one or more modes (Box 69.2). The principal mode is defined by the device's location on either the spine's flexion or extension side and by the principal mechanism of loading. The degree to which a stabilization mode is "needed" depends on the spine's mechanical deficits. For example, an anterior cervical plate's role varies depending on the quality of the interbody grafting. When the spine

BOX 69.2 Functional Modes of Spinal Implants

Tension banding
Buttressing
Neutralization
Lag screw
Deformity correction

Modified from Aebi M, Thalgott JS, Webb JK. *AO ASIF Principles in Spine Surgery.* Berlin: Springer; 1998:243.

remains unable to sustain compressive forces, a strong, rigid, bridging implant, applied to either the anterior or posterior columns, serves as the weight-bearing column. The most common cervical bridging implants are multilevel, segmental, rigid posterior screw-rod systems compensating for multilevel anterior metastatic disease or difficult-to-reach, anterior cervicothoracic or occipitocervical lesions.[108] Posterior lateral mass plates or rods are more typically used in neutralization mode. To decrease strains across bone healing surfaces, the neutralization implant shields flexion and axial loading forces while minimizing torsional bending and shearing loads.

The buttress principle is designed to prevent axial deformity. In the appendicular skeleton, a buttress plate holds impacted or depressed fragments once they have been elevated back into anatomic position. Anterior cervical surgery often includes restoration of disc height with an interbody device. Here, the plate, placed on the side of load application, "buttresses" the spine, minimizing compression, torque and shear forces. The buttress effect requires close surface contact between the implant and the bone surface. The implant and bone surface should be carefully contoured before fixation. Any osteophytes that cause the plate to "ride up" should be resected. In buttress mode, the middle screws should be inserted first, moving away afterward in both directions.

A tension band is also applied to the extensor side but requires competent load-bearing ability. A typical example is posterior wiring used to encourage fusion in anterior cervical discectomy and fusion (ACDF) with delayed union. This wire resists tensile and bending forces only if the anterior spinal column can bear weight. In the pseudarthrosis setting, this limitation confers an advantage because it encourages fusion by dynamically compressing the anterior weight-bearing column. In most cases, additional posterior bone graft is not required.

Only 36% of cervical axial loads are borne anteriorly while 32% is borne by each of the posterior articular pillars.[109] Despite the relative importance of the articular pillars, the mobility and heavy weight of the head relative to the small size of the cervical bony elements underscores the anterior column's critical role in construct stability. When comparing "loose" with "tight" grafts, graft status predicted overall construct stability and plate effectiveness.[110] On the other hand, excessive anterior distraction decreases posterior column load transmission and thereby subjects the anterior graft and vertebral bodies to excessive loads.[111,112] In trauma cases, for stability, cover at least 30% of the endplate area.[113] Similarly, endplate preparation affects graft support and axial loads.[114,115]

Cervical stabilization is achieved with bone screws used independently or with plates, rods, or cages. Name screws by describing their major diameters, intended bone type and thread proportion (partially or fully threaded), thread pitch, lead, and length. A screw's minor (root or shaft) diameter determines its tensile strength and breakage resistance. The distance between adjacent threads is a screw's pitch. Increasing pitch increases bone between threads but decreases number of threads over the length of the screw. Pullout strength is determined by its root area and the host bone's composition. Root area, the total surface of thread contact to bone, is primarily determined by the screw's major (outside or thread) diameter.

Cortical screws typically exhibit a smaller major diameter, decreased pitch, and a shallower thread than cancellous screws. Pretapping the hole prior to screw insertion reduces thread-bone interface microfracture and improves holding power, but requires an extra step. Self-tapping cortical screws confer similar holding power and have become standard.[101,116] However, the cutting flute at the screw's tip limits thread contact and may require 1-2 mm increased depth of penetration. Cancellous screws, on the other hand, provide more surface area for bone purchase by increasing major diameter and pitch. As insertion compacts trabecular bone, cancellous screws are not tapped.

Torque applied through the screwdriver rotates the screw clockwise, advancing it along its predrilled path. Screw advancement creates an axial compression force against the cortex or plate. On average, insertion applies 2500 to 3000 N.[117] Over time, living bone remodels, slowly decreasing compressive force. External forces magnify this innate loss of holding power.

Individual screws may also be placed in one of several "modes." Positional or neutralization screws hold the implant, such as an anterior plate, to the spine via compressive forces. For neutralization screws, use a centering guide to drill a pilot hole of equal diameter to its root. Lag screws provide compression across two surfaces. Overdrill the proximal bone to the screw's outer diameter. The distal piece is drilled to the inner diameter. The torque differential pulls the distal bone to the proximal. Cervical cages with predrilled screw paths utilize this principle. Lag techniques offer little protection against axial loading and rotation. Thus, in the spine, they are best used with cages or plates.

In rigid, locking plates, the screw head is locked to the plate through either secondary metal-on-metal threads, a Morse taper, or an external blocking system. In that these screws function mechanically more like a bolt than a screw implies that the axial force generated during insertion is not critical. The simplest of these designs act like internal external fixators.[93,118] Longer screws improve fixation.[119]

Anterior Spinal Instrumentation

Unlike the posterior cervical spine, all anterior implants are constrained by limited purchase sites, sagittal profile concerns, and the limited extensibility of most surgical approaches. Anterior fixation points are limited to the vertebral body and endplates. Anterior cervical pedicle and occipital condyle screws have been described, but are technically challenging and infrequently performed.[21] Bulky implants may cause swallowing difficulty or respiratory compromise. Currently, anterior reconstruction options can be divided into direct dens fracture fixation, anterior load-bearing implants, and plates. Load bearing implants, including disc replacements, bone struts and cages, reconstruct defects created by discectomy and corpectomy procedures.

Anterior Screw Stabilization of the Upper Cervical Spine

In the cervical spine, stand-alone screw fixation is used most frequently to provide rigid internal fixation of unstable dens fractures while preserving C1–C2 motion and avoiding extensor muscle dissection and graft harvest morbidity. Dens screw fixation is indicated mainly in widely displaced type II fractures.[120] Before C1 lateral mass fixation, dens screw fixation was specifically recommended in patients with concomitant C1 ring fractures to avoid posterior fusion to the occiput. Direct anterior stabilization is associated with decreased blood loss, postoperative pain, and morbidity relative to posterior fusion operations.[121] In patients with incomplete reduction from traction, an attempt at direct, open anterior reduction may be undertaken. These maneuvers are performed with fluoroscopic guidance from an entry point significantly caudal to the injury. This technical challenge sways surgeons with only limited anterior open reduction internal fixation (ORIF) experience to treat incompletely reduced fractures posteriorly.

Contraindications to dens screw fixation include transverse atlantal ligament (TAL) disruption and fractures more than 18 months old.[120,122-124] Horizontal and posterior oblique fracture lines are much more likely to heal in anatomic position than anterior oblique.[120] Some "high" type III fractures have enough bone in the body inferiorly to maintain purchase of the base of the screw. But, in "low" type III dens fractures, the screws may break out of the inferior aspect of the C2 body.

The utility of stand-alone dens screw fixation in osteoporotic and elderly patients continues to be controversial.[125] In one retrospective study, 102 of 110 achieved fracture healing.[126] The nonunion rate was 4% and 12% in those under and over age 65, respectively. However, in a comparison study of 29 odontoid fracture patients older than age 65, all posteriorly fused patients healed uneventfully. Only 8 of the 11 dens screw patients healed. Interestingly, 7 of the 10 treated nonoperatively healed and only after long and complicated courses. The authors concluded that, in the elderly, posterior C1–C2 fusion was superior to both anterior fixation and nonoperative treatment.[88]

Dens screws are placed using an anteromedial approach. Before surgery, reduce the fracture with traction. The transverse incision is made just above the level of the cricoid cartilage. Split the platysma muscle longitudinally and the carotid sheath is identified. Blunt dissection extends the approach cranially. The prevertebral fascia and anterior longitudinal ligament (ALL) are split in the midline over the axis. Expose the fracture site only if open reduction is needed.[121] Once the fracture is reduced, place two 2.0 mm K-wires into the anterior inferior C2 body with biplanar fluoroscopy guidance. Optimal access typically requires resection of the anterior anulus of the C2-C3 disc space. One maintains rotational stability as the other is tapped. A 3.5-mm cortical screw is placed after which the second wire is removed. Some surgeons continue to recommend dual-screw placement. Recently, percutaneous dens screw fixation has been reported using a cannulated system.[127]

Dens screws average 40 mm in length. While single screw fixation is sufficient, the tip of the screw must penetrate the apical cortex. Postoperative immobilization regimens vary among surgeons from either soft collar to halo vest immobilization for 2 months. Direct osteosynthesis of acute dens fractures is associated with an 88% union rate as soon as 6 weeks postoperatively.[120,121] Remote fractures healed at a significantly lower rate of fusion (25%). Overall, hardware failure occurs in 10%.

Other anterior screw fixation techniques into axis and occiput have also been described.[21,128] Early, anatomic feasibility studies of an endoscopic, endonasal approach to atlantoaxial transarticular screw fixation have been reported.[129] To date, these techniques appear to be used rarely in clinical situations in which posterior fixation techniques are not possible or have already failed. Here, anterior screw fixation may add stability to augment continued attempts at posterior arthrodesis.

Anterior Cervical Plating

In the early 1990s, as cervical plates became safer and easier to implant, their use exploded in tandem with interbody allograft over structural autograft.[130,131] Benefits include decreased rates of: pseudarthrosis, graft extrusion, and graft subsidence (Fig. 69.3).[132] Plating allows the patient to avoid postoperative bracing and begin early rehabilitation.[113,133] While the benefits of plating may justify application, this does not imply that a plate is "needed" in most degenerative conditions. Good outcomes have been reported without instrumentation and there is little proof that routine anterior cervical plating improves surgical outcomes.[5,134-137] With proper graft carpentry and immobilization, even unplated corpectomies heal.[138] Yet, one series of 97 tricortical autogenous iliac crest ACDFs reported pseudarthrosis rates of 11% and 28% in one- and two-level cases, respectively, despite 2 months of collar immobilization.[139] The reduction in pseudarthrosis and graft extrusion rates associated with plating justifies multilevel anterior procedures.[6,133,135,140-142]

The drawbacks of cervical plating include implant cost and bulk and the possibility of late soft tissue injury. Previous concerns over stress shielding of the plated bone and graft appear to have minimal clinical relevance.[143-145] Esophageal erosion secondary to screw or plate loosening, while rare, may be fatal.[146] Additionally, if adjacent-segment surgery is indicated, the approach may require a more extensive dissection to remove the old plate. "Extension" plates and all-in-one screw-cage designs may allow previous implant retention without significant biomechanical compromise.[147,148]

The least controversial indications for anterior cervical plating include stabilization after major anterior bone resections after corpectomy for tumor or fracture. Anterior plates are also used, with or without supplementary, posterior instrumentation in:

- Multilevel discectomy
- Most cervical corpectomy procedures
- Irreducible locked facets with cervical disc herniation
- Anterior cervical pseudarthrosis
- Trauma with loss of anterior load-bearing ability

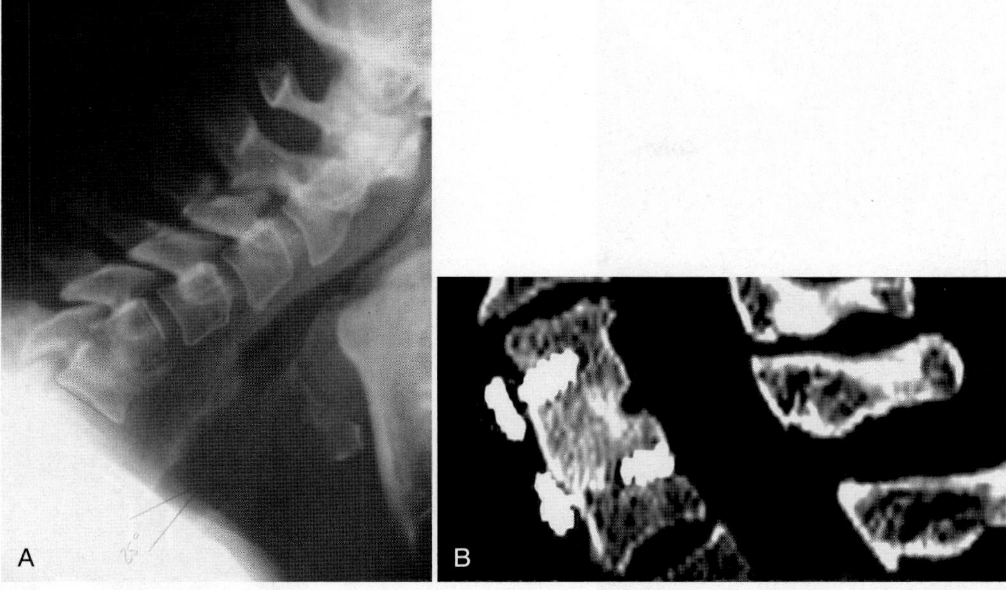

FIG. 69.3 (A) Lateral radiograph of patient with painful C5–C6 pseudarthrosis after uninstrumented anterior cervical discectomy and fusion. (B) After revision with a plate, the bone graft healed, as confirmed by sagittal computed tomography. Note plate prominence proximally.

After posterior instrumentation, anterior plating does not appear to confer additional mechanical benefits.[149-151] Thus, if an immediate posterior approach with screw and rod placement is to be performed, anterior grafting or cages are helpful, but the plate is probably not needed.

Evolution and Mechanics of Anterior Cervical Plates

Most anterior cervical plates are placed in a buttress mode. As such, they do not eliminate all motion. The more levels included in the construct, the more motion, including plate bending and screw-bone and screw-plate interface toggling is expected.[152] In many loading modes, anterior plating is inferior to a rigid, posterior construct. As a stabilization method, therefore, it fills a role somewhere between "too stable to need an implant" and "too unstable to survive plating alone."

Without a plate, spinal flexion loads the graft, and extension unloads it. With a rigid anterior plate, these forces reverse. Flexion unloads the graft and extension loads the strut more than similar degrees of flexion in the unplated state.[153] Taller grafts magnify this effect by disc space distraction and diminished posterior column loading.[111]

Initially, small fragment appendicular plating was used. The Caspar plate was among the first specifically for the cervical spine. Its parallel screw slots allowed settling, making the Caspar also the first axially dynamic plate. At that time, settling was considered undesirable and plate was modified by replacing half of its slots with round holes. These screws were not locked to the plate. After cycling, all unlocked unicortical constructs lose significant rigidity.[93] Bicortical purchase was required to decrease back-out.

Second-generation cervical plating systems, such as the Cervical Spine Locking Plate (CSLP, Synthes, Inc.), added rigidity and locking mechanisms. Many of these plates force a medial screw convergence to resist pullout through the triangulation effect. Advantages of locking the screw-plate interface:

- allows unicortical fixation
- prevent screw back-out
- improve fatigue life (loss of rigidity after cycling)

Typically, differences in grafting technique yield greater differences in overall construct rigidity than plate choice.[154] For most degenerative indications, nonrigid plates are mechanically similar to locking plates.[155] In multilevel and more unstable constructs, however, failures, including plate and screw fracture, construct pullout, and delayed or nonunions were reported even with second-generation plates.[133,135,140,142] Designers responded with thicker and stronger implants.

Even with highly rigid third-generation plates, pseudarthroses continued to occur. Benzel and others observed fracture of rigid plates in patients with solid arthrodesis and hypothesized that plate failure allowed construct dynamization similar to a sliding hip screw.[156] Sliding hip-nail constructs permit deformation along the femoral neck axis, subjecting the fracture to optimal compression forces. Several cervical plates seek to control subsidence and bone graft load sharing.

Today, cervical plates can be placed into three groups. *Rigid* plates remain popular. Recent mechanical studies, often in destabilized cadaveric models, continue to support their use over nonlocking and dynamic implants.[157,158] *Dynamic* plates could allow oversettling, resulting in kyphosis, foraminal narrowing, and lower fusion rates.[159-161] Dynamic plate advocates argue that late rigid plate nonunions are under-recognized.[156,162] *Intermediate* designs allow variable screw angulation in an otherwise rigid plate. Some plates offer both fixed and variable screw insertion methods. Interestingly, variable screw plates

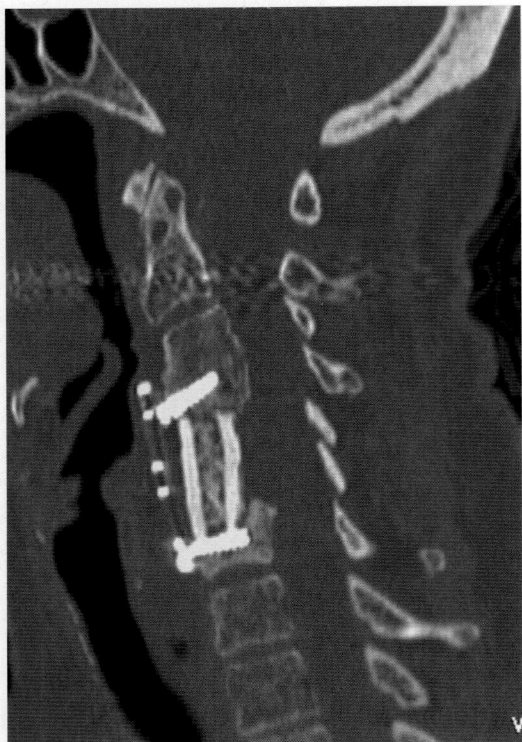

FIG. 69.4 Sagittal postoperative computed tomographic image showing subsidence of a fibular strut after anterior cervical corpectomy. Note the dynamization of plate with telescoping superiorly and the near absence of the normal vertebral body trabecular pattern. The loss of horizontal trabeculae should alert the surgeon to osteoporosis and a higher risk of implant failure, especially with fixation in the anterior, mostly cancellous spine.

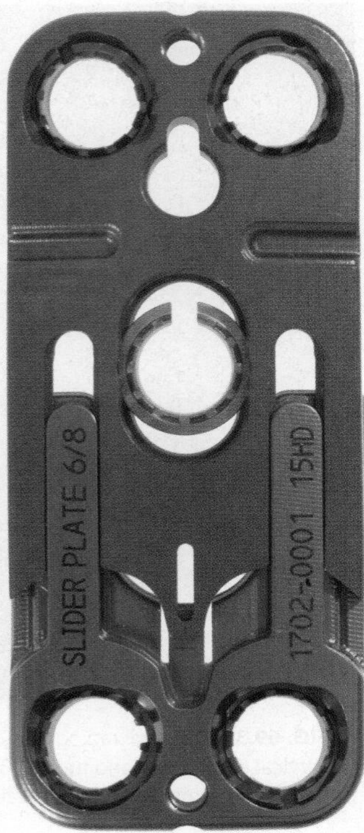

FIG. 69.5 Anterior cervical dynamic plate (Ant-Cer Plate) allowing controlled collapse. (Courtesy Zimmer Biomet, Warsaw, IN.)

have detractors from both the rigid and "fully" dynamic camps. One mechanical study found that variable-angled plates had more favorable pullout characteristics no matter what angle for screw insertion was used.[163]

In general, locked cervical plates and dynamic plates are similar in flexion-extension, lateral bending, and torsional stiffness. All plates effectively share load with a full-length graft. As normal graft resorption occurs, a rigid anterior cervical plate may prevent graft load sharing by maintaining a gap between the graft and the host bone.[164] However, if graft subsidence (or controlled impaction) occurs, dynamic plates share load more effectively than locked plates (Fig. 69.4).[165-168] The degree of load shielding engendered by rigid plating is controversial.[169,170] Another cadaveric study reported that dynamic and static plates offered similar overall stabilization, but the dynamic plate performed better in extension and after endplate removal.[171] Whether dynamic plates are appropriate in trauma and other highly unstable situations continues to be debated.[157,171]

Dynamic systems offer significant design variability, but typically incorporate implant telescoping features or movement along the spine itself. For example, the ABC slotted plate design allows up to 10 mm each of cephalad and caudad plate migration. While telescoping implants may be more elegant, one study found them less stiff than slotted designs.[165] Some allow graft preloading (Fig. 69.5).[112,167]

While several studies have been released over the last 15 years, no clear clinical evidence of the superiority of one plate over another has been identified. In a series of 34 DOC plate system cases, 85% of plates subsided and 61% impacted more than 3 mm but mean lordosis changed only 0.4 degree.[142] Anterior cervical reconstruction employing dense cancellous grafts and dynamic plates reported a 1-year fusion rate of 96%.[172] Average subsidence for single-level and two-level fusions were 2.0 and 3.2 mm, respectively. In a prospective analysis of 50 consecutive patients, either a rigid or a load-sharing plate (Orion and Premier, respectively) was placed.[173] After 12 to 35 months, there was no difference in the fusion rates. Interestingly, significant differences in pain and functional impairment favored the load-sharing system. Other studies have reported similar or lower fusion rates with dynamic plates (16% vs. 5% with the static plate).[160,174]

At the time of the last edition of this text, anterior cervical plates constructed from bioresorbable polymers had been introduced.[175,176] Their rationale was function as graft containment devices while reducing or eliminating complications such as implant migration and failure, imaging degradation, and stress shielding of the fusion mass. The implants theoretically dissolve after their mechanical function has been fulfilled and before long-term problems occur. Ultimately, however, the mixed quality of fixation offered (with early, dramatic failures), the variable speed to resorption, and the occurrence of inflammatory reactions led to a marked decline in investigations in that direction.[177,178]

Similarly, while still available, the popularity of plates with single screw fixation per level has waned. These devices were produced to reduce thickness and operating room time; however, few appreciable benefits were realized and higher pseudarthrosis rates encountered.[179]

Cervical Plating: Indications and Rationale

After multilevel reconstruction and high-energy trauma, stand-alone anterior plating is controversial. After multilevel strut grafting, anterior plates significantly increased global spinal stiffness and decreased segmental motion.[153] However, while excellent radiographic outcomes are reported after single- or two-level plated constructs, with additional levels, the risk of graft failure increases substantially, even with a plate.[134,180]

However, ongoing screw-vertebral motion is seen after three-level corpectomy and 4 level discectomy cases.[150] While two motion segment constructs are acceptably immobilized, lateral mass screw systems are significantly more rigid in longer constructs.[149,170,181,182] After cycling, range of motion at the lower end of the construct increased 171% in flexion, 164% in extension, 153% in lateral bending, and 115% in axial rotation. This fatigue failure explains caudal loosening of long anterior plate constructs.[150] In multilevel reconstructions, consider longer and larger diameter screws, or supplementary, posterior instrumentation.[183]

Rather than perform multilevel corpectomies, many surgeons prefer hybrid corpectomy/discectomy decompressions to allow improved restoration of lordosis and additional, mid-construct anchors. Whether the spared ligamentous and bony interconnections justify the additional time and fusion surfaces that must heal remains unclear.[110,184-187] In a cadaveric study segmental fixation afforded by three-level discectomy and hybrid discectomy and corpectomy yielded significantly more flexion-extension and lateral bending stiffness than the two-level corpectomy.[188] In two small studies of four- and five-level hybrid anterior reconstructions, all patients ultimately fused.[189,190] The authors concluded that adjunctive, posterior stabilization was not needed when hybrid techniques are used.

Historically, stabilization of the traumatized cervical spine required either posterior stabilization or halo immobilization.[191] More recently, in patients with a flexion-distraction injury and disc herniations, anterior plate fixation was reported to obviate a posterior approach.[192] Some recommend this approach only in patients with good bone quality, utilizing wedged grafts and external immobilization until radiographic fusion is evident.[193] In a mechanical study, anterior fixation was "adequate" to stabilize the traumatized segment, but lateral mass plating was even more effective.[194]

Failure rates increase with age and medical comorbidities.[195] In that front-back surgeries are difficult to recommend to older, sicker patients, halo bracing has been tried instead. Unfortunately, halo-vests poorly immobilize the lower cervical segments at most risk for construct failure. Halos confer additional pulmonary and other medical morbidity.[196] As such, formal anterior-posterior reconstructions must be considered. After posterior instrumentation, anterior plating does not confer additional mechanical benefits.[149-151]

Cervical Plating: Technique

Anterior plates are typically applied through a standard anteromedial approach. A transverse incision generally suffices. In some cases, a longitudinal incision along the anterior border of the sternocleidomastoid is required. Optimal screw trajectories may be limited by tension from the midline viscera, especially in males with a large thyroid cartilage. In this setting, adequate fascial release improves implant alignment and decreases retractor pressure.[146] Inadequate exposure risks aberrant screw trajectories into the adjacent (usually superior) disc space. Some authors recommend intraoperative fluoroscopy or K-wire placement into adjacent disc spaces to guide subsequent plate and screw trajectory planning.[197] On the other hand, unnecessary dissection or incorrect needle localization may increase adjacent-segment degeneration (ASD) risk.[198]

Select a plate of appropriate size. Depending on the intended screw angulation, the plate should extend no further than the midportions of the superior and inferior vertebrae. Adjacent-level ossification disorder (ALOD), an early form of ASD, increases with plate impingement on the cranial adjacent segment. In one series of 330 ACDFs, Caspar pins, plate impingement, and ALL stripping were all risk factors for ALOD, which was seen in the 6 to 12 months after surgery.[199]

With longer constructs holding pins maintain plate alignment while drilling the screw tracts. Otherwise, drilling may dislodge or rotate the plate. In long constructs, malangulation may translate into poor fixation at the opposite end of the construct. On the other hand, in a series of 200 patients undergoing one-, two-, and three-level ACDFs, frontal plane angulation and lateral displacement were not significantly associated with outcomes.[200]

Close plate contouring increases effective buttressing, may decrease swallowing difficulties, and increases the number of screw threads in the vertebral body.[201] Overcontouring may risk plate fracture.[202] Prior to plate application, ensure proper alignment, especially neck rotation and remove any externally applied traction.

Many surgeons universally use 14 mm screws. Optimally, base screw depth on the anterior-posterior depth of the adjacent intact vertebrae should be 12 to 20 mm. If measuring from CT, confirm that the gantry angle simulates the ultimate screw trajectory. Consider bicortical purchase in osteoporotic bone or more unstable situations.[89] Bicortical screws may better "lever" the spine into lordosis, but may also decrease graft-plate alignment prevent load sharing, and increase force on the bone-implant interface.[156,201] The biggest disadvantage to bicortical screw fixation lies in the danger of cord or root injury.[118,170] If bicortical screws are to be placed, use a screw-tap method under image intensification control. Palpate the posterior cortex with a thin, blunt K-wire or ball-tipped probe.

Some plates strictly fix the screw trajectory. Others allow a "cone" of variable screw placement. Variable angle plates have been recommended as a means of "dynamizing" the construct.[158] Angulation may allow longer screws to be placed with triangulation to enhance pullout strength. Most commonly, an "up and in" trajectory is recommended. Others recommend the screws be angled into the dense, subchondral bone plate. More recently, a trajectory 90 degrees to the plate has been recommended.[163] Proper screw placement in anterior cervical plating cases is often suboptimal if done without radiographic guidance.[203] When possible, redirect screws that enter adjacent disc spaces.

Typically, the plate supplements the more critical portions of the procedure. Emphasize any necessary canal and foraminal decompression, sagittal alignment correction, and subsequent grafting. Cervical plates will not compensate for poor grafting technique.[74,77] Traditionally, patients undergoing anterior cervical plating procedures were placed in rigid braces postoperatively. More recently, a strong trend toward soft collar or nonbracing has emerged. In a 257-patient randomized, multicenter trial, the nonbraced patients had a higher, but not statistically different, fusion rate.[204]

Cervical Plating: Outcomes and Complications

Anterior cervical plate outcomes and complications vary most by the underlying indication for placement. On the other hand, a general sense of these risks and benefits assists the surgeon when deciding what types of implants are rational in a given clinical situation.

Given that plating is often recommended to improve fusion rates, our limited ability to identify a solid fusion, "stable pseudarthrosis", or symptomatic nonunion must be clear. Plain films do not always reveal subtle clefts or inducible displacement on flexion and extension.[205] Fine-cut CT scans better define bridging trabecular bone, but with significant radiation exposure. Further, implants, particularly stainless steel plates or "trabecular metal" cages cause scatter.

The advantage of anterior plates for single-level cervical fusions continues to be debated.[139,206,207] When comparing reoperation rates before and after they began routinely plating ACDFs, Bose et al.[207] reported 48 unplated cases, in which three developed early graft extrusions and two had symptomatic pseudarthrosis. In comparison, one of the 35 plated one-level ACDFs developed displacement and three exhibited symptomatic pseudarthrosis.[207] Others found little advantage in outcomes or fusion rates after plating one-level cases.[140,208] Unplated patients more often drifted into kyphosis.[208] Another series of single-level discectomies reported pseudarthrosis rates of 4.5% and 8.3% with and without plate fixation, respectively.[134] Based on Odom's criteria, good or excellent results were reported in 91% and 88% of the plated and nonplated patients, respectively. Single-level plating is associated with few complications.[6,132] After one-level ACDF, routine radiographic assessment may not be warranted in asymptomatic patients.[209] Only 2% of the asymptomatic patients had construct abnormalities compared with 25% of the symptomatic patients.

Fusion rates decrease with increasing levels and the advantages of plating become more apparent. In a two-level ACDF cohort, pseudarthrosis rates were 0% for plated patients and 25% for those with no plating.[135] In three-level fusions, better clinical outcomes and an 18% pseudarthrosis rate were reported in the plated group versus a 37% pseudarthrosis rate in the nonplated group.[136]

After ACDF and corpectomy, bone graft collapse or settling into the adjacent endplates commonly results in a kyphotic deformity. Plating is superior to nonplating in maintenance of segmental lordosis, though the impact of that lordosis on long-term clinical outcomes continues to be debated.[210-213] In Wang et al.'s series, the 0.75 mm of graft collapse in plated patients compared with 1.5 mm for nonplated patients.[134] In 93 patients undergoing cervical corpectomy without instrumentation, there was a mean loss of 10.4 degrees of lordosis. Sagittal contour was not associated with neurologic decline or functional outcome.[211]

The complications of instrumented procedures include all of those associated with noninstrumented procedures, with the addition of:

- Metal sensitivity
- Disruption of imaging
- Bulk of instrumentation/soft tissue impingement
- Elimination of space for bone graft
- Late hematogenous seeding of infection
- Increased morbidity of any revision surgeries

A number of authors have reported that cervical plating is "permissive" and over the last 15 years, complications have become similar to those for nonplated fusions.[135,214,215] In large, society-wide reports, cervical instrumentation complications included a 2% to 3% neurologic injury rate, 3% to 45% reoperation rate for implant failure, and 5% to 10% infection rate.[216] Today, neurologic injuries and infections from plate application are rare.[215,217]

Unfortunately, implant failures are reported more frequently (1-4%) and may result from osteoporosis, multiple insertion attempts, inadequate postoperative immobilization, or excessive postoperative loading.[215,217] Often, the implant failure rate is proportional to the number of multilevel cases. Plate rigidity and bicortical screw fixation also impact failure rates.[95,170]

In osteoporotic patients, avoid Caspar pins (which may pull through the bone and disrupt plate anchorage), consider bicortical fixation, and, for those patients with significant cervical deformities, plan a back-front-back approach to serially release and correct alignment.[99] In one recent biomechanical investigation of 12 cadaveric spines, the addition of posterior screws and rods always increased stiffness and resistance to cyclic loading from the anterior plate alone. An especially large difference was noted for fixation of three or more levels.[218]

Unicortical screws may break their plate retention mechanism and back out, or may take the plate with them. Bicortical screws tend to fail in the middle from three-point bending loads after graft settling. When screws enter the neighboring disc space, they may accelerate ASD. The impact of well-performed ACDF on the incidence of degeneration at adjacent levels remains controversial. One cadaveric study found no difference in adjacent-segment motion or pressures between a grafted fusion with and without plate fixation.[219]

Screw displacement may cause esophageal injury.[220,221] Vascular complications arise from over-retraction on carotid sheath or direct injury to the vertebral artery.[29] Retraction is especially problematic in older patients with atherosclerosis and may lead to strokes. Vertebral artery injury is rare with anterior procedures and is thought to occur with excessive lateral dissection.

Dysphonia and dysphagia have received more attention in the recent literature. While rates vary from 2% to 60% (which may depend on whether and how the question is asked), both are more common in women.[222-224] Rates increase with revision and more cranial levels.[222-224] The degree to which plate placement and thickness affect dysphagia remains controversial.[223,225,226] If there is a plating effect, it may arise from plate thickness, texture, or merely the increased exposure necessary to place one. One study compared final construct height with preoperative osteophyte height.[224] No differences in rates of dysphagia were noted. When comparing 156 consecutive patients undergoing ACDF with either the thinner, smoother Zephir plate or the thicker and rougher Atlantis plate, dysphagia gradually decreased over 2 years to 0% and 14% in the Zephir and Atlantis groups, respectively.[225] Plate removal improved dysphagia in 17 of 31 patients.[226] In those improving after plate removal, adhesions were found between the plate and surrounding fascial structures.

Anterior Cervical Cages

Along with plating, cervical cages have evolved as increasingly complex cervical reconstruction efforts were carried out anteriorly. Structural grafting historically required tricortical iliac crest or autologous fibula harvest. In some countries, allograft bone banks have obviated the morbid structural bone harvest. In other parts of the world, allograft is not readily available and axially stable implants were sought to eliminate structural graft harvest.[227]

Mechanics and Rationale

Initially, mesh cages were developed for corpectomy indications. Over time, cage materials and geometries have rapidly expanded. Now, there are interbody devices for ACDF procedures, struts to reconstruct corpectomy defects, expandable cages, and cages with built-in plating or screw-in mechanisms. Cage materials include machined allograft, titanium, polyetheretherketone (PEEK), carbon fiber, and trabecular metal (among others) (Fig. 69.6). The ideal cage provides the following benefits[228]:

- Immediate structural support to resist axial compression and maintain anterior column distraction
- An adequate "footprint" to resist subsidence
- Small enough size to prevent stress shielding of the graft material
- Decreased surgical morbidity by obviating structural autograft harvest
- Avoidance of structural allograft complications (interspecimen quality variability, microfracture, collapse, and the possibility of viral transmission)

Theoretical disadvantages of anterior cage placement include the following [229]:

- Variable modulus of elasticity mismatch with host bone (depending on cage material)
- Increased cost
- Sharp edges causing soft tissue injury with displacement (mainly titanium mesh)
- Difficulty with postoperative imaging and confirmation of fusion (metallic implants)
- Limited true fusion (spot welding of small graft area inside the cage to host bone)
- Limitations in "sculpting" of material after insertion

As with cervical plates, many design philosophies have evolved that attempt to maximize cage advantages while minimizing their limitations. As with other implants, no best cage has been identified. Some implants are better suited for some patients or indications than others.

Cervical cages come in two main geometries: vertical and horizontal. Typically, vertical implants fill corpectomy defects and horizontal implants reconstruct postdiscectomy gaps. For the latter group, the mechanical goal is of distraction-compression via restoration of annular tension.[230,231] Implantation technique varies but is not significantly different than bone graft placement. The metallic tines of vertical cages and threads or texturing of horizontal cages allow better torsion and displacement resistance than an equivalently sized, smooth bone graft.

Cages are further subdivided by shape and material. Horizontal cage designs, for example, include screw-in, box, or mesh. Screw-in cages are threaded cylinders (e.g., BAK/C; Zimmer Biomet). The use of these implants has declined since the last edition of this text due to the excessive endplate violation required for insertion. Box cages are rectangular with textured bearing surfaces. The titanium implants developed initially gave way to carbon fiber and then PEEK designs (Fig. 69.7). One recent comparative study found no difference in the mechanical properties or fusion potential of PEEK vs. titanium ACDF spacers.[232]

Several mechanical studies have been undertaken to better understand the relative merits of different cage materials and geometries. In one, multiple cage types and autologous iliac crest grafts were tested in flexion, extension, axial rotation, and lateral bending in 80 sheep spines. Compared with an intact segment, cages increased flexion but decreased rotational stiffness. Mesh designs provided greater extension and bending stiffness than screw-in designs.[233] When compared with standard Smith-Robinson ACDF, single BAK/C offered significantly lower stiffness and failure loads.[234] Cage size and placement in the disc space are more important than differences in pore size or materials.[235] A fully open cylinder transferred loads more effectively than a central pore in a box design.[236]

The mechanical benefits of cages over bone graft are small. A cage does not supplant the additional stability afforded by plating.[90,228,237-239] A finite element model compared four implantation methods and found that stand-alone cages offered the least stabilization. The cage with a locking plate was very stiff in all directions. Two dynamic plate configurations reduced flexibility in all directions compared with intact cage but left significant mobility.[240]

One disadvantage of cage implantation is difficulty assessing radiographic fusion status; radiolucent carbon fiber and PEEK interfere less.[229] Even more important is the expense;

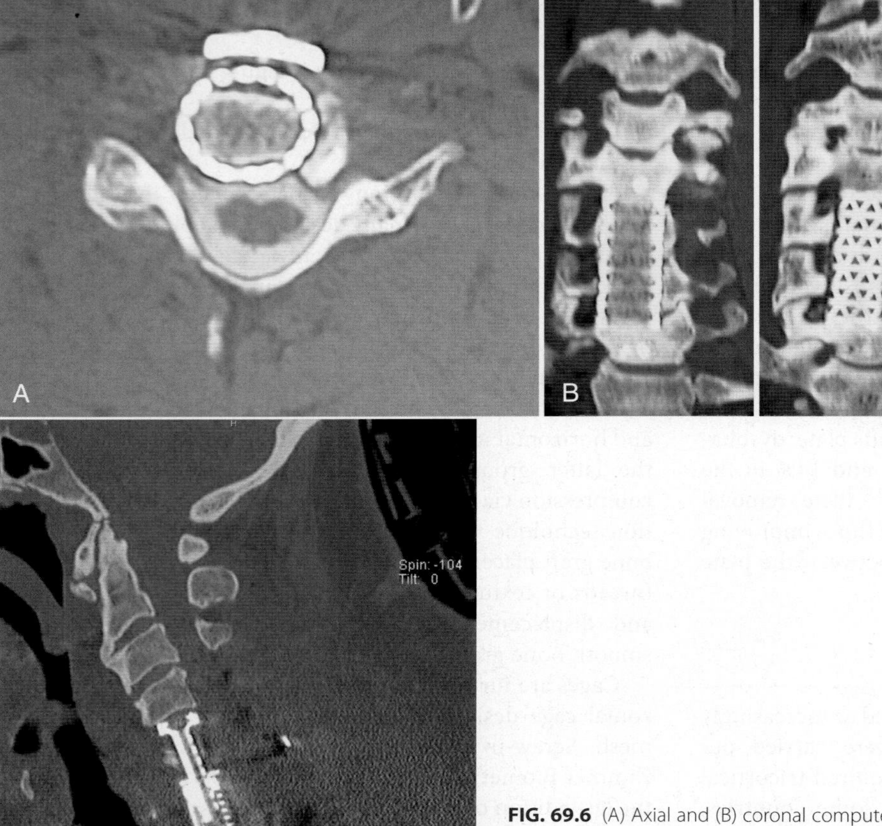

FIG. 69.6 (A) Axial and (B) coronal computed tomographic (CT) scan of structural vertical mesh cage with autogenous bone graft placed inside cage. The cage was placed too far to the right (best seen in A), and the patient reported right-sided radicular symptoms. (C) Sagittal CT image of patient in whom reconstruction of a three-level corpectomy for ossification of the posterior longitudinal ligament was attempted with an expandable cage. Despite the presence of fusion with segmental instrumentation, cage subsidence into the T1 superior endplate led to anterior displacement. This cage was ultimately replaced with a custom-cut mesh cage.

in most cases, cages are used with, rather than in lieu of, plating.

As with traditional grafting, subsidence has been seen with cages, but less with wide endplate coverage.[238,241] For example, cylindrical implants subside significantly further than plate and graft or rectangular cage constructs.[228,242] Endplate preservation and graft pegging or limited endplate perforation for vascular ingrowth decrease subsidence.[114,243]

Expandable cages, initially used in tumor reconstruction cases, have recently received increased attention in reconstruction of the degenerative cervical spine. Proponents argue that traditional cages require segmental overdistraction to place the cage and achieve tight endplate contact.[244] Distraction in situ allows the cage to be precisely adjusted to the defect.

Thus, these cages may also be easier to place in anatomically challenging regions such as the occipitocervical and cervicothoracic junctions. Alternatively, more extensive jaw-splitting or submandibular approaches may be used to place mesh cages. Anterior occipitocervical implants continue to be described, typically for post–tumor resection cases and usually with posterior, rigid, adjunctive instrumentation. Recently, a biomechanical study of anterior mesh cage placement with screws into the clivus demonstrated stable fixation for reconstruction of extensive ventral upper cervical spine defects.[245]

In a retrospective review of 20 corpectomy patients reconstructed with a distractible cage with an attached plate, stability was achieved in all cases. One subsidence and 75% good or excellent outcomes were reported.[246] In anatomic regions with limited anterior access (e.g., cervicothoracic and occipitocervical junctions), formal anterior plating may be difficult. Custom cages decrease the need for perpendicular access to the spine.[247] Detractors argue that expandable cages limit bone graft area, add significant cost, and generate high forces that precipitate adjacent-segment fractures.[248]

Newer hybrid cage devices incorporate plates or screw recesses.[229,249] These anchored spacers integrate screws to provide immediate fixation while maintaining low implant profile. This approach may decrease procedure time and allow decreased morbidity of approach by limiting anterior soft tissue disruption, particularly for surgery adjacent to a previous fusion, in that it may obviate the need for plate removal. However, a stiff fusion mass may overtax the holding power of these devices. While one biomechanical comparison of an anchored spacer to predicate cage-plate constructs found no significant differences, the same authors more recently found

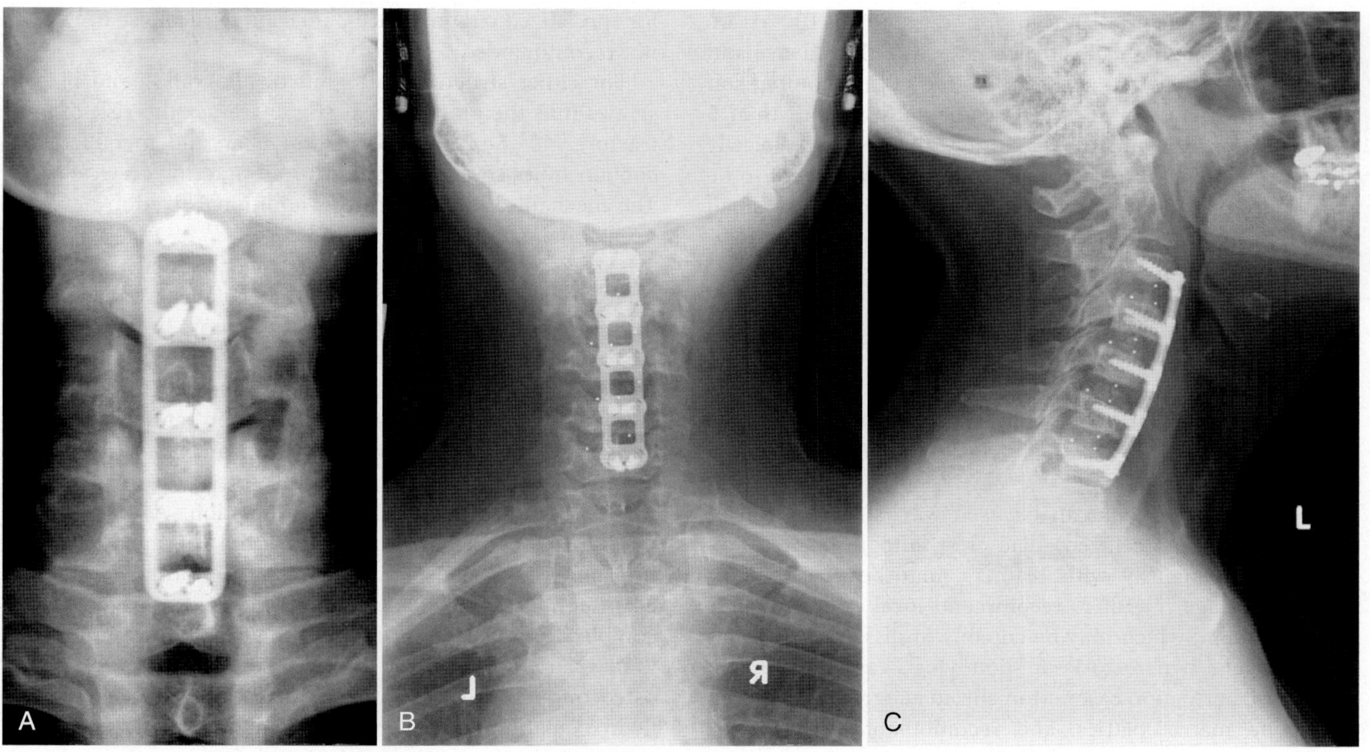

FIG. 69.7 (A–B) Anteroposterior and (C) lateral radiographs showing multilevel C3–C7 anterior-only reconstruction with anterior cervical plate. Local autograft was used to fill polyetheretherketone cages, and full healing was documented on computed tomography. The patient later reported painful subjacent degeneration at C7–T1.

that separate plate and graft constructs were stiffer than integrated devices in all testing modes.[148,250] The difference increased with the number of levels performed. On the other hand, one recent cadaveric biomechanical study concluded that the anchored spacer "showed stabilizing potential at the operated level statistically similar to that of the standard revision with a two-level plate."[251]

In a recent clinical study, 63 patients underwent either stand-alone cage or more typical cage-plate reconstruction.[252] At 1-year follow-up, similar overall clinical outcomes were achieved, but the stand-alone device was associated with a lower risk of dysphagia, procedure time, and estimated blood loss. Other small series have also reported good clinical results.[253]

As with anterior plating, interbody bioresorbable polymers have been studied. Results have been mixed.[76,177,254] At this point, these devices cannot be recommended for implantation outside of carefully controlled trials.

Implant Selection and Technique Notes

Cervical cages are used to reconstruct anterior spinal column defects. As such, they may be used after discectomy procedures or to fill in corpectomy defects after surgery for degenerative, traumatic, or neoplastic indications. Use of nonbiologic materials in the face of active infection remains controversial.[255] Allograft struts are just as susceptible to glycocalyx or biofilm formation as metal or PEEK implants.

Ideally, structural autograft would be used in patients with osteomyelitis. However, because the autograft harvest adds morbidity in already frail patients, several authors have used titanium and PEEK implants and have reported successful reconstructions.[255-257] At follow-up intervals of 20 to 54 months, these authors reported greater than 90% fusion rates and no recurrent infections. However, "radical" anterior debridement is recommended along with posterior screw-rod stabilization and 8 to 12 weeks of intravenous antibiotics. As an exception, one series reported two recurrences in a group of 36 patients with vertebral bone destruction treated with expandable cages caused by infections ranging from *Staphylococcus aureus* to tuberculosis.[258]

Restoration of stability may be more critical than avoiding implants. Full debridement of cervical osteomyelitis often requires two-level corpectomy. Typically, surgical indications include neurologic compromise, vertebral body destruction with kyphosis, segmental instability, failure of medical treatment, and epidural or paravertebral abscess.

As with plating, anterior cage procedures are mechanically most vulnerable when carried over multiple levels, risking extrusion and subsidence. Cage subsidence is associated with neck pain, plate failure, significantly lower Japanese Orthopedic Association score recovery, and late neurologic deterioration.[227] As with plating, hybrid approaches and multilevel discectomy are more stable than corpectomy.[259]

Stand-alone cages (e.g., without anterior plating or a posterior rod-screw construct) are also controversial. Typically, good clinical outcomes and fusion rates (93.3–100%) are described despite high subsidence rates.[260,261] Subsidence and segmental kyphosis are worst at C6–C7.[262] In a comparison study, 44% of stand-alone cage segments lost more than 5 degrees of lordosis and subsided more than 3 mm, typically by 3 months after surgery.[263] Outcomes do not appear to be affected by these radiographic findings.[263,264] However, small series have reported successful use of stand-alone cages adjacent to previous ACDF constructs.[265]

Bone Graft Selection

Particularly in areas without allograft banks, cages provide structural support, thereby avoiding the chronic donor site pain seen in up to 31% of patients undergoing structural autograft harvest.[139,266-268]

Several graft options can be used with structural cages. Nonstructural (morcellized) iliac crest autograft, often collected percutaneously with reamers, may be placed in or around the cage.[269] Others recommend local bone from the decompression, which may be copious in disseminated idiopathic skeletal hyperostosis or spondylosis cases but limited in soft disc herniation cases. Morcellized allograft, demineralized bone matrix patties, and recombinant human bone morphogenetic protein 2 (BMP-2)–containing sponges have also been used. A few series report excellent results after implanting "empty" cages.[270–273]

Machined allograft cages may not require additional grafting and have compared favorably to autograft in one- and two-level anterior procedures.[274] A number of allograft options are available. For discectomy procedures, tricortical iliac crest wedges and small fibular rings predominate. Dense cancellous allograft (e.g., patellar wedge) has been recommended for its open-matrix structure. This structure imparts axial stability comparable to tricortical iliac crest and more fully cortical fibular grafts while maintaining a porous structure that promotes vascularization and cellular penetration.[275] In one series of 98 patients, dense cancellous allograft was used with one- and two-level dynamic plating. At 12 months, the fusion rate was 96%. While there were no allograft or hardware complications, mean subsidence was 2.0 and 3.2 mm for the single- and double-level constructs, respectively.[172]

In a multilevel ACDF study in alpine goats, threaded intervertebral fusion cages filled with BMP demonstrated a much higher arthrodesis rate and accelerated bone formation compared with either autogenous bone-filled BAK/C or autogenous bone grafts.[276] In humans, enthusiasm for anterior cervical BMP placement has been tempered by postoperative swallowing and breathing problems in nearly one-fourth of patients implanted.[277] BMPs may also stimulate the resorptive phase of bone healing, leading to endplate resorption and increased cage migration.[278] Another series of 200 retrospectively reviewed one- to three-level ACDF patients found a 100% fusion rate using CT and dynamic radiographs.[279] Soft tissue problems included 14 (7%) with clinically significant dysphagia and four (2%) who required repeated operation for hematoma or seroma. Outside of very low doses implanted for specialized circumstances, anterior cervical use of BMP is not recommended.

For either structural autograft or allograft, avoid placing screws into the graft itself as this increases the risk of graft fracture.[280,281] Some PEEK, carbon fiber, and metallic cages contain holes to allow fixation to an anterior cervical plate. The mechanical benefits of this additional fixation have not been convincingly demonstrated.

Cages constructed entirely of osteoconductive materials such as tricalcium phosphate or trabecular metal have come into use. The crystalline grafts may be more brittle, but they have better imaging characteristics than their metallic counterparts. Small studies using coralline interbody implants have reported variable clinical outcomes, fusion rates around 45%, and high rates of graft fragmentation and subsidence.[282-284] Tantalum interbody implants are far less brittle but add considerable scatter even with CT evaluation. A recent study randomized 61 patients to ACDF with a tantalum interbody implant or autologous iliac bone graft and plating.[285] Although 24-month radiologic and clinical outcomes were similar, complications were considerably higher in the autologous graft group. Some hybrid PEEK or metal cages incorporate osteoconductive cores of tricalcium phosphate, coralline hydroxyapatite, or similar materials.[286] Use of these implant types remains limited.

Technique

Wider endplate coverage allows the cage to better resist axial compression forces. Therefore, especially at lower cervical levels, choose the widest cage that will fit in the defect.[235,262,287] For some multilevel procedures, different cages may be optimal at different levels.[262] Some recommend anterior osteophytes be retained to increase load-bearing area.[261] It is unclear whether the axial load-bearing benefits of osteophyte retention exceed detrimental effects on plate prominence or buttressing.

To decrease extrusion rates, achieve a tight interference fit. Excessive traction unloads the articular pillars posteriorly.[112] Increasing cage height also increases segmental lordosis, but this may decrease adjacent-segment motion.[288] When selecting and implanting a cervical cage, observe the following:

- Maximize endplate coverage, especially at lower cervical levels
- Avoid excessive traction before insertion
- Avoid excessive endplate violation
- Add a plate for discectomies of more than one level and all corpectomies
- Consider supplementary posterior fixation for two or more level corpectomies

In the absence of specialized indications, avoid radiopaque and expensive, cylindrical, and poorly modulus-matched implants.

Outcomes and Complications

Several studies examine the impact of cages after anterior cervical reconstruction. Most typically, outcomes vary far more by the indications for surgery than by the implant selected. On the other hand, some studies have compared various instrumentation types.

Initial favorable reports in 80 and 135 patients receiving BAK/C cage implants reported high fusion rates.[289,290] These initial reports were followed by prospective, randomized, FDA trials comparing BAK/C cages with uninstrumented ACDF in 344 radiculopathy patients. Virtually all outcome measures were similar in both groups and maintained over 2 years. The authors concluded that threaded fusion cage outcome are the same as those of a conventional uninstrumented ACDF with iliac crest autograft.[291] With longer, 4.8-year follow-up in 103 patents, 95% good-to-excellent outcomes were reported with a 98.9% fusion rate.[292] Lordosis was maintained in 93.8% and increased in 6.2%.

Other, smaller studies have compared rectangular carbon fiber and titanium cages with iliac crest autograft. High fusion rates and equivalent outcomes were reported in all groups. Significant donor site pain was reported in 20% to 33% of the structural autograft patients.[269,293,294] An economic comparison found that costs between mesh cages and autograft were not significantly different because of the iliac crest harvest morbidity.[267] Another prospective, randomized study of 42 cervical interbody fusions found similar results with either an autologous tricortical graft or a cage and that tricortical graft was cheaper.[295]

Fewer studies report cage outcomes after corpectomy surgery. Most are retrospective reports of 26 to 100 patients reporting titanium mesh or PEEK packed with local autograft or allograft chips.[256,296,297] Successful use of stand-alone cages in one-level corpectomies is reported, whereas three or more corpectomy levels use adjunctive posterior stabilization. Fusion rates from 97% to 100% are reported, but so too are occasional cage extrusions, kyphotic collapse, and postoperative radiculopathy. Most authors concluded that titanium cages provide immediate strong anterior column support with minimal hardware complications and avoid bone graft site morbidity.

Other prospective, randomized studies have been somewhat less enthusiastic about the cage outcomes. In three studies with approximately 100 patients randomized to ACDF with a carbon fiber cage or a traditional Cloward procedures, overall pain and disability were similar for both groups.[298-301] Although donor site pain was significantly less in the cage group, the fusion rate was significantly lower as well (85%, 86%, and 81% vs. 55%, 62%, and 74%, respectively). In both studies, patients with pseudarthrosis reported more severe neck pain than those solidly fused.

Anterior cervical reconstruction with cages conveys the same risks as surgery without cages.[238] Complications such as displacement or subsidence with foraminal stenosis occur more frequently in multilevel procedures (up to 33%) and in osteopenic or spastic patients. In these settings, adjunctive posterior stabilization should be considered.[302-304]

Cervical Disc Arthroplasty

As of this writing, only three cervical implant strategies seek to preserve segmental motion: direct screw osteosynthesis, laminoplasty with plates, and cervical disc replacement. Although there is longer clinical experience with lumbar disc arthroplasty, cervical total disc replacement (TDR) is more commonly offered in most countries.[305,306]

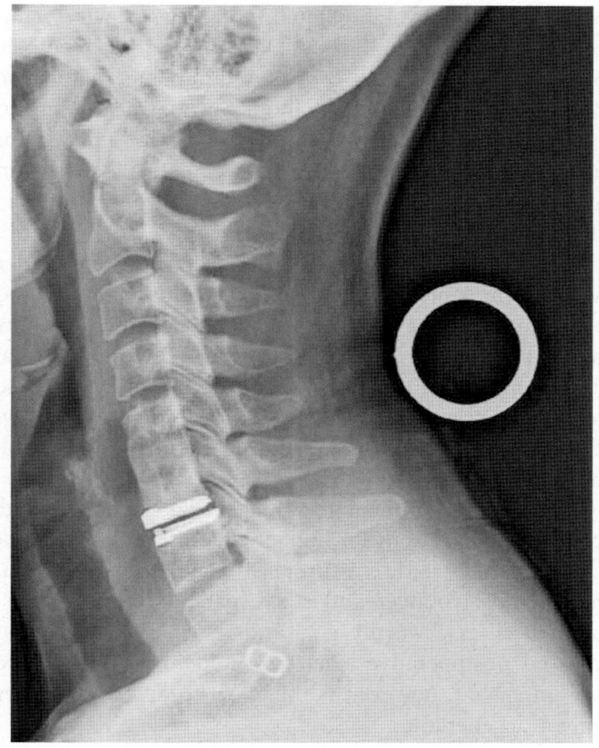

FIG. 69.8 Lateral radiograph of a patient who underwent cervical disc replacement at C6–C7 below a previous C5–C6 anterior cervical discectomy and fusion.

Relative to the lumbar spine, differences between fusion and nonfusion stabilization methods are more pronounced in cervical applications. The cervical lateral masses have a much larger role in axial load bearing than the lumbar posterior elements. The smaller cervical bony endplates challenge endplate fixation.[307] The anterior airway and posterior cord amplify the risks associated with cervical TDR relative to their lumbar counterparts (Fig. 69.8).

A wide variety of materials have been incorporated into TDR systems, including cobalt-chrome, titanium, and high-molecular-weight polyethylene; optimal biomaterials have not been identified.[308,309] The cobalt-chrome devices affect postoperative MRI imaging to a much greater degree than the titanium-based devices.[309] The likelihood and effects of wear debris do not appear to be significant concerns in early follow-up studies or in experimental models, but these particles clearly migrate into the periprosthetic and epidural spaces.[310] The long-term inflammatory potential of metal-on-metal appendicular prosthesis debris has led to the removal of both spinal and appendicular arthroplasty systems from the market.[311,312]

Even within material groups (e.g., metal-on-polyethylene), many design questions remain unanswered.[307,313] Some systems rely on a midline keel to achieve fixation; others use spikes or endplate texturing. Keels may risk sagittal split fractures, especially in multilevel implantations.[314] These devices vary in terms of the constraint they place on normal segmental motion.[313] Typically, more constrained implants require more elaborate endplate fixation methods but may also offer more protection of the facets.[315] No current device fully restores normal segmental kinematics.[307,316] Even suitable device kinematics require perfect midline positioning and rotation to provide proper motion.

Unlike lumbar applications, cervical disc replacements have been implanted in the treatment of spondylotic radiculopathy and myelopathy, not axial pain syndromes.[317] Contraindications include active infection, osteoporosis, and radiographic evidence of mechanical instability or absent motion. The prevalence of contraindications in patients with cervical degenerative disease is lower than in similar lumbar cohorts.

Given the perception of traditional ACDF surgery as highly successful, expectations for implementation of expensive new technology such as disc arthroplasty have been very high.[317] First, in most younger and active patients, preservation of motion itself is a worthy goal and may be associated with decreased postoperative axial pain and improved function. More important, however, is the effort to decrease adjacent-segment degeneration.[318]

As of this writing, cervical arthroplasty continues to slowly gather proponents. Certainly, patient selection for arthroplasty is far more selective than for predicate anterior discectomy and fusion procedures.[317] Most randomized trials show outcomes that favor TDR; an analysis of outcome predictors shows that patient factors such as work status and pending litigation have a far greater impact on outcomes than the disc spacer utilized.[319,320] Most recent reports detail FDA trials of newer implants or two-level placement. For example, a recent report detailed the 4-year outcomes of a two-level implantation of the Mobi-C (Zimmer Biomet).[321] The device maintained motion, and no device failures were reported. In this study, and most others, arthroplasty patients had better outcomes in terms of Neck Disability Index and Short Form-12 scores while having a lower rate of secondary surgeries compared with ACDF. Favorable 10-year outcomes have been reported.[322,323] Interestingly, strong evidence favoring arthroplasty in terms of adjacent-segment degeneration has not yet emerged.[324,325]

Posterior Cervical Instrumentation

Posterior cervical instrumentation can be categorized by location into occipitocervical and subaxial implants. Functional categorization includes rigid segmental systems versus nonrigid wiring systems. Posterior implants may be used in a motion-sparing capacity when stabilizing a laminoplasty door. Recently, spacers have also been introduced for placement in the cervical facets.

Occipitocervical Instrumentation

As with other types of spinal instrumentation, nonrigid wire constructs have given way to screw-based rigid constructs. Still, the heterogeneous mix of pathologies and patient age requiring occipitocervical stabilization ensure the older methods remain relevant.

Nonrigid Occipitocervical Systems

Initially, occipitocervical stabilization involved onlay fusion with morcellized graft followed by prolonged halo immobilization.[34,326] Fusion rates from 75% to 89% were reported. Subsequently, to allow early mobilization without a halo, occipitocervical stabilization using sublaminar wires and PMMA was reported.[327] Although excellent clinical results were reported, fusion rates were not and this technique has been largely abandoned.

Wertheim and Bohlman reported good results using a structural bone grafting technique with sublaminar wires.[328] To improve stiffness, subsequent authors incorporated bent Steinmann pins, Kirschner wires, curved rods, and malleable loops and rods into sublaminar wire or cable constructs.[329-334] These constructs often use cancellous rather than structural autograft. While these rods confer additional stability over wired structural bone, they are semirigid and typically require halo immobilization.[335-337] Fusion rates vary from 90% to 100%.[328,337]

Typically, semirigid constructs achieve occipital fixation with burr holes. Segmental spinal fixation is obtained with interspinous or sublaminar wires. Interspinous wires decrease risk to neurovascular structures and offer less-restrictive placement options. Wire-graft and wire-loop constructs have disadvantages, including limited utility in patients requiring decompression, decreased fatigue life, and the need for postoperative immobilization. Rods wired to the bone may piston through the wires, reducing vertical stability.[338-341] In patients with poor healing potential, the increased fatigue susceptibility of wired constructs favors rigid fixation.[342] Similarly, rigid stabilization should be considered when bulky external bracing is contraindicated, as in spinal cord or pulmonary-injured patients, or when compliance may be limited.[331] Luque rectangle and two rigid plating systems conferred similar compression and flexion stiffness in one study, but the plates were far more stiff against extension and torsion.[341]

Sublaminar and suboccipital wire passage can be technically challenging, especially in patients with axial collapse or stenosis. These difficulties stimulated interest in rigid systems, which evolved from contoured appendicular trauma reconstruction plates. These implants stabilize without canal incursion or postoperative halo immobilization.[337,339] Whether wiring or screws offer better fixation in the osteoporotic cervicocranium remains controversial.[329,330]

Rigid systems are recommended in cases of deformity correction or with multiplanar, particularly vertical, instability.[339] Specifically, screw-rod constructs are indicated in patients undergoing decompressive laminectomy, dens resection, or multiple-level fixation from the occiput to the lower cervical spine.[343] Ostensibly, rigid stabilization allows shorter constructs, saving fusion levels.[337,339] Historically, occipitocervical fusion was utilized in dens fracture malunion or nonunion.[344] Today, C1 lateral mass screw fixation avoids extension to the occiput in many cases.

There are no specific contraindications to occipitocervical fusion. In fact, for patients with clear occipitocervical instability, few alternatives exist. In some patients, medical issues provide a relative contraindication. Unfortunately, external stabilization is relatively ineffective in patients with higher degrees of instability. Typically, contraindications imply safety of one technique over another. Aberrance in vertebral artery anatomy, for example, increases risks of C2 pars fixation.

Autogenous iliac crest bone grafting remains standard for occipitocervical fusions. If possible, cable a strut down to bridge the bleeding surfaces of the host bone.[345] Allograft bone has been less successful.[346] BMP has been used and results have varied, but they may approach autograft.[347] Complications, including neurologic decline, have been reported.[348]

Occipitocervical fusion requires rigid head control with either a Mayfield head clamp or an open halo ring. The articulation's large flexion and extension arc requires careful attention to alignment. On lateral fluoroscopy, assess the occipitocervical angle.[349,350] In neutral, the intersection of McRae's line and a line through the superior endplate of C3 should be 44 degrees. Of three techniques used to measure occipitocervical alignment, McGregor's line was more reproducible and reliable than Chamberlain's and McRae's lines.[351] Improper alignment may increase subsequent subaxial degeneration.[352] Shallow postoperative occiput–C2 angles, which decrease oropharynx cross-sectional area, predict postoperative dyspnea and dysphagia.[349,352]

Until the 1990s, the semirigid Wertheim and Bohlman technique was the most common form of occipitocervical fusion.[328] Expose the posterior elements from the EOP to C4. Create a trough on both sides of the EOP 2 cm above the foramen magnum with a high-speed burr. Use a towel clip to create a hole in the ridge and pass an 18-gauge wire through the hole. Twist the wire over the ridge. Then, pass a second, sublaminar loop around the C1 arch. Pass a third loop through and around the base of the C2 spinous process. Harvest a thick, 3 × 5 cm corticocancellous graft from the posterior iliac crest. Divide the graft longitudinally into two parts and drill three evenly spaced holes into each graft. Decorticate the occiput, C1 ring, and C2 laminae. Thread the more lateral arm of the wire at each level through the corresponding holes. Maneuver the graft down the wires until it is apposed to the decorticated bone. Bring the second arm of each wire medially around the graft and tighten the wires sequentially. Pack additional cancellous bone between the two grafts. If fixation is secure and bone quality is good, use a skull-occiput-mandibular immobilization or Minerva brace postoperatively. If fixation is poor, maintain the patient in a halo vest for 6 to 12 weeks.

Alternatively, obtain safe bicortical wire passage by enlarging the foramen magnum and thinning the occiput with a burr in a 5- to 7-mm semicircle. Then resect the remaining inner table piecemeal with a 2-mm Kerrison rongeur to remove the posterior lip of the foramen magnum. Create two to four occipital holes with a 4-mm burr approximately 1 cm lateral to the inion and approximately 7 mm cranial to the foramen magnum. Elevate the dura off the inner table toward the burr holes and from the foramen magnum with a 4-0 curved curette. Pass a looped, double-twisted, 24-gauge wire or braided cables through the holes on both sides. If a C1 laminectomy has been performed, drill a small hole through the remnant of the lamina on either side, if there is sufficient remaining bone, and pass a single 24-gauge wire through.

In the presence of neurologic compression, do not attempt sublaminar wire passage. Instead, pass a wire through the C2 spinous process by drilling transversely approximately one-third of the length up the spinous process. On each side, perforate the cortex with a 2-mm burr and connect those holes with a towel clip. Then pass a 20-gauge wire through the hole, loop it under the spinous process, and pass it a second time.

Occipitocervical fusion with a Luque or Ransford loop uses similar wiring positions and requires a template and fluoroscopy to ensure appropriate rod contouring. The rod profile must exactly match the skull and cervical laminae to prevent wire or cable cut-through. The wires are used to hold both the rod and the bone graft, or the rod alone, with nonstructural bone graft placed around the rod.

Rigid Occipitocervical Instrumentation

Rigid occipital fixation has been achieved with unicortical and bicortical 3.5-mm screws, inside-out, and screw-nut techniques.[353-355] The original, rigid, longitudinal connectors between the cervical spine and skull were dual pelvic reconstruction plates extending laterally from cervical spine lateral masses to lateral positions on the occiput.[356,357] Because the occiput is thickest and pullout strength greatest at the EOP, Y-plates, utilizing the stronger midline occipital keel, were developed (Table 69.1).[358] Histologically, this 9.7 to 15.1 mm thick, dense bone is ideal for screw fixation but decreases radially from the inion.[359,360] The midline bone between the inion and the foramen magnum remains thicker than laterally. Newer modular systems with occiput-specific plates optimize skull fixation by placing screws in the thick, midline keel.[361]

In some children or when adequate bone anchorage is not available in the midline keel, hooks may be placed in the occipital squama.[362] Alternatively, occipital screws may be placed into the condyles instead. The clinical and mechanical pros and cons of this technique have not yet been elucidated.[363]

The mobile locking mechanisms found in newer systems require less meticulous rod contouring, but all are technically demanding and require a thorough knowledge of occipitocervical anatomy.[356] These rod-plate hybrids allow more room for bone graft and increased intraoperative flexibility with no fixed hole-to-hole distances but are more expensive.[364] Many of these plates allow additional perimedian screw placement to improve rotational control.[365]

The various occipital constructs can be combined with a variety of cervical fixation methods. Most commonly, C1 lateral mass screws alone or with C2 pedicle screws, C2 pedicle screws alone, or C1–C2 transarticular screws are described.[108] When plated to six occipital screws, C1–C2 transarticular screws are either the most rigid form of occipitocervical fusion or are equivalent to C2 pedicle screws.[330,366-368] Occiput–C1 transarticular screws have been described but are technically demanding to place and require additional Magerl screw stabilization. These screws may not be appropriate in patients with distracting injuries.[369]

At surgery, place the distal anchoring screws first. With the cervical fixation in place, template the skull. Match both contour and the cervical screws' position. The need for coronal and sagittal plane contouring has increased the popularity of rod-plate hybrids. Occipital fixation should be as close to midline as possible and close to, but not over, the EOP. Plating over the inion causes painful occipital prominence. Caudally, avoid the foramen magnum because the bone is thin and the trajectory difficult. Screw lengths range from 6 to 14 mm, average 10 mm, and become longer toward the EOP. Use a set-depth drill bit at 8 to 10 mm. Drill, palpate the inner cortex, deepen the depth setting 1 to 2 mm, and redrill until the cortex is breached. Because the occipital bone is hard, these screws should be tapped. The smaller threads on self-tapping screws may not be adequate in younger patients with good bone stock. Constructs incorporating a bone strut with the plate allow longer screws to be used but add construct bulk.

The weakness of the skull's inner table and the proximity of the venous sinuses argue for unicortical fixation.[24,359,370] Bicortical screw pullout strength is 50% greater than unicortical screws, whose holding power is similar to wiring.[360] Usually, bicortical purchase is recommended because unicortical screws strip on contact with the inner cortex. Vascular injury and dural leak can be avoided with a careful drill-tapping technique. In older patients, the dura may be adherent to the skull's inner surface. Stop the ensuing cerebrospinal fluid leak by placing the screw.[330,356]

Once the plate is in place, fashion a corticocancellous graft to lie between the two plates. Notch the graft to straddle the C2 spinous process and cover the posterior arch of C1 and the occiput. Hold the graft in place using heavy suture or wire. Alternatively, place a screw in the midline of the skull and wrap wire or cable around the screw, then over the graft and around the C2 spinous process. Denuding the C1–C2 facet joint cartilage allows additional bone to be packed directly. Immobilize rigidly stabilized patients in a collar for 4 to 12 weeks. Before discharge from care, verify union with flexion-extension radiographs.

Outcomes and Complications

Occipitocervical fusion patients are often acutely ill from high-energy trauma, neoplasm, systemic infection, or advanced rheumatoid arthritis. Modern anesthetic and perioperative management has reduced the mortality rate from 10% to 1.7%.[326,371,372] Complication rates vary widely based on underlying comorbidities. For example, perioperative complications were historically common with occipitocervical fusion in rheumatoid patients.[373,374] Complication rates decrease when patients are treated earlier in the disease.[375] Children have rarer but still significant complication rates. Although some series describe "minimal" complications using contoured plating systems, others report complication rates up to 30%, including transient quadriplegia, pneumonia, hydrocephalus, cerebrospinal fluid leak, and traumatic fusion fracture.[326,333,356,376]

Irrespective of the construct used, with autograft occipitocervical arthrodesis rates are high, at 85% to 100%.[108,328,337,377,378] However, one study reported 100% failure of seven fusions performed with cadaveric bone. Subsequent autogenous iliac crest graft achieved fusion in all seven.[346] In children, 100% fusion rates have been reported without internal fixation.[379] Even rheumatoid patients, perceived as poor healers, demonstrated 94% to 100% fusion rates with rigid occipitocervical fixation.[326,339,380,381]

The construct failure rate, with loss of fixation and recurrence of deformity, is proportional to the fusion rate. The rate and mode of failure depend on the surgical technique and postoperative immobilization. Wiring constructs fail by cut-through of the wire through the bone or by fatigue failure of the wires themselves. Rigid systems fail by fracture through the inferior lateral mass or pedicle.[341] Construct failures also increase in patients with osteoporosis and neuromuscular disorders. With constructs ranging from the Ransford loop to modern, rigid systems, failure rates of 0% to 5% are reported.[337,357,372,382-386] In a recent study using CT assessment of final fusion, 27 occipitocervical fusion patients were assessed at a mean 7.2 years.[387] In this series, failures were seen at a mean of 31.2 months. The authors emphasized the importance of "sufficient bone grafting, proper decortication of the bone bed, use of thicker and high stiffness rods, and ultra-high molecular weight polyethylene tape" reinforcement to minimize implant failure.

Of course, successful osteointegration does not guarantee a favorable clinical outcome. Occipitocervical fusion limits postoperative motion, an effect compounded by postoperative halo. In one report, neck stiffness caused half the patients to make lifestyle changes.[383] A series of cancer patients reported 75% excellent or good outcomes.[377] Children exhibit far less range-of-motion loss after occipitocervical fusion and have overall favorable outcomes.[379,388]

In children, the possibility of an occipitocervical "crankshaft" phenomenon remains controversial.[389] In children younger than 6 years, postoperative increases in occipitocervical junction lordosis have been reported. Fixation in a neutral or slight flexion may counteract this increase.[382] Spontaneous fusion extension occurs in adults but is more common, at up to 38%, in younger patients.[333,390] In a 17-year follow-up study, 90% of children and adolescent patients had reported excellent or good results with a low complication rate despite an overall increase in osteoarthritis changes in unfused segments and a decrease in mobility.[390] In another study, the rate of adjacent-level degeneration at 5 years was 7%.[326] Late subaxial subluxations can occur in any patient group but are more common in patients with active rheumatoid arthritis.[384]

The subcutaneous nature of the occiput also risks wound infection and dehiscence, especially in rheumatoid, less-mobile, and older patients.[384] In a heterogeneous patient population, a 5% wound infection rate was recorded.[326] Older series report pin site infections and skin breakdown under the halo vest.[333] Even patients immobilized by collars should be observed closely for occipital ulcerations, especially those with greater occipital nerve anesthesia.

While more rigid constructs have higher theoretical risk of neurovascular injury, the reported rate of these injuries has been low.[356,376] In a series by Sasso and colleagues, a total of 78 occipital screws were placed. No patient deteriorated neurologically and no complications resulted from any of these screws.[381] Abumi and colleagues' series included subaxial pedicle screws, and no neurovascular complications were seen.[391]

In most series, the risk of postoperative neurologic deterioration and the prognosis for recovery are inversely proportional preoperative deficits.[392] In a Ransford loop study by Malcolm and colleagues, of seven patients who deteriorated neurologically after surgery, none had been neurologically normal.[383] In rheumatoid patients, more severe neurologic involvement is associated with lower recovery rates.[372,393] In most series, surgical intervention reliably prevents further neurologic decline.[372,385,393-395] The literature demonstrates less reliability in neurologic improvement.[372,385,393] In Huckell and colleagues' series, for example, no patients experienced neurologic decline, and average neurologic improvement was one Nurick grade.[378] In a Dutch series, 35% improved dramatically—one whole Nurick grade.[396]

Atlantoaxial Instrumentation

Atlantoaxial instrumentation is indicated for segmental instability, often from trauma (e.g., transverse atlantal ligament rupture or dens fracture), rheumatoid arthritis, or congenital or metabolic anomalies.[397-399] Radiographically, abnormal C1–C2 motion is expressed as an increase in the anterior atlanto-dens interval (AADI). The AADI passes from the midposterior margin of the anterior ring of C1 to the anterior dens surface. In adults, the AADI is normally less than 3 mm; in children, it should be less than 4 mm. Acute increases in the interval usually signal instability. With chronic joint destruction, greater motion may be well tolerated.

Gallie and Brooks Techniques

Historically, the Gallie technique has been used to stabilize C1–C2.[372,400,401] This technique offers good resistance to flexion and is indicated in flexion-unstable situations such as transverse atlantal ligament rupture or, occasionally, dens fracture with anterior displacement. Gallie fusion requires C1 sublaminar wire passage and should be avoided in patients with arch fracture or cord swelling. At C2, the wire is simply passed around the spinous process. This wiring offers little rotational or extension stability and should therefore be avoided in posteriorly displaced dens fractures, for example. Despite its limitations, this technique or one of its many reported modifications is still routinely used because of ease and safety (Fig. 69.9).

Upper cervical stabilization requires rigid fixation to the operating frame. Immediately after positioning, assess the reduction and visibility of the upper cervical levels on open-mouth views. Next, make a midline incision from occiput to C3 and expose the tips of spinous processes. Carry a subperiosteal dissection along the C2 lamina, which preserves the suboccipital triangle muscular insertions for subsequent repair. Carry the subperiosteal dissection around the arch superiorly and inferiorly to allow passage of a doubled, U-shaped 18- to 20-gauge (1.2 mm) wire or equivalent titanium cable in a caudal to cranial direction. Harvest an H-shaped bone block from the iliac crest bone block and

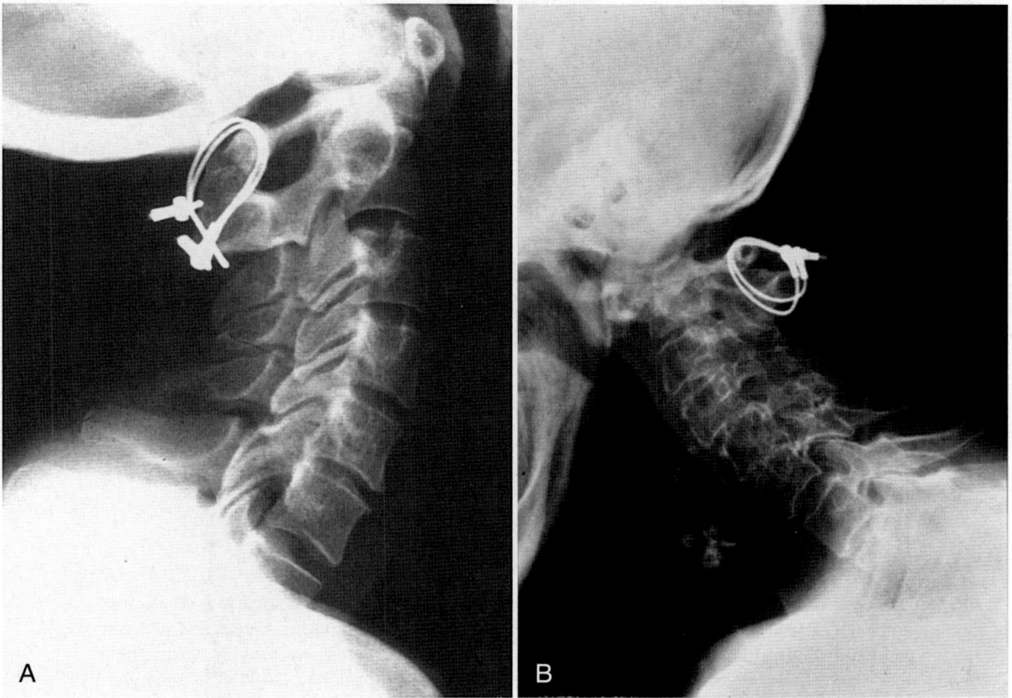

FIG. 69.9 Lateral radiographs of (A) Gallie and (B) Brooks posterior C1–C2 wiring constructs.

shape it to fit the C1–C2 laminae and interlaminar space. Notch the inferior part to fit over the C2 spinous process. Decorticate the posterior elements and pass the loop over the bone block and around the C2 spinous process. Pack open areas with cancellous graft.

One common Gallie modification is the wedge compression, or Brooks, technique.[402,403] With this method, bone blocks are fashioned to fit between the C1 arch and the C2 lamina, providing additional rotational and extension stability. Sublaminar wiring is undertaken at both levels. This technique cannot be used when the posterior elements have been compromised. Most authors recommend halo immobilization after Brooks fusion.

The indications for a Brooks fusion are like those for a Gallie. Gallie fusion is adequate for most flexion injuries. Consider Brooks technique for extension injuries and when more rigid fixation is deemed necessary.[137] A Brooks fusion is performed much as a Gallie but requires additional exposure of the inferior C2 lamina. Carefully preserve the atlantoaxial membrane. Doubled cables are passed under the C1 arch, then under the lamina of C2. Two rectangular iliac crest bone grafts approximately 1.25 × 3.5 cm are harvested and beveled to fit the interval between the C1 arch and the C2 lamina. The posterior elements are decorticated and the wires or cables are tightened to secure the grafts in position.

Various modifications to the Brooks method include passing the wires or cables through the grafts themselves. Avoid C2 sublaminar wire placement by passing two 18-gauge stainless-steel wires beneath the posterior arch of the atlas and around a threaded Steinmann pin, which is drilled through the base of the axis spinous process.[404]

Magerl Transarticular Screws

In 1987, Magerl described a rigid C1–C2 transarticular screw fixation technique. Intact posterior elements are required.[405] These screws offer greater rigidity, especially in rotation, and better maintenance of reduction than wired fusions.[403] On the other hand, screw placement is technically more challenging and risks vertebral and internal carotid artery injury.[27] Consider Magerl screws in acute or chronic atlantoaxial instability, when revising C1–C2 pseudarthroses, as part of occipitocervical stabilization, or in patients who cannot tolerate halo immobilization. Irreducible fractures and aberrant vertebral artery anatomy may contraindicate transarticular screws (Figs. 69.10 and 69.11).

To achieve the cranial trajectory required to place Magerl screws, extend a standard upper cervical midline approach more distally. Alternatively, augment a small C1–C2 incision with more distal stabs for drill placement. The screws enter C2 at its inferior aspect and exit at the posterior aspect of the upper articular process. On their way into the C1 lateral masses, the screws pass through the C1–C2 facet, which is considerably more anterior than C1–C2. Magerl recommends direct exposure of the C1–C2 facet joint. He uses Kirschner wires to retract the soft tissues containing the greater occipital

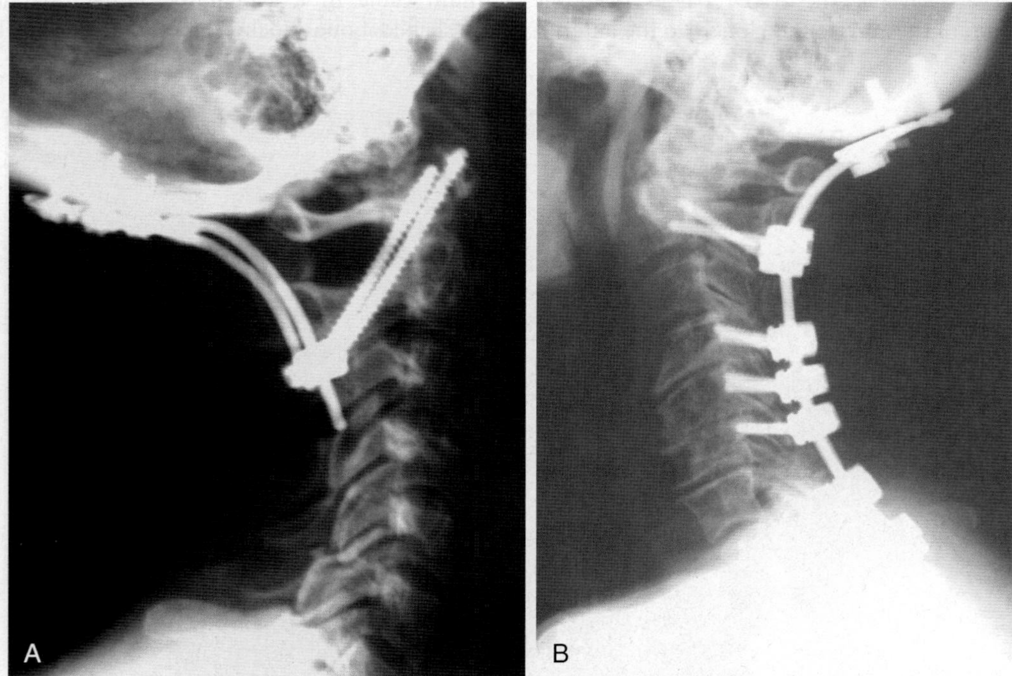

FIG. 69.10 Lateral postoperative images of two patients after occipitocervical fusion. (A) A young man underwent skull–C2 fixation after ejection from a motor vehicle led to traumatic occipitocervical dissociation. Magerl technique was used caudally. (B) A 72-year-old woman with long history of rheumatoid arthritis experienced basilar invagination, multilevel stenosis, and subaxial subluxation at C7–T1. She underwent an occiput–T2 decompression and fusion using a midline occipital keel plate, C2 pedicle fixation, C4–C6 lateral mass screws, and pedicle screws in T1 and T2.

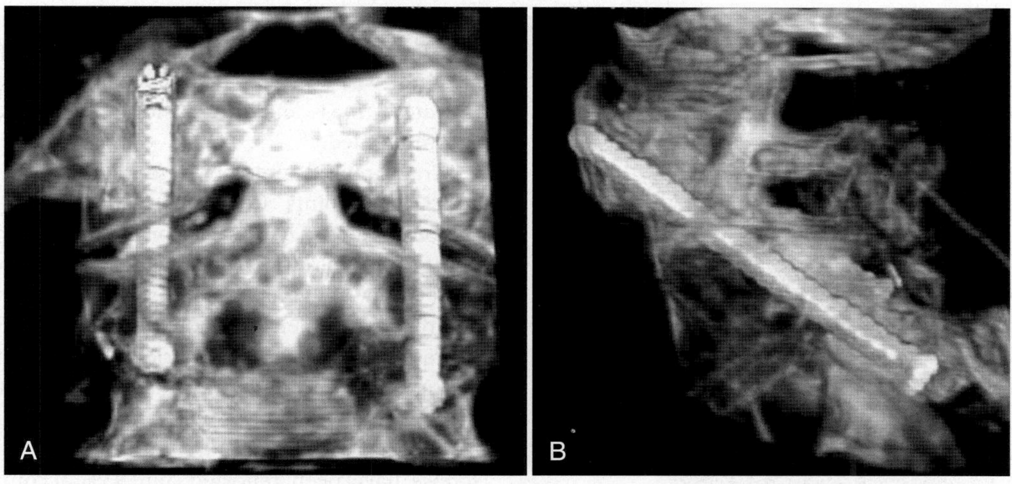

FIG. 69.11 This patient underwent Magerl transarticular C1–C2 screw fixation for atlantoaxial instability. (A) Anteroposterior and (B) lateral three-dimensional reconstructed images are presented.

nerve and its accompanying venous plexus.[405] As with the Harms technique described later, the plexus of thin-walled vessels lying on the C1–C2 facet capsule is typically injured with posterior exposure. The rich venous plexus can bleed profusely, and serial attempts to reach the joint with interval packing are often needed. The risk of these injuries can be reduced by bluntly dissecting the soft tissues in a caudal to rostral direction along the C2 pedicle. The consequences of plexus disruption are not significant.

Start the screw on the medial side of the inferior facet of the axis, aiming for the exposed isthmus cranially. Proceed toward the middle of the C1–C2 facet on the AP view and the anterior C1 ring on the lateral. To avoid the vertebral artery, direct the screws 25 degrees *toward* midline, and 25 degrees cranial. Navigation assistance decreases breach rates, but screw revisions were not required in unguided surgeries.[406] Some advocate cannulated drills to reposition the guide wire for optimal orientation. To stabilize the segment during the first screw's passage, place both guide wires before drilling. The hard subchondral bone at the joint level may deflect the guide wires. Tap past the facet joint to prevent screw deflection. The screws should just reach the inferior edge of the anterior C1 ring on the lateral view. Bicortical purchase is typically recommended but may not be necessary in all cases. In patients with satisfactory bone quality, no significant differences in pullout strength were seen.[407] Avoid overpenetration, which risks structures running vertically along the anterior C1 lateral mass, including the hypoglossal nerve and the internal carotid artery.[27,408]

With the C1–C2 facet exposed, decorticate the joint and impact bone graft. The rich venous plexus and anterior positioning of the joint have prompted many spine surgeons to skip this step, apparently without increased pseudarthrosis. Others, to restore segmental height, aggressively expose this area, sacrificing the greater occipital nerve and placing allograft shims in the joint.[409] Magerl augments the screws with Gallie wiring and fusion. In addition, a looped sublaminar wire at C1 improves reduction and allows motion segment stabilization during guide wires, drills, and screw passage. Others have reported 100% fusion rates without concomitant Gallie fusion.[410] Overall, transarticular screw fixation is associated fusion rates between 85% and 98%.[381,411] In comparative studies, transarticular screw fixation was associated with fewer complications and up to 21 times fewer nonunions than atlantoaxial wiring and halo.[412,413] Still, the advantages of Magerl screws must be weighed against the procedure's potential morbidity, particularly for surgeons who rarely perform C1–C2 posterior stabilization. If one vertebral artery is injured, do not attempt to place the opposite screw.

C1 Lateral Mass Screws and the Goel-Harms Technique

Beginning in 2000, screw fixation into the C1 lateral mass, described initially by Goel, was popularized by Harms.[414,415] Although Harms' technique shares indications with Magerl, over time it has become more frequently performed. This technique tolerates imperfect C1–C2 reduction and aberrant vertebral artery trajectories. Thus, the Harms technique is feasible in many cases that are inappropriate for Magerl screws.

Today, C1 lateral mass screws may be used as interval anchors in long occipitocervical constructs or end anchors in occiput–C1, C1–C2, or longer C1 to subaxial cervical constructs. Single-level implant placement without fusion to achieve fracture healing without necessitating later implant removal has long been described for C1 ring fractures using C1 lateral mass screws and transverse plating.[416]

The atlantoaxial complex is exposed posteriorly. The C2 dorsal primary ramus (greater occipital nerve) passes inferolateral to the joint and can be pulled sideways out of the C1 screw's trajectory. As with C1–C2 facet exposure, the rich venous plexus around the greater occipital nerve may require successive attempts at dissection with interval packing. Blood loss ranges widely from 50 to 1500 mL (mean, 540 mL).[417] Postoperative greater occipital nerve dysfunction is common.[418] Some authors routinely sacrifice this nerve to improve visualization and hemostasis.[409] The relative risks and benefits of resection of the C2 root have been debated.

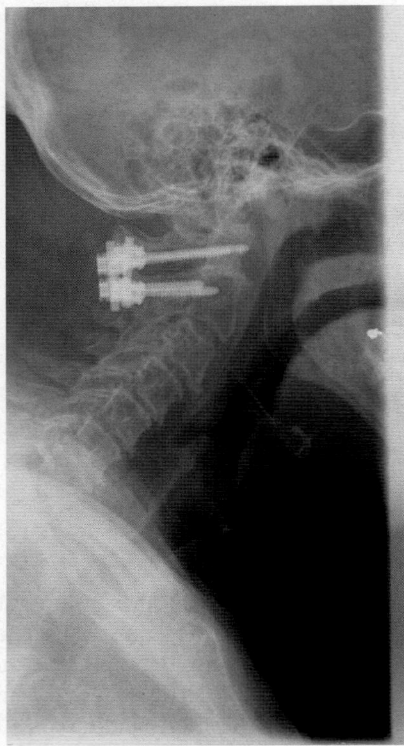

FIG. 69.12 This patient shows healing of type II odontoid fracture after a Goel-Harms construct including screw fixation into lateral mass of C1 and pars of C2.

Resection of the root allows easier and more accurate placement of C1 screws. It also allows greater access to the C1–C2 facet for direct fusion or reconstruction of collapsed C1–C2 segments. One recent study found that preservation of the C2 root was associated with higher rates of occipital neuralgia (Fig. 69.12).[419]

Most begin just below the C1 posterior ring, "flushing" any overhanging bone with a burr or Kerrison rongeur. The large size of the atlanto-lateral mass makes screw placement forgiving.[420] Mean C1 lateral mass is 11.6 ± 1.4 mm wide and 12.7 ± 1.0 mm high.[418] The large size of the lateral mass and the variety of angulation options may allow this step to be skipped in up to 50% of cases.[421] If performed, be very careful laterally because the vertebral artery passes directly over an increasingly thin C1 ring.

Placement through the C1 posterior ring avoids the plexus around the C2 dorsal primary ramus but may risk injury to the vertebral artery. In one recent series, a starting point on the C1 arch was associated with fracture in one case, which was addressed with sublaminar wiring.[422] The authors concluded that the technique was justified but that careful review of the preoperative imaging was critical. A recent literature review assessed the impact of starting point on C1 lateral mass fixation. High success rates in terms of arthrodesis were reported with each of the reported entry points.[423]

Select the midpoint of the lateral mass by palpation or fluoroscopic control.[424] From this central starting point, straight-ahead and 10 to 15 degrees of medialized trajectories have been recommended. While medialization avoids the internal carotid artery laterally, avoid more than 25 degrees.[418,420,425] An anatomic study found that although optimal screw medialization was about 21 degrees, when there was variation in C1 lateral mass anatomy customized surgical planning was recommended.[426]

Craniocaudal angulation seeks to avoid the occiput–C1 and C1–C2 joints. Recommendations vary, but a safe zone surrounds a 20-degree superior inclination or the 20% to 40% point of the anterior C1 arch.[418,427] Preoperative planning with axial CT or MRI images helps select the safest angle. Look for an arcuate foramen, an anomaly seen in 15.5% of patients.[428] If present, the arcuate's posterior aspect (ponticulus posticus) is occasionally mistaken for the C1 screw entry point.

Use polyaxial screws with an average length within the lateral mass of 22 mm.[418,420] Most often 3.5-mm diameter screws have been reported, but 93% accommodate 4.0-mm screws.[421] To reach the posterior C1 ring, add a mean 11.4 mm (range, 6.9–17 mm) to the screw length outside the bone.[420] Partially unthreaded screw shanks may decrease greater occipital nerve irritation.[418] Even in children, less than 1% of atlases are unable to accommodate a 3.5-mm screw.[429] Screw depth averaged 20.3 mm and arch overhang 6.3 mm (range, 2.1–12.4 mm).

The 1800-N pullout force of C1 lateral mass screws is significantly lower than occipital screws but similar to C2 pedicle screws.[418] Both unicortical and bicortical C1 lateral mass screws are stronger than subaxial lateral mass screws.[430] Although bicortical screws are significantly stronger than unicortical, this additional holding power might not be needed. The C1 lateral mass screws, once locked to their inserting drivers, can be used to improve the reduction. When compared with Magerl screws, the Harms technique provides identical stabilization, except in extension.[431] If significant extension instability is encountered, consider an interspinous graft. Most reports have included 28 to 102 patients and concluded the Harms technique is safe and effective.[409,417,432] Fusion rates from 98% to 100% have been reported. Although screw protrusion into the vertebral artery canal is occasionally seen, no clinically significant neurovascular compromise has been reported.

A recent study of 26 patients reported 100% C1–C2 fusion rate for the Goel-Harms technique, even including previous nonunion of other treatment modalities. There were no neurovascular complications and the authors recommended that this approach be considered first.[433]

Elliott and others reported a meta-analysis comparing Magerl vs. Goel-Harms technique for C1–C2 rigid stabilization.[434,435] They examined 69 class III studies incorporating 3146 patients. They concluded the Goel-Harms technique was associated with higher fusion rates and lower vertebral artery injury rates.[434] The same authors found that the vertebral artery injury rate was higher with Magerl transarticular screws than with C2 pedicle screws.[435]

C2 Fixation Options

As an alternative to the Magerl technique, screws may be placed into C2 alone. C2 fixation includes true pedicle, pars,

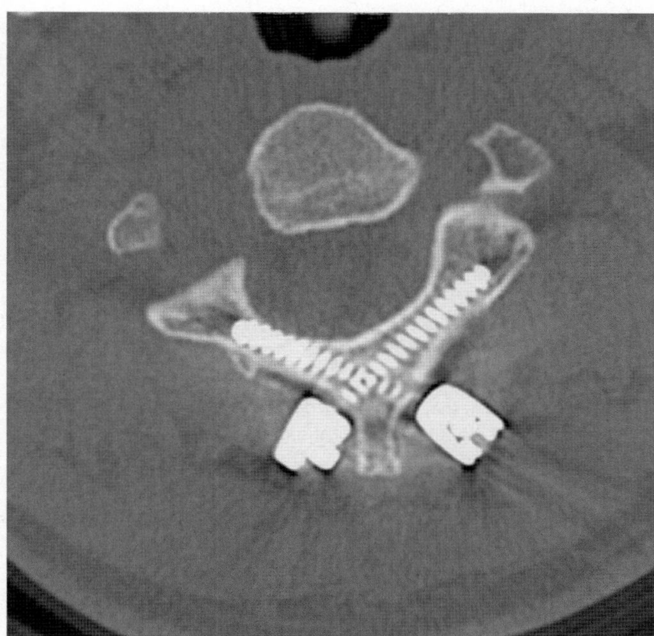

FIG. 69.13 Axial computed tomographic cut showing crossed C2 translaminar screws. (From Wright NM. Posterior C2 fixation using bilateral, crossing C2 laminar screws: case series and technical note. *J Spinal Disord Tech*. 2004;17:158–162.)

and intralaminar screws. Most of what are commonly termed C2 pedicle screws are, in fact, pars screws. Only screws passing beyond the very anterior C1–C2 facet and into the small C2 vertebral body are true pedicle screws.

The relative vertebral artery and neurologic risks of C2 pedicle and Magerl screws continue to be debated.[436,437] In a retrospective analysis of 341 C2 pedicle screws placed in 181 patients, postoperative CT scans demonstrated a 17.3% breach rate.[437] Lateral breaches were more common than medial breaches. No neurologic sequelae resulted.

In most studies, C2 pedicle screws are mechanically equivalent to C1–C2 transarticular screws and are stronger than intralaminar screws, which are stronger than pars screws.[368,438,439] Intralaminar screws are less effective at reducing lateral bending range of motion and thus may be suboptimal in dens fractures (Fig. 69.13).

Occasionally C2 screws are described for direct osteosynthesis of C2 pars fractures (hangman's fracture). Most authors agree that hangman's fractures without significant angulation, translation, or C2–C3 disc injury do not require operative intervention. Therefore, isolated use of C2 pedicle screws for osteosynthesis is rare. On the other hand, temporary rigid C1–C2 instrumentation without fusion is increasingly common in Asia in patients with odontoid fractures not amenable to dens screw fixation.[440,441] The screws are removed once the fracture has healed.

Pars screws are inserted in a manner like that described for Magerl screws earlier. The same entry site is used. The screw is angled less cranially, and mediolateral angulation mimics the easily palpated pars angle. Typically, these screws are angled 10 to 15 degrees medially and 35 degrees superiorly to avoid injury to the vertebral artery. Start true C2 pedicle screws in a far lateral position on the C2 lateral mass, just superior to the C2–C3 facet. This lateral starting point and the 40- to 45-degree medial direction required to pass all the way into the body may require a percutaneous stab. Before placement, carefully assess preoperative axial images. About 20% of the time, local anatomic conditions preclude true pedicle screws.[409]

Crossed C2 laminar screws decrease vertebral artery injury risk and allow segmental C2 fixation in patients with a narrow isthmus.[442] Technique modifications include a bony window in the lateral lamina to ensure that the screws have not entered the canal.[443] Occasionally a deeply furrowed spinous process or underdeveloped C2 midline posterior ring mandates parallel, rather than crossing, screw placements.[444] Good clinical performance of this anchorage method continues to be reported.[445,446]

Other C1–C2 Stabilization Options

In the 1980s, Halifax clamps enjoyed a period of favor because canal intrusive instrumentation could be avoided.[447] These devices were easy to use and more rigid than the available alternatives. These devices were among the first titanium implants in the cervical spine and therefore offered less interference with postoperative MRI. Unfortunately, Halifax clamps were prone to arch fracture, implant slippage, difficulties with graft placement, and a nearly 25% pseudarthrosis rate.[448,449] PMMA has been recommended for patients with rheumatoid arthritis (due to the poor iliac crest bone quality) and for immediate stabilization in patients with metastases.[450] The long-term results of PMMA used with wiring or alone have been poor. More recently, some authors have recommended midline PMMA for immediate stability and lateral bone grafting for long-term stability.[451]

Posterior Subaxial Instrumentation

Mid-cervical posterior instrumentation offers an array of wiring and more rigid rod-screw techniques like that in the upper cervical spine. The merits of each approach in terms of ease of insertion, cost, and mechanics are analogous. The more homogeneous mid-cervical anatomy simplifies level-to-level fixation decisions.

Posterior Wiring

The oldest, and simplest, form of cervical instrumentation is spinous process wiring. A variety of wiring strategies have been reported. All function as a nonrigid tension band. As in the upper cervical spine, wiring affords good flexion stability but less stability in other planes of motion, especially extension and rotation. The degree to which wires stabilize the spine varies by route of wire passage, quality of bone against which the wires pull, and wire tension.

To resist flexion and extension, the wire must be tensioned to 22 N. At 50 N, rotation resistance begins. Unfortunately, augmented tension also increased the chance of cut-through.[452]

Previously, wiring techniques were used in the stabilization of facet dislocations, teardrop fractures, postlaminectomy instabilities, and neoplastic collapse. Today, routine wiring has given way to rigid, lateral mass fixation. Most frequently, posterior cervical wiring is used to treat anterior interbody fusion pseudarthroses. Still, wiring continues to offer spine surgeons a back-up to supplement or replace an inadequate lateral mass construct. Wiring remains a low-profile, cost-effective solution in cases of limited flexion instability.[453] Avoid wiring in patients with movement disorders or torsional or axial instability.[454] Over time, bone graft, Steinmann pins, or Luque rectangles have been added to increase extension stability.[455,456] Even these modified wiring techniques remain unstable to axial load.

As with all posterior spine procedures, prone positioning requires careful attention to alignment and ocular pressure. The skin and subcutaneous tissue are dissected down to the midline fascia. Subperiosteal dissection is then completed to expose the spinous processes, laminae, and facet joints at the level of interest. To prevent inadvertent fusion extension, limit dissection to the intended levels and protect adjacent facet capsules. Drill a 3-mm burr hole in the base of the spinous process on both sides. Aim the holes toward the proximal aspect of the cephalic spinous process and distal aspect of the caudal spine. Run a nerve hook along the inferior lamina border to identify the canal; low holes may injure the dura or posterior cord.

To create a tunnel for the wires, pass a towel clip gently through the holes. Pass a single 18- or 20-gauge wire through both spinous processes. In a single-level fusion, this wire can be tensioned and tightened. When fusing more than one level, incorporate intervening spinous processes with a figure-of-eight wiring pattern. To maintain tension, avoid wiring fractured posterior elements. A variation, the Dewar technique improves the wire's holding power by spooling it over Kirschner wires inserted through the spinous process bases.[457]

For most uses, the Bohlman triple wiring has supplanted the Rogers technique. This procedure begins with a simple wiring but adds second and third wires through the cephalic and caudal holes in the bases of the spinous processes, respectively. Carefully decorticate the laminae and facets with a burr. Harvest two corticocancellous grafts of appropriate length from the outer table of the iliac crest. The grafts are drilled for wire passage, ensuring firm contact with the underlying lamina. Place the graft's posterior cortical edge just under the spinous process to enhance stability and maximize graft-lamina contact. Simultaneously tighten the wires on each side of the spine (Fig. 69.14). Place additional cancellous chips on the exposed lamina or facets. As a function of construct stability and patient compliance, a cervicothoracic orthosis or halo vest may be used for 6 weeks. This technique has been shown to be safe, effective, and biomechanically superior to many other wired constructs.[458,459]

The smaller subaxial canal compounds risk associated with sublaminar wiring below C2. More typically, interfacet wiring and fusion are performed after laminectomy or when the spinous process is fractured.[460] Additionally, adding an oblique interfacet wire to a simple midline technique improves

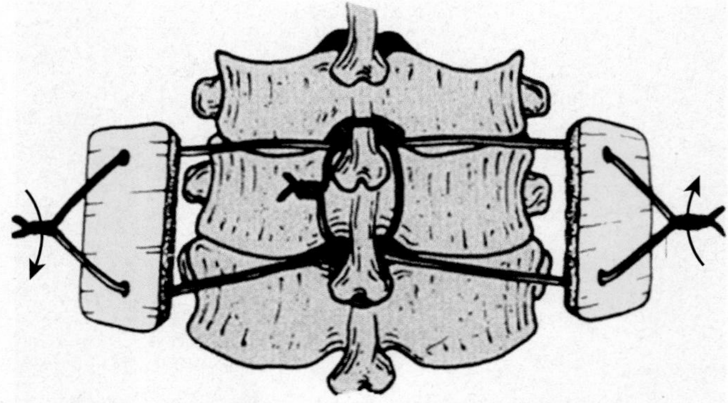

FIG. 69.14 Schematic showing Bohlman's triple-wire technique for posterior fixation of the subaxial cervical spine.

rotational stability.[461] To place an oblique wire, insert a Penfield No. 4 dissector into the facet joint. Direct a 2-mm drill inferiorly into the facet. For single-level fusion, pass a 20-gauge wire through this hole and loop it around the inferior spinous process. For multiple-level and postlaminectomy facet stabilization, extend facet wires to adjacent facets. Tie facet wires to structural bone grafts or metallic rods for additional stability.

Multistrand, braided cables are stronger, more flexible, and more fatigue resistant than monofilament wire. Cable utilization increased after reports of frequent fatigue failure, loosening, and bone cut-through with monofilament wires.[452] On the other hand, cables are more expensive than wires and cable memory may lead to gradual loss of reduction or canal intrusion. If wires or cables break, the strands may penetrate the dura, leading to cerebrospinal fluid leak or direct neurologic injury.[462] Stainless steel, titanium, and polyethylene offer similar mechanical properties.[452,463] Titanium and polyethylene cables are more imaging friendly than stainless steel wires. Cable systems often come with sophisticated tensioners. These constructs lack sagittal axis control, and overtensioning may induce retrolisthesis. Recent outcome reports are limited but favorable for both wires and cables.[464,465]

Rigid Posterior Mid-Cervical Instrumentation

Rigid subaxial instrumentation options include hooks and lateral mass, pedicle, and transarticular screws. Rigid fixation implies both a tight interface with the host bone and a rigid locking mechanism between the anchor and the longitudinal member (a plate or rod). These systems more effectively maintain sagittal alignment than wiring and remain effective after laminectomy or posterior element fracture.[466,467]

Initially, reconstruction plates were used. Today, plates continue to be used because they are cheaper and lower profile than rod systems. On the other hand, interfacet distances vary widely among individuals (9–16 mm; mean, 13 mm), and a plate's hole spacing limits optimal screw placement.[468,469] Oblong holes better accommodate variable interfacet distances at the cost of rigid axial control of the screw. Rods are more easily contoured and allow greater freedom in lateral mass screw placement. Newer rod constructs offer rigid locking and cross-linking.[468] Screw-rod systems are more easily extended to the occiput and across the cervicothoracic junction. Finally, screw-rod systems permit the application of compression, distraction, and reduction forces within the construct.[469] Both plating and rodding systems tend to fail with superior screw loosening and pullout. In cadaveric testing, plate failure occurred earlier and more likely fractured the superior lateral mass.[84] Posterior lateral mass constructs are more rigid than either anterior plating or posterior wiring systems.[470,471]

Cervical Hooks

Hooks, although not as rigid as screws, have relatively simple placement. There are several types: Halifax clamps (discussed earlier), laminar (canal intrusive) hooks, and the hybrid hook-plate. Cervical hooks were initially used at the cranial end of long deformity constructs. Other indications include tumors and upper thoracic trauma. The need to extend thoracic constructs into the low cervical spine has decreased with the increased utilization of thoracic pedicle screws. Utilization for cervical pathologies has decreased with improved lateral mass systems and dedicated cervicothoracic junction constructs. Hook-plates provide one-level stabilization in which the screw is placed into the superior lateral mass and the hook captures the inferior lamina. Hook-plate designs remain practical for C6–C7 instabilities because they avoid screw placement in the thin C7 lateral mass.[472] More commonly, C7 pedicle screws are placed.

Few outcome studies are available describing utilization of cervical hooks. Most describe atlantoaxial placement.[473] Particular risks of hooks include dural penetration, iatrogenic neurologic injury, or late hook disengagement.[474] Laminar hooks must be avoided at levels with cord edema canal stenosis. Biomechanical testing reveals that hook constructs are comparable to lateral mass screws in flexion and extension loading but less rigid in lateral bend and rotation.[475] All posterior systems resist lateral bending better than anterior plates.

Lateral Mass Screws

Most typically, rigid subaxial fixation relies on placement of lateral mass screws into C3–C6. Lateral mass screw fixation is indicated when more rigid fixation than wiring is necessary (Figs. 69.15 and 69.16). Polytrauma patients typically benefit from the earlier mobilization and decreased bracing engendered by rigid stabilization. More rigid fixation should be considered in any patient in whom healing may be delayed, compliance is suspect, or multilevel fusion is required.

Safe lateral mass screw placement requires familiarity with the articular pillar anatomy. Expose to the lateral edge of the pillar. Do not pass over the edge as bleeders in this region retract anteriorly and are difficult to control. Remove the osteophytes to better delineate the articular pillar's margins. Sagittal alignment of the neck varies with each case. Pass a Penfield No. 4 dissector into the facet to ascertain its angulation. Locate the center of the lateral mass by defining the notch between the lamina and the lateral mass. Several trajectories have been described. The Roy-Camille technique describes screw insertion at the apex of convexity of the lateral mass. Aim 10 degrees laterally to decrease the risk of nerve root injury. To decrease facet violation, Magerl recommended an entry point 2 to 3 mm medial and superior to the apex. He described a 25-degree lateral drill angle and a superior trajectory parallel to the facet (typically 45 degrees). Anderson,[472] An,[466] and others[469] have described variations of entry site and angulation. An and colleagues[137] suggested lateral mass entry 1 mm medial to its center. The drill is angled 30 degrees lateral and 15 degrees cranially.

When these trajectories were assessed in cadavers, the Roy-Camille technique frequently violated neurovascular structures below C3, especially, with more lateral screw angulation, the nerve root.[472] The Magerl technique was safe at the standard 25 degrees and modified positions of 20 degrees and 30 degrees. The Anderson technique was safe at 20- and 30-degree modified positions. At C7, only the modified Anderson technique (20–30 degrees of lateral angulation) was safe.

Bicortical penetration improves failure resistance by 20% but increases root injury risk. Consider bicortical screws in the presence of osteoporotic bone, few acceptable anchor points, unstable spines and, particularly, in those with anterior column collapse and decreased axial load-bearing capability. To place a bicortical screw, gradually increase the drill's set depth. Palpate the opposite cortex. To avoid stripping the threads, be sure to tap the full screw depth.

Lateral mass screw placement risks canal intrusion and vertebral artery or nerve root injury.[51,476] Typically, overly long screws or poor drilling technique precipitated the complication. Occasionally, poor plate or rod contouring compresses the root from foraminal stenosis engendered by a lag screw effect when the screw pulls the lateral mass up to the plate or rod. Adjacent facet joint violation may accelerate adjacent-segment degeneration.

Lateral mass screws have recently been reclassified and are now approved as adjuncts to cervical fusion. Despite their late reclassification, they remain among the safest implants in spine surgery.[477] In one series, despite coronal and sagittal plane deformities and lateral mass abnormalities, 212 lateral mass screws were safely implanted. There were no cord or vertebral artery injuries, cerebrospinal fluid leaks, screw malposition or back-out, loss of alignment, or implant failure.[469] Iatrogenic radiculopathy (usually transient) risk is less than 1.8% per screw, even in children as young as 6 years.[478,479] Unlike wiring, loss of fixation and reduction are rare, even when no formal autogenous grafting is performed.[480-482] Failure in kyphosis is occasionally seen in patients with incompetent anterior column load bearing (e.g., C5 burst fracture).[481] One study compared anterior or posterior stabilization in 52 patients with unstable cervical spine injuries and spinal cord injuries.[483] Neurologic improvement was seen in 70% and 57% of the anterior and posterior groups, respectively. There were two nonunions in the anterior group and none in the posterior. There were no statistically significant differences in fusion rates, alignment, neurologic recovery, or long-term pain complaints. A recent series of 2500 lateral mass screws placed in 430 patients found that only three patients needed revision for implant-related reasons.[484]

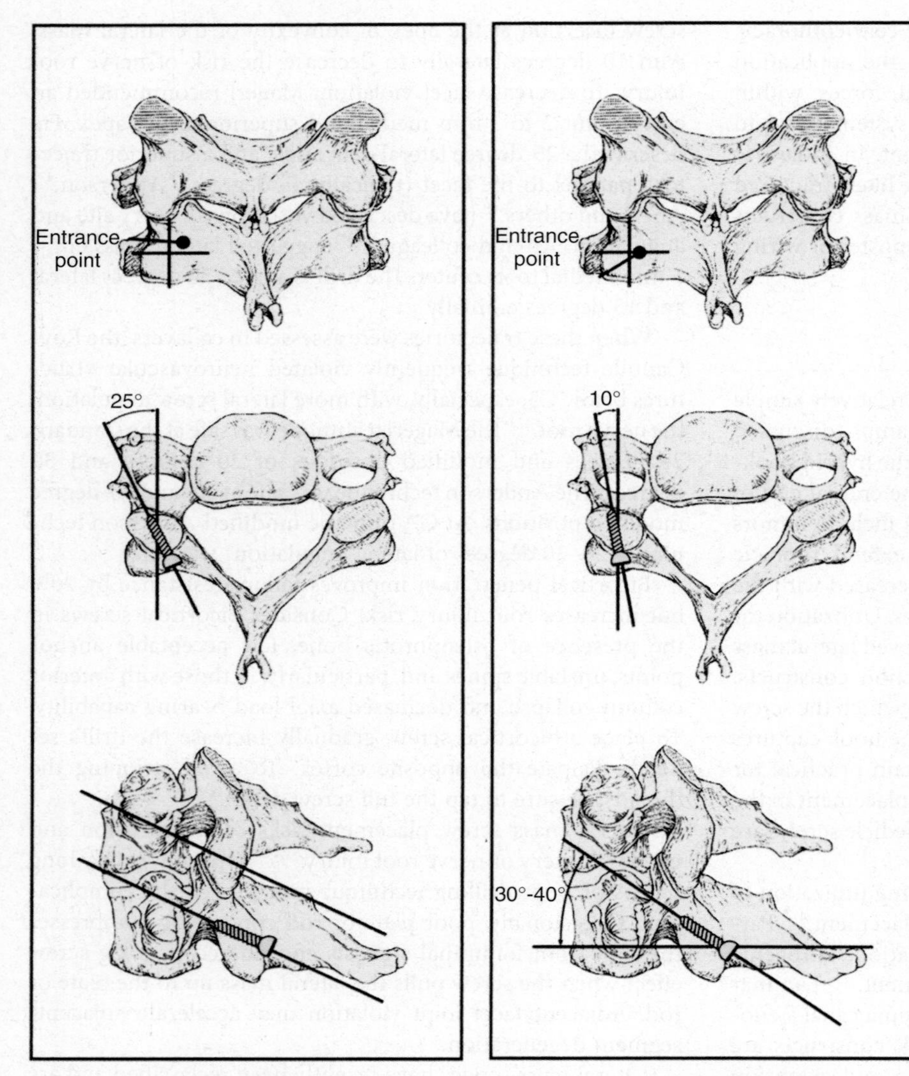

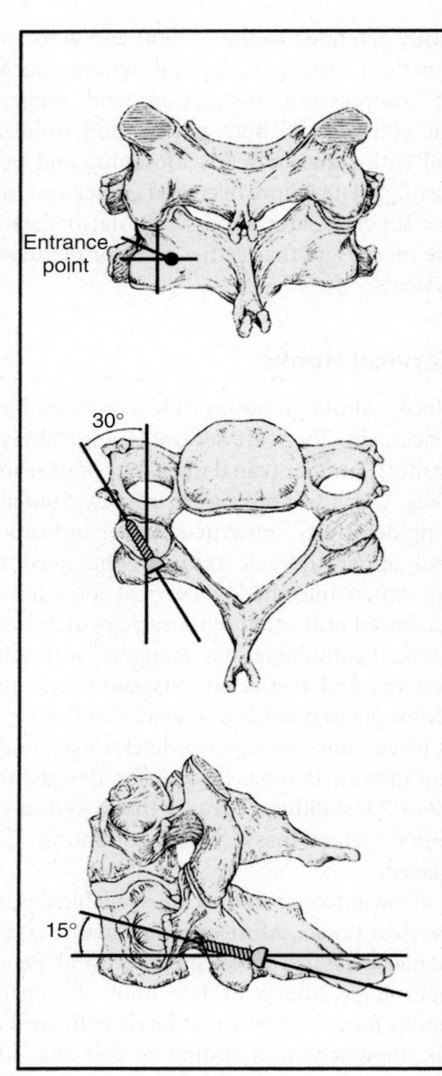

FIG. 69.15 Various lateral mass screw placement options. (From Xu R, Haman S, Ebraheim N, et al. The anatomic relation of lateral mass screws to the spinal nerves: a comparison of the Magerl, Anderson, and An techniques. *Spine [Phila Pa 1976]*. 1999;24:2057.)

Ongoing concerns with lateral mass screw fixation include the muscle dissection required for insertion and the increased profile associated with polyaxial systems and rods. A number of systems have been introduced with decreased bulk and "favored angle" geometries to allow closer apposition to the bone.[485] The degree of constraint at the screw-rod interface varies between systems. Loose connections or flexible rods may allow a drift into kyphosis. On the other hand, overcorrection of kyphosis may increase postoperative nerve traction injury risk. One series reported that, in a series of myelopathy patients undergoing decompression, half of those instrumented with lateral mass screws and rods (five of 10) had a postoperative C5 palsy.[486] In five of 63 (8%) of the uninstrumented patients with C5 palsy, the deltoid weakness was not as severe as in the instrumented patients.

Increasingly, lateral mass screws are inserted through tubular retractors or percutaneous cannulated routes. These approaches preserve muscle and ligament integrity, thereby maintaining the posterior tension band. With most systems, up to two levels can be treated.[487] The real benefits of this approach are not yet clear.

Salvage of failed lateral mass screws can include 4.0-mm revision screws in the same trajectory, redirection to a Roy-Camille technique, and conversion to pedicle screw placement. In a cadaveric evaluation, no significant differences were seen between a larger Magerl lateral mass screw versus a Roy-Camille revision.[488] Pedicle screw revision offers significantly greater pullout strength (566 N) compared with either the Magerl (382 N) or Roy-Camille (351 N) revision. At the cranial and caudal ends of a decompression and fusion construct, or at intervening levels in nonlaminectomy cases, laminar hooks and transarticular and translaminar screws can also be considered.[489] One clinical study concluded translaminar screws were technically simpler and offered adequate stability.

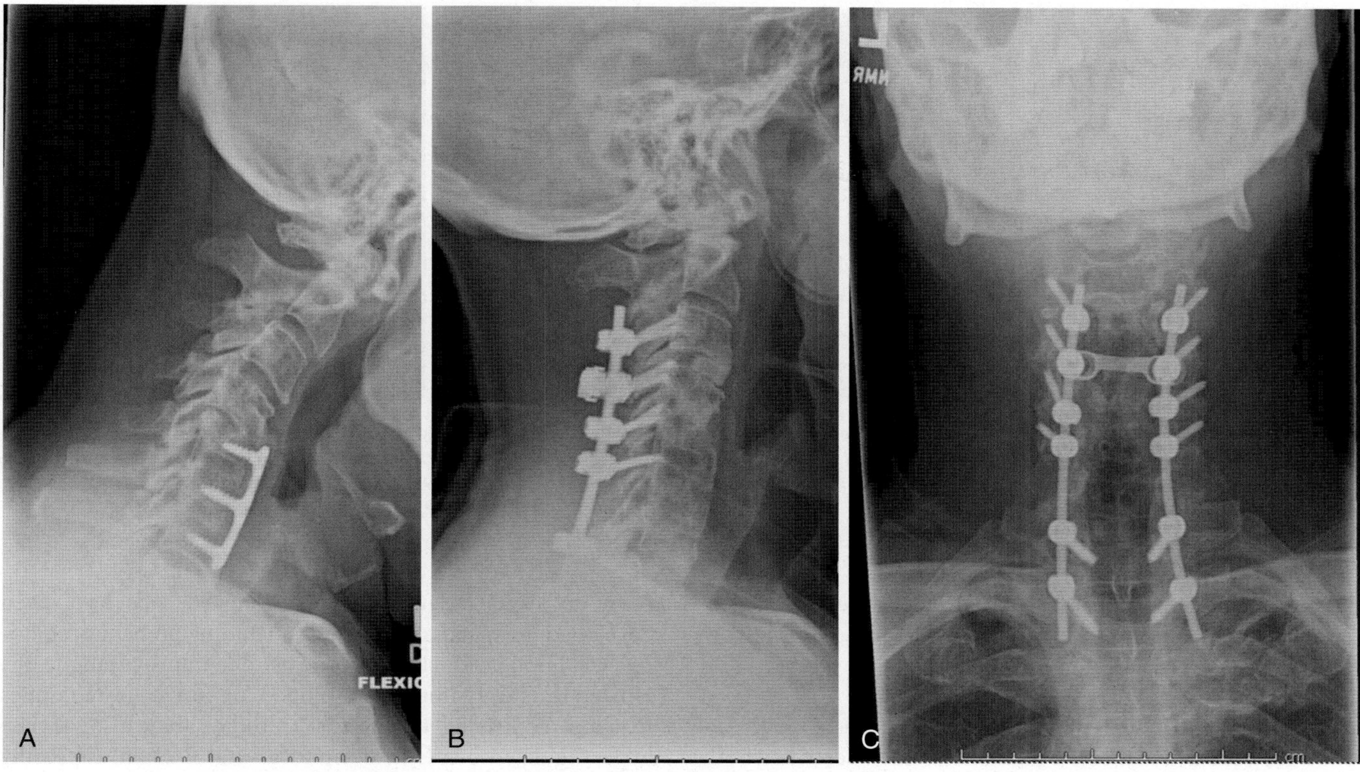

FIG. 69.16 (A) A 56-year-old man who had undergone previous C5–C7 anterior cervical discectomy and fusion (ACDF) presented with adjacen-segment (C4–C5) degeneration, kyphosis, stenosis, and increasing myelopathy. The anterior plate was removed and ACDF performed at C3–C4 and C4–C5, and a posterior stabilization was performed with lateral mass screws from C3 to C6 and pedicle screws at T1. Postoperative (B) lateral and (C) anteroposterior views are also shown.

Mid and Lower Cervical Pedicle Screws

Pedicle screws offer three-column fixation and have greater pullout strength than lateral mass screws.[22,117,490] A single C7 pedicle screw approximates the stability provided by lateral mass screws at both C6 and C7.[491] While single-screw pullout and fatigue resistance are higher with pedicle fixation, whole-construct strength differences may be minimal.[475] The small mid-cervical pedicles and the proximity of the cord, vertebral arteries, and nerve roots limit enthusiasm for routine screw fixation. Most frequently, C3–C6 pedicle screw placement is recommended in posterior-only corrections of markedly unstable three-column injury or maintenance of correction after cervical osteotomy or postlaminectomy kyphosis.

The standard pedicle screw placement method uses an entry point 3 mm below the superior facet joint (Fig. 69.17).[22] The drill is angled 45 degrees medially and advanced in a vertical line parallel to the endplate. Alternatively, a line parallel to the contralateral lamina provides a 3-mm safe corridor for sagittal plane angulation.[492] Alternatively, Abumi recommends burr removal of the lateral mass to provide a direct view of the pedicle introitus.[490] The pedicle is then probed and tapped and a 3.5-mm cortical screw inserted. Mean pullout resistances are similar. Unfortunately, standard angulations and entry points may be dangerous because, between C4 and C6, pedicle anatomy surface topography is highly variable.[64] Avoidance of pedicles smaller than 4.5 mm, a laminoforaminotomy technique to directly palpate the pedicle, and navigation assistance improve safety.[20] Some have reported safe placement with patient-specific, rapid-prototype drill guides.[493,494]

A number of studies report safe utilization of mid-cervical pedicle screws and cite high fusion rates and excellent correction of cervical deformity with this technique.[391,495] More recent series reported a 20% malposition rate with an 8% symptomatic breach rate and 3.4% vertebral artery injury rate.[496,497] Both groups concluded that mid-cervical pedicle screws posed significant additional risks and should be used by very experienced spine surgeons for destructive lesions only.

The large C7 pedicle size and absence of the vertebral artery in the foramen transversarium encourage more routine placement.[498,499] C7 pedicle screws can be inserted with any of the techniques described for mid-cervical screws. Close assessment of preoperative axial CT and MRI images is recommended to ensure that the foramen transversarium does not contain the vertebral artery, to measure the patient's medial angulation and pedicle diameter, and to familiarize the surgeon with the surface bone topography. Intraoperatively, a C6–C7 laminotomy allows direct palpation of the pedicle. Adequate fascial release prevents undermedialization.

With any posterior cervical screw placement, intraoperative electromyographic assessment may be helpful. To reduce scatter, test the screws before placing the connecting rod. Stimulation thresholds correlate with screw position, and

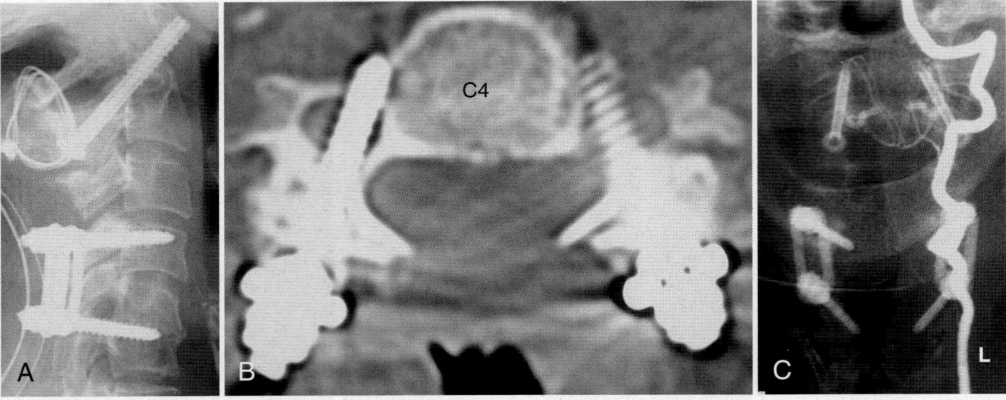

FIG. 69.17 (A) Lateral radiograph demonstrating placement of subaxial cervical pedicle screws during posterior cervical fusion. (B) Axial computed tomographic image of subaxial cervical pedicle screw within the foramen transversarium at C4. (C) Angiogram demonstrating flow through left vertebral artery with no flow on the right side. (From Abumi K, Shono Y, Ito M, et al. Complications of pedicle screw fixation in reconstructive surgery of the cervical spine. *Spine (Phila Pa 1976)*. 2000;25:962–969.)

values greater than 15 mA reliably predict acceptable screw position.[51]

Lower Cervical Transarticular Screws

Subaxial transarticular screw fixation has been described both alone and with rods.[500] Unisegmental bone screws traverse four cortices for excellent holding power; their lack of polyaxial heads or rods reduces implant costs and profile. At C7, the limitations of fixation to the thin lateral mass and difficulty of pedicle screws favor 8- to 10-mm screws placed perpendicular to the facet.[501] Multilevel transfacet screw constructs compare favorably to the more typical lateral mass screw and rod technique.[502,503] One recent finite element model found that downward-angled, transarticular screws were stronger than either pedicle or lateral mass screws in the treatment of a three-column mid-cervical injury.[504]

In clinical studies, multilevel transfacet screw constructs compare favorably to the more typical lateral mass screw and rod technique.[500,502,503] A recent study compared direct sagittal placement with a 30-degree lateralized placement that would theoretically convey less risk to the cervical roots.[505] A total of 95 screws were placed in 18 consecutive patients. One complication, nerve root irritation due to screw malposition, was reported. Lateralized positioning was reported to significantly increase four-cortex placement and decrease loosening (29% vs. 5% and 24% vs. 2%, respectively). Although the authors supported the technique, they noted that "extensive cranial exposure is required to align the instruments in the proper sagittal trajectory." In fact, the occiput can block screw placement, especially in the upper cervical spine.

Posterior Cervical Rods and Cross-Links

A variety of "longitudinal members" are available for posterior cervical spine surgery. Titanium rods from 3.0 to 4.0 mm are the most frequently used. Stainless steel implants remain available and may be preferable when durability and deformity correction are sought. Overbending, especially in titanium rods, decreases fatigue life.[506] Customized rods have been developed for specific indications, including prebent occipitocervical implants thickened at the bend to improve fatigue life. Hinged rods were initially developed for cervical osteotomies to allow controlled osteoclasis.[507] Today, they also obviate hyperangulated bends in occipitocervical fixation, especially in patients with rheumatoid arthritis and occipitocervical impaction.

A variety of specialized cervical cross-links are available. With decompression procedures, the posterior cord drift may lead to cross-link impingement. Precurved cross-links arch over the canal. Cervical cross-links are indicated in the presence of coronal instability, to compensate for limited fixation points, and to contain structural grafts.[98] Also consider cross-links for increased torsional stability, to reconstruct axial bursting injuries, in longer constructs, and in osteoporotic bone.[508]

Facet Spacers

Spacers made of allograft bone, PEEK, and other materials, typically around 2 mm thick, have been described to restore alignment or improve foraminal volume. Many have a large osteoconductive surface. When implanted, compression across the implant may enhance the fusion process. One recent biomechanical study found that these spacers alone did not adequately reduce spinal motion, however, and adjunctive screw and rod fixation had to be used.[509] Another study found that the devices were easy to implant and did not increase kyphosis.[510]

Laminoplasty Implants

Laminoplasty implants seek to contain hinge bone grafts and to prevent closure. A wide variety of implants support the many described laminoplasty techniques. Most common are sutures, spacers, precut bone grafts and miniplates for the Hirabayashi open-door technique. Because the facet capsules are often thinned or stripped during exposure, 2-mm metallic

TABLE 69.1 Occipital Bone Thickness

Skull Location	Midline (mm)	1 cm off Midline (mm)	2 cm off Midline (mm)
EOP	10–15	9–11	7.5–9
1 cm below EOP	9–11	5–7	4.5–6
2 cm below EOP	8–9	4–6	3.5–4.5
3 cm below EOP	6–7	4–5	3.5–4.5

EOP, external occipital protuberance.

suture anchors inserted along the standard lateral mass screw trajectory augment the initially described suture.[511,512] In two series of 15 and 42 patients, respectively, low complication rates, ease of use, and closure avoidance were reported.[513,514] Over the last few years, laminoplasty miniplates have been offered to more rigidly stabilize the hinge and to allow more aggressive decompression. These devices are FDA approved only as graft containment systems. Custom-shaped allograft plugs further assist in "propping" the laminoplasty door and offer biologic healing over time. Late displacement leading to tetraparesis has been reported.[515] A recent study compared laminoplasty plates with suture suspension fixation. The authors concluded that "miniplate fixation preserved more cervical range of motion and better cervical alignment, maintained cervical spine canal expansive stability, and effectively avoided lamina reclosure" than suture fixation.[516]

Conclusions

Cervical instrumentation options are rapidly evolving. On one hand, the explosion in the number and variety of implants available offers the spinal surgeon choices heretofore never imagined. On the other, choosing the optimal approach for the patient has become increasingly difficult.

As both more sophisticated stabilization and fusion devices and motion-sparing techniques evolve, the surgeon will require a clear understanding of cervical spine biomechanics. Appropriate surgical strategies will arise from the patient's specific anatomic and pathomechanical needs.

Today, the wealth of conflicting data points out limits of our current mechanical models. Aside from the most common procedures (e.g., ACDF), there are very few direct comparisons of available techniques. However, large database studies may help us.

Since the last edition of this text, lateral mass screw placement in the posterior cervical spine has been approved for most common indications. This labeling change, and increasing attention on sagittal spinal balance, has continued to push rigid segmental instrumentation in the cervical spine. Cervical disc replacement has become more commonplace, but utilization varies significantly and it is likely appropriate only in a fraction of patients for whom anterior cervical fusion techniques can be considered.

The pressure for surgeons to consider the costs of implant choices has only increased. New "bundling" models of reimbursement are on the horizon that will require surgeons to more clearly delineate how much surgery is "enough." A clear understanding of spinal biomechanics and reconstruction options will allow the surgeon to decrease immediate costs through pragmatic implant selection as well as long-term costs through a reduction in surgical failure and revision. The patient will benefit in several ways, not least of which is the avoidance of the morbidity of excessive reconstruction. Anterior cervical implantation of BMP has proven to be an example of this phenomenon.

KEY POINTS

1. Patient positioning:
   - Intraoperative alignment is critical, especially in long fusions.
   - Appropriate alignment allows safer placement of the implants.
   - If in doubt, check radiographs and examine rotation (midline spinous processes).
2. Adequate exposure:
   - Accurate placement requires clear delineation of the relevant anatomy.
   - In anterior procedures, release fascia, undercut platysma, remove retractors regularly, and decrease endotracheal cuff pressure to decrease soft tissue complications.
3. Closely inspect the preoperative imaging studies; individual anatomy varies widely.
4. Preoperative planning: list the types and sizes of implants required before scrubbing in.
5. Have a back-up plan; familiarity with multiple techniques is useful if a screw backs out or proves difficult to place.
6. New products: carefully evaluate the data yourself; there is little advantage to the patient for their surgeon to be the "first on the block."

KEY REFERENCES

1. Benzel E. *Biomechanics of Spine Stabilization: Principles and Clinical Practice*. New York: McGraw-Hill; 1995.
   This short, well-illustrated text provides an excellent overview of the mechanical principles that inform rational implant selection and placement. This book describes the various stabilization modes in greater detail than this chapter allows.
2. White AA 3rd, Panjabi M. *Clinical Biomechanics of the Spine*. Philadelphia: Lippincott; 1990.
   This short text describes normal and pathologic mechanics of the spine. Without a solid understanding of how disease disrupts normal spinal stability, instrumentation becomes a rote or knee-jerk process. Instead, the surgeon should consider the deficiencies and postoperative needs of the individual patient when planning reconstruction.
3. Steinmetz MP, Benzel EC, Apfelbaum RI. Axially dynamic implants for stabilization of the cervical spine. *Neurosurgery*. 2006;59(4 suppl 2):ONS378-ONS388.
   This article provides an excellent overview of the evolution of anterior plates. Although the overt bias here favors axially dynamic implants, given the frequency with which anterior cervical plates are used, the surgeon should have a clear understanding of the relative merits of different design philosophies.
4. Dvorak MF, Pitzen T, Zhu Q, et al. Anterior cervical plate fixation: a biomechanical study to evaluate the effects of plate design, endplate preparation, and bone mineral density. *Spine*. 2005;30:294-301.
   This well-done biomechanical study addresses some of the challenges to anterior cervical plate fixation. Spinal surgeons

SECTION IX

increasingly are encountering patients with osteoporosis, for example. The authors describe the positive and negative effects of varied endplate preparation methods and plate designs.

5. Wang JC, McDonough PW, Kanim LE, et al. Increased fusion rates with cervical plating for three-level anterior cervical discectomy and fusion. *Spine*. 2001;26:643-646.
This is one of a series of articles published from 1999 to 2001 outlining the University of California–Los Angeles experience with anterior cervical discectomy and fusion procedures. Fusion rates and other radiographic parameters were assessed with and without plating in one-, two-, and three-level procedures. Plates offer increasing advantages over nonplated constructs with increasing number of levels treated. Failure rates increase with additional levels of surgery, however, even with plates.

6. Wertheim SB, Bohlman HH. Occipitocervical fusion: indications, technique, and long-term results in thirteen patients. *J Bone Joint Surg Am*. 1987;69:833-836.
This classic article details Bohlman's modification of cervical wiring. In the occipitocervical and the subaxial applications, additional wires were used to apply structural grafts to the spine. These structural grafts increased extension stiffness over previous simple wiring. Although rigid fixation is currently more common, variable bone quality and anatomy continue to make these approaches relevant.

7. Ebraheim NA, Lu J, Biyani A, et al. An anatomic study of the thickness of the occipital bone: implications for occipitocervical instrumentation. *Spine*. 1996;21:1725-1729.
This is one of several key anatomic studies assessing occipital bone thickness and the proximity of the cranial sinuses. These studies and clinical experience led to a gradual migration away from off-midline plates to modular designs that fix to the thick midline keel.

8. Harms J, Melcher RP. Posterior C1-C2 fusion with polyaxial screw and rod fixation. *Spine*. 2001;26:2467-2471.
Use of upper cervical fixation techniques has changed markedly since Harms' popularization of C1 lateral mass screw placement. With rigid C1 fixation, extension of cervical fusions to the occiput has been limited to the rare, true occipitocervical instability only. This procedure is technically simpler than Magerl's transarticular screw fixation and is not as limited by incomplete reductions and anatomic abnormalities. As a result, more surgeons have chosen to exploit this approach than either transarticular screws or wiring. Increased use of C2 crossed laminar screws has furthered this trend.

REFERENCES

1. Albert T, et al. Spinal instrumentation. In: Herkowitz HN, et al., eds. *Rothman-Simeone: The Spine*. Philadelphia: WB Saunders; 1999:1641-1660.
2. Hadra B. Wiring of the spinous process in Pott's disease. *Trans Am Orthop Assoc*. 1891;4:206.
3. Rogers W. Treatment of fracture dislocation of the cervical spine. *J Bone Joint Surg Am*. 1942;24:254-258.
4. Bohlman HH. Surgical management of cervical spine fractures and dislocations. *Instr Course Lect*. 1985;34:163-187.
5. Robinson R, Smith G. Anterolateral cervical disc removal and interbody fusion for cervical disc syndrome. *Bull Johns Hopkins Hosp*. 1955;96:223-224.
6. Kostuik JP, et al. Anterior cervical plate fixation with the titanium hollow screw plate system. *Spine*. 1993;18(10):1273-1278.
7. Emstad E, et al. The VariLift Interbody Fusion System: expandable, standalone interbody fusion. *Med Devices (Auckl)*. 2015;8:219-230.
8. Weber MH, et al. Graft subsidence and revision rates following anterior cervical corpectomy: a clinical study comparing different interbody cages. *Clin Spine Surg*. 2016. Epub ahead of print.
9. Elder BD, et al. A systematic review of the use of expandable cages in the cervical spine. *Neurosurg Rev*. 2016;39(1):1-11.
10. Goel VK, et al. Ligamentous laxity across C0-C1-C2 complex. Axial torque-rotation characteristics until failure. *Spine*. 1990;15(10):990-996.
11. Puttlitz CM, et al. Stability analysis of craniovertebral junction fixation techniques. *J Bone Joint Surg Am*. 2004;86-A(3):561-568.
12. Werne S. Studies in spontaneous atlas dislocation. *Acta Orthop Scand*. 1957;23(suppl):1.
13. Panjabi M, et al. Three dimensional movements of the upper cervical spine. *Spine*. 1988;13:726.
14. Apple J, Kirks D, Merten D. Cervical spine fractures and dislocations in children. *Pediatr Radiol*. 1987;17:45.
15. Penning L, Wilmink J. Rotation of the cervical spine: a CT study in normal subjects. *Spine*. 1987;12:732.
16. Dickman CA, Locantro J, Fessler RG. The influence of transoral odontoid resection on stability of the craniovertebral junction. *J Neurosurg*. 1992;77(4):525-530.
17. Jarrett P, Whitesides TJ. Injuries of the cervicocranium. In: Browner BD, Levine AM, et al., eds. *Skeletal Trauma: Fractures, Dislocations, Ligamentous Injuries*. Philadelphia.: WB Saunders; 1992:668.
18. Levine A, Edwards C. Treatment of injuries in the Cl-C2 complex. *Orthop Clin North Am*. 1986;17:31.
19. Kwon B, et al. Morphologic evaluation of cervical spine anatomy with computed tomography: anterior cervical plate fixation considerations. *J Spinal Disord*. 2004;17(2):102-107.
20. Ludwig SC, et al. Placement of pedicle screws in the human cadaveric cervical spine: comparative accuracy of three techniques. *Spine*. 2000;25(13):1655-1667.
21. Dvorak MF, et al. Anterior occiput-to-axis screw fixation. Part I: a case report, description of a new technique, and anatomical feasibility analysis. *Spine*. 2003;28(3):E54-E60.
22. Kotani Y, et al. Biomechanical analysis of cervical stabilization systems. An assessment of transpedicular screw fixation in the cervical spine. *Spine*. 1994;19(22):2529-2539.
23. Kaneda K, McAfee P. The role of anteromedial foraminotomy and the uncovertebral joints in the stability of the cervical spine. A biomechanical study. *Spine*. 1998;23(14):1559-1565.
24. Nadim Y, et al. Occipital screws in occipitocervical fusion and their relation to the venous sinuses: an anatomic and radiographic study. *Orthopedics*. 2000;23(7):717-719.
25. Currier BL, et al. Relationship of the internal carotid artery to the anterior aspect of the C1 vertebra: implications for C1-C2 transarticular and C1 lateral mass fixation. *Spine*. 2008;33(6):635-639.
26. Bogaerde MV, Viaene P, Thijs V. Iatrogenic perforation of the internal carotid artery by a transarticular screw: an unusual case of repetitive ischemic stroke. *Clin Neurol Neurosurg*. 2007;109(5):466-469.
27. Currier B, et al. *Relationship of the internal carotid artery to the anterior aspect of the C1 vertebra: implications of C1-2 transarticular and C1 lateral mass screw fixation*. Presented at the 30th Annual Meeting of the CSRS; 2002, Miami Beach, Fla.
28. Miyata M, et al. Is rheumatoid arthritis a risk factor for a high-riding vertebral artery? *Spine*. 2008;33(18):2007-2011.

29. Peng CW, et al. Vertebral artery injury in cervical spine surgery: anatomical considerations, management, and preventive measures. *Spine J.* 2009;9(1):70-76.
30. Huang MJ, Glaser JA. Complete arcuate foramen precluding C1 lateral mass screw fixation in a patient with rheumatoid arthritis: case report. *Iowa Orthop J.* 2003;23:96-99.
31. Bloch O, et al. Effect of frameless stereotaxy on the accuracy of C1-2 transarticular screw placement. *J Neurosurg.* 2001; 95(1 suppl):74-79.
32. Paramore C, Dickman C, Sonntag V. The anatomic suitability of the C1-C2 complex for transarticular screw fixation. *J Neurosurg.* 1996;85:221.
33. Nassr AN, et al. Aberrant posterior inferior cerebellar artery injury with C1 lateral mass screw placement: a case report and review of the literature. *Spine J.* 2014;14(9):e7-e14.
34. Elia M, Mazzara JT, Fielding JW. Onlay technique for occipitocervical fusion. *Clin Orthop.* 1992;280:170-174.
35. Helenius I, et al. Rigid fixation improves outcomes of spinal fusion for C1-C2 instability in children with skeletal dysplasias. *J Bone Joint Surg Am.* 2015;97(3):232-240.
36. Geck MJ, et al. Feasibility of rigid upper cervical instrumentation in children: tomographic analysis of children aged 2-6. *J Spinal Disord Tech.* 2014;27(3):E110-E117.
37. Singh B, Cree A. Laminar screw fixation of the axis in the pediatric population: a series of eight patients. *Spine J.* 2015;15(2):e17-e25.
38. Schultz KD Jr, et al. Pediatric occipitocervical arthrodesis. A review of current options and early evaluation of rigid internal fixation techniques. *Pediatr Neurosurg.* 2000;33(4): 169-181.
39. Brockmeyer D, et al. Pediatric cervical spine instrumentation using screw fixation. *Pediatr Neurosurg.* 1995;22(3): 147-157.
40. Li V, Lopes DK, Bennett GJ. Use of a craniofacial miniplate for internal fixation in a young child with cervical instability. Case report. *J Neurosurg.* 2001;95(1 suppl):128-131.
41. Gieger M, Roth PA, Wu JK. The anterior cervical approach to the cervicothoracic junction. *Neurosurgery.* 1995;37(4): 704-709.
42. Kaya R, et al. A perspective for the selection of surgical approaches in patients with upper thoracic and cervicothoracic junction instabilities. *Surg Neurol.* 2006;65:454-463.
43. Sharan AD, Przybylski GJ, Tartaglino L. Approaching the upper thoracic vertebrae without sternotomy or thoracotomy: a radiographic analysis with clinical application. *Spine.* 2000;25(8):910-916.
44. Luk KD, Cheung KM, Leong JC. Anterior approach to the cervicothoracic junction by unilateral or bilateral manubriotomy. A report of five cases. *J Bone Joint Surg Am.* 2002;84-A(6):1013-1017.
45. Fraser JF, et al. Preoperative magnetic resonance imaging screening for a surgical decision regarding the approach for anterior spine fusion at the cervicothoracic junction. *Spine.* 2002;27(7):675-681.
46. Teng H, et al. Surgery in the cervicothoracic junction with an anterior low suprasternal approach alone or combined with manubriotomy and sternotomy: an approach selection method based on the cervicothoracic angle. *J Neurosurg Spine.* 2009;10(6):531-542.
47. Hashizume H, et al. A clinical case of endoscopically assisted anterior screw fixation for the type II odontoid fracture. *Spine.* 2003;28(5):E102-E105.
48. Wang MY, et al. Minimally invasive lateral mass screws in the treatment of cervical facet dislocations: technical note. *Neurosurgery.* 2003;52(2):444-447.
49. Rodriguez-Catarino M, et al. Percutaneous vertebroplasty at C2: case report of a patient with multiple myeloma and a literature review. *Eur Spine J.* 2007;16(suppl 3):242-249.
50. McLain RF. Salvage of a malpositioned anterior odontoid screw. *Spine.* 2001;26(21):2381-2384.
51. Djurasovic M, et al. A prospective analysis of intraoperative electromyographic monitoring of posterior cervical screw fixation. *J Spinal Disord Tech.* 2005;18(6):515-518.
52. Giordano BD, et al. Cervical spine imaging using standard C-arm fluoroscopy: patient and surgeon exposure to ionizing radiation. *Spine.* 2008;33(18):1970-1976.
53. Yukawa Y, et al. Cervical pedicle screw fixation in 100 cases of unstable cervical injuries: pedicle axis views obtained using fluoroscopy. *J Neurosurg Spine.* 2006;5(6):488-493.
54. Roche S, et al. Posterior cervical screw placement without image guidance: a safe and reliable practice. *J Spinal Disord Tech.* 2006;19(6):383-388.
55. Dickerman RD, et al. Lateral mass screws: anatomy is the key, not image guidance! *J Spinal Disord Tech.* 2007;20(1):109.
56. Ondra SL, et al. Safety and efficacy of C2 pedicle screws placed with anatomic and lateral C-arm guidance. *Spine.* 2006;31(9):E263-E267.
57. Cha SH, et al. C-arm assessment of cervical pedicle screw: screw coaxial fluoroscopy and oblique view. *Spine.* 2007; 32(16):1721-1727.
58. Kotil K, Bilge T. Accuracy of pedicle and mass screw placement in the spine without using fluoroscopy: a prospective clinical study. *Spine J.* 2008;8(4):591-596.
59. Kouyoumdjian P, et al. Centering of cervical disc replacements: usefulness of intraoperative anteroposterior fluoroscopic guidance to center cervical disc replacements: study on 20 discocerv (scient'x prosthesis). *Spine.* 2009;34(15): 1572-1577.
60. Mao GP, et al. Design of cervical pedicle locator and three-dimensional location of cervical pedicle. *Spine.* 2005;30(9):1045-1050.
61. Hott JS, et al. Intraoperative Iso-C C-arm navigation in craniospinal surgery: the first 60 cases. *Neurosurgery.* 2004;54(5):1131-1136.
62. Deinsberger R, Regatschnig R, Ungersbock K. Intraoperative evaluation of implants in anterior cervical spine surgery by three-dimensional fluoroscopy. *J Spinal Disord Tech.* 2005; 18(3):216-218.
63. Abumi K, Kaneda K. Pedicle screw fixation for nontraumatic lesions of the cervical spine. *Spine.* 1997;22(16):1853-1863.
64. Ludwig SC, et al. Cervical pedicle screws: comparative accuracy of two insertion techniques. *Spine.* 2000;25(20):2675-2681.
65. Schlenzka D, Laine T, Lund T. Computer-assisted spine surgery. *Eur Spine J.* 2000;9(suppl 1):S57-S64.
66. Lang Z, et al. Minimally invasive pedicle screw fixation using intraoperative three-dimensional fluoroscopy-based navigation (CAMISS Technique) For hangman's fracture. *Spine.* 2016;41(1):39-95.
67. Ma X, et al. The application of atlantoaxial screw and rod fixation in revision operations for postoperative re-dislocation in children. *Arch Orthop Trauma Surg.* 2015;135(3):313-319.
68. Takahashi J, et al. Computer-assisted screw insertion for cervical disorders in rheumatoid arthritis. *Eur Spine J.* 2007;16(4):485-494.

SECTION IX

69. Guppy KH, Chakrabarti I, Banerjee A. The use of intraoperative navigation for complex upper cervical spine surgery. *Neurosurg Focus*. 2014;36(3):E5.
70. Luther N, et al. Comparison of navigated versus non-navigated pedicle screw placement in 260 patients and 1434 screws: screw accuracy, screw size, and the complexity of surgery. *J Spinal Disord Tech*. 2015;28(5):E298-E303.
71. Rath SA, et al. Accuracy of pedicle screw insertion in the cervical spine for internal fixation using frameless stereotactic guidance. *J Neurosurg Spine*. 2008;8(3):237-245.
72. Arand M, et al. Spinal navigation in cervical fractures—a preliminary clinical study on Judet-osteosynthesis of the axis. *Comput Aided Surg*. 2001;6(3):170-175.
73. Aebi M, Thalgott JS, Webb JK. *AO ASIF Principles in Spine Surgery*. Berlin: Springer; 1998:243.
74. Benzel E. *Biomechanics of Spine Stabilization. Principles and Clinical Practice*. 1st ed. New York: McGraw-Hill; 1995:278.
75. White AA 3rd, Panjabi M. *Clinical Biomechanics of the Spine*. Philadelphia: Lippincott; 1990.
76. Shikinami Y, Okuno M. Mechanical evaluation of novel spinal interbody fusion cages made of bioactive, resorbable composites. *Biomaterials*. 2003;24(18):3161-3170.
77. Benzel EC. Biomechanics of cervical spine surgery for tumor and degenerative diseases. *Neurol Med Chir (Tokyo)*. 1997;37(8):583-593.
78. Bagby GW. Compression bone-plating: historical considerations. *J Bone Joint Surg Am*. 1977;59(5):625-631.
79. Evans CH. John Hunter and the origins of modern orthopaedic research. *J Orthop Res*. 2007;25(4):556-560.
80. Roguski M, et al. Postoperative cervical sagittal imbalance negatively affects outcomes after surgery for cervical spondylotic myelopathy. *Spine*. 2014;39(25):2070-2077.
81. White AA 3rd, et al. Biomechanical analysis of clinical stability in the cervical spine. *Clin Orthop*. 1975;109: 85-96.
82. Shedid D, Benzel EC. Cervical spondylosis anatomy: pathophysiology and biomechanics. *Neurosurgery*. 2007;60(1 Suppl 1):S7-S13.
83. Aghayev K, et al. Biomechanical comparison of a two-level anterior discectomy and a one-level corpectomy, combined with fusion and anterior plate reconstruction in the cervical spine. *Clin Biomech (Bristol, Avon)*. 2014;29(1):21-25.
84. Grubb MR, et al. Biomechanical evaluation of posterior cervical stabilization after a wide laminectomy. *Spine*. 1997; 22(17):1948-1954.
85. McCall T, Fassett D, Brockmeyer D. Cervical spine trauma in children: a review. *Neurosurg Focus*. 2006;20(2):E5.
86. Natarajan R, et al. Anterior cervical fusion: a finite element model study on motion segment stability including the effect of osteoporosis. *Spine*. 2000;25(8):955-961.
87. Hilibrand AS, et al. Impact of smoking on the outcome of anterior cervical arthrodesis with interbody or strut-grafting. *J Bone Joint Surg Am*. 2001;83-A(5):668-673.
88. Andersson S, Rodrigues M, Olerud C. Odontoid fractures: high complication rate associated with anterior screw fixation in the elderly. *Eur Spine J*. 2000;9(1):56-59.
89. Ryken TC, et al. Biomechanical analysis of bone mineral density, insertion technique, screw torque, and holding strength of anterior cervical plate screws. *J Neurosurg*. 1995; 83(2):325-329.
90. Pitzen TR, et al. Initial stability of cervical spine fixation: predictive value of a finite element model. Technical note. *J Neurosurg*. 2002;97(1 suppl):128-134.
91. Pitzen T, et al. Screw fixation to the posterior cortical shell does not influence peak torque and pullout in anterior cervical plating. *Eur Spine J*. 2002;11(5):494-499.
92. Maiman DJ, et al. Pull-out strength of Caspar cervical screws. *Neurosurgery*. 1992;31(6):1097-1101.
93. Spivak JM, Chen D, Kummer FJ. The effect of locking fixation screws on the stability of anterior cervical plating. *Spine*. 1999;24(4):334-338.
94. Gallagher MR, et al. Biomechanical evaluation of Caspar cervical screws: comparative stability under cyclical loading. *Neurosurgery*. 1993;33(6):1045-1050.
95. Chen IH. Biomechanical evaluation of subcortical versus bicortical screw purchase in anterior cervical plating. *Acta Neurochir (Wien)*. 1996;138(2):167-173.
96. Chen IH, Yang RS, Chen PQ. Plate fixation for anterior cervical interbody fusion. *J Formos Med Assoc*. 1991;90(2):172-175.
97. Muffoletto AJ, et al. Cervical stability with lateral mass plating: unicortical versus bicortical screw purchase. *Spine*. 2003;28(8):778-781.
98. Papagelopoulos PJ, et al. Biomechanical evaluation of posterior screw fixation in cadaveric cervical spines. *Clin Orthop Relat Res*. 2003;411:13-24.
99. Mattei TA, et al. Surgical challenges in the management of cervical kyphotic deformity in patients with severe osteoporosis: an illustrative case of a patient with Hajdu-Cheney syndrome. *Eur Spine J*. 2015;24(12):2746-2753.
100. Pitzen T, et al. Insertion torque and pullout force of rescue screws for anterior cervical plate fixation in a fatigued initial pilot hole. *J Neurosurg Spine*. 2004;1(2):198-201.
101. Hitchon PW, et al. Factors affecting the pullout strength of self-drilling and self-tapping anterior cervical screws. *Spine*. 2003;28(1):9-13.
102. Panjabi M. The stabilizing system of the spine: II. Neutral zone and instability hypothesis. *J Spinal Disord*. 1992;5: 390-396.
103. Patwardhan A, et al. Load-carrying capacity of the human cervical spine in compression is increased under a follower load. *Spine*. 2000;25:1548-1554.
104. Lang Z, et al. Minimally invasive pedicle screw fixation using intraoperative 3-dimensional fluoroscopy-based navigation (CAMISS Technique) for hangman fracture. *Spine*. 2016;41(1):39-45.
105. Sakaura H, et al. Preservation of the nuchal ligament plays an important role in preventing unfavorable radiologic changes after laminoplasty. *J Spinal Disord Tech*. 2008;21(5):338-343.
106. Sasai K, et al. Cervical curvature after laminoplasty for spondylotic myelopathy: involvement of tallow ligament, semispinalis cervicis muscle, and nuchal ligament. *J Spinal Disord*. 2000;13:26-30.
107. Danis MR. The operative treatment of fractures. 1947. *Clin Orthop Relat Res*. 1993;292:10-12.
108. Abumi K, et al. Posterior occipitocervical reconstruction using cervical pedicle screws and plate-rod systems. *Spine*. 1999;24(14):1425-1434.
109. Pal G, Sherk H. The vertical stability of the cervical spine. *Spine*. 1988;13:447-449.
110. Wang JL, Panjabi MM, Isomi T. The role of bone graft force in stabilizing the multilevel anterior cervical spine plate system. *Spine*. 2000;25(13):1649-1654.
111. Olsewski JM, Garvey TA, Schendel MJ. Biomechanical analysis of facet and graft loading in a Smith-Robinson type cervical spine model. *Spine*. 1994;19(22):2540-2544.

112. Truumees E, et al. Effects of disc height and distractive forces on graft compression in an anterior cervical discectomy model. *Spine*. 2002;27(22):2441-2445.
113. Aebi M, Zuber K, Marchesi D. Treatment of cervical spine injuries with anterior plating. Indications, techniques, and results. *Spine*. 1991;16(3 suppl):S38-S45.
114. Truumees E, et al. Failure of human cervical endplates: a cadaveric experimental model. *Spine*. 2003;28(19):2204-2208.
115. Lim TH, et al. Effect of endplate conditions and bone mineral density on the compressive strength of the graft-endplate interface in anterior cervical spine fusion. *Spine*. 2001;26(8): 951-956.
116. Conrad BP, et al. Biomechanical evaluation of the pullout strength of cervical screws. *J Spinal Disord Tech*. 2005;18(6): 506-510.
117. Johnston TL, et al. Cervical pedicle screws vs. lateral mass screws: uniplanar fatigue analysis and residual pullout strengths. *Spine J*. 2006;6(6):667-672.
118. Omeis I, et al. History of instrumentation for stabilization of the subaxial cervical spine. *Neurosurg Focus*. 2004;16(1):E10.
119. Johnston FG, Crockard HA. One-stage internal fixation and anterior fusion in complex cervical spinal disorders. *J Neurosurg*. 1995;82(2):234-238.
120. Apfelbaum RI, et al. Direct anterior screw fixation for recent and remote odontoid fractures. *J Neurosurg*. 2000;93(2 suppl):227-236.
121. Bohler J. Anterior stabilization for acute fractures and non-unions of the dens. *J Bone Joint Surg Am*. 1982;64(1): 18-27.
122. Song KJ, Lee KB, Kim KN. Treatment of odontoid fractures with single anterior screw fixation. *J Clin Neurosci*. 2007;14(9): 824-830.
123. Borm W, et al. Anterior screw fixation in type II odontoid fractures: is there a difference in outcome between age groups? *Neurosurgery*. 2003;52(5):1089-1092.
124. Kriskovich MD, Apfelbaum RI, Haller JR. Vocal fold paralysis after anterior cervical spine surgery: incidence, mechanism, and prevention of injury. *Laryngoscope*. 2000;110(9):1467-1473.
125. Joaquim AF, Patel AA. Surgical treatment of Type II odontoid fractures: anterior odontoid screw fixation or posterior cervical instrumented fusion? *Neurosurg Focus*. 2015;38(4):E11.
126. Platzer P, et al. Anterior screw fixation of odontoid fractures comparing younger and elderly patients. *Spine*. 2007;32(16):1714-1720.
127. Sucu HK, et al. Percutaneous anterior odontoid screw fixation. *Minim Invasive Neurosurg*. 2008;51(2):106-108.
128. Reindl R, Sen M, Aebi M. Anterior instrumentation for traumatic C1-C2 instability. *Spine*. 2003;28(17):E329-E333.
129. Mendes GA, et al. Endoscopic endonasal atlantoaxial transarticular screw fixation technique: an anatomical feasibility and biomechanical study. *J Neurosurg Spine*. 2015;22(5):470-477.
130. Zeidman SM, Ducker TB, Raycroft J. Trends and complications in cervical spine surgery: 1989-1993. *J Spinal Disord*. 1997;10(6):523-526.
131. Tippets RH, Apfelbaum RI. Anterior cervical fusion with the Caspar instrumentation system. *Neurosurgery*. 1988; 22(6 Pt 1):1008-1013.
132. Bose B. Anterior cervical instrumentation enhances fusion rates in multilevel reconstruction in smokers. *J Spinal Disord*. 2001;14(1):3-9.
133. Vaccaro AR, Balderston RA. Anterior plate instrumentation for disorders of the subaxial cervical spine. *Clin Orthop Relat Res*. 1997;335:112-121.
134. Wang JC, et al. The effect of cervical plating on single-level anterior cervical discectomy and fusion. *J Spinal Disord*. 1999;12(6):467-471.
135. Wang JC, et al. Increased fusion rates with cervical plating for two-level anterior cervical discectomy and fusion. *Spine*. 2000;25(1):41-45.
136. Wang JC, et al. Increased fusion rates with cervical plating for three-level anterior cervical discectomy and fusion. *Spine*. 2001;26(6):643-646.
137. An HS. Internal fixation of the cervical spine: current indications and techniques. *J Am Acad Orthop Surg*. 1995; 3(4):194-206.
138. Bohlman HH, Anderson PA. Anterior decompression and arthrodesis of the cervical spine: long-term motor improvement. Part 1: improvement in incomplete traumatic quadriparesis. *J Bone Joint Surg Am*. 1992;74(5):671-682.
139. Wright IP, Eisenstein SM. Anterior cervical discectomy and fusion without instrumentation. *Spine*. 2007;32(7):772-774.
140. Connolly PJ, Esses SI, Kostuik JP. Anterior cervical fusion: outcome analysis of patients fused with and without anterior cervical plates. *J Spinal Disord*. 1996;9(3):202-206.
141. Shapiro S. Banked fibula and the locking anterior cervical plate in anterior cervical fusions following cervical discectomy. *J Neurosurg*. 1996;84(2):161-165.
142. Steinmetz MP, et al. Preliminary experience with the DOC dynamic cervical implant for the treatment of multilevel cervical spondylosis. *J Neurosurg*. 2002;97(3 suppl):330-336.
143. Stromberg L, Dalen N. Atrophy of cortical bone caused by rigid internal fixation plates. *Acta Orthop Scand*. 1978;49: 448-456.
144. Hanci M. Pharyngo-cutaneous fistula following anterior cervical fusion. *Br J Neurosurg*. 2000;14(1):68.
145. Smith M, Bolesta M. Esophageal perforation after anterior cervical plate fixation. A report of two cases. *J Spinal Disord*. 1992;5:357-362.
146. Tortolani PJ, et al. A comparison of retraction pressure during anterior cervical plate surgery and cervical disc replacement: a cadaveric study. *J Spinal Disord Tech*. 2006;19(5):312-317.
147. Fassett DR, et al. Biomechanical analysis of a new concept: an add-on dynamic extension plate for adjacent-level anterior cervical fusion. *Spine*. 2005;30(22):2523-2529.
148. Scholz M, et al. A new stand-alone cervical anterior interbody fusion device: biomechanical comparison with established anterior cervical fixation devices. *Spine*. 2009;34(2):156-160.
149. Singh K, et al. Biomechanical comparison of cervical spine reconstructive techniques after a multilevel corpectomy of the cervical spine. *Spine*. 2003;28(20):2352-2358.
150. Panjabi MM, Isomi T, Wang JL. Loosening at the screw-vertebra junction in multilevel anterior cervical plate constructs. *Spine*. 1999;24(22):2383-2388.
151. Dahdaleh NS, et al. Biomechanical rigidity of cadaveric cervical spine with posterior versus combined posterior and anterior instrumentation. *J Neurosurg Spine*. 2009;10(2): 133-138.
152. Mourning D, et al. Initial intervertebral stability after anterior cervical discectomy and fusion with plating. *Spine J*. 2007;7(6):643-646.
153. DiAngelo DJ, et al. Anterior cervical plating reverses load transfer through multilevel strut-grafts. *Spine*. 2000;25(7): 783-795.

154. Yang S, Wang LW. Biomechanical comparison of the stable efficacy of two anterior plating systems. *Clin Biomech (Bristol, Avon)*. 2003;18(6):S59-S66.
155. Lehmann W, et al. Biomechanical analysis of anterior cervical spine plate fixation systems with unicortical and bicortical screw purchase. *Eur Spine J*. 2004;13(1):69-75.
156. Steinmetz MP, Benzel EC, Apfelbaum RI. Axially dynamic implants for stabilization of the cervical spine. *Neurosurgery*. 2006;59(4 suppl 2):ONS378-ONS388.
157. Lehmann W, et al. Biomechanical comparison of anterior cervical spine locked and unlocked plate-fixation systems. *Eur Spine J*. 2005;14(3):243-249.
158. DiPaola CP, et al. Screw pull-out force is dependent on screw orientation in an anterior cervical plate construct. *J Spinal Disord Tech*. 2007;20(5):369-373.
159. Rhee JM, Riew KD. Dynamic anterior cervical plates. *J Am Acad Orthop Surg*. 2007;15(11):640-646.
160. DuBois CM, et al. Static versus dynamic plating for multilevel anterior cervical discectomy and fusion. *Spine J*. 2007;7(2):188-193.
161. Campos RR, Botelho RV. Systematic review of the effect of dynamic fixation systems compared with rigid fixation in the anterior cervical spine. *Eur Spine J*. 2014;23(2): 298-304.
162. Nunley PD, et al. Choice of plate may affect outcomes for single versus multilevel ACDF: results of a prospective randomized single-blind trial. *Spine J*. 2009;9(2): 121-127.
163. Dipaola CP, et al. Screw orientation and plate type (variable- vs. fixed-angle) effect strength of fixation for in vitro biomechanical testing of the Synthes CSLP. *Spine J*. 2008;8(5):717-722.
164. Paramore CG, Dickman CA, Sonntag VK. Radiographic and clinical follow-up review of Caspar plates in 49 patients. *J Neurosurg*. 1996;84(6):957-961.
165. Brodke DS, et al. Dynamic cervical plates: biomechanical evaluation of load sharing and stiffness. *Spine*. 2001;26(12): 1324-1329.
166. Foley KT, et al. The in vitro effects of instrumentation on multilevel cervical strut-graft mechanics. *Spine*. 1999;24(22): 2366-2376.
167. Truumees E, et al. Effects of a cervical compression plate on graft forces in an anterior cervical discectomy model. *Spine*. 2003;28(11):1097-1102.
168. Reidy D, et al. Cervical spine loading characteristics in a cadaveric C5 corpectomy model using a static and dynamic plate. *J Spinal Disord*. 2004;17(2):117-122.
169. Rapoff AJ, et al. Anterior cervical graft and plate load sharing. *J Spinal Disord*. 1999;12(1):45-49.
170. Clausen JD, et al. Biomechanical evaluation of Caspar and Cervical Spine Locking Plate systems in a cadaveric model. *J Neurosurg*. 1996;84(6):1039-1045.
171. Dvorak MF, et al. Anterior cervical plate fixation: a biomechanical study to evaluate the effects of plate design, endplate preparation, and bone mineral density. *Spine*. 2005;30(3):294-301.
172. Balabhadra R, Zhang H. Anterior cervical fusion using dense cancellous allografts and dynamic plating. *Neurosurgery*. 2004;1405-1412.
173. Saphier PS, et al. Stress-shielding compared with load-sharing anterior cervical plate fixation: a clinical and radiographic prospective analysis of 50 patients. *J Neurosurg Spine*. 2007; 6(5):391-397.
174. Goldberg G, et al. Short-term comparison of cervical fusion with static and dynamic plating using computerized motion analysis. *Spine*. 2007;32(13):E371-E375.
175. Vaccaro AR, et al. Use of a bioabsorbable anterior cervical plate in the treatment of cervical degenerative and traumatic disk disruption. *Orthopedics*. 2002;25(10 suppl):s1191-s1199.
176. Thomas KA, et al. Bioresorbable polylactide interbody implants in an ovine anterior cervical discectomy and fusion model: three-year results. *Spine*. 2008;33(7):734-742.
177. Cahill DW, et al. Suitability of bioresorbable cages for anterior cervical fusion. *J Neurosurg*. 2003;98(2 suppl):195-201.
178. Brkaric M, et al. Early failure of bioabsorbable anterior cervical fusion plates: case report and failure analysis. *J Spinal Disord Tech*. 2007;20(3):248-254.
179. Dumont TM, et al. Pseudarthrosis failures of anterior subaxial cervical spine fusion using a plate with a single screw per vertebral body: a case series. *World Neurosurg*. 2014;82(1-2):225-230.
180. Wang JC, et al. A comparison of fusion rates between single-level cervical corpectomy and two-level discectomy and fusion. *J Spinal Disord*. 2001;14(3):222-225.
181. Griffith SL, et al. Biomechanical comparison of anterior instrumentation for the cervical spine. *J Spinal Disord*. 1995;8(6):429-438.
182. Schmidt R, et al. Pedicle screws enhance primary stability in multilevel cervical corpectomies: biomechanical in vitro comparison of different implants including constrained and nonconstrained posterior instumentations. *Spine*. 2003;28(16):1821-1828.
183. Dogan S, et al. Biomechanical consequences of cervical spondylectomy versus corpectomy. *Neurosurgery*. 2008;63(4 suppl 2):303-308.
184. Bolesta MJ, Rechtine GR 2nd, Chrin AM. Three- and four-level anterior cervical discectomy and fusion with plate fixation: a prospective study. *Spine*. 2000;25(16): 2040-2044.
185. Fessler RG, Steck JC, Giovanini MA. Anterior cervical corpectomy for cervical spondylotic myelopathy. *Neurosurgery*. 1998;43(2):257-265.
186. Mayr MT, et al. Cervical spinal stenosis: outcome after anterior corpectomy, allograft reconstruction, and instrumentation. *J Neurosurg*. 2002;96(1 suppl):10-16.
187. Swank ML, et al. Anterior cervical allograft arthrodesis and instrumentation: multilevel interbody grafting or strut graft reconstruction. *Eur Spine J*. 1997;6(2):138-143.
188. Singh K, et al. Enhancement of stability following anterior cervical corpectomy: a biomechanical study. *Spine*. 2004;29(8):845-849.
189. Koller H, et al. 4- and 5-level anterior fusions of the cervical spine: review of literature and clinical results. *Eur Spine J*. 2007;16(12):2055-2071.
190. Ashkenazi E, et al. Anterior decompression combined with corpectomies and discectomies in the management of multilevel cervical myelopathy: a hybrid decompression and fixation technique. *J Neurosurg Spine*. 2005;3(3): 205-209.
191. Fisher CG, et al. Comparison of outcomes for unstable lower cervical flexion teardrop fractures managed with halo thoracic vest versus anterior corpectomy and plating. *Spine*. 2002;27(2):160-166.
192. Harrington JF Jr, Park MC. Single level arthrodesis as treatment for midcervical fracture subluxation: a cohort study. *J Spinal Disord Tech*. 2007;20(1):42-48.

193. Paxinos O, et al. Anterior cervical discectomy and fusion with a locked plate and wedged graft effectively stabilizes flexion-distraction stage-3 injury in the lower cervical spine: a biomechanical study. *Spine*. 2009;34(1):E9-E15.
194. Duggal N, et al. Unilateral cervical facet dislocation: biomechanics of fixation. *Spine*. 2005;30(7):E164-E168.
195. Cloyd JM, Acosta FL Jr, Ames CP. Effect of age on the perioperative and radiographic complications of multilevel cervicothoracic spinal fusions. *Spine*. 2008;33(26):E977-E982.
196. Majercik S, et al. Halo vest immobilization in the elderly: a death sentence? *J Trauma*. 2005;59(2):350-356.
197. Ball PA, Benzel EC, Baldwin NG. A simple method to ensure proper screw position and plate size selection using the Morscher cervical spine locking plate. Technical note. *J Neurosurg*. 1994;80(4):748-749.
198. Nassr A, et al. Does incorrect level needle localization during anterior cervical discectomy and fusion lead to accelerated disc degeneration? *Spine*. 2009;34(2):189-192.
199. Yang JY, et al. Adjacent level ossification development after anterior cervical fusion without plate fixation. *Spine*. 2009;34(1):30-33.
200. Ipsen BJ, et al. Effect of plate position on clinical outcome after anterior cervical spine surgery. *Spine J*. 2007;7(6):637-642.
201. Jea A, Vanni S. Anterior correction of cervical spine lordosis using an adjustable depth tap: technical note. *J Spinal Disord Tech*. 2005;18(2):178-181.
202. Baldwin NG, et al. Failure of a titanium anterior cervical plate implant: microstructural analysis of failure. Case report. *J Neurosurg*. 1995;83(4):741-743.
203. Heidecke V, Rainov NG, Burkert W. Anterior cervical fusion with the Orion locking plate system. *Spine*. 1998;23(16):1796-1802.
204. Campbell MJ, et al. Use of cervical collar after single-level anterior cervical fusion with plate: is it necessary? *Spine*. 2009;34(1):43-48.
205. Zoega B, Karrholm J, Lind B. Mobility provocation radiostereometry in anterior cervical spine fusions. *Eur Spine J*. 2003;12(6):631-636.
206. Epstein NE. Reoperation rates for acute graft extrusion and pseudarthrosis after one-level anterior corpectomy and fusion with and without plate instrumentation: etiology and corrective management. *Surg Neurol*. 2001;56(2):73-80.
207. Bose B. Anterior cervical arthrodesis using DOC dynamic stabilization implant for improvement in sagittal angulation and controlled settling. *J Neurosurg*. 2003;98(1 suppl):8-13.
208. Zoega B, Karrholm J, Lind B. One-level cervical spine fusion. A randomized study, with or without plate fixation, using radiostereometry in 27 patients. *Acta Orthop Scand*. 1998;69(4):363-368.
209. Ugokwe KT, et al. A review of the utility of obtaining repeated postoperative radiographs following single-level anterior cervical decompression, fusion, and plate placement. *J Neurosurg Spine*. 2008;9(2):175-179.
210. Troyanovich SJ, et al. Does anterior plating maintain cervical lordosis versus conventional fusion techniques? A retrospective analysis of patients receiving single-level fusions. *J Spinal Disord Tech*. 2002;15(1):69-74.
211. Rajshekhar V, Arunkumar MJ, Kumar SS. Changes in cervical spine curvature after uninstrumented one- and two-level corpectomy in patients with spondylotic myelopathy. *Neurosurgery*. 2003;52(4):799-804.
212. Zoega B, Karrholm J, Lind B. Plate fixation adds stability to two-level anterior fusion in the cervical spine: a randomized study using radiostereometry. *Eur Spine J*. 1998;7(4):302-307.
213. Burkhardt JK, et al. The influence of cervical plate fixation with either autologous bone or cage insertion on radiographic and patient-rated outcomes after two-level anterior cervical discectomy and fusion. *Eur Spine J*. 2015;24(1):113-119.
214. Kasimatis GB, et al. Complications of anterior surgery in cervical spine trauma: an overview. *Clin Neurol Neurosurg*. 2009;111(1):18-27.
215. Shapiro SA, Snyder W. Spinal instrumentation with a low complication rate. *Surg Neurol*. 1997;48(6):566-574.
216. Graham JJ. Complications of cervical spine surgery. A five-year report on a survey of the membership of the Cervical Spine Research Society by the Morbidity and Mortality Committee. *Spine*. 1989;14(10):1046-1050.
217. Lambiris E, et al. Treatment of unstable lower cervical spine injuries by anterior instrumented fusion alone. *J Spinal Disord Tech*. 2008;21(7):500-507.
218. Hartmann S, et al. Biomechanical testing of circumferential instrumentation after cervical multilevel corpectomy. *Eur Spine J*. 2015;24(12):2788-2798.
219. Rao RD, et al. Does anterior plating of the cervical spine predispose to adjacent segment changes? *Spine*. 2005;30(24):2788-2792.
220. Witwer BP, Resnick DK. Delayed esophageal injury without instrumentation failure: complication of anterior cervical instrumentation. *J Spinal Disord Tech*. 2003;16(6):519-523.
221. Pompili A, et al. Asymptomatic esophageal perforation caused by late screw migration after anterior cervical plating: report of a case and review of relevant literature. *Spine*. 2002;27(23):E499-E502.
222. Yue WM, Brodner W, Highland TR. Persistent swallowing and voice problems after anterior cervical discectomy and fusion with allograft and plating: a 5- to 11-year follow-up study. *Eur Spine J*. 2005;14(7):677-682.
223. Lee MJ, et al. Risk factors for dysphagia after anterior cervical spine surgery: a two-year prospective cohort study. *Spine J*. 2007;7(2):141-147.
224. Chin KR, Eiszner JR, Adams SB Jr. Role of plate thickness as a cause of dysphagia after anterior cervical fusion. *Spine*. 2007;32(23):2585-2590.
225. Lee MJ, et al. Influence of anterior cervical plate design on dysphagia: a 2-year prospective longitudinal follow-up study. *J Spinal Disord Tech*. 2005;18(5):406-409.
226. Fogel GR, McDonnell MF. Surgical treatment of dysphagia after anterior cervical interbody fusion. *Spine J*. 2005;5(2):140-144.
227. Chen Y, et al. Subsidence of titanium mesh cage: a study based on 300 cases. *J Spinal Disord Tech*. 2008;21(7):489-492.
228. Wilke HJ, Kettler A, Claes L. Primary stabilizing effect of interbody fusion devices for the cervical spine: an in vitro comparison between three different cage types and bone cement. *Eur Spine J*. 2000;9(5):410-416.
229. Samandouras G, Shafafy M, Hamlyn PJ. A new anterior cervical instrumentation system combining an intradiscal cage with an integrated plate: an early technical report. *Spine*. 2001;26(10):1188-1192.
230. Riew KD, Rhee JM. The use of titanium mesh cages in the cervical spine. *Clin Orthop Relat Res*. 2002;394:47-54.
231. Vaccaro AR, Cirello J. The use of allograft bone and cages in fractures of the cervical, thoracic, and lumbar spine. *Clin Orthop Relat Res*. 2002;394:19-26.

232. Pelletier MH, et al. PEEK versus Ti interbody fusion devices: resultant fusion, bone apposition, initial and 26-week biomechanics. *Clin Spine Surg*. 2016;29(4):E208-E214.
233. Kandziora F, et al. Biomechanical comparison of cervical spine interbody fusion cages. *Spine*. 2001;26(17): 1850-1857.
234. Hart R, et al. Comparison of stiffness and failure load of two cervical spine fixation techniques in an in vitro human model. *J Spinal Disord Tech*. 2005;18(suppl):S115-S118.
235. Teo E, et al. Effects of cervical cages on load distribution of cancellous core: a finite element analysis. *J Spinal Disord Tech*. 2004;17(3):226-231.
236. Epari DR, Kandziora F, Duda GN. Stress shielding in box and cylinder cervical interbody fusion cage designs. *Spine*. 2005;30(8):908-914.
237. Greene DL, et al. Biomechanical comparison of cervical interbody cage versus structural bone graft. *Spine J*. 2003;3(4): 262-269.
238. Gercek E, et al. Subsidence of stand-alone cervical cages in anterior interbody fusion: warning. *Eur Spine J*. 2003;12(5): 513-516.
239. Shimamoto N, et al. Biomechanical evaluation of stand-alone interbody fusion cages in the cervical spine. *Spine*. 2001; 26(19):E432-E436.
240. Galbusera F, et al. Anterior cervical fusion: a biomechanical comparison of 4 techniques. Laboratory investigation. *J Neurosurg Spine*. 2008;9(5):444-449.
241. Zdeblick TA, Phillips FM. Interbody cage devices. *Spine*. 2003;28(15 suppl):S2-S7.
242. Eysel P, et al. [Initial instability of different cages for fusion of the cervical spine]. *Zentralbl Neurochir*. 2000;61(4):171-176.
243. Ordway NR, et al. Anterior cervical interbody constructs: effect of a repetitive compressive force on the endplate. *J Orthop Res*. 2012;30(4):587-592.
244. Truumees E, et al. Effects of disc height and distractive forces on graft compression in an anterior cervical corpectomy model. *Spine*. 2008;33(13):1438-1441.
245. Ji W, et al. A clivus plate fixation for reconstruction of ventral defect of the craniovertebral junction: a novel fixation device for craniovertebral instability. *Eur Spine J*. 2015;24(8):1658-1665.
246. Woiciechowsky C. Distractable vertebral cages for reconstruction after cervical corpectomy. *Spine*. 2005;30(15): 1736-1741.
247. Puttlitz CM, et al. A biomechanical analysis of C2 corpectomy constructs. *Spine J*. 2007;7(2):210-215.
248. Chou D, et al. Adjacent-level vertebral body fractures after expandable cage reconstruction. *J Neurosurg Spine*. 2008;8(6):584-588.
249. Keogh A, Hardcastle P, Ali SF. Anterior cervical fusion using the IntExt combined cage/plate. *J Orthop Surg (Hong Kong)*. 2008;16(1):3-8.
250. Scholz M, et al. A zero-profile anchored spacer in multilevel cervical anterior interbody fusion: biomechanical comparison to established fixation techniques. *Spine*. 2015;40(7):E375-E380.
251. Healy AT, et al. Zero-profile hybrid fusion construct versus 2-level plate fixation to treat adjacent-level disease in the cervical spine. *J Neurosurg Spine*. 2014;21(5):753-760.
252. Wang Z, et al. The application of zero-profile anchored spacer in anterior cervical discectomy and fusion. *Eur Spine J*. 2015;24(1):148-154.
253. Grasso G, et al. Anterior cervical discectomy and fusion with ROI-C peek cage: cervical alignment and patient outcomes. *Eur Spine J*. 2014;23(suppl 6):650-657.
254. Totoribe K, et al. Comparative biomechanical analysis of a cervical cage made of an unsintered hydroxyapatite particle and poly-L-lactide composite in a cadaver model. *Spine*. 2003;28(10):1010-1015.
255. Suess O, et al. Debridement and spinal instrumentation as a single-stage procedure in bacterial spondylitis/ spondylodiscitis. *Zentralbl Neurochir*. 2007;68(3):123-132.
256. Aryan HE, et al. Corpectomy followed by the placement of instrumentation with titanium cages and recombinant human bone morphogenetic protein-2 for vertebral osteomyelitis. *J Neurosurg Spine*. 2007;6(1):23-30.
257. Acosta FL Jr, et al. Long-term biomechanical stability and clinical improvement after extended multilevel corpectomy and circumferential reconstruction of the cervical spine using titanium mesh cages. *J Spinal Disord Tech*. 2008;21(3):165-174.
258. Lu DC, Wang V, Chou D. The use of allograft or autograft and expandable titanium cages for the treatment of vertebral osteomyelitis. *Neurosurgery*. 2009;64(1):122-129.
259. Bucciero A, Zorzi T, Piscopo GA. Peek cage-assisted anterior cervical discectomy and fusion at four levels: clinical and radiographic results. *J Neurosurg Sci*. 2008;52(2):37-40.
260. Kulkarni AG, Hee HT, Wong HK. Solis cage (PEEK) for anterior cervical fusion: preliminary radiological results with emphasis on fusion and subsidence. *Spine J*. 2007;7(2):205-209.
261. Barsa P, Suchomel P. Factors affecting sagittal malalignment due to cage subsidence in standalone cage assisted anterior cervical fusion. *Eur Spine J*. 2007;16(9):1395-1400.
262. van Jonbergen HP, et al. Anterior cervical interbody fusion with a titanium box cage: early radiological assessment of fusion and subsidence. *Spine J*. 2005;5(6):645-649.
263. Fujibayashi S, Neo M, Nakamura T. Stand-alone interbody cage versus anterior cervical plate for treatment of cervical disc herniation: sequential changes in cage subsidence. *J Clin Neurosci*. 2008;15(9):1017-1022.
264. Dai LY, Jiang LS. Anterior cervical fusion with interbody cage containing beta-tricalcium phosphate augmented with plate fixation: a prospective randomized study with 2-year follow-up. *Eur Spine J*. 2008;17(5):698-705.
265. Arnold P, Boswell S, McMahon J. Threaded interbody fusion cage for adjacent segment degenerative disease after previous anterior cervical fusion. *Surg Neurol*. 2008;70(4):390-397.
266. Hacker RJ. A randomized prospective study of an anterior cervical interbody fusion device with a minimum of 2 years of follow-up results. *J Neurosurg*. 2000;93(2 suppl):222-226.
267. Castro FP Jr, et al. A cost analysis of two anterior cervical fusion procedures. *J Spinal Disord*. 2000;13(6):511-514.
268. Schnee CL, et al. Analysis of harvest morbidity and radiographic outcome using autograft for anterior cervical fusion. *Spine*. 1997;22(19):2222-2227.
269. Brooke NS, et al. Preliminary experience of carbon fibre cage prostheses for treatment of cervical spine disorders. *Br J Neurosurg*. 1997;11(3):221-227.
270. Krayenbuhl N, et al. Use of an empty, Plasmapore-covered titanium cage for interbody fusion after anterior cervical microdiscectomy. *J Clin Neurosci*. 2008;15(1):11-17.
271. Frederic S, Benedict R, Payer M. Implantation of an empty carbon fiber cage or a tricortical iliac crest autograft after cervical discectomy for single-level disc herniation: a

prospective comparative study. *J Neurosurg Spine*. 2006;4(4): 292-299.

272. Payer M, et al. Implantation of an empty carbon fiber composite frame cage after single-level anterior cervical discectomy in the treatment of cervical disc herniation: preliminary results. *J Neurosurg*. 2003;98(2 suppl):143-148.
273. Ryu SI, Mitchell M, Kim DH. A prospective randomized study comparing a cervical carbon fiber cage to the Smith-Robinson technique with allograft and plating: up to 24 months follow-up. *Eur Spine J*. 2006;15(2):157-164.
274. Samartzis D, et al. Is autograft the gold standard in achieving radiographic fusion in one-level anterior cervical discectomy and fusion with rigid anterior plate fixation? *Spine*. 2005;30(15):1756-1761.
275. Ryu SI, et al. Comparison of the biomechanical stability of dense cancellous allograft with tricortical iliac autograft and fibular allograft for cervical interbody fusion. *Eur Spine J*. 2006;15(9):1339-1345.
276. Zdeblick TA, et al. Cervical interbody fusion cages. An animal model with and without bone morphogenetic protein. *Spine*. 1998;23(7):758-765.
277. Shields LB, et al. Adverse effects associated with high-dose recombinant human bone morphogenetic protein-2 use in anterior cervical spine fusion. *Spine*. 2006;31(5):542-547.
278. Vaidya R, et al. Complications in the use of rhBMP-2 in PEEK cages for interbody spinal fusions. *J Spinal Disord Tech*. 2008;21(8):557-562.
279. Tumialan LM, et al. The safety and efficacy of anterior cervical discectomy and fusion with polyetheretherketone spacer and recombinant human bone morphogenetic protein-2: a review of 200 patients. *J Neurosurg Spine*. 2008;8(6):529-535.
280. Meding JB, Stambough JL. Critical analysis of strut grafts in anterior spinal fusions. *J Spinal Disord*. 1993;6(2):166-174.
281. McKoy BE, et al. Fibular allograft after anterior cervical corpectomy: long term follow-up. *Iowa Orthop J*. 2002;22: 42-46.
282. Cosar M, et al. The results of beta-tricalcium phosphate coated hydroxyapatite (beta-TCP/HA) grafts for interbody fusion after anterior cervical discectomy. *J Spinal Disord Tech*. 2008;21(6):436-441.
283. Ramzi N, et al. Long term outcome of anterior cervical discectomy and fusion using coral grafts. *Acta Neurochir (Wien)*. 2008;150(12):1249-1256.
284. McConnell JR, et al. A prospective randomized comparison of coralline hydroxyapatite with autograft in cervical interbody fusion. *Spine*. 2003;28(4):317-323.
285. Fernandez-Fairen M, et al. Anterior cervical fusion with tantalum implant: a prospective randomized controlled study. *Spine*. 2008;33(5):465-472.
286. Agrillo U, Mastronardi L, Puzzilli F. Anterior cervical fusion with carbon fiber cage containing coralline hydroxyapatite: preliminary observations in 45 consecutive cases of soft-disc herniation. *J Neurosurg*. 2002;96(3 suppl):273-276.
287. Truumees E, et al. Compression load of human cervical vertebral endplates: a cadaveric experimental model. *Spine*. 2003;28(19):2204-2208.
288. Hwang SH, et al. Biomechanical comparison of adjacent segmental motion after ventral cervical fixation with varying angles of lordosis. *Spine J*. 2007;7(2):216-221.
289. Matge G. Anterior interbody fusion with the BAK-cage in cervical spondylosis. *Acta Neurochir (Wien)*. 1998;140(1):1-8.
290. Matge G, Leclercq TA. Rationale for interbody fusion with threaded titanium cages at cervical and lumbar levels. Results on 357 cases. *Acta Neurochir (Wien)*. 2000;142(4):425-433.
291. Hacker RJ, et al. A prospective randomized multicenter clinical evaluation of an anterior cervical fusion cage. *Spine*. 2000;25(20):2646-2654.
292. Caroli E, et al. Anterior cervical fusion with interbody titanium cage containing surgical bone site graft: our institution's experience in 103 consecutive cases of degenerative spondylosis. *J Spinal Disord Tech*. 2007;20(3):216-220.
293. Thome C, Krauss JK, Zevgaridis D. A prospective clinical comparison of rectangular titanium cages and iliac crest autografts in anterior cervical discectomy and fusion. *Neurosurg Rev*. 2004;27(1):34-41.
294. Hwang SL, et al. Anterior corpectomy with iliac bone fusion or discectomy with interbody titanium cage fusion for multilevel cervical degenerated disc disease. *J Spinal Disord Tech*. 2007;20(8):565-570.
295. Siddiqui AA, Jackowski A. Cage versus tricortical graft for cervical interbody fusion. A prospective randomised study. *J Bone Joint Surg Br*. 2003;85(7):1019-1025.
296. Majd ME, Vadhva M, Holt RT. Anterior cervical reconstruction using titanium cages with anterior plating. *Spine*. 1999;24(15):1604-1610.
297. Thalgott JS, Xiongsheng C, Giuffre JM. Single stage anterior cervical reconstruction with titanium mesh cages, local bone graft, and anterior plating. *Spine J*. 2003;3(4):294-300.
298. Vavruch L, et al. A prospective randomized comparison between the Cloward procedure and a carbon fiber cage in the cervical spine: a clinical and radiologic study. *Spine*. 2002;27(16):1694-1701.
299. Thome C, et al. A prospective randomized comparison of rectangular titanium cage fusion and iliac crest autograft fusion in patients undergoing anterior cervical discectomy. *J Neurosurg Spine*. 2006;4(1):1-9.
300. Peolsson A, Vavruch L, Hedlund R. Long-term randomised comparison between a carbon fibre cage and the Cloward procedure in the cervical spine. *Eur Spine J*. 2007;16(2): 173-178.
301. Kasliwal MK, O'Toole JE. Clinical experience using polyetheretherketone (PEEK) intervertebral structural cage for anterior cervical corpectomy and fusion. *J Clin Neurosci*. 2014;21(2):217-220.
302. Daubs MD. Early failures following cervical corpectomy reconstruction with titanium mesh cages and anterior plating. *Spine*. 2005;30(12):1402-1406.
303. Celik SE, Kara A, Celik S. A comparison of changes over time in cervical foraminal height after tricortical iliac graft or polyetheretherketone cage placement following anterior discectomy. *J Neurosurg Spine*. 2007;6(1):10-16.
304. Hee HT, et al. Complications of multilevel cervical corpectomies and reconstruction with titanium cages and anterior plating. *J Spinal Disord Tech*. 2003;16(1):1-8.
305. Guyer RD, Ohnmeiss DD. Intervertebral disc prostheses. *Spine*. 2003;28(15):S15-S23.
306. Baaj AA, et al. History of cervical disc arthroplasty. *Neurosurg Focus*. 2009;27(3):E10.
307. Puttlitz CM, DiAngelo DJ. Cervical spine arthroplasty biomechanics. *Neurosurg Clin N Am*. 2005;16(4):589-594, v.
308. Hallab N, Link HD, McAfee PC. Biomaterial optimization in total disc arthroplasty. *Spine*. 2003;28(20):S139-S152.

309. Sekhon LH, et al. Magnetic resonance imaging clarity of the Bryan, Prodisc-C, Prestige LP, and PCM cervical arthroplasty devices. *Spine*. 2007;32(6):673-680.
310. Anderson P, et al. Wear analysis of the Bryan Cervical Disc prosthesis. *Spine*. 2003;28(20):S186-S194.
311. Cavanaugh DA, et al. Delayed hyper-reactivity to metal ions after cervical disc arthroplasty: a case report and literature review. *Spine*. 2009;34(7):E262-E265.
312. Gornet MF, et al. Serum metal concentrations in subjects with titanium ceramic composite cervical disc replacements. *Spine*. 2017;42(6):366-371.
313. Beaurain J, et al. Intermediate clinical and radiological results of cervical TDR (Mobi-C) with up to 2 years of follow-up. *Eur Spine J*. 2009;18(6):841-850.
314. Datta JC, et al. Sagittal split fractures in multilevel cervical arthroplasty using a keeled prosthesis. *J Spinal Disord Tech*. 2007;20(1):89-92.
315. Lin CY, et al. Stress analysis of the interface between cervical vertebrae end plates and the Bryan, Prestige LP, and ProDisc-C cervical disc prostheses: an in vivo image-based finite element study. *Spine*. 2009;34(15):1554-1560.
316. Rousseau MA, Bonnet X, Skalli W. Influence of the geometry of a ball-and-socket intervertebral prosthesis at the cervical spine: a finite element study. *Spine*. 2008;33(1):E10-E14.
317. Denaro V, et al. Cervical spinal disc replacement. *J Bone Joint Surg Br*. 2009;91(6):713-719.
318. Sasso RC, Best NM. Cervical kinematics after fusion and Bryan disc arthroplasty. *J Spinal Disord Tech*. 2008;21(1):19-22.
319. Anderson PA, Subach BR, Riew KD. Predictors of outcome after anterior cervical discectomy and fusion: a multivariate analysis. *Spine*. 2009;34(2):161-166.
320. Kan SL, et al. Cervical disc arthroplasty for symptomatic cervical disc disease: traditional and Bayesian meta-analysis with trial sequential analysis. *Int J Surg*. 2016;35:111-119.
321. Davis RJ, et al. Two-level total disc replacement with Mobi-C cervical artificial disc versus anterior discectomy and fusion: a prospective, randomized, controlled multicenter clinical trial with 4-year follow-up results. *J Neurosurg Spine*. 2015;22(1):15-25.
322. Dejaegher J, et al. 10-year follow-up after implantation of the Bryan Cervical Disc Prosthesis. *Eur Spine J*. 2017;26(4):1191-1198.
323. Sasso WR, et al. Long-term clinical outcomes of cervical disc arthroplasty: a prospective, randomized, controlled trial. *Spine*. 2016. Epub ahead of print.
324. Chang KE, Pham MH, Hsieh PC. Adjacent segment disease requiring reoperation in cervical total disc arthroplasty: A literature review and update. *J Clin Neurosci*. 2017;37:20-24.
325. Zhu Y, et al. Cervical disc arthroplasty versus anterior cervical discectomy and fusion for incidence of symptomatic adjacent segment disease: a meta-analysis of prospective randomized controlled trials. *Spine*. 2016;41(19):1493-1502.
326. Deutsch H, et al. Occipitocervical fixation: long-term results. *Spine*. 2005;30(5):530-535.
327. Brattstrom H, Granholm L. Atlanto-axial fusion in rheumatoid arthritis. A new method of fixation with wire and bone cement. *Acta Orthop Scand*. 1976;47(6):619-628.
328. Wertheim SB, Bohlman HH. Occipitocervical fusion. Indications, technique, and long-term results in thirteen patients. *J Bone Joint Surg Am*. 1987;69(6):833-836.
329. McAfee PC, et al. Fusion of the occiput to the upper cervical spine. A review of 37 cases. *Spine*. 1991;16(10 suppl): S490-S494.
330. Grob D, et al. The role of plate and screw fixation in occipitocervical fusion in rheumatoid arthritis. *Spine*. 1994;19(22):2545-2551.
331. Higo M, et al. Occipitocervical fusion by Luque loop rod instrumentation in Down syndrome. *J Pediatr Orthop*. 1995;15(4):539-542.
332. Sonntag V, Dickman C. Craniocervical Stabilization. *Clin Neurosurg*. 1993;40:243.
333. Rodgers WB, et al. Occipitocervical fusions in children. Retrospective analysis and technical considerations. *Clin Orthop Relat Res*. 1999;364:125-133.
334. Fehlings MG, et al. Occipitocervical fusion with a five-millimeter malleable rod and segmental fixation. *Neurosurgery*. 1993;32(2):198-207.
335. Thompson GH, et al. Atlantoaxial rotatory subluxation, congenital absence of the posterior arch of the atlas, and cerebral palsy: an unusual triad. *J Pediatr Orthop*. 1985;5(2):232-235.
336. Singh SK, et al. Occipitocervical reconstruction with the Ohio Medical Instruments Loop: results of a multicenter evaluation in 30 cases. *J Neurosurg*. 2003;98(3 suppl):239-246.
337. Apostolides PJ, et al. Threaded Steinmann pin fusion of the craniovertebral junction. *Spine*. 1996;21(14):1630-1637.
338. Naderi S, Pamir MN. Further cranial settling of the upper cervical spine following odontoidectomy. Report of two cases. *J Neurosurg*. 2001;95(2 suppl):246-249.
339. Vale FL, Oliver M, Cahill DW. Rigid occipitocervical fusion. *J Neurosurg*. 1999;91(2 suppl):144-150.
340. Oda I, et al. Biomechanical evaluation of five different occipito-atlanto-axial fixation techniques. *Spine*. 1999;24(22): 2377-2382.
341. Sutterlin CE 3rd, et al. Biomechanical evaluation of occipitocervical fixation devices. *J Spinal Disord*. 2001;14(3): 185-192.
342. Hurlbert R, et al. A biomechanical evaluation of occipitocervical instrumentation: screw compared with wire fixation. *J Neurosurg*. 1999;90(1 suppl):84-90.
343. Smith MD, Biel M, Falconer D. Anterior occipital cervical reconstruction with a free vascularized osteocutaneous graft: a case report. *J Spinal Disord*. 1993;6(5):371-379.
344. Dai LY, et al. Surgical treatment of nonunited fractures of the odontoid process, with special reference to occipitocervical fusion for unreducible atlantoaxial subluxation or instability. *Eur Spine J*. 2000;9(2):118-122.
345. Jain VK, et al. Posterior occipitoaxial fusion for atlantoaxial dislocation associated with occipitalized atlas. *J Neurosurg*. 1996;84(4):559-564.
346. Stabler CL, et al. Failure of posterior cervical fusions using cadaveric bone graft in children. *J Bone Joint Surg Am*. 1985;67(3):371-375.
347. Stone JG, et al. Evaluation of occipitocervical arthrodesis rates with screw-based fixation and osteoinductive fusion adjuncts. *J Neurol Surg A Cent Eur Neurosurg*. 2015;76(5):361-368.
348. Shahlaie K, Kim KD. Occipitocervical fusion using recombinant human bone morphogenetic protein-2: adverse effects due to tissue swelling and seroma. *Spine*. 2008;33(21):2361-2366.
349. Phillips FM, et al. Occipitocervical neutral position. Possible surgical implications. *Spine*. 1999;24(8):775-778.
350. Nagashima S, et al. A new method of measuring the occipitocervical angle that could be applied as an intraoperative indicator during occipitocervical fusion. *Clin Spine Surg*. 2016. Epub ahead of print.

351. Shoda N, et al. Measurement of occipitocervical angle. *Spine*. 2004;29(10):E204-E208.
352. Matsunaga S, Onishi T, Sakou T. Significance of occipitoaxial angle in subaxial lesion after occipitocervical fusion. *Spine*. 2001;26(2):161-165.
353. Pait TG, et al. Inside-outside technique for posterior occipitocervical spine instrumentation and stabilization: preliminary results. *J Neurosurg*. 1999;90(1 suppl):1-7.
354. Faure A, et al. Inverted-hook occipital clamp system in occipitocervical fixation. Technical note. *J Neurosurg*. 2002;97(1 suppl):135-141.
355. Paquis P, et al. Occipitocervical fixation using hooks and screws for upper cervical instability. *Neurosurgery*. 1999;44(2):324-330.
356. Smith MD, Anderson P, Grady MS. Occipitocervical arthrodesis using contoured plate fixation. An early report on a versatile fixation technique. *Spine*. 1993;18(14):1984-1990.
357. Heywood AW I., Learmonth D, Thomas M. Internal fixation for occipito-cervical fusion. *J Bone Joint Surg Br*. 1988;70(5):708-711.
358. Grob D. Posterior occipitocervical fusion in rheumatoid arthritis and other instabilities. *J Orthop Sci*. 2000;5(1): 82-87.
359. Ebraheim NA, et al. An anatomic study of the thickness of the occipital bone. Implications for occipitocervical instrumentation. *Spine*. 1996;21(15):1725-1729.
360. Haher TR, et al. Occipital screw pullout strength. A biomechanical investigation of occipital morphology. *Spine*. 1999;24(1):5-9.
361. Richter M, et al. Biomechanical evaluation of a new modular rod-screw implant system for posterior instrumentation of the occipito-cervical spine: in-vitro comparison with two established implant systems. *Eur Spine J*. 2000;9(5):417-425.
362. Odent T, et al. Internal fixation with occipital hooks construct for occipito-cervical arthrodesis. Results in 14 young or small children. *Eur Spine J*. 2015;24(1):94-100.
363. El-Gaidi MA, Eissa EM, El-Shaarawy EA. Free-hand placement of occipital condyle screws: a cadaveric study. *Eur Spine J*. 2014;23(10):2182-2188.
364. Jeanneret B. Posterior rod system of the cervical spine: a new implant allowing optimal screw insertion. *Eur Spine J*. 1996;5(5):350-356.
365. Frush TJ, et al. Biomechanical evaluation of parasagittal occipital plating: screw load sharing analysis. *Spine*. 2009; 34(9):877-884.
366. Eismont F, Bohlman H. Posterior atlanto-occipital dislocation with fractures of the atlas and odontoid process. *J Bone Joint Surg Am*. 1978;60:397.
367. Grob D, et al. Posterior occipitocervical fusion. A preliminary report of a new technique. *Spine*. 1991;16(3 suppl):S17-S24.
368. Puttlitz CM, et al. A finite element investigation of upper cervical instrumentation. *Spine*. 2001;26(22):2449-2455.
369. Grob D. Transarticular screw fixation for atlanto-occipital dislocation. *Spine*. 2001;26(6):703-707.
370. Zipnick RI, et al. Occipital morphology. An anatomic guide to internal fixation. *Spine*. 1996;21(15):1719-1724.
371. Boden SD. Rheumatoid arthritis of the cervical spine. Surgical decision making based on predictors of paralysis and recovery. *Spine*. 1994;19(20):2275-2280.
372. Ranawat CS, et al. Cervical spine fusion in rheumatoid arthritis. *J Bone Joint Surg Am*. 1979;61(7):1003-1010.
373. Ferlic DC, et al. Surgical treatment of the symptomatic unstable cervical spine in rheumatoid arthritis. *J Bone Joint Surg Am*. 1975;57(3):349-354.
374. Hamblen DL. Occipito-cervical fusion. Indications, technique and results. *J Bone Joint Surg Br*. 1967;49(1):33-45.
375. Grob D, et al. Posterior occipito-cervical fusion in rheumatoid arthritis. *Arch Orthop Trauma Surg*. 1990;110(1):38-44.
376. Grob D, Schutz U, Plotz G. Occipitocervical fusion in patients with rheumatoid arthritis. *Clin Orthop Relat Res*. 1999;366:46-53.
377. Sanpakit S, Mansfield TL, Liebsch J. Role of onlay grafting with minimal internal fixation for occipitocervical fusion in oncologic patients. *J Spinal Disord*. 2000;13(5):382-390.
378. Huckell CB, et al. Functional outcome of plate fusions for disorders of the occipitocervical junction. *Clin Orthop Relat Res*. 1999;359:136-145.
379. Letts M, Slutsky D. Occipitocervical arthrodesis in children. *J Bone Joint Surg Am*. 1990;72(8):1166-1170.
380. Zygmunt SC, et al. Occipito-cervical fixation in rheumatoid arthritis—an analysis of surgical risk factors in 163 patients. *Acta Neurochir (Wien)*. 1995;135(1-2):25-31.
381. Sasso RC, et al. Occipitocervical fusion with posterior plate and screw instrumentation. A long-term follow-up study. *Spine*. 1994;19(20):2364-2368.
382. Rodgers WB, et al. Increasing lordosis of the occipitocervical junction after arthrodesis in young children: the occipitocervical crankshaft phenomenon. *J Pediatr Orthop*. 1997;17(6):762-765.
383. Malcolm GP, Ransford AO, Crockard HA. Treatment of non-rheumatoid occipitocervical instability. Internal fixation with the Hartshill-Ransford loop. *J Bone Joint Surg Br*. 1994;76(3):357-366.
384. Peppelman WC, et al. Cervical spine surgery in rheumatoid arthritis: improvement of neurologic deficit after cervical spine fusion. *Spine*. 1993;18(16):2375-2379.
385. Clark CR. Occipitocervical fusion for the unstable rheumatoid neck. *Orthopedics*. 1989;12(3):469-473.
386. Santavirta S, et al. Ten-year results of operations for rheumatoid cervical spine disorders. *J Bone Joint Surg Br*. 1991;73(1):116-120.
387. Ando K, et al. Minimum 5-year follow-up results for occipitocervical fusion using the screw-rod system in craniocervical instability. *Clin Spine Surg*. 2016. Epub ahead of print.
388. Dormans JP, et al. Occipitocervical arthrodesis in children. A new technique and analysis of results. *J Bone Joint Surg Am*. 1995;77(8):1234-1240.
389. Nakagawa T, et al. Occipitocervical fusion with C1 laminectomy in children. *Spine*. 1997;22(11):1209-1214.
390. McGrory BJ, Klassen RA. Arthrodesis of the cervical spine for fractures and dislocations in children and adolescents. A long-term follow-up study. *J Bone Joint Surg Am*. 1994;76(11):1606-1616.
391. Abumi K, et al. Correction of cervical kyphosis using pedicle screw fixation systems. *Spine*. 1999;24(22):2389-2396.
392. Ransford AO, et al. Occipito-atlanto-axial fusion in Morquio-Brailsford syndrome. A ten-year experience. *J Bone Joint Surg Br*. 1996;78(2):307-313.
393. Boden SD, et al. Rheumatoid arthritis of the cervical spine. A long-term analysis with predictors of paralysis and recovery. *J Bone Joint Surg Am*. 1993;75(9):1282-1297.
394. Matsunaga S, Ijiri K, Koga H. Results of a longer than 10-year follow-up of patients with rheumatoid arthritis treated by occipitocervical fusion. *Spine*. 2000;25(14):1749-1753.

395. Omura K, et al. Evaluation of posterior long fusion versus conservative treatment for the progressive rheumatoid cervical spine. *Spine*. 2002;27(12):1336-1345.
396. Alt V, et al. Gesundheitsokonomische Uberlegungen fur den Einsatz des Knochenwachstumsfaktors BMP-2 in der Wirbelsaulenchirurgie fur das Deutsche Gesundheitssystem. *Z Orthop Ihre Grenzgeb*. 2006;144(6):577-582.
397. Tokuhashi Y, et al. C1-C2 intra-articular screw fixation for atlantoaxial posterior stabilization. *Spine*. 2000;25(3):337-341.
398. Stevens JM, et al. The odontoid process in Morquio-Brailsford's disease. The effects of occipitocervical fusion. *J Bone Joint Surg Br*. 1991;73(5):851-858.
399. Shirasaki N, et al. Os odontoideum with posterior atlantoaxial instability. *Spine*. 1991;16(7):706-715.
400. Farey ID, Nadkarni S, Smith N. Modified Gallie technique versus transarticular screw fixation in C1-C2 fusion. *Clin Orthop Relat Res*. 1999;359:126-135.
401. Richter M, et al. Posterior atlantoaxial fixation: biomechanical in vitro comparison of six different techniques. *Spine*. 2002;27(16):1724-1732.
402. Brooks AL, Jenkins EB. Atlanto-axial arthrodesis by the wedge compression method. *J Bone Joint Surg Am*. 1978;60(3):279-284.
403. Montesano PX, et al. Odontoid fractures treated by anterior odontoid screw fixation. *Spine*. 1991;16(3 suppl):S33-S37.
404. Aprin H, Harf R. Stabilization of atlantoaxial instability. *Orthopedics*. 1988;11(12):1687-1693.
405. Magerl F, Grob D, Seeman P. Stable dorsal fusion of the cervical spine (C2-T1) using hook plates. In: Kehr P, Weidner A, eds. *Cervical Spine*. New York: Springer-Verlag; 1987:217-221.
406. Lee JH, Jahng TA, Chung CK. C1-2 transarticular screw fixation in high-riding vertebral artery: suggestion of new trajectory. *J Spinal Disord Tech*. 2007;20(7):499-504.
407. Cyr SJ, et al. Fixation strength of unicortical versus bicortical C1-C2 transarticular screws. *Spine J*. 2008;8(4):661-665.
408. Ebraheim NA, et al. The optimal transarticular C1-2 screw length and the location of the hypoglossal nerve. *Surg Neurol*. 2000;53(3):208-210.
409. Aryan HE, et al. Stabilization of the atlantoaxial complex via C-1 lateral mass and C-2 pedicle screw fixation in a multicenter clinical experience in 102 patients: modification of the Harms and Goel techniques. *J Neurosurg Spine*. 2008;8(3):222-229.
410. Wang C, et al. Atlantoaxial transarticular screw fixation with morselized autograft and without additional internal fixation: technical description and report of 57 cases. *Spine*. 2007;32(6):643-646.
411. Magerl F, Seemann P. Stable posterior fusion of the atlas and axis by transarticular screw fixation. In: Kehr P, Weidner A, eds. *Cervical Spine*. Berlin: Springer-Verlag; 1986:322.
412. Reilly TM, Sasso RC, Hall PV. Atlantoaxial stabilization: clinical comparison of posterior cervical wiring technique with transarticular screw fixation. *J Spinal Disord Tech*. 2003;16(3):248-253.
413. Taggard D, et al. Case-control study comparing the efficacy of surgical techniques for C1 C2 arthrodesis. *J Spinal Disord Tech*. 2004;17(3):189-194.
414. Goel A, Desai KI, Muzumdar DP. Atlantoaxial fixation using plate and screw method: a report of 160 treated patients. *Neurosurgery*. 2002;51(6):1351-1356.
415. Harms J, Melcher RP. Posterior C1-C2 fusion with polyaxial screw and rod fixation. *Spine*. 2001;26(22):2467-2471.
416. He B, et al. Self-designed posterior atlas polyaxial lateral mass screw-plate fixation for unstable atlas fracture. *Spine J*. 2014;14(12):2892-2896.
417. Stulik J, et al. Atlantoaxial fixation using the polyaxial screw-rod system. *Eur Spine J*. 2007;16(4):479-484.
418. Hong X, et al. Posterior screw placement on the lateral mass of atlas: an anatomic study. *Spine*. 2004;29(5):500-503.
419. Dewan MC, et al. C2 nerve root transection during C1 lateral mass screw fixation: does it affect functionality and quality of life? *Neurosurgery*. 2014;74(5):475-480.
420. Wang MY, Samudrala S. Cadaveric morphometric analysis for atlantal lateral mass screw placement. *Neurosurgery*. 2004;54(6):1436-1439.
421. Rocha R, et al. Working area, safety zones, and angles of approach for posterior C-1 lateral mass screw placement: a quantitative anatomical and morphometric evaluation. *J Neurosurg Spine*. 2007;6(3):247-254.
422. Menger RP, et al. Placement of C1 pedicle screws using minimal exposure: radiographic, clinical, and literature validation. *Int J Spine Surg*. 2015;9:43.
423. Elliott RE, et al. Impact of starting point and bicortical purchase of C1 lateral mass screws on atlantoaxial fusion: meta-analysis and review of the literature. *J Spinal Disord Tech*. 2015;28(7):242-253.
424. Liu G, et al. The feasibility of microscope-assisted "free-hand" C1 lateral mass screw insertion without fluoroscopy. *Spine*. 2008;33(9):1042-1049.
425. Murakami S, et al. Relationship between screw trajectory of C1 lateral mass screw and internal carotid artery. *Spine*. 2008;33(24):2581-2585.
426. Hu Y, et al. An anatomic study to determine the optimal entry point, medial angles, and effective length for safe fixation using posterior C1 lateral mass screws. *Spine*. 2015;40(4):E191-E198.
427. Yeom JS, et al. Lateral fluoroscopic guide to prevent occipitocervical and atlantoaxial joint violation during C1 lateral mass screw placement. *Spine J*. 2009;9(7):574-579.
428. Young JP, et al. The ponticulus posticus: implications for screw insertion into the first cervical lateral mass. *J Bone Joint Surg Am*. 2005;87(11):2495-2498.
429. Chamoun RB, et al. Computed tomography morphometric analysis for C-1 lateral mass screw placement in children. Clinical article. *J Neurosurg Pediatr*. 2009;3(1):20-23.
430. Eck JC, et al. Biomechanical comparison of unicortical versus bicortical C1 lateral mass screw fixation. *J Spinal Disord Tech*. 2007;20(7):505-508.
431. Hott JS, et al. Biomechanical comparison of C1-2 posterior fixation techniques. *J Neurosurg Spine*. 2005;2(2):175-181.
432. Harms J, Melcher RP. Posterior C1-C2 fusion with polyaxial screw and rod fixation. *Spine*. 2001;26(22):2467-2471.
433. Bourdillon P, et al. C1-C2 stabilization by Harms arthrodesis: indications, technique, complications and outcomes in a prospective 26-case series. *Orthop Traumatol Surg Res*. 2014;100(2):221-227.
434. Elliott RE, et al. Outcome comparison of atlantoaxial fusion with transarticular screws and screw-rod constructs: meta-analysis and review of literature. *J Spinal Disord Tech*. 2014;27(1):11-28.
435. Elliott RE, et al. Comparison of screw malposition and vertebral artery injury of C2 pedicle and transarticular screws: meta-analysis and review of the literature. *J Spinal Disord Tech*. 2014;27(6):305-315.

436. Yoshida M, et al. Comparison of the anatomical risk for vertebral artery injury associated with the C2-pedicle screw and atlantoaxial transarticular screw. *Spine*. 2006;31(15):E513-E517.
437. Bydon M, et al. Accuracy of C2 pedicle screw placement using the anatomic freehand technique. *Clin Neurol Neurosurg*. 2014;125:24-27.
438. Dmitriev AE, et al. Acute and long-term stability of atlantoaxial fixation methods: a biomechanical comparison of pars, pedicle, and intralaminar fixation in an intact and odontoid fracture model. *Spine*. 2009;34(4):365-370.
439. Lehman RA Jr, et al. Salvage of C2 pedicle and pars screws using the intralaminar technique: a biomechanical analysis. *Spine*. 2008;33(9):960-965.
440. Han B, et al. Motion preservation in type II odontoid fractures using temporary pedicle screw fixation: a preliminary study. *Eur Spine J*. 2015;24(4):686-693.
441. Ni B, et al. Posterior reduction and temporary fixation for odontoid fracture: a salvage maneuver to anterior screw fixation. *Spine*. 2015;40(3):E168-E174.
442. Wright NM. Translaminar rigid screw fixation of the axis. Technical note. *J Neurosurg Spine*. 2005;3(5):409-414.
443. Jea A, et al. Translaminar screw fixation in the subaxial pediatric cervical spine. *J Neurosurg Pediatr*. 2008;2(6):386-390.
444. Sciubba DM, et al. Laminar screw fixation of the axis. *J Neurosurg Spine*. 2008;8(4):327-334.
445. Mendelsohn D, et al. Bilateral pedicle and crossed translaminar screws in C2. *Asian Spine J*. 2015;9(5):783-788.
446. Dorward IG, Wright NM. Seven years of experience with C2 translaminar screw fixation: clinical series and review of the literature. *Neurosurgery*. 2011;68(6):1491-1499.
447. Cybulski GR, et al. Use of Halifax interlaminar clamps for posterior C1-C2 arthrodesis. *Neurosurgery*. 1988;22(2):429-431.
448. Aldrich EF, et al. Use of MR imaging-compatible Halifax interlaminar clamps for posterior cervical fusion. *J Neurosurg*. 1991;74(2):185-189.
449. Aldrich EF, Weber PB, Crow WN. Halifax interlaminar clamp for posterior cervical fusion: a long-term follow-up review. *J Neurosurg*. 1993;78(5):702-708.
450. Stambough JL, Balderston RA, Grey S. Technique for occipito-cervical fusion in osteopenic patients. *J Spinal Disord*. 1990;3(4):404-407.
451. Awasthi D, Voorhies RM. Posterior cervical fusion with methylmethacrylate, wire, and bone: technical note. *Surg Neurol*. 1994;42(3):259-264.
452. Weis JC, et al. In vitro biomechanical comparison of multistrand cables with conventional cervical stabilization. *Spine*. 1996;21(18):2108-2114.
453. Epstein NE. An argument for traditional posterior cervical fusion techniques: evidence from 35 cases. *Surg Neurol*. 2008;70(1):45-51.
454. Wong AS, Massicotte EM, Fehlings MG. Surgical treatment of cervical myeloradiculopathy associated with movement disorders: indications, technique, and clinical outcome. *J Spinal Disord Tech*. 2005;18(suppl):S107-S114.
455. Garfin SR, Moore MR, Marshall LF. A modified technique for cervical facet fusions. *Clin Orthop*. 1988;230:149-153.
456. Murphy MJ, Daniaux H, Southwick WO. Posterior cervical fusion with rigid internal fixation. *Orthop Clin North Am*. 1986;17(1):55-65.
457. Davey JR, et al. A technique of posterior cervical fusion for instability of the cervical spine. *Spine*. 1985;10(8):722-728.
458. Weiland DJ, McAfee PC. Posterior cervical fusion with triple-wire strut graft technique: one hundred consecutive patients. *J Spinal Disord*. 1991;4(1):15-21.
459. Abdu WA, Bohlman HH. Techniques of subaxial posterior cervical spine fusions: an overview. *Orthopedics*. 1992;15(3):287-295.
460. Callahan RA, et al. Cervical facet fusion for control of instability following laminectomy. *J Bone Joint Surg Am*. 1977;59(8):991-1002.
461. Cahill DW, Bellegarrigue R, Ducker TB. Bilateral facet to spinous process fusion: a new technique for posterior spinal fusion after trauma. *Neurosurgery*. 1983;13(1):1-4.
462. Blacklock JB. Fracture of a sublaminar stainless steel cable in the upper cervical spine with neurological injury. Case report. *J Neurosurg*. 1994;81(6):932-933.
463. Yonezawa I, et al. Atlantoaxial transarticular screw fixation and posterior fusion using ultra-high-molecular-weight polyethylene cable. *J Spinal Disord Tech*. 2005;18(5):392-395.
464. al Baz MO, Mathur N. Modified technique of tension band wiring in flexion injuries of the middle and lower cervical spine. *Spine*. 1995;20(11):1241-1244.
465. Arslantas A, et al. Instrumentation for posterior stabilisation of cervical traumatic and degenerative disorders: bullet-shaped implant and titanium cable. *J Neurosurg Sci*. 2001;45(4):202-204.
466. Ebraheim NA, et al. Internal fixation of the unstable cervical spine using posterior Roy-Camille plates: preliminary report. *J Orthop Trauma*. 1989;3(1):23-28.
467. Savini R, Parisini P, Cervellati S. The surgical treatment of late instability of flexion-rotation injuries in the lower cervical spine. *Spine*. 1987;12(2):178-182.
468. Gargano FP. Transverse axial tomography of the spine. *CRC Crit Rev Clin Radiol Nucl Med*. 1976;8(3):279-328.
469. Deen HG, et al. Lateral mass screw-rod fixation of the cervical spine: a prospective clinical series with 1-year follow-up. *Spine J*. 2003;3(6):489-495.
470. Coe JD, et al. Biomechanical evaluation of cervical spinal stabilization methods in a human cadaveric model. *Spine*. 1989;14(10):1122-1131.
471. Ulrich C, et al. Comparative study of the stability of anterior and posterior cervical spine fixation procedures. *Arch Orthop Trauma Surg*. 1987;106(4):226-231.
472. Merola AA, et al. Anatomic consideration for standard and modified techniques of cervical lateral mass screw placement. *Spine J*. 2002;2(6):430-435.
473. Maciejczak A, Wolan-Nieroda A, Jablonska-Sudol K. Comparison of fusion rates between rod-based laminar claw hook and posterior cervical screw constructs in Type II odontoid fractures. *Injury*. 2015;46(7):1304-1310.
474. Hildingsson C, Jonsson H. Posterior stabilization of the cervical spine with hooks and screws. A clinical evaluation of 26 patients with traumatic, degenerative or metastatic lesions, using a new implant system. *Eur Spine J*. 2001;10(1):50-54.
475. Espinoza-Larios A, et al. Biomechanical comparison of two-level cervical locking posterior screw/rod and hook/rod techniques. *Spine J*. 2007;7(2):194-204.
476. Onibokun A, et al. Anatomical considerations for cervical pedicle screw insertion: the use of multiplanar computerized tomography measurements in 122 consecutive clinical cases. *Spine J*. 2009;9(9):729-734.

477. Kurd MF, et al. Lateral mass fixation in the subaxial cervical spine. *J Spinal Disord Tech*. 2015;28(7):259-263.
478. Graham AW, et al. Posterior cervical arthrodesis and stabilization with a lateral mass plate. Clinical and computed tomographic evaluation of lateral mass screw placement and associated complications. *Spine*. 1996;21(3):323-328.
479. Hedequist D, Hresko T, Proctor M. Modern cervical spine instrumentation in children. *Spine*. 2008;33(4):379-383.
480. Cooper PR, et al. Posterior stabilization of cervical spine fractures and subluxations using plates and screws. *Neurosurgery*. 1988;23(3):300-306.
481. Fehlings MG, Cooper PR, Errico TJ. Posterior plates in the management of cervical instability: long-term results in 44 patients. *J Neurosurg*. 1994;81(3):341-349.
482. Pateder DB, Carbone JJ. Lateral mass screw fixation for cervical spine trauma: associated complications and efficacy in maintaining alignment. *Spine J*. 2006;6(1):40-43.
483. Brodke DS, et al. Comparison of anterior and posterior approaches in cervical spinal cord injuries. *J Spinal Disord Tech*. 2003;16(3):229-235.
484. Al Barbarawi MM, Allouh MZ. Cervical lateral mass screw-rod fixation: surgical experience with 2500 consecutive screws, an analytical review, and long-term outcomes. *Br J Neurosurg*. 2015;29(5):699-704.
485. Sehati N, Khoo LT. Minimally invasive posterior cervical arthrodesis and fixation. *Neurosurg Clin N Am*. 2006;17(4):429-440.
486. Takemitsu M, et al. C5 nerve root palsy after cervical laminoplasty and posterior fusion with instrumentation. *J Spinal Disord Tech*. 2008;21(4):267-272.
487. Scheufler KM, Kirsch E. Percutaneous multilevel decompressive laminectomy, foraminotomy, and instrumented fusion for cervical spondylotic radiculopathy and myelopathy: assessment of feasibility and surgical technique. *J Neurosurg Spine*. 2007;7(5):514-520.
488. Hostin RA, et al. A biomechanical evaluation of three revision screw strategies for failed lateral mass fixation. *Spine*. 2008;33(22):2415-2421.
489. Hong JT, et al. Significance of laminar screw fixation in the subaxial cervical spine. *Spine*. 2008;33(16):1739-1743.
490. Kowalski JM, et al. Cervical spine pedicle screws: a biomechanical comparison of two insertion techniques. *Spine*. 2000;25(22):2865-2867.
491. Ames CP, et al. Biomechanics of stabilization after cervicothoracic compression-flexion injury. *Spine*. 2005;30(13):1505-1512.
492. Hacker AG, Molloy S, Bernard J. The contralateral lamina: a reliable guide in subaxial, cervical pedicle screw placement. *Eur Spine J*. 2008;17(11):1457-1461.
493. Ryken TC, et al. Engineering patient-specific drill templates and bioabsorbable posterior cervical plates: a feasibility study. *J Neurosurg Spine*. 2009;10(2):129-132.
494. Reinhold M, et al. Cervical pedicle screw placement: feasibility and accuracy of two new insertion techniques based on morphometric data. *Eur Spine J*. 2007;16(1):47-56.
495. Abumi K, et al. Indirect posterior reduction and fusion of the traumatic herniated disc by using a cervical pedicle screw system. *J Neurosurg*. 2000;92(1 suppl):30-37.
496. Kast E, et al. Complications of transpedicular screw fixation in the cervical spine. *Eur Spine J*. 2006;15(3):327-334.
497. Hasegawa K, et al. Indications for cervical pedicle screw instrumentation in nontraumatic lesions. *Spine*. 2008;33(21):2284-2289.
498. Richter M, Mattes T, Cakir B. Computer-assisted posterior instrumentation of the cervical and cervico-thoracic spine. *Eur Spine J*. 2004;13(1):50-59.
499. Jeanneret B, Gebhard JS, Magerl F. Transpedicular screw fixation of articular mass fracture-separation: results of an anatomical study and operative technique. *J Spinal Disord*. 1994;7(3):222-229.
500. Takayasu M, et al. Transarticular screw fixation in the middle and lower cervical spine. Technical note. *J Neurosurg*. 2003;99(1 suppl):132-136.
501. Horn EM, et al. Transfacet screw placement for posterior fixation of C-7. *J Neurosurg Spine*. 2008;9(2):200-206.
502. Miyanji F, et al. Biomechanical differences between transfacet and lateral mass screw-rod constructs for multilevel posterior cervical spine stabilization. *Spine*. 2008;33(23):E865-E869.
503. DalCanto RA, et al. Biomechanical comparison of transarticular facet screws to lateral mass plates in two-level instrumentations of the cervical spine. *Spine*. 2005;30(8):897-1002.
504. Duan Y, et al. Finite element analysis of posterior cervical fixation. *Orthop Traumatol Surg Res*. 2015;101(1):23-29.
505. Aota Y, Honda A, Saito T. Clinical and computed tomographic evaluation of safety and efficacy of facet screw fixation in the subaxial cervical spine. *J Spinal Disord Tech*. 2014;27(3):136-143.
506. Lindsey C, et al. The effects of rod contouring on spinal construct fatigue strength. *Spine*. 2006;31(15):1680-1687.
507. Khoueir P, Hoh DJ, Wang MY. Use of hinged rods for controlled osteoclastic correction of a fixed cervical kyphotic deformity in ankylosing spondylitis. *J Neurosurg Spine*. 2008;8(6):579-583.
508. Tessitore E, Momjian A, Payer M. Posterior reduction and fixation of an unstable Jefferson fracture with C1 lateral mass screws, C2 isthmus screws, and crosslink fixation: technical case report. *Neurosurgery*. 2008;63(1 suppl 1):ONSE100-ONSE101.
509. Maulucci CM, et al. Cortical bone facet spacers for cervical spine decompression: effects on intervertebral kinetics and foraminal area. *J Neurosurg Spine*. 2016;24(1):69-76.
510. Tan LA, Straus DC, Traynelis VC. Cervical interfacet spacers and maintenance of cervical lordosis. *J Neurosurg Spine*. 2015;22(5):466-469.
511. Chen HC, et al. Lateral mass anchoring screws for cervical laminoplasty: preliminary report of a novel technique. *J Spinal Disord Tech*. 2008;21(6):387-392.
512. Yang SC, et al. Open-door laminoplasty with suture anchor fixation for cervical myelopathy in ossification of the posterior longitudinal ligament. *J Spinal Disord Tech*. 2007;20(7):492-498.
513. Yang SC, et al. Open-door laminoplasty for multilevel cervical spondylotic myelopathy: good outcome in 12 patients using suture anchor fixation. *Acta Orthop*. 2008;79(1):62-66.
514. Lee JY, et al. Use of small suture anchors in cervical laminoplasty to maintain canal expansion: a technical note. *J Spinal Disord Tech*. 2007;20(1):33-35.
515. Kanemura A, et al. Delayed dural laceration by hydroxyapatite spacer causing tetraparesis following double-door laminoplasty. *J Neurosurg Spine*. 2008;8(2):121-128.
516. Chen H, et al. Clinical and radiography results of mini-plate fixation compared to suture suspensory fixation in cervical laminoplasty: A five-year follow-up study. *Clin Neurol Neurosurg*. 2015;138:188-195.

CHAPTER 70

Thoracic and Lumbar Instrumentation: Anterior and Posterior

Eeric Truumees*

Introduction

The spinal column functions mechanically to support the load of the body, allow controlled motion, and protect the neural elements. Diseases of the spinal column affect its performance and ability to function normally. A vertebral body tumor disrupts the load-bearing capability, and aggressive decompression for stenosis can lead to instability and kyphotic collapse.

In most cases, spinal implants are combined with segmental fusion as part of a treatment strategy to restore the mechanical functions disrupted by trauma, tumor, deformity, infection, or degenerative disease or by the surgical management of these disorders. In each etiologic subgroup, the particular indications for thoracolumbar instrumentation may be different, but the goals remain the same: to increase or maintain stability, prevent or reduce deformity, help bear the loads of the spine, and encourage the healing of bone graft.

Thoracolumbar implant constructs are used to prevent further collapse by neutralizing a deforming force or by holding the spine in a mechanically more favorable position. In some cases, deformity correction may be beneficial and may decompress the canal. Either way, an understanding of spinal pathomechanics is crucial. In addition, spine surgeons must be aware of the available implants and how they can be best used to optimize treatment, help ensure a good surgical outcome, and minimize the risks associated with surgery.

Overview and History

Internal fixation of the thoracolumbar spine has been used for the past century.[1] Many implants were developed to treat specific spinal conditions in specific populations, with use broadening later. For example, the "Hong Kong procedure" gave rise to modern anterior thoracolumbar surgery in an effort to treat the deformity associated with spinal tuberculosis.[2]

*The editors sincerely thank Dr. Truumees for his work on this chapter in the sixth edition of this text, for which he was not credited.

In other cases, the concepts behind new spinal implants were borrowed from other fields. Artificial disc replacement arose from low-friction total knee arthroplasty designs. Kyphoplasty to treat painful osteoporotic fractures evolved from angioplasty balloons.[3,4]

From their initial incarnations, each generation of implants evolves to broaden applications, reduce the difficulty of application, or address unintended consequences of previous procedures. One of the most dramatic examples of this iterative phenomenon is the development of segmental instrumentation in the correction of spinal deformity and its role in preventing the flat back deformity engendered by previous hook-rod constructs.

When considering an implant, the spine surgeon needs to understand its US Food and Drug Administration (FDA) status. Although the FDA may not dictate or interfere with medical care, they do place medical devices into one of three categories (Box 70.1).

In early 2017, the FDA announced the results of a 2-year review process of thoracolumbosacral pedicle screw systems. Although individual companies still need to apply to downgrade their implant's classification, overall rigid pedicle screw systems have been downgraded from class III to class II.

Off-label use of thoracolumbar instrumentation occurs in two settings, each of which makes different demands on the physician. First, the common practice of using a device for an indication other than that for which it was assessed by the FDA is termed "practice of medicine." The second off-label use involves experimental or investigational devices. On a practical level, these devices have been used widely for years. However, the downgrade allows expanded, company-directed education efforts and decreases the regulatory burden associated with system development.

For a commercially available and marketed device, the physician is legally allowed to use the device in any manner, according to his or her best knowledge and judgment. When the treatment regimen is not included in labeling, however, the physician should be able to document device efficacy from the scientific literature. Outside of individual hospital rules, no investigational device exemption or institutional review board review is needed.

BOX 70.1 US Food and Drug Administration (FDA) Medical Device Classifications

Class I: Neither Standard nor Premarket Approval Warranted

- Present little risk to public
- General controls sufficient to ensure safety and efficacy
- Subject to minimal FDA regulation

Examples: cast materials, crutches, wheelchairs

Class II: Higher Risk, General Regulatory Controls *Not* Sufficient

- Enough data exist to develop a performance standard
- May present some additional risk to public
- Individual performance standards developed by FDA

Examples: intramedullary nails, bone screws, plates, cemented total hip arthroplasty

Class III: Highest Risk, Requires FDA Premarket Approval

- Not enough information exists to ensure safety and efficacy or to establish a performance standard
- May present a substantial risk to the public
- Not enough information to establish performance standard
- Not cleared for marketing for a particular purpose by FDA

A device that has not received market approval for any indication is deemed experimental. Experimental devices may be used only in accordance with an approved protocol derived from an investigational device exemption submission. It is unreliable to depend on a textbook or sales representative for this changing classification. Instead, it is prudent to review the product's labeling on the FDA's website (www.fda.gov).

The emphasis in this chapter is on currently available thoracolumbar instrumentation systems used to maintain alignment and to decrease motion while awaiting solid bony fusion of the treated spinal segments. Implants used for direct fracture repair are rarely used in thoracolumbar spine surgery. One exception is for direct repair of spondylolysis without segmental fusion.

Implants developed to improve segmental stability without fusion, such as physeal staples, disc arthroplasty, and interspinous process devices, are briefly discussed. Dynamic pedicle screw systems are now included in an FDA subtype of semi-rigid systems, including polyetheretherketone (PEEK) rods. These systems were also downgraded to class II, but only as an adjunct to fusion.

Relevant Anatomy

A firm grasp of thoracolumbar anatomy is required to understand the implications of disease on anatomy and allow safe placement of implants.

The thoracolumbar spine can be divided into five regions: the cervicothoracic junction, the mid-thoracic spine, the thoracolumbar junction, the mid-lumbar spine, and the lumbosacral junction. Each region has distinct anatomic and biomechanical characteristics that must be considered when planning reconstructive and instrumentation surgery. The anatomy typically serves the biomechanics. For example, facet orientation predicts motion segment direction and range of motion. Facet orientation also "couples" motion so that flexion necessitates translation.[5]

Surgical approaches and implant placement affect the local spinal anatomy directly or indirectly. Direct anterior lumbar interbody approaches require sacrifice of the anterior longitudinal ligament. In disc replacement procedures, to achieve more parallel distraction, the posterior longitudinal ligament may need to be resected.

The thoracic spine's articulation with the rib cage increases its rigidity.[6] Before proceeding with a transthoracic approach and spinal reconstruction, the surgeon must be familiar with the articulations between the rib and vertebral body. There are two sets of demifacets: one at the disc level and the other at the transverse process. Radiate ligaments stabilize the articulation further. The rib attaches to the transverse process and the superior aspect of the same-number vertebra (at the level of the pedicle). For example, to reach the T9–T10 disc, one can follow the T10 rib to the superior aspect of the T10 body.

The rib–pedicle–transverse process junction is critical in posterior approaches as well. Because the pedicles of the mid-thoracic spine are quite narrow, some authors have recommended an in-out-in approach for pedicle screw insertion. With this technique, the pedicle screw trajectory begins dorsally, but as the pedicle narrows, the screw passes laterally into the space between the rib and the pedicle. This space, containing only ligamentous tissues, does not jeopardize neurologic structures or the lung parenchyma.[7]

The thoracolumbar junction represents a straight segment and a mechanical transition zone between the lordosis of the mobile, lumbar spine and the kyphosis of the more rigid, thoracic spine. As such, it is vulnerable to injury and loss of fixation with externally applied forces.

The lumbar spine permits significant flexion and extension across all levels. There is a sharp increase in the amount of lateral bending exhibited at L3–L4. There is less lateral bending at L2–L3 and L4–L5. In the lumbar spine, axial rotation is limited by the vertical orientation of the facets.

Successful spinal fixation requires a stable bone-implant interface. The proximity of the neural elements limits the bone surfaces available for spinal instrumentation. In addition, the bone's size and shape influence which implants can be used. For example, larger pedicles accommodate larger screws. Larger screws increase the stability of fixation and increase holding strength.

There is significant anatomic variation among patients. Modern imaging systems allow preoperative measures of optimal screw length and diameter.

The spinal cord typically ends at the L1–L2 disc space. Below the conus, the nerve roots pass from the central thecal sac through the neuroforamen into the pelvis. Several cadaveric and imaging studies have described the proximity of the bony elements to nearby neural structures. One cadaveric study measured the average distance from lumbar pedicle to the dural sac medially. From cranial to caudal in the lumbar canal, the range was 1.29 to 1.56 mm; clinically, this means that a medical pedicle breach greater than 1.29 mm has a significant chance of contacting or injuring the dura.[8]

It is important to understand the relationship of the pedicle and the exiting nerve root. In the thoracolumbar spine, a given root exits the central canal into the foramen just below the

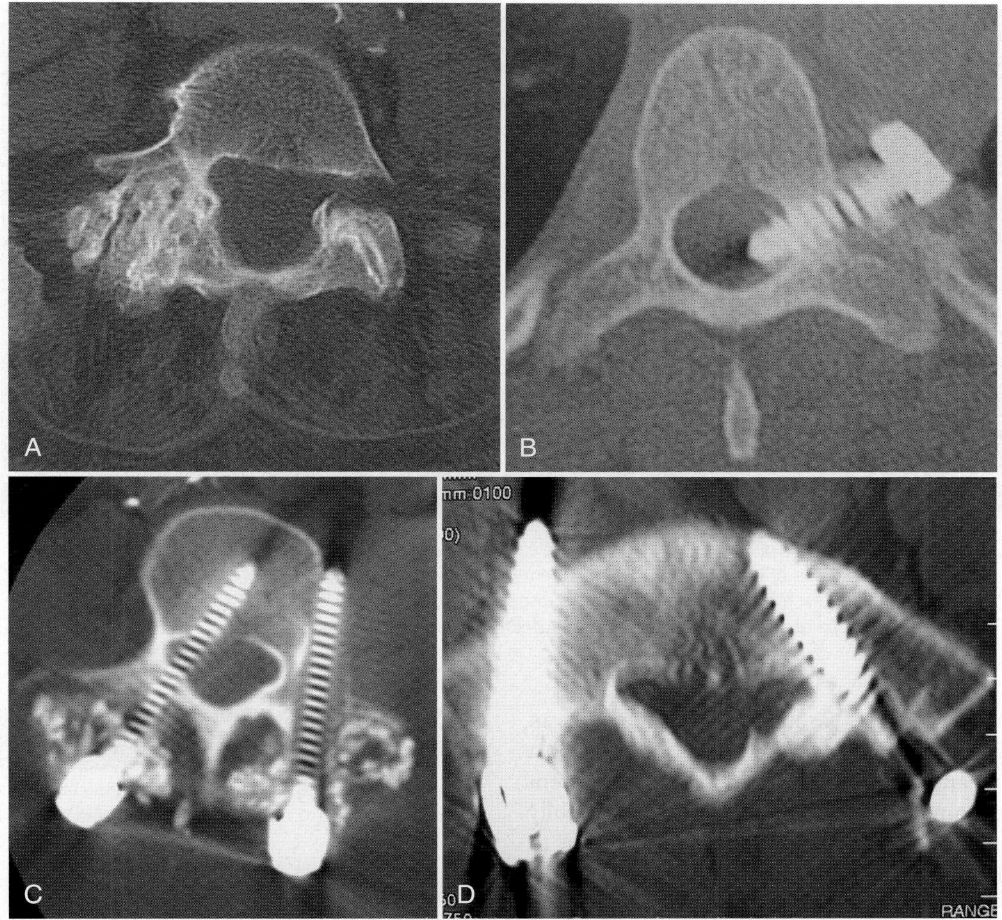

FIG. 70.1 Importance of good exposure. (A) Axial computed tomographic (CT) scan of a patient with marked facet hypertrophy. In most cases, complete takedown of the soft tissue around the lateral pars and medial transverse process provides enough anatomic clues for appropriate positioning of the pedicle probe. In cases such as this, resection of the facet osteophytes significantly improves identification of normal anatomic landmarks, improving pedicle screw placement accuracy. (B) Anteriorly, soft tissues must be reflected posteriorly enough to palpate the posterior vertebral body margin. This gives the surgeon a markedly improved three-dimensional sense of the position of the spine in space and can avoid inadvertent penetration of the spinal canal with a screw, as shown here. Proper positioning of the patient is critical. If the patient is rotated, the surgeon's orientation to the spine may be confused. That may have contributed to the misplacement shown here. (C) Adequate exposure also requires adequate soft tissue release. Particularly in patients with a narrow pelvis, if the thoracodorsal fascia remains tight, the surgeon has to struggle to achieve proper medialization of the screws. (D) Postoperative axial CT scan shows S1 screws. The left-sided screw is in acceptable position, whereas the trajectory of the right-sided screw is not medialized enough. The screw penetrates the anterior sacrum and impinges on the L5 root anteriorly.

pedicle of the same numbered vertebra. For example, at the T11–T12 level, the T11 root exits beneath the 11th pedicle. After the L5 nerve root exits the neuroforamen, it travels anterior to the sacral ala. An S1 pedicle screw that is placed too far lateral or is too long places the L5 nerve root at risk for injury. The pedicle is farther from the superior nerve root at 4.12 to 5.52 mm but closer to the inferior root, where distances ranged from 1.10 to 1.06 mm. The nerve roots and dura are statistically further from the L5 pedicle than from other pedicles, making the L5 pedicle safer than other lumbar pedicles for screw insertion (Fig. 70.1).

Knowledge of the intimate relationship of the major vessels to the spine is crucial to avoid life-threatening complications during anterior and posterior thoracolumbar instrumentation. The surgical goals, local anatomic realities, and implant size and mechanical features must be considered together. For example, when addressed anteriorly, a scoliotic curve is typically approached from its convexity to allow a more complete release. However, in the upper thoracic spine, the approach is typically from the right to avoid the arch of the aorta.

The lumbar spine is typically approached from the left for several reasons. First, the liver is on the right and is more difficult to mobilize. Second, a left-sided approach brings the surgeon into contact with the aorta before the vena cava. The aorta is more easily recognized and is more durable. This decreases the risk of sudden, catastrophic blood loss (Fig. 70.2).

Placing anterior thoracolumbar implants requires preoperative evaluation of the vascular structures and detection of

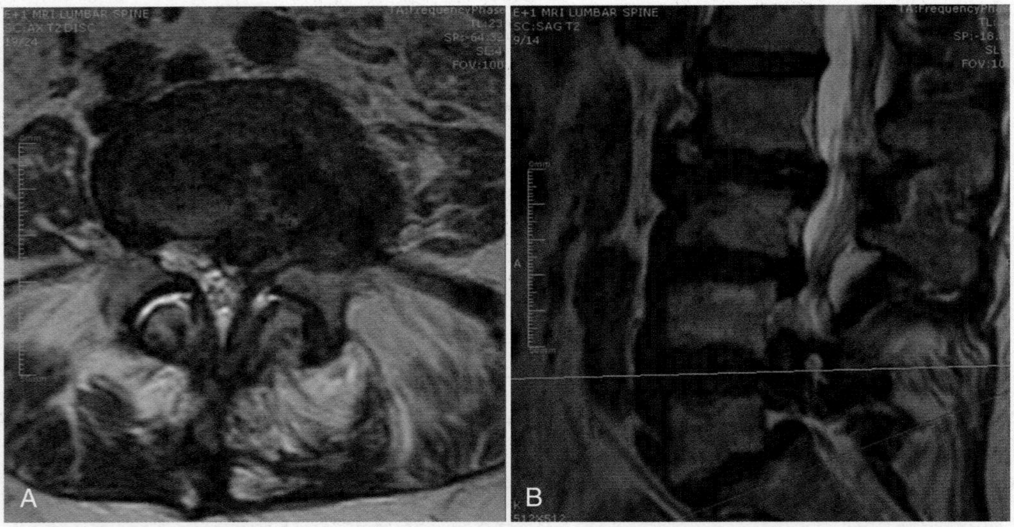

FIG. 70.2 Preoperative planning is crucial when selecting the implants or the angle of the approach to the spine. In certain cases, one implant may suit a patient better than another. (A) Cross-sectional and (B) parasagittal magnetic resonance images of L4–L5 disc space. Note the right iliac vessels are more lateral than expected. This type of anatomy may preclude the use of a transpsoas approach.

potential vascular anomalies. Vascular calcifications in an older patient may limit retraction of the vessels and may be a contraindication to anterior surgery. In addition, any patient with previous abdominal or hernia surgery must be carefully evaluated because scar tissue may be a contraindication to abdominal surgery.

In posterior approaches, the heart-shaped thoracic vertebral bodies allow thoracic pedicle screws to breach the vertebral cortex and endanger the aorta. This distance can vary with scoliosis but may be as little as 2 mm.[9] Placement of interbody devices from a posterior approach may also endanger the anterior vascular structures.

BOX 70.2 Important Factors in the Selection of Thoracolumbar Implants

Pathoanatomy: mechanism of injury and direction of instability
Mode of failure (e.g., in trauma, direction, and magnitude of injury vector)
Direction of instability
Degree of instability
Compromised stabilizing structure
Number of levels
Number of spinal columns per level
Bone vs. ligament (anticipated healing)
Host bone quality
Graft bone quality
Expected level of patient loading
Availability of postoperative immobilization
Surgeon familiarity with techniques
Availability of implants

Biomechanics of Thoracolumbar Instrumentation

Understanding disease state pathomechanics and implant biomechanics is crucial to successful construct design. Occasionally, implants fail because they are misplaced. More commonly, implants fail due to a judgment error (Box 70.2). Typically, the surgeon fails to understand fully one or more of the following factors:

1. Forces to which the spine is subjected
2. How the implants counteract those forces
3. Planes in which the spine is unstable
4. How instrumentation affects forces passing through structural grafts
5. Destabilizing effects of the operative procedure itself
6. Nature and extent of postoperative muscular forces
7. Time course of bone and soft tissue healing

The third factor, that of instability, remains controversial and difficult to predict. In trauma, understanding the mechanism of injury and direction of instability allows the surgeon to attempt to reverse that direction and those forces to affect a reduction and provide stability. Although not always clear in trauma, these factors become more opaque with etiologies such as inflammatory, neoplastic, and degenerative disease. Overestimation of the degree of instability present may lead to unnecessarily large surgeries or, in some cases, surgery without an indication. On the other hand, failure to appreciate clinically relevant instability may lead to inadequate treatment.

In general, the degree of anatomic disruption, as depicted by magnetic resonance imaging (MRI) or by abnormal angulation or translation on plain radiographs, should direct the surgeon toward the type of stabilization.

Implants are used to exert forces on the spine (e.g., to effect a reduction or scoliosis correction) or to resist forces (e.g., to prevent postoperative kyphosis). To select spinal implants properly, the surgeon must understand the size and direction of the forces to be applied. The surgeon must have an idea of how well the bone and soft tissue elements of the spine would respond to these forces (e.g., would the screws hold).

TABLE 70.1 Factors Used to Select Thoracolumbar Instrumentation Strategy

Internal Factors	External Factors
Compromised stabilizing structures (e.g., an injured anterolateral ligament may render the spine less able to resist extension forces)	Anticipated stresses exerted by the patient
Tissue type of the compromised stabilizer (healing time will vary)	Appropriateness and effectiveness of postoperative immobilization (e.g., external bracing may do little to shield the lumbosacral junction; patients with spinal cord injury may not be the best candidates for postoperative bracing)
Number of levels involved	Surgeon familiarity with relevant technique
Number of spinal columns involved	Availability of implants
Biologic and biomechanical quality of the host bone; consider preoperative dual-energy x-ray absorptiometry scan in at-risk patients	Effect of the surgery on adjacent levels
Biologic and biomechanical quality of the bone graft used. Because allograft will have longer incorporation times than autograft, a construct with greater fatigue resistance may be required.	Morbidity of the approach

Finally, the change in these forces during healing, including the effects of bone fusion, muscle healing, and implant fatigue, should be considered to minimize the risk of late implant failure. The more completely the surgeon understands these factors, the better able he or she is to choose the appropriate type of implant, appropriate implant material, optimal number and position of anchor points, and duration of postoperative immobilization.

Regardless of the etiology, delineating a few characteristics of the disease state is always useful (Table 70.1).

Implant Materials and Fusion Characteristics

Most posterior thoracolumbar fixation systems are made of stainless steel, pure titanium or, most commonly, titanium-aluminum-vanadium alloy. Metallic implants are also used in anterior column surgery as both screw-plate/screw-rod systems as well as rigid structural spacers to maintain or restore anterior load-carrying capacity.

Surgical stainless steel is very strong, with yield strength of 700 MPa. It is also stiff, having a modulus of elasticity 12 times that of normal bone. Steel implants usually have cobalt-chromium alloy and molybdenum to enhance corrosion resistance. Titanium alloys tend to have greater native biocompatibility and corrosion resistance. Titanium has a modulus of elasticity only six times greater than bone, which makes it easier to bend and insert than steel. These characteristics allow titanium-based devices to transfer load effectively to the vertebral body, partly shielding the implant from some stresses.

Two types of titanium are typically used. Pure titanium is recommended only when very low strength is needed because it has a low yield strength of only 170 to 485 MPa. More typically, a titanium-aluminum-vanadium alloy, with yield strength of 800 MPa, is used. Its greater strength does not change the favorable modulus of pure titanium (110 GPa).[10]

Cobalt-chrome rods are often used in deformity surgery, where some reports suggest long fatigue life and better maintenance of coronal plane correction.[11,12] However, one recent series reported a significantly higher rod fracture rate when cobalt-chrome rods were used to stabilize pedicle subtraction osteotomies.[13]

A reduction in stress shielding allows bone grafts to respond to more load appropriately. Use of titanium alloys has increased because of improved imaging characteristics, high strength/weight ratio, enhanced ductility, and increased fatigue life. Even with titanium, one of the disadvantages of metal cage implantation lies in plain radiographic assessment of fusion.[14]

Increasingly, nonmetallic implant materials have been used in thoracolumbar implants. Common materials include machined allograft bone, carbon fiber, or PEEK. Typically, these materials are used as cages, spacers, and graft containment systems rather than as fixation systems. Advantages of radiolucent materials such as PEEK include easier radiographic assessment of graft integration. For some nonmetallic implants, the modulus of elasticity is closer to that of host bone, allowing greater load sharing.[15] Mechanical testing showed acceptable mechanical and fatigue characteristics for PEEK as a load-bearing implant material.

Rods made of PEEK were briefly used for similar load-sharing reasons. Cadaveric tests compared the impact of PEEK versus titanium rods on adjacent-segment motion and intradiscal pressure.[16] No significant benefits of PEEK rod placement were noted. Furthermore, high failure and implant mobility rates have diminished their popularity.[17,18]

Although allograft bone spacers may be used alone, similar to their metal counterparts, they are typically filled with bone graft or bone morphogenetic protein. Radiographic assessment of bone healing may be improved when nonmetallic biomaterials are used. Even with radiolucent cages, differentiation of bone adherence versus through-growth (true fusion) is difficult, however. Bridging bone anterior (sentinel sign) or lateral to the cage is often used to signal fusion.

In a biologic environment, fretting and corrosion can occur between the modular components of a spine construct. Kirkpatrick and colleagues[19] subjected 48 spinal implant constructs to surface analysis stereomicroscopy. Titanium alloy implants (n = 25) showed no significant corrosion, but three of the constructs showed fatigue failure of the anchoring screws. The cobalt alloy construct showed no evidence of corrosion. Semirigid stainless steel implants had mild surface alteration, whereas rigid constructs showed moderate to severe corrosion. Based on their findings, the authors recommended avoiding rigid stainless steel implants or constructs with different surface finishes between rods and connectors.

The surgeon must use caution when combining implants made of different metals.[20] Mixing stainless steel with titanium could lead to a galvanic response and early corrosion, although titanium has been used with cobalt-chromium alloy without significant corrosion or complications.

In the early 2000s, there was quite of bit of interest in resorbable spine implants. At that time, numerous absorbable polymers, such as polylactic acid, were undergoing testing. With resorbable cages, the graft is gradually loaded to a greater and greater degree as the cage is enzymatically digested.[21,22] Each interbody device had different mechanical characteristics, such as modulus of elasticity and different resorption times. Implant failures and heterogeneity in implant performance in different patients have curbed enthusiasm, although new materials may revitalize this area of research.

The material properties of implants are also affected by manufacturing variables, such as drill holes, structural imperfections, and surface irregularities. Ultimate tensile strength—the maximum stress a material can sustain without changing shape—may be altered during surgery. Titanium rods are particularly sensitive to notching. If a complex rod contour is required, a template should be used to minimize the amount of rod bending. In some patients with rigid dual-curve deformities, it may be more effective to use separate rods in the thoracic and lumbar spine, employing rod-to-rod connectors ("dominoes") to complete the construct.

Implant fatigue is an important cause of failure. The average spine cycles 3 million times per year.[23-25] Current implants are overengineered for their designated function; therefore implant failure is more likely to occur from improper selection than from mechanical properties.[26] If bone healing is delayed or incomplete, the implant or construct ultimately fails, so meticulous attention to bone grafting technique is imperative.

Although newer rod materials, such as Ti6Al-4V alloy, allow better deformity correction with lower rod fracture rates, notch sensitivity continues to be reported.[27,28] Recently, nitinol rods have shown improved wear resistance compared with titanium and similar wear resistance to cobalt-chrome.[29]

Spinal implants are designed to provide segmental stability to facilitate bone healing. However, the type of fusion also affects the construct selected. For example, improved spinal implants have fostered a trend away from autogenous bone graft to allograft. Although allograft requires longer incorporation times, rigid instrumentation increases the rate of maturation.

A number of factors may impact the rate of bone healing and the chance of nonunion. For example, postoperative wound infections may affect fusion rates, especially in areas vulnerable to cyclic loading.[30] Other factors include motion, loading, muscle status, medical comorbidities, nutritional status, and tobacco use.

For fusions expected to heal slowly, more robust forms of instrumentation, possibly with additional anchor points, should be used. For example, lower fusion rates in smokers may justify instrumentation in settings in which in situ fusion would otherwise be appropriate. When clinical or mechanical circumstances increase the risk of pseudarthrosis, use of bone morphogenetic protein (BMP), on the other hand, may accelerate healing and may permit use of less fatigue-resistant constructs.[13] Other steps, such as addition of L5–S1 interbody fusion below a long posterolateral fusion, can be considered.[31]

Along the same lines, the anticipation of increased postoperative loading, poor patient compliance, or inadequate postoperative immobilization may warrant more rigid forms of operative stabilization. Examples include patients with neurologic or motion disorders who are subject to increased spinal loads and patients with spinal cord injury or a colostomy for whom brace immobilization is impractical.

The type of fusion achieved has implications on regional spinal mechanics as well and the advisability of subsequent implant removal. Historically, the most common fusion technique was the posterior fusion. The primary advantage of this approach was easy surgical access to the midline posterior elements (spinous processes and lamina). Disadvantages included its limited utility in laminectomy patients. Also, the graft material lies distant from the center of rotation and experiences significant tensile forces with spine flexion. This distance increases tensile stress and motion on the graft that could lead to migration, excessive motion, or graft resorption and ultimate nonunion.

Over time, direct posterior fusion was replaced by intertransverse fusion. For an intertransverse (posterolateral) fusion, the facet joints, lateral pars, and transverse processes are decorticated and grafted, leaving the lamina accessible for decompression. Intertransverse graft material is closer to the center of vertebral rotation. The disadvantage is a poor vascular bed and a decreased area for fusion.

Interbody fusion provides significant mechanical advantages in terms of graft compression and a large, well-vascularized fusion surface. The anterior column fusion spans the neutral zone and, when healed, represents the strongest mechanical block to segmental motion.[32,33] Even a solid intertransverse fusion may fracture or elongate if excessive or repeated load is placed across the motion segment.

The stability of this type of fusion has implications on subsequent implant removal. A report of 75 patients who underwent implant removal for late operative site pain, infection, or hardware failure, with a minimum of 2-year follow-up, found that the average loss of curve correction was 23.1 degrees.[34] Only 40% of those with operative site pain reported postoperative relief, and indolent infections were found in 37%.

Thoracolumbar implants share applied loads with the spine until a stable fusion occurs. If a construct bears most of the load, stress shielding of the spine results and may lead to device-related osteopenia.[35,36] The clinical sequelae of this shielding theoretically include graft resorption and possible implant failure, although emphasis on this phenomenon has declined over the last few years.

Temporary screw-and-rod fixation of spinal fractures to allow near-anatomic healing without arthrodesis have increasingly been described.[37] In a recent series, a cohort of 45 consecutive trauma patients who underwent implant removal after fracture healing were compared with 45 patients whose implants were retained. In most cases, a long-segment instrumentation and short-segment fusion had been performed. At 2-year follow-up, the implant removal group was found to have better visual analog pain scale and Oswestry Disability Index (OSI) scores as well as better range of motion.[38] A recent retrospective study of 104 patients found that minimally invasive surgery (MIS) with these principles was as effective as open surgery, while reducing procedure time and hospital stay.[39] Successful use in patients with ankylosing spondylitis and disseminated idiopathic skeletal hyperostosis has also been reported.[40]

In addition, temporary percutaneous stabilization of thoracolumbar trauma in patients with other major systemic injuries has been reported. In this setting, the initial construct is converted to formal fusion when the patient has stabilized medically. Mechanically, this damage control approach was evaluated in five cadavers. At least two levels of fixation above and below the level of injury were required to restore adequate rotational stability for log-rolling and sitting up.[41]

Demand Matching, Improving Fixation, and the Implications of Osteoporosis

The number of fixation points required of a spine construct depends on the demand placed on the construct, the fixation strength of the anchor, and the time required for bone healing. The most common, and increasing, challenge to thoracolumbar fixation comes from osteoporosis. Osteoporosis is the most common metabolic bone disorder and results from loss of both the crystalline (inorganic) and collagenous (organic) portions of bone.[42] Similar difficulties may be encountered in patients with spinal neoplasia or inflammatory arthritides.[43]

Throughout life, the body constantly remodels bone by removing old bone and creating new bone. Osteoporosis occurs when the rate of bone resorption exceeds the rate of bone formation. Lower rates of bone formation result in a decline in overall mineral density of bone. Unbalanced osteoclast activity results in disruption of the normal connectivity between bony trabeculae. Osteoporotic bone is weakened in the material and architectural sense.[42]

At least 40 million people are at risk for osteoporosis in North America. With the aging of the population, this number is likely to triple over the next 3 decades. Management of spinal disorders in an osteoporotic spine will thus be an increasing challenge. These bone quality issues are also noteworthy when treating patients with metastatic disease or inflammatory spinal arthritides.[44]

Implant failure in osteoporotic bone is common. Even if healing occurs uneventfully, patients with osteoporosis are at risk for compression fractures and spondylolisthesis adjacent to rigid constructs.[45]

For many patients, the diagnosis of osteoporosis and initiation of appropriate management are delayed. Because the consequences of the failure to recognize osteoporosis are so high, the spine surgeon must screen at-risk patients. Because at least 30% bone mass loss is needed to identify osteopenia reliably on plain radiographs, dual-energy x-ray absorptiometry (DEXA) and serum vitamin D levels are better screening tools.[46,47]

Results of DEXA scans are given in T and Z scores. The T score compares the patient's bone mineral density (BMD) with mean values for healthy, same-gender young adults. For each standard deviation below the norm, fracture risk increases 1.5- to 3-fold. A T score of −1 implies a 30% chance of fracture. As the T score decreases from −1 to −2, the risk of instrumentation failure increases significantly. The Z score compares BMD with age-matched controls. A Z score less than −1.5 warrants a more extensive workup for osteomalacia or neoplasm. DEXA values are falsely increased with scoliosis, compression fractures, spondylosis, extraosseous calcification, and vascular disease. In many spine patients, the T score at the femoral neck hip may be more predictive of implant holding power than the spine value.[48]

Depending on the patient's activity level, the nature of the intended surgery, and the severity of the osteoporosis, preoperative initiation of antiosteoporotic management and delay of elective spine procedures may be warranted.[42] Bisphosphonates dramatically suppress bone resorption and decrease hip and spine fractures. These agents inhibit osteoclast activity and directly stabilize the bone crystal, making it more resistant to osteoclastic bone resorption. Parathyroid hormone (Forteo) is anabolic to bone and leads to early, dramatic increases in bone mass. Preoperative Forteo programs, typically for 6 months, have been increasingly reported and may accelerate spinal fusion as well.[49]

When planning a spinal reconstruction procedure in an osteoporotic patient, it is important to recognize the differing vulnerabilities of various spinal structures. Trabecular bone represents 20% of the total bone mass and comprises the larger part of the vertebral body. Because trabecular bone exhibits eight times greater metabolic activity than cortical bone, osteoporosis affects trabecular bone earlier and to a greater degree than cortical bone.[50] The threshold BMD for successful anterior spinal instrumentation has been reported at 0.22 g/cm (as measured by quantitative computed tomography [CT]).[51]

The cortical bone of the pedicle and laminae is preserved longer in patients with early or moderate osteoporosis. As a result, posterior fixation is typically recommended. Initially, the relative holding power of pedicle screws versus infralaminar pedicle hooks was debated. While the pullout strength of hooks appears to be less sensitive to osteoporosis than screws, screws still offer greater fixation strength.[52]

Because of the difficulty achieving a stable anterior column reconstruction in an osteoporotic patient, combined anterior and posterior surgeries are often recommended to achieve adequate fixation. Other strategies to improve fixation in this patient population include augmentation of screw tracts with polymethylmethacrylate (PMMA), use of laminar hooks to protect inferior pedicle screws, expansion of screw designs, triangulated screw placement, increased use of transverse connectors, and bicortical vertebral body purchase.

BMD is linearly related to screw insertion torque and pullout strength.[53] The surgeon's tactile sense of purchase when placing the screw relates to construct strength. On the other hand, a recent study measured screw placement force and torque in 76 cadaveric pedicles.[54] Proper cannulation axial force was a mean 48 N. Medial and lateral breach required 129 and 86 N, respectively. The authors noted that "A large range of cannulation and breach forces and torques were measured due to variations in bone quality and geometry."

PMMA may be added to screw tracts to increase pullout strength (Fig. 70.3).

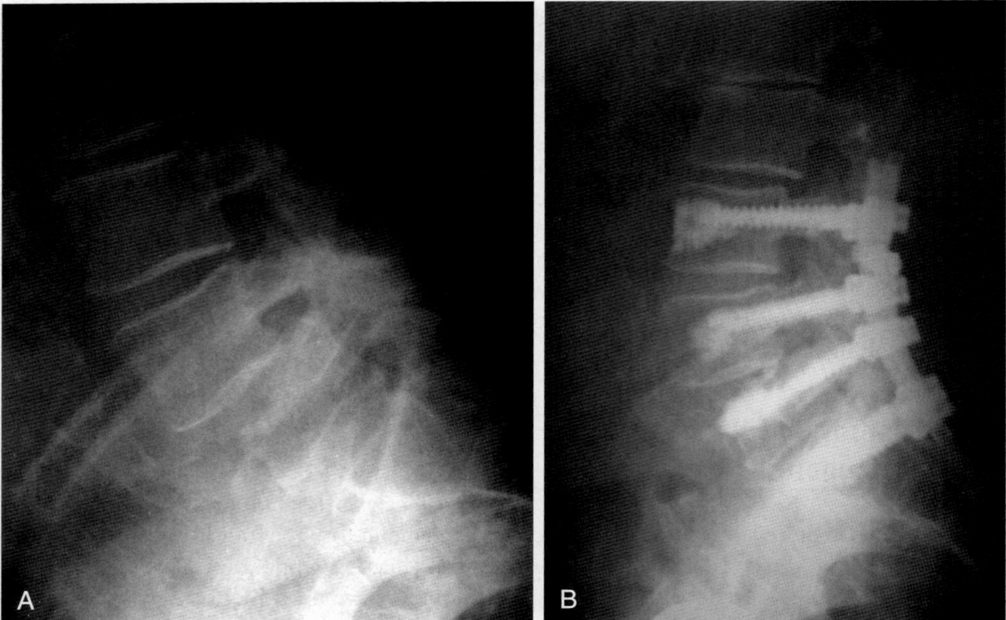

FIG. 70.3 (A) Preoperative and (B) postoperative lateral lumbar radiographs demonstrate the surgical strategy used in an osteoporotic patient with long-standing spinal stenosis associated with an L4–L5 spondylolisthesis as well as back pain from a nonhealing L5 superior endplate compression fracture. A facet-sparing laminectomy was performed as well as a three-level fusion from L3–S1. To improve fixation in the osteoporotic bone, cement augmentation (vertebroplasty) of the anterior cancellous bone was performed before screw insertion. At L5, balloon-assisted augmentation was undertaken to improve anterior load-bearing capacity. Additional fixation points, including L3 and L5, were also used.

Use of calcium sulfate and PMMA augmentation of the vertebral body continues to be reported to restore anterior column stability in combination with posterior transpedicular screw placement in trauma, tumor, and other indications. Typically, good outcomes with minimal cement leak rates and without associated complications are reported.[55,56] In addition to kyphoplasty and vertebroplasty techniques, a vertebral body stenting approach has also been described.[57]

Cannulated screws with ports for PMMA injection have been reported with reasonable results. Other surgeons simply place the PMMA before placing the screw, arguing that a doughier PMMA can be placed if not requiring extrusion through small holes in the screw.[58] PMMA augmentation has also been used in the reconstruction of pathologic fractures from neoplastic disease, including those in which the pedicle itself has been compromised.[59]

Although bicortical purchase increases the screw's pullout strength and resistance to cyclic loading, BMD has an overall greater impact.[60] Improved unicortical screw strength can be achieved with triangulated and subchondral placement.[61-63]

If bilateral screws are placed in a triangulated pattern, use of a transverse or cross connector further increases fixation strength. Mechanically, stability is improved by the presence of bone between the screws rather than merely by the bone within the threads of each screw individually. Avoid parallelogram (four-bar linkage) constructs in which the screws and longitudinal members form a perfect square or rectangle. These constructs resist lateral loads less well than a triangulated pedicle screw placement.[64] In anterior dual-rod constructs, a trapezoidal short-short/long-long construct is typically recommended.

Screw length is linearly related to pullout strength. Little difference is seen between self-drilling or self-tapping designs; if tapping is performed, undertapping by 1 mm leads to greater pullout strength than undertapping by 0.5 mm.[65,66] For sacral screws, especially in long constructs, bicortical screws improve holding power and sagittal plane correction. Some authors have recommended aiming the screw upward into the disc space or through the sacral promontory.[67,68]

Another option lies in transdiscal screw placement. Here, lumbar pedicle screws are aimed cranially through the superior endplate, across the disc space, and into the vertebral body above. Most typically, this approach has been used in spondylolisthesis. Depending on pedicle size, this can add holding power to screws across even sagittally aligned segments.[69]

The implants themselves may also be modified to address a given patient's clinical needs. For example, maximizing the diameter of typical pedicle screws improves pullout strength and decreases the risk of fatigue failure of the screw. Other, newer approaches include hydroxyapatite (HA) screw coatings to improve screw-bone integration. One recent study found that the HA shank prevented triggered electromyographic responses.[70] Increasingly, surface roughness and nanostructural surfaces are being studied to improve osseointegration of screws and other spine implants.[71] Drug- and chemotherapy-eluting implants have recently been devised for specific clinical situations. One recent study described successful use of pedicle screws with iodine surfaces to decrease concerns about bacterial adherence and biofilm formation.[72]

Posterior Thoracolumbar Instrumentation

Modern, posterior, rigid, segmental spine stabilization systems arose in response to kyphoscoliosis deformity occurring in patients surviving polio and tuberculosis.[73] Internal stabilization began in the early 1900s by Lange, but it was not until the 1950s and 1960s that Harrington, Moe, and others developed the first generation of modern spinal instrumentation.[74] In the 1980s, Cotrel and Dubousset first popularized rigid, segmental hook-based fixation.[75]

Currently, rigid, segmental, posterior transpedicular constructs represent the most common form of thoracolumbar instrumentation. Despite the dominance and versatility of transpedicular constructs, instrumentation failure is by no means rare. The implants below are orgnanized by the bone elements to which they anchor.

The midline posterior approach remains the most common access route for placement of thoracolumbar instrumentation. This extensile approach is applicable from the occiput to the sacrum. Below L2–L3, the dural sac may be safely retracted to afford enough exposure to the posterior disc space for performance of a posterior lumbar interbody fusion. In the upper lumbar spine, the risk of neural injury with dural retraction increases, and more oblique approaches to the disc space, such as transforaminal lumbar interbody fusion (TLIF), are safer. Practically, however, these oblique posterior approaches to the thoracolumbar disc space have become more common at every level.

In the thoracic spine, a midline posterior approach is considered dangerous for decompression of anterior compressive pathology. The lateral extracavitary or costotransversectomy approach allows access to thoracic vertebral bodies from a posterior approach without violation of the pleura or takedown of the diaphragm.[76] While this approach allows a one-step approach to decompression and long, rigid, posterior stabilization, anterior column visualization and access are inferior to that afforded by a transthoracic approach. Significantly more bone resection (including the rib, costotransverse joint, facets, and pedicle) is required to achieve that visualization. Costotransversectomy is associated with increased blood loss, longer operative time, increased paraspinal muscle disruption, and chest wall numbness from intercostal nerve resection. Occasionally, anterolateral cord compression can be addressed with a compromise approach between a standard laminectomy and a formal costotransversectomy. These transpedicular decompressions are known by various names, such as pediculofacetectomy, and are particularly useful in patients with tumors in whom the neoplasm has already destroyed most of the pedicle.[77,78] In this case, the decompression is mainly soft tissue removal, and the anterior compressive elements can be removed indirectly by pulling them away. Although this approach confers limited visualization, even relative to costotransversectomy, it reduces operative time, blood loss, and iatrogenic destabilization. An angled microscope or 70-degree endoscope may improve visualization of the anatomy anterior to the dura.[79]

Most thoracolumbar instrumentation requires a relatively wide exposure beyond the facet and out into the transverse process. The powerful retractor systems affording this wide exposure create extremely high levels of intramuscular pressure.[80] Over time, this pressure can cause muscle necrosis similar to a compartment syndrome. For longer cases, the retractors should be removed every 2 hours to allow muscle recovery. This recovery time is particularly important because preoperative muscle abnormalities may exist in some conditions, which can be accentuated by the trauma of extended muscle retraction.

Over time, a variety of less invasive approaches to the posterolateral lumbar spine have evolved. For example, the Wiltse paramedian approach, although initially described for resection of far-lateral disc herniations, has been used for interbody and posterolateral fusions.[81] A bilateral paramedian trajectory in the intermuscular plane between the longissimus and multifidus muscles is best when no midline decompression is needed. In addition, this approach could be considered for posterolateral pseudarthrosis revision to avoid midline scar. A variant of the Wiltse paramedian approach is used in most MIS fusions using tubular retractors, microscopic dissection, and fluoroscopic guidance. Iatrogenic muscle injury can result from denervation of the primary motor branch of the dorsal primary ramus when the muscle is stripped from the midline beyond the facets.[82]

Interspinous Process Stabilization

A variety of interspinous process devices have been introduced for varying indications. Most share a minimally invasive concept in that they can be inserted with the patient under local or limited anesthesia through small incisions. However, some devices require formal, open exposure of the posterior elements to attach or wrap "artificial ligaments" or other outriggers.

In North America, the most familiar of these interspinous process devices is the X-STOP (Medtronic). Marketed as a less-invasive alternative to laminectomy, the X-STOP is used to distract the spinous processes in patients with symptomatic spinal stenosis. Subtle segmental flexion or prevention of extension is said to increase canal diameter and relieve neural compression.

In 2005, a randomized, controlled, prospective, multicenter trial of 191 patients with neurogenic claudication compared outcomes of patients treated with X-STOP with outcomes of patients receiving nonoperative care. At 2 years, the symptom severity score of patients treated with X-STOP improved by 45.4% over mean baseline. The control group had only 7.4% improvement. Physical function improved 44.3% in the X-STOP group but declined in the controls. The authors concluded that the X-STOP provided effective treatment for patients with spinal stenosis (Fig. 70.4).[83]

Subsequently, studies have compared less-invasive decompression with X-STOP surgery. Similar clinical outcomes were achieved, but the interspinous process device has a higher rate

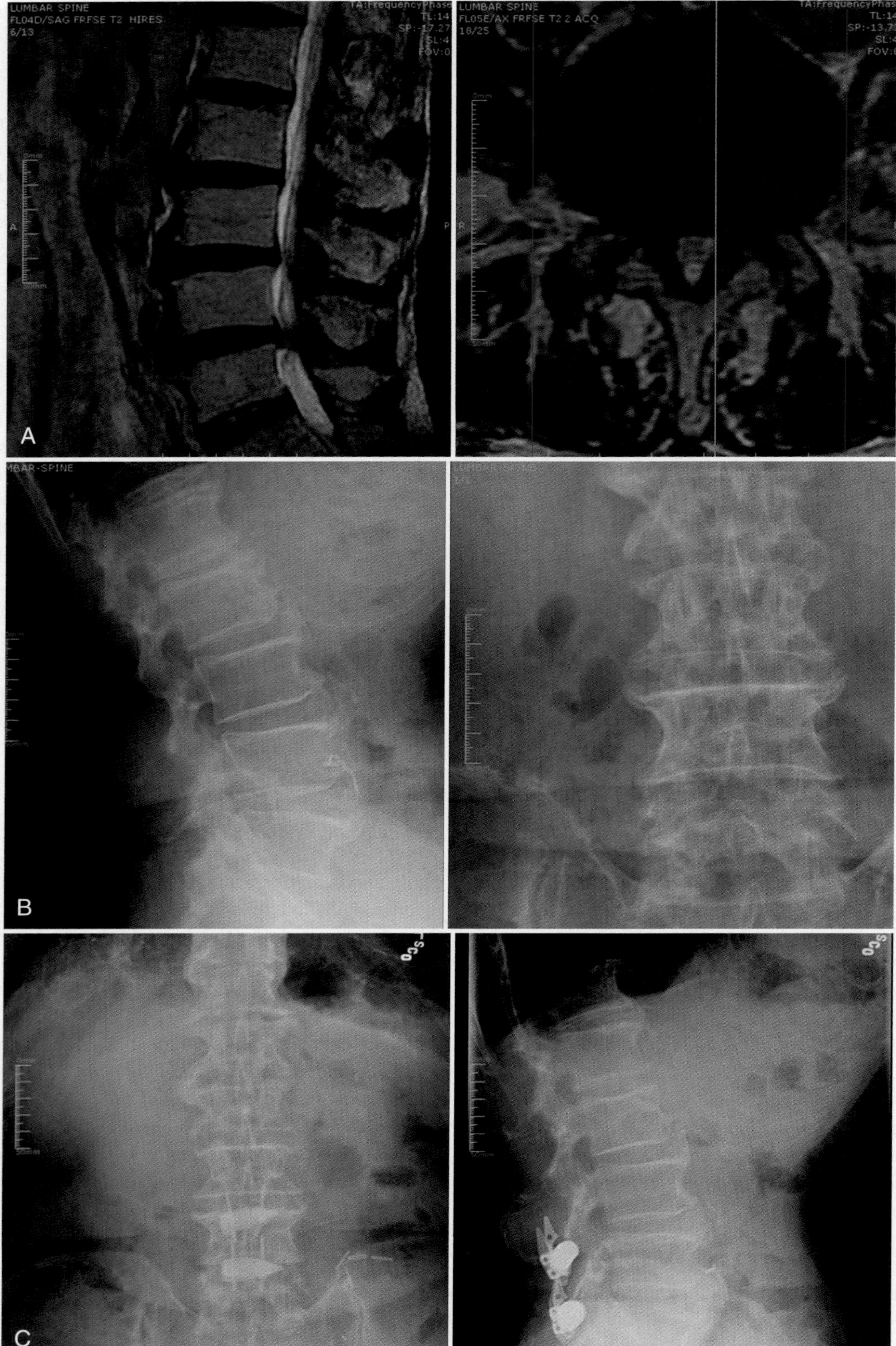

FIG. 70.4 As a less-invasive alternative to laminectomy, an interspinous spacer is used to distract the spinous processes in patients with symptomatic spinal stenosis. Subtle segmental flexion or prevention of extension is said to increase canal diameter and relieve neural compression. (A) Preoperative magnetic resonance image showing multilevel stenosis. (B) Preoperative radiographs. (C) Postoperative radiographs showing placement of interspinous spacers placed at L4–L5 and L3–L4.

of secondary surgery and a much higher cost of care.[84,85] Use of this device appears to be declining, however, and reasonable outcomes with newer study devices have been reported.[86,87]

Other interspinous process devices are used to stabilize the segment rather than decompress the canal. Some of these are meant to be used after decompression and in lieu of or as a means of achieving segmental fusion.[88]

One of the devices intended to treat mechanical low back pain through either distraction or restriction of motion was the Wallis implant (Zimmer Biomet), in which a semielastic blocker dampens forces passing through the posterior elements while decreasing the neutral zone.[89] The first-generation implant, with a titanium blocker and an artificial ligament made of Dacron, was developed in 1986. More than 300 patients were implanted from 1988 to 1993. Subsequently, a PEEK version of the Wallis implant was developed. Without permanent fixation into the vertebral bone, the "floating" design of the Wallis and similar implants seeks to avoid the risk of loosening encountered with pedicle screw–based and facet replacement–based dynamic stabilization systems. According to a more recent review of the Wallis implant, significant improvements in back pain were seen "without serious complications." The Wallis system was recommended for (1) discectomy when massive fragment leads to substantial loss of disc material, (2) first disc herniation recurrence, (3) discectomy for herniation of a transitional disc with sacralization of L5, (4) degenerative disc disease at a level adjacent to a previous fusion, and (5) isolated endplate lesions leading to chronic low back pain.

A recent study reported 2-year outcomes of posterior tension band placement after laminectomy and in lieu of fusion in patients with degenerative stenosis and spondylolisthesis. Good clinical outcomes, no progressive instability, and only one reoperation were reported.[90]

Spinous process fixation may also be used during fusion procedures as a posterior tension band. Because of the limited stability afforded by the spinous process, these devices were initially recommended to "back up" anterior lumbar interbody fusion (ALIF) procedures. Recently, a biomechanical study was undertaken to compare the utility of such a device with transpedicular instrumentation in stabilizing the spine after insertion of a lateral interbody cage in six cadavers.[91] The authors found that posterior supplementary fixation increased stability but that pedicle screws offered additional coronal plane stability. At this point, little long-term data or biomechanical data under multiple load cycles are available. In another biomechanical study, the interspinous process device improved flexion-extension stability compared with ALIF alone, but demonstrated little lateral bending or rotational stability when compared with a bilateral pedicle screw construct.[92]

One recent review concluded that although the wide variety of designs and materials for interspinous process devices was generally safe, the clinical benefits declined over the long term.[93] Spinous process–based devices have limited utility at L5–S1 due to the small size of the S1 spinous process. A recent study found that the sacral spines were highly variable in their morphology but had a similar load to failure of lumbar spinous processes.[94] In addition, spinous process erosion or fracture can occur with either the motion-preserving or fusion devices.

Facet-Based Stabilization

Numerous methods of facet fixation have been proposed. Historically, small screws were placed directly through the facet joint. Although these screws were able to lock the facets, their short length produced too small of a lever arm to counteract the forces to which the lumbar facet is exposed, and many of these implants failed. Techniques at the present time are exploring additional methods of bony purchase. The most common of these is the Magerl technique, in which 4.5-mm, fully threaded cortical screws, usually 50 to 60 mm in length, are passed from the opposite side of the spinous process through the ipsilateral lamina and across the facet.[95] The Boucher technique is similar but incorporates a greater degree of pedicle penetration.[96] In both of these techniques, the screws are not placed in lag mode.

These translaminar facet screws are indicated for one- or two-level fixation when reduction is not needed. Most often, they have been used as posterior column stabilization after ALIF procedures. The advantages of these screws include minimally invasive insertion via a 4-cm percutaneous approach. Translaminar facet screws are much less expensive than transpedicular constructs and offer less impingement on surrounding musculature.

Using contemporary techniques, fusion rates are high and cases of screw failure are rare. Recently, facet screws were compared with pedicle screws in 62 patients undergoing circumferential single-level lumbar fusion.[97] Facet screw utilization was associated with less blood loss, cost and, at long-term follow-up, less back pain and adjacent-segment degeneration than pedicle screw placement.

Disadvantages to translaminar facet fixation include absence of the three-column purchase afforded by transpedicular instrumentation. Patients may therefore need postoperative immobilization. Contraindications to translaminar facet screws include absence of adequate lamina or facet joints. These screws may be placed after laminotomy procedures but not typically after full laminectomy.

Recently, focus on direct facet and translaminar facet screws has declined due to increased use of spinous process fixation and cortical screws. That said, as a means of posterior tension band reconstruction after ALIF, though, they continue to have a longer track record than the newer techniques mentioned.[98]

Over the last 10 years, a number of percutaneously placed allograft dowels and other facet joint implants have been marketed as adjuncts to fusion. Reports of clinical effectiveness remain sparse. A recent biomechanical study of six cadaveric specimens compared two facet bone dowels.[99] One offered little stability at any time point. The other did restrict flexion-extension motion but lost fixation after 5000 cycles. The authors concluded that these devices were not mechanically effective and warned that "considerable magnitudes of device migration were detected."

When the previous edition of this text was published, study of facet arthroplasty systems was underway. These systems were not intended to treat facet-mediated axial low back pain, but rather to restore stability after laminectomy without necessitating spinal fusion. They fit into a narrow treatment window between clearly unstable spines (e.g., spines with scoliosis or a dynamic spondylolisthesis) that require concomitant fusion and cases in which a narrow decompression can be performed that would not jeopardize postoperative stability.

Creation of a functional facet replacement system is a complex undertaking. Four main components, the superior and inferior right and left facets, have to be sized to the individual. Different designs rely on varying forms of attachment, but fixation through the pedicle is generally required. Various outriggers, cross-links, or other devices hold the system together and balance tension to maintain stability while maintaining segmental motion. Although a 7-year follow-up study of 10 patients treated internationally for spinal stenosis and spondylosis revealed reasonable results, it appears that clinical study of these devices in North America has been abandoned.[100]

Laminar Wires, Ribbons, and Hooks

Posterior thoracolumbar instrumentation has traditionally been divided into rigid and nonrigid implants. The earliest constructs incorporated the spinous processes or other posterior elements alone or with slabs of structural iliac crest autograft. Although simple wiring techniques are no longer used in the thoracolumbar spine, many wire-rod techniques continue to be routinely used. The most common technique—Luque wiring—uses sublaminar wires as anchors. These wires are wrapped around rods to form a segmental, nonrigid spine construct. Such techniques are nonrigid because they allow "pistoning" of the spine in a craniocaudal direction. Luque's construct was the first segmental system that used multiple wire attachment points.[73,101]

In North America, Luque constructs are currently preferentially used in the thoracic spine. Common indications include neuromuscular scoliosis, scoliosis with thoracic lordosis, and occasional cases of idiopathic scoliosis. Hybrid constructs using Luque wires with pedicle screws and other bone anchors are more commonly used. Contraindications to sublaminar fixation include absence of laminae. In addition, there is a danger of passing the wire through the spinal canal, particularly in patients with kyphosis or canal stenosis.[102] Because wiring techniques do not provide axial stability, they are a poor choice for stabilization of pathologic processes with anterior column insufficiency. For example, sublaminar wires should not be used as primary fixation in patients with vertebral fractures or tumors.

In response to the risk of sublaminar wire passage, Drummond proposed a technique, commonly referred to as the Wisconsin method, in which the rod is wired to the spinous processes.[103,104] This method has been used with Harrington rods and other rod systems to provide additional stability by segmental fixation.[105] A button may be used to decrease wire cut-through of the spinous process. Although this technique is rarely used alone anymore, it may be useful in hybrid constructs, particularly when limitations of bony anatomy or breakout of prior instrumentation renders the pedicles and other posterior elements unusable.

The next evolutionary step after wiring in thoracolumbar instrumentation came with simple, hook-based distraction devices intended to assist in the correction of scoliosis. After Harrington's initial ground-breaking design, several other modified designs were developed. Harrington rods were used in thoracic curves and for thoracolumbar burst fractures.[106] In trauma cases, the Harrington system provided quick and easy stabilization compared with the earlier devices. This construct could be combined with a rod sleeve to provide a three-point fixation and was particularly advantageous in polytrauma patients. Because Harrington rods produced distraction, they often led to flat back deformities that resulted in persistent pain and fatigue. When the importance of sagittal plane balance was understood, and as newer, more powerful systems became available, Harrington rods fell out of use.

Early hook-based segmental thoracolumbar spine constructs allowed lordosis to be contoured into the rod and held with segmental bone anchorage. These constructs were significantly more rigid than their predecessors. This increased rigidity improved fusion rates and sometimes obviated the need for postoperative bracing or cast immobilization. This was particularly advantageous for children and adolescents undergoing surgical correction of idiopathic scoliosis.

Disadvantages of this construct, as with rigid implants elsewhere, included the effect of fusion on adjacent segments. In contrast to pedicle screw constructs, which use the concept of three-column spine fixation, hooks anchor to the posterior elements alone and do not have the same power to reduce scoliosis.[107] Although misplaced pedicle screws can produce catastrophic neurologic or vascular injury, hooks by their very nature are canal intrusive. Volumetric studies suggest that mildly misplaced screws produce less canal encroachment than hooks.[108]

In a comparison of pullout strength, thoracic pedicle screws were found to be significantly stronger than hooks and were recommended for rigid curves.[109] Another study, in children with idiopathic scoliosis, found no differences in operative time or curve correction achieved with hook or screw constructs.[110]

Various hooks with different characteristics are available. Each of these is suited to a particular mode of placement and loading. Pedicle hooks, resting on the lamina of the instrumented vertebra and the superior articular process of the next distal vertebra, are the strongest. They are always directed cephalad so that their U-shaped tip captures the pedicle and provides maximal stability for rotation and translation maneuvers. Because of their configuration and their dependence on facet joint anatomy, these implants can be placed from T1 to T10 or T11.[111] There are subtle variations in hook shape, including short-throated and long-throated configurations and straight or offset collars. Contemporary anatomic hook designs give better bony contact.

Laminar hooks are available in various designs. Variation in blade width and style and the relationship of the blade to the body of the hook allow for optimal hook-bone interface. Between T3–T10 or T11, lamina hooks may also be placed on the superior surface of the transverse process. Here the transverse process hook is combined with a pedicle hook to yield a pedicle-transverse grip or "claw." Although such claws may be constructed over one or two levels, two-level claws are easier to insert and mechanically stronger.[112] Claws are used mainly at the ends of a construct. Above T3, the transverse process becomes more horizontal, and transverse process hooks do not align with the pedicle hook. The claws must be pedicle–supralaminar hook combinations.

A supralaminar hook enters the spinal canal in a cranial to caudal direction and, while providing the second strongest anchorage, risks iatrogenic cord injury if the hook pistons in and out of the canal during rod manipulation. Thus, careful selection of the hook shape is mandatory. Moreover, one should consider avoiding periapical placement or utilization of supralaminar hooks in the correction of hyperkyphosis. Finally, infralaminar hooks are placed in a cephalad direction. These anchors are rarely necessary in the thoracic spine because pedicle hooks provide proximally directed forces. Usually, these implants are used inferiorly, along with pedicle screws in hybrid constructs. Occasionally, they are added to transpedicular constructs to protect the screws from pullout.[113]

In younger patients with painful pars defects and minimal segmental degeneration, a screw-hook combination can be used for direct osteosynthesis of the spondylolysis.[114]

While wired, semirigid constructs are no longer frequently used as a stand-alone in lumbar spine surgery, these tools are occasionally used in osteoporotic patients or in deformity or trauma surgery to improve reduction or provide temporary or adjunctive fixation before transpedicular implants are used.[115]

For some indications, sublaminar wires have given way to polyester bands. The possible advantages of these bands include their radiolucency and the wider surface area through which to grip osteoporotic bone (which may mean less cut-through compared with sublaminar wires).[116] Sublaminar and transverse process polyester band fixation has been reported to successfully aid the reduction of scoliosis.[117]

A recent report of 115 neuromuscular scoliosis cases included 29 patients treated with a hybrid pedicle screw, polyester clamp and band technique.[118] At a mean of 29 months' follow-up, a 69% correction had been achieved and sagittal balance was corrected to within 2 cm of the C7 plumb line in 97% of the patients. The authors believed these results compared favorably to sublaminar wire and all pedicle screw cases. In particular, they wrote "Sublaminar bands utilized in a hybrid construct appear to be safe, can achieve corrections equivalent to all-pedicle screw constructs, and may decrease the potential complications associated with every level transpedicular fixation in the patient with a highly dysmorphic and osteoporotic spine."

Unfortunately, sublaminar implant passage may still subject the patient to iatrogenic neurologic injury. In one recent series of 21 patients with neuromuscular scoliosis, two neurologic injuries occurred.[116] Although successful radiographic outcomes were achieved, the authors suggested tempered enthusiasm for this technique.

Although these bands are typically placed in a sublaminar trajectory, subtransverse bands have also been reported.[119] Superelastic cables have recently been tested under the theory that they would provide constant stabilization during various loading modes.[120]

Pedicle Screws

Pedicle screws continue to offer the only three-column fixation available in the thoracolumbar spine. Because they are inserted from the posterior elements into the vertebral body, they allow the surgeon to apply distraction, compression, lordosis, rotation, or translatory forces selectively.[121]

Pedicle screw systems have been studied in Europe since the early 1980s. Modern attempts at pedicle fixation were popularized in North America by Steffee. Their use temporarily declined after a series of television exposés and high-profile lawsuits. Subsequently, many of the available systems received FDA class II status. This approval stopped many of the lawsuits and led to a rapid escalation in the number of systems available and the extent of their use.[122] Advantages of transpedicular fixation spine include:

- Rigid segmental fixation
- Improved fusion rates
- Reduction of deformity and maintenance of correction
- Earlier rehabilitation
- Minimized use of postoperative bracing

Disadvantages and complications of pedicular screw fixation include:

- Increased operative time and risk of infection
- Increased cost
- Risk of pedicle fracture
- Increased complication rates, particularly with regard to implant soft tissue impingement and screw malposition
- Dural tear
- Nerve toot or spinal cord injury
- Anterior vascular injury
- Stress shielding and device-related osteopenia
- Risk of adjacent-level degeneration

Adjacent-segment degeneration issues continue to plague lumbar fusion patients. Park and colleagues found that pedicle screw placement, more than the actual number of levels fused, was the strongest predictor of adjacent-segment degeneration.[123] This review reported a 12.2% to 18.5% incidence of symptomatic adjacent-segment degeneration during the follow-up period compared with a 5.2% to 5.6% rate in patients fused with other forms of instrumentation or no instrumentation. Damage to the adjacent unfused facet by the screw was thought to be a potentially significant factor producing adjacent-level degeneration. Unintended adjacent-level fusion may also be encountered more frequently in patients undergoing transpedicular instrumentation. One prospective, randomized trial of 130 patients undergoing either instrumented or uninstrumented fusion found that inadvertent fusion had occurred in 19 cases (14%). There was a higher risk of unintended fusion with pedicle screw instrumentation, although functional outcomes were not affected.[124]

The role of stress shielding in patient outcomes is controversial. The concept was introduced by McAfee and colleagues in 1991.[125] Subsequent studies have failed to show osteoporotic collapse within a fusion construct. Transpedicular screw fixation does not affect the postoperative reduction of fusion mass.[126] The indications for and contraindications to pedicle screw placement remain controversial. Pedicle screw constructs are widely indicated in cases with clearly defined instability, particularly in the setting of trauma and tumor. In particular, they provide stability where prior laminectomy has been performed.

Pedicle screw systems may also be divided by the type of longitudinal member or the connection between the anchor and the longitudinal member. Plating systems are one such system and are generally less expensive than modular, polyaxial screw-and-rod systems. Typically, plate-screw systems require that the screws function as bolts that are rigidly affixed to the plates with nuts and washers. Contemporary polyaxial systems have a U-shaped saddle in the head of the screw into which the rod can be secured. Polyaxial systems fare better under static and cyclic compressive loads. Because higher rod manipulation forces are possible, these connections serve to increase stresses at the end levels of the construct. Although theoretically their increased freedom of motion should make polyaxial screw constructs less stiff, this has not been borne out in cadaveric testing.[127] Rods are discussed in greater detail below.

Clinical failure of transpedicular constructs occurs in one of two ways: through loosening with fixation failure or through failure to fuse. Loosening occurs as repetitive loading persists beyond the tolerance of bone. This is usually the result of delayed union or motion at a screw-bone interface, often from excessive activity. The screw is exposed to a combination of cantilever bending and axial pullout loads (Fig. 70.5).

Subacute or acute bending failure and implant breakage result from cantilever bending loads in excess of the yield point of the screws. Even severely degenerated and collapsed discs undergo cyclic axial displacement during axial loading. These cyclic displacements may lead to significant cantilever loads and bending moments. These are most pronounced around the screw hub, inside the pedicle.

This effect is multiplied when the screw-rod construct operates in a bridging mode and bears most or all of the anterior column axial loads, as with burst fractures. If a deformity reduction maneuver is performed during surgery, this subjects the screws to increased load. Typically, the end vertebrae are affected. Various techniques for correction, such as derotation maneuvers, have been described. A strategy that emphasizes correction in the middle segments of the construct with decreased corrective force at the terminal levels is associated with good reduction, while limiting axial tensile forces at the cranial end screw.[128,129] After bony healing, fatigue failure of the implants may still theoretically occur but should no longer be of clinical concern.

A number of studies sought to retrospectively quantify pedicle screw–related complications. Significant variability was seen among studies, with overall complications of varying severity reported up to 54%. Rates of deep infections, screw misplacement, and screw breakage ranged from 5% to 10% but appeared to be decreasing in more recent studies.[130-133]

Spondylolisthesis may be stabilized with or without an attempt at slip reduction. Reduction maneuvers include rod contouring with an additional cranial fixation point with screws with an extended head into which the rod can be forcibly delivered, translating the slipped segment posteriorly.[134,135] Some screw-rod systems have been designed solely for slip reduction. With reduction of an L5–S1 spondylolisthesis, there is increased risk of a postoperative L5 root palsy.[136] Although slip reduction has not been shown to improve outcomes, more recent series also report very low rates of L5 root injury.[137,138] Pedicle screw constructs are also routinely used to increase the likelihood of fusion in the surgical management of junctional stenosis, degenerative spondylolisthesis or scoliosis, isthmic spondylolisthesis, prior pseudarthrosis, and more than a three-level fusion (Fig. 70.6).

Typically, pedicle screw fixation is avoided in the presence of overt infection, but it may be considered in cases of significant instability. Relative contraindications to pedicle screw fixation include very small pedicles, marked osteoporosis, and inadequate anterior column support.

The question of when to add pedicle screw fixation remains unanswered. Although pedicle screw instrumentation enhances the rate of spinal fusion in degenerative

FIG. 70.5 When posterior thoracolumbar instrumentation fails, it is usually at the screw-bone interface. (A) If fusion fails to occur, the screws may loosen, as demonstrated by the lucency around the pedicle screws. Various techniques have been reported to improve screw pullout strength of the construct. (B) One technique uses screw insertion into the endplate of the level above for additional purchase. (C–D) This elderly, osteoporotic patient had had a previous long fusion to L5. Subsequently he developed an isthmic spondylolisthesis at L5–S1 with a progressive slip. He returned to the operating room for extension of fusion to the pelvis. The Bohlman technique of posterior fibular strut placement from S1 to L5 was undertaken using a reamer over the guide wire shown in the (C) lateral fluoroscopic image. (D) Postoperative axial computed tomographic image shows the fibular strut in good position. Short iliac screws were also placed. (E) In patients with poor bone quality, polymethylmethacrylate may be used in the vertebral body to improve screw pullout strength. Another concern is the appropriate number of fixation points; the more unstable the spine or the poorer the quality of the patient's bone, the more fixation points are required for a successful construct. (F) Failure of a long scoliosis construct presumably because too much force was concentrated at the base, where all the inferior anchors were crowded together.

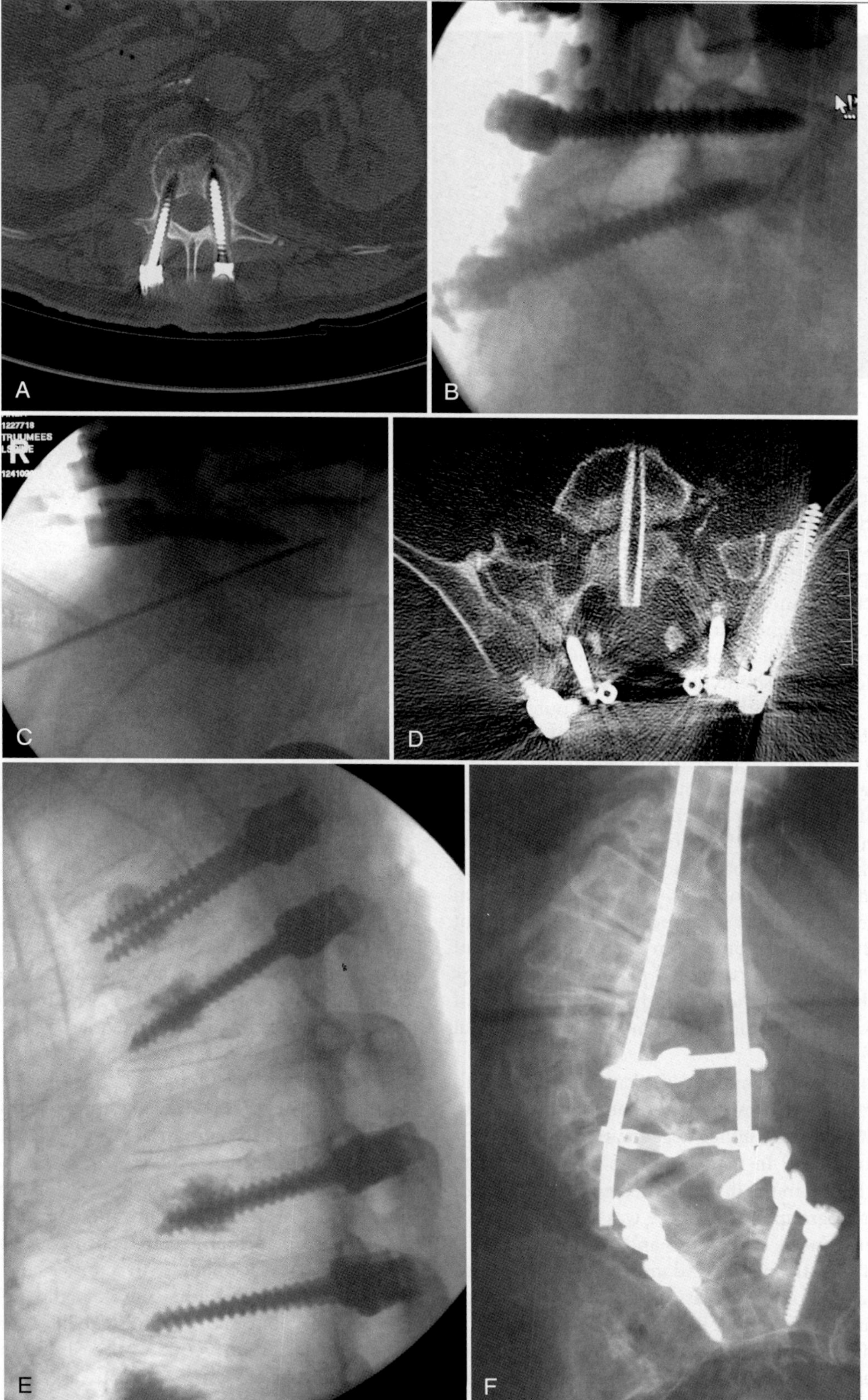
A
B
C
D
E
F

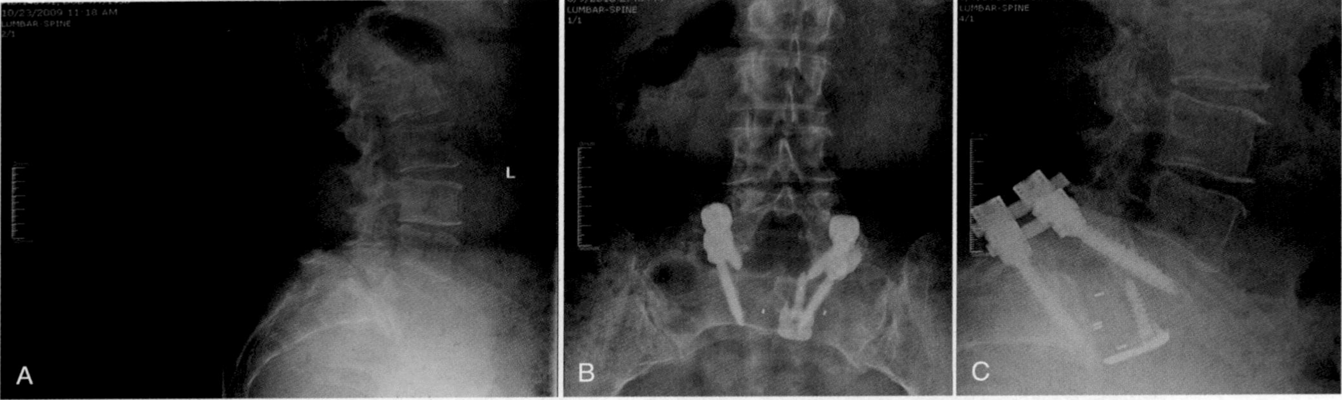

FIG. 70.6 A 65-year-old woman with L5–S1 isthmic spondylolisthesis who underwent anterior L5–S1 anterior lumbar interbody fusion with instrumentation followed by posterior instrumentation and fusion. (A) Lateral preoperative standing radiograph. Postoperative (B) anteroposterior and (C) lateral standing radiographs.

conditions of the lumbar spine, such fusion does not always correlate with clinical outcomes. Conversely, patients may report excellent symptomatic improvement even in the setting of radiographic pseudarthrosis.[139]

One prospective, randomized, controlled trial of 130 patients evaluated supplementary pedicle screw fixation in posterolateral lumbar spinal fusion and found that fusion rates were not significantly different between instrumented and uninstrumented groups. Although functional outcome, as assessed by the Dallas Pain Questionnaire, improved significantly in uninstrumented and instrumented groups, there were no significant differences in outcome between the two groups. A trend toward higher patient satisfaction was noted in the instrumented group (82%) versus the uninstrumented group (74%). The addition of pedicle screws significantly increased operative time, blood loss, and early reoperation rate. The two infections in that series occurred in the implant group, and significant symptoms from screw misplacement were seen in 4.8% of the instrumented patients. The authors concluded that these results did not justify the general use of pedicle screw fixation as a routine adjunct to posterolateral lumbar fusion.[140]

A similar prospective, randomized, controlled trial with 5-year follow-up was performed in 129 patients with severe chronic low back pain from either degenerative instability or isthmic spondylolisthesis. In that series, the reoperation rate was significantly higher in the instrumented group (25%) than the uninstrumented group (14%). There was no difference in work capacity between the two groups and no significant difference between the instrumented and uninstrumented groups in regard to functional outcome, as measured by the Dallas Pain Questionnaire and Low Back Pain Rating Scale. When the subgroups of isthmic and degenerative spondylolisthesis were analyzed separately, patients with isthmic spondylolisthesis had a significantly better outcome after posterolateral fusion without supplemental instrumentation compared with instrumented fusion ($P < .03$). Patients with primary degenerative spondylolisthesis had more significant improvement with instrumented posterolateral fusion ($P < .02$).[141]

In a recent American Association of Neurological Surgeons guideline, use of pedicle screws as an adjunct to lumbar fusion in degenerative disease was recommended to be "reserved for those patients in whom there is an increased risk of nonunion when treated with only PLF."[142]

Once a decision has been made to use transpedicular screw fixation, the numbers of levels of fixation should also be considered. Historically, internal spine fixators were applied to the cranial and caudal fusion levels. This approach was associated, in the lumbar spine, with flat back deformity. These systems are also less rigid than segmental fixation, in which one or more bone anchors are placed in every or most intervening levels of long fusions as well.

Classically, additional segmental fixation may benefit patients undergoing deformity correction or trauma stabilization. In a recent finite element analysis of an adolescent idiopathic scoliosis model (with data taken from 20 real patients), fixation was simulated over a mean 8.9 segments with a mean 45-degree Cobb angle correction.[27] Using a simultaneous double-rod rotation technique, a 160-N pullout force was measured at the apical concave screw. Forces on the convex side were lower at about 35 N. Push forces on the lower and upper instrumented vertebrae were 305.1 N on the concave side and 86.4 N on the convex side. The authors concluded that these forces were within safe margins for a segmental construct; however, to protect from implant failure or pedicle fracture, appropriate soft tissue release and facetectomy were required.

Another recent study compared consecutive-level screw fixation with interval fixation and found better corrections in all three planes and better cosmetic results with higher density screw placement.[143] In another study, planned screw dropout at the periapical convexity did not decrease curve correction.[144] One study found that full screw placement did not afford better correction of the rib hump than interval or hybrid constructs.[145]

In posterior-only treatment of Scheuermann kyphosis, the correction and outcomes of a mean of 25 screws placed in 10 patients were compared with 16.8 screws placed in 11 patients.[146] Similar corrections were achieved, but complications and costs were higher in the high screw density group (19% vs. 9% and 32%, respectively) In one recent study, levels fused had a greater impact on outcomes than pedicle screw density, which was most closely correlated, as expected, with costs.[147]

Posttraumatic spinal instability raises similar questions about the number of levels to incorporate in a surgical construct. One recent biomechanical study found that, with the exception of lateral bending, short-segment fixation with fracture-level screws was equivalent to two-level above and below constructs.[148]

A retrospective review of 32 patients with comminuted burst fractures reported excellent clinical and radiographic outcomes with short-segment fixation incorporating the injured vertebra.[149] In a 70-patient comparative study of short-segment instrumentation for burst fracture with and without fracture-level screw placement, additional screws were associated with better kyphosis and anterior vertebral height correction.[150] The clinical significance of these radiographic findings was not clear. The utility of this six-screw construct has been confirmed in other recent reports.[151]

The ability of posterior implants to function in a bridging mode to stabilize patients with major defects in anterior column stability (such as a burst fracture or tumor) is diminished in osteoporosis. In this setting, formal anterior column support through PMMA augmentation or corpectomy and cage reconstruction may be preferred, even in medically frail patients. One recent study recommended anterior column support through a formal corpectomy approach followed by posterior transpedicular instrumentation over screws and kyphoplasty for anterior column support.[152]

Here, too, it is important to recognize the planes of instability. Although PMMA augmentation may improve axial stiffness, it will do little to compensate for posterior tension band disruption. In a recent biomechanical study, kyphoplasty alone was not effective in stabilizing high-energy burst fractures.[153]

Just as modifications to increase implant hold are needed in patients with poor bone quality, increased rigidity will be needed in patients with additional stress on the construct, such as those of a greater size or with movement disorders.[154]

Certainly, less-robust constructs are required in patients with degenerative spinal conditions. Here, for one-level fusions for degenerative indications, the potential benefits of unilateral instrumentation include decreased surgical time, blood loss, muscle trauma, and cost. In two recent meta-analyses, these conclusions were supported, as were equivalent clinical and radiographic outcomes.[155,156] Other recent studies have supported this conclusion.[157] On the other hand, in one study of 80 patients undergoing single-level lumbar TLIF for degenerative disease, the pseudarthrosis rate was significantly higher in the unilateral fixation group (17.5%) compared with the bilateral fixation group (2.5%).[158] The authors concluded that bilateral fixation was likely biomechanically superior. A 2014 meta-analysis incorporated five prospective studies with 407 patients to compare the outcomes of unilateral and bilateral pedicle screw placement in lumbar degenerative disease.[159] The authors concluded that there were no differences in fusion rates or outcomes, but that operative time and blood loss were lower in the unilateral group.

In a biomechanical study, a translaminar facet screw contralateral to unilateral pedicle screw placement was found to improve stability to the level of bilateral screw-rod placement.[160] A similar group of authors did not find any clinical benefits of adding a contralateral transfacet screw in a comparative study of 58 patients.[161]

Cortical Screws

Laterally directed, cortical screws have been increasingly used in the lumbar spine (Fig. 70.7). Potential advantages of these screws are a near-midline placement, thereby decreasing the muscle dissection required. One biomechanical study argued that a cortical screw trajectory would be more effective in osteoporotic patients, although mixed results with pullout and toggle tests were noted.[162] In one recent biomechanical study, the stabilizing impact of cortical screws as rescue screws after pedicle screw placement was tested in 10 cadaveric spines.[163] L3 pedicle screws were pulled out. Cortical screws were then placed and exhibited 60% of the original pedicle screw pullout strength. The construct's stability in flexion-extension, lateral bending, and axial rotation was similar to the original pedicle screw.

Two small studies reported failure of cortical screws that required revision for pseudarthrosis, pars fracture, and caudal adjacent-segment failure. The authors recommended caution when using this technique clinically, despite the favorable biomechanical studies.[164,165] Other retrospective studies have offered more favorable outcomes.[166]

Pelvic Fixation

Overall, the use of pelvic fixation has increased as authors have recommended greater efforts at correcting or maintaining sagittal balance. In many cases, though, the exact indications for this extension are not always clear. For example, one 2014 study compared the outcomes and complications associated with primary long fusion to the pelvis with revision procedures, including extension to the pelvis.[167] Although the revision procedures offered the "same expectation of radiographic and clinical success," the complication rate was similar to that of the primary procedure, including pelvic fixation. It is not clear how many of those procedures could avoid pelvic fixation.

As with the thoracolumbar spine, the variety of bone anchors used in the pelvis has gradually given way to increased use of screws. For example, the use of intrasacral fixation, such as Jackson intrasacral rods, has continued to decline due to problems with loosening and the improved holding power of segmental fixation to the pelvis.[168]

In addition, when comparing iliac screws to unit rods or the Luque-Galveston technique, screw-based rigid fixation, while costing more at $15,488 versus $3128 for the nonrigid group, offered significantly greater curve and pelvic obliquity correction while decreasing pseudarthrosis and the need for anterior release.[169] A maximal-width sacropelvic fixation technique allows greater correction of pelvic obliquity in neuromuscular scoliosis.[170,171]

A variety of iliac screw placement techniques have been described, but iliac screws placed either under or through the

SECTION IX

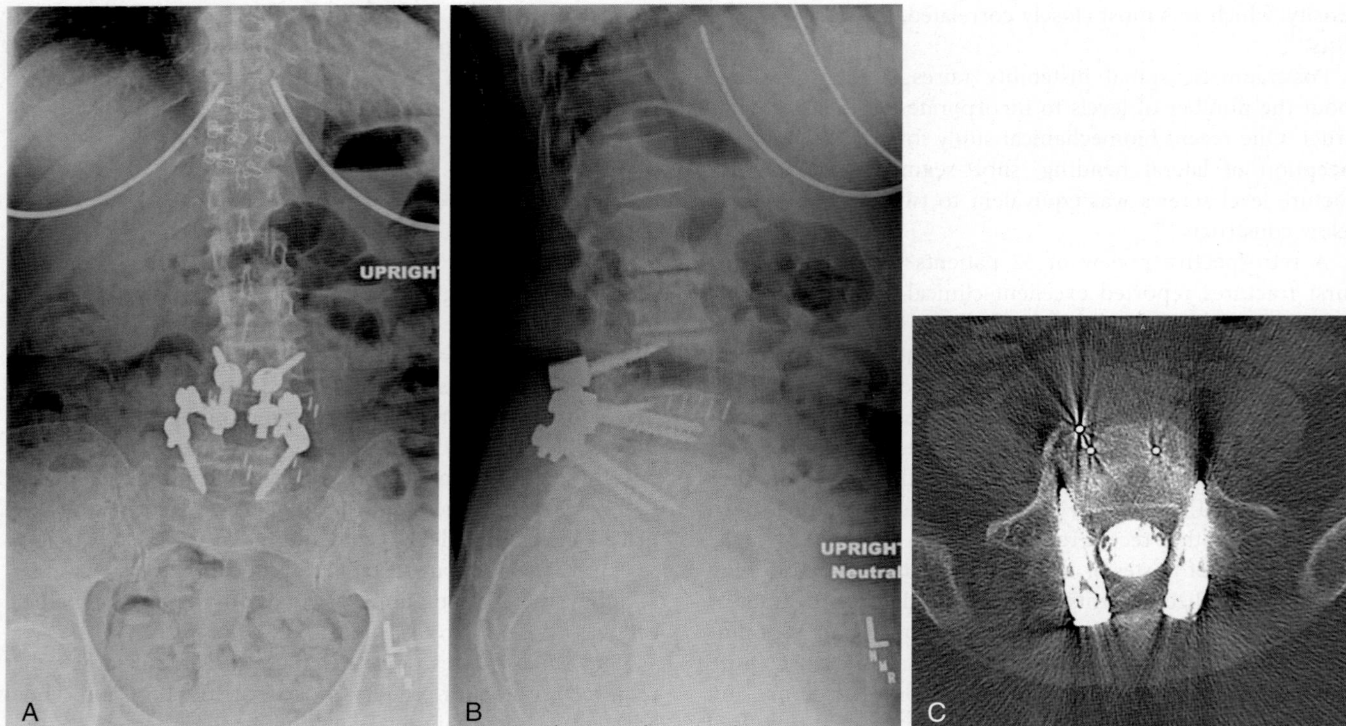

FIG. 70.7 (A) Anteroposterior and (B) lateral views of an initial transpedicular stabilization at L4–L5 was revised and extended to L3–L4 using cortical screws at the more cranial levels. Note the lateral positioning of the interbody cages. (C) Axial computed tomographic view at the L4 pedicle level. These cortical screws were found to be loose and re-re-revision with transpedicular grafting was performed.

posterior sacroiliac spine with transverse connectors to the midline rods and S2 alar iliac fixation are the most common.[172] S2 alar fixation has a number of potential advantages in terms of decreased soft tissue dissection and in-line placement. However, in one recent study, a higher rate of failure was associated with this technique compared with more typical iliac fixation with lateral connectors (25% vs. 12%).[173] The same authors noted a higher rate of failure in patients in whom sagittal balance had not been restored and in patients in whom S2 iliac screws were placed (over more traditional iliac bolts with lateral connectors).[173] In contrast, another study of 60 patients, 23 of whom had received S2 alar-iliac screws, found a lower rate of wound-related complications and instrumentation failures compared with more typical iliac bolts.[174]

Here, too, the number of anchors should match the patient's individual characteristics. In neuromuscular scoliosis, for example, a 30% rate of pelvic screw failure was noted when bilateral L5 and S1 screws were not placed.[175] In other settings, S2 alar or buttress screws may be used in lieu of iliac fixation to neutralize long thoracolumbar fixation to the sacrum.[168] Placement of sacral screws and use of sacroiliac screws reduce the stress on iliac screw fixation.[176]

Access and Guidance

As mentioned in other sections, the degree of soft tissue dissection required to place these implants has been decreasing over time. However, screw placement continues to be challenged by malpositioning, which could result in neurologic injury. A variety of imaging and guidance systems have been developed to decrease this risk.

For example, although intraoperative fluoroscopy remains a standard technique to assess implant trajectories, pelvic fixation may benefit from fluoroscopic views not typically exploited by spine surgeons, such as the pelvic inlet view. One recent series of 14 neuromuscular scoliosis patients had safe placement of iliac screw fixation by identification of the posterior sacroiliac spine and the inlet view.[177] Another study found that anteroposterior images were effective in patients with rotational deformities.[178]

For the last 10 years, cone-beam imaging systems (O-Arm [Medtronic] and Orbic [Siemens]), and now true intraoperative CT scanners, have been available to assess implant placement prior to leaving the operating room or to mate with navigation systems to guide that placement. In one recent study, intraoperative true CT–based navigation guidance with a portable 32-slice scanner was reported in 85 cases.[179] The authors found that the imaging quality allowed a 99.13% accuracy rate in placement of 571 screws regardless of the patient's body habitus or positioning at the time of surgery. Another study reviewed 1148 screws placed in 203 patients utilizing intraoperative CT.[180] Intraoperative CT increased the rate of immediate screw revision but did not affect the rates of reoperation for misplaced screws. The authors concluded that intraoperative CT lowered the threshold for intraoperative screw revision.

Robotic guidance has also become available for thoracolumbar implant placement, although data remain sparse at this point.[181,182] Custom-printed screw guides and the built-in gyroscopes in modern smart phones can be used to assist screw placement.[183]

Use of percutaneous transpedicular constructs has been increasing. These systems may be used to stabilize an ALIF or lateral lumbar interbody fusion (LLIF) or provide contralateral-side stabilization after a minimally invasive TLIF. Occasionally, a limited facet fusion is included with this less-invasive approach.[184]

Some systems use a rod-insertion device that links to the screw extension sleeves and allows a precut contoured rod to be placed through the screw saddles via a small stab wound and a muscle-splitting technique. A remote engagement of the screw-locking mechanism is then used. Long-term outcomes for these techniques are sparse, but short-term success has been reported in small numbers of patients. Proponents of this technique believe that paraspinous tissue trauma is minimized without compromising the quality of spinal fixation. Techniques reporting safe placement without guidewires have recently been reported.[185]

Because MIS screw placement requires less local soft tissue disruption, the idea that MIS placement of cranial screws in adult deformity surgery would decrease proximal junctional kyphosis was proposed, but it was not supported in a propensity-matched cohort analysis of 136 patients.[186]

Intraoperative monitoring can also be used to assess the safe placement of thoracolumbar implants. One recent study used a unique four-pulse stimulus train within the pedicle screw tract with a ball-tipped probe. Lower extremity electromyography correctly detected 100% of 32 medially breached thoracic screws out of 802 total screws placed.[187,188]

Rods and Cross-Links

In patients with complex deformity, correct rod bending may be quite difficult. The rod should not be contoured in more than one plane at a time. In children and patients with flexible deformities, the rod can be contoured to fit the screws and rotated into proper sagittal balance. Alternatively, a series of force vectors and direct rotational maneuvers may be undertaken. In patients with rigid curves and most adults, accurate rod contouring to fit into the screws can be difficult. It is often helpful to use lateral connectors between the rod and screw instead. Some surgeons, in an effort to maximize correction power, use separate rods in the upper and lower portions of a stiff, dual-curve deformity and connect them with a domino on one side and use a neutralization rod on the opposite side.[189]

When bending rods for hook-based constructs, slight deviation from perfect contour puts a moment on the hook. In the thoracic spine, a kyphotic moment pulls the hook away from the cord. In general, the aim is for a 30-degree thoracic kyphosis with its apex at T7 or T8. The lumbar lordosis should be 45 degrees with an apex at the L2–L3 interspace. The rod should change from kyphosis to lordosis at the T12–L1 interspace. After placement of the hooks, the convex rod is placed first. The more mobile the hooks, the more easily the rod engages. Hook mobility is a function of the amount of bone resection during hook placement. The ease of rod insertion improves with spine mobility, which is a function of facet resection.

Dynamic Rods

Numerous coils, springs, jointed rods, and semielastic cords have been devised to replace rigid rods as pedicle screw connectors. Some of these devices are intended to be used as less-rigid fusion devices. Others are meant to "top off" the most cranial level of a long fusion construct, theoretically to decrease the risk of adjacent-segment degeneration because less-rigid fixation is believed to be associated with reduced adjacent-segment motion compared with rigid fixation.[138] Biomechanical studies continue to assess various dynamic systems. Most show decreased stress on the adjacent segments.[190] In a recent clinical study of 36 patients undergoing the Isobar semirigid dynamic posterior stabilization system, disc degeneration continued despite the dynamic stabilization at 24-month follow-up.[191]

Still other dynamic systems were used without attempt at fusion as motion-preserving spinal stabilization. In this setting, dynamic rod devices were intended to treat mechanical back pain associated with lumbar degenerative disease. These systems varied architecturally and materially. Ideally, each design was logically constructed to "fix" a clearly delineated problem in the painful or degenerated spine. Each system apparently relies on a different theory of pain generation and uses different mechanical means to address the pain. In some cases, a clear hypothesis as to the source of the pain is not evident.

For example, one of the first dynamic posterior instrumentation systems was the Graf ligament, an inelastic cord wrapped around two pedicle screws. The goal was to lock the motion segment into full lordosis, restricting flexion and preventing rotation.[192] There was no experimental basis for this design concept, but clinical results were acceptable. Limitations of the Graf ligament included the increase in posterior anulus load it engendered. This increase led to late failure with back pain or earlier failure resulting from the marked lateral recess and foraminal stenosis the system caused.[193]

The Dynesys implants (Zimmer Biomet) received FDA approval as stabilization devices adjunctive to fusion. As a result, this was the only system available in the United States, but they were typically used in an off-label manner as a fusionless, dynamic construct. As with the Graf system, the Dynesys system connects pedicle screws with a nonelastic ligament. In this case, a plastic cylinder surrounds the ligament and prevents hyperlordosis. At surgery, the ligament is threaded through the cylinder and pulled with a set 300-N force. This force approximates the two screw heads with the interposed cylinder. Active extension opens the anulus anteriorly without compressing it posteriorly. The Dynesys system limits full flexion and extension. The developers of the system claim it decreases pain by eliminating "parasitic" or "abnormal" movement. In addition to restricting the range of movement, it may also unload the disc, however, if the patient achieves a position of lordosis, so that the plastic cylinder becomes weight bearing.[194,195] Limitations of the Dynesys system include the

SECTION IX

unpredictable degree to which it unloads the disc and the need for strong extensor musculature to maintain lordosis. Lordosis and load sharing by the plastic cylinder vary markedly with implant placement.[196]

There are common contraindications to use of these nonrigid devices, including significant preoperative instability, osteoporosis, and anterior column insufficiency.

Concerns about the possibility of long-term screw loosening led to modifications with HA-coated or plasma-sprayed screws. Some systems required the screws to be cemented into the pedicle. That said, one recent study compared pedicle screw–based dynamic stabilization systems with more tradition screw-rod fusion constructs in elderly patients with degenerative scoliosis.[197] Although the fusion patient achieved better deformity corrections, operative time, blood loss, and complication rates were lower in the dynamic stabilization group. At a mean follow-up of 64 months, clinical outcomes were similar. Still, among deformity specialists, the current, countervailing trend incorporates larger surgical constructs to effect greater correction of sagittal plane alignment, even in patients undergoing surgery for degenerative disease.[198]

All dynamic systems require perfect screw placement because a pedicle breach risks screw loosening and ultimate dislodgment. A highly medialized trajectory is sought to avoid facet violation and subsequent painful facet degeneration.

Unfortunately, the promise of these systems has not been realized. Screw loosening and other implant failures were common, and use of these systems has markedly declined in North America. In recent reviews, although the idea remains promising, no clear benefits of dynamic systems were uncovered.[199,200] Dynamic systems were associated with a higher rate of loss of lordotic correction.

Variable Stiffness Rods

Several generations of low- or variable-stiffness implants have been developed to improve load sharing with the spine and, perhaps, to decrease stress on the adjacent segments.[201] With partial annealing, a rod's flexural stiffness can be varied.[202] Recently, rods with decreased end stiffness have been assessed biomechanically. In this setting, decreased stress on the anchors and greater load sharing of the instrumentation with the spine were noted.[203] The real mechanical utility of these systems has yet to be conclusively demonstrated.[204]

Larger, stiffer 6.35-mm rods are often recommended for better maintenance of correction in long deformity and trauma surgeries. In one series of 93 patients undergoing surgery for adolescent idiopathic scoliosis, rod size did not affect radiographic outcomes at a minimum of 2 years.[205] Of note, these patients were Taiwanese children; different results could be reported in larger adult patients.

In other cases, a more rigid longitudinal connector is required. For example, in long adult deformity surgery, particularly in the case of pedicle subtraction osteotomy, rod fractures are common. Use of two additional, "outrigger" rods to span the high-risk area (the pedicle subtraction osteotomy level or the thoracolumbar junction) significantly decreased implant failure and symptomatic pseudarthrosis rates.[206,207] In very unstable cases, such as en bloc tumor resections, orthogonal anterior and posterior implants may more effectively restore spinal stability.[208]

Growing Rods

A vertical expandable prosthetic titanium rib (VEPTR; DePuy Synthes) provides an internal, nonrigid brace for spinal or thoracic cage deformity to allow further thoracic cage growth.[209] A recent report described 10 children with arthrogryposis who underwent VEPTR placement at 5 years of age.[210] At a mean 4.2-year follow-up, the scoliosis decreased from 67 to 43 degrees and kyphosis decreased from 65 to 48 degrees. During the treatment period, spinal growth from T1 to S1 increased 4.2 cm. Six complications were reported in four patients: three infections, two rib failures, and one implant failure. Proximal junctional kyphosis greater than 45 degrees was reported in six patients.

More traditionally, "growing rods" have been used to provide temporary, internal bracing of rapidly progressive curves in young children and to allow additional axial growth before a formal fusion is performed. In an effort to prevent long-term pulmonary restriction, these modalities seek to allow maximal chest cavity development.

The first of these techniques, the Shilla growth guidance technique, avoided repeat surgery by performing a short-segment, periapical fusion with sliding pedicle screws cephalad and caudad. In a report of 40 patients with a mean age just below 7 years and 7-year follow-up, a mean 69- to 38.4-degree correction was reported.[211] Although a high 73% complication rate was reported (with 24 of 40 having instrumentation-related complications), it was believed to be acceptable compared with predicate procedures.

A recent porcine study attempted to refute the idea that growing rods were kyphogenic by demonstrating distribution of the distracting force across multiple levels of the spine.[212] Other works have examined use of side-to-side connectors used as gliding connections.[213] As might be expected, dual rods and additional apical and intermediate anchors are likely to improve correction.[214,215]

Two small, early series of magnetically controlled growing rods found that implant-related complications were not uncommon, including rod fracture and apical hook pullout, but "the avoidance of multiple surgeries following implantation is beneficial compared with traditional growing rod systems."[216,217]

Cross-Links

The relative merits of cross-link placement in longer, posterior thoracolumbar constructs continue to be debated. Traditionally, these implants were used to improve torsional stability of anterior and posterior dual-rod constructs.[218,219] Depending on the number of motion segments instrumented, the degree of instability of the spine, and the strength of the bone-implant interface, placement of one to three cross-links has been recommended. Classically, if two cross-links are used, one should be as proximal as possible and the other as distal as possible. If the instrumentation exceeds 30 cm in length, a third transverse connector should be considered in the middle. The addition of a cross-link may mechanically compensate for a missing pedicle screw in a polysegmental construct.

Various cadaveric biomechanical studies of transpedicular fixation across the thoracolumbar junction found that rotational stiffness increased significantly with the number of cross-links placed; some found improved bending stiffness as well.[220] Another study compared constructs using no, one, or two cross-links. This study found that two cross-links were no more effective than one in significantly increasing axial, flexion, and lateral stiffness, although additional cross-links significantly improved the torsional stiffness of the construct.[219] When comparing different types of cross-links, larger cross-sectional area and diagonal geometries are associated with greater increases in stiffness.[221,222]

Three recent studies concluded that cross-link placement improved construct torsional rigidity and holding power.[223,224] Earlier concerns over cross-link connector bulk affecting the area available for bone grafting and "excessive" stiffness inhibiting fusion through stress shielding have not been borne out. That said, the real utility of cross-links continues to be debated in various clinical contexts. While initially recommended in long deformity and trauma surgery, some surgeons use cross-links in tumor and degenerative cases with spinal rotational stiffness or when a screw site has been compromised.

Anterior Thoracolumbar Instrumentation

Modern forms of anterior thoracolumbar instrumentation were initially developed for deformity surgery separately by Zielke and Dwyer in the late 1960s to mid-1970s.[73] Their techniques of anterior release and fixation allowed better deformity correction, necessitating fewer fused segments. These deformity techniques were adapted to traumatic conditions by Kaneda, Dunn, and others. Use of these early-generation devices began to wane due to reports of catastrophic vascular erosions.

In the 1990s, next-generation, soft tissue–friendly anterior plate-and-rod constructs became more common. As with posterior fixation constructs, anterior systems are used to provide stability, attain or maintain alignment, or improve or accelerate fusion. Over the last 10 years, however, use of anterior surgery has varied. Introduction of lateral lumbar interbody approaches has stimulated interest in less-invasive adult deformity corrections with anterior cages and posterior, often percutaneous, screw-rod constructs. In pediatric deformity, stronger posterior implants and improved correction techniques have decreased the use of anterior release and fusion procedures.[225]

Today, the least controversial indications for anterior thoracolumbar surgery include reconstruction of tumors or vertebral body fractures. These indications include (Fig. 70.8):

- Corpectomy defects (after burst fracture or tumor)
- Marked anterior canal compression
- Marked loss of the spine's ability to support axial loading
- Discectomy defects
- Painful disc in low-grade isthmic spondylolisthesis or degenerative disc disease
- Pseudarthrosis after multilevel fusion
- Anterior support in long fusion constructs (particularly at L5–S1)
- Anterior release procedures (in patients with coronal or sagittal deformity and loss of spinal balance)

The indications for interbody fusion after a posterior decompression and stabilization remain unclear. In many

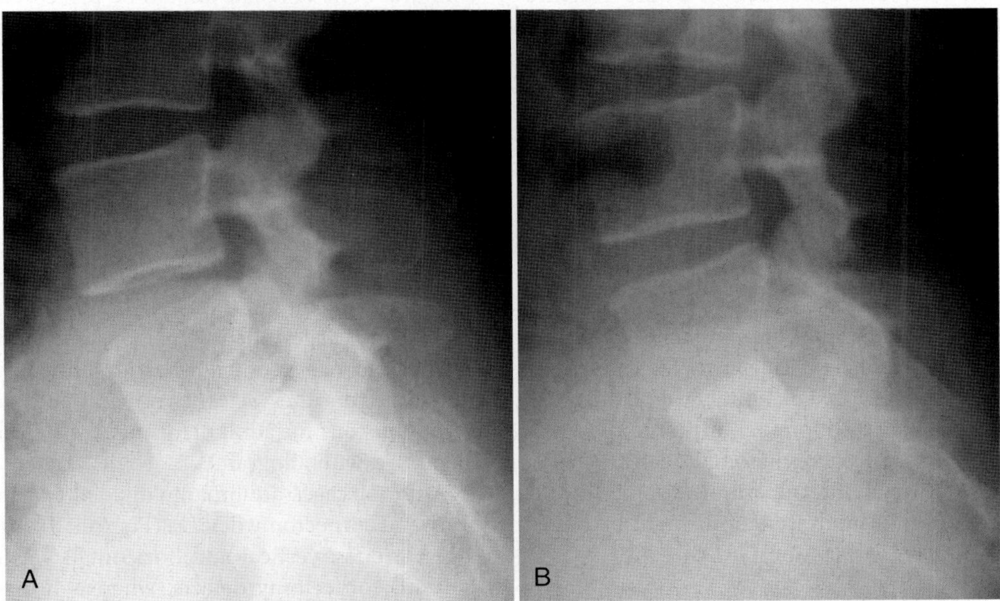

FIG. 70.8 Stand-alone anterior lumbar interbody fusion continues to be performed, albeit with more limited indications, such as patients with markedly collapsed disc spaces. (A) Preoperative and (B) postoperative lateral radiographs in a patient undergoing a tapered cage anterior lumbar interbody fusion with bone morphogenetic protein within the cage.

clinical scenarios such as degenerative or isthmic spondylolisthesis, better radiographic results in terms of slip and, possibly, lordosis correction, are reported but no measurable improvement in clinical outcomes follows.[226] The most controversial indication for anterior surgery is for the treatment of discogenic pain.[227]

In some settings, however, one-stage circumferential approaches from the back have supplanted separate anterior surgery. In tumor and trauma surgery, wide posterior approaches have allowed corpectomy with (often expandable) cage reconstruction without a separate anterior incision.

A number of recent studies have examined the role of multilevel, rigid posterior implants in obviating separate anterior release and instrumentation procedures. For example, in 30 patients with Scheuermann kyphosis, posterior fusion surgery offered similar radiographic and clinical outcomes to an anterior-posterior approach.[228] In right thoracic adolescent idiopathic scoliosis, a recent study compared 18 patients undergoing an anterior and 24 undergoing a posterior approach.[229] Clinical and coronal plane results were similar between the groups. Posterior surgery more effectively addressed sagittal plane deformity.

In most cases, however, the procedural goals remain the same. Anterior surgeries are indicated to release and stabilize thoracolumbar deformity correction (scoliosis, spondylolisthesis, kyphosis), remove anteriorly based tumors and infections, decompress anterior canal compression, and restore the anterior load-bearing column through strut grafting (Fig. 70.9).[230]

Relative contraindications for anterior procedures include osteoporosis. Anterior systems rely on softer cancellous vertebral body bone with thin cortices as opposed to posterior pedicle screw systems that rely on cortical pedicle bone.

On the other hand, osteoporotic patients may be in greater need of anterior column load sharing. Gurwitz and colleagues assessed the stability of several constructs in a burst fracture model.[231] Axial stiffness and torsional rigidity were measured before and after posterior instrumentation alone, posterior instrumentation with anterior strut grafting, and anterior instrumentation with anterior strut grafting. They found that posterior instrumentation alone was associated with 76% less axial stiffness. The addition of an anterior strut rendered the construct as stiff as the intact spine. Anterior struts with anterior instrumentation were as strong as the intact spine in axial loading. All these constructs were 30% less rigid in torsion compared with the intact spine.

The less-expansile nature of anterior approaches decreases their utility in patients with multisegmental pathologic processes (e.g., multiple spine metastases) in which multilevel exposure is required. Contraindications to abdominal or thoracic surgery also limit the utility of these procedures in some patients. Patients with multiple prior abdominal or retroperitoneal surgeries and patients with severe pulmonary dysfunction might be better treated with a posterior reconstruction.

Cages and Struts

Although most anterior column spacers are used to improve the alignment and rate of spinal fusion, some are used without attempted fusion. Traditionally, PMMA was one of the first and simplest constructs for reconstruction of corpectomy defects. It is currently rarely used, but it may be considered in patients with limited life expectancy and is best limited to one-level or two-level corpectomies only. The stability of this construct is improved by the use of Steinmann pins that can be placed through the PMMA construct and embedded into the vertebral endplates above and below the defect.[232] C-clamps and other devices have been used to improve endplate support. In an open total spondylectomy model, PMMA can be packed into the anterior defect from a posterior approach. As with all interbody procedures, endplate coverage is important in avoiding subsequent subsidence. A mechanical assessment of this construct in cadaveric spines found that only combined approaches with posterior screws and anterior PMMA restored the spine to its previous state. With the posterior elements removed, use of PMMA and anterior instrumentation or anterior pins was unable to restore the motion segment stability.[233]

Although morcellized graft material has been used alone, a structural graft or morcellized graft material within an interbody cage is more typically selected. Options for interbody grafts include various types of structural autogenous grafting (e.g., rib or tricortical iliac crest) or allograft struts (e.g., rings or dowels). No mechanical advantage of supplemental screw placement into the graft or cage has been shown.

Regardless of which strut graft, spacer, or cage is placed, a few rules governing endplate and fusion bed preparation must be followed. First, as much disc material as possible should be removed because residual disc material actively discourages fusion. This is more easily and completely attained by a direct anterior approach than a posterior approach via a posterior lumbar interbody fusion or TLIF. Second, the endplate cartilage should be removed down to bleeding bone, but the subchondral bone endplate should be preserved. Some surgeons advocate endplate perforation to facilitate bone ingrowth from the vertebral body into the graft. Because loads and, consequently, the risk of implant subsidence are much higher in the thoracolumbar spine than in the cervical spine, the endplate must be carefully protected, particularly in osteoporotic and obese patients.

In one recent series of 116 patients treated for thoracolumbar trauma, all received posterior instrumentation followed by anterior grafting.[234] When assessed by CT, tricortical iliac crest healed 66% of the time versus 90% of the time for rib grafts and 98% for cages filled with cancellous bone from the fractured vertebra. Another study described successful use of autograft from the adjacent vertebral body to fill ALIF cages in long fusions for adult deformity.[235] The vertebral body was then filled with allograft.

Anterior cages are broadly divided by purpose into interbody and corpectomy devices (Fig. 70.10). There are two main cage varieties: vertical and horizontal. Vertical devices typically fill corpectomy defects, whereas horizontal (cylindric) cages are used in discectomy procedures. For the latter, the mechanical goal is interspace distraction and restoration of annular tension.[236] A wide variety of allografts are available for use in either vertical or horizontal modes. These may be "off-the-shelf" sections of femur, tibia, humerus, or fibula, which the surgeon cuts into the desired size and shape, or one of myriad machined bone products. Commercial bone implants are typically prefabricated to specific sizes and may have special surface textures to resist extrusion. The rationale behind machined allograft and manufactured cages includes the following:

- Immediate structural support to resist axial compression and maintain distraction
- Adequate contact area with adjacent vertebrae to resist subsidence without stress shielding of bone growing in the cage
- Avoidance of structural autograft harvest

Nonallograft cages have the additional potential advantages of avoidance of structural allograft complications (microfracture, collapse, and potential viral transmission).

The shape of horizontal interbody cage devices has evolved over time to reflect differing methods of insertion and

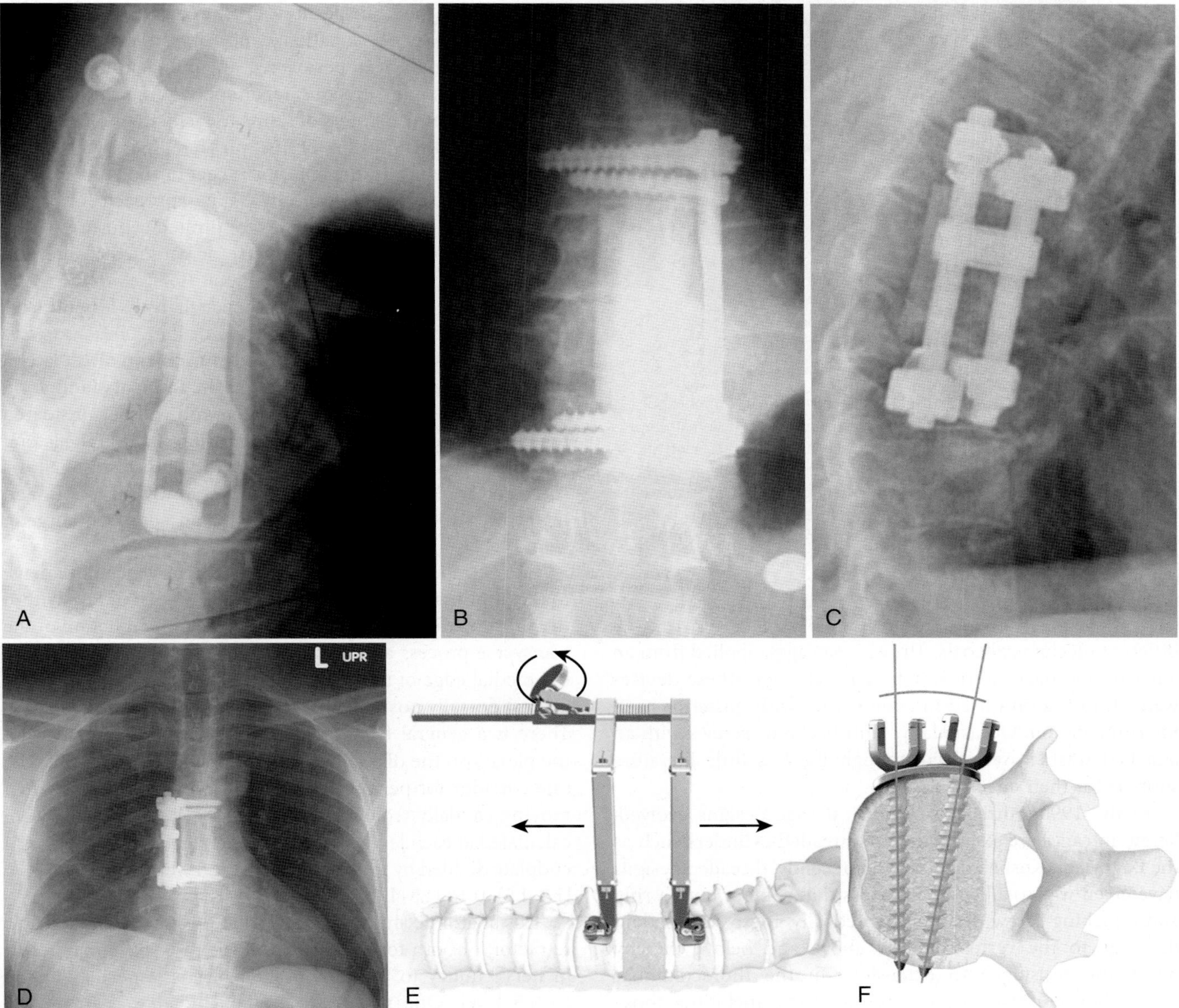

FIG. 70.9 Thoracolumbar corpectomy operations may be performed with or without anterior or posterior instrumentation. When possible, additional posterior procedures should be avoided. In many burst fracture models, anterior column instrumentation may be biomechanically adequate. There are many options, but the most common are plate-and-rod systems. (A–B) Plating systems are said to be easier to implant and have a lower profile. (C–D) Rod-based systems confer greater mechanical strength in that the longitudinal member (in this case the rods) lies farther from the spine's instant axis of rotation. This advantage is also a disadvantage, however, in that it increases implant bulk and profile. (E) Most rigid anterior instrumentation systems allow distraction of the interspace for safe canal decompression and subsequent compression to improve immediate construct stability. (F) For virtually all of these systems, triangulated, bicortical placement of the screws improves holding power in osteoporotic bone.

Continued

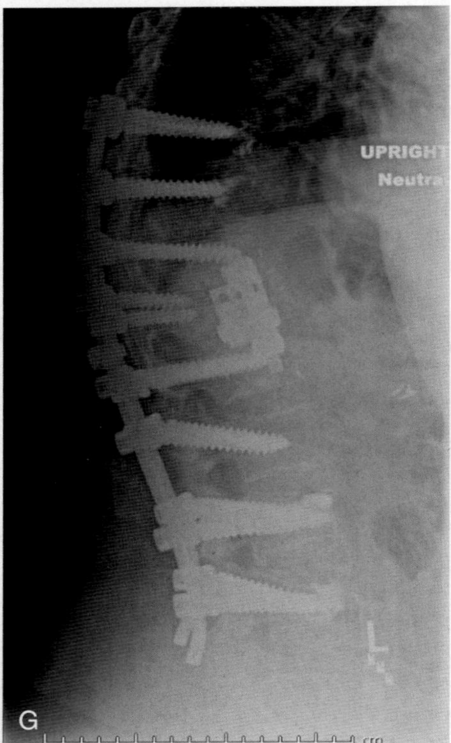

FIG. 70.9, cont'd (G) Use of an expandable cage to treat a chronic burst fracture in a patient who had two previous failed posterior fusion attempts. To reduce the focal kyphosis, the anterolateral ligament was resected and bicortical screws were placed in the bone above and below the fracture. The screws and interbody distraction were used sequentially to restore height. The loose posterior instrumentation was revised with larger diameter screws, polymethylmethacrylate augmentation, and short screws in the fractured vertebrae. (E–F, Courtesy Stryker, Kalamazoo, MI.)

different mechanical goals. The earliest cages, applied from an anterior approach, were simple femoral rings. These devices were almost always used in conjunction with posterior rigid instrumentation. Occasionally, "anti-backout" screws with an attached washer were used, though there is little literature support for their effectiveness.

In the 1990s, threaded cylindrical cage designs evolved. Screw-in cages are exemplified by threaded cylinders such as the Bagby and Kuslich device. More recently, threaded designs have given way to all-in-one devices that contain both a ring and a locking screw design. Theoretically, these screws hold the cage to the vertebral body above and below, thereby improving resistance to extension. In the thoracolumbar spine, they are available in several forms, including those optimized for ALIF and lateral placement. Interestingly, the most common horizontal anterior cage has returned to a ring configuration.

Horizontal cages are typically used in anterior lumbar fusion procedures and had been virtually exclusively used in the lumbar spine. More recently, transforaminal approaches to the disc space have been reported even in thoracic level procedures. A recent randomized, controlled study compared transforaminal thoracic interbody fusion with anterior-posterior fusion in 57 patients with thoracolumbar trauma.[237] Similar fusion, loss of correction, and clinical outcomes were reported. Formal posterior-anterior surgery was associated with greater blood loss and perioperative complications.

Transperitoneal approaches enjoyed a short burst of popularity in the mid-1990s when endoscopic techniques were used for threaded cage placement. This attempt at less-invasive fusion surgery has given way to miniopen retroperitoneal approaches, which offer similar recovery and morbidity rates with decreased operative time and retrograde ejaculation.[238]

Currently, the transperitoneal approach is occasionally used in markedly obese patients and when prior retroperitoneal exposure has been performed. In approaching the sacral promontory, some surgeons recommend infiltration of the tissue with a few milliliters of saline to facilitate the dissection and aid in identification of the presacral parasympathetic fibers. More typically, the anterior aspect of the lumbar spine is approached retroperitoneally. This approach improves access to the upper lumbar spine. For limited exposures to the low lumbar spine, a short transverse or paramedian incision is made.

To replace the long flank incision, relatively less-invasive transpsoas lateral approaches evolved in the 2000s and were marketed as extreme lateral interbody fusion and direct lateral fusion by their manufacturers. From the implant standpoint, however, these approaches are similar and will be considered together as lateral lumbar interbody fusion (LLIF). The lateral retroperitoneal, transpsoas approach to the disc space allows sufficient access for a complete discectomy, distraction, and interbody fusion without the need for an approach surgeon (Fig. 70.11).

Complications associated with LLIF surgery include damage to the lumbosacral plexus. The lumbosacral plexus lays within the substance of the psoas muscle between the junction of the transverse process and vertebral body. The nerves exit along the medial edge of the psoas distally. The lumbosacral plexus is most dorsally positioned at the posterior endplate of L1–L2. There is a general trend of progressive ventral migration of the plexus on the disc space from L2–L3 through L4–L5. The safe corridor for performing LLIF procedures narrows when moving caudally from L1–L2 to L4–L5. Average ratios were calculated at each level (distance of the plexus from the dorsal endplate divided by total disc length) and were 0 (L1–L2), 0.11 (L2–L3), 0.18 (L3–L4), and 0.28 (L4–L5).[238a]

This anatomic study suggested that positioning the dilator, retractor, or both too posteriorly at the disc space may result in nerve injury to the lumbosacral plexus, especially at the L4–L5 level. One recent review concluded that there was anatomic justification for lateral cage placement from L1–L2 to L4–L5.[239] Another review confirmed the utility of this approach in improving coronal and sagittal balance in patients with degenerative scoliosis.[240]

These findings have led to newer approaches that access the disc space anterior to the psoas muscle. For example, the oblique lumbar interbody fusion is another variant of LLIF and has been promoted as less likely to irritate the lumbar plexus during cage insertion. A small 12-patient series of kyphoscoliosis patients undergoing anterior-posterior corrections

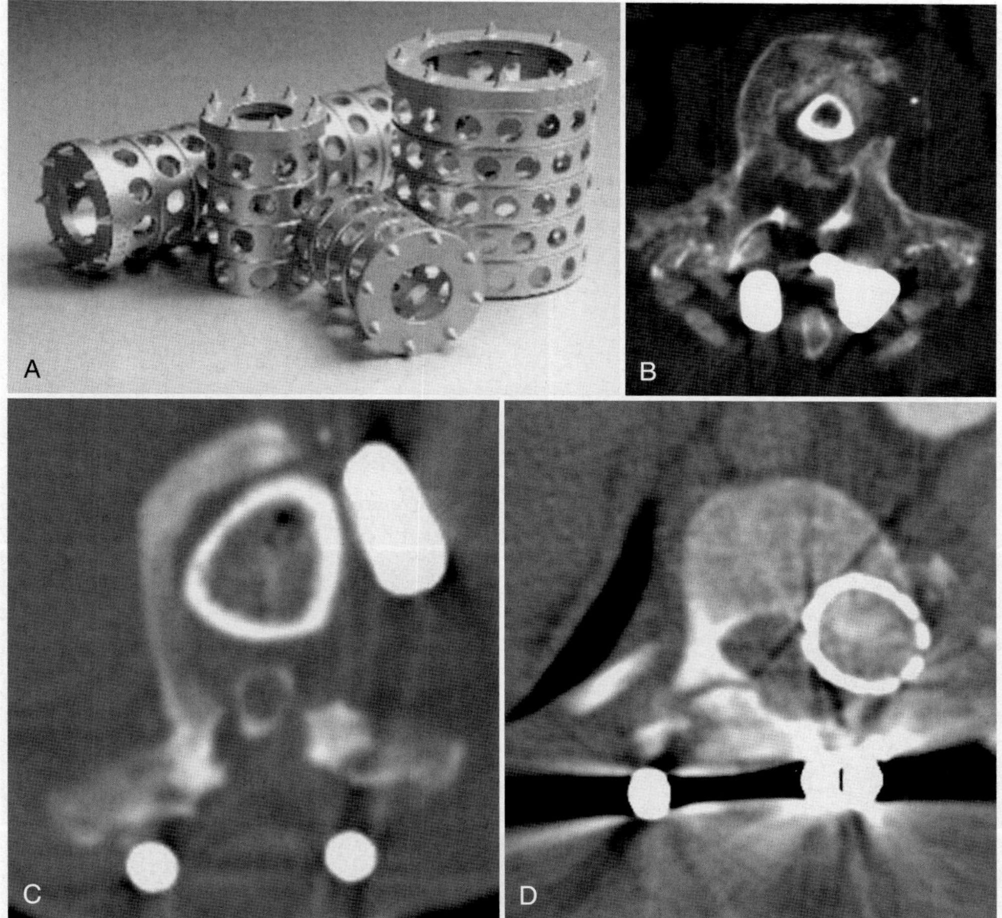

FIG. 70.10 When an anterior corpectomy is performed, various materials are available to reconstruct the defect. (A) Example of vertical mesh cage. These devices offer end caps that engage the host bone, improving rotational stability of the construct. Various allograft materials may be used as well. (B) Use of a single fibular shaft. Graft geometry should match as much as possible that of the host endplate. Particularly in patients with osteoporosis, small corpectomy struts penetrate the endplate, and all axial stability is lost. Disengagement of the hooks posteriorly is noted here. (C) Postoperative axial computed tomographic myelogram in a case in which a tibial shaft has been used. The graft fills most of the corpectomy. As with all other forms of instrumentation, careful attention to positioning of the implant is crucial with corpectomy devices. (D) Grossly malpositioned cage in a patient with postoperative radicular symptoms. (A, Courtesy Stryker, Kalamazoo, MI.)

was reported with a 90% fusion rate and no neurovascular injuries.[241]

However, reasonable results have been reported for LLIF procedures thus far. Stand-alone LLIF outcomes were reported in 59 patients,[242] with a fusion rate of 93%. A recent biomechanical study found that posterior implants improved stability after LLIF.[91] Pedicle screw constructs provided more stability in lateral bending than interspinous process fixation, but the authors concluded that interspinous process devices were likely adequate. Another study found that a lateral plate with an interspinous process device provided similar stiffness to LLIF with pedicle screw-rod constructs.[243]

A recent cohort controlled study concluded that LLIF improved lumbar lordosis more than ALIF.[244] In another recent study of 145 levels in 90 patients, at a mean 12.6-month follow-up 5.3-degree restoration of lordosis was noted but, with subsidence, 2.9 degrees of final correction were noted.[245] A mix of stand-alone cages, lateral plates, and transpedicular instrumentation was used. New postoperative thigh numbness and weakness were noted in 4.4% and 2.2% of the patients, respectively. Good clinical outcomes were also reported. On the other hand, a recent systematic review was unable to establish superiority of LLIF over TLIF in adults with lumbar degenerative conditions.[246]

This MIS lateral transpsoas approach may also be used for corpectomy and anterior release in burst fractures and kyphotic deformity. In a study comparing this approach with an all-posterior approach, similar rates of complications and correction were noted.[247]

By providing disc space distraction, interbody devices and procedures restore foraminal height. Interbody techniques can also provide indirect reduction of central canal compression. One cadaveric CT study found that anteriorly or laterally placed interbody devices can reduce anterior listhesis and increase canal and foraminal volume in a degenerative spondylolisthesis model.[248] One clinical study followed a series of 56 patients with back pain, neuroclaudication, or both from degenerative spondylolisthesis and spinal stenosis

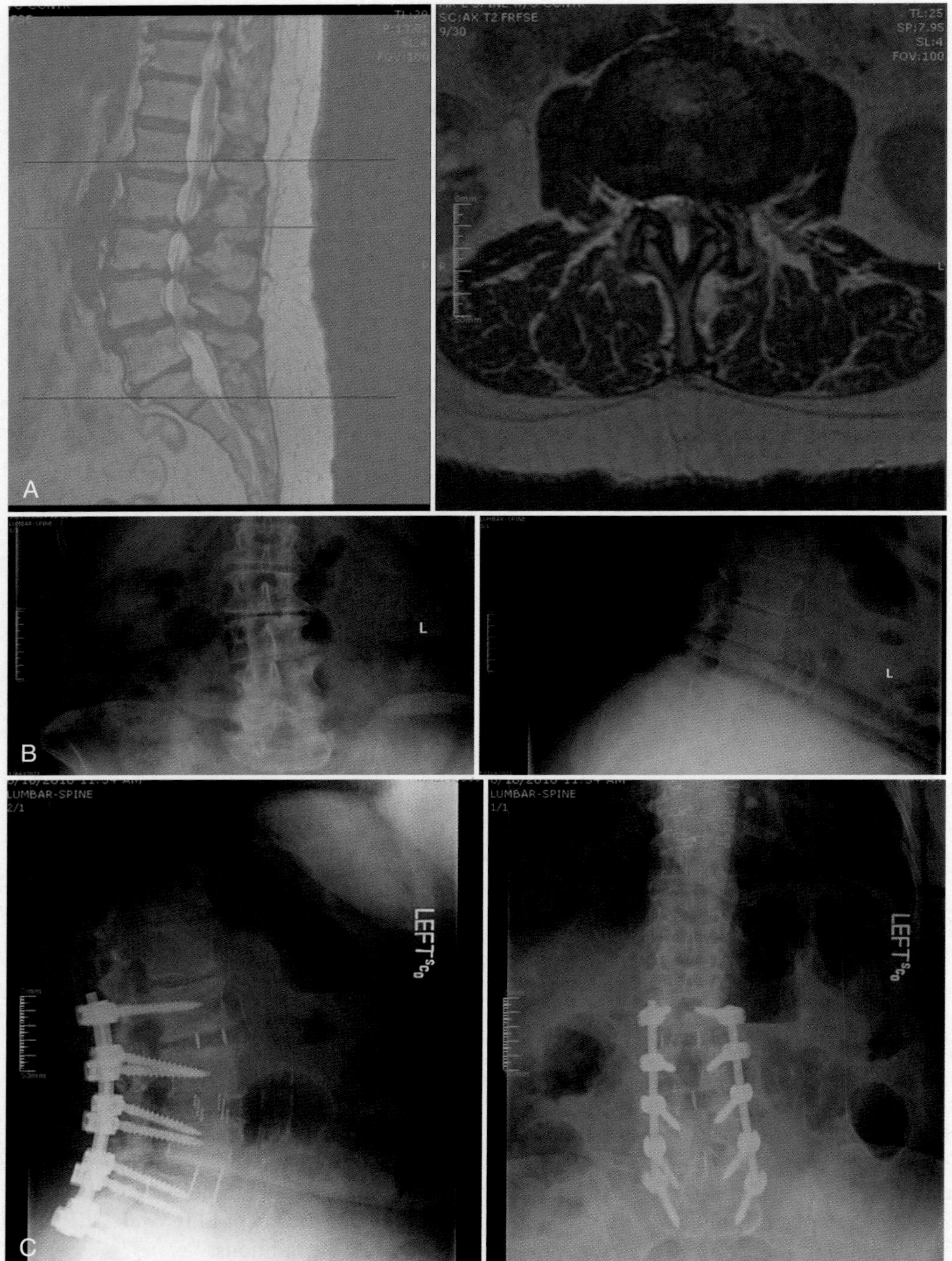

FIG. 70.11 Extreme lateral interbody fusion (XLIF) device minimal access spinal approaches have certain advantages over open procedures, including decreased postoperative pain and narcotic requirements, shorter hospital stay, less blood loss, and smaller incisions. This patient underwent L2–L3, L3–L4, and L4–L5 XLIF instrumentation followed by posterior stabilization. (A) Preoperative magnetic resonance image showing multilevel stenosis and disc degeneration. (B) Preoperative radiographs showing multilevel disc degeneration, spondylolisthesis, and lumbar scoliosis. (C) Postoperative radiographs.

who underwent ALIF for reduction and fusion. Outcomes were comparable to the published outcomes of in situ fusion after formal laminectomy, avoiding the risk of epidural fibrosis and "fusion disease" associated with posterior decompression and fusion.[249]

Vertical cages are most frequently used in the context of thoracolumbar corpectomy procedures. Historically, this procedure was performed in the thoracic spine via a lateral, transthoracic approach and in the lumbar spine via a retroperitoneal approach. The transthoracic approach is a modification of the standard approach to aortic aneurysms and offers excellent exposure to the anterior and lateral aspects of the thoracic and upper lumbar spine. Although double-lumen intubation and postoperative chest tube placement are often required, this approach provides a safe avenue for decompression of bony stenosis of the thoracic canal. Approaches to the thoracolumbar junction often require partial diaphragmatic takedown. For patients with marked anterior column disruption and axial instability, the anterior approach allows the most stable reconstruction.

The lateral approach used in the thoracolumbar approach limits subsequent instrumentation placement options. A laterally placed plate is less able to prevent segmental spine extension than a plate on the anterior vertebral surface. When approaching the lower lumbar spine anteriorly, the retroperitoneal approach is generally preferred.

In the lumbar spine, oblique flank incision may be used for multilevel and corpectomy procedures. For single-level, low lumbar approaches, a midline or a Pfannenstiel incision may be used.

Numerous miniopen modifications of the standard retroperitoneal exposure have been described and have become commonplace over the last 10 years. These modifications rely chiefly on the experience of the access surgeon and powerful retractor systems to minimize the incision length. In one retrospective 2-year follow-up, 28 patients underwent ALIF via a 6- to 10-cm left lower quadrant transverse skin incision.[250] A paramedian anterior rectus fascial Z-plasty allowed access to the retroperitoneal space for placement of various implants. No vascular, visceral, or urinary tract injuries occurred, but a mild ileus was noted in three cases. Another report described similar use of a 5-cm left flank incision in 25 patients. No injury to the great vessels or neurologic deterioration was noted.[251] This approach is safe, uses a small skin incision, avoids cutting the abdominal wall musculature, allows various interbody fusion techniques, and does not require peritoneal violation or endoscopic instrumentation. Other advantages include fewer radiographs with reduced radiation exposure during surgery and a shortened learning curve because the approach is similar to the anterior open lumbar technique.

As with pedicle screws, vertical cages can be placed through the vertebral body instead of on the endplates. The Bohlman technique used a fibular strut between the sacrum and the L5 vertebral body in high-grade spondylolisthesis. Over time, this approach has been modified to use vertical mesh cages. In high-grade slips, various modifications of the Bohlman technique continue to be reported with high success and low rates of L5 radiculopathy.[252]

The most recent change to these devices, both horizontal and vertical, has been the addition of gears or threads that allow vertical expansion in situ. For corpectomy defects reconstructed with expandable cages, adequate anterior column restoration may be achieved through smaller anterior exposures or through wide posterior approaches. In one recent series, 85 thoracolumbar fracture patients underwent anterior corpectomy with expandable cage and bilateral pedicle screw placement.[253] Impaction into the endplates of the neighboring levels was seen in 35%. The fusion rate was 100%. Reasonable achievement and maintenance of alignment were reported.

Posterior extracavitary resections of tumors using expandable cages in a single-stage posterior approach with adjunctive, rigid, segmental screw-rod stabilization are also being reported. Recent 34- and 46-patient series reported neurologic improvement and excellent early radiographic outcomes with "acceptable" complication rates.[254,255] Use in multilevel corpectomies in metastatic disease has also been reported, albeit with a high complication rate.[256]

In a biomechanical study, expandable cages were superior to femoral strut allografts and more typical cage struts from the ilium to the L5 vertebral body.[257] MIS techniques have increasingly been reported for placement of these cages as well.[258]

In a biomechanical study of expandable cages used in lateral interbody fusions, the stability of the expandable and static changes was similar, but the authors cautioned that "there may be a greater chance of endplate collapse by over-distracting the disc space because of the minimal haptic feedback from the expansion."[259]

In fact, all strut grafts, disc replacements, cages, and other anterior spacers are subject to subsidence and extrusion.[236,260] The rate and degree of this subsidence are related to cage geometry and sizing, endplate coverage, and preparation.

Several studies have shown excellent early interspace distraction but gradual collapse with further follow-up. One clinical study of dual rectangular cages found that 76% of patients developed subsidence, more often into the superior than the inferior endplate, although it did not appear to affect fusion rates or clinical outcomes.[261] A number of studies have shown that increasing cage footprint, either with multiple cages, larger cages, or expandable cages, decreases the risk of subsidence.[240,243,245,246,255]

Faizan et al.[262] describe this subsidence as typically occurring by 4 months postoperatively. In that study, mean preoperative intervertebral disc height was 11.6 ± 3.1 mm, immediate postoperative height was 16.9 ± 2.0 mm, and final follow-up disc height was 13.2 ± 2.4 mm.

The frequency of use of posterior cylindrical implants has decreased due to their higher rates of nerve injury. Anterior use has declined due to greater subsidence than plate-and-graft constructs and rectangular cages.[263-265]

Lateral positioning on the endplate is associated with decreased rates of subsidence. Ultimately, cage size and placement in the disc space are more important than implant design.[266,267] Placement of the cage anteriorly in the disc space gives the construct a better moment arm and therefore better segmental stabilization when compared with more posterior placement.[266] A recent biomechanical study found that cages with rectangular endplates had a lower subsidence rate than those with round endcaps.[268] By their nature, LLIF procedures offer the ability to place very wide cages that cover a large portion of the vertebral endplate. While these cages have a greater surface area than TLIF or PLIF cages, they are still susceptible to subsidence, particularly in osteopenic patients.[46]

For similar reasons, subsidence is a major concern for disc replacement procedures. In contrast to fusion procedures, there is no point at which the construct can be said to be healed in position. Implant sizing is crucial. Because an overly large implant is virtually impossible to insert into a degenerated and collapsed disc space, an undersized implant is more commonly inserted owing to difficulty in adequately distracting the collapsed disc space. Because small implants cover very little of the vertebral endplate and offer virtually no end bearing, central positioning of the device risks endplate subsidence. Finally, if the patient subsequently develops osteoporosis, endplate support itself may decrease.

Anterior Plates and Screw-Rod Systems

Purported benefits of anterior fixation include decreased rates of pseudarthrosis (particularly in smokers), graft extrusion, postoperative kyphosis, and graft subsidence. Anterior plating reduces the need for postoperative bracing and allows early rehabilitation. Mechanically, anterior devices function in a neutralization mode. The implant partly shields axial stress and minimizes torsional bending and shearing and also provides resistance to vertebral extension.

Anterior thoracolumbar implants are chosen as part of a complete reconstruction strategy. Depending on whether a discectomy or corpectomy is performed, the decision of whether to include anterior or posterior instrumentation is made in conjunction with the decision about the type of interbody device or graft.

Anterior fixation systems can be classified as either unconstrained or constrained. The earliest attempts at anterior fixation used dynamic compression plates, originally designed for the appendicular skeleton, across disc spaces. Most unconstrained constructs are single-rod systems used in the anterior management of scoliosis.[269,270]

The advantage of an unconstrained system is its ease of insertion. The disadvantage is its poor rotational stability.[269] Most unconstrained systems provide no fixed angle between the bone anchor (typically a screw) and the longitudinal member, which increases the risk of screw backout, especially if placed unicortically. Unconstrained anterior systems are often used in deformity surgery and are augmented with bracing. In more unstable settings involving trauma or tumor, their role is best limited to the mid-thoracic spine with an intact rib cage and sternum.[271] The greater stresses associated with the thoracolumbar or lumbar spine limit the usefulness of unconstrained systems there to cases in which supplemental posterior instrumentation would be used.

Constrained systems include rigid fixation between the anchor point and the longitudinal member, be it a plate or a rod. Constrained systems can be divided into plate systems and dual-rod systems. Plating systems are generally considered easier to place and lower profile than dual-rod systems. Anterior plates are not quite as rigid as dual plating systems, particularly with regard to torsional stability.[272]

Advantages of constrained systems include the ability to apply compression across the graft. The fixed angle between the screw and the plate or rod allows maintenance of sagittal balance. A fixed angle can also be a disadvantage because it limits screw placement options, such as in hemicorpectomy, in which screws may need to be placed close together. Other potential disadvantages include implant bulk. Lateral, rather than anterolateral, placement is key in avoiding the great vessels and risk of vascular erosion.

Application of dual-rod systems involves placing screws through spiked plates into the lateral vertebral body. The plates decrease axial load through the screws by distributing axial load across the vertebral body. Distribution of this load is helpful because of the thinness of the lateral vertebral cortices. Without the plates, the screws could tear through the lateral vertebral body wall.[273] In some systems, individual screw plates are available. These single-screw plates spread vertical loads over a smaller area but have increased placement options.

Plates designed to stabilize the lower lumbar spine after ALIFs have been offered by various manufacturers.[274] These devices seek to provide extension stability to the fused segment while obviating the need for a supplementary posterior construct. At this time, biomechanical or clinical support for these devices remains limited, though they may have a role in avoiding posterior surgery in certain degenerative conditions.[275,276] That said, there is renewed interest in anterior plating when combined with LLIF surgery.

Some anterior thoracolumbar implants are placed more to contain graft material than to control segmental motion. Numerous resorbable implants have been developed for this purpose.[277] More common are screw-washer constructs or various small plates that attach to one vertebral body and span the intervertebral disc space. Such "anti-backout" systems have little biomechanical support for their use.

Recently, there has been an increase in the number of all-in-one devices available. These implants integrate the cage with a plate or locking screws. In one recent biomechanical study, integrated lateral cage-plate devices offered similar restriction of motion to a separate plate and cage construct and more restriction than the cage alone.[278] This construct was not as rigid as cage plus posterior pedicle screws or facet screw placement.

In one recent biomechanical study in nine cadaveric spines, an integrated ALIF spacer performed especially well in patients with higher sacral slopes.[279] The authors surmised that this advantage arose from the angulation of the integrated plate screws. They suggested that increasing sacral slope reduced the stiffness of most typical reconstructions and that "more aggressive fixation techniques" be used. Use of an integrated cage-screw construct was reported in 65 patients for degenerative conditions at three spine centers.[280] The fusion rate was 96.3% with a 2.0% subsidence rate.

The drawbacks of anterior thoracolumbar instrumentation include cost, lack of familiarity with the approach, the occasional need for an access surgeon, and space available for the implant. Hardware loosening may be the result of osteoporosis with insufficient bone purchase or inadequate postoperative immobilization. Potential complications, as with all types of spinal fixation, include deep infection, implant failure, and vascular and neurologic injury. Specific risks include parenchymal injuries to the lungs and erosion into the vessels. The exact risk of vascular erosion is unknown. There are no reported cases of late vascular injury reported with contemporary systems, although some earlier anterior fixation systems were discontinued because of this risk. Current recommendations are to keep metal components more than 1 cm away from the great vessels.

Lumbar Disc Arthroplasty, Nuclear Replacement, and Other Motion-Sparing Approaches

Disc-level anterior motion-preserving implants (disc and nuclear replacement systems) are also available, although their use has decreased markedly.

The historical precursor to total disc replacement and nuclear replacement was the stainless steel Fernström ball. This spherical endoprosthesis was developed and implanted in the 1950s and 1960s as a spacer that allowed motion of the adjacent vertebrae.[281] The shape of the device concentrated the loads on a small portion of the implant and vertebral endplate surface. Normal load distribution could not be recovered; because of concerns about device migration and subsidence, the device was subsequently abandoned.[282]

Later efforts at nuclear replacement sought to use less-stiff, preferably viscoelastic materials. These devices included preformed implants and injected polymers that cure in situ. The ideal nuclear replacement restores disc mechanics with much less normal tissue ablation than total disc arthroplasty. These devices sought to offer shock absorption not seen with lumbar disc arthroplasty designs.[283]

These implants were intended for use as a primary treatment of early, painful lumbar disc degeneration or for placement at the time of discectomy in a patient with radicular symptoms. In the latter case, the nuclear replacement was intended to maintain or restore disc height and function. It was hoped that in the short term this restoration of disc mechanics would decrease postoperative back pain. Ideally, nuclear replacement would prevent further motion-segment degeneration, decreasing the likelihood of more invasive and destructive surgeries such as fusion or disc arthroplasty.[283,284]

Contraindications for a nucleus prosthesis include disc height less than 5 mm, anular incompetence (in the form of major tears), grade II or greater spondylolisthesis, and Schmorl nodes.[285]

The most studied device was Ray's prosthetic disc nucleus (PDN), consisting of a hydrogel core encased in a polyethylene jacket and first developed in 1988. The hydrogel absorbs water and expands to fill the nuclear cavity. The jacket prevents the hydrogel from overexpansion. Initially, two devices were implanted at each operated level. After extrusion problems were encountered, a larger, single PDN was designed. Although the device was initially inserted solely through a large posterolateral annulotomy, the consequences of device extrusion into the canal led to anterolateral insertions.[285]

Minimally invasive delivery of injectable materials can be accomplished with small anular windows, decreasing the risk of implant extrusion. Preformed implants may have the advantage of improved mechanical strength and fatigue life, but several designs have been associated with high extrusion rates. In many of these devices, intense, inflammatory endplate reactions were reported as were high rates of explantation and conversion to fusion.[286]

After the Fernström ball, the evolution of total disc and nuclear replacement diverged. Unlike cervical disc arthroplasty, which is typically indicated to restore stable and segmental height after anterior decompression, lumbar disc replacement is indicated for reduction of axial low back pain and to avoid the morbidity associated with fusion. Disc replacement seeks to remove the pain generator while preserving motion. In avoiding fusion, bone graft donor site morbidity is avoided, as is the possibility of pseudarthrosis. Theoretical benefits include decreased rates of adjacent-segment degeneration and improved sagittal balance.

In 1982, in what was then East Germany, Büttner-Janz and Schellnack initiated development of their artificial disc at the Charité Hospital in Berlin.[287] They based their design on the "low-friction" principle used in total knee and total hip arthroplasty. In particular, they placed a polyethylene sliding core between two highly polished metal endplates. This sliding core was to mimic the movement of nucleus within its annular containment. Their initial effort was frustrated by endplate and device fractures as well as insufficient instrumentation for implantation. The large European medical device manufacturer Helmut Link took over production in 1987 and funded an FDA trial in the United States. Eventually, this device was purchased by DePuy Johnson & Johnson (now DePuy Synthes).

The next disc arthroplasty system was the Prodisc, two titanium endplates with a fixed polyethylene core between them. Motion occurs by articulation of only the upper plate on the convex superior surface of the constrained core. This device was designed and implanted into a group of patients, after which the designer, Thierry Marnay, refrained from further implantations for 8 years. Subsequently, Marnay reported 8- to 10-year follow-up results on a group of 44 patients who received this prosthesis. He reported 78% good to excellent results. Synthes brought this device to the North American market and funded an FDA trial. After Depuy and Synthes merged, the Charité was discontinued.[288] Current indications for lumbar disc replacement are as follows:

- One- or two-level (L5–S1 or L4–L5, or both) lumbar disc degeneration (Fig. 70.12)
- Postdiscectomy mechanical back pain
- Degeneration of levels adjacent to a former lumbar fusion

Contraindications for disc arthroplasty are more controversial. Although subtle retrolisthesis related to disc collapse is acceptable, disc replacement with greater degrees of translational instability or spinal deformity should be avoided. Disc arthroplasty should not be performed in patients with marked facet osteoarthritis.[289] The ideal arthroplasty patient presents with a single painful level with more than 4 mm of remaining disc height at that level. This ideal patient has intact posterior elements and no facet or adjacent-level degeneration. Certainly, the percentage of patients who might be candidates for total disc arthroplasty is much smaller than those who could be considered for fusion surgery.

Over the previous decade, many differing lumbar disc arthroplasty designs have been under study. Proponents of constrained versus semiconstrained implants and differing bearing surfaces, such as metal-on-metal versus metal-on-polyethylene, debated at meetings and in the literature.[290-292] Proponents of metal-on-metal designs cite the increased rate at which polyethylene wears. Polyethylene particles could lead to osteolytic reactions and loss of bone stock. Thin polyethylene

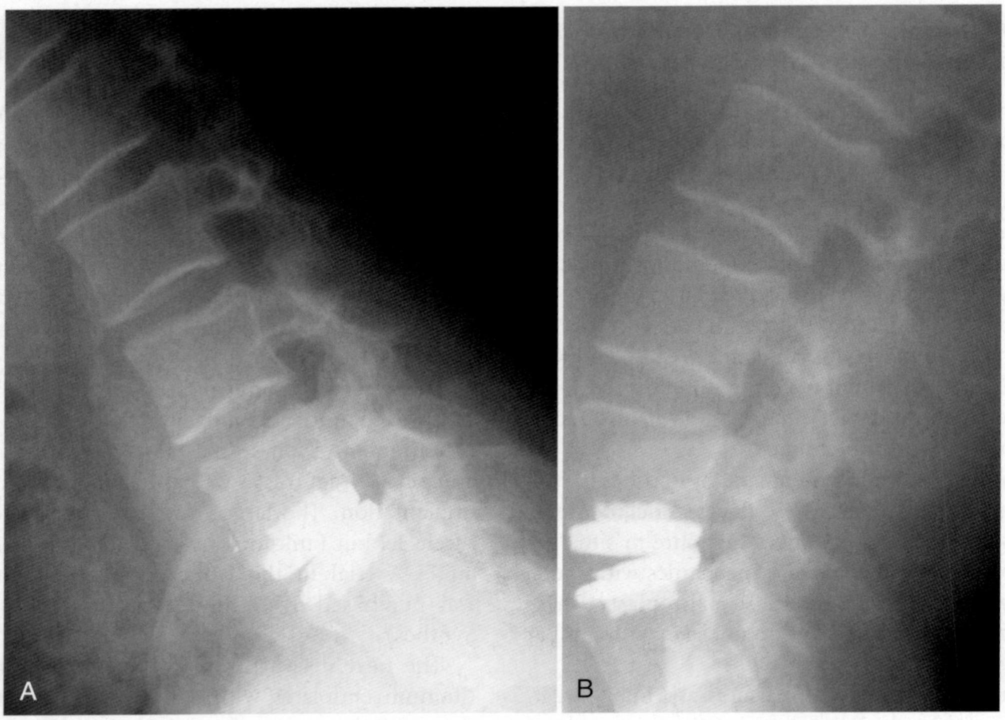

FIG. 70.12 Anterior lumbar disc replacement. All disc replacement systems seek to decrease pain while maintaining motion, eliminating some of the morbidity of fusion such as adjacent-segment disease or graft harvest pain. (A–B) Flexion-extension radiographs obtained 1 year postoperatively in a pain-free patient.

is subject to creep and cracking. However, initial polyethylene wear rate studies suggest excellent prospects for long-term viability.[20]

Metal-on-metal, although more durable, is approached suspiciously by some spine surgeons because of concerns about metal ions leaching into the bloodstream. Currently available data are inadequate to compare these risks. Given the concerns around metal-on-metal hip prostheses, those designs have largely disappeared from the market.[293,294]

The issue of device constraint remains unresolved as well. Proponents of unconstrained devices state that these are most capable of restoring the normal, coupled motion of the lower lumbar spine. Supporters of semiconstrained designs cite occasional polyethylene liner extrusions as evidence that more constraint is needed. The concept of "semiconstrained" is elusive: How much is enough? How much is too much? In particular, do these values hold over various levels of the lumbar spine? The instantaneous axis of rotation of the lumbar spine is not constant, and changes depend on the joint position.[295,296]

If disc replacement systems restore motion, critics worry that improper motion may be worse than no motion. Disc degeneration rarely occurs in isolation. More typically, at least some facet degeneration coexists. One concern is that maintenance of motion would precipitate further facet degeneration. Given that the facets guide segmental motion, further facet degeneration may further disrupt normal kinematics.[297] In a prospective, clinical study of 64 patients, low-grade facet arthrosis did not influence outcomes after implantation of a semiconstrained metal-on-metal total disc replacement.[297a] At 2-year follow-up, the preoperative ODI score of 43.8 had improved to 23.1. Visual analog scale back pain score had decreased from 7.6 to 3.2.

More constrained implants require more elaborate fixation methods to the host vertebral body.[298] Several of the semiconstrained implants in the first generation of devices include keels. Although it is unclear if the keel offers a net advantage to the patient in terms of long-term stability, it would complicate any attempt to remove the implant. Two deep keels at adjacent levels of disc arthroplasty may subject the vertebral body to sagittal split fracture. For all but the tallest degenerated discs, current lumbar disc arthroplasty designs require marked disc space distraction. Too much distraction seems to decrease motion at the adjacent segment. Too little distraction risks implant extravasation.

Finally, critics of the current total disc arthroplasty systems have cited the suboptimal outcomes reported in the published articles. In particular, the actual amount of motion preserved may be very low, and rates of adjacent-segment degeneration have not been definitively affected by arthroplasty over fusion procedures.[299,300]

The final category of anterior implants are staples used for fusion or epiphysiodesis in pediatric scoliosis surgery. Physeal staples, which may be inserted thoracoscopically, are being used to halt growth selectively on the convex side of the deformity.[301] Some seek to cross the disc space, others just cross the epiphysis to compress the growth plate, allowing further growth on the convex side.

A recent computer simulation reported for such a device suggested that properly placed in time (relative to the patient's growth) and space, the device could control the progression of scoliosis without fusion.[302] Posterior screw placement for posterior convex growth arrest has also been described in congenital scoliosis surgery.[303]

Summary

The use of instrumentation in the thoracolumbar spine greatly increases the surgeon's ability to provide stability to the spine. Enhanced posture and healing of the spine often result. Improved functional outcome for degenerative conditions is more difficult to assess, however. Functional outcome is frequently related more to patient selection, decompression, and patient comorbidities.

At this writing, attempts to restore stability without fusion remain under study, but are limited.

Successful use of thoracolumbar instrumentation requires a detailed knowledge of spinal anatomy and the biomechanics. The intended patient's biologic and pathomechanical factors must also be considered in relationship to the implant's ability to address the identified deficits.

KEY REFERENCES

1. Sugiura T, Kashii M, Matsuo Y, et al. Intermittent administration of teriparatide enhances graft bone healing and accelerates spinal fusion in rats with glucocorticoid-induced osteoporosis. *Spine J.* 2015;15(2):298-306.
2. Lonne G, Johnsen LG, Rossvoll I, et al. Minimally invasive decompression versus X-STOP in lumbar spinal stenosis: a randomized controlled multicenter study. *Spine.* 2015;40(2):77-85.
3. Wray S, Mimran R, Vadapalli S, et al. Pedicle screw placement in the lumbar spine: effect of trajectory and screw design on acute biomechanical purchase. *J Neurosurg Spine.* 2015;22(5):503-510.
4. Calvert GC, Lawrence BD, Abtahi AM, Bachus KN, Brodke DS. Cortical screws used to rescue failed lumbar pedicle screw construct: a biomechanical analysis. *J Neurosurg Spine.* 2015;22(2):166-172.
5. Palumbo MA, Shah KN, Eberson CP, Hart RA, Daniels AH. Outrigger rod technique for supplemental support of posterior spinal arthrodesis. *Spine J.* 2015;15(6):1409-1414.

REFERENCES

1. Kostuik JP, Errico TJ, Gleason TF. Techniques of internal fixation for degenerative conditions of the lumbar spine. *Clin Orthop Relat Res.* 1986;203:219-231.
2. Boachie-Adjei O, Squillante RG. Tuberculosis of the spine. *Orthop Clin North Am.* 1996;27(1):95-103.
3. Bono CM, Garfin SR. History and evolution of disc replacement. *Spine J.* 2004;4(6 suppl):145S-150S.
4. Truumees E, Hilibrand A, Vaccaro A. Percutaneous vertebral augmentation. *Spine J.* 2004;4(2):218-229.
5. Steffen T, Rubin RK, Baramki HG, et al. A new technique for measuring lumbar segmental motion in vivo. Method, accuracy, and preliminary results. *Spine.* 1997;22(2):156-166.
6. Perry TG, Mageswaran P, Colbrunn RW, et al. Biomechanical evaluation of a simulated T-9 burst fracture of the thoracic spine with an intact rib cage. *J Neurosurg Spine.* 2014;21(3):481-488.
7. Husted DS, Yue JJ, Fairchild TA, Haims AH. An extrapedicular approach to the placement of screws in the thoracic spine: an anatomic and radiographic assessment. *Spine.* 2003;28(20):2324-2330.
8. Soyuncu Y, Yildirim FB, Sekban H, et al. Anatomic evaluation and relationship between the lumbar pedicle and adjacent neural structures: an anatomic study. *J Spinal Disord Tech.* 2005;18(3):243-246.
9. Maruyama T, Takeshita K, Nakamura K, Kitagawa T. Spatial relations between the vertebral body and the thoracic aorta in adolescent idiopathic scoliosis. *Spine.* 2004;29(18):2067-2069.
10. Dick JC, Bourgeault CA. Notch sensitivity of titanium alloy, commercially pure titanium, and stainless steel spinal implants. *Spine.* 2001;26(15):1668-1672.
11. Lamerain M, Bachy M, Delpont M, et al. CoCr rods provide better frontal correction of adolescent idiopathic scoliosis treated by all-pedicle screw fixation. *Eur Spine J.* 2014;23(6):1190-1196.
12. Nguyen TQ, Buckley JM, Ames C, Deviren V. The fatigue life of contoured cobalt chrome posterior spinal fusion rods. *Proc Inst Mech Eng H.* 2011;225(2):194-198.
13. Smith JS, Shaffrey E, Klineberg E, et al. Prospective multicenter assessment of risk factors for rod fracture following surgery for adult spinal deformity. *J Neurosurg Spine.* 2014;21(6):994-1003.
14. Cook SD, Patron LP, Christakis PM, et al. Comparison of methods for determining the presence and extent of anterior lumbar interbody fusion. *Spine.* 2004;29(10):1118-1123.
15. Rao PJ, Pelletier MH, Walsh WR, Mobbs RJ. Spine interbody implants: material selection and modification, functionalization and bioactivation of surfaces to improve osseointegration. *Orthop Surg.* 2014;6(2):81-89.
16. Abode-Iyamah K, Kim SB, Grosland N, et al. Spinal motion and intradiscal pressure measurements before and after lumbar spine instrumentation with titanium or PEEK rods. *J Clin Neurosci.* 2014;21(4):651-655.
17. Tsouknidas A. The effect of pedicle screw implantation depth and angle on the loading and stiffness of a spinal fusion assembly. *Biomed Mater Eng.* 2015;25(4):425-433.
18. Mavrogenis AF, Vottis C, Triantafyllopoulos G, Papagelopoulos PJ, Pneumaticos SG. PEEK rod systems for the spine. *Eur J Orthop Surg Traumatol.* 2014;24(suppl 1):S111-S116.
19. Kirkpatrick J, Venugopalan R, Beck P, Lemons J. Corrosion on spinal implants. *J Spinal Disord Tech.* 2005;18(3):247-251.
20. Serhan H, Slivka M, Albert T, Kwak SD. Is galvanic corrosion between titanium alloy and stainless steel spinal implants a clinical concern? *Spine J.* 2004;4(4):379-387.
21. Krijnen MR, Mullender MG, Smit TH, Everts V, Wuisman PI. Radiographic, histologic, and chemical evaluation of bioresorbable 70/30 poly-L-lactide-CO-D, L-lactide interbody fusion cages in a goat model. *Spine.* 2006;31(14):1559-1567.
22. Lazennec JY, Madi A, Rousseau MA, Roger B, Saillant G. Evaluation of the 96/4 PLDLLA polymer resorbable lumbar interbody cage in a long term animal model. *Eur Spine J.* 2006;15(10):1545-1553.
23. Cunningham BW, Sefter JC, Shono Y, McAfee PC. Static and cyclical biomechanical analysis of pedicle screw spinal constructs. *Spine.* 1993;18(12):1677-1688.
24. Goel VK, Winterbottom JM, Weinstein JN. A method for the fatigue testing of pedicle screw fixation devices. *J Biomech.* 1994;27(11):1383-1388.
25. Kummer FJ, Neuwirth M, Yabut S. Cyclic loading of segmental spinal instrumentation. *Bull Hosp Jt Dis Orthop Inst.* 1988;48(2):204-206.

26. Ashman RB, Birch JG, Bone LB, et al. Mechanical testing of spinal instrumentation. *Clin Orthop Relat Res.* 1988;227: 113-125.
27. Abe Y, Ito M, Abumi K, et al. Scoliosis corrective force estimation from the implanted rod deformation using 3D-FEM analysis. *Scoliosis.* 2015;10(suppl 2):S2.
28. Yamanaka K, Mori M, Yamazaki K, et al. Analysis of the fracture mechanism of Ti-6Al-4V alloy rods that failed clinically after spinal instrumentation surgery. *Spine.* 2015; 40(13):E767-E773.
29. Lukina E, Kollerov M, Meswania J, et al. Analysis of retrieved growth guidance sliding LSZ-4D devices for early onset scoliosis and investigation of the use of nitinol rods for this system. *Spine.* 2015;40(1):17-24.
30. Weiss LE, Vaccaro AR, Scuderi G, McGuire M, Garfin SR. Pseudarthrosis after postoperative wound infection in the lumbar spine. *J Spinal Disord.* 1997;10(6):482-487.
31. Kuklo TR, Bridwell KH, Lewis SJ, et al. Minimum 2-year analysis of sacropelvic fixation and L5-S1 fusion using S1 and iliac screws. *Spine.* 2001;26(18):1976-1983.
32. Bono CM, Khandha A, Vadapalli S, et al. Residual sagittal motion after lumbar fusion: a finite element analysis with implications on radiographic flexion-extension criteria. *Spine.* 2007;32(4):417-422.
33. Esses SI, Doherty BJ, Crawford MJ, Dreyzin V. Kinematic evaluation of lumbar fusion techniques. *Spine.* 1996;21(6):676-684.
34. Alpert HW, Farley FA, Caird MS, et al. Outcomes following removal of instrumentation after posterior spinal fusion. *J Pediatr Orthop.* 2014;34(6):613-617.
35. Craven TG, Carson WL, Asher MA, Robinson RG. The effects of implant stiffness on the bypassed bone mineral density and facet fusion stiffness of the canine spine. *Spine.* 1994;19(15):1664-1673.
36. Goel VK, Kim YE, Lim TH, Weinstein JN. An analytical investigation of the mechanics of spinal instrumentation. *Spine.* 1988;13(9):1003-1011.
37. Dahdaleh NS, Smith ZA, Hitchon PW. Percutaneous pedicle screw fixation for thoracolumbar fractures. *Neurosurg Clin N Am.* 2014;25(2):337-346.
38. Jeon CH, Lee HD, Lee YS, Seo JH, Chung NS. Is it beneficial to remove the pedicle screw instrument after successful posterior fusion of thoracolumbar burst fractures? *Spine.* 2015;40(11):E627-E633.
39. Fitschen-Oestern S, Scheuerlein F, Weuster M, et al. Reduction and retention of thoracolumbar fractures by minimally invasive stabilisation versus open posterior instrumentation. *Injury.* 2015;46(suppl 4):S63-S70.
40. Nayak NR, Pisapia JM, Abdullah KG, Schuster JM. Minimally invasive surgery for traumatic fractures in ankylosing spinal diseases. *Global Spine J.* 2015;5(4):266-273.
41. Pekmezci M, Herfat S, Theologis AA, et al. Integrity of "damage control" posterior spinal fusion constructs for poly-trauma patients: a biomechanical investigation. *Spine.* 2015;40(23):E1219-E1225.
42. Goldstein CL, Brodke DS, Choma TJ. Surgical management of spinal conditions in the elderly osteoporotic spine. *Neurosurgery.* 2015;77(suppl 4):S98-S107.
43. Harel R, Doron O, Knoller N. Minimally invasive spine metastatic tumor resection and stabilization: new technology yield improved outcome. *Biomed Res Int.* 2015;2015:948373.
44. Jang JS, Lee SH, Rhee CH, Lee SH. Polymethylmethacrylate-augmented screw fixation for stabilization in metastatic spinal tumors. Technical note. *J Neurosurg.* 2002;96(1 suppl):131-134.
45. Tu CW, Huang KF, Hsu HT, et al. Zoledronic acid infusion for lumbar interbody fusion in osteoporosis. *J Surg Res.* 2014;192(1):112-116.
46. Tempel ZJ, Gandhoke GS, Okonkwo DO, Kanter AS. Impaired bone mineral density as a predictor of graft subsidence following minimally invasive transpsoas lateral lumbar interbody fusion. *Eur Spine J.* 2015;24(suppl 3):414-419.
47. Ravindra VM, Godzik J, Guan J, et al. Prevalence of vitamin D deficiency in patients undergoing elective spine surgery: a cross-sectional analysis. *World Neurosurg.* 2015;83(6):1114-1119.
48. Leslie WD, Ward LM. Bone density monitoring with the total hip site: time for a re-evaluation? *J Clin Densitom.* 2004;7(3):269-274.
49. Sugiura T, Kashii M, Matsuo Y, et al. Intermittent administration of teriparatide enhances graft bone healing and accelerates spinal fusion in rats with glucocorticoid-induced osteoporosis. *Spine J.* 2015;15(2):298-306.
50. Myers E, Wilson S. Biomechanics of osteoporosis and vertebral fracture. *Spine.* 1997;22:255-315.
51. Knoller SM, Meyer G, Eckhardt C, et al. Range of motion in reconstruction situations following corpectomy in the lumbar spine: a question of bone mineral density? *Spine.* 2005;30(9):E229-E235.
52. Hackenberg L, Link T, Liljenqvist U. Axial and tangential fixation strength of pedicle screws versus hooks in the thoracic spine in relation to bone mineral density. *Spine.* 2002;27(9):937-942.
53. Ryken TC, Clausen JD, Traynelis VC, Goel VK. Biomechanical analysis of bone mineral density, insertion technique, screw torque, and holding strength of anterior cervical plate screws. *J Neurosurg.* 1995;83(2): 325-329.
54. Blair-Pattison A, Hu RW, Swamy G, Anglin C. Forces in spinal cannulation and breaches ex vivo. *Proc Inst Mech Eng H.* 2014;228(7):693-702.
55. Chen C, Lv G, Xu B, Zhang X, Ma X. Posterior short-segment instrumentation and limited segmental decompression supplemented with vertebroplasty with calcium sulphate and intermediate screws for thoracolumbar burst fractures. *Eur Spine J.* 2014;23(7):1548-1557.
56. Chen SH, Lee CH, Huang KC, Hsieh PH, Tsai SY. Postoperative wound infection after posterior spinal instrumentation: analysis of long-term treatment outcomes. *Eur Spine J.* 2015;24(3):561-570.
57. Disch AC, Schmoelz W. Cement augmentation in a thoracolumbar fracture model: reduction and stability after balloon kyphoplasty versus vertebral body stenting. *Spine.* 2014;39(19):E1147-E1153.
58. Dai F, Liu Y, Zhang F, et al. Surgical treatment of the osteoporotic spine with bone cement-injectable cannulated pedicle screw fixation: technical description and preliminary application in 43 patients. *Clinics (Sao Paulo).* 2015;70(2):114-119.
59. Moussazadeh N, Rubin DG, McLaughlin L, et al. Short-segment percutaneous pedicle screw fixation with cement augmentation for tumor-induced spinal instability. *Spine J.* 2015;15(7):1609-1617.
60. Pitzen T, Barbier D, Tintinger F, Steudel WI, Strowitzki M. Screw fixation to the posterior cortical shell does not

influence peak torque and pullout in anterior cervical plating. *Eur Spine J*. 2002;11(5):494-499.
61. Ruland CM, McAfee PC, Warden KE, Cunningham BW. Triangulation of pedicular instrumentation. A biomechanical analysis. *Spine*. 1991;16(6 suppl):S270-S276.
62. Hadjipavlou AG, Nicodemus CL, al-Hamdan FA, Simmons JW, Pope MH. Correlation of bone equivalent mineral density to pull-out resistance of triangulated pedicle screw construct. *J Spinal Disord*. 1997;10(1):12-19.
63. Lowe T, O'Brien M, Smith D, et al. Central and juxta-endplate vertebral body screw placement: a biomechanical analysis in a human cadaveric model. *Spine*. 2002;27(4):369-373.
64. Carson WL, Duffield RC, Arendt M, Ridgely BJ, Gaines RW Jr. Internal forces and moments in transpedicular spine instrumentation. The effect of pedicle screw angle and transfixation—the 4R-4bar linkage concept. *Spine*. 1990;15(9):893-901.
65. Kuklo TR, Lehman RA Jr. Effect of various tapping diameters on insertion of thoracic pedicle screws: a biomechanical analysis. *Spine*. 2003;28(18):2066-2071.
66. Hitchon PW, Brenton MD, Coppes JK, From AM, Torner JC. Factors affecting the pullout strength of self-drilling and self-tapping anterior cervical screws. *Spine*. 2003;28(1):9-13.
67. Robertson PA, Plank LD. Pedicle screw placement at the sacrum: anatomical characterization and limitations at S1. *J Spinal Disord*. 1999;12(3):227-233.
68. Lehman RA Jr, Kuklo TR, Belmont PJ Jr, Andersen RC, Polly DW Jr. Advantage of pedicle screw fixation directed into the apex of the sacral promontory over bicortical fixation: a biomechanical analysis. *Spine*. 2002;27(8):806-811.
69. Aghayev K, Gonzalez-Blohm SA, Doulgeris JJ, et al. Feasibility and biomechanical performance of a novel transdiscal screw system for one level in non-spondylolisthetic lumbar fusion: an in vitro investigation. *Spine J*. 2014;14(4):705-713.
70. Davis TT, Tadlock S, Bernbeck J, Fung DA, Molinares DM. Can triggered electromyography be used to evaluate pedicle screw placement in hydroxyapatite-coated screws: an electrical examination. *J Clin Neurophysiol*. 2014;31(2):138-142.
71. Gittens RA, Olivares-Navarrete R, Schwartz Z, Boyan BD. Implant osseointegration and the role of microroughness and nanostructures: lessons for spine implants. *Acta Biomater*. 2014;10(8):3363-3371.
72. Demura S, Murakami H, Shirai T, et al. Surgical treatment for pyogenic vertebral osteomyelitis using iodine-supported spinal instruments: initial case series of 14 patients. *Eur J Clin Microbiol Infect Dis*. 2015;34(2):261-266.
73. Mohan AL, Das K. History of surgery for the correction of spinal deformity. *Neurosurg Focus*. 2003;14(1):e1.
74. Harrington PR. Treatment of scoliosis. Correction and internal fixation by spine instrumentation. *Am J Orthop*. 1962;44-A:591-610.
75. Cotrel Y, Dubousset J. [A new technic for segmental spinal osteosynthesis using the posterior approach]. *Rev Chir Orthop Reparatrice Appar Mot*. 1984;70(6):489-494.
76. Cybulski GR, Stone JL, Opesanmi O. Spinal cord decompression via a modified costotransversectomy approach combined with posterior instrumentation for management of metastatic neoplasms of the thoracic spine. *Surg Neurol*. 1991;35(4):280-285.
77. Chacko AG, Moorthy RK, Chandy MJ. The transpedicular approach in the management of thoracic spine tuberculosis: a short-term follow up study. *Spine*. 2004;29(17):E363-E367.
78. Viale GL, Silvestro C, Francaviglia N, et al. Transpedicular decompression and stabilization of burst fractures of the lumbar spine. *Surg Neurol*. 1993;40(2):104-111.
79. McLain RF. Endoscopically assisted decompression for metastatic thoracic neoplasms. *Spine*. 1998;23(10):1130-1135.
80. Lu K, Liang CL, Cho CL, et al. Oxidative stress and heat shock protein response in human paraspinal muscles during retraction. *J Neurosurg*. 2002;97(1 suppl): 75-81.
81. Wiltse LL, Spencer CW. New uses and refinements of the paraspinal approach to the lumbar spine. *Spine*. 1988;13(6):696-706.
82. Khoo LT, Palmer S, Laich DT, Fessler RG. Minimally invasive percutaneous posterior lumbar interbody fusion. *Neurosurgery*. 2002;51(5 suppl):S166-S181.
83. Zucherman J, Hsu K, Hartjen C, et al. A multicenter, prospective, randomized trial evaluating the X STOP interspinous process decompression system for the treatment of neurogenic intermittent claudication: two-year follow-up results. *Spine*. 2005;30(12):1351-1358.
84. Lonne G, Johnsen LG, Aas E, et al. Comparing cost-effectiveness of X-STOP with minimally invasive decompression in lumbar spinal stenosis: a randomized controlled trial. *Spine*. 2015;40(8):514-520.
85. Lonne G, Johnsen LG, Rossvoll I, et al. Minimally invasive decompression versus X-STOP in lumbar spinal stenosis: a randomized controlled multicenter study. *Spine*. 2015;40(2):77-85.
86. Patel VV, Whang PG, Haley TR, et al. Superior interspinous process spacer for intermittent neurogenic claudication secondary to moderate lumbar spinal stenosis: two-year results from a randomized controlled FDA-IDE pivotal trial. *Spine*. 2015;40(5):275-282.
87. Alexandre A, Alexandre AM, De Pretto M, Coro L, Saggini R. One-year follow-up of a series of 100 patients treated for lumbar spinal canal stenosis by means of HeliFix interspinous process decompression device. *Biomed Res Int*. 2014;2014:176936.
88. Galarza M, Gazzeri R, De la Rosa P, Martinez-Lage JF. Microdiscectomy with and without insertion of interspinous device for herniated disc at the L5-S1 level. *J Clin Neurosci*. 2014;21(11):1934-1939.
89. Sénégas J. Mechanical supplementation by non-rigid fixation in degenerative intervertebral lumbar segments: the Wallis system. *Eur Spine J*. 2002;11(suppl 2):S164-S169.
90. Gibson JN, Depreitere B, Pflugmacher R, et al. Decompression and paraspinous tension band: a novel treatment method for patients with lumbar spinal stenosis and degenerative spondylolisthesis. *Spine J*. 2015;15(3 suppl): S23-S32.
91. Doulgeris JJ, Aghayev K, Gonzalez-Blohm SA, Lee WE 3rd, Vrionis FD. Biomechanical comparison of an interspinous fusion device and bilateral pedicle screw system as additional fixation for lateral lumbar interbody fusion. *Clin Biomech (Bristol, Avon)*. 2015;30(2):205-210.
92. Gonzalez-Blohm SA, Doulgeris JJ, Aghayev K, et al. Biomechanical analysis of an interspinous fusion device as a stand-alone and as supplemental fixation to posterior expandable interbody cages in the lumbar spine. *J Neurosurg Spine*. 2014;20(2):209-219.
93. Gazzeri R, Galarza M, Alfieri A. Controversies about interspinous process devices in the treatment of degenerative

lumbar spine diseases: past, present, and future. *Biomed Res Int.* 2014;2014:975052.

94. Wang T, Fielding LC, Parikh A, Kothari M, Alamin T. Sacral spinous processes: a morphologic classification and biomechanical characterization of strength. *Spine J.* 2015;15(12):2544-2551.
95. Shim CS, Lee SH, Jung B, et al. Fluoroscopically assisted percutaneous translaminar facet screw fixation following anterior lumbar interbody fusion: technical report. *Spine.* 2005;30(7):838-843.
96. Margulies JY, Seimon LP. Clinical efficacy of lumbar and lumbosacral fusion using the Boucher facet screw fixation technique. *Bull Hosp Jt Dis.* 2000;59(1):33-39.
97. Buttermann GR, Thorson TM, Mullin WJ. Outcomes of posterior facet versus pedicle screw fixation of circumferential fusion: a cohort study. *Eur Spine J.* 2014;23(2):347-355.
98. Chin KR, Seale J, Cumming V. Mini-open or percutaneous bilateral lumbar transfacet pedicle screw fixation: a technical note. *J Spinal Disord Tech.* 2015;28(2):61-65.
99. Cook DJ, Yeager MS, Oh MY, Cheng BC. Lumbar intrafacet bone dowel fixation. *Neurosurgery.* 2015;76(4):470-478, discussion 478.
100. Anekstein Y, Floman Y, Smorgick Y, et al. Seven years follow-up for total lumbar facet joint replacement (TOPS) in the management of lumbar spinal stenosis and degenerative spondylolisthesis. *Eur Spine J.* 2015;24(10):2306-2314.
101. Luque ER. Segmental spinal instrumentation for correction of scoliosis. *Clin Orthop Relat Res.* 1982;163:192-198.
102. Zdeblick TA, Becker PS, McAfee PC, et al. Neuropathologic changes with experimental spinal instrumentation: transpedicular versus sublaminar fixation. *J Spinal Disord.* 1991;4(2):221-228.
103. Drummond D, Guadagni J, Keene JS, Breed A, Narechania R. Interspinous process segmental spinal instrumentation. *J Pediatr Orthop.* 1984;4(4):397-404.
104. Drummond DS. Harrington instrumentation with spinous process wiring for idiopathic scoliosis. *Orthop Clin North Am.* 1988;19(2):281-289.
105. Jeng CL, Sponseller PD, Tolo VT. Outcome of Wisconsin instrumentation in idiopathic scoliosis. Minimum 5-year follow-up. *Spine.* 1993;18(12):1584-1590.
106. Moe JH. Complications of scoliosis treatment. *Clin Orthop.* 1967;53:21-30.
107. Rohlmann A, Richter M, Zander T, et al. Effect of different surgical strategies on screw forces after correction of scoliosis with a VDS implant. *Eur Spine J.* 2005;S0940-6719.
108. Polly DW Jr, Potter BK, Kuklo T, et al. Volumetric spinal canal intrusion: a comparison between thoracic pedicle screws and thoracic hooks. *Spine.* 2004;29(1):63-69.
109. Liljenqvist U, Hackenberg L, Link T, Halm H. Pullout strength of pedicle screws versus pedicle and laminar hooks in the thoracic spine. *Acta Orthop Belg.* 2001;67(2):157-163.
110. Storer SK, Vitale MG, Hyman JE, et al. Correction of adolescent idiopathic scoliosis using thoracic pedicle screw fixation versus hook constructs. *J Pediatr Orthop.* 2005;25(4):415-419.
111. Cheung KM, Luk KD, Leong JC. Radiographic assessment of pedicle hook placement. *Spine.* 1997;22(18):2106-2111.
112. Roach JW, Ashman RB, Allard RN. The strength of a posterior element claw at one versus two spinal levels. *J Spinal Disord.* 1990;3(3):259-261.
113. Hilibrand AS, Moore DC, Graziano GP. The role of pediculolaminar fixation in compromised pedicle bone. *Spine.* 1996;21(4):445-451.
114. Roca J, Iborra M, Cavanilles-Walker JM, Alberti G. Direct repair of spondylolysis using a new pedicle screw hook fixation: clinical and CT-assessed study: an analysis of 19 patients. *J Spinal Disord Tech.* 2005;18(suppl):S82-S89.
115. Hasankhani EG, Omidi-Kashani F. Posterior tension band wiring and instrumentation for thoracolumbar flexion-distraction injuries. *J Orthop Surg (Hong Kong).* 2014;22(1):88-91.
116. Desai SK, Sayama C, Vener D, et al. The feasibility and safety of using sublaminar polyester bands in hybrid spinal constructs in children and transitional adults for neuromuscular scoliosis. *J Neurosurg Pediatr.* 2015;15(3):328-337.
117. Hirsch C, Ilharreborde B, Fournier J, Mazda K, Bonnard C. Adolescent idiopathic scoliosis correction achieved by posteromedial translation using polyester bands: a comparative study of subtransverse process versus sublaminar fixation. *Orthop Traumatol Surg Res.* 2014;100(7):791-795.
118. Albert MC, LaFleur BC. Hybrid fixation with sublaminar polyester bands in the treatment of neuromuscular scoliosis: a comparative analysis. *J Pediatr Orthop.* 2015;35(2):172-177.
119. Strickland BA, Sayama C, Briceno V, et al. Use of subtransverse process polyester bands in pediatric spine surgery: a case series of 4 patients with a minimum of 12 months' follow-up. *J Neurosurg Pediatr.* 2015;1-7.
120. Tremblay J, Mac-Thiong JM, Brailovski V, Petit Y. Braided tubular superelastic cables provide improved spinal stability compared to multifilament sublaminar cables. *Proc Inst Mech Eng H.* 2015;229(9):645-651.
121. Chang KW, Dewei Z, McAfee PC, et al. A comparative biomechanical study of spinal fixation using the combination spinal rod-plate and transpedicular screw fixation system. *J Spinal Disord.* 1988;1(4):257-266.
122. Orthopedic devices: classification and reclassification of pedicle screw spinal systems; technical amendment. Final rule; technical amendment. *Fed Regist.* 2001;66(99):28051-28053.
123. Park P, Garton HJ, Gala VC, Hoff JT, McGillicuddy JE. Adjacent segment disease after lumbar or lumbosacral fusion: review of the literature. *Spine.* 2004;29(17):1938-1944.
124. Thomsen K, Christensen FB, Eiskjaer SP, et al. The effect of pedicle screw instrumentation on functional outcome and fusion rates in posterolateral lumbar spinal fusion: a prospective, randomized clinical study. *Spine.* 1997;22(24):2813-2822.
125. McAfee PC, Farey ID, Sutterlin CE, et al. The effect of spinal implant rigidity on vertebral bone density. A canine model. *Spine.* 1991;16(6 suppl):S190-S197.
126. Lim TH, Goel VK, Winterbottom JM, et al. A comparison of stress-induced porosity due to conventional and a modified spinal fixation device. *J Spinal Disord.* 1994;7(1):1-11.
127. Shepard MF, Davies MR, Abayan A, Kabo JM, Wang JC. Effects of polyaxial pedicle screws on lumbar construct rigidity. *J Spinal Disord Tech.* 2002;15(3):233-236.
128. Rohlmann A, Bergmann G, Graichen F, Weber U. Comparison of loads on internal spinal fixation devices measured in vitro and in vivo. *Med Eng Phys.* 1997;19(6):539-546.
129. Rohlmann A, Riley LH 3rd, Bergmann G, Graichen F. In vitro load measurement using an instrumented spinal fixation device. *Med Eng Phys.* 1996;18(6):485-488.
130. Faraj AA, Webb JK. Early complications of spinal pedicle screw. *Eur Spine J.* 1997;6(5):324-326.

131. Tang H, Zhu J, Ji F, et al. Risk factors for postoperative complication after spinal fusion and instrumentation in degenerative lumbar scoliosis patients. *J Orthop Surg Res.* 2014;9(1):15.
132. Mummaneni PV, Dhall SS, Eck JC, et al. Guideline update for the performance of fusion procedures for degenerative disease of the lumbar spine. Part 11: interbody techniques for lumbar fusion. *J Neurosurg Spine.* 2014;21(1):67-74.
133. Jutte PC, Castelein RM. Complications of pedicle screws in lumbar and lumbosacral fusions in 105 consecutive primary operations. *Eur Spine J.* 2002;11(6):594-598.
134. Aota Y, Kumano K, Hirabayashi S, Ogawa Y. Reduction of lumbar spondylolisthesis using a CDI pedicle screw system. *Arch Orthop Trauma Surg.* 1995;114(4):188-193.
135. Hu SS, Bradford DS, Transfeldt EE, Cohen M. Reduction of high-grade spondylolisthesis using Edwards instrumentation. *Spine.* 1996;21(3):367-371.
136. Ogilvie JW. Complications in spondylolisthesis surgery. *Spine.* 2005;30(6 suppl):S97-S101.
137. Lian XF, Hou TS, Xu JG, et al. Single segment of posterior lumbar interbody fusion for adult isthmic spondylolisthesis: reduction or fusion in situ. *Eur Spine J.* 2014;23(1):172-179.
138. Spruit M, Pavlov PW, Leitao J, et al. Posterior reduction and anterior lumbar interbody fusion in symptomatic low-grade adult isthmic spondylolisthesis: short-term radiological and functional outcome. *Eur Spine J.* 2002;11(5):428-433.
139. Kim DH, Albert TJ. Update on use of instrumentation in lumbar spine disorders. *Best Pract Res Clin Rheumatol.* 2002;16(1):123-140.
140. Ekman P, Moller H, Hedlund R. The long-term effect of posterolateral fusion in adult isthmic spondylolisthesis: a randomized controlled study. *Spine J.* 2005;5(1): 36-44.
141. Kimura I, Shingu H, Murata M, Hashiguchi H. Lumbar posterolateral fusion alone or with transpedicular instrumentation in L4–L5 degenerative spondylolisthesis. *J Spinal Disord.* 2001;14(4):301-310.
142. Groff MW, Dailey AT, Ghogawala Z, et al. Guideline update for the performance of fusion procedures for degenerative disease of the lumbar spine. Part 12: pedicle screw fixation as an adjunct to posterolateral fusion. *J Neurosurg Spine.* 2014;21(1):75-78.
143. Ketenci IE, Yanik HS, Demiroz S, Ulusoy A, Erdem S. Three-dimensional correction in patients with Lenke 1 adolescent idiopathic scoliosis: comparison of consecutive versus interval pedicle screw instrumentation. *Spine (Phila Pa 1976).* 2016;41(2):134-138.
144. Le Naveaux F, Aubin CE, Larson AN, et al. Implant distribution in surgically instrumented Lenke 1 adolescent idiopathic scoliosis: does it affect curve correction? *Spine.* 2015;40(7):462-468.
145. Soultanis KC, Stavropoulos NA, Grivas TB, et al. Rib hump deformity assessment using the rib index in adolescent idiopathic scoliotics treated with full screw or hybrid constructs: aetiological implications. *Scoliosis.* 2015;10 (suppl 2):S10.
146. Behrbalk E, Uri O, Parks RM, et al. Posterior-only correction of Scheuermann kyphosis using pedicle screws: economical optimization through screw density reduction. *Eur Spine J.* 2014;23(10):2203-2210.
147. Gebhart S, Alton TB, Bompadre V, Krengel WF. Do anchor density or pedicle screw density correlate with short-term outcome measures in adolescent idiopathic scoliosis surgery? *Spine.* 2014;39(2):E104-E110.
148. Bartanusz V, Harris J, Moldavsky M, Cai Y, Bucklen B. Short segment spinal instrumentation with index vertebra pedicle screw placement for pathologies involving the anterior and middle vertebral column is equally effective as long segment stabilization with cage reconstruction: a biomechanical study. *Spine (Phila Pa 1976).* 2016;41(1):46-52.
149. Kanna RM, Shetty AP, Rajasekaran S. Posterior fixation including the fractured vertebra for severe unstable thoracolumbar fractures. *Spine J.* 2015;15(2):256-264.
150. Okten AI, Gezercan Y, Ozsoy KM, et al. Results of treatment of unstable thoracolumbar burst fractures using pedicle instrumentation with and without fracture-level screws. *Acta Neurochir (Wien).* 2015;157(5):831-836.
151. Pellise F, Barastegui D, Hernandez-Fernandez A, et al. Viability and long-term survival of short-segment posterior fixation in thoracolumbar burst fractures. *Spine J.* 2015;15(8):1796-1803.
152. Nakashima H, Imagama S, Yukawa Y, et al. Comparative study of 2 surgical procedures for osteoporotic delayed vertebral collapse: anterior and posterior combined surgery versus posterior spinal fusion with vertebroplasty. *Spine.* 2015;40(2):E120-E126.
153. Wong EK, Whyne CM, Singh D, Ford M. A biomechanical assessment of kyphoplasty as a stand-alone treatment in a human cadaveric burst fracture model. *Spine.* 2015;40(14):E808-E813.
154. Ha Y, Oh JK, Smith JS, et al. Impact of movement disorders on management of spinal deformity in the elderly. *Neurosurgery.* 2015;77(suppl 4):S173-S185.
155. Li X, Lv C, Yan T. Unilateral versus bilateral pedicle screw fixation for degenerative lumbar diseases: a meta-analysis of 10 randomized controlled trials. *Med Sci Monit.* 2015;21:782-790.
156. Molinari RW, Saleh A, Molinari R Jr, Hermsmeyer J, Dettori JR. Unilateral versus bilateral instrumentation in spinal surgery: a systematic review. *Global Spine J.* 2015;5(3):185-194.
157. Liang Y, Shi W, Jiang C, et al. Clinical outcomes and sagittal alignment of single-level unilateral instrumented transforaminal lumbar interbody fusion with a 4 to 5-year follow-up. *Eur Spine J.* 2015;24(11):2560-2566.
158. Gologorsky Y, Skovrlj B, Steinberger J, et al. Increased incidence of pseudarthrosis after unilateral instrumented transforaminal lumbar interbody fusion in patients with lumbar spondylosis: Clinical article. *J Neurosurg Spine.* 2014;21(4):601-607.
159. Ding W, Chen Y, Liu H, Wang J, Zheng Z. Comparison of unilateral versus bilateral pedicle screw fixation in lumbar interbody fusion: a meta-analysis. *Eur Spine J.* 2014;23(2):395-403.
160. Luo B, Yan M, Huang J, et al. Biomechanical study of unilateral pedicle screw combined with contralateral translaminar facet screw in transforaminal lumbar interbody fusion. *Clin Biomech (Bristol, Avon).* 2015;30(7):657-661.
161. Luo P, Chen YH, Wu YS, et al. Comparison of transforaminal lumbar interbody fusion performed with unilateral pedicle screw fixation or unilateral pedicle screw-contralateral percutaneous transfacet screw fixation. *Br J Neurosurg.* 2015;1-5.
162. Wray S, Mimran R, Vadapalli S, et al. Pedicle screw placement in the lumbar spine: effect of trajectory and screw design on acute biomechanical purchase. *J Neurosurg Spine.* 2015;22(5):503-510.

163. Calvert GC, Lawrence BD, Abtahi AM, Bachus KN, Brodke DS. Cortical screws used to rescue failed lumbar pedicle screw construct: a biomechanical analysis. *J Neurosurg Spine*. 2015;22(2):166-172.
164. Glennie RA, Dea N, Kwon BK, Street JT. Early clinical results with cortically based pedicle screw trajectory for fusion of the degenerative lumbar spine. *J Clin Neurosci*. 2015;22(6):972-975.
165. Cheng WK, Akpolat YT, Inceoglu S, Patel S, Danisa OA. Pars and pedicle fracture and screw loosening associated with cortical bone trajectory: a case series and proposed mechanism through a cadaveric study. *Spine J*. 2016;16(2):e59-e65.
166. Snyder LA, Martinez-Del-Campo E, Neal MT, et al. Lumbar spinal fixation with cortical bone trajectory pedicle screws in 79 patients with degenerative disease: perioperative outcomes and complications. *World Neurosurg*. 2016;88:205-213.
167. Fu KM, Smith JS, Burton DC, et al. Revision extension to the pelvis versus primary spinopelvic instrumentation in adult deformity: comparison of clinical outcomes and complications. *World Neurosurg*. 2014;82(3-4):e547-e552.
168. Fukuda K, Takemitsu M, Machida M, Asazuma T. Lumbosacral fixation using sacroiliac buttress screws: a modification to the Jackson technique with intrasacral rods. *Scoliosis*. 2014;9:8.
169. Funk S, Lovejoy S, Mencio G, Martus J. Rigid instrumentation for neuromuscular scoliosis improves deformity correction without increasing complications. *Spine (Phila Pa 1976)*. 2015;40(22):1729-1736.
170. Awwad W, Al-Ahaideb A, Jiang L, et al. Correction of severe pelvic obliquity using maximum-width segmental sacropelvic screw fixation: an analysis of 20 neuromuscular scoliosis patients. *Eur J Orthop Surg Traumatol*. 2015;25(suppl 1): S233-S241.
171. Bouyer B, Bachy M, Zahi R, et al. Correction of pelvic obliquity in neuromuscular spinal deformities using the "T construct": results and complications in a prospective series of 60 patients. *Eur Spine J*. 2014;23(1):163-171.
172. Jain A, Hassanzadeh H, Strike SA, et al. Pelvic fixation in adult and pediatric spine surgery: historical perspective, indications, and techniques: AAOS exhibit selection. *J Bone Joint Surg Am*. 2015;97(18):1521-1528.
173. Guler UO, Cetin E, Yaman O, et al. Sacropelvic fixation in adult spinal deformity (ASD): a very high rate of mechanical failure. *Eur Spine J*. 2015;24(5):1085-1091.
174. Mazur MD, Ravindra VM, Schmidt MH, et al. Unplanned reoperation after lumbopelvic fixation with S-2 alar-iliac screws or iliac bolts. *J Neurosurg Spine*. 2015;23(1):67-76.
175. Myung KS, Lee C, Skaggs DL. Early pelvic fixation failure in neuromuscular scoliosis. *J Pediatr Orthop*. 2015;35(3):258-265.
176. Desrochers-Perrault F, Aubin CE, Wang X, Schwend RM. Biomechanical analysis of iliac screw fixation in spinal deformity instrumentation. *Clin Biomech (Bristol, Avon)*. 2014;29(6):614-621.
177. Gressot LV, Patel AJ, Hwang SW, Fulkerson DH, Jea A. Iliac screw placement in neuromuscular scoliosis using anatomical landmarks and uniplanar anteroposterior fluoroscopic imaging with postoperative CT confirmation. *J Neurosurg Pediatr*. 2014;13(1):54-61.
178. Ahmad FU, Wang MY. Use of anteroposterior view fluoroscopy for targeting percutaneous pedicle screws in cases of spinal deformity with axial rotation. *J Neurosurg Spine*. 2014;21(5):826-832.
179. Barsa P, Frohlich R, Benes V 3rd, Suchomel P. Intraoperative portable CT-scanner based spinal navigation—a feasibility and safety study. *Acta Neurochir (Wien)*. 2014;156(9):1807-1812.
180. Bydon M, Xu R, Amin AG, et al. Safety and efficacy of pedicle screw placement using intraoperative computed tomography: consecutive series of 1148 pedicle screws. *J Neurosurg Spine*. 2014;21(3):320-328.
181. Barzilay Y, Schroeder JE, Hiller N, et al. Robot-assisted vertebral body augmentation: a radiation reduction tool. *Spine*. 2014;39(2):153-157.
182. Kim HJ, Lee SH, Chang BS, et al. Monitoring the quality of robot-assisted pedicle screw fixation in the lumbar spine by using a cumulative summation test. *Spine*. 2015;40(2):87-94.
183. Chen X, Xu BN, Yu XG. iPod touch-assisted instrumentation of the spine: is it accurate and reliable? *Neurosurgery*. 2014;75(6):E734-E736.
184. Miyashita T, Ataka H, Kato K, Tanno T. Good clinical outcomes and fusion rate of facet fusion with a percutaneous pedicle screw system for degenerative lumbar spondylolisthesis: minimally invasive evolution of posterolateral fusion. *Spine*. 2015;40(9):E552-E557.
185. Beckman JM, Murray G, Bach K, Deukmedjian A, Uribe JS. Percutaneous minimally invasive (MIS) guide wire-less self-tapping pedicle screw placement in the thoracic and lumbar spine: safety and initial clinical experience: technical note. *Oper Neurosurg*. 2015;11(4):530-536.
186. Mummaneni PV, Park P, Fu KM, et al. Does minimally invasive percutaneous posterior instrumentation reduce risk of proximal junctional kyphosis in adult spinal deformity surgery? A propensity-matched cohort analysis. *Neurosurgery*. 2016;78(1):101-108.
187. Calancie B, Donohue ML, Harris CB, et al. Neuromonitoring with pulse-train stimulation for implantation of thoracic pedicle screws: a blinded and randomized clinical study. Part 1. Methods and alarm criteria. *J Neurosurg Spine*. 2014;20(6):675-691.
188. Calancie B, Donohue ML, Moquin RR. Neuromonitoring with pulse-train stimulation for implantation of thoracic pedicle screws: a blinded and randomized clinical study. Part 2. The role of feedback. *J Neurosurg Spine*. 2014; 20(6):692-704.
189. Lee SM, Suk SI, Chung ER. Direct vertebral rotation: a new technique of three-dimensional deformity correction with segmental pedicle screw fixation in adolescent idiopathic scoliosis. *Spine*. 2004;29(3):343-349.
190. Erbulut DU, Kiapour A, Oktenoglu T, Ozer AF, Goel VK. A computational biomechanical investigation of posterior dynamic instrumentation: combination of dynamic rod and hinged (dynamic) screw. *J Biomech Eng*. 2014;136(5):051007.
191. Fu L, France A, Xie Y, et al. Functional and radiological outcomes of semi-rigid dynamic lumbar stabilization adjacent to single-level fusion after 2 years. *Arch Orthop Trauma Surg*. 2014;134(5):605-610.
192. Graf H. Lumbar instability. Surgical treatment without Fusion. *Rachis*. 1992;412:123-137.
193. Grevitt MP, Gardner AD, Spilsbury J, et al. The Graf stabilisation system: early results in 50 patients. *Eur Spine J*. 1995;4(3):169-175.
194. Stoll TM, Dubois G, Schwarzenbach O. The dynamic neutralization system for the spine: a multi-center study

of a novel non-fusion system. *Eur Spine J*. 2002;11(suppl 2):S170-S178.
195. Grob D, Benini A, Junge A, Mannion AF. Clinical experience with the Dynesys semirigid fixation system for the lumbar spine: surgical and patient-oriented outcome in 50 cases after an average of 2 years. *Spine*. 2005;30(3):324-331.
196. Sengupta DK, Mulholland RC. Fulcrum assisted soft stabilization system: a new concept in the surgical treatment of degenerative low back pain. *Spine*. 2005;30(9):1019-1029, discussion 1030.
197. Di Silvestre M, Lolli F, Bakaloudis G. Degenerative lumbar scoliosis in elderly patients: dynamic stabilization without fusion versus posterior instrumented fusion. *Spine J*. 2014;14(1):1-10.
198. Diebo BG, Henry J, Lafage V, Berjano P. Sagittal deformities of the spine: factors influencing the outcomes and complications. *Eur Spine J*. 2015;24(suppl 1):S3-S15.
199. Botelho RV, Bastianello R Jr, Albuquerque LD, Bernardo WM. Dynamic compared to rigid fixation in lumbar spine: a systematic review. *Rev Assoc Med Bras*. 2014;60(2):151-155.
200. Prud'homme M, Barrios C, Rouch P, et al. Clinical outcomes and complications after pedicle-anchored dynamic or hybrid lumbar spine stabilization: a systematic literature review. *J Spinal Disord Tech*. 2015;28(8):E439-E448.
201. Melnyk AD, Chak JD, Singh V, et al. Characterization of the behavior of a novel low-stiffness posterior spinal implant under anterior shear loading on a degenerative spinal model. *Eur Spine J*. 2015;24(4):775-782.
202. Facchinello Y, Brailovski V, Petit Y, Mac-Thiong JM. Monolithic superelastic rods with variable flexural stiffness for spinal fusion: modeling of the processing-properties relationship. *Med Eng Phys*. 2014;36(11):1455-1463.
203. Facchinello Y, Brailovski V, Petit Y, et al. Biomechanical assessment of the stabilization capacity of monolithic spinal rods with different flexural stiffness and anchoring arrangement. *Clin Biomech (Bristol, Avon)*. 2015;30(10):1026-1035.
204. Reichl M, Kueny RA, Danyali R, et al. Biomechanical effects of a dynamic topping off instrumentation in a long rigid pedicle screw construct. *J Spinal Disord Tech*. 2017;30(4):E440-E447.
205. Huang TH, Ma HL, Wang ST, et al. Does the size of the rod affect the surgical results in adolescent idiopathic scoliosis? 5.5-mm versus 6.35-mm rod. *Spine J*. 2014;14(8):1545-1550.
206. Hyun SJ, Lenke LG, Kim YC, Koester LA, Blanke KM. Comparison of standard 2-rod constructs to multiple-rod constructs for fixation across 3-column spinal osteotomies. *Spine*. 2014;39(22):1899-1904.
207. Palumbo MA, Shah KN, Eberson CP, Hart RA, Daniels AH. Outrigger rod technique for supplemental support of posterior spinal arthrodesis. *Spine J*. 2015;15(6):1409-1414.
208. Zaidi HA, Awad AW, Dickman CA. Complete spondylectomy using orthogonal spinal fixation and combined anterior and posterior approaches for thoracolumbar spinal reconstruction: technical nuances and clinical results. *J Spinal Disord Tech*. 2017;30(4):E466-E474.
209. Odent T, Ilharreborde B, Miladi L, et al. Fusionless surgery in early-onset scoliosis. *Orthop Traumatol Surg Res*. 2015;101(6 suppl):S281-S288.
210. Astur N, Flynn JM, Flynn JM, et al. The efficacy of rib-based distraction with VEPTR in the treatment of early-onset scoliosis in patients with arthrogryposis. *J Pediatr Orthop*. 2014;34(1):8-13.
211. McCarthy RE, McCullough FL. Shilla growth guidance for early-onset scoliosis: results after a minimum of five years of follow-up. *J Bone Joint Surg Am*. 2015;97(19):1578-1584.
212. Mahar A, Kabirian N, Akbarnia BA, et al. Effects of posterior distraction forces on anterior column intradiscal pressure in the dual growing rod technique. *J Orthop Sci*. 2015;20(1):12-16.
213. Dede O, Demirkiran G, Yazici M. Self-growing instrumentation with gliding connectors for collapsing spine deformities in children: a novel technique. *J Pediatr Orthop*. 2015;35(4):367-373.
214. Akgul T, Dikici F, Sar C, Talu U, Domanic U. Growing rod instrumentation in the treatment of early onset scoliosis. *Acta Orthop Belg*. 2014;80(4):457-463.
215. Enercan M, Kahraman S, Erturer E, Ozturk C, Hamzaoglu A. Apical and intermediate anchors without fusion improve Cobb angle and thoracic kyphosis in early-onset scoliosis. *Clin Orthop Relat Res*. 2014;472(12):3902-3908.
216. Hickey BA, Towriss C, Baxter G, et al. Early experience of MAGEC magnetic growing rods in the treatment of early onset scoliosis. *Eur Spine J*. 2014;23(suppl 1):S61-S65.
217. La Rosa G, Oggiano L, Ruzzini L. Magnetically controlled growing rods for the management of early-onset scoliosis: a preliminary report. *J Pediatr Orthop*. 2017;37(2):79-85.
218. Dick JC, Jones MP, Zdeblick TA, Kunz DN, Horton WC. A biomechanical comparison evaluating the use of intermediate screws and cross-linkage in lumbar pedicle fixation. *J Spinal Disord*. 1994;7(5):402-407.
219. Dick JC, Zdeblick TA, Bartel BD, Kunz DN. Mechanical evaluation of cross-link designs in rigid pedicle screw systems. *Spine*. 1997;22(4):370-375.
220. Lazaro BC, Deniz FE, Brasiliense LB, et al. Biomechanics of thoracic short versus long fixation after 3-column injury. *J Neurosurg Spine*. 2011;14(2):226-234.
221. Alizadeh M, Kadir MR, Fadhli MM, et al. The use of X-shaped cross-link in posterior spinal constructs improves stability in thoracolumbar burst fracture: a finite element analysis. *J Orthop Res*. 2013;31(9):1447-1454.
222. Valdevit A, Kambic HE, McLain RF. Torsional stability of cross-link configurations: a biomechanical analysis. *Spine J*. 2005;5(4):441-445.
223. Chen ZH, Chen X, Zhu ZZ, et al. Does addition of crosslink to pedicle-screw-based instrumentation impact the development of the spinal canal in children younger than 5 years of age? *Eur Spine J*. 2015;24(7):1391-1398.
224. Lehman RA Jr, Kang DG, Wagner SC, et al. Biomechanical stability of transverse connectors in the setting of a thoracic pedicle subtraction osteotomy. *Spine J*. 2015;15(7):1629-1635.
225. Ferrero E, Pesenti S, Blondel B, et al. Role of thoracoscopy for the sagittal correction of hypokyphotic adolescent idiopathic scoliosis patients. *Eur Spine J*. 2014;23(12):2635-2642.
226. Macki M, Bydon M, Weingart R, et al. Posterolateral fusion with interbody for lumbar spondylolisthesis is associated with less repeat surgery than posterolateral fusion alone. *Clin Neurol Neurosurg*. 2015;138:117-123.
227. Anderson PA, Schwaegler PE, Cizek D, Leverson G. Work status as a predictor of surgical outcome of discogenic low back pain. *Spine*. 2006;31(21):2510-2515.
228. Etemadifar M, Ebrahimzadeh A, Hadi A, Feizi M. Comparison of Scheuermann's kyphosis correction by combined anterior-posterior fusion versus posterior-only procedure. *Eur Spine J*. 2016;25(8):2580-2586.

229. Rushton PR, Grevitt MP, Sell PJ. Anterior or posterior surgery for right thoracic adolescent idiopathic scoliosis (AIS)? A prospective cohorts' comparison using radiologic and functional outcomes. *J Spinal Disord Tech.* 2015;28(3):80-88.
230. Gurr KR, McAfee PC, Shih CM. Biomechanical analysis of anterior and posterior instrumentation systems after corpectomy. A calf-spine model. *J Bone Joint Surg Am.* 1988;70(8):1182-1191.
231. Gurwitz GS, Dawson JM, McNamara MJ, Federspiel CF, Spengler DM. Biomechanical analysis of three surgical approaches for lumbar burst fractures using short-segment instrumentation. *Spine.* 1993;18(8):977-982.
232. Heller JG, Zdeblick TA, Kunz DA, McCabe R, Cooke ME. Spinal instrumentation for metastatic disease: in vitro biomechanical analysis. *J Spinal Disord.* 1993;6(1): 17-22.
233. Shannon FJ, DiResta GR, Ottaviano D, et al. Biomechanical analysis of anterior poly-methyl-methacrylate reconstruction following total spondylectomy for metastatic disease. *Spine.* 2004;29(19):2096-12.
234. Antoni M, Charles YP, Walter A, Schuller S, Steib JP. Fusion rates of different anterior grafts in thoracolumbar fractures. *J Spinal Disord Tech.* 2015;28(9):E528-E533.
235. Ni J, Zheng Y, Liu N, et al. Radiological evaluation of anterior lumbar fusion using PEEK cages with adjacent vertebral autograft in spinal deformity long fusion surgeries. *Eur Spine J.* 2015;24(4):791-799.
236. Zdeblick TA, Phillips FM. Interbody cage devices. *Spine.* 2003;28(15 suppl):S2-S7.
237. Hao D, Wang W, Duan K, et al. Two-year follow-up evaluation of surgical treatment for thoracolumbar fracture-dislocation. *Spine.* 2014;39(21):E1284-E1290.
238. Kleeman TJ, Michael Ahn U, Clutterbuck WB, Campbell CJ, Talbot-Kleeman A. Laparoscopic anterior lumbar interbody fusion at L4-L5: an anatomic evaluation and approach classification. *Spine.* 2002;27(13):1390-1395.
238a. Benglis DM, Vanni S, Levi AD. An anatomical study of the lumbosacral plexus as related to the minimally invasive transpsoas approach to the lumbar spine. Laboratory investigation. *J Neurosurg Spine.* 2009;10(20):139-144.
239. Lehmen JA, Gerber EJ. MIS lateral spine surgery: a systematic literature review of complications, outcomes, and economics. *Eur Spine J.* 2015;24(suppl 3):287-313.
240. Phan K, Rao PJ, Scherman DB, Dandie G, Mobbs RJ. Lateral lumbar interbody fusion for sagittal balance correction and spinal deformity. *J Clin Neurosci.* 2015;22(11):1714-1721.
241. Ohtori S, Mannoji C, Orita S, et al. Mini-Open Anterior retroperitoneal lumbar interbody fusion: oblique lateral interbody fusion for degenerated lumbar spinal kyphoscoliosis. *Asian Spine J.* 2015;9(4):565-572.
242. Ahmadian A, Bach K, Bolinger B, et al. Stand-alone minimally invasive lateral lumbar interbody fusion: multicenter clinical outcomes. *J Clin Neurosci.* 2015;22(4):740-746.
243. Fogel GR, Parikh RD, Ryu SI, Turner AW. Biomechanics of lateral lumbar interbody fusion constructs with lateral and posterior plate fixation: laboratory investigation. *J Neurosurg Spine.* 2014;20(3):291-297.
244. Baghdadi YM, Larson AN, Dekutoski MB, et al. Sagittal balance and spinopelvic parameters after lateral lumbar interbody fusion for degenerative scoliosis: a case-control study. *Spine.* 2014;39(3):E166-E173.
245. Alimi M, Hofstetter CP, Cong GT, et al. Radiological and clinical outcomes following extreme lateral interbody fusion. *J Neurosurg Spine.* 2014;20(6):623-635.
246. Barbagallo GM, Albanese V, Raich AL, et al. Lumbar lateral interbody fusion (LLIF): comparative effectiveness and safety versus PLIF/TLIF and predictive factors affecting LLIF outcome. *Evid Based Spine Care J.* 2014;5(1):28-37.
247. Akbarnia BA, Mundis GM Jr, Moazzaz P, et al. Anterior column realignment (ACR) for focal kyphotic spinal deformity using a lateral transpsoas approach and ALL release. *J Spinal Disord Tech.* 2014;27(1):29-39.
248. Vamvanij V, Ferrara LA, Hai Y, et al. Quantitative changes in spinal canal dimensions using interbody distraction for spondylolisthesis. *Spine.* 2001;26(3):E13-E18.
249. Bednar DA. Surgical management of lumbar degenerative spinal stenosis with spondylolisthesis via posterior reduction with minimal laminectomy. *J Spinal Disord Tech.* 2002;15(2):105-109.
250. Dewald CJ, Millikan KW, Hammerberg KW, Doolas A, Dewald RL. An open, minimally invasive approach to the lumbar spine. *Am Surg.* 1999;65(1):61-68.
251. Huang TJ, Hsu RW, Chen SH, Lee YY. Minimal access surgery in managing anterior lumbar disorders. *Clin Orthop.* 2001;387:140-147.
252. Hart RA, Domes CM, Goodwin B, et al. High-grade spondylolisthesis treated using a modified Bohlman technique: results among multiple surgeons. *J Neurosurg Spine.* 2014;20(5):523-530.
253. Graillon T, Rakotozanany P, Blondel B, et al. Circumferential management of unstable thoracolumbar fractures using an anterior expandable cage, as an alternative to an iliac crest graft, combined with a posterior screw fixation: results of a series of 85 patients. *Neurosurg Focus.* 2014;37(1):E10.
254. Joubert C, Adetchessi T, Peltier E, et al. Corpectomy and vertebral body reconstruction with expandable cage placement and osteosynthesis via the single stage posterior approach: a retrospective series of 34 patients with thoracic and lumbar spine vertebral body tumors. *World Neurosurg.* 2015;84(5):1412-1422.
255. Chandra SP, Ramdurg SR, Kurwale N, et al. Extended costotransversectomy to achieve circumferential fusion for pathologies causing thoracic instability. *Spine J.* 2014;14(9):2094-2101.
256. de Ruiter GC, Lobatto DJ, Wolfs JF, Peul WC, Arts MP. Reconstruction with expandable cages after single- and multilevel corpectomies for spinal metastases: a prospective case series of 60 patients. *Spine J.* 2014;14(9):2085-2093.
257. Clark AJ, Tang JA, Leasure JM, et al. Gait-simulating fatigue loading analysis and sagittal alignment failure of spinal pelvic reconstruction after total sacrectomy: comparison of 3 techniques. *J Neurosurg Spine.* 2014;20(4):364-370.
258. Lau D, Chou D. Posterior thoracic corpectomy with cage reconstruction for metastatic spinal tumors: comparing the mini-open approach to the open approach. *J Neurosurg Spine.* 2015;23(2):217-227.
259. Gonzalez-Blohm SA, Doulgeris JJ, Aghayev K, et al. In vitro evaluation of a lateral expandable cage and its comparison with a static device for lumbar interbody fusion: a biomechanical investigation. *J Neurosurg Spine.* 2014;20(4):387-395.
260. Choi JY, Sung KH. Subsidence after anterior lumbar interbody fusion using paired stand-alone rectangular cages. *Eur Spine J.* 2006;15(1):16-22.

261. Choi J, Sung K. Subsidence after anterior lumbar interbody fusion using paired stand-alone rectangular cages. *Eur Spine J*. 2005;S940-S6719.
262. Faizan A, Kiapour A, Kiapour AM, Goel VK. Biomechanical analysis of various footprints of transforaminal lumbar interbody fusion devices. *J Spinal Disord Tech*. 2014;27(4):E118-E127.
263. Fan CY, Hsu CC, Chao CK, Lin SC, Chao KH. Biomechanical comparisons of different posterior instrumentation constructs after two-level ALIF: a finite element study. *Med Eng Phys*. 2010;32(2):203-211.
264. Kim Y. Finite element analysis of anterior lumbar interbody fusion: threaded cylindrical cage and pedicle screw fixation. *Spine*. 2007;32(23):2558-2568.
265. Scaduto AA, Gamradt SC, Yu WD, et al. Perioperative complications of threaded cylindrical lumbar interbody fusion devices: anterior versus posterior approach. *J Spinal Disord Tech*. 2003;16(6):502-507.
266. Hueng DY, Chung TT, Chuang WH, et al. Biomechanical effects of cage positions and facet fixation on initial stability of the anterior lumbar interbody fusion motion segment. *Spine*. 2014;39(13):E770-E776.
267. Sohn MJ, Kayanja MM, Kilincer C, Ferrara LA, Benzel EC. Biomechanical evaluation of the ventral and lateral surface shear strain distributions in central compared with dorsolateral placement of cages for lumbar interbody fusion. *J Neurosurg Spine*. 2006;4(3):219-224.
268. Deukmedjian AR, Manwaring J, Le TV, Turner AW, Uribe JS. Corpectomy cage subsidence with rectangular versus round endcaps. *J Clin Neurosci*. 2014;21(9):1632-1636.
269. Wattenbarger JM, Herring JA, Bronson D, Ashman RB. Mechanical testing of a single rod versus a double rod in a long-segment animal model. *J Spinal Disord*. 2001;14(3):232-236.
270. Wattenbarger JM, Richards BS, Herring JA. A comparison of single-rod instrumentation with double-rod instrumentation in adolescent idiopathic scoliosis. *Spine*. 2000;25(13):1680-1688.
271. Kaneda K, Taneichi H, Abumi K, et al. Anterior decompression and stabilization with the Kaneda device for thoracolumbar burst fractures associated with neurological deficits. *J Bone Joint Surg Am*. 1997;79(1):69-83.
272. Faro FD, White KK, Ahn JS, et al. Biomechanical analysis of anterior instrumentation for lumbar corpectomy. *Spine*. 2003;28(22):E468-E471.
273. Kaneda K, Shono Y, Satoh S, Abumi K. New anterior instrumentation for the management of thoracolumbar and lumbar scoliosis. Application of the Kaneda two-rod system. *Spine*. 1996;21(10):1250-1261, discussion 1261-1252.
274. Aryan HE, Lu DC, Acosta FL Jr, Ames CP. Stand-alone anterior lumbar discectomy and fusion with plate: initial experience. *Surg Neurol*. 2007;68(1):7-13.
275. Snyder LA, Kalb S, Kakarla UK, et al. Effects of anterior plating on clinical outcomes of anterior lumbar interbody fusion. *J Spinal Disord Tech*. 2016;29(7):300-304.
276. Beaubien BP, Derincek A, Lew WD, Wood KB. In vitro, biomechanical comparison of an anterior lumbar interbody fusion with an anteriorly placed, low-profile lumbar plate and posteriorly placed pedicle screws or translaminar screws. *Spine*. 2005;30(16):1846-1851.
277. Vaccaro AR, Singh K, Haid R, et al. The use of bioabsorbable implants in the spine. *Spine J*. 2003;3(3): 227-237.
278. Basra S, Bucklen B, Muzumdar A, Khalil S, Gudipally M. A novel lateral lumbar integrated plate-spacer interbody implant: in vitro biomechanical analysis. *Spine J*. 2015;15(2): 322-328.
279. Drazin D, Hussain M, Harris J, et al. The role of sacral slope in lumbosacral fusion: a biomechanical study. *J Neurosurg Spine*. 2015;23(6):1-9.
280. Allain J, Delecrin J, Beaurain J, et al. Stand-alone ALIF with integrated intracorporeal anchoring plates in the treatment of degenerative lumbar disc disease: a prospective study on 65 cases. *Eur Spine J*. 2014;23(10):2136-2143.
281. Fernstrom U. Arthroplasty with intercorporal endoprosthesis in herniated disc and in painful disc. *Acta Chir Scand*. 1966;355:154-159.
282. Klara PM, Ray CD. Artificial nucleus replacement: clinical experience. *Spine*. 2002;27(12):1374-1377.
283. Bao Q, Yuan H. New technologies in spine: nucleus replacement. *Spine*. 2002;27:1245-1247.
284. Eysel P, Rompe J, Schoeymaye R, et al. Biomechanical behaviour of a prosthetic lumbar nucleus. *Acta Neurochir (Wien)*. 1999;141:1083-1087.
285. Bertagnoli R, Vazquez RJ. The anterolateral transpsoatic approach (ALPA): a new technique for implanting prosthetic disc-nucleus devices. *J Spinal Disord Tech*. 2003;16(4):398-404.
286. Shim CS, Lee SH, Park CW, et al. Partial disc replacement with the PDN prosthetic disc nucleus device: early clinical results. *J Spinal Disord Tech*. 2003;16(4):324-330.
287. Büttner-Janz K, Schellnack K. Bandscheibenendoprothetik, Entwick-Lungsweg und Gegenwärtiger Stand. *Beitr Orthop Traumatol*. 1990;3:137-147.
288. Tropiano P, Huang RC, Girardi FP, Marnay T. Lumbar disc replacement: preliminary results with ProDisc II after a minimum follow-up period of 1 year. *J Spinal Disord Tech*. 2003;16(4):362-368.
289. Bertagnoli R, Kumar S. Indications for full prosthetic disc arthroplasty: a correlation of clinical outcome against a variety of indications. *Eur Spine J*. 2002;11(suppl 2):S131-S136.
290. Hallab N, Link HD, McAfee PC. Biomaterial optimization in total disc arthroplasty. *Spine*. 2003;28(20):S139-S152.
291. Hallab NJ, Cunningham BW, Jacobs JJ. Spinal implant debris-induced osteolysis. *Spine*. 2003;28(20): S125-S138.
292. Veruva SY, Lanman TH, Isaza JE, et al. UHMWPE wear debris and tissue reactions are reduced for contemporary designs of lumbar total disc replacements. *Clin Orthop Relat Res*. 2015;473(3):987-998.
293. Gornet MF, Burkus JK, Harper ML, et al. Prospective study on serum metal levels in patients with metal-on-metal lumbar disc arthroplasty. *Eur Spine J*. 2013;22(4):741-746.
294. Wang MY. Metal-on-metal lumbar total disc arthroplasty: ready for prime time? *World Neurosurg*. 2012;78(3-4):247.
295. Pearcy MJ. Stereo radiography of lumbar spine motion. *Acta Orthop Scand Suppl*. 1985;212:1-45.
296. Pearcy MJ, Whittle MW. Movements of the lumbar spine measured by three-dimensional X-ray analysis. *J Biomed Eng*. 1982;4(2):107-112.
297. Gunzburg R, Mayer H, Szpalski M, Aebi M. Arthroplasty of the spine: the long quest for mobility. *Eur Spine J*. 2002;11(suppl 2):S63-S64.
297a. Le Huec JC, Basso Y, Aunoble S, et al. Influence of facet and posterior muscle degeneration on clinical results of lumbar

total disc replacement: two-year follow-up. *J Spinal Disord Tech*. 2005;18(3):219-223.

298. Huang RC, Girardi FP, Cammisa FP Jr, Wright TM. The implications of constraint in lumbar total disc replacement. *J Spinal Disord Tech*. 2003;16(4):412-417.
299. Trincat S, Edgard-Rosa G, Geneste G, Marnay T. Two-level lumbar total disc replacement: functional outcomes and segmental motion after 4 years. *Orthop Traumatol Surg Res*. 2015;101(1):17-21.
300. Saavedra-Pozo FM, Deusdara RA, Benzel EC. Adjacent segment disease perspective and review of the literature. *Ochsner J*. 2014;14(1):78-83.
301. Wall EJ, Bylski-Austrow DI, Kolata RJ, Crawford AH. Endoscopic mechanical spinal hemiepiphysiodesis modifies spine growth. *Spine*. 2005;30(10):1148-1153.
302. Clin J, Aubin CE, Parent S. Biomechanical simulation and analysis of scoliosis correction using a fusionless intravertebral epiphyseal device. *Spine*. 2015;40(6):369-376.
303. Demirkiran G, Yilmaz G, Kaymaz B, et al. Safety and efficacy of instrumented convex growth arrest in treatment of congenital scoliosis. *J Pediatr Orthop*. 2014;34(3):275-281.

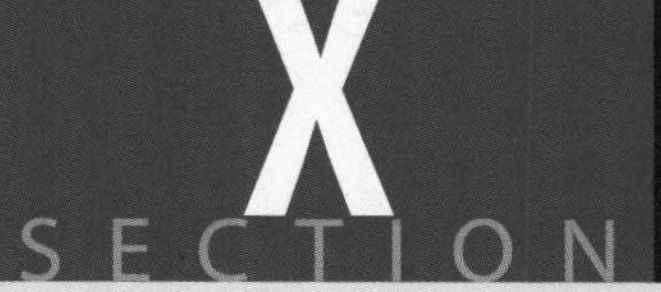

SECTION X

ADULT DEFORMITY

CHAPTER 71 Adult Isthmic Spondylolisthesis

Brian Kwon
Neel Shah
David H. Kim

Introduction

Spondylolisthesis is the ventral (or anterior) displacement of one vertebra relative to the subjacent vertebra. Spondylolysis is a defect in the pars interarticularis due to congenital, traumatic, dysplastic, or neoplastic etiologies. It is generally considered to occur prior to appearance of spondylolisthesis, as the anterior column of the vertebra is no longer in continuity with the posterior column. Over time, the vertebral body then displaces ventrally once the disc and supporting soft tissues are no longer able to maintain the structural integrity and anatomic alignment of the vertebrae.

Classification

Spondylolisthesis can be classified by the severity of slippage as described by Meyerding.[1] It is measured as a percentage using the length of slip of the cranial vertebra compared to the length of superior endplate of the caudal vertebra (Fig. 71.1). The classification is based on slip percentage: grade 1, less than 25%; grade 2, 26% to 50%; grade 3, 51% to 75%, grade 4, 76% to 100%, grade 5, greater than 100% or spondyloptosis. An etiologic classification system was described by Wiltse,[2] which includes dysplastic, isthmic, degenerative, traumatic, and neoplastic types. Isthmic spondylolisthesis is the subject of this chapter.

Natural History/Incidence

Fredrickson et al.[3] reported a prospective, population-based study of 500 schoolchildren from northern Pennsylvania in the 1950s. They reported an incidence of lumbar spondylolysis of 4.4% and spondylolisthesis of 2.6% in children younger than 6 years. At adulthood, the incidence of lumbar spondylolysis was found to be 5.4% and spondylolisthesis was 4%. Furthermore, they reported that pars defects did not typically heal, and slippage occurred throughout the follow-up period. Fredrickson also reported that two-thirds of the spondylolysis cases were found in males, and greater than 90% occurred at L5–S1. Spondylolisthesis was found in 74% of patients with bilateral pars defects at L5–S1, but not in patients with unilateral defects or pars defects at other levels. Females had a lower incidence of defects but a higher rate of slip progression.[3]

A more recent study by Urrutia et al.[4] found a similar incidence of isthmic spondylolisthesis in a non-US adult population of 3.8% (range, 1.7–6.8%). The incidence appeared not to change into adulthood, and the authors concluded spondylolysis is more likely an acquired disorder. A 45-year follow-up study on Fredrickson's initial sample population was conducted by Beutler et al.[5] They reported that low back pain (LBP) in patients with pars defects follows a clinical course like that of the general population. Patients with unilateral spondylolysis never experienced slippage throughout the study and half of the patients with bilateral defects did not go on to have any spondylolisthesis. The half who did slip had a mean slippage of 24%.

Kalichman et al.[6] studied spondylolysis on abdominal computed tomography (CT) scans obtained to assess aortic calcification in patients enrolled in the Framingham Heart Study. They reported the incidence of spondylolysis in their sample to be 11.5% and did not find an association with LBP within the previous 12 months of the study. It is notable that this is more than double the incidence reported by radiographically based studies, as CT has been recognized as the most accurate imaging modality for isthmic spondylolisthesis.[7] This suggests that isthmic spondylolisthesis may be more prevalent than initially reported but also that it may be a largely indolent condition with a benign natural history in many, if not most, individuals.

Pathophysiology

The primary pathologic entity in isthmic spondylolisthesis is a defect in the pars interarticularis, a critical structural component of the posterior element of the vertebra. The pars is the intersection of the lamina, inferior and superior articular

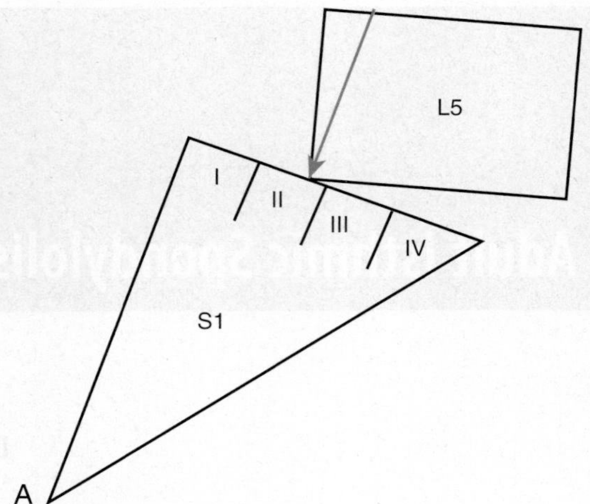

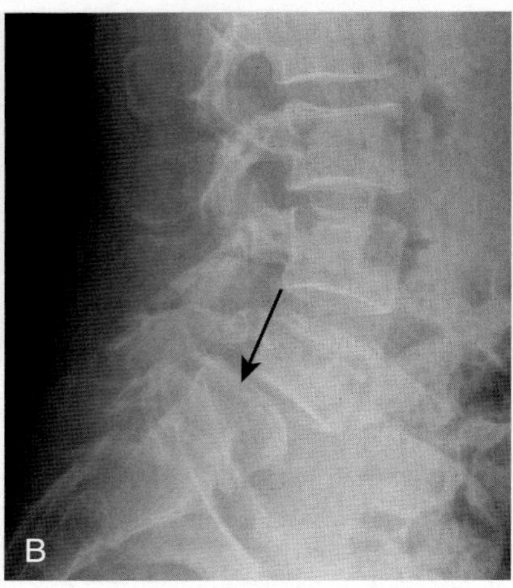

FIG. 71.1 The Meyerding classification measures severity of spondylolisthesis by using a ratio of the amount of anterior listhesis compared to the length of the superior end plate of the S1 vertebra measured in quartiles. Grade 1 = 0–25%; grade 2 = 26–50%; grade 3 = 51–75%; grade 4 = 75–100%; grade 5 = >100% or spondyloptosis. (A) Schematic showing how the measurements for the Meyerding classification are made. This example shows a grade 2 slip, 25–50%. (B) Lateral radiograph showing where the measurement on the S1 end plate is made for Meyerding slip severity.

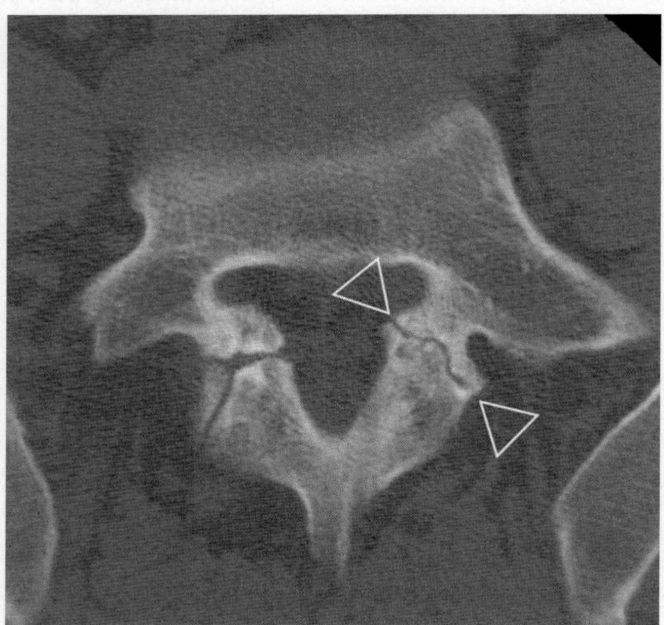

FIG. 71.2 Axial computed tomographic image showing spondylolysis (*open triangles*). Note the undulating course of lucency, making it distinct from a facet joint.

processes, and pedicle. A spondylolysis essentially divides the neural arch (Fig. 71.2). Wiltse divided these defects into three subtypes: A, B, and C. Type A refers to the classic stress fracture of the pars. Type B refers to an intact, but elongated, isthmus due to repeated cycles of trauma and repair. Type C is an acute fracture of the pars interarticularis due to trauma.[8]

Etiologies for spondylolysis are numerous but many believe that the vast majority are due to stress fractures of the pars interarticularis. Biomechanical studies have shown this region is exposed to the highest extension forces in the lumbar spine.[9] It has also been suggested that this region of bone is the weakest structural component of the posterior neural arch.[10] Repetitive lumbar extension loading appears to result in a localized stress reaction in the vulnerable bone of the pars region, and if the stress is sustained or excessive and if the bone is unable to heal, then a spondylolysis develops. Rosenberg et al.[11] support this hypothesis, reporting their observation that spondylolysis does not occur in nonambulatory individuals. Additional support for the relationship between extension stress and spondylolysis is the observation that a high incidence of pars defects are observed in athletes such as wrestlers, football linemen, and gymnasts—who frequently undergo repetitive hyperextension loads.[12–14]

The most common level for spondylolysis is L5, and isthmic spondylolisthesis at L5–S1 accounts for 90% of those who present with the condition.[15,16] Don and Robertson evaluated facet joint orientation in individuals with and without isthmic spondylolisthesis. Due to previous data suggesting that sagittally oriented facet joints predispose individuals to *degenerative* spondylolisthesis, they analyzed facet joint orientation in an *isthmic* spondylolisthesis group. The group with isthmic spondylolisthesis had significantly more coronal orientation of the facets of L3–L4 and L4–L5, that is, above the affected level. They concluded that facet joints with more coronal—less sagittal—orientation allow for less dorsal-ventral translation of cranial motion segments, which leads to greater extension stresses on the L5 pars and results in spondylolysis.[17] Ward and Latimer[18] evaluated the intrafacet distances of lumbar vertebrae in individuals with and without spondylolysis and found an increase in cranial-to-caudal intrafacet distance in nonaffected individuals, which they concluded allowed for overlap of lamina during lordosis. Individuals in whom spondylolysis was found showed relatively lower intrafacet distances, potentially resulting in impingement of the L4 inferior articular process on the pars of L5 (Fig. 71.3).[18]

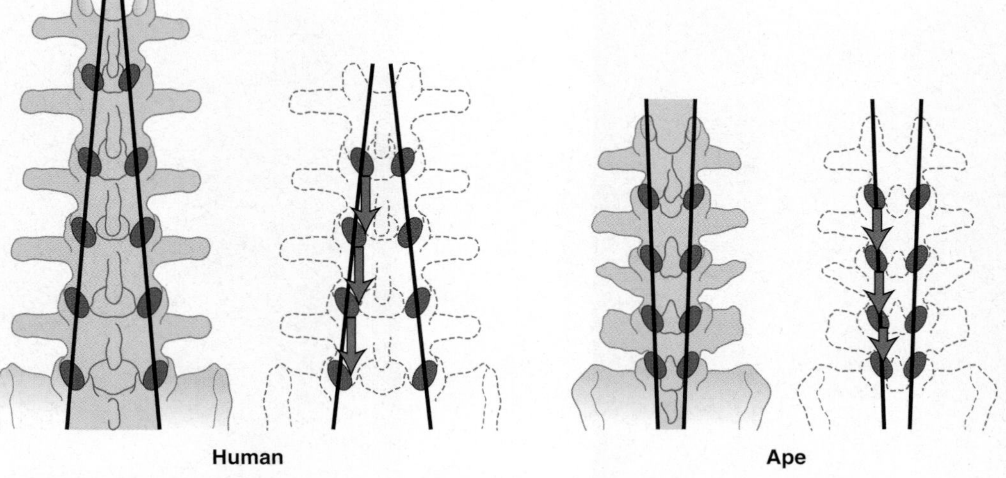

FIG. 71.3 Ward and Latimer's measurement of intrafacet distances. They found that individuals with spondylolysis had a statistically smaller increase in this distance. (From Ward CV, Latimer B. Human evolution and the development of spondylolysis. *Spine*. 2005;30(16):1809.)

Biomechanics

The biomechanical environment at the lumbosacral junction is a complex one that normally functions as a harmonious linkage between the trunk and pelvis. During radiographic assessment of patients, lumbar lordosis (LL), pelvic incidence (PI), sacral slope (SS), and pelvic tilt (PT) are most commonly measured (Fig. 71.4). PI is considered a fixed anatomic measurement and does not change for any given individual through adulthood. LL, SS, and PT are measurements of the relative position of the lumbosacral spine in space. Sagittal spinopelvic parameters have been found to correlate significantly with spondyloptosis[19] as well as the severity of isthmic spondylolisthesis.[20] Labelle et al.[21] show in a sample of 214 young adults (ages 10–40 years) that PI is significantly greater in individuals with isthmic spondylolisthesis and correlates linearly with higher (Meyerding) slip severities. They also showed that PI strongly correlates with the other parameters: LL, SS, and PT. They concluded that individuals with isthmic spondylolisthesis stand with increased SS, PT, and LL. Moreover, these increased values—in particular, LL—are an important factor in the amount of shear stress on the L5 lamina and pars.

Diagnosis

History

Most individuals with spondylolysis are asymptomatic. While it is the most common cause of LBP in children, the same does not hold true in the adult population.[22-24] Andrade et al.[25] recently reported a review of observational studies on the association of spondylolysis and isthmic spondylolisthesis with LBP. They reported that only 1 of 15 eligible studies found an association and 11 did not. In fact, they found that LBP was significantly more prevalent in individuals without spondylolysis/isthmic spondylolisthesis.

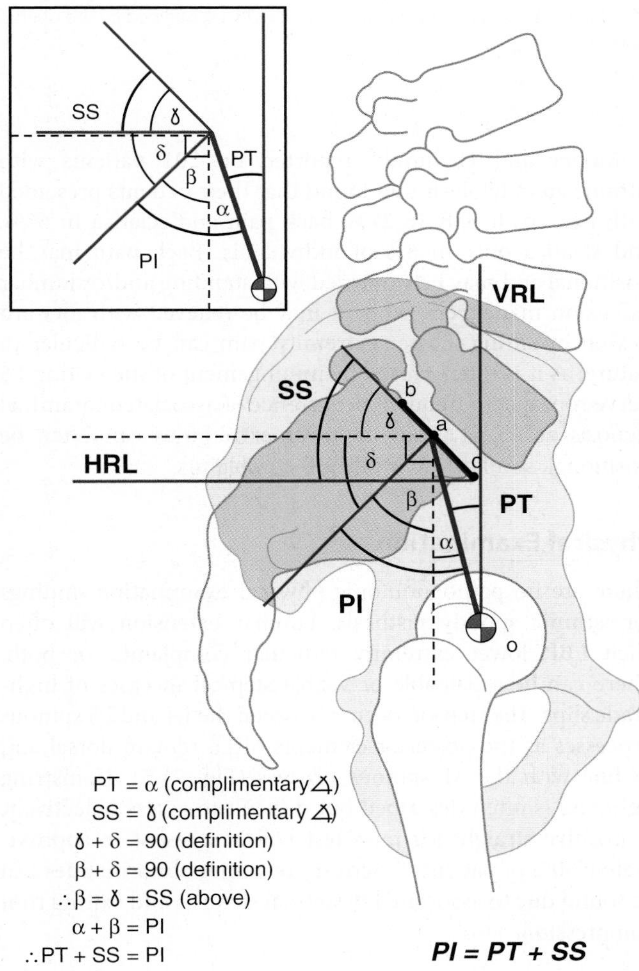

FIG. 71.4 Commonly measured pelvic parameters are altered in individuals with isthmic spondylolisthesis. HRL, horizontal reference line; PI, pelvic incidence; PT, pelvic tilt; SS, sacral slope; VRL, vertical reference line. (From O'Brien MF, Kuklo TR, Blanke KM, et al, eds. *Spinal Deformity Study Group Radiographic Measurement Manual.* Medtronic Sofamor Danek, 2004.)

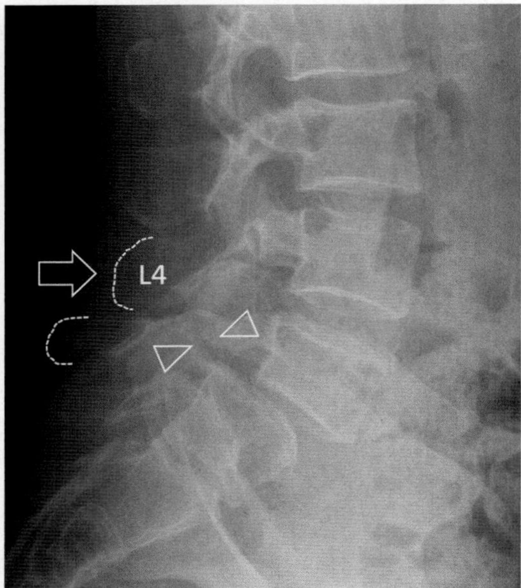

FIG. 71.5 Lateral radiograph showing step-off of the L4 spinous process from the L5 spinous process (*arrow*). Spondylolysis is outlined by the open triangles.

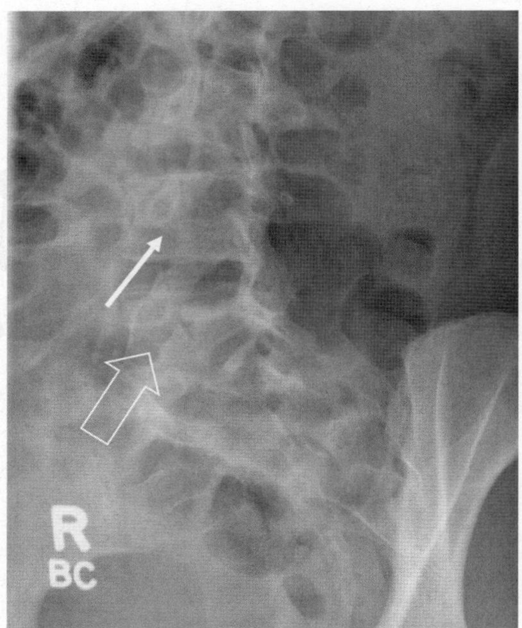

FIG. 71.6 Radiographs of 45-degree oblique image showing the "Scotty dog." Open arrow shows a lucency at pars of L5 commonly referred to as a "break in the neck of the Scotty dog." Solid arrow shows normal pars of L4.

Moller and Hedlund[26] reported on 201 patients with isthmic spondylolysis and found that their patients presented with back pain only in 27%, back pain and sciatica in 65%, and sciatica only in 8% of individuals. Back pain may be positional and may be worsened with standing and/or lumbar extension maneuvers, while it may be relieved with forward flexion or sitting. Lower extremity pain can be radicular in nature, as it is often caused by impingement of the exiting L5 nerve root due to frequent occurrence of associated foraminal stenosis at L5–S1. Pain in lower extremities can often be positional, similar to typical LBP complaints.

Physical Examination

There are no pathognomonic physical examination findings for isthmic spondylolisthesis. Lumbar extension will often elicit LBP, lower extremity radicular complaints, or both. There can be a palpable or visible step-off in cases of high-grade slips. The step-off occurs between the L4 and L5 spinous processes as the posterior elements of L5 remain dorsal and in line with the S1 spinous process (Fig. 71.5). Hamstring tightness is often described but difficult to assess objectively. A positive straight-leg raise test will be present in approximately 50% of patients.[27] Sensory or motor abnormalities can be found due to associated foraminal stenosis and exiting root compression.

Imaging

Routine radiographic images can detect spondylolysis, especially if spondylolisthesis is present, and slip severity can be measured on lateral images. Additionally, standing images that include flexion and extension positioning should be evaluated. If spondylolysis is suspected but not visualized, oblique radiographic images 45 degrees to the sagittal plane can be obtained that can detect up to 96% of pars defects.[28] Abnormalities in the "neck of the Scotty dog" is the hallmark radiographic finding (Fig. 71.6); complete defects are most common, but pars dysplasia and hypoplasia can also be observed.

Computed tomography (CT) scans are the best imaging modality to clearly visualize and define a spondylolysis. On axial images, spondylolysis appears as discontinuity of the posterior neural arch and can be differentiated from the adjacent facet joints. Sagittal reformatted images best show the pars defect as being distinct from facet joints (Fig. 71.7) and are the definitive finding in spondylolysis. One limitation of CT is the lower sensitivity for soft tissue densities, especially the internal anatomy of the neural foramen and the extent of any associated nerve root compression (see Fig. 71.7).

Magnetic resonance imaging (MRI) is increasingly used as the primary imaging modality in patients with LBP with or without radiculopathy. However, compared to CT scans, routine MRI sequences used for lumbar imaging may be less accurate for detecting spondylolysis, especially if no spondylolisthesis is present.[29–31] Sagittal T1-weighted images provide the greatest level of contrast between hyperintense bone marrow and the signal void of bony cortex at the pars defect[32] (Fig. 71.8).

Single-photon emission computed tomography can be used in the evaluation of suspected acute or impending spondylolysis. However, single-photon emission computed tomography has been reported to have notable false-positive and false-negative results in spondylolysis and thus should be used with caution, although it may be of particular value in cases in which MRI is contraindicated.[33]

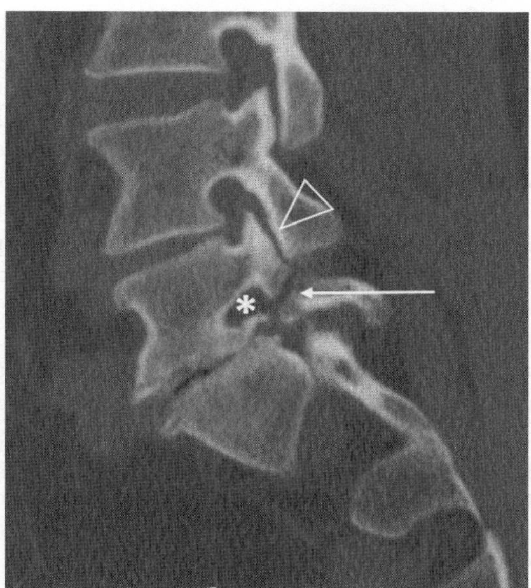

FIG. 71.7 Sagittal reformatted computed tomographic image of L5–S1 foramen. The open triangle shows the L4–L5 facet joint and the arrow highlights the pars defect. Note the difference in orientation. The asterisk shows the usual location of L5 nerve root but no further details of soft tissues within the neuroforamen.

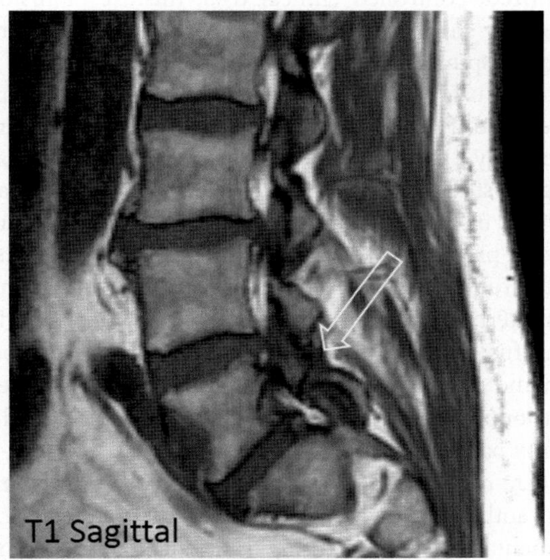

FIG. 71.8 T1-weighted sagittal magnetic resonance image showing subtle sign of pars defect (*open arrow*). Note the difference in orientation from the L4–L5 facet joint just cranial to it.

Differential Diagnosis

The differential diagnoses for isthmic spondylolisthesis are those of its clinical presentations: LBP and sciatica. First, spinal trauma, tumors, and infections should be ruled out. Next, degenerative disc disease, spondylosis, spinal stenosis, or disc herniation should be considered. Other causes include systemic diagnoses, such as rheumatoid arthritis and spondyloarthropathies, and other nonspinal, musculoskeletal etiologies, such as sacroiliac joint arthrosis, hip arthritis, and more. Finally, abdominal/visceral considerations would include renal, gastrointestinal, and vascular disorders.

Treatment

Nonoperative Treatment

Initial treatment for patients presenting with acute LBP should be nonoperative. The mainstays are patient education, activity modification, and medications such as nonsteroidal antiinflammatory drugs. The addition of physical therapy and exercise can be considered when early treatments fail and LBP becomes more long-standing. Other alternative pain management modalities—such as chiropractic care, acupuncture, and massage—have been widely utilized, with reported improvements in pain and function. The short-term use of narcotic analgesics should be considered with caution. A minor neurologic deficit, such as radicular numbness or paresthesias, but excluding severe motor weakness, can also be managed nonoperatively but may benefit from corticosteroid injection via injection therapies, such as fluoroscopically guided selective nerve root blocks.[34]

Operative Treatment

Indications

Severe, persistent back and/or lower extremity pain that is associated with functional limitations or that significantly impacts quality of life—with or without flexion–extension instability on radiographs, progressive motor weakness, or cauda equina syndrome—are all generally accepted indications for operative intervention. Patients should complete a rigorous course of nonoperative treatment prior to considering surgery unless a significant neurologic deficit exists.

Contraindications

Contraindications for surgery outside of absolute surgical ones—such as active infection, life-threatening medical conditions, and a broad range of relative contraindications related to an increased potential for perioperative complications or poor outcomes—include morbid obesity, cigarette smoking, worker's compensation, and active litigation.

Surgery

The goals of operative intervention in isthmic spondylolisthesis are to decompress neural elements and stabilize the affected motion segment. Uncommonly, decompression alone can be performed in certain circumstances when fusion is not necessary. More typically, surgery involves stabilization traditionally performed with posterior in situ fusion techniques with or without pedicle screw instrumentation and sometimes without decompression. Supplemental anterior column support using interbody fusion techniques approached posteriorly (posterior lumbar interbody fusion [PLIF]) or anteriorly (anterior lumbar interbody fusion) has been recently popularized and may currently represent the most popular form of surgical treatment in the United States.

Decompression

Decompression without fusion can be performed on individuals who have only radicular symptoms and stable spondylolisthesis on dynamic radiographs or a bony fusion seen on CT scans. Low-demand individuals or those with significant medical comorbidities may be reasonable candidates. Gill laminectomy entails removal of the entire posterior arch and the hypertrophied fibrocartilaginous tissue at the pars, as well as partial facetectomies to decompress the nerve root.[35,36] Long-term results of laminectomy alone have not been favorable, leading most experts to believe that addition of fusion is required in most cases to obtain good clinical outcomes.

Direct Pars Repair

Direct pars repair is a potential option in younger patients with no evidence of disc degeneration or spondylolisthesis and in whom pain is believed to arise mainly from the pars defect. Because of the high rate of clinical success with nonoperative treatment in this setting, patients should have failed a rigorous course of nonoperative treatment. The key operative principles are debridement of the defect, bone grafting, and providing adequate compression and stability of the defect for osteosynthesis. In small retrospective studies, this technique has been shown to yield good clinical outcomes in greater than 80% of patients.[37,38] Supplemental fixation is most often used; methods include translaminar screws, translaminar wires, and pedicle screw/sublaminar hook constructs.

Fusion

The primary operative intervention in isthmic spondylolisthesis is segmental fusion. While there are no definitive studies proving superior results of fusion over nonoperative care, spinal fusion at the level of the isthmic spondylolisthesis is a widely accepted treatment option. Several questions remain, however.

Is fusion better than nonoperative treatment? High-level evidence that surgery performs better than nonoperative treatments for isthmic spondylolisthesis has not been established. However, in general practice, most spinal surgeons believe that lumbar fusion is the treatment of choice for an individual with isthmic spondylolisthesis who has severe back or radicular pain, functional disability, and failed nonoperative treatments. Moller and Hedlund[26] evaluated 111 patients randomized to operative versus exercise treatment arms. They found that, at 2 years, patients who underwent posterolateral fusion had significantly better pain and functional outcomes compared to the exercise group. Laminectomy was performed in only those individuals who also complained of sciatica.[26]

Using the same cohort in a long-term study, Ekman et al.[39] reported results after a mean follow-up period of 9 years (range, 5–10 years). They used similar outcome measurements with the addition of the Oswestry Disability Index (ODI) and the Short-Form-36 to capture more disease-specific and quality-of-life data. They found no significant differences in pain and disability scores when comparing operative to nonoperative groups. However, global outcome score was significantly better in the operative group. The authors concluded that posterior lumbar fusion provided superior clinical improvement at 2 years, but at 9 years some of the measured clinical differences were lost. They did make note that no radiographic studies were done and therefore adjacent-level conditions could not be accounted for. Because global patient-reported outcomes were significantly better, spinal fusion appears to have long-lasting, positive effects in a patient with isthmic spondylolisthesis. In 2012, Turunen et al.[40] reported on a long-term, retrospective study of patients who had instrumented spinal fusion performed for degenerative spondylolisthesis, isthmic spondylolisthesis, and failed back surgery. The group with isthmic spondylolisthesis showed statistically significant improvements in pain and ODI scores as well as satisfaction scores of 70% at an average of 11 years after surgery.[40]

Surgical treatment, specifically spinal fusion, for the management of painful isthmic spondylolisthesis provides long-term benefits for pain, disability, and global quality-of-life measures. While this has not been demonstrated using a randomized, controlled clinical trial, the use of fusion has been widely supported in the literature and general practice patterns of spinal surgeons in the United States.

Indeed, fusion without decompression has been reported to yield good if not better outcomes compared to fusion with laminectomy.[41] There are two likely explanations for this finding. First, Gill laminectomy reduces the bone available to participate in the biologic fusion process. The remaining L5 transverse process and sacral ala can be small and act as poor hosts for robust fusion. Additionally, use of instrumentation and an interbody device may further bolster construct rigidity and the fusion process. Second, fusion eliminates repetitive flexion and extension motions at the pars defect and reduces nerve root trauma, which may be sufficient for back and lower extremity pain relief in most patients.

Is there a benefit to use of pedicle screw instrumentation? Several authors have reported on the use of pedicle screw instrumentation supplementing in situ fusion for treatment of isthmic spondylolisthesis and have found no clinical advantages associated with their use.[42,43] Previous papers on the use of pedicle screws in spinal fusions (not necessarily for isthmic spondylolisthesis) have shown no significant clinical advantage with their use.[44,45]

Another claimed benefit of pedicle screw use is lower pseudarthrosis rates, specifically for fusion in isthmic spondylolisthesis. Deguchi et al.[46] reported a retrospective series of 83 consecutive patients with isthmic spondylolisthesis treated with a Gill laminectomy and posterior fusion; 69 received pedicle screw instrumentation. They showed no difference in fusion rates for one-level fusion with or without instrumentation. However, in fusions that were more than one level, rigid posterior instrumentation did lead to higher fusion rates. The series is small and retrospective and likely underpowered to detect a difference between the two groups. Jacobs et al.[47] in 2006 reported a systematic literature review on best fusion techniques for isthmic spondylolisthesis. Their conclusion, using pooled data analysis, was that any potential advantage of using pedicle screws was not shown and, in two studies, worse fusion rates were reported. While it appears that use of instrumentation in posterior spinal fusion is commonly used in surgical practice, there is little to no definitive evidence that technical or clinical outcomes are necessarily improved with their use.

The use of pedicle screw instrumentation may be relevant due to the demanding fusion environment at L5–S1. Anatomically, the sacral ala is small, as is often the L5 transverse process, and the posterolateral gutter, especially with a spondylolisthesis, is also not a uniform fusion bed. Additionally, following a Gill laminectomy, the vertebral segment is unstable. This can lead to early motion, which challenges the fusion process and can be painful for the patient. Last, rigid internal fixation may lead to better and earlier postoperative pain reduction, resulting in shorter hospital stay and length of disability.

Does the use of interbody fusion result in better outcomes? Anterior column support can be approached posteriorly using transforaminal or posterior lumbar interbody fusion (T/PLIF), lateral lumbar interbody fusion (LLIF), or anterior lumbar interbody fusion techniques. In the review by Jacobs et al.,[47] they found that there was no data to support the superiority of interbody fusion over posterior lumbar fusion (PLF). Although fusion rates were high, 80% to 95% based on their analysis, they could not designate a distinctly superior technique for treatment of isthmic spondylolisthesis. Ye et al.[48] performed a meta-analysis of five studies on the operative treatment of isthmic spondylolisthesis using PLF versus PLIF. There was a total of 389 participants, 188 adults treated with PLF and 201 treated with PLIF. They found that there were no significant differences in pain relief, functional improvement, or infection rate. While fusion rates are significantly higher, it appears that anterior column support using posterior approaches does not yield better clinical outcomes.

Kwon et al.[49] analyzed the literature on surgical approaches for isthmic spondylolisthesis. While the reports and patients reported on varied, the patients were pooled and chi-square analysis was performed to determine the relationship between surgical approach and patient outcome. They found that combined (anteroposterior) approaches versus posterior-only procedures had significantly higher fusion rates and better clinical outcomes. Other notable findings were that use of pedicle screws led to better fusion rates and clinical outcomes, while laminectomy did not influence outcomes. Swan et al.[50] compared clinical outcomes in 92 patients who underwent posterior-alone versus anteroposterior fusion. They measured pain relief, improvement in ODI scores, medication use, and work status. Patients in the combined fusion group had significantly better clinical outcomes at all follow-up intervals except at 2 years, when the difference was not statistically significant. Additionally, fusion rate was higher in the combined group, which had only one nonunion, while the PLF group had three.

There appears to be debate in the literature regarding the ideal operative procedure for the treatment of isthmic spondylolisthesis. A critical goal in treatment of isthmic spondylolisthesis, particularly at L5–S1, is to achieve fusion; the literature supports anteroposterior fusion techniques in the treatment of isthmic spondylolisthesis. The use of an interbody device in the anterior column provides a second, much larger fusion bed compared to posterolateral gutter as well as early postoperative stability, which theoretically should increase short- and long-term segmental rigidity and fusion rates. An interbody device can increase foraminal dimensions and arrest the repeated flexion and extension movements on the nerve root, which should reduce radicular pain. Additionally, because 40% of lumbar lordosis occurs at L5–S1 and 67% occurs at L4–S1, the restoration or maintenance of lumbar lordosis is critical to avoid sagittal plane deformities and the need for future complex surgical reconstruction. This cannot be more emphatically stated, particularly in a group known to have high pelvic incidence and sacral slope.

Reduction of High-Grade Spondylolisthesis

Reduction of high-grade spondylolisthesis has been performed for improved sagittal balance and cosmesis. However, its routine use does not lead to significant improvements in clinical outcomes, may increase the risk of nerve injury, and is not recommended.[51] Clinical outcomes should take priority over radiographic ones and it appears that reduction of high-grade spondylolisthesis compromises clinical outcomes for improved radiographic ones.

PEARLS

1. Isthmic spondylolisthesis is prevalent in approximately 5% to 6% of adults in the United States.
2. Individuals with isthmic spondylolisthesis are rarely symptomatic, but those who do develop severe back pain, radiculopathy, or both can be effectively treated without surgery.
3. Significant evidence exists that isthmic spondylolisthesis develops in adolescence as a result of an extension stress injury. The spondylolisthesis develops as the soft tissues around the vertebral motion segment become incompetent.
4. Isthmic spondylolisthesis in symptomatic individuals who fail nonoperative treatment is commonly treated with a spinal fusion.
5. The ideal treatment technique has not been agreed upon and often involves use of pedicle screw instrumentation and interbody techniques.

PITFALLS

1. Failure to identify spondylolysis on imaging studies is common; if high suspicion exists, further imaging should be considered.
2. Because spinal fusion is the mainstay of treatment, individuals with high risk of nonunion should be approached with caution.
3. Decompression alone should be reserved in individuals who are low demand and poor operative candidates.
4. Nerve root involvement occurs at the level of the foramen and should correlate with clinical symptoms at presentation.
5. Reduction of high-grade slips can increase risk of nerve injuries.

KEY POINTS

1. Spondylolysis is a common radiographic finding that likely arises from a physiologic stress on the pars and occurs sometime during adolescence.
2. When symptomatic, isthmic spondylolisthesis can be managed nonoperatively in many cases, as most cases of low back pain are treated.
3. While spinal fusion is the most common treatment option, the literature is not clear on whether surgery is superior to nonoperative care. Moreover, which surgical techniques lead to the best clinical outcomes are not yet established.

KEY REFERENCES

1. Urrutia J, Zamora T, Cuellar J. Does the prevalence of spondylolysis and spina bifida occulta observed in pediatric patients remain stable in adults? *Clin Spine Surg*. 2016. Epub ahead of print.
2. Kalichman L, et al. Spondylolysis and spondylolisthesis: prevalence and association with low back pain in the adult community-based population. *Spine*. 2009;34:199-205.
3. Don AS, Robertson PA. Facet joint orientation in spondylolysis and isthmic spondylolisthesis. *J Spinal Disord Tech*. 2008;21: 112-115.
4. Andrade NS, Ashton CM, Wray NP, Brown C, Bartanusz V. Systematic review of observational studies reveals no association between low back pain and lumbar spondylolysis with or without isthmic spondylolisthesis. *Eur Spine J*. 2015;24: 1289-1295.
5. Möller H, Hedlund R. Surgery versus conservative management in adult isthmic spondylolisthesis–a prospective randomized study: part 1. *Spine*. 2000;25:1711-1715.
6. Carragee EJ. Single-level posterolateral arthrodesis, with or without posterior decompression, for the treatment of isthmic spondylolisthesis in adults. A prospective, randomized study. *J Bone Joint Surg Am*. 1997;79:1175-1180.
7. Ekman P, Möller H, Tullberg T, Neumann P, Hedlund R. Posterior lumbar interbody fusion versus posterolateral fusion in adult isthmic spondylolisthesis. *Spine*. 2007;32:2178-2183.
8. Jacobs WCH, Vreeling A, De Kleuver M. Fusion for low-grade adult isthmic spondylolisthesis: a systematic review of the literature. *Eur Spine J*. 2006;15:391-402.

REFERENCES

1. Meyerding H. Spondylolisthesis: surgical treatments and results. *Surg Gyn Obstet*. 1932;54:371-377.
2. Wiltse LL, Newman PH, Macnab I. Classification of spondylolisis and spondylolisthesis. *Clin Orthop*. 1976; 23-29.
3. Fredrickson BE, Baker D, McHolick WJ, Yuan HA, Lubicky JP. The natural history of spondylolysis and spondylolisthesis. *J Bone Joint Surg Am*. 1984;66:699-707.
4. Urrutia J, Zamora T, Cuellar J. Does the prevalence of spondylolysis and spina bifida occulta observed in pediatric patients remain stable in adults? *Clin Spine Surg*. 2016. Epub ahead of print.
5. Beutler WJ, et al. The natural history of spondylolysis and spondylolisthesis: 45-year follow-up evaluation. *Spine*. 2003;28:1027-1035.
6. Kalichman L, et al. Spondylolysis and spondylolisthesis: prevalence and association with low back pain in the adult community-based population. *Spine*. 2009;34:199-205.
7. Leone A, Cianfoni A, Cerase A, Magarelli N, Bonomo L. Lumbar spondylolysis: a review. *Skeletal Radiol*. 2011;40: 683-700.
8. Wiltse LL, Newman PH, Macnab I. Classification of spondylolysis and spondylolisthesis. *Clin Orthop*. 1976;23-29.
9. Cyron BM, Hutton WC. The fatigue strength of the lumbar neural arch in spondylolysis. *J Bone Joint Surg Br*. 1978;60B: 234-238.
10. Troup JD. Mechanical factors in spondylolisthesis and spondylolysis. *Clin Orthop*. 1976;59-67.
11. Rosenberg NJ, Bargar WL, Friedman B. The incidence of spondylolysis and spondylolisthesis in nonambulatory patients. *Spine*. 1981;6:35-38.
12. Herman MJ, Pizzutillo PD, Cavalier R. Spondylolysis and spondylolisthesis in the child and adolescent athlete. *Orthop Clin North Am*. 2003;34:461-467.
13. Lundin DA, Wiseman DB, Shaffrey CI. Spondylolysis and spondylolisthesis in the athlete. *Clin Neurosurg*. 2002;49: 528-547.
14. Jackson DW, Wiltse LL, Cirincoine RJ. Spondylolysis in the female gymnast. *Clin Orthop*. 1976;68-73.
15. Wiltse LL, Rothman S. Spondylolisthesis: classification, diagnosis, and natural history. *Semin Spine Surg*. 1989;1:78.
16. Saraste H. Long-term clinical and radiological follow-up of spondylolysis and spondylolisthesis. *J Pediatr Orthop*. 1987;7: 631-638.
17. Don AS, Robertson PA. Facet joint orientation in spondylolysis and isthmic spondylolisthesis. *J Spinal Disord Tech*. 2008;21: 112-115.
18. Ward CV, Latimer B. Human evolution and the development of spondylolysis. *Spine*. 2005;30:1808-1814.
19. Curylo LJ, Edwards C, DeWald RW. Radiographic markers in spondyloptosis: implications for spondylolisthesis progression. *Spine*. 2002;27:2021-2025.
20. Hanson DS, Bridwell KH, Rhee JM, Lenke LG. Correlation of pelvic incidence with low- and high-grade isthmic spondylolisthesis. *Spine*. 2002;27:2026-2029.
21. Labelle H, et al. Spondylolisthesis, pelvic incidence, and spinopelvic balance: a correlation study. *Spine*. 2004;29: 2049-2054.
22. Vaccaro AR, Martyak GG, Madigan L. Adult isthmic spondylolisthesis. *Orthopedics*. 2001;24:1172-1179.
23. Bunnell WP. Back pain in children. *Orthop Clin North Am*. 1982;13:587-604.
24. Turner RH, Bianco AJ. Spondylolysis and spondylolisthesis in children and teen-agers. *J Bone Joint Surg Am*. 1971;53:1298-1306.
25. Andrade NS, Ashton CM, Wray NP, Brown C, Bartanusz V. Systematic review of observational studies reveals no association between low back pain and lumbar spondylolysis with or without isthmic spondylolisthesis. *Eur Spine J*. 2015; 24:1289-1295.
26. Möller H, Hedlund R. Surgery versus conservative management in adult isthmic spondylolisthesis–a prospective randomized study: part 1. *Spine*. 2000;25:1711-1715.
27. Markwalder TM, Saager C, Reulen HJ. "Isthmic" spondylolisthesis—an analysis of the clinical and radiological presentation in relation to intraoperative findings and surgical results in 72 consecutive cases. *Acta Neurochir (Wien)*. 1991; 110:154-159.
28. Amato M, Totty WG, Gilula LA. Spondylolysis of the lumbar spine: demonstration of defects and laminal fragmentation. *Radiology*. 1984;153:627-629.

29. Dunn AJ, Campbell RSD, Mayor PE, Rees D. Radiological findings and healing patterns of incomplete stress fractures of the pars interarticularis. *Skeletal Radiol.* 2008;37:443-450.
30. Jinkins JR, Matthes JC, Sener RN, Venkatappan S, Rauch R. Spondylolysis, spondylolisthesis, and associated nerve root entrapment in the lumbosacral spine: MR evaluation. *AJR Am J Roentgenol.* 1992;159:799-803.
31. Jinkins JR, Rauch A. Magnetic resonance imaging of entrapment of lumbar nerve roots in spondylolytic spondylolisthesis. *J Bone Joint Surg Am.* 1994;76:1643-1648.
32. Johnson DW, Farnum GN, Latchaw RE, Erba SM. MR imaging of the pars interarticularis. *AJR Am J Roentgenol.* 1989;152:327-332.
33. Payne WK, Ogilvie JW. Back pain in children and adolescents. *Pediatr Clin North Am.* 1996;43:899-917.
34. Dagenais S, Gay RE, Tricco AC, Freeman MD, Mayer JM. NASS contemporary concepts in spine care: spinal manipulation therapy for acute low back pain. *Spine J.* 2010;10:918-940.
35. Gill GG, Manning JG, White HL. Surgical treatment of spondylolisthesis without spine fusion; excision of the loose lamina with decompression of the nerve roots. *J Bone Joint Surg Am.* 1955;37A:493-520.
36. Gill GG. Long-term follow-up evaluation of a few patients with spondylolisthesis treated by excision of the loose lamina with decompression of the nerve roots without spinal fusion. *Clin Orthop.* 1984;215-219.
37. Giudici F, Minoia L, Archetti M, Corriero AS, Zagra A. Long-term results of the direct repair of spondylolisthesis. *Eur Spine J.* 2011;20(suppl 1):S115-S120.
38. Pedersen AK, Hagen R. Spondylolysis and spondylolisthesis. Treatment by internal fixation and bone-grafting of the defect. *J Bone Joint Surg Am.* 1988;70:15-24.
39. Ekman P, Möller H, Hedlund R. The long-term effect of posterolateral fusion in adult isthmic spondylolisthesis: a randomized controlled study. *Spine J.* 2005;5:36-44.
40. Turunen V, et al. Lumbar instrumented posterolateral fusion in spondylolisthetic and failed back patients: a long-term follow-up study spanning 11-13 years. *Eur Spine J.* 2012;21:2140-2148.
41. Carragee EJ. Single-level posterolateral arthrodesis, with or without posterior decompression, for the treatment of isthmic spondylolisthesis in adults. A prospective, randomized study. *J Bone Joint Surg Am.* 1997;79:1175-1180.
42. Möller H, Hedlund R. Instrumented and noninstrumented posterolateral fusion in adult spondylolisthesis—a prospective randomized study: part 2. *Spine.* 2000;25:1716-1721.
43. Ekman P, Möller H, Tullberg T, Neumann P, Hedlund R. Posterior lumbar interbody fusion versus posterolateral fusion in adult isthmic spondylolisthesis. *Spine.* 2007;32:2178-2183.
44. Bridwell KH, Sedgewick TA, O'Brien MF, Lenke LG, Baldus C. The role of fusion and instrumentation in the treatment of degenerative spondylolisthesis with spinal stenosis. *J Spinal Disord.* 1993;6:461-472.
45. France JC, et al. A randomized prospective study of posterolateral lumbar fusion. Outcomes with and without pedicle screw instrumentation. *Spine.* 1999;24:553-560.
46. Deguchi M, Rapoff AJ, Zdeblick TA. Posterolateral fusion for isthmic spondylolisthesis in adults: analysis of fusion rate and clinical results. *J Spinal Disord.* 1998;11:459-464.
47. Jacobs WCH, Vreeling A, De Kleuver M. Fusion for low-grade adult isthmic spondylolisthesis: a systematic review of the literature. *Eur Spine J.* 2006;15:391-402.
48. Ye Y-P, Xu H, Chen D. Comparison between posterior lumbar interbody fusion and posterolateral fusion with transpedicular screw fixation for isthmic spondylolisthesis: a meta-analysis. *Arch Orthop Trauma Surg.* 2013;133:1649-1655.
49. Kwon BK, et al. A critical analysis of the literature regarding surgical approach and outcome for adult low-grade isthmic spondylolisthesis. *J Spinal Disord Tech.* 2005;18(suppl):S30-S40.
50. Swan J, et al. Surgical treatment for unstable low-grade isthmic spondylolisthesis in adults: a prospective controlled study of posterior instrumented fusion compared with combined anterior-posterior fusion. *Spine J.* 2006;6:606-614.
51. Hanson DS, Bridwell KH, Rhee JM, Lenke LG. Dowel fibular strut grafts for high-grade dysplastic isthmic spondylolisthesis. *Spine.* 2002;27:1982-1988.

CHAPTER 72 Adult Scoliosis

David Nelles
Kamran Majid

Introduction

It has been estimated that adult scoliosis may be present in anywhere from 1.4% to 68% of adults, based on a variety of studies using various definitions of scoliosis and various methods of studying the population.[1–6] In our aging population, the clinical, financial, and societal impact of this condition cannot be underestimated. Clinically, patients with this condition can range from asymptomatic to severely debilitated. A recent study calculated an average cost of $72,034 for adult scoliosis surgery.[7] In a separate study, patients were found to have improved health-related quality of life (HRQOL) measures with surgery compared with no such improvement in patients treated nonsurgically.[8] These studies highlight the importance of a thorough understanding of this disease state, including the natural history, treatment options, surgical considerations, and potential complications and pitfalls encountered when treating these patients.

Adolescent scoliosis can result in radiographic images not dissimilar to those in adult scoliosis patients, with similar coronal spinal profiles. However, there are many important differences between these two disease processes, and only fairly recently has this understanding begun to be thoroughly addressed in the literature. Differences include symptoms, progression, treatment options, and outcomes. In adolescent scoliosis, patients are typically asymptomatic or have very mild symptoms. Treatment goals emphasize stopping progression of the deformity to prevent further deterioration and symptoms while maintaining as much motion and function as possible. In contradistinction, adult scoliosis patients often present to the physician due to significant spine-related symptoms, including functional deficits, back pain, severe radicular symptoms, and symptoms related to stenosis. Treatment goals emphasize alleviating these symptoms in a manner that is as conservative as possible while still decreasing the likelihood of recurrent or new issues.

Adult scoliosis can be very broadly divided into two groups: adult idiopathic scoliosis, resulting as the natural progression of preexisting adolescent idiopathic scoliosis, and adult degenerative scoliosis, arising de novo from a relatively straight spine as a result of degenerative processes. Degenerative curves tend to be of a lower magnitude than idiopathic ones; lumbar curves predominate in this population.[9]

Terminology

Adult scoliosis can create a deformity that exists in three dimensions, as well as rotational abnormality. Patients with severe deformities can be relatively pain free, and some with comparatively smaller deformities can have debilitating pain and functional limitations. Add to this varying degrees of inflexibility of the deformity and countless other patient factors, and adult scoliosis is by definition a very complex issue. As expected, it comes with a correspondingly large and steadily increasing vocabulary of descriptive terms to help define and quantify it. Table 72.1 provides a cursory glossary of terms used in the treatment of scoliosis.

Current Understanding of Spinal Alignment

The concept of the "cone of economy" was popularized by Jean Dubousset in the 1990s (Fig. 72.1). The cone of economy basically describes the concept of centering our pelvis, torso, and head above our feet and knees. If an individual is able to optimize balance and posture and maintain the majority of the body weight over the feet, or very near to it, the individual is able to maintain this position with minimal effort. However, as deformity causes a person to deviate outside of this energetically economical zone, significantly more energy is required to maintain a standing posture. A supportive device, such as a cane or walker, may be required, and eventually pain and disability may result.[10] This model of alignment emphasizes the underlying importance of the ability to maintain an upright posture and has formed the basis for our current thoughts on spinal alignment.

Scoliosis has classically been defined by deformity in the coronal plane, but it is in reality a three-dimensional deformity that can result in curves in the coronal plane, lordotic or kyphotic (or both) sagittal imbalance, and rotational issues.

TABLE 72.1 Glossary of Descriptive Terms for Adult Spinal Deformity

Term	Definition
Scoliosis	Lateral curvature of the spine on coronal imaging
Kyphosis	Posterior or convex angulation of the spine on lateral view with the patient facing rightward. The terms hyperkyphosis and hypokyphosis refer to conditions in which the kyphosis is greater or less than the normal range, respectively.
Lordosis	Anterior convex angulation of the spine on lateral view with the patient facing rightward. The terms hyperlordosis and hypolordosis refer to conditions in which the lordosis is greater or less than the normal range, respectively.
Kyphoscoliosis	Scoliosis accompanied by a true hyperkyphosis
Lordoscoliosis	Scoliosis accompanied by a true hyperlordosis
Major curve	Curve with the largest Cobb angle measurement on upright long cassette radiograph of the spine
Minor curve	Any curve that does not have the largest Cobb angle measurement on upright long cassette radiograph of the spine
Structural curve	Measured spinal curve in the coronal plane in which the Cobb measurement fails to correct on supine maximal voluntary lateral side-bending radiograph
Compensatory curve	Minor curve above or below a major curve that may or may not be structural
End vertebrae	Vertebrae that define the ends of a curve in a coronal or sagittal projection. The cephalad end vertebra is the first vertebra in the cephalad direction from a curve apex whose superior surface is tilted maximally toward the concavity of the curve. The caudal end vertebra is the first vertebra in the caudal direction from a curve apex whose inferior surface is tilted maximally toward the concavity of the curve.
Neutral vertebra	Vertebra without axial rotation in reference to the most cephalad and caudal vertebrae that are not rotated in a curve
Apical vertebra	In a curve, the vertebra most deviated laterally from the vertical axis that passes through the patient's sacrum (CSVL)
Apical disc	In a curve, the disc most deviated laterally from the vertical axis of the patient that passes through the sacrum (CSVL)
Stable vertebra	Thoracic or lumbar vertebra cephalad to scoliosis that is most closely bisected by a vertically directed CSVL, assuming the pelvis is level. Alternatively, both pedicles of this vertebra should lie between vertical reference lines drawn from the sacroiliac joints.
CSVL	Vertical line in a coronal radiograph that passes through the center of the sacrum.
C7 plumb line	Vertical line drawn starting from the center of the C7 vertebral body and dropped straight downward. If drawn on a coronal view, the horizontal distance from this line to the central sacral line is a measure of the Cobb angle (coronal "balance"), with rightward and leftward deviations designated as positive and negative values, respectively. If drawn on a sagittal view, the horizontal distance from this line to the posterosuperior corner of S1 reflects a measure of the sagittal alignment (SVA), with positive values assigned for C7 plumb lines anterior to the sacrum and negative values assigned for C7 plumb lines that fall behind the sacrum.

CSVL, central sacral vertical line; SVA, sagittal vertical alignment.
From Smith J, Shaffrey C, Kai-Ming G, et al. Clinical and radiographic evaluation of the adult spinal deformity patient. *Neurosurg Clin North Am*. 2013;24:143–156.

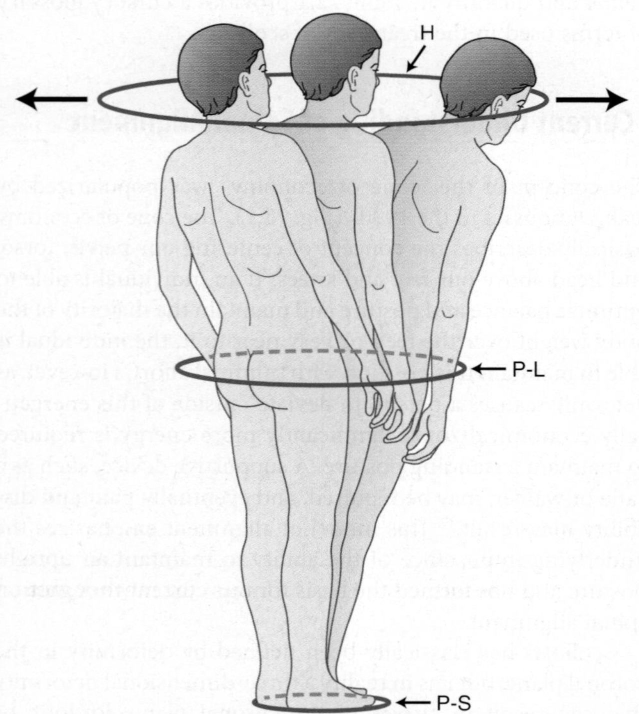

FIG. 72.1 Cone of economy.

Coronal deformities are typically described using the Cobb method. Earlier classification systems (King-Moe) and treatment methods (Harrington-style nonsegmental fixation) focused on the coronal plane, sometimes to the detriment of the other facets of the disorder. However, steady progress has been made in understanding complex deformities and in our ability to simultaneously address deformity in multiple planes using segmental instrumentation.

In recent years, the focus of spinal alignment has shifted toward the pelvis. Thanks in large part to the works of the International Spine Study Group (ISSG), a large multicenter group pooling dedicated resources with the goal of furthering knowledge of adult spinal deformity (ASD), as well as other groups and individuals,[11–19] we are now beginning to understand the complex interaction between sagittal spinal deformity and pelvic morphology/alignment. A brief description follows of each of the various pelvic and spinopelvic parameters that are currently being used or are being studied as useful measurements in ASD. In the following descriptions, assume a lateral radiograph in which the femoral heads are perfectly superimposed (Figs. 72.2 and 72.3 and Table 72.2)

- **Pelvic incidence (PI)[11]:** This parameter describes the angle between a line perpendicular to the sacral endplate and a line from the center of the femoral heads to the center of

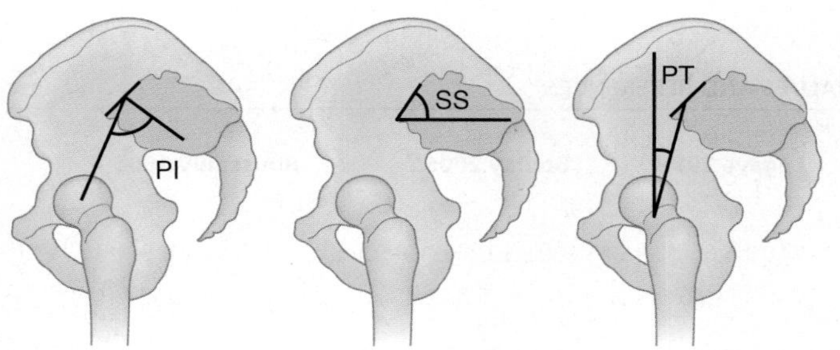

FIG. 72.2 Angles of pelvic incidence (PI), sacral slope (SS), and pelvic tilt (PT).

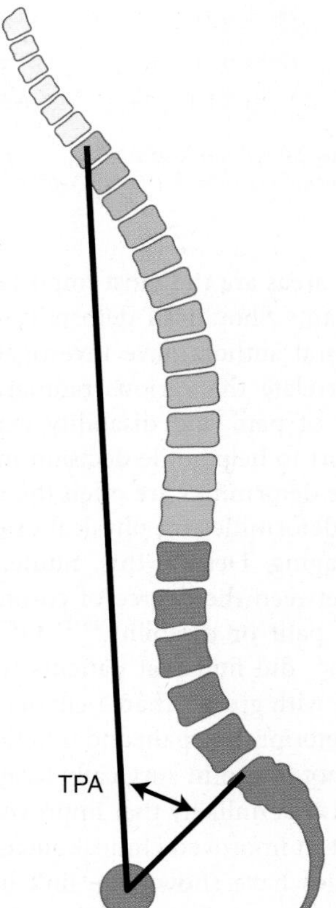

FIG. 72.3 T2 pelvic angle (TPA), a novel radiographic parameter that accounts for both global malalignment and compensation through pelvic retroversion. TPA is defined as the angle between the line from the femoral head axis to the centroid of T1 and the line from the femoral head axis to the middle of the S1 endplate. (From Ryan D, et al. T1 pelvic angle [TPA] effectively evaluates sagittal deformity and assesses radiographical surgical outcomes longitudinally. *Spine*. 2014;39[15]:1203-1210.)

the sacral endplate. This is an individual morphologic characteristic and does not change. It is related intimately with lumbar lordosis, as will be described in the following text. Normal values are considered from 50 to 55, although this can vary substantially.

- **Pelvic tilt (PT)**[20]: This parameter describes the angle between a vertical line through the center of the femoral heads and a line from the center of the femoral heads to the center of the sacral endplate. This angle can be physiologically altered via pelvic retroversion/translation. This can be seen as a compensatory mechanism, as described in the following text.
- **Sacral slope (SS)**[20]: This parameter describes the angle between the horizontal and the sacral endplate. It indicates the sacral inclination. Importantly, these three parameters have a relationship such that **PI = PT + SS.** As PI is a static morphologic parameter, this relationship ensures that changing one SS or PT will affect the other parameter accordingly.
- **Sagittal vertical axis (SVA)**: This parameter is commonly referred to as global sagittal alignment. A line is drawn straight down from the center of the C7 body on a full-length standing lateral radiograph. The SVA is the distance between this line and the posterior superior aspect of the sacral endplate. A positive number indicates that the C7 plumb line is anterior to the sacrum. Normal is considered less than 5 cm.
- **T1/T9 spinopelvic inclination (SPI):** This parameter describes the angle between a line drawn from the center of the femoral heads to the center of the T1/T9 body and a plumb line drawn from the center of the body.
- **T1 pelvic angle (TPA)**[21]: This parameter describes the angle between a line drawn from the center of the T1 body to the center of the femoral heads and the line from the center of the femoral heads and the midpoint of the sacral endplate. Both the TPA and T1 SPI are true spinopelvic parameters that describe the relationship between the spine and the pelvis.

The SVA is the simplest and most primitive means of describing the sagittal alignment. It is referred to as the global sagittal alignment because it gives a broad illustration of the sum of lordosis and kyphosis of the thoracolumbar spine. However, it fails to take into account pelvic parameters and any compensatory mechanisms at work.

Pelvic inclination is a discrete morphologic parameter that changes minimally with aging.[22] Described in Legaye's works, it has formed the basis for other pelvic and spinopelvic measurements. In the work by Boulay,[23] it was linked with the degree of lumbar lordosis, which makes anatomic sense. Assuming minimal to no movement through the SI joints, a large PI indicates a more vertical sacrum, which would require more lumbar lordosis to maintain balance for a given amount of thoracic kyphosis. Conversely, a smaller PI means a horizontal sacrum and a smaller lordosis to balance a given amount of thoracic kyphosis (TK). Schwab et al.[24] investigated this relationship and established the formula for lumbar lordosis (LL) = PI + 9 degrees (±9 degrees) or, put more simply, LL should be within about 10 degrees of PI.

PT is a parameter that changes with time, body position, and shape of the spine.[22] An individual can attempt to alter pelvic tilt by retroverting the pelvis and rotating about the hip joint. This can be done in an attempt to maintain an upright posture in the face of improper spinal balance. This parameter is one of the main reasons that simply looking at SVA to gauge sagittal alignment can be misleading. Depending on the range of motion (ROM) of the hip joints and the flexibility of the soft tissues around the hips, extending through the hips and increasing pelvic tilt can be used to compensate for a net positive balance. This can become important as we get older, and degenerative disc disease leads to a loss of LL.[25] Other factors that occur as

TABLE 72.2 Radiographic Norms of Various Spinopelvic Parameters

	NORMATIVE VALUES AND REFERENCES					
Parameter	**Schwab 2006[28]**	**Berthonnaud 2005[14]**	**Vialle 2005**	**Legaye 1998[11]**	**Boulay 2006[23]**	**Roussouly 2006**
No. subjects	75	160	300	49	149	153
Age	49.3 y (18–80)	25.7 ± 5.5 y (20–70)	35 y (20–70)	24.0 ± 5.8 y (19–50)	30.8 ± 6.0 y (19–50)	27 y (18–48)
Male/female ratio	0.56	0.95	0.63	0.56	0.52	0.52
SVA	−20 ± 30	—	—	—	—	35.2 ± 19.4 (−18.1 to 80.8)
T1–SPI	—	—	−1.4 ± 2.7 (−9.2 to 7.1)	—	—	—
TK (T4–T12)	41 ± 12	47.5 ± 4.8 (22.5–70.3)	40.6 ± 10.0 (0–69)	~43.0 ± 13.0	53.8 ± 10.1 (33.2–83.5)	46.3 ± 9.5 (23.0–65.9)
LL (L1–S1)	60 ± 12	42.7 ± 5.4 (16–71.9)	60.2 ± 10.3 (30–89)	~60.0 ± 10.0	66.4 ± 9.5 (44.8–87.2)	61.2 ± 9.4 (39.9–83.7)
PI	52 ± 10	51 ± 5.3 (33.7–83.7)	54.7 ± 10.6 (33–82)	~52.0 ± 10.0	53.1 ± 9.0 (33.7–77.5)	50.6 ± 10.2 (27.9–82.8)
PT	15 ± 7	12.1 ± 3.2 (−5.1 to 30.5)	13.2 ± 6.1 (−4.5 to 27)	~11.0 ± 5.5	12.0 ± 6.4 (−2 to 30)	11.1 ± 5.9 (−2.8 to 23.7)
SS	30 ± 9	39.7 ± 4.1 (21.2–65.9)	41.2 ± 8.4 (17–63)	~40.0 ± 8.5	41.2 ± 7.0 (0.6–19.7)	39.6 ± 7.6 (17.5–63.4)

From Schwab F, et al. Radiographical spinopelvic parameters and disability in the setting of adult spinal deformity. *Spine*. 2013;38(13):E803-E812.
LL, lumbar lordosis; PI, pelvic inclination; PT, pelvic tilt; SS, sacral slope; SVA, sagittal vertical alignment; T1-SPI, T1 spinopelvic inclination; TK, thoracic kyphosis.

we age, such as hip arthritis and soft tissue contracture, can limit an individual's ability to use PT to compensate.

Sacral slope is a parameter that refers to how horizontal the sacral endplate is. It coexists with the two parameters discussed earlier in a geometric relationship such that PT + SS = PI. Accordingly, when an individual increases pelvic tilt, the sacral slope is decreased, and the sacral endplate gets closer to the horizontal.

TPA is a parameter that was more recently described by LaFage et al.[21] This measurement was developed in an attempt to establish a single parameter that could take into account spinal alignment and pelvic compensatory mechanisms (PT). It describes the angle between a line drawn from the sacral endplate to the femoral head axis and a line from the T1 pelvic body to the femoral head axis. This single measure combines the SVA and PT information. Further advantages include the lack of needing to calibrate imaging due to being an angular measure (and thus standardized across all magnifications) and the ability to be measured intraoperatively using fluoroscopic images. In their study describing this parameter, the ISSG compared using TPA to classify the degree of deformity with the Scoliosis Research Society (SRS)-Schwab Classification system (to be described shortly), and found that TPA was very often similar, and at times better, than the SRS-Schwab system. They proposed a target TPA of 10 degrees, thus allowing for some degree of error or loss of correction before reaching the severe deformity threshold of 20 degrees.

Similarly, T1/T9 SPI includes information from both SVA and PT, thus taking into account pelvic compensatory mechanisms.

Spinopelvic Parameters and Health-Related Quality of Life Measures

When faced with a complex ASD case—in patients with deformity in multiple planes, multiple comorbidities, and multiple complaints—a surgeon is faced with a difficult set of decisions: which areas are the most important and which are the least important? Should all deformity be corrected and how much? Several authors have investigated this area and attempted to correlate the various radiographic parameters with the degree of pain and disability experienced by the patient in an effort to help guide decision making.

Coronal plane deformities are often the most striking and obvious patient deformities on physical examination and on radiographic imaging. Despite this, numerous studies have found no link between the degree of coronal deformity and patient-reported pain or disability.[26–29] Of note, one of the Glassman studies[27] did find that patients who had not been treated surgically with greater than 4 cm of coronal imbalance were at risk for deteriorating pain and function scores, but this correlation was not found in surgically treated patients. They concluded that it was unlikely that improved coronal correction would result in improved clinical outcomes.

Multiple studies have shown the link between SVA and patient-reported pain and disability scales. Lafage et al.[15] quantified pain and disability in 125 adult patients with deformity using the Oswestry Disability Index (ODI), 12-Item Short Form Health Survey (SF-12), and SRS 23 Patient Questionnaire (SRS-23), and then compared their scores over a variety of spinopelvic parameters. They found strong correlations between SVA and SRS-23 scores and the ODI "standing disability" score. Glassman et al.[26] also described a statistical correlation between SVA and pain/disability measures, albeit a weaker correlation. Lafage attributed this difference in strength to the fact that SVA is a measurement requiring calibration of magnification of radiographs, which is difficult to take into account in multicenter studies such as the Glassman one.

In a pilot study,[30] and again in a follow-up study,[31] Schwab et al. established a correlation between self-reported pain and disability and several radiographic measures. Spondylolisthesis, endplate obliquity, and loss of LL were all correlated with worse patient-reported outcomes.

The Lafage study[15] investigated many of the spinopelvic parameters. They found a strong correlation between LL and the walking and standing portions of the ODI, as well as the bodily pain and Physical Composite Scale (PCS) of the SF-12. Other regional sagittal profiles (thoracolumbar, thoracic) were studied, but no such correlation was noted. The strongest correlations between patient-reported disability and radiographic parameters was with the T1-SPI. This measure correlated strongly with SF-12 PCS, SRS total score, SRS activity score, and the ODI standing disability score.

This study also took a rigorous look at PT as it relates to patient-reported outcomes. They reported that this has the second strongest correlation with disability, particularly with walking disability. The investigators concluded that this illustrates the inadequacy of PT as a compensatory mechanism. Patients with a high PT, who were retroverting their pelvis and extending their hips to make up for a positive sagittal balance, were not walking well, including the subgroup that was able to completely compensate (high PT, but normal SVA). At some point, these compensatory mechanisms become a detriment in their own right, and walking with fully extended hips and bent knees may not be efficient or well tolerated. They emphasized the importance of assessing pelvic parameters as well as spinal ones, as this group had significant disability despite an SVA within norms. They also noted a subgroup in this population that had a high SVA but normal PT, thus were not compensating for poor sagittal balance at all. They recommend a careful assessment of hip and knee motion in this subgroup.

In a study of patients treated with lumbosacral fusions, Lazennec et al.[29] also found a correlation between PT and pain postoperatively.

In 2013, the ISSG published a study in which they prospectively enrolled 492 consecutive adult deformity patients.[32] Multiple radiographic parameters were measured, and correlations between these and the ODI, SF-36, and SRS-22 forms were investigated. They determined that the strongest correlations with patient-reported disability were the PT, SVA, and PI-LL mismatch (this parameter having the strongest correlation). They noted a strong correlation between PT and PI-LL mismatch, highlighting the roll that PT plays as a compensatory mechanism for sagittal spinal malalignment, as illustrated by the PI-LL mismatch. They then conducted linear regression analysis for these three parameters to establish equations for predicting ODI scores based on these radiographic measurements. Based on an ODI greater than 40 indicating severe disability, they used these equations to predict severe disability from radiographs. They determined that PT greater than 21, SVA greater than 46 mm, and PI-LL greater than 10 would correlate with severe disability.

Ideal Values for Spinopelvic Parameters

A variety of studies have investigated spinopelvic alignment parameters and anatomic considerations in asymptomatic adults. These investigations have helped us to establish a range of normative values in the "normal" adult population (see Table 72.2). Using these values and an extensive review of the literature to determine the correlations between alignment parameters and HRQOL outcomes, Schwab et al.[32] attempted to establish a set of "target" values for several of these parameters. These are values that a surgeon should hope to obtain postoperatively in order to maximize HRQOL values for the patient.

An SVA less than 50 mm has been identified as a cutoff value for this parameter. Similarly, a T1-SPI of less than 0 degrees is also desirable. Both of these numbers indicate an anatomic position where the patient's C7 plumb line is behind or directly above the femoral heads. This position can help to maximize efficiency of movement for the patient, help to level the gaze, and avoid the common subjective complaint of "falling forward."

PT should be less than 20 degrees. It is important to recognize that this is not an anatomic parameter that can be adjusted surgically. PT represents the individual's response to an existing degree of spinal malalignment. The extent of pelvic retroversion exhibited by the patient should be carefully considered *preoperatively*. A large amount of PT likely indicates an attempt at compensating for a positive sagittal balance, *even in the context of a normal, or near normal, SVA*. If sagittal balance is considered without taking into account PT, this can easily result in surgical undercorrection and continued pain and disability for the patient. PT has been shown to normalize following normalization of the sagittal spinal profile.[33]

Finally, PI-LL should be less than 10. As mentioned earlier, a value greater than 10 can be considered a "spinopelvic mismatch," in which the amount of LL has not been appropriately matched to the individual patient's spinopelvic anatomy.

Classification Systems for Adult Spinal Deformity

As has been stated previously, ASD is a quite complex entity, and our understanding of it is constantly changing and growing. Several attempts have been made at classifying spinal deformity (although most have focused on pediatric deformity, until recently). Classification systems should ideally meet several requirements in order to be clinically useful. They should (1) identify different severities of disease state, (2) facilitate communication between health care providers in order to ensure accuracy and reproducibility in describing the disease state, (3) allow comparison of different treatment methods, and (4) call for creation of accurate treatment recommendations.[34]

The Terminology Committee of the SRS introduced the earliest classification for scoliosis in 1969. It was an entirely nominal classification system, describing the cause of the spinal deformity. Although this was easily reproducible and did give some clinical information regarding the patient's disease state and associated illness, it failed to describe any radiologic parameters or specific symptomatology.

The King-Moe classification was introduced as a guideline for the treatment of thoracic curves in adolescents.[35] It was useful for establishing fusion levels in these patients, but it was not intended for use in patients with complex adult deformities. Similarly, the Lenke Classification system[36] was presented as a means of predicting appropriate arthrodesis levels in

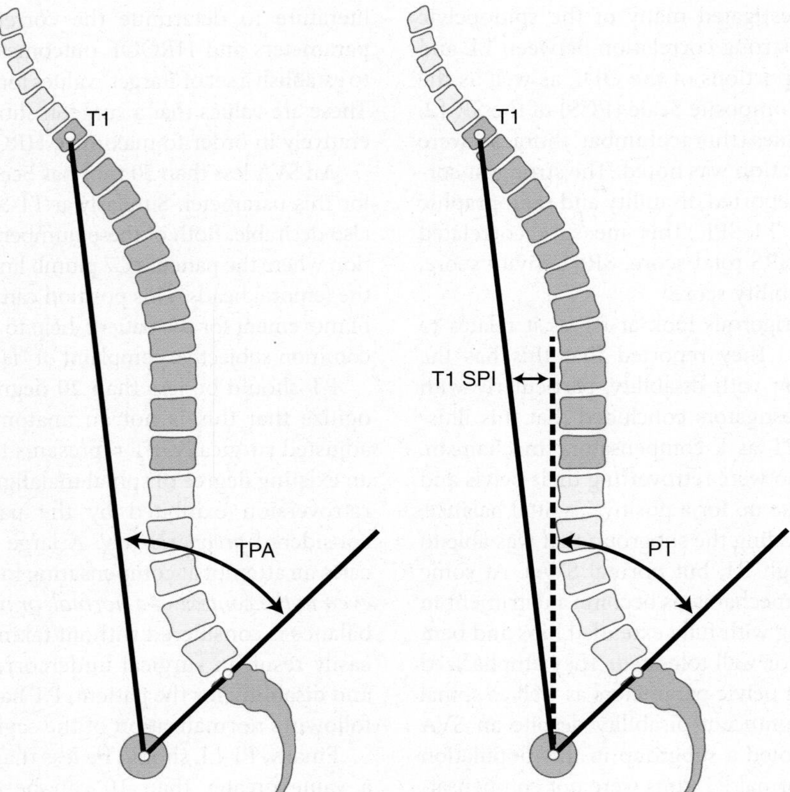

FIG. 72.4 T1 and T9 spinopelvic inclination (SPI). PT, pelvic tilt; TPA, T2 pelvic angle.

patients with adolescent idiopathic scoliosis. This was a far more comprehensive and descriptive system than was previously available and was met with great success in its use in the target population. However, attempts to apply the Lenke system to adult deformity were a mistake in several ways. Most importantly, the fundamental differences in treatment goals between the two disease entities made a combined classification system difficult, if not impossible. Adolescent idiopathic scoliosis is primarily treated to prevent *future* disability, while pain and disability are the primary complaints in adult deformity (with, as has been discussed, sagittal imbalance being the primary driving force of pain).

In 2006, Schwab et al. introduced a clinically oriented classification system based on existing studies linking certain spinal alignment parameters (though not pelvic parameters at this point) with HRQOL data.[28] They described five types of scoliosis based on the apex of the curve in the coronal plane: type I thoracic only, type II upper thoracic major (apex T4–T8), type III lower thoracic major (apex T9–T10), type IV thoracolumbar major (apex T11–L1), and type V lumbar major (apex L2–L4). They then added two modifiers to the classification, LL and intervertebral subluxation. Both of these radiographic findings were linked with poor HRQOLscores. Shortly after its introduction, a third modifier was added, the global balance modifier. This was added in response to new data indicating that SVA was a strong predictor of HRQOL.

This Schwab Clinical Impact Classification system was comprehensive and fairly reproducible. In addition, it was an evidence-based system that focused on parameters shown to correlate with poor patient-reported outcomes. However, in the years following its introduction, multiple studies began to show the importance of pelvic alignment parameters in spinal disorders and linking these parameters with poor HRQOL scores.[11,14–17,19]

In response to the relatively recent findings showing the pivotal role that the pelvis plays in ASD, the Schwab classification was updated and combined with works done through the SRS to become the SRS–Schwab Adult Spinal Deformity Classification[37] (Fig. 72.4 and Box 72.1). This system continues in the path of the Schwab Clinical Impact system in that it focuses on parameters that have been shown in the literature to correlate the most poor patient-reported outcomes and now includes the pelvic parameters that appear to be intimately related with pain and disability related to spinal deformity.

In the SRS–Schwab Adult Spinal Deformity Classification system, coronal deformity is divided into four groups: (1) T, thoracic only (lumbar curve <30 degrees), (2) L, TL/lumbar only (thoracic curve <30 degrees), (3) D, double curve (both curves >30 degrees), and (4) N, no major coronal deformity (all curves <30 degrees). The simplified coronal scheme reflects the mounting evidence that coronal malalignment is not related to pain or disability in ASD.

Similar to the Schwab Clinical Impact system, the sagittal modifiers were based on evidence indicating which parameters had the strongest correlation with poor HRQOL scores. All three of the modifiers are divided into three subgroups such that a score of 0 indicates a normal parameter, + indicates moderate

BOX 72.1 SRS-Schwab Classification System

Coronal Curve Types

Thoracic (T): Lumbar curve <30 degrees
Thoracolumbar/Lumbar (L): Thoracic curve <30 degrees
Double Curve (D): T and TL/L curves >30 degrees
No Major Coronal Deformity (N): All coronal curves <30 degrees

Sagittal Modifiers

PI – LL

0: <10 degrees
+: moderate 10–20 degrees
++: marked >20 degrees

Global Alignment

0: SVA <4 cm
+: SVA 4–9.5 cm
++: SVA >9.5 cm

Pelvic Tilt

0: PT <20 degrees
+: PT 20–30 degrees
++: PT >30 degrees

LL, lumbar lordosis; PI, pelvic incidence; PT, pelvic tilt; SVA, sagittal vertical alignment.

deformity, and ++ indicates a severe deformity likely associated with poor HRQOL scores. The first modifier is PI – LL: 0 is within 10 degrees, + (moderate) is from 10 to 20 degrees, and ++ (marked) is greater than 20 degrees. The second modifier is global alignment: 0 indicates an SVA less than 4 cm, + is an SVA from 4 to 9.5 cm, and ++ is an SVA greater than 9.5 cm. The third modifier is PT: 0 is a PT less than 20 degrees, + is a PT of 20 to 30 degrees, and ++ is a PT greater than 30 degrees.

The investigators' initial validation study indicated good to excellent intrarater and interrater reliability, showing that its use as a classification system is reproducible among and between users and should thus facilitate ease of communication.[37] Another independent group investigated the reliability and ease of use of this system, reporting excellent intraobserver reliability and substantial interobserver reliability, with most disagreements occurring while differentiating between thoracic and thoracolumbar curves in the coronal plane.[38] They concluded that the system was comprehensive, user friendly, and had sufficient reliability. Investigators have since used the system to prospectively analyze a group of ASD patients, who were then treated operatively or nonoperatively at the surgeon's discretion. The operatively treated group had worse HRQOL and worse sagittal modifier scores in all categories than those treated nonoperatively.[39] In addition, it has been shown that, following surgical correction of ASD, changes in SRS-Schwab sagittal modifier scores accurately predicted changes in HRQOL scores.[40]

Clinical Presentation of Adult Spinal Deformity Patients

The first step in evaluating a complex disease process such as ASD in typically complex older patients with significant comorbidities is a thorough history and physical examination. Presenting complaints from ASD patients can range from incidentally noted deformity or mild back pain to severe pain or near-total disability associated with their spinal deformity. It is important to establish early on the reason that the patient has sought medical treatment and the patient's future goals pertaining to health care. Having a clear discussion with the patient regarding these issues can avoid potential miscommunications that could damage the physician–patient relationship.

As has been demonstrated in several studies, pain and disability are both common reasons for a patient with ASD to present to a surgeon.[41–43] Both leg pain and back pain are common in this patient population. Smith et al. looked at a series of patients evaluated at a surgical clinic and found that 99% complained of back pain, 85% complained of some radicular pain, and 10% had complaints that were neurologic in nature. As there is significant overlap, it is important to attempt to quantify the amount that each of these complaints contributes to overall patient disability. Any aggravating or ameliorating factors should be investigated as well, as these could help guide treatment. Any history of subjective weakness, altered sensation, or other neurologic deficits should be carefully explored. Bowel or bladder dysfunction or claudicatory symptoms could indicate lumbar stenosis, and any upper extremity complaints or gait disturbances should elicit an assessment of the neck for cervical stenosis. Other complaints may include cosmetic ones, feeling of "falling over," or difficulty in maintaining eye contact due to an overall kyphotic alignment.

A history of past treatments—including but not limited to prior surgeries, medications, physical therapy, steroid injections, and activity modifications—should be obtained. It is not uncommon for ASD patients to present to a surgeon's office with a prior history of back surgeries, either to address the deformity or for other spine issues.[44] The purpose, extent, and clinical results of these surgeries should be discussed. In addition, an effort should be made to obtain old operative notes and office notes in order to fully understand both technical details of the surgery and the decision-making process involved.

Clinical Evaluation

The clinical evaluation of an ASD patient should begin with careful visual observation.[45] Patients should be observed in the supine, sitting, and standing positions. They should be observed during their normal gait to reveal any gait disturbances. Visual assessment of the patient's back in standing and bending positions may reveal spinal deformity, waist asymmetry, or rib humps, but smaller curves may not be easily appreciable. Clavicle or shoulder asymmetry can help provide clues to the nature of the deformity.

Careful ROM examinations should be done of the knees, hips, and spine. Chronic spine deformity may lead to a crouched knee gait, which can eventually lead to hip or knee flexion contractures. Upon evaluation of the patient in the standing position, the patient should be instructed to fully extend the knees. This can help assess knee ROM and reveal the true extent of the patient's sagittal imbalance, which had been obscured by the crouched posture. The patient should also be assessed for any real or perceived limb-length inequality.

The true incidence and severity of comorbidities in the ASD population is not known. It is likely highly variable, but the older patient population frequently associated with some types of adult deformity (e.g., degenerative deformity) often has a concomitant increase in number of comorbidities. Fu et al.[46] examined a large multicenter database of 22,857 ASD cases and stratified them by American Society of Anesthesiologists (ASA) classification. They found that the rate of perioperative complications increased with ASA grade from 1 to 5. This study highlights the importance of careful perioperative management to understand the risks associated with surgery and minimize them as much as possible.

Some basic preoperative laboratory work should be done to assess for and address any overt metabolic or hematologic abnormalities. Laboratory work should include an assessment of patient nutrition. Adogwa et al.[47] reviewed 136 cases of patients undergoing spine fusion (including deformity and nondeformity, elective and nonelective cases). They found that, in elective cases, preoperative hypoalbuminemia (serum albumin <3.5 g/dL) was a significant risk factor for postoperative complication. Close attention should be paid to the patient's nutritional status perioperatively to maximize outcomes.

Some controversy exists regarding appropriate blood loss management. ASD surgeries are frequently large surgeries with considerable blood loss and often require blood transfusion.[48] A recent study retrospectively reviewed a large multicenter database of patients who had undergone deformity surgery and divided them into two groups based on whether or not they had donated blood preoperatively. They found that preoperative donation was not protective against allogeneic transfusion, was associated with a higher overall transfusion rate, and often went unused. They concluded that, at this time, preoperative donation was not supported in the literature. Red blood cell salvage methods (e.g., Cell Saver) are increasingly popular blood loss management techniques. Similar to preoperative donation, these devices are designed to use the patient's own blood in order to obviate the need for allogeneic transfusion. There are currently conflicting studies in the literature regarding how effective it is for that purpose.

There is a current trend toward using antifibrinolytic therapy in adult deformity spine surgery. Agents such as tranexamic acid and epsilon-aminocaproic acid are lysine analogs that act by inhibiting the formation of plasmin by plasminogen, thereby blocking the fibrinolytic pathway.[49] They have well-accepted use, specifically in the joint replacement literature, indicating a lower blood loss as well as lower transfusion rates when used either intravenously or topically.[50] According to a recent meta-analysis[51] of the current spine literature regarding the topic, as well as a separate review of the literature,[52] the use of tranexamic acid in adult deformity surgery decreases intraoperative, postoperative, and total blood loss, as well as decreasing transfusion rates, while not increasing cardiac or thromboembolic risks. Epsilon-aminocaproic acid has had similar results, and there does not appear to be any consensus on the superiority of one agent over the other.[53]

Imaging Evaluation

The first and essential step in the radiographic evaluation of ASD patients begins with posteroanterior (PA) and lateral 36-inch radiographs. These images should be taken freestanding, with knees fully extended, elbow flexed approximately 45 degrees, with fingers on contralateral clavicles. It is important that these films extend at least as high as C7 and at least as far down as the femoral heads in order to accurately obtain measurements for all of the important parameters that were previously discussed.

The PA image should be viewed with the heart on the left side. Coronal alignment and pelvic obliquity can be measured on this image, as can curve angle. Pelvic obliquity can indicate potential limb-length discrepancy; if it is noted, lower extremity scanograms should be taken to assess for this. Any limb-length discrepancy detected should be corrected with blocks under the shorter leg until pelvic obliquity is normalized in order to get a true sense of the spinal alignment. Scoliosis curve angles should be measured using the standard Cobb method.

Lateral radiographs should be viewed with the patient facing to the right. The full-length lateral is useful for assessing both global and regional alignment parameters.[54] Regional parameters, such as LL and TK, should be documented. Global alignment in the form of the SVA should be measured. This film can also be used to measure spinopelvic parameters, such as TPA, T1-SPI, PT, sacral slope, and PI. As indicated earlier, accurate assessment of these parameters is instrumental in appropriately understanding and treating the patient's spinal deformity.

Flexibility of curves can be measured using a variety of different techniques. Side-bending PA films, traction films, and bolster films can all help improve the understanding of complex deformities. Curves that decrease to less than 25 degrees can be considered compensatory curves, not structural curves that would have to be addressed with any planned surgical procedure. In addition, comparing weight-bearing and supine films can also give information regarding flexibility.[44]

Although a considerable amount of information can be gleaned from the 36-inch PA and lateral films, advanced imaging has become standard in evaluating ASD cases. Considering the large amount of patients presenting with radicular symptoms, magnetic resonance imaging (MRI) is often utilized to evaluate individual nerve roots for compression. MRI is also useful for assessing the degree of disc degeneration and any areas of significant stenosis. Thin-slice computed tomography scans are excellent for assessing bony anatomy, including the location of any significant osteophyte formation, pedicle size, and location. Any patient with a condition precluding MRI (such as some implantable defibrillators) should have a computed tomography myelogram.

Treatment of Adult Scoliosis

When considering various options for scoliosis correction treatment, surgeons need to discuss the various pros and cons with their patients. The variability of management when considering adult scoliosis depends on the type of pathology and the surgeon's experience and comfort levels. There is also a lack of evidence-based medicine to help decision making. Options include nonoperative management, decompression alone, local decompression and fusion, regional decompression and fusion, and global decompression and fusion. Approach options vary from anterior, anterior/posterior, lateral/posterior, and all posterior.

Nonoperative Management

Nonoperative treatment should be focused on improving quality of life by decreasing the pain and disability in patients with adult scoliosis. This may include physical therapy, epidural steroid injections, acupuncture, massage, aquatics-based programs, and chiropractic manipulation.[55–57] Analgesics, including nonsteroidal antiinflammatory drugs and nerve stabilizers (e.g., gabapentin, pregabalin), may be beneficial; however, these should be used judiciously due to their potential respective side-effect profiles. For acute exacerbations of symptoms, narcotics can be considered, but their long-term use is not routinely recommended due to short- and long-term side effects, including overdose, tolerance, and addiction. There is limited evidence to support nonoperative management with adult scoliosis patients.[58–60]

The cost of nonoperative management has been studied by Glassman et al.[61] They looked at 123 adults with scoliosis who underwent nonoperative management consisting of medications, physical therapy, exercise, injections/blocks, chiropractic care, pain management, bracing, and bed rest. After 2 years, with a mean cost of $10,815, there was no improvement of pain or disability.

Recent studies have focused on identifying the predictors of reaching a minimally clinically important difference in patients who undergo nonoperative treatment.[62] Their retrospective review of a prospective, multicenter database studied 215 nonoperative patients with a minimum of 2-year follow-up. They concluded that nonoperative patients who achieved a minimal clinically important difference in SRS Activity or Pain scores had a lower baseline SRS Pain Score and less coronal deformity in the thoracolumbar region. They proposed that patients with greater baseline pain offered more room for potential improvement. In addition, patients with coronal deformities in the thoracolumbar region with associated vertebral obliquity may not do well with nonoperative management.

Operative Management

With the advancing age of patients with adult scoliosis and our ability to handle more complex deformities, the number of surgeries on adult scoliosis patients is increasing.[63] The goals of surgery on patients with adult scoliosis include nerve decompression, deformity correction (both in the sagittal and coronal planes), and reduction of axial back pain.[64] When discussing the options with patients who present with adult scoliosis, indications for surgery would include pain that has not improved with nonoperative management, inability to do activities of daily living, worsening of their deformity, and/or nerve compression causing radicular or neurogenic symptoms.

Improvements in surgical techniques and perioperative care have expanded our ability to care for adults with significant comorbidities, including pulmonary and cardiac disease, osteoporosis, and nutritional deficiency. The unique aspect of care in adult patients with scoliosis is the frequent presence of associated medical comorbidities. The long duration of surgery, resultant blood loss, and perioperative complications that can arise are factors that need to be considered and discussed in preoperative counseling sessions. The incidence of medical comorbidities in patients with adult scoliosis has been studied. An increasing rate of complications is seen in patients with comorbidities, leading to higher levels of physical status deterioration. Fu et al.[46] reported on a multicenter, multisurgeon Scoliosis Research Society Morbidity and Mortality database of 22,857 cases, stratified by the ASA physical status classification. A progressively increasing rate of complications was found in patients with ASA grade 1 (5.4%) to grade 5 (50%). Medical comorbidities that lead to physical status deterioration have a significant impact on the complications in the perioperative period in this patient population.

Patients with a history of coronary artery disease or other significant cardiac risk factors should undergo preoperative stress testing followed by optimization of cardiac function before scoliosis surgery. Perioperative use of beta blockers in these patients has been shown to cause significant reduction in cardiac events at 30 days after the surgery and decline in the 1- and 2-year mortality rates.[65] In addition, there is a reduction in postoperative pulmonary complication rate following smoking cessation a minimum of 6 to 8 weeks prior to surgery.[66] Diabetes has been implicated in a wide variety of postoperative complications, including reoperation,[67] infection,[68,69] and recurrent disc herniation.[70] Every attempt should be made to control blood sugars preoperatively and perioperatively; consultation with a medical doctor or endocrinologist to aid in the management of this condition may be beneficial. In addition to physical health, the surgeon may consider social, financial, and psychological well-being of the patient because spinal deformity surgery and subsequent recovery will surely affect all of these areas.

Patients with concurrent scoliosis and osteoporosis represent a significant management challenge. Osteoporosis can compromise the interface between bone and instrumentation, which may lead to pedicle screw loosening and graft subsidence.[71] Patients considering surgery should be referred to a bone endocrinologist for evaluation and treatment preoperatively to optimize their bone quality. In general, medical management can include bisphosphonates, nonbisphosphonate antiresorptive agents, and parathyroid hormone analogs. For patients who elect surgery, several important principles should be followed, including the use of multiple sites of fixation; meticulous preparation of endplates for interbody graft placement, making sure not to violate the vertebral endplates; use of bicortical screw fixation where safe; and possibly accepting lesser degrees of deformity correction. Adjuncts to improve fixation include the use of specialized pedicle screws, cement augmentation of pedicles with polymethylmethacrylate, and the use of anterior column support to reduce the stress on posterior instrumentation.[72]

Perioperative Considerations

The effect of general anesthetic agents and muscle relaxants on intraoperative neuromonitoring potentials warrants consideration. Halogenated inhalational agents and nitrous oxide produce a dose-dependent decrease in amplitude and increase in latency of somatosensory evoked potentials.[73] Benzodiazepines can also cause significant depression of motor potentials. The use of muscle relaxants precludes proper acquisition of motor evoked potentials (MEPs), and their action should be reversed before proceeding with MEP testing again. Ketamine and etomidate, on the other hand, cause increases in cortical amplitudes of somatosensory evoked potentials and MEPs, making them agents of choice when monitoring responses to stimulation are difficult.[74]

Placement of an arterial line facilitates more accurate monitoring of blood pressure throughout the procedure. Monitoring of core body temperature is also essential in addition to blood pressure, pulse oximetry, and urine output monitoring.

The importance of proper intraoperative patient positioning, especially in the backdrop of the long duration of corrective surgeries, cannot be underestimated. Attention should be paid to padding the eyes properly and keeping them free from any source of external compression when placing the patient prone. In patients undergoing surgery in the prone position, abducting the arms greater than 90 degrees or placing them in extension or external rotation should be avoided to prevent excessive stretch on the brachial plexus.[75] Consideration should be given for intraoperative monitoring of upper extremities to help ensure appropriate positioning and brachial plexus function.

Significant blood loss and transfusion requirements are associated with adult scoliosis surgery. Elgafy et al.[76] conducted a review of the literature on reduction of blood loss in major spine surgery and found a high level of evidence supporting the use of antifibrinolytics (e.g., tranexamic acid, aprotinin, and epsilon- aminocaproic acid). Intraoperative red blood cell salvage devices are also popular in the field of spinal deformity correction. The potential to reduce or obviate allogeneic blood transfusions, elimination of risk of alloimmunization and viral disease transmission, and preservation of the normal oxygen-carrying capacity of salvaged red blood cells are some of the major advantages of cell salvage techniques.[77] In a prospective randomized study involving 110 scoliosis patients undergoing posterior instrumented spinal fusion, Liang et al.[78] reported reduced mean intraoperative red blood cell transfusion requirement and a lower perioperative allogeneic blood transfusion rate in the cell saver group (14.5% vs. 32.7%; P = .025). However, several other studies do not support its efficacy in reducing the requirements of allogeneic blood transfusions in spine surgeries.[79,80]

Operative Decision Making

There exists tremendous variability in the operative management of adult scoliosis, with little consensus on surgical strategy regarding approach and levels.[81–83] Debate between selective decompression versus decompression and fusion versus limited fusion, identification of proximal fusion levels, and choosing distal fusion levels—including fusion to the pelvis—all remain sources of controversy.

Decompression

Selective decompression in the setting of adult scoliosis involves decompression of neurologic compression without fusion or correction of coronal, axial, or sagittal alignment. Radicular pain and neural symptoms are important clinical presentations of adult scoliosis. Limited decompression of stenotic levels may offer significant improvement of clinical symptoms while limiting surgical risks associated with a larger reconstructive operation. The negative of doing only a decompression is that there may be progression of the deformity, possibly requiring a secondary procedure in the future.[84] Indications for a selective decompression operation would include patients who present with primarily radicular pain, patients with a stable deformity with bridging osteophytes or ankylosis, patients with radicular symptoms from compression of nerve roots from the convexity of the curvature as opposed to foraminal stenosis from the concavity of the curve, and patients with central or lateral recess stenosis.

Decompression With Limited Fusion

As with selective decompression alone, selective decompression and limited fusion has a role in a specific patient population. Patients who cannot undergo long thoracic and lumbar fusions may be candidates for limited fusion. The ideal candidate for limited fusion is a patient whom the surgeon desires to treat with decompression only for the reasons stated earlier; however, radiographs reveal apical progression or a symptomatic lumbosacral fractional curve. The lumbosacral or fractional curve in adults with scoliosis may be a localized source of symptomatic neural compression and pain, even in the presence of more generalized deformity. When performing selective decompressions, transforaminal lumbar interbody fusion or posterior lumbar interbody fusion can be used as a posterior-only approach, with the placement of the intervertebral cage on the concavity of the deformity to allow some deformity correction.[85]

There is little consensus on the proximal fusion level in patients with adult scoliosis once the decision has been made to proceed with decompression and fusion. The proximal fusion should not be stopped at the thoracolumbar junction and, at a minimum, the apex of the deformity should be included in the fusion levels.[86] It is important to consider the proximal and distal levels beyond the ending point of the fusion, as the amount of stability and degeneration at an adjacent vertebral segment to the fusion will predict the stability of the adjacent level after fusion. Intraoperatively, efforts should also be made to preserve the supra-adjacent facet, the intraspinous ligaments, and the supraspinous ligaments, thus preserving the normal intravertebral ligamentous relationships.[87] In thoracic and lumbar double-curve degenerative scoliosis, the proximal construct should include the thoracic curve and should not stop distal to any portion of the curve.[88] Stopping at the physiologic apex of thoracic kyphosis (T5–T6) should be avoided due to the increased risk of proximal junctional kyphosis.[89] Thus constructs typically end either at or below T10 or between T2 and T4.

The decision to continue the distal fusion level from L5 to S1 is controversial and heavily debated. A fusion that extends to the sacrum provides greater stability, but with the increased stability comes increased risks and complications. Stopping the fusion at L5 may reduce the magnitude of the procedure and may limit perioperative complications. However, this advantage may come at the cost of a loss of deformity correction over time and a possible need for future surgery with extension of arthrodesis to the sacrum. When comparing fusion to S1 and fusion to L5, studies have shown increased coronal balance and lateral listhesis with fusion to S1.[90–93]

The biomechanical forces of the sacrum allow for implant prominence, implant loosening, and instrument-related issues when fusing to the pelvis.[94] Common techniques to minimize sacropelvic fixation prominence complications include the use of S2 iliac screws and S2 alar screws, which allows for reduced implant prominence and allows the use of a single rod, reducing the number of required connections. Kebaish et al.[95] prospectively reviewed the use of S2AI screws in 52 consecutive patients with mean 2.5-year follow-up, concluding that the method is easy, safe, and effective for achieving sacropelvic fixation in long posterior constructs, with minimal complications and low revision rate.

Clear indications to extend instrumentation and fusion to the level of the sacrum include a spondylolisthesis at L5–S1, stenosis requiring decompression at L5–S1, fixed obliquity of the L5–S1 motion segment, incomplete correction of global sagittal balance, and symptomatic degenerative changes at L5–S1.

Surgical Approaches in Adult Scoliosis Surgery

The choice of surgical approach to the spine in adult deformity has an important effect on the morbidity of surgery and on the efficacy of deformity correction and clinical outcomes. Spinal reconstruction can be performed via anterior, posterior, and combined approaches, with or without staging of the procedures. The optimal method must take into consideration the patient's sagittal alignment, bone quality, nutritional status, need for fusion across the lumbosacral junction, anterior column mobility, and the surgeon's technical expertise.

Anterior surgery to treat adult thoracolumbar scoliosis was originally described by Dwyer et al. in 1969.[96] These anterior-only reconstructions were typically utilized for thoracolumbar curvature; they were able to achieve effective correction, especially in the sagittal plane, because of the release of the anterior longitudinal ligament. Distal lumbar motion segments were often able to be spared, a distinct advantage in comparison to the posterior approach options. In addition, anterior-only correction maintains the integrity of the posterior ligamentous complex. The major disadvantage of anterior approaches to the spine is the morbidity of the dissection, with risks to the lung, diaphragm, sympathetic chain, and major vascular structures in the thoracic and thoracolumbar spine, as well as the genitofemoral nerve, kidney and ureter, and the peritoneal contents in the lumbar spine. Smith and colleagues[97] reported excellent clinical outcomes with limited complications in a series of 15 consecutive adult patients treated with rigid single-rod anterior surgery for thoracolumbar scoliosis.

Through an anterior approach, stiff spinal deformities caused by degenerative disc collapse via discectomy can be released by sectioning the anterior longitudinal ligament, allowing for significant correction of segmental sagittal malalignment. This is particularly useful in reestablishing lordosis of the lumbar spine. Correction achieved through anterior column reconstruction may eliminate the need for more aggressive posterior-based osteotomies. Anterior approaches also allow for placement of bone graft within the anterior column that is under a compressive load and the large bony surface area leads to higher fusion rates. Especially at the lumbosacral junction, an interbody fusion is important to mitigate the risk of pseudarthrosis.[98]

Bradford et al.[99] demonstrated that a combined anterior and posterior approach to Scheuermann kyphosis resulted in significantly better deformity correction and better fusion rates and maintenance of correction over the instrumented segments than posterior-only surgery with nonsegmental instrumentation. Similarly, in adult scoliosis, a combined anterior and posterior approach has been advocated for improvement of lumbar lordosis and improvement of fusion rates, especially at the lumbosacral junction.[100,101] Berven et al.[102] studied the outcomes of combined anterior and posterior surgery for the management of fixed sagittal plane deformity. They noted that patient satisfaction with surgery and overall clinical outcomes were best in cases that resulted in an increase in lumbar lordosis. Patients with preoperative regional hypolordosis (≥30 degrees) had the most reliable improvement of health status and had better clinical outcomes than those with lumbar lordosis in the physiologic range. The authors noted that 40% of patients in the study had major complications, including pneumonia, dural tears, wound infection, and pseudarthrosis. Relative indications for combined anterior and posterior fusion include planned arthrodesis across the lumbosacral junction, lumbar pseudarthrosis, correction of a fixed lumbosacral obliquity, lumbar hypolordosis, posterior-element deficiency, and osteoporosis. These rates of complications from combined anterior-posterior approaches have been detailed in several studies in the literature.[103–105]

When a decision for a combined approach for treatment of spinal deformity has been made, the options of doing the anterior and posterior surgery on the same day versus on two separate days must be considered. Staged procedures are well tolerated by many patients, but they may be associated with a higher risk of infection and blood transfusion. For fused, rigid deformities, patients may be served better with a two-stage surgery with two periods of anesthesia. During the first anesthetic, anterior discectomies and interbody placement with temporary fixation may be performed. At the next stage, done approximately 4 to 6 weeks later, posterior releases, instrumentation, and deformity correction can be performed. This allows ample time to recover from the first surgery before undergoing the second.

The role of minimally invasive approaches to the anterior column, including direct lateral approaches, has expanded the indications and use of anterior surgery for adult scoliosis.[106] Although initially used primarily for foraminal stenosis with loss of disc height and for adjacent-segment degeneration in the lumbar spine, more attention has been paid recently to using various forms of the direct lateral retroperitoneal approach for correcting and stabilizing adult deformity cases. The use for lateral interbody fusion in obtaining indirect decompression of neuroforamina and obviating the need for direct decompression has been well documented,[107] and now it has increasing use in deformity correction. A recent review of the literature[108] on using a specific form of lateral interbody fusion indicated that ODI and visual analog scale scores improved comparatively with other forms of lumbar interbody fusion and that coronal alignment and balance were both corrected, but minimal LL and sagittal balance correction was obtained. A more recent innovation involves release of the anterolateral ligament via the minimally invasive lateral approach, allowing for significant segmental correction (in some cases approaching 30 degrees) in an effort to avoid having to perform the more morbid posterior osteotomy. There has been evidence to support the use of minimally invasive surgery techniques in ASD surgery, particularly in symptomatic elderly patients without significant sagittal imbalance.[109]

Posterior-only approaches for the correction of spinal deformity have become increasingly more common. Three-column segmental transpedicular instrumentation and the development of posterior osteotomy techniques enable greater curve correction without the need for anterior apical releases.[110] Posterior-based osteotomies, including posterior column osteotomies (e.g., Ponte osteotomies), pedicle subtraction osteotomies, and vertebral column resections, allow for significant coronal and sagittal deformity correction from the posterior approach. Posterior column osteotomies typically allow 10 degrees of sagittal correction per level or about 1 degree of correction for every millimeter of bone resected. The pedicle subtraction osteotomy, which is a V-shaped wedge resection of the vertebral body including both pedicles and posterior elements, can achieve a correction of between 30 and 40 degrees at a single level.[111] Vertebral column resection can deliver much greater coronal and sagittal plane correction.[112] The use of osteobiologics may improve fusion rates in adult scoliosis surgery and preclude the need for circumferential fusion at the lumbosacral junction.[113]

Kim et al.[114] analyzed the radiographic and functional outcomes after posterior segmental spinal instrumentation and fusion with and without anterior apical release of the lumbar curve in adult scoliosis patients. Their study showed superior clinical outcome scores (SRS) and subscales in self-image and function in the group with posterior-only surgery as compared to the group with the combined approach, without a difference in radiographic parameters. Perioperative morbidity and complications were higher in the group of patients treated with combined anterior and posterior surgery.

Multiple studies[115–117] have compared outcomes and complications in adults with thoracolumbar scoliosis. Overall, the authors demonstrated similar radiographic correction of deformity for each group. However, patients with staged anterior and posterior surgery had significantly more perioperative complications.

One challenge in treating patients with a posterior-only approach is the risk for pseudarthrosis. Kim et al.[118] reported a 17% incidence (nearly 1 in 5) of pseudarthrosis after long primary arthrodesis with the use of modern segmental spinal instrumentation for the treatment of adult idiopathic scoliosis. Some authors contend that risk for pseudarthrosis in the posterior-only approach can be mitigated with recombinant human bone morphogenetic protein-2. Luhmann et al.[119] have reported a high rate of fusion for both anterior-only (96%) and posterior-only (93%) surgery with the use of rhBMP-2 for ASD. A subsequent long-term follow-up study on the same patients showed significant fusion rates for anterior (91%), posterior (97%), and high-dose posterior (100%) spinal fusion.[120]

For severe spinal deformity, vertebral column resection is a useful technique to permit spinal column shortening and trunk translation. O'Neill et al.[121] recently published their 5-year follow-up on 120 patients who underwent three-column osteotomies. They showed radiographic alignment improvement but were negatively affected by prior surgery and complications requiring revision surgeries. Major complications occurred in 27%, with major reoperations in 25%. A posterior-only vertebral column resection may be effective for spinal deformity that is focal and in which the apex of coronal and sagittal deformity is matched. The combined anterior and posterior approach may be more effective in treating the patient with a deformity that extends across multiple segments; deformity that involves multiple apices, including different apices in the coronal and sagittal planes; and in the spine with hypokyphosis or lordosis across the thoracic spine.

Complications of Adult Scoliosis Surgery

Spinal deformity is one of the oldest conditions known to humankind. Its correction is inherently complicated and has certain risks involved. Neurologic injury during spine surgery can have devastating consequences for the patient; the surgeon being aware of the causes of these complications can help dissipate and potentially prevent them from occurring. The risk of neurologic injury depends on the surgical procedure performed, the amount of manipulation of the spinal cord, the use of spinal instrumentation, and the degree of preoperative spinal deformity and stability. The spinal cord is more sensitive to manipulation than the nerve roots. The pathophysiology of spinal cord injury is extremely complex and can involve physiologic processes such as inflammation, edema, hemorrhage, and ischemia.

The SRS used the largest known database of adult scoliosis to determine the rate of complications of adult scoliosis surgery.[122] Looking at their data from 2004 to 2007, complications were identified and analyzed on the type of scoliosis, age, use of osteotomy, revision surgery status, and surgical approach. Each group was stratified to age 60 years or younger versus older than 60 years. Surgical approach was divided into anterior, posterior, or combined anterior/posterior. Looking at a total of 4980 cases, there were 521 patients with complications (10.5%) and a total of 669 complications (13.4%). The most common complications were dural tear, 142 (2.9%); superficial wound infection, 46 (0.9%); deep wound infection, 73 (1.5%); implant complication, 80 (1.6%); acute neurologic deficits, 49 (1.0%); delayed neurologic deficits, 41 (0.5%); epidural hematoma, 12 (0.2%); wound hematoma, 22 (0.4%); pulmonary embolus, 12 (0.2%); and deep venous thrombosis, 9 (0.2%). There were also 17 deaths (0.3%). In their study, age was not associated with complication rate ($P = .32$). Significantly higher complication rates were identified in osteotomies, revision surgery, and combined anterior/posterior surgery.

As noted by Schwab et al.,[6] surgical complications were prevalent in 60% of patients older than 60 years. Surgical complications can be further differentiated into mechanical in nature, such as radiographic complications from proximal junctional kyphosis, and implant-related complications, such as pullout and implant failure. Complications may also be nonmechanical in nature, such as neurologic, dural injury, and wound healing.

Soroceanu et al.[123] recently looked at the radiographic and implant-related complications seen in adults undergoing spinal deformity surgery. With 2-year follow-up, the radiographic and implant complication rate was 31.7%, with half of these patients requiring a revision operation. These mechanical complications affected HRQOL by decreasing the rate of improvement over time after adjacent-segment disease surgery.

Several techniques have been proposed to reduce the risk of proximal junctional kyphosis. These include strategies to reduce the stiffness of the instrumentation, such as selecting rods of smaller diameter, transitional rods, and/or less stiff composite metals, and using hooks[124] or sublaminar wires in place of pedicle screws at the upper instrumented vertebra. Other authors have advocated the use of cement to augment the upper instrumented vertebra.[125,126] Percutaneous placement of pedicle screws in the upper one or two levels of the construct to minimize injury to the facet complex and supporting soft tissue structures is currently being evaluated. The best strategy to prevent proximal junctional kyphosis is the subject of much debate and an area of active research.[127]

The effect of advancing age on postoperative complications and revision surgery following fusion for scoliosis has been investigated recently.[128] In a retrospective cohort study examining 8432 patients with the average age at 53.3 years, there was an increase in risk of hemorrhage, pulmonary embolism, infection, and refusion associated with age.

The impact of obesity on complication rate infection and patient-reported outcomes in patients undergoing surgery for ASD has been examined by the International Spine Study Group.[129] Their retrospective processed active database of patients with ASD who are surgically treated included 2-year follow-up on 241 patients. This study reported that obese patients had higher overall major complications and wound infections. Obesity did not increase the number of minor complications, radiographic complications, neurologic complications, or the need for revision surgery. Despite these increased major complications, obese patients also benefited from surgical intervention; however, their HRQOL is less than that of nonobese patients.

The use of bone morphogenetic protein (BMP)-2 in ASD surgery has been investigated, most recently by a multicenter prospective study by Bess et al.[130] They reviewed a total of 279 patients, with a mean follow-up of 28.8 months. The BMP group had similar age, smoking history, previous spine surgery, total spinal levels fused, estimated blood loss, and duration of hospital stay as the no-BMP group. The BMP group had greater comorbidity, greater scoliosis, longer operative times, osteotomies per patient, and greater percentage of anterior/posterior surgery. The BMP group had more complications per patient and more minor complications per patient than the non-BMP group. The non-BMP group had more complications requiring surgery per patient than the BMP group. Major, neurologic, wound, and infectious complications were similar for both groups. Their conclusion was that BMP use and location did not increase acute major, neurologic, or wound complications.

Summary

Adult scoliosis is characterized by malalignment in the sagittal and/or coronal planes and can present with pain and disability. Clinical evaluation involves a thorough history, a complete physical examination, and radiographic evaluation with a particular focus on overall balance. Nonoperative management is recommended for patients with mild, nonprogressive symptoms. However, the evidence of its efficacy is limited. Operative management seeks to restore spinal alignment, decompress neural elements as indicated, obtain a solid fusion, and to minimize complications. A variety of surgical approaches and techniques are available to achieve these goals. In well-selected patients, surgery yields excellent outcomes in terms of reduction in pain and disability.

Case Studies

Figs. 72.5 through 72.12 provide several case studies for reference.

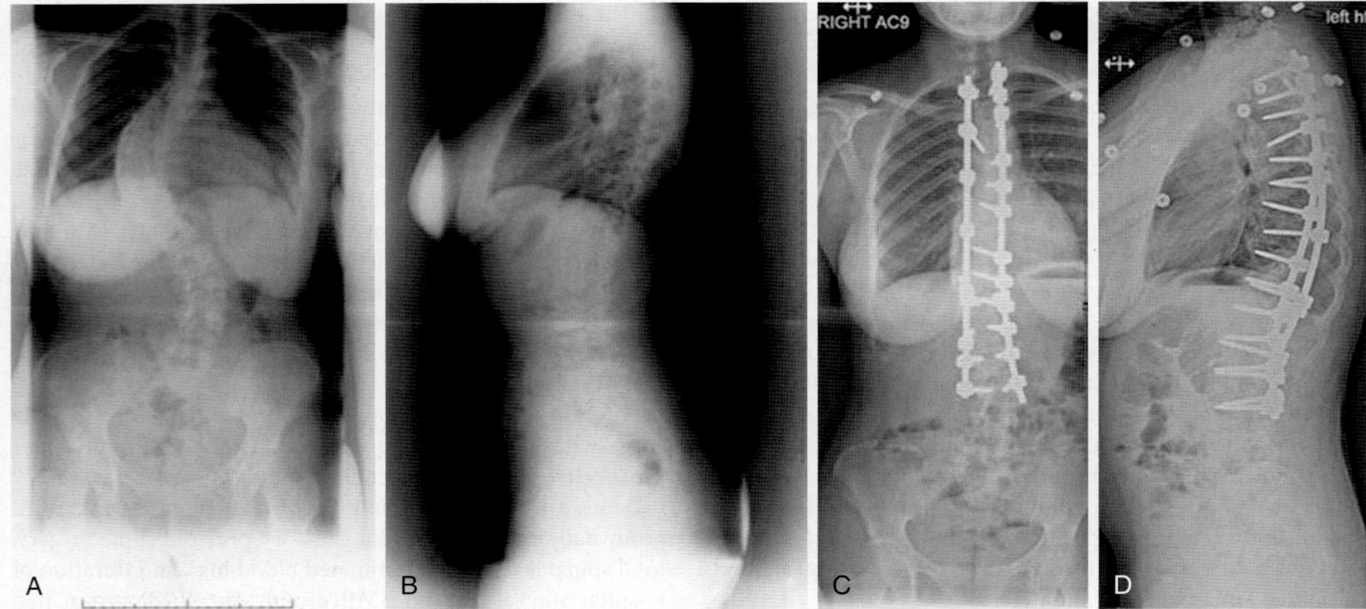

FIG. 72.5 (A–B) Radiographs of a 23-year-old woman with a history of untreated adolescent idiopathic scoliosis. (C–D) The patient underwent posterior spinal fusion of T2–L3 with instrumentation, autograft, and allograft.

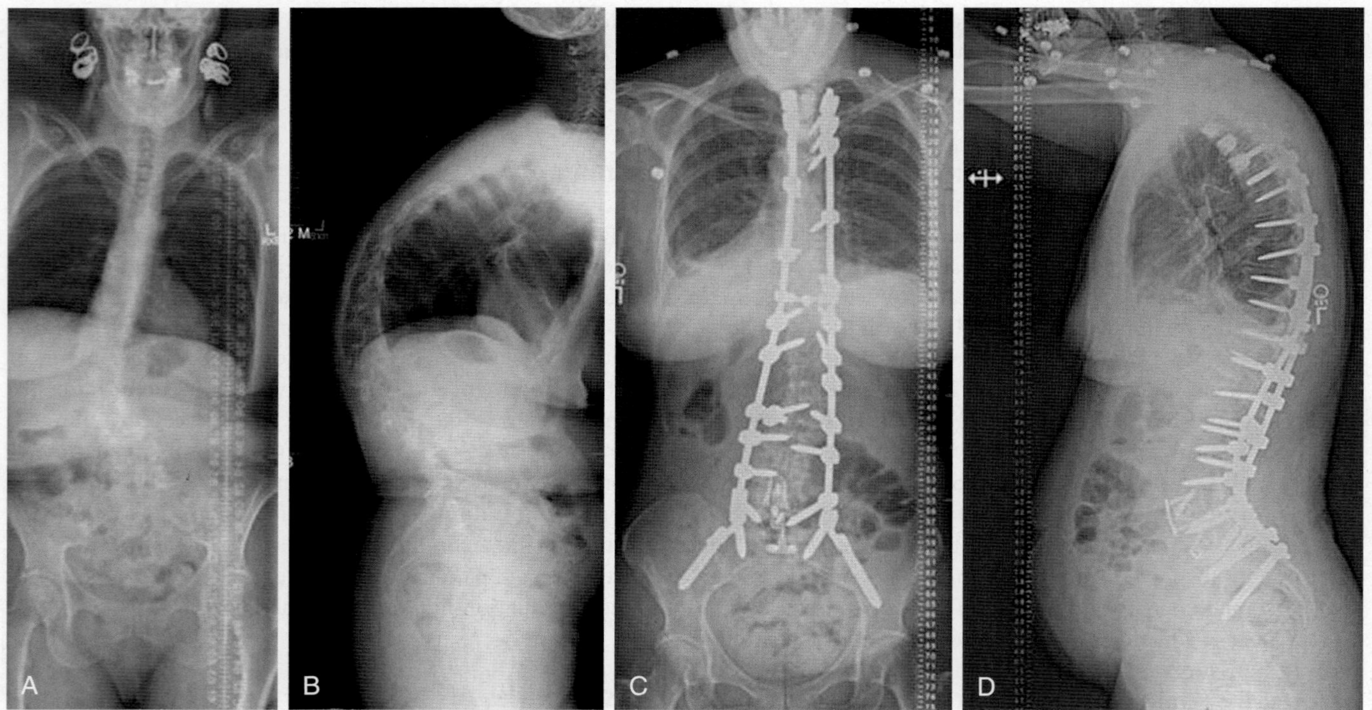

FIG. 72.6 (A–B) Radiographs of a 63-year-old woman with kyphoscoliosis who reported back pain and sagittal alignment issues. (C–D) The patient had an anterior lumbar interbody fusion done at L4–L5 and L5–S1, followed by posterior spinal fusion from T4 to pelvis done about 8 weeks later. At that time, she had Ponte osteotomies done from T9 to L3 to enhance the correction in the sagittal plane.

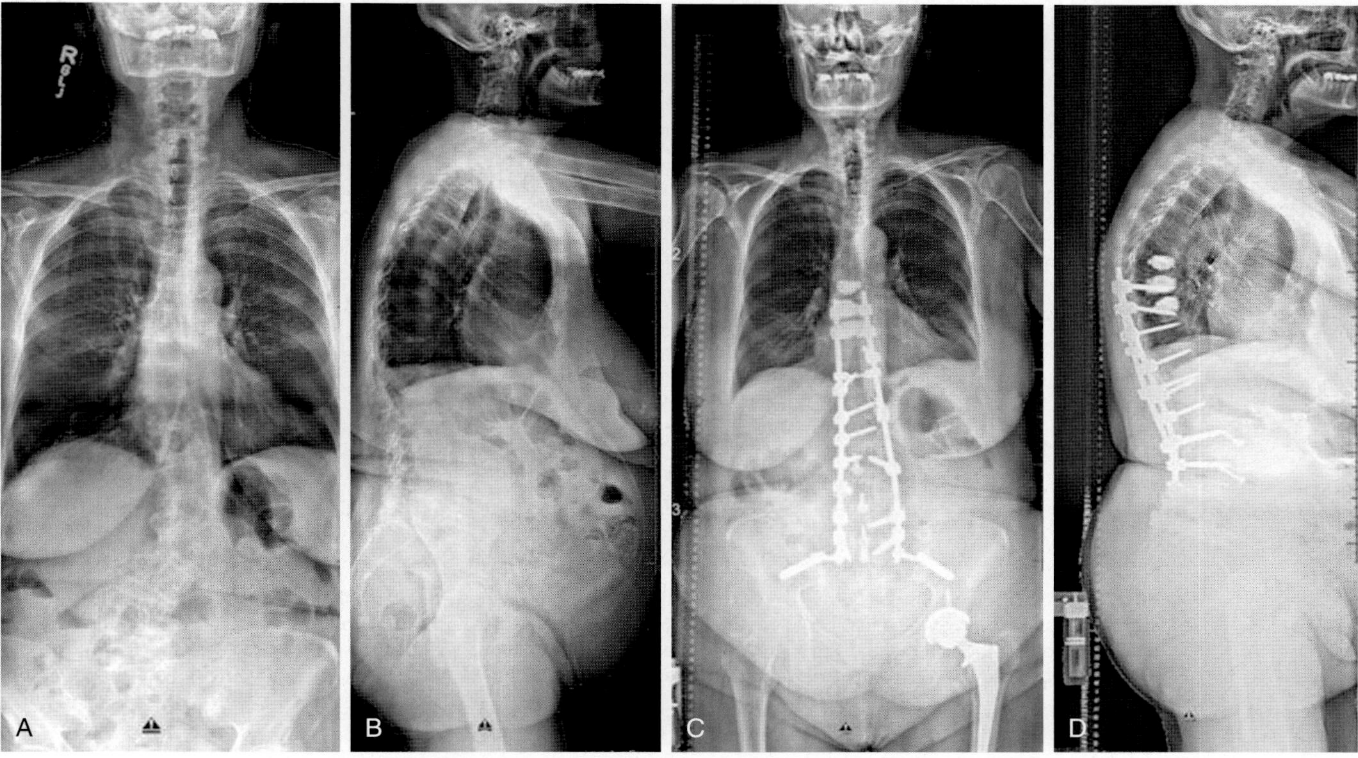

FIG. 72.7 (A–B) Radiographs of a 79-year-old woman with back and leg pain. The patient had an anterior/posterior procedure done at the same setting. (C–D) Anteriorly, she had an anterior lumbar interbody fusion at L3–L4, L4–L5, and L5–S1. Posteriorly, she had a posterior spinal fusion from T9 to S1, with laminectomies at L3–L4 and L4–L5 2/2 lumbar stenosis. Preoperatively, she had vertebroplasties done at three levels at the superior end of the construct, leaving the top level of vertebroplasty uninstrumented.

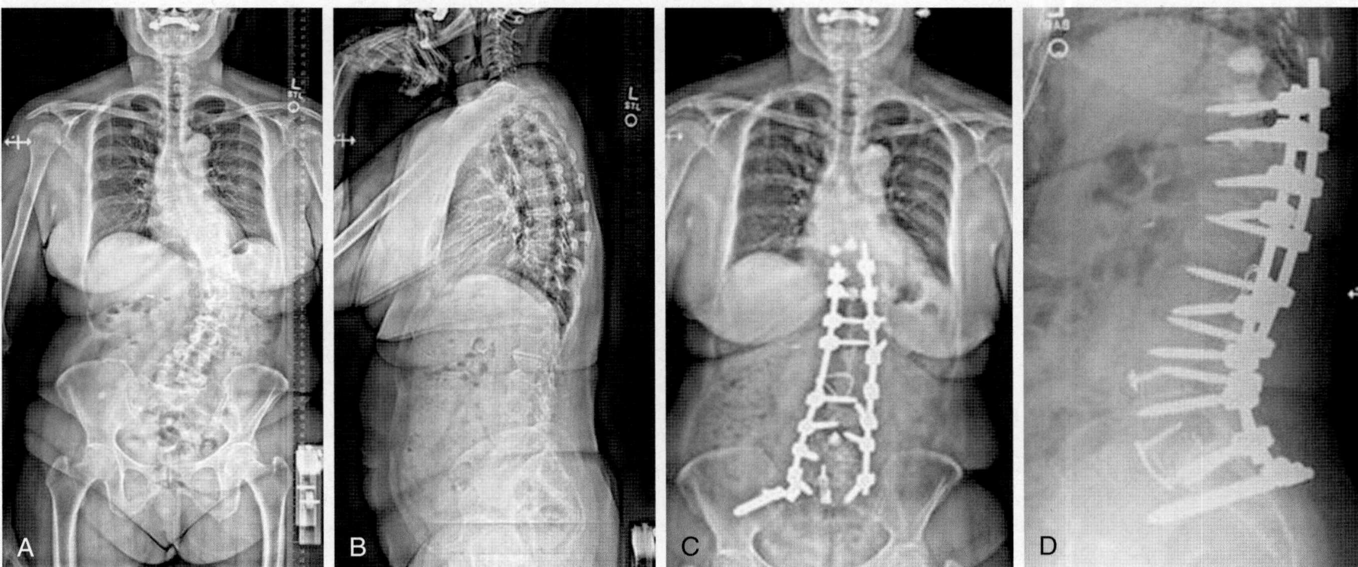

FIG. 72.8 (A–B) Radiographs of a 67-year-old woman who reported back and leg pain as well as issues with coronal imbalance. She had an anterior/posterior procedure done in the same setting. (C–D) She had an anterior lumbar interbody fusion at L4–L5 and L5–S1, followed by a posterior spinal fusion from T10 to pelvis, as well as laminectomies from L1 to L4. Preoperatively, she had vertebroplasties done at three levels at the superior end of the construct, leaving the top level of vertebroplasty uninstrumented.

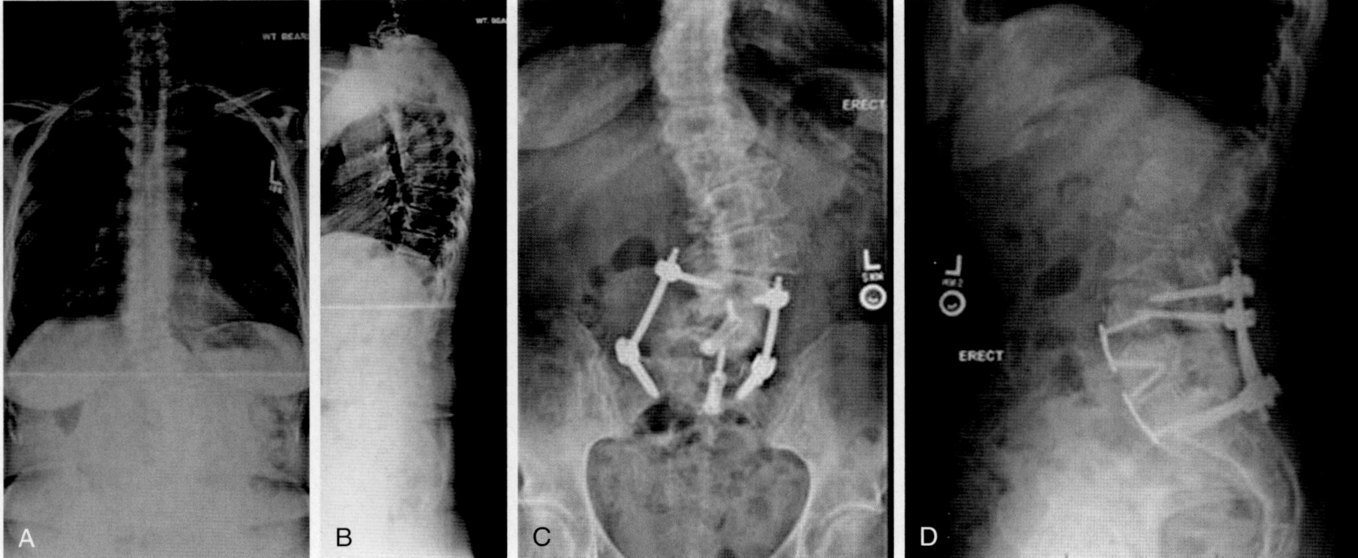

FIG. 72.9 (A–B) Radiographs of a 65-year-old woman with degenerative scoliosis who reported radicular symptoms associated with foraminal stenosis at the L4–L5 and L5–S1 levels. She had an anterior/posterior procedure done at the same setting. (C–D) Anteriorly, she had an anterior lumbar interbody fusion at L4–L5 and L5–S1. Posteriorly, she had percutaneous pedicle screw fixation from L4 to S1.

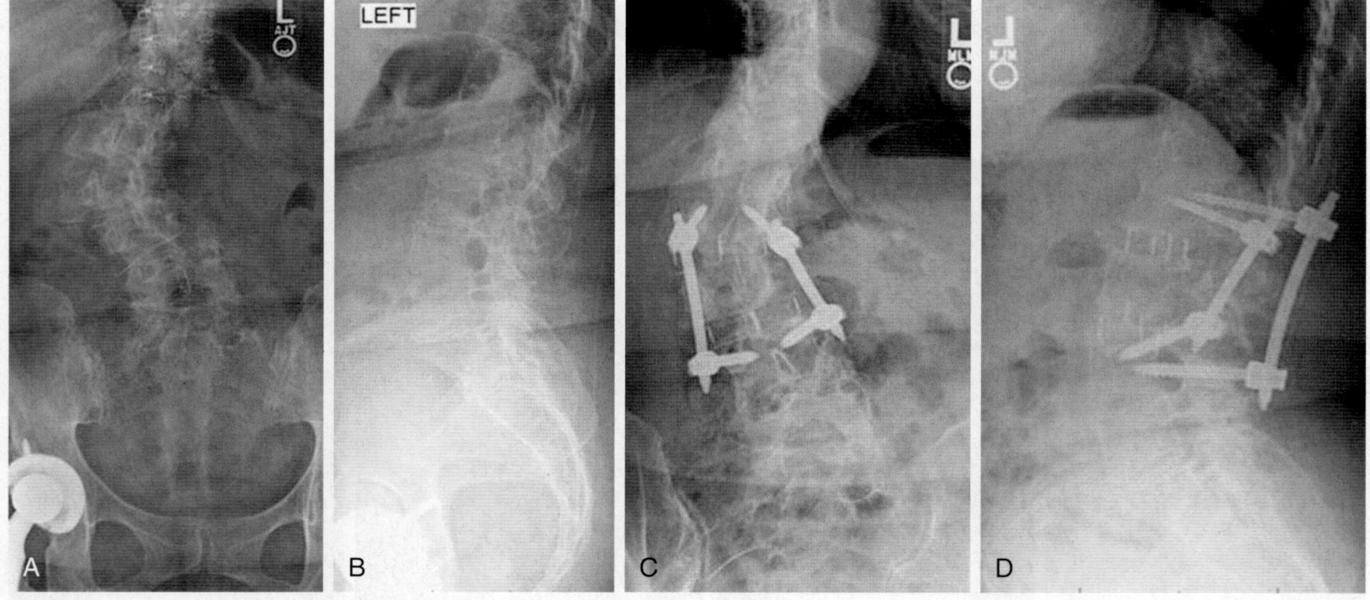

FIG. 72.10 (A–B) Radiographs of a 68-year-old woman with degenerative scoliosis who reported left lower extremity pain in the L2 and L3 distribution. She had minimal back pain and her symptoms improved in a recumbent position. (C–D) The patient had interbody cages placed at L2–L3 and L3–L4 via a direct lateral approach, followed by pedicle screws placed at L2 and L4 percutaneously.

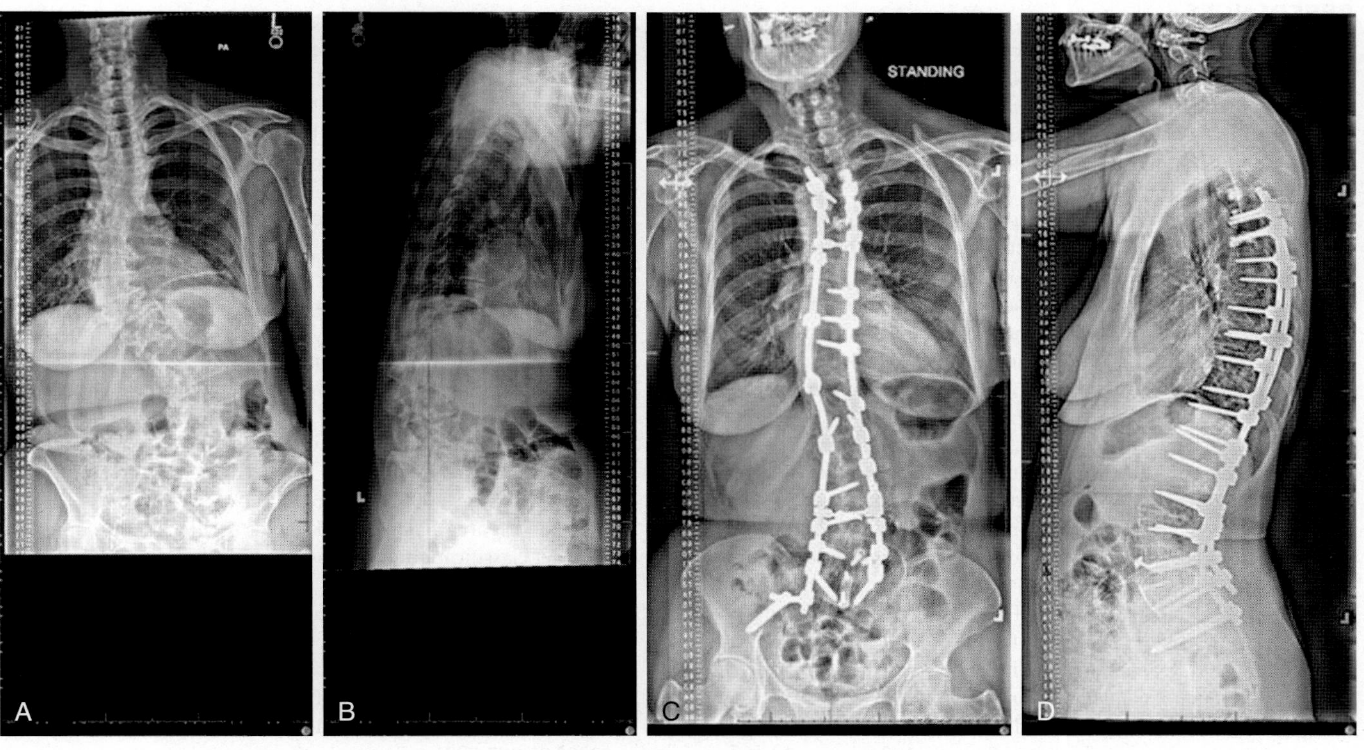

FIG. 72.11 (A–B) Radiographs of a 58-year-old woman with kyphoscoliosis who reported back pain and had sagittal alignment issues. (C–D) The patient had an anterior lumbar interbody fusion done at L4–L5 and L5–S1, followed by a posterior spinal fusion from T4 to pelvis done about 8 weeks later. She underwent preoperative vertebroplasties at the upper end of the construct.

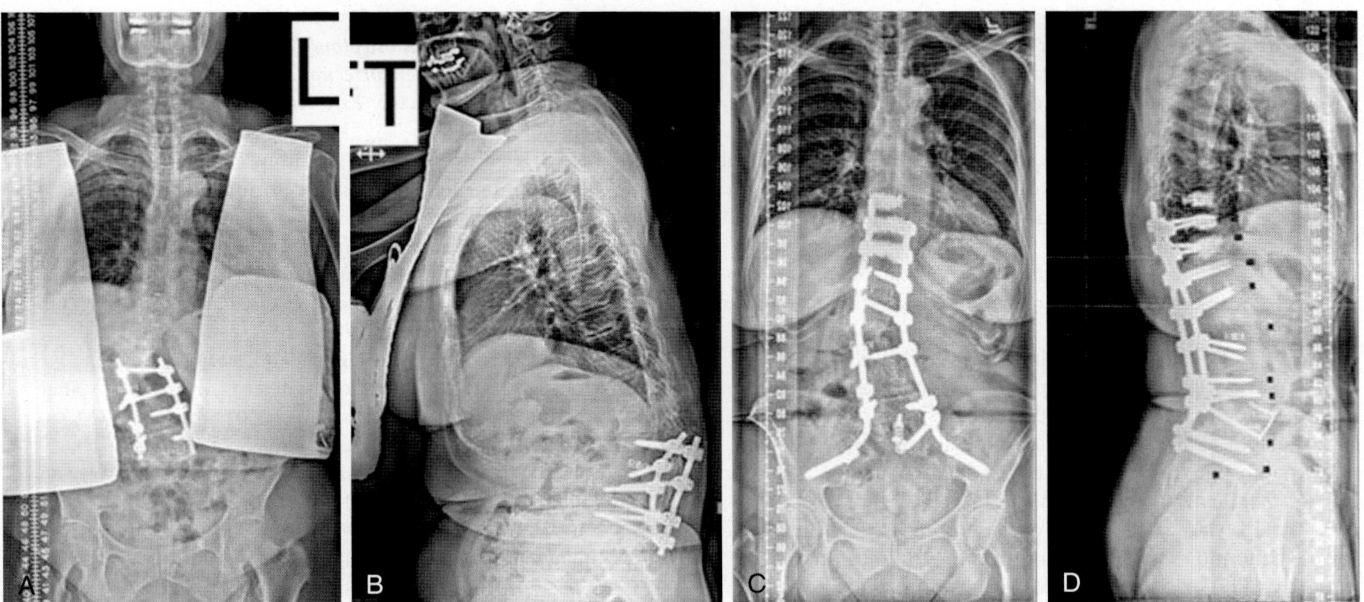

FIG. 72.12 (A–B) Radiographs of a 65-year-old woman with prior L2–L5 fusion who had worsening back and leg pain. She had lumbar lordosis/pelvic incidence mismatch. (C–D) The patient underwent an anterior lumbar interbody fusion at L5–S1 with a 30-degree spacer, anterior instrumentation, spinal implant removal at L3–L5, Smith-Petersen osteotomy at L5–S1, pedicle subtraction osteotomy at L2, transforaminal lumbar interbody fusion at T12–L1 and L1–L2, spinopelvic instrumentation with fixed iliac screws, revision instrumentation at T10–pelvis, and posterior spinal fusion at T10–L2 and L5–S1. She also underwent preoperative T9, T10, and T11 vertebroplasty.

REFERENCES

1. Carter O, Haynes S. Prevalence rates for scoliosis in US adults: results from the first National Health and Nutrition Examination Survey. *Int J Epidemiol.* 1987;16:537-544.
2. Pappou I, Girardi F, Sandhu H, et al. Discordantly high spinal bone mineral density values in patients with adult lumbar scoliosis. *Spine.* 2006;31:1614-1620.
3. Perennou D, Marcelli C, Herisson C, et al. Adult lumbar scoliosis: epidemiologic aspects in a low-back pain population. *Spine.* 1994;19:123-128.
4. Urratia J, Ledezma C, Espinosa J, et al. Lumbar scoliosis in postmenopausal women: Prevalence and relationship with bone density, age, and body mass index. *Spine.* 2011;36(9):737-740.
5. Robin G, Span Y, Steinberg R, et al. Scoliosis in the elderly: a follow-up study. *Spine.* 1982;7:335-359.
6. Schwab F, Dubey A, Gamez L, et al. Adult scoliosis: prevalence, SF-36, and nutritional parameters in an elderly volunteer population. *Spine.* 2005;30:1082-1085.
7. McCarthy I, Hostin R, O'brien M, et al. Analysis of the direct cost of surgery for four diagnostic categories of adult spinal deformity. *Spine J.* 2013;13:1843-1848.
8. Paulus M, Kalantar S, Radcliff K. Cost and value of spinal deformity surgery. *Spine.* 2014;39:388-393.
9. Gupta MC. Degenerative scoliosis: options for surgical management. *Orthop Clin North Am.* 2003;34:269-279.
10. Dubousset J. Weinstein SL, ed. *The Pediatric Spine: Principles and Practice.* New York: Raven Express; 1994.
11. Legaye J, Duval-Beaupere G, Hecquet J, et al. Pelvic Incidence: a fundamental pelvic parameter for three-dimensional regulation of spinal sagittal curves. *Eur Spine J.* 1998;7:99-103.
12. Gottfried ON, Daubs MD, Patel AA, Dailey AT, Brodke DS. Spinopelvic parameters in postfusion flatback deformity patients. *Spine J.* 2009;9:639-647.
13. Labelle H, Roussouly P, Chopin D, et al. Spinopelvic alignment after surgical correction for developmental spondylolisthesis. *Eur Spine J.* 2008;17:1170-1176.
14. Labelle H, Roussouly P, Berthonnaud E, et al. The importance of spino-pelvic balance in L5-S1 developmental spondylolisthesis: a review of the pertinent radiologic measurements. *Spine.* 2005;17:S27-S34.
15. Lafage V, Schwab F, Patel A, Hawkinson N, Farcy J. Pelvic tilt and truncal inclination: two key radiographic parameters in the setting of adults with spinal deformity. *Spine.* 2009;34: E599-E606.
16. Lafage V, et al. Standing balance and sagittal plane spinal deformity: analysis of spinopelvic and gravity line parameters. *Spine.* 2008;33:1572-1578.
17. Rajnics P, Templier A, Skalli W, Levaste F, Illes T. The importance of spinopelvic parameters in patients with lumbar disk lesions. *Int Orthop.* 2002;26:104-108.
18. Vidal J, Marnay T. Morphology and anteroposterior body equilibrium in spondylolisthesis L5-S1 [in French]. *Rev Chir Orthop Reparatrice Appar Mot.* 1983;69:17-28.
19. Vidal J, Marnay T. Saggital deviations of the spine, and trial classification as a function of the pelvic balance [in French]. *Rev Chir Orthop Reparatrice Appar Mot.* 1984;70:124-126.
20. Roussouly P, Berthonnaud E, Dimnet J. Geometrical and mechanical analysis of lumbar lordosis in an asymptomatic population: proposed classification [in French]. *Rev Chir Orthop Reparatrice Appar Mot.* 2003;89:632-639.
21. Ryan D, et al. T1 pelvic angle (TPA) effectively evaluates sagittal deformity and assesses radiographical surgical outcomes longitudinally. *Spine.* 2014;39(15):1203-1210.
22. Mac-Thiong JM, Berthonnaud E, Dimar J, et al. Sagittal alignment of the spine and pelvis during growth. *Spine.* 2004;29(15):1642-1647.
23. Boulay C, Tardieu C, Hecquet J, et al. Sagittal alignment of spine and pelvis regulated by pelvic incidence: standard values and prediction of lordosis. *Eur Spine J.* 2006;15(4): 415-422.
24. Schwab F, Lafage V, Patel A, et al. Sagittal plane considerations and the pelvis in the adult patient. *Spine.* 2009;34(17):1828-1833.
25. Klineberg E, Schwab F, Smith J, et al. Sagittal spinal pelvic alignment. *Neurosurg Clin N Am.* 2013;24:157-162.
26. Glassman SD, Bridwell K, Dimar JR, et al. The impact of positive sagittal balance in adult spinal deformity. *Spine.* 2005;30:2024-2029.
27. Glassman SD, Berven S, Bridwell K, et al. Correlation of radiographic parameters and clinical symptoms in adult scoliosis. *Spine.* 2005;30:682-688.
28. Schwab F, Farcy JP, Bridwell K, et al. A clinical impact classification of scoliosis in the adult. *Spine.* 2006;31:2109-2114.
29. Lazennec JY, Ramare S, Arafati N, et al. Sagittal alignment in lumbosacral fusion: relations between radiological parameters and pain. *Eur Spine J.* 2009;9:47-55.
30. Schwab F, Smith V, Biserni M, et al. Adult scoliosis: a quantitative radiographic and clinical analysis. *Spine.* 2002;27:387-392.
31. Schwab F, et al. Radiographical spinopelvic parameters and disability in the setting of adult spinal deformity. *Spine.* 2013;38(13):E803-E812.
32. Schwab F, Patel A, Ungar B, Farcy JP, Lafage V. Adult spinal deformity—postoperative standing imbalance: How much can you tolerate? An overview of key parameters in assessing alignment and planning corrective surgery. *Spine.* 2010;35(25):2224-2231.
33. Schwab F, Lafage V, Patel A, et al. *Does vertebral level of pedicle subtraction osteotomy correlate with degree of spinopelvic parameter correction.* Presented at the North American Spine Society 23rd Annual Meeting, Austin, TX, Sept 10-13, 2008.
34. Bess S, Schwab F, Lafage V, Shaffrey C, Ames C. Classifications for adult spinal deformity and use of the Scoliosis Research Society- Schwab adult spinal deformity classification. *Neurosurg Clin N Am.* 2013;24:185-193.
35. King H, Moe J, Bradford DS, et al. The selection of fusion levels in thoracic idiopathic scoliosis. *J Bone Joint Surg Am.* 1983;65:1302-1313.
36. Lenke L, Betz R, Harms J, et al. Adolescent idiopathic scoliosis: a new classification to determine extent of spinal arthrodesis. *J Bone Joint Surg Am.* 2001;83A:1169-1181.
37. Schwab F, Ungar B, Blondel B, et al. Scoliosis Research Society–Schwab adult spinal deformity classification: a validation study. *Spine.* 2012;37:1077-1082.
38. Liu Y, Liu Z, Zhu F, et al. Validation and reliability analysis of the new SRS-Schwab classification for adult spinal deformity. *Spine.* 2013;38(11):902-908.
39. Terran J, Lafage V, Shaffrey C, et al. The SRS-Schwab adult spinal deformity classification: assessment and clinical correlations based on a prospective operative and non-operative cohort. *Neurosurgery.* 2013;73(4):559-568.
40. Smith J, Klineberg E, Schwab F, et al. Change in classification grade by the SRS-Schwab ASD classification predicts impact on health related quality of life (HRQOL) measures:

prospective analysis of operative and nonoperative treatment. *Spine*. 2013;38(19):1663-1671.
41. Smith J, Shaffrey C, Berven S, et al. Operative vs. non-operative treatment of leg pain in adults with scoliosis: a retrospective review of a prospective multicenter database with two-year follow-up. *Spine*. 2009;34(16):1693-1698.
42. Smith J, Shaffrey C, Berven S, et al. Improvement of back pain with operative and non-operative treatment in adults with scoliosis. *Neurosurgery*. 2009;65(1):86-93.
43. Smith J, Shaffrey C, Berven S, et al. Risk-benefit assessment of surgery for adult scoliosis: an analysis based on patient age. *Spine*. 2011;36(10):817-824.
44. Kasilwal M, Smith J, Shaffrey C, et al. Does prior short-segment surgery for adult scoliosis impact perioperative complication rates and clinical outcome among patients undergoing scoliosis correction. *J Neurosurg Spine*. 2012;17(2): 128-133.
45. Smith J, Shaffrey C, Kai-Ming G, et al. Clinical and radiographic evaluation of the adult spinal deformity patient. *Neurosurg Clin N Am*. 2013;24:143-156.
46. Fu K-MG, Smith JS, Polly DW, et al. Correlation of higher preoperative American Society of Anesthesiology grade and increased morbidity and mortality rates in patients undergoing spine surgery. *J Neurosurg Spine*. 2011;14:470-474.
47. Adogwa O, Martin JR, Huang K, et al. Preoperative serum albumin level as a predictor of postoperative complication after spine fusion. *Spine*. 2014;39(18):1513-1519.
48. Yoshihara H, Yoneoka D. Trends in the utilization of blood transfusions in spinal fusion in the United States from 2000 to 2009. *Spine*. 2014;39:297-303.
49. Henry DA, et al. Anti-fibrinolytic use for minimising perioperative allogeneic blood transfusion. *Cochrane Database Syst Rev*. 2011;(3):CD001886.
50. May JH, et al. The assessment of blood loss during total knee arthroplasty when comparing intravenous vs intracapsular administration of tranexamic acid. *J Arthroplasty*. 2016;31(11):2452-2457.
51. Cheriyan T, et al. Efficacy of tranexamic acid on surgical bleeding in spine surgery: a meta-analysis. *Spine J*. 2015;15(4):752-761.
52. Winter SF, et al. Systemic and topical use of tranexamic acid in spinal surgery: a systematic review. *Global Spine J*. 2016;6(3):284-295.
53. Soroceanu A, et al. Effect of antifibrinolytic therapy on complications, thromboembolic events, blood product utilization, and fusion in adult spinal deformity surgery. *Spine*. 2016;41(14):E879-E886.
54. Ailon T, Smith J, Shaffrey C, et al. Degenerative spinal deformity. *Neurosurgery*. 2015;77(4):S75-S91.
55. Winter RB, Lonstein JE. Adult scoliosis. *Instr Course Lect*. 1983;32:170-191.
56. Fast A. Low back disorders: conservative management. *Arch Phys Med Rehabil*. 1988;69:880-891.
57. Cummins J, Lurie JD, Tosteson TD, et al. Descriptive epidemiology and prior healthcare utilization of patients in the Spine Patient Outcomes Research Trial (SPORT) three observational cohorts: disc herniation, spinal stenosis, and degenerative spondylolisthesis. *Spine*. 2006;31:806-814.
58. Bridwell KH, Glassman S, Horton W, et al. Does treatment (nonoperative and operative) improve the two-year quality of life in patients with adult symptomatic lumbar scoliosis: a prospective multicenter evidence-based medicine study. *Spine*. 2009;34:2171-2178.
59. van Dam BE. Nonoperative treatment of adult scoliosis. *Orthop Clin North Am*. 1988;19:347-351.
60. Smith JS, Shaffrey CI, Berven S, et al. Spinal Deformity Study Group: improvement of back pain with operative and nonoperative treatment in adults with scoliosis. *Neurosurgery*. 2009;65:86-93.
61. Glassman SD, Carreon LY, Shaffrey CI, et al. The costs and benefits of nonoperative management for adult scoliosis. *Spine*. 2010;35:578-582.
62. Liu S, Diebo B, Henry J, et al. The benefit of nonoperative treatment for adult spinal deformity: identifying predictors for reaching a minimal clinically important difference. *Spine J*. 2016;16(2):210-218.
63. Deyo RA, Mirza SK, Martin BI, et al. Trends, major medical complications, and charges associated with surgery for lumbar spinal stenosis in older adults. *JAMA*. 2010;303:1259-1265.
64. Albert TJ, Purtill J, Mesa J, et al. Health outcome assessment before and aft er adult deformity surgery. A prospective study. *Spine*. 1995;20:2002-2004.
65. Hu SS, Berven SH. Preparing the adult deformity patient for spinal surgery. *Spine*. 2006;31:S126-S131.
66. Warner MA, Offord KP, Warner ME, et al. Role of preoperative cessation of smoking and other factors in postoperative pulmonary complications: a blinded prospective study of coronary artery bypass patients. *Mayo Clin Proc*. 1989;64:609-616.
67. Miller JA, et al. Association between hemoglobin a1c and reoperation following spine surgery. *Neurosurgery*. 2016;63(suppl 1):193.
68. Hikata T, et al. High preoperative hemoglobin A1c is a risk factor for surgical site infection after posterior thoracic and lumbar spinal instrumentation surgery. *J Orthop Sci*. 2014;19(2):223-228.
69. Chen S, et al. Diabetes associated with increased surgical site infections in spinal arthrodesis. *Clin Orthop Relat Res*. 2009;467:1670-1673.
70. Huang W, et al. Risk factors for recurrent lumbar disc herniation: a systematic review and meta-analysis. *Medicine (Baltimore)*. 2016;95(2):e2378.
71. Birknes JK, Harrop JS, White AP, Albert TJ. Adult degenerative scoliosis: a review. *Neurosurgery*. 2008;63 (3 suppl):94-103.
72. Ailon T, Smith JS, Shaffrey CI, et al. Degenerative Spinal Deformity. *Neurosurgery*. 2015;77(suppl 4):S75-S91.
73. Sloan TB, Heyer EJ. Anesthesia for intraoperative neurophysiologic monitoring of the spinal cord. *J Clin Neurophysiol*. 2002;19:430-443.
74. Glassman SD, Shields CB, Linden RD, et al. Anesthetic effects on motor evoked potentials in dogs. *Spine*. 1993;18:1083-1089.
75. Uribe JS, Kolla J, Omar H, et al. Brachial plexus injury following spinal surgery. *J Neurosurg Spine*. 2010;13:552-558.
76. Elgafy H, Bransford RJ, McGuire RA, Dettori JR, Fischer D. Blood loss in major spine surgery: are there effective measures to decrease massive hemorrhage in major spine fusion surgery? *Spine*. 2010;35(9 suppl):S47-S56.
77. Bélisle S, Hardy JF. Hemorrhage and the use of blood products after adult cardiac operations: myths and realities. *Ann Thorac Surg*. 1996;62:1908-1917.
78. Liang J, Shen J, Chua S, et al. Does intraoperative cell salvage system effectively decrease the need for allogeneic transfusions in scoliotic patients undergoing posterior spinal fusion? A prospective randomized study. *Eur Spine J*. 2015;24(2):270-275.

79. Gause PR, Siska PA, Westrick ER, et al. Efficacy of intraoperative cell saver in decreasing postoperative blood transfusions in instrumented posterior lumbar fusion patients. *Spine*. 2008;33:571-575.
80. Reitman CA, Watters WC, Sassard WR. The Cell Saver in adult lumbar fusion surgery: a cost-benefit outcomes study. *Spine*. 2004;29:1580-1583.
81. Lenke LG, Betz RR, Haher TR, et al. Multisurgeon assessment of surgical decision-making in adolescent idiopathic scoliosis: curve classification, operative approach, and fusion levels. *Spine*. 2001;26:2347-2353.
82. Berven SH, Deviren V, Mitchell B, et al. Operative management of degenerative scoliosis: an evidence-based approach to surgical strategies based on clinical and radiographic outcomes. *Neurosurg Clin N Am*. 2007;18: 261-272.
83. Akbarnia BA, Ogilvie JW, Hammerberg KW. Debate: Degenerative scoliosis: to operate or not to operate. *Spine*. 2005;31(19 suppl):S195-S201.
84. Kelleher MO, Timlin M, Persaud O, Rampersaud YR. Success and failure of minimally invasive decompression for focal lumbar spinal stenosis in patients with and without deformity. *Spine*. 2010;35:E981-E987.
85. Birknes JK, White AP, Albert TJ, Shaffrey CI, Harrop JS. Adult degenerative scoliosis: a review. *Neurosurgery*. 2008;63:94-103.
86. Shufflebarger H, Suk SI, Mardjetko S. Debate: determining the upper instrumented vertebra in the management of adult degenerative scoliosis: stopping at T10 versus L1. *Spine*. 2006;31(19 suppl):S185-S194.
87. Kwon BK, Elgafy H, Keynan O, et al. Progressive junctional kyphosis at the caudal end of lumbar instrumented fusion: etiology, predictors, and treatment. *Spine*. 2006;31:1943-1951.
88. Kim HJ, Boachie-Adjei O, Shaffrey CI, et al. International Spine Study Group. Upper thoracic versus lower thoracic upper instrumented vertebrae endpoints have similar outcomes and complications in adult scoliosis. *Spine*. 2014;39: E795-E799.
89. Bernhardt M, Bridwell KH. Segmental analysis of the sagittal plane alignment of the normal thoracic and lumbar spines and thoracolumbar junction. *Spine*. 1989;14(7):717-721.
90. Eck KR, Bridwell KH, Ungacta FF, et al. Complications and results of long adult deformity fusions down to L4, L5, and the sacrum. *Spine*. 2001;26:E182-E192.
91. Edwards CC 2nd, Bridwell KH, Patel A, et al. Long adult deformity fusions to L5 and the sacrum. A matched cohort analysis. *Spine*. 2004;29:1996-2005.
92. Swamy G, Berven S, Bradford DS. The selection of L5 versus S1 in long fusions for adult idiopathic scoliosis. *Neurosurg Clin N Am*. 2007;18:281-288.
93. Edwards CC 2nd, Bridwell KH, Patel A, et al. Thoracolumbar deformity arthrodesis to L5 in adults: the fate of the L5-S1 disc. *Spine*. 2003;28:2122-2131.
94. Youssef JA, Orndorff DO, Patty CA, et al. Current status of adult spinal deformity. *Global Spine J*. 2013;3:51-62.
95. Kebaish K, Gunne APT, Mohamed A, et al. A new low profile sacro-pelvic fixation technique using S2 ALAR Iliac (S2AI) screws in adult deformity fusion to the sacrum: a prospective study with minimum 2-year follow-up. *Spine J*. 2009;9(suppl 10):56S-57S.
96. Dwyer AF, Newton NC, Sherwood AA. An anterior approach to scoliosis: a preliminary report. *Clin Orthop Relat Res*. 1969;62:192-202.
97. Smith JA, Deviren V, Berven S, Bradford DS. Does instrumented anterior scoliosis surgery lead to kyphosis, pseudarthrosis, or inadequate correction in adults? *Spine*. 2002;27:529-534.
98. Kim YJ, Bridwell KH, Lenke LG, et al. Pseudarthrosis in primary fusions for adult idiopathic scoliosis: incidence, risk factors, and outcome– analysis. *Spine*. 2005;30:468-474.
99. Bradford DS, Ahmed KB, Moe JH, et al. The surgical management of patients with Scheuermann's disease: a review of twenty-four cases managed by combined anterior and posterior spine fusion. *J Bone Joint Surg Am*. 1980;62:705-712.
100. Kostuik JP. Treatment of scoliosis in the adult thoracolumbar spine with special reference to fusion to the sacrum. *Orthop Clin North Am*. 1988;19:371-381.
101. Johnson JR, Holt RT. Combined use of anterior and posterior surgery for adult scoliosis. *Orthop Clin North Am*. 1988;19:361-370.
102. Berven S, Diveren V, Smith J, Hu S, Bradford D. Management of fixed sagittal plane deformity: outcome of combined anterior and posterior surgery. *Spine*. 2003;28:1710-1776.
103. Shapiro GS, Taira G, Boachie-Adjei O. Results of surgical treatment of adult idiopathic scoliosis with low back pain and spinal stenosis: a study of long-term clinical radiographic outcomes. *Spine*. 2003;28:358-363.
104. Lapp MA, Bridwell KH, Lenke LG, et al. Long-term complications in adult spinal deformity patients having combined surgery a comparison of primary to revision patients. *Spine*. 2001;26:973-983.
105. Kim YB, Lenke LG, Kim YJ, et al. The morbidity of an anterior thoracolumbar approach: adult spinal deformity patients with greater than five-year follow-up. *Spine*. 2009;34:822-826.
106. Anand N, Baron EM, et al. Minimally invasive multilevel percutaneous correction and fusion for adult lumbar degenerative scoliosis: a technique and feasibility study. *J Spinal Disord Tech*. 2008;21:459-467.
107. Pawar A, et al. Lateral lumbar interbody fusion. *Asian Spine J*. 2015;9(6).
108. Phan K, et al. Lateral lumbar interbody fusion for sagittal balance correction and spinal deformity. *J Clin Neurosci*. 2015;22(11):1714-1721.
109. Haque RM, Mundis GM, Ahmed Y. Comparison of radiographic results after minimally invasive, hybrid, and open surgery for adult spinal deformity: a multicenter study of 184 patients. *Neurosurg Focus*. 2014;36:E13.
110. Dorward IG, Lenke LG. Osteotomies in the posterior-only treatment of complex adult spinal deformity: a comparative review. *Neurosurg Focus*. 2010;28:E4.
111. Ames CP, Smith JS, Scheer JK, Bess S. Impact of spinopelvic alignment on decision making in deformity surgery in adults: a review. *J Neurosurg Spine*. 2012;16(6):547-564.
112. Lenke LG, Sides BA, Koester LA, et al. Vertebral column resection for the treatment of severe spinal deformity. *Clin Orthop Relat Res*. 2010;468:687-699.
113. Maeda T, Buchowski JM, Kim YJ, et al. Long adult spinal deformity fusion to the sacrum using rhBMP-2 versus autogenous iliac crest bone graft. *Spine*. 2009;34:2205-2212.
114. Kim Y, Lenke L, Kim Y, et al. Surgical treatment of adult scoliosis: is anterior apical release and fusion necessary for the lumbar curve? *Spine*. 2008;33:1125-1132.
115. Burton DC, Sama AA, Asher MA, et al. The treatment of large (>70 degrees) thoracic idiopathic scoliosis curves with posterior instrumentation and arthrodesis: when is anterior release indicated? *Spine*. 2005;30:1979-1984.

116. Suk SI, Kim JH, Cho KJ, et al. Is anterior release necessary in severe scoliosis treated by posterior segmental pedicle screw fixation? *Eur Spine J*. 2007;16:1359-1365.
117. Pateder DB, Kebaish KM, Cascio BM, et al. Posterior only versus combined anterior and posterior approaches to lumbar scoliosis in adults: a radiographic analysis. *Spine*. 2007;32:1551-1554.
118. Kim YJ, Bridwell KH, Lenke LG, et al. Pseudarthrosis in primary fusions for adult idiopathic scoliosis: incidence, risk factors, and outcome analysis. *Spine*. 2005;30:468-474.
119. Luhmann SJ, Bridwell KH, Cheng I, et al. Use of bone morphogenetic protein-2 for adult spinal deformity. *Spine*. 2005;30:S110-S117.
120. Mulconrey DS, Bridwell KH, Flynn J, et al. Bone morphogenetic protein (rhBMP-2) as a substitute for iliac crest bone graft in multi-level adult spinal deformity surgery: minimum two-year evaluation of fusion. *Spine*. 2008;33:2153-2159.
121. O'Neill KR, Lenke LG, Bridwell KH, et al. Factors associated with long-term patient-reported outcomes after three-column osteotomies. *Spine J*. 2015;15(11):2312-2318.
122. Sansur CA, Smith JS, Coe JD, et al. Scoliosis research society morbidity and mortality of adult scoliosis surgery. *Spine*. 2011;36(9):E593-E597.
123. Soroceanu A, Diebo BG, Burton D, et al. for the International Spine Study Group. Radiographical and implant-related complications in adult spinal deformity surgery: incidence, patient risk factors, and impact on health-related quality of life. *Spine*. 2015;40(18):1414-1421.
124. Helgeson MD, Shah SA, Newton PO, et al. Evaluation of proximal junctional kyphosis in adolescent idiopathic scoliosis following pedicle screw, hook, or hybrid instrumentation. *Spine*. 2010;35(2):177-181.
125. Kebaish KM, Martin CT, O'Brien JR, LaMotta IE, Voros GD. Belkoff SM. Use of vertebroplasty to prevent proximal junctional fractures in adult deformity surgery: a biomechanical cadaveric study. *Spine J*. 2013;13(12):1897-1903.
126. Hart RA, Prendergast MA, Roberts WG, Nesbit GM, Barnwell SL. Proximal junctional acute collapse cranial to multi-level lumbar fusion: a cost analysis of prophylactic vertebral augmentation. *Spine J*. 2008;8(6):875-881.
127. Arlet V, Aebi M. Junctional spinal disorders in operated adult spinal deformities: present understanding and future perspectives. *Eur Spine J*. 2013;22(suppl 2):S276-S295.
128. Verla T, Adogwa O, Toche U, et al. Impact of increasing age on outcomes of spinal fusion in adult scoliosis. *World Neurosurg*. 2016;87:591-597.
129. Soroceanu A, Diebo BG, Burton D, et al. for the International Spine Study Group. Impact of obesity on complications, infection, and patient-reported outcomes in adult spinal deformity surgery. *J Neurosurg Spine*. 2015;1-9.
130. Bess S, Line BG, Lafage V, et al. for the International Spine Study Group ISSG. Does recombinant human bone morphogenetic protein-2 use in adult spinal deformity increase complications and are complications associated with location of rhBMP-2 use? A prospective, multicenter study of 279 consecutive patients. *Spine*. 2014;39(3):233-242.

SECTION X

CHAPTER 73

Fixed Sagittal Imbalance

Evan J. Smith
Christine Piper
Joseph R. O'Brien

Introduction

Fixed sagittal imbalance refers to the condition in which there is a loss of global spine alignment and an inability to compensate for it through flexibility in the lumbar or thoracic spine. This condition eventually leads to a pitched-forward posture for the patient. The etiology of fixed sagittal imbalance can be diverse, resulting from both natural disease processes, such as ankylosing spondylitis (Fig. 73.1), and iatrogenically after spinal surgery (Fig. 73.2). Fixed imbalance often leads to diminished quality of life and significant patient distress. Patients may experience pain, difficulty with horizontal gaze, difficulty with ambulation, and poor endurance as a result of altered kinematics. Compensation may occur through the hips and knees (increased pelvic tilt), which is a high-energy state leading to rapid fatigue. Treatment of symptomatic sagittal imbalance has traditionally relied on correction of the deformity through spinal osteotomy. Spinal osteotomy may be performed posteriorly or anteriorly; modern spinal fixation is a crucial element of these surgeries.

Etiology

Sagittal imbalance, also known as "flatback syndrome," has a variety of etiologies. The most common presentation is the elderly patient presenting with degenerative imbalance in the setting of previous spine surgery, including lumbar fusion(s). The use of Harrington distraction instrumentation to treat scoliosis deformity in the 1970s to 1980s is often regarded as the main iatrogenic cause of fixed imbalance.[1–4] This surgery involved implanting straight distraction rods posteriorly into the spine, thereby disrupting the normal sagittal curves. When this instrumentation involved the thoracolumbar junction, patients were often left with a proximal lumbar hyperlordosis; the patient would then compensate for this with the remaining lumbar discs.[1-4] Over time and with degeneration, however, the ability to compensate for this imbalance is lost, and deformity ensues (see Fig. 73.2). After prior fusion, there is a progression of degeneration at adjacent levels. The patient progressively loses lumbar lordosis (LL) or increases thoracic kyphosis, making it difficult to stand fully erect.[1] Last, some authors have implicated anterior decompression instrumentation when used with an interbody graft as well as posterior lumbar fusion without structural grafting as a potential cause of sagittal imbalance.[5]

Spinal trauma can also lead to fixed deformity. Any fracture along the length of the spinal column may contribute, but especially those near the thoracolumbar junction can result in a kyphotic deformity, causing pain and loss of natural sagittal curvature.[6] The most commonly encountered example of this would be a compression fracture (Fig. 73.3). Increased stress is then applied to the adjacent segments and their associated discs, transferring load and stress that the fractured level cannot support.

Last, inflammatory and rheumatologic conditions are an often-cited source of sagittal imbalance. Ankylosing spondylitis is a frequently discussed cause of fixed sagittal imbalance. This disease results in a stiffness that allows for little variation in balance before deformity occurs. LL is often greatly decreased in these patients, frequently resulting in a concomitant increase in thoracic and/or cervical kyphosis[7] (see Fig. 73.1). Other disorders leading to flatback deformity include postinfectious kyphosis and congenital kyphosis or scoliosis, the latter being caused by a failure in formation of either the anterior/lateral segments or vertebral segmentation.[8]

Evaluation

The assessment of a patient with sagittal imbalance goes beyond just looking at the spinal deformity—a thorough history is paramount. Patients may present with a variety of symptoms; it is important to understand the etiology of these symptoms. Patients may present with focal back pain around the deformity or neurologic symptoms extending into the lower extremities, suggestive of concomitant stenosis or nerve compression. These patients may require a concurrent revision decompression at the time of corrective surgery, or they may have had previous spine surgeries that will affect future procedures. Others may present with little pain but have significant fatigue, poor endurance, difficulty with horizontal gaze, and

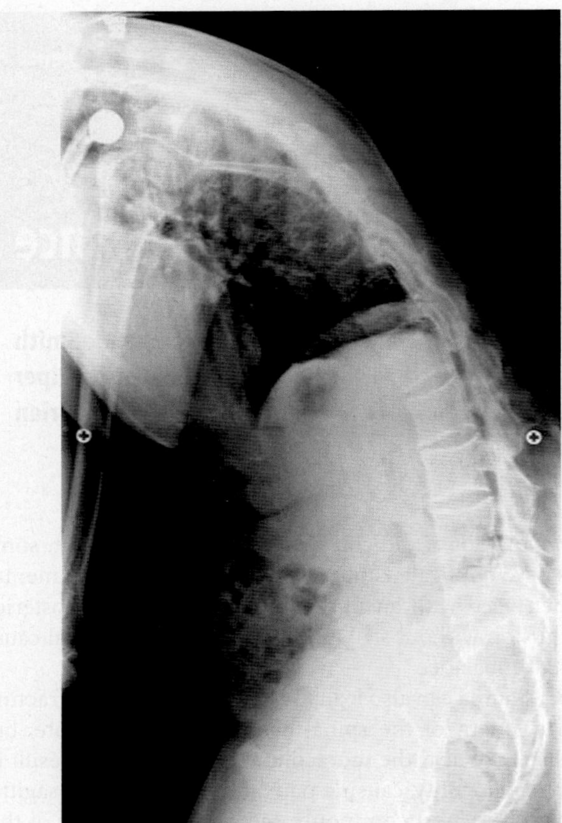

FIG. 73.1 Standing radiograph of a patient with ankylosing spondylitis showing severe loss of natural lordosis in the lumbar spine, leading to a rigid bent-forward posture. This patient also had cervical kyphosis, leading to further deformity and disability.

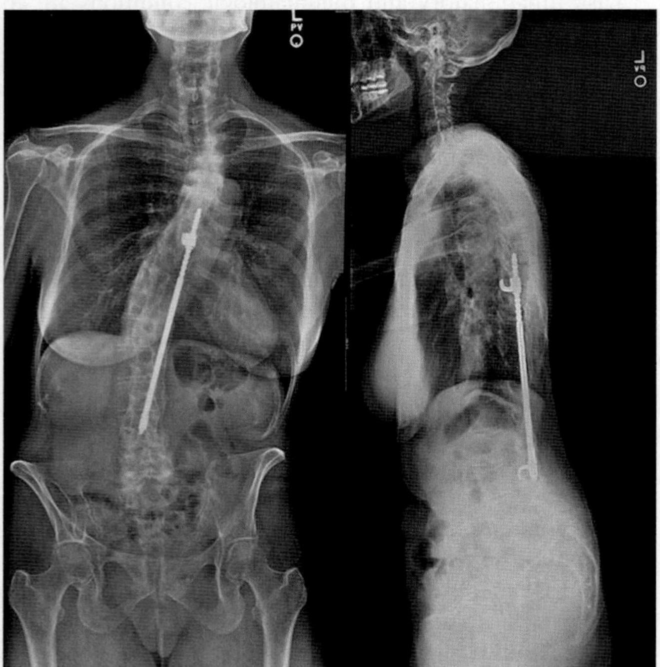

FIG. 73.2 Standing radiographs of a patient with Harrington rods implanted to treat adolescent scoliosis. The lateral image shows the loss of curvature at the thoracolumbar junction and the general loss of lumbar lordosis and sagittal balance as a result of the combination of the rigid rods and the natural degenerative changes that lead to loss of lumbar lordosis.

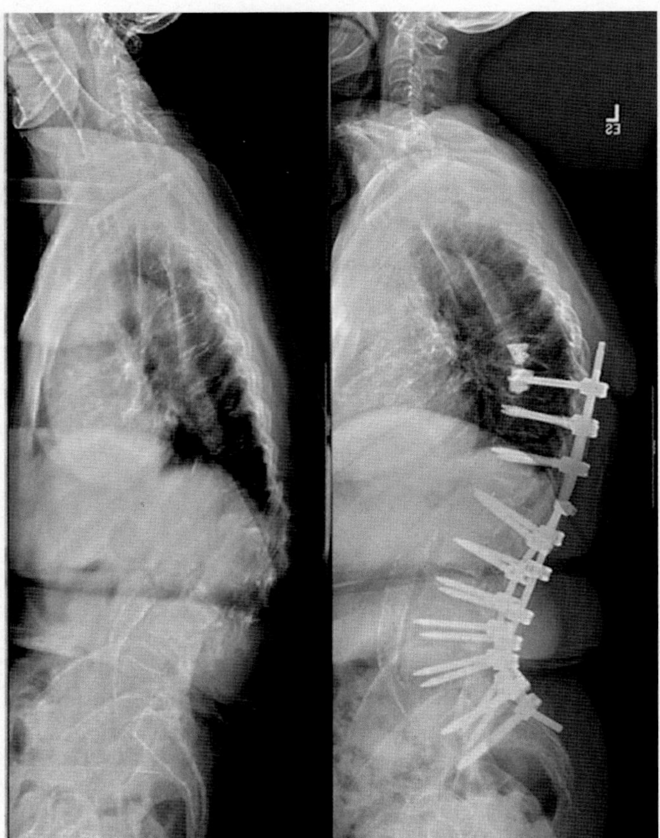

FIG. 73.3 Standing lateral radiographs of a patient who had compression fractures at the thoracolumbar levels, leading to significant fixed kyphosis. The patient underwent Smith-Petersen osteotomies at T9, T10, L1, L2, L3, and L4, as well as fusion from T9 to S1. The patient also underwent laminectomy at T12–L1, three-column osteotomy at T12, and vertebroplasty augmentation at T8 and T9.

an inability to perform activities of daily living. It is important to ask about comorbidities in this older population. The effect of osteoporosis, diabetes, congestive heart failure, and chronic obstructive pulmonary disease on the postoperative course should be discussed prior to surgery to establish realistic expectations and understand the significant risks of surgery. The enthusiasm for a technically well-executed surgery must be tempered with the risk of death and disability.

On physical examination, it is important to perform a thorough neurologic exam in addition to an assessment of balance and gait. One must observe the patient with and without assistive devices, such as canes or walkers. As mentioned previously, there are multiple mechanisms to compensate for sagittal imbalance. A patient may be able to maintain an upright posture (i.e., keeping the pelvis under the spine) by extending the hips and flexing at the knees. Because of this compensation mechanism, the examiner should ask the patient to stand erect with the knees straight to truly visualize the patient's posture. Additionally, the examination should be done sitting and supine to isolate the deformity and to assess flexibility of the deformity. A neurologic exam should be done to confirm any nerve compression resulting in sensory or motor deficit. If the deformity is in spinal cord territory (generally above L1), one should pay particular attention to reflex and pathologic reflex testing.

Radiographic Assessment

Understanding the normal variation in spine alignment allows an individualized appraisal of spinal deformity and the potential for correction in a patient with symptomatic sagittal imbalance. However, many of the radiographic measures have large ranges of normal values; therefore, it can be difficult to reach conclusions about sagittal balance from these measures in isolation. Instead, one must assess these measures in relation to each other. The treating surgeon must understand the idea of spinopelvic harmony, which refers to the interaction of these myriad radiographic measures to assess a patient's pathology. Initial imaging should include standing long cassette radiographs (36 inches) to assess global alignment and to establish the sagittal vertical axis (SVA), as well as regional imaging of the thoracic and lumbar spine and imaging of the pelvis and sacrum to assess thoracic kyphosis (TK) and LL, as well as sacral parameters pelvic incidence (PI), pelvic tilt (PT), and sacral slope (SS), respectively (Fig. 73.4). Flexibility of the deformity can be assessed by comparing standing and supine radiographs. Often, computed tomography (CT) is utilized to assess partial or complete fusion of the spinal deformity. Additionally, magnetic resonance imaging (MRI) is crucial for assessment of neural, vascular, and ligamentous anatomy.

The SVA is the most often cited method to assess sagittal balance. The measurement can be achieved on a standing sagittal cassette of the spine by extending a vertical line from the vertebral body of C7 and measuring its relationship to the vertebral body at S1. In patients with normal sagittal balance, this line should lie within the vertebral body at S1. Negative values indicate an SVA behind the posterior superior edge of S1, while positive values indicate anterior location. Normal ranges for this parameter have varied depending on which study is cited. In a series on asymptomatic patients, Jackson reported that SVA offset greater than 2.5 cm was beyond the normal range. However, generally, a value greater than 5 cm anterior is considered detrimental to quality of life[9] (Table 73.1). It is important to note that SVA has been found to vary with age, with recent studies showing that SVA moves anteriorly as a result of degenerative changes, resulting in loss of LL.[10] Clinically, SVA has shown the strongest correlation with quality-of-life measures.[11]

Regional curvature is also helpful in understanding patient-specific deformity. The normal range of LL varies between studies, and like many of the radiographic measures of the spine, there appears to be a wide range of normal values. Bernhardt and Bridwell found a range of LL of −14 to −69 degrees (standard deviation, ±12 degrees) in a series of 102 asymptomatic adolescent patients.[12] In a series on 100 healthy French volunteers, Stagnara et al. found values ranging from −32 to −84, with an average of −50 degrees of LL.[13] Jackson compared asymptomatic and symptomatic patients, noting a statistical difference in the amount of LL from 60.9 to 56.3, respectively.[9]

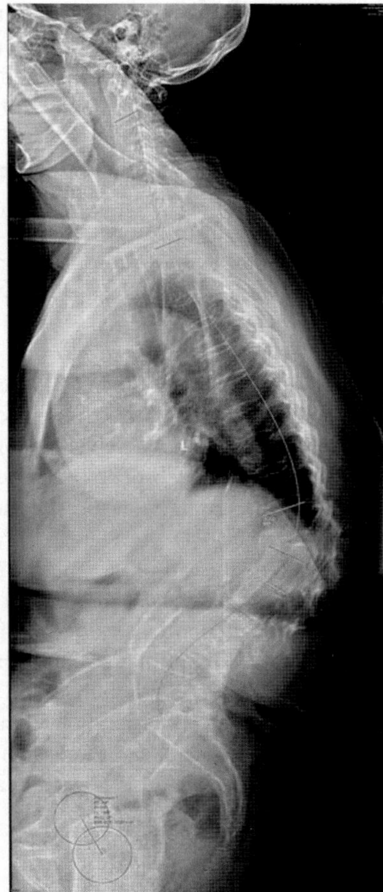

FIG. 73.4 Standing lateral radiograph of a patient with a significant fixed kyphotic deformity to the thoracolumbar spine who presented with fatigue, pain, and neurologic symptoms. Radiographic analysis of the sagittal curves found a normal sagittal vertical axis of 1.7 cm, a lumbar lordosis of −48 degrees, and a pelvic incidence of 50 degrees but a pelvic tilt of 29 degrees, suggesting some compensatory posturing in the pelvis.

TABLE 73.1 Radiographic Measurements to Assess Curvature in the Sagittal Plane*

Parameter	Balanced Value
SVA	<5 cm
Cervical SVA	<1.5 cm
T1 tilt	<13 degrees
Pelvic tilt	<25 degrees
Proportional balance	Lumbar lordosis = pelvic incidence ± 9 degrees
Proportional balance	Pelvic incidence + lumbar lordosis + thoracic kyphosis ≤45 degrees

*Based on review of the current literature.
SVA, sagittal vertebral axis.

Pelvic incidence has emerged as an objective measure to better understand ideal LL. Roussouly et al. studied 160 healthy volunteers, demonstrating that the variability seen in LL in normal patients may be the result of natural variations in PI.[14] PI is defined as the angle between a line drawn perpendicular to the surface of the superior endplate of the sacrum and a line connecting the midpoint of the superior endplate of the sacrum to the center of the femoral head. Often, this angle is used preoperatively to define different pelvic morphologies and understand the ideal LL for a given morphotype.

Last, one can examine at the amount of TK present. TK is defined as the Cobb angle between T1 and T12. These values have been found to range from about 20 to 70 degrees in normal individuals.[14] As with other radiographic parameters, there is a large range of normal values. Ideally, TK values compensate for LL to maintain a normal SVA.

Compensatory mechanisms can develop to maintain a normal SVA despite significant disability. As the spine moves forward with rigid spinal deformity, there is an increased onus on the musculature of the hips and pelvis to compensate to maintain vertical alignment. Much of this compensation can be identified through radiographic measures of the pelvis. The often-studied angles include PT, PI (Fig. 73.5), and SS. The measures are interrelated; the simple formula PI = PT + SS describes their relationship. However, in contrast to the fixed PI, SS and PT are posture-dependent values. SS is defined as the angle between the superior endplate of the sacrum and the horizontal. PT is defined as the angle between a vertical line and a line from the midpoint of the sacral plate and the center of the femoral head. An individual can increase his or her PT to compensate for a rigid deformity by increasing pelvic retroversion, hip hyperextension, and knee flexion, centering the spine over the pelvis and maintaining a normal SVA. These altered postural measures require increased energy for ambulation and limit effective ambulation. Furthermore, there is a positive correlation between PT values and worsening pain and disability scores.[15]

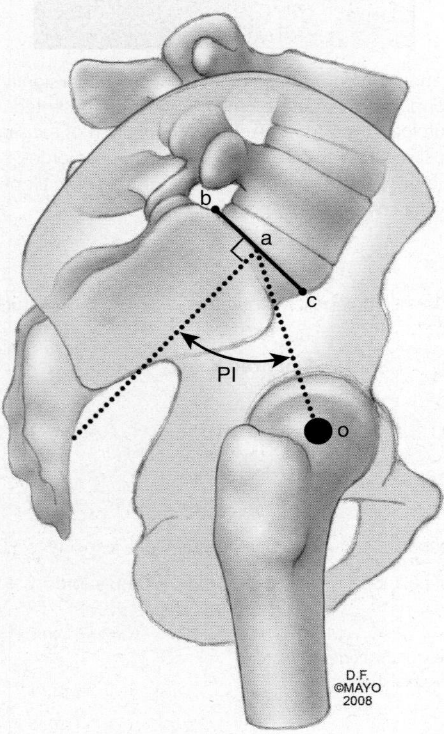

FIG. 73.5 Method of measuring pelvic incidence (PI). PI is the angle subtended by a line perpendicular from the cephalad endplate of S1 and a line connecting the center of the femoral head to the center of the cephalad endplate of S1. (From Rose PS, Bridwell KH, Lenke LG, et al. Role of pelvic incidence, thoracic kyphosis, and patient factors on sagittal plane correction following pedicle subtraction osteotomy. *Spine [Phila Pa 1976]*. 2009;34:785–791.)

Recent attention has focused on cervical sagittal alignment. The SVA of the cervical spine is measured from the centroid of the dens (C2) to the posterior superior corner of C7. Less than 1.5 cm is desired (see Table 73.1). Additionally, T1 tilt has been examined in cervical deformity. Because T1 is the foundation of the cervical spine, one may consider excessive TK as tantamount to a high pelvic incidence. In cases of cervical deformity, one may have to consider normalization of T1 tilt to correct the deformity and therefore extend surgery into the thoracic spine. In addition to cervical SVA and T1 tilt, the chin-brow angle is used to measure horizontal gaze and deformity in fixed cervical or cervicothoracic deformity.

Surgical Management

The decision to pursue operative versus nonoperative treatment often depends on the severity of symptoms. In patients with mild symptoms or significant comorbidities, undertaking a large corrective procedure with significant morbidity may not be prudent. These individuals can benefit from physical therapy, occupational therapy, antiinflammatory medication, targeted injections for neurologic symptoms, and lifestyle modifications. However, patients with significant distress from debilitating symptoms may be better served by corrective surgery.

The goal of surgery is to restore normal spinal balance and alignment in the sagittal and coronal planes. The surgeon should aim to establish normal spinopelvic harmony. SVA has the strongest correlation with quality-of-life measures.[16] The surgeon should attempt to restore SVA to less than 5 cm.[16] However, one should also examine the PT and PI. Normalized PT (<25 degrees) is crucial for efficient ambulation. Last, the surgeon should assess the LL. The relationship between LL and PI is related to natural spinopelvic morphology. The surgeon must assess these values to establish patient-specific alignment. The formula LL = PI ± 9 degrees allows the surgeon a rough idea of the amount of LL to gain to match the normal patient's spinopelvic morphotype.[17] Rose et al. used TK in conjunction with PI and LL as preoperative measures to determine what amount of LL correction was necessary to provide adequate correction at 2 years in patients undergoing pedicle subtraction osteotomy (PSO).[17] They found that a value of PI + LL + TK less than or equal to 45 (where LL is a negative number) had a 91% specificity for predicting adequate correction at 2 years (see Table 73.1).

Surgical Technique

Open corrective procedures are the workhorse of rigid deformity surgery. These are extensile procedures that aim to

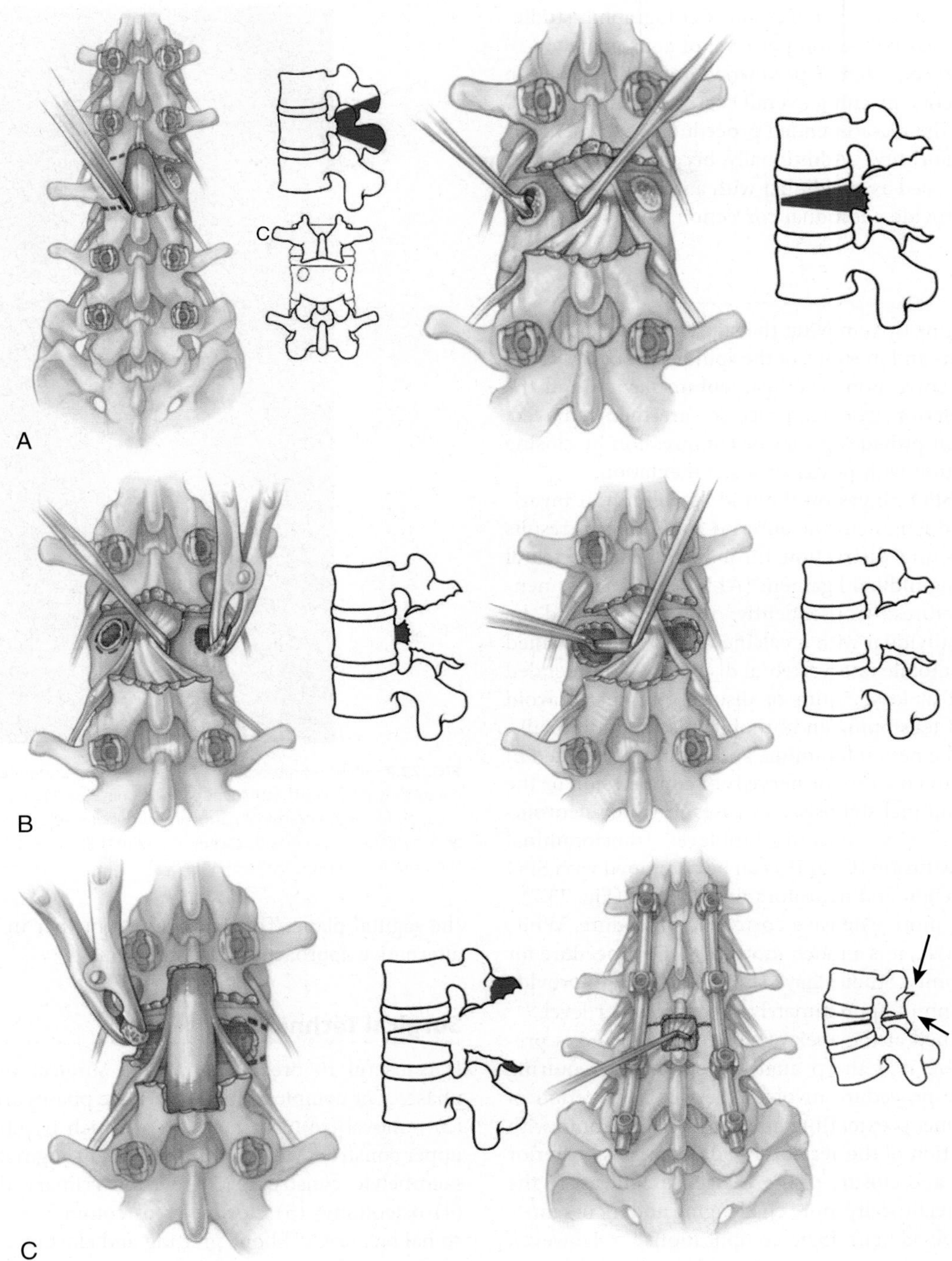

FIG. 73.6 Surgical technique for pedicle subtraction osteotomy. (A) *Left,* Initial resection of the posterior elements and surrounding pedicles. *Right,* Decancellation of the pedicles and the vertebral body. (B) *Left,* Resection of the pedicles flush to the posterior vertebral body. *Right,* Greensticking and resecting of the posterior vertebral cortex. (C) *Left,* Resection of the lateral walls. Note the V-shaped wedge. *Right,* Central canal enlargement. Closure of the osteotomy and final instrumentation. (From Bridwell KH, Lewis SJ, Rinella A, et al. Pedicle subtraction osteotomy for the treatment of fixed sagittal imbalance: Surgical technique. *J Bone Joint Surg Am* 2004;86A:44-50.)

correct deformity primarily by shortening the posterior column. These include the Smith-Petersen osteotomy (SPO), PSO, extensile PSO (Fig. 73.6), and the vertebral column resection (VCR). Invariably, greater correction is gained by removing increasing amounts of posterior bony and ligamentous tissue.

The SPO has evolved to be a corrective procedure for restoring small amounts of LL. The procedure was described in 1945 for the treatment of rigid deformity in ankylosing spondylitis and rheumatoid arthritis.[18] It involves the wedge resection of the posterior components without violation of the posterior longitudinal ligament or vertebral body with posterior closure by either gravity or posterior fixation. Radiographic studies have shown lordosis correction per level of approximately 10 to 15 degrees and can often be performed in multiple levels in appropriate patients, reaching overall correction as high as 40 degrees.[15,19] It is the recommended procedure when there is a long, smooth deformity.[20] Additionally, because of its relative ease, it has been used as an adjunct with anterior lengthening procedures to provide additional correction.

Technique

The surgeon begins by removing the supraspinous and interspinous ligaments and portions of the spinous processes at the desired level of correction. The ligamentum flavum and the superior and inferior articular processes are then removed. Next, the surgeon provides posterior compression by closing the wedge resection with posterior instrumentation.

Because the SPO hinges on the middle column, it invariably tensions and lengthens the anterior column. This results in anterior structure distraction through the intervertebral disc, anterior longitudinal ligament (ALL), and anterior neurovascular structures. Consequently, the SPO should be avoided in an individual with a calcified, rigid ALL, calcified vessels, or an immobile intervertebral disc. It is recommended that a height of at least 5 mm of disc be present to avoid complications of tensioning an immobile disc.[20] Additionally, the SPO closes the neural foramina, and should be avoided in an individual with concern for nerve root compression or the potential for foraminal stenosis.[20] In cases in which neuroforaminal stenosis is a concern, cantilever transforaminal lumbar interbody fusion (C-TLIF) can be combined with SPO to restore disc height and neuroforaminal height (Fig. 73.7).

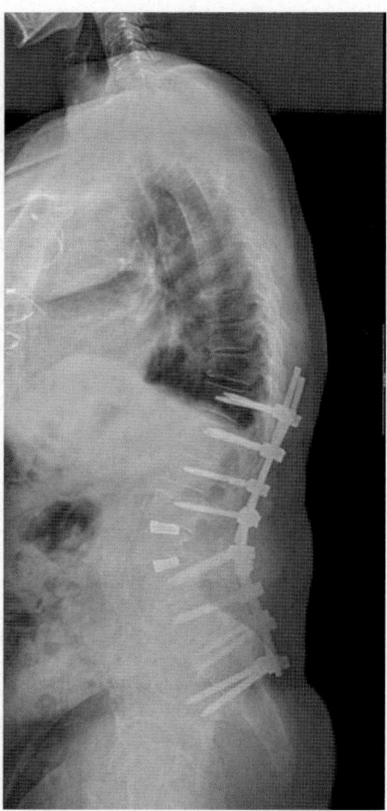

FIG. 73.7 Standing radiograph of a patient who underwent Smith-Petersen osteotomy (SPO) with cantilever transforaminal interbody fusion. There was concern for neuroforaminal narrowing preoperatively; the interbody cage allows distraction across the anterior and middle columns, as opposed to the normal compression seen after SPO.

The PSO is a more extensive corrective procedure. While incurring more risk, it is a much more versatile procedure for correcting deformity. Studies have shown the PSO to provide lordosis correction of approximately 30 degrees per level.[21,22] It is best performed at the apex of the deformity and is preferred when there is a sharp angle of deformity requiring correction.[20] The procedure involves the wedge resection of the posterior elements extending into the middle column with removal of a portion of the vertebral body as well as posterior instrumentation and closure of the wedge. In contrast to the SPO, the PSO is technically more challenging and incurs more blood loss, as well as neurologic complications.[19,23] However, the PSO does not tension the anterior column, and does not require the same considerations regarding flexible discs and calcified anterior ligaments and vessels (see Fig. 73.6).

Additionally, the PSO does not result in foraminal narrowing, and can be modified to provide coronal plane correction. This can be accomplished by performing asymmetrical resection of the posterior vertebral body. A greater amount of resection should be taken at the convexity of the deformity; this resection often extends into the vertebral discs above and below.[24]

Like the SPO, surgeons have begun to combine anterior and posterior procedures to increase the degree of correction. The combination of anterior ligament releases with interbody cages and posterior osteotomy has shown to improve correction in the sagittal plane. This is discussed further in the section on alternative approaches for correction.

Surgical Technique

It is useful to break down large surgical procedures into phases. For complex osteotomies, the phases are (1) exposure; (2) removal/(re)instrumentation, which is subdivided to the upper construct with or without cement augmentation and the sacropelvic construct; (3) revision/primary decompression; (4) osteotomy; (5) closure of osteotomy; (6) assessment of spinal balance; (7) bone grafting and closure; and (8) postoperative avoidance of complications.

Exposure

For exposure, it is crucial to limit blood loss. It is also important to keep the dissection close to the old laminectomy sites to facilitate revision decompression. Antifibrinolytic agents, such as tranexamic acid, have proved to be valuable in limiting blood loss in adult spinal deformity surgery.[24–26]

Removal/(Re)Instrumentation

For cases with removal of hardware, it is imperative to have the operative notes of the patient's former surgery and a list of what hardware is currently present. During (re)instrumentation, one may consider the upper construct and sacropelvic base separately. For lower thoracic stopping points (i.e., T10), we prefer to cement augment the upper screws and the uninstrumented level above. Such methods have been shown biomechanically and clinically to result in less proximal junctional kyphosis.[27,28] After the upper construct is built, the sacropelvic base is built. It has been our preference to utilize pelvic fixation in *all cases* and not choose L5 as a stopping point for lumbar osteotomies. S2AI screws are used preferentially, and show a lower unplanned revision rate as compared to iliac fixation.[29]

Revision/Primary Decompression

This step is often the most onerous phase. Primary decompression is performed as though one would be performing open TLIF two levels above and two levels below the osteotomy site. One seeks to skeletonize the pedicles, and visualize the nerve roots in the extraforaminal zone. Revision decompression can be difficult. It may be approached by doing the following. Identify the margin of the old laminectomy site. Generally, the pars will be present. If transforaminal interbody fusion (TLIF) has been performed previously, consider another level for osteotomy due to extensive anterior scarring. Karlin curettes can be utilized to mobilize above the pedicle, which is a safe neural zone in most cases.

Osteotomy and Closure

Surprisingly, this portion can be as easy as a TLIF once the proper preparation has been completed. A number of manufacturers have supplied osteotomy sets with specialized instruments to facilitate this phase. One should be sure that the exiting and traversing nerve roots are mobile, as is the thecal sac. It is our preference to isolate the pedicle prior to starting removal. This setup requires that the prior posterolateral fusion mass must be fractured and taken down first. The pedicle then is quartered with a 7-mm osteotome. The osteotome is sunk into the pedicle 1 cm and rotated to allow for a controlled fracture. The quarters are then removed. At this point, the pedicle should be flush with the posterior vertebral wall. Conical shavers and wedge paddle shavers are used to remove a wedge of bone. After bilateral pedicle removal, the posterior wall is removed with down-going tamps or a Woodson elevator in osteoporotic bone. A single rod is compressed to close the osteotomy. For cervical cases, the head is moved into lordosis. In cases of pancaking of the vertebra, the osteotomy is opened and a 10- to 20-mm TLIF cage is placed anteriorly in the vertebral body; the osteotomy may be closed over the cage.

Assessment of Spinal Balance and Bone Grafting

At this juncture, a lateral radiograph is taken to determine if the desired correction has been achieved. Instrumentation is visualized at each level to check for proper placement. Intraoperative CT scanning may be considered to check placement as well. The osteotomy site is a potential site for pseudarthrosis. One may consider the use of fusion accelerators, such as recombinant human bone morphogenetic protein, at the site or TLIF at the discs above and below. Lateral surgery and multiple rod use is also a consideration to decrease the incidence of pseudarthrosis at the osteotomy site.

Avoidance of Complications

As with all major blood loss surgeries, management is crucial to success.[30] Intraoperatively, the use of crystalloid should be limited to less than 4 L. Blood products and those that remain intravascular are to be utilized. Use of the intensive care unit should follow the patient's international normalized ratio (INR) and electrolyte levels. Calcium should be replenished. Postoperatively, anticoagulation may be started once the INR is below 1.2 and the platelets are above 100.[31] It is our preference to utilize enoxaparin (Lovenox) 40 mg once daily to avoid deep vein thrombosis. Studies examining postoperative epidural hematoma have shown risk factors to be the following: greater than five-level laminectomy, INR greater than 2.0 in the first 48 hours, and blood loss greater than 1 L. Anticoagulation was not shown to be a risk factor.[31]

Cervical/Cervicothoracic Posterior Osteotomies

While the PSO has a durable track record of providing correction in the lumbar spine, it is also being used to provide correction in the cervical spine outside the territory of the vertebral artery (generally <C6). Initially, attempts to correct rigid deformity in the cervical spine were seen only in patients with ankylosing spondylitis. The techniques used were similar to the SPO, involving removal of the posterior elements at C7 with controlled fracture of the anterior spine and closure of the wedge using a halo orthosis. This procedure has undergone some modifications, as described by Simmons in 1972 and later amended in 2006, including a more extensive bone resection and posterior instrumentation.[32] Recent publications on cervical PSO have shown strong correction potential with an average increase in cervical lordosis of 24 to 50 degrees with no intraoperative or postoperative neurologic complications and improvement in patient outcome measures.[33,34] However, the studies are limited by small patient groups. Reports of long-term outcomes are limited.

Surgical Technique

As with PSO, it is useful to divide the procedure into phases. The setup is quite important in cervical osteotomy cases. We have moved away from the Mayfield holder to a floating setup with traction (Fig. 73.8). This setup is also used for cranial settling cases.[35] For osteotomy closure, we change the traction vector to facilitate the head and neck position. Preoperative planning should consider T1 tilt prior to correction of neck position. For cases with extensive TK, the surgeon should consider extension of the distal aspect of the surgery to T6 or L1. Proximally, one needs to ensure pedicular fixation, and the revision nature of the surgery may limit fixation. Navigation

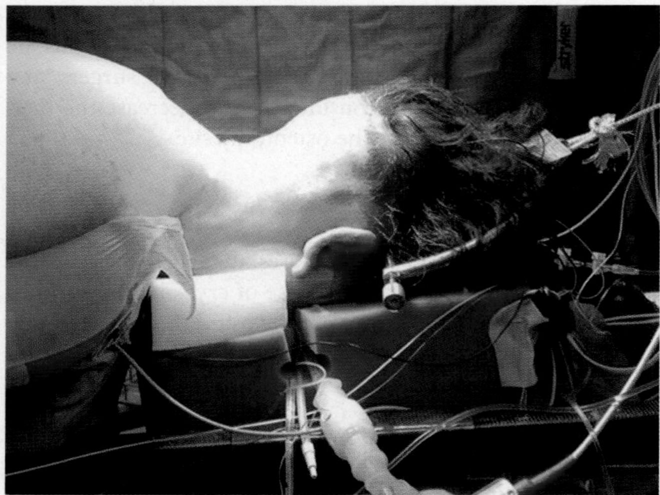

FIG. 73.8 The senior author (J.R.O.), when performing cervical osteotomy, uses the floating setup with traction as pictured.

has been used to safely place midcervical pedicle screws[36]; it is important to consider that one level of pedicle fixation is equivalent to two levels of cervical lateral mass fixation.[37] The C2 level is a reasonable stopping point. In cases of poor bone stock, we have utilized the occiput as a temporary fixation point without bone graft applied to the occipital-cervical junction. The rods may be cut at a later date or pseudarthrosis and rod fracture at the occiput may be expected. The surgeon begins by placing pedicle screws for fusion from the level of C2 to three levels below the osteotomy site: T3. If the patient had a large amount of TK, then the fusion can be extended lower to include the apex of the deformity. Osteotomies begin by removal of the facets and lateral masses at C6–C7 and C7–T1. The nerve roots are then identified and the C7 pedicles are isolated. Next, the pedicles are taken down and the posterior vertebral body is decancellated. The walls of the vertebral body are then removed and the neck is extended to close the osteotomy site. We prefer to use a traction setup to do so.[32]

Midcervical Osteotomy for Fixed Sagittal Imbalance

In some cases, midcervical osteotomy may be required. Generally, in the territory of the vertebral artery (C2–C6), anterior and posterior approaches are utilized. In this segment, our preferred technique will be outlined.

It is our preference to open the posterior portion of the neck only once. As such, our approach begins anteriorly. The anterior cervical spine is exposed broadly. The longus colli is striped laterally, as is done in typical anterior cervical discectomy and fusion. The center of the spine is found either with C-arm fluoroscopy or by placing Penfield dissectors laterally and marking the midline. Corpectomy is performed, as is standard. A width of 16 mm is utilized in all but the smallest-stature patients. The intraoperative use of a ruler from midline facilitates a straight corpectomy trough. After standard corpectomy and spinal decompression, the Penfield retractor is placed laterally around the vertebral body. A burr is then used to remove the lateral wall until the desired cut is obtained. At this point, a cage and plate are placed. If surgical planning does not include returning to the anterior neck, only cephalad screws are placed into the plate spanning the osteotomy site to allow for correction of kyphosis. The patient is then repositioned for posterior surgery. The neck is exposed and decompressed as needed. The fusion mass (if present) is cut and a Cobb elevator or wedge osteotome is placed into the neo-facet joint and twisted until fracture occurs. The neck can then be repositioned into lordosis. Instrumentation is performed as needed. Surgeons may then elect to perform anterior definitive fixation as needed.

Vertebral Column Resection

As the name implies, this procedure removes the posterior elements entirely and all but an anterior cortical shell of the vertebral body. Circumferential removal of the spinal column allows for powerful deformity correction, but is also the most technically demanding. Consideration for robust neuromonitoring must be made. Multimodal neuromonitoring is crucial, as is neurology input at the time of surgery. It is important to realize that both spinal decompression and realignment may impair the function of the spinal cord. As such, when changes in neuromonitoring occur, the context is very important—if a decline in signals occurs just after correction of the spinal alignment, one must reverse the maneuver.

VCR is best used where there is severe malalignment in the thoracolumbar spine, as opposed to focal rigid lumbar deformity. The lumbar deformity is more amenable to PSO. Examples of scenarios in which to use VCR include individuals with sharp, angular kyphosis in the thoracic spine or a severe thoracic or thoracolumbar kyphoscoliosis. During VCR, the surgeon performs complete resection of one or more vertebral levels either from a posterior or combined anteroposterior approach. This is a technically demanding procedure that should be performed by surgeons at centers experienced with deformity surgery. Using this technique, correction can be gained in both the coronal and sagittal plane by a combination of compression and translation of the column. The use of interbody cages and grafts is required, as the spinal column invariably shortens with vertebral body resection. Establishing fusion is critical given the degree of circumferential destabilization.[38]

Surgical Technique

As with pedicle subtraction osteotomy, it is useful to divide the procedure into phases. Once again, for complex osteotomies, the phases are (1) exposure; (2) removal/(re)instrumentation, which is subdivided to the upper construct with or without cement augmentation and the sacropelvic construct; (3) revision/primary decompression; (4) osteotomy; (5) closure of osteotomy; (6) assessment of spinal balance; (7) bone grafting and closure; and (8) postoperative avoidance of complications. See the earlier section to review the preparatory phases of surgery. Differences are highlighted later in this chapter.

The procedure is centered over the deformity and involves resection of the posterior elements. The adjacent-level laminae and facets are removed as well as the pedicles, vertebral body, and cephalad and caudal discs. Initial efforts to perform VCR may utilize a combined anterior and posterior approach—especially in the lumbar spine, where nerve root sacrifice is not routinely done. Anterior approaches, whether open or minimally invasive, focus on disc removal and mobilization of the great vessels. Alternatively, an osteotomy through the vertebral body in the coronal plane to leave an anterior cortical shell may be performed. A Silastic sheet may be implanted to help find the plane of the cut/mobilization. Posterior instrumentation allows manipulation in the sagittal and coronal planes before final correction. In the thoracic spine, the rib heads may be disarticulated to visualize the vertebral body.

Complication rates increase with the extent of surgery and complexity of the osteotomy. While open procedures have a strong history of providing correction, they may also impart significant morbidity to the patient: blood loss, neurologic complications and postoperative disability, posttraumatic stress disorder, and death.[19,20,39] The Scoliosis Research Society (SRS) in 2011 published results on patients with rigid deformity undergoing corrective surgery. They noted increasing complication rates from SPO (28.1%), to PSO (39.1%), to VCR (61.1%).[23] The complication rates observed in the VCR group were much higher than previously reported rates of 20% to 30%.[38,40] The complications included dural tears, neurologic deficits, deep wound infections, hematomas, pulmonary emboli, and malpositioned implants. Generally, the neurologic deficits were mostly nerve root injuries (82%), while the remaining were incomplete spinal cord injuries. Despite neuromonitoring, only 2 of 18 nerve root injuries were detected. Half of the patients with nerve root injuries had complete recovery, and half had partial recovery at 9 months. Naturally, surgeons have looked for less morbid alternatives to these procedures.

Minimally Invasive Surgery

Minimally invasive approaches to the spine have gained popularity over the last 2 decades. Much of this interest was bolstered by studies demonstrating less morbidity when compared to open posterior procedures.[41–43] These include anterior lumbar interbody fusion (ALIF), TLIF, lateral lumbar interbody fusion (LLIF), direct lateral interbody fusion (DLIF), and extreme lateral interbody fusion (XLIF). The improved complication rates are presumed to be the result of less tissue dissection. Invariably, this improved complication profile has inspired surgeons to apply minimally invasive techniques to treating spinal deformity. In contrast with posterior procedures, these techniques aim to perform primarily anterior elongation through placement of interbody cages and release of anterior restraints.

ALIF has been used with mixed results. Hsieh et al. found that ALIF was superior to TLIF at improving LL.[44] However, the improvement was minimal. This difference may be due to the ALL release required for anterior exposure. There are few studies looking at the stand-alone effect of ALIF on sagittal balance, as it is often combined with posterior osteotomies to provide circumferential correction. In contrast to other minimally invasive approaches, the ALIF procedure allows unimpeded access to the lowest lumbar levels. However, there are significant complications to this technique. These include neurologic complications from injury to hypogastric plexuses, resulting in sexual dysfunction, retrograde ejaculation, and bowel and bladder dysregulation. The most devastating complications include injury to the great vessels, which occur at rates from 1% to 24%.[45] Nevertheless, experienced practitioners have success when combining this approach with posterior osteotomies.[44]

More recently, there has been a progression to using LLIF (DLIF/XLIF) approaches for correcting the anterior column and placement of interbody cages. These approaches utilize a lateral retroperitoneal, transpsoas corridor to access the lateral vertebral body with minimal soft tissue dissection. When compared to ALIF, this approach avoids the need for an access surgeon, and avoids complications related to damage to the anterior neurovascular structures or abdominal or genitourinary viscera. Additionally, this approach avoids the complications frequently seen in posterior procedures: extensive muscle stripping and manipulation of the thecal sac. Preliminary reports have confirmed the lower complication profile when compared to traditional posterior procedures.[46] However, in a systematic review by Phan et al., there was weak and inconsistent correction in the sagittal plane using standard cages with these lateral techniques.[47] XLIF and DLIF have their own set of complications related to psoas muscle injury and genitofemoral nerve injury, including thigh pain, hip flexor weakness, and groin pain.

LLIF has also been used to improve sagittal plane correction. Uribe et al., in an initial cadaveric study, assessed the potential of 20-degree and 30-degree hyperlordotic cages to provide sagittal plane correction with positive results.[48] Subsequently, Marchi et al.[49] examined eight cases using a DLIF approach with 30-degree hyperlordotic cages on patients with sagittal imbalance. These authors noted markedly improved LL with average gains of 10 degrees per level, which was higher than that seen with standard XLIF.[49] They also noted an improvement in SVA from 24 to 9 cm. However, they noted an increase in anterior cage subsidence as well, particularly where there was a tight ALL, making cage placement difficult. As a follow-up, Deukmedjian et al. proposed a minimally invasive technique involving the release of the ALL to decrease tension on the anterior column.[50] Called anterior column release (ACR), this technique allows easier insertion of the hyperlordotic cages, especially where a narrow disc space may result in endplate damage, cage subsidence, and limitation to lordotic correction. In initial follow-up studies, these authors found improvement in sagittal balance by 4.9 cm from 9 to 4.1 cm and a per-level improvement of 17 degrees in segmental LL. They noted that the procedure could be technically challenging, particularly when avoiding sympathetic and neurovascular structures during ALL release, and advocated for curved retractors to protect these structures. With diligence, they reported no neurovascular complications in their initial cohort.[51]

Other groups have examined the addition of posterior procedures to minimally invasive correction. Manwaring et al., in a follow-up study of early outcomes, studied correction provided by the addition of posterior instrumentation to standard LLIF procedures.[52] These authors found that posterior instrumentation did not provide additional correction with or without the use of hyperlordotic cages or ACR. However, the ACR with hyperlordotic cages did provide a correction similar to that previously seen and similar to the SPO per level, and patients with multilevel procedures had correction similar to that reported for PSO. Berjano et al. examined the effect on sagittal balance with the addition of posterior osteotomies to the ACR.[53] They found that the addition of the SPO provided 24 degrees of correction on average per level. This was similar to correction provided by the PSO in the literature. In a multicenter analysis, Turner et al. confirmed this further improvement offered by posterior SPO. They reported a modest correction of 12 to 15 degrees.[54]

Summary

Fixed sagittal imbalance is a cause of significant disability and distress to patients. It is important for the surgeon to understand the disease process that leads to fixed sagittal imbalance and understand the changes in thoracolumbar and spinopelvic alignment that occur. In patients undergoing surgery, restoring spinopelvic harmony is paramount. Radiographic measures of sagittal balance can be assessed through radiographic measures of the spine. However, surgery to treat this disorder is not without significant morbidity; it is important for the surgeon to understand the risks and benefits of surgery when discussing treatment with patients. Recently, there has been more effort into using minimally invasive approaches for deformity correction with less morbidity when compared to the traditional open posterior osteotomies that have long been the traditional approaches to deformity surgery.

KEY REFERENCES

1. Booth KC., et al. Complications and predictive factors for the successful treatment of flatback deformity (fixed sagittal imbalance). *Spine*. 1999;24(16):1712.
2. Schwab F, Patel A, Ungar B, Farcy J-P, Lafage V. Adult spinal deformity—postoperative standing imbalance: how much can you tolerate? An overview of key parameters in assessing alignment and planning corrective surgery. *Spine*. 2010;35(25):2224-2231.
3. Cho KJ, Bridwell KH, Lenke LG, et al. Comparison of Smith-Petersen versus pedicle subtraction osteotomy for the correction of fixed sagittal imbalance. *Spine*. 2005;30:2030-2037.
4. Bridwell KH. Decision making regarding Smith-Petersen vs. pedicle subtraction osteotomy vs. vertebral column resection for spinal deformity. *Spine*. 2006;31:S171-S178.
5. Rose PS, et al. Role of Pelvic incidence, thoracic kyphosis, and patient factors on sagittal plane correction following pedicle subtraction osteotomy. *Spine*. 2009;34(8):785-791.

REFERENCES

1. Booth Kevin C, et al. Complications and predictive factors for the successful treatment of flatback deformity (fixed sagittal imbalance). *Spine*. 1999;24(16):1712.
2. Doherty JH. Complications of fusion in lumbar scoliosis: proceedings of the Scoliosis Research Society. *J Bone Joint Surg Am*. 1973;55:438.
3. Bradford DS, Tribus CB. Current concepts and management of patients with mixed decompensated spinal deformity. *Clin Orthop*. 1994;306:64-72.
4. Denis F. The iatrogrenic loss of lumbar lordosis. The flat back and flat buttock syndromes. In: Farcy J-P, ed. *Complex spinal deformities. Spine: State of the Art Reviews*. Philadelphia: Hanley & Belfus, Inc.; 1994:659-680.
5. Hsieh PC, Koski TR, O'Shaughnessy BA, et al. Anterior lumbar interbody fusion in comparison with transforaminal lumbar interbody fusion: implications for the restoration of foraminal height, local disc angle, lumbar lordosis, and sagittal balance. *JNS*. 2007;7(4):379-386.
6. Bridwell KH, Lewis SH, Rinella A, et al. Pedicle subtraction osteotomy for the treatment of fixed sagittal imbalance: surgical technique. *J Bone Joint Surg Am*. 2004;86A(suppl 1):44-50.
7. Bradford DS, Schumacher WL, Lonstein JE, et al. Ankylosing spondylitis: experience and surgical management of 21 patients. *Spine*. 1987;12:238-243.
8. Wang Y, et al. A single posterior approach for multilevel modified vertebral column resection in adults with severe rigid congenital kyphoscoliosis: a retrospective study of 13 cases. *Eur Spine J*. 2008;17.
9. Jackson RP, McManus AC. Radiographic analysis of sagittal plane alignment and balance in standing volunteers and patients with low back pain matched for age, sex, and size. A prospective controlled clinical study. *Spine*. 1994;19: 1611-1618.
10. El Fagoun AB, Schwab F, Gamez L, et al. Center of gravity and radiographic posture analysis: a preliminary review of adult volunteers and adult patients affected by scoliosis. *Spine*. 2005;30:1535-1540.
11. Glassman SD, Bridwell K, Dimar JR, et al. The impact of positive sagittal balance in adult spinal deformity. *Spine*. 2005;30(18):2024-2029.
12. Bernhardt M, Bridwell KH. Segmental analysis of the sagittal plane alignment of the normal thoracic and lumbar spines and thoracolumbar junction. *Spine*. 1989;14(7):717-721.
13. Stagnara P, DeMauroy JC, Dran G, et al. Reciprocal angulation of vertebral bodies in a sagittal plane: approach to references for the evaluation of kyphosis and lordosis. *Spine*. 1982;7(4):335-342.
14. Roussouly P, et al. Classification of the normal variation in the sagittal alignment of the human lumbar spine and pelvis in the standing position. *Spine*. 2005;30(3):346-353.
15. Lafage V, Schwab F, Patel A, et al. Pelvic tilt and truncal inclination: two key radiographic parameters in the setting of adults with spinal deformity. *Spine*. 2009;34(17): E599-E606.
16. Schwab F, Patel A, Ungar B, et al. Adult spinal deformity—postoperative standing imbalance: how much can you tolerate? An overview of key parameters in assessing alignment and planning corrective surgery. *Spine*. 2010;35(25):2224-2231.
17. Rose PS, et al. Role of pelvic incidence, thoracic kyphosis, and patient factors on sagittal plane correction following pedicle subtraction osteotomy. *Spine*. 2009;34(8):785-791.

18. Smith-Petersen MH, Larson CB. Aufranc OE: Osteotomy of the spine for the correction of flexion deformity in rheumatoid arthritis. *J Bone Joint Surg Am*. 1945;27:1-11.
19. Cho KJ, Bridwell KH, Lenke LG, et al. Comparison of Smith-Petersen versus pedicle subtraction osteotomy for the correction of fixed sagittal imbalance. *Spine*. 2005;30:2030-2037.
20. Bridwell KH. Decision making regarding Smith-Petersen vs. pedicle subtraction osteotomy vs. vertebral column resection for spinal deformity. *Spine*. 2006;31:S171-S178.
21. Chen IH, Chien JT, Yu TC. Transpedicular wedge osteotomy for correction of thoracolumbar kyphosis in ankylosing spondylitis: experience with 78 patients. *Spine*. 2001;26:E354-E360.
22. Bridwell KH, Lewis SJ, Lenke LG, et al. Pedicle subtraction osteotomy for the treatment of fixed sagittal imbalance. *J Bone Joint Surg Am*. 2003;85-A:454-463.
23. Smith, Justin S, et al. Short-term morbidity and mortality associated with correction of thoracolumbar fixed sagittal plane deformity: a report from the Scoliosis Research Society Morbidity and Mortality Committee. *Spine*. 2011;36(12):958-964.
24. Elwatidy S, Jamjoom Z, Elgamal E, et al. Efficacy and safety of prophylactic large dose of tranexamic acid in spine surgery: a prospective, randomized, double-blind, placebo-controlled study. *Spine*. 2008;33(24):2577-2580.
25. Wong J, El Beheiry H, Rampersaud YR, et al. Tranexamic acid reduces perioperative blood loss in adult patients having spinal fusion surgery. *Anesth Analg*. 2008;107(5):1479-1486.
26. Urban MK, Beckman J, Gordon M, Urquhart B, Boachie-Adjei O. The efficacy of antifibrinolytics in the reduction of blood loss during complex adult reconstructive spine surgery. *Spine*. 2001;26(10):1152-1156.
27. Kebaish KM, Martin CT, O'Brien JR, et al. Use of vertebroplasty to prevent proximal junctional fractures in adult deformity surgery: a biomechanical cadaveric study. *Spine J*. 2013;13(12):1897-1903.
28. Martin CT, Skolasky RL, Mohamed AS, Kebaish KM. Preliminary results of the effect of prophylactic vertebroplasty on the incidence of proximal junctional complications after posterior spinal fusion to the low thoracic spine. *Spine Deformity*. 2013;1(2):132-138.
29. Mazur MD, Ravindra VM, Schmidt MH, et al. Unplanned reoperation after lumbopelvic fixation with S-2 alar-iliac screws or iliac bolts. *J Neurosurg Spine*. 2015;23(1):67-76.
30. Nahtomi-Shick O, Kostuik JP, Winters BD, et al. Does intraoperative fluid management in spine surgery predict intensive care unit length of stay. *J Clin Anesth*. 2001;13(3):208-212.
31. Awad JN, Kebaish KM, Donigan J, et al. Analysis of the risk factors for the development of post-operative spinal epidural haematoma. *J Bone Joint Surg Br*. 2005;87(9):1248-1252.
32. Simmons EH. The surgical correction of flexion deformity of the cervical spine in ankylosing spondylitis. *Clin Orthop Relat Res*. 1972;86:132-143.
33. Deviren V, Scheer JK., Ames CP. Technique of cervicothoracic junction pedicle subtraction osteotomy for cervical sagittal imbalance: report of 11 cases. *J Neurosurg Spine*. 2011;15(2):174-181.
34. Tokala DP, Lam KS, Freeman BJ, Webb JK. C7 decancellisation closing wedge osteotomy for the correction of fixed cervico-thoracic kyphosis. *Eur Spine J*. 2007;16:1471-1478.
35. Young RM, et al. Treatment of craniocervical instability using a posterior-only approach: report of 3 cases. *J Neurosurg Spine*. 2014;21(2):239-248.
36. Richter M, Cakir B, Schmidt R. Cervical pedicle screws: conventional versus computer-assisted placement of cannulated screws. *Spine*. 2005;30(20):2280-2287.
37. Jones EL, Heller JG, Silcox DH, Hutton WC. Cervical pedicle screws versus lateral mass screws: anatomic feasibility and biomechanical comparison. *Spine*. 1997;22(9):977-982.
38. Suk SI, Kim JH, Kim WJ, et al. Posterior vertebral column resection for severe spinal deformities. *Spine*. 2015;27(21):2374-2382.
39. Kim YJ, Bridwell KH, Lenke LG, et al. Results of lumbar pedicle subtraction osteotomies for fixed sagittal imbalance: a minimum 5-year follow up study. *Spine*. 2007;32: 2189-2197.
40. Wang Y, Zhang Y, Zhang X, et al. A single posterior approach for multilevel modified vertebral column resection in adults with severe rigid congenital kyphoscoliosis: a retrospective study of 13 cases. *Eur Spine J*. 2008;17(3):361-372.
41. Smith JS, Shaffrey CI, Glassman SD, et al. Risk-benefit assessment of surgery for adult scoliosis: an analysis based on patient age. *Spine*. 2011;36:817-824.
42. Le TV, Vivas AC, Dakwar E, Baaj AA, Uribe JS. The effect of the retroperitoneal transpsoas minimally invasive lateral interbody fusion on segmental and regional lumbar lordosis. *Scientific World Journal*. 2012;2012:516706.
43. Wang MY, Mummaneni PV. Minimally invasive surgery for thoracolumbar spinal deformity: initial clinical experience with clinical and radiographic outcomes. *Neurosurg Focus*. 2010;28(3):E9.
44. Hsieh MK, Chen LH, Niu CC, et al. Combined anterior lumbar interbody fusion and instrumented posterolateral fusion for degenerative lumbar scoliosis: indication and surgical outcomes. *BMC Surg*. 2015;15(1):26.
45. Garg J, Woo K, Hirsch J, Bruffey JD, Dilley RB. Vascular complications of exposure for anterior lumbar interbody fusion. *J Vasc Surg*. 2010;51:946-950.
46. Phillips FM, Isaacs RE, Rodgers WB, et al. Adult degenerative scoliosis treated with XLIF: clinical and radiographical results of a prospective multicenter study with 24-month follow-up. *Spine*. 2013;38:1853-1861.
47. Phan K, Rao PJ, Scherman DB, Dandie G, Mobbs RJ. Lateral lumbar interbody fusion for sagittal balance correction and spinal deformity. *J Clin Neurosci*. 2015;22(11):1714-1721.
48. Uribe JS, Smith DA, Dakwar E, et al. Lordosis restoration after anterior longitudinal ligament release and placement of lateral hyperlordotic interbody cages during the minimally invasive lateral transpsoas approach: a radiographic study in cadavers: laboratory investigation. *J Neurosurg Spine*. 2012;17(5):476-485.
49. Marchi L, Oliveira L, Amaral R, et al. Anterior elongation as a minimally invasive alternative for sagittal imbalance—a case series. *HSS J*. 2012;8:122-127.
50. Deukmedjian AR, Le TV, Baaj AA, et al. Anterior longitudinal ligament release using the minimally invasive lateral retroperitoneal transpsoas approach: a cadaveric feasibility study and report of 4 clinical cases. *J Neurosurg Spine*. 2012;17:530-539.
51. Deukmedjian AR, Dakwar E, Ahmadian A, et al. Early outcomes of minimally invasive anterior longitudinal ligament release for correction of sagittal imbalance in

patients with adult spinal deformity. *Scientific World Journal.* 2012;2012:789698.

52. Manwaring JC, Bach K, Ahmadian AA, et al. Management of sagittal balance in adult spinal deformity with minimally invasive anterolateral lumbar interbody fusion: a preliminary radiographic study. *J Neurosurg Spine.* 2014;20:515-522.
53. Berjano A. Pedicle subtraction osteotomies (PSO) in the lumbar spine for sagittal deformities. *Eur Spine J.* 2015;24 (suppl 1):S49-S57.
54. Turner JD, Akbarnia BA. Radiographic outcomes of anterior column realignment for adult sagittal plane deformity: a multicenter analysis. *Eur Spine J.* 2015;24(3): 427-432.

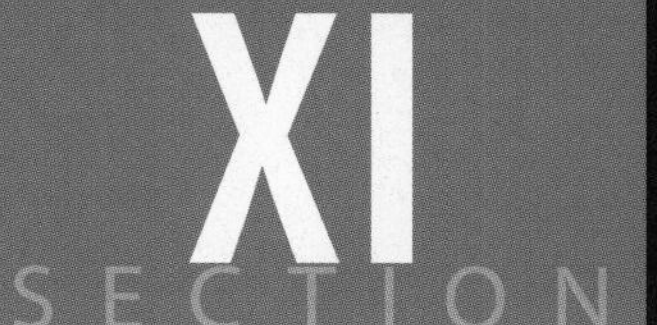

SECTION XI

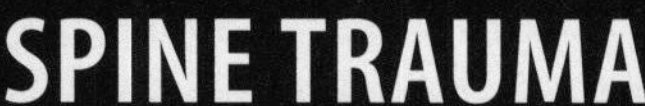

SPINE TRAUMA

CHAPTER 74 Basic Science of Spinal Cord Injury

Alexandre Rasouli

There is still no cure for spinal cord injury (SCI). Recovery in the spinal cord is thwarted by two fundamental obstacles: the inherently weak regenerative ability of central nervous system (CNS) axons and a powerfully inhibitive—and often deleterious—postinjury milieu of physical and chemical factors. These factors are intertwined in a so-called secondary response of tremendous complexity that ironically does more to injure the spinal cord further than to heal it. Years of research have slowly elucidated the pathophysiologic processes that follow a traumatic insult to the spinal cord. This chapter reviews the biochemical and physiologic features of the SCI response and establishes a foundation on which the latest therapeutic strategies can be understood.

The first section discusses the inflammatory cascade that occurs in the moments after an assault to the spinal cord. The second section reviews current understanding of the inhibitory extracellular environment that results from the injury response and that ultimately prevents axonal regeneration. The chapter concludes with a review of the biochemical processes that can be targeted by candidate therapies.

Pathophysiologic Response to Spinal Cord Injury

The acutely traumatized spinal cord is subjected to multiple physical and chemical mediators that cause additional (secondary) injury.[1,2] This concept of secondary injury has been validated in both animal and clinical studies, and secondary injury mechanisms have been the target of the bulk of pharmacologic interventions to date. These processes begin immediately following the injury and continue for weeks (Fig. 74.1).

Hemorrhage and Circulatory Collapse

Upon injury, the blood–spinal cord barrier is disrupted and intraparenchymal hemorrhage occurs, the extent of which depends on the force of the initial trauma. Microcirculatory insufficiency follows.[3,4] Vascular hypoperfusion due to capillary loss, capillary spasm, thrombosis, systemic hypotension, and autonomic regulatory interruption lead to cellular ischemia at the epicenter of cord injury. The neuronal cell bodies in the gray matter are highly vulnerable to ischemia. The resultant shift in pH renders neuronal cell body and axonal membranes highly vulnerable to subsequent injury.

Oxidative Damage

Reperfusion and oxidative stress follow the transient period of hypoperfusion. The introduction of oxygen to the compromised cell membranes produces a highly toxic environment in which the membrane lipid fatty acids undergo oxidation.[5] This membrane lipid peroxidation produces several varieties of free radicals that, in turn, drive even further lipid peroxidation and free radical production. Some of the free radicals accumulate within the cell and denature deoxyribonucleic acid, mitochondrial proteins, and eventually bring energy production to a halt, resulting in irreversible damage and cell death.

Excitotoxicity

Disruption of the neuronal cellular membrane undermines one of the crucial features of cellular equilibrium—ionic regulation.[6] The destabilized neurons undergo an influx of sodium ions that eventually alters cellular pH and leads to cytotoxicity. The ionic balance is perturbed by, and will cause neuronal destruction via, an additional important mechanism: the cellular release of the ubiquitous neurotransmitter glutamate changes the extracellular space into a hostile extracellular milieu.[6] Glutamate activates various cell surface receptors that, in turn, mediate a large variety of intracellular processes. Excessive glutamate will drive these processes to the point of fatal overload to the cell. The most studied of the glutamic receptors is the *N*-methyl-D-aspartate receptor, which mediates entry of Ca^{2+} into cellular cytoplasm from both extracellular and intracellular stores. While calcium in physiologic amounts is the necessary component for many important enzyme-mediated cellular processes, pathophysiologic quantities of calcium lead to the persistent activity of destructive enzymes, including lipoxygenases and phospholipases. These

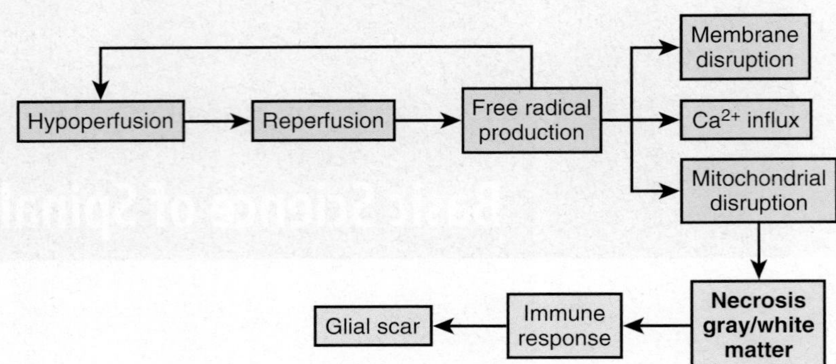

FIG. 74.1 The self-perpetuating injury cascade begins with a sequence of hypoperfusion and reperfusion. The ensuing oxidative damage leads to tissue necrosis and an immune response that culminates in the inhibitory glial scar.

enzymes will target the beleaguered cell membrane again to generate free radicals from lipid oxidation. The radicals will disrupt cellular proteins, in particular, those that mediate the ability of mitochondria, the chief source of cellular energy, to drive oxidative phosphorylation.

Mitochondrial Collapse and Cytotoxicity

The aforementioned free radical formation and glut of Ca^{2+} ions abolish mitochondrial integrity by activating mitochondrial permeability transition pores.[6] The opening of these pores leads to a massive increase in mitochondrial membrane permeability. The organelle loses its electrochemical gradient, adenosine triphosphate production ceases, and the outer membrane swells until it ruptures. The damage is far-reaching. Calcium ions, free radicals, and cytochrome c, once sequestered within the mitochondria, are now free to escape into the neuronal cytoplasm where they immediately activate necrosis and apoptosis.

Neuroimmunologic Response

The cells of the immune system are eventually attracted to the neuronal self-destruction. Over the next hours to weeks, they will lay the foundations for an extracellular environment that will inhibit axonal regeneration. The first of these cells to appear at the site of injury are circulating neutrophils. Once active, neutrophils will secrete cytokines that stimulate production of phospholipases and cyclooxygenase.[7] The former will consume neural membranes to produce arachidonic acid, which the latter (cyclooxygenase) uses to produce prostaglandins and thromboxanes. Prostaglandins (PGE_2, PGD_2, $PGF_{2\alpha}$, PGI_2) serve (1) to amplify the inflammatory response by increasing capillary permeability to allow additional inflammatory cell influx; (2) to increase neuronal calcium concentration, thus promoting excitotoxicity; and (3) to activate other inflammatory cells.[1] Thromboxanes promote platelet aggregation within capillaries and thus worsen local tissue ischemia.

Macrophages, local microglia, and astrocytes eventually appear and begin secreting the two most important factors of the cytotoxic inflammatory response: interleukin-1 and tumor necrosis factor α. Interleukin-1 stimulates the expression of adhesion factors on endothelial cells, which will allow circulating lymphocytes to penetrate the blood–brain barrier. Tumor necrosis factor α serves to recruit activated cytotoxic lymphocytes to first adhere to endothelial cells and then to the site of injury. The recruited lymphocytes, which target myelin basic protein, are particularly adept at causing disruption of the all-important myelin sheath—a critical component of nerve conductivity and axonal regeneration. The epicenter of traumatic injury thus becomes an inflammatory tangle of necrosis, apoptosis, and demyelination. Over the coming weeks, the cellular debris will first liquefy into a posttraumatic cyst and then organize into the notorious astroglial scar, which will inhibit axonal regeneration.

Astroglial Scar

The most significant factor in the inhibition of axonal regeneration after SCI is the glial scar that develops.[8–11] The glial scar is a collection of reactive cells (astrocytes, microglia, oligodendrocyte precursors, meningeal fibroblasts) that express cell-surface and matrix molecules, which surround the area of injury and ultimately repel the advancement of regenerating axons (Fig. 74.2).

The scar features a core zone of meningeal cells and oligodendrocyte precursors, and a lesion-surround zone of astrocytes, oligodendrocyte precursors, and microglia. The core zone is separated from the surround zone by a basement membrane composed mostly of type IV collagen.[12] While some axons may regenerate through the surround zone, no axon can penetrate the core zone without some form of experimental manipulation.[13]

The inhibitory effects of the scar are conferred by three classes of molecules, all of which are expressed by one or more of the reactive cells in the glial scar. These include the chondroitin sulfate proteoglycans (CSPGs; NG2, brevican, phosphacan, neurocan, versican), semaphorin 3 proteins, and eph/ephrin tyrosine kinases. Although the precise mechanisms of their actions are unclear, the molecules exert their inhibitory effects either by directly or indirectly binding to the axon cell

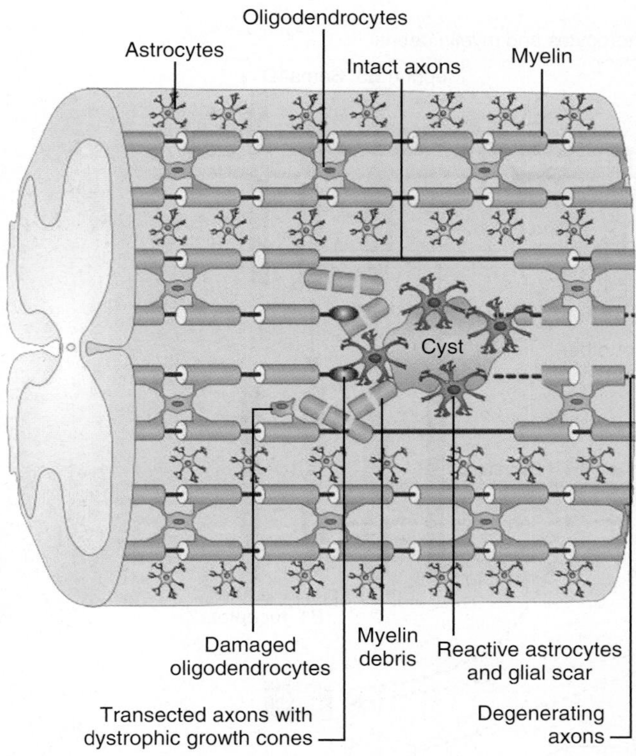

FIG. 74.2 The astroglial scar presents nonpermissive cues to regeneration. These nonpermissive cues include deprivation of trophic support, lack of permissive cues at the axonal growth cones, progressive demyelination, decreased cyclic adenosine monophosphate levels, and a strong inhibitory environment established by extracellular matrix molecules (keratin sulfate proteoglycans and chondroitin sulfate proteoglycans NG2, neurocan, brevican, versican, phosphacan), and by glial and myelin components.

surface or by binding and deactivating trophic factors, cell adhesion molecules, and extracellular matrix molecules that are a requisite for axonal growth and regeneration.[14] The ultimate effect of the gliotic response to injury is the inhibition of successful axonal regeneration and remyelination by both physical and chemical means[15] (Fig. 74.3).

There is tremendous therapeutic potential in the ability to modulate the gliotic scarring response to CNS injury. In vitro and in vivo studies to date, though relatively limited, have demonstrated enhancement of axonal regeneration and functional recovery after inhibition of specific glial scar constituents. Enzymatic digestion of the glycosoaminoglycan chains of CSPGs, for instance, stimulates axonal regeneration through the site of injury.[16] Function-blocking antibodies to semaphorin receptors have allowed sensory axons to regenerate into the formidable core zone of the scar.[17] Chelating agents that prevent collagen IV synthesis around the core zone have also allowed successful axonal regeneration in some animal models.[18] Animals with clonal deletions of a certain eph molecule have almost no astroglial scar response and demonstrate unimpeded regeneration of motor axons through the zone of injury.[19]

Despite its multifaceted inhibitory influence, several recent studies suggest that the glial scar must offer some protective benefit to the injured spinal cord. The role of the gliotic response in mitigating the extension of cord injury beyond the initial site of trauma, for instance, has been proposed.[20] In a study of transgenic mice, selective ablation of reactive astrocytes in the glial scar after both contusion and penetrating spinal cord injury led to markedly increased tissue disruption, cellular degeneration, cystic changes, and profound and persistent motor deficits relative to nonablated controls.[21] It is likely that both the cellular and extracellular matrix elements of the gliotic scar play a critical role in biochemical protection and structural stabilization of cord integrity, and thus function, after SCI.

The duality of the inflammatory response after spinal cord trauma, both inhibitory to axonal regeneration and protective against further injury, is perhaps the most perplexing aspect of SCI and a key reason that a cure has proven so challenging.

BOX 74.1 Classification of Treatment Strategies

Neuroprotective

Methylprednisolone
Ganglioside
Thyrotropin-releasing hormone
Calcium channel blockers

Regenerative

Activated macrophages
Rho antagonists
Anti-Nogo antibodies
Peripheral nerve/Schwann cell transplantation
Olfactory ensheathing
Cell transplantation

Basic Science of a Cure

Consistent with their basic science foundations, the human acute SCI therapies have one of two ambitions: (1) to limit secondary injury (neuroprotection, acute surgical intervention, rehabilitation) and (2) to reverse injury (Box 74.1).

Methylprednisolone

The first randomized, controlled multicenter trial of a neuroprotective agent was the National Acute Spinal Cord Injury (NASCIS) I Study, which attempted to establish the clinical efficacy of methylprednisolone.[22,23] Though its precise mechanism of action is still unclear, methylprednisolone was thought to exert either a cell-stabilizing effect via the glucocorticoid receptor or a cord-stabilizing effect via free-radical inhibition.[24–26] The trial was based on several animal studies that suggested improved neurologic recovery when the corticosteroid was administered promptly after experimental injury.[27] Published in 1984, NASCIS I included 330 patients with acute SCI (defined as any loss of sensation or motor function below the level of injury), who were randomized into two groups within 48 hours of injury: a "low-dose group" receiving 100 mg IV methylprednisolone bolus and then 25 mg every 6 hours for 10 days; and a "high-dose" group receiving bolus and maintenance doses 10 times those of the low-dose group every 6 hours for 10 days. Outcome measures consisted of motor

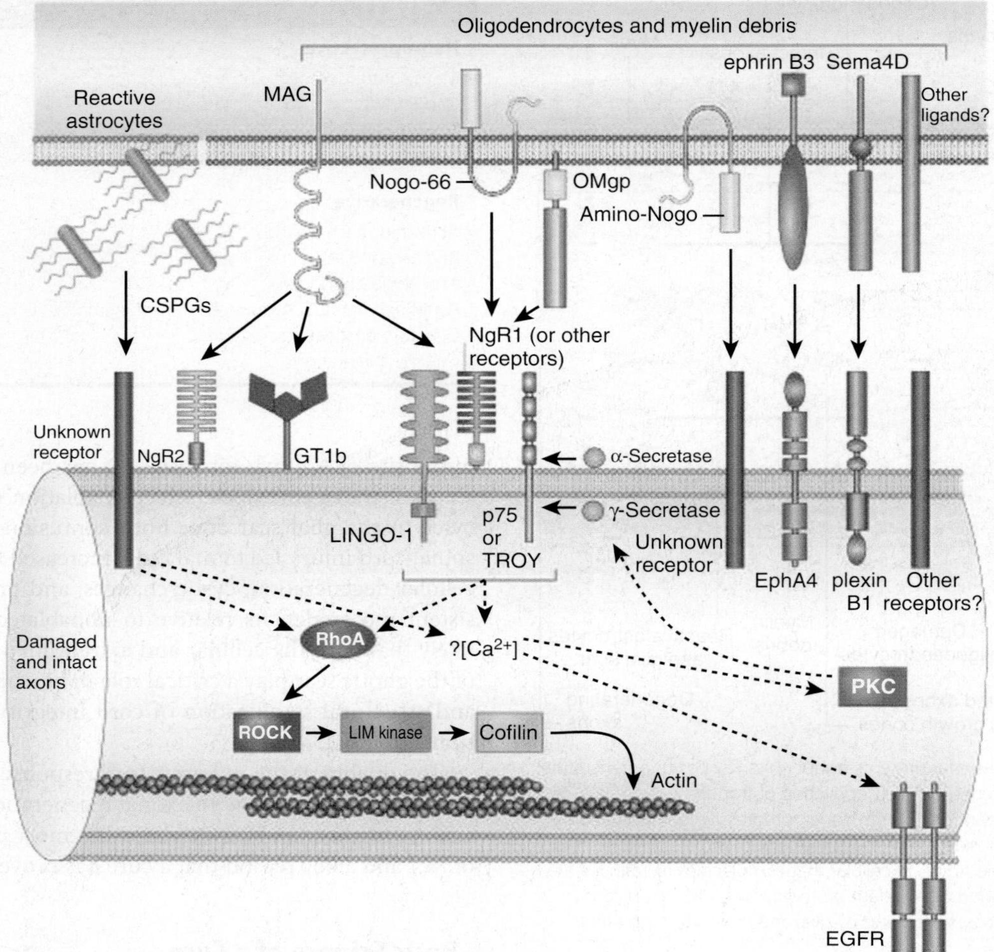

FIG. 74.3 Although the precise mechanisms of their actions are unclear, the molecules of the glial scar exert their inhibitory effects either by directly or indirectly binding to the axon cell surface or by binding and deactivating trophic factors, cell adhesion molecules, and extracellular matrix molecules that are requisite for axonal growth and regeneration. The ultimate effect of the gliotic response to injury is an embarrassment of axonal regeneration *and* remyelination by both physical and chemical means. CSPGs, chondroitin sulfate proteoglycans; EGFR, epidermal growth factor receptor; LINGO1, Nogo receptor-interacting protein; MAG, myelin-associated glycoprotein; NgR1, Nogo-66 receptor 1; NgR2, Nogo-66 receptor 2; Nogo, neurite outgrowth inhibitor; OMgp, oligodendrocyte myelin glycoprotein; PKC, protein kinase C; ROCK, rho-associated kinase; sema4D, semaphorin-4D.

and sensory indices of 14 muscle groups and 29 dermatomes. The follow-up periods were 6 weeks and 6 months. Though there was no difference between the two groups in terms of neurologic outcome, there was an increased incidence of wound infection and even fatality in the higher-dose group, with the former achieving statistical significance.

One year later, NASCIS II was launched as the first randomized, prospective, placebo-controlled trial of a candidate therapy for SCI.[28,29] It was devised to address the lack of a placebo control in NASCIS I and to incorporate new basic-science findings regarding effective methylprednisolone dosing and mechanisms of action. The study involved 487 patients who were randomized into three groups within 12 hours of sustaining either complete or incomplete SCI: a methylprednisolone group receiving an unprecedented 30 mg/kg IV bolus, followed by a maintenance infusion of 5.4 mg/kg/h over 23 hours; a placebo group; and a third group consisting of a 5.4 mg/kg bolus and 4.0 mg/kg/h maintenance infusion of the opioid antagonist naloxone, whose neuroprotective effects had also been suggested by animal studies.[30] The outcome methodology was similar to that in NASCIS I.

When all members of the methylprednisolone group were compared to placebo, there were no statistically significant improvements in sensory or motor function at 6 weeks. However, when the steroid group was stratified according to timing of administration, patients receiving treatment within 8 hours of injury demonstrated a significant improvement in sensory and motor function by 6 weeks versus placebo. The relative improvement was sustained through the 6-month follow-up point. Within the steroid group treated within 8 hours, further subgroup analysis with respect to ASIA scale injury severity revealed that class A patients had the greatest statistically significant improvement in motor and sensory measures versus placebo. Additionally, American Spinal

Injury Association (ASIA) class C and D patients had only motor improvement, whereas class B patients had neither sensory nor motor improvement that reached statistical significance.[28,31] The complication of wound infection was more frequent but statistically insignificant in the steroid group despite the heavy dosing. There were no differences in motor or sensory outcomes between the naloxone and placebo group at either of the follow-up points. NASCIS II established the now ubiquitous "steroid protocol," despite controversies regarding possible nontransparency, data misinterpretation, and near-normal function of some participants.

The objective of the third and final NASCIS was to investigate the interplay between timing of steroid administration and duration of therapy and to evaluate the efficacy of the 21-aminosteroid tirilazad mesylate, which purportedly had a better safety profile than methylprednisolone. A total of 499 patients were randomized into three treatment groups within 6 hours of injury: the first group received methylprednisolone according to the NASCIS II dosing for 24 hours, the second group received this dosing for 48 hours, and the third group received a methylprednisolone bolus of 5.4 mg/kg/h followed by a maintenance infusion of tirilazad at 2.5 mg/kg IV every 6 hours for 48 hours.[32] With outcome measures including motor function, sensory function, and functional independence, the NASCIS III revealed that increased duration of steroid administration (48 hours) resulted in statistically significant benefit only if treatment was initiated between 3 and 8 hours of injury. Infectious complications were more common in the 48-hour corticosteroid group but were statistically insignificant. There were no differences between the tirilazad group and the 24-hour methylprednisolone group.

Ganglioside GM-1

Trials of the glycosphingolipid ganglioside GM-1 followed closely on the heels of the methylprednisolone studies. Gangliosides are mammalian neuronal cell membrane constituents and play a substantial role in neuronal plasticity, axonal recovery after experimental SCI, and cell preservation after ischemia.[33–36] The Maryland GM-1 ganglioside trial was a prospective, randomized, placebo-controlled pilot study of 37 patients with SCI who were assigned to one of two groups: GM-1 100 mg IV per day for 30 days versus placebo.[35] Outcome measures were in terms of motor scores and Frankel grades, and the follow-up point was at 6 months. By 6 months, the authors demonstrated a 2-grade improvement on the Frankel scale in 50% of patients receiving GM-1 but only in 7% of patients receiving placebo, a difference that was statistically significant. The pilot study was then expanded into the largest clinical trial of SCI therapy, known as the Sygen Multicenter Acute Spinal Cord Injury Study (SMASCIS).[37] SMASCIS randomized 797 patients with SCI into two groups receiving GM-1 (300 mg IV bolus + 100 mg IV daily for 56 days versus 600 mg IV bolus + 200 mg IV daily for 56 days) and NASCIS II protocol. Outcome measures included ASIA sensory and motor scores and the ASIA impairment scale rating. At 8 weeks, patients exhibited dose-related, statistically significant improvements in impairment scale ratings relative to placebo; but by the 6-month endpoint, there were no differences in the number of patients achieving improvement (defined as at least a 2-grade improvement in the impairment index) between any of the groups. SMASCIS had revealed that GM-1 ganglioside was ultimately no better than placebo in the setting of acute SCI.

Thyrotropin-Releasing Hormone

Thyrotropin-releasing hormone (TRH) and its analogs have been shown in multiple animal models of acute SCI to improve functional recovery by acting as a neuroprotective partial opioid antagonist.[29,38–40] The prospective trial evaluating its efficacy in human subjects involved 20 patients with acute SCI who were randomly assigned within 12 hours of injury into one of two groups: a TRH group receiving 0.2 mg/kg bolus IV dose followed by 0.2 mg/kg/h infusion for 6 hours and a placebo group.[41] NASCIS motor and sensory indices and the Sunnybrook system were used as outcome measures. Follow-up time points were at 24 hours, 72 hours, 7 days, 1 month, and 4 months, and 1 year after injury. Patients with complete injuries did not demonstrate a benefit from TRH administration relative to placebo group patients; patients with incomplete injuries did show statistically significant improvement in outcome measure after TRH treatment versus placebo. However, the authors were cautious with their conclusions due to sample size issues and the number of patients lost to follow-up. A larger clinical trial of the hormone has not been completed.

Nimodipine and Gacyclidine

In a number of animal models of SCI, the calcium channel blocker nimodipine has been reported to improve neurologic recovery by increasing spinal cord blood flow and limiting vasospasm, ischemia, and secondary infarction.[42,43] The prospective clinical trial of the antihypertensive involved 106 patients with complete or incomplete SCI who were randomized to one of four groups: nimodipine 0.015 mg/kg/h IV loading dose for 2 hours + 0.03 mg/kg/h infusion for 7 days, methylprednisolone according to NASCIS II protocol, both agents, and placebo.[43] Outcome was measured with the ASIA grade and ASIA motor and sensory scores. At 1 year follow-up, none of the treatment groups demonstrated efficacy over placebo. Interestingly, 80 of the 106 patients were surgically treated within 24 hours of injury; a subgroup analysis revealed that surgery within 8 hours of injury and between 8 to 24 hours of injury yielded identical outcomes.

Posttraumatic glutamate toxicity is the target of the novel *N*-methyl-D-aspartate receptor antagonist gacyclidine, which has been shown to enhance recovery after contusive SCI in rat models.[44] In a prospective, controlled clinical trial, 272 patients were randomized to one of four groups within 2 hours of SCI: gacyclidine at 0.005 mg/kg IV within 2 hours of trauma and once again at 6 hours after trauma, gacyclidine at 0.001 mg/kg IV × 2 doses, gacyclidine at 0.02 mg/kg × 2 doses, and placebo. Outcome measures included the ASIA motor and sensory scores. At 1 year follow-up, there were no statistical differences in outcomes between any of the groups.

Regeneration Strategies

While neuroprotective strategies are directed primarily at limiting secondary neural injury, regeneration strategies involve repair of the damaged tissues. The prerequisite for these therapeutic strategies is the modification of the nonideal local milieu of the injured cord as biochemical, cellular, and extracellular matrix perturbations may limit the potential for axonal repair.[6,45,46]

Rho Antagonist

Several inhibitors of nerve regeneration have been identified, including Nogo, myelin-associated glycoprotein, and myelin-oligodendrocyte glycoprotein. These factors act commonly through the GTPase Rho, an enzyme that orchestrates a potent inhibitory cascade after injury that culminates in growth cone disintegration, neurite sprouting inhibition, and neuronal and glial cell apoptosis.[47,48] The naturally occurring inhibitor of the Rho enzyme, C3 transferase from *Clostridium botulinum*, has been shown to effect remarkably rapid functional recovery in hemisection SCI rats.[49] Histologic analysis of C3-treated rats treated within 24 hours of injury showed increased neuronal sprouting and functional analysis revealed enhanced locomotor recovery and limb coordination.

A recombinant pharmaceutical version of C3 transferase known as Cethrin, in which the enzyme is linked to a protein that facilitates blood-brain barrier penetration, has undergone phase I/IIa trials at nine North American centers to establish safety and efficacy. Preliminary results of this trial have been discussed at scientific meetings and published in abstract form.[50] The study included 37 patients with complete (ASIA class A) SCI at either the cervical or thoracic level who were given increasing doses of extradurally applied Cethrin (0.3, 1.0, 3.0, and 6.0 mg). Outcome measures (ASIA International Standards) were collected at 1.5, 3, 6, and 12 months. The investigators documented no adverse effects of the treatment and by the 1.5-month follow-up period observed improvement of at least one ASIA Impairment Scale grade in 30% of patients. Initial data from the 6-month follow-up period suggest similar rates of recovery.

A phase II/III multicenter clinical trial of the drug Cethrin is planned. The study is anticipating enrollment of complete SCI (ASIA class A) patients to undergo surgery for epidural application of the soluble enzyme antagonist at the time of early surgical decompression.[24] Study enrollment will incorporate a Bayesian trial design in an effort to determine optimal dosing while keeping sample numbers to a minimum.

Anti-Nogo Antibody

Nogo is an oligodendrocyte-expressed soluble factor that is potent in its ability to inhibit axonal regeneration. Investigators have been able to restore corticospinal axonal regeneration and locomotion in rat and primate SCI models in which Nogo was neutralized with the monoclonal antibody IN-1.[51,52] A phase I clinical trial of intrathecally administered Nogo-A antibody in acute, complete (ASIA class A) SCI is currently underway in European SCI centers with expansion of the trial to Canadian centers anticipated.

Peripheral Nerve and Schwann Cell Transplantation

Inducing the CNS to mimic the natural regenerative ability of the peripheral nervous system is a pillar of current SCI research. The injured peripheral nerve expresses a permissive environment for axonal regrowth that is engendered primarily by its myelin-forming cell, the Schwann cell and its basal lamina. Schwann cells secrete trophic factors, express cell adhesion molecules, and produce extracellular matrix molecules that are requisite for axonal growth and regeneration.[53,54] The permissive features of Schwann cells may prove valuable in the treatment of SCI. Several groups have demonstrated improved axonal regeneration and functional recovery after Schwann cell transplantation to the site of SCI in rats.[55] Furthermore, the grafting of peripheral nerves with varying combinations of growth factors in SCI rats has resulted in significant axonal and functional recovery.[56] Most of the ongoing clinical studies involving peripheral nerve grafts that are used to bridge lesional sites in the spinal cord are phase 1 trials and currently involve very few patients. Some have shown neurologic improvement while others have not; none of these yet are prospective, randomized trials.[57] Other studies have involved the injection of Schwann cells and oligodendrocyte precursor cells to the area of cord lesion.[4]

Olfactory Ensheathing Glial Cell Transplantation

The olfactory ensheathing glial (OEG) cell spans both the peripheral nervous system and CNS and thus has a unique role in regenerative SCI therapy; several preclinical studies have shown the OEG to have permissive capabilities similar to that of the Schwann cell.[58] A nonrandomized, noncontrolled clinical trial of OEG transplantation in 171 patients with SCI showed modest improvement in ASIA motor and sensory scores after 8 weeks.[59] The study was criticized for its short duration, potential for bias, and lack of control. Neurologic outcomes in the first seven chronic (> 6 months postinjury) SCI patients treated with surgical implantation of olfactory mucosal autograft in an ongoing surgical case series in Lisbon, Portugal were recently published.[60] The investigators claimed to show a modest improvement in ASIA motor and sensory scores in the treated patients. Preliminary safety results of a small Australian controlled clinical trial of surgical implantation of cultured autologous olfactory cells in patients with chronic SCI has recently been published.[61] The investigators report no significant safety concerns at 1 year postimplant and plan to report efficacy outcomes.

Stem Cell Strategies

The ability of stem cells to differentiate into spinal cord tissue carries significant implications for SCI repair. The classic study by Keirstead et al. involved the use of human embryonic stem cell–derived oligodendrocyte progenitor cells to remyelinate the area of contusion injury.[62] In the study, human embryonic stem cells were differentiated in vitro into oligodendrocyte progenitor cells which, in turn, were injected onto rat thoracic cord contusion sites both acutely (7 days) and latently (10 months after injury). The oligodendroglial cells that were acutely transplanted led to enhanced remyelination of axons and to enhanced hindlimb locomotor recovery, whereas latent transplants and control groups did not. There have been at least two attempts to translate these findings into human subjects with some preliminary success.

Genetic Modification Strategies

Despite the promising results of Schwann cell transplantation, the strategy is limited by the fact the regenerated axons do not leave the graft to incorporate with the contiguous native tissue rostral and caudal to the graft. The ability of regenerated axons to migrate out of the graft and into surrounding tissue would improve both locomotor and sensory recovery after injury.[62] The main barrier to axonal incorporation is, of course, the astroglial scar. Golden et al.[63] devised a model in which transplanted Schwann cells are first transduced with lentiviral vectors containing deoxyribonucleic acid encoding for chondroitinase ABC, which degrades CSPGs, the previously discussed component of glial scars, and for D15A, a powerful neurotrophic factor. The modified cells were then transplanted into the site of contusion injury. Relative to previous models with nonmodified Schwann cells, this led to (1) enhanced regeneration of axons both within the graft and into the surrounding tissue, (2) enhanced locomotor recovery in subjects, and (3) enhanced recovery of allodynia. This therapy combines strategies for defeating both of the chief obstacles in SCI recovery: the weak CNS reparative capacity and the stultifying effects of the glial scar. It will likely hold great promise.

As the cellular and molecular components of the injury response continue to be characterized, it will be possible to specifically neutralize the inhibitory constituents while preserving its proregenerative protective elements. The ability to modulate the behavior of the inflammatory response can enhance almost every existing modality of SCI treatment, from transplantation to gene therapy. SCI remains a challenging clinical problem. Ultimately, the plethora of promising interventions being studied in the laboratory will have to be validated in the clinical setting; thus, the creation of a streamlined and financially feasible mechanism for clinical trials will be necessary. Ultimately, combination therapies incorporating interventions to limit secondary injury, surgical treatment, regenerative therapies, and rehabilitation will likely be necessary to impact the outcome of this devastating disease.

KEY POINTS

1. A cascade of events following spinal cord injury can both inhibit recovery and cause additional neural damage.
2. The glial scar is a product of the inflammatory response to injury. It is a collection of reactive cells (astrocytes, microglia, oligodendrocyte precursors, meningeal fibroblasts) that express cell-surface and matrix molecules, which surround the area of injury and ultimately repel the advancement of regenerating axons.
3. Future treatment strategies are based on either neuroprotective or regenerative modalities that capitalize on our current understanding of the biochemical processes after injury.

PEARLS AND PITFALLS

1. There is currently no cure for SCI in human beings.
2. Some of the same processes that are involved in wound healing elsewhere in the body prevent healing of SCI.
3. NASCIS II/III results must be interpreted and applied with caution.

REFERENCES

1. Ramón y Cajal S, May RM. *Degeneration and Regeneration of the Nervous System*. New York: Hafner Publishing; 1928.
2. Kwon BK, Tetzlaff W, Grauer JN, Beiner J, Vaccaro AR. Pathophysiology and pharmacologic treatment of acute spinal cord injury. *Spine J*. 2004;4(4):451-464.
3. Tator CH, Fehlings MG. Review of the secondary injury theory of acute spinal cord trauma with emphasis on vascular mechanisms. *J Neurosurg*. 1991;75(1):15-26.
4. Whetstone WD, et al. Blood-spinal cord barrier after spinal cord injury: relation to revascularization and wound healing. *J Neurosci Res*. 2003;74(2):227-239.
5. Basu S, Hellberg A, Ulus AT, Westman J, Karacagil S. Biomarkers of free radical injury during spinal cord ischemia. *FEBS Lett*. 2001;508(1):36-38.
6. Vialle RL, Fehlings MG, Weidner N. *AOSpine Masters Series: Spinal Cord Injury and Regeneration*. New York: Thieme; 2016.
7. Popovich PG, Wei P, Stokes BT. Cellular inflammatory response after spinal cord injury in Sprague-Dawley and Lewis rats. *J Comp Neurol*. 1997;377(3):443-464.
8. Fawcett JW. Overcoming inhibition in the damaged spinal cord. *J Neurotrauma*. 2006;23(3-4):371-383.
9. Bahr M, Przyrembel C, Bastmeyer M. Astrocytes from adult rat optic nerves are nonpermissive for regenerating retinal ganglion cell axons. *Exp Neurol*. 1995;131(2):211-220.
10. Davies SJ, Goucher DR, Doller C, Silver J. Robust regeneration of adult sensory axons in degenerating white matter of the adult rat spinal cord. *J Neurosci*. 1999;19(14):5810-5822.
11. Hermanns S, Klapka N, Muller HW. The collagenous lesion scar—an obstacle for axonal regeneration in brain and spinal cord injury. *Restor Neurol Neurosci*. 2001;19(1-2):139-148.
12. Stichel CC, Muller HW. The CNS lesion scar: new vistas on an old regeneration barrier. *Cell Tissue Res*. 1998;294(1):1-9.
13. Rasouli A, Bhatia N, Suryadevara S, Cahill K, Gupta R. Transplantation of preconditioned Schwann cells in peripheral nerve grafts after contusion in the adult spinal cord. Improvement of recovery in a rat model. *J Bone Joint Surg Am*. 2006;88(11):2400-2410.
14. Li Y, Raisman G. Schwann cells induce sprouting in motor and sensory axons in the adult rat spinal cord. *J Neurosci*. 1994;14(7):4050-4063.
15. Fawcett JW, Asher RA. The glial scar and central nervous system repair. *Brain Res Bull*. 1999;49(6):377-391.
16. Smith-Thomas LC, Stevens J, Fok-Seang J, et al. Increased axon regeneration in astrocytes grown in the presence of proteoglycan synthesis inhibitors. *J Cell Sci*. 1995;108(Pt 3):1307-1315.
17. Shearer MC, Niclou SP, Brown D, et al. The astrocyte/meningeal cell interface is a barrier to neurite outgrowth which can be overcome by manipulation of inhibitory

molecules or axonal signalling pathways. *Mol Cell Neurosci.* 2003;24(4):913-925.

18. Klapka N, Hermanns S, Straten G, et al. Suppression of fibrous scarring in spinal cord injury of rat promotes long-distance regeneration of corticospinal tract axons, rescue of primary motoneurons in somatosensory cortex and significant functional recovery. *Eur J Neurosci.* 2005;22(12): 3047-3058.
19. Goldshmit Y, Galea MP, Bartlett PF, Turnley AM. EphA4 regulates central nervous system vascular formation. *J Comp Neurol.* 2006;497(6):864-875.
20. Yiu G, He Z. Glial inhibition of CNS axon regeneration. *Nat Rev Neurosci.* 2006;7(8):617-627.
21. Faulkner JR, Herrmann JE, Woo MJ, et al. Reactive astrocytes protect tissue and preserve function after spinal cord injury. *J Neurosci.* 2004;24(9):2143-2155.
22. Bracken MB, Shepard MJ, Hellenbrand KG, et al. Methylprednisolone and neurological function 1 year after spinal cord injury. Results of the National Acute Spinal Cord Injury Study. *J Neurosurg.* 1985;63(5):704-713.
23. Ducker TB, Hamit HF. Experimental treatments of acute spinal cord injury. *J Neurosurg.* 1969;30(6):693-697.
24. Campbell JB, DeCrescito V, Tomasula JJ, et al. Experimental treatment of spinal cord contusion in the cat. *Surg Neurol.* 1973;1(2):102-106.
25. Hall ED, Braughler JM. Glucocorticoid mechanisms in acute spinal cord injury: a review and therapeutic rationale. *Surg Neurol.* 1982;18(5):320-327.
26. Lammertse DP. Update on pharmaceutical trials in acute spinal cord injury. *J Spinal Cord Med.* 2004;27(4):319-325.
27. Bracken MB. Treatment of acute spinal cord injury with methylprednisolone: results of a multicenter, randomized clinical trial. *J Neurotrauma.* 1991;8(suppl 1):S47-S50.
28. Bracken MB, Shepard MJ, Collins WF, et al. A randomized, controlled trial of methylprednisolone or naloxone in the treatment of acute spinal-cord injury. Results of the Second National Acute Spinal Cord Injury Study. *N Engl J Med.* 1990;322(20):1405-1411.
29. Faden AI, Jacobs TP, Holaday JW. Thyrotropin-releasing hormone improves neurologic recovery after spinal trauma in cats. *N Engl J Med.* 1981;305(18):1063-1067.
30. Bracken MB, Shepard MJ, Collins WF Jr, et al. Methylprednisolone or naloxone treatment after acute spinal cord injury: 1-year follow-up data. Results of the Second National Acute Spinal Cord Injury Study. *J Neurosurg.* 1992;76(1):23-31.
31. Otani K, Abe H, Kadoya S, et al. Beneficial effect of methylprednisolone sodium succinate in the treatment of acute spinal cord injury. *Sekitsui Sekizui J.* 1994;7:633-647.
32. Bracken MB, Shepard MJ, Holford TR, et al. Administration of methylprednisolone for 24 or 48 hours or tirilazad mesylate for 48 hours in the treatment of acute spinal cord injury. Results of the Third National Acute Spinal Cord Injury Randomized Controlled Trial. National Acute Spinal Cord Injury Study. *JAMA.* 1997;277(20):1597-1604.
33. Agnati LF, Fuxe K, Calza L, et al. Further studies on the effects of the GM1 ganglioside on the degenerative and regenerative features of mesostriatal dopamine neurons. *Acta Physiol Scand Suppl.* 1984;532:37-44.
34. Bose B, Osterholm JL, Kalia M. Ganglioside-induced regeneration and reestablishment of axonal continuity in spinal cord-transected rats. *Neurosci Lett.* 1986;63(2): 165-169.
35. Toffano G, Agnati LF, Fuxe KG. The effect of the ganglioside GM1 on neuronal plasticity. *Int J Dev Neurosci.* 1986;4(2):97-100.
36. Toffano G, Savoini G, Moroni F, et al. GM1 ganglioside stimulates the regeneration of dopaminergic neurons in the central nervous system. *Brain Res.* 1983;261(1):163-166.
37. Geisler FH, Coleman WP, Grieco G, Poonian D. The Sygen multicenter acute spinal cord injury study. *Spine.* 2001;26(24 suppl):S87-S98.
38. Faden AI. New pharmacologic approaches to spinal cord injury: opiate antagonists and thyrotropin-releasing hormone. *Cent Nerv Syst Trauma.* 1985;2(1):5-8.
39. Faden AI. Opiate antagonists and thyrotropin-releasing hormone. II. Potential role in the treatment of central nervous system injury. *JAMA.* 1984;252(11):1452-1454.
40. Vink R, McIntosh TK, Faden AI. Treatment with the thyrotropin-releasing hormone analog CG3703 restores magnesium homeostasis following traumatic brain injury in rats. *Brain Res.* 1988;460(1):184-188.
41. Pitts LH, Ross A, Chase GA, Faden AI. Treatment with thyrotropin-releasing hormone (TRH) in patients with traumatic spinal cord injuries. *J Neurotrauma.* 1995;12(3): 235-243.
42. Guha A, Tator CH, Piper I. Effect of a calcium channel blocker on posttraumatic spinal cord blood flow. *J Neurosurg.* 1987;66(3):423-430.
43. Pointillart V, Gense D, Gross C, et al. Effects of nimodipine on posttraumatic spinal cord ischemia in baboons. *J Neurotrauma.* 1993;10(2):201-213.
44. Lepeintre JF, D'Arbigny P, Mathe JF, et al. Neuroprotective effect of gacyclidine. A multicenter double-blind pilot trial in patients with acute traumatic brain injury. *Neurochirurgie.* 2004;50(2-3 Pt 1):83-95.
45. Dinh P, Bhatia N, Rasouli A, et al. Transplantation of preconditioned Schwann cells following hemisection spinal cord injury. *Spine.* 2007;32(9):943-949.
46. Rasouli A, Bhatia N, Dinh P, et al. Resection of glial scar following spinal cord injury. *J Orthop Res.* 2009;27(7): 931-936.
47. Dubreuil CI, Winton MJ, McKerracher L. Rho activation patterns after spinal cord injury and the role of activated Rho in apoptosis in the central nervous system. *J Cell Biol.* 2003;162(2):233-243.
48. Sung JK, Miao L, Calvert JW, et al. A possible role of RhoA/Rho-kinase in experimental spinal cord injury in rat. *Brain Res.* 2003;959(1):29-38.
49. Dergham P, Ellezam B, Essagian C, et al. Rho signaling pathway targeted to promote spinal cord repair. *J Neurosci.* 2002;22(15):6570-6577.
50. Lehmann M, Fournier A, Selles-Navarro I, et al. Inactivation of Rho signaling pathway promotes CNS axon regeneration. *J Neurosci.* 1999;19(17):7537-7547.
51. Chen MS, Huber AB, van der Haar ME, et al. Nogo-A is a myelin-associated neurite outgrowth inhibitor and an antigen for monoclonal antibody IN-1. *Nature.* 2000;403(6768):434-439.
52. Weinmann O, Schnell L, Ghosh A, et al. Intrathecally infused antibodies against Nogo-A penetrate the CNS and downregulate the endogenous neurite growth inhibitor Nogo-A. *Mol Cell Neurosci.* 2006;32(1-2):161-173.
53. Bixby JL, Lilien J, Reichardt LF. Identification of the major proteins that promote neuronal process outgrowth on Schwann cells in vitro. *J Cell Biol.* 1988;107(1):353-361.

54. Bryan DJ, Wang KK, Chakalis-Haley DP. Effect of Schwann cells in the enhancement of peripheral-nerve regeneration. *J Reconstr Microsurg.* 1996;12(7):439-6.
55. Bunge MB. Bridging the transected or contused adult rat spinal cord with Schwann cell and olfactory ensheathing glia transplants. *Prog Brain Res.* 2002;137:275-282.
56. Keirstead HS, Morgan SV, Wilby MJ, Fawcett JW. Enhanced axonal regeneration following combined demyelination plus Schwann cell transplantation therapy in the injured adult spinal cord. *Exp Neurol.* 1999;159(1):225-236.
57. Tadie M, Liu S, Robert R, et al. Partial return of motor function in paralyzed legs after surgical bypass of the lesion site by nerve autografts three years after spinal cord injury. *J Neurotrauma.* 2002;19(8):909-916.
58. Pearse DD, Sanchez AR, Pereira FC, et al. Transplantation of Schwann cells and/or olfactory ensheathing glia into the contused spinal cord: survival, migration, axon association, and functional recovery. *Glia.* 2007;55(9):976-1000.
59. Huang H, Chen L, Wang H, et al. Influence of patients' age on functional recovery after transplantation of olfactory ensheathing cells into injured spinal cord injury. *Chin Med J.* 2003;116(10):1488-1491.
60. Lima C, Pratas-Vital J, Escada P, et al. Olfactory mucosa autografts in human spinal cord injury: a pilot clinical study. *J Spinal Cord Med.* 2006;29(3):191-203.
61. Mackay-Sim A, Féron F, Cochrane J, et al. Autologous olfactory ensheathing cell transplantation in human paraplegia: a 3-year clinical trial. *Brain.* 2008;131(9): 2376-2386.
62. Keirstead HS, et al. Human embryonic stem cell-derived oligodendrocyte progenitor cell transplants remyelinate and restore locomotion after spinal cord injury. *J Neurosci.* 2005;25(19):4694-4705.
63. Golden KL, et al. Transduced Schwann cells promote axon growth and myelination after spinal cord injury. *Exp Neurol.* 2007;207(2):203-217.

75 CHAPTER Injuries of the Upper Cervical Spine

Bobby K.-B. Tay
Frank J. Eismont

The upper cervical spine consists of the occiput, atlas, and axis. These three structures, along with their strong ligamentous attachments, are often referred to as the craniocervical junction (CCJ). This osseoligamentous complex that surrounds and protects the upper cervical spinal cord, the brain stem, and lower cranial nerves is anatomically and functionally distinct from the motion segments in the subaxial cervical spine (C3–C7). These differences also are responsible for the distinct patterns of injury that occur at the CCJ. The prevalence of injuries to the upper cervical spine has a bimodal distribution—they are most often encountered in children and in those older than 60 years of age. In the pediatric population, motor vehicle accidents and pedestrians hit by cars are the predominant mechanisms of injury. In the elderly, falls are the most common mechanism. Adults between these two age groups tend to suffer more injuries to the subaxial cervical spine. Upper cervical injuries occurring in these pediatric and intermediate age groups are often caused by high-energy trauma (vehicular accidents and falls) and are associated with a high rate of neurologic injury and mortality. Improvements in emergency medical care, trauma care, and imaging modalities have been beneficial in reducing both the mortality and morbidity of these injuries. Early detection and treatment significantly decreases mortality and improves overall outcomes.

As with internal fixation of extremity fractures, internal fixation of spine fractures has allowed early mobilization and rehabilitation of the patient, resulting in improved overall functional outcomes. The stability of internal fixation of the CCJ has also improved significantly over the past 15 years. Early plate/screw designs have evolved to rod/screw designs and plate–rod/screw hybrid designs, providing more versatility and improved fixation to the occiput using multiple points of fixation and the ability to place screws in the midline on the occiput, where the bone is thickest. Methods to obtain segmental fixation of the atlas and axis through the lateral masses, pars, pedicle, and lamina have improved the spinal surgeon's ability to correct deformity and decompress the neural elements without jeopardizing bony fixation and stability. Advances in the rehabilitation of patients with high cervical spinal cord injuries (SCIs) have improved the overall functional abilities of these patients.

Demographics

Traumatic injuries to the upper cervical spine are most often encountered in children and in people older than 60 years of age. Fortunately, they are still rare occurrences in children. Motor vehicle accidents are the cause of pediatric cervical spine trauma in about 38% of cases.[1–3] Cervical spine injuries in children account for 1% to 9% of all reported pediatric spinal trauma.[4,5] Upper cervical spine injuries are responsible for the majority of these, accounting for 56% to 73% of all cervical spine injuries in children.[2,6] Head injury occurs in conjunction with cervical spine injuries in up to 53% of these cases. When these two entities are concurrent, the overall mortality is very high (41%).[7]

Upper cervical spine injuries constitute a large proportion of cervical spine trauma in people older than 60 years of age. Injuries to the C1–C2 complex account for up to 69.8% of all cervical spine trauma in those older than 60 years.[8] Odontoid fractures alone can constitute up to 57% of all cervical spine injuries in this age group. Unlike the pediatric and young adult populations, upper cervical spine trauma in the elderly often occurs from minor trauma. Falls are often the predominant cause of injury. Any fall greater than 3 feet or 5 stairs requires cervical spine clearance with appropriate imaging. Many explanations for this phenomenon include the presence of weakened bone at the CCJ owing to osteoporosis/osteopenia, higher stresses on the upper cervical spine owing to spondylosis and deformity of the lower cervical spine (leading to compensatory hyperextension at the CCJ), and an increased propensity to fall from deterioration in locomotor response and balance control due to age and cervical spinal stenosis. The lower energy of the trauma is directly correlated to the lower rate of neurologic injury seen in this age group after injury as compared with the pediatric and young adult populations. However, when neurologic deficits occur, they can have devastating consequences. A 26% to 28% mortality for upper cervical level SCI has been reported for this population, with a dismal 59% survival at 2 years.[9–12]

In the young adult population, the majority of patients with spinal column injury are young males (up to 30% are males in their 30s).[13] The most common mechanism in this age group is vehicular accidents, followed by falls, gunshot injuries, and sports injuries. Most of the cervical spine trauma in this age group occurs in the subaxial spine, and is often associated with a high-energy mechanism, severe head injury, or a focal neurologic deficit.[14] Trauma to the CCJ in this population is often associated with severe neurologic injury and head trauma, with relatively high rates of mortality and morbidity.

Anatomy of the Upper Cervical Spine (Craniocervical Junction)

The upper cervical spine is a complex three-unit joint that includes the bones of the occiput, atlas, and axis; their synovial articulations; and the associated ligamentous structures. The six synovial joints in this complex include the paired occipitoatlantal joints, the anterior and posterior median atlanto-odontoid joints, and the paired atlantoaxial joints. These joints allow for a significant amount of motion at the CCJ. The occiput–C1 articulation supplies approximately 50% of total cervical flexion and extension, and the C1–C2 articulations supply 50% of total cervical rotation.[15] Corresponding to this, the majority of the mechanical stability at the CCJ is provided by the investing ligamentous structures. An understanding of the anatomy of the CCJ is necessary to appreciate the spectrum of injuries that occur in the upper cervical spine and the strategies that have been devised to treat them. The specific articulations, ligamentous restraints, and neurovascular structures at risk for injury are addressed here in a systematic fashion.

The occiput articulates with the atlas through paired occipitoatlantal joints. The occipital condyle is oval and sloped inferiorly from lateral to medial in the coronal plane, making a 25- to 28-degree angle with the midsagittal plane. The convex occipital condyles articulate with the concave superior articular facets of C1 in a "cup-and-saucer" type fashion. In the coronal plane, the joint slopes medially toward the foramen magnum. The shape of the occipitoatlantal joint allows significant flexion and extension and some lateral bending, but minimal axial rotation. Flexion is limited by the bony impingement of the anterior portion of the foramen magnum on the odontoid process; extension is limited by the posterior arch of the atlas impinging on the posterior aspect of the skull. The anterior atlanto-odontoid joint lies between the anterior arch of the atlas and the anterior aspect of the dens. The posterior atlanto-odontoid articulation lies between the posterior aspect of the dens and the anterior portion of the transverse ligament. The paired atlantoaxial joints are situated between the inferior articular facets of the atlas and the superior articular facets of the axis. These joints are fairly shallow to allow for a significant amount of motion at the CCJ. The ligamentous restraints provide the necessary stability to prevent injury to the enclosed brain stem and spinal cord (Fig. 75.1).

The anterior longitudinal ligament (ALL) attaches to the anterior body of the axis, the anterior arch of the atlas, and the anteroinferior edge of the foramen magnum. The cruciform ligament is composed of vertical and transverse portions. The vertical portion attaches to the anterior edge of the foramen magnum and the posterior aspect of the body of the axis. The transverse component of the cruciform ligament is commonly referred to as the transverse ligament. This important structure is made entirely of relatively nonelastic collagen fibers, and extends between the osseous tubercles on the medial aspects of the lateral masses of the atlas. The tectorial membrane is the broad cephalic extension of the posterior longitudinal ligament (PLL) and runs from the posterior surface of the body and dens of the axis to the anterolateral edge of the foramen magnum. This structure is a primary stabilizer of the occipitoatlantal articulation[15] and helps to limit extension at this joint. The nuchal ligament extends from the posterior border of the occiput to the spinous processes of the cervical vertebrae

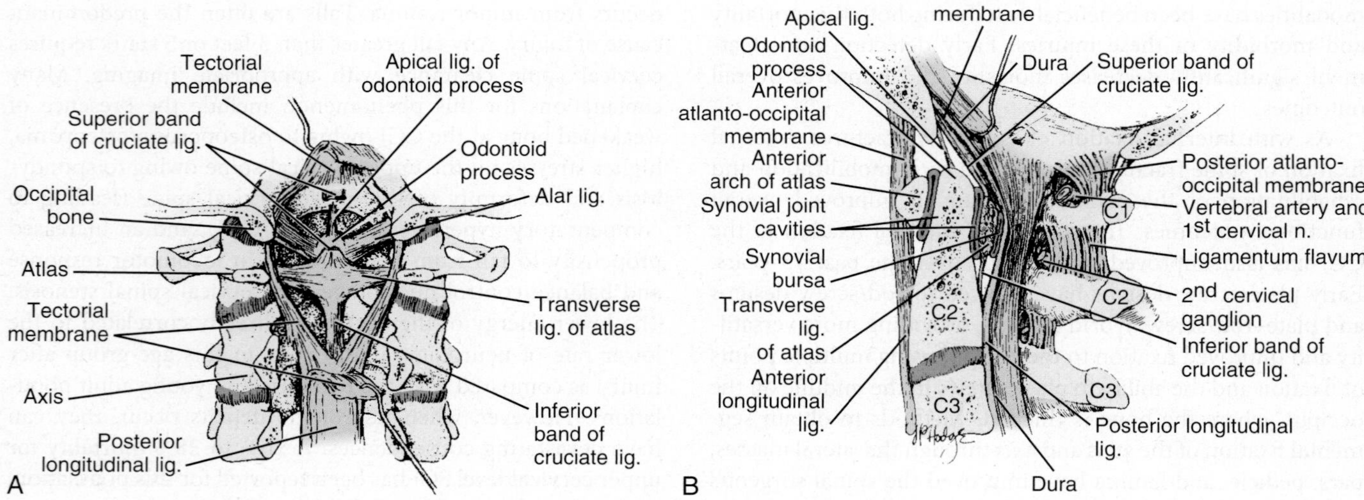

FIG. 75.1 The ligaments at the occipitocervical junction. (A) Coronal view shows the two alar ligaments extending from the superior tip of the odontoid process and extending to the medial aspect of the occipital condyles. (B) Midsagittal view shows the tectorial membrane, which is continuous with the posterior longitudinal ligament. (From Martel W. The occipital-atlanto-axial joints in rheumatoid arthritis and ankylosing spondylitis. *AJR Am J Roentgenol.* 1961;86:223–240.)

to C7 and the intervening interspinous ligaments. The anterior occipitoatlantal membrane, part of the ALL, extends from the cephalad portion of the anterior arch of the atlas to the anterior edge of the foramen magnum. The atlanto-odontoid ligament runs from the anterior surface of the odontoid process and the caudal portion of the anterior arch of the atlas. The apical ligament of the dens lies between the vertical band of the cruciform ligament and the anterior occipitoatlantal ligament. This structure connects the apex of the dens with the anterior edge of the foramen magnum. The alar ligaments are paired structures that arise from the dorsolateral aspect of the dens and run obliquely to connect with the inferomedial aspect of the occipital condyles and the lateral masses of the atlas. These ligaments are very important stabilizers of the occipitoatlantal joint, limiting axial rotation and lateral bending.[16] Like the transverse ligament, the alar ligaments are also made entirely of collagen fibers, and failure occurs at 10% stretch.[17] These ligaments are most vulnerable in whiplash-type injuries.[18] The posterior occipitoatlantal membrane attaches to the posterior margin of the foramen magnum and the posterior arch of the atlas. The posterior atlantoaxial membrane runs between the posterior arches of the atlas and the axis.

The vertebral artery and the internal carotid artery lie in close proximity to the osseous structures of the CCJ. Within the atlas and the axis, the paired vertebral arteries typically lie in the foramen transversarium. At this level, the artery is susceptible to injury by shearing forces with rotation and flexion or extension. At the upper atlantal surface, the artery curves posteriorly into a transverse groove in the atlas behind the superior atlantal articular facet. It then enters the subarachnoid space by piercing the posterior occipitoatlantal membrane and dura mater just medial to the occipital condyle. The vertebral artery can often take an aberrant course around or within the C1 ring. In computed tomography (CT) studies, arcuate foramen was present in 24% of patients and a high-riding vertebral artery, ponticulus posticus, was present in 34% of patients.[19] The internal carotid artery is adjacent to the anterior surface of the lateral mass of C1. This position renders it susceptible to injury by a forward thrust of the lateral mass as the head is forcefully rotated to the contralateral side.[19]

The neurologic structures protected by the osseoligamentous components of the CCJ include the medulla oblongata, lower cranial nerves, upper cervical spinal cord, and the C1 and C2 nerve roots. The medulla oblongata is bounded by the foramen magnum. The hypoglossal nerves (CN XII) traverse through the base of the occipital condyles within the anterior condyloid canals. With these nerves travel a meningeal branch of the ascending pharyngeal artery and an emissary vein. The nerve then descends ventrally and vertically 2 to 3 mm lateral to the center of the lateral mass of C1. At this point, it is at risk for iatrogenic injury by bicortical C1–C2 transarticular screws and C1 lateral mass screws. The jugular foramen (posterior foramen lacerum) is located lateral to the occipital condyle and the hypoglossal canal and posterior to the carotid canal. The glossopharyngeal nerves (CN IX) and the Jacobson nerves (branch of CN IX) pass through the anteromedial portion of the jugular foramen (pars nervosa). The vagus nerves (CN X), the Arnold nerves (branch of CN X), and the spinal accessory nerves (CN XI) pass through the posterolateral portion of the jugular foramen (pars vascularis) along with the internal jugular veins, posterior meningeal arteries, and small meningeal branches of the ascending pharyngeal artery. The proximity of these neurologic structures to the bony anatomy of the CCJ places them at risk for injury in the presence of ligamentous instability or fracture.

Clinical Evaluation

The treatment of a patient with a cervical spine injury regardless of location is initiated at the scene of the injury. Without exception, all victims of trauma are suspected to have a cervical injury until proven otherwise. Cervical spine injury has been closely linked to the presence of severe head injury (odds ratio [OR] = 8.5), a high-energy mechanism (OR = 11.6), or a focal neurologic deficit (OR = 58).[14] In suspected injuries of the upper cervical spine, an adequate airway and ventilation must be established because upper SCI can lead to diaphragmatic and intercostal paralysis with respiratory failure. In addition, large retropharyngeal hematomas can cause upper airway obstruction. Nasotracheal intubation or cricothyroidotomy is safest in the acute setting because it causes less cervical spine motion than direct oral intubation techniques.[19–21] Improvements in fiberoptic imaging have resulted in technologies such as the Glidescope. This videolaryngoscope allows oral–tracheal intubation without the need for significant neck manipulation and is technically easier than the traditional method of fiberoptic-assisted intubation. Once the patient's airway, breathing, and circulation are stabilized, initial stabilization of the cervical spine begins with the application of a rigid cervical collar, a spine board, and sandbags.

In general, noncontiguous spinal injuries can occur in 6% of patients. These fractures can be easily missed in the presence of head injury, upper cervical injury, or cervicothoracic injury. Atlas fractures, specifically, are associated with up to a 50% incidence of concurrent cervical spine fractures.[22] Facial and head injuries are also commonly seen in conjunction with fractures and ligamentous disruptions of the CCJ. Upper cervical injuries are also more frequently seen in patients with trauma to the lower third of the face.[23] In addition, up to 50% of patients with cervical spine injuries, SCIs, or both have associated head trauma. Brain damage is more associated with upper cervical injuries than with injuries to the subaxial spine.[24] Subarachnoid hemorrhages, subdural hemorrhages, and cerebral contusions must be diagnosed and treated expeditiously because they are the most common cause of mortality in these patients.

In addition to spinal trauma, other injuries should be assessed because they may influence the treatment of the spinal lesion and could significantly affect the outcome of the patient. In cervical spine trauma, much attention has been paid to the evaluation of these patients for vertebral artery injury (see Chapter 73). Friedman and colleagues reported a 24% overall incidence of vertebral artery injury in 37 cases of nonpenetrating cervical spine trauma.[25] Vaccaro and associates noted a 19.7% incidence of vertebral artery injury found by magnetic resonance angiography in 61 patients.[26] In Cothren and coworkers' series, 18% of 69 patients with vertebral artery injury and cervical spine trauma sustained injuries to the CCJ.[27] The incidence of vertebral artery injury increases if the fracture extends into the foramen transversarium.[28] Bilateral or dominant vertebral artery injury can cause fatal ischemic damage to the brain stem and cerebellum.[29] Delayed cortical blindness and recurrent quadriparesis can also occur from occult vertebral artery injury after cervical trauma.[30] Despite the high incidence of vertebral artery injury with cervical trauma as well as the potential morbidity and mortality associated with vertebral artery injury, the great majority of these injuries are clinically silent.

Neurologic evaluation of injuries to the CCJ can be difficult because there is no specific myotomal or dermatomal distributions of motor and sensory loss, and it is further confounded by the frequent coexistence of facial and head trauma. Injuries to the C1 and C2 roots generally result in sensory deficits to the occiput and posterior scalp. A complete SCI at this level can result in ventilator-dependent quadriplegia. Incomplete SCI syndromes can also occur. At the occipitocervical junction, a peculiar syndrome of incomplete paralysis can develop as a result of compression/injury of the pyramidal decussation on the anterior aspect of the brain stem where the corticospinal tracts cross from one side to the other. The tracts to the arms cross cephalad to the tracts to the legs. If the primary injury is to the upper decussation, the arms can be more affected and give the appearance of a central cord syndrome. More caudal injury will affect the legs more than the arms. It is even possible to affect crossed arm fibers and uncrossed leg fibers, the so-called cruciate paralysis as described by Bell.[31] These patients can also have large variations in heart rate, blood pressure, and respiratory rate owing to injuries to the cardiovascular and respiratory centers in the brain stem.[32] Dysfunction of the lower cranial nerves (CN IX, X, XI, XII) is often seen with severe injuries to the occipitoatlantal joint and the skull base.

Imaging

Plain radiography is used as the first imaging modality for the upper cervical spine. The standard series includes anteroposterior (AP), lateral, and open-mouth views. In general, about 85% of all significant injuries to the cervical spine will be detected on the lateral view of the cervical spine. In the upper cervical spine, the lateral view and the open-mouth view are the most useful. Flexion and extension views will be inadequate to assess for ligamentous injury owing to voluntary guarding in 33% of cases.[33]

Evaluation of the lateral cervical view should include assessment for prevertebral soft tissue swelling, sagittal alignment, and instability. The soft tissue shadow should be less than 10 mm at C1, 5 mm at C3, and 15 to 20 mm at C6. Although this measure may be nonspecific for cervical injury, prevertebral soft tissue swelling may be the only evidence of severe ligamentous injury to the upper cervical spine. The sagittal alignment of the spine should be assessed by evaluation of four imaginary lines: (1) a line formed by the anterior margins of the vertebral bodies, (2) a line formed by the posterior margins of the vertebral bodies, (3) a line formed by the anterior cortical margins of the lamina, and (4) a line formed by the tips of the spinous processes. In the upper cervical spine, the relationships of these imaginary lines to the basion and opisthion also should be evaluated.

CT remains the most sensitive imaging modality to evaluate fractures of the upper cervical spine, subaxial spine, and cervicothoracic junction. In a prospective study of polytrauma patients, CT used as a primary screening tool had a sensitivity of 84% in detecting upper cervical injury.[14] CT is also cost-effective as a primary screening tool, especially in high- and moderate-risk patients.[34] With the added benefit of sagittal and coronal reconstructed images, CT has immense power to demonstrate complex fracture patterns not easily seen on standard radiography and on the axial images, especially at the occipitocervical junction.[35]

The availability of intraoperative CT scanning, such as the O-arm (Medtronic) and the Iso-C (Siemens), combined with better image guidance software allows real-time assessment of fracture displacement and reduction. This technology is especially useful in patients who are difficult to image due to size or associated injuries. When combined with intraoperative image guidance software, internal fixation can be more precisely and safely placed than with traditional fluoroscopic imaging.

Magnetic resonance imaging (MRI) is not as good as CT or plain radiographs in the identification and evaluation of cervical fractures. Klein and coworkers showed that MRI had only a 11.5% sensitivity for posterior fractures and a 36.7% sensitivity for anterior fractures.[36] Katzberg and colleagues reported that, for acute fractures, MRI had a weighted average sensitivity of 43%, compared with 48% for conventional radiography.[13] Vaccaro and associates also noted that MRI is not cost-effective as a screening device in patients without a neurologic deficit.[37]

Despite its inadequacies in evaluating bony detail, MRI is unsurpassed for the assessment of the soft tissue elements in the cervical spine. These structures include the intervertebral disc, ligamentous structures, and the spinal cord itself.[13] MRI is much more sensitive and specific than plain radiographs for the evaluation of a prevertebral hematoma. MRI is also useful for the detection of spinal cord hemorrhage, which, if present, carries a poor prognosis for neurologic recovery.[38] Acute hemorrhage has a low signal intensity on T2-weighted images (secondary to intracellular deoxyhemoglobin) and becomes hyperintense over the next several days after it becomes converted to extracellular methemoglobin. MRI diffusion studies allow a more accurate assessment of the degree of spinal stenosis. These diffusion studies assess the flow of cerebrospinal fluid (CSF) around the spinal cord at an area of constriction. If the degree of spinal stenosis is severe, the CSF flow is significantly compromised.[39]

Newer magnets that can produce field strengths over 3 Tesla are able to image individual tracts within the spinal cord itself, providing a more accurate assessment of the neurologic injury after cervical trauma.

MRI neurography provides detailed visualization of individual nerve roots as they exit the brain stem, the CCJ, and the subaxial cervical spine. This MRI modality can help distinguish root-level injuries from more peripheral injuries as well as double-crush-type nerve damage.[40]

Bedside fluoroscopic flexion and extension views have shown some diagnostic value in clearing the cervical spine in obtunded patients. In one report, it was noted that 30% of these patients could not be adequately evaluated by this technique.[41] Other researchers, however, have found this helpful, using a combination of initial inline traction followed by flexion and extension views only if the traction views are normal.[42] Due to the space constraints of most intensive care units and the lack of appropriate built-in shielding for the extensive use of fluoroscopic imaging, bedside fluoroscopy is relatively impractical in most hospitals. In addition, the use of both CT and MRI may provide sufficient information to allow removal of the cervical collar in an obtunded patient without the need for manipulation of the neck.

Initial Stabilization

In general, reduction and stabilization of the cervical spine in the acute setting is usually accomplished by Gardner-Wells tong traction in a rotating bed. The only contraindications to the use of traction in injuries of the CCJ include type II occipitoatlantal dislocations and type IIA hangman's fractures, in which the application of traction can result in significant distraction at the injury site and increased neurologic deficit. The use of a rotating bed minimizes the incidence of pulmonary complications, decubitus ulcers, and deep vein thrombosis. Carbon fiber Gardner-Wells tongs are often sufficient for injuries of the upper cervical spine, because gentle traction is adequate in most cases to achieve and maintain a closed reduction.

Specific Injuries to the Upper Cervical Spine

Occipital Condyle Fractures

Most injuries to the occipital condyles are caused by high-energy trauma to the head and neck. Bell reported the first case of occipital condylar fracture in 1817. The incidence of occipital condyle fractures is reported to range from 3% to 16%.[42,43]

The clinical presentation of these injuries can range from minimal deficits to frank quadriparesis. Patients may complain of high cervical pain, torticollis, headaches, and impaired mobility. The most severe neurologic deficits are often seen with concurrent head injury. Up to 31% of these patients may exhibit acute lower cranial nerve deficits.

Although radiographs may show some abnormal soft tissue swelling in the presence of an occipital condyle fracture, these injuries are often extremely difficult to detect with conventional radiography (Fig. 75.2).[44]

CT with reconstruction is the imaging modality of choice in the diagnosis and classification of these fractures. MRI can be used to assess for damage to the alar and tectorial membranes, but is less useful than CT from a treatment perspective.

The most utilized classification system for occipital condyle injuries was described by Anderson and Montesano (Fig. 75.3).[45] The injuries are categorized into three types according to morphology and mechanism of injury. Type I injuries are impaction fractures of the condyle from axial loading. These fractures tend to be comminuted. The tectorial membrane and the alar ligaments are usually intact. Unilateral type I lesions are stable, but bilateral lesions may be unstable. Type II injuries are part of a more extensive basioccipital fracture that involves one or both occipital condyles. The common mechanism of injury is a direct blow to the skull. The tectorial and alar ligaments are intact, and the fracture is usually stable. Type III

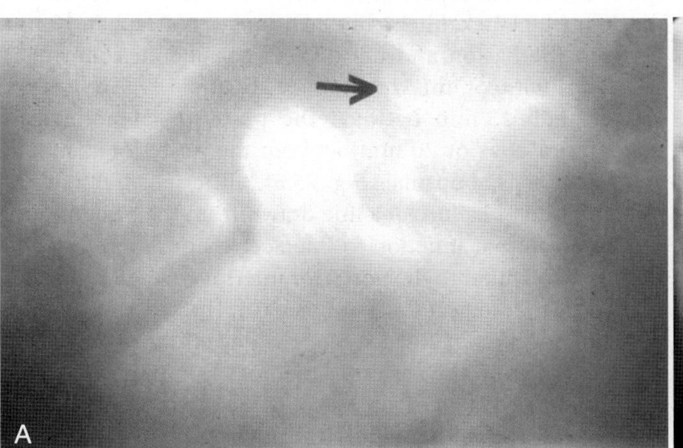

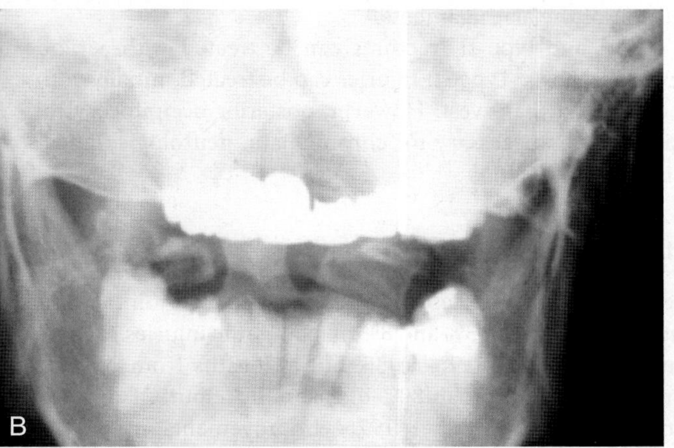

FIG. 75.2 Images of a patient who had fallen on his head and complained of a persistent pain in his upper neck as well as persistent headaches. (A) Open-mouth view shows an asymmetry between the plane of the skull and the plane of the C2 vertebra (*arrow*). The head appears tipped to one side. (B) Anteroposterior tomogram of the occipitocervical junction shows that the patient had sustained a type I impaction fracture of the occipital condyle. This would be expected to cause laxity of the alar ligament on that side. He was treated with a rigid cervical collar for 8 weeks, with gradual improvement of his pain. (From Eismont FJ, Frazier DD. Cranial cervical trauma. In: Levine AM, Eismont FJ, Garfin SR, Zigler JE [eds]. *Spine Trauma*. Philadelphia: WB Saunders; 1998:207.)

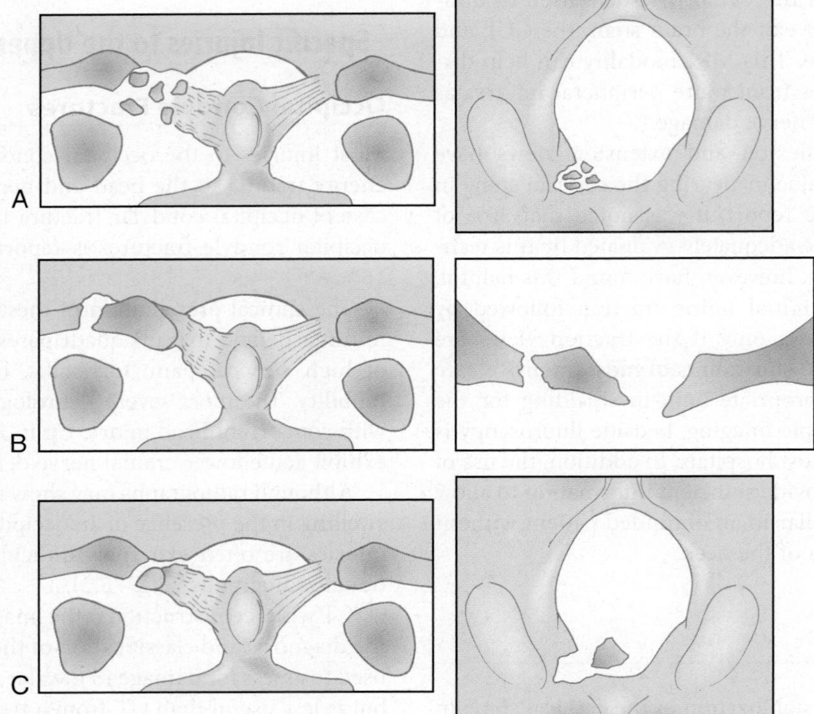

FIG. 75.3 The best available classification for fractures involving the occipital condyles. (A) Impacted occipital condyle fracture. In most cases, this would be a stable injury and can be treated with a collar. (B) This occipital condyle fracture is associated with a basilar skull fracture. In most cases, this would be stable. (C) This condyle fracture destabilizes the origin of the alar ligament, and may be associated with significant occipitocervical instability. (From Anderson PA, Montesano PX. Morphology and treatment of occipital condyle fractures. *Spine*. 1988;13:731–736.)

injuries are avulsion fractures near the alar ligament insertion that result in medial displacement of the condylar fracture fragment from the inferomedial aspect of the occipital condyle into the foramen magnum. The mechanism of injury is a forced rotation of the head combined with lateral bending. Type III fractures are potentially unstable injuries owing to avulsion of the alar ligaments.

Type I and type II fractures can be treated with a rigid cervical orthosis. Type III injuries can be treated initially with an orthosis or halo vest. However, posterior occipitocervical fusion may be necessary for chronic pain, neurologic deficit, or instability.

Atlanto-Occipital Injuries

The incidence of injuries to the atlanto-occipital joint is estimated to be between 5% and 8% of fatal traffic injuries.[46] These injuries account for 19% to 35% of all deaths from cervical spine trauma. More than 80% of cases of occiput-C1 dislocations were reported after 1975. Improvements in on-site resuscitation and emergency transportation have increased the number of patients who survive this catastrophic injury, which is typically the result of a motor vehicle accident. In a review of 146 traffic fatalities, Alker and associates found a 5% incidence of occipitoatlantal dislocations.[47] Children younger than 12 years of age are uniquely predisposed to this injury because their occipitoatlantal joints are flatter and because their head weight to body weight ratio is significantly greater than in adults.

Radiographically, significant retropharyngeal soft tissue swelling at C3 will be seen (Fig. 75.4). Multiple anatomic lines mark the normal relationship of occiput to C1. A line drawn down the cranial aspect of the clivus should be tangential to the dens (the Wackenheim line). Distance greater than 10 mm between the basion and the dens is considered abnormal.[48] The sensitivity of this method is about 50%. An interval greater than 13 mm between the posterior mandible and the anterior atlas or 20 mm between the posterior mandible and the dens is abnormal (Fig. 75.5).[49] The sensitivity of this method is 25%. Failure of a line drawn from the basion to the axis spinolaminar junction to intersect C2 or failure of a line from the opisthion to the posterior inferior corner of the body of the axis to intersect C1 is abnormal.[50] The sensitivity of this method ranges from 20% to 75%. The Powers ratio, the ratio of the distance from the basion to the posterior arch of the atlas divided by the distance from the opisthion to the anterior arch of the atlas, should be 1.0 or less in the absence of anterior occipitoatlantal dislocation (Fig. 75.6).[51] Another method to diagnose occipitoatlantal subluxation or dislocation on plain radiographs was described by Harris and colleagues.[52,53] They described a posterior axial line as the cranial extent of the posterior cortex of the axis body. If the distance between the basion and the posterior axial line (the basion–axial interval) is greater than 12 mm, or if the basion-dental interval is greater

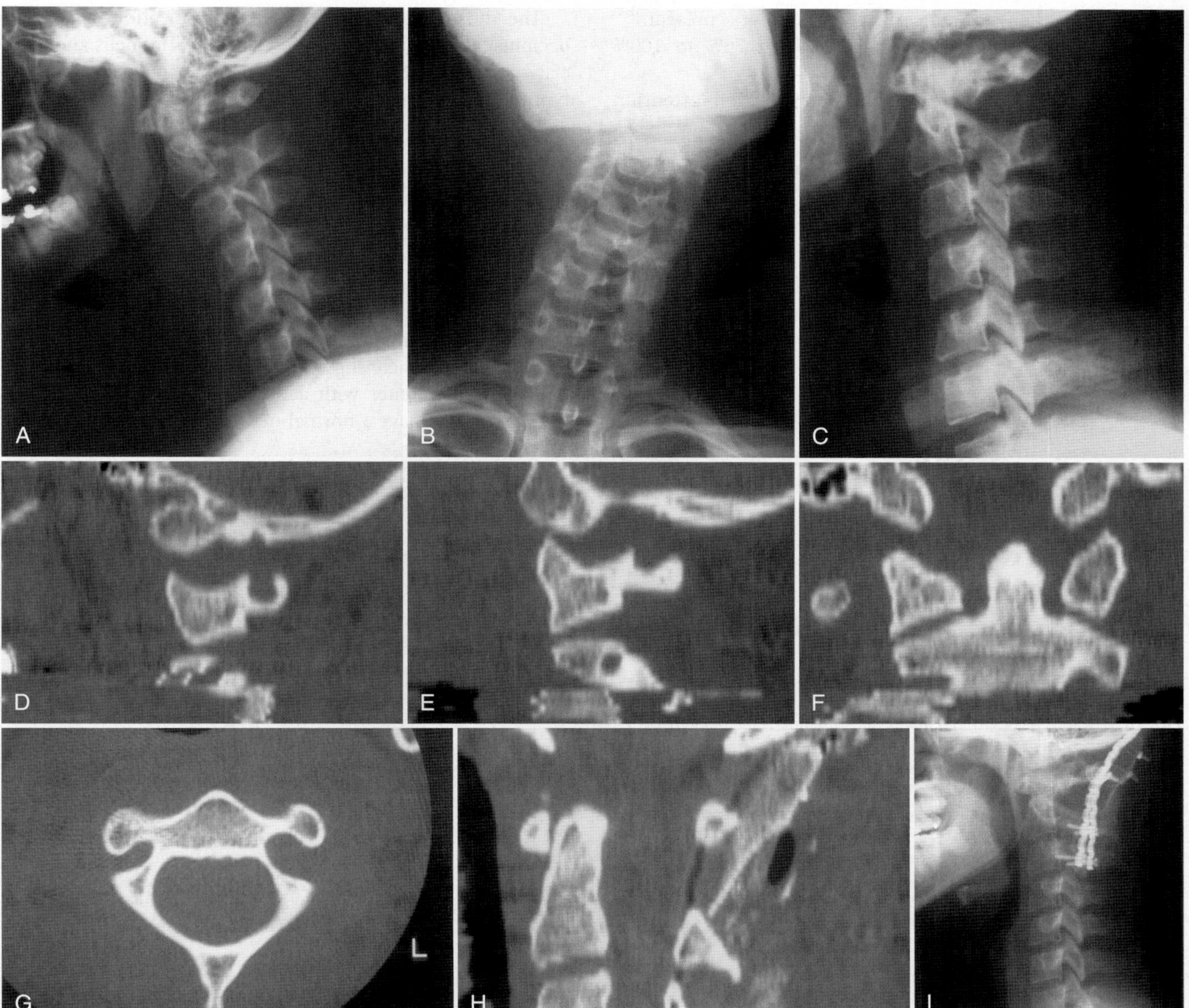

FIG. 75.4 This patient was involved in a motor vehicle accident with an unrecognized occipitocervical injury. (A) Radiograph taken when the patient originally presented to the emergency department shows more than 2 cm of soft tissue swelling in front of C3. His injury was not recognized and he was discharged from the hospital. He was neurologically normal. (B) Ten days later, when the patient returned to the emergency department, he had an obvious occipitocervical deformity. He was still neurologically normal. (C) When the patient was placed in 5 lb of traction, it was apparent that he had separation between his occiput and C1 vertebra. (D) Computed tomography (CT) shows that he has anterior displacement of his occipital condyle in relation to his C1 lateral mass as well as approximately 1 cm distraction of his occipitocervical joint. At the C2 level, he also has a fracture extending into the lateral mass of C2. (E) On the opposite side, the same type of anterior subluxation of the occiput on C1 can be seen as well as separation of the occipitocervical joint. (F) Coronal reconstructed CT scan shows the pathologic distraction between the occiput and C1. Only a 2-mm joint space would be expected at this level. (G) Transverse CT scan shows that the patient has a vertebral artery course that is more medial than usual on each side and prohibited passage of C1–C2 transarticular screws. (H) Midsagittal reconstructed CT scan shortly after surgery shows the large structural bone graft placed centrally between the occiput and C2. This was wired independently to the skull and spine, and is necessary in addition to the plates and screws to ensure adequate healing and stability. (I) Lateral radiograph of the spine taken approximately 2 years after the patient's injury. His spine has maintained normal alignment at the occipitocervical junction and stability has been restored. (From Eismont FJ, Frazier DD. Cranial cervical trauma. In: Levine AM, Eismont FJ, Garfin SR, Zigler JE [eds]. *Spine Trauma*. Philadelphia: WB Saunders; 1998: 205-206.)

than 12 mm, then occipitocervical instability is present.[52,53] The sensitivity of this method varies from 76% to 100% (Fig. 75.7).

Because this is a very unstable injury, flexion–extension views are not recommended. However, if they are available, there should be less than 1 mm of translation seen at the occipitoatlantal articulation. In children, more than 5 mm widening of the occipitoatlantal joints should raise the suspicion of this injury.

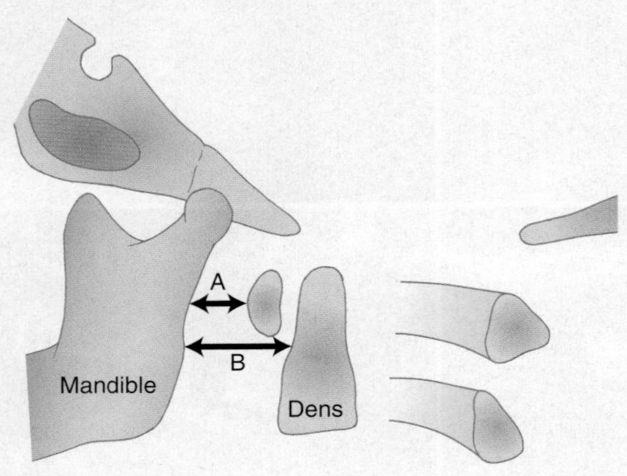

FIG. 75.5 Normal relationship of the posterior ramus of the mandible in relation to the anterior ring of C1 and the dens. Radiographs were taken of 23 normal patients, and distance A averaged 2 mm with a range from −10 to +9 mm. The average for distance B was 10 mm, with a range from 2 to 17 mm. Distances significantly greater than these averages denote anterior occipitocervical dislocation; distances significantly smaller indicate likely posterior occipitocervical dislocation. All radiographs must be done with the patient's mouth closed. (From Dublin AB, Marks WM, Weinstock D, Newton TH. Traumatic dislocation of the atlanto-occipital articulation [AOA] with short-term survival—with a radiographic method of measuring the AOA. *J Neurosurg.* 1980;52:541–546.)

The most commonly employed classification system for occiput-C1 dislocations was described by Traynelis and associates (Fig. 75.8), who categorized these injuries into three types.[54] In type I injuries, there is anterior displacement of the occiput on the atlas. Type II injuries are the result of longitudinal distraction. Any traction applied to a type II injury can result in progression of the existing neurologic deficit. Type III injuries involve a posterior subluxation or dislocation. Very light traction of about 5 pounds applied to type I and type III injuries will help to reduce the dislocation and may improve the neurologic deficit. Radiographs should be taken immediately to ensure that there is no overdistraction.

As noted earlier, the mortality from head-on-neck dislocation is extremely high. Only 20% of patients presenting to the trauma center with acute traumatic atlanto-occipital dislocation will have a normal neurologic examination.[55] The

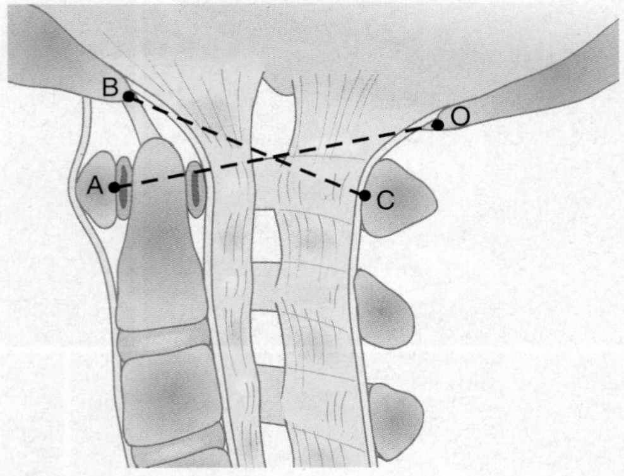

FIG. 75.6 Midsagittal section through the craniocervical junction. B, basion; O, opisthion; A, anterior arch of the atlas; C, posterior arch of the atlas. The ratio of BC/OA should always be ≤1. If it is >1, the patient most likely has an anterior occipitocervical subluxation or dislocation. (From Powers B, Miller MD, Kramer RS, et al. Traumatic anterior atlanto-occipital dislocation. *Neurosurgery.* 1979;4:12–17.)

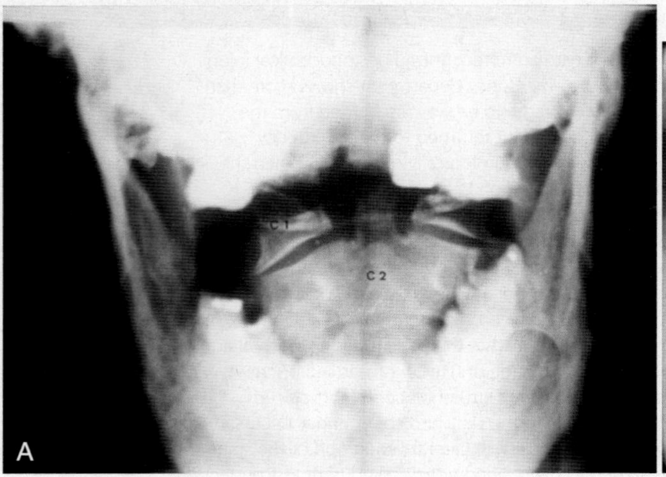

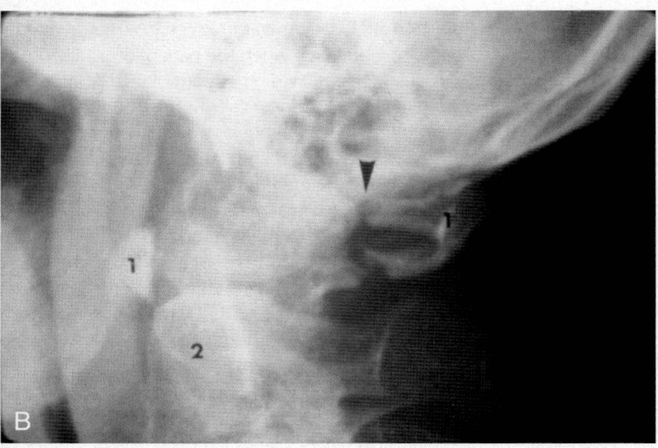

FIG. 75.7 This 68-year-old man was involved in a high-speed motor vehicle accident and was ejected from the vehicle. He complained of neck pain and had a fracture of his femur. He was initially neurologically normal; he was placed in a soft cervical collar and his femur was immobilized. (A) Anteroposterior radiograph of the upper cervical spine looks relatively normal. (B) Cone-down lateral radiograph of the upper cervical spine reveals a fracture of the posterior arch of C1 (*arrowhead*). It also appears that his basion is slightly more posterior than normal. There is significant soft tissue swelling in the retropharyngeal space at C1 and C2.

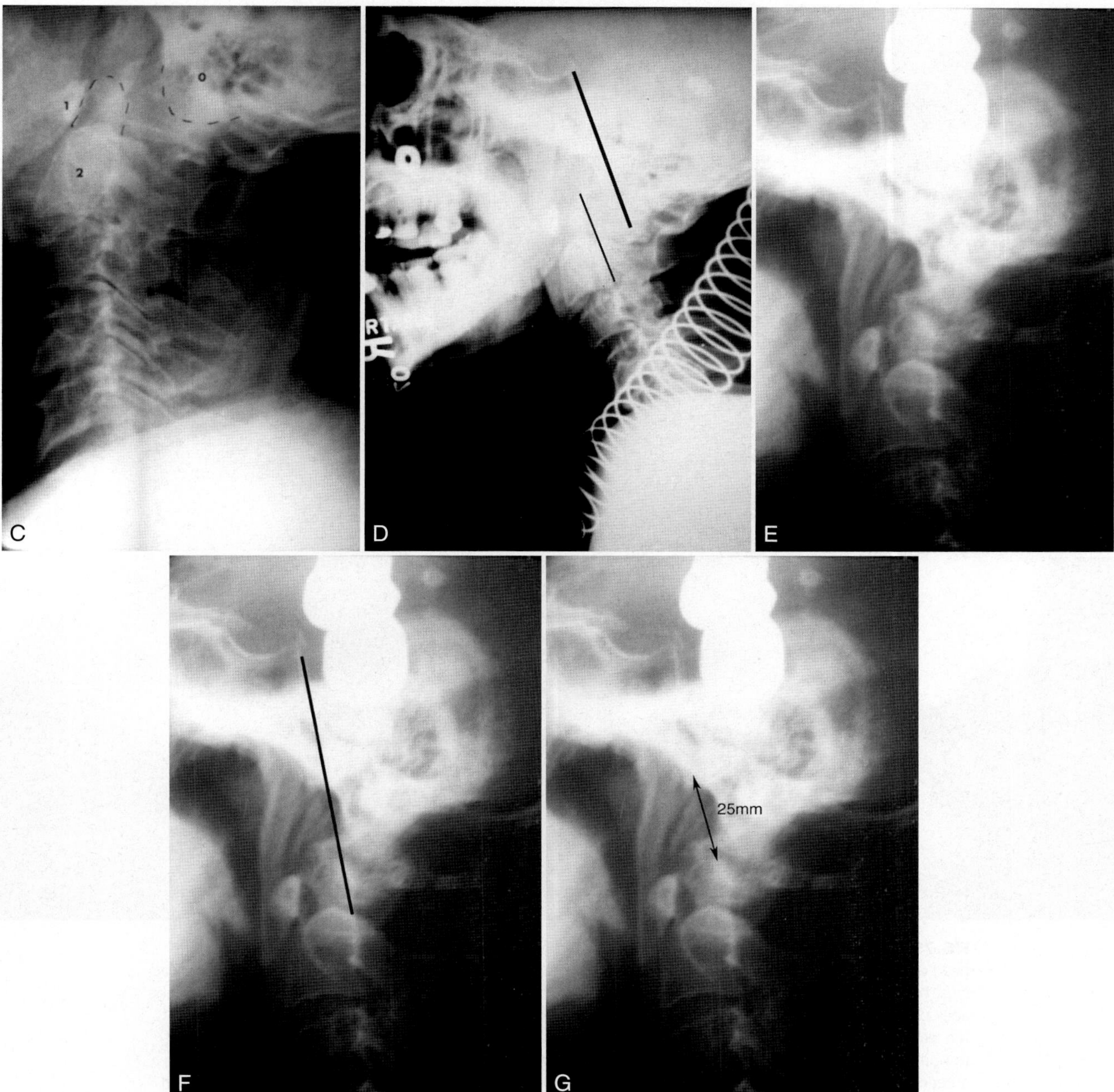

FIG. 75.7, cont'd (C) At 10 days postinjury, the *dotted lines* mark occipital condyles and the odontoid process. It is apparent that his head is posteriorly displaced on the atlas. At this time, he was in a soft cervical collar. He was experiencing problems with hypertension and paroxysmal atrial tachycardia and respiratory distress associated with a spastic quadriparesis. His head-on-neck dislocation was diagnosed at this time, and he was placed in skull tong traction of 4.6 kg. (D) Lateral radiograph shows a posterior dislocation also. The *thick dark line* demonstrates the Wackenheim line extending from the posterior sella turcica down the clivus and over the basion. This line should normally be tangential to the posterior aspect of the odontoid. In this case, there is almost 2 cm of posterior subluxation. It can also be noted that the posterior aspect of the ramus of the mandible also significantly overlaps the anterior arch of the atlas, which, according to Dublin's criteria, denotes posterior occipitocervical dislocation. (E) Lateral radiograph of the upper cervical spine shows that the occiput is correctly located over the atlas and odontoid, but that there is moderate overdistraction. At this time, the weight was reduced to 2.3 kg of traction. The patient's quadriparesis resolved over several hours, and his spasticity subsided over approximately 6 weeks. (F) The Wackenheim line is now drawn and is almost perfectly tangential to the posterior aspect of the odontoid as it would normally be seen. This shows that the posterior occipital subluxation has been corrected. (G) This measurement from the basion to the tip of the odontoid measures 25 mm. This line of Harris should normally be ≤12 mm. Thus, this line demonstrates the overdistraction that is present.

Continued

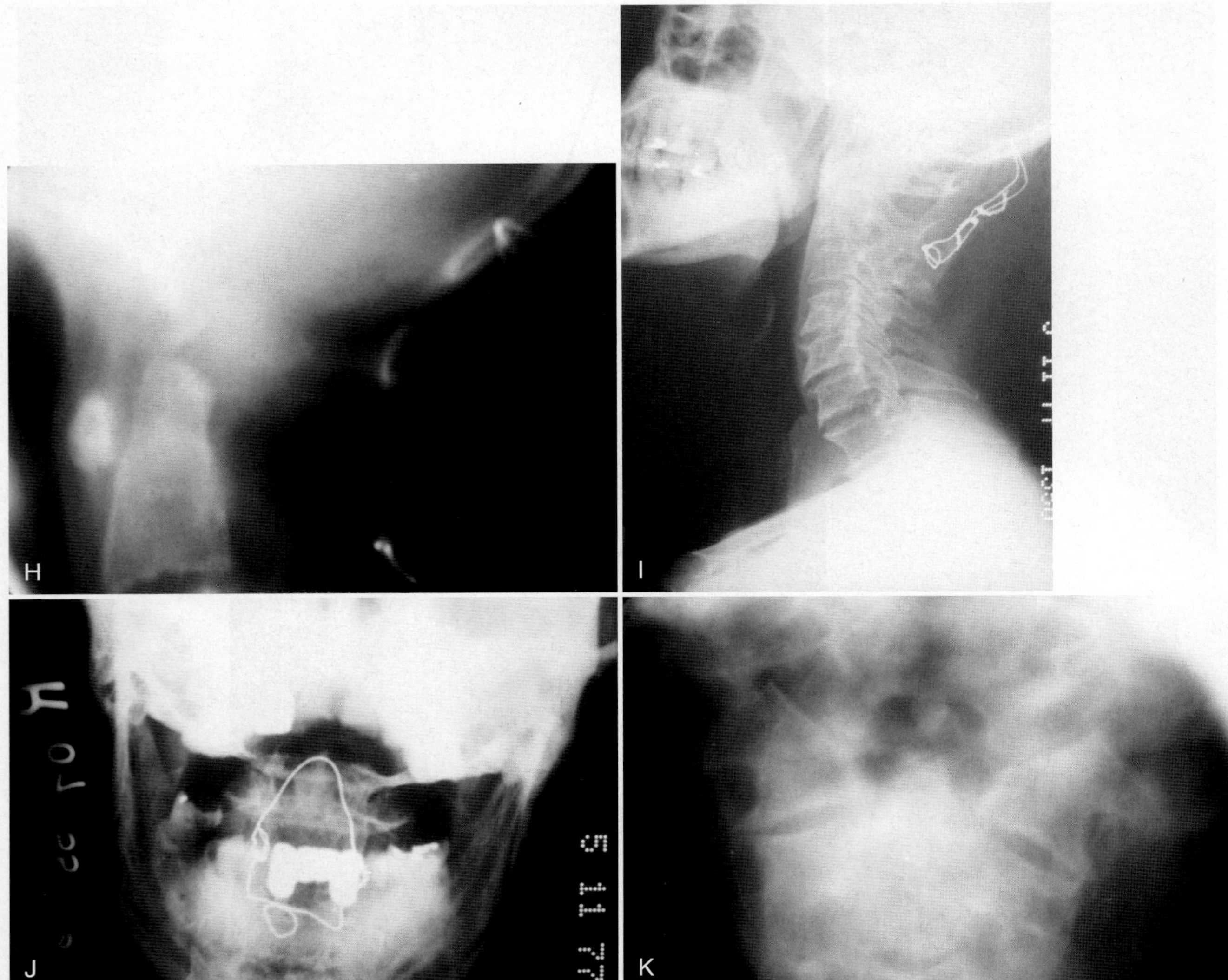

FIG. 75.7, cont'd (H) At 6 weeks after injury, a halo and body cast were applied to immobilize the patient's head on his neck. Twelve weeks after injury, a posterior fusion from the occiput to C3 was performed with iliac crest bone graft wired in place. This lateral tomogram taken 10 weeks after fusion demonstrates avulsion of the apex of the odontoid process, which is a type I odontoid fracture. This probably includes bone attachment of the alar ligaments. This film also shows that the relationship of the basion to the odontoid has been restored to normal and that the posterior laminar line is now again normal. In addition, there is spontaneous fusion anteriorly extending from the basion down to the anterior arch of C1. (I) Anteroposterior tomogram obtained 10 months after fusion reveals that the tip of the odontoid process is avulsed and is a type I odontoid fracture. The occipital condyles are again congruous. (J) Lateral radiograph obtained 14 months after the original injury shows a solid posterior occiput to C3 fusion with good alignment of the occipitocervical junction. (K) Anteroposterior radiograph 14 months after injury shows that normal alignment of the occipitocervical junction has been maintained. (From Eismont FJ, Bohlman HH. Posterior atlanto-occipital dislocation with fractures of the atlas and odontoid process. *J Bone Joint Surg Am.* 1978;60:397–399.)

remainder will suffer deficits of the cranial nerves, brain stem, and upper cervical spinal cord. Vertebral artery injury may accompany the dislocation. The most common mechanism is from an extension-rotation force. Patients with vertebral artery insufficiency at this level may exhibit Wallenberg syndrome, consisting of ipsilateral defects of cranial nerves V, IX, X, and XI; ipsilateral Horner syndrome; dysphagia; and cerebellar dysfunction.

All occipitocervical dislocations should be treated initially by immediate application of a halo vest. Because the majority of these injuries are unstable, posterior occipitocervical fusion is the procedure of choice (Fig. 75.9).[32,56] This can be done using a variety of techniques, including posterior wiring and structural grafting (Fig. 75.10), Ransford loop fixation with wiring, and plate and rod and screw fixation with structural grafting (Fig. 75.11). The first technique will require the use of postoperative halo immobilization; the latter two techniques will usually only need collar immobilization as external support. Improvements in occipital plate designs allow multiple points of fixation in the occiput, especially in the midline,

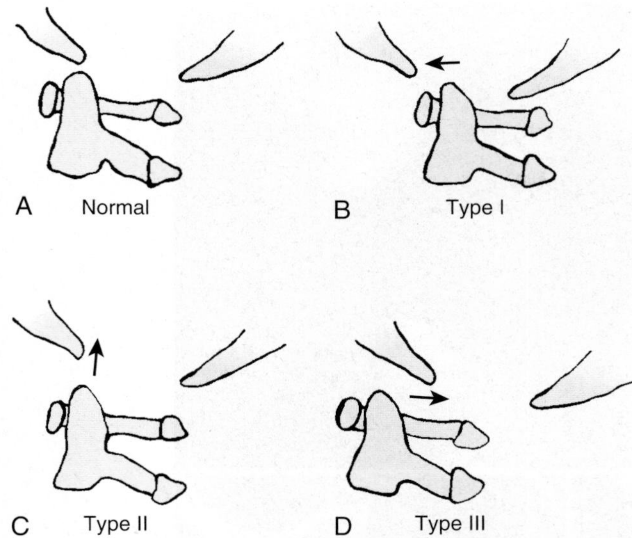

FIG. 75.8 Classification system of Traynelis and coworkers, which describes occipitocervical subluxation and dislocation. (Modified from Traynelis VC, Marano GC, Dunker RO, et al. Traumatic atlanto-occipital dislocation. *J Neurosurg*. 1986;65:863–870.)

where the occipital bone is thicker, providing significantly better initial fixation than off-midline plate-rod constructs.[57]

Fractures of the Atlas

Fractures of the atlas were first described by Jefferson in 1921. They usually occur in the anterior and posterior arches, which are the weakest points on the C1 ring. These injuries comprise 2% to 13% of all cervical spine fractures and approximately 25% of all injuries to the atlantoaxial complex.[22] They are often seen in the younger age groups (mean age, 30 years) and are most commonly the result of vehicular accidents or a fall on the top of the head.

These fractures are caused by axial loading. Because of this mechanism, these fractures commonly accompany head injuries in the polytrauma patient. In addition, there is an extremely high association (up to 50%) of atlas fractures with other cervical spine fractures. These include dens fractures, hangman's fractures, teardrop fractures of C2, cervical burst fractures, and lateral mass fractures.[22]

Patients will often complain of severe suboccipital discomfort and a sense of instability. Neurologic injury is uncommon in the case of isolated fractures of the atlas, but, when it occurs, the greater occipital nerve is most frequently injured, followed by the lower cranial nerves.[58]

Retropharyngeal soft tissue swelling greater than 5 mm at C3 in combination with a fracture of the posterior arch of C1 is highly suggestive of a burst-type injury. A combined lateral mass displacement on the open-mouth AP view exceeding 6.9 mm is indicative of transverse ligament insufficiency (Fig. 75.12),[59] but this measurement may not be sensitive enough to detect all unstable injuries. MRI can be used to help assess the continuity of the transverse ligament in those cases in which ligament status is unclear.[60]

Fine-cut CT in the plane of the axis will clearly delineate the fracture pattern. Common fracture patterns include isolated posterior arch fractures, lateral mass fractures, and burst fractures with combined anterior and posterior arch fractures. Isolated posterior arch fractures (Fig. 75.13) most commonly occur at the vertebral artery groove at the junction of the lateral mass and posterior arch. These are stable fractures that can be treated in a cervical collar for comfort. Lateral mass fractures can be either displaced or nondisplaced. Nondisplaced injuries can be treated with a cervical collar. Fractures that are displaced more than 5 mm can be treated with immediate halo vest application. A variation of the C1 lateral mass fracture, a unilateral C1 lateral mass sagittal split fracture, has a propensity to cause late deformity and pain if not treated with either C1–C2 fusion or direct osteosynthesis.[61] Burst fractures of the C1 ring are often referred to as Jefferson fractures. These injuries have one or two fractures in the posterior arch and one or two fractures in the anterior arch. Minimally displaced fractures (<7 mm) can be treated in a cervical collar.[61,62] Treatment of fractures with a combined diastasis of more than 6.9 mm consists of immobilization in a halo vest for 3 months (Fig. 75.14). After the halo vest is removed, flexion and extension radiographs are taken to test for C1–C2 instability, which, if significant, can be treated by C1–C2 posterior fusion.

Treatment of Jefferson fractures with greater than 6.9 mm of separation is controversial. Levine and Edwards advocate initial reduction of the fracture with skeletal traction for up to 6 to 8 weeks, followed by another 6 weeks of halo vest treatment.[63] Other series have found that immediate treatment with a halo vest can result in an acceptable outcome and avoids the morbidity associated with prolonged bed rest.[64,65] Traction reduction followed by early C1–C2 fusion using C1–C2 transarticular screws has also been described,[66] but intraoperative difficulty may be found owing to gross instability of the C1 lateral masses and the loose C1 posterior arch.

Most surgeons would agree that operative treatment is indicated if more than 5 mm of C1–C2 instability exists on flexion and extension radiographs once the halo is removed. If the posterior arch of C1 is healed, a posterior C1–C2 fusion is indicated. In the case of nonunion of the posterior arch of C1 or significant injury to the occipital condyles, occiput–C2 fusion can be performed. Another indication for surgery is neck and/or occipital nerve pain in a patient with a nonunion of the atlas ring fractures. The recommended treatment would then be a posterior occiput–C2 fusion.[67]

Atlantoaxial Subluxation and Dislocation

Conservative care of atlantoaxial rotatory subluxation in children, also known as Grisel syndrome, is most effective when treatment is instituted early. Most children who have had symptoms for less than 1 week will improve with a soft cervical collar and close observation. When symptoms have been present for 2 to 4 weeks, hospital admission and head-halter traction is usually successful in achieving reduction. For patients who present 1 month after the subluxation occurs, skull traction can be instituted and continued for up to 3

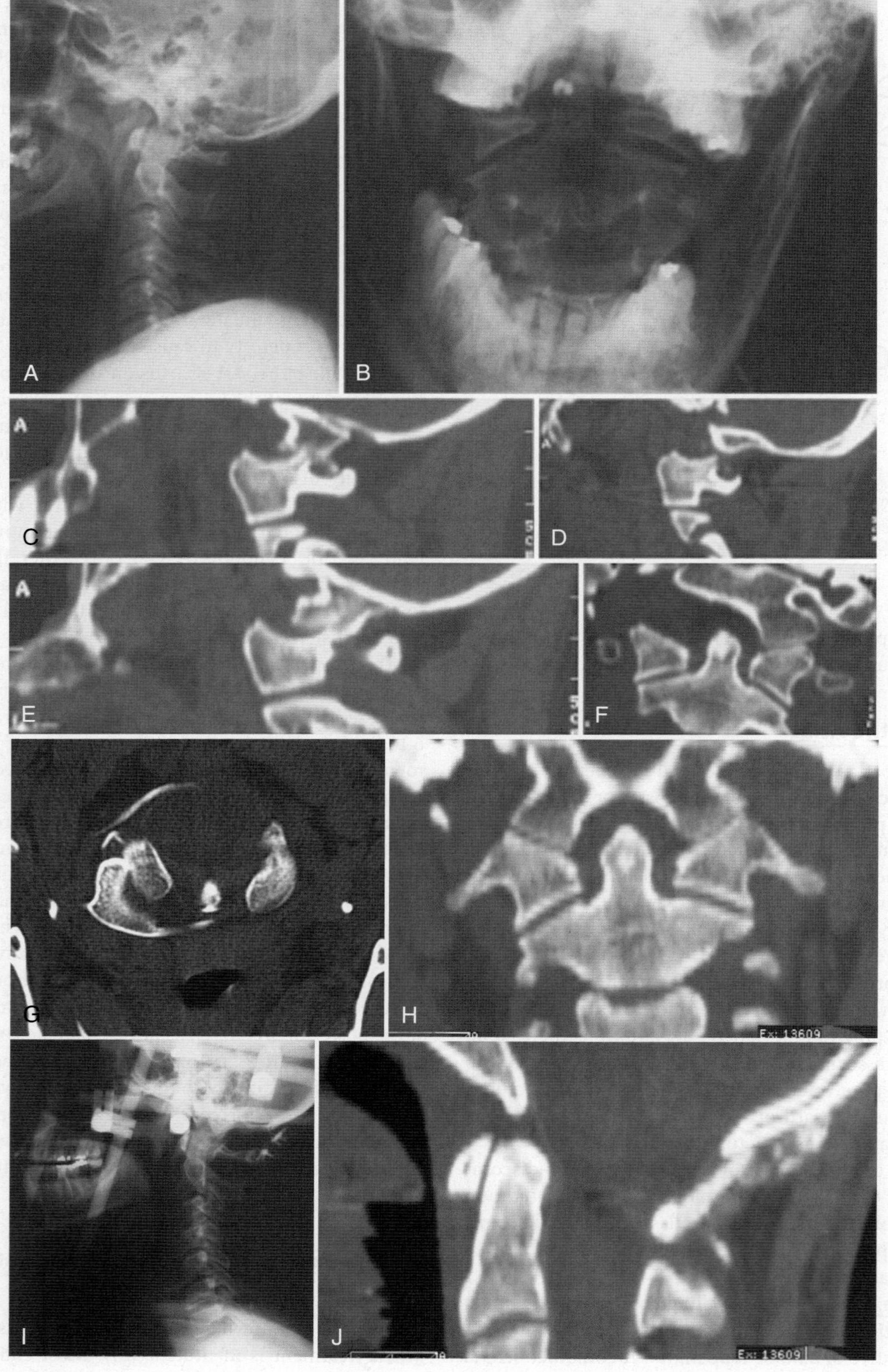
A
B
C
D
E
F
G
H
Ex: 13609
I
J
Ex: 13609

FIG. 75.9 This man was injured when his car struck a tree. He had an immediate onset of pain in his upper cervical spine, with radiation to the back of his head. (A) Lateral radiograph shows normal alignment of the upper cervical spine and the occipitocervical junction. There is no abnormal soft tissue swelling. The basion appears to be directly over the tip of the odontoid and is less than 1 cm from the tip. The Wackenheim line is not drawn here, but the bony line down the clivus and the posterior aspect of the basion appears to be tangential to the posterior aspect of the odontoid. (B) Open-mouth view of the odontoid is abnormal. The patient's right lateral mass of C1 appears smaller than the lateral mass of C1 on the left side. There is also some asymmetry, with the distance from the lateral mass of C1 to the odontoid being shorter on the right side than on the left side. (C) Parasagittal CT reconstruction shows that his occipital condyle on the right side is posterior to the lateral mass of C1. (D) This computed tomographic (CT) image is slightly more medial than that in (C) and shows that the occipital condyle is impacted into the posterior aspect of the posterior lip of the right lateral mass of C1. (E) This view is even more medial, and again shows the occipital condyle to be posteriorly displaced and impacted into the posterior lip of the lateral mass of C1. (F) Coronal reconstruction of the CT scan shows that the left-sided occipitoatlantal joint is normal. On the right side, the occipital condyle is posterior to the lateral mass of C1; thus, it is not seen on this view. (G) This transverse axial image shows the abnormal appearance of the right-sided occipitoatlantal joint. (H) The patient was initially placed in skull tong traction, but the occipitoatlantal dislocation could not be reduced. The patient was then taken to surgery. At the time of surgery, with a combination of skull tong traction and manual manipulation with a cable passed under the posterior arch of C1, the occiput–C1 dislocation was reduced with an audible "clunk." Fusion was performed using titanium cables to fasten autograft bone to the base of the skull posteriorly and to the posterior arch of C1. This postoperative coronal CT reconstruction shows complete reduction of the occipitoatlantal joints bilaterally. (I) Lateral radiograph shows the bone graft and cables in place. Because rigid internal fixation was not utilized, the patient was immobilized in a halo vest postoperatively. (J) Midsagittal reconstructed CT scan shows the bone graft healing at 3 months from the time of surgery.

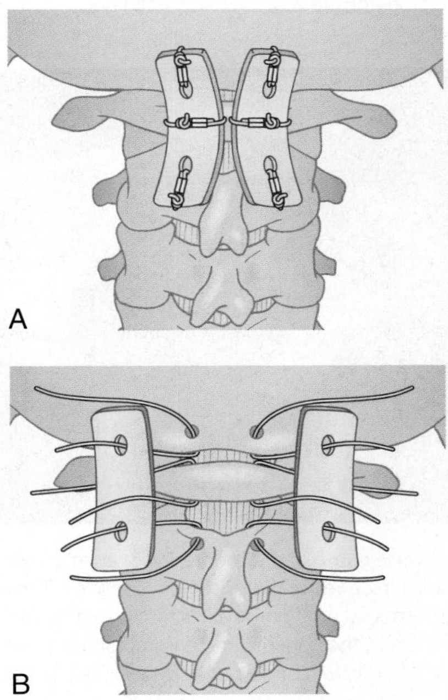

FIG. 75.10 Classic wiring technique for occipitocervical fusion. The titanium cables fastening the bone graft to the skull are passed through two burr holes just posterior to the foramen magnum. The cables are also passed bilaterally under the posterior arch of C1 and under the lamina of C2. Drill holes are made in the iliac crest bone graft to allow passage of the wires as shown. The cables under C2 are passed all the way around the graft. It is imperative that the graft be a thick structural iliac bone graft. If the bone graft is not solid enough, a combination of cortical structural allograft bone graft superficially and the patient's autogenous iliac bone graft beneath this would be used to provide a combination of structural stability and autogenous factors to promote bone healing. If rigid instrumentation (plates or rods combined with screws) is not used, then the patient would be placed in a halo vest until the construct was completely healed. This would usually require a period of 3 months. (From Eismont FJ, Frazier DD. Cranial cervical trauma. In: Levine AM, Eismont FJ, Garfin SR, Zigler JE [eds]. *Spine Trauma*. Philadelphia: WB Saunders; 1998:203.)

weeks. Initial traction should be 7 pounds and gradually increased to 15 pounds. If traction fails to reduce the deformity, open reduction and C1–C2 fusion is recommended.[68]

Traumatic rotatory subluxation or dislocation in adults is most commonly caused by vehicular trauma. Like children, adults will present with a "cock robin" appearance with the head tilted toward and rotated away from the side of the dislocation.

Radiographs will show asymmetry of the lateral masses on the open-mouth view. A "wink sign" may be appreciated; it is caused by overriding of the C1–C2 joint on one side with a normally aligned joint on the contralateral side. Dynamic CT is the best means of demonstrating the condition. Cervical spine CT scans are done in a neutral position and then repeated with the head maximally rotated to one side and then the other side.

Fielding and Hawkins presented the most commonly used classification scheme for these injuries (Fig. 75.15).[69] Type I dislocations are pure rotational injuries. Type II injuries have both rotatory malalignment with anterior displacement of the atlas less than 3 to 5 mm, suggesting only a mild deficiency of the transverse ligament. Type III injuries combine rotatory subluxation with greater than 5 mm of displacement, suggesting complete deficiency of the transverse ligament. Type IV injuries have both rotational malalignment and posterior displacement.

In adults, reduction of the rotational deformity can usually be achieved by skull tong traction. Topical anesthetic in the posterior pharynx may be helpful. The reduction can be palpated through the mouth. If it was difficult to obtain the reduction, then halo vest immobilization may be needed. For most cases, a rigid cervical collar is adequate.

If closed reduction fails, open reduction is performed and a posterior C1–C2 fusion is used to stabilize the reduction. Many methods to achieve fusion of the C1–C2 complex have

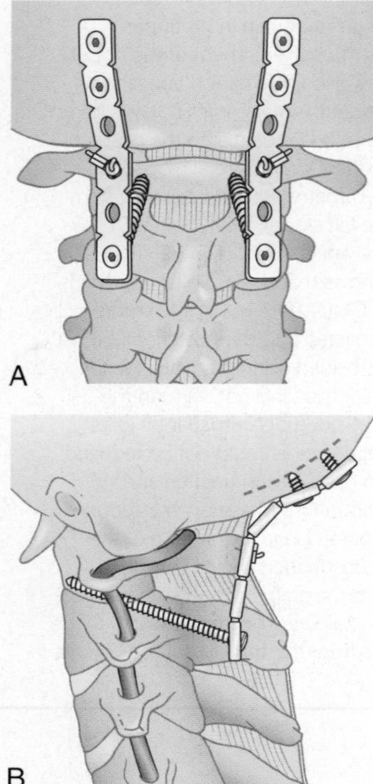

FIG. 75.11 (A) Anteroposterior and (B) lateral views of the occipital cervical plating technique using C1–C2 transarticular screws and titanium reconstruction plates with bicortical skull screws. Because the transarticular C1–C2 screw is the most critical in terms of its positioning, the C1–C2 transarticular screw is always the first screw to be placed in this construct. The path would initially be drilled and tapped. A plate would then be bent to accommodate the local anatomy. The plate must fit flush against the skull, fit against the posterior arch of C1, and fit the contour of the posterior arch of C2. The C1–C2 transarticular screw is then placed through the plate and tightened to within two turns of its final position. The plate is then held against the skull, and two or three screws are placed into the skull. The screws in the skull are always bicortical. The thickness in this area of the bone ranges from 4 to 6 mm. A cable is also usually passed under the posterior arch of C1 and around the plate, then tightened. These cables contribute significantly to the rigidity of the construct. After one side is secured, the second side is similarly instrumented. The C1–C2 screws are placed under lateral fluoroscopic guidance. The pedicle of C2 is dissected so that it can be visualized directly during screw insertion. The starting point for the C1–C2 screw is usually 3 to 4 mm cephalad to the C2–C3 facet joint. The distal tip of the screw should be just to the anterior cortex of C1. It can also protrude slightly through the anterior cortex, but it should be kept in mind that the internal carotid artery lies within a few millimeters of the usual anterior exit point for these screws. (From Eismont FJ, Frazier DD. Cranial cervical trauma. In: Levine AM, Eismont FJ, Garfin SR, Zigler JE [eds]. *Spine Trauma*. Philadelphia: WB Saunders; 1998:204.)

been described, including the Gallie technique, the Brooks technique, C1–C2 transarticular screws supplemented with a posterior fusion, and C1 lateral mass and C2 pedicle (or translaminar) screw construct. The use of transarticular screws and screw–rod constructs provides sufficient fixation to obviate the need for postoperative halo vest immobilization. The other methods of stabilizing C1–C2 may be rigid enough to permit mobilization in a rigid collar or may require use of a halo vest to supplement the fixation, especially if it is difficult to achieve the reduction or if the bone quality is poor.

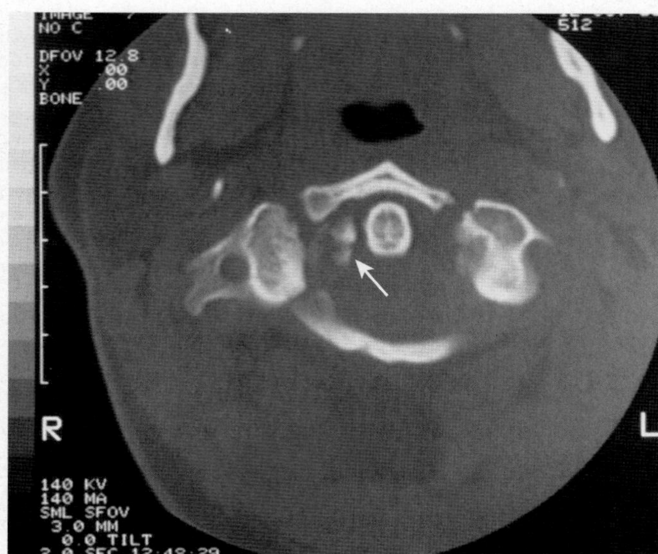

FIG. 75.12 Transverse computed tomographic scan at the C1 level showing a Jefferson fracture with significant spreading of the lateral masses of C1. This has resulted in the avulsion of the origin of the transverse ligament from the right lateral mass of C1 (*arrow*). The usual treatment for this would be a halo vest and mobilization for 3 months, followed by flexion and extension radiographs to assess C1–C2 stability.

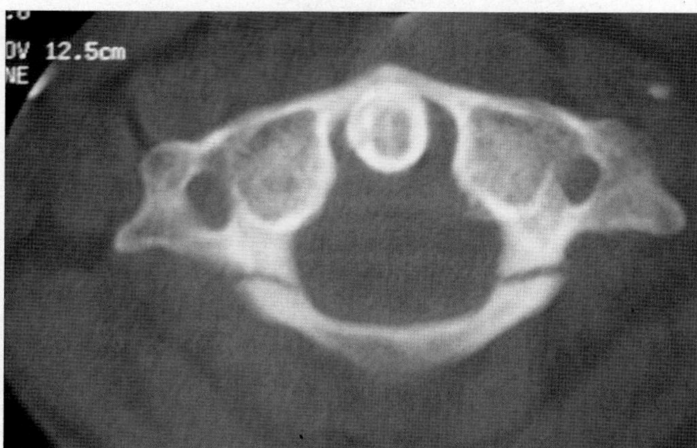

FIG. 75.13 Transverse computed tomographic scan at C1 showing minimally displaced fractures of the posterior arch of C1. This always occurs at the site of the vertebral artery groove. Provided that no other fractures are associated with this, the patient can be immobilized in a cervical collar for a short period of time, for comfort only. By itself, this is a stable injury.

Rupture of the Transverse Ligament

The transverse ligament is the major ligamentous stabilizing structure for the atlantoaxial articulation. It is composed primarily of collagen fibers, which render it stiff and inelastic.[70] When torn or disrupted, it is incapable of repair, and its original strength and function cannot be restored.

Insufficiency of the transverse ligament and subsequent C1–C2 instability is suspected if the atlantodens interval is greater than 3.5 mm in adults and greater than 5 mm in children on lateral radiographs and in atlas fractures when the combined overhang of the C1 lateral masses on C2 is greater than 6.9 mm on an AP open-mouth view of the upper cervical spine.[59,60] Plain radiographs, however, are often inadequate to

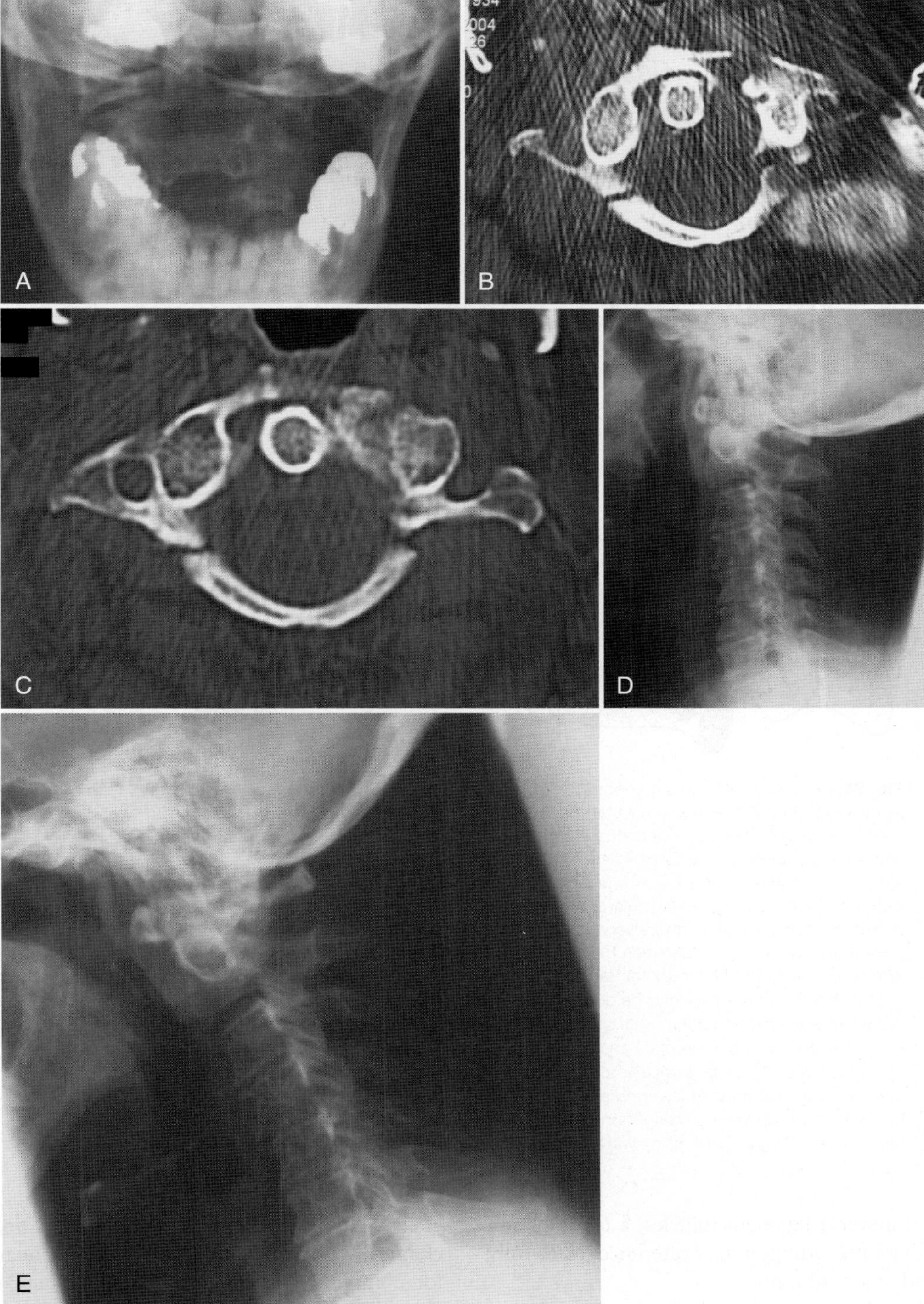

FIG. 75.14 This patient sustained a moderately displaced Jefferson fracture in an accident. He was treated with a halo vest with no initial reduction. (A) Open-mouth view of the C1–C2 joints shows a 2-mm overhang on the right and an 8-mm overhang on the left. (B) Computed tomographic (CT) scan at C1 shows the 8-mm lateral displacement of the left C1 lateral mass. (C) Final CT scan shows that the lateral mass displacement is unchanged, but there is now copious callus anteriorly between the anterior C1 arch, the C1 lateral mass, and the odontoid. (D–E) Flexion and extension radiographs 1 year after the injury show no evidence of instability at C1–C2 or at the occipitocervical joints. He has had no pain since removal of the halo vest and is gradually resuming his preinjury activities with no restrictions.

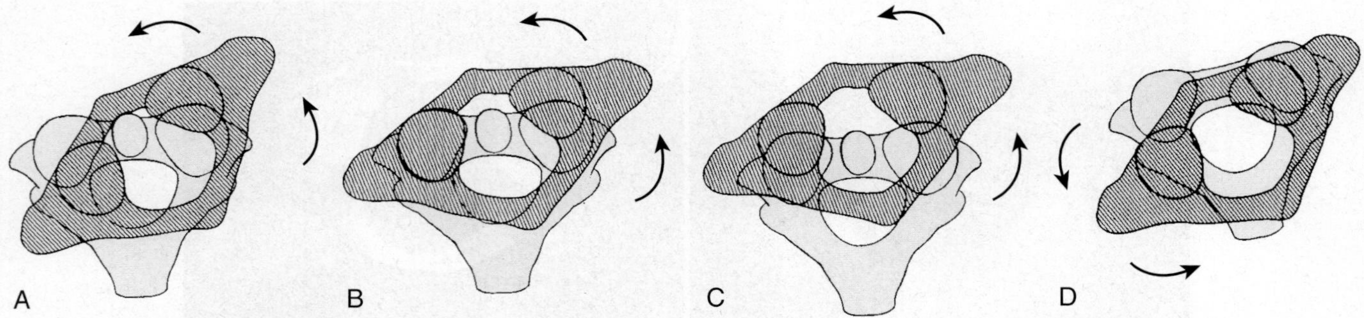

FIG. 75.15 Four types of C1–C2 rotatory fixation. (A) Type I: rotatory fixation with no anterior displacement and the odontoid acting as the pivot. (B) Type II: rotatory fixation with anterior displacement of 3 to 5 mm, with one lateral articular process acting as the pivot. (C) Type III: rotatory fixation with anterior displacement of >5 mm. (D) Type IV: rotatory fixation with posterior displacement. (From Fielding JW, Hawkins RJ. Atlanto-axial rotatory fixation. *J Bone Joint Surg Am*. 1977;59:37–44.)

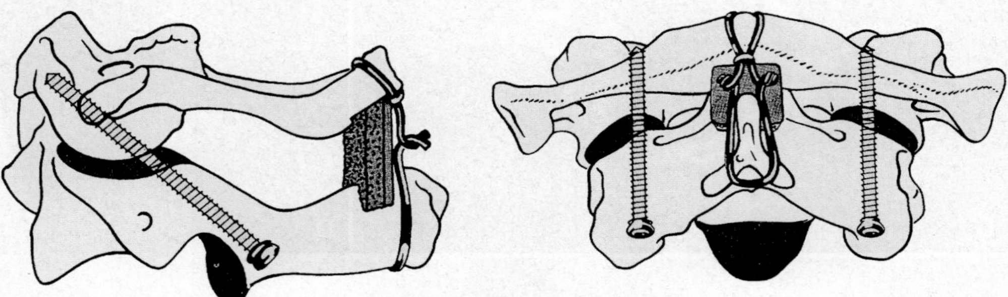

FIG. 75.16 Lateral (*left*) and anteroposterior (*right*) illustrations show the technique described by Grob and associates.[82] They advise having the start point 3 to 4 mm cephalad to the C2–C3 facet joint and having it as medial as possible without penetrating the medial wall of the C2 pedicle. They emphasize seeing the medial and superior aspects of the C2 pedicle as well as the C1–C2 joint. The anterior aspect of the screw should be either to the anterior cortex of C1 or just through it. The internal carotid artery lies just anterior to the usual exit point for the C1–C2 transarticular screw; it is therefore extremely important that the screw tip either not protrude anteriorly at all or only a very minimal distance. The illustration also demonstrates placement of an autogenous bone graft between the arches of C1 and C2 and adequately tightening the wires or cables, which, together with the C1–C2 transarticular screws, makes this an extremely strong construct. Packing bone graft within the C1–C2 joint may be done, but it adds considerably greater risk to the procedure and does not seem to be needed under the usual circumstances. It is necessary to perform fine-cut computed tomographic sagittal reconstruction views of C1 and C2 from side to side to be certain that there is adequate room for placement of a C1–C2 transarticular screw without compromising the vertebral artery. In approximately 15% of cases, local anatomy of the vertebral artery precludes placement of two screws. Placement of one screw in combination with the posterior bone graft seems to be adequate. (From Grob D, Jeanneret B, Aebi M, Markwalder T. Atlanto-axial fusion with transarticular screw fixation. *J Bone Joint Surg Br*. 1991;73:972–981.)

assess suspected transverse ligament injuries; a combination of MRI, CT, and dynamic radiographs is often needed to fully assess the type and extent of injury.[60]

Dickman and colleagues classified transverse ligament injuries into two types.[60] Type I injuries encompass intrasubstance ruptures. Type IA injuries occur in the midportion of the ligament. Type IB injuries occur at the periosteal insertion of the ligament onto the atlas. Type II injuries occur when there is an avulsion of the tubercular insertion of the transverse ligament from the C1 lateral mass. Type IIA injuries occur if the lateral mass is comminuted, and type IIB injuries occur if the lateral mass is intact.

Type I injuries should be treated surgically with C1–C2 fusion. The most common way to achieve this is posteriorly. Wiring techniques, such as Brooks and Gallie fusions, are effective more than 90% of the time,[71] but are the least biomechanically stable,[72] and a rigid cervical collar is usually used for 3 months postoperatively. Transarticular screw fixation (Fig. 75.16) provides sufficient additional stability to allow the immobilization time to be reduced to 6 weeks in a rigid collar or even to allow the patient to be immobilized in a soft cervical collar. There is, however, risk to the vertebral artery when instrumentation is done across the pars interarticularis of C2. C1 lateral mass screw and C2 pedicle screw constructs provide comparable biomechanical rigidity to transarticular screws with less risk to the vertebral artery but with more risk to the internal carotid artery. If necessary, sacrificing the C2 nerve root provides direct visualization of the C1 lateral mass and the C1–C2 joint. The structures can then be instrumented, reduced, and fused under direct visualization. The combination of C1 lateral mass screws connected to C2 translaminar screws is another alternative fixation option that provides the same degree of stability of the C1–C2 complex. C1–C2 fusion can also be achieved by an anterior approach with anteriorly placed C1–C2 screws.[73] Proponents of this technique note that there is less soft tissue dissection involved as compared with posterior approaches.[74] We, however, recommend the posterior approach in order to provide better supplemental bone grafting and to minimize postoperative swallowing and airway problems.

Type II fractures can be treated with external immobilization for 3 months. Up to 74% of these type II injuries will heal with nonoperative care.[60]

Fractures of the Odontoid

Fractures of the dens constitute 7% to 13% of all cervical spine injuries.[75] They are frequently missed because of the paucity of clinical symptoms other than for neck pain. In addition, if the patient suffers from head trauma and is intoxicated or obtunded, the injury can be easily missed. Both flexion and extension mechanisms can cause fractures of the dens. Hyperflexion results in anterior displacement of the dens fracture; hyperextension results in posterior displacement of the dens fracture.

The fracture can usually be seen on open-mouth and lateral radiographs of the cervical spine, although nondisplaced fractures can easily be missed. Classification of these fractures is based on their location in the odontoid. The most commonly used classification scheme was described by Anderson and D'Alonzo (Fig. 75.17).[76] Type I fractures consist of avulsion injuries at the tip of the dens. Type II fractures occur through the base of the dens at the junction of the dens and the central body of the axis. Type III fractures extend into the body of the axis.

Type I injuries can be treated nonoperatively with a rigid cervical collar, but the possibility of occipital cervical instability must first be ruled out because the bone avulsion always means that at least one alar ligament is incompetent. After 3 months of immobilization, flexion and extension radiographs are taken to assess for healing and residual ligamentous instability.

Type II odontoid fracture is the most problematic type of odontoid fracture. In a prospective study of 144 odontoid fractures reported by the Cervical Spine Research Society[77] there were 96 type II and 48 type III fractures. The incidence of spinal cord–level neurologic deficits was 14 of 96 (14%) of type II fractures and 4 of 48 (8%) of type III fractures. Two of the 14 patients with type II fractures and cord deficits presented with upper extremity monoplegia, which probably represents the cruciate paralysis described earlier in this chapter.

In this same prospective study, of the 38 patients with type II fractures treated primarily in a halo vest, only 66% had a successful result, with seven patients (18%) having nonunions, three having malunions, two having fracture displacement, and one dying before union. Of the 16 patients with type III odontoid fractures treated primarily in a halo vest, 13 (81%) had a successful outcome, with one nonunion, one fracture

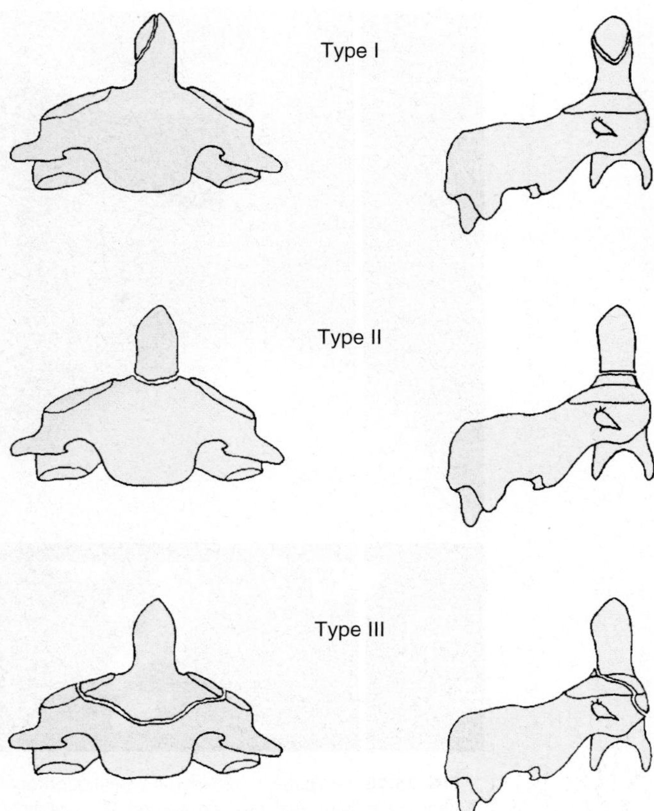

FIG. 75.17 Three types of odontoid fractures. Type I is an oblique fracture at the tip of the odontoid process. It is usually an avulsion of bone at the insertion of the alar ligament. This is normally taught to be a benign injury, but it can be seen in significant occipitocervical injuries. Type II is a fracture at the neck or base of the odontoid, but before it goes down into the body of the axis. This area has a poor blood supply and the smallest cross-sectional area; thus, it has a lower potential for healing. A type III fracture extends down into the body of the axis. It therefore has a larger surface area compared with a type II fracture; in addition, there is a much greater ratio of cancellous bone to cortical bone. Type III fractures have a better healing potential than type II fractures. (From Anderson LD, D'Alonzo RT. Fractures of the odontoid process of the axis. *J Bone Joint Surg Am.* 1974;56:1663–1674.)

displacement, and one death, which occurred 1 day after injury due to cardiac arrest. Of the 30 patients (including both type II and type III fractures) treated primarily with a posterior C1–C2 fusion, 96% had a successful outcome, with only one nonunion.

In a retrospective review of 322 consecutive patients with type II odontoid fractures treated at three level 1 trauma centers, surgically treated patients had improved 30-day and long-term survival advantage over patients treated nonoperatively even when adjusting for age, sex, and comorbidities.[78] The results of this retrospective review were further supported by a subgroup analysis of a prospective multicenter study. Fifty-eight elderly patients with type II odontoid fractures treated nonoperatively showed worse functional outcomes and higher mortality (14%) at 12 months than their surgically treated cohorts.[79]

The overall nonunion rate for type II odontoid fractures is reported to be about 32%. There is an increased nonunion rate

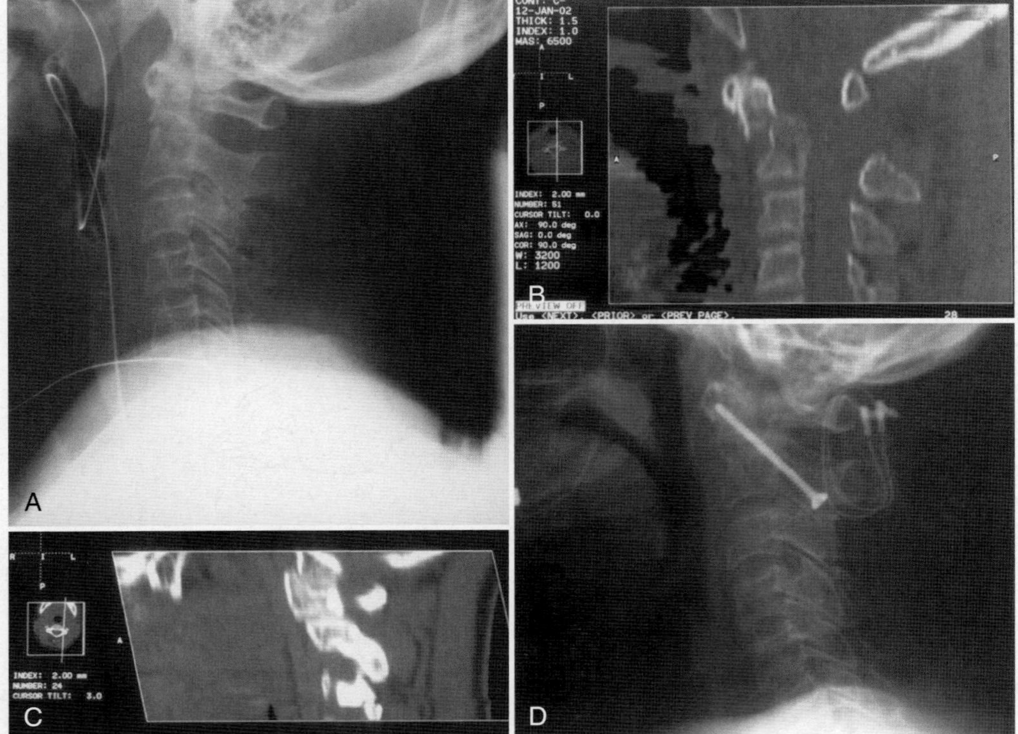

FIG. 75.18 This patient sustained a type II odontoid fracture in a motor vehicle collision. She was neurologically normal, but complained of neck pain. (A) Initial lateral radiograph shows a minimally displaced type II odontoid fracture. There is a slight gap anteriorly at the fracture site. The patient was kept immobilized in a rigid collar and was sent for a computed tomographic (CT) evaluation. (B) Midsagittal reconstruction of the CT scan shows that the fracture has displaced 12 mm anteriorly. This fracture obviously was more unstable than it initially appeared. (C) Parasagittal CT reconstruction is necessary to be certain that there is an adequate path for the C1–C2 transarticular screw. In this patient, the path was adequate on one side, as seen on this image. (D) The patient was placed in skull tong traction and reduced. She was then taken to surgery for fixation using one C1–C2 transarticular screw combined with sublaminar cables from C1 to C2 combined with autogenous structural iliac bone graft. The patient's fracture healed satisfactorily. (From Eismont FJ, Currier BL, McGuire RA Jr. Cervical spine and spinal cord injuries: recognition and treatment. In Helfet DL, Greene WB [eds]. *Instructional Course Lectures, vol 53*. Rosemont, IL: American Academy of Orthopaedic Surgeons; 2003:346.)

associated with fractures with greater than 5 mm of displacement, angulation greater than 10 degrees, age older than 40 years, and posterior displacement.[80] Hadley showed a 78% nonunion rate for type II fractures displaced more than 6 mm in comparison to a 10% nonunion rate when the displacement was less than 6 mm.[81]

Treatment options need to be individualized for each patient. Halo vest treatment may be a good option for a patient with an undisplaced type II odontoid fracture or an undisplaced/minimally displaced type III odontoid fracture in a patient with few or no risk factors for nonunion. The patient needs to understand, however, that even with 3 months of halo vest treatment, there is still a risk of at least 10% that surgery will be needed to treat the fracture. As the amount of displacement and angulation increases and as the number of other risk factors such as more advanced age and smoking increases, then the chance of failing to heal appropriately in a halo vest becomes significantly large.

As the risk factors for nonunion increase, surgical treatment with a C1–C2 fusion or anterior odontoid screw fixation becomes a better option. If primary C1–C2 fusion is selected, the patient should understand that he or she will lose 50% of neck rotation. Many options exist for fixation and fusion of C1–C2. C1–C2 transarticular screws (Fig. 75.18),[82] C1 lateral mass/C2 pedicle screw constructs (Fig. 75.19), and C1 lateral mass/C2 translaminar screw constructs offer a biomechanical advantage over traditional wiring techniques and should minimize the chance of losing the fracture reduction and maximize the chance of having a solid fusion. A fusion rate and fracture union rate of 98% should be expected. If wiring techniques are used, a fusion rate of 94% to 96% can be expected, but there will be a higher chance of losing reduction. Gallie-type constructs are biomechanically advantageous for anteriorly displaced fractures; Brooks constructs are advantageous for posteriorly displaced fractures.

Primary osteosynthesis of the dens (Fig. 75.20) has the theoretical advantage of preserving rotation at the atlantoaxial joint, but the amount of motion that is preserved over a C1–C2 fusion may not be significant.[83] To achieve successful anterior fracture fixation, the fracture needs to be transverse, noncomminuted, and reducible. The patient's chest anatomy and odontoid anatomy must also be amenable to this technique.

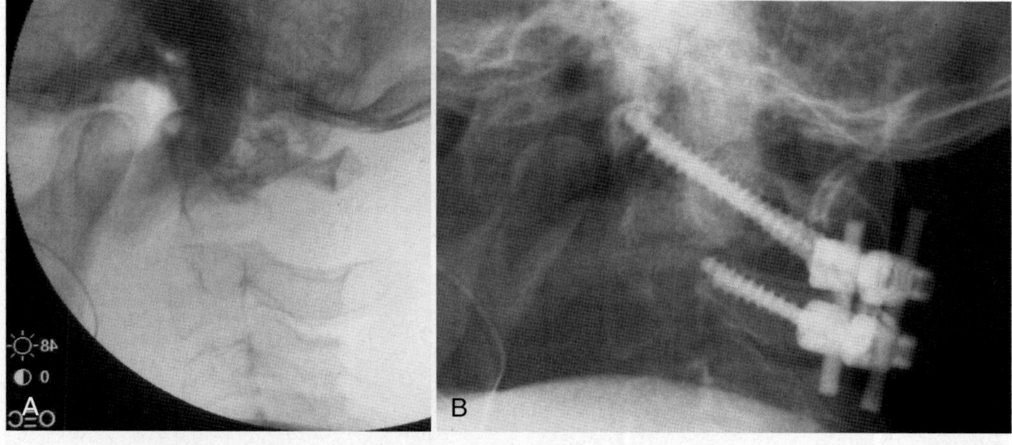

FIG. 75.19 This patient was involved in a motor vehicle collision and sustained multiple trauma with multiple fractures, including this type II odontoid fracture. (A) Postinjury lateral radiograph shows a type II odontoid fracture, which appears well aligned but to have a significant gap in the posterior cortex of the odontoid. With this type of gap present between C1 and C2, it would usually not be possible to insert C1–C2 transarticular screws and obtain adequate purchase. (B) This patient's odontoid fracture was stabilized with C1 lateral mass screws combined with C2 pedicle screws. The starting point for the C1 lateral mass screw is just beneath the posterior arch of C1, and the anterior endpoint is the same as for C1–C2 transarticular screws. This screw-rod construct combined with C1–C2 wiring is able to provide adequate compression across the fracture site to achieve reduction and provide the best opportunity for fracture healing.

In the elderly, the use of odontoid screws is associated with a high complication rate.[84] Two large series of anterior odontoid screw fixation show failure rates of 13% to 17%.[85,86]

Biplanar fluoroscopy or intraoperative CT with image guidance is essential for this technique.

Traumatic Spondylolisthesis of the Axis

Traumatic spondylolisthesis of the axis, also known as a hangman's fracture, can be caused by a variety of mechanisms, including combinations of extension, flexion, distraction, and axial loading of the cervical spine. The fracture line passes through the neural arch of the axis. These fractures are best classified using the modification of the Effendi classification system (Fig. 75.21).[87] Type I fractures occur through the pars interarticularis bilaterally with less than 3 mm translation and no angulation. This fracture usually results from hyperextension and axial load. The neural arch fractures, but the intervertebral disc and anterior longitudinal ligament are still intact (Fig. 75.22). This fracture is associated with other extension-type injuries, including C1 posterior arch fractures and dens fractures.

Type II fractures are bipedicular fractures with greater than 3 mm of displacement and angulation of C2 on C3. This fracture results from an initial axial load, with hyperextension of the neck causing a fracture of the neural arch followed by a flexion moment that results in disruption of the C2–C3 intervertebral disc. This is often accompanied by a compression fracture of the anterosuperior corner of C3 or the posteroinferior body of C2.[87] Two variants of type II fractures have been described. The type IIA fracture shows significant angulation but has minimal (rarely exceeding 2–3 mm) translation and includes significant disruption of the disc and posterior longitudinal ligament. Gross disc space distraction occurs after the application of minimal amounts of traction (Fig. 75.23). This injury usually results from a flexion–distraction injury. In a type II variant described by Starr and Eismont, the fracture line propagates through the posterior aspect of the vertebral body with unilateral or bilateral continuity of the posterior cortex, and is associated with a 33% incidence of neurologic deficit (Fig. 75.24).[88]

Type III hangman's fractures are unstable injuries with severe displacement and angulation, associated with unilateral or bilateral facet dislocations of C2 on C3. Disruption of the posterior longitudinal ligament and the C2–C3 intervertebral disc occurs in these injuries. These injuries are commonly associated with neurologic injuries. Type III injuries occur in three basic patterns: bilateral neural arch fractures anterior to the facet joints with bilateral facet dislocations posterior to it; a rotational injury with fracture of the neural arch on one side anterior to the facet joint and on the second side in the area of the facet joint, causing a unilateral facet dislocation; and a bilateral facet dislocation with fractures of the neural arch just posterior to the facet joints. Type III injuries are usually the result of flexion–distraction followed by hyperextension.

Isolated type I fractures can be treated in a rigid cervical collar for 8 to 12 weeks. Type II fractures are treated with initial traction in extension followed by immobilization in a halo vest. Type IIA fractures are treated with immediate application of a halo vest. Traction is avoided in patients with type IIA injuries because even minimal traction can cause severe overdistraction. All type III fractures should be treated with surgical reduction and posterior C2–C3 fusion. Internal fixation can be achieved with posterior pedicle screws at C2 into the C2 vertebral body and lateral mass screws at C3.

Nonunions of type II or IIA injuries are uncommon,[89] but if they occur and are symptomatic, they can be treated with either a posterior C1–C3 fusion or an anterior C2–C3 fusion.

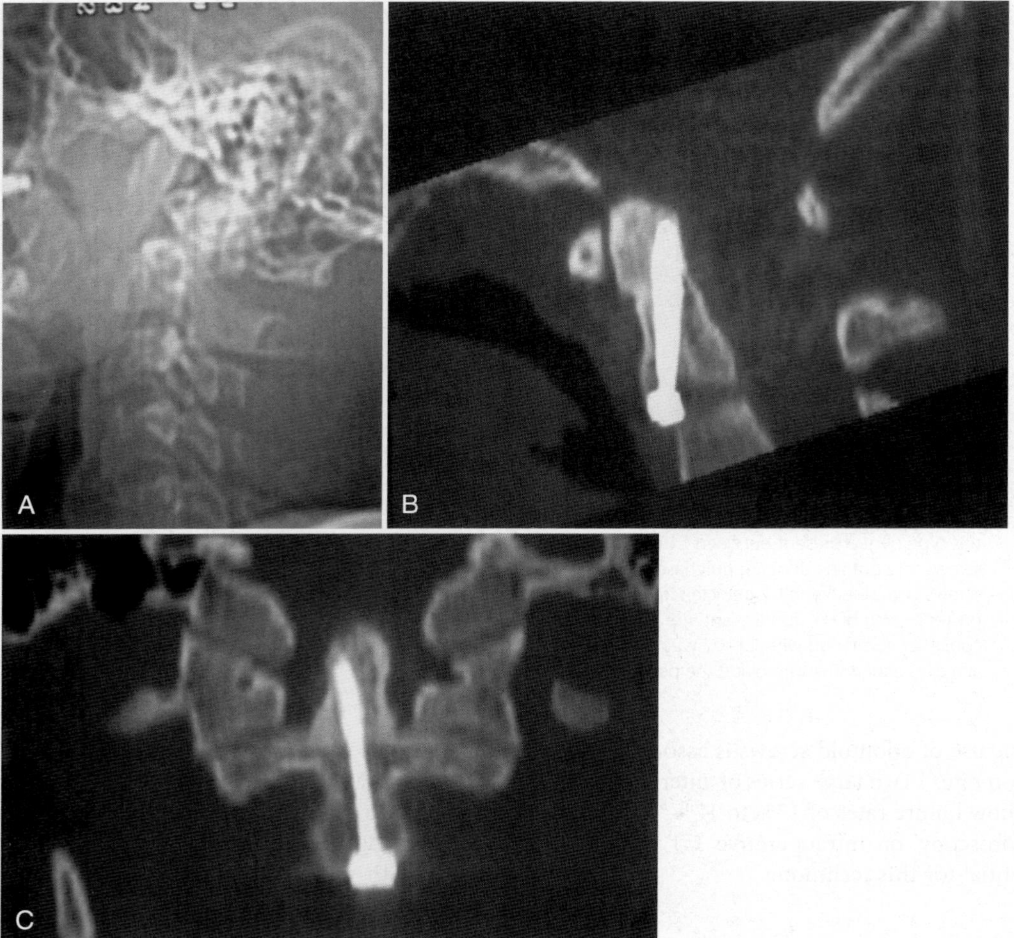

FIG. 75.20 This patient fell from a moving vehicle and sustained a type II odontoid fracture. (A) Scout film from the computed tomographic (CT) scan shows that his odontoid process is displaced posteriorly >1 cm. The patient's young age made anterior odontoid fracture fixation preferable to a posterior C1–C2 fusion. (B–C) Midsagittal and coronal CT reconstruction images were taken at 3 months from the time of surgery. It can be seen that the fracture was well reduced and is now well healed. It is important that the cephalad portion of the screw penetrates through the cortex to gain optimal fixation.

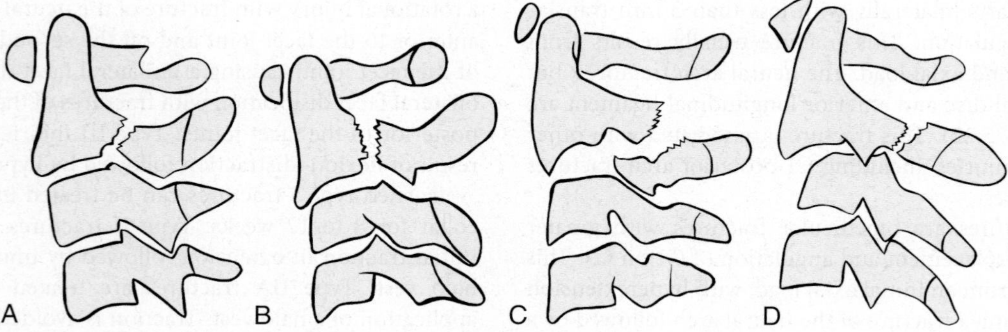

FIG. 75.21 Classification of traumatic spondylolisthesis of the axis. (A) Type I hangman's fracture has fractures of the C2 pedicles bilaterally with no angulation and with as much as 3 mm of displacement. (B) Type II fractures have both significant angulation and significant displacement. (C) Type IIA fractures show minimum displacement, but there is severe angulation, apparently hinging from the anterior longitudinal ligament. These fractures have disruption through the disc space and are easily overdistracted with even small amounts of traction. (D) Type III hangman's fracture combines bilateral facet dislocations between the second and third cervical vertebra with the fracture of the neural arch. This group of patients will always require surgery to reduce the dislocated facets. (From Levine AM, Edwards CC. The management of traumatic spondylolisthesis of the axis. *J Bone Joint Surg Am.* 1985;67:217–226.)

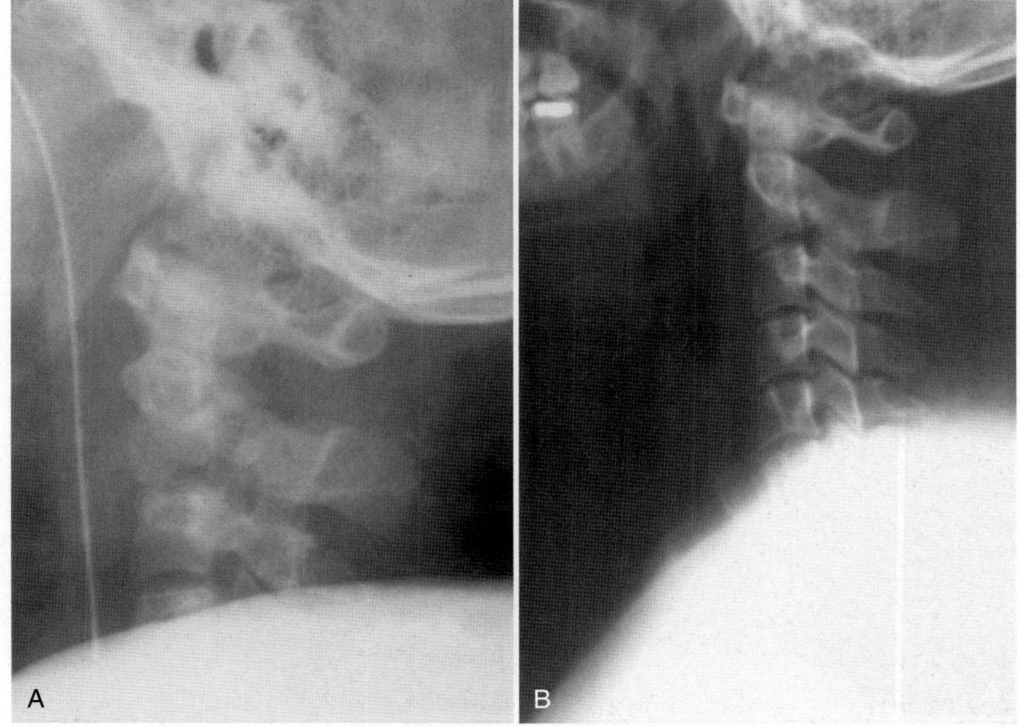

FIG. 75.22 This patient was involved in a motor vehicle accident and sustained a type I fracture of the pedicles of C2. He had no other injuries. (A) Lateral radiograph taken immediately after injury shows minimal angulation and no significant displacement at the fracture site. The patient was treated in a rigid cervical collar for 8 weeks. (B) There is adequate healing of the C2 fracture with good alignment of the spine. (From Eismont FJ, Currier BL, McGuire RA Jr. Cervical spine and spinal cord injuries: recognition and treatment. In Helfet DL, Greene WB [eds]. *Instructional Course Lectures, vol. 53.* Rosemont, IL: American Academy of Orthopedic Surgeons; 2003:343.)

Summary

The unique anatomy of the craniocervical junction results in unique patterns of injuries from typical mechanisms of trauma. In this area, ligamentous structures are as important as or more important than the bony constraints in providing stability and mobility. Luckily, the majority of trauma to the upper cervical spine does not result in neurologic deficit. However, unrecognized injuries may result in severe and permanent injury to the brain stem, upper spinal cord, and lower cranial nerves. A high index of suspicion and meticulous evaluation of the patient, mechanism of injury, and imaging studies will allow early diagnosis and proper treatment of these potentially devastating injuries.

PEARLS AND PITFALLS

1. Use of traction in type IIA hangman's fractures and in occipitoatlantal dislocations can lead to worsening neurologic deficit. In these cases, a small amount of traction can be applied during radiographic imaging under direct supervision to detect the presence of gross longitudinal instability. These patients are best managed with immediate application of a halo vest in compression.
2. Odontoid screw fixation is best accomplished in patients with good bone stock and fractures that reduce in neck extension. Beware of patients with a large chest, as this will compromise the angulation necessary for accurate placement of the odontoid screw. Biplanar fluoroscopy or intraoperative CT scanning is important for safe and accurate placement of internal fixation.
3. Beware of associated injuries and noncontiguous spinal injuries. Patients with multiple bony cervical injuries without neurologic deficit can be managed initially with application of a halo vest to allow the majority of the bony injuries to heal, then with delayed surgical stabilization and fusion of the remaining unstable areas.
4. Prior to placing a halo on patients with head and facial injuries, evaluate the head CT scan to rule out potential skull fractures that may lie in an area of halo pin placement.
5. If the C2 nerve root needs to be sacrificed for exposure of the C1–C2 joint, make sure that it is ligated proximal to the spinal ganglion. Failure to do so can result in severe occipital neuritis.
6. Assess preoperative imaging carefully in placement of any screw fixation into C1 and C2, especially looking for aberrant courses of the vertebral artery.

KEY POINTS

1. Patients who have sustained severe trauma to the head or face caused by a high-energy mechanism have a high incidence of upper cervical spine injuries.
2. Brain damage is more associated with upper cervical injuries than with injuries to the subaxial spine. These intracranial injuries must be diagnosed and treated expeditiously because they are the most common cause of mortality in these patients.

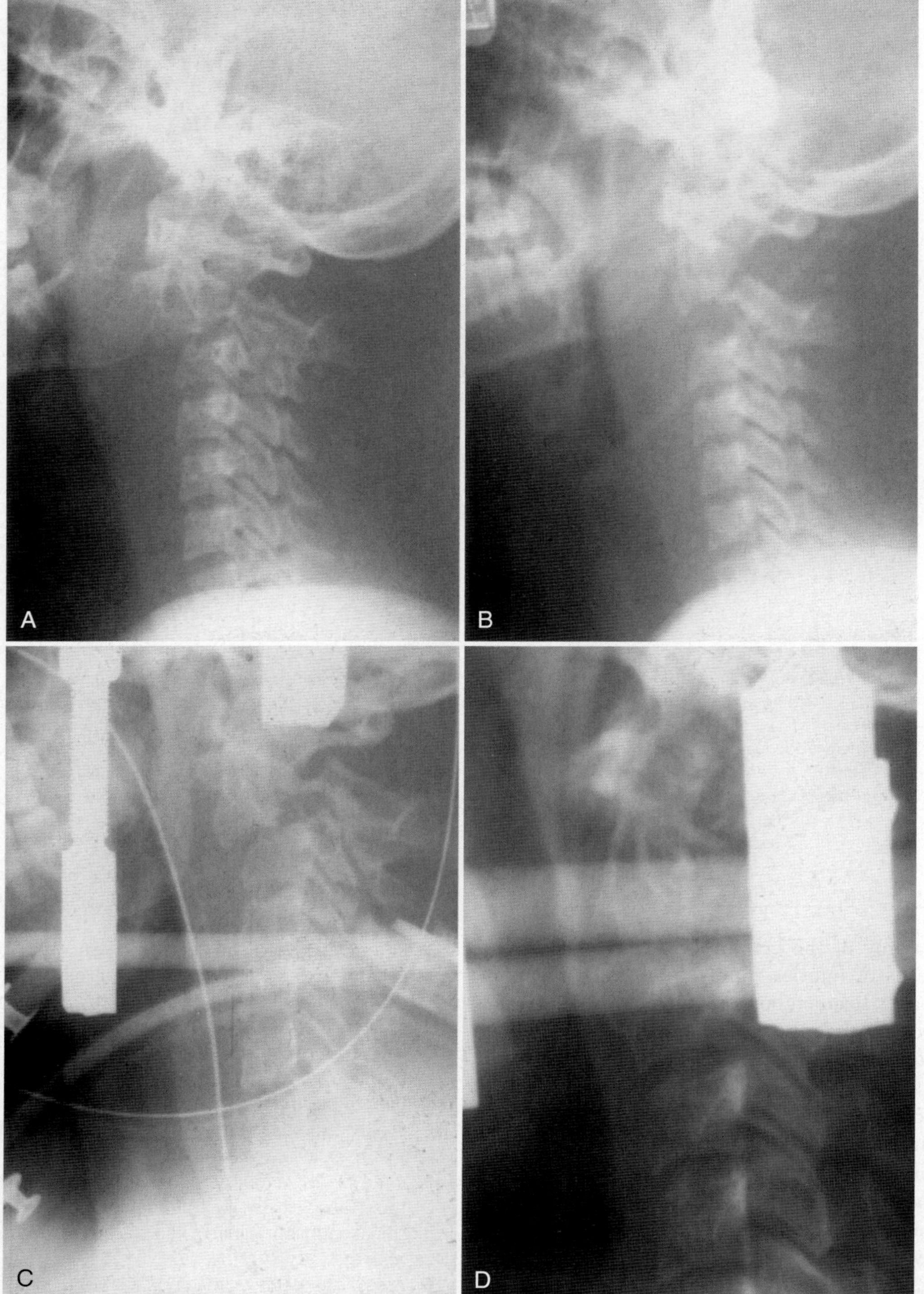

FIG. 75.23 This patient was involved in a motor vehicle collision and sustained a fracture of the pedicles of C2. She had no other significant injuries and was neurologically intact. (A) Lateral radiograph shows approximately 8 mm anterior subluxation with C2 anteriorly displaced on C3. The angulation of C2 on C3 is quite minimal. One would suspect that the disc at C2–C3 is completely disrupted, however, because of the severe degree of displacement. This is also consistent with the very large amount of anterior soft tissue swelling in front of C3, which measures 40 mm. (B) The patient was placed in 5 lb of traction. Overdistraction at the C2–C3 disc space is apparent. The patient remained neurologically intact. (C) The patient's traction was discontinued, and a halo vest was applied. Reduction was achieved under fluoroscopy. The patient remained neurologically normal. She was mobilized more slowly than most patients because of the instability that was present. (D) Lateral radiograph taken 3 months after her injury shows that the soft tissue swelling is completely resolved. There is calcification anteriorly at the C2–C3 disc space. This is often seen with these injuries owing to the significant amount of anterior striping of the anterior longitudinal ligament from the anterior aspect of the C3 vertebral body. With an anterior C2–C3 spontaneous fusion, posterior healing at the pedicles is unimportant.

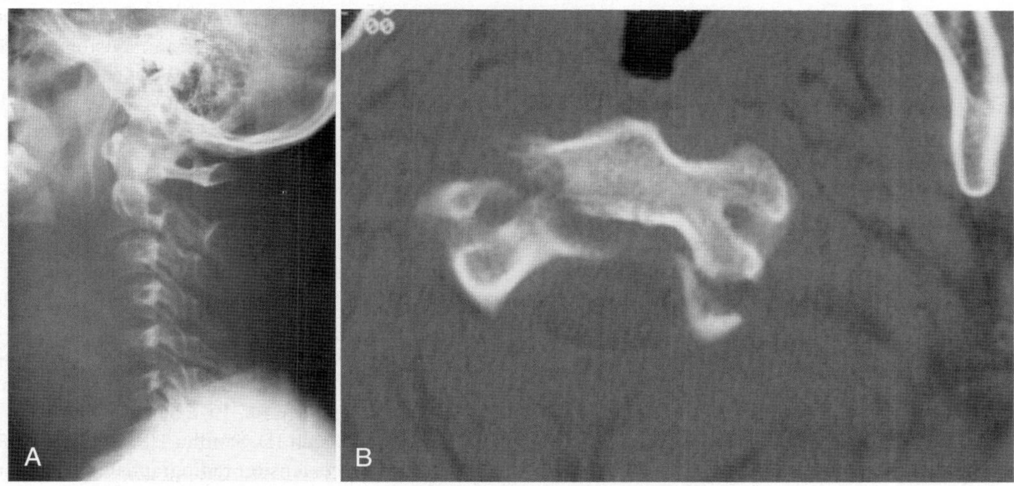

FIG. 75.24 This patient sustained a C2 pedicle fracture as a pedestrian when struck by a car. He had sustained an incomplete quadriplegia noted at the time of the accident. (A) Lateral radiograph shows mild to moderate anterior displacement of C2 on C3. By looking at the posterior aspect of the C2 vertebral body, it is apparent that there is a fracture with part of the C2 vertebral body staying in line with the C3 vertebral body, but there is also a fracture line just above this showing anterior displacement of the more cephalad aspect of the axis. (B) Computed tomography scan shows that the fracture line involved the posterior aspect of the vertebral body on the right side. This patient was treated in a halo vest and had complete resolution of his paralysis, and his C2 fractures healed. His spine was stable when seen at follow-up.

3. Dysfunction of the lower cranial nerves (CN IX, X, XI, XII) implicates severe injuries to the occipitoatlantal joint and the skull base.
4. CT remains the most sensitive imaging modality to evaluate fractures of the upper cervical spine, subaxial spine, and the cervicothoracic junction. CT is also cost effective as a primary screening tool, especially in high- and moderate-risk patients.[11]
5. Reduction and stabilization of the cervical spine is usually accomplished by Gardner-Wells tong traction in a rotating bed. The only contraindications to the use of traction in injuries of the CCJ are occipitoatlantal dislocations and type IIA hangman's fractures in which the application of traction can result in pathologic distraction and increased neurologic deficit.

KEY REFERENCES

1. Anderson LD, D'Alonzo RT. Fractures of the odontoid process of the axis. *J Bone Joint Surg Am.* 1974;56:1663-1674.
   The authors describe the most utilized classification system for odontoid fractures. The study also provides treatment recommendations based on fracture type and displacement.
2. Anderson PA, Montesano PX. Morphology and treatment of occipital condyle fractures. *Spine.* 1988;13:76.
   This article describes the three most common injury patterns seen in occipital condyle fractures. The authors describe a classification scheme that allows determination of the most efficacious methods of treatment.
3. Chapman J, Smith JS, Kopjar B, et al. *The AOSpine North America Geriatric Odontoid Fracture Mortality Study: a retrospective review of mortality outcomes for operative versus nonoperative treatment of 322 patients with long-term follow-up. Spine.* 2013;38(13):1098-1104.
   This study has become the main reference regarding the surgical and nonsurgical treatment of type II odontoid fractures in patients over the age of 65 years.
4. Dickman CA, Greene KA, Sonntag VK. Injuries involving the transverse atlantal ligament: classification and treatment guidelines based upon experience with 39 injuries. *Neurosurgery.* 1997;40:886-887.
   This classic article provides the most useful classification scheme for transverse ligament injuries based on CT and MRI evaluation. Evaluation and classification of specific injury types allows the practitioner to predict with high probability the likelihood of late instability. Treatment recommendations are also provided.
5. Harris JH Jr, Carson GC, Waganer LK, Kerr N. Radiologic diagnosis of traumatic occipitovertebral dissociation: II. Comparison of three methods of detecting occipitovertebral relationships on lateral radiographs of supine subjects. *AJR Am J Roentgenol.* 1994;162:887-892.
   This article evaluates the various radiographic methods of detecting occipital-cervical subluxation and dislocation with an assessment of the sensitivity and specificity of each of the available tests.
6. Levine AM, Edwards CC. The management of traumatic spondylolisthesis of the axis. *J Bone Joint Surg Am.* 1985;67:217-226.
   This classic article provides the most useful and utilized classification scheme for hangman's fractures along with treatment guidelines.

REFERENCES

1. McGrory BJ, Klassen RA, Chao EY, et al. Acute fractures and dislocations of the cervical spine in children and adolescents. *J Bone Joint Surg Am.* 1993;75:988-995.
2. Sherk HH, Nicholson JT, Chung SM. Fractures of the odontoid process in young children. *J Bone Joint Surg Am.* 1978;60:921-924.
3. Alker GJ Jr, Oh YS, Leslie EV. High cervical spine and craniocervical junction injuries in fatal traffic accidents: a radiological study. *Orthop Clin North Am.* 1978;9:1003-1010.
4. Hachen HJ. Spinal cord injury in children and adolescents: diagnostic pitfalls and therapeutic considerations in the acute stage [Proceedings]. *Paraplegia.* 1977;15:55-64.
5. Bohlman HH. Acute fractures and dislocations of the cervical spine: an analysis of three hundred hospitalized patients and review of the literature. *J Bone Joint Surg Am.* 1979;61:1119-1142.

6. Birney TJ, Hanley EN Jr. Traumatic cervical spine injuries in childhood and adolescence. *Spine*. 1989;14:1277-1282.
7. Givens TG, Polley KA, Smith GF, Hardin WD Jr. Pediatric cervical spine injury: a three-year experience. *J Trauma*. 1996;41:310-314.
8. Spivak JM, Weiss MA, Cotler JM, Call M. Cervical spine injuries in patients 65 and older. *Spine*. 1994;19:2302-2306.
9. Michaleff ZA, Maher CG, Verhagen AP, Rebbeck T, Lin CW. Accuracy of the Canadian C-spine rule and NEXUS to screen for clinically important cervical spine injury in patients following blunt trauma: a systematic review. *CMAJ*. 2012;184(16):E867-E876.
10. Kiwerski JE. Injuries to the spinal cord in elderly patients. *Injury*. 1992;23:397-400.
11. Weingarden SI, Graham PM. Falls resulting in spinal cord injury: patterns and outcomes in an older population. *Paraplegia*. 1989;27:423-427.
12. DeVivo MJ, Kartus PL, Rutt RD, et al. The influence of age at time of spinal cord injury on rehabilitation outcome. *Arch Neurol*. 1990;47:687-691.
13. Katzberg RW, Benedetti PF, Drake CM, et al. Acute cervical spine injuries: prospective MR imaging assessment at a level 1 trauma center. *Radiology*. 1999;213:203-212.
14. Blackmore CC, Emerson EE, Mann FA, Koepsell TD. Cervical spine imaging in patients with trauma: determination of fracture risk to optimize use. *Radiology*. 1999;211:759-765.
15. White AA III, Panjabi MM. *Clinical Biomechanics of the Spine*. Philadelphia: JB Lippincott; 1978.
16. Werne S. Studies in spontaneous atlas dislocation. *Acta Orthop Scand Suppl*. 1957;23:1-150.
17. Dvorak J, Schneider E, Saldinger P, Rahn B. Biomechanics of the craniocervical region: the alar and transverse ligaments. *J Orthop Res*. 1988;6:452-461.
18. Saldinger P, Dvorak J, Rahn BA, Perren SM. Histology of the alar and transverse ligaments. *Spine*. 1990;15:257-261.
19. Elgafy H, Pompo F, Vela R, Elsamaloty HM. Ipsilateral arcuate foramen and high-riding vertebral artery: implication on C1-C2 instrumentation. *Spine J*. 2014;14(7):1351-1355.
20. Lyness SS, Simeone FA. Vascular complications of upper cervical spine injuries. *Orthop Clin North Am*. 1978;9:1029-1038.
21. Fitzgerald RD, Krafft P, Skrbensky G, et al. Excursions of the cervical spine during tracheal intubation: blind oral intubation compared with direct laryngoscopy. *Anaesthesia*. 1994;49:111-115.
22. Levine AM, Edwards CC. Fractures of the atlas. *J Bone Joint Surg Am*. 1991;73:680-691.
23. Lalani Z, Bonanthaya KM. Cervical spine injury in maxillofacial trauma. *Br J Oral Maxillofac Surg*. 1997;35:243-245.
24. Iida H, Tachibana S, Kitahara T, et al. Association of head trauma with cervical spine injury, spinal cord injury, or both. *J Trauma*. 1999;46:450-452.
25. Friedman DP, Tartaglino LM, Fisher AR, Flanders AE. MR imaging in the diagnosis of intramedullary spinal cord diseases that involve specific neural pathways or vascular territories. *AJR Am J Roentgenol*. 1995;165:515-523.
26. Vaccaro AR, Klein GR, Flanders AE, et al. Long-term evaluation of vertebral artery injuries following cervical spine trauma using magnetic resonance angiography. *Spine*. 1998;23:789-794.
27. Cothren CC, Moore EE, Biffl WL, et al. Cervical spine fracture patterns predictive of blunt vertebral artery injury. *J Trauma*. 2003;55:811-813.
28. Weller SJ, Rossitch E Jr, et al. Detection of vertebral artery injury after cervical spine trauma using magnetic resonance angiography. *J Trauma*. 1999;46:660-666.
29. Wirbel R, Pistorius G, Braun C, et al. Bilateral vertebral artery lesion after dislocating cervical spine trauma: a case report. *Spine*. 1996;21:1375-1379.
30. Vaccaro AR, Urban WC, Aiken RD. Delayed cortical blindness and recurrent quadriplegia after cervical trauma. *J Spinal Disord*. 1998;11:535-539.
31. Bell HS. Paralysis of both arms from injury of the upper portion of the pyramidal decussation: "cruciate paralysis". *J Neurosurg*. 1970;33:376-380.
32. Eismont FJ, Bohlman HH. Posterior atlanto-occipital dislocation with fractures of the atlas and odontoid process. *J Bone Joint Surg Am*. 1978;60:397-399.
33. Wang JC, Hatch JD, Sandhu HS, Delamarter RB. Cervical flexion and extension radiographs in acutely injured patients. *Clin Orthop*. 1999;365:111-116.
34. Blackmore CC, Ramsey SD, Mann FA, Deyo RA. Cervical spine screening with CT in trauma patients: a cost-effectiveness analysis. *Radiology*. 1999;212:117-125.
35. Katz MA, Beredjiklian PK, Vresilovic EJ, et al. Computed tomographic scanning of cervical spine fractures: does it influence treatment? *J Orthop Trauma*. 1999; 13:338-343.
36. Klein GR, Vaccaro AR, Albert TJ, et al. Efficacy of magnetic resonance imaging in the evaluation of posterior cervical spine fractures. *Spine*. 1999;24:771-774.
37. Vaccaro AR, Kreidl KO, Pan W, et al. Usefulness of MRI in isolated upper cervical spine fractures in adults. *J Spinal Disord*. 1998;11:289-293.
38. Cotler HB, Kulkarni MV, Bondurant FJ. Magnetic resonance imaging of acute spinal cord trauma: preliminary report. *J Orthop Trauma*. 1988;2:1-4.
39. Lee KH, Chung TS, Jeon TJ, et al. Application of spatial modulation of magnetization to cervical spinal stenosis for evaluation of the hydrodynamic changes occurring in cerebrospinal fluid. *Korean J Radiol*. 2000;1(1):11-18.
40. Du R, Auguste KI, Chin CT, Engstrom JW, Weinstein PR. Magnetic resonance neurography for the evaluation of peripheral nerve, brachial plexus, and nerve root disorders. *J Neurosurg*. 2010;112(2):362-371.
41. Sees DW, Rodriguez Cruz LR, Flaherty SF, Ciceri DP. The use of bedside fluoroscopy to evaluate the cervical spine in obtunded trauma patients. *J Trauma*. 1998;45:768-771.
42. Blacksin MF, Lee HJ. Frequency and significance of fractures of the upper cervical spine detected by CT in patients with severe neck trauma. *AJR Am J Roentgenol*. 1995;165:1201-1204.
43. Bloom AI, Neeman Z, Slasky BS, et al. Fracture of the occipital condyles and associated craniocervical ligament injury: incidence, CT imaging and implications. *Clin Radiol*. 1997;52:198-202.
44. Mariani PJ. Occipital condyle fracture presenting as retropharyngeal hematoma. *Ann Emerg Med*. 1990;19:1447-1449.
45. Anderson PA, Montesano PX. Morphology and treatment of occipital condyle fractures. *Spine*. 1998;13:731-736.
46. Bucholz RW, Burkhead WZ, Graham W, Petty C. Occult cervical spine injuries in fatal traffic accidents. *J Trauma*. 1979;19:768-771.
47. Alker GJ, Oh YS, Leslie EV, et al. Postmortem radiology of head and neck injuries in fatal traffic accidents. *Radiology*. 1975;114:611-617.

48. Wholey MH, Bruwer AJ, Baker HL Jr. The lateral roentgenogram of the neck; with comments on the atlanto-odontoid-basion relationship. *Radiology*. 1958;71:350-356.
49. Dublin AB, Marks WM, Weinstock D, Newton TH. Traumatic dislocation of the atlanto-occipital articulation (AOA) with short-term survival: with a radiographic method of measuring the AOA. *J Neurosurg*. 1980;52:541-546.
50. Lee C, Woodring JH, Goldstein SJ, et al. Evaluation of traumatic atlantooccipital dislocations. *AJNR Am J Neuroradiol*. 1987;8:19-26.
51. Powers B, Miller MD, Kramer RS, et al. Traumatic anterior atlanto-occipital dislocation. *Neurosurgery*. 1979;4:12-17.
52. Harris JH, Carson GC, Wagner LK. Radiologic diagnosis of traumatic occipitovertebral dissociation: I. Normal occipitovertebral relationships on lateral radiographs of supine subjects. *AJR Am J Roentgenol*. 1994;162:881-886.
53. Harris JH Jr, Carson GC, Wagner LK, Kerr N. Radiologic diagnosis of traumatic occipitovertebral dissociation: II. Comparison of three methods of detecting occipitovertebral relationships on lateral radiographs of supine subjects. *AJR Am J Roentgenol*. 1994;162:887-892.
54. Traynelis VC, Marano GD, Dunker RP, Kaufman HH. Traumatic atlanto-occipital dislocation: case report. *J Neurosurg*. 1986;65:863-870.
55. Hadley MN. Management of pediatric cervical spine and spinal cord injuries. *Neurosurgery*. 2002;50(3 suppl):S85-S99.
56. Montane I, Eismont FJ, Green BA. Traumatic occipitoatlantal dislocation. *Spine*. 1991;16:112-116.
57. Frush TJ, Fisher TJ, Ensminger SC, Truumees E, Demetropoulos CK. Biomechanical evaluation of parasagittal occipital plating: screw load sharing analysis. *Spine*. 2009;34(9):877-884.
58. Connolly B, Turner C, DeVine J, Gerlinger T. Jefferson fracture resulting in Collet-Sicard syndrome. *Spine*. 2000;25:395-398.
59. Spence KF Jr, Decker S, Sell KW. Bursting atlantal fracture associated with rupture of the transverse ligament. *J Bone Joint Surg Am*. 1970;52:543-549.
60. Dickman CA, Greene KA, Sonntag VK. Injuries involving the transverse atlantal ligament: classification and treatment guidelines based upon experience with 39 injuries. *Neurosurgery*. 1996;38:44-50.
61. Bransford R, Chapman JR, Bellabarba C. Primary internal fixation of unilateral C1 lateral mass sagittal split fractures: a series of 3 cases. *J Spinal Disord Tech*. 2011;24(3):157-163.
62. Lee TT, Green BA, Petrin DR. Treatment of stable burst fractures of the atlas (Jefferson fracture) with rigid cervical collar. *Spine*. 1998;23:1963-1967.
63. Levine AM, Edwards CC. Treatment of injuries in the C1-C2 complex. *Orthop Clin North Am*. 1986;17:31-44.
64. Fowler JL, Sandhu A, Fraser RD. A review of fractures of the atlas vertebra. *J Spinal Disord*. 1990;3:19-24.
65. Hadley MN, Dickman CA, Browner CM, Sonntag VK. Acute traumatic atlas fractures: management and long term outcome. *Neurosurgery*. 1988;23:31-35.
66. McGuire RA Jr, Harkey HL. Primary treatment of unstable Jefferson's fractures. *J Spinal Disord*. 1995;8:233-236.
67. Segal LS, Grimm JO, Stauffer ES. Bursting atlantal fracture associated with rupture of the transverse ligament. *J Bone Joint Surg Am*. 1987;69:1423-1434.
68. Phillips WA, Hensinger RN. The management of rotatory atlanto-axial subluxations in children. *J Bone Joint Surg Am*. 1989;71:664-668.
69. Fielding JW, Hawkins RJ. Atlanto-axial rotatory fixation (fixed rotatory subluxation of the atlanto-axial joint). *J Bone Joint Surg Am*. 1977;59:37-44.
70. Fielding JW, Cochran GB, Lawsing JF 3rd, Hohl M. Tears of the transverse ligament of the atlas: a clinical and biomechanical study. *J Bone Joint Surg Am*. 1974;56:1683-1691.
71. Brooks AL, Jenkins EB. Atlanto-axial arthrodesis by the wedge compression method. *J Bone Joint Surg Am*. 1978;60:279-284.
72. Crawford NR, Hurlbert RJ, Choi WG, Dickman CH. Differential biomechanical effects of injury and wiring at C1-C2. *Spine*. 1999;24:1894-1902.
73. Lesoin F, Autricque A, Franz K, et al. Transcervical approach and screw fixation for upper cervical spine pathology. *Surg Neurol*. 1987;27:459-465.
74. Reindl R, Sen M, Aebi M. Anterior instrumentation for traumatic C1-C2 instability. *Spine*. 1993;28:E329-E333.
75. Amyes EW, Anderson FM. Fracture of the odontoid process; report of sixty-three cases. *AMA Arch Surg*. 1956;72:377-393.
76. Anderson LD, D'Alonzo RT. Fractures of the odontoid process of the axis. *J Bone Joint Surg Am*. 1974;56:1663-1674.
77. Clark CR, White AA. Fractures of the dens: a multicenter study. *J Bone Joint Surg Am*. 1985;67:1340-1348.
78. Chapman J, Smith JS, Kopjar B, et al. The AOSpine North America Geriatric Odontoid Fracture Mortality Study: a retrospective review of mortality outcomes for operative versus nonoperative treatment of 322 patients with long-term follow-up. *Spine*. 2013;38(13):1098-1104.
79. Smith JS, Kepler CK, Kopjar B, et al. Effect of type II odontoid fracture nonunion on outcome among elderly patients treated without surgery: based on the AOSpine North America geriatric odontoid fracture study. *Spine*. 2013;38(26): 2240-2246.
80. Roberts A, Wickstrom J. Prognosis of odontoid fractures. *Acta Orthop Scand*. 1973;44:21-30.
81. Hadley MN, Dickman CA, Browner CM, Sonntag VK. Acute axis fractures: a review of 229 cases. *J Neurosurg*. 1989;71 (5 Pt 1):642-647.
82. Grob D, Jeanneret B, Aebi M, Markwalder TM. Atlanto-axial fusion with transarticular screw fixation. *J Bone Joint Surg Br*. 1991;73:972-976.
83. Jeanneret B, Vernet O, Frei S, Magerl F. Atlantoaxial mobility after screw fixation of the odontoid: a computed tomographic study. *J Spinal Disord*. 1991;4:203-211.
84. Andersson S, Rodrigues M, Olerud C. Odontoid fractures: high complication rate associated with anterior screw fixation in the elderly. *Eur Spine J*. 2000;9:56-59.
85. Chiba K, Fujimura Y, Toyama Y, et al. Treatment protocol for fractures of the odontoid process. *J Spinal Disord*. 1996;9:267-276.
86. Vieweg U, Meyer B, Schramm J. Differential treatment in acute upper cervical spine injuries: a critical review of a single-institution series. *Surg Neurol*. 2000;54:203-210.
87. Levine AM, Edwards CC. The management of traumatic spondylolisthesis of the axis. *J Bone Joint Surg Am*. 1985;67:217-226.
88. Starr JK, Eismont FJ. Atypical hangman's fractures. *Spine*. 1993;18:1954-1957.
89. Francis WR, Fielding JW, Hawkins RJ, et al. Traumatic spondylolisthesis of the axis. *J Bone Joint Surg Br*. 1981;63:313-318.

76 CHAPTER

Lower Cervical Spine Injuries

Paul A. Anderson

Introduction

Cervical spine injuries occur in 3% to 6% of patients presenting for evaluation and should be considered in all blunt trauma patients.[1-3] The subaxial spine from C3 to C7 accounts for two-thirds of all cervical injuries.[4] Spinal cord injuries are present in 0.8% to 1.2% of cases.[1,5] The incidence increases in patients over the age of 65 years and is less common in children. Males predominate and are twice as likely as females to sustain cervical spine injury. The mechanism of injury is from vehicular trauma in up to 50%, while falls account for 40% of injuries, especially in the elderly.[6] Over the past 15 years, the incidence of spinal cord injury and death associated with cervical spine injury has decreased by more than half due to a lower incidence of vehicular trauma.[1]

This chapter reviews the evaluation and management of subaxial trauma patients, focusing on using new classification systems to aid the decision treatment process.

Anatomy

Bony Anatomy

The lower cervical spine normally has a lordotic alignment, which decreases with age. Vertebrae from C3 to T1 have similar shapes, but are increasingly larger caudally, with C7 and T1 having large spinous processes due to attachments of the nuchal ligaments. On the superior surface of each vertebral body, a bony protrusion extends laterally and cranially, called the uncinate process. With age, these may hypertrophy and cause foraminal stenosis. Short pedicles connect the body with the lateral masses. The pedicles are oriented outward relative to the body from 10 to 45 degrees. The lateral masses viewed laterally are rhomboid in shape. Each lateral mass has cranial and caudal articular surfaces; the superior and inferior facet joints form the zygoapophyseal joints. The articular surfaces are flat in the coronal plane and are oriented upward 30 to 45 degrees. The laminae are bony plates connecting the lateral masses posteriorly. The spinous processes are dorsal midline projections from the lamina. From C2 to C5 or C6, the spinous process is bifid. The transverse process extends from the anterior body and connects with bony projections from the lateral masses to form the foramen transversarium.

The subaxial vertebrae articulate with each other through the intervertebral disc and the paired facet joints. The disc is composed of the anulus fibrosus, nucleus, and vertebral endplates. The anulus has approximately 20 layers of type I collagen fibers. The collagen layers are alternatively oriented 40 degrees from the long axis and insert in the outer ring of the endplate. The vertebral endplates are thickened bony plate structures lined with cartilage. The nucleus is a viscoelastic cartilaginous structure containing cells, water, type II collagen, and proteoglycans. The normal disc has 70% to 80% water content, which is bound by the proteoglycans, giving the disc its mechanical properties.

Ligamentous Anatomy

The spinal ligaments are essential to function; assessment of their integrity is critical when evaluating injuries. The anterior longitudinal ligaments (ALL) and posterior longitudinal ligaments (PLL) are continuous, broad, bandlike structures extending from C2 to the sacrum along the anterior and posterior vertebral surfaces, respectively. At each disc, the ALL and PLL can blend with the anulus and span each intervertebral disc. The ALL ends at C2; the PLL continues above C2 as the tectorial membrane, which attaches at the basion at the foramen magnum. Posterior ligaments are essential to stability and include the ligamenta flava, facet joint capsules, and the nuchal ligaments. The ligamentum flavum is largely composed of elastin and spans between laminae. It is not continuous and is elastic, and rupture of it indicates that significant displacement has occurred. The facet capsules are redundant to allow motion of zygapophyseal joints. The nuchal ligaments include the ligamentum nuchae, supraspinous, and interspinous ligaments. The nuchal ligament is strongly attached at C7, T1, and C2 and is essential to maintaining an upright head position.

Neurovascular Anatomy

The spinal cord lies within the spinal canal. It is remarkably similar in dimensions among humans, with an average of about an 8-mm midsagittal diameter in adults. The spinal canal diameter should be a minimum of 13 mm; when less than 10 mm, spinal stenosis is present. Smaller spinal canals correlate with increased risk and severity of spinal cord injury.[7]

At each level, the dorsal and ventral rootlets form a spinal nerve in the neuroforamina. The spinal nerve root lies above each pedicle, behind the disc and posterolateral body, and in front of the lateral masses.

The spinal cord blood supply is from the two posterior and single ventral spinal arteries. In addition, there are several radicular arteries that provide important segmental blood flow, which are variable in number and location. The second part of the vertebral artery passes into the foramen transversarium between C6 and C7 and ascends to C2. Fractures of the transverse processes or lateral masses or subluxations may injure these vessels.

Mechanism of Injury

The cervical spine supports the cranium and is rigidly attached to the thoracic cavity at the cervicothoracic junction; thus, any forces applied to the cranium will be transmitted to the cervical spine. In addition to downward or axially directed forces, bending moments can lead to combinations of compression and distraction injuries. An example is the flexion–axial loading injury or teardrop fracture, in which comminution of the body occurs from compression and tensile failure of the posterior osteoligamentous complex from distraction. Finally, less common, but often the most severe, are injuries from acceleration-deceleration forces. Because the bone and ligamentous tissues have viscoelastic properties, short loading times on the order of 5 to 8 ms create large accelerations/decelerations (which occur during vehicular trauma) and cause proportionally greater damage, especially to ligamentous tissues.

Compression forces are generally downward, centrally, onto the vertebral bodies, but also can be projected laterally onto the lateral masses or posteriorly to the spinous processes. The injury type will be determined by the location of the axial load relative to the vertebrae and the position of the vertebrae at the time of impact. Since the cranium is mobile and may be relatively flexed or extended, the same force can produce a variety of fracture types.[8] In addition, during loading from the cranium, segmental motion occurs, known as snaking, so that one vertebra may be subject to direct compressive forces while another level is subject to distractive forces.

Distraction forces occur from bending moments or from rapid head acceleration-deceleration. Ligamentous injuries with or without bony avulsions can result. This is most commonly seen in hyperflexion, in which facet dislocations and posterior ligamentous injuries occur. Extension-distraction is being seen more commonly, especially in geriatric patients who fall onto their heads or faces. These injuries can result in discoligamentous injuries combined with posterior element fractures.

Increasingly seen as the population ages are patients who have hyperextension injuries and sustain spinal cord injury without significant bony abnormalities. The spinal column may have subtle signs of injury, such as a discoligamentous injury, gaps in the facet joints, or isolated spinous process or laminar fracture. The spinal cord injury occurs due to transient compression of the spinal cord between bulging discs and an infolded ligamentum flavum. The patient will usually have a narrow spinal canal and have ongoing spinal cord compression.

Assessment of the Spine-Injured Patient

Initial Evaluation

Patients sustaining blunt trauma should be assumed to have a potential spinal column injury. During transport, patients are placed on a backboard and immobilized in a hard extraction collar. The immediate primary care is to evaluate airway, breathing, and cardiovascular functions, and begin resuscitation. The secondary exam includes visual examination of the spinal column by log rolling the patient and palpation to determine tenderness, crepitus, and gaps or step-offs between spinous processes. Hemorrhage, contusion, and abrasion on the face, head, or dorsal spine should raise suspicion of spinal injury. The goal of spinal evaluation is to identify patients who require further imaging and to critically measure neurologic function.

Clearing the Cervical Spine

The goal of this evaluation is to identify patients who have significant cervical injury after trauma. Patients can be divided into four categories: asymptomatic, temporarily not evaluable, symptomatic, and obtunded. Asymptomatic patients are those who have no pain, tenderness to palpation, normal cognitive function, and no distracting injuries. Distracting injuries are other sources of trauma that may decrease or eliminate cervical spine signs or symptoms. Examples of distracting injuries are fracture-dislocations, long-bone fractures, burns, shock, chest trauma, and craniofacial trauma.

Asymptomatic Patients

Asymptomatic adult patients can be cleared of cervical spine injury without any radiologic imaging. The National Emergency X-Radiography Utilization Study (NEXUS) screened 34,068 patients using the criteria and identified 99.8% of all injuries.[9] Six of the eight missed cases were trivial fractures and two were significant (odontoid fractures) that did not develop a neurologic injury. The specificity was low (12.8%), indicating that many patients still required imaging, which was negative. A simple modification is the Canadian Cervical Spine Rule (CCR), which adds 45 degrees of pain-free rotation of the head to the examination.[10] Stiell reported a 100% sensitivity using this method and improved specificity over the NEXUS method.[10] Both of these protocols are not applicable to children and are less accurate in geriatric patients.[11]

Temporarily Not Evaluable

These patients are less well defined. However, they could be cleared using the asymptomatic criteria, but have distracting injuries or impaired cognitive function, such as intoxication, that will clear or be corrected within 24 to 48 hours.[12] Initially, they are immobilized in an orthosis, then later reevaluated based on NEXUS or CCR criteria. If negative at that time, they may be cleared with further imaging. If clearance is required immediately, then they should be evaluated as described later for obtunded patients.

Symptomatic Patients

All symptomatic patients following blunt trauma are at high risk for cervical spine injury, thus require radiologic imaging.[9] Computed tomography (CT) in adults is highly sensitive and preferred over plain radiography.[13] Magnetic resonance imaging (MRI) is not recommended as a screening examination due to its cost and high rate of false positives.[14] MRI is indicated in patients who have unexplained neurologic deficits (such as central cord syndrome), for patients for whom there is suspected ligamentous injury, in patients with significant degenerative or postsurgical changes, as well as to aid surgical decision making. A negative MRI, however, does accurately exclude the presence of a cervical spine injury.[14]

Obtunded Patients

The clearance of obtunded patients remains controversial. Maintaining spine precautions and cervical immobilization in this patient population is associated with reduced pulmonary function, increased intracranial pressure, and risk of skin decubitus. Thus, timely clearance is important. Two options are available in obtunded patients: utilize results of CT or include MRI.[12] Modern helical CT is highly sensitive and rarely have significant injuries been reported following CT. Most cases are results of misreading by radiologists. MRI, however, has been shown to identify more injuries than CT and, in some studies, resulted in need for surgical treatment. Like investigations regarding CT, these studies are small retrospective studies without adequate statistical power. I recommend that each institution utilize its own protocol and continue to monitor effectiveness.

Neurologic Examination

A complete neurologic examination is performed, including cognitive function, cranial nerve, motor sensory function in the extremities, reflexes, and pathologic reflexes. In addition, in patients with any neurologic deficits, careful evaluation of perineal function is performed. Patients' neurologic function should be reported per American Spinal Injury Association (ASIA) standards (Fig. 76.1).[15] The ASIA motor score is the summation of motor function of 10 key muscle groups, five in the upper and five in the lower extremities, bilaterally; each is graded from 0 to 5. Summation of these scores defines the ASIA motor score and the total ranges from 0 to 100. Sensory examination of each dermatome is recorded as intact, hypoesthesia, or absent. Perianal examination is essential, as patients may have only sacral root sparing, which can dramatically change the prognosis.

Perianal rectal function is determined by digital rectal examination, assessing the initial tone and asking the patient to perform voluntary rectal contractions. The bulbocavernosus reflex and the anal wink are spinal cord–mediated reflexes at the level of the conus medullaris. The anal wink is obtained by brushing the paraspinal area with a pin and observing for an anal contraction. The bulbocavernosus reflex is best obtained during digital rectal examination by placing tension on a Foley catheter and observing for a rectal contraction. These reflexes are present in intact patients. Although they are typically absent in acute spinal cord–injured patients, they may return early (within 7 to 10 days after spinal cord injury). Intact perianal function in injuries at the conus medullaris, such as L1 or T12 fractures, or for cauda equina injuries is a good prognostic sign, as it indicates that the afferent and efferent neurons and the conus are functional.

Deep tendon reflexes, including biceps, triceps, patella, and Achilles, are assessed. In acute spinal cord injuries, the reflexes below the level of injury are usually absent due to spinal shock, but will return in 10 to 21 days when they will become hyperreflexic. In addition, pathologic reflexes—such as Hoffman, Babinski, and clonus—should be recorded. Priapism, if present, is a sign of acute spinal cord injury.

Spinal Cord Injury Classification

Spinal cord injuries are classified at the level and extent of injury. ASIA defines the level as the lowest segment with at least antigravity (grade ≥3) motor function.[15] The extent of spinal cord injuries is how much of the cross-sectional area of the cord is injured. Complete cord injuries are defined as complete loss of motor and sensory function; incomplete cord injuries have some retained motor and/or sensory function below the zone of injury. Special attention needs to be focused in the perineal area, as this may be the only area distinguishing complete from incomplete injuries. Incomplete cord injuries are important to recognize and have a much better prognosis. The anterior cord syndrome represents loss of the anterior two-thirds of the spinal cord, where there is paralysis of distal motor function and loss of pain and temperature sensation. These patients have retained dorsal column function, so that they may experience light touch, proprioception, and vibratory sensation, but no pinprick or motor function.

Central cord syndrome is a common cord injury in which there is loss of gray matter and central white matter. The white matter tracts are laminated, with cervical tracts positioned more centrally and lumbar and sacral tracts located toward the periphery. Because of the relative sparing of these laterally located tracts, the central cord syndrome is manifested by greater loss of upper than lower extremity function. The prognosis for central cord syndrome is good, with an expectation for ambulation, but hand function may be chronically impaired. The posterior cord syndrome is the loss of the posterior column with sparing of the anterior cord. These injuries produce loss of vibration, light touch, and position sense, but maintain pain, temperature, and motor functions. Brown-Séquard syndrome is a hemicord injury with ipsilateral motor paralysis and loss of dorsal column function as well as

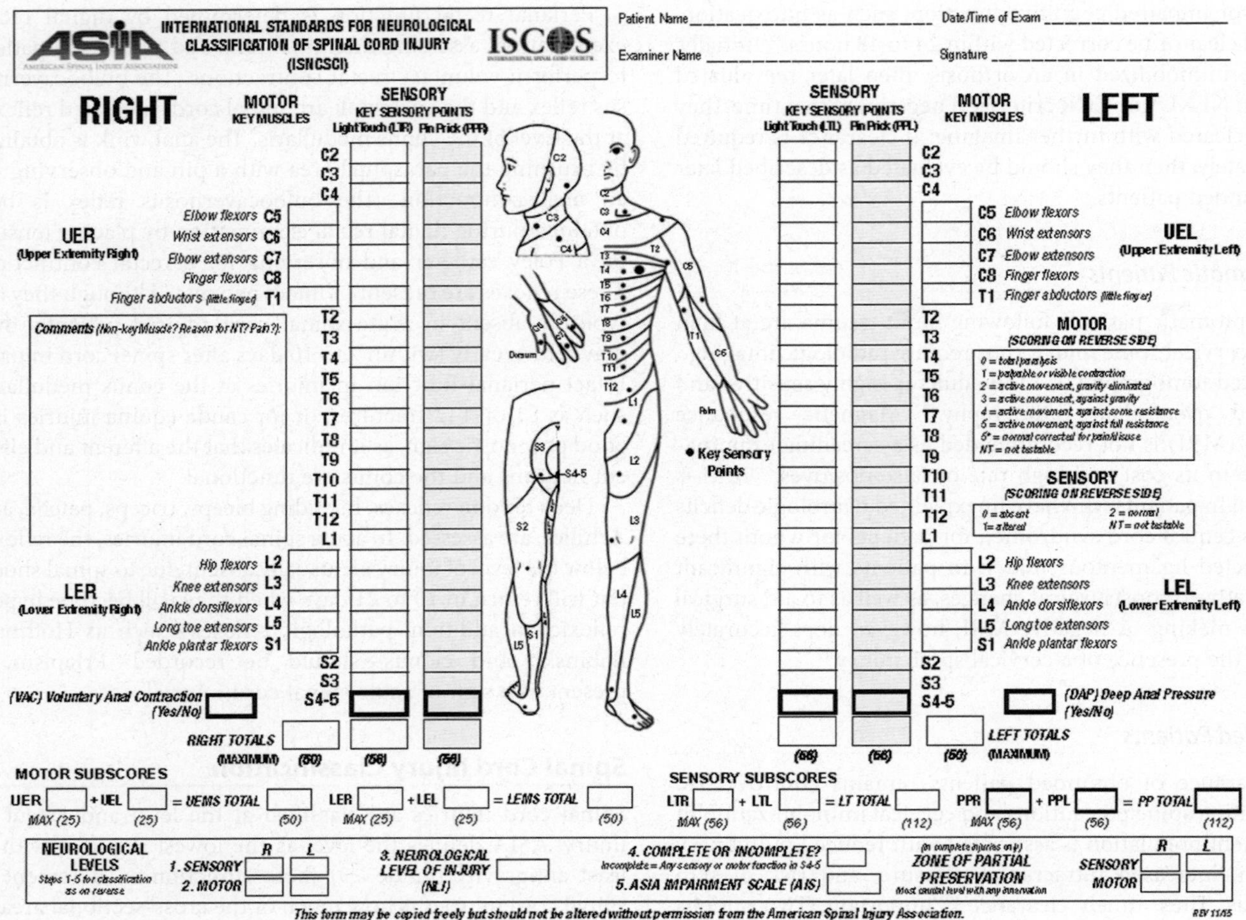

ASIA — INTERNATIONAL STANDARDS FOR NEUROLOGICAL CLASSIFICATION OF SPINAL CORD INJURY (ISNCSCI) — ISCOS

Patient Name ______ Date/Time of Exam ______
Examiner Name ______ Signature ______

RIGHT — MOTOR KEY MUSCLES — SENSORY KEY SENSORY POINTS Light Touch (LTR) Pin Prick (PPR)

C2, C3, C4

UER (Upper Extremity Right): Elbow flexors C5; Wrist extensors C6; Elbow extensors C7; Finger flexors C8; Finger abductors (little finger) T1

T2, T3, T4, T5, T6, T7, T8, T9, T10, T11, T12, L1

Comments (Non-key Muscle? Reason for NT? Pain?):

LER (Lower Extremity Right): Hip flexors L2; Knee extensors L3; Ankle dorsiflexors L4; Long toe extensors L5; Ankle plantar flexors S1

S2, S3, S4-5

(VAC) Voluntary Anal Contraction (Yes/No)

RIGHT TOTALS (MAXIMUM) (50) (56) (56)

LEFT — SENSORY KEY SENSORY POINTS Light Touch (LTL) Pin Prick (PPL) — MOTOR KEY MUSCLES

C2, C3, C4

UEL (Upper Extremity Left): C5 Elbow flexors; C6 Wrist extensors; C7 Elbow extensors; C8 Finger flexors; T1 Finger abductors (little finger)

T2, T3, T4, T5, T6, T7, T8, T9, T10, T11, T12, L1

LEL (Lower Extremity Left): L2 Hip flexors; L3 Knee extensors; L4 Ankle dorsiflexors; L5 Long toe extensors; S1 Ankle plantar flexors

S2, S3, S4-5

(DAP) Deep Anal Pressure (Yes/No)

LEFT TOTALS (MAXIMUM) (56) (56) (50)

• Key Sensory Points

MOTOR (SCORING ON REVERSE SIDE)
0 = total paralysis
1 = palpable or visible contraction
2 = active movement, gravity eliminated
3 = active movement, against gravity
4 = active movement, against some resistance
5 = active movement, against full resistance
5* = normal corrected for pain/disuse
NT = not testable

SENSORY (SCORING ON REVERSE SIDE)
0 = absent 2 = normal
1 = altered NT = not testable

MOTOR SUBSCORES
UER ___ + UEL ___ = UEMS TOTAL ___ LER ___ + LEL ___ = LEMS TOTAL ___
MAX (25) (25) (50) MAX (25) (25) (50)

SENSORY SUBSCORES
LTR ___ + LTL ___ = LT TOTAL ___ PPR ___ + PPL ___ = PP TOTAL ___
MAX (56) (56) (112) MAX (56) (56) (112)

NEUROLOGICAL LEVELS (Steps 1-5 for classification as on reverse) R L
1. SENSORY
2. MOTOR
3. NEUROLOGICAL LEVEL OF INJURY (NLI)
4. COMPLETE OR INCOMPLETE? Incomplete = Any sensory or motor function in S4-5
5. ASIA IMPAIRMENT SCALE (AIS)
ZONE OF PARTIAL PRESERVATION (In complete injuries only) Most caudal level with any innervation — SENSORY R L; MOTOR R L

This form may be copied freely but should not be altered without permission from the American Spinal Injury Association. REV 11/15

A

ASIA Impariment Scale (AIS)

A = Complete. No sensory or motor function is preserved in the sacral segments S4-5.

B = Sensory Incomplete. Sensory but not motor function is preserved below the neurological level and includes the sacral segments S4-5 (light touch or pin prick at S4-5 or deep anal pressure) AND no motor function is preserved more than three levels below the motor level on either side of the body.

C = Motor Incomplete. Motor function is preserved at the most caudal sacral segments for voluntary anal contraction (VAC) OR the patient meets the criteria for sensory incomplete status (sensory function preserved at the most caudal sacral segments (S4-S5) by LT, PP or DAP), and has some sparing of motor function more than three levels below the ipsilateral motor level on either side of the body.
(This includes key or non-key muscle functions to determine motor incomplete status.) For AIS C – less than half of key muscle functions below the single NLI have a muscle grade ≥ 3.

D = Motor Incomplete. Motor incomplete status as defined above, with at least half (half or more) of key muscle functions below the single NLI having a muscle grade ≥ 3.

E = Normal. If sensation and motor function as tested with the ISNCSCI are graded as normal in all segments, and the patient had prior deficits, then the AIS grade is E. Someone without an initial SCI does not receive an AIS grade.

Using ND: To document the sensory, motor and NLI levels, the ASIA Impairment Scale grade, and/or the zone of partial preservation (ZPP) when they are unable to be determined based on the examination results.

B

FIG. 76.1 (A) American Spinal Injury Association (ASIA) system to grade the neurologic function of spinal-injured patients. (B) ASIA Impairment Scale. (Courtesy of the American Spinal Injury Association.)

contralateral loss of pain and temperature. The prognosis for Brown-Séquard syndrome is excellent.

The ASIA Impairment Scale (AIS) assesses the extent of injury and is highly predictive of outcomes (Fig. 76.1B).[15] Complete cord injuries with absence of distal and sensory motor function are ASIA A. The ASIA B patient has some sensation, but no motor function below the zone of injury. ASIA C patients have both motor and sensory function below the zone of injury, but the motor function is less than grade 3. ASIA D patients, like ASIA C patients, have both motor and sensory function, but motor function is grade 4 or 5. ASIA E patients are intact.

Patients with neurologic deficits should have neurologic exams at least every 2 hours, which are documented in the record. Neurologic function may change in the initial stages after spinal cord injury, which will be an important determinant of treatment. Therefore, accurate reporting of the neurologic exams is essential. The ASIA classification is useful for a comprehensive report of the neurologic examination (see Fig. 76.1A).

Classification of Injuries

Many classification systems of lower cervical spine injuries have been described, with none being universally accepted. These systems are based on fracture morphology, presumed mechanism, force vectors of injury, or ratings of severity, such as stable versus unstable. These all have shortcomings, including poor reliability, high complexity, utilization of out-of-date imaging, lack of inclusion of neurologic deficits, and poor prediction of surgical indications and prognosis. One important determinant of treatment is severity of injury, which is difficult to quantify.

Fracture Stability

Determining fracture stability is essential for determination of the best course of treatment. Stability has been defined as the ability to maintain alignment and protect the neural tissues, resulting in a long-term painless spine under physiologic loads. This simple concept is difficult to apply in individual patients even by experienced practitioners. Stability thus defined is binary: stable or unstable. However, in reality, stability is a continuum. Also, stability may be time dependent, usually worse initially but may recover at later points in time depending on the healing potential of the tissues involved and of the patient. Newer systems apply this concept of assessing stability along a continuing scale rather than present or absent.

Cervical Spine Injury Severity Score

More recent systems have been developed to resolve these shortcomings. The Cervical Spine Injury Severity Score (CSISS) divides the spine into four columns: anterior, each lateral column, and the posterior osteoligamentous complex.[16] The severity of injury to each column is assessed using an analog scale from 0 to 5. A 0 is given for no injury and 5 for the most severe injury possible to that column. The scale is continuous, and each column is graded independently. The scores from each of the four columns are summed, resulting in the CSISS, and ranges from 0 (no injury) to 20 (most severe injury). The reliability of the CSISS is excellent. In one study, a score of 7 or greater was associated with surgery in 100% of cases and a score less than 5 indicated nonoperative treatment.[16]

TABLE 76.1 Subaxial Cervical Injury Classification System (SLIC)[17]

	Points
Fracture Morphology	
Compression	1
Burst	2
Distraction	3
Translation/rotation	4
Osteoligamentous Complex	
Intact	0
Intermediate	1
Disrupted	2
Neurologic	
Intact	0
Root injury	1
Complete spinal cord injury	2
Incomplete spinal cord injury	3
Ongoing cord compression in setting of neurologic deficit	+1
Total SLIC	**0–9**

Subaxial Cervical Injury Classification System

The Subaxial Cervical Injury Classification System (SLIC) was developed to include both severity of injury and the neurologic state to aid in surgical decision making.[17] Three domains are assessed and graded independently: fracture morphology, the osteoligamentous complex, and neurologic function (Table 76.1). The morphology is graded based on a general description of the fracture mechanism: compression, burst, distraction, and translation/rotation. The osteoligamentous complex has long been felt to be essential to maintain spine stability. In the SLIC system, this is assessed as intact, intermediate, and injured. The intermediate grade is allowed, as in many cases it is impossible, even with MRI, to know the state of the osteoligamentous complex. Neurologic function is graded as intact, radiculopathy, complete spinal cord injury, and incomplete spinal cord injury. The incomplete spinal cord injury is given the higher score compared to complete, as the urgency in surgical indications are greater in this injury pattern. Each of the three domains are scored and summed, giving a SLIC score ranging from 0 to 9. Scores of 3 or less are treated nonoperatively, and scores of greater than 5 are treated surgically. Scores of 4 or 5 may be treated either nonoperatively or operatively. In many cases, an orthosis is attempted and upright serial radiographs are obtained to assess maintenance of alignment. If neurologic symptoms or progressive kyphosis or subluxation develops, then surgery is warranted.

AO Cervical Spine Classification

The AO group has been a leader in developing classification systems for all skeletal traumas. Their spine classification system is based on three basic morphologies: compression, distraction, and translation. However, this system lacked reliability and was too complex for clinical use. Recently, an updated AO classification system has been developed.[18] The AO system uses four criteria: injury morphology, facet injury, neurologic status, and case-specific modifiers. When using the system, the user should record level, morphology type, and secondary injuries. In addition, modifiers such as facet injury, neurologic status, and case-specific variants are placed in parentheses.

The modified AO classification system has been updated to simplify its use, promote better direction for treatment, and is based on modern imaging, including MRI.[18] Three basic categories describe the primary injury (Table 76.2). Type A occurs from compressive forces with intact posterior tension band. Type B is distractive injuries of the posterior or anterior tension bands. Type C is injuries in which there is translational displacement in any of the primary axes, including anteroposterior (AP), lateral, rotational, or vertical. If multiple types of injuries are present, then the fracture is graded with its highest score.

AO Type A Injuries

AO type A compressive lesions are vertebral body injuries that occur under axial loading forces with loss of vertical height.

TABLE 76.2 Modified AO Classification Cervical Spine Injuries

Type A	A0	No bony or trivial injury
	A1	Compression fracture of only single endplate
	A2	Compression fracture involving two endplates
	A3	Burst fracture with bone retropulsion involving only single endplate
	A4	Burst fracture with bone retropulsion involving both endplates
Type B	B1	Bony injury of either anterior or posterior tension bands
	B2	Posterior ligamentous distractive injury with or without fracture
	B3	Anterior discoligamentous disruption
Type C	C	Translation or rotational injury along any axis
Facet injuries	F1	Nondisplaced facet injury with low potential for subluxation (<1 cm and <40% facet)
	F2	Nondisplaced facet injury with low potential for subluxation (>1 cm and >40% facet)
	F3	Fracture separation of lateral mass
	F4	Perched facets
Neurologic	N0	Intact
	N1	Transient neurologic deficit
	N2	Root injury or radiculopathy
	N3	Incomplete spinal cord injury
	N4	Complete spinal cord injury
Case-specific modifiers	M1	Possible ligamentous injury
	M2	Traumatic disc herniation
	M3	Fracture in ankylosed spine
	M4	Vertebral artery injury

Similarly, impaction of the spinous processes can cause fracturing under compression. Compression injuries are subcategorized into five types. Type A0 has no bony or trivial injuries, such as fractures of the spinous process or transverse process and patients who have spinal cord injuries without bony fracture. Type A1 fractures are compression fractures of a single endplate without involvement of the posterior vertebral body wall. Type A2 are fractures that include both superior and inferior endplates without fracture of the posterior vertebral body wall. Type A3 are burst fractures when there is fracture of one endplate and the posterior vertebral body wall with retropulsion of bone into the spinal canal. Type A4 injuries are comminuted burst fractures that involve both superior and inferior endplates and sagittal split fractures that also involve both endplates.

AO Type B Injuries

The AO type B are distractive lesions and can include disruptions of either the anterior or posterior tension bands. These injuries do not have associated translation. Type B1 are bony injuries of the posterior or the anterior tension band. Type B2 are distractive injuries involving posterior ligaments, with or without fracture. These lesions may include nuchal ligaments, facet capsules, and ligamenta flava. Type B3 are anterior tension band injuries with distraction injuries to the discoligamentous complex and the ALL. The posterior tension band is intact, which acts as a tether or center for rotation. There may be bony avulsion fractures along the bodies.

AO Type C Injuries

Type C are translational injuries along any axis, resulting in displacement of one vertebral body relative to the other.

Facet Fractures

Facet injuries are difficult to classify in traditional systems. The AO system grades each facet independently. For bilateral facet injuries, the right side is annotated before the left. If the type of facet injury is identical between sides, BL is designated. Injuries that are isolated to the facet articulations—without a type A, B, or C injury—are classified as facet injuries. F1 are nondisplaced, inferior, or superior facet fractures that have low potential for displacement (<1 cm, <40% of lateral mass). F2 are inferior and superior facet fractures that involve a larger area of the facet with increased likelihood of displacement (>1 cm, >40% of lateral mass). Type F3 is a fracture separation of the lateral mass, where there is an ipsilateral fracture of the lamina and pedicle, which creates a free-floating lateral mass.[19] If this subluxes or rotates anteriorly, then vertebral subluxation can occur at both the cranial and caudal level. Type F4 are facet injuries, where the inferior edge of the cranial facet lies in the perched position at the tip of the facet. Another pathologic subluxation includes posterior diastasis of the facets.

In the AO system, the neurologic status is graded similarly to the SLIC. N0 is neurologically intact. N1 is a transient neurologic deficit that has resolved. N2 is a radiculopathy or nerve root injury. N3 is an incomplete spinal cord injury, and N4 is a complete spinal cord injury.

Case-specific modifiers are important, as they can alter treatment. M1 is an incomplete posterior tension band injury. CT or plain radiographs may indicate a possible ligamentous disruption, but MRI shows that the nuchal ligament, interspinous/supraspinous ligaments are intact, although they may have edema. M2 is traumatic herniation of the intervertebral disc behind the vertical line drawn along the posterior wall of the caudal vertebrae. M3 are fractures in patients with ankylosed spine. M4 is an associated vertebral artery injury.

General Approach to Treatment of Injuries

Each patient is assessed clinically for signs of injury by palpation, checking for tenderness, and by a detailed neurologic examination. A patient with tenderness or signs and symptoms of neurologic injury should have a CT to identify injury patterns. If any ligamentous injury is suspected or unexplained neurologic deficits are present, an MRI scan is indicated. At this point, the injury is classified morphologically using the AO system. The severity is then graded using CSISS or SLIC. Patients who have a score greater than 5 SLIC or greater than 7 CSISS are treated surgically. In patients with less severe injuries, nonoperative treatment in orthosis is attempted.

Nonoperative Care of Subaxial Cervical Injuries

Nonoperative care is indicated for those with stable fractures or those who are not otherwise surgical candidates. For most lower cervical spine injuries, patients are managed in an orthosis. Choices include soft collar, hard collar (e.g., Miami J [Össur]; Aspen collar [Aspen Medical Products], or CervMax [PMT Corporation]), cervicothoracic brace, and halo vest. The general approach in all orthotic management is similar (Box 76.1). The orthosis is fitted by a trained orthotist. Pads that wick fluids away from the skin can help to prevent skin breakdown. The brace needs to control head-mandible motion relative to the thorax. No brace, including the halo vest, will completely prevent segmental motion in a fractured cervical spine, as the spinal column can easily assume snakelike intervertebral motions.[20] Twice-daily skin checks are ordered while the patient is hospitalized or in a rehabilitation facility. Training of patients and family is essential to ensure proper use and to avoid complications of the orthosis. In patients older than 65 years, a swallow consult is obtained to assess aspiration risk prior to institution of diet. Occupational therapy trains patients to use the brace and in the activities of daily living while immobilized.

BOX 76.1 Principles of Nonoperative Treatment

- Appropriate indication for fracture type and patient condition
- Orthotic placement by certified orthotist
- In patients >65 years, a swallow study before feeding
- Twice-daily skin check
- Removable pads
- Proper training of patient, family, and nursing staff
- Check alignment initially and at regular intervals

Upright radiographs are obtained after brace placement and scrutinized for increasing kyphosis and/or subluxation. Any change in these, or new or worsening neurologic symptoms indicates instability, and surgery is recommended. Follow-up radiographs are obtained at 2, 6, and 10 weeks. In most subaxial injuries, healing will occur by 10 to 12 weeks or earlier. Patients are initially informed that their orthosis is a test of stability and that about 5% to 10% of patients will fail and may require surgery. In patients without clear surgical indication (such as SLIC scores of 4 or 5 and CSISS scores of 5 to 7), either approach can be chosen. In general, I recommend a trial of nonoperative therapy with orthosis in these cases. In such cases, shared decision making should occur, taking into account the patient's preferences.

Soft Collar

Soft collars provide little stability and are used for comfort but also to alert medical personnel that injury is present. These are indicated for frail elderly patients with minimal or stable fractures or in patients who cannot tolerate even a hard collar.

Hard Collar

Many forms of hard collar are available. Use of extraction collars and Philadelphia collars should be avoided, as these fit poorly and can lead to skin breakdown. It does not appear that the stabilization effect among well-fitting hard collars varies by manufacturer. It is best that the orthotist use a single brand so that personnel can become familiar with their use and maintenance. Hard collars do not provide sufficient stability for unstable fractures, but are effective, in my experience, in stable SLIC score less than 3 and CSISS score less than 5.

Cervicothoracic Orthosis

The cervicothoracic orthosis (CTO) has anterior and posterior chest pads that are connected by straps under the axilla and over the shoulder. Vertically, they are connected to occipital and mandibular pads rigidly. The CTO brace provides greater stability than hard collars, especially at the cervicothoracic junction. The CTO places increasing pressure on the occiput and chin, and should be used with caution. I do not recommend its use in spinal cord–injury patients who lack body control or any patient with cognitive impairment due to the risk of skin ulcerations. I recommend the CTO for patients with injuries at the cervicothoracic junction, those with multilevel spine fractures where multilevel fusions might be otherwise utilized, and cervical spine injuries combined with upper thoracic injuries. An alternative treatment for this injury pattern is the thoracolumbosacral orthosis with chin piece (cervical-thoraco-lumbosacral orthosis). I have abandoned its use due to risk for skin ulceration and poor patient acceptance.

Halo Vest

The halo vest is the most rigid external orthosis, although segmental motion can still occur at the fracture site. Anderson reported in patients with unstable fractures treated in the halo vest that 1.8 mm of translation and 7 degrees of angulation fracture site motion occur during position change from supine to upright.[20] The use of the halo vest has declined and is rarely used today in my experience for subaxial injuries. It is indicated for unstable fractures in which fusion is a poor alternative, such as young patients who are neurologically intact or those with multilevel injuries. For these cases, the halo vest may provide the best nonoperative approach, thereby avoiding multilevel fusions.

Treatment of Acute Spinal Cord Injury

The goals of treatment of spinal cord–injury patients are to protect the neural tissues from further injury, reduce and stabilize fracture-dislocations, and provide a stable long-term painless spine.

Transport

Patients presumed to have spinal cord injuries should be transferred to institutions that are experienced in their management, have advanced imaging available, and can provide intensive care and urgent surgical services. Treatment of spinal cord injuries in Level 1 trauma centers is shown to reduce rates of complication as well as shorten the length of hospitalization and rehabilitation time.[21] Spinal cord–injury patients require intensive care to monitor neurologic state and provide hemodynamic support, assess pulmonary function (which often deteriorates over time), and prevent adverse events, such as skin breakdown.

Immediate Care of the Spinal-Injured Patient

Once a subaxial fracture is diagnosed, consideration of immediate treatment is entertained. All patients with spinal cord and nerve root injury as well as those with unstable fractures are candidates for immediate intervention. This includes hemodynamic support, further diagnostic testing, administration of neuroprotective agents, reduction using tong traction, and urgent surgery. While the decision-making process for resuscitation is taking place, patients with subaxial fractures should be immobilized in a hard collar and maintained flat on a bed or stretcher. Although the backboard is an excellent aid for transport to and within the hospital, it should be removed as soon as possible to reduce the risk of skin breakdown. In addition, backboards can be associated with fracture displacement, especially in children or in patients with thoracic kyphosis.

Hemodynamic Support

The injured or compressed spinal cord is ischemic, which can further exacerbate the spinal cord injury. If spinal cord injury is present, there is a loss of vasomotor tone, with resultant hypotension and bradycardia, causing a condition known as neurogenic shock. In addition, the spinal cord, like the traumatized brain, loses its ability to autoregulate blood flow. Therefore, intramedullary blood flow becomes related to the systemic arterial pressure. Any hypotension, either from loss of vasomotor control or from blood loss, can worsen or exacerbate the spinal cord injury. Guidelines recommend resuscitation of a spinal cord–injured patient to a systolic blood pressure greater than 120 mm Hg (usually with pressor agents) and maintaining the mean arterial pressure at 85 mm Hg.[22] A high FiO_2 should be administered to maintain O_2 saturation greater than 95%. Ventilatory failure may be present or develop over time and requires intubation and mechanical support. Intubation needs to be performed carefully so that fracture displacement is minimized. It is best that the surgical team assist in this task by holding the head while maintaining traction.

Magnetic Resonance Imaging in Acute Spinal Cord Injuries

Early treatment decisions may require further imaging by MRI. Urgent MRI is indicated for unexplained neurologic deficits, neurologic deterioration, to evaluate ligamentous structures, or in patients with no or minimal deficits who have facet dislocations to determine the presence of a traumatic disc herniation. In these cases, neurologic worsening has been reported after open reduction when the disc lies behind the vertebral body compressing the spinal cord after reduction. Several case reports have documented that disc herniation behind the vertebral body remains in that location after reduction, causing significant neurologic deficits.[23] In addition, MRI is useful for preoperative planning.

Neuroprotection

To address the secondary spinal cord injury caused by vascular, molecular, biochemical, and/or inflammatory changes, early treatment using neuroprotective agents has been proposed. Many pharmacologic and cellular agents show promise in laboratory animals. However, only methylprednisolone is approved for current use. Methylprednisolone, when given within 8 hours of injury, has an antioxidant effect by reducing lipid peroxidation that occurs as part of the secondary injury pathophysiology. The clinical evidence for use of methylprednisolone is based on the National Acute Spinal Cord Injury Study 2 (NACISC2). In this randomized control trial, 454 patients with blunt traumatic spinal cord injuries were randomized to naloxone, methylprednisolone, and placebo.[24] All patients had randomization and administration of drugs within 8 hours of injury. Naloxone was thought to have neuroprotective properties at the time. Patients receiving methylprednisolone had a statistically significant improvement of 5 points of ASIA motor level. The impact of the NACISC2 study was significant; subsequently, almost all spinal cord injuries were treated using the NACISC2 protocols. However, critical analysis of the statistical methodology, identification of potential harms, including death, and the minimal perceived benefits have led many to abandon or limit the use of methylprednisolone for spinal cord injury. Recent guidelines by the American Academy of Neurological Surgeons and the Congress of Neurological Surgeons recommend against the use of methylprednisolone in acute spinal cord injury.[25]

Unfortunately, the data from the NACISC2 study included mostly patients who did not have surgery or even reduction of fracture dislocations within 24 hours. Further, hemodynamic support was not utilized routinely at the time of the original study. Thus, there is a knowledge gap as to whether methylprednisolone may have a beneficial effect when combined with other current standard practices in care. My current recommendations are to administer methylprednisolone in select patients with cervical cord injuries, both complete and incomplete, and in incomplete thoracic cord injuries. Methylprednisolone is recommended only in patients without other significant traumatic injuries or comorbidities. I do not recommend its use in geriatric patients with spinal cord injuries. When used, methylprednisolone is administered as a 30-mg/kg loading bolus over 1 hour and a continuous infusion of 5.4 mg/kg per hour for 23 hours.

Fracture-Dislocation Reduction

Early fracture-dislocation reduction is important to remove neural compression and reestablish blood flow to ischemic tissue to prevent deterioration and maximize the chance of neurologic recovery. This can be achieved by two methods: cranial tong traction and surgery. Cranial tong traction is a useful and generally safe method to stabilize the spine and to achieve realignments of fractures and dislocations.[26] Indications for cranial tong traction vary and are being supplanted by immediate surgery where reduction by traction is avoided. In a study to evaluate the timing of surgery on the outcomes of spinal cord injury, the authors found that only one-third of patients were ever treated with tong traction before surgery.[27] Cranial tong traction is a fast method to reestablish spinal cord blood flow through reduction. In low-energy facet dislocations, such as from sporting accidents, early reduction within 4 hours of injury in patients with quadriplegia was shown to have a reversible effect in 80% of cases.[28]

Timing of Surgery

The timing of surgery in humans remains controversial, despite a large volume of animal data that demonstrates early surgery correlates with greater neurologic recovery. Because of difficulties with study design, heterogeneity, and severity of injury, these benefits of early surgery have not been proven in humans. A recent observational study, Surgical Timing in Acute Spinal Cord Injury Study (STASCIS), compared neurologic improvement at 6 months based on ASIA impairment scale between early (≤24 hours) and late (>24 hours).[27] Patients were stratified according to whether surgery was performed before or after 24 hours. There was no difference for the chance of improving one ASIA level; however, there was a statistically significant and better chance of improving 2 ASIA levels if surgery was performed within 24 hours. In patients with spinal cord injuries, the potential for neurologic deterioration caused by early surgery has been a concern. The mechanics of this are unclear, but likely are due to hemodynamic changes that occur during surgery. In the STASCIS study, only one patient deteriorated neurologically; the authors believe that early surgery was feasible and safe in patients treated at centers with experience in managing spinal cord injuries.

Cranial Tong Technique

Cranial tongs have a metal or carbon fiber arc, two pins which are inserted into the skull, and a hook for traction rope. The pins are disposable, and one pin has a compression spring that acts to measure the applied force of the pins into the skull. Both MRI-compatible and non–MRI-compatible devices are available. Unless heavy weights are anticipated, I recommend the use of MRI-compatible devices.

Guidelines for Initial Closed Reduction of Subaxial Cervical Fractures

Gelb reported guidelines based on a systematic review of the use of closed reduction with tong traction in subaxial fractures and dislocations.[26] Based on a retrospective case series, he recommends early reduction with cranial tong traction for subaxial injuries in awake patients without more rostral injuries. Prereduction MRI should be obtained in patients who cannot be examined during closed reduction or if closed reduction fails. MRI will identify disc disruptions in up to 50% of cases, but does not appear to influence outcomes in awake patients; therefore, their utility is questioned.

Cranial Tong Insertion

The location of tong insertion is 1 cm above the pin and in line with the external auditory meatus. Placement more anteriorly or posteriorly can change the force vectors, which may theoretically aid reduction. For consistency, I recommend placement in line with the exterior auditory meatus. The skin is prepared with chlorhexidine and the subcutaneous tissue and periosteum is infiltrated with local anesthetic. No shaving of the scalp is required. The surgeon holds the tongs with pins located just above the correct starting point, which are then symmetrically tightened into the skin and skull. The pin containing the compression spring is scrutinized until it protrudes 1 mm out from the surface of the pin. Jam nuts along the side of the pins are tightened to prevent inadvertent further tightening of the pins. If the traction is to be continued (unusual today), the pins may be retightened one time at 24 hours. The rope is attached to the tongs and connected to weights by a pulley at the head of the bed. I prefer to raise the head of the bed 20 to 30 degrees while keeping the angle of the rope at the same slope.

Reduction Technique

Reduction of fractures and dislocations requires a rigid protocol to maintain safety. The initial weight is selected depending on many factors, including body weight, level of injury, age, and fracture pattern. For midcervical and lower cervical spine injuries, it is recommended starting with 10 kg (20–25 lb). After the weight has been attached (and after any increase or decrease of weight), a radiograph is obtained and a neurologic examination is performed and documented in the medical record. The radiograph is assessed to determine if reduction has been achieved and for signs of overdistraction. Overdistraction is assessed by examination of the disc space and facet joints. Overdistraction may cause excess traction on the spinal cord and vertebral arteries, which could result in neurologic deterioration. However, to reduce a facet dislocation in the absence of fractures, overdistraction of 3 to 5 mm may be required. The neurologic examination assesses any change in perceived sensations, increasing pain, or paresthesia in the extremities, or deterioration of sensory or motor function.

If reduction is not achieved, 5 to 7 kg of additional weight is added as long as no neurologic deficits or radiologic signs of overdistraction occur. A C-arm with the patient on a stretcher or Jackson-type table can reduce the time required to obtain the reduction. In general, once the reduction is achieved, weights may be decreased. However, for unstable fractures, reducing weight can result in displacement and neurologic injury. Therefore, if weights are decreased, it is essential to repeat the neurologic examination and examine new radiographs. Some manipulation may be required to achieve reduction, which should only be done by experienced surgeons. In facet dislocations, slight flexion may be required to unlock the impacted dislocated facets. This is accomplished by adding bolsters underneath the occiput to create neck flexion. Another method is to manually manipulate the spine while in traction. For bilateral facet dislocations, an attempt to reduce each facet independently is preferred. The tongs are grasped and a lateral bending movement and forward flexion is applied, ideally reducing one facet. The same movements are performed on the contralateral side.

In several conditions, cranial tong traction reduction may lead to neurologic deficits. Distractive lesions, although uncommon in the subaxial cervical spine, lack any longitudinal running ligaments, which provide the potential for ligamentotaxis that controls reductions. Facet dislocations have a disrupted disc complex in almost all cases. In a few cases, however, the intervertebral disc may be herniated behind the cranial vertebral body. The disc may not reduce when the spinal column is realigned and the disc behind the vertebral body may increase compression on the spinal cord, resulting in neurologic deficit. This appears to be a rare condition and almost exclusively occurs during closed reductions with patients under general anesthesia.[23] Most surgeons agree that cervical tong traction in awake patients using the method described earlier is much safer. In patients with significant neurologic deficits, I believe that the benefit of immediate reduction exceeds the potential for worsening due to disc herniation, and I proceed with rapid reduction when indicated. In patients who are intact or have mild deficits, it is usually possible to obtain an MRI scan prior to reduction. If a traumatic disc herniation behind the body of the cranial vertebra is present, the patient should undergo anterior discectomy and then reduction using direct vertebral manipulation or intraoperative tong traction. If reduction is achieved, then anterior interbody fusion with a plate is performed. If reduction is not achieved, the patient is turned prone on a turning frame and open posterior reduction is performed. Lateral mass fixation and bone graft is applied. The wound is closed and the patient is repositioned supine and anterior body fusion performed with or without addition of an anterior plate.

Another contraindication to traction reduction is ankylosing spondylitis. These are highly unstable injuries in which the ALL and PLL are absent and thus do not provide ligamentotaxis. Traction in these cases can lead to loss of alignment, overdistraction, and neurologic deficits.

Surgical Treatment of Subaxial Cervical Spine Injuries

Surgical Goals

The goals of surgery are to decompress neural elements when warranted, realign the spine by reduction and correction of kyphosis, provide stabilization while minimizing the number of segments permanently arthrodesed, minimize orthotic use postoperatively, and to provide a long-term painless spine (Box 76.2). In addition, patients should be able to be mobilized as soon as possible and the surgical procedure should avoid adverse events.

Indications

The indications for surgical treatment are unstable injuries that have poor potential for healing, the need to decompress the neurologic elements in the presence of neurologic deficits, or failure of conservative treatment. In general, injuries that have SLIC scores of 5 or greater and CSISS of 7 or greater are treated with surgery.

Surgical Approach

The subaxial cervical spine can be approached by anterior, posterior, or combined approaches. Many factors determine which approach will be used, but often are related to surgeon preference. I recommend identifying the goals of surgery and choosing an approach that best matches those goals. Surgical fixation should meet the biomechanical requirements of the injured segments.

BOX 76.2 Goals of Surgical Treatment

- Decompress spinal cord and nerve roots
- Reduce fractures and dislocations, and correct kyphosis
- Stabilization
- Minimize number of levels fused
- Rapid mobilization of the patient
- Minimize orthotic use
- Avoid adverse events

The advantages of the anterior approach are direct decompression of the spinal cord, ease of positioning, familiarity of the approach by most surgeons, less blood loss, lower risk of infection, and better ability to correct kyphosis, if present. Disadvantages are that biomechanical strength of fixation is less than posterior fixation techniques, higher rates of nonunion, and postoperative dysphagia with aspiration risk and airway compromise. The advantages of a posterior approach are the ability to extend to more cranial and caudal levels, greater ease of reduction, improved biomechanical strength, and avoidance of anterior soft tissue complications. A combined approach provides maximum fixation, the chance for circumferential decompression, and less need for postoperative immobilization. However, the combined approach is associated with more complications and longer operative times.

Anterior Decompression and Fusion

Anterior decompression and fusion is performed using the Smith-Robinson approach. After confirmation of the correct level, the disc anulus is sectioned and discectomy performed. If needed, the canal is decompressed directly. The endplates are prepared by removal of cartilage and flattening. In cases requiring corpectomy, such as burst fracture, the discs cranially and caudally are removed, the vertebral body is removed piecemeal, and the posterior wall is removed with a burr. A trough a minimum of 15 mm wide should be created. Reconstructive options for discectomies include allograft or autograft. After corpectomy, I prefer radius allograft strut graft, although satisfactory results have been obtained using cages filled with autogenous graft material from the corpectomy. Stabilization is achieved with a plate and screws, either static or dynamic. Final radiographs are obtained to assess alignment and instrumentation.

Posterior Approach

The posterior approach requires prone positioning, which is done by either log rolling the patient onto an operating table or use of a turning frame. In the former, the neck can be stabilized with a collar and with the surgeon holding the head. If traction is already applied, I prefer the turning frame, in which traction can be maintained. After positioning and taping the arms caudally, the alignment is confirmed radiographically. A midline incision is used and the spinous processes and laminae out to the edges of the lateral masses are exposed. When dissecting, the nuchal ligamentous complex needs to be preserved to avoid adjacent segment kyphosis.

If reduction of facet dislocation is needed, the spinous processes may be grasped as levers and manipulated to gain realignment. In some cases, an elevator may be placed into the dislocated facet joint and used as a lever to achieve reduction. Alternatively, 3 to 5 mm of the superior facet can be removed with a burr, allowing clearing of the inferior facet into position. Kyphosis can be reduced, if present, by use of an interspinous wire fixation.

Optimal fixation is achieved with lateral mass screw and rod constructs.[29] The borders of the lateral mass are exposed and the center identified. A starting point is placed 2 mm medial to the center of the lateral mass with a burr. A drill or Kirschner wire (K-wire) with a stopped drill guide creates a pilot hole. The screw orientation is upward (parallel to facet joint) and laterally away from the vertebral artery, 15 to 20 degrees. The hole is drilled and checked for far cortex perforation. If not perforated, the drill guide is adjusted to allow 2 mm more length, and the process is repeated. This continues until the far cortex is reached, a length of 16 to 20 mm. Variable head screws are inserted and rods of appropriate length are placed into screw heads, then set screws are tightened. The posterior third of the facet joint is decorticated and packed with bone graft. The nuchal ligaments are reconstructed and vancomycin powder applied to the wound.

Anteroposterior Approach

Combined AP approaches are occasionally needed when injuries have total ligamentous disruption, are highly comminuted, when compression is located both anteriorly and posteriorly, or when reduction cannot be achieved preoperatively or by only one approach. It is best if the patient is hemodynamically stable to accomplish this under one session of anesthesia.

Treatment of Specific Fracture Types

AO Compression Injuries Type A1 and A2

These compression-type injuries rarely require surgical treatment. The important determinate is whether the posterior ligamentous complex is intact. Several authors have noted that compression fractures can be associated with posterior ligamentous injury, resulting in progressive kyphosis, so-called "hidden flexion injury."[30] Careful scrutiny of CT images and plain radiographs for disruption of facet articulations and widening between spinous processes are clues to possible ligamentous injury. Fat-suppressed MRI is the best method to determine the status of those ligaments. If there is associated ligamentous injury, then this is an AO type B injury and treated surgically, as described later.

AO Compression Injuries Type A3 and Type 4

These are burst fractures without disruption of the posterior ligaments and, in the absence of neurologic injury, can be treated nonoperatively. A cervical orthosis for 10 weeks is recommended. These commonly occur at C7, where a CTO should be considered. The posterior ligamentous complex needs to be assessed as described earlier for A1 and A2 injuries. In cases of neurologic injury, reduction using cranial tong traction reduction can be achieved. Surgically, these are best treated by anterior corpectomy and fusion with plate instrumentation. In cases in which reduction has been achieved, posterior fusion is also an option. The type A4 fracture has greater comminution of the vertebral body and, therefore, is more likely to develop progressive kyphosis, which might require surgery.

AO Distractive Injuries Type B1

These are rare bony distractive lesions from either flexion or extension forces that often occur in patients with an ankylosed spine. Nonoperative treatment can be attempted in nonankylosed patients, but any change in alignment should be treated surgically. Patients with ankylosed spines with these injuries are best treated surgically. Posterior lateral mass fixation is the preferred technique, as this provides the best fixation strength and it is easier to include more levels if needed.

AO Distractive Injuries Type B2

This injury is a posterior ligamentous disruption often associated with a minimal compression fracture. These are inherently unstable and have a SLIC score of 5 or greater and, except in the young, are best treated surgically (Fig. 76.2). Either an anterior or posterior approach can be used if bony structures are intact. During surgery, attention to achieving correction of the kyphotic deformity is important. When performing anterior fusion, lordosis is achieved by positioning in extension using blanket rolls placed behind the shoulders and by placing distraction pins, which initially converge and, when distracted, tend to lordose the spine. Posteriorly, if reduction does not reduce kyphosis, either compression of the lateral mass screws or use of an interspinous wire can be performed to correct kyphosis.

Posterior ligamentous injuries are associated with various anterior column injuries, such as compression or burst fractures. These injuries are best treated surgically; I prefer a posterior fusion if reduction is achieved preoperatively. A special case is the flexion–axial loading fracture in which the body splits, leaving a small triangular fragment at the anterior longitudinal ligament, and the remaining body translates posteriorly into the spinal canal (Fig. 76.3). Associated with this injury are varying degrees of posterior ligamentous disruption, facet fracturing, and subluxation. The fracture can be reduced but may require large weight, up to 50% to 70% of body weight. Definitive treatment is by anterior corpectomy and plate fixation. An additional posterior fusion may be indicated in the more displaced and comminuted injuries.

AO Distractive Injuries Type B3

These are discoligamentous injuries resulting from hyperextension and may be associated with central cord syndromes. They often also occur in patients with ankylosed spines. The discoligamentous injury is often not apparent on initial radiographs and may be hard to differentiate from degenerative changes (Fig. 76.4). The potential for late deformity is less than in posterior ligamentous injuries, but these injuries can result in posterior translation (retrolisthesis) of the cranial vertebral body. Discoligamentous injuries without neurologic injury can be treated in a cervical orthosis. When associated with central cord syndrome, early decompression—either by anterior or posterior approach—and fusion is recommended. Discoligamentous injuries in patients with ankylosed spines should be treated surgically, usually with a posterior fusion, although anterior discectomy and fusion in patients with excellent bone quality can be considered.

AO Translational/Rotational Injuries Type C

Many forces can result in translational and rotational deformities in the subaxial spine. Most common are unilateral and bilateral facet dislocations with or without facet fractures. In addition, bilateral pars fractures can result in traumatic spondylolisthesis, which occurs most commonly at C7. Extension forces, when severe, can cause complete disc and facet joint disruptions and posterior translational injuries.

Unilateral Facet Dislocations

Unilateral facet dislocation occurs when the inferior facet is translated over the superior facet, and is often associated with facet fracture. Radiographically, there will be up to 25% vertebral body subluxation. Biomechanical studies suggest that significant posterior ligamentous and disc anulus injury is required for this injury to occur. The ipsilateral neuroforamen is narrowed and may be associated with a radiculopathy. Disc disruptions occur universally and disc herniation is present in 56% of patients.[31]

The treatment of these injuries remains controversial. Most agree that closed reduction should be performed. In the presence of a facet fracture, especially if it involves more than 40% of the facet, displacement may recur.[32] One treatment after reduction is orthotic management with an orthosis or halo vest. Alternatively, surgery, either anterior or posterior, can be performed. When reduction has been achieved, anterior discectomy and fusion is recommended. Posterior fusion is indicated when vertebral body fractures are present and when open reduction is required. Long-term outcomes have been shown to be improved with surgical rather than nonoperative treatment.

Bilateral Facet Dislocations

Bilateral facet dislocations are highly unstable and result in a minimum of 50% vertebral subluxation. Spinal cord injuries occur frequently. In addition to the facet dislocations, the posterior osteoligamentous complex and disc anulus are disrupted. Fractures of the lamina and spinous process also occur frequently, which may affect treatment decisions. Further, the intervertebral disc is always disrupted and may appear displaced into the spinal canal. The disc is located in the normal position relative to the caudal vertebra but posterior to the cranial vertebra. In some cases, free disc fragments are located behind the cranial vertebral body wall and may remain after reduction, causing increased cord compression.[23]

All bilateral facet dislocations should be reduced and undergo spinal fusion (Fig. 76.5). In spinal cord–injured patients, it is urgent that reduction is achieved to allow restitution of vascular supply and is best done by traction or early surgery.

In intact patients, there is a small incidence of neurologic worsening from intervertebral disc herniation behind the vertebral body after reduction. If possible, an MRI before

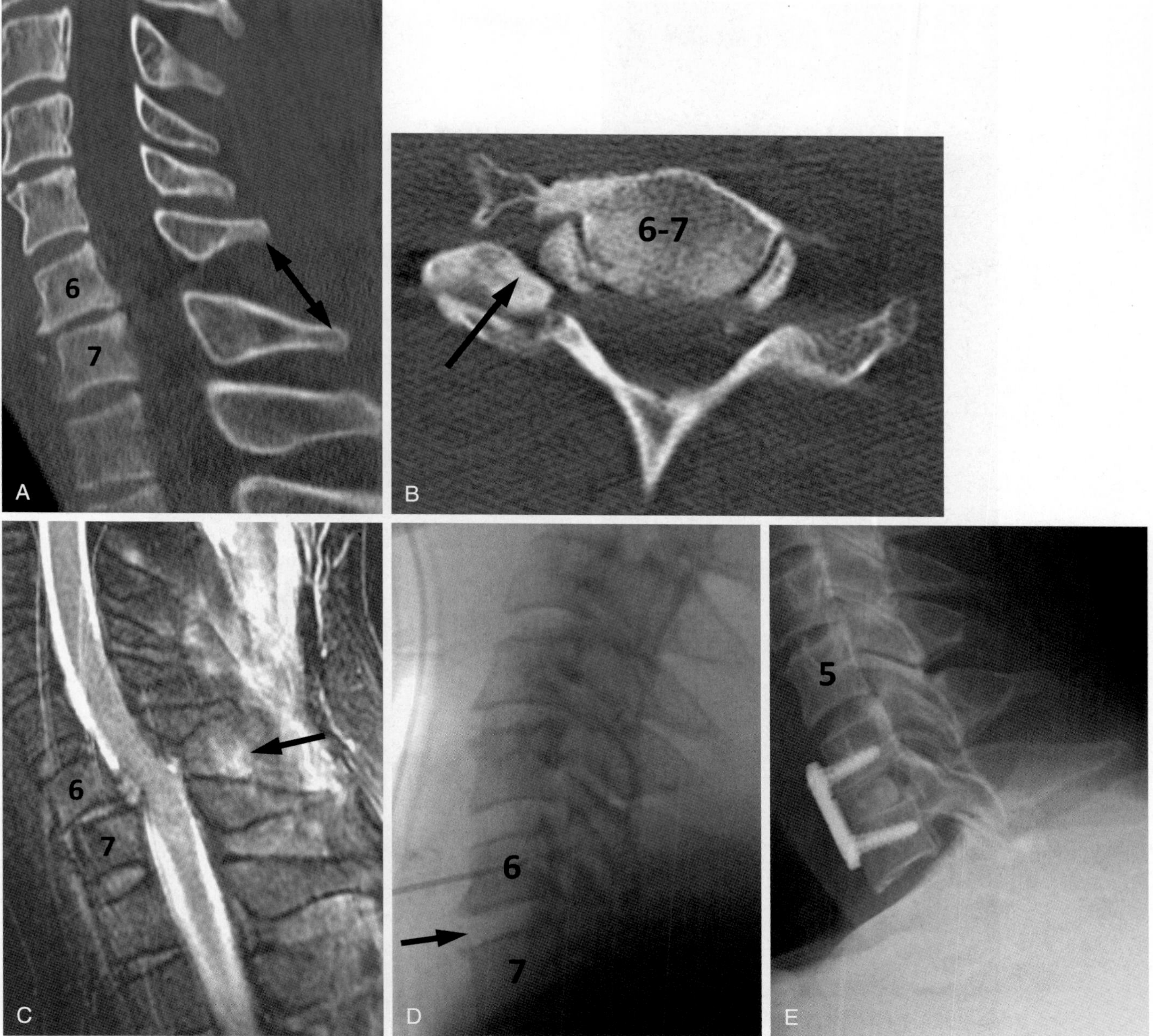

FIG. 76.2 (A) Sagittal computed tomographic (CT) image showing posterior ligamentous injury at C6–C7 in a 52-year-old man who presented with American Spinal Injury Association quadriplegia. Wide separation is noted (*arrow*) between spinous processes. The disc is narrow, with suspicion of herniation into the canal. (B) Axial CT at C6–C7 shows a right facet fracture and a displaced superior facet fracture in the neuroforamina (*arrow*). (C) Magnetic resonance image showing disc herniation with significant cord compression. The spinal cord is deformed and had signal changes within. The arrow points to disrupted posterior ligaments. (D) Intraoperative fluoroscopic image after placement of 20 lb of traction and extension with a roll behind the shoulders. Note overall excellent alignment and disc distraction relative to preoperative CT. At surgery, the anterior and posterior longitudinal ligaments and disc were disrupted. (E) The patient was treated by anterior discectomy and fusion with dynamic plating.

reduction is recommended. If the disc appears behind the body, then anterior discectomy and fusion is performed prior to reduction. Then, reduction can be obtained by manipulation and interbody fusion with placement of bone graft and plate. If reduction cannot be achieved, the patient can be turned prone and an open reduction and posterior fusion performed. Finally, an anterior interbody fusion is performed. Alternatively, a closed reduction can be attempted if the patient is awake and cooperative by carefully monitoring the neurologic function as increasing weight is added. This protocol can be done safely and has not been associated with neurologic deficits in awake patients.[33]

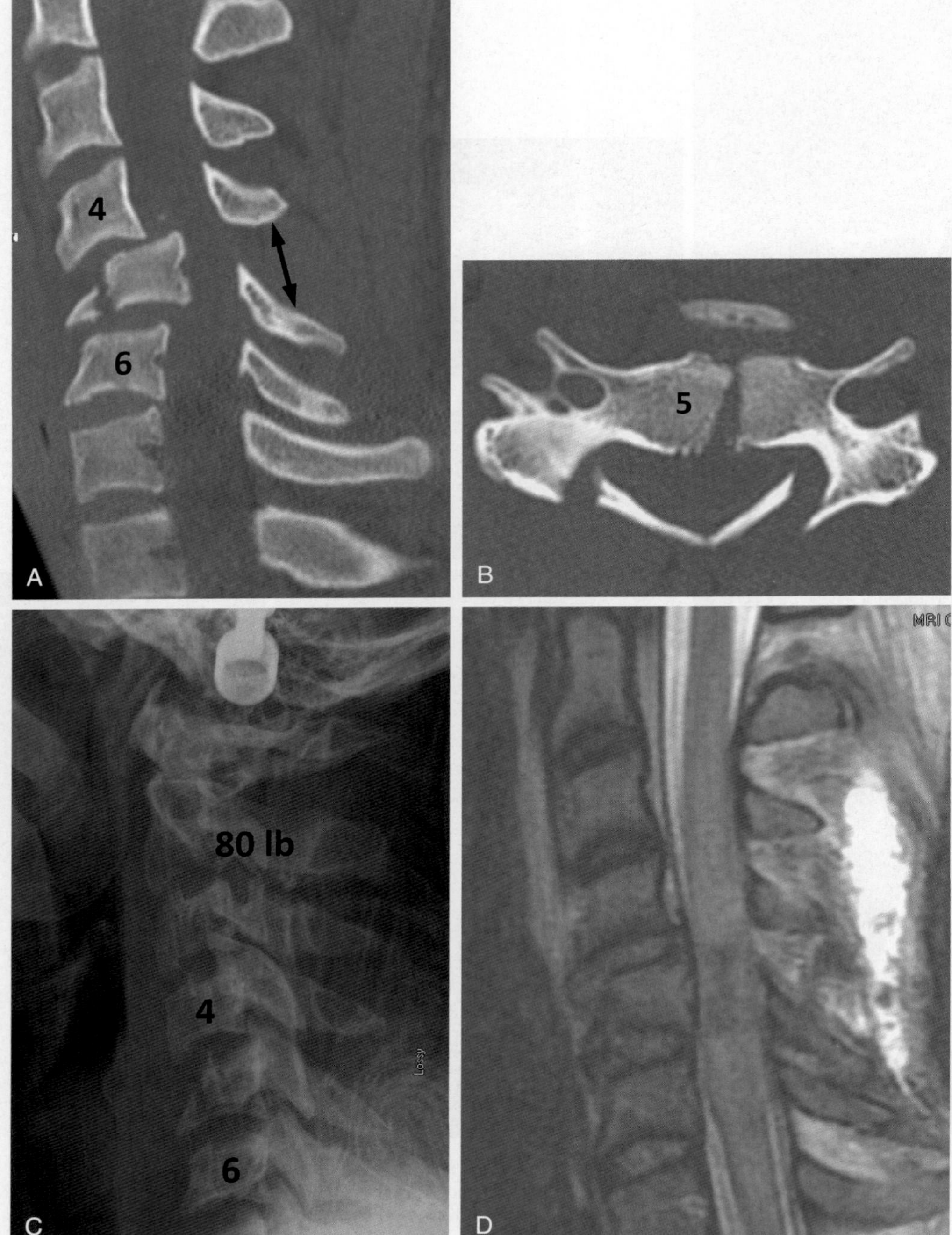

FIG. 76.3 (A) A 20-year-old man was a C5 complete quadriplegic from a diving accident. The sagittal computed tomographic (CT) image shows a flexion–axial loading injury (AO B2). There is a teardrop fracture of the anterior-inferior corner of C5, and the posterior aspect of C5 is rotated into the spinal canal. The posterior osteoligamentous complex is disrupted (*arrow*). The fracture is unstable and has a Subaxial Cervical Injury Classification System score of 9. (B) Axial CT demonstrating comminuted body and posterior element fracture with narrowing of the spinal canal. (C) After application of 80 lb of traction, excellent reduction was achieved. (D) The patient was treated with a posterior fusion of C4–C6. The postoperative magnetic resonance image shows severe cord edema, hematoma at the site of the injury, and posterior ligamentous disruption.

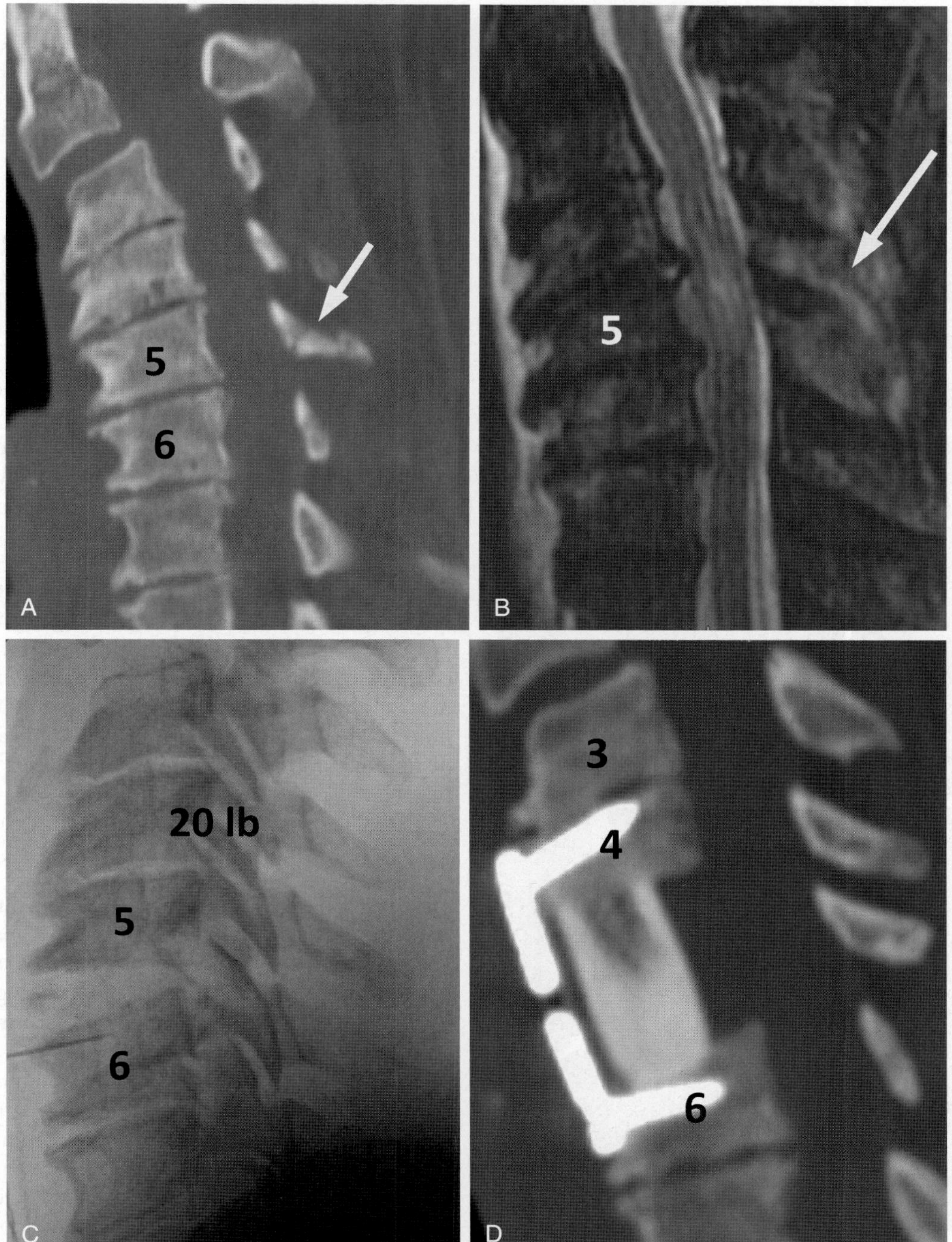

FIG. 76.4 (A) A 56-year woman had a hyperextension injury from a fall. She presented to an outside hospital complaining of weakness in both arms. Twelve hours later, she deteriorated and was transferred with central cord syndrome. Sagittal computed tomography (CT) showed multilevel degenerative disease, cervical kyphosis, and nondisplaced fracture of C5 (*arrow*). (B) Short tau inversion recovery magnetic resonance imaging showed spinal cord edema opposite C5 and edema in posterior osteoligamentous structures (*arrow*). No evidence of discoligamentous injury was present. (C) The patient was positioned in neutral alignment in 20 lb of traction. The lateral radiograph shows significant C5–C6 disc distraction. The traction weight was reduced and an anterior C5 corpectomy was performed. (D) Postoperative CT after corpectomy at C5 and reconstruction with radius allograft and plate.

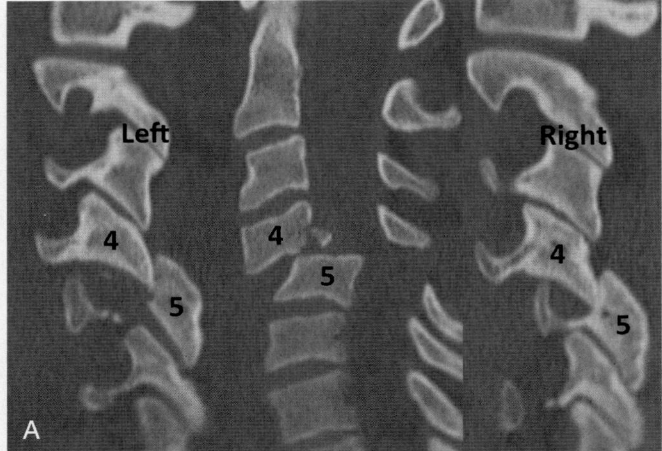

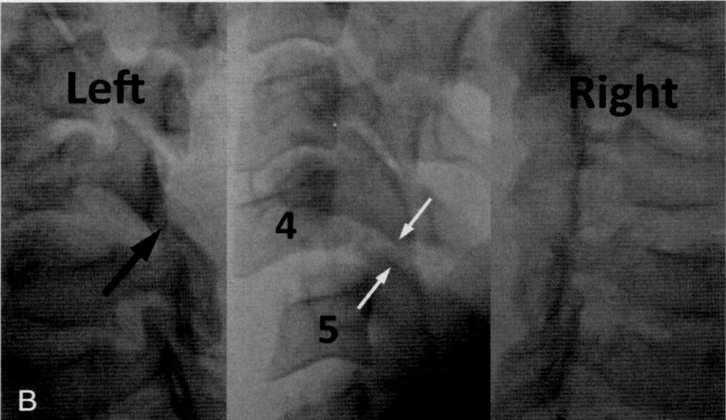

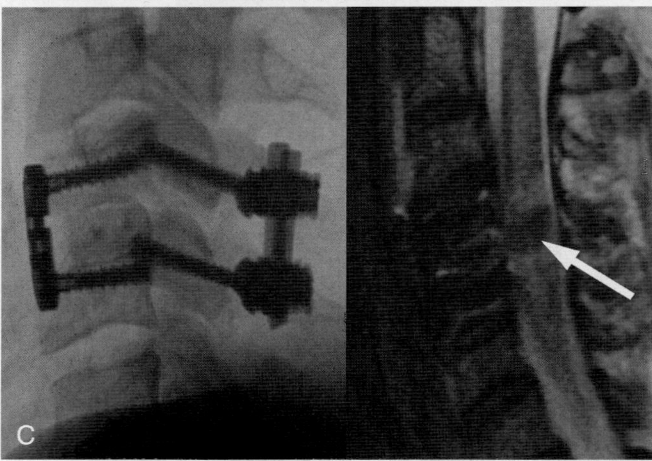

FIG. 76.5 (A) A 22-year-old man rated as a complete quadriplegic sustained bilateral facet dislocations from a diving accident. The left and right sagittal computed tomographic sections show facet dislocations. There is 80% anterior translation of C4 on C5, with a fracture of the posterior inferior corner of C4 displaced into the spinal canal. (B) Cranial tong traction of 50 lb reduced the right facet, but the left facet (*black arrow*) remained dislocated. In the center panel, the vertebral bodies realigned with only 25% residual subluxation, and reduction of one of the facet dislocations is seen (*white arrows*). The patient underwent posterior open reduction and lateral mass fixation. The patient was turned supine, and anterior decompression and fusion were performed. (C) Postoperative lateral radiograph (*left*) demonstrating excellent reduction from combined anterior-posterior fusion. The MRI (*right*) confirms excellent canal decompression. Unfortunately, the cord appears to be transected (*arrow*) and spinal cord edema is seen from C2–C5.

In patients who do not require decompression, either anterior or posterior fusion can be performed.[34] Despite the high degree of instability, anterior fusion with instrumentation provides adequate stability without the need for additional posterior surgery unless vertebral body fractures are present.

Traumatic Spondylolisthesis

Hyperextension forces can result in bilateral pedicle or pars fractures. With continued forces, the disc anulus is disrupted and vertebral subluxation occurs. The spinal canal becomes larger despite subluxation and spinal cord injuries are less frequent. This injury is unstable, requiring reduction and stabilization. Traction reduction is attempted, but complete reduction is difficult to obtain. Either an anterior or posterior approach can be utilized; in some cases, a combined approach is required. Instrumentation of two levels will be required.

Hyperextension Subluxations

Hyperextension forces can cause disruption of the disc anulus, facet capsules, and even posterior ligaments, resulting in posterior vertebral body subluxation. The spinal cord may be compressed and exiting nerve roots are compressed. Treatment may be traction initially but may result in overdistraction, as these injuries may have significant ligamentous disruptions. Definitive treatment is anterior discectomy and fusion.

AO Facet Fractures F1 and F2

The cervical facets are essential to prevent anterior projection translation due to their upward coronal plane orientation. When incompetent from injury, anterior translation may result, with the potential for pain and neurologic injury. Stability models such as the SLIC and CSISS scoring systems often fail to predict behavior.[35]

The treatment goals are to maintain alignment and prevent late instability. Better clinical and radiographic outcomes appear to be associated with surgery.[35] Aarabi studied 25 patients with unilateral nondisplaced facet fractures.[35] In the 10 surgical patients, alignment was maintained and no further treatment was required. Nine of the 15 nonoperatively treated patients developed increased subluxation or kyphosis and needed surgical repair. In a systematic review, Kepler found that 88% of operative compared to 43% of nonoperatively treated patients maintained reduction.[36] Anterior instrumentation had a higher success rate, 92% compared to only 64%, with posterior fusion. However, many posterior fusion patients were treated with outdated wire fixation. Brodke et al.[34] and Kwon et al.[37] noted no difference in results between anterior and posterior fusion.

The treatment of F1 and F2 isolated facet fractures without initial displacement is attempted nonoperatively with a collar or CTO. If subluxation or kyphosis develops, then anterior fusion is recommended. Posterior fusion is an alternative and occasionally needed if there is a displaced facet fracture causing radiculopathy requiring foraminotomy.

AO Facet Fractures F3

This fracture, called "fracture separation of the lateral mass," occurs when the pedicle and lamina are fractured, creating a free-floating lateral mass.[19] The lateral mass can rotate forward and lead to anterior subluxation of both the cranial and caudal vertebral levels. Often, the foramen is narrowed and radiculopathy is present. Sufficient anterior subluxation can cause spinal cord compression. Manoso reviewed 60 cases and found that 38% had radiculopathy and 18% had spinal cord injury.[38]

Nondisplaced F3 injuries can initially be treated nonoperatively with an orthosis. However, fracture separations are likely to develop subluxation, and careful follow-up is required. In Manoso's study, two-thirds of patients treated nonoperatively developed subluxation.[38]

Those patients with initial displacement should be reduced and undergo arthrodesis. An important consideration is whether both segments should undergo fusion or just the level with subluxation. If alignment of the facets can be achieved, then a single-level arthrodesis can be attempted with either the anterior or posterior approach. However, failure can occur when the nonfused segment develops subluxation. Alternatively, a two-level arthrodesis can be performed.

AO Facet Fractures F4

Hyperflexion causes disruption of the posterior osteoligamentous complex from the posterior to the anterior direction. As the vertebra rotates in flexion, the cranial inferior facets slide upward and may become perched in an almost dislocated position. Perched facets indicate substantial injury to the nuchal ligaments, ligamenta flava, and likely the disc anulus, thus should be considered unstable.

Most patients with perched facets should be treated surgically with either anterior or posterior fusion. In younger patients, nonoperative treatment can be attempted with a collar.

Special Cases

Fractures in Patients With Ankylosed Spines

An increasing number of patients who have ankylosed spines due to ankylosing spondylitis, diffuse idiopathic skeletal hyperostosis, severe degenerative disease, or from surgical fusion are sustaining cervical fractures.[39,40] These injuries usually occur from hyperextension and are highly unstable. The most common injury patterns are hyperextension through the disc space.

Displacement, neurologic deterioration, and progressive deformity occur with nonoperative treatment; therefore, surgery is recommended in most cases (Fig. 76.6). Caron et al. reviewed 122 cases and found that delay in diagnosis was common, resulting in neurologic deficits in 81% of those cases.[39] They found that posterior instrumentation three levels above and below was most successful. Fusion of additional levels is immaterial, as these patients are already fused by their disease.

Vertebral Artery Injury

Vertebral artery injuries are common, and may occur in up to 11% of cervical trauma patients.[41] Indications for screening with CT angiography specific to the subaxial cervical spine injury are fractures involving the foramen transversarium, lateral mass fractures, and fracture dislocations. The treatment remains controversial since the majority of patients are asymptomatic. Patients with documented vertebral artery injuries are to be treated with antiplatelet therapy.[21] Symptomatic patients or those who have strokes related to vertebral artery injury may need endovascular repair or revascularization.

Central Cord Syndrome

There is an increasing incidence of patients sustaining hyperextension injuries from falls who present with central cord syndrome. At the time of injury, there is transient compression of the spinal cord, resulting in a central cord injury. Clinically, patients present with worse neurologic deficits in their arms compared to the legs. Bony injury may be absent, but fractures of spinous processes and laminae, disc distraction, and retrolisthesis of vertebral bodies are often present. MRI shows spinal stenosis, often at multiple levels, and spinal cord edema.

The treatment of central cord injuries remains controversial. Nonoperative treatment may be appropriate in patients making rapid recovery. Decompression is warranted in patients with significant deficits, instability, or progressive worsening.

The surgical approach will depend on the degree of skeletal injury, number of levels requiring decompression, and location of cord compression. I often recommend laminoplasty for patients with normal or lordotic alignment and multilevel compression (Fig. 76.7). The timing of decompression of central cord syndrome has been recently evaluated in a systematic review.[42] Anderson reported that patients having decompression within 25 hours of injury had better neurologic outcomes than those decompressed after 72 hours.[42]

Traumatic Disc Herniation

Rarely, a patient with head or neck trauma sustains a traumatic disc herniation with spinal cord compression. These are often the result of sporting accidents in younger patients. Treatment can be nonoperative in the absence of neurologic deficits. Those with spinal cord injury are best treated by early anterior cervical discectomy and fusion.

Adverse Events

Adverse events are common in patients with cervical spine trauma. A commitment to patient safety at all stages of care is required to minimize the chance and severity of complications.

Neurologic Deterioration

Delay in diagnosis and subsequent neurologic deterioration is still frequent, occurring in 0.21% of patients presenting to

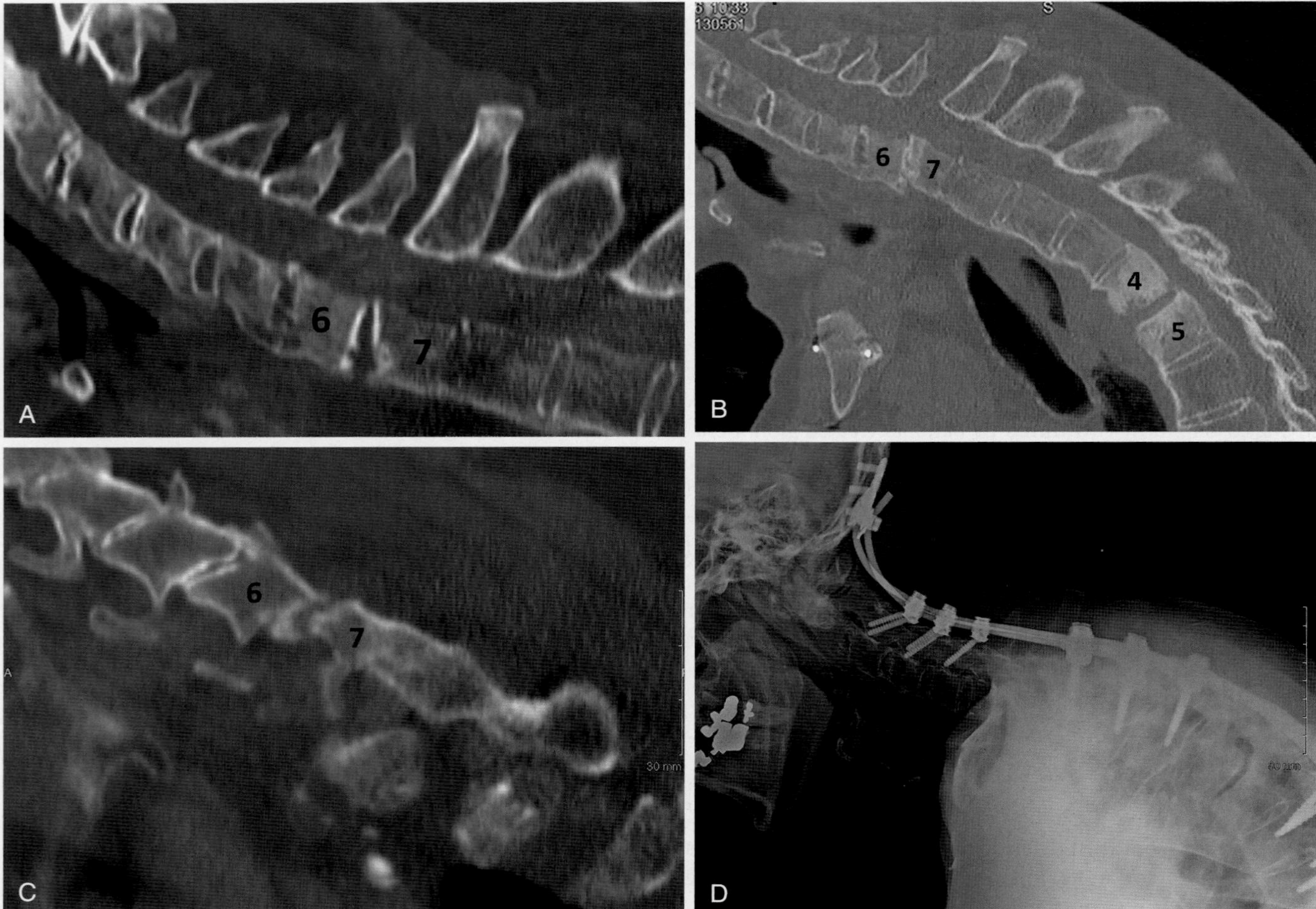

FIG. 76.6 (A) A 58-year-old man with ankylosing spondylitis fell and was seen in an outside hospital complaining of back pain. Computed tomography (CT) showed ankylosing spondylitis with opening across the C6–C7 disc space, indicating hyperextension injury. There is preexisting kyphosis. The diagnosis of injury was missed. (B) Sagittal CT 1 month later showed displacement of the C6–C7 injury, and increased kyphosis (*double arrow*) between the C6–C7 spinous processes. At T4–T5, there is chronic spondylodiscitis (chronic nonfusion). (C) Parasagittal CT demonstrating C6–C7 facet fracture. (D) The patient was treated by posterior instrumentation occiput–T6, as seen on lateral radiograph. His C1–C2 segment was also unstable, requiring extension to the occiput.

trauma centers.[2] The most common cause is insufficient imaging or misreading of images. Careful attention to screening criteria described earlier and critical review of all images by an experienced radiologist can minimize these changes. At-risk groups are the elderly, unconscious, or those with impaired mentation and patients with ankylosed spines.[2]

Neurologic deterioration after hospitalization occurs in 2% to 3% of patients with known spinal fractures.[2] Patients with complete spinal cord injury are at higher risk, reported by Harrop et al. as 6% neurologic deterioration in 186 cord-injured patients.[43] The early cause of deterioration was instability and fracture displacement, deterioration occurring in 2 to 7 days likely being from hypotension, with later deterioration from vertebral artery injury.

Wound Infections

Posterior cervical fusion in trauma patients has a high incidence of surgical site infection (SSI). Cooper reported 4%, while Caroom reported a 15% incidence of SSI. Efforts to minimize these risks include avoiding the use of methylprednisolone and using intrawound vancomycin powder. In studies specific to posterior cervical wound, the use of vancomycin powder can reduce infection by 50% to 75%.[44,45]

Loss of Reduction

The use of modern fixation methods has significantly reduced the cases of loss of reduction. In nonoperatively treated patients, I estimate that 5% of cases will develop increased

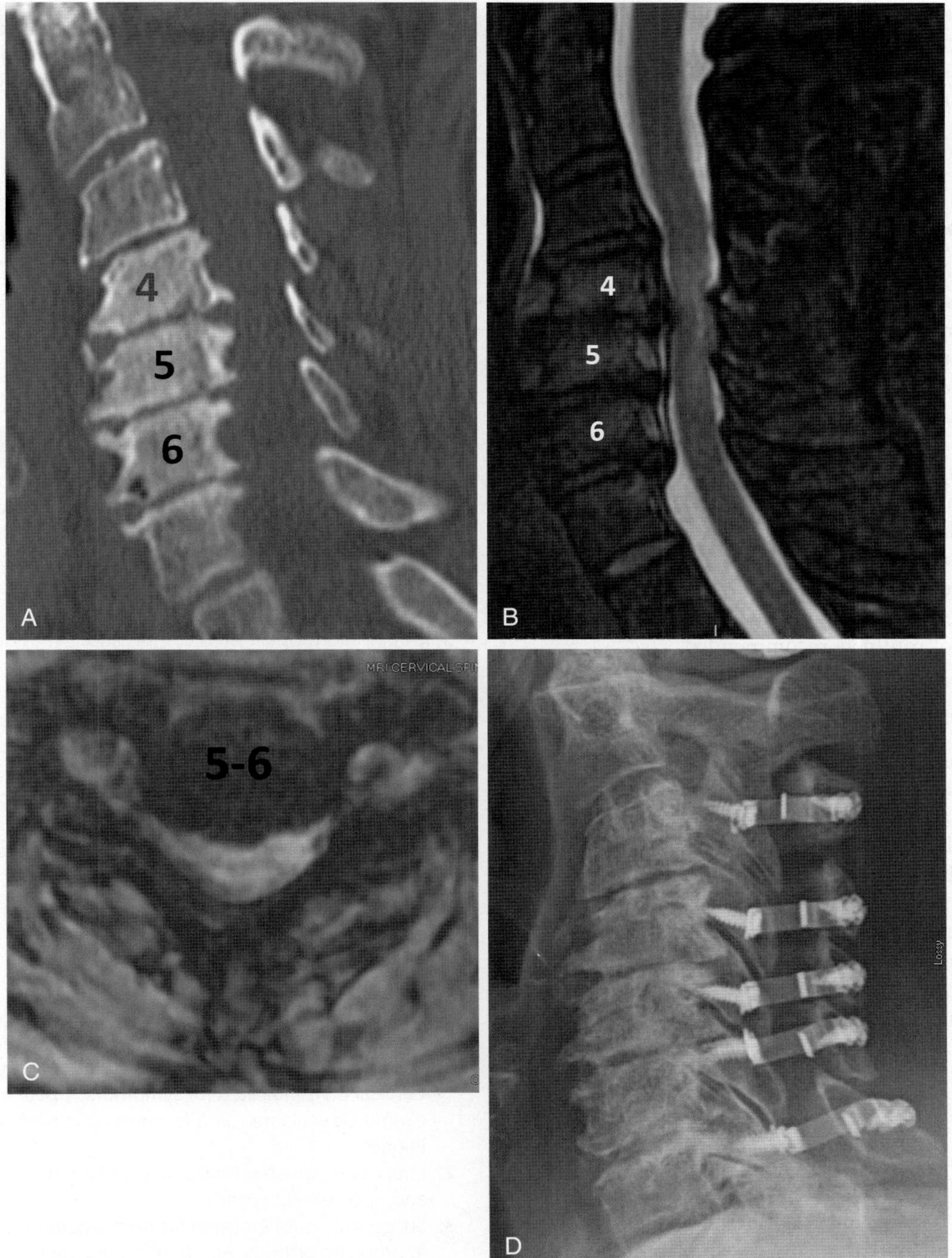

FIG. 76.7 (A) A 58-year-old woman sustained central cord syndrome after a ground-level fall. Sagittal computed tomography shows severe degenerative disc disease with larger osteophytes projecting into the spinal canal causing canal narrowing from C4–C7. (B) Sagittal short tau inversion recovery magnetic resonance imaging (MRI) demonstrated severe cord compression at C4–C6 with cord signal changes. There was no evidence of acute ligamentous or disc injury. She was treated by C3–C7 laminoplasty. (C) Axial MRI at C5–C6 showed severe cord compression. (D) Laminoplasty of C3–C7 was performed with reconstruction with laminoplasty plates.

subluxation or kyphosis requiring fusion. Therefore, careful attention to upright radiographs and follow-up is needed to identify these cases and treat them surgically before neurologic changes. Matching the construct to the biomechanical requirements and rigid methods of fixation reduce the risk of loss of reduction.

Venous Thromboembolism

Venous thromboembolism (VTE), including DVT and pulmonary injuries, are known complications associated with spinal cord injury that often result in death. The combination of stasis from muscle paralysis, intimal damage, and hypercoagulable state increases the risk of VTE in patients with spinal cord injury. Guidelines recommended that all spinal cord–injured patients receive anticoagulant prophylaxis, although the optimal method is not clear.[46] Patients treated with fractionated heparin are four times less likely to develop VTE than without prophylaxis. Treatment should start within 72 hours of injury. It is not clear whether the risk of VTE in neurologically intact patients is sufficient to warrant anticoagulation, but, given the risk of epidural hematoma, anticoagulation prophylaxis is not routinely recommended.

Pulmonary Events

Pulmonary adverse events occur frequently in spinal cord–injured patients as a result of impaired ventilation, poor cough, and absence of accessory muscles for respiration, leading to atelectasis and fluid collection. Early surgery reduces pulmonary complications, length of hospitalization, and overall complications.[47] Prolonged traction and bed rest should be avoided. Respiratory therapy and pulmonary toilet should be routine in spinal cord–injured patients. A swallow study should be performed before feeding quadriplegics to assess the risk of aspiration.

Summary

Cervical spine injuries occur in 3% to 5% of all blunt trauma patients. Assessment in all patients must include determination of whether significant cervical spine injury is present utilizing evidence-based protocols. Essential to the determination of treatment is neurologic function and fracture stability. Initially, patients are immobilized in collars; then, injury is classified for stability and fracture type using systems such as SLIC and the modified AO cervical spine system. The more stable injuries are treated nonoperatively with an orthosis. An important component is to critically assess efficacy using upright radiographs to identify maintenance of alignment. Surgical care is warranted for injuries having SLIC grade 5 or greater and most AO types B and C. In addition, surgery is indicated when decompression is required in neurologically impaired patients, for progressive neurologic deterioration, and for failure of nonoperative treatment. Either anterior or posterior approaches may be utilized but depend on the goals of treatment. Rarely is a combined AP approach warranted.

PEARLS

1. Determine stability of injuries based on CT and MRI, then tailor surgery or orthotic management to the biomechanical needs of the injury pattern.
2. Early reduction and surgery is warranted for patients with spinal cord injury or highly unstable fractures.
3. The choice of surgical approach depends on the morphology of injury and should provide excellent stabilization while minimizing the number of spinal segments permanently fused.
4. Decompression is required in neurologically impaired patients when the neural elements are compressed.
5. Early mobilization of spinal-injured patients reduces risk of complications.
6. Regardless of treatment choice, monitor spinal alignment with upright radiographs on a regular basis.

PITFALLS

1. Delay in diagnosis secondary to inadequate interpretation or misinterpretation of radiologic imaging of spinal injury is associated with significant risk for neurologic deterioration.
2. When attempting nonoperative treatment, fracture displacement may occur in 5% to 10% of patients, who may require surgical treatment.
3. Diminish orthosis-related complications with optimal fitting by a certified orthotist and by using the most appropriate orthosis for the patient and the patient's injury pattern.
4. Fracture comminution may weaken the surgical construct. Consider using an alternative approach in areas with adequate bone stock.
5. Avoid posterior cervical surgical wound infections by meticulous aseptic technique, intravenous antibiotics, and possibly by intrawound administration of vancomycin powder.
6. Vertebral artery injuries should be investigated by CT angiography when fractures involve the foramen transversarium, fracture dislocations, and lateral mass fractures. If present, antiplatelet treatment is recommended.

KEY POINTS

1. Critical evaluation by history and physical examination is needed to identify trauma patients with potential cervical injury. Cervical CT is indicated for symptomatic patients, those who cannot be evaluated, and for those who have distracting injuries.
2. Injuries are assessed for stability and classified using the SLIC and updated AO system.
3. Successful nonoperative treatment requires selection of an appropriate orthosis. An upright radiograph is assessed to determine efficacy of treatment. Progressive deformity, translation, or neurologic change warrants surgical consideration.
4. Surgery is indicated for unstable injuries, those with SLIC >4, or for most B and C type AO lesions.
5. Early reduction with tong traction in quadriplegic patients with facet dislocations and burst-type fractures should be considered.
6. Fractures in patients with ankylosed spines should be treated with posterior instrumentation.

KEY REFERENCES

1. Kirshblum SC, Waring W, Biering-Sorensen F, et al. Reference for the 2011 revision of the International Standards for Neurological Classification of Spinal Cord Injury. *J Spinal Cord Med*. 2011;34(6):547-554.

2. Vaccaro AR, Hulbert RJ, Patel AA, et al. The subaxial cervical spine injury classification system: a novel approach to recognize the importance of morphology, neurology, and integrity of the disco-ligamentous complex. *Spine*. 2007;32(21):2365-2374.
3. Vaccaro AR, Koerner JD, Radcliff KE, et al. AOSpine subaxial cervical spine injury classification system. *Eur Spine J*. 2016;25(7):2173-2184.
4. Fehlings MG, Vaccaro A, Wilson JR, et al. Early versus delayed decompression for traumatic cervical spinal cord injury: results of the Surgical Timing in Acute Spinal Cord Injury Study (STASCIS). *PLoS One*. 2012;7(2):e32037.
5. Caron T, Bransford R, Nguyen Q, et al. Spine fractures in patients with ankylosing spinal disorders. *Spine*. 2010;35(11):E458-E464.
6. Hurlbert RJ, Hadley MN, Walters BC, et al. Pharmacological therapy for acute spinal cord injury. *Neurosurgery*. 2013;72(suppl 2):93-105.
7. Kwon BK, Fisher CG, Boyd MC, et al. A prospective randomized controlled trial of anterior compared with posterior stabilization for unilateral facet injuries of the cervical spine. *J Neurosurg Spine*. 2007;7(1):1-12.
8. Brodke DS, Anderson PA, Newell DW, Grady MS, Chapman JR. Comparison of anterior and posterior approaches in cervical spinal cord injuries. *J Spinal Disord Tech*. 2003;16(3):229-235.

REFERENCES

1. Oliver M, Inaba K, Tang A, et al. The changing epidemiology of spinal trauma: a 13-year review from a Level I trauma centre. *Injury*. 2012;43(8):1296-1300.
2. Levi AD, Hurlbert RJ, Anderson P, et al. Neurologic deterioration secondary to unrecognized spinal instability following trauma—a multicenter study. *Spine*. 2006;31(4):451-458.
3. Milby AH, Halpern CH, Guo W, Stein SC. Prevalence of cervical spinal injury in trauma. *Neurosurg Focus*. 2008;25(5):E10.
4. Goldberg W, Mueller C, Panacek E, et al. Distribution and patterns of blunt traumatic cervical spine injury. *Ann Emerg Med*. 2001;38(1):17-21.
5. Tee JW, Chan CH, Fitzgerald MC, Liew SM, Rosenfeld JV. Epidemiological trends of spine trauma: an Australian level 1 trauma centre study. *Global Spine J*. 2013;3(2):75-84.
6. Hasler RM, Exadaktylos AK, Bouamra O, et al. Epidemiology and predictors of cervical spine injury in adult major trauma patients: a multicenter cohort study. *J Trauma Acute Care Surg*. 2012;72(4):975-981.
7. Post MJ, Green BA, Quencer RM, et al. The value of computed tomography in spinal trauma. *Spine*. 1982;7(5):417-431.
8. Nightingale RW, McElhaney JH, Richardson WJ, Best TM, Myers BS. Experimental impact injury to the cervical spine: relating motion of the head and the mechanism of injury. *J Bone Joint Surg Am*. 1996;78(3):412-421.
9. Hoffman JR, Mower WR, Wolfson AB, Todd KH, Zucker MI. Validity of a set of clinical criteria to rule out injury to the cervical spine in patients with blunt trauma. National Emergency X-Radiography Utilization Study Group. *N Engl J Med*. 2000;343(2):94-99.
10. Stiell IG, Clement CM, McKnight RD, et al. The Canadian C-spine rule versus the NEXUS low-risk criteria in patients with trauma. *N Engl J Med*. 2003;349(26):2510-2518.
11. Goode T, Young A, Wilson SP, et al. Evaluation of cervical spine fracture in the elderly: can we trust our physical examination? *Am Surg*. 2014;80(2):182-184.
12. Anderson PA, Gugala Z, Lindsey RW, Schoenfeld AJ, Harris MB. Clearing the cervical spine in the blunt trauma patient. *J Am Acad Orthop Surg*. 2010;18(3):149-159.
13. McCulloch PT, France J, Jones DL, et al. Helical computed tomography alone compared with plain radiographs with adjunct computed tomography to evaluate the cervical spine after high-energy trauma. *J Bone Joint Surg Am*. 2005;87(11):2388-2394.
14. Muchow RD, Resnick DK, Abdel MP, Munoz A, Anderson PA. Magnetic resonance imaging (MRI) in the clearance of the cervical spine in blunt trauma: a meta-analysis. *J Trauma*. 2008;64(1):179-189.
15. Kirshblum SC, Waring W, Biering-Sorensen F, et al. Reference for the 2011 revision of the International Standards for Neurological Classification of Spinal Cord Injury. *J Spinal Cord Med*. 2011;34(6):547-554.
16. Anderson PA, Moore TA, Davis KW, et al. Cervical spine injury severity score. Assessment of reliability. *J Bone Joint Surg Am*. 2007;89(5):1057-1065.
17. Vaccaro AR, Hulbert RJ, Patel AA, et al. The Subaxial Cervical Spine Injury Classification System: a novel approach to recognize the importance of morphology, neurology, and integrity of the disco-ligamentous complex. *Spine*. 2007;32(21):2365-2374.
18. Vaccaro AR, Koerner JD, Radcliff KE, et al. AOSpine subaxial cervical spine injury classification system. *Eur Spine J*. 2016;25(7):2173-2184.
19. Levine AM, Mazel C, Roy-Camille R. Management of fracture separations of the articular mass using posterior cervical plating. *Spine*. 1992;17(10 suppl):S447-S454.
20. Anderson PA, Budorick TE, Easton KB, Henley MB, Salciccioli GG. Failure of halo vest to prevent in vivo motion in patients with injured cervical spines. *Spine*. 1991;16(10 suppl): S501-S505.
21. Theodore N, Aarabi B, Dhall SS, et al. Transportation of patients with acute traumatic cervical spine injuries. *Neurosurgery*. 2013;72(suppl 2):35-39.
22. Ryken TC, Hurlbert RJ, Hadley MN, et al. The acute cardiopulmonary management of patients with cervical spinal cord injuries. *Neurosurgery*. 2013;72(suppl 2):84-92.
23. Eismont FJ, Arena MJ, Green BA. Extrusion of an intervertebral disc associated with traumatic subluxation or dislocation of cervical facets: case report. *J Bone Joint Surg Am*. 1991;73(10):1555-1560.
24. Bracken MB, Shepard MJ, Collins WF, et al. A randomized, controlled trial of methylprednisolone or naloxone in the treatment of acute spinal-cord injury. Results of the Second National Acute Spinal Cord Injury Study. *N Engl J Med*. 1990;322(20):1405-1411.
25. Hurlbert RJ, Hadley MN, Walters BC, et al. Pharmacological therapy for acute spinal cord injury. *Neurosurgery*. 2013;72(suppl 2):93-105.
26. Gelb DE, Hadley MN, Aarabi B, et al. Initial closed reduction of cervical spinal fracture-dislocation injuries. *Neurosurgery*. 2013;72(suppl 2):73-83.
27. Fehlings MG, Vaccaro A, Wilson JR, et al. Early versus delayed decompression for traumatic cervical spinal cord injury: results of the Surgical Timing in Acute Spinal Cord Injury Study (STASCIS). *PLoS One*. 2012;7(2):e32037.
28. Newton D, England M, Doll H, Gardner BP. The case for early treatment of dislocations of the cervical spine with cord involvement sustained playing rugby. *J Bone Joint Surg Br*. 2011;93(12):1646-1652.

29. Anderson PA, Henley MB, Grady MS, Montesano PX, Winn HR. Posterior cervical arthrodesis with AO reconstruction plates and bone graft. *Spine*. 1991;16(3 suppl):S72-S79.
30. Webb JK, Broughton RB, McSweeney T, Park WM. Hidden flexion injury of the cervical spine. *J Bone Joint Surg Br*. 1976;58(3):322-327.
31. Vaccaro AR, Madigan L, Schweitzer ME, et al. Magnetic resonance imaging analysis of soft tissue disruption after flexion-distraction injuries of the subaxial cervical spine. *Spine*. 2001;26(17):1866-1872.
32. Spector LR, Kim DH, Affonso J, et al. Use of computed tomography to predict failure of nonoperative treatment of unilateral facet fractures of the cervical spine. *Spine*. 2006;31(24):2827-2835.
33. Vaccaro AR, Falatyn SP, Flanders AE, et al. Magnetic resonance evaluation of the intervertebral disc, spinal ligaments, and spinal cord before and after closed traction reduction of cervical spine dislocations. *Spine*. 1999;24(12):1210-1217.
34. Brodke DS, Anderson PA, Newell DW, Grady MS, Chapman JR. Comparison of anterior and posterior approaches in cervical spinal cord injuries. *J Spinal Disord Tech*. 2003;16(3):229-235.
35. Aarabi B, Mirvis S, Shanmuganathan K, et al. Comparative effectiveness of surgical versus nonoperative management of unilateral, nondisplaced, subaxial cervical spine facet fractures without evidence of spinal cord injury: clinical article. *J Neurosurg Spine*. 2014;20(3):270-277.
36. Kepler CK, Vaccaro AR, Chen E, et al. Treatment of isolated cervical facet fractures: a systematic review. *J Neurosurg Spine*. 2015;1-8.
37. Kwon BK, Fisher CG, Boyd MC, et al. A prospective randomized controlled trial of anterior compared with posterior stabilization for unilateral facet injuries of the cervical spine. *J Neurosurg Spine*. 2007;7(1):1-12.
38. Manoso MW, Moore T, Agel J, Bellabarba C, Bransford RJ. Floating lateral mass fractures of the cervical spine. *Spine (Phila Pa 1976)*. 2016;41(18):1421-1427.
39. Caron T, Bransford R, Nguyen Q, et al. Spine fractures in patients with ankylosing spinal disorders. *Spine*. 2010;35(11):E458-E464.
40. Bransford RJ, Koller H, Caron T, et al. Cervical spine trauma in diffuse idiopathic skeletal hyperostosis: injury characteristics and outcome with surgical treatment. *Spine*. 2012;37(23):1923-1932.
41. Harrigan MR, Hadley MN, Dhall SS, et al. Management of vertebral artery injuries following non-penetrating cervical trauma. *Neurosurgery*. 2013;72(suppl 2):234-243.
42. Anderson KK, Tetreault L, Shamji MF, et al. Optimal timing of surgical decompression for acute traumatic central cord syndrome: a systematic review of the literature. *Neurosurgery*. 2015;77(suppl 4):S15-S32.
43. Harrop JS, Sharan AD, Vaccaro AR, Przybylski GJ. The cause of neurologic deterioration after acute cervical spinal cord injury. *Spine*. 2001;26(4):340-346.
44. Cooper K, Glenn CA, Martin M, et al. Risk factors for surgical site infection after instrumented fixation in spine trauma. *J Clin Neurosci*. 2016;23:123-127.
45. Caroom C, Tullar JM, Benton EG Jr, Jones JR, Chaput CD. Intrawound vancomycin powder reduces surgical site infections in posterior cervical fusion. *Spine*. 2013;38(14):1183-1187.
46. Dhall SS, Hadley MN, Aarabi B, et al. Deep venous thrombosis and thromboembolism in patients with cervical spinal cord injuries. *Neurosurgery*. 2013;72(suppl 2):244-254.
47. Fehlings MG, Wilson JR. Timing of surgical intervention in spinal trauma: what does the evidence indicate? *Spine*. 2010;35(21 suppl):S159-S160.

CHAPTER 77 Thoracic and Lumbar Spinal Injuries

Joseph P. Gjolaj
Seth K. Williams

The treatment goals for patients with injuries to the thoracic, thoracolumbar, or lumbar spine are primarily to maintain or restore spinal alignment and stability, preserve neurologic function, assist appropriate management of other injuries, and mobilize the patient as soon as possible. Controversy persists over the choice of operative versus nonoperative treatment of certain fractures, but there is agreement on the basic principles in the diagnosis and management of thoracic and lumbar spinal injuries.

Incidence

The thoracolumbar junction is the most common injury site for thoracic and lumbar trauma. Most patients are young males involved in high-energy accidents. More than half of fractures occur between T11 and L1, and another 30% occur between L2 and L5.[1–3] More than 50% of injuries are sustained in motor vehicle accidents, and another 25% are sustained in a fall from greater than 6 feet. Complete neurologic injuries occur in about 20%, and incomplete neurologic injuries occur in about 15% of patients. Associated injuries—including fractures, head trauma, pulmonary injuries, and intraabdominal injuries—occur more than 50% of the time. Noncontiguous spine injuries remote from the site of the primary injury occur in 5% of patients.[1–3]

Anatomic Considerations

Considerable anatomic differences exist throughout the thoracolumbar spine, contributing to the differences in spinal injury patterns in the thoracic spine, thoracolumbar junction (T11–L2), and lower lumbar spine. The thoracic spine is kyphotic and has the greatest amount of intrinsic stability because of the rib cage, but it also has a relatively narrow canal that gives little reserve for neural element protection after spine trauma.[4] Axial rotation is greater in the thoracic spine than the lumbar spine because of the coronal alignment of the facets. The lower lumbar spine is lordotic and has the greatest amount of flexion and extension capabilities due to the sagittal facet joint orientation.[5,6] The human body's center of gravity is anterior to the thoracic and thoracolumbar spine, which places compressive forces on the vertebral bodies and tensile forces on the posterior ligamentous structures in the upright position. The center of gravity is located more posteriorly in the lower lumbar spine, in part due to the greater degree of regional lordosis; the posterior elements, in particular the osseous components, experience significant compressive rather than tensile forces in the upright position.[7–10] The posterior osteoligamentous complex consists of the lamina, facets, facet joint capsules, and interspinous ligaments. These structures are commonly referred to as the posterior ligamentous complex (PLC), reflecting the key role of the ligaments in maintaining spinal stability when there is injury to the vertebral body and intervertebral discs. The lower lumbar spine is inherently stable and somewhat protected from injury due to its lordotic configuration, distribution of compressive forces across the vertebral bodies and posterior elements, and relatively large vertebral bodies. The thoracolumbar junction is the transition zone from the rigid, stable kyphotic thoracic spine to the mobile, lordotic, relatively stable lower lumbar spine. Therefore, it is particularly susceptible to injury.

Mechanisms of Injury

Thoracic and lumbar spinal injury patterns can usually be explained by the application of one or two force vectors. These forces cause relatively consistent injury types that serve as the basis for the main classification schemes, which are described later. The most common primary forces are axial compression, lateral compression, flexion, extension, distraction, shear, and rotation (Fig. 77.1A–E). The most common force combinations are flexion-rotation and flexion-distraction (Fig. 77.1F–G).

Initial Evaluation and Management

Any patient with a known or suspected spine injury should be evaluated in a systematic fashion, starting with assessment of the airway, breathing, and circulation as per standard Acute Trauma Life Support protocol. Spine injury precautions are

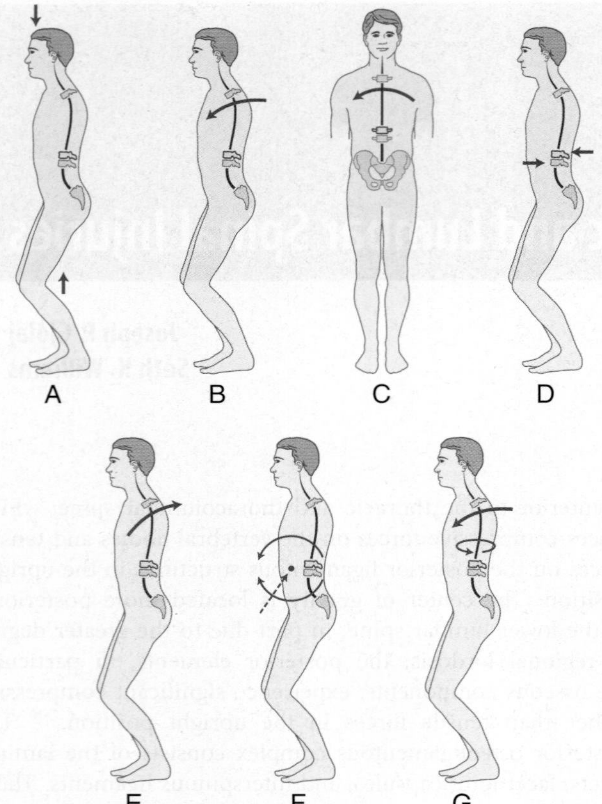

FIG. 77.1 (A) Axial compression forces usually result in compression or burst fractures. (B) Flexion forces may result in compression or burst fractures or, if the force is severe, Chance injuries. (C) Lateral compression forces usually result in lateral wedge fractures, which are asymmetrical compression and burst fractures. (D) Shear forces tend to produce unstable injuries, such as fracture-dislocations. (E) Extension forces usually cause injuries in ankylosed spines, but occasionally may cause injuries in patients with normal spinal anatomy. (F) Flexion-distraction combined forces cause Chance fractures and Chance variant injuries. (G) Flexion-rotation forces cause a variety of fracture patterns involving vertebral body fracture and disruption of the posterior elements. (From Eismont FJ, Garfin SR, Abitbol JJ. Thoracic and upper lumbar spine injuries. In Browner B, Jupiter J, Levine A, et al. [eds]. *Skeletal Trauma: Basic Science, Management, and Reconstruction.* 4th ed. St. Louis: Elsevier; 2009.)

usually instituted in the field by emergency medical personnel and should be continued as long as there is suspicion of spine injury. The patient is maintained in the supine position on a rigid backboard, and the cervical spine is immobilized with a prefabricated collar. The airway is secured, hemodynamic status is addressed, and extremity injuries are splinted. A team of three or more people should roll the patient to the lateral decubitus position, with the lead physician immobilizing the cervical spine and the other two controlling the torso to move the body as a unit to prevent any displacement of the spine injury. The back is then inspected for any signs of trauma such as lacerations, ecchymosis, localized tenderness, swelling, and deformity, such as a step-off between adjacent spinous processes. The patient is then rolled back to the supine position. If additional transfers are necessary for computed tomography (CT) scans or magnetic resonance imaging (MRI) scans, the patient may be left on the backboard until the trauma evaluation is complete. Subsequent spinal immobilization depends on the severity of the spine injury; it may be necessary to place the patient in a rotating bed and institute measures to prevent skin breakdown.

In patients with spinal cord injuries, attention must be made to minimizing the secondary cascade of injury caused by hypoperfusion. Hypotension may occur secondary to hemorrhagic or neurogenic shock. It should be treated aggressively with fluid and blood replacement and vasopressive medication or interventions if necessary.

Associated injuries are common, which can include chest and abdominal injuries, as well as orthopaedic injuries, including pelvis and extremity fractures, head trauma, and contiguous and noncontiguous spine injuries.[11,12] The potential for these injuries must be kept in mind and reassessed periodically, especially in the early stages and in obtunded or severely injured patients who cannot direct attention to their injuries. The initial assessment and subsequent surveys should be systematic and thorough from head to toe, realizing that even in the highest volume and most experienced trauma centers, injuries in the spine and elsewhere sometimes go undetected and can have significant functional consequences.[3,13–15]

The use of pharmacologic agents in spinal cord injury as part of the initial resuscitative protocol has been extensively studied and debated. The rationale is to minimize the harmful secondary cascade of events, such as the inflammatory response and oxidative cell injury that occurs after mechanical injury to the spinal cord. The National Acute Spinal Cord Injury Studies (NASCIS II and III) examined methylprednisolone, naloxone, and tirilazad for this purpose. If administered within 8 hours of injury, there may be improvement in long-term neurologic function with high-dose methylprednisolone. The study dose was a bolus of 30 mg/kg, followed by a 5.4 mg/kg per hour infusion for 23 hours if therapy is initiated within 3 hours of injury or 48 hours if initiated at 3 to 8 hours after injury. There are significant potential complications—such as pneumonia, postoperative wound infection, gastrointestinal bleeding, and sepsis—with the use of steroids.[16–18] Steroids have not been shown to be effective in purely lower motor neuron lesions. GM-1 ganglioside has been studied as well.[19] The use of steroids has not been universally accepted and remains controversial, but can be considered as a treatment option, as can GM-1 ganglioside.[20] There is interest in systemic hypothermia after spinal cord injury, but clinical data are limited.[21]

Initial Neurologic Evaluation

Neurologic injury may have a profound effect on a patient's ultimate function, and the presence or absence of a neurologic deficit often guides subsequent injury management, including operative versus nonoperative treatment. A detailed neurologic examination is therefore critical. It consists of testing both motor and sensory function as well as reflexes in a sequential and systematic manner. Findings should be carefully documented to enable accurate assessment of neurologic deterioration or recovery. Motor function is assessed in the main muscle groups in the upper and lower extremities, which can sometimes be difficult in an injured extremity, but every attempt should be made under these circumstances. Motor function should be graded on a 0 to 5 scale. A score of 5 is normal, with full range of motion (ROM) against gravity and resistance; 4 is full ROM against gravity and slight resistance; 3 is full ROM against gravity only; 2 is full ROM only with gravity eliminated; 1 is palpable or visible contraction of a muscle without joint motion; and 0 is a muscle without any function. Rectal sphincter tone and volitional control should be tested as well. Sensory function should be assessed in a dermatomal distribution. This should include testing of the perineal region because sparing of the sacral dermatomes may provide an indicator for functional recovery in patients sustaining a spinal cord injury. Temperature, pain, and light touch are spinothalamic tract functions that can be assessed with a sterile needle and an alcohol swab. Vibration and position sense are posterior column functions that can be assessed with a tuning fork and limb or digit positioning. Reflexes include superficial abdominal (stroking of the abdominal skin causes the umbilicus to be drawn toward the stimulated area, above the umbilicus T7–T10, below the umbilicus T11–L1); cremasteric (in males, stroking of the inner thigh causes the scrotum to be drawn upward, T12–L1); patellar tendon (quadriceps reflex or knee jerk, L3–L4); Achilles tendon (ankle jerk, S1); anal wink (anal sphincter contraction with stimulation of the perineal skin, S2–S4); and bulbocavernosus reflex (described later, S2–S4). Pathologic reflexes indicating an upper motor neuron lesion include clonus and an abnormal Babinski test. The Babinski test is normal when a stroke along the lateral plantar aspect of the foot results in down-going toes and is abnormal with up-going toes. Paralysis may be secondary to spinal shock, which is a physiologic disruption of spinal cord–mediated function and is characterized by absence of all motor and sensory function and reflexes below the level of spinal cord injury. It is only after spinal shock has resolved that an accurate neurologic assessment can be made because some patients will have spontaneous recovery of function. Spinal shock resolves within 24 to 48 hours in almost all cases, heralded by the return of spinal cord–mediated reflexes below the level of injury. The bulbocavernosus reflex is the first to return because it is the lowest cord-mediated reflex. Brief traction on the Foley catheter or placing pressure on the clitoris or penis should result in contraction of the anal sphincter around the examiner's gloved finger. When this bulbocavernosus reflex occurs, there is an intact reflex arc, spinal shock is not present, and the degree of neurologic injury can be accurately assessed. If the bulbocavernosus reflex is absent, spinal shock is present and spinal cord injury severity cannot yet be accurately determined.

Spinal shock should not be confused with abolition of the bulbocavernosus reflex with injury at the level of the conus medullaris and cauda equina. These involve injury to the lower motor neurons that are part of the reflex arc; thus, the bulbocavernosus reflex may be permanently extinguished. It is important to recognize that patients in this condition are not in spinal shock.

Neurologic Injury Classification

The most basic delineation of neurologic injury is a complete versus an incomplete lesion. A complete neurologic injury is a total lack of sensory and motor function below the level of injury once spinal shock has resolved. An incomplete neurologic injury means that there is some residual spinal cord and/or nerve root function below the level of injury. Incomplete lesions involving the spinal cord usually manifest in distinct patterns that are a reflection of the specific anatomic region of the spinal cord that is affected and are named accordingly, with one exception (central, anterior, and posterior cord syndromes and Brown-Séquard syndrome). Because the spinal cord typically transitions at the thoracolumbar junction to the lower motor neurons of the cauda equina, these four incomplete injury patterns apply to injuries in the cervical and thoracic spine. Injuries involving the conus medullaris and cauda equina (or lumbosacral nerve roots) may be complete or incomplete, and are usually classified descriptively according to the level of nerve roots involved.

Central cord syndrome usually involves an injury to the cervical spine in older patients. It is characterized by upper extremity weakness, with relative sparing of the lower extremities and sacral nerves. Although this injury pattern usually applies to cervical spine injuries because of the upper extremity involvement, Bohlman described a central cord injury pattern in thoracic spine trauma with a greater degree of muscle weakness in the trunk and proximal muscle groups, with relative sparing of the distal muscle groups and preserved bowel and bladder function.[22] Although central cord syndrome is the most common of the incomplete patterns when considering all spinal cord injuries, it is rare when cervical injuries are excluded and thoracic injuries alone are considered. Anterior cord syndrome is the most common incomplete pattern in thoracic spine injury, characterized by loss of all motor and most sensory function below the level of the lesion, with sparing of the vibratory and position sense via the posterior columns.[22] This has a poor prognosis for recovery and is a debilitating injury pattern. Posterior cord syndrome is rare and involves loss of vibratory and position sense. Patients cannot rely on tactile lower extremity feedback for spatial orientation and must use visual cues when ambulatory. They have preserved bowel and bladder function. Brown-Séquard syndrome is usually a result of cord hemisection by penetrating trauma and is characterized by ipsilateral loss of motor function and contralateral loss of pain, temperature, and light touch sensation. Patients typically have preserved bowel and bladder function, are ambulatory but may require assistive devices, and have the best prognosis for recovery from incomplete spinal cord injury syndromes. The conus medullaris marks the anatomic transition from the upper motor neurons of the spinal cord to the lower motor neurons of the cauda equina, and is usually found at the T12–L1 levels. The conus medullaris injury pattern is characterized by flaccid paralysis, loss of reflexes, and sensory loss of the lower extremities with bowel, bladder, and sexual dysfunction. Injury to the cauda equina below the conus medullaris is a purely lower motor neuron injury and presents with the same types of findings as with conus medullaris injury, except that there is a higher incidence of asymmetric involvement and can occur at any level below the conus medullaris. These injuries may be complete or incomplete.[23,24]

Radiologic Evaluation

Suspected spine trauma requires radiologic evaluation. The primary goal is to detect a spine injury, with the secondary goal to determine the stability of the injury pattern in order to guide subsequent treatment. The main imaging modalities are conventional radiography, CT, and MRI.

Anteroposterior (AP) and lateral conventional radiographs of the thoracic and lumbar spine are the most basic imaging modalities available. A swimmer's view of the upper thoracic spine may be necessary to visualize the vertebral bodies through the shoulder region. The lateral radiograph is used to examine the height, width, and alignment of the vertebral bodies, pedicles, spinal canal, neural foramina, facets, and spinous processes. The cortical margins of the vertebral bodies should be smooth and contiguous and, when viewed in conjunction with adjacent vertebral bodies, should form a gently arcing line both at the anterior margin (anterior vertebral body line) and posterior margin (posterior vertebral body line). The AP radiograph allows assessment of coronal alignment, interpedicular distance, and alignment of the spinous processes, and best visualizes the ribs and transverse processes. Anterior wedging of the vertebral body with a break in the anterior cortical margin signifies a compression fracture. Loss of posterior vertebral body height, a break in the posterior vertebral body cortical margin, spinal canal narrowing, and widening of the interpedicular distance signifies a burst fracture.[25] The posterior vertebral body angle can also be used to distinguish subtle burst fractures from compression fractures.[26] Facet widening; spinous process splaying or malalignment; fracture lines in the pedicle, lamina, facets, and spinous processes; and vertebral body translation signify injury to the posterior elements, including possible ligamentous injury, and are radiographic markers of potential instability.[27] Conventional radiography of the thoracolumbar spine has technical, logistical, and diagnostic limitations; therefore, CT has become a key modality in evaluating thoracolumbar trauma.

Many trauma centers now use screening spiral CT of the chest, abdomen, and pelvis as part of the standard trauma evaluation. These images include collateral thoracic and lumbar spine information. As a result, some centers are adopting CT protocols as the initial screening radiologic modality for spine trauma.[28–30] Studies have shown that CT scans have a higher sensitivity than conventional radiographs in the detection of thoracic and lumbar spine fractures, although this applies mainly to stable rather than unstable fractures.[31–33] CT is better than conventional radiography at discerning compression fractures from burst fractures; misdiagnosis may occur in up to 25% of injuries when relying on conventional radiography alone.[34–36] Screening CT scans may decrease the incidence of missed, delayed, or incorrect diagnoses of thoracic and lumbar trauma, especially in obtunded and multiply injured patients, but the clinical significance of this has not been determined. Thus, it is not standard in all trauma centers to obtain screening CT scans. The typical protocol for a trauma-screening CT scan consists of sequential 5-mm axial images with or without reconstructions, whereas a dedicated spine CT protocol consists of 2- to 3-mm axial images with sagittal and coronal reconstructions. It may be necessary to obtain a dedicated spine protocol CT scan if it seems that some important detail may not have been imaged during the screening examination. If the thoracic or lumbar spine injury is initially diagnosed on conventional radiographs alone and a high-energy mechanism is known or suspected, a dedicated spine protocol CT scan should be considered. The main limitation of CT is the limited ability to visualize the soft tissues, for which an MRI scan may be useful.

MRI allows for high-resolution imaging of soft tissues, making it particularly important in the evaluation of spinal cord injury because the neural elements can be visualized. This helps to delineate the presence of edema, hemorrhage, hematoma, compression, and transection of the neural elements. MRI findings may contribute to the understanding of injury severity, including the potential for spinal instability and the need for surgical intervention, and may be useful for predicting the potential for neurologic recovery.[37] Hemorrhage within the spinal cord and edema extending over multiple cord levels are correlated with poor prognosis for neurologic recovery.[38–40] The posterior ligamentous structures can be reliably evaluated with MRI.[41–44] Unless contraindicated, MRI should be considered in all cases with neurologic injury and in cases for which further evaluation of the PLC is necessary in deciding between operative versus nonoperative treatment. The main limitations for MRI are logistics, cost, and the inferior visualization of the bony elements; thus, MRI is usually complementary to CT rather than a substitute.

Concept of Spinal Stability and Its Role in Fracture Classification Systems

Spinal mechanical stability refers to the structural integrity of the spinal column. In its simplest form, it is the ability to resist physiologic loads without progressive deformity or damage to the neural elements.[45] Spinal neurologic stability refers to the presence or absence of a neurologic deficit. The concept of mechanical stability serves as the basis for the main recognized fracture classifications; more recently, attempts have been made to incorporate neurologic stability into the classification schema. Classification systems are potentially useful for communication, research, determining prognosis, and guiding treatment. With respect to thoracic and lumbar spine injuries, certain fracture patterns and associated injury mechanisms have been recognized. As a result, terminology has evolved to form a core group of specific injuries with relatively consistent nomenclature, even though there is not a universally accepted classification system. The majority of fractures can be grouped into these main well-recognized categories, but some injuries are of a mixed pattern and are not readily classifiable. The underlying theme of modern classification systems is to determine whether or not an injury is mechanically stable; the lack of universal acceptance of one classification system reflects the great difficulty in assessing stability in some cases. As the injury severity increases, so does the degree of instability. This occurs along a continuum, however; thus, it is not always possible to determine the point where the transition from a stable injury to an unstable injury occurs. Despite intense work in this area, assessment of mechanical stability remains a judgment call at times. This mainly explains the disparity in treatment approach for certain injuries (especially burst fractures) from one surgeon to the next.

Fracture Classification Systems

Classifications have evolved since their introduction in the mid-twentieth century. Descriptions of thoracic and lumbar injuries first appeared in print publications in the mid-1900s.[46–48] Nicoll[49] credited these early authors and classified injuries as anterior wedge fractures, lateral wedge fractures, fracture-dislocations, and isolated neural arch fractures in 1949. Holdsworth[50] expanded on this classification and detailed the traumatic forces causing distinct fracture patterns, described as flexion, flexion and rotation, extension, and compression. He conceptualized the two-column theory of spinal stability, with the anterior column resisting compressive loads and the posterior ligamentous complex resisting tensile forces. Wedge compression and compression burst fractures were considered stable due to preservation of PLC integrity, whereas dislocations, extension fractures and dislocations, and rotational fracture-dislocations were considered unstable. Kelly and Whitesides[51] built on Holdsworth's work and formally presented the two-column theory as a conceptualization of spinal stability as it relates to spine trauma. These classification systems did not incorporate the extent of neurologic injury; other authors focused on this aspect of the injury.[52,53] The application of CT to spine imaging marked a major change in the understanding of the various fracture patterns, contributing to the evolution of the modern classification systems. Denis[54] analyzed 412 thoracic and lumbar spine injuries with CT scans, classifying major injuries as compression fractures, burst fractures, flexion-distraction injuries, and fracture-dislocations (Figs. 77.2 to 77.5). He proposed a three-column theory of spinal stability and delineated the concepts of mechanical instability and neurologic instability. In this scheme, the anterior column is composed of the anterior longitudinal ligament (ALL), anterior anulus, and the anterior portion of the vertebral body. The middle column is composed of the posterior vertebral body, posterior anulus, and posterior longitudinal ligament. The posterior column is composed of the ligamentum flavum, neural arch, facet joints and facet capsules, and the PLC. Mechanical instability begins to occur with failure of two of the three columns.[54,55] The three-column theory was later validated with biomechanical cadaver studies.[56] Injuries with neurologic deficit were deemed by Denis to have neurologic instability. Neurologic instability was felt to be an important concept because injuries severe enough to cause neurologic injury are usually also mechanically unstable. Subsequent classification systems and current treatment algorithms are based on the perceived mechanical stability of the injured spine and the presence or absence of neurologic injury. Mechanical stability is a continuum—great controversy exists in determining at what point a "stable" injury becomes "unstable." This controversy is most evident with burst fractures.

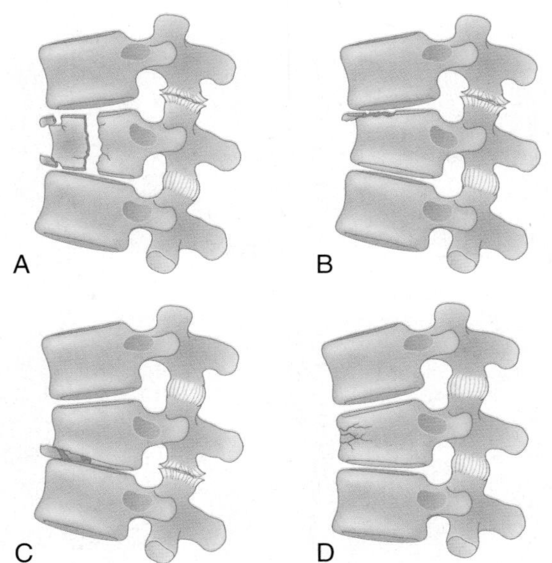

FIG. 77.2 Denis classification of thoracolumbar compression fractures. These injuries may involve (A) both endplates, (B) the superior endplate only, (C) the inferior endplate only, or (D) a buckling of the anterior cortex, with both endplates intact.

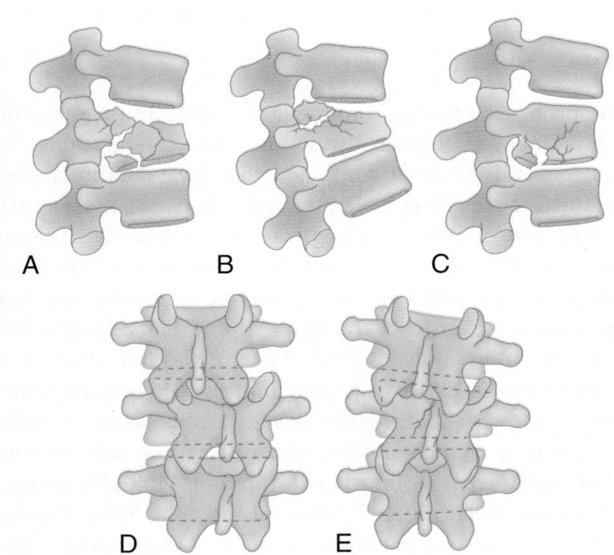

FIG. 77.3 Denis classification of thoracolumbar burst fractures. The fracture may involve (A) both endplates, (B) the superior endplate only, or (C) the inferior endplate only. (D) A combination of a burst fracture with rotational forces, with vertebral body translation best appreciated in the coronal plane. (E) An eccentrically loaded fracture, also best appreciated in the coronal plane.

McAfee described a classification based on analysis of the CT scan appearance of 100 fractures. Six basic injury patterns

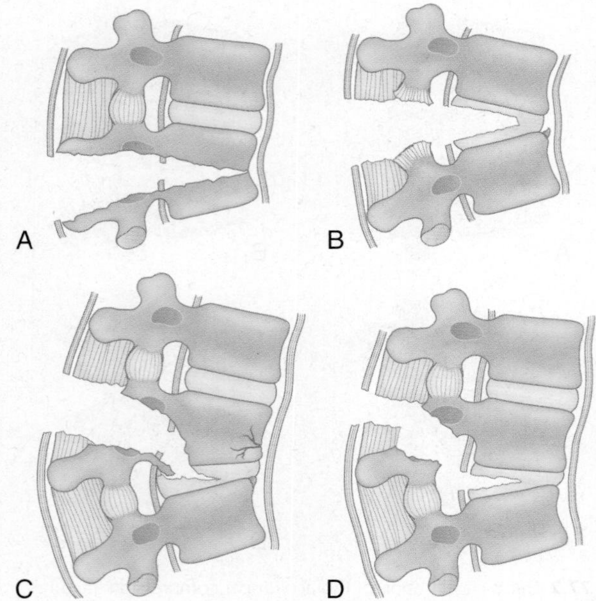

FIG. 77.4 Denis classification of flexion-distraction injuries. These may occur (A) at one level through bone; (B) at one level through ligaments and disc; (C) at two levels, with the middle column injured through bone; or (D) at two levels, with the middle column injured through disc.

were proposed: wedge-compression, stable burst, unstable burst, Chance, flexion-distraction, and translational.[57,58] Ferguson and Allen[59,60] combined the three-column theory with the forces causing the injury and proposed a mechanistic classification. Fracture types included compressive flexion, distractive flexion, lateral flexion, translational, torsional flexion, vertical compression, distractive extension, and isolated transverse process fractures. The Arbeitsgemeinschaft für Osteosynthesefragen (AO) system was an attempt at comprehensively classifying spine injuries. Three main injury types were recognized: vertebral body compression, anterior and posterior element injury with distraction, and anterior and posterior element injury with rotation. Multiple subtypes exist within each group.[61,62] Most recently, the Spine Trauma Study Group has integrated key concepts of these various classification systems to create a more simple and reproducible schema. Neurologic status is included in the classification, with the goal of generating a more standardized thoracic and lumbar spine injury treatment approach. The Thoracolumbar Injury Classification and Severity Score (TLICSS) is based on three categories: injury morphology, integrity of the PLC, and neurologic status. Injuries are analyzed and point values assigned to subgroups within each category. More severe injuries receive higher injury scores; therefore, treatment theoretically may be guided by calculating the injury score.[63–67]

Description and Diagnosis of Specific Fracture Types

There is no universally accepted classification system, but these design efforts over the years have resulted in the development of relatively consistent terminology used in the literature and among spine surgeons to describe the main fracture types. The pathoanatomy and diagnosis of these injury types are described in this section, with treatment described in the following sections.

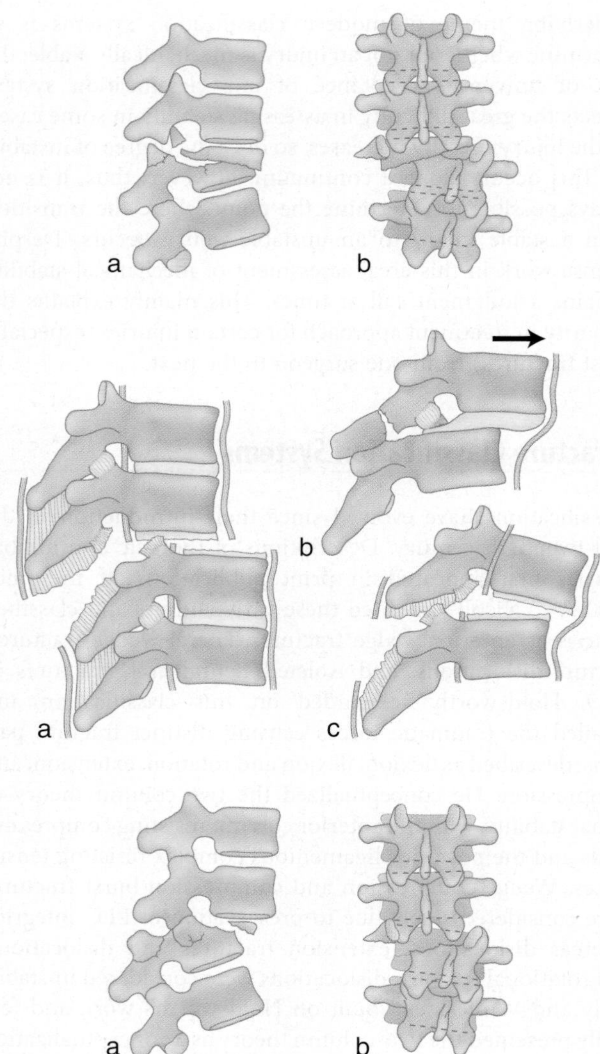

FIG. 77.5 Denis classification of fracture-dislocations. These may occur at one level through bone (*top*, a–b); at one level through ligaments and disc (*middle*, a–c); or at two levels, with the middle column injured through the bone or through the disc (*bottom*, a–b).

Sprains

Injuries to the spinal column involving the ligaments and musculotendinous units that do not cause facet joint subluxation, fracture, or listhesis are considered sprains and are stable.[68] This tends to be a diagnosis of exclusion based on the history, physical examination, and imaging studies. With a reliable history, mild physical examination findings, and otherwise normal spine anatomy, plain radiographs may be sufficient to rule out spinal instability and diagnose a sprain. If there is a high-energy mechanism, unreliable history, significant physical examination findings (such as obvious swelling or neurologic injury), or abnormal anatomy (such as with ankylosing spondylitis or congenital anomaly), advanced imaging studies are warranted. CT followed by MRI are often necessary under these circumstances to diagnose a sprain rather than a more significant injury.

Disc Herniations

Traumatic disc herniations caused by high-energy mechanisms are relatively rare as an isolated injury. Fractures are often associated with disc disruption, and the displaced disc material may contribute to neurologic injury. The category of injury described here, however, refers to an otherwise intact spinal column in association with a disc herniation that appears to be traumatic on the basis of the patient's history, symptoms, and physical examination combined with correlating imaging studies. Disc herniations are commonly associated with minor trauma such as that which occurs with lifting a heavy object, but the disc herniations considered here are due to high-energy trauma such as motor vehicle accidents that also caused or had the potential to cause other significant injuries. Diagnosis is made with MRI. There may be other imaging or clinical evidence of injury to the spinal column, such as a soft tissue injury that would otherwise be called a sprain. However, in order to be considered an isolated disc injury, there must not be any facet subluxation or traumatic listhesis. The classification scheme is anatomically descriptive and identical to that used in atraumatic disc herniations: bulging, protruded, extruded, or sequestered.[69,70] It may be difficult to definitively establish a disc herniation as traumatic rather than preexisting because disc herniations are common in the asymptomatic population and it is a rare luxury to have the availability of preinjury magnetic resonance images. From a clinical perspective, it is not so important to establish a disc herniation as traumatic or preexisting because management of the disc herniation depends primarily on the presence or absence of neurologic symptoms (radicular pain), the physical examination findings (sensory and motor deficits), and the apparent temporal sequence in which these signs and symptoms developed. The spinal column itself is usually stable, with isolated disc injuries.

Minor Fractures

Transverse process fractures and spinous process fractures usually represent an avulsion injury due to indirect trauma, but they are also caused by direct trauma and can occur as a single fracture or as multiple fractures. Transverse process fractures are best visualized on AP radiographs; spinous process fractures are more readily detected on lateral radiographs, though CT will show these fractures clearly. Isolated pars fractures, lamina fractures, and articular process fractures can also be considered minor injuries and are best detected by CT. These fractures are stable provided that they are not associated with significant ligamentous injury. This can be demonstrated by maintenance of spinal alignment on upright radiographs once the patient has mobilized. L5 transverse process fractures may be associated with vertical-shear sacral fractures; CT images should extend through the pelvis when an L5 transverse process fracture is detected.

Compression Fractures

Compression fractures result from axial compression through the vertebral body, with failure through the anterior column. The fracture may involve the superior or inferior endplate alone, both endplates, or buckling of the anterior cortex with endplate preservation. The posterior column is usually not involved, but occasionally is. When this is the case, what appears to be a compression fracture may be a more significant flexion-distraction injury, described later as a Chance fracture (Fig. 77.6). The main distinguishing feature of the compression fracture is predominant failure of the anterior column in compression, whereas the flexion-distraction injury is characterized by predominant failure of the posterior column in tension. Plain radiographs are usually diagnostic, but CT scans may be necessary to confirm the diagnosis because extension into the middle column may be subtle and burst fractures may be misdiagnosed as compression fractures 25% of the time on the basis of plain radiographs alone.[36]

Burst Fractures

Burst fractures, like compression fractures, are caused by axial compression through the vertebral body. The fracture may involve the superior or inferior endplate alone, both endplates, or rarely with preservation of the endplates. Lateral compression forces may cause an injury variant that is asymmetrical in the coronal plane. The posterior column may or may not be involved, though more frequently it is involved when compared with compression fractures. In more severe injuries, the distinction between a burst fracture and a compression fracture is clear, with retropulsion of the fractured middle column fragments into the spinal canal being the hallmark of a burst fracture. In less severe injuries, the distinction between compression and burst fractures is less clear and practically speaking may be in nomenclature alone, such as when the middle column fracture is minimally displaced and barely extends into the posterior cortex and there is minimal retropulsion of the middle column fragments (Fig. 77.7). The generally accepted differentiation between compression and burst fractures occurs at the middle column, which is spared in compression fractures and involved with burst fractures. Practically speaking, the transition from compression fracture to burst fracture represents a continuum of injury rather than distinct injury patterns because the same force vector is responsible. Plain radiographs are often diagnostic, but CT scans are usually necessary to distinguish compression fractures from subtle burst fractures.[36] For classification and descriptive purposes, if CT confirms that the fracture extends into the posterior cortex of the vertebral body, regardless of the degree of displacement, it is referred to as a *burst fracture*.

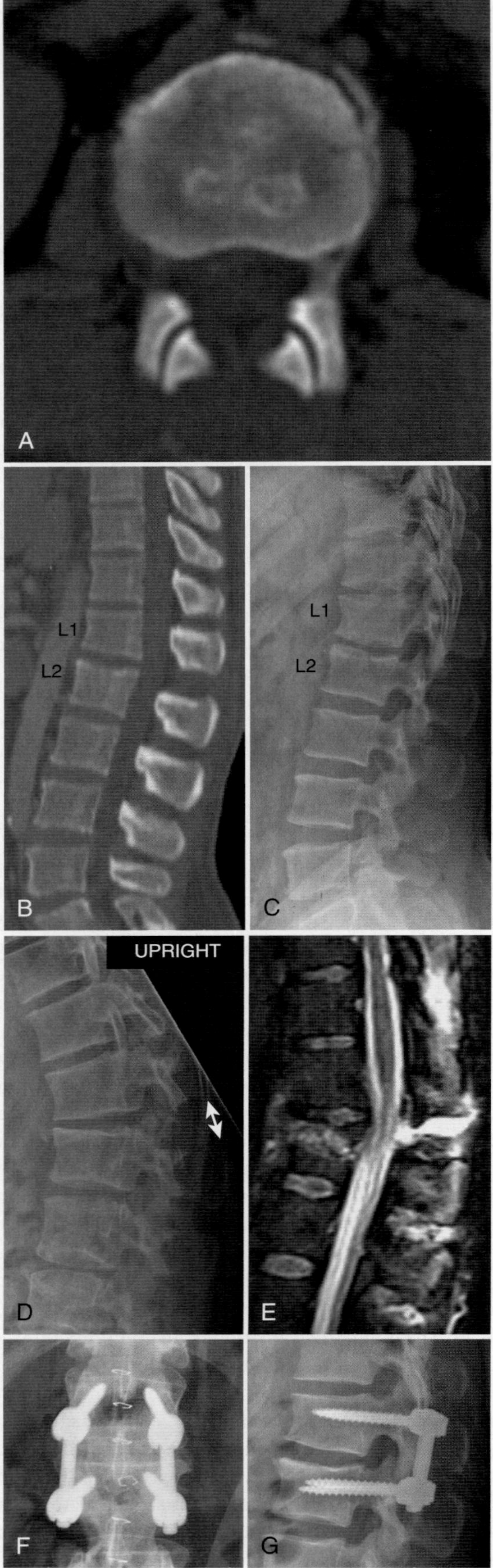

FIG. 77.6 Unstable ligamentous Chance injury variant masquerading as a compression fracture. (A–B) Computed tomography cuts and (C) a lateral radiograph showing what appears to be a compression fracture. There is subtle splaying of the spinous processes of L1 with respect to L2 in (B), but minimal focal kyphosis and L2 height loss. (D) Upright radiograph in a brace shows an obvious increased distance between the spinous processes of L1 and L2 with focal kyphosis. (E) Subsequent magnetic resonance imaging demonstrates the ligamentous injury through L1–L2 posteriorly. (F–G) The deformity was reduced, and the posterior tension band was restored with short-segment posterior instrumented fusion.

Flexion-Distraction Injuries (Chance Fractures and Chance Variants)

Flexion-distraction injuries are characterized by primary distractive forces on the spine, rather than crushing forces as seen with compression and burst fractures. These distractive forces cause tension failure of the PLC and associated injuries to the anterior and middle column, either involving the disc or vertebral body. The axis of rotation is within or just in front of the anterior column, and at times the height of the anterior column can be relatively well maintained. The injury may be entirely osseous or entirely discoligamentous, or a combination of osseous and ligamentous (Fig. 77.8). Chance described the purely osseous lesion as a horizontal fracture extending through the spinous process, through the lamina and pedicles, and into the vertebral body.[57] These injuries are commonly referred to as *Chance fractures.* Variants of this injury involve disc and ligamentous disruption with or without fracture. Anterior column disruption occurs through the disc space, not the vertebral body, and posterior column disruption is manifested as facet dislocation and ligamentous rupture, rather than fracture through the pedicle. These discoligamentous injuries are commonly referred to as *Chance variants.* If the axis of rotation is anterior to the spine, the vertebral body may be completely intact without fracture; if such an injury is severe, all the spine ligaments including the ALL may be disrupted, resulting in a severely unstable injury. If the axis of rotation is within the anterior column, there may be a vertebral body fracture with radiographic findings consistent with a compression or burst fracture If attention is not paid to the posterior elements and the distractive nature of the injury is not appreciated, underdiagnosis as a compression or burst fracture may occur.

The diagnosis of a flexion-distraction injury may be made with plain radiographs, but CT is helpful in defining the precise anatomy of the osseous injury and identifies minimally displaced and nondisplaced injuries. Facet dislocations have a characteristic appearance on axial CT images, known as the "naked facet" or "empty facet" sign.[71] This was first described in Chance variant injuries but is probably seen more commonly with fracture-dislocations.[72] MRI is particularly good at detailing the extent of ligament and disc involvement with Chance fractures and Chance variants.

Fracture-Dislocations

Fracture-dislocations may be caused by a variety of mechanisms, including shear, rotation, distraction, flexion, and

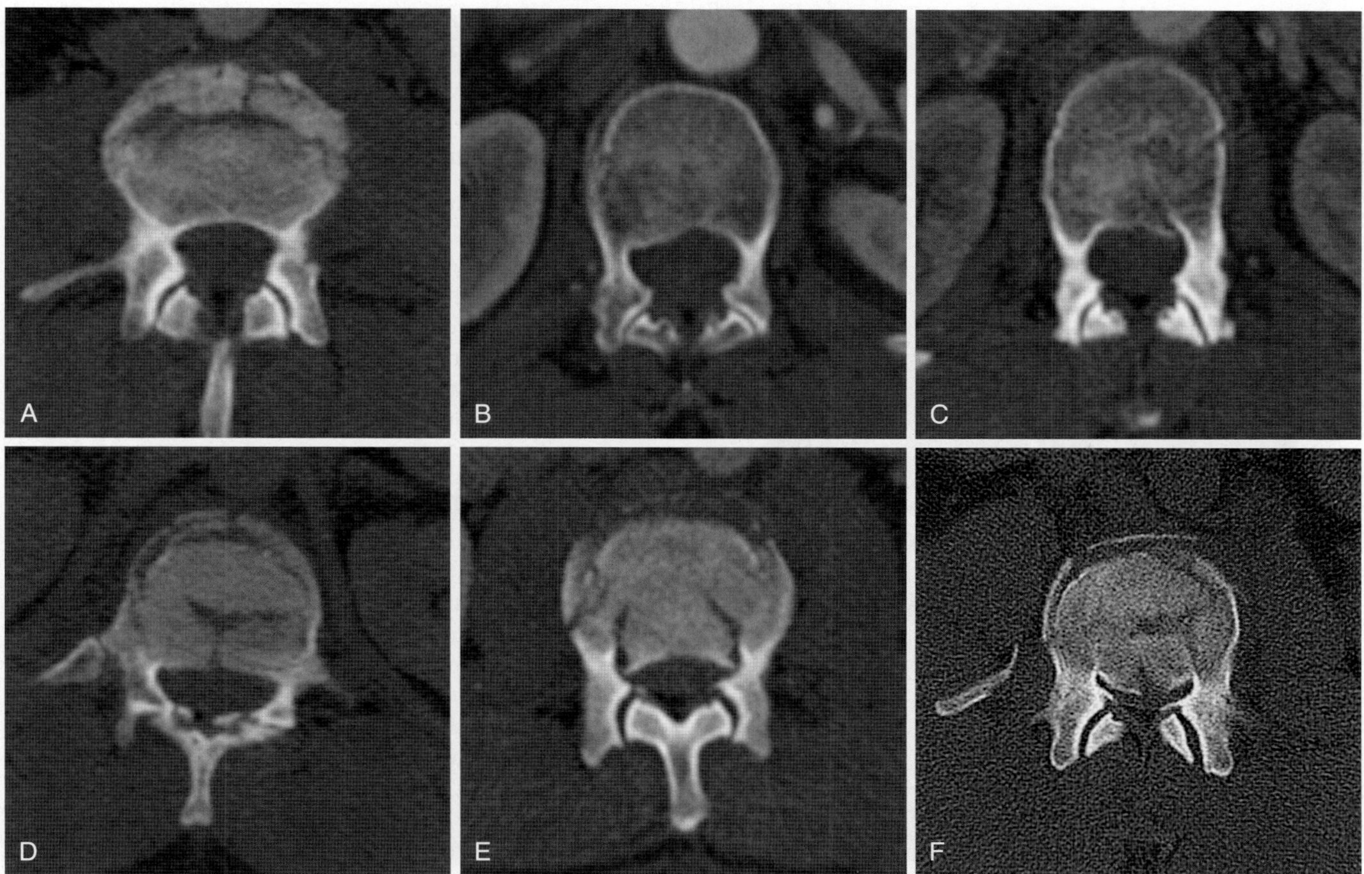

FIG. 77.7 Axial compression injury continuum. These axial computed tomography images show increasing injury severity and the transition from compression fracture to mild burst fracture to severe burst fracture. (A) A compression fracture, with maintained integrity of the posterior wall of the vertebral body. (B–F) Burst fractures. (B) Minimal retropulsion of one side of the posterior vertebral body is seen. (C–F) Increasing retropulsion is apparent, with almost complete obliteration of the spinal canal (F).

extension. Often, the injury mechanism involves a combination of these force vectors; thus, it is difficult—if not impossible—to discern the precise nature of the injury. The unifying theme with this fracture pattern is a high degree of spinal instability. All three spinal columns are disrupted via some combination of fracture, disc disruption, and ligamentous injury. The hallmark is unilateral or bilateral facet disruption due to fracture, subluxation, or dislocation, with anterior, posterior, or lateral translation of the cephalad vertebral body on the adjacent caudal vertebral body. When facet dislocation and vertebral body listhesis are present, this diagnosis may be readily apparent. Sometimes, there has been spontaneous reduction of the listhesis and the main clue to the extent of the injury is subtle facet subluxation. This type of injury is particularly dangerous in a neurologically intact patient because the degree of instability may be overlooked and neurologic deterioration may occur during routine patient care. Any time there is subluxation of one facet or both facets and/or vertebral body translation, this diagnosis must be strongly considered.

Diagnosis can often be made on plain radiographs. The AP view may show lateral translation, whereas the lateral view may show anterior or posterior translation. CT scans will better quantify the bony injury and often demonstrate the "naked facet" or "empty facet" sign (Fig. 77.9).[71,72] MRI should also be performed to assess the degree of disc and ligament injury and to visualize the neural elements.

Extension and Extension-Distraction Injuries

Injuries caused by an extension mechanism are relatively rare and are most commonly seen in patients with an ankylosed spine such as ankylosing spondylitis (AS) or diffuse idiopathic skeletal hyperostosis (DISH). The ankylosed spine is immobile and often demonstrates a kyphotic deformity. The discs and ligaments are ossified; thus, the spine acts as a single contiguous segment. Fractures do not follow typical patterns and come to resemble long-bone fractures more than vertebral fractures (Fig. 77.10). These fractures are usually unstable. Extension injuries can also occur in the otherwise normal spine.

Conventional radiography provides the first clue to the diagnosis, not necessarily because the fracture is readily identified, but because AS and DISH should be readily apparent. If there is displacement, the cephalad segment may be

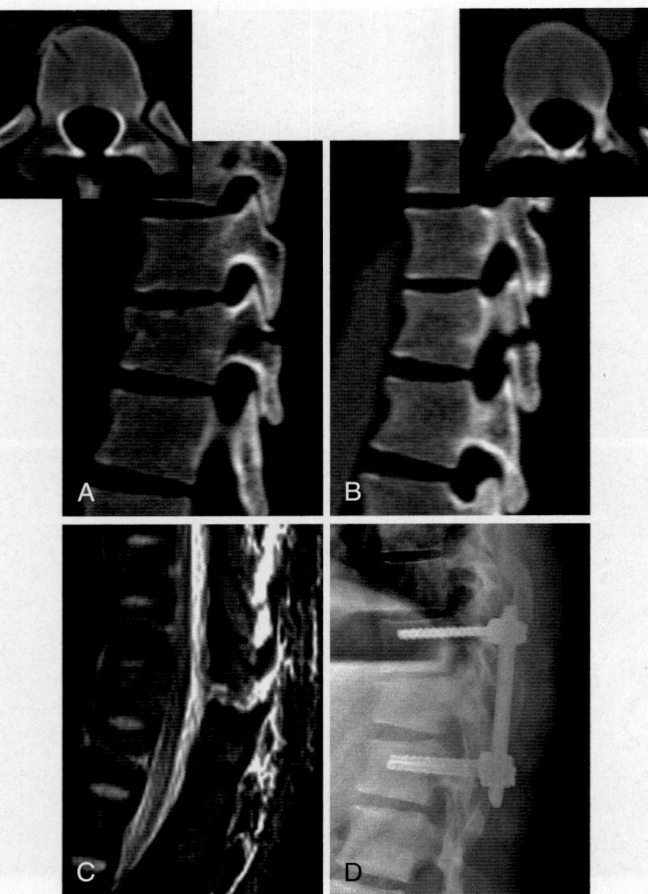

FIG. 77.8 Chance fracture. (A–B) Axial and sagittal computed tomography images of a fracture involving the vertebral body extending through the right pedicle and the left pars interarticularis. (C) Magnetic resonance image showing the increased signal intensity through the posterior ligaments of the involved level. (D) The fracture was stabilized with posterior pedicle screws.

located posterior to the caudal segment due to the extension nature of the injury. Fractures in the AS and DISH population must be treated with caution because of the high degree of instability associated with these injuries, even if there is minimal displacement and the plain radiographs appear relatively innocuous. Therefore, any patient who presents with trauma and the potential for spine injury with evidence of AS or DISH on conventional radiographs must be treated with a high index of suspicion and CT scans must be obtained. CT scans will identify and characterize the injury. Because the discs and ligaments are ossified and this injury is purely osseous in nature, MRI is used primarily to visualize the neural elements. It is also useful for detecting epidural hematomas, which occur more frequently in this group of patients.

In those circumstances in which an extension injury is evident radiographically but AS or DISH is not present and the spine is otherwise normal, MRI is helpful to characterize the disc and ligamentous injury. These injuries are typically due to an extension-distraction mechanism and are rare, identified by gapping in the anterior and middle spinal columns rather than the more typical gapping in the posterior column seen in flexion and axial-load type injuries.[73] The facets may be dislocated with the axial CT images, demonstrating the "naked facet" sign.[72]

Penetrating Injuries

Gunshot injuries to the spine are the most common form of penetrating injury. These injuries are almost always inherently stable. Radiographs and CT scans are usually sufficient to characterize the injury. The use of MRI when the bullet is in the spinal canal is controversial because of the potential risk of neurologic deterioration if the bullet migrates due to the pull of the MRI magnet. Bullet migration has been reported, but appears to be quite rare.[74–77]

General Treatment Principles: Operative and Nonoperative

The decision to treat a fracture surgically with internal fixation with or without neural element decompression, or nonsurgically with a brace, depends on several factors. Indications for surgery are clear in some cases but controversial in others and include spinal mechanical instability, neurologic deficit, significant spinal deformity, and multiple injuries complicating the ability to brace.

A nonoperative treatment option that is less commonly considered in the era of modern spinal fixation systems is prolonged bed rest.[52,78,79] This is a consideration in the setting of a spinal injury that is too mechanically unstable to treat with a brace, but surgery is contraindicated or refused by the patient. This approach is most likely to be successful when the injury is primarily bony in nature and is not associated with significant deformity. However, prolonged bed rest is often associated with complications such as deep vein thrombosis (DVT), pulmonary embolism, pneumonia, and decubitus ulcers. Because this treatment approach is so rarely employed and is usually a result of necessity rather than surgeon preference, the discussion hereafter centers on bracing principles and surgical principles.

Bracing Principles

Fractures that are mechanically stable in neurologically intact patients without significant spinal deformity can usually be treated successfully by bracing. Bracing helps stabilize the spine by providing relative immobilization above and below the level of injury. For upper lumbar and mid-to-low thoracic injuries, a standard thoracolumbar orthosis is appropriate. This may consist of a Jewett-type hyperextension brace for sagittal-plane injuries or a custom-molded, total-contact brace for injuries with coronal or rotational components. Lower lumbar injuries are more difficult to immobilize because the lumbosacral junction must be incorporated in the brace in order to stabilize the spinal segment below the level of injury. Options include a thoracolumbosacral orthosis, possibly with incorporation of one of the thighs to maximize stability in fractures below L3. Similarly, fractures above T6 usually require a cervicothoracic

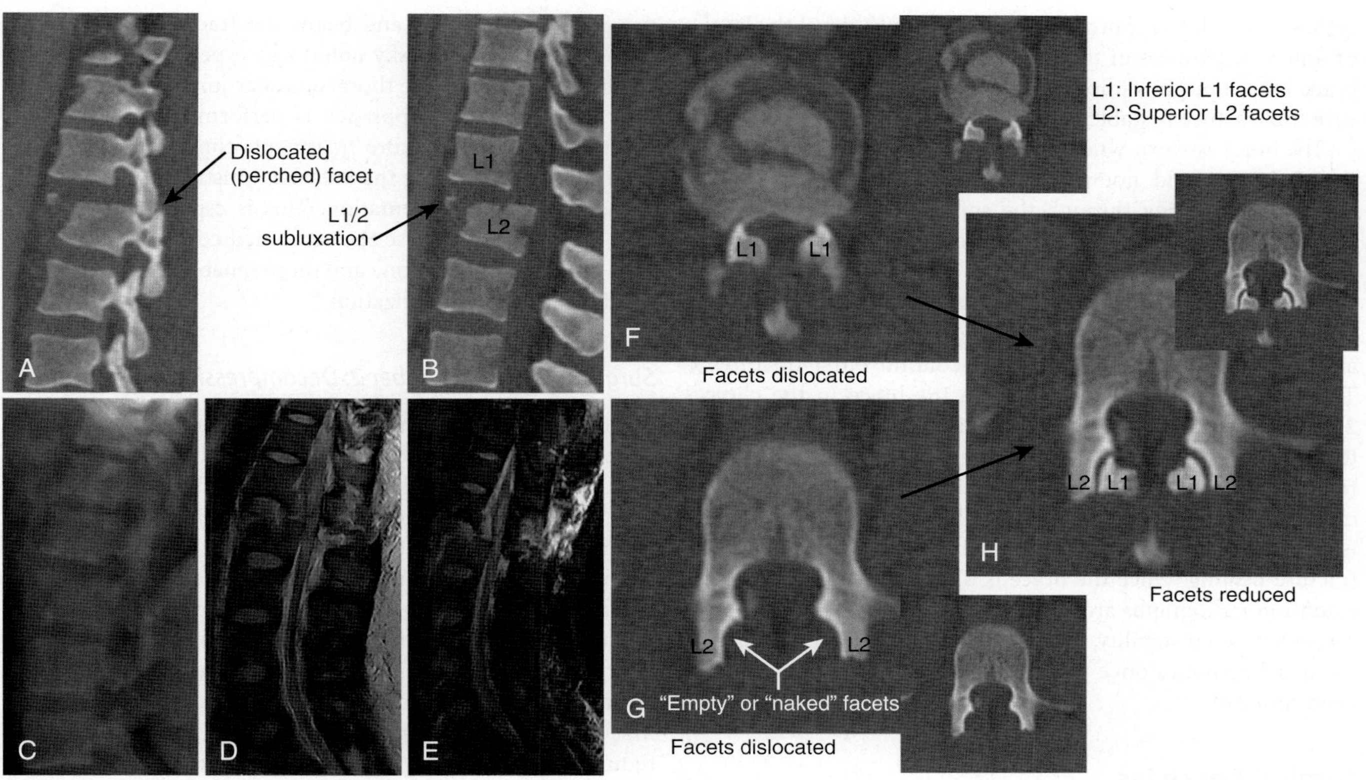

FIG. 77.9 Fracture-dislocation. (A–B) Sagittal computed tomography (CT) images showing listhesis of L1 on L2, with dislocation of the facets. (C) Lateral radiograph showing the listhesis of L1 on L2. (D–E) Sagittal magnetic resonance images (T2-weighted and short tau inversion recovery [STIR], respectively) clearly demonstrate the injury, including the involvement of the posterior ligamentous complex, which is particularly evident on the STIR images. (F–G) Axial CT images showing the dislocated facets, which are shown in their reduced anatomic position (H). (G) "Empty facet" or "naked facet" sign.

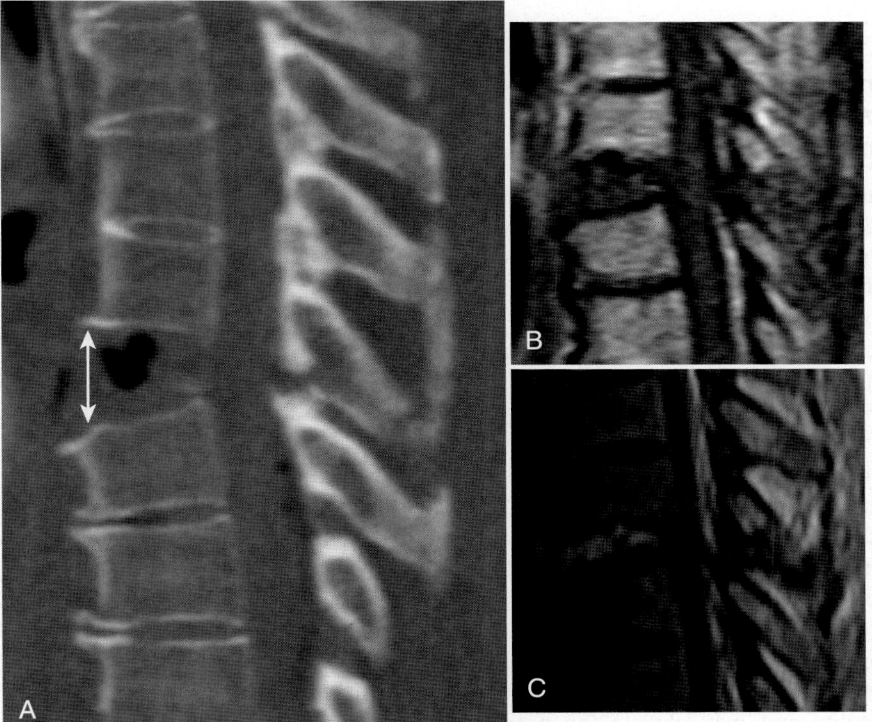

FIG. 77.10 Extension-distraction injury. (A) Sagittal computed tomography image showing an ankylosed spine with distraction across adjacent vertebral bodies (*white arrow*). (B) Sagittal T1-weighted magnetic resonance image through the level of injury. (C) Sagittal T2-weighted magnetic resonance image through the level of injury.

orthosis in order to control the spinal segment above the level of injury. Regardless of the level and type of injury, once the brace is fit, upright radiographs should be obtained to make sure the fracture is stable in the brace.

The brace is worn whenever the patient is out of bed, and the patient should not perform any activities that involve bending or twisting through the spine or lifting more than 10 pounds. This may be a relatively conservative regimen and under certain circumstances may be modified, but only with caution. The typical brace duration is approximately 3 months, perhaps somewhat shorter with mild compression fractures and up to 4 to 6 months for three-column burst fractures. Typically, the patient is evaluated in the brace in the clinic 2 weeks and 6 weeks after injury with upright radiographs, to make sure that the brace is being properly worn and the fracture remains stable. After the second visit, subsequent clinic visits are made at 6- to 8-week intervals. Brace weaning is initiated once there is clinical and radiographic evidence of fracture healing. Once the brace is discontinued, flexion and extension radiographs are obtained. Provided that these show no evidence of instability, the patient can slowly start to resume the usual activities once pain-free motion and strength have been restored.

Surgical Principles

Injuries that are not believed to be amenable to bracing should be treated surgically. The goals of surgery are to achieve and maintain anatomic reduction, minimize construct length while providing sufficient stability to allow for early mobilization, achieve neural element decompression when indicated, avoid complications, and proceed within the most appropriate time frame.

Surgical Principle Number 1: Achieving and Maintaining Anatomic Reduction and Stability—Surgical Approach and Instrumentation Choice

In order to achieve and maintain anatomic reduction, the forces that caused the injury must be counteracted by the instrumentation construct, which should be robust enough to withstand physiologic loads until the injury heals. Posterior pedicle screw and rod constructs are more rigid than anterior constructs, thus have become the mainstay of spinal instrumentation in thoracic and lumbar trauma.[80] The posterior approach is quite versatile, allowing for powerful reduction techniques. However, the anterior spine performs the majority of the axial load bearing, which must be taken into consideration. Anterior approaches are primarily used for neural element decompression and structural restoration of the anterior column. The integrity of the anterior column may be restored by performing a corpectomy of a highly comminuted vertebral body fracture followed by reconstruction with structural bone grafting or a structural device, such as a titanium cage.[81] Anterior internal fixation devices may provide additional stability and may obviate the need for additional posterior instrumentation. This requires further exposure to place the internal fixation device in the intact vertebral bodies above and below the fractured level, which may be difficult and risky anteriorly, especially in the lower lumbar spine and at the thoracolumbar junction.[82–85] In cases in which an anterior approach is performed as the primary component of the fracture treatment, consideration may be given to supplementing the anterior construct with posterior pedicle screw instrumentation. This is especially true if the PLC is disrupted because the combined construct is stronger than either construct alone and more reliably handles the load demands of early mobilization.[86]

Surgical Principle Number 2: Decompression

Neural element decompression is generally reserved for patients with neurologic deficits, irrespective of the degree of spinal canal compromise. Neurologically intact patients with significant canal compromise of 50% or more do not benefit from decompression. It has been shown that resorption of retropulsed bone occurs naturally, and late spinal stenosis has not been shown to be a problem provided that there is maintenance of spinal alignment.[87–90] Patients with neurologic deficit may benefit from decompression, either indirectly or directly. Indirect decompression is best achieved within the first 48 hours after injury and relies on ligamentotaxis to reduce retropulsed fragments as the fracture is reduced and spinal alignment restored.[91–94] Direct decompression may be performed anteriorly or posteriorly. Posterior decompression via laminectomy is useful when a piece of fractured lamina or infolded ligamentum flavum is protruding into the canal or a single nerve root requires decompression. Retropulsed vertebral body fragments in the spinal canal cause most neurologic deficits; these require a direct decompression. Because the compression is anterior to the thecal sac, an anterior approach is the most direct method to effect the decompression. In some instances, the decompression may be achieved via a posterolateral transpedicular approach, especially in the lumbar spine at the nerve root level, where the dural tube may be retracted more safely than at cord level.[95] The offending bone fragments are identified and either removed or tamped anteriorly. Posterior pedicle screw instrumentation is then performed to achieve stability.

Surgical Principle Number 3: Minimization of Construct Length

Minimization of construct length is more important in the mobile lumbar spine than the thoracic spine. Classically, long-segment constructs consisted of instrumentation 2 or 3 levels above and below the injured level.[96,97] With the advent of modern pedicle screw systems, constructs now typically include one or two levels above and below the injured level, provided that the bone quality is normal. The addition of sublaminar hooks at the same level as the terminal screws may improve the biomechanical performance of the construct while minimizing the construct length.[98–100] Short-segment fixation is the term used to describe a construct limited to one level above and below the injury. Initial reports with this technique were disappointing due to relatively high rates of instrumentation failure and loss of reduction.[101–104] As techniques, implants, and indications have been refined, short-segment fixation may be used with a similar success rate as long-segment fixation in certain injury patterns, which maintains as much native spinal motion as possible.[105,106] Placement of screws in the injured level when technically possible may provide enough additional rigidity to allow for short-segment fixation in cases that would have been traditionally treated with long-segment fixation.[107–109] The surgeon may choose to support the instrumentation construct with an orthosis depending on individual patient factors such as screw purchase and patient compliance.

Surgical Principle Number 4: Appropriate Surgical Timing

The optimal timing for surgical decompression and stabilization in patients with neurologic injury is not well established.[110–112] The potential benefit of early decompression must be weighed against other factors, such as medical optimization, management of coexisting injuries, and operating room conditions, such as availability of neurophysiologic monitoring and the appropriate anesthesia team and operating room personnel. Those patients with a progressive neurologic deficit should certainly be taken to surgery as quickly as possible.

Surgical Principle Number 5: Avoidance of Complications

The main complications associated with surgery include dural tear, iatrogenic neural injury, pseudarthrosis, failure of fixation, iatrogenic flat back, infection, and medical complications. Burst fractures with associated lamina fractures have a high incidence of dural tear, especially in the setting of a neurologic deficit.[113] The surgeon must be aware of the possibility of nerve roots entrapped in the lamina fracture and must be prepared to repair dural tears or place a cerebrospinal fluid drain, if needed. Iatrogenic neural injuries may occur during prone patient positioning or from direct injury during surgery. Great care must be taken when positioning patients with unstable injuries. Consideration should be given to performing awake positioning in patients with severe spinal instability and intact neural function or incomplete neural injuries. The patient may be able to self-protect the spine to some degree with muscle tone, and the surgeon can directly and continuously monitor the patient's neurologic function.

If neurophysiologic monitoring deteriorates during surgery, standard measures—such as the reversal of any recently performed reductions, assessment of potential implant malpositioning, and treatment of hypotension—are employed. If the patient emerges from surgery with a new neurologic deficit, the decision must be made whether to immediately reoperate if the deficit is believed to be a result of hematoma or screw malpositioning or proceed directly to MRI or CT myelography to try to determine the cause.

Infection, pseudarthrosis, instrumentation failure, and iatrogenic flat back are related to patient factors and surgical technique. The surgeon should take the necessary steps to minimize the risk of these complications while achieving the primary goals of reduction, decompression, and stabilization. Medical problems may occur due to unfamiliarity with the patient's medical and social history, associated injuries, and the lack of a preoperative outpatient medical evaluation to identify and optimize any medical conditions. Extra effort must be exerted in ascertaining the patient's history and involving other medical and surgical disciplines to help identify and manage these potential problems.

Contemporary Concepts in Surgical Treatment of Thoracolumbar Spine Injuries

Spinal Stabilization Without Fusion

The concept of spine fracture stabilization without fusion has theoretical advantages, such as the ability to achieve and maintain fracture reduction and healing without permanent stiffening associated with spinal fusion. This technique is most often used with minimally invasive surgery but has its origin in traditional open techniques.[106,114–117] The preservation of joint motion by avoiding fusion is a widely accepted notion in orthopaedic extremity fracture care and increasingly adopted in the treatment of spinal fractures. Before pedicle screw instrumentation, Harrington rods were used to instrument the spine two to three levels above and below the injured segment. To avoid long-segment fusions, the "rod long fuse short" method was utilized, which involved local fusion limited to the injured levels and subsequent rod removal 1 year later.[118] Dekutoski and colleagues retrospectively studied this method, noting that the unfused segments regained 5 to 6 degrees of flexion-extension motion after instrumentation removal, with good-to-excellent overall results in all study patients. However, they noted that kyphosis increased by an average of 9 degrees by final follow-up.[119] Another study by Ko et al.[120] reported on 60 patients who underwent fusionless instrumentation for unstable thoracolumbar burst fractures and noted maintenance of spinal motion and alignment after instrumentation removal. There are select fracture types that have excellent bony healing potential, thus should be considered for fusionless instrumentation. Patients with fractures through an ankylosed spine, most commonly with AS or DISH, have a clear indication for fusionless instrumentation, especially percutaneous pedicle screws and rods, due to the fact that the fracture can be stabilized without concern about the effect on adjacent spine segments because the spine is immobile. Chance variant fractures with the posterior element injury through the spinous process also have excellent primary bony healing potential and are particularly well suited to fusionless techniques. The role of fusionless instrumentation is not as clear in flexion-distraction injuries, burst fractures, compression fractures, and multilevel spine fractures. In the case of AS or DISH, fractures through ankylosed spine segments have been noted to heal rapidly once adequately stabilized.[121,122] If instrumentation is solely performed across ankylosed segments, there is no role for performing a fusion; in actuality, the concept of a fusion does not apply because the spine is already fused. Because of this, there is no need to remove the instrumentation once the fracture has healed unless the instrumentation is prominent, which is unusual.

Flexion-distraction and Chance variant (bony Chance type) fractures also heal rapidly, in particular if the posterior element injury is predominantly bony, thus should be considered for fusionless instrumentation. Grossbach and colleagues found no difference in clinical and radiographic outcomes when treating flexion-distraction injuries with fusionless technique versus open fusion.[133] They identified advantages, including shortened operative time and less blood loss with the fusionless technique. This technique may also have a larger role in pediatric patients who more promptly heal posterior ligamentous complex (PLC) injuries.[122–124] Fusionless instrumentation in adults with flexion-distraction injuries and Chance fractures with a posterior element injury that is predominantly ligamentous depends on ligamentous healing. The role of this technique is still being established.

Regarding burst fractures treated with the fusionless instrumentation technique, Dai and colleagues reported minimal difference in clinical and radiographic outcomes in their randomized trial of short-segment posterior instrumentation with or without fusion for stable burst fractures at the thoracolumbar junction.[106] A meta-analysis by Tian and colleagues[117] comparing fusion to nonfusion for thoracolumbar burst fractures found that patients treated without fusion had shorter operative times and less blood loss, but the second procedure of hardware removal was not included in their analysis. They found no differences in radiographic results besides greater vertebral height loss after instrumentation in the fusion group and no differences in clinical outcomes or instrumentation failure rates.

The disadvantages of fusionless surgery include recurrent kyphosis after instrumentation removal, instrumentation failure (loosening or breakage), possible need for removal of instrumentation, and/or facet arthrosis. Gardner and colleagues found autofusion (facet arthrosis) in only 2 of 75 facet joints traversed by rods but not fused after utilizing "rod long fuse short" treatment of lumbar burst fractures.[124] In contrast, Kahanovitz found that stabilization using Harrington rods across a mobile facet joint might lead to facet arthrosis based on a canine study and biopsy of eight human facet joints obtained during instrumentation removal.[125,126] However, it is not known whether these findings apply to pedicle screw fixation and timely instrumentation removal, nor if the development of facet joint arthrosis is clinically relevant. Additional disadvantages include the theoretical need for hardware removal with fusionless instrumentation treatment and the associated costs of a second procedure. However, some advocate that instrumentation removal is unnecessary in certain circumstances, such as when performed in the thoracic spine across relatively immobile segments, and more obviously in cases of AS or DISH, as discussed previously. Despite these disadvantages, our experience shows that patients tolerate instrumentation removal well with a low complication rate, and that it can usually be performed on an outpatient basis.

Minimally Invasive Stabilization Using Percutaneous Instrumentation

The concept of fusionless spine surgery for thoracolumbar fracture treatment and the technique of percutaneous pedicle screw placement certainly have a synergistic relationship. Although percutaneous pedicle screw placement was initially applied to degenerative spinal conditions, this technique has more recently been increasingly utilized in spine trauma care. The construct is biomechanically analogous to those placed in open techniques, but the percutaneous approach relies on muscle splitting rather than muscle stripping, as is typical of the open approach. Minimally invasive stabilization can be performed either with paired parasagittal Wiltse-style approaches or through multiple small incisions large enough to accommodate the pedicle screws. The overall goals are to stabilize the spinal injury while minimizing blood loss, surgical time, and complications, such as surgical site infection, while decreasing the physiologic burden of surgery. While percutaneous instrumentation is most often placed without the addition of a fusion, in cases in which arthrodesis is felt to be necessary, a facet arthrodesis can be performed through the same percutaneous incisions that are utilized for pedicle screw placement.

The indications for percutaneous stabilization and the necessary construct length are similar to open instrumentation, with potential contraindications including incomplete neurologic injury that necessitates direct decompression of the spinal cord or nerve roots, fracture-dislocations in the neurologically intact patient who may have a risk for neurologic deterioration without an open direct reduction, and in cases of delayed fixation in which postural reduction is not expected to restore adequate spinal alignment. As with open fusionless techniques, percutaneous instrumentation is ideally suited to fractures through ankylosed spine segments (Fig. 77.11) and flexion-distraction injuries with a primarily bony component (see Fig. 77.8). Additional indications include unstable burst fractures in the neurologically intact patient (Figs. 77.12 to 77.14) and multiple-level fractures (Figs. 77.12 to 77.15) in which percutaneous instrumentation over multiple segments are possible with much less blood loss and surgical time compared to open procedures, while avoiding a long fusion and the potentially long-term deleterious consequences associated with fusion, including loss of spine flexibility and adjacent-segment degeneration. The polytrauma patient with stable thoracolumbar fractures can be difficult to manage with orthoses, especially when pelvic, abdominal, and/or chest trauma makes bracing impractical. Percutaneous stabilization may facilitate immediate patient mobilization and the avoidance of skin breakdown from the orthosis or prolonged bed rest. Percutaneous stabilization can also be considered for spine fracture-dislocation patients with complete neurologic injury, with the intention to restore stability and indirectly decompress the spinal canal. Furthermore, a focal direct decompression through a small midline incision can be performed in tandem with percutaneous instrumentation placement several levels above and below the level of injury in those cases in which decompression is necessary. This is particularly useful in cases of ankylosing spondylitis with neurologic compression related to fracture displacement and/or epidural hematoma. Percutaneous instrumentation can also be used to provide additional stability after an anterior or anterolateral corpectomy and arthrodesis, a technique that is

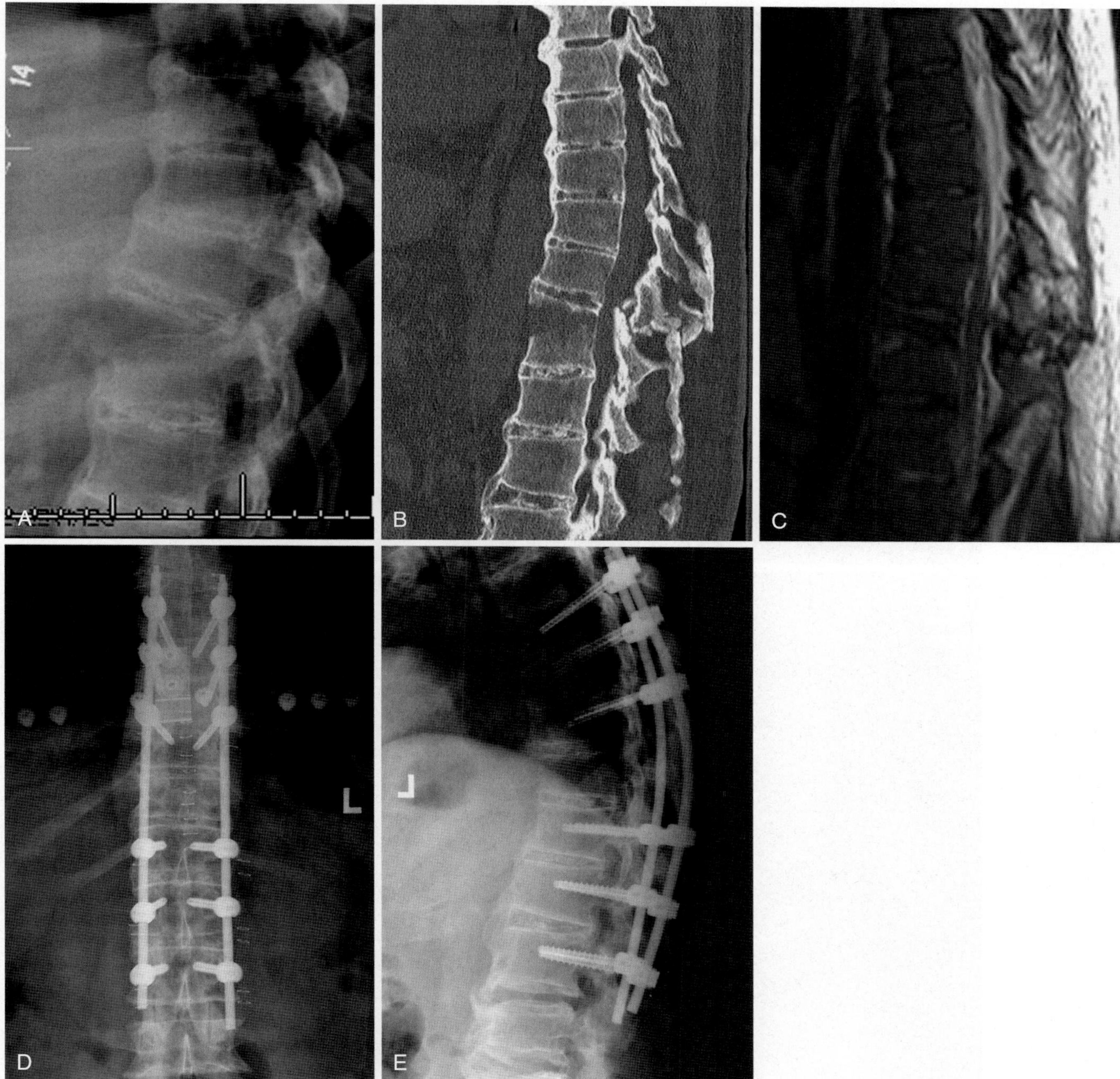

FIG. 77.11 Extension injury through an ankylosed spine stabilized with posterior percutaneous instrumentation placement. (A) Lateral radiograph shows an ankylosed spine with a fracture gap anteriorly, also seen on (B) sagittal computed tomography imaging and (C) magnetic resonance imaging. (D–E) The fracture was reduced with intraoperative positioning, a focal decompression was performed, and the fracture was stabilized with posterior percutaneous pedicle screw instrumentation.

most commonly performed in patients with a thoracolumbar burst fracture and neurologic injury.

Multiple authors have shown that percutaneous stabilization techniques can be performed safely and efficiently with a low rate of complications compared to open techniques.[127–132] Percutaneous stabilization may also have the added benefit of avoiding the need for or an alternative to brace immobilization in certain patients.[133] Grossbach et al. retrospectively compared open versus percutaneous techniques for treatment of flexion-distraction injuries and found similar clinical and radiographic outcomes but shorter operative times and less blood loss in the percutaneous group.[133] Furthermore, no difference in the rate of adverse events was found between the two groups. Other authors have reported comparable findings.[134–137] Ni et al. successfully treated 36 burst fracture patients using percutaneous instrumentation, with an average operative time of 78 minutes and an average blood loss of 75 mL.[138] Additionally, percutaneous pedicle screw placement

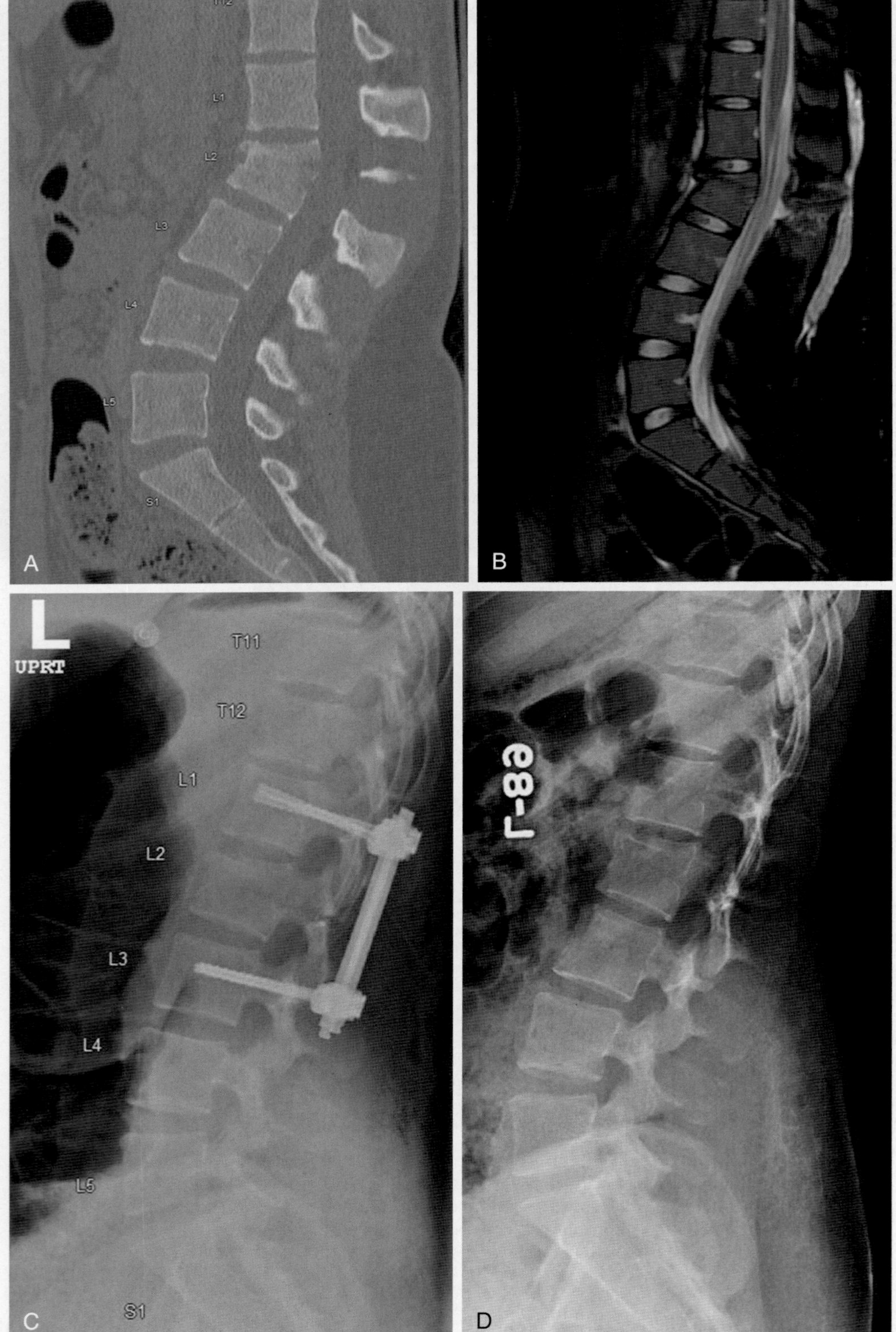

FIG. 77.12 Flexion-distraction injuries with a primarily bony component stabilized with posterior percutaneous instrumentation placement. (A) Sagittal computed tomography image and (B) T2-weighted magnetic resonance image show a flexion-distraction injury associated with vertebral body compression. (C–D) The fracture was successfully reduced intraoperatively and was stabilized with posterior percutaneous pedicle screw instrumentation.

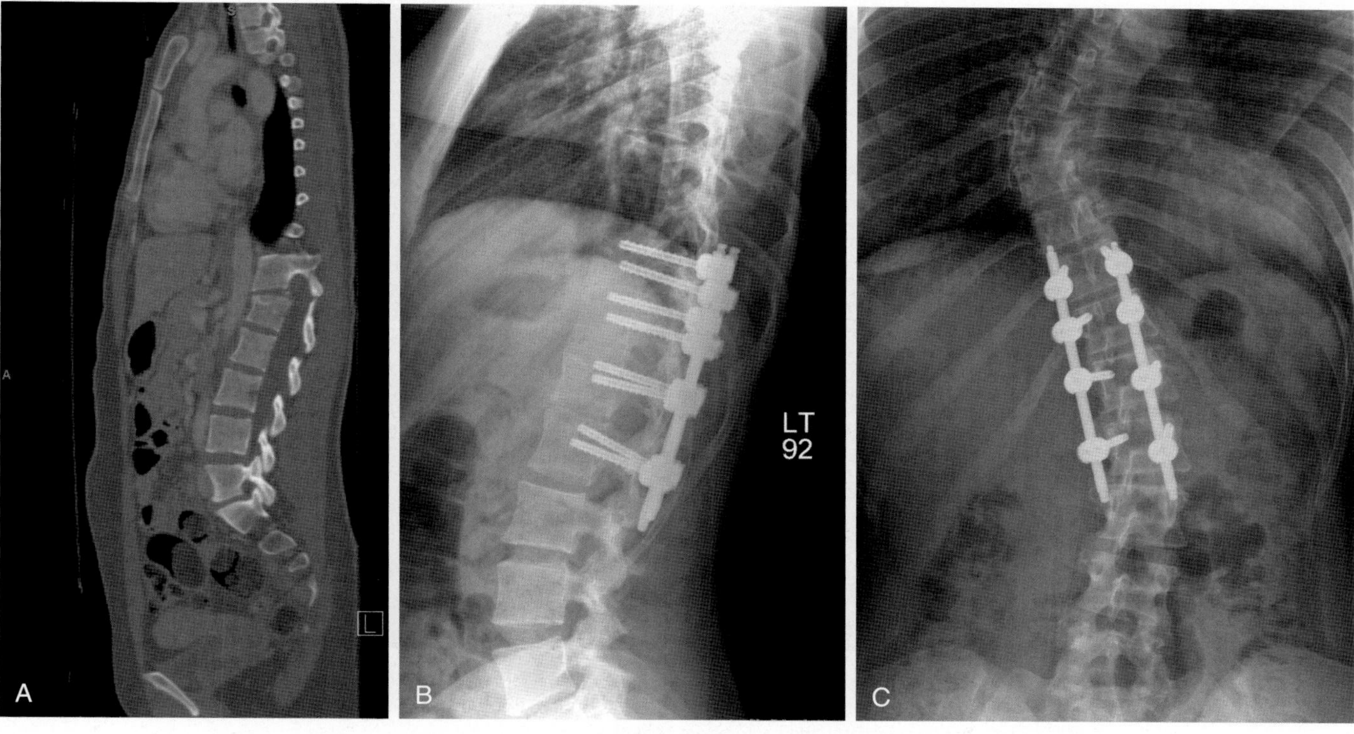

FIG. 77.13 Unstable burst fracture in a neurologically stable patient with idiopathic scoliosis. (A) Sagittal computed tomography image shows an L1 burst fracture with unilateral perched facet. Note that the spinal deformity complicates the imaging interpretation. Surgical stabilization with posterior percutaneous instrumentation placement is shown on (B) lateral and (C) anteroposterior radiographic images.

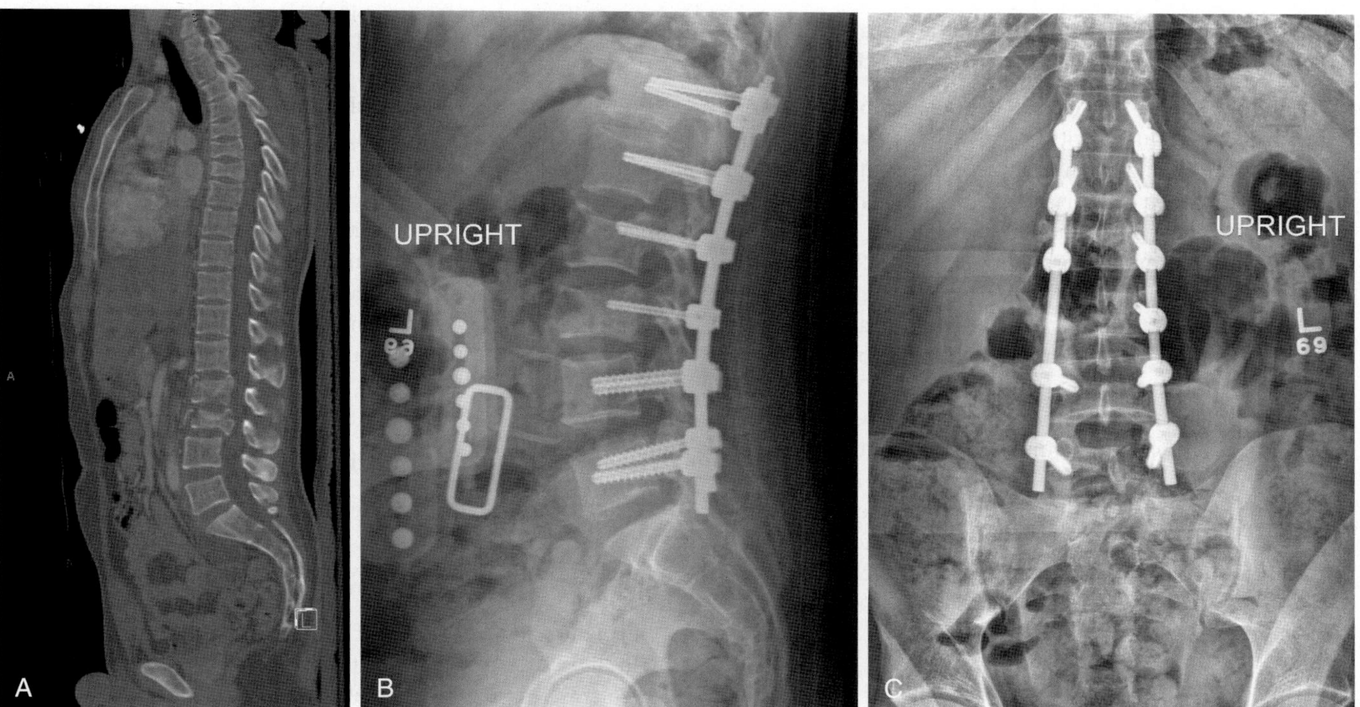

FIG. 77.14 Multiple-level burst fractures treated surgically with posterior percutaneous instrumentation placement. (A) Sagittal computed tomography shows consecutive burst fractures at L2 and L3, with the patient unable to tolerate mobilization using a thoracolumbar brace. Surgical stabilization with posterior percutaneous pedicle screw instrumentation is shown on (B) lateral and (C) anteroposterior radiographic images.

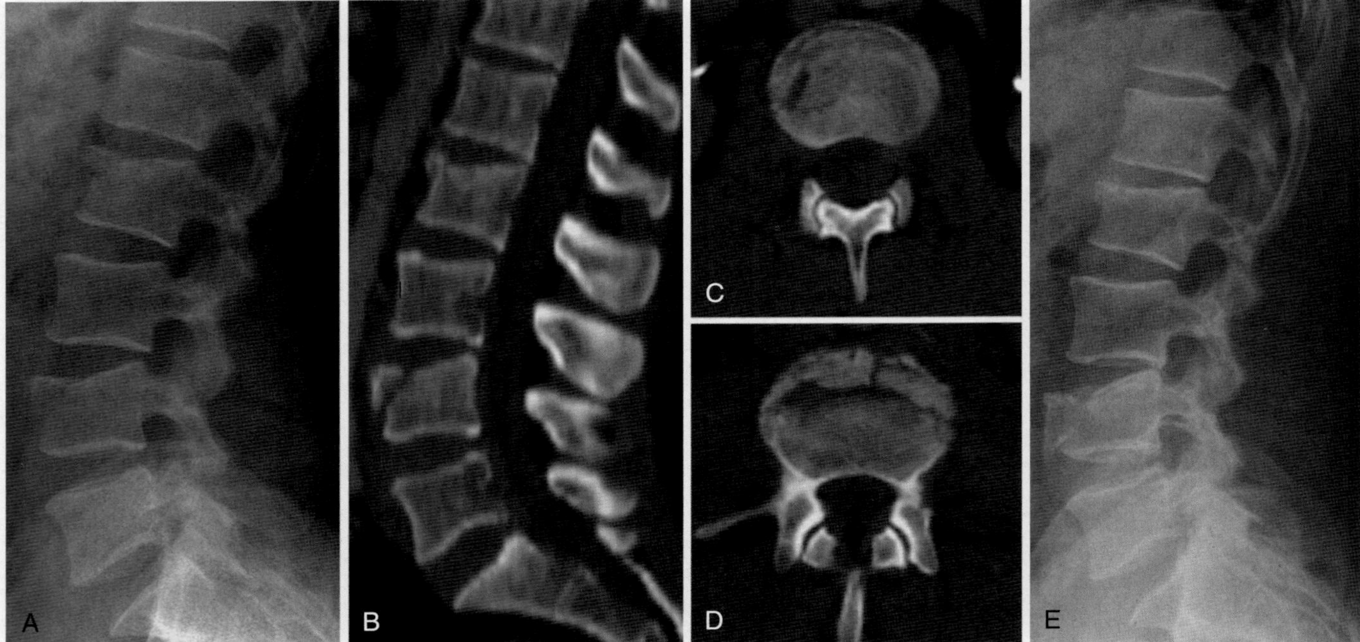

FIG. 77.15 Compression fractures treated in a brace. The compression fractures of L2 and L4 are shown in (A) the lateral radiograph, (B) sagittal computed tomography images, and axial computed tomographic images (C is L2 and D is L4). (E) Two years later, the fractures are healed.

using conventional fluoroscopic techniques has been shown to be highly accurate in the trauma setting.[139–141]

Balloon-Assisted Reduction and Cement Augmentation of Thoracolumbar Fractures

Several authors have reported percutaneous balloon-assisted reduction techniques with or without vertebral body augmentation.[142–151] This technique can be utilized in combination with open surgery or percutaneous pedicle screw instrumentation. The theoretical advantages include aiding in fracture reduction and providing anterior column support through a minimally invasive approach, avoiding the added surgical physiologic burden associated with an open reduction, which would typically require an anterior or combined AP approach. Using the balloon-assisted reduction and cement augmentation technique combined with percutaneous stabilization for thoracolumbar spine fractures, Zairi et al. have shown the technique to be a viable option associated with stable long-term clinical and radiographic results.[152] Singer et al. reported similar results when applied to the pediatric population.[153] Overall, the role of this technique is not yet clear.

Treatment of Specific Injuries

Sprains and Minor Fractures

Sprains and isolated minor fractures are not associated with neurologic deficits or spinal instability; they can usually be treated symptomatically, with or without bracing.[154,155] If a brace is chosen for comfort, it need not be rigid. The main concern with these injuries is misdiagnosis and undertreatment of a more serious spinal injury, such as with disruption of the PLC, or sacral fracture associated with an L5 transverse process fracture. Consideration must be given to the mechanism of injury and clinical examination; if there is doubt, advanced imaging techniques should be used to assess for more significant occult injury. It should also be kept in mind that patients with minor spine fractures may have more significant intraabdominal injuries.[156] Patients with isolated sprains and minor fractures should be able to mobilize readily, and full recovery is expected over a 6-week to 6-month period depending on the extent of the injury, with most patients returning to unrestricted activities within 6 to 12 weeks.

Traumatic Disc Herniations

Isolated disc herniations secondary to high-energy trauma are sufficiently rare that it is not possible to comment on the rate of neurologic injury, appropriate treatment, or long-term outcomes. Terhaag[157] found only four traumatic disc herniations in his series of 1771 patients with disc lesions. The literature is scarce on this subject.[158–160] Treatment protocols are similar to that of nontraumatic disc herniations, with an initial trial of nonoperative management and early mobilization. Bracing is not necessary. Preference may be given to early surgical intervention if there is severe radiculopathy or a dense nerve root motor deficit caused by the disc herniation. Emergency surgery would be indicated if the patient presented with or developed a cauda equina syndrome.

Compression Fractures

Compression fractures are usually intrinsically stable and rarely cause neurologic deficits. They occur most frequently due to a low-energy mechanism in elderly osteopenic patients, but also occur due to higher-energy mechanisms in patients with normal bone. This discussion is directed toward fractures in patients with normal bone—osteoporotic compression fracture treatment is discussed in more detail in Chapter 89. Compression fractures were classically treated with postural reduction and plaster cast immobilization.[161,162] The use of plaster casts gave way to less cumbersome brace treatment; these fractures can be reliably treated with bracing the vast majority of the time, using either a three-point hyperextension type or a custom-molded orthosis (see Fig. 77.15).[163,164]

The prognosis is generally favorable, though some patients will complain of persistent back pain long after the fracture has healed. Several clinical reviews did not find a correlation between the initial injury severity and the degree of residual pain.[49,165,166] Other studies, however, have shown a correlation between the severity of injury and back pain.[167–172] It is from these studies that the degrees of vertebral body height loss and traumatic kyphosis became criteria for surgical treatment in a small proportion of these fractures.

Surgical stabilization may be considered when there is significant traumatic kyphosis and/or vertebral body height loss, especially in the setting of PLC compromise. It is difficult to say with certainty at what point the degree of deformity is deemed significant and the transition should be made from brace to surgical treatment, but commonly cited numbers are 30 degrees of traumatic kyphosis and 50% vertebral body height loss, with these fractures thus deemed unstable.[169] Individual patient factors and overall spinal alignment need to be considered as well. Posterior pedicle screw instrumentation with fusion is the usual mode of surgical treatment, either short-segment or long-segment depending on the circumstances. Provided that the fracture is treated surgically within the first 7 to 10 days of injury, significant reduction can usually be achieved posturally and additional correction may be achieved with distraction through the pedicle screws with the intact ALL preventing overdistraction. An anterior approach is not necessary for decompression because there is no retropulsion into the canal, but it may be considered when there is a residual bone void anteriorly after the fracture is reduced or in delayed fracture treatment when an anterior release is necessary to achieve a reduction. Fractures treated surgically generally have a good prognosis, similar to stable compression fractures treated in a brace. There are no meaningful randomized trials comparing surgery with brace treatment in these "unstable" high-energy compression fractures. Osteoporotic compression fractures are generally stable and may be treated in a brace, although persistent pain may be an indication for vertebroplasty or kyphoplasty. The efficacy of vertebroplasty is a source of controversy, which is discussed more thoroughly in Chapter 89.[173,174]

Burst Fractures

Burst fractures range in severity from those that are barely distinguishable from stable compression fractures to devastating unstable injuries causing paralysis. Although the three-column theory of spinal stability proposes that all burst fractures are by definition mechanically unstable because two of the three columns are disrupted, in reality, this is not always the case. Stability is a continuum; thus, the concept of "stable burst fractures" and "unstable burst fractures" has evolved. Stable burst fractures are treated with bracing, and unstable burst fractures are treated with surgery, but considerable controversy surrounds the transition from a "stable" fracture pattern to an "unstable" fracture pattern. The factors guiding treatment are the presence or absence of a neurologic deficit, extent of spinal canal compromise, degree of deformity (vertebral body height loss and angular kyphosis) at the site of injury, and integrity of the posterior osteoligamentous complex.

As with compression fractures, there is controversy regarding the role of imaging measurements in guiding operative versus brace treatment. The commonly cited radiographic measurements are the degree of kyphotic deformity, percent of vertebral body height loss, and percent of canal compromise. It is unclear as to the role that these variables play in actual fracture stability. The historical significance of these measurements dates to the pre-MRI era and is based on their association with posterior ligamentous injury. Investigators postulated three radiographic parameters that were associated with posterior osteoligamentous complex disruption and thus were unstable injuries: kyphosis greater than 30 degrees, vertebral body height loss of 50%, and canal compromise of 50%. As MRI was introduced and the PLC could be more reliably imaged, it became clear that this was not necessarily true. Canal compromise in particular has not been associated with adverse long-term outcomes in the absence of a neurologic deficit, especially because we know that significant resorption of retropulsed bone occurs over time. High degrees of canal compromise, well in excess of 50%, can be asymptomatic neurologically below the level of the conus. It is possible to have even 80% of the spinal canal filled with bone fragments yet have the patient remain intact neurologically. Similarly, vertebral body height loss of greater than 50% can be tolerated, provided that there is no neurologic injury and no significant traumatic kyphosis. Of these classic three parameters, the one that seems to be best associated with instability and may be the best indication for surgical treatment is the degree of traumatic kyphosis.

Brace treatment has been established as appropriate for neurologically intact patients with less than 30 degrees of traumatic kyphosis, less than 50% vertebral body height loss, and no or minimal injury to the posterior ligamentous complex.[175–181] A few authors have even advocated brace treatment for burst fractures with greater than 50% height loss and in some instances when kyphosis exceeds 30 degrees, provided that the injury is otherwise stable.[177] Another group of authors have suggested that a subset of stable burst fractures (AO type A3) without neurologic injury may even be treated without brace immobilization.[180] However, it is important to consider

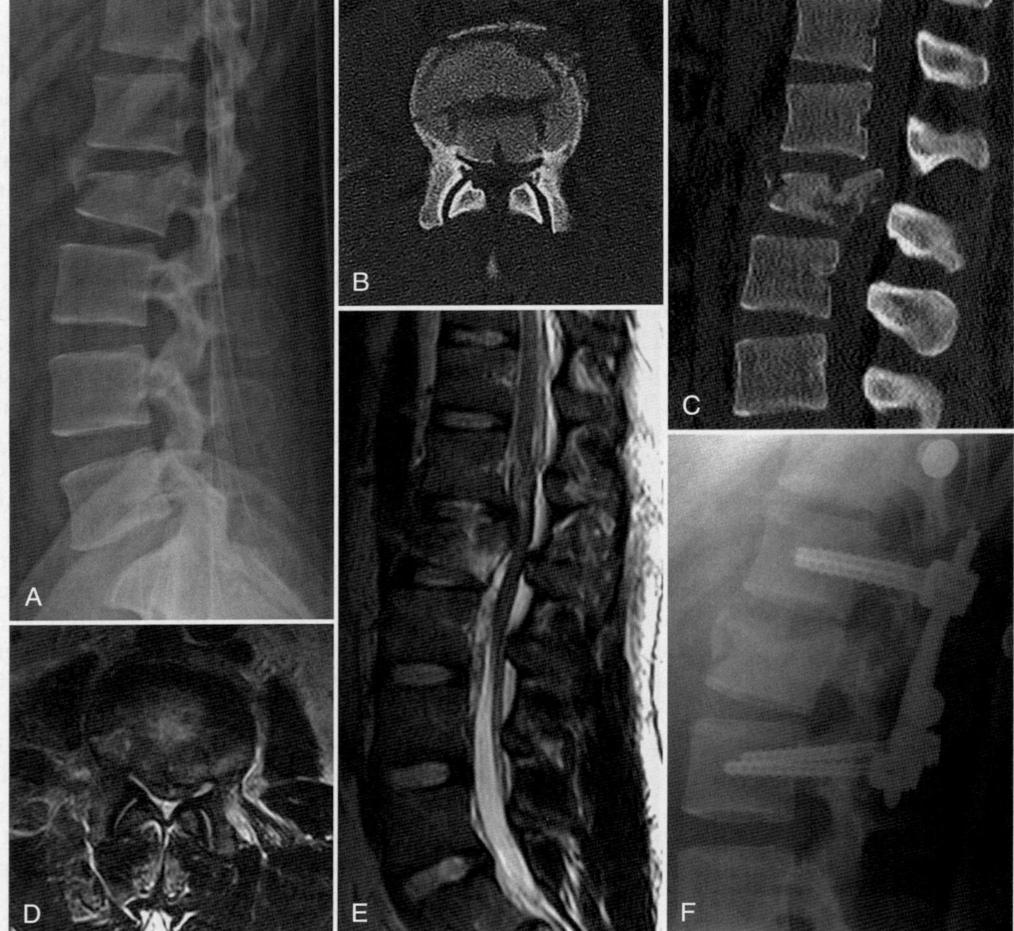

FIG. 77.16 Burst fracture treated surgically. (A) Lateral radiograph. (B) Axial computed tomography (CT) image showing canal compromise of approximately 75%. The patient was neurologically intact. (C) Sagittal CT image. (D) Axial and (E) sagittal T2-weighted magnetic resonance images showing compression of the neural elements. (F) Lateral postoperative radiograph showing short-segment pedicle screw instrumentation.

individual patient factors and overall sagittal alignment in deciding on operative versus nonoperative management with or without bracing, rather than relying on strict radiographic criteria to make the decision.

Burst fractures with a neurologic deficit are defined as unstable because of the neurologic injury, regardless of the extent of deformity or the integrity of the posterior elements, and are best treated surgically. This gives the best chance of neurologic recovery and prevents neurologic deterioration in incomplete injuries by stabilizing the fracture, as well as allowing early mobilization of the patient with paralysis. Exceptions can be made for mild isolated nerve root injuries in an otherwise mechanically stable fracture pattern, with a high rate of neurologic recovery under these circumstances.[181] The dorsally displaced fragments from the vertebral body usually cause the neural element injury, typically necessitating direct decompression. Laminectomy alone is contraindicated because it tends to be destabilizing and does not effectively decompress the neural elements.[22,164] Direct decompression is most reliably accomplished via an anterior approach, but it can also be performed via a posterior transpedicular approach.[94,182–185]

Burst fractures with PLC disruption are mechanically unstable, thus are best treated with surgery. Posterior pedicle screw instrumentation, either open with fusion or percutaneously without fusion, restores the posterior ligament tension-band effect and is the treatment of choice in neurologically intact patients (Fig. 77.16).[186,187]

In cases with a highly comminuted vertebral body and/or loss of greater than 50% of the vertebral body height, consideration may be given to performing anterior surgery to restore the integrity of the anterior column (Fig.77.17).

Exceptions to surgical management of burst fractures with posterior column injury should be made when the posterior injury consists of isolated sagittal lamina fractures, minimally displaced facet or spinous process fractures, and minimal facet opening. Under these circumstances, the PLC may retain its integrity; these injuries are therefore potentially stable. Consideration should be given to nonoperative treatment. True disruption of the PLC means that the tension-band stabilizing effect of the posterior elements is lost, as may occur with facet subluxation, dislocation, and fracture-dislocation. This leads to progressive instability; surgery is therefore indicated for

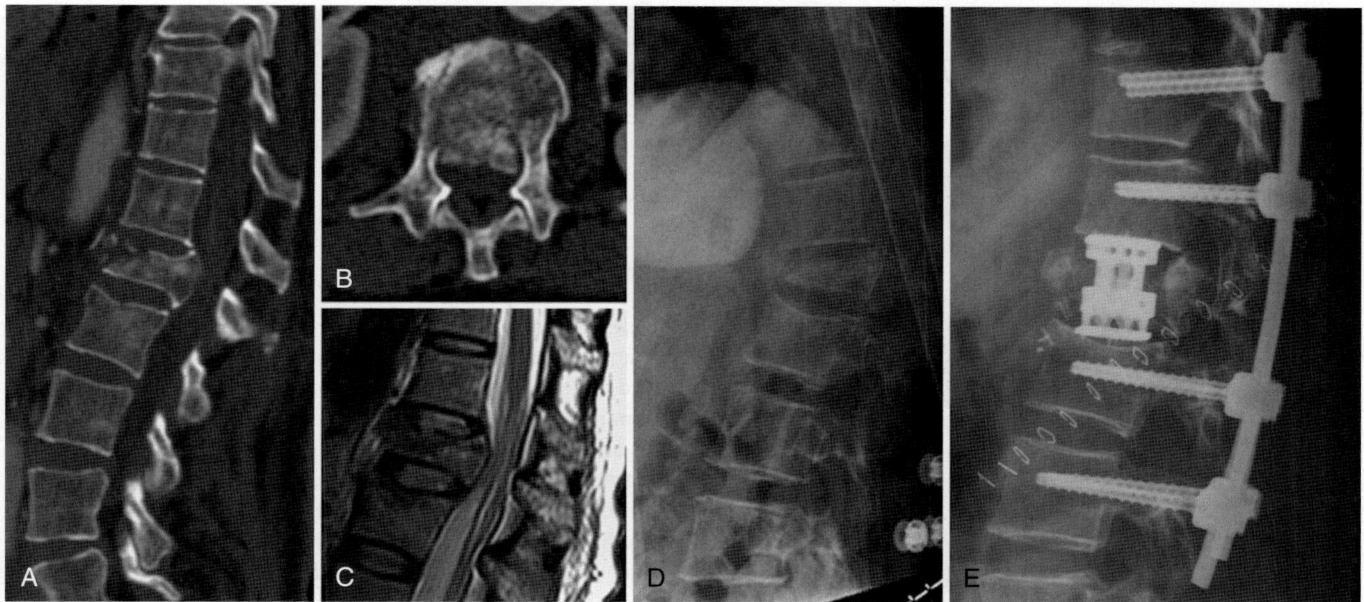

FIG. 77.17 Burst fracture treated surgically, with a staged anteroposterior procedure. It was believed that the degree of vertebral body height loss and angular kyphosis was best treated with restoration of the anterior column followed by posterior pedicle screw instrumentation. (A–D) Injury films. (A) Sagittal computed tomography. (B) Axial computed tomography. (C) Sagittal T2-weighted magnetic resonance image. (D) Lateral radiograph. (E) Postoperative radiograph.

stabilization purposes. In those fractures with posterior element injury, the difficulty lies in discerning the extent and significance of this component of the injury and its implications on stability. When the significance of a posterior element injury is borderline, it is usually safe to carefully mobilize a neurologically intact patient in a brace and closely assess for progressive instability with serial upright radiographs.

Long-term outcomes are mainly related to the extent of neurologic injury. For patients who are neurologically intact, the prognosis is generally favorable.[188–192] Rates of residual pain and disability as well as the ability to return to vigorous work are similar in surgically and nonsurgically treated patients. There are few prospective randomized studies on these rates, however, which show conflicting results.[188,190] If a kyphotic deformity reduction is performed surgically or with bracing, some loss of correction can be expected on long-term follow-up.[191,192] Radiographic parameters—including residual kyphosis, vertebral body height loss, and canal compromise—have not been definitively shown to be associated with long-term outcomes (Fig. 77.18).[177,178,188,190,192]

Of these three measurements, kyphosis greater than 30 degrees is the least desirable and is probably most commonly believed to be a predictor of long-term back pain.[1]

Flexion-Distraction Injuries (Chance Fractures and Chance Variants)

The incidence of neurologic deficit in flexion-distraction injuries is relatively low, perhaps 10% to 15%.[193,194] The injury classically occurs with lap-belt car restraints and is associated with a high incidence of intraabdominal injury.[195] The deforming forces occur in the sagittal plane, with displacement manifesting as focal kyphosis due to gapping of the posterior elements. Injuries through bone may be acutely unstable, but tend to heal reliably via primary osteosynthesis. Injuries through the PLC do not heal as well and carry a more guarded prognosis. Brace treatment therefore is more likely to be successful in stable bony injuries. Minimally angulated bony injuries may be treated in a brace. Minimally angulated ligamentous injuries may also be considered for brace treatment, but need to be followed closely to make sure healing occurs. Ligamentous injuries are more likely to require surgery than a purely osseous injury. Caution should be used when declaring these injures minimally angulated because the kyphotic deformity may reduce with gravity when the patient is imaged in the typical supine position. Swelling and tenderness over the spinous processes is potentially indicative of such a situation. MRI will show the extent of posterior injury in questionable cases. Unstable injuries of both the bony and ligamentous types are best treated surgically. The main difficulty with this type of injury is determining stability. Although a minimally angulated fracture may be obviously stable, and a large focal kyphotic deformity may be obviously unstable, it is the cases that fall between these extremes that pose a dilemma. LeGay et al.'s series of 18 patients showed an association of initial kyphotic deformity greater than 17 degrees with a poor prognosis.[195] Glassman et al.'s series of 12 cases in children showed that brace treatment failed when the initial kyphotic deformity was greater than 20 degrees.[196] These numbers are consistent with biomechanical studies that show substantial structural injury, with potential instability occurring somewhere between 12 and 17 degrees of traumatic focal kyphosis, and definite instability beyond 19 to 22 degrees of focal kyphosis.[197–200] These numbers are helpful in guiding treatment in borderline

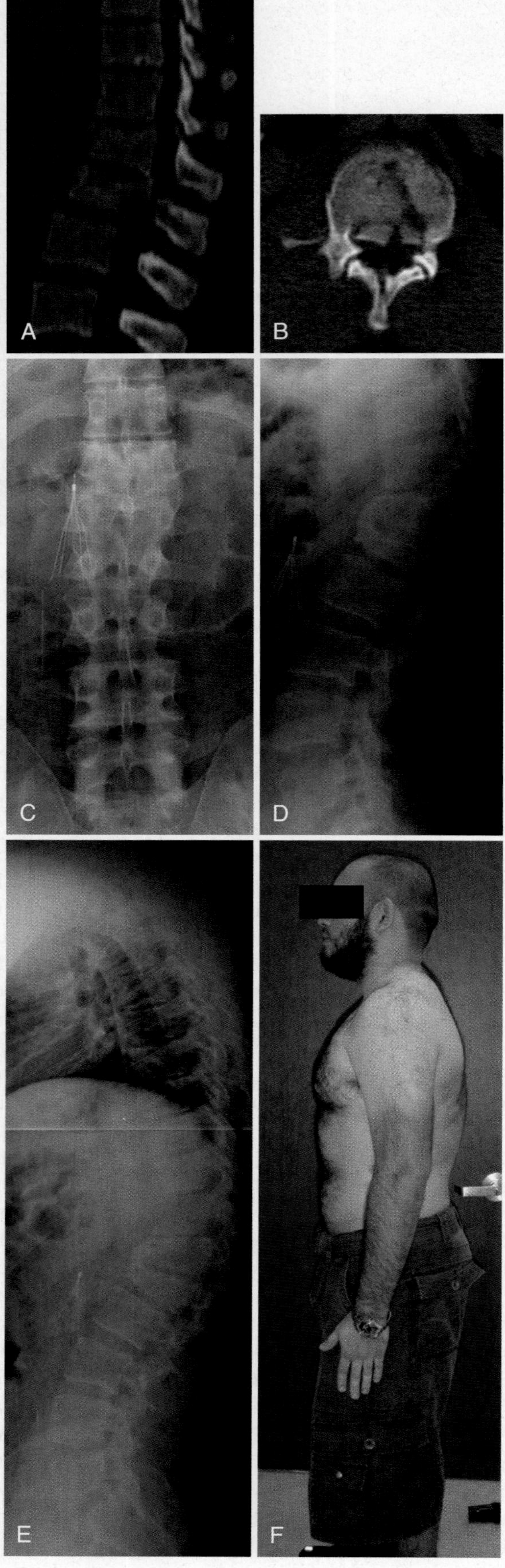

FIG. 77.18 This burst fracture was treated with bed rest and bracing because the patient was unable to undergo surgery. (A) Injury sagittal computed tomography image. (B) Axial computed tomography image. (C–E) Radiographs almost 2 years after the injury. The fractures have healed, and there is spontaneous fusion across T12–L1 anteriorly. (F) Though there is residual kyphosis of greater than 30 degrees on the lateral radiograph, the patient's clinical appearance is normal. He has no back pain and has returned to full activities.

cases. It is also reasonable under borderline circumstances to brace and cautiously mobilize the neurologically intact patient and obtain serial radiographs to see if instability becomes apparent.

Surgery typically consists of posterior pedicle screw instrumentation and fusion across the injured level (Fig. 77.19). This serves as a tension band and effectively counteracts the distractive forces across the posterior elements. Instrumentation may cross two or three levels depending on the anatomy of the injury. Consideration may be given to performing percutaneous pedicle screw instrumentation without fusion in a primarily bony injury, allowing the fractures to heal, then removing the instrumentation 6 to 9 months after injury. It should be noted, however, that this technique has not been proven. Whatever technique is chosen, the goal is to achieve anatomic reduction and stabilization, which under most circumstances is readily achieved because this injury occurs as a result of tensile forces, thus tends to be less destructive than those injuries that occur secondary to compressive forces. Careful intraoperative patient positioning on a standard spine frame with support under the hips and chest usually results in excellent reduction of the injury, and the native anatomy is restored. Long-term prognosis therefore tends to be favorable in neurologically intact patients.[195,196,201,202]

Fracture-Dislocations

Fracture-dislocations are highly unstable injuries and result in neurologic injury in 75% or more of patients.[1,54] There is no role for bracing. Surgical treatment should proceed as soon as possible. If surgery must be delayed, the patient should be carefully transferred to a rotating bed. Awake positioning is usually well tolerated with proper patient coaching before surgery and may be considered in patients with a normal neurologic examination or incomplete neurologic injury. This allows the patient to maintain muscle tone and self-protect against further spinal subluxation. It also allows for real-time monitoring of neurologic status. Posterior pedicle screw instrumentation and fusion can usually be limited to two levels above and below the injury, though longer constructs may be required (Fig. 77.20).

Anterior procedures are usually not necessary. Prognosis depends primarily on neurologic status.

Extension and Extension-Distraction Injuries

Extension injuries are rare, thus it is difficult to comment on the incidence of neurologic deficit, but it is high, perhaps

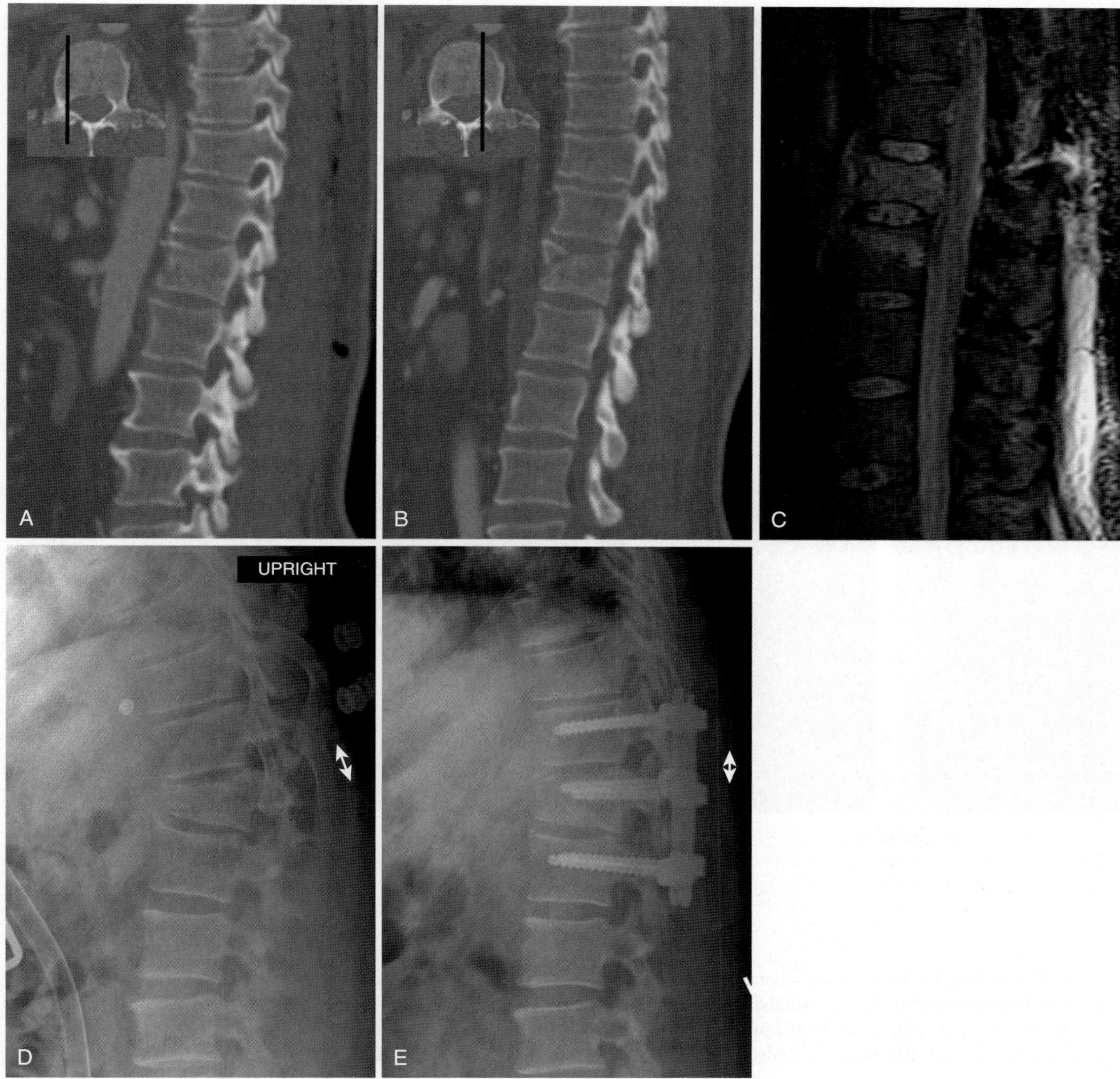

FIG. 77.19 Flexion-distraction injury (Chance fracture). (A–B) Computed tomography images showing the vertebral body compression fracture component of the injury. (A) A subtle minimally displaced fracture through the pedicle is seen. (B) A possible subtle nondisplaced pars fracture can be appreciated. (C) Sagittal T2-weighted magnetic resonance imaging shows disruption of the posterior ligamentous complex. Because the injury films showed normal spinal alignment, bracing was attempted. (D) Subsequent upright radiograph shows loss of vertebral body height, distraction posteriorly (*arrow*), and focal kyphosis. (E) Alignment was restored with posterior pedicle screw instrumentation, and the posterior element distraction is reduced, as shown by the arrow.

75%.[73,160] These injuries tend to be unstable, especially in the AS and DISH populations, but also when there is posterior element disruption in an otherwise normal spine. Brace treatment may be considered when the injury is minimally displaced in an otherwise normal spine, but this injury pattern is unusual. Otherwise, surgery is indicated. The spine should be assumed to be highly unstable and consideration given to awake positioning. In the ankylosed spine, multiple points of fixation are necessary because of poor bone quality, usually three levels above and below the injury. Percutaneous pedicle screw instrumentation is ideal because the spine is immobile and fusion is not necessary (see Fig. 77.11), but may be

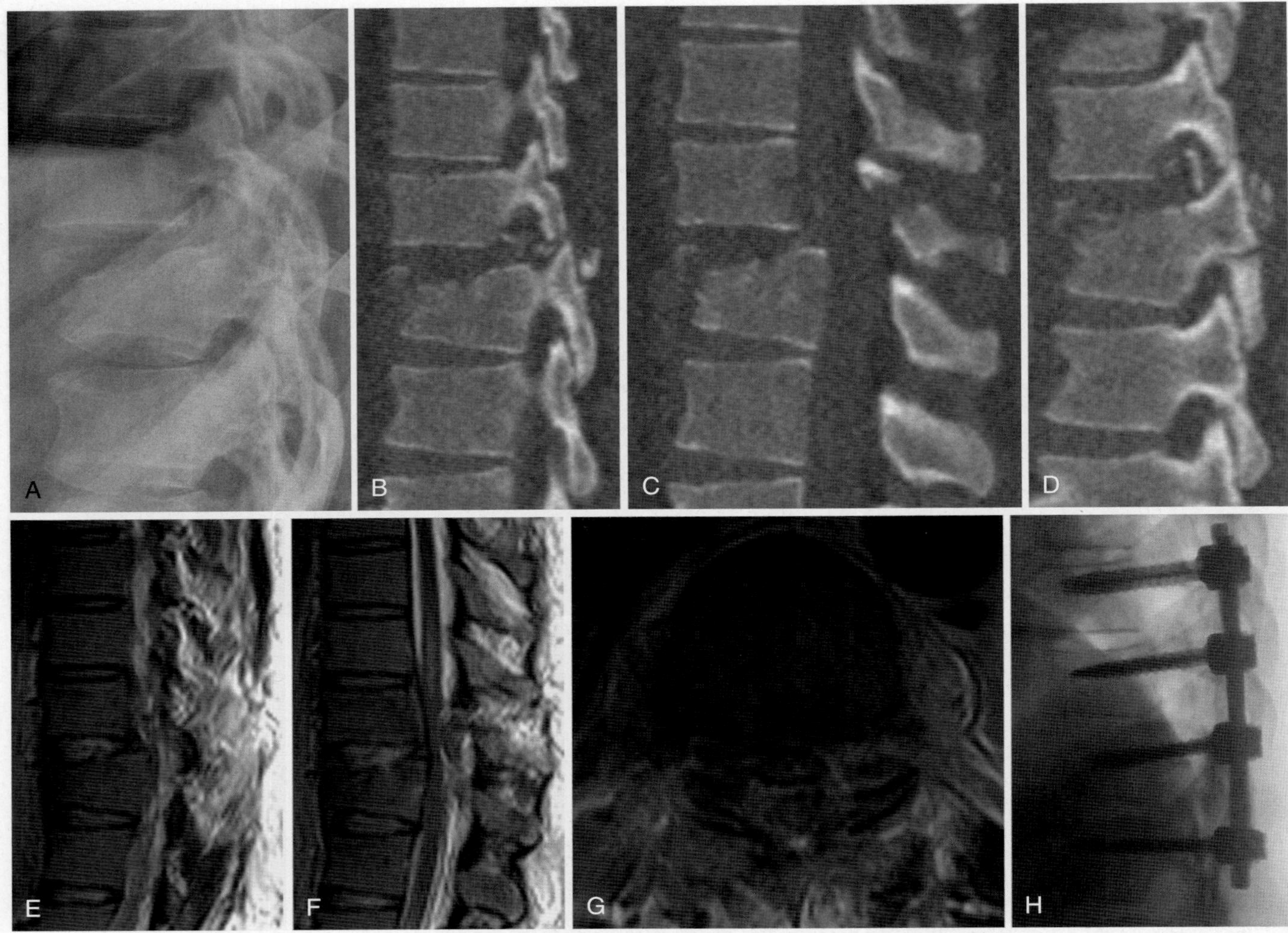

FIG. 77.20 Fracture-dislocation. (A) Lateral radiograph showing listhesis and facet dislocation, better demonstrated by the (B–D) sagittal computed tomography images. (E–F) Sagittal T2-weighted magnetic resonance images. (G) Axial T2-weighted magnetic resonance image. (H) The dislocation was reduced intraoperatively, and a posterior instrumented fusion was performed.

technically challenging for a variety of reasons, including the degree of kyphosis and difficulty visualizing the pedicles on fluoroscopy. Healing reliably occurs via primary osteosynthesis. Prognosis depends primarily on neurologic status.

Penetrating Injuries: Gunshot Wounds

Penetrating injuries are usually secondary to gunshot wounds and are rarely mechanically unstable, even in the setting of a neurologic deficit. Neurologic injury is common, with gunshot wounds being the third leading cause of spinal cord injury after motor vehicle accidents and falls.[203] Injuries involving a single spinal column do not require bracing, but those involving two or three columns should be braced for 6 to 12 weeks. Instability is seen in those rare cases with significant comminution of the vertebral body with extension of the injury through the posterior elements. This is the rare type of gunshot wound to the spine that may require surgical stabilization. Low-velocity (handgun) wounds are the most common type of injury in the civilian population; local wound care in this population can usually be performed in the emergency department. High-velocity (rifle) gunshot wounds are less common in the civilian population, for which debridement should be performed in the operating room.

Surgery may be indicated to remove a bullet from the spinal canal if it is causing compression of the neural elements and there is a neurologic deficit. Below the level of the conus, significant motor improvement may be seen, although this does not seem to be the case above T12.[204] With a stable neurologic deficit, surgery should be performed at 7 to 10 days after injury to allow the dura and surrounding soft tissues to heal, thus simplifying the operation.[205] Cerebrospinal fluid cutaneous fistulas occur 6% of the time after laminectomy to remove the bullet, but delaying surgery 7 to 10 days after injury may decrease the incidence.[205] With a progressive neurologic deficit, surgery should be performed as soon as it is safe to proceed. Instrumentation is usually not required unless instability is created during decompression to remove the bullet. Surgery may also be considered to remove a bullet from the disc space if mechanical symptoms occur and to avoid potential lead poisoning. Lead toxicity may result from a bullet bathed in synovial fluid, which may also be true with a bullet in the disc space.[206]

Spine infections following gunshot wounds are well recognized, most commonly following injury to a hollow viscus, such as the colon. For gunshots not involving visceral injury, prophylactic parenteral antibiotics should be administered for 72 hours, with a low incidence of subsequent spine infection. For gunshots involving contaminated visceral injury, broad-spectrum parenteral antibiotics should be administered for 7 to 10 days, although a shorter course may be adequate.[207] Infection rates may range from 5% to 10% with these regimens.[205,207,208]

It is common for patients with spinal cord injuries secondary to a gunshot wound to experience local and referred pain radiating into the paralyzed extremities. Surgical decompression does not seem to help.[204,206] Pain usually slowly resolves with time; medications such as nonsteroidal antiinflammatory drugs, amitriptyline, carbamazepine, gabapentin, or pregabalin may be of benefit.

Summary

Treatment of thoracic and lumbar spine injuries should be guided by an understanding of spinal anatomy, the biomechanics of spinal stability, neurologic status, and overall medical condition of the patient, including other injuries. The goal is to achieve neural element decompression in the case of a neurologic deficit, maintain or restore spinal stability and alignment, and mobilize the patient expeditiously while minimizing the risk of complications. The majority of thoracic and lumbar injuries in the neurologically intact patient can be managed nonoperatively with bracing. The most common exception to this is the unstable Chance fracture, which has a low incidence of neurologic injury but is often mechanically unstable. Most injuries with an associated neurologic deficit are best treated surgically. Unstable spine fractures, with or without neurologic deficit, are usually best treated surgically. The management of certain injuries continues to be controversial, especially burst fractures of moderate severity in the neurologically intact patient. It is difficult to determine the degree of instability with these fractures; consequently, they may be treated operatively in one surgeon's hands and nonoperatively in another's. Across all thoracic and lumbar spine injury types, the greatest difficulty in decision making occurs in neurologically intact patients with radiographic parameters that fall in the transition zone between what are classically considered to be stable and unstable injuries. It is uncertain what is the best approach in these cases; multiple factors must be considered in determining the most appropriate course of action.

PEARLS

1. Thoracic and lumbar burst fractures without significant posterior column disruption can usually be treated nonoperatively with bracing and early mobilization in neurologically intact patients. Significant posterior column disruption may be directly diagnosed with bilateral facet joint widening and should be suspected when there is focal kyphosis of greater than 30 degrees, 50% loss of vertebral body height, or interspinous process widening.
2. Traditional radiographic indicators of spinal instability are not strongly supported by the literature. Consideration may be given to treatment with a brace on a case-by-case basis in the neurologically intact patient with radiographic measurements in excess of 50% canal compromise and/or 50% vertebral body height loss.
3. Surgical decompression and stabilization are usually indicated in thoracic and lumbar spine injuries associated with a neurologic deficit attributable to the injured level.
4. Percutaneous pedicle screw stabilization is promising (but unproven) in the treatment of thoracic and lumbar spine fractures, especially in cases of ankylosing spondylitis and Chance fractures because healing of these injuries occurs by direct osseous union.
5. Intravenous methylprednisolone is an option, but not a guideline, in cases of blunt spinal cord injury and may be dosed in accordance with the NASCIS protocol. There are risks associated with administration of high-dose steroids, which must be balanced with the potential benefits on a case-by-case basis.

PITFALLS

1. Spine injuries are noncontiguous in 5% or more of cases; radiographic investigations should therefore usually include the entire spine once a significant spine injury is diagnosed.
2. Spine injuries are often missed on initial examination, especially noncontiguous injuries in patients with multiple injuries.
3. Short-segment pedicle screw fixation is effective in some cases and has the benefit of sparing fusion levels. The literature is mixed, with relatively high rates of failure reported in some series. These constructs should be used with caution, especially when there is loss of anterior or middle column support.
4. Contemporary techniques, such as percutaneous pedicle screw stabilization, have an increasingly important role in the treatment of thoracolumbar fractures associated with spinal ankylosis for which arthrodesis is arguably not necessary. However, their role in stabilization of thoracolumbar fractures in a nonankylosed spine is still evolving.
5. Neurologic injury in burst fractures is typically caused by anterior neural element compression from the retropulsed vertebral body. In these cases, laminectomy alone as a decompressive procedure is not effective and may further destabilize the spine. The offending vertebral body fragment must be directly addressed, which may be done reliably from an anterior or lateral approach, or in some cases via a posterior approach.
6. In patients with neurologic injury, an accurate assessment of neurologic status can only be made after the patient has recovered from spinal shock. This almost always occurs within 48 hours of injury.

KEY POINTS

1. The most controversy in the management of thoracic and lumbar spine injuries involves surgical versus nonsurgical treatment of burst fractures.
2. Thoracic and lumbar spine burst fractures in neurologically intact patients can usually be treated nonoperatively with bracing.

3. Surgery is usually appropriate in patients with neurologic injury and/or significant spinal instability.
4. The goal of surgery is to achieve neural element decompression in the case of a neurologic deficit, restore spinal stability and alignment, and allow for patient mobilization while minimizing the risk of complications.
5. The entire spine should be imaged when a spine fracture is detected, especially when a neurologic deficit is present, because noncontiguous spine injuries occur up to 5% of the time.

KEY REFERENCES

1. Bohlman HH, Kirkpatrick JS, Delamarter RB. Anterior decompression for late pain and paralysis after fractures of the thoracolumbar spine. *Clin Orthop Relat Res*. 1994;300:24-29.
This study demonstrated the benefit of late decompression in thoracolumbar fractures with persistent neural element compression. Forty-five patients underwent anterior decompression for chronic pain or paralysis at an average of 4.5 years after injury. Pain was improved in 41 of 45 patients. Twenty-one of 25 patients with neurologic deficit showed improvement.
2. Cantor JB, Lebwohl NH, Garvey T, Eismont FJ. Nonoperative management of stable thoracolumbar burst fractures with early ambulation and bracing. *Spine*. 1993;19:1731-1740.
Eighteen neurologically intact patients with burst fractures at the thoracolumbar junction were treated with bracing and early mobilization. This treatment was effective, and there were no cases of neurologic deterioration. CT scans obtained on eight patients after the fractures had healed demonstrated spontaneous resorption of much of the retropulsed bone.
3. Denis F. The three-column spine and its significance in the classification of acute thoracolumbar spinal injuries. *Spine*. 1983;8:817-831.
This sentinel work is commonly quoted to describe the basic biomechanics of thoracolumbar fracture stability. Denis broke from the traditional two-column theory of spine stability by introducing the concept of the middle column on the basis of a retrospective review of 412 thoracolumbar injuries.
4. Bracken MB, Shepard MJ, Collins WF, et al. A randomized, controlled trial of methylprednisolone or naloxone in the treatment of acute spinal-cord injury. Results of the Second National Acute Spinal Cord Injury Study. *N Engl J Med*. 1990;322(20):1405-1411.
The NASCIS II trial was a multicenter, randomized, double-blind, placebo-controlled trial in patients with spinal cord injuries. Methylprednisolone was administered as a bolus of 30 mg/kg, followed by infusion at 5.4 mg/kg per hour for 23 hours. Patients treated with methylprednisolone within 8 hours of injury had a small but significant improvement compared with placebo in motor and sensory recovery. This study led to the adoption of the high-dose methylprednisolone protocol in many countries. However, many spine surgeons feel the potential risks of steroid administration outweigh the potential benefits, and the use of steroids in spinal cord injury remains controversial.
5. Wood K, Buttermann G, Mehbod A, et al. Operative compared with nonoperative treatment of a thoracolumbar burst fracture without neurological deficit. A prospective, randomized study. *J Bone Joint Surg Am*. 2003;85-A(5):773-781.
Forty-seven neurologically intact patients with stable burst fractures (intact posterior ligamentous complex) were randomized to operative treatment with posterior instrumentation or nonoperative treatment with casting or bracing. There was no benefit demonstrated from surgery. The degree of canal compromise ranged as high as 75% and improved at long-term follow-up in both operative and nonoperative cases via canal remodeling.

REFERENCES

1. Gertzbein SD. Scoliosis Research Society. Multicenter spine fracture study. *Spine*. 1992;17:528-540.
2. Riggins RS, Kraus JF. The risk of neurologic damage with fractures of the vertebrae. *J Trauma*. 1977;17:126-133.
3. Calenoff L, Chessare JW, Rogers LF, et al. Multiple level spinal injuries: importance of early recognition. *AJR Am J Roentgenol*. 1978;130:665-669.
4. Stagnara P, De Mauroy JC, Dran G, et al. Reciprocal angulation of vertebral bodies in a sagittal plane: approach to references for the evaluation of kyphosis and lordosis. *Spine*. 1982;7:335-342.
5. White AA 3rd, Panjabi MM. The basic kinematics of the human spine. A review of past and current knowledge. *Spine*. 1978;3:12-20.
6. Vialle R, Levassor N, Rillardon L, et al. Radiographic analysis of the sagittal alignment and balance of the spine in asymptomatic subjects. *J Bone Joint Surg Am*. 2005;87:260-267.
7. Panjabi MM, Brand RA Jr, White AA 3rd. Three-dimensional flexibility and stiffness properties of the human thoracic spine. *J Biomech*. 1976;9:185-192.
8. Roussouly P, Gollogly S, Noseda O, et al. The vertical projection of the sum of the ground reactive forces of a standing patient is not the same as the C7 plumb line: a radiographic study of the sagittal alignment of 153 asymptomatic volunteers. *Spine*. 2006;31:E320-E325.
9. Roussouly P, Gollogly S, Berthonnaud E, Dimnet J. Classification of the normal variation in the sagittal alignment of the human lumbar spine and pelvis in the standing position. *Spine*. 2005;30:346-353.
10. Kuntz C 4th, Levin LS, Ondra SL, et al. Neutral upright sagittal spinal alignment from the occiput to the pelvis in asymptomatic adults: a review and resynthesis of the literature. *J Neurosurg Spine*. 2007;6:104-112.
11. Saboe LA, Reid DC, Davis LA, et al. Spine trauma and associated injuries. *J Trauma*. 1991;31:43-48.
12. Henderson RL, Reid DC, Saboe LA. Multiple noncontiguous spine fractures. *Spine*. 1991;16:128-131.
13. Reid DC, Henderson R, Saboe L, Miller JD. Etiology and clinical course of missed spine fractures. *J Trauma*. 1987;27:980-986.
14. Bohlman HH. Acute fractures and dislocations of the cervical spine. An analysis of three hundred hospitalized patients and review of the literature. *J Bone Joint Surg Am*. 1979;61:1119-1142.
15. Anderson S, Biros MH, Reardon RF. Delayed diagnosis of thoracolumbar fractures in multiple-trauma patients. *Acad Emerg Med*. 1996;3:832-839.
16. Bracken MB, Shepard MJ, Collins WF, et al. A randomized, controlled trial of methylprednisolone or naloxone in the treatment of acute spinal-cord injury. Results of the Second National Acute Spinal Cord Injury Study. *N Engl J Med*. 1990;322:1405-1411.
17. Bracken MB, Shepard MJ, Holford TR, et al. Administration of methylprednisolone for 24 or 48 hours or tirilazad mesylate for 48 hours in the treatment of acute spinal cord injury. Results of the Third National Acute Spinal Cord Injury Randomized Controlled Trial. National Acute Spinal Cord Injury Study. *JAMA*. 1997;277:1597-1604.

18. Bracken MB, Shepard MJ, Holford TR, et al. Methylprednisolone or tirilazad mesylate administration after acute spinal cord injury: 1-year follow up. Results of the third National Acute Spinal Cord Injury randomized controlled trial. *J Neurosurg*. 1998;89:699-706.
19. Geisler FH, Coleman WP, Grieco G, et al. The Sygen multicenter acute spinal cord injury study. *Spine*. 2001;26(24 suppl):S87-S98.
20. Pharmacological therapy after acute cervical spinal cord injury. *Neurosurgery*. 2002;50(suppl):S63-S71.
21. Levi AD, Green BA, Wang MY, et al. Clinical application of modest hypothermia after spinal cord injury. *J Neurotrauma*. 2009;26:407-415.
22. Bohlman HH, Freehafer A, Dejak J. The results of treatment of acute injuries of the upper thoracic spine with paralysis. *J Bone Joint Surg Am*. 1985;67:360-369.
23. Kingwell SP, Curt A, Dvorak MF. Factors affecting neurological outcome in traumatic conus medullaris and cauda equina injuries. *Neurosurg Focus*. 2008;25:E7.
24. Harrop JS, Hunt GE Jr, Vaccaro AR. Conus medullaris and cauda equina syndrome as a result of traumatic injuries: management principles. *Neurosurg Focus*. 2004; 16:E4.
25. Harris JH Jr. Radiographic evaluation of spinal trauma. *Orthop Clin North Am*. 1986;17:75-86.
26. McGrory BJ, VanderWilde RS, Currier BL, Eismont FJ. Diagnosis of subtle thoracolumbar burst fractures. A new radiographic sign. *Spine*. 1993;18:2282-2285.
27. Atlas SW, Regenbogen V, Rogers LF, Kim KS. The radiographic characterization of burst fractures of the spine. *AJR Am J Roentgenol*. 1986;147:575-582.
28. Berry GE, Adams S, Harris MB, et al. Are plain radiographs of the spine necessary during evaluation after blunt trauma? Accuracy of screening torso computed tomography in thoracic/lumbar spine fracture diagnosis. *J Trauma*. 2005;59:1410-1413.
29. Epstein O, Ludwig S, Gelb D, et al. Comparison of computed tomography and plain radiography in assessing traumatic spinal deformity. *J Spinal Disord Tech*. 2009;22:197-201.
30. Diaz JJ Jr, Cullinane DC, Altman DT, et al. Practice management guidelines for the screening of thoracolumbar spine fracture. *J Trauma*. 2007;63:709-718.
31. Hauser CJ, Visvikis G, Hinrichs C, et al. Prospective validation of computed tomographic screening of the thoracolumbar spine in trauma. *J Trauma*. 2003;55:228-234.
32. Sheridan R, Peralta R, Rhea J, et al. Reformatted visceral protocol helical computed tomographic scanning allows conventional radiographs of the thoracic and lumbar spine to be eliminated in the evaluation of blunt trauma patients. *J Trauma*. 2003;55:665-669.
33. Inaba K, Munera F, McKenney M, et al. Visceral torso computed tomography for clearance of the thoracolumbar spine in trauma: a review of the literature. *J Trauma*. 2006;60:915-920.
34. Campbell SE, Phillips CD, Dubovsky E, et al. The value of CT in determining potential instability of simple wedge-compression fractures of the lumbar spine. *AJNR Am J Neuroradiol*. 1995;16:1385-1392.
35. Bagley LJ. Imaging of spinal trauma. *Radiol Clin North Am*. 2006;44:1-12.
36. Ballock RT, Mackersie R, Abitbol JJ, et al. Can burst fractures be predicted from plain radiographs? *J Bone Joint Surg Br*. 1992;74:147-150.
37. Lammertse D, Dungan D, Dreisbach J, et al. Neuroimaging in traumatic spinal cord injury: an evidence-based review for clinical practice and research. *J Spinal Cord Med*. 2007;30:205-214.
38. Flanders AE, Spettell CM, Tartaglino LM, et al. Forecasting motor recovery after cervical spinal cord injury: value of MR imaging. *Radiology*. 1996;201:649-655.
39. Miyanji F, Furlan JC, Aarabi B, et al. Acute cervical traumatic spinal cord injury: MR imaging findings correlated with neurologic outcome - prospective study with 100 consecutive patients. *Radiology*. 2007;243:820-827.
40. Flanders AE, Spettell CM, Friedman DP, et al. The relationship between the functional abilities of patients with cervical spinal cord injury and the severity of damage revealed by MR imaging. *AJNR Am J Neuroradiol*. 1999;20:926-934.
41. Oner FC, van Gils AP, Dhert WJ, Verbout AJ. MRI findings of thoracolumbar spine fractures: a categorisation based on MRI examinations of 100 fractures. *Skeletal Radiol*. 1999;28:433-443.
42. Lee HM, Kim HS, Kim DJ, et al. Reliability of magnetic resonance imaging in detecting posterior ligament complex injury in thoracolumbar spinal fractures. *Spine*. 2000;25:2079-2084.
43. Lee JY, Vaccaro AR, Schweitzer KM Jr, et al. Assessment of injury to the thoracolumbar posterior ligamentous complex in the setting of normal-appearing plain radiography. *Spine J*. 2007;7:422-427.
44. Vaccaro AR, Lee JY, Schweitzer KM Jr, et al. Assessment of injury to the posterior ligamentous complex in thoracolumbar spine trauma. *Spine J*. 2006;6:524-528.
45. White AA, Panjabi MM. *Clinical Biomechanics of the Spine*. Philadelphia: JB Lippincott; 1978.
46. Bohler L. *The Treatment of Fractures*. 4th ed. Baltimore: W. Wood; 1935.
47. Watson-Jones R. *Fractures and Joint Injuries*. 3rd ed. Edinburgh: E & S Livingstone; 1943.
48. Key JA, Conwell HE. *The Management of Fractures, Dislocations, and Sprains*. 4th ed. St Louis: CV Mosby & Co; 1946.
49. Nicoll EA. Fractures of the dorso-lumbar spine. *J Bone Joint Surg Am*. 1949;31:376-394.
50. Holdsworth F. Fractures, dislocations, and fracture-dislocations of the spine. *J Bone Joint Surg Am*. 1970;52:1534-1551.
51. Kelly RP, Whitesides TE Jr. Treatment of lumbodorsal fracture-dislocations. *Ann Surg*. 1968;167:705-717.
52. Bedbrook GM. Treatment of thoracolumbar dislocation and fractures with paraplegia. *Clin Orthop Relat Res*. 1975;(112):27-43.
53. Lucas JT, Ducker TB. Motor classification of spinal cord injuries with mobility, morbidity and recovery indices. *Am Surg*. 1979;45:151-158.
54. Denis F. The three column spine and its significance in the classification of acute thoracolumbar spinal injuries. *Spine*. 1983;8:817-831.
55. Denis F. Spinal instability as defined by the three-column spine concept in acute spinal trauma. *Clin Orthop Relat Res*. 1984;(189):65-76.
56. Panjabi MM, Oxland TR, Kifune M, et al. Validity of the three-column theory of thoracolumbar fractures. A biomechanic investigation. *Spine*. 1995;20: 1122-1127.

57. Chance GQ. Note on a type of flexion fracture of the spine. *Br J Radiol.* 1948;21:452.
58. McAfee PC, Yuan HA, Fredrickson BE, Lubicky JP. The value of computed tomography in thoracolumbar fractures. An analysis of one hundred consecutive cases and a new classification. *J Bone Joint Surg Am.* 1983;65:461-473.
59. Ferguson RL, Allen BL Jr. A mechanistic classification of thoracolumbar spine fractures. *Clin Orthop Relat Res.* 1984;189:77-88.
60. Ferguson RL, Allen BL Jr. An algorithm for the treatment of unstable thoracolumbar fractures. *Orthop Clin North Am.* 1986;17:105-112.
61. Gertzbein SD. Classification of thoracic and lumbar fractures. In: Gertzbein SD, ed. *Fractures of the Thoracic and Lumbar Spine.* Baltimore: Williams and Wilkins; 1992.
62. Magerl F, Aebi M, Gertzbein SD, et al. A comprehensive classification of thoracic and lumbar injuries. *Eur Spine J.* 1994;3:184-201.
63. Vaccaro AR, Lehman RA Jr, Hurlbert RJ, et al. A new classification of thoracolumbar injuries: the importance of injury morphology, the integrity of the posterior ligamentous complex, and neurologic status. *Spine.* 2005;30:2325-2333.
64. Patel AA, Dailey A, Brodke DS, et al. Thoracolumbar spine trauma classification: the Thoracolumbar Injury Classification and Severity Score system and case examples. *J Neurosurg Spine.* 2009;10:201-206.
65. Rihn JA, Anderson DT, Harris E, et al. A review of the TLICS system: a novel, user-friendly thoracolumbar trauma classification system. *Acta Orthop.* 2008;79:461-466.
66. Whang PG, Vaccaro AR, Poelstra KA, et al. The influence of fracture mechanism and morphology on the reliability and validity of two novel thoracolumbar injury classification systems. *Spine.* 2007;32:791-795.
67. Patel AA, Vaccaro AR, Albert TJ, et al. The adoption of a new classification system: time-dependent variation in interobserver reliability of the thoracolumbar injury severity score classification system. *Spine.* 2007;32:E105-E110.
68. Fast A, Sosner J, Begeman P, et al. Lumbar spinal strains associated with whiplash injury: a cadaveric study. *Am J Phys Med Rehabil.* 2002;81:645-650.
69. Costello RF, Beall DP. Nomenclature and standard reporting terminology of intervertebral disk herniation. *Magn Reson Imaging Clin N Am.* 2007;15:167-174.
70. Milette PC. Classification, diagnostic imaging, and imaging characterization of a lumbar herniated disk. *Radiol Clin North Am.* 2000;38:1267-1292.
71. Gellad FE, Levine AM, Joslyn JN, et al. Pure thoracolumbar facet dislocation: clinical features and CT appearance. *Radiology.* 1986;161:505-508.
72. O'Callaghan JP, Ullrich CG, Yuan HA, Kieffer SA. CT of facet distraction in flexion injuries of the thoracolumbar spine: the "naked" facet. *AJR Am J Roentgenol.* 1980;134:563-568.
73. Denis F, Burkus JK. Shear fracture-dislocations of the thoracic and lumbar spine associated with forceful hyperextension (lumberjack paraplegia). *Spine.* 1992;17:156-161.
74. Bono CM, Heary RF. Gunshot wounds to the spine. *Spine J.* 2004;4:230-240.
75. Moon E, Kondrashov D, Hannibal M, et al. Gunshot wounds to the spine: literature review and report on a migratory intrathecal bullet. *Am J Orthop.* 2008;37:E47-E51.
76. Finitsis SN, Falcone S, Green BA. MR of the spine in the presence of metallic bullet fragments: is the benefit worth the risk? *AJNR Am J Neuroradiol.* 1999;20:354-356.
77. Gjolaj JP, Eismont FJ. Gunshot injuries to the spine. *JBJS Rev.* 2015;3(11):e3.
78. Jacobs RR, Asher MA, Snider RK. Thoracolumbar spinal injuries. A comparative study of recumbent and operative treatment in 100 patients. *Spine.* 1980;5:463-477.
79. Frankel HL, Hancock DO, Hyslop G, et al. The value of postural reduction in the initial management of closed injuries of the spine with paraplegia and tetraplegia. *Paraplegia.* 1969;7:179-192.
80. Kallemeier PM, Beaubien BP, Buttermann GR, et al. In vitro analysis of anterior and posterior fixation in an experimental unstable burst fracture model. *J Spinal Disord Tech.* 2008;21:216-224.
81. Kaneda K, Abumi K, Fujiya M. Burst fractures with neurologic deficits of the thoracolumbar-lumbar spine. Results of anterior decompression and stabilization with anterior instrumentation. *Spine.* 1984;9:788-795.
82. An HS, Lim TH, You JW, et al. Biomechanical evaluation of anterior thoracolumbar spinal instrumentation. *Spine.* 1995;20:1979-1983.
83. Sasso RC, Renkens K, Hanson D, et al. Unstable thoracolumbar burst fractures: anterior-only versus short-segment posterior fixation. *J Spinal Disord Tech.* 2006;19:242-248.
84. Oskouian RJ Jr, Johnson JP. Vascular complications in anterior thoracolumbar spinal reconstruction. *J Neurosurg.* 2002;96 (1 suppl):1-5.
85. Fantini GA, Pappou IP, Girardi FP, et al. Major vascular injury during anterior lumbar spinal surgery: incidence, risk factors, and management. *Spine.* 2007;32:2751-2758.
86. Gurwitz GS, Dawson JM, McNamara MJ, et al. Biomechanical analysis of three surgical approaches for lumbar burst fractures using short-segment instrumentation. *Spine.* 1993;18:977-982.
87. Chakera TM, Bedbrook G, Bradley CM. Spontaneous resolution of spinal canal deformity after burst-dispersion fracture. *AJNR Am J Neuroradiol.* 1988;9:779-785.
88. Dai LY. Remodeling of the spinal canal after thoracolumbar burst fractures. *Clin Orthop Relat Res.* 2001;382:119-123.
89. de Klerk LW, Fontijne WP, Stijnen T, et al. Spontaneous remodeling of the spinal canal after conservative management of thoracolumbar burst fractures. *Spine.* 1998;23:1057-1060.
90. Sjöström L, Jacobsson O, Karlström G, et al. Spinal canal remodeling after stabilization of thoracolumbar burst fractures. *Eur Spine J.* 1994;3:312-317.
91. Crutcher JP Jr, Anderson PA, King HA, Montesano PX. Indirect spinal canal decompression in patients with thoracolumbar burst fractures treated by posterior distraction rods. *J Spinal Disord.* 1991;4:39-48.
92. Doerr TE, Montesano PX, Burkus JK, Benson DR. Spinal canal decompression in traumatic thoracolumbar burst fractures: posterior distraction rods versus transpedicular screw fixation. *J Orthop Trauma.* 1991;5:403-411.
93. Harrington RM, Budorick T, Hoyt J, et al. Biomechanics of indirect reduction of bone retropulsed into the spinal canal in vertebral fracture. *Spine.* 1993;18:692-699.
94. Edwards CC, Levine AM. Early rod-sleeve stabilization of the injured thoracic and lumbar spine. *Orthop Clin North Am.* 1986;17:121-145.
95. Garfin SR, Mowery CA, Guerra J Jr, Marshall LF. Confirmation of the posterolateral technique to decompress and fuse thoracolumbar spine burst fractures. *Spine.* 1985;10:218-223.

96. Sasso RC, Cotler HB. Posterior instrumentation and fusion for unstable fractures and fracture-dislocations of the thoracic and lumbar spine. A comparative study of three fixation devices in 70 patients. *Spine*. 1993;18:450-460.
97. Tasdemiroglu E, Tibbs PA. Long-term follow-up results of thoracolumbar fractures after posterior instrumentation. *Spine*. 1995;20:1704-1708.
98. de Peretti F, Hovorka I, Cambas PM, et al. Short device fixation and early mobilization for burst fractures of the thoracolumbar junction. *Eur Spine J*. 1996;5:112-120.
99. Chiba M, McLain RF, Yerby SA, et al. Short-segment pedicle instrumentation. Biomechanical analysis of supplemental hook fixation. *Spine*. 1996;21:288-294.
100. Farcy JP, Weidenbaum M, Glassman SD. Sagittal index in management of thoracolumbar burst fractures. *Spine*. 1990;15:958-965.
101. Kramer DL, Rodgers WB, Mansfield FL. Transpedicular instrumentation and short-segment fusion of thoracolumbar fractures: a prospective study using a single instrumentation system. *J Orthop Trauma*. 1995;9:499-506.
102. Tezeren G, Kuru I. Posterior fixation of thoracolumbar burst fracture: short-segment pedicle fixation versus long-segment instrumentation. *J Spinal Disord Tech*. 2005;18:485-488.
103. McLain RF, Burkus JK, Benson DR. Segmental instrumentation for thoracic and thoracolumbar fractures: prospective analysis of construct survival and five-year follow-up. *Spine J*. 2001;1:310-323.
104. Scholl BM, Theiss SM, Kirkpatrick JS. Short segment fixation of thoracolumbar burst fractures. *Orthopedics*. 2006;29:703-708.
105. Parker JW, Lane JR, Karaikovic EE, Gaines RW. Successful short-segment instrumentation and fusion for thoracolumbar spine fractures: a consecutive 4 1/2-year series. *Spine*. 2000;25:1157-1170.
106. Dai LY, Jiang LS, Jiang SD. Posterior short-segment fixation with or without fusion for thoracolumbar burst fractures. A five to seven-year prospective randomized study. *J Bone Joint Surg Am*. 2009;91:1033-1041.
107. McLain RF. The biomechanics of long versus short fixation for thoracolumbar spine fractures. *Spine*. 2006;31(11 suppl):S70-S79.
108. Norton RP, Milne EL, Kaimrajh DN, et al. Biomechanical analysis of four- versus six-screw constructs for short-segment pedicle screw and rod instrumentation of unstable thoracolumbar fractures. *Spine J*. 2014;14(8):1734-1739.
109. Mahar A, Kim C, Wedemeyer M, et al. Short-segment fixation of lumbar burst fractures using pedicle fixation at the level of the fracture. *Spine*. 2007;32:1503-1507.
110. Vaccaro AR, Daugherty RJ, Sheehan TP, et al. Neurologic outcome of early versus late surgery for cervical spinal cord injury. *Spine*. 1997;22:2609-2613.
111. Fehlings MG, Perrin RG. The role and timing of early decompression for cervical spinal cord injury: update with a review of recent clinical evidence. *Injury*. 2005;36(suppl 2):B13-B26.
112. La Rosa G, Conti A, Cardali S, et al. Does early decompression improve neurological outcome of spinal cord injured patients? Appraisal of the literature using a meta-analytical approach. *Spinal Cord*. 2004;42:503-512.
113. Cammisa FP Jr, Eismont FJ, Green BA. Dural laceration occurring with burst fractures and associated laminar fractures. *J Bone Joint Surg Am*. 1989;71:1044-1052.
114. Sanderson PL, et al. Short segment fixation of thoracolumbar burst fractures without fusion. *Eur Spine J*. 1999;8(6):495-500.
115. Wang ST, et al. Is fusion necessary for surgically treated burst fractures of the thoracolumbar and lumbar spine? A prospective, randomized study. *Spine*. 2006;31(23):2646-2652.
116. Yang H, et al. Outcome of thoracolumbar burst fractures treated with indirect reduction and fixation without fusion. *Eur Spine J*. 2011;20(3):380-386.
117. Tian NF, et al. Fusion versus nonfusion for surgically treated thoracolumbar burst fractures: a meta-analysis. *PLoS One*. 2013;8(5):e63995.
118. Broom MJ, Jacobs RR. Update-1988. Current status of internal fixation of thoracolumbar fractures. *J Orthop Trauma*. 1989;3(2):148-155.
119. Dekutoski MB, Conlan ES, Salciccioli GG. Spinal mobility and deformity after Harrington rod stabilization and limited arthrodesis of thoracolumbar fractures. *J Bone Joint Surg Am*. 1993;75(2):168-176.
120. Ko SB, et al. Result of posterior instrumentation without fusion in the management of thoracolumbar and lumbar unstable burst fracture. *J Spinal Disord Tech*. 2012;27(4):189-195.
121. Caron T, et al. Spine fractures in patients with ankylosing spinal disorders. *Spine*. 2010;35(11):E458-E464.
122. Westerveld LA, Verlaan JJ, Oner FC. Spinal fractures in patients with ankylosing spinal disorders: a systematic review of the literature on treatment, neurological status and complications. *Eur Spine J*. 2009;18(2):145-156.
123. Daniels AH, Sobel AD, Eberson CP. Pediatric thoracolumbar spine trauma. *J Am Acad Orthop Surg*. 2013;21(12):707-716.
124. Gardner VO, Armstrong GW. Long-term lumbar facet joint changes in spinal fracture patients treated with Harrington rods. *Spine*. 1990;15(6):479-484.
125. Kahanovitz N, et al. The effects of internal fixation on the articular cartilage of unfused canine facet joint cartilage. *Spine*. 1984;9(3):268-272.
126. Kahanovitz N, Bullough P, Jacobs RR. The effect of internal fixation without arthrodesis on human facet joint cartilage. *Clin Orthop Relat Res*. 1984;189:204-208.
127. Cappuccio M, Amendola L, Paderni S, et al. Complications in minimally invasive percutaneous fixation of thoracic and lumbar spine fractures. *Orthopedics*. 2013;36(6):e729-e734.
128. Giorgi H, Blondel B, Adetchessi T, et al. Early percutaneous fixation of spinal thoracolumbar fractures in polytrauma patients. *Orthop Traumatol Surg Res*. 2014;100(5):449-454.
129. Wang H, Zhou Y, Li C, Liu J, Xiang L. Comparison of open versus percutaneous pedicle screw fixation using the sextant system in the treatment of traumatic thoracolumbar fractures. *J Spinal Disord Tech*. 2014. Epub ahead of print.
130. Krüger A, Frink M, Oberkircher L, et al. Percutaneous dorsal instrumentation for thoracolumbar extension-distraction fractures in patients with ankylosing spinal disorders: a case series. *Spine J*. 2014;14(12):2897-2904.
131. Vanek P, Bradac O, Konopkova R, et al. Treatment of thoracolumbar trauma by short-segment percutaneous transpedicular screw instrumentation: prospective comparative study with a minimum 2-year follow-up. *J Neurosurg Spine*. 2014;20(2):150-156.
132. Medici A, Meccariello L, Falzarano G. Non-operative vs. percutaneous stabilization in Magerl's A1 or A2 thoracolumbar spine fracture in adults: is it really advantageous for a good alignment of the spine? Preliminary

data from a prospective study. *Eur Spine J*. 2014;23(suppl 6): 677-683.

133. Grossbach AJ, et al. Flexion-distraction injuries of the thoracolumbar spine: open fusion versus percutaneous pedicle screw fixation. *Neurosurg Focus*. 2013;35(2):E2.
134. Wang HW, et al. Percutaneous pedicle screw fixation through the pedicle of fractured vertebra in the treatment of type A thoracolumbar fractures using Sextant system: an analysis of 38 cases. *Chin J Traumatol*. 2010;13(3):137-145.
135. Wild MH, et al. Five-year follow-up examination after purely minimally invasive posterior stabilization of thoracolumbar fractures: a comparison of minimally invasive percutaneously and conventionally open treated patients. *Arch Orthop Trauma Surg*. 2007;127(5):335-343.
136. Palmisani M, et al. Minimally invasive percutaneous fixation in the treatment of thoracic and lumbar spine fractures. *Eur Spine J*. 2009;18(suppl 1):71-74.
137. Lee JK, et al. Percutaneous short-segment pedicle screw placement without fusion in the treatment of thoracolumbar burst fractures: is it effective? Comparative study with open short-segment pedicle screw fixation with posterolateral fusion. *Acta Neurochir (Wien)*. 2013;155(12):2305-2312.
138. Ni WF, et al. Percutaneous pedicle screw fixation for neurologic intact thoracolumbar burst fractures. *J Spinal Disord Tech*. 2010;23(8):530-537.
139. Heintel TM, Berglehner A, Meffert R. Accuracy of percutaneous pedicle screws for thoracic and lumbar spine fractures: a prospective trial. *Eur Spine J*. 2013;22(3):495-502.
140. Park DK, et al. Percutaneous lumbar and thoracic pedicle screws: a trauma experience. *J Spinal Disord Tech*. 2014;27(3):154-161.
141. Yang WE, et al. Percutaneous pedicle screw fixation for thoracolumbar burst fracture: a Singapore experience. *Singapore Med J*. 2012;53(9):577-581.
142. Bironneau A, et al. Percutaneous internal fixation combined with kyphoplasty for neurologically intact thoracolumbar fractures: a prospective cohort study of 24 patients with one year of follow-up. *Orthop Traumatol Surg Res*. 2011;97(4):389-395.
143. Blondel B, et al. Percutaneous management of thoracolumbar burst fractures: evolution of techniques and strategy. *Orthop Traumatol Surg Res*. 2011;97(5):527-532.
144. Fuentes S, et al. Percutaneous kyphoplasty and pedicle screw fixation for the management of thoraco-lumbar burst fractures. *Eur Spine J*. 2010;19(8):1281-1287.
145. Jung HJ, et al. Bone cement-augmented short segment fixation with percutaneous screws for thoracolumbar burst fractures accompanied by severe osteoporosis. *J Korean Neurosurg Soc*. 2012;52(4):353-358.
146. Korovessis P, Hadjipavlou A, Repantis T. Minimally invasive short posterior instrumentation plus balloon kyphoplasty with calcium phosphate for burst and severe compression lumbar fractures. *Spine*. 2008;33(6):658-667.
147. Marco RA, Kushwaha VP. Thoracolumbar burst fractures treated with posterior decompression and pedicle screw instrumentation supplemented with balloon-assisted vertebroplasty and calcium phosphate reconstruction. *J Bone Joint Surg Am*. 2009;91(1):20-28.
148. Oner FC, et al. Cement augmentation techniques in traumatic thoracolumbar spine fractures. *Spine*. 2006;31(11 suppl):S89-S95.
149. Charles YP, et al. Thoracolumbar fracture reduction by percutaneous in situ contouring. *Eur Spine J*. 2012;21(11): 2214-2221.
150. de Falco R, Bocchetti A. Balloon kyphoplasty for pure traumatic thoracolumbar fractures: retrospective analysis of 61 cases focusing on restoration of vertebral height. *Eur Spine J*. 2014;23(suppl 6):664-670.
151. Maestretti G, Sutter P, Monnard E, et al. A prospective study of percutaneous balloon kyphoplasty with calcium phosphate cement in traumatic vertebral fractures: 10-year results. *Eur Spine J*. 2014;23(6):1354-1360.
152. Zairi F, Aboukais R, Marinho P, Allaoui M, Assaker R. Minimally invasive percutaneous stabilization plus balloon kyphoplasty for the treatment of type A thoracolumbar spine fractures: minimum 4 years' follow-up. *J Neurosurg Sci*. 2014;58(3):169-175.
153. Singer G, Wegmann H, Kraus T, et al. Balloon kyphoplasty and percutaneous fixation of lumbar fractures in pediatric patients. *Eur Spine J*. 2014;25(2):651-656.
154. Homnick A, Lavery R, Nicastro O, et al. Isolated thoracolumbar transverse process fractures: call physical therapy, not spine. *J Trauma*. 2007;63:1292-1295.
155. Bradley LH, Paullus WC, Howe J, Litofsky NS. Isolated transverse process fractures: spine service management not needed. *J Trauma*. 2008;65:832-836.
156. Miller CD, Blyth P, Civil ID. Lumbar transverse process fractures—a sentinel marker of abdominal organ injuries. *Injury*. 2000;31:773-776.
157. Terhaag D, Frowein RA. Traumatic disc prolapses. *Neurosurg Rev*. 1989;12(suppl 1):588-594.
158. Vazquez D, Solano I, Pages E, et al. Thoracic disc herniation, cord compression, and paraplegia caused by electrical injury: case report and review of the literature. *J Trauma*. 1994;37:328-332.
159. Ando T, Mimatsu K. Traumatic lumbar disc herniation. A case report. *Spine*. 1993;18:2355-2357.
160. Martin G. The role of trauma in disc protrusion. *N Z Med J*. 1978;87:208-211.
161. Birch-Jensen A. Fracture of the spine; conservative treatment with plaster jacket without preceding reduction; a follow-up examination of 42 patients with isolated fractures of the vertebral body. *Acta Chir Scand*. 1955;109:377-383.
162. Davis AG. Fractures of the spine. *J Bone Joint Surg*. 1929;11:133-156.
163. Jewett EL. Fracture of the spine; new treatment without plaster casts. *J Int Coll Surg*. 1950;13:407-414.
164. Bohlman HH. Treatment of fractures and dislocations of the thoracic and lumbar spine. *J Bone Joint Surg Am*. 1985;67:165-169.
165. Hazel WA Jr, Jones RA, Morrey BF, Stauffer RN. Vertebral fractures without neurological deficit. A long-term follow-up study. *J Bone Joint Surg Am*. 1988;70:1319-1321.
166. Young MH. Long-term consequences of stable fractures of the thoracic and lumbar vertebral bodies. *J Bone Joint Surg Br*. 1973;55:295-300.
167. Westerborn A, Olsson O. Mechanics, treatment and prognosis of fractures of the dorso-lumbar spine. *Acta Chir Scand*. 1951;102:59-83.
168. Baab OD, Howorth MB. Fractures on the dorsal and lumbar vertebrae. *J Am Med Assoc*. 1951;146:97-100.
169. Day B, Kokan P. Compression fractures of the thoracic and lumbar spine from compensable injuries. *Clin Orthop Relat Res*. 1977;(124):173-176.
170. Härkönen M, Kataja M, Lepistö P, et al. Fractures of the thoracic spine. Clinical and radiological results in 98 patients. *Arch Orthop Trauma Surg*. 1979;94:179-184.

171. Härkönen M, Kataja M, Keski-Nisula L, et al. Fractures of the lumbar spine. Clinical and radiological results in 94 patients. *Arch Orthop Trauma Surg*. 1979;94:43-48.
172. Härkönen M, Kataja M, Keski-Nisula L, et al. Injuries of the thoracolumbar junction. Clinical and radiological results in 149 patients. *Arch Orthop Trauma Surg*. 1979;94:35-41.
173. Kallmes DF, Comstock BA, Heagerty PJ, et al. A randomized trial of vertebroplasty for osteoporotic spinal fractures. *N Engl J Med*. 2009;361:569-579.
174. Buchbinder R, Osborne RH, Ebeling PR, et al. A randomized trial of vertebroplasty for painful osteoporotic vertebral fractures. *N Engl J Med*. 2009;361:557-568.
175. Cantor JB, Lebwohl NH, Garvey T, Eismont FJ. Nonoperative management of stable thoracolumbar burst fractures with early ambulation and bracing. *Spine*. 1993;18:971-976.
176. Mumford J, Weinstein JN, Spratt KF, Goel VK. Thoracolumbar burst fractures. The clinical efficacy and outcome of nonoperative management. *Spine*. 1993;18:955-970.
177. Moller A, Hasserius R, Redlund-Johnell I, et al. Nonoperatively treated burst fractures of the thoracic and lumbar spine in adults: a 23- to 41-year follow-up. *Spine J*. 2007;7:701-707.
178. Weinstein JN, Collalto P, Lehmann TR. Thoracolumbar "burst" fractures treated conservatively: a long-term follow-up. *Spine*. 1988;13:33-38.
179. Chow GH, Nelson BJ, Gebhard JS, et al. Functional outcome of thoracolumbar burst fractures managed with hyperextension casting or bracing and early mobilization. *Spine*. 1996;21:2170-2175.
180. Bailey CS, Urquhart JC, Dvorak MF, et al. Orthosis versus no orthosis for the treatment of thoracolumbar burst fractures without neurologic injury: a multicenter prospective randomized equivalence trial. *Spine J*. 2014;14(11):2557-2564.
181. Dai LY, Jiang LS, Jiang SD. Conservative treatment of thoracolumbar burst fractures: a long-term follow-up results with special reference to the load sharing classification. *Spine*. 2008;33:2536-2544.
182. Kaneda K, Taneichi H, Abumi K, et al. Anterior decompression and stabilization with the Kaneda device for thoracolumbar burst fractures associated with neurological deficits. *J Bone Joint Surg Am*. 1997;79:69-83.
183. McAfee PC, Bohlman HH, Yuan HA. Anterior decompression of traumatic thoracolumbar fractures with incomplete neurological deficit using a retroperitoneal approach. *J Bone Joint Surg Am*. 1985;67:89-104.
184. McNamara MJ, Stephens GC, Spengler DM. Transpedicular short-segment fusions for treatment of lumbar burst fractures. *J Spinal Disord*. 1992;5:183-187.
185. Kaya RA, Aydin Y. Modified transpedicular approach for the surgical treatment of severe thoracolumbar or lumbar burst fractures. *Spine J*. 2004;4:208-217.
186. McLain RF, Burkus JK, Benson DR. Segmental instrumentation for thoracic and thoracolumbar fractures: prospective analysis of construct survival and five-year follow-up. *Spine J*. 2001;1:310-323.
187. Danisa OA, Shaffrey CI, Jane JA, et al. Surgical approaches for the correction of unstable thoracolumbar burst fractures: a retrospective analysis of treatment outcomes. *J Neurosurg*. 1995;83:977-983.
188. Wood K, Buttermann G, Mehbod A, et al. Operative compared with nonoperative treatment of a thoracolumbar burst fracture without neurological deficit. A prospective, randomized study. *J Bone Joint Surg Am*. 2003;85:773-781.
189. Seybold EA, Sweeney CA, Fredrickson BE, et al. Functional outcome of low lumbar burst fractures. A multicenter review of operative and nonoperative treatment of L3-L5. *Spine*. 1999;24:2154-2161.
190. Siebenga J, Leferink VJ, Segers MJ, et al. Treatment of traumatic thoracolumbar spine fractures: a multicenter prospective randomized study of operative versus nonsurgical treatment. *Spine*. 2006;31:2881-2890.
191. Tropiano P, Huang RC, Louis CA, et al. Functional and radiographic outcome of thoracolumbar and lumbar burst fractures managed by closed orthopaedic reduction and casting. *Spine*. 2003;28:2459-2465.
192. Willén J, Anderson J, Toomoka K, Singer K. The natural history of burst fractures at the thoracolumbar junction. *J Spinal Disord*. 1990;3:39-46.
193. Eismont FJ, Cuartas E. Flexion-distraction injuries of the thoracic and lumbar spine. In: Zigler JE, Eismont FJ, Garfin SR, Vaccaro AR, eds. *Spine Trauma 2*. Rosemont, IL: AAOS; 2011:515-534.
194. Gertzbein SD, Court-Brown CM. Flexion-distraction injuries of the lumbar spine. Mechanisms of injury and classification. *Clin Orthop Relat Res*. 1988;227:52-60.
195. LeGay DA, Petrie DP, Alexander DI. Flexion-distraction injuries of the lumbar spine and associated abdominal trauma. *J Trauma*. 1990;30:436-444.
196. Glassman SD, Johnson JR, Holt RT. Seatbelt injuries in children. *J Trauma*. 1992;33:882-886.
197. Neumann P, Nordwall A, Osvalder AL. Traumatic instability of the lumbar spine. A dynamic in vitro study of flexion-distraction injury. *Spine*. 1995;20:1111-1121.
198. Neumann P, Osvalder AL, Nordwall A, et al. The mechanism of initial flexion-distraction injury in the lumbar spine. *Spine*. 1992;17:1083-1090.
199. Osvalder AL, Neumann P, Lövsund P, Nordwall A. A method for studying the biomechanical load response of the (in vitro) lumbar spine under dynamic flexion-shear loads. *J Biomech*. 1993;26:1227-1236.
200. Nagel DA, Koogle TA, Piziali RL, Perkash I. Stability of the upper lumbar spine following progressive disruptions and the application of individual internal and external fixation devices. *J Bone Joint Surg Am*. 1981;63:62-70.
201. Gumley G, Taylor TK, Ryan MD. Distraction fractures of the lumbar spine. *J Bone Joint Surg Br*. 1982;64:520-525.
202. Levine AM, Bosse M, Edwards CC. Bilateral facet dislocations in the thoracolumbar spine. *Spine*. 1988;13:630-640.
203. Graham B, Van Peteghem PK. Fractures of the spine in ankylosing spondylitis. Diagnosis, treatment, and complications. *Spine*. 1989;14:803-807.
204. Waters RL, Adkins RH. The effects of removal of bullet fragments retained in the spinal canal. *Spine*. 1991;16:934-939.
205. Stauffer ES, Wood RW, Kelly EG. Gunshot wounds of the spine: the effects of laminectomy. *J Bone Joint Surg Am*. 1979;61:389-392.
206. Grogan DP, Bucholz RW. Acute lead intoxication from a bullet in an intervertebral disk space. *J Bone Joint Surg Am*. 1981;63:1180-1182.
207. Rabinowitz RP, Tabatabai A, Stein DM, Scalea TM. Infectious complications in GSW's through the gastrointestinal tract into the spine. *Injury*. 2012;43(7):1058-1060.
208. Roffi RP, Waters RL, Adkins RH. Gunshot wounds to the spine associated with a perforated viscus. *Spine*. 1989;14:808-811.

78 CHAPTER Sacral Fractures

Carlo Bellabarba
Richard A. Lindtner
Richard J. Bransford

The sacrum acts as a keystone at the junction of the pelvis and the spinal column. It protects lumbosacral neurologic function and maintains pelvic and spinal column alignment. Accordingly, sacral fractures can potentially compromise stability of the pelvic ring, the spinopelvic junction, or both. Injuries to the sacrum may result in deformity, chronic pain, and loss of lower extremity, bowel, bladder, and sexual function. Consequently, treatment of sacral fractures needs to optimize both structural and neurologic outcome and requires a thorough understanding of neural decompression and skeletal reconstruction techniques. The severity of sacral fractures varies widely from insufficiency fractures in osteopenic patients to complex fracture patterns seen in high-energy injury mechanisms, such as motor vehicle collisions or falls from significant heights. Care of these patients must take into consideration the associated injuries in the trauma patient and the underlying medical conditions in patients with metabolic bone disease. Coordination of diagnostic and treatment efforts between the spine surgeon and other surgical, medical, critical care, and rehabilitation specialists is necessary to obtain optimal results.

Anatomic and Biomechanical Considerations

The sacrum is the lowest functional portion of the spinal column and provides an anchor for the mobile lumbar spine. Lumbosacral motion occurs through the lumbosacral intervertebral disc and the paired zygapophyseal (facet) joints. In addition to the usual intervertebral stabilizing structures, the lumbosacral articulation is further stabilized by the iliolumbar ligaments connecting the L5 transverse processes to the crest of the ilium and the sacrolumbar ligaments that have an origin contiguous with the iliolumbar ligament and insert into the anterosuperior aspect of the sacrum and sacroiliac joint.[1] These structures make the L5–S1 motion segment inherently more stable than the more cephalad lumbar motion segments.

The sacrum has an inclination that is balanced by a cascade of lumbar lordosis, thoracic kyphosis, and cervical lordosis so that a plumb line from C7 typically passes through the posterior aspect of the L5–S1 intervertebral disc. The sacral inclination angle, defined as the angle between a tangent to the dorsal surface of the sacrum and a vertical reference line, varies between 10 and 90 degrees and is usually between 45 and 60 degrees.[2,3] Pelvic incidence measures the orientation of the lumbosacral junction relative to the pelvis and approximates 50 degrees in the general population.[4] It is normally referred to in the context of sagittal plane deformities and is valuable in determining sagittal alignment when treating sacral fractures. Sacral fractures that significantly alter spinal sagittal alignment, usually by shifting the C7 plumb line anteriorly, may result in difficulty in maintaining an erect posture, compensatory hyperlordosis, and associated functional deficits[5] (Fig. 78.1).

The sacrum forms the posterior segment of the pelvic ring through the sacroiliac joints. Forces transmitted through the lumbosacral articulation into the upper sacrum propagate laterally across the sacroiliac joints to the pelvis (Fig. 78.2). Because of these load-transferring properties, the sacrum has been described as the keystone of the pelvic ring.[6] More specifically, the sacrum functions as a "true keystone" in the pelvic outlet plane, in which the orientation of the sacrum relative to the ilium is such that axial forces lock the sacrum into the pelvic ring and further stabilize the sacroiliac articulation. In the pelvic inlet plane, the sacrum is shaped like a "reverse keystone" and its position in this plane is inherently unstable, permitting pelvic ring motion (Fig. 78.3). This pelvic ring instability necessitates substantial intrinsic and extrinsic ligamentous stabilization of the sacroiliac joints. Intrinsic stability is provided by the substantial interosseous ligaments and posterior sacroiliac ligaments as well as the relatively weaker anterior sacroiliac ligaments. Extrinsic stability is provided by the sacrospinous and sacrotuberous ligaments of the pelvic floor.[7]

The sacrum itself is composed of five kyphotically aligned vertebral segments. The upper two sacral segments are similar in size to the lumbar vertebrae, whereas the lower three sacral segments rapidly diminish in size.[8] Intersegmental fusion begins between the lowest two segments around the age of 15 years and proceeds in a cephalad direction until the sacrum is

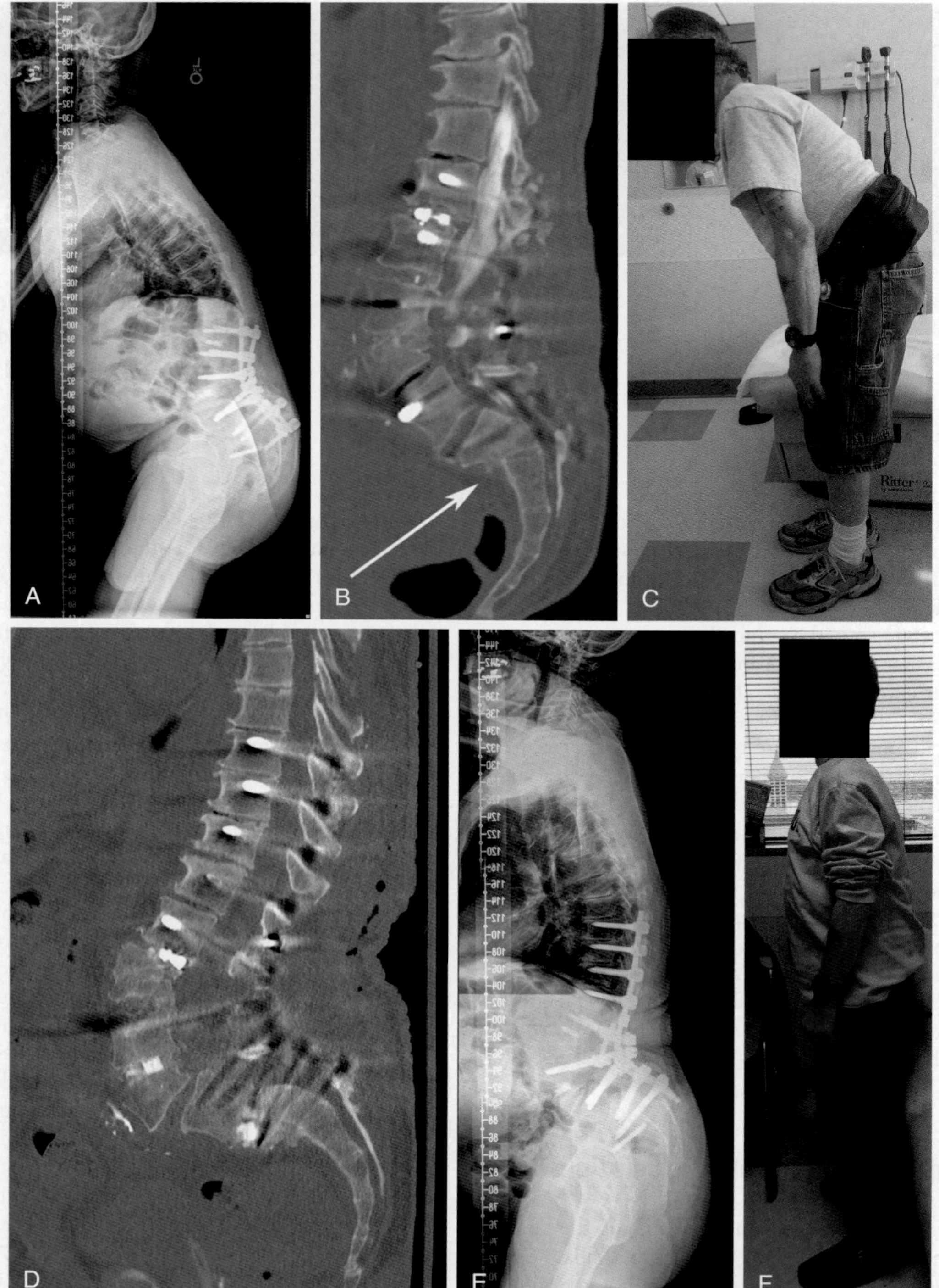

FIG. 78.1 Sagittal plane malalignment after malunited AO type C3 sacral fracture. Because of its caudal location, malunited fractures of the sacrum can have highly deleterious effects on spinal alignment. (A) Lateral spine radiograph and (B) sagittal computed tomographic (CT) image of the lumbosacral spine after L4 pedicle subtraction osteotomy had been done in an unsuccessful attempt at treating severe sagittal malalignment due to kyphotically malunited AO type C3 sacral U fracture (*arrow*). (C) Persistent, severely positive sagittal plane deformity. (D) Sagittal CT image and (E) lateral radiograph after L2 pedicle subtraction osteotomy largely restored physiologic sagittal plane alignment (F). Stabilizing sacral fractures in acceptable alignment helps prevent the need for more complex and risky reconstructive operations in the future.

completely fused by 25 to 30 years of age. Significant variability in upper sacral anatomy can exist in the form of transitional vertebrae and sacral dysplasia. Forms of transitional vertebrae include a sacralized lumbar segment, an incomplete congenital fusion of L5 to the sacrum that is usually unilateral, and a lumbarized sacrum identified by a persistent articulation between the S1 and S2 segments.[9] Complete or bilateral sacralization may result in dysplastic sacral morphology with the upper sacrum located cephalad relative to the iliac crests. Because upper sacral variability results in significant alteration in the relationships among the sacrum, pelvis, and spinal column, as well as their adjacent neurovascular structures, anatomic variations must be recognized during the evaluation and treatment of sacral fractures, particularly if surgical treatment is considered.[10]

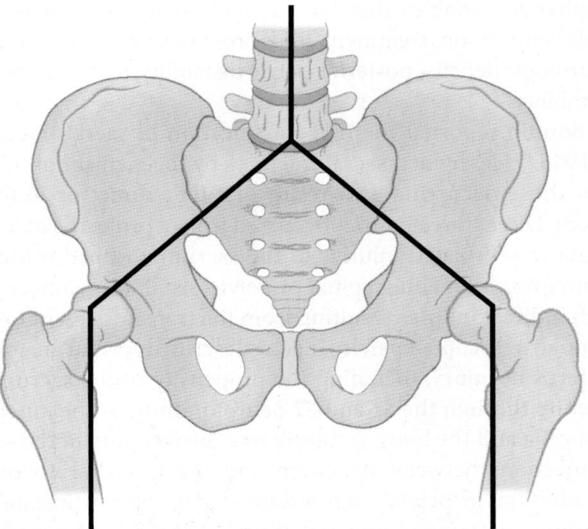

FIG. 78.2 Weight-bearing axis of the spinal column and pelvic ring.

The upper sacral body, which constitutes the base of the mobile spine, consistently has the highest density of cancellous bone, with the S1 segment adjacent to the superior endplate having the greatest density overall. The ventral aspect of the upper S1 body that projects anteriorly and superiorly into the pelvis is termed the *sacral promontory.* The sacral ala, the lateral portion of the sacrum that articulates with the ilium through the sacroiliac joints, is largely cancellous and is formed by the coalescence of the sacral transverse processes. There is wide variability in sacral alar morphology among individuals, and the ala can be substantial broad shoulders of bone or narrow, partially segmented structures. The cancellous alar bone is hypodense, particularly in older individuals, and an alar void is a consistent finding in middle-aged and older adults.[11,12] The relative difference in bone density between the upper and lower sacral body predisposes this transitional area to fracture. The hypodense ala are predisposed, particularly in the older and osteopenic person, to fracture line propagation. This effect is accentuated by the relative strength of the sacroiliac joint ligaments that stabilize and prevent their displacement or disruption. Similarly, younger individuals injured before complete ossification of the sacrum are predisposed to disruption at the S1–S2 level owing to relative weakness at that interval. The relatively sparse alar bone density must also be taken into consideration when planning reconstructive procedures.

The posterior surface of the sacrum is convex and is formed by the coalescence of posterior elements. Accordingly, the middle sacral crest corresponds to the spinous processes, the intermediate sacral crests correspond to the zygapophyseal joints, and the area in between corresponds to the laminae. The lowest one or two sacral segments have incompletely formed bony posterior elements, resulting in an aperture into the sacral spinal canal known as the sacral hiatus. Enlargement of the sacral hiatus may relatively weaken the sacrum and predispose it to fracture.[13]

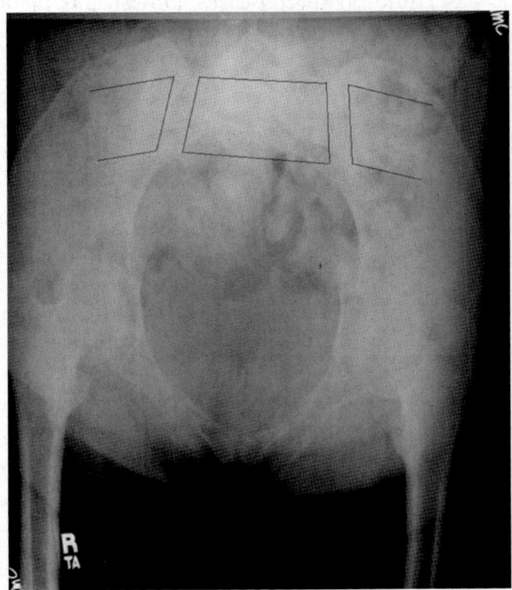

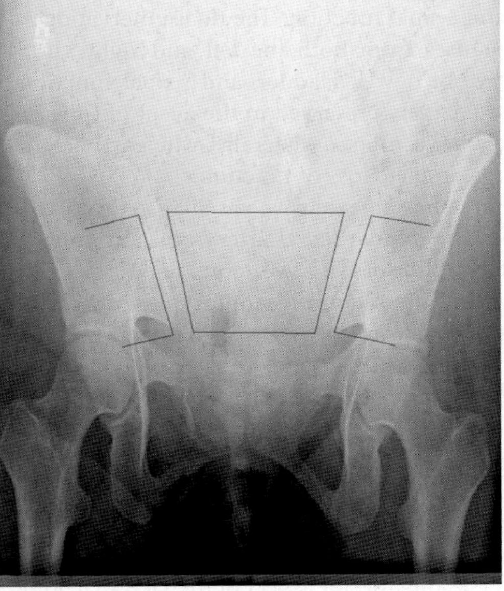

FIG. 78.3 Keystone and reverse keystone configuration of the sacrum in the pelvic ring.

Sacral pedicles and laminae form the lateral and posterior borders of the spinal canal as it tapers in size distally from a triangular cross-section at the S1 level to a flat and narrow cross-section at the most caudal segments. The dural sac typically ends at the S2 level and the filum terminale attaches its caudal end to the coccyx. At the junction of the body and the sacral ala are four paired ventral and dorsal neuroforamina through which the ventral and dorsal sacral nerve root rami pass, respectively. The relative space available to the sacral nerve roots in the ventral foramina is lowest at the S1 and S2 levels, where the nerve roots occupy one-third to one-fourth of the foraminal area compared with the S3 and S4 levels, where the nerve roots occupy one-sixth of the available foraminal space. It follows that the lower sacral roots are less likely to be impinged upon in injuries involving displacement and narrowing of the neuroforamina.[14]

Numerous structures positioned adjacent to the sacrum may be injured in sacral fracture-dislocations. The majority are neurovascular structures, with the rectum being the only visceral structure in close proximity. Below the rectosigmoid junction, located at the S3 level, the mesentery disappears and the rectum lies directly adjacent to the sacrum.[15]

The dorsal nerve roots exit through their respective posterior neuroforamina to supply motor branches to the paraspinous muscles and cutaneous sensory branches that form the cluneal nerves. Anteriorly, the L5 nerve root is intimately associated with the sacrum as it passes underneath the inferior edge of the sacrolumbar ligament and drapes over the anterosuperior aspect of the sacral ala. It anastomoses with the L4 ventral ramus and, in passing caudally, adjacent to the sacral ala, is joined by the exiting ventral sacral nerve roots to form the sacral plexus.[16] Branches of the sacral plexus include the sciatic nerve, pudendal nerve, superior gluteal nerve, and inferior gluteal nerve. In addition, the sympathetic chain lies directly on the ventral sacrum immediately medial to the neuroforamina. At each level, it distributes a gray ramus communicans to the ventral nerve root. Therefore, the sacral plexus mediates major lower extremity function, as well as bowel, bladder, and sexual function. The dual innervation of the perineal structures from both the left and right sacral plexus is protective of bowel, bladder, and sexual function. These functions are largely preserved in the event of transection of the sacral nerve roots unilaterally, whereas bilateral transection causes complete loss of function.[17]

The presacral area has an extensive vascular network that is highly variable. The middle sacral artery typically courses ventrally along the midline of the L5 vertebral body, across the L5–S1 disc space and the sacral promontory and down the sacrum after branching from the aorta at the common iliac bifurcation. The common iliac arteries subsequently give rise to the internal iliac arteries that lie anterior to the sacroiliac joints and give off both superior and inferior lateral sacral arteries. The superior lateral sacral artery traverses the upper sacroiliac joint and proceeds caudally just lateral to the sacral foramina, giving off spinal arteries that pass through the S1 and S2 ventral foramina to the spinal canal. The inferior lateral sacral artery traverses the inferior aspect of the sacroiliac joint before anastomosing with the middle sacral artery and giving off spinal arteries that pass through the S3 and S4 ventral foramina.[9] The internal iliac veins lie posteromedial to the internal iliac arteries and course caudally. They are located medial to the sacroiliac joint directly adjacent to the sacral ala.[15] The internal iliac veins are the repository of an extensive presacral venous plexus. This plexus is formed by extensive anastomoses between the lateral and middle sacral veins and receives transforaminal veins that communicate with epidural veins in the spinal canal.[1,8,18] This extensive vascular network renders anterior exposures to the sacrum impractical and perilous.

History and Classification

Sacral fracture classifications have prioritized several different features over time and have evolved over the past 70 years to emphasize variables that are currently believed to have the most impact on treatment and prognosis: the presence of neurologic deficits, posterior pelvic instability, and spinopelvic instability.

Bonnin reported the first classification of sacral fractures in 1945.[19] He divided sacral fractures by mechanism of injury into those occurring as a result of either direct or indirect forces. Direct force injuries occurred from a projectile or a fall. These were isolated injuries to the sacrum and had minimal or no impact on either spinal or pelvic instability. Conversely, with indirect injuries resulting from the transmission of forces through a disrupted pelvic ring, he described several anatomic patterns of injury, including the propensity of the sacrum to fracture through the S1 and S2 neuroforamina at the junction of the ala and the body, resulting in a "broken link in the solid connections between the ilium and the vertebral column." In addition to pelvic ring and/or spinal column instability, anatomic patterns of injury that included the neuroforamina or spinal canal were noted to be associated with possible neurologic deficit. Specifically, S1 or S2 nerve root injury was common in his cases. Bowel and bladder dysfunction as a result of lower sacral nerve root injury was sometimes also seen.[19]

Several other classification schemes based on the identification of additional injury patterns were subsequently proposed.[20,21] None was widely adopted until 1988, when Denis and colleagues,[14] based on a series of 236 sacral fractures, formulated a simplified anatomic classification that correlates fracture location with the incidence of neurologic injury. This classification divides the sacrum into three zones (Fig. 78.4). In zone 1, or the alar zone, fractures remain lateral to the neuroforamina throughout their course. In zone 2, or the foraminal zone, fractures are located in the transition area between the sacral ala and body and involve one or more neuroforamina while remaining lateral to the spinal canal. In zone 3, or the central zone, fractures involve the spinal canal. The key relationship is that the incidence and the severity of neurologic injury increases as fractures are more centrally located. Accordingly, in the series of Denis and colleagues, zone 1 fractures had a 5.9% incidence of neurologic injury, primarily to the L5 nerve root as it coursed over the ala. Zone

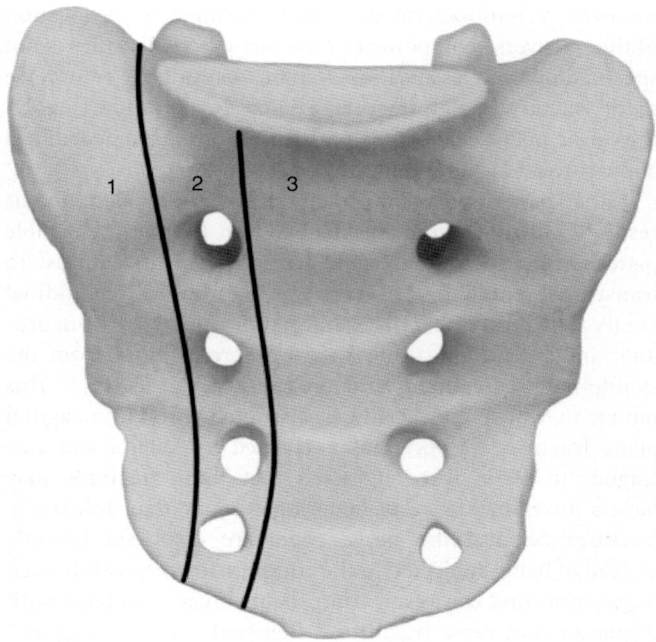

FIG. 78.4 Denis and coauthors[14] categorized sacral fractures according to the location of fractures relative to the sacral foramina (zones 1, 2, and 3). More medially located fractures have a higher risk of neurologic deficits and a worse prognosis.

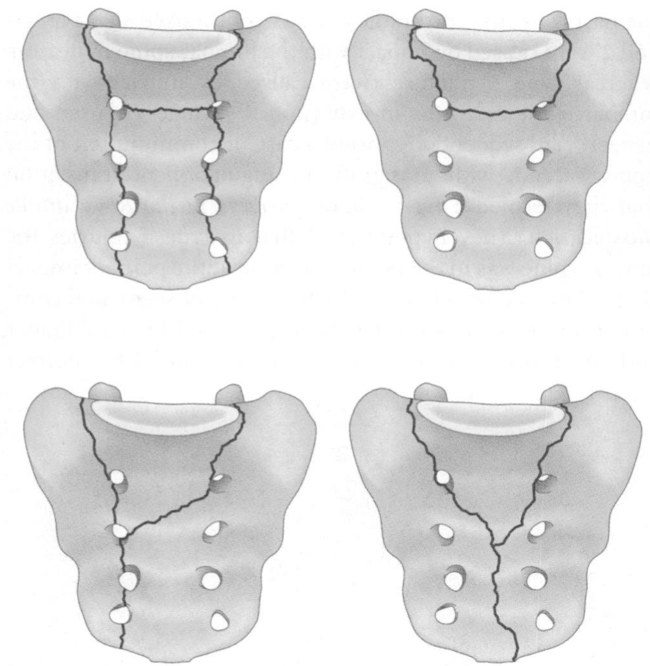

FIG. 78.5 Descriptive classification of sacral fractures: Sacral U variants with spinopelvic instability include (clockwise from top left) H, U, Y, and lambda fractures.

2 fractures had a 28.4% incidence of associated neurologic injury occurring as a result of either foraminal displacement and resulting impingement on the exiting nerve root or of the "traumatic far-out syndrome," in which the L5 nerve root is caught between the L5 transverse process and the displaced sacral ala. Zone 3 fractures had a 56.7% incidence of neurologic injury resulting from injury at the level of the spinal canal, with 76.1% of these individuals having bowel, bladder, and sexual dysfunction. Denis and colleagues[14] noted a spectrum of zone 3 sacral fracture-dislocations, including both transverse and longitudinal fracture line orientations, and described a subtype that they termed a *sacral burst fracture*, consisting of retropulsion of the sacral body with intact sacral laminae.

Gibbons and colleagues[22] subsequently considered 44 cases of sacral fracture according to the Denis classification system. They found a 34% incidence of neurologic injury overall. Six of 25 patients (24%) with zone 1 injuries had L5 and/or S1 nerve root injuries. Two of seven patients with zone 2 injuries similarly had L5 and S1 deficits. No patient with zone 1 or 2 injuries had bowel or bladder dysfunction. Three of five patients with zone 3 injuries had neurologic injury, two with bladder dysfunction. Gibbons and colleagues[22] used these findings as a basis for a classification of neurologic injury from sacral fractures. Neurologic injuries were classified as follows: 1, no injury; 2, lower extremity paresthesias only; 3, lower extremity motor deficit with intact bowel and bladder function; or 4, impaired bowel and/or bladder control. They also noted that significant neurologic deficit is rare in transverse sacral fractures below the S4 level. This classification system, while simple, does not address incomplete injuries or sexual function.

Huittinen,[23] in a postmortem study of 42 individuals with posterior pelvic ring disruptions, studied the incidence and anatomic basis of nerve injuries. A total of 40 lumbosacral nerve injuries were identified in 20 of the autopsies. A total of 53% were traction injuries and 38% were ruptures. Compression injuries, the most amenable to surgical intervention, were present in only 20% of the nerve injuries.

Because of the high potential for neurologic injury, as well as spinal column instability, sacral body (Denis zone 3) fractures have been specifically considered by several investigators. Early case reports often characterized the injury pattern as solely a transverse fracture, possibly owing to imaging limitations.[24–26] Computed tomography (CT) demonstrates that most transverse fractures of the upper sacrum have complex fracture patterns. The majority of these injuries are now understood to consist of a transverse fracture of the sacrum with associated longitudinal or "vertical" injury components, usually in the form of bilateral transforaminal fractures that extend as far rostrally as the lumbosacral junction, the so-called sacral "U" fracture. Variations in fracture line propagation include the "H," "Y," and "lambda" fracture patterns (Fig. 78.5). There is also a high incidence of L5 transverse process fractures, indicating disruption of the iliolumbar ligament.[27]

Roy-Camille and colleagues[28] reviewed their experience of 13 patients with transverse sacral fractures, 11 as a result of attempted suicide by jumping. They classified the fractures as type 1, flexion deformity of upper sacrum (angulation alone); type 2, flexion deformity with posterior displacement of the upper sacrum on the lower sacrum (angulation and posterior translation); and type 3, anterior displacement of the upper sacrum without angulation (anterior translation alone). On the basis of cadaveric studies, they hypothesized that types 1 and 2 were caused by impact with the lumbar spine in flexion, whereas type 3 fractures were caused by impact with the lumbar spine and hips in extension.[28] Strange-Vognsen and Lebech[29] subsequently reported a case of comminution of the upper sacrum without significant angulation or translation that they termed a *type 4 injury relative to the Roy-Camille classification.* They hypothesized that in type 4 injuries the lumbar spine was in the neutral position at the point of impact (Fig. 78.6). A type 5 injury, which consists of segmental comminution of the sacrum, has been proposed by Schildhauer and coauthors.[30] All of these injuries are caused by indirect forces to the lumbosacral junction. Unfortunately, the location of the transverse component of the sacral body fracture is not specified by this classification system. Defining the transverse sacral fracture as high (involving S2 or above) or low (involving S3 or below) can be helpful from both a biomechanical and neurologic standpoint.[24]

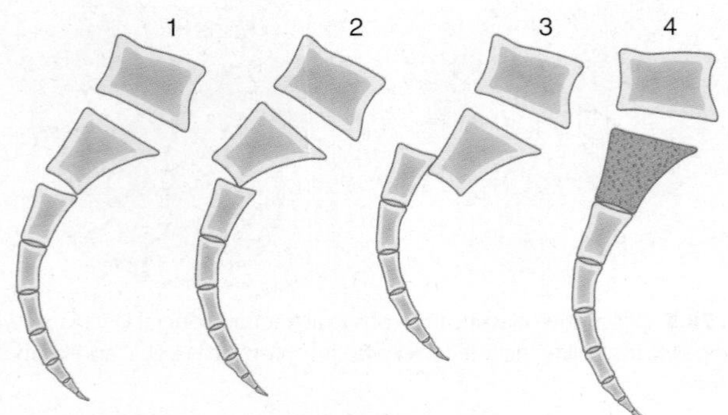

FIG. 78.6 Roy-Camille classification of sacral fractures. The Roy-Camille classification,[28] as modified by Strange-Vognsen and Lebech,[29] categorizes AO type C3[45] fractures according to sagittal plane angulation and displacement.

Other patterns of sacral fractures have been identified as resulting from specific mechanisms or having predictable patterns of associated injuries. In particular, in contrast to transverse Denis zone 3 sacral fractures, midline longitudinal Denis zone 3 sacral fractures have a low incidence of neurologic injury and constitute a very different injury from the standpoint of treatment and prognosis (Fig. 78.7).[31-33] This injury, in which the sacrum is disrupted through a sagittal plane fracture, was originally reported by Wiesel and colleagues in 1979, who suggested that these fractures may have a lower incidence of neurologic injury than transverse fractures because the nerve roots are displaced laterally instead of being subjected to the compression or possibly even transection that can result from shear forces associated with displaced transverse fractures.[33] Bellabarba and colleagues[31] subsequently described this injury as a variant of the anteroposterior compression pelvic ring injury. In their series of 10 patients, none had neurologic deficits in contradistinction to the high incidence of neurologic injury reported in patients with predominantly transverse sacral fractures through the spinal canal.[31]

Even in the absence of a transverse fracture line, sacral fractures can be associated with spinal column instability. Isler

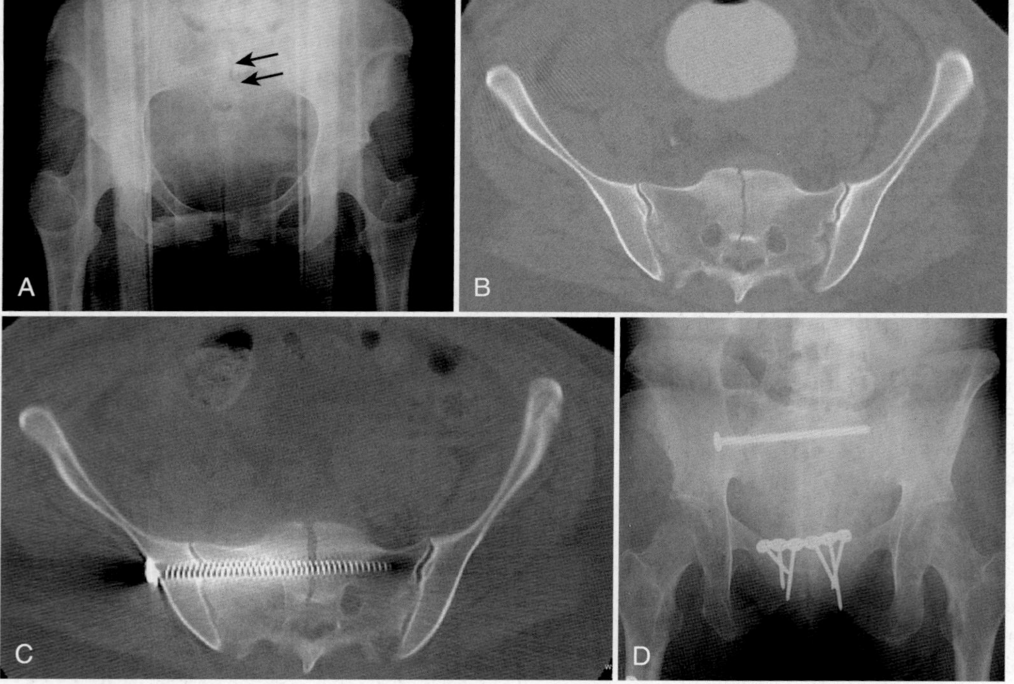

FIG. 78.7 (A–B) An unusual Denis zone 3 variant that is usually not accompanied by neurologic deficits consists of a longitudinal fracture of the sacral vertebral bodies that does not extend into the neuroforamina (arrows). Because this is typically the most benign of the longitudinal sacral fracture patterns, it has been designated as AO type B1. (C–D) After treatment with iliosacral screw fixation and symphyseal plating.

described variations of longitudinal sacral fractures through the S1 and S2 neuroforamina that result in L5–S1 motion segment instability owing to facet joint disruption (Fig. 78.8).[34] Injuries with the fracture line lateral to the S1 articular process are not associated with instability of the lumbosacral articulation because the L5–S1 articulation remains continuous with the stable fracture component of the sacrum. Fracture that extends into or medial to the S1 articular process, however, may disrupt the associated facet joint and potentially destabilize the lumbosacral junction (Fig. 78.9). Complete displacement of the facet joint can cause a locked facet joint, making sacral fracture reduction difficult with closed methods alone. Facet disruption may also cause posttraumatic arthrosis and late lumbosacral pain.

In contrast to sacral fractures that occur as a result of high-energy mechanisms of injury, the precipitating event in sacral insufficiency fractures is often not identifiable or may be related to a fall onto the buttocks from a standing or sitting position. Insufficiency fractures occur in weakened bone, and these injuries typically occur in postmenopausal women due to osteoporosis. Conditions contributing to the suboptimal bone quality, such as chronic corticosteroid use or a history of radiation therapy to the pelvis, are often present (Fig. 78.10).[35] The presenting symptoms are often vague and frequently consist of poorly localized low back pain that may be exacerbated by sitting and standing, possibly with lumbosacral radiculopathy. These fractures are typically oriented vertically and occur through the ala adjacent to the sacroiliac joint. There may also be a transverse component resulting in more complex sacral "U"-fracture variants. Because of the predisposition of these patients to osteoporotic fractures, there is high association with insufficiency fractures at other sites, most commonly the pubis and thoracolumbar vertebrae. Neurologic deficits are uncommon in most series.[36,37] Cauda

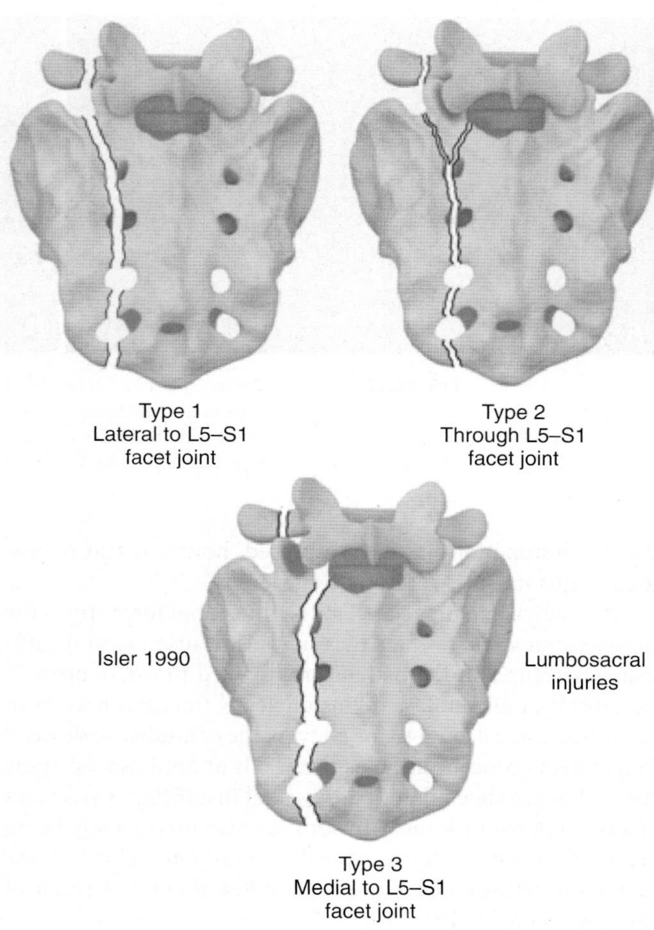

FIG. 78.8 Isler classification of sacral fractures.[34] Isler classified vertical sacral fractures according to the location of the fracture relative to the L5–S1 facet joint. Fracture patterns that extend medial to the L5–S1 facet joint (types 2 and 3) result in spinopelvic instability.

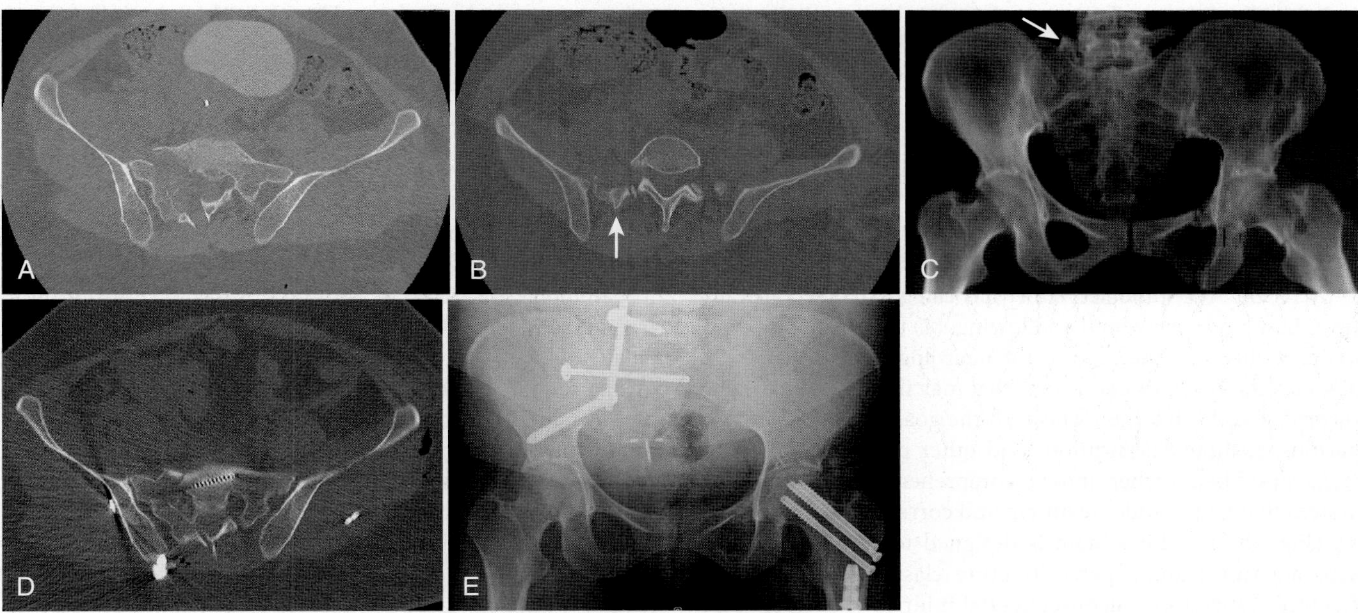

FIG. 78.9 (A) Displaced Denis zone 2 sacral fracture associated with (B–C) dislocation of the L5–S1 facet joint, Isler type 3. (D–E) After open reduction and triangular osteosynthesis.

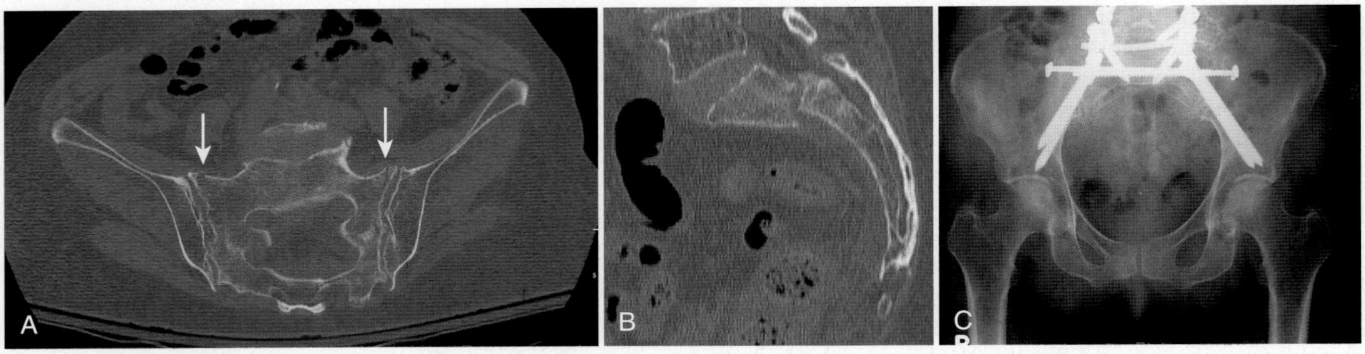

FIG. 78.10 (A–B) Sacral U insufficiency fracture in a patient with a history of radiation therapy to the pelvis for cervical cancer who had recently developed severe low back pain and progressive loss of bowel and bladder function. (C) After treatment with decompression and lumbopelvic fixation, her bowel and bladder function returned and she was able to resume pain-free normal activity.

equina dysfunction has been reported, however, and neurologic status must be carefully considered.[38]

Mechanical factors related to the transfer of forces from the lumbosacral spine to the pelvis may also cause sacral insufficiency fractures in the patient predisposed to osteoporosis.[29] Specifically, unilateral sacral insufficiency fractures have been identified contralateral to the convex side of lumbar scoliosis.[36] Pelvic stress concentration as the result of lumbosacral spine fusion has also been described[39]; sacral insufficiency fractures caudal to previous lumbar fusions are also increasingly being reported. These fractures probably represent failure of the sacrum to withstand forces concentrated there as a result of the large cephalad lever arm.[40–44]

Stress fractures of the sacrum, as opposed to insufficiency fractures, occur in bone that is not weakened by a pathologic process. They are seen in individuals whose activity level causes repetitive stress that exceeds the bone's reparative ability. High-demand individuals, such as endurance athletes and military recruits, are particularly susceptible. As with individuals with insufficiency fractures, these patients may present with vague and nonspecific low back pain. Other areas of stress fracture may cause additional symptomatic areas; femoral neck fractures, in particular, must be considered in the instance of groin pain. In some instances, the etiology of low-energy sacral fractures may be related to both repetitive stress and insufficiency. In particular, sacral fractures in female athletes with amenorrhea may result from both overuse and osteopenia.

A recent AO Spine–led effort has categorized sacral fractures based primarily on the following: (1) the extent and type of instability; (2) the severity of neurologic injury; and (3) associated injuries or conditions that may influence treatment or prognosis.[45] This was done with the goal of combining the various existing classifications and other published observations described earlier into a comprehensive classification system that helps guide treatment and correlates with prognosis (Fig. 78.11). This system is designed to complement the separate AO Trauma pelvic fracture classification. Type A fractures range from inconsequential injuries to severely displaced transverse fractures that occur below the sacroiliac joint, and therefore result in neither posterior pelvic nor spinopelvic instability. Type B fractures are longitudinal or "vertical" fracture patterns that result in posterior pelvic instability without compromise of the spinopelvic junction. Type C injuries result in spinopelvic instability with or without posterior pelvic instability. Type A and type B fractures are each divided into three subtypes, and type C injuries are divided into four subtypes, categorized according to injury severity based on greater risk of neurologic deficit or of instability. Neurologic injury is classified according to the same system used by the AO Spine classification throughout the entire spine: NX, patient not examinable; N0, no neurologic deficit; N1, transient neurologic deficit; N2, nerve root injury; N3, incomplete spinal cord injury or cauda equina syndrome (either complete or incomplete); N4, complete spinal cord injury. Because sacral fractures do not occur at the spinal cord level, they cannot cause neurologic injuries more severe than N3. Modifiers that may affect treatment or prognosis include the following: M1, soft tissue injury (either an open or a closed degloving injury); M2, metabolic bone disease; M3, anterior pelvic or acetabular fracture; M4, sacroiliac joint injury.

Evaluation

Sacral fractures occur in two distinctly different patient groups. Most commonly, sacral fractures are the result of high-energy trauma. As noted previously, they are also increasingly being seen in patients with metabolic bone disorders that predispose to pathologic fractures. In both groups of patients, but more frequently in patients with insufficiency fractures, diagnosis is frequently delayed, which may result in further displacement or neurologic deterioration. In their retrospective analysis of 236 patients with sacral fractures, Denis and colleagues[14] found that in neurologically intact patients, the diagnosis of sacral fractures was made during the initial hospitalization only 51% of the time. The presence of a neurologic deficit increased the diagnostic accuracy to only 70%. As in most cases of diagnostic delay, the etiology of missed sacral fractures is multifactorial and ranges from the relative difficulty in identifying these fractures on screening anteroposterior pelvis radiographs combined with the presence of associated injuries

TYPE	General Description		Specific (Injury Types)	Images
A.	Lower Sacral (Coccygeal) Injuries (Below SI Joint)	No Impact on Pelvic Ring or Spinopelvic Instability	A1. Coccygeal or Lower Sacral Compression or Ligamentation Avulsion Injury	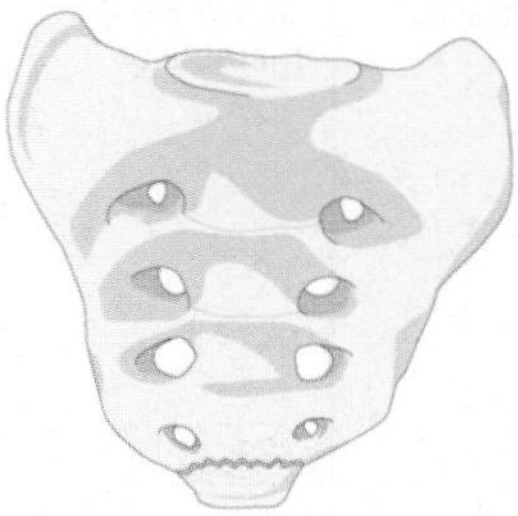
			A2: Nondisplaced Transverse Fractures Below SI Joint	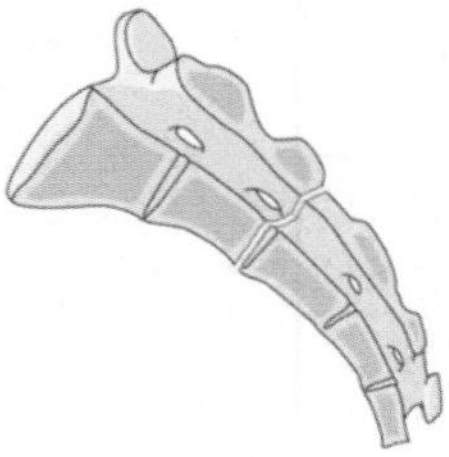
			A3: Displaced Transverse Fractures Below SI Joint	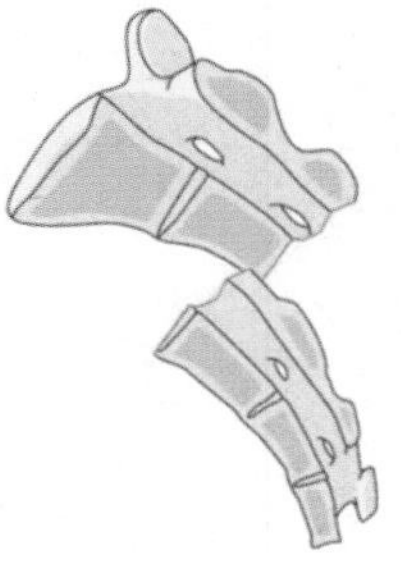
B.	Posterior Pelvic Injuries	Posterior Pelvic Ring Instability Without Spino-Pelvic Instability	B1: Central Longitudinal Sacral Fracture Without Foraminal Involvement	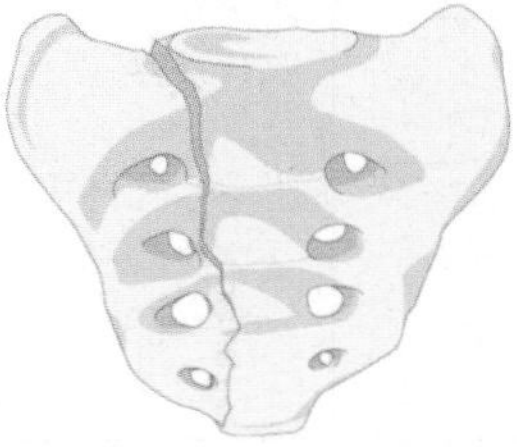
			B2: Unilateral Longitudinal Transalar Fracture Without Foraminal Involvement	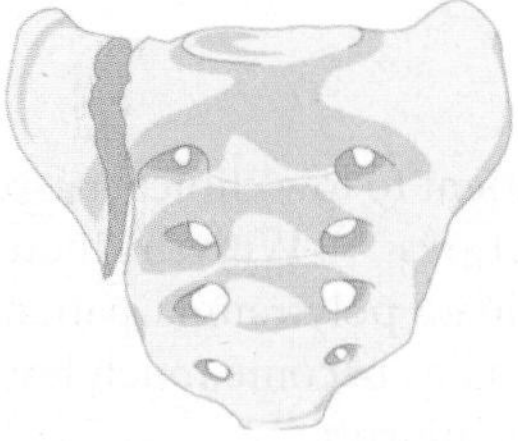
			B3: Unilateral Transforaminal Fracture	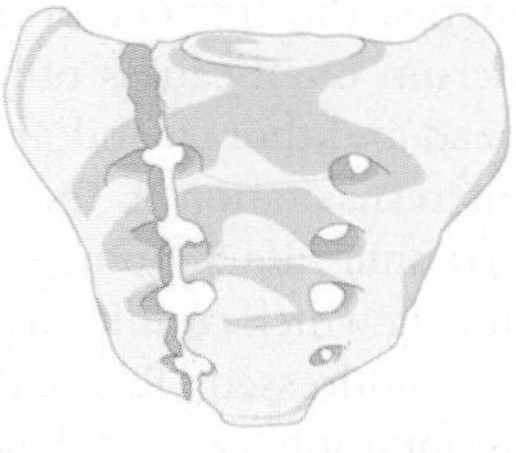

FIG. 78.11 AO Spine sacral fracture classification. SI, sacroiliac. In addition to the morphologic classification shown in the figure, neurologic status is indicated according to the AO Spine Neurologic Injury Scale. NX, unable to assess neurologic status; N0, no neurologic deficits; N1, transient neurologic deficits; N2, nerve root injury; N3, cauda equina syndrome or incomplete spinal cord injury; N4, complete spinal cord injury (does not apply to sacral fractures). Modifiers are also added for specific conditions that may affect treatment or prognosis as follows: M1, significant soft tissue injury; M2, metabolic bone disease; M3, anterior pelvic ring injury; M4, sacroiliac joint injury; M5, transitional lumbosacral segmentation; M6, lumbosacral spine fusion above sacral fracture.

Continued

C.	Spino-Pelvic Injuries	Spino-Pelvic Instablility	C0: Sacral U-Type Insufficiency Fracture	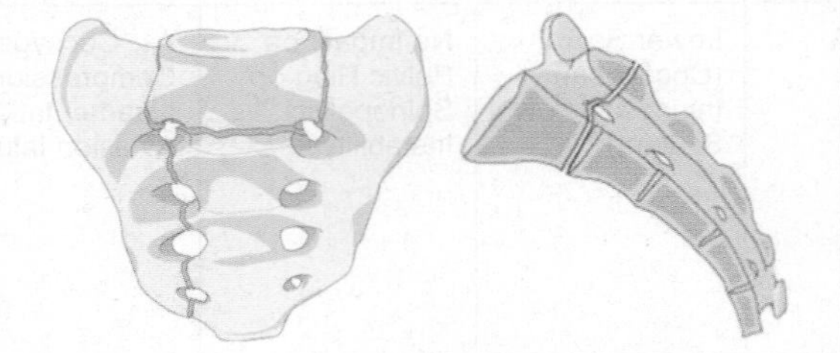
			C1: Unilateral B-Type Fracture That Detaches SI Superior Facet	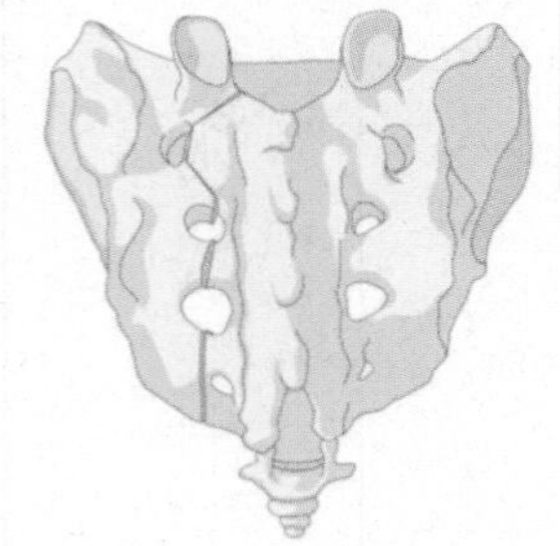
			C2: Bilateral Type B Injuries Without Transverse Fracture	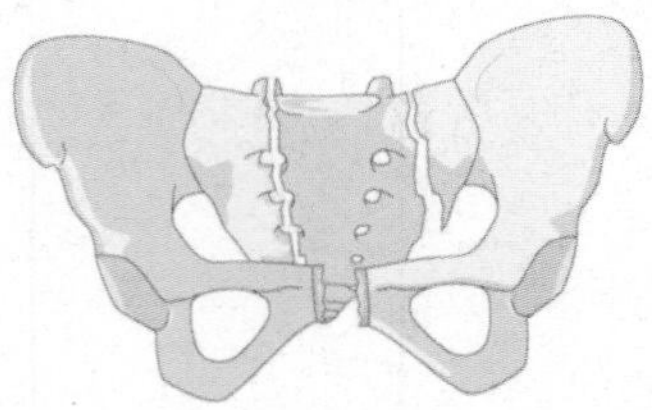
			C3: Displaced High-Energy U-Type Fracture	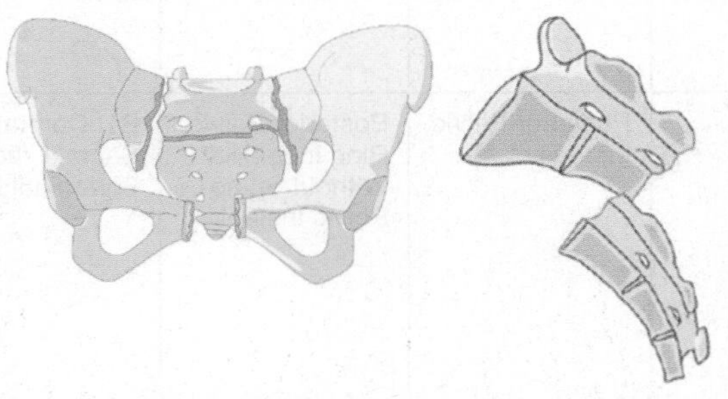

FIG. 78.11, cont'd

in the trauma patient to low clinical suspicion in patients with insufficiency fractures.[14,46] With the increased use of full-body CT scans to evaluate polytrauma patients, delayed diagnosis of sacral fractures has become much less common in patients with high-energy injuries.

In trauma patients, the transfer of energy resulting in a fracture of the sacrum often causes other injuries, including life-threatening head and thoracoabdominal trauma. In these patients, emergent resuscitation is the top priority. Accordingly, Advanced Trauma Life Support protocol begins with a primary survey during which conditions that are immediately life threatening are addressed. Resuscitation is focused on maintaining cardiopulmonary and hemodynamic stability. Only after this primary goal has been achieved should the secondary survey be completed, composed of examination of the patient to identify additional injuries.[47]

The secondary survey includes screening evaluation of both the spinal column and pelvic ring. Precautions to maintain spinal column integrity are necessary; patients should be initially maintained on a flat surface and log-rolled side to side to prevent spinal column displacement. Evaluation includes inspection and palpation of the patient's back from the occiput to the coccyx. Sacral fractures commonly have overlying skin discoloration or lacerations, palpable step-offs or crepitus, localized tenderness, and hematomas, any of which can indicate the presence of a sacral fracture. Significant soft tissue contusion or internal degloving, analogous to Morel-Lavallee lesions seen with acetabular fractures, can have implications on subsequent treatment.[48] Manual compression over the iliac crests, both anteroposteriorly and laterally, may also help identify a sacral fracture. Perforations of the rectum or vagina can represent open sacral fractures, which can be detected with rectal and vaginal digital examination as well as the use of a speculum and proctoscope.

Because pelvic ring disruption may be associated with significant intrapelvic hemorrhage, temporary methods of pelvic ring stabilization may be necessary to reduce pelvic volume and provide provisional stability. These methods include the application of a circumferential pelvic antishock sheet,[10] pelvic clamp, anterior external fixator, or skeletal traction, depending on the pelvic ring fracture pattern. Associated vascular injury, particularly to the hypogastric arterial system, may require embolization to adequately control arterial hemorrhage.[49]

Determining the patient's neurologic status is of paramount importance in patients with sacral fractures.[50–52] A rectal examination is performed early in the workup of all multiply injured patients, even in the absence of obvious sensorimotor deficits in the extremities, to evaluate perianal sensation, anal sphincter tone, and voluntary perianal contraction and to assess for presence of anal wink and the bulbocavernosus reflex. The bulbocavernosus is a polysynaptic reflex that is generally useful in testing for spinal shock and gaining information about the state of spinal cord injuries, but is particularly useful in evaluating sacral root function. The test involves monitoring anal sphincter contraction in response to squeezing the glans penis or clitoris, or tugging on an indwelling Foley catheter. The reflex is spinal mediated and will be absent with injury to the S2–S4 spinal nerves. The absence of the reflex without sacral root or conus medullaris trauma indicates spinal shock. A straight-leg raise test may be useful in the cognitively unimpaired patient to assess for entrapment of the lumbosacral plexus. Overall severity of neurologic injury is graded according to the American Spinal Injury Association modification of the Frankel grading system. Extremity motor function is further graded on a scale of 0 to 5 to establish the American Spinal Injury Association motor score, and a sensory level is obtained. Neurologic examination can only distinguish injuries to the L5 and S1 levels, however, and injuries to the lower sacral roots cannot be more specifically identified beyond obtaining a perianal sensory level.

Fracture displacement can cause neurologic injury from a variety of mechanisms, including angulation, translation, and direct compression by displaced bone fragments. Potentially reversible injuries include contusion, compression, and traction. Recovery of transected or avulsed nerve roots cannot be expected. Delayed neurologic deficit can occur from epidural hematoma, late fracture displacement, or callus formation[19] and should be promptly reinvestigated to determine its cause.

There are multiple adjunctive methods for the evaluation of the neurologic status in a patient with a sacral fracture. Electrodiagnostic studies may be of value in the evaluation of cognitively impaired patients and in differentiating upper motor neuron injuries or spinal cord injury from cauda equina injury in patients with head or more rostral spinal column injury, in the evaluation of patients with urinary tract injury, and for intraoperative monitoring.[53] Conventional electromyography (EMG) and somatosensory-evoked potentials may be useful for the evaluation of L5 and S1 function, while pudendal somatosensory-evoked potentials and anal sphincter EMG can be used to evaluate the sacral roots below the S1 level. These electrodiagnostic techniques are typically not used in the setting of acute injuries, however.[54–57] EMG is particularly limited in the acute setting because abnormalities may take weeks to develop. Possible abnormalities on sphincter EMG include detrusor areflexia, uninhibited sphincter relaxation, or denervation. For patients with neurogenic bladder, serial postvoid residuals or cystometrography are useful diagnostic aids.

Careful scrutiny of the anteroposterior pelvic radiograph, if available, allows for a majority of sacral fractures to be identified. Nevertheless, with the use of plain radiographs alone, sacral fractures can be easily missed, owing to a variety of circumstances. Because of its sagittal inclination and the juxtaposition of the iliac wings, sacral fractures can be difficult to visualize on the anteroposterior radiograph. This is particularly true of injuries with less obvious deformity of the pelvic ring that present mainly with displacement of the transverse sacral component and spinopelvic instability. Osteopenic bone and sacral dysmorphism can also obscure landmarks, making the identification of fractures more challenging.

The increasingly routine use of more sophisticated imaging techniques in the initial assessment of the trauma patient's visceral injuries, such as CT of the abdomen and pelvis, has facilitated the detection of previously under-recognized sacral fractures. The identification of a sacral fracture on these studies mandates complete radiographic evaluation, including a dedicated CT scan of the sacrum with 2-mm or less axial cuts and sagittal and coronal reformations to allow the detail required for determining the fracture configuration, resulting instability pattern, and extent of sacral canal and neuroforaminal compromise (Fig. 78.12).[58] Three-dimensionally reformatted CT scans may add insight into fracture morphology for less experienced clinicians or in the case of highly complex fracture configurations.

Several additional plain radiographic projections can yield important information. The pelvic inlet and outlet views, obtained with 45-degree caudal and 60-degree cephalad tilt, respectively, are standard techniques for evaluating pelvic ring injuries. The Ferguson view, a coned-down true anteroposterior view of the sacrum, is obtained with a 30-degree cranially inclined projection. A lateral radiograph is useful in evaluating sacral inclination and the presence of a transverse fracture. Useful radiographic indicators of sacral injuries include abnormalities in the contour of the sacral foramina and sacral arcuate lines and the presence of a "paradoxical inlet" view of the sacrum on the anteroposterior pelvic view. Their presence strongly suggests a sacral fracture, and further investigation should be done. These radiographic projections can also be obtained from three-dimensional reconstruction of the initial posttraumatic CT image, limiting the need for additional imaging studies.

Magnetic resonance imaging is not usually helpful except in cases of unclear neurologic deficits or discrepancies between skeletal and neurologic levels of injury, although it may provide early evidence of lumbosacral nerve root avulsion.[59] Recent advances in magnetic resonance imaging neurography allowing for visualization of lumbosacral plexus injuries may be of some help in their evaluation, although at this point it is neither a reliably effective nor a practical diagnostic tool.

General Principles

Decision making in sacral fracture treatment is primarily based on the fracture pattern and location and neurologic

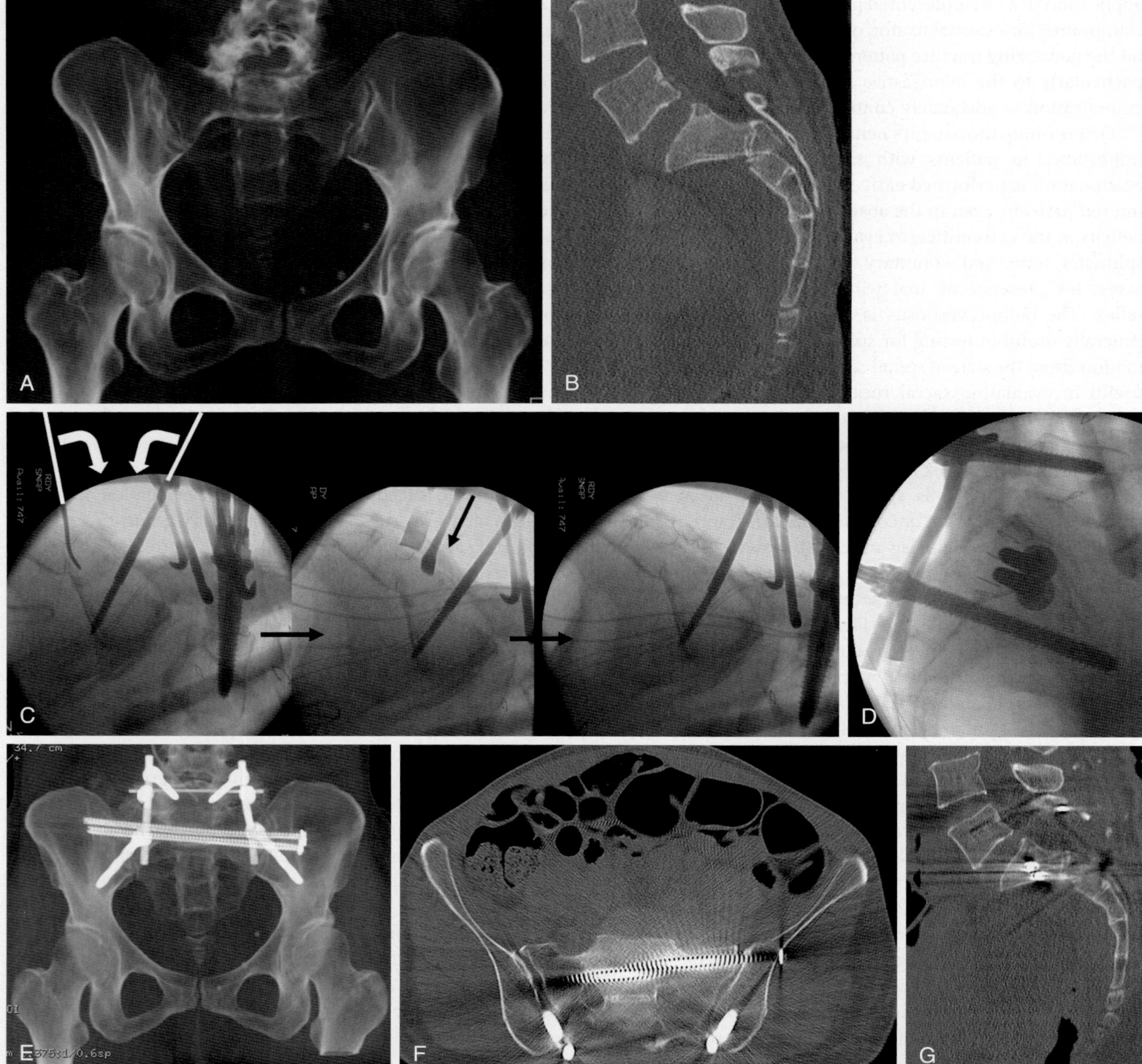

FIG. 78.12 Reduction and stabilization of AO type C3, Roy-Camille type 2 sacral fracture. (A) Despite severe sacral fracture displacement with cauda equina syndrome after a 10-foot fall, this anteroposterior view of the pelvis appears deceptively benign in the absence of pelvic ring deformity. (B) This sagittal computed tomographic (CT) image illustrates kyphosis, retrolisthesis, and spinal canal compromise consistent with Roy-Camille type 2 variant of AO type C3 fracture. Note the distended urinary bladder due to loss of sacral root function. (C) Intraoperative radiographs demonstrate reduction techniques, which include mobilization of impacted fracture fragments with an elevator and direct manipulation of the fracture fragments with Schanz pin joystick placed in the upper sacral fracture fragment. (D) After acceptable fracture reduction, provisional stabilization is achieved with transiliac-transsacral screw fixation, which is then supported by spinopelvic fixation. (E) Postoperative anteroposterior reconstruction of the pelvis. (F) Axial CT image, and (G) sagittal CT reformation of the sacrum demonstrate restoration of acceptable alignment and decompression of the sacral spinal canal and foramina. This patient regained sacral root function.

status. Surgical indications include the presence of instability, malalignment, and neurologic deficit. Other key factors are the patient's general medical condition and additional injuries, particularly in the trauma patient. Hemodynamic instability or compromised pulmonary function may preclude early surgical stabilization in critically injured patients. Conversely, the benefits of early mobilization in trauma patients with pulmonary injuries may make early surgical stabilization advisable.[60,61] Surgical timing in patients with closed-head injuries in particular is controversial, and skilled perioperative management is essential to prevent secondary brain injury.[62,63] Isolated sacral fractures in the patient who is otherwise healthy may be amenable to a period of recumbency followed by protected weight bearing. Chronic medical conditions also need to be considered and may require an initial period of nonoperative stabilization before surgical intervention while medical conditions are optimized.

Careful examination of the fracture pattern is essential in determining if the sacral fracture is associated with instability of the weight-bearing axis and whether this involves posterior pelvic instability, spinopelvic instability, or a combination of the two. Unilateral longitudinal fractures through the ala (AO type B2) or foraminal (AO type B3) zone maintain continuity of the contralateral weight-bearing axis, allowing weight bearing on that side (Fig. 78.13; also see Fig. 78.9). Bilateral displaced longitudinal fractures (AO type C2), as well as transverse fractures with associated bilateral longitudinal fractures through the upper sacrum (AO type C3), dissociate the spinal column from the pelvic ring and represent complete disruption of the weight-bearing axis.[28,64–66] Weight bearing on either lower extremity may cause displacement in these instances. Conversely, transverse fractures below the sacroiliac joint (AO type A) have no implication on the weight-bearing axis and therefore on either posterior pelvic or spinopelvic instability, as long as they are not associated with secondary fracture lines extending rostrally.[67]

Neurologic deficit needs to be correlated with fracture anatomy. Residual compression of nerve roots at the level of the spinal canal or neuroforamina due to impingement by bony fragments or malalignment of the spinal canal at the fracture site with the cauda equina draping over a kyphotic ridge should be identified. Possible neurologic deterioration from persistent fracture instability should also be considered. Although the presence of a neurologic deficit is an indication for operative intervention, the effectiveness of surgery in improving neurologic outcomes after fracture of the sacrum remains unproven since the literature on this topic consists primarily of small, heterogeneous case series without consistent grading and definitions of neurologic dysfunction.[14,20–22,24,26,27] Therefore, each case needs to be individually considered; our opinion is that surgical decompression, which usually can also be achieved with fracture reduction and stabilization, should be considered in the presence of a potentially reversible neurologic injury.

Functional outcome studies have demonstrated that a minority of sacral fracture patients returned to their preinjury vocational status over a year after injury. Although the vast majority of patients sustained long-term physical and mental

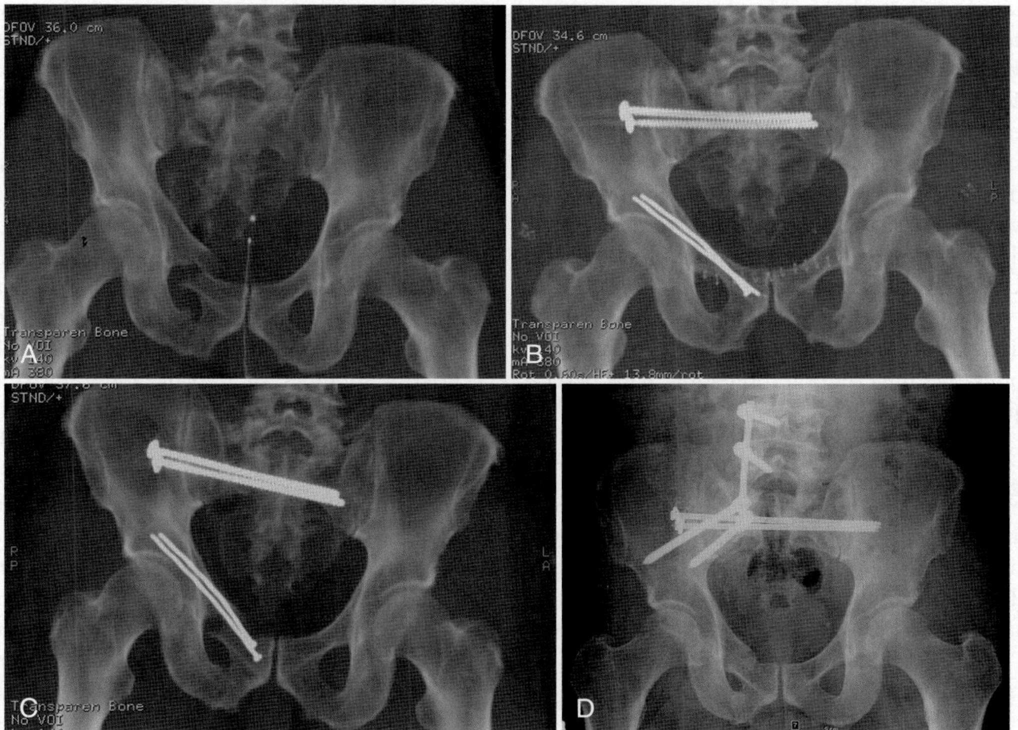

FIG. 78.13 (A) Right AO type B3 (Denis zone 2) sacral fracture treated with (B) closed reduction and percutaneous iliosacral screw and superior pubic ramus fixation. (C) Early fracture displacement required (D) revision with the triangular osteosynthesis variant of lumbopelvic fixation.

impairment, the severity of these impairments did not correlate directly with fracture characteristics but was more a function of associated injuries and sacral root function.[68,69]

Nonoperative Treatment

The traditional treatment of sacral fractures was by nonoperative means. Nonoperative treatment consists of a period of recumbency followed by protected weight bearing and possibly bracing to minimize load transfer to the sacrum. The period of recumbency varies considerably, depending on the extent of fracture instability. Recumbency is usually required in insufficiency fractures for pain control; in unstable fractures, it is required to allow for callus formation and to decrease the possibility of displacement. Displaced fractures are treated with skeletal traction to improve alignment and bifemoral traction has been used to improve alignment in complex sacral fractures with bilateral involvement.

Nonoperative treatment in displaced, high-energy sacral fractures can be problematic, however, and contradicts modern trauma principles of early mobilization of patients with multiple injuries. Although surgical complications can be avoided by using closed treatment methods, potential disadvantages include life-threatening pulmonary and thromboembolic events that are associated with prolonged recumbency in patients with multiple injuries, the development of decubitus ulcers, the inability to reliably relieve sacral canal and neuroforaminal compression, and the potential for late instability causing neurologic deficits and fixed deformities that are difficult to correct (see Fig. 78.1).[70]

Nonoperative treatment is most attractive in patients with minimally displaced, unilateral sacral fractures without associated neurologic deficits. Mobilization is usually with a walker or crutches enabling toe-touch weight bearing on the injured side. These patients must be followed carefully for fracture displacement, which may warrant surgical stabilization. Insufficiency or stress fractures are also usually amenable to nonoperative treatment in spite of frequent bilateral involvement. Along with activity modification and correction of underlying metabolic conditions, nonoperative treatment has a high likelihood of success in the majority of insufficiency and stress fractures and is usually the treatment of choice in these fractures. However, if patient mobility or pain control is sufficiently compromised, operative intervention, preferably with percutaneous techniques, may be the better option (Fig. 78.14).[38]

Operative Treatment

The goals of surgical treatment are twofold: (1) neurologic decompression in cases of neurologic deficit and (2) realignment and stabilization of the bony architecture in cases of significant displacement or instability. The timing of surgical intervention is dictated by many factors. The presence of an open fracture, either externally or into the alimentary or genital tracts, requires expeditious operative intervention with irrigation and debridement followed by surgical stabilization in cases with the potential for recurrent or persistent fracture displacement through the open wound. Neurologic deficit also suggests the need for immediate surgical decompression, though associated injuries and the patient's physiologic state may dictate the feasibility of doing so, given that decompression within 2 weeks of injury appears to be an acceptable time frame. Severe angulation of a transverse sacral fracture may also tent the overlying soft tissues and cause skin breakdown, particularly in patients whose body habitus or general physical condition predisposes them to pressure sores. In many cases, the multiply injured patient's physiologic status is the main determinant in the timing of operative intervention.

Neurologic Decompression

Decompression of the neural elements can be achieved by either direct or indirect means. Indirect decompression can sometimes be achieved simply with fracture reduction. An attempt at indirect decompression is best accomplished before consolidation of the fracture hematoma.[71] If neural impingement persists and is associated with a neurologic deficit, direct decompression should be considered.

In patients with sacral root deficits, direct decompression alone by laminectomy and removal of compressive bone fragments without stabilization has been advocated as a method for providing sacral root decompression, therefore theoretically enhancing the possibility of neurologic recovery while minimizing the potential for complications associated with more extensive dissection and surgical stabilization.[24] Whereas unilateral injuries can be approached with a parasagittal exposure, the surgical exposure for bilateral injuries is preferably through a posterior midline approach. The parasagittal approach is not recommended for anything more than percutaneous spinopelvic fixation of bilateral injuries because it limits exposure to the spine and may result in the need for bilateral parasagittal exposures, which are even less desirable owing to the potential for soft tissue necrosis. Intraoperative fluoroscopy is useful for orientation and to assess alignment and decompression of the spinal canal. Decompression can be performed focally for selective ventral foraminal impingement or to achieve a more comprehensive decompression of the S1–S4 neural elements. In the instance of L5 root entrapment between the L5 transverse process and an alar bone fragment, decompression is performed by following the root laterally onto the shoulder of the ala and removing the offending fragment.

The possibility of significant epidural bleeding during direct decompression requires experience with techniques of epidural hemostasis. Similarly, experience with neural element repair is essential and dural tears that are encountered should be repaired if possible. The dura at the sacral level is often relatively thin and friable, and direct repair is often best performed with fine (e.g., 6-0) monofilament suture. Augmentation with fibrin glue may be used to increase the strength of the repair. Often, a direct repair is not possible owing to the severity of the disruption, in which case a patch may be required. In many cases, the disruption is through individual nerve roots caudal to the termination of the dural sac at the S2 level and is irreparable.

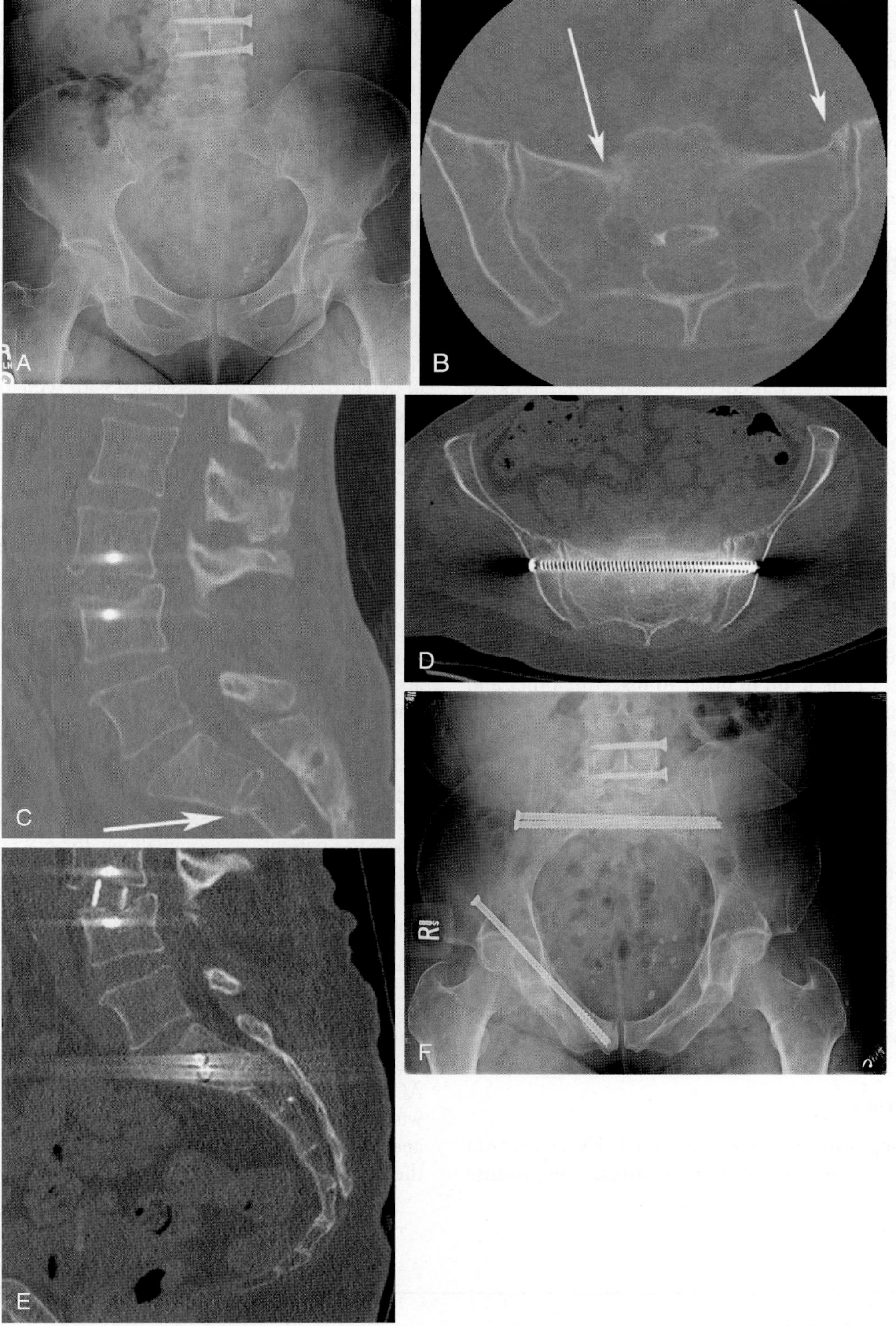

FIG. 78.14 AO type C0 sacral insufficiency fracture with right pubic ramus fracture treated by supine closed percutaneous transiliac-transsacral screw fixation. (A) Preoperative anteroposterior radiograph of the pelvis plus (B) axial and (C) sagittal lumbosacral spine computed tomographic (CT) images demonstrate minimally displaced sacral U insufficiency fracture (*arrows*) and right pubic ramus fracture in a patient with severe acute low back pain and sciatica whose symptoms were initially attributed to nonunion of a previous L3–L4 arthrodesis. (D) Postoperative axial and (E) sagittal CT images and (F) pelvic inlet radiograph after percutaneous fixation with two percutaneous transiliac-transsacral screws and a right percutaneous pubic ramus screw.

The utility of posterior decompression without fracture reduction and stabilization is limited, however, in cases of neural impingement caused by fracture displacement and is generally not recommended. In situations in which fracture displacement contributes significantly to nerve root compression, decompression is difficult to achieve solely with laminectomy and foraminotomy, and it is usually necessary to realign and stabilize the fracture.

Fracture Reduction Techniques

Unilateral Injuries

Unilateral, vertical AO type B sacral fractures are most commonly treated with closed reduction using distal femoral traction and percutaneous iliosacral or transiliac-transsacral screw fixation in the supine position. In more highly displaced fractures in which an acceptable closed reduction cannot be achieved, or if foraminal compression requires an open decompression and open reduction can be performed, typically prone through a posterior paramedian approach is appropriate. Exposure is typically performed as far medially as the spinous process of the sacrum, on which a reduction clamp can be hooked to provide medial-lateral fracture compression. A small soft tissue window can also be made along the lateral aspect of the ilium in order to place the other end of the clamp. Once the fracture is exposed, the fracture edges are debrided of soft tissue and foraminal debris can often be removed through the fracture surface. Reduction is then achieved by identifying fracture lines that correspond to each other. This can be particularly challenging in more comminuted fractures, but usually appropriate length can be assessed at the sciatic notch by either palpation or direct visualization. Once appropriate length has been established, the fracture is realigned and reduction is achieved with clamps placed between the sacral spinous processes and the ilium. Fixation is then undertaken percutaneously, usually with iliosacral or transiliac-transsacral screws. Decompression is performed if still deemed necessary.

Bilateral Injuries

When considering displaced sacral “U” fracture variants (AO type C3 injuries), spinal canal and foraminal compromise due to translation and angulation are often the main cause of nerve root compromise. In these cases, decompression, realignment, and stabilization are required. Realignment and stabilization of these fractures can be difficult, typically involving the following: (1) restoration of fracture length, (2) mobilization of impacted fracture fragments, (3) fracture reduction by direct manipulation, (4) provisional fracture stabilization with iliosacral or transiliac-transsacral screws, and (5) definitive fracture stabilization with spinopelvic fixation (Figs. 78.12 and 78.15). Fracture length can be obtained through distal bifemoral traction or direct manipulation with various instruments, including the universal distractor secured to the L5 pedicle and ipsilateral ilium (Fig. 78.16). The use of specialized fracture reduction tables designed for the treatment of pelvic fractures may also assist with reduction. Once length is obtained and access to the anterior column of the transverse fracture has been achieved by laminectomy and sacral root retraction, elevators or a lamina spreader can be used to pry the impacted fracture fragments apart (see Figs. 78.12 and 78.15). A combination of instruments can then be used to reduce the fracture, such as a threaded Schanz pin placed into the upper sacral body, which can be used as a joystick to help realign the fracture (see Figs. 78.12 and 78.15). The kyphotic segment may further be reduced by retracting the upper sacral nerve roots and using a bone impactor to directly reduce the apex of angulation. Reduction of the bilateral vertical sacral fracture components can be performed in a manner similar to that described earlier for unilateral sacral fractures. Once reduction is achieved, provisional stabilization can be obtained with either iliosacral or transiliac-transsacral screw fixation (see Figs. 78.12 and 78.15). In some situations, particularly when the patient’s anatomy allows for placement of multiple screws, this may provide enough stability. However, as will be described later, spinopelvic fixation provides additional stability and is typically used for definitive fixation of AO types C1 through C3 injuries. The typical reduction techniques are illustrated for Roy-Camille type 2 (see Fig. 78.12) and type 3 (see Fig. 78.15) sacral fractures. In situations in which anatomic reduction of the sacral kyphosis cannot be achieved or maintained, as is common with Roy-Camille type 2 variants of AO type C3 fractures in particular, sacral root decompression within the sacral canal can be enhanced by resection of the apex of the kyphosis along the anterior spinal canal, over which the sacral roots would otherwise be draped (see Fig. 78.12B).

FIG. 78.15 AO type C3 (Roy-Camille type 3). Reduction and stabilization of AO type C3, Roy-Camille type 3 sacral fracture. (A) Anteroposterior computed tomographic (CT) reconstruction of the pelvis and (B) sagittal CT image of the sacrum demonstrate Roy-Camille type 3 variant of AO type C3 sacral fracture with anterior pelvic ring injury and severe urinary bladder distention caused by sacral root dysfunction. (C) The sequence of fracture reduction is illustrated, involving prying open the transverse fracture with elevators, followed by fracture manipulation with a Schanz pin inserted as a joystick into the upper sacral body, and direct pressure applied to the posterior lower sacrum by a spike-pusher. Once the fracture had been reduced, a transiliac-transsacral screw was placed for provisional stability, followed by spinopelvic fixation, as illustrated on postoperative (D) anteroposterior and (E) inlet reconstructions. (F) Postoperative sagittal CT image of the sacrum demonstrates restoration of sagittal plane alignment and decompression of the spinal canal. Anatomic reduction is typically easier to achieve with Roy Camille type 2 fractures.

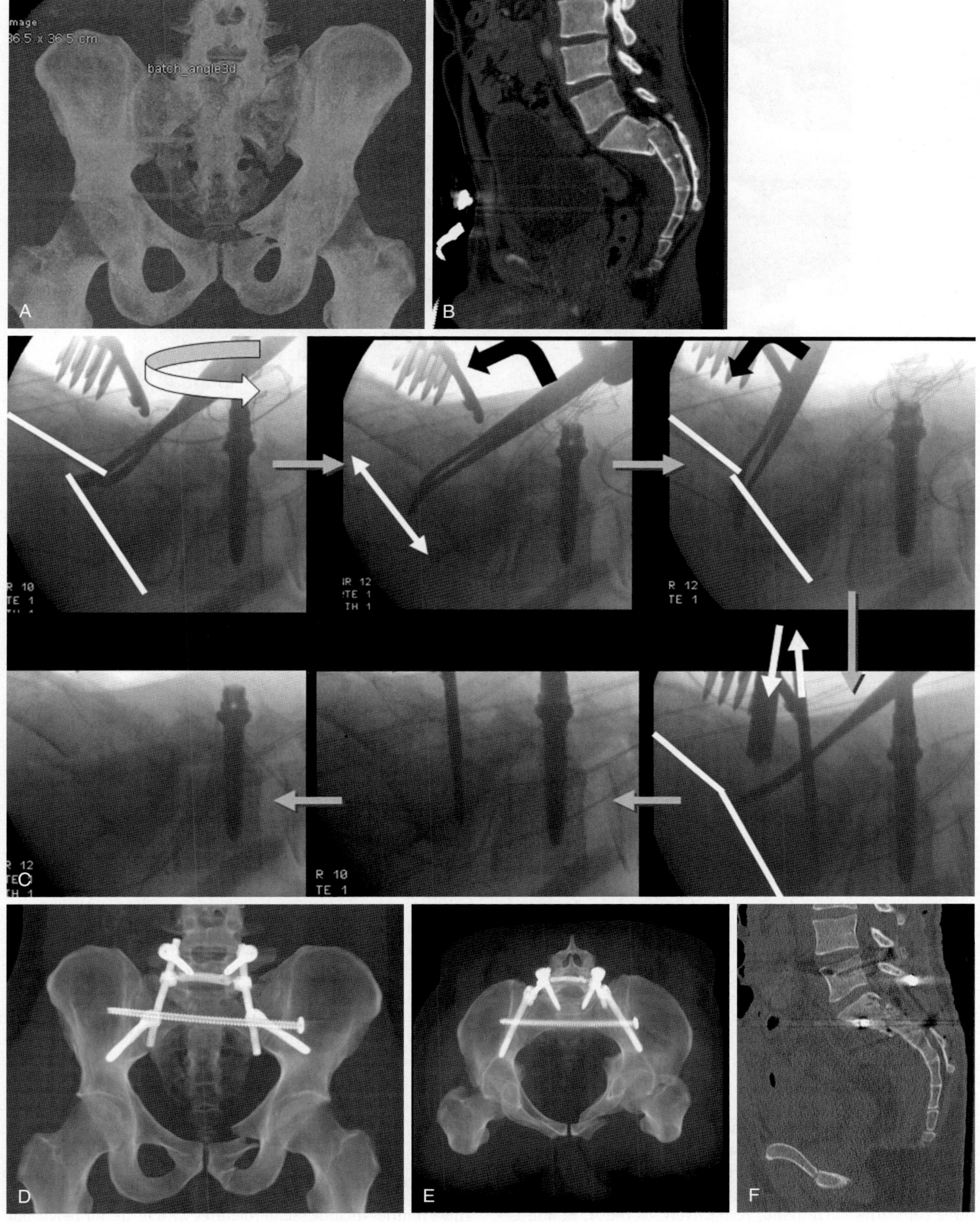
mage
36.5 x 36.5 cm
batch_angle3d
A
B
R 10
TE 1
IR 12
TE 1
IH 1
R 12
TE 1
R 12
TE
TH 1
C
R 10
TE 1
D
E
F

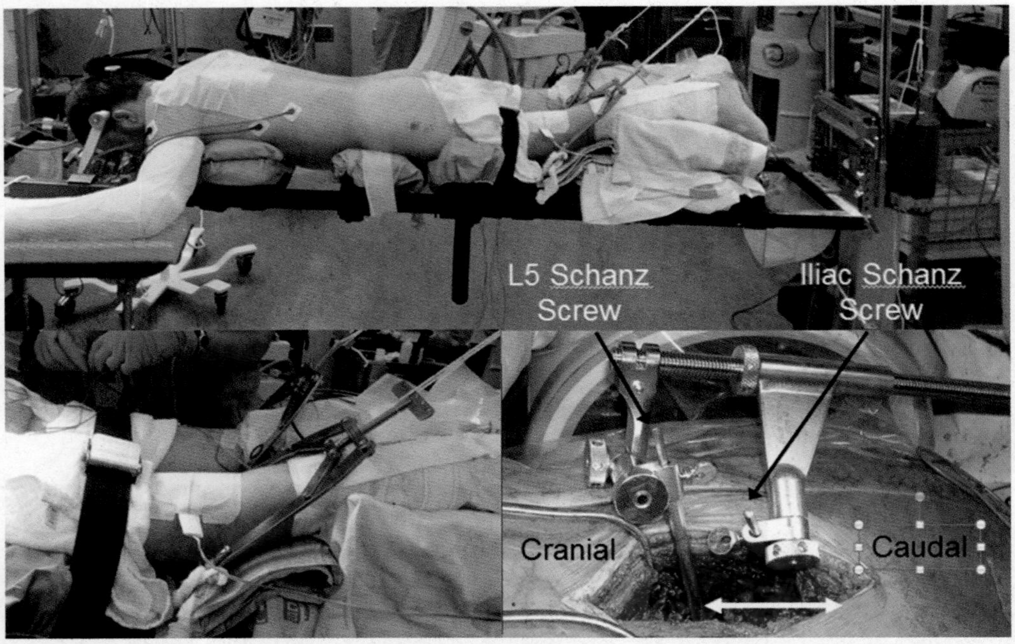

FIG. 78.16 Restoration of fracture length can be the most challenging step in reducing complex sacral fractures. Several techniques can be used to restore fracture length at the spinopelvic junction, including distal femoral traction and the use of a femoral distractor anchored to the lumbar pedicles and the ipsilateral iliac wing.

Surgical Stabilization Techniques

The goal of surgical fixation is to avoid prolonged recumbency and to correct and prevent fracture displacement and malalignment, which may lead to postural difficulties, chronic pain, and nerve compression. Hart et al. reported that restoration of appropriate sagittal alignment of sacral fractures decreases pain by preventing compensatory lumbar hyperlordosis, allowing for a more physiologic alignment of the lumbar spine (see Fig. 78.1).[5] Therefore, pelvic incidence can be used as an intraoperative guide to lumbopelvic alignment and adequacy of reduction.

There are three broad categories of fixation types for sacral fractures: (1) direct osteosynthesis of the sacrum, (2) posterior pelvic ring stabilization, and (3) spinopelvic fixation. The appropriate fixation type is based on the fracture pattern and location. Optimal stabilization may require use of multiple sacral fixation techniques. The three situations most commonly encountered in this decision-making process involve the following: (1) low transverse sacral fracture below the sacroiliac joint, in which there are no implications of either posterior pelvic or spinopelvic instability; (2) vertical sacral fracture with unilateral pelvic instability (and intact spinopelvic junction); and (3) complex sacral fracture with spinopelvic and usually also posterior pelvic instability (e.g., sacral "U" fracture variant or bilateral vertical sacral fracture). These three categories correspond, respectively, to the A, B, and C fracture types proposed in the new AO spinopelvic injury classification (see Fig. 78.11).

AO Sacral Fracture Classification Type A Injuries

These injuries include sacral fractures without posterior pelvic or spinopelvic instability. A few fixation options have been described to treat isolated transverse or oblique sacral fractures without pelvic involvement. Roy-Camille[28] described a technique for direct osteosynthesis of sacral fractures with sacral alar plates. The plates are placed lateral to the dorsal foramina and oriented vertically. The orientation of these plates is theoretically optimal to allow for compression loading across a transverse fracture. Although not recommended for stabilization of spinopelvic dissociation injuries, direct plating alone may be useful in maintaining alignment of transverse sacral fractures below the sacroiliac joints because these fractures are not subject to the high loads seen with fractures involving the weight-bearing axis, and the goal of their treatment is primarily to avoid pain due to prominence or nonunion.[67] It can be combined with spinopelvic fixation techniques if there is a need to maintain alignment of the lower sacrum while having to stabilize a contiguous spinopelvic dissociation injury. Sacral alar plating alone therefore has few clinical applications. Its utility is usually in combination with other methods of surgical stabilization in the treatment of sacral fractures involving the weight-bearing axis.[72]

AO Sacral Fracture Classification Type B Injuries

These injuries include sacral fractures with posterior pelvic but not spinopelvic instability. Displaced unilateral vertical sacral fractures are generally treated with posterior stabilization.

Sacral bars, tension band plating, iliosacral screws and, most recently, transiliac-transsacral screws have all been described as a means of stabilizing the posterior pelvic ring.[53,73,74] Simonian and Routt,[75] in a biomechanical study of cadaveric specimens, found no difference in the resulting pelvic ring stability between the various constructs. Sacral bars and tension band plating are both predisposed to soft tissue problems owing to their location superficial to the nearly subcutaneous dorsal sacrum.[73] The potential for dorsal soft tissue compromise is minimized by the use of iliosacral or transiliac-transsacral screw fixation; these methods have become the most widely used for posterior pelvic ring fixation. In all methods of posterior pelvic ring stabilization, however, fixation is perpendicular to the weight-bearing axis and does not provide adequate stabilization for immediate weight bearing.[74,76,77]

Iliosacral and transiliac-transsacral screw fixation are usually performed in a percutaneous manner, with minimal blood loss. The success of percutaneous fixation depends on the surgeon's ability to achieve an anatomic reduction under fluoroscopic visualization; otherwise, in addition to the problem of malreduction, a safe trajectory for iliosacral/transiliac-transsacral screw placement cannot be reliably established.[61,78] These techniques can be performed with the patient in either a supine or prone position depending in part on surgeon preference and on the potential need for either concurrent anterior pelvic ring stabilization or open posterior reduction or decompression of foraminal debris. In spite of its advantages, iliosacral and transiliac-transsacral screw fixation have several potential pitfalls. In the instance of comminuted longitudinal fractures through the neuroforamina (AO type B3), overcompression of the foramina can occur if the screws are placed using interfragmentary compression, which can potentially lead to nerve root injury.[79] However, in experienced centers, the reported rate of neurologic injury is low even without the use of electrodiagnostic monitoring.[80] Like other methods of closed reduction and posterior pelvic ring stabilization alone, percutaneous iliosacral and transiliac-transsacral screw fixation carry the disadvantage of not allowing for reduction of sacral angulation. Combining these techniques with open reduction can provide the necessary kyphocorrection, but may not provide the adequate stability for preventing failure of fixation and recurrent deformity. In the case of sacral comminution or osteoporosis, transiliac-transsacral screws should be used in lieu of iliosacral screws since fixation into the contralateral ilium is likely to provide far better stability than fixation of an iliosacral screw into the compromised bone of the sacrum. As mentioned previously, the orientation of the screw perpendicular to the fracture's deforming forces may also contribute to a higher likelihood of fixation failure (see Fig. 78.13). Nevertheless, iliosacral and transiliac-transsacral screw fixation have been shown to be effective in the stabilization of unstable longitudinal sacral fractures.[81] A 3-month period of protected weight bearing is recommended with iliosacral and transiliac-transsacral screw fixation.

AO Sacral Fracture Classification Type C Injuries

These injuries include sacral fractures with spinopelvic instability. Contrary to sacral bars and posterior tension band plating, which are largely ineffective in stabilizing multiplanar sacral fractures with a transverse component, iliosacral and transiliac-transsacral screws can also be used successfully in patients with minimally displaced sacral "U" fracture variants, whether AO type C0 or C3, as well as in bilateral vertical sacral fractures (AO type C2). In a series of 13 patients who had fractures with minimal sacral angulation and displacement allowing for in situ screw placement, Nork and colleagues[82] found bilateral percutaneous iliosacral screw fixation to be safe and effective in treating minimally displaced sacral U-type fracture patterns. In our experience, this technique has been particularly well suited for treatment of AO type C0 sacral U variant insufficiency fractures (see Fig. 78.14). However, this minimally invasive method does not allow for reduction of fracture angulation. Moreover, if a near-anatomic reduction cannot be achieved, the safe zone for iliosacral and transiliac-transsacral screw trajectory may be small or absent, thus also precluding its use in more complex and highly displaced injuries.[78] Iliosacral or transiliac-transsacral screw fixation alone is therefore not generally recommended for patients with displaced AO type C3 (sacral U) fractures and their variants if they are irreducible by closed manipulation or if neural decompression is required.

Lumbopelvic fixation provides the biomechanically strongest fixation of sacral fractures.[83] This technique was derived from the Galveston method of anchoring the caudal end of long thoracolumbar rod constructs into the ilium. Sacral fracture fixation is obtained rostrally by pedicle screw fixation in the lumbosacral spine and caudally by long screw fixation in the ilium.[84–94] The construct spans the sacrum and restores the integrity of load transfer from the lumbar spine to the pelvis.[44,83] Lumbopelvic fixation can be applied unilaterally (triangular osteosynthesis) to add more stability to iliosacral/transiliac-transsacral screw fixation for highly displaced or comminuted unilateral AO type B or AO type C1 longitudinal sacral fractures, or bilaterally for AO type C2 and C3 spinopelvic dissociation injuries and occasionally AO type C0 injuries. The strength of the construct permits immediate weight bearing without the use of external bracing (see Figs. 78.12 and 78.15).

Bilateral lumbopelvic fixation is most commonly indicated for AO types C2, C3, and some C0 injuries and is performed through a midline longitudinal dorsal approach with the patient in the prone position. Screw placement may be performed under fluoroscopic guidance or some other form of navigation to ensure correct screw orientation. A thorough understanding of pelvic anatomy is necessary for verification of correct iliac screw placement. Screw malposition can be catastrophic, potentially injuring neurovascular structures in the sciatic notch or the pelvic viscera or penetrating the acetabulum. Choice of a more anterior iliac screw starting point, such as along the medial (rather than posterior) surface of the posterior ilium or on the dorsolateral surface of the sacrum, can help prevent excessive prominence of the iliac screw heads. Infection and wound-related problems are common, however, and have been found to approach 20%.[85,90] In situations in which formal open reduction is not required but iliosacral/transiliac-transsacral screw fixation is considered to be insufficient, percutaneous lumbopelvic fixation can be used to provide enhanced stability while mitigating the risk of wound-related complications. Formal lumbosacral arthrodesis is not typically performed in the absence of preexisting pathology (e.g., spondylolisthesis) or injury to the lumbosacral facet joints. Hardware removal is generally performed 6 months postoperatively after imaging studies have confirmed healing of the sacral fracture. Hardware removal is not performed in patients who have had lumbosacral arthrodesis. In these cases, because formal sacroiliac joint arthrodesis is not usually performed, in many instances the rod will break from fatigue failure, an expected consequence of continued sacroiliac joint motion. Late rod fracture is asymptomatic in the majority of cases, and the need for routine hardware removal in all circumstances is questionable.[85,90]

The optimal stabilization of complex sacral fractures may require the use of a combination of the three categories of fixation described earlier. For instance, sacral U or H fractures can be stabilized with the use of iliosacral or transiliac/transsacral screw fixation combined with lumbopelvic fixation to obtain optimal fixation in the "horizontal" direction to stabilize the posterior pelvic ring and in the "vertical" direction along the weight-bearing axis to neutralize spinopelvic instability.[83,89] Lumbopelvic fixation of sacral fractures requiring neural decompression may also benefit from adjunctive sacral plating, which, in this case, is used solely to fine-tune fracture realignment and to prevent recurrent displacement and resulting nerve root compression, allowing the lumbopelvic fixation to neutralize the bulk of the loads being transferred across the sacrum.

Summary

Sacral fractures have emerged from relatively underappreciated entities to injuries whose optimal treatment is recognized to have profound consequences on the patient's functional outcome. Advances in diagnostic imaging continue to provide additional insights into the structural and neurologic aspects of the injured sacrum, allowing comprehensive injury assessment even in the cognitively impaired and polytraumatized patient. In cases of neurologic deficit, excessive malalignment or instability, surgical intervention involves neurologic decompression, fracture realignment, and surgical fixation in order to optimize long-term outcomes. The timing of surgical intervention is determined by several factors, including the patient's associated injuries, overall physiologic condition, and the presence of neurologic deficits, open fractures, or soft tissue compromise that places skin at risk of necrosis. Surgical options continue to expand as new stabilization methods and implants are developed. Surgeons now have a wide spectrum of procedures at their disposal, ranging from minimally invasive to comprehensive stabilization techniques. Many issues concerning evaluation and treatment remain controversial and, in the absence of comparative treatment trials, conclusions are currently based largely on anecdotal reports and observations. The benefits of any proposed treatment need to be weighed carefully against the potential risks and must be individualized to the patient and specific injury. Treatment decisions continue to be based on a substantial degree of intuition and foresight gained from experience. The challenge to the spine surgeon remains to implement the available resources effectively as our understanding of the pathophysiology of these injuries grows.

PEARLS

1. The evaluation of sacral root function is paramount in patients with sacral fractures and should include assessment of anal sphincter tone, voluntary anal contraction, sharp/dull perineal sensation, and reflexes, such as the anal wink and bulbocavernosus reflex.
2. Intraoperative bilateral distal femoral traction and the universal distractor applied across the spinopelvic junction can help achieve the fracture length required for reduction in complex AO type C3 sacral U fractures.
3. In patients with associated anterior pelvic ring or acetabular fractures, fixing the anterior pelvic injury first facilitates reduction of complex sacral fractures and, in some acetabular fractures, decreases the risk of articular malreduction.
4. Accurate placement of iliac screws can be facilitated and confirmed with a true lateral C-arm trajectory that allows superimposition of the sciatic notches and the obturator outlet (teardrop) view.
5. When placing spinopelvic fixation, a starting point along the medial aspect of the posterior ilium or within the sacrum allows for iliac screw heads to be buried as deep as possible relative to the posterior ilium, which minimizes the risk of screw prominence that might require reoperation.

PITFALLS

1. Spontaneous partial fracture reduction can lead to the deceptively innocuous radiographic appearance of an inherently unstable injury.
2. A fracture–dislocation in this region can lead to critical blood loss.
3. The subcutaneous nature of the sacrum exposes any open surgical approach in this region to higher risk of infection.
4. Sacral root decompression is typically not successfully achieved when there is significant residual fracture malreduction.
5. Diagnostic delay may increase the risk of prolonged neurologic deficit and fixed spinal deformity that is difficult and risky to correct.

KEY POINTS

1. The sacrum is a keystone structure that is important to the structural integrity of the base of the spinal column and posterior pelvic ring. Therefore, depending on the fracture pattern, fracture of the sacrum may have implications on posterior pelvic or spinopelvic stability.
2. Sacral fracture classifications are based on fracture location, pattern of instability, and risk of neurologic deficits.
3. Sacral fractures generally occur as the result of either high-energy injuries, in which associated injuries will likely have an impact on treatment decisions, or low-energy injuries due to sacral insufficiency, in which associated medical comorbidities are likely to influence treatment decisions.
4. Multidimensional (CT) imaging of the sacrum is essential for evaluating fracture patterns and determining the extent of instability.

5. Various options exist for the treatment of sacral fractures. Minimally displaced fractures can often be treated nonoperatively. Displaced, unilateral longitudinal (AO type B1–3) fracture patterns result in posterior pelvic instability and are generally treated with reduction and iliosacral or transiliac-transsacral screw fixation. Unilateral lumbopelvic fixation provides additional stability for widely displaced injuries, those requiring a decompression procedure, or those involving the L5–S1 facet joint (AO type C1). Bilateral lumbopelvic fixation is the most stable construct for complex sacral fractures with bilateral involvement and spinopelvic dissociation (AO types C2 and C3). In situations with neural compromise, decompression usually requires excision of bony fragments causing nerve root compression, as well as fracture realignment and stabilization. Multiplanar, minimally displaced sacral insufficiency fractures (AO type C0) may require surgical treatment, in which case iliosacral or transiliac-transsacral screw fixation is most commonly used.

KEY REFERENCES

1. Denis F. Sacral fractures. An important problem—a retrospective analysis of 236 cases. *Clin Orthop*. 1988;227:67-81.
This is arguably the seminal publication on sacral fractures to date. Despite limitations of being retrospective with a multicenter, mail-in response study design and using outdated workup and surgical management options, this publication provides a comprehensive review of the entire severity spectrum of sacral fractures and an unsurpassed clinical experience perspective on this subject.
2. Gibbons KJ, Soloniuk DS, Razack N. Neurological injury and patterns of sacral fractures. *J Neurosurg*. 1990;72:889-893.
The subject of sacral neurologic injury is frequently overlooked. This publication provides a meaningful sacral root injury severity classification and provides class 3 data supporting the concept of decompression surgery.
3. Huittinen VM. Lumbosacral nerve injury in fracture of the pelvis. *Acta Chir Scand Suppl*. 1972;429:7-43.
This seminal publication provided the foundation for an improved understanding of sacral root function and prevalence of transection and the possibility for recovery. It also underscored the potential for patients with unilateral preservation of S2 and S3 roots to have meaningful bowel and bladder control.
4. Peretz AM, Hipp JA, Heggeness MH. The internal bony architecture of the sacrum. *Spine*. 1998;23:971-974.
These authors provide an important review of the structural idiosyncrasies of the sacrum. On the basis of these findings, the relevance of the S1 segment in transferring the lumbar loads to the iliac wings is underscored. Furthermore, the foundations for ideal fixation points for sacral promontory, alar, and iliac screw placement are provided.
5. Routt MLC, Nork SE, Mills WJ. Percutaneous fixation of pelvic ring disruptions. *Clin Orthop*. 2000;375:15-29.
The authors provide a retrospective review of minimally invasive stabilization strategies for posterior pelvic ring disruption. This technique has strongly influenced the treatment of patients with pelvic ring injuries.
6. Schildhauer TA, Ledoux WR, Chapman JR, et al. Triangular osteosynthesis and iliosacral screw fixation for unstable sacral fractures: a cadaveric and biomechanical evaluation under cyclic loads. *J Orthop Trauma*. 2003;17:22-31.
These authors provide biomechanical data for the stiffness of lumbopelvic stabilization techniques using simple current segmental spine fixation components over posterior sacroiliac screw fixation for vertically unstable sacral fractures.
7. Bellabarba C, Schildhauer TA, Vaccaro AR, Chapman JR. Complications associated with surgical stabilization of high-grade sacral fracture dislocations with spino-pelvic instability. *Spine*. 2006;31(suppl 11):S80-S88.
These authors provide an analysis of morbidity associated with high-grade sacral fracture-dislocations and their treatment. They identified traumatic dural tears or root avulsions in 74% of patients. Wound-healing problems including postoperative infection or draining seroma or hematoma were present in 26% of patients, with no cases of chronic osteomyelitis. Hardware prominence was problematic, particularly early in the series. There was a notable absence of nonunion, malunion, and failure of fixation.
8. Schildhauer TA, Bellabarba C, Nork SE, et al. Decompression and lumbopelvic fixation for sacral fracture-dislocations with spino-pelvic dissociation. *J Orthop Trauma*. 2006;20:447-457.
These authors provide a retrospective review of a series of patients with high-grade sacral fracture-dislocations and cauda equina injuries who were treated with lumbopelvic fixation. They noted that this method of fixation reliably achieved the goal of correction of sacral kyphosis and provided adequate stabilization, thereby preventing fracture malunion or nonunion. Neurologic improvement occurred in 83% of patients and depended primarily on completeness of the injury and continuity of sacral roots. The majority of complications were wound related or associated with hardware prominence.
9. Gardner MJ, Routt ML Jr. Transiliac-transsacral screws for posterior pelvic stabilization. *J Orthop Trauma*. 2011;25:378-384.
These authors provide a comprehensive assessment of the use of transiliac-transsacral screw fixation, which provides a more stable alternative to iliosacral screw fixation, particularly in the presence of extensive comminution or osteopenia of the upper sacral bodies.
10. Bellabarba C, Bransford RJ. Spinopelvic fixation. In: Vialle LR, Bellabarba C, Kandziora F, eds. *AOSpine Masters Series. Vol 6: Thoracolumbar Spine Trauma*. New York: Thieme; 2016:152-183.
These authors describe a new, comprehensive classification of sacral fractures that categorizes the injuries based on their implications on posterior pelvic and spinopelvic stability, neurologic function, and presence of additional factors that may affect treatment or prognosis.

REFERENCES

1. Williams PL, Warwick R, Dyson M, et al., eds. *Gray's Anatomy*. New York: Churchill Livingstone; 1989.
2. Jackson RP, McManus AC. Radiographic analysis of sagittal plane alignment and balance in standing volunteers and patients with low back pain matched for age, sex, and size. *Spine*. 1994;19:1611-1618.
3. Wiltse LL, Winter RB. Terminology and measurement of spondylolisthesis. *J Bone Joint Surg Am*. 1983;65:768-772.
4. Legaye J, Duval-Beaupere G, Hecquet J, et al. Pelvic incidence: a fundamental pelvic parameter for three dimensional regulation of spinal sagittal curves. *Eur Spine J*. 1998;7:99-103.
5. Hart RA, Badra MI, Madala A, Yoo JU. Use of pelvic incidence as a guide to reduction of H-type spino-pelvic dissociation injuries. *J Orthop Trauma*. 2007;21:369-374.
6. Schmidek HH, Smith D, Kristiansen TK. Sacral fractures: issues of neural injury, spinal stability, and surgical management. In: Dunsker SB, et al., eds. *The Unstable Spine*. New York: Harcourt; 1986.
7. Tile M. *Fractures of the Pelvis and Acetabulum*. 2nd ed. Baltimore: Williams & Wilkins; 1995.

8. Morris H, Lond MB, eds. *Human Anatomy*. Philadelphia: P. Blakiston's Son & Co; 1989.
9. Williams P, Warwick R, Dyson M, et al., eds. *Gray's Anatomy*. 37th ed. Edinburgh: Churchill Livingstone; 1989.
10. Routt ML, Simonian PT, Agnew SG, Mann FA. Radiographic recognition of the sacral alar slope for optimal placement of iliosacral screws: a cadaveric and clinical study. *J Orthop Trauma*. 1996;10:171-177.
11. Peretz AM, Hipp JA, Heggeness MH. The internal bony architecture of the sacrum. *Spine*. 1998;23:971-974.
12. Smith SA, Abitbol JJ, Carlson GD, et al. The effects of depth of penetration, screw orientation and bone density on sacral screw fixation. *Spine*. 1993;18:1006-1010.
13. Carter SR. Stress fracture of the sacrum: brief report. *J Bone Joint Surg*. 1987;69:843-884.
14. Denis F, Davis S, Comfort T. Sacral fractures: an important problem-a retrospective analysis of 236 cases. *Clin Orthop*. 1988;227:67-81.
15. Mirkovic S, Abitbol JJ, Steinman J, et al. Anatomic consideration for sacral screw placement. *Spine*. 1991;16:S289-S294.
16. Esses SI, Botsford DJ, Huler RJ, Rauschning W. Surgical anatomy of the sacrum: a guide for rational screw fixation. *Spine*. 1991;16:S283-S288.
17. Gunterberg B. Effects of major resection of the sacrum. *Acta Orthop Scand Suppl*. 1976;162:1-38.
18. *Grant's Atlas of Anatomy*. 8th ed. Baltimore: Williams & Wilkins; 1983.
19. Bonnin JG. Sacral fractures. *J Bone Joint Surg Am*. 1945;27: 113-127.
20. Sabiston CP, Wing PC. Sacral fractures: classification and neurologic implications. *J Trauma*. 1986;26:1113-1115.
21. Schmidek HH, Smith DA, Kristiansen TK. Sacral fractures. *Neurosurgery*. 1984;15:735-746.
22. Gibbons KJ, Soloniuk DS, Razack N. Neurological injury and patterns of sacral fractures. *J Neurosurg*. 1990;72:889-893.
23. Huittinen VM. Lumbosacral nerve injury in fracture of the pelvis. *Acta Chir Scand Suppl*. 1972;429:7-43.
24. Fountain SS, Hamilton RD, Jameson RM. Transverse fractures of the sacrum: a report of six cases. *J Bone Joint Surg Am*. 1977;59:486-489.
25. Rao SH. Traumatic transverse fracture of sacrum with cauda equina injury: a case report and review of literature. *J Postgrad Med*. 1998;44:14-15.
26. Phelan ST, Jones DA, Bishay M. Conservative management of transverse fractures of the sacrum with neurological features: a report of four cases. *J Bone Joint Surg Br*. 1991;73:969-971.
27. Fisher RG. Sacral fracture with compression of cauda equina: Surgical treatment. *J Trauma*. 1998;28:1678-1680.
28. Roy-Camille R, Saillant G, Gogna G, Mazel C. Transverse fracture of the upper sacrum: suicidal jumper's fracture. *Spine*. 1985;10:838-845.
29. Strange-Vognsen HH, Lebech A. An unusual type of fracture in the upper sacrum. *J Orthop Trauma*. 1991;5:200-203.
30. Schildhauer TA, Chapman JR, Mayo KA. Multisegmental open sacral fracture due to impalement: a case report. *J Orthop Trauma*. 2005;19:134-139.
31. Bellabarba C, Stewart JD, Ricci WM, et al. Midline sagittal sacral fractures in anterior-posterior compression ring injuries. *J Orthop Trauma*. 2003;17:32-37.
32. Hatem SF, West OC. Vertical fracture of the central sacral canal: plane and simple. *J Trauma*. 1996;40:138-140.
33. Wiesel SW, Zeide MS, Terry RL. Longitudinal fracture of the sacrum: case report. *J Trauma*. 1979;19:70-71.
34. Isler B. Lumbosacral lesions associated with pelvic ring injuries. *J Orthop Trauma*. 1990;4:1-6.
35. Herman MP, Kopetz S, Bhosale PR, et al. Sacral insufficiency fractures after preoperative chemoradiation for rectal cancer: incidence, risk factors, and clinical course. *Int J Radiat Oncol Biol Phys*. 2009;74:818-823.
36. Gotis-Graham I, McGuigan L, Diamond T, et al. Sacral insufficiency fractures in the elderly. *J Bone Joint Surg Br*. 1994;76:882-886.
37. Weber M, Haster P, Gerber H, et al. Insufficiency fractures of the sacrum: twenty cases and review of the literature. *Spine*. 1993;18:2507-2512.
38. Jacquot JM, Finiels H, Fardjad S, et al. Neurological complications in insufficiency fractures of the sacrum: three case reports. *Rev Rhum Engl Ed*. 1999;66:109-113.
39. Wood KB, Geissele AE, Ogilvie JW. Pelvic fractures after long lumbosacral spine fusions. *Spine*. 1996;21:1357-1362.
40. Elias WJ, Shaffrey ME, Whitehill R. Sacral stress fracture following lumbosacral arthrodesis: case illustration. *J Neurosurg*. 2002;96(suppl 1):135.
41. Fourney DR, Prabhu SS, Cohen ZR, et al. Early sacral stress fractures after reduction of spondylolisthesis and lumbosacral fixation: case report. *Neurosurgery*. 2002;51:1510-1511.
42. Klineberg E, McHenry T, Bellabarba C, et al. Sacral insufficiency fractures caudal to instrumented posterior lumbosacral arthrodesis. *Spine*. 2008;33:1806-1811.
43. Mathews V, McCance SE, O'Leary PF. Early fracture of the sacrum or pelvis: an unusual complication after multilevel instrumented lumbosacral fusion. *Spine*. 2001;26:E571-E575.
44. Wood KB, Schendel MJ, Ogilvie JW, et al. Effect of sacral and iliac instrumentation on strains in the pelvis. *Spine*. 1996;21:1185-1191.
45. Bellabarba C, Bransford RJ. Spinopelvic Fixation. In: Vialle LR, Bellabarba C, Kandziora F, eds. *AOSpine Masters Series. Vol 6: Thoracolumbar Spine Trauma*. New York: Thieme; 2016:152-183.
46. Laasonen EM. Missed sacral fractures. *Ann Clin Res*. 1977;9: 84-87.
47. Course ATLS. *Manual: Advanced Trauma Life Support*; 2012. American College of Surgeons.
48. Kellam JF, McMurtry RY, Paley D, Tile M. The unstable pelvic fracture: operative treatment. *Orthop Clin North Am*. 1987;18:25-41.
49. Ben-Menachem Y, Coldwell DM, Young JW, Burgess AR. Hemorrhage associated with pelvic fractures: causes, diagnosis, and emergent management. *AJR Am J Roentgenol*. 1991;157:1005-1014.
50. Byrnes DP, Russo GL, Duckert TB, Cowley RA. Sacrum fractures and neurological damage: report of two cases. *J Neurosurg*. 1977;47:459-462.
51. Goodell CL. Neurological deficits associated with pelvic fractures. *J Neurosurg*. 1966;24:837-842.
52. Lam CR. Nerve injury in fractures of the pelvis. *Ann Surg*. 1936;104:945-951.
53. Routt ML Jr, Simonian PT. Closed reduction and percutaneous skeletal fixation of sacral fractures. *Clin Orthop*. 1996;329:121-128.
54. Cohen BA, Major MR, Huizenga BA. Pudendal nerve evoked potential monitoring in procedures involving low sacral fixation. *Spine*. 1991;16:S375-S378.
55. Helfet DL, Koval KJ, Hissa EA, et al. Intraoperative somatosensory evoked potential monitoring during acute pelvic fracture surgery. *J Orthop Trauma*. 1995;9:28-34.

56. Kothbauer K, Schmid UD, Seiler RW, Eisner W. Intraoperative motor and sensory monitoring of the cauda equina. *Neurosurgery*. 1994;34:702-707.
57. Slimp JC. Electrophysiologic intraoperative monitoring for spine procedures. *Phys Med Rehabil Clin N Am*. 2004;15: 85-105.
58. Kuklo TR, Potter BK, Ludwig SC, et al. Spine Trauma Study Group: radiographic measurement techniques for sacral fractures consensus statement of the Spine Trauma Study Group. *Spine*. 2006;31:1047-1055.
59. Sasaka KK, Phisitkul P, Boyd JL, et al. Lumbosacral nerve root avulsions: MR imaging demonstration of acute abnormalities. *AJNR Am J Neuroradiol*. 2006;27:1944-1946.
60. Bone LB, Johnson KD, Weigelt J, Scheinberg R. Early versus delayed stabilization of femoral fractures: a prospective randomized study. *J Bone Joint Surg Am*. 1989; 71:336-340.
61. Johnson KD, Cadambi A, Seibert GB. Incidence of adult respiratory distress syndrome in patients with multiple musculoskeletal injuries: effect of early operative stabilization of fractures. *J Trauma*. 1985;25:375-384.
62. Jaicks RR, Cohn SM, Moller BA. Early fracture fixation may be deleterious after head injury. *J Trauma*. 1977;42:1-5.
63. Scalea TM, Scott JD, Brumback RJ, et al. Early fracture fixation may be "just fine" after head injury: no difference in central nervous system outcomes. *J Trauma*. 1999;46:839-846.
64. Marcus RE, Hansen ST. Bilateral fracture-dislocation of the sacrum: a case report. *J Bone Joint Surg Am*. 1984;66: 1297-1299.
65. Pennal GF, Tile M, Waddell JP, Garside H. Pelvic disruption: assessment and classification. *Clin Orthop*. 1980;151:12-21.
66. Wild J, Hanson GW, Tullas HS. Unstable fractures of the pelvis treated by external fixation. *J Bone Joint Surg Am*. 1982;64:1010-1020.
67. Sommer C. Fixation of transverse fractures of the sternum and sacrum with the locking compression plate system: two case reports. *J Orthop Trauma*. 2005;19:487-490.
68. Tötterman A, Glott T, Søberg HL, et al. Pelvic trauma with displaced sacral fractures: functional outcome at one year. *Spine*. 2007;32:1437-1443.
69. Tötterman A, Glott T, Madsen JE, Røise O. Unstable sacral fractures: associated injuries and morbidity at 1 year. *Spine*. 2006;31:E628-E635.
70. Latenser BA, Gentilello LM, Tarver AA, et al. Improved outcome with early fixation of skeletally unstable pelvic fractures. *J Trauma*. 1991;31:28-31.
71. Pohlemann T, Angst A, Schneider E, et al. Fixation of transforaminal sacrum fractures: a biomechanical study. *J Orthop Trauma*. 1993;2:107-117.
72. Templeman D, Goulet J, Dawelius PJ, et al. Internal fixation of displaced fractures of the sacrum. *Clin Orthop*. 1996;329:180-185.
73. Suzuki T, Hak DJ, Ziran BH, et al. Outcome and complications of posterior transiliac plating for vertically unstable sacral fractures. *Injury*. 2009;40:405-409.
74. Gardner MJ, Routt ML Jr. Transiliac-transsacral screws for posterior pelvic stabilization. *J Orthop Trauma*. 2011;25: 378-384.
75. Simonian PT, Routt ML Jr. Biomechanics of pelvic fixation. *Orthop Clin North Am*. 1997;28:351-368.
76. Suzuki K, Mochida J. Operative treatment of a transverse fracture-dislocation at the S1-S2 level. *J Orthop Trauma*. 2001;15:363-367.
77. Taguchi T, Kawai S, Kaneko K, Yugue D. Operative management of displaced fractures of the sacrum. *J Orthop Sci*. 1999;4:347-352.
78. Reilly MC, Bono CM, Litkouhi B, et al. The effect of sacral fracture malreduction on the safe placement of iliosacral screws. *J Orthop Trauma*. 2003;17:88-94.
79. Routt MLC, Simonian PT, Swiontkowski MF. Stabilization of pelvic ring disruptions. *Orthop Clin North Am*. 1997;28:369-388.
80. Gardner MJ, Farrell ED, Nork SE, et al. Percutaneous placement of iliosacral screws without electrodiagnostic monitoring. *J Trauma*. 2009;66:1411-1415.
81. Routt MLC, Nork SE, Mills WJ. Percutaneous fixation of pelvic ring disruptions. *Clin Orthop*. 2000;375:15-29.
82. Nork SE, Jones CB, Harding SP, et al. Percutaneous stabilization of U-shaped sacral fractures using iliosacral screws: technique and early results. *J Orthop Trauma*. 2001;15:238-246.
83. Schildhauer TA, Ledoux WR, Chapman JR, et al. Triangular osteosynthesis and iliosacral screw fixation for unstable sacral fractures: a cadaveric and biomechanical evaluation under cyclic loads. *J Orthop Trauma*. 2003;17:22-31.
84. Acharya NK, Bijukachhe B, Kumar RJ, Menon VK. Ilio-lumbar fixation–the Amrita technique. *J Spinal Disord Tech*. 2008;21: 493-499.
85. Bellabarba C, Schildhauer TA, Vaccaro AR, Chapman JR. Complications associated with surgical stabilization of high-grade sacral fracture dislocations with spino-pelvic instability. *Spine*. 2006;31(suppl 11):S80-S88.
86. O'Brien JR, Yu WD, Bhatnagar R, Sponseller P, Kebaish KM. An anatomic study of the S2 iliac technique for lumbopelvic screw placement. *Spine*. 2009;34:E439-E442.
87. Sagi HC. Technical aspects and recommended treatment algorithms in triangular osteosynthesis and spinopelvic fixation for vertical shear transforaminal sacral fractures. *J Orthop Trauma*. 2009;23:354-360.
88. Schildhauer TA, McCullough P, Chapman JR, Mann FA. Anatomic and radiographic considerations for placement of transiliac screws in lumbopelvic fixations. *J Spinal Disord Tech*. 2002;15:199-205.
89. Schildhauer TA, Josten C, Muhr G. Triangular osteosynthesis of vertically unstable sacrum fractures: a new concept allowing early weight-bearing. *J Orthop Trauma*. 1998;12:307-314.
90. Schildhauer TA, Bellabarba C, Nork SE, et al. Decompression and lumbopelvic fixation for sacral fracture-dislocations with spino-pelvic dissociation. *J Orthop Trauma*. 2006;20:447-457.
91. Schildhauer TA, Bellabarba C, Selznick HS, et al. Unstable pediatric sacral fracture with bone loss caused by a high-energy gunshot injury. *J Trauma*. 2007;63:E95-E99.
92. Strange-Vognsen HH, Kiaer T, Tondevold E. The Cotrel-Dubousset instrumentation for unstable sacral fractures: report of 3 patients. *Acta Orthop Scand*. 1994;65:219-220.
93. Vilela MD, Gelfenbeyn M, Bellabarba C. U-shaped sacral fracture and lumbosacral dislocation as a result of a shotgun injury: case report. *Neurosurgery*. 2009;64:E193-E194.
94. Lebwohl NH, Cunningham BW, Dmitriev A, et al. Biomechanical comparison of lumbosacral fixation techniques in a calf spine model. *Spine*. 2002;27:2312-2320.

CHAPTER 79 Acute Treatment of Patients With Spinal Cord Injury

Rajiv Saigal
Matthew F. Gary
Allan D. Levi

Introduction

In spite of many decades of active research, traumatic spinal cord injury (SCI) is a devastating disease that still lacks good treatment options. It can dramatically impact a patient's quality of life, lessens life expectancy, and is most common in adolescents and young adults with many years left to live.[1] The emotional and financial burdens placed on these patients and their families are immense. Likewise, the societal costs from long-term care and lost productivity of this mostly young population are vast. Much knowledge of SCI pathophysiology has been gained, yet translating preclinical successes in the laboratory to human patients remains challenging. Current treatments for the acute SCI patient are far from a cure. However, progress has been made in ensuring the best possible long-term recovery. A multidisciplinary approach to treating these patients in high-volume centers using evidence-based guidelines is the ultimate goal.

Epidemiology

There are approximately 17,000 new cases of SCI in the United States each year and 282,000 people living with an SCI.[1] The prevalence of SCI patients has been increasing due to improved survival in both the acute and chronic phases of the disease process. Due to their higher incidence of trauma, males are approximately 4 times more likely to have SCIs than females.[1] The average age at injury (42 years)[1] has climbed substantially over the last 5 decades from the age of 29 years in the 1970s. Pediatric SCIs, aged 15 years or younger, are exceedingly rare (3.5%); in contrast, injuries in the elderly are on the rise, particularly due to falls.

Patients may present with any degree of neurologic impairment. Nationwide, 45% present as incomplete tetraplegic, 21% present as incomplete paraplegic, 20% as complete paraplegic, and 13% as complete tetraplegic.[1] Given comorbidities, the mortality in the first year after injury is significantly higher in older (>60 years) patients who sustain a spinal cord injury.[2] The racial distribution of individuals with an SCI are 66.5% white, 26.8% black, 8.3% Hispanic, and 2.0% Asian.

The financial burden of SCI treatment is high. The first-year cost per patient ranges from approximately $350,000 in American Spinal Injury Association (ASIA) D classified patients (see Initial Evaluation section) to over $1 million for C1 to C4–injured tetraplegic patients.[1] Estimated lifetime costs for a 25-year-old SCI patient ranges from $1.6 to $4.7 million. Direct medical costs for these patients in the United States are estimated to be over $14.5 billion per year. In addition, another $5.5 billion is relinquished in lost productivity.[3] This cost is directly related to the affected level, severity of deficits, and age at the time of injury.

Motor vehicle accidents (38%) and falls (30.5%) account for the vast majority of SCIs.[1] A total of 13.5% are the result of violence, including gunshot wounds and stabbings; 9% are caused by sports-related trauma. Medical or surgical causes, including iatrogenic injury, account for another 5%. The remaining 4% have other etiologies.

Initial Evaluation

The initial evaluation of the suspected SCI patient follows that of acute trauma. Securing the airway, ensuring voluntary or mechanical ventilation, and maintaining circulation take highest precedence, as with all trauma patients. Patients should be immobilized on a backboard with straps and with a cervical collar from initial encounter until at least when definitive imaging is obtained; less rigid immobilization is not recommended.[4] In patients with penetrating trauma, resuscitation should be prioritized over immobilization due to worse mortality rates when the former is delayed.[4] For patients requiring intubation, the neck should be maintained in a neutral posture. Patients should be moved with log roll precautions until thoracic and lumbar injuries have been ruled out. Patients must be assessed for any concomitant injuries. Polytrauma and associated traumatic brain injury are common in SCI patients.

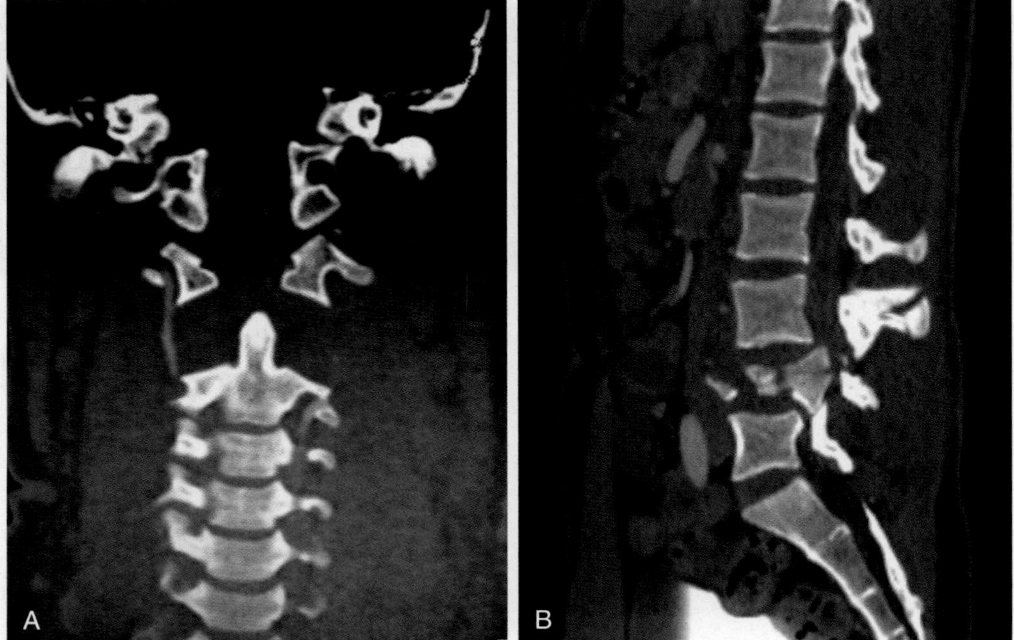

FIG. 79.1 (A) Coronal thin-cut computed tomography scan reconstruction, demonstrating a severe nonsurvivable C1–C2 distraction injury along with an occipital cervical dislocation. (B) Severe L4 burst fracture with retro portion into the spinal canal. The scan demonstrates the bony features of the injury with exquisite quality.

Once the patient is stabilized, a detailed neurologic assessment should follow, including testing all major upper and lower extremity motor groups and dermatomal sensation. Examination of rectal tone and sensation are part of the routine spine trauma assessment of distal sacral nerve root function. Otherwise neurologically complete SCI patients who maintain rectal tone and/or sensation have improved prognosis compared to those who do not. Based on the motor and sensory exam, the ASIA impairment scale (AIS) grade should be determined. The AIS includes five scoring grades ranging from A (neurologically complete injury) to E (neurologically intact). These divisions are important for prognosis.

In major trauma centers, computed tomography (CT) images with sagittal and coronal reconstructions are completed for all suspected SCI patients (Fig. 79.1). Cervical spine fractures through the transverse foramina may be associated with injury to the vertebral arteries; CT angiography or traditional catheter-based angiography may be completed to rule out such vascular injuries, including dissection, pseudoaneurysm, or occlusion (Fig. 79.2). Clearing the unconscious patient with high-resolution CT scans of the spine has greater than a 99.9% sensitivity and specificity; thus, modern CT alone is sufficient in detecting unstable cervical spine injuries in trauma patients.[5] Magnetic resonance imaging (MRI) is not always necessary but may be a useful adjunct in assessing the degree of spinal cord or nerve root compression and any ligamentous injury (Fig. 79.3). The degree of canal compromise in relation to the spinal cord and nerve roots is best assessed with this imaging modality. MRI can also assess the severity of SCI, including the extent of signal change and associated intraparenchymal blood, which carries a worse prognosis for neurologic recovery.[6] Fortunately, significant hematomas, which compress the spinal cord after trauma, are uncommon except in the setting of ankylosing spondylitis, where it should be diligently sought.[7]

A high-quality CT scan will identify nearly all unstable fractures. In a level 1 trauma center retrospective study of 690 patients, all acute traumatic cervical spine injuries seen on MRI were already identified on CT.[8] Thus, even the comatose or obtunded patient may be cleared of cervical spine injury by CT-based imaging.[8] In the absence of imaging, cervical immobilization is not necessary in neurologically intact, awake, alert, nonintoxicated patients without neck pain.[4] Upon completion of initial workup, admission to an intensive care unit (ICU) is recommended.

Blood Pressure Management

Optimizing spinal cord perfusion is a critical consideration in the acute management of traumatic SCI. The acute traumatic patient frequently presents in a hypovolemic state; the SCI patient is at added risk of neurogenic shock. The latter may occur from injury onset up until approximately 6 weeks due to unopposed parasympathetic output in the setting of interrupted sympathetic pathways.[9] As mentioned earlier, the priorities of trauma resuscitation take early precedence in management. The circulation focus also has indirect benefit to the spinal cord in maintaining an adequate perfusion pressure. In order to maintain adequate blood pressure, SCI patients should be given intravenous (IV) volume resuscitation and pressors, as needed. Hypotonic solutions should be avoided

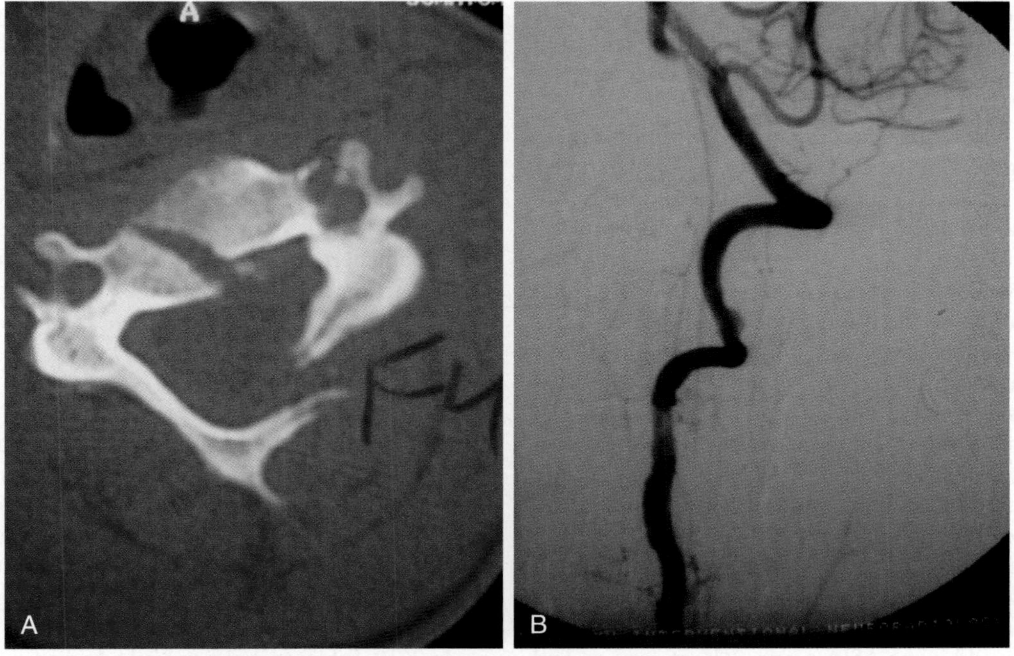

FIG. 79.2 (A) Complex cervical fracture through the body and lamina with an associated fracture of the vertebral artery foramen. (B) Associated injury to the vertebral artery with dissection and pseudoaneurysm seen on catheter-based angiogram.

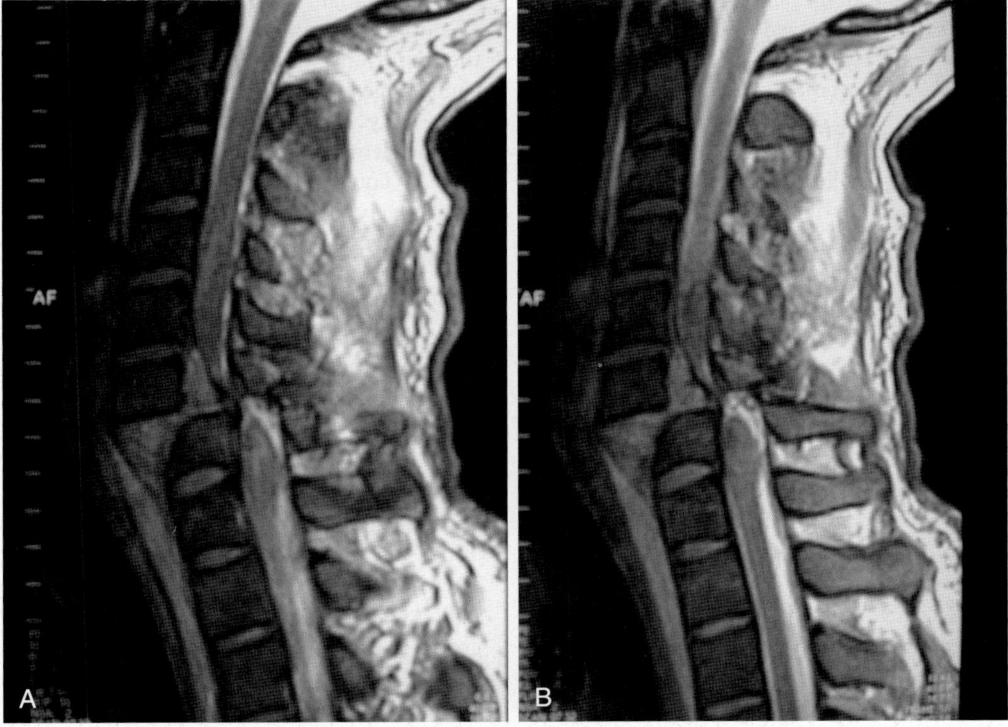

FIG. 79.3 Sequential sagittal magnetic resonance images C6–C7 vertebral body dislocation with associated tearing of the disc and severe compression of the spinal cord at that level. The posterior ligament complex is also disrupted.

in order to minimize risk of cerebral edema. Immediate resuscitation generally is achieved with crystalloid solutions with a transition toward colloids and/or blood transfusions in anemic patients.[9] Intravascular volume should be restored prior to pressor use in order to avoid adverse medication effects when possible and to maximize their efficacy when necessary.[9]

Recent guidelines make level 3 recommendations to avoid episodes of hypotension (defined as systolic blood pressure <90 mm Hg) and maintain mean arterial pressure (MAP) greater than 85 to 90 mm Hg for 7 days after injury.[10] In order to achieve these goals, admission to an ICU and placement of appropriate monitoring devices, such as an arterial line, are recommended.[10]

There are no randomized clinical studies to support these blood pressure goals, and such trials may never materialize due to a lack of perceived equipoise. Nonetheless, preclinical and clinical studies provide a limited basis for empirical support of this practice.[11]

Animal models show evidence of decreased spinal cord blood flow after SCI. In a feline contusion model of SCI, white matter blood flow decreased by 50% in placebo-treated animals.[12] In a nonhuman primate clip compression model of SCI, there was a 5.6-fold decrease in blood flow to gray matter and 4.8-fold decrease to white matter, emphasizing the importance of restoring more normal perfusion; blood transfusion nearly doubled spinal cord blood flow.[13] A study of 77 cervical and thoracic SCI patients managed with aggressive resuscitation and MAP maintenance above 85 mm Hg for 7 days in addition to surgical decompression/stabilization and IV methylprednisolone (MP) showed that 60% of cervical and 33% of thoracic ASIA A patients improved by one ASIA grade; 30% of cervical and 10% of thoracic patients regained the ability to walk.[14] The 7-day target was chosen in order to exceed the 3- to 5-day window during which maximal spinal cord edema occurs in animal studies.[15] A study of 50 cervical SCI patients treated with a MAP goal of 90 mm Hg showed no AIS improvement in motor-complete patients with a "severe hemodynamic deficit" compared to 45% improvement in those with adequate hemodynamics.[16] Hemodynamic deficit was defined based on pulmonary vascular resistance and systemic vascular resistance.[16] In a recent analysis of high-resolution ICU vital sign data on SCI patients, a higher proportion of recorded MAPs below the target of 85 mm Hg was associated with poorer outcomes.[17] A systematic review found no difference in outcome between 85 and 90 mm Hg as the therapeutic MAP target.[9]

The choice of pressor for maintaining MAPs above 85 or 90 mm Hg may have an impact on adverse events. Although dopamine is a common first-line agent in SCI management, it may be associated with higher risk. A study in shock patients showed greater arrhythmia risk and greater risk of death after treatment of cardiogenic shock with dopamine versus phenylephrine.[18] A retrospective study found a 69.2% medical complication rate with dopamine compared with 46.5% with phenylephrine administration after SCI.[19] Complications included troponin leak, atrial fibrillation, ventricular tachycardia, severe tachycardia (heart rate >130 beats/min) or bradycardia (heart rate <50 beats/min).[19] Thus, there is reason to question use of dopamine as a first-line pressor after SCI and need for renewed study on optimal vasopressor choice. With isolated peripheral vasoconstrictor effects via α-adrenergic agonism, phenylephrine may be a good pressor choice in low thoracic or lumbar injuries, but some have suggested using phenylephrine with caution in cervical and high thoracic injuries.[9,20] When sympathetic output is disrupted in such lesions, resulting in neurogenic shock, there is generally a need for both α- and β-adrenergic stimulation. Dopamine and norepinephrine can accomplish this.[9,21] Dobutamine is used infrequently due to vasodilatory effects and risk of bradycardia.[22] Vasopressin, isoproterenol, and milrinone are generally avoided in SCI, the former due to diuretic effects and risk for hyponatremia and the latter two due to lack of efficacy.[9,23]

Of note, while there is a greater availability of data to support use of MAP goals for nonpenetrating injury, this is less true for penetrating injuries, such as stab or gunshot wounds through the spinal cord. A small retrospective series suggested that induced hypertension via a MAP goal of 85 mm Hg may have no impact on functional outcome after penetrating SCI.[24]

Surgical Timing

There is a growing body of literature to support early surgical intervention in SCI. The definition of early surgery for traumatic SCI in the past has varied from 8 to 72 hours; this should be kept in mind in an evaluation of the literature.[25] In general, there appears to be a trend to decreased hospital length of stay and shortened ICU stays when surgical decompression is offered within 72 hours.[26–32]

In 2012, Fehlings et al.[33] published a well-designed, prospective cohort study of 313 patients with cervical traumatic spinal cord injury (tSCI) comparing early and late decompressive surgery using a 24-hour cutoff. The study was nonrandomized and patient selection for the early versus the late group was up to the surgeon based on clinical factors. This stresses the importance of assessing whether the two groups are truly comparable. It is important to note that the mean time to surgery in the early and late groups was 14.2 and 48.3 hours, respectively. Patients demonstrated a 19.8% and 8.8% improvement of greater than or equal to 2 AIS grades in the early and late groups, respectively, corresponding to 2.8 times higher odds in the early group. Follow-up was conducted at 6 months after injury. This trial represents the largest prospective trial specifically addressing the question of early versus late decompression in acute tSCI. Despite its importance, this study has major limitations that must be considered. First, were the two groups, early versus late surgery, comparable? In the early surgery group, there were 57.7% of patients with AIS A and B injury versus 38.2% in the late surgery group ($P < .01$). This is a problem in that patients with AIS C and D type injuries have a ceiling on the degree of improvement that they can achieve, and it is impossible for AIS D–injured patients to improve 2 AIS grades. There were 35.9% of patients in the late surgery group with AIS D classification versus only 24.7% in the early surgery group. Another potential confounding variable is whether spinal shock played a role, masking the neurologic exam in the early surgery group. Patients in the early surgery group were significantly younger (45.0 vs. 50.7 years old; $P < .01$) and a greater proportion received steroids ($P = .04$). Although this was a prospective study, the decision to offer early surgery was left to the discretion of the attending surgeon.[33] Some have suggested that an even earlier time point for decompression may be more beneficial. A recent retrospective study showed improved spinal cord independence measures, ASIA impairment scale, and motor function for cervical decompressions performed within 8 hours of injury.[34] Preclinical animal data suggested that early decompression is effective in improving neurologic outcomes with or without concomitant administration of MP.[35]

Neuroprotective Strategies

There are a number of neuroprotective strategies that are in various phases of investigation. Steroids, gangliosides, and spinal cord cooling will be discussed later. More recent pharmacologic strategies for tSCI include riluzole, a sodium channel blocker that is approved by the US Food and Drug Administration (FDA) for treatment of amyotrophic lateral sclerosis, and minocycline, an antibiotic that is a tetracycline analog, that are in phase II/III studies.

Steroids

There remains no clearly beneficial pharmacotherapy for acute traumatic SCI, although many have been studied. Administration of IV MP is the most highly studied, perhaps the most controversial therapeutic option, and the subject of three National Acute Spinal Cord Injury Studies (NASCIS). MP was chosen due to effects on reduction of membrane lipid peroxidation with possible beneficial effects on blood flow and neuronal excitability.[36] The first NASCIS trial assessed two doses of MP.[37] The high-dose MP consisted of a 1000-mg IV bolus, followed by 250 mg IV every 6 hours given over 10 days. The standard dose was 100 mg IV bolus, followed by 25 mg IV every 6 hours for 10 days. The primary outcome was motor and sensory examinations at 6 weeks and 6 months. No difference in motor function, pinprick, or light touch was found between the low dose and high dose of MP. There were higher early fatalities with high-dose MP (relative risk [RR], 3.1 deaths ≤14 days; RR, 1.9 deaths 15–28 days) and higher wound infections with high-dose MP (RR, 3.6).[37] Important limitations were the lack of a nontreatment control group and only 54% patient availability at final follow-up.

After NASCIS I, preclinical data suggested that a higher (30 mg/kg) MP loading dose might be optimal after SCI.[36,38–40] Following these studies, NASCIS II was planned to compare a higher-dose MP to naloxone and placebo.[41] The three study arms were (1) MP: 30 mg/kg IV bolus + 5.4 mg/kg/h × 23 hours; (2) naloxone: 5.4 mg/kg IV bolus + 4 mg/kg/h × 23 hours; and (3) placebo. The primary outcome was again motor and sensory examination at 6 weeks and 6 months. Naloxone, an opioid antagonist, was included in the study due to functional utility seen in preclinical animal studies, possibly due to effects on blood pressure and/or cord perfusion.[12,42] In NASCIS II, naloxone and MP given more than 8 hours after injury did not lead to neurologic improvement. When given within 8 hours of injury, MP led to increased change in motor (16 vs. 11.2 placebo; $P = .03$), pinprick (11.4 vs. 6.6; $P = .02$), and touch (8.9 vs. 4.3; $P = .03$) scores. Important limitations to interpreting these data were the post-hoc application of the 8-hour limit and reporting of only unilateral results.

NASCIS III consisted of three study arms: (1) 24-hour MP: 30 mg/kg IV bolus + 5.4 mg/kg/h × 24 hours; (2) 48-hour MP: 30 mg/kg bolus + 5.4 mg/kg/h × 48 hours, and (3) tirilizad: 2.5 mg/kg every 6 hours × 48 hours.[43] Tirilizad was chosen due to its expected effects on decreasing peroxidation of the neuronal membrane. There was no nontreatment control. The primary outcome was motor function and change in Functional Independence Measure (FIM) at 6 weeks and 6 months. Compared to 24-hour MP, 48-hour MP led to a nonsignificant trend toward neurologic improvement. In the subset of patients with 48-hour MP initiated 3 to 8 hours after treatment, the neurologic improvement was significant relative to 24-hour MP. However, the 48-hour MP group had significantly higher rates of severe sepsis and pneumonia.

Given modest and questionable benefits from MP in the NASCIS trials combined with higher rates of adverse events in these and other studies, the most recent American Association of Neurological Surgeons/Congress of Neurological Surgeons (AANS/CNS) guidelines changed MP from a treatment option to a level 1 recommendation against utilization.[44] The guidelines change was highly controversial, with leading experts arguing that there were no new data since the prior guidelines to support the downgraded MP recommendation.[45] Experts agree that MP should not be administered in patients who lack a neurologic deficit.[21]

In the setting of mixed recommendations, one important consideration is the patient's desire for treatment. A recent study showed that 69.6% of chronic SCI patients favored selective use of MP and 29% felt that all acute SCI patients should receive it; only 1.4% were against administration in all circumstances.[46] A total of 59.4% thought that even small motor or sensory improvement would be "extremely important" to them. However, only 4% of patients who arrived within the MP window and were able to communicate were asked about their preference. Given the controversial nature of MP, treating physicians might consider discussing risks and benefits with patients and involving them in the treatment decision. Additionally, when considering MP treatment, the balance of risks and benefits may be improved by judicious patient selection toward those with lesser risk of adverse events, such as the younger, previously healthy patient.

GM-1 Ganglioside

GM-1 ganglioside forms a component of the central nervous system (CNS) membrane. It had been shown in preclinical studies to facilitate regeneration and regrowth and to promote neuroprotection. In a small randomized, controlled single-center trial in SCI, a 100-mg IV daily dose of GM-1 for 18 to 32 days after 72 hours of MP (250 mg IV bolus followed by 125 mg every 6 hours) led to significant improvement in Frankel grade, with a 50% rate of at least one grade improvement versus 28% in MP-only treated patients.[47] There was also significantly better 1-year improvement in ASIA motor score of 39.6 in MP plus GM-1 patients versus 21.6 in MP-only patients.[47] However, a larger multicenter randomized control trial was not able to validate the results.[48] There were three therapeutic arms: (1) GM-1 low dose (LD): 300 mg IV bolus + 100 mg daily × 56 days; (2) GM-1 high dose (HD): 600 mg bolus + 200 mg daily × 56 days; and (3) MP only. All patients also received IV MP according to the NASCIS II protocol. The primary outcome was the percentage of patients with greater than or equal to 2-grade AIS improvement at 26 weeks. Overall, 70.2% of MP plus GM-1–treated patients (69.8% LD vs. 71.7% HD) achieved this goal, but 71.2% MP-only treated patients did as well. There was a 5.8% death rate in GM-1 patients compared to 5.5% for MP only.[48] Neither GM-1 trial included a placebo group with no pharmacologic treatment. Given the lack of clear therapeutic benefit, AANS/CNS guidelines also recommend against treatment with GM-1 ganglioside.[44]

Hypothermia

Induced local or systemic hypothermia is a treatment option for tSCI and a current topic of active research. Initially, multiple preclinical studies showed neuroprotective effects of induced hypothermia in traumatic brain and animal studies.[49,50] Hypothermia has been utilized successfully in other domains, such as reducing hypoxic-ischemic encephalopathy after cardiac arrest and reducing incidence of SCI after aortic aneurysm surgery.[51] In traumatic brain injury clinical trials, induced hypothermia was associated with decreases in intracranial pressure but mixed functional outcome.[52–55]

Attempts at local cooling in human SCI patients began in the 1970s.[56–60] Using an epidural cooling system during the time of surgical decompression for cervical or thoracic ASIA A patients, 65% improved at least one ASIA grade.[61] Of 14 patients in the cervical cohort, five patients converted to ASIA B, three to ASIA C, and one to ASIA D.[61] Of six patients in the thoracic cohort, one converted to ASIA B, two to ASIA C, and one to ASIA D.[61]

Systemic modest hypothermia, defined as cooling to 32°C to 34°C via a central venous catheter, has recently been the focus of several clinical studies in SCI (Fig. 79.4).[51,62,63] Of 35 neurologically complete cervical ASIA A adult patients who received 48 hours of cooling starting at a mean of 5.8 hours after injury, 43% improved at least one AIS grade by last follow-up.[64] A total of 23% regained some motor function and 11% improved to AIS D or better. The most common associated adverse events were atelectasis (83%), pleural effusion (54%), anemia, pulmonary edema (43%), electrolyte disturbance, and urinary tract infection (37%). There was an associated 14% rate of thromboembolic events. There were several exclusionary criteria, including cardiac history, Raynaud disease, bleeding, pregnancy, thrombocytopenia, pancreatitis, blood dyscrasia, hyperthermia on admission, penetrating injury, and patients showing neurologic improvement within 12 hours.[64] Given the high conversion rate for initially complete SCI patients, hypothermia is an area of interest for future study but requires prospective, randomized validation.

Managing Body Systems Complications Related to Spinal Cord Injury

Pulmonary

SCI patients are at high risk for pulmonary complications. A total of 11% of early mortality is due to atelectasis, pulmonary

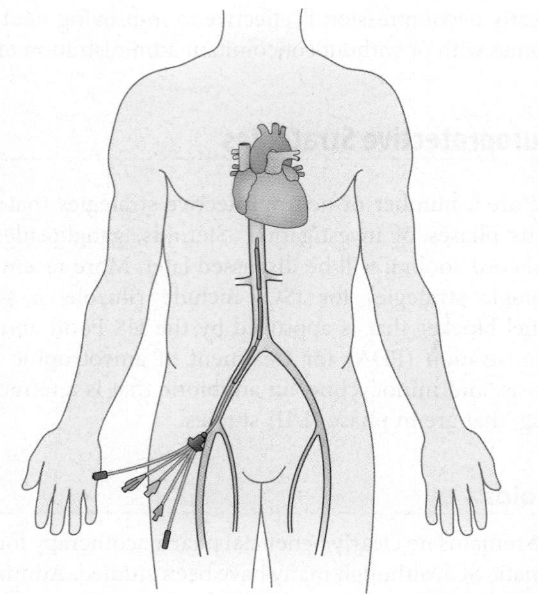

FIG. 79.4 Hypothermia catheter with several ports. The balloon catheter resides within the inferior vena cava. A closed-loop system exists in which cold saline circulates at a rate to achieve the desired systemic temperature by cooling the blood rushing by the catheter.

embolism, edema, pneumonia, or aspiration.[11] Vital capacity is often restricted, especially in high cervical injuries. Of SCI patients, 70% have some degree of respiratory insufficiency.[65] Thoracic spine injuries are frequently associated with rib fractures and/or hemothorax as a contributing factor. Aside from continuous pulse oximetry, the SCI patient should be monitored with arterial blood gas measurements to assess for early signs of respiratory failure.

Integument

Wound and skin complications, including decubitus ulcers, are of high concern in SCI patients. Acute management should include steps to decrease the likelihood of their development. Between 30% and 50% of SCI patients will develop a pressure ulcer to some degree in the first month postinjury.[21] Patients should be transferred from a rigid backboard as soon as it is deemed safe. When available, specialized, pressure-controlled hospital beds should be used in patients with limited mobility.[21] Nursing care should include patient repositioning every 2 hours to limit the shear stress on dependent skin.[21] Once spine injuries are stabilized with surgery and/or bracing, as indicated, patients should be mobilized early. Thus, early surgical stabilization also has indirect benefits on skin protection.

Thromboembolic

Venous thromboembolic complications, including deep vein thrombosis (DVT) and pulmonary embolism, occur frequently in SCI patients. Scientific literature shows wide-ranging incidence rates, from 7% to 100% in SCI patients with inadequate prophylaxis.[66–79] Level 1 evidence exists to support chemical and mechanical prophylaxis.[66] Chemical prophylaxis may consist of subcutaneous low-molecular-weight heparin or LD heparin combined with sequential compression devices on the lower extremities. Appropriate prophylaxis reduces the incidence of venous thromboembolism below 5% in the first weeks after SCI.[74] Level 2 recommendations support commencing chemical prophylaxis upon admission or within 72 hours and continuing for a 3-month duration.[66] Such therapy is generally held for 24 hours before and after surgery. Inferior vena cava filters should be used judiciously when other prophylactic mechanisms are not possible.

Urinary

Many acute SCI patients require placement of a Foley catheter. Patients may initially present with urinary retention from an atonic bladder in the acute setting of spinal shock. Documentation of initial bladder volume on presentation or of postvoid residual volume in patients who are able to urinate is helpful in assessing the degree of neurologic dysfunction. The placement of an indwelling catheter puts patients at risk for the development of urinary tract infection. Thus, if voluntary bladder function does not resume after the acute phase, patients should be transitioned to a system of intermittent catheterization every 4 to 6 hours. Bladder distention is a leading cause of autonomic dysreflexia in the SCI population. Thus, vigilant bladder care is necessary to avoid potentially life-threatening complications.

Nutrition

Similar to trauma, and particularly CNS injury, the acute SCI patient may present in a hypercatabolic state.[80] Such patients require a nutritional source to meet high metabolic demands. Indirect calorimetry may help assess the patient's nutritional needs.[80] There are level 3 recommendations to support early enteral nutrition. However, there is no clear evidence that early nutrition leads to improved neurologic outcome or decreased length of stay.[80]

Rehabilitation

Ultimately, intense inpatient rehabilitation is critical to maximize functional returns (Fig. 79.5).

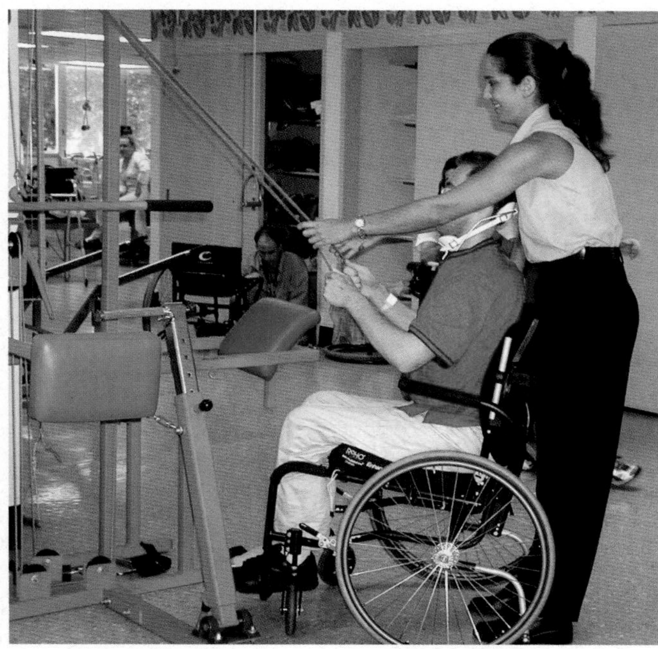

FIG. 79.5 A patient in rehabilitation after a cervical spinal cord injury shown increasing upper extremity strength and performance.

Summary

Acute management of the SCI patient is a complex undertaking, requiring dedicated multidisciplinary care. Admission to an ICU or dedicated SCI unit is recommended. Hypotension should be avoided and MAP maintained above 85 mm Hg for 7 days. In patients with ongoing spinal cord compression from their trauma, early surgical decompression and stabilization should occur, at least within 24 hours. There is no clear clinical benefit from pharmacotherapy. MP is the most widely prescribed, based on the NASCIS II protocol, although its use is waning due to controversial guidelines changes and potential risks. Induced hypothermia is under active study as a treatment option. The treating provider should anticipate associated medical risks of SCI, including respiratory compromise, infection, DVT, and development of decubitus ulcers, with steps taken to mitigate their development. Clinical attention to each of these areas helps maximize neurologic function and minimize the chance of death from associated complications.

PEARLS

1. Current guidelines provide level 3 recommendations to avoid episodes of hypotension (defined as systolic blood pressure <90 mm Hg) and maintain MAP greater than 85 to 90 mm Hg for 7 days after injury.
2. There is a growing body of literature to support early (<24 hours) surgical intervention in SCI.
3. New neuroprotective strategies under investigation for SCI include hypothermia, riluzole, and minocycline.

PITFALLS

1. The average age at time of SCI has increased substantially over the last 5 decades, from the age of 29 years in the 1970s to 42 years currently.
2. The most recent AANS/CNS guidelines changed MP from a treatment option to a level 1 recommendation against utilization. Use of MP remains controversial and most experts would agree that there is no role for its use in complete (AIS A) thoracic SCI.
3. SCI has systemic effects that affect every organ system, especially pulmonary, cardiovascular, integument, and urinary.

KEY POINTS

1. CT images with sagittal and coronal reconstructions are completed for nearly all suspected SCI patients.

2. Early surgery, particularly for cervical SCI, is routinely accepted as safe, with the most recent studies suggesting improved long-term neurologic outcomes.
3. While steroid use for SCI remains controversial, there are a number of neuroprotective strategies that are being investigated for safety and efficacy, including hypothermia, riluzole, and minocycline.
4. Health care providers of SCI patients should anticipate associated complications of SCI, including respiratory compromise, infection, DVT, and development of decubitus ulcers, with steps taken to mitigate their development.

KEY REFERENCES

1. Panczykowski DM, Tomycz ND, Okonkwo DO. Comparative effectiveness of using computed tomography alone to exclude cervical spine injuries in obtunded or intubated patients: meta-analysis of 14,327 patients with blunt trauma. *J Neurosurg.* 2011;115(3):541-549.
2. Vale FL, Burns J, Jackson AB, Hadley MN. Combined medical and surgical treatment after acute spinal cord injury: results of a prospective pilot study to assess the merits of aggressive medical resuscitation and blood pressure management. *J Neurosurg.* 1997;87(2):239-246.
3. Fehlings MG, Vaccaro A, Wilson JR, et al. Early versus delayed decompression for traumatic cervical spinal cord injury: results of the Surgical Timing in Acute Spinal Cord Injury Study (STASCIS). *PLoS One.* 2012;7(2):e32037.
4. Hurlbert RJ, Hadley MN, Walters BC, et al. Pharmacological therapy for acute spinal cord injury. *Neurosurgery.* 2013;72(suppl 2):93-105.
5. Dididze M, Green BA, Dietrich WD, et al. Systemic hypothermia in acute cervical spinal cord injury: a case-controlled study. *Spinal Cord.* 2013;51(5):395-400.

REFERENCES

1. National Spinal Cord Injury Statistical Center. *Facts and Figures at a Glance*. Birmingham, AL: University of Alabama; 2016.
2. Prusmack C. The effect of age on survival following traumatic spinal cord injury. *Top Spinal Cord Inj Rehabil.* 2006;12(1):49-57.
3. Berkowitz M, O'Leary PK, Kruse DL, et al. *Spinal Cord Injury: An Analysis of Medical and Social Costs*. New York: Demos Medical Publishing; 1998.
4. Theodore N, Hadley MN, Aarabi B, et al. Prehospital cervical spinal immobilization after trauma. *Neurosurgery.* 2013;72(suppl 2):22-34.
5. Panczykowski DM, Tomycz ND, Okonkwo DO. Comparative effectiveness of using computed tomography alone to exclude cervical spine injuries in obtunded or intubated patients: meta-analysis of 14,327 patients with blunt trauma. *J Neurosurg.* 2011;115(3):541-549.
6. Schaefer DM, Flanders AE, Osterholm JL, Northrup BE. Prognostic significance of magnetic resonance imaging in the acute phase of cervical spine injury. *J Neurosurg.* 1992;76(2):218-223.
7. Foo D, Rossier AB. Post-traumatic spinal epidural hematoma. *Neurosurgery.* 1982;11(1 Pt 1):25-32.
8. Tomycz ND, Chew BG, Chang YF, et al. MRI is unnecessary to clear the cervical spine in obtunded/comatose trauma patients: the four-year experience of a level I trauma center. *J Trauma.* 2008;64(5):1258-1263.
9. Ploumis A, Yadlapalli N, Fehlings MG, Kwon BK, Vaccaro AR. A systematic review of the evidence supporting a role for vasopressor support in acute SCI. *Spinal Cord.* 2010;48(5):356-362.
10. Ryken TC, Hurlbert RJ, Hadley MN, et al. The acute cardiopulmonary management of patients with cervical spinal cord injuries. *Neurosurgery.* 2013;72(suppl 2):84-92.
11. Casha S, Christie S. A systematic review of intensive cardiopulmonary management after spinal cord injury. *J Neurotrauma.* 2011;28(8):1479-1495.
12. Young W, Flamm ES, Demopoulos HB, Tomasula JJ, DeCrescito V. Effect of naloxone on posttraumatic ischemia in experimental spinal contusion. *J Neurosurg.* 1981;55(2):209-219.
13. Dolan EJ, Tator CH. The effect of blood transfusion, dopamine, and gamma hydroxybutyrate on posttraumatic ischemia of the spinal cord. *J Neurosurg.* 1982;56(3):350-358.
14. Vale FL, Burns J, Jackson AB, Hadley MN. Combined medical and surgical treatment after acute spinal cord injury: results of a prospective pilot study to assess the merits of aggressive medical resuscitation and blood pressure management. *J Neurosurg.* 1997;87(2):239-246.
15. Yashon D, Bingham WG Jr, Faddoul EM, Hunt WE. Edema of the spinal cord following experimental impact trauma. *J Neurosurg.* 1973;38(6):693-697.
16. Levi L, Wolf A, Belzberg H. Hemodynamic parameters in patients with acute cervical cord trauma: description, intervention, and prediction of outcome. *Neurosurgery.* 1993;33(6):1007-1016.
17. Hawryluk G, Whetstone W, Saigal R, et al. Mean arterial blood pressure correlates with neurological recovery after human spinal cord injury: analysis of high frequency physiologic data. *J Neurotrauma.* 2015;32(24):1958-1967.
18. De Backer D, Biston P, Devriendt J, et al. Comparison of dopamine and norepinephrine in the treatment of shock. *N Engl J Med.* 2010;362(9):779-789.
19. Inoue T, Manley GT, Patel N, Whetstone WD. Medical and surgical management after spinal cord injury: vasopressor usage, early surgeries, and complications. *J Neurotrauma.* 2014;31(3):284-291.
20. Blood pressure management after acute spinal cord injury. *Neurosurgery.* 2002;50(suppl 3):S58-S62.
21. Consortium for Spinal Cord Medicine. Early acute management in adults with spinal cord injury: a clinical practice guideline for health-care professionals. *J Spinal Cord Med.* 2008;31(4):403-479.
22. Ball PA. Critical care of spinal cord injury. *Spine.* 2001;26(suppl 24):S27-S30.
23. Stratman RC, Wiesner AM, Smith KM, Cook AM. Hemodynamic management after spinal cord injury. *Orthopedics.* 2008;31(3):252-255.
24. Readdy WJ, Saigal R, Whetstone WD, et al. Failure of mean arterial pressure goals to improve outcomes following penetrating spinal cord injury. *Neurosurgery.* 2016;79(5):708-714.
25. Furlan JC, Noonan V, Cadotte DW, Fehlings MG. Timing of decompressive surgery of spinal cord after traumatic spinal cord injury: an evidence-based examination of pre-clinical and clinical studies. *J Neurotrauma.* 2011;28(8):1371-1399.
26. Vaccaro AR, Daugherty RJ, Sheehan TP, et al. Neurologic outcome of early versus late surgery for cervical spinal cord injury. *Spine.* 1997;22(22):2609-2613.
27. Mirza SK, Krengel WF 3rd, Chapman JR, et al. Early versus delayed surgery for acute cervical spinal cord injury. *Clin Orthop Relat Res.* 1999;359:104-114.

28. McKinley W, Meade MA, Kirshblum S, Barnard B. Outcomes of early surgical management versus late or no surgical intervention after acute spinal cord injury. *Arch Phys Med Rehabil*. 2004;85(11):1818-1825.
29. Kerwin AJ, Frykberg ER, Schinco MA, et al. The effect of early spine fixation on non-neurologic outcome. *J Trauma*. 2005;58(1):15-21.
30. Croce MA, Bee TK, Pritchard E, Miller PR, Fabian TC. Does optimal timing for spine fracture fixation exist? *Ann Surg*. 2001;233(6):851-858.
31. Chipman JG, Deuser WE, Beilman GJ. Early surgery for thoracolumbar spine injuries decreases complications. *J Trauma*. 2004;56(1):52-57.
32. Schinkel C, Frangen TM, Kmetic A, et al. Timing of thoracic spine stabilization in trauma patients: impact on clinical course and outcome. *J Trauma*. 2006;61(1):156-160.
33. Fehlings MG, Vaccaro A, Wilson JR, et al. Early versus delayed decompression for traumatic cervical spinal cord injury: results of the Surgical Timing in Acute Spinal Cord Injury Study (STASCIS). *PLoS One*. 2012;7(2):e32037.
34. Grassner L, Wutte C, Klein B, et al. Early decompression (< 8 h) after traumatic cervical spinal cord injury improves functional outcome as assessed by spinal cord independence measure after one year. *J Neurotrauma*. 2016;33(18):1658-1666.
35. Rabinowitz RS, Eck JC, Harper CM Jr, et al. Urgent surgical decompression compared to methylprednisolone for the treatment of acute spinal cord injury: a randomized prospective study in beagle dogs. *Spine*. 2008;33(21):2260-2268.
36. Hall ED, Braughler JM. Glucocorticoid mechanisms in acute spinal cord injury: a review and therapeutic rationale. *Surg Neurol*. 1982;18(5):320-327.
37. Bracken MB, Collins WF, Freeman DF, et al. Efficacy of methylprednisolone in acute spinal cord injury. *JAMA*. 1984;251(1):45-52.
38. Hall ED, Wolf DL, Braughler JM. Effects of a single large dose of methylprednisolone sodium succinate on experimental posttraumatic spinal cord ischemia. Dose-response and time-action analysis. *J Neurosurg*. 1984;61(1):124-130.
39. Braughler JM, Hall ED. Lactate and pyruvate metabolism in injured cat spinal cord before and after a single large intravenous dose of methylprednisolone. *J Neurosurg*. 1983;59(2):256-261.
40. Braughler JM, Hall ED. Pharmacokinetics of methylprednisolone in cat plasma and spinal cord following a single intravenous dose of the sodium succinate ester. *Drug Metab Dispos*. 1982;10(5):551-552.
41. Bracken MB, Shepard MJ, Collins WF, et al. A randomized, controlled trial of methylprednisolone or naloxone in the treatment of acute spinal-cord injury. Results of the Second National Acute Spinal Cord Injury Study. *N Engl J Med*. 1990;322(20):1405-1411.
42. Faden AI, Jacobs TP, Holaday JW. Opiate antagonist improves neurologic recovery after spinal injury. *Science*. 1981;211(4481):493-494.
43. Bracken MB, Shepard MJ, Holford TR, et al. Administration of methylprednisolone for 24 or 48 hours or tirilazad mesylate for 48 hours in the treatment of acute spinal cord injury. Results of the Third National Acute Spinal Cord Injury Randomized Controlled Trial. National Acute Spinal Cord Injury Study. *JAMA*. 1997;277(20):1597-1604.
44. Hurlbert RJ, Hadley MN, Walters BC, et al. Pharmacological therapy for acute spinal cord injury. *Neurosurgery*. 2013;72(suppl 2):93-105.
45. Fehlings MG, Wilson JR, Cho N. Methylprednisolone for the treatment of acute spinal cord injury: counterpoint. *Neurosurgery*. 2014;61(suppl 1):36-42.
46. Bowers CA, Kundu B, Rosenbluth J, Hawryluk GW. Patients with spinal cord injuries favor administration of methylprednisolone. *PLoS One*. 2016;11(1):e0145991.
47. Geisler FH, Dorsey FC, Coleman WP. Recovery of motor function after spinal-cord injury—a randomized, placebo-controlled trial with GM-1 ganglioside. *N Engl J Med*. 1991;324(26):1829-1838.
48. Geisler FH, Coleman WP, Grieco G, Poonian D, Sygen Study Group. The Sygen multicenter acute spinal cord injury study. *Spine*. 2001;26(suppl 24):S87-S98.
49. Dietrich WD, Atkins CM, Bramlett HM. Protection in animal models of brain and spinal cord injury with mild to moderate hypothermia. *J Neurotrauma*. 2009;26(3):301-312.
50. Albin MS, White RJ, Acosta-Rua G, Yashon D. Study of functional recovery produced by delayed localized cooling after spinal cord injury in primates. *J Neurosurg*. 1968;29(2):113-120.
51. Ahmad FU, Wang MY, Levi AD. Hypothermia for acute spinal cord injury—a review. *World Neurosurg*. 2014;82(1-2):207-214.
52. Clifton GL. A review of clinical trials of hypothermia treatment for severe traumatic brain injury. *Ther Hypothermia Temp Manag*. 2011;1(3):143-149.
53. Clifton GL, Coffey CS, Fourwinds S, et al. Early induction of hypothermia for evacuated intracranial hematomas: a post hoc analysis of two clinical trials. *J Neurosurg*. 2012;117(4):714-720.
54. Clifton GL, Miller ER, Choi SC, et al. Hypothermia on admission in patients with severe brain injury. *J Neurotrauma*. 2002;19(3):293-301.
55. Clifton GL, Valadka A, Zygun D, et al. Very early hypothermia induction in patients with severe brain injury (the National Acute Brain Injury Study: Hypothermia II): a randomised trial. *Lancet Neurol*. 2011;10(2):131-139.
56. Bricolo A, Ore GD, Da Pian R, Faccioli F. Local cooling in spinal cord injury. *Surg Neurol*. 1976;6(2):101-106.
57. Demian YK, White RJ, Yashon D, Kretchmer HE. Anaesthesia for laminectomy and localized cord cooling in acute cervical spine injury. Report of three cases. *Br J Anaesth*. 1971;43(10):973-979.
58. Koons DD, Gildenberg PL, Dohn DF, Henoch M. Local hypothermia in the treatment of spinal cord injuries. Report of seven cases. *Cleve Clin Q*. 1972;39(3):109-117.
59. Meacham WF, McPherson WF. Local hypothermia in the treatment of acute injuries of the spinal cord. *South Med J*. 1973;66(1):95-97.
60. Negrin J Jr. Spinal cord hypothermia in the neurosurgical management of the acute and chronic post-traumatic paraplegic patient. *Paraplegia*. 1973;10(4):336-343.
61. Hansebout RR, Hansebout CR. Local cooling for traumatic spinal cord injury: outcomes in 20 patients and review of the literature. *J Neurosurg Spine*. 2014;20(5):550-561.
62. Levi AD, Casella G, Green BA, et al. Clinical outcomes using modest intravascular hypothermia after acute cervical spinal cord injury. *Neurosurgery*. 2010;66(4):670-677.
63. Levi AD, Green BA, Wang MY, et al. Clinical application of modest hypothermia after spinal cord injury. *J Neurotrauma*. 2009;26(3):407-415.
64. Dididze M, Green BA, Dietrich WD, et al. Systemic hypothermia in acute cervical spinal cord injury: a case-controlled study. *Spinal Cord*. 2013;51(5):395-400.
65. Hachen HJ. Idealized care of the acutely injured spinal cord in Switzerland. *J Trauma*. 1977;17(12):931-936.

66. Dhall SS, Hadley MN, Aarabi B, et al. Deep venous thrombosis and thromboembolism in patients with cervical spinal cord injuries. *Neurosurgery*. 2013;72(suppl 2):244-254.
67. Burns GA, Cohn SM, Frumento RJ, Degutis LC, Hammers L. Prospective ultrasound evaluation of venous thrombosis in high-risk trauma patients. *J Trauma*. 1993;35(3):405-408.
68. El Masri WS, Silver JR. Prophylactic anticoagulant therapy in patients with spinal cord injury. *Paraplegia*. 1981;19(6):334-342.
69. Frisbie JH, Sasahara AA. Low dose heparin prophylaxis for deep venous thrombosis in acute spinal cord injury patients: a controlled study. *Paraplegia*. 1981;19(6):343-346.
70. Green D, Lee MY, Ito VY, et al. Fixed- vs adjusted-dose heparin in the prophylaxis of thromboembolism in spinal cord injury. *JAMA*. 1988;260(9):1255-1258.
71. Gunduz S, Ogur E, Mohur H, et al. Deep vein thrombosis in spinal cord injured patients. *Paraplegia*. 1993;31(9):606-610.
72. Kulkarni JR, Burt AA, Tromans AT, Constable PD. Prophylactic low dose heparin anticoagulant therapy in patients with spinal cord injuries: a retrospective study. *Paraplegia*. 1992;30(3):169-172.
73. Lamb GC, Tomski MA, Kaufman J, Maiman DJ. Is chronic spinal cord injury associated with increased risk of venous thromboembolism? *J Am Paraplegia Soc*. 1993;16(3):153-156.
74. Merli GJ, Crabbe S, Doyle L, Ditunno JF, Herbision GJ. Mechanical plus pharmacological prophylaxis for deep vein thrombosis in acute spinal cord injury. *Paraplegia*. 1992;30(8):558-562.
75. Myllynen P, Kammonen M, Rokkanen P, et al. Deep venous thrombosis and pulmonary embolism in patients with acute spinal cord injury: a comparison with nonparalyzed patients immobilized due to spinal fractures. *J Trauma*. 1985;25(6):541-543.
76. Perkash A, Prakash V, Perkash I. Experience with the management of thromboembolism in patients with spinal cord injury: Part I. Incidence, diagnosis and role of some risk factors. *Paraplegia*. 1978;16(3):322-331.
77. Powell M, Kirshblum S, O'Connor KC. Duplex ultrasound screening for deep vein thrombosis in spinal cord injured patients at rehabilitation admission. *Arch Phys Med Rehabil*. 1999;80(9):1044-1046.
78. Tator CH, Duncan EG, Edmonds VE, Lapczak LI, Andrews DF. Comparison of surgical and conservative management in 208 patients with acute spinal cord injury. *Can J Neurol Sci*. 1987;14(1):60-69.
79. Waring WP, Karunas RS. Acute spinal cord injuries and the incidence of clinically occurring thromboembolic disease. *Paraplegia*. 1991;29(1):8-16.
80. Dhall SS, Hadley MN, Aarabi B, et al. Nutritional support after spinal cord injury. *Neurosurgery*. 2013;72(suppl 2):255-259.

Vertebral Artery Injuries Associated With Cervical Spine Trauma

SECTION XI

Adam L. Shimer
Alexander R. Vaccaro

Vertebral artery injury (VAI) due to blunt cervical trauma is often initially asymptomatic; however, potentially devastating sequelae—including embolism, arterial dissection, and stroke—make this condition a diagnostic challenge and treatment dilemma. Recent improvements in diagnostic imaging have led to a higher rate of VAI detection, but the optimal treatment of VAI in the setting of cervical spinal trauma remains controversial. Although treatment of symptomatic VAI is prudent in nearly all settings, the treating physician must balance the treatment of asymptomatic patients with the complications of anticoagulation therapy and possibly the delay of surgical intervention when a diagnosis of vertebral arterial disruption is encountered.

Anatomy

The right vertebral artery (VA) arises from the right subclavian artery distal to the origin of the common carotid artery. On the left side, the VA usually arises directly from the subclavian artery. In 3% to 6% of cases, however, it may arise from the arch of the aorta as a separate vessel. From the vessel's origin at the subclavian to its intracranial termination, the VA can be divided into four anatomic segments. The first portion (V1) extends from the subclavian take-off to the foramen transversarium of C6 as it travels between the longus colli and anterior scalene muscles. The second portion (V2) of the artery then courses cephalad through successive transverse foramina until the level of C2, where the arteries diverge and then course superiorly to enter the more laterally situated foramen transversarium of the C1 vertebral body. The third segment (V3) begins on exiting the C1 foramen transversarium, where it lies in a groove along the superior margin of the posterior arch of the atlas. It then turns anteromedially and passes through the foramen magnum, lying anterior to the medulla oblongata. The fourth and final segment (V4) is intracranial after it pierces the dura mater. The VA then joins with the contralateral artery to form the basilar artery, which feeds the circle of Willis and contributes to the posterior circulation of the brain. This confluence is the anatomic basis of unilateral VA occlusion often being asymptomatic.

Epidemiology

As improved, higher-resolution imaging protocols have been developed and instituted, the incidence of detectable VAIs has increased. Although VAI has been reported as a result of low-energy movements—such as chiropractic manipulation,[1,2] yoga, and sudden head turning[3-5]—discussion of incidence is most appropriate for consideration in high-energy cervical spine trauma, such as motor vehicle collisions and falls.

Investigation into incidence of VAI began as reports on small cohort groups and then later matured into larger prospective studies. Louw and colleagues[6] were the first to investigate VAI in bilateral facet dislocation in a prospective fashion using digital subtraction angiography (DSA) and detected arterial occlusion in 9 of 12 (75%) patients. Willis and colleagues[7] defined "high-risk" groups as those with criteria of either cervical spine fracture involving the transverse foramen or bilateral facet dislocations and, using DSA, detected VAI in 12 of 26 (46%) patients. Miller and colleagues[8] described a broader definition of "high-risk" criteria, including (1) cervical spine fracture–dislocation, (2) neurologic findings not explained by brain imaging, (3) Horner syndrome, (4) Le Fort II or III fracture, (5) skull base fracture, or (6) expanding neck soft tissue injury. Of 216 patients who met the criteria, they found 49 (22.7%) VAIs. Biffl and colleagues'[9] selection criteria were even more inclusive and found 92 VAIs among 605 patients (15.2%). Using magnetic resonance angiography (MRA), Vaccaro and colleagues[10] noted a 37% rate of VAI with unilateral and bilateral cervical facet dislocations. In a follow-up study, Vaccaro found a 20% (12/61) incidence of VA occlusion in patients with subaxial cervical spine fractures.[11]

Later epidemiologic studies have used large level I trauma registries to more accurately define overall incidence of VAI in blunt trauma admissions. The incidence of VAI among total blunt trauma admissions ranged from 0.075% to 0.77%.[8,12,13] The studies had inherent variations due to location and referral pattern of the center and different imaging modalities used, including DSA, computed tomography (CT) angiogram, and magnetic resonance arteriography. Despite the relatively low overall incidence of blunt VAI in the overall trauma population, this small population of patients has a substantial risk of

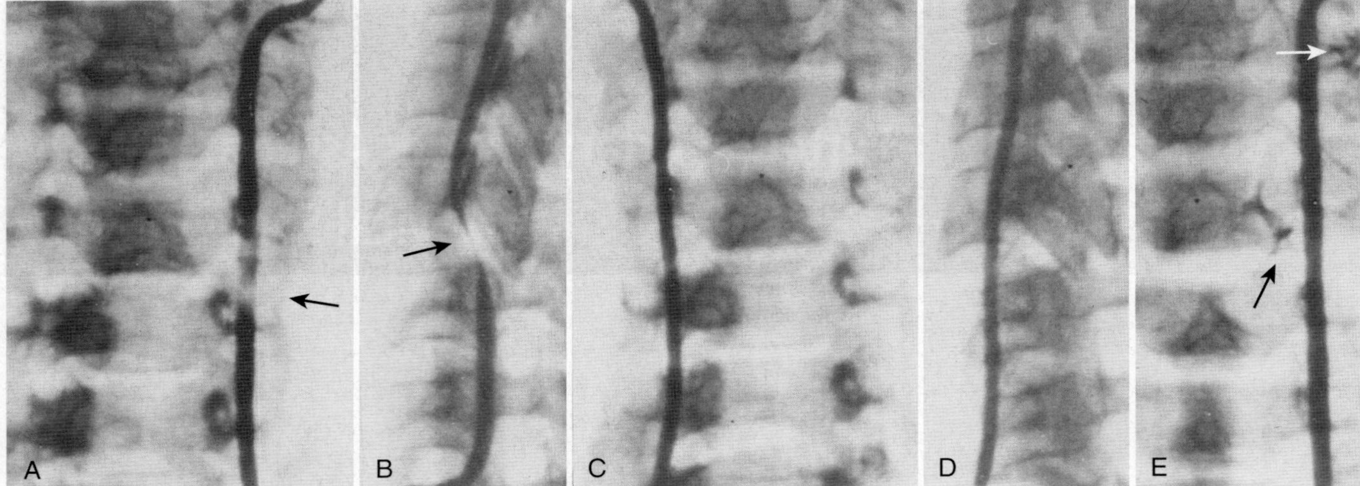

FIG. 80.1 Flexion-distraction stage II injury (lordotic position). A unilateral facet dislocation has been created at C4–C5. The (A) anteroposterior and (B) lateral projections show an hourglass-like stenosis of the left vertebral artery (*arrows*). The contralateral vessel (*right*) has a normal course in the (C) anteroposterior and (D) lateral projections. (E) Contrast extravasation by rupture of a local radicular artery (*black arrow*) and loosening of a muscular arterial ligature (*white arrow*) is demonstrated at dye injection into the left vertebral artery. (From Sim E, Vaccaro AR, Berzianovich A, Simon P. The effects of staged static cervical flexion–distraction deformities on the patency of the vertebral arterial vasculature. *Spine*. 2002;25:2180–2186.)

stroke and mortality,[14] thereby demanding screening criteria and structured protocols for detection of clinically silent lesions.

Mechanism and Types of Arterial Injury

Although VAI has been described at all levels, the V2 segment is the most commonly cited level of injury due to its confinement and tethering within the foramen transversarium, making it susceptible to shear forces during forceful cervical rotation or direct injury from fracture fragments.[15,16] Although less common, the tortuous V3 segment is vulnerable to injury due to its tethering between the foramen transversarium of the atlas and the atlanto-occipital membrane.[17]

Cervical flexion-distraction fracture patterns most commonly result in VAIs, followed by flexion-compression injuries (Figs. 80.1 and 80.2).[11] A review of the literature suggests that a rotational component to the cervical spine may also be a risk factor for VA occlusion.

In an attempt to better refine patient screening criteria for VAI, Cothren and colleagues[13] reviewed 17,007 blunt trauma patients, 125 of whom had cerebral vascular injuries associated with cervical spine injuries. The injuries were characterized as subluxations in 56 (48%) patients, C1 to C3 cervical spine fractures in 42 (36%), and extension of the fracture through the foramen transversarium in 19 (16%). Cervical spine fractures were the sole indication for screening in 90% of the study population. Screening yield of all patients admitted with one of these three fracture patterns was 37%. Therefore, they recommended focused screening for patients with cervical subluxations, fractures through the transverse foramen, or fractures of C1 through C3.

Injury to the VA in the setting of nonpenetrating cervical trauma is most likely due to a stretching mechanism.[18] Sim and colleagues[19] demonstrated in a cadaveric cervical spine model that the static deformity of a flexion-distraction stage II to stage IV subaxial cervical injury resulted in significant compression/stretch of the vertebral arterial vasculature (Figs. 80.3 to 80.5). Initially, the vessel, or a portion of its intimal lining, is injured through excessive distraction in a flexion-distraction injury owing to the soft tissue attachments of the vessel in the foramina transversaria. Secondary events, such as thrombus formation, may then lead to occlusion of the vessel lumen. Recanalization over time after blunt injury to the VA was not a feature observed in a long-term follow-up study reported by Vaccaro and colleagues[10] of image-confirmed vertebral vessel disruption. The lack of recanalization suggests that significant vessel intimal disruption occurs and that thrombus formation is not the only factor involved in vessel occlusion.

The intima of the VA is highly sensitive to shear forces experienced during high-energy blunt trauma. Because the vessel adventitia is more resilient, isolated intimal disruption can lead to a spectrum of clinical entities, including an intimal flap with resultant thrombus formation or a dissection as the intima and adventitia separate cranially. Thrombus and dissection can lead to occlusion. If the energy transmitted is high enough, the adventitia can fail, leading to a pseudoaneurysm formation[20] or transection if complete.

DSA provides the most anatomic detail of arterial injuries. A dissection of the VA has been shown to be the most common pattern of VAI, followed by occlusion. Multiple studies have demonstrated that dissections tend to resolve, whereas occlusions, as a rule, do not recanalize regardless of therapeutic attempts.[10,21,22]

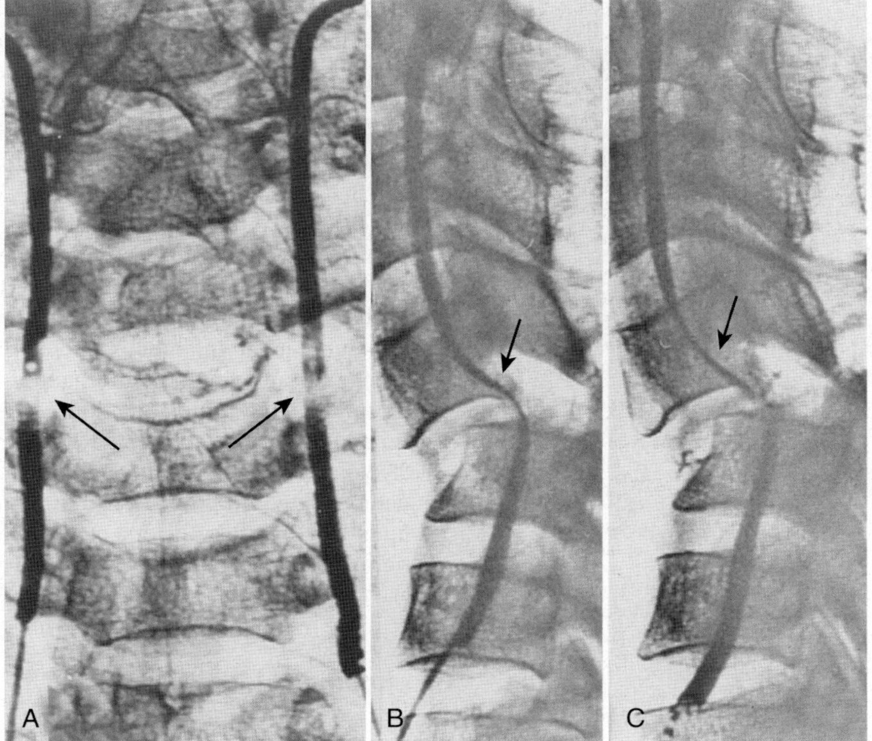

FIG. 80.2 Flexion-distraction stage III injury. A bilateral facet dislocation has been created at C4–C5. The (A) anteroposterior and lateral projections (B, *right*, and C, *left vertebral artery*) reveal excessive thinning of dye flow without complete obstruction (*arrows*) in both the vertebral vessels. (From Sim E, Vaccaro AR, Berzianovich A, Simon P. The effects of staged static cervical flexion–distraction deformities on the patency of the vertebral arterial vasculature. *Spine*. 2002;25:2180–2186.)

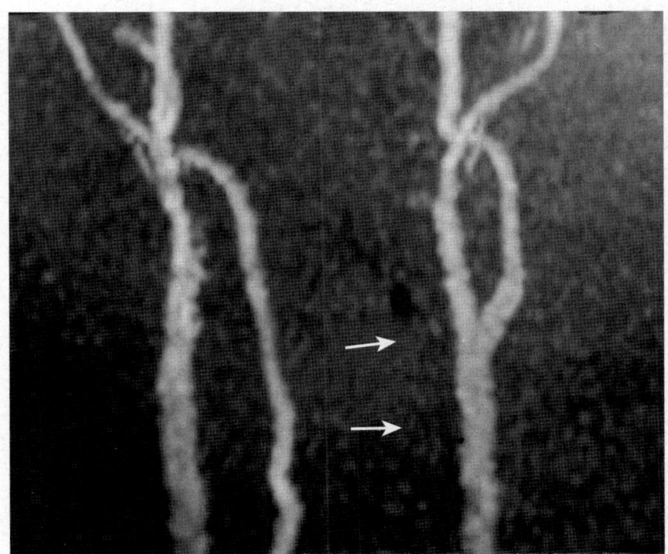

FIG. 80.3 A 73-year-old woman incurred a flexion-distraction injury at C5–C6 after a fall. A magnetic resonance angiography coronal projection image from a two-dimensional time-of-flight dataset shows evidence of normal antegrade flow in the common carotid arteries bilaterally and the right vertebral artery. There is absence of flow in the expected course of the left vertebral artery (*arrows*). (From Vaccaro AR, Gregg KR, Flanders AE, et al. Long-term evaluation of vertebral artery injuries following cervical spine trauma using magnetic resonance angiography. *Spine*. 1998;23:789–794.)

Clinical Diagnoses

Abundant collateral circulation feeding the vertebrobasilar system and posterior circulation of the brain often allows unilateral disruption of the VA to remain asymptomatic. When this collateral circulation is diminished in situations of atherosclerosis or anatomic variations, patients may initially present with symptoms of vertebrobasilar insufficiency (VBI). Symptoms of VA insufficiency may manifest as dizziness, dysarthria, dysphagia, diplopia, blurred vision, and tinnitus.[17]

Initially, asymptomatic patients can have progression of symptoms either acutely or delayed due to embolism, thrombus extension, or dissection. Heros and colleagues[23] described a patient who sustained a VAI with a resultant cerebellar infarction despite having a normal contralateral artery. To explain the infarction, the authors postulated that the thrombosis had extended distally to the intracranial portion of the VA. Interestingly, Six and colleagues[24] reported a case of an asymptomatic posttraumatic bilateral VA occlusion. Angiography demonstrated occlusion of both VAs but with the presence of blood flow through the intramuscular collateral vessels of the thyrocervical trunk and by collaterals from the superficial occipital artery. In fact, Blam and colleagues[25] conducted a retrospective review of 1283 patients

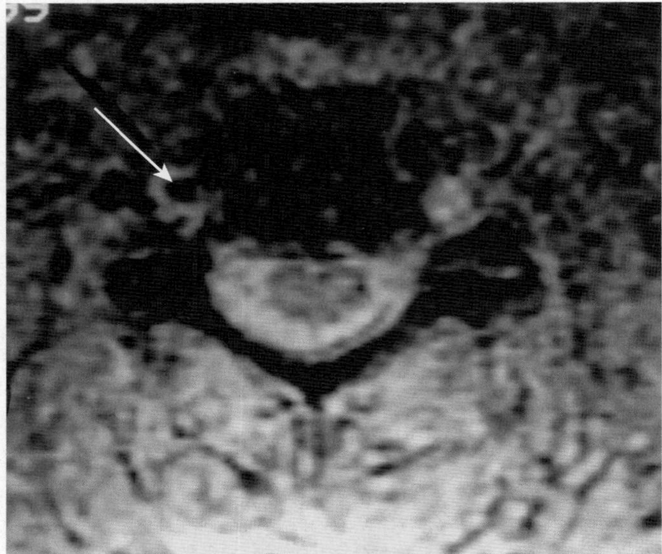

FIG. 80.4 A 51-year-old woman sustained a C4–C5 flexion-distraction injury after a motor vehicle accident. This patient underwent a posterior cervical fusion. Magnetic resonance imaging revealed a C4–C5 central herniated disc, resulting in spinal cord compression. Cord edema was seen from C3 to C5. An axial magnetic resonance angiography gradient-echo image obtained at the mid-C4 level shows a hypointense focus (compared with the normal [hyperintense] left foramen transversarium) contained within the right foramen transversarium (*arrow*) that is consistent with acute thrombosis of the right vertebral artery. (From Vaccaro AR, Gregg KR, Flanders AE, et al. Long-term evaluation of vertebral artery injuries following cervical spine trauma using magnetic resonance angiography. *Spine*. 1998;23:789–794.)

with cervical spine trauma and determined that a normal neurologic examination is not predictive of VA patency after significant cervical spine trauma. These authors also noted that VAI was observed in similar frequency in both neurologically intact and motor incomplete patients (American Spinal Injury Association [ASIA] classifications C and D).[25]

The interval between spinal injury and the development of vertebrobasilar symptoms varies greatly from immediately after trauma to up to 3 months later.[17,26] The late onset of symptoms suggests a process of vertebral vessel thrombus formation at the injury site with clot propagation or embolism and subsequent infarction. Therefore, clinicians should be aware that late symptoms and signs of VBI after cervical spine trauma may be a manifestation of VAI that occurred at the time of trauma.[11] Vaccaro and colleagues[10] demonstrated that 83% of patients with a known traumatic vertebral vessel injury demonstrated no flow reconstitution after an average follow-up of 25.8 months. The one patient who did show reconstitution of flow was thought to have a resolution of vertebral arterial spasm that initially compromised flow.

Imaging Modalities

DSA is a type of fluoroscopy technique used in interventional radiology to clearly visualize blood vessels in a bony or dense soft tissue environment. Images are produced using contrast medium by subtracting a "precontrast image," or the mask from

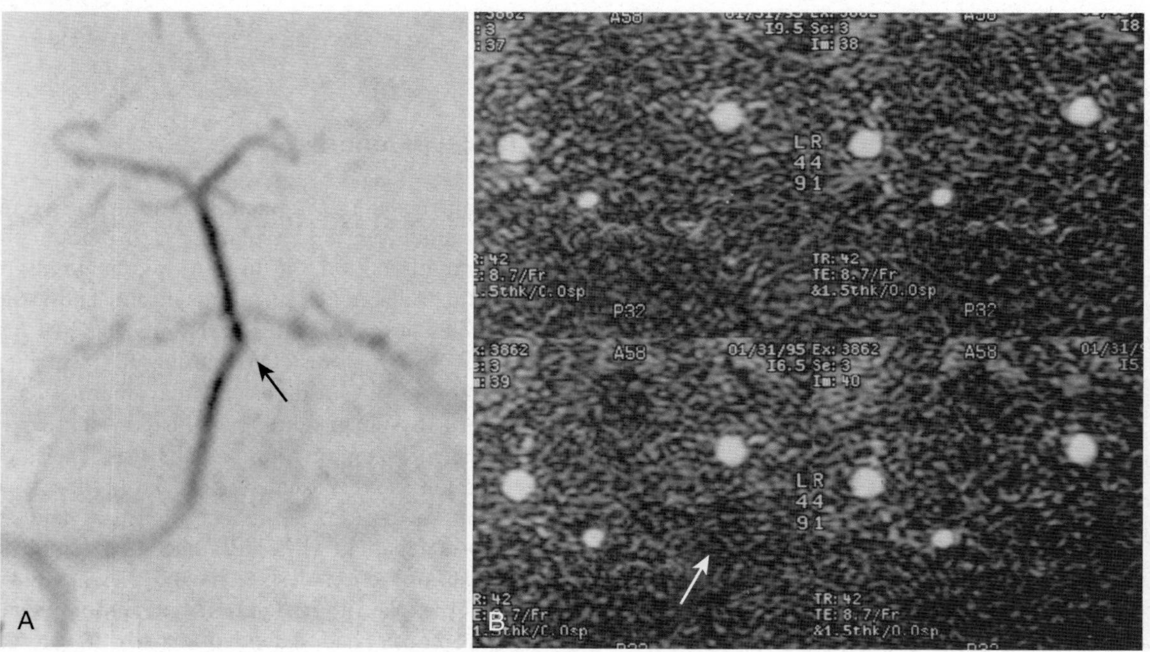

FIG. 80.5 A 28-year-old man sustained a flexion-distraction injury at the C5–C6 level following a motor vehicle accident. (A) Coronal projection image from a two-dimensional time-of-flight magnetic resonance angiography dataset shows the junction of the right vertebral artery with the basilar artery at the expected location of the vertebrobasilar junction. The distal left vertebral artery is absent (*arrow*). (B) Four transaxial contiguous images from a two-dimensional time-of-flight dataset show absence of flow-related enhancement in the left foramen transversarium, which is consistent with occlusion of the left vertebral artery. (From Vaccaro AR, Gregg KR, Flanders AE, et al: Long-term evaluation of vertebral artery injuries following cervical spine trauma using magnetic resonance angiography. *Spine*. 1998;23:789–794.)

later images, once the contrast medium has been introduced into a structure. DSA has routinely been described as the gold standard for detection of VA abnormalities. It is the only imaging technique that can reproducibly detect subtle intimal abnormalities. DSA is also the only technique that allows an interventional neuroradiologist to perform interventions if deemed necessary and appropriate. DSA, however, is time demanding, technique dependent, and invasive, with inherent risks including iatrogenic arterial perforation, puncture-site hematoma/false aneurysm, and dye toxicity. Because of this, DSA may not be a suitable screening tool, leading to development of alternate tests including computed tomography angiography (CTA) and MRA. However, neither of these techniques has proven to match the sensitivity or specificity of DSA.

CTA is a technique that combines precisely timed high-speed, multidetector CT imaging shortly after a bolus of contrast dye through a peripheral intravenous line. Using bolus tracking, a specific anatomic site—in this example, the vertebral arteries—can be imaged without the need for cannulating a catheter directly to the site, thereby eliminating many possible complications associated with DSA. In addition, the amount of dye used in CTA is substantially less than that used in DSA. The majority of high-energy trauma patients require head and cervical spine scans; therefore, this imaging modality can be done in the same clinical setting as other required trauma-specific imaging studies. The previous-generation four-detector CT scanner was widely found to be inadequate for VAI injury. Newer high-speed 16-detector CT scanner imaging is far superior in resolution and in its ability to bolus track. Therefore, this technique has experienced near-universal acceptance within the radiology community as a replacement for DSA. Eastman and colleagues[27] found that CTA was nearly identical to DSA for detection of VAI in 162 patients determined to be at risk of injury. As imaging technology continues to improve, subsequent studies utilizing 32- and 64-channel multidetector CT have found that DSA can confidently and effectively be replaced with CTA.[28]

Although these less-invasive imaging techniques are attractive for the reasons stated earlier and despite wide acceptance in the radiology literature, some trauma surgeons remain skeptical of CTA accuracy. Biffl and colleagues[21] have questioned their ability to detect all vascular lesions when compared with the gold standard DSA. The investigators developed a grading scale to evaluate the performance of MRA and CTA: grade I, dissection with less than 25% luminal narrowing; grade II, dissection with more than 25% luminal narrowing; grade III, pseudoaneurysm; grade IV, occlusion; and grade V, transection. Forty-six consecutive patients underwent CTA or MRA in conjunction with DSA. Although adequate for dramatic lesions, the more subtle grades I, II, and III lesions were routinely missed by CTA or MRA.

Malhotra and colleagues[29] also noted that, increasingly, CTA has been replacing DSA in suspected VAI injuries and selected 119 patients who met screening criteria (facial/cervical–spinal fractures; unexplained neurologic deficit; anisocoria; lateral neck soft tissue injury; clinical suspicion) out of 7000 level I blunt trauma admissions and performed DSA and CTA. In agreement with Biffl's study, they found an alarming rate of missed VAIs using CTA that were visualized using DSA. The authors went as far as to say that using CTA was dangerous due to the risk of missed injuries. Miller and colleagues' study also found CTA and MRA to be inadequate screening tools.[8] Although many investigators have shown failures of CTA to detect subtle lesions, Berne and colleagues[30] have asserted that CTA is sufficient for detection of clinically relevant injuries (i.e., high-grade injuries). Although screening criteria may be employed to direct a dedicated CTA of the cerebrovascular system, another consideration is to integrate a CTA of the VA into the standard CT trauma series protocol. Langner and colleagues[31] developed such a protocol and found that an optimized craniocervical CTA can be easily integrated into a whole-body CT protocol for polytrauma patients. They assert that no additional screening technique is necessary to identify clinically relevant vascular injuries. This type of protocol could lead to a more liberalized screening of all trauma patients, as recommended by some investigators.[32]

MRA uses magnetic resonance imaging (MRI) with specifically designed sequences or gadolinium dye to image arterial blood flow. Similar to CTA, MRA offers a minimally invasive alternative to DSA. In addition, MRA is nonionizing. MRA can be performed in the same clinical setting as a spine or brain MRI. Although many studies have compared CTA to the gold standard DSA, there are relatively fewer studies comparing the sensitivity and specificity of MRA in detecting VAI.

The most common noncontrast, flow-based method is inflow angiography, or "time-of-flight" (TOF), which is simply ordinary MRI using settings that make flowing blood much brighter than stationary tissue.

MRA based on an injected contrast medium (usually containing gadolinium) is currently the most common form of MRA. The contrast medium is injected into a vein, and images are acquired during the first pass of the agent through the arteries. Provided that the timing is correct, this may result in images of high quality. An alternative is to use a contrast agent that does not, as most agents do, leave the vascular system within a few minutes but remains in the circulation up to an hour (a "blood-pool agent"). Because longer time is available for image acquisition, higher-resolution imaging is possible. A problem, however, is the fact that both arteries and veins are enhanced at the same time.

Veras and colleagues[33] performed a retrospective review of patients with VAI to determine the ideal MRA imaging sequence. They noted that two-dimensional TOF sequencing was a more effective imaging sequence than the three-dimensional time-of-flow because of a reduced false-positive signal dropout. Axial T1-weighted MRI was useful because of its ability to delineate the absence of flow from an intimal occlusion, including an intraluminal clot. In a dog model, Ren and colleagues[34] found that MRA was comparable with DSA for evaluation of VAI.

Screening

As discussed in the previous section, many studies have demonstrated the convenience, low risk, and reliability of modern multidetector CTA to detect blunt cerebrovascular injury (BCVI), including vertebral artery injury. Determining which patients are at a high risk of BCVI and who should have a CTA is an important aspect of the detection and treatment algorithm. The most often used criteria are that set forth by the Denver group. The "Denver" criteria include (1) an injury mechanism compatible with severe cervical hyperextension with rotation or hyperflexion; (2) Lefort II or III midface fractures; (3) basilar skull fractures involving the carotid canal; (4) closed head injury consistent with diffuse axonal injury with Glasgow Coma Scale score less than 6; (5) cervical vertebral body or transverse foramen fracture, subluxation, or ligamentous injury at any level, or fracture at the level of C1–C3; (6) near-hanging resulting in cerebral anoxia; or (7) seat belt or other clothesline-type injury with significant cervical pain or swelling.[35] The "Denver" criteria have been widely adopted, but more recent studies have asserted that the screening be more focused[36] or more relaxed.[37]

Treatment

Treatment considerations should be divided into (1) symptomatic with evidence of stroke, (2) symptomatic without evidence of stroke, and (3) asymptomatic VAI.

Several different methods of therapy have been used to treat symptomatically occluded VAs. The American Association of Neurological Surgeons/Congress of Neurological Surgeons Guidelines consensus concluded that patients with posterior circulation stroke and VAI have a better outcome when treated with intravenous heparin than patients who do not receive this treatment.[38] Fibrinolysis with streptokinase has also been described to successfully restore flow with varied results.[39]

Although the exact mechanism is ill defined, be it ischemia or embolic, the outcome of patients who develop symptoms of posterior circulation ischemia without stroke and are treated with intravenous heparin[1,40–42] is similar to that of patients receiving no treatment.[6,43] In the symptomatic patient, Schellinger and colleagues[41] advocated the initial use of heparin with a target-activated partial thromboplastin time of at least twice the baseline value followed by oral anticoagulation (warfarin) for at least 3 to 6 months as a secondary prophylaxis.

Complications associated with anticoagulation in the trauma population range from 25% to 54%.[44] Bleeding complications include intracranial hemorrhage, gastrointestinal bleeding, retroperitoneal hemorrhage, and excessive surgical site bleeding. In fact, in a study by Eachempati and colleagues,[45] only 14% of trauma patients were deemed candidates for full anticoagulation. These facts have led physicians to focus more on antiplatelet therapy as opposed to heparinization.

In appropriately selected candidates with a symptomatic dissecting VA, surgical intervention may include vertebral vessel resection followed by grafting. Another method of arresting vessel flow is through the use of catheter embolization with Guglielmi detachable coils.[46–48] Today, the gold standard surgical procedure for a symptomatic vertebral dissection remains ligation of the injured VA proximal and distal to the site of the lesion rather than primary repair.[47] As mentioned previously, ligation is well tolerated if there is adequate collateral flow.

The treatment of asymptomatic VAIs has been controversial in the past. In the previous edition of this text, in the majority of level I trauma centers, formal treatment was not recommended for a patient with an asymptomatic VAI after trauma.[24,48] Multiple groups have since endorsed the use of aspirin (acetylsalicylic acid [ASA]) for treatment of all VAI. The use of ASA has been shown to prevent stroke and potentially increase the chance of arterial injury healing and flow abnormality resolution.

Because of the risk of rupture and embolic source, a pseudoaneurysm of the VA is usually aggressively treated most commonly with coil embolization or stenting.

Transection of the VA is a life-threatening emergency due to hemorrhagic shock and/or airway compromise. Treatment is airway management, resuscitation, and emergent interventional neuroradiology embolization.[49] An additional reason to routinely evaluate for the presence of a vertebral vessel disruption in an asymptomatic patient is to ensure safety of the intact vessel if surgical intervention with implants that may put the vertebral vasculature at risk are to be used.

Summary

Despite its controversial treatment, the diagnosis of VAIs after blunt cervical trauma is beneficial in that it may alter or modify the proposed surgical procedure and may explain late onset of symptoms consistent with VBI. The potential risk for injury to the uninjured VA should be known to the surgeon when operating on the cervical spine, especially when performing procedures that may place the uninjured artery at risk (i.e., lateral mass plating or cervical pedicle screw placement). The physician must realize that the injured VA is a potential source for thrombus propagation and embolization with resultant neurologic injury. Imaging should be considered in all patients who present with signs and symptoms of VBI, especially in the presence of a cervical dislocation, high cervical spine (C1–C3) fracture, or fracture involving the foramen transversarium. Multiple societies have published practice management guidelines for the screening and treatment of BCVI. The Eastern Association for the Surgery of Trauma[50] and Western Trauma Association[51] reported guidelines very similar to those described in this chapter in 2010 and 2009, respectively. The consensus statement from the American Association of Neurological Surgeons/Congress of Neurological Surgeons recommends anticoagulation for VAI with evidence of posterior circulation stroke and recommends consideration for anticoagulation in symptomatic VAI without evidence of stroke. Vertebral artery injury without symptoms should be treated with aspirin when deemed safe from a bleeding risk perspective. These recommendations in general have continued to be supported by the majority of contemporary studies. Fortunately, because of adequate collateral circulation, most VAIs remain asymptomatic.

PEARLS

1. Most VAIs are asymptomatic because of sufficient collateral blood flow through the contralateral vertebral artery.
2. VAIs should be suspected after blunt cervical trauma when patients present with neurologic deficits, such as dysarthria, dizziness, diplopia, and dysphagia.
3. Flexion-distraction injuries are most commonly associated with VAIs, followed by flexion-compression injuries.
4. Imaging should be considered in the setting of specific cervical spine injuries, such as cervical dislocations, fracture involving the foramen transversarium, and injuries to the upper cervical spine (C1–C3) to rule out VAI.
5. Anticoagulation with intravenous heparin is recommended for patients with VAI who have evidence of posterior circulation stroke. Aspirin should be utilized for all other VAIs if no contraindication exists.

PITFALLS

1. DSA provides the most detailed, highest-resolution imaging of the vertebral artery pathoanatomy but is an invasive procedure with potential risks.
2. CT and magnetic resonance arteriograms may be acceptable screening tools for clinically relevant VAIs but may fail to detect more subtle lesions. CTA sensitivity and specificity continues to improve with higher-number detector channels.
3. Anticoagulation treatment is associated with potentially significant complications, such as hemorrhage, stroke propagation, and neural ischemia.
4. Surgeons should be cognizant of prior cervical spine trauma and possible VAI when performing procedures that may place the uninjured vertebral artery at risk (i.e., lateral mass plating).
5. Most VA occlusions do not reconstitute their blood flow, and late neurologic deterioration may occur from extension of the arterial thrombus, emboli formation, and resultant infarction.

KEY POINTS

1. VAIs are most commonly seen in cervical spine fractures involving the foramen transversarium, upper cervical spine (C1–C3), and cervical subluxations/dislocations. Intimal disruption and secondary thrombus formation is the most common pattern of vascular injury seen in cervical spine fractures. Most VAIs are asymptomatic due to sufficient collateral blood flow through the contralateral VA.
2. In the previously shown fracture patterns, it is suggested that advanced imaging (MRA or CT arteriography) of the VAs is performed to evaluate for injury. DSA provides the most detailed, highest-resolution imaging of the VA pathoanatomy but is an invasive procedure with potential risks. CT and magnetic resonance arteriograms may be acceptable screening tools for clinically relevant VAIs but may fail to detect more subtle lesions.
3. Key neurologic signs and symptoms of vertebrobasilar (posterior/cerebellar) insufficiency can be subtle and include dysarthria, dizziness, diplopia, and dysphagia.
4. Anticoagulation with intravenous heparin is recommended for patients with VAI who have evidence of posterior circulation stroke. Aspirin should be utilized for all other VAIs if no contraindication exists.

KEY REFERENCES

1. Giacobetti F, Vaccaro A, Bos-Giacobetti M, et al. Vertebral artery occlusion associated with cervical spine trauma: a prospective analysis. *Spine*. 1997;22:188-192.
   The authors noted an alarmingly high rate of vertebral artery injury (19.7%), particularly with flexion-distraction and flexion-compression injuries and suggested selective magnetic resonance angiography evaluation of these patients.
2. Vaccaro AR, Klein GR, Flanders AE, et al. Long-term evaluation of vertebral artery injuries following cervical spine trauma using magnetic resonance angiography. *Spine*. 1998;23:789-796.
   A prospective study determined at 25.8-month follow-up that the majority of patients (83%) who sustained a vertebral artery injury secondary to cervical spinal trauma did not reconstitute the occluded vertebral artery.
3. Cothren CC, Moore EE, Biffl WL, et al. Cervical spine fracture patterns predictive of blunt vertebral artery injury. *J Trauma*. 2003;55:811-813.
   Blunt cerebrovascular injury is associated with complex cervical spine fractures that include subluxation, extension into the foramen transversarium, or upper C1 to C3 fractures. One of these three injury patterns was observed in 90% (subluxations in 48%, C1 to C3 cervical spine fractures in 36%, or extension of the fracture through the foramen transversarium in 16%) of blunt cerebrovascular injuries associated with cervical spine trauma at one institution. Patients sustaining such cervical fractures should undergo prompt screening.
4. Biffl WL, Ray CE Jr, Moore EE, et al. Noninvasive diagnosis of blunt cerebrovascular injuries: a preliminary report. *J Trauma*. 2002;53:850-856.
   This is the first description of a VAI grading system from I to V in order of severity (partial occlusion to transection). CT and MR angiography can identify VAI, but they regularly miss more subtle grade I, II, and III injuries. Future technical modifications may improve their accuracy, but in the interim, arteriography remains the gold standard for diagnosis. If arteriography is not available, CT or MR angiography should be used to screen for VAI in patients at risk.
5. American Association of Neurological Surgeons/Congress of Neurological Surgeons Joint Section of Disorders of the Spine and Peripheral Nerves. Management of vertebral artery injuries after nonpenetrating cervical trauma. *Neurosurgery*. 2002;50(3 suppl):S173-S178.
   Anticoagulation with intravenous heparin is recommended for patients with vertebral artery injury who have evidence of posterior circulation stroke. Either observation or treatment with antiplatelet agents in patients with vertebral artery injuries who clinically demonstrate vertebrobasilar insufficiency without evidence of posterior circulation stroke is recommended. Observation in patients with vertebral artery injuries and no evidence of posterior circulation ischemia is recommended.

REFERENCES

1. Lee KP, Carlini WG, McCormick GF, Albers GW. Neurologic complications following chiropractic manipulation: a survey of California neurologists. *Neurology*. 1995;45:1213-1215.
2. Oehler J, Gandjour J, Fiebach J, Schwab S. Bilateral vertebral artery dissection after chiropractic treatment. *Orthopade*. 2003;32:911-915. [in German].
3. Traflet RF, Babaria AR, Bell RD, et al. Vertebral artery dissection after rapid head turning. *AJNR Am J Neuroradiol*. 1989;10:650-651.
4. DeBehnke DJ, Brady W. Vertebral artery dissection due to minor neck trauma. *J Emerg Med*. 1994;12:27-31.
5. McCrory P. Vertebral artery dissection causing stroke in sport. *J Clin Neurosci*. 2000;7:298-300.
6. Louw JA, Mafoyane NA, Small B, Neser CP. Occlusion of the vertebral artery in cervical spine dislocations. *J Bone Joint Surg Br*. 1990;72:679-681.

7. Willis BK, Greiner F, Orrison WW, Benzel EC. The incidence of vertebral artery injury after midcervical spine fracture or subluxation. *Neurosurgery*. 1994;34:435-442.
8. Miller PR, Fabian TC, Croce MA, et al. Prospective screening for blunt cerebrovascular injuries: analysis of diagnostic modalities and outcomes. *Ann Surg*. 2002;236:386-395.
9. Biffl WL, Moore EE, Elliott JP, et al. The devastating potential blunt vertebral arterial injuries. *Ann Surg*. 2000;231:672-681.
10. Vaccaro AR, Klein GR, Flanders AE, et al. Long-term evaluation of vertebral artery injuries following cervical spine trauma using magnetic resonance angiography. *Spine*. 1998;23:789-794.
11. Giacobetti FB, Vaccaro AR, Bos-Giacobetti MA, et al. Vertebral artery occlusion associated with cervical spine trauma: a prospective analysis. *Spine*. 1997;22:188-192.
12. Berne JD, Norwood SH, McAuley CE, Villareal DH. Helical computed tomographic angiography: an excellent screening test for blunt cerebrovascular injury. *J Trauma*. 2004;57:11-19.
13. Cothren CC, Moore EE, Biffl WL, et al. Cervical spine fracture patterns predictive of blunt vertebral artery injury. *J Trauma*. 2003;55:811-813.
14. Berne JD, Norwood SH, McAuley CE, et al. The high morbidity of blunt cerebrovascular injury in an unscreened population: more evidence of the need for mandatory screening protocols. *J Am Coll Surg*. 2001;192:314-321.
15. Parent AD, Harkey HL, Touchstone DA, et al. Lateral cervical spine dislocation and vertebral artery injury. *Neurosurgery*. 1992;31:501-509.
16. Biffl WL, Ray CE Jr, Moore EE, et al. Treatment-related outcomes from blunt cerebrovascular injuries: importance of routine follow-up arteriography. *Ann Surg*. 2002;235:699-707.
17. Deen HG Jr, McGirr SJ. Vertebral artery injury associated with cervical spine fracture. *Spine*. 1992;17:230-234.
18. Bula WI, Loes DJ. Trauma to the cerebrovascular system. *Neuroimaging Clin North Am*. 1994;4:753-772.
19. Sim E, Vaccaro AR, Berzlanovich A, Pienaar S. The effects of staged static cervical flexion-distraction deformities on the patency of the vertebral arterial vasculature. *Spine*. 2000;25:2180-2186.
20. Saito T, Kamisawa O, Kaminishi Y, et al. Isolated traumatic vertebral pseudoaneurysm: report of a case. *Surg Today*. 2003;33:145-147.
21. Biffl WL, Ray CE Jr, Moore EE, et al. Noninvasive diagnosis of blunt cerebrovascular injuries: a preliminary report. *J Trauma*. 2002;53:850-856.
22. Miller PR, Fabian TC, Bee TK, et al. Blunt cerebrovascular injuries: diagnosis and treatment. *J Trauma*. 2001;51:279-286.
23. Heros RC. Cerebellar infarction resulting from traumatic occlusion of a vertebral artery. *J Neurosurg*. 1979;51:111-113.
24. Six EG, Stringer WL, Cowley AR, Davis CH. Posttraumatic bilateral vertebral artery occlusion: case report. *J Neurosurg*. 1981;54:814-817.
25. Blam O, Torina P, Vaccaro AR, et al. *Incidence of vertebral artery thrombosis in cervical spine trauma. Unpublished data.* Miami Beach, FL: Submitted to Cervical Spine Research Society; 2002 December 5-7.
26. Quint DJ, Spickler EM. Magnetic resonance demonstration of vertebral artery dissection: report of two cases. *J Neurosurg*. 1990;72:964-967.
27. Eastman AL, Chason DP, Perez CL, et al. Computed tomographic angiography for the diagnosis of blunt cervical vascular injury: is it ready for primetime? *J Trauma*. 2006;60:925-929.
28. Paulus EM, Fabian TC, Savage SA, et al. Blunt cerebrovascular injury screening with 64-channel multidetector computed tomography: more slices finally cut it. *J Trauma Acute Care Surg*. 2014;76(2):279-283.
29. Malhotra AK, Camacho M, Ivatury RR, et al. Computed tomographic angiography for the diagnosis of blunt carotid/vertebral artery injury: a note of caution. *Ann Surg*. 2007;246:632-642.
30. Berne JD, Reuland KS, Villarreal DH, et al. Sixteen-slice multi-detector computed tomographic angiography improves the accuracy of screening for blunt cerebrovascular injury. *J Trauma*. 2006;60:1204-1209.
31. Langner S, Fleck S, Kirsch M, et al. Whole-body CT trauma imaging with adapted and optimized CT angiography of the craniocervical vessels: do we need an extra screening examination? *AJNR Am J Neuroradiol*. 2008;29:1902-1907.
32. Kerwin AJ, Bynoe RP, Murray J, et al. Liberalized screening for blunt carotid and vertebral artery injuries is justified. *Neurosurgery*. 2002;50(3 suppl):S173-S178.
33. Veras L, Gutierrez S, Castellanos J, et al. Vertebral artery occlusion after acute cervical spine trauma. *Spine*. 2000;25:1171-1177.
34. Ren X, Wang W, Zhang X, et al. Clinical study and comparison of magnetic resonance angiography (MRA) and angiography diagnosis of blunt vertebral artery injury. *J Trauma*. 2007;63:1249-1253.
35. Cothren CC, Moore EE, Ray CE Jr, et al. Screening for blunt cerebrovascular injuries is cost-effective. *Am J Surg*. 2005;190(6):845-849.
36. Lockwood MM, Smith GA, Tanenbaum J, et al. Screening via CT angiogram after traumatic cervical spine fractures: narrowing imaging to improve cost effectiveness. Experience of a Level I trauma center. *J Neurosurg Spine*. 2016;24(3):490-495.
37. Jacobson LE, Ziemba-Davis M, Herrera AJ. The limitations of using risk factors to screen for blunt cerebrovascular injuries: the harder you look, the more you find. *World J Emerg Surg*. 2015;10:46.
38. American Association of Neurological Surgeons/Congress of Neurological Surgeons Joint Section of Disorders of the Spine and Peripheral Nerves. Management of vertebral artery injuries after nonpenetrating cervical trauma. *Neurosurgery*. 2002;50(3 suppl):S173-S178.
39. Schwarz N, Buchinger W, Gaudernak T, et al. Injuries to the cervical spine causing vertebral artery trauma: case reports. *J Trauma*. 1991;31:127-133.
40. Prabhu V, Kizer J, Patil A, et al. Vertebrobasilar thrombosis associated with nonpenetrating cervical spine trauma. *J Trauma*. 1996;40:130-137.
41. Schellinger PD, Schwab S, Krieger D, et al. Masking of vertebral artery dissection by severe trauma to the cervical spine. *Spine*. 2001;26:314-319.
42. Thibodeaux LC, Hearn AT, Peschiera JL, et al. Extracranial vertebral artery dissection after trauma: a five year review. *Br J Surg*. 1997;84:94.
43. Schwarz N, Buchinger W, Gaudernak T, et al. Injuries to the cervical spine causing vertebral artery trauma: case reports. *J Trauma*. 1991;31:127-133.
44. Biffl WL, Moore EE, Ryu RK, et al. The unrecognized epidemic of blunt carotid arterial injuries: early diagnosis improves neurologic outcome. *Ann Surg*. 1998;228:462-470.
45. Eachempati SR, Vaslef SN, Sebastian MW, Reed RL 2nd. Blunt vascular injuries of the head and neck: is heparinization necessary? *J Trauma*. 1998;45:997-1004.

46. Alexander JJ, Glagov S, Zarins CK. Repair of a vertebral artery dissection. *J Neurosurg*. 1986;64:662-666.
47. Blickenstaff KL, Weaver FA, Yellin AE, et al. Trends in the management of traumatic vertebral arteries injuries. *Am J Surg*. 1989;158:101-106.
48. Bose B, Northrup BE, Osterholm JL. Delayed vertebrobasilar insufficiency following cervical spine injury. *Spine*. 1985;18:108-110.
49. Willis BK, Greiner F, Orrison WW, Benzel EC. The incidence of vertebral artery injury after midcervical spine fracture or subluxation. *Neurosurgery*. 1994;34:435-442.
50. Bromberg WJ, Collier BC, Diebel LN, et al. Blunt cerebrovascular injury practice management guidelines: the Eastern Association for the Surgery of Trauma. *J Trauma*. 2010;68(2):471-477.
51. Biffl WL, Cothren CC, Moore EE, et al. Western Trauma Association critical decisions in trauma: screening for and treatment of blunt cerebrovascular injuries. *J Trauma*. 2009;67(6):1150-1153.

81

CHAPTER

Spinal Orthoses for Traumatic and Degenerative Disease

SECTION XI

Michael J. Vives

Braces have played an integral role in the management of spinal pathologic processes for thousands of years. Smith, in his 1908 article "The Most Ancient Splints," described brace use in ancient Egypt more than 2500 years ago.[1] Much of the early literature focused on treatment of spinal deformities, including Galen's chest-strapping method and Paré's leather-lined metal jacket, popular in the late 16th century.[2] Nicholas Andry developed the "iron cross" in the early 18th century for cervical immobilization, consisting of a straight metal upright with a cross and metal ring attached to the top for support of the head.[3] Today, spinal bracing continues to be a mainstay of treating deformity (covered elsewhere in this text) and the management of traumatic and degenerative spinal disorders. In medical terms, spinal braces are referred to as orthoses, which are defined as externally applied devices that restrict motion, correct deformity, or improve function in a particular body segment.[4]

Spinal orthoses can be broadly categorized based on the body segment that they are employed to immobilize: cervical (CO), cervicothoracic (CTO), thoracolumbosacral (TLSO), lumbosacral (LSO), and sacroiliac (SIO). This chapter focuses on the biomechanics, laboratory studies, and the classic and recent clinical results of commonly used commercially available spinal orthoses. The US Food and Drug Administration (FDA) has classified spinal orthoses as class I devices. As a result, they have not been subject to the strict regulations and scrutiny applied to implantable devices. The currently available knowledge on these devices is the product of observations of varying degrees of scientific merit. Additionally, many commercially available products do not have peer-reviewed data to support their purported effectiveness. The prosthetics and orthotics community has produced numerous publications in print and online trade journals regarding their products and design developments, but comparatively little is published in medical journals familiar to practicing spine specialists. A PubMed search using the key words "spinal orthoses" will result in a fraction of the results that an Internet search will yield. The paucity of readily available peer-reviewed literature has presumably contributed to the variability of prescribing patterns among spine specialists. Bible and colleagues illustrated this point using a questionnaire study of the postoperative bracing preferences among spine surgeons.[5] Most of the respondents braced their patients postoperatively, but there was no consensus on the type, duration, or indications for bracing. In this chapter, therefore, we have attempted to discuss the available data and review design features of various orthoses rather than make specific recommendations on the superiority of one commercial product versus another. Hopefully, the information provided can help clinicians choose the appropriate orthoses to meet their patients' needs.

Biomechanics and Biomaterials

An improved understanding of spinal biomechanics has led to advances in spinal bracing. Conceptually, the spine can be thought of as a series of semirigid bodies interconnected by viscoelastic linkages. Spinal kinematics involves motion in six degrees of freedom, with rotation about three axes and translation along the three coordinates.[6] For clinical considerations, testing (particularly involving human subjects) has generally been confined to three planes of motion: flexion-extension, axial rotation, and lateral bending.

The efficacy of a particular orthosis to limit spinal motion has been tested using various methods, including radiography and goniometry. Standard radiography, typically utilizing flexion-extension views, has been commonly employed. Cineradiography evaluates motion through the use of fluoroscopy. Goniometry utilizes external devices attached to the subject to measure spinal motion. It has been demonstrated to correlate fairly well with radiographic techniques[7] and avoids exposing subjects to radiation. However, there is some decreased accuracy and lack of information on motion at any particular segment. Motion analysis systems that permit spinal motion to be measured in three dimensions have been utilized more recently to study the efficacy of orthoses.[8,9]

Because bracing attempts to control the position of the spine through the application of external forces, orthotic design must account for regional variations of the surrounding anatomy and accommodate vulnerable structures. This includes the vital soft tissue about the anterior neck, the rigid thoracic rib cage, the compressible abdomen, and the bony pelvis at the base of the lumbar spine. The surrounding soft tissue envelope has a substantial effect on the ability of an externally applied force to control spinal movement. Pressure measurements on the soft tissues may be an objective way to

BOX 81.1 Commonly Used Materials in the Fabrication of Orthoses[a]

Ionomer (Thermovac Surlyn)
Oliphin (polypropylene)
Polycarbonate (Lexan)
Polyethylene (Vitrathene)
Polyethylene foam (Plastazote, Aliplast)
Acrylic–polyvinyl chloride (Kydex)
Resins (epoxy, polyester)

[a]Common product names are in parentheses.

assess the fit of a spinal orthosis. The role of soft tissue pressure measurement as an index of applied corrective or stabilizing force, however, remains unclear.[10,11] The intervening soft tissue envelope is also an area of potential complications: problems include breakdown, local pain, decreased vital capacity, and increased lower extremity venous pressure.[12]

Along with our improved understanding of the biomechanics of spinal bracing, improvements in the materials available for brace manufacture have led to dramatic advances in their design. During the 18th century, braces were generally constructed of leather, iron, and wood. German developments in the 19th and early 20th centuries led to many new brace designs, with paper cellulose and glue being added to wooden or iron frames.[4] Newer composite materials, polymer resins, and thermoplastics have led to a proliferation of commercially available orthoses that are lightweight and comfortable without sacrificing the stability afforded by the heavier, more cumbersome designs of the past. New low-density polyethylene shells have considerable flexibility off the body, facilitating donning and doffing, but once strapped have comparable vertical stiffness to other rigid designs. Commonly used materials in the fabrication of orthoses are listed in Box 81.1.

Beyond the advances in our understanding of biomechanics and biomaterials, advances in computer engineering have led to innovative methods for customized production of orthoses with decreased time requirements. At our institutions, efforts to limit the length of inpatient admissions have necessitated a close working relationship between the treating physicians and the orthotists. A computerized database of key measurements that have been recorded over the years has allowed our orthotists to develop digitized models of various sizes and body types utilizing computer-aided design/computer-aided manufacturing technology (CAD/CAM). Using this approach, simple measurement at the sternal notch, xiphoid, and waist along with linear measurements can be performed and integrated with CAD/CAM technology to rapidly design a precision-fit orthosis in a fraction of the time needed for standard mold-based orthoses. Researchers have evaluated this approach for bracing patients with idiopathic scoliosis. Braces comparable to those made using traditional mold techniques (in comfort and curve correction) could be produced in roughly one-third of the time previously required.[13] Continuing advances in this area include the development of handheld three-dimensional laser imagers that utilize reflectors placed on the patient to capture shape information. This technology is already frequently used in limb applications and is becoming more commonly employed for spinal applications.

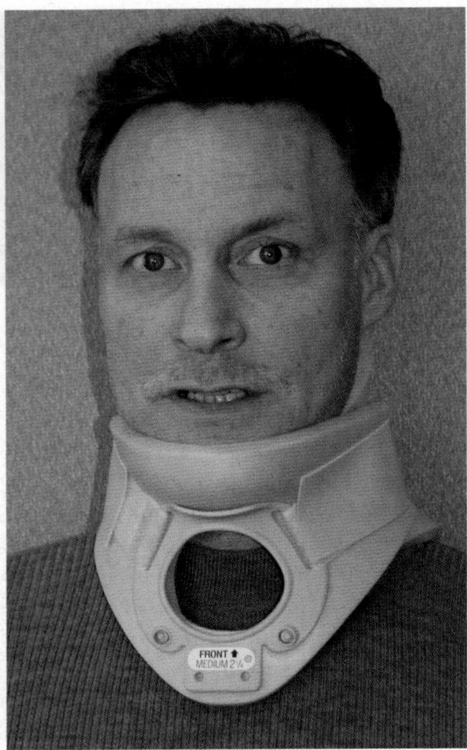

FIG. 81.1 Philadelphia collar. The design includes anterior and posterior shells that are fastened with Velcro straps. The anterior hole is for a tracheostomy tube.

Cervical Orthoses

The cervical region provides a challenge for externally applied spine immobilization due to the soft tissue structures about the neck and high level of mobility of the spine segments. COs can be divided into two broad categories: soft and rigid. Soft collars provide comfort and proprioception but little immobilization, decreasing flexion and extension by 5% to 15%, lateral bending by 5% to 10%, and axial rotation by 10% and 17%.[14] They are often used in the treatment of whiplash-type injuries or muscular strains about the neck, where proprioceptive feedback helps "remind" a patient to voluntarily restrict motion. Such proprioception appears to be reasonably effective in the course of everyday living. Miller and colleagues evaluated the amount of motion recorded by 10 subjects during various functional tasks of everyday living. They found that the amount of motion was not significantly different whether soft or rigid COs were used.[15]

Rigid COs are available in several forms, but all forms must be able to accommodate the vital soft tissue structures in the neck while simultaneously providing rigid immobilization of the mobile cervical spine. This is generally accomplished by firm seatings about the base of the skull and upper thorax connected by a rigid column. Most include an anterior opening to accommodate a tracheostomy tube. Rigid COs are generally used to provide stabilization to the midcervical spine. Examples of COs include the Philadelphia collar (Fig. 81.1), the Miami J collar (Ossur; Fig. 81.2), the Aspen CO (Aspen; Fig. 81.3), and the Malibu collar (Fig. 81.4).

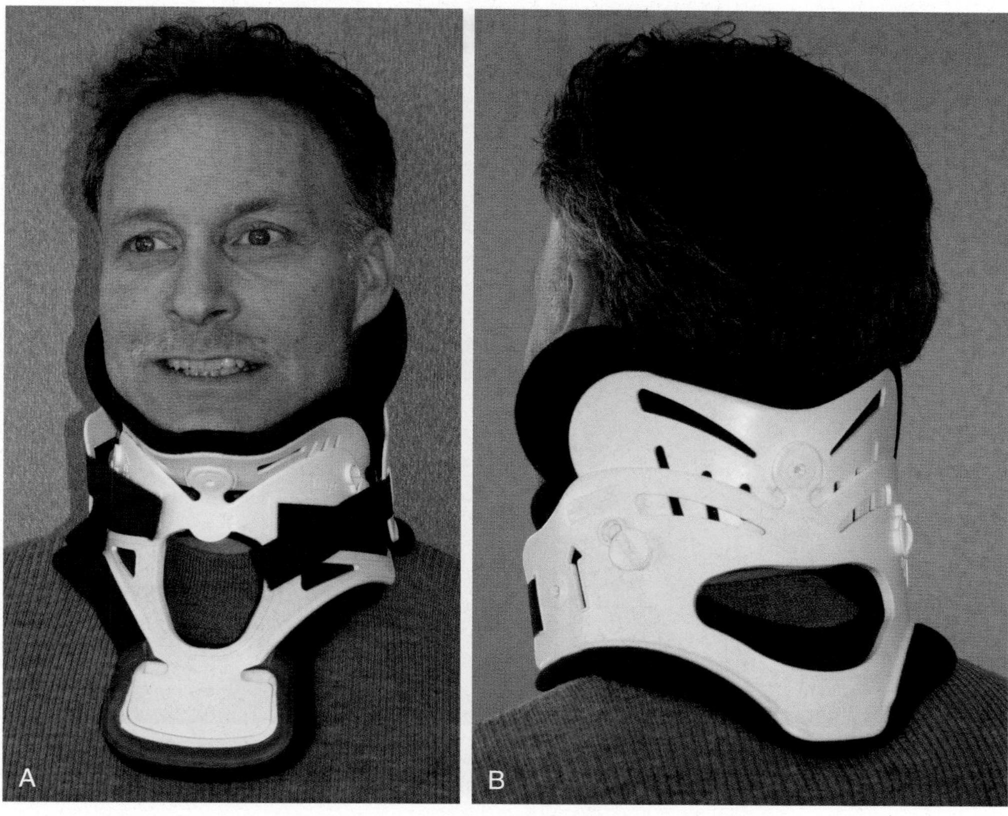

FIG. 81.2 Miami J cervical orthosis. (A) Anterior view. (B) Posterior view. The design includes anterior and posterior shells with a soft lining that can be changed for hygiene purposes.

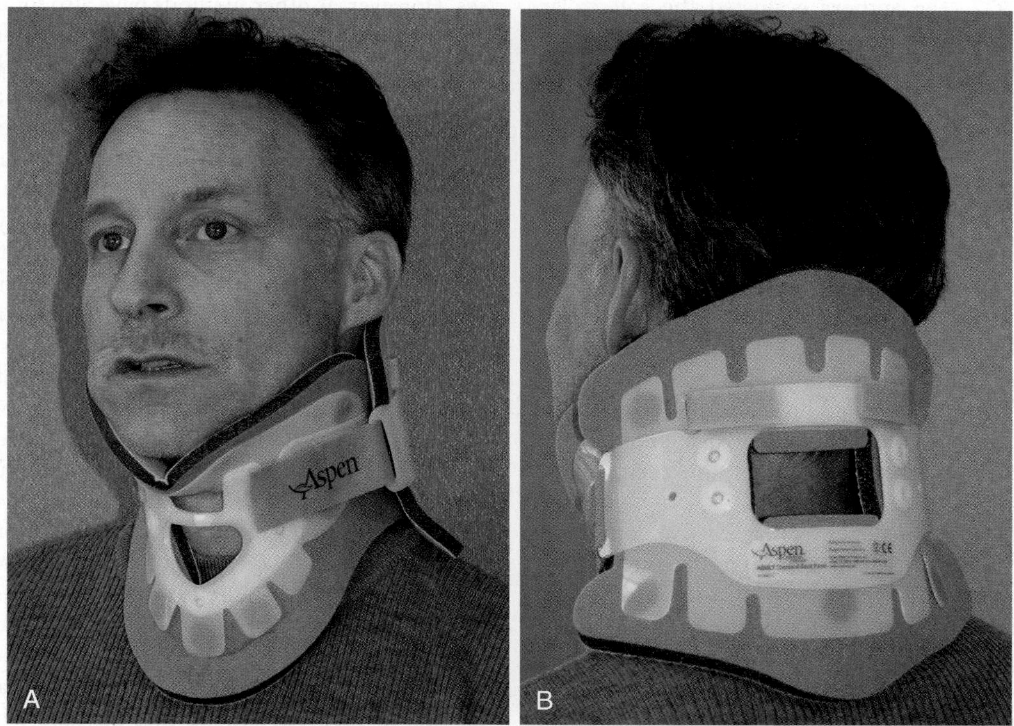

FIG. 81.3 Aspen cervical collar. (A) Anterior view. (B) Posterior view. The design includes patented tabs that allow the collar to better conform to the patient when tightened.

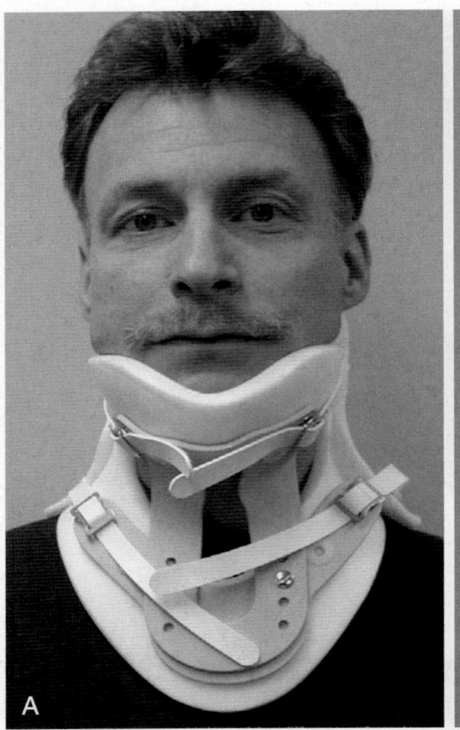

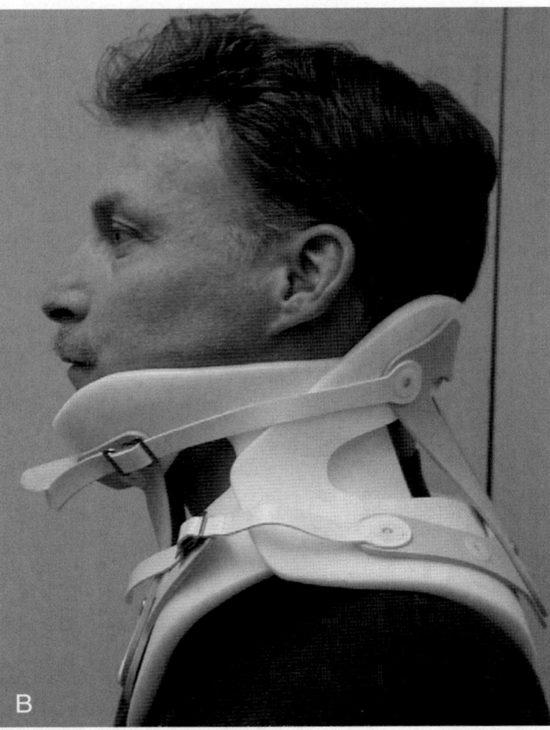

FIG. 81.4 Malibu collar. (A) Anterior view. (B) Lateral view. The design features include tight-fitting chin and occipital rests and more anterior and posterior extension onto the thorax than the Philadelphia collar.

The landmark study evaluating the effectiveness of various orthoses in immobilizing the cervical spine was performed by Johnson and colleagues.[16] The methods of this study have often been emulated and its results frequently quoted since its publication in 1977. The authors evaluated the soft collar, Philadelphia collar, four-poster orthosis, sterno-occipito-mandibular immobilizer (SOMI), and a cervicothoracic orthosis. They utilized radiographs and overhead photographs taken at the extremes of motion in flexion-extension, rotation, and lateral bending. They quantified sagittal plane motion for each brace at every level of the cervical spine (Fig. 81.5). As others had demonstrated, they found that a soft collar offered no restriction of motion in any plane. They found that increasing the length of the orthosis (extending it onto the thorax) and increasing the rigidity of the connection improved flexion control, but lateral bending and total flexion and extension were less controlled. They also demonstrated increased motion between the occiput and C1 in all braces compared with the unbraced state. This "snaking," or paradoxical motion, has subsequently been described throughout the cervical and thoracolumbar spine.[17–19]

Another study by Askins et al. compared five commonly used COs in terms of their efficacy in restricting cervical motion.[20] Radiographic and goniometric measurements found the NecLoc (Ossur) orthosis to be superior to the Miami J, Philadelphia, Aspen, and Stifneck (Laerdal) orthoses in terms of flexion-extension, rotation, and lateral bending. The Miami J collar was also found to be significantly superior to the Philadelphia and Aspen orthoses in extension and combined flexion-extension. Motion analysis systems have been used in recent studies, which typically measure gross rather than segmental movement of the cervical spine.[8,9] Interestingly, these have reported findings different from the aforementioned studies in comparing efficacy among commonly used orthoses. However, as other methods have also found, these studies reported that flexion-extension and rotational movements were more effectively restricted than lateral bending among all of the collars. Separate studies in children have also demonstrated differing performance among commercially available pediatric collars, with the Miami J and NecLoc demonstrating better motion limitation than the Philadelphia collar.[21]

Many hospitals have an in-house inventory of COs so that they are readily available without the need for an orthotist. Predicting the appropriately sized collar can be somewhat imprecise, however. A study by Bell et al. investigated the adverse effects of an ill-fitting Miami J CO using electromagnetic sensors.[22] The authors compared motion in healthy subjects using a Miami J of correct size to one that was too small and one that was too big, among other orthoses. They found that the ill-fitting COs allowed a significant increase in motion in multiple planes when compared to the correctly sized Miami J. The authors reiterated the importance of correct fitting of a CO to avoid the potentially detrimental effects of excessive motion. In an effort to provide customized fitting with decreased inventory, some manufacturers offer adjustable COs. Gao compared the motion restriction of adjustable COs to standard COs in healthy participants across a range of loading levels.[23] They found that the adjustable COs were as effective as standard COs. In our institution, we have found that nursing and nonspine clinicians can have difficulty in adjusting such collars despite educational efforts. Hands-on involvement of the spine specialist or orthotist may be necessary to ensure appropriate fit of the adjustable COs.

Known complications of COs include skin breakdown over bony prominences, such as the occiput, mandible, and sternum. Skin breakdown is especially prevalent in multitrauma patients with prolonged recumbency and in patients with altered sensorium. One study reported orthosis-related decubiti in 38% of patients with associated severe closed-head injuries.[24] Molano Alvarez et al. reported a 23.9% incidence of pressure sores in their series of patients with acute cervical spine injury placed in a cervical collar.[25] The pressure sores were found at day 7, on average, and were most frequently noted over the chin, occipital, and suprascapular areas. The authors found that pressure sores were associated with a higher injury severity score, longer time on mechanical ventilation, longer stays, and a greater percentage of catheter carriers of intracranial pressure. In addition, days spent in a cervical collar and presence of edema are thought to be significant predictors of skin breakdown.[26] Plaisier and colleagues compared the skin pressure associated with the use of the Stifneck, Philadelphia, Miami J, and Aspen/Newport collars in supine patients.[27] They found that the Miami J and the Aspen collars produced the lowest chin and occiput pressures, both being below the mean capillary closing pressure. Tescher et al.[28] assessed the effects of four commercially available cervical collars on mandibular and occipital tissue-interface pressure using custom-sized pads from a proprietary capacitive pressure-sensing transducer system. These authors found that the Miami J collar, with and without Occian back, had

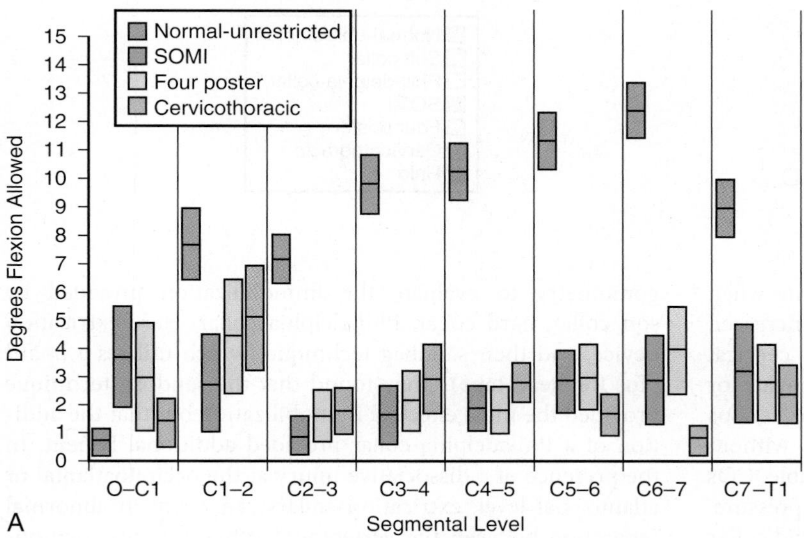

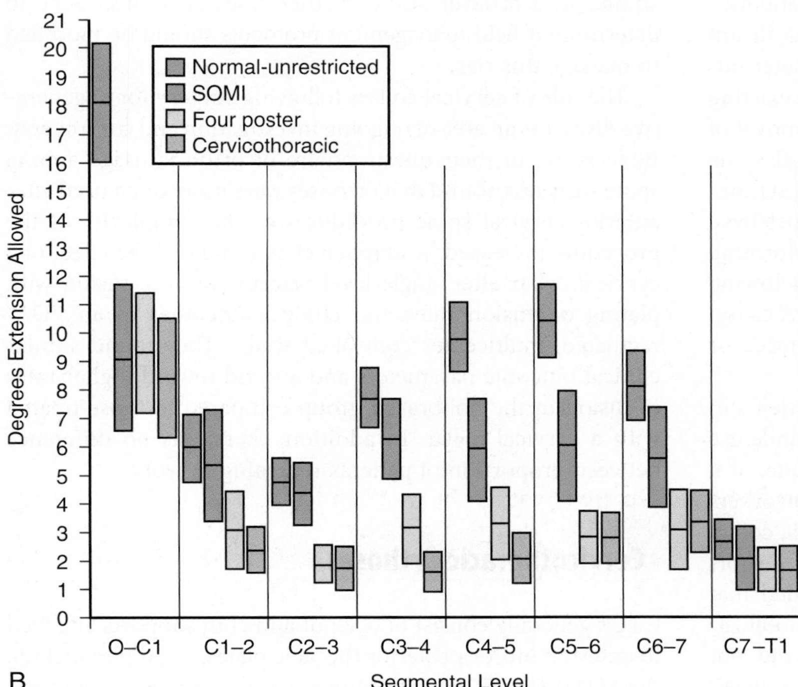

FIG. 81.5 Graphs demonstrating motion allowed in the normal cervical spine compared with cervical orthoses. (A) Degrees of flexion permitted in sterno-occipito-mandibular immobilizer (SOMI), four-poster, and cervicothoracic braces compared with the normal unrestricted cervical spine. (B) Degrees of extension permitted in SOMI, four-poster, and cervicothoracic braces compared with the normal unbraced cervical spine.

Continued

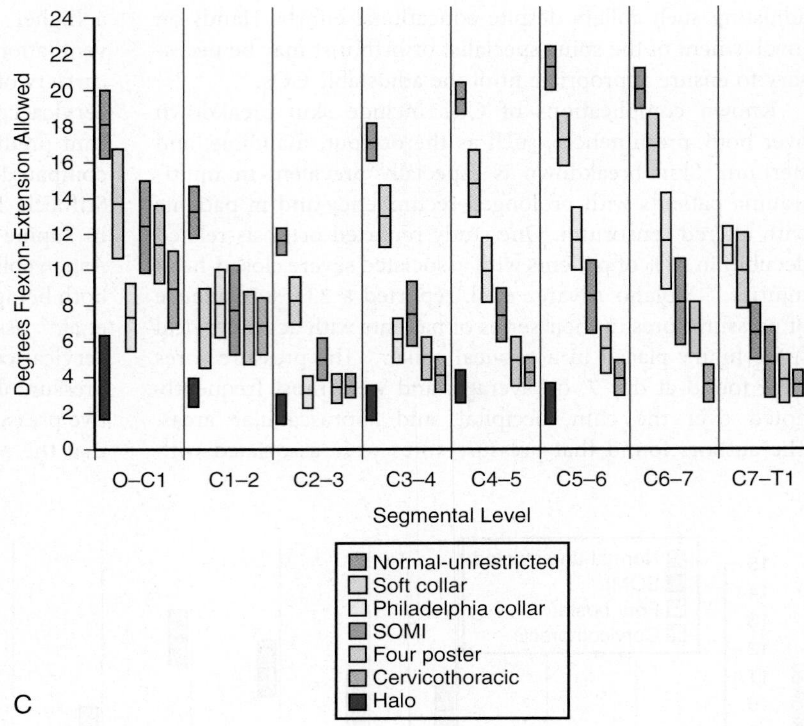

FIG. 81.5, cont'd (C) Degrees of flexion-extension allowed at each cervical segment in a variety of orthoses compared with the normal unrestricted cervical spine. (From Johnson RM, Hart DL, Simmons EF, et al. Cervical orthoses: a study comparing their effectiveness in restricting cervical motion in normal subjects. *J Bone Joint Surg Am.* 1977;59:332–339.)

the lowest levels of mandibular and occipital pressure when compared to the Aspen and Philadelphia collars. Increased intracranial pressure as a consequence of rigid cervical orthotic immobilization has been described. As a surrogate for intracranial pressure, Karason et al. measured jugular venous pressure by catheter in healthy subjects with and without COs.[29] They found that most commercially available COs resulted in a significant increase in jugular venous pressure. Hunt and colleagues directly studied the effects of rigid collar placement on intracranial pressure in head-injured patients.[30] They found that rigid collars cause a small but significant increase in intracranial pressure, which may have deleterious effects in patients with severe head injuries and preexisting intracranial hypertension. They recommend early removal of rigid collars from head-injured patients once cervical spine injury has been excluded. Aspiration and dysphagia are at times anecdotally attributed to cervical collar use, but studies have been inconclusive. When using healthy volunteers performing swallowing studies, some mechanical changes in swallowing physiology were noted, but no aspirations occurred.[31] A causal link between cervical collar use and aspiration in injured or elderly patients has been suggested but not proven.

Methods for immobilizing the cervical spine of patients in the field have also been extensively studied. These include use of a cervical collar, a short board or sandbag technique, or a combination of a collar and short board. Cline and coworkers compared the Hare extrication collar, the Philadelphia collar, and their immobilization protocol, which consists of a short board with forehead and chin straps.[32] They concluded that the short board with straps provided the best immobilization and that the addition of a Philadelphia collar did not provide additional benefit. Podolsky and colleagues[33] utilized goniometry to evaluate the immobilization provided by soft collar, hard collar, Philadelphia collar, Hare extrication device, and their sandbag technique (which utilizes a board plus forehead tape). They found that the sandbag technique provided the most effective immobilization but that the addition of a Philadelphia collar provided additional benefit. In the presence of a dissociative injury at the occipitoatlantal or atlantoaxial level, extrication collars can result in abnormal separation between the vertebrae.[34] While this was demonstrated in a cadaver study, further research is necessary to determine if field management protocols should be modified to manage this risk.

The role of cervical collars following surgery for degenerative disease is an area of ongoing investigation and controversy. Bible at al., in their questionnaire of orthosis usage among spine surgeons, found that orthoses were more often used after anterior cervical spine procedures as the complexity of the procedure increased.[5] Campbell et al. evaluated the effect of a cervical collar after single-level anterior cervical fusion with plating on fusion rates and clinical outcomes in an FDA-regulated, multicenter controlled trial.[35] They found similar clinical outcome parameters and a trend toward higher rates of fusion in the nonbraced group compared to those treated with a cervical collar. In addition, there was no difference between proportion of patients returning to work.

Cervicothoracic Orthoses

CTOs generally consist of occiput and chin supports attached to anterior and/or posterior thoracic plates. Examples include the SOMI (Fig. 81.6), the Minerva brace (Fig. 81.7), and the

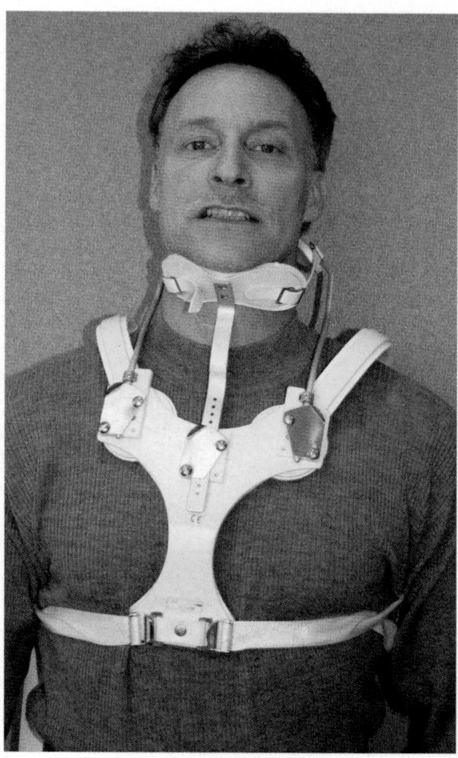

FIG. 81.6 Sterno-occipito-mandibular immobilizer (SOMI). The three upright rods that extend from the mandibular and occipital rests all connect on the anterior thoracic plate.

Yale brace (Fig. 81.8). Compared with COs, these devices improve control in all planes of motion and are particularly suited for immobilization of the middle to lower cervical spine and upper thoracic spine. This improved rigidity, however, comes at the expense of patient comfort. Some of the earlier authors distinguished between the two/four-poster designs and those with more extensive connections between the head and thoracic components.[16] The more recent standardized classification system, however, categorizes the poster braces as CTOs along with the other designs. The traditional four-poster brace was shown to limit 79% of overall cervical flexion-extension and limit midcervical flexion to a comparable degree as the more rigid CTOs.[4,36] Because of their heavy design and high resting pressures on the chin and occiput,[7] this brace is less commonly used today.

The SOMI (see Fig. 81.6) utilizes metal uprights to connect occipital and mandibular rests to a sternal plate that is secured to the thorax by padded metal "over-the-shoulder" straps and additional circumferential straps that cross in the back. Because there is no posterior thoracic plate, the occipital rests are supported by uprights from the sternal piece. This results in adequate control of flexion but deficient control of extension throughout the cervical spine.[16,36] These braces are fairly comfortable to patients but also are associated with high resting pressures at the chin and occiput.[7]

The original Minerva brace consisted of a heavy custom plaster jacket that created difficulties in maintaining patient

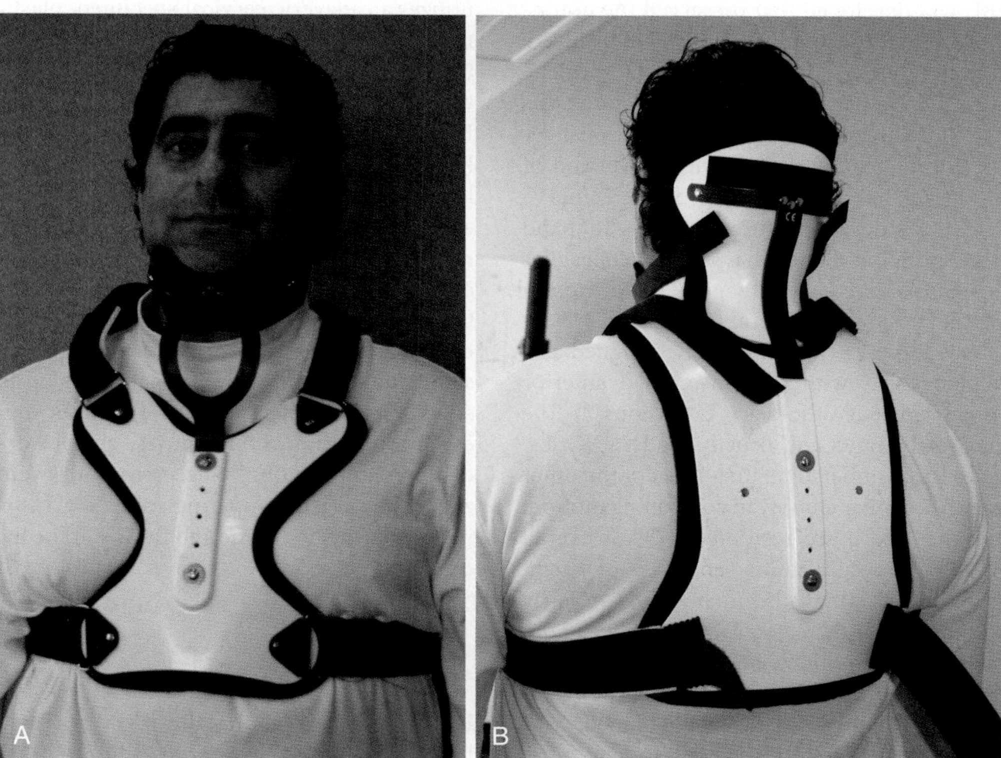

FIG. 81.7 Minerva cervicothoracic orthosis. (A) Anterior view. (B) Posterior view. This design has an expansive occipital flare to help limit rotation.

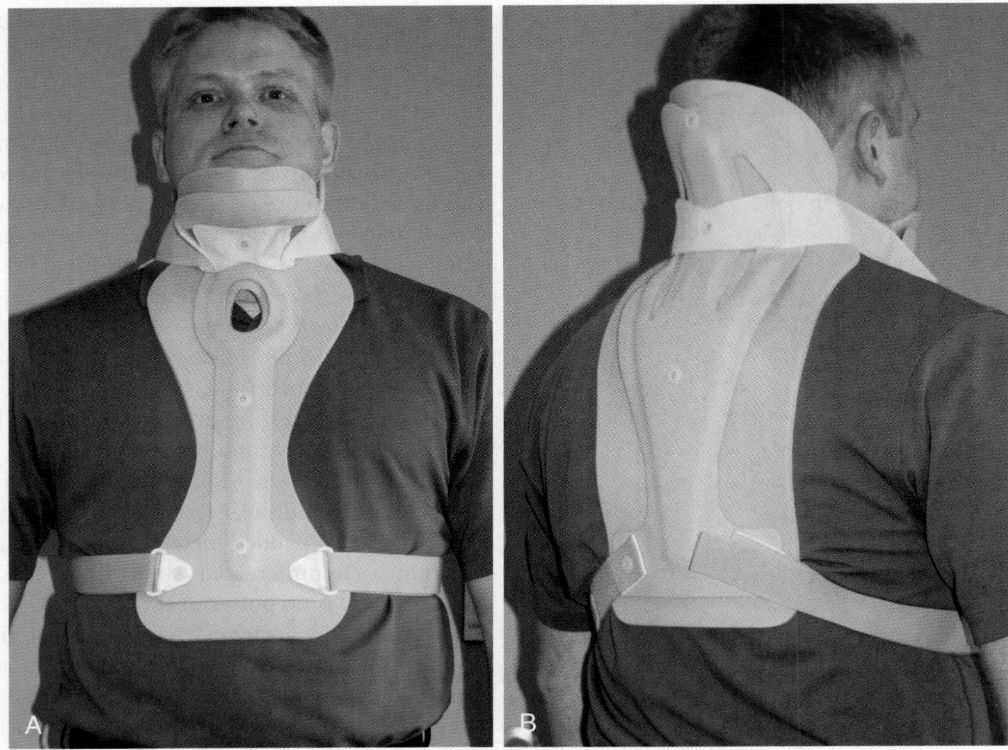

FIG. 81.8 Yale brace. (A) Anterior view. (B) Posterior view. Note the similarities of the head rest to a Philadelphia collar, from which the early version was originally adapted.

hygiene and obtaining radiographs.[37] As a result of the difficulties encountered in managing patients with this device, the halo came into popular use. Later, the thermoplastic Minerva body jacket (TMBJ) was developed that preserved the noninvasive nature of the original concept. Its lightweight, bivalved, polyform shell allowed improved patient comfort and hygiene and interfered less with follow-up radiographs.[38] Donning this brace is somewhat complex, often requiring an orthotist for proper application. More recently, a prefabricated version of the Minerva body jacket has been developed, the Minerva CTO (see Fig. 81.7). Its design features a forehead band attached to a large occipital flare. Sharpe and colleagues reported that this orthosis limits overall sagittal plane motion by 79%, axial rotation by 88%, and lateral bending by 51%.[39]

The Yale brace (see Fig. 81.8) was originally designed as a modified Philadelphia collar with custom-molded anterior and posterior polypropylene thoracic extensions.[40] The modern version is prefabricated and usually made of Kydex. Although lighter and less cumbersome than most of the other CTOs, the Yale brace has similar efficacy in controlling motion. In Johnson's study, the Yale brace restricted 87% of overall flexion-extension, 75% of axial rotation, and 61% of lateral bending.[41] Whereas the CTOs have been shown to be fairly effective at limiting motion of the cervical spine, they should not be expected to rigidly immobilize below the C7–T1 level despite their thoracic components. The use of any of the CTOs in bedbound patients can be problematic, as the tendency for cephalad migration of the brace in the semirecumbent position increases the likelihood of pressure phenomena on the chin or occiput.

Ivancic recently devised a novel skull-neck-thorax model to study the effectiveness of both COs and CTOs, given the limitations inherent in using live human subjects.[42] This model utilizes a cadaveric cervical specimen, plastic skull, and mannequin thorax and load input flexibility testing to determine three-dimensional load-displacement properties. Braced and unbraced states in uninjured models were initially compared. He demonstrated that cervical orthoses effectively immobilized the entire cervical spine in flexion-extension and the lower cervical spine in lateral bending. They appeared least effective at restricting lateral bending of the upper cervical region and axial rotation of all spinal levels, except C1–C2. As other researchers had demonstrated, CTOs improved immobilization of the lower cervical spine compared to standard collars. He subsequently performed further study using the same approach in experimentally created injuries, including atlas fractures, type 3 dens fractures, midregion subaxial extension-compression injuries, and lower cervical flexion-compression injuries.[43] Successive improvement in immobilization was noted comparing collar to CTO in extension at the injured midregion spine and flexion at the injured lower cervical spine.

Halo Vest

It is generally agreed that the halo vest provides the most rigid immobilization of the cervical spine of all the currently used orthoses and is particularly effective in the upper cervical spine. Originally inspired by a device used by Bloom to treat facial fractures in pilots with overlying burns during World War II, modified versions were used by Nickel and Perry to immobilize patients with polio who had undergone posterior cervical fusion.[44,45] The early halo devices consisted of a circumferential stainless steel ring with four pins for skull fixation. The ring was attached to a plaster jacket by upright posts.[46] Numerous improvements have been made to the various components of the halo vest, but the overall design principles remain the same. A ring is fixed to the skull with multiple pins. The ring is then attached to a vest by four connecting rods. Newer rings are made of composite materials, which have the beneficial properties of light weight, radiolucency, and compatibility with magnetic resonance imaging. There does not appear to be a difference in fixation strength between newer radiolucent graphite rings and the earlier titanium ones.[47] Rings that are open posteriorly or have crown-type designs allow for ease in placement since the head of the patient does not need to be passed through the ring. Additionally, because the patient is not lying on the back of the ring, there is less risk of cervical spine fracture displacement through ring manipulation.

The initial halo vest was fashioned from heavy plaster of Paris. With the development of plastic technology, lightweight, easily applied vests of various sizes based on chest circumference have been fabricated (Fig. 81.9). Adjustable straps and supports help customize the fit. The connecting rods have been anodized to prevent seizing of the metal during tightening. The connecting rods in many designs are made of carbon fiber for their radiographic lucency as well as for compatibility with magnetic resonance imaging. Torque wrenches are included in the application sets to prevent overtightening of the bolts that connect the rods to the vest and ring. Mirza and colleagues[48] found that most commercially available vests provide comparable immobilization. Factors associated with decreased motion include increasing vest snugness, decreasing the deformability of the vest, and appropriate fit and application.

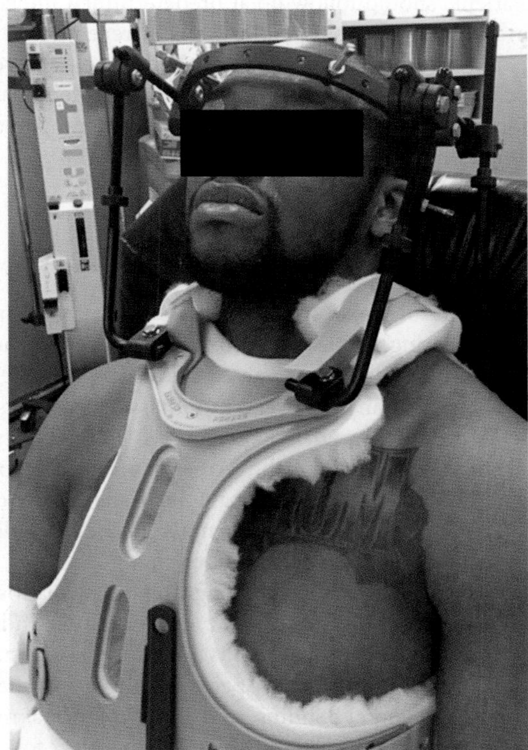

FIG. 81.9 Halo vest (Bremer). This crown-type design allows easier placement in the supine position.

Technological advances have also been made in the field of halo pin materials and pin design. The popular pin composition at this time is stainless steel. Different pin-tip designs have been studied to determine which may provide the greatest resistance to shear frequently encountered at the pin-bone interface. Interest has arisen regarding a bullet-type tip that may be able to withstand higher shear forces.[49,50] Some systems have torque wrenches that break off at a set torque.[51] These wrenches are made to be low profile, allowing for ease of use in cramped areas, such as the posterior aspect of the skull.

Application Principles

Because many of the complications of halo fixation are related to inappropriate site selection or technique, a thorough understanding of pin insertion principles is essential. Many years of clinical data have fine-tuned the optimal location of halo pin placement. To minimize pin complications but maximize the rigidity of the halo-vest frame, two anterior and two posterior pins are usually placed. The standard position of the two anterior pins is 1 cm superior to the orbital rim, over the lateral two-thirds of the orbit, below the level of the greatest circumference of the skull (Fig. 81.10). This is considered the safe zone. In a cadaveric study, it was found that the skull thickness in this region averaged approximately 2 mm for the outer cortical table and 3 mm for the intercalvarial space or inner diploë. A more recent study demonstrated that skull thickness in these areas gradually increases with age.[52] Pins placed too medial may damage the supraorbital or supratrochlear nerves. Also, the frontal sinus has a varied position in the midline. The outer table of the frontal sinus is often very thin,

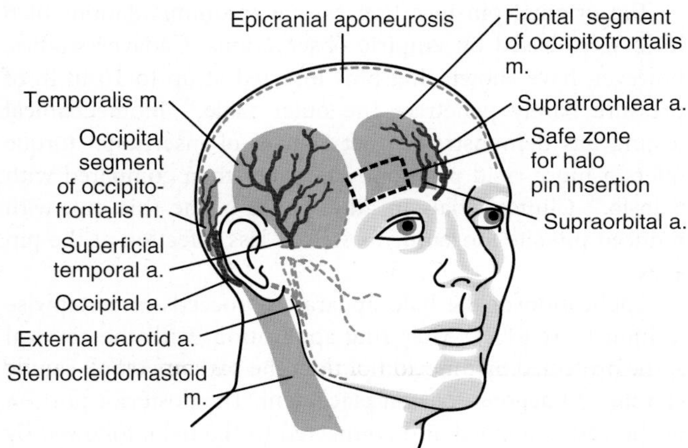

FIG. 81.10 Diagram of the safe zone for placement of anterior halo fixator pins. (From Ballock RT, Botte MJ, Garfin SR. Complications of halo immobilization. In: Garfin SR, ed. *Complications of Spine Surgery*. Baltimore: Williams & Wilkins; 1989:376.)

which can lead to perforation with medial pin placement. Laterally placed anterior pins over the temporalis fossa have been suggested to avoid unsightly scarring over the anterior forehead. At this location, however, the zygomaticotemporal nerve may be injured, which provides sensation to the area over the temple. Also, by entering through the temporalis muscle, the pin often causes irritation during mandibular motion (e.g., eating). Additionally, in cadaveric studies, in this region the skull was found to have a thin outer and inner table with minimal cancellous diploë.[53] An alternative frontolateral pin site has been described as just in front of the temporalis muscle, several centimeters below the equator in or near a triangular forward projection of the temporal hairline.[54] Skull thickness in this region was similar to the standard supraorbital position when measured by computed tomography (CT). The investigators suggested this as a safe alternative with better cosmesis.

Placement of posterior pins is less critical than for anterior pin location. There are no neuromuscular structures at risk and the skull has a near-uniform thickness, with the thickest section being straight posterior. Direct posterior pin placement is avoided, however, because the patient would lie on this pin when supine. The pins are usually placed diagonally opposite to the anterior pins, approximately 1 cm superior to the upper helix of the ear. Care must be taken to avoid any contact between the ring/pin and ear while remaining inferior enough to the equator of the skull to prevent superior pin migration.

Because skull shapes differ, placing pins perpendicular to the tangent of the skull may be difficult. Because the halo is not a static unidirectional device, shear forces act at each of the pin sites. Triggs and associates,[55] in a biomechanical study, evaluated the transverse shear forces to failure of pins placed in decremental angles from 90 degrees, 75 degrees, and 60 degrees. The load to deformity and failure was substantially higher for pins inserted perpendicular to the outer cortex of the skull as compared with 60 degrees. To minimize the incidence of pin loosening, it is important to try to place pins as perpendicular to the skull as possible to provide the most strength at the pin-bone interface.

The original pin-insertion torque recommendations of 6 in-lb were based on empiric observations. Cadaver studies, however, have shown that pins inserted at up to 10 in-lb of pressure barely penetrate the outer table.[51] Biomechanical testing has demonstrated that 8 in-lb of insertional torque offers a more rigid pin-bone interface when compared with 6 in-lb.[50] Clinical trials in adults have borne this out, with reduced pin site loosening as well as less infection at the pin sites.[51]

Application of the halo apparatus proceeds in a stepwise fashion (Box 81.2). After ring application, with the cervical spine protected by manual traction, the patient's trunk can be elevated 30 degrees for vest placement. The posterior portion of the vest is applied and connected to the halo, followed by the anterior portion. Alternative methods include log rolling the patient, although it may be difficult to maintain cervical alignment. In rare instances of a stable fracture pattern, or after surgical internal fixation, the patient can be instructed to sit upright and the vest can be applied. All the vest locking bolts are then tightened to 28 in-lb of torque preset on the screwdriver. Once all the bolts are tightened, cervical spine alignment should be confirmed radiographically. The pins should be retightened 24 to 48 hours after placement. Baum and colleagues have documented an immediate drop of 2 to 4 in-lb in pin fixation purchase after vest placement.[56] A commonly used pin-care regimen consists of daily cleansing with dilute hydrogen peroxide (50/50 with water) on a cotton swab. Patients should follow up at predetermined intervals to confirm lack of halo-vest complications. A recent study compared a new pin-care regimen using chlorhexidine and regular torque checking as a standard protocol.[57] They demonstrated a pronounced reduction of pin-site infection compared to a saline regimen for pin care.

BOX 81.2 Application of the Halo Skeletal Fixator

1. Determine ring or crown size (hold ring or crown over head to visualize size).
2. Determine vest size (from chest circumference measurement).
3. Identify pin site locations.
4. Shave hair at posterior pin sites.
5. Prepare pin sites with povidone-iodine solution.
6. Apply local anesthesia.
7. Advance sterile pins to level of skin.
8. Have patient close eyes.
9. Tighten pins at 2-in/lb increments in diagonal fashion.
10. Tighten pins to 8-in/lb torque.
11. Apply lock nuts to pins.
12. Maintain cervical traction and raise patient trunk to 30 degrees.
13. Apply posterior portion of vest.
14. Apply anterior portion of vest.
15. Connect anterior and posterior portions of vest.
16. Apply upright posts and attach ring to vest.
17. Recheck fittings, screws, and nuts.
18. Tape vest-removing tools to vest.
19. Obtain cervical spine radiographs.

From Botte MJ, Garfin SR, Byrne TP, et al. The halo skeletal fixator: principles of application and maintenance. *Clin Orthop Relat Res.* 1989;239:12–18.

Biomechanical Analysis

The skull pins of most commonly used halo systems can withstand shearing forces of approximately 100 N in normal physiologic motion.[58,59] Although compressive pin forces may decrease by more than 80% over 3 months, shearing resistance may be better preserved.[53] Experiments on cadavers and physical models following the American Society for the Testing of Materials (ASTM) indicate that a shear force on the order of 1100 N is needed to abruptly dislodge skull pins inserted through an open carbon fiber ring.[60]

Whereas the halo is the most rigid external orthosis for immobilization of the cervical spine, some motion and force transmission to the cervical elements do occur. In early studies, the halo device was found to permit only 4% of flexion-extension, 4% of lateral bending, and 1% of rotational motion of the normal native cervical spine.[16] However, follow-up studies have shown that such significant immobilization is not routinely accomplished. One study has demonstrated up to 51 degrees of motion with halo immobilization.[19] Segmentally, the greatest motion was observed at the occiput-C1 level (11.5 degrees). The least motion was observed at C2–C3 (6.7 degrees). Interestingly, when flexion was observed at one segment of the spine, extension was observed at another level, the phenomenon known as "snaking." Motion of the cervical spine was observed with patient position changes from supine to prone or from supine to sitting. However, there was no increased motion at the level of injury. In contrast, Anderson and collaborators reported in a clinical series greater than 3 degrees of angulation and 1 mm of translation at the fracture site in 77% of the patients evaluated.[61] A more recent study evaluated the effect of cyclic physiologic loading on halo performance in a mannequin model.[62] The investigators found that after a few cycles of loading, analogous to a few steps taken by a patient, the support provided by a halo orthosis becomes nonlinear. When analyzed through straightforward structural modeling, they found that the nonlinearity permitted mild head motion while severely restricting larger motion. They speculated that halo design could be optimized to permit mild spinal loading to foster bony healing while neutralizing pathologic loads.

Studies have also examined the directional force generated by the halo device. Maximal forces appear to be exerted in the mediolateral plane. However, in daily activities, anteroposterior and vertical forces are much larger. This was confirmed by Lind and colleagues, who observed no horizontal motion in the halo device.[19] They reported significant differences in distractive forces between the supine and upright positions that can be attributed to the added weight of the head. Distractive forces were most increased with deep breathing, shoulder shrugging, and arm elevation, although no patient experienced any discomfort. These high distractive forces were most elevated in patients with tight-fitting vests. It was noted that the halo vest can be elevated by the sternum and the scapulae. They recommended that there be at least 30 mm of space between the sternum and the vest to prevent gross motion of the vest with daily activities. Conversely, a recent study evaluated motion of the injured cervical spine while moving from upright to supine and prone positions.[63] The investigators used composite models (surrogate head, cadaveric cervical specimen, and mannequin torso) comparing properly applied and loose-fitting vests. Snaking motion was again observed, but was significantly more in loose-fitting vests. Another study using the same model found that a loose suprastructure displayed increased lateral bending motion at C6–C7.[64] As such, there appears to be a window of proper vest fit, outside of which immobilization is compromised. Patients should be cautioned regarding exercises that involve twisting and bending, because these tend to transmit undesirable forces to the cervical spine through the halo.

Complications

Although clinical studies have clearly demonstrated the efficacy of the halo device, complications with its use are not infrequent. Absolute contraindications to halo usage include cranial fracture, infection, and severe soft tissue injury at the proposed pin sites.[65] Awareness of the most commonly seen complications can help minimize their severity and avoid catastrophic sequelae. Pin loosening has been identified as one of the most common problems with the halo device.[66] In two large studies, pin loosening was observed in 36% and 60% of patients.[67,68] The hypothesized decrease in compressive pin forces with time was confirmed in a biomechanical study utilizing instrumented halos in three patients. Pin force values at the time of halo-vest application and at subsequent clinical visits were compared by Fleming and associates.[69] They measured an 83% drop in torque pressure by the time of halo removal. They believed that the mechanism of pin loosening was through bone resorption at the pin tip. To help decrease loss of the halo because of loosening, if there is no sign of infection, the pins may be retightened to 8 in-lb of torque as long as resistance is met on the first few turns of the pin. If no resistance is met, then a new pin should be placed in another position. The old pin should be kept in place until the new pin has been rigidly placed to keep the correct orientation of the ring on the skull.

Halo-pin infection rates have been documented to occur in approximately 20% of cases.[67,68] If drainage and erythema continue at a pin site even with aggressive pin care, bacterial cultures should be obtained and appropriate oral antibiotics started. If cellulitis persists or an abscess forms, the pin should be removed and placed in another position. The patient may require incision and drainage of the abscess with parenteral antibiotics.[67]

Skull and dural penetration by a halo pin are rare complications. It is often related to patient falls. Clinically, the patient may present with a headache, malaise, or visual disturbances if symptomatic pin penetration has occurred. Radiographs taken tangential to the skull may demonstrate whether pin perforation of the inner table has occurred. Clear cerebrospinal fluid leakage from the pin site is a definitive sign that dural puncture has occurred. In these circumstances, a new pin should be placed in another region and the old pin removed.[68] Elevation of the head decreases intracerebral pressure and facilitates closure of the dural tear. These tears usually heal in 4 to 5 days. If the tear does not heal or an infection is suspected (subdural abscess), formal surgical intervention may be necessary.[70]

Patients may report difficulty swallowing during halo immobilization. Deglutition dysfunction leading to aspiration has been reported.[71] In a study performed at a level 1 trauma center, Bradley et al. reported a 66% prevalence of dysphagia that resulted in longer intensive care unit and hospital stays.[72] The authors recommended formal swallowing evaluation for all such patients to reduce the risks of aspiration. Many instances of swallowing difficulty are a result of the cervical spine being immobilized in the extended position. Efforts to flex the cervical spine while maintaining cervical reduction may assist in resolution of dysphagia.[70]

Pressure sores have been reported in 4% to 11% of patients during halo immobilization.[67] These sores frequently develop underneath the vest or cast vest secondary to pressure against prominent bony surfaces, or due to insufficient padding or incorrect sizing of the vest. Principles of pressure sore prevention include frequent turning, adequate vest padding, and routine skin inspections. Pressure sores are more prevalent in patient populations using a cast vest rather than the padded prefabricated plastic vest. This is especially important in patients with neurologic deficits who may not have normal sensation over their trunk. Alternative strategies to halo immobilization, such as rigid internal fixation, should be considered in this patient population (spinal cord injury). Pressure sore treatment may require split-thickness skin grafting and/or employing rotational muscle flaps for coverage.[68]

A prospective study by van Middendorp et al. investigated the incidence and risk factors associated with complications during halo-vest immobilization over a 5-year period in 239 patients.[73] There was a 6% incidence of death, although only one was directly related to the immobilization. There was a 5% incidence of pneumonia; however, elderly patients did not have an increased risk of pneumonia. There was also a 12% incidence of pin-site infection, which was significantly related to pin penetration through the outer table of the skull. The authors reiterated that, although there were relatively low rates of major complications, awareness of the substantial rates of minor complications is necessary to prevent further morbidity.

Halo-vest immobilization in the elderly is an area of increasing concern due to reports of significant morbidity and mortality. Tashjian et al. investigated the morbidity and mortality of halo usage in patients over the age of 65 years in treating odontoid fractures compared to a rigid cervical orthosis or operative fixation.[74] Of the patients treated with a halo vest, 42% died compared to 20% in the nonhalo group. This difference was statistically significant. There was also a significantly increased rate of major complications in the halo-vest group. The authors concluded that treatment of odontoid fractures in the elderly with a halo are associated with significant morbidity and mortality. Other authors have evaluated the treatment of elderly patients with type 2 odontoid fracture with cervical collars and found that fracture stability by either osseous or fibrous union could be achieved with acceptable clinical results.[75]

Pediatric Considerations

Halo immobilization has been successful in the treatment of children and infants after both unstable cervical injuries and congenital abnormalities.[76,77] The recommended pin torque pressure in children is 2 to 5 in-lb owing to the skull being thinner and more pliable than the adult skull.[76] In patients younger than 3 years, a multiple low-torque pin-insertion technique is recommended to achieve maximal stability.[78]

In young children, up to 12 pins can be inserted at 2 in-lb of torque pressure under general anesthesia. Halo pins should be placed under the largest diameter of the skull, with care to avoid the frontal sinus and temporal regions. Some authors recommend a computed tomogram of the head to identify the location of suture lines and bone fragments (in congenital cases) before placement of the halo.[65] Furthermore, in the presence of open suture lines and fontanelles, vigilant care must be taken to make sure that equal pressure is placed symmetrically on the skull through the halo pins to prevent skull deformity.

Owing to sizing issues in this age group, a custom-made ring and vest are often required. Once the halo is placed, the vest is applied in normal fashion and connected to the halo. Children require the same pin care as adults. Baum and colleagues observed that children have a higher rate of pin loosening than adults.[56] Children with halo fixators should have close parental and medical supervision.

Noninvasive Halo

A noninvasive halo (NIH) has been investigated as an alternative that avoids invasive pin placement while potentially providing more immobilization than a CTO. This orthosis consists of a halo mask that encircles the patient's head over the forehead and the chin and attaches to a rigid anterior vest. DiPaola et al. performed a biomechanical evaluation of conventional and noninvasive halos in cadaveric C1–C2 and C5–C6 instability models using various maneuevers.[79] The authors found less cervical spine motion during application of the NIH compared to the conventional halo. The conventional halo, however, did provide superior immobilization during the log roll maneuver, although the halos were similar during the sit-up maneuver. Skaggs et al. treated 30 children with stable spines in an NIH postoperatively and found only one complication.[80] Sawers et al. retrospectively reviewed the use of an NIH to treat 19 patients for cervical trauma.[81] All fractures healed in acceptable alignment without neurologic deterioration; there was one case of occipital ulceration and two cases of noncompliance. Although NIH is a tempting option to avoid the potential complications associated with traditional halo usage, there is insufficient data to recommend its usage as an equivalent alternative.

Thoracolumbar and Sacral Orthoses

SIOs, LSOs, and TLSOs are available in flexible and rigid variations. The flexible versions have a similar design to their rigid counterparts but provide only mild immobilization. SIOs generally encircle the pelvis, spanning the tops of the iliac crests to the trochanters. These may provide relief in traumatic postpartum separation of the sacroiliac joints. LSOs extend from the pelvis to the xiphoid anteriorly and the inferior angle of the scapula posteriorly. TLSOs extend higher, generally to the midscapular level.

Flexible Thoracolumbosacral and Lumbosacral Orthoses

Flexible LSOs and TLSOs are prescribed by some for the treatment of low back pain. These corset-style devices are adjustable by means of laces, hooks, or Velcro straps. Some authors have reported that these types of orthoses decrease the myoelectric activity of the paraspinal muscles and increase intraabdominal pressure, possibly resulting in decreased loads on the intervertebral discs.[82,83] Others have reported increased myoelectric activity, as measured through surface electrodes on the paraspinal muscles, when certain tasks are performed in braced subjects.[84] Less controversy surrounds the effect on the abdominal muscles, with several authors reporting decreased measured myoelectric activity with brace wear.[83,85] Design modifications to improve brace effectiveness have included the use of pneumatic lifters designed to transfer some of the patient's upper body weight from the lumbar spine to the iliac crests (Fig. 81.11). In a survey of 44 patients who completed an 8-week regimen using the Orthotrac Pneumatic Vest (Orthofix, Inc.), 59% reported moderate to significant improvement of mechanical back pain symptoms.[86] The role of lumbar supports for prevention and treatment of low back pain continues to be an area of controversy because clinical studies on their efficacy are conflicting. Jellema and colleagues performed a systematic review of the literature to assess this issue.[87] They searched the Medline, Cinahl, and Current Contents databases, the Cochrane Controlled Trials Register, and the Embase database. Two reviewers independently assessed methodologic quality and performed data review. In performing a quantitative analysis, they classified the strength of evidence as strong, moderate, limiting or conflicting, or no evidence. Only four of the 13 studies identified were believed to be high quality. They determined that, based on the literature available, there is no strong evidence to support the use of lumbar supports for prevention or treatment of low back pain.

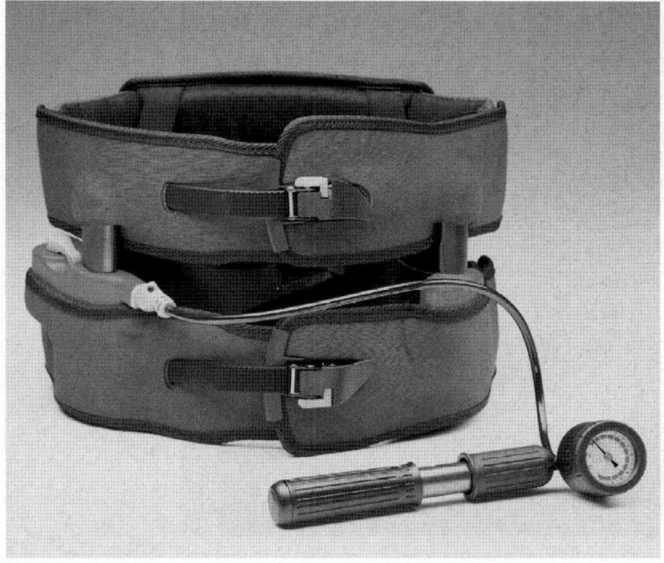

FIG. 81.11 Orthotrac Pneumatic Vest. The design includes patented patient-controlled pneumatic lifts designed to transfer some of the body weight from the lumbar spine to the iliac crests. (Courtesy Orthofix, Inc., McKinney, TX.)

Rigid Thoracolumbosacral and Lumbosacral Orthoses

Most conventional TLSOs are more effective in limiting motion in the sagittal plane than in controlling rotation or lateral bending. The Jewett hyperextension brace is an example of a non–custom-molded TLSO brace (Fig. 81.12).

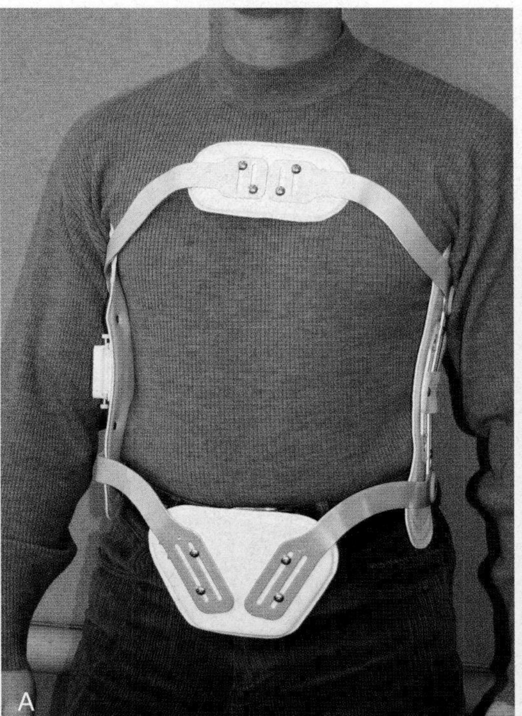

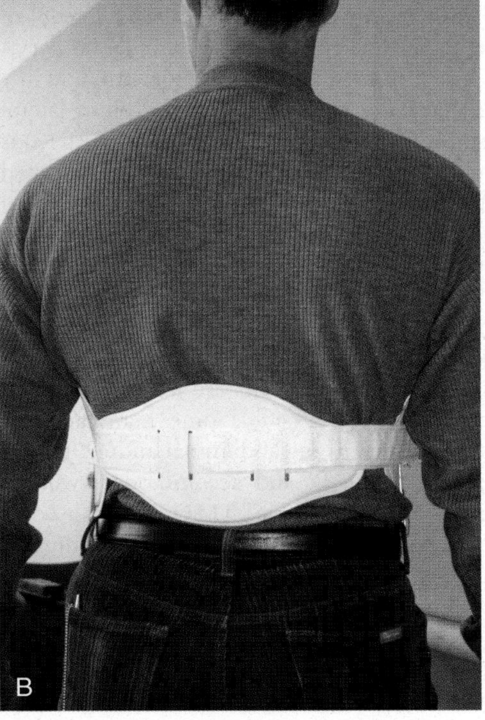

FIG. 81.12 Jewett brace. (A) Anterior view. (B) Posterior view. The anterior pads cross the sternum and pubic symphysis. The posterior pad crosses the upper lumbar spine. The design attempts to provide extension with three-point fixation.

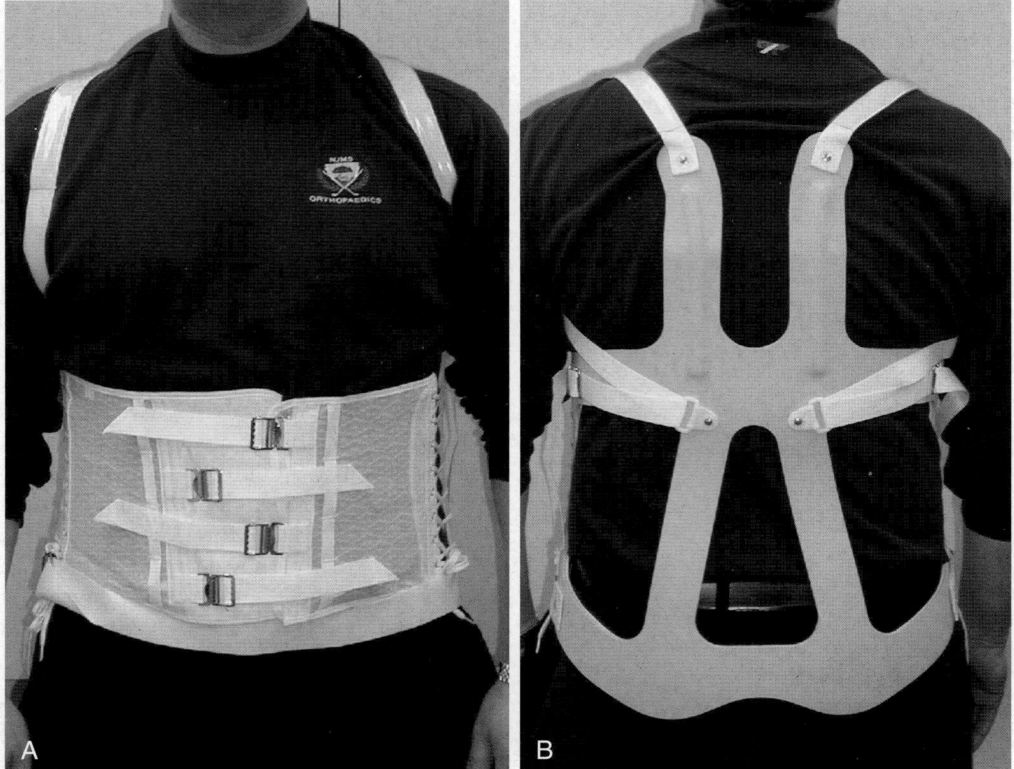

FIG. 81.13 Knight-Taylor orthosis. (A) Anterior view. (B) Posterior view. Control of thoracic sagittal plane motion is achieved through axillary straps attached to posterior thoracic uprights.

It applies three-point fixation to the torso through anterior pads on the symphysis pubis and sternum and a posterior pad midway between the anterior pads. This arrangement of forces places the spine in slight extension. Similar to cervical collars, this brace is best in controlling motion in the flexion-extension plane and less effective in controlling lateral bending and rotation. The Knight-Taylor brace (Fig. 81.13) is another commonly prescribed TLSO and can be prefabricated or custom molded. It has a corset-style front for abdominal compression and lateral and posterior uprights attached to over-the-shoulder straps for thoracic control. Prefabricated TLSOs often consist of clamshell-style braces that can be ordered to measurements and usually are fabricated of $\frac{1}{8}$- to $\frac{3}{16}$-inch low-density polyethylene with a full $\frac{1}{4}$-inch foam liner. The anterior and posterior shells are fastened in place with three Velcro closures per side. Some manufacturers include pneumatic bladders in the abdominal and/or lumbar areas to help customize the fit and accommodate volume changes. Prefabricated "customizable" TLSOs are also commercially available with apron-style fronts that can be adjusted with Velcro straps and telescoping sternal pads (Fig. 81.14). These braces provide good control in all three planes, but once again the major restriction is in the flexion-extension plane. For optimal control in all three planes between T5 and L4, a fully custom-molded TLSO (Fig. 81.15) should be used. These are often formed from high-temperature thermoplastic that is custom fitted from a plaster cast formed from the patient. When immobilization proximal to T5 is required, a cervical

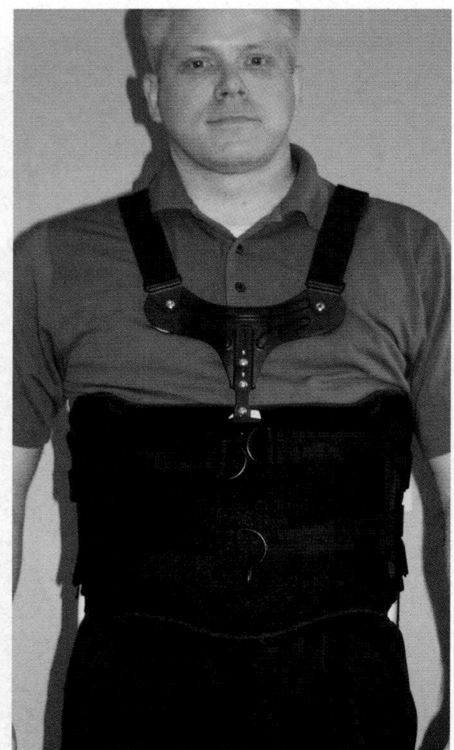

FIG. 81.14 Prefabricated "customizable" thoracolumbosacral orthosis. This particular design (Orthomerica) has an apron-style front with an adjustable sternal pad to help customize the fit.

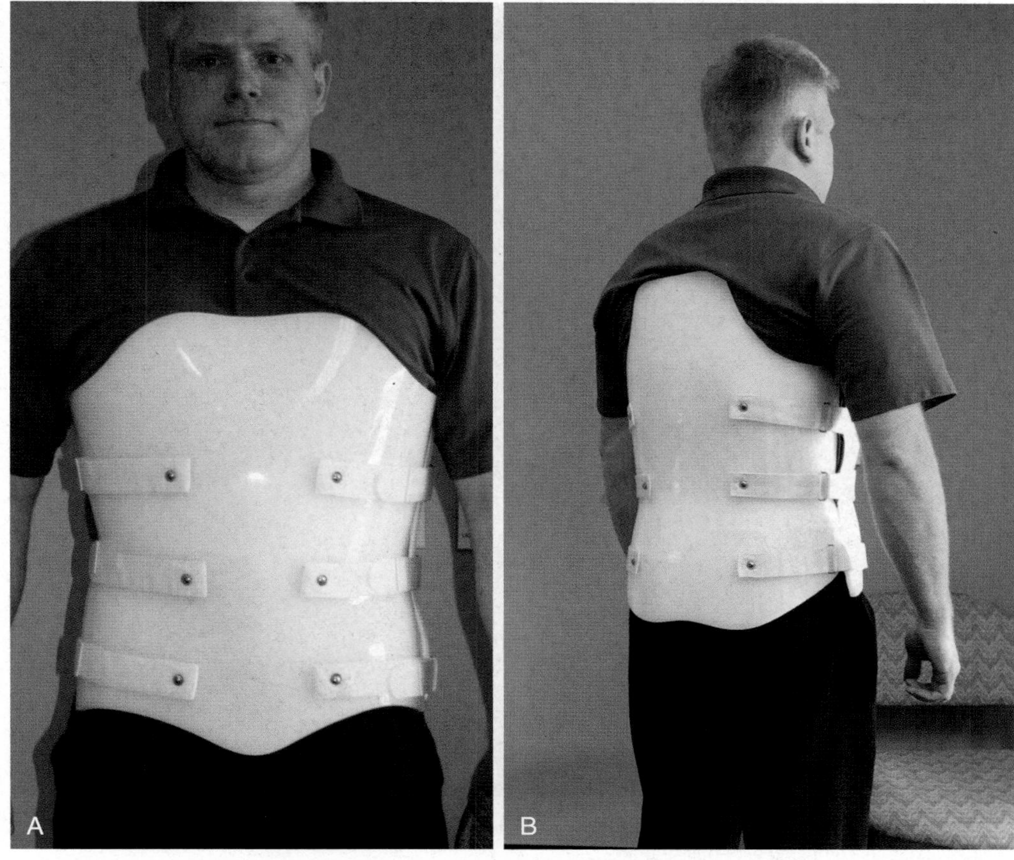

FIG. 81.15 Custom-molded thoracolumbosacral orthosis. (A) Anterior view. (B) Posterior view. This bivalve design can be made from a plaster cast of the patient or created with an algorithm based on key measurements.

extension should be included.[88] If immobilization distal to L4 is needed, a thigh cuff should be added to the orthosis to control pelvic motion.[89,90]

Compared with COs, few studies have been performed to scientifically evaluate the ability of external orthoses to immobilize the thoracolumbosacral spine. In one study, a molded TLSO provided 94% restriction in lateral bending and 69% restriction of flexion-extension in the lumbar spine.[91] The amount of restriction in lumbar rotation was inconsequential because of the limited rotation of the lumbar spine under unbraced normal conditions. In the thoracic spine, the device restricted flexion-extension by 49%, lateral bending by 38%, and total rotation by 60%. Brown and Norton conducted one of the most referenced studies on motion restriction with lumbar external supports.[89] They evaluated three rigid LSOs, one flexible LSO, and a TLSO. Kirschner wires were inserted into the spinous processes of volunteers. The angles between the wires were measured to determine the amount of motion. Radiographic evaluation was also performed. Of note, they reported increased motion across the lumbosacral junction in all of the braces. Increased motion at L4–L5 was also noted while the subjects were sitting. Compared with the unbraced state, all of the braces resulted in some flexion at L4–L5 and L5–S1 while standing. Lumsden and Morris[92] reported similar findings when they studied lumbosacral rotational motion in subjects wearing either a chairback brace or an LSO corset. Volunteers had Steinmann pins placed in their posterior superior iliac spines. Motion was determined by radiographs and measurement of pin rotation. In each case, they found that the braces increased motion at the lumbosacral level. Fidler and Plasmans[90] used radiographs to compare the effect on lumbosacral motion of a corset, a brace, and a plaster jacket with and without a thigh cuff. They found that the custom-molded plaster jacket provided the best immobilization at the L1–L3 level. The mean percentage of motion allowed at L4–L5 and L5–S1 was 32% and 70%, respectively, in a lumbar brace without a thigh extension. The addition of a unilateral thigh extension decreased allowable motion at these levels to 12% and 8%, respectively. To improve immobilization at the L4–S1 levels, they recommended adding a thigh cuff to the orthosis. Other authors have reported similar findings, noting an additional 15% to 30% reduction in motion at L4–L5 and L5–S1 with the addition of a unilateral thigh extension.[93,94] To study the ability of orthoses to restrict motion in the injured spine, Rubery and colleagues created experimental burst fractures in cadaver spines and utilized an electromagnetic motion tracking and analysis system to track angular and linear displacement during routine "patient maneuvers."[95] Both prefabricated and custom-molded TLSOs were found to diminish, but not eliminate, angular motion at the fracture site. Their effect on linear translation was minimal, however.

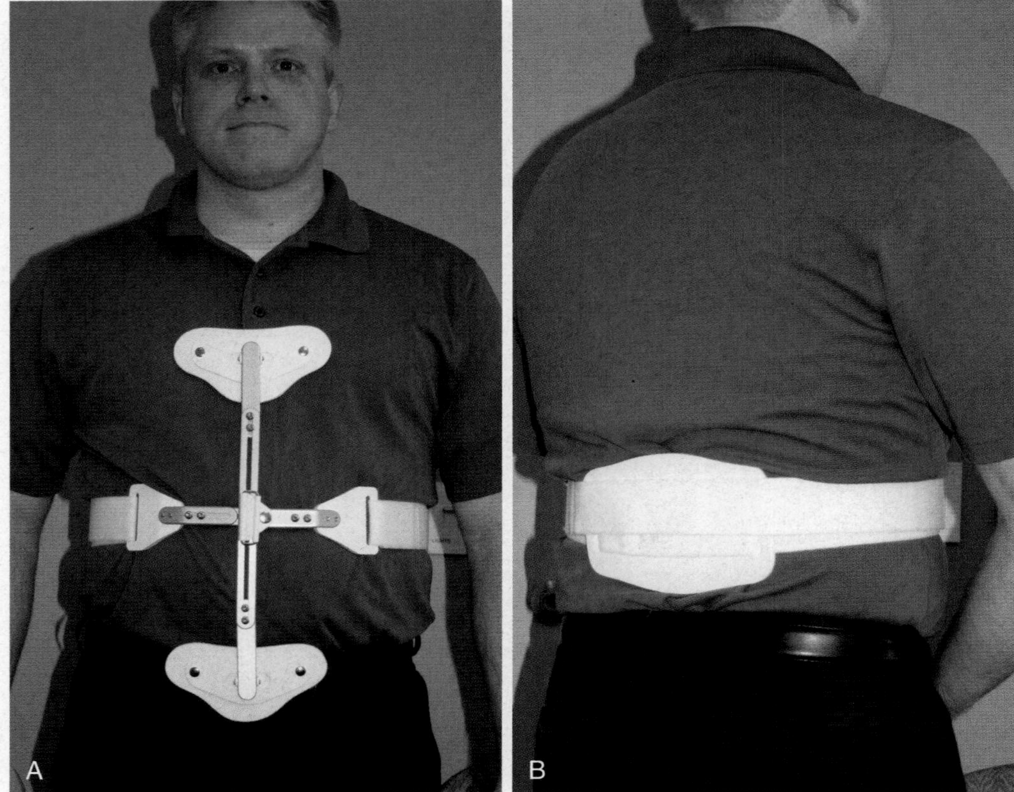

FIG. 81.16 CASH brace. (A) Anterior view. (B) Posterior view. The lightweight design is better tolerated by elderly patients compared with bulkier braces.

Indications for TLSOs are less well defined than for COs. Bracing for compression fractures of the thoracolumbar spine is not tolerated well by the elderly. Treatment in these patients usually consists of early mobilization and close follow-up. A soft binder or corset may provide support and symptomatic relief. The CASH brace (Patterson Medical; Fig. 81.16) is another lightweight alternative that may be reasonably tolerated. A recent study by Kim et al. compared treatment outcomes of patients with osteoporotic compression fractures treated using a rigid brace, soft brace, and no brace in a randomized controlled trial.[96] The Oswestry Disability Index scores for the patients treated without a brace were not inferior to those with soft or rigid braces. Furthermore, the improvement in back pain and progression of anterior body compression were similar among the three groups.

In younger patients, however, anterior column fractures are often the result of greater energy than their osteoporotic counterparts; therefore, a more cautious approach is often favored. These patients are commonly treated with a rigid Jewett or Knight-Taylor brace. However, the need for rigid bracing of these fractures is still a matter of debate. Ohana and associates[97] retrospectively reviewed the outcome of 129 young patients with mild compression fractures who were treated with or without a Jewett hyperextension brace. They found that one-column fractures of the thoracolumbar spine with as much as 30% compression can be safely treated without bracing, instead prescribing early ambulation, hyperextension exercises, and close follow-up. In addition, there is no consensus on the use of TLSOs after lumbar spine surgery for degenerative disease. In one questionnaire study, 49% of spine surgeons stated that they utilize braces after lumbar spine surgery, with no statistically different frequency of use between instrumented and noninstrumented fusions.[5]

Burst fractures comprise another entity in the spectrum of thoracolumbar injuries. Historically, neurologically intact patients with burst fractures were treated with bed rest for 4 to 12 weeks, followed by progressive mobilization. Today, controversy exists as to which injuries require surgical stabilization and which can be treated with bracing and early mobilization. Any neurologic deficit is often an indication for operative management. Other commonly mentioned criteria for surgery, rather than bracing, include canal compromise of 50% or more, kyphotic deformity of greater than 30 degrees, and posterior column involvement. The final determination, however, often remains a case-by-case judgment on the part of the treating specialist. Chow and colleagues[98] retrospectively studied functional outcomes in 24 patients treated with hyperextension body casts and/or Jewett hyperextension braces for thoracolumbar burst fractures. None of these patients had posterior column fractures, significant kyphosis, or neurologic deficit. Patients were initially treated with bed rest and log roll precautions until the predictable ileus and abdominal distention resolved 2 to 3 days later. At that point, patients were placed in a cast or brace and progressively mobilized. Patients were followed for a minimum of 1 year. They concluded that hyperextension casting or bracing with early mobilization

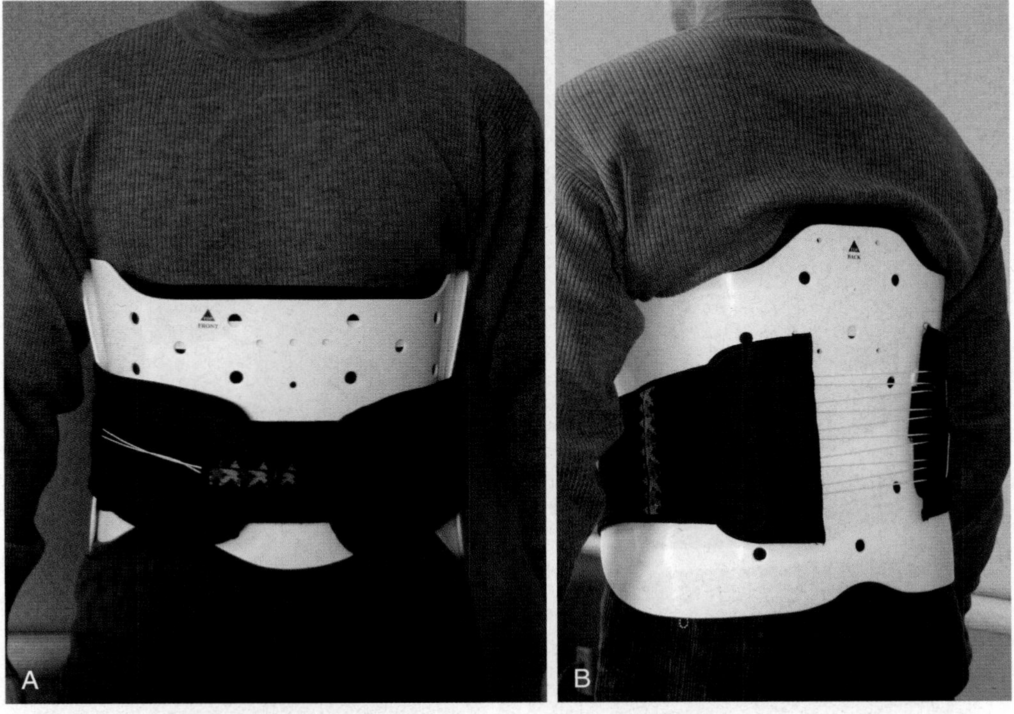

FIG. 81.17 Prefabricated lumbosacral orthosis. (A) Anterior view. (B) Posterior view. This design (California Compression Jacket, Orthomerica) has a patented "rip cord" used to help adjust the snugness of the fit.

reduced hospital time, avoided costs and risks of surgery, and allowed patients a relatively early return to work. Additionally, the authors mentioned that patients treated nonoperatively tended to experience moderate back pain up to a year after the injury and that this pain eventually diminished over time. Other more recent studies have also suggested that, in the absence of a neurologic deficit, operative and nonoperative treatment have comparable results. In a restricted cohort study, Stadhouder and colleagues found similar pain scores, disability indices, and general health outcomes at midterm follow-up.[99] A recent meta-analysis pooling patients from four trials made similar observations, again suggesting that nonoperative treatment in a brace has similar results to operative treatment but with lower costs and complications.[100]

LSOs (Figs. 81.17 and 81.18) are often prescribed for treatment after arthrodesis for degenerative conditions. As discussed earlier, several studies demonstrate little or no immobilizing effect from wearing LSOs and possibly an increase in L4–L5 and L5–S1 motion after application of these orthoses. The point continues to be debated. Post–lumbar fusion bracing is believed by some to help relieve pain and decrease the risk of pseudarthrosis and fixation failure; therefore, it is prescribed by some surgeons for up to 12 weeks postoperatively. Others believe that lumbosacral orthoses do little to immobilize the lumbar spine beyond the stabilization provided by rigid operative fixation.[101] Yee et al. recently performed a randomized controlled trial to assess the benefit of wearing a lumbar corset for 8 weeks after lumbar fusion for degenerative conditions.[102] Complication rates and rate of revision surgery were not different between the groups. Rohlmann and colleagues[103] evaluated the effect of a brace on loads on internal spinal fixation devices. The implant loads were measured using telemeterized fixators in six patients for several positions and activities, including sitting, standing, walking, bending forward, and lifting an extended leg in a supine position. They found that none of the braces tested was able to markedly reduce the loads on the fixators. They observed that higher fixator loads were often observed while wearing a brace. The same research group more recently studied the effect of an orthosis on the loads acting on a vertebral body replacement.[104] Telemeterized vertebral body replacements were implanted in five patients undergoing lumbar corpectomy. They found that the average resultant force on the vertebral body for 26 common daily activities was reduced by 19% with a hyperextension orthosis, particularly activities performed in a sitting position.

While many studies have examined the ability of spinal orthoses to immobilize the spine during daily activities, others have examined the impact of wearing them on such essential functions. Frownfelter et al. examined the effect of TLSOs on pulmonary function in healthy adults.[105] They found that wearing the brace had a significant effect on forced vital capacity and forced expiratory volume in 1 second both at rest and with exertion. Furthermore, they demonstrated that an abdominal cutout in the brace improved pulmonary function, especially with activity. They postulated that this was due to reduced restraint on abdominal expansion and suggested that this modification be considered in patients with compromised pulmonary function. Hofmann and colleagues studied the effect of LSOs on driving. Braking parameters in 30 healthy volunteers were measured with and without bracing using a custom-made automobile simulator.[106] They found that the spinal orthoses led to a significant increase in brake reaction time, which could lead to lengthening the total

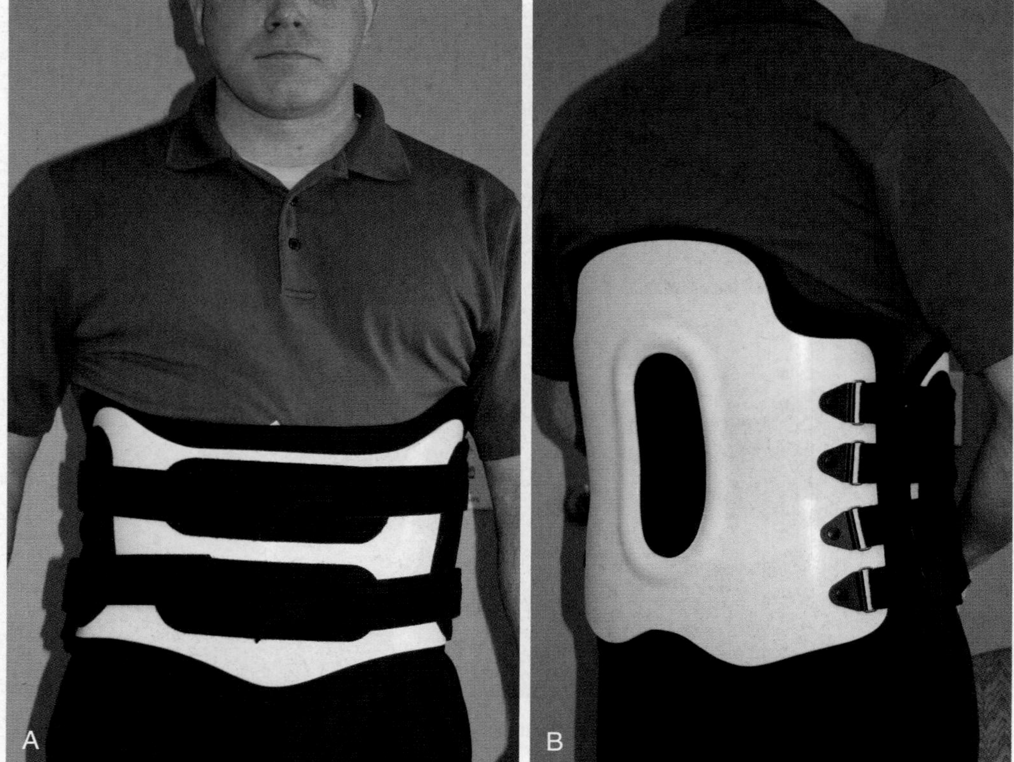

FIG. 81.18 Prefabricated lumbosacral orthosis. (A) Anterior view. (B) Posterior view. This design (Aspen) has a posterior cutout window that avoids direct pressure over a midline incision.

stopping distance. Patients should therefore be counseled on this potential effect when they seek to resume driving.

Summary

Spinal orthoses continue to be commonly prescribed for the management of both traumatic and degenerative conditions. There are many different types commercially available. The scientific evidence to document their effectiveness is variable. Despite the potential for complications, the halo remains the most rigid of external cervical immobilizers. A thorough appreciation of the biomechanics of spinal orthoses and their potential complications can help maximize their utility and minimize associated morbidity. Ongoing collaboration between the medical and prosthetics/orthotics communities is necessary as new technology continues to emerge.

Acknowledgment

Unless noted otherwise, the orthoses in the figures were supplied by Precision Orthotics and Prosthetics, Linden, NJ. The models are Paul Goodman, CO, Ryan, CPO, and David Sussman, CPO, all of Precision Orthotics and Prosthetics. We greatly appreciate their contribution to this chapter.

PEARLS

1. Halo pins should be retightened 24 to 48 hours after placement since fixation purchase decreases after vest placement.
2. In infants younger than 3 years, a multiple low-torque pin insertion technique is recommended to achieve maximal stability given decreased skull thickness and increased pliability.
3. When external immobilization is desired cephalad to T5, a cervical extension should be added to the TLSO.
4. When external immobilization is desired caudal to L3, a thigh cuff may improve the stability offered by a TLSO.

PITFALLS

1. A properly sized and fitted orthosis is essential to provide desired support and avoid soft tissue complications.
2. While commercially available collars come in a range of sizes, predicting appropriate fit can be difficult. Spine specialists may need to give direction to ancillary staff in determining and confirming the appropriate size.
3. Rigid cervical collars may exacerbate intracranial hypertension in patients with severe head injuries; therefore, early efforts to exclude coexistent cervical injuries should be pursued.
4. Excessive extension may precipitate swallowing difficulty in patients immobilized in halo vests.
5. Halo-vest immobilization in the elderly has been associated with substantial morbidity and mortality; thus, operative treatment of selected injuries in this age group may actually offer more favorable risk-benefit profiles.

KEY POINTS

1. Spinal orthoses are externally applied devices that serve to restrict motion in that particular body segment. They can be broadly categorized based on the region they are employed to immobilize: cervical (CO), cervicothoracic (CTO), thoracolumbosacral (TLSO), lumbosacral (LSO), and sacroiliac (SIO).

2. The indications and usage of spinal orthoses is a subject of ongoing investigation, and there is a lack of consensus among spine surgeons on their use in postoperative patients.
3. Improved flexion control of the cervical spine may be obtained by increasing the length of the orthosis (extending it onto the thorax) and increasing the rigidity of the connections between the proximal (submandibular and occipital) and distal (thoracic) rests.
4. The halo vest provides the most rigid immobilization of the cervical spine of all the currently used orthoses. However, complications are not uncommon and halo usage in the elderly can be associated with significant morbidity and mortality.
5. Most conventional TLSOs are more effective in limiting motion in the sagittal plane than in controlling rotation or lateral bending.
6. Several studies demonstrate little or no immobilizing effect from wearing LSOs and possibly an increase in L4–L5 and L5–S1 motion after application of these orthoses. Their utility for the treatment of back pain or as postfusion adjuncts is therefore debatable.

KEY REFERENCES

1. Botte MJ, Garfin SR, Byrne TP, et al. The halo skeletal fixator: principles of application and maintenance. *Clin Orthop.* 1989;239:12-18.
   The authors provide a detailed description of the specific steps for application of the halo skeletal fixator and their suggestions for maintenance.
2. Garfin SR, Botte MJ, Waters RL, Nickel VL. Complications in the use of halo fixation device. *J Bone Joint Surg Am.* 1986;68:320-325.
   The authors report the complications observed with their extensive use of the halo device.
3. Jellema P, van Tulder MW, van Poppel MNM. Lumbar supports for prevention and treatment of low back pain: a systematic review within the framework of the Cochrane Back Review Group. *Spine.* 2001;26:377-386.
   In this systematic review of therapeutic trials, the authors report only limited evidence that lumbar supports are more effective than no treatment.
4. Johnson RM, Hart DL, Simmons EF, et al. Cervical orthoses: a study comparing their effectiveness in restricting cervical motion in normal subjects. *J Bone Joint Surg Am.* 1977;59:332-339.
   This classic study evaluated the effect of various orthoses in immobilizing the cervical spine, utilizing radiographs and overhead photographs.
5. Norton PL, Brown T. The immobilizing efficacy of back braces. *J Bone Joint Surg Am.* 1957;39:111-138.
   The earliest report on motion restriction with external lumbar supports; the authors noted increased motion across the lumbosacral junction in all of the braces, demonstrating the difficulty of immobilizing this area without more distal control.

REFERENCES

1. Smith G. The most ancient splints. *BMJ.* 1908;1:732-734.
2. Peltier L. *Orthopedics, a History and Iconography.* San Francisco: Norman Publishing; 1993.
3. Edwards J. *Orthopaedic Appliance Atlased.* St. Louis: American Academy of Orthopaedic Surgeons; 1952.
4. American Academy of Orthopaedic Surgeons. *Atlas of Orthotics.* St. Louis: CV Mosby; 1975.
5. Bible JE, Biswas D, Whang PG, et al. Postoperative bracing after spine surgery for degenerative conditions—a questionnaire study. *Spine J.* 2009;9(4):309-316.
6. White A, Panjabi M. Physical properties and functional biomechanics of the spine. In: White A, Panjabi M, eds. *Clinical Biomechanics of the Spine.* 2nd ed. Philadelphia: JB Lippincott; 1990.
7. Fisher SV, Bowar JF, Awad EA, et al. Cervical orthoses effect on cervical spine motion: roentgenographic and goniometric method of study. *Arch Phys Med Rehabil.* 1977;58:109-115.
8. Schneider AM, Hipp JA, Nguyen L, et al. Reduction in head and intervertebral motion provided by 7 contemporary cervical orthoses in 45 individuals. *Spine.* 2007;32(1):E1-E6.
9. Evans NR, Hooper G, Edwards R, et al. A 3D motion analysis study comparing the effectiveness of cervical spine orthoses at restricting motion through physiologic ranges. *Eur Spine J.* 2013;22:S10-S15.
10. Chase AP, Bader DL, Houghton GR. The biomechanical effectiveness of the Boston brace in the management of adolescent idiopathic scoliosis. *Spine.* 1989;14:636-642.
11. Wilner F. The effect of the Boston brace on the frontal sagittal curves of the spine. *Acta Orthop Scand.* 1984;55:457-460.
12. Sypert GW. External spinal orthotics. *Neurosurgery.* 1987;20:642-649.
13. Wong MS, Cheng JC, Lo KH. A comparison of treatment effectiveness between the CAD/CAM method and the manual method for managing adolescent idiopathic scoliosis. *Prosthet Orthot Int.* 2005;29:105-111.
14. Hsu JD, Michael JW, Fisk JR. *AAOS Atlas of Orthoses and Assistive Devices.* 4th ed. Philadelphia: Elsevier; 2008.
15. Miller CP, Bible JE, Jegede KA, et al. Soft and rigid collars provide similar restriction in cervical range of motion during fifteen activities of daily living. *Spine.* 2010;35(13):1271-1278.
16. Johnson RM, Hart DL, Simmons EF, et al. Cervical orthoses. A study comparing their effectiveness in restricting cervical motion in normal subjects. *J Bone Joint Surg Am.* 1977;59:332-339.
17. Colachis SC Jr, Strohm BR. Radiographic studies of cervical spine motion in normal subjects: flexion and hyperextension. *Arch Phys Med Rehabil.* 1965;46:753-760.
18. Hartman JT, Palumbo F, Hill BJ. Cineradiography of the braced normal cervical spine. A comparative study of five commonly used cervical orthoses. *Clin Orthop Relat Res.* 1975;109:97-102.
19. Lind B, Sihlbom H, Nordwall A. Forces and motions across the neck in patients treated with halo-vest. *Spine.* 1988;13:162-167.
20. Askins V, Eismont FJ. Efficacy of five cervical orthoses in restricting cervical motion. A comparison study. *Spine.* 1997;22:1193-1198.
21. Assi A, Yazbeck P, Massaad A, et al. Kimematic evaluation of 4 pediatric collars and distribution of cervical movement between them in primary and coupled angles. *J Pediatr Orthop.* 2014;34(5):496-502.
22. Bell KM, Frazier EC, Shively CM, et al. Assessing range of motion to evaluate the adverse effects of ill-fitting cervical orthoses. *Spine J.* 2009;9:225-231.
23. Gao F. Effectiveness of adjustable cervical orthoses and modular cervical thoracic orthoses in restricting neck motion. *Spine.* 2015;40(19):E1046-E1051.

SECTION XI

24. Chendrasekhar A, Moorman DW, Timberlake GA. An evaluation of the effects of semirigid cervical collars in patients with severe closed head injury. *Am Surg.* 1998;64:604-606.
25. Molano Alvarez E, Murillo Perez Mdel A, Salobral Villegas MT, et al. [Pressure sores secondary to immobilization with cervical collar: a complication of acute cervical injury]. *Enferm Intensiva.* 2004;15:112-122.
26. Powers J, Daniels D, McGuire C, et al. The incidence of skin breakdown associated with use of cervical collars. *J Trauma Nurs.* 2006;13:198-200.
27. Plaisier B, Gabram SG, Schwartz RJ, et al. Prospective evaluation of craniofacial pressure in four different cervical orthoses. *J Trauma.* 1994;37:714-720.
28. Tescher AN, Rindflesch AB, Youdas JW, et al. Range-of-motion restriction and craniofacial tissue-interface pressure from four cervical collars. *J Trauma.* 2007;63:1120-1126.
29. Karason S, Reynisson K, Sigvaldason K, et al. Evaluation of clinical efficacy and safety of cervical trauma collars: differences in immobilization, effect on jugular venous pressure and patient comfort. *Scand J Trauma Resusc Emerg Med.* 2014;22(37):1-7.
30. Hunt K, Hallworth S, Smith M. The effects of rigid collar placement on intracranial and cerebral perfusion pressures. *Anaesthesia.* 2001;56:511-513.
31. Stambolis V, Brady S, Klos D, et al. The effects of cervical bracing upon swallowing in young, normal, healthy volunteers. *Dysphagia.* 2003;18:39-45.
32. Cline JR, Scheidel E, Bigsby EF. A comparison of methods of cervical immobilization used in patient extrication and transport. *J Trauma.* 1985;25:649-653.
33. Podolsky S, Baraff LJ, Simon RR, et al. Efficacy of cervical spine immobilization methods. *J Trauma.* 1983;23:461-465.
34. Ben-Galim P, Dreiangel N, Mattox KL, et al. Extrication collars can result in abnormal separation between vertebrae in the presence of a dissociative injury. *J Trauma.* 2010;69:447-450.
35. Campbell MJ, Carreon LY, Traynelis V, et al. Use of cervical collar after single-level anterior cervical fusion with plate: is it necessary? *Spine.* 2009;34:43-48.
36. Johnson RM, Owen JR, Hart DL, et al. Cervical orthoses: a guide to their selection and use. *Clin Orthop Relat Res.* 1981;154:34-45.
37. Benzel EC, Larson SJ, Kerk JJ, et al. The thermoplastic Minerva body jacket: a clinical comparison with other cervical spine splinting techniques. *J Spinal Disord.* 1992;5:311-319.
38. Millington PJ, Ellingsen JM, Hauswirth BE, et al. Thermoplastic Minerva body jacket—a practical alternative to current methods of cervical spine stabilization. A clinical report. *Phys Ther.* 1987;67:223-225.
39. Sharpe KP, Rao S, Ziogas A. Evaluation of the effectiveness of the Minerva cervicothoracic orthosis. *Spine.* 1995;20:1475-1479.
40. Zelenik R, Chapin W, Hart D, et al. Yale cervical orthosis. *Phys Ther.* 1978;58:861-864.
41. Johnson RM, Hart DL, Owen JR, et al. The Yale cervical orthosis: an evaluation of its effectiveness in restricting cervical motion in normal subjects and a comparison with other cervical orthoses. *Phys Ther.* 1978;58:865-871.
42. Ivancic PC. Effects of orthoses on three-dimensional load displacement properties of the cervical spine. *Eur Spine J.* 2013;22:169-177.
43. Ivancic PC. Do cervical collars and cervicothoracic orthoses effectively stabilize the injured cervical spine? *Spine.* 2013;38:E767-E774.
44. Perry J, Nickel V. Total cervical spine fusion for neck paralysis. *J Bone Joint Surg Am.* 1959;41:37-60.
45. Botte M, Garfin S, Byrne T, et al. The halo skeletal fixator: principles of application and maintenance. *Clin Orthop Relat Res.* 1989;239:12-18.
46. Botte MJ, Byrne TP, Abrams RA, et al. Halo skeletal fixation: techniques of application and prevention of complications. *J Am Acad Orthop Surg.* 1996;4:44-53.
47. Lerman JA, Haynes RJ. Open versus closed halo rings: comparison of fixation strengths. *Spine.* 2001;26:2102-2104.
48. Mirza SK, Moquin RR, Anderson PA, et al. Stabilizing properties of the halo apparatus. *Spine.* 1997;22:727-733.
49. Voor MJ, Khalily C. Halo pin loosening: a biomechanical comparison of experimental and conventional designs. *J Biomech.* 1998;31:397-400.
50. Garfin SR, Lee TQ, Roux RD, et al. Structural behavior of the halo orthosis pin-bone interface: biomechanical evaluation of standard and newly designed stainless steel halo fixation pins. *Spine.* 1986;11:977-981.
51. Botte MJ, Byrne TP, Garfin SR. Application of the halo device for immobilization of the cervical spine utilizing an increased torque pressure. *J Bone Joint Surg Am.* 1987;69:750-752.
52. Chavasiri C, Chavasiri S. The thickness of the skull at the halo pin insertion site. *Spine.* 2011;36(22):1819-1823.
53. Garfin SR, Botte MJ, Centeno RS, et al. Osteology of the skull as it affects halo pin placement. *Spine.* 1985;10:696-698.
54. Stone JL, Gulabani A, Gorelick G, et al. Frontolateral pins for halo ring placement: reassessment of a common neurosurgical procedure with CT measurements of skull thickness. *J Neurosurg Spine.* 2013;19:744-749.
55. Triggs KJ, Ballock RT, Lee TQ, et al. The effect of angled insertion on halo pin fixation. *Spine.* 1989;14:781-783.
56. Baum JA, Hanley EN Jr, Pullekines J. Comparison of halo complications in adults and children. *Spine.* 1989;14: 251-252.
57. Kazi HA, de Matas M, Pillay R. Reduction of halo pin site morbidity with a new pin care regimen. *Asian Spine J.* 2013;7(2):91-95.
58. Ersmark H, Kalen R, Lowenhielm P. A methodical study of force measurements in three patients with odontoid fractures treated with a strain gauge equipped halo-vest. *Spine.* 1988; 13:433-435.
59. Walker PS, Lamser D, Hussey RW, et al. Forces in the halo-vest apparatus. *Spine.* 1984;9:773-777.
60. Kuester WM, Stamper RE, Ordway NR. Analysis of pin force distributions of halo orthoses. *Biomed Sci Instrum.* 2002;38:221-226.
61. Anderson PA, Budorick TE, Easton KB, et al. Failure of halo vest to prevent in vivo motion in patients with injured cervical spines. *Spine.* 1991;16:S501-S505.
62. Genin GM, Rosenberg SP, Seger LM, et al. The freedom to heal: nonrigid immobilization by a halo orthosis. *J Neurosurg Spine.* 2014;21:811-816.
63. Ivancic PC, Telles CJ. Neck motion due to the halo-vest in prone and supine positions. *Spine.* 2010;35:E400-E406.
64. Ivancic PC, Beauchman NN, Tweardy L. Effect of halo-vest components on stabilizing the injured cervical spine. *Spine.* 2009;34:167-175.
65. Bono CM. The halo fixator. *J Am Acad Orthop Surg.* 2007;15:728-737.

66. Glaser JA, Whitehill R, Stamp WG, et al. Complications associated with the halo-vest. A review of 245 cases. *J Neurosurg*. 1986;65:762-769.
67. Lind B, Sihlbom H, Nordwall A. Halo-vest treatment of unstable traumatic cervical spine injuries. *Spine*. 1988;13:425-432.
68. Garfin SR, Botte MJ, Waters RL, et al. Complications in the use of the halo fixation device. *J Bone Joint Surg Am*. 1986;68:320-325.
69. Fleming BC, Krag MH, Huston DR, et al. Pin loosening in a halo-vest orthosis: a biomechanical study. *Spine*. 2000;25:1325-1331.
70. Garfin SR, Botte MJ, Triggs KJ, et al. Subdural abscess associated with halo-pin traction. *J Bone Joint Surg Am*. 1988;70:1338-1340.
71. Kelly P, Beregin D, Cunningham U, et al. Deglutition dysfunction in cervical orthosis. *J Bone Joint Surg Br*. 2002;84(suppl).
72. Bradley JF, Jones MA, Farmer EA, et al. Swallowing dysfunction in trauma patients with cervical spine fractures treated with halo-vest fixation. *J Trauma*. 2011;70(1):46-48.
73. van Middendorp JJ, Slooff WB, Nellestein WR, et al. Incidence of and risk factors for complications associated with halo-vest immobilization: a prospective, descriptive cohort study of 239 patients. *J Bone Joint Surg Am*. 2009;91:71-79.
74. Tashjian RZ, Majercik S, Biffl WL, et al. Halo-vest immobilization increases early morbidity and mortality in elderly odontoid fractures. *J Trauma*. 2006;60:199-203.
75. Koech F, Ackland HM, Varma DK, et al. Nonoperative management of type II odontoid fractures in the elderly. *Spine*. 2008;33:2881-2886.
76. Kopits SE, Steingass MH. Experience with the “halo-cast” in small children. *Surg Clin North Am*. 1970;50:935-943.
77. Osenbach RK, Menezes AH. Pediatric spinal cord and vertebral column injury. *Neurosurgery*. 1992;30:385-390.
78. Mubarak SJ, Camp JF, Vuletich W, et al. Halo application in the infant. *J Pediatr Orthop*. 1989;9:612-614.
79. DiPaola CP, Sawers A, Conrad BP, et al. Comparing cervical spine motion with different halo devices in a cadaveric cervical instability model. *Spine*. 2009;34:149-155.
80. Skaggs DL, Lerman LD, Albrektson J, et al. Use of a noninvasive halo in children. *Spine*. 2008;33:1650-1654.
81. Sawers A, DiPaola CP, Rechtine GR 2nd. Suitability of the noninvasive halo for cervical spine injuries: a retrospective analysis of outcomes. *Spine J*. 2009;9:216-220.
82. Nachemson A, Schultz A, Andersson G. Mechanical effectiveness studies of lumbar spine orthoses. *Scand J Rehabil Med Suppl*. 1983;9:139-149.
83. Waters RL, Morris JM. Effect of spinal supports on the electrical activity of muscles of the trunk. *J Bone Joint Surg Am*. 1970;52:51-60.
84. Lantz SA, Schultz AB. Lumbar spine orthosis wearing. II. Effect on trunk muscle myoelectric activity. *Spine*. 1986;11:838-842.
85. Morris JM, Lucas DB. Biomechanics of spinal bracing. *Ariz Med*. 1964;21:170-176.
86. Loguidice V, Polaski E. Patient satisfaction with the Orthotrac pneumatic vest for low back pain. *Care Manage*. 2002;8:4.
87. Jellema P, van Tulder MW, van Poppel MN, et al. Lumbar supports for prevention and treatment of low back pain: a systematic review within the framework of the Cochrane Back Review Group. *Spine*. 2001;26:377-386.
88. White A, Panjabi M. *Clinical Biomechanics of the Spine*. Toronto: JB Lippincott; 1978.
89. Brown T, Norton PL. The immobilizing efficiency of back braces; their effect on the posture and motion of the lumbosacral spine. *J Bone Joint Surg Am*. 1957;39-A:111-139.
90. Fidler MW, Plasmans CM. The effect of four types of support on the segmental mobility of the lumbosacral spine. *J Bone Joint Surg Am*. 1983;65:943-947.
91. Buchalter D, Kahonovitz N, Viola K, Dorsky S, Nordin M. Three dimensional spinal motion measurements: part 2. A noninvasive assessment of lumbar brace immobilization of the spine. *J Spinal Disord*. 1988;1:284-286.
92. Lumsden RM 2nd, Morris JM. An in vivo study of axial rotation and immobilization at the lumbosacral joint. *J Bone Joint Surg Am*. 1968;50:1591-1602.
93. Nahemson AL. Orthotic treatment for injuries and diseases of the spinal column. *Phys Med Rehabil*. 1987;1:11-24.
94. Vander Kooi D, Abad G, Basford JR, et al. Lumbar spine stabilization with a thoracolumbosacral orthosis: evaluation with video fluoroscopy. *Spine*. 2004;29:100-104.
95. Rubery PT, Brown R, Prasarn M, et al. Stabilization of 2-column thoracolumbar fractures with orthoses. A cadaver model. *Spine*. 2013;38:E270-E275.
96. Kim HJ, Cho HG, Chang BS, et al. Comparative study of the treatment outcomes of osteoporotic compression fractures without neurologic injury using a rigid brace, a soft brace, and no brace. *J Bone Joint Surg Am*. 2014;96:1959-1966.
97. Ohana N, Sheinis D, Rath E, et al. Is there a need for lumbar orthosis in mild compression fractures of the thoracolumbar spine?: a retrospective study comparing the radiographic results between early ambulation with and without lumbar orthosis. *J Spinal Disord*. 2000;13:305-308.
98. Chow GH, Nelson BJ, Gebhard JS, et al. Functional outcome of thoracolumbar burst fractures managed with hyperextension casting or bracing and early mobilization. *Spine*. 1996;21:2170-2175.
99. Stadhouder A, Buskens E, de Klerk LK, et al. Traumatic thoracic and lumbar spinal fractures: operative or nonoperative treatment. *Spine*. 2008;33:1006-1017.
100. Gnanenthiran S, Adie S, Harris IA. Nonoperative versus operative treatment for thoracolumbar burst fractures without neurologic deficit. A meta-analysis. *Clin Orthop Relat Res*. 2012;470:567-577.
101. Connolly PJ, Grob D. Bracing of patients after fusion for degenerative problems of the lumbar spine—yes or no? *Spine*. 1998;23:1426-1428.
102. Yee AJ, Yoo JU, Marsolais EB, et al. Use of a postoperative lumbar corset after lumbar spinal arthrodesis for degenerative conditions of the spine. A prospective randomized trial. *J Bone Joint Surg Am*. 2008;90:2062-2068.
103. Rohlmann A, Bergmann G, Graichen F, et al. Braces do not reduce loads on internal spinal fixation devices. *Clin Biomech (Bristol, Avon)*. 1999;14:97-102.
104. Rohlmann A, Zander T, Graichen F, et al. Effect of an orthosis on the loads acting on a vertebral body replacement. *Clin Biomech (Bristol, Avon)*. 2013;28(5):490-494.
105. Frownfelter D, Stevens K, Massery M, et al. Do abdominal cutouts in thoracolumbosacral orthoses increase pulmonary function? *Clin Orthop Relat Res*. 2014;472:720-726.
106. Hofmann UK, Thumm S, Jordan M, et al. The effects of hip and spine orthoses on braking parameters: a simulated study with healthy subjects. *PM R*. 2016;8(1):35-44.

CHAPTER 82

Spinal Cord Injury Rehabilitation

Andrew L. Sherman
Kevin L. Dalal

Spinal cord injury (SCI) is a catastrophic event that results in impairments that impact various aspects of the patient's bodily function. SCI is not only devastating to the individual, it also imposes a burdensome cost to society. These injuries typically affect young and previously healthy individuals who now require urgent and comprehensive emergency care, frequently involving medical and surgical stabilization. The SCI patient then arrives on the rehabilitation unit and must learn to manage basic bodily functions despite seeing slow or no neurologic recovery. Finally, the SCI patient is expected to learn to perform once simple and now complex tasks of daily living independently with the goal of returning home. The amount of time available for recovery in the inpatient setting prior to discharge is continually shrinking in the current medical climate.

SCI is defined as an injury to the spinal cord that partially or completely interrupts its main functions: motor, sensory, and reflex activities. Egyptian physicians long ago labeled SCI as an ailment not to be treated at all[1] because they feared that the pharaoh would kill them if they let a patient die under their care. Prior to World War I, SCI typically resulted in early death. Significant advances in treatment began during World War II and have continued to progress, allowing many individuals with SCI to live far longer than previously expected. Today, many patients with SCI can expect to live a normal or almost normal lifespan. As a result, the numbers of persons alive today in the United States with SCI has increased to over 200,000.[2]

Epidemiology

In 1970, the first federally funded Spinal Cord Injury Model Systems (SCIMSs) were developed. Currently, 14 such centers have received this designation by the National Institute on Disability, Independent Living, and Rehabilitation Research (NIDILRR). Each center is a comprehensive interdisciplinary service that integrates all aspects of care for the SCI patient, from the initial injury to lifelong follow-up. The model center's guiding principles were set forth by Sir Ludwig Guttman, a British physician who pioneered these advances in the care of SCI patients during World War II:[1]

1. Transfer of the SCI patient to a specialized unit as soon after injury as possible.
2. Unit management by a physician who is knowledgeable and dedicated to spinal care.
3. A team of allied health professionals who are trained in the intricacies of spinal cord problems.
4. A commitment to vocational pursuits.
5. An emphasis on psychosocial and recreational needs.
6. Provision for follow-up care for the lifetime of the individual.

The 14 current Model Spinal Cord Injury Care System (MSCICS) centers (and eight previously designated centers) have been contributing clinical information to the National Spinal Cord Injury Statistical Center (NSCISC) database following a jointly agreed upon protocol. They have been able to report results based on an estimated 13% of all SCI injuries in the United States occurring since 1973. The database contains information on approximately 25,000 spinal cord injured persons.[3] The end result is a wealth of information regarding injury trends from 1973 to 1998 and some updates that include information through the year 2004. The data not only allows physicians to know the current status of SCI patients but also has given physicians insight into trends in the demographic data. These changes in the demographics of SCI have allowed rehabilitation programs and centers to adapt to reduce costs and ultimately improve the quality of medical rehabilitative care for their patients with SCI.[4]

Incidence, Race, Age, and Gender

According to the NSCISC database, there are approximately 11,000 new cases (40 per million in the US population) each year. However, this number is based on older data from the 1970s. The prevalence is estimated to be 225,000 to 296,000 persons and growing.[3] The recently updated national SCI Statistical Center statistics estimates the prevalence at 255,702.

Between 1973 and 2004, 66% of patients were white, 21% were African-American, and 9.7% were Hispanic.[3]

Cervical injuries resulting in tetraplegia occur in 54% of SCI patients. Lumbar and thoracic injuries causing paraplegia comprise the rest (45%). A few (1%) were discharged as "normal" or indeterminate. Since 1990, the number of patients with complete SCI has exceeded the incomplete injuries (56% vs. 44%).[3] Since 2000, however, the most common injury has been incomplete tetraplegia (34.7%), followed by incomplete paraplegia (23.0%), complete tetraplegia (18.5%), and complete paraplegia (18.5%).

SCI most commonly affects young adults. Population-based data shows that the highest incidence of injuries (51.6%) occurs in the 16- to 30-year-old group.[3] However, the most recent trends suggest that SCI is occurring with increasing frequency in older persons. The result is that the fastest growing population of new SCI patients is over 60 years old at onset. Since 1990, the incidence of SCI in persons older than 60 years has increased from 4.5% in the 1970s to 12%.[3] As of 2007, the average age at the time of injury has increased from 28.7 years to 38.9 years. Additionally, while SCI is an injury that occurs primarily in males (81.6% since 1973), some centers are reporting increasing numbers of females sustaining SCI.

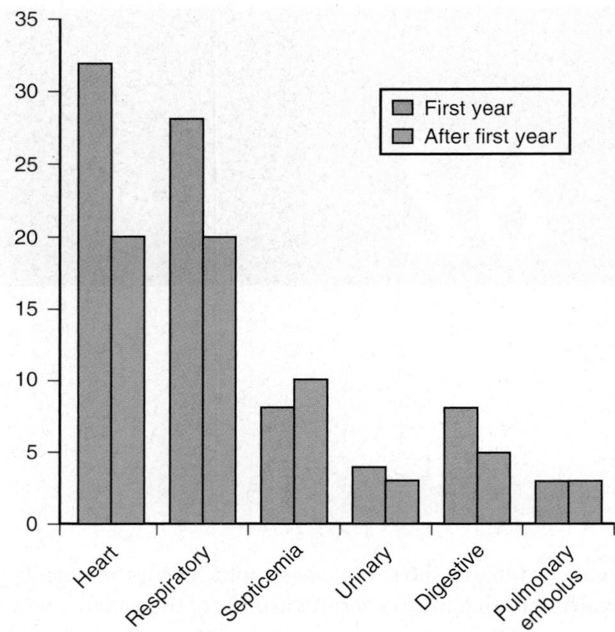

FIG. 82.1 Causes of death after spinal cord injury.

Life Expectancy

Life expectancies for persons with SCI have continued to steadily increase over time. Mortality rates, however, while improving, continue to be highest during the first year after injury. Complete injuries still have lower ultimate survival rates than incomplete injuries. The degree of neurologic impairment as measured by the Frankel Grade or the American Spinal Injury Association (ASIA) Impairment Scale and the level of injury were significantly correlated with mortality risk. For example, the average life expectancy of a 20-year-old who sustains complete paraplegia is 66 years. This compares to 61 years for a C5–C8 injury, 57 years for a C1–C4 injury, and 43 years for a ventilator-dependent patient. This compares to the normal life expectancy in the general population of 77 years and in a patient with an incomplete SCI of 72 years.[5] The factors that can increase life expectancy are favorable circumstances for good health, community integration, and higher income.[6]

Mortality

Many years ago, the leading cause of death among persons with SCI was renal failure. Pulmonary embolism (PE), usually in the first few weeks after injury and usually associated with a deep vein thrombosis (DVT), was another frequent cause of death. Advances in urologic management, DVT and PE prevention, and early mobilization have reduced the number of early deaths in SCI patients. Today, renal failure rarely occurs in the acute SCI setting. Because more SCI patients live not only through first year after injury but also survive to old age, cardiovascular disease has become a more frequent cause of death (Fig. 82.1). Nash and colleagues[7] demonstrated that SCI is an independent risk factor for developing multiple risks for cardiovascular disease, such as elevated cholesterol levels. Respiratory illness, particularly pneumonia, is now the leading cause of death among older SCI patients with cervical injuries.[8] The cause of death in persons with paraplegia is more varied. In addition to heart disease, cancer, suicide, and septicemia are the leading causes.

Etiology

The causes of SCI are typically divided into traumatic and nontraumatic. The top five causes of traumatic SCI in males are auto accidents, falls, gunshot wounds, diving, and motorcycle accidents.[3] The top three causes remain the same in women but the final two are medical complications and diving (Fig. 82.2).[3]

The major trend is that violent injuries have decreased from 20% in the 1990s to 9.8% in 2004.[3] Geographic variations occur depending on the state or city. In the older SCI patients, in addition to falls, nontraumatic causes of SCI—such as cancer, vascular injuries, and infection—make up a larger proportion of injuries. Etiology is also reported in terms of major groups. Fig. 82.3 illustrates the frequency of various causes of SCI.

Classification of SCI

There are three basic physiologic functions of the spinal cord. The ascending tracts in the cord receive sensory information from the somatic and visceral receptors through dorsal root ganglia and transmit this information to higher centers. The descending tracts receive signals from higher centers and ultimately transmit these signals to target sites via the ventral roots. The other basic function of the spinal cord is to modulate these signals via a variety of local mechanisms.

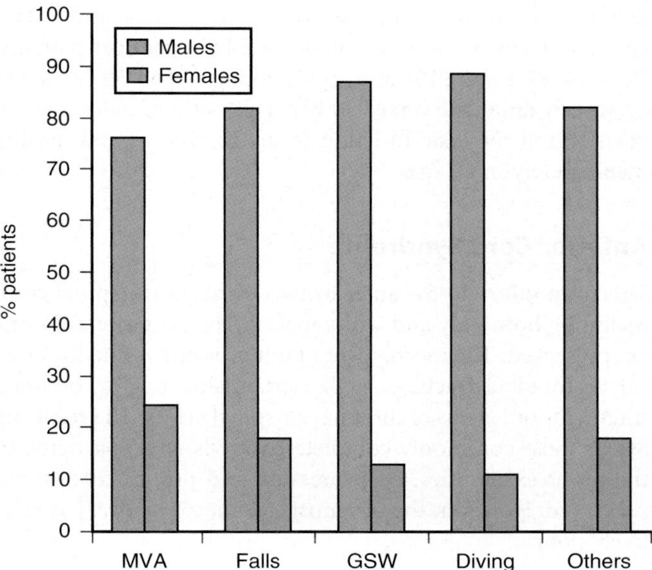

FIG. 82.2 Causes of spinal cord injury by gender of patients. GSW, gunshot wound; MVA, motor vehicle accident. (Modified from Jackson AB, Dijkers M, DeVivo MJ, Poczatek RB. A demographic profile of new traumatic spinal cord injuries: change and stability over 30 years. *Arch Phys Med Rehab.* 2004;85:1740–1748.)

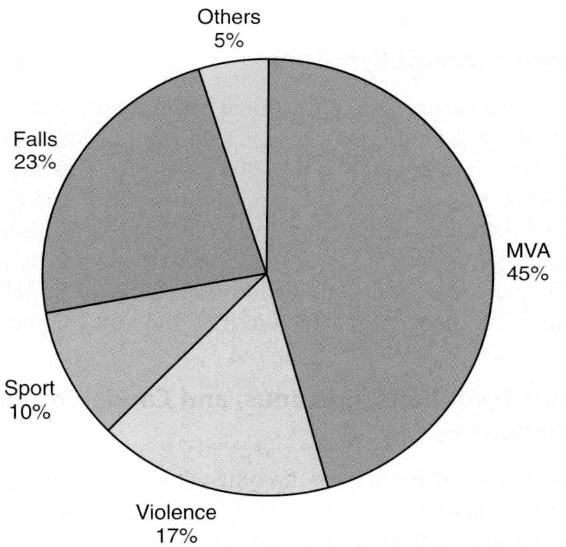

FIG. 82.3 Etiology of causes of spinal cord injury overall for both genders. MVA, motor vehicle accident. (Modified from Jackson AB, Dijkers M, DeVivo MJ, Poczatek RB. a demographic profile of new traumatic spinal cord injuries: change and stability over 30 years. *Arch Phys Med Rehab.* 2004;85:1740–1748.)

Assessment, treatment, and classification of SCI flow directly from the anatomy, physiology, and topography of the spinal cord. Classification or grouping of patients allows the rehabilitation physician to predict the outcome and ultimate function in a majority of patients based on others with similar injuries. This allows the rehabilitation team to design a rehabilitation program appropriate for each SCI patient to provide the best opportunity to maximize the patient's potential functional outcome.

TABLE 82.1 American Spinal Injury Association (ASIA) Impairment Scale

Scale Grade	Description
A	Complete—No motor or sensory function is preserved in the sacral segments S4–S5.
B	Incomplete—Sensory but not motor function is preserved below the neurologic level and includes the sacral segments S4–S5.
C	Incomplete—Motor function is preserved below the neurologic level and more than half of key muscles below the neurologic level have a muscle grade <3.
D	Incomplete—Motor function is preserved below the neurologic level and at least half of key muscles below the neurologic level have a muscle grade of ≥3.
E	Normal—Motor and sensory function is normal.

There are two assessment tools used in the evaluation of patients after SCI.[9] One is the neurologic classification of SCI using the ASIA impairment scale. The other is the functional score or Functional Independence Measure (FIM) score. The most accurate way to assess a patient who has suffered an SCI is to perform a standardized physical examination as outlined by the ASIA. The neurologic examination includes two key components—the motor and sensory exam with required and optional elements. The result allows the clinician to compile a score and determine the completeness of injury. The neurologic level is also determined by rules set forth in the ASIA examination. From these data, a functional classification is assigned to each patient. This information can then be used to design each patient's rehabilitation program and predict the patient's functional outcome based on previous patients with similar injury classifications.

The ASIA impairment scale measures the degree of completeness of injury using categories from A to E (Table 82.1). Complete paralysis is defined as the absence of sensory and motor function below the level of injury, including the lowest sacral segments, and incomplete paralysis as preservation of sensation below the level of the injury, including the lowest sacral segments. Sacral sparing is defined as voluntary anal contraction or the presence of dull touch and pinprick sensation in the rectal and perianal area.

The motor component of the ASIA impairment scale measures the strength of each muscle on a 6-point scale (0–5) and sensation for pinprick and dull touch on a three-point scale (0–2). The motor level of SCI is defined as the lowest normal motor segment that has a grade 3 or more, provided that the muscles above that level are graded as a 5. The motor level best reflects the severity of impairment and disability during rehabilitation.

The FIM score is a widely accepted functional assessment tool and is currently used as an indicator of function in patients with SCI. The FIM is an 18-item scale. There are two categories of items, motor and cognitive. Individual items in each category score from 1 to 7, ranging from "total assistance" to "complete independence." There are 13 items of motor scoring important in determination of self-care, sphincter control, and mobility (Box 82.1). Scores falling below 6

BOX 82.1 Functional Independence Measure (FIM) Scale

Motor Items

Self-care
Seating
Grooming
Bathing
Dressing upper body
Dressing lower body
Toileting

Sphincter Control

Bladder management
Bowel management

Mobility

Bed, chair transfer
Toilet transfer
Tub, shower transfer
Walking/wheelchair
Locomotion
Stairs

FIM Scale Level of Function Scoring

Independent
7—Complete independence
6—Modified independence

Modified Dependence

5—Supervision
4—Minimal assist
3—Moderate assist

Complete Dependence

2—Maximal assist
1—Total assist

indicate that the patient requires another person for assistance. Many rehabilitation units now use FIM scores to measure patient outcomes. Quality assurance units use this data from groups of patients to draw inferences on the effectiveness of the rehabilitation unit.

Clinical Syndromes

Many patients, especially those with complete SCIs, can be precisely described strictly based on their neurologic level, However, there are certain clinical syndromes describing variations in incomplete SCIs. Principal among these named syndromes include central cord, anterior cord, posterior cord, Brown-Séquard, conus medullaris, and cauda equina syndromes.[10,11]

Central Cord Syndrome

The most common type of incomplete SCI in the elderly is the central cord syndrome. It also carries with it a relatively favorable prognosis for recovery. The mechanism of injury is usually hyperextension of an already stenotic cervical canal, producing central hematomyelia.[12] Because the lumbar and sacral motor tracts are located in the periphery of the white matter, the syndrome is characterized by motor weakness of the upper extremities greater than the lower extremities and sacral sparing. Recovery occurs more favorably in younger patients. Between 87% and 97% of patients younger than 50 years will eventually ambulate versus 31% to 41% of those older than 50 years. Hand intrinsic function is last to recover and usually incompletely in all ages.

Anterior Cord Syndrome

This is an injury to the anterior two-thirds of the spinal cord, including both gray and white matter. The posterior columns are preserved. The mechanism of injury is either due to cervical or thoracic fractures with retropulsion of disc or bone fragments or lesions of the anterior spinal artery. The resulting SCI is most commonly complete paralysis with spasticity. In the lower extremities, deep pressure and proprioception are preserved. However, the prognosis for motor recovery is relatively poor.

Posterior Cord Syndrome

Posterior cord syndrome is the least common incomplete SCI and is characterized by absence of position sense. There is usually preservation of pain, temperature, and touch. Motor function is impaired to variable extents.

Brown-Séquard Syndrome

This injury occurs with a functional hemisection of the spinal cord. The most common cause is a gunshot or knife wound. The classic presentation is ipsilateral loss of motor function, ipsilateral loss of dorsal column sensation, and contralateral loss of pain and temperature below the level of the lesion. Overall, these patients have the greatest potential for functional outcome and ambulation (75–90%).[13] Bowel and bladder continence is regained in 82% and 89%, respectively.

Conus Medullaris, Epiconus, and Cauda Equina Syndromes

Patients with these lesions present with similar motor and sensory deficits but can also be differentiated. Patients typically present with patchy lower extremity weakness, saddle anesthesia, and incontinence of stool. Urinary retention is more common than incontinence. Lesions of the cauda equina exhibit lower motor neuron signs, including decreased lower extremity motor tone, absent lower extremity and bulbocavernosus reflexes, flaccid bladder, and asymmetric weakness. High conus (epiconus) lesions may have upper motor neuron findings mixed with the lower motor neuron findings.

Cauda equina lesions carry a much more favorable prognosis for functional motor and sensory recovery, especially when surgical/medical treatment occurs promptly. Bowel, bladder, and sexual function return less frequently, however, often leading to adjustment and psychological difficulties. The long-term outcomes in patients with cauda equina injuries are compounded by a very high incidence of severe neuropathic lower extremity pain not usually seen in conus injuries. Thus, patients recovering from cauda equina injuries may have long-term physical and emotional disabilities despite their seemingly "normal" outward appearance even after successful physical rehabilitation.

Therapy Approaches

The rehabilitation of the SCI patient should begin from the moment of injury. An immediate response—transfer to a level I trauma center—and prompt medical and surgical treatment helps mitigate medical complications and facilitates preservation of neurologic function. In the acute hospital setting, consultation with an SCI specialist should be done immediately for recommendations regarding treatment of neurogenic bowel and bladder, prophylaxis of DVT and PE, prophylaxis of gastric ulcer, preventing atelectasis and pneumonia via proper pulmonary management, and preventing skin ulcers with proper positioning in bed and turning every 2 hours. Physical and occupational therapies are initiated in the acute hospital unit once the spine is stabilized. Range of motion (ROM) is performed on the shoulders, hips, elbows, and heel cords. ROM should be performed twice daily to prevent joint contractures and can be taught to family members. Splints are made for the upper extremities for the same reason. The patient begins to build tolerance to out-of-bed sitting and is taught weight shifting to prevent pressure ulcers.

Once the acute treatment is completed and the patient deemed medically stable, the patient can be transferred to an acute inpatient rehabilitation unit.[14] As economic pressures accelerate the transfer process from postoperative care to acute inpatient rehabilitation, patients with high tetraplegia may achieve medical stability while the patient is still on a ventilator. The weaning process can be improved by ramping up exercise demand and tolerance in the ventilator-dependent patient.

An accelerated path through their hospital stay to rehabilitation may have negative consequences as well. Patients may not have a chance to fully psychologically adjust to their injury. Additionally, the length of stay (LOS) on the rehab service has become progressively shorter as well. Such shorter LOSs may necessitate that the patient may not fully plateau in their physical, psychological, and functional recovery until they are transitioned to the outpatient setting. Therefore, it is imperative that the rehabilitation be focused and aggressive to accomplish as much as possible in a shorter amount of time. The challenge is to provide SCI patients with the highest quality rehabilitative care despite these imposed constraints so that they leave the hospital with the best possible outcome.

On the rehabilitation unit, the SCI patient begins a new journey. The basic skills of mobility, self-care, and bladder/bowel management must be learned to the maximum degree of independence that the injury and recovery allows. Often, this can be a slow, frustrating process. Though total independence is the ultimate goal, often, modified or various degrees of assistance is the more realistic objective. The level of neurologic injury best predicts the level of independence and mobility that each patient can achieve,[15] even though individual variability occurs. In addition to their therapy, patients on an SCI unit can utilize other resources, such as computer programs and handbooks, to supplement their understanding of their disease process. Many patients also receive counseling for emotional and psychological adjustment, discover initial vocational options for their future, and participate in recreational and leisure activities that ease their reintegration into society. SCI patients who suffer concurrent head trauma receive cognitive testing and retraining. SCI patients who remain on ventilators receive more advanced respiratory and speech therapy. Finally, each patient is discharged to the most independent living situation possible. During the rehabilitation stay, the therapy team can perform a home evaluation to determine any necessary home modifications to maximize independent living with the appropriate adaptive equipment.

The rehabilitation process involves multiple different organ systems, care teams, and longitudinal planning. The complex acute and chronic interplay between these services requires a dedicated interdisciplinary team to properly manage comprehensive rehabilitation and maximize outcome.[16] Historically, the leader of the team has been the rehabilitation physician, or physiatrist, who would delineate the rehabilitation goals, lead weekly team meetings, and decide when the program is complete. More recently, most rehabilitation programs have shifted to a more patient-centered approach, with the interdisciplinary team working toward goals set together with the patient.[17] With this approach, the patient, often the family, is intimately involved in deciding the direction of the rehabilitation and the date of discharge. The individual disciplines are listed in Table 82.2.[18]

TABLE 82.2 Interdisciplinary Team for Spinal Cord Injury Patients

Discipline	Role
Psychiatrist	Medical care, coordination of rehabilitation, team leader
Rehabilitation nurse	Daily care, medication, education, reinforce skills, transfers
Physical therapist	Gross motor skills, transfers, mobility (wheelchair, standing, ambulation)
Occupational therapist	Fine motor skills, activities of daily living (e.g., feeding, dressing, bathing)
Recreational therapist	Leisure activities, community reintegration, assistive technology use
Social worker	Obtain community resources; assist with disposition planning; communicate with insurance companies
Speech therapist	Assess cognitive status; provide communication, swallowing, and cognitive training
Respiratory therapist	Manage patients on respirator; provide respiratory treatments
Prosthetist/orthotist	Design and fabricate upper/lower extremity braces and prosthesis; fit spine braces
Vocational counselor	Test skills and interest; recommend training and assist with placement
Vendor	Wheelchair procurement and fitting, adaptive equipment

Recent advances in rehabilitation techniques have led to both increased functional outcomes and decreased LOSS. The Spinal Cord Injury Rehabilitation project, led by the Rocky Mountain Regional Spinal Injury System, used practice-based evidence research to identify the rehabilitation interventions most strongly associated with positive outcomes.[19] This would not necessarily correlate to shorter LOSs but could offer clinicians more evidence-based outcomes by which to base their treatments. Ultimately, what they found was that patient characteristics drove the outcomes more than the type of rehabilitation obtained. Thus, a patient with more severe injuries received more rehabilitation interventions and thus it was difficult to compare and contrast the types of therapy offered.[20]

Over the years, another one of the most influential advances to quickening the pace of rehabilitation has been in surgical stabilization. Historically, large, bulky cervical braces that included halos dominated rehabilitation units. Now, more advanced internal fixation has allowed patients to come onto the rehabilitation units almost immediately after surgery, usually with only a hard collar.[21] The less intrusive bracing allows patients to progress more quickly in their mobility training. A recent study touted the benefits of early surgical decompression on patient outcomes, including neurologic improvement of two levels more often.[22]

Medications have also allowed SCI patients to recover more quickly. Patients who were having difficulty with postural hypotension now can get upright sooner and for longer time periods. Other medications have decreased the incidence of DVT, PE, and spasticity. Those SCI patients slowed by neuropathic pain benefit from improved pain medications, specifically antiepileptics and serotonin-norepinephrine reuptake inhibitors (SNRIs). Aggressive percussive lung treatments have also decreased the incidence of pneumonia and "down time" on the unit. The functional rehabilitation program begins with an initial comprehensive assessment of the medical impairments, functional deficits, and environmental setup. Then, based on the findings, appropriate goals can be set and a treatment approach to reach those goals can be initiated and completed. Persons with complete SCI will typically plateau sooner, and their impairments can remain chronic and lifelong.

Therapists may choose from a number of treatment approaches to achieve the goal of functional independence and achieving maximum function. More than one different type of approach may also be used if felt appropriate by the therapist. Additionally, although therapy sessions and tasks are divided by discipline (e.g., transfer training by physical therapy, activities of daily living (ADLs) by occupational therapy), all therapists must utilize expertise from other specialists on the team to maximize functional restoration and treatment. Within that framework, treatment can be either restorative or compensatory. The goal of restorative treatment is simply to reverse the disability despite the impairment present even though the impairment cannot be reversed. In this case, the individual is encouraged to perform the ADL task the same way as before the injury, despite the impairment. Compensatory treatments aim to reverse the disability and the handicap by finding other means of traversing the divide created by the impairment without directly restoring the function. One example is utilizing equipment with special adaptations to eat or bathe. Either way, the function can be accomplished with modified independence or at least with the least setup or assistance possible at the time of discharge.

The choice of which method to use depends on the underlying condition of the patient. Most persons with complete SCI may regain one or two levels of neurologic function but are unlikely to regain any more neurologic return in the acute phase of recovery. Therefore, therapists most often utilize compensatory strategies to create independent function. However, persons with incomplete SCI may see tremendous neurologic recovery over time and are more appropriate for restorative therapy immediately. Therefore, therapists must carefully observe their patient and try to project the amount and speed of the recovery. If the patient's recovery is more rapid, restorative treatment strategies are more appropriate. One example would be employing standing balance strategies at the kitchen even when the patient cannot yet ambulate but should be able to in the near future. Areas of focus on the inpatient rehabilitation stay include the following:

- Bed mobility
- Transfer training
- Wheelchair training
- Functional mobility
- Self-dressing
- Self-feeding
- Bathing and grooming
- Neurogenic bladder management
- Neurogenic bowel management
- Assistive devices
- Home and environment modifications

Many advances in therapy techniques have improved treatment offered to SCI patients in rehabilitation. Functional electrical stimulation has been applied to patients both in the acute rehabilitation setting and later in the outpatient setting to upper and lower extremities.[23] Assisted or weighted standing and walking, even with patients with complete injuries, is now being tried in a few centers with promising early results.[24] One rehabilitation modality that does seem promising for SCI patients, especially those with paraplegia, and later in rehabilitation is exoskeleton ambulation assist devices.[25]

Technology and equipment innovation has greatly influenced the quality of care that SCI patients receive. Power wheelchairs can be equipped with standing options, wheels for outside use, the ability to navigate stairs, and automatic pressure relief. Manual chairs are now fitted with more advanced cushions, sport options, and "power assist" wheels. Power assist wheels allow the patient to contribute a variable amount of push force and were found to reduce energy costs of propulsion and decrease shoulder pain.[26] Most cars and vans can be outfitted with hand controls. Finally, computerized environmental control units and voice-activated systems have improved independence and freedom for patients with high-level tetraplegia.

Because shorter LOSs have moved patients home sooner, the majority of rehabilitation gains often occur in the outpatient setting. Patients with chronic SCI some years after their injury may benefit from renewed or prolonged rehabilitation. Jacobs et al.[27] showed improvements in cardiovascular status after circuit strength training in SCI patients. Competitive sports for patients with disabilities offer not only physical but also psychological benefits. Technology has also fueled growth in the rehabilitative treatment of SCI patients long after injury. Tendon transfers had been coupled with a "freehand" implant to improve hand function in many tetraplegic patients.[28] Bladder implants or injections of botulinum toxin may reduce incontinence,[29] intrathecal baclofen pumps reduce malignant spasticity,[30] and functional electrical stimulation implants have allowed for limited amounts of standing and ambulation.[31] All of these devices can increase functional independence in the appropriate SCI candidate, but also require post-placement rehabilitation training.[32]

Medical Management

Rehabilitation should begin as soon as possible after SCI. The most important medical aspects in the acute period of rehabilitation include neurogenic bowel and bladder care, pulmonary management, thromboembolic and gastric ulcer prevention, and proper positioning in bed. If early medical complications can be prevented, the rehabilitation course is facilitated and the cost of care is significantly reduced.

Neurogenic Bowel Dysfunction

Neurogenic bowel dysfunction is common after SCI and has the potential to influence the social, emotional, and physical well-being of patients. Establishment of an effective bowel program during rehabilitation can minimize the development of disability related to neurogenic bowel. The goal is to control severe constipation, promote regularity, and prevent involuntary bowel movements. There are two types of neurogenic bowel dysfunction after SCI: reflexic and areflexic.[33]

Reflexic or upper motor neuron (UMN) bowel dysfunction is seen in patients with SCI above the conus medullaris. Voluntary control of bowel is lost in these patients but conus-mediated reflex activity and intestinal peristalsis are intact. The external anal sphincter becomes spastic due to spasticity of the pelvic floor, preventing stool evacuation. Stool accumulates in the colon unless reflex defecation is triggered. Bowel care in these patients may include[34]: (1) nutritional changes with increased fiber and fluid intake, (2) oral medication (lubricants and cathartics), (3) rectal chemical stimulation (suppositories or enema), and (4) mechanical digital stimulation.

Areflexic or lower motor neuron (LMN) bowel dysfunction is a result of lesions at or below the conus medullaris. Voluntary control of bowel is lost as well as sacral reflex activity. The external anal sphincter becomes atonic and flaccid, which increases the risk of fecal incontinence. Management of LMN bowel dysfunction includes[34]: (1) diet with fiber and some fluid restriction, (2) oral medication (bulk-forming agent), and (3) mechanical digital removal of stool.

Neurogenic Bladder Dysfunction

Urosepsis was the leading cause of death prior to introduction of intermittent catheterization (IC).[35] Urologic problems are the most common complications of SCI. The rate of urinary tract infections is 50% to 80% in the first year postinjury. The goal of bladder management during rehabilitation is to establish an effective and safe method of emptying the bladder and avoiding incontinence. There are two types of neurogenic bladder dysfunction: reflexic and areflexic.

Reflexic or UMN bladder is secondary to lesions above conus medullaris. It is characterized by (1) incontinence secondary to conus-mediated reflex contractions of bladder detrusor muscle, (2) spastic external urethral sphincter, and (3) detrusor/sphincter dyssynergia.

Areflexic or LMN bladder occurs in lesions below the conus medullaris. This condition is characterized by (1) denervated external urethral sphincter and (2) flaccid detrusor muscle, leading to overflow or stress incontinence.

Management of neurogenic bladder after SCI is similar for both types. The routine recommendations are based on clinical practice guidelines prepared by the Consortium for Spinal Cord Medicine[36]:

- Management of fluid intake to maintain daily urine output between 1.5 and 2 L
- Intermittent catheterization using clean or sterile technique
- Indwelling catheter for patients with poor hand control and lack of attendant care
- Suprapubic catheter for, most commonly, patients with urethral lesions
- External (condom) catheter for male patients with UMN bladder with reflex voiding
- Surgery

The two circumstances when surgery is indicated in the management of neurogenic bladder after SCI is to correct the failure to store or the failure to empty urine. The most commonly performed corrective procedures are augmentation of small capacity bladder with intestine, and sphincterotomy. The most frequent method of bladder management at discharge from SCI rehabilitation centers is intermittent catheterization (59%). However, a relatively high number of patients were discharged with indwelling catheters (13%).[4] A newer treatment for upper motor neuron neurogenic bladder when detrusor/sphincter dyssynergia is the problem is detrusor injections of botulinum toxin. This will relax the bladder and/or sphincter to allow catheterization to occur.[37]

Spasticity

Spasticity is seen frequently in patients after SCI. In 37% of patients, the spasticity is significant and requires chronic therapy. Spasticity may interfere with function, daily activities, and sleep. The severity of spasticity during rehabilitation in SCI patients varies. It has been reported that patients with cervical and upper thoracic injuries have a higher incidence of spasticity than patients with lower spine injuries.[38] The underlying processes involved in pathogenesis of hyperactive reflexes are multifactorial and involve both inhibitory and excitatory neurotransmitters. The role of neurotransmitters in spasticity is not fully understood; therefore, the therapy is generally symptomatic. Immediately after SCI, there is a short period (2–3 weeks) of areflexia that is followed by a gradual occurrence of increased muscle tone below the level of injury. In mild to moderately severe cases, ROM and static stretching can be used to treat spasticity during rehabilitation.

Medication is usually indicated for severe and chronic spasticity. The different drugs that can be used for spasticity are, in order: (1) baclofen, (2) benzodiazepines, (3) tizanidine, and (4) dantrolene. Baclofen is a γ-aminobutyric acid (GABA) agonist, a major inhibitory neurotransmitter in the central nervous system (CNS). The starting dose is 10 mg 2 to 3 times daily with a total daily dose of 80 mg. Benzodiazepines facilitate the effect of endogenous GABA, and they are second-choice medication in treatment of spasticity since their sedative CNS side effects exceed that of baclofen. Tizanidine is an α-adrenergic receptor agonist with effects similar to noradrenaline. Noradrenaline belongs to the group of inhibitory neurotransmitters that prevent release of excitatory amino acids from nerve terminals. Tizanidine blocks hyperactive spinal reflexes and, similar to other antispastic medication, has a sedative effect on the CNS. Dantrolene has no effects on the CNS; it acts directly on skeletal muscle cells, where it inhibits contraction of myofibrils. The inhibitory effect of dantrolene is due to blockade of endoplasmatic release of calcium. Neurolytic nerve blocks and surgery (dorsal rhizotomy) are additional therapeutic modalities in the treatment of spasticity. These therapies are not frequently used, but may be indicated for severe spasticity unresponsive to medication. More often for refractory cases, SCI patients can benefit from baclofen being delivered directly to the spinal cord via an implant. When baclofen can be given by intrathecal pump, it can reduce the therapeutic dose 100 times, thus markedly decreasing the sedative side effects of the drug on the CNS. One recent study found reduced spasm frequency and severity with greater dose stability with intrathecal compared with oral baclofen. However, they found no difference in fatigue, quality of life, or function.[39]

Cardiovascular Complications

The primary mechanisms underlying cardiovascular abnormalities are related to the disruption of sympathetic control located in the cervical cord. The most frequent symptoms are orthostatic hypotension (68%) and bradycardia (71%).[40] Autonomic dysreflexia develops in patients with SCI above the T6 spinal segment.

Orthostatic hypotension after SCI is caused by passive vasodilatation below the level of injury, while bradycardia is due to uninhibited parasympathetic tone. Frequent associated clinical findings are weakness, dizziness, blurred vision, and fainting during positional changes. The majority of patients gradually develop adaptation to hypotension and may tolerate orthostasis for an extended period of time. During the period of rehabilitation, different measures can be effective, such as elastic stockings, abdominal binders, and slow mobilization from the bed. Also, in early periods after SCI, medication may be indicated. There are two oral agents with different mechanisms of action that can be used, midodrine and fludrocortisone. Midodrine is an α-1 adrenergic agonist (ProAmatine); it is the first-choice drug. Fludrocortisone (Florinef), a mineralocorticosteroid, enhances renal resorption of sodium and may be used as an alternative.

Autonomic dysreflexia (AD) is a serious complication after SCI.[41] It is characterized by a sudden onset of pounding headache, increase of blood pressure, and bradycardia. AD occurs in patients with SCI above the T6 spine segment. These patients have interrupted central inhibitory control of the thoracic sympathetic system. Therefore, various peripheral noxious stimuli below the injury (e.g., bladder distension, pressure ulcers, ingrown toenails, urinary tract infection, constipation) may lead to overstimulation of the sympathetic system. AD may have different causes; however, it is most commonly related to bladder or bowel distension.[41] Treatment of AD includes immediate repositioning of the patient in a sitting position and loosening of clothing or constrictive devices to allow a pooling of blood into the lower extremities. The placement of an indwelling catheter should be performed early because the most common cause of AD is bladder distension. If after the catheterization systolic blood pressure remains elevated over 150 mm Hg, an antihypertensive agent with rapid onset and short duration (nitrates or nifedipine) is recommended.[41] If bowel distension or impaction is suspected, antihypertensive medication needs to be administered prior to rectal examination for stool.

The incidence of thromboembolism is high in the acute stage of SCI. The routine screening for DVT showed positive results in 47% to 100% of patients.[42] Studies based on clinical parameters estimated lower incidence of DVT in acute SCI. The incidence of clinically diagnosed DVT was 11.4% in 1996, which was significantly reduced to 5.2% in 1998. The decline in the incidence of DVT is most likely the result of the introduction of low-molecular-weight heparin (LMWH).[43] Prevention of thromboembolism starts after injury and continues throughout rehabilitation. Current methods for prevention of thromboembolism used in SCI patients are mechanical (compression hose, boots, pneumatic devices), pharmacologic (unfractionated heparin, LMWH, warfarin), and inferior vena cava filter. A consortium organized by Paralyzed Veterans of America in 1997[42] recommended mechanical prevention for the first 2 weeks following injury. In patients with motor complete SCI, pharmacologic prevention with unfractionated heparin or LMWH is recommended for a minimum of 8 weeks or until discharge from the rehabilitation center. Patients with motor complete injuries and risk factors such as obesity, heart failure, cancer, lower extremity fractures, previous DVT, or age greater than 70 years may need their prevention extended after discharge. Recommendations for the prevention of thromboembolism in the rehabilitation phase of patients with SCI is based on the 6th American College of Clinical Pharmacy consensus in 2001.[44] LMWH or full-dose oral anticoagulation with warfarin was the initial recommended method, with inferior vena cava filter recommended in patients who failed or have contraindications to anticoagulation. A meta-analysis of 13 studies showed strong evidence

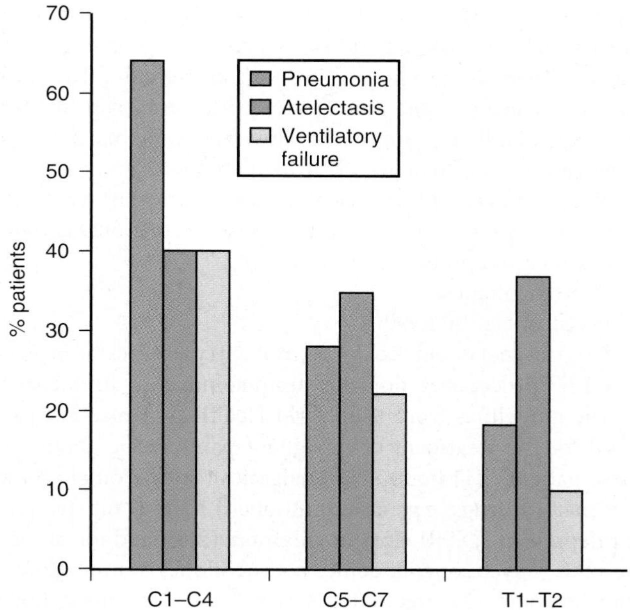

FIG. 82.4 Respiratory complications after spinal cord injury. (Modified from Jackson AB, Grooms TE. Incidence of respiratory complications following spinal cord injury. *Arch Phys Med Rehab.* 1994;75:270–275.)

to support the use of LMWH in reducing venous thrombosis events.[45] A higher adjusted dose of unfractionated heparin was also found to be more effective than 5000 units administered every 12 hours, although bleeding complication was more common. Treatment of thromboembolism in patients with SCI does not differ from treatment currently used in non-SCI patients.

Respiratory Complications

Respiratory complications are the most common early and late cause of death after SCI. Fig. 82.4 shows the most common respiratory complications in patients with different levels of SCI.[46] Pneumonia is the most common complication in high-level injuries, while atelectasis is seen in all groups of patients in similar frequency regardless of level of injury. Smith and coworkers found in over 18,000 veterans with SCI a steady rate of visits for acute respiratory infection, without a declining trend in frequency.[47]

There are several factors important in the pathophysiology of ventilatory abnormalities after SCI,[48] such as (1) restrictive ventilatory dysfunction as a result of muscle paralysis; (2) inability to cough, which is due primarily to paralysis of abdominal and intercostal muscles; and (3) hypersecretion of mucus. Overproduction of mucus (about 1 L/day) is due to absent sympathetic outflow and unopposed parasympathetic tone, which also leads to bronchoconstriction.

The neurologic level of injury mainly determines the management of respiratory complications after SCI. Patients with cervical injuries from C1 to C3 frequently need mechanical ventilation. These patients may benefit from diaphragmatic pacing in order to give them some freedom from the ventilator for periods of time and is becoming more common with the improvement of minimally invasive surgical techniques.[49] Patients with C4 to C7 and upper thoracic injuries often require the following treatments during rehabilitation: bronchodilators (β-adrenergic agonists and /or anticholinergics), mucolytic agents, and chest physiotherapy.

Later in the phase of rehabilitation and with the return of peripheral sympathetic tone, there is a decrease of mucus production. At this stage, respiratory treatments are focused on assisted cough and prevention of respiratory complications. All patients with cervical and high thoracic injuries need yearly vaccination for influenza and vaccination every five years for pneumonia.

Pressure Ulcers

Spinal cord injury causes profound changes in the structure and physiology of the skin, which leaves patients susceptible to the development of pressure ulcers. The incidence of pressure sores after SCI is high, with approximately 50% of chronic patients with SCI developing a pressure ulcer in their lifetime. Pressure ulcers are seen on the sacrum in 26%, on the ischium in 23%, on the heel in 12%, and on the trochanter in 10% of chronic SCI patients.[50] Several factors are responsible for the development of pressure ulcers after SCI but most important is prolonged pressure over a bone prominence. The cornerstones in the prevention of pressure ulcers are regular daily inspection of the skin and the performance of pressure relief techniques.

The management of pressure ulcers requires a multidisciplinary team approach. It is also important to provide sufficient nutritional support, treatment of comorbid conditions, and special support surfaces (cushions and mattresses). Two types of mattresses, static (foam, gel, air, or water) and dynamic (air pump with alternating pressure) are used to reduce pressure on the ulcer. Basic medical treatment used to include enzymatic debridement and moist wound dressing changes. More recently, ulcers have been treated with various growth factors and products such as transparent membranes, hydrogels, foams, alginates, and hyularonase.[51] Surgical repair is recommended when the ulcers are too large and only if nutritional and medical conditions of the patient are satisfactory.

Heterotopic Ossification

Heterotopic ossification (HO) is another early complication after SCI. Often occurring in the first month of rehabilitation, HO is often a cause of "fever of unknown origin." The incidence of HO after SCI is about 50%.[52,53] The etiology of HO is unknown. The pathology of HO is characterized by bone growth in extraarticular tissue of paralyzed extremities. Clinically, in the acute stage of HO, the most common findings are swelling, fever, and reduction in ROM of affected joint(s). The level of creatine phosphokinase in serum in the early stage may indicate the severity of muscle involvement. In the chronic stage, HO may limit the functional status of the patient. Diagnosis of HO in the early stages is based on a positive three-phase bone scintigraphy with technetium-99m diphosphonate. Prevention of HO with indomethacin in patients with SCI is effective if started early (3 to 4 weeks) after

SECTION XI

injury.[54] Etidronate is first-line treatment for management of HO in the acute stage along with aggressive joint motion by physical therapy. Only when the heterotopic bone is mature up to 1 year after the onset can surgical resection be considered.

Osteoporosis and Fractures

In patients with SCI, there is significant bone loss in paralyzed limbs in the early period after injury. The most severely involved skeletal regions are the distal femur and proximal tibia. Bone densitometric studies showed that patients with complete paralysis might have bone loss of 30% in the first 3 months.[55] In later periods, bone loss will continue at a slower rate, reaching a new steady state after 2 years. At the final stages, bone mineral loss can be about 30% in the femoral shaft and 50% in the proximal tibia.[56] Patients who actually suffer fractures were found to have even higher bone loss: approximately 40% in femoral shaft and 70% in proximal tibia. Presently, there is no cure for osteoporosis after SCI. Many different preventive programs for bone loss have been evaluated. So far, all preventive measures have shown some positive effect on bone mass, but the effects are transient and the bone loss resumes as soon as the intervention stops. The incidence of lower extremity fractures after SCI is about 1% to 2% per year. Lower limb fractures are most often treated using a nonsurgical approach with the goal of maintaining functional independence. Use of splints and early mobilization are generally allowed initially in a supervised setting.

Pain

Pain prevalence is stable over time, ranging from 81% at 1 year after injury to 83% at 25 years.[57] Approximately 90% of patients with SCI have a delayed onset of pain and many are not finding adequate pain relief from commonly used medication.[58] Nepomuceno and coworkers[59] described the negative impact of pain on the life of patients with SCI. A total of 37% of patients with cervical injuries and 23% of patients with a lower level of SCI reported that if they had the chance, they would trade pain for loss of bladder, bowel, or sexual function. The majority of patients describe pain as stable or controlled, while others report that pain increased their disability. Of the different classifications of pain after SCI, the most commonly described are central neuropathic and musculoskeletal pain.[60,61] Clinical differentiation between central neuropathic and musculoskeletal pain is shown in Table 82.3.

Several mechanisms have been proposed in the pathophysiology of central pain, but the causes still remain uncertain. In contrast, musculoskeletal pain is most commonly due to spine injury or overuse of joint, tendon, or ligament structures. Treatment measures depend on which type of pain is being treated. There is no known cure for central pain. The most effective strategy in the management of central pain involves an interdisciplinary approach. However, only partial pain relief can be expected. The treatment strategies are:

1. Nonpharmacologic (transcutaneous electrical nerve stimulation, aerobic and anaerobic exercise, recreational activity, massage, acupuncture, heat or cold)
2. Pharmacologic
3. Psychosocial/biofeedback
4. Surgical (nerve blocks, dorsal root entry zone lesioning [the DREZ procedure], dorsal column spinal cord stimulator)

The guidelines from the World Health Organization proposal for the treatment of malignant pain can be applied in these patients: (1) nonopioid analgesics (nonsteroidal antiinflammatory drugs, e.g., acetaminophen) ± adjuvant (tricyclic antidepressants, SSRI, anticonvulsants); (2) opioid for moderate pain (oxycodone, codeine, hydrocodone) ± nonopioid ± adjuvant; and (3) opioid for severe pain (hydromorphone, morphine, fentanyl) ± nonopioid ± adjuvant. Caution should be employed in the use of opioids for chronic nonmalignant pain, especially neuropathic pain, as any efficacy could prove short-lived due to tolerance and dependence.[62] Another recent meta-analysis showed anticonvulsants to be of the most value in treating neuropathic pain of SCI.[63]

Musculoskeletal pain can be treated with mild analgesic, nonsteroidal antiinflammatory drugs, passive ROM, and trigger point injections.

TABLE 82.3 Characteristics of Pain After Spinal Cord Injury

	Pain	Activity	Location
Central	Burning, tingling, sharp, shooting	Not related	Anesthetic area
Musculoskeletal	Dull, aching	Aggravated	Above level of injury

Outcomes of Rehabilitation

Length of Stay

In general, patients with tetraplegia need a longer period for rehabilitation than patients with paraplegia. Similarly, patients with complete paralysis require a longer stay at rehabilitation centers than with incomplete paralysis. Statistical analysis showed that time needed for acute care has not changed during the past 20 years; however, significant changes were found in the LOS at the rehabilitation centers. Fig. 82.5 illustrates results from a database derived from the NSCISC database.[5] A dramatic reduction of LOS was documented at rehabilitation centers across the country from 1977 to 2000. The average LOS was 106 days in 1977, 90 days in 1987, 51 days in 1997, and 39 in 2004. The changes in the LOS of patients after SCI can mainly be attributed to measures that managed care instituted in the early 1990s.[64]

Discharge Disposition

The changes in the LOS of patients at rehabilitation centers had some effect on the discharge disposition of these patients. The results from the NSCISC database[4] obtained in 1997 showed that the majority of patients were still discharged home (91.2%); however, the percent of patients discharged to skilled nursing homes also increased (5.3%) as compared to 2.8% in 1990.

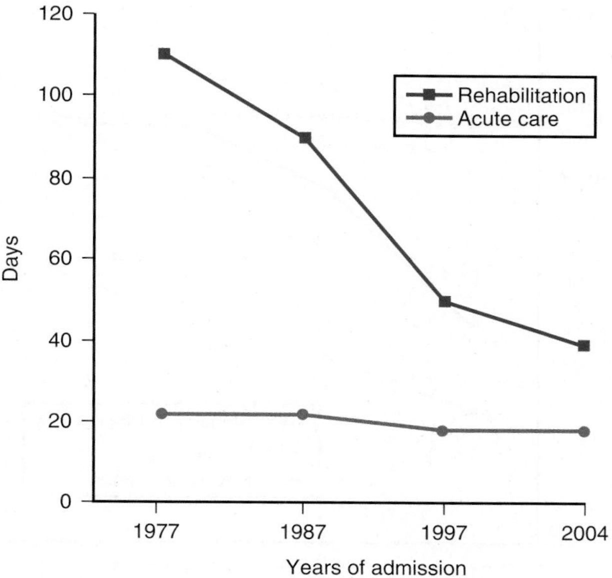

FIG. 82.5 Length of stay in rehabilitation centers after spinal cord injury. (Modified from Fiedler IG, Laud PW, Maiman DJ, Apple DF. Economics of managed care in spinal cord injury. *Arch Phys Med Rehab.* 1999;80:1441–1449.)

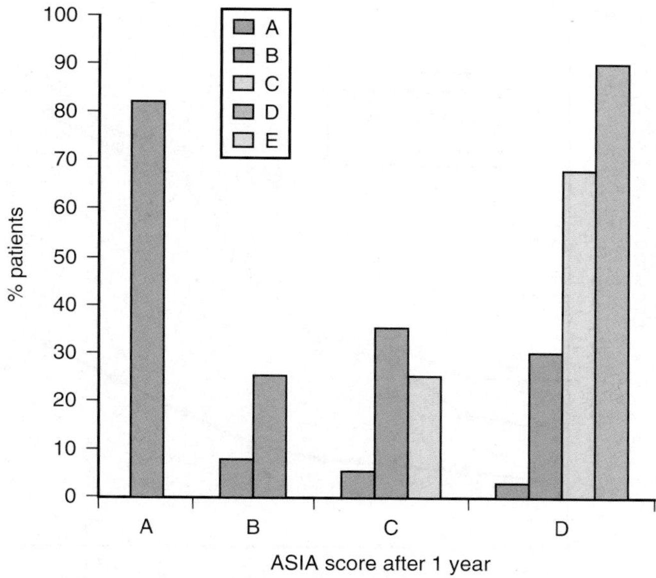

FIG. 82.6 Changes in motor function after spinal cord injury. The American Spinal Injury Association (ASIA) scale is used to grade motor function (see text for explanation of scale). (Modified from Marino RJ, Ditunno J, Donovan WH, Maynard F. Neurological recovery after spinal cord injury. *Arch Phys Med Rehab.* 1999;80:1031–1396.)

Gain of Motor Function

The outcomes of motor function are determined by the ASIA standardized evaluation previously discussed by using the ASIA examination and the data obtained from the NSCISC database.[65] The outcomes of motor function were related to rehabilitation and neurologic recovery and shown in Fig. 82.6. As illustrated in Fig. 82.6, about 10% to 15% of patients diagnosed as complete, or ASIA Impairment Scale classification AIS-A, will convert in 1 year to incomplete AIS-B, -C, or -D. Typically, neurologic return of motor function starts in the first month after injury but may continue for up to 24 months. Despite recent advances in pharmacologic treatment of SCI, prognosis for recovery of patients with an initial classification of AIS-A remains poor. The prognosis for motor function recovery of patients with AIS-B designation is intermediate. One-third of these patients remain unchanged, one-third converts to AIS-C, and one-third to AIS-D or -E. In the group of patients with the AIS-C designation, 70% will convert to AIS-D. Patients with an initial AIS-D designation showed functional improvement to AIS-E in 4%, while 96% of these patients remained in D category. Even after 5 years from traumatic SCI, results are not very different. Kirshblum et al. found that only 4.5% of patients with motor complete paralysis regained some motor or sensory recovery.[66]

Functional Independence (Charting ADL Improvement Objectively)

Currently, the most widely used, validated ADL evaluation scale is the Functional Independence Measure (FIM).[67] The FIM instrument evaluates nine areas of self-care, and can be applied multiple times throughout the course of treatment not only to provide a baseline of function but also to chart improvement in these key areas. The areas that the FIM reports on are self-feeding, grooming, bathing, dressing upper and lower body, toileting, and transfer to the toilet, tub, or shower. The FIM has demonstrated a high degree of interrelater reliability.[68] After the SCI patient leaves the hospital, the FIM can be continued in a self-reporting form (FIM-SR). Masedo et al. found the FIM-SR motor scales and total FIM-SR score are reliable and valid measures of perceived functional independence in individuals with SCI.[67]

Fig. 82.7 shows the results from the NSCISC database on FIM scores.[69] The data were obtained on admission and discharge from rehabilitation and at the followup after 1 year. There is a marked difference in FIM motor scores from admission to discharge from rehabilitation in all neurologic groups of patients. The greatest improvements are seen in patients with lower cervical and thoracolumbar injuries. There was very little change in FIM scores in all categories of patients beyond discharge from rehabilitation. Fig. 82.7 illustrates mean FIM motor scores for each neurologic group of patients and indicates that a score of 78 (13 motor items with scores of 6), correlating with functional independence, is reached only in patients with thoracolumbar injuries.

Despite the advantages that using a validated comprehensive ADL measure creates, there are significant limitations. Specifically, the FIM is not specific to SCI but is a general measure of any rehabilitation diagnosis. Thus, some aspects critical to SCI function, such as mastery of the environment and respiratory function, are not charted.

Therefore, the Spinal Cord Independence Measure (SCIM III), created a new, more comprehensive measure applicable to persons with paraplegia and tetraplegia, complete and incomplete.[70] Itzkovich et al. found that total agreement between raters was above 80% in most SCIM III tasks.[9,71] They also found

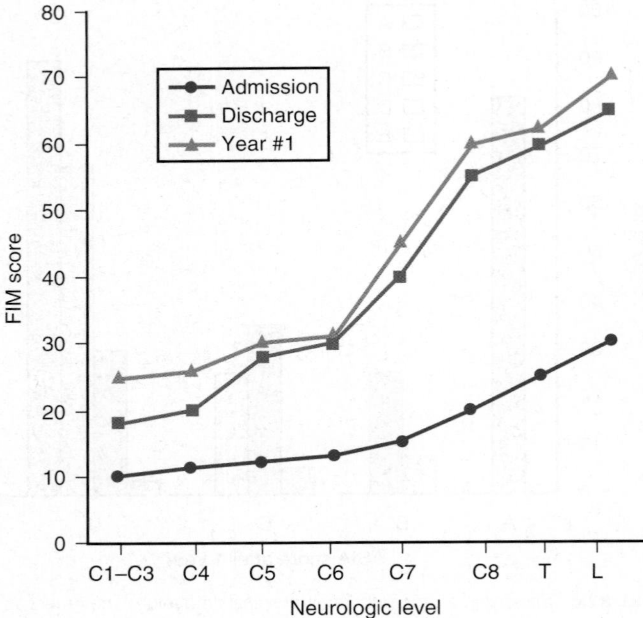

FIG. 82.7 Functional Independence Measure (FIM) of spinal cord injury patients at admission and discharge from rehabilitation center and 1 year thereafter (see text for explanation of score). (Modified from Hall KM, Cohen ME, Wright J, et al. Characteristics of the functional independence measure in traumatic spinal cord injury. *Arch Phys Med Rehab.* 1999;80:1471–1476.)

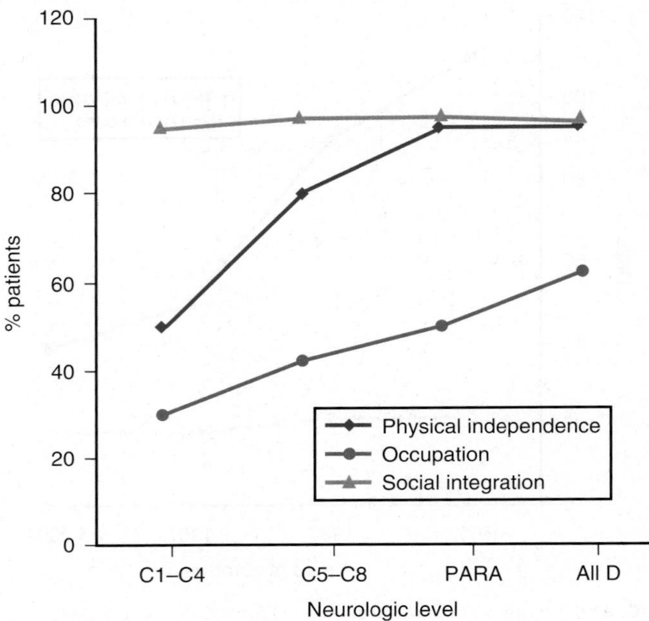

FIG. 82.8 Community integration after spinal cord injury. Each neurologic group included patients with American Spinal Injury Association scale A, B, and C (see text for explanation of scale). PARA, paraplegia. (Modified from Whiteneck G, Tate D, Charlifue S: Predicting community integration after spinal cord injury from demographic and injury characteristics. *Arch Phys Med Rehab.* 1999;80:1485–1491.)

that the SCIM III was more responsive to changes than FIM in the subscales of respiration and sphincter management and mobility indoors and outdoors. The measure is now undergoing final studies to see if it is more sensitive or specific for SCI patients than other measures while maintaining the practicality of the FIM. A new measure, called the SCI Functional Index, is currently in development and being validated as a potentially more specific measure than the FIM.[72] Functional ability level development and validation provides clinical meaning for the Spinal Cord Injury Functional Index scores.

Employment

More than half (57.4%) of those persons with SCI admitted to a Model System reported being employed at the time of their injury. The postinjury employment picture is better among persons with paraplegia than among their tetraplegic counterparts. By postinjury year 10, 32.4% of persons with paraplegia are employed, while 24.2% of those with tetraplegia are employed during the same year. National data from Model System Spinal Cord Centers revealed that the rate of employment of SCI patients is approximately 27% after rehabilitation.[73] Similar results were found for both genders: 24.1% in female patients and 27.7% in male patients. Important factors in obtaining employment after SCI were age, severity of injury, and educational level prior to injury.

Community Integration

Community integration of patients with SCI starts during inpatient rehabilitation and continues after discharge from the rehabilitation center. The involvement of human services plays a major role in assisting patients in the community. Fig. 82.8 depicts the three aspects of community integration after SCI: functional independence, social integration, and occupation. Data are obtained from the NSCISC database[74] indicate very high levels of social integration in all neurologic groups of patients after SCI. The lowest median score of community integration was found in occupation, as just mentioned. Community and athletic groups increase the levels of community integration. Activities that injured persons used to participate in can be modified for the wheelchair athlete or participant, increasing the quality of life for those injured. Sports for SCI patients include sailing programs, diving programs, wheelchair basketball teams, skiing, rugby, marathon racing, and Paralympic competitions.

In general, analysis of demographic data indicates that survivors of SCI with less severe neurologic injury, of younger age, of White race, and more education will achieve greater community integration.

Reintegration Into the Environment

As a part of most inpatient rehabilitation treatment programs, the home evaluation and the home visit are highly anticipated. The home visit can serve as a motivator for the SCI patient to reach his or her goals and participate fully. However, evaluating the home environment as early as possible in the rehabilitation process is also important so that appropriate goals can be set and needed modifications can begin earlier.[75]

The environmental evaluation begins with a family history (who is in the home), vocational history, and leisure history.

These are the components of the patient's lifestyle that allow the therapist to create a roadmap of where the injured patient was and where the patient needs to get back to, and even beyond, to maximize function. In certain cases, the therapist may find that the SCI patient was not functioning at optimal levels even before the injury due to psychiatric illness or other disorders.

The second component of the evaluation concerns the home structure itself. The therapist must create a picture of the home and environment that will allow for an understanding of what impediments might exist that will pose a barrier to maximizing function. Through knowing the individual limitations of their patient, the therapist can set therapy goals that may also involve making modifications to the home and environment to maximize function.[76] Ultimately, by marrying the functional abilities of injured patients to the environment that they are going to live within, the interdisciplinary rehabilitation team can help to maximize the quality of life of their SCI patients while minimizing cost to the patients and health care system.[75]

In summary, the key points to be gleaned from this section include the following. The rehabilitation of SCI patients begins from the moment of initiation into the health care system rather than when they are admitted to rehabilitation. Acute care treatment, including surgical choices, affects the rehabilitation methods chosen and speed of progress. Once in rehabilitation, close monitoring by the physiatrist is necessary to prevent medical complications of immobility. Finally, the entire rehabilitation interdisciplinary team must be involved in the treatment and goal setting to maximize outcome and minimize cost.

Acknowledgments

We thank Kresimir Banovac, MD, retired rehabilitation and endocrine medicine physician who coauthored the original manuscript, for his years of dedication to the field. We also thank Marine Dididze MD, SCI research physician, who assisted in the formatting of the chapter.

PEARLS

1. Rehabilitation of the SCI patient begins from the moment of injury and continues throughout the life of the patient.
2. The life expectancy of SCI patients continues to increase with improved medical and rehabilitative care.
3. Surgical advances have resulted in SCI patients being transferred more quickly to rehabilitation with improved functional abilities.
4. Shorter LOS in the rehabilitation unit has reduced inpatient cost but led to an increased need for prolonged outpatient rehabilitation.
5. Technological advances have impacted SCI patients by improving their mobility, function, and fitness.

PITFALLS

1. As patients with SCI live longer, the probability of developing cardiovascular and other medical problems associated with aging is increasing.
2. On average, patients with SCI have higher cholesterol levels and reduced levels of fitness compared to able-bodied persons of similar age. This can be improved with exercise training.
3. The increase in elderly patients with multiple comorbidities suffering SCI has led to an increase in medical complexity seen on rehabilitation units.
4. Many patients who suffer SCI do not have adequate insurance coverage to meet their complex medical, rehabilitation, and equipment needs.
5. Much of the new technology designed for treatment of SCI is expensive and not available currently for the majority of patients who could benefit.

SECTION XI

KEY POINTS

1. *Timing of rehabilitation.* Rehabilitation and rehabilitation planning should start immediately when the patient arrives into the acute care system. Accurate assessment of neurologic level and an ASIA motor and sensory score facilitates initiation of treatment that can minimize deficits and allow for maximum functional recovery.
2. *Minimize medical complications.* As early as possible, rehabilitation should be started to prevent complications of immobility and provide the patient with the tools to succeed later in rehabilitation when the medical condition fully stabilizes.
3. *Optimize teamwork.* Rehabilitation of the SCI patient requires all members of the interdisciplinary team to work together in a coordinated fashion. This includes members of physical therapy, occupational therapy, specialized nursing, recreation therapy, the orthotics team, respiratory therapists, psychologists, social workers, and the vocational team. Creating achievable short-term and long-term goals will allow patients to work to achieve their optimum function.
4. *Demographics.* As more patients suffer SCIs who are elderly, many from nontraumatic causes, specialized rehabilitation programs will need to be created to address their unique medical and functional needs.
5. *Pain.* Chronic pain—neuropathic related to SCI or musculoskeletal related to acute or repetitive trauma—is often the chief identified problem that SCI patients identify. Optimal treatment of pain improves rehabilitation participation and optimizes function and quality of life.
6. *Future of rehabilitation.* Two trends are being seen that will continue into the future. The first is shorter length of inpatient stays, leading to increased importance and focus on outpatient rehabilitation. The second is the introduction of neurotechnology to supplement general strength rehabilitation, improve function, and even allow assisted ambulation.

KEY REFERENCES

1. Kirshblum S, Campangnolo DL, DeLisa JA, eds. *Spinal Cord Medicine*. Philadelphia: Lippincott, Williams & Wilkins; 2002.
   An excellent comprehensive textbook written specifically for physicians specializing in SCIs.
2. *Archives of Physical Medicine and Rehabilitation*. Vol. 80. November 1999.
   This entire issue is devoted to reviewing SCI Model Systems data and outcomes in patients with SCI.
3. Geerts WH, Heit JA, Clagett GT, et al. Prevention of venous thromboembolism. *Chest*. 2001;119:132S-175S.
   This article presents the most recent consensus definition of DVT prevention after SCI.
4. Consortium for Spinal Cord Medicine. Acute management of acute autonomic dysreflexia. *J Spinal Cord Med*. 2002;25: S67-S88.
   This article is considered a guideline in the management of AD.

5. Consortium Spinal Cord Consensus:. Pressure ulcer prévention and treatment following spinal cord injury. *J Spinal Cord Med.* 2001;24:S39-S101.
This provides an excellent source of recommendations for prevention and treatment of pressure ulcers.

REFERENCES

1. Apple DF Jr. Spinal cord injury rehabilitation. In: Rothman RH, Simeone FA, eds. *The Spine*. Philadelphia: WB Saunders; 1998:1225-1246.
2. DeVivo MJ. Epidemiology of traumatic spinal cord injury. In: Kirshblum S, Campagnolo DL, DeLisa JA, eds. *Spinal Cord Medicine*. Philadelphia: Lippincott, Williams & Wilkins; 2002:69-81.
3. Jackson AB, Dijkers M, DeVivo MJ, Poczatek RB. A demographic profile of new traumatic spinal cord injuries: change and stability over 30 years. *Arch Phys Med Rehabil.* 2004;85:1740-1748.
4. Lammertse DP, Jackson AB, Sipski ML. Research from model spinal cord injury systems: findings from the current 5-year grant cycle. *Arch Phys Med Rehabil.* 2004;85:1737-1739.
5. Fiedler IG, Laud PW, Maiman DJ, et al. Economics of managed care in spinal cord injury. *Arch Phys Med Rehabil.* 1999;80:1441-1449.
6. Krause JS, DeVivo MJ, Jackson AB. Health status, community integration, and economic risk factors for mortality after spinal cord injury. *Arch Phys Med Rehabil.* 2004;28:1764-1773.
7. Nash MS, Jacobs PL, Mendez AJ, et al. Circuit resistance training improves the atherogenic lipid profiles of persons with chronic paraplegia. *J Spinal Cord Med.* 2001;24:2-9.
8. Frankel HL, Coll JR, Charlifue SW, et al. Long term survival in spinal cord injury: a fifty-year investigation. *Spinal Cord.* 1998;36:266-274.
9. Kirshblum S, Donovan WH. Neurologic assessment and classification of traumatic spinal cord injury. In: Kirshblum S, Campagnolo DL, DeLisa JA, eds. *Spinal Cord Medicine*. Philadelphia: Lippincott, Williams & Wilkins; 2002:82-95.
10. Bing R. *Compendium of Regional Diagnosis in Affection of the Brain and Spinal Cord*. 2nd ed. New York: Rebman; 1911.
11. Schneider RC, Cherry GR, Patek H. Syndrome of acute central cervical spinal cord injury with special reference to mechanisms involved in hyper-extension injuries of the cervical spine. *J Neurosurg.* 1954;11:546-577.
12. Quencer RM, Bunge RP, Egnor M, et al. Acute traumatic central cord syndrome: MRI pathological correlations. *Neuroradiology*. 1992;34:85-94.
13. Roth EJ, Park T, Pang T, et al. Traumatic cervical Brown-Sequard and Brown-Sequard plus syndromes: the spectrum of presentations and outcomes. *Paraplegia.* 1991;29:582-589.
14. Ditunno JF, Cardenas DD, Formal C, et al. Advances in the rehabilitation management of acute spinal cord injury. *Handb Clin Neurol.* 2012;109:181-195.
15. Kirshblum SC, O'Connor KC. Predicting neurologic recovery in traumatic cervical spinal cord injury. *Arch Phys Med Rehabil.* 1998;79:1456-1466.
16. Ragnarsson KT, Gordon WA. Rehabilitation after spinal cord injury: the team approach. *Phys Med Rehabil Clin N Am.* 1992;3:853-878.
17. Zigler JE, Atkins MS, Resnik CD, et al. Rehabilitation. In: Levie AM, Eismont FJ, Garfin SR, Zigler JE, eds. *Spine Trauma*. Philadelphia: WB Saunders; 1998:567-596.
18. Banovac K, Fertel D, Bauerlein J. Principles of rehabilitation medicine. In: Humes D, ed. *Kelly's Textbook of Internal Medicine*. 4th ed. Philadelphia: Lippincott Williams & Wilkins; 2000:308-313.
19. Whiteneck G, Gassaway J. The SCIRehab project: what rehabilitation interventions are most strongly associated with positive outcomes after spinal cord injury? *J Spinal Cord Med.* 2012;35(6):482-483.
20. Teeter L, Gassaway J, Taylor S, et al. Relationship of physical therapy inpatient rehabilitation interventions and patient characteristics to outcomes following spinal cord injury: the SCIRehab project. *J Spinal Cord Med.* 2012;35(6):503-526.
21. Askins V, Eismont FJ. Efficacy of five cervical orthoses in restricting cervical motion: a comparison study. *Spine.* 1997;22:1193-1198.
22. Fehlings MG, Vaccaro A, Wilson JR, et al. Early versus delayed decompression for traumatic cervical spinal cord injury: results of the Surgical Timing in Acute Spinal Cord Injury Study (STASCIS). *PLoS ONE.* 2012;7(2):e32037.
23. Stein RB, Chong SL, James KB, et al. Electrical stimulation for therapy and mobility after spinal cord injury. *Prog Brain Res.* 2002;137:27-34.
24. Field-Foote EC, Tepavac D. Improved intralimb coordination in people with incomplete spinal cord injury following training with body weight support and electrical stimulation. *Phys Ther.* 2002;82:707-715.
25. Hartigan C, Kandilakis C, Dalley S, et al. Mobility outcomes following five training sessions with a powered exoskeleton. *Top Spinal Cord Inj Rehabil.* 2015;21(2):93-99.
26. Nash MS, Koppens D, van Haaren M, et al. Power-assisted wheels ease energy costs and perceptual responses to wheelchair propulsion in persons with shoulder pain and spinal cord injury. *Arch Phys Med Rehabil.* 2008;89(11):2080-2085.
27. Jacobs PL, Nash MS, Rusinowski JW. Circuit training provides cardiorespiratory and strength benefits in persons with paraplegia. *Med Sci Sports Exerc.* 2001;33:711-717.
28. Kilgore KL, Peckham PH, Keith MW, et al. An implanted upper-extremity neuroprosthesis follow-up of five patients. *J Bone Joint Surg.* 1997;79A:533-541.
29. Creasey GH. Electrical stimulation of sacral roots for micturition after spinal cord injury. *Urol Clin North Am.* 1993;20:505-515.
30. Coffey RJ, Cahill D, Steers W, et al. Intrathecal baclofen for intractable spasticity of spinal origin: results of a long term multi-center study. *J Neurosurg.* 1993;78:226-232.
31. Yarkony GM, Roth EJ, Cybulski GR, et al. Neuromuscular stimulation in spinal cord injury: restoration of functional movement of the extremities. *Arch Phys Med Rehabil.* 1992;73:78-86.
32. Moynahan M, Mullin C, Cohn J, et al. Home use of a functional electrical stimulation system for standing and mobility in adolescents with spinal cord injury. *Arch Phys Med Rehabil.* 1996;77:1005-1013.
33. Stiens SA, Bergman SB, Goetz LL. Neurogenic bowel dysfunction after spinal cord injury: clinical evaluation and rehabilitation management. *Arch Phys Med Rehabil.* 1997;78:S86-S102.
34. Consortium for Spinal Cord Medicine. *Neurogenic Bowel Management in Adults With Spinal Cord Injury*. Washington, DC: Paralyzed Veterans of America; 1998.
35. Guttman L, Frankel H. The value of intermittent catheterization in the early management of traumatic paraplegia and tetraplegia. *Paraplegia.* 1966/1967;4:63-84.
36. Consortium for spinal cord medicine. Bladder management for adults with SCI. *J Spinal Cord Med.* 2006;29:532-567.

37. Chen YC, Kuo HC. The therapeutic effects of repeated detrusor injections between 200 or 300 Units of onabotulinumtoxin A in chronic spinal cord injured patients. *Neurourol Urodyn*. 2014;33(1):129-134.
38. Maynard FM, Karunas R, Waring WW. Epidemiology of spasticity following traumatic spinal cord injury. *Arch Phys Med Rehabil*. 1990;71:566-569.
39. McCormick ZL, Chu SK, Binler D, et al. Intrathecal versus oral baclofen: a matched cohort study of spasticity, pain, sleep, fatigue, and quality of life. *PM R*. 2016;8(6):553-562.
40. Lehman KG, Lane JG, Piepmeier JM, Batsford WP. Cardiovascular abnormalities accompanying acute spinal cord injury in humans: incidence, time course and severity. *J Am Coll Cardiol*. 1987;10:46-52.
41. Consortium for Spinal Cord Medicine. Acute management of acute autonomic dysreflexia. *J Spinal Cord Med*. 2002;25:S67-S88.
42. Consortium for Spinal Cord Medicine. *Prevention of Thromboembolism in Spinal Cord Injury*. Washington, DC: Paralyzed Veterans of America; 1997.
43. Chen D, Apple DF, Hudson LM, Bode R. Medical complications during acute rehabilitation following spinal cord injury–current experience of the model systems. *Arch Phys Med Rehabil*. 1997;80:1397-1402.
44. Geerts WH, Heit JA, Clagett GT, et al. Prevention of venous thromboembolism. *Chest*. 2001;119:132S-175S.
45. Teasell RW, et al. Venous thromboembolism following spinal cord injury. *Arch Phys Med Rehabil*. 2016;2009:232-245.
46. Jackson AB, Grooms TE. Incidence of respiratory complications following spinal cord injury. *Arch Phys Med Rehabil*. 1994;75:270-275.
47. Smith BM, Evans CT, Kurichi JE, et al. Acute respiratory tract infection visits of veterans with spinal cord injury and disorders: rates, trends, and risk factors. *J Spinal Cord Med*. 2007;30:355361.
48. Lanig IS, Peterson WP. The respiratory system in spinal cord injury. *Phys Med Rehabil Clin N Am*. 2000;11:29-37.
49. Tedde ML, et al. Diaphragmatic pacing stimulation in spinal cord injury: anesthetic and perioperative management. *Clinics (Sao Paulo)*. 2012;67(11):1265-1269.
50. Consortium Spinal Cord Consensus. Pressure ulcer prevention and treatment following spinal cord injury. *J Spinal Cord Med*. 2001;24:S39-S101.
51. Sunn G. Spinal cord injury pressure ulcer treatment: an experience-based approach. *Phys Med Rehabil Clin N Am*. 2014;25(3):671-680.
52. Banovac K, Renfree KJ, Hornicek FJ. Heterotopic ossification after brain and spinal cord injuries. *Clin Rev Phys Rehab Med*. 1998;10:223-256.
53. Van Kuijuk AA, Geuts ACH, van Kupperelt HJM. Neurogenic heterotopic ossification after spinal cord injury. *Spinal Cord*. 2002;40:313-326.
54. Banovac K, Williams JM, Patrick LD, et al. Prevention of heterotopic ossification after spinal cord injury with indomethacin. *Spinal Cord*. 2001;39:370-374.
55. Garland DE, Stewart CA, Adkins RH, et al. Osteoporosis after spinal cord injury. *J Orthop Res*. 1992;10:371-378.
56. Biering-Sorensen F, Bohr H, Schaadt O. Bone mineral content of the lumbar spine and lower extremities years after spinal cord lesion. *Paraplegia*. 1988;26:293-301.
57. Cardenas DD, Bryce TN, Shem K, et al. Gender and minority differences in the pain experience of people with spinal cord injury. *Arch Phys Med Rehabil*. 2004;85:1774-1781.
58. Cardenas DD, Jansen MP. Treatment of chronic pain in persons with spinal cord injuries: a survey study. *J Spinal Cord Med*. 2006;29:109-117.
59. Nepomuceno C, Fine PR, Scott Richards J, et al. Pain in-patients with spinal cord injury. *Arch Phys Med Rehabil*. 1979;60:605-609.
60. Siddal PJ, Taylor DA, Cousins MJ. Classification of pain following spinal cord injury. *Spinal Cord*. 1997;35:69-75.
61. Cardenas DD, Turner JA, Warms CA, Marshall HM. Classification of chronic pain associated with spinal cord injuries. *Arch Phys Med Rehabil*. 2002;83:1708-1714.
62. Siddall PJ, Middleton JW. Spinal cord injury-induced pain: mechanisms and treatments. *Pain Manag*. 2015;5(6): 493-507.
63. Mehta S, McIntyre A, Janzen S. A systematic review of pharmacological treatments of pain after spinal cord injury: an update. *Arch Phys Med Rehabil*. 2016;12:S9993-S9998.
64. Facts and figures at a glance. *J Spinal Cord Med*. 2008; 31(3):357.
65. Marino RJ, Ditunno J, Donovan WH, Maynard F. Neurological recovery after spinal cord injury. *Arch Phys Med Rehabil*. 1999;80:1031-1396.
66. Kirschblum S, Millis S, McKinley W, et al. Late neurologic recovery after traumatic spinal cord injury. *Arch Phys Med Rehabil*. 2004;85(11):1811-1817.
67. Masedo AI, Hanley M, Jensen MP, et al. Reliability and validity of a self-report FIM (FIMSR) in persons with amputation or spinal cord injury and chronic pain. *Am J Phys Med Rehabil*. 2005;84(3):167-176.
68. Ottenbacher KJ, Hsu Y, Granger CV, Fiedler RC. The reliability of the functional independence measure: a quantitative review. *Arch Phys Med Rehabil*. 1996;77(12): 1226-1232.
69. Hall KM, Cohen ME, Wright J, et al. Characteristics of the functional independence measure in traumatic spinal cord injury. *Arch Phys Med Rehabil*. 1999;80:1471-1476.
70. Catz A, Greenberg E, Itzkovich M, et al. A new instrument for outcome assessment in rehabilitation medicine: Spinal cord injury ability realization measurement index. *Arch Phys Med Rehabil*. 2004;85:399-404.
71. Itzkovich M, Gelernter I, Biering-Sorensen F, et al. The Spinal Cord Independence Measure (SCIM) version III: reliability and validity in a multi-center international study. *Disabil Rehabil*. 2007;29:1926-1933.
72. Sinha R, Slavin MD, Kisala PA, et al. Functional ability level development and validation: providing clinical meaning for Spinal Cord Injury Functional Index scores. *Arch Phys Med Rehabil*. 2015;96(8):1448-1457.
73. Stuart Krause J, Kewman D, DeVivo MJ, et al. Employment after spinal cord injury. *Arch Phys Med Rehabil*. 1999;80:1492-1500.
74. Whiteneck G, Tate D, Charlifue S. Predicting community integration after spinal cord injury from demographic and injury characteristics. *Arch Phys Med Rehabil*. 1999;80:1485-1491.
75. Culler KH. Home management. In: Crepeau EB, Cohn ES, Schell BAB, eds. *Willard and Spackman's Occupational Therapy*. Philadelphia: Lippincott Williams & Wilkins; 2003:534-541.
76. Cooper BA, Cohen U, Hasselkus BR. Barrier free design: a review and critique of the occupational therapy perspective. *Am J Occup Ther*. 1991;45:344-350.

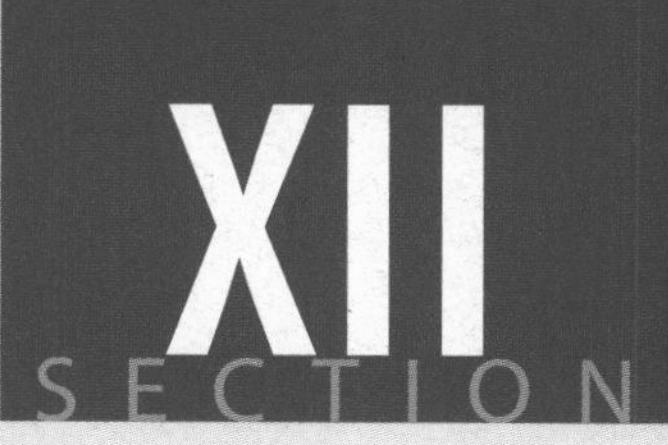

AFFLICTIONS OF THE VERTEBRAE

83 CHAPTER Arthritic Disorders

David G. Borenstein

Rheumatologic disorders of the axial skeleton are an important cause of spinal pain. These inflammatory disorders affect the bones, joints, ligaments, tendons, and muscles that are anatomic components of the spine. The most important rheumatic disorders that cause inflammation of the joints of the axial skeleton are the seronegative spondyloarthropathies and rheumatoid arthritis (RA). The spondyloarthropathies are characterized by damage of the sacroiliac joints, axial skeleton, and peripheral large joints and the absence of rheumatoid factor. The seronegative spondyloarthropathies include ankylosing spondylitis (AS), reactive arthritis, psoriatic arthritis, and enteropathic arthritis. Genetic factors predispose patients to these illnesses. Environmental factors play a role as triggers of the inflammatory response in genetically predisposed individuals, but these factors have been only partially identified.

RA, a disease that causes chronic inflammation of the synovial lining of the joints, affects the cervical spine at the atlantoaxial junction and the subaxial apophyseal joints. These changes occur most commonly in patients with diffuse disease of long duration. Cervical spine involvement in RA is associated with a wide range of symptoms and signs, from mild neck pain and headaches to severe neurologic dysfunction consisting of radiculopathy, paresthesias, incontinence, quadriplegia, and sudden death.

In the seronegative spondyloarthropathies and RA, joint pain is most severe in the morning and improves with activity. Physical examination reveals localized tenderness with palpation and limitation of motion in all planes of motion of the axial skeleton. Laboratory abnormalities are consistent with systemic inflammatory disease but are nonspecific except for the presence of rheumatoid factor in 80% of patients with RA. Radiographic evaluation identifies characteristic joint space narrowing, sclerosis, and fusion in the sacroiliac joints; vertebral body squaring; and ligamentous calcification that may help in the differential diagnosis of a patient with spinal arthritis. Magnetic resonance imaging (MRI) is a valuable tool identifying individuals with sacroiliac or axial joint inflammation prior to radiographic alterations. This joint modification related to early inflammation identifies individuals with nonradiographic axial spondyloarthritis.

Although there are no cures for these illnesses, medical therapy consisting of nonsteroidal antiinflammatory drugs (NSAIDs), and disease-modifying antirheumatic drugs (DMARDs) can be effective in controlling symptoms and improving function, particularly with RA. Newer biologic therapies in the form of tumor necrosis factor (TNF)-α, interleukin (IL)-1, IL-6, and B-cell inhibitors, among others, offer the potential to prevent joint inflammation and destruction to a greater degree than with prior therapies.

The prognosis and course of these rheumatic conditions are rarely related to the extent of spine disease alone. Occasionally, atlantoaxial subluxation secondary to RA or the spondyloarthropathies may result in catastrophic neurologic dysfunction. In most circumstances, the status of disease in other areas of the musculoskeletal system and the severity of constitutional symptoms have a greater effect on the patient's daily existence.

Ankylosing Spondylitis

AS is a chronic inflammatory disease characterized by a variable symptomatic course and progressive involvement of the sacroiliac and axial skeletal joints. It is the prototype of the seronegative spondyloarthropathies. This disease complex is characterized by axial skeletal arthritis; the absence of rheumatoid factor in serum (seronegative); the lack of rheumatoid nodules; and the presence of a tissue factor on host cells, human leukocyte antigen (HLA)-B27.

Epidemiology

AS affects 0.9% to 1.4% of whites, which is equal to the prevalence for RA.[1] A strikingly high association between HLA-B27 and AS has been shown. HLA-B27 is present in more than 90% of white patients with AS compared with a frequency of 7% to 8% in a normal white population.[2] In North American whites, with a prevalence of HLA-B27 of 7%,.[3] A positive family history of AS or related spondyloarthropathy increases the risk to 30% among HLA-B27–positive first-degree relatives compared with HLA-B27–positive control subjects (1%–4%).[4]

The male-to-female ratio is reported in the range of 2:1.[5] Women tend to be less symptomatic, however, and develop less severe disease. Women may also present more often with cervical spine disease with minimal lumbar spine symptoms or more peripheral joint involvement. The overall pattern of illness may be similar in men and women.[6]

Pathogenesis

The pathogenesis of AS is unknown. A genetic predisposition to AS and to the seronegative spondyloarthropathies in general exists. A genetically determined host response to an environmental factor in genetically susceptible individuals seems to be the most likely basis for the pathogenesis of the spondyloarthropathies. The presence of HLA-B27 is not sufficient to develop AS; this is supported by the facts that not all individuals with HLA-B27 develop disease, that HLA-B27 even in a homogeneous form does not cause disease, and that a few patients with AS do not have HLA-B27.[7]

Enthesitis (inflammation of an enthesis—attachment of tendon to bone) is the hallmark that distinguishes the spondyloarthropathies from other forms of arthritis.[8] An enthesis is a dynamic structure undergoing constant modification in response to applied stress. This area is a target for inflammation by the activation of resident IL-23–sensitive T cells. Subsequent downstream activation of IL-17 and IL-22 results in characteristic spondyloarthritic modification of skeletal structures.[9] Although entheses are primarily affected in the spondyloarthropathies, inflammation of these structures is insufficient to explain the alterations that occur in (sacroiliac) joints. Synovitis plays an important role. Synovitis may be a secondary event, however, after initiation with an enthesitis.[10]

AS is a disease of the synovial and cartilaginous joints of the axial skeleton, including sacroiliac joints, spinal apophyseal joints, and symphysis pubis. The large appendicular joints, hips, shoulders, knees, elbows, and ankles are also affected in 30% of patients. The inflammatory process is characterized by chondritis (inflammation of cartilage) or osteitis (inflammation of bone) at the junction of the cartilage and bone in the spine. As opposed to RA, which is associated with osteoporosis as an early manifestation of disease, the inflammation of AS is characterized by ankylosis of joints and ossification of ligaments surrounding the vertebrae (syndesmophytes) and other musculotendinous structures, such as the heels and pelvis.

Clinical History

The classic AS patient is a man 15 to 40 years old with intermittent dull low back pain. The associated stiffness is slowly progressive, measured in months to years. AS rarely occurs in individuals older than 50 years. Patients with spondyloarthropathy initiated after age 50 years are more likely to have a non-AS spinal inflammatory disorder, such as psoriatic spondylitis.[11] Back pain, which occurs throughout the disease in 90% to 95% of patients, is greatest in the morning and is increased by periods of inactivity. Patients may have difficulty sleeping because of pain and stiffness; they may awaken at night and find it necessary to leave bed and move about for a few minutes before returning to sleep. Fatigue can be a major symptom and correlates with level of disease activity, functional ability, global well-being, and mental health status.[12]

Back pain improves with exercise. The mode of onset is variable, with most patients developing pain in the lumbosacral region. Peripheral joints (hips, knees, and shoulders) are initially involved in a few patients; occasionally, acute iridocyclitis (eye inflammation) or heel pain may be the first manifestation of disease. Occasionally, individuals older than 50 years may present with mild symptoms despite extensive spinal involvement.[13] Conversely, back pain may be severe, with radiation into the lower extremities, mimicking acute lumbar disc herniation. Patients have symptoms related to the piriformis syndrome. The belly of the piriformis muscle crosses over the sciatic nerve. Inflammation in the sacroiliac joint, where the muscle attaches, results in muscle spasm and nerve compression. There are no abnormal, persistent neurologic signs associated with the sciatic pain. The symptoms are reversible with medical therapy that relieves joint inflammation. This symptom complex of radicular pain is referred to as *pseudosciatica*.

Patients usually have a moderate degree of intermittent aching pain localized to the lumbosacral area. Paraspinal musculoskeletal spasm may also contribute to the discomfort. With progression of the disease, pain develops in the dorsal and cervical spine and rib joints.

Flattening of the lumbar spine and loss of normal lordosis are consistent with spinal involvement. Thoracic spine disease causes decreased motion at the costovertebral joints, reduced chest expansion, and impaired pulmonary function. In 81% of patients, the initial symptoms are back pain; back stiffness; thigh, hip, or groin pain; and sciatica. Pain in peripheral joints is the initial complaint in 13% of patients, pain in the chest is the initial complaint in 2%, and generalized aches are the initial complaint in 1%.

Cervical spine disease occurs less frequently than lumbosacral involvement in AS and at a later time in the course of the illness. Studies of large groups of AS patients report cervical spine involvement to range from 0% to 53.9%. The primary symptom of cervical spine disease is neck stiffness and pain. Patients may develop intermittent episodes of torticollis. Involvement of the cervical spine causes the head to protrude forward, making it difficult to look straight ahead.

Peripheral joint arthritis (hips, knees, ankles, shoulders, and elbows) occurs in 30% of patients within the first 10 years of disease. Hip disease is the most frequent limiting factor in mobility rather than spinal stiffness. Ankylosis may also occur in cartilaginous joints, such as the symphysis pubis, sternomanubrial, and costosternal joints. Erosions of the plantar surface of the calcaneus at the attachment of the plantar fascia result in an enthesitis. This inflammation causes a fasciitis and periosteal reaction, which causes heel pain and the formation of heel spurs. Achilles tendinitis is another enthesitis associated with heel pain and AS.

Neurologic Complications

Atlantoaxial Subluxation

Neurologic complications of AS are secondary to nerve impingement or trauma to the spinal cord. In a study of 33 patients with AS and neurologic complications, cervical abnormalities were the most common cause of neurologic compromise.[14] Atlantoaxial subluxation occurs in the setting of AS but less often than in RA.[15] In a study of 103 AS patients, 21% had atlantoaxial subluxations. Vertical subluxation is a rare complication. About one-third of patients have progression of subluxations. Five of the 22 patients with subluxation required surgical fusion.[16] Rarely, symptoms of atlantoaxial subluxation may be the presenting manifestation of AS.[17] Significant instability may occur without symptoms in RA because of generalized ligamentous laxity and erosion of bone. AS patients have symptoms and signs of nerve impingement more frequently in the setting of instability secondary to the immobilized state of the calcified structures surrounding the spine. Spinal cord compression is associated with myelopathic symptoms, including sensory deficits, spasticity, paresis, and incontinence. AS patients who are at increased risk are those with elevated C-reactive protein (CRP), peripheral arthritis, and lack of response to NSAIDs.[18]

Spinal Fracture

The other change is the loss of normal flexibility because of ankylosis of the spinal joints and ligaments. The spine in this ankylosed state is much more brittle and is prone to fracture, even with minimal trauma. The most common location for fracture is the cervical spine, although dorsal and lumbar spine fractures have also been described.[19,20] The occurrence of traumatic cervical spine injury is 3.5 times greater in AS patients than in the normal population.[21] The risk for fracture may be present within the first 2.5 years of diagnosis.[22] The lower cervical spine (C6–C7) is the most frequent location for fracture, which is often associated with a fall. Patients who develop fractures may complain of nothing more than localized pain and decreased or increased spinal motion, but severe sensory and motor functional loss corresponding to the location of the lesion may develop. The onset of neurologic dysfunction may be delayed for weeks after initial trauma.

The diagnosis of fracture may be delayed because of the difficulty of detecting fractures in osteoporotic bone with plain radiographs. Computed tomography (CT) may be needed to identify the location of the fracture.[23] Neurologic deficits may persist despite surgical intervention in 85.7% of patients.[24] A mortality rate of 35% to 50% may be found, particularly in AS patients who are elderly, who have complete cord lesions, or who develop pulmonary complications after fracture.[25]

Spondylodiscitis

Another complication of AS is spondylodiscitis, a destructive lesion of the disc and its surrounding vertebral bodies. These lesions occur in individuals with younger age at disease onset.[26] This lesion may be associated with new onset of localized pain in the spine, which uncharacteristically for a patient with AS is improved with bed rest. The cause of these lesions may be localized inflammation or minor trauma.[27] MRI evaluation reveals increased activity in the central portion of the vertebral endplate, confirming this area as an area of enthesitis. In most cases, external immobilization is effective in controlling symptoms; thus, surgical fusion is reserved for more severely affected patients.

Extraarticular Manifestations

AS is also associated with many nonarticular abnormalities. Constitutional manifestations of disease—such as fever, fatigue, and weight loss—are seen in a few patients with active disease, particularly patients with peripheral joint manifestations. Iritis, inflammation of the anterior uveal tract of the eye, may be the presenting complaint of 25% of patients with AS and is present in 40% of patients over the course of the disease. Cardiac involvement occurs in 10% of patients, with disease durations of 30 years or longer. A fibrosing lesion causes the aortic valve and proximal root to thicken. Aortic disease may be more common in patients with peripheral arthritis. Mild features include tachycardia, conduction defects, and pericarditis. AS causes cardiac conduction disturbances, particularly bradyarrhythmias. The most serious cardiac abnormality is proximal aortitis, which results in aortic valve insufficiency, heart failure, and death. Prosthetic valve replacement may forestall cardiac deterioration. Pulmonary involvement is manifested by decreased chest expansion, which limits lung capacity, particularly with severely kyphotic individuals.

Physical Examination

A careful musculoskeletal examination is necessary, particularly of the lumbosacral spine, to discover the early findings of limitation of motion of the axial skeleton, which is especially noticeable with lateral bending or hyperextension. Percussion over the sacroiliac joints elicits pain in most circumstances. Other tests that may be helpful in identifying sacroiliac joint dysfunction place stress on the joint. The tests to be considered include a FABER (flexion abduction and external rotation of the hip) maneuver, Gaenslen test (pressure on a hyperextended thigh with a contralateral flexed hip), Yoeman test (hyperextension of the thigh with a prone patient), and distraction of the pelvic wings anteriorly and posteriorly.

Measurements of spinal motion, including the Schober test (lumbar spine motion), lateral bending of the lumbosacral spine, occiput to wall (cervical spine motion), and chest expansion, are important in ascertaining limitations of motion and following the progression of the disease. Paraspinous muscles may be tender on palpation and in spasm, resulting in limitation of back motion. Finger-to-floor measurements should be done but are more to determine flexibility, which is more closely associated with hip motion than with back mobility. Rotation may be checked with the patient seated. This position fixes the pelvis, limiting pelvic rotation. Chest expansion is measured at the fourth intercostal space in men and below the breasts in women or at the xiphoid process. Patients raise their hands over their head and are asked to take a deep inspiration. Normal expansion is 2.5 cm or greater. Cervical spine evaluation includes measurement of all planes of motion. Peripheral joint examination is also indicated. Careful hip examination is necessary to determine the potential loss of function involved with simultaneous arthritis of the back and hip. Examination of the eyes, heart, lungs, and nervous system may uncover unsuspected extraarticular disease.

Laboratory Data

Laboratory results are nonspecific and add little to the diagnosis of AS. Mild anemia is present in 15% of patients. The erythrocyte sedimentation rate is increased in 80% of patients with active disease. Patients with normal sedimentation rates with active arthritis may have elevated levels of CRP.[28] Rheumatoid factor and antinuclear antibody are characteristically absent. Histocompatibility testing (for HLA) is positive in 90% of AS patients but is also present in an increased percentage of patients with other spondyloarthropathies (reactive arthritis, psoriatic spondylitis, and spondylitis with inflammatory bowel disease). It is not a diagnostic test for AS. HLA testing may be useful in a young patient with early disease for whom the differential diagnosis may be narrowed by the presence of HLA-B27.

Radiographic Evaluation

Characteristic changes of AS in the sacroiliac joints and lumbosacral spine are helpful in making a diagnosis but may be difficult to determine in the early stages of the disease.[29] The areas of the skeleton most frequently affected include the sacroiliac, apophyseal, discovertebral, and costovertebral joints. The disease affects the sacroiliac joints initially and then appears in the upper lumbar and thoracolumbar areas. Subsequently, in ascending order, the lower lumbar, thoracic, and cervical spine are involved. The radiographic progression of disease may be halted at any stage, although sacroiliitis alone is a rare finding except in some women with spondylitis or in men in the early stage of disease.

The European League Against Rheumatism (EULAR) has issued guidelines for the evaluation of spondyloarthritis.[30] Evaluation of the sacroiliac joints should be with a conventional anteroposterior supine view of the pelvis and should be the first imaging method to diagnose sacroiliitis.[30] Other conventional radiographic views do not offer greater sensitivity for the increased exposure to radiation.

Sacroiliitis is a bilateral, symmetrical process in AS. During the next stage, the articular space becomes "pseudowidened" secondary to joint surface erosions. With continued inflammation, the area of sclerosis widens and is joined by proliferative bony changes that cross the joint space. In the final stages of sacroiliitis, complete ankylosis with total obliteration of the joint space occurs (Fig. 83.1). Ligamentous structures surrounding the sacroiliac joint may also calcify. The radiographic changes associated with sacroiliitis may be graded from 0 (normal) to 4 (complete ankylosis).

In the lumbar spine, osteitis affecting the anterior corners of vertebral bodies is an early finding. The inflammation associated with osteitis causes loss of the normal concavity of the anterior vertebral surface, resulting in a "squared" body (Fig. 83.2).

While osteopenia of the bony structures appears, calcification of disc and ligamentous structures emerges. Thin, vertically oriented calcifications of the anulus fibrosus and anterior and posterior longitudinal ligaments are termed *syndesmophytes*. *Bamboo spine* is the term used to describe the spine of a patient with AS with extensive syndesmophytes encasing the axial skeleton (Fig. 83.3).

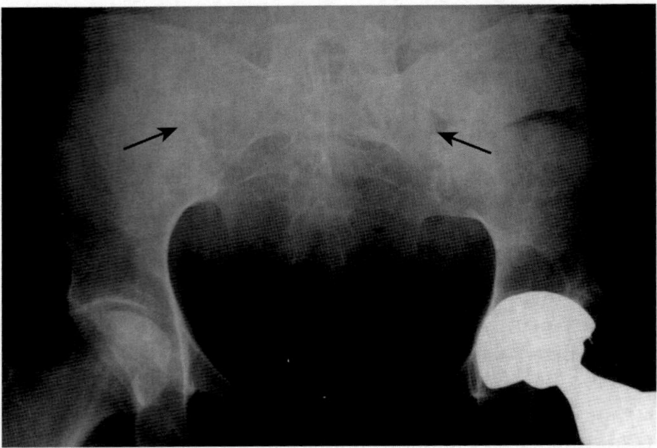

FIG. 83.1 Ankylosing spondylitis. Anteroposterior view of the pelvis of a 38-year-old woman with a 15-year history of ankylosing spondylitis shows bilateral fused sacroiliac joints (*arrows*). She underwent hip replacement because of destructive disease secondary to spondyloarthropathy.

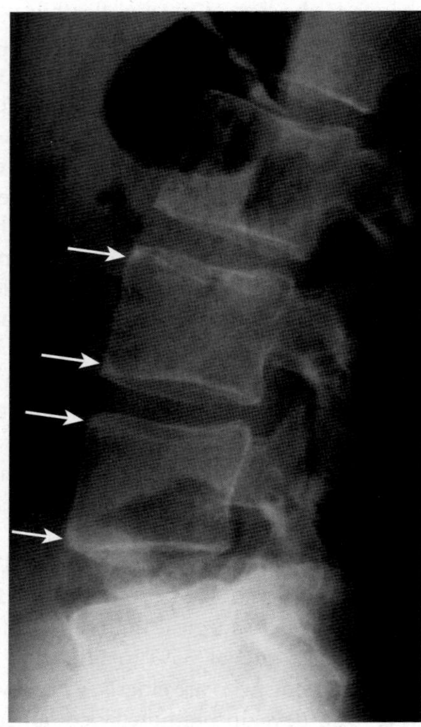

FIG. 83.2 Ankylosing spondylitis. Lateral view of the lumbosacral spine shows "squaring" of all lumbar vertebral bodies (*arrows*).

The apophyseal joints are also affected in the illness. As the disease progresses, fusion of the apophyseal joints occurs. Radiographs of the spine may show the loss of joint space and complete fusion of the joints. Cervical spine ankylosis may be particularly severe (Fig. 83.4). Complete obliteration

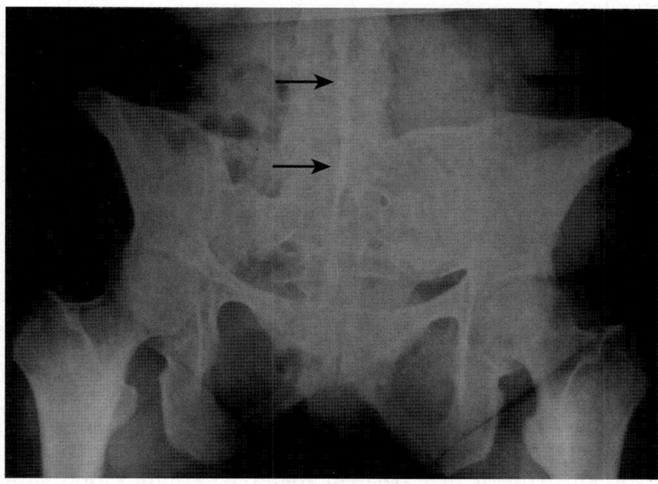

FIG. 83.3 Ankylosing spondylitis. Anteroposterior view of the pelvis of a 64-year-old man with 40 years of ankylosing spondylitis and bamboo spine. Sacroiliac joints are fused and interspinous ligaments are calcified (*arrows*).

BOX 83.1 Modified New York Diagnostic Criteria for Ankylosing Spondylitis

Clinical Criteria

1. Limitation of motion of lumbar spine in anterior flexion, lateral flexion, and extension
2. History of or presence of pain at dorsolumbar junction or in lumbar spine
3. Limitation of chest expansion to ≤1 inch

Radiologic Criteria (Sacroiliitis)

Grade 3: Unequivocal abnormality, moderate or advanced sacroiliitis with one or more erosions, sclerosis, widening, narrowing, or partial ankylosis

Grade 4: Severe abnormality, total ankylosis

Diagnosis

Definite grade 3-4: Bilateral sacroiliitis + one clinical criterion

Grade 3-4: Unilateral or grade 2 bilateral sacroiliitis with clinical criterion 1 or 2 and 3

Probable grade 3-4: Bilateral sacroiliitis alone

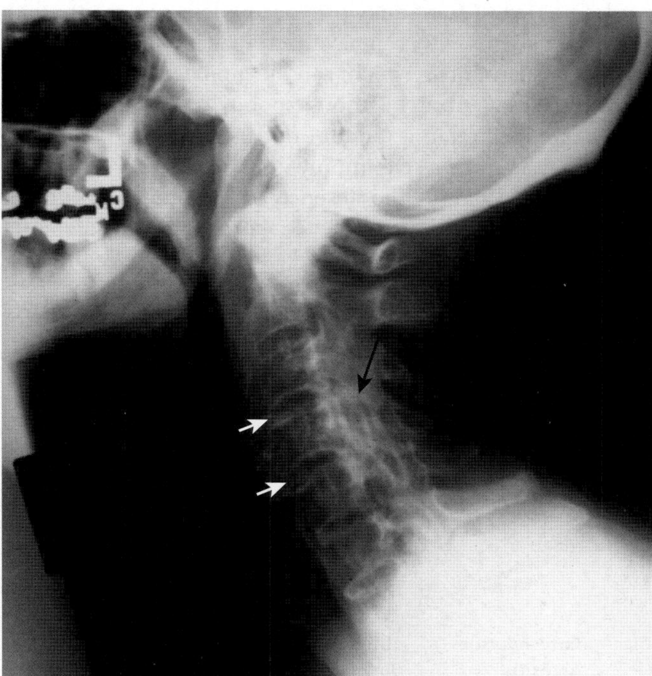

FIG. 83.4 Ankylosing spondylitis. Lateral view of the cervical spine of the patient in Fig. 83.3. Radiograph shows anterior syndesmophytes (*white arrows*) and fusion of posterior zygapophyseal joints (*black arrow*).

of articular spaces between the posterior elements of C2–C7 results in a column of solid bone. Patients with complete ankylosis of the apophyseal joints and syndesmophytes may develop extensive bony resorption of the anterior surface of the lower cervical vertebrae late in the course of the illness. Bone under the ligaments connecting the spinous processes may also be eroded in the setting of apophyseal joint ankylosis.

The C1–C2 joints may become eroded and partially dislocated. Synovial tissue around the dens may cause erosion of the odontoid process. Further damage of the surrounding ligaments results in instability that is measured by the movement of the odontoid process from the posterior aspect of the atlas with flexion and extension views of the cervical spine. Widening of the space is indicative of a dynamic subluxation. No movement of the distance between the atlas and axis suggests a fixed subluxation. In addition to atlantoaxial subluxation, migration of the odontoid into the foramen magnum and rotary subluxation may occur. Subaxial subluxation is more characteristic of RA than AS.

MRI with fat saturation or contrast medium–enhanced images are able to detect early inflammatory lesions in the sacroiliac joints and the lumbar spine before conventional radiographs.[31] MRI is able to identify this group, which has been classified as suffering from nonradiographic spondyloarthritis. From a diagnostic and clinical perspective, plain radiographs normally provide adequate information at a reasonable cost. Plain radiographs remain the usual radiographic technique used for the diagnosis of AS. MRI is a good choice for young women with suspected sacroiliitis as a means of decreasing radiographic exposure and detection of earlier lesions.

Differential Diagnosis

Diagnostic criteria exist for the diagnosis of AS. The modified New York criteria require alterations in the sacroiliac joints (Box 83.1). The criteria include a grading system for radiographs of the sacroiliac joints in addition to limited spine motion, chest expansion, and back pain.[32] Although these criteria are used mostly for studies of patient populations, they are helpful in the office setting. The Assessment of Spondyloarthritis International Society has proposed classification criteria based on clinical or imaging findings (Table 83.1).[33]

Although spondyloarthropathies are a common inflammatory musculoskeletal disorder, this group of illnesses is frequently overlooked by nonrheumatologists. A delay in diagnosis from the onset of symptoms and referral to a rheumatologist ranged from 6 to 264 months. Individuals who are misdiagnosed by primary care physicians have mild to moderate disease, with atypical presentations, and are women.[34] The differential diagnosis of spinal pain includes other spondyloarthropathies, rheumatoid arthritis, and herniated intervertebral disc. Characteristics of these specific diseases are listed in Table 83.2. The inflammatory disorders are discussed briefly here.

Psoriatic Arthritis

Patients with psoriasis who develop a characteristic pattern of joint disease have psoriatic arthritis.[35] The prevalence of psoriasis is 1% to 3% of the population. Classic psoriatic arthritis is described as involving distal interphalangeal joints and associated nail disease alone.[36] This pattern occurs in 5% of patients. The most common form of the disease, affecting 70% of patients with psoriatic arthritis, is an asymmetrical oligoarthritis; a few large or small joints are involved. Dactylitis, diffuse swelling of a digit, is most closely associated with this form of the disease. Skin activity and joint symptoms do not correlate, and patients with little skin activity may experience continued joint pain and stiffness.

Psoriatic spondyloarthropathy is found in 5% to 23% of patients with psoriatic arthritis. Patients who develop axial skeletal disease, sacroiliitis, or spondylitis are usually men who have onset of psoriasis later in life. HLA-B27 is more common in individuals with axial disease. Sacroiliac involvement may be unilateral or bilateral. Percussion over the sacroiliac joints can elicit symptoms over the affected side. Patients may develop spondylitis in the absence of sacroiliitis, which has maximal tenderness with percussion over the spine above the sacrum. In the cervical spine, limitation of motion is a primary manifestation of neck involvement. Rarely, patients with psoriatic arthritis may develop atlantoaxial subluxation with evidence of cervical myelopathy. Fracture after minor trauma may be overlooked for an extended period.[37]

Spondylitis on radiographs is characterized by asymmetrical involvement of the vertebral bodies and nonmarginal syndesmophytes. Joint ankylosis occurs less commonly than in AS. Of patients, 25% can have sacroiliac involvement manifested by sacroiliitis, which can be unilateral or bilateral. Sacroiliitis may occur without spondylitis. Spinal disease progression occurs in a random rather than orderly fashion, ascending the spine as commonly noted in AS. Cervical spine disease may occur in the absence of sacroiliitis or lumbar spondylitis. Alterations in the cervical spine include joint space sclerosis and narrowing and anterior ligamentous calcification (Fig. 83.5).

The Classification of Psoriatic Arthritis study group proposed classification criteria for psoriatic arthritis. These criteria include the presence of psoriasis, nail changes, dactylitis, juxtaarticular new bone formation, and the absence of rheumatoid factor. These criteria have excellent sensitivity in early and late disease.[38]

TABLE 83.1 ASAS Criteria for Axial Spondyloarthritis (SpA) in Patients With Chronic Back Pain and Age of Onset of Back Pain <45 Years

Sacroiliitis on Imaging Plus ≥1 SpA Feature	*or*	HLA-B27 Plus ≥2 Other SpA Features
Active (acute) inflammation on MRI highly suggestive of sacroiliitis associated with SpA		Inflammatory back pain
Definite radiographic sacroiliitis according to New York criteria		Arthritis
		Enthesitis (heel)
		Uveitis
		Dactylitis
		Psoriasis
		Crohn disease
		Good response to NSAIDs
		Family history of SpA
		HLA-B27
		Elevated CRP

ASAS, Assessment of Spondyloarthritis International Society; CRP, C-reactive protein; HLA, human leukocyte antigen; NSAIDs, nonsteroidal antiinflammatory drugs.

TABLE 83.2 Differential Diagnosis of Ankylosing Spondylitis

	Ankylosing Spondylitis	Psoriatic Arthritis	Reactive Arthritis	Enteropathic Arthritis	Rheumatoid Arthritis	Herniated Disc
Sacroiliitis	Symmetrical	Asymmetrical	Asymmetrical	Symmetrical	–	–
Axial skeleton	+	±	±	+	–	–
Peripheral joints	Lower	Upper	Lower	Lower	Upper and lower	–
Enthesopathy	+	+	+	–	–	–
ESR	Elevated	Elevated	Elevated	Elevated	Elevated	Normal
Rheumatoid factor	–	–	–	–	+	–
HLA-B27	90%	60%	90%	50%	8%	8%
Course	Continuous	Continuous	Self-limited	Continuous	Continuous	Episodic or continuous
Therapy	NSAIDs, DMARDs	NSAIDs/DMARDs, NSAIDs/antibiotics	NSAIDs	Steroids	NSAIDs, DMARD	NSAIDs
		TNF	Biologics	Biologics	Biologics	Epidural steroids
Disability		Hip	Lower extremity	Lower extremity	Extremities	Radiculopathy

DMARDs, disease-modifying antirheumatic drugs; ESR, erythrocyte sedimentation rate; HLA, human leukocyte antigen; NSAIDs, nonsteroidal antiinflammatory drugs; TNF, tumor necrosis factor.

Treatment of psoriatic arthritis is directed at reducing inflammation and preventing structural damage with early intervention. The EULAR has published recommendations for the pharmacologic therapy of psoriatic arthritis.[39] Immunosuppressive agents and TNF-α inhibitors are listed in Table 83.3. Treatments are used indefinitely.

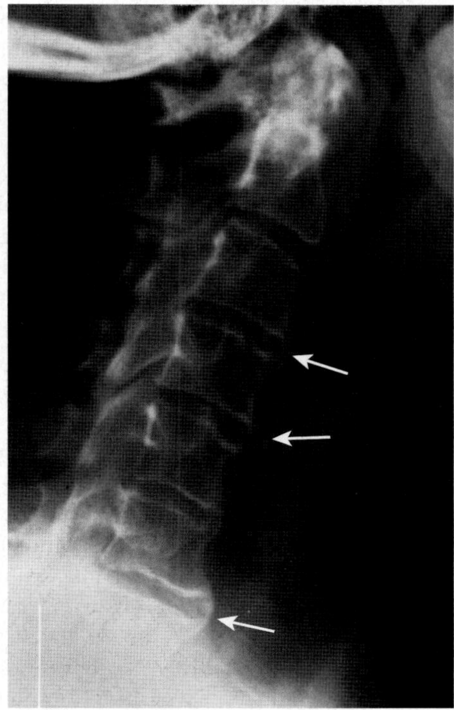

FIG. 83.5 Psoriatic arthritis. Lateral view of the cervical spine of a 45-year-old woman with psoriasis shows anterior syndesmophytes at levels C3–C4, C4–C5, and C6–C7 (*arrows*).

Reactive Arthritis

Reactive arthritis is associated with an infectious agent causing an aseptic inflammation in joints and other organs. This disorder has been associated with the triad of urethritis (inflammation of the lower urinary tract), arthritis, and conjunctivitis formerly referred to as *Reiter syndrome,* a form of reactive arthritis. Reactive arthritis is the most common cause of arthritis in young men and primarily affects the lower extremity joints and the low back. Involvement of the cervical spine is rare. The disease results from the interaction of an environmental factor, usually a specific infection, and a genetically predisposed host. Approximately 3% of patients with the common infection nongonococcal urethritis develop the syndrome. The syndrome develops in 0.2% to 15% of all patients with enteric infections secondary to *Shigella, Salmonella, Campylobacter,* and *Yersinia*. The male-to-female ratio in venereal infection is 10 : 1, and the ratio is 1 : 1 in large outbreaks secondary to enteric infection.

Reactive arthritis is associated with HLA-B27 in 60% to 80% of individuals. The classic patient with reactive arthritis is a young man about 25 years old who develops urethritis and a mild conjunctivitis, followed by the onset of a predominantly lower extremity oligoarthritis. The conjunctivitis is usually mild and is manifested by an erythema (redness) and crusting of the lids. Arthritis may occur 1 to 3 weeks after the initial infection. In many patients, arthritis is the only manifestation of disease.[40] Back pain is a frequent symptom of patients with reactive arthritis. During the acute course, 31% to 92% of patients may develop pain in the lumbosacral region. Occasionally, the pain radiates into the posterior thighs but rarely below the knees; it may be unilateral. Spondylitis affecting the lumbar, thoracic, and cervical spine occurs less commonly than sacroiliitis, with 23% of patients with severe disease showing such involvement.[41]

TABLE 83.3 Disease-Modifying and Biologic Antirheumatic Drugs

Drug	Availability (mg)	Dose (mg)	Toxicities	Comment
Disease Modifying				
Hydroxychlorcquine	200	200–400	Retinopathy	Requires 6 mo to work
Sulfasalazine	500	1000–2000	Gastrointestinal, anemia	Sulfa allergy
Methotrexate	2.5, 5, 7.5	5–25	Hepatitis, anemia	Requires 6 wk to work
Azathioprine	50	50–300	Hepatitis, leukopenia	Requires 3 mo to work
Leflunomide	10, 20, 100	20	Diarrhea, alopecia	100 × 3 initially; onset at 4 wk
Biologics				
Etanercept	25, 50	50 (IM)	Injection pain, infections	Requires 6 wk to work
Adalimumab	40	40 every 1–2 wk (IM)	Injection pain, infections	Requires 6 wk to work
Infliximab	100	3–10 mg/kg 4–8 wk (IV)	Infusion reactions, infections	Best with methotrexate
Certolizumab	200	200 every 2 wk or 400 every 4 wk (IM)	Infections	Less injection pain
Golimumab	50	50 IM monthly, 50 IV monthly	Infections	Best with methotrexate
Tocilizumab	4, 8, 162 (SQ)	4 or 8 mg/kg IV or 162 mg IM every 2 wk	Infections	Monotherapy
Abatacept	500, 750, 1000 IV, 125 SQ	Depending on weight, every 4 wk or 125 SQ weekly	Infections	Not to be used with TNF inhibitors
Rituximab	500	1000 for 2 doses 2 wk apart, repeated at 6 mo	Infusion reaction	May be repeated
Anakinra	100	100, daily injection	Injection pain	Given same time every day
Toficitanib	5	5 twice daily	Infections, hyperlipidemia	With or without methotrexate

IM, intramuscular; IV, intravascular; SQ, subcutaneous; TNF, tumor necrosis factor.

Neck pain is a rare symptom of patients with reactive arthritis. Constitutional symptoms occur in about one-third of patients and include fever, anorexia, weight loss, and fatigue.

On examination, men tend to have involvement in the knees, ankles, and feet; women have more upper extremity disease. Percussion tenderness over the sacroiliac joints may be unilateral, correlating with asymmetrical involvement in reactive arthritis. The mobility of the lumbosacral and cervical spine should be measured in all planes of motion. Evaluation for enthesopathy, heel pain, or Achilles tendon tenderness is also required.

Sacroiliac involvement may mimic AS (symmetrical disease) or may be asymmetrical in severity of joint changes. Unilateral sacroiliac disease occurs early in the disease process. Variable amounts of sclerosis are associated with erosions. The progression of radiographic changes shows widening of the joint (erosion), then narrowing (fusion). Fusion of the joints occurs less frequently than in AS. Sacroiliitis may be detected in 5% to 10% of individuals early in the illness and in 60% in prolonged illness. Spondylitis is discontinuous in its involvement of the axial skeleton (skip lesions) and is characterized by nonmarginal bony bridging of vertebral bodies. These vertebral hyperostoses are markedly thickened compared with the thin syndesmophytes of AS. Cervical spine disease is associated with hyperostoses at the anteroinferior corners of one or more cervical vertebrae.

The joint and enthesopathic manifestations of reactive arthritis respond to NSAIDs. The drugs are continued as long as the patient remains symptomatic. Oral corticosteroids have some efficacy. The role of antibiotic therapy in the acute phase of reactive arthritis is controversial. Antibiotics may be ineffective for *Chlamydia*-associated reactive arthritis.[41] Sulfasalazine has been reported to improve spinal pain and swollen joints in patients with reactive arthritis. The usual dose of sulfasalazine is 2 g/day in divided doses. The immunosuppressive methotrexate is reserved for patients with uncontrolled progression of joint disease and unresponsive, extensive skin involvement. The dose of methotrexate ranges from 7.5 to 25 mg/week. The role of anti-TNF drugs remains controversial in an illness that is associated with infection as its initiating factor.[41]

The course of the illness is unpredictable. A self-limited illness, lasting 3 months to 1 year, occurs in 30% to 40% of patients. Another 30% to 50% develop a relapsing pattern of illness with periods of complete remission. The final 10% to 25% develop chronic, unremitting disease associated with significant disability.

Enteropathic Arthritis

Ulcerative colitis and Crohn disease are inflammatory bowel diseases. Ulcerative colitis is limited to the colon; Crohn disease, or regional enteritis, may involve any part of the gastrointestinal tract.[42] Inflammation of the gut results in numerous gastrointestinal symptoms, including abdominal pain, fever, and weight loss. These inflammatory diseases are also associated with extraintestinal manifestations, including arthritis. Articular involvement in inflammatory bowel disease includes peripheral and axial skeleton joints. Peripheral arthritis is generally nondeforming and follows the activity of the underlying bowel disease.[43] Axial skeleton disease is similar to AS and follows a course independent of activity of bowel inflammation.

Symptomatic ulcerative colitis usually occurs in adults 25 to 45 years old. Crohn disease occurs in all races and is distributed worldwide. In the United States, the annual incidence of the disease is 4 per 100,000. The disease occurs most often in individuals 15 to 35 years old. The frequency of peripheral arthritis is 11% in ulcerative colitis and 20% in Crohn disease. Spondylitis occurs in 3% to 4% of both diseases, and radiographic sacroiliitis occurs in 10%. Axial arthritis of inflammatory bowel disease may be a hereditary accompaniment of the disease and not a manifestation of activity of bowel disease itself. Non–HLA-related factors and HLA-B27 may play a role.

Early symptoms of ulcerative colitis are frequent bowel movements with blood or mucus. Mild disease is associated with some abdominal pain and a few bowel movements per day. Severe disease is characterized by fatigue, weight loss, fever, and extracolonic involvement. Crohn disease is frequently an indolent illness characterized by generalized fatigue, mild nonbloody diarrhea, anorexia, weight loss, and cramping lower abdominal pain. Patients may have symptoms for years before the diagnosis is made.

Articular involvement in inflammatory bowel disease is divided into two forms: peripheral and spondylitic. Axial skeleton involvement in ulcerative colitis and Crohn disease is similar. Spondylitis antedates bowel disease in about one-third of patients. This interval may be 10 to 20 years. Of patients, 70% are HLA-B27 positive, 68% have radiographic changes of spondylitis, and 25% have iritis. The spondylitis of inflammatory bowel disease has a course totally independent of the course of the bowel disease. The clinical and radiographic findings are similar to findings of AS, including involvement of shoulders and hips.

On examination, patients with spondyloarthropathy may have decreased motion of the spine in all planes and percussion tenderness over the sacroiliac joints. Rarely, chest expansion is diminished. Patients with more extensive disease have limitation of motion of the cervical spine. Occiput-to-wall measurements document the immobility of the entire axial skeleton, including the cervical spine.

The radiographic changes of spondylitis in inflammatory bowel disease are indistinguishable from classic AS (Fig. 83.6). Findings include squaring of vertebral bodies; erosions; widening and fusion of the sacroiliac joints; symmetrical involvement of sacroiliac joints; and marginal syndesmophytes involving the lumbar, thoracic, or cervical spine.

The factors that help make the diagnosis of enteropathic spondyloarthropathy are the pattern of peripheral arthritis if present (upper extremity disease is uncommon in AS and reactive arthritis; bilateral ankle arthritis is uncommon in psoriatic disease), erythema nodosum, and iritis. Therapy for enteropathic spondylitis is similar to therapy for classic AS. TNF-α inhibitors are effective agents for bowel and articular disease.[44]

The ultimate course and outcome of these patients depend on the severity of bowel disease. Patients with severe ulcerative

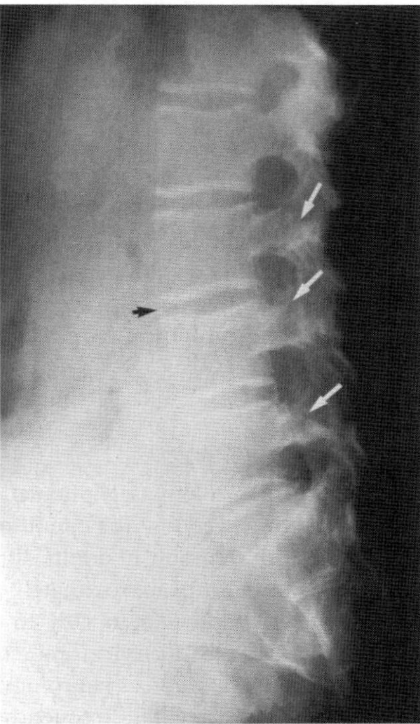

FIG. 83.6 Enteropathic spondylitis: a lateral view of the lumbar spine demonstrates loss of lumbar lordosis, fusion of the facet joints (*white arrows*), and early syndesmophyte formation (*black arrow*) in a 25-year-old woman with a 9-year history of Crohn disease. (From Borenstein DG, Weisel SW, Boden SD. *Low Back and Neck Pain: Comprehensive Diagnosis and Management*. 3rd ed. Philadelphia: Saunders; 2004.)

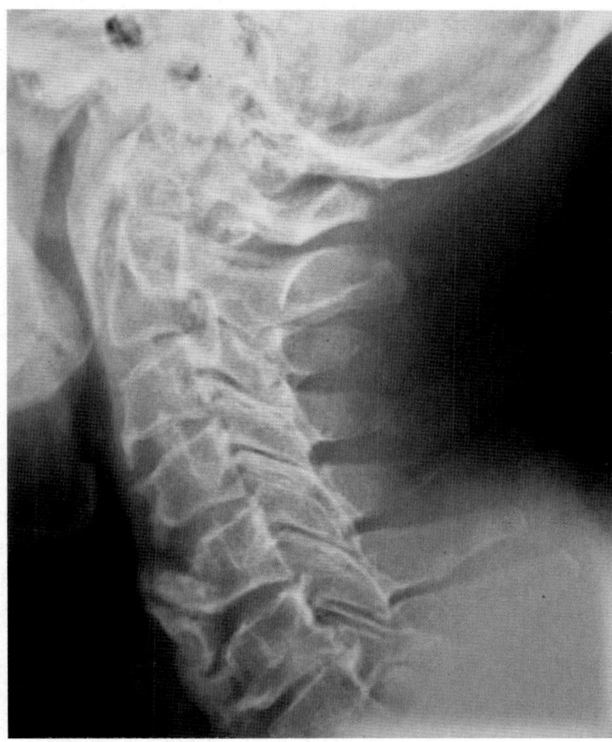

FIG. 83.7 Diffuse idiopathic skeletal hyperostosis. Lateral view of the cervical spine shows large anterior, horizontally oriented osteophytes characteristic of this illness.

colitis have a mortality rate of 10% to 20% over 5 years. Patients with a severe initial attack, continuous clinical activity, involvement of the entire colon, and disease for 10 years or longer have a higher risk of developing cancer of the colon. These patients may require colectomy. Although Crohn disease is associated with frequent recurrences, the overall mortality rate of 5% for the first 5 years of disease is much less than in ulcerative colitis.

Diffuse Idiopathic Skeletal Hyperostosis

Diffuse idiopathic skeletal hyperostosis (DISH) is another disease that may occur in the setting of spondylitis. Patients with AS and DISH should be easily differentiated by careful radiographic evaluation.[45] DISH may cause alterations of the sacroiliac joints.[46] CT of the sacroiliac joints differentiates the hyperostotic joint changes from changes associated with joint erosion and fusion (Fig. 83.7). Also of note is the occurrence of fracture in patients with DISH and patients with AS. The convergence of two common diseases in the same host, a middle-aged man, is likely. The occurrence of AS and DISH of the cervical spine has been reported.[47]

Treatment

The goals of therapy for AS, as with other forms of inflammatory arthritis, are to control pain and stiffness, reduce inflammation, maintain function, and prevent deformity with avoidance of undue toxicity. Patients require a comprehensive program of education, physiotherapy, medications, and other measures. In 2015, the American College of Rheumatology (ACR) published recommendations for the treatment of AS.[48] The publication lists nonpharmacologic and pharmacologic therapies and the strength of evidence for the recommendations. Nonpharmacologic recommendations include land-based active physical therapy interventions. Use of braces, splints, and corsets should be avoided.

Nonsteroidal Antiinflammatory Drugs

Medications to control pain and inflammation are useful to patients with AS. NSAIDs possess antipyretic, analgesic, and antiinflammatory characteristics. They are antiinflammatory and analgesic when given long term in larger doses. NSAIDs are effective at decreasing pain and improving movement but have not been proven to slow the progression of disease.

Cyclooxygenase-2 inhibitors are another class of NSAIDs with less gastrointestinal toxicity. These drugs should be used continuously in AS patients with high activity of disease.

Muscle Relaxants

Patients with acute AS may develop severe muscle spasm with associated limited motion that may hinder their return to normal daily activities. In these patients, the addition of muscle relaxant to NSAIDs helps decrease muscle pain and muscle spasm and improve back motion. Muscle relaxants, such as cyclobenzaprine, at low dosages (5–10 mg/day) are helpful while limiting possible drug toxicity. The sleepiness associated with muscle relaxants with long half-lives can be limited by giving the medication 2 hours before bedtime.

Corticosteroids

Systemic corticosteroids are rarely needed and are ineffective for the spinal articular disease of AS. The ACR publication recommends against the use of systemic steroids.[48]

Anti–Tumor Necrosis Factor-α Inhibitors

TNF-α, an inflammatory cytokine, is associated with the inflammatory process that results in the phenotypic expression of AS. Anti–TNF-α therapies are available in the form of infliximab, etanercept, certolizumab, golimumab, and adalimumab, which inhibit the inflammatory effects of TNF-α.[49] Table 83.3 contains information about these biologic drugs and their use in rheumatic disease, including AS. Studies have demonstrated the greater efficacy of each of these agents in comparison to placebo in the treatment of AS patients.[49]

The full benefits of anti–TNF-α therapy in AS remain to be determined. The efficacy of these agents in disease of long duration is less certain. These agents are expensive and their availability is limited. Toxicities are associated with their use, including the activation of latent tuberculosis. Questions remain in regard to the potency of TNF drugs to inhibit calcification of the spine in active disease. Also, the ability of these agents to produce a remission and the opportunity to discontinue treatment remains an active area of research.

Prognosis

The general course of AS is benign and is characterized by exacerbations and remissions. Many patients with AS may have sacroiliitis with mild involvement of the lumbosacral spine alone. Limitation of lumbosacral motion may be mild. The disease can become quiescent at any time. Patients who go on to develop total fusion of the spine may feel better because ankylosis of the spinal joints is associated with decreased pain. In a study of 1492 patients for 2 years, the frequency of patients with a total remission of disease was less than 2%.[50]

Rheumatoid Arthritis

RA is a chronic, systemic inflammatory disease that causes pain, heat, swelling, and destruction in synovial joints. The joints characteristically affected by RA are small joints of the hands and feet, wrists, elbows, hips, knees, ankles, and cervical spine. Most patients with RA have cervical spine disease manifested as neck pain, headaches, or arm numbness. Signs of cervical spine disease include decreased neck motion with stiffness; undue prominence of the spinous process of the axis (C2); and neurologic dysfunction, including paresthesias, spasticity, incontinence, and quadriplegia. The diagnosis of RA is made in the setting of a history of persistent joint inflammation in the appropriate joints and the presence of specific serum antibodies (rheumatoid factor). The degree of cervical spine destruction in RA does not always correlate with patient complaints and is detected by radiographic evaluation. RA of the cervical spine responds to the same therapy that is effective for the peripheral joints. Surgical intervention with stabilization of the cervical spine is required for persistent neurologic abnormalities.

Epidemiology

The prevalence of RA is 1% of the US population.[51] RA is found in all racial and ethnic groups. The condition occurs in all age groups but is most common in adults 40 to 70 years old.[52] The male-to-female ratio is approximately 1:3. Symptoms of cervical spine disease occur in 40% to 80% of RA patients. Radiographic evidence of cervical spine involvement is found in 86% of RA patients, whereas neurologic symptoms from cervical spine disease occur less frequently in 10% of patients with radiographic changes. Cervical spine disease usually occurs in the setting of active peripheral disease; however, occasionally, neck symptoms may be the initial or predominant symptom without clinical signs of RA in other locations. The lumbar spine is rarely involved in the rheumatoid process. One study suggested that 5% of men and 3% of women with RA have lumbar spine involvement.[53]

Pathogenesis

RA is a chronic immune-mediated disease whose initiation and perpetuation are dependent on T-lymphocyte response to unknown antigens.[54] The interaction of genetic factors, the shared epitope in the HLA-DRB1 region, with environmental factors, such as smoking, periodontitis, and the gut microbiome, increase the risk for disease. Increased numbers of $CD4^+$ lymphocytes that activate B lymphocytes to produce immunoglobulin are frequently found in synovium from RA patients. The activation of macrophages results in the production of monokines, including TNF-α, interleukins, and intracellular signaling and transcription factors. These factors attract additional lymphocytes and neutrophils. Angiogenesis factors result in the growth of new capillaries. Synovial cells cause tissue destruction by release of activated metalloproteinases, including procollagenase and progelatinase. The inflammatory response is also enhanced by the production of arachidonic acid metabolites.

Clinical History

Patients with RA develop joint pain, heat, swelling, and tenderness. The joint involvement is additive and symmetrical. The joints at greatest risk of being affected by the disease process include the proximal interphalangeal, metacarpocarpal, wrist, elbow, hip, knee, ankle, and metatarsophalangeal joints. In the axial skeleton, the cervical spine is most frequently affected. Patients have joint pain and stiffness, which are most severe in the morning. Activity improves symptoms. The phenomenon of stiffness of a joint with rest occurs frequently with active disease. As a component of systemic inflammation, afternoon fatigue, anorexia, and weight loss are common complaints.

Neck movement frequently precipitates or aggravates neck pain that is aching and deep in quality. Atlantoaxial disease is experienced in the upper part of the cervical spine; pain radiates over the occiput into the temporal and frontal regions with increasing disease of the C1–C2 joint. Occipital headaches are frequently associated with active rheumatoid involvement of the cervical spine. Other symptoms of C1–C2 subluxation include a sensation of the head falling forward with flexion of the neck, loss of consciousness or syncope, incontinence, dysphagia, vertigo, convulsions, hemiplegia, dysarthria, nystagmus, or peripheral paresthesias.[55] Peripheral joint erosion is a harbinger of C1–C2 subluxation. Development of cervical subluxation occurs in patients who have joint erosions of hands and feet, serum rheumatoid factor, and subcutaneous nodules.

Pain associated with RA in the subaxial segments of the cervical spine is located in the lateral aspects of the neck and clavicles (C3–C4) and over the shoulders (C5–C6). Neurologic symptoms include paresthesias and numbness. Paresthesias have a burning quality that may be attributed to an entrapment neuropathy (carpal tunnel syndrome) but is sufficiently different not to be confused with joint pain. Patients with sensory symptoms alone may have their symptoms ascribed to arthritis, delaying the diagnosis of cervical myelopathy.[56]

The appearance of spasticity, gait disturbance, muscular weakness, and incontinence (urinary or rectal) indicates significant compression of the spinal cord. Symptoms suggesting vertebrobasilar artery insufficiency include visual disturbances, dizziness, paresthesias of the face, ataxia, and dysarthria.

Cervical Subluxation

In the cervical spine, the structures lined with synovial membrane may be involved in RA. These structures include the atlantoaxial joint. This joint connects the atlas (C1) with the axis (C2) and is responsible for rotation of the skull on the cervical spine. Synovial tissue is located between the atlas and axis and between the ligaments and atlas. Other synovial joints include the zygapophyseal and uncovertebral joints.

RA causes disease in the cervical spine by causing chronic inflammatory changes to occur in the atlanto-occipital, atlantoaxial, zygapophyseal, and uncovertebral joints along with the discs and ligamentous and bursal structures. At the level of the atlantoaxial joint, synovial inflammation of the bursae and ligaments results in laxity of the transverse ligament that holds the atlas and axis together. Normally, the distance between the bones does not exceed 2.5 to 3 mm in adults. The relaxation of supporting ligaments results in excess motion of the axis in relation to the atlas-atlantoaxial subluxation.

Luxation of the atlantoaxial joint may occur anteriorly, posteriorly, superiorly or vertically, or laterally. Anterior subluxation is the most common form and results from insufficiency of the transverse ligament or fracture of the odontoid and occurs in 49% of patients.[57] Posterior subluxation occurs when C1 moves posteriorly on C2 and results from erosion or fracture of the odontoid; this occurs in 7% of patients. Vertical or superior subluxation results from destruction of the lateral atlantoaxial joints around the foramen magnum and is found in 38% of patients. Lateral subluxation occurs in 20%, with erosion of the lateral mass and odontoid. Abnormal motion of this joint in any direction may result in compression of the cervical spinal cord or medulla oblongata, resulting in the development of neurologic symptoms and signs of myelopathy, including paresthesias, muscle weakness, reflex changes, spasticity, and incontinence. Subluxation of the atlantoaxial joint by the odontoid process of the axis and the posterior arch of the atlas may compress the vertebral arteries. The vertebral arteries are compressed as they travel through the foramina in the transverse processes of C1 and C2. Vertebral artery compression may cause tetraplegia, coma, or sudden death.[56]

Subluxation may occur between cervical vertebrae below the atlantoaxial joint. Common levels include C3–C4 and C4–C5. Inflammation in the zygapophyseal joints and surrounding bursae undermines the stability of these joints, resulting in excessive motion and angulation of the cervical spine.[58] Intervertebral discs may be invaded by growing synovial tissue, resulting in disc space narrowing. The reported frequency of subaxial subluxation ranges from 7% to 29% of RA patients.[59]

Myelopathy may also occur in patients without atlantoaxial or cervical spine subluxation. The 10-year incidence of RA-associated cervical myelopathy in Olmsted County, Minnesota, was 0.7%.[60] In these patients, synovitis from the zygapophyseal joints along with intervertebral disc lesions may compromise the blood supply to the spinal cord through stenosis of vertebral vessels that feed the anterior spinal artery. Ischemic myelopathy is the result. Sudden death may also be a consequence of thrombosis of vertebral vessels.[61]

Physical Examination

Physical examination of a patient with RA with cervical spine disease reveals diffuse peripheral joint involvement characterized by heat, swelling, bogginess, tenderness, and loss of motion. Nodules over the extensor surfaces are noted in 20% of RA patients. Examination of the cervical spine may show tenderness with palpation over the bony skeleton and limitation of all spinal movements. Inspection may show fixation of the head tilted down and to one side. This lateral tilt is caused by the asymmetrical destruction of the lateral atlantoaxial joints. Normal cervical lordosis may also be absent. With the neck flexed, the spinous process of the axis may be prominent in the midline of the neck of a patient with atlantoaxial subluxation. Patients with subaxial subluxation may show abnormalities in the upper extremities. Compression of C6–C8 segments causes distinctive numb, clumsy hands and tactile agnosia.[62] Neurologic abnormalities are seen in approximately 7% of RA patients.

Laboratory Data

Abnormal laboratory findings include anemia, elevated erythrocyte sedimentation rate, and increases in serum globulin levels. Thrombocytosis is found in patients with active RA. Rheumatoid factors (antibodies directed against host antibodies) are present in up to 80% of patients with RA. Citrullination alters arginine and occurs in inflammatory environments, such as the gingiva and the lung.[63] Measurement of antibodies directed against cyclic citrullinated protein has specificity for RA in the range of 95%.[64] Antinuclear antibodies are present in 30% of RA patients. C-reactive protein, an acute-phase reactant, may be helpful when obtained in a serial manner to predict individuals who are at increased risk for joint deterioration and as a measure of response to therapy. Individuals with persistent elevations in C-reactive protein are at risk of progressive cervical spine subluxations.[65] Synovial fluid analysis shows inflammatory fluid characterized by poor viscosity, increased numbers of white blood cells, decreased glucose level, and increased protein level.

Radiographic Evaluation

Characteristic radiographic changes of RA in peripheral joints include soft tissue swelling, bony erosion without reactive sclerotic bone, joint space narrowing, and periarticular osteopenia. Radiographic evaluation of the cervical spine includes anteroposterior, lateral with flexion and extension, oblique, and open-mouth frontal projections.

The radiographic criteria for the diagnosis of RA cervical spine disease as proposed by Bland and colleagues[66] are (1) atlantoaxial subluxation of 2.5 mm or more; (2) multiple subluxation of C2–C3, C3–C4, C4–C5, and C5–C6; (3) narrow disc spaces with little or no osteophytosis; (4) erosion of vertebrae, especially vertebral plates; (5) odontoid, small, pointed, eroded loss of cortex; (6) basilar impression; (7) apophyseal joint erosion and blurred facets; (8) cervical spine osteoporosis; (9) wide space (>5 mm) between posterior arch of the atlas and spinous process of the axis (flexion to extension); and (10) secondary osteosclerosis of the atlantoaxial-occipital complex, which may indicate local degenerative change. The normal distance between the odontoid and atlas is 2.5 mm in women and 3 mm in men as measured from the posteroinferior aspect of the tubercle of C1 to the nearest point on the odontoid (Fig. 83.8).[67] The posterior atlanto-odontoid interval is the remaining distance between the posterior surface of the odontoid process and the anterior edge of the posterior ring of the atlas. RA patients with a posterior interval of more than 14 mm did not have neurologic deficits. Posterior subluxation may also occur if the atlas "jumps" over the axis, resting in a dorsal position resulting in posterior subluxation. Vertebrobasilar artery insufficiency associated with neurologic dysfunction is a manifestation of this form of subluxation.

Upward translocation occurs when the bony and ligamentous integrity of the atlanto-occipital articulations is disrupted. Disease of the occipital condyles, lateral masses of the atlas, and lateral articulations of the axis results in bony erosions or collapse. Erosion of the lateral apophyseal joints allows for a

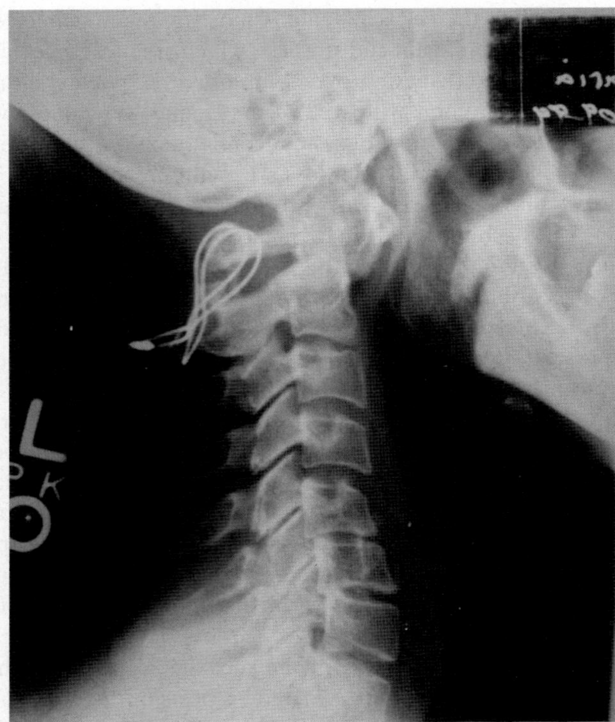

FIG. 83.8 Rheumatoid arthritis. Lateral view of the cervical spine in a 56-year-old woman with more than 20 years of disease. She developed increasing neck pain and dysesthesias in the arms. She had significant dynamic subluxations. C1–C2 spinous processes were wired together; she has had resolution of her symptoms for the subsequent 5 years. (Reproduced with permission from Borenstein DG, Weisel SW, Boden SD. *Low Back and Neck Pain: Comprehensive Diagnosis and Management*. 3rd ed. Philadelphia: Saunders; 2004.)

rotational head tilt. The open-mouth view may show narrowing of the atlanto-occipital and atlantoaxial joints and erosion of the odontoid. Subluxation occurs when the lateral masses of the atlas are displaced more than 2 mm with respect to masses of the axis. Bony erosion is the most important factor in the development of severe lateral subluxation.

In addition to changes in the upper cervical spine, radiographic abnormalities—including subaxial subluxation, apophyseal joint narrowing, and disc space narrowing—occur in the lower cervical spine. Subaxial subluxation is present in instances of malalignment of more than 3.5 mm. The stability of flexion and extension of the lower cervical spine depends on the integrity of the anterior and posterior longitudinal ligaments. Greater than 3.5 mm of malalignment is indicative of a mechanically unstable spine. Multiple subluxations may occur, producing a "staircase" appearance on lateral radiographs. Anterior subluxation is more frequent than posterior subluxation. Subaxial subluxation is most notable on a lateral flexion view of the cervical spine (Fig. 83.9). Apophyseal joint disease includes narrowing, erosions, and sclerosis. Disc destruction in the cervical spine is associated with disc space narrowing and is caused by extension of erosive disease from uncovertebral joints or by ongoing trauma to vertebral endplates secondary to instability. The final stage of apophyseal disease is fibrous ankylosis of one or more levels, which may rarely simulate the appearance of AS.

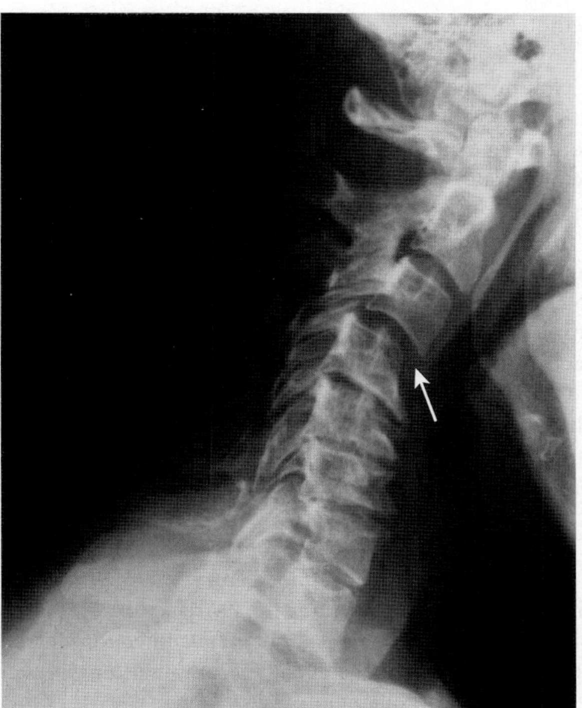

FIG. 83.9 Rheumatoid arthritis. Lateral view of the flexed cervical spine of a 45-year-old woman with 15 years of disease. She has neck and shoulder pain. The neck has anterior subluxation at C3–C4 (*arrow*). Cervical lordosis is reversed.

CT is a useful imaging technique for detecting the extent of bony destruction of structures that may not be easily visualized with plain radiographs. CT detects the position of an eroded odontoid process that may not be seen on open-mouth view radiographs.

MRI is a noninvasive method that is useful in detecting soft tissue abnormalities in the cervical spine of RA patients. It is able to detect pannus around the odontoid and alterations in the substance of the spinal cord. MRI may also be useful in documenting the response of pannus to therapy or the status of the spinal cord in the postoperative state. Compared with CT and plain radiographs, MRI with plain radiographs shows lytic lesions and odontoid erosions and vertical atlantoaxial subluxations more often, shows anterior subluxations as often, and shows lateral subluxations less often.[68]

Differential Diagnosis

RA is a clinical diagnosis based on history of joint pain, distribution of joint involvement, and characteristic laboratory abnormalities (rheumatoid factor). New classification criteria for RA were published by the ACR in partnership with the EULAR in 2010 (Table 83.4).[69] The focus of the new criteria is to identify individuals with earlier stages of disease. In the setting of generalized active disease, the finding of neck pain associated with multiple abnormalities—including atlantoaxial subluxation, apophyseal joint erosion without sclerosis, disc space narrowing without osteophytes, and multiple subluxations—is most appropriately attributed to RA. The cervical spine abnormalities of AS, psoriatic arthritis, reactive

TABLE 83.4 American College of Rheumatology/European League Against Rheumatism Classification Criteria for RA

Criteria	Score
A. Joint Involvement	
1 large joint	0
2–10 large joints	1
1–3 small joints (with or without large joints)	2
4–10 small joints (with or without large joints)	3
>10 joints (at least 1 small joint)	5
B. Serology (At Least 1 Test Result Is Needed for Classification)	
Negative RF and negative ACPA	0
Low-positive RF or low-positive ACPA	2
High-positive RF or high-positive ACPA	3
C. Acute-Phase Reactants (At Least 1 Test Result for Classification)	
Normal CRP and normal ESR	0
Abnormal CRP or abnormal ESR	1
D. Duration of Symptoms	
<6 wk	0
>6 wk	1
TOTAL (score of ≥6/10 = definite RA diagnosis)	

ACPA, anti-citrullinated protein antibody; CRP, C-reactive protein; ESR, erythrocyte sedimentation rate; RA, rheumatoid arthritis; RF rheumatoid factor.
From Aletaha D, Neogi T, Silman AJ et al. 2010 Rheumatoid Arthritis classification criteria: an American College of Rheumatology/European League Against Rheumatism collaborative initiative. *Arthritis Rheum*. 2010;62:2569-2581.

arthritis, enteropathic arthritis, osteoarthritis, and DISH are associated with new bone formation or ligamentous calcification that differentiate them from RA. Occasionally, atlantoaxial subluxation may occur alone in the setting of little peripheral disease. In those circumstances, other disease processes that may cause subluxation include AS, psoriatic arthritis, reactive arthritis, trauma, or local infection.

Treatment

The treatment of RA has undergone a paradigm shift with the advent of new drug therapies directed at control of the factors that mediate the immunologic destruction of joints. The ACR has reviewed all the available therapies and has proposed new options for the treatment of RA.[69,70] These new guidelines include data supporting the use of biologic agents in the therapy for RA.

Nonsteroidal Antiinflammatory Drugs

NSAIDs are medications that control pain and inflammation and are useful in patients with RA for symptomatic relief. However, NSAIDs do not prevent joint destruction and should be discontinued when disease activity is controlled with other forms of drug therapy.

Disease-Modifying Antirheumatic Drugs

Patients who have joint inflammation or damage (joint space narrowing, bony erosions, or cysts) are candidates for remittive therapy. Remittive agents have a delayed onset of action compared with NSAIDs. Table 83.3 lists DMARDs used for the treatment of RA. Methotrexate at doses of 7.5 to 25 mg/week is effective in decreasing the inflammation of RA and may slow disease progression. Methotrexate may be given all at once during the week. It is effective over a long duration of therapy.

Leflunomide is an oral pyrimidine inhibitor used to treat RA.[71] The dose is 100 mg for 3 days, then 20 mg or 10 mg daily as tolerated. Toxicities include abnormal liver function tests and diarrhea. Leflunomide and methotrexate can be used together. Patients taking this combination need to be monitored closely for potential hepatotoxicity.[52]

Systemic corticosteroids are effective in controlling the inflammatory components of RA. Corticosteroids are the most powerful and predictable remedy, inducing immediate relief of joint inflammation in RA. Corticosteroids at low doses (5–10 mg) have a modest effect on reducing the rate of radiologically detected joint destruction. A prospective trial showed disease-modifying properties of 10 mg of prednisone over a 2-year period.[72] Corticosteroids are also associated with a wide range of toxicities, from hypertension and diabetes to cataracts and obesity.

Biologic Therapies, Including Anti–Tumor Necrosis Factor-α Inhibitors

A variety of biologic therapies are available for the treatment of RA (see Table 83.3).[70] No category of biologic therapy is clearly superior in efficacy compared to another. The decision to use one agent as opposed to another involves a number of issues, including the preferred method of administration (oral, injection, or infusion).

TNF therapies are efficacious in decreasing inflammatory signs and slowing joint damage. TNF drugs indicated for the therapy for RA include infliximab, etanercept, adalimumab, certolizumab, and golimumab. Infliximab is partly humanized mouse monoclonal antibody directed against TNF-α. It is administered intravenously. Infliximab is added to methotrexate to limit the production of neutralizing antibodies to the mouse component of the agent. In a 30-week trial, combined infliximab and methotrexate was more effective than methotrexate alone in patients with active RA.[73] In a 54-week study, infliximab, 3 mg/kg or 10 mg/kg, and a stable dose of methotrexate prevented radiographic progression to a greater degree than methotrexate alone.[74]

Etanercept is a recombinant form of the p75 TNF receptor fusion protein. Etanercept 25 mg is administered by subcutaneous injection twice weekly or 50 mg once a week. Etanercept is more effective than placebo in limiting joint activity in RA.[75] It is also effective and safe when added to methotrexate.[76] This drug is also effective over a 12-month period.[77]

Adalimumab is a fully human monoclonal TNF-α antibody given by subcutaneous injection every 2 weeks at a dose of 40 mg. This anti–TNF-α factor is effective with methotrexate in decreasing joint activity.[78]

Certolizumab pegol is a recombinant, humanized Fc-free, polyethylene glycol anti-TNF monoclonal antibody. Certolizumab 200 mg every 2 weeks or 400 mg every 4 weeks is administered by subcutaneous injection. Certolizumab with methotrexate is more effective than methotrexate and placebo in limiting joint destruction in active RA.[79]

Golimumab is a fully humanized monoclonal antibody to anti-TNF. Golimumab is administered 50 mg subcutaneously monthly or 2 mg/kg infused every 8 weeks. Golimumab plus methotrexate decreases signs and symptoms of RA to a greater degree than methotrexate alone.[80]

The concern with anti–TNF-α therapies are the toxicities. Blocking TNF-α increases the risk for serious infection. TNF-α helps to maintain containment of organisms in granulomas. Inhibition of TNF-α has been associated with the reactivation of tuberculosis.[81,82]

Other biologic therapies include inhibitors of interleukins, inhibitors of cellular stimulation, cell-directed therapies, and intracellular signal inhibitors. These therapies affect different components of the immune process that result in joint damage in RA.

Anakinra is a recombinant, nonglycosylated form of human IL-1 receptor antagonist. This agent works by competitively inhibiting IL-1 from binding to its receptor site. Anakinra 100 mg is given as a daily subcutaneous injection. It has been shown to be an effective agent in combination with methotrexate in the improvement of RA.[83]

Tocilizumab is a recombinant, fully humanized monoclonal antibody against IL-6 receptor, inhibiting IL-6 functioning. Tocilizumab is administered by infusion at a dose between 4 mg/kg to 8 mg/kg on a 4-week basis. Tocilizumab plus methotrexate inhibits joint damage to a greater degree than methotrexate alone.[84]

Abatacept is a soluble fusion protein composed of the extracellular domain of human cytotoxic T lymphocyte antigen 4 and a fragment of the Fc portion of human immunoglobulin G1. Abatacept is a selective costimulation modulator that functions to inhibit T-cell activation by preventing binding of CD86 to CD28 on the surface of T lymphocytes. Abatacept is administered as 10 mg/kg intravenously on a 4-week basis or 125 mg subcutaneously on a weekly basis. Abatacept plus methotrexate is more effective than methotrexate alone in decreasing disease symptoms and joint destruction that can be sustained.[85]

Rituximab is a genetically engineered, chimeric monoclonal antibody directed against the CD20 transmembrane protein on B cells, resulting in subsequent cell death and depletion of B cells. Rituximab is administered intravenously at a dose of 1000 mg separated by 15 days repeated at 6-month intervals. Rituximab is effective in controlling RA in patients who have failed TNF therapy.[86]

Tofacitinib is a small-molecule chemical inhibitor of Janus kinase 3, which is an activator of transcription molecules that upregulates immune function. Tofacitinib is an oral agent given as a 5-mg dose twice daily. Tofacitinib is effective in controlling active RA in comparison to placebo.[87]

Immunosuppressive Agents

Immunosuppressive agents are associated with severe toxicities (aplastic anemia and cancer), which limits their benefit to severely affected patients. Only a few patients with RA require this therapy. Immunosuppressive agents used in RA include azathioprine, cyclophosphamide, and cyclosporine. A combination of cyclosporine and methotrexate may be effective for therapy of patients with severe disease.

Cervical Spine Therapy

Conservative treatment of RA of the cervical spine is supportive. Early aggressive medical management is important to prevent joint destruction. Early DMARD therapy results in better outcomes. Combination therapy used early in the course of RA can limit the development of atlantoaxial and vertical subluxations. Sulfasalazine, methotrexate, hydroxychloroquine, and prednisolone were more effective than a single DMARD with prednisolone in preventing cervical subluxation.[88] Soft cervical collars offer comfort but do not protect against progressive subluxations. Rigid collars can limit anterior subluxations but do not allow reduction of the subluxations in extension. They are poorly tolerated by RA patients with temporomandibular disease.[89]

Prognosis

The course of RA cannot be predicted at time of onset. Some patients develop sustained disease that is associated with joint destruction and resistance to therapy. Patients who are older with seropositive generalized disease with nodules are at greater risk of developing cervical spine disease. Not all patients develop subluxation. In a 5- to 14-year follow-up study, 25% of patients had an increase in subluxation, 50% had no change, and 25% had improvement. In a 5-year study of 106 RA patients, the prevalence of cervical spine subluxation increased from 43% to 70%. In subaxial disease, myelopathy was associated with narrowing of the canal, destruction of spinous processes, axial shortening, younger age of patient, longer duration of disease, higher dose of corticosteroids, and higher stage of disease. Sudden death remains a complication of RA cervical spine disease, particularly in patients with vertical subluxation. Individuals with subluxations had eight times the mortality as RA patients without subluxations.[90] In those RA patients who do develop neurologic deficits with cervical spine disease, surgical repair to relieve nerve compression and spinal stability is appropriate.[91]

PEARLS

1. Most HLA-B27–positive individuals (98%) do not have an inflammatory arthropathy of the spine.
2. Enthesopathy is a frequent mechanism of axial and peripheral arthritis in spondyloarthropathies.
3. Plain radiographs are the preferred imaging technique for identification of sacroiliitis.
4. New biologic therapies for treatment of RA and spondyloarthropathies may offer an opportunity to control inflammation before skeletal damage occurs in individuals who fail disease-modifying drug therapy.
5. AS and enteropathic arthritis share common clinical findings that differ from findings associated with reactive arthritis and psoriatic arthritis.

PITFALLS

1. Patients with spondyloarthropathy may have significant axial disease without pain.
2. A minimal amount of trauma can cause devastating fracture in a patient with a fused spine.
3. Atlantoaxial subluxation may occur without significant degrees of peripheral disease in RA.
4. Inflammatory arthropathies of the axial skeleton are chronic illnesses that do not have a cure.
5. A patient with stable AS of long duration may develop spondylodiscitis with spinal instability that is difficult to treat.

KEY POINTS

1. Inflammatory spinal arthritis is an important, relatively common form of specific low back and neck pain.
2. Most patients with inflammatory spinal arthritis may be identified based on historical and physical examination findings along with plain radiographs.
3. New biologic therapies directed at specific cytokines can control the signs and symptoms of inflammatory arthritis and may slow progression of the disease.

KEY REFERENCES

1. Robinson PC, Brown MA. Genetics of ankylosing spondylitis. *Mol Immunol.* 2014;57:2-11.
   This article provides a lucid discussion of the role of genetics in the predisposition and pathogenesis of inflammatory arthropathies of the spine.
2. Singh JA, Saag KG, Bridges SL Jr, et al. 2015 American College of Rheumatology Guideline for the Treatment of Rheumatoid Arthritis. *Arthritis Rheumatol.* 2016;68(1):1-26.
   This current listing of new therapies for rheumatoid arthritis highlights the importance of early aggressive therapy.
3. Mandl P, Navarro-Compan V, Terslev L, et al. Recommendation for the use of imaging in the diagnosis and management of spondyloarthritis in clinical practice. *Ann Rheum Dis.* 2015;74:1327-1339.
   This is an excellent review of the radiologic methods needed to discover inflammatory alterations of the axial skeleton and the pathologic mechanisms that cause them.
4. Ward MW, Deodhar A, Akl E. American College of Rheumatology/Spondylitis Association of America/Spondyloarthritis Research and Treatment Network 2015 recommendations for the treatment of ankylosing spondylitis and nonradiographic axial spondyloarthritis. *Arthritis Rheum.* 2016;68(2):282-298.
   This is an excellent synopsis of current studies for the treatment of spondyloarthropathies.
5. Reiter MF, Boden SD. Inflammatory disorders of the cervical spine. *Spine.* 1998;23:2755-2766.
   The epidemiology, pathogenesis, and surgical considerations of inflammatory arthropathies that damage the cervical spine are reviewed.

REFERENCES

1. Revielle JD, Witter JP, Weisman MH. Prevalence of axial spondyloarthritis in the United States: estimates from a cross-sectional survey. *Arthritis Care Res (Hoboken).* 2012;64:905-910.
2. Schlosstein L, Terasaki PI, Bluestone R, et al. High association of an HL antigen, W27, with ankylosing spondylitis. *N Engl J Med.* 1973;288:704-706.

3. Lawrence RC, Helmick CG, Arnett FC, et al. Estimates of the prevalence of arthritis and selected musculoskeletal disorders in the United States. *Arthritis Rheum*. 1998;41:58-67.
4. Reveille JD, Ball EJ, Khan MA. HLA-B27 and genetic predisposing factors in spondyloarthropathies. *Curr Opin Rheumatol*. 2001;13:265-272.
5. Sieper J. Developments in the scientific and clinical understanding of the spondyoloarthritides. *Arthritis Res Ther*. 2009;11:208.
6. Gran JT, Ostensen M. Spondyloarthritides in females. *Ballieres Clin Rheumatol*. 1998;12:695-715.
7. Robinson PC, Brown MA. Genetics of ankylosing spondylitis. *Mol Immunol*. 2014;57:2-11.
8. Braun J, Khan MA, Siepper J. Enthesitis and ankylosis in spondyloarthropathy: what is the target of the immune response? *Ann Rheum Dis*. 2000;59:985-994.
9. Lories RJ, McInnes IB. Primed for inflammation: enthesis-resident T cells. *Nature Med*. 2012;18:1018-1019.
10. McGonagle D, Gibbon W, Emery P. Classification of inflammatory arthritis by enthesitis. *Lancet*. 1998;352:1137-1140.
11. Caplanne D, Tubach F, Le Parc JM. Late onset spondyloarthropathy: clinical and biological comparison with early onset patients. *Ann Rheum Dis*. 1997;56:176-179.
12. Van Tubergen A, Coenen J, Landewe R, et al. Assessment of fatigue in patients with ankylosing spondylitis: a psychometric analysis. *Arthritis Rheum*. 2002;47:8-16.
13. Mader R. Atypical clinical presentations of ankylosing spondylitis. *Semin Arthritis Rheum*. 1999;29:191-196.
14. Fox MW, Onofrio BM, Kilgore JE. Neurological complications of ankylosing spondylitis. *J Neurosurg*. 1993;78:871-878.
15. Sorin S, Askari A, Moskowitz RW. Atlantoaxial subluxation as a complication of early ankylosing spondylitis. *Arthritis Rheum*. 1979;22:273-276.
16. Ramos-Remus C, Gomez-Vargas A, Hernandez-Chavez A, et al. Two-year follow-up of anterior and vertical atlantoaxial subluxations in ankylosing spondylitis. *J Rheumatol*. 1997;24:507-510.
17. Hamilton MG, MacRae ME. Atlantoaxial dislocation as the presenting symptom of ankylosing spondylitis. *Spine*. 1993;18:2344-2346.
18. Lee JS, Lee S, Bang SY, et al. Prevalence and risk factors of anterior atlantoaxial subluxation in ankylosing spondylitis. *J Rheumatol*. 2012;39:2321-2326.
19. Broom MJ, Raycroft JF. Complications of fractures of the cervical spine in ankylosing spondylitis. *Spine*. 1988;13:763-766.
20. Klingberg E, Geijer M, Gothlin J, et al. Vertebral fractures in ankylosing spondylitis are associated with lower bone mineral density in the central and peripheral skeleton. *J Rheumatol*. 2012;39:1987-1995.
21. Detwiler KN, Loftus CM, Godersky JC, et al. Management of cervical spine injuries in patients with ankylosing spondylitis. *J Neurosurg*. 1990;72:210-215.
22. Prieto-Alhambra D, Munoz-Ortego J, De Vries F, et al. Ankylosing spondylitis confers substantially increased risk of clinical spine fractures: a nationwide case-control study. *Osteoporosl Int*. 2015;26:85-91.
23. Harrop JS, Sharan A, Anderson G, et al. Failure of standard imaging to detect a cervical fracture in a patient with ankylosing spondylitis. *Spine*. 2005;30:E417-E419.
24. Rowed DW. Management of cervical spinal cord injury in ankylosing spondylitis: the intervertebral disc as a cause of cord compression. *J Neurosurg*. 1992;77:241-246.
25. Foo D, Sarkarati M, Marcelino V. Cervical spinal cord injury complicating ankylosing spondylitis. *Paraplegia*. 1985;23:358-365.
26. Kabasakal Y, Garrett SL, Calin A. The epidemiology of spondylodiscitis in ankylosing spondylitis—a controlled study. *Br J Rheumatol*. 1996;35:660-663.
27. Rasker JJ, Prevo RL, Lanting PJ. Spondylodiscitis in ankylosing spondylitis, inflammation or trauma? A description of six cases. *Scand J Rheumatol*. 1996;25:52-57.
28. Spoorenberg A, van der Heijde D, de Klerk E, et al. Relative value of erythrocyte sedimentation rate and C-reactive protein in assessment of disease activity in ankylosing spondylitis. *J Rheumatol*. 1999;26:980-984.
29. McEwen C, DiTata D, Ling GC, et al. Ankylosing spondylitis and spondylitis accompanying ulcerative colitis, regional enteritis, psoriasis, and Reiter's disease: a comparative study. *Arthritis Rheum*. 1971;14:291-318.
30. Mandl P, Navarro-Compan V, Terslev L, et al. EULAR recommendation for the use of imaging in the diagnosis and management of spondyloarthritis in clinical practice. *Ann Rheum Dis*. 2015;74:1327-1339.
31. Ostergaard M, Lambert RG. Imaging in ankylosing spondylitis. *Ther Adv Muscuoloskelt Dis*. 2012;301-311.
32. van der Linden S, Valkenburg HA, Cats A. Evaluation of diagnostic criteria for ankylosing spondylitis: a proposal for modification of the New York criteria. *Arthritis Rheum*. 1984;27:361-368.
33. Rudwaleit M, van der Heijde D, Landewe R, et al. The development of Assessment of Spondyloarthritis International Society classification criteria for axial spondyloarthritis (part II): validation and final selection. *Ann Rheum Dis*. 2009;68:777-783.
34. Boyer GS, Templin DW, Bowler A, et al. A comparison of patients with spondyloarthropathy seen in specialty clinics with those identified in a communitywide epidemiologic study. *Arch Intern Med*. 1997;157:2111-2117.
35. Cohen MR, Reda DJ, Clegg DO. Baseline relationships between psoriasis and psoriatic arthritis: analysis of 221 patients with active psoriatic arthritis. *J Rheumatol*. 1999;26:1752-1756.
36. Gladman DD. Psoriatic arthritis. *Rheum Dis Clin North Am*. 1998;24:829-844.
37. Sosner J, Fast A, Kahan BS. Odontoid fracture and C1-C2 subluxation in psoriatic cervical spondyloarthropathy. *Spine*. 1996;21:519-521.
38. Taylor W, Gladman D, Helliwell P, et al. Classification criteria for psoriatic arthritis; development of new criteria from a large internation study. *Arthritis Rheum*. 2006;54:2665-2673.
39. Gossec L, Smolen JS, Gaujoux-Viala C, et al. European League Against Rheumatism recommendations for the management of psoriatic arthritis with pharmacological therapies. *Ann Rheum Dis*. 2012;71:4-12.
40. Arnett FC, McClusky E, Schacter BZ, et al. Incomplete Reiter's syndrome: discriminating features and HLA-W27 in diagnosis. *Ann Intern Med*. 1976;84:8-12.
41. Carter JD, Hudson AP. Reactive arthritis: clinical aspects and medical management. *Rheum Dis Clinics North Am*. 2009;35::21-44.
42. Abraham C, Cho JH. Inflammatory bowel disease. *N Engl J Med*. 2009;361:2066-2078.
43. Bourikas LA, Papadakis KA. Musculoskeletal manifestations of inflammatory bowel disease. *Inflamm Bowel Dis*. 2009;15:1915-1924.
44. Ford AC, Sandborn WJ, Khan KJ, et al. Efficacy of biological therapies in inflammatory bowel disease: systematic review

and meta-analysis. *Am J Gastroenterol.* 2011;106: 644-659.

45. Yagan R, Khan MA. Confusion of roentgenographic differential diagnosis of ankylosing hyperostosis (Forestier's disease) and ankylosing spondylitis. *Spine State Art Rev.* 1990;4:561-572.
46. Durback MA, Edelstein G, Schumacher HR Jr. Abnormalities of the sacroiliac joints in diffuse idiopathic skeletal hyperostosis: demonstration by computed tomography. *J Rheumatol.* 1988;15:1506-1511.
47. Williamson PK, Reginato AJ. Diffuse idiopathic skeletal hyperostosis of the cervical spine in a patient with ankylosing spondylitis. *Arthritis Rheum.* 1984;27:570-573.
48. Ward MW, Deodhar A, Akl E. American College of Rheumatology/Spondylitis Association of America/ Spondyloarthritis Research and Treatment Network 2015 recommendations for the treatment of ankylosing spondylitis and nonradiographic axial spondyloarthritis. *Arthritis Rheum.* 2016;68(2):282-298.
49. Callhoff J, Sieper J, Weib A, et al. Efficacy of TNF alpha blockers in patients with ankylosing spondylitis and non-radiographic axial spondyloarthritis: a meta-analysis. *Ann Rheum Dis.* 2015;74:1241-1248.
50. Kennedy LG, Edmunds L, Calin A. The natural history of ankylosing spondylitis: does it burn out? *J Rheumatol.* 1993;20:688-692.
51. Helmick CG, Felson DT, Lawrence RC, et al. Estimates of the prevalence of arthritis and other rheumatic conditions in the United States. Part 1. *Arthritis Rheum.* 2008;58:15-25.
52. Lee DM, Weinblatt ME. Rheumatoid arthritis. *Lancet.* 2001;358:903-911.
53. Lawrence JS, Sharp J, Ball J, et al. Rheumatoid arthritis of the lumbar spine. *Ann Rheum Dis.* 1964;23:205-217.
54. McInnes IB, Schett G. The pathogenesis of rheumatoid arthritis. *N Engl J Med.* 2011;365:2205-2219.
55. Gordon DA, Hastings DE. Clinical features of rheumatoid arthritis. In: Hochberg MC, Silman AJ, Smolen JS, et al., eds. *Rheumatology*. 3rd ed. Edinburgh: Mosby; 2003:765-780.
56. Zeidman SM, Ducker TB. Rheumatoid arthritis: neuroanatomy, compression, and grading of deficits. *Spine.* 1994;19:2259-2266.
57. Reiter MF, Boden SD. Inflammatory disorders of the cervical spine. *Spine.* 1998;23:2755-2766.
58. Yonezawa T, Tsuji H, Matsui H, Hirano N. Subaxial lesions in rheumatoid arthritis: radiographic factors suggestive of lower cervical myelopathy. *Spine.* 1995;20:208-215.
59. Halla JT, Hardin JG, Vitek J, et al. Involvement of the cervical spine in rheumatoid arthritis. *Arthritis Rheum.* 1989;32:652-659.
60. Myasoedova E, Crowson CS, Turesson C, et al. Incidence of extraarticular rheumatoid arthritis in Olmsted County, Minnesota, in 1995-2007 versus 1985-1994: a population-based study. *J Rheumatol.* 2011;38:983-989.
61. Webb F, Hickman J, Brew D. Death from vertebral artery thrombosis in rheumatoid arthritis. *BMJ.* 1968;2:537-538.
62. Chang MH, Liao KK, Cheung SC, et al. "Numb, clumsy hands" and tactile agnosia secondary to high cervical spondylotic myelopathy: a clinical and electrophysiological correlation. *Acta Neurol Scand.* 1992;86:622-625.
63. Klareskog L, Ronnelid J, Lundberg K, et al. Immunity to citrullinated proteins in rheumatoid arthritis. *Annu Rev Immunol.* 2008;26:651-675.
64. Schellekens GA, Visser H, de Jong BA, et al. The diagnostic properties of rheumatoid arthritis antibodies recognizing a cyclic citrullinated peptide. *Arthritis Rheum.* 2000;43:155-163.
65. Fujiwara K, Fujimoto M, Owaki H, et al. Cervical lesions related to the systemic progression in rheumatoid arthritis. *Spine.* 1998;23:2052-2056.
66. Bland JH, Van Buskirk FW, Tampas JP, et al. A study of roentgenographic criteria for rheumatoid arthritis of the cervical spine. *AJR Am J Roentgenol.* 1965;95:949-954.
67. Komusi T, Munro T, Harth M. Radiologic review: the rheumatoid cervical spine. *Semin Arthritis Rheum.* 1985;14:187-195.
68. Oostveen JCM, van de Laar MAFJ. Magnetic resonance imaging in rheumatic disorders of the spine and sacroiliac joints. *Semin Arthritis Rheum.* 2000;30:52-69.
69. Aletha D, Neogi T, Silman AJ, et al. 2010 Rheumatoid arthritis classification criteria: an American College of Rheumatology/ European League Against Rheumatismn collaborative initiative. *Arthritis Rheum.* 2010;62:2569-2981.
70. Singh JA, Saag KG, Bridges SL Jr, et al. 2015 American College of Rheumatology Guideline for the Treatment of Rheumatoid Arthritis. *Arthritis Rheum.* 2016;68(1):1-26.
71. Kremer JM. Rational use of new and existing disease-modifying agents in rheumatoid arthritis. *Ann Intern Med.* 2001;134:695-706.
72. Van Everdingen AA, Jacobs JWG, van Reesema DRS, et al. Low-dose prednisone therapy for patients with early active rheumatoid arthritis: clinical efficacy, disease-modifying properties, and side effects. *Ann Intern Med.* 2002; 136:1-12.
73. Maini R, St. Clair EW, Breedveld F, et al. Infliximab (chimeric anti-tumor necrosis factor α monoclonal antibody) versus placebo in rheumatoid arthritis patients receiving concomitant methotrexate: a randomized phase III trial. *Lancet.* 1999;354:1932-1939.
74. Lipsky PE, van der Heijde DMFM, St. Clair EW, et al. Infliximab and methotrexate in the treatment of rheumatoid arthritis. *N Engl J Med.* 2000;343:1594-1602.
75. Moreland LW, Schiff MH, Baumgartner SW, et al. Etanercept therapy in rheumatoid arthritis: a randomized controlled trial. *Ann Intern Med.* 1999;130:478-486.
76. Weinblatt ME, Kremer JM, Bankhurst AD, et al. A trial of etanercept, a recombinant tumor necrosis factor: Fc fusion protein in patients with rheumatoid arthritis receiving methotrexate. *N Engl J Med.* 1999;340:253-259.
77. Bathon JM, Martin RW, Fleischmann RM, et al. A comparison of etanercept and methotrexate in patients with early rheumatoid arthritis. *N Engl J Med.* 2000;343:1586-1593.
78. Weinblatt ME, Keystone EC, Furst DE, et al. Adalimumab, a fully human anti-tumor necrosis factor alpha monoclonal antibody, for the treatment of rheumatoid arthritis in patients taking concomitant methotrexate: the ARMADA trial. *Arthritis Rheum.* 2003;48:35-45.
79. Smolen J, Landewe RB, Mease P, et al. Efficacy and safety of certolizumab pegol plus methotrexate in active rheumatoid arthritis: the RAPID 2 study. A randomized controlled trial. *Ann Rheum Dis.* 2009;68:797-804.
80. Golimumab, a human antibody to tumour necrosis factor (alpha) given by monthly subcutaneous injections in active rheumatoid arthritis despite methotrexate therapy: the Go-Forward Study. *Ann Rheum Dis.* 2009;68:789-796.
81. Keane J, Gershon S, Wise RP, et al. Tuberculosis associated with infliximab, a tumor necrosis factor α-neutralizing agent. *N Engl J Med.* 2001;345:1098-1104.
82. Baghai M, Osmon DR, Wolk DM, et al. Fatal sepsis in a patient with rheumatoid arthritis treated with etanercept. *Mayo Clin Proc.* 2001;76:653-656.

83. Cohen S, Hurd E, Cush J, et al. Treatment of rheumatoid arthritis with anakinra: a recombinant human interleukin-1 receptor antagonist, in combination with methotrexate: results of a twenty-four-week, multicenter, randomized, double-blind, placebo-controlled trial. *Arthritis Rheum*. 2002;46:614-624.
84. Kremer JM, Blanco R, Brzosko M, et al. Tocilizumab inhibits structural joint damage in rheumatoid arthritis patients with inadequate responses to methotrexate: results from the double-blind treatment phase of a randomized placebo-controlled trial of tocilizumab safety and prevention of structural joint damage at one year. *Arthritis Rheum*. 2011;63:609-621.
85. Kremer JM, Genant HK, Moreland LW, et al. Results of a two-year followup study of patients with rheumatoid arthritis who received a combination of Abatacept and methotrexate. *Arthritis Rheum*. 2008;58:953-963.
86. Cohen SB, Emery P, Greenwald MW, et al. Rituximab for rheumatoid arthritis refractory to anti-tumor necrosis factor therapy: results of a multicenter, randomized, double-blind, placebo-controlled, phase III trial evaluating primary efficacy and safety at twenty-four weeks. *Arthritis Rheum*. 2006;54:2793-2806.
87. Fleischmann R, Kremer J, Cush J, et al. Placebo-controlled trial of tofacitinib monotherapy in rheumatoid arthritis. *N Engl J Med*. 2012;367:495-507.
88. Neva MH, Kauppi MJ, Kautiainen H, et al. Combination drug therapy retards the development of rheumatoid atlantoaxial subluxations. *Arthritis Rheum*. 2000;43:2397-2401.
89. Kauppi M, Anttila P. A stiff collar can restrict atlantoaxial instability in rheumatoid atlantoaxial subluxations. *Br J Rheumatol*. 1996;35:771-774.
90. Riise T, Jacobsen BK, Gran JT. High mortality in patients with rheumatoid arthritis and atlantoaxial subluxations. *J Rheumatol*. 2001;28:2425-2429.
91. Cha TD, An HS. Cervical spine manifestations in patients with inflammatory arthritides. *Nature Rev Rheumatol*. 2013;9:423-432.

84 CHAPTER Surgical Management of Rheumatoid Arthritis

Shari Cui
Scott D. Daffner
Sanford E. Emery

Rheumatoid arthritis (RA) is a chronic, progressive, systemic disease with widespread involvement of connective tissues, primarily synovial joints. Females are affected two to three times more often than males, with the majority of cases presenting in the fourth or fifth decades. Improvements in medical management have correlated with a decrease in hospitalizations for severe rheumatoid disease over the years.[1] The effect of biologic medications and other disease-modifying antirheumatic drugs (DMARDs) on the incidence of cervical spine surgery, however, varies in literature, with some studies showing decreased incidence and others no significant change.[2,3] The cervical spine is involved in 25% to 90% of patients with RA, making it the most commonly affected site after the metatarsophalangeal and metacarpophalangeal joints.[4,5] In contrast to RA of the thoracic and lumbar spine, cervical spine involvement carries significant risks of spinal cord, medullary, and vertebral artery compromise, which can lead to sudden death.[6–8]

Patients with cervical instability may be asymptomatic or present with pain and/or neurologic complaints. Neva et al. attempted to define the prevalence of cervical subluxation in this population.[9] They evaluated 154 Finnish patients with RA who were awaiting an orthopaedic procedure and found that 44% of patients had radiographic evidence of cervical subluxation or prior surgical fusion. Excluding patients with fusions, 69% of the patients with radiographic subluxation reported neck pain compared to 65% of patients without subluxation. Rates of occipital, temporal, retro-orbital, and upper extremity radicular pain were similar, with or without cervical instability. Nazarinia et al. studied 100 asymptomatic rheumatoid patients and found cervical subluxation in 17% on dynamic radiographs.[10] The only meaningful correlation found was with elevated C-reactive protein (CRP). Unfortunately, a large proportion of patients with significant cervical involvement may be overlooked by the treating physician due to the lack of clear findings on physical examination. The physician must therefore be cognizant of the natural history, pathophysiology, clinical presentation, radiologic findings, and treatment options to avoid potentially significant consequences of rheumatoid disease of the cervical spine.

Historical Perspective

There is some evidence that RA was described in the 17th and 18th centuries.[11,12] However, a more concrete description was reported around 1800 by Landré-Beauvais, a French medical student, in his doctoral thesis.[13] Rheumatoid involvement of the cervical spine was described much later (in 1890) by A. E. Garrod.[14]

Reports on cervical instability increased in the 1950s and 1960s[15–18] and articles on its surgical treatment followed in the 1960s and 1970s.[19–23] For the most part, C1–C2 fusion with Gallie-type[24] wiring and graft techniques were utilized early on and later modified by Brooks,[25] Wertheim and Bohlman,[26] and Clark et al.[27] Other types of C1–C2 fixation emerged with the use of the Halifax interlaminar clamp,[28] Magerl transarticular screw,[29–34] and posterior C1 lateral mass–C2 pedicle screw fixation.[35]

Occipitocervical procedures were originally described by Foerster in 1927[36] and modified to include iliac crest bone graft by Kahn and Yglesias in 1935.[37] The addition of wiring by Hamblen in 1967 was described in four rheumatoid patients.[21] Brattström and Granholm modified the wiring technique for occipitocervical fusion by adding methylmethacrylate in a 1976 report.[19] Evolution of techniques continued in the 1980s with the emergence of the looped rod with iliac crest bone graft as described by Ransford et al.[38] and Flint et al[39] and later by occipitocervical plating, described by Grob et al.[29,40] and Smith et al.[41] Current use of plate or rod fixation extends to the subaxial spine, especially with fixation of the lateral masses as described by Magerl and Roy-Camille.[30,31,33]

Pathophysiology

The inflammatory process in the cervical spine mirrors that in other sites of the body and consists predominantly of T lymphocytes, macrophages, and plasma cells in a hypervascular synoviocytic pannus.[42,43] The inflammatory reaction has a predilection for synovial joints; as such, the facets, uncovertebral, atlanto-occipital, and atlantodens joints are preferably affected over the discoligamentous structures in the cervical spine.[44] This is in contrast to the traditional pattern of age-related degenerative changes. The cervical spine relies heavily on ligaments and joint congruency for stability and thus is at greater risk for instability than the thoracic or lumbar spine. Cervical instability can result from inflammatory changes that cause pannus formation and erosion of joint surfaces and capsular structures. These manifest as atlantoaxial (C1–C2) subluxation (AAS), subaxial subluxation, cranial settling (also known as basilar invagination or atlantoaxial impaction), or a combination of these. Although biologic pharmaceuticals and other DMARDs have been credited with lowering the prevalence of cervical spine instability, modern medical treatment cannot prevent progression of preexisting damage.[45–48] Rheumatoid discitis may also occur at the discovertebral junctions with noninfectious erosion of the endplates.[6]

Atlantoaxial instability is the most common instability pattern in the rheumatoid cervical spine and associated with the development of a periodontoid pannus and progressive inflammatory joint destruction.[44,49,50] Pannus formation localizes around the synovial joint formed between the transverse ligament, the posterior arch of the atlas, and the base of the odontoid. The soft tissue may compress the spinal cord and often distends and erodes the surrounding periodontoid-ligamentous structures (alar, apical, and transverse ligaments), the odontoid process (dens), and the lateral articular masses between C1 and C2.[51] Erosion of the dens may even lead to the development of occult, atraumatic dens fractures.[52] Subsequent static or dynamic instability or subluxation occurred historically in 50% to 70% of patients.[23,53] Most often, the subluxation is anterior (70%), but lateral, posterior, and rotational subluxations can also occur.[54,55] Anterior subluxation of 0 to 3 mm is normal in adults, 3 to 6 mm suggests instability with disruption of the transverse ligament, and 9 mm or more suggests disruption of the entire periodontoid-ligamentous and capsular structures with gross instability.[23,56,57]

The combination of periodontoid pannus buildup and instability may cause spinal cord and root impingement leading to myeloradiculopathy and potentially sudden death. Delamarter and Bohlman[58] conducted postmortem studies suggesting that paralysis can be due to both mechanical neural compression and/or vascular impairment of the neural structures. Henderson et al.[59] reported that diffuse axonal injury with or without frank necrosis may irreversibly affect the spinal cord due to mechanical damage. These findings may partly explain the smaller diameter and cross-sectional area of the spinal cord found in patients with severe disease.[60] Surgical stabilization can result in pannus regression.[49,61]

Posterior atlantoaxial subluxation is rare and should raise the possibility of an anterior arch defect of the atlas or erosion, or fracture, of the odontoid.[57] Patients usually present with myelopathy and posterior kinking of the cord without radiographic compression.[62] Lateral subluxation is defined as more than 2 mm of lateral displacement of the C1–C2 lateral masses, occurs in up to 21% of atlantoaxial subluxations,[57] and is often accompanied by rotational deformity.[63]

Subaxial subluxation is the second most common instability pattern and results from destruction of the facet joints, interspinous ligaments, and discovertebral joints.[53,64] These pathologic changes can lead to longitudinal collapse, bony erosion, soft tissue hypertrophy, and multisegmental sagittal plane instability, causing a "step ladder" type of deformity pattern. Patients can demonstrate significant preoperative neurologic deficits, and improvements from surgical intervention are at times short lived. Worsening rheumatoid disease and complications can result in deterioration of outcome and mortality rates as high as 20% and 33% at 5 and 10 years, respectively, even after surgery.[65] Cranial settling is the least common, yet most ominous, form of instability and occurs primarily due to bone and cartilage destruction at the atlantoaxial and occipitoatlantal joints. Caudad settling of the cranium and apparent cranial migration of the odontoid are characteristic. As a result, there is an increased risk of sudden death from either static or dynamic stenosis of the foramen magnum and compression of the brain stem. Other sequelae include obstructive hydrocephalus or syringomyelia, presumably from obstructing the normal flow of cerebrospinal fluid. In some cases, fixed rotation of the head may occur due to unilateral joint destruction.

Natural History

It is difficult to study the natural history of RA since patients are usually treated at some stage of the disease. Studies have shown that inflammatory processes in the cervical spine begin early after the onset of RA and progress along with peripheral involvement. Atlantoaxial instability may be detected within 2 to 10 years of disease onset,[66] and there is a strong correlation between cervical spine subluxation and peripheral erosions of the hands and feet.[66] Although the spine is commonly affected, only approximately 10% of patients with cervical spine involvement will eventually require surgery.[67] The natural history of RA of the spine without surgical intervention, especially in patients with myelopathy, is one of progressive disability and risk of sudden death. Vertebral artery injury and positional occlusion can also result from progressive instability.[8,68] In one study of 21 rheumatoid patients treated medically, 76% showed deterioration at an average of 6 years of follow-up.[69] All patients in the study became bedridden within 3 years of developing myelopathy and all died within 7 years, with one-third dying suddenly for unknown reasons. Risk factors for progression include mutilating articular disease, history of high-dose corticosteroid use, high seropositivity (rheumatoid factor), rheumatoid subcutaneous nodules, vasculitis, and male gender. Other potential risk factors for cervical involvement include high serum CRP level and HLA-Dw2 or -B27 positivity.[70,71] As the disease progresses, pain, neurologic deficits, and sudden death are the primary risks.

Clinical Presentation

Neck pain is the most common symptom in patients with cervical spine involvement. Peripheral erosive changes similarly occur along the apophyseal joints and surrounding soft tissues and may be a source of pain. Cervical instability may cause secondary impingement of the posterior rami of the lesser and greater occipital nerves, which may lead to occipital headaches. In general, pain in the suboccipital region suggests atlantoaxial pathology or cranial settling. Middle or lower cervical pain should suggest subaxial subluxation. Subaxial involvement may also lead to painful neck deformity with loss of sagittal plane supporting structures, which may later become fixed due to postinflammatory ankylosis. Patients may complain of a "clunking" sensation in the neck with neck motion. This condition/symptom is most common with C1–C2 instability due to spontaneous reduction of the subluxation with neck extension (Sharp-Purser test).[72]

Progressive instability can lead to decreased canal diameter and brain stem or cord compression. Myelopathy and vertebrobasilar dysfunction may result due to mechanical and ischemic damage to the white and gray matter evidenced on histologic specimens by long tract demyelinization, lateral column necrosis, and focal gliosis.[58] According to Bell,[73] C1–C2 instability may lead to a phenomenon termed "cruciate paralysis," characterized by upper motor neuron dysfunction of the upper extremities and normal lower extremities, similar to a mild central cord syndrome after trauma. Pathologically, there is selective injury to the decussating corticospinal tracts of the upper extremities at the level of the cervicomedullary junction with sparing of the uncrossed lower extremity pyramidal and extrapyramidal tracts.

Additional neurovascular changes may occur due to vertebral artery occlusion with decreased flow into the posterior inferior cerebellar artery and cephalad brain stem circulation. Without adequate collateral blood flow, these patients may develop Wallenberg syndrome or lateral medullary infarction. These clinical syndromes are characterized by ipsilateral cranial nerve palsies (cranial nerves V, IX, X, and XI), cerebellar ataxia, Horner syndrome (ptosis, miosis, anhidrosis, and enophthalmos), facial pain, and contralateral loss of pain and temperature sensation.[74] In rare instances, patients may develop quadriplegia, quadriplegia with facial muscle paralysis (locked-in syndrome),[75] and sudden death.[43,69]

Unlike pain symptoms, neurologic signs are less straightforward. Patients must be assessed keeping their global disease in mind. Progressive myelopathy may not be evident by loss of fine motor control, gait imbalance, or global numbness of the hands, but rather by the slow onset of deteriorating independence and becoming wheelchair bound. Often, hand deformities will mask motor deficits in the upper extremities and the patients' deteriorating ambulatory status may be attributed to large joint involvement rather than myelopathy. Progression of myelopathy, especially early disease, may be misinterpreted as progression of their peripheral disease. Therefore, a high index of suspicion is necessary to diagnose myelopathy, as these patients do poorly without early surgical intervention.[43,69]

The Ranawat grading system may provide some useful clinical information in assessing patients with neurologic deficits[76] (Table 84.1). This system classifies pain as none (grade 0), mild (1), moderate (2), or severe (3). Neurologic function falls into three classes: Class I has no neurologic deficit; class II has subjective weakness, dysesthesia, and hyperreflexia; and class III has objective weakness and long-tract signs. Class III is further subdivided into ambulatory patients (A) and quadriparetic nonambulatory patients (B). Casey et al. reported that only 25% of Ranawat IIIB patients who underwent surgical decompression and stabilization had a favorable outcome. The mortality rate was 13% after 30 days and 60% by 4 years.[77]

TABLE 84.1 Ranawat Criteria for Pain and Neural Assessment

Grade/Class	Description
Pain Assessment	
Grade 0	None
Grade 1	Mild, intermittent, requiring only aspirin analgesia
Grade 2	Moderate; a cervical collar is needed
Grade 3	Severe; pain could not be relieved by either aspirin or collar
Neural Assessment	
Class I	No neural deficit
Class II	Subjective weakness with hyperreflexia and dysesthesias
Class IIIA	Objective findings of paresis and long tract signs, but walking possible
Class IIIB	Quadriparesis with resultant inability to walk or feed oneself

From Ranawat CS, O'Leary P, Pellici P, et al. Cervical spine fusion in rheumatoid arthritis. *J Bone Joint Surg Am.* 1979;61A:1003–1010.

Radiologic Evaluation

Plain radiographs are an effective screening tool for identifying patients with atlantoaxial instability, cranial settling, or subaxial subluxations. Standard anterior-posterior (AP), open mouth (odontoid view), lateral, and controlled flexion-extension plain views should suffice. The flexion–extension views are the most important in detecting whether there is dynamic or static instability in the upper or lower cervical spine and allow for measurement of the anterior atlantodental interval (AADI) and posterior atlantodental interval (PADI). The AADI is the transverse distance from the anterior surface of the dens to the posterior margin of the anterior ring of C1, while the PADI is the distance between the posterior surface of the dens and the anterior margin of the posterior ring of the atlas. Historically, the AADI was used to screen patients who required surgical stabilization for atlantoaxial instability based on an AADI greater than 9 mm, with 0 to 6 mm suggesting instability and 0 to 3 mm being normal.[57] The AADI is limited by the occasional difficulty of obtaining accurate measurements in some patients because of erosive changes that distort anatomy and because there is some variation in the size of the C1 ring. In contrast, Boden et al.[78] showed that the PADI more reliably predicts neurologic outcome since it represents the space available for the cord. Patients with a PADI of at least 14 mm were more likely to have neurologic recovery after surgical stabilization, while those with a PADI less than 10 mm had no neurologic recovery. Anatomically, this correlates to the dura taking up 1 mm on the anterior and posterior sides, 2 mm of cerebrospinal fluid, and 10 mm for the cord for a total of 14 mm.[79] Neither measurement on plain films takes into account possible pannus formation with mass effect on the cord, which requires advanced imaging.

The open-mouth view is useful to identify lateral subluxation.[57,63] Erosive changes of the dens and C1–C2 articulations may also be visualized. Taniguchi et al. defined the atlanto-dental lateral shift (ADLS) as a means of assessing lateral atlantoaxial instability.[80] Utilizing dynamic open-mouth odontoid views (taken in maximal left and right lateral bending), the ADLS is calculated by dividing the distance from the center of the dens to the medial edge of the C1 lateral mass (in the direction of lateral bending) by the distance between the medial borders of the bilateral C1 lateral masses and is expressed as a percentage. In rheumatoid patients, the ADLS averaged 14.8% compared to 6.1% in control patients. Among patients with increased AADI, the ADLS averaged 20.6% versus 12.7% in patients without anterior atlantoaxial instability.

Posterior subluxation, though rare, may be seen on lateral radiographs of the cervical spine and should be suspected in patients with an absent or fractured odontoid process.[62] It is important to note that the AADI will decrease with worsening cranial settling as the arch of the atlas approaches the wider base of the odontoid process and is a potential source of mistaken radiographic improvement.

Cranial settling carries the greatest risk of neurologic deficits and sudden death, especially when superimposed on atlantoaxial instability. As a consequence, several measurement techniques have been utilized with varying sensitivity and specificity, based on lateral plain radiographs of the upper cervical spine[81] (Fig. 84.1). The majority of these techniques assess the relationship between the tip of the odontoid, the hard palate, and the base of the skull. Traditionally, the McGregor line (drawn from the posterior-superior tip of the hard palate to the caudad base of the occiput) has been widely used for its simplicity. Cranial settling occurs when the tip of the dens is more than 4.5 mm above this line. Erosive changes in the odontoid anatomy may make it difficult to analyze many of the measurement techniques; thus, Redlund-Johnell and Pettersson[82] described a technique that measured the vertical line from the midpoint of the caudad margin of C2 to the McGregor line. Cranial settling occurs when the distance is less than 34 mm in males or 29 mm in females. Ranawat et al.[76] described a similar technique in which the distance along the odontoid was measured from the C2 pedicle to the transverse axis of the ring of C1. This technique avoided problems with changes in odontoid anatomy and identifying the bony landmarks at the base of the skull and hard palate. Cranial settling was positive if the distance was less than 15 mm in males or 13 mm in females. Clark et al.[27] (Fig. 84.2) defined the "station of the atlas," which indicates the position of the anterior ring of C1 to parts of the body of the axis divided into thirds. Normally, the atlas is adjacent to the upper third (station I) of the axis. Riew et al.[81] noted that none of the current radiographic measurements alone had a high sensitivity, specificity, or negative or positive predictive value greater than 90% and therefore recommended the combination of the Clark station, Redlund-Johnell, and the Ranawat criteria with sensitivity and negative predictive values of 94% and 91%, respectively.

Subaxial subluxation can be evaluated on AP and lateral static and dynamic radiographs. White and Panjabi[83] defined radiographic cervical instability as 3.5 mm or more of vertebral translation and greater than 11 degrees of angular changes between adjacent motion segments, although their study is more representative of acute conditions. The space available for the cord should also be considered since critical stenosis may be present with or without instability. Boden et al.[78] correlated anatomic measurements with neurologic findings and reported that a sagittal diameter less than 14 mm is considered critically stenotic in the rheumatoid subaxial spine. This is in contrast to 13 mm in cervical spondylotic patients who do not have pannus in the canal.

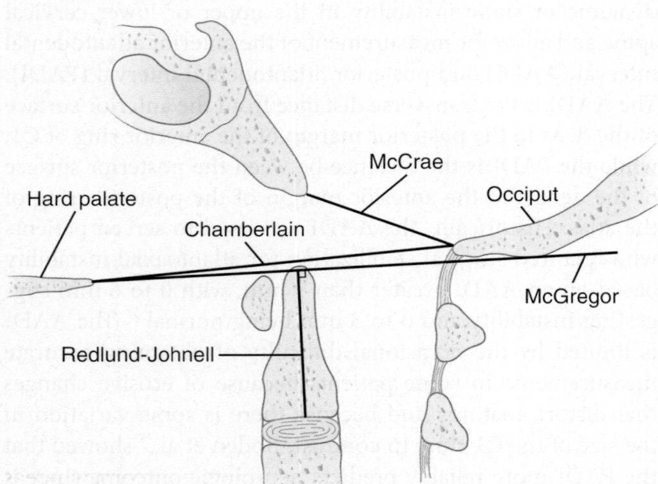

FIG. 84.1 Various measurements of basilar invagination. Chamberlain line: odontoid tip >6 mm above the line. McCrae line: odontoid tip above this line. McGregor line: males, odontoid tip >8 mm above the line; females, odontoid tip >9.7 mm above the line. Redlund-Johnell distance: males, <34 mm; females, <29 mm.

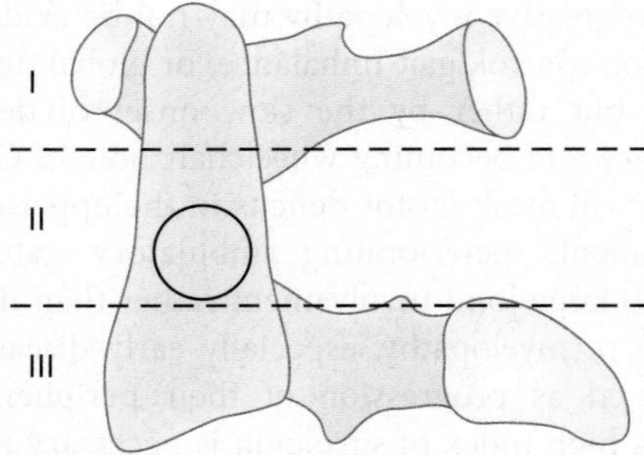

FIG. 84.2 The station of the atlas is determined by dividing the odontoid process into thirds in the sagittal plane. Normally, the anterior ring of the atlas should be adjacent to the cephalad third of the axis (station I). If the ring of the atlas is adjacent to the middle third of the axis, mild cranial settling is indicated (station II). If the anterior ring of the atlas is adjacent to the base of the axis, it is considered evidence of severe cranial settling (station III). (From Clark CR, Goetz DD, Menezes AH. Arthrodesis of the cervical spine in rheumatoid arthritis. *J Bone Joint Surg Am*. 1989;71:381-392.)

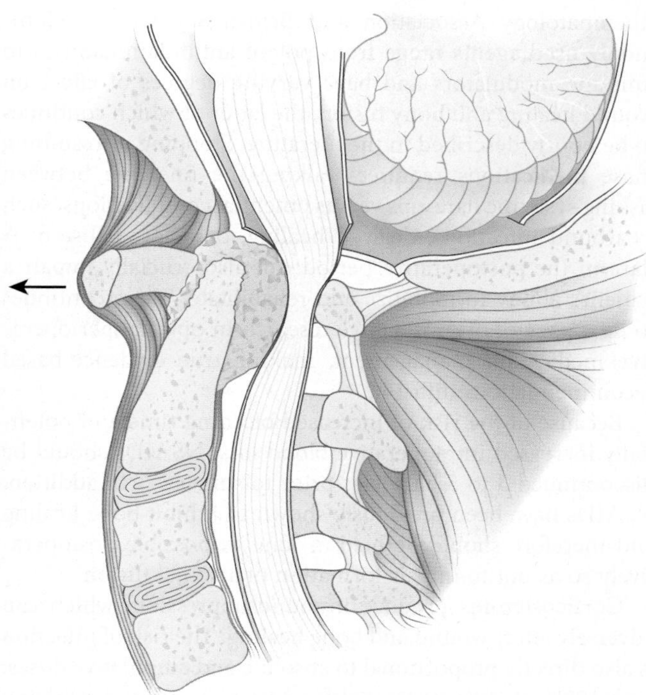

FIG. 84.3 Forward subluxation of the atlas on the axis, pannus formation around the odontoid process, and osseous erosions. There is severe compression of the spinal cord between the pannus anteriorly and the arch of the atlas posteriorly. (From Boden SD, Dodge LD, Bohlman HH, et al. Rheumatoid arthritis of the cervical spine: a long term analysis with predictors of paralysis and recovery. *J Bone Joint Surg Am*. 1993; 75:1282-1297.)

Patients with any radiographic instability, with or without symptoms or neurologic deficits, should be followed closely as existing instability of any subgroup (AAS, vertical subluxation, or subaxial subluxation) is at risk for accelerated progression to severe instability within 5 years.[84]

Computed tomography (CT), especially with intrathecal contrast, is a valuable addition to plain radiographs in delineating the bony anatomy and identifying cord compression and cranial settling. The degree of medullary compression on CT scans has been shown to correlate with myelopathy.[49] Static or dynamic magnetic resonance imaging (MRI), however, is the best option to assess the soft tissues and to look for the presence of periodontoid pannus (Fig. 84.3) and spinal cord or brain stem compression.[49,61,85–87] Myelopathic signs correlate with MRI findings[87] of a cervicomedullary angle of less than 135 degrees (normal, 135–175 degrees). This angle measures the intersection of vertical lines drawn along the anterior surface of the brain stem and the cord on a sagittal MRI.

Nonsurgical Treatment

Although life expectancy is lower in rheumatoid patients, many are living longer with advances in medical therapy that has slowed disease progression with fewer side effects.[70] Only a minority of these patients will eventually need surgical stabilization. Patients with early cervical disease and intermittent pain without radiographic instability or myelopathy can be managed with a soft cervical orthosis or trials of physical therapy. Medication options include nonsteroidal antiinflammatory drugs (NSAIDs), oral steroids (prednisone), and DMARDs such as methotrexate, gold, sulfasalazine, hydroxychloroquine, D-penicillamine, and azathioprine. Biologic agents such as tumor necrosis factor-α (TNF-α) and interleukin-1 (IL-1) antagonists have become more common. The addition of antiresorptive osteoporosis therapy may improve vertebral bone strength in rheumatoid patients.[88] Patients should be followed closely for neurologic or radiographic changes. Cervical collars provide support, warmth, some pain relief, and a feeling of stability; however, rigid collars are often poorly tolerated, especially in patients with temporomandibular disease, dental problems, and skin sensitivity and may have further detrimental effects by blocking spontaneous reduction of anterior atlantoaxial subluxation in extension.

Surgical Management

Indications

Patients with any one or more of the instability patterns described earlier—with or without associated pain, myelopathy, or neurologic deficits—should consider early surgery. Presence of mild or moderate instability should be followed closely due to high risk of progression to severe symptomatic instability.[84] As noted previously, radiographic indicators for surgery include an AADI of 9 mm or more, PADI of less than 14 mm, mobile subaxial subluxation greater than 3.5 mm, cord compression or space available for the cord of less than 14 mm, and cranial settling measured most accurately by the combination of the Clark station, Redlund-Johnell, and Ranawat criteria.[81] Computed tomographic myelograms and MRI demonstrating cord compression or a cervicomedullary angle of less than 135 degrees are suggestive of impending neurologic deficits and should be weighed heavily as an indication for surgery within the context of the remaining clinical picture. Patients with headaches in the distribution of the greater or lesser occipital nerve are likely to have atlantoaxial instability and may need C1–C2 arthrodesis for pain relief.

Timing of surgical intervention is crucial. In a retrospective review of 110 patients who underwent cervical spine fusion for RA, only three of 55 patients (5.5%) with early C1–C2 fusion for isolated AAS developed subaxial subluxation requiring surgery an average of 9 years later.[44] In contrast, 36% of patients who were stabilized for more progressive instability (atlantoaxial with cranial settling) developed recurrent cervical instability at a mean of 2.6 years. These authors recommended early surgery before cranial settling to decrease the risks of recurrent instability. In a series of 28 patients, Schmitt-Sody et al.[89] reported that seven of 10 patients who were Ranawat class II improved to class I following surgery, whereas only one of 11 class III patients improved (class IIIA to class II), and two patients deteriorated (class IIIA to class IIIB) postoperatively. Similarly, these authors recommended early surgical stabilization prior to the development of neurologic symptoms.

Preoperative Assessment

The goals of surgery should be pain relief, restoration of spinal alignment, decompression of neurologic deficits, and stabilization of the involved motion segments.

Thorough preoperative assessment is a prerequisite to good outcome in this often-fragile patient population. The quality of bone stock, presence of irreducible subluxations, and the overall medical condition of the patients should guide the preoperative decision-making process, including the potential need for awake fiberoptic nasal or endotracheal intubation.[90]

Patients with severe basilar invagination should be considered for preoperative skeletal traction using a halo ring (which can be incorporated into a halo vest after surgery) or cranial tongs. Preoperative traction can improve alignment and the resultant indirect decompression can improve neurologic symptoms and pain. Traction may be required for 3 to 7 days or longer, with wheelchair-halo configurations available to allow the patient greater mobility and avoid secondary problems, such as decubitus ulcers and pulmonary issues, associated with prolonged bed rest.[62,91,92] Gentle traction along the midline longitudinal axis with approximately 7 to 12 pounds, while avoiding hyperflexion or hyperextension, is recommended. Patients are monitored with frequent neurologic examinations (every 1–2 hours), and plain radiographs should be obtained to avoid overdistraction during the process. We have not felt the need to routinely use preoperative traction in atlantoaxial instability or subaxial subluxation. Many of these instabilities that moved little on preoperative flexion-extension views are better reduced when the patient is under general anesthesia positioned with the head holder (with concomitant use of neurophysiologic monitoring).

Once in the operating room, obtaining baseline neurophysiologic data, including somatosensory evoked potentials (SSEPs) and motor evoked potentials (MEPs), before and after positioning a myelopathic patient may alert the surgeon to impending spinal cord injury during or after positioning of the head and neck. Finally, the surgical approach should be determined by the underlying pathology and its location, in part analogous to the approach for compressive lesions in cervical spondylotic patients.[93,94]

Perioperative Management of Rheumatoid Medication

Approximately 80% of rheumatoid patients undergoing elective joint arthroplasty surgery are on corticosteroid therapy and 75% to 84% are on either traditional or biologic (anti-TNF-α) DMARDs.[95] Patients with rheumatoid spinal disease, in comparison, are typically older with greater disease progression, thereby making the possibility of medication complications even higher. Despite this potential, perioperative management of rheumatoid medications continues to be debated. Recommendations differ between rheumatologists and vary widely even among the rheumatology organizations; for example, anti-TNF-α discontinuation ranges from >1 week before surgery (American College of Rheumatology), to 2, 3, or up to 5 times the half-life of the drug (Canadian Rheumatology Association and British Society).[96–99] Commonly used agents range from potent antiinflammatories to immune modulators and have varying degrees of effect on wound healing and bony fusion, the latter of which continues to be poorly described in the literature. Stopping or resuming these medications requires walking the fine line between risking systemic flare-ups versus potential complications, such as wound infections, delayed healing, or delayed fusion. A flare in the postoperative period can also crucially impair a patient's ability to mobilize and rehabilitate. There continues to be a paucity of prospective research in optimal perioperative medication management, making true evidence-based recommendations difficult.

Because of the risk of increased bleeding time and potentially increased intraoperative blood loss, NSAIDs should be discontinued 3 to 5 half-lives prior to surgery.[100] In addition, NSAIDs have been previously shown to inhibit bone healing and therefore should be held as long as possible postoperatively so as not to impair formation of a spinal fusion.

Corticosteroids produce immunosuppression, which can adversely affect wound and bone healing. The risk of infection is also directly proportional to absolute and cumulative doses, with 100% of patients treated for 3 years or more developing an infection.[101] In addition, sudden stoppage of chronic corticosteroids may lead to adrenal insufficiency and hypotension, and patients are frequently given stress dosing. Several studies indicate, however, that patients receiving their usual dose of steroids responded to surgery (major and minor) with an increase in serum cortisol levels without signs of hemodynamic instability.[102–105] Most *spinal* procedures for this patient population, however, would be considered highly stressful, and patients on chronic moderate- to high-dose regimens (>20 mg/day of prednisone) should receive stress dose steroids on the day of surgery with rapid tapering over 1 to 2 days to their usual chronic dosage.[100,106]

Continued use of methotrexate in the perioperative period has not been shown to increase infection rates.[107] Previous studies linked methotrexate with nonunion following osteotomy of the extremities[108]; however, this result has not been found to be true in the existing spine literature.[109] Although withholding methotrexate may increase the likelihood of a flare-up of rheumatoid symptoms, we routinely discontinue its use 1 week preoperatively, and recommend that patients remain off of methotrexate postoperatively as long as symptomatology allows, up to 6 to 8 weeks.

Few studies exist to direct perioperative management of biologic agents such as TNF-α and IL-1 antagonists. Because of their strong immunoregulatory effects, these agents may predispose patients for opportunistic infections.[100,106] Early innate immune response to infection, particularly in the presence of orthopaedic implants, is heavily dependent on cellular defense mechanisms and activation by cytokines, such as TNF-α and IL-6.[110] In a recent meta-analysis of rheumatoid patients undergoing major orthopaedic surgery (the majority were joint arthroplasties), 3681 patients had a history of preoperative treatment by TNF-α inhibitors and 4310 patients did not. Exposure to an anti-TNF-α agent preoperatively was shown to favor infection. Odds ratios were 3.16 for studies

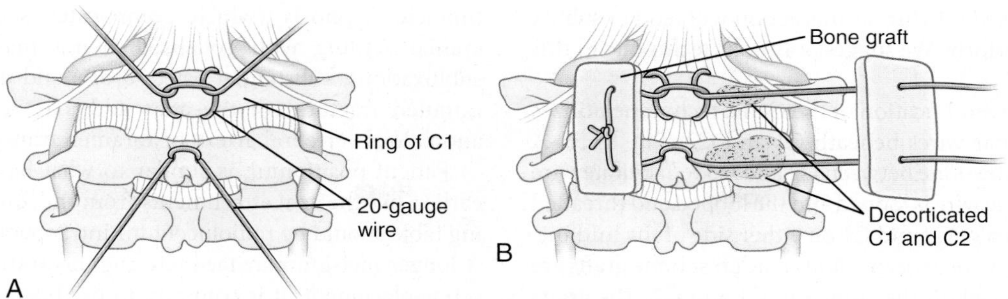

FIG. 84.4 Modified Gallie-type wiring for a posterior C1–C2 arthrodesis.

with confirmed rheumatoid diagnoses and 3.01 for studies meeting Centers for Disease Control and Prevention (CDC) criteria for infection. All studies included were retrospective. There are no data on these agents' effects on bone fusion; however, anti-TNF-α agents may allow expedited postoperative hemoglobin recovery.[111] Duration of discontinuation lacks high-quality evidence and control in the available literature, as cohorts are comprised of a heterogeneous mix of surgical procedures and variable arbitrary time intervals selected for withholding treatment.[112,113] Current recommendations are to discontinue biologic agents preoperatively (for 1.5 times the dosing interval),[114] and restart 10 to 14 days postoperatively at wound healing.

It is our practice to confer with the treating rheumatologist and individualize the duration of drug holiday, before and after surgery, based on patient factors (disease severity, duration, quality of disease control) and the extent of surgery required. As treatment with anti-TNF-α agents has been linked with neurologic adverse events such as demyelinating lesions and peripheral neuropathy, nontraditional manifestation of spinal disease should be worked up prior to surgery.[115,116] Postoperatively, patients should be monitored with daily laboratory tests due to baseline myelosuppression and placed on a regimen for nutritional optimization and vitamin/mineral supplementation.

Operative Procedures

Atlantoaxial (C1–C2) Instability

Posterior fusion is considered the standard treatment for C1–C2 instability.[35,117–119] The Gallie[24] and Brooks[25] wiring techniques require the presence of the posterior arch of C1, supplemental bone graft, and external immobilization. Claw-type constructs such as the Halifax clamp are rarely used today because of biomechanical limitations and better options. Transarticular screw fixation is popular because of its multidirectional rigidity, but it requires intraoperative fluoroscopy and preoperative axial imaging to visualize the vertebral artery anatomy. Direct screw fixation of the C1 lateral masses and C2 pedicles, pars, or lamina has become the most common and effective technique.[35,117–120]

Wire Techniques

Stand-alone wiring techniques have largely fallen by the wayside in favor of transarticular screw or direct screw-rod fixation techniques. Wiring techniques are frequently used as adjuncts to other fixation, particularly for securing bone graft material to help facilitate fusion or as a "bailout" in patients with anatomy unfavorable to other techniques. Sublaminar wire fixation is obtained on the C1 ring and around the C2 spinous process (Fig. 84.4). However, we recommend a modification of the Gallie technique. The patient's head is placed in a tong-type holder for rigid positioning with reduction checked by intraoperative imaging. The chin should be tucked to open the space between the occiput and C1 to facilitate passage of sublaminar wire. Note that an occiput–C2 fusion may be safer with or without a C1 laminectomy in cases of an inadequate posterior space available for safe wire passage of an unreducible C1 ring.

A posterior exposure is utilized, remaining close to the midline with approximately 1.5 cm lateral dissection in each direction on the C1 ring to avoid the vertebral artery and the venous plexus between C1 and C2. Cobb elevators are utilized to subperiosteally expose the base of the occiput to the caudad aspect of the C2 lamina at a minimum. Small curettes can be used to develop the plane under the C1 ring for wire passage. Loop a 20-gauge wire with the tip contoured for safe passage under the C1 ring. A nerve hook is used to engage the loop and pull it through approximately 2 cm. The free ends of the 20-gauge wire are then fed through the loop and the wire is cinched down tightly onto the C1 ring at the midline. Alternatively, sutures may be passed underneath C1 with a Mayo needle placed in a reverse manner with the blunt end from caudad to cephalad. Wires are then placed within the suture loops and passed underneath the lamina as the sutures are withdrawn caudally. A burr hole is made at the base of the C2 spinous process and a second 20-gauge wire is passed through the hole and looped beneath the spinous process and through the hole again to provide stress distribution. Two rectangular blocks of corticocancellous iliac crest bone graft can be harvested and placed over the laminae of C1 and C2 on either side of the midline. The grafts should be near full thickness to allow for tightening of the wires with less risk of breaking through the fragile bone. The wires are tightened over the graft while watching closely to prevent wire breakthrough. Cancellous chips can be placed around the bone blocks, especially on the ring of C1, where nonunions tend to occur. A drain is typically used and the wound closed in layers. If no supplemental internal fixation is used, a halo vest may be needed postoperatively to help maintain reduction. Care must be taken when tightening the wires in the unusual case of a posteriorly subluxed C1 ring, as this action will tend to sublux the C1 ring posteriorly. We suggest a Brooks technique in this situation.

A Brooks-type modification of the Gallie technique utilizes bilateral sublaminar wires beneath C1 and C2 (Fig. 84.5). A laminotomy may be done between C2 and C3 to facilitate wire passage; a 20-gauge wire is looped and the looped end threaded beneath the lamina of C2 and C1 on either side of the midline. Near full-thickness corticocancellous iliac crest bone grafts are harvested and placed on the lamina of C1 and C2. The grafts should be contoured to fit snugly to reduce the risk of graft slippage. Alternatively, a full bone block may be used with a caudad notch to fit around the C2 spinous process. Decortication is not necessary and risks weakening the lamina. The wires are then tightened down in a longitudinal fashion over the bone block on either side. This fixation may provide more rotational stability over the Gallie technique because of fixation on both sides of the midline. A halo vest may be used at the discretion of the surgeon based on the need for maintaining reduction and the adequacy of intraoperative fixation.

Transarticular Screw Fixation

This technique provides rigid fixation for atlantoaxial fusion and can be used in conjunction with wire techniques to provide three-point fixation.[33] (Figs. 84.6 and 84.7) It rigidly fixes the C1 and C2 facets, minimizing the need for postoperative external immobilization. Preoperative CT scan is necessary to adequately define the vertebral artery anatomy. It also ensures that the C2 isthmus is wide enough to accept at least a 3.5-mm screw and that the lateral mass of C1 is reduced and aligned with the superior facet of C2. Other considerations that may preclude the use of this technique include significant thoracic kyphosis (which complicates screw placement), cranial settling with collapsed lateral masses, irreducible subluxations, substantial osteoporosis and osteopenia, comminuted fractures of the atlas and axis vertebrae, and an anomalous vertebral artery or foramen transversarium.

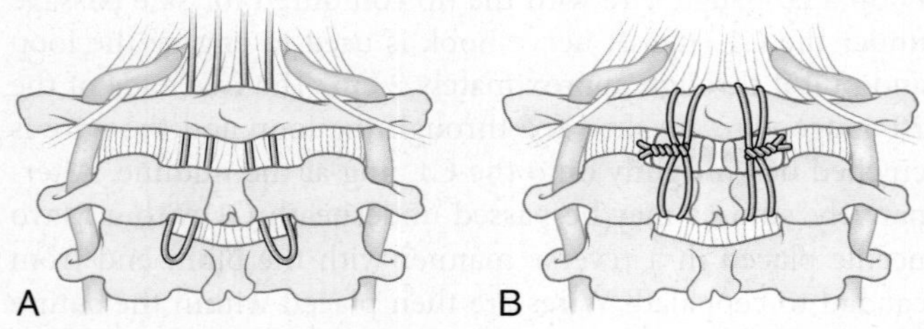

FIG. 84.5 Brooks-type wiring for a posterior C1–C2 arthrodesis. (A) Sublaminar wires are passed under both C1 and C2 and are tightened down over wedge-shaped, sculpted corticocancellous grafts. (B) The shaping of the grafts minimizes the chance of graft displacement into the canal.

Patient positioning is similar to what has been described earlier, but the arm attachments from the tongs to the operating table should be radiolucent for intraoperative fluoroscopy. A longer incision may facilitate angling of the drill guide and screw placement. It is common to use bilateral percutaneous stab wounds about the level between the T2–T6 spinous process to achieve the correct angle for screw placement. The starting point for drill placement is 3 mm above the C2–C3 facet articulation and 2 to 3 mm lateral to the medial border of the C2 facet. The drill guide should be aimed 0 to 10 degrees medially and toward the dorsal cortex of the anterior arch of C1. Consider palpating the medial wall of the pedicle with a nerve hook or a small blunt elevator through a laminotomy between C1 and C2. Biplanar fluoroscopic images should be obtained prior to inserting the starting Kirschner wire and during drilling to ensure that the wire hugs the superior cortex of the isthmus to avoid the vertebral artery inferiorly. The vertebral artery is inferior on lateral views and parallel or slightly lateral to the cord on AP views. The tip of the wire should end about 3 mm short of the anterior cortex of C1 to avoid passing the drill into the oropharynx. Instrumentations are cannulated, which makes it easier to place screws. Usually, a 3.5- or 4.5-mm cannulated screw measuring 40 to 44 mm is adequate. Ideally, guide wires are drilled on both sides prior to placing the screws bilaterally. A Gallie-type posterior fixation technique with autologous iliac crest bone graft can be used to supplement the fixation. External immobilization devices should be prescribed based on the strength of the construct and bone quality. In many cases, a soft collar is all that is required.

Posterior C1–C2 Intraarticular Screw Fixation

A variation of this concept is the use of a C1–C2 intraarticular interference screw, as described by Tokuhashi et al.[121] In this technique, posterior dissection exposes the C1–C2 joints bilaterally. The joint capsule is dissected off the bone and retracted superiorly with the greater occipital nerve. When placing a screw on one side, atlantoaxial subluxation is reduced and maintained by application of a Halifax interlaminar clamp to the contralateral side. A 1-mm Kirschner wire is inserted

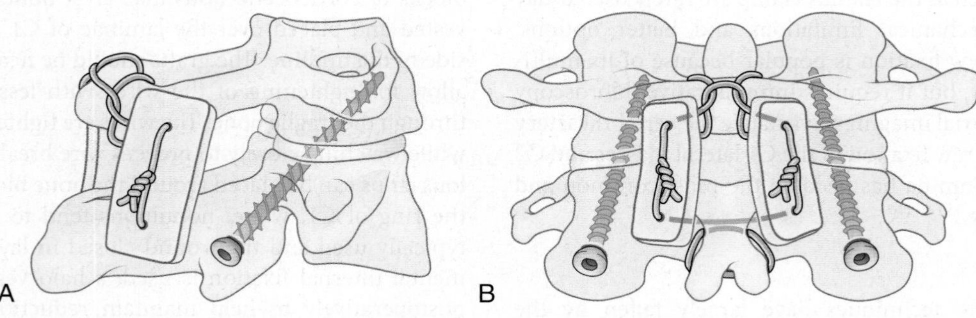

FIG. 84.6 Transarticular screw technique for C1–C2 arthrodesis.

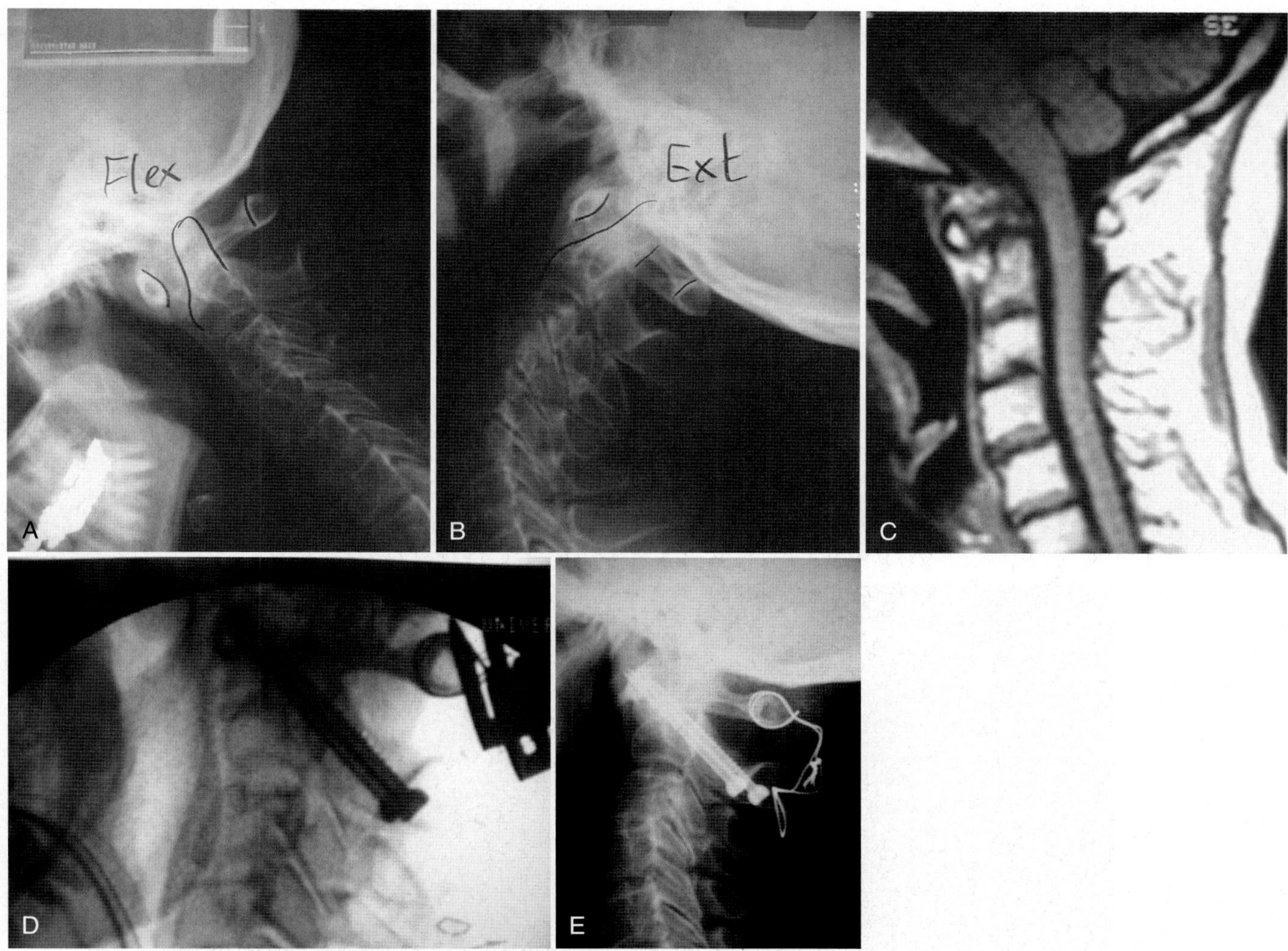

FIG. 84.7 A 52-year-old woman with long-standing rheumatoid arthritis had neck pain without evidence of frank myelopathy. (A–B) Flexion and extension lateral cervical spine radiographs show C1–C2 instability. There is incomplete reduction in extension. (C) A sagittal magnetic resonance image shows pannus around the dens. This is likely blocking complete reduction in extension. There is still enough space available for the spinal cord, however, as visualized on this image. (D–E) A lateral intraoperative fluoroscopic view of C1–C2 and postoperative lateral radiographic view following transarticular screw placement, modified Gallie-type wiring with bone grafting for posterior C1–C2 arthrodesis.

directly into the C1–C2 joint and a cannulated tap is used to prepare the site for insertion of the cannulated 5.6- or 6.5-mm titanium interference screw. These screws are typically 8 mm or 10 mm long. The procedure is then performed on the opposite side. Finally, corticocancellous bone graft is fashioned to fit the intralaminar space and is secured beneath bilateral Halifax clamps. Patients are placed in a cervical collar postoperatively. Tokuhashi et al.[121] used this technique in 22 rheumatoid patients, all of whom reported significant improvement in pain, and all patients who were Ranawat class IIIA or above improved neurologically by 2-year follow-up. Atlantoaxial reduction was maintained and bony fusion was noted in all patients; although four patients developed subaxial pathology, none required surgical intervention.

Posterior C1–C2 Screw-Rod Constructs

Several methods of posterior C1–C2 rigid instrumentation have been described. Harms and Melcher[35] reported a technique involving placement of 3.5-mm polyaxial screws directly into the lateral mass of C1 and into the pars interarticularis or pedicle of C2 bilaterally (Fig. 84.8). Vertical rods are then attached to these screws, followed by bone grafting for arthrodesis. Recently, the use of posterior C1–C2 screw-rod constructs has become the most commonly employed technique.[122] This method allows for direct manipulation and reduction of C1 on C2 as needed. The advantages of this technique includes rigid three-column fixation, high fusion rates (97.5%), low rates of implant failure, and the theoretical decreased risk to the vertebral artery compared to C1–C2 transarticular screws.[122,123] Bleeding from the venous lakes covering the C1 lateral masses can easily be encountered and is a disadvantage. This bleeding is usually minimized by meticulous subperiosteal dissection and can typically be controlled by hemostatic agents. Either technique requires an intimate knowledge of the anatomy by the operating surgeon aided by good fluoroscopic technique.

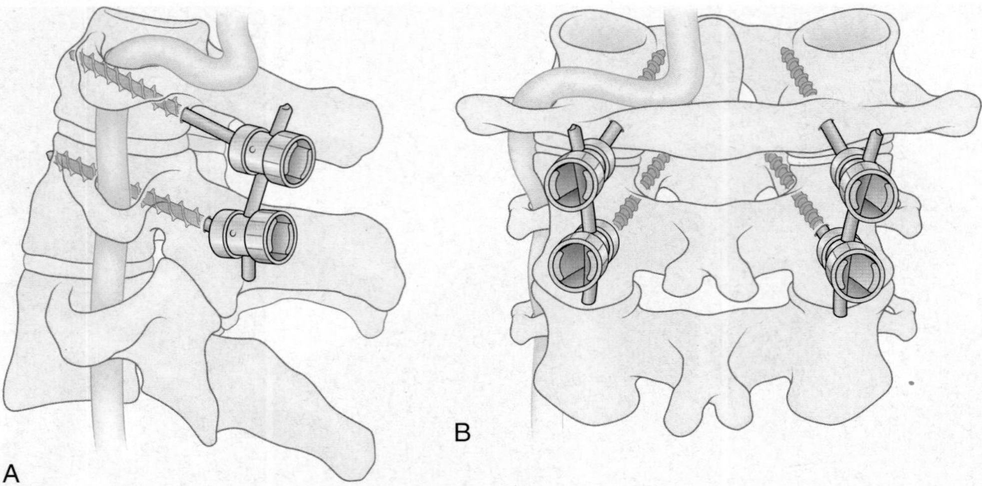

FIG. 84.8 Posterior C1–C2 fixation technique with polyaxial screws and rods. Screws are placed into the lateral masses of C1 and into the pedicles of C2.

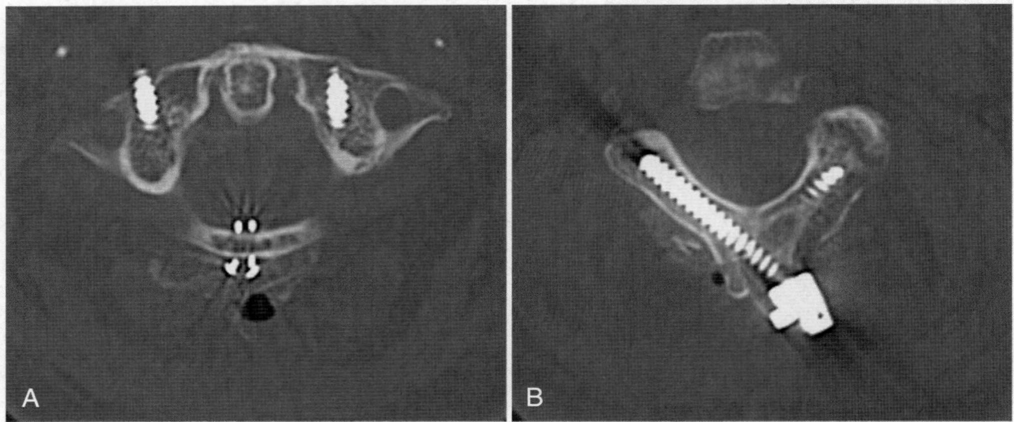

FIG. 84.9 Posterior C1–C2 fixation with placement of C1 lateral mass screws and C2 intralaminar screws. (A) Axial computed tomographic (CT) scan through C1 demonstrating location of lateral mass screws. (B) Axial CT through C2 laminae showing bilateral intralaminar screws. Note that because of the technique required for insertion, the screws are not in exactly the same axial plane.

After exposure, the C1–C2 joint is identified since this serves as the anatomic landmark for accurate placement of the C1 lateral mass screw. Removing a small amount of the caudal part of the C1 posterior arch with a burr will aid in visualizing the C1 screw starting point. The C2 nerve root can be gently retracted caudally for visualization or sacrificed, which has been shown to result in less neuralgia, decreased operative time, and decreased blood loss in studies. However, patients should be warned of postoperative numbness.[122,124] The screw is placed in the center of the lateral mass, first using a high-speed burr to create a dimple so that the drill bit does not skid while drilling. The pilot hole is drilled straight or slightly convergent and parallel to the C1 posterior arch in the sagittal direction. The drill hole is typically 18 to 22 mm, which should be confirmed with fluoroscopy. A longer screw than this will be needed since the polyaxial screw head will need to be elevated off of the cortex of the lateral mass in order to accommodate rod fixation. Typically, partially threaded screws are used, which allow the threads to remain within the bone of the lateral mass, while the nerve root then lies against the smooth shaft of the screw. The entry point for the C2 pedicle screw is in the upper and medial quadrants of the isthmus surface. The direction of the pilot hole is approximately 20 to 30 degrees in a convergent and cephalad direction. The medial border of the C2 pars interarticularis can initially be palpated with a small elevator or the edge of a nerve hook to help with accurate placement of C2 screws. A typical length for C2 pedicle screws is 22 to 28 mm, which should be confirmed with fluoroscopy. In their study, Harms and Melcher did not wire in grafts for their fusion technique[35]; however, this technique is certainly an option to augment the stability of the screw–rod construct and to help ensure a successful arthrodesis (see Fig. 84.7).

An alternative to the C2 pedicle or pars screw is placement of an intralaminar C2 screw (Fig. 84.9). As described by Wright, this technique provides excellent fixation of C2 with virtually no risk of injury to neurovascular structures.[117] Exposure is as described earlier for the placement of C1 lateral mass and C2 pedicle screws. Placement of the C1 lateral mass screws is performed by the previously described technique. For placement of the C2 intralaminar screws, a high-speed burr is used to open a small cortical window at the cranial end of the junction of the C2 spinous process and lamina. A hand drill is then used to drill the intercortical space of the contralateral lamina to a depth of approximately 30 mm while maintaining alignment of the drill with the exposed dorsal aspect of the lamina. After palpation of the drill tract with a ball-tip probe, a 4.0 × 30 mm polyaxial screw is inserted. A starting hole is then burred in the contralateral side at the caudal junction of the spinous process and lamina and, using the same technique, an intralaminar screw is inserted. Care must be taken when inserting the screws to maintain the angle of insertion slightly shallower than the angle of the lamina; this technique will ensure that any cortical breach occurs dorsally rather than ventrally into the spinal canal. The polyaxial screw heads from C1 and C2 are then connected with a rod. In some instances, because of the angle of the screws relative to one another, offset connectors may need to be used to facilitate rod insertion. The laminae of C1 and C2 may then be decorticated and corticocancellous bone graft applied (and wired into place if desired).

A biomechanical study examined the relative stability of several C1–C2 screw-rod constructs in an odontoid fracture model.[125] Using cadaveric specimens, C1 lateral mass screws were placed and connected to either C2 intralaminar screws, C2 pars screws, or C2 pedicle screws. Insertional torque for C2 pedicle screws and intralaminar screws was similar, and both of these screw types were significantly higher than pars screws. Pullout strength was greatest for pedicle screws. In intact models, intralaminar screws provided superior resistance to axial rotation compared to pars screws and similar resistance to pedicle screws. After experimentally induced odontoid fracture, both pars and pedicle screws were superior in resisting lateral bending. Pedicle screws overall provided the greatest stability of C1–C2 in all planes, particularly after experimental odontoid fracture. Lapiswala et al.[126] noted similar results, with C2 intralaminar screws providing less resistance to lateral bending than C2 pedicle screws or C2–C1 transarticular screws. All posterior constructs, when supplemented with posterior cable fixation, provided similar stiffness in flexion–extension and axial rotation.

Cranial Settling or Atlantoaxial Subluxation With C1 Stenosis

Occipitocervical Fusion

The technique of choice to treat patients with cranial settling or fixed AAS with posterior cord impingement from the ring of C1 is occipitocervical fusion.[62,92,127] In the latter case, an occiput to C2 fusion with a C1 laminectomy is preferred. Patient positioning is same as with wire techniques. Particular care must be taken to ensure neutral alignment of the head in the sagittal and axial planes. Excess flexion or extension can lead to chronic pain, dysphagia, breathing problems, and functional impairment due to disruption of forward gaze. The skin incision extends proximally to the external occipital protuberance (EOP). Historical techniques include direct wiring of bone graft to the skull or the use of looped rods wired into place. Presently, rigid fixation with occipital plate-screw constructs is the standard treatment.

Wiring and Graft Technique

This technique utilizes corticocancellous bone blocks wired to the occiput and laminae[62,92,127] (Fig. 84.10). The prominent bony protuberance (inion) that is present approximately 2 cm below the EOP is the site of wire fixation (approximately 5–7 cm from the base of the skull). A 2-mm diamond burr is used to make unicortical holes to form a tunnel with a bridge of superficial cortical bone on each side of the midline. The holes are connected with a towel clamp between the inner and outer tables of the skull. A 20-gauge wire is passed through the tunnel and looped back under and out again to wrap around the bony bridge. A second wire is passed beneath the C1 lamina (if it has not been removed) and looped onto itself to cinch down on the lamina. A wire is passed transversely through the base of the C2 spinous process and looped around and passed back through to distribute stress. Other interspinous or sublaminar wires can be used in more caudad segments as needed. Long, thick corticocancellous posterior iliac crest grafts are harvested, typically 9 mm to 10 cm in length and 1.5 cm wide. For occiput to C2 fusions, a single block of graft may be used with the caudad end fashioned to fit around the C2 spinous process. A 1.5-mm drill bit is used to place holes through the graft. The wires are threaded through the graft with the cancellous side facing the exposed skull and laminae. The concavity of the central part of the iliac crest facilitates excellent contact between the occiput and the laminae. In severely osteopenic patients, a wire mesh may be placed over the cortical side of the graft to prevent the wires from cutting through the graft.[62] The wires are tightened down cautiously to prevent breakage or cutting through the graft. Cancellous bone chips may be added to the construct. A drain is typically used and the wound closed in layers. Without adjuvant fixation, most patients are managed in a halo vest postoperatively, but a two-poster brace or other cervical orthosis may be used based on the stability of the construct.

Occipitocervical Plating

This technique provides more rigid fixation compared with wiring techniques,[40,41,128,129] even in patients with significant osteoporosis. Current implants incorporate plate-rod hybrid constructs (Fig. 84.11). It may be technically challenging to produce the correct amount of contour required at the base of the skull. In longer fusions, it is recommended that fixation is achieved in and below C2 before fixation into the skull, since the distal fixation points require more precise placement. C2 fixation can be done with pedicle screws, transarticular screws, or intralaminar screws. Due to inferior pullout strength, C2 pars screws should not be used unless the fusion will be carried down into the subaxial cervical spine.

Fixation to the skull requires knowledge of the venous sinus anatomy to avoid bleeding complications. Screws should be placed distal to the transverse sinus, which lies at the level of the EOP. The thickness of the skull decreases laterally away

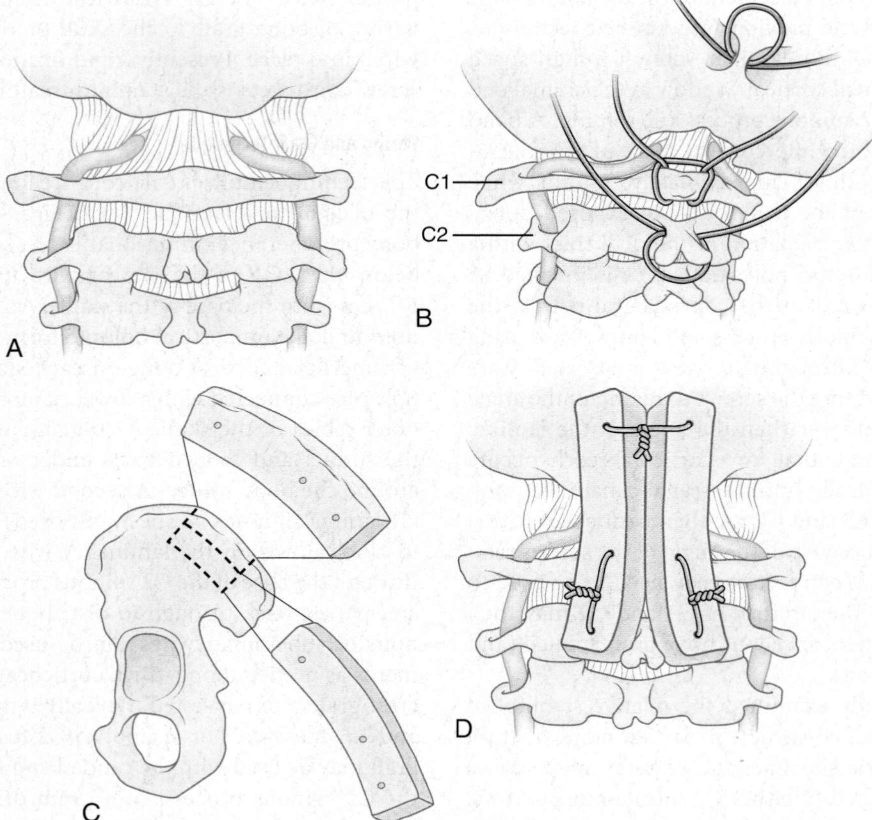

FIG. 84.10 Technique of posterior occipitocervical fusion. (A) A burr hole is made in the nuchal bony ridge, staying between the cortical table. (B) Twenty-gauge wires are passed down; looping the wire through a second time improves the grip and distributes the stress. (C) Near-full-thickness corticocancellous grafts are harvested from the ilium. (D) The grafts are wired in place as shown. Cancellous bone is also packed in the crevices. (Modified from Werthein SB, Bohlman HH. Occipitocervical fusion: indications, technique, and long-term results in thirteen patients. *J Bone Joint Surg Am.* 1987;69A:833–836.)

from the midline and closer to the foramen magnum.[130] Unicortical fixation is adequate in the thicker areas of the skull, but bicortical fixation can be performed safely. Two to three screws should be used on each side of the midline. A 2-mm diamond burr is used to minimize the chance of a spinal fluid leak common when using more aggressive carbide burrs. The holes are tapped and 3.5- to 4.5-mm screws between 6 and 12 mm in length are placed. In case of a spinal fluid leak, bone wax may be sufficient to stop the leak; otherwise, placing the screw usually tamponades the leak. There does not appear to be any adverse effect from breaching the inner table. Structural bone graft may be wired in or around the construct and augmented with cancellous bone. The head and neck are immobilized in a two-poster brace or a halo vest in osteoporotic patients with questionable fixation; in other patients, a hard cervical collar may be used. Patients are typically changed to a soft collar for comfort after 8 weeks.

Contoured Loop/Rod Techniques

This technique was first proposed by Ransford and colleagues[38] in 1986 and is used with segmental wiring to provide occipitocervical fixation.[38,131–133] The exposure is similar to that described earlier for plate fixation. Wires are placed in the occiput and beneath the lamina of C1 and the subaxial vertebrae. Earlier constructs relied on a horseshoe-shaped loop of 5/32 threaded stainless steel rods. The horizontal limb should be approximately 3.5 to 4 cm wide and the length of the occipital portion of the loop should be 2.5 to 3 cm. More recent constructs utilize a custom-contoured threaded titanium loop with titanium-threaded cables, which allows for postoperative MRI.

Resection of the Odontoid

Mild to moderate cervicomedullary compression can be treated with posterior C1 laminectomy and occipitocervical fusion as described earlier. The pannus will resorb with stabilization.[49] However, anterior decompression may be needed to treat an irreducible anterior extradural compression of the cervicomedullary junction by pannus or a severely migrated odontoid.[134,135] The transoral approach is associated with an increased risk of infection with mouth flora; the high retropharyngeal approach is a good alternative in many patients.[136] Supplemental posterior fusion is required unless there is a solid prior posterior fusion mass, in which case resection of the odontoid without grafting will suffice. In cases without prior posterior fusion, anterior strut grafting with iliac crest

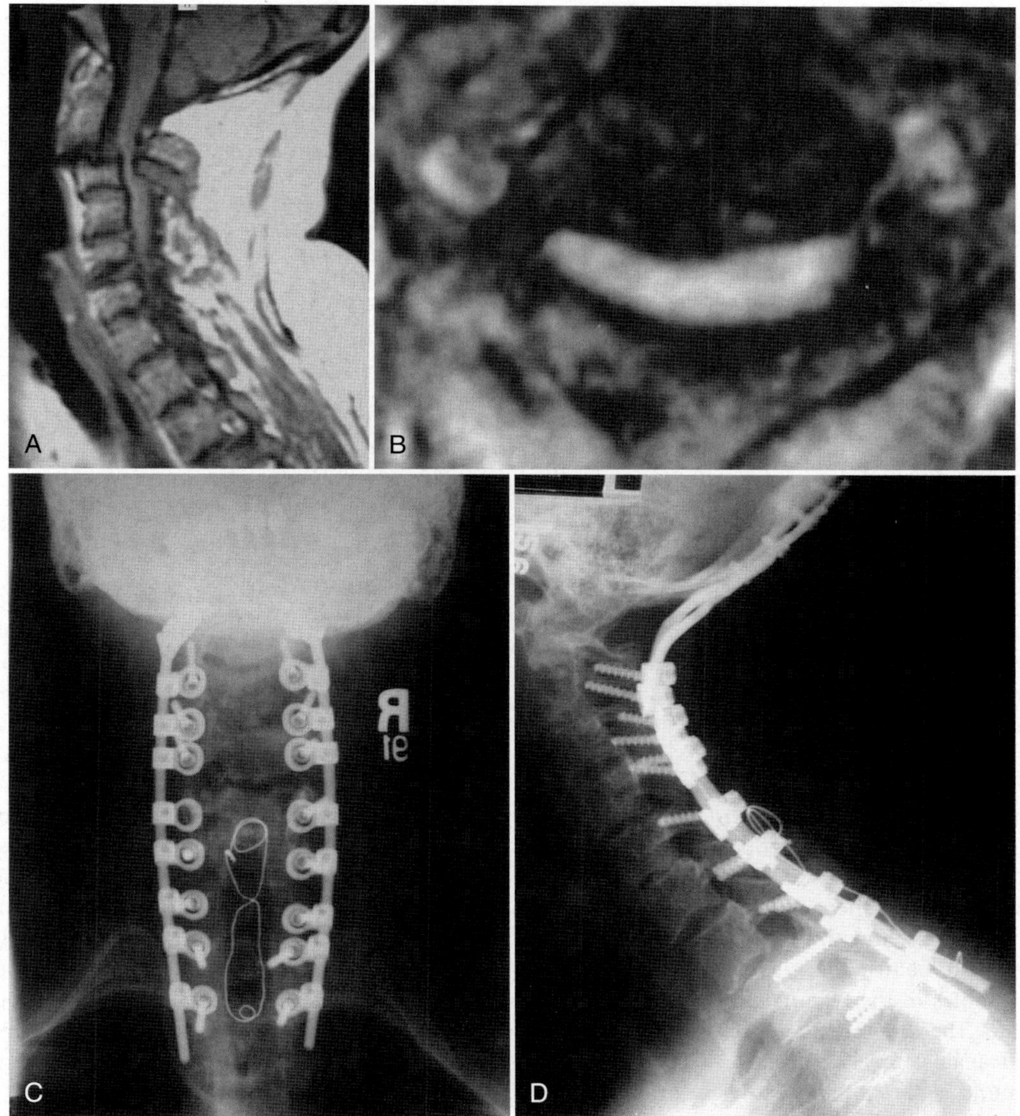

FIG. 84.11 This 46-year-old woman had a long history of rheumatoid arthritis since she was a young girl. She had chronic neck pain but developed worsening neck pain over the previous 6 weeks with increasing numbness of her arms and some truncal numbness. Some weakness of her upper extremities was evident on physical examination. (A–B) Magnetic resonance imaging showed severe cord compression, primarily at the C2–C3 level. She had multiple levels of subluxation in the subaxial spine, including C7–T1. (C–D) Anteroposterior and lateral postoperative plain films after a posterior decompression at C2–C3 followed by a long occipitocervical fusion with bone grafting and posterior instrumentation. Screws were placed in the pedicles of C7 and T1 for maximum fixation and osteoporotic bone.

or fibula is required between C2 or C3 and the clivus, followed by posterior occipitocervical fusion. Thorough preoperative assessment is necessary, which includes swallowing and respiratory function considerations, dental assessment, and the presence of a mobile temporomandibular joint to allow about 2.5 to 3 cm of opening.

Subaxial Subluxation

Subaxial subluxations may be fixed or mobile. The fixed types may be best treated with anterior decompression and fusion and strongly considered for supplemental posterior fixation since anterior column instability may occur from graft resorption or settling into the osteoporotic vertebral bodies. Mobile subluxations are best treated with traction to realign the spine and posterior instrumented fusion. Better reduction may be obtained after anesthesia when positioning of the head is done gently with neuromonitoring.

Anterior Fusion

Anterior decompression and fusion may be utilized for treatment of fixed cervical kyphosis or when needed to decompress

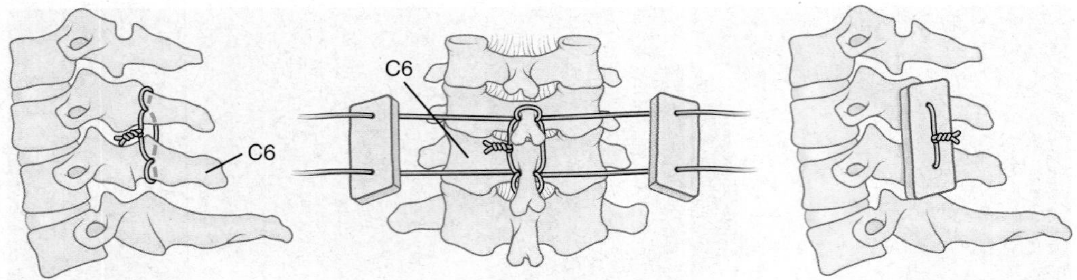

FIG. 84.12 Bohlman triple-wire technique for posterior cervical arthrodesis.

stenotic segments. These techniques may be performed as described for treatment of spondylotic disease elsewhere in this text. Because patients with RA frequently require multilevel procedures and because of the risk for graft settling into osteoporotic bone, consideration must be given to a supplemental posterior fusion.

Wiring Techniques

Posterior wiring and autogenous bone grafting may provide stable fixation at a high fusion rate. The preferred method for wire stabilization is the triple-wire technique described by Bohlman[136] (Fig. 84.12). The first 20-gauge wire is woven in a figure-of-eight fashion through holes burred into the base of the spinous processes of the involved vertebrae. This wire tethers the midline and is typically looped onto itself after passing through the spinous process to help distribute stress. Twenty-two-gauge wires can then individually pass through the same holes to loop around the spinous processes at the ends of the segments to be fused. The ends of these wires will pass through drill holes in the rectangular corticocancellous iliac crest autografts. The wires are tightened down on the graft to force the graft against the laminae. Decortication is not necessary; the wound is closed in layers over a drain. A two-poster cervical brace or halo is used for 6 to 8 weeks to allow solid fusion.

Lateral Mass Fixation

This treatment provides rigid fixation of the subaxial spine. Several modifications exist in the way the screws are angled in the lateral mass.[30–33] According to An,[30] 15 degrees of superior angulation and 30 degrees of lateral angulation best avoids violating the facet joints and nerve roots. All the techniques avoid the vertebral artery, which lies anterior to the lateral mass. The starting point is 1 mm medial to the center of the lateral mass. The screws average between 12 and 16 mm, depending on the size of the patient. The C7 lateral mass is thin and may require pedicle screw placement or supplemental posterior wiring between the C6 and C7 spinous processes, as described earlier. Fluoroscopy is helpful in placing C7 pedicle screws if the shoulders are not in the way, but a C7 laminotomy provides direct palpation of the medial wall of the pedicle for safer screw placement. A 25- to 30-degree medial angulation is recommended.[30] Pedicle screw fixation of all involved levels of the cervical vertebrae has been described frequently in other patient populations but has limitations of pedicle size and risks to the vertebral artery.[137] Because of the risk of subluxation with a long cervical fusion, consideration should be given to extending the fusion across the cervicothoracic junction.

Complications

Complications of cervical spine surgery in rheumatoid patients include dural tears, quadriplegia, infection, wound dehiscence, skin problems from external immobilization devices, nonunion, and subaxial subluxation above or below a fused segment. Anterior fusion procedures are at risk for graft resorption and anterior column collapse due to the inflammatory process and secondary osteoporosis of the vertebral bodies and may benefit from adjunctive posterior stabilization. The progressive nature of rheumatoid disease of the spine demands long-term follow-up to assess for the development of new symptoms in previously asymptomatic segments (see Fig. 84.12). In a study of 51 rheumatoid patients undergoing cervical fusion for instability, Clarke et al. reported that 39% of patients undergoing C1–C2 fixation developed subaxial subluxation at an average of 8 years.[138] No patient who underwent long posterior fusions (C1–C6 through T1) for combined atlantoaxial and subaxial instability required secondary procedures. In contrast, Tanouchi et al.[139] noted a 26% incidence of adjacent-level failures in 35 rheumatoid patients after occipitothoracic fusion. All failures were due to fracture at the distal junction. Including all involved unstable levels in the initial fusion procedure may reduce the risk of subsequent adjacent-level subluxation; however, fusion length and stress of the lever arm must be considered in these fragile patients. Age, presence of atlantoaxial instability, and perioperative complications are independent predictors of long-term mortality following cervical surgery in this population.[140]

Thoracolumbar Disease

Unlike the cervical spine, rheumatoid disease of the thoracic and lumbar spine less frequently leads to severe neurologic symptoms, thus has received less attention. Yet cases of thoracic myelopathy, lumbar radiculopathy, and cauda equina syndrome have been reported and appear to be due to bony destruction leading to instability and subluxation with or without the presence of pannus or nodules.[141–143] Radiographic findings include poorly defined margins of the vertebral endplates and a relative lack of osteophytes.[6,7] Involvement of the facet joints may lead to spondylolisthesis and instability on flexion-extension films. Heywood and Meyers postulated that the pathologic process in the lumbar spine begins with synovitis of the facet joints causing functional incompetence, allowing AP and lateral translation.[6] This step is followed by discitis, which may start as an enthesopathy at the junction of the endplate and disc, resulting in loss of disc height and further contributing to instability. In the thoracic spine, the disease may also spread directly into the spine via the costovertebral joints. Nerve root impingement may be due to spinal instability as well as direct impingement from rheumatoid pannus.[6] To correlate radiographic findings with clinical symptoms, Kawaguchi et al. studied 106 rheumatoid patients and found a 40% rate of back pain, 18% had leg pain, and 12% exhibited symptoms of neurogenic claudication.[7] They reported abnormal radiographic findings in 57% of patients, most commonly disc space narrowing (37%), followed by coronal plane deformity (28%), spondylolisthesis (23%), and endplate or facet erosion (20%). They noted a high percentage of osteoporosis related to steroid therapy. Using MRI, Sakai et al.[144] reported a 45.2% incidence of lumbar involvement in RA and described two distinct patterns of disc destruction: narrowing, in which the disc space progressively collapsed, and ballooning, in which endplate changes gave the illusion of increasing disc height. Additionally, they found that the degree of lumbar involvement related to the severity of peripheral joint involvement.

Surgical treatment of the rheumatoid lumbar spine is tailored to the specific pathology involved; outcomes are similar to nonrheumatoid patients with similar pathology.[145] Complications, however, are more common and comprise screw loosening and cut-out, likely due to the relative osteoporosis of the population, and a greater risk of wound infections related to immune modulators used to treat the disease. Junctional breakdown can also occur.

Summary

The majority of patients with RA of the cervical spine can be managed nonoperatively. These patients, however, should be monitored closely since the progression of disease may be silent and the clinical findings nonspecific. Screening flexion and extension lateral radiographs should be done periodically before neurologic symptoms develop as well as prior to any planned surgical procedure that may require general anesthesia, intubation, or manipulation of the cervical spine. The benefits of early detection and surgical intervention in patients with progressive cervical instability cannot be overemphasized and should be done before the development of cranial settling or frank neurologic symptoms.[44,60,92] Otherwise, mortality and morbidity significantly increase as patients become less functional and fall under Ranawat class III criteria.[60,69,76,91,136] Although surgery in patients with quadriparesis may provide some neurologic and functional recovery, the results are not as predictable as with early surgery.

PEARLS

1. The periodontoid pannus begins to resorb as early as 6 weeks after atlantoaxial fusion.
2. Radiographic AADI 9 mm or greater confirms AAS and is a relative indication for cervical fusion.
3. A PADI less than 14 mm has a high sensitivity of predicting paralysis and is a more reliable radiographic criterion for cervical fusion than the AADI. A PADI less than 10 mm is associated with poor motor recovery after fusion, while a PADI greater than 14 mm has a higher likelihood of recovery.
4. A cervicomedullary angle of less than 135 degrees (normal, 135–175 degrees) correlates with myelopathic signs and suggests AAS as the source of myelopathy.
5. Patients with AAS have better outcomes if surgery is done prior to neurologic impairment.

PITFALLS

1. Anterior fusion procedures are at risk for graft resorption and anterior column collapse due to the inflammatory process and secondary osteoporosis of the vertebral bodies. Patients may therefore benefit from adjunctive posterior stabilization.
2. Radiologic improvement of AAS is a "radiographic illusion" and is due to worsening cranial settling of the anterior arch of C1 onto the base of the odontoid in reality.
3. Rheumatoid patients are at risk for late segmental instability below a previous fusion; therefore, they should be followed long term.
4. Myelopathy patients are at high risk for progression and sudden death if treated nonoperatively.
5. Perioperative upper airway complications are 14 times higher if intubation is done without fiberoptic assistance in rheumatoid patients undergoing posterior cervical fusion.
6. Attempts should not be made to pass sublaminar wires beneath a severely stenotic or unreduced C1 arch. Consider occipitocervical fusion with or without C1 laminectomy.
7. Commonly used rheumatic medications potentially place patients at risk for postoperative wound infections and their effects on spinal fusion are unknown. Most should be stopped preoperatively and held for as long as possible postoperatively. Close collaboration with the patient's rheumatologist is essential in balancing the need to minimize perioperative complications while preventing flares of rheumatoid symptoms.
8. Patients on chronic steroids may require perioperative stress dosing.

KEY POINTS

1. The cervical spine is involved in 25% to 90% of rheumatoid patients. Because cervical instability may be asymptomatic in many rheumatoid patients, the clinician must be vigilant in evaluating the cervical spine, especially preoperatively, for spinal or nonspinal procedures.
2. RA has a predilection for synovial joints, including the facet, occipitoatlantal, and atlantoaxial joints. The resulting joint erosion can lead to instability, of which the most common pattern is atlantoaxial, followed by subaxial and occipitoatlantal instability. Patients frequently present with pain but may also present with neurologic symptoms.
3. Surgical indications include the presence of myelopathy. Radiographic indicators include an AADI 9 mm or greater, PADI less than 14 mm, mobile subaxial subluxation greater than 3.5 mm, space available for the cord less than 14 mm, and cranial settling. A cervicomedullary angle less than 135 degrees

SECTION XII

suggests impending neurologic deficit. Surgical intervention performed early, before clinically significant impairment, has the best functional outcomes.

4. Rheumatoid medications should be managed carefully in the perioperative period, as many mechanisms of action can increase the risk of infection, delayed wound healing, or affect fusion.
5. Modern rigid internal fixation should be used for surgical stabilization whenever possible. Because of variations in patient anatomy, the surgeon must be aware of different fixation options, such as C2 pedicle screws, C2 interlaminar screws, transarticular screws, or classical fixation techniques (e.g., wiring), as these may be the only available options at times. A clear understanding of the individual patient's anatomy and pathology is necessary to perform safe, effective surgery.

KEY REFERENCES

1. Boden SD, Dodge LD, Bohlman HH, Rechtine GR. Rheumatoid arthritis of the cervical spine. *J Bone Joint Surg Am.* 1993;75A:1282-1297.
   The authors showed that the PADI may be more reliable in predicting neurologic outcome since it is a more accurate indicator of the space available for the cord. Patients with a PADI of at least 14 mm were more likely to have neurologic recovery after surgical stabilization, whereas those with a PADI less than 10 mm had no neurologic recovery. The critical space available for the cord in the subaxial spine was also shown to be 14 mm.
2. Bundschuh C, Modic MT, Kearney F, Morris R, Deal C. Rheumatoid arthritis of the cervical spine: surface-coil MR imaging. *AJNR Am J Neuroradiol.* 1988;9:565-571.
   The authors determined that patients with a cervicomedullary angle less than 135 degrees (normal, 135–175 degrees) were likely to have evidence of brain stem compression, cervical myelopathy, or C2 root pain.
3. Larsson E-M, Holtås S, Zygmunt S. Pre- and postoperative MR imaging of the craniocervical junction in rheumatoid arthritis. *AJNR Am J Neuroradiol.* 1989;152:561-566.
   The authors noted reduction of the periodontoid pannus as early as 6 weeks after surgical stabilization of the atlantoaxial instability.
4. Ranawat CS, O'Leary P, Pellici P, et al. Cervical spine fusion in rheumatoid arthritis. *J Bone Joint Surg Am.* 1979;61A:1003-1010.
   The authors studied 33 patients with cervical instability and devised a classification of pain and neurologic dysfunction that is widely used to assess the functional capacity of rheumatoid patients with cervical disease. An improved method to measure the amount of cranial settling was also presented.
5. Riew KD, Hilibrand A, Palumbo MA, Sethi N, Bohlman HH. Diagnosing basilar invagination in the rheumatoid patient. *J Bone Joint Surg Am.* 2001;83A:194-200.
   The authors noted that none of the traditional radiographic measurements alone had a high sensitivity, specificity, or negative or positive predictive value greater than 90% but that the combination of the Clark station, Redlund-Johnell, and the Ranawat criteria had a sensitivity and negative predictive value of 94% and 91%, respectively.
6. Harms J, Melcher R. Posterior C1-C2 fusion with polyaxial screw and rod fixation. *Spine.* 2001;26:2467-2471.
   The authors describe the surgical technique for posterior C1 lateral mass and C2 pedicle screw fixation, which has become the preferred method of atlantoaxial fixation.

REFERENCES

1. Ward MM. Decreases in rates of hospitalizations for manifestations of severe rheumatoid arthritis, 1983-2001. *Arthritis Rheum.* 2004;50(4):1122-1131.
2. Stein BE, et al. Changing trends in cervical spine fusions in patients with rheumatoid arthritis. *Spine.* 2014;39(15):1178-1182.
3. Sugita S, et al. Clinical characteristics of rheumatoid arthritis patients undergoing cervical spine surgery: an analysis of National Database of Rheumatic Diseases in Japan. *BMC Musculoskelet Disord.* 2014;15:203.
4. Bland JH. Rheumatoid arthritis of the cervical spine. *J Rheumatol.* 1974;3:319-341.
5. da Corte FC, Neves N. Cervical spine instability in rheumatoid arthritis. *Eur J Orthop Surg Traumatol.* 2014;24(suppl 1):S83-S91.
6. Heywood AW, Meyers OL. Rheumatoid arthritis of the thoracic and lumbar spine. *J Bone Joint Surg Br.* 1986;68(3):362-368.
7. Kawaguchi Y, et al. Radiologic findings of the lumbar spine in patients with rheumatoid arthritis, and a review of pathologic mechanisms. *J Spinal Disord Tech.* 2003;16(1):38-43.
8. Mahajan R, Huisa BN. Vertebral artery dissection in rheumatoid arthritis with cervical spine disease. *J Stroke Cerebrovasc Dis.* 2013;22(7):e245-e246.
9. Neva MH, et al. High prevalence of asymptomatic cervical spine subluxation in patients with rheumatoid arthritis waiting for orthopaedic surgery. *Ann Rheum Dis.* 2006;65(7):884-888.
10. Nazarinia M, et al. Asymptomatic atlantoaxial subluxation in rheumatoid arthritis. *Acta Med Iran.* 2014;52(6): 462-466.
11. Hansen SE. The recognition of rheumatoid arthritis in the eighteenth century. The contribution of Linne and Boissier de la Croix de Sauvages. *Scand J Rheumatol.* 1993;22(4): 178-182.
12. Short CL. The antiquity of rheumatoid arthritis. *Arthritis Rheum.* 1974;17(3):193-205.
13. Snorrason E. Landre-Beauvais and his "goutte asthenique primitive." *Acta Med Scand Suppl.* 1952;266:115-118.
14. Garrod AE. *A Treatise on Rheumatism and Rheumatoid Arthritis.* London: Griffin; 1890.
15. Lourie H, Stewart WA. Spontaneous atlantoaxial dislocation. A complication of rheumatoid disease. *N Engl J Med.* 1961;265:677-681.
16. Pratt TL. Spontaneous dislocation of the atlanto-axial articularion occurring in ankylosing spondylitis and rheumatoid arthritis. *J Fac Radiol.* 1959;10(1):40-43.
17. Werne S. Spontaneous dislocation of the atlas as a complication in rheumatoid arthritis. *Acta Rheumatol Scand.* 1956;2(4):101-107.
18. Wilson PD Jr, Dangelmajer RC. The problem of atlanto-axial dislocation in rheumatoid arthritis. *J Bone Joint Surg Am.* 1963;45:1780.
19. Brattstrom H, Granholm L. Atlanto-axial fusion in rheumatoid arthritis. A new method of fixation with wire and bone cement. *Acta Orthop Scand.* 1976;47(6):619-628.
20. Ferlic DC, et al. Surgical treatment of the symptomatic unstable cervical spine in rheumatoid arthritis. *J Bone Joint Surg Am.* 1975;57(3):349-354.
21. Hamblen DL. Occipito-cervical fusion. Indications, technique and results. *J Bone Joint Surg Br.* 1967;49(1):33-45.
22. McGraw RW, Rusch RM. Atlanto-axial arthrodesis. *J Bone Joint Surg Br.* 1973;55(3):482-489.
23. Rana NA, et al. Atlanto-axial subluxation in rheumatoid arthritis. *J Bone Joint Surg Br.* 1973;55(3):458-470.
24. Gallie WE. Fractures and dislocations of the cervical spine. *Am J Surg.* 1939;46:495-499.

25. Brooks AL, Jenkins EB. Atlanto-axial arthrodesis by the wedge compression method. *J Bone Joint Surg Am.* 1978;60(3):279-284.
26. Wertheim SB, Bohlman HH. Occipitocervical fusion. Indications, technique, and long-term results in thirteen patients. *J Bone Joint Surg Am.* 1987;69(6):833-836.
27. Clark CR, Goetz DD, Menezes AH. Arthrodesis of the cervical spine in rheumatoid arthritis. *J Bone Joint Surg Am.* 1989;71(3):381-392.
28. Cybulski GR, et al. Use of Halifax interlaminar clamps for posterior C1-C2 arthrodesis. *Neurosurgery.* 1988;22(2):429-431.
29. Grob D, et al. Posterior occipitocervical fusion. A preliminary report of a new technique. *Spine.* 1991;16(3 suppl): S17-S24.
30. An HS, Gordin R, Renner K. Anatomic considerations for plate-screw fixation of the cervical spine. *Spine.* 1991;16(10 suppl):S548-S551.
31. Heller JG, et al. Anatomic comparison of the Roy-Camille and Magerl techniques for screw placement in the lower cervical spine. *Spine.* 1991;16(10 suppl):S552-S557.
32. Anderson PA, et al. Posterior cervical arthrodesis with AO reconstruction plates and bone graft. *Spine.* 1991;16(3 suppl):S72-S79.
33. Magerl F, Seeman PS. Stable posterior fusion of the atlas and axis by transarticular screw fixation. In: Weidner A, Kehr P, eds. *Cervical Spine.* Berlin: Springer-Verlag; 1986:322-327.
34. Grob D, et al. Atlanto-axial fusion with transarticular screw fixation. *J Bone Joint Surg Br.* 1991;73(6):972-976.
35. Harms J, Melcher RP. Posterior C1-C2 fusion with polyaxial screw and rod fixation. *Spine.* 2001;26(22):2467-2471.
36. Foerster O. *Die Leitungsbahnen des Schmerzgefuhls.* Berlin und Wein: Urgan und Schwarzenburg; 1927:266.
37. Kahn EA, Yglesias L. Progressive atlanto-axial dislocation. *JAMA.* 1935;105:348-352.
38. Ransford AO, et al. Craniocervical instability treated by contoured loop fixation. *J Bone Joint Surg Br.* 1986;68(2):173-177.
39. Flint GA, et al. A new method of occipitocervical fusion using internal fixation. *Neurosurgery.* 1987;21(6):947-950.
40. Grob D, et al. The role of plate and screw fixation in occipitocervical fusion in rheumatoid arthritis. *Spine.* 1994;19(22):2545-2551.
41. Smith MD, Anderson P, Grady MS. Occipitocervical arthrodesis using contoured plate fixation. An early report on a versatile fixation technique. *Spine.* 1993;18(14):1984-1990.
42. Konttinen YT, et al. Inflammatory involvement of cervical spine ligaments in patients with rheumatoid arthritis and atlantoaxial subluxation. *J Rheumatol.* 1987;14(3):531-534.
43. Mikulowski P, et al. Sudden death in rheumatoid arthritis with atlanto-axial dislocation. *Acta Med Scand.* 1975;198(6):445-451.
44. Agarwal AK, et al. Recurrence of cervical spine instability in rheumatoid arthritis following previous fusion: can disease progression be prevented by early surgery? *J Rheumatol.* 1992;19(9):1364-1370.
45. Joaquim AF, Appenzeller S. Cervical spine involvement in rheumatoid arthritis—a systematic review. *Autoimmun Rev.* 2014;13(12):1195-1202.
46. Takahashi S, et al. Current prevalence and characteristics of cervical spine instability in patients with rheumatoid arthritis in the era of biologics. *Mod Rheumatol.* 2014;24(6):904-909.
47. Alcala JM, et al. Radiographic changes of cervical spine in rheumatoid arthritis. *Rev Bras Reumatol.* 2013;53(5):388-393.
48. Kaito T, et al. Effect of biological agents on cervical spine lesions in rheumatoid arthritis. *Spine.* 2012;37(20): 1742-1746.
49. Larsson EM, Holtas S, Zygmunt S. Pre- and postoperative MR imaging of the craniocervical junction in rheumatoid arthritis. *AJR Am J Roentgenol.* 1989;152(3):561-566.
50. Toolanen G, Larsson SE, Fagerlund M. Medullary compression in rheumatoid atlanto-axial subluxation evaluated by computerized tomography. *Spine.* 1986;11(3):191-194.
51. Chen TY, Lin KL, Ho HH. Morphologic characteristics of atlantoaxial complex in rheumatoid arthritis and surgical consideration among Chinese. *Spine.* 2004;29(9):1000-1004.
52. Lewandrowski KU, et al. Atraumatic odontoid fractures in patients with rheumatoid arthritis. *Spine J.* 2006;6(5):529-533.
53. Smith PH, Benn RT, Sharp J. Natural history of rheumatoid cervical luxations. *Ann Rheum Dis.* 1972;31(6):431-439.
54. Bogduk N, Major GA, Carter J. Lateral subluxation of the atlas in rheumatoid arthritis: a case report and post-mortem study. *Ann Rheum Dis.* 1984;43(2):341-346.
55. Rana NA. Natural history of atlanto-axial subluxation in rheumatoid arthritis. *Spine.* 1989;14(10):1054-1056.
56. Papadopoulos SM, Dickman CA, Sonntag VK. Atlantoaxial stabilization in rheumatoid arthritis. *J Neurosurg.* 1991;74(1):1-7.
57. Weissman BN, et al. Prognostic features of atlantoaxial subluxation in rheumatoid arthritis patients. *Radiology.* 1982;144(4):745-751.
58. Delamarter RB, Bohlman HH. Postmortem osseous and neuropathologic analysis of the rheumatoid cervical spine. *Spine.* 1994;19(20):2267-2274.
59. Henderson FC, Geddes JF, Crockard HA. Neuropathology of the brainstem and spinal cord in end stage rheumatoid arthritis: implications for treatment. *Ann Rheum Dis.* 1993;52(9):629-637.
60. Casey AT, et al. Surgery on the rheumatoid cervical spine for the non-ambulant myelopathic patient—too much, too late? *Lancet.* 1996;347(9007):1004-1007.
61. Bydon M, et al. Regression of an atlantoaxial rheumatoid pannus following posterior instrumented fusion. *Clin Neurol Neurosurg.* 2015;137:28-33.
62. Lipson SJ. Cervical myelopathy and posterior atlanto-axial subluxation in patients with rheumatoid arthritis. *J Bone Joint Surg Am.* 1985;67(4):593-597.
63. Burry HC, et al. Lateral subluxation of the atlanto-axial joint in rheumatoid arthritis. *Ann Rheum Dis.* 1978;37(6):525-528.
64. Kudo H, Iwano K. Surgical treatment of subaxial cervical myelopathy in rheumatoid arthritis. *J Bone Joint Surg Br.* 1991;73(3):474-480.
65. Miyamoto H, Sumi M, Uno K. Outcome of surgery for rheumatoid cervical spine at one institute over three decades. *Spine J.* 2013;13(11):1477-1484.
66. Winfield J, et al. A prospective study of the radiological changes in the cervical spine in early rheumatoid disease. *Ann Rheum Dis.* 1981;40(2):109-114.
67. Pellicci PM, et al. A prospective study of the progression of rheumatoid arthritis of the cervical spine. *J Bone Joint Surg Am.* 1981;63(3):342-350.
68. Takeshima Y, et al. Rheumatoid arthritis-induced lateral atlantoaxial subluxation with multiple vertebrobasilar infarctions. *Spine.* 2015;40(3):E186-E189.
69. Sunahara N, et al. Clinical course of conservatively managed rheumatoid arthritis patients with myelopathy. *Spine.* 1997;22(22):2603-2607.

70. Paimela L, et al. Progression of cervical spine changes in patients with early rheumatoid arthritis. *J Rheumatol.* 1997;24(7):1280-1284.
71. Young A, et al. A prognostic index for erosive changes in the hands, feet, and cervical spines in early rheumatoid arthritis. *Br J Rheumatol.* 1988;27(2):94-101.
72. Sharp J, Purser DW. Spontaneous atlanto-axial dislocation in ankylosing spondylitis and rheumatoid arthritis. *Ann Rheum Dis.* 1961;20(1):47-77.
73. Bell HS. Paralysis of both arms from injury of the upper portion of the pyramidal decussation: "cruciate paralysis". *J Neurosurg.* 1970;33(4):376-380.
74. Gurley JP, Bell GR. The surgical management of patients with rheumatoid cervical spine disease. *Rheum Dis Clin North Am.* 1997;23(2):317-332.
75. Rana NA, et al. Upward translocation of the dens in rheumatoid arthritis. *J Bone Joint Surg Br.* 1973;55(3): 471-477.
76. Ranawat CS, et al. Cervical spine fusion in rheumatoid arthritis. *J Bone Joint Surg Am.* 1979;61(7):1003-1010.
77. Casey AT, et al. Predictors of outcome in the quadriparetic nonambulatory myelopathic patient with rheumatoid arthritis: a prospective study of 55 surgically treated Ranawat class IIIb patients. *J Neurosurg.* 1996;85(4):574-581.
78. Boden SD, et al. Rheumatoid arthritis of the cervical spine. A long-term analysis with predictors of paralysis and recovery. *J Bone Joint Surg Am.* 1993;75(9):1282-1297.
79. Koehler PR, et al. MR measurement of normal and pathologic brainstem diameters. *AJNR Am J Neuroradiol.* 1985;6(3):425-427.
80. Taniguchi D, et al. Evaluation of lateral instability of the atlanto-axial joint in rheumatoid arthritis using dynamic open-mouth view radiographs. *Clin Rheumatol.* 2008;27(7):851-857.
81. Riew KD, et al. Diagnosing basilar invagination in the rheumatoid patient. The reliability of radiographic criteria. *J Bone Joint Surg Am.* 2001;83-A(2):194-200.
82. Redlund-Johnell I, Pettersson H. Radiographic measurements of the cranio-vertebral region. Designed for evaluation of abnormalities in rheumatoid arthritis. *Acta Radiol Diagn (Stockh).* 1984;25(1):23-28.
83. White AA, Panjabi MM. *Clinical Biomechanics of the Spine.* 2nd ed. Philadelphia: JB Lippincott; 1990.
84. Yurube T, et al. Accelerated development of cervical spine instabilities in rheumatoid arthritis: a prospective minimum 5-year cohort study. *PLoS One.* 2014;9(2):e88970.
85. Dvorak J, et al. Functional evaluation of the spinal cord by magnetic resonance imaging in patients with rheumatoid arthritis and instability of upper cervical spine. *Spine.* 1989;14(10):1057-1064.
86. Bell GR, Stearns KL. Flexion-extension MRI of the upper rheumatoid cervical spine. *Orthopedics.* 1991;14(9):969-973.
87. Bundschuh C, et al. Rheumatoid arthritis of the cervical spine: surface-coil MR imaging. *AJR Am J Roentgenol.* 1988;151(1):181-187.
88. Mawatari T, et al. Vertebral strength changes in rheumatoid arthritis patients treated with alendronate, as assessed by finite element analysis of clinical computed tomography scans: a prospective randomized clinical trial. *Arthritis Rheum.* 2008;58(11):3340-3349.
89. Schmitt-Sody M, et al. Timing of cervical spine stabilisation and outcome in patients with rheumatoid arthritis. *Int Orthop.* 2008;32(4):511-516.
90. Wattenmaker I, et al. Upper-airway obstruction and perioperative management of the airway in patients managed with posterior operations on the cervical spine for rheumatoid arthritis. *J Bone Joint Surg Am.* 1994;76(3):360-365.
91. van Asselt KM, et al. Outcome of cervical spine surgery in patients with rheumatoid arthritis. *Ann Rheum Dis.* 2001;60(5):448-452.
92. Peppelman WC, et al. Cervical spine surgery in rheumatoid arthritis: improvement of neurologic deficit after cervical spine fusion. *Spine.* 1993;18(16):2375-2379.
93. Emery SE, et al. Anterior cervical decompression and arthrodesis for the treatment of cervical spondylotic myelopathy. Two to seventeen-year follow-up. *J Bone Joint Surg Am.* 1998;80(7):941-951.
94. Chin KR, Ozuna R. Options in the surgical treatment of cervical spondylotic myelopathy. *Current Opinions Orthop.* 2000;11:151-157.
95. Goodman SM, et al. Patients with rheumatoid arthritis are more likely to have pain and poor function after total hip replacements than patients with osteoarthritis. *J Rheumatol.* 2014;41(9):1774-1780.
96. Saag KG, et al. American College of Rheumatology 2008 recommendations for the use of nonbiologic and biologic disease-modifying antirheumatic drugs in rheumatoid arthritis. *Arthritis Rheum.* 2008;59(6):762-784.
97. Ledingham J, Deighton C. Update on the British Society for Rheumatology guidelines for prescribing TNFalpha blockers in adults with rheumatoid arthritis (update of previous guidelines of April 2001). *Rheumatology (Oxford).* 2005;44(2):157-163.
98. Bombardier C, et al. Canadian Rheumatology Association recommendations for the pharmacological management of rheumatoid arthritis with traditional and biologic disease-modifying antirheumatic drugs: part II. Safety. *J Rheumatol.* 2012;39(8):1583-1602.
99. Johnson BK, et al. Patterns and associated risk of perioperative use of anti-tumor necrosis factor in patients with rheumatoid arthritis undergoing total knee replacement. *J Rheumatol.* 2013;40(5):617-623.
100. Howe CR, Gardner GC, Kadel NJ. Perioperative medication management for the patient with rheumatoid arthritis. *J Am Acad Orthop Surg.* 2006;14(9):544-551.
101. Dixon WG, Suissa S, Hudson M. The association between systemic glucocorticoid therapy and the risk of infection in patients with rheumatoid arthritis: systematic review and meta-analyses. *Arthritis Res Ther.* 2011;13(4):R139.
102. Friedman RJ, Schiff CF, Bromberg JS. Use of supplemental steroids in patients having orthopaedic operations. *J Bone Joint Surg Am.* 1995;77(12):1801-1806.
103. Yong SL, et al. Supplemental perioperative steroids for surgical patients with adrenal insufficiency. *Cochrane Database Syst Rev.* 2009;(4):CD005367.
104. Glowniak JV, Loriaux DL. A double-blind study of perioperative steroid requirements in secondary adrenal insufficiency. *Surgery.* 1997;121(2):123-129.
105. Marik PE, Varon J. Requirement of perioperative stress doses of corticosteroids: a systematic review of the literature. *Arch Surg.* 2008;143(12):1222-1226.
106. Scanzello CR, et al. Perioperative management of medications used in the treatment of rheumatoid arthritis. *HSS J.* 2006;2(2):141-147.
107. Grennan DM, et al. Methotrexate and early postoperative complications in patients with rheumatoid arthritis

undergoing elective orthopaedic surgery. *Ann Rheum Dis.* 2001;60(3):214-217.

108. Gerster JC, Bossy R, Dudler J. Bone non-union after osteotomy in patients treated with methotrexate. *J Rheumatol.* 1999;26(12):2695-2697.
109. Khanna R, et al. The impact of steroids, methotrexate, and biologics on clinical and radiographic outcomes in patients with rheumatoid arthritis undergoing fusions at the craniovertebral junction. *J Craniovertebr Junction Spine.* 2015;6(2):60-64.
110. Zimmerli W, Moser C. Pathogenesis and treatment concepts of orthopaedic biofilm infections. *FEMS Immunol Med Microbiol.* 2012;65(2):158-168.
111. Hirano Y, et al. Influences of anti-tumour necrosis factor agents on postoperative recovery in patients with rheumatoid arthritis. *Clin Rheumatol.* 2010;29(5):495-500.
112. den Broeder AA, et al. Risk factors for surgical site infections and other complications in elective surgery in patients with rheumatoid arthritis with special attention for anti-tumor necrosis factor: a large retrospective study. *J Rheumatol.* 2007;34(4):689-695.
113. Ruyssen-Witrand A, et al. Complication rates of 127 surgical procedures performed in rheumatic patients receiving tumor necrosis factor alpha blockers. *Clin Exp Rheumatol.* 2007;25(3):430-436.
114. Goodman SM. Rheumatoid arthritis: perioperative management of biologics and DMARDs. *Semin Arthritis Rheum.* 2015;44(6):627-632.
115. Kaltsonoudis E, et al. Neurological adverse events in patients receiving anti-TNF therapy: a prospective imaging and electrophysiological study. *Arthritis Res Ther.* 2014;16(3):R125.
116. Fromont A, et al. Inflammatory demyelinating events following treatment with anti-tumor necrosis factor. *Cytokine.* 2009;45(2):55-57.
117. Wright NM. Posterior C2 fixation using bilateral, crossing C2 laminar screws: case series and technical note. *J Spinal Disord Tech.* 2004;17(2):158-162.
118. Payer M, Luzi M, Tessitore E. Posterior atlanto-axial fixation with polyaxial C1 lateral mass screws and C2 pars screws. *Acta Neurochir (Wien).* 2009;151(3):223-229.
119. Sinha S, et al. Occiput/C1-C2 fixations using intra-laminar screw of axis—a long-term follow-up. *Br J Neurosurg.* 2015;29(2):260-264.
120. Chieng LO, Madhavan K, Vanni S. Pooled data analysis on anterior versus posterior approach for rheumatoid arthritis at the craniovertebral junction. *Neurosurg Focus.* 2015;38(4):E18.
121. Tokuhashi Y, et al. C1-C2 intra-articular screw fixation for atlantoaxial subluxation due to rheumatoid arthritis. *Orthopedics.* 2009;32(3):172.
122. Elliott RE, et al. Atlantoaxial fusion with screw-rod constructs: meta-analysis and review of literature. *World Neurosurg.* 2014;81(2):411-421.
123. Okamoto T, et al. Mechanical implant failure in posterior cervical spine fusion. *Eur Spine J.* 2012;21(2):328-334.
124. Squires J, Molinari RW. C1 lateral mass screw placement with intentional sacrifice of the C2 ganglion: functional outcomes and morbidity in elderly patients. *Eur Spine J.* 2010;19(8):1318-1324.
125. Dmitriev AE, et al. Acute and long-term stability of atlantoaxial fixation methods: a biomechanical comparison of pars, pedicle, and intralaminar fixation in an intact and odontoid fracture model. *Spine.* 2009;34(4):365-370.
126. Lapsiwala SB, et al. Biomechanical comparison of four C1 to C2 rigid fixative techniques: anterior transarticular, posterior transarticular, C1 to C2 pedicle, and C1 to C2 intralaminar screws. *Neurosurgery.* 2006;58(3):516-521.
127. McAfee PC, et al. Fusion of the occiput to the upper cervical spine. A review of 37 cases. *Spine.* 1991;16(10 suppl):S490-S494.
128. Huckell CB, et al. Functional outcome of plate fusions for disorders of the occipitocervical junction. *Clin Orthop Relat Res.* 1999;359:136-145.
129. Sasso RC, et al. Occipitocervical fusion with posterior plate and screw instrumentation. A long-term follow-up study. *Spine.* 1994;19(20):2364-2368.
130. Roberts DA, Doherty BJ, Heggeness MH. Quantitative anatomy of the occiput and the biomechanics of occipital screw fixation. *Spine.* 1998;23(10):1100-1107.
131. Fehlings MG, et al. Occipitocervical fusion with a five-millimeter malleable rod and segmental fixation. *Neurosurgery.* 1993;32(2):198-207.
132. Matsunaga S, Ijiri K, Koga H. Results of a longer than 10-year follow-up of patients with rheumatoid arthritis treated by occipitocervical fusion. *Spine.* 2000;25(14):1749-1753.
133. Moskovich R, et al. Occipitocervical stabilization for myelopathy in patients with rheumatoid arthritis. Implications of not bone-grafting. *J Bone Joint Surg Am.* 2000;82(3):349-365.
134. Kerschbaumer F, et al. Transoral decompression, anterior plate fixation, and posterior wire fusion for irreducible atlantoaxial kyphosis in rheumatoid arthritis. *Spine.* 2000;25(20):2708-2715.
135. Crockard HA, Calder I, Ransford AO. One-stage transoral decompression and posterior fixation in rheumatoid atlanto-axial subluxation. *J Bone Joint Surg Br.* 1990;72(4):682-685.
136. McAfee PC, Bohlman HH. One-stage anterior cervical decompression and posterior stabilization with circumferential arthrodesis. A study of twenty-four patients who had a traumatic or a neoplastic lesion. *J Bone Joint Surg Am.* 1989;71(1):78-88.
137. Kast E, et al. Complications of transpedicular screw fixation in the cervical spine. *Eur Spine J.* 2006;15(3):327-334.
138. Clarke MJ, et al. Long-term incidence of subaxial cervical spine instability following cervical arthrodesis surgery in patients with rheumatoid arthritis. *Surg Neurol.* 2006;66(2):136-140.
139. Tanouchi T, et al. Adjacent-level failures after occipito-thoracic fusion for rheumatoid cervical disorders. *Eur Spine J.* 2014;23(3):635-640.
140. Ronkainen A, et al. Cervical spine surgery in patients with rheumatoid arthritis: longterm mortality and its determinants. *J Rheumatol.* 2006;33(3):517-522.
141. Nakamura C, et al. Upper thoracic myelopathy caused by vertebral collapse and subluxation in rheumatoid arthritis: report of two cases. *J Orthop Sci.* 2004;9(6):629-634.
142. Hirohashi N, et al. Lumbar radiculopathy caused by extradural rheumatoid nodules. Case report. *J Neurosurg Spine.* 2007;7(3):352-356.
143. Kawaji H, et al. A case report of rapidly progressing cauda equina symptoms due to rheumatoid arthritis. *J Nippon Med Sch.* 2005;72(5):290-294.
144. Sakai T, et al. Radiological features of lumbar spinal lesions in patients with rheumatoid arthritis with special reference to the changes around intervertebral discs. *Spine J.* 2008;8(4):605-611.
145. Crawford CH 3rd, et al. Lumbar fusion outcomes in patients with rheumatoid arthritis. *Eur Spine J.* 2008;17(6):822-825.

CHAPTER 85 Ankylosing Spondylitis

Dheera Ananthakrishnan
Serena S. Hu

Ankylosing spondylitis (AS) was first described in the late 1800s by a group of French neurologists. It is currently classified as one of the spondyloarthritides. The hallmark of the disease is pain and stiffness of joints, mainly in the axial skeleton, with early inflammation in the sacroiliac joints and the spine and later findings of increased bone formation, leading to global and regional stiffness. The disease usually is diagnosed in men in their second and third decades of life. There is some debate about the true male-to-female ratio. It was previously thought that the ratio was almost 10 : 1. It is now accepted that the ratio is much lower, probably about 4 : 1. The disease affects males predominantly, with a 2 : 1 ratio. The disease in women is usually less severe, possibly leading to what may be perceived as a decreased incidence. AS is an autoimmune condition that often results in chronic pain, disability, deformity, and fractures, much of which is of a spinal etiology. In addition, large joints—most notably the hips, knees, and shoulders—develop early arthritic changes.

Pathophysiology

The association between the major histocompatibility complex antigen HLA-B27 and AS has been well established.[1–6] Approximately 90% of AS patients are positive for the HLA-B27 antigen, although less than 10% of patients who are HLA-B27 positive manifest the signs and symptoms of AS. First-degree relatives of AS patients who are HLA-B27 positive who are also positive for the antigen have a 30% risk of having AS in contrast to the prevalence in the general population, which is 1% to 2%. The exact mechanism of the AS and HLA-B27 connection is unknown, although a bacterial association has been proposed. Recent research has revealed complex associations of AS with cytokines, such as the interleukins and tumor necrosis factor; this research has led to new treatment algorithms for disease modification.

AS is an inflammatory disease in which joints become arthritic and eroded, followed by autofusion (ankylosis). Microscopic evaluation of early lesions shows lymphocytic infiltrates, plasma cells, and macrophages. The first joints to be affected are usually the sacroiliac joints, followed by the vertebral apophyses, followed by the costovertebral joints. When the costovertebral joints have been fused, chest expansion is much reduced, leading to a decrease in pulmonary function. Enthesopathies are also common, leading to inflammation and erosions of the junction of the anulus and the vertebral endplate. Subchondral marrow edema is a classic finding in enthesopathies associated with AS. Erosions lead to ossification of the endplates, which is manifested by the bridging syndesmophytes seen on plain radiographs. Ankylosis of the facet joints leads to the “bamboo spine” seen on plain radiographs. During the progression of facet ankylosis, patients tend to assume a kyphotic posture to unload the joints and relieve the pain. With time, this compensatory mechanism leads to the fixed deformities of cervicothoracic, thoracic, and lumbar kyphosis commonly seen in AS patients who present to spinal surgeons. These deformities lead to difficulty with horizontal gaze, ambulation, and activities of daily living.

When the spine has become completely ankylosed, it functions as a rigid, brittle beam, leading to an increased incidence of fracture with even minor trauma. These fractures represent the second pressing issue that spine surgeons must deal with when treating patients with AS. Osteoporosis also plays an important role in AS.[1,7–10] The greatest decrease in bone mass occurs early in the course of the disease, although the reason for this is unknown. Decreased bone density in AS patients is multifactorial: it results from the uncoupling of bone formation and resorption, stress shielding in the vertebral bodies, and decreased activity and decreased muscle mass.

AS affects peripheral joints as well. The most common joint involved is the hip joint, where protrusio acetabuli can be seen. Hip involvement is often bilateral and often occurs early in the course of the disease. In addition, the presence of thoracic and lumbar kyphosis compounds the problems seen with hip flexion contractures because these conditions contribute to an inability to stand upright. The shoulders, knees, wrists, and hands are also affected but to a much lesser degree.

Disease modifying antirheumatic drugs are currently being researched for treatment of AS.[10–12] In particular, tumor necrosis factor blocking agents such as infliximab have been shown to improve clinical symptoms as well as decrease inflammatory markers and decrease appearance of inflammation on magnetic resonance imaging (MRI), all in the axial skeleton. These drugs have been promising, particularly when compared with traditional agents such as sulfasalazine, methotrexate, and nonsteroidal antiinflammatory drugs (NSAIDs), which have not been shown to be very effective in the axial skeleton, although they have been shown to help in the appendicular skeleton.

Nonorthopaedic Manifestations

Although it is the musculoskeletal system that is mainly affected by AS, there are other serious effects of the disease. The most common extraskeletal abnormality is anterior uveitis (approximately 25% of patients), which is usually treated with topical agents and rarely leads to vision loss. Ankylosis in the thoracic spine and at the costovertebral joints leads to markedly diminished chest wall expansion, resulting in restrictive lung disease with decreased lung volumes (vital capacity and total lung volume) and increased dependence on diaphragmatic excursion. Preoperative pulmonary function tests are recommended as is smoking cessation and aggressive postoperative pulmonary toilet. Some AS patients (25–30%) also have a component of ileitis or colitis, or both; regardless, all patients for whom surgery is being contemplated should have a preoperative nutritional assessment and should be considered for perioperative nutritional supplementation. The incidence of aortic stenosis and aortic valve insufficiency is increased in these patients as well; a preoperative echocardiogram is recommended routinely.

Physical Examination and Diagnosis

A patient with AS is most often a young man who gives a history of vague nonlocalizing back pain, morning stiffness, and possibly increasing difficulty with activities of daily living. Although women are affected with AS, men often present earlier or with more advanced disease. Upon physical examination, diminished spinal mobility, especially in the sagittal plane, is usually present. The Schober test is used to evaluate lumbar spinal motion: points 10 cm above and 5 cm below the lumbosacral junction in the midline are marked on the patient in the fully upright position. With full forward flexion, there should be at least 5 cm of excursion between these two points. Chest expansion is commonly limited to less than 2.5 cm of excursion and is typically measured at the fourth intercostal space. The modified New York diagnostic criteria for AS were outlined in 1984 and are as follows[13]:

1. Sacroiliitis confirmed by radiographs
2. Persistent low back pain greater than 3 months in duration
3. Diminished chest expansion (as just described)
4. Limited range of motion of the lumbar spine in the sagittal and coronal planes

The presence of sacroiliac inflammation and one of the other three criteria are generally considered enough to establish the diagnosis of AS.

Sacroiliitis is usually identified on an anteroposterior pelvis film (with or without a Ferguson view). It is widely accepted that the presence of sacroiliitis is crucial for the diagnosis of AS. Sacroiliac joint destruction is the earliest manifestation of AS. The earliest stages of sacroiliitis show some blurring of the cortical margins; this progresses to subcortical erosions (more commonly on the iliac side because it is less robust than the sacral side). In advanced stages, the sacroiliac joints become completely fused and the cortical erosions disappear. Sacroiliac joint involvement usually is symmetrical and bilateral. Studies have suggested that the use of bony pelvis computed tomography (CT) or MRI in conjunction with plain radiographs may lead to earlier diagnosis of AS.[8] It has yet to be determined whether this early diagnosis favorably affects clinical outcomes.

Management of Acute Injury

The spinal surgeon is usually not the physician making the initial diagnosis of AS but rather is called on to address spinal deformity caused by AS in the clinic and spinal trauma in an AS patient in an emergency setting. A trauma patient with AS also presents a great challenge to the spinal surgeon. The spine in AS functions as a long rigid beam, acting much like a long bone. This altered biomechanical state, plus the presence of osteoporosis and the lack of ligamentous constraints, significantly decreases the fracture threshold of the ankylosed spine. The key to detecting fractures in these patients is having a high index of suspicion, especially after minor trauma. Delay in diagnosis is common and is associated with secondary neurologic injury. The cervical and cervicothoracic regions are the most commonly affected, followed by the thoracolumbar junction. Plain radiography is neither sensitive nor specific in these instances; in many trauma centers, plain radiography has been replaced by CT as the initial radiographic evaluation for a suspected spinal injury. Epidural hematoma, spinal cord injury, and disc injury can be visualized with MRI as a secondary evaluation. The physician making the initial evaluation should keep in mind that often CT scan is not sensitive enough to pick up an occult fracture; given the high cost of missing these fractures, an MRI should be obtained in cases of clinically suspected fracture not visualized on CT scan.

A patient with AS may present with a progressive neurologic deficit without obvious bony injury or with progression of the spinal deformity and increased pain. This may be a missed spinal column injury that presents at a later time to the clinic or the emergency department with progressive neurologic deficit or worsening of deformity, or both. The evaluating clinician must also be aware of possible hyperextension through a fracture at a kyphotic segment, which may result in relatively normal sagittal alignment. Attempts to determine the patient's preexisting deformity from history and prior radiographs should always be made. There have been reports of neurologic injury in patients strapped to spine boards in a position of hyperextension when compared with their preinjury alignment.[14,15] Because of the stiff and osteoporotic spine, minor trauma may result in acute angulation or moderately rapid deformity progression. One should refrain from attempting acute correction through such a fracture. The patient should be initially immobilized in a halo vest in the preinjury alignment. Every attempt to maintain the patient's preinjury posture while performing the evaluation should be made.

For a patient with a neurologic deficit, MRI is imperative. MRI may reveal an epidural hematoma, buckling of the ligamentum flavum, or a disc herniation. Hematomas can occur in these patients from minor trauma from the osteoporotic bone or from scarred epidural vessels adjacent to a fracture. Evacuation of a hematoma is essential in the presence of progressive neurologic deficit. The decompression required may significantly destabilize the AS patient; thus, the surgeon should be prepared to stabilize the spine at the same setting. Usually, rigid instrumentation is required, although rarely halo immobilization may be sufficient for some cervical cases. As with instrumentation for elective cases, the screw-bone interface is compromised because of osteoporosis and the overall spinal column can be extremely unstable in these situations. Both of these concerns warrant aggressive stabilization with multiple fixation points above and below the fracture site.

The incidence of neurologic injuries in these patients is quite high (58–65%) owing to excessive bleeding at the fracture site leaking into the confined epidural space and translation (displacement) at the fracture site. The translation causes direct injury to the spinal cord and persistent bleeding due to motion, resulting in an enlarging compressive hematoma. Most spinal injuries in AS patients are three-column injuries (because of the stiffness of the load-absorbing structures). These injuries are highly unstable because there are two long lever arms hinging at the fracture site. In addition, the presence of preinjury kyphosis increases the likelihood of translation at the level of the injury, which subsequently increases the likelihood of neurologic injury. Last, poor bone stock and difficult radiographic evaluation can lead to a delay in diagnosis and a secondary neurologic decline. Most of these injuries (60–75%) are at the cervicothoracic junction, which is notoriously difficult to evaluate with plain radiographs. If the surgeon uses lateral mass screws in the cervical spine, these constructs should generally be supplemented by external support, such as with a halo vest. Laminar hooks may be more rigid in many patients, but external bracing should still be considered.

It is generally accepted that AS patients sustain more spinal fractures and dislocations than individuals without AS, anywhere from 4 to 7 times the fracture rate of those unaffected by AS.[10–12,16–20] Carbone and colleagues[2] retrospectively looked at 158 patients in Rochester, Minnesota, with AS and found a sevenfold increase in the incidence of spinal fractures over that of a cohort of patients without AS. They found no such increase in extremity fractures. The patients with spinal fractures tended to be older and had a greater preinjury involvement of the spine than patients without fractures. Cooper and colleagues[16] also noted that this higher incidence was mainly during the first 5 years after diagnosis and suggested that this was due to a greater percentage of bone density loss during this period, resulting in a decreased fracture threshold. In addition, the dampening structures present in a normal spine have lost their load-absorbing qualities in the ankylosed spine. The intervertebral discs are stiff, as are the ligamentous structures, and the facet joints are ankylosed.

Whang and colleagues[21] compared a cohort of 12 patients with AS who sustained spinal injuries with 18 patients with diffuse idiopathic skeletal hyperostosis (DISH) who sustained spinal injuries. The DISH group represents a group of patients of similar age whose spinal condition results in stiff segments above and below any spinal fracture. Falls from a standing position were the most common mechanism of injury. There was a greater likelihood that the DISH patients did not incur any neurologic deficit (44.4%) compared with AS patients (25% of whom did not have a neurologic deficit). Complication rates were higher in the AS group (42% vs. 33% in the DISH group). There were two deaths in each group related to the injury or its treatment, all of which were considered to be related to the use of the halo vest (aspiration [two deaths], respiratory failure, and multisystem organ failure). Several patients died of unrelated causes during the follow-up period; however, all surviving patients were contacted and were classified as having excellent or good outcomes.

Caron et al.[22] looked retrospectively at 112 patients with AS and DISH who sustained 122 fractures. The majority of these were extension-type injuries, most at the C6–C7 disc level. Nearly 60% had a spinal cord injury. Nineteen percent of the patients had a delayed fracture diagnosis. Subgroup analysis noted no significant differences between the AS group and the DISH group (28 and 74, respectively). Two-thirds of the patients underwent surgery, which usually consisted of a posterior fusion with a minimum of three levels of fixation above and below the injury level. There was a high rate of complications (84%) as well as a high rate of mortality (32%), the latter of which correlated with advanced age (>70 years old). However, 34% of the patients with a spinal cord injury improved neurologically, and these authors did feel that surgery could be beneficial, though difficult, in these patients.

Westerveld et al.[12] did a literature review of fractures in patients with AS and DISH. Ninety-three articles were reviewed, with 345 ankylosing spondylitis patients and 55 DISH patients. They noted that most of the injuries were as a result of a low-energy insult (65–69%) and that most were cervical spine fractures (60–81%). Of the AS patients, 17% had a delay in diagnosis, with 14% of patients sustaining a secondary neurologic decline. Of the patients, 54% underwent surgery; the majority of these surgeries were posterior spinal fusions. They did note some unusual complications after surgery, such as aortic dissection, pseudoaneurysm, and tracheal rupture; however, the patients treated nonoperatively had a similar mortality rate compared to the surgically treated patients (11–13% vs. 6–7%, not significantly different from a statistical standpoint).

Finkelstein and colleagues[23] looked retrospectively at 21 AS patients with a diagnosis of spinal trauma. One-third of these patients had a delay in diagnosis; three had complete spinal cord injuries on presentation, and three experienced neurologic deterioration to complete spinal cord injuries after admission. These authors recommended quick-screening cervical and thoracic MRI (one film) and screening lumbosacral spine MRI (one film) for diagnosis, in addition to minimal transfers and immediate stabilization. They did not comment on their definitive protocol for treatment of these patients (operative vs. nonoperative).

Hitchon and colleagues[24] retrospectively reviewed 11 patients with AS and thoracic and lumbar fractures. They found that 10 of these patients had sustained three-column injuries; 9 patients had extension-type injuries. More than half of these patients had a neurologic deficit (the specifics of which the study authors did not mention); half of these neurologically injured patients had some improvement in function. These authors recommended surgical intervention for stabilization of thoracic and lumbar three-column injuries because of their inherent instability.

The relatively recent adoption of minimally invasive techniques has been looked at in the AS population. Nayak et al.[25] looked at 11 consecutive patients with AS and/or DISH treated with minimally invasive surgery stabilization after hyperextension injuries of the thoracolumbar spine. The mean age was 77 years and the mean American Society of Anesthesiologists grade was 3. An average of 7 segments were instrumented. Of note is that the authors did not comment on whether they attempted a fusion in these patients or not. There were no revisions, and the clinical outcomes were similar to those of elective lumbar degenerative surgery.

Graham and van Peteghem[26] looked retrospectively at 15 patients over 6 years (1978–84) comparing types of injuries and treatments. Of the patients, 12 had cervical spine injuries; 9 of these had spinal cord injuries. The two patients with thoracic injuries had anterior cord syndromes. There were no compression-type injuries; most injuries resulted from a flexion-extension type of mechanism. The only patient treated with operative intervention was the patient with the lumbar injury, who had hardware failure and had to undergo revision. Two patients died, and three patients had pulmonary complications.

Apple and Anson[27] reviewed AS patients with spinal fracture and spinal cord injury, comparing operative versus nonoperative treatments. This study was a retrospective, multicenter study of 59 patients. In the operative group, 37 patients were treated with a variety of procedures. Patients in the nonoperative group were placed in halo traction followed by halo vests and placed on bed rest. There were no significant differences between the two groups with regard to motor recovery, fusion complications, or mortality rate (22% in both groups). The nonoperative group did have significantly shorter hospital stays. No analysis of the patients according to type of injury or treatment was done, and no discussion of the deaths was presented.

Hunter and Dubo[17] reviewed the cases of 19 AS patients who had sustained cervical spine fractures. Five of these patients had a complete spinal cord injury, and all of these patients died after their injury without having had any surgical intervention. All of these patients were treated nonoperatively. No patient developed neurologic deterioration, and all of the patients with incomplete cord injury regained some function. The authors concluded that nonoperative treatment worked well in these patients, although they suggested that surgery be considered in patients with grossly unstable injuries.

In a classic article, Bohlman[28] retrospectively reviewed 300 patients with cervical spine injuries.[28] He found only eight patients who carried a preinjury diagnosis of AS. Five of these patients died of pulmonary or gastrointestinal causes. Clinically significant epidural hematomas were found only in the AS patients. Bohlman recommended decompression for patients with progressive neurologic deficit. There was a delay in diagnosis in four patients, all of whom developed spinal cord injuries.

The generally accepted protocol with respect to the management of spine trauma in AS patients is as follows. If the clinician has even the slightest suspicion of spinal injury, the patient should be immobilized in the preinjury position. Plain radiography and fine-cut CT with reconstructions should be obtained. If the patient has a neurologic injury, MRI should be considered, looking for an epidural hematoma. If a fracture is detected and displacement or gross instability is noted, low-weight inline traction should be used in an attempt to facilitate a reduction to the preinjury alignment. If a reduction is obtained, the patient should be placed in a halo vest for definitive treatment. If a reduction cannot be obtained, internal fixation is recommended, with or without decompression if indicated by the patient's neurologic status. Postoperative immobilization in the form of a halo vest is then recommended. In a patient with a progressive neurologic deficit, MRI is likely to reveal the presence of a hematoma. In a patient with a stable deficit and no hematoma, the cord injury likely occurred at the time of injury; as long as the spine is stable, management of the neurologic injury should be expected. If the spine is unstable, reduction and stabilization either with traction followed by a halo vest or with surgery is recommended if the patient is medically able to tolerate surgery. If not, external immobilization, such as a halo vest or rigid thoracolumbar orthosis, can be used to manage these injuries, but in general the clinical outcomes are better with surgical intervention due to the high rate of unstable injuries. Despite some case reports to the contrary,[12,14] the standard of care for the AS patient with a spinal fracture is *not* to attempt a deformity correction at the same sitting as fracture stabilization. Rather, the two issues should be dealt with separately, allowing the patient to recover from the fracture and the surgery, then planning an elective deformity correction if it is warranted and the patient is able to tolerate it.

Complications can arise at the time of injury and from treatment of the injury. Deformity and neurologic injury can occur as a result of the injury; treatment with decompression and internal fixation carries risks of nonunion, hardware failure, failure of the bone-screw interface that results in loss of fixation, and infection. Halo management carries its own risk of complications. Skull fractures, pin tract infections, intracerebral hemorrhage, and intracranial air all have been reported with halo immobilization in these patients.[14,29] Taggard and Traynelis[30] described a posterior cervical fusion (lateral mass plating) that they used in seven AS patients who had sustained fractures. The fusions were supplemented with autologous rib grafts. Postoperatively, the patients were immobilized in collars only, with the exception of one, who was placed in a sternal-occipital-mandibular immobilizer. Fusion occurred in all patients; there were two deaths in quadriplegic patients. The authors recommended operative intervention as a means of avoiding postoperative halo immobilization. Other complications that have been reported include cardiac issues, aortic rupture, postoperative dysphagia, and infection, to name a few.

Deformity

The deformities seen in AS are a result of excessive kyphosis throughout the spine and excessive flexion at the hip joints. All areas of the spine can be affected, with the lumbar spine affected most often, followed by the thoracic and cervical spine. If the physical examination and radiographic examinations indicate that the hip flexion contracture plays a significant role in the overall deformity, hip arthroplasty should be performed before spinal surgical intervention. In this manner, the less morbid operation is performed first; in addition, the spine surgeon can better assess the actual amount of sagittal imbalance attributable to the spine.

The spine surgeon must carefully examine the patient in the standing, seated, and supine positions to determine the major component of the deformity. If a major portion of the deformity corrects on moving from a standing to a seated position, the deformity is most likely arising from the hip joints or the lumbar spine and arthroplasty should be performed first. If the deformity persists on sitting but corrects in the supine position, the deformity is arising from the thoracic, thoracolumbar, or lumbar spine, and a lumbar osteotomy is usually indicated. If the deformity persists even in the supine position, the deformity is in the cervicothoracic area, and an osteotomy in this area is indicated.

From a radiographic standpoint, a full spine lateral radiograph with the neck in a neutral position and the hips in a fully extended position is crucial for surgical planning. This radiograph allows measurement of the chin-brow angle, which is formed by a line from the chin-brow to the floor vertical angle. This measurement is helpful when planning any osteotomy. Ideally, the chin-brow angle should be zero. Suk and colleagues[31] looked at the significance of the chin-brow measurement in assessing the success of surgical intervention. These investigators evaluated 34 AS patients undergoing lumbar or thoracolumbar osteotomies for correction of sagittal imbalance. Preoperative and postoperative chin-brow angles were measured. Clinical outcome assessment involved the Modified Arthritis Impairment Scales (AIMS). This questionnaire consists of three simple questions plus numerous subscales: function, indoor activity, outdoor activity, psychosocial activity, pain, and overall subjectivity. The authors found improved postoperative AIMS scores for questions involving looking forward, going up stairs, and going down stairs. There was a negative correlation between chin-brow angles and correction obtained but no correlation between chin-brow angle and clinical outcome. The patients who were overcorrected (to an angle <10 degrees) had worse scores with regard to looking forward and going down stairs; these results were found to be statistically significant.

Song et al.[32] investigated the optimal chin-brow angle for AS patients. They looked at 25 patients with AS who underwent surgical intervention for deformity correction, evaluating the final chin-brow angle as well as visual field–related life quality measurement scales and subjective appearance. In addition, they evaluated a number of indoor and outdoor activities. They found that the optimal chin-brow angle for best function and appearance was between 10 and 20 degrees.

When the location of the primary spine deformity is determined, the surgeon must decide what type of osteotomy would be most appropriate. It is preferable to place the osteotomy at the apex of the deformity, but this is not always possible. Thoracic and thoracolumbar osteotomies are limited by the rib cage, the spinal cord, and the conus medullaris. Deformities in these areas are often almost always treated with a lumbar osteotomy. By moving the osteotomy more caudally, one can obtain more sagittal plane alignment correction owing to a longer lever arm. By overcorrecting at the lumbar level, one can address the thoracic kyphosis and lumbar kyphosis. If overcorrection is to be performed, the surgeon should take into account what portion of the deformity is cervicothoracic because the patient's horizontal gaze would be affected and may not be restored. Of note, however, is that lumbar osteotomies present their own assortment of problems, such as difficulty with visualization and fewer points of fixation available distal to the osteotomy. These issues may lead the surgeon to perform an osteotomy or vertebral body resection in the thoracic spine, which carry their own set of risks and potential complications.

Preoperative Assessment

A careful history should yield information about the patient's lifestyle, habits, and medications. Smoking cessation is imperative in these patients; many surgeons do not undertake the operation while a patient is actively smoking. NSAIDs should be discontinued at least 2 weeks before surgery. Preoperative pulmonary function tests are indicated because most of these patients have restrictive lung disease. Preoperative echocardiography may also be indicated, as previously mentioned, although cardiac intervention is not often needed. Results of renal function tests should be obtained before surgery; an awareness of tenuous renal function would benefit intraoperative and postoperative fluid management. Many AS patients have a component of renal dysfunction because of long-term use of NSAIDs. Cervical spine flexibility should be assessed by the orthopedist and the anesthesia service before the procedure; fiberoptic intubation is usually needed because of concomitant ankylosis of the cervical spine.

Historically, most osteotomies in AS patients were performed with the patient awake or using a Stagnara wake-up test for evaluation of spinal cord function before, during, and after a correction. Somatosensory evoked potentials and motor evoked potentials (epidural or transcranial) have become more reliable so that the wake-up test is less frequently needed. The anterior tracts are better monitored by motor evoked potentials. These tracts can be preferentially affected during an extension maneuver when addressing kyphotic deformities, either by direct compression or by impairing the vascular supply to the spinal cord. Of note is that in 2006, Simmons presented his 36 years of experience with his classically described cervicothoracic osteoclasis procedure performed in the seated position under local anesthesia alone.[61] He noted a slight change in technique in the latter years, with a larger area of bony resection laterally, but the anesthesia and surgical position remained the same. No instrumentation was used; rather, all patients were placed in a halo vest for 4 months. He reviewed 131 cases and noted three cases of intraoperative paraplegia, one of which resolved after the dura was split, one of which was thought to be related to a carotid artery distraction. The third did not recover significantly after splitting of the dura. Sixteen patients developed a C8 radiculopathy. Four patients died within 3 months of surgery from pulmonary and cardiac complications. Also noted were few complications of pseudarthrosis, pneumonia, deep vein thrombosis, and halo pin infections.

A preoperative nutritional assessment (albumin, prealbumin, total protein) should be performed; perioperative nutritional supplementation (tube feedings or parenteral nutritional assessment) may be indicated. Klein and colleagues[33] noted a significant increase in complications, such as deep wound infection in patients undergoing lumbar spinal fusion who were malnourished by nutritional parameters preoperatively. Hu and colleagues[34] and Lapp and colleagues[35] showed that supplementation in the form of parenteral nutrition is beneficial in reducing complication rates after reconstructive spine surgery.

Lumbar Osteotomies

The first lumbar osteotomy was described in 1945 by Smith-Petersen for use in the rheumatoid patient.[36] This osteotomy is an opening osteotomy, meaning that the apex of the wedge lies posteriorly, opening up the anterior column during correction (osteoclasis through ossified disc space and anterior longitudinal ligament). Smith-Petersen and colleagues performed multilevel osteotomies in six patients. These osteotomies were V-shaped in the coronal plane, with the point of the "V" at the midline in the interlaminar space. The osteotomies are carried out through the articular processes bilaterally at two or three levels. It is imperative that adequate amounts of lamina and flavum are resected before correction so that compression of the neural elements on closure does not occur.

Cauda equina syndrome has been reported by Simmons[37] as a result of a decrease in canal dimensions. The posteriorly based closing wedge type of osteotomy results in an anterior opening at the level of the disc space. This anterior opening can be better achieved in an AS patient than a patient without AS because of the stiffness of the disc space. Complications of an opening wedge osteotomy include superior mesentery artery syndrome and aortic rupture owing to stretching of the abdominal vasculature.[38,39] Vascular complications are rare and tend to occur in older patients with calcific, adherent abdominal vessels.

Lichtblau and Wilson[38] described a patient who underwent closed osteoclasis followed by cast placement. This patient died in the immediate postoperative period of an aortic rupture. His history was significant for a large dose of radiation that was used to treat the ankylosed spine. Fazl and colleagues[39] described an AS patient who sustained a fracture through the T12–L1 disc space. He was treated with Harrington rod instrumentation and fusion but died 2 days postoperatively from an aortic rupture at the level of the injury. Aortic necrosis was present at autopsy, as were adhesions of the vessels to the spine. More common complications reported include ileus, pneumonia, and root traction injury. Cauda equina syndrome with flaccid paralysis below the level of injury, although rare, was reported in these studies as well.

Patients originally were immobilized in plaster; segmental instrumentation currently is indicated for these patients. Many investigators have reported their results after multilevel Smith-Petersen osteotomies.[36,40,41] Nonunion rates resulting in recurrence and progression of deformity were significant. Soon after the original description of this technique, reports of "plugging up" the open disc spaces with interbody fusions showed increased fusion rates and decreased complications.[42] The complications associated with opening wedge osteotomies led to modifications of Smith-Petersen's techniques. In 1949, Wilson and Turkell[43] described a procedure similar to the Smith-Petersen procedure in which less bone is removed but more osteotomies are created. The anterior longitudinal ligament is not ruptured; the anterior column length is not changed. In 1985, McMaster[41] described the addition of Harrington compression instrumentation to Smith-Petersen osteotomies in 14 patients. This instrumentation was used to close the wedges produced after osteotomy. Postoperatively, the patients were placed in casts for 9 months. Mean correction was 33 degrees at final follow-up. Subjective improvement was found in horizontal gaze and height and posture. The author suggested that a slow controlled osteotomy closure was beneficial in terms of overall stability and protection of neural elements. Püschel and Zielke[44] also performed multiple wedge-shaped Smith-Petersen type osteotomies and used Zielke instrumentation to close the osteotomies. They also recommended a slow correction with a gradual lordosis.

After reports of nonunions and concerns about stretching of the abdominal vasculature and viscera, Thomasen[45] described a closing wedge osteotomy. He reported on 11 patients in whom he performed a complete laminectomy at L2, transected the transverse processes, and resected the ankylosed facets at L2–L3. The pedicles of L2 were removed in their entirety down to the posterior aspect of the vertebral body. The entire vertebral body was decancellated, followed by removal of the posterior cortex and osteotomies of both lateral cortices. After careful mobilization of the dura above and below L2, Thomasen[45] closed the wedge by gradual flexion of the table. Internal fixation (plates and wiring) was used in six patients; all patients were placed in casts. One patient had a fracture-dislocation above the level of the osteotomy, resulting in a cauda equina syndrome. This patient had almost complete return of neurologic function after revision decompression and internal fixation. Correction ranged from 12 to 50 degrees. All patients had subjective improvement of posture and horizontal gaze.

Heinig's eggshell procedure[45a] was described in 1984 as a monosegmental osteotomy to be used in the same situations in which one would use Thomasen's procedure. Thomasen leaves the anterior vertebral body cortex intact, whereas Heinig actually describes fracturing this cortex, which decreases the length of the anterior column and the posterior column. As long as more bone is removed posteriorly, restoration of lordosis occurs.

Bradford and colleagues[46] reported in 1987 on a series of 21 patients with AS who underwent single-level or multilevel lumbar or thoracic osteotomies with or without anterior discectomies. All patients had internal fixation posteriorly with a thoracolumbosacral orthosis. Average corrections ranged from 9 to 36 degrees. Complications were noted more frequently in the closing wedge-type osteotomies (neurapraxias and fracture during hook placement). Wake-up tests were used in all patients. In addition, these authors recommended closing-type osteotomies to avoid traction on the spinal cord, wide decompression, and internal fixation to avoid neurologic complications.

In 1990, Hehne and colleagues[47] reported on 177 patients with AS in whom multisegmental opening wedge lumbar and thoracolumbar osteotomies were performed. These authors were the first to report on the use of pedicle screw fixation. Casting and bracing were used postoperatively. Average correction at follow-up (18–42 months) was 43 degrees, with horizontal gaze subjectively restored in all cases. Complications included deaths, transient paresis, transient and permanent nerve root injuries, implant failures, and infections. These authors suggested that pedicle screw fixation with multisegmental osteotomies can produce a smoother lordosis than that produced by a monosegmental osteotomy.

In 1992, Jaffray and colleagues[48] presented three patients in whom a decancellation closing wedge osteotomy was performed. They did not remove the entire pedicle; rather, the inferior aspect of the pedicle was preserved to ensure protection for the exiting nerve root. Pedicle screw fixation plus a postoperative cast was used. These authors recommended two-level osteotomies (L2 and L4) for patients who needed more correction. Horizontal gaze was corrected in two patients; one patient required a cervicothoracic osteotomy for complete gaze correction. Complications were not discussed.

The technique for lumbar osteotomy, whether via an opening wedge osteotomy or a closing wedge three-column osteotomy, begins similarly. The patient is positioned in the prone position on an operative table with the abdomen free to decrease venous congestion and bleeding. Often, an operative table that can be extended to facilitate correction is useful for these patients. Standard exposure of the areas to be instrumented is performed. Fixation points, usually pedicle screws at least three levels above and below the intended apex of the correction, are attained. Smith-Petersen osteotomies are performed as desired, gaining correction at each level, which can be facilitated by extending the operative table. A rod of the desired and intended configuration should be contoured in preparation for the correction. If a three-column osteotomy is needed, the laminectomy is performed at the desired level. This is most often L3 or L4, since the more distal correction will allow more improvement of the sagittal vertical axis but still allow three levels of fixation distally. The pedicle is skeletonized and then removed; the vertebral body is then decancellated in a wedge configuration. Often, a temporary rod is needed to prevent the osteotomy from collapsing prematurely. Decancellation of the osteoporotic spongy bone can result in significant bleeding and intermittent packing of the site with hemostatic agents is usually needed. Once the vertebra has been resected, the lateral body wall can be divided and the posterior body wall imploded into the defect. Placement of the contoured rod, supplemented by extension of the table, usually facilitates excellent correction. Once the spine has been stabilized, radiographs are taken to assess correction; if additional correction is needed, more bone can be removed or the rod or table further adjusted.

More recently, Van Royen and De Gast[49] mathematically analyzed the sagittal plane corrections of two patients and determined that the amount of correction needed depends on three parameters: sacral endplate angle, C7 plumb line, and chin-brow angle. The sacral endplate angle reflects the amount of sagittal plane deformity that can be attributed to the hip joints: as the flexion contracture at the hip increases, the pelvis must rotate posteriorly to keep the body center of mass over the pelvis, decreasing the sacral endplate angle. The chin-brow angle has been shown to be a quantifiable parameter that reflects the restoration of horizontal gaze.[40] A mathematical formula was found that determines the ideal location and angle for each particular patient for a closing wedge-type osteotomy centered on the anterior longitudinal ligament.

There have been many retrospective reviews of AS patients treated with various osteotomies for sagittal imbalance. Van Royen and De Gast[49] performed a meta-analysis of 856 AS patients. They found three different techniques described: multisegment (two to three levels) opening wedge osteotomies with rupture of the anterior longitudinal ligament (i.e., Smith-Petersen), multisegment closing wedge osteotomies (Wilson-Turkell), and closing wedge-type osteotomy with pedicle resection and an anterior hinge (Thomasen). After a thorough and careful review, the authors concluded that, although no single technique was clearly superior to the others, the complications associated with closing wedge osteotomies were less serious than the complications associated with the other two groups. In addition, loss of correction was more prevalent in patients treated with opening wedge and polysegmental wedge osteotomies and the closing wedge types.

A few studies have attempted to quantify results in terms of patient outcomes using a standardized grading system. In 1995, Halm and colleagues[50] used the modified AIMS questionnaire to evaluate 175 patients retrospectively after lumbar osteotomy. Treatment groups were multisegment Smith-Petersen with Harrington compression instrumentation (n = 34), multisegment Smith-Petersen with transpedicular fixation (n = 136), and monosegmental Thomasen with segmental fixation (n = 4). The investigators found statistically significant improvement in 47 of 60 items. Kim and colleagues[51] used the AIMS questionnaire prospectively in 45 patients with AS who were treated with Thomasen osteotomies at one or two levels. Osteotomies were mainly performed in the lumbar spine (usually L3). Average increase in lumbar lordosis was 34 degrees, with no significant increase in thoracic kyphosis. All parameters measured were significantly improved. Clinical outcome scores were significantly improved in all five categories; no correlation was found between the amount of radiographic correction obtained and clinical outcome as measured by the questionnaire.

Berven and colleagues[52] looked at 13 patients undergoing transpedicular wedge resection. Three of these patients had AS and were having spine surgery for the first time. These investigators also used outcome measures (modified Scoliosis Research Society questionnaire) in a retrospective manner. After 2 years, most of these patients were satisfied and would have the surgery again. The changes in C7 plumb line and lumbar lordosis were statistically significant. Complications included dural tear, transient nerve root injury, pulmonary embolus, and loss of sagittal balance. None of the AS patients showed a loss of sagittal balance at follow-up.

Bridwell and colleagues[53] looked at 27 patients undergoing pedicle subtraction osteotomy, also in a retrospective fashion. Two of these patients had AS. Outcome data (Oswestry Disability Index [ODI] and Scoliosis Research Society 24-item questionnaire [SRS-24]) were also obtained retrospectively. These authors found a significant improvement in sagittal balance and lumbar lordosis and a high level of patient satisfaction. Complications included deep vein thrombosis, myocardial infarction, compartment syndrome, visual field loss, pseudarthrosis, loss of correction, urinary retention, and neurologic deficits (root lesions). The patients with the latter two complications all responded to a central canal decompression.

Liu et al.[54] looked retrospectively at 53 AS patients who had complex spinal reconstruction surgery for kyphosis. In addition to standard outcome measures of the ODI and the Scoliosis Research Society 22-item questionnaire [SRS-22], they looked at gastrointestinal function as measured by abdominal measurements from CT scans as well as bowel habits. They found significant clinical improvements in gastrointestinal function after pedicle subtraction osteotomy in addition to improvement in spinal outcomes.

Zhang et al.[55] evaluated lung volume changes after pedicle subtraction osteotomies in 26 patients with AS. They noted improved lung volumes (measured on CT scans) after osteotomy, and noted that the magnitude of improvement correlated with the improvement in sagittal balance.

Hu et al.[56] retrospectively compared single pedicle subtraction osteotomy (PSO) to dual PSO in 60 patients with AS. They looked at radiographic parameters as well as outcome scores and operative parameters such as operating room time, estimated blood loss (EBL), and complications. They found increased EBL and operative time for the two-level cases but no differences in the other parameters. They did make note of the inherent selection bias with this study, as the patients selected to have the two-level PSOs were those whose imbalance was worse and that the more unhealthy patients did not undergo surgery.

Liu and colleagues[57] performed a meta-analysis of AS patients undergoing deformity correction via a posterior column extension osteotomy versus pedicle subtraction osteotomy. Twenty-three studies were evaluated, with 979 patients total; 441 of those had an extension osteotomy (posterior column osteotomy [PCO]), 538 underwent a PSO. Most patients had a one-level osteotomy between T11 and L5; there were no significant differences in any of the group characteristics, including the pelvic parameters. The review noted no significant differences in correction between the two groups and no significant differences in terms of complications, but the PSO patients had a longer average operating room time and higher than average EBL. Also of interest is that aortic rupture occurred infrequently but exclusively in the PCO group; the authors recommended avoidance of this technique in patients over 50 years old and in those who have radiographic evidence of abdominal aortic plaques/calcifications.

In extreme situations, two-level osteotomies have been performed. Zheng et al.[58] looked at 48 patients who underwent two lumbar osteotomies. All of these patients had single-stage interrupted PSOs. There were no major complications and no pseudarthroses. All patients had significant improvements in their clinical outcome scores, and chin-brow angles and sagittal balance were significantly improved. The authors recommended this approach in the severely deformed patient, but cautioned against inexperienced surgeons performing the procedure.

Thoracic Osteotomies

Even when the deformity has been localized primarily to the thoracic spine, lumbar osteotomies are usually recommended. These can be performed below cord and conus level, and they have the advantage of large degrees of correction of the sagittal vertical axis with a long lever arm. Osteotomies performed in the thoracic spine are usually Smith-Petersen, although closing wedge osteotomies and vertebral column resections may be indicated in the thoracic and thoracolumbar spine.

Kawahara and colleagues[59] described a closing-opening wedge osteotomy in the thoracic and thoracolumbar spine. They used this procedure on seven patients with sagittal imbalance. The osteotomy consisted of a partial vertebrectomy with a large posterior wedge that is performed in a manner similar to a costotransversectomy. After bony resection, pedicle screw instrumentation plus temporary correction rods are used to facilitate a closing wedge correction of about 30 degrees. An opening wedge-type maneuver is facilitated, again through the instrumentation, and a spacer or allograft is inserted. The authors noted good improvement in kyphosis, lordosis, and plumb line. They had no neurologic complications, no nonunions, and no loss of correction (follow-up, 2.2–7.5 years).

Cervicothoracic Osteotomy

If the primary deformity has been determined to be in the cervical spine, an osteotomy at the cervicothoracic junction can be performed. Patients with these deformities, in addition to the problems with horizontal gaze, also can experience dysphagia and problems related to poor oral intake. The chin-brow angle is of paramount importance when planning a corrective osteotomy in the cervicothoracic region. A key point is not to overcorrect the horizontal gaze because this can lead to inability of patients to see the floor ahead of them. These patients may function better when corrected to a chin-brow angle of about 10 degrees. In 1958, Urist[60] described an osteotomy in the cervicothoracic region, noting that the canal at this level is quite large and that the C8 nerve root is quite mobile compared with the upper cervical roots. In addition, potential loss of the lower cervical roots is less morbid than loss of the upper cervical roots. Last, the vertebral arteries are typically extraosseous at these levels, making resection of the lateral masses less risky.

Careful preoperative planning with radiographic studies is of paramount importance when performing a cervicothoracic osteotomy. Full-length standing lateral spine radiographs are needed to measure the chin-brow angle. Lateral tomography or fine-cut CT with sagittal and coronal reconstructions is performed to delineate the anatomy.[37,60] Axial CT scans can be very helpful in characterizing the distorted anatomy often seen in patients with AS, especially with regard to placement of instrumentation. MRI can help to rule out occult fractures, which should be suspected if there is recent onset of pain or rapid progression of deformity; MRI should be obtained if there is any neurologic deficit. In addition, flexion and extension lateral cervical spine radiographs should be obtained to look for any instability occurring at the occipitocervical and atlantoaxial levels. A subset of AS patients develop instability in these areas as a result of excessive stiffness of the entire spinal column because the stress placed on these upper cervical areas can be quite high. Although the number of AS patients who have occipitocervical or atlantoaxial instability is not as high as the number of AS patients with rheumatoid arthritis, missing this instability can be catastrophic.

The surgeon must carefully examine the preoperative radiographs and CT scans to determine the amount of correction needed. The measured chin-brow angle should be transposed onto a neutral cervicothoracic film, with the apex of the angle centered on the posterior longitudinal ligament at the C7–T1 level. By extrapolation, the extent of posterior elements to be resected can be determined.

As originally described by Urist and popularized by Simmons, the procedure was performed under local anesthesia only, with the patient awake in a seated position, in seated halo traction. The seated position carries with it the risk of air embolus in a patient with a patent foramen ovale so that continuous cardiac monitoring is indicated during the procedure. With the widespread use of neurophysiologic monitoring, the awake seated position is almost never used for these procedures at the present time except in the case in which the severe spinal deformity precludes prone positioning. A baseline set of somatosensory evoked potentials and motor evoked potentials is obtained, and the patient's head is placed in a rigid head holder (three-pin Mayfield). After the flip, a repeat run of neurophysiologic monitoring is obtained.

After a wide and lengthy exposure, a wide cervical decompression at C7 and T1 is performed, including a dorsal unroofing of bilateral C8 nerve roots. The lateral masses at C7 are also resected; in addition, the pedicles at C7 are partially removed to ensure that the C8 nerve roots are not compressed after the correction. Sometimes, a portion of the superior aspect of the T1 pedicles must be removed as well. Before the widespread use of instrumentation, postoperative immobilization consisted of a halo vest or cast that was custom measured or fitted to the patient's torso preoperatively. Currently, sublaminar hooks or lateral mass and pedicle screw instrumentation can be used for rigid stabilization, which greatly reduces the likelihood of translation at the osteoclasis level and subsequent neurologic injury. Lateral mass screws generally do not hold well in these patients due to underlying osteoporosis and can be supplemented by halo vest immobilization if the surgeon prefers to use it, keeping in mind that this orthosis carries its own risks of complications. Instrumentation is placed three levels above and three levels below C7–T1 after the decompression but before osteoclasis.

After the instrumentation has been placed, a temporary rod is prepared. One surgeon breaks scrub and manipulates the head and neck via the halo ring, facilitating the osteoclasis. The neck is slowly extended about the C7–T1 level, while the scrubbed surgeon watches the decompression site for excessive dural compression. Neurophysiologic signals are carefully monitored during the correction. An audible crack is often heard; the manipulating surgeon should appreciate a decrease in resistance when the osteoclasis has been completed. If the decompression has been planned and executed properly, any residual lateral mass of C7 should be opposed to T1, the C8 nerve roots should be free, and the dura should not be excessively compressed. The halo or Mayfield is resecured to the operative table in the corrected position. The rods are secured into position.

Even with neurophysiologic monitoring, a wake-up test is often performed after correction. Adjustments can be made intraoperatively after the main correction has been obtained. After the instrumentation has been secured, the local bone resected during the osteotomy is used for grafting, supplemented by allograft if the surgeon believes this is indicated, and the wound is closed. The anterior soft tissues are usually tight after being in a shortened position for a long time. The patient is usually kept intubated until the soft tissue edema and the postoperative anterior hematoma lessen. Even with rigid segmental instrumentation, the patient's osteopenia may necessitate placement in a rigid halo vest for the duration of the healing period. Dysphagia is common and usually resolves with time. If the patient's caloric intake is borderline, as is common, it is imperative that the patient receive nutritional supplementation during the healing period in the form of either tube feedings or parenteral supplementation (Fig. 85.1).

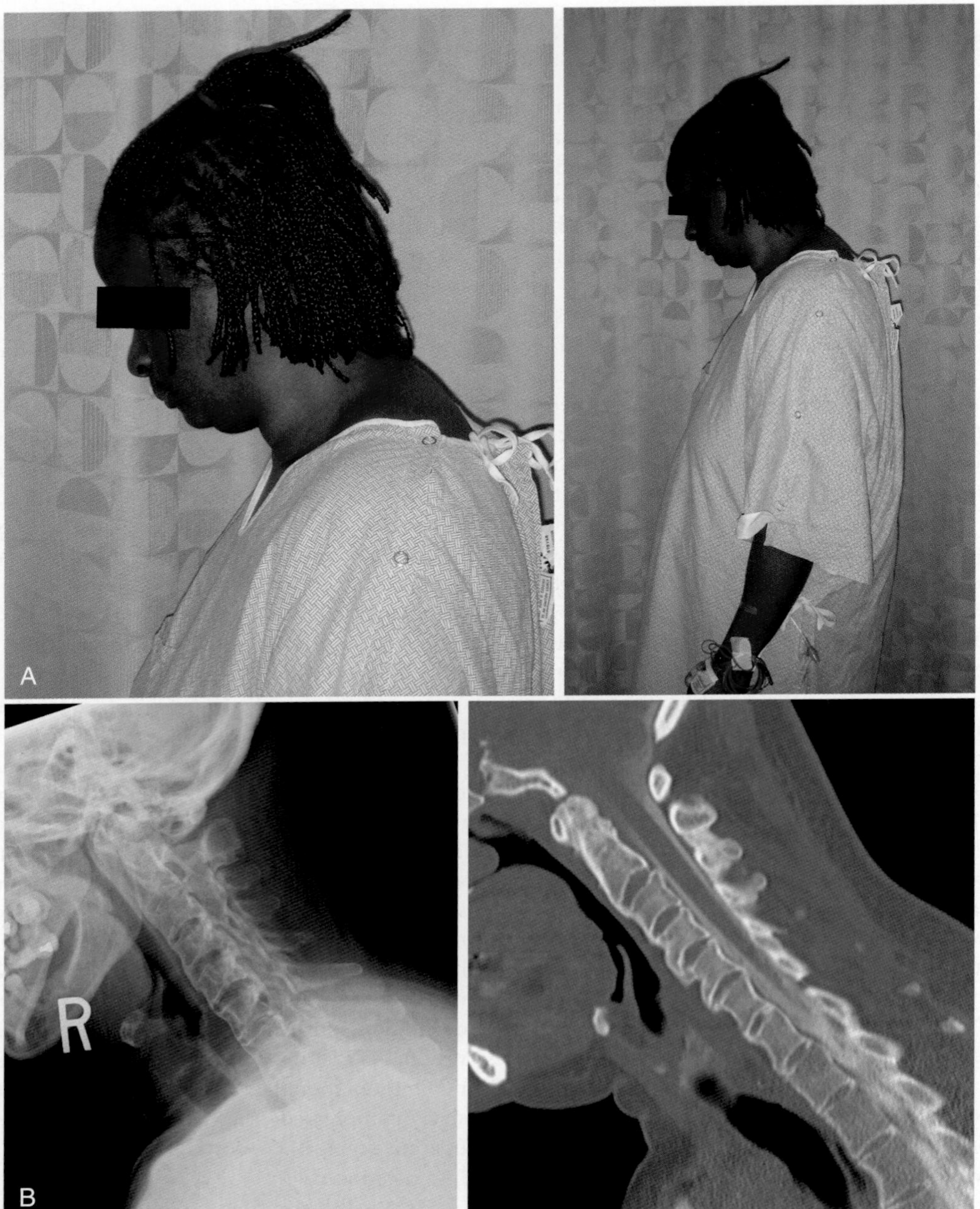

FIG. 85.1 (A) Photographs of a 45-year-old female with known ankylosing spondylitis, difficulty with activities of daily living and horizontal gaze, chin-brow to vertical angle (CBVA) of 40 degrees, and mildly positive sagittal balance. She had no neurologic complaints. (B) Lateral radiograph and sagittal computed tomography (CT) myelogram showing flowing syndesmophytes in the cervical spine; no significant central stenosis noted.

The literature concerning cervicothoracic osteotomies in AS patients is not robust. Simmons in his original article[37] reported on 42 patients who underwent cervicothoracic osteotomy as described by Urist. The operations were performed in the seated position under local anesthesia, and postoperative immobilization consisted of a halo vest. Simmons reported two nonunions successfully treated with anterior fusion, one pulmonary embolus, two myocardial infarctions (one fatal), and one root injury treated with repeat decompression. The patients who did not experience complications all were quite satisfied with their outcomes and had their horizontal gaze restored.

In 2006, Simmons and colleagues[61] reported on 36 years of experience in performing cervicothoracic osteotomies. They looked retrospectively at 131 cases, 114 of which had the "conventional" technique, with the remainder undergoing the "current" technique. Both techniques include local anesthesia with the patient awake during the procedure in a seated position, with halo fixation alone (no internal fixation). The difference in the two techniques is in regard to the amount of bone resected. The current technique resects all of the C7 posterior arch, including the pedicles as well as some resection of the posterolateral portions of C6 and T1. The conventional technique does not remove the pedicle or any portions of C6

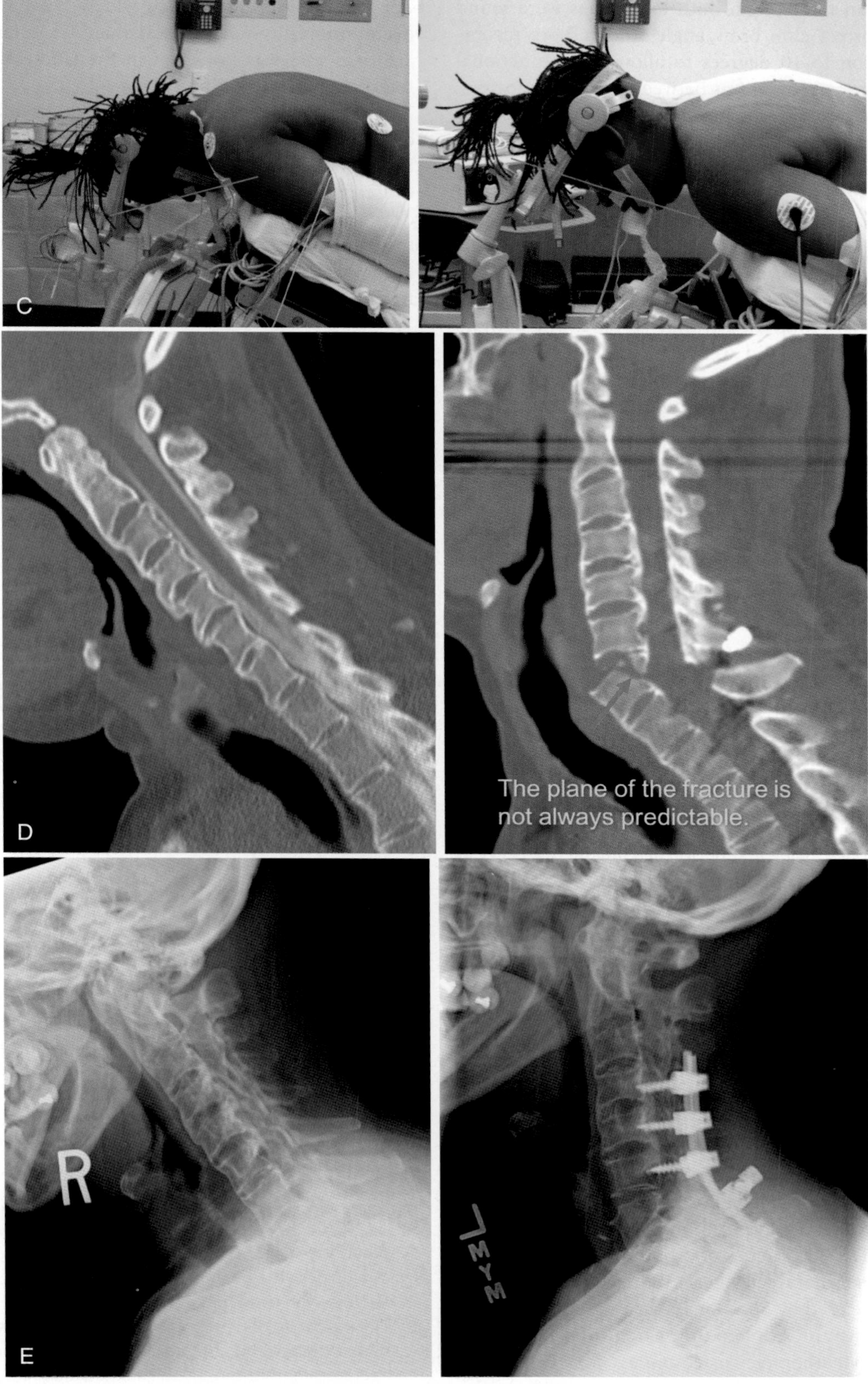

FIG. 85.1, cont'd (C) Patient positioned on the operating table preoperatively and postoperatively. Once the patient was in the final position on the operating table, the CBVA was recorded with radiographs and photographs. This allowed for a reasonable assessment of the degree of correction. Note that the position and angle of the operating table during surgery were not changed. (D) Preoperative and postoperative sagittal CT myelogram. Note fracture through the superior-posterior portion of the C7 vertebral body. (E) Preoperative and postoperative lateral cervical radiographs after C6–C7 osteoclasis and C4–T2 posterior cervical fusion with instrumentation.

and T1 other than the lamina. Both techniques were found to adequately correct chin-brow angle (the authors recommended correction to 10 degrees to allow for a functional position). Average correction was between 49 and 56 degrees. Two patients in the conventional group had intraoperative neurologic complications that did not resolve. There were 16 transient C8 radiculopathies in the conventional group, with two noted in the current group. Sixteen patients went on to nonunion in the conventional group, with none in the current group. There were four cases of deep vein thrombosis resulting in pulmonary embolism in the conventional group; none were noted in the current group. Four patients in the conventional group died within 90 days. The authors noted that most patients did well with these surgeries and were able to tolerate the awake seated procedure, but they cautioned against the average surgeon performing this type of procedure.

McMaster[61a] reported retrospectively on 15 patients with abnormal horizontal gaze who were treated with an extension osteotomy at the cervicothoracic junction. These surgeries were performed in the prone position with a halo jacket in place before the osteotomy. Only three patients had internal fixation. All patients had their horizontal gaze restored. Complications included one patient with delayed postoperative quadriparesis, two nonunions, a C8 nerve root lesion, and subluxation at the osteotomy site. McMaster also treated their nonunions with anterior fusion with subsequent good results.

Mummaneni et al.[62] described a “front-back-front” approach to cervical deformity, which they presented as a more controlled osteotomy than an osteoclasis. The violent maneuver of fracture for correction of the deformity is avoided, although the difficulty with intubation and anterior approach in the setting of cervical kyphosis is mentioned. They first performed an anterior cervical release, then a posterior instrumentation with resection of all posterior elements, followed by anterior instrumentation and grafting.

Hoh et al.[63] performed an extensive review of the literature regarding cervical deformity in the setting of ankylosing spondylitis. The authors looked at 183 patients who had extension osteotomies of the cervical spine, most of which were at the C7–T1 level due to the vertebral artery anatomy and the capacious spinal canal at this level. Five patients had a spinal cord injury, and 35 patients had postoperative issues related to the C8 nerve root, most temporary. Their conclusions were that the chin-brow angle should not be corrected to less than −10 degrees of flexion, usually a posterior-only approach was enough, multilevel segmental fixation avoided halo fixation, and that the modern techniques of propofol and neuromonitoring allowed for general anesthesia rather than local anesthesia as recommended by Simmons.

Etame et al.[64] also did a literature search to evaluate outcomes after cervicothoracic osteotomies for ankylosing spondylitis. They evaluated 227 patients (6 articles); the majority of these patients had a loss of horizontal gaze, causing severe limitations of activities of daily living. Total neurologic risk across these 6 studies was 23%, mainly related to the C8 nerve root. A majority of the root injuries were transient, resulting in a low incidence of permanent injury. The complication rate varied widely (27–88%), although the overall mortality rate was less than 3%. Interestingly, pseudarthrosis rate was low even in the studies that did not use internal instrumentation.

The remainder of the literature dealing with cervicothoracic osteotomies in AS patients is in the form of case reports. Sengupta and colleagues[65] addressed the complication of overcorrection resulting in the inability of the patient to look down. They performed a same-day, four-stage procedure in the lateral decubitus position with transparent drapes and reported restoration of horizontal gaze in one patient. They recommended this procedure only in extreme cases.

Summary

Spinal reconstructive surgery in patients with AS is a complex and high-risk procedure. These patients have significant disability from their spinal deformities, however, and can experience significant benefit from correction of their alignment and sagittal imbalance. Careful preoperative planning, a clear understanding of the characteristics of the spines of AS patients, and meticulous intraoperative and postoperative care can lead to measurable improvement in quality of life for these patients.

PEARLS

1. The progression of facet spondylosis causes compensatory kyphosis, which can lead to the fixed deformities of cervicothoracic, thoracic, and lumbar kyphosis commonly seen in AS. These deformities lead to difficulty with horizontal gaze, ambulation, and activities of daily living.
2. Initial immobilization of a patient with AS who has a spinal column fracture should be in the preinjury position because of the potential for injury to the spinal cord if hyperextension from the prior position is performed.
3. Determining the major component of the deformity requires examining the patient in the standing, seated, and supine positions. A truncal forward-flexed deformity that corrects when changing from a standing to a seated position is usually due to hip flexion contracture or lumbar deformity. If the deformity persists on sitting but corrects in the supine position, the deformity is arising from the thoracic, thoracolumbar, or lumbar spine, and a lumbar osteotomy is usually indicated. If the deformity persists in the supine position, the deformity is in the cervicothoracic area.

PITFALLS

1. When the spine has become completely ankylosed, it functions as a rigid, brittle beam, leading to an increased incidence of fracture with even minor trauma.
2. The incidence of neurologic injuries in these patients is quite high, owing to the potential for translation (displacement) at the fracture site. This translation causes direct injury to the spinal cord and persistent bleeding secondary to motion, resulting in an enlarging compressive hematoma.
3. Balancing the achievement of horizontal gaze with the improvement of sagittal balance requires proper planning and staging of lumbar osteotomies relative to cervicothoracic osteotomies when both are needed.

KEY POINTS

1. Recommended corrective lumbar osteotomies in AS patients are Smith-Petersen osteotomies if disc spaces are still mobile and PSOs if disc spaces are fully autofused.
2. Correction at the time of lumbar osteotomy can be facilitated by positioning the patient so that when the osteotomy is completed, the table can be extended, resulting in the controlled extension of the patient's spine. The use of a supporting frame where the trunk and shoulders are supported separately from the pelvis may be required.
3. For cervicothoracic osteotomy, the patient's head must be held rigidly in a halo or tongs, which can be manipulated to a corrected position after the osteotomy is completed. Osteotomy is best performed at C7 for maximum canal size, mobility of the nerve roots at this level, and the advantageous vertebral artery position.

KEY REFERENCES

1. Graham B, van Peteghem PK. Fractures of the spine in ankylosing spondylitis. *Spine*. 1989;14:803-807.
   This is a retrospective review of spinal injuries in AS patients from 1978 to 1984. The authors reviewed 15 patients and noted a preponderance of cervical injuries and a high rate of neurologic injury.
2. Halm H, Metz-Stavenhagen P, Zielke K. Results of surgical correction of kyphotic deformities of the spine in ankylosing spondylitis on the basis of the modified Arthritis Impact Measurement Scales. *Spine*. 1995;20:1612-1619.
   This is a retrospective review of 175 AS patients who underwent surgical correction of flexion deformities from 1979 to 1988. The modified AIMS was used as an outcome measure; 47 of 60 items showed significant increases; pain, mobility, depression, and anxiety items were particularly improved.
3. Hehne H, Zielke K, Bohm H. Polysegmental lumbar osteotomies and transpedicled fixation for correction of long-curved kyphotic deformities in ankylosing spondylitis. *Clin Orthop Relat Res*. 1990;(258):49-55.
   This is a review of 177 patients with AS in whom segmental pedicle screw fixation and Smith-Petersen osteotomies were performed in the lumbar spine for correction of kyphotic deformities. Harmonious lordosis was obtained, and all patients had restoration of horizontal gaze.
4. Simmons EH. Kyphotic deformity of the spine in ankylosing spondylitis. *Clin Orthop Relat Res*. 1977;128:65-77.
   This was the first report in the literature of the use of fixation for correction of kyphosis in AS. The technique of cervicothoracic osteotomy at the C7-T1 level was described; 48 patients who underwent this osteotomy were presented.
5. Thomasen E. Vertebral osteotomy for correction of kyphosis in ankylosing spondylitis. *Clin Orthop Relat Res*. 1985;194:142-153.
   This classic article introduced the technique of Thomasen closing wedge pedicle subtraction osteotomy. The author reviewed 11 patients who underwent the osteotomy, six of whom had internal fixation as supplementation.

REFERENCES

1. Calin A. Ankylosing spondylitis. *Clin Rheum Dis*. 1985;11(1):41-60.
2. Carbone LD, Cooper C, Michet CJ, et al. Ankylosing spondylitis in Rochester, Minnesota, 1935–1989. Is the epidemiology changing? *Arthritis Rheum*. 1992;35(12):1476-1482.
3. Kahn MF, Chamot AM. SAPHO syndrome. *Rheum Dis Clin North Am*. 1992;18(1):225-246.
4. Brewerton DA, Hart FD, Nicholls A, et al. Ankylosing spondylitis and HL-A 27. *Lancet*. 1973;301(7809):904-907.
5. Reveille JD. HLA-B27 and the seronegative spondyloarthropathies. *Am J Med Sci*. 1998;316(4):239-249.
6. Schlosstein L, Terasaki PI, Bluestone R, Pearson CM. High association of an HL-A antigen, W27, with ankylosing spondylitis. *N Engl J Med*. 1973;288(14):704-706.
7. Magrey M, Khan MA. Osteoporosis in ankylosing spondylitis. Curr Rheumatol Rep. *Curr Sci*. 2010;12(5):332-336.
8. Devogelaer JP, Maldague B, Malghem J, Nagant de Deuxchaisnes C. Appendicular and vertebral bone mass in ankylosing spondylitis. A comparison of plain radiographs with single- and dual-photon absorptiometry and with quantitative computed tomography. *Arthritis Rheum*. 1992;35(9):1062-1067.
9. Vasdev V, Bhakuni D, Garg MK, et al. Bone mineral density in young males with ankylosing spondylitis. *Int J Rheum Dis*. 2011;14(1):68-73.
10. Leone A, Marino M, Dell'Atti C, et al. Spinal fractures in patients with ankylosing spondylitis. *Rheumatol Int*. 2016;36(10):1335-1346.
11. Chaudhary SB, Hullinger H, Vives MJ. Management of acute spinal fractures in ankylosing spondylitis. *ISRN Rheumatol*. 2011;2011(5):150484-150489.
12. Westerveld LA, Verlaan JJ, Oner FC. Spinal fractures in patients with ankylosing spinal disorders: a systematic review of the literature on treatment, neurological status and complications. *Eur Spine J*. 2009;18(2):145-156.
13. van der Linden S, Valkenburg HA, Cats A. Evaluation of diagnostic criteria for ankylosing spondylitis. A proposal for modification of the New York criteria. *Arthritis Rheum*. 1984;27(4):361-368.
14. Moreau APM, Willcox N, Brown MF. Immobilisation of spinal fractures in patients with ankylosing spondylitis. *Injury*. 2003;34(5):372-373.
15. Podolsky SM, Hoffman JR, Pietrafesa CA. Neurologic complications following immobilization of cervical spine fracture in a patient with ankylosing spondylitis. *Ann Emerg Med*. 1983;12(9):578-580.
16. Hanson JA, Mirza S. Predisposition for spinal fracture in ankylosing spondylitis. *AJR Am J Roentgenol*. 2000;174(1):150.
17. Hunter T, Dubo HI. Spinal fractures complicating ankylosing spondylitis. A long-term followup study. *Arthritis Rheum*. 1983;26(6):751-759.
18. Verlaan JJ, Diekerhof CH, Buskens E, et al. Surgical treatment of traumatic fractures of the thoracic and lumbar spine: a systematic review of the literature on techniques, complications, and outcome. *Spine*. 2004;29(7):803-814.
19. Wade W, Saltzstein R, Maiman D. Spinal fractures complicating ankylosing spondylitis. *Arch Phys Med Rehabil*. 1989;70(5):398-401.
20. Westerveld LA, van Bemmel JC, Dhert WJA, Oner FC, Verlaan JJ. Clinical outcome after traumatic spinal fractures in patients with ankylosing spinal disorders compared with control patients. *Spine J*. 2014;14(5):729-740.
21. Whang PG, Goldberg G, Lawrence JP, et al. The Management of spinal injuries in patients with ankylosing spondylitis or diffuse idiopathic skeletal hyperostosis. *J Spinal Disord Tech*. 2009;22(2):77-85.
22. Caron T, Bransford R, Nguyen Q, et al. Spine fractures in patients with ankylosing spinal disorders. *Spine*. 2010;35(11):E458-E464.

23. Finkelstein JA, Chapman JR, Mirza S. Occult vertebral fractures in ankylosing spondylitis. *Spinal Cord.* 1999;37(6):444-447.
24. Hitchon PW, From AM, Brenton MD, Glaser JA, Torner JC. Fractures of the thoracolumbar spine complicating ankylosing spondylitis. *J Neurosurg.* 2002;97(2 suppl):218-222.
25. Nayak NR, Pisapia JM, Abdullah KG, Schuster JM. Minimally invasive surgery for traumatic fractures in ankylosing spinal diseases. *Global Spine J.* 2015;5(4):266-273.
26. Graham B, van Peteghem PK. Fractures of the spine in ankylosing spondylitis. *Spine.* 1989;14(8):803-807.
27. Apple DF, Anson C. Spinal cord injury occurring in patients with ankylosing spondylitis: a multicenter study. *Orthopedics.* 1995;18(10):1005-1011.
28. Bohlman HH. Acute fractures and dislocations of the cervical spine. An analysis of three hundred hospitalized patients and review of the literature. *J Bone Joint Surg Am.* 1979;61(8):1119-1142.
29. Schröder J, Liljenqvist U, Greiner C, Wassmann H. Complications of halo treatment for cervical spine injuries in patients with ankylosing spondylitis—report of three cases. *Arch Orthop Trauma Surg.* 2003;123(2-3):112-114.
30. Taggard DA, Traynelis VC. Management of cervical spinal fractures in ankylosing spondylitis with posterior fixation. *Spine.* 2000;25(16):2035-2039.
31. Suk K-S, Kim K-T, Lee S-H, Kim J-M. Significance of chin-brow vertical angle in correction of kyphotic deformity of ankylosing spondylitis patients. *Spine.* 2003;28(17):2001-2005.
32. Song K, Su X, Zhang Y, et al. Optimal chin-brow vertical angle for sagittal visual fields in ankylosing spondylitis kyphosis. *Eur Spine J.* 2016;25(8):2596-2604.
33. Klein JD, Hey LA, Yu CS, et al. Perioperative nutrition and postoperative complications in patients undergoing spinal surgery. *Spine.* 1996;21(22):2676-2682.
34. Hu SS, Fontaine F, Kelly B, Bradford DS. Nutritional depletion in staged spinal reconstructive surgery. The effect of total parenteral nutrition. *Spine.* 1998;23(12):1401-1405.
35. Lapp MA, Bridwell KH, Lenke LG, et al. Long-term complications in adult spinal deformity patients having combined surgery a comparison of primary to revision patients. *Spine.* 2001;26(8):973-983.
36. Smith-Petersen MN, Larson CB, Aufranc OE. Osteotomy of the spine for correction of flexion deformity in rheumatoid arthritis. *Clin Orthop Relat Res.* 1969;66:6-9.
37. Simmons EH. The surgical correction of flexion deformity of the cervical spine in ankylosing spondylitis. *Clin Orthop Relat Res.* 1972;86:132-143.
38. Lichtblau PO, Wilson PD. Possible mechanism of aortic rupture in orthopaedic correction of rheumatoid spondylitis. *J Bone Joint Surg Am.* 1956;38-A(1):123-127.
39. Fazl M, Bilbao JM, Hudson AR. Laceration of the aorta complicating spinal fracture in ankylosing spondylitis. *Neurosurgery.* 1981;8(6):732-734.
40. Law WA. Osteotomy of the spine. *Clin Orthop Relat Res.* 1969;66(1):70-76.
41. McMaster MJ. A technique for lumbar spinal osteotomy in ankylosing spondylitis. *J Bone Joint Surg Br.* 1985;67(2):204-210.
42. Herbert JJ. [Technique and results of vertebral osteotomy in 26 cases]. *Acta Orthop Scand.* 1952;22(1):36-58.
43. Wilson MJ, Turkell JH. Multiple spinal wedge osteotomy its use in a case of Marie-Strumpell spondylitis. *Am J Surg.* 1949;77(6):777-782.
44. Püschel J, Zielke K. Korrekturoperation bei Bechterew-Kyphose -Indikation, Technik, Ergebnisse. *Z Orthop Ihre Grenzgeb.* 2008;120(3):338-342.
45. Thomasen E. Vertebral osteotomy for correction of kyphosis in ankylosing spondylitis. *Clin Orthop Relat Res.* 1985;194:142-152.
45a. Heinig CF. Eggshell procedure. In: Luque ER, ed. *Segmental Spinal Instrumentation.* Thorofare, NJ: Slack; 1984.
46. Bradford DS, Schumacher WL, Lonstein JE, Winter RB. Ankylosing spondylitis: experience in surgical management of 21 patients. *Spine.* 1987;12(3):238-243.
47. Hehne HJ, Zielke K, Böhm H. Polysegmental lumbar osteotomies and transpedicled fixation for correction of long-curved kyphotic deformities in ankylosing spondylitis. *Clin Orthop Relat Res.* 1990;258:49-55.
48. Jaffray D, Becker V, Eisenstein S. Closing wedge osteotomy with transpedicular fixation in ankylosing spondylitis. *Clin Orthop Relat Res.* 1992;279:122-126.
49. Van Royen BJ, De Gast A. Lumbar osteotomy for correction of thoracolumbar kyphotic deformity in ankylosing spondylitis. A structured review of three methods of treatment. *Ann Rheum Dis.* 1999;58(7):399-406.
50. Halm H, Metz-Stavenhagen P, Zielke K. Results of surgical correction of kyphotic deformities of the spine in ankylosing spondylitis on the basis of the modified arthritis impact measurement scales. *Spine.* 1995;20(14):1612-1619.
51. Kim K-T, Suk K-S, Cho Y-J, Hong G-P, Park B-J. Clinical outcome results of pedicle subtraction osteotomy in ankylosing spondylitis with kyphotic deformity. *Spine.* 2002;27(6):612-618.
52. Berven SH, Deviren V, Smith JA, et al. Management of fixed sagittal plane deformity: results of the transpedicular wedge resection osteotomy. *Spine.* 2001;26(18):2036-2043.
53. Bridwell KH, Lewis SJ, Lenke LG, Baldus C, Blanke K. Pedicle subtraction osteotomy for the treatment of fixed sagittal imbalance. *J Bone Joint Surg Am.* 2003;85-A(3):454-463.
54. Liu C, Zheng G, Zhang Y, et al. The radiologic, clinical results and digestive function improvement in patients with ankylosing spondylitis kyphosis after pedicle subtraction osteotomy. *Spine J.* 2015;15(9):1988-1993.
55. Zhang G, Fu J, Zhang Y, et al. Lung volume change after pedicle subtraction osteotomy in patients with ankylosing spondylitis with thoracolumbar kyphosis. *Spine.* 2015;40(4):233-237.
56. Hu X, Thapa AJ, Cai Z, et al. Comparison of Smith-Petersen osteotomy, pedicular subtraction osteotomy, and poly-segmental wedge osteotomy in treating rigid thoracolumbar kyphotic deformity in ankylosing spondylitis a systematic review and meta-analysis. *BMC Surg.* 2016;16(1):4.
57. Liu H, Yang C, Zheng Z, et al. Comparison of Smith-Petersen osteotomy and pedicle subtraction osteotomy for the correction of thoracolumbar kyphotic deformity in ankylosing spondylitis: a systematic review and meta-analysis. *Spine.* 2015;40(8):570-579.
58. Zheng G-Q, Song K, Zhang Y-G, et al. Two-level spinal osteotomy for severe thoracolumbar kyphosis in ankylosing spondylitis. Experience with 48 patients. *Spine.* 2014;39(13):1055-1058.
59. Kawahara N, Tomita K, Baba H, et al. Closing-opening wedge osteotomy to correct angular kyphotic deformity by a single posterior approach. *Spine.* 2001;26(4):391-402.
60. Urist MR. Osteotomy of the cervical spine. *J Bone Joint Surg Am.* 1958;40(4):833-843.

61. Simmons ED, DiStefano RJ, Zheng Y, Simmons EH. Thirty-six years experience of cervical extension osteotomy in ankylosing spondylitis: techniques and outcomes. *Spine*. 2006;31(26):3006-3012.
61a. McMaster MJ. Osteotomy of the cervical spine in ankylosing spondylitis. *J Bone Joint Surg Br*. 1997;79(2): 197-203.
62. Mummaneni PV, Mummaneni VP, Haid RW, Rodts GE, Sasso RC. Cervical osteotomy for the correction of chin-on-chest deformity in ankylosing spondylitis. Technical note. *Neurosurg Focus*. 2003;14(1):e9.
63. Hoh DJ, Khoueir P, Wang MY. Management of cervical deformity in ankylosing spondylitis. *Neurosurg Focus*. 2008;24(1):E9.
64. Etame AB, Than KD, Wang AC, La Marca F, Park P. Surgical management of symptomatic cervical or cervicothoracic kyphosis due to ankylosing spondylitis. *Spine*. 2008;33(16):E559-E564.
65. Sengupta DK, Khazim R, Grevitt MP, Webb JK. Flexion osteotomy of the cervical spine: a new technique for correction of iatrogenic extension deformity in ankylosing spondylitis. *Spine*. 2001;26(9):1068-1072.

CHAPTER 86 Tumors of the Spine

Umesh Metkar
Swamy Kurra
William F. Lavelle

Introduction

Involvement of the spinal column by a tumor may lead to catastrophic outcomes. Thorough knowledge of the imaging and histologic characteristics of the tumor is of the utmost importance to obtain favorable outcomes. Spinal tumors are classified based on the location of the occurrence and the nature of the disease. Tumors that occur in the spine are termed primary spinal tumors. If the primary tumor origin is extraspinal and metastasized to the spine through a hematogenous or lymphatic route, these tumors are considered metastatic spinal tumors. Primary spinal tumors can be benign or malignant based on the growth rate and surrounding tissue expansion. Primary spinal tumors are far less common than metastatic tumors. Benign tumors are usually smaller in size and have well-defined sclerotic margins on radiographs. However, locally aggressive benign spine tumors, such as osteoblastomas, giant cell tumors, and aneurysmal bone cysts, have rapid growth rates, poorly defined borders, and aggressive cortex destruction and sometimes extend to surrounding soft tissues. Aggressive benign spinal tumors can grow to a significant extent, and the larger tumor size and aggressive cortex destruction can lead to pathologic fractures and/or compression of surrounding neurologic structures. Primary malignant spinal tumors are rare but can cause significant morbidity and mortality. Malignant tumors most commonly metastasize to the lungs. Metastatic spine tumors have a higher incidence than primary spine tumors.

Radiographs, computed tomography (CT), and magnetic resonance imaging (MRI) are common imaging modalities used to determine size, location, staging, type, surrounding soft tissue expansion, and pathologic fractures. Imaging studies are used in the diagnostic process of the tumor. Diagnosis can be confirmed only through a tissue biopsy. This combined approach is used to manage tumors.

Various treatments are available for spinal tumors. The optimal treatment is determined by the location of the tumor, staging, and type of tumor. Radiation therapy, chemotherapy, embolization, and surgical resection are common treatments in the management of spinal tumors. Local control of the spinal tumor can be achieved through surgical resection. The type of excision and surgical approach are determined based on the nature of the tumor and its location. Spinal instability and neurologic compromise are potential complications associated with spinal tumors. Aggressive decompression helps achieve neurologic improvement. Spinal instrumentation is used with instability of the spine. Primary benign tumors have a good prognosis after surgical resection. For aggressive benign and malignant tumors, a good prognosis requires complete resection of the tumor, the preservation of neurologic function, adequate decompression of the neural elements, and avoidance of local and systemic metastases. All these factors depend on the size of the tumor and responsiveness of the tumor to treatment. Metastatic spinal lesions have a worse prognosis, which depends on the number of skeletal metastases, the presence of visceral metastases, the primary site of origin, and the overall health of the patient.

Imaging Techniques

Imaging modalities are essential for diagnosing the tumor and evaluating the extent of the tumor. Plain radiographs, CT scans, bone scans, and MRIs are the most commonly used imaging modalities for detecting the location of the tumor and its nature (benign vs. malignant primary vs. metastatic). Recent advancements in spine imaging studies aid in staging the tumors for optimal surgical treatment.

Although a plain radiograph is the first recommended imaging study for the diagnosis of spinal pathologies, radiographs have a limited contribution in the detection of spinal lesions. At least a 50% loss of the trabecular bone is required to visualize spinal bone lesions in plain radiographs. The classic presentations that can be seen on plain radiographs are osteolytic and osteoblastic lesions, mixed lesions, and fractures. Plain radiographs are also useful in determining the stability of the spinal column and assessing the overall alignment of the spinal column in an upright position. Pathologic compression fractures can also be easily diagnosed on plain radiographs. However, radiographs have limited use in detecting latent lesions or skip lesions.

A bone scan (bone scintigraphy) is another diagnostic procedure performed by using radioisotopes. These scans detect the uptake of the radioisotope by bone-forming osteoblastic activity. Bone scans can identify lesions in symptomatic patients whose plain radiographs are negative or suspicious. Bone scans have a high sensitivity in diagnosing osteoblastic activity but have a low specificity because nonneoplastic conditions, like osteoarthritis, can produce an increase in the uptake of the radioisotope. The ability to scan the entire body makes bone scans advantageous to determine the extent of dissemination in patients with a known systemic disease and to define the most accessible lesion to biopsy in patients with an unknown primary malignancy. More recently, intraoperative bone scans have been used for osteoid osteomas to ensure complete resection and avoid recurrence.[1]

CT scans have a high sensitivity for abnormal bone mineralization compared with plain radiographs. CT scans can detect early osseous lesions, unlike radiographs. With the ability to obtain three-dimensional reconstructive imaging of the tumor mass, to detect minor variations in bone mineralization as well as soft tissue extent of the tumor mass, CT imaging has been an important tool in decision making for tumor surgery. CT scans are also important in defining the stability of the spinal column based on three-dimensional measurements of the tumor mass. With the advent of portable CT scanners, intraoperative CT scan imaging has become widely used in spine surgery. Because CT imaging provides excellent visualization of osseous pathology, it can be extremely helpful in the evaluation of tumor resections during complex spinal operations.

Myelography, once the only reliable way to assess spinal cord and nerve root compression, has now given way to MRI in most instances. In combination with CT, myelography remains a valuable tool for detecting neural compression due to bony impingement in patients unable to undergo MRI due to pacemakers or other metallic devices.

MRI scans have superior sensitivity and specificity for spinal lesions and can be done without any radiation exposure to the patient. MRI is the best imaging modality in spine oncology because of its ability to delineate the borders between the tumor and surrounding normal tissues. MRI is equally useful in detecting the extent of neural compression. Gadolinium contrast-enhanced MRI scans are helpful in distinguishing between intradural and extradural tumors as well as intramedullary and extramedullary tumors.[2] Gadolinium is also beneficial for assessing the extent of tumor necrosis present initially as well as tumor necrosis as a response to chemotherapy.

Summary of Imaging Appearance

The imaging appearance of primary bony tumors of the spine and simulating lesions of the spine have been described recently. Benign bone tumors are usually well circumscribed. As slow-growing lesions, they may present with a calcified or sclerotic matrix. Malignancy, on the other hand, is often characterized by permeative margins with bone destruction, cortical erosion, and associated soft tissue masses. CT is helpful in the characterization of the tumor matrix, exact location and extension of the tumor, and osseous changes. MRI is best for evaluation of the associated soft tissue mass, bone marrow infiltration, and intraspinal extension.[3]

Biopsy Techniques

Obtaining a tissue diagnosis is the next step in the treatment of spinal tumors. A biopsy is needed to obtain a tissue sample to diagnose an unknown spinal lesion or confirm the provisional diagnosis obtained through clinical and imaging workups. The tissue sample can be obtained through a fine-needle, core, incisional, or excisional biopsy.

Fine-needle aspiration and core biopsies allow percutaneous extraction of the tissue sample. The use of image guidance (fluoroscopy, CT, or MRI) has significantly improved the ability to obtain the tissue sample from the desired tumor region. CT-guided biopsy by an interventional radiologist has become a common practice at many cancer treatment centers. In certain instances, tissue diagnosis can only be obtained through a surgical procedure. In those situations, a tissue sample is sent for immediate tissue diagnosis, and followed by the complete excisional biopsy of the tumor with appropriate margin selection based on the nature of the tumor.

If definitive excision is considered after incisional biopsy, a new set of instruments and drapes is mandatory to prevent accidental tumor seeding. Similar precautions should be followed when harvesting graft material from another site.[4]

Primary Tumors

Primary tumors in the spine constitute less than 10% of all spinal tumors. Patients with spinal tumors usually present with pain, which can be local and/or radicular and is often worse at night. Other patients present with weakness from spinal cord or nerve root compression. Some tumors are incidental findings discovered in the imaging studies performed for other problems. Radiographs, CT, and MRI are used to determine the location, type of lesion (osteoblastic/osteolytic), soft tissue extension, fluid levels, and spine instability. Evolving imaging modalities have improved the ability to make a diagnosis of the tumor type without the need for biopsy; however, most tumors can only be definitively diagnosed through biopsy based on the histologic appearance. Only a few tumors can be diagnosed by combining clinical symptoms and imaging studies. Management of primary tumors in the spine varies and depends on whether they are benign or malignant, indolent or aggressive, and their location relative to the spinal cord and nerve roots. Follow-up observation, symptomatic treatment, chemotherapy, radiation therapy, embolization, and surgical resection with or without instrumentation are all commonly used modalities in the management and treatment of primary tumors.

Benign Tumors

Osteochondroma

An osteochondroma is the cartilaginous exostosis arising from a parent bone, containing a cartilaginous cap at the end. The growth of the tumor ends with skeletal maturity. These are the most common type of bone tumors, but they constitute only 4% of the primary benign tumors of the spine. In the spine, osteochondromas are either solitary or multiple (multiple hereditary exostosis). Multiple hereditary exostosis (MHE) occurs in an autosomal dominant fashion; the majority of patients have mutations in the exostosin-1 and exostosin-2 genes.[5,6] Osteochondromas are predominantly diagnosed in the third and fourth decades of life and have a higher incidence in males, but patients with MHEs most commonly present in adolescence. Within the spinal column, osteochondromas are most commonly seen in the cervical spine,[7] more commonly in C2 due to the presence of an osteocartilaginous growth plate (Fig. 86.1). Microtrauma to this growth plate leads to the displacement and subsequent growth of small cartilaginous remains, thus resulting in a predominance of cervical lesions.[8]

Patients with spinal osteochondromas usually present with pain over the affected areas, especially if the lesion is in the posterior elements. Osteochondromas originating from the lamina can grow into the spinal canal and can lead to spinal cord compression or nerve root compression and present with neurologic deficits and with local back pain.[8]

Radiographs have limited utility in diagnosing osteochondromas due to the predominant presence of cartilaginous elements and the typically small size of the lesions. CT scans can demonstrate the presence of a sessile or pedunculated mass arising from a parent bone with calcification. MRI aids in the assessment of the cartilaginous cap and its size. The cartilaginous cap can be seen as a hypointense structure on T1-weighted images and as hyperintense on T2-weighted images. MRI determination of the thickness of this cartilaginous cap also has prognostic significance. A cartilaginous cap thickness more than 3 cm signifies a malignant transformation of the osteochondroma. Studies have reported that the intracanal osteochondroma rate (20–27%) is greater in children with MHE; routine axial screening (MRI or CT) is recommended in this population for early detection of intracanal osteochondromas to prevent potential neurologic consequences.[8,9]

Histologically, the cartilaginous cap consists of hyaline cartilage, which continues through the process of endochondral ossification until skeletal maturity.

Treatment of osteochondromas mainly involves a complete surgical excision (Fig. 86.2) at the point of the cortical and marrow junction to the parent bone. A complete resection is usually curative, and recurrence is rare.[10] Approximately 10% of osteochondromas may undergo a malignant transformation to an osteosarcoma.[9,11]

Hemangioma

Hemangiomas are mostly asymptomatic, benign vascular tumors primarily located inside the vertebral bodies. Vertebral hemangiomas (VHs) are mostly incidental findings on MRIs performed for other pathologies. They are most commonly seen in the thoracic spine, and the estimated occurrence is greater than 10% in autopsy studies.[12,13] However, hemangiomas that extend into the posterior elements and surrounding soft tissues can become symptomatic. Clinical symptoms of symptomatic VH are pain and neurologic deficits from expansion. Pregnancy is a risk factor for symptomatic VH, and the thoracic vertebrae are most commonly affected.[14] VHs can also weaken the vertebral body and present as a pathologic compression fracture. Aggressive VHs can present with

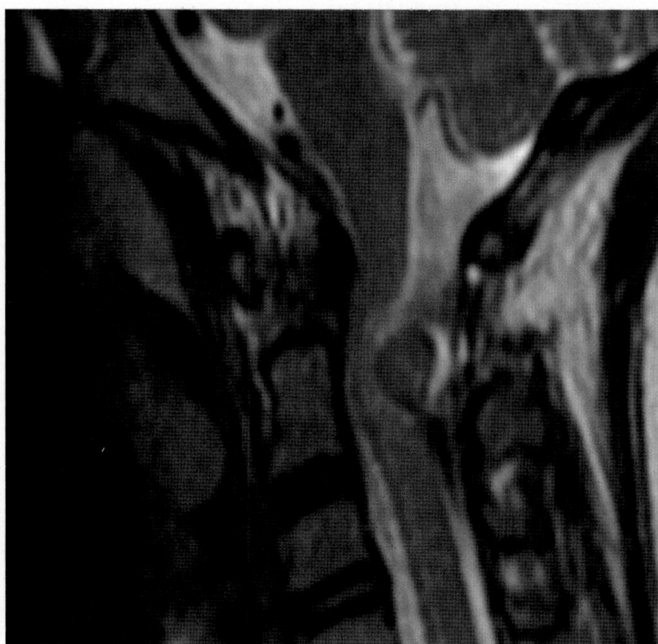

FIG. 86.1 Sagittal T2-weighted magnetic resonance image demonstrating C2 osteochondroma.

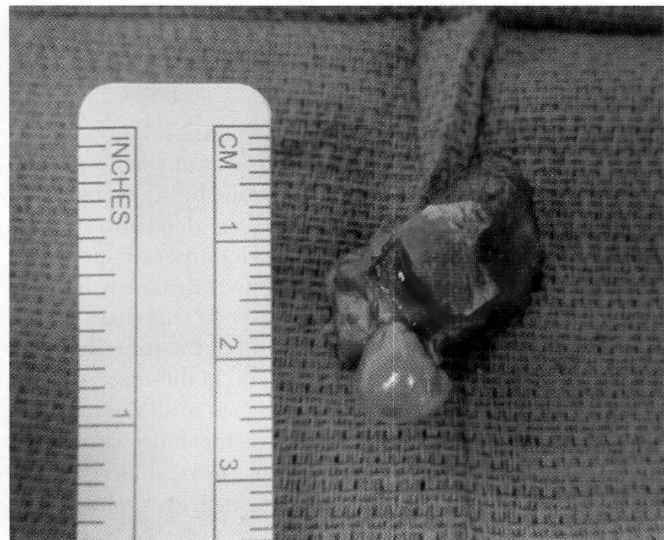

FIG. 86.2 Gross specimen showing en bloc removal of compressive C2 osteochondroma.

neurologic symptoms caused by canal compromise or nerve root impingement.

VHs can be diagnosed on radiographs, where they show a peculiar "corduroy pattern" with vertical striations. Axial CT images show a punctate, or "polka dot," appearance. MRI shows the presence of a hyperintense signal on both T1- and T2-weighted images.

Histologically, VHs appear as blood-filled, dilated vascular loops lined by endothelial cells. The loops are separated by trabecular bone. VHs can be capillary or cavernous according to the type of vessels involved.

Most VHs are asymptomatic and do not need to be followed clinically. Symptomatic VHs are rare and can be treated with endovascular embolization,[15-18] intralesional ethanol injections,[19-23] radiation therapy,[24] surgical intralesional resection, and vertebroplasty or kyphoplasty.[25-27] Embolization is used to treat painful VH or preoperatively to reduce intraoperative blood loss.[28,29] Vertebroplasty and kyphoplasty have been shown to potentially provide improvements in painful VH. Patients with pathologic compression fractures may be treated with either vertebroplasty or kyphoplasty. Patients presenting with neurologic symptoms caused by compressive VHs need surgical treatment based on the type and severity of the compression.

There is no consensus regarding the management of symptomatic VH in pregnant women. Chi et al[30] proposed a treatment algorithm for symptomatic VHs in pregnant women based on the week of gestation. At 36 weeks of gestation, observation is recommended and symptoms can be resolved after delivery or with postpartum treatment. If neurologic deterioration is seen, a cesarean section can be performed or labor can be induced followed by surgery with or without radiation, embolization, and/or sclerotherapy. Between 32 and 36 weeks of gestation, expectant observation may also be considered. If symptoms are severe and progressive, embolization or surgery without preterm delivery may be considered. For less than 32 weeks of gestation, observation is recommended for mild symptoms and surgery and/or embolization for severe neurologic deficits.

Eosinophilic Granuloma

Eosinophilic granulomas present as multifocal or unifocal lytic bony lesions. They commonly occur in children and adolescents. These lesions are formed due to the benign proliferation of Langerhans histiocytosis (dendritic cells).[31] Hand-Schüller-Christian disease (skull lesions, exophthalmos, and diabetes insipidus) and Letterer-Siwe disease (malignant) are two other systemic diseases affected by Langerhans histiocytosis (LCH) proliferation.[32] The skull is the most frequent site for occurrence in the skeletal system. In the spine, eosinophilic granulomas account for 6.5% to 25% of all skeletal LCH cases, and the thoracic vertebrae are the most commonly involved sites. Clinical presentation of eosinophilic granulomas includes back pain, rare neurologic deficits, kyphosis, and torticollis.

On radiographs, the lytic lesion in the vertebral bodies rarely extends to the posterior elements. Flattening of the vertebra (vertebra plana) is a typical radiographic feature of eosinophilic granulomas. On MRI, lesions appear as low to intermediate signal in T1-weighted images and as hyperintense in T2-weighted images.

CT scans show the lytic destruction of the involved vertebra. Osteomyelitis, aneurysmal bone cysts, neuroblastomas, chondromas, Ewing sarcomas, osteosarcomas, leukemia, and lymphoma comprise the differential diagnoses for eosinophilic granulomas. MRI is used to identify a paravertebral soft tissue mass, peridural compression, or edematous zone around the lesions. On MRI, the vertebra plana presents as a "dumbbell" and may be considered a feature of spinal LCH. A technetium bone scan or positron emission tomography/CT scan is recommended for multiple bony lesions or disseminated disease.

Clinical and radiographic findings are often enough to confirm the diagnosis. In a typical LCH, classic radiographic findings include vertebral collapse, maintenance of disc spaces, lack of extraspinal spread, and lack of a soft tissue mass. These findings provide sufficient evidence to avoid an unnecessary biopsy and the risk of inadvertently damaging the vertebral growth plates during biopsy. A biopsy is essential, however, in suspected cases of spinal Langerhans cell histiocytosis only if there are any atypical features such as a soft tissue mass, disc space involvement, or neurologic symptoms.[31,33]

Histologically, in immunohistochemical staining, tennis racquet–shaped Birbeck granules appear in the cytoplasm and are characteristic of eosinophilic granulomas. Significant eosinophilic infiltration can be seen in the lesion. Birbeck granules are plentiful in aggressive eosinophilic granulomas.[13]

Various modalities are used to treat eosinophilic granulomas, which often improve spontaneously and frequently reconstitute the lost vertebral height. These patients are managed with pain medications and rest and are followed clinically with radiographs. Systemic chemotherapy can be used for management of systemic or disseminated lesions. CT-guided corticosteroid injections may be helpful in symptomatic solitary eosinophilic granulomas. Most patients with spinal instability can be supported in an orthosis until sufficient reconstitution has occurred to restore stability. Surgery is the procedure of choice in patients who have an unstable spine segment that cannot be stabilized with an orthosis or have neurologic symptoms due to the compression of the neural elements from the collapsed vertebrae.

Osteoblastoma/Osteoid Osteoma

Osteoid osteomas are benign tumors frequently seen in children. These tumors have a slight male predominance and have a higher predilection for the posterior elements of the vertebrae. Osteoid osteomas are smaller in size, measuring less than 2 cm.

Patients with an osteoid osteoma typically present with back pain at the site of the lesion. The pain gradually worsens over a period of weeks and has a characteristic nighttime exacerbation. The pain responds well to nonsteroidal antiinflammatory drugs (NSAIDs), mainly salicylates. Patients with severely painful lesions may also present with scoliosis with an osteoid osteoma in the concavity of the curve. Due to the

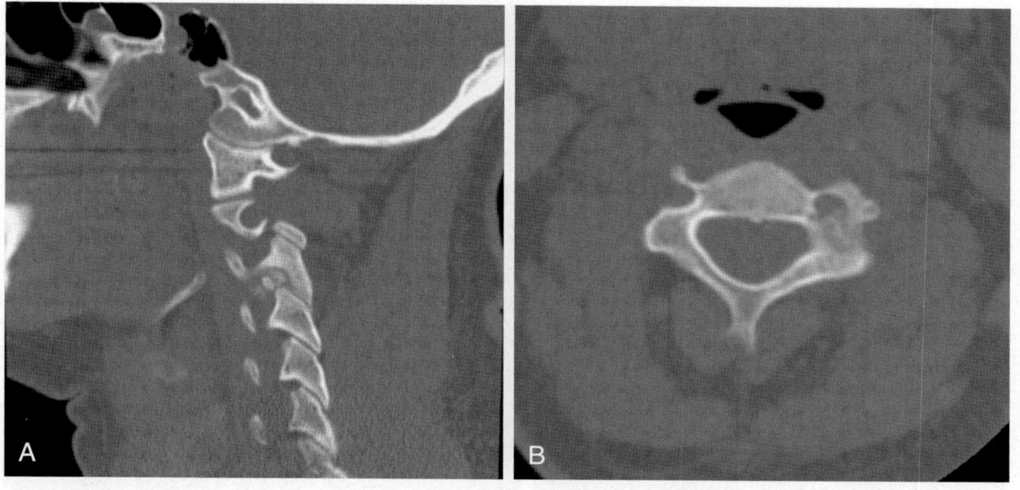

FIG. 86.3 (A) Sagittal and (B) axial computed tomographic views demonstrating discrete nidus consistent with osteoid osteomas.

smaller size of these lesions, they rarely cause significant bone destruction that would produce instability or neurologic deficits.

Osteoid osteomas are difficult to diagnose on plain radiographs unless there is a high suspicion of this diagnosis. The smaller size, radiolucency of the lesion, and common posterior element occurrence makes radiographic diagnosis challenging. On plain radiographs, they appear as radiolucent lesions in the posterior elements most commonly found in the lumbar spine with a calcified nidus. CT is considered to be essential in the diagnosis of these lesions. On CT scans, these lesions present as radiolucent lesions with or without a central calcified nidus (Fig. 86.3). Surrounding cortical thickening or sclerosis is also evident on these images. On MRI, osteoid osteomas present as a low- to intermediate-density lesion on T1-weighted images and as intermediate- to high-intensity lesions on T2-weighted images. MRI can be used to rule out canal compromise and for preoperative planning.[2]

Histologically, osteoid osteomas consist of a reddish nidus of woven bone with interconnected trabeculae. Intertrabecular spaces contain hypocellular fibrovascular tissue. The lesion may be surrounded by reactive bone with sclerosis.

Osteoid osteomas usually respond to NSAIDs, especially salicylates. For tumors that have not responded to conservative treatment or in patients with severe disabling pain, image-guided percutaneous thermal ablation (radiofrequency or laser ablation) has been shown to significantly reduce pain.[34-37] Surgeons have limited the use of thermal ablation techniques in the spine due to the risk of thermal injury to the proximal neural structures. With a minimum distance of 10 mm between the periosteum and neural elements, an intact thick cortex and thermal protection techniques can reduce thermal neural injury.[38,39] A complete resection is recommended for patients with neurologic compromise and those with secondary scoliosis. Surgical resection is also recommended for patients with severe refractory pain who are at risk of thermal injury from thermal ablation procedures (Fig. 86.4).[35,40]

Osteoblastomas are benign bone tumors and are histologically similar to osteoid osteomas; however, they are larger in size (>2 cm). They are usually found in the second and third decades of life, with a higher incidence in males. Osteoblastomas are more aggressive and often have a cortical breach and soft tissue extension and can undergo malignant transformation. Unlike other primary osseous tumors, osteoblastomas have a predilection for the spinal column and constitute about 32% to 45% of all osteoblastomas. Osteoblastomas commonly occur in the posterior elements, mainly the lamina and pedicles, and have a higher predilection for the lumbar spine.[41] Aggressive osteoblastomas can expand into the vertebral bodies; however, anterior vertebral body involvement is rare.[41] Osteoblastomas are usually slow-growing tumors, and malignant transformation to osteosarcoma is rare.[42] Due to their aggressive growth pattern, osteoblastomas have a higher risk of recurrence after excision. More aggressive lesions have an approximately 50% recurrence rate after excision.

Patients with osteoblastomas present with a dull, aching pain. However, the pain does not increase at night, and NSAIDs are not as effective in alleviating the pain as in the case of osteoid osteomas. More aggressive lesions may present with neurologic symptoms caused by the compression of neural structures.

On plain radiographs, osteoblastomas present as a radiolucent nidus with a surrounding sclerotic rim. They are more than 2 cm in size and are differentiated from osteoid osteomas based on their size and aggressive growth pattern. The nidus may have varying amounts of calcification. More aggressive lesions may show variable matrix calcifications, have an expansile appearance, and cause extensive destruction along with growth into the surrounding paraspinal soft tissues. Approximately 10% to 15% of osteoblastomas have an associated aneurysmal bone cyst. CT is the investigative method of choice and helps identify the multifocal calcifications in the nidus and the thin surrounding rim of sclerosis. MRI is considered helpful in preoperative planning to assess the soft tissue involvement and compression of the neural elements.[43]

Histologically, osteoblastomas are similar in appearance to an osteoid osteoma. The osteoblastoma has a characteristic

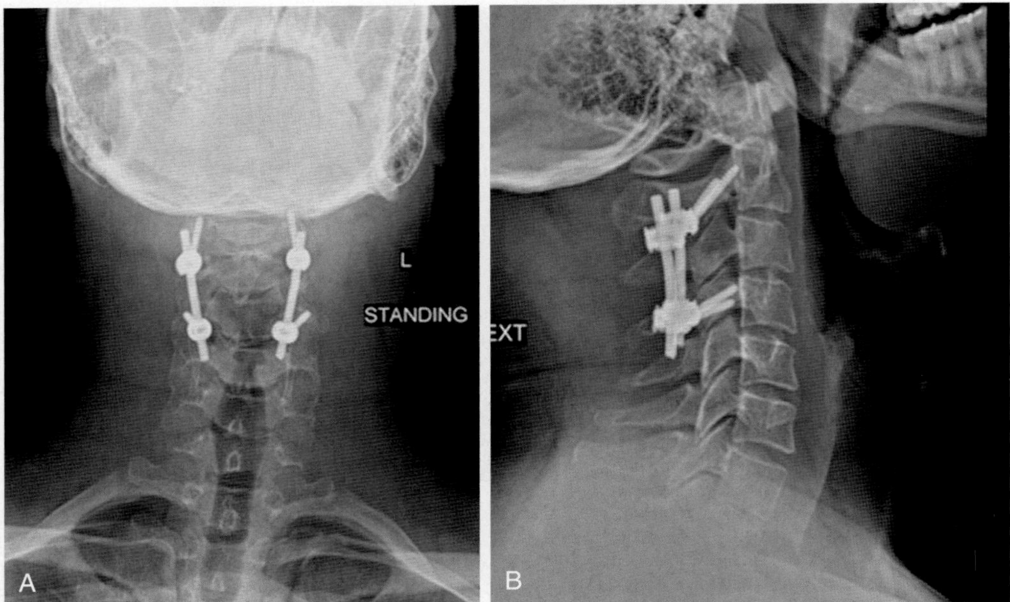

FIG. 86.4 (A) Anteroposterior and (B) lateral radiographs demonstrating posterior decompression and fusion of the osteoid osteoma.

reddish appearance due to the rich vasculature and consists of woven bone containing bone-forming osteoblasts.

Complete resection is the treatment of choice. A total en bloc resection is recommended whenever possible. The extensive resection necessary to completely remove these aggressive lesions usually causes significant spinal instability and requires fusion with instrumentation. In some cases, due to the location of the lesion, en bloc resection may not be feasible. In such cases intralesional curettage and cementing or bone grafting may be considered.[44] Postoperatively, patients need a close follow-up, every 3 months for the first 2 years, to detect recurrence. Approximately 10% to 15% of patients present with a recurrence of the tumor.[43,45] However, malignant transformation is rare.

Aneurysmal Bone Cyst

Aneurysmal bone cysts (ABCs) are benign cystic lesions affecting the bone. ABCs are peculiar in their pathologic appearance of an expansile bony lesion containing blood-filled cavities separated by fibrous septae or trabecular bone. Approximately 8% to 30% of ABCs occur in the spine, most commonly the lumbar spine. ABCs are more common in females. ABCs constitute approximately 15% of the primary benign tumors of the spine and are most commonly diagnosed in the second and third decades of life. ABCs are mainly seen in the posterior elements; however, they may extend into the vertebral bodies.

Patients with ABCs usually present with progressively worsening local pain. Patients with expansile lesions that cause neural compression may present with neurologic deficits. A palpable mass may be felt in a few patients.

Diagnosis of an ABC involves plain radiographs, CT, and contrast-enhanced MRI. ABCs show an expansile lytic lesion or "blown out" appearance on plain radiographs. They typically involve the posterior elements of thoracolumbar spine with expansion to the vertebral body. On CT, ABCs appear as multiloculated lytic lesions with a "soap bubble" appearance. Fluid-filled levels may occasionally be seen on CT scans. A pathologic fracture may be apparent on CT scans. Contrast-enhanced MRI is useful to detect soft tissue involvement and the status of neural structures, which are assessed in axial scans. Fluid levels can be seen on these axial scans. ABCs show increased signal intensity on both T1- and T2-weighted images, which can be attributed to the high concentration of methemoglobin in the fluid. The presence of a fluid level in a lytic expansile lesion aids in the confirmation of the diagnosis and also allows the physician to look for the presence of associated solid tumors to rule out a secondary ABC.

Differential diagnosis of ABCs includes other lytic lesions of the spine, namely giant cell tumors, malignant fibrous histiocytomas, and eosinophilic granulomas. ABCs can be secondary to the presence of a giant cell tumor or osteoblastoma. Histologically, ABCs show the presence of blood-filled cavities separated by septae, which consist of fibrous tissue, giant cells, and reactive trabecular bone.

The treatment of ABCs depends on the level of the tumor in the spinal column, the anatomic location of the lesion in the vertebra, the magnitude of bony destruction, the degree of instability of the spinal column, and the presence or absence of neurologic compromise. Treatment options for ABCs include local intralesional curettage with or without bone grafting, cryotherapy, radiotherapy, embolization, and an en bloc resection. An en bloc resection is the highest degree of cure; however, it is difficult to perform in many cases of ABCs. A complete piecemeal intralesional resection is the most commonly performed surgical treatment of ABCs. Aggressive curettage of the cyst wall using a high-speed burr is highly recommended to minimize the risk of recurrence. Preoperative embolization of the tumor is also highly recommended.

Giant Cell Tumor

A giant cell tumor (GCT) is a locally aggressive benign tumor; approximately 7% to 15% of all GCTs are found in the spine. GCTs have a peak incidence in the second to fourth decades of life and are more commonly seen in females. GCTs are rare before skeletal maturity and are most commonly seen in the sacrum.

Clinically, pain is the most common symptom on presentation.[46] The expansion of a GCT can further lead to the development of neurologic deficits caused by either nerve root or spinal cord compression.

GCTs present radiographically as an expansile lytic lesion arising from the vertebral body that may involve the posterior elements. Expansion of the lesion can cause canal encroachment leading to spinal cord or thecal sac compression. The expansile lesion lacks a surrounding sclerotic rim and has a characteristic "soap bubble" appearance on radiographs. The lesion can spread to the paraspinal areas as well as the adjacent discs and/or vertebral bodies. On MRI, the majority of GCTs appear to have low to moderate intensity on both T1- and T2-weighted images. The presence of a fluid level on the MRI suggests presence of an accompanying ABC.[2]

A biopsy aids in confirmation of the diagnosis. Histologically, GCTs show the presence of osteoclast-like giant cells surrounded by mononuclear cells (Fig. 86.5). There is an absence of mineralization of the matrix, which is interspersed with hemorrhagic areas.[47]

Traditionally, GCTs are considered benign tumors. However, locally aggressive expansile lesions may cause significant destruction of the vertebral body and encroachment of surrounding soft tissue structures, including canal compromise. A malignant transformation rarely develops, leading to the formation of metastatic lesions. Such malignant lesions may metastasize hematogenously, predominantly to the lungs.[48,49]

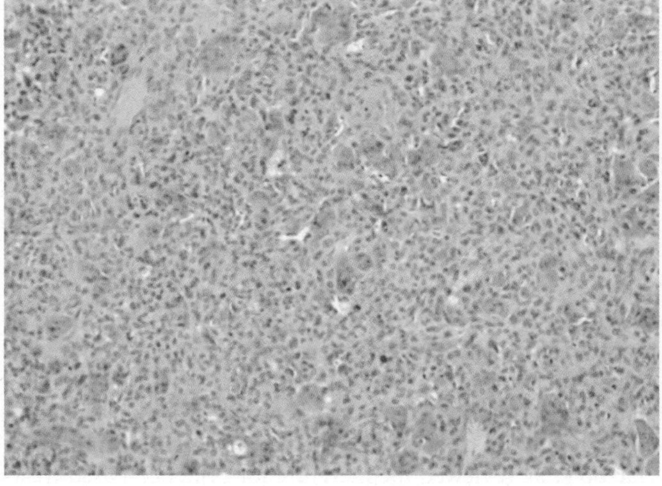

FIG. 86.5 Histologic appearance of a giant cell tumor.

An en bloc excision with a wide marginal resection is the treatment of choice for GCTs. An en bloc resection is recommended for patients with stage 3 Enneking GCTs.[50] Even with an en bloc resection with wide margins, the local recurrence rate is 0 to 14% (Fig. 86.6).[46] Although an en bloc resection may be feasible in the lumbar and thoracic spine, it may not be possible in lesions located in the cervical spine or sacrum. In such cases, intralesional curettage with phenol and cementing can be considered. Postoperatively, the local area can be treated with radiation to prevent local recurrence. Intralesional resections have higher recurrence rates even with adjuvant treatments (up to 71%).[2,51] An intralesional resection is recommended for Enneking stage 2 GCTs.[50] Radiation has been studied as a treatment for an incomplete resection or local resection. However, radiation poses a risk of malignant transformation in up to 25% of the patients.[52] The recurrence rate is higher in patients who undergo incomplete resection, which necessitates revision surgery or additional systemic treatment.

In the sacrum, resections must be stabilized whenever there is a suspicion for instability of the spine (Fig. 86.7). En bloc resection in the sacrum has been found to have a high incidence of postoperative neurologic deficits, especially with more proximal levels of tumor occurrence. Preoperative embolization followed by an intralesional resection has been shown to have a lower postoperative morbidity than en bloc resections.[46,53,53a] Serial arterial embolization has also been found to be an effective treatment modality in sacral lesions.[54,55] It can be considered in patients who are at risk for potential morbidities from other treatments. Preoperative embolization, followed by intralesional resection, should be the treatment of choice for patients with sacral GCTs that are too large for en bloc excision.[46]

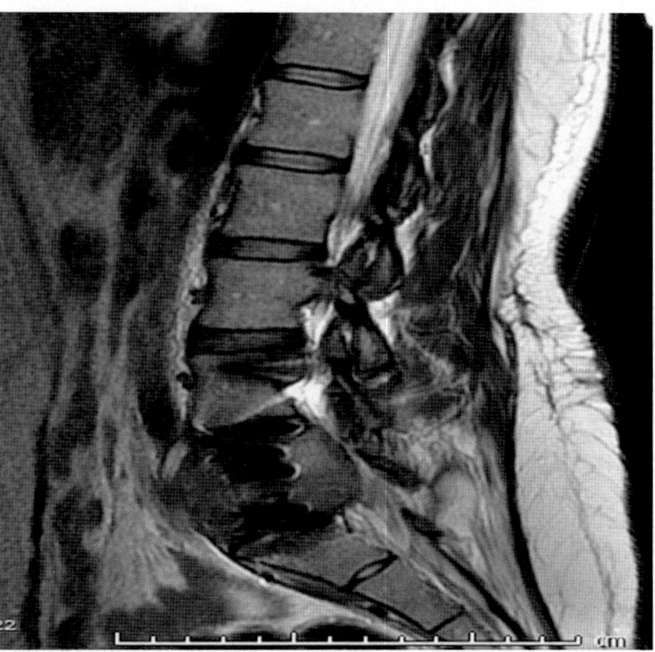

FIG. 86.6 Sagittal T2-weighted magnetic resonance image demonstrating giant cell tumor recurrence.

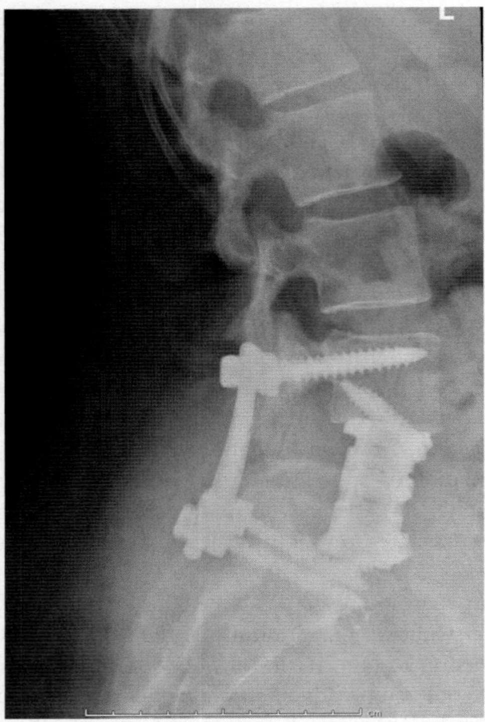

FIG. 86.7 Lateral plain radiograph demonstrating fusion construct for stabilization before recurrence.

The treatment paradigm for patients with GCTs of the spine has been changed recently with the advent of monthly injections with denosumab, which is a fully human monoclonal antibody that targets and binds with high affinity and specificity to the receptor activator of nuclear factor-κB ligand. There is experience using it in recurrent GCTs of the spine, GCTs thought to be inoperative because of tumor size or location, and GCTs in patients who refuse surgery. A recent study showed a clinically beneficial radiologic response and an impressive histologic response in most, but not all, patients.[56–58] It will be important to keep this new treatment modality in mind as more studies become available, allowing better evaluation of the current GCT treatment algorithm.

Malignant Tumors

Osteosarcoma

Osteosarcomas (osteogenic sarcomas) are the most common primary malignant tumor of the bone; however, only 3% to 5% of these tumors are seen in the spine. An osteosarcoma of the spine is usually seen in the fourth decade of life. Osteosarcomas are slightly more common in males and are most commonly located in the thoracic and lumbar spine. Osteosarcomas are high-grade aggressive tumors that may present secondary to radiation therapy after the treatment of a primary tumor. They may also occur in patients with Paget disease, enchondromatosis, or fibrous dysplasia. Patients with a history of retinoblastoma also have a high probability of developing an osteosarcoma later in life.

Patients with an osteosarcoma present with local pain, a palpable mass, or a neurologic deficit caused by spinal cord or nerve root compression from growth of the tumor. Some patients may also present with metastatic lesions, mainly in the lungs, liver, or bone, at the time of diagnosis.

Osteosarcomas are predominantly osteosclerotic lesions. On plain radiographs they appear as a heterogeneous mass with mixed lytic and sclerotic components. This appearance is caused by the presence of ossified and nonossified parts of the tumor. A pathologic fracture may be visible. CT shows a permeative bone lesion with significant bone destruction, involvement of the surrounding soft tissue, and the presence of canal compromise. The appearance of the tumor on MRI depends on the amount of mineralization within the tumor. The mineralized part of the tumor appears hypointense in both T1- and T2-weighted images, whereas the nonmineralized part of the tumor gives a hyperintense appearance on T2-weighted images. MRI is useful in presurgical planning to determine the extent of soft tissue involvement, extent of canal compromise, and severity of compression of neural structures. Technetium and gallium scanning may be used to determine the presence of skip lesions, whereas positron emission tomography scans are the most effective tools to monitor the effects of the treatment and staging of the tumor.

Grossly, the tumor has a reddish granular appearance caused by the presence of calcifications. Histologic evaluation shows the presence of a woven bone formation by malignant osteoblasts. The woven bone masses are haphazardly present in a richly vascular stroma. Typical palisading of the osteoblasts seen in normal bone is characteristically absent. The osteoblasts are dispersed in the background of the spindle cell stroma. Hemorrhagic and necrotic areas are also present within the tumor. If osteoblasts are not seen in the histologic appearance, a diagnosis of malignant fibrous histiocytoma or fibrosarcoma should be considered.

Treatment of an osteosarcoma involves a multimodal approach. Significant advancements have occurred in the treatment of osteosarcomas of the long bones; these advances have been extrapolated to the treatment of osteosarcomas of the spine. The treatment of spinal osteosarcomas starts with imaging investigations to determine the presence of metastatic lesions and the staging of the tumor. The presence of micrometastasis is common in cases of osteosarcomas. Neoadjuvant chemotherapy has been an important tool in the treatment of osteosarcomas. The addition of neoadjuvant chemotherapy aids in the treatment of systemic micrometastases, prevention of further systemic spread, and reduction of the size of the primary tumor. Histologic studies of surgically resected primary tumors obtained after neoadjuvant chemotherapy help determine the effectiveness of chemotherapy on the primary tumor. These data can then be used to plan the postoperative chemotherapy regimen. In summary, an osteosarcoma of the axial skeleton can be effectively treated with a total spondylectomy or a wide marginal excision completed after neoadjuvant chemotherapy. Local external-beam radiotherapy is reserved for palliative treatment purposes. Harrop et al. reviewed the literature for evidence-based treatment of spinal osteosarcomas.[59] They studied the effect of chemotherapy on local recurrence and the 5-year survival of patients and determined if the extent of surgical resection mattered when chemotherapy was used as part of the multimodal therapy. The authors found six studies that addressed these questions. Based on their review, they concluded that there was moderate evidence to support neoadjuvant chemotherapy and low evidence supporting en bloc resections. The authors strongly recommended the use of neoadjuvant chemotherapy as a multimodal treatment in addition to en bloc resection of the tumor. Despite recent advances, an osteosarcoma still has one of the lowest survival rates in pediatric cancers.

Ewing Sarcoma

Ewing sarcoma is a primary malignant tumor of neuroectodermal origin in the spine found in children and young adults.[60] Approximately 3% to 10% of all Ewing sarcomas arise in the spinal column.[61] Metastatic involvement of the spinal column from a primary tumor in an appendicular skeleton is much more common than a primary Ewing sarcoma in the spine. Ewing sarcoma is the most common nonlymphoproliferative malignant tumor of the spine. The tumor has a predilection for the sacrococcygeal region; however, it may also be seen in the lumbar and thoracic spine. Ewing sarcoma of the cervical spine is extremely rare. The tumors are most commonly seen in the pediatric age group (5–15 years of age).[62] The most common clinical symptoms in these patients include local pain and the presence of a neurologic deficit. Patients may also present with a soft tissue mass. Like other pediatric malignant tumors, systemic constitutional symptoms of weight loss and fever are also commonly seen. Sacral tumors may grow to a significant extent before becoming symptomatic.

On plain radiographs, Ewing sarcoma shows a moth-eaten appearance with surrounding concentric layers of reactive bone formation, giving it a classic "onion ring" appearance. However, this appearance is not seen in the spine. Most patients show aggressive vertebral destruction and lysis with a large paraspinal soft tissue mass on plain radiographs. Defining margins are absent, and vertebra plana may be seen. CT is helpful in detecting the amount of bony destruction. MRI is used to study the extent of soft tissue involvement as well as any neurologic compromise. The tumor shows intermediate signal intensity on T1-weighted images and high signal intensity on T2-weighted images.

Approximately 20% of patients present with a symptomatic metastasis, and the presence of micrometastasis is seen in a majority of the patients. The most common sites for metastasis are the lungs, long bones, and bone marrow. Bone scanning is used to detect the presence of metastatic lesions. The suspicious lesions should be confirmed with a biopsy.

On gross examination, the tumor appears as a firm, gray, friable mass with areas of hemorrhage and necrosis. Histological examination shows the presence of characteristic small round cells that form large sheets separated by septae. There is an abundance of collagen in the tumors. Patients with Ewing sarcoma or other types of peripheral neuroectodermal tumors of the bone have a translocation mutation. The diagnostic workup should include investigations into immunohistochemistry, cytogenetic, and molecular genetic testing.

Initial treatment of Ewing sarcoma involves chemotherapy. The survival rate with six-drug chemotherapy has been shown to be as high as 80%, which is significantly higher than four-drug chemotherapy. The cure rate with a multimodal treatment has been shown to be more than 50%. Patients with systemic metastatic disease do not respond favorably to chemotherapy and pose a therapeutic challenge to the treating physician. The 5-year survival rate is only 20% despite advances in treatment. Treatment of the local tumor can be done with surgical resection or radiation. The size of the tumor, older age at onset, and presence of systemic metastatic lesions have been thought to be poor prognostic signs. A review of literature by Harrop et al.[59] considered the evidence-based recommendations for the treatment for Ewing sarcoma. The authors studied the effects of neoadjuvant chemotherapy in local control, long-term survival of patients with Ewing sarcoma, and how the extent of a local surgical resection affects local control and long-term survival. The authors strongly recommended neoadjuvant chemotherapy as a first-line treatment modality but only had moderate evidence to support this line of treatment. The authors also recommended the use of surgical resections for local control of the tumor with low-quality supporting evidence. Radiation was believed to be a useful treatment modality in the cases of incomplete resections.

Chordoma

Chordomas are primary malignant tumors arising from the notochordal remnants in the spinal segments from the clivus to the coccyx and account for 2% to 4% of primary malignant bone tumors. They are the most common primary malignant tumor affecting the sacrum. The tumor is most frequently seen in the sacrococcygeal location (50%) followed by the spheno-occipital location (35–40%). Chordomas can be seen at almost any age; however, they are most commonly found in the fifth to sixth decades of life. It is the most common nonlymphoproliferative primary malignant tumor of the spine in adults. The tumor is more common in men than women, with a ratio of 2 : 1. Chordomas are considered to be slow-growing, locally aggressive tumors and may arise from the vertebral bodies and grow posteriorly, causing compression of the neurologic structures. They may also grow anteriorly into the paraspinal soft tissues. Within the sacrum, the tumor most commonly affects the fourth and fifth sacral segments and protrudes into the pelvis as it grows. Involvement of the pelvic bones is rare. Metastatic lesions can be seen in approximately 30% of sacrococcygeal chordomas.

Patients with chordomas that affect the sacrococcygeal region present with an insidious onset of back pain. The pelvis and sacral canal can accommodate the enormous growth of the tumor before it becomes symptomatic. Patients most often present with low back pain or sciatic pain, constipation from compression of the rectum, or a neurologic deficit caused by compression of the sacral nerve roots. Patients may also present with a gluteal or sacral mass. Chordomas of the mobile spinal column present earlier with a neurologic

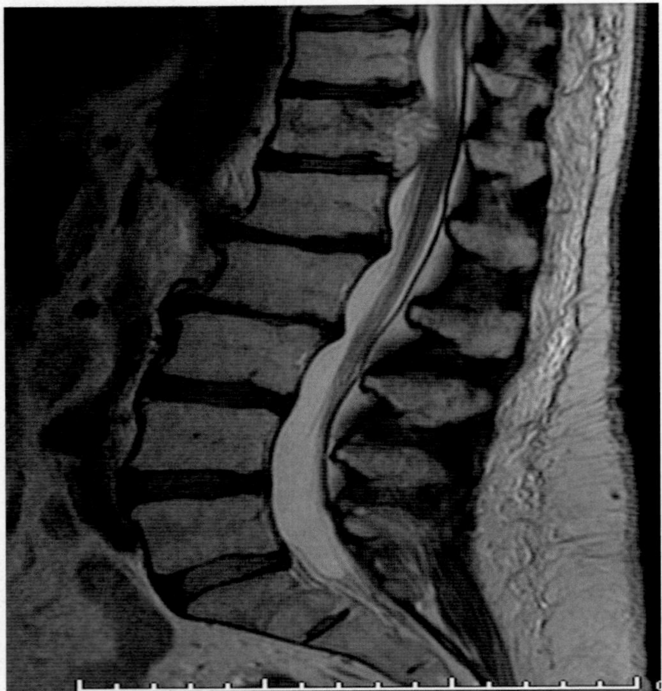

FIG. 86.8 Sagittal magnetic resonance image demonstrating expansile thoracic tumor proven by biopsy to be a chordoma.

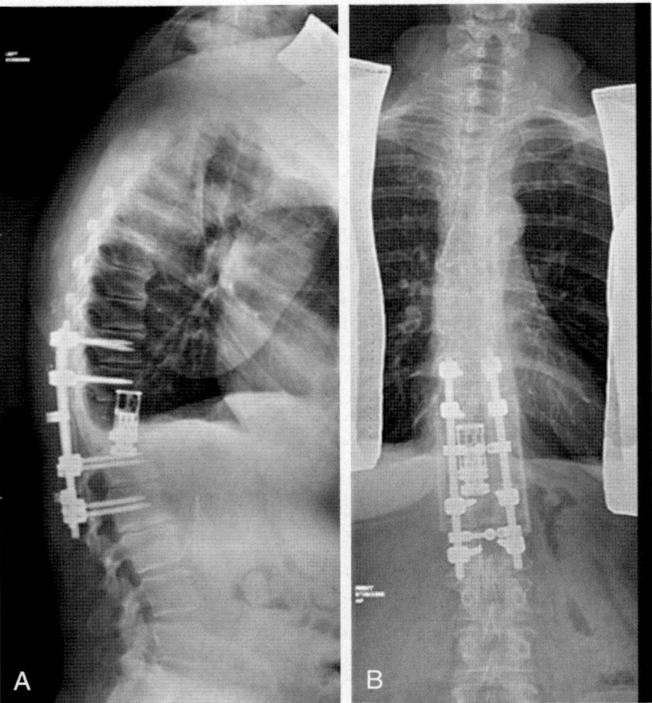

FIG. 86.9 (A) Posteroanterior and (B) lateral long standing films demonstrating postoperative reconstruction after an en bloc spondylectomy.

deficit compared with sacrococcygeal tumors. Chordomas in the cervical region may present with symptoms of dysphagia, breathing difficulty, or neurologic deficits.

Chordomas usually appear as lytic lesions with a large associated soft tissue mass. The majority of chordomas present with calcifications throughout the tumor. Unlike other malignant tumors of the vertebral bodies, chordomas (along with GCTs) are the only tumors that involve the adjacent intervertebral disc as they spread to the adjacent vertebral bodies. Chordomas give a uniform appearance of the soft tissue mass with the occasional presence of lucencies indicating the areas of necrosis. Sacral chordomas often show the presence of mottled densities/calcific debris within the tumor mass. MRI helps delineate the tumor extent, especially on T2-weighted images (Fig. 86.8). It also aids in defining the presence or absence of the plane of separation between the tumor and the rectum. Tumors appear hyperintense to the surrounding muscles on T2-weighted images. On gadolinium-enhanced images, the tumor shows signal enhancement with areas of attenuation around the calcifications.

Workup should involve investigations to diagnose the presence of local and systemic spread of the tumor. CT scans of the chest, abdomen, and pelvis and a bone scan may aid in determining the spread of the tumor. The tumor usually shows normal or a decreased uptake on the bone scans. Tissue diagnosis is equally important and requires a biopsy. Chordomas are notoriously known to spread along the biopsy needle tracks, and care should be taken to avoid other body cavities while doing the biopsy. The tissue sample allows for the diagnosis and determination of the tumor's aggressiveness.

On gross examination, the tumor appears as a gray, soft to firm mass with a lobulated structure and a translucent surface. The tumors are well circumscribed due to the presence of a pseudocapsule formation. Within the bone, the tumor appears as a lytic lesion with a clear margin of reactive bone. Histologically, the tumor shows the presence of a lobular architecture with signet ring cells separated by fibrous septae. The septae are densely infiltrated with lymphocytes.

Effective treatment of a chordoma requires en bloc resection of the tumor with the resection of the circumferential margin of normal tissue. Resection with a wide margin is important to decrease the risk of local recurrence. For sacral chordomas, complete resection of the sacrum is occasionally required. Due to the complex anatomy of the sacrum and surrounding structures, surgical treatment involves a combined approach with the assistance of multiple specialties. A resection of the chordoma involves a combination of various surgical approaches. Usually, posterior elements are resected through the posterior approach. The anterior tumor mass is separated from the thecal sac. Posterior stabilization is carried out using instrumentation to the pelvis if the entire sacrum or all of the sacrum distal to S1 is resected. This is followed by an anterior resection of the vertebral body. The anterior column is then reconstructed using an expandable titanium biomechanical device with or without allograft (Fig. 86.9). Resection of sacral chordomas may necessitate the sacrifice of the sacral nerve roots, resulting in a postoperative neurologic deficit and the loss of bowel, bladder, and sexual function. Preservation of at least one of the S2 nerves allows the patient to retain control of the bowel or bladder function. Resection of the sacrum at or above S1 leads to significant neurologic deficits and the need for a specialized postoperative treatment plan. Adjuvant treatment with radiation is reserved for palliative treatment for local recurrences. Chordomas are thought to be radioresistant tumors. Due to the slow-growing nature of the tumor, chemotherapy has a limited role in the treatment of chordomas.

Chondrosarcoma

Chondrosarcomas are cartilage-forming malignant tumors that affect the spinal column. Tumor osteoid formation is characteristically absent. Spinal chondrosarcomas are extremely rare. Chondrosarcomas can present de novo or can develop secondary to a preexisting benign tumor of the spine. They can also be associated with multiple hereditary osteochondromatosis. Chondrosarcomas are more common in males, with a ratio of 2 to 4 : 1. The average age at diagnosis is between the fourth and fifth decades of life, but they can be seen at any age. The tumor is more commonly found in the posterior elements than anterior elements. The most common location in the spinal column is the thoracic spine.

Patients with a chondrosarcoma present with an insidious-onset pain over the tumor site. Neurologic deficits in the form of radiculopathy or myelopathy are commonly seen and present in up to 50% of patients. Patients with posterior element involvement may also have a palpable mass as the tumor grows in size.

Lytic lesions with occasional calcifications (arc and ring patterns) are common presentations in radiographs and CT scans. A lobulated soft tissue mass has low signal intensity on T1-weighted images and high signal intensity on T2-weighted images (Fig. 86.10). CT and MRI studies demonstrate the tumor's extension and are helpful for preoperative planning.[63-65] Because chondrosarcomas are avascular in nature, they are resistant to chemotherapy and radiation. Chondrosarcomas show cortical destruction and soft tissue extension. Most of these tumors are low grade and slow growing, but once metastatic they have a poor prognosis. Chondrosarcomas are classified based on origin (intramedullary and periosteal) and histologic appearance (conventional and variant types). Variant subtypes seen are clear cell, dedifferentiated, mesenchymal, and myxoid. Conventional chondrosarcomas have a higher incidence rate than variant chondrosarcomas.[66]

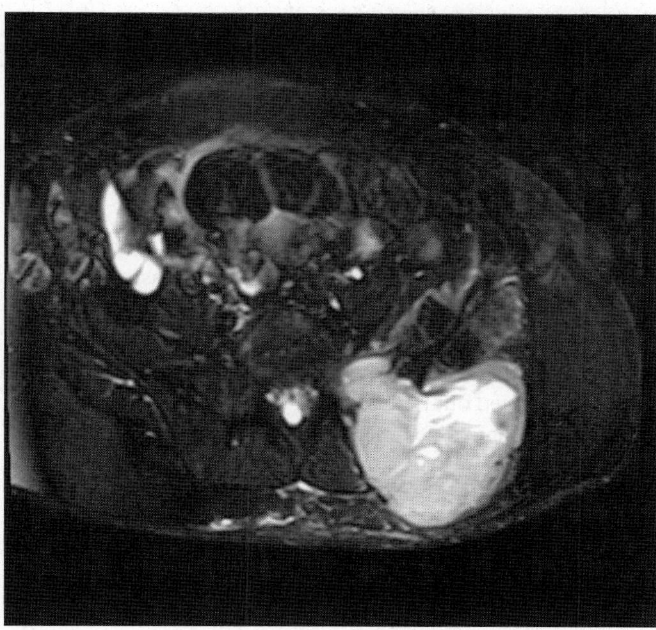

FIG. 86.10 T2-weighted axial magnetic resonance image showing chondrosarcoma involvement of the left sacrum and ilium.

Chondrosarcomas are primarily managed by en bloc excision with wide margins. A wide marginal resection is sometimes impossible due to the size and extension of the tumor into the surrounding important structures and risks the stability of the spine. Stener pioneered en bloc excision of the chondrosarcoma of the spine in 1971.[67] Since then, all subsequent series have demonstrated the importance of obtaining negative margins in an en bloc fashion to increase disease-free survival.[68] The prognosis of the tumor depends on histologic grading and surgical resection.[68] Incomplete surgical resection results in local recurrence and a much worse prognosis. Although chondrosarcomas are resistant to radiation therapy, Harwood et al.[69] reported that high radiation dosage (5000 cGy) for 4 to 5 weeks is helpful for long-term control of the local disease. They recommended radiation therapy only in patients in whom surgical resection was impossible. Negative marginal resections are uncommon in en bloc excision, and adjuvant radiation therapy is recommended to control local recurrence.[70]

When the management of sacral tumors requires partial or complete sacrectomy (Fig. 86.11), reconstruction of the lumbosacral junction is necessary. A staged anterior/posterior en bloc sacrectomy with a Galveston L-rod pelvic ring reconstruction or more modern variation is often required. Understanding the anatomy and biomechanics of the spinopelvic apparatus and the lumbosacral junction, as well as having a familiarity with the various techniques available for carrying out sacrectomy and pelvic ring reconstruction, enables the spine surgeon to effectively manage sacral tumors.[1]

Multiple Myeloma and Solitary Plasmacytoma

Multiple myeloma is a hematologic malignancy with a primary bone origin constituting multifocal plasma cell neoplasms that commonly involve the spine. The plasma cells undergo a malignant transformation, producing an excess amount of immunoglobulin. This leads to the activation of osteoclasts and inhibition of osteoblastic activity, which also leads to the formation of multiple lytic lesions throughout the skeletal system. Multiple myeloma constitutes approximately 1% of all malignant diseases. The most common age of presentation is in the sixth decade of life. Skeletal involvement is a very common mode of presentation. More than 70% of patients have bone involvement and pain at the time of presentation. Patients with multiple myeloma present with multiple lytic lesions in the spine as well as the appendicular skeleton. They have bone pain and a vertebral compression fracture, but rarely have neurologic symptoms or deficits. However, patients with extension of the tumor to the epidural space or compression fractures with severe canal compromise may present with neurologic deficits. They may have associated

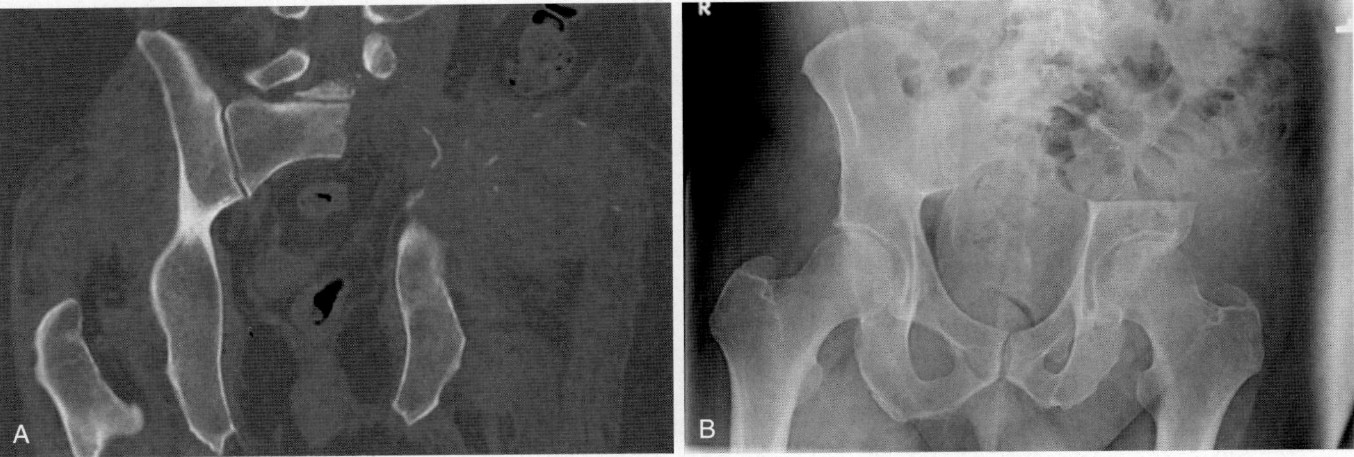

FIG. 86.11 (A) Coronal computed tomography and (B) plain radiograph demonstrating hemisacrectomy and hemipelvectomy without reconstruction.

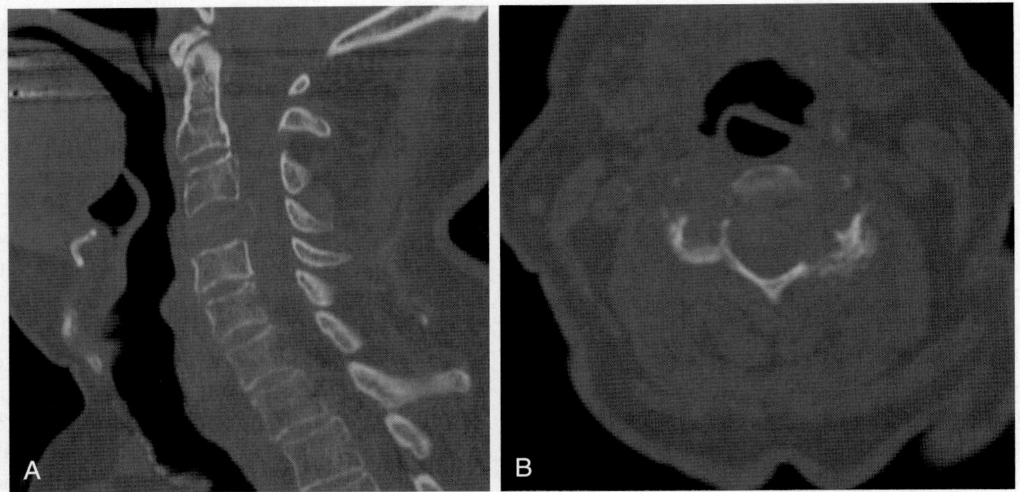

FIG. 86.12 (A) Sagittal and (B) axial computed tomographic images of C4 vertebra showing complete destruction of the vertebral body with infiltration of the posterior elements.

systemic symptoms in the form of fatigue, recurrent infections, and severe life-threatening anemia.

Plain radiographs are used for a skeletal survey when multiple myeloma is suspected. The radiographs show the typical lytic lesions, with a sharp zone of transition and lack of reactive bone formation giving the appearance of "punched out" lesions. Pathologic compression fractures are most commonly seen in the thoracolumbar region. Due to the suppression of osteoblastic activity, a bone scan has a very limited role in the diagnosis of multiple myeloma lesions. CT scans are used to detect the amount of bony destruction and assess spinal stability (Fig. 86.12). CT scans are useful when the lesions are not well visualized on radiographs. Typical CT findings include classic lytic lesions, a soft tissue mass, pathologic fracture, or an epidural mass. MRI is useful to assess the extent of neurologic compression (Fig. 86.13). The tumor appears as hypointense on T1-weighted images and hyperintense on T2-weighted images. Fluorodeoxyglucose positron emission tomography (FDG-PET) scan has become the investigative tool of choice and has replaced MRI as a tool in the early detection and staging of multiple myeloma. Schirrmeister et al. reported these scans to be 92% sensitive in the early detection of lesions that were not seen on radiographs.[71] MRI or FDG-PET scans are also important to look for other skeletal lesions when the diagnosis of a solitary plasmacytoma is considered.

The treatment of multiple myeloma involves a thorough investigation to assess the severity of the disease. These assessments are carried out to determine the neurologic status of the patient, oncologic assessment, assessment of mechanical stability, and systemic disease assessment. These fundamental assessments help in deciding the most appropriate treatment modality (radiotherapy, chemotherapy, or surgery) for the patient. Thorough assessment of the neurologic status is important to determine the presence of radiculopathy or myelopathy and the extent of canal compromise. An oncologic assessment is necessary to determine the tumor's response to radiotherapy or chemotherapy. Mechanical stability can be

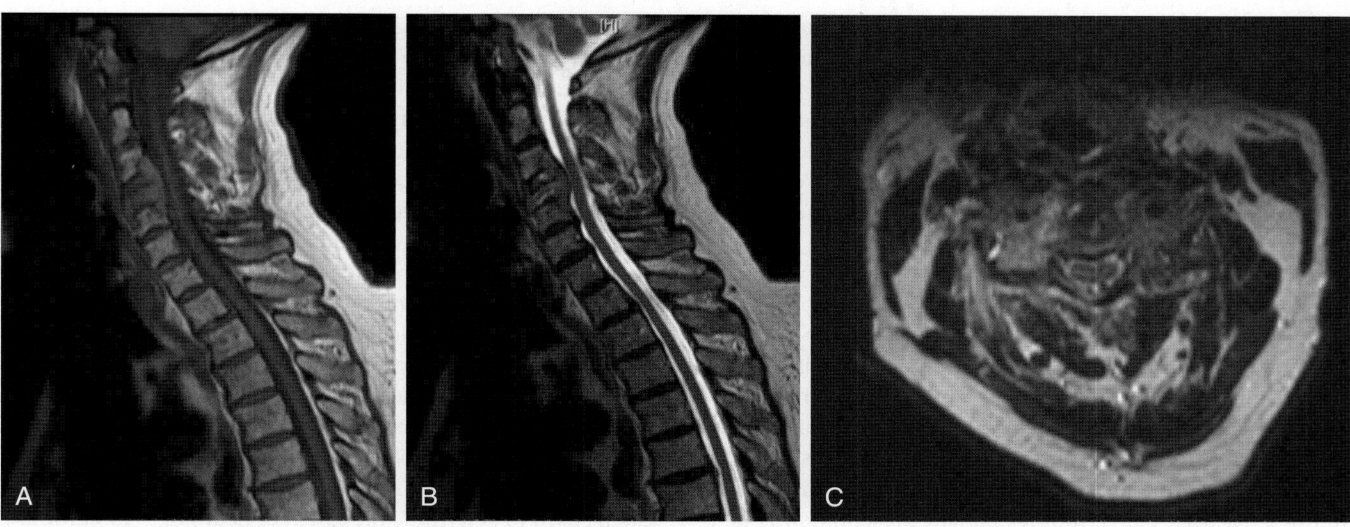

FIG. 86.13 (A) T1-weighted and (B) T2-weighted sagittal images and (C) T2-weighted axial magnetic resonance images of a solitary plasmacytoma presenting as a lytic lesion of the C4 vertebra.

assessed based on the extent of bone destruction. A systemic assessment involves the determination of the extent of the disease and other medical comorbidities.

Radiation therapy, in addition to surgery, has been shown to increase the long-term survival rate. It has been the frontline treatment modality for multiple myelomas. Patients with minimal epidural canal compromise with or without neurologic symptoms can be treated with image-guided, intensity-modulated radiation therapy. However, patients with severe canal compromise or the presence of neurologic deficits are initially treated with radiation therapy. Patients who present with compression or burst fractures are treated with vertebroplasty or kyphoplasty. These procedures should be avoided in patients with a breach in the posterior vertebral cortex or significant epidural disease. Cement augmentation procedures have been shown to improve pain and the functionality of patients with multiple myeloma.[72] Patients with significant spinal instability need surgical treatment. Due to accompanying osteopenia/osteoporosis, a stabilization and reconstruction procedure often involves anterior column reconstruction as well as posterior instrumented spinal fusion (Fig. 86.14).

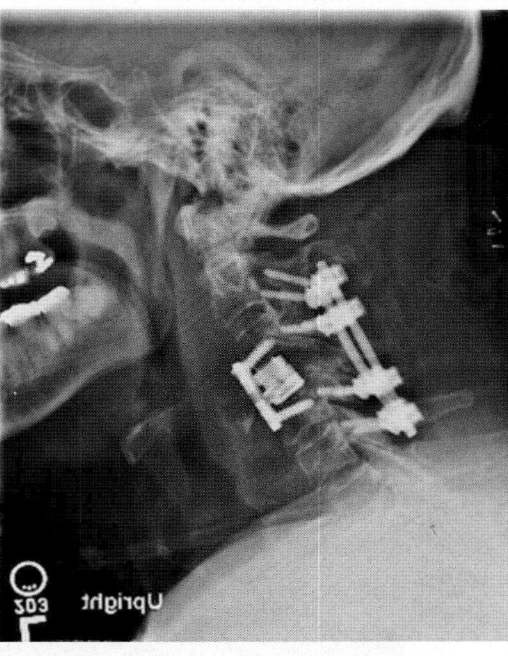

FIG. 86.14 Postoperative upright radiograph showing spinal column reconstruction after a cervical corpectomy and excision of tumor.

Metastatic Tumors

Metastatic lesions are the most commonly seen malignant tumors of the spine, and symptomatic metastatic lesions are the initial manifestation in up to 20% of patients with malignancy. The spinal column is the third most common site of malignancy after the lungs and liver and is the most common site of skeletal metastasis. With an increase in the life span of the current population, the incidence of cancer and spinal metastatic lesions is on the rise. The most common primary tumors that metastasize to the spine are breast, prostate, lung, kidney, and thyroid. Within the spinal column, the thoracic spine is the most common site for metastasis (70%) followed by lumbosacral (16–22%) and cervical (8–15%).

Pathophysiology of Metastasis

The process of metastasis involves the dissociation of tumor cells from the primary tumor, the penetration of the surrounding matrix, followed by the invasion of vascular or lymphoreticular channels. Tumor cells act as emboli and travel to the distant organ site where they invade through the walls of the blood or lymphatic vessels and eventually adhere to the extracellular matrix. Various chemical modulators secreted by the tumor cells then promote neoangiogenesis. In the skeletal system, the tumors most often stimulate osteoclasts, leading to lytic lesion formation, or less commonly stimulate osteoblasts, leading to an osteoblastic lesion. Spinal metastasis most frequently occurs through a hematogenous route either through the segmental vessels or the retrograde spread through the valveless Batson's venous plexus. Lung tumors spread to the vertebral column through the segmental arteries, whereas breast, gastrointestinal, and prostate carcinomas spread through the Batson's venous plexus. The expression of surface protein and receptors has also shown to contribute to the selectivity of tissues for metastatic lesions.

Clinical Presentation

Axial pain is the most frequently reported symptom in patients with a spinal metastasis. The pain caused by the metastatic lesion is usually nonmechanical in nature and is associated with a characteristic nighttime aggravation. Patients may also present with pathologic compression fractures with aggravation of axial back pain. Another patient presentation is neurologic symptoms that may include the presence of radiculopathy or myelopathy. The symptoms may be caused by a direct extension of the tumor to the epidural space or compression of the neurologic structures caused by retropulsed fragments and deformity created by the pathologic fractures. Spinal metastatic lesions can also be asymptomatic and may only be detected in a general workup for a visceral malignant tumor.[73]

Diagnosis

Evaluation of the patient with metastatic lesions should begin with a thorough clinical examination. Patients should be evaluated for the presence of local tenderness, deformity, neurologic deficits, and instability. A thorough neurologic examination is very important to diagnose spinal cord or nerve root compression. Signs of myelopathy commonly seen in these patients are exaggerated reflexes, a positive Babinski sign, and gait disturbances.

The next step in the management of metastatic lesions involves imaging investigations to determine the extent of local involvement and the source of the primary tumor.

The imaging investigations start with a series of biplanar plain radiographs. The images should be evaluated for the presence of spinal stability, alignment, pathologic compression fractures, as well as any lytic or sclerotic lesions. However, plain radiographic evaluations have limitations posed by the location in the spinal column as well the overall bone quality of the patient. Fifty percent of the trabecular bone must be lost before the lesion can be diagnosed as a lytic lesion on a plain radiograph. Lytic lesions involving the pedicle may give the appearance of a "winking owl" sign. CT or MRI is necessary to diagnose metastatic lesions. CT scans provide information about the extent of bony destruction caused by the lesion (Fig. 86.15). CT scans can assess the bone destruction in the sagittal, coronal, and axial planes, which aids in the determination of potential spinal instability. CT scans also show involvement of surrounding paraspinal structures. In addition, CT myelogram can be used to determine the extent of neurologic compromise. MRI is routinely used in the evaluation of spinal metastatic lesions. MRI of patients with metastatic lesions involves T1- and T2-weighted images and short tau inversion recovery sequences. MRI is useful in differentiating metastatic compression fractures from osteoporotic compression fractures. T2-weighted images show hyperintense signal in both types of fractures (Fig. 86.16), whereas T1-weighted images of metastatic lesions show diminished signal due to marrow involvement by the tumor. Osteoporotic fractures appear isointense on T1-weighted images (Fig. 86.17). Gadolinium contrast-enhanced imaging sequences help evaluate soft tissue involvement and epidural space involvement. MRI is a very important tool when surgical treatment is contemplated. It aids in the evaluation of adjacent and distant vertebrae so that a reliable point of fixation can be obtained. MRI of the entire spine is conducted to detect the presence of metastatic lesions. It has a high specificity in diagnosing noncontiguous multiple foci of metastatic lesions and a very high specificity and a low false-positive rate. Bone scans may also be used for a similar purpose due to their high sensitivity, but they have a higher false-positive rate.

Obtaining a tissue diagnosis is of the utmost importance in differentiating a primary tumor from a metastatic lesion.

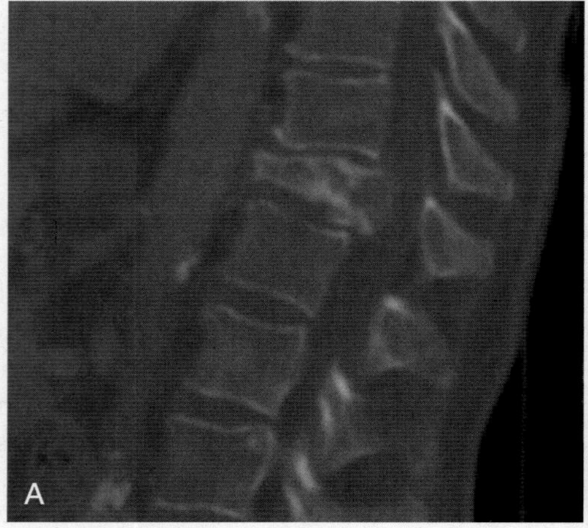

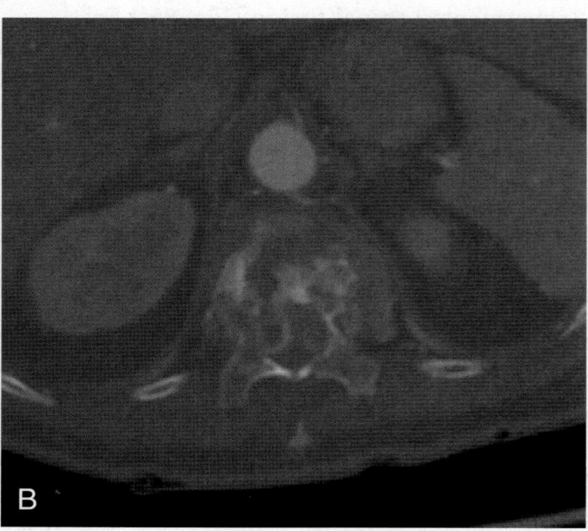

FIG. 86.15 (A) Sagittal and (B) axial computed tomographic images showing a lytic lesion in the T12 vertebra with pathologic fracture, retropulsion, and canal compromise.

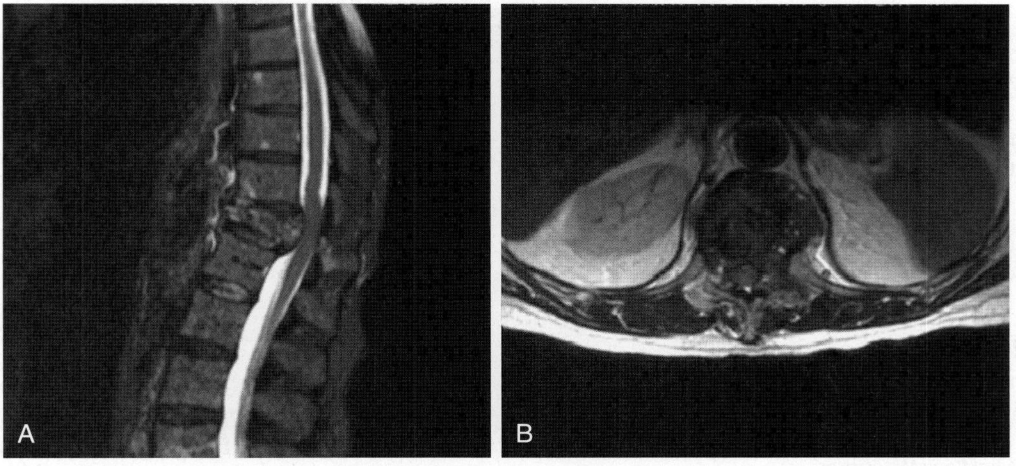

FIG. 86.16 (A) Sagittal and (B) axial T2-weighted images showing a hypointense lesion causing spinal cord compression and infiltration of the pedicle and vertebral body along with posterior elements by the metastatic lesion.

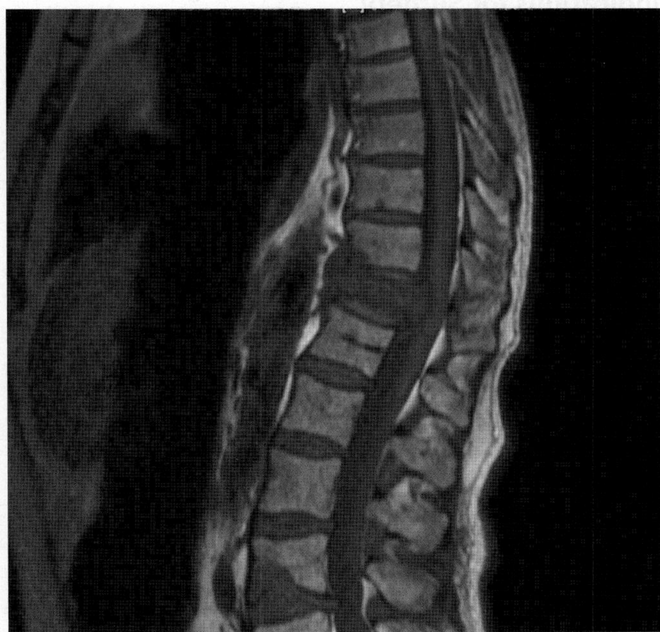

FIG. 86.17 T1-weighted image showing presence of marrow infiltration by the lesion appearing as hypointense signal intensity compared with surrounding bone marrow.

CT-guided biopsy usually provides an adequate sample for tissue diagnosis in 93% of lytic and 76% of sclerotic lesions and has obviated the need for an open biopsy.

Treatment

Most surgeons agree that metastatic spine tumor surgery should be limited to patients who have an estimated life expectancy of greater than 3 months. Treatment outcomes are highly dependent on the prognosis of the primary tumor. An early study estimated the average survival for patients with metastatic spinal cord compression to be between 3 and 7 months, with a 36% probability of survival to 12 months.[74] In an effort to better determine a patient's life expectancy, Tokuhashi et al.[75] presented a scoring system to be used in the preoperative evaluation of patients with metastatic spine tumors. Scores of 0 to 2 points are assigned to each of six parameters. The patient's general health condition, number of extraspinal skeletal metastases, number of metastases to the spine, status of metastases to internal organs, site of primary tumor, and the patient's neurologic status are all weighted parameters. The same study group later published a revised system of scoring that slightly increased the weight of the primary site of cancer,[76] which is commonly used as an indication for patient survivability (Table 86.1). Regardless of the type of scoring system used, spine surgeons are encouraged to consult with the patient's medical and radiation oncologists because multimodal treatment may offer the patient even longer survival than otherwise predicted.

The treatment of metastatic spinal tumors requires a multidisciplinary approach that integrates surgery, radiation and medical oncology, and interventional radiology. Recently, a multidisciplinary team at Memorial Sloan Kettering Cancer Center established the NOMS decision framework to incorporate four fundamental assessments: neurologic, oncologic, mechanical instability, and systemic disease. This framework established guidelines in the decision-making process to administer conventional external-beam radiation, stereotactic radiosurgery, surgical intervention, separation surgery, or a combination of these treatment modalities based on the most recent advancements in technology and outcomes based on the literature. In NOMS, the neurologic consideration is an assessment of the degree of epidural spinal cord compression, myelopathy, and/or functional radiculopathy. The degree of epidural spinal cord compression is based on a 6-point scale that incorporates gradations of the thecal sac impingement. A grade of 0 indicates only bone disease. Grade 1a indicates epidural impingement without deformation of the thecal sac; grade 1b indicates deformation of the thecal sac without spinal cord abutment; and grade 1c indicates deformation of the thecal sac with spinal cord abutment but without cord compression. A grade of 2 indicates spinal cord compression but with visible cerebrospinal fluid around the cord; grade 3 indicates spinal cord compression with no cerebrospinal fluid visible around the cord.[77] The oncologic consideration is predicated on the expected tumor response and the durability of the response to available treatments. Mechanical instability takes into account the integrity of the spinal column and the extent of pathologic fractures to determine whether to use conservative management with a brace or surgical intervention. The final consideration of systemic disease and medical comorbidities is to evaluate the ability of the patient to tolerate a proposed treatment and the overall survival based on tumor histology and extent of disease. Table 86.2 provides a guide to the current NOMS decision framework.

TABLE 86.1 Tokuhashi Scoring System for Preoperative Evaluation of Patients With Metastatic Spinal Tumors

Parameter	Score
General Condition	
Poor	0
Moderate	1
Good	2
Number of Extraspinal Bone Metastases	
>3	0
1 or 2	1
0	2
Number of Metastases in the Spine	
>3	0
2	1
1	2
Metastases to Major Internal Organs	
Irremovable	0
Removable	1
None	2
Primary Site of Cancer	
Lung, osteosarcoma, stomach, bladder, esophagus, pancreas	0
Liver, gallbladder, unidentified	1
Others	2
Kidney, uterus	3
Rectum	4
Thyroid, breast, prostate, carcinoid tumor	5
Myelopathy	
Complete	0
Incomplete	1
None	2

Data from Tokuhasi T, Matsuzaki H, Oda H, et al. A revised scoring system for preoperative evaluation of metastatic spine tumor prognosis. *Spine (Phila Pa 1976)*. 2005;30: 2186-2191.

Treatment

The goal of treatment for patients with spinal tumors is to provide a possible cure, palliation, and early return to activity. If this is not possible, the goal is to provide a stable spinal column and normal or improved neurologic function. Table 86.3 provides a general outline for the treatment of spinal tumors.

Indications for Surgery

Not all patients with spinal tumors require surgery. Patients with clearly benign tumors and those with diffuse metastases in which the primary tumor is known can simply be observed. With the acceptance of more aggressive surgical methods, surgical indications have been expanded to include (1) isolated primary or metastatic lesion or a solitary site of relapse, (2) pathologic fracture or deformity with bony impingement producing neurologic symptoms or pain, (3) radioresistant tumor (metastatic or primary), (4) tumor progression despite or after radiotherapy, (5) segmental instability with significant pain or impending neurologic injury, and (6) inability to obtain tissue diagnosis by other means. All these presume a patient who is healthy enough to survive surgery but are not incumbent on a long-expected survival.

Staging

The initial diagnostic workup allows spine surgeons to determine the nature, extent of the tumor, extent of soft tissue

TABLE 86.2 NOMS Decision Framework

Neurologic	Oncologic	Mechanical	Systemic	Decision
Low-grade ESCC + no myelopathy	Radiosensitive	Stable		cEBRT
	Radiosensitive	Unstable		Stabilization followed by cEBRT
	Radioresistant	Stable		SRS
	Radioresistant	Unstable		Stabilization followed by SRS
High-grade ESCC + myelopathy	Radiosensitive	Stable		cEBRT
	Radiosensitive	Unstable		Stabilization followed by cEBRT
	Radioresistant	Stable	Able to tolerate surgery	Decompression/stabilization followed by SRS
	Radioresistant	Stable	Unable to tolerate surgery	cEBRT
	Radioresistant	Unstable	Able to tolerate surgery	Decompression/stabilization followed by SRS
	Radioresistant	Unstable	Unable to tolerate surgery	Stabilization followed by cEBRT

Low-grade ESCC is defined as grade 0 or 1 in the Spine Oncology Study Group scoring system. High-grade ESCC is defined as grade 2 or 3 in the Spine Oncology Study Group scoring system. cEBRT, conventional external-beam radiation therapy; ESCC, epidural spinal cord compression; SRS, stereotactic radiosurgery.
Modified from Laufer I, Rubin DG, Lis E, et al. The NOMS framework: approach to the treatment of spinal metastatic tumors. *Oncologist*. 2013;18(6):744-751.

TABLE 86.3 General Treatment Approach for Spine Tumors

Therapy	Indication
Observation	Indolent and clearly benign tumors (hemangioma, osteochondroma, bone island, bone infarct)
Radiotherapy	Metastatic lesions from a known radiosensitive primary (multiple myeloma, breast carcinoma)
Chemotherapy	Metastatic lesions from a known chemosensitive primary (thyroid)
Intralesional excision, curettage	Benign tumors with limited potential for recurrence (aneurysmal bone cyst, osteoblastoma), radiosensitive metastatic lesions with adjuvant radiation therapy
Marginal excision ± adjuvant cryotherapy or radiotherapy	Locally aggressive benign lesions (giant cell tumor), radiosensitive primary and metastatic lesions (plasmacytoma, breast and prostate carcinoma), low-grade malignancies
Wide excision	All primary malignancies without known metastases (osteosarcoma, chondrosarcoma, chondroma); solitary metastases with likelihood of prolonged survival (breast, prostate, renal cell carcinoma); locally aggressive benign tumors (giant cell tumor)

involvement, stability of the spinal column, and extent of neurogenic compromise. This information can then be used to stage the tumor. Boriani et al. published a novel system for staging primary spinal tumors.[78] According to the Weinstein-Boriani-Biagini staging system, the affected vertebra is divided into 12 radiating zones, numbered 1 to 12 in a clockwise manner starting from the left side of the spinous process, and five concentric layers (labeled A to E) starting from the paravertebral extraosseous region to the dural involvement. Layer A corresponds to the extraosseous soft tissues, B is the intraosseous superficial layer, C is the intraosseous deep layer, D is the extraosseous extradural layer, and E is the extraosseous intradural layer.[78,79] CT, MRI, and angiography techniques are used to stage the tumor. These investigations also help determine the longitudinal extent of the tumor.

Surgical Approach

The primary goals of surgery are local control of the tumor, neurologic improvement, and maintenance of spinal stability. The surgical approach must provide sufficient access for both tumor excision and stabilization of the spine. A complete radiographic evaluation should be performed to determine the accurate location of the tumor and its extension to the surrounding tissues. Additional laboratory and screening studies should focus on further differentiation, allowing the surgeon to plan an operation that will adequately treat the tumor without exposing the patient to needless risks. The approach and extent of surgery depend on the location of tumor in the vertebrae and the extent of the disease. General approaches for spinal tumors are described below.

A dorsal approach is recommended for a dorsal element tumor (lamina and spinous process) or lesions in radiating zones 10 to 3. Studies have reported that an aggressive dorsal decompressive laminectomy provides more neurologic improvement than a simple decompressive laminectomy.[80,81] At all vertebral levels, dorsal elements can be accessed through a midline incision.

Lesions that involve the posterior elements and pars (zones 2 to 5 and 7 to 11) can be excised through a dorsal or dorsolateral approach. Most tumors need both a ventral and dorsal approach. In such cases, a dorsolateral approach is considered to avoid a two-stage surgery. In the upper thoracic and thoracolumbar junction, lateral vertebrae are exposed through a costotransversectomy approach for both ventral and dorsal decompression and segmental dorsal fixation.[81] This approach exposes half of the ventral body. For dorsal decompression, concomitant thoracic laminectomy and resection of the facet joints and pedicles are needed. The surgeon may consider sacrificing at least one single nerve for extensive ventral decompression and spinal instrumentation. Care should be taken to protect the underlying pleural structures, and the patient's mean arterial pressure should be maintained at greater than 75 mm Hg to protect the spinal cord from ischemia during the procedure.

Lesions involving the anterior and posterior halves of the vertebral body (zones 5 to 9 and 4 to 8) are resected using anterior approach techniques, especially for benign tumors. However, dual-approach techniques are needed in cases of malignant lesions. The majority of malignant tumors affecting this region require a vertebrectomy, which is performed with a dual approach. The standard surgical approach is determined according to which vertebral levels are involved. For the upper cervical lesions, transoral and extraoral ventral approaches are used.[82,83] For lower cervical tumors, most surgeons use the Southwick-Robinson anterior approach.[84] In the thoracic region, a right- or left-sided approach is usually determined by the area of the compressed tumor. If neither side is more involved, the spine is often approached from the right side at or above T5 to avoid the arch of the aorta. Below T5, the spine is approached from the left to minimize retraction on the liver. Surgeons typically select the intercostal space one or two segments above the targeted vertebral body approach. The upper part of the thoracic spine from the first to the third thoracic vertebrae can be exposed using a thoracoplasty approach by mobilizing the scapula ventrally and resecting the second vertebra. As described by Harrington, the major advantage of a ventral approach is the surgeon's ability to resect the tumor directly, decompress the neurologic structures from the side of their compromise, and "jack" open the collapsed vertebral space, thereby correcting the typical kyphotic deformity at its source.[85,86] In the thoracolumbar junction, both a thoracotomy and lumbar retroperitoneal approach must be completed for a ventral approach.[87,88] The most common approach is through the rib just proximal to the area of interest. Lumbar spine tumors can be accessed ventrally through a retroperitoneal approach.[89] Care should be taken to protect the genitofemoral nerve and ureter from injury during the procedure.

Resections

En bloc and intralesional resections are the two general types of surgical resections classified based on the type of margin achieved during surgery. In intralesional resections, the surgeon removes the tumor from within the tumor mass. An intralesional resection has a high recurrence rate compared with en bloc resections. The high recurrence rate is due to the presence of the residual tumor or an incomplete resection. Radiation therapy is often used after intralesional resections to facilitate local control. En bloc resection is the surgical removal of the tumor in a single piece, fully encased within a layer of healthy tissue. En bloc resections can be marginal, wide, or radical. Marginal resection means the removal of the entire tumor with or without a thin healthy tissue layer. En bloc resection in the spine may still have recurrences from positive tumor margins. A wide margin resection means the complete removal of the tumor with the continuous shell of healthy tissue. Wide resections are not always possible in the spine and often lead to spine instability and morbidities. Wide resections have a lower recurrence rate. A radical resection is the removal of an entire organ along with the blood and lymph supply to the organ and is almost always impossible in the spine.[90]

Decompression

Metastatic tumors of the spine cause more spinal cord compression than primary benign and malignant tumors. Spinal metastasis is seen in 70% of cancer patients, and up to 10% of cancer patients develop metastatic cord compression.[91] Spinal cord compression may result from one of four types of processes: (1) direct compression from an enlarging soft tissue mass, (2) pressure due to fracture and retropulsion of bony fragments into the canal, (3) severe kyphosis after vertebral collapse, and (4) pressure due to intradural metastases. The most common cause of cord compression is mechanical pressure from the tumor tissue or bone extruded from the collapsing vertebral body.

Primary tumor compression is often effectively addressed during resection of the tumor by decompression techniques. Spinal cord decompression can provide dramatic improvement in neurologic function, even in advanced states. Decompression can be achieved through radiation therapy, surgical decompression or, occasionally, serial arterial embolization.

Radiation therapy alone can be used to treat spinal cord impingement, especially for spinal metastatic tumors. Studies have reported positive neurologic outcomes and retained ambulatory status in patients who underwent radiation therapy after surgical decompression compared with radiation therapy alone.[92,93] Recent advancements such as stereotactic radiosurgery have been effective in treating radioresistant solid spinal metastatic tumors.[94] One prospective study demonstrated the safety and effectiveness of spinal stereotactic radiosurgery as a first-line therapy for spinal metastasis in the absence of significant spinal cord compression.[95]

Surgical decompression is necessary for progressive neurologic deficits. Surgical decompression can be achieved either by dorsal or ventral approaches.[96] Studies reported that neurologic status, ambulatory status, and functional status improved in patients who underwent ventral surgical decompression.[97-100]

Posterior decompression and stabilization for metastatic spinal cord compression in the cervical spine is less likely to improve or maintain motor function compared with metastatic spinal cord compression in the thoracic and lumbar spine after posterior decompression and spine stabilization.[101]

Important factors in determining the prognosis for the neurologic outcome include tumor biology, pretreatment neurologic status, and tumor location within the spinal canal.

Spine Stability

Aggressive tumor resections, aggressive decompression techniques, severe bone destruction by the tumor, and associated pathologic fractures predispose the vertebral column to mechanical instability and the risk of neurologic injury. Planning for tumor surgery should include optimal reconstruction techniques to maintain the stability of the spinal column. The Spine Oncology Study Group created a novel classification to study spinal stability in neoplastic spinal lesions.[102] The spine instability neoplastic score (SINS) created by the group aids in the assessment of spinal stability and the determination of the need for a surgical consult. This classification system is primarily useful with metastatic involvement of the spine compared with primary or benign tumors of the spine. However, the classification system provides a thorough insight into key elements of spinal stability. Surgical treatment of aggressive benign lesions or primary malignant lesions involves resection of a majority of the vertebral body and stabilizing structures. In such cases, surgical treatment involves reconstruction techniques that use expandable biomechanical devices that help restore the sagittal alignment of the patient and anterior column reconstruction. However, stand-alone anterior column reconstruction is considered suboptimal when aggressive resections are contemplated. In most cases anterior column resections are reinforced with posterior instrumentation of the spinal column using various fixation techniques depending on the level of involvement in the spinal column.

Assessment of any potential spinal instability can be achieved by looking at key elements of the SINS classification system. The scoring system grades stability based on six parameters: tumor location within the spinal column (junctional, mobile, rigid, or semirigid part of the spinal column), pain-related response from the mechanical loading and unloading of the spinal column (alleviation of pain on recumbency and reproduction in upright posture), quality of the bone lesion (lytic, mixed, or blastic), radiographic spinal alignment (subluxation, kyphosis/scoliosis versus normal), percentage of vertebral body collapse, and the involvement of posterolateral spinal elements (pars, pedicle, and facet joints). Scores of 0 to 6 denote stability, 7 to 12 denote indeterminate or impending instability, and 13 to 18 denote definite instability of the spinal column.

A minimally invasive spine stabilization technique can be an alternative to conventional open surgery for metastatic spine tumor patients with a short life expectancy.[103]

Summary

Primary and metastatic lesions of the spinal column present a unique challenge to the treating surgeon. The treatment of these complex pathologies requires a team approach and expertise. A thorough clinical evaluation and a high suspicion for a tumor are very important to achieve early detection and better outcomes. Advances in imaging technologies have also promoted early tumor detection and the accurate assessment of tumor extent in spinal tumors, but the treatment of primary malignant tumors continues to pose a challenge to spine surgeons.

Development of newer chemotherapy medications and advancements in radiotherapy delivery mechanisms have also improved survival rates in these patients. Due to the increased survival in these patients, preservation of neurologic function and spinal stability is of utmost importance to maintain the functional independence and dignity of the patient.

Advancements in rehabilitative technologies allow patients with residual deficits to be independent as well. Surgery should be offered to the patients who can tolerate surgery.

Advances in surgical techniques and instrumentation systems have considerably decreased the morbidity of the surgical procedures. These newer techniques also provide correction and prevention of deformity. The widespread use of posterior-only vertebral column resection techniques has negated the need for multistage procedures and the morbidities that came with it. The widespread use of percutaneous fixation techniques as well as robotic- and navigation-guided surgical techniques will further improve the outcomes of tumor surgery and fusion in these patients.

Advances in interventional radiology techniques have allowed preoperative embolization of hypervascular tumors. This has been beneficial for spinal surgeons and has significantly reduced the perioperative morbidity of tumor surgery. With all these advances, vertebrectomy has become a common procedure and has improved the outlook of tumor surgery.

KEY POINTS

1. Spinal surgery, if well planned, properly executed, and combined with contemporary radiotherapy and chemotherapy, can reduce pain, improve neurologic function, greatly enhance survival, and provide greater opportunity for a curative treatment in patients with spinal tumors. Hence it is imperative that physicians recognize the presence of spinal neoplasia with early detection and carefully observe the principles of tumor staging and management.
2. A diagnostic workup should include imaging investigations to study the extent of the tumor as well as its distant spread. Tissue diagnosis is equally important and can be completed with CT-guided biopsy at a facility equipped to perform spine tumor surgery and by a surgeon who will ultimately do the surgical resection.
3. Treatment of primary benign or malignant tumors involving the spinal column is aimed at obtaining a tissue diagnosis, preserving neurologic function, and maintaining or restoring spinal alignment and stability.
4. MRI has become a key imaging tool to define tumor characteristics. It has a superior sensitivity and specificity in defining the extent of the tumor, soft tissue involvement, and extent of canal compromise. MRI is also useful in detecting noncontiguous lesions in metastatic lesions.
5. Tissue diagnosis is of the utmost importance and forms the basis of the treatment algorithm. CT-guided biopsy has become the procedure of choice to obtain tissue samples. The adequacy of the tissue sample should always be verified. A frozen section, taken at the time of biopsy, can help obtain the most diagnostic sample from the tumor. A biopsy should be performed by the surgeon who will perform the final excision. Biopsy needles should not cross any body cavities. The tumor biopsy should be approached in an optimal way.
6. Benign tumors of the spinal column can be treated with resection of the tumor and reconstruction of the spinal column in cases of instability. However, GCTs are locally aggressive tumors and may have an associated large soft tissue mass that rarely metastasizes to the lungs. They are associated with a high local recurrence rate of en bloc resection is not possible due to location. Aggressive surgical resection is important to prevent local recurrence. Patients with a local recurrence have associated poor outcomes. New medical modalities such as serial intravenous denosumab injections show evidence of radiologic and histologic improvement in these patients and may change the current algorithms for treatment of GCTs.
7. Primary malignant tumors are very rare but need an extensive planning and team approach to prevent recurrence. Primary osteogenic sarcomas are associated with aggressive local growth and metastasis. They are most commonly seen in the vertebral body. Secondary osteosarcomas can present in patients with long-standing Paget disease or patients who have had radiation for treatment of benign tumors such as GCTs. A multimodal approach and neoadjuvant chemotherapy have decreased the incidence of local recurrences and have improved the disease-free survival rate.
8. Locally aggressive benign tumors such as GCTs and malignant tumors such as chordomas are associated with a high local recurrence rate. Aggressive local resection with wide margins is of utmost importance. En bloc resection has been shown to decrease the risk of local recurrence and is thought to be curative if a wide marginal resection can be obtained. Local recurrence is associated with poor outcome.
9. Metastatic tumors are the most common type of malignant tumors that affect the spinal column. Tumors that commonly metastasize to the spine include breast, lung, kidney, and prostate tumors. Treatment of the metastatic lesion depends on the overall prognosis of the patient. Radiation therapy is the mainstay of treatment. However, surgical treatment may be necessary in patients who have the potential for spinal instability or neurologic compression.
10. Multiple myeloma is a plasma cell disorder that commonly affects the spinal column. The lesions have a characteristic "punched out" lytic appearance on plain radiographs. The tumors are highly radiosensitive, and radiotherapy can be curative. However, surgical treatment may be needed when there is neurologic compromise or the potential for spinal instability after radiotherapy.
11. Surgical treatment is necessary in spine tumor patients mainly to obtain local control of the lesion. Surgical treatment helps obtain a definitive tissue diagnosis, allows thorough decompression of the neural structure, and helps maintain or restore spinal stability.

12. Neurologic compromise can lead to catastrophic outcomes and warrants prompt treatment. Compromise most commonly results from retropulsed fragments from a pathologic compression fracture or the presence of an epidural mass causing direct compression of the neural structures. Radiotherapy is the initial treatment of choice if the tumor is radiosensitive and the neural progression is gradual; however, surgical treatment may eventually be needed in the presence of potential spinal instability. Surgical treatment is necessary if progression is rapid, if the tumor is known to be radioresistant, and/or the neural compression is caused by retropulsed bone fragments.

KEY REFERENCES

1. Orguc S, Arkun R. Primary tumors of the spine. *Semin Musculoskelet Radiol*. 2014;18(3):280-299.
2. Ropper AE, Cahill KS, Hanna JW, et al. Primary vertebral tumors: a review of epidemiologic, histological, and imaging findings. Part I: benign tumors. *Neurosurgery*. 2011;69(6):1171-1180.
3. Thakur NA, Daniels AH, Schiller J, et al. Benign tumors of the spine. *J Am Acad Orthop Surg*. 2012;20(11):715-724.
4. Boriani S, Bandiera S, Casadel R, et al. Giant cell tumor of the mobile spine: a review of 49 cases. *Spine*. 2012;37(1):E37-E45.
5. Harrop JS, Schmidt MH, Boriani S, et al. Aggressive "benign" primary spine neoplasms: osteoblastoma, aneurysmal bone cyst, and giant cell tumor. *Spine*. 2009;34(22 suppl):S39-S47.
6. Tokuhashi Y, Matsuzaki H, Toriyama S, et al. Scoring system for the preoperative evaluation of metastatic spine tumor prognosis. *Spine*. 1990;15(11):1110-1113.
7. Tokuhashi Y, Matsuzaki H, Oda H, et al. A revised scoring system for preoperative evaluation of metastatic spine tumor prognosis. *Spine*. 2005;30(19):2186-2191.
8. Fisher CG, DiPaola CP, Ryken TC, et al. A novel classification system for spinal instability in neoplastic disease: an evidence-based approach and expert consensus from the Spine Oncology Study Group. *Spine*. 2010;35(22):E1221-E1229.

REFERENCES

1. Ciftdemir M, Kaya M, Selcuk E, et al. Tumors of the spine. *World J Orthop*. 2016;7(2):109-116.
2. Orguc S, Arkun R. Primary tumors of the spine. *Semin Musculoskelet Radiol*. 2014;18(3):280-299.
3. Abdel Razek AA, Castillo M. Imaging appearance of primary bony tumors and pseudo-tumors of the spine. *J Neuroradiol*. 2010;37(1):37-50.
4. Donthineni R. Diagnosis and staging of spine tumors. *Orthop Clin North Am*. 2009;40(1):1-7.
5. Gunay C, Atalar H, Yildiz Y, et al. Spinal osteochondroma: a report on six patients and a review of the literature. *Arch Orthop Trauma Surg*. 2010;130(12):1459-1465.
6. Ishimaru D, Gotoh M, Takayama S, et al. Large-scale mutational analysis in the EXT1 and EXT2 genes for Japanese patients with multiple osteochondromas. *BMC Genet*. 2016;17:52.
7. Albrecht S, Crutchfield JS, SeGall GK. On spinal osteochondromas. *J Neurosurg*. 1992;77(2):247-252.
8. Ashraf A, Larson AN, Ferski G, et al. Spinal stenosis frequent in children with multiple hereditary exostoses. *J Child Orthop*. 2013;7(3):183-194.
9. Roach JW, Klatt JW, Faulkner ND. Involvement of the spine in patients with multiple hereditary exostoses. *J Bone Joint Surg Am*. 2009;91(8):1942-1948.
10. Chin KR, Kharrazi FD, Miller BS, et al. Osteochondromas of the distal aspect of the tibia or fibula. Natural history and treatment. *J Bone Joint Surg Am*. 2000;82(9):1269-1278.
11. Altay M, Bayrakci K, Yildiz Y, et al. Secondary chondrosarcoma in cartilage bone tumors: report of 32 patients. *J Orthop Sci*. 2007;12(5):415-423.
12. Barzin M, Maleki I. Incidence of vertebral hemangioma on spinal magnetic resonance imaging in Northern Iran. *Pak J Biol Sci*. 2009;12(6):542-544.
13. Ropper AE, Cahill KS, Hanna JW, et al. Primary vertebral tumors: a review of epidemiologic, histological, and imaging findings. Part I: benign tumors. *Neurosurgery*. 2011;69(6):1171-1180.
14. Moles A, Hamel O, Perret C, et al. Symptomatic vertebral hemangiomas during pregnancy. *J Neurosurg Spine*. 2014;20(5):585-591.
15. Acosta FL Jr, Sanai N, Chi JH, et al. Comprehensive management of symptomatic and aggressive vertebral hemangiomas. *Neurosurg Clin N Am*. 2008;19(1):17-29.
16. Jayakumar PN, Vasudev MK, Srikanth SG. Symptomatic vertebral haemangioma: endovascular treatment of 12 patients. *Spinal Cord*. 1997;35(9):624-628.
17. Smith TP, Koci T, Mehringer CM, et al. Transarterial embolization of vertebral hemangioma. *J Vasc Interv Radiol*. 1993;4(5):681-685.
18. Hekster RE, Endtz LJ. Spinal-cord compression caused by vertebral haemangioma relieved by percutaneous catheter embolisation: 15 years later. *Neuroradiology*. 1987;29(1):101.
19. Doppman JL, Oldfield EH, Heiss JD. Symptomatic vertebral hemangiomas: treatment by means of direct intralesional injection of ethanol. *Radiology*. 2000;214(2):341-348.
20. Goyal M, Mishra NK, Sharma A, et al. Alcohol ablation of symptomatic vertebral hemangiomas. *AJNR Am J Neuroradiol*. 1999;20(6):1091-1096.
21. Munk PL, Marotta TR. Intralesional injection of absolute alcohol into vertebral hemangiomas: a new treatment option? *AJNR Am J Neuroradiol*. 1999;20(6):959-960.
22. Bas T, Aparisi F, Bas JL. Efficacy and safety of ethanol injections in 18 cases of vertebral hemangioma: a mean follow-up of 2 years. *Spine*. 2001;26(14):1577-1582.
23. Niemeyer T, McClellan J, Webb J, et al. Brown-Sequard syndrome after management of vertebral hemangioma with intralesional alcohol. A case report. *Spine*. 1999;24(17):1845-1847.
24. Miszczyk L, Tukiendorf A. Radiotherapy of painful vertebral hemangiomas: the single center retrospective analysis of 137 cases. *Int J Radiat Oncol Biol Phys*. 2012;82(2):e173-e180.
25. Guarnieri G, Ambrosanio G, Vassallo P, et al. Vertebroplasty as treatment of aggressive and symptomatic vertebral hemangiomas: up to 4 years of follow-up. *Neuroradiology*. 2009;51(7):471-476.
26. Yu B, Wu D, Shen B, et al. Noncontiguous lumbar vertebral hemangiomas treated by posterior decompression, intraoperative kyphoplasty, and segmental fixation. *J Neurosurg Spine*. 2014;20(1):60-66.
27. Moore JM, Poonnoose S, McDonald M. Kyphoplasty as a useful technique for complicated haemangiomas. *J Clin Neurosci*. 2012;19(9):1291-1293.
28. Asumu TO, Williamson B, Hughes DG. Symptomatic spinal hemangiomas in association with cutaneous hemangiomas. A case report. *Spine*. 1996;21(9):1082-1084.
29. Raco A, Ciappetta P, Artico M, et al. Vertebral hemangiomas with cord compression: the role of embolization in five cases. *Surg Neurol*. 1990;34(3):164-168.

30. Chi JH, Manley GT, Chou D. Pregnancy-related vertebral hemangioma. Case report, review of the literature, and management algorithm. *Neurosurg Focus*. 2005;19(3):E7.
31. Garg S, Mehta S, Dormans JP. Langerhans cell histiocytosis of the spine in children. Long-term follow-up. *J Bone Joint Surg Am*. 2004;86-A(8):1740-1750.
32. Schajowicz F, Slullitel J. Eosinophilic granuloma of bone and its relationship to Hand-Schuller-Christian and Letterer-Siwe syndromes. *J Bone Joint Surg Br*. 1973;55(3):545-565.
33. Huang WD, Yang XH, Wu ZP, et al. Langerhans cell histiocytosis of spine: a comparative study of clinical, imaging features, and diagnosis in children, adolescents, and adults. *Spine J*. 2013;13(9):1108-1117.
34. Weber MA, Sprengel SD, Omlor GW, et al. Clinical long-term outcome, technical success, and cost analysis of radiofrequency ablation for the treatment of osteoblastomas and spinal osteoid osteomas in comparison to open surgical resection. *Skeletal Radiol*. 2015;44(7):981-993.
35. Vanderschueren GM, Obermann WR, Dijkstra SP, et al. Radiofrequency ablation of spinal osteoid osteoma: clinical outcome. *Spine*. 2009;34(9):901-904.
36. Tsoumakidou G, Thenint MA, Garnon J, et al. Percutaneous image-guided laser photocoagulation of spinal osteoid osteoma: a single-institution series. *Radiology*. 2016;278(3):936-943.
37. Hadjipavlou AG, Tzermiadianos MN, Kakavelakis KN, et al. Percutaneous core excision and radiofrequency thermo-coagulation for the ablation of osteoid osteoma of the spine. *Eur Spine J*. 2009;18(3):345-351.
38. Rybak LD, Gangi A, Buy X, et al. Thermal ablation of spinal osteoid osteomas close to neural elements: technical considerations. *AJR Am J Roentgenol*. 2010;195(4):W293-W298.
39. Bitsch RG, Rupp R, Bernd L, et al. Osteoid osteoma in an ex vivo animal model: temperature changes in surrounding soft tissue during CT-guided radiofrequency ablation. *Radiology*. 2006;238(1):107-112.
40. Thakur NA, Daniels AH, Schiller J, et al. Benign tumors of the spine. *J Am Acad Orthop Surg*. 2012;20(11):715-724.
41. Maharajan K, Hallinan JT, Sitoula P, et al. Unusual presentation of osteoblastoma as vertebra plana - a case report and review of literature. *Spine J*. 2017;17(1):e1-e5.
42. Dorfman HD, Weiss SW. Borderline osteoblastic tumors: problems in the differential diagnosis of aggressive osteoblastoma and low-grade osteosarcoma. *Semin Diagn Pathol*. 1984;1(3):215-234.
43. Kroon HM, Schurmans J. Osteoblastoma: clinical and radiologic findings in 98 new cases. *Radiology*. 1990;175(3):783-790.
44. Berry M, Mankin H, Gebhardt M, et al. Osteoblastoma: a 30-year study of 99 cases. *J Surg Oncol*. 2008;98(3):179-183.
45. McLeod RA, Dahlin DC, Beabout JW. The spectrum of osteoblastoma. *AJR Am J Roentgenol*. 1976;126(2):321-325.
46. Martin C, McCarthy EF. Giant cell tumor of the sacrum and spine: series of 23 cases and a review of the literature. *Iowa Orthop J*. 2010;30:69-75.
47. Cohen DM, Dahlin DC, Maccarty CS. Vertebral giant-cell tumor and variants. *Cancer*. 1964;17:461-472.
48. Siebenrock KA, Unni KK, Rock MG. Giant-cell tumour of bone metastasising to the lungs. A long-term follow-up. *J Bone Joint Surg Br*. 1998;80(1):43-47.
49. Tubbs WS, Brown LR, Beabout JW, et al. Benign giant-cell tumor of bone with pulmonary metastases: clinical findings and radiologic appearance of metastases in 13 cases. *AJR Am J Roentgenol*. 1992;158(2):331-334.
50. Boriani S, Bandiera S, Casadel R, et al. Giant cell tumor of the mobile spine: a review of 49 cases. *Spine*. 2012;37(1): E37-E45.
51. Pazionis TJ, Alradwan H, Deheshi BM, et al. A systematic review and meta-analysis of en-bloc vs intralesional resection for giant cell tumor of bone of the distal radius. *Open Ortho J*. 2013;7:103-108.
52. Sanjay BK, Sim FH, Unni KK, et al. Giant-cell tumours of the spine. *J Bone Joint Surg Br*. 1993;75(1):148-154.
53. Guo W, Ji T, Tang X, et al. Outcome of conservative surgery for giant cell tumor of the sacrum. *Spine*. 2009;34(10): 1025-1031.
53a. Randall RL. Giant cell tumor of the sacrum. *Neurosurg Focus*. 2003;15(2):E13.
54. Lin PP, Guzel VB, Moura M, et al. Long-term follow-up of patients with giant cell tumor of the sacrum treated with selective arterial embolization. *Cancer*. 2002;95(6): 1317-1325.
55. Lackman RD, Khoury LD, Esmail A, et al. The treatment of sacral giant-cell tumours by serial arterial embolisation. *J Bone Joint Surg Br*. 2002;84(6):873-877.
56. Goldschlager T, Dea N, Boyd M, et al. Giant cell tumors of the spine: has denosumab changed the treatment paradigm? *J Neurosurg Spine*. 2015;22:526-533.
57. Xu SF, Adams B, Yu XC, Xu M. Denosumab and giant cell tumour of bone – a review and future management considerations. *Curr Oncol*. 2013;20:e442-e447.
58. Rodrigo Alves de Carvalho Cavalcante, Romulo Alberto Silva Marques, Yvens Barbosa Fernandes: Spondylectomy for giant cell tumor after denosumab therapy. *Spine*. 2016;41:E178-E182.
59. Harrop JS, Schmidt MH, Boriani S, et al. Aggressive "benign" primary spine neoplasms: osteoblastoma, aneurysmal bone cyst, and giant cell tumor. *Spine*. 2009;34(22 suppl):S39-S47.
60. Giner J, Isla A, Cubedo R, et al. Primary epidural lumbar Ewing sarcoma: case report and review of the literature. *Spine*. 2016;41(6):E375-E378.
61. Venkateswaran L, Rodiriquez-Galindo C, Merchant TE, et al. Primary Ewing tumor of the vertebrae: clinical characteristics, prognostic factors, and outcome. *Med Pediatr Oncol*. 2001; 37(1):30-35.
62. Leeson MC, Smith A, Carter JR, et al. Eosinophilic granuloma of bone in the growing epiphysis. *J Pediatr Orthop*. 1985;5(2):147-150.
63. Adimonye A. A rare and interesting case of a massive secondary spinal chondrosarcoma and review of the literature. *Case Rep Ortho*. 2015;2015:ID 386482.
64. Strike SA, McCarthy EF. Chondrosarcoma of the spine: a series of 16 cases and a review of the literature. *Iowa Orthop J*. 2011;31:154-159.
65. Shives TC, McLeod RA, Unni KK, et al. Chondrosarcoma of the spine. *J Bone Joint Surg Am*. 1989;71(8):1158-1165.
66. Katonis P, Alpantaki K, Michail K, et al. Spinal chondrosarcoma: a review. *Sarcoma*. 2011;2011:ID 378957.
67. Stener B. Total spondylectomy in chondrosarcoma arising from the seventh thoracic vertebra. *J Bone Joint Surg Br*. 1971;53(2):288-295.
68. Boriani S, De Iure F, Bandiera S, et al. Chondrosarcoma of the mobile spine: report on 22 cases. *Spine*. 2000;25(7):804-812.
69. Harwood AR, Krajbich JI, Fornasier VL. Radiotherapy of chondrosarcoma of bone. *Cancer*. 1980;45(11):2769-2777.

70. Schoenfeld AJ, Hornicek FJ, Pedlow FX, et al. Chondrosarcoma of the mobile spine: a review of 21 cases treated at a single center. *Spine*. 2012;37(2):119-126.
71. Schirrmeister H, Buck AK, Bergmann L, et al. Positron emission tomography (PET) for staging of solitary plasmacytoma. *Cancer Biother Radiopharm*. 2003;18(5):841-845.
72. Dudeney S, Lieberman IH, Reinhardt MK, et al. Kyphoplasty in the treatment of osteolytic vertebral compression fractures as a result of multiple myeloma. *J Clin Oncol*. 2002;20(9):2382-2387.
73. White AP, Kwon BK, Lindskog DM, et al. Metastatic disease of the spine. *J Am Acad Orthop Surg*. 2006;14(11):587-598.
74. Sutcliffe P, Connock M, Shyangdan D, et al. A systematic review of evidence on malignant spinal metastases: natural history and technologies for identifying patients at high risk of vertebral fracture and spinal cord compression. *Health Technol Assess*. 2013;17(42):1-274.
75. Tokuhashi Y, Matsuzaki H, Toriyama S, et al. Scoring system for the preoperative evaluation of metastatic spine tumor prognosis. *Spine*. 1990;15(11):1110-1113.
76. Tokuhashi Y, Matsuzaki H, Oda H, et al. A revised scoring system for preoperative evaluation of metastatic spine tumor prognosis. *Spine*. 2005;30(19):2186-2191.
77. Bilsky MH, Lauger I, Fourney DR, et al. Reliability analysis of the epidural spinal cord compression scale. *J Neurosurg Spine*. 2010;13(3):324-328.
78. Boriani S, Weinstein JN, Biagini R. Primary bone tumors of the spine. Terminology and surgical staging. *Spine*. 1997; 22(9):1036-1044.
79. Weinstein JN, McLain RF. Primary tumors of the spine. *Spine*. 1987;12(9):843-851.
80. Nicholls PJ, Jarecky TW. The value of posterior decompression by laminectomy for malignant tumors of the spine. *Clin Orthop Relat Res*. 1985;201:210-213.
81. Bauer HC. Posterior decompression and stabilization for spinal metastases. Analysis of sixty-seven consecutive patients. *J Bone Joint Surg Am*. 1997;79(4):514-522.
82. de Andrade JR, Macnab I. Anterior occipito-cervical fusion using an extra-pharyngeal exposure. *J Bone Joint Surg Am*. 1969;51(8):1621-1626.
83. Salas E, Sekhar LN, Ziyal IM, et al. Variations of the extreme-lateral craniocervical approach: anatomical study and clinical analysis of 69 patients. *J Neurosurg*. 1999;90(2 suppl): 206-219.
84. Southwick WO, Robinson RA. Surgical approaches to the vertebral bodies in the cervical and lumbar regions. *J Bone Joint Surg Am*. 1957;39-A(3):631-644.
85. Harrington KD. Metastatic disease of the spine. *J Bone Joint Surg Am*. 1986;68(7):1110-1115.
86. Harrington KD. Anterior decompression and stabilization of the spine as a treatment for vertebral collapse and spinal cord compression from metastatic malignancy. *Clin Orthop Relat Res*. 1988;233:177-197.
87. Gokaslan ZL, York JE, Walsch Gl, et al. Transthoracic vertebrectomy for metastatic spinal tumors. *J Neurosurg*. 1998;89(4):599-609.
88. Kim MP, Nolan P, Finkelstein JA. Evaluation of 11th rib extrapleural-retroperitoneal approach to the thoracolumbar junction. Technical note. *J Neurosurg*. 2000;93(1 suppl): 168-174.
89. Muhlbauer M, Pfisterer W, Eyb R, et al. Minimally invasive retroperitoneal approach for lumbar corpectomy and anterior reconstruction. Technical note. *J Neurosurg*. 2000;93(1 suppl): 161-167.
90. Yamazaki T, McLoughlin GS, Patel S, et al. Feasibility and safety of en bloc resection for primary spine tumors: a systematic review by the Spine Oncology Study Group. *Spine*. 2009;34(22 suppl):S31-S38.
91. Schmidt MH, Klimo P Jr, Vrionis FD. Metastatic spinal cord compression. *J Natl Compr Canc Netw*. 2005;3(5):711-719.
92. Sundaresan N, Rothman A, Manhardt K, et al. Surgery for solitary metastases of the spine: rationale and results of treatment. *Spine*. 2002;27(16):1802-1806.
93. Patchell RA, Tibbs PA, Regine WF, et al. Direct decompressive surgical resection in the treatment of spinal cord compression caused by metastatic cancer: a randomised trial. *Lancet*. 2005;366(9486):643-648.
94. Moussazadeh N, Laugfer I, Yamada Y, et al. Separation surgery for spinal metastases: effect of spinal radiosurgery on surgical treatment goals. *Cancer Control*. 2014;21(2): 168-174.
95. Garg AK, Shiu AS, Yang J, et al. Phase 1/2 trial of single-session stereotactic body radiotherapy for previously unirradiated spinal metastases. *Cancer*. 2012;118(20): 5069-5077.
96. Hall AJ, Mackay NN. The results of laminectomy for compression of the cord or cauda equina by extradural malignant tumour. *J Bone Joint Surg Br*. 1973;55(3):497-505.
97. Siegal T, Tiqva P, Siegal T. Vertebral body resection for epidural compression by malignant tumors. Results of forty-seven consecutive operative procedures. *J Bone Joint Surg Am*. 1985;67(3):375-382.
98. Kostuik JP, Errico TJ, Gleason TF, et al. Spinal stabilization of vertebral column tumors. *Spine*. 1988;13(3):250-256.
99. Riley LH 3rd, Frassica DA, Kostuik JP, et al. Metastatic disease to the spine: diagnosis and treatment. *Instr Course Lect*. 2000;49:471-477.
100. Onimus MP, Papin P, Gangloff S. Results of surgical treatment of spinal thoracic and lumbar metastases. *Eur Spine J*. 1996; 5(6):407-411.
101. Lei M, Liu Y, Yan L, et al. Posterior decompression and spine stabilization for metastatic spinal cord compression in the cervical spine. A matched pair analysis. *Eur J Surg Oncol*. 2015;41(12):1691-1698.
102. Fisher CG, DiPaola CP, Ryken TC, et al. A novel classification system for spinal instability in neoplastic disease: an evidence-based approach and expert consensus from the Spine Oncology Study Group. *Spine*. 2010;35(22):E1221-E1229.
103. Hikata T, Isogai N, Shiono Y, et al. A retrospective cohort study comparing the safety and efficacy of minimally invasive versus open surgical techniques in the treatment of spinal metastases. *Clin Spine Surg*. 2016. Epub ahead of print.

87 CHAPTER Infections of the Spine

Jason C. Eck
Choll W. Kim
Bradford L. Currier
Frank J. Eismont

Infections of the Spine

Historically, spine infections were devastating diseases with exceedingly high morbidity and mortality rates. With the advent of new diagnostic techniques, multidrug antimicrobial chemotherapy, and improvements in surgical techniques, the prognosis has improved dramatically in recent years. Successful management of spine infections requires a high level of diagnostic acuity to avoid delays in diagnosis, use of appropriate antibiotic therapy as directed by biopsy results, and institution of appropriate surgical intervention when indicated.

There are numerous ways to classify spine infections. The most basic is by the histologic response of the host to the specific organism. Most bacteria cause a pyogenic response, whereas *Mycobacterium,* fungi, *Brucella,* and syphilis induce granulomatous reactions. Infections may be classified by their primary anatomic location—vertebral osteomyelitis, discitis, or epidural abscess. Another way to categorize spine infections is by cause; the main routes of infection are hematogenous, direct inoculation (postoperative and traumatic), and spread from a contiguous source. Finally, age may be the determinant and infections may be classified as occurring in pediatric or adult populations. Each of these classifications has implications with regard to evaluation, treatment, and prognosis.

Historic Perspective

The first recorded descriptions of spine infections were those in the Hippocratic texts on tuberculous spondylitis written between the 4th century BC and the 1st century AD. Sir Percival Pott's description of paralysis in association with tuberculosis of the spine in the 18th century led to the eponym "Pott paraplegia." His frustration with the inadequate treatment options available to him was shared by physicians for another 150 years: "To attend to a distemper from its beginning through a long and painful course, to its last fatal period, without even the hope of being able to do anything which shall be really serviceable, is of all tasks the most unpleasant."[1]

Before the advent of antimicrobial therapy, the treatment of tuberculosis of the spine was based on bed rest, often in a plaster cast, with attention to diet and exposure to fresh air and sunlight. Laminectomy was the mainstay of surgical treatment in the late 1800s and the early part of the 20th century but was later condemned by Seddon and others because it did not address the anterior disease and led to further instability.[2] In 1911, Hibbs[3] and Albee[4] independently described the use of posterior fusion to hasten the recovery. The idea evolved from the demonstration that ankylosis of peripheral joints led to remission of local disease. Unfortunately, posterior fusion did not prevent progressive kyphosis or address the lesion that was causing paralysis, and the technique was later abandoned. The mortality rate for children treated by these various techniques was 40%.[5] In 1894, Menard described a series of patients with Pott paraplegia successfully treated with decompression by costotransversectomy.[6] The technique fell into disfavor because of a high rate of secondary infection; it did not gain acceptance until Girdlestone reintroduced it in 1931 with aseptic technique.[7]

Ito and colleagues[8] described the anterior approach to the lumbar spine in 1934, demonstrating that it provided wider exposure and allowed more radical debridement and fusion. Hodgson and colleagues[9,10] popularized the anterior approach for the management of tuberculosis of the spine and stressed radical excision and strut-graft fusion to prevent kyphosis and late-onset paraplegia.

Antituberculous chemotherapy became available in 1945 and was found to be capable of curing the disease even without surgery.[11–15] Faced with a number of widely divergent regimens for the treatment of the disease, a group of investigators formed the British Medical Research Council Working Party on Tuberculosis of the Spine. This group set out to perform a number of large-scale, controlled prospective trials of treatment methods. These studies, as well as others to be described later, helped to determine the current treatment recommendations for this disease.

The first recorded description of a pyogenic spine infection was by Lannelongue in 1897.[16] Although pyogenic spine infections differ in many ways from tuberculous spondylitis, the surgical treatment of the former has been influenced a great deal by the developments in the management of tuberculosis. The introduction of penicillin and streptomycin revolutionized the treatment of all spine infections. As more powerful antimicrobial agents were developed and combinations and dosages were refined, the relative effectiveness of surgical treatment decreased.

The introduction of needle biopsy of the spine obviated the need for open biopsy in many cases. Greater awareness of spine infections and greater availability of better diagnostic modalities have shortened the delay in diagnosis and have diminished the role of surgery in prevention or treatment of deformity. However, patients with a neurologic deficit and/or progressive deformity are still managed best with surgical debridement and reconstruction. In this area as well, significant advances in surgical techniques, development of specialized implants, and application of biologic adjuncts have significantly improved the treatment outcomes for patients with severe spinal infections.

Pyogenic Infections

Postoperative Wound Infections

See Chapter 99.

Spinal Intradural Infections

See Chapter 91.

Vertebral Osteomyelitis

Epidemiology

Although the incidence of tuberculous spondylitis has decreased dramatically in recent years, the incidence of pyogenic vertebral osteomyelitis appears to have increased.[17,18] Various reports have stated that vertebral osteomyelitis represents 2% to 7% of all cases of osteomyelitis.[19–22] The disease may occur from infancy to old age but has a predilection for the elderly.[17,21,23–32] Approximately one-half of the patients with spine infections are more than 50 years old and two-thirds are male.[31] The mean age is 66 years, but the incidence may be higher in younger patients who are intravenous (IV) drug abusers.[2] There is a median length of stay of 31.5 days with increased mortality associated with elevated C-reactive protein (CRP), advanced age, and a Charlson Comorbidity index greater than 2.[33]

Etiology

Any condition that causes a bacteremia may lead to hematogenous vertebral osteomyelitis. Approximately 50% of cases are thought to seed the vertebral column through arterial or venous conduits at the intervertebral disc or endplates. Another 40% are from direct inoculation, such as after a spine procedure. The remaining cases are from local extension from adjacent areas of infection.[34] The most frequent sources are urinary tract infections and the transient bacteremia caused by genitourinary procedures.[18,24,26,30,35–37] Of 198 cases in the literature in which the probable source of infection was noted, it was the genitourinary tract in 29%, soft tissue infections in 13%, and respiratory tract infections in 11%; 1.5% of the infections occurred in IV drug abusers,[31] but this association is being reported with increasing frequency.[31,38–43] Vertebral osteomyelitis may also be caused by direct inoculation of bacteria into the spine by penetrating wounds, spine surgery, chemonucleolysis, or discography.[31,44–53] The source of infection could not be identified in 37% of cases.[31] Immunocompromised hosts appear to be particularly susceptible to spine infections.[24,31,35,37] In particular, diabetic patients have a high incidence of vertebral osteomyelitis.[18,23,35,54] Those who are human immunodeficiency virus (HIV) positive are also predisposed to develop spinal infections even when IV drug users are eliminated from the study group.[55] In a recent series of 253 patients from the Cleveland area, 33% of infections were acquired in the hospital. In total, 51% of patients had predisposing extravertebral infections with most due to hematogenous spread from urinary tract, skin and subcutaneous tissues, infected vascular access sites, endocarditis, and bursitis of septic arthritis.[56] Kulowski thought that trauma was a predisposing factor in pyogenic vertebral osteomyelitis.[29] More recent studies have not supported that association.[2,30,35] In Sapico and Montgomerie's[31] review of 207 literature cases in which the presence or absence of blunt trauma was discussed, in only 5% was there a history of trauma.

Bacteriology

In 1931, Hatch reviewed the literature and reported that the causative organism was almost exclusively *Staphylococcus aureus*.[57] There has been an increase in the number of gram-negative bacillary infections.[26] In the series from Cleveland, gram-negative bacilli accounted for 23% of infections.[56] From data reported in the postantibiotic era, Sapico and Montgomerie[31] found that 67% of 222 patients were infected with gram-positive aerobic cocci; *S. aureus* constituted 55% of the total. The emergence of tolerant *S. aureus* is a concern, and such strains may become more prevalent with the widespread use of antibiotics.[58] Gram-negative organisms are responsible for approximately 13% of cases. The most frequently isolated gram-negative organisms are *Escherichia coli, Pseudomonas* species, *Haemophilis influenzae*, *Klebsiella pneumoniae*, and *Proteus* species.[59] These are frequently found in association with genitourinary tract infection.[26,35,36,60–62] *Pseudomonas aeruginosa* is frequently isolated from heroin abusers.[38,40,42,63–65] In a review of 67 reported cases, gram-negative aerobic bacilli were isolated in 82% of the cases and *Pseudomonas* was the pathogen in 66%.[42] However, one series included 15 IV drug abusers with pyogenic vertebral osteomyelitis; all 11 with positive cultures were infected with *S. aureus*.[24] Isolating an organism in the blood is most likely when fever is present. In the absence of a fever, bacteremia can be detected in only 21% of patients.[56]

Salmonella osteomyelitis is uncommon. It generally occurs after an acute intestinal infection, but the interval between the gastroenteritis and the onset of osteomyelitis may be quite long[66]; in some cases, no previous infection can be identified.[67] *Salmonella* has a strong tendency to localize in tissues where there is preexisting disease.[66,68] Infection with anaerobic bacteria is unusual and is generally associated with foreign bodies, open fractures, infected wounds, diabetes, or human bites.[31,69]

Infection caused by multiple organisms is encountered in up to 8% of cases.[31,70] Infection with *Haemophilus* species has been reported but is extremely rare in adults.[71,72] Low-virulence organisms, such as diphtheroids and coagulase-negative staphylococci, may cause indolent infections with delayed diagnosis.[73] These organisms may grow slowly; thus, cultures should be held for 10 days before they are considered to be negative. Low-virulence organisms should not be dismissed as contaminants in patients suspected clinically to have vertebral osteomyelitis.[73] In one series of 111 cases of pyogenic vertebral osteomyelitis, low-virulence organisms caused 48% of the infections in the 61 patients who were 60 years of age or older and 55% of the 44 patients who had an impaired immune system.[24]

Pathogenesis/Pathology

Although the nucleus pulposus is an avascular tissue, it is relatively active metabolically.[74] It receives its nutrition via diffusion across the endplates and from blood vessels at the periphery of the anulus fibrosus.[74] In the developing spine, orderly arranged cartilage canals within the endplate contain vascular organs resembling glomeruli.[75,76] Earlier studies suggested that blood vessels penetrate the nucleus pulposus in human fetuses and neonates.[77] However, elegant studies by Whalen and colleagues[76] demonstrated that the nucleus pulposus is always avascular. Coventry and colleagues[78] demonstrated that, after birth, the cartilage endplates become progressively thinner and the vessels within the cartilage canals become obliterated. Some persist up to age 30 years, but by adulthood, most of the vessels within the endplate itself have disappeared.[78]

Wiley and Trueta[79] demonstrated the rich arterial anastomosis within the vertebral body, with end arterioles in the metaphyseal region. Spinal arteries enter the canal through the intervertebral foramen at the level of the disc. Branches ascend and descend, supplying the vertebral bodies above and below. Through their injection studies, Wiley and Trueta demonstrated how bacteria could easily spread hematogenously to the metaphyseal region of adjacent vertebrae. The infection may also start in the metaphyseal region of one vertebra and either spread across the avascular disc by lysosomal destruction of the nucleus pulposus or through vessels anastomosing on the periphery of the anulus fibrosus.[79]

It has been suggested that Batson's plexus may be the route of hematogenous spread of infection. Batson demonstrated, in injection studies, that dye flows into the valveless vertebral venous plexus when pressure is applied to the lower abdominal wall.[80] The distribution of veins within the vertebral body is an arborization of vessels. Minute tributaries draining the metaphyseal region empty into large, valveless, venous channels that drain into the loose plexus lining the canal. Wiley and Trueta demonstrated that it takes considerable force to fill the small metaphyseal vessels in a retrograde fashion compared with the ease of injection of the metaphyseal arterioles; this suggests that the former is an unlikely route of hematogenous seeding.[79]

Once microorganisms lodge in the low-flow vascular arcades in the metaphysis, infection spreads. The disc is destroyed by bacterial enzymes in a manner similar to the destruction of cartilage in septic arthritis. This is in contrast to tuberculous infections (described later), in which the endplates and bone are destroyed, but the disc is frequently better preserved.[81] In children, the cartilage canals allow microorganisms nearly direct access to the disc, which probably explains the clinical differences between spine infections in children and adults. In adults, disc space infection may occur by direct inoculation of the disc as a result of surgery, chemonucleolysis, or discography but is less likely to occur spontaneously.[82,83]

Some authors have suggested that discitis in adults is a separate entity from vertebral osteomyelitis.[28,84] Ghormley and colleagues[84] stressed the benign nature of this variation, but in Kemp and colleagues'[28] series, the disease was quite severe, with a high rate of irreversible paralysis. It is conceivable that adult discs could receive blood directly through persistent vascular channels in the endplate, degenerative defects in the endplate, or vessels anastomosing on the peripheral anulus fibrosus and perhaps gaining access through rents in the anulus. When adult discitis occurs, it appears that hematogenous involvement of the metaphysis is far and away the most common mechanism and, whether the infection begins in the metaphysis and spreads across the disc or vice versa, the clinical manifestations and treatment are the same.

The upper cervical spine has a peculiar blood supply. Parke and colleagues[85] have demonstrated a venous plexus around the odontoid, called the "pharyngeal vertebral vein," which frequently has lymphovenous anastomoses. This venous plexus may be responsible for hematogenous spread to the upper cervical spine.[85,86] Abscesses may drain into the soft tissues surrounding the spine or into the spinal canal itself. In the cervical spine, a retropharyngeal abscess may invade the mediastinum.[29,87] In the thoracic spine, an abscess may be paraspinous or retromediastinal.[29] Infection in the lumbar spine may cause a psoas abscess or, less commonly, an abscess pointing through the Petit triangle.[29] Occasionally, an abscess may create a tract through the greater sciatic foramen and appear in the buttock beneath the piriformis fascia, in the perirectal region, or even in the popliteal fossa.[29] The more virulent organisms may not follow fascial planes and may extend into visceral structures. They also are more likely to produce spinal deformity. An abscess that enters the spinal canal is considered to be an epidural abscess and is discussed later. Infection may cross the dura, causing a subdural or intradural abscess or meningitis.[29,88]

The pathogenesis of neural compromise may be related to direct compression by epidural pus, granulation tissue, or bone and disc from the development of spinal deformity and instability. In addition, the cord or nerve roots may suffer ischemic damage from septic thrombosis or may be damaged by inflammatory infiltration of the dura (Figs. 87.1 and 87.2).[28,29,31]

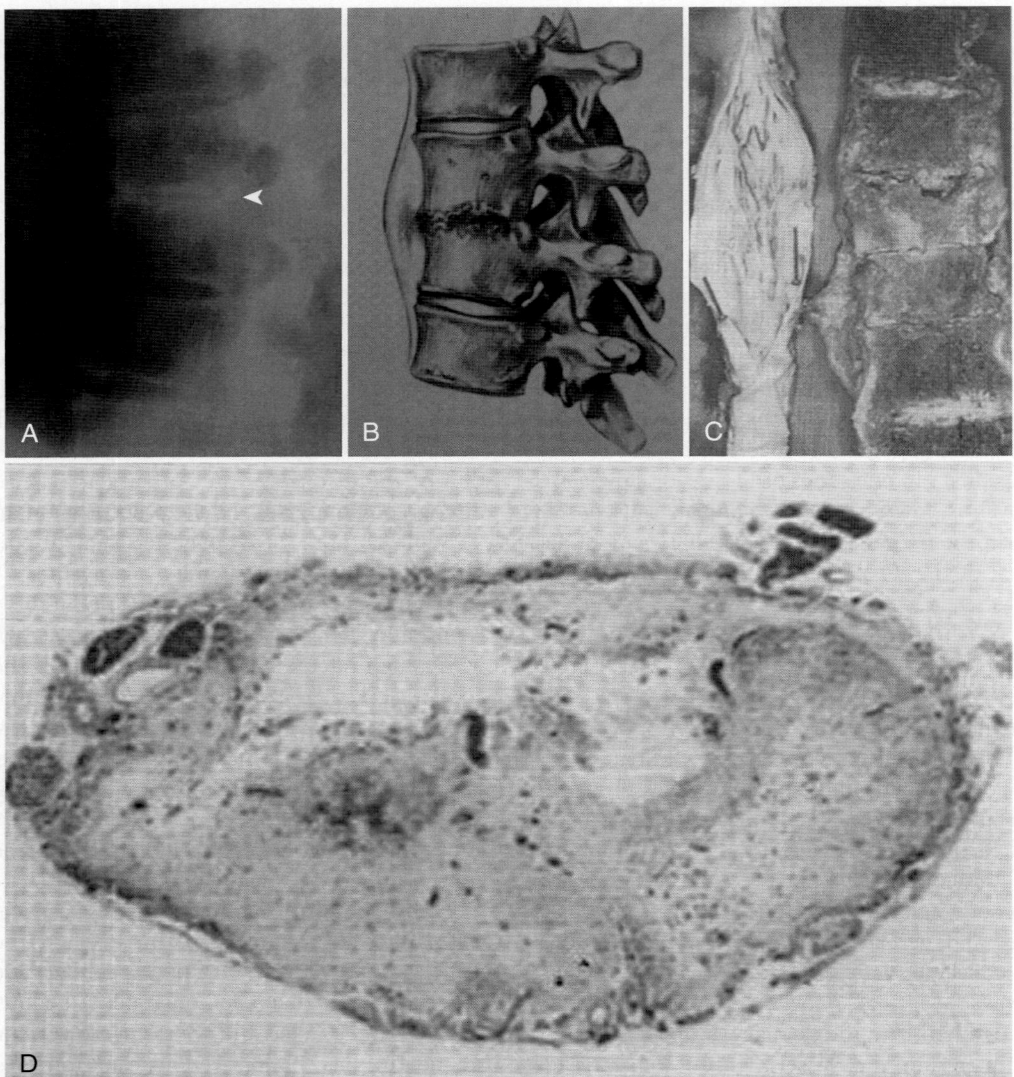

FIG. 87.1 This patient with a T7–T8 disc space infection with associated vertebral osteomyelitis developed progressive paraplegia and died as a result of overwhelming sepsis associated with antibiotic-induced neutropenia. (A) Lateral radiograph showing marked narrowing and sclerosis at the T7–T8 interspace (*arrowhead*). (B) Artist's rendition of the pathology shows the collapse centered at the T7–T8 interspace and associated paraspinal abscess. (C) Two months later, infection spread down to the T9–T10 interspace, with marked narrowing at that level. Gross destruction of the disc can be seen on this gross pathology specimen at the T7–T8, T8–T9, and T9–T10 levels. (D) This microscopic section of the spinal cord has been taken at 11.5 times normal magnification. The dorsal aspect of the spinal cord is at the top of this figure. The patient was completely paraplegic. This is consistent with the changes seen within the spinal cord. (Courtesy Dr. H.H. Bohlman, Cleveland, Ohio.)

An unusual association between vertebral osteomyelitis and compression fractures secondary to osteoporosis has been described. It is theorized that the osteomyelitis may develop as a complication of the fracture because the fracture creates a favorable environment for the hematogenous infection. Alternatively, the osteomyelitis may develop within the central portion of an osteoporotic vertebral body, perhaps because the bone is more hyperemic or because of vascular stasis. Infection may then lead to a pathologic fracture of the vertebra without the usual involvement of the disc space.[89]

Clinical Presentation

The clinical manifestations of spine infection are determined by the virulence of the organism and the resistance of the host. The presentation may be acute, subacute, or chronic.[28,29] Before the antibiotic era, most patients had acute osteomyelitis, and in 68% of the cases the disease was fulminant with severe toxemia.[57] The mortality rate ranged from 25% to 71%.[29,57] A literature review in 1979 found that only 20% of the patients had symptoms for less than 3 weeks before presentation, 30%

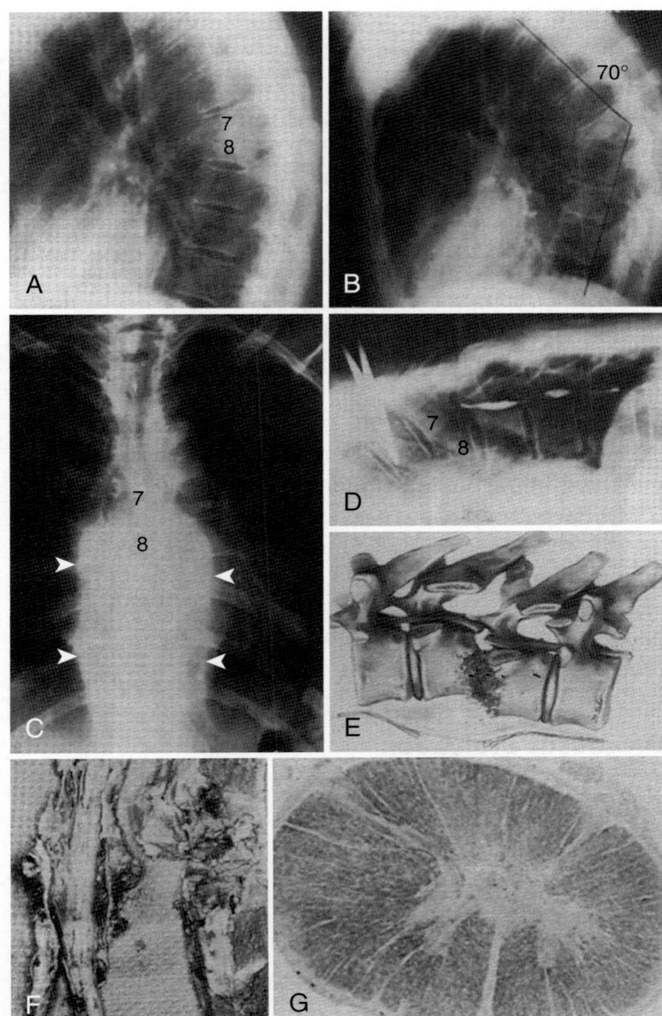

FIG. 87.2 This patient died with thoracic vertebral osteomyelitis secondary to overwhelming meningitis associated with the spine infection. (A) The patient developed a T7–T8 disc space infection with associated vertebral osteomyelitis following a urologic operation with associated postoperative sepsis. He was treated initially with oral antibiotics. (B) One month later, there is an obvious increasing kyphosis secondary to the spine infection. The patient is still being mobilized despite this deformity. (C) This anteroposterior radiograph at the time of transfer to our institution reveals a large paraspinous abscess (*arrowheads*). At this time, the patient had an incomplete paraplegia. (D) This lateral intraoperative radiograph demonstrates gross instability of the thoracic spine with the T7 vertebra 50% retrolisthesed on the T8 vertebra. At this time, the patient still had an incomplete paraplegia. Surgery was undertaken in order to drain the paraspinal abscess. (E) Extent of destruction at the T7–T8 interspace. The retrolisthesis of T7 on T8 is well demonstrated. The paraspinous abscess is also clearly shown. (F) The gross destruction of the anterior vertebral column is well demonstrated in this pathology specimen. (G) This transverse section of the spinal cord has been magnified 11.5 times. Although there are significant changes within the neural tissue, this patient had an incomplete paraplegia at the time of death. (Courtesy Dr. H.H. Bohlman, Cleveland, Ohio.)

had symptoms for 3 weeks to 3 months, and 50% had symptoms for longer than 3 months.[31] Greater awareness of the disease and improved diagnostic modalities (especially magnetic resonance imaging [MRI]) have shortened the delay in diagnosis. In one series reported in 1997, 68 of 111 patients were diagnosed within 28 days of the onset of their symptoms and only 8 patients were diagnosed more than 3 months after their symptoms began.[24] In an urban setting, the infection is discovered within 1 month in only 28% and the median time to diagnosis is 1.8 months.[5] More recently, the mean time from onset of symptoms until diagnosis was 30.2 days in culture-positive cases and 72.2 days in culture-negative cases.[90,91]

Fever is present in only 52% of the patients overall, 85% in culture-positive and 32% of culture-negative patients. Pain in the back or neck is a much more common finding, occurring in approximately 90% of patients.[31,91] Concomitant infections are found in 47% of culture-positive cases and 4% of culture-negative cases.[90] Patients with acute infection commonly present with fever, local spine pain, severe muscle spasm, and limitation of motion of the spine. With lumbar spine involvement, there may be a positive straight-leg raise test, reluctance to bear weight, and hip flexion contracture due to psoas irritation. Hamstring tightness and loss of lumbar lordosis may be noted. Torticollis and fever may be the only presenting signs with cervical osteomyelitis.[86,92]

Subacute and chronic infections may be much more insidious, and these patients have a vague history. Pain may be the only symptom, especially with an occult infection by a low-virulence organism.[73] Approximately 15% of the patients have atypical symptoms such as chest pain, abdominal pain, hip pain, radicular symptoms, or meningeal irritation.[18,31,93] These unusual and often vague complaints have led to unnecessary exploratory laparotomies before the diagnosis has been made.[31,93] A significant delay in diagnosis is common with chronic infections.[18,23,25–27,31,94,95]

Vertebral osteomyelitis is more common in the lumbar region. In Sapico and Montgomerie's[31] literature review, in 48% of 294 cases the involvement was lumbar, in 35% thoracic, in 6.5% cervical, and in approximately 5% thoracolumbar and lumbosacral. Vertebral osteomyelitis at noncontiguous levels is uncommon, occurring in approximately 3% (Fig. 87.3).[91] With the advent of antibiotics, significant spine deformity is not as common as it was in the past, but significant kyphosis still may occur.[26,29] Bacterial infection in the vertebral body can lead to increased intraosseous pressures and impede blood flow to the vertebrae and discs, leading to ischemic necrosis and subsequent deformity. Additionally, production of hyaluronidase by certain bacteria can invade the anulus fibrosus and cause proteolytic breakdown and subsequent biomechanical instability and deformity.[96]

Abscesses are not encountered as frequently now as they were before the antibiotic era but should still be sought in the paraspinous region, psoas region, and in remote areas.[29] A tender or pulsatile abdominal mass may be caused by a mycotic aneurysm, a dilatation of the wall of an artery resulting from an infection.[97] In the lumbar spine, abscesses in the psoas muscle are common and help to distinguish spinal infections from other lesions, such as tumors or trauma (Fig. 87.4).

Approximately 17% of the patients present with a neurologic deficit secondary to nerve root or spinal cord involvement.[31] Eismont and colleagues identified several factors that predisposed patients to paralysis, including diabetes,[18,29,54,98] rheumatoid arthritis,[98] increased age,[98,99] and a more cephalad

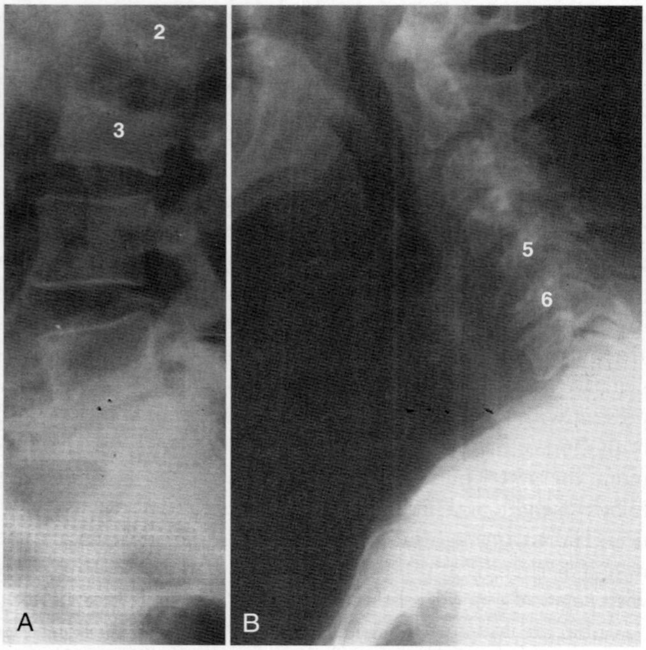

FIG. 87.3 Although uncommon, some patients present with vertebral osteomyelitis at noncontiguous levels. This diabetic patient had an infection of the cervical spine as well as the lumbar spine secondary to *Staphylococcus aureus.* (A) The patient has an obvious disc space infection at L2–L3, with an associated vertebral osteomyelitis. (B) This lateral radiograph of the cervical spine demonstrates a disc space infection at C5–C6 with destruction of the adjacent bone. The patient had a quadriparesis as a result of this infection.

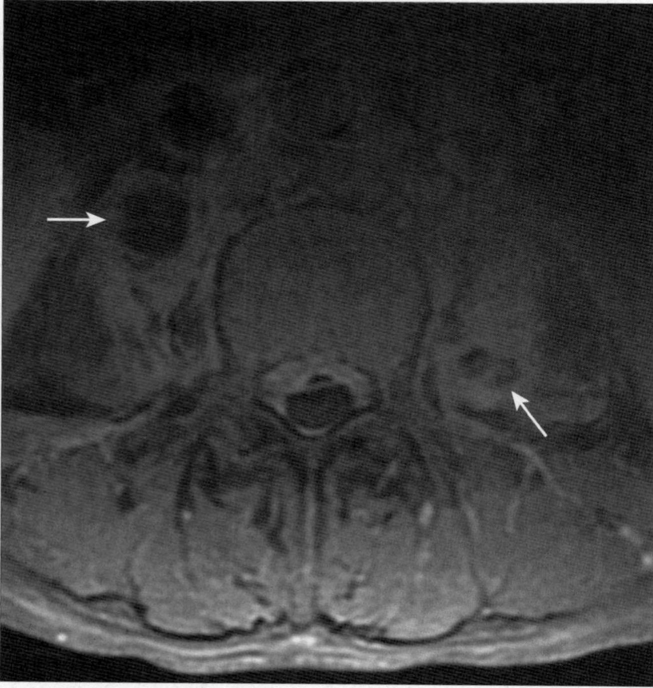

FIG. 87.4 T1-weighted contrast-enhanced magnetic resonance axial image through lumbar spine. Increased signal intensity can be seen diffusely in the psoas muscle bilaterally with low signal intensity abscess pockets (*arrows*).

level of infection.[41,98] Patients on systemic steroid therapy are more likely to be paralyzed, and those infected with *S. aureus* seem to have the most severe degree of paralysis.[98] Some authors have noted that neurologic involvement is uncommon in patients infected with *Pseudomonas.*[63,65]

Infants and IV drug abusers are two subsets of patients who have slightly different presentations. Infants generally present acutely with high temperature, septicemia, and generalized signs of systemic illness.[99,100] The radiographic findings of vertebral osteomyelitis in infants is striking, with almost complete dissolution of the involved vertebral bodies and nearly normal adjacent endplates. The late radiographic appearance may be identical to that of congenital kyphosis (Fig. 87.5). Heroin abusers also present earlier than most patients. In a review of the literature, 81% of heroin abusers presented within 3 months after the onset of their symptoms, compared with 50% in the general population with vertebral osteomyelitis.[31,42,99,100] The authors postulated that the earlier presentation may be related to infection with more virulent organisms or the fact that their patients have less tolerance to pain or may be using their back pain as an excuse to receive more narcotics (Fig. 87.6).[42]

Diagnostic Evaluation

Laboratory Evaluation

The erythrocyte sedimentation rate (ESR) and Gram stain and culture are commonly used laboratory tests in the diagnosis of pyogenic spine infections.[25,31,35,82] The leukocyte count is increased on presentation in only 42% of cases and is usually normal in patients with chronic disease.[31,35,82] Conversely, the sedimentation rate was increased in 92% of 184 patients reported in the literature.[31] It is a nonspecific test, however, and the rate may be increased in pregnancy, malignancy, other infections, dysproteinemias, and connective tissue diseases. In addition, it is influenced by serum levels of fibrinogen and globulin.[31] The sedimentation rate may be normal in occult infections with low-virulence organisms.[73]

CRP has been shown to be helpful in the diagnosis of postoperative discitis[101] and has supplanted ESR as the laboratory study of choice for assessing the presence of infection. CRP was discovered in 1930 by Tillett and Francis in their studies of pneumonia. This acute-phase protein is a 187 amino peptide that can precipitate the C-fraction polysaccharide from *Streptococcus pneumoniae.*[102] With the onset of an infection or other inflammatory process, the CRP level increases within 4 to 6 hours, doubling every 8 hours and peaking at about 36 to 50 hours.[102] The half-life of CRP is 24 to 48 hours. The degree of increase can be up to 10,000-fold higher than normal, while ESR increases only 10- to 100-fold.[103] The ESR begins to increase only several days after onset of infection and peaks at 7 to 8 days.[102] An additional limitation of the ESR is the long period of recovery. The ESR has been useful in follow-up to assess the response to treatment.[17,25,26,28,31,104,105] In one small series, the sedimentation rate decreased to at least two-thirds of the original value at the completion of successful antibiotic therapy in all patients and decreased to half of the

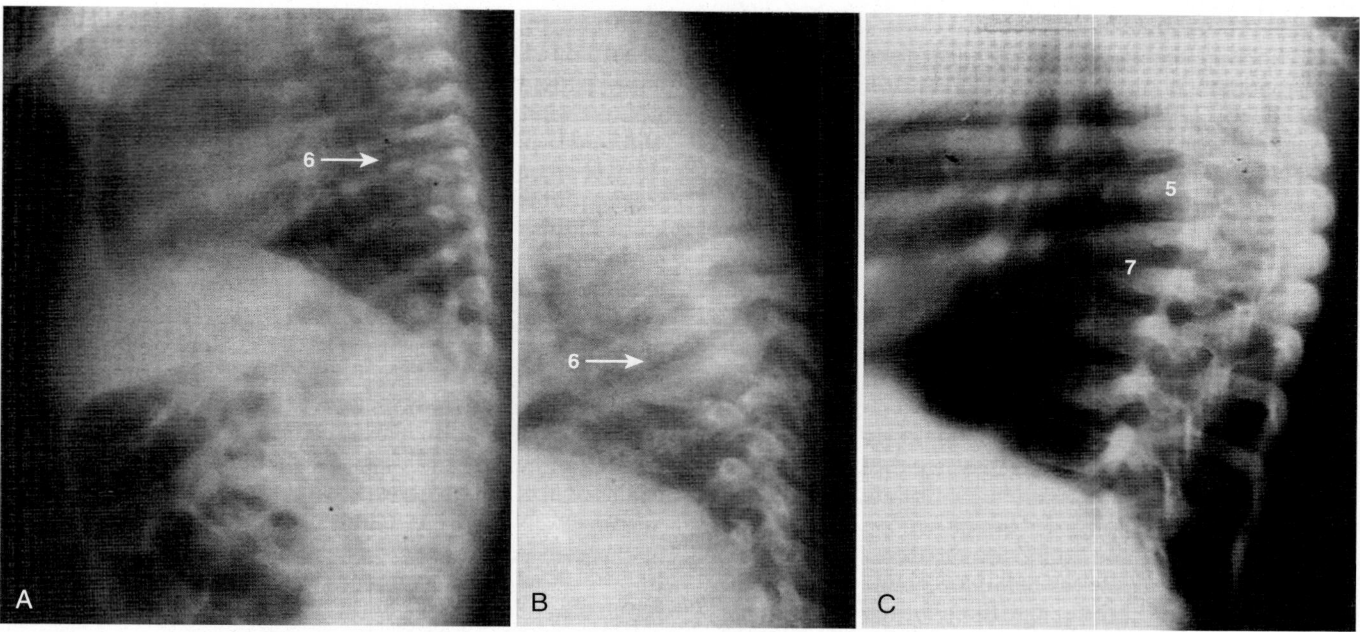

FIG. 87.5 This infant developed a vertebral osteomyelitis and life-threatening sepsis. Unlike the relatively benign disc space infection of childhood, this infection of infancy follows a much more destructive course. (A) At the time that the infant became septic, the T6 vertebral body could be clearly visualized (*arrow*). (B) Two months later, despite aggressive antibiotic treatment, there is gross destruction of the T6 vertebral body (*arrow*). (C) This lateral radiograph taken 2.5 years after the spine infection reveals that the patient has a kyphotic deformity from T5 to T7. This deformity behaves much like an anterior failure of formation of the T6 vertebral body. (From Eismont FJ, Bohlman HH, Soni PL, et al. Vertebral osteomyelitis in infants. *J Bone Joint Surg Br.* 1982;64[1]:32–35.)

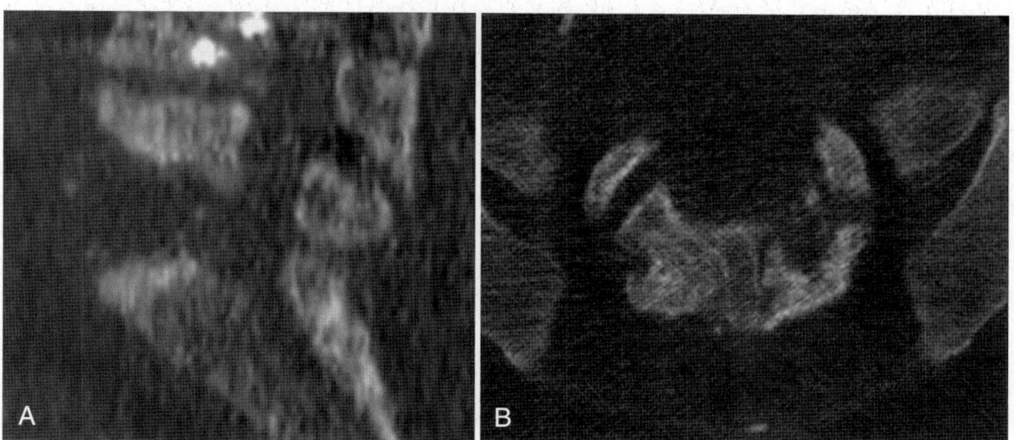

FIG. 87.6 Computed tomography scan with (A) sagittal and (B) axial images of the lumbar spine of an active intravenous drug abuser. Severe destruction of L5 can be seen. The patient presented with severe back pain, bilateral dorsiflexor weakness, and fever. The L5 vertebral body and the inferior portion of L4 have been destroyed by infection. Cultures revealed *Staphylococcus aureus.*

original value in the majority.[31] In another series of 30 cases, the sedimentation rate returned to normal after resolution of the infection.[25] However, the ESR remains elevated for more than 3 weeks after infection.[106] The CRP, in contrast, decreases more rapidly and returns to normal levels in 10 days. In cardiac patients, elevated preoperative CRP increases the risk of postoperative infectious complications.[107] Similar to the ESR, the CRP unfortunately suffers from low specificity because any infectious or inflammatory process will elevate these values.[108] After routine spinal surgery, the CRP returns to normal in 5 to 14 days, whereas the ESR takes 21 to 42 days to return to normal.[109] Thus, an abnormal increase in CRP 1 to 2 weeks after spinal surgery may represent onset of postoperative infection. In all cases, a blood culture should be obtained because it remains a convenient, readily accessible means of identifying an organism. Blood cultures may only be positive in about 30% of cases.[91] In most cases, the identification of the offending organism correlates well with biopsy results.

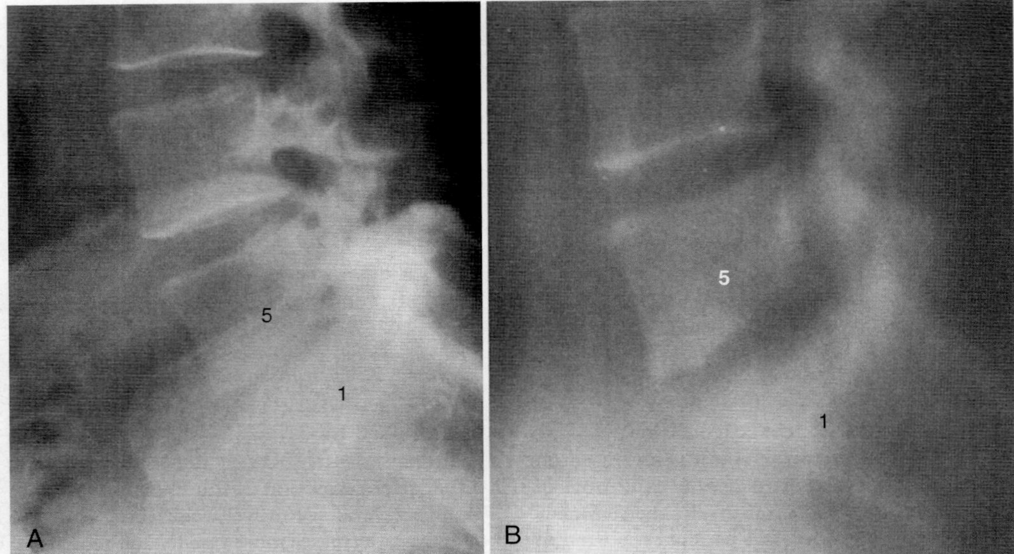

FIG. 87.7 This patient presented with an idiopathic disc space infection at L5–S1 with an associated vertebral osteomyelitis. His main complaint was low back pain. (A) This lateral radiograph demonstrates marked narrowing of the disc space at L5–S1; however, nothing is seen on this radiograph that would clearly demonstrate this to be a spine infection. (B) This lateral tomogram better demonstrates the destruction of the endplates at L5–S1 and the rarefaction of the adjacent bone. The only diagnosis consistent with these findings is a disc space infection with associated vertebral osteomyelitis.

In a study of 29 cases of pyogenic spondylitis, O'Daly and colleagues[110] found a 100% correlation between blood cultures and vertebral cultures when both were positive. In patients who are medically stable, antibiotics should be helpful until a biopsy can be obtained since the yield decreases from 80% to 48% in patients receiving antibiotic treatment.[111]

Imaging Studies

The findings on plain radiographs are characteristic but do not appear for at least 2 to 4 weeks.[25,30,32,35,61,81] The earliest and most constant radiographic finding, narrowing of the disc space, is present in 74% of patients at presentation.[31] Other findings include endplate destruction, osteolysis, and vertebral collapse. Plain radiographs also provide valuable information regarding alignment and mechanical stability.[112] Tomograms show abnormalities earlier than plain radiographs (Fig. 87.7) and may show local osteopenia of the endplates at 10 to 14 days, but tomography has largely been supplanted by computed tomography (CT).[35] Widening of the retropharyngeal space in the cervical spine, enlargement of the paravertebral shadow in the thoracic spine, or changes in the psoas shadow in the lumbar spine may indicate either abscess or granulation tissue surrounding the infection. After 3 to 6 weeks, destructive changes in the body can be noted, usually beginning as a lytic area in the anterior aspect of the body adjacent to the disc and diffusely in the endplate.

Reactive bone formation and sclerosis are present in 11% of patients on presentation; most patients will have sclerosis when the disease heals.[31] Depending on the virulence of the organism and the response to treatment, progressive bony destruction, collapse, and kyphosis may develop. The radiographic findings generally lag behind the clinical response by 1 to 2 months. With healing, new bone formation and hypertrophic changes at the vertebral margins eventually may produce spontaneous fusion. Fusion occurs in just over 50% of the cases[31,113] but may take up to 5 years.[114] If a solid fusion does not occur, a fibrous ankylosis may be achieved.[26,113]

Although the radiographic findings are characteristic, they are not specific; a definite diagnosis is possible only by biopsy.[113] An unusual radiographic finding that may help with the diagnosis is gas in the disc space; this may represent infection with a gas-forming organism (Fig. 87.8).[70] However, the most common cause of gas in the disc space in adults is due to degenerative disease.

An atypical presentation of vertebral osteomyelitis was reported by McHenry and colleagues.[89] They described a series of six patients with osteomyelitis in an osteoporotic vertebral compression fracture. The vertebral endplates were intact on the initial plain radiographs.[89] This presentation occurred in 13% of all hospitalized patients with vertebral osteomyelitis and 2.4% of inpatients with osteoporotic compression fractures at one institution over a 5-year period.[115] Chest radiographs may reveal atelectasis, pleural effusion, and soft tissue masses that may be confused with a tumor.[94]

Radionuclide studies are useful for early detection and localization of infection before plain films become positive.[26,28,32,95,105,116-118] Clinical studies have suggested that gallium scans become positive before technetium scans do,[116] which has been confirmed in experimental studies.[119] Technetium scans show increased uptake diffusely in the region of the infection, whereas gallium scans may show increased uptake in a butterfly area around the infected spine.[120] Gallium scanning has been found to have a sensitivity of 89%, a specificity

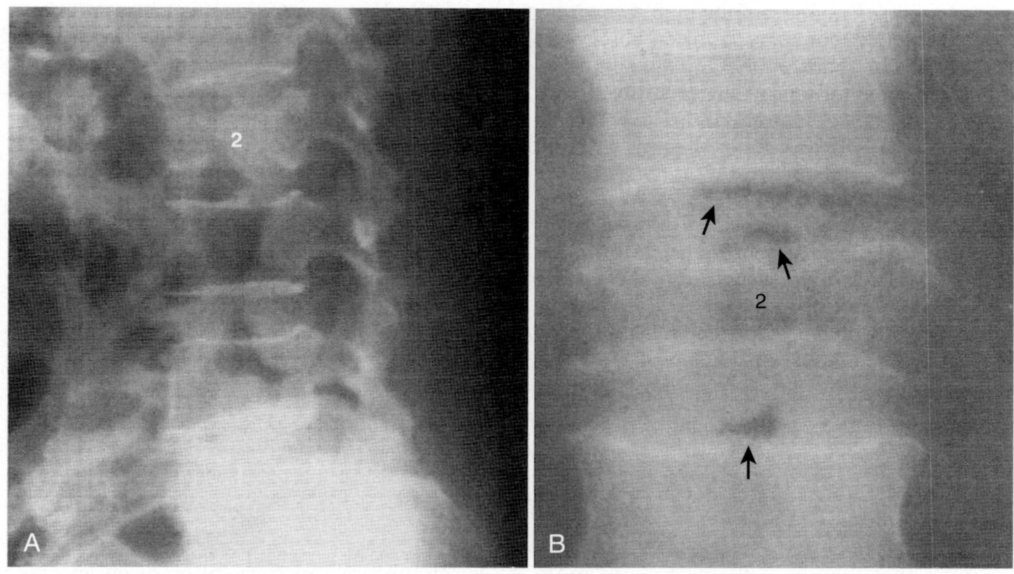

FIG. 87.8 This patient presented with a significant paraparesis and associated sepsis. (A) This lateral radiograph demonstrates marked diminution in the height of the L2 vertebral body. It is surprising that the disc heights at L1–L2 and L2–L3 appear to be relatively normal. (B) Tomograms of the lumbar spine reveal gas shadows (*arrows*) within the disc spaces at L1–L2 and L2–L3. At the time of surgical debridement, *Escherichia coli* was cultured.

of 85%, and an accuracy of 86% in the diagnosis of disc space infections.[116] In a separate study,[117] technetium scans were found to have a sensitivity of 90%, a specificity of 78%, and an accuracy of 86%. The accuracy of combined technetium and gallium scans was 94%.[117] These two scans combined are currently our preferred nuclear medicine studies.

In experimental disc space infection, bone scans were positive in 23% at 3 to 5 days, in 29% at 6 to 8 days, and in 71% at 13 to 15 days.[121] The probability of technetium bone scans becoming abnormal increases with the duration of symptoms, to almost 100%, but false-negative scans have been reported in young children and in the elderly. This has been postulated to be the result of regional ischemia.[73]

The major mechanism of gallium localization is thought to be neutrophil labeling followed by migration to the inflammatory focus. False-negative gallium scans have been reported in leukopenic patients.[118] Both technetium and gallium scans may be negative with occult infection by low-virulence organisms.[73] Two cases have been reported in which the technetium scan was negative but the gallium scan was positive; the authors postulated that this represented pyogenic discitis without vertebral osteomyelitis.[122] Technetium scans remain positive for a long time after resolution of the disease, whereas gallium scans become normal during healing and, therefore, may be useful in following the response to treatment.[123]

Indium-111-labeled leukocyte imaging has been found to be helpful in the evaluation of sepsis in the appendicular skeleton.[124] Unfortunately, it is not sensitive in the spine.[125–127] This may be related to the fact that most cases of vertebral osteomyelitis are chronic by the time the patients are studied, and the inflammatory response may have fewer leukocytes. The overall sensitivity of indium scanning for infections of the spine is 17%, the specificity is 100%, and the accuracy is only 31%.[126] A correlation was found between prior antibiotic therapy and false-negative indium scans and photon-deficient indium uptake.[126] Photon-deficient lesions may be detected by indium-111-labeled leukocyte imaging in many other conditions, including previous surgery, radiation therapy, or metastatic disease.[128] Palestro and colleagues[129] reported that the specificity was 52% and the sensitivity was 54% when decreased activity was the criteria for osteomyelitis with indium-111 scanning. Single-photon emission computed tomography (SPECT) is a sensitive bone scintigraphic modality for early detection of spondylitis. It is more sensitive than planar scintigraphy and has the advantage of increased contrast resolution and the capability of three-dimensional localization.[130] Scintigraphy with technetium and gallium are now often performed with SPECT. Love and colleagues[131] compared three-phase bone technetium SPECT with gallium SPECT and MRI in 11 patients with spinal infections. Gallium SPECT and MRI were comparable in accuracy and superior to technetium SPECT. Thus, gallium SPECT may be useful in patients in whom MRI is contraindicated or in cases in which the diagnosis is uncertain. A positive technetium SPECT in the setting of a negative gallium scan points toward noninfectious causes of back pain such as degenerative disease or pseudarthrosis.[132]

CT may show cystic changes in the bone as well as soft tissue masses, gas in the soft tissues or within the bone and disc, and, later, lytic destruction of the body.[133–135] The prevertebral soft tissue involvement seen on CT usually completely surrounds the spine anteriorly, and the destruction of the vertebra is generally an osteolytic process around the disc space (see Fig. 87.6). This is in contrast to neoplasms, which are characterized by no or only partial paravertebral soft tissue

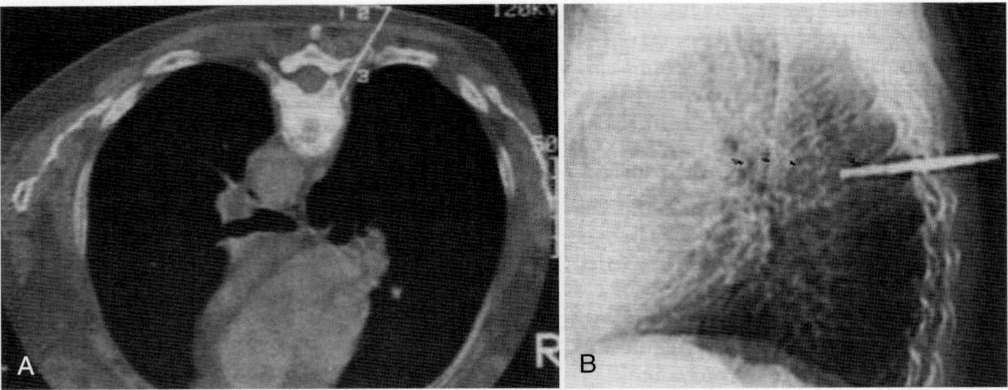

FIG. 87.9 Craig needle biopsy in the thoracic spine. (A) The course of the needle is determined by the measurements obtained on the scout computed tomography (CT) scan. The distance from midline and the angle from the vertical position can be accurately determined. (B) The lateral scout film from the CT scan should be used to determine the exact level to be sampled.

swelling and by changes that may be osteoblastic and more likely to involve the posterior elements than in infection.[136]

CT is valuable in differentiating pyogenic spondylitis from a tuberculous or fungal infection; in the latter, the soft tissue components tend to be more prominent.[137] The finding of disc hypodensity on CT is relatively specific for infection in the lumbar spine but is less useful in the thoracic and cervical region.[135] A relatively unique feature of tuberculous infection is vertebral fragmentation and paraspinal calcifications.[138,139] The destruction tends to extend into the pedicle, which is uncommon in pyogenic infections. CT with contrast medium is helpful to delineate the boundary between abscesses and swollen paravertebral muscles.[133–135] CT after intrathecal administration of a water-soluble, nonionic contrast agent provides exquisite detail of the spinal canal.[137] CT-guided biopsies of the spine have been shown to be safe and can be done at all levels of the spine (Fig. 87.9).[133,140–142] Myelography and postmyelography CT are indicated in cases of neurologic deficit and radicular pain to rule out epidural and subdural abscesses and are always used when an MRI scan is contraindicated. Cerebrospinal fluid (CSF) should also be examined to rule out meningitis whenever the myelogram is done with suspicion of a spine infection.[88]

The imaging modality of choice for the evaluation of spine infections is MRI. MRI permits early diagnosis of infection and recognition of paravertebral or intraspinal abscesses without the risk associated with myelography.[143,144] In a prospective study of 37 patients suspected clinically of having vertebral osteomyelitis, MRI was found to be at least as accurate and as sensitive as gallium and bone scanning combined: MRI had a sensitivity of 96%, a specificity of 93%, and an accuracy of 94%.[117] MRI has the advantage of providing more anatomic information than radionuclide studies and is capable of differentiating degenerative and neoplastic disease from vertebral osteomyelitis.[145] The changes on MRI occur at about the same time as the changes on gallium scans.[117]

Disadvantages of MRI are that it is more sensitive to motion degradation, and there are problems with patient positioning and claustrophobia. MRI has a limited field of view, whereas radionuclide scans can image the entire skeleton. MRI may be falsely negative in cases of epidural abscess without involvement of the adjacent bone because the signal intensity of the inflammatory exudate is similar to that of CSF.[117,146]

The MRI changes in vertebral osteomyelitis are characteristic (Fig. 87.10). On T1-weighted sequences, there is a confluent decreased signal intensity of the vertebral bodies and adjacent disc, making the margin between the two structures indistinct. On T2-weighted sequences, the signal intensity of the vertebral bodies and the involved disc is higher than normal, and there is generally an absence of the intranuclear cleft normally seen within the adult disc.[117,143] The extent of the infection is best seen, however, using gadolinium contrast enhancement. The disc and the involved portions of the vertebral bodies reveal a marked increased signal intensity that delineates the margins of the infection (see Fig. 87.10C).[147] The typical T1 changes in the vertebral body and endplates and the T2 changes in the disc space were seen in 95% of the 37 cases of vertebral osteomyelitis described by Dagirmanjian and colleagues.[148] Only 56% of their cases had typical T2 vertebral body changes. Isointense or decreased signal in the vertebral body on T2-weighted images is consistent with infection if the other typical findings are present. In a more recent study by Ledermann and colleagues,[149] 46 patients with culture or histologic-positive spinal infections were systematically evaluated with gadolinium-enhanced MRI. The most sensitive MRI criterion was the presence of paraspinal or epidural inflammation (97.7% sensitivity), followed by disc enhancement (95.4% sensitivity). Hyperintensity or fluid-equivalent disc signal intensity on T2-weighted MRI was 93.2% sensitive, erosion or destruction of at least one vertebral endplate was 84.1% sensitive, and effacement of the nuclear cleft was 83.3% sensitive. When the infection is confined to a single vertebral body, spread of infection occurs in a subligamentous path.[150] Interestingly, the spread of infection tends to be more commonly in a cephalad direction, affecting the superior disc space more commonly than the inferior disc space. The cause of the signal intensity changes seen in vertebral osteomyelitis is uncertain but is thought to parallel the pathogenesis of the disease. The earliest changes are thought to be related to ischemia and the increased water content of the inflammatory

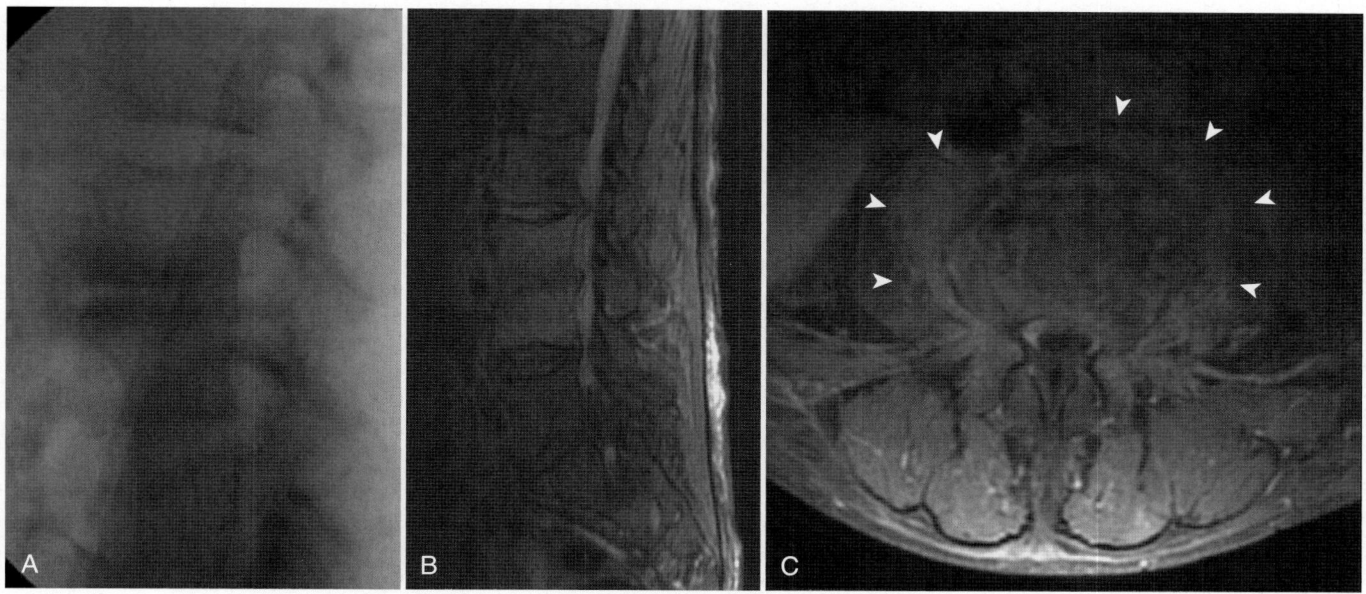

FIG. 87.10 (A) Preoperative imaging studies show L3–L4 disc height loss and irregular endplate sclerosis on lateral radiographs. (B) Contrast-enhanced magnetic resonance image shows involvement of the L2–L3 disc space along with increased signal of the L3 and L4 vertebral bodies. (C) Axial image shows enhancement of the anterior soft tissues (*arrowheads*).

process. As the infection crosses the endplate, a confluent signal intensity occurs on MRI. The normal finding of an intranuclear cleft within adult discs is thought to be related to fibrous tissue within the nucleus pulposus. This cleft is lost at the time of inflammatory involvement of the disc.[117]

In an elegant study comparing MRI findings of pyogenic vertebral osteomyelitis with tuberculous osteomyelitis, Chang and colleagues[151] identified five key distinguishing features that help to differentiate between the two disease entities. A retrospective study of 33 patients with confirmed tuberculous spondylitis were compared with 33 randomly selected patients with known pyogenic osteomyelitis. The key distinguishing features were (1) degree of bone destruction; (2) degree of disc preservation; (3) paraspinal abscess appearance; (4) abscess with postcontrast rim enhancement; and (5) postcontrast enhancement pattern of the vertebral body. As expected, the degree of vertebral body and disc destruction were the two most distinguishing differences found. Most patients in the tuberculous (TB) group (82%) had near-complete destruction of at least one vertebral body, whereas less than one-third (30%) in the pyogenic group had severe vertebral body destruction. Conversely, the disc was preserved in more than one-half (57%) of the TB group, whereas only 3% of the pyogenic group had a preserved disc space. Thus, the credo that TB spondylitis "skips the disc space" is relatively well supported. However, a more accurate distinguishing feature would be better stated that pyogenic vertebral osteomyelitis differs from TB spondylitis by severe disc space destruction with relative preservation of the vertebral body.

Chang and colleagues went on to further show that there were marked differences in the imaging pattern of the vertebral body itself.[151] In the TB group, the enhancement pattern of the vertebral body was always focal and heterogeneous, with rim-enhancing abscesses. In contrast, the enhancement pattern of the vertebral body in the pyogenic group was nearly always (94%) diffuse and homogeneous. A discrete rim enhancement intraosseous abscess was never observed in the pyogenic group. The paraspinal soft tissue imaging patterns provide further distinguishing features. In the TB group, the paraspinal soft tissues revealed well-defined rim-enhancing lesions. In contrast, the pyogenic infections tended to show more diffuse, ill-defined areas of enhancement.

In a comparison of MRI, bone scans, and plain radiographic evaluations in an animal model of disc space infection, MRI was found to have a sensitivity of 93%, a specificity of 97%, and an accuracy of 95%, corresponding well to results of clinical studies in humans.[117,121] The findings are time related. In one study, scans of rabbits made 3 to 5 days after injection of bacteria all showed a decreased signal from the nucleus pulposus on both T1-weighted and short T1-inversion recovery (STIR) sequences. Scans at 6 to 8 days also showed increased signal from the adjacent endplates on the STIR sequence and blurring of the disc margins on the T1 image. Scans at 13 to 18 days showed more florid endplate changes, and in several scans at 21 days there was increased signal from the vertebral endplates and the disc on STIR sequences.[121] The MRI findings slowly return to normal after successful treatment of vertebral osteomyelitis.[117] Gallium scans revert to normal much more rapidly and are better indications of appropriate therapy. Post and colleagues[147] noted that abnormal gadolinium enhancement of the disc, vertebral bodies, and paraspinal soft tissues progressively decreases with successful treatment of the infection. Gillams and colleagues[152,153] described some patients who were improving clinically and had stable or increasing enhancement patterns and concluded that such findings should not be interpreted as treatment failure.

Unfortunately, even MRI may be negative in surgically documented occult infections by low-virulence organisms.[73] Despite the accuracy of MRI, an absolute diagnosis must be based on bacteriologic or microscopic examination of the tissue.[29,154,155] The only situation in which the diagnosis can be made without a tissue biopsy is when a positive blood culture is obtained from a patient with signs and symptoms of spondylitis. Blood cultures are positive in 24% to 59% of patients with pyogenic spine infections.[24,28] Urine cultures are less reliable because patients with vertebral osteomyelitis may have a coexistent urinary tract infection with a different organism.[24,26]

Finally, a transesophageal echocardiogram should be considered to rule out bacterial endocarditis.[156]

Biopsy

Needle biopsy of the spine was first reported by Ball in 1934. In 1956, Craig described a set of instruments designed to increase the percentage of successful closed-needle biopsies, especially in sclerotic or softened bone, discs, or fibrous tissue.[157] Needle biopsies have been shown to be safe in the cervical and thoracic spine as well as in the lumbar spine.[158,159] A definite diagnosis is possible by closed-needle biopsy in 68% to 86% of cases.[31,35,142,159,160] CT-guided closed biopsy of the spine should provide a margin of safety and allow biopsy of the area most likely to yield the diagnosis. In a series of 22 patients with a mass or destructive lesion who underwent this procedure, 17 biopsies provided a definite diagnosis; only one was false negative and in four cases the specimens were insufficient. All areas of the spine were sampled, including one lesion at C2. The patient with the C2 lesion had a transient increase in quadriparesis but returned to baseline, and no other complications were reported.[140]

Closed biopsies of the spine are often false negative in patients who are being treated with antibiotics at the time of the biopsy. If a biopsy is nondiagnostic, it would be reasonable to observe the patient off the antibiotic regimen and repeat the biopsy if the clinical situation allows such a delay. If the second closed biopsy is also nondiagnostic, an open biopsy should be considered. This will provide larger tissue samples and selection of grossly pathologic tissue and should have a lower false-negative rate. In their review of the literature, Sapico and Montgomerie[31] found that 30% of needle biopsy specimens and aspirates were sterile, compared with only 14% of surgical specimens. The technique of transpedicular biopsy allows for larger bony samples to be obtained. The transpedicular approach is safely performed with either fluoroscopy or CT. For general biopsies, including tumor, the accuracy rate is over 92%.[161–163] In the setting of infection, this technique yields better results than traditional needle biopsy. Hadjipavlou and colleagues[164] examined 28 patients with suspected spinal infections diagnosed by a combination of laboratory test, MRI, and scintigraphy. Positive cultures were obtained in 71% of the biopsies.[164]

The differential diagnosis of pyogenic vertebral osteomyelitis includes tuberculosis, fungal infections, metastatic carcinoma, multiple myeloma, localized Scheuermann disease, trauma, degenerative disease, epidural abscess, and fractures associated with osteoporosis.[17,31,89,165] Less common disorders in the differential diagnosis are leukemia, perinephric abscess, neuropathic spinal arthropathy, and sarcoidosis, as well as erosive arthritides in rare cases of facet joint involvement.[30,82,100,166–168] With such a wide variety of diseases that can present with signs and symptoms similar to those of vertebral osteomyelitis, diagnostic acuity is important. As Kulowski said in 1936, "Knowledge of the disease is the primary factor in the diagnosis."[29]

Management

Before the advent of antibiotic therapy, treatment of pyogenic vertebral osteomyelitis involved drainage of abscesses, rest on a frame or plaster bed, and attention to nutrition and general hygiene. The mortality rate with this approach was between 25% and 70%.[29,57] The use of antibiotics has drastically changed the prognosis with this disease, but attention to good general medical care is still a vital part of the treatment. Associated conditions that compromise wound healing or immune response should be managed aggressively. Attention to proper nutrition and the reversal of metabolic deficits and hypoxia are essential. Diabetes and other systemic illnesses should be brought under control.[98] Any underlying focus of infection in the urinary tract, lungs, skin, or elsewhere must be treated concurrently with the spine infection.[169]

The goals of treatment are to establish tissue and bacteriologic diagnoses, prevent or reverse neurologic deficits, relieve pain, establish spinal stability, correct symptomatic spinal deformity, eradicate the infection, and prevent relapses. Biopsy, by either a closed or an open method, is mandatory in any case of spine infection before the institution of antibiotic therapy. The only exceptions to this rule are straightforward cases of pediatric discitis and cases with positive blood cultures in association with strong clinical evidence of spine infection.

Changes in patterns of pathogenic organisms and antimicrobial agents necessitate an accurate bacteriologic diagnosis. If possible, treatment should be withheld until an organism is identified in case a second biopsy is necessary. However, patients who are systemically toxic should be treated with maximal doses of broad-spectrum antibiotics as soon as the biopsy has been completed. Most patients with vertebral osteomyelitis are not septic and will not be harmed by a delay in treatment for several days. Conversely, if the biopsy is nondiagnostic and antibiotic therapy has been started, a second biopsy may not yield the organism. Patients with clinical evidence of vertebral osteomyelitis but negative cultures from open biopsy should be treated with a full course of broad-spectrum antibiotics. When possible, the choice of antibiotics should be based on the culture and sensitivity test results so that more specific and less toxic agents can be used.

Daly and colleagues[170,171] have demonstrated that antibiotic penetration of osteomyelitic bone parallels serum concentrations for all classes of antibiotics. The penetration of antibiotics into inflammatory exudates and the intervertebral disc is less certain.[172–177] Vancomycin, gentamicin, tobramycin, clindamycin, and teicoplanin all penetrate the nucleus pulposus reasonably well.[172,178] The data regarding cephalosporins are inconclusive, but if penetration does occur, it appears to be at a relatively low level.[173,176,177] The penetration of cephalosporins into inflammatory exudates appears to be inversely proportional to the degree of serum protein binding.[174] Riley and colleagues[179] have shown that the penetration and distribution of antibiotics into the nucleus pulposus is significantly influenced by the charge of the antibiotic, with positively charged molecules penetrating the best.

The route of administration of the antibiotics and the duration of therapy are somewhat empiric because little research has been done to clarify these topics. At present, it is recommended that parenteral antibiotic therapy be used in maximal dosage for 6 weeks and followed with an oral course of antibiotics until resolution of the disease. It may be reasonable to switch from parenteral to oral therapy at 4 weeks.[26] Parenteral therapy for less than 4 weeks results in a higher rate of failure.[31] Oral ciprofloxacin therapy has been used successfully in the management of patients with chronic osteomyelitis of the tibia or femur.[180] It is possible that ciprofloxacin and other new agents for oral use may supplant parenteral treatment of vertebral osteomyelitis in the future, but general use of these agents should await evidence of their effectiveness.

The ESR has been found to be a reasonable guide to the response to therapy[17,25,26,28,31,104,105] and can be expected to decrease to one-half to two-thirds of pretherapy levels by the completion of successful treatment.[31] If the sedimentation rate does not decrease with treatment, consideration should be given to a repeat biopsy. CRP is a more useful laboratory test to follow resolution of the infection, as described earlier. However, it is still unclear at what point to discontinue antibiotics on the basis of CRP levels. Further studies are necessary to correlate CRP levels with the duration of antibiotic treatment. Currently, at least 6 weeks of parenteral antibiotics is used empirically. Antibiotic administration must be carefully monitored to avoid toxicity, especially in diabetics and others who might have impaired renal function.[54] Risk factors for failure of conservative treatment include ESR greater than 55 mm/h and CRP greater than 2.75 μg/mL after 4 weeks of IV antibiotic therapy.[181,182]

Patients should be immobilized for pain control and prevention of deformity or neurologic deterioration. The length of time that a patient should rest, the type of orthosis, and the duration of its use all depend on the location of the infection in the spine, the degree of bone destruction and deformity, and the response to treatment. In rare cases, thoracic and thoracolumbar lesions may require bed rest on a RotoRest or similar device if there is undue pain. Rigid bracing with a thoracolumbosacral orthosis (TLSO) suffices in most cases to allow mobilization of the patient. Thoracic and thoracolumbar lesions are more likely to cause deformity and, if neurologic deficits occur, the prognosis is worse with these lesions than with lumbar spine involvement.[26,98]

Cervical and cervicothoracic lesions may be immobilized with a halo device if there is significant instability or deformity. In most cases, external bracing is sufficient and is always better tolerated by the patient. Upper thoracic lesions are best immobilized in a TLSO device with a chin piece; lower thoracic and lumbar lesions should be immobilized in a TLSO device without a chin piece. Frederickson and colleagues[26] found that immobilization was most important in those patients with destruction of greater than 50% of a vertebra and recommended immobilization for the first 3 months. In 5 of their 17 cases, significant deformity developed in the first 6 to 8 weeks, all at the thoracolumbar junction or above. Those patients with the greatest deformity had 50% or more vertebral body destruction at presentation.[116] Most authors recommend bracing for at least 3 to 4 months. Garcia and Grantham[35] recommended that the duration of immobilization should be individualized and based on the response to treatment.

Surgical Treatment

Surgery is indicated in the following circumstances: (1) to obtain a bacteriologic diagnosis when closed biopsy is negative or deemed unsafe; (2) when a clinically significant abscess is present (spiking temperatures and septic course); (3) in cases refractory to prolonged nonoperative treatment, in which the ESR and/or CRP remain high or pain persists; (4) in cases with spinal cord compression causing a neurologic deficit; and (5) in cases with significant deformity or with significant vertebral body destruction, especially in the cervical spine.[98,183,184] Upper cervical osteomyelitis is rare but generally requires fusion because of the associated instability.[86]

In cases of lumbar lesions with root deficits, the final outcome is satisfactory with or without surgical treatment, but patients with spinal cord compression have a better prognosis with surgery.[98] Surgery should be carried out as soon as possible in these cases, but when doubt exists regarding the chances of a reversible spinal cord lesion, decompression should be carried out because recovery has been noted in patients with paralysis who underwent decompression as late as 5 months after the onset of weakness.[98]

In most cases, the spine should be approached anteriorly because this allows direct access to the infected tissues and adequate debridement. Anterior exposure allows stabilization of the spine by bone grafting, which promotes rapid healing without collapse and assists rehabilitation (Fig. 87.11).[98,185–189] Laminectomy without anterior debridement and reconstruction is contraindicated in most cases because it may lead to neurologic deterioration and increased instability.[98,186,190] The situation is similar to that in acute trauma.[191] Laminectomy may be performed in the lumbar spine below the level of the conus provided that there is no psoas abscess or extensive anterior destruction of the bodies that would require debridement.

Anterior approaches to the spine have been described elsewhere[187,192] and are reviewed in Chapters 17, 18, and 19. For lesions in the thoracic or thoracolumbar spine, the transthoracic approach has the advantage of better exposure, allowing more extensive debridement and better decompression of the cord and more effective bone grafting.[185,189,193,194] The disadvantage is the potential increased morbidity after a thoracotomy in the presence of a purulent infection. After debridement of the infected focus, anterior strut grafting can be performed during the same procedure. The graft should extend from healthy bone above to healthy bone below.[185,189,193,194] Autogenous bone

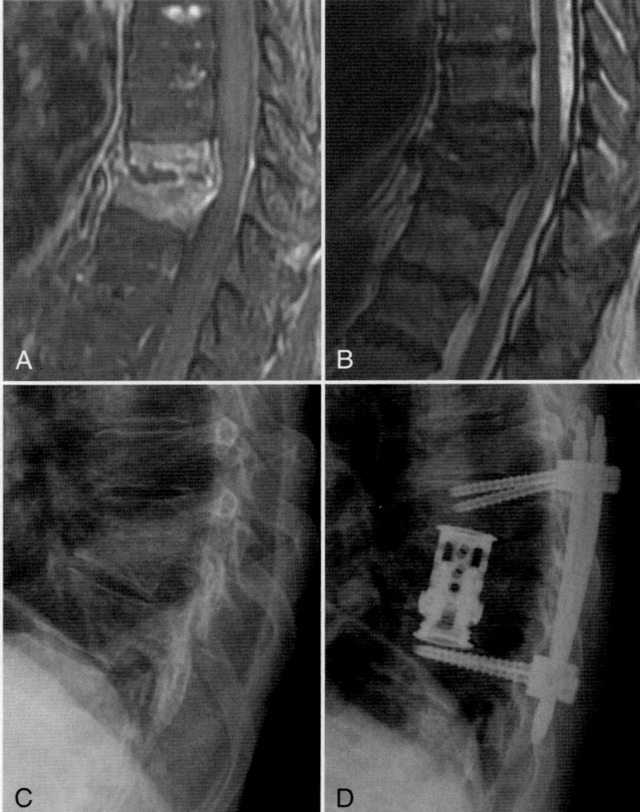

FIG. 87.11 T8–T9 discitis with osteomyelitis. Magnetic resonance imaging showing enhancement with (A) gadolinium and (B) corresponding T2-weighted image showing bony destruction. (C) Preoperative lateral radiograph shows focal kyphosis, which is treated with anterior mini-open direct lateral thoracotomy with T8 and T9 corpectomies and strut fusion with a titanium expandable cage (D). Posterior stabilization was achieved by percutaneous pedicle screw fixation at the same stage.

grafting after vertebral body resection in the presence of active infection was first reported by Wiltberger in 1952 and has since been demonstrated to be safe and effective regardless of the causative organism.[32,195] Grafting with iliac crest is generally better than grafting with rib.[185,188,196] If a good-quality rib is excised in the process of a transthoracic approach, however, it is often adequate as long as a large segment does not need to be spanned and there is no significant kyphotic deformity.[196] Revascularization of a cortical graft may not be complete even after 1 year.[197] Vascularized rib grafts have been used with good success for the stabilization of kyphosis.[198] Louw has reported successful fusions in 95% of cases at 6 months and 100% at 1 year when vascularized rib grafts were used for TB kyphosis.[199] Fibular grafts have been shown to be effective for reconstruction of multiple-level anterior decompressions of the cervical spine[200]; however, the large amount of cortical bone in fibular grafts makes them less ideal in the presence of infection. In cases with significant kyphotic deformity, anterior reconstruction with autogenous bone grafts after debridement should be carried out as a first stage.[185,189,196] Posterior stabilization and fusion can be performed in a second-stage procedure if necessary (see Fig. 87.11D).[185,186,196,197,201] Posterior instrumentation has been shown to be safe and effective after anterior debridement and fusion.[24,202] The use of titanium mesh cages may provide better anterior column support because their structural integrity is not affected by degradative enzymes present in an infected environment.[203] The addition of posterior instrumentation provides even better deformity correction and faster rates of fusion.[203] The addition of posterior instrumentation does not appear to increase the risk of infection.[181,204] The anterior and posterior surgeries can be performed on the same day with good results. Safran and colleagues[205] reported on 10 consecutive patients with lumbar osteomyelitis treated with same-day anterior decompression and strut fusion with posterior instrumented fusion. All 10 patients achieved solid fusion with eradication of infection. Single-stage anterior and posterior surgery has been shown to be safe and effective using titanium implants. Interestingly, bacteria have a lower propensity to adhere to titanium compared with stainless steel.[206–210] Kuklo and colleagues[211] retrospectively reviewed 21 consecutive patients with pyogenic vertebral osteomyelitis treated with anterior and posterior surgery on a single day with titanium mesh cages. Most patients (16 of 21) had a significant reduction of pain. Radiographically, they averaged 12 degrees of improvement in segmental kyphosis (preoperatively 11.5 degrees to 0.8 degrees postoperatively) with an average of 2.2-mm cage settling (range, 0–5 mm) on latest follow-up. There were no instrumentation failures, signs of chronic infection, or rejection, but two patients required a second surgery during the same admission for persistent wound drainage at the posterior wound. Both patients were successfully treated with irrigation and debridement. These findings are supported by previous studies showing the safety and efficacy of single-stage surgical debridement and reconstruction.[205,212,213]

In the past, cervical spine vertebral osteomyelitis was managed effectively without bone grafting by drainage, antibiotics, and skull traction for 6 to 12 weeks.[41] Prolonged hospitalization can be avoided by debridement, bone grafting, halo immobilization, and outpatient antibiotics. Posterior stabilization performed as a second stage may be reasonable in order to avoid a halo. Today, most cervical spine infections refractory to nonoperative treatment are treated with anterior plate fixation at the time of debridement and strut grafting.[214]

When vertebral osteomyelitis occurs in a patient who has undergone a surgical procedure on the spine or sustained a penetrating trauma of the spine, a fistula should be suspected. Depending on the level of the spine infection, the appropriate imaging study (barium swallow or gastrointestinal series) or endoscopic examination should be ordered to rule out a fistula. If a fistula is identified, it must be repaired along with treatment of the spine infection (Fig. 87.12).

Costotransversectomy or the slightly more extensive lateral rachiotomy described by Capener is recommended when a spine biopsy or minimal decompression with limited grafting is necessary or when gross purulence is expected.[215] This approach is being used more frequently with the advent of improved spinal reconstruction devices, such as expandable cages. Lu and colleagues[216] reported on 36 patients with known vertebral osteomyelitis treated with anterior debridement and reconstruction with an expandable titanium cage. In four of

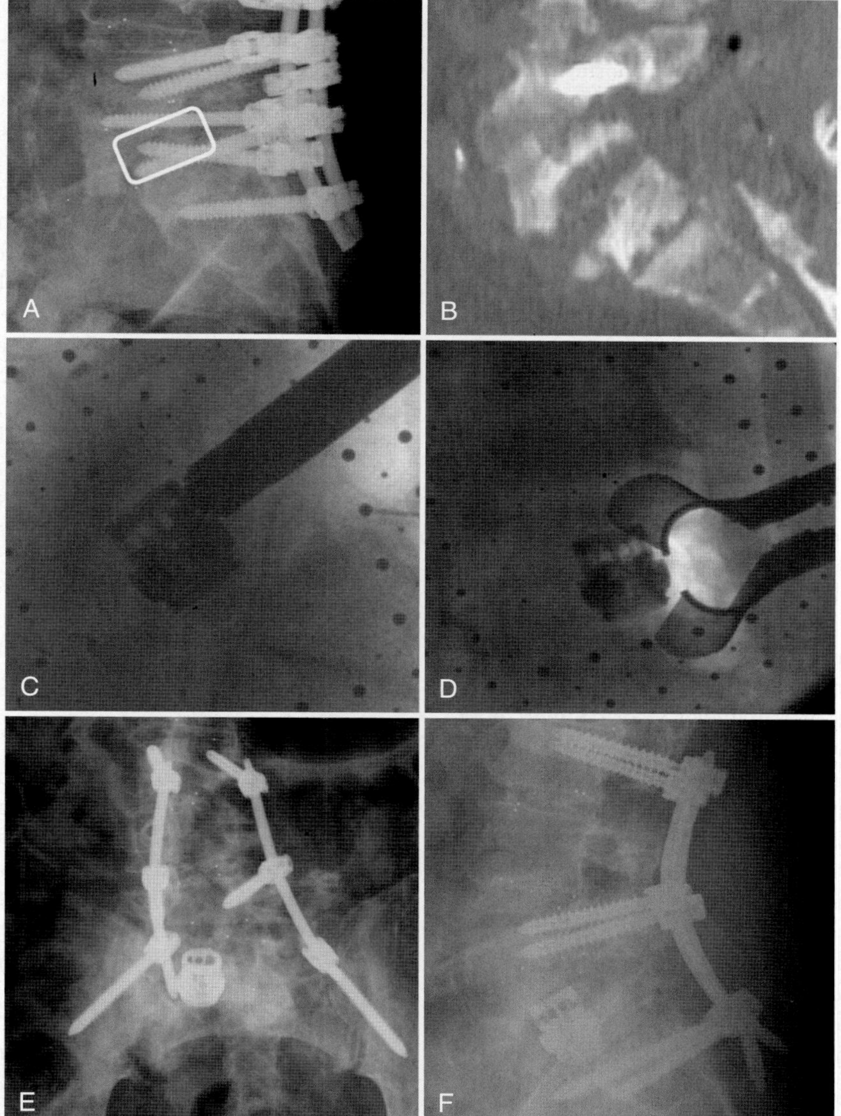

FIG. 87.12 (A) Mini-open posterior transpedicular corpectomy and reconstruction of L5 vertebral osteomyelitis. Preoperative radiograph of a 57-year-old man with a history of multiple previous operations and progressively worsening back pain showing destruction of the L5 vertebral body. The white square outlines the expected location of L5. (B) Sagittal computed tomography image shows complete destruction of L5 and partial destruction of L4 and S1. A posterior, mini-open corpectomy was performed through a paramedian approach with insertion of an expandable titanium cage. (C) Anteroposterior view of the retractor system used. (D) Removal of instrumentation was achieved through separate mini-open approaches using tubular retractors. (E, F) Posterior stabilization was achieved with reinsertion of pedicle screws into L2 and L4 with insertion of iliac screws through the mini-open, paramedian exposure.

those cases, a transpedicular approach was used to perform debridement anteriorly, followed by insertion of an expandable cage from the same posterior exposure. All four patients had an excellent clinical result. The transpedicular approach has several advantages. First, the entire surgery can be completed in a single stage. In the treatment of burst fractures, single-stage surgery leads to shortened total operative time and decreased total blood loss.[217] Mochida and colleagues[218] described the treatment of osteoporotic compression fractures through a transpedicular approach. This strategy is better described in the treatment of metastatic spinal tumors.[219] Senel and colleagues[220] described good results with transpedicular tumor resection in seven patients with spinal metastases from breast, prostate, and thyroid cancer. Similarly, Bilsky and colleagues[221] described 25 patients who underwent posterior-only transpedicular procedures when comorbidities precluded an anterior approach or when the tumor was likely inaccessible entirely from an anterior approach. More recently, this technique has been used by Lee and colleagues[222] for the correction of late traumatic thoracic and thoracolumbar kyphotic spinal deformities in 28 patients. In light of the advantages of single-stage surgery, it appears that anterior-only single-stage surgery may be less advantageous. In the study by Lu and colleagues,[223] there was a difference in terms of postoperative pain among various procedures. Only 60% of the patients who underwent an anterior-only approach reported being pain free as compared with 81% of patients who had anteroposterior surgery and 100% of the patients who had a transpedicular approach. Furthermore, one of two recurrent infections at the site of previous debridement occurred in the anterior-only patient.[216] Historically, much concern for the fate of the hardware has prompted removal of the retained instrumentation once a fusion is obtained. However, in our experience, the need for instrumentation removal due to recurrent infection at the original site of infection is uncommon. Routine removal of retained spinal instrumentation placed for vertebral osteomyelitis is not recommended.

Recent advances in minimally invasive spine (MIS) techniques offer alternative methods of surgical treatment. Staatz and colleagues[223] reported on 21 patients treated with catheters inserted into abscess cavities adjacent to the vertebral body via CT guidance. Two patients went on to surgery; however, the remainder were successfully treated with catheter drainage and parenteral antibiotics. Percutaneous suction-irrigation systems combined with posterior external fixation have also been shown as effective minimally invasive treatment.[224] However, the use of external fixators in the spine has not gained wide acceptance. Percutaneous debridement of the infected disc, such as via automated percutaneous lumbar discectomy[225] or endoscopic discectomy,[226–228] holds promise as a means of hastening antibiotic treatment when infection is identified before significant bony collapse, abscess formation, and deformity develops. Such techniques would be used when antibiotic treatment alone is likely to be insufficient but the infection is not severe enough to warrant major spinal surgery. Korovessis and colleagues[229] showed in a small number of patients that anterior debridement and reconstruction with titanium mesh cages followed by posterior MIS screw fixation led to decreased blood loss and shortened operative time. In a series of 24 consecutive patients, the last 8 cases were treated with posterior fixation and intertransverse fusion using bilateral paramedian intermuscular approaches. Intraoperative blood loss for their initial open posterior surgeries was 540 mL (range, 350–750 mL). With the MIS technique, blood loss averaged only 70 mL (range, 50–100 mL). This difference was statistically significantly ($P < .001$).

The combined use of expandable titanium cages and a minimally invasive posterior transpedicular approach provides another method of surgical treatment. Kim and colleagues[230] have described a unilateral paramedian (Wiltse-type) approach to expose the posterior aspect of the involved vertebral body. A subtotal vertebrectomy can then be performed using the transpedicular technique, followed by insertion of an expandable cage that can be placed in a smaller collapsed form and thereafter expanded to the proper size in situ (see Fig. 87.12). Similarly, the use of MIS direct lateral interbody fusion/extreme lateral interbody fusion (DLIF/XLIF) techniques shows promise for the treatment of frail patients with vertebral osteomyelitis (Fig. 87.13).[230a]

The recent advent and commercialization of bone morphogenetic proteins (BMPs) provides another adjunctive treatment. In both human and animal studies of infected long bone defects, the use of BMP led to improved bone healing in the presence of active infection.[231,232] Several studies in humans show similar efficacy in the treatment of vertebral osteomyelitis. Garfin and colleagues[233] reported on 14 patients treated by anterior reconstruction using structural allograft or titanium cages filled with BMP-2. Despite the presence of active infection, all 14 patients went on to solid fusion and eradication of infection. In 8 of the 14 cases, treatment was successful even when the anterior and posterior surgeries were performed on the same day. Similar results have been reported by other groups. O'Shaughnessy and colleagues[234] reported on the successful treatment of 20 patients with at least 2-year follow-up. Aryan and colleagues[235] showed successful treatment in 15 patients. On the basis of the mechanism of action and histologic studies of BMP in animal models, it is hypothesized that BMP increases vascular ingrowth and recruitment of immunologic cells to the site of infection.[233] BMP has not been proven to be safe or effective in large-scale studies of infection, and its use in this setting would be considered to be a physician-directed (off-label) use by the US Food and Drug Administration.

Prognosis

Relapse of infection is uncommon if antibiotics are administered for more than 28 days.[31,98] Nonoperative treatment has a higher failure rate in patients with an impaired immune system.[24] The mortality rate is less than 5% to 16% depending on the average age and comorbidities of patients in the series. Death is much more likely in the elderly and in those with an underlying disease.[24,31,35,98] In one series, *S. aureus* infection was associated with a higher mortality rate than infection with other pathogens.[24]

Factors that have been found to predispose a patient to paralysis include increased age, a more cephalic level of infection, and a history of diabetes mellitus or rheumatoid arthritis.[98] In one series, a neurologic deficit occurred in 45% of the 44 patients who had an impaired immune system, whereas only 19% of the remaining 67 patients developed a deficit.[24] Less than 7% to 15% of patients overall have residual neurologic deficits.[24,31] Diabetics are more likely to have permanent neurologic deficits, and patients with thoracic involvement are the least likely to recover.[31,98] Eismont and colleagues[98] described the results of operation in 14 patients with spinal cord paralysis. Three of the seven patients who underwent a laminectomy deteriorated, and four remained unchanged. In contrast, half of the patients treated by an anterior procedure recovered normal or nearly normal function, and no patient was made worse by the procedure. The patients with root lesions alone had an excellent outcome with or without operation.

In selected patients who require surgical treatment for pyogenic osteomyelitis, the prognosis is very good after the anterior debridement and primary bone grafting in conjunction with a full course of antibiotics. In a series of 21 patients, 6 of whom had neurologic deficits, there were no deaths and no relapses and all of the patients with neurologic deficit recovered. All but one of the patients who underwent fusion had a solid fusion, and one of the two patients who did not

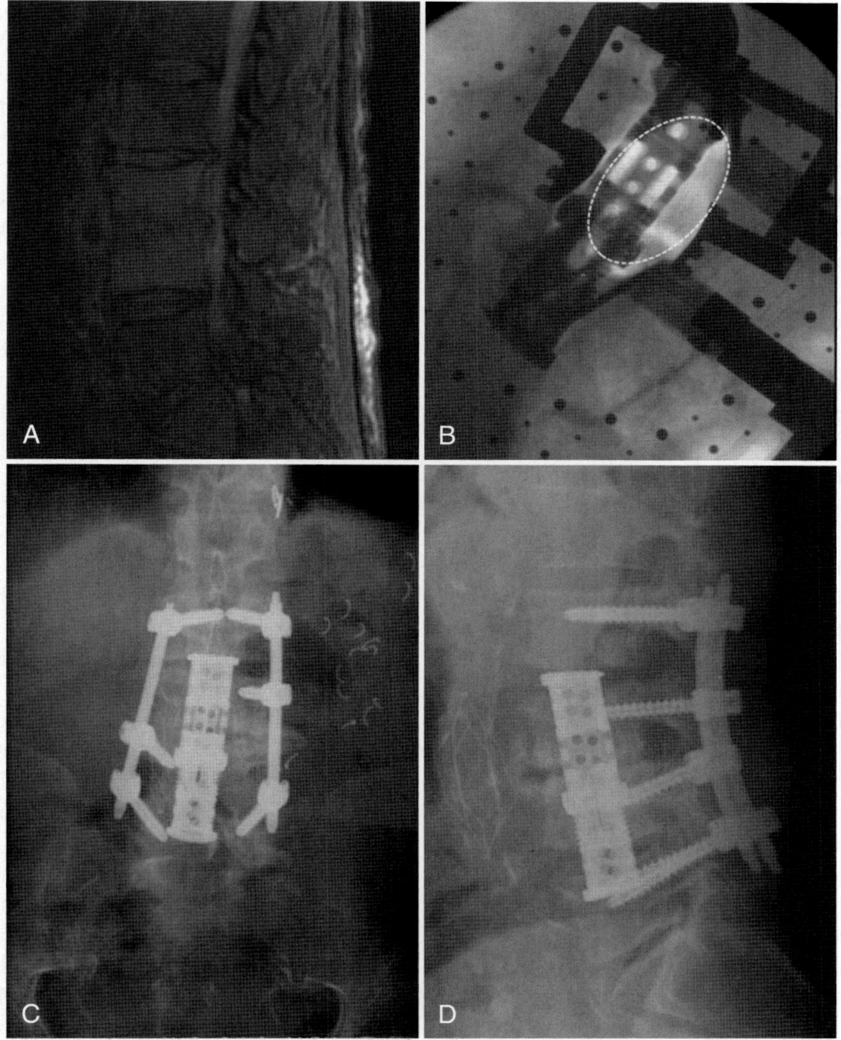

FIG. 87.13 Mini-open direct lateral lumbar corpectomy and reconstruction with expandable cages. A 67-year-old man presented with an infected pacemaker, sepsis, and severe intractable low back pain. (A) Gadolinium-enhanced magnetic resonance imaging shows disc space destruction and increased signal intensity at L3 and L4. (B) Direct lateral, mini-open, transpsoas exposure for L3 and L4 corpectomies, with insertion of expandable titanium cage filled with bone morphogenetic protein 2. (C) Anteroposterior and (D) lateral radiographs following posterior percutaneous pedicle screw fixation.

have a graft had spontaneous fusion. The mean increase in kyphosis was 3 degrees.[183]

Garcia and Grantham[35] found that spontaneous interbody fusion was the rule, which occurred in less than 1 year in most patients and in 2 years in almost all other cases. Some studies have found that the chance of spontaneous fusion in patients treated nonoperatively is 50% or less.[26,31,113] Fortunately, those who do not develop a bony union achieve a fibrous ankylosis, which is generally painless.[26,35,113,114] Occasionally, a patient complains of persistent back pain from localized degenerative changes at the site of previous infection.[26,35,113]

The more cephalad the level of infection, the higher the rate of spontaneous fusion; almost all cases of cervical infection will fuse spontaneously.[17,41] In one series, 6 of 6 cervical lesions went on to solid interbody fusion compared with 22 of 29 thoracic lesions and 5 of 21 lumbar lesions.[17] One of the patients with cervical infection and one with thoracic involvement had undergone posterior fusion. Fifteen of the patients with thoracic disease underwent costotransversectomy, and five patients with lumbar involvement had anterior debridement without fusion.[17]

Although deformities are much less common with pyogenic infection than with tuberculosis infection, they still may occur.[26,236] Deformities have been reported to occur in the cervical spine[236] but are more common in the thoracic and thoracolumbar areas and in those cases with involvement of more than 50% of one or more vertebral bodies.[26] Interestingly, IV drug abusers have an excellent prognosis. Ninety-two percent responded to parenteral antibiotic therapy for 4 weeks or more, and relapses responded to a second course. In 67 cases reported in the literature, there were no deaths or permanent neurologic sequelae.[42]

Overall, the long-term outcome of patients with vertebral osteomyelitis is relatively poor compared with the normal population. O'Daly and colleagues assessed the long-term functional outcome of patients with pyogenic spinal infection using the Oswestry Disability Index (ODI) and the Short-Form 36 questionnaire (SF-36) survey to measure health-related quality of life (HRQOL).[110] Twenty-nine patients with a median follow-up of 61 months (range, 37–104 months) were examined. IV drug use was not reported in the study population. Eight patients (28%) underwent operative treatment and 21 (72%) were managed nonoperatively with antibiotics alone. "Recovery" was classified as survival and disappearance of all signs and symptoms of active infection, with no residual disability. "Adverse outcome" was classified as survival and disappearance of all signs and symptoms of infection but persistence of clinically significant residual disability or pain, or death caused by or associated with persistent infection at any time before follow-up. Nineteen patients (66%) had an "adverse outcome" as defined by this study. As expected, there were marked differences in SF-36 scores between these patients and the normative population. However, the "recovery" group patients had SF-36 physical function scores and ODI scores that were comparable with the normative values. There was no correlation between SF-36 bodily pain and general health measures and the ODI. Forty-eight percent of patients reported being pain free. Due to the small number of patients, no statistically significant difference was found between patients who underwent surgery compared with patients treated nonoperatively. Delay in diagnosis (>8 weeks) and neurologic deficit at diagnosis were independent risk factors for an "adverse outcome." Advanced age was a risk factor for acute death, and previous surgery at the site of initial infection was a risk factor for recurrent infection.

Woertgen and colleagues[237] compared the outcome of operative and nonoperative treatment using the SF-36. The authors retrospectively investigated 62 patients suffering from pyogenic spinal infections: 28 patients (45%) underwent nonoperative treatment and 34 (55%) underwent surgery. As seen in the study by O'Daly and colleagues,[110] most patients continued to suffer some sort of pain and various SF-36 measures did not reach normative levels. Despite different indications, the surgically treated patients experienced a slightly better HRQOL, self-reported satisfaction levels, and better clinical outcomes than patients treated nonoperatively. These results support the current recommendations that surgery should be pursued in those patients with progressive neurologic deficits, in those with obvious spinal instability, and in cases in which medical therapy has failed.

Epidural Abscess

Epidemiology

An epidural abscess is a bacterial infection of the spine that results in the accumulation of purulent fluid or infected granulation tissue in the epidural space. Most cases occur in adults (mean age, 57 years; range, 2–81 years).[238] Occurrence in children younger than age 12 years is rare.[239] The male/female ratio is approximately 1 : 1.[238] The incidence of the disease is 0.2 to 1.2 per 10,000 hospital admissions per year with an incidence of 1.8 per 100,000 population annually.[240,241] At the University of Miami/Jackson Memorial Hospital Medical Center, 137 spine infections were treated by the orthopaedic service over an 8-year period; of these, epidural abscess occurred in 10 (7.3%).[146] Approximately 50% of patients are initially misdiagnosed (range, 11%–75%).[242,243]

Danner and Hartman[238] noted an increased frequency at their hospital between 1971 and 1982. This increase was disproportionate to the small increase in admissions and laminectomies performed at that hospital. The authors' proposed explanations were an increased use of medical instrumentation, an increase in frequency of IV drug abuse, and an aging population.[238] Other investigators have also documented an increasing incidence in the condition.[244,245]

Etiology

Spinal epidural abscess occurs from a collection of purulent material between the dura and the osseous-ligamentous structures of the spine and was first described by Morgagni in 1761.[246] The primary source of infection can be identified in approximately 60% of the cases.[238] Infection may occur by hematogenous spread from a remote focus of infection,[238,240,247–250] by spread from a contiguous focus of vertebral osteomyelitis or a disc space infection,[146,238,240,249,251] or from direct inoculation at the time of operation, epidural steroid injection, lumbar puncture, or epidural catheterization.[44,238,240,249,252–254] In 136 cases compiled from five series in the literature, skin and soft tissue infections were thought to be the source in 21%, bone or joint infections in 13% (up to 28% if vertebral osteomyelitis is included), spine surgery or other procedures in 10%, upper respiratory tract infection in 6%, abdominal sources in 4%, urinary tract infection in 2%, and IV drug abuse in 4%.[3,238,240,248,250] The incidence of epidural abscess after catheter insertion is about 0.001%.[255] Although this risk is low, the increased use of epidural analgesia as a method of postoperative pain control is increasing.

Factors that may be associated with a higher incidence of infection include diabetes mellitus, human immunodeficiency virus (HIV) infection, IV drug abuse, prior back trauma, renal failure, liver disease, alcoholism, and pregnancy.[55,146,238,240,251] Between 12% and 30% of patients reported an episode of trauma preceding the infection.[238,240,251] A review of 75 patients from Baltimore revealed an increase in the incidence of epidural abscess over the prior 10-year period.[256] This increase may be due in part to better diagnostic techniques, particularly with gadolinium-enhanced MRI. This study population may be at higher risk of this disease. In this series of 75 patients, 33% had a history of IV drug abuse.

Bacteriology

In 1948, Heusner reported on 20 patients with an epidural abscess; *S. aureus* was the pathogen in all of the cases in which the organism was known.[249] In more recent series, *S. aureus* accounts for approximately 60% of cases in which the organism is known.[238,240,250] From the results in 166 patients from five series, *S. aureus* accounted for 62%, aerobic streptococci for 8%, *Staphylococcus epidermidis* for 2%, aerobic gram-negative rods for 18%, anaerobes for 2%, and other bacteria for 1%; 6% of the organisms were unidentified.[238,240,248–250] Gram-negative organisms have been reported with increasing frequency.[240,247,250] One study found that IV drug abusers were frequently infected with gram-negative organisms[250]; in another series, 12 of 18 IV drug abusers were infected with *S. aureus* and only one with *Pseudomonas*.[39] A meta-analysis of 915 patients by Reihsaus and colleagues[257] showed that *S. aureus* accounted for 73%, other staphylococcal species 9.3%, aerobic streptococci for 7.7%, Enterobacteriaceae (mainly *E. coli*) 4.9%, *Pseudomonas* species 4.9%, mixed bacterial infections 3.6%, and fungi 1.7%.

Pathogenesis/Pathology

The epidural space is filled with fat and loose areolar tissue containing numerous veins.[258] The size and shape of this space is determined by the variations in size of the spinal cord. In the cervical region, this is a potential space with almost no fat between bone and dura. The epidural space exists only dorsal to the origin of the spinal nerves. Ventrally, the dura is closely applied to the canal from C1 to S2. Posteriorly, the space begins to appear at C7 and gradually deepens along the thoracic vertebrae to a depth of 0.5 to 0.75 cm between T4 and T8. The space tapers again and becomes shallow between T11 and L2 and attains its greatest depths below L2. Below S2, the epidural space surrounds the dura on all sides.[259] The epidural space communicates with the retroperitoneal and posterior mediastinal spaces through the intervertebral foramina.[260] As would be expected by this description of the anatomy, most epidural abscesses are in the thoracic and lumbar spine and are generally posterior.[238,240,248–250,261–263]

In several series, the thoracic spine was involved in 51% of cases, the lumbar spine in 35%, and the cervical spine in 14%.[238,240,249,250,261,262] The abscess was anterior in 21% and posterior in 79% of the 133 patients from four series in which the location was recorded.[238,240,248,249] An abscess is more likely to be located anteriorly if the infection is in the lumbar spine and if it is secondary to vertebral osteomyelitis.[238,248] Because there is no anatomic boundary within the space, the infection may extend the entire length of the canal but generally covers only three or four segments.[146,238,239,249,250,262]

The pathogenesis of the neurologic manifestations is related either to direct compression from epidural pus or granulation tissue or to disruption of the intrinsic circulation of the cord.[240,249,251,258] A microangiographic study in a rabbit model demonstrated that the initial neurologic deficit is related to compression rather than to ischemia. The spinal arteries and epidural venous plexus remained patent in cases of mild to moderate spinal cord compression. The vessels became occluded only with extreme spinal cord compression.[264] On the basis of postmortem examinations, Russell and colleagues[263] identified thrombosis and thrombophlebitis of the veins of the cord and epidural space without involvement of the arteriolar supply. However, others have found thrombosis of the arteriolar supply and veins.[240]

Several authors have identified a correlation between the duration of infection and the gross appearance at operation or postmortem examination. Corrandini and colleagues described an early presuppurative phase in which the inflammatory lesion was characterized by an epidural mass of swollen, red, friable fat without any gross pus.[265] In patients who have had symptoms for less than 2 weeks, gross pus with varying amounts of red granulation tissue has been identified.[238,240,251,263,265] Above and below the level of the pus, the epidural fat may undergo reactive changes and appear swollen and necrotic.[251] In patients with symptoms of longer duration, granulation tissue is often identified on the dura. Small beads of pus embedded in the granulation tissue are frequently observed.[238,240,263,265] In delayed cases with symptoms for 150 days or longer, grayish-white granulation tissue or maturing fibrous tissue has been found.[263] Some authors have thought that it is not always possible to predict whether pus or granulation tissue is likely to be found at operation.[248–250] Hancock described patients in whom granulation tissue was found 1 day after the onset of symptoms and other patients who had had symptoms for up to 4 weeks and had no granulation tissue at operation.[248] Subdural extension of infection is possible but uncommon.[88,240] With spinal cord involvement, there may be evidence of vessel thrombosis, inflammatory response of glial cells, and myelomalacia with liquefaction and vacuolization of the white matter.[251,258]

Clinical Presentation

Patients with an epidural abscess have a highly variable presentation, which causes initial misdiagnosis in approximately 50% of cases.[238] The difficulty in making the correct diagnosis frequently leads to significant delays between presentation and definitive treatment.[238,240,248-250,258,261,262,266,267] Patients who present acutely and who have had symptoms for less than 2 to 3 weeks generally have a better-defined syndrome than do patients with chronic disease. The differentiation between acute and chronic disease is somewhat arbitrary and probably relates to the virulence of the organism, the resistance of the host, and the type of treatment received before definitive diagnosis. Most patients with an acute epidural abscess present with fever, back pain, and spine tenderness. These signs and symptoms may be lacking in patients with chronic disease.[146,248,249,251,261–263] The most common presenting symptoms are spinal pain (89%), neurologic deficit (80%), and fever/chill (67%). Local tenderness (48%) and paresthesia (28%) are less common.[242] Patients with a history of IV drug use, diabetes, or multiple medical problems are particularly susceptible.[256]

Without treatment, the disease frequently progresses through four stages. The patients complain of local spine pain initially, followed by radicular pain and weakness and, finally, by paralysis. Heusner is frequently given credit for defining these stages of progression; however, Browder described the same syndrome in 1937, and a number of other authors reiterated the pattern before Heusner's report in 1948.[249,251,265,267,268] The transition from one stage to another is highly variable, and weakness or paralysis may not develop for many months or may occur suddenly and unpredictably in a matter of hours.[146,238,262] Neurologic symptoms occur with motor weakness in 30% of cases, and 19% of cases involve paralysis.[269] The location of the pain depends on the site of disease; therefore, pain is more common in the thoracic than in the lumbar or cervical spine.

If the abscess penetrates the dura, a subdural abscess or meningitis may result.[88,240] Many patients with an epidural abscess have nuchal rigidity; this sign is not helpful in differentiating an epidural abscess from meningitis.[240] Fraser and colleagues[88] suggested that a patient with a subdural abscess presents exactly like one with an epidural abscess, except that often there is no spinal percussion tenderness. Butler and colleagues[270] reviewed 16 patients with subdural abscesses described in the literature and found that only four had spinal tenderness. Unfortunately, this feature is not pathognomonic because not all patients with an epidural abscess have spine tenderness.[248,261]

Heusner thought that it was possible to differentiate patients with acute hematogenous epidural abscess from those whose abscess developed secondary to vertebral osteomyelitis: the latter patients had a predictable delay between the phases of spine pain and radicular pain followed by rapid progression of the illness.[249]

Diagnostic Evaluation

Patients with an acute epidural abscess generally have more systemic illness than those with vertebral osteomyelitis. Despite this, the initial diagnosis is incorrect in most cases.[242] The leukocyte count and the ESR are generally increased. In a meta-analysis of 915 patients, the ESR was 77 mm/h (range, 1–150 mm/h) and the mean leukocyte count was 15,700/μL (range, 1500–42,000/μL).[257] Patients with chronic disease usually have less systemic illness and display leukocyte counts that are often normal.[240]

CRP is a sensitive marker for infection. In a study of 26 patients with epidural abscesses treated without surgery, the initiation of antibiotic therapy led to a rapid drop in CRP within 5 to 10 days.[271] CRP values returned to normal at 25.5 days, on average. The definitive diagnosis is based on identification of the organism. Pus from the abscess is positive in approximately 90% of the cases, blood cultures are positive in 60%, and cultures of spinal fluid yield the organism in approximately 17%.[238,240,248–250]

Imaging Studies

Plain radiographs are frequently normal unless vertebral osteomyelitis or disc space infection is present and enough time has elapsed for the radiograph to become positive.[39,263] Radionuclide studies are often helpful but nonspecific and may be falsely negative.[39] The gallium scan may be slightly more sensitive than the technetium scan.[39]

In the past, myelography was the standard imaging tool for the diagnosis of an epidural abscess, but now it is used only if the patient is unable to undergo MRI or if spinal fluid is necessary for diagnostic testing. The puncture should be performed at a level remote from the expected area of infection. It may be necessary to perform injections at two sites in order to demonstrate both the cranial and caudal extents of compression. The findings are those of an extradural mass, and generally there is a high-grade or complete block. The lateral myelogram will demonstrate whether the abscess is anterior or posterior.[240,250,263] In one series, myelography was accurate to within one vertebral level in both the cephalic and caudal extents of the abscess in 10 of 12 cases compared with findings at operation.[146]

The needle should be inserted slowly and, if pus is encountered, a specimen should be taken for culture without entering the thecal sac. Myelography can then be performed at a different level. At the time of myelography, CSF should be studied for cell total and differential counts, glucose, protein, and culture and sensitivities. The CSF findings generally reflect a parameningeal infection with markedly increased protein content and no bacteria unless there is an associated subdural abscess or meningitis.[240,250,263] If a CT scan can be done expeditiously after the myelogram is performed, the degree of neural compression will be defined more accurately.

Plain CT scans may be helpful if they demonstrate an extradural mass.[39] Plain CT has a high false-negative rate, and in one study it was diagnostic in only four of nine cases.[238] The CT scan may demonstrate hypodense tissue in the epidural space.[252] If gas-forming organisms are present, gas may be seen within the epidural space.[272] When positive, CT could be useful to guide epidural puncture for isolation of the organism.[273] Contrast-enhanced CT has been found to be helpful by some authors.[273–276] Positive findings include the loss of physiologic epidural fat and fixation of contrast at the level of the dura surrounded by an area of higher density between the bone and the dura.[273] One major limitation of CT without a preceding myelogram is that the area of interest may be missed unless a large number of cuts are taken.

MRI has proved extremely useful and is the imaging study of choice.[146,274,277,278] It is noninvasive and safe and is able to visualize the degree of cord compression and extent of abscess in all directions. In addition, it has the capability of diagnosing disc space infection or vertebral osteomyelitis. Areas of infection have characteristically high signal intensity on T2-weighted images (Fig. 87.14). One potential disadvantage of MRI is that the CSF also has high signal intensity on T2-weighted images; therefore, there is little contrast between the CSF and the epidural abscess. This has led to false-negative MRI results, especially with long abscesses that do not have a discrete abnormality.[148] MRI may also be falsely negative in patients with concomitant epidural abscess and meningitis because the signal changes in the abscess may not be distinct from those in the infected CSF.[144]

The sensitivity of MRI at detecting an epidural abscess is increased by administration of gadolinium.[147,256,279] The pus in the epidural space will enhance with gadolinium, whereas the CSF will have a low signal intensity on the T1-weighted sequence. Patients who have abundant epidural lipomatous tissue may have false-negative scans because fat has a bright signal on T1-weighted images before administration of gadolinium and the contrast enhancement of the epidural pus may

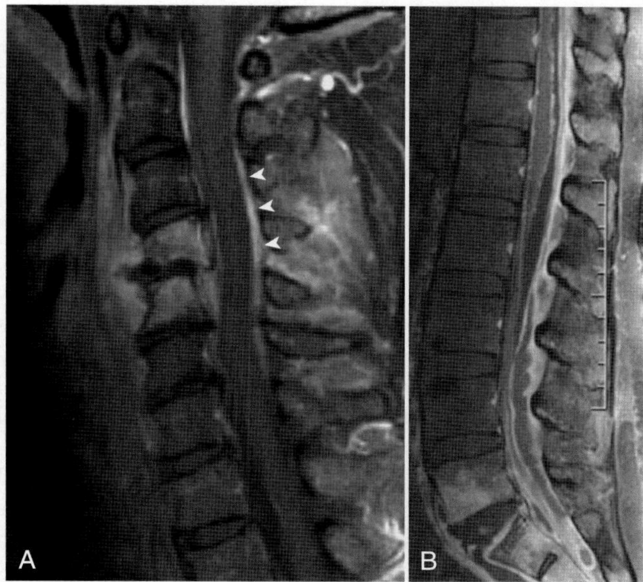

FIG. 87.14 Use of gadolinium-enhanced magnetic resonance imaging to detect epidural abscess. (A) Posterior epidural abscess in the cervical spine (*arrowheads*). (B) Multiloculated epidural abscess spanning entire lumbar spine.

be obscured.[279] The epidural venous plexus normally enhances with gadolinium administration and may be mistaken for an epidural abscess.[279] The plexus is characteristically more prominent in the cervical spine, and it should be symmetrical and extend into the neural foramina. The presence of concurrent noncontiguous spinal epidural abscess lesions, or skip lesions, should be conserved. Patients with a delay in diagnosis greater than 7 days, a concomitant area of infection outside of the spine or paraspinous region, and ESR greater than 95 mm/h have greater risk of a skip lesion. The predictive value was 73% for patients with all three characteristics, 13% with two, 2% with one, and 0% with zero.[280]

Myelography followed by CT should be performed in patients with negative MRI scans if they are suspected clinically to have an epidural abscess.[144] Injection of contrast via a lateral C1–C2 approach has been advocated as a means of avoiding the abscess pocket.[256] A repeat MRI with gadolinium enhancement may also detect an infection missed on the first study because there is a short time delay between the onset of clinical symptoms and the MRI appearance of an abnormality on MRI.[152,279]

Two other conditions to consider in the differential diagnosis of an epidural abscess are epidural metastasis and subdural abscess. It is much more critical to make the appropriate diagnosis in the case of epidural metastasis because the treatment of the two disorders is distinctly different. Subdural abscesses are uncommon. A review of the literature in 1988 revealed only 16 reported cases.[270] Myelography will reveal an intradural extramedullary filling defect, usually with a complete spinal block, and may demonstrate defects at several levels.[88,270,281,282] CT with intrathecal contrast provides better definition of the process than does myelography alone.[39,282] The definitive diagnosis is based on identification of the organism. Pus from the abscess is positive in approximately 90% of the cases, blood cultures are positive in 60%, and cultures of spinal fluid yield the organism in approximately 17%.[238,250]

Management

An epidural abscess accompanied by a neurologic deficit is a medical and surgical emergency. The goals of treatment are eradication of infection, preservation or improvement of the neurologic status, relief of pain, and preservation of spinal stability. The standard approach to an epidural abscess in the early part of the 20th century was immediate laminectomy for spinal decompression. In 1941, Browder and Meyers[258] suggested that chemotherapy might be a helpful adjunct to surgery. Heusner[249] found survival rates of 63% in patients managed surgically without antibiotics and 90% in those who received antibiotics in addition. A review of the literature from 1970 to 1990[283] revealed 37 cases of epidural abscess that had been treated conservatively. Of these cases, 63% had a successful result; however, some of the patients had poor outcomes.[238,240,249,266,268] Nonoperative management of epidural abscesses is recommended only in selected cases: (1) poor surgical candidates, (2) abscess involves a considerable length of the vertebral canal, (3) no significant neurologic deficit, and (4) complete paralysis for more than 3 days.[284,285] Surgical decompression and debridement is strictly recommended when there is emerging or worsening neurologic deficit or sepsis. The following factors are reported to predict a failure of medical management alone: diabetes, CRP greater than 155 μg/mL, WBC greater than $\times 10^9$/L and bacteremia.[286]

Nonoperative Treatment in the Neurologically Intact Patient

With increased use of MRI and a heightened awareness of this disorder, more patients are diagnosed early in the course of the disease. Recent reports show many patients present with no neurologic deficits. In this subset of patients, nonoperative treatment appears to be efficacious. In a retrospective review of 30 cases, Sorensen showed that all 8 patients without neurologic deficit were successfully treated with antibiotic therapy alone.[271] Liem and colleagues[287] reported on 21 patients with thoracic epidural abscesses. Three patients had no neurologic deficit. These patients were treated with antibiotics alone with good results. Mampalam and colleagues[285] showed good results in six patients without neurologic deficit treated with 4 to 6 weeks of IV antibiotics. The causative organism was identified by blood cultures. All patients became afebrile within 48 hours after initiation of antibiotic therapy. Most patients also noticed a marked diminution in pain. In most series, antibiotic therapy lasted at least 4 weeks and up to 12 weeks.

Siddiq and colleagues[288] compared the outcomes of patients treated with antibiotics alone (25 patients), antibiotics with percutaneous CT-guided drainage (7 patients), or surgery (28 patients). Nearly half of the nonsurgical group had neurologic deficits. Despite this, the overall treatment outcome was comparable with the surgical group. The only predictor of outcome was neurologic abnormality at the time of hospital admission. This is consistent with previous findings, in which patients with little or no neurologic deficit had good overall results with nonoperative treatment.[283] To date, no randomized study directly comparing prophylactic surgery and medical therapy has been performed. However, it is clear that once neurologic deficits appear, surgical decompression and debridement must be timely. When surgery is performed within 24 hours after the onset of neurologic symptoms, overall good results can be obtained in 53% to 80% of cases.[256,287] If surgery is performed after 24 hours, the success rate is 10%.

Thus, nonoperative treatment should be pursued with extreme caution. If an epidural abscess is discovered before the onset of neurologic symptoms, the patient should be hospitalized for close clinical follow-up. Identification of the organism is a critical step in the treatment regimen. Often, this can be done through blood cultures. If the infection begins in the disc space or vertebral body, a percutaneous biopsy in that area can be performed along with drainage. Once cultures are obtained, IV antibiotics should be initiated promptly and serial physical examination and daily CRP values should be assessed.[289] The fever curve and CRP levels should trend downward within 24 to 48 hours. Pain may decrease to some extent. If the baseline leukocyte count was elevated, a downward trend will also be appreciated. In approximately 5 to 10 days, the CRP should be dramatically decreased and is often near normal ranges. Antibiotic therapy should be started immediately on the basis of the Gram stain results and the known bacteriologic basis of the disease. Gram-negative organisms should be suspected if there is a history of a spinal procedure or in IV drug abusers. *S. epidermidis* should also be considered after spinal procedures.[238] The definitive antibiotic therapy should be based on the culture and sensitivity results. Antibiotics should be given in maximal dosages for at least 2 weeks; most authors recommend 3 to 4 weeks of parenteral therapy.[238,240] Antibiotics must be administered parenterally for at least 6 to 8 weeks for coexistent vertebral osteomyelitis.[238,240]

If the patient remains neurologically intact and afebrile, outpatient treatment can be instituted in the reliable patient. Initially, weekly follow-up examinations and laboratory studies should be performed. Such outpatient therapy is reserved for patients who can reliably return to appointments and can readily respond to changes in their symptoms. In our institution, we typically treat with IV antibiotics for at least 6 weeks. Surgical treatment in this patient population is pursued for the following indications: (1) lack of response to medical treatment, (2) onset of systemic infection (sepsis), and/or (3) development of neurologic signs and symptoms. A lack of response to medical treatment often follows a relatively slow course. There is a lack of decline in the fever curve and CRP levels. Pain may persist or increase. Often, this is evident after 5 to 10 days of medical treatment.[289] When systemic infection (sepsis) or neurologic deficits emerge, surgical treatment becomes urgent because the time point when a neurologic injury becomes irreversible is unknown.[290]

Surgical Treatment

It is clear that, in a small proportion of patients, a rapid neurologic decline can occur despite the initiation of appropriate antibiotics.[283] This can be a devastating event; for this reason, surgical decompression and debridement remain the treatment of choice in nearly all patients.[291–293] Up to 75% of patients are reported to fail medical management alone.[294] The surgical approach depends on the location of the abscess. Because the abscess is posterior in most cases, laminectomy is generally the treatment of choice.[240,249] The facet joints should be left intact for spinal stability. Intraoperative ultrasonography after laminectomy allows localization of epidural masses and differentiation of them from the adjacent spinal cord.[144] When the abscess is secondary to vertebral osteomyelitis, it may be necessary to perform both anterior and posterior decompression. Instrumentation and fusion may be necessary in those cases in which spinal stability has been compromised by the decompression. Such extensive reconstruction can be staged at a time subsequent to an initial decompression and debridement in patients who have active comorbidities.

The wound may be closed over drains.[238,240,249] Garrido and Rosenwasser[295] recommended closure of the wound and continuous suction-irrigation for 5 days after decompressive laminectomy. Baker and colleagues[240] recommended open-wound treatment in cases with gross purulence followed by closure of the wound only when granulation tissue is identified. If the wound is left open, delayed closure may be carried out when the leukocyte count, sedimentation rate, and temperature return to normal and the wound shows good granulation tissue.[249] Closure with wound vacuum-assisted closure therapy (Kinetic Concepts Inc.) may be considered, although no series have been reported to our knowledge on the safety or efficacy of the technique.

In children, an extensive laminectomy is undesirable because of the risk of postoperative spinal deformity.[170,266] Hulme and Dott[266] suggested two limited procedures for children. They recommended first a laminoplasty type of en bloc removal of the lamina and ligaments with replacement after drainage. Alternatively, they advised exploration of the canal through a small fenestration made by removing the ligamentum flavum and portions of the adjacent lamina and insertion of thin rubber catheters. They thought that this technique was appropriate when gross purulence was encountered but recommended laminectomy if granulation tissue was found to be compressing the dura.[266] de Villiers and Cluver[260] reported on four children successfully managed by a modification of Hulme's second technique. A single-level laminectomy was performed, catheters were passed cranially and caudally, and the epidural space was irrigated with antibiotic solution. None of the children required reoperation, and no sinus tract developed with this technique.[260]

A variation of Hulme's technique was reported by Cardan and Nanulescu in 1987.[296] A 2.5-year-old boy with an extensive epidural abscess was treated by epidural lavage using Mancao needles. Three hundred milliliters of isotonic saline was flushed through the epidural space over a 30-minute period while the patient was under general anesthesia. A multiple-hole catheter was then inserted from the sacral hiatus to the midthoracic spine, and a gentamicin isotonic saline solution was administered. The patient improved clinically and, at 18 months postoperatively, was neurologically intact without any sequelae.

A modification of this technique has been employed in adults with good initial outcome. Schultz and colleagues[297] reported on two patients with extensive epidural abscesses. Both patients had abscesses extending from the cervical to the lumbar spine. Rather than performing full-length laminectomies, limited approaches above and below the levels of involvement were used to pass Fogarty catheters through the areas of the abscesses. Once the catheters reached to the opposite opening, the balloon was inflated and carefully pulled back through the canal, effectively "milking" the purulent material out of the canal. Usually, two passes were required. Both patients had resolution of the infection. One patient had near full recovery of motor function; the other patient had moderate improvement of motor function. This technique is promising as an alternative to complete laminectomies, particularly when there is extensive involvement over many levels or when a minimally invasive approach is warranted due to a fragile medical condition of the patient.

Prognosis

The natural history of an untreated epidural abscess is relentless progression of symptoms and eventual paralysis and possibly death. Before the advent of antibiotics, the overall mortality rate was between 55% and 70%.[251,258,298] Mixter and Smithwick[298] reported on 10 cases; all 3 patients treated nonoperatively died. With surgery, the mortality rate decreased to between 30% and 57%[258,298]; 50% of the survivors were left with residual neurologic deficit.[258] From the data on 168 patients reported in six early series since the introduction of antibiotics, 38% made a complete recovery, 29% had residual weakness, 21% were paralyzed, and 12% died.[238,240,248,250,258,261,262] The data from five series published since 1990[244,245,299–302] indicated that 78% of patients undergoing surgery recover fully or with minimal weakness. The prognosis is similar for patients with acute or with chronic disease as long as they are managed appropriately.[240]

The prognosis for neurologic recovery depends on the duration and severity of the neurologic deficit.[238,249,250,261,262] Heusner found that most patients with paresis of less than 36 hours' duration had a complete recovery. No patient with complete paralysis for more than 36 to 48 hours recovers significant neurologic function.[249,261,303] Complete sensory loss is also a poor prognostic factor.[261] Patients who have an acute progressive syndrome with complete paraplegia occurring within the first 12 hours have a poor prognosis; it is postulated that these patients have spinal cord infarction rather than mechanical compression as the pathogenesis of the neurologic deficit.[39] Rigamonti and colleagues[256] reported more recently on 75 patients with spinal epidural abscesses. In patients with severe neurologic deficit, treatment after 24 hours had a 47% poor outcome, whereas those treated before 24 hours had a 10% poor outcome. Thus, they recommend early surgical intervention in patients with neurologic deficit.

Other associated conditions thought to be poor prognostic factors are diabetes, advanced age, female gender, HIV infection, and associated vertebral osteomyelitis.[39,55,249] Furthermore, patients with thoracic-level involvement and those with severe deficits preoperatively also have significantly worse outcomes.[304] The prognosis with subdural abscess is relatively similar—two-thirds of the patients in reported cases made a complete or good recovery after surgical treatment in association with antibiotic therapy.[281,305]

Granulomatous Infections

Granulomatous infections may be caused by fungi, certain bacteria, and spirochetes. If a granuloma is identified on the frozen section, appropriate studies should be initiated to assist an accurate diagnosis.[306] The most common granulomatous spine infection in the world is tuberculosis (TB). TB spondylitis will be described in detail; the fungal and other granulomatous infections will be briefly reviewed by outlining the differences between them and TB infection. Bacteria in the order Actinomycetales cause chronic infections. This order includes the following families of pathogens: Mycobacteriaceae (genus: *Mycobacterium*), Actinomycetaceae (genera: *Actinomyces, Arachnia*), and Nocardiaceae (genus: *Nocardia*).[307]

Tuberculosis

The incidence of TB spondylitis varies considerably throughout the world and is usually proportional to the quality of public health services available. It is extremely common in underdeveloped countries where malnutrition and overcrowding are major problems. In affluent countries, the incidence has decreased dramatically in the past 30 years, and it now is uncommon.[17] Bone and joint involvement develops in approximately 10% of patients with TB[308]; half of these affected patients have TB of the spine.[309,310] A neurologic deficit will develop in 10% to 47% of those with TB spondylitis.[5,201,310–319] In developing countries, the disease is still a significant source of morbidity and mortality and remains the most common cause of nontraumatic paraplegia.[320]

In North America, Europe, and Saudi Arabia, the disease primarily affects adults; in Asia and Africa, a large percentage of the patients are children.[312,313,318,321–327] These patterns are changing, and a decrease in the incidence of infection in infants and young children has been noted in Hong Kong.[324] The age incidence of paraplegia corresponds with the general age incidence of TB of the spine, except for the first decade, in which the incidence of paraplegia is significantly less.[315]

In the United States, it is estimated that 10% of all TB cases occurred in HIV-positive patients.[328] Although it can occur in patients with any range of CD4 count, disseminated and extrapulmonary disease is more common in patients with CD4 counts less than 200 cells/μL and is an acquired immunodeficiency syndrome (AIDS)-defining condition.[328] Weinstein and Eismont[55] showed that patients with HIV had a

SECTION XII

higher rate of osseous spinal TB than the general public. Their data indicated that HIV-positive patients were 11 times more likely to be admitted for spinal TB than HIV-negative patients. HIV-positive patients represented 24% of the patients admitted with spinal TB. Among their patients with spinal TB, the average CD4 count was 75.7 cells/mm^3.[55]

Etiology

Spinal TB may occur from hematogenous spread from well-established foci outside the spine. The pulmonary and genitourinary systems are the most frequent sources, but spinal TB may also arise from other skeletal lesions.[81,312] At presentation, the primary focus of infection may be quiescent. Spinal involvement may develop from visceral lesions by direct extension.[81]

Bacteriology

Infection is most commonly caused by *Mycobacterium tuberculosis,* but any species of *Mycobacterium* may be responsible.[329]

Pathogenesis/Pathology

The pathogenesis of the early stages of spinal TB is similar to that of pyogenic infections of the spine and may result from hematogenous spread or from direct extension of disease.[81] One study has suggested that the venous or lymphatic routes may be more important than the arterial system for dissemination of this disease. Blacklock was unable to produce spinal disease by injection of mycobacteria into a vertebra or into the left ventricle of experimental animals.[330]

There are three major types of spinal involvement: paradiscal, central, and anterior.[331] In one series of 914 cases, the disease was paradiscal in 33%, central in 11.6%, and anterior in 2.1%; in 52.8%, the disease was too widespread at presentation for identification of the primary focus.[314] Atypical forms of spinal TB include those with neural arch involvement only and rare cases in which granulomas occur in the spinal canal without bony involvement.[314,332,333] A similar classification system along with specific MRI findings have recently been described by Moorthy and Prabhu.[334] The actual incidence of TB primarily involving the posterior elements is unknown but is probably between 2% and 10%.[332,333,335] MRI shows a homogeneous hyperintense T2-weighted signal in the posterior elements and associated paraspinal abscess.[334]

With paradiscal disease, the infection begins in the metaphyseal area and spreads under the anterior longitudinal ligament to involve the adjacent bodies. In contrast to pyogenic infections, the disc is relatively resistant to infection and may be preserved, even with extensive bone loss.[81] Disc space narrowing has been postulated to occur either as a result of extension of disease or from dehydration of the disc secondary to the altered functional capacities of the endplate. MRI shows low signal on T1-weighted images and high signal on T2-weighted images in the endplate, with disc space narrowing and large paraspinal and occasional epidural abscesses.[334]

In cases with primarily anterior involvement, the infection spreads beneath the anterior longitudinal ligament and may extend over several segments. The radiographic features include scalloped anterior erosion of several vertebral bodies. This pattern is said to result from aortic pulsations transmitted via a prevertebral abscess beneath the anterior longitudinal ligament.[336] However, similar changes have been seen in the cervical spine, and another hypothesis is that the scalloping may be due to changes in local vertebral body blood supply.[201] A combination of pressure and ischemia caused by this pus may produce anterior scalloping. MRI reveals subligamentous abscesses, preservation of disc space, and abnormal signal of multiple vertebral bodies.[334]

In cases classified as central involvement, the disease begins within the middle of the vertebral body and remains isolated to one vertebra. These lesions are frequently mistaken for a tumor. They tend to lead to vertebral collapse and therefore are the most likely type to produce significant spinal deformity.[331] Such pathologic fractures may mimic the more common osteoporotic compression fracture.[337] MRI in central lesions shows signal abnormality of the vertebral body with preservation of the disc space and may also mimic lymphoma or metastases.[334] The pathologic features of TB spondylitis may be altered by secondary pyogenic infection, which may occur through sinus tracts or after debridement procedures.[81]

The pathologic findings in TB spondylitis differ in several ways from those in pyogenic infections. The disc is relatively resistant to TB infection. The pathologic changes generally take longer to develop and are frequently associated with greater deformity. Large paraspinal abscesses are more common with TB infections.[25,30,81,319]

There are numerous mechanisms by which a neurologic deficit may develop in a patient with TB spondylitis. The focus of disease may be within the bone or, occasionally, within the spinal canal without osseous involvement.[322,332,333,338–341] Seddon recognized that neurologic deficits may occur either acutely or chronically.[2] He classified acute disease as "paraplegia of active disease" and recognized that this was due to either external pressure or invasion of the dura. Pressure on the spinal cord may arise from an epidural granuloma or abscess, from sequestered bone and disc, or from pathologic subluxation or dislocation of the vertebra. The paraplegia in chronic cases is related to pressure on the cord from epidural granulomas or fibrosis or from a ridge of bone anteriorly caused by a progressive kyphotic deformity. Several other authors have confirmed these pathogenetic mechanisms at operation or postmortem examination.[10,201,308,341–344]

An epidural granuloma is analogous to a pyogenic epidural abscess. Most frequently, the granuloma arises by spread from the adjacent bone. Because the primary bony lesion is anterior in the majority of cases, spinal cord compression occurs anteriorly. With posterior arch involvement, however, the cord may be compressed from behind.[333,335,345] Although isolated involvement of the neural arch is uncommon, posterior compression from arch involvement occurs in approximately 10% of cases associated with paralysis.[14]

Rarely, an epidural granuloma may occur directly by hematogenous seeding without any bony involvement.[48,273,322,332,333,340,341]

Other lesions that may cause a neurologic deficit without bony involvement are intradural tuberculomas and TB arachnoiditis.[322,338,340] Paraplegia from extraosseous disease occurs in no more than 5% of cases.[322] Transdural extension of TB inflammation was first described by Michod in 1871.[343] Since then, it has been described by other authors.[201,319,340,341,343] Presumably, transdural extension can occur regardless of whether or not the process originates within the bone. TB meningitis is characterized by a granulomatous reaction in the subarachnoid space.[346] Intradural extramedullary mycobacterial disease is the least common presentation of spinal TB. In 2005, Roca reviewed 22 cases in the literature over the past 25 years.[346] Only 3 (14%) were HIV positive and had CD4 counts of 137 to 228/μL.[346] Roca reported that the majority of patients (82%) with intradural extramedullary tuberculomas required operative intervention. At surgery, pathologic tissue revealed granulomatous reaction secondary to a persistent inflammatory reaction. Although organisms may be absent in the specimen, immunohistochemical staining reveals TB antigen (Fig. 87.15).

Clinical Presentation

The clinical presentation of TB spondylitis is variable and depends on many factors. In the classic presentation, the patient complains of spine pain and exhibits manifestations of chronic illness such as weight loss, malaise, and intermittent fever. The physical findings include local tenderness, muscle spasm, and restricted motion. The patient may also have a spinal deformity and neurologic deficit. The duration of symptoms before a definitive diagnosis is made varies from months to years; most cases are diagnosed in less than 2 years.[201] In affluent countries, presentation is generally early. In underdeveloped countries, the complications of neglected disease—such as paraplegia, kyphosis, and draining sinuses—may be the presenting complaints.[319,326,347]

The location of the pain corresponds to the site of the disease, which is most frequent in the thoracic region, less common in the lumbar region, and rare in the cervical spine and sacrum.[201,314,317] Patients may present with an abscess in any one of many locations, including the groin and buttocks.[331]

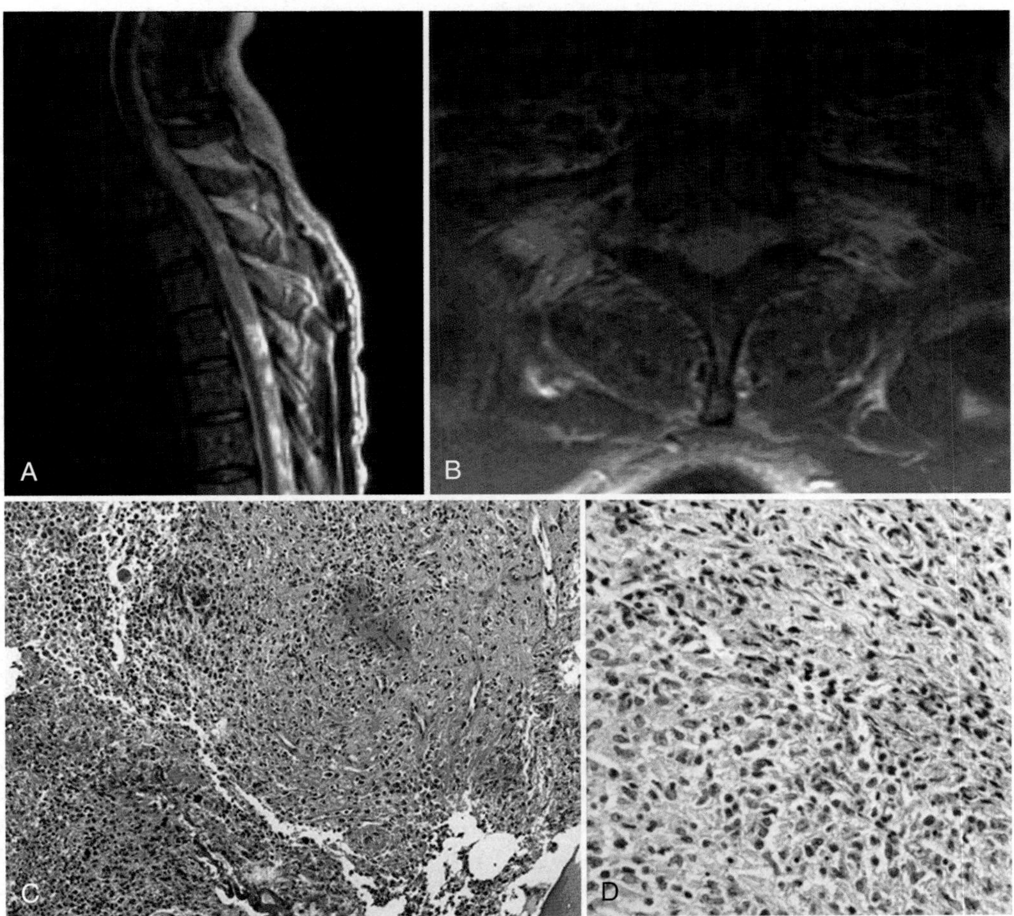

FIG. 87.15 (A) Sagittal T2-weighted magnetic resonance image (MRI) demonstrating a diffuse posterior mass displacing the spinal cord anteriorly. (B) Axial T2-weighted MRI demonstrating a diffuse posterior mass displacing the spinal cord anteriorly. (C) Hematoxylin and eosin–stained tissue of the pathologic specimen removed at surgery. This ×10 magnification view demonstrates a poorly formed granuloma. (D) Antituberculosis immunohistochemical stain at ×40 magnification. The immunohistochemical stain is directed against tuberculosis antigen and is brown in the pathologic specimen. This brown staining indicates the presence of tuberculosis antigen.

In 10% to 47% of patients, neurologic deficits develop during the course of their disease.[5,201,310–312,314–319] The incidence of paraplegia is higher with spondylitis in the thoracic and the cervical spine.[314,348] The most common complications occurring prior to diagnosis include abscesses (69%), neurologic deficits (40%), spinal instability (21%), and spinal deformity (16%).[349]

The manifestations of cervical spine involvement vary with the age of the patient. Children younger than age 10 years usually have extensive disease, with large abscesses and a relatively low (17%) incidence of paralysis. In older patients, the disease is more localized with less pus, but the incidence of paraplegia is 81%.[348] A distinct syndrome has been reported in heroin addicts with TB spondylitis. All five patients in one series had an acute toxic reaction with fever, back pain, weight loss, night sweats, and rapidly evolving neurologic deficits. All patients had disseminated TB with involvement of extravertebral sites.[350]

Diagnostic Evaluation

The sedimentation rate is generally increased with TB spondylitis, but this is nonspecific. The tuberculin purified protein derivative skin test is usually positive and indicates either past or present exposure to *Mycobacterium*.[322] Cultures of early morning urine samples may be helpful in cases of renal involvement, and sputum specimens and gastric washings may be positive with active pulmonary disease. These laboratory findings are helpful in the diagnosis, but an absolute diagnosis can be made only by biopsy of the spine lesion.[189] Aspiration of a subcutaneous abscess on occasion may reveal the organism and obviate the need for spine biopsy.

Isolation of *Mycobacterium* from clinical specimens takes 6 to 8 weeks, and the sensitivity of culture may be as low as 50%.[351] In the past, the most rapid method of detecting mycobacteria was the staining and smear microscopy of acid-fast bacilli. However, the acid-fast bacilli smear technique requires 5000 to 10,000 bacilli per milliliter of sputum for detection, with only 50% to 80% of specimens testing positive.[352] Polymerase chain reaction (PCR) has been used to rapidly identify the presence of mycobacteria in formaldehyde solution–fixed, paraffin-embedded tissue specimens.[353] Over the past several years, a number of commercially available molecular detection systems have been introduced. All of these systems use detection of *Mycobacterium* DNA or RNA, using the publication of the *M. tuberculosis* genome.[352] These extremely sensitive detection systems require great care in minimizing contaminants in the sample specimens and thus are relatively expensive. Molecular detection systems are also able to test for genes known to be associated with drug resistance, including rifampin, isoniazid, pyrazinamide, ethambutol, and streptomycin. The specificity of molecular detection techniques is approximately 98%, the sensitivity 85%, the positive predictive value 95%, and the negative predictive value 93%.[354]

The findings on plain radiographs of the spine will vary depending on the pathologic type and chronicity of the infection. The earliest finding may be bone rarefaction, regardless of type. With peridiscal involvement, disc space narrowing is followed by bone destruction, similar to pyogenic infections. With anterior multilevel spine involvement, the anterior aspect of several adjacent vertebrae may be eroded in a scalloped fashion. Central body involvement resembles a tumor, with central rarefaction and bone destruction followed by collapse. The initial radiographs often show far advanced bony changes in contrast to pyogenic infections, in which radiographs may be normal on first presentation. The central type is more common in the thoracic area, and the peridiscal variant is more common in the lumbar region. The central type causes greater and earlier bone collapse than the peridiscal type.[331] Although these radiographic changes are characteristic, a diagnosis based on radiologic changes alone is inadequate in 10% of cases.[355]

Chest radiographs are helpful in demonstrating pulmonary involvement and may show a paraspinal abscess. It is not possible to differentiate fibrosis and paravertebral edema from abscess formation on the basis of plain radiographs.[201] Occasionally, lumbar spine radiographs will demonstrate calcification in the psoas muscle in cases with a long-standing abscess.[201] Sclerotic reactive bone formation occurs with healing of TB infection but is seen much later and is less marked than with pyogenic infection.[93] Heroin addicts with Pott disease may have atypical radiographs. In one study, four of five patients had atypical radiographs, including two with an ivory vertebra.[350] Radionuclide scanning with technetium or gallium may help to define the extent of disease.[356] Gallium scanning has been recommended for diagnosing extrapulmonary TB and also to monitor the response to treatment.[356] Unfortunately, radionuclide scans are not sensitive for TB infection; technetium bone scans are negative in 35% of cases, and gallium scans are negative in 70%.[322] CT is useful to delineate soft tissue changes around the spine and in the canal but is not capable of differentiating an abscess from granulation tissue.

MRI is the imaging modality of choice because it demonstrates both bony and soft tissue involvement. The MRI findings in TB spondylitis may be indistinguishable from pyogenic infections, but there are some differences that are characteristic of TB and reflect the different pathologic types described earlier.[357] The intervertebral disc may have normal height and a normal signal on MRI, reflecting the resistance of the disc to TB infection (Fig. 87.16). Involvement of the anterior aspect of several contiguous vertebral bodies or involvement of posterior elements suggests a diagnosis of TB spondylitis. Paraspinal masses tend to be longer in TB spondylitis than in pyogenic infections and can be imaged well with plain or gadolinium-enhanced MRIs. Enhanced scans can distinguish abscesses from granulation tissue (Fig. 87.17). A mass with near-total enhancement is generally granulation tissue, whereas a mass with enhancement only at the periphery is generally an abscess.[358] As the infection resolves, the T1-weighted images of the vertebral body characteristically have progressively greater signal intensity.[115] Even the MRI findings are not completely characteristic; thus, a biopsy is necessary in all cases. Central body TB closely resembles a neoplasm[357,359]; an epidural TB granuloma without osseous involvement cannot be differentiated from an epidural neoplastic metastatic lesion. The distinction between

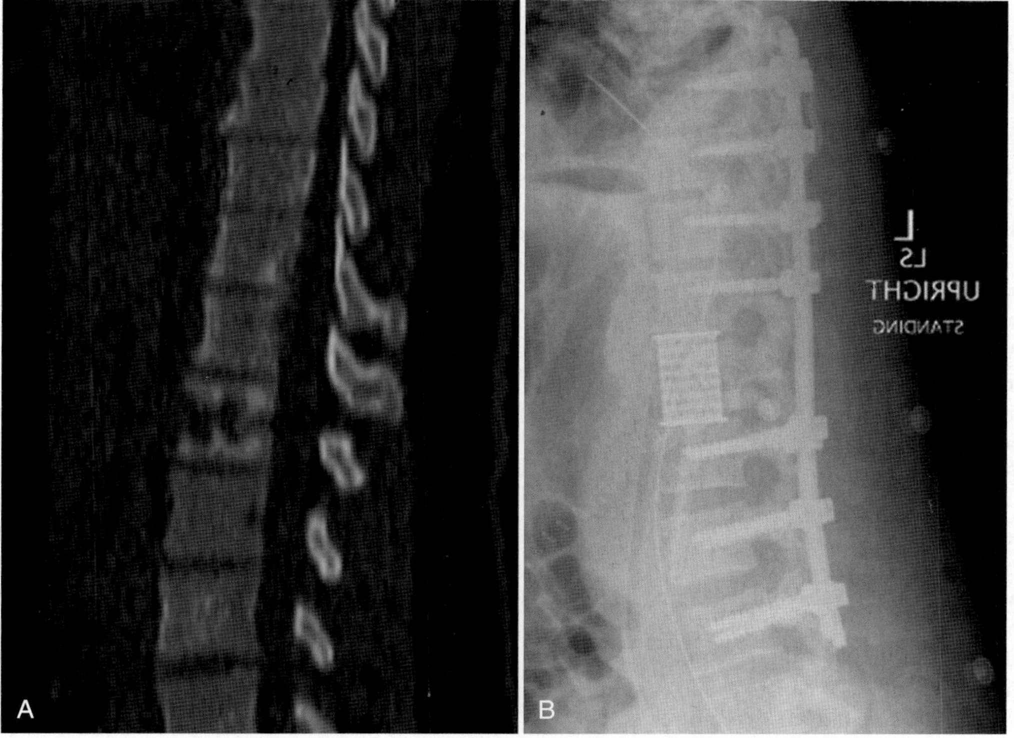

FIG. 87.16 Tuberculous vertebral osteomyelitis. In contrast to pyogenic infections, the disc tends to be spared relative to the vertebral body. (A) Computed tomography scan showing tuberculous infection of the vertebral body and relative preservation of the disc spaces above and below. (B) Radiograph of anterior corpectomy and strut fusion with posterior instrumented fusion.

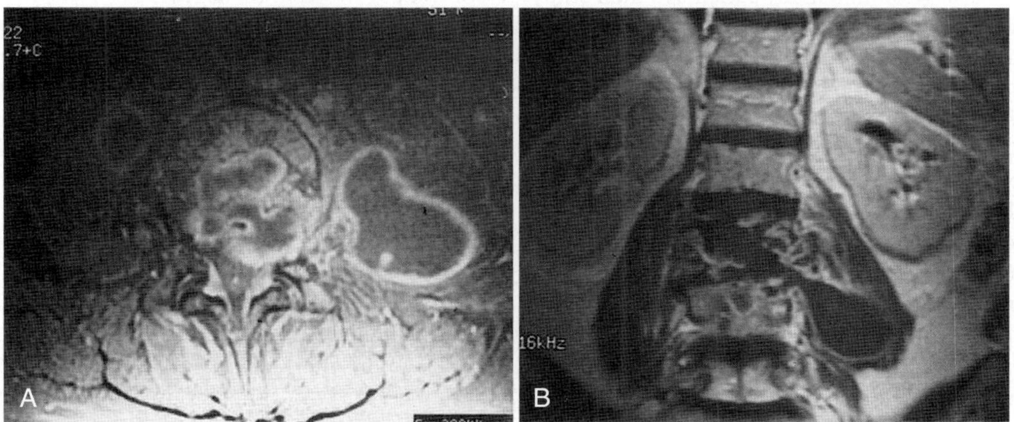

FIG. 87.17 (A) Axial and (B) coronal images of an abscess in the left psoas muscle in association with L3 and L4 tuberculous vertebral osteomyelitis. The periphery of the abscess enhances after administration of gadolinium, suggesting that the mass is an abscess rather than granulation tissue. The psoas abscess was found to be a sterile loculation of pus.

these conditions can be made only at operation.[332] Two MRI findings shown to significantly identify TB versus pyogenic infection are the presence of abscesses with thin and smooth walls (75% with TB vs. 0% in pyogenic spondylitis; $P < .001$) and well-defined paraspinal soft tissue (66.7% in TB vs. 11.1% in pyogenic spondylitis; $P = .007$).[360]

The differential diagnosis should include other bacterial and fungal infections as well as sarcoidosis and neuropathic spine disease. Sarcoidosis rarely involves the spine but may produce paraspinal masses and circumscribed lytic spine lesions with or without a sclerotic rim. Purely sclerotic lesions occur less frequently.[82] Neuropathic disease of the spine is usually limited to one to three contiguous vertebrae and is characterized by marked reactive sclerosis or destruction. Sclerosis associated with neuropathic disease of the spine parallels the base of the vertebral body and commonly involves the posterior arch. It is associated with paraspinal debris but not masses.[82]

Management

The goals of management are to eradicate the infection and to prevent or treat neurologic deficits and spinal deformity. The modern era in the treatment of spinal TB began in 1943 with the discovery of streptomycin by Waxmin. The first major description on the use of streptomycin in TB bone and joint lesions was published by Bosworth and colleagues[361] in 1950. The drug had a tremendous influence on the mortality rate from TB. Between the 5 years before streptomycin was used and the 5 years after its introduction, the mortality rate at Sea View Hospital in New York decreased by 72.5%.[275] Kondo and Yamada[362] reported a decrease in the mortality rate from 42.9% to 9.3% with the addition of streptomycin to the regimen for patients treated nonoperatively. In patients undergoing Albee fusion, the mortality rate was 32% without streptomycin and none with streptomycin. In patients undergoing focal debridement, the mortality rate decreased from 71.4% without streptomycin to 2.1% with streptomycin.[362]

In 1952, Bosworth and associates published a preliminary report showing encouraging results with the use of isoniazid.[363] These drugs and others eliminated the risk of dissemination of disease and the development of chronic sinuses after surgical debridement and allowed radical procedures to be performed in relative safety.[9,364] Both drugs were found to be effective without surgery when the patients were kept immobilized in the hospital for long periods.[365]

In Nigeria, a shortage of medical beds and poor medical facilities forced Konstam and Konstam[12,13] to use chemotherapy on an ambulatory basis. Although many patients in their study were lost to follow-up, 96% of those returning were thought to be healed and free of disease. Spinal deformity was found to be a problem with this form of treatment; only 75% developed a bony fusion, 49% had between 0 and 10 degrees of increased kyphosis, and 18% had 30 degrees or more of kyphosis.[12] Other authors found reasonably good results with chemotherapy alone.[9,312,366]

Hodgson and Stock[9,10] had excellent results with their procedure of radical debridement and anterior strut graft fusion in association with chemotherapy (the Hong Kong operation). In 1963, the Medical Research Council Committee for Research on Tuberculosis in the Tropics began to investigate these widely divergent forms of treatment. A subcommittee was established that later became known as the Working Party on Tuberculosis of the Spine. This group initiated a number of large-scale controlled, prospective trials of treatment methods. The design of each study was based on the available resources in areas where TB was endemic. The first studies, carried out in Korea and Rhodesia, established that chemotherapy is highly effective in ambulatory patients.[325,347,367] These investigations showed that there was no advantage to an initial period of bed rest in the hospital,[325] application of a plaster of Paris jacket,[367] or addition of streptomycin to the chemotherapy regimen.[325,347,367] These results were maintained after 5 years[368] and 10 years[369] of follow-up. Other studies comparing the effectiveness of debridement with that of more radical resection and bone grafting were carried out at three different centers. In Hong Kong, where the radical procedure was popularized, resection and fusion were found to have advantages in terms of less deformity and earlier bony fusion.[370] Patients with extensive disease and neurologic deficit were excluded from that study. In two concurrent studies in Africa, in which patients with more severe disease were included, there was no significant difference between the two surgical approaches.[326] Most of the patients in the three centers were doing well by the 3-year follow-up, and these results were maintained with up to 5 years of follow-up.[327] No changes were found at 10 years in the Hong Kong series.[371] The Medical Research Council then set out to determine whether short courses of chemotherapy would be as effective as the standard 18-month regimen (used in all previous studies). In Hong Kong, patients underwent the radical operation and either a 6- or 9-month chemotherapy regimen of isoniazid and rifampin supplemented with streptomycin for 6 months. The 6- and 9-month courses were equally effective and at least as successful as the standard 18-month regimen when assessed at 3 years.[372] In South India, ambulatory chemotherapy alone with 6- or 9-month regimens was compared with radical surgery plus 6 months of chemotherapy.[373] Of the patients treated by the 9-month regimen, 97% achieved a favorable status at 3 years compared with 93% for the patients in the 6-month ambulatory group. Surprisingly, only 85% of the patients in the surgical series achieved a favorable status. The conclusion of the Medical Research Council was that the treatment of choice for spinal TB in developing countries is ambulatory chemotherapy with 6- or 9-month regimens of isoniazid and rifampin. Surgery should be considered only for biopsy or the management of myelopathy, abscesses, and sinuses. Even in technically advanced countries, they advised against surgery in all cases. When surgery is felt to be necessary, the Hong Kong operation was recommended.[371,372] Although the results of the studies in Hong Kong and Africa on radical debridement and fusion versus debridement alone were at variance, the overall conclusion was that the Hong Kong operation allows anterior bony fusion to occur earlier and in a higher percentage of patients. Kyphotic deformity was less common and not progressive in those patients undergoing the more radical procedure.[371] Other independent studies have demonstrated the effectiveness of debridement and fusion and support the recommendation of the Medical Research Council.[185,189,374–377] The group in Hong Kong has written extensively on this approach and is responsible for its popularity.[9,10,188,319,323,348,378] Another advantage of anterior decompression and fusion compared with nonoperative treatment that has been demonstrated by a number of authors is the higher recovery rate in patients with neurologic deficit.[201,316,318,322]

Refinements in antituberculosis chemotherapy have permitted a more selective approach to the surgical management of spinal TB. Many mild cases respond well to standard chemotherapy without the need for surgery.[378a] Rather than operate in every case, Tuli described a "middle-path" regimen of operating only when medical management failed.[14,309] The first line of treatment was drug therapy; operation was considered for the following: decompression in patients with neurologic deficit who failed to respond to conservative therapy, posterior spinal lesions, failure of response after 3 to

6 months of nonoperative treatment, doubtful diagnosis, instability after healing, or recurrence of disease or of neurologic complications. In cases without neurologic involvement, healing occurred in 94% with antibiotics alone. In 200 cases with neurologic involvement, 38% of the patients recovered with drugs alone; of those patients requiring operation, 69% recovered completely. The overall success rate in patients with neurologic complications treated by this regimen was 78.5%.[14]

The indications for operation outlined by Tuli are similar to our current recommendations, except that patients with a neurologic deficit would be operated on urgently rather than after a delay to see if drug therapy alone would be effective. In general, the indications for operation are the same as with pyogenic infection. Lifeso and colleagues[322] think that patients with mild neurologic deficits should not undergo operation because medical therapy alone with close observation is safe. Two of their 23 patients became worse with conservative treatment; both recovered completely after anterior decompression and fusion. They also thought that patients with slight kyphosis could be treated with medical therapy alone because the increase in kyphosis and in the number of affected vertebral bodies reported in children was not found in adults treated medically.[322]

When an operation is indicated, it is easier to do it early because abscesses tend to dissect along tissue planes. If operation is delayed, fibrosis makes the procedure technically much more difficult. Hodgson and Stock[188] found a direct correlation between the duration of neurologic symptoms before the operation and the time for recovery from paraplegia. Others have confirmed this finding.[316] Operation also is advised in late-onset paralysis associated with cord compression by a hard bony ridge in association with kyphosis. Hsu and colleagues[342] think that, in patients with mild or moderate paraplegia, stabilization alone may be indicated, with decompression reserved for those patients with severe paralysis.

Regardless of whether an operation is performed or not, chemotherapy is an integral part of the management of spinal TB. The only cases in which chemotherapy is not indicated are those in which late-onset paraplegia from progressive deformity has occurred in a patient with healed inactive disease. Drug therapy is usually started preoperatively but may be started after operation if a biopsy is necessary. The first line of drugs currently in use include isoniazid (INH), rifampin (RMP), pyrazinamide (PZA), streptomycin (STM), and ethambutol (EMB). A number of second-line agents that occasionally are used in special circumstances include ethionamide, cycloserine, kanamycin, capreomycin, prothionamide, and para-aminosalicylic acid.[379] The choice of agents, dosages, and duration of therapy should be directed by an infectious disease expert.

Multiple drugs are used because of the potential for resistance to a single agent. Selection of rational combinations of drugs is based on the mechanism of action and toxicity of the agents.[379] The organisms may be in several different environments and therefore not accessible to all agents. They may reside in the extracellular space, either in the hyperoxic neutral environment of the pulmonary cavity or in the hypoxic acidic environment of caseous material in the spine. They also may exist in the highly suppressive acidic environment inside the activated macrophage. INH and RMP are bactericidal against both intracellular and extracellular organisms.[380] RMP may have an advantage against bacilli with low metabolic activity, as are present in caseous material. PZA is bactericidal only in an acidic environment and therefore is effective against intracellular organisms or within caseous lesions. Conversely, STM is active only in the extracellular space and therefore is often used to complement PZA. EMB is bacteriostatic against both intracellular and extracellular organisms and often is used in multiple-drug regimens in place of the once-popular para-aminosalicylic acid. All of these agents have the potential for significant toxicity. Hepatitis may be caused by both INH and RMP and is four times more common in patients receiving both agents than in those receiving INH alone. INH can also cause dose-dependent peripheral neuritis. The major toxicity of STM is nerve VIII damage; that of EMB is optic neuritis.

Antimicrobial resistance may occur from the multiplication of resistant mutants under the selective pressure of single-drug therapy. Resistance developing during the course of treatment in a patient with an initially drug-sensitive infection is termed "secondary resistance." "Primary resistance," defined as infection with drug-resistant organisms in a previously untreated patient, may be transmitted to other patients. The prevalence of primary resistance rose from less than 3% in the United States during the 1970s to approximately 9% by 1986.[381] Resistance is much more common in certain urban areas and in patients who are homeless, drug abusers, or infected with HIV. The patterns of drug resistance are variable throughout the world, reemphasizing the need for close follow-up during treatment.[12,188,322,372] Resistance is generally not a problem with multiple-drug regimens as long as the patient is in compliance.

A 6-month, three-drug regimen including INH, RMP, and PZA is used for most cases of drug-sensitive infection in Western nations. Atypical mycobacterial species are often resistant to standard drug regimens.[329] Because spinal TB carries a significant risk, maximal chemotherapy should be used. In a study of lumbar and lumbosacral spine involvement, triple antibiotic therapy with INH, EMB, and RMP yielded excellent results.[382] All patients healed the original site of infection with little change in spinal alignment. At 36 months' follow-up, the kyphosis angle improved slightly by 2.2 degrees and the Cobb angle increased slightly by 5.4 degrees.[382] Spontaneous bony union occurred in 87.5% of patients. Purtuiset and colleagues[383] reported on their experience of 103 cases of spinal TB occurring in a developed country. Most of their patients (74%) were treated with medical therapy alone and the remainder with surgery. Overall, there were two TB-related deaths. Their mean duration of medical treatment was 14 months. These results are similar to those observed in less developed countries, such as India.[384]

Surgical Treatment

An operation may be performed to drain abscesses, to debride sequestered bone and disc, to decompress the spinal cord, or to stabilize the spine for the prevention or correction of deformity. In 1779, Pott described the drainage of a TB abscess: "The remedy for this most dreadful disease consists merely in procuring a large discharge of matter, by suppuration from underneath the membrana adiposa on each side of the curvature, and in maintaining such discharge until the patient shall have perfectly recovered the use of his legs."[1] His statement was rather optimistic—many patients did not recover neurologic function after this procedure, and many others died of secondary pyogenic infection. In general, abscess drainage is indicated only if the patient is septic from the abscess or has a neurologic deficit from an epidural abscess or when the abscess is extremely extensive. After drainage of an abscess, the tissues may be closed in layers or the wound may be packed open. Paravertebral abscesses in the thoracic spine can be drained effectively by a costotransversectomy.[215] Large psoas abscesses may be drained by a retroperitoneal approach.[385]

Simple debridement of the spine without fusion is advocated by some surgeons.[326,362] However, most authors agree with the conclusions of the Medical Research Council that the Hong Kong procedure of anterior radical debridement and strut graft fusion is superior.[10,185,188,189,201,319,375–377,386] Surgery performed when the disease is active is safer, and the response is faster and better than that performed in patients with healed disease.[342]

In the Hong Kong procedure, the spine is approached anteriorly so that the affected area may be dealt with most directly. The sequestered bone and caseous material must be debrided back to bleeding bone above and below and back to the posterior longitudinal ligament. The decompression should go back to the dura in cases of neurologic deficit when spinal cord decompression is necessary.[327] The angular deformity is corrected by insertion of a strut graft. The anterior approach produces statistically better kyphosis correction and less correction loss, but it has been reported to be clinically insignificant.[387] Autogenous bone grafting at the time of the primary debridement is reliable in both adults and children.[10,185,188,189,194,201,316,319,323,371,375,377,388–390] The incidence of fusion with a bone graft is 97% at 10 years compared with 90% with debridement alone. Medical management with chemotherapy alone may yield a solid fusion in 65% to 79% of cases.[11,12,113]

The choice of graft material is based on considerations of graft incorporation and structural support. The grafts used most frequently are iliac crest and ribs. Fibular grafts provide good structural support, but the large amount of cortical bone is undesirable in cases of infection. In addition, long segments of fibula are likely to fracture. In a study of 4-cm-long canine fibular grafts, the grafts were markedly weakened between 6 weeks and 6 months after implantation. The total incorporation may take several years; at 48 weeks, approximately 60% of the necrotic matrix had been remodeled. Despite that, the strength of the graft is nearly normal at 1 year.[197] Bradford and Daher[198] described the use of vascularized rib grafts for stabilization of kyphosis. Incorporation of the grafts occurred between 4 weeks and 16 weeks (mean, 8.5 weeks). They described three patients in whom the graft was placed 4 cm or more anterior to the apical vertebra for mechanical advantage; none of these grafts fractured.[198] High fusion rates have been reported when vascularized rib grafts are used in the treatment of TB kyphosis.[199]

Kemp and colleagues[185] found that rib grafting was inadequate in adults. They reported a 32% incidence of graft fracture and a mean increase in kyphosis of 20 degrees. Partial collapse occurred in some cases because the ribs penetrated the endplate. The overall fusion rate was 62% with rib grafts and 94.5% when autogenous, full-thickness iliac crest grafts were inserted as long as they crossed the coronal diameter of the vertebra.[185] Iliac crest may be preferable to rib, especially in patients with large defects.[185,188,196]

McCuen described the first case of TB spondylitis treated by laminectomy in 1882. In the early part of the twentieth century, it had become a common procedure for patients with Pott paraplegia. In 1935, Seddon condemned the procedure, claiming that "laminectomy is futile" because it removes the integrity of the posterior arch and may lead to instability and further neurologic damage.[190] The opinion that laminectomy is contraindicated is shared by many authors.[186,315,316,319,341,364,375,391] Patients actually may improve considerably immediately after laminectomy. As Bosworth and colleagues[361] noted, however, paraplegia inevitably recurs unless fusion is performed both anteriorly and posteriorly. They described 14 patients who had had laminectomies: all died except 4, who had "circumduction" fusions.[361] Currently, the only indication for laminectomy in the treatment of Pott paraplegia is atypical disease involving the neural arch and causing posterior spinal cord compression.[155,186,190,314,333] It is also reasonable in rare circumstances with posterior epidural tuberculoma without bony involvement.[332]

Debridement, decompression, and fusion in the thoracic spine may be performed through a transthoracic approach, through a costotransversectomy, or by an extrapleural anterolateral approach. The last has the theoretical benefit of avoiding the TB empyema.[375] However, no studies have demonstrated any actual advantage of an extrapleural approach over a standard thoracotomy. Kirkaldy-Willis and Thomas[189] demonstrated that the transthoracic approach is more successful than lateral rachiotomy (modified costotransversectomy). The fusion rate was 95% in the former and 78% in the latter; the mortality was 3% and 8%, respectively.[189] They recommended thoracotomy in cases of early TB, with lateral rachiotomy reserved for late-onset paraplegia associated with a large kyphotic deformity requiring lateral exposure of the dura.[189] Kemp and colleagues[185] support this concept.

With TB, the periosteum is generally thicker and frequently adherent to the pleura. Therefore, it is often necessary to dissect in a subperiosteal plane for exposure. If a lung abscess is found at the time of thoracotomy, the abscess may be debrided by scooping out the necrotic material. Yau and Hodgson[392] rarely found an air leak in this situation and had good success by insufflating the cavity with streptomycin and suturing the visceral pleura. Because of the potential for wound dehiscence in these patients, who are frequently immunocompromised and have poor wound-healing potential, the wounds should be closed in layers with interrupted nonabsorbable sutures. In patients with lesions involving

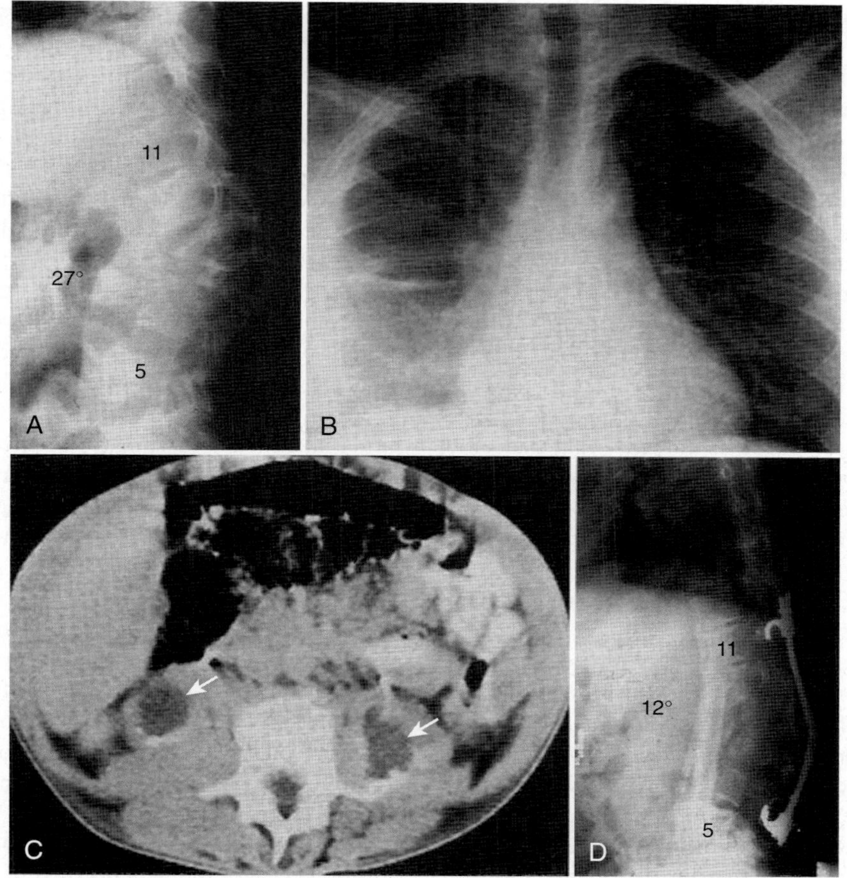

FIG. 87.18 This patient presented with intermittent fevers and spine deformity. He complained only of relatively minor spine pain. He was neurologically intact. Tuberculosis was suspected and confirmed by culture. (A) This lateral radiograph shows a 27-degree kyphosis from the inferior portion of T12 to the superior endplate of L5. The intervening vertebrae are grossly destroyed. (B) An anteroposterior chest radiograph reveals chronic changes in the right lung and an effusion, which are also consistent with tuberculosis. (C) Computed tomography (CT) scan of the lumbar spine reveals bilateral psoas abscesses (*arrows*). There is also a significant paraspinal mass, which is most likely granulation tissue. This was later verified at surgery. (D) This postoperative lateral radiograph reveals that the kyphosis at the thoracolumbar spine has been reduced to 12 degrees. The intervening neural elements have been decompressed with complete corpectomies from T12 through L4. The patient's fibula was used for an autogenous bone graft and supplemented with autogenous cancellous iliac bone graft. The patient remained neurologically intact. At the time of surgery, gross purulence was found, which corresponded with the psoas abscesses identified on the CT scan.

more than two vertebral bodies, a period of bed rest followed by external support in a TLSO is recommended until the fusion becomes consolidated if instrumentation is not used.[196]

Posterior fusion alone, without instrumentation, does not control progressive kyphosis,[393] but it may be performed in addition to anterior strut grafting for added stability (Fig. 87.18).[196,201] If a laminectomy is performed for posterior neural compression, a fusion should also be performed if any of the facets are removed.[186] Progressive kyphosis may occur in the immature spine in spite of a solid anterior fusion. Some authors recommend that a posterior fusion should be performed in addition to an anterior fusion in order to eliminate the risk of increasing deformity.[186,366] Fountain and colleagues[386] found that progressive kyphosis developed in only 3 of 31 children with solid anterior fusions. They recommended performing a supplementary posterior fusion only if progressive deformity is noted.

Anterior grafts may not provide stable fixation, especially in cases in which the graft spans more than two disc spaces.[196] To prevent loss of correction, some authors recommend a two-stage procedure with an instrumented posterior fusion followed by anterior debridement and fusion.[358,394,395] Moon and colleagues[394] reported on 39 adults undergoing the two-stage procedure in the same operative setting or in a delayed fashion. The infection was cured in all cases, and they achieved excellent deformity correction without a prior anterior release. The loss of correction did not exceed 3 degrees. Similarly good results have been reported by other groups from various countries, such as Taiwan, South Africa, India, Kuwait, and Turkey.[396–400]

Güven and colleagues[401] recommend a single-stage posterior approach without any anterior procedure in cases without paralysis, multisegmental involvement, or large abscesses. They reported on 10 patients who underwent the procedure.

All patients had resolution of the infection and the mean loss of correction was only 3.4 degrees. Mehta and Bhojraj[402] have proposed a reasonable classification system for surgical treatment of patients with thoracic spine infection. They propose four treatment groups on the basis of the location of the infection. Group A patients, who had paradiscal or central involvement with no deformity, were treated with transthoracic debridement and strut fusion with no further instrumentation. Group B patients, who had paradiscal or central involvement along with deformity, were treated with transthoracic debridement and strut fusion with posterior instrumentation. Group C patients were similar to group A patients but were too ill to tolerate a transthoracic approach. These patients were treated via a posterior transpedicular decompression and posterior instrumentation. Group D patients, who had only posterior element involvement but no deformity were treated with posterior decompression alone with no fusion or instrumentation. With these treatment guidelines, all their patients did well.[402]

Oga and colleagues[403] studied the risk of using spinal instrumentation despite active TB infection. All 11 of their patients had resolution of the infection and none developed a kyphotic deformity after operation. They also evaluated the adherence properties of *Mycobacterium tuberculosis* and *S. epidermidis* to stainless steel. The *Staphylococcus* heavily colonized the rods and was covered with a thick biofilm, whereas only a few biofilm-covered colonies of *M. tuberculosis* were seen. These findings have prompted the use of anterior instrumentation at the time of initial anterior debridement. Three recent reports reveal that this single-stage technique is efficacious. Benli and colleagues[404] reported on 63 patients from Turkey with involvement of the thoracic and lumbar spines. All patients underwent anterior debridement and decompression with autogenous iliac crest strut grafting. In the same setting, a lateral plate was applied. Kyphosis was corrected by 89% and maintained at an average follow-up of 51 months. Of the patients who had neurologic deficit, 80% had full recovery and 16% had partial recovery. No recurrence of infection was found. Govender reported on 41 patients from South Africa.[405] In these patients, the anterior strut was fresh-frozen allograft. Compared with autogenous rib graft, the fusion rate was slower with allograft. Fusion and remodeling was seen in 33 of 41 patients and partial remodeling with fusion in 8 patients at a mean follow-up of 6.4 years. There were no cases of fracture or late sepsis. Yilmaz and colleagues[406] reported on 22 patients from Turkey with similar results.

The incidence of cord compression with cervical TB spondylitis is more than 40% overall and much higher in adults[348]; therefore, an infection in this region requires aggressive treatment. Hsu and Leong[348] reported excellent results from using the Hong Kong procedure via a Southwick-Robinson approach in conjunction with medical management. With C1–C2 involvement, drainage may be performed by the transoral route with or without a supplementary posterior occiput-to-C2 fusion.[378] Isolated involvement of the arch of the atlas has been treated successfully in one case by chemotherapy, needle aspiration of an abscess, and halo-brace immobilization.[407] Lesions at the craniocervical junction are rare, occurring in only 0.3% to 1% of patients with TB spondylitis.[408] Behari and colleagues[408] reported on 25 patients treated variably for craniocervical infection. They classified patients as grade I, defined by neck pain only and no pyramidal signs; grade II, defined by a neurologic status of independent but with minor disability; grade III, defined by partial disability requiring assistance with activities of daily living; and grade IV, defined by severe disability, including respiratory compromise. Grade I and grade II patients were treated with brace immobilization and medical therapy. Grade III and grade IV patients underwent anterior decompression followed by posterior fusion. Significant improvements in all grades were seen with this strategy.

Lesions between C3 and C7 may be approached through either the anterior triangle[187] or the posterior triangle. The latter may be preferable in some cases because pus often tracks and points in the posterior triangle, making dissection easier.[409] When cervical disease is complicated by kyphosis, staged procedures may be necessary. Strut grafting may be performed at the time of debridement if the deformity can be reduced. If the deformity is too great, traction may be necessary before final anterior grafting. Anterior reconstruction should be followed by posterior stabilization and fusion.[378] Laminectomies are contraindicated in the cervical spine because subluxation and further neurologic deficits may occur.[348]

Complications of surgical treatment are frequent. The operative risk is greatest in elderly patients with extensive disease. In one series, the operative mortality was 2.9% and an additional 1% of the patients died of the disease later.[10] Early complications include wound sepsis, pleural effusion, pulmonary embolism, CSF fistula into the pleural cavity, ileus, progressive neurologic deficit, damage to the ureter, loss of graft fixation or graft fracture, atelectasis, pneumonia, air leak, Horner syndrome, and injury to one of the great vessels.[194] When streptomycin is placed directly on exposed dura, convulsions may occur.[194] Late complications include graft resorption, graft fracture, nonunion, and progressive kyphosis.[185,196,410] Adrenal insufficiency may occur secondary to TB involvement of the adrenal glands. Adrenal suppression should be suspected, especially if calcification is noted on radiographic studies.[316]

Prognosis

With TB spondylitis, the prognosis depends on the age and general health of the patient, the severity and duration of the neurologic deficit, and the treatment selected.

Mortality

Before the advent of chemotherapy, the mortality rate in patients treated nonoperatively was 12% to 43%.[5,314,317,362] The rate in patients with a neurologic deficit was close to 60%.[315] In one study, the mortality rate was found to be linked directly to associated pulmonary involvement: 9.4% of the patients with spine infections and inactive pulmonary TB died in contrast to 51.3% of those who had active pulmonary disease or metastatic spread to other organs.[310] Attempted debridement of the spine without antibiotic coverage was associated with a mortality rate as high as 71%.[362] With the chemotherapeutic regimens now available, the mortality rate should be less than 5% if the disease is diagnosed early, the patients comply with the regimen, and follow-up is close.[321,322] The mortality rate in patients treated with the Hong Kong procedure in addition to antibiotics is directly proportional to the severity of the neurologic deficit. In one study, among patients undergoing operation, the mortality rate was 2% in those with mild to moderate neurologic deficit, 6% in those with moderate neurologic deficit, and 11% in those with a severe deficit.[321]

Relapse

The relapse rate in patients treated with the antibiotics available between 1952 and 1962 was 21%.[312] With current medical regimens and close follow-up, the rate should approach zero.[322]

Kyphosis

Progressive kyphosis is a significant cosmetic deformity, but more important is the fact that it may cause a neurologic deficit or respiratory and cardiac failure due to restriction of pulmonary function (Fig. 87.19). Rajasekaran and Soundarapandian reported the results of a prospective controlled study performed in collaboration with the Medical Research Council.[196] The treatment groups included chemotherapy alone for either 6 or 9 months or radical surgery in combination with 6 months of chemotherapy. Ninety patients (98% of the study group) were followed for a minimum of 6 years. Those who underwent nonoperative treatment had a statistically significant higher rate of kyphotic deformity than those treated surgically. There was a direct correlation between the final angle of the deformity and the amount of initial loss of vertebral body. The angle increased severely in 10% of the surgical group and in 32% of the nonsurgical group. Severe deformity in the surgical group was related to graft failure.

To predict the angle of deformity expected, the researchers devised a formula[410]; $Y = a + bX$, in which Y is the final angle of the deformity, X is the amount of initial loss of vertebral body, and a and b are constants (5.5 and 30.5, respectively). With their formula, the final angle of the gibbus was predictable, with 90% accuracy in the patients treated nonsurgically.[410] If the predicted angle is excessive, early operation should be considered.

Rajasekaran and Soundarapandian[196] provided additional information on 81 patients treated by the Hong Kong operation and followed for a minimum of 8 years; 19% of these patients had an increase in the gibbus angle of up to 20 degrees, and in 22% it was more than 20 degrees. The major risk factor for increasing deformity was extensive involvement of the vertebral bodies, which resulted in a large defect after debridement and necessitated a graft spanning more than two disc spaces. Patients with lesions of the thoracic vertebrae and those with marked kyphosis preoperatively were also more likely to have progression. These authors concluded that when the length of the graft exceeds two disc spaces, surgical treatment should be augmented by prolonged bed rest, bracing, or posterior arthrodesis. Rib strut grafts were used in many of the patients with progressive deformities, and it was proposed that iliac crest graft may be preferable in patients with large defects.[196] Iliac crest grafts were used exclusively by Hodgson and Stock[188] and may explain the low incidence of progressive kyphosis in their series. Others also have recommended the use of iliac crest grafts rather than

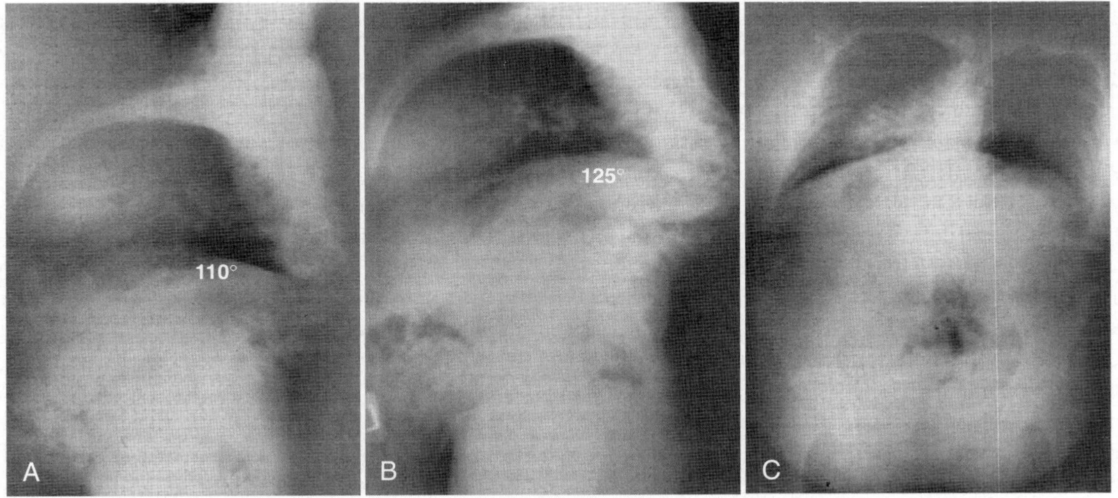

FIG. 87.19 This young adult patient was known to have had tuberculosis of the spine as a child. At this time, she presented with a history of spine pain that was relieved with bed rest and aggravated by increasing activities. (A) At the time of first presentation, the patient was seen to have a kyphosis of 110 degrees. It is apparent that she has had extreme shortening of the trunk due to the combination of kyphosis and vertebral body destruction. (B) Over a period of 5 years, it can be seen that the patient has had an increase in the kyphosis from 110 degrees to 125 degrees. At this point, she remained neurologically normal. (C) This anteroposterior radiograph of the thoracic and lumbar spine is consistent with the gross deformity seen on the lateral radiographs and obvious on clinical inspection. This is the type of deformity that is best prevented with surgical intervention.

rib struts.[185] In patients with small defects, however, the availability of rib graft and avoidance of additional donor site problems make rib grafts a more attractive alternative.

In addition to graft failure, children are at risk of progressive deformity after anterior debridement and fusion because of persistent growth posteriorly and growth retardation anteriorly. Close follow-up is necessary and a supplementary posterior fusion should be performed if progressive kyphosis occurs.[201,386] A study comparing the radiographs of 117 children operated on for spinal tuberculosis at the age of 2 to 6 years showed that anterior fusion alone leads to greater kyphotic angulation than a posterior fusion, a combined anterior and posterior fusion, or anterior debridement alone.[411]

Neurologic Deficit

Patients with neurologic deficit may improve spontaneously without surgery or chemotherapy[317,341] or with chemotherapy alone,[12,14,312] but in general the prognosis is improved with early surgery.[201,285,322] In one study, 94% of neurologically impaired patients recovered normal function after anterior decompression; only 79% totally recovered after nonoperative management.[322] When patients with a neurologic deficit were operated on only if they failed to respond to an initial course of antibiotics, the overall success rate was 78.5%.[14] As expected, patients with less severe neurologic deficit and those who were treated early after the development of neurologic signs had a better outcome.[14,308,311,319,321,412] In one study of 64 patients, only 48% of those with severe neurologic deficits recovered, whereas 83% of patients with moderate deficits recovered; only 4 of 10 patients with late-onset paraplegia had a satisfactory recovery.[321]

Patients with paraplegia of long duration should be treated aggressively. Hodgson and colleagues[319] found that the chances of complete recovery are good after surgical treatment, although it may take longer for them to recover. They documented recovery in a patient who had had a neurologic deficit for 5 years.[319] In patients with late-onset paraplegia, the response to operation is faster, better, and safer in patients who have active disease than in those with healed disease and a hard, bony ridge compressing the cord.[342] Overall, most patients with a neurologic deficit recover within 6 months, but those who have direct involvement of the meninges (pachymeningitis) may recover more slowly.[319] Govender and colleagues[308] found that patients who have an atrophic cord as seen on CT myelography preoperatively usually do poorly after decompression. Patients with cervical spine involvement are at high risk of neurologic deficit but do well after anterior debridement and fusion.[348]

The only indication for laminectomy is posterior cord involvement. In 19 patients with posterior element disease undergoing laminectomy, 16 had good results and 3 had fair results in one series. Six of 10 patients undergoing laminectomy for epidural tuberculomas without bony involvement had good results, 3 patients had fair results, and 1 had a poor result.[332] The overall prognosis with posterior spinal TB is better in those patients who have less severe neurologic deformity of shorter duration, slower progression, and are younger and in good general health.[335] In general, children have a better prognosis than adults.[185,201,318,319]

Fusion

Bosworth and colleagues[315] thought that a solid fusion was essential for permanent recovery from TB spondylitis. They described five patients who initially recovered but became paralyzed again with the development of pseudarthrosis. These patients recovered once again after repair of the pseudarthrosis.[315]

Spontaneous bony fusion occurred in 27% of patients treated with bed rest in a plaster shell, without surgery or chemotherapy.[314] With chemotherapy alone, spontaneous fusion occurred in 24% at 18 months and in 36% at 36 months.[366] In the prospective study by the Medical Research Council, the fusion rate in patients treated by the Hong Kong procedure was 28% by 6 months, 70% by 12 months, 85% by 18 months, and 92% at 5 years. The corresponding values for the patients undergoing debridement without fusion were 3%, 23%, 52%, and 84%, and the fusion rates in patients treated by ambulatory chemotherapy alone were 9%, 26%, 50%, and 85%, respectively.

Actinomycosis

Actinomyces israelii is an anaerobic, slowly growing, filamentous, gram-positive bacterium. *Actinomyces* was originally discovered in 1877 as a genus containing the causative agent of actinomycosis in cattle. Thereafter, in 1891, *A. israelii* was first isolated from a lung abscess by Wolff and Israel.[413] Since then, other *Actinomyces* species and related bacteria have been isolated and are believed to be involved in a wide variety of human infections, most commonly linked to *A. israelii*. A number of other species have also been involved in human infections. These include *Actinomyces meyeri, Actinomyces graevenitzii, Actinomyces turicensis, Actinomyces gerencseriae, Actinomyces odontolyticus, Actinomyces cardiffensis, Actinomyces radingae, Actinomyces naeslundii*, other *Actinomyces* species, and a closely related species, *Varibaculum cambriensis*.[413] It is postulated that the coexistence of other organisms may assist anaerobic growth by reducing the oxygen tension in the local environment.

The diseases it causes mimic those produced by fungi. The organism, an endogenous, oral saprophyte, requires trauma, surgery, or other infection to penetrate the mucosa. Once *Actinomyces* invades the tissue of a disrupted mucus membrane, it slowly expands and develops into an abscess. It is noted for causing chronic suppurative infections with external sinuses that discharge distinctive aggregates of organisms ("sulfur granules").[306,414] Infections involving *Actinomyces* frequently are polymicrobic, including *Fusobacterium, Bacteroides, Capnocytophaga, Eikenella, Staphylococcus, Streptococcus,* and *Enterococcus* species.[414]

The lesions are characterized by hard, fibrotic walls with granulation tissue surrounding loculations of pus. Sinus tracts extending to the skin or into other organs are commonly seen in more chronic infections.[414] Classic actinomycosis presents as an oral-cervicofacial lesion, known as "lumpy jaw" lesion, which occurs in approximately 55% of actinomycosis cases.[415] Infection occurs at other sites and is manifest as thoracic (15%), abdominal and pelvic (20%), musculoskeletal (rare), and central nervous system (rare) disease.[82]

Several risk factors for the development of actinomycosis exist. It occurs more commonly in males, but there is no clear explanation for this. Other risk factors may include poor oral hygiene and the use of intrauterine devices. In addition, immunocompromise and other conditions such as diabetes, alcoholism, infections with immunosuppressive agents (e.g., HIV), and steroid use are thought to predispose individuals to the development of actinomycosis.[413,417]

Before 1950, vertebral actinomycosis was the most common form of osseous involvement. Vertebral involvement is usually secondary to an infection at an adjacent tissue. Hematogenous spread is less common for actinomycosis. Vertebral infection occurs by extension from retropharyngeal, mediastinal, or retroperitoneal soft tissue abscesses. Unlike *M. tuberculosis,* the organism has a predilection for the cervical and thoracic spine from retropharyngeal or pulmonary spread.[418,419]

Actinomycosis may be difficult to differentiate from mycobacterial and nocardial infections. Accurate diagnosis is essential because the treatment regimens differ markedly from these other organisms. The organism must be isolated from an anaerobic culture, which may take up to 21 days for positive culture growth. As in tuberculosis, the radiographs may demonstrate prominent paraspinal abscesses and involvement of several vertebral bodies. Distinctive features include simultaneous vertebral body and posterior element involvement, spread to adjacent ribs, periosteal new bone formation outlining the vertebra, and a mixture of lytic and sclerotic changes that may produce a honeycomb appearance of the bone.[82] The vertebral body collapse and disc space narrowing that are common in TB are uncommon in actinomycosis.[82]

Epidural abscesses may occur by extension from a vertebral source or through an intervertebral foramen from a cervical, pulmonary, or abdominal focus.[414] The dura generally resists penetration, but neurologic deficit may occur by epidural compression.[414] Before the introduction of penicillin, most cases of actinomycosis were fatal. The current treatment is still penicillin in large doses given over extended periods in association with abscess drainage and excision of sinus tracts when necessary.[414] Other first-line antibiotics that are effective are tetracycline, erythromycin, clindamycin, and the cephalosporins.[420,421] Long-term treatment for up to 6 months is common.[419] When response to penicillin is poor, the possible reasons include an undrained abscess, polymicrobial infection, and perhaps bacterial resistance. Overall, the treatment of actinomycosis infection results in good outcomes, even when there is extensive involvement. In a recent case report of a patient with severe mediastinal, paraspinal, and thoracic epidural involvement, limited debridement and laminectomy combined with antibiotics yielded excellent results.[422]

Nocardiosis

Nocardia asteroides is the most common human pathogen in this family of aerobic, weakly gram-positive bacteria. It is a natural soil saprophyte often found in decaying organic matter.[307] Infection most commonly occurs through the respiratory tract, although other modes of infection may occur. This infection is now seen most frequently in immunocompromised hosts. The predisposing factors are long-term corticosteroid use, chronic lung disease, hematologic malignancies, and organ transplant patients. Renal transplant patients are particularly susceptible, with a reported incidence as high as 5%.[423,424] Nocardiosis may initiate a chronic granulomatous response, but more frequently the histologic features are suppurative necrosis and abscess formation, typical of pyogenic infections.[414]

The most frequent primary site is the pulmonary system, but dissemination occurs frequently to the central nervous system, skin and subcutaneous tissues, eyes (especially the retina), kidneys, joints, and heart in up to 56% of cases.[425,426] Dissemination to the brain, meninges, and spinal cord occurs in 23%, but hematogenous involvement of the vertebrae is uncommon.[427] In a recent literature review and case report, Graat and colleagues[428] found only 11 cases of *Nocardia* spinal osteomyelitis reported in 40 years. Epidural spinal cord compression from vertebral osteomyelitis has been reported.[429,430]

Diagnosis of nocardiosis can be difficult because there are no pathognomonic signs or symptoms. Historically, phenotypic characteristics in conjunction with antibiotic susceptibility patterns have been used for diagnosis. These tests suffered from poor reliability. Current methods of identification rely on gene sequencing, particularly of the 16S rRNA gene, which has become the gold standard.[431] Rapidly growing bacteria in mixed cultures may obscure the growth of *Nocardia* species, and the laboratory should be alerted if *Nocardia* infection is suspected.

Sulfonamides, in conjunction with appropriate surgery, have been the mainstay of treatment since 1944. Many other antibiotics—including minocycline, trimethoprim-sulfamethoxazole, amikacin, imipenem, ceftriaxone, cefuroxime, and cefotaxime—have been used either alone or in combination. The most common first-line therapy is cotrimoxazole, with imipenem and amikacin as second-line therapies.[432,433] The optimal duration of therapy is uncertain but, because of the possibility of relapse, treatment is often continued for many months after apparent cure. A poor response to treatment may be related to the presence of a second pathogen.

Brucellosis

Human brucellosis remains an important public health problem in most developing countries, including those of the Mediterranean, Balkans, Middle East, Central Asia, and Central and South America. The occurrence is high when there is ineffective eradication of brucellosis in animals.[434–436] Brucellosis is caused by an aerobic, gram-negative coccobacillus commonly found in domestic animals and transmitted to humans by direct contact, by ingestion of contaminated products, and possibly, by inhalation of aerosols.[306,437,438] The disease affects approximately 500,000 persons per year worldwide. Its incidence is decreasing throughout the United States, primarily because of pasteurization of milk. In 1976,

$75.6 million were spent to maintain the brucellosis control program and the incidence in the United States is now less than 0.5 cases per 100,000 population.[439] The causative organisms include *Brucella abortus* (cattle), *Brucella melitensis* (goats), *Brucella suis* (swine), and *Brucella canis* (dogs).

Brucellosis mainly affects the musculoskeletal system, with the spine as the most common location.[440,441] The infection spreads via lymphatics and blood vessels and produces acute systemic infection, as well as chronic relapsing disease (undulant fever). Involvement in joints tends to occur during acute infections, whereas spinal manifestations tend to occur during chronic infections.[436,442,443]

The clinical presentation of patients with brucellosis varies widely. After an incubation period of days to several weeks, low-grade fever, weakness, headaches, lymphadenopathy, hepatosplenomegaly, and generalized musculoskeletal complaints may develop insidiously.[306,444] Approximately one-third of the patients have a more fulminant illness with acute onset of systemic toxicity.[445] Some infections are asymptomatic initially. After the initial illness, which may last for several days to weeks, relapses occur in about 5% of patients. Relapses seldom occur in patients who receive appropriate treatment and are often the result of focal suppurative complications, such as spondylitis.[445] The classic feature of an undulating fever is not present in most cases.[437,445] Late complications may affect almost any organ system and include septic arthritis, central nervous system involvement, osteomyelitis, and spine infection. The statistics on brucellosis vary widely depending on the source of the information. Between 11% and 80% of patients with brucellosis have bone and joint involvement and, of these, 6% to 54% have spinal column involvement,[438,444–447] most commonly in the lumbar spine.[306,437] Localized spine pain is the earliest sign of spondylitis.[437] Of those with spondylitis, between 10% and 43% have some degree of neurologic compromise,[438,444] and in 10% to 20%, a paraspinal abscess develops. This may occur with other system signs such as fever, hepatomegaly, and splenomegaly. Osteoarticular infections have a genetic predisposition and are associated with HLA-B39.[436,442,443]

In one series of 593 patients with brucellosis, neurologic deficits occurred in five of the patients with cervical spondylitis, two of the patients with thoracic involvement, and nine of the patients with lumbar disease. The patients with cervical and thoracic disease had significantly more paraspinal and epidural abscesses than the patients with lumbar infection. Patients with cervical spine involvement had a much worse prognosis than those with disease in other areas.[446]

Blood cultures are positive in less than half the cases overall but are positive in 70% of patients with acute *B. melitensis* infection.[437,438] An agglutination reaction with a *Brucella* antibody titer of 1:160 or greater is presumptive evidence of infection, but an increasing titer is a more helpful sign of active infection.[437,438] If *B. canis* infection is suspected, a specific agglutination test must be used because the standard test does not react with antibodies against *B. canis*. When blood cultures are combined with serologic tests, the diagnostic yield is high. Colmenero and colleagues[448] reported on 105 cases of brucellar spondylitis. In only five cases (4%) was a bone biopsy necessary for diagnosis. This is in contrast to pyogenic and TB spondylitis, for which bone biopsies were required in 50% and 75%, respectively, to confirm the diagnosis.

The characteristic radiologic features of brucellar spondylitis include predilection for the lower lumbar spine, intact vertebral architecture despite evidence of diffuse vertebral osteomyelitis, disc space involvement, minimal associated paraspinal soft tissue involvement, and absence of gibbus deformity.[438,449,450] The facet joints are often involved in brucellar infections, which can be readily seen on gadolinium-enhanced MRI.[451] Bone destruction is less severe than in TB spondylitis.[452] Bone scintigraphy is not helpful in differentiating brucellar from tubercular spondylitis. The MRI findings are similar in the two, except that tuberculosis often produces more severe changes with more deformity and abscess formation.[450]

The current World Health Organization treatment of choice for brucellosis is doxycycline at 200 mg/day and rifampin at 600 to 900 mg/day for at least 6 weeks.[445] A randomized, double-blind study comparing doxycycline plus rifampin with doxycycline plus streptomycin for 45 days showed that the latter was more effective for treatment of spondylitis.[453] Some authors recommend that treatment should be continued for at least 3 months in cases of spondylitis because high relapse rates have been reported with shorter courses.[438] After single-agent therapy with tetracycline, streptomycin, rifampin, or trimethoprim-sulfamethoxazole, the relapse rates are between 5% and 40%.[445] Response to treatment is monitored with repeated agglutination tests. Lifeso and colleagues[438] recommend continuing antibiotic therapy until the titer is 1:160 or less and there is clinical and radiographic evidence of resolution. Surgery is usually unnecessary.[438] However, Nas and colleagues[454] reported on 11 cases from Turkey: 8 patients required surgical decompression to alleviate neural compression.

Fungal Infections

Some fungi are normal commensals of the body and cause opportunistic infections (e.g., *Candida* and *Aspergillus*). Other fungi are endemic and are limited to specific geographic areas. The two most common endemic fungi that give rise to spinal infections are *Coccidioides immitis* and *Blastomyces dermatitidis*. The former is endemic to parts of the southwestern United States (especially the San Joaquin Valley in central California), Central America, and parts of South America.[306,455] The fungus exists in its mycelial phase in the soil of desert areas. Humans become infected most commonly by inhalation of the spores (conidia) or, less commonly, through abrasions of the skin. Person-to-person transmission is rare. *Blastomyces dermatitidis* is a dimorphic fungus endemic in the southeastern and south central states, especially those bordering the Mississippi and Ohio River basins, and in the Midwestern states that border the Great Lakes. Cases have also been reported in Central and South America, Africa, and the Middle East.[306] *B. dermatitidis* is considered to be an inhabitant of soil, and infection occurs by inhalation of conidia.

Cryptococcus, *Candida*, and *Aspergillus* are found worldwide. *Cryptococcus neoformans* is found in the soil and in pigeon feces. The disease is the fourth most common infection in HIV-infected patients and is found in 1% to 5% of organ transplant recipients. *Candida* species are part of the normal flora and are commonly found on the skin and in the gastrointestinal (GI) tract. These sites are believed to be the most likely ports of entry into the bloodstream. *Candida* species are also commonly found in sputum, the female genital tract, and the urine of patients with indwelling urinary catheters. Human-to-human transmission is possible, but most infections are endogenous.[456–458] *Aspergillus* species are ubiquitous saprophytic fungi that produce numerous small spores (2–4 μm in diameter). The small size of the spores allows for ready dispersion onto air currents from contaminated air-handling systems and deposition into human lung alveoli.[459] Spores are frequently found in water, soil, decaying vegetation, hay, and grains.

Fungal infections of the spine are uncommon. They frequently occur in immunosuppressed hosts with multiple medical problems. Often, there is a long delay in diagnosis, mainly because other medical conditions may mask the diagnosis and because fungal spondylitis characteristically runs an indolent course.[460] In one series of 11 cases, the source of infection was hematogenous seeding from septic episodes in five, postoperative osteomyelitis in three, local extension from an adjacent fungal infection in two, and direct traumatic implantation in one.[460] The incidence of fungal infections has risen markedly in recent years. Several factors have contributed to this increase. These include greater use of immunosuppressive drugs, prolonged use of broad-spectrum antibiotics, widespread use of indwelling catheters, and AIDS.

Because presenting features can be nonspecific, mycotic spine infections can be difficult to recognize in the early stages. In addition, diagnostic and susceptibility testing methods for fungi have not progressed as quickly as those for bacteria. As such, institution of appropriate treatment is often delayed, which can lead to poor patient outcome. Definitive diagnosis rests on the evaluation of a tissue specimen. Biopsies must be evaluated with fungal stains as well as cultures because the latter may be negative or take several weeks or months before identification is possible. Closed biopsy was reported to be positive in only 50% of cases, whereas open biopsy was positive in all cases in the series of Campbell and colleagues.[460]

Laboratory Studies

A rise in inflammatory markers—such as white cell count, ESRs, and CRP levels—can alert the physician to the possibility of a spinal infection. However, these are not specific for fungal infections. Antibody tests are seldom helpful in the diagnosis of spinal infections due to ubiquitous fungi such as *Candida* and *Aspergillus.* Because these are sometimes normal commensals, previous exposures can elicit antibody formation and reduce the sensitivity and specificity of these tests. Several tests are commercially available. The Platelia *Aspergillus* assay (Bio-Rad, Marnes-la-Coquette, France) is a commercial kit with relatively high sensitivity to *Aspergillus* galactomannan antigen.[461] This test is one of the most sensitive methods currently available for detection of this fungus. The Platelia *Aspergillus* assay, however, has a false-positive rate ranging from 1% to 18%.[462] Several commercial kits are also available for detection of *Candida* species antigens. These also have limitations in sensitivity or specificity, or both.[462] In general, repeated serum sampling can improve sensitivity for antigen detection tests.[463] Detection of cryptococcal capsular polysaccharide antigen by latex agglutination procedure is a rapid serodiagnostic test. Rheumatoid factor, however, can also cause agglutination, leading to a false-positive result. The PREMIER Cryptococcal antigen assay (Meridian Diagnostics) does not react with rheumatoid factor, gives fewer false-positive reactions, and is helpful in diagnosis of the disease.[464]

The detection of fungal nucleic acid via PCR holds promise as a diagnostic tool. So far, the technology has demonstrated high sensitivity and specificity for detecting isolates of *Candida* and *Aspergillus.*[465,466] The technology not only allows for the rapid identification and subtyping of fungi but it also enables monitoring of clinical progress.[467–470] Disadvantages include the inability to distinguish between normal colonization and active infection. A false-positive result can also be obtained from specimen contamination due to the high sensitivity of the PCR assay.[462]

Histology

Biopsy and histopathologic assessments are critical in the diagnosis of fungal infections. Accurate diagnosis is dependent on the skill of the pathologist and adequacy of organisms received in aspirates or tissue biopsies. Further identification can be aided by other methods, such as the carbohydrate-assimilation test for *Candida* and the phenol oxidase reaction for *Cryptococcus.* It is important that microscopic appearances are correlated with microbiology findings as well as other tests for specific host antibodies, fungal antigens, and fungal nucleic acids.

Imaging Studies

Radiographic findings in mycotic spinal infections resemble those of TB: relative sparing of the disc, anterior involvement of the vertebral body, and development of large abscesses (Fig. 87.20). There may be less frequent invasion of adjacent ribs or involvement of the posterior elements and formation of draining sinuses.[82,306] Certain patterns do occur more commonly with certain fungal infections. For instance, paravertebral soft tissue swelling with involvement of the posterior structures is more common in late *Coccidioides* infections (Fig. 87.21).[471] With *Blastomyces,* collapse and gibbus deformity tend to be seen more commonly.[82,306,472] In *Cryptococcus,* lytic lesions within vertebral bodies can resemble those in coccidioidomycosis or the cystic form of TB with discrete margins and surrounding abscess formation (Fig. 87.22). The infection may also appear as a permeative lesion of a single vertebra with collapse.[82] The degree of bone involvement is often advanced compared with a patient's symptoms.

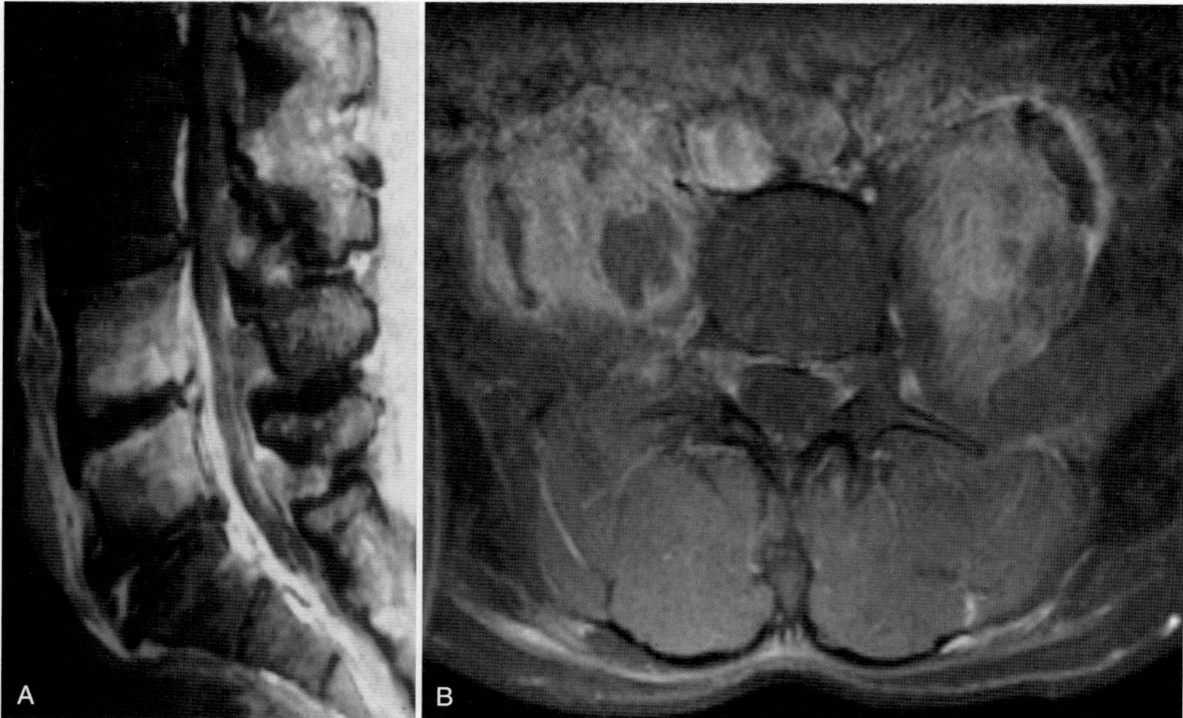

FIG. 87.20 (A) Sagittal and (B) axial gadolinium-enhanced magnetic resonance images of L4–L5 *Aspergillus* infection.

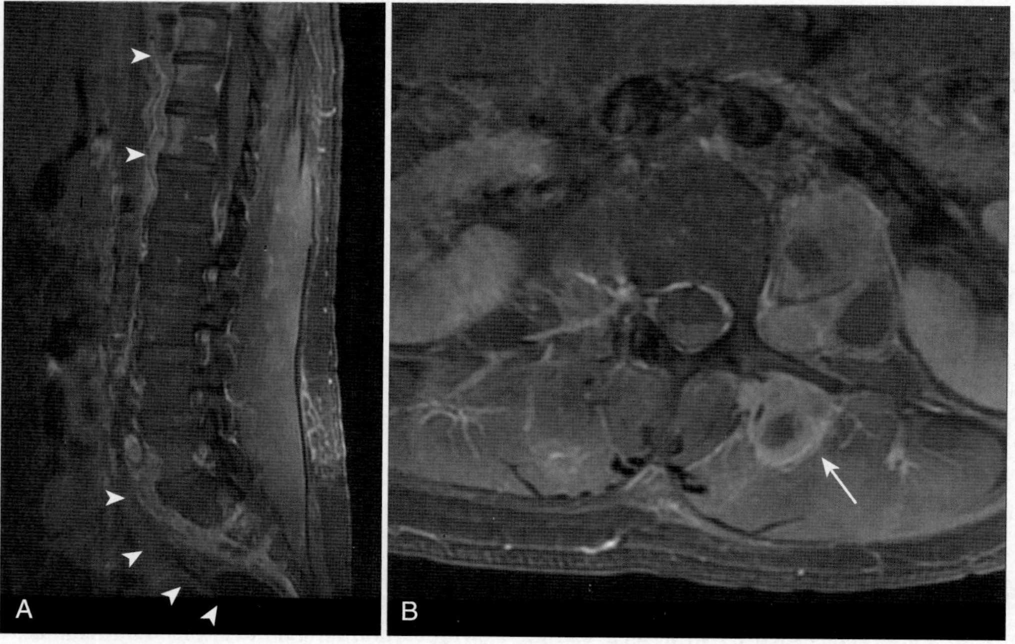

FIG. 87.21 (A) Sagittal and (B) axial gadolinium-enhanced magnetic resonance images showing diffuse, multifocal infection of the lower thoracic spine and sacral region (*arrowheads*) along with large paraspinal abscesses of *Coccidioides immitis* infection. The arrow shows extension into posterior compartment.

In fungal vertebral osteomyelitis, CT and MRI are effective in determining the extent of disease spread. In contrast to pyogenic vertebral osteomyelitis, fungal infections often spare the disc.[473] These changes, however, can be seen in other causes of nonpyogenic vertebral osteomyelitis, such as TB, and are not specific to fungal vertebral osteomyelitis. The CT appearance is often one with holes in the bone, punctuated with small irregular bone islands, contrasted with tumors where bone is completely gone over segments of the vertebra.

Scintigraphic studies can also be helpful in identifying regions of infection, but they cannot differentiate among the various causes of vertebral osteomyelitis. Radionuclide scans

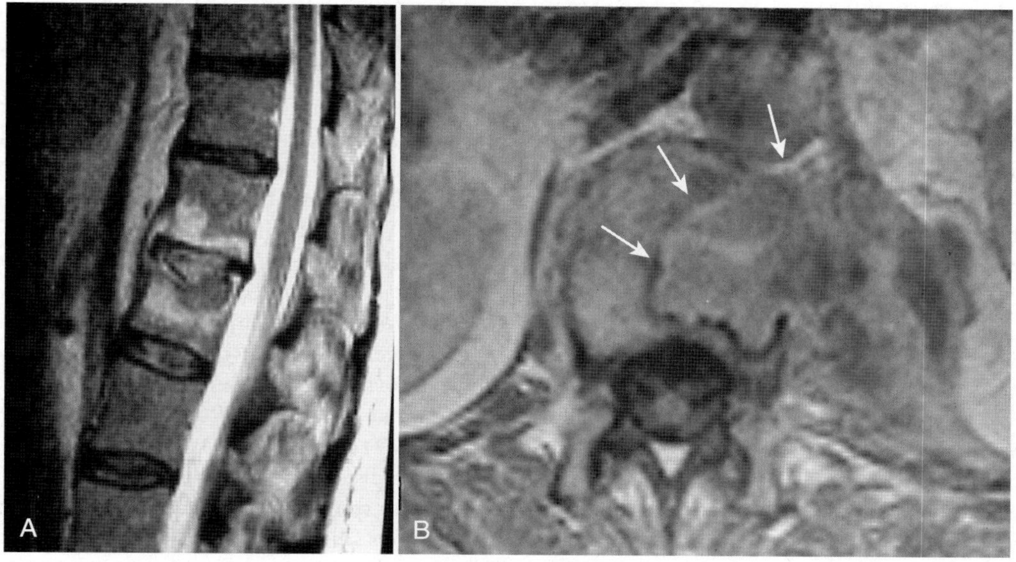

FIG. 87.22 (A) Sagittal and (B) axial gadolinium-enhanced magnetic resonance images of T12–L1 *Cryptococcus neoformans* infection. Vertebral body involvement shows discrete margins along with paraspinal abscess formation (*arrows*).

with technetium-99m compounds are frequently abnormal before changes are seen on plain radiographs and may be useful in the early stages of infection. Isotope uptake occurs in any bone-forming process and is nonspecific for infection. Indium-111-labeled white blood cells are more specific for infection and can be used to differentiate tumor from abscess. These tests are less important since the advent of MRI.

Treatment

The treatment of fungal infection involves correcting any underlying medical conditions that may compromise wound healing or immune defense capabilities. Antifungal agents are the mainstay of treatment, but surgery is often necessary in cases of abscess formation, spinal instability, developing neurologic deficits, or sepsis. The use of newer antifungal medications, including azoles, has improved patient survival rates.[474] The approach should be based on the pathologic features encountered, but in general anterior debridement and stabilization are preferred.[460] The prognosis for patients with fungal vertebral osteomyelitis depends on the organism and the host. As with bacterial infections, it appears that patients with diabetes mellitus or neurologic deficits have a poorer prognosis.[460]

Nonoperative Treatment

Historically, nonsurgical treatment has been met with varied success in the management of fungal spinal infections. Successfully treated patients experience resolution of spine pain and often fuse spontaneously. Nonoperative treatment includes the institution of antifungals, spinal immobilization (cast or bracing), and early ambulation. Consulting an infectious disease specialist is advised because treatment is often prolonged and antifungal agents may be toxic. It has been shown, however, in a rabbit model that both amphotericin B and the lipid formulations of amphotericin B have poor penetration into the intervertebral disc when given IV.[475]

Amphotericin B is a broad-spectrum antifungal that is often used as a first-line agent for fungal spinal infections.[476] It is also recommended in cases of *Blastomyces* that are nonresponsive to oral azoles. It must be administered intravenously, which can be inconvenient, and it possesses nephrotoxicity. The newer lipid formulations are significantly less toxic.

The azoles (e.g., itraconazole, ketoconazole, fluconazole, miconazole) are alternative agents for fungal osteomyelitis.[476–480] In the same rabbit model study discussed earlier, fluconazole had excellent penetration into the intervertebral disc.[475] On the basis of these data, fluconazole might be a better first-choice antifungal agent when a fungus is sensitive to both amphotericin B and fluconazole. The potential side effects of fluconazole are also significantly less than amphotericin B.[475] Itraconazole and ketoconazole are the first-line agents for spinal infections due to *Blastomyces.*[481] Echinocandin and caspofungin are newer promising drugs that are capable of providing higher availability at infected sites with better long-term tolerability.[482,483]

Surgical Treatment

Indications for surgical intervention include relief of spinal cord or nerve root compression, correction of instability and/or deformity, and management of overwhelming infection. Lack of identification of organisms on blood culture, serology, and needle aspirates may necessitate open surgical biopsy. Due to the relative scarcity of reported cases in the literature, the optimal method of surgical treatment is difficult to define. In general, it is accepted that infected tissue should be thoroughly debrided and existing or anticipated spinal instability addressed.

Posterior Decompression Without Fusion

This method of treatment may be advisable only in isolated posterior epidural collections without anterior vertebral element involvement. This is relatively uncommon. In general, when the pathology is located in the anterior vertebral elements, posterior decompression fails to address the problem and may further contribute to instability by removing uninvolved supporting tissue.

Posterior Decompression With Fusion and Instrumentation

Aggressive vertebrectomy via a posterior approach can be challenging and has the potential for anterior column instability. Debridement of the anterior vertebral elements may be accomplished posteriorly through variations of the extracavitary or costotraversectomy approaches. An important advantage of this approach is that it avoids entering the thoracic cavity. The disadvantages are the limited exposure and visualization of the anterior thecal sac.[460] There is also the risk of rupturing a mycotic aneurysm, with little or no ability to control it. Anterior graft placement can also be difficult. Additionally, there is the dilemma of placing instrumentation during the initial surgical debridement close to a contaminated wound. If there is adequate anterior column support, posterior instrumentation and autograft fusion will provide spinal stability and prevent sagittal plane deformity.

Anterior Decompression and Fusion With Posterior Stabilization

Successful vertebrectomy and fusion using anterior strut grafts and posterior instrumentation for fungal vertebral osteomyelitis has been described.[484,485] This can be performed under the same anesthetic, with little risk of infection from the fungal infection posteriorly. The anterior approach also provides the best opportunity of a thorough debridement. In most cases, posterior stabilization is required (Fig. 87.23). This type of treatment is highly successful in the treatment of pyogenic and mycobacterial spinal infections. The effectiveness for the treatment of fungal infections appears to be modest on the basis of the limited information available to date.

Percutaneous Techniques

Percutaneous suction/irrigation systems with adjunctive percutaneous external spinal fixation have been described for the treatment of bacterial vertebral osteomyelitis.[224] These procedures may be alternatives to open instrumentation for disease located between T3 and S1. At present, there are no published cases of fungal spinal infections treated in this manner. Percutaneous techniques in fungal spinal infections have been limited to tissue sampling and for performing therapeutic aspiration.[486,487]

Coccidioidomycosis

Coccidioides immitis infection was first described in 1892 by an Argentinian medical student, Alejandro Posadas.[488] The disease, often referred to as “valley fever,” is localized to geographic regions with arid soil due to high temperatures and low humidity.[489] *C. immitis* is endemic in parts of the southwestern United States (especially the San Joaquin Valley in central California), Central America, and parts of South America.[306,455] Disease prevalence is increasing with the rise in tourism to those countries. The fungus exists in its mycelial phase in the soil of desert areas. The saprophytic cycle includes the formation of spores that become airborne. Humans become infected most commonly by inhalation of the spores or, less commonly, through abrasions of the skin. The spores swell and become spherules, which reproduce by the formation of internal spores known as “endospores.” When the spherule ruptures, endospores are released and each may develop into a new spherule, completing the parasitic cycle. The saprophytic cycle can begin again only when the spores are returned to the soil. The disease is not contagious because person-to-person transmission can occur only in rare circumstances when the fungus reverts from its tissue phase to its airborne form in contaminated secretions.[490]

The primary focus of disease is the lung, but infection may become disseminated in 0.5% of the cases; osseous manifestations occur in 10% to 50% of those with disseminated disease.[491] Histologically, coccidioidomycosis causes a granulomatous tissue reaction resembling TB. Extrapulmonary disease is uncommon if the infection has been quiescent in the year after the initial pulmonary infection, unless the host is immunocompromised.[490] Bone lesions are multifocal in 40% of cases overall and in most cases of vertebral involvement. The bones most commonly involved are the skull, metacarpals, metatarsals, spine, and tibia. Spine infection occurs in 10% to 60% of patients with osseous involvement.[82]

Serum immunoglobulin M precipitins can be detected by a variety of methods. These antibodies occur in 75% of cases 1 to 3 weeks after onset of symptoms of primary infection, and they disappear within 4 months. Skin tests with coccidioidal antigens are positive within 3 weeks after the onset of symptoms. Anergy is common in disseminated coccidioidomycosis; therefore, skin testing is unreliable in systemic disease. A negative skin test in a patient with a primary infection suggests that dissemination will occur.[490] An increased complement-fixing antibody titer indicates disseminated disease. Sixty-one percent of patients with disseminated disease have titers of at least 1:32, and 41% have titers of at least 1:64. In contrast, 95% of patients without disseminated disease have titers below 1:32, and 99% have titers below 1:64.[490]

Spine lesions are frequently multiple (Fig. 87.24) and generally lytic.[82,306,492] Filipinos, African Americans, pregnant women in their third trimester, young children, and elderly individuals are at higher risk of developing disseminated disease.[493] The entire vertebra including the arch is often involved, but the disc is usually spared. Paraspinal masses are frequent, and contiguous rib involvement may be seen.[492] Vertebral collapse occurs late.[492] MRI of coccidioidal spondylitis is nonspecific. Infection may involve a single level, multiple levels, the surrounding soft tissues, and the disc space.[494] The disc may become narrowed; however, the extent of disc space

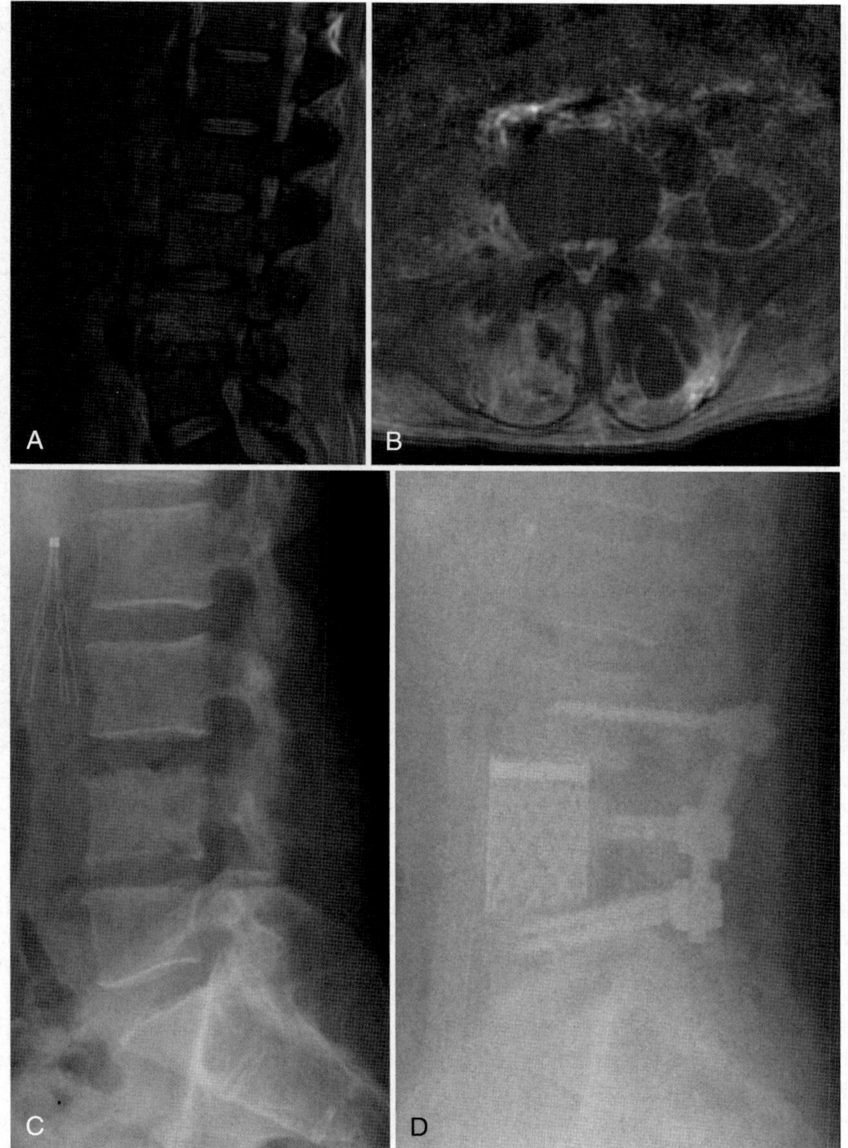

FIG. 87.23 (A) Sagittal and (B) axial gadolinium-enhanced magnetic resonance images of L4 fungal infection showing relative sparing of the disc space along with large multiloculated abscesses in both the anterior psoas compartment and posterior spinous erectae compartment. (C) Plain radiograph shows bony changes of the L4 vertebral body. (D) Surgical treatment included staged debridement of the posterior paraspinal abscesses followed by debridement of the left psoas abscesses, L4 corpectomy, and strut grafting with posterior instrumented fusion.

changes is disproportionately less than the extensive vertebral body and adjacent soft tissue involvement.

Although most patients with primary, localized infection recover without therapy, a small subgroup of patients (<0.5% of cases) will develop severe primary infection with dissemination, which will often involve the spine. Coccidioidomycosis of the spine is a highly aggressive disease that, if not managed appropriately, can lead to significant morbidity and mortality. Treatment regimens limited to systemic antifungal therapy alone, percutaneous drainage of lesions, or limited open debridement have led to poor outcomes with chronic recurrence of disease.[495] The standard treatment of coccidioidomycosis has been a total dose of 1 to 2.5 g of amphotericin B intravenously. Alternative agents include miconazole, an azole available for IV therapy, or the oral azole ketoconazole. The oral triazole drugs, itraconazole and fluconazole, are under evaluation in clinical trials.[490] Itraconazole is now available in both parenteral and oral formulations.[496–499] Reliable absorption of the itraconazole oral solution has been demonstrated in patients with HIV infection, neutropenic patients with hematologic malignancies, bone marrow transplantation patients, and neutropenic children. In clinical trials, the oral form of itraconazole is more effective than the oral forms of fluconazole and amphotericin B.[479,480] In chronic granulomatous disease of childhood, itraconazole is effective as a prophylactic treatment against recurrent fungal infections.[500]

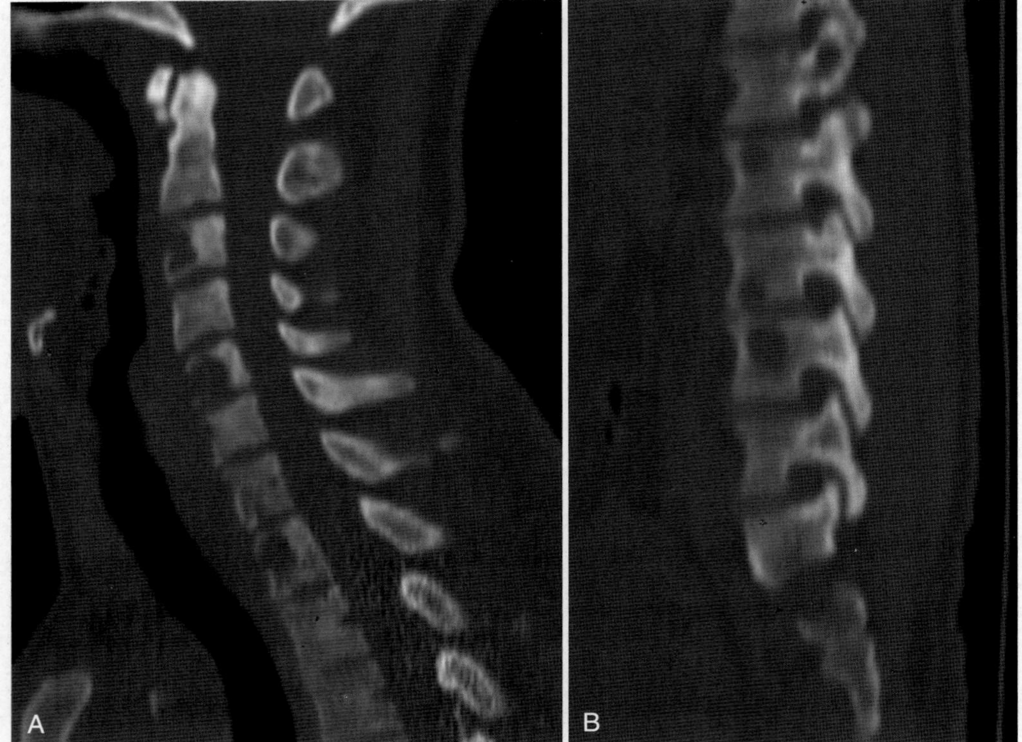

FIG. 87.24 Computed tomography (CT) scan of a 35-year-old man with fevers, weight loss, neck pain, and low back pain. (A) Sagittal CT of the cervical spine shows lytic lesions within C3, C5, and T1. (B) Similar lytic lesions are present in L1–L3. There is no disc involvement. Surgical specimens revealed coccidioidomycosis infection.

However, its prophylactic effect in neutropenic patients due to hematologic malignancy was not shown.[501] Relapse rates are high and azole therapy should probably be continued for 6 months after the disease is inactive.[490]

The response to treatment may be followed by measuring complement-fixing antibody titers. The treatment program should be reassessed if the titers are increasing.[490] The indications for surgery are the same as in other spine infections.[455] In established spinal disease, surgery is often required to eradicate infection.[502] The local use of antifungal agents may be added by depositing amphotericin B with bone cement or calcium sulfate cements.[495]

Blastomycosis

Blastomyces dermatitidis is a dimorphic fungus endemic in areas bordering the Mississippi and Ohio Rivers, the Great Lakes, and the St. Lawrence River.[503] Cases have also been reported in Central and South America, Africa, and the Middle East.[82,306] The organism exists in warm, moist soil rich in organic debris.

Primary infection in humans occurs by inhalation of conidia, which then converts to the yeast phase at body temperature. Infection occurs by inhalation of the conidia, a product from the hyphae in the mycelia form, which, in turn, causes pneumonia.[504] The inflammatory response resembles coccidioidomycosis, with clusters of neutrophils and noncaseating granulomas. The incubation period for acute pulmonary infection is 30 to 45 days. The symptoms are nonspecific, and acute infection may go unrecognized. Dissemination by hematogenous spread occurs frequently. Direct invasion from adjacent tissues is also common. The skin is the most common extrapulmonary site, being affected in 40% to 80% of the patients. Skeletal blastomycosis is seen in 10% to 50% of cases; the long bones, vertebrae, and ribs are the most common sites of osseous involvement.[82]

The radiographic findings in vertebral blastomycosis resemble those in TB: disc space narrowing, anterior involvement of the vertebral body, and development of large abscesses. Collapse and gibbus deformity are more common with blastomycosis than with the other fungal diseases.[82,472] The thoracic and lumbar regions are more commonly involved than the cervical spine.[505] Unlike the situation in TB, lesions frequently invade adjacent ribs, cause draining sinuses, and involve the posterior elements.[82,306,472]

Unfortunately, serum complement-fixation tests are not sensitive or specific. An immunodiffusion test is more sensitive and more specific and is more likely to be positive in patients with disseminated disease. A radioimmunoassay and an enzyme immunoassay are available and are quite sensitive but lack specificity. An enzyme-linked immunosorbent assay is commercially available and is often used for initial screening.

Before the availability of effective antimicrobial therapy, the mortality rate exceeded 60%.[506] The drug of choice for mild to moderate disease is itraconazole, an oral broad-spectrum antifungal, which has a 90% to 95% cure rate in such cases.[504] In severe cases, the drug of choice is amphotericin B, which can be converted to an oral azole such as itraconazole, ketoconazole, fluconazole, and miconazole.[507] Itraconazole has less toxicity and is at least as effective as ketoconazole. Some authors consider itraconazole to be the oral azole of choice.[506] Fluconazole has been compared to ketoconazole with comparable cure rates, but with less toxicity.[504] Miconazole is only moderately active and must be administered intravenously; thus, it has been widely used. Ketoconazole cannot be used in patients with central nervous system blastomycosis because it does not cross the blood-brain barrier.[506] Chemotherapy should be continued for 6 months, although the optimal duration of treatment has not been determined. A reasonable regimen is amphotericin B given intravenously for 4 weeks, followed by 6 months of itraconazole.[508] The role of surgery in blastomycosis is the same as in other spine infections. Successful anterior instrumentation at the time of initial debridement and strut grafting has been reported.[507]

Cryptococcosis

Cryptococcus neoformans, a yeastlike fungus, is surrounded by a thick, gelatinous capsule. It is found throughout the world, most commonly in pigeon feces and soil.[509] The disease is more common in males, whites, and immunocompromised hosts. Cryptococcosis is the fourth most common life-threatening infection in patients with AIDS. In the parts of Africa where there is a high HIV seroprevalence, *Cryptococcus neoformans* is the leading cause of adult meningitis, and infection accounts for a high proportion of deaths in HIV-infected cohorts.[510–513] Infection is acquired by inhalation after the organism is aerosolized. There are no known instances of direct human-to-human or animal-to-human transmission.[306,509] The inflammatory response is variable and generally made up of chronic inflammatory cells, but neutrophils may predominate. The cellular reaction usually is minimal, and there is little suppuration and necrosis.[306] The exudate in cryptococcal lesions is quite mucoid, giving the granuloma a gelatinous appearance so that it may be mistaken for a myxomatous tumor.[306] Well-formed granulomas are uncommon.[509]

Cryptococcosis may be localized to the lung or generalized. Central nervous system involvement is common in the disseminated form. Osseous involvement occurs in approximately 5% to 10% of patients and resembles cold abscesses, similar to TB.[509] Unlike the findings in other fungal infections, sinus tracts and abscess formation are rare.[82] Radiographically, the lesions resemble those of coccidioidomycosis. Lucent lesions of the vertebral bodies and posterior elements are sharply defined but lack reactive sclerosis or periosteal new bone formation.[82] The disc spaces are frequently spared, but involvement of the posterior elements is common.[82]

A latex agglutination procedure for the detection of cryptococcal polysaccharide capsular antigen is available. Both serum and CSF should be tested. The tests detect antigen in 90% of patients with cryptococcal meningitis, but antigen is much less sensitive in patients without central nervous system involvement.[509] Rheumatoid factor also causes agglutination in this procedure, necessitating a test for rheumatoid factor as a control on all samples.[509] Definitive diagnosis is made by culture of the organism.

The current recommended medical treatment of cryptococcosis is a combination of amphotericin B (0.3 mg/kg/day, intravenously) and flucytosine (37.5 mg/kg every 6 hours by mouth) for 6 weeks. The dose of flucytosine can be adjusted on the basis of serum levels to reduce the risk of drug accumulation. Alternatively, amphotericin B alone in doses of 0.5 to 0.7 mg/kg/day for at least 10 weeks can be given. Flucytosine is limited by the development of drug resistance when used alone. Ketoconazole and itraconazole both penetrate CSF poorly and therefore cannot be used in cases of central nervous system involvement. Of the patients initially cured of the disease, 20% to 25% have a relapse. Patients who also have AIDS are rarely cured of the cryptococcal infection; the goal of treatment in these patients is suppression of disease.[509] Recently, Bicanic and colleagues[514] performed a randomized control trial of higher-dose amphotericin B in HIV-infected patients. Higher-dose amphotericin B at 1 mg/kg/day with flucytosine showed improved fungicidal activity with 2-week and 10-week mortality rates of 6% and 24%, respectively. Surgical treatment with decompression and strut grafting in cases of neurologic compression progresses to successful fusion in most cases.[471]

Candidiasis

Ten species of *Candida* are regarded as pathogens for humans. *Candida* organisms are small, thin-walled yeast cells that reproduce by budding. The organisms are normal commensals of humans and are found throughout the gastrointestinal tract, in sputum, in the female genital tract, on diseased skin, and in the urine of patients with indwelling catheters. Human-to-human transmission is possible, but most infections are endogenous.[515] For *Candida* organisms to become pathogenic, the host must be immunocompromised. *Candida* may gain access to the vascular system of susceptible patients via IV lines or monitoring devices and the implantation of prosthetic materials. IV drug abusers are also at risk.[515–517] Although there are 10 species of *Candida* that are pathogenic to humans, 62% of cases of vertebral osteomyelitis are caused by *Candida albicans,* 19% by *Candida tropicalis,* and 14% by *Candida glabrata* (formerly called *Torulopsis glabrata*).[518] Infection caused by *C. glabrata,* however, is becoming more common. This may be secondary to the general trend of increasing *Candida* infections and widespread use of azole antifungals.[519]

The initial cellular reaction is by polymorphonuclear leukocytes. Chronic inflammatory cells appear early, causing a granulomatous response. In severely immunocompromised patients, the reaction may be minimal.[515] Spinal involvement (Fig. 87.25) is rare. Overall, *Candida* is responsible for approximately 0.7% to 2.7% of cases of spinal infections.[56,458,520] The lower thoracic or lumbar spine is most frequently involved (95% of patients) with only a few reported cases occurring at a higher spinal level and one published case involving the sacrum.[518,521] At presentation, 83% of patients complain of back pain of more than 1 month's duration. Only 32% of cases have fever. Most of these patients had complex multisystem

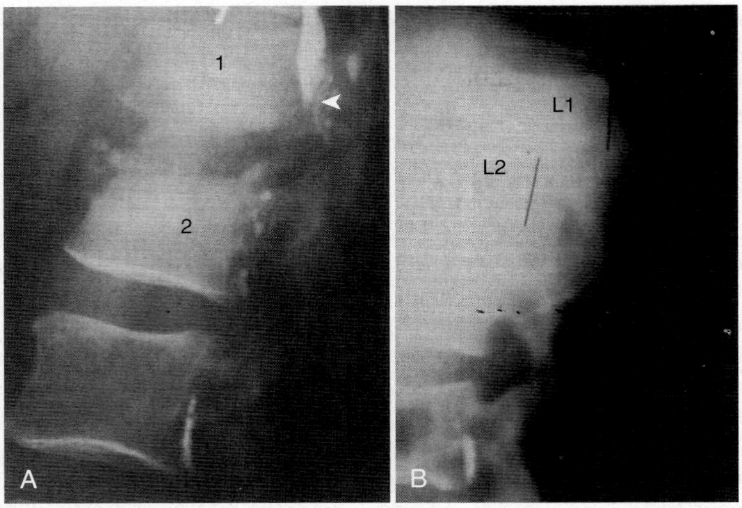

FIG. 87.25 This patient, who had been chronically ill, developed a *Candida* disc space infection at the L1–L2 interspace. (A) This lateral radiograph reveals erosion of the endplates at the inferior portion of L1 and superior portion of L2 vertebral bodies, which is consistent with a standard disc space infection and adjacent vertebral osteomyelitis. This cannot be differentiated from a standard pyogenic disc space infection. (B) The patient was inappropriately treated with a wide laminectomy posteriorly and subsequently developed retrolisthesis of L1 on L2. The paraparesis never improved. He subsequently died of a gastrointestinal hemorrhage while still under treatment for this spinal condition. (From Eismont FJ, Bohlman HH, Soni PL, et al. Pyogenic and fungal vertebral osteomyelitis with paralysis. *J Bone Joint Surg Am.* 1983;65[1]:19–29.)

medical problems, and the disease occurred after prolonged hospitalization.[516]

The treatment of choice is amphotericin B; a total dose of 1 to 1.2 g may be adequate. Flucytosine and ketoconazole are alternative agents in selected patients, but comparative studies with amphotericin B have not been done.[516] Patients who have persistent back pain should undergo another biopsy to confirm resolution of the disease. Most cases reported in the literature of candidal spinal osteomyelitis have undergone surgery combined with medical therapy with good results.[522–524] When making treatment choices for treating patients with *Candida* intervertebral disc space infection, it is important to understand that, in a rabbit model, both amphotericin B and its lipid complex formulation have poor penetration into the disc and fluconazole has excellent penetration.[475]

Aspergillosis

Aspergillus is a mold found throughout the world. There are more than 350 known species of *Aspergillus.* The organism is pathogenic only in immunocompromised hosts.[353,484,525] The one report of aspergillosis occurring in a previously healthy young man without immunocompromise is an enigma.[526] The most frequently isolated species in humans are *Aspergillus fumigatus* and *Aspergillus flavus.* Patients with AIDS and chronic granulomatous disease, those on long-term antibiotics, and IV drug abusers are especially at risk of developing the disseminated form.[527,528] Infection occurs by inhalation of small spores (conidia). Vascular invasion is common in immunosuppressed patients and leads to necrosis of tissues with abundant hyphae from proliferation of the organism. In patients with chronic granulomatous disease, vascular invasion is uncommon and hyphae are sparse.[525]

Osseous involvement may occur by direct extension from the lung or by hematogenous spread.[253,525] It has also been reported as a complication after lumbar discectomy.[525] Spine involvement with *Aspergillus* is uncommon, with only 45 cases in the literature to date.[529–532] The lumbar region is the main area (63%) of osseous involvement followed by the tibia, ribs, wrist, sternum, pelvis, and knee.[533] Advances in imaging and a greater awareness of the severity of this disease have led to a higher rate of diagnosis. *Aspergillus* vertebral osteomyelitis shares several features in common with other causes of pyogenic vertebral osteomyelitis. These include bimodal age distribution, male preponderance, predominance of lumbar involvement, and back pain.[31,530,534] Back pain has been reported almost consistently as the initial complaint with this infection.

The radiographic findings are similar to those in TB of the spine. Disc space narrowing, involvement of adjacent vertebrae, and the presence of paraspinal abscesses are characteristic.[82] Dense new bone formation with small lytic lesions without sequestration may be seen.[253] Clinically, sinus tract formation is characteristic. The incidence of epidural abscess formation in association with neurologic deficits is quite high.[253] The diagnosis is made by microscopic examination of tissue and by culture. *Aspergillus* may be isolated in culture due to contamination or colonization; thus, the culture results must be correlated with the clinical situation.

The drug of choice for the treatment of aspergillosis is amphotericin B, although the response may be poor in markedly immunosuppressed patients.[525] Itraconazole has been effective in some of the more indolent cases of aspergillosis.[525,535] The prognosis of patients with *Aspergillus* spondylitis is guarded. Surgery has been used in the past in almost all cases. In 10 cases in adults reported in the literature, all were treated by posterior decompression and antifungal therapy; four recovered and two died. The four patients with epidural abscess and paraplegia did not improve, and one died. Of five children with aspergillosis but without paraplegia, four died.[253] There have been several reports of successful treatment with antifungal agents alone, without surgery.[253,532] If surgery is thought to be indicated, the principles of treatment outlined for TB should be followed.[484,536] Posterior segmental instrumentation and fusion may be necessary in some cases of spinal instability.[484] With surgical treatment, including posterior instrumentation, the overall recovery rate is 68%.[530]

Syphilitic Disorders of the Spine

The spirochete *Treponema pallidum,* the organism responsible for syphilis, causes two types of spine lesions. The incidence of syphilis has decreased significantly with the advent of penicillin, but another rise has been observed with the appearance of AIDS.[537] The central nervous system is most commonly involved in tertiary syphilis. Tabes dorsalis is the most well-known spinal form of neurosyphilis. Other spinal manifestations include meningomyelitis, pachymeningitis, spastic paraparesis, and myotrophy.[538,539] Establishing the diagnosis is based on a positive antitreponemal antibody test such as the Venereal Disease Research Laboratory (VDRL) test, *Treponema pallidum* hemagglutination antibody (TPH), and fluorescent treponemal antibody (FTA) tests. The VDRL test of the CSF is highly specific for active neurosyphilis but suffers from a relatively low sensitivity of 27%.[540]

Charcot spine is the most common lesion and tends to occur in the thoracolumbar or lumbar spine.[82,541] It may be detected coincidentally or may produce low back pain or root involvement if destruction and hypertrophic changes are severe. The pathophysiology of the lesion is a manifestation of posterior column involvement of the spinal cord and not a primary lesion of the bone itself. It is related to defective protective sensation. The treatment should be bracing to limit excessive movement and to prevent further injury. The role of fusion is undetermined.

Infection of the spine causes syphilitic granulomas due to the local reaction of the tissues to the organism and its products. Granulomas are destructive and usually symptomatic, causing collapse and neurologic deficits. When infection occurs in the spinal cord, termed *syphilitic meningomyelitis,* MRI reveals diffuse spinal cord swelling that mimics transverse myelitis, sarcoidosis, tumor, demyelinating disease, or spinal cord ischemia.[542] The involvement of the dorsal column is characteristic in neurosyphilis, whereas in spinal cord infarction the anterior cord is affected when the anterior spinal artery of Adamkiewicz is occluded.[543] Syphilis is the "great imitator" and must be differentiated from a host of other disorders, including TB of the spine. It is difficult to distinguish the clinical features of spinal disease from coincident neuropathy that is frequently present, and biopsy is necessary for the diagnosis.[541]

The combination of penicillin and prednisolone is the treatment of choice for syphilitic myelitis. The use of prednisolone is to reduce spinal cord edema or ischemia.[539] Ceftriaxone and doxycycline can be used in patients who are allergic to penicillin. For neurosyphilis, 2.4 million units of procaine penicillin daily with probenecid 500 mg four times a day or IV benzyl penicillin 12 to 24 million units daily can achieve treponemicidal levels in the CSF. A 10-day course is adequate for early syphilis, but late-stage disease should be treated for 21 to 28 days.[544]

PEARLS

1. For every spine biopsy, send tissue for appropriate cultures and pathologic study. Uncommon infections, such as TB and fungal infections, will often be identified first by microscopic evaluation.
2. Delay antibiotic treatment for a suspected spine infection in an adult until culture results are positive except in cases in which there are clinically significant signs of systemic infection (sepsis) or undue risk of neurologic deterioration.
3. Antibiotics with a positive charge—such as vancomycin, aminoglycosides, and clindamycin—penetrate into the nucleus pulposus better than negatively charged antibiotics, such as penicillin, oxacillin, and cephalosporins.
4. Surgery for disc space infection with associated osteomyelitis at spinal cord level is usually best done anteriorly and should include a fusion.
5. A high index of suspicion for a spinal infection should be maintained for patients presenting with worsening nonmechanical back pain (e.g., worse at night, not relieved with rest) in immunocompromised patients, such as transplant patients, AIDS, intravenous drug abusers, and frail patients with significant malnutrition.

PITFALLS

1. In adult patients with discitis and associated vertebral osteomyelitis, laminectomy alone is associated with a high rate of clinical deterioration.
2. For an established disc space infection at L4–L5, the blood vessels are usually adherent to the spine, which can make surgical treatment challenging due to risk of blood vessel injury.
3. The granulation tissue associated with discitis and vertebral osteomyelitis often resembles an abscess on MRI.
4. Although more than 50% of spine infections are due to *Staphylococcus,* many are due to uncommon organisms.
5. Relapse often occurs when the course of antibiotics is discontinued before 6 weeks and/or the sedimentation rate and C-reactive protein levels are abnormal.

KEY POINTS

1. *Diagnosis:* Nonspecific complaints, such as back pain without fever or constitutional symptoms, often lead to delayed diagnosis of spinal infection. A high index of suspicion should be maintained for patients at risk for spinal infection, including diabetics, frail and elderly patients with malnutrition, IV drug abusers, immunocompromised patients, and patients with travel history to endemic areas. MRI together with biopsy remains the most reliable method of accurate diagnosis and treatment.
2. *Initial treatment:* Identification of the offending organism, together with antibiotic sensitivity profiles, provides a means of successful nonoperative treatment in patients without undue instability or neurologic compromise. The CRP profiles are useful to monitor the activity of most infections and can guide duration of antibiotic therapy, especially pyogenic infections.

Serial MRI is not recommended because improvements in the appearance on MRI tend to lag significantly behind clinical improvement.

3. *Surgical treatment:* Surgical treatment is indicated when there is clinically significant instability (such as worsening deformity), neurologic deterioration (due to epidural abscess or bony nerve compression), or severe infection (such as sepsis or persistent infection after trial of nonoperative treatment). When infection affects the anterior column, marked with bony destruction and deformity, circumferential reconstruction with anterior support and posterior instrumented fusion remains the standard of care. Single-stage anteroposterior reconstruction is viable when sufficient debridement and stabilization can be achieved.
4. *Postoperative management:* Appropriate antibiotic therapy is required after surgical treatment. Selective antibiotics based on biopsy results should be used according to the specific disease entity. For most pyogenic infections, 4 to 6 weeks of antibiotics are recommended, whereas fungal, granulomatous, and especially mycobacterial infections require longer periods of postoperative antibiotic treatment.

KEY REFERENCES

1. Carragee EJ. Pyogenic vertebral osteomyelitis. *J Bone Joint Surg Am*. 1997;79:874-880.
   This retrospective review of 111 patients with pyogenic vertebral osteomyelitis reviews the diagnosis, optimal treatment, and clinical outcomes of patients with spinal discitis/osteomyelitis.
2. McHenry MC, Easley KA, Locker GA. Vertebral osteomyelitis: long-term outcome for 253 patients from 7 Cleveland-area hospitals. *Clin Infect Dis*. 2002;34:1342-1350.
   This retrospective study described 253 patients with vertebral osteomyelitis and the independent risk factors for long-term outcome.
3. Eismont FJ, Bohlman HH, Soni PL, et al. Pyogenic and fungal vertebral osteomyelitis with paralysis. *J Bone Joint Surg Am*. 1983;65:19-29.
   This study describes factors that affect neurologic outcomes in 31 patients with vertebral osteomyelitis.
4. Kuklo TR, Potter BK, Bell RS, et al. Single-stage treatment of pyogenic spinal infection with titanium mesh cages. *J Spinal Disord Tech*. 2006;19:376-382.
   Modern surgical management of pyogenic spinal infections is described in a consecutive series of 21 patients undergoing single-stage anterior-posterior reconstruction using titanium mesh cages.
5. Dai LY, Jiang LS, Wang W, Cui YM. Single-stage anterior autogenous bone grafting and instrumentation in the surgical management of spinal tuberculosis. *Spine*. 2005;30:2342-2349.
   This prospective study reviewed 39 patients treated with single-stage anterior radical debridement, autogenous bone grafting, and instrumentation.

REFERENCES

1. Pott P. *Remarks on That Kind of Palsy of the Lower Limbs Which Is Frequently Found to Accompany a Curvature of the Spine and Is Supposed to Be Caused by it. Together With Its Method of Cure*. London: J Johnson; 1779:1-84.
2. Musher DM, Thorsteinsson SB, Minuth JN, Luchi RJ. Vertebral osteomyelitis. Still a diagnostic pitfall. *Arch Intern Med*. 1976;136:105-110.
3. Hibbs RA. An operation for progressive spinal deformities. *N Y State Med J*. 1911;93:1013-1016.
4. Albee FH. Transplantation of a portion of the tibia into the spine for Pott's disease: a preliminary report 1911. *Clin Orthop Relat Res*. 2007;460:14-16.
5. Adams ZB. Tuberculosis of the spine in children. A review of sixty-three cases from the Lakeville State Sanatorium. *J Bone Joint Surg Am*. 1940;22:860-861.
6. Menard V. Causes de paraplégie dans le mal de Pott. Son traitement chirurgical par l'ouverture directe du foyer tuberculeux des vertébres. *Revue d'Orthopedie*. 1894;5:47-64.
7. Girdlestone GR. The operative treatment of Pott's paraplegia. *Br J Surg*. 1931;9:121-141.
8. Ito H, Tsuchiya J, Asami G. A new radical operation for Pott's disease: a report of ten cases. *J Bone Joint Surg*. 1934;16:499-515.
9. Hodgson AR, Stock FE. Anterior spinal fusion. A preliminary communication on the radical treatment of Pott's disease and Pott's paraplegia. *Br J Surg*. 1956;44:266-275.
10. Hodgson AR, Stock FE, Fang HS, Ong GB. Anterior spinal fusion. The operative approach and pathological findings in 412 patients with Pott's disease of the spine. *Br J Surg*. 1960;48:172-178.
11. Dickson JA. Spinal tuberculosis in Nigerian children. A review of ambulant treatment. *J Bone Joint Surg Br*. 1967;49:682-694.
12. Konstam PG, Blesovsky A. The ambulant treatment of spinal tuberculosis. *Br J Surg*. 1962;50:26-38.
13. Konstam PG, Konstam ST. Spinal tuberculosis in Southern Nigeria with special reference to ambulant treatment of thoracolumbar disease. *J Bone Joint Surg Br*. 1958;40-B:26-B32.
14. Tuli SM. Results of treatment of spinal tuberculosis by "middle-path" regime. *J Bone Joint Surg Br*. 1975;57:13-23.
15. Friedman B, Kapur VN. Newer knowledge of chemotherapy in the treatment of tuberculosis of bones and joints. *Clin Orthop Relat Res*. 1973;97:5-15.
16. Lannelongue O. *On Acute Osteomyelitis, Miscellaneous, Pathological, and Practical Medicine Tracts*. Paris: 1897.
17. Collert S. Osteomyelitis of the spine. *Acta Orthop Scand*. 1977;48:283-290.
18. Stone DB, Bonfiglio M. Pyogenic vertebral osteomyelitis. A diagnostic pitfall for the internist. *Arch Intern Med*. 1963;112:491-500.
19. Kulowski J. Management of hematogenous pyogenic osteomyelitis. *Surgery*. 1956;40:1094-1104.
20. Robinson BH, Lessof MH. Osteomyelitis of the spine. *Guys Hosp Rep*. 1961;110:303-318.
21. Waldvogel FA, Medoff G, Swartz MN. Osteomyelitis: a review of clinical features, therapeutic considerations and unusual aspects. *N Engl J Med*. 1970;282:198-206.
22. Wilensky AO. Osteomyelitis of the vertebrae. *Ann Surg*. 1929;89:561-570.
23. Bonfiglio M, Lange TA, Kim YM. Pyogenic vertebral osteomyelitis. Disk space infections. *Clin Orthop Relat Res*. 1973;96:234-247.
24. Carragee EJ. Pyogenic vertebral osteomyelitis. *J Bone Joint Surg Am*. 1997;79:874-880.
25. Digby JM, Kersley JB. Pyogenic non-tuberculous spinal infection: an analysis of thirty cases. *J Bone Joint Surg Br*. 1979;61:47-55.
26. Frederickson B, Yuan H, Olans R. Management and outcome of pyogenic vertebral osteomyelitis. *Clin Orthop*. 1978;131:160-167.
27. Griffiths HE, Jones DM. Pyogenic infection of the spine. A review of twenty-eight cases. *J Bone Joint Surg Br*. 1971;53:383-391.

28. Kemp HB, Jackson JW, Jeremiah JD, Hall AJ. Pyogenic infections occurring primarily in intervertebral discs. *J Bone Joint Surg Br.* 1973;55:698-714.
29. Kulowski J. Pyogenic osteomyelitis of the spine. An analysis and discussion of 102 cases. *J Bone Joint Surg.* 1936;18:343-364.
30. Ross PM, Fleming JL. Vertebral body osteomyelitis: spectrum and natural history. A retrospective analysis of 37 cases. *Clin Orthop Relat Res.* 1976;118:190-198.
31. Sapico FL, Montgomerie JZ. Pyogenic vertebral osteomyelitis: report of nine cases and review of the literature. *Rev Infect Dis.* 1979;1:754-776.
32. Waldvogel FA, Papageorgiou PS. Osteomyelitis: the past decade. *N Engl J Med.* 1980;303:360-370.
33. Loibl M, Stoyanov L, Doenitz C, et al. Outcome-related co-factors in 105 cases of vertebral osteomyelitis in a tertiary care hospital. *Infection.* 2014;42:503-510.
34. Sans N, Faruch M, Lapegue F, et al. Infections of the spinal column—spondylodiscitis. *Diagn Interven Imaging.* 2012;93:520-529.
35. Garcia A Jr, Grantham SA. Hematogenous pyogenic vertebral osteomyelitis. *Am J Orthop.* 1960;42-A:429-436.
36. Genster HG, Andersen MJ. Spinal osteomyelitis complicating urinary tract infection. *J Urol.* 1972;107:109-111.
37. Wedge JH, Oryschak AF, Robertson DE, Kirkaldy-Willis WH. Atypical manifestations of spinal infections. *Clin Orthop Relat Res.* 1977;123:155-163.
38. Holzman RS, Bishko F. Osteomyelitis in heroin addicts. *Ann Intern Med.* 1971;75:693-696.
39. Koppel BS, Tuchman AJ, Mangiardi JR, et al. Epidural spinal infection in intravenous drug abusers. *Arch Neurol.* 1988;45:1331-1337.
40. Kurtzman RS. Complications of narcotic addiction. *Radiology.* 1970;96:23-30.
41. Messer HD, Litvinoff J. Pyogenic cervical osteomyelitis. Chondro-osteomyelitis of the cervical spine frequently associated with parenteral drug use. *Arch Neurol.* 1976;33:571-576.
42. Sapico FL, Montgomerie JZ. Vertebral osteomyelitis in intravenous drug abusers: report of three cases and review of the literature. *Rev Infect Dis.* 1980;2:196-206.
43. Selby RC, Pillay KV. Osteomyelitis and disc infection secondary to *Pseudomonas aeruginosa* in heroin addiction. *Case report. J Neurosurg.* 1972;37:463-466.
44. Bergman I, Wald ER, Meyer JD, Painter MJ. Epidural abscess and vertebral osteomyelitis following serial lumbar punctures. *Pediatrics.* 1983;72:476-480.
45. Dripps RD, Vandam LD. Hazards of lumbar puncture. *J Am Med Assoc.* 1951;147:1118-1121.
46. El-Gindi S, Aref S, Salama M, Andrew J. Infection of intervertebral discs after operation. *J Bone Joint Surg Br.* 1976;58:114-116.
47. Lindholm TS, Pylkkanen P. Discitis following removal of intervertebral disc. *Spine.* 1982;7:618-622.
48. Pilgaard S. Discitis. Closed-space infection after lumbar discus prolapse operation. *Acta Orthop Scand.* 1969;40:681.
49. Puranen J, Makela J, Lahde S. Postoperative intervertebral discitis. *Acta Orthop Scand.* 1984;55:461-465.
50. Rawlings CE 3rd, Wilkins RH, Gallis HA, et al. Postoperative intervertebral disc space infection. *Neurosurgery.* 1983;13:371-376.
51. Schaefer SD, Bucholz RW, Jones RE, Carder HM. The management of transpharyngeal gunshot wounds to the cervical spine. *Surg Gynecol Obstet.* 1981;152:27-29.
52. Sullivan CR, Bickel WH, Svien HJ. Infections of vertebral interspaces after operations on intervertebral disks. *J Am Med Assoc.* 1958;166:1973-1977.
53. Thibodeau AA. Closed space infection following removal of lumbar intervertebral disc. *J Bone Joint Surg Am.* 1968;50:400-410.
54. Cooppan R, Schoenbaum S, Younger MD, et al. Vertebral osteomyelitis in insulin-dependent diabetics. *S Afr Med J.* 1976;50:1993-1996.
55. Weinstein MA, Eismont FJ. Infections of the spine in patients with human immunodeficiency virus. *J Bone Joint Surg Am.* 2005;87:604-609.
56. McHenry MC, Easley KA, Locker GA. Vertebral osteomyelitis: long-term outcome for 253 patients from 7 Cleveland-area hospitals. *Clin Infect Dis.* 2002;34:1342-1350.
57. Hatch ES. Acute osteomyelitis of the spine: report of case with recovery. Review of the literature. *N Orleans Med Surg J.* 1931;83:861-873.
58. Musher DM, Fletcher T. Tolerant *Staphylococcus aureus* causing vertebral osteomyelitis. *Arch Intern Med.* 1982;142: 632-634.
59. Graham SM, Fishlock A, Millner P, et al. The management of gram-negative bacterial haematogenous vertebral osteomyelitis: a case series of diagnosis, treatment and therapeutic outcomes. *Eur Spine J.* 2013;22:1845-1853.
60. Henriques CQ. Osteomyelitis as a complication in urology; with special reference to the paravertebral venous plexus. *Br J Surg.* 1958;46:19-28.
61. Henson SW Jr, Coventry MB. Osteomyelitis of the vertebrae as the result of infection of the urinary tract. *Surg Gynecol Obstet.* 1956;102:207-214.
62. Redfern RM, Cottam SN, Phillipson AP. *Proteus* infection of the spine. *Spine.* 1988;13:439-441.
63. Jabbari B, Pierce JF. Spinal cord compression due to pseudomonas in a heroin addict. Case report. *Neurology.* 1977;27:1034-1037.
64. Lewis R, Gorbach S, Altner P. Spinal *Pseudomonas* chondro-osteomyelitis in heroin users. *N Engl J Med.* 1972;286:1303.
65. Wiesseman GJ, Wood VE, Kroll LL, Linda L. *Pseudomonas* vertebral osteomyelitis in heroin addicts. Report of five cases. *J Bone Joint Surg Am.* 1973;55:1416-1424.
66. Carvell JE, Maclarnon JC. Chronic osteomyelitis of the thoracic spine due to *Salmonella typhi:* a case report. *Spine.* 1981;6:527-530.
67. Miller ME, Fogel GR, Dunham WK. *Salmonella* spondylitis. A review and report of two immunologically normal patients. *J Bone Joint Surg Am.* 1988;70:463-466.
68. Sandiford JA, Higgins GA, Blair W. Remote salmonellosis: surgical masquerader. *Am Surg.* 1982;48:54-58.
69. Incavo SJ, Muller DL, Krag MH, Gump D. Vertebral osteomyelitis caused by *Clostridium difficile.* A case report and review of the literature. *Spine.* 1988;13:111-113.
70. Charles RW, Mody GM, Govender S. Pyogenic infection of the lumbar vertebral spine due to gas-forming organisms. A case report. *Spine.* 1989;14:541-543.
71. Oill PA, Chow AW, Flood TP, Guze LB. Adult *Haemophilus influenzae* type B vertebral osteomyelitis: a case report and review of the literature. *Clin Orthop Relat Res.* 1978;136: 253-256.
72. Petty BG, Burrow CR, Robinson RA, Bulkley GB. *Hemophilus aphrophilus* meningitis followed by vertebral osteomyelitis and suppurative psoas abscess. *Am J Med.* 1985;78:159-162.

73. Schofferman L, Schofferman J, Zucherman J, et al. Occult infections causing persistent low-back pain. *Spine*. 1989; 14:417-419.
74. Brown MD, Tsaltas TT. Studies on the permeability of the intervertebral disc during skeletal maturation. *Spine*. 1976;1:240-244.
75. Crock HV, Goldwasser M. Anatomic studies of the circulation in the region of the vertebral end-plate in adult Greyhound dogs. *Spine*. 1984;9:702-706.
76. Whalen JL, Parke WW, Mazur JM, Stauffer ES. The intrinsic vasculature of developing vertebral end plates and its nutritive significance to the intervertebral discs. *J Pediatr Orthop*. 1985;5:403-410.
77. Hassler O. The human intervertebral disc: a microangiographical study on its vascular supply at various ages. *Acta Orthop Scand*. 1970;40:765-772.
78. Coventry MB, Ghormley RK, Kernohan JW. The intervertebral disc: its microscopic anatomy and pathology. Part I: anatomy, development, and physiology. *J Bone Joint Surg*. 1945;27:105-112.
79. Wiley AM, Trueta J. The vascular anatomy of the spine and its relationship to pyogenic vertebral osteomyelitis. *J Bone Joint Surg Br*. 1959;41-B:796-809.
80. Batson OV. The function of the vertebral veins and their role in the spread of metastasis. *Ann Surg*. 1940;112: 138-149.
81. Compere EL, Garrison M. Correlation of pathologic and roentgenologic findings in tuberculosis and pyogenic infections of the vertebrae: the fate of the intervertebral disk. *Ann Surg*. 1936;104:1038-1067.
82. Goldman AB, Freiberger RH. Localized infectious and neuropathic diseases. *Semin Roentgenol*. 1979;14:19-32.
83. Stauffer RN. Pyogenic vertebral osteomyelitis. *Orthop Clin North Am*. 1975;6:1015-1027.
84. Ghormley RK, Bickel WH, Dickson DD. A study of acute infectious lesions of the intervertebral discs. *South Med J*. 1940;33:347-352.
85. Parke WW, Rothman RH, Brown MD. The pharyngovertebral veins: an anatomical rationale for Grisel's syndrome. *J Bone Joint Surg Am*. 1984;66:568-574.
86. Zigler JE, Bohlman HH, Robinson RA, et al. Pyogenic osteomyelitis of the occiput, the atlas, and the axis. A report of five cases. *J Bone Joint Surg Am*. 1987;69:1069-1073.
87. Nyberg DA, Jeffrey RB, Brant-Zawadzki M, et al. Computed tomography of cervical infections. *J Comput Assist Tomogr*. 1985;9:288-296.
88. Fraser RA, Ratzan K, Wolpert SM, Weinstein L. Spinal subdural empyema. *Arch Neurol*. 1973;28:235-238.
89. McHenry MC, Duchesneau PM, Keys TF, et al. Vertebral osteomyelitis presenting as spinal compression fracture. Six patients with underlying osteoporosis. *Arch Intern Med*. 1988;148:417-423.
90. Lora-Tamayo J, Euba G, Navraez JA, et al. Changing trends in the epidemiology of pyogenic vertebral osteomyelitis: the impact of cases with no microbiologic diagnosis. *Semin Arthritis Rheum*. 2011;41:247-255.
91. Mylona E, Samarkos M, Kakalou E, et al. Pyogenic vertebral osteomyelitis: a systematic review of clinical characteristics. *Semin Arthritis Rheum*. 2009;39:10-17.
92. Visudhiphan P, Chiemchanya S, Somburanasin R, Dheandhanoo D. Torticollis as the presenting sign in cervical spine infection and tumor. *Clin Pediatr (Phila)*. 1982;21: 71-76.
93. Guri JP. Pyogenic osteomyelitis of the spine: differential diagnosis through clinical and roentgenographic observations. *J Bone Joint Surg*. 1946;28:29-39.
94. Bloom R, Yeager H Jr, Garagusi VF. Pleuropulmonary complications of thoracic vertebral osteomyelitis. *Thorax*. 1980;35:156-157.
95. Kern RZ, Houpt JB. Pyogenic vertebral osteomyelitis: diagnosis and management. *Can Med Assoc J*. 1984;130:1025-1028.
96. Srinivasan D, Terman SW, Himedan M, et al. Risk factors for the development of deformity in patients with spinal infections. *Neurosurg Focus*. 2014;37:E2.
97. Rubery PT, Smith MD, Cammisa FP, Silane M. Mycotic aortic aneurysm in patients who have lumbar vertebral osteomyelitis. A report of two cases. *J Bone Joint Surg Am*. 1995;77:1729-1732.
98. Eismont FJ, Bohlman HH, Soni PL, et al. Pyogenic and fungal vertebral osteomyelitis with paralysis. *J Bone Joint Surg Am*. 1983;65:19-29.
99. Eismont FJ, Bohlman HH, Soni PL, et al. Vertebral osteomyelitis in infants. *J Bone Joint Surg Br*. 1982;64:32-35.
100. Pritchard AE, Thompson WA. Acute pyogenic infections of the spine in children. *J Bone Joint Surg Br*. 1960;42-B:86-89.
101. Schulitz KP, Assheuer J. Discitis after procedures on the intervertebral disc. *Spine*. 1994;19:1172-1177.
102. Jaye DL, Waites KB. Clinical applications of C-reactive protein in pediatrics. *Pediatr Infect Dis J*. 1997;16:735-746; quiz 46-7.
103. Saez-Llorens X, Lagrutta F. The acute phase host reaction during bacterial infection and its clinical impact in children. *Pediatr Infect Dis J*. 1993;12:83-87.
104. Kersley JB. Nontuberculous infection of the spine. *Proc R Soc Med*. 1977;70:176-181.
105. McCain GA, Harth M, Bell DA, et al. Septic discitis. *J Rheumatol*. 1981;8:100-109.
106. Khachatourians AG, Patzakis MJ, Roidis N, Holtom PD. Laboratory monitoring in pediatric acute osteomyelitis and septic arthritis. *Clin Orthop Relat Res*. 2003;409:186-194.
107. Fransen EJ, Maessen JG, Elenbaas TW, et al. Enhanced preoperative C-reactive protein plasma levels as a risk factor for postoperative infections after cardiac surgery. *Ann Thorac Surg*. 1999;67:134-138.
108. Lin ZY, Chuang WL, Dai CY, et al. Clinical application of serum C-reactive protein measurement in the detection of bacterial infection in patients with liver cirrhosis. *Kaohsiung J Med Sci*. 2002;18:121-126.
109. Thelander U, Larsson S. Quantitation of C-reactive protein levels and erythrocyte sedimentation rate after spinal surgery. *Spine*. 1992;17:400-404.
110. O'Daly BJ, Morris SF, O'Rourke SK. Long-term functional outcome in pyogenic spinal infection. *Spine*. 2008;33:E246-E253.
111. Kim CJ, Kang SJ, Yoon D, et al. Factors influencing culture positivity in pyogenic vertebral osteomyelitis patients with prior antibiotic exposure. *Antimicrob Agents Chemother*. 2015;59:2470-2473.
112. Corentt CA, Vincent SA, Crow J, Hewlett A. Bacterial spine infections in adults: evaluation and management. *J Am Acad Orthop Surg*. 2016;24:11-18.
113. King DM, Mayo KM. Infective lesions of the vertebral column. *Clin Orthop Relat Res*. 1973;96:248-253.
114. Ambrose GB, Alpert M, Neer CS. Vertebral osteomyelitis. A diagnostic problem. *JAMA*. 1966;197:619-622.

115. Dagirmanjian A. Spinal osteomyelitis. *Semin Spine Surg.* 1997;9:38-50.
116. Bruschwein DA, Brown ML, McLeod RA. Gallium scintigraphy in the evaluation of disk-space infections: concise communication. *J Nucl Med.* 1980;21:925-927.
117. Modic MT, Feiglin DH, Piraino DW, et al. Vertebral osteomyelitis: assessment using MR. *Radiology.* 1985;157:157-166.
118. Staab EV, McCartney WH. Role of gallium 67 in inflammatory disease. *Semin Nucl Med.* 1978;8:219-234.
119. Norris S, Ehrlich MG, McKusick K. Early diagnosis of disk space infection with 67Ga in an experimental model. *Clin Orthop Relat Res.* 1979;293-298.
120. Haase D, Martin R, Marrie T. Radionuclide imaging in pyogenic vertebral osteomyelitis. *Clin Nucl Med.* 1980;5:533-537.
121. Szypryt EP, Hardy JG, Hinton CE, et al. A comparison between magnetic resonance imaging and scintigraphic bone imaging in the diagnosis of disc space infection in an animal model. *Spine.* 1988;13:1042-1048.
122. Dux S, Halevi J, Pitlik S, Rosenfeld JB. Early diagnosis of infective spondylitis with Gallium-67. *Isr J Med Sci.* 1981;17:451-452.
123. Onofrio BM. Intervertebral discitis: incidence, diagnosis, and management. *Clin Neurosurg.* 1980;27:481-516.
124. Merkel KD, Fitzgerald RH Jr, Brown ML. Scintigraphic evaluation in musculoskeletal sepsis. *Orthop Clin North Am.* 1984;15:401-416.
125. Fernandez-Ulloa M, Vasavada PJ, Hanslits ML, et al. Diagnosis of vertebral osteomyelitis: clinical, radiological and scintigraphic features. *Orthopedics.* 1985;8:1144-1150.
126. Whalen JL, Brown ML, McLeod R, Fitzgerald RH Jr. Limitations of indium leukocyte imaging for the diagnosis of spine infections. *Spine.* 1991;16:193-197.
127. Wukich DK, Van Dam BE, Abreu SH. Preoperative indium-labeled white blood cell scintigraphy in suspected osteomyelitis of the axial skeleton. *Spine.* 1988;13:1168-1170.
128. Brown ML, Hauser MF, Aznarez A, Fitzgerald RH. Indium-111 leukocyte imaging. The skeletal photopenic lesion. *Clin Nucl Med.* 1986;11:611-613.
129. Palestro CJ, Kim CK, Swyer AJ, et al. Radionuclide diagnosis of vertebral osteomyelitis: indium-111-leukocyte and technetium-99m-methylene diphosphonate bone scintigraphy. *J Nucl Med.* 1991;32:1861-1865.
130. Swayne LC, Dorsky S, Caruana V, Kaplan IL. Septic arthritis of a lumbar facet joint: detection with bone SPECT imaging. *J Nucl Med.* 1989;30:1408-1411.
131. Love C, Patel M, Lonner BS, et al. Diagnosing spinal osteomyelitis: a comparison of bone and Ga-67 scintigraphy and magnetic resonance imaging. *Clin Nucl Med.* 2000;25:963-977.
132. Gates GF, McDonald RJ. Bone SPECT of the back after lumbar surgery. *Clin Nucl Med.* 1999;24:395-403.
133. Golimbu C, Firooznia H, Rafii M. CT of osteomyelitis of the spine. *AJR Am J Roentgenol.* 1984;142:159-163.
134. Kattapuram SV, Phillips WC, Boyd R. CT in pyogenic osteomyelitis of the spine. *AJR Am J Roentgenol.* 1983;140:1199-1201.
135. Larde D, Mathieu D, Frija J, et al. Vertebral osteomyelitis: disk hypodensity on CT. *AJR Am J Roentgenol.* 1982;139:963-967.
136. Van Lom KJ, Kellerhouse LE, Pathria MN, et al. Infection versus tumor in the spine: criteria for distinction with CT. *Radiology.* 1988;166:851-855.
137. Brant-Zawadzki M, Burke VD, Jeffrey RB. CT in the evaluation of spine infection. *Spine.* 1983;8:358-364.
138. De Backer AI, Mortele KJ, Vanschoubroeck IJ, et al. Tuberculosis of the spine: CT and MR imaging features. *JBR-BTR.* 2005;88:92-97.
139. LaBerge JM, Brant-Zawadzki M. Evaluation of Pott's disease with computed tomography. *Neuroradiology.* 1984;26:429-434.
140. Adapon BD, Legada BD Jr, Lim EV, et al. CT-guided closed biopsy of the spine. *J Comput Assist Tomogr.* 1981;5:73-78.
141. Hoffer FA, Strand RD, Gebhardt MC. Percutaneous biopsy of pyogenic infection of the spine in children. *J Pediatr Orthop.* 1988;8:442-444.
142. Ghelman B. Percutaneous CT guided biopsy of the thoracic and lumbar spine. *Orthop Trans.* 1990;14:635.
143. Bruns J, Maas R. Advantages of diagnosing bacterial spondylitis with magnetic resonance imaging. *Arch Orthop Trauma Surg.* 1989;108:30-35.
144. Post MJ, Quencer RM, Montalvo BM, et al. Spinal infection: evaluation with MR imaging and intraoperative US. *Radiology.* 1988;169:765-771.
145. Abram SR, Tedeschi AA, Partain CL, Blumenkopf B. Differential diagnosis of severe back pain using MRI. *South Med J.* 1988;81:1487-1492.
146. Gardner RD. Nongranulomatous spinal epidural abscesses. *Orthop Trans.* 1989;13:562-563.
147. Post MJ, Sze G, Quencer RM, et al. Gadolinium-enhanced MR in spinal infection. *J Comput Assist Tomogr.* 1990;14:721-729.
148. Dagirmanjian A, Schils J, McHenry M, Modic MT. MR imaging of vertebral osteomyelitis revisited. *AJR Am J Roentgenol.* 1996;167:1539-1543.
149. Ledermann HP, Schweitzer ME, Morrison WB, Carrino JA. MR imaging findings in spinal infections: rules or myths? *Radiology.* 2003;228:506-514.
150. Shih TT, Huang KM, Hou SM. Early diagnosis of single segment vertebral osteomyelitis—MR pattern and its characteristics. *Clin Imaging.* 1999;23:159-167.
151. Chang MC, Wu HT, Lee CH, et al. Tuberculous spondylitis and pyogenic spondylitis: comparative magnetic resonance imaging features. *Spine.* 2006;31:782-788.
152. Carragee EJ. The clinical use of magnetic resonance imaging in pyogenic vertebral osteomyelitis. *Spine.* 1997;22:780-785.
153. Gillams AR, Chaddha B, Carter AP. MR appearances of the temporal evolution and resolution of infectious spondylitis. *AJR Am J Roentgenol.* 1996;166:903-907.
154. Eismont FJ, Green BA, Brown MD, Ghandur-Mnaymneh L. Coexistent infection and tumor of the spine. A report of three cases. *J Bone Joint Surg Am.* 1987;69:452-458.
155. Nagel DA, Albright JA, Keggi KJ, Southwick WO. Closer look at spinal lesions: open biopsy of vertebral lesions. *JAMA.* 1965;191:975-978.
156. Koslow M, Kuperstein R, Eshed I, et al. The unique clinical features and outcome of infectious endocarditis and vertebral osteomyelitis coinfection. *Am J Med.* 2014;127:669.e9-669.e15.
157. Craig FS. Vertebral-body biopsy. *J Bone Joint Surg Am.* 1956;38-A:93-102.
158. Ottolenghi CE. Aspiration biopsy of the spine. Technique for the thoracic spine and results of twenty-eight biopsies in this region and over-all results of 1050 biopsies of other spinal segments. *J Bone Joint Surg Am.* 1969;51:1531-1544.
159. Ottolenghi CE, Schajowicz F, Deschant FA. Aspiration biopsy of the cervical spine. Technique and results in thirty-four cases. *J Bone Joint Surg Am.* 1964;46:715-733.

160. Armstrong P, Chalmers AH, Green G, Irving JD. Needle aspiration/biopsy of the spine in suspected disc infection. *Br J Radiol.* 1978;51:333-337.
161. Ashizawa N, Yano K. Tuberculous pericarditis. *Ryoikibetsu Shokogun Shirizu.* 1999;(24 Pt 2):198-200.
162. Jelinek J, Pearl AB, Kominsky SJ, Schultz PM. Magnetic resonance imaging of the foot. Rheumatologic disorders mimicking osteomyelitis. *J Am Podiatr Med Assoc.* 1996;86:228-231.
163. Renfrew DL, Whitten CG, Wiese JA, et al. CT-guided percutaneous transpedicular biopsy of the spine. *Radiology.* 1991;180:574-576.
164. Hadjipavlou AG, Crow WN, Borowski A, et al. Percutaneous transpedicular discectomy and drainage in pyogenic spondylodiscitis. *Am J Orthop.* 1998;27:188-197.
165. Cohn SL, Akbarnia BA, Luisiri A, Sundaram M. Disk space infection versus lumbar Scheuermann's disease. *Orthopedics.* 1988;11:330-335.
166. Kalen V, Isono SS, Cho CS, Perkash I. Charcot arthropathy of the spine in long-standing paraplegia. *Spine.* 1987;12: 42-47.
167. Park YH, Taylor JA, Szollar SM, Resnick D. Imaging findings in spinal neuroarthropathy. *Spine.* 1994;19:1499-1504.
168. Piazza MR, Bassett GS, Bunnell WP. Neuropathic spinal arthropathy in congenital insensitivity to pain. *Clin Orthop Relat Res.* 1988;236:175-179.
169. Scherbel AL, Gardner WJ. Infections involving the intervertebral disks. Diagnosis and management. *JAMA.* 1960;174:370-374.
170. Fischer EG, Greene CS Jr, Winston KR. Spinal epidural abscess in children. *Neurosurgery.* 1981;9:257-260.
171. Daly RC, Fitzgerald RH, Washington JA. Penetration of cefazolin into normal and osteomyelitic canine cortical bone. *Antimicrob Agents Chemother.* 1982;22:461-469.
172. Currier BL, Banovac K, Eismont FJ. Gentamicin penetration into normal rabbit nucleus pulposus. *Spine.* 1994;19:2614-2618.
173. Fraser RD, Osti OL, Vernon-Roberts B. Iatrogenic discitis: the role of intravenous antibiotics in prevention and treatment. An experimental study. *Spine.* 1989;14:1025-1032.
174. Guerrero IC, MacGregor RR. Comparative penetration of various cephalosporins into inflammatory exudate. *Antimicrob Agents Chemother.* 1979;15:712-715.
175. Hall WH, Gerding DN, Schierl EA. Penetration of tobramycin into infected extravascular fluids and its therapeutic effectiveness. *J Infect Dis.* 1977;135:957-961.
176. Eismont FJ. Antibiotic penetration into rabbit nucleus pulposus. *Spine.* 1987;12:254-256.
177. Gibson MJ. The penetration of antibiotics into the normal intervertebral disc. *J Bone Joint Surg.* 1987;69B:784-786.
178. Scuderi GJ, Greenberg SS, Banovac K, et al. Penetration of glycopeptide antibiotics in nucleus pulposus. *Spine.* 1993;18:2039-2042.
179. Riley LH 3rd, Banovac K, Martinez OV, Eismont FJ. Tissue distribution of antibiotics in the intervertebral disc. *Spine.* 1994;19:2619-2625.
180. Mader JT, Cantrell JS, Calhoun J. Oral ciprofloxacin compared with standard parenteral antibiotic therapy for chronic osteomyelitis in adults. *J Bone Joint Surg Am.* 1990;72:104-110.
181. Bydon M, De la Garza-Ramos R, Macki M, et al. Spinal instrumentation in patients with primary spinal infections does not lead to greater recurrent infection rates: an analysis of 118 cases. *World Neurosurg.* 2014;82:e807-e814.
182. Yoon SH, Chung SK, Kim KJ, et al. Pyogenic vertebral osteomyelitis: identification of microorganism and laboratory markers used to predict clinical outcome. *Eur Spine J.* 2010;19:575-582.
183. Emery SE, Chan DP, Woodward HR. Treatment of hematogenous pyogenic vertebral osteomyelitis with anterior debridement and primary bone grafting. *Spine.* 1989;14:284-291.
184. Forsythe M, Rothman RH. New concepts in the diagnosis and treatment of infections of the cervical spine. *Orthop Clin North Am.* 1978;9:1039-1051.
185. Kemp HB, Jackson JW, Jeremiah JD, Cook J. Anterior fusion of the spine for infective lesions in adults. *J Bone Joint Surg Br.* 1973;55:715-734.
186. Kemp HB, Jackson JW, Shaw NC. Laminectomy in paraplegia due to infective spondylosis. *Br J Surg.* 1974;61:66-72.
187. Southwick WO, Robinson RA. Surgical approaches to the vertebral bodies in the cervical and lumbar regions. *J Bone Joint Surg Am.* 1957;39-A:631-644.
188. Hodgson AR, Stock FE. Anterior spine fusion for the treatment of tuberculosis of the spine: the operative findings and results of treatment in the first one hundred cases. *J Bone Joint Surg.* 1960;42A:295-310.
189. Kirkaldy-Willis WH, Thomas TG. Anterior approaches in the diagnosis and treatment of infections of the vertebral bodies. *J Bone Joint Surg.* 1965;47A:87-110.
190. Seddon HJ. Pott's paraplegia: prognosis and treatment. *Br J Surg.* 1934-1935;22:769-799.
191. Bohlman HH, Freehafer A, Dejak J. The results of treatment of acute injuries of the upper thoracic spine with paralysis. *J Bone Joint Surg Am.* 1985;67:360-369.
192. Bohlman HH, Eismont FJ. Surgical techniques of anterior decompression and fusion for spinal cord injuries. *Clin Orthop Relat Res.* 1981;154:57-67.
193. Fountain SS. A single-stage combined surgical approach for vertebral resections. *J Bone Joint Surg Am.* 1979;61:1011-1017.
194. Hodgson AR, Yau ACMC. Anterior surgical approaches to the spinal column. *Recent Adv Orthop.* 1969;1:289-323.
195. McGuire RA, Eismont FJ. The fate of autogenous bone graft in surgically treated pyogenic vertebral osteomyelitis. *J Spinal Disord.* 1994;7:206-215.
196. Rajasekaran S, Soundarapandian S. Progression of kyphosis in tuberculosis of the spine treated by anterior arthrodesis. *J Bone Joint Surg Am.* 1989;71:1314-1323.
197. Enneking WF, Burchardt H, Puhl JJ, Piotrowski G. Physical and biological aspects of repair in dog cortical-bone transplants. *J Bone Joint Surg Am.* 1975;57:237-252.
198. Bradford DS, Daher YH. Vascularized rib grafts and stabilization of kyphosis. *J Bone Joint Surg.* 1986;68B:357-361.
199. Louw JA. Spinal tuberculosis with neurologic deficit. Treatment with vascularized rib grafts, posterior osteotomies and fusion. *J Bone Joint Surg.* 1990;72B:686-693.
200. Whitecloud TS, LaRocca H. Fibular strut graft in reconstructive surgery of the cervical spine. *Spine.* 1976;1:33-43.
201. Bailey HL, Gabriel M, Hodgson AR, Shin JS. Tuberculosis of the spine in children. Operative findings and results in one hundred consecutive patients treated by removal of the lesion and anterior grafting. *J Bone Joint Surg Am.* 1972;54:1633-1657.
202. Graziano GP, Sidhu KS. Salvage reconstruction in acute and late sequelae from pyogenic thoracolumbar infection. *J Spinal Disord.* 1993;6:199-207.

203. Hee HT, Majd ME, Holt RT, Pienkowski D. Better treatment of vertebral osteomyelitis using posterior stabilization and titanium mesh cages. *J Spinal Disord Tech*. 2002;15: 149-156.
204. Carragee EJ. Instrumentation of the infected and unstable spine: a review of 17 cases from the thoracic and lumbar spine with pyogenic infections. *J Spinal Disord*. 1997;10: 317-324.
205. Safran O, Rand N, Kaplan L, Sagiv S, Floman Y. Sequential or simultaneous, same-day anterior decompression and posterior stabilization in the management of vertebral osteomyelitis of the lumbar spine. *Spine*. 1998;23:1885-1890.
206. Ha KY, Chung YG, Ryoo SJ. Adherence and biofilm formation of *Staphylococcus epidermidis* and *Mycobacterium tuberculosis* on various spinal implants. *Spine*. 2005;30:38-43.
207. Barth E, Myrvik QM, Wagner W, Gristina AG. In vitro and in vivo comparative colonization of *Staphylococcus aureus* and *Staphylococcus epidermidis* on orthopaedic implant materials. *Biomaterials*. 1989;10:325-328.
208. Gracia E, Fernandez A, Conchello P, et al. Adherence of *Staphylococcus aureus* slime-producing strain variants to biomaterials used in orthopaedic surgery. *Int Orthop*. 1997;21:46-51.
209. Gristina AG, Hobgood CD, Webb LX, Myrvik QN. Adhesive colonization of biomaterials and antibiotic resistance. *Biomaterials*. 1987;8:423-426.
210. Oga M, Sugioka Y, Hobgood CD, et al. Surgical biomaterials and differential colonization by *Staphylococcus epidermidis*. *Biomaterials*. 1988;9:285-289.
211. Kuklo TR, Potter BK, Bell RS, Moquin RR, Rosner MK. Single-stage treatment of pyogenic spinal infection with titanium mesh cages. *J Spinal Disord Tech*. 2006;19:376-382.
212. Przybylski GJ, Sharan AD. Single-stage autogenous bone grafting and internal fixation in the surgical management of pyogenic discitis and vertebral osteomyelitis. *J Neurosurg Spine*. 2001;94:1-7.
213. Liljenqvist U, Lerner T, Bullmann V, et al. Titanium cages in the surgical treatment of severe vertebral osteomyelitis. *Eur Spine J*. 2003;12:606-612.
214. Young WF, Weaver M, Snyder B, Narayan R. Reversal of tetraplegia in patients with cervical osteomyelitis—epidural abscess using anterior debridement and fusion. *Spinal Cord*. 2001;39:538-540.
215. Capener N. The evolution of lateral rhachiotomy. *J Bone Joint Surg Br*. 1954;36B:173-179.
216. Lu DC, Wang V, Chou D. The use of allograft or autograft and expandable titanium cages for the treatment of vertebral osteomyelitis. *Neurosurgery*. 2009;64:122-129.
217. Korovessis P, Baikousis A, Zacharatos S, et al. Combined anterior plus posterior stabilization versus posterior short-segment instrumentation and fusion for mid-lumbar (L2-L4) burst fractures. *Spine*. 2006;31:859-868.
218. Mochida J, Toh E, Chiba M, Nishimura K. Treatment of osteoporotic late collapse of a vertebral body of thoracic and lumbar spine. *J Spinal Disord*. 2001;14:393-398.
219. Snell BE, Nasr FF, Wolfla CE. Single-stage thoracolumbar vertebrectomy with circumferential reconstruction and arthrodesis: surgical technique and results in 15 patients. *Neurosurgery*. 2006;58:ONS-263-8.
220. Senel A, Kaya AH, Kuruoglu E, Celik F. Circumferential stabilization with ghost screwing after posterior resection of spinal metastases via transpedicular route. *Neurosurg Rev*. 2007;30:131-137.
221. Bilsky MH, Lis E, Raizer J, et al. The diagnosis and treatment of metastatic spinal tumor. *Oncologist*. 1999;4:459-469.
222. Lee MC, Wang MY, Fessler RG, et al. Instrumentation in patients with spinal infection. *Neurosurg Focus*. 2004;17:E7.
223. Staatz G, Adam GB, Keulers P, et al. Spondylodiskitic abscesses: CT-guided percutaneous catheter drainage. *Radiology*. 1998;208:363-367.
224. Jeanneret B, Magerl F. Treatment of osteomyelitis of the spine using percutaneous suction/irrigation and percutaneous external spinal fixation. *J Spinal Disord*. 1994;7:185-205.
225. Onik G. Automated percutaneous biopsy in the diagnosis and treatment of infectious discitis. *Neurosurg Clin N Am*. 1996;7:145-150.
226. Tsou PM, Yeung AT. Transforaminal endoscopic decompression for radiculopathy secondary to intracanal noncontained lumbar disc herniations: outcome and technique. *Spine J*. 2002;2:41-48.
227. Yeung AT, Tsou PM. Posterolateral endoscopic excision for lumbar disc herniation: surgical technique, outcome, and complications in 307 consecutive cases. *Spine*. 2002;27:722-731.
228. Corpataux JM, Halkic N, Wettstein M, Dusmet M. The role of laparoscopic biopsies in lumbar spondylodiscitis. *Surg Endosc*. 2000;14:1086.
229. Korovessis P, Repantis T, Iliopoulos P, Hadjipavlou A. Beneficial influence of titanium mesh cage on infection healing and spinal reconstruction in hematogenous septic spondylitis: a retrospective analysis of surgical outcome of twenty-five consecutive cases and review of literature. *Spine*. 2008;33:E759-E767.
230. Gottschalk L, Regev G, Taylor W, et al.: *The use of posterior minimally invasive approach for corpectomy*. Poster presentation at SAS 9 Annual Meeting. London, April 28, 2009.
230a. Madhavan K, Vanni S, Williams SK. Direct lateral retroperitoneal approach for the surgical treatment of lumbar discitis and osteomyelitis. *Neurosurg Focus*. 2014;37(2):E5.
231. Chen X, Kidder LS, Lew WD. Osteogenic protein-1 induced bone formation in an infected segmental defect in the rat femur. *J Orthop Res*. 2002;20:142-150.
232. Southwood LL, Frisbie DD, Kawcak CE, et al. Evaluation of Ad-BMP-2 for enhancing fracture healing in an infected defect fracture rabbit model. *J Orthop Res*. 2004;22:66-72.
233. Allen RT, Lee YP, Stimson E, Garfin SR. Bone morphogenetic protein-2 (BMP-2) in the treatment of pyogenic vertebral osteomyelitis. *Spine*. 2007;32:2996-3006.
234. O'Shaughnessy BA, Kuklo TR, Ondra SL. Surgical treatment of vertebral osteomyelitis with recombinant human bone morphogenetic protein-2. *Spine*. 2008;33:E132-E139.
235. Aryan HE, Lu DC, Acosta FL Jr, Ames CP. Corpectomy followed by the placement of instrumentation with titanium cages and recombinant human bone morphogenetic protein-2 for vertebral osteomyelitis. *J Neurosurg Spine*. 2007;6:23-30.
236. Malik GM, Crawford AH, Halter R. Swan-neck deformity secondary to osteomyelitis of the posterior elements of the cervical spine. Case report. *J Neurosurg*. 1979;50:388-390.
237. Woertgen C, Rothoerl RD, Englert C, Neumann C. Pyogenic spinal infections and outcome according to the 36-Item Short Form Health Survey. *J Neurosurg Spine*. 2006;4:441-446.
238. Danner RL, Hartman BJ. Update on spinal epidural abscess: 35 cases and review of the literature. *Rev Infect Dis*. 1987;9:265-274.
239. Baker CJ. Primary spinal epidural abscess. *Am J Dis Child*. 1971;121:337-339.

240. Baker AS, Ojemann RG, Swartz MN, Richardson EP Jr. Spinal epidural abscess. *N Engl J Med.* 1975;293:463-468.
241. Zimmerer SM, Conen A, Muller AA, et al. Spinal epidural abscess: aetiology, predispondent factors and clinical outcomes in a 4-year prospective study. *Eur Spine J.* 2011;20:2228-2234.
242. Tang HJ, Lin HJ, Liu YC, Li CM. Spinal epidural abscess—experience with 46 patients and evaluation of prognostic factors. *J Infect.* 2002;45:76-81.
243. Davis DP, Wold RM, Patel RJ, et al. The clinical presentation and impact of diagnostic delays on emergency department patients with spinal epidural abscess. *J Emerg Med.* 2004;26:285-291.
244. Hlavin ML, Kaminski HJ, Ross JS, Ganz E. Spinal epidural abscess: a ten-year perspective. *Neurosurgery.* 1990;27:177-184.
245. Nussbaum ES, Rigamonti D, Standiford H, et al. Spinal epidural abscess: a report of 40 cases and review. *Surg Neurol.* 1992;38:225-231.
246. Feldenzer JA, McKeever PE, Schaberg DR, et al. Experimental spinal epidural abscess: a pathophysiological model in the rabbit. *Neurosurgery.* 1987;20:859-867.
247. Guerrero IC, Slap GB, MacGregor RR, et al. Anaerobic spinal epidural abscess. Case report. *J Neurosurg.* 1978;48:465-469.
248. Hancock DO. A study of 49 patients with acute spinal extradural abscess. *Paraplegia.* 1973;10:285-288.
249. Heusner AP. Nontuberculosis spinal epidural infections. *N Engl J Med.* 1948;239:845-854.
250. Kaufman DM, Kaplan JG, Litman N. Infectious agents in spinal epidural abscesses. *Neurology.* 1980;30:844-850.
251. Browder J, Meyers R. Infection of the spinal epidural space. *Am J Surg.* 1937;37:4-26.
252. Chan ST, Leung S. Spinal epidural abscess following steroid injection for sciatica. Case report. *Spine.* 1989;14:106-108.
253. Ferris B, Jones C. Paraplegia due to aspergillosis. Successful conservative treatment of two cases. *J Bone Joint Surg Br.* 1985;67:800-803.
254. Rangell L, Glassman F. Acute spinal epidural abscess as a complication of lumbar puncture. *J Nerv Ment Dis.* 1945;102:8-18.
255. Wang LP, Hauerberg J, Schmidt JF. Incidence of spinal epidural abscess after epidural analgesia: a national 1-year survey. *Anesthesiology.* 1999;91:1928-1936.
256. Rigamonti D, Liem L, Sampath P, et al. Spinal epidural abscess: contemporary trends in etiology, evaluation, and management. *Surg Neurol.* 1999;52:189-196.
257. Reihsaus E, Waldbaur H, Seeling W. Spinal epidural abscess: a meta-analysis of 915 patients. *Neurosurg Rev.* 2000;23:175-204.
258. Browder J, Meyers R. Pyogenic infections of the spinal epidural space. A consideration of the anatomic and physiologic pathology. *Surgery.* 1941;10:296-308.
259. Dandy WE. Abscesses and inflammatory tumors in the spinal epidural space (so-called pachymeningitis externa). *Arch Surg.* 1926;13:477-494.
260. de Villiers JC, Cluver PF. Spinal epidural abscess in children. *S Afr J Surg.* 1978;16:149-155.
261. Hakin RN, Burt AA, Cook JB. Acute spinal epidural abscess. *Paraplegia.* 1979;17:330-336.
262. Phillips GE, Jefferson A. Acute spinal epidural abscess. Observations from fourteen cases. *Postgrad Med J.* 1979;55:712-715.
263. Russell NA, Vaughan R, Morley TP. Spinal epidural infection. *Can J Neurol Sci.* 1979;6:325-328.
264. Feldenzer JA, McKeever PE, Schaberg DR, et al. The pathogenesis of spinal epidural abscess: microangiographic studies in an experimental model. *J Neurosurg.* 1988;69:110-114.
265. Corradini EW, Turney MF, Browder EJ. Spinal epidural infection. *N Y State J Med.* 1948;48:2367-2370.
266. Hulme A, Dott NM. Spinal epidural abscess. *Br Med J.* 1954;4853:64-68.
267. Rankin RM, Flothow PG. Pyogenic infection of the spinal epidural space. *West J Surg Obstet Gynecol.* 1946;54:320-323.
268. Grant FC. Epidural spinal abscess. *J Am Med Asoc.* 1945;128:509-511.
269. Schoenfeld AJ, Wahlquist TC. Mortality, complication risk, and total charges after the treatment of epidural abscess. *Spine J.* 2015;15:249-255.
270. Butler EG, Dohrmann PJ, Stark RJ. Spinal subdural abscess. *Clin Exp Neurol.* 1988;25:67-70.
271. Sorensen P. Spinal epidural abscesses: conservative treatment for selected subgroups of patients. *Br J Neurosurg.* 2003;17:513-518.
272. Kirzner H, Oh YK, Lee SH. Intraspinal air: a CT finding of epidural abscess. *AJR Am J Roentgenol.* 1988;151:1217-1218.
273. Leys D, Lesoin F, Viaud C, et al. Decreased morbidity from acute bacterial spinal epidural abscesses using computed tomography and nonsurgical treatment in selected patients. *Ann Neurol.* 1985;17:350-355.
274. Angtuaco EJ, McConnell JR, Chadduck WM, Flanigan S. MR imaging of spinal epidural sepsis. *AJR Am J Roentgenol.* 1987;149:1249-1253.
275. Arnott G, Delfosse JM. Acute spinal epidural abscess. *J Neurol.* 1985;213:343-344.
276. Bouchez B, Arnott G, Delfosse JM. Acute spinal epidural abscess. *J Neurol.* 1985;231:343-344.
277. Bertino RE, Porter BA, Stimac GK, Tepper SJ. Imaging spinal osteomyelitis and epidural abscess with short TI inversion recovery (STIR). *AJNR Am J Neuroradiol.* 1988;9:563-564.
278. Erntell M, Holtas S, Norlin K, et al. Magnetic resonance imaging in the diagnosis of spinal epidural abscess. *Scand J Infect Dis.* 1988;20:323-327.
279. Kuker W, Mull M, Mayfrank L, Topper R, Thron A. Epidural spinal infection. Variability of clinical and magnetic resonance imaging findings. *Spine.* 1997;22:544-550.
280. Ju KL, Kim SD, Melikian R, et al. Predicting patients with concurrent noncontiguous spinal epidural abscess lesions. *Spine J.* 2015;15:95-101.
281. Lownie SP, Ferguson GG. Spinal subdural empyema complicating cervical discography. *Spine.* 1989;14:1415-1417.
282. Theodotou B, Woosley RE, Whaley RA. Spinal subdural empyema: diagnosis by spinal computed tomography. *Surg Neurol.* 1984;21:610-612.
283. Wheeler D, Keiser P, Rigamonti D, Keay S. Medical management of spinal epidural abscesses: case report and review. *Clin Infect Dis.* 1992;15:22-27.
284. Lang IM, Hughes DG, Jenkins JP, et al. MR imaging appearances of cervical epidural abscess. *Clin Radiol.* 1995;50:466-471.
285. Mampalam TJ, Rosegay H, Andrews BT, et al. Nonoperative treatment of spinal epidural infections. *J Neurosurg.* 1989;71:208-210.
286. Patel AR, Alton TB, Bransford RJ, et al. Spinal epidural abscesses: risk factors, medical versus surgical management,

a retrospective review of 128 cases. *Spine J*. 2014;14: 326-330.

287. Liem LK, Rigamonti D, Wolf AL, et al. Thoracic epidural abscess. *J Spinal Disord*. 1994;7:449-454.
288. Siddiq F, Chowfin A, Tight R, et al. Medical vs surgical management of spinal epidural abscess. *Arch Intern Med*. 2004;164:2409-2412.
289. Kim CW, Garfin SR. The management of cervical and thoracic epidural abscess in the neurologically asymptomatic patient. *Semin Spine Surgery*. 2004;16:188-194.
290. Tuchman A, Pham M, Hsieh PC. The indications and timing for operative management of spinal epidural abscess: literature review and treatment algorithm. *Neurosurg Focus*. 2014; 37:E8.
291. Ghobrial GM, Beygi S, Viereck MJ, et al. Timing in the surgical evacuation of spinal epidural abscesses. *Neurosurg Focus*. 2014;37:E1.
292. Connor DR Jr, Chittiboina P, Caldito G, Nanda A. Comparison of operative and nonoperative management of spinal epidural abscess: a retrospective review of clinical and laboratory predictors of neurologic outcome. *J Neurosurg Spine*. 2013;19:119-127.
293. Ghobrial GM, Viereck MJ, Margiotta PJ, et al. Surgical management in 40 consecutive patients with cervical spinal epidural abscesses. Shifting toward circumferential treatment. *Spine*. 2015;40:E949-E953.
294. Alton TB, Patel AR, Bransford RJ, et al. Is there a difference in neurologic outcome in medical versus early operative management of cervical epidural abscesses? *Spine J*. 2015;15:10-17.
295. Garrido E, Rosenwasser RH. Experience with the suction-irrigation technique in the management of spinal epidural infection. *Neurosurgery*. 1983;12:678-679.
296. Cardan E, Nanulescu M. Epidural lavage for extensive epidural suppuration. *Anaesthesia*. 1987;42:1023.
297. Schultz KD Jr, Comey CH, Haid RW Jr. Technical note. Pyogenic spinal epidural abscess: a minimally invasive technique for multisegmental decompression. *J Spinal Disord*. 2001;14:546-549.
298. Mixter WJ, Smithwick RH. Acute intraspinal epidural abscess. *N Engl J Med*. 1932;207:126-131.
299. Corboy JR, Price RW. Myelitis and toxic, inflammatory, and infectious disorders. *Curr Opin Neurol Neurosurg*. 1993;6:564-570.
300. McGee-Collett M, Johnston IH. Spinal epidural abscess: presentation and treatment. A report of 21 cases. *Med J Aust*. 1991;155:14-17.
301. Redekop GJ, Del Maestro RF. Diagnosis and management of spinal epidural abscess. *Can J Neurol Sci*. 1992;19:180-187.
302. Curling OD, Gower DJ, McWhorter JM. Changing concepts in spinal epidural abscess: a report of 29 cases. *Neurosurgery*. 1990;27:185.
303. Yang SY. Spinal epidural abscess. *N Z Med J*. 1982;95:302-304.
304. Wang LP, Hauerberg J, Schmidt JF. Long-term outcome after neurosurgically treated spinal epidural abscess following epidural analgesia. *Acta Anaesthesiol Scand*. 2001;45: 233-239.
305. Levy ML, Wieder BH, Schneider J, et al. Subdural empyema of the cervical spine: clinicopathological correlates and magnetic resonance imaging. Report of three cases. *J Neurosurg*. 1993;79:929-935.
306. Pritchard DJ. Granulomatous infections of bones and joints. *Orthop Clin North Am*. 1975;6:1029-1047.
307. Lerner PI. *Nocardia Species*. New York: Churchill Livingstone; 1995:2273-2280.
308. Govender S, Charles RW, Naidoo KS, Goga IE. Results of surgical decompression in chronic tuberculous paraplegia. *S Afr Med J*. 1988;74:58-59.
309. Tuli SM, Srivastava TP, Varma BP, Sinha GP. Tuberculosis of spine. *Acta Orthop Scand*. 1967;38:445-458.
310. Cleveland M. Tuberculosis of the spine. A clinical study of 203 patients from Sea View and St. Luke's Hospital. *Am Rev Tuberculosis*. 1940;41:215-321.
311. Adendorff JJ, Boeke EJ, Lazarus C. Pott's paraplegia. *S Afr Med J*. 1987;71:427-428.
312. Friedman B. Chemotherapy of tuberculosis of the spine. *J Bone Joint Surg Am*. 1966;48:451-474.
313. Martin NS. Tuberculosis of the spine. A study of the results of treatment during the last twenty-five years. *J Bone Joint Surg Br*. 1970;52:613-628.
314. Dobson J. Tuberculosis of the spine; an analysis of the results of conservative treatment and of the factors influencing the prognosis. *J Bone Joint Surg Br*. 1951;33-B: 517-531.
315. Bosworth DM, Della Pietra A, Rahilly G. Paraplegia resulting from tuberculosis of the spine. *J Bone Joint Surg Am*. 1953;35-A:735-740.
316. Fellander M. Paraplegia in spondylitis: results of operative treatment. *Paraplegia*. 1975;13:75-88.
317. Kaplan CJ. Pott's disease in South African Bantu children; an analysis of results and comparison with Lancashire figures. *Br J Tuberc Dis Chest*. 1952;46:209-213.
318. Martin NS. Pott's paraplegia: a report of 120 cases. *J Bone Joint Surg*. 1971;53B:596-608.
319. Hodgson AR, Yau AC, Kwon JS. A clinical study of one hundred consecutive cases of Pott's paraplegia. *Clin Orthop Relat Res*. 1964;36:128-150.
320. Scrimgeour EM, Kaven J, Gajdusek DC. Spinal tuberculosis—the commonest cause of non-traumatic paraplegia in Papua New Guinea. *Trop Geogr Med*. 1987;39:218-221.
321. Adendorff JJ, Boeke EJ, Lazarus C. Tuberculosis of the spine: results of management of 300 patients. *J R Coll Surg Edinb*. 1987;32:152-155.
322. Lifeso RM, Weaver P, Harder EH. Tuberculous spondylitis in adults. *J Bone Joint Surg Am*. 1985;67:1405-1413.
323. Hodgson AR. Report of the findings and results in 300 cases of Pott's disease treated by anterior fusion of the spine. *J West Pacific Orthop Assoc*. 1964;1:3.
324. Moodie AS. Tuberculosis in Hong Kong. *Tubercle*. 1963;4:334-345.
325. A controlled trial of ambulant out-patient treatment and in-patient rest in bed in the management of tuberculosis of the spine in young Korean patients on standard chemotherapy: a study in Masan, Korea. First Report of the Medical Research Council Working Party on Tuberculosis of the Spine. *J Bone Joint Surg Br*. 1973;55:678-697.
326. A controlled trial of anterior spinal fusion and debridement in the surgical management of tuberculosis of the spine in patients on standard chemotherapy: a study in two centres in South Africa. Seventh Report of the Medical Research Council Working Party on Tuberculosis of the Spine. *Tubercle*. 1978;59:79-105.
327. Five-year assessments of controlled trials of ambulatory treatment, debridement and anterior spinal fusion in the management of tuberculosis of the spine. Studies in Bulawayo (Rhodesia) and in Hong Kong. Sixth Report of the Medical

Research Council Working Party on Tuberculosis of the Spine. *J Bone Joint Surg Br*. 1978;60-B:163-177.

328. Benson CA, Kaplan JE, Masur H, et al. Treating opportunistic infections among HIV-infected adults and adolescents: recommendations from CDC, the National Institutes of Health, and the HIV Medicine Association/Infectious Diseases Society of America. *MMWR Recomm Rep*. 2004;53:1-112.
329. Pirofsky JG, Huang CT, Waites KB. Spinal osteomyelitis due to *Mycobacterium avium-intracellulare* in an elderly man with steroid-induced osteoporosis. *Spine*. 1993;18:1926-1929.
330. Blacklock JWS. Injury as an aetiological factor in tuberculosis: president's address. *Proc R Soc Med*. 1957;50:61-68.
331. Doub HP, Badgley CE. The roentgen signs of tuberculosis of the vertebral body. *Am J Radiol*. 1932;27:827-837.
332. Babhulkar SS, Tayade WB, Babhulkar SK. Atypical spinal tuberculosis. *J Bone Joint Surg Br*. 1984;66:239-242.
333. Naim Ur R, Al-Arabi KM, Khan FA. Atypical forms of spinal tuberculosis. *Acta Neurochir (Wien)*. 1987;88:26-33.
334. Moorthy S, Prabhu NK. Spectrum of MR imaging findings in spinal tuberculosis. *AJR Am J Roentgenol*. 2002;179:979-983.
335. Kumar K. A clinical study and classification of posterior spinal tuberculosis. *Int Orthop*. 1985;9:147-152.
336. Ghormley RK, Bradley JI. Prognostic signs in the x-rays of tuberculous spines in children. *J Bone Joint Surg*. 1928;10:796-804.
337. Dass B, Puet TA, Watanakunakorn C. Tuberculosis of the spine (Pott's disease) presenting as 'compression fractures'. *Spinal Cord*. 2002;40:604-608.
338. Mathuriya SN, Khosla VK, Banerjee AK. Intradural extramedullary tuberculous spinal granulomas. *Clin Neurol Neurosurg*. 1988;90:155-158.
339. Postacchini F, Montanaro A. Tuberculous epidural granuloma simulating a herniated lumbar disk: a report of a case. *Clin Orthop Relat Res*. 1980;148:182-185.
340. Freilich D, Swash M. Diagnosis and management of tuberculous paraplegia with special reference to tuberculous radiculomyelitis. *J Neurol Neurosurg Psychiatry*. 1979;42:12-18.
341. Garceau GJ, Brady TA. Pott's paraplegia. *J Bone Joint Surg Am*. 1950;32A:87-96.
342. Hsu LC, Cheng CL, Leong JC. Pott's paraplegia of late onset. The cause of compression and results after anterior decompression. *J Bone Joint Surg Br*. 1988;70:534-538.
343. Hodgson AR, Skinsnes OK, Leong CY. The pathogenesis of Pott's paraplegia. *J Bone Joint Surg Am*. 1967;49:1147-1156.
344. Scully RE, Mark EJ, McNeely BU. Case records of the Massachusetts General Hospital. *N Engl J Med*. 1982;306:729-737.
345. Azzam NI, Tammawy M. Tuberculosis spondylitis in adults: diagnosis and treatment. *Br J Neurosurg*. 1988;2:85-91.
346. Roca B. Intradural extramedullary tuberculoma of the spinal cord: a review of reported cases. *J Infect*. 2005;50:425-431.
347. A controlled trial of debridement and ambulatory treatment in the management of tuberculosis of the spine in patients on standard chemotherapy. A study in Bulawayo, Rhodesia. *J Trop Med Hyg*. 1974;77:72-92.
348. Hsu LC, Leong JC. Tuberculosis of the lower cervical spine (C2 to C7). A report on 40 cases. *J Bone Joint Surg Br*. 1984;66:1-5.
349. Batirel A, Erdem H, Sengoz G, et al. The course of spinal tuberculosis (Pott disease): results of the multinational, multicenter Backbone-2 study. *Clin Microbiol Infect*. 2015;21:1008.e9-1008.e18.
350. Forlenza SW, Axelrod JL, Grieco MH. Pott's disease in heroin addicts. *JAMA*. 1979;241:379-380.
351. Daniel TM. The rapid diagnosis of tuberculosis: a selective review. *J Lab Clin Med*. 1990;116:277-282.
352. Huggett JF, McHugh TD, Zumla A. Tuberculosis: amplification-based clinical diagnostic techniques. *Int J Biochem Cell Biol*. 2003;35:1407-1412.
353. Berk RH, Yazici M, Atabey N, et al. Detection of *Mycobacterium tuberculosis* in formaldehyde solution-fixed, paraffin-embedded tissue by polymerase chain reaction in Pott's disease. *Spine*. 1996;21:1991-1995.
354. Albay A, Kisa O, Baylan O, Doganci L. The evaluation of FASTPlaqueTB test for the rapid diagnosis of tuberculosis. *Diagn Microbiol Infect Dis*. 2003;46:211-215.
355. Roaf R, Kirkaldy Willis WH. *Surgical Treatment of Bone and Joint Tuberculosis*. Edinburgh: Churchill Livingstone; 1959.
356. Sarkar SD, Ravikrishnan KP, Woodbury DH, et al. Gallium-67 citrate scanning—a new adjunct in the detection and follow-up of extrapulmonary tuberculosis: concise communication. *J Nucl Med*. 1979;20:833-836.
357. Smith AS, Weinstein MA, Mizushima A, et al. MR imaging characteristics of tuberculous spondylitis vs vertebral osteomyelitis. *AJR Am J Roentgenol*. 1989;153:399-405.
358. Kim NH, Lee HM, Suh JS. Magnetic resonance imaging for the diagnosis of tuberculous spondylitis. *Spine*. 1994;19:2451-2455.
359. Singer J, Sundaram M. Radiologic case study. Tuberculosis of the vertebra. *Orthopedics*. 1988;11:1220-1224.
360. Thammaroj J, Kitkuandee A, Sawanyawisuth K. Differences of MRI features between tuberculosis and bacterial spondylitis in a TB-endemic area. *Southeast Asian J Trop Med Public Health*. 2015;46:71-79.
361. Bosworth DM, Pietra AD, Farrell RF. Streptomycin in tuberculous bone and joint lesions with mixed infection and sinuses. *J Bone Joint Surg Am*. 1950;32A:103-108.
362. Kondo E, Yamada K. End results of focal debridement in bone and joint tuberculosis and its indications. *J Bone Joint Surg*. 1957;39A:27-31.
363. Bosworth DM, Wright HA, Fielding JW. The treatment of bone and joint tuberculosis; effect of 1-isonicotinyl-2-isopropylhydrazine; a preliminary report. *J Bone Joint Surg Am*. 1952;34 A:761-771. passim.
364. Johnson RW Jr, Hillman JW, Southwick WO. The importance of direct surgical attack upon lesions of the vertebral bodies, particularly in Pott's disease. *J Bone Joint Surg Am*. 1953;35-A:17-25. passim.
365. Kaplan CJ. Conservative therapy in skeletal tuberculosis: an appraisal based on experience in South Africa. *Tubercle*. 1959;40:355-368.
366. Moon MS, Kim I, Woo YK, Park YO. Conservative treatment of tuberculosis of the thoracic and lumbar spine in adults and children. *Int Orthop*. 1987;11:315-322.
367. A controlled trial of plaster-of-Paris jackets in the management of ambulant outpatient treatment of tuberculosis of the spine in children on standard chemotherapy. A study in Pusan, Korea. Second Report of the Medical Research Council Working Party on Tuberculosis of the Spine. *Tubercle*. 1973;54:261-282.
368. A five-year assessment of controlled trials of in-patient and out-patient treatment and of plaster-of-Paris jackets for tuberculosis of the spine in children on standard chemotherapy. Studies in Masan and Pusan, Korea. Fifth Report of the Medical Research Council Working

Party on tuberculosis of the spine. *J Bone Joint Surg Br.* 1976;58-B:399-411.

369. A 10-year assessment of controlled trials of inpatient and outpatient treatment and of plaster-of-Paris jackets for tuberculosis of the spine in children on standard chemotherapy. Studies in Masan and Pusan, Korea. Ninth Report of the Medical Research Council Working Party on Tuberculosis of the Spine. *J Bone Joint Surg Br.* 1985;67:103-110.
370. A controlled trial of anterior spinal fusion and debridement in the surgical management of tuberculosis of the spine in patients on standard chemotherapy: a study in Hong Kong. *Br J Surg.* 1974;61:853-866.
371. A 10-year assessment of a controlled trial comparing debridement and anterior spinal fusion in the management of tuberculosis of the spine in patients on standard chemotherapy in Hong Kong. Eighth Report of the Medical Research Council Working Party on Tuberculosis of the Spine. *J Bone Joint Surg Br.* 1982;64:393-398.
372. A controlled trial of six-month and nine-month regimens of chemotherapy in patients undergoing radical surgery for tuberculosis of the spine in Hong Kong. Tenth Report of the Medical Research Council Working Party on Tuberculosis of the Spine. *Tubercle.* 1986;67:243-259.
373. Medical Research Council Working Party on Tuberculosis of the Spine. A comparison of 6 or 9 month course regime of chemotherapy in patients receiving ambulatory treatment or undergoing radical surgery for tuberculosis of the spine. *Indian J Tuberculosis (Suppl).* 1989;36:1-21.
374. Arct W. Operative treatment of tuberculosis of the spine in old people. *J Bone Joint Surg Am.* 1968;50:255-267.
375. Guirguis AR. Pott's paraplegia. *J Bone Joint Surg Br.* 1967;49:658-667.
376. Wiltberger BR. Resection of vertebral bodies and bone-grafting for chronic osteomyelitis of the spine; a case report. *J Bone Joint Surg Am.* 1952;34-A:215-218.
377. Shaw NE, Thomas TG. Surgical treatment of chronic infective lesions of the spine. *Br Med J.* 1963;1:162-164.
378. Yau ACMC, Hsu LCS, O'Brien JP. Tuberculous kyphosis: correction with spinal osteotomy, halo-pelvic distraction, and anterior posterior fusion. *J Bone Joint Surg.* 1974;56A: 1419-1434.
378a. Zheng Z, Lou F, Zhou Q. The outcomes of chemotherapy only treatment on mild spinal tuberculosis. *J Orthop Surg Res.* 2016;11:49.
379. Haas DW. *Mycobacterium Tuberculosis.* New York: Churchill Livingstone; 1995:2213-2243.
380. Barclay WR, Ebert RH, Le Roy GV, et al. Distribution and excretion of radioactive isoniazid in tuberculous patients. *J Am Med Assoc.* 1953;151:1384-1388.
381. Snider DE Jr, Cauthen GM, Farer LS, et al. Drug-resistant tuberculosis. *Am Rev Respir Dis.* 1991;144:732.
382. Moon MS, Moon YW, Moon JL, et al. Conservative treatment of tuberculosis of the lumbar and lumbosacral spine. *Clin Orthop Relat Res.* 2002;398:40-49.
383. Pertuiset E. Medical therapy of bone and joint tuberculosis in 1998. *Rev Rhum Engl Ed.* 1999;66:152-157.
384. Bhojraj S, Nene A. Lumbar and lumbosacral tuberculous spondylodiscitis in adults. Redefining the indications for surgery. *J Bone Joint Surg Br.* 2002;84:530-534.
385. Weinberg JA. The surgical excision of psoas abscesses resulting from spinal tuberculosis. *J Bone Joint Surg Am.* 1957;39-A:17-27.
386. Fountain SS, Hsu LC, Yau AC, Hodgson AR. Progressive kyphosis following solid anterior spine fusion in children with tuberculosis of the spine. A long-term study. *J Bone Joint Surg Am.* 1975;57:1104-1107.
387. Assaghir YM, Rafae HH, Alam-Eddin M. Anterior versus posterior debridement fusion for single-level dorsal tuberculosis: the role of graft type and level of fixation on determining the outcome. *Eur Spine J.* 2016;25(12):3884-3893.
388. Allen AR, Stevenson AW. The results of combined drug therapy and early fusion in bone tuberculosis. *J Bone Joint Surg.* 1957;39A:32-42.
389. Allen AR, Stevenson AW. Follow-up notes on articles previously published in the Journal: a ten-year follow-up of combined drug therapy and early fusion in bone tuberculosis. *J Bone Joint Surg Am.* 1967;49A:1001-1003.
390. Ito M, Abumi K, Kotani Y, et al. Clinical outcome of posterolateral endoscopic surgery for pyogenic spondylodiscitis: results of 15 patients with serious comorbid conditions. *Spine.* 2007;32:200-206.
391. Rand C, Smith MA. Anterior spinal tuberculosis: paraplegia following laminectomy. *Ann R Coll Surg Engl.* 1989;71:105-109.
392. Yau AC, Hodgson AR. Penetration of the lung by the paravertebral abscess in tuberculosis of the spine. *J Bone Joint Surg Am.* 1968;50:243-254.
393. Halpern AA, Rinsky LA, Fountain S, Nagel DA. Coccidioidomycosis of the spine: unusual roentgenographic presentation. *Clin Orthop Relat Res.* 1979;140:78-79.
394. Moon MS, Woo YK, Lee KS, et al. Posterior instrumentation and anterior interbody fusion for tuberculous kyphosis of dorsal and lumbar spines. *Spine.* 1995;20:1910-1916.
395. Lee EY, Hahn MS. A study of influences of the anterior intervertebral fusion upon the correct ability of kyphosis in tuberculous spondylitis. *J Korena Orthop Assoc.* 1968;3: 31-40.
396. Chen WJ, Wu CC, Jung CH, et al. Combined anterior and posterior surgeries in the treatment of spinal tuberculous spondylitis. *Clin Orthop Relat Res.* 2002;398:50-59.
397. Govender S, Parbhoo AH. Support of the anterior column with allografts in tuberculosis of the spine. *J Bone Joint Surg Br.* 1999;81:106-109.
398. Sundararaj GD, Babu N, Amritanand R, et al. Treatment of haematogenous pyogenic vertebral osteomyelitis by single-stage anterior debridement, grafting of the defect and posterior instrumentation. *J Bone Joint Surg Br.* 2007;89:1201-1205.
399. Mukhtar AM, Farghaly MM, Ahmed SH. Surgical treatment of thoracic and lumbar tuberculosis by anterior interbody fusion and posterior instrumentation. *Med Princ Pract.* 2003;12:92-96.
400. Turgut M. Spinal tuberculosis (Pott's disease): its clinical presentation, surgical management, and outcome. A survey study on 694 patients. *Neurosurg Rev.* 2001;24:8-13.
401. Göven O, Kumano K, Yalcin S, et al. A single stage posterior approach and rigid fixation for preventing kyphosis in the treatment of spinal tuberculosis. *Spine.* 1994;19:1039-1043.
402. Mehta JS, Bhojraj SY. Tuberculosis of the thoracic spine. A classification based on the selection of surgical strategies. *J Bone Joint Surg Br.* 2001;83:859-863.
403. Oga M, Arizono T, Takasita M, Sugioka Y. Evaluation of the risk of instrumentation as a foreign body in spinal tuberculosis. Clinical and biologic study. *Spine.* 1993;18:1890-1894.

404. Benli IT, Acaroglu E, Akalin S, et al. Anterior radical debridement and anterior instrumentation in tuberculosis spondylitis. *Eur Spine J*. 2003;12:224-234.
405. Govender S. The outcome of allografts and anterior instrumentation in spinal tuberculosis. *Clin Orthop Relat Res*. 2002;398:60-66.
406. Yilmaz C, Selek HY, Gurkan I, et al. Anterior instrumentation for the treatment of spinal tuberculosis. *J Bone Joint Surg Am*. 1999;81:1261-1267.
407. Corea JR, Tamimi TM. Tuberculosis of the arch of the atlas. Case report. *Spine*. 1987;12:608-611.
408. Behari S, Nayak SR, Bhargava V, et al. Craniocervical tuberculosis: protocol of surgical management. *Neurosurgery*. 2003;52:72-80.
409. Hodgson AR. An approach to the cervical spine (C-3 to C-7). *Clin Orthop Relat Res*. 1965;39:129-134.
410. Rajasekaran S, Shanmugasundaram TK. Prediction of the angle of gibbus deformity in tuberculosis of the spine. *J Bone Joint Surg Am*. 1987;69:503-509.
411. Schulitz KP, Kothe R, Leong JC, Wehling P. Growth changes of solidly fused kyphotic bloc after surgery for tuberculosis. Comparison of four procedures. *Spine*. 1997;22:1150-1155.
412. Kohli SB. Radical surgical approach to spinal tuberculosis. *J Bone Joint Surg Br*. 1967;49:668-673.
413. Smego RA Jr, Foglia G. Actinomycosis. *Clin Infect Dis*. 1998;26:1255-1261.
414. Russo TA. *Agents of Actinomycosis*. New York: Churchill Livingstone; 1995:2280-2288.
415. Bennhoff DF. Actinomycosis: diagnostic and therapeutic considerations and a review of 32 cases. *Laryngoscope*. 1984;94:1198-1217.
416. Deleted in review.
417. Apotheloz C, Regamey C. Disseminated infection due to *Actinomyces meyeri:* case report and review. *Clin Infect Dis*. 1996;22:621-625.
418. Cope VZ. Actinomycosis of bone with special reference to infection of vertebral column. *J Bone Joint Surg Br*. 1951;33B:205-214.
419. Honda H, Bankowski MJ, Kajioka EH, et al. Thoracic vertebral actinomycosis: *Actinomyces israelii* and *Fusobacterium nucleatum*. *J Clin Microbiol*. 2008;46:2009-2014.
420. Lerner PI. Susceptibility of pathogenic actinomycetes to antimicrobial compounds. *Antimicrob Agents Chemother*. 1974;5:302-309.
421. Martin MV. Antibiotic treatment of cervicofacial actinomycosis for patients allergic to penicillin: a clinical and in vitro study. *Br J Oral Maxillofac Surg*. 1985;23: 428-434.
422. Yung BC, Cheng JC, Chan TT, et al. Aggressive thoracic actinomycosis complicated by vertebral osteomyelitis and epidural abscess leading to spinal cord compression. *Spine*. 2000;25:745-748.
423. Leaker B, Hellyar A, Neild GH, et al. *Nocardia* infection in a renal transplant unit. *Transplant Proc*. 1989;21:2103-2104.
424. Wilson JP, Turner HR, Kirchner KA, Chapman SW. Nocardial infections in renal transplant recipients. *Medicine (Baltimore)*. 1989;68:38-57.
425. Patel R, Paya CV. Infections in solid-organ transplant recipients. *Clin Microbiol Rev*. 1997;10:86-124.
426. Torres OH, Domingo P, Pericas R, et al. Infection caused by *Nocardia farcinica:* case report and review. *Eur J Clin Microbiol Infect Dis*. 2000;19:205-212.
427. Yanoff DB, Church ML. Nocardial vertebral osteomyelitis. *Clin Orthop Relat Res*. 1983;175:223-226.
428. Graat HC, Van Ooij A, Day GA, McPhee IB. *Nocardia farcinica* spinal osteomyelitis. *Spine*. 2002;27:E253-E257.
429. Awad I, Bay JW, Petersen JM. Nocardial osteomyelitis of the spine with epidural spinal cord compression—a case report. *Neurosurgery*. 1984;15:254-256.
430. Siao P, McCabe P, Yagnik P. Nocardial spinal epidural abscess. *Neurology*. 1989;39:996.
431. Clarridge JE 3rd. Impact of 16S rRNA gene sequence analysis for identification of bacteria on clinical microbiology and infectious diseases. *Clin Microbiol Rev*. 2004;17:840-862. table of contents.
432. Lerner PI. Nocardiosis. *Clin Infect Dis*. 1996;22:891-903.
433. Saubolle MA, Sussland D. Nocardiosis: review of clinical and laboratory experience. *J Clin Microbiol*. 2003;41:4497-4501.
434. Pappas G, Papadimitriou P, Akritidis N, et al. The new global map of human brucellosis. *Lancet Infect Dis*. 2006;6:91-99.
435. Pappas G, Papadimitriou P, Christou L, Akritidis N. Future trends in human brucellosis treatment. *Expert Opin Investig Drugs*. 2006;15:1141-1149.
436. Pappas G, Solera J, Akritidis N, Tsianos E. New approaches to the antibiotic treatment of brucellosis. *Int J Antimicrob Agents*. 2005;26:101-105.
437. Keenan JD, Metz CW Jr. *Brucella* spondylitis. A brief review and case report. *Clin Orthop Relat Res*. 1972;82:87-91.
438. Lifeso RM, Harder E, McCorkell SJ. Spinal brucellosis. *J Bone Joint Surg Br*. 1985;67:345-351.
439. Wiseman J, McHenry C. Focal marrow replacement in intervertebral disc space infection. Demonstrated by Tc-99m sulfur colloid imaging. *Clin Nucl Med*. 1984;9:291-292.
440. Franco MP, Mulder M, Gilman RH, Smits HL. Human brucellosis. *Lancet Infect Dis*. 2007;7:775-786.
441. Franco MP, Mulder M, Smits HL. Persistence and relapse in brucellosis and need for improved treatment. *Trans R Soc Trop Med Hyg*. 2007;101:854-855.
442. Pappas G, Akritidis N, Bosilkovski M, Tsianos E. Brucellosis. *N Engl J Med*. 2005;352:2325-2336.
443. Pappas G, Akritidis N, Tsianos E. Effective treatments in the management of brucellosis. *Expert Opin Pharmacother*. 2005;6:201-209.
444. Mousa AR, Muhtaseb SA, Almudallal DS, et al. Osteoarticular complications of brucellosis: a study of 169 cases. *Rev Infect Dis*. 1987;9:531-543.
445. Young EJ. *Brucella Specia*. New York: Churchill Livingstone; 1995:2053-2060.
446. Colmenero JD, Cisneros JM, Orjuela DL, et al. Clinical course and prognosis of *Brucella* spondylitis. *Infection*. 1992;20: 38-42.
447. Ganado W, Craig AJ. Brucellosis myelopathy. *J Bone Joint Surg Am*. 1958;40-A:1380-1388.
448. Colmenero JD, Jimenez-Mejias ME, Sanchez-Lora FJ, et al. Pyogenic, tuberculous, and brucellar vertebral osteomyelitis: a descriptive and comparative study of 219 cases. *Ann Rheum Dis*. 1997;56:709-715.
449. al-Shahed MS, Sharif HS, Haddad MC, et al. Imaging features of musculoskeletal brucellosis. *Radiographics*. 1994;14:333-348.
450. Sharif HS, Aideyan OA, Clark DC, et al. Brucellar and tuberculous spondylitis: comparative imaging features. *Radiology*. 1989;171:419-425.
451. Ozaksoy D, Yucesoy K, Yucesoy M, et al. Brucellar spondylitis: MRI findings. *Eur Spine J*. 2001;10:529-533.

452. Alp E, Doganay M. Current therapeutic strategy in spinal brucellosis. *Int J Infect Dis*. 2008;12:573-577.
453. Ariza J, Gudiol F, Pallares R, et al. Treatment of human brucellosis with doxycycline plus rifampin or doxycycline plus streptomycin. A randomized, double-blind study. *Ann Intern Med*. 1992;117:25-30.
454. Nas K, Gur A, Kemaloglu MS, et al. Management of spinal brucellosis and outcome of rehabilitation. *Spinal Cord*. 2001;39:223-227.
455. Winter WG Jr, Larson RK, Zettas JP, Libke R. Coccidioidal spondylitis. *J Bone Joint Surg Am*. 1978;60:240-244.
456. Shaikh BS, Appelbaum PC, Aber RC. Vertebral disc space infection and osteomyelitis due to *Candida albicans* in a patient with acute myelomonocytic leukemia. *Cancer*. 1980;45:1025-1028.
457. Cone LA, Byrd RG, Potts BE, Wuesthoff M. Diagnosis and treatment of *Candida* vertebral osteomyelitis: clinical experience with a short course therapy of amphotericin B lipid complex. *Surg Neurol*. 2004;62:234-237.
458. Rodriguez D, Pigrau C, Almirante B, et al. Vertebral osteomyelitis due to *Candida* spp. *Enferm Infecc Microbiol Clin*. 2003;21:568-570.
459. Lutz BD, Jin J, Rinaldi MG, Wickes BL, Huycke MM. Outbreak of invasive *Aspergillus* infection in surgical patients, associated with a contaminated air-handling system. *Clin Infect Dis*. 2003;37:786-793.
460. Frazier DD, Campbell DR, Garvey TA, et al. Fungal infections of the spine. Report of eleven patients with long-term follow-up. *J Bone Joint Surg Am*. 2001;83-A:560-565.
461. Stynen D, Goris A, Sarfati J, Latge JP. A new sensitive sandwich enzyme-linked immunosorbent assay to detect galactofuran in patients with invasive aspergillosis. *J Clin Microbiol*. 1995;33:497-500.
462. Yeo SF, Wong B. Current status of nonculture methods for diagnosis of invasive fungal infections. *Clin Microbiol Rev*. 2002;15:465-484.
463. Sendid B, Tabouret M, Poirot JL, et al. New enzyme immunoassays for sensitive detection of circulating *Candida albicans* mannan and antimannan antibodies: useful combined test for diagnosis of systemic candidiasis. *J Clin Microbiol*. 1999;37:1510-1517.
464. Gade W, Hinnefeld SW, Babcock LS, et al. Comparison of the PREMIER cryptococcal antigen enzyme immunoassay and the latex agglutination assay for detection of cryptococcal antigens. *J Clin Microbiol*. 1991;29:1616-1619.
465. Kirby A, Chapman C, Hassan C, Burnie J. The diagnosis of hepatosplenic candidiasis by DNA analysis of tissue biopsy and serum. *J Clin Pathol*. 2004;57:764-765.
466. Montone KT, Litzky LA. Rapid method for detection of *Aspergillus* 5S ribosomal RNA using a genus-specific oligonucleotide probe. *Am J Clin Pathol*. 1995;103:48-51.
467. Rementeria A, Vivanco AB, Cadaval A, et al. Typing fungal isolates: molecular methods and computerized analysis. *Methods Mol Biol*. 2004;268:117-125.
468. Einsele H, Hebart H, Roller G, et al. Detection and identification of fungal pathogens in blood by using molecular probes. *J Clin Microbiol*. 1997;35:1353-1360.
469. Loffler J, Hebart H, Sepe S, et al. Detection of PCR-amplified fungal DNA by using a PCR-ELISA system. *Med Mycol*. 1998;36:275-279.
470. Rappelli P, Are R, Casu G, et al. Development of a nested PCR for detection of *Cryptococcus neoformans* in cerebrospinal fluid. *J Clin Microbiol*. 1998;36:3438-3440.
471. Govender S, Mutasa E, Parbhoo AH. Cryptococcal osteomyelitis of the spine. *J Bone Joint Surg Br*. 1999;81:459-461.
472. Gehweiler JA, Capp MP, Chick EW. Observations on the roentgen patterns in blastomycosis of bone. A review of cases from the Blastomycosis Cooperative Study of the Veterans Administration and Duke University Medical Center. *Am J Roentgenol Radium Ther Nucl Med*. 1970;108:497-510.
473. Williams RL, Fukui MB, Meltzer CC, et al. Fungal spinal osteomyelitis in the immunocompromised patient: MR findings in three cases. *AJNR Am J Neuroradiol*. 1999;20:381-385.
474. Ganesh D, Gottlieb J, Chan S, et al. Fungal infections of the spine. *Spine*. 2015;40:E719-E728.
475. Conaughty JM, Khurana S, Banovac K, et al. Antifungal penetration into normal rabbit nucleus pulposus. *Spine*. 2004;29:E289-E293.
476. Stevens DA, Kan VL, Judson MA, et al. Practice guidelines for diseases caused by *Aspergillus*. Infectious Diseases Society of America. *Clin Infect Dis*. 2000;30:696-709.
477. Rex JH, Walsh TJ, Sobel JD, et al. Practice guidelines for the treatment of candidiasis. Infectious Diseases Society of America. *Clin Infect Dis*. 2000;30:662-678.
478. Saag MS, Graybill RJ, Larsen RA, et al. Practice guidelines for the management of cryptococcal disease. Infectious Diseases Society of America. *Clin Infect Dis*. 2000;30:710-718.
479. Galgiani JN, Ampel NM, Catanzaro A, et al. Practice guideline for the treatment of coccidioidomycosis. Infectious Diseases Society of America. *Clin Infect Dis*. 2000;30:658-661.
480. Galgiani JN, Catanzaro A, Cloud GA, et al. Comparison of oral fluconazole and itraconazole for progressive, nonmeningeal coccidioidomycosis. A randomized, double-blind trial. Mycoses Study Group. *Ann Intern Med*. 2000;133:676-686.
481. Chapman SW, Bradsher RW Jr, Campbell GD Jr, et al. Practice guidelines for the management of patients with blastomycosis. Infectious Diseases Society of America. *Clin Infect Dis*. 2000;30:679-683.
482. Arikan S, Lozano-Chiu M, Paetznick V, Rex JH. In vitro synergy of caspofungin and amphotericin B against *Aspergillus* and *Fusarium* spp. *Antimicrob Agents Chemother*. 2002;46:245-247.
483. Stone EA, Fung HB, Kirschenbaum HL. Caspofungin: an echinocandin antifungal agent. *Clin Ther*. 2002;24:351-377.
484. Bridwell KH, Campbell JW, Barenkamp SJ. Surgical treatment of hematogenous vertebral *Aspergillus* osteomyelitis. *Spine*. 1990;15:281-285.
485. Broner FA, Garland DE, Zigler JE. Spinal infections in the immunocompromised host. *Orthop Clin North Am*. 1996;27:37-46.
486. Muller EJ, Russe OJ, Muhr G. Osteomyelitis of the spine. *Orthopade*. 2004;33:305-315.
487. Yu WY, Siu C, Wing PC, et al. Percutaneous suction aspiration for osteomyelitis. Report of two cases. *Spine*. 1991;16:198-202.
488. Campins H. Coccidioidomycosis in South America. A review of its epidemiology and geographic distribution. *Mycopathol Mycol Appl*. 1970;41:25-34.
489. Ogiso A, Ito M, Koyama M, et al. Pulmonary coccidioidomycosis in Japan: case report and review. *Clin Infect Dis*. 1997;25:1260-1261.

490. Stevens DA. *Coccidioides Immitis*. New York: Churchill Livingstone; 1995:2365-2375.
491. McGahan JP, Graves DS, Palmer PE. Coccidioidal spondylitis: usual and unusual radiographic manifestations. *Radiology*. 1980;136:5-9.
492. Dalinka MK, Dinnenberg S, Greendyk WH, Hopkins R. Roentgenographic features of osseous coccidioidomycosis and differential diagnosis. *J Bone Joint Surg Am*. 1971;53:1157-1164.
493. Crum NF, Lederman ER, Stafford CM, et al. Coccidioidomycosis: a descriptive survey of a reemerging disease. Clinical characteristics and current controversies. *Medicine (Baltimore)*. 2004;83:149-175.
494. Olson EM, Duberg AC, Herron LD, et al. Coccidioidal spondylitis: MR findings in 15 patients. *AJR Am J Roentgenol*. 1998;171:785-789.
495. Lewicky YM, Roberto RF, Curtin SL. The unique complications of coccidioidomycosis of the spine: a detailed time line of disease progression and suppression. *Spine*. 2004;29:E435-E441.
496. Boogaerts M, Maertens J. Clinical experience with itraconazole in systemic fungal infections. *Drugs*. 2001;61(suppl 1):39-47.
497. Boogaerts M, Maertens J, van Hoof A, et al. Itraconazole versus amphotericin B plus nystatin in the prophylaxis of fungal infections in neutropenic cancer patients. *J Antimicrob Chemother*. 2001;48:97-103.
498. Boogaerts M, Winston DJ, Bow EJ, et al. Intravenous and oral itraconazole versus intravenous amphotericin B deoxycholate as empirical antifungal therapy for persistent fever in neutropenic patients with cancer who are receiving broad-spectrum antibacterial therapy. A randomized, controlled trial. *Ann Intern Med*. 2001;135:412-422.
499. Boogaerts MA, Maertens J, Van Der Geest R, et al. Pharmacokinetics and safety of a 7-day administration of intravenous itraconazole followed by a 14-day administration of itraconazole oral solution in patients with hematologic malignancy. *Antimicrob Agents Chemother*. 2001;45:981-985.
500. Gallin JI, Alling DW, Malech HL, et al. Itraconazole to prevent fungal infections in chronic granulomatous disease. *N Engl J Med*. 2003;348:2416-2422.
501. Kaptan K, Ural AU, Cetin T, et al. Itraconazole is not effective for the prophylaxis of fungal infections in patients with neutropenia. *J Infect Chemother*. 2003;9:40-45.
502. Wrobel CJ, Chappell ET, Taylor W. Clinical presentation, radiological findings, and treatment results of coccidioidomycosis involving the spine: report on 23 cases. *J Neurosurg Spine*. 2001;95:33-39.
503. Chapman SW, Dismukes WE, Proia LA, et al. Clinical practice guidelines for the management of blastomycosis: 2008 update by the Infectious Diseases Society of America. *Clin Infect Dis*. 2008;46:1801-1812.
504. Bradsher RW, Chapman SW, Pappas PG. Blastomycosis. *Infect Dis Clin North Am*. 2003;17:21-40, vii.
505. Saccente M, Abernathy RS, Pappas PG, et al. Vertebral blastomycosis with paravertebral abscess: report of eight cases and review of the literature. *Clin Infect Dis*. 1998;26:413-418.
506. Chapman SW. *Blastomyces Dermatitidis*. New York: Churchill Livingstone; 1995:2353-2365.
507. Hadjipavlou AG, Mader JT, Nauta HJ, et al. Blastomycosis of the lumbar spine: case report and review of the literature, with emphasis on diagnostic laboratory tools and management. *Eur Spine J*. 1998;7:416-421.
508. Gottlieb JR, Eismont FJ. Nonoperative treatment of vertebral blastomycosis osteomyelitis associated with paraspinal abscess and cord compression. A case report. *J Bone Joint Surg Am*. 2006;88:854-856.
509. Diamond RD. *Cryptococcus Neoformans*. New York: Churchill Livingstone; 1995:2331-2340.
510. Corbett EL, Churchyard GJ, Charalambos S, et al. Morbidity and mortality in South African gold miners: impact of untreated disease due to human immunodeficiency virus. *Clin Infect Dis*. 2002;34:1251-1258.
511. French N, Gray K, Watera C, et al. Cryptococcal infection in a cohort of HIV-1-infected Ugandan adults. *AIDS*. 2002;16:1031-1038.
512. Hakim JG, Gangaidzo IT, Heyderman RS, et al. Impact of HIV infection on meningitis in Harare, Zimbabwe: a prospective study of 406 predominantly adult patients. *AIDS*. 2000;14:1401-1407.
513. Okongo M, Morgan D, Mayanja B, et al. Causes of death in a rural, population-based human immunodeficiency virus type 1 (HIV-1) natural history cohort in Uganda. *Int J Epidemiol*. 1998;27:698-702.
514. Bicanic T, Wood R, Meintjes G, et al. High-dose amphotericin B with flucytosine for the treatment of cryptococcal meningitis in HIV-infected patients: a randomized trial. *Clin Infect Dis*. 2008;47:123-130.
515. Edwards JE. *Candida Species*. New York: Churchill Livingstone; 1995:2289-2306.
516. Friedman BC, Simon GL. *Candida* vertebral osteomyelitis: report of three cases and a review of the literature. *Diagn Microbiol Infect Dis*. 1987;8:31-36.
517. O'Connell CJ, Cherry AV, Zoll JG. Letter: osteomyelitis of cervical spine: *Candida guilliermondii*. *Ann Intern Med*. 1973;79:748.
518. Miller DJ, Mejicano GC. Vertebral osteomyelitis due to *Candida* species: case report and literature review. *Clin Infect Dis*. 2001;33:523-530.
519. Fidel PL Jr, Vazquez JA, Sobel JD. *Candida glabrata:* review of epidemiology, pathogenesis, and clinical disease with comparison to *C. albicans*. *Clin Microbiol Rev*. 1999;12:80-96.
520. Calvo JM, Ramos JL, Garcia F, et al. Pyogenic and non-pyogenic vertebral osteomyelitis: descriptive and comparative study of a series of 40 cases. *Enferm Infecc Microbiol Clin*. 2000;18:452-456.
521. Armstrong N, Schurr M, Helgerson R, Harms B. Fungal sacral osteomyelitis as the initial presentation of Crohn's disease of the small bowel: report of a case. *Dis Colon Rectum*. 1998;41:1581-1584.
522. El-Zaatari MM, Hulten K, Fares Y, et al. Successful treatment of *Candida albicans* osteomyelitis of the spine with fluconazole and surgical debridement: case report. *J Chemother*. 2002;14:627-630.
523. Derkinderen P, Bruneel F, Bouchaud O, Regnier B. Spondylodiscitis and epidural abscess due to *Candida albicans*. *Eur Spine J*. 2000;9:72-74.
524. Dwyer K, McDonald M, Fitzpatrick T. Presentation of *Candida glabrata* spinal osteomyelitis 25 months after documented candidaemia. *Aust N Z J Med*. 1999;29: 571-572.
525. Bennett JE. *Aspergillus Species*. New York: Churchill Livingstone; 1995:2306-2311.
526. McKee DF, Barr WM, Bryan CS, Lunceford EM Jr. Primary aspergillosis of the spine mimicking Pott's paraplegia. *J Bone Joint Surg Am*. 1984;66:1481-1483.

527. Govender S, Rajoo R, Goga IE, Charles RW. *Aspergillus* osteomyelitis of the spine. *Spine*. 1991;16:746-749.
528. Meyohas MC, Roux P, Poirot JL, et al. Aspergillosis in acquired immunodeficiency syndrome. *Pathol Biol (Paris)*. 1994;42:647-651.
529. Kim CW, Perry A, Currier B, et al. Fungal infections of the spine. *Clin Orthop Relat Res*. 2006;444:92-99.
530. Vinas FC, King PK, Diaz FG. Spinal *Aspergillus* osteomyelitis. *Clin Infect Dis*. 1999;28:1223-1229.
531. van Ooij A, Beckers JM, Herpers MJ, Walenkamp GH. Surgical treatment of *Aspergillus* spondylodiscitis. *Eur Spine J*. 2000;9:75-79.
532. Holmes PF, Osterman DW, Tullos HS. *Aspergillus* discitis. Report of two cases and review of the literature. *Clin Orthop Relat Res*. 1988;226:240-246.
533. Hummel M, Schuler S, Weber U, et al. Aspergillosis with *Aspergillus* osteomyelitis and diskitis after heart transplantation: surgical and medical management. *J Heart Lung Transplant*. 1993;12:599-603.
534. Perronne C, Saba J, Behloul Z, et al. Pyogenic and tuberculous spondylodiskitis (vertebral osteomyelitis) in 80 adult patients. *Clin Infect Dis*. 1994;19:746-750.
535. Denning DW, Stevens DA. Antifungal and surgical treatment of invasive aspergillosis: review of 2,121 published cases. *Rev Infect Dis*. 1990;12:1147-1201.
536. Nasca RJ, McElvein RB. *Aspergillus fumigatus* osteomyelitis of the thoracic spine treated by excision and interbody fusion. *Spine*. 1985;10:848-850.
537. Tien RD, Gean-Marton AD, Mark AS. Neurosyphilis in HIV carriers: MR findings in six patients. *AJR Am J Roentgenol*. 1992;158:1325-1328.
538. Harris DE, Enterline DS, Tien RD. Neurosyphilis in patients with AIDS. *Neuroimaging Clin N Am*. 1997;7:215-221.
539. Simon RP. Neurosyphilis. *Arch Neurol*. 1985;42:606-613.
540. MacLean S, Luger A. Finding neurosyphilis without the Venereal Disease Research Laboratory test. *Sex Transm Dis*. 1996;23:392-394.
541. Johns D. Syphilitic disorders of the spine. Report of two cases. *J Bone Joint Surg Br*. 1970;52:724-731.
542. Kikuchi S, Shinpo K, Niino M, Tashiro K. Subacute syphilitic meningomyelitis with characteristic spinal MRI findings. *J Neurol*. 2003;250:106-107.
543. Tsui EY, Ng SH, Chow L, et al. Syphilitic myelitis with diffuse spinal cord abnormality on MR imaging. *Eur Radiol*. 2002;12:2973-2976.
544. Goldmeier D, Hay P. A review and update on adult syphilis, with particular reference to its treatment. *Int J STD AIDS*. 1993;4:70-82.
545. Zhang Z, Luo F, Zhou Q, et al. The outcomes of chemotherapy only treatment on mild spinal tuberculosis. *J Orthop Surg Res*. 2016;11:49.

CHAPTER 88 Metabolic Bone Disorders of the Spine

Joseph M. Lane
Matthew R. Cohn
Tyler Kreitz
Mark F. Kurd

Metabolic bone diseases are a group of disorders that occur as a result of changes in osteoblast and osteoclast function. Because the spine represents a significant portion of the skeletal bone mass, contains the largest quantity of metabolically active (cancellous) bone, and loads this bone in compression during upright posture, metabolic bone diseases often affect the spine primarily.

Bone fulfills its role as a metabolically active homeostatic organ. As in all bones, the component cells of the spine are physiologically active and responsive to numerous metabolic and mechanical stimuli. The bony skeleton actively performs three main roles: (1) a biochemical role of mineral balance (through storage and release of Ca^{2+}, Mg^{2+}, HPO_4^{2-}, and H^+); (2) a structural role, responding to the skeletal demands for remodeling and repair; and (3) protection of the spinal cord.

Metabolic bone diseases result when bone constituents (cells and matrices) behave abnormally, when the stimuli to which bone responds are inappropriately interpreted, or when systemic processes disturb the bone's environment, leading to impairment of either its biochemical or structural tasks.

Accordingly, this chapter begins with an understanding of the normal bone physiology: the characteristic interplay of cells, ions, and proteins and the role of bone in maintaining skeletal and mineral homeostasis. Next, abnormal metabolic bone pathology and pathophysiology are considered. Finally, for the two most common metabolic bone diseases of the spine—osteoporosis and Paget disease—the epidemiology, clinical manifestations, and prevention and treatment strategies are discussed.

Cellular Biology

Bone Cells

Four families of cells combine to create bone tissue that is biomechanically functional and structurally sound. These include the osteoprogenitor cell from the mesenchymal stem cell lineage; its derivative, the osteoblast; the incorporated mature form, the osteocyte; and, finally, the osteoclast. Together, these cells produce new osseous tissue. This tissue is maintained through resorption and remodeling. In short, the cells determine mechanical stability and mineral homeostasis. Healthy bone metabolism results from equilibrating these competing forces. Therefore, some forms of metabolic bone disease can be viewed as the pathologic imbalance—in number, power, or degree of differentiation—of bone-forming and bone-resorbing cells.[1,2]

The osteoprogenitor cells are components of the bone marrow stromal system, approximating the surfaces of bone (periosteum and endosteum) and the adjacent bone marrow environment.[3] These potentially mitotic cells, under appropriate stimulation and conditions, give rise to either the bone-forming osteoblast or the cartilage-producing chondroblast. The natural history of these osteoprogenitor cells and the precise signals for their differentiation and modulation are not yet fully elucidated.

Osteoblasts sit on the metabolically active surface of bone in an adherent row, where they synthesize and release unmineralized bone matrix called osteoid.[4–7] They subsequently participate in the mineralization of the osteoid by releasing packets of ions and by synthesizing regulatory and crystal-nucleating noncollagenous proteins. These cells are characterized by high levels of alkaline phosphatase, the ability to manufacture type I collagen and osteocalcin, and the presence of numerous receptor sites for parathyroid hormone (PTH), estrogen, vitamin D, and other growth factors and extracellular matrix proteins. Osteoblasts are also thought to govern the actions of osteoclasts (described later), thus regulating and coupling bone formation and bone resorption.

The osteocyte, the terminal cell of the osteogenic cell line, is derived from osteoblasts.[4,5] As the osteoblast synthesizes bone matrix, it becomes embedded within its mineralized product. Once embedded, the cell is termed an *osteocyte* and the space in which it sits is termed a *lacuna.* Despite being surrounded by bone matrix, the osteocyte communicates with other cells via slender cell processes that it extends for some distance into canaliculi in the surrounding matrix. The surface area covered by the canaliculi is greater than the surface area of osteoblasts; the total volume is comparable to the brain.[8] Thus, osteocytes are not completely isolated in their lacunae from other cells but appear to communicate with one another and with surface cells via these cell-to-cell junctions. In this way, osteocytes maintain the matrix that envelops them, regulate local ionic concentrations, and govern the degree of mineralization. In addition, they monitor the local mechanical load and signal changes in the matrix, translating these forces into biologic activity. One crucial mechanism through which the osteocytes regulate bone formation is by the secretion of the glycoprotein sclerostin.[9,10] Sclerostin reduces osteoblast proliferation and the formation of bone by inhibiting the canonical Wnt/β-catenin signaling pathway.[11] Antibodies that bind sclerostin increase bone mineral density (BMD) and show promise in treating osteoporosis.[12] Romosozumab, an anti-sclerostin antibody, has shown efficacy in increasing BMD and reducing risk of vertebral fractures.[12,13]

Osteoclasts resorb bone.[14,15] Unlike the mesenchymally derived osteoblast lineage, osteoclasts arise from hematopoietic progenitor cells of the monocyte line. These large multinucleated cells are found on the resorbing surfaces of bone, where they bind to a bone-specific integrin and form an isolated macrocavity. At this attachment cavity site, an acidic microenvironment causes the dissolution of the hydroxyapatite mineral and releases acidic proteases that degrade the organic collagen matrix. The resultant resorption cavity is called a *Howship lacuna*. Thus, by remodeling formed bone and delivering calcium into the circulation, the osteoclasts participate in both the mechanical and biochemical roles of bone tissue. The coordinated activity of osteoclast resorption and osteoblast bone formation is most prominent during periods of growth, fracture repair, and periosteal bone widening.

Neighboring osteoblasts and osteocytes influence osteoclast differentiation as well as osteoclast activity. Osteoclast precursors are stimulated to differentiate by osteoblast lineage cells and bone marrow stromal cells that express receptor activator of nuclear factor-κβ ligand (RANKL), also known as osteoprotegerin-ligand (OPGL), and macrophage colony-stimulating factor (M-CSF). M-CSF primarily induces osteoclast progenitor cell replication, whereas RANKL promotes differentiation.[11] Osteoclasts are devoid of PTH receptors, even though they functionally respond to this hormone. On stimulation by PTH, osteoblasts produce RANKL, leading to differentiation and activation of mature osteoclasts. Osteoprotegerin (OPG, also known as osteoclastogenesis inhibitory factor [OCIF]) is a soluble decoy receptor for RANKL that blocks this pathway. RANKL, reeptor activator of NF-κβ (RANK) and OPG are the key regulators for the development and activation of mature osteoclasts (Fig. 88.1). Agents that inhibit RANKL via OPG or anti-RANKL antibodies can be used for the treatment of osteopenic disorders such as osteoporosis as well as bone loss associated with bone metastases.[16–19]

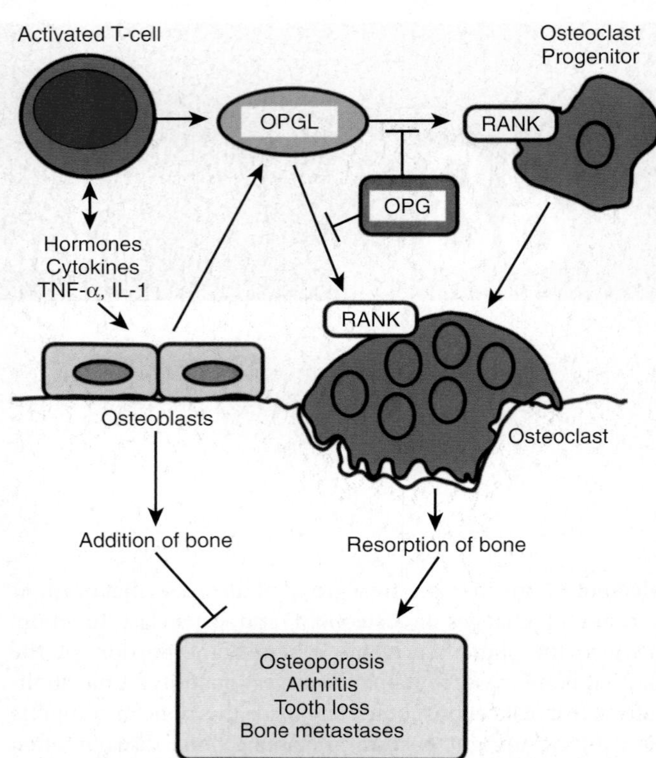

FIG. 88.1 The relationship between RANKL (also known as OPGL), RANK, and the decoy receptor OPG in bone formation and bone resorption. Activated T cells lead to expression of RANKL on osteoblasts by two pathways: (1) They produce cytokines that lead to RANKL expression and (2) they directly express and produce RANKL. OPG, the decoy receptor for RANKL, blocks both of these pathways. RANKL induces osteoclast formation and activation, thereby increasing bone resorption. Inhibition of RANKL via OPG may prove useful in the pharmacologic treatment of osteopenic disorders, including osteoporosis and Paget disease. IL-1, interleukin-1; OPG, osteoprotegerin; OPGL, osteoprotegerin ligand; RANKL, receptor activator of nuclear factor-κβ ligand; TNF-α, tumor necrosis factor-α. (From Theill LE, Boyle WJ, Penninger JM. RANK-L and RANK: T cells, bone loss, and mammalian evolution. *Annu Rev Immunol.* 2002;20:795–823.)

Bone Matrix

In addition to the cellular component, two matrices—an organic matrix and an inorganic matrix—constitute the remainder of bone tissue (Fig. 88.2). Whereas the inorganic matrix consists of bone mineral, the organic matrix consists of collagenous fibers embedded in a ground substance.

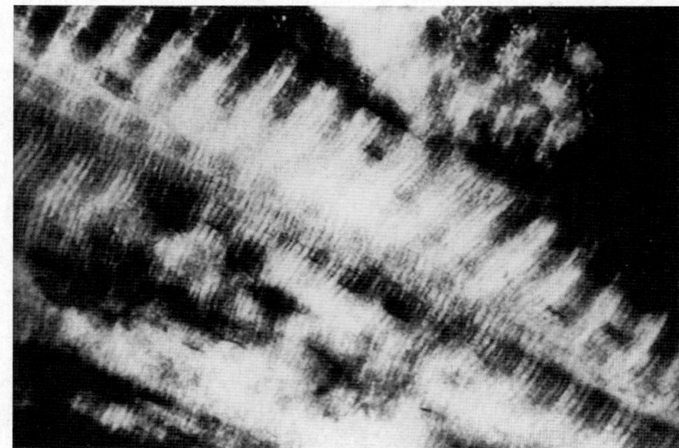

FIG. 88.2 Collagen-mineral relationship. The hydroxyapatite forms in the hole zone between collagen molecules. (From Anatomy II. Orthop. Science. Park Ridge, IL: American Academy of Orthopaedic Surgeons; 1986.)

Bone Mineral

The inorganic matrix represents two-thirds of the dry weight of bone and primarily consists of calcium phosphate,[16] which exists in three forms: (1) crystalline hydroxyapatite [$Ca_{10}(PO_4)_6(OH)_2$], the most abundant; (2) octacalcium phosphate [$Ca_8H_2(PO_4)_6 \cdot 5H_2O$)], a rarer form; and (3) brushite [$CaHPO_4 \cdot 2H_2O$]. The hydroxyapatite forms platelike crystals 40 nm in length and 3 nm in thickness. Occasional contaminants, including carbonate substituted for a phosphate or a fluoride for a hydroxy group (as well as the potential inclusion of lead or arsenic), disrupt the purity of the crystals. These contaminants alter the physical properties of the matrix and may also affect the biologic characteristics. The mineral crystal closely associates with the organic matrix, initially deposited in the hole zones of the collagen fibril. Later, it surrounds itself with ground substance (proteoglycan), as well as with water and other ions.

The initial formation of hydroxyapatite is under the control of osteoblasts, which contain abundant alkaline phosphatase. This enzyme catalyzes reactions that, among others, release phosphate from pyrophosphate. The conversion of pyrophosphate has two effects: (1) it increases the local concentration of phosphate to a level that permits calcium and phosphate to precipitate; and (2) it destroys pyrophosphate, an inhibitor of calcification. Vitamin D and adequate calcium are critical for mineral deposition.

Collagen

Concentrations of calcium and phosphate alone do not dictate mineral deposition. An organic matrix, consisting of collagenous fibers embedded in ground substance, assists with and regulates mineralization.[20] The organic matrix of bone is primarily composed of proteins, approximately 95% of which is collagen in adult humans. Collagen, a rigid macromolecule, employs tropocollagen as its basic structural unit. Tropocollagen, in turn, is composed of three polypeptide chains, each comprising approximately 1000 amino acids.[21] In bone collagen (type I), two of these chains share an identical amino acid sequence; a third chain (α_2) has a similar, but not identical, sequence. All three chains contain unusually high concentrations of glycine, proline, alanine, hydroxyproline, and hydroxylysine and are wound into right-handed helices.

Type I collagen synthesis occurs in osteoblasts. It is formed as a precursor "procollagen" molecule in the cytoplasm and then extruded from the osteoblast after cleavage of signal sequences. Numerous additional modifications are subsequently made to the secreted procollagen molecule. Notably, extensive nonhelical regions are removed from both its amino and carboxy terminals, and key proline and lysine residues are hydroxylated by an iron-containing enzyme. (The iron in this hydroxylase functions only in the ferrous state; therefore, ascorbic acid, functioning as a reducing agent, is necessary.) The hydroxylation of proline and lysine occurs after these amino acids are incorporated into the chain; therefore, free hydroxyproline in the serum signifies lysis of collagen or its precursors. Accordingly, measurements of urinary hydroxyapatite excretion provide a qualitative measure of bone turnover. The hydroxylation of proline and lysine assists cross-linking, which, in turn, lowers the solubility of collagen and increases its tensile strength. Collagen is one of the strongest components of bone; the tensile strength of bone collagen exceeds the compressive strength of the bone mineral by 2000 N/cm^2. Pyridinoline, deoxypyridinoline, C-telopeptides, and N-telopeptides are cross-link breakdown products that all provide better markers of bone resorption than hydroxyproline.[22,23] They are elevated in high-turnover osteoporosis and Paget disease, and they decline rapidly with successful antiresorptive therapy (discussed later). Adequate nutrition and vitamin C (ascorbic acid) are required for collagen maintenance.

Type I collagen is found not only in the bones of the spine but also in the intervertebral discs, where it coexists with type II collagen. These homologous molecules differ only in the chains that compose their triple helices. Within the disc, each type of collagen maintains a separate anatomic domain: type I collagen is more abundant in the anulus fibrosus, whereas type II predominates in the nucleus pulposus.[24]

Collagen derives its mechanical strength from covalent collagen cross-links between helical and nonhelical domains of neighboring collagen molecules. Cross-links between collagen molecules are formed by one of two mechanisms: (1) enzymatic cross-linking, which occurs via lysine hydroxylase and lysyl oxidase; and (2) nonenzymatic cross-linking, which occurs via glycation or oxidation. The latter mechanism occurs when states of hyperglycemia, oxidative stress, or aging induce spontaneous formation of advanced glycation end products (AGEs) within collagen fibers. These AGEs undergo nonenzymatic cross-linking within collagen matrix and undermine bone quality. This mechanism is believed to contribute to elevated fracture risk in patients with diabetes and advanced age. In addition, AGE-related collagen cross-links have been shown to be a significant risk factor for vertebral fracture in clinical samples[25,26] and suppression of bone turnover by bisphosphonates leads to continued addition of nonenzymatic cross-links. Long-term bisphosphonate users may have less plasticity and reduced toughness in certain regions of bone, which may contribute to the occurrence of atypical femoral fractures in this population.[27]

Ground Substance

Proteoglycans form the ground substance of bone. A proteoglycan monomer is composed of two kinds of glycosaminoglycans—keratin sulfate and chondroitin sulfate—joined to a core protein. Keratin and chondroitin sulfate form through the polymerization of disaccharide units, one sugar of which is always a hexosamine possessing an anionic group. This negatively charged group binds water, expanding the tissue volume and imparting resilience to the ground substance. In addition, the presence of water in the ground substance allows for the diffusion of metabolites in the organic matrix. Thus, the proteoglycans in bone exert regulatory and structural forces. When the bone mineralizes, the water content is reduced, leading to denser, more compact tissue. The intervertebral discs also contain proteoglycans, which comprise 30% to 60% of the dry weight of the nucleus pulposus. With age, proteoglycan concentration (and, consequently, water concentration) declines. However, even with decreased proteoglycan concentration, osmotic forces allow the proteoglycans to remain somewhat hydrated.[28]

Osteocalcin is a bone-specific protein that, like type I collagen, is synthesized by osteoblasts.[29] Osteocalcin comprises only 2% of the organic matrix by weight. Vitamin D enhances the synthesis of osteocalcin but is not an absolute requirement for synthesis. Osteocalcin prefers to bind to calcium within hydroxyapatite. The precise function of this prevalent osseous protein is currently being explored, although its levels are correlated with bone mineral content. Possible roles include the attraction of osteoclasts to sites of bone resorption, regulation of the rate of mineral turnover, and determination of the morphology of the mineral crystal. Osteocalcin also functions as a bone-derived hormone that exerts systemic effects. These actions include stimulation of insulin secretion by the pancreatic beta cells, promotion of insulin receptor sensitivity, and stimulation of testosterone production in the Leydig cells of the testes.[30] Through a feed-forward loop, insulin also stimulates secretion of osteocalcin by osteoblasts, which, in turn, increases insulin release. Osteocalcin production is halted by the hormone leptin. Through this interplay with osteocalcin, insulin, and leptin, bone remodeling is linked to energy metabolism and may be involved in the development of osteoporosis in patients with inflammatory bowel disease.[31]

Osteonectin, a 32-kd phosphoprotein secreted by osteoblasts, is the second most prevalent protein in bone. It binds to both collagen and hydroxyapatite[32] as well as to carbohydrate moieties. Putative roles for osteonectin include calcium phosphate nucleation and stabilization of the newly formed crystal.

Bone morphogenetic protein (BMP), as the name implies, induces osteoprogenitor cells to form bone.[25,33] A small protein, BMP accounts for only 0.1% of the total bone protein mass in cortical bone, and even less in the spine. More than 15 BMPs exist, some of which are related to the transforming growth factors. Experimentally, BMP implanted in ectopic sites (in the absence of bone collagen) induces perivascular mesenchymal cells to become bone-forming osteoprogenitor cells. The absence of BMPs (or the inhibition of their activity) may contribute to the pathogenesis of diseases of decreased bone mass or impaired bone remodeling or repair. The genes for the expression of BMPs have been cloned,[33,34] and the protein has proven to possess a pharmacologic role in repairing bone and inducing spinal arthrodesis.[35] Recombinant human bone morphogenetic protein-2 has been used clinically as a bone graft substitute in anterior interbody lumbar fusion, posterolateral lumbar fusion, posterior lumbar interbody fusion, and anterior cervical discectomy and fusion. However, early industry-sponsored reports may have overestimated the decreased need for revision surgery with recombinant human bone morphogenetic protein-2 use and underestimated serious adverse events such as osteolysis, subsidence, graft migration, cyst formation, wound problems, and others.[36]

Skeletal Homeostasis

Bone growth occurs during all phases of life.[4,5] Functionally, this growth can be divided into two processes: modeling and remodeling. The deposition of new bone in regions not first cleared by resorption or the resorption of old bone without deposition of new tissue is termed *modeling*. Modeling results in changes to the external shape, mass, or volume of existing bone. Alternatively, remodeling retains approximately the external form of bones. During remodeling, bone replaces itself by balancing synthesis in some places with lysis in others. This balanced turnover releases ions into the circulation and prevents accumulation of aged or fatigued bone.

In the remodeling cycle, osteoclasts work as much as four times faster than osteoblasts. Although the clastic phase in the typical remodeling unit requires approximately 20 days, the blastic phase requires 80 days. After this period elapses, the tissue is restored, notably with younger, newly mineralized bone. The preferential remodeling of older tissue leads to an overall younger skeleton, one better suited to constant mechanical demands.

Remodeling, a process that ordinarily prevents structural collapse by repairing old or damaged regions in bone, can be responsible for eroding the bones' mechanical integrity. This may result in any of several ways. First, the remodeling can occur too frequently, magnifying what would ordinarily be an inconsequential net loss. Second, the remodeling can be poorly focused, inappropriately replacing young, healthy bone instead of weaker, older tissue. Finally, the remodeling can be unbalanced if the formation cycle does not fully replace the bone lost during resorption. After the age of 40 years, the remodeled bone unit rarely fully reconstitutes itself. High turnover states lead to net bone loss, and the younger matrix has a lower modulus until the crystals can fully mature.

Mineral Homeostasis

Calcium

Bone exchanges calcium, magnesium, and phosphate and participates in acid–base balance. Of all of these, calcium homeostasis is the most important to both the skeletal and metabolic functions of bone.[37–40] Calcium fulfills its skeletal role in the hydroxyapatite mineral crystal, where it provides mechanical strength. It serves its metabolic function as a free divalent cation. These functions include transducing hormonal signals within the cytoplasm ("second messenger" function), coupling neural excitation with muscular contraction, and effecting homeostasis by interacting with both vascular smooth muscle and platelets.

Body stores of calcium in the typical, 70-kg male total approximately 1300 g, more than 98% of which resides in the teeth and bones. The remainder is divided between the cytoplasmic and extracellular fluids. The normal serum calcium concentration centers around 9 mg/dL and is found in three states: (1) free (ionized and diffusible); (2) complexed to citrate and other anions (i.e., nonionized but diffusible); and

(3) bound to proteins (i.e., neither ionized nor diffusible). Only the free ion (normally about 45% of the total) possesses physiologic activity. At normal body pH, albumin and other anionic proteins bind 50% of the total body calcium. The proportion of protein-bound calcium increases with alkalinity. Accordingly, as the pH rises, the individual becomes effectively hypocalcemic, even though the total amount of calcium, and, importantly, the amount typically reported by standard laboratory tests, remains within normal range. Conversely, in states of liver and kidney failure, when albumin is either not synthesized or lost in the urine, even though the absolute levels of total serum calcium may be depressed, the effective physiologic calcium concentration may be near normal. Calcium-anion complexes account for the remaining 5% of serum calcium. Abnormal levels of these anions may also cause a physiologic calcium disturbance, one not necessarily obvious from the serum calcium concentration. Thus, unless ionic calcium is directly measured, attention should be directed at albumin levels and pH state before inferring functional calcium levels from the total serum measurement.

Maintenance of calcium concentration is the responsibility of three organ systems: the gut, to absorb calcium; the bone, to store it; and the kidney, to excrete it. Each of these systems can alter the magnitude of the calcium contribution in response to a number of regulatory substances.

The gut (duodenum and jejunum, specifically) absorbs calcium from the diet, ingested primarily from dairy products. Despite the critical need for calcium absorption, the gut performs this duty with surprising inefficiency: of the recommended daily allowance of 800 mg, only half will ever cross the luminal border; of that fraction, more than half will be returned to the lumen with the secretion of intestinal fluids.[41] Thus, less than one-fourth of the daily intake (or only about 150 mg) enters the system.

Active absorption in the duodenum takes place by means of a protein-dependent transport system[32] that is activated by 1,25-dihydroxyvitamin D [1,25$(OH)_2$D]. In the jejunum, passive diffusion accounts for the remainder of the calcium absorbed. Clearly, the jejunal phase depends more on concentration gradients and intestinal transit times. In addition, dietary composition affects absorption: diets high in fiber and oxalate (both found in green vegetables) allow for less calcium absorption. In times of increased calcium demand—such as the growth years, or during pregnancy—the duodenal fractional absorption can be augmented by increased carrier protein synthesis, which is, in turn, stimulated by the active vitamin D metabolite (discussed later). The efficiency of calcium absorption decreases with aging and is adversely affected with bariatric surgery.[40]

The bone stores calcium. The bone tissue constantly exchanges calcium with the plasma, even when intake matches excretion. This daily 400-mg exchange results from the nearly balanced remodeling activity of osteoclasts and osteoblasts as well as the movement of ions between intracellular and extracellular compartments at the osteocyte plasma membrane.

The kidneys are the prime organs of calcium excretion. The glomerular load of calcium is almost 10,000 mg. Most of it is resorbed proximally, following sodium-driven bulk flow. Some calcium remains in the lumen until the distal nephron, where it can be selectively resorbed by calcium-specific transport processes. It follows not only the dictates of calcium-regulating agents but also the demands of salt and water balance and acid-base control. For example, when volume depletion demands increased sodium resorption, proportionally more calcium will be retained proximally, regardless of the serum levels. Diet can also affect renal calcium handling, with both high-protein and high-carbohydrate loads increasing urine calcium excretion. Under normal conditions, the kidneys resorb 98% of the filtered load, with excretion commensurate with intake or resorption from bone. One deleterious consequence of the renal response to high calcium is the formation of stones. Although there is no precise threshold at which stones will form (because other factors, such as urinary flow rate, influence the process) the risk of stone formation increases with hypercalciuria. Most diuretics (with the exception of the thiazides) induce renal calcium loss. Patients with low calcium levels should be evaluated for excessive calcium excretion.

Phosphate

The second important ion in bone metabolism is phosphate.[42] Like calcium, phosphate serves multiple functions throughout the body. As a component of adenosine triphosphate, phosphate participates in the interconversion of the energy of metabolism; as a constituent of nucleotides, phosphate partakes in the transmission and expression of genetic information; and in 2,3-diphosphoglycerate, it regulates the oxygen affinity of hemoglobin.

Phosphate is found in two forms: $H_2PO_4^-$ and PO_4^{3-}. The ratio of this dissociation, like that of any acid, depends on the pKa of the system, a constant, and the local pH, which can vary. In the extracellular fluid, where the pH is 7.4, the ratio of $H_2PO_4^-$ to PO_4^{3-} is about 4:1, whereas in the slightly less alkaline cytosol, the ratio is closer to 2.5:1. Unlike calcium, which is physiologically sensed as the free ion, phosphate is internally measured as a sum of both forms. Phosphate's role outside of bone is also less dependent on concentration; therefore, alterations in its level cause few immediate effects. Nevertheless, the quantity of phosphate, normally about 4 mg/dL, is regulated.

Similarly to calcium, serum phosphorus concentration is determined by the degree of intestinal phosphate absorption in the gut, storage of phosphate in bone, and phosphate excretion by the kidney. Regulatory mechanisms for calcium and phosphate are intertwined, as PTH and vitamin D are key regulators. However, fibroblast growth factor-23 (FGF-23) is also critical for phosphate control and is secreted by osteoblasts and osteocytes.[43] The body stores of phosphate sum to 700 g, about half that of calcium. As with calcium, the majority of phosphate (perhaps 85% of the total) resides in bone. The typical dietary intake is about 1000 mg/day, of which about two-thirds is absorbed. The presence of substances in the gut that can bind phosphate, such as aluminum salts, largely determines the amount of phosphate absorbed. Under normal circumstances, the amount absorbed increases linearly with intake. As with calcium, the kidney is responsible for maintaining phosphate balance,[45] and it does so by a similar mechanism: proximal sodium bulk-driven flow and distal control. When phosphate intake is high, the kidney excretes increasing amounts by spilling the excess phosphate into the urine. When serum phosphate concentrations are low, the kidney can avidly conserve phosphate by implementing vitamin D–mediated changes in calcium concentration. In addition to calcium balance, dietary load, volume status, and acid–base balance also affect renal phosphate handling

Regulators of Bone and Mineral Metabolism

Parathyroid Hormone

PTH is an 84-amino-acid polypeptide secreted by the chief cells of the parathyroid glands in response to low serum calcium.[46] Its physiologic role is to restore a normal calcium concentration by stimulating all three organs of calcium homeostasis. The kidney and the bone are affected directly,[47] whereas the intestine is affected only indirectly, by means of the synthesis of the active vitamin D metabolite 1,25$(OH)_2D_3$.

PTH promotes calcium conservation in the kidney.[48] There, increased serum calcium is achieved through a twofold mechanism; both steps depend on stimulation of adenylate cyclase, the enzyme that forms cyclic adenosine monophosphate. First, PTH increases calcium resorption in the distal nephron. It also promotes the loss of phosphate. This phosphaturic effect prevents the recently resorbed calcium from being deposited into the bone hydroxyapatite or into ectopic calcium-phosphate deposits. Moreover, the excretion of phosphate lowers the levels of circulating calcium-anion complexes, causing more of the serum calcium to remain in the physiologically useful free form.

In the kidney, PTH further promotes elevation of calcium level by stimulating additional synthesis of 1α-hydroxylase, a key enzyme in the formation of 1,25$(OH)_2$ vitamin D, which, in turn, enhances calcium absorption in the digestive system. In this manner, PTH indirectly affects gut handling of calcium as well.

In the bone, PTH affects calcium metabolism by increasing the surface resorption of the mineral by osteoclasts, by promoting ion flux by osteocytes, and by decreasing their bone synthetic activity through the inhibition of calcium "consumption" by osteoblasts. PTH increases the number of resorptive surfaces in bone and, within them, the density of osteoclasts. However, the effects of intermittent and continuous PTH stimulations on bone differ. Low-dose, intermittent PTH stimulation exerts anabolic properties, which is believed to be through direct effects on osteoblasts and inhibition of sclerostin—a promoter of bone resorption.[43,49] Conversely, continuous PTH stimulation of osteoblasts causes expression of RANKL. Osteoclasts respond to RANKL by resorbing bone and release of calcium and phosphate into the systemic circulation. The most commonly used laboratory test to measure PTH clinically is intact PTH, which detects levels of both the 84-amino-acid polypeptide and the C-terminal PTH fragments.[28]

Vitamin D

Unlike the polypeptide hormone PTH, vitamin D is a steroid.[47] As such, it defies rapid proteolytic inactivation and thus functions best as a longer-acting regulator of calcium homeostasis. The principal effect of this hormone is to increase intestinal absorption of calcium from the diet, a process that is usually only 25% efficient. Secondarily, it complements PTH in the promotion of calcium resorption from the bone, again by promoting transport across cell membranes (in this case, bone cells rather than intestinal cells).

Cholecalciferol (inactive vitamin D_3) forms in the skin from the ultraviolet light activation of 7-dehydrocholesterol, an intermediate of cholesterol synthesis.[50] 7-Dehydrocholesterol can degrade and re-form cholecalciferol; therefore, once formed, cholecalciferol is removed from the local environment by a transport protein, thus favoring further formation. As little as 15 minutes of sunlight exposure allows the synthesis of a fair-skinned individual's vitamin D_3 requirement. The total need for sunlight increases with melanin concentration. In the absence of sun exposure, cod liver oil and enriched milk and cereals can provide usable precursors of the hormone.

In the liver, vitamin D_3 undergoes 25-hydroxylation,[51] forming the prehormone 25-hydroxyvitamin D [25(OH)D]. Subsequent 1-hydroxylation to the active form, 1,25$(OH)_2D_3$, takes place in the kidney and is promoted by PTH. In the presence of low PTH or FGF-23, an alternative hydroxylation occurs at the 24 position, yielding 24,25$(OH)_2$ D_3, an inactive form of the hormone. Unlike PTH, which is functionally regulated at the level of secretion (calcium levels do not cause minute-to-minute changes in messenger RNA activity but rather control the release of PTH), vitamin D is regulated at the level of biosynthesis. The 1-hydroxylation reaction is the rate-limiting step and is regulated by feedback inhibition as well as by PTH levels.

Active vitamin D, also known as *calcitriol,* promotes increased transport across cell borders. As a steroid maturation hormone, vitamin D works by crossing the cell membrane and subsequently entering the nucleus. There, it binds to DNA via the vitamin D receptor to promote DNA translation, thus increasing the synthesis of the target proteins. Vitamin D receptor is most highly expressed in the intestinal enterocytes, osteoblasts, and renal distal tubules, where it mediates expression of calcium-transport proteins.[52] In the gut, 1,25$(OH)_2D_3$ causes increased calcium and phosphate absorption. In the bone, 1,25$(OH)_2D_3$ complements the action of PTH by increasing calcium transport across bone cell membranes, thus assisting with the mobilization of calcium from the bone and into the circulation. As such, it functions as an agent of bone resorption. It can indirectly assist with bone formation as well because the tasks of mineral homeostasis and skeletal homeostasis are not always at odds with each other. Vitamin D also functions as a maturation hormone by increasing the villous membrane of the gut and augmenting PTH recruitment of macrophage stem cells, the bone-resorbing osteoclast precursors. Accordingly, vitamin D, which promotes the uptake of dietary calcium, typically also serves as an agent of bone maintenance. In addition, vitamin D has been associated with decreased cancer rates, improved muscle function, and a more normal immune system.[53]

Fibroblast Growth Factor-23 (FGF-23)

The major sources of fibroblast growth factor-23 (FGF-23) in the body are osteocytes and osteoblasts. This protein is a potent regulator of serum phosphate and contributes to vitamin D and PTH homeostasis.[54] After FGF-23 is released into the systemic circulation, it acts synergistically with PTH in promoting renal phosphate excretion.[55] This is done by suppressing expression of the sodium phosphate cotransporter in the proximal tubule.[44] However, unlike PTH, FGF-23 inhibits conversion of 25-(OH)D to the active form, 1,25-$(OH)_2D$[56] and promotes its conversion to the inactive form.[54] The net result is a decrease in serum phosphate. Primary elevation of FGF-23 leads to conditions characterized by hypophosphatemia, decreased 1,25$(OH)_2D$, and rickets/osteomalacia. These include autosomal-dominant hypophosphatemic rickets, tumor-induced osteomalacia, and X-linked hypophosphatemic rickets.[57] This interplay between FGF-23, PTH, and vitamin D in controlling calcium and phosphate handling is often described as the bone-parathyroid-kidney axis.

Calcitonin

Calcitonin is a 32-amino-acid polypeptide secreted by the parafollicular cells in the thyroid in response to increased serum calcium concentration. Calcitonin lowers serum calcium levels by its actions in the bone and the kidney. Still, its precise physiologic role awaits determination.[58,59]

In the bone, calcitonin rapidly inhibits osteoclastic action at pharmacologic doses. Direct calcitonin-binding sites are present on osteoclasts. Calcitonin decreases the number and activity of osteoclasts. Specifically, it decreases the adherence of osteoclasts to bone resorptive surfaces and diminishes their activity once they adhere. Calcitonin also affects osteocytes, causing decreased calcium ion flux across their cell membranes. In the kidney, calcitonin blocks the reuptake from the glomerular fluid of calcium and phosphate, as well as that of other ions, notably sodium (which influences calcium uptake by the passive mechanisms described earlier). Calcitonin may also influence calcium handling in the gut and, at pharmacologic doses, may alter other intestinal processes (such as water balance).[60]

High levels of calcitonin may cause transient hypocalcemia without causing any residual skeletal effects. In patients with medullary carcinoma of the thyroid (a malignancy of the parafollicular cells), calcitonin levels are several orders of magnitude higher than in healthy patients. Nevertheless, such patients demonstrate neither long-term derangements of calcium metabolism nor loss of skeletal integrity. Furthermore, patients who have had a complete thyroidectomy, and are thus completely calcitonin deficient, show no persistent hypercalcemia. Both examples bolster the hypothesis of a small physiologic role for calcitonin.

Despite a perhaps minor physiologic role, calcitonin is important medically. First, in patients with medullary carcinoma of the thyroid, measurement of serum calcitonin level provides an assessment of tumor burden. Calcitonin levels can be measured as a screening test in those patients at risk for medullary carcinoma, namely, relatives of patients with multiple endocrine neoplasia type II. Finally, calcitonin (most often as a salmon-derived analog) is also used as a drug to inhibit osteoclasts, as in Paget disease and osteoporosis, or to quell the hypercalcemia accompanying a variety of malignancies. In addition, it has analgesic properties that enhance its therapeutic use.

Osteoporosis

Osteoporosis is a metabolic bone disease characterized by low bone mass and microarchitectural deterioration of bone tissue, leading to increased bone fragility and a consequent increase in fracture risk. In the United States, osteoporosis affects an estimated 10 million adults. An additional 43 million are estimated to have low bone mass, placing them at increased risk for osteoporosis.[61] It is the most prevalent metabolic bone disease, affecting 10.3% of those over the age of 50.[61] The direct medical costs of osteoporosis are substantial, accounting for an estimated 17 to 20 billion dollars in 2005, expected to increase 50% by 2025.[62] Among the elderly, especially postmenopausal women, osteoporosis is a major cause of pathologic fractures, specifically fractures of the hip, spine, pelvis, proximal humerus, and wrist.[63] In 2005, osteoporosis accounted for approximately 2 million fractures, 27% of those occurring in the vertebrae. The number of fractures is estimated to grow to over 3 million annually by 2025.[62]

Like all metabolic bone diseases, osteoporosis is not limited to the spine. While 27% of postmenopausal women will develop a vertebral compression fracture, an additional 15% will experience a hip fracture.[64] In the elderly, hip fractures, most caused by osteoporosis, result in death, disability, and dependency: the in-hospital mortality rate in patients with hip fractures exceeds 5%[65]; up to 50% require long-term nursing home care, and more than half do not regain their prefracture level of mobility in the first postoperative year.[66,67]

Among the vertebral fractures, two-thirds are clinically silent; however, these patients have lower quality-of-life function.[68] Of women with scoliosis older than 65 years of age, 75% have at least one osteopenic wedge fracture. Although primary osteoporosis is a common cause of osteopenia in the elderly, it is only one of many possible causes. Medicare patients with vertebral compression fractures have a mortality rate approximately twice that of age-matched controls.[69]

Generally, osteoporosis is classified as either primary or secondary. Primary osteoporosis is further subdivided on the basis of its pathogenesis. Type I, or postmenopausal osteoporosis, is related to the abrupt decline of estrogen levels that occurs in menopausal women. Type II osteoporosis, known as senile or age-related osteoporosis, is due to the progressive decrease of BMD that occurs with aging.

Several risk factors for osteoporosis have been identified. Nonmodifiable risk factors include age greater than 50 years, female sex, family history of fragility fractures, and white or

Asian ethnicity.[70–72] A typical patient is a slim, white, postmenopausal woman of northwestern European descent.[50] She may have a history of premature menopause, cigarette or excessive alcohol use,[37] an eating disorder (e.g., anorexia nervosa), a sedentary lifestyle, use of anticonvulsants,[52] or lifelong low calcium intake.

Secondary osteoporosis results from any medical condition or medication that contributes to accelerated bone loss. A secondary cause of osteoporosis is found in about 30% of postmenopausal women, 40% to 50% of premenopausal women, and 50% to 55% of men. The most common causes are glucocorticoid use, hypogonadism, alcohol abuse, and malnutrition.[73] Corticosteroid-induced osteoporosis is the most common cause of drug-related osteoporosis and is associated with a high fracture rate. Corticosteroid therapy causes bone loss and fractures because it suppresses bone formation and inhibits intestinal calcium absorption, which leads to secondary hyperparathyroidism and increased osteoclastic bone resorption.[74] Less common causes include hematologic and neoplastic diseases, such as multiple myeloma and lymphoma; inflammatory diseases, such as inflammatory bowel disease and rheumatoid arthritis; endocrine conditions, including hyperthyroidism and adrenal insufficiency; human immunodeficiency virus (HIV); renal osteodystrophy; and nutritional deficiencies resulting from bariatric surgery or celiac disease, among others.[73] Endogenous hyperthyroidism increases cortical bone loss and may accelerate skeletal deterioration.[75] Inflammatory bowel disease (i.e., Crohn disease or ulcerative colitis) can cause osteoporosis both from the disease itself and its treatment. Autoimmune disorders and malignancies that destroy localized regions of bone, resulting in isolated areas of low BMD, include rheumatoid arthritis, periodontal disease, myeloma bone disease, and osteolytic bone metastases. These are associated with overexpression of RANKL at the site of pathology. In addition, osteomalacia (vitamin D deficiency) may mask itself as osteoporosis. The distinction is important because antiresorptive medications for osteoporosis are not appropriate choices to treat osteomalacia. Many secondary causes of osteoporosis are treatable and may necessitate a different management course than primary osteoporosis.

Pathology

Osteoporosis is defined as low bone strength. The two components of bone strength are bone mass and bone quality. Osteoporosis results from decreased overall bone mass with normal bone mineralization. Cortical and cancellous bone differ in their microarchitecture but maintain the same molecular composition. In addition, inadequate mineralization, poor-quality collagen, and microfractures all result in diminished bone quality.[76] Bone is remodeled throughout our lives in response to stress, up to 10% of bone mass may be remodeling at any one time. Peak bone mass is attained in the mid-30s for both sexes. Gender, nutrition, race, exercise habits, and overall health all influence bone mass. Peak bone mass is higher in men than in women and higher in African Americans than in whites.[77] After the fourth decade, both men and women lose bone mass from the skeleton (Fig. 88.3). Two phases of this loss have been identified: slow and accelerated. The slow phase, related to a bone remodeling imbalance with less bone formation than resorption, leads to trabecular thinning and subsequently destruction of connections between trabeculae. It results in an annual basal slow-phase rate of bone loss of 0.3% to 0.5%.[78] The accelerated phase that occurs with estrogen deficiency—a phenomenon found exclusively in women—is responsible for cortical bone mass loss of 2% to 3% per year. This loss is in addition to the slow-phase losses, which continue during the accelerated phase. The accelerated phase begins after surgical or natural menopause and lasts for approximately 5 years.[78] Thereafter, bone loss continues at the basal slow-phase rate.

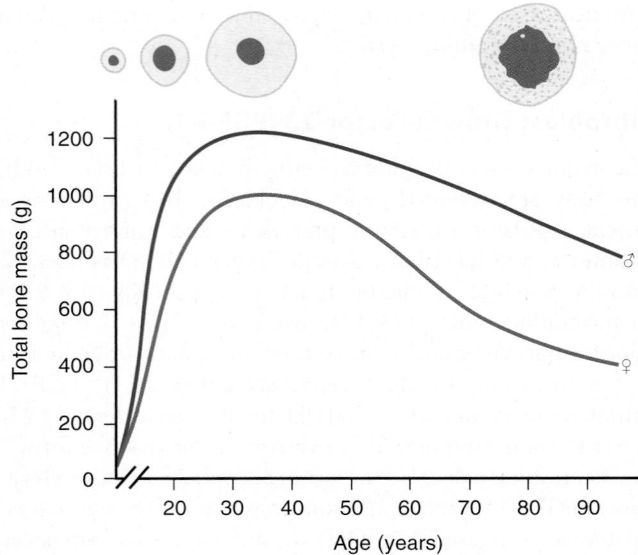

FIG. 88.3 Bone mass as a function of age in men *(blue)* and women *(purple)*. The images above the graph depict a cross-section of bone as maturation occurs over time. Mass is accumulated until peak bone mass is reached and then decreases and becomes more porous in advanced age. (From American Academy of Orthopaedic Surgeons, Park Ridge, IL: 1986.)

Multiple studies have shown the importance of estrogen deficiency in the causation of the accelerated phase.[79,80] Estrogen is thought to play a critical role in maintaining bone mass in adult women by suppressing cancellous bone remodeling and maintaining remodeling balance between osteoblastic and osteoclastic activity. At the molecular level, RANKL expression by bone marrow stromal cells and lymphocytes increases during the acute phase of estrogen deficiency.[81] In addition, estrogen stimulates production of OPG in premenopausal women, which binds RANKL and prevents bone resorption. As estrogen decreases in menopause, the net result of both of these mechanisms is enhanced osteoclast activity and bone loss.[82] Estrogen is also implicated in calcium metabolism through its effects on the kidney and intestine.[83] Others contend that estrogen antagonizes PTH activity[84] or stimulates calcitonin release. Decreased calcitonin levels have been found in oophorectomized and postmenopausal patients. Estrogen likely acts on a multitude of pathways affecting bone metabolism. The administration of estrogen to women during this period of rapid bone loss can decrease the loss in all bones, especially

TABLE 88.1 Type I vs. Type II Osteoporosis

	Type I	Type II
Female/male ratio	6:1	2:1
Calcium deficiency	No	Yes
Estrogen deficiency	Yes	No
Bone loss	Disproportionate loss of trabecular bone	Proportionate loss of both cortical and trabecular bone

From Riggs BL, Melton LJ 3rd. Evidence for two distinct syndromes of involutional osteoporosis. *Am J Med.* 1983;75:899.

those rich in trabecular bone (e.g., the vertebral bodies, the pelvis and other flat bones, in the ends of long bones).[85]

Riggs and Melton[78] have subclassified primary osteoporosis on the basis of patterns of bone loss and fracture (Table 88.1). Type I osteoporosis primarily affects trabecular bone sites and is characterized by fractures of the vertebral bodies and wrist. In patients with type I osteoporosis, the rate of trabecular bone loss is three times above normal, but the rate of cortical bone loss is only slightly above normal. In contrast, type II osteoporosis occurs in both men and women aged 75 years and older and involves areas of predominantly cortical bone. Clinically, fractures of the hip, pelvis, proximal humerus, and proximal tibia are seen. The causes of senile osteoporosis are the aging process itself and chronic calcium deficiency. Senile osteoporosis may also involve decreased vitamin D and increased PTH activity or impaired bone formation. Osteoporosis in women between the ages of 66 and 74 years may represent a combination of these two syndromes.

Metabolic remodeling occurs on the surface of bones and affects primarily trabecular bone. Due to their shape and trabecular pattern, vertebral bodies are preferentially resorbed in times of bone mass loss.[86] Osteoporosis is thus characterized by trabeculae of decreased size and number. Work by Dempster and colleagues[87] has demonstrated that osteoporosis involves a thinning of the cortex and a change in the shape of the trabecular bone from plates to narrow bars. The trabecular bone contains areas in which osteoclasts create a loss of connectivity, leading to a significant and localized weakening of the bone.[87,88] Vertebral body density declines before a similar loss is detected in cortical areas.

The body accommodates bone loss by redistribution. As people grow older, the diameter of the long bones gradually increases in both women and in men. Concurrently, the medullary diameter also increases, leading to a net thinning of the cortical bone. A 10% shift of bone mass outward from the epicenter through an enlargement of the bone diameter will compensate for a 30% decrease in the bone mass against applied bending and torque stresses but not against axial loading. This differential resorption explains the timing and patterns of the fracture syndromes seen in osteoporosis.[66] The incidence of vertebral compression fractures rises immediately after menopause, whereas the hip (with its higher proportion of cortical bone) fractures later in life, when cortical bone loss accumulates over the next 1 to 2 decades. The distal forearm, like the spine, has high trabecular content; thus, the incidence of Colles fractures also increases in menopause.

Deficiencies in dietary calcium cause decreased peak bone mass.[89] White women, on average, have less bone than either white men or African Americans of either sex.[90] Thus, the risk of clinically significant osteoporosis depends on hereditary factors, gender, race, and nutrition, which all contribute to peak bone mass, and aging, which causes progressive bone loss. Although the formation of good bone in sufficient quantity in young adulthood is clearly important, the aging process remains the most important cause of involutional osteoporosis.

Aging leads to bone loss independent of menopause, but the rapid decline of skeletal mass after estrogen deficiency implies that this hormone prevents the dissolution of the skeleton.[91] Nonetheless, its precise mechanism is unclear. Some investigators believe that the action is mediated by estrogen receptors on osteoblasts.[92] Others contend that estrogen antagonizes PTH activity[93] or stimulates endogenous calcitonin release. Decreased calcitonin levels have been found in oophorectomized and postmenopausal patients, and increased calcitonin levels are noted after estrogen administration. Regardless of the mechanism, estrogen deficiency leads to bone loss and plays a major role in the pathogenesis of type I osteoporosis.

The age-related ("slow-phase") bone loss is not affected by estrogen; rather, it likely represents impaired vitamin D metabolism. As an individual ages, the kidney gradually loses its ability to hydroxylate vitamin D into its active form, $1,25(OH)_2D$.[94] This active vitamin D is necessary to transport calcium in the gut; therefore, decreased hydroxylation, often coupled with poor dietary intake, leads to lowered serum calcium levels and, in turn, to elevated secretion of PTH. In addition to secondary hyperparathyroidism, elderly people are also more likely to take medications (e.g., diuretics) that further contribute to calcium losses. Furthermore, there is some evidence that the mechanism in remodeling that couples the actions of osteoclasts and osteoblasts functions suboptimally in old age: after the fourth decade, at a given site of remodeling, less bone is laid down than is resorbed.[90] Accordingly, normal bone turnover in the elderly leads to calcium depletion as well.

Clinical Course

End-stage osteoporosis culminates in fracture.[37,38,95] Still, for most of its course, osteoporosis is a silently progressive disease. Patients typically present to the physician late in the course, following one of three general scenarios. In the first of these, the patient presents with an acute painful fracture, usually of the spine (Fig. 88.4), but possibly of the rib, wrist, or hip. In the spine, normal activity (even minimal activity) may exceed the depleted bones' stress tolerance and result in fracture. The acute fracture can be severely painful, with the pain remaining over the affected area or radiating across the thorax. The pain from a vertebral fracture does not radiate down the legs. Symptoms such as leg pain suggest involvement of the spinal cord and obligate the physician to search for another or concomitant process to explain the pain. Osteoporosis, even if established in such a case, is probably not the only disease present. The acute pain usually abates when the fracture heals.

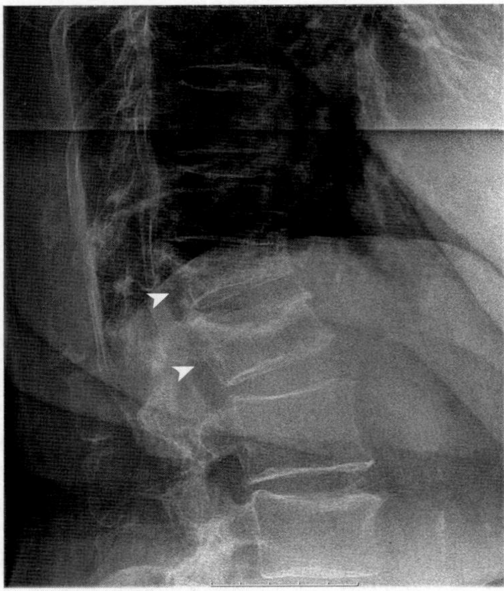

FIG. 88.4 Lateral radiograph of the lumbar spine showing vertebral compression fractures at L1 and L2 levels (*arrowheads*).

Nonetheless, the patient rarely returns to prefracture status. At a minimum, there may be point tenderness over the fracture site. The patient may note constant abdominal pain, often brought about by the constraining forces on the viscera in the now smaller abdominal cavity. Other patients complain of generalized backache. The backache may be due to changing muscular demands brought on by altered spinal curvature. Furthermore, some patients fear reinjury and strictly limit their activities. Others develop chronic pain syndromes, dysthymic states, or even overt clinical depression. Osteoporosis, therefore, often has a profound effect beyond the acute fracture episode. The incidence of vertebral compression fractures (highly trabecular bone) rises after menopause, whereas hip fractures occur 1 to 2 decades after menopause from progressive loss of cortical bone. Evidence suggests that these patients have a 15% increase in 5-year mortality risk.[96]

Not every patient has an acute episode. In an alternate scenario, an asymptomatic thoracic wedge or lumbar compression fracture of the spine may be noted on a radiographic examination performed for an unrelated purpose. These compression fractures may present subacutely, with twinge pain noted on minimal strain or exercise over a period of time, or the patient may even have no complaints at all. The macroscopic fracture observed on radiography, then, represents integration over time of a series of small, individually insignificant microfractures.

In the thoracic spine, both asymptomatic and painful fractures have a predilection for the anterior aspect of the bone. Progressive fracture thus leads to progressive shortening of the anterior height of the vertebral body relative to the posterior. The resultant shape of the body suggests the name of this process: wedge fracture. The wedge shape of the body, when summed over two or more vertebrae, causes dorsal kyphosis. In the lumbar region, the fractures are usually distributed equally throughout the vertebral body. No wedge is formed in this situation, and the process is thus termed

TABLE 88.2 Definition of Osteoporosis Based on Total Hip Bone Mass Density

Group	T Score
Normal	≥–1.0 SD
Osteopenia (low bone mass)	Between –1.0 and –2.5 SD
Osteoporosis	≤–2.5 SD
Severe osteoporosis	≤ –2.5 SD and fragility fracture

SD, standard deviation.
Modified from Kanis JA, Glüer CC. An update on the diagnosis and assessment of osteoporosis with densitometry. Committee of Scientific Advisors, International Osteoporosis Foundation. *Osteoporos Int.* 2000;11:192–202.

compression or *collapse fracture.* The combined effects of compression and wedge fractures lead to an unfortunate, but common, skeletal deformity: lost height coupled with excessive dorsal kyphosis. A vertebral body deformation due to an osteoporotic fracture can be difficult to determine.

Finally, generalized osteopenia without fracture may be noted on plain radiographs. This is not a different disease but, rather, an earlier phase of the same process that leads to fracture and deformity. These patients suffer from bone loss but have not yet crossed the critical point of stress tolerance.

Diagnosis

Though osteoporosis is characterized by low bone mass as well as poor bone quality, which includes microarchitectural deterioration, the only readily available test for osteoporosis focuses on the bone mass. BMD measured via dual-energy x-ray absorptiometry (DEXA) remains the clinical standard for diagnosing osteoporosis. The World Health Organization (WHO) defines osteoporosis by the T score, or number of standard deviations (SD) below peak bone mass of healthy adults (Table 88.2). A T score within 1 SD (T score ≥–1) of the mean is considered normal bone density. A T score between 1 and 2.5 SDs below the mean (T score <–1 but –2.5) is defined as osteopenia. Osteoporosis is diagnosed with a T score greater than 2.5 SDs below the mean (T score <–2.5). Concomitant fragility fracture denotes severe osteoporosis.[97]

DEXA also provides a Z score, a value for BMD relative to those of the same age, sex, and ethnicity. The Z score cannot be used to diagnose osteoporosis but is useful for screening for secondary causes of osteoporosis. Patients with a Z score 1.5 SDs below the mean for their age, sex, and ethnicity (Z < –1.5) should be evaluated for secondary causes of osteoporosis.[98] In addition, the Z score less than 1.5 is an indicator of osteoporosis in patients under the age of 40 years old.[99] DEXA is a fast and noninvasive means to determine BMD. It is produced by penetration of a low-energy and high-energy x-ray beam aimed at the posteroanterior spine and hip.

Wrist BMD is measured if the spine/hip measurement cannot be determined, if the patient is obese, or if the patient has hyperparathyroidism.[100] The spine is a useful site for BMD measurement because it predicts the risk of any fracture as well as or better than hip BMD in the perimenopausal population in which hip fracture risk is low. With advancing age, however, spine measurements are confounded by osteoarthritis and soft tissue calcification to a greater degree than the hip.[101,102] For this reason, the hip is the preferred site, especially in women older than 60 years. Based on the WHO diagnostic threshold, 15% to 20% of postmenopausal women can be identified as having osteoporosis when measurements using DEXA are made at the spine or hip.[95] The US Preventive Services Task Force recommends that all women aged 65 years should receive a DEXA scan. They conclude that there is insufficient evidence to suggest screening in men,[103] but the National Osteoporosis Foundation recommends DEXA screening in men aged 70 years or those older than 50 years with risk factors.[104]

The Fracture Risk Assessment Tool (FRAX) provides physicians a means to determine 10-year fracture risk in at-risk populations. The FRAX model was developed by the WHO by studying population-based cohorts around the world. This was created to broaden the evaluation beyond bone density alone. Factors evaluated by FRAX include age, sex, height and weight, previous fracture, parent with fractured hip, smoking and alcohol use, glucocorticoid use, rheumatoid arthritis, secondary osteoporosis, and BMD at the femoral neck. An individual with a 20% chance of a long bone fracture or a 3% chance of a hip fracture within 10 years is deemed of sufficient risk to warrant antiosteoporotic drug intervention.

While BMD is an indispensable tool in evaluating for osteoporosis, the National Bone Health Alliance issued a statement that osteoporosis may be diagnosed clinically based on the presence of hip fracture; osteopenia-associated vertebral, proximal humerus, pelvis, or low-trauma distal forearm fracture; or FRAX scores with more than 3% (hip) or 20% (major) 10-year fracture risk.[63]

The trabecular bone score is a newly developed tool that estimates trabecular microarchitecture using gray-level texture measurements of DEXA images. The diagnostic utility of this tool is under continuing investigation, but reports show that low lumbar spine trabecular bone score is associated with both history of fracture and incidence of new fracture. This tool has shown greatest utility in patients who are close to an intervention threshold based on BMD. Notably, it is unclear at this time whether trabecular bone score continues to reflect fracture risk once osteoporosis treatment is initiated.[105]

Evaluation for Osteoporosis

Once diagnosed with osteoporosis, a complete medical history should be obtained with particular attention to the risk factors for osteoporosis. These include age of 65 years or older, a history of vertebral fracture or any fracture during childhood, a family history of hip fracture, low body weight (body mass index [BMI] <21 or weight <127 pounds), cigarette smoking, and use of corticosteroids for more than 3 months.[106] Assessment of fall risk in the elderly should also be performed by evaluating orthostatic hypotension, cognitive impairment, sedating medications, and loss of vision/hearing. Physical examination for vertebral injuries should be included as up to two-thirds of osteoporotic compression fractures are asymptomatic.[107] Examination includes height, excessive deformity, and tenderness over the spinous process.

Laboratory Investigations for Osteoporosis

Generally, laboratory investigations other than bone mass density measurement are not required for the diagnosis of osteoporosis. Some routine tests, however, should be performed to obtain baseline values as part of the initial workup. These include complete blood count with differential, urinalysis, and blood chemistry profiles with serum calcium and phosphate. Although vitamin D deficiency is common among the elderly, with a prevalence of approximately 50%, many patients are asymptomatic. In addition, serum calcium and phosphate levels in this group of patients may not necessarily be abnormal. All older individuals, therefore, should be tested for vitamin D deficiency by measuring levels of 25(OH)D. If low, adequate vitamin D supplementation is encouraged. Performance speed and proximal muscle strength were markedly improved when 25(OH)D levels increased from 4 to 16 ng/mL and continued to improve as the levels increased to more than 40 ng/mL.[108]

Notably, blacks consistently have lower levels of 25(OH)D than whites, and are frequently labeled as having vitamin D deficiency. However, this population also has significantly lower levels of vitamin D–binding protein due to high prevalence of a common genetic variant. The low level of vitamin D–binding protein results in levels of bioactive 25(OH)D that are equivalent to those in whites. Indeed, black patients with measured 25(OH)D levels below the threshold used to diagnose vitamin D deficiency do not typically have the associated clinical manifestations. Therefore, low vitamin D levels in this population should be interpreted with caution and future workups may incorporate vitamin D–binding protein levels as well.[109]

Some special laboratory tests are available to measure the balance between bone resorption and bone formation from serum and urine samples. These assays are called *biochemical bone markers*. Biochemical bone markers can be classified into two groups: bone formation and bone resorption markers (Table 88.3). Although BMD is a critical measurement used

TABLE 88.3 Biochemical Markers of Bone Turnover

Bone Formation Markers	Bone Resorption Markers
Serum	*Serum*
• Bone-specific alkaline phosphatase • Osteocalcin • Carboxyterminal propeptide of type I collagen • Aminoterminal propeptide of type I collagen	• Tartrate-resistant acid phosphatase • NTXs • CTXs
	Urine
	• Free and total pyridinolines • Free and total deoxypyridinolines • NTXs • CTXs

CTX, C-telopeptide of collagen cross-link; NTX, N-telopeptide of collagen cross-link. Modified from Camacho P. Biochemical markers of bone turnover. In Favus MJ, ed. *Primer on the Metabolic Bone Diseases and Disorders of Mineral Metabolism*, ed 6. Washington, DC: American Society for Bone and Mineral Research; 2006.

to evaluate patients for osteoporosis, it represents a static parameter that provides no information regarding the rate of bone turnover in a given patient. Biochemical bone markers are generally noninvasive, widely available, quickly performed, and relatively inexpensive. Unlike DEXAs, they can be used repeatedly over short intervals to assess the dynamic process of bone turnover. In principle, they can be used (along with BMD) to predict future risk of fracture.

Biochemical Markers of Bone Turnover

During bone formation, osteoblasts produce type I collagen, which is their major synthetic product. Carboxy-terminal propeptide and amino-terminal propeptide of type I collagen, known as *PICP* and *PINP*, respectively, are cleaved from the newly formed collagen molecule and therefore can be used as the indices to indicate type I collagen biosynthesis. Osteoblasts also secrete a variety of noncollagenous proteins, two of which are used clinically as markers of osteoblast activity: bone-specific alkaline phosphatase and osteocalcin. It is these noncollagenous products that are most useful as markers for bone formation. Although alkaline phosphatase is derived from several tissues, the two most common sources are from liver and bone. Utilization of tissue-specific monoclonal antibodies enables differentiation between liver and bone isoform; however, the bone isoform has 10% to 20% cross-reactivity with the liver isoform.[110]

During osteoclast-mediated bone resorption, the collagen structure within bone is degraded. This collagen degradation product is used as an indicator for bone resorption. In general, collagen molecules in bone matrix are staggered to form collagen fibrils by covalent cross-links.[111] These cross-links consist of pyridinolines (Pyds) and deoxypyridinolines (Dpds). Pyd and Dpd cross-links occur at two intermolecular sites in the collagen molecule: amino-terminal-telopeptide (NTX) and carboxy-terminal-telopeptide (CTX). As part of this degradation process, cross-linked collagen peptides from both the NTX and CTX are released and achieve measurable concentrations in both serum and urine. Therefore, when osteoclasts resorb bone, they release a variety of collagen breakdown products into the circulation that are further metabolized by the liver and kidney. These include free Pyds, free Dpds, NTX, and CTX.

Despite the popularity of urine NTX, there are limitations to its use as a dynamic measure of bone resorption. As with other urine biochemical bone markers, NTX must be normalized for creatinine clearance. The urine assay loses reliability with impaired renal function, and the serum markers are then preferred. Biochemical bone markers are also subject to technical and biologic variability. Unlike BMD measurements for osteopenia and osteoporosis, there are currently no accepted criteria for what constitutes a high turnover rate.

The use of bone biochemical markers to determine therapy effectiveness is their best established clinical use. Several studies indicate that, within 4 to 6 weeks, there is significant reduction in biochemical markers of bone resorption after initiation of antiresorptive therapy.[112–114] Lack of marker reduction may indicate noncompliance or the need to change the dosage or the therapeutic agent. Serial BMD tests should be at least 12 (and possibly 24) months apart; therefore, more frequent measurements of biochemical markers offer a significant advantage.

Evaluation for Secondary Osteoporosis

When secondary osteoporosis is suspected on the basis of clinical findings or because the patient is relatively young and presented with a fragility fracture, specific tests should be considered to evaluate contributing causes that may require additional medical attention. These include basic laboratory investigation of a complete blood count with differential, erythrocyte sedimentation rate, serum calcium and phosphate levels, liver function tests, thyroid-stimulating hormone level, testosterone level in men, and a serum protein electrophoresis if myeloma is considered (Table 88.4). When abnormalities are detected, the patient should be referred to a specialist for further evaluation and specific treatment (see Table 88.4).

TABLE 88.4 Laboratory Investigations for Secondary Osteoporosis

Medical Diseases	Diagnostic Study
Endocrine	
Hyperparathyroidism	Serum calcium, serum phosphate, parathyroid hormone level
Hyperthyroidism	TSH, T3, free T4
Hypogonadism	LH, FSH, estrogen, testosterone (men)
Diabetes	Blood glucose
Gastrointestinal Disorders	
Crohn disease, ulcerative colitis	CBC, ESR, CRP, serum albumin, colonoscopy
Liver Disease	
Primary biliary cirrhosis, chronic active hepatitis	Liver function test, antimitochondrial antibody, antibody for hepatitis A, B, and C
Bone Marrow Disorders	
Multiple myeloma, leukemia, lymphoma	CBC with differential, serum calcium, serum protein electrophoresis
Collagen Vascular Disease	
Osteogenesis imperfecta, Ehlers-Danlos syndrome, Marfan syndrome	Genetic testing for collagen defects
Inflammatory Disease	
Rheumatoid arthritis	CBC, ESR, CRP, rheumatoid factor
Other	
Renal failure	BUN, creatinine
Osteomalacia	Serum 25-hydroxy-vitamin D, parathyroid hormone level

BUN, blood urea nitrogen; CBC, complete blood count; CRP, C-reactive protein; ESR, erythrocyte sedimentation rate; FSH, follicle-stimulating hormone; LH, luteinizing hormone; TSH, thyroid-stimulating hormone.

Data from Unnanuntana A, Gladnick BP, Lane JM: Osteoporosis and the aging spine: diagnosis and treatment. In: Yue JJ, Guyer RD, Hochschuler SH, et al., eds. *The Comprehensive Treatment of the Aging Spine: Minimally Invasive and Advanced Techniques.* Philadelphia: Elsevier; 2011.

Prevention and Treatment

Osteoporosis is a silent disease with a multitude of causes and risk factors. Patients may not present until they experience a fall and painful fracture; even those patients may not present with fracture pain, which often abates without intervention. First and foremost, treatment aims at prevention of osteoporosis and associated morbidity. Building strong bones begins in childhood and adolescence. Up to 90% of peak bone mass occurs at age 18 years in girls and 20 years in boys and may continue to climb until age 30 years. At this point, peak bone mass is achieved.[115] Adequate peak bone mass is achieved through proper nutrition, including calcium and vitamin D, exercise, and avoidance of smoking and alcohol abuse. Inadequate calcium intake during adolescence can account for a 10% reduction in peak bone mass.[115] Smoking one pack per day throughout adult life is associated with a 5% to 10% reduction in bone density,[116] and cigarette smoking is also associated with accelerated metabolism of estrogen.[117] It is recommended that clinicians strongly encourage smoking cessation when initiating osteoporosis treatment.

Nutrition, Calcium, and Vitamin D Supplementation

First-line treatment of osteoporosis includes adequate dietary intake of calories, protein, calcium, and vitamin D. Calcium and vitamin D supplementation is the cornerstone of all treatment modalities for osteoporosis. Literature has clearly shown that adequate calcium and vitamin D intake reduces the risk of fractures.[118] Adequate calcium and vitamin D intake reduces fracture risk.[118] A diet balanced with fruit, vegetables, and low-fat dairy can provide the majority of calcium needs. The National Osteoporotic Foundation (NOF) and Institute of Medicine recommend that men age 50 to 70 years consume 1000 mg per day of calcium and that women age 51 years and older and men age 71 years and older consume 1200 mg per day.[119–122] To maximize the absorption of calcium across the small bowels, no more than 500 to 600 mg of elemental calcium should be taken at any given time.[123] A patient's PTH level is used to adjust the dose of calcium to the individual patient. Generally, a PTH greater than 50 pg/mL indicates inadequate calcium, while a PTH less than 25 pg/mL suggests oversupplementation of calcium. Among all calcium formulations, calcium citrate is the preferred form because it can be readily absorbed in patients taking proton pump inhibitors or H_2 blockers, and it does not lead to kidney stone formation.[124]

The current recommended dosages of vitamin D_3 from the Institute of Medicine are 600 to 800 IU per day,[120] whereas the NOF recommends 800 to 1000 international units (IU) of vitamin D per day for adults aged 50 years and older.[119] However, many experts consider these recommendations to be too low and suggest that the minimum adult intake should be 1000 to 2000 IU/day.[125] The appropriate amount of vitamin D intake should be evaluated by monitoring 25(OH)D level and serum PTH. Experts suggest that 25(OH)D concentration be maintained at a minimum of 50 nmol or 20 ng/mL.[126] The upper limit of safety is estimated to be 125 nmol/L. Toxicity is rare even if a dosage of 10,000 IU/day is given for up to 5 months.[126,127]

Protein is also a significant contributor to bone health. A randomized prospective study that studied hip fractures in 82 elderly women demonstrated that those who took protein supplementation in addition to calcium and vitamin D supplements had an attenuation of the loss of bone at 1 year compared with those who received nonprotein supplements.[128] However, high dietary protein and sodium increase urinary calcium excretion and have also been shown to decrease the calcium available to the skeleton.[129]

Exercise

Those diagnosed with osteoporosis are recommended to engage in exercise 3 to 5 times per week for at least 45 minutes.[119] Regular physical activity reduces the risk for osteoporosis and osteoporotic fractures.[130,131] Weight-bearing exercise has beneficial effects on BMD, including that of the spine in both premenopausal and postmenopausal women.[130,132-135] In one study, young women (aged 20 to 35 years) were randomized into groups of exercise and calcium supplementation for 2 years and bone density at various sites was evaluated. The group randomized to the aerobics and weight-training program had a 2.5% increase in their spine density compared with the calcium and stretching program.[136] Muscle mass is significantly correlated to bone mass,[40] suggesting that increased skeletal loading leads to increased bone mass. As little as 1 hour of exercise two or three times per week can increase vertebral bone mass in postmenopausal women, whereas inactivity results in continued bone loss and increased risk for hip fracture.[137]

Immobilization results in decreased bone mass through increased activation at remodeling sites and decreased osteoblast stimulation.[138] Bone loss with complete immobilization can reach 40% in 1 year but can be prevented with upright positioning and daily postural shifting for 30 minutes.[139] Permanent bone loss can be prevented by instituting exercise within the first months of immobilization.[138] Therefore, although the gains in bone mass with exercise may be small, the decline in bone mass and subsequent increased fracture risk with inactivity can be substantial and irreversible.

Regular physical activity also improves muscle strength and balance, thus reducing the risk of falls.[140-143] Recommended exercises include resistance training, walking/jogging, Tai Chi, yoga, and Pilates. These programs significantly improve balance,[144] mitigate the fear of falling, and reduce falls in the elderly by more than 47%.[140]

Conservative management of osteoporotic patients should include an exercise program to minimize the effects of a more sedentary lifestyle common in the elderly. The prescribing physician should tailor the exercise regimen to the patient's overall fitness, most specifically cardiac tolerance. Accordingly, exercises that deliver high impact for a given aerobic effort, such as walking, are preferable to those that have less effect, such as swimming. Nevertheless, general muscle-strengthening therapy prevents falls.

A comprehensive general rehabilitation program that stresses spine extension and abdominal-strengthening exercises without flexion, as well as impact-loading activities such as walking, should be part of the treatment plan for every osteoporotic patient. Persistent participation in the exercise program is important because the benefits of exercise are quickly lost with cessation of the exercise regimen.[134]

Pharmacologic Treatment

Current pharmacotherapies aim to improve BMD and halt osteoporosis progression.

The NOF recommends pharmacologic treatment in postmenopausal women and men aged 50 years or older who have a hip or vertebral fracture, T score of −2.5 with secondary causes ruled out, or a T score between −1.0 and −2.5 with 10-year hip fracture risk of at least 3% or 10-year risk of osteoporotic fracture of 20%.[119] Current US Food and Drug Administration (FDA)-approved pharmacotherapies for osteoporosis include bisphosphonates, estrogen agonists, calcitonin, PTH, and the RANKL inhibitor denosumab. According to the American Association of Clinical Endocrinology, the bisphosphonates—alendronate, risedronate, and zoledronic acid—and denosumab are first-line therapies. Second-line agents include ibandronate and raloxifene. Calcitonin is a last-line agent and teriparatide is reserved for high fracture risk patients in whom bisphosphonates have failed or anabolic agents are indicated.[145] Before beginning pharmacologic treatment, all patients should take calcium and vitamin D supplements and participate in an exercise regimen.

Estrogen

Hormone replacement therapy, including estrogen, was once considered first-line treatment for osteoporosis. Postmenopausal osteoporosis results from loss of estrogen; its replacement has been shown to increase bone mass and reduce the risk of vertebral and hip fractures by 30% to 40%.[146] Hormone replacement therapy is no longer considered first-line therapy for osteoporosis because of its association with breast cancer, myocardial infarction, stroke, and venous thromboembolism.[146] Rather, it is used for management of postmenopausal symptoms in a tapered fashion.[146]

Selective Estrogen Receptor Modulators (SERMs)

Selective estrogen receptor modulators (SERMs) were developed for their beneficial effects of estrogen while limiting the adverse side effects described earlier. Raloxifene (Evista) is FDA approved for both the prevention of breast cancer, decreasing the risk by 70%, and for osteoporosis through its effects on bone estrogen receptors.[147] Raloxifene has been shown to reduce the risk of vertebral fracture but has no significant effect on nonvertebral fractures.[148] Its beneficial effects must be weighed with increased risk of venous thromboembolism and exacerbation of postmenopausal symptoms.[148,149] In 2013, the FDA approved the use of bazedoxifene combined with conjugated estrogens for the treatment of osteoporosis and vasomotor menopausal symptoms. This combination has increased BMD of the spine and hip significantly greater than raloxifene alone.[150] The benefit of SERMs should be weighed against their potential harmful side effects before initiation of treatment.

Bisphosphonates

Bisphosphonates are the most commonly used antiresorptive agents in the treatment of osteoporosis and are available in both oral and intravenous forms. Several bisphosphonates have been approved by the FDA for the treatment and prevention of osteoporosis: alendronate (Fosamax), risedronate (Actonel), ibandronate (Boniva), and zoledronic acid (Reclast). Bisphosphonates exist as nitrogen-containing and non-nitrogen-containing forms. Nitrogen-containing bisphosphonates inhibit osteoclast GTPase synthesis via farnesyl pyrophosphate synthase enzyme, inactivating these cells. Non-nitrogen-containing bisphosphonates form an ATP analog, preventing DNA synthesis and ultimately osteoclast apoptosis.[151] These drugs differ in their potency, administration, and dosing schedules. All bisphosphonates bind to bone and reside within the bone mineral for periods of up to 60 years. Alendronate and risedronate are given orally, zoledronic acid intravenously, and ibandronate is available in both oral and intravenous formulations. Bone turnover rate significantly slows within 6 weeks in those taking oral formulations and within 3 days with intravenous formulations.

Several clinical trials have shown that oral bisphosphonates —alendronate (Fosamax), risedronate (Actonel, Atelvia), and ibandronate (Boniva)—reduce the risk of osteoporotic fractures of the spine by 70% and hip up to 50% over 1 to 3 years after previous fracture.[152–154] Intravenous zoledronic acid is the most potent bisphosphonate available, increasing BMD of the spine by 4.3% to 5.1% and BMD of the hip by 3.1% to 3.5% compared with placebo. It also reduced the incidence of vertebral fractures by 70%, hip fractures by 41%, and nonvertebral fractures by 25% over 3 years.[152] It reduces cardiac mortality by more than 20% when given within 3 months of hip fracture without affecting fracture healing.[155]

The most common side effects of bisphosphonates include difficulty swallowing and dyspepsia from mucosal irritation. All bisphosphonates can affect renal function and are contraindicated in patients with a glomerular filtration rate less than 30 mL/min.[119] Acute renal failure requiring dialysis has been reported with zoledronic acid use; therefore, the FDA recommends serum creatinine testing before administration.[156] Long-term use of bisphosphonates beyond 5 years is associated with osteonecrosis of the jaw (ONJ), although this is more common with high doses used to treat bone cancers.[157] ONJ is characterized by exposed bone in the musculofascial region that fails to heal after 8 weeks. Prolonged use of bisphosphonates can lead to adynamic fragile bone, resulting in atypical fractures of the femur. Atypical subtrochanteric and femoral shaft fractures appear radiographically as a transverse pattern with beaking of the cortex and occur with minimal trauma. Any patient presenting with groin pain should be evaluated with radiographs of both hips and potentially MRI or bone scan if suspicion persists. The absolute risk of atypical subtrochanteric or femoral shaft fracture after 5 years of bisphosphonate use is 0.13% during the subsequent year and 0.22% within 2 years.[158] The American Association of Clinical Endocrinology recommends a drug holiday after 4 to 5 years of bisphosphonate therapy in mild osteoporosis.[145] While effective, the use of bisphosphonates requires the prescribing physician to be vigilant for the potentially severe side effects.

Calcitonin

Calcitonin (Fortical, Miacalcin) works by inhibiting osteoclastic bone resorption. Evidence suggests a reduction of vertebral fractures with modest effect on BMD.[159,160] Calcitonin may offer an analgesic effect in vertebral fractures, thought to be mediated by increased beta endorphins.[161] A postmarketing analysis by the FDA revealed increased risk of malignancy, 4.1% versus 2.9% in placebo groups, although a causal relationship has not been identified.[70] It is available as injection or nasal spray and is indicated only in postmenopausal women with reduced BMD in whom other agents have failed.

Anabolic Agents

Teriparatide (Forteo), recombinant human parathyroid hormone (1–34), is the only anabolic agent available for the treatment of osteoporosis. It is indicated for postmenopausal women or hypogonadal men who are at high risk for fracture and intolerant to or failed other treatment options. It is contraindicated in patients with hypercalcemia, renal impairment, pregnancy, breastfeeding, skeletal malignancy, Paget disease, or elevated alkaline phosphatase.[162] When given continuously, it results in increased bone turnover and net bone loss; however, when given intermittently, it leads to an anabolic phase and increased bone mass. It has been shown to increase bone mass up to 13% over 2 years[163] with reduction of vertebral and nonvertebral fractures by 65% and 53%, respectively.[164] Evidence suggests benefits of teriparatide on fracture healing through accelerated callus formation and proliferation of osteoprogenitor cells. Studies have shown promotion of healing in atypical subtrochanteric fractures associated with bisphosphonate use[165] as well as treatment of ONJ.[166] Prolonged exposure to high doses of teriparatide in rodents has been associated with increased risk of osteosarcoma.[167] Patients should be monitored using serum calcium, PTH levels, and 25(OH) vitamin D levels and treatment discontinued after 2 years.

Denosumab

Denosumab (Prolia) is approved for the treatment of men and postmenopausal women with osteoporosis at high risk for fracture. It is a human monoclonal antibody that acts as a RANKL inhibitor, dosed every 6 months by subcutaneous injection. Over 3 years, denosumab reduces the risk of vertebral fractures by 68%, hip fractures by 40%, and nonvertebral fractures by 20%.[168] Denosumab is associated with hypocalcemia, skin rash, and, less commonly, ONJ and atypical femur fractures. It does not bind to bone and is not measurable within the body after 2 months.

Pharmacologic Agents and Spinal Fusion

The effect of bisphosphonates on spinal fusion rates in animal models has provided inconsistent results. Several studies have shown no effect on fusion rates in porcine and rabbit models receiving alendronate postoperatively.[169–172] Others have shown increased size of fusion mass, new bone formation, and improved adherence at the screw-bone interface in rat models.[172,173] Nagahama et al.[174] performed a prospective randomized controlled trial in humans with osteoporosis undergoing lumbar interbody fusion. They demonstrated greater 1-year fusion rates (95%) in those receiving alendronate compared to control groups receiving vitamin D (65%). They also demonstrated decreased rates of cage subsidence, pseudarthrosis, and adjacent-level compression fractures in those taking alendronate.[174] Intermittent administration of teriparatide in both rat and rabbit models significantly enhanced spinal fusion rates and increased the fusion mass.[175,176] Clinically, in randomized trials, PTH enhanced distal radius fracture and pelvic fracture fusion rates over controls. A recent series of randomized blinded trials of PTH, risedronate, and controls were tested in 1-level and 2-level spine fusions by Ohtori and his colleagues.[177] PTH decreased fusion failure by 50% and pedicle screw pullout by 50%. Risedronate, a bisphosphonate, was undistinguished from controls. Presently, the use of calcium and vitamin D supplements, bisphosphonates, teriparatide, and anabolic agents appears to enhance spinal fusion rates in the perioperative period.[178]

Strategies for Treatment of the Osteoporosis Spine Patient

Patients considered for spine surgery with a diagnosis of osteopenia or osteoporosis should optimize nutrition status with adequate protein intake, calcium, and vitamin D supplementation. If a patient is under consideration and has significant osteoporosis, consider presurgical treatment with an anabolic agent to increase trabecular bone for 3 to 6 months. At surgery, in line with Ohtori data, place on anabolic PTH until fusion is united, usually for 1 to 2 years. If there is prior bisphosphonate exposure and low bone turnover (NTX <20), pretreat with PTH until NTX is over 20 and then continue for 2 years postoperatively. If the patient has osteopenia, hold bisphosphonate until fusion takes, then start bisphosphonate.

Spinal cord injury (SCI) results in unique and significant loss of BMD in its distribution, rate, and mechanism. In patients with complete SCI, sublesional BMD loss may approach 1% per week during the initial postinjury period. This rate is significantly higher than disuse osteopenia seen in nonparalytic conditions, such as bed rest. Proposed mechanisms include loss of sensory and sympathetic osteoanabolic innervation and catabolic effects of muscle atrophy. The rate of sublesional fracture in complete SCI patients is 1% for the first year and then 4.6% for each additional year.[179] Given the accelerated bone loss in these patients, an aggressive approach is recommended, including optimizing calcium and vitamin D intake, the use of antiosteoclastic medications such as bisphosphonates, teriparatide, or denosumab, correction of hypogonadal states, and weight-bearing movements, such as gait training.

Future Directions

Current pharmacologic agents for the treatment of osteoporosis have unique mechanisms, benefits, and side effects. These factors must be considered for each patient given each individual's diagnosis and associated risk factors. Current developmental treatments focus on monoclonal antibodies targeting specific metabolites and enzymes involved in bone homeostasis. Research in rare genetic diseases—sclerosteosis and Van Buchem disease—has led to the discovery of the protein sclerostin. This protein inhibits the Wnt signaling pathway and formation of new bone. Current trials using rosozumab and blosozumab, monoclonal antibodies against sclerostin, demonstrate superiority to placebo.[12,181] Emerging pharmacologic agents should aim to reduce resorptive activity while promoting bone formation in a way that maintains the structural integrity of the bone and limits side effects of the drugs.

Strontium ranelate is an agent that has both antiresorptive and anabolic action. Treatment of postmenopausal osteoporotic women with strontium ranelate has been shown to decrease fracture risk and increase bone mineral density.[182,183] The long-term effects, however, remain unknown. The development of new formulations of teriparatide (noninjectable forms) or development of alternative PTH analogs that possess longer half-life, leading to less frequent dosing, are also under investigation.[184,185]

Paget Disease of Bone (Osteitis Deformans)

Paget disease of the bone is the second most prevalent metabolic bone disease. The overall incidence of Paget disease is decreasing, however.[186,187] The pelvis is the most frequently affected site, but the disease in the pelvis is most often asymptomatic. When Paget disease is clinically apparent, spinal complaints, notably pain, are the most common.[188] Paget disease primarily affects older individuals; in the United States, it occurs in 2% to 3% of people older than the age of 60 years.[189] Paget disease affects men and women equally and has a distinctive geographic distribution. It is found more commonly in the United Kingdom, North America, Australia, New Zealand, France, and Germany. It is rarely encountered in Scandinavia, China, Japan, India, Africa, or the Middle East.[103,190]

Pathology

Paget disease is a focal disorder of accelerated skeletal remodeling that usually involves a single bone (monostotic) or several bones (polyostotic) and rarely affects numerous bones. Initially, there is an increase in the rate of bone resorption at areas of bone remodeling (Fig. 88.5). Pagetic osteoclasts are abnormal in several ways: they are greater in size and number and highly multinucleate, with up to 100 nuclei.[191,192] In response to this increased resorptive activity, additional osteoblasts are recruited to remodeling sites, with increased production of qualitatively poor new bone matrix that is deposited in a disorganized woven pattern. The result is increased bone formation and a disruption of the normally organized lamellar collagen architecture.[191] Over time, this woven bone is incompletely replaced by more organized bone, as is the case with a fracture callus.

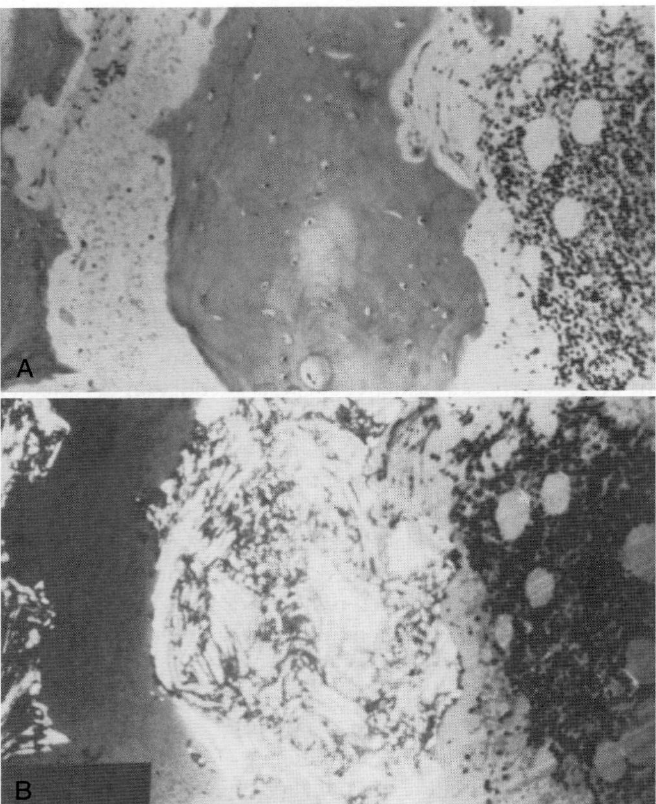

FIG. 88.5 Histologic appearance of Paget disease. (A) Mosaic pattern. (B) Polarized view of disorganized collagen. (From Disorders of Bone 20. Orthop. Science. Park Ridge, IL: American Academy of Orthopaedic Surgeons; 1986.)

The etiology of Paget disease remains unknown. Evidence exists for both viral and hereditary causes. Genetic factors seem to play a role, as evidenced by the epidemiology of British migrants being affected more frequently. Familial clusters of Paget disease have been documented.[193,194] A positive family history has been reported in up to 40% of patients.[189] A first-degree relative has 7 times greater risk of developing Paget disease.[194] Genetic studies have identified several possible loci for Paget disease.[195–197] Sequestosome 1 (*SQSTM1*) is the best studied and encodes for a scaffold protein (p62) in the nuclear factor κ1 (NF κ1) signaling pathway.[198] The common area of interruption is the region encoding the binding site for ubiquitin. The loss of the ubiquitin site leads to dysregulation of the protein, which is thought to lead to activation of the RANKL pathway and subsequent increased osteoclast activity.[45] There is currently a large clinical trial investigating if zolendronate may prevent or delay the onset of Paget disease in patients with *SQSTM1* gene mutations.[199]

Environmental factors also may play a role in Paget disease. Initial enthusiasm for a viral etiology was stimulated by the nuclear and cytoplasmic inclusion bodies, similar to paramyxovirus nucleocapsids, detected in affected osteoclasts by numerous methods in several studies.[200–203] Several syncytial viruses and canine distemper virus have also been postulated to play a role in the etiology of Paget disease.[200,201] A characteristic feature of these viruses is their ability to persist at low levels and invade the host immune system.

Despite decades of research, a pure viral cause for Paget disease has not been proven. No virus has ever been cultured from pagetic cells. Polymerase chain reaction studies have had mixed results attempting to isolate measles virus and canine distemper virus from blood and osteoblasts of patients with the disease.[204,205] Also, unlike the distinctive geographic distribution of paget disease, measles has a similar incidence worldwide and occurs in young patients, whereas Paget disease generally occurs in the elderly.[206] Furthermore, similar viral nuclear inclusion bodies have been identified in other skeletal disorders; thus, the virus may be a nonetiologic cotraveler in an osteoclast altered by some other mechanism.

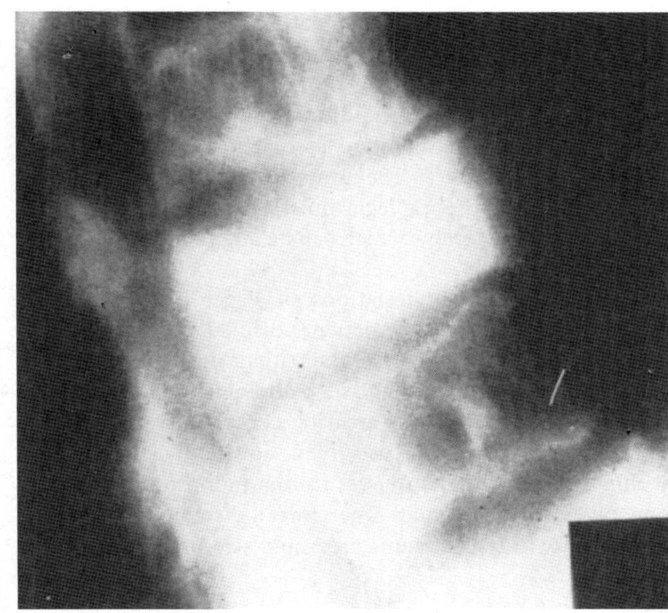

FIG. 88.6 Spinal involvement in Paget disease. The vertebral body is squared and enlarged.

Clinical Course

Most patients with Paget disease are asymptomatic. In fact, 22% of patients diagnosed with Paget disease are asymptomatic. The disease is often detected when the patient has a radiograph taken or serum alkaline phosphatase measured for an unrelated reason. In the majority of patients with Paget disease, one or several bones are involved. In decreasing order, the most commonly involved bones include the pelvis, lumbar spine, femur, thoracic spine, skull, tibia, humerus, and cervical spine; however, any bone may be affected. The lumbar, thoracic, and cervical vertebrae are affected in 58%, 45%, and 14% of patients, respectively.[204,207]

Clinical manifestations, when present, cover a wide spectrum. In order of decreasing frequency, symptomatic individuals may present with pain, bone deformity, deafness, and pathologic fractures.[208] Patients who are symptomatic most often present with back pain,[209] although other areas, especially the hip, can be involved. The skull can be implicated in the disease, and when it is the woven bone, expansion can encroach on the cranial nerves, most typically the eighth nerve. Both the acoustic and the vestibular branches can be affected; thus, the initial presentation of Paget disease might be decreased hearing or difficulty with gait or balance.[210]

In the spine, the pain is infrequently due to primary pagetic involvement alone but rather represents related secondary changes (Fig. 88.6).[211] These include osteoarthritis of the spinal facets; encroachment on the spinal cord; or, in the case of intense pain, pathologic fracture. When the spinal column is involved, most often it is the thoracolumbar regions that are affected, but cervical disease may also contribute.[212] Involvement of the spinal cord may be secondary to a mechanical or vascular complication. Of the mechanical causes, vertebral collapse, osteophytic overgrowth, or bony volume expansion in the osteosclerotic phase (discussed later) can all impinge on neural elements.[213] The spinal cord's vascular supply can likewise be disrupted by bone compression of afferent arteries, leading to neural ischemia. In addition, Paget disease causes a reactive vasodilation near diseased areas. This may lead to shunting of blood and ischemia of the deprived areas. In the spine, increased blood flow around pagetic lesions may result in a diversion of blood destined for the cord, causing the so-called arterial steal phenomenon and leading to neurologic signs. In summary, spinal Paget disease can cause not only bone pain and arthritis or pathologic fractures but also, through its effect on nerves, headaches, hearing or vision loss, cerebellar deficits, and even fecal and urinary incontinence.

A hallmark of Paget disease is skeletal deformity, which may be manifest as an increase in bone size or an abnormality in bone shape. Bone is resorbed and replaced rapidly in Paget disease, and the replacement bone is necessarily less organized and weaker. In weight-bearing bones, this can cause skeletal deformities.[214] Although this problem is more common in the femur and tibia, it can occur in the spine, leading to significant kyphotic changes.

Paget disease can also cause high-output cardiac failure. This rare occurrence is not due to increased blood flow within the pagetic bone but rather to reactive vasodilatation of the tissue adjacent to the involved bone. This increased vascular flow explains the skin warmth felt over the involved bone and, as discussed earlier, may cause ischemia in regions where the blood normally flows.

The most serious clinical complication of Paget disease heralded by the acute onset of pain or sharp increase in the intensity of chronic pain is osteosarcoma or other types of sarcoma. Although the incidence of osteosarcoma is less than 1% of patients with Paget disease, it is 1000 times higher than in the general population for this age group.[215] Moreover, the tumors that do form are particularly aggressive. Fortunately, sarcomatous degeneration is especially infrequent in spinal Paget disease. An unusual form of tumorous degeneration in Paget disease is the giant cell tumor. The lesion is frequently multifocal and has a unique association with individuals from Avellino, Italy.[216] The tumor frequently involves the spine and leads to paraplegia unless treated. It responds to dexamethasone therapy, which can be augmented by selective radiation.

Other clinical manifestations of Paget disease may be related to the phase of the patient's disease. During the early osteolytic phase, for example, the patient may suffer the consequences of bone loss, such as a pathologic fracture, whereas in the late sclerotic phase, arthritic complaints predominate. Furthermore, Paget disease may advance geographically within a bone or may progress from a monostotic disease to one involving many bones. Therefore, a mixed picture may be observed, with lysis in some areas and sclerosis in others.

Diagnosis

Radiographic Assessment

Paget disease is nearly always diagnosed radiographically. Although the osteoclastic lesion is readily apparent on histologic section, because the radiologic presentation is classic and generally unambiguous, there is rarely a need to progress beyond radiographs. Paget disease occurs in three phases, each of which has a distinct appearance on radiographs. In the earliest phase of the disease (lytic phase) when osteoclast resorption predominates, a well-demarcated, circular region of decreased bone density may be seen in the affected bone. This lesion has been termed *osteoporosis circumscripta*. Later, in the lytic-blastic phase, when osteoblasts begin to replace resorbed bone, radiographs demonstrate both osteolytic and sclerotic changes in the same bone. In the spine, this mixed picture is seen with expanded, radiodense regions in the periphery of the vertebral bodies (cortical thickening) and heightened radiolucency centrally. In the final phase of the disease, when osteoblastic bone formation outpaces osteolysis and primarily sclerotic changes are seen on radiographs, the affected bones appear dense, enlarged, and often deformed. The differentials for osteoblastic vertebrae include lymphoma, Paget disease, and osteoblastic metastases. Only Paget disease increases the size of the vertebrae.

Biochemical Markers

The increase in bone resorption and bone formation is reflected in an increase in biochemical markers of bone turnover. Bone resorption releases fragments of the collagen matrix, as evidenced by an elevated urinary excretion of hydroxyproline and hydroxylysine. Although these provide reasonably accurate measures of bone collagen resorption, more specific tests are used routinely. Serum total alkaline phosphatase is a bone formation marker; its elevation in Paget disease is the most common index of disease activity. A measure of bone-specific alkaline phosphatase may be preferred in a subset of patients with hepatic disease or monostotic involvement, in which 15% of patients have a normal alkaline phosphatase level[207] but appears to offer no advantage in the average patient.[217] In all patients, however, changes in total serum alkaline phosphatase activity are adequate to monitor changes in overall disease activity. Urinary and serum markers of bone resorption—including deoxypyridinoline, N-telopeptide, and C-telopeptide—provide more immediate measures of response to therapy than bone formation markers.

Biopsy

Although radiographic and biochemical indices are usually diagnostic, if uncertainty remains, a bone biopsy can definitively diagnose the disease. However, early Paget disease cannot always be distinguished with sufficient confidence from a metastatic tumor in the spine (a frequent site of metastasis). In such a case, a biopsy of the lesion (not of the iliac crest, the typical location of biopsy in metabolic bone disease) may be performed.

Treatment

Calcium and Vitamin D

Calcium and vitamin D deficiency should be corrected before the use of any bisphosphonates or treatments for Paget disease. Hypocalcemia is a significant risk, especially with the use of any of the intravenous bisphosphonates.[218]

Bisphosphonates

The emergence of newer, more potent bisphosphonates has resulted in a major change in the treatment of Paget disease over the past several years. Bisphosphonates, which inhibit osteoclast-mediated bone resorption and induce osteoclast apoptosis,[219] are the mainstay of drug treatment for Paget disease. Studies have demonstrated that bisphosphonates are effective in reducing bone turnover,[220–222] decreasing pain,[220,222] and promoting healing of osteolytic lesions.[223] On the other hand, studies have yet to demonstrate the long-term efficacy of bisphosphonates to prevent complications of the disease. There is debate as to whether to treat only symptomatic patients or to treat all patients with the goal of normalizing bone turnover markers. While there is some evidence from a large randomized clinical trial that there is no difference in outcomes between the two approaches, other studies have shown that treating to normalization of bone turnover markers leads to healing of lytic radiologic lesions, pain relief, and improved quality of life.[220,223–225] Availability of more potent bisphosphonates in recent years also supports an early intervention approach. In order of decreasing potency, the FDA-approved bisphosphonates for the treatment of Paget disease are zoledronic acid, risedronate, alendronate, pamidronate, tiludronate, and etidronate. Zoledronic acid was recently shown to be more efficacious than risedronate in controlling pain, decreasing bone turnover markers, and maintenance of suppression after treatment.[220]

Calcitonin

Calcitonin, the first widely used therapy for Paget disease, also inhibits osteoclastic bone resorption.[226] In addition, calcitonin has analgesic properties that can benefit patients with significant pain. Salmon calcitonin is available in injectable and nasal-spray forms, but only the injectable form is FDA approved for the treatment of Paget disease. Compared with bisphosphonates, calcitonin is less powerful and does not suppress the disease activity for as long after cessation. Calcitonin use today is largely limited to those patients who are unable to tolerate bisphosphonates.[227]

Surgery

Finally, some patients with Paget disease benefit from surgery. Although operative intervention cannot cure the basic lesion of the disease, surgery may relieve symptoms caused by secondary changes, including fractures, bone deformities, arthritis, and spinal stenosis. Before surgery, pretreatment with a potent oral bisphosphonate (or pamidronate infusion if time is limited) quiets the operative field, helps prevent postoperative hypercalcemia, and fosters better healing and hemostasis.

Summary

Metabolic bone diseases are a group of disorders that occur as a result of changes in osteoblast and osteoclast function. The osteoblast and osteoclast play a major role in maintaining the structure and material properties of bone, controlling the synthesis of bony matrix, and regulating mineral metabolism and the mineralization process. Thus, an alteration of these cells' function results in a variety of clinical disorders. An understanding of the pathogenesis of such diseases and an attempt to define the cause of a patient's acute problem is the key for treatment. This requires a thorough medical history, physical examination, imaging studies, and appropriate laboratory investigations. In general, appropriate care includes adequate replacement of calcium, vitamin D, and initiation of antiosteoporotic agents, including bisphosphonates for high-turnover state and teriparatide for low-turnover state. Anabolic agents are the preferred drugs in the setting of operative spinal fusion for osteoporotic patients. Orthopaedic surgeons should be aware of these biologic and biochemical disorders and familiar with their clinical presentation.

PEARLS

1. An approach combining assessment of BMD, bone turnover rate, and tissue properties may allow improved prediction of fracture risk.
2. Osteoporosis has been divided into high-turnover and low-turnover osteoporosis. Antiresorptive agents, such as bisphosphonates, have been developed to address the high-turnover state, while an anabolic agent, PTH, provides active building of bone mass and treats the low-turnover state. Clinical trials suggest that the anti-sclerostin antibody romosozumab has significant potential to increase BMD and reduce risk of vertebral and nonvertebral fractures.
3. In the setting of spinal fusion and fracture healing, an anabolic agent may be advantageous in the early phases to enhance appropriate biologic healing responses.
4. The treatment of metabolic bone diseases of the spine, including osteoporosis and Paget disease, requires a multidisciplinary approach. An understanding of the pathogenesis of such diseases and an attempt to define the cause of a patient's acute problem is the key for treatment.

PITFALLS

1. Failure to recognize metabolic bone disease preoperatively in patients may lead to inferior postsurgical outcomes.
2. BMD and bone quality are the major determinants of bone strength. An alteration in either BMD or bone quality results in osteoporotic vertebral compression fractures.
3. Prolonged treatment with bisphosphonates may result in oversuppression of bone turnover, leading to adynamic, fragile bone.
4. Bisphosphonates should be discontinued following spinal fusion or acute vertebral fracture in order to reduce the possible adverse effects to the early biologic processes of fracture healing.
5. Teriparatide is contraindicated in Paget disease, unexplained elevations of alkaline phosphatase, history of skeletal irradiation, and children with open physes.

KEY POINTS

1. Metabolic bone diseases are a group of disorders that occur as a result of changes in osteoblast and osteoclast function. Among all disorders of the spine, osteoporosis is the most common metabolic bone disease affecting the spine.
2. BMD and bone quality are the major predictors for osteoporotic vertebral compression fractures. An approach combining assessment of BMD, bone turnover rate, and tissue properties may allow improved prediction of fracture risk.
3. Osteoporosis has been divided into high-turnover and low-turnover osteoporosis. Antiresorptive agents, such as bisphosphonates, have been developed to address the high-turnover state, while an anabolic agent, PTH, provides active building of bone mass and treats the low-turnover state.
4. In the setting of spinal fusion and fracture healing, clinicians should discontinue bisphosphonates at the time of surgery. An anabolic agent, such as teriparatide, may be advantageous in the early steps to enhance appropriate biologic healing responses.
5. The treatment of metabolic bone diseases of the spine, including osteoporosis and Paget disease, requires a multidisciplinary approach. An understanding of the pathogenesis of such diseases and an attempt to define the cause of a patient's acute problem are the keys for treatment.

KEY REFERENCES

1. Ohtori S, Inoue G, Orita S, et al. Comparison of teriparatide and bisphosphonate treatment to reduce pedicle screw loosening after lumbar spinal fusion surgery in postmenopausal women with osteoporosis from a bone quality perspective. *Spine*. 2013;38(8):487-492.
This prospective study evaluates the efficacy of teriparatide and risedronate in preventing pedicle screw loosening after lumbar

posterolateral fusion in female patients with osteoporosis. It concludes that teriparatide (daily subcutaneous injection of 20 μg) significantly reduces the incidence of pedicle screw loosening compared with risedronate and the control group. Use of risedronate was not associated with decreased loosening compared with controls. The authors recommend administration of teriparatide to improve the quality of lumbar spine bone marrow and pedicle cortex.

2. McClung MR, Grauer A, Boonen S, et al. Romosozumab in postmenopausal women with low bone mineral density. *N Engl J Med.* 2014;370(5):412-420.
This randomized controlled trial assesses the safety and efficacy of romosozumab, a monoclonal antibody that increases bone formation by binding sclerostin. Results indicate that romosozumab significantly increases bone mineral density in the lumbar spine. An 11.3% increase in bone mineral density was observed with the 210-mg dose at 12-month follow-up. Adverse events were limited to mild injection-site reactions. It concludes that romosozumab is a robust stimulator of bone formation in postmenopausal women with osteoporosis.

3. Cosman F, Crittenden DB, Adachi JD, et al. Romosozumab treatment in postmenopausal women with osteoporosis. *N Engl J Med.* 2016;375(16):1532-1543.
This large, randomized controlled trial evaluates the rates of new vertebral and nonvertebral fractures in patients treated with romosozumab versus placebo. Patients on romosozumab had a 73% lower risk of vertebral fractures and a 36% lower risk of nonvertebral fractures compared with those on placebo.

4. Kanis JA. FRAX and the assessment of fracture probability in men and women from the UK. *Osteoporos Int.* 2008;19:385-397.
This study reports the use of an assessment tool to determine the absolute risk of a hip fracture or osteoporotic fracture within the next 10 years on the basis of the patient information, including BMD, body mass index, a prior history of fracture, a parental history of hip fracture, use of oral glucocorticoids, rheumatoid arthritis and other secondary causes of osteoporosis, current smoking, and alcohol intake.

5. Vieth R. Why the optimal requirement for Vitamin D3 is probably much higher than what is officially recommended for adults. *J Steroid Biochem Mol Biol.* 2004;89-90:573-579.
This review article provides a concise summary of the current evidence from animal studies, epidemiologic studies, and randomized, controlled clinical trials of fracture prevention using vitamin D. It concludes that the optimal 25(OH)D concentration in osteoporotic patients should exceed 70 nmol/L, which requires an average vitamin D intake of 800 to 1000 IU per day. The author further suggests that optimal vitamin D levels for other aspects of human health are probably higher still.

6. Lyles KW, Colon-Emeric CS, Magaziner JS, et al. Zoledronic acid and clinical fractures and mortality after hip fracture. *N Engl J Med.* 2007;357:1799-1809.
This randomized controlled trial found that the administration of zoledronic acid after a hip fracture decreased fracture risk and mortality rate compared with placebo.

7. Huang RC, Khan SN, Sandhu HS, et al. Alendronate inhibits spine fusion in a rat model. *Spine.* 2005;30:2516-2522.
This study investigates the effects of alendronate on posterolateral lumbar fusion in a rat model. The investigators concluded that alendronate inhibits spine fusion in rats. The fusion masses in rats treated with alendronate were radiographically larger and denser than those in control animals despite lower fusion rates. Alendronate was also shown to inhibit bone graft resorption and incorporation. The authors recommend that patients undergoing spine arthrodesis should not take alendronate until fusion is achieved.

8. O'Loughlin PF, Cunningham ME, Bukata SV, et al. Parathyroid hormone (1-34) augments spinal fusion, fusion mass volume, and fusion mass quality in a rabbit spinal fusion model. *Spine.* 2009;34:121-130.
The aim of this study was to assess whether intermittent parathyroid hormone (PTH) would improve spinal fusion outcomes in the Boden rabbit posterolateral spinal fusion model. The investigators found that PTH increased posterolateral fusion success in rabbits. Fusion bone mass and histologic determinants were also improved with PTH treatment. The authors conclude that PTH has promise for use as an adjunctive agent to improve spinal fusion in clinical medicine.

REFERENCES

1. Bruder SP, Fink DJ, Caplan AI. Mesenchymal stem cells in bone development, bone repair, and skeletal regeneration therapy. *J Cell Biochem.* 1994;56(3):283-294.
2. Lazarus H, et al. Ex vivo expansion and subsequent infusion of human bone marrow-derived stromal progenitor cells (mesenchymal progenitor cells): implications for therapeutic use. *Bone Marrow Transplant.* 1995;16(4):557-564.
3. Owen M. Lineage of osteogenic cells and their relationship to the stromal system. *Bone Mineral Res.* 3:1-25.
4. Buckwalter JA, et al. Bone biology. I. Structure, blood supply, cells, matrix, and mineralization. *Instr Course Lect.* 1996;45:371.
5. Buckwalter JA, et al. Bone biology. II. Formation, form, modeling, remodeling, and regulation of cell function. *J Bone Joint Surg Am.* 1995;77(8):1276-1289.
6. Nijweide PJ, Burger EH, Feyen JH. Cells of bone: proliferation, differentiation, and hormonal regulation. *Physiol Rev.* 1986;66(4):855-886.
7. Stein GS, Lian JB. Molecular mechanisms mediating proliferation/differentiation interrelationships during progressive development of the osteoblast phenotype. *Endocr Rev.* 1993;14(4):424-442.
8. Teitelbaum SL, Abu-Amer Y, Ross FP. Molecular mechanisms of bone resorption. *J Cell Biochem.* 1995;59(1):1-10.
9. Poole KES, et al. Sclerostin is a delayed secreted product of osteocytes that inhibits bone formation. *FASEB J.* 2005;19(13):1842-1844.
10. Winkler DG, et al. Osteocyte control of bone formation via sclerostin, a novel BMP antagonist. *EMBO J.* 2003;22(23):6267-6276.
11. O'Brien CA, Nakashima T, Takayanagi H. Osteocyte control of osteoclastogenesis. *Bone.* 2013;54(2):258-263.
12. McClung MR, et al. Romosozumab in postmenopausal women with low bone mineral density. *N Engl J Med.* 2014;370(5):412-420.
13. Cosman F, Crittenden DB, Adachi JD, et al. Romosozumab treatment in postmenopausal women with osteoporosis. *N Engl J Med.* 2016;375(16):1532-1543.
14. Chambers TJ. The origin of the osteoclast. *Bone Mineral Res.* 1989;6:1-25.
15. Bartkiewicz M, et al. Characterization of the osteoclast vacuolar H(+)-ATPase B-subunit. *Gene.* 1995;160(2):157-164.
16. Theill LE, Boyle WJ, Penninger JM. RANK-L and RANK: T cells, bone loss, and mammalian evolution. *Annu Rev Immunol.* 2002;20(1):795-823.
17. Body J-J, et al. A study of the biological receptor activator of nuclear factor-kappaB ligand inhibitor, denosumab, in

patients with multiple myeloma or bone metastases from breast cancer. *Clin Cancer Res*. 2006;12(4):1221-1228.

18. Brown JP, et al. Comparison of the effect of denosumab and alendronate on BMD and biochemical markers of bone turnover in postmenopausal women with low bone mass: a randomized, blinded, phase 3 trial. *J Bone Miner Res*. 2009;24(1):153-161.
19. McClung MR, et al. Denosumab in postmenopausal women with low bone mineral density. *N Engl J Med*. 2006;354(8): 821-831.
20. Raisz LG, Kream BE. Regulation of bone formation. *N Engl J Med*. 1983;309(1):29-35.
21. Prockop DJ, et al. The biosynthesis of collagen and its disorders. *N Engl J Med*. 1979;301(1):13-23.
22. Price CP, Thompson PW. The role of biochemical tests in the screening and monitoring of osteoporosis. *Ann Clin Biochem*. 1995;32(3):244-260.
23. Sanchez CP, Salusky IB. Biochemical markers in metabolic bone disease. *Curr Opin Orthop*. 1994;5(5):43-49.
24. Bullough PA, Boachie-Adjei O. *Atlas of Spinal Disease*. New York: Gower Medical Publishing; 1988.
25. Shiraki M, et al. Nonenzymatic collagen cross-links induced by glycoxidation (pentosidine) predicts vertebral fractures. *J Bone Miner Metab*. 2008;26(1):93-100.
26. Saito M, Marumo K. Collagen cross-links as a determinant of bone quality: a possible explanation for bone fragility in aging, osteoporosis, and diabetes mellitus. *Osteoporos Int*. 2010;21(2):195-214.
27. Ettinger B, Burr DB, Ritchie RO. Proposed pathogenesis for atypical femoral fractures: lessons from materials research. *Bone*. 2013;55(2):495-500.
28. Kondo H, Guo J, Bringhurst FR. Cyclic adenosine monophosphate/protein kinase A mediates parathyroid hormone/parathyroid hormone-related protein receptor regulation of osteoclastogenesis and expression of RANKL and osteoprotegerin mRNAs by marrow stromal cells. *J Bone Miner Res*. 2002;17(9):1667-1679.
29. Price PA. Osteocalcin. *Bone Mineral Res Annu*. 157-190.
30. Karsenty G, Ferron M. The contribution of bone to whole-organism physiology. *Nature*. 2012;481(7381):314-320.
31. Miheller P, Lőrinczy K, Lakatos PL. Clinical relevance of changes in bone metabolism in inflammatory bowel disease. *World J Gastroenterol*. 2010;16(44):5536.
32. Whyte MP. Physiological role of alkaline phosphatase explored in hypophosphatasia. *Ann N Y Acad Sci*. 2010; 1192(1):190-200.
33. Gazdag AR, et al. Alternatives to autogenous bone graft: efficacy and indications. *J Am Acad Orthop Surg*. 1995; 3(1):1-8.
34. Wozney JM, et al. Novel regulators of bone formation: molecular clones and activities. *Science*. 1988;242(4885):1528-1534.
35. Hoffmann A, et al. Perspectives in the biological function, the technical and therapeutic application of bone morphogenetic proteins. *Appl Microbiol Biotechnol*. 2001;57(3):294-308.
36. Carragee EJ, Hurwitz EL, Weiner BK. A critical review of recombinant human bone morphogenetic protein-2 trials in spinal surgery: emerging safety concerns and lessons learned. *Spine J*. 2011;11(6):471-491.
37. Mohler DG, et al. Skeletal failure in osteoporosis. *Diagnosis and Management of Pathologic Fractures*. 1993;13-36.
38. Boden SD, Kaplan FS. Calcium homeostasis. *Orthop Clin North Am*. 1990;21(1):31-42.
39. Minaire P, et al. Quantitative histological data on disuse osteoporosis. *Calcif Tissue Res*. 1974;17(1):57-73.
40. Lane JM, Riley EH, Wirganowicz PZ, et al. Osteoporosis: diagnosis and treatment. *J Bone Joint Surg Am*. 1996;78(4):618-632.
41. Johnston CC Jr, Slemenda CW. Peak bone mass, bone loss and risk of fracture. *Osteoporos Int*. 1994;4(1):S43-S45.
42. Marcus R. Endocrine control of bone and mineral metabolism. In Manolagas SC, Olefsky JM, eds. *Metabolic Bone and Mineral Disorders*. New York: Churchill Livingstone; 1988:13.
43. Bonewald LF. The amazing osteocyte. *J Bone Miner Res*. 2011;26(2):229-238.
44. Bergwitz C, Jüppner H. Regulation of phosphate homeostasis by PTH, vitamin D, and FGF23. *Annu Rev Med*. 2010;61:91-104.
45. Klahr S, Hruska K. Effects of parathyroid hormone on the renal reabsorption of phosphorus and divalent cations. *Bone Mineral Res Annu*. 1983;2(65):125.
46. Wong GL. Skeletal effects of parathyroid hormone. *Bone Mineral Res*. 1986;4:103-129.
47. Norman AW, Roth JR, Orci L. The vitamin D endocrine system: steroid metabolism, hormone receptors, and biological response (calcium binding proteins). *Endocr Rev*. 1982;3(4):331-366.
48. Potts JT, Kronenberg HM, Rosenblatt M. *Parathyroid Hormone: Chemistry, Biosynthesis, and Mode of Action*. Academic Press; 1982.
49. Lombardi G, et al. The roles of parathyroid hormone in bone remodeling: prospects for novel therapeutics. *J Endocrinol Invest*. 2011;34(7 suppl):18-22.
50. Bell NH. Vitamin D-endocrine system. *J Clin Invest*. 1985; 76(1):1.
51. Compston JE. Hepatic osteodystrophy: vitamin D metabolism in patients with liver disease. *Gut*. 1986;27(9):1073.
52. Wang Y, Zhu J, DeLuca HF. Where is the vitamin D receptor? *Arch Biochem Biophys*. 2012;523(1):123-133.
53. Holick MF. Vitamin D deficiency. *N Engl J Med*. 2007;357(3):266-281.
54. Shimada T, et al. FGF-23 is a potent regulator of vitamin D metabolism and phosphate homeostasis. *J Bone Miner Res*. 2004;19(3):429-435.
55. Jüppner H. Phosphate and FGF-23. *Kidney Int*. 2011;79: S24-S27.
56. Quarles LD. Skeletal secretion of FGF-23 regulates phosphate and vitamin D metabolism. *Nat Rev Endocrinol*. 2012;8(5):276-286.
57. Liu S, Quarles LD. How fibroblast growth factor 23 works. *J Am Soc Nephrol*. 2007;18(6):1637-1647.
58. Hurley DL, et al. Axial and appendicular bone mineral density in patients with long-term deficiency or excess of calcitonin. *N Engl J Med*. 1987;317(9):537-541.
59. Tiegs RD, et al. Calcitonin secretion in postmenopausal osteoporosis. *N Engl J Med*. 1985;312(17):1097-1100.
60. Austin LA, Heath H 3rd. Calcitonin: physiology and pathophysiology. *N Engl J Med*. 1981;304(5):269.
61. Wright NC, et al. The recent prevalence of osteoporosis and low bone mass in the United States based on bone mineral density at the femoral neck or lumbar spine. *J Bone Miner Res*. 2014;29(11):2520-2526.
62. Burge R, et al. Incidence and economic burden of osteoporosis-related fractures in the United States, 2005–2025. *J Bone Miner Res*. 2007;22(3):465-475.

63. Siris ES, et al. The clinical diagnosis of osteoporosis: a position statement from the National Bone Health Alliance Working Group. *Osteoporos Int.* 2014;25(5):1439-1443.
64. Jensen GF, et al. Epidemiology of postmenopausal spinal and long bone fractures. *Clin Orthop Relat Res.* 1982;166: 75-81.
65. Neuman MD, et al. Survival and functional outcomes after hip fracture among nursing home residents. *JAMA Intern Med.* 2014;174(8):1273-1280.
66. Riggs BL, Melton LJ. Evidence for two distinct syndromes of involutional osteoporosis. *Am J Med.* 1983;75(6):899-901.
67. Vochteloo AJH, et al. More than half of hip fracture patients do not regain mobility in the first postoperative year. *Geriatr Gerontol Int.* 2013;13(2):334-341.
68. Silverman SL. Quality-of-life issues in osteoporosis. *Curr Rheumatol Rep.* 2005;7(1):39-45.
69. Lau E. Mortality following the diagnosis of a vertebral compression fracture in the Medicare population. *J Bone Joint Surg Am.* 2008;90(7):1479.
70. Kanis JA, et al. The diagnosis of osteoporosis. *J Bone Miner Res.* 1994;9(8):1137-1141.
71. Fink HA, et al. Association of Parkinson's disease with accelerated bone loss, fractures and mortality in older men: the Osteoporotic Fractures in Men (MrOS) study. *Osteoporos Int.* 2008;19(9):1277-1282.
72. Lyles KW, Schenck AP, Colón-Emeric CS. Hip and other osteoporotic fractures increase the risk of subsequent fractures in nursing home residents. *Osteoporos Int.* 2008;19(8):1225-1233.
73. Walker-Bone K. Recognizing and treating secondary osteoporosis. *Nat Rev Rheumatol.* 2012;8(8): 480-492.
74. Lukert BP. Glucocorticoid-induced osteoporosis: pathogenesis and management. *Ann Intern Med.* 1990;112(5):352.
75. Ben-Shlomo A, et al. Early postmenopausal bone loss in hyperthyroidism. *Maturitas.* 2001;39(1):19-27.
76. Donnelly E, Lane JM, Boskey AL. Research perspectives: the 2013 AAOS/ORS research symposium on Bone Quality and Fracture Prevention. *J Orthop Res.* 2014;32(7):855-864.
77. National Institutes of Health, National Resource Center. *Information for patients about Paget's disease of bone.* Available at: https://www.niams.nih.gov/Health_info/Bone/Pagets/patient_info.asp.
78. Riggs BL, Melton LJ I. Involutional osteoporosis. *N Engl J Med.* 1986;314(26):1676-1686.
79. Richelson LS, et al. Relative contributions of aging and estrogen deficiency to postmenopausal bone loss. *N Engl J Med.* 1984;311(20):1273-1275.
80. Klibanski A, et al. Decreased bone density in hyperprolactinemic women. *Obstet Gynecol Surv.* 6(5):3.
81. Eghbali-Fatourechi G, et al. Role of RANK ligand in mediating increased bone resorption in early postmenopausal women. *J Clin Invest.* 2003;111(8):1221.
82. Hofbauer LC, et al. Estrogen stimulates gene expression and protein production of osteoprotegerin in human osteoblastic cells. *Endocrinology.* 1999;140(9):4367-4370.
83. Manolagas SC. From estrogen-centric to aging and oxidative stress: a revised perspective of the pathogenesis of osteoporosis. *Endocr Rev.* 2010;31(3):266-300.
84. Lane JM, et al. Orthopedic management of osteoporosis: effects of nutrition and exercise on the skeleton. In: Uhthoff HK, Stahl E, eds. *Current Concepts of Bone Fragility.* Berlin: Springer; 1986:429-447.
85. Lane JM, Nydick M. Osteoporosis: current modes of prevention and treatment. *J Am Acad Orthop Surg.* 1999;7(1):19-31.
86. Riggs BL, et al. Effect of fluoride treatment on the fracture rate in postmenopausal women with osteoporosis. *N Engl J Med.* 1990;322(12):802-809.
87. Mellish RWE, et al. A new manual method for assessing two-dimensional cancellous bone structure: comparison between iliac crest and lumbar vertebra. *J Bone Miner Res.* 1991;6(7):689-696.
88. Compston JE. Connectivity of cancellous bone: assessment and mechanical implications. *Bone.* 1994;15(5):463-466.
89. Matković V, et al. Bone status and fracture rates in two regions of Yugoslavia. *Am J Clin Nutr.* 1979;32(3):540-549.
90. Lips P, Courpron P, Meunier PJ. Mean wall thickness of trabecular bone packets in the human iliac crest: changes with age. *Calcif Tissue Res.* 1978;26(1):13-17.
91. Meema S, Bunker ML, Meema HE. Preventive effect of estrogen on postmenopausal bone loss: a follow-up study. *Arch Intern Med.* 1975;135(11):1436-1440.
92. Eriksen EF, et al. Evidence of estrogen receptors in normal human osteoblast-like cells. *Science.* 1988;241(4861): 84-86.
93. Lane JM, et al. Orthopedic management of osteoporosis: effects of nutrition and exercise on the skeleton. In: Uhthoff HK, Stahl E, eds. *Current Concepts of Bone Fragility.* Berlin: Springer; 1986:429-447.
94. Tsai K-S, et al. Impaired vitamin D metabolism with aging in women. Possible role in pathogenesis of senile osteoporosis. *J Clin Invest.* 1984;73(6):1668.
95. Kanis JA, Adami S. Bone loss in the elderly. *Osteoporos Int.* 1994;4(1):S59-S65.
96. Cooper C, et al. Population-based study of survival after osteoporotic fractures. *Am J Epidemiol.* 1993;137(9):1001-1005.
97. Czerwiński E, et al. Current understanding of osteoporosis according to the position of the World Health Organization (WHO) and International Osteoporosis Foundation. *Ortop Traumatol Rehabil.* 2006;9(4):337-356.
98. Stein E, Shane E. Secondary osteoporosis. *Endocrinol Metab Clin North Am.* 2003;32(1):115-134.
99. Mazess RB, et al. Bone density of the radius, spine, and proximal femur in osteoporosis. *J Bone Miner Res.* 1988;3(1):13-18.
100. Schousboe JT, et al. Executive Summary of the 2013 International Society for Clinical Densitometry Position Development Conference on Bone Densitometry. *J Clin Densitom.* 2013;16(4):455-466.
101. Marshall D, Johnell O, Wedel H. Meta-analysis of how well measures of bone mineral density predict occurrence of osteoporotic fractures. *BMJ.* 1996;312(7041):1254-1259.
102. Masud T, et al. Effect of spinal osteophytosis on bone mineral density measurements in vertebral osteoporosis. *BMJ.* 1993;307(6897):172-173.
103. Screening for osteoporosis: U.S. Preventive Services Task Force Recommendation Statement. *Ann Intern Med.* 2011;154(5):356.
104. National Osteoporosis Foundation. *Clinician's Guide to Prevention and Treatment of Osteoporosis.* Washington, DC: National Osteoporosis Foundation; 2008.
105. Harvey NC, et al. Trabecular bone score (TBS) as a new complementary approach for osteoporosis evaluation in clinical practice. *Bone.* 2015;78:216-224.

106. Kaufman JD, Cummings SR. Osteoporosis and prevention of fractures: practical approaches for orthopaedic surgeons. *Instr Course Lect*. 2002;51:559.
107. Kanis JA, et al. FRAX™ and the assessment of fracture probability in men and women from the UK. *Osteoporos Int*. 2008;19(4):385-397.
108. Bischoff-Ferrari HA, et al. Estimation of optimal serum concentrations of 25-hydroxyvitamin D for multiple health outcomes. *Am J Clin Nutr*. 2006;84(1):18-28.
109. Powe CE, et al. Vitamin D–binding protein and vitamin D status of black Americans and white Americans. *N Engl J Med*. 2013;369(21):1991-2000.
110. Camacho P, Kleerekoper M, Favus MJ. *Biochemical Markers of Bone Turnover. Primer on the Metabolic Bone Diseases and Disorders of Mineral Metabolism*. 6th ed. Washington, DC: American Society for Bone and Mineral Research; 2006:127-133.
111. Calvo MS, Eyre DR, Gundberg CM. Molecular basis and clinical application of biological markers of bone turnover. *Endocr Rev*. 1996;17(4):333-368.
112. Chesnut CH, et al. Hormone replacement therapy in postmenopausal women: urinary N-telopeptide of type I collagen monitors therapeutic effect and predicts response of bone mineral density. *Am J Med*. 1997;102(1):29-37.
113. Prestwood KM, et al. The short-term effects of conjugated estrogen on bone turnover in older women. *J Clin Endocrinol Metab*. 1994;79(2):366-371.
114. Garnero P, et al. Comparison of new biochemical markers of bone turnover in late postmenopausal osteoporotic women in response to alendronate treatment. *J Clin Endocrinol Metab*. 1994;79(6):1693-1700.
115. Reid DM. Pathophysiology. In: Reid DM, ed. *Handbook of Osteoporosis*. London: Springer; 2011:13-19.
116. Hopper JL, Seeman E. The bone density of female twins discordant for tobacco use. *N Engl J Med*. 1994;330(6):387-392.
117. Byrjalsen I, Haarbo J, Christiansen C. Role of cigarette smoking on the postmenopausal endometrium during sequential estrogen and progestogen therapy. *Obstet Gynecol*. 1993;81(6):1016-1021.
118. Larsen ER, Mosekilde L, Foldspang A. Vitamin D. and calcium supplementation prevents osteoporotic fractures in elderly community dwelling residents: a pragmatic population-based 3-year intervention study. *J Bone Miner Res*. 2003;19(3):370-378.
119. Cosman F, et al. Clinician's guide to prevention and treatment of osteoporosis. *Osteoporos Int*. 2014;25(10):2359-2381.
120. Institute of Medicine Committee to Review Dietary Reference Intakes for Vitamin D and Calcium; Ross AC, Taylor CL, Yaktine AL, et al, editors. *Dietary Reference Intakes for Calcium and Vitamin D*. Washington, DC: National Academies Press; 2011. Available at: https://www.ncbi.nlm.nih.gov/books/NBK56070/.
121. Institute of Medicine Standing Committee on the Scientific Evaluation of Dietary Reference Intakes. *Dietary Reference Intakes for Calcium, Phosphorus, Magnesium, Vitamin D, and Fluoride*. Washington, DC: National Academies Press; 1997. Available at: https://www.ncbi.nlm.nih.gov/books/NBK109825/.
122. Del Valle HB, et al. *Dietary Reference Intakes for Calcium and Vitamin D*. Washington, DC: National Academies Press; 2011.
123. Levine JP. Pharmacologic and nonpharmacologic management of osteoporosis. *Clin Cornerstone*. 2006;8(1):40-53.
124. Lin JT, Lane JM. Osteoporosis: a review. *Clin Orthop Relat Res*. 2004;425:126-134.
125. Gehrig L, Lane J, O'Connor MI. Osteoporosis: management and treatment strategies for orthopaedic surgeons. *J Bone Joint Surg Am*. 2008;90(6):1362-1374.
126. Rizzoli R, et al. Vitamin D supplementation in elderly or postmenopausal women: a 2013 update of the 2008 recommendations from the European Society for Clinical and Economic Aspects of Osteoporosis and Osteoarthritis (ESCEO). *Curr Med Res Opin*. 2013;29(4):305-313.
127. Vieth R. Why the optimal requirement for vitamin D_3 is probably much higher than what is officially recommended for adults. *J Steroid Biochem Mol Biol*. 2004;89:575-579.
128. Schurch M-A. Protein supplements increase serum insulin-like growth factor-I levels and attenuate proximal femur bone loss in patients with recent hip fracture. *Ann Intern Med*. 1998;128(10):801.
129. Massey LK. Dietary salt, urinary calcium, and kidney stone risk. *Nutr Rev*. 1995;53(5):131-134.
130. Nelson ME. Effects of high-intensity strength training on multiple risk factors for osteoporotic fractures. *JAMA*. 1994;272(24):1909.
131. Ernst E. Exercise for female osteoporosis. *Sports Med*. 1998;25(6):359-368.
132. Kerr D, et al. Resistance training over 2 years increases bone mass in calcium-replete postmenopausal women. *J Bone Miner Res*. 2001;16(1):175-181.
133. Dalsky GP, et al. Weight-bearing exercise training and lumbar bone mineral content in postmenopausal women. *Ann Intern Med*. 1988;108(6):824-828.
134. Kohrt WM, et al. Additive effects of weight-bearing exercise and estrogen on bone mineral density in older women. *J Bone Miner Res*. 1995;10(9):1303-1311.
135. Layne JE, Nelson ME. The effects of progressive resistance training on bone density: a review. *Med Sci Sports Exerc*. 1999;31(1):25-30.
136. Friedlander AL, et al. A two-year program of aerobics and weight training enhances bone mineral density of young women. *J Bone Miner Res*. 1995;10(4):574-585.
137. Cummings SR, et al. Risk factors for hip fracture in white women. *N Engl J Med*. 1995;332(12):767-774.
138. Minaire P. Immobilization osteoporosis: a review. *Clin Rheumatol*. 1989;8(2):95-103.
139. Whalen RT, Carter DR, Steel CR. The relationship between physiological activity and bone density. *Trans Orthop Res Soc*. 1987;12:464-470.
140. Wolf SL, et al. Reducing frailty and falls in older persons: an investigation of Tai Chi and computerized balance training. *J Am Geriatr Soc*. 1996;44(5):489-497.
141. Campbell AJ, et al. Randomised controlled trial of a general practice programme of home based exercise to prevent falls in elderly women. *BMJ*. 1997;315(7115):1065-1069.
142. Lord SR, Ward JA, Williams P. Exercise effect on dynamic stability in older women: a randomized controlled trial. *Arch Phys Med Rehabil*. 1996;77(3):232-236.
143. Lord SR, et al. The effect of a 12-month exercise trial on balance, strength, and falls in older women: a randomized controlled trial. *J Am Geriatr Soc*. 1995;43(11):1198-1206.
144. Hain TC, et al. Effects of T'ai Chi on balance. *Arch Otolaryngol Head Neck Surg*. 1999;125(11):1191-1195.
145. Watts N, et al. American Association of Clinical Endocrinologists Medical Guidelines for Clinical Practice

for the Diagnosis and Treatment of Postmenopausal Osteoporosis. *Endocr Pract.* 2010;16(suppl 3):1-37.

146. Anderson GL, et al.; Women's Health Initiative Steering Committee. Effects of conjugated equine estrogen in postmenopausal women with hysterectomy: the Women's Health Initiative randomized controlled trial. *JAMA.* 2004;291(14):1701-1712.
147. Cauley JA, et al. Continued breast cancer risk reduction in postmenopausal women treated with raloxifene: 4-year results from the MORE trial. *Breast Cancer Res Treat.* 2001;65(2):125-134.
148. Siris ES, et al. Skeletal effects of raloxifene after 8 years: results from the continuing outcomes relevant to Evista (CORE) study. *J Bone Miner Res.* 2005;20(9):1514-1524.
149. Barrett-Connor E, et al. Effects of raloxifene on cardiovascular events and breast cancer in postmenopausal women. *N Engl J Med.* 2006;355(2):125-137.
150. Lindsay R, et al. Efficacy of tissue-selective estrogen complex of bazedoxifene/conjugated estrogens for osteoporosis prevention in at-risk postmenopausal women. *Fertil Steril.* 2009;92(3):1045-1052.
151. Weinstein RS, Roberson PK, Manolagas SC. Giant osteoclast formation and long-term oral bisphosphonate therapy. *N Engl J Med.* 2009;360(1):53-62.
152. Black DM, et al. Once-yearly zoledronic acid for treatment of postmenopausal osteoporosis. *N Engl J Med.* 2007;356(18):1809-1822.
153. Chesnut CH, et al. Effects of oral ibandronate administered daily or intermittently on fracture risk in postmenopausal osteoporosis. *J Bone Miner Res.* 2004;19(8):1241-1249.
154. Reginster JY, et al. Randomized trial of the effects of risedronate on vertebral fractures in women with established postmenopausal osteoporosis. *Osteoporos Int.* 2000;11(1):83-91.
155. Lyles KW, et al. Zoledronic acid and clinical fractures and mortality after hip fracture. *N Engl J Med.* 2007;357(18):1799-1809.
156. US Food and Drug Administration. *FDA Drug Safety Communication: New Contraindication and Updated Warning on Kidney Impairment for Reclast (Zoledronic Acid).* 2011. Available at: https://www.fda.gov/Drugs/DrugSafety/ucm270199.htm.
157. Khosla S, et al. Bisphosphonate-associated osteonecrosis of the jaw: report of a task force of the American Society for Bone and Mineral Research. *J Bone Miner Res.* 2007;22(10):1479-1491.
158. Park-Wyllie LY. Bisphosphonate use and the risk of subtrochanteric or femoral shaft fractures in older women. *JAMA.* 2011;305(8):783.
159. Chesnut CH, et al. A randomized trial of nasal spray salmon calcitonin in postmenopausal women with established osteoporosis: the prevent recurrence of osteoporotic fractures study. *Am J Med.* 2000;109(4):267-276.
160. Muñoz-Torres M, Alonso G, Raya PM. Calcitonin therapy in osteoporosis. *Treat Endocrinol.* 2004;3(2):117-132.
161. Gennari C. Analgesic effect of calcitonin in osteoporosis. *Bone.* 2002;30(5):67-70.
162. Quattrocchi E, Kourlas H. Teriparatide: a review. *Clin Ther.* 2004;26(6):841-854.
163. Neer RM, et al. Effect of parathyroid hormone (1-34) on fractures and bone mineral density in postmenopausal women with osteoporosis. *N Engl J Med.* 2001;344(19):1434-1441.
164. Dempster DW, et al. Effects of daily treatment with parathyroid hormone on bone microarchitecture and turnover in patients with osteoporosis: a paired biopsy study. *J Bone Miner Res.* 2001;16(10):1846-1853.
165. Saleh A, et al. Management strategy for symptomatic bisphosphonate-associated incomplete atypical femoral fractures. *HSS J.* 2012;8(2):103-110.
166. Lau AN, Adachi JD. Resolution of osteonecrosis of the jaw after teriparatide [recombinant human PTH-(1-34)] therapy. *J Rheumatol.* 2009;36(8):1835-1837.
167. Vahle JL, et al. Bone neoplasms in F344 rats given teriparatide [rhPTH (1-34)] are dependent on duration of treatment and dose. *Toxicol Pathol.* 2004;32(4):426-438.
168. Cummings SR, et al. Denosumab for prevention of fractures in postmenopausal women with osteoporosis. *N Engl J Med.* 2009;361(8):756-765.
169. Xue Q-Y, et al. Alendronate treatment does not inhibit bone formation within biphasic calcium phosphate ceramics in posterolateral spinal fusion: an experimental study in porcine model. *Chin Med J.* 2009;122(22):2770-2774.
170. Bae H, et al. Alendronate influences bone volume in rabbit posterolateral spine fusion. *Spine J.* 2002;2(5):98-99.
171. Lehman RA, et al. The effect of alendronate sodium on spinal fusion: a rabbit model. *Spine J.* 2004;4(1):36-43.
172. Xue Q, et al. Alendronate treatment improves bone–pedicle screw interface fixation in posterior lateral spine fusion: an experimental study in a porcine model. *Int Orthop.* 2010;34(3):447-451.
173. Nakao SI, et al. The influence of alendronate on spine fusion in an osteoporotic animal model. *Spine.* 2011;36(18):1446-1452.
174. Nagahama K, et al. Does alendronate disturb the healing process of posterior lumbar interbody fusion? A prospective randomized trial. *J Neurosurg Spine.* 2011;14(4):500-507.
175. O'Loughlin PF, et al. Parathyroid hormone (1-34) augments spinal fusion, fusion mass volume, and fusion mass quality in a rabbit spinal fusion model. *Spine.* 2009;34(2):121-130.
176. Abe Y, et al. Enhancement of graft bone healing by intermittent administration of human parathyroid hormone (1–34) in a rat spinal arthrodesis model. *Bone.* 2007;41(5):775-785.
177. Ohtori S, Inoue G, Orita S, et al. Comparison of teriparatide and bisphosphonate treatment to reduce pedicle screw loosening after lumbar spinal fusion surgery in postmenopausal women with osteoporosis from a bone quality perspective. *Spine.* 2013;38(8):487-492.
178. Kalb S, et al. Pharmacophysiology of bone and spinal fusion. *Spine J.* 2013;13(10):1359-1369.
179. Bauman WA, Cardozo CP. Osteoporosis in individuals with spinal cord injury. *PM R.* 2015;7(2):188-201.
180. Deleted in review.
181. Recker RR. A randomized, double-blind phase 2 clinical trial of blosozumab, a sclerostin antibody, in postmenopausal women with low bone mineral density. *J Bone Miner Res.* 2015;30:216-224.
182. Reginster J-Y, et al. Strontium ranelate reduces the risk of nonvertebral fractures in postmenopausal women with osteoporosis: Treatment of Peripheral Osteoporosis (TROPOS) study. *J Clin Endocrinol Metab.* 2005;90(5):2816-2822.
183. Burlet N, Reginster J-Y. Strontium ranelate: the first dual acting treatment for postmenopausal osteoporosis. *Clin Orthop Relat Res.* 2006;443:55-60.

184. Morley P. Delivery of parathyroid hormone for the treatment of osteoporosis. *Expert Opin Drug Deliv*. 2005;2(6):993-1002.
185. Kostenuik PJ, et al. Infrequent delivery of a long-acting PTH-Fc fusion protein has potent anabolic effects on cortical and cancellous bone. *J Bone Miner Res*. 2007;22(10):1534-1547.
186. Poor G, et al. Epidemiology of Paget's disease in Europe: the prevalence is decreasing. *J Bone Miner Res*. 2006;21(10):1545-1549.
187. Cooper C, et al. The epidemiology of Paget's disease in Britain: is the prevalence decreasing? *J Bone Miner Res*. 1999;14(2):192-197.
188. Altman RD, Collins B. Musculoskeletal manifestations of Paget's disease of bone. *Arthritis Rheum*. 1980;23(10):1121-1127.
189. Siris ES. Paget's disease of bone. *J Bone Miner Res*. 1998;13(7): 1061-1065.
190. Barker DJP. The epidemiology of Paget's disease of bone. *Br Med Bull*. 1984;40(4):396-400.
191. Meunier PJ, et al. Bone histomorphometry in Paget's disease quantitative and dynamic analysis of pagetic and nonpagetic bone tissue. *Arthritis Rheum*. 1980;23(10):1095-1103.
192. Rasmussen H, Bordier P. The cellular basis of metabolic bone disease. *N Engl J Med*. 1973;289(1):25-32.
193. Barry HC. *Paget's Disease of Bone*. Philadelphia: Churchill Livingstone; 1969.
194. Siris ES. Epidemiological aspects of Paget's disease: family history and relationship to other medical conditions. *Semin Arthritis Rheum*. 1994;23(4):272.
195. Cody JD, et al. Genetic linkage of Paget disease of the bone to chromosome 18q. *Am J Hum Genet*. 1997;61(5):1117-1122.
196. Haslam SI, et al. Paget's disease of bone: evidence for a susceptibility locus on chromosome 18q and for genetic heterogeneity. *J Bone Miner Res*. 1998;13(6):911-917.
197. Lucas GJA, Daroszewska A, Ralston SH. Contribution of genetic factors to the pathogenesis of Paget's disease of bone and related disorders. *J Bone Miner Res*. 2006;21(S2):P31-P37.
198. Layfield R, et al. p62 mutations, ubiquitin recognition and Paget's disease of bone. *Biochem Soc Trans*. 2006;34(Pt 5):735-737.
199. Wat WZM. Current perspectives on bisphosphonate treatment in Paget's disease of bone. *Ther Clin Risk Manag*. 2014;10:977.
200. Gordon MT, Anderson DC, Sharpe PT. Canine distemper virus localised in bone cells of patients with Paget's disease. *Bone*. 1991;12(3):195-201.
201. Mills BG, Singer FR. Critical evaluation of viral antigen data in Paget's disease of bone. *Clin Orthop Relat Res*. 1987;217:16-25.
202. Rebel A, Malkani K, Basle M. [Nuclear anomalies in osteoclasts in Paget's bone disease]. *Nouv Presse Med*. 1974;3(20): 1299-1301.
203. Reddy SV, et al. Detection of measles virus nucleocapsid transcripts in circulating blood cells from patients with Paget disease. *J Bone Miner Res*. 1996;11(11):1602-1607.
204. Ralston SH, et al. Multicenter blinded analysis of RT-PCR detection methods for paramyxoviruses in relation to Paget's disease of bone. *J Bone Miner Res*. 2007;22(4):569-577.
205. Matthews BG, et al. Failure to detect measles virus ribonucleic acid in bone cells from patients with Paget's disease. *J Clin Endocrinol Metab*. 2008;93(4):1398-1401.
206. Rota JS, et al. Molecular epidemiology of measles virus: identification of pathways of transmission and implications for measles elimination. *J Infect Dis*. 1996;173(1):32-37.
207. Schneider D, Hofmann MT, Peterson JA. Diagnosis and treatment of Paget's disease of bone. *Am Fam Physician*. 2002;65(10):2069-2072.
208. Tan A, Ralston SH. Paget's disease of bone. *QJM*. 2014;hcu075.
209. Altman RD, Brown M, Gargano F. Low back pain in Paget's disease of bone. *Clin Orthop Relat Res*. 1987;217: 152-161.
210. Ralston SH, Langston AL, Reid IR. Pathogenesis and management of Paget's disease of bone. *Lancet*. 2008;372(9633):155-163.
211. Dinneen SF, Buckley TF. Spinal nerve root compression due to monostotic Paget's disease of a lumbar vertebra: a case report. *Spine*. 1987;12(9):948-949.
212. Rosen HN, et al. Serum CTX: a new marker of bone resorption that shows treatment effect more often than other markers because of low coefficient of variability and large changes with bisphosphonate therapy. *Calcif Tissue Int*. 2000;66(2):100-103.
213. Hadjipavlou A, et al. Pagetic spinal stenosis with extradural pagetoid ossification: a case report. *Spine*. 1988;13(1): 128-130.
214. Barry HC. Orthopedic aspects of Paget's disease of bone. *Arthritis Rheum*. 1980;23(10):1128-1130.
215. Reddy SV, et al. Paget's disease of bone: a disease of the osteoclast. *Rev Endocrinol Metab Disord*. 2001;2(2):195-201.
216. Cabot RC, et al. Case 1-1986: A 67-year-old man with Paget's disease and progressive leg weakness. *N Engl J Med*. 1986;314(2):105-113.
217. Lyles KW, et al. A clinical approach to diagnosis and management of Paget's disease of bone. *J Bone Miner Res*. 2001;16(8):1379-1387.
218. Reid IR, et al. Intravenous zoledronic acid in postmenopausal women with low bone mineral density. *N Engl J Med*. 2002;346(9):653-661.
219. Hughes DE, et al. Bisphosphonates promote apoptosis in murine osteoclasts in vitro and in vivo. *J Bone Miner Res*. 1995;10(10):1478-1487.
220. Reid IR, et al. Comparison of a single infusion of zoledronic acid with risedronate for Paget's disease. *N Engl J Med*. 2005;353(9):898-908.
221. Altman RD, et al. Influence of disodium etidronate on clinical and laboratory manifestations of Paget's disease of bone (osteitis deformans). *N Engl J Med*. 1973;289(26): 1379-1384.
222. Fraser WD, et al. A double-blind, multicentre, placebo-controlled study of tiludronate in Paget's disease of bone. *Postgrad Med J*. 1997;73(862):496-502.
223. Reid IR, et al. Biochemical and radiologic improvement in Paget's disease of bone treated with alendronate: a randomized, placebo-controlled trial. *Am J Med*. 1996;101(4):341-348.
224. Langston AL, et al. Randomized trial of intensive bisphosphonate treatment versus symptomatic management in Paget's disease of bone. *J Bone Miner Res*. 2010;25(1):20-31.
225. Miller PD, et al. A randomized, double-blind comparison of risedronate and etidronate in the treatment of Paget's disease of bone. *Am J Med*. 1999;106(5):513-520.
226. Kallio DM, Garant PR, Minkin C. Ultrastructural effects of calcitonin on osteoclasts in tissue culture. *J Ultrastruct Res*. 1972;39(3):205-216.
227. Reginster JY, Lecart MP. Efficacy and safety of drugs for Paget's disease of bone. *Bone*. 1995;17(5):S485-S488.

CHAPTER 89 Osteoporosis: Surgical Strategies

Frank M. Phillips
Mark F. Kurd
Gregory D. Schroeder
Tyler Kreitz

Osteoporosis is a metabolic bone disease characterized by low bone mass, microarchitectural deterioration, and skeletal fragility resulting in an increased risk of fracture. Osteoporosis and low bone mass affects more than 50 million adults in the United States; with a prevalence of 10.3%, it is the most common metabolic bone disease in those over 50 years of age.[1,2] Among the elderly, especially postmenopausal women, osteoporosis is a major cause of pathologic fractures predominantly of the hip, spine, and wrist. In 2005, osteoporosis accounted for approximately 2 million fractures and approximately 27% occurred in the spine. This number is expected to continue to grow to over 3 million total fractures annually by 2025.[2] Fragility fractures are most common in postmenopausal women with approximately half of all postmenopausal women experiencing an osteoporosis-related fracture. While these fractures are common, up to two-thirds of osteoporotic vertebral fractures are undiagnosed, despite the fact that these injuries have been clearly shown to lead to a decrease in the patient's quality of life[3] and a mortality rate twice that of age-matched controls. The survival rates following a fracture diagnosis were 53.9%, 30.9%, and 10.5% at 3, 5, and 7 years, respectively.[4]

The World Health Organization defines osteoporosis as having bone mineral density (BMD) more than 2.5 standard deviations below that of the average peak bone mass as measured by dual-energy x-ray absorptiometry.[5] Type I osteoporosis results from loss of estrogen and occurs abruptly in women at the time of menopause. Immediately after menopause, women may lose up to 2% to 3% of their trabecular bone mass per year for approximately 5 years, resulting in an increased risk of vertebral and distal radius fractures. Type II, or senile osteoporosis, is an age-related process occurring in both men and women. It affects predominantly cortical bone, resulting in a 0.3% to 0.5% rate of annual bone loss, and increased risk of hip and spine fracture.

With an aging population that desires to remain active, a spine surgeon must be knowledgeable of the strategies for treating the sequelae of osteoporosis of the spine. This includes managing painful osteoporotic fractures and the late sequelae, such as kyphotic deformities. Additionally, spine surgeons must understand the effect of low BMD on spine reconstructive procedures. Recognizing osteoporosis prior to surgical intervention is critical so that osteoporotic patients undergoing spine surgery can be appropriately treated and optimized from a medical perspective.

Osteoporotic Vertebral Compression Fractures

Osteoporotic vertebral compression fractures (VCFs) are a major cause of morbidity in the elderly. These injuries may lead to chronic pain from a nonunion, a significant deformity that results in sagittal imbalance and even depression. Fractures are often painful in the acute setting, but they also may result in chronic pain from a pseudarthrosis or altered kinematics with progressive deformity leading to sagittal imbalance. A kyphotic deformity from a thoracolumbar compression fracture shifts the center of gravity anteriorly, resulting in an increased bending moment about the apex. This deformity creates an environment favorable to additional fractures, which can lead to a progressive deformity.[6] The risk of a new vertebral fracture within 1 year of a VCF is 5 to 25 times above baseline risk.[4,7] Therefore, treatment strategies for osteoporotic vertebral fractures should not only focus on pain management but also on overall bone health to prevent subsequent fractures. Additionally, if a significant deformity is present, correcting sagittal alignment can lead to improved health-related quality-of-life (HRQOL) metrics.

Nonsurgical Treatment

Conventional management of osteoporotic VCFs includes pain management, activity modification, physical therapy, and bracing.[8] Acute pain management using antiinflammatory medications and narcotics should be limited to the short term, as these medications increase risk of confusion, falls, and gastrointestinal complications in the elderly. Physical therapy and an exercise regimen focused on axial muscle strengthening may improve deformity and prevent further injury.[9] Early mobilization is preferred to bed rest as immobilization results in disuse osteopenia, muscle atrophy, and

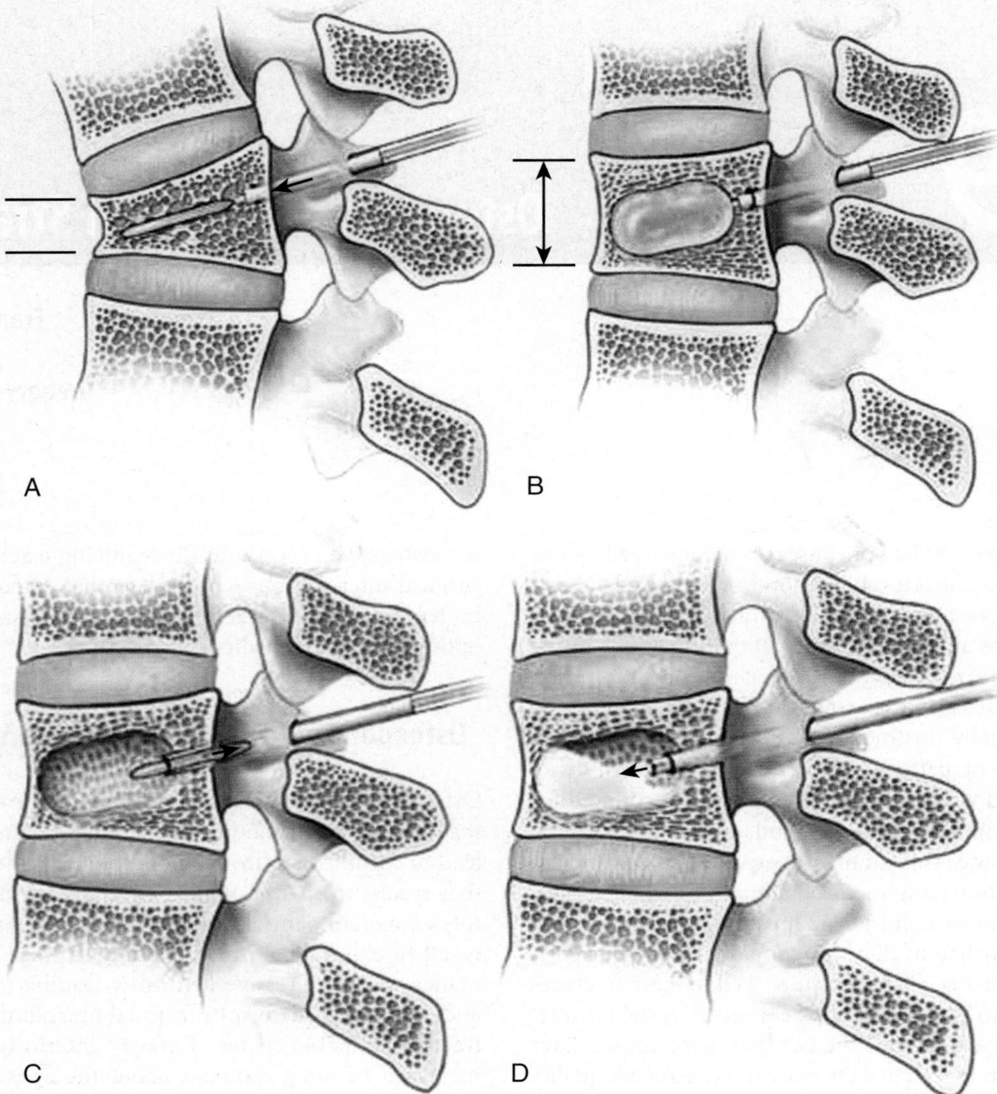

FIG. 89.1 (A) During kyphoplasty, the fractured vertebral body is percutaneously cannulated with an inflatable bone tamp. (B) The tamp is inflated, which elevates the vertebral body endplates and restores vertebral body height. (C) The tamp is withdrawn, leaving a cavity to be filled with bone void filler. (D) Bone void filler is placed into the vertebral body under low pressure.

deconditioning. Bracing may improve pain and posture but is expensive, often not tolerated in the elderly due to poor fit and compliance, and may result in further restriction in severely debilitated patients.[8] Appropriate nonoperative management involves pain control, prevention of secondary complications, maintenance of endurance, and optimized medical management of osteoporosis, as discussed in Chapter 88.

Cement Augmentation: Vertebroplasty and Kyphoplasty

Orthopaedic fracture care emphasizes restoring anatomy, correcting deformity, and preserving function. Cement augmentations in the form of vertebroplasty and kyphoplasty have been used as minimally invasive procedures to address pain and deformity in osteoporotic spine fractures. Both involve percutaneous fluoroscopic or computed tomography (CT)-guided injection of polymethylmethacrylate (PMMA) into a fractured vertebral body. Vertebroplasty involves percutaneous cement injection into a fractured vertebral body without any attempt at reduction. Kyphoplasty involves the percutaneous insertion of an inflatable bone tamp into a fractured vertebral body. Inflation of the tamp elevates the endplate and restores the vertebral body height while creating a cavity to be filled with PMMA (Fig. 89.1). Indications for cement augmentation in VCFs include painful osteoporotic VCFs refractory to nonsurgical management, patients requiring hospitalization for pain or medical complications secondary to VCFs,[10] and VCFs with progressive kyphotic deformity.[11] Suggested mechanisms for pain improvement with cement augmentation include fracture immobilization, cortical support by cement, and thermal deafferentation of the vertebra by

PMMA polymerization.[12] In 2009, the American Academy of Orthopaedic Surgeons recommended strongly against the use of vertebroplasty in osteoporotic VCFs and gave kyphoplasty a weak recommendation for use in pain relief in osteoporotic VCFs.[13] Their recommendations were based primarily on two randomized control trials (RCTs) comparing vertebroplasty and kyphoplasty to sham procedures.[14,15] Buchbinder et al. performed a multicenter double-blinded RCT evaluating overall pain in patients undergoing vertebroplasty versus a sham procedure. They found no difference in pain improvement between vertebroplasty and the sham procedure group at all intervals during the 6-month follow-up.[14] Kallmes et al.[15] performed a multicenter RCT assigning patients with osteoporotic compression fractures to either a vertebroplasty or a simulated procedure. They found improvements in pain and pain-related outcomes in patients treated with vertebroplasty that were similar to improvements in the simulated procedure group. These studies, however, had significant methodological flaws, including inconsistent inclusion criteria, inability to determine that radiographically identified fractures were the source of the patient's pain, validity of sham procedure in control groups, and inability to complete enrollment targets at busy centers, suggesting that those patients in most pain with acute fractures may have been unwilling to undergo randomization.[16]

Since that time, there have been numerous RCTs and meta-analyses published regarding the efficacy of cement augmentation for VCFs.[17–29] Wardlaw et al.[17] performed a large multicenter RCT comparing outcomes of kyphoplasty versus nonsurgical care in patients with one to three acute VCFs. They demonstrated significant improvement in the Short-Form 36 questionnaire physical component summary at 1 month in the kyphoplasty group, 7.2 points, compared to the nonsurgical care group, 2 points ($P < .0001$), with no difference in frequency of adverse events. This suggested that kyphoplasty is an effective and safe procedure in the management of acute VCFs. Anderson et al.[26] performed a meta-analysis of six RCTs evaluating pain, function, and HRQOL outcomes of vertebroplasty compared to conservative management in VCFs in both short-term (<12 weeks) and long-term (6–12 months) follow-up. They demonstrated superior pain relief, functional recovery, and greater HRQOL in vertebroplasty compared to conservative management or sham procedure at both early and late time points.[26] More recently, Li et al.[27] performed a meta-analysis of 8 RCTs comparing vertebroplasty to conservative management or sham procedure with regard to pain relief, function, and quality of life. The results of their analysis demonstrated improved pain relief, especially with fracture age less than 3 months, greater spine function, and quality of life at early, middle, and late time points in those treated with cement augmentation compared to control. Conversely, Buchbinder et al.[28] published a Cochrane Review evaluating outcomes and complications of vertebroplasty compared to sham procedure (two trials), conservative or usual care (six trials), and vertebroplasty versus kyphoplasty (three trials). The results of their review demonstrated no difference in pain, disability, or quality of life at any time point between those treated with vertebroplasty compared to sham procedure. Compared to nonoperative care, vertebroplasty resulted in improved pain outcomes at all time points.

Given the conflicting results in the literature, it is likely that there is a select group of patients who will benefit from cement augmentation for acute painful VCFs; however, the ideal indications are still unclear.

Vertebroplasty Versus Kyphoplasty

Although similar to vertebroplasty, kyphoplasty allows for improvement in vertebral body height and kyphotic deformity in addition to cement augmentation. Han et al.[30] performed a meta-analysis of RCTs and nonrandomized trials comparing vertebroplasty to kyphoplasty. Their results demonstrated greater improvement in pain with vertebroplasty in the first 7 days, greater improvement with kyphoplasty at 3 months, and no difference in long-term pain relief or functional outcomes between the two techniques.[30] Papanastassiou et al.[31] performed a systematic review of nonrandomized trials and RCTs comparing efficacy and safety of vertebroplasty, kyphoplasty, and nonsurgical management (NSM). Superior pain reduction was seen in vertebroplasty (−4.55/10; $P < .01$) and kyphoplasty (−5.07/10 points; $P < .01$) compared to NSM (−2.17/10). Subsequent fracture rate was greater in the NSM group (22%) compared to both vertebroplasty and kyphoplasty (11%). Comparison of cement augmentation techniques demonstrated greater kyphosis correction (4.8 vs. 1.7 degrees; $P < .01$; Fig. 89.2) and quality-of-life improvement ($P = .04$) with a lower rate of cement extravasation ($P = .01$) in kyphoplasty compared to vertebroplasty. This review suggests superior outcomes with cement augmentation techniques and a preference for kyphoplasty in reduction of kyphotic deformity and disability. Omidi-Kashani et al.[11] showed improvement in baseline visual analog scale and the Short-Form 36 questionnaire with both vertebroplasty and kyphoplasty but demonstrated no difference between the two in single-level osteoporotic VCFs. There was a 3.1-degree improvement in focal kyphosis associated with kyphoplasty, although the clinical significance of this improvement is unknown. More recently, Gu et al.[32] performed a systematic review and meta-analysis of RCTs and nonrandomized studies comparing vertebroplasty to kyphoplasty. They demonstrated no difference between the two methods of cement augmentation with regard to pain and disability outcomes in the short and long term. Significant heterogeneity exists in the literature comparing outcomes of kyphoplasty to vertebroplasty in the treatment of VCFs, though kyphoplasty may be preferable in the setting of significant kyphotic collapse.

Indications and Contraindications

Cement augmentation has historically been used for many vertebral disorders, including the treatment of acute painful VCF, pain due to vertebral metastasis and myeloma, vertebral hemangiomas, and Kummell disease, which is avascular necrosis of the vertebrae after VCF. Recent clinical evidence supports its use in the management of acute pain associated with VCFs that have failed to improve with nonsurgical

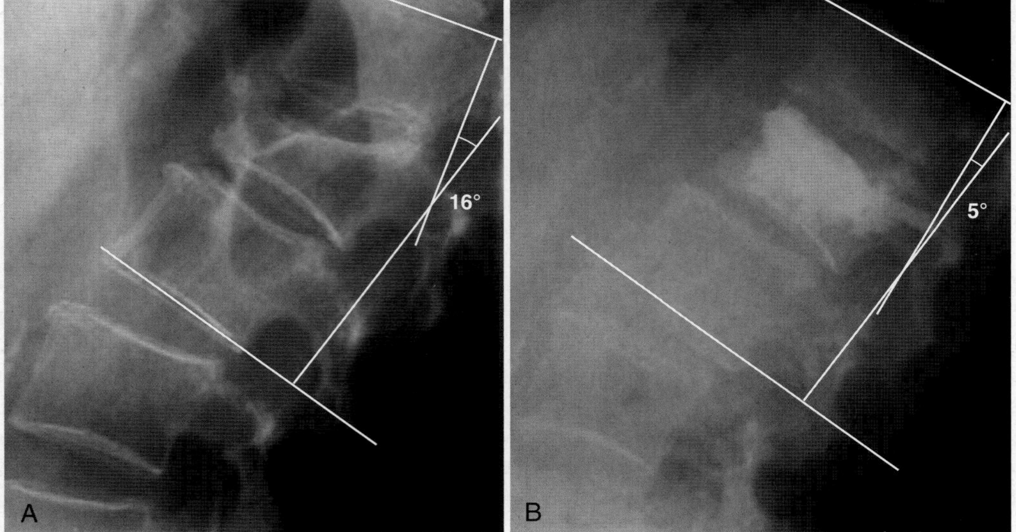

FIG. 89.2 A 73-year-old woman with an L1 vertebral compression fracture was treated with kyphoplasty 6 weeks after the injury occurred. The focal kyphosis was corrected from (A) 16 degrees to (B) 5 degrees.

management and patients requiring hospitalization for pain or medical complications secondary to VCFs.[10] In addition to pain relief, kyphoplasty may also aid in reduction of fractured vertebrae and improvement of sagittal alignment with kyphotic deformity.[11] Contraindications include subacute or chronic injuries, neurologic compromise, radicular symptoms, loss of integrity of the posterior vertebral cortex, and osteomyelitis. Considerations include bleeding disorders and cardiopulmonary compromise that may preclude safe performance of the procedure. When considering cement augmentation as treatment for a painful VCF, a clinician must ensure that the fracture is the source of the patient's back pain. This requires careful correlation of the patient's history and clinical examination with radiographic documentation of an acute VCF.[33] Magnetic resonance imaging (MRI) may be useful in detecting vertebral edema, suggesting an acute fracture as well as ruling out infection or tumor as potential causes of fracture. Acute VCFs will show bony edema characterized by increased signal on T2-weighted MRI and short tau inversion recovery imaging sequences and decreased signal on T1-weighted MRI. Subacute and chronic fractures will not show increased signal on T2-weighted and short tau inversion recovery MRI images.

Techniques

Vertebroplasty

Vertebroplasty is performed on an outpatient basis with the use of mild sedation and local anesthesia. The patient is positioned prone with the spine extended by chest and pelvic bolsters. Under fluoroscopic or CT guidance, an 11- to 13-gauge needle is advanced toward the center of the affected vertebral body using a transpedicular or peripedicular approach. If concern exists for metastatic or metabolic disease, a biopsy may be obtained before cement injection. PMMA cement is mixed with barium for fluoroscopic opacification. Antibiotics may also be added to the cement mixture if concern exists for infection, such as when operating on immunocompromised patients. Once reaching appropriate consistency, 2 to 10 mL of cement is injected into the vertebral body under live fluoroscopy until complete opacification or evidence of extravasation occurs. The patient is maintained in the prone position until the cement has cured. Patients rest supine under observation for at least 4 hours before discharge.

Kyphoplasty

Kyphoplasty is similar to vertebroplasty, but it also involves reconstitution of lost vertebral height using 1 or 2 inflatable bone tamps in addition to cement augmentation. When inflated, the percutaneous bone tamp elevates the depressed vertebral body endplate(s), thereby restoring vertebral body height and pushing remaining trabecular bone to the periphery, creating a cavity within the vertebral body that is then filled with bone cement. The patient is positioned prone on a radiolucent table. As with vertebroplasty, percutaneous needle placement into the affected vertebrae is performed under fluoroscopic or CT guidance using a transpedicular or peripedicular technique. Once accurate placement within the vertebrae is confirmed, a working channel is created within the vertebrae. The balloon tamp is inserted into the canal and inflated within the vertebrae. The balloon tamp is expanded using visual (fluoroscopy), volume, and pressure (digital manometer) controls. The inflation continues until (1) adequate fracture reduction is achieved, (2) the maximal balloon pressure is reached, or (3) cortical wall contact occurs. The balloon is then deflated and removed. Prepared thickened cement is injected through the cannula into the expanded void within the vertebrae under low pressure. The cement volume should approximate that of the intravertebral cavity. The patient is maintained in the prone position until the cement has solidified.

Complications

There is a low incidence of clinically significant complications reported for vertebral cement augmentation. Most complications result from cement extravasation, embolization, and adjacent vertebral fractures. Asymptomatic cement extravasation has been observed clinically in up to 72% of patients[22] and by postprocedure CT in 88% of patients undergoing vertebroplasty. The most common site of leakage is the endplate or disc (45%), paravertebral (35%), epidural (20%), and prevertebral (18%).[34] Leakage has been correlated with lower-viscosity cement, greater injected volume, and more severe fracture.[35] One meta-analysis demonstrated no difference in the rates of cement extravasation and subsequent fracture between vertebroplasty and kyphoplasty.[30] Two systematic reviews demonstrated reduced rate of cement extravasation[31,32] and reduced rate of subsequent fracture in kyphoplasty compared to vertebroplasty.[32] The cavity created during kyphoplasty allows for use of low-pressure, high-viscosity PMMA, resulting in controlled filling and possibly reduced rate of cement extravasation. Accounts of neurologic dysfunction from cement extravasation have been reported in the literature. The majority of dysfunction resolves with prompt surgical intervention, although permanent dysfunction has been reported.[36] Asymptomatic venous extravasation of cement toward the lungs has been reported in 2.9% of patients.[37] A systematic review reported the incidence of cement pulmonary embolism from 2% to 26%, with severity ranging from asymptomatic embolus to transient hemodynamic instability and death.[38] Bone marrow fat embolus may also occur with vertebroplasty.

There is concern that the increased stiffness of vertebrae after cement augmentation may result in increased load across adjacent vertebrae and increased risk of adjacent-level VCF. However, the meta-analysis by Anderson at al. demonstrated roughly a 20% risk of new fracture within 12 months of index VCF treated with either vertebroplasty or conservative management.[26] Zhang et al. reported a similar rate, 21%, of new VCF after vertebroplasty and correlated low BMD, low body mass index, and intradiscal cement leakage as significant risk factors for a subsequent fracture.[39] An RCT comparing outcomes and complications of vertebroplasty to kyphoplasty demonstrated no difference in rate of new fracture between the treatment groups at 12 and 24 months of follow-up.[40]

Novel Implants

Tutton et al.[41] have recently published initial outcomes of the Kiva Safety and Effectiveness Trial. The Kiva system involves deployment of small-coiled implants with a single transpedicular approach allowing for directed and controlled insertion of PMMA into the fractured vertebrae. They demonstrated noninferiority of the Kiva system compared to balloon kyphoplasty for pain reduction and functional outcomes at 12 months in patients with VCFs. This multicenter industry-sponsored trial randomized 300 patients with one or two VCFs to receive Kiva system or balloon kyphoplasty. They demonstrated a similar improvement in the mean visual analog pain scale (70.8 vs. 71.8) and in the Oswestry Disability Index (38.1 vs. 42.2) in patients undergoing either Kiva or kyphoplasty, respectively. Additionally, they demonstrated no difference in adverse device-related events or adjacent-level fracture rate at 12 months between the two groups (20.9% vs. 22.3%, respectively). Benefits of the Kiva group included use of approximately 50% less PMMA cement with more direct injection and significant reduction of cement extravasation in the Kiva group, 16.9%, compared to kyphoplasty, 25.8%.[41]

Instrumentation of the Osteoporotic Spine

As the population ages, there will be greater demand for spine procedures in patients with significant comorbidities, including osteoporosis. In those aged 50 years or older who required spine surgery, the reported incidence of osteoporosis was 14.5% and 51.3% for men and women, respectively.[42] Osteoporosis of the spine places patients at elevated risk of pathologic fracture, progressive deformity, and spinal stenosis. Loss of microarchitectural integrity makes successful instrumentation of osteoporotic bone a challenge. Selection of spinal instrumentation must take into account the fragility of osteoporotic bone, the stability of the spine, and the likely failure mechanisms of applied instrumentation.

Early postoperative complications (<3 months) in patients older than 65 years with poor bone quality include instrumentation failure, pedicle fracture, and VCFs. Late complications (>3 months) include pseudarthrosis, graft subsidence, proximal junctional kyphosis, and progressive deformity.[43] Optimal screw orientation, multiple points of fixation, combined anterior and posterior procedures, cement augmentation, and the use of novel implants are all proposed strategies for reducing the risk of complications.

Regardless of the increased risk due to medical comorbidities and instrumentation failure, evidence suggests considerable benefit for spinal fusion in this patient population.[44–47] One retrospective study demonstrated a successful fusion rate of 93% and no correlation between BMD and fusion and complication rates in adults undergoing spinal fusion for deformity correction, suggesting that a high frequency of successful outcomes can be achieved in this population.[45] Kim et al.[46] retrospectively reviewed 40 patients with low BMD who underwent lumbar fusion for degenerative kyphosis. They demonstrated good correction of deformity and no association between low BMD and rate of pseudarthrosis or adjacent-level vertebral fractures. Rather, they demonstrated correlation between postoperative spinopelvic parameters and sagittal decompensation, suggesting that correction of sagittal balance in this population can result in successful outcome. Recent analysis of the Spine Patient Outcomes Research Trial data compared outcomes of patients older than 80 years to those younger than 80 years who underwent surgical treatment of lumbar stenosis and degenerative spondylolisthesis.[47] Those patients older than 80 years had greater baseline prevalence of medical comorbidities, including osteoporosis. Those in the octogenarian cohort treated surgically had significant improvement in all primary outcome measures compared to those treated nonsurgically without an increase in complication or mortality rates compared to younger patients. Clinical outcomes suggest substantial benefit of spine surgery in older patients with lower BMD. The preoperative workup for these patients should include evaluation for the severity of osteoporosis as well as optimized medical and pharmacologic management, as described previously.

Posterior Spinal Instrumentation

Posterior instrumentation may be used to stabilize the spine after decompression of neural elements in combination with anterior procedures for increased stability and enhanced fusion or primarily for deformity correction. Pedicle screws, sublaminar wires, and hooks may be used in conjunction with rods or plates to achieve posterior spinal fusion. Failure of posterior thoracolumbar instrumentation has been shown to correlate with BMD.[48] Instrumentation failure may occur at physiologic loads in the osteoporotic spine, resulting in failure of fusion and recurrence of deformity. Modes of failure of all devices most commonly occur at the implant-bone interface through implant pullout or cutout. Therefore, recognition of poor purchase and optimization of bone implant fixation at the time of insertion is of paramount importance for successful outcome.[49,50]

Strategies for improved purchase and reduced risk of screw cutout include increased length and diameter of screws, optimal screw trajectory, cement augmentation, expandable pedicle screws, and hybrid constructs. Previous studies focused on improving fixation through increased screw length and diameter, though these techniques were limited by risk of anterior cortical breach and pedicle fracture. Newer techniques advocate optimal screw trajectory, cement augmentation, and screw design to improve bone purchase.

Optimal screw trajectory can improve fixation at the bone-implant interface by capturing robust subchondral bone, resulting in enhanced stability in the osteoporotic spine. In the sagittal plane, screw threads engaging subchondral bone may provide superior fixation over thread engagement of cancellous bone centrally within the vertebrae. Biomechanical analysis has demonstrated that pedicle screws oriented cephalad 23 degrees to the vertebral endplate resulted in a 100% increase in pullout strength compared to standard anatomic placement.[51] In the axial plane, medialization of the screw vector and triangulation of bilateral screws have been demonstrated to increase pullout strength by 121%.[52] A bilateral triangulated pedicle effectively holds all of the bone between the screws rather than just the bone within the threads of each screw. Bony anatomy limits triangulation of pedicle screws; lower lumbar levels allow for more medialization, whereas upper lumbar and thoracic pedicles allow for less. In the thoracic spine, maximal insertional torque and implant fixation may be better achieved through straightforward orientation of pedicle screws rather than anatomic orientation.[53] The technique of screw "hubbing" has been used in the thoracic spine in an attempt to provide a load-sharing effect by providing additional aperture purchase of the dorsal lamina with the screw head. Biomechanical analysis has demonstrated decreased pullout strength of thoracic pedicle screws that are "hubbed" with this technique compared to standard anatomic insertion. In addition, this technique may predispose to iatrogenic fracture of the lamina[54] and is therefore not recommended.

Subchondral purchase strategies may also be used in instrumentation of the sacrum. Sacral screws should be directed toward the promontory for tricortical bone purchase. Sacral screws inserted in this manner have been shown to have twice the insertional torque as bicortical screws.[55] Divergent screws placed in the sagittal plane may also increase pullout strength and by improving load-bearing capacity in the sacrum.[50]

Pretapped pedicle screws provide several advantages in the osteoporotic spine by providing tactile feedback, improved screw orientation, and maximizing diameter. Tapping insertion torque has been shown to directly predict pullout strength; therefore, tactile feedback can be used to optimize bone purchase and screw size.[49] Using this technique, care should be taken to not aggressively tap or oversize the screw, which would result in pedicle fracture. Biomechanical analysis demonstrates that undertapping pedicle screws by 1 mm increases maximal insertional torque by 47% compared to undertapping by 0.5 mm.[56] Undertapping improves pullout strength by compacting preserved cancellous bone between screw threads.

Pedicle screw augmentation with PMMA bone cement is used to enhance the strength of the bone-implant interface.[57–59] Cement augmentation may lead to higher fusion rates and decreased loss of deformity correction in patients with osteoporosis undergoing posterior instrumentation. In a retrospective analysis of patients undergoing posterior spinal fusion for pseudarthrosis after VCF, those with cement augmentation of pedicle screws demonstrated higher fusion rate (94.1% vs. 76.1%) and decreased correction loss (3 vs. 7.2 degrees) compared to nonaugmented screws with at least 2 years' follow-up.[59] Cement augmentation may be combined with other strategies. Biomechanical analysis demonstrates that pretapping cement-augmented screws improves fixation strength by 54% compared to cement augmentation alone.[51] Risks of this technique include cement extravasation outside the vertebra, spinal canal, or neural foramen. This risk may be reduced by screw design, with fenestrated screws reducing extravasation.[57] Non-PMMA augments, such as calcium phosphate, may also be used to enhance the implant-bone interface.[60]

Expandable pedicle screws have been designed to enhance bone purchase and spinal fixation. In these screws, the distal two-thirds of the screw is split lengthwise by two perpendicular slots to form four anterior fins when expanded. An expansion peg is threaded into the inner core of the pedicle screw, resulting in fin expansion. Biomechanical studies demonstrate superior fixation with expandable pedicle screws compared to standard screws with a twofold increase in pullout strength. Cement augmentation of expandable screws resulted in a 250% increase in pullout strength.[61,62] Wu et al.[63] demonstrated a decreased rate of screw loosening and greater fusion rates at 24 months postoperatively in osteoporotic patients undergoing lumbar spine fusion with expandable compared to conventional pedicle screw fixation. The use of expandable pedicle screws is recommended for use in the osteoporotic spine and may be combined with other strategies for improved bone purchase.

Increasing the number of fixation points to the spine improves stability of the construct by distributing deforming forces and reducing risk of segmental or junctional failure. The levels of the construct should address the underlying pathology and maintain sagittal alignment while avoiding termination at transition zones and at the apex of deformity. Risk of kyphotic collapse of the instrumented osteoporotic spine can be limited by fixation at three levels above and below the apex of kyphosis.[50] Hybrid constructs using pedicle screws with sublaminar wires or hooks may provide additional stability and reduce the risk of failure in osteoporotic bone.[64] Evidence suggests increased risk of proximal junctional kyphosis with larger deformity correction in patients older than 60 years[65] (Fig. 89.3). Accepting incomplete correction of sagittal balance in this population may be needed in order to improve successful fusion rates and reduced complications caused by proximal junctional kyphosis. The extent of deformity correction needs to be determined based on an individual patient's comorbidities and degree of disability. Extension of the instrumentation construct to the pelvis may also reduce the risk of instrumentation failure in this population.[66] The advantages of additional points of fixation must be weighed against the risks and morbidity associated with the additional-level surgery and potential long-term consequences of a longer fusion construct.

As described previously, failure of posterior instrumentation in the osteoporotic spine typically occurs through loss of fixation by screw toggling, loosening, and eventually pulling out. This may result in a relatively large void around the loose screw that can preclude reusing the same pedicle for revision screw fixation. If revision instrumentation is required, all previously mentioned strategies for enhancing posterior fixation should be considered. In addition, consideration should be given to including anterior column structural support and fusion as part of the revision strategy. Anterior column support will increase load sharing and reduce flexion-bending moments on the posterior instrumentation (Fig. 89.4).

Interbody Fusion

Interbody fusion techniques are often used in this population for the treatment of degenerative spondylolisthesis, deformity, and discogenic back pain. Interbody fusion may be performed through an anterior, lateral, posterior, or transforaminal approach. It typically involves the use of bone graft with or without cage support, and is often used in combination with pedicle screw or plate fixation. With this technique, the bone graft or cage is placed under compression and acts as a load-sharing construct with adjacent vertebral endplates. Solid fusion and successful clinical outcomes may be reliably achieved with interbody techniques in the osteoporotic spine.[67,68]

Failure of interbody fusion techniques in osteoporotic bone most commonly occurs as a result of graft subsidence into weakened cancellous bone of adjacent vertebrae, adjacent vertebral fracture, or screw loosening as described previously. Interbody graft and cage subsidence results from poor structural support by weakened adjacent vertebral endplates, graft pistoning, and modulus mismatch. Subsidence may result in recurrent deformity and stenosis. Maintaining the integrity of adjacent vertebral endplates during preparation for graft insertion may reduce the risk of graft subsidence. Oh et al.[68] demonstrated a correlation between cage subsidence and BMD in patients undergoing posterior lumbar interbody fusion. All patients, including those with cage subsidence, demonstrated improvement in clinical outcomes compared to preoperative scores, without deterioration in those with subsidence in the postoperative period. Their data suggests that, although subsidence may occur, posterior lumbar interbody fusion may be used to treat lumbar degenerative disease in osteoporotic patients with good outcome.

Larger-diameter struts and cages should be used preferentially in osteoporotic patients, as smaller implants tend to cut into and piston against weakened adjacent endplates. Avoiding stiff, high-modulus implants may also reduce the risk of subsidence.[69] Autologous corticocancellous grafts with wide and uniform surfaces may best accomplish this goal. Finally, low BMD is also a risk factor for adjacent vertebral fracture after interbody fusion requiring revision fusion surgery.[70,71] Supplementation with previously described techniques to improve screw fixation are recommended to reduce the risk of graft subsidence and adjacent vertebrae fracture in this patient population.

Considerations in the Cervical Spine

Decompression and fusion of the cervical spine is frequently performed to address pathologic degenerative changes in the elderly and is performed through an anterior, posterior, or combined approach. As with posterior instrumentation in the lumbar and thoracic spine, biomechanical analysis has demonstrated a linear relationship between decreased BMD and a decreased plate/screw cutout strength in the anterior cervical spine.[72] Increasing anterior screw length, diameter, and bicortical fixation are strategies that may be used to achieve superior bony purchase and limit excessive implant-vertebral motion in anterior cervical constructs. Cement augmentation may also be used to improve pullout strength and fatigue resistance.[73]

Graft subsidence into adjacent vertebral endplates may also occur when used after anterior discectomy or corpectomy. This risk is accentuated with multilevel anterior cervical plating and corpectomy as a result of increased construct stiffness and excessive graft extension load. When using multilevel anterior instrumentation in osteoporotic bone, the points of fixation should be maximized and strong consideration given to combined posterior stabilization to augment strength of the construct.[74] As with interbody fusion of the lumbar spine, care should be taken to maintain the viability of the adjacent vertebral endplate to reduce the risk of graft subsidence.

Novel techniques may provide adequate construct stability in osteoporotic bone while avoiding a combined approach. Anterior transpedicular screw fixation allows for improved

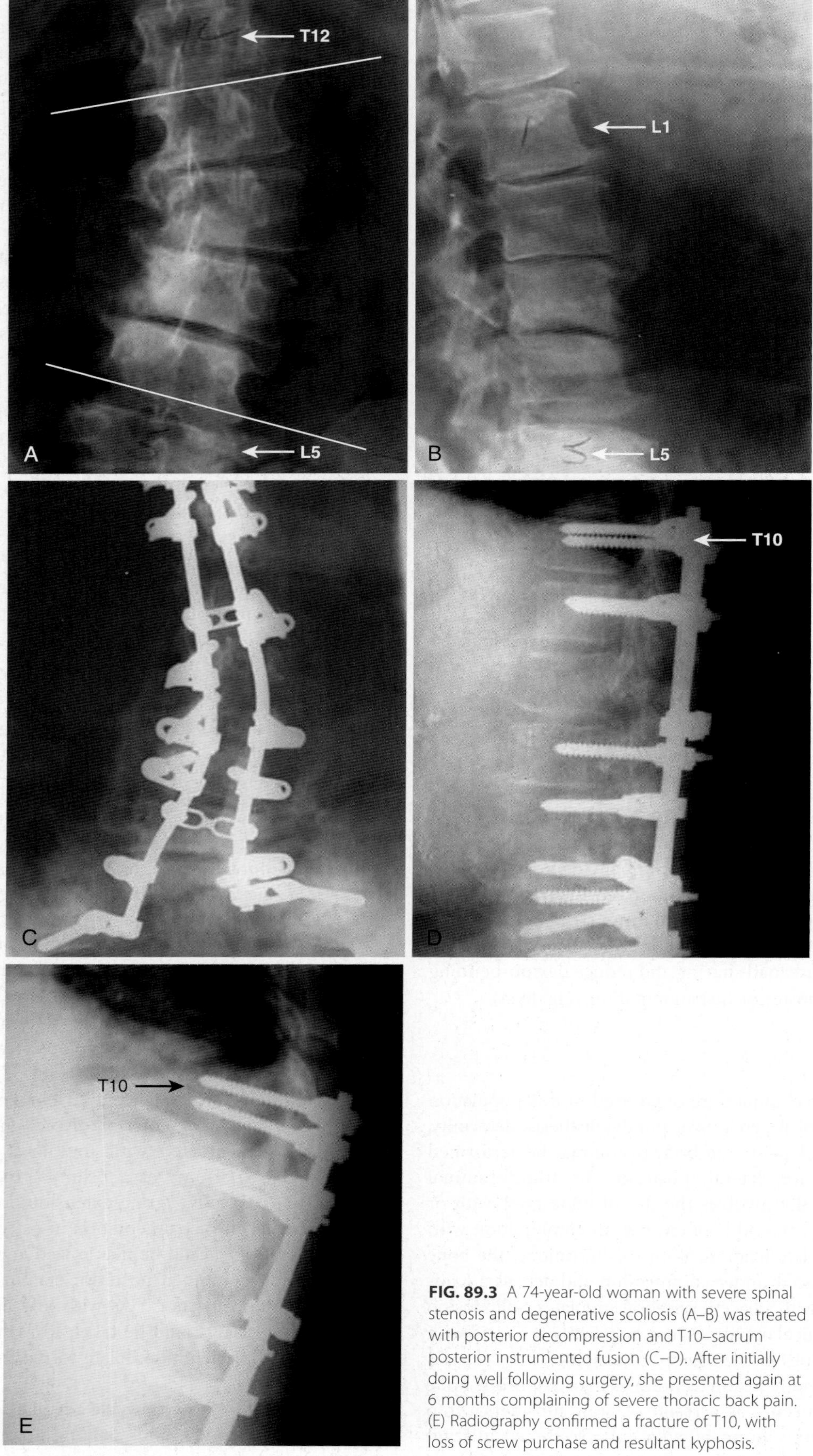

FIG. 89.3 A 74-year-old woman with severe spinal stenosis and degenerative scoliosis (A–B) was treated with posterior decompression and T10–sacrum posterior instrumented fusion (C–D). After initially doing well following surgery, she presented again at 6 months complaining of severe thoracic back pain. (E) Radiography confirmed a fracture of T10, with loss of screw purchase and resultant kyphosis.

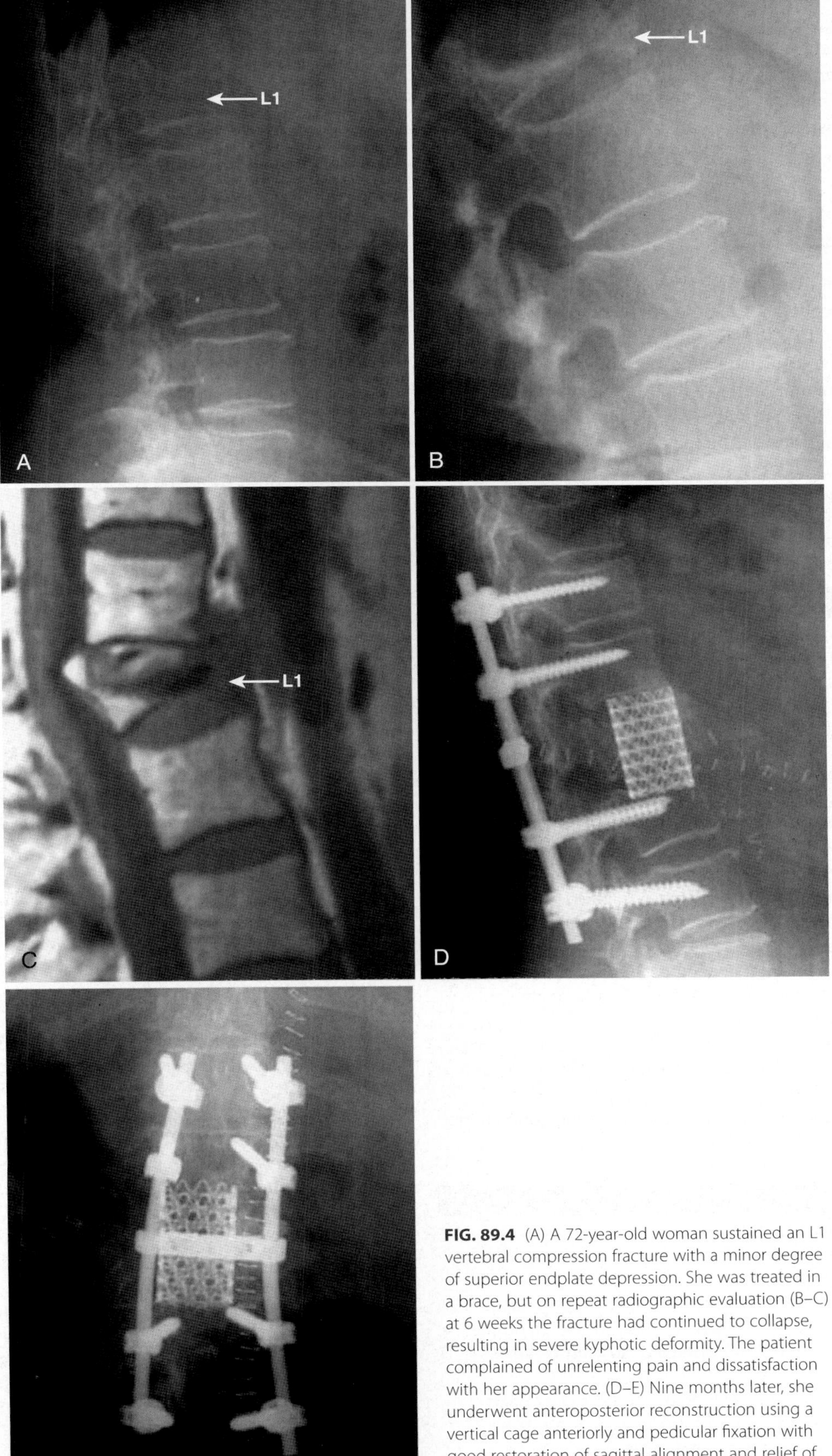

FIG. 89.4 (A) A 72-year-old woman sustained an L1 vertebral compression fracture with a minor degree of superior endplate depression. She was treated in a brace, but on repeat radiographic evaluation (B–C) at 6 weeks the fracture had continued to collapse, resulting in severe kyphotic deformity. The patient complained of unrelenting pain and dissatisfaction with her appearance. (D–E) Nine months later, she underwent anteroposterior reconstruction using a vertical cage anteriorly and pedicular fixation with good restoration of sagittal alignment and relief of pain.

fixation in patients undergoing multilevel anterior cervical spine discectomy or corpectomy through an anterior-only approach.[75] This technique involves use of fluoroscopic-guided wires for placement of anterior pedicle screws. Biomechanical analysis demonstrates smaller reduction in peak pullout force with anterior transpedicular screw (24%) compared to control (48%).[76]

Summary

With an aging population, the spine surgeon must appreciate the effects of osteoporosis on the spine. Osteoporotic VCFs may be associated with significant morbidity. The spine surgeon should be knowledgeable regarding the indications for vertebral augmentation for reduction of pain and improved sagittal balance. Reconstructive surgery in the osteoporotic spine may offer substantial benefit for patients but requires specific consideration of approach, implant use and design, augmentation, and length of construct in order to maximize the likelihood of fusion and reduce the potential of construct failure.

PEARLS

1. The spine surgeon may be required to treat direct sequelae of osteoporosis in the form of painful spinal fractures or resultant deformity or to consider osteoporosis as it relates to spinal reconstructive surgery in the older patient.
2. Osteoporotic VCFs and resultant spinal kyphosis are a leading cause of disability and morbidity in the elderly.
3. Treatment of osteoporotic vertebral fractures with vertebroplasty or kyphoplasty, although controversial, likely results in pain relief in a select patient population with acute fracture.
4. When neurogenic symptoms can be isolated to a particular level or nerve root, limited decompression in elderly osteoporotic patients is favored.
5. Surgical strategies that include improving screw purchase in bone and combining anterior and posterior stabilization should be considered to reduce the likelihood of instrumentation failure in the osteoporotic spine.
6. Consider improving pedicle screw fixation in the osteoporotic spine by increasing screw diameter, achieving bicortical fixation (at the sacrum), obtaining multiple points of fixation, use of expandable pedicle screws, hybrid constructs, and augmenting screw fixation with bone cement.

PITFALLS

1. Consider the patient's nutritional status and medical comorbidities before embarking on large spinal reconstructive surgeries in elderly patients.
2. Patients undergoing vertebroplasty or kyphoplasty for acute painful VCFs should be carefully selected while weighing the risks and benefits of these procedures versus conservative management.
3. Instrumented fusion should extend beyond the apex of any deformity to reduce risks of implant failure or progressive deformity adjacent to the fusion construct.
4. Avoid stand-alone interbody implants with modulus mismatch with bone in the osteoporotic spine.
5. Avoid excessive correction of rigid deformity that would place extreme forces on instrumentation.
6. Combined anterior/posterior circumferential fusion constructs should be considered for patients with osteoporotic bone.

KEY POINTS

1. When performing reconstructive spinal surgery in the elderly patient, the surgeon must consider the fragility of osteoporotic bone, the stability of the spine, and the potential failure mechanisms of any applied instrumentation.
2. Selective decompression and fusion should be performed based on the patient's symptoms and with consideration of potential for construct failure.
3. Increasing pedicle screw length and/or diameter can be the first-line in improving pedicle screw construct rigidity.
4. A twofold to threefold increase in screw pullout can be achieved with the use of PMMA injected into the vertebral body around the screws.
5. Combined anterior/posterior procedures may reduce the risk of instrumentation failure in patients with osteoporotic bone. This benefit must be weighed against the morbidity associated with additional surgery.

KEY REFERENCES

1. Rihn JA, Hilibrand AS, et al. Effectiveness of surgery for lumbar stenosis and degenerative spondylolisthesis in the octogenarian population: analysis of the Spine Patient Outcomes Research Trial (SPORT) data. *J Bone Joint Surg Am*. 2015;97(3):177-185.
   This analysis of SPORT data suggests substantial benefit of spine surgery in older patients with lower BMD similar to their younger cohort.
2. Lehman RAJ, Kang DG, Wagner SC. Management of osteoporosis in spine surgery. *J Am Acad Orthop Surg*. 2015;23(4):253-263.
   This review article discusses important considerations and options for patients who have osteoporosis and require spinal surgery.
3. Li L, Ren J, Liu J, et al. Results of vertebral augmentation treatment for patients of painful osteoporotic vertebral compression fractures: a meta-analysis of eight randomized controlled trials. *PLoS One*. 2015;10(9).
   This meta-analysis demonstrated improved pain relief, especially with fracture age less than 3 months, improved spine function, and quality of life in patients undergoing vertebroplasty compared to conservative management for VCFs.
4. Buchbinder R, Golmohammadi K, Johnston RV, et al. Percutaneous vertebroplasty for osteoporotic vertebral compression fracture. *Cochrane Database Syst Rev*. 2015;(4):CD006349.
   This Cochrane Review demonstrated no difference in pain, disability, or quality of life at any time point between those treated with vertebroplasty compared with sham procedure.
5. Sawakami K, Yamazaki A, Ishikawa S, et al. Polymethylmethacrylate augmentation of pedicle screws increases the initial fixation in osteoporotic spine patients. *J Spinal Disord Tech*. 2012;25(2):E28-E35.
   This retrospective analysis demonstrated higher fusion rates in patients undergoing posterior spinal fusion using cement-augmented pedicle screws compared to nonaugmented screws.
6. Oh KW, Lee JH, Lee J-H, Lee D-Y, Shim HJ. The correlation between cage subsidence, bone mineral density, and clinical results in posterior lumbar interbody fusion. *Clin Spine Surg*. 2016; [Epub ahead of print].
   This retrospective analysis demonstrated correlation between cage subsidence and BMD in osteoporotic patients undergoing PLIF;

these patients demonstrated improved clinical outcomes from preoperative examination, suggesting benefit of interbody fusion in this population.

REFERENCES

1. Wright NC, Looker AC, Saag KG, et al. The recent prevalence of osteoporosis and low bone mass in the United States based on bone mineral density at the femoral neck or lumbar spine. *J Bone Miner Res.* 2014;29(11):2520-2526.
2. Watts NB, Lewiecki EM, Miller PD, Baim S. National Osteoporosis Foundation 2008 clinician's guide to prevention and treatment of osteoporosis and the World Health Organization Fracture Risk Assessment Tool (FRAX): what they mean to the bone densitometrist and bone technologist. *J Clin Densitom.* 2008;11(4):473-477.
3. Silverman SL. Quality-of-life issues in osteoporosis. *Curr Rheumatol Rep.* 2005;7(1).
4. Lau E, Ong K, Kurtz S, Schmier J, Edidin A. Mortality following the diagnosis of a vertebral compression fracture in the Medicare population. *J Bone Joint Surg Am.* 2008;90(7):1479-1486.
5. Czerwinski E, Badurski JE, Marcinowska-Suchowierska E, Osieleniec J. Current understanding of osteoporosis according to the position of the World Health Organization (WHO) and International Osteoporosis Foundation. *Ortop Traumatol Rehabil.* 2007;9(4):337-356.
6. Belmont PJJ, Polly DWJ, Cunningham BW, Klemme WR. The effects of hook pattern and kyphotic angulation on mechanical strength and apical rod strain in a long-segment posterior construct using a synthetic model. *Spine.* 2001;26(6):627-635.
7. Haczynski J, Jakimiuk A. Vertebral fractures: a hidden problem of osteoporosis. *Med Sci Monit.* 2001;7(5):1108-1117.
8. Prather H, Watson JO, Gilula LA. Nonoperative management of osteoporotic vertebral compression fractures. *Injury.* 2007;38(suppl 3):S40-S48.
9. Sinaki M, Itoi E, Wahner HW, et al. Stronger back muscles reduce the incidence of vertebral fractures: a prospective 10 year follow-up of postmenopausal women. *Bone.* 2002;30(6):836-841.
10. Rollinghoff M, Zarghooni K, Schluter-Brust K, et al. Indications and contraindications for vertebroplasty and kyphoplasty. *Arch Orthop Trauma Surg.* 2010;130(6):765-774.
11. Omidi-Kashani F, Samini F, Hasankhani EG, et al. Does percutaneous kyphoplasty have better functional outcome than vertebroplasty in single level osteoporotic compression fractures? A comparative prospective study. *J Osteoporos.* 2013; Jul 18 [Epub ahead of print].
12. Belkoff SM, Maroney M, Fenton DC, Mathis JM. An in vitro biomechanical evaluation of bone cements used in percutaneous vertebroplasty. *Bone.* 1999;25(2 suppl):23S-26S.
13. Esses SI, McGuire R, Jenkins J, et al. The treatment of symptomatic osteoporotic spinal compression fractures. *J Am Acad Orthop Surg.* 2011;19(3):176-182.
14. Buchbinder R, Osborne RH, Ebeling PR, et al. A randomized trial of vertebroplasty for painful osteoporotic vertebral fractures. *N Engl J Med.* 2009;361(6):557-568.
15. Kallmes DF, Comstock BA, Heagerty PJ, et al. A randomized trial of vertebroplasty for osteoporotic spinal fractures. *N Engl J Med.* 2009;361(6):569-579.
16. Bono CM, Heggeness M, Mick C, Resnick D, Watters WC 3rd. North American Spine Society: Newly released vertebroplasty randomized controlled trials: a tale of two trials. *Spine J.* 2010;10(3):238-240.
17. Wardlaw D, Cummings SR, Van Meirhaeghe J, et al. Efficacy and safety of balloon kyphoplasty compared with non-surgical care for vertebral compression fracture (FREE): a randomised controlled trial. *Lancet.* 2009;373(9668):1016-1024.
18. Grafe IA, Da Fonseca K, Hillmeier J, et al. Reduction of pain and fracture incidence after kyphoplasty: 1-year outcomes of a prospective controlled trial of patients with primary osteoporosis. *Osteoporos Int.* 2005;16(12):2005-2012.
19. Van Meirhaeghe J, Bastian L, Boonen S, et al. A randomized trial of balloon kyphoplasty and nonsurgical management for treating acute vertebral compression fractures: vertebral body kyphosis correction and surgical parameters. *Spine.* 2013;38(12):971-983.
20. Boonen S, Van Meirhaeghe J, Bastian L, et al. Balloon kyphoplasty for the treatment of acute vertebral compression fractures. *J Bone Miner Res.* 2011;26(7):1627-1637.
21. Farrokhi MR, Alibai E, Maghami Z. Randomized controlled trial of percutaneous vertebroplasty versus optimal medical management for the relief of pain and disability in acute osteoporotic vertebral compression fractures. *J Neurosurg Spine.* 2011;14(5):561-569.
22. Klazen CAH, Lohle PNM, de Vries J, et al. Vertebroplasty versus conservative treatment in acute osteoporotic vertebral compression fractures (Vertos II): an open-label randomised trial. *Lancet.* 2010;376(9746):1085-1092.
23. Rousing R, Andersen MO, Jespersen SM, Thomsen K, Lauritsen J. Percutaneous vertebroplasty compared to conservative treatment in patients with painful acute or subacute osteoporotic vertebral fractures: three-months follow-up in a clinical randomized study. *Spine.* 2009;34(13):1349-1354.
24. Rousing R, Hansen KL, Andersen MO, et al. Twelve-months follow-up in forty-nine patients with acute/semiacute osteoporotic vertebral fractures treated conservatively or with percutaneous vertebroplasty: a clinical randomized study. *Spine.* 2010;35(5):478-482.
25. Blasco J, Martinez-Ferrer A, Macho J, et al. Effect of vertebroplasty on pain relief, quality of life, and the incidence of new vertebral fractures: a 12-month randomized follow-up, controlled trial. *J Bone Miner Res.* 2012;27(5):1159-1166.
26. Anderson PA, Froyshteter AB, Tontz WLJ. Meta-analysis of vertebral augmentation compared with conservative treatment for osteoporotic spinal fractures. *J Bone Miner Res.* 2013;28(2):372-382.
27. Li L, Ren J, Liu J, et al. Results of vertebral augmentation treatment for patients of painful osteoporotic vertebral compression fractures: a meta-analysis of eight randomized controlled trials. *PLoS One.* 2015;10(9).
28. Buchbinder R, Golmohammadi K, Johnston RV, et al. Percutaneous vertebroplasty for osteoporotic vertebral compression fracture. *Cochrane Database Syst Rev.* 2015;(4):CD006349.
29. Savage JW, Schroeder GD, Anderson PA. Vertebroplasty and kyphoplasty for the treatment of osteoporotic vertebral compression fractures. *J Am Acad Orthop Surg.* 2014;22(10):653-664.
30. Han S, Wan S, Ning L, et al. Percutaneous vertebroplasty versus balloon kyphoplasty for treatment of osteoporotic vertebral compression fracture: a meta-analysis of randomised and non-randomised controlled trials. *Int Orthop.* 2011;35(9):1349-1358.
31. Papanastassiou ID, Phillips FM, Van Meirhaeghe J, et al. Comparing effects of kyphoplasty, vertebroplasty, and

non-surgical management in a systematic review of randomized and non-randomized controlled studies. *Eur Spine J*. 2012;21(9):1826-1843.

32. Gu CN, Brinjikji W, Evans AJ, Murad MH, Kallmes DF. Outcomes of vertebroplasty compared with kyphoplasty: a systematic review and meta-analysis. *J Neurointerv Surg*. 2016;8(6):632-642.
33. Postacchini R, Paolino M, Faraglia S, Cinotti G, Postacchini F. Assessment of patient's pain-related behavior at physical examination may allow diagnosis of recent osteoporotic vertebral fracture. *Spine J*. 2013;13(9):1126-1133.
34. Martin DJ, Rad AE, Kallmes DF. Prevalence of extravertebral cement leakage after vertebroplasty: procedural documentation versus CT detection. *Acta Radiol*. 2012;53(5):569-572.
35. Verlaan J-J, Dhert WJA, Verbout AJ, Oner FC. Balloon vertebroplasty in combination with pedicle screw instrumentation: a novel technique to treat thoracic and lumbar burst fractures. *Spine*. 2005;30(3):E73-E79.
36. Sidhu GS, Kepler CK, Savage KE, et al. Neurological deficit due to cement extravasation following a vertebral augmentation procedure. *J Neurosurg Spine*. 2013;19(1).
37. Chen D, An Z-Q, Song S, Tang J-F, Qin H. Percutaneous vertebroplasty compared with conservative treatment in patients with chronic painful osteoporotic spinal fractures. *J Clin Neurosci*. 2014;21(3):473-477.
38. Wang L, Yang H, Shi Y, Jiang W, Chen L. Pulmonary cement embolism associated with percutaneous vertebroplasty or kyphoplasty: a systematic review. *Orthop Surg*. 2012;4(3):182-189.
39. Zhang Z, Fan J, Ding Q, Wu M, Yin G. Risk factors for new osteoporotic vertebral compression fractures after vertebroplasty: a systematic review and meta-analysis. *J Spinal Disord Tech*. 2013;26(4):E150-E157.
40. Dohm M, Black CM, Dacre A, Tillman JB, Fueredi G. A randomized trial comparing balloon kyphoplasty and vertebroplasty for vertebral compression fractures due to osteoporosis. *AJNR Am J Neuroradiol*. 2014;35(12): 2227-2236.
41. Tutton SM, Pflugmacher R, Davidian M, et al. KAST Study: The Kiva system as a vertebral augmentation treatment—a safety and effectiveness trial: a randomized, noninferiority trial comparing the Kiva system with balloon kyphoplasty in treatment of osteoporotic vertebral compression fractures. *Spine*. 2015;40(12):865-875.
42. Chin DK, Park JY, Yoon YS, et al. Prevalence of osteoporosis in patients requiring spine surgery: incidence and significance of osteoporosis in spine disease. *Osteoporos Int*. 2007;18(9):1219-1224.
43. DeWald CJ, Stanley T. Instrumentation-related complications of multilevel fusions for adult spinal deformity patients over age 65: surgical considerations and treatment options in patients with poor bone quality. *Spine*. 2006;31(19 suppl):S144-S151.
44. Glassman SD, Carreon L, Dimar JR. Outcome of lumbar arthrodesis in patients sixty-five years of age or older. Surgical technique. *J Bone Joint Surg Am*. 2010;92(suppl 1 Pt 1).
45. Yagi M, King AB, Boachie-Adjei O. Characterization of osteopenia/osteoporosis in adult scoliosis: does bone density affect surgical outcome? *Spine*. 2011;36(20):1652-1657.
46. Kim KT, Chan CYW, Lee SH, Huh DS, Son ES. Surgical correction in patients with lumbar degenerative kyphosis who had low bone mineral density: an analysis of 40 patients with a minimum follow-up of two years. *Asian Spine J*. 2015;9(1):65-74.
47. Helgeson M, Formby P. Surgery for octogenarians is supported by SPORT data: commentary on an article by Jeffrey A. Rihn, MD, et al. Effectiveness of surgery for lumbar stenosis and degenerative spondylolisthesis in the octogenarian population. Analysis of the Spine Patient Outcomes Research Trial (SPORT) data. *J Bone Joint Surg Am*. 2015;97(3):e17.
48. Lehman RAJ, Kang DG, Wagner SC. Management of osteoporosis in spine surgery. *J Am Acad Orthop Surg*. 2015;23(4):253-263.
49. Helgeson MD, Kang DG, Lehman RAJ, Dmitriev AE, Luhmann SJ. Tapping insertional torque allows prediction for better pedicle screw fixation and optimal screw size selection. *Spine J*. 2013;13(8):957-965.
50. Dodwad S-NM, Khan SN. Surgical stabilization of the spine in the osteoporotic patient. *Orthop Clin North Am*. 2013;44(2):243-249.
51. Kuhns CA, Reiter M, Pfeiffer F, Choma TJ. Surgical strategies to improve fixation in the osteoporotic spine: the effects of tapping, cement augmentation, and screw trajectory. *Global Spine J*. 2014;4(1):47-54.
52. Ono A, Brown MD, Latta LL, Milne EL, Holmes DC. Triangulated pedicle screw construct technique and pull-out strength of conical and cylindrical screws. *J Spinal Disord*. 2001;14(4):323-329.
53. Lehman RAJ, Polly DWJ, Kuklo TR, et al. Straight-forward versus anatomic trajectory technique of thoracic pedicle screw fixation: a biomechanical analysis. *Spine*. 2003;28(18):2058-2065.
54. Paik H, Dmitriev AE, Lehman RAJ, et al. The biomechanical effect of pedicle screw hubbing on pullout resistance in the thoracic spine. *Spine J*. 2012;12(5):417-424.
55. Lehman RAJ, Kuklo TR, Belmont PJJ, Andersen RC, Polly DWJ. Advantage of pedicle screw fixation directed into the apex of the sacral promontory over bicortical fixation: a biomechanical analysis. *Spine*. 2002;27(8):806-811.
56. Carmouche JJ, Molinari RW, Gerlinger T, Devine J, Patience T. Effects of pilot hole preparation technique on pedicle screw fixation in different regions of the osteoporotic thoracic and lumbar spine. *J Neurosurg Spine*. 2005;3(5):364-370.
57. Choma TJ, Pfeiffer FM, Swope RW, Hirner JP. Pedicle screw design and cement augmentation in osteoporotic vertebrae: effects of fenestrations and cement viscosity on fixation and extraction. *Spine*. 2012;37(26):E1628-E1632.
58. Chen L-H, Tai C-L, Lee D-M, et al. Pullout strength of pedicle screws with cement augmentation in severe osteoporosis: a comparative study between cannulated screws with cement injection and solid screws with cement pre-filling. *BMC Musculoskelet Disord*. 2011;12:33.
59. Sawakami K, Yamazaki A, Ishikawa S, et al. Polymethylmethacrylate augmentation of pedicle screws increases the initial fixation in osteoporotic spine patients. *J Spinal Disord Tech*. 2012;25(2):E28-E35.
60. Hashemi A, Bednar D, Ziada S. Pullout strength of pedicle screws augmented with particulate calcium phosphate: an experimental study. *Spine J*. 2009;9(5):404-410.
61. Cook SD, Salkeld SL, Stanley T, Faciane A, Miller SD. Biomechanical study of pedicle screw fixation in severely osteoporotic bone. *Spine J*. 2004;4(4):402-408.
62. Gazzeri R, Roperto R, Fiore C. Litanium expandable pedicle screw for the treatment of degenerative and traumatic spinal diseases in osteoporotic patients: preliminary experience. *Surg Technol Int*. 2012;22:320-325.

63. Wu Z, Gong F, Liu L, et al. A comparative study on screw loosening in osteoporotic lumbar spine fusion between expandable and conventional pedicle screws. *Arch Orthop Trauma Surg*. 2012;132(4):471-476.
64. Kebaish KM. Sacropelvic fixation: techniques and complications. *Spine*. 2010;35(25):2245-2251.
65. Kim HJ, Bridwell KH, Lenke LG, et al. Patients with proximal junctional kyphosis requiring revision surgery have higher postoperative lumbar lordosis and larger sagittal balance corrections. *Spine*. 2014;39(9):E576-E580.
66. Kwon BK, Elgafy H, Keynan O, et al. Progressive junctional kyphosis at the caudal end of lumbar instrumented fusion: etiology, predictors, and treatment. *Spine*. 2006;31(17):1943-1951.
67. Wu W-J, Liang Y, Zhang X-K, Cao P, Zheng T. Complications and clinical outcomes of minimally invasive transforaminal lumbar interbody fusion for the treatment of one- or two-level degenerative disc diseases of the lumbar spine in patients older than 65 years. *Chin Med J*. 2012;125(14):2505-2510.
68. Oh KW, Lee JH, Lee J-H, Lee D-Y, Shim HJ. The correlation between cage subsidence, bone mineral density, and clinical results in posterior lumbar interbody fusion. *Clin Spine Surg*. 2016; [Epub ahead of print].
69. Galbusera F, Schmidt H, Wilke H-J. Lumbar interbody fusion: a parametric investigation of a novel cage design with and without posterior instrumentation. *Eur Spine J*. 2012;21(3):455-462.
70. Tempel ZJ, Gandhoke GS, Bolinger BD, Okonkwo DO, Kanter AS. Vertebral body fracture following stand-alone lateral lumbar interbody fusion (LLIF): report of two events out of 712 levels. *Eur Spine J*. 2015;24(suppl 3):409-413.
71. Dua K, Kepler CK, Huang RC, Marchenko A. Vertebral body fracture after anterolateral instrumentation and interbody fusion in two osteoporotic patients. *Spine J*. 2010;10(9):e11-e15.
72. Reitman CA, Nguyen L, Fogel GR. Biomechanical evaluation of relationship of screw pullout strength, insertional torque, and bone mineral density in the cervical spine. *J Spinal Disord Tech*. 2004;17(4):306-311.
73. Chen C, Zhao W, Liu D, et al. A biomechanical study to evaluate the effect of PMMA augmentation and restoration of the strength of cervical vertebral screws inserted in an osteoporotic vertebral body. *J Spinal Disord Tech*. 2014;27(4):224-231.
74. Koller H, Hempfing A, Ferraris L, et al. 4- and 5-level anterior fusions of the cervical spine: review of literature and clinical results. *Eur Spine J*. 2007;16(12):2055-2071.
75. Koktekir E, Toktas ZO, Seker A, et al. Anterior transpedicular screw fixation of cervical spine: Is it safe? Morphological feasibility, technical properties, and accuracy of manual insertion. *J Neurosurg Spine*. 2015;22(6):596-604.
76. Wu C, Chen C, Wu W, et al. Biomechanical analysis of differential pull-out strengths of bone screws using cervical anterior transpedicular technique in normal and osteoporotic cervical cadaveric spines. *Spine (Phila Pa 1976)*. 2015;40(1):E1-E8.

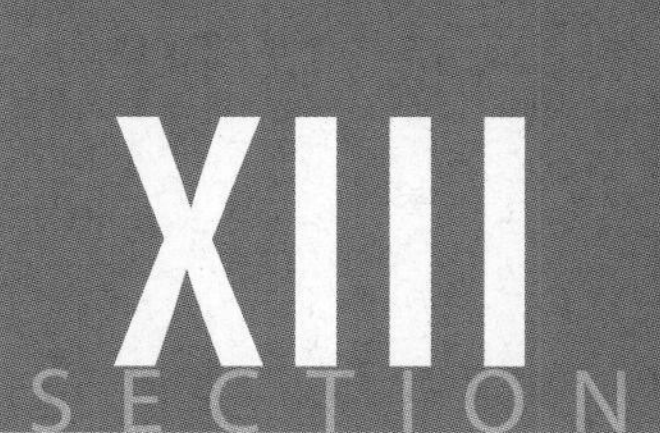
XIII
SECTION

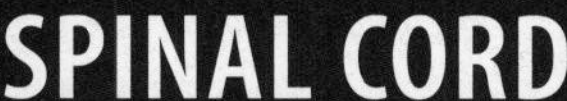
SPINAL CORD

CHAPTER 90 Intradural Tumors

Ashish H. Shah
Jeremiah N. Johnson
Barth A. Green

Intradural Tumors

The era of spinal tumor surgery began in London in 1887 when the influential surgeon Dr. Victor Horsley removed a thoracic intradural extramedullary tumor from a 42-year-old British Army General at the urging of the neurologist Dr. William Gowers.[1] The patient presented with a 4-year history of progressive symptoms that had culminated in urinary incontinence, spasticity, and paraplegia. Dr. Gowers diagnosed the lesion as a thoracic compressive lesion on the basis of a history and clinical examination and proposed surgery. After a thoracic laminectomy and removal of a compressive fibromyxoma, the patient made a remarkable recovery, regained the ability to walk, returned to work, and lived 20 additional years without recurrence. As a result, Dr. Horsley became a proponent of surgery as a viable treatment option for spinal tumors.

The next advancement in spinal tumor surgery was the first successful intramedullary spinal cord tumor removal in 1907 by Dr. Anton von Eiselsberg in Austria. However, the first published report of a successful intramedullary tumor removal is credited to Dr. Charles Elsberg in 1911 at the New York Neurological Institute.[2,3] Soon thereafter, in 1916, Elsberg published his influential book *Diagnosis and Treatment of Surgical Diseases of the Spinal Cord and Its Membranes*. He later published the first large series of intradural spinal cord tumor resections in 1925.[4] In his early writings, Elsberg advocated a two-stage surgery for intramedullary tumors: a laminectomy and myelotomy followed 1 week later by removal of the tumor that had delivered through the myelotomy. However, as his experience grew, he transitioned into performing single-stage operations for intramedullary tumor removal. For these significant early contributions, he is remembered as an important figure in spinal cord surgery.

Over the ensuing decades, the widespread practice of intraspinal tumor surgery was hindered by difficulty with tumor localization, infections, neurologic morbidity, and poor outcomes. Throughout the mid-20th century, intradural—especially intramedullary—tumors were treated with decompressive laminectomy, biopsy, and palliative radiation.[5] In the 1960s, technological advances—such as loupe magnification, widespread use of myelography, and bipolar cautery—began making good outcomes after surgery feasible and there was a renewed interest in aggressive surgical management.[6] Even in the past 30 years, the evolution of technologies such as the operating microscope, microsurgical instruments, magnetic resonance imaging (MRI), ultrasonic cavitation, and electrophysiologic monitoring has made aggressive surgical resection a low-morbidity mainstay of spinal tumor treatment.

Epidemiology

The incidence of intradural spinal tumors is reported to be between 1 and 2 per 100,000 population, and they account for 5% to 10% of central nervous system tumors.[7–9] In adults, extramedullary tumors predominate, accounting for 60% to 75% of intradural masses with intramedullary tumors accounting for the remainder. In children, however, intramedullary tumors are more common, accounting for greater than 35% of intradural masses.[8,10] Intradural tumors occur with equal frequency in both sexes, with the exception of a higher incidence of meningiomas in women. The most frequent intradural extramedullary tumors are nerve sheath tumors and meningiomas, with filum terminale ependymomas being a distant third.[10,11] Ependymomas and astrocytomas are the most common intramedullary lesions, followed by hemangioblastomas and cavernous malformations.[8,10,12] One institution's large experience is summarized in Box 90.1.

Clinical Presentation

Intradural tumors are typically slow-growing, benign lesions that may be asymptomatic or minimally symptomatic for years before presentation. The most common presenting symptoms for intramedullary tumors are sensory deficits, motor weakness, gait ataxia, and pain.[10] Pain is often worse at night and awakens the patient from sleep, but pain from a tumor may

BOX 90.1 Incidence of Tumors in Adults

Extramedullary (Two-Thirds of Cases)

Nerve sheath tumor: 40%
Meningioma: 40%
Filum ependymoma: 15%
Miscellaneous[a]: 5%

Intramedullary (One-Third of Cases)

Ependymoma: 45%
Astrocytoma[b]: 40%
Hemangioblastoma: 5%
Miscellaneous[c]: 10%

From Schwartz TH, McCormick PC. Spinal cord tumors in adults. In: Winn HR, ed. *Youmans Neurological Surgery*. 5th ed. Philadelphia, PA: Saunders; 2004.
[a]Includes paraganglioma, drop metastases, and granuloma.
[b]Includes oligodendroglioma, ganglioglioma, neurocytoma, and subependymoma.
[c]Includes metastatic tumor; inclusion tumor (e.g., lipoma); inflammation (e.g., abscess, tuberculosis, sarcoid); and vascular condition (e.g., cavernous malformation, aneurysm).

be difficult to differentiate from common degenerative back pain.[13] In patients harboring slow-growing tumors, there is an indolent progression of symptoms from nonspecific pain and sensory disturbance to loss of balance, motor weakness, and other signs of myelopathy.[14,15] Patients may present with symptoms at any point along this continuum; however, since the advent of the MRI, tumors are being discovered earlier, resulting in less severe deficits at presentation. Intramedullary tumors can be associated with a suspended dissociated sensory loss.[7,16] This pattern of sensory disturbance is attributable to dilatation of the central cord by the tumor or an associated spinal cord syrinx causing an interruption of the pain and temperature fibers crossing in the anterior commissure. In fact, spinal axis imaging with contrast is an important step in the workup of an unexplained spinal cord syrinx in order to rule out an underlying spinal cord tumor.

The most common presenting symptoms for extramedullary tumors are as follows: pain, sensory disturbances, motor deficits, and gait ataxia. Schwannomas are derived from the nerve root sleeve and are more likely to present as unilateral radiculopathy; meningiomas, derived from the dura, are more likely to present with diffuse pain or symptoms of cord compression.[17,18] Yet, these symptoms are not mutually exclusive and patients often present with a mixture of nonspecific signs and symptoms.

The presenting signs and symptoms of intradural tumors are also influenced by the tumor's spinal level.[19] Both cervical and thoracic tumors can enlarge or compress the cord, resulting in cord impairment with prominent motor weakness and myelopathy. Cervical tumors are more likely to present with occipitocervical pain, arm pain, hand clumsiness, and sensory disturbances. Thoracic tumors often present with myelopathy and sensory disturbances in the lower body but can also produce pain that is mistakenly attributed to the heart and visceral organs. Tumors of the cauda equina typically cause back and leg pain that is classically worse while lying down and relieved by standing. This is thought to be due to positional pressure fluctuations in the epidural venous plexus.[20]

Radiologic Diagnosis

In the treatment of intradural tumors, the advent of MRI has allowed earlier tumor discovery, superior lesion characterization, precise localization, and improved surgical planning. MRI has supplanted computed tomography (CT) and contrast myelography as the imaging modality of choice in the diagnosis of intradural tumors. In most cases, MRI is now a stand-alone imaging modality with CT for certain tumors, and CT myelogram is reserved for use in patients with contraindications to undergoing an MRI (e.g., those with implanted ferromagnetic objects).[21] Plain radiographs are rarely important in the setting of intradural tumors but are useful when looking for abnormal alignment or structural instability in patients who have undergone a previous tumor resection.

In the evaluation of spinal tumors, MRI with gadolinium greatly increases the ability to identify a mass, show its relationship to the spinal cord, identify surrounding vascular structures, and give clues as to the pathologic diagnosis. Additionally, it can help differentiate tumors from less ominous lesions, such as arachnoid cysts, lipomas, and neurenteric cysts. On T1-weighted images, intradural tumors are typically isointense or slightly hypointense to the spinal cord. In T2-weighted sequences, cerebrospinal fluid (CSF) has a high signal and intramedullary tumors are often hyperintense. Spinal cord edema and syrinx associated with tumors are best identified with T2 images.[22] After the intravenous administration of gadolinium (paramagnetic ions), T1-weighted MRI detects contrast that leaks through the compromised blood–spinal cord barrier at the tumor interface. The subsequent delay in T1 relaxation time by the gadolinium within the tumor is interpreted as enhancement. Most intradural tumors display some degree of contrast enhancement. In certain cases in which multiple intradural lesions are discovered, the use of a positron emission tomography/CT (PET/CT) may be helpful to determine the degree of metabolic activity within the tumor. Certain tumors—such as chondrosarcomas, renal cell carcinomas, and lymphomas—may be hypermetabolic on PET/CT imaging; PET/CT becomes especially useful for patients with a previous history of treated cancer.[23–25]

Intramedullary tumors are generally contrast enhancing, can be either well circumscribed or diffuse, may have associated cysts, and can expand the spinal cord. Extramedullary lesions are usually well rounded, contrast enhancing, and compress the cord rather than expand it. Cauda equina tumors and nerve sheath tumors are usually heterogeneously enhancing with areas of cystic degeneration, hemorrhage, or necrosis. Imaging characteristics of specific tumors are discussed in the subsequent sections.

Extramedullary Tumors

Meningiomas

Intraspinal meningiomas are the most common type of intradural extramedullary tumors and occur predominantly in

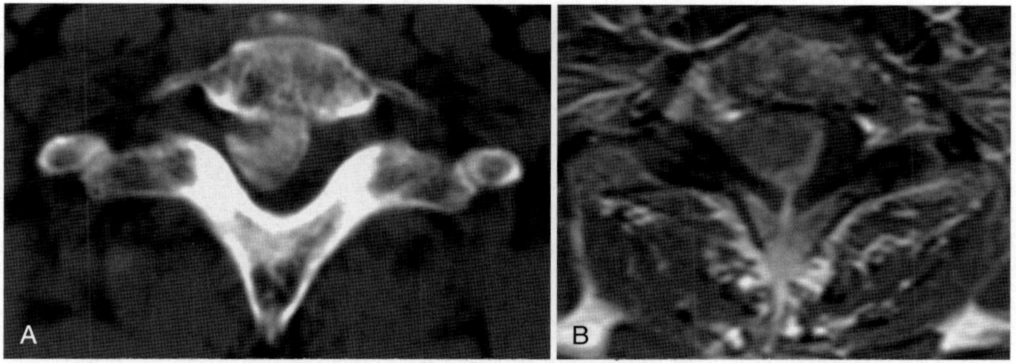

FIG. 90.1 (A) Axial computed tomographic image of a tumor showing homogeneous calcification and the ventral dural attachment. (B) Axial gadolinium-enhanced magnetic resonance image of the same tumor shows an enhancing ventral cervical meningioma with the spinal cord displaced laterally.

women (75% to 85%). They typically present in the fifth to seventh decades of life with pain, paresthesias, weakness, and long tract signs.[26,27] Meningiomas are homogeneously enhancing, smooth-bordered masses on MRI and can contain calcifications that help differentiate them from nerve sheath tumors (Fig. 90.1). With suspected meningiomas, preoperative CT scans are helpful to determine the presence and extent of tumor calcification, which can significantly affect surgical strategy. Seventy-five percent of intraspinal meningiomas arise in the thoracic spine and are typically dorsolateral to the cord; however, cervical tumors (20%) do occur and are frequently located in the upper cervical region and ventral to the cord.[20,28] Lumbar meningiomas are the least common. Spinal meningiomas are thought to arise from arachnoid cap cells in the dura near the nerve root sleeve laterally but may also grow from dural fibroblasts or pial cells, explaining their occasional ventral or dorsal location.[29] Meningiomas invariably arise and derive their blood supply from a broad dural base that is often visible as a dural tail on MRI. These tumors are typically benign, encapsulated, slow-growing masses, but other growth patterns are seen, including en plaque, atypical, and invasive malignant meningiomas.[10,30] Treatment for symptomatic tumors is surgical, with the goal of gross total resection; however, total removal may not be possible with en plaque or ventral calcified tumors.[28,30] Overall, spinal meningiomas are amenable to surgical removal and have low recurrence rates after complete resection.

Nerve Sheath Tumors

Tumors of the nerve sheath account for up to 30% of spinal neoplasms and are categorized as either schwannomas or neurofibromas.[31] They typically arise from the posterior sensory nerve root near its entrance into the neural foramen. Although both tumors are thought to be of Schwann cell origin, their significant histologic, epidemiologic, and biologic differences warrant discussing them separately.

Schwannomas are common intradural extramedullary neoplasms that make up 85% of nerve sheath tumors.[18] They occur equally in men and women, with a peak age of presentation between the fourth and sixth decades. Most appear as solitary tumors and occur equally throughout the spinal canal. Although rare, there are patients with multiple schwannomas but nearly always in the setting of neurofibromatosis 2 (NF2) and schwannomatosis.[32] Radiographically, schwannomas are well-demarcated masses associated with a nerve root, intensely enhance, can include cystic areas, and may grow along the root into the extraspinal space (Fig. 90.2A). Up to 30% of schwannomas grow through the neural foramen, giving the classic "dumbbell" shape on imaging (Fig. 90.2B).[18] At surgery, schwannomas are smooth, well-demarcated tumors that are discretely attached to an intact nerve root and can usually be separated from the root without nerve injury. The goal of surgery should be complete tumor removal and can usually be achieved. However, if complete resection is not possible, aggressive debulking with preservation of the root can relieve symptoms and the patient can be monitored radiographically for recurrence.

Neurofibromas are less common than schwannomas, accounting for approximately 15% of nerve sheath tumors, and more than half are associated with neurofibromatosis 1 (NF1).[18,33] Patients with NF1 can harbor single or multiple neurofibromas and are more likely to have malignant tumors.[34] Neurofibromas typically, but not exclusively, arise from the sensory root. Consequently, patients most commonly present with pain. Radiographically, neurofibromas are similar to schwannomas but are solid, not cystic. Yet they, too, can extend through the dural root sleeve as a dumbbell tumor (Fig. 90.3). Tumor cells characteristically arise from central nerve root fibers and expand the root, making dissection of the tumor from the root unrealistic. Optimal treatment for symptomatic neurofibromas includes total surgical removal of tumor, often necessitating the sacrifice of the nerve root.[31]

Ependymomas of the Filum Terminale

Ependymomas of this region are slow-growing tumors that arise from the filum terminale near the junction with the conus. At the terminal filum, ependymomas are thought to arise from ependymal rests ectopically deposited during development. They typically present in the third to fourth decades of life with slowly progressive low back pain, sensory

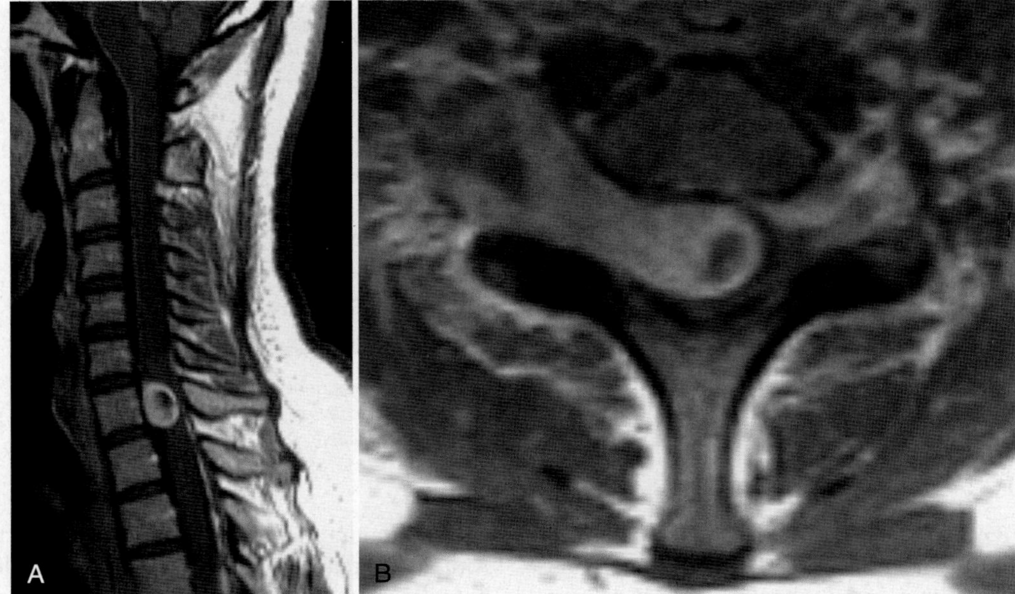

FIG. 90.2 (A) Sagittal T1-weighted gadolinium-enhanced magnetic resonance imaging (MRI) scan showing heterogeneously enhancing, well-demarcated, extradural schwannoma. (B) Axial T1-weighted gadolinium-enhanced MRI of the same cervical schwannoma showing dumbbell-shaped tumor extending through the right neural foramen.

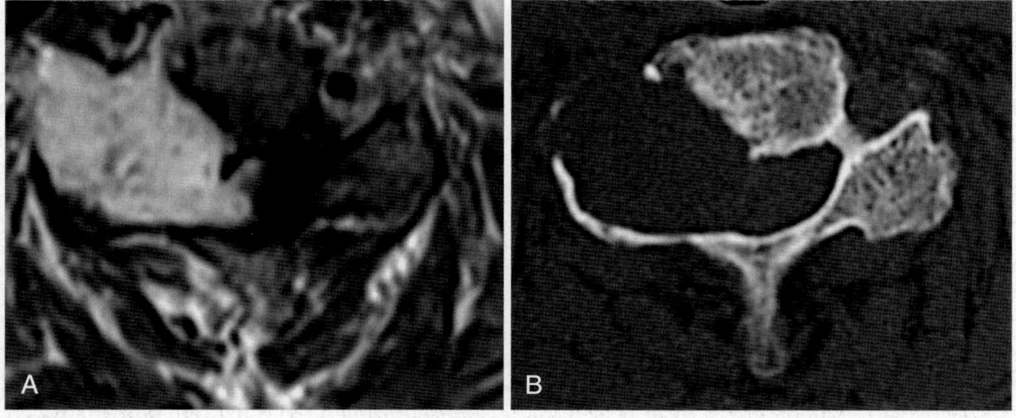

FIG. 90.3 (A) Axial T1-weighted gadolinium-enhanced magnetic resonance image of a malignant neurofibroma expanding the right neural foramen and extending into the extraspinal space. (B) Axial computed tomography of the same mass showing the extensive bony erosion caused by the tumor.

deficits, and even sphincter and sexual disturbances.[10] Histologically, filum terminale ependymomas are overwhelmingly of the benign myxopapillary pathologic subtype, but cellular and papillary histiotypes do occur.[35] On MRI, these tumors exhibit intense contrast uptake and can be anywhere on a spectrum from small, well-circumscribed tumors at the inferior tip of the conus to massive septated tumors filling the spinal canal (Fig. 90.4). An MRI of the neural axis should be obtained because cauda region ependymomas can disseminate along the neural axis via CSF or can be the result of intracranial cranial tumor seeding to the spine. Therapy is surgical, with a goal of gross total resection; however, this is often not achievable with massive tumors that are adherent to neural structures. Even after gross total resection of larger tumors, the recurrence rate is up to 20% and patients may need multiple surgeries for recurrences.[36,37]

Less Common Extramedullary Tumors

Paragangliomas

Paragangliomas are benign, well-circumscribed vascular tumors that typically arise from the filum terminale or cauda equina. They are clinically and radiographically similar to filum terminale ependymomas but are thought to arise from sympathetic nerve cells. Histologically, they resemble

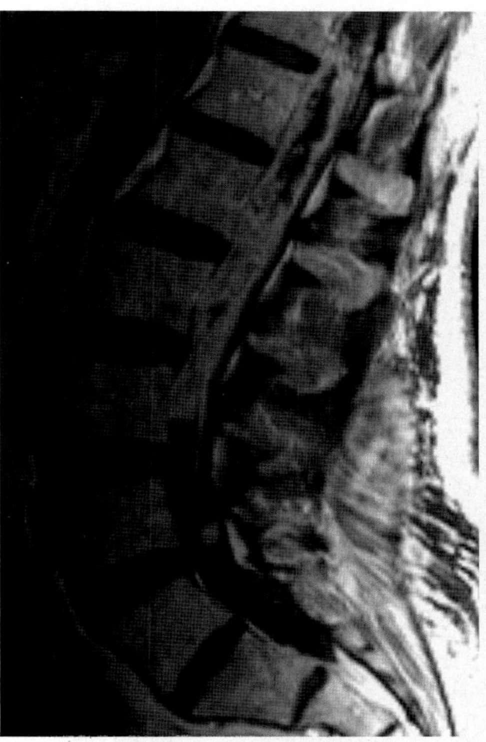

FIG. 90.4 Sagittal T1-enhanced magnetic resonance image demonstrating a large filum terminale ependymoma filling the lower thoracic–upper lumbar spinal canal and encasing the cauda equina. Note the more inferior tumor nodule at the L4 level junction representing a drop metastasis.

the parasympathetic tumors of the carotid body and glomus region. Despite their sympathetic origin, they are nonsecreting tumors. Some of these tumors can be locally aggressive, with a penchant for recurrence. Optimal treatment is complete surgical excision, and radiotherapy may be indicated for incompletely removed tumors or recurrences.

Lipomas

Spinal lipomas have many forms, but the most common type arises in the lumbosacral region in the setting of occult spinal dysraphism. Most types of lipomas present during childhood, but intradural tumors can present in adults. They are considered benign but are often intimately associated with nerves of the cauda equina. When indicated to relieve symptomatic compression, surgery should be conservative because aggressive attempts to clear neural elements of tumor can lead to neurologic injury.

Arachnoid Cysts

Although not tumors, these structures can appear as a cystic mass compressing the spinal cord on MRI. They are composed of arachnoid membranes that have become loculated with CSF under pressure. The most common place for symptomatic arachnoid cysts is in the thoracic region. They typically present with pain and signs of myelopathy. Surgical excision relieves spinal cord compression and is the mainstay of treatment for symptomatic lesions.[38]

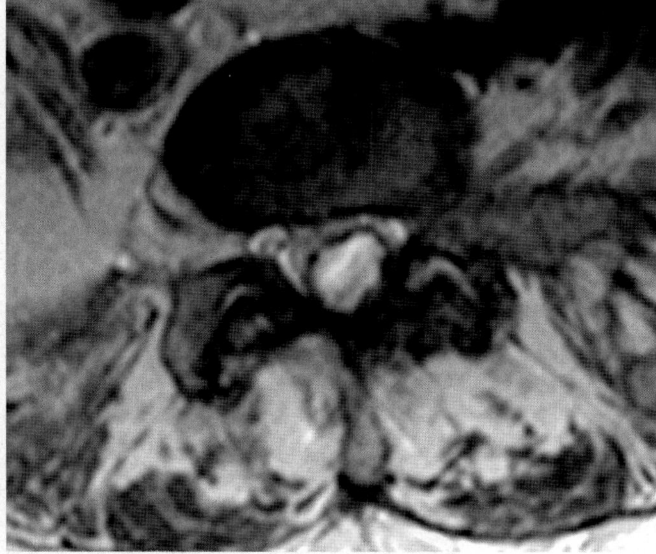

FIG. 90.5 Axial T2-weighted magnetic resonance image sequence of a large left L4 synovial cyst expanding from the facet into the spinal canal. These lesions can mimic spinal tumors.

Synovial Cysts

These extradural structures are cystic enlargements of the facet capsule that can enlarge to displace the thecal sac, compress the cord, or impinge nerve roots, causing radiculopathy. They are most common in the lumbar region, especially at L4–L5, but have been reported in the cervical spine.[39] These cysts are thought to result from excess motion at a vertebral level, leading to facet capsule hypertrophy and cystic enlargement. These lesions are filled with synovial fluid and can mimic intradural lesions on plain MRI (Fig. 90.5). Large or persistently symptomatic lesions can be managed with image-guided percutaneous drainage or more definitively with surgical removal.[40,41]

Intramedullary Tumors

Ependymomas

Intramedullary tumors of the spinal cord are rare, accounting for 15% to 30% of intradural spinal lesions. Ependymomas are the most common type of intramedullary spinal cord tumor and usually present in the middle-age years with pain, mild sensory changes, motor weakness, and signs of myelopathy.[42] There is a curious association of intramedullary ependymomas and NF2. A significant portion of NF2 patients harbor intramedullary ependymomas, and genetic studies on tumor cells have shown NF2 gene mutations in spontaneous intramedullary ependymomas.[43–45] Ependymomas of the cord are typically solitary tumors that arise from the ependymal lining of the central canal, cause a diffuse enlargement of the cord over several levels, and have an associated syrinx in up to 50% of cases.[45] Among the four ependymoma histologic subtypes, all are considered benign.[12,46,47] On MRI, intramedullary ependymomas are sharply demarcated lesions that are isointense on

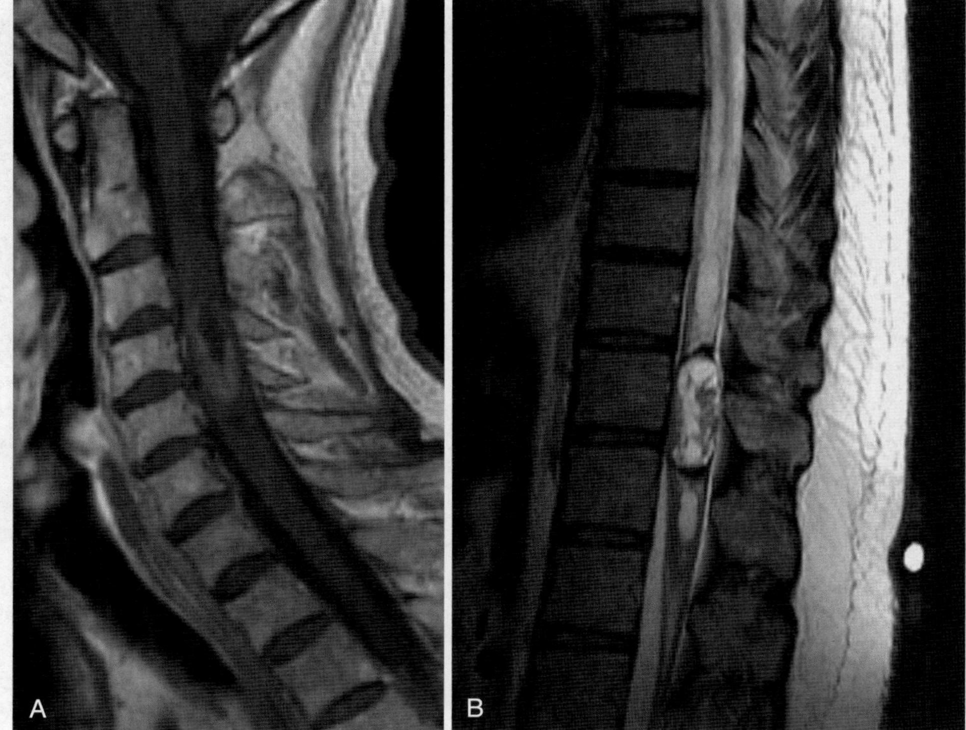

FIG. 90.6 (A) Sagittal T1-weighted gadolinium-enhanced magnetic resonance image (MRI) showing a midcervical enhancing ependymoma with a central cystic component. (B) T2-weighted thoracic MRI of a different spinal cord ependymoma showing a tumor with a large cystic component and a syrinx extending rostral and caudal to the lesion.

plain T1 sequences and enhance homogeneously with gadolinium (Fig. 90.6A). Classic radiographic features of spinal cord ependymomas include a distinct tumor–spinal cord border, an associated syrinx, cysts within or adjacent to the mass, and hemosiderin deposits or "caps" near the poles of the tumor on T1- and T2-weighted images (Fig. 90.6B).[48] The treatment of choice is gross total surgical resection. In contrast to intracranial ependymomas, intramedullary spinal cord ependymomas have a good prognosis and a low rate of local recurrence after complete resection, but cases of malignant transformation after resection have been reported.[49–51]

Astrocytomas

Astrocytomas are the second most common intramedullary spinal cord tumor in adults, representing 6% to 8% of intradural tumors. In children, they are the most common histologic type of intramedullary tumors, accounting for 60% to 90% of these lesions.[8,52] Patients harboring astrocytomas present most commonly with pain, motor weakness, and gait ataxia that can either be of long duration or of relatively brief onset before presentation.[10,53] The average symptom duration before presentation is between 12 and 29 months. Astrocytomas of the spinal cord are infiltrative tumors that are often eccentrically located dorsal or lateral to the central canal. Large tumors can expand and rotate the cord, making identification of landmarks difficult during surgery.[12] On MRI, astrocytomas have intermediate T1 signal intensity, can demonstrate heterogeneous or homogeneous T1-weighted contrast enhancement, often contain cystic areas, and can rarely grow exophytically into the extramedullary space. The tumor boundaries may be better identified on T2 sequences (Fig. 90.7). In contrast to ependymomas, spinal astrocytomas infiltrate functional cord, have ill-defined borders with normal cord, and are consequently more difficult to remove successfully. Fortunately, intramedullary astrocytomas in adults are largely low grade (WHO grade I and II) with approximately 25% considered high grade (Kernohan grade III and IV). In children, in whom pilocytic astrocytomas predominate, high-grade lesions are even less common, occurring at a rate of 10% to 15%.

Hemangioblastomas

Hemangioblastomas represent 2% to 6% of intramedullary spinal cord tumors and approximately one-third are associated with von Hippel-Lindau disease (VHL).[54,55] Spontaneous hemangioblastomas are usually solitary, but patients with VHL can harbor multiple hemangioblastomas, especially in the posterior fossa.[55] Patients who present with hemangioblastoma in the spinal column should be evaluated for lesions associated with VHL including the presence of other hemangioblastomas in the neural axis, retinal hemangioblastoma, renal/adrenal lesions, and less commonly endolymphatic sac tumors. Hemangioblastomas have a 2 : 1 male-to-female predominance and usually become symptomatic in the third to fourth decades of life. Because of their predilection for the dorsal cord, numerous patients present with posterior column dysfunction or experience it after surgery. Histologically, these tumors consist of a vascular tuft surrounded by pale stromal cells, and there is often an associated cyst that accounts for much of the tumor volume. Radiographically, the tumors can be predominantly cystic masses with a small enhancing nodule of tumor cells located on the cyst wall or a solid homogeneously enhancing mass (Fig. 90.8). They are predominantly dorsal or dorsolaterally located and often grow to and expand the pial surface of the cord. Up to 89% have an associated syrinx that always resolves after tumor removal.[45,55] Treatment of spinal hemangioblastomas is surgical resection. Removal of these tumors carries the lowest surgical morbidity and best neurologic outcomes of all the intramedullary tumors.

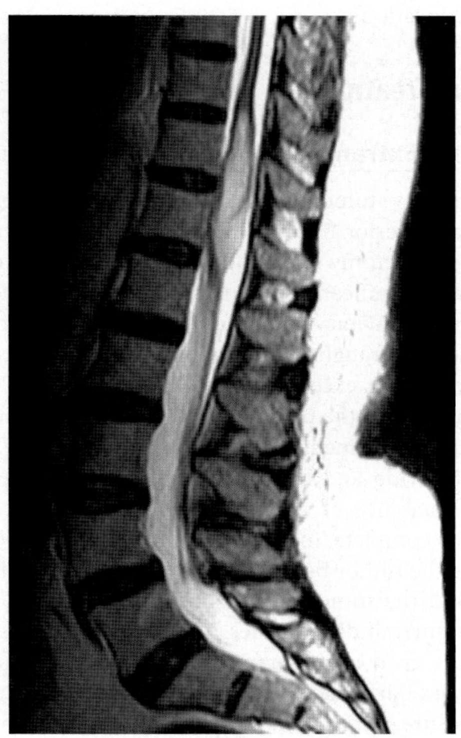

FIG. 90.7 Sagittal T2-weighted magnetic resonance image showing an astrocytoma with high signal expanding the spinal cord and conus medullaris.

Less Common Intramedullary Lesions

Lipomas

True intramedullary lipomas are rare lesions composed of metabolically normal fat cells ectopically deposited within the cord during embryologic development. Patients typically present in their 20s to 40s complaining of indolent neurologic symptoms that can rapidly progress over several months.[56] MRI is diagnostic, and the tumor signal follows that of normal fat. Treatment of symptomatic lesions is internal debulking to relieve symptoms.[57] Complete excision is difficult due to poor dissection planes, and delayed recurrence is common.

An expansile duraplasty may be helpful during dural closure to create more room in the spinal canal around the tumor site and delay compressive symptoms in the event of tumor recurrence.

Dermoid and Epidermoid Cysts

These tumors arise from an anomalous deposition of ectodermal cells during embryonic neural tube closure, but some cases have been linked to epidural cells implanted into the lumbar canal during lumbar puncture.[58] Patients present in the second to fourth decades with typical neurologic complaints of intramedullary masses; however, acute presentations secondary to aseptic

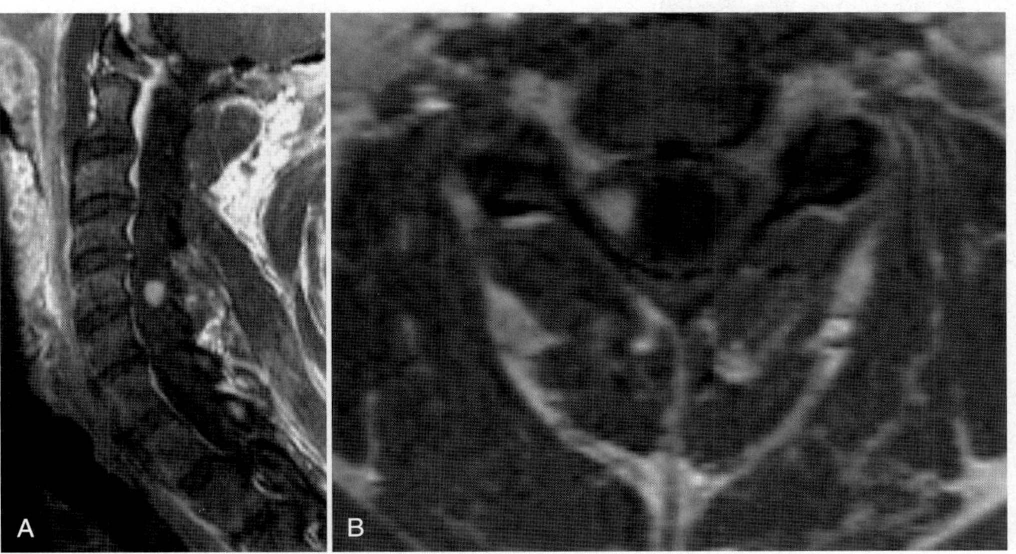

FIG. 90.8 (A) Sagittal T1-weighted contrast-enhanced image of a cervical hemangioblastoma showing a well-defined homogeneously enhancing mass. (B) An axial T1-weighted, contrast-enhanced MRI sequence of the same tumor revealing a large central cyst with a typical small, enhancing peripheral nodule.

meningitis or abscess formation have been reported.[59,60] Optimal treatment is complete surgical excision, but the cyst wall is often adherent to the spinal cord substance and incomplete resections are often performed with low recurrence rates.[61,62] Again, expansile duraplasty can be helpful after resection to delay symptoms in the event of a recurrence.

Cavernous Angiomas

These lesions are not tumors but rather are angiographically occult vascular malformations composed of tightly packed venous-like channels without intervening neural tissue. They represent 1% to 3% of intramedullary spinal cord lesions. Spinal cord cavernomas can be asymptomatic, present with slow stepwise decline of neurologic function due to small hemorrhages, or present as an acute neurologic deterioration from a larger bleed.[61] Most cavernomas are well-defined single lesions, some have ectopic portions nearly invisible under the pial surface, and rarely they are multiple. Cavernomas are best seen on T2-weighted MRI sequences, often have a mulberry-like appearance, and do not enhance (Fig. 90.9). Patients with symptomatic lesions should undergo surgical excision to prevent neurologic morbidity from future bleeds.[63]

Metastasis

The spinal cord parenchyma is a rare site of metastasis for systemic cancer and may occur in patients with extensive disseminated disease. The most common tumors that metastasize to the spinal cord are lung cancer (54%), breast cancer (14%), and melanoma (9%).[64,65] These patients generally have a grim prognosis related to their primary disease; however, surgical excision of cord lesions should be considered in those with radioresistant tumors and in those with a low systemic burden of disease who have symptomatic, surgically accessible solitary lesions.[66] Surgical excision of these lesions is also indicated in cases in which there is rapid neurologic decline in a surgically accessible location.

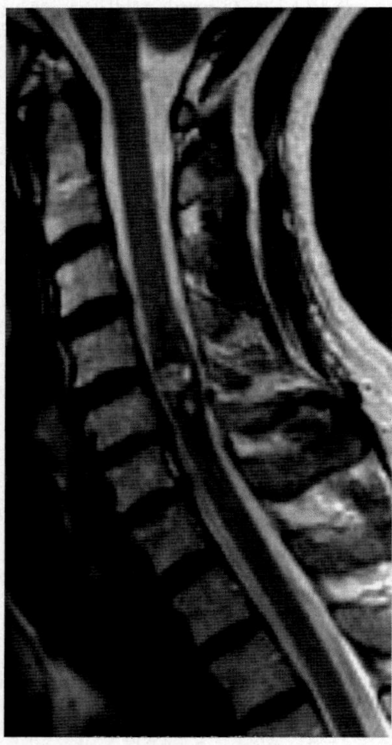

FIG. 90.9 Sagittal T2-weighted magnetic resonance image of a cervical cavernoma with heterogeneous signal characteristics and suggestion of a surrounding hemosiderin ring (low T2 signal).

Surgical Treatment

Intradural Extramedullary Tumors

Extramedullary tumors are almost exclusively approached through a posterior midline approach. Anterior tumors may require a facetectomy for adequate tumor exposure; dumbbell tumors with significant extraspinal extension may necessitate a lateral extracavitary approach.[67] Purely anterior surgical approaches are fraught with high complication rates and are necessary only in exceptional cases. To perform a posterior midline approach, the patient is positioned prone and a laminectomy is performed. The laminectomy usually does not need to be wide and the facets are spared to preserve the structural stability of that bony segment. When the bony exposure is complete, intraoperative ultrasound can be useful to localize the tumor before dural opening.[68] Once the dura is opened and the tumor is visualized, the tumor is dissected from the surrounding tissues. Care must be taken not to damage the cord parenchyma by excessive manipulation or damage vascular structures compromising cord blood flow. After exposure, removal may be performed en bloc, piecemeal, or with ultrasonic cavitation for internal debulking and, finally, capsule removal. After tumor resection, the spinal cord should be carefully dissected from arachnoid adhesions to the dura that often develop with chronic cord compression and local inflammation. In general, the goal of surgery is maximal tumor removal without neurologic injury. However, some extramedullary tumors force a decision between sacrificing the parent nerve root for complete tumor removal versus subtotal resection with root preservation. This decision is usually based on function of the involved root, tumor pathology, and tumor characteristics.

Meningiomas are abnormal dural outgrowths that push the spinal cord away from the dural attachment zone. These tumors are usually removed by cautery of the capsule, internal debulking, release of the dural attachment to free the tumor, and, finally, excision of the dural attachment zone. En plaque, infiltrating, and calcified tumors may be more challenging to remove due to cord adherence, heavy calcification, and involvement of tumor with cord blood supply. These tumors may not be amenable to complete resection. Complete tumor removal requires excision of the dural attachment zone and application of a dural patch graft. However, when complete removal is not possible, the surgeon may perform a partial dural dissection or coagulation of the attachment zone to maximize tumor cell removal in the setting of a subtotal resection. Recent series suggest that Simpson grade II/III resection in high-risk settings should be considered to avoid morbidity from aggressive surgical resection.[69–71]

Nerve sheath tumor removal is dependent on tumor location and characteristics. Most schwannomas are dorsolateral and easily accessed, but more anteriorly located or dumbbell tumors with paraspinal extension may require extended posterolateral exposures.[67] Most nerve sheath tumor capsules are adherent to the arachnoid of the nerve root, and this layer must be incised to reach the lesion. The capsule is generally cauterized to shrink and decrease vascular input to the tumor; then, the tumor–nerve root attachment can be visualized. Piecemeal tumor removal or internal debulking with an ultrasonic aspirator should be used with large tumors. Nerve root sacrifice may be required due to tumor inside the root of large tumors encasing it. However, the incidence of permanent neurologic deficit from transection of a tumor-enveloped root is lower than might be expected, usually due to poor preoperative function of the root secondary to the tumor.[72,73] Care must be taken to carefully assess root function and weigh the benefit of complete tumor removal against loss of function before and during surgery.

Ependymomas of the filum terminale are variable in size and degree of involvement with the cauda equina. Smaller ependymomas should be resected in toto if possible to avoid CSF tumor seeding. Larger encapsulated tumors should be carefully debulked with CSF suction and surgical adjuncts placed around the tumor to decrease tumor dissemination. Tumors filling the lumbosacral spinal canal usually lack a discernable capsule and tend to infiltrate the conus and cauda equina nerve roots, making complete resection difficult. In these cases, care should be taken to maximally debulk the tumor without injuring the enveloped neural structures. Expansile duraplasty can be useful, especially in these extensive tumors, to enlarge the spinal canal and delay symptom recurrence if the tumor regrows. If a postoperative CSF leak is anticipated or encountered, a C1–C2 CSF diversion drain can be placed with fluoroscopic guidance and prevent the need for lumbar drain placement at the surgical site.

Intramedullary Tumors

The role of surgery in the treatment of intramedullary spinal cord tumors has expanded considerably in recent decades. With the advent of the operative microscope, MRI, ultrasonic aspiration, and electrophysiologic monitoring, experienced surgeons can now safely remove or greatly debulk most intramedullary lesions. Neuroprotection is an important consideration during spinal cord tumor surgery, and perioperative steroids are commonly employed. Recently, intraoperative hypothermia using intravenous cooling catheter systems has emerged as a potential neuroprotective adjunct during spinal tumor surgery. Our 4-year experience with intraoperative hypothermia has found it to be safe (unpublished data), but randomized controlled trials will ultimately be necessary to judge its efficacy. Surgery is nearly always performed through a posterior midline approach with laminectomy at the tumor level as well as one level above and one below. Ultrasound can be useful to confirm the tumor location and confirm that it is within the limits of the bony exposure.[68,74] Then, a midline dural incision is made. With the aid of an operative microscope, the midline is identified and a myelotomy is made in the posterior median sulcus. Of note, the midline is often difficult to identify with larger tumors due to an expanded and often rotated cord, but the midpoint between dorsal root entry zones can be used as a rough estimate of the midline in such cases. The myelotomy is deepened until the tumor is identified; then, the resection is guided by the presence or absence of a dissection plane between the tumor and cord parenchyma. Intraoperative frozen sections can be helpful if suspicion is high for an unusual diagnosis, such as demyelinating disease or metastasis; however, frozen sections can be unreliable in differentiating between astrocytomas and ependymomas. Tumor resection is performed to the maximal extent possible while avoiding neurologic injury.

Ependymomas are centrally located, smooth, red-gray, well-demarcated lesions that often have cystic areas at their superior and inferior limits. When the cord is exposed, small blood vessels are commonly seen running across the tumor surface. There is usually a good cleavage plane between tumor and cord, and they can be removed completely in 70% to 95% of cases.[75,76] Smaller tumors can often be removed in one piece by gentle capsule dissection and light bipolar coagulation to shrink the mass. Larger tumors must be internally decompressed and then the capsule carefully dissected from the cord. The final removal is often achieved by gentle retraction of the superior tumor pole and cauterization of the last arterial feeders. At this point, a common surgical error is to aggressively resect a layer of slightly discolored but ultimately functional tissue that can surround the tumor at the parenchyma-tumor interface. Resection should not continue past obvious tumor into the glial tissue to avoid unnecessary neurologic injury.

Astrocytomas are generally low-grade infiltrating tumors that tend to be asymmetrically located in the spinal cord. Intraoperatively, the tumor appears grossly different than cord parenchyma, but most often tumor cells infiltrate functional cord tissue, preventing the development of a safe dissection plane. This makes complete tumor resection hazardous. Some authors have argued for aggressive resection of low-grade astrocytomas, but there is an unclear relationship between extent of resection and survival. Therefore, resection of obvious tumor without risking neurologic deterioration is recommended.[10,51,74,77] Patients harboring high-grade astrocytomas have poor prognosis regardless of the degree of tumor removal, and resection of high-grade lesions is typically conservative. Several long-term survivals have been reported in grade IV astrocytoma patients with tumors below T1, including two patients in the senior author's (B.A.G.) personal series.[74,78]

Hemangioblastomas are highly vascular, well-demarcated, often cystic lesions that can rise to the dorsal surface of the spinal cord. These tumors are extremely vascular; thus, the superficial and deep arterial supply should always be interrupted and the capsule shrunken away from the cord with bipolar coagulation before the tumor is entered or removed. Entering the capsule before interrupting the tumor arterial feeders risks a large hemorrhage. Hemangioblastomas should be completely resected because residual tumors will lead to a recurrence. Preoperative embolization has been advocated by some authors but is not commonly performed because most feeders are surgically accessible.[79]

Radiation/Chemotherapy/Adjuvant Treatments

Intradural Extramedullary Tumors

Surgical excision is first-line therapy for extramedullary intradural tumors, with radiation and chemotherapy being rarely indicated for benign pathologies. Adjunctive radiation therapy and chemotherapy is typically reserved for World Health Organization grades III and IV extramedullary tumors. Radiotherapy for spinal atypical meningiomas (WHO grade II) also should be reserved for tumor progression/ recurrence as gross total resection only seems to provide adequate tumor control.[80] Fractionated radiation is not routinely used for extramedullary low-grade lesions, but some authors advocate radiation for residual or recurrent large filum terminale ependymomas.[81] Radiosurgery, however, has recently been proposed as an alternative to surgery for poor surgical candidates harboring low-grade lesions.[82] The studies are small, and follow-up is brief. Delayed radiation-induced spinal cord toxicity is a feared complication of spinal cord radiotherapy; more follow-up data are necessary to determine its safety, which is of vital importance when treating benign pathologies.[82,83]

Recently, image-guided laser interstitial thermal therapy has also been proposed to control epidural metastases. Laser interstitial thermal therapy (LITT) works by introducing a catheter into the lesion that delivers controlled thermal energy into the lesion to allow for tumor necrosis prior to adjuvant stereotactic radiosurgery.[84] However, theoretically, LITT may pose more risks in the spinal cord than the brain; LITT ablates the tumors in close proximity to the spinal cord and does not reduce tumor mass effect immediately. Nevertheless, LITT remains a potential option for metastatic epidural disease and may be tested for malignant intradural pathologies in the near future.

Intramedullary Tumors

Gross total resection is the treatment of choice for most common intramedullary pathologies, with radiation and chemotherapy having limited roles. Chemotherapy regimens are generally reserved for high-grade lesions and typically mirror the regimens given for intracranial tumors of the same pathology. New-generation intrathecal pumps can deliver measured doses of chemotherapy directly to the intrathecal space, and intrathecal chemotherapy regimens are being explored.

Ependymomas are generally amenable to safe, complete removal with low recurrence rates. MRI is a noninvasive method for monitoring for tumor regrowth or seeding of the subarachnoid space and can obviate the need for early radiation after surgery. Radiation may be indicated in the setting of a malignant ependymoma or when a significant portion of a tumor cannot be resected.[85,86]

Intramedullary astrocytomas are typically low-grade tumors treated by surgical resection and monitored for recurrence by clinical and radiographic follow-up. In the setting of subtotal tumor removal, some authors have advocated radiation to the residual tumor, but there is no compelling evidence that radiotherapy alters the natural history.[74,87] Patients with grade III astrocytomas may be candidates for adjunctive radiation and chemotherapy.[88] Malignant astrocytomas of the spinal cord, however, have a poor prognosis and radical resection results in high morbidity; therefore, conservative tumor removal for tissue diagnosis followed by radiation therapy is common practice.[74,89] Alternatively, one group has reported extended survival times for malignant astrocytoma patients treated with radiocordectomy, and long-term survival for spinal cord grade IV astrocytomas has been reported after surgical cordectomy, including two long-term survivals in the senior author's personal series (unpublished).[78,90]

Stereotactic radiosurgery for intramedullary tumors has been described in small studies with brief follow-up.[91,92] In the future, this treatment strategy may prove useful in select cases in which complete surgical excision is not possible or after multiple recurrences. However, more studies are necessary to determine safety and long-term efficacy, especially in light of the proven success of surgery and the low-grade pathologies of most intramedullary tumors.

Outcomes

Intradural Extramedullary Tumors

The surgical morbidity and mortality in the removal of extramedullary tumors is low while the neurologic prognosis is generally good. Postoperative neurologic function is generally predicted by the preoperative neurologic status, patient age, and duration of symptoms.[20,26,31] In one large series of intradural extramedullary tumors, there was a 12.3% rate of postoperative neurologic worsening, but most deficits were transient and only 2.3% of the patients had a permanent postoperative loss of function.[10] Overall, intradural extramedullary tumors have a recurrence rate of 8.9% to 32% at 5 years, with the strongest predictors of recurrence being histologic grade and previous surgical resection.[93] Meningiomas have a 4% to 8% long-term recurrence rate after gross total resection with higher-grade tumors recurring more frequently. After surgery, recovery of neurologic deficits is common, with 80% to 90% of patients showing improvement of preoperative neurologic deficits.[28] In the absence of NF2, the recurrence rate for schwannomas is 6% to 12%, but in patients with neurofibromatosis, it is increased fourfold.[93,94] Completely resected neurofibromas recur in approximately 12% of patients.[95] Intradural malignant nerve sheath tumors are rare but must be managed aggressively, as outcomes are generally poor with a 5-year survival rate of 44%. Tumors that stain negative for S-100 tend to be more aggressive and recur more quickly.[96] A recent review suggests that extent of resection in patients with intradural spinal nerve sheath tumors remains one of the most important prognostic factors for patients, while presence of neurofibromatosis and cervical tumors was associated with higher rates of recurrence.[97] Large filum terminale ependymomas have a high recurrence rate. Even after gross total resection, the recurrence rate is up to 20% and patients may need multiple operations for revision debulking.[37,67]

Intramedullary Tumors

The neurologic morbidity for intramedullary tumor removal is significantly higher than for extramedullary tumors. Preoperative neurologic status is the number one predictor of postoperative functional status, but other factors—such as aggressive tumor pathology and thoracic location—also portend worse functional outcomes.[98,99] Up to 57% of postsurgical patients experience a transient neurologic worsening, but only 10% to 20% are left with a new permanent deficit.[10,51] Dorsal column dysfunction is common after midline myelotomy.[42] Despite the new deficits, however, most patients recover to baseline functional status within 1 year.[10]

After complete resection, ependymomas have good neurologic outcomes, low recurrence rates, and long survival times.[47,85] Tumors that are not completely resected tend to have less improvement in function and higher recurrence rates.[10,75,93,100] Survival rates at 5 years are reported to be between 83% and 95% for postoperative intramedullary ependymoma patients.[51,101]

Astrocytomas are more difficult to completely remove surgically and have a higher recurrence rate. Astrocytoma patients have shorter survival times than those harboring ependymomas. Extent of tumor resection seems to modestly affect local recurrence rates, but this has not been conclusively demonstrated in the literature.[10,12,98] The 5-year survival rate has been reported to be 63% to 77% for grade I and II tumors and 27% for grade III and IV tumors.[74] Median survival for high-grade lesions is around 1 year, with grade IV tumors having a particularly poor prognosis.[102–104]

Hemangioblastomas are amenable to complete resection, have low surgical morbidity, and have low recurrence rates.[105–107] The presence or absence of VHL seems to have little impact on outcomes. Intramedullary hemangioblastoma patients experience the lowest surgical morbidity and the best neurologic prognosis of all the common intramedullary spinal cord tumors.

Summary

Technical advances in diagnostic modalities—such as MRI and operative adjuncts such as the operating microscope, bipolar cautery, neurophysiologic monitoring, intraoperative ultrasound, and ultrasonic cavitation—have ushered in the modern renaissance of surgical treatment of spinal tumors. In the near future, advances in the area of intraoperative neuroprotection—including meticulous intraoperative blood pressure control, steroids, and modest hypothermia (33°C)—may prove to lower surgical morbidity. The goal of surgery for intradural tumors is maximal tumor removal with minimal neurologic morbidity. Yet, even after gross total removal, a cure is not guaranteed and recurrences are common. The continued evolution of surgical tools, emergence of new biologic therapies, and development of adjunctive technologies will undoubtedly shape the future of the diagnosis and treatment of intradural spinal cord tumors. However, it remains the surgeon's careful preoperative assessment, tailored surgical strategies for each individual patient, and a well-executed tumor removal that define effective spinal tumor surgery.

PEARLS

1. A patient's postoperative neurologic status is most strongly predicted by his or her preoperative neurologic status.
2. MRI with and without contrast is the preferred imaging technique for investigating intradural tumors.
3. When assessing an intradural tumor on imaging, first determine if it is intramedullary or extramedullary by noting whether it displaces the spinal cord or is within and expands it. Then, create a differential diagnosis on the basis of imaging characteristics of the lesion, age of the patient, and clinical history and physical examination.
4. Patients with multiple neurofibromas or multiple hemangioblastomas should be investigated for the presence of NF1 and VHL disease, respectively.
5. Complete removal of a hemangioblastoma will be followed by resolution of the associated syrinx.

PITFALLS

1. Schwannomas arise from the nerve root, whereas neurofibromas infiltrate it; therefore, nerve root sacrifice is necessary for complete removal of neurofibromas but rarely for schwannomas.
2. Intramedullary astrocytoma tumor cells typically infiltrate functional nervous tissue, creating an indistinct tumor-cord border. Achieving true gross total resection can result in neural injury.
3. When removing a cystic hemangioblastoma, always completely remove the enhancing nodule or the tumor will recur.
4. Care should be taken not to create an unnecessarily wide laminectomy to prevent postoperative kyphosis.
5. Patients with spinal metastasis often have disseminated primary cancer and carry a poor overall prognosis.

KEY POINTS

1. Preoperative MRI with contrast is essential for formulating a differential diagnosis and an appropriate surgical plan.
2. Intradural extramedullary tumors account for approximately two-thirds of intradural tumors, are typically benign, and can usually be completely excised. With nerve sheath tumors, functional status of the involved nerve root function is important if root sacrifice might be necessary for complete resection.
3. Intramedullary tumors are less common and usually benign but carry a greater risk of iatrogenic neurologic morbidity with surgical excision. Intraoperatively, careful observance of the tumor-parenchyma border is important for safe removal of intramedullary tumors.
4. Intradural spinal tumors are nearly always approached via a standard posterior midline approach. However, intradural extramedullary tumors with extensive lateral extraspinal growth may require an extended posterolateral approach.

5. Survival and recurrence rates for intraspinal tumors are heavily influenced by tumor grade and extent of resection.
6. Surgical resection is the preferred treatment for intradural tumors. Radiation and chemotherapy are used in a secondary role to aid in the treatment of recurrence or residual tumor that is not amenable to resection.

KEY REFERENCES

1. Horsley V, Gowers WR. A case of tumors of the spinal cord: removal-recovery. *Med Chir Trans.* 1888;71:377-428.
   This is the first description of a successful intradural tumor removal.
2. Elsberg CA, Beer E. The operability of intramedullary tumors of the spinal cord: a report of two operations with remarks upon the extrusion of intraspinal tumors. *Am J Med Sci.* 1911;142:636-647.
   Early published cases of successful intramedullary spinal cord tumor removal with discussion of safe surgical techniques and second-stage surgery.
3. Elsberg CA. Tumors of the spinal cord and the symptoms of irritation and compression of the spinal cord and nerve roots. In: Elsberg CA, ed. *Pathology, Symptomatology, Diagnosis and Treatment.* New York: Paul B. Hoeber; 1925:206-239.
   A landmark book describing Elsberg's large early spinal tumor removal experience.
4. Greenwood J Jr. Intramedullary tumors of spinal cord. A follow-up study after total surgical removal. *J Neurosurg.* 1963;20:665-668.
   A follow-up of a series of successfully removed spinal cord tumors with an argument for the feasibility, safety, and efficacy of careful tumor removal.
5. Klekamp J, Samii M. *Surgery of Spinal Tumors.* New York: Springer; 2007.
   A detailed description and analysis of a large modern spinal tumor surgical experience.

REFERENCES

1. Gowers WR, Horsley V. A case of tumour of the spinal cord. removal; recovery. *Med Chir Trans.* 1888;71(1):377-428.
2. von Eiselsberg AF, Ranzi E. Über die chirurgische Behandlung der Hirnund Rückenmarkstumoren. *Arch Klin Chir.* 1913;102:309-468.
3. Elsberg CA, Beer E. A report of two operations, with remarks upon the extrusion of intraspinal tumors. *Am J Med Sci.* 1911;142(5):636-647.
4. Elsberg CA. Tumors of the spinal cord. The symptoms of irritation and compression of the spinal cord and nerve roots. Pathology, symptomatology, diagnosis and treatment. *JAMA.* 1925;85(6):460.
5. Wood EH, Berne AS, Taveras JM. The value of radiation therapy in the management of intrinsic tumors of the spinal cord. *Radiology.* 1954;63(1):11-24.
6. Greenwood J. Intramedullary tumors of spinal cord. *J Neurosurg.* 1963;20(8):665-668.
7. Cooper PR, Epstein F. Radical resection of intramedullary spinal cord tumors in adults. *J Neurosurg.* 1985;63(4):492-499.
8. Helseth A, Mørk SJ. Primary intraspinal neoplasms in Norway, 1955 to 1986. *J Neurosurg.* 1989;71(6):842-845.
9. Sasanelli F, Beghi E, Kurland LT. Primary intraspinal neoplasms in Rochester, Minnesota, 1935–1981. *Neuroepidemiology.* 1983;2(3-4):156-163.
10. Klekamp J. *Surgery of Spinal Tumors.* New York: Springer; 2007.
11. Miller DC. Surgical pathology of intramedullary spinal cord neoplasms. *J Neurooncol.* 2000;47(3):189-194.
12. Cooper PR. Outcome after operative treatment of intramedullary spinal cord tumors in adults: intermediate and long-term results in 51 patients. *Neurosurgery.* 1989;25(6):855-859.
13. McGuire RA, Brown MD, Green BA. Intradural spinal tumors and spinal stenosis. *Spine.* 1987;12(10):1062-1066.
14. El-Mahdy P, et al. Spinal intradural tumours: part I-extramedullary. *Br J Neurosurg.* 1999;13(6):550-557.
15. Kane WE, et al. Spinal intradural tumours: part II-intramedullary. *Br J Neurosurg.* 1999;13(6):558-563.
16. Quintero-Wolfe S, Green BA, Wang MY. Surgical treatment of non-traumatic myelopathies. In: Lin VW, ed. *Spinal Cord Medicine: Principles and Practice.* 2nd ed. Demos Medical Publishing; 2010.
17. Gezen F, Kahraman S, Çanakci Z, Bedük A. Review of 36 cases of spinal cord meningioma. *Spine.* 2000;25(6):727-731.
18. Seppälä MT, Haltia MJJ, Sankila RJ, Jääskeläinen JE, Heiskanen O. Long-term outcome after removal of spinal schwannoma: a clinicopathological study of 187 cases. *J Neurosurg.* 1995;83(4):621-626.
19. Green BA, Eismont FJ, Klose KJ. Management of cervical cord lesions including advances in rehabilitative engineering. In: Camins MB, O'Leary PF, eds. *Disorders of the Cervical Spine.* Baltimore: Williams & Wilkins; 1992.
20. McCormick PC, Post KD, Stein BM. Intradural extramedullary tumors in adults. *Neurosurg Clin N Am.* 1990;1(3):591-608.
21. Green BA, Diaz RD, Post MJ. The diagnosis of spinal column and spinal cord tumors with emphasis on the value of computed tomography. In: Post J, ed. *Computed Tomography of the Spine.* Baltimore: Williams & Wilkins; 1984.
22. Jea A, Green BA. Syringomyelia. In: Herkowitz RS, ed. *The Spine.* Philidelphia: Elsevier; 2007.
23. Gaetani P, Di Ieva A, Colombo P, et al. Intradural spinal metastasis of renal clear cell carcinoma causing cauda equina syndrome. *Acta Neurochir (Wien).* 2004;146(8):857-861.
24. Lee E, Lee HY, Choe G, et al. Extraskeletal intraspinal mesenchymal chondrosarcoma; 18F-FDG PET/CT finding. *Clin Nucl Med.* 2014;39(1):e64-e66.
25. Nguyen BD, Fletcher GP, Patel AC. PET/CT imaging of conus medullaris metastasis from lung cancer. *Clin Nucl Med.* 2005;30(4):253-256.
26. Roux F-X, Nataf F, Pinaudeau M, et al. Intraspinal meningiomas: review of 54 cases with discussion of poor prognosis factors and modern therapeutic management. *Surg Neurol.* 1996;46(5):458-464.
27. Solero CL, Fornari M, Giombini S, et al. Spinal meningiomas: review of 174 operated cases. *Neurosurgery.* 1989;25(2):153-160.
28. Levy WJ, Bay J, Dohn D. Spinal cord meningioma. *J Neurosurg.* 1982;57(6):804-812.
29. Nittner K. Spinal meningiomas, neurinomas, and neurofibromas and hourglass tumors. In: Vinken P, Bruyn B, eds. *Handbook of Clinical Neurology.* New York: Elsevier; 1976:177-322.
30. Caroli E, Acqui M, Roperto R, et al. Spinal en plaque meningiomas: a contemporary experience. *Neurosurgery.* 2004;1275-1279.
31. Levy WJ, Latchaw J, Hahn JF, et al. Spinal neurofibromas: a report of 66 cases and a comparison with meningiomas. *Neurosurgery.* 1986;18(3):331-334.
32. McClatchey AI. Neurofibromatosis. *Annu Rev Pathol Mech Dis.* 2007;2(1):191-216.

33. McCormick PC. Surgical management of dumbbell tumors of the cervical spine. *Neurosurgery*. 1996;38(2):294-300.
34. Seppälä MT, Haltia MJJ. Spinal malignant nerve-sheath tumor or cellular schwannoma? A striking difference in prognosis. *J Neurosurg*. 1993;79(4):528-532.
35. Celli P, Cervoni L, Cantore G. Ependymoma of the filum terminale: treatment and prognostic factors in a series of 28 cases. *Acta Neurochir (Wien)*. 1993;124(2-4):99-103.
36. Schweitzer JS, Batzdorf U. Ependymoma of the cauda equina region. *Neurosurgery*. 1992;30(2):202-207.
37. Sonneland PRL, Scheithauer BW, Onofrio BM. Myxopapillary ependymoma. A clinicopathologic and immunocytochemical study of 77 cases. *Cancer*. 1985;56(4):883-893.
38. Kumar K, Malik S, Schulte PA. Symptomatic spinal arachnoid cysts: report of two cases with review of the literature. *Spine*. 2003;28(2):E25-E29.
39. Song JK, Musleh W, Christie SD, Fessler RG. Cervical juxtafacet cysts: case report and literature review. *Spine J*. 2006;6(3):279-281.
40. Boviatsis EJ, Staurinou LC, Kouyialis AT, et al. Spinal synovial cysts: pathogenesis, diagnosis and surgical treatment in a series of seven cases and literature review. *Eur Spine J*. 2008;17(6):831-837.
41. Lyons MK, Atkinson JLD, Wharen RE, et al. Surgical evaluation and management of lumbar synovial cysts: the Mayo Clinic experience. *J Neurosurg Spine*. 2000;93(1):53-57.
42. Manzano G, Green BA, Vanni S, Levi AD. Contemporary management of adult intramedullary spinal tumors—pathology and neurological outcomes related to surgical resection. *Spinal Cord*. 2008;46(8):540-546.
43. Ebert C, von Haken M, Meyer-Puttlitz B, et al. Molecular genetic analysis of ependymal tumors. *Am J Pathol*. 1999;155(2):627-632.
44. Lee M, Rezai AR, Freed D, Epstein FJ. Intramedullary spinal cord tumors in neurofibromatosis. *Neurosurgery*. 1996;38(1):32-37.
45. Samii M, Klekamp J. Surgical results of 100 intramedullary tumors in relation to accompanying syringomyelia. *Neurosurgery*. 1994;35(5):865-873.
46. Epstein FJ, Farmer J-P, Freed D. Adult intramedullary spinal cord ependymomas: the result of surgery in 38 patients. *J Neurosurg*. 1993;79(2):204-209.
47. McCormick PC, Torres R, Post KD, Stein BM. Intramedullary ependymoma of the spinal cord. *J Neurosurg*. 1990;72(4):523-532.
48. Lowe GM. Magnetic resonance imaging of intramedullary spinal cord tumors. *J Neurooncol*. 2000;47(3):195-210.
49. Mørk SJ, Løken AC. Ependymoma. A follow-up study of 101 cases. *Cancer*. 1977;40(2):907-915.
50. Nadeem SQ, Feun LG, Bruce-Gregorios JH, Green B. Post radiation sarcoma (malignant fibrous histiocytoma) of the cervical spine following ependymoma (a case report). *J Neurooncol*. 1991;11(3):263-268.
51. Raco A, Esposito V, Lenzi J, et al. Long-term follow-up of intramedullary spinal cord tumors: a series of 202 cases. *Neurosurgery*. 2005;56(5):972-981.
52. Reimer R, Onofrio BM. Astrocytomas of the spinal cord in children and adolescents. *J Neurosurg*. 1985;63(5):669-675.
53. Kim MS, Chung CK, Choe G, Kim IH, Kim HJ. Intramedullary spinal cord astrocytoma in adults: postoperative outcome. *J Neurooncol*. 2001;52(1):85-94.
54. Lee DK, Choe WJ, Chung CK, Kim HJ. Spinal cord hemangioblastoma: surgical strategy and clinical outcome. *J Neurooncol*. 2003;61(1):27-34.
55. Lonser RR, Weil RJ, Wanebo JE, Devroom HL, Oldfield EH. Surgical management of spinal cord hemangioblastomas in patients with von Hippel–Lindau disease. *J Neurosurg*. 2003;98(1):106-116.
56. Lee M, Rezai AR, Abbott R, Coelho DH, Epstein FJ. Intramedullary spinal cord lipomas. *J Neurosurg*. 1995; 82(3):394-400.
57. Dyck P. Intramedullary lipoma. *Spine*. 1992;17(8):979-980.
58. Halcrow SJ, Crawford PJ, Craft AW. Epidermoid spinal cord tumour after lumbar puncture. *Arch Dis Child*. 1985;60(10):978-979.
59. Çokça F, Meço O, Arasil E, Ünlü A. An intramedullary dermoid cyst abscess due to *Brucella abortus* biotype 3 at T11-L2 spinal levels. *Infection*. 1994;22(5):359-360.
60. de Baecque C, Snyder DH, Suzuki K. Congenital intramedullary spinal dermoid cyst associated with an Arnold-Chiari malformation. *Acta Neuropathol*. 1977;38(3):239-242.
61. Deutsch H, Jallo GI, Faktorovich A, Epstein F. Spinal intramedullary cavernoma: clinical presentation and surgical outcome. *J Neurosurg Spine*. 2000;93(1):65-70.
62. Lunardi P, Missori P, Gagliardi FM, Fortuna A. Long-term results of the surgical treatment of spinal dermoid and epidermoid tumors. *Neurosurgery*. 1989;25(6):860-864.
63. Ojemann RG, Crowell RM, Ogilvy CS. Management of cranial and spinal cavernous angiomas (honored guest lecture). *Clin Neurosurg*. 1993;40:98-123.
64. Mut M, Schiff D, Shaffrey ME. Metastasis to nervous system: spinal epidural and intramedullary metastases. *J Neurooncol*. 2005;75(1):43-56.
65. Post MJ, Quencer RM, Green BA, et al. Intramedullary spinal cord metastases, mainly of nonneurogenic origin. *AJR Am J Roentgenol*. 1987;148(5):1015-1022.
66. Connolly ES Jr, Winfree CJ, McCormick PC, Cruz M, Stein BM. Intramedullary spinal cord metastasis: report of three cases and review of the literature. *Surg Neurol*. 1996;46(4):329-337.
67. Steck JC, Dietze DD, Fessler RG. Posterolateral approach to intradural extramedullary thoracic tumors. *J Neurosurg*. 1994;81(2):202-205.
68. Quencer RM, Montalvo BM, Green BA, Eismont FJ. Intraoperative spinal sonography of soft-tissue masses of the spinal cord and spinal canal. *AJR Am J Roentgenol*. 1984;143(6):1307-1315.
69. Kim CH, Chung CK, Lee SH, et al. Long-term recurrence rates after the removal of spinal meningiomas in relation to Simpson grades. *Eur Spine J*. 2015;25(12):4025-4032.
70. Bostrom A, Burgel U, Reinacher P, et al. A less invasive surgical concept for the resection of spinal meningiomas. *Acta Neurochir (Wien)*. 2008;150(6):551-556.
71. Tsuda K, Akutsu H, Yamamoto T, et al. Is Simpson grade I removal necessary in all cases of spinal meningioma? Assessment of postoperative recurrence during long-term follow-up. *Neurol Med Chir (Tokyo)*. 2014;54(11):907-913.
72. Lot G, George B. Cervical neuromas with extradural components: surgical management in a series of 57 patients. *Neurosurgery*. 1997;41(4):813-822.
73. McCormick PC. Anatomic principles of intradural spinal surgery. *Clin Neurosurg*. 1994;41:204-223.

74. Epstein FJ, Farmer J-P, Freed D. Adult intramedullary astrocytomas of the spinal cord. *J Neurosurg.* 1992;77(3):355-359.
75. Chang UK, Choe WJ, Chung SK, Chung CK, Kim HJ. Surgical outcome and prognostic factors of spinal intramedullary ependymomas in adults. *J Neurooncol.* 2002;57(2):133-139.
76. Ferrante L, Mastronardi L, Celli P, et al. Intramedullary spinal cord ependymomas—a study of 45 cases with long-term follow-up. *Acta Neurochir (Wien).* 1992;119(1-4):74-79.
77. Minehan KJ, Shaw EG, Scheithauer BW, Davis DL, Onofrio BM. Spinal cord astrocytoma: pathological and treatment considerations. *J Neurosurg.* 1995;83(4):590-595.
78. Marchan EM, Sekula RF, Jannetta PJ, Quigley MR. Long-term survival enhanced by cordectomy in a patient with a spinal glioblastoma multiforme and paraplegia. *J Neurosurg Spine.* 2007;7(6):656-659.
79. Lee DK, Choe WJ, Chung CK, Kim HJ. Spinal cord hemangioblastoma: surgical strategy and clinical outcome. *J Neurooncol.* 2003;61(1):27-34.
80. Sun SQ, Cai C, Ravindra VM, et al. Simpson grade I-III resection of spinal atypical (World Health Organization grade II) meningiomas is associated with symptom resolution and low recurrence. *Neurosurgery.* 2015;76(6):739-746.
81. Whitaker SJ, Bessell EM, Ashley SE, et al. Postoperative radiotherapy in the management of spinal cord ependymoma. *J Neurosurg.* 1991;74(5):720-728.
82. Gerszten PC, Burton SA, Ozhasoglu C, McCue KJ, Quinn AE. Radiosurgery for benign intradural spinal tumors. *Neurosurgery.* 2008;62(4):887-896.
83. Dodd RL, Ryu M-R, Kamnerdsupaphon P, et al. CyberKnife radiosurgery for benign intradural extramedullary spinal tumors. *Neurosurgery.* 2006;58(4):674-685.
84. Tatsui CE, Stafford RJ, Li J, et al. Utilization of laser interstitial thermotherapy guided by real-time thermal MRI as an alternative to separation surgery in the management of spinal metastasis. *J Neurosurg Spine.* 2015;23(4):400-411.
85. Lee TT, Gromelski EB, Green BA. Surgical treatment of spinal ependymoma and post-operative radiotherapy. *Acta Neurochir (Wien).* 1998;140(4):309-313.
86. Lin Y-H, Huang C-I, Wong T-T, et al. Treatment of spinal cord ependymomas by surgery with or without postoperative radiotherapy. *J Neurooncol.* 2005;71(2):205-210.
87. Jyothirmayi R, Madhavan J, Nair MK, Rajan B. Conservative surgery and radiotherapy in the treatment of spinal cord astrocytoma. *J Neurooncol.* 1997;33(3):205-211.
88. Vaillant B, Loghin M. Treatment of spinal cord tumors. *Curr Treat Options Neurol.* 2009;11(4):315-324.
89. Cristante L, Herrmann H-D. Surgical management of intramedullary spinal cord tumors. *Neurosurgery.* 1994;35(1):69-76.
90. Shirato H, Kamada T, Hida K, et al. The role of radiotherapy in the management of spinal cord glioma. *Int J Radiat Oncol Biol Phys.* 1995;33(2):323-328.
91. Moss JM, Choi CYH, Adler JR, et al. Stereotactic radiosurgical treatment of cranial and spinal hemangioblastomas. *Neurosurgery.* 2009;65(1):79-85.
92. Ryu SI, Kim DH, Chang SD. Stereotactic radiosurgery for hemangiomas and ependymomas of the spinal cord. *Neurosurg Focus.* 2003;15(5):1-5.
93. Schick U, Marquardt G, Lorenz R. Recurrence of benign spinal neoplasms. *Neurosurg Rev.* 2001;24(1):20-25.
94. Klekamp J, Samii M. Surgery of spinal nerve sheath tumors with special reference to neurofibromatosis. *Neurosurgery.* 1998;42(2):279-289.
95. Seppälä MT, Haltia MJJ, Sankila RJ, Jääskeläinen JE, Heiskanen O. Long-term outcome after removal of spinal neurofibroma. *J Neurosurg.* 1995;82(4):572-577.
96. Wang T, Yin H, Han S, et al. Malignant peripheral nerve sheath tumor (MPNST) in the spine: a retrospective analysis of clinical and molecular prognostic factors. *J Neurooncol.* 2015;122(2):349-355.
97. Safaee M, Parsa AT, Barbaro NM, et al. Association of tumor location, extent of resection, and ncurofibromatosis status with clinical outcomes for 221 spinal nerve sheath tumors. *Neurosurg Focus.* 2015;39(2):E5.
98. Innocenzi G, Salvati M, Cervoni L, Delfini R, Cantore G. Prognostic factors in intramedullary astrocytomas. *Clin Neurol Neurosurg.* 1997;99(1):1-5.
99. Nakamura M, Ishii K, Watanabe K, et al. Surgical treatment of intramedullary spinal cord tumors: prognosis and complications. *Spinal Cord.* 2007;46(4):282-286.
100. Rawlings CE, Giangaspero F, Burger PC, Bullard DE. Ependymomas: a clinicopathologic study. *Surg Neurol.* 1988;29(4):271-281.
101. Lonjon M, Goh KYC, Epstein FJ. Intramedullary spinal cord ependymomas in children: treatment, results and follow-up. *Pediatr Neurosurg.* 1998;29(4):178-183.
102. Ciappetta P, Salvati M, Capoccia G, et al. Spinal glioblastomas: report of seven cases and review of the literature. *Neurosurgery.* 1991;28(2):302-306.
103. Cohen AR, Wisoff JH, Allen JC, Epstein F. Malignant astrocytomas of the spinal cord. *J Neurosurg.* 1989;70(1):50-54.
104. Santi M, Mena H, Wong K, et al. Spinal cord malignant astrocytomas. *Cancer.* 2003;98(3):554-561.
105. Murota T, Symon L. Surgical management of hemangioblastoma of the spinal cord: a report of 18 cases. *Neurosurgery.* 1989;25(5):699-708.
106. Pietilä TA, et al. Surgical treatment of spinal hemangioblastomas. *Acta Neurochir (Wien).* 2000;142(8):879-886.
107. Van Velthoven V, Reinacher PC, Klisch J, Neumann HPH, Glasker S. Treatment of intramedullary hemangioblastomas, with special attention to von Hippel-Lindau disease. *Neurosurgery.* 2003;53(6):1306-1313.

CHAPTER 91 Spinal Intradural Infections

Walter J. Jermakowicz
Samuel H. Cass
Allan D. Levi

Introduction

The spinal cord and subdural space are the regions of the central nervous system (CNS) least likely to harbor infections. Since the first description of a spinal subdural infection in 1927,[1] cumulative knowledge of these infections has been limited to sparse case reports and small series due to their low prevalence, their variable presentation and outcomes, and inaccurate diagnostic methods. Despite the rarity of spinal subdural infections, the reported incidence has been on the rise due to improved imaging techniques and an increase in spinal infections linked to immunocompromise and invasive spine procedures. In 2013, spinal infections hit the mainstream media after a string of aspergillosis infections linked to contaminated epidural steroid injections from a common manufacturer affected more than 700 patients and killed 61.[2] As drug resistance among common microbes evolves, rates of diabetes mellitus (DM) and intravenous (IV) drug use increase, and the number of invasive spinal procedures performed continues to increase, it is clear that a greater understanding of these infections is necessary. This chapter focuses on the presentation, diagnosis, and treatment of the most common spinal intradural infections. Emphasis is placed on advances in imaging for the diagnosis of spinal subdural infections as well as on lessons learned from the recent epidural steroid injection–related epidemic.

Bacterial Pathogens

Spinal Subdural Abscess

Background and Demographics

Infections of the spinal subdural space are the rarest localized infections of the CNS. Since their initial description by Sittig in 1927,[1] there have been only 86 cases of spinal subdural abscess (SSA) reported in the literature, namely, in case reports and small case series; thus, their incidence remains unclear. However, reporting of these infections is on the rise due to a suspected increase in their incidence and due to improvements in imaging tools that help identify SSAs earlier and guide their management.[3–13]

Apart from the rarity of SSAs, understanding of their natural history and pathophysiology has been hindered by their variable clinical course. Age of presentation varies from the fourth week to the eighth decade of life, with roughly 50% of patients reported presenting in the fifth to seventh decades of life. In adults, SSAs have a predilection for the lumbar spine, with a slight predominance of females over males; in pediatric patients, the infections tend to occur in the thoracic spine, with males outnumbering females 2 : 1.[4,5,13] Of the 86 reported cases of SSA, only two are considered idiopathic and the rest have been linked to immunocompromise (DM, IV drug use, alcoholism, cancer, human immunodeficiency virus [HIV]), anatomic abnormalities (dermal sinuses, cysts, degenerative disc disease, trauma) or prior intervention (epidural injections, catheters, surgical implants).[3–13]

Pathophysiology

Advances in the understanding of the anatomy of the subdural space have helped explain the relative paucity of SSAs compared to epidural or intramedullary spinal infections.[11,14,15] Contrary to the classic view of the subdural space existing as a potential space between the dura and the arachnoid, several cytoarchitectural studies have shown that the dura and arachnoid are bridged by specialized fibroblasts called dural border cells that eliminate this potential space, making formation of an abscess less likely. This dural border layer, however, is thought to be structurally weaker than the dura or arachnoid, occasionally allowing a hematoma or infection to dissect through the border cells and form a pathologic subdural extramedullary collection.[11] In addition, the subdural space is relatively avascular compared to the epidural space and spinal cord, which reduces the risk of seeding from a distant infection.[14,15] The significantly lower incidence of SSAs compared to cranial subdural abscesses has been explained by (1) centripetal blood flow in the spine compared to centrifugal in the cranium; (2) the lack of air sinuses in the spine that may directly spread infection to the subdural space of the cranium; and (3) the lack of an open epidural space in the cranium, unlike in the spine, where the epidural space filters out pathogens before they reach the dura.[4,11,14,15]

The pathogenesis of SSAs has been historically classified into four main categories. The first, and considered most common, is seeding of bacteria from a distant primary infection.[16–18] Many different primary infection sources have been described, such as urinary tract infections, endocarditis, upper respiratory tract infections, and septic abortions. However, Bartels et al. found skin ulcers and cellulitis to be the most common primary site.[4] The second category, which is growing in frequency as the number of invasive spine procedures increases, is iatrogenic. This includes lumbar punctures, epidural injections, and incidental durotomies during spine surgery.[4,7,17] Unlike the recent US outbreak of fungal intradural infections after injection of contaminated methylprednisone during epidural steroid injections, only three bacterial subdural infections have been attributed to epidural injections: two from epidural steroid injections and one from epidural anesthesia.[2,4] The third category involves direct extension of infection into the subdural space. This extension is mostly considered to be due to dermal sinus tracts or destruction of dura by local infection or trauma.[5,7,11,19–22] A recent report by Usoltseva et al.[12] describes direct seeding of an SSA from a decubitus ulcer in a 55-year-old paraplegic male with an acutely worsened motor examination. Cultures from the SSA and ulcer both grew *Bacteroides fragilis* and *Enterobacter cloacae*, but blood cultures were negative. In the pediatric population, over half of SSAs have been attributed to spinal dysraphism or other congenital anomalies.[11,19,22,23] The fourth and least common category is idiopathic subdural infections, for which no primary source can be identified.[18,24–26]

Whereas the anatomic location of an SSA along the spine largely determines the neurologic deficits that will be present, other important pathologic features include the presence of a capsule and the rate of growth of the abscess. Review of prior literature on spinal subdural infections reveals the often interchangeable use of the words "abscess," which describes the accumulation of purulent material in a fibrous capsule, and "empyema," which is the accumulation of this material in a preexisting space. Despite the pathologic distinction between abscesses and empyemas, studies do not indicate a significant difference in the treatment or prognosis of these disease entities. The age of an SSA also affects the clinical picture. Chronic SSAs have less specific features than acute SSAs. Clinical features of chronic SSAs are less focal and of slower onset, and laboratory markers are usually normal. Chronic SSAs are also more difficult to identify by imaging than acute SSAs and have been frequently confused with tumors[3–13] (Box 91.1).

BOX 91.1 Spinal Subdural Empyema Organisms

Staphylococcus aureus
Staphylococcus species
Streptococcus species
Escherichia coli
Pseudomonas aeruginosa
Streptococcus pneumoniae
Peptococcus magnus

Clinical Presentation

The diagnosis and treatment of SSAs has historically been made difficult by their diverse clinical presentation. The classic triad of symptoms was initially described by Fraser et al. in 1973 and includes fever, neck/back pain, and symptoms of cord or cauda equina compression.[14] Bartels et al. in 1992 suggested three stages to the temporal progression of SSAs.[4] Stage 1 includes fever with possible neck/back pain. Stage 2 shows symptoms of compression resulting in motor, sensory, or bowel/bladder deficits. Stage 3 shows complete motor and sensory loss below the lesion. In practice, however, it is unclear how many SSA patients fit this clinical picture. In their study, Bartels et al. found 87% of SSA patients with fever, 84% had neck/back pain, and 82% had neurologic deficits.[4] Other reports suggest a more variable presentation, however. Levy at al. found only 18 of 47 patients in their study to fit the classic triad.[27–31] Sandler et al.[11] found in their review of the pediatric literature that 50% present with fever, 34% with urinary dysfunction, 56% with motor weakness, and only 21% with neck/back pain. A total of 37% of the pediatric patients also presented with symptoms of meningismus. The lack of spine tenderness was previously considered a distinguishing feature of SSAs from spinal epidural abscesses but has since been commonly reported in patients with SSAs. Levy et al. found 14 of 47 patients with spine tenderness[31] and the pediatric review by Sandler et al. found 10% of patients with tenderness.[11]

The onset of SSA symptoms in cases linked to epidural injections also appears to be variable. The two patients with SSAs after epidural steroid injections presented 5 days and 11 weeks after the injections. The patient with SSA following epidural anesthesia for delivery presented 1 week after the treatment.[2,4,7]

Laboratory Evaluation

Obtaining labs and cultures is an important component of the workup for SSAs, but results are usually nonspecific and of little therapeutic value.[4] Blood leukocyte count, erythrocyte sedimentation rate, and C-reactive protein are usually mildly elevated but may also be normal. Lumbar puncture is generally not recommended since the clinical utility is low and there is risk of spreading infection from the subdural space into deeper meningeal layers or of causing cord herniation if an obstruction of cerebrospinal fluid (CSF) flow is present. Even when a CSF sample is obtained, results are usually more suggestive of a parameningeal process rather than meningitis due to frequent encapsulation of the pathogens, generally showing moderately increased pleocytosis and protein content, normal to low glucose, and negative cultures. Blood cultures are generally recommended for all spine infection patients. Whereas the concordance between spinal epidural abscesses and blood cultures is near 100%, the concordance between SSAs and blood cultures is unknown but presumed to be significantly lower due to the sparse vasculature of the spinal subdural space.[11,16,18,32]

Imaging

Whereas findings on computed tomography (CT) are generally nonspecific,[33–35] magnetic resonance imaging (MRI) has remained the most important imaging modality for diagnosis of SSAs.[36,37] Generally, a subdural collection or mass that is hypointense on T1 and hyperintense on T2 with a thin, variable-thickness, contrast-enhancing rim points toward an SSA. The abscesses are usually crescentic in shape and the overlying dura may be thickened and subarachnoid space narrowed or obliterated in severe cases. Differentiating SSAs and epidural abscesses remains difficult in certain cases. Compared to epidural abscesses, SSAs tend to have preserved epidural fat on the MRI. In addition, whereas SSAs are confined to the spinal canal, epidural abscesses may extend further laterally and into the neural foramina. Distinguishing subdural and epidural spine infections is further complicated by their occasional co-occurrence.[4,11,16]

Recent advances in MRI have improved preoperative characterization of SSAs.[36,37] Fat suppression techniques that remove effects from epidural fat and bone marrow allow for better definition of SSAs. Diffusion-weighted imaging has emerged as an important sequence for showing the extent and multiplicity of spinal abscesses. This aids not only in diagnosis but also in planning surgical treatments for these abscesses. Restricted diffusion for the diagnosis of SSAs becomes especially crucial in cases in which gadolinium contrast cannot be administered[37] (Fig. 91.1).

Treatment and Prognosis

Nearly all prior reports of SSAs advocated for immediate surgical decompression followed by 4 to 6 weeks of antibiotics tailored to the cultures. Conservative measures have been advocated in cases in which patients may not tolerate surgery or in which infectious organism is known, but the unpredictable progression of these infections makes delaying surgery very risky.[3–13] When surgery is performed, the exposure should encompass the entire extent of the abscess and copious irrigation needs to be used.[37] The use of drains following surgery is inconsistent and has not been shown to be of benefit. Since obtaining a definitive organism to treat is usually a major indication of the surgery, antibiotics should be withheld until intraoperative cultures have been collected. When empiric antibiotics are given, coverage of gram-positive cocci is of highest priority both in adult and pediatric populations. It has been argued that antibiotics prior to surgery may reduce inflammation at the time of the surgery, but this has not been adopted into practice. The administration of dexamethasone prophylactically to prevent thrombophlebitis has been previously advocated but also lacks support in the literature.[14,16,24,27,37]

The sparse incidence and variable nature of these infections makes outcomes difficult to predict. Generally, however, early diagnosis with preserved neurologic function is correlated with better postoperative outcomes. In a review of 45 patients by Bartels and colleagues,[4] 82% of patients who underwent surgery had a complete recovery or improvement in symptoms and 18% died. In a group of 5 conservatively treated patients they analyzed, only one survivor was found. Likely as a result of improved diagnosis and treatment of these infections, deaths from SSAs are rarely reported in the modern literature and, when reported, are usually the result of multiple comorbidities.[4] The three previously reported cases of SSAs associated with epidural injections all had complete or near-complete recovery of their symptoms after surgical decompression and antibiotic treatment.[2,4,7]

As expected, pediatric SSA patients have lower mortality and greater recovery of neurologic function compared to their adult counterparts.[11,19,22,23] In a review of 72 pediatric cases with SSAs for which decompression was performed, Sandler et al.[11] found complete recovery in 52% of patients and residual disability in 37%. No deaths were reported in their review. Functional outcomes were highly correlated with underlying pathology. In 51 children with dysraphic or abnormal spines, only 16 (31%) showed a complete recovery. In addition, children infected with *Mycobacterium tuberculosis* or *Echinococcosis granulosus* had better functional outcomes generally (59% complete recovery) than children who cultured other organisms.

Intramedullary Spinal Cord Abscesses

Background and Demographics

Intramedullary spinal cord abscesses (ISCAs) are suppurative infections similar to pyogenic brain abscesses but with much lower incidence. The incidence of ISCAs reported in the literature is on par with SSAs; similarly, knowledge of this entity is restricted to case reports and small retrospective reviews.[38–42] Since the initial description of an ISCA in 1830 by Hart, there have been fewer than 150 reported cases. In 1944, Arzt reviewed all cases of the preantibiotic era.[27] Then, in 1977, Menezes et al.[41] and DiTullio et al.[40] independently published the first reviews of these infections in the postantibiotic era. Although these and more recent reports suggest that the incidence and severity of ISCAs dropped after the advent of antibiotics, there continue to be cases reported, mostly in association with immunocompromise, IV drug use, DM, invasive spine procedures, and trauma.[41] Very few ISCAs have been considered idiopathic.[43,44]

Compared to the subdural abscesses described earlier, ISCAs have a different demographic. First, ISCAs tend to occur in younger patients. Although there is a broad age range (1 month to 72 years), it has been reported that roughly 25% of all cases involve patients younger than 10 years.[45–50] In a recent review of 45 pediatric cases, the mean age of presentation was 27 months.[50] Among adult patients, cases tend to present in the fourth decade of life.[38–42] Second, ISCAs tend to occur in males over females, both in the pediatric (78%)[51] and adult populations (60%–70%).[38] Third, compared to subdural abscesses, ISCAs have less of a predilection for the lumbar spine. Byrne et al. found that, of reported ISCAs, 36% involve the cervical cord, 29% the thoracic cord, and 36% are in the conus.[52] These abscesses may be multiple in 26% of the cases.[44]

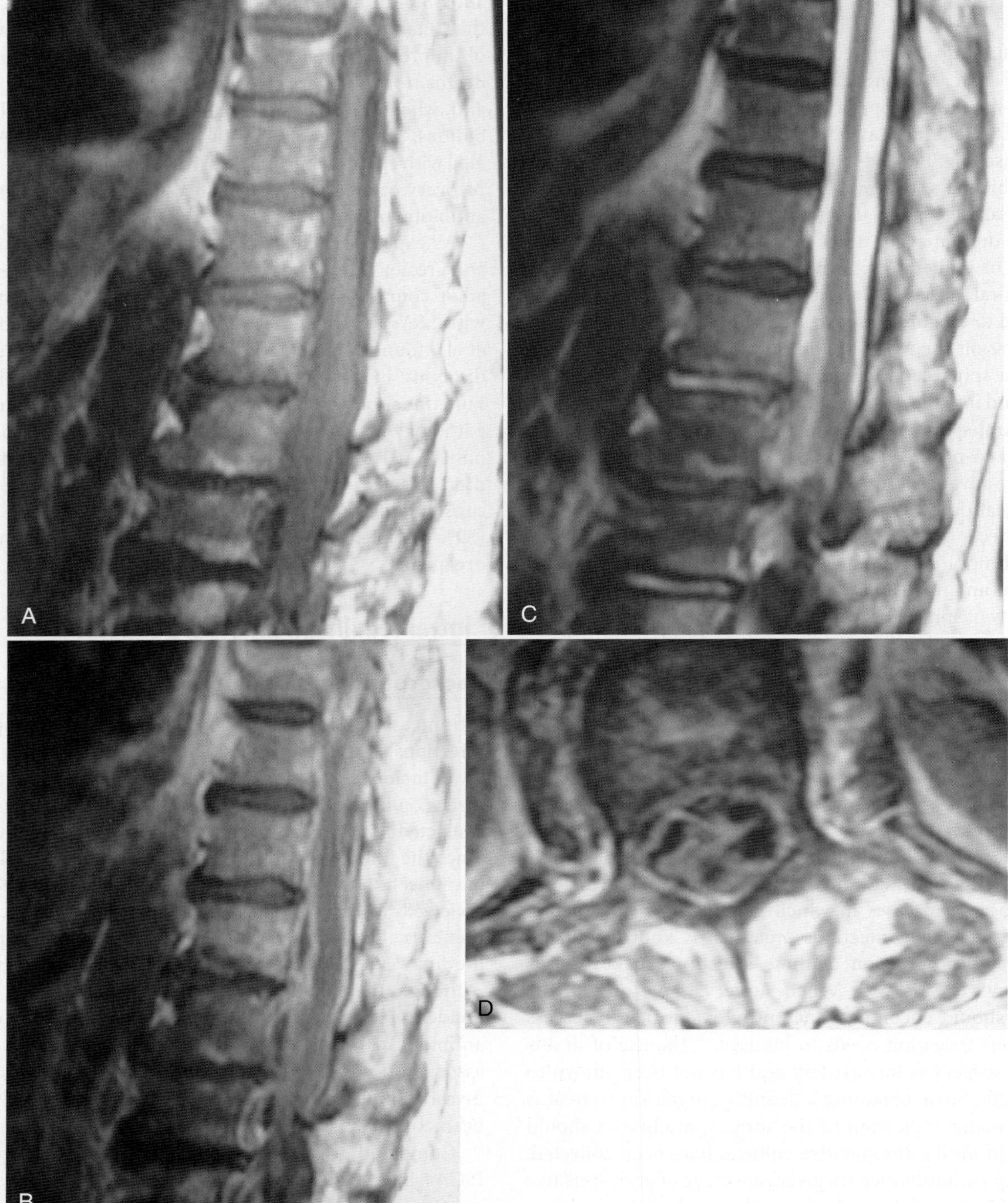

FIG. 91.1 Spinal subdural empyema secondary to *Escherichia coli*. An 86-year-old woman with a history of intractable lower back pain was treated with epidural corticosteroid injections. She presented 2 months after her last epidural injection with increasing lower back pain, fever, paraparesis, and altered mental status. She underwent T12–L1 decompressive laminectomy and intradural exploration. Intraoperative cultures grew *E. coli*. Significant improvement in lower extremity strength was achieved after surgery. Magnetic resonance imaging showed an intradural infection extending from T11 to L4, which was isointense on T1-weighted image (A), isointense to hyperintense on T2 weighting with associated edema of the spinal cord (C), and homogeneously enhancing with gadolinium (B, D).

Pathophysiology

ISCAs are suppurative infections similar to brain abscesses with purulent myelitis surrounding a region of central necrosis. They are thought to begin in the central gray matter with peripheral extension into the white matter. ISCAs initially develop as microscopic nodules with an abundance of polymorphonuclear cells with enzymes that induce liquefactive necrosis in surrounding tissue. These necrotic areas are walled off by a capsule produced by fibroblasts. These abscesses are usually in proximity to blood vessels, and organisms can usually be identified both in the abscess and the vessel. Small punctate areas of hemorrhage are usually observed in the vicinity of these infections, and surrounding veins may become thrombosed. The surrounding meninges are often inflamed and infiltrated with polymorphonuclear cells and lymphocytes.[53,54] Chronic abscesses typically have three well-defined layers. The center primarily contains collagen fibers and polymorphonuclear cells. The middle layer consists of fibroblasts, capillaries, histiocytes, and plasma cells; the outer layer is a connective tissue capsule. The abscesses grow caudad and cephalad separating the fiber tracts and may extend from medulla to the conus medullaris, but significant compression is not caused until later in the disease.[38–42]

In adults, ISCAs are historically thought to occur through the spread of pathogens through one of three mechanisms: direct extension, hematogenous seeding, or via lymphatics. Direct extension leading to the formation of ISCAs has been described with epidural abscesses, discitis, dermal sinus tracts, spine trauma, meningitis, and with invasive spine procedures.[54–59] Several reports have also described the formation of ISCAs in association with preexisting masses.[60,61] The tumors most frequently associated with ISCAs have been ependymomas and epidermoid tumors; however, recent papers describe the co-occurrence of acute ISCAs with astrocytomas, typically resulting in disastrous consequences despite aggressive management.[60]

The hematogenous route remains a common mechanism of pathogen spread leading to the formation of ISCAs, even in the postantibiotic era.[38–42] The arterial network of the spinal cord contains many collaterals with various feeders, while the venous system of the spine is a low-pressure system that communicates with the venous systems of the chest and abdomen. Thus, with changes in intraabdominal pressure, retrograde flow of blood may seed pathogens from the chest and abdomen in the spine. This sluggish flow of blood combined with the watershed zone of the thoracic cord have been used to explain the increased incidence of ISCAs in thoracic cord relative to other types of spine infection. The most common sites of origin for metastatic ISCA are the lung, heart, and urinary tract, but many different sources have been reported.[38–42,62–64] Applebee et al.[43] described a 47-year-old woman who developed complete paralysis at the T3 level 1 week after a dental cleaning. An ISCA was discovered upon imaging and oral flora were cultured intraoperatively.

Despite the rich vasculature of the spine and the low-pressure venous flow, the spinal cord is very resistant to infections compared to other organ systems. Although the reason for this is not understood, early work by Hoche[65] helped shed light on the mechanism of abscess formation in the CNS. In his experiments, when bacterial pathogens were injected into the arterial supplies of the brain or spinal cord, abscesses did not develop. However, abscesses did form when he injected either septic emboli or aseptic emboli later followed by bacteria. These data suggest that for an ISCA to occur not only does a microbial pathogen have to be present but there has to be structural pathology that allows the organism to seed. This is likely why, in adults, nearly all cases of ISCAs are associated with preexisting pathology (trauma, discitis, tumor, and so on).[38–59] The study also suggests a mechanism by which subclinical bacterial infections can lead to ISCAs that are later classified as cryptogenic.

The spread of bacterial pathogens to the spinal cord by the lymphatic system has been suggested but is less clearly understood than the other routes. Experiments by Galkin in the 1930s[66] demonstrated that lymphatic channels that drain the chest, abdomen, and retroperitoneum have connections with the Virchow-Robin spaces of the spinal cord. Thus, infections may potentially spread directly into the cord via the lymphatics. Although several case reports have suggested lymphatics as a possible route for ISCA formation, this has never been demonstrated definitively in the laboratory or clinical setting.[38–40]

Ultimately, the majority of cases in adults are cryptogenic, possibly a result of transient bacteremia from mucosal surfaces or clinically unrecognized extraspinal infections. Most reviews from the antibiotic era categorize 50% to 64% of ISCA cases as cryptogenic.[38–42] Chan and Gold[39] compared 25 of their patients treated during the antibiotic era (1977–1997) to 42 ISCA patients from the preantibiotic era (1830–1944) that were reviewed by Arzt.[27] They found a trend toward increases in cryptogenic cases in the postantibiotic group. They attributed this to the effectiveness of antibiotics in treating primary infections since in the preantibiotic group, 45% of abscesses were attributed to hematogenous spread from an extraspinal source but in the postantibiotic group, only 8% of abscesses were associated with hematogenous spread.

The pathogens responsible for ISCAs reflect the mechanism of abscess formation and source of primary infection. A causative organism was identified in 64% of cases reviewed by Chan and Gold[39] and 60% of cases reviewed by Bartels et al.[67] Whereas cultures of ISCAs caused by hematogenous spread typically reflect cultures of the primary infection site, cases of cryptogenic ISCA are usually associated with *Listeria monocytogenes*, viridans streptococci, *Haemophilus* species, *Actinomyces*, or oral flora. The high association of *L. monocytogenes* with ISCAs is attributed to its tropism for the CNS.[39,67–69] Postsurgical cases, however, are most frequently associated with *Staphylococcus epidermidis*, *S. aureus*, Enterobacteriaceae, and *Pseudomonas aeruginosa*.[38–42]

Contrary to adults, in the pediatric population only about a quarter of ISCAs are cryptogenic. Instead, they are typically caused by spinal cord developmental abnormalities that allow direct extension of the organisms into the cord.[45–50] In a recent review of pediatric cases of ISCA, 53% were associated with anatomic defects, such as dermal sinuses, myelomeningoceles,

BOX 91.2 Intramedullary Spinal Cord Abscess Organisms

Staphylococcus epidermidis
Staphylococcus aureus
Streptococcus spp.
Actinomyces meyeri
Proteus mirabilis
Listeria monocytogenes
Haemophilus species
Escherichia coli

bony lumbar malformations, and sacral decubitus ulcers. Dermal sinuses are epithelialized tracts formed as a result of imperfect separation of cutaneous and neural ectoderm early in fetal life and are considered the leading cause of ISCAs in the postantibiotic era. Only 1% of dermal sinus tracts are located in the cervical area, 10% are in the thoracic area, 41% in the lumbar area, and 35% in the lumbosacral area.[49] Dermal sinuses account for about half of the ISCAs reported in children but only account for about a quarter of ISCAs in adults.[44] Bacterial flora associated with dermal sinus tracts include *S. epidermidis*, *S. aureus*, Enterobacteriaceae, *B. fragilis*, and *Proteus mirabilis*[45–50] (Box 91.2).

Clinical Presentation

The classic presentation of ISCAs includes fevers, back pain, and compromise of neurologic function at and below the level of spine affected. In practice, however, there is great variability. Studies of ISCAs from the postantibiotic era report that, at the time of diagnosis, 83% to 94% of patients have some degree of motor weakness, 60% to 78% have sensory loss, and 51% to 56% have loss of sphincter control. The percentage of spinal patients that are febrile at the time of diagnosis is 25% to 50%, and 36% to 60% report pain in the affected area at some point prior to diagnosis.[38–42] Presentation of ISCAs after invasive procedures is also variable. Four cases of ISCA after lumbar puncture have been reported, each presenting with lower extremity weakness, with time to presentation of symptoms varying from 12 hours to 27 days.[51] Less frequently, ISCAs have been reported to present with hydrocephalus, brain stem findings, and Horner syndrome.[39,70,71]

The neurologic deterioration caused by an ISCA is related to its mass effect and rate of expansion. ISCAs were categorized by Foley[72] into three clinical groups with significant prognostic indications based on the severity and chronicity of symptoms. Acute abscesses typically present with more severe neurologic compromise and are more likely associated with fever and leukocytosis. The subacute group has symptoms for up to 6 weeks and the chronic group beyond 6 weeks. The presentation of ISCAs in these latter two groups more closely mirrors the presentation of an intramedullary tumor and patients are usually afebrile.

Laboratory Evaluation

Laboratory studies are usually of little diagnostic value in the diagnosis of ISCAs, though cultures may be important for tailoring treatment, especially in conservatively managed cases. Leukocytosis and elevations in erythrocyte sedimentation rate and C-reactive protein are more likely in acute ISCAs but may also be present in the subacute and chronic groups. CSF analyses are usually normal; if abnormal, they usually show elevated white blood cell (WBC) counts and mildly elevated protein, consistent with a likely parameningeal process.[38–42] Reports of ISCAs in pediatric patients suggest that abnormal CSF studies are more common than in adults in as many as 78% of cases with positive cultures obtained in 64% of patients[51]; however, these studies have been of little diagnostic significance in the recent published literature.

Imaging

Together with clinical presentation, imaging usually provides the most valuable information for the diagnosis of ISCAs. While ISCAs are rare and often difficult to distinguish radiographically from tumors, infarcts, resolving hematomas, or demyelinating disease, a degree of suspicion for these lesions needs to be maintained given the acuity of treatment required with ISCAs. Plain radiographs will not detect ISCAs but often show associated conditions, such as osteomyelitis, trauma, or dysraphism.[73–77] Myelography was the early method of choice for diagnosis of ISCAs prior to the advent of the MRI. The contrast of a myelogram shows symmetrical thickening of the spinal cord with partial or complete obstruction of CSF flow in the region of the abscess. CT scans of the spine are an integral component in the evaluation of any decline in motor function but are usually nonremarkable in the case of ISCAs. Plain CT may reveal widening of the spinal cord and when used with intravenous contrast can show an intramedullary process. Postmyelographic CT scans are more likely to show the cord widening and blocked CSF flow characteristic of ISCAs; however, the use of this modality has become obsolete together with conventional myelography.[40,41]

Since its widespread use, MRI has remained the gold standard in the diagnosis of ISCAs. Typical MRI features of these abscesses include widening of the spinal cord, hypointensity on T1-weighted images, hyperintensity on T2 images, and peripheral enhancement after administration of gadolinium. However, it has become clear that MRI features vary depending on stage of the ISCA and often reflect changes observed in the evolution of cerebral abscesses. Early stages have greater hyperintensity on T2-weighted images but less contrast enhancement on T1 images compared to later stages. The well-defined ring enhancement classically described with abscesses has been reported to occur around 7 days after initial presentation. After capsule formation, however, this is also variable. The T2 signal becomes less intense with time and usually resolves over several weeks after treatment of the lesion.[73–77]

Several recent studies have shown the value of diffusion-weighted imaging (DWI) in diagnosing ISCAs and initiating prompt treatment. The purulent fluid of abscesses impairs the diffusion of water molecules, which is observed as a hyperintense signal on DWI with reduced apparent diffusion coefficient values compared to surrounding tissues.[74–76] Hood et al.[44] described the case of a 57-year-old physician transferred from an outside hospital several days after developing hemiparesis and dysesthesias. He had been afebrile, CSF studies were negative, and MRI with contrast from the outside hospital (without DWI) showed an enhancing lesion but could not distinguish intramedullary tumor from ISCA. Urgent DWI posttransfer showed restricted diffusion consistent with abscess and the patient was emergently decompressed on the basis of this finding with subsequent good neurologic recovery. It is noteworthy that ISCAs have been diagnosed that possessed no findings on DWI, likely reflecting the dependence of these findings on age of the lesion and stage of encapsulation.[74–76]

Treatment and Prognosis

The two factors that most closely correlate with good outcomes in the management of ISCAs are clinical presentation and administration of antibiotics. Menezes et al.[41] showed in their review of 55 cases from 1830 to 1977 that chronicity is a particularly important component of the clinical presentation. In their review, mortality was 90% in patients presenting acutely, 66% in subacute patients, and 53% for those with chronic symptoms. Seventeen patients reported in their study were treated in the antibiotic era and had only 23% mortality. Chan and Gold,[39] in their comprehensive review of ISCAs from the pre- and postantibiotic eras, suggested 90% mortality without use of antibiotics (1830–1944) and only 8% mortality with antibiotics (after 1944). Deaths from ISCAs in the modern era are rare and generally occur due to the presence of multiple CNS abscesses or other related comorbidities. Even in the modern era, however, around 70% of adult patients retain some degree of neurologic disability. Antibiotic therapy usually starts empiric but is then tailored to cultures, if available. There are no guidelines for duration of antibiotic therapy; however, most studies use a 4- to 6-week course. The recurrence rate of ISCAs is reported to be around 25%.[38–42]

The standard of therapy for ISCAs is urgent surgical decompression and administration of antibiotics.[38,39] Very few reports of conservatively managed ISCAs exist in the modern era since any change in motor examination associated with imaging findings generally warrants decompression. Because ISCAs extend rostrally and caudally, displacing fiber tracts, the goal of surgery is not only to preserve viable tissue in the area of the abscess but also to prevent its spread through the cord. Most authors advocate that surgery should include laminectomies at least at the levels involved, intradural exploration, midline myelotomy, and washout of the abscess cavity.[78,79] Focused surgical exposure and drainage, however, have been advocated in cases with focal imaging findings and presentation.[44] Permanent CSF shunting has been used for hydrocephalus caused by ISCAs.[39]

Since around half of ISCAs in children are associated with dermal sinus tracts (DSTs), experts advocate for thorough screening and complete resection of DSTs prophylactically.[38,45–51] When an abscess is associated with the DST, the current recommendation is for limited laminectomy and myelotomy.[38] In their extensive review of pediatric ISCA cases, da Silva et al. report 20% mortality, residual neurologic deficits in 60%, and full recovery in 60% of patients.[51]

Mycobacterial Pathogens

Spinal Intradural Tuberculosis

Background

Tuberculosis (TB) is an infectious disease caused by *M. tuberculosis*, an acid-fast bacillus that typically infects alveolar macrophages, leading to focal granulomatous lesions of the lungs. While Robert Koch first identified its causative agent in 1882, TB continued to be a plight to society until the 1945 discovery of streptomycin's anti-TB effects.[80] TB remains a leading infectious disease killer, especially among the immunodeficient. Although TB is predominantly described in the lungs, organisms can disseminate hematogenously and reactivation of latent infections can arise in nearly any tissue.

The first mention of spinal TB was in 1779, when Percivall Pott described treatment of a patient with paraplegia by surgically draining a spinal abscess.[81] Neurologic involvement of this infectious mycobacterium can present in four ways: Pott disease (tuberculous spondylitis), nonosseous spinal tuberculoma, tuberculous arachnoiditis, and tuberculous meningitis.[82] Because Pott disease presents as a vertebral infection and tuberculous meningitis primarily presents as intracranial dysfunctions, these will not be discussed in this chapter.

Since the development of anti-TB drugs, the worldwide incidence has declined in both developing and developed countries; the incidence has declined, on average, 1.5% per year since 2000, according to the World Health Organization.[83] Regardless of this success, TB still remains a leading cause of death worldwide alongside HIV. In 2014, there were 1.5 million TB-related deaths and 1.2 million HIV deaths.[83] Tuberculosis is transmitted from person to person via respiratory droplets. Thus, the populations at risk include those who live in crowded conditions, the malnourished, and the immunocompromised. Those especially at risk are the HIV infected and patients who undergo solid organ transplants (SOT).[84] In 2015, 1 in 3 HIV deaths worldwide was due to TB. Furthermore, SOT patients are 20 to 74 times more likely to be infected with TB.[83]

In 2013, there were 5.4 million new cases of TB, 800,000 of which were extrapulmonary in nature. In the United States, among 253,299 new cases, 18.7% were extrapulmonary and 5.4% were specifically meningeal.[85] No statistics were available for intradural spinal cases, which is consistent with the rare nature of these findings. There are currently no standardized guidelines for the treatment of spinal intradural TB.

Two numbers have been reported for the incidence of CNS TB involvement. One claim is that 10% of patients with TB experience some sort of CNS involvement, though this statistic may not truly represent the number of cases of brain and spinal cord infection.[86,87] A more likely analysis puts the prevalence of CNS TB at 0.5% to 2%, most of which occurs as intracranial lesions.[84,88,89] Among these cases, infections of the spine are very rare. When TB does involve the spine, the incidence of associated pathologies is as follows: 64% Pott disease, 20% arachnoiditis, 8% intramedullary tuberculomas, and 8% are other presentations, including extramedullary tuberculomas and abscesses.[90]

Spinal arachnoiditis frequently precipitates from intracranial TB meningitis. The incidence is slightly higher in females than males, with a ratio of 1.3 : 1; the median age of infection is between 27 and 28 years of age.[85] Spinal intramedullary tuberculomas are much rarer than their intracranial counterpart, at a ratio of 1 : 42. Spinal intramedullary tuberculomas are more common in males than in females (3.25 : 1), while extramedullary tuberculomas present at equal frequencies. The median age for the development of spinal tuberculomas is in the 20s and 30s.[88] Furthermore, MacDonnell et al. in their review found that 39 of 43 cases presented in developing nations, with only 4 cases coming from the United States and Italy.[91]

Pathophysiology

Occurrences of TB in the intradural space are secondary infections, usually originating from primary sites in the pulmonary system. *M. tuberculosis* is a species of aerobic acid-fast bacillus, most commonly transmitted via respiratory droplets and for which humans are the only natural reservoirs. Infections at secondary sites are the result of bacteremia, in this case, involving the formation of meningeal TB granulomas.[85] Granuloma formation arises from a delayed type IV hypersensitivity reaction, in which recruitment of lymphocytes by infected macrophages results in encapsulation and caseous necrosis by giant cells. Tuberculous foci can remain latent for an extended period of time, potentially leading to subacute presentation; it has been hypothesized that strains have evolved resistance to macrophage-mediated elimination, which has allowed them to induce this method of dormancy.[81,92] When immunity wanes, the granuloma can discharge the bacilli into the intradural space, leading to tuberculous meningitis, tuberculomas, arachnoiditis, and tuberculous abscesses.[93–95] For this reason, HIV-infected patients are at higher risk for intradural expression of TB.

The manifestation of TB in the CNS has been shown to critically depend on tumor necrosis factor-α (TNF-α) from microglial cells. The role of this cytokine seems to be important for granuloma formation and increasing permeability of the blood-brain barrier, critical for the development of infections in the spinal cord. The role of TNF-α is not entirely understood, though low levels of the cytokine are linked to TB overgrowth and high levels are linked to an overreactive immune response.[96]

The development of spinal TB is derived from three routes of dissemination. First, the intradural infections can represent the first manifestation within the CNS via direct dissemination from the primary site.[97] While direct hematogenous dissemination to the spinal cord is rare, intradural tuberculomas, along with intracranial tuberculomas, are often seen in conjunction with miliary TB. The second route is downward extension of exudate from intracranial infection; descent from intracranial tuberculous meningitis is the most common cause of intradural arachnoiditis.[97,98] Last, the most rare route involves the infection of intradural space via adjacent vertebral disease.[99]

TB meningitis is the most commonly recorded intradural TB infection but is seen in the brain much more often than the spine. Overall, the incidence of spinal cord involvement compared to brain involvement is represented by an overall ratio of 1 : 42, which reflects the weights of spinal cord to brain (1 : 47).[84,88,91] Spinal arachnoiditis is frequently the direct result of intracranial TB meningitis, but can also arise from meningeal TB lesions or spread from adjacent vertebrae, as previously indicated. A literature review from 1966 to 2003 indicated 78 cases of spinal arachnoiditis from the inferior extension of TB meningitis.[86] Thoracic cord involvement is most frequently cited; the thoracic region contains 45% of spinal volume, which is believed to be responsible for these rates.[85,86,93] Arachnoiditis results in collagen deposition from proliferating fibroblasts, causing subsequent matting of nerve roots as pia and arachnoid are adhered. A more severe case has been described as adhesive arachnoiditis when this results in the encapsulation of atrophied nerve roots.[85,95,96,99]

Tuberculomas appear in the intradural spinal cord as either intramedullary or extramedullary. Intramedullary tuberculomas directly involve infection of the spinal cord, while extramedullary tuberculomas involve the subdural space.[84,86–88] Intradural tuberculomas, tuberculous abscesses, and arachnoiditis can all lead to the encasement of emerging nerve roots by exudate. This compression of the spinal cord and its roots can also coincide with edema, inflammation, and potentially even spinal cord infarction due to thrombosis of spinal vessels.[87]

Finally, paradoxical reactions leading to extrapulmonary TB infections are not uncommon in literature reviews. A paradoxical reaction is the escalation or reappearance of granulomas in response to a seemingly effective anti-TB treatment regimen.[85,96] In a 2013 study, 76 HIV-negative patients with extrapulmonary TB were studied and 19 (25%) demonstrated paradoxical reactions.[96] The pathogenesis of this has been hypothetically linked to regulatory T cells, whose levels are shown to increase in patients with active TB. These regulatory lymphocytes modulate tolerance and prevent autoimmunity through inhibition of interleukin 10 (IL-10) and interferon γ (IFN-γ) production. Although the mechanism of action is unknown, dysfunction of regulatory T cells has been linked to the promotion of paradoxical reactions.[96]

Clinical Presentation

The clinical symptoms of intradural tuberculomas most commonly present as subacute or acute spinal cord compression syndromes.[90] Therefore, the presentation mimics spinal cord neoplasms. The most frequently affected age group are young adults in their 20s and 30s. Development in pediatric patients has been presented, though the incidence of this is rare.[88] In a review of patients with spinal intradural tuberculomas, 94% were implicated with myelopathy that progressed over several months.[91] Symptoms vary depending on location, from upper cervical spine to the cauda equina. Lower limb weakness and progressive paresthesia are among the most prevalent manifestations; headaches, fever, rigidity, altered sensation and seizures have also been recorded.[84,86–88,100,101] The second most common indication is bowel and bladder dysfunction, with a prevalence of 67% among those affected.[91] Finally, 33% experienced back pain, representing the third most common manifestation of the spinal tuberculomas.[86–88,91,97,102] Many of these symptoms are due to spinal cord cavitation and edema caused by the tuberculoma. Many deficits can arise from spinal cord compression syndromes. Intradural tuberculoma patients, especially those positive for tuberculous meningitis, may present with abscesses in the brain; due to this location, cerebral ischemia and hydrocephalus can be serious developments.[96]

Arachnoiditis presents in a similar fashion, though with variable rates. Both develop most commonly in the thoracic spine but with various frequencies. Intramedullary tuberculomas are more prevalent in males, with the ratio of male to female at 3.25 : 1; extramedullary tuberculomas have equal frequencies. Arachnoiditis is more common in females, with a ratio of 1.3 : 1.[85] The median age of spinal arachnoiditis is similar to that of tuberculomas, with a median age between 27 and 28 years of age.[85] The clinical presentation of spinal arachnoiditis is repeatedly described in reviews as monoradicular and polyradicular pain syndromes that correspond with progressive deficits in the sensorimotor system.[93] There are many recurring and relevant symptoms, many of which overlap with the development of intradural spinal tuberculomas: subacute paraparesis with reflex deficits, paresthesias, radiculopathies, hypotonia of the lower limbs, and bladder dysfunction. Among patients with arachnoiditis of the spine, paraparesis is the most frequent clinical presentation, occurring 58.8% of the time.[85,93,103] Spinal arachnoiditis has also been reported to be asymptomatic, though this is rare and dependent on location.

Tuberculous exudate presenting around lumbosacral nerve roots leading to cauda equina syndrome has also been described. Unlike classic cauda equina—characterized by asymmetrical paraplegia, loss of perineal sensation, and bladder dysfunction—a common motor deficit among patients with tuberculous lesions on the cauda equina is the absence of ankle reflexes, though extensor plantar reflexes remain intact.[85]

Imaging Studies

Upon recognition of the aforementioned clinical presentations and evidence of TB, imaging of the patients should begin with chest radiographs. Recognition of active or prior pulmonary TB in the patient is crucial for understanding the risk of spinal intradural TB infection. After physical examination for sensorimotor deficits, spinal radiographs can be performed in the appropriate locations. Plain radiographs are generally useless for tuberculomas, but a negative result can remove suspicion of Pott disease.[91,97,104,105] Axial CT scans can show growth in the spinal column, but the most informative and thorough radiographic method is the MRI.[84–86,88,89,96]

Intradural tuberculomas are undetectable by myelography. Through investigation by MRI, intradural tuberculomas are detectable at three stages of development.[85,88,90] Initial development begins as a noncaseating granuloma. At this level, inflammation and edema within the subdural space is evident, while a collagen capsule is not. On T1- and T2-weighted images, lesions appear isointense and are homogeneously enhanced. The second stage takes the form of a caseating granuloma with a solid center; as the capsule enriches with collagen, a reduction or outright disappearance of edema is often seen. T1-weighted images will remain isointense. Lesions will also show isointense to hypointense signal intensity on T2-weighted images and ring enhancement with hypointense centers at this stage. The third and most developed stage is a caseating granuloma with a liquid necrotic center. At this point, T2-weighted images demonstrate diverse findings, from a hypointense target to a hyperintense rim. Spinal cord edema can also be demonstrated by surrounding hyperintensity of T2-weighted images.[84–86]

In 2014, Chittem et al. demonstrated the "precipitation sign" as a new MRI diagnostic sign for spinal intramedullary tuberculomas.[106] This term refers to a mass of precipitated tubercular pus. Initial MRI images in their study showed an intradural mass at the conus equina that demonstrated hypointensity at T1-weighted images and hypointensity to isointensity at T2-weighted images, which did not enhance with contrast. Their hypothesis of precipitation of tubercular pus along the spinal canal via gravity was confirmed intraoperatively. Thus, a precipitation sign paired with hyperintensity on T2-weighted images can be indicative of intramedullary tuberculomas.[106]

Spinal arachnoiditis should also be imaged using MRI, though images can demonstrate variable findings.[85] Depending on staging and location, images can show clumping of roots, subarachnoid space destruction, and loss of spinal cord outline. Irregular cord surface and CSF loculation are also frequently seen. Absence of spinal cord border can be the result of increased protein in the CSF.[84–86,96] Variation in signal intensity can also be explained by edema, myelitis, or ischemia. Postcontrast studies can be used for clarification. Arachnoiditis can be confirmed by smooth and linear enhancements of the spinal cord or its emerging nerve roots. Last, meningeal enhancement is the most prevalent MRI finding for arachnoiditis, occurring among 80% of confirmed patients.[85,86]

Treatment and Prognosis

Due to the rarity of intradural spinal tuberculosis, standardized treatments are controversial. Medical treatment rather than surgical intervention is considered curative and, thus, the frontline approach.[82,84,87,88,91,96] However, in one-third of patients demonstrating spinal cord compression syndrome, systemic TB is not diagnosed and surgical intervention is warranted for treatment and diagnosis.[88]

As soon as a TB diagnosis is made, anti-TB therapies should be initiated and continued for at least 9 months.[85,96] At least four anti-TB drugs should be used, such as isoniazid, rifampin, pyrazinamide, streptomycin, and ethambutol; four of these drugs constitute the initial intensive phase that should last 2 months.[96] A continuation phase should be used for the duration of the treatment; this phase administers a two-drug regimen.[85,88,96]

Corticosteroids are also routinely used in treatment protocols, though the mechanism of action is not fully understood.[85,81,96] However, in tuberculous meningitis patients with spinal cord involvement, high-dose corticosteroid use has demonstrated effectiveness in treatment. The steroids have been shown to reduce death as well as reduce lasting neurologic deficits in patients with eliminated infections.[85] Nonetheless, these are not universally used.

A study using nonrandomized patients demonstrated that the use of intrathecal hyaluronidase can be valuable in the treatment of tuberculous spinal arachnoiditis; hyaluronidase enzymatically degrades hyaluronic acid and other mucopolysaccharides in connective tissue.[85] This treatment, however, is still under investigation and not frequently used.

Surgical approaches are not considered to be the frontline treatment but are commonly used due to the mysterious nature of these infections. There are two indications for surgical intervention.[84] The first is simply an uncertain diagnosis; this is common with spinal cord compression in the absence of evidence of TB. The second is a failed response to medical treatment. This can include three forms of its own. First, the patient may experience a poor response to the medical management of the infection. Next, if neurologic assessments show progressive deterioration in mental status, surgery is indicated. Finally, lesion enlargement on imaging following medical treatment indicates the need for surgical removal.[84,85,96]

The most common surgery involves the excision of an intradural tuberculoma. Typically, the tuberculomas are encapsulated and, thus, well circumscribed; surgical removal can be performed effectively without compromising the neurologic system. The most common surgical approach for spinal arachnoiditis involves decompressive laminectomy.[85,96]

Overall, the prognosis for patients presenting with isolated forms of intradural spinal TB is good. MacDonnell et al. found that 65% of these patients demonstrated neurologic improvements.[91] Furthermore, there is no significant difference in outcomes between those treated medically and those treated surgically.[91] However, because intradural TB occurs more often in the immunocompromised or those with concurrent tuberculous infections in other organs, the prognosis is generally unpredictable.

Fungal Pathogens

Spinal Intradural Fungal Infections

Background

Fungal infections of the CNS are very rare and historically have been limited to immunocompromised patients. However, recent outbreaks associated with epidural anesthesia injections have brought much attention to the disease.[2,107–110] In 2005, five cases of fungal meningitis resulted in Sri Lanka after medical equipment contaminated by damp conditions from the recent tsunami was used for spinal anesthesia during cesarean sections. *Aspergillus fumigatus* was identified in all five cases. Three of the cases ultimately resulted in death.[107] Then, in 2012, a fungal outbreak associated with preservative-free methylprednisolone acetate for spinal epidural anesthesia was noted in Tennessee and soon spread to 20 other states. Several vials linked to the infections were tied to a single compounding pharmacy; soon after initiation of the investigation, government agencies had recovered *Exserohilum rostratum* from unopened vials of the same lot. One year later, over 749 cases of infection had been reported, leading to death in 61 patients (8%). Although paraspinal and epidural abscesses were the most common fungal infections associated with this outbreak, intradural infection was reported in 17% to 26% of cases and these were the patients who most frequently succumbed to death.[108,109] Through a quick concerted response from the government, hospitals, and laboratories, this outbreak was identified and addressed quickly. Since then, several reports have been published that elaborate on the CNS findings associated with the outbreak, increasing our understanding of spinal intradural fungal infections.[2,108–110]

Fungi are ubiquitous organisms that are generally of low virulence and can be divided into two groups. True pathogens, which cause infections in patients with normal immune systems, include *Coccidioides immitis*, *Cryptococcus neoformans*, *Blastomyces dermatitidis*, and *Histoplasma capsulatum*. The other group, opportunistic pathogens, cause infections in immunocompromised hosts and include *Candida albicans*, *A. fumigatus*, *Nocardia asteroides*, and *Mucor* (Zygomycetes class).[111,112] Typical causes of immunosuppression in these patients include HIV/acquired immunodeficiency syndrome (AIDS), immunosuppression after transplants, chronic steroid use, chemotherapy, DM, IV drug use, and congenital diseases of cellular immunity.[112–114]

Pathophysiology

Although the pathogenic mechanism of CNS fungal infections is not clear, it is evident that these organisms have evolved features that make the infections elusive and difficult to treat. Some of these properties include the presence of a capsule in some species, ability to grow at 37°C, and dimorphism, which allows the fungus to change between mycelial and unicellular morphologies when invading host tissues.[111,112] Spread to the spinal cord is usually by direct extension or via systematic spread. Direct extension is usually caused by osteomyelitis, discitis, epidural abscess, trauma, or iatrogenic causes. Most cases involving systematic spread originate from the lungs.[108,109,111,112]

Spinal intradural fungal infections may be extramedullary and/or intramedullary. Extramedullary infections typically involve arachnoiditis with chronic fibrosis and granulomatous processes containing giant cells.[108–111] A specific pathology unique to intradural extramedullary fungal infections of the spine is septic thromboemboli to the arterial supply of the spine, resulting in strokes. These strokes may also be caused by direct extension from acute purulent arachnoiditis. A common finding on microscopy is occlusion of arteries by fibrinoid thromboemboli containing fungal elements.[115] The associated spinal cord infarct also typically shows evidence of fungal invasion. Intramedullary fungal infections of the spine, on the other hand, manifest as granulomas of the spinal cord. Similar to other fungal infections of the CNS, these lesions are

BOX 91.3 Subdural Fungal Infection Organisms

Exserohilum rostratum
Aspergillus spp.
Candida albicans
Histoplasma capsulatum
Rhizopus spp.
Cryptococcus neoformans

necrotic, noncaseating, and highly cellular with Langerhans multinucleated giant cells.[116,117]

The organisms most frequently associated with intradural fungal infections of the spine have been the *Aspergillus* species, both for immunocompetent and immunodeficient patients.[111,116] Incidence of *Exserohilum* has greatly increased recently as a result of the recent spinal epidural injection–associated outbreak. Another common iatrogenic cause of these infections is the *Candida* species.[2,108–110] *Candida* gains access to blood vessels by means of intravenous lines, urinary catheters, surgical implants, or during surgeries (mostly abdominal) and then may spread to the spinal cord[111,116] (Box 91.3).

Presentation

The classic presentation of spinal intradural fungal infections is a focal neurologic deficit secondary to spinal cord compression, infarction, or both. Localized neck or back pain often precedes the deficit and the rapidity of symptom onset is variable, ranging from a few days to over a year. Other conditions typically high on the differential include neurosarcoidosis, meningeal carcinomatosis, or bacterial infection.[118] Systemic manifestations associated with intradural fungal infections of the spine include malaise, anorexia, and weight loss. Most focal intradural fungal infections are localized to the thoracic cord followed by the cervical cord. Disseminated infections of the entire spine have also been reported.[108,112,116]

The epidural analgesia–associated epidemic of 2012 further shows us the diversity of the presentation of spinal intradural fungal infections.[2,108–110] Although reported infections occurred due to a similar iatrogenic mechanism and had a common source, the natural course and imaging findings were very diverse. In a report published a year after the outbreak, Smith et al. reported that, of 13,534 potentially exposed persons, there were 749 reported cases of fungal CNS infection.[110] The median age of patients was 64 years (range, 15–97 years) and the median incubation period was 47 days (range, 0–249 days). In these patients, 43% had spinal or paraspinal infections only, 31% had meningitis only, 20% had meningitis with spinal infection, 5% had peripheral joint infections, and 1% presented with stroke (likely from meningitis).[109] During this outbreak, factors associated with a significantly increased risk of developing an intradural fungal infection in patients who received the drug from contaminated lots included multiple epidural injections, female sex, translaminar (vs. transforaminal) epidural approach, and methylprednisolone lot age above 50 days.[2]

Interestingly, these iatrogenic fungal infections were initially associated with meningitis, but after about 6 weeks, the meningitis became less prevalent and spinal and paraspinal abscesses became the primary manifestation of the contaminated epidural steroid injections.[108] For patients with spinal or paraspinal infection, back pain was the predominant symptom (70%) followed by headache (35%). Neurologic deficits were rare presenting symptoms and included numbness (6%) and incontinence (2%). The back pain was often described as typical chronic back pain but more severe and unrelenting at the injection site. For patients who presented with fungal meningitis, headache (73%), neck pain (32%), light sensitivity (32%), nausea (44%), and vomiting (22%) were the most common presenting symptoms. Fever was noted in 17% of patients presenting with solely meningitis and in only 4% of patients presenting with spinal or paraspinal infection.[109]

Laboratory Evaluation

Serum WBC count, erythrocyte sedimentation rate, and C-reactive protein are rarely elevated in cases of spinal intradural fungal infections. Analysis of CSF is the most important component of the laboratory evaluation. The CSF profile is suggestive of a parameningeal inflammatory process rather than meningitis. Mild to moderate leukocytosis is usually associated with increased protein. Glucose levels are typically normal and cultures most often negative.[112,116] In their analysis of all 749 cases of fungal infections caused by the 2012 epidural injection–associated outbreak (64% of whom had spinal or paraspinal infection), Smith et al. reported that median CSF WBC count was 83 (interquartile range, 12–850), protein was 84 (interquartile range, 47–141), and glucose was 53 (interquartile range, 12–850).[110] Fungal CSF cultures are usually positive in 10% to 30% of reported patients.[109–110]

For patients presenting with progressive focal neurologic symptoms who are immunocompromised, have implanted medical devices, or previous interventional procedures and have equivocal initial CSF results, a degree of suspicion must be maintained for fungal infection of the spine and further analysis of the CSF is warranted. Such tests include CSF cytology, polymerase chain reaction (PCR), analysis and antigen testing. Cytology is typically negative but can provide a quick result. Experienced pathologists with knowledge of the clinical picture should be consulted. Antigen detection tests used for detecting certain fungal infections (e.g., *Cryptococcus, Aspergillus*) have shown success recently but they are still being refined and their utility remains unknown. CSF PCR analysis has become an important tool in diagnosis of fungal genetic sequences.[112,116] During the epidural injection–associated outbreak, PCR analysis of CSF samples detected *E. rostratum* in roughly half the patients eventually diagnosed with a fungal infection of the spine.[108,109]

Imaging

Many patients with spinal cord pathology are usually first evaluated by radiograph or CT. In most published reports, these radiographs are typically normal. They may reveal evidence of osteomyelitis/discitis, however, which are often

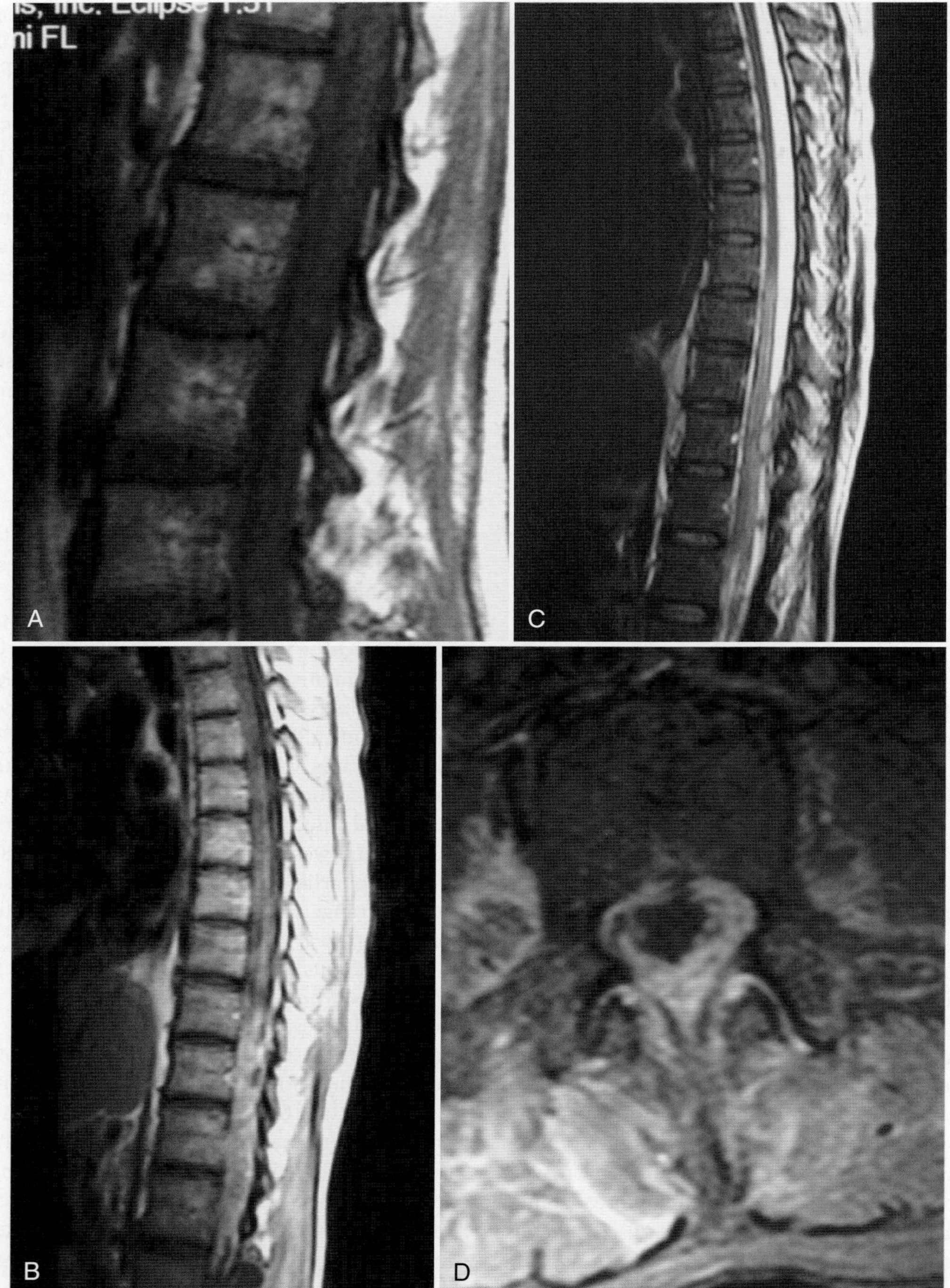

FIG. 91.2 Spinal intradural fungal infection secondary to *Aspergillus fumigatus.* A 31-year-old woman had a history of intractable lower back pain after minor trauma. She was treated with epidural injections and intradiscal thermal electrocoagulation without relief. She then underwent an L5–S1 discectomy without relief. She eventually had epiduroscopy. One month postepiduroscopy, she developed increasing lower back pain, tenderness to palpation, bowel/bladder dysfunction, and paraparesis. She required a T12 decompressive laminectomy and intradural exploration; intraoperative cultures grew *A. fumigatus.* Her paraparesis improved, but she was left with neuropathic pain and neurogenic bowel and bladder. Magnetic resonance imaging showed an intradural infection centered at T11 and epidural abscess from T11 to S1 with associated T2-weighted hyperintensity of the spinal cord. The lesion is isointense on T1 weighting (A), isointense to hyperintense on T2 weighting (C), and homogeneously enhancing (B) with loculated collections surrounding the spinal cord (D).

considered a common source of intradural fungal infections, but this is usually of little prognostic value. In the pre-MRI era, myelography was frequently used, which occasionally identified varying degrees of contrast block in the spinal canal, especially in cases in which the fungal infection was a result of intramedullary granulomatous disease. This was useful for localizing the level of lesion in the spinal cord but was not particularly specific for identifying infectious pathologies.[109,116]

Since its advent, MRI has been the method of choice for evaluating spine infections and recent advances continue to increase its utility. Because of the rarity of spinal intradural fungal infections, little was known about their MRI characteristics until recently, but the epidural anesthesia–associated outbreak gave us a better understanding of their MRI features. In certain patients, initial MRI results were negative but then were found to have intradural phlegmon or abscesses on repeat imaging. In their characterization of MRI findings associated with the outbreak, Kainer et al. identified MRI abnormalities in 30% of exposed patients when an MRI of the head was obtained and in 46% of patients in whom an MRI of the spine was obtained.[2] MRI abnormalities of the spine included arachnoiditis, neuritis, epidural abscess, psoas or paraspinal muscle abscess, or subarachnoid hemorrhage. Fat-suppressed postcontrast MRIs are considered particularly sensitive and effective at distinguishing these infections from other sources of enhancement.[108]

Malani et al.[108] provided even further characterization of MRI findings associated with the epidural anesthesia–associated outbreak by analyzing imaging findings in 172 patients from a pain clinic who had been exposed to the contaminated lots but had not yet presented with symptoms. All patients received an MRI with and without contrast within 1 year of exposure to the drug. The MRIs were abnormal in 35 (21%) of the patients. Findings included spinal or paraspinal abscess or phlegmon, arachnoiditis, osteomyelitis, or discitis. Of those 36 patients with spine MRI findings, 35 met Centers for Disease Control and Prevention criteria for probably or confirmed fungal spine or paraspinal infection and underwent therapy. All those patients received antibiotic therapy and 24 received surgical debridement. Interestingly, 17 of the 24 patients, including five who denied symptoms prior to surgery, had laboratory evidence of fungal infection of the spine at the time of surgery (Fig. 91.2).

Treatment and Prognosis

Treatment strategies and outcomes for fungal infections of the CNS depend on both host and pathogen factors. A medication's ability to cross the blood-brain barrier and activity in the CNS are also important factors to consider. In most early reports of intradural fungal infection of the spine, patients were treated with 3 to 9 months of amphotericin B, with 5-fluorocytosine or rifampicin often used as adjuvant therapies.[109,116,119] In the case of CNS aspergillosis, the Infectious Diseases Society of America recommends 6 to 8 weeks of treatment with voriconazole in immunocompetent patients and potentially indefinite treatment in patients with chronic immunosuppression.[117]

In patients in whom there is suspicion of an infections process of the spine, as was the case with the epidural anesthesia–associated outbreak of 2012, positive cultures should not be mistaken for contamination. Early antibiotic therapy and aggressive surgical debridement may reduce disease burden and improve patient outcomes. During the 2012 outbreak, nearly all patients were treated with voriconazole and most patients (53%–75%) also received amphotericin B.[2,109]

There are generally two reasons for decompressing the spine in a patient with suspected intradural fungal infection. The first is to provide decompression in the case of a space-occupying mass causing neurologic deficits. The second reason is to obtain samples for diagnosis, which is usually obtained by means of direct tissue culture or histopathology. In cases that involve granulomas (intramedullary or extramedullary), the surgery may involve resection of a discrete lesion.[118–121] During the 2012 outbreak, the most common intraoperative findings identified in patients who had MRI evidence of arachnoiditis were foci of purulent material and clumping of nerve roots encased in inflammatory tissue.[109]

Once intramedullary extension occurs, appropriate pharmacologic and surgical therapies are often unable to control the ensuing spread of infection, often resulting in death. Prior to the 2012 outbreak, 14 cases of intradural fungal infection had been described, resulting in 10 deaths. All 4 survivors, 3 of whom made complete recoveries, were treated with aggressive decompression and antifungal medications. Only three of the 10 mortalities had been treated with surgery and antibiotics.[2,112,119] During the 2012 outbreak, roughly 10% of patients died from the disease. Half of those patients who died had evidence of intradural extension of the infection, although only 17% to 26% of all patients involved in the outbreak had intradural spread. The lower mortality rates from intradural fungal infections associated with the outbreak have been attributed to the quick public health response and thorough screening of all patients exposed to the infected methylprednisolone lots.[110]

PEARLS AND PITFALLS

1. Intradural infections remain rare entities; thus, high clinical suspicion is essential to early diagnosis.
2. Aggressive surgical therapy combined with an antibiotic regimen is the most effective treatment for bacterial infections.
3. Medical therapy with judicious use of surgical intervention (diagnosis and decompression) is the most effective approach for management of spinal intradural infections.
4. One must look for the primary site of infection, especially in mycobacterial and fungal infections. Bacterial infections are often cryptogenic, but fungal and mycobacterial infections are often secondary infections that begin in the lungs. For mycobacterial infections, the genitourinary tract must also be investigated.
5. Good recovery is possible with all pathogens, although fungal infections remain the most difficult to cure.

KEY POINTS

Spinal Subdural Empyema

1. Pathogenesis: Hematogenous, iatrogenic, direct extension, and cryptogenic (most common).
2. For more than 50% of cases, the organism is *S. aureus*.

3. Classic triad: Fever, pain, and spinal cord/cauda equina compression
4. Primary treatment is surgical drainage followed by long-term antibiotic therapy.
5. Conservative therapy results in 80% mortality and 20% recovery. Surgical therapy results in 17.9% mortality and 82.1% recovery.

Intramedullary Spinal Cord Abscess

1. Pathogenesis: Hematogenous (arterial/anterograde flow or venous/retrograde flow), direct inoculation (neuroectodermal defects), and cryptogenic (most common)
2. For hematogenous spread, septic embolus or aseptic embolus is needed, followed by bacteremia; bacteremia alone is insufficient.
3. Organisms: *Staphylococcus* species followed by *Streptococcus* species
4. Presentation: Acute (<2 weeks), subacute (2 to 6 weeks), or chronic (>6 weeks)
5. Primary treatment is surgical drainage followed by long-term antibiotic therapy.
6. Prognosis depends on chronicity: Acute presentation = worse outcome; chronic presentation = better outcome.

Mycobacterial Pathogens

1. Four categories: Subdural tuberculomas, intramedullary tuberculomas, arachnoiditis, and meningitis
2. Rare occurrence but increased incidence since 1985 due to HIV/AIDS
3. Demographics: Developing countries = younger patients, developed countries = older and HIV/AIDS patients
4. Pathogenesis: Secondary site of infection, with primary being respiratory or genitourinary
5. Presentation: Most common is spinal cord dysfunction. Only one-third will have constitutional symptoms or pain.
6. Medical management is primary treatment modality with anti-TB regimen for 1 year. Surgery is frequently necessary for diagnosis or for spinal decompression.
7. Prognosis: Generally good neurologic recovery

Fungal Pathogens

1. Two primary manifestations: Extramedullary disease (arachnoiditis) and intramedullary disease (granulomas)
2. Pathogens: True (immunocompetent patients) and opportunistic (immunocompromised patients)
3. Presentation: Pain and spinal cord dysfunction
4. Pathogenesis: Cryptogenic. If hematogenous, then the primary site is pulmonary.
5. Treatment: Long-term antifungals with surgery necessary for diagnosis and decompression
6. Prognosis remains poor.

KEY REFERENCES

1. Bartels RH, de Jong TR, Grotenhuis JA. Spinal subdural abscess: case report. *J Neurosurg*. 1992;76:307-311.
Spinal subdural abscesses are rare. A review of previous reports describes the clinical course of symptoms, which include initial findings of fever and spinal pain, progression to motor and sensory deficits, and ultimately paralysis and total sensory loss. A staging system is proposed from stages 1 to 3 describing the progression of symptoms.
2. DiTullio MV Jr. Intramedullary spinal abscess: a case report with a review of 53 previously described cases. *Surg Neurol*. 1977;7:351-354.
Intramedullary spinal cord abscesses are diseases of the young with a higher prevalence in males. Bacterial infections of the spinal cord occur most frequently in the thoracic spinal cord. Early surgical intervention resulted in improved functional outcome, mandating early diagnosis and aggressive treatment.
3. MacDonnell AH, Baird RW, Bronze MS. Intramedullary tuberculomas of the spinal cord: case report and review. *Rev Infect Dis*. 1990;12:432-439.
Reported cases of intramedullary tuberculomas of the spine originate predominantly from developing countries with a higher prevalence in females and the young. Presenting signs and symptoms are consistent with compression of the spinal cord. The presence of tuberculoid disease outside the vertebral canal was common. Medical intervention is favored, with surgical excision and drainage suggested for failure of medical management.
4. Menezes AH, Graf CJ, Perret G. Spinal cord abscess: a review. *Surg Neurol*. 1977;8:461-467.
Case reports of spinal cord abscesses are reviewed, and pathophysiologic mechanisms for spinal cord inoculation are proposed. Direct inoculation of the spinal cord can occur, such as in trauma. In addition, hematogenous spread via venous backflow from shifts in intraabdominal pressure and lymphatic spread to spinal cord have been proposed as potential routes.
5. Smith RM, et al. Fungal infections associated with contaminated methylprednisolone injections. *N Engl J Med*. 2013;369(17):1598-1609.
This is a review of the epidemiology, treatment, and outcomes associated with the spinal epidural anesthesia outbreak that began in 2013. From 17% to 26% of patients showed intradural infection, and these patients were associated with worse outcomes. Radiographic and laboratory features of the outbreak are presented in great detail.

REFERENCES

1. Sittig O. Metastatischer Rückenmarksabsceß bei septischem Abortus. *Z Gesamte Neurol Psy*. 1927;107(1):146-151.
2. Kainer MA, et al. Fungal infections associated with contaminated methylprednisolone in Tennessee. *N Engl J Med*. 2012;367(23):2194-2203.
3. Agarwal N, et al. Presentation of cauda equina syndrome due to an intradural extramedullary abscess: a case report. *Spine J*. 2014;14(2):e1-e6.
4. Bartels RH, de Jong TR, Grotenhuis JA. Spinal subdural abscess. Case report. *J Neurosurg*. 1992;76(2):307-311.
5. Harris LF, et al. Subdural empyema and epidural abscess: recent experience in a community hospital. *South Med J*. 1987;80(10):1254-1258.
6. Ko MW, et al. Papilledema as a manifestation of a spinal subdural abscess. *J Neurol Sci*. 2007;260(1-2):288-292.
7. Kraeutler MJ, et al. Spinal subdural abscess following epidural steroid injection. *J Neurosurg Spine*. 2015;22(1):90-93.
8. Lim HY, et al. Chronic spinal subdural abscess mimicking an intradural-extramedullary tumor. *Eur Spine J*. 2013;22(suppl 3):S497-S500.
9. Martin RJ, Yuan HA. Neurosurgical care of spinal epidural, subdural, and intramedullary abscesses and arachnoiditis. *Orthop Clin North Am*. 1996;27(1):125-136.
10. Nadkarni T, et al. An intradural-extramedullary gas-forming spinal abscess in a patient with diabetes mellitus. *J Clin Neurosci*. 2010;17(2):263-265.

11. Sandler AL, et al. Infections of the spinal subdural space in children: a series of 11 contemporary cases and review of all published reports. A multinational collaborative effort. *Childs Nerv Syst*. 2013;29(1):105-117.
12. Usoltseva N, et al. Spinal subdural abscess: a rare complication of decubitus ulcer. *Clin Med Res*. 2014;12(1-2):68-72.
13. Velissaris D, et al. Spinal subdural *Staphylococcus aureus* abscess: case report and review of the literature. *World J Emerg Surg*. 2009;4:31.
14. Fraser RA, et al. Spinal subdural empyema. *Arch Neurol*. 1973;28(4):235-238.
15. Schiller F, Shadle OW. Extrathecal and intrathecal suppuration: report of two cases and discussion of the spinal subdural space. *Arch Neurol*. 1962;7(1):33-36.
16. Hirson C. Spinal subdural abscess. *Lancet*. 1965;286(7424): 1215-1217.
17. Krauss WE, McCormick PC. Infections of the dural spaces. *Neurosurg Clin North Am*. 1992;3(2):421-433.
18. Kumar S, Gulati DR. Spinal abscesses. A report on 22 cases. *Neurol India*. 1978;26(4):193-195.
19. Chen CY, et al. Dermoid cyst with dermal sinus tract complicated with spinal subdural abscess. *Pediatr Neurol*. 1999;20(2):157-160.
20. Lownie SP, Ferguson GG. Spinal subdural empyema complicating cervical discography. *Spine*. 1989;14(12):1415-1417.
21. Harries-Jones R, et al. Meningitis and spinal subdural empyema as a complication of sinusitis. *J Neurol Neurosurg Psychiatry*. 1990;53(5):441.
22. Walker AE, Bucy PC. Congenital dermal sinuses: a source of spinal meningeal infection and subdural abscesses. *Brain*. 1934;57(4):401-421.
23. Schneider P, Givens TG. Spinal subdural abscess in a pediatric patient: a case report and review of the literature. *Pediatr Emerg Care*. 1998;14(1):22-23.
24. Hlavin ML, et al. Spinal epidural abscess: a ten-year perspective. *Neurosurgery*. 1990;27(2):177-184.
25. Olson DP, Soares S, Kanade SV. Community-acquired MRSA pyomyositis: case report and review of the literature. *J Trop Med*. 2011;2011:970848.
26. Reddy DR, Rao GN, Krishnamurthy D. Pneumococcal spinal subdural abscess (a case report). *J Postgrad Med*. 1973;19(4):190-192.
27. Arzt PK. Abscess within the spinal cord: review of the literature and report of three cases. *Arch Neurol Psychiatry*. 1944;51(6):533-543.
28. Baker AS, et al. Spinal epidural abscess. *N Engl J Med*. 1975;293(10):463-468.
29. Dus V. Spinal peripachymeningitis (epidural abscess). Report of 8 cases. *J Neurosurg*. 1960;17:972-983.
30. Schnegg JF, Glauser M, de Tribolet N. Infection of a lumbar dermoid cyst by an anaerobic peptococcus. *Acta Neurochir (Wien)*. 1981;58(1-2):127-129.
31. Levy ML, et al. Subdural empyema of the cervical spine: clinicopathological correlates and magnetic resonance imaging. Report of three cases. *J Neurosurg*. 1993;79(6):929-935.
32. Sathi S, et al. Spinal subdural abscess: successful treatment with limited drainage and antibiotics in a patient with AIDS. *Surg Neurol*. 1994;42(5):424-427.
33. Knudsen LL, Voldby B, Stagaard M. Computed tomographic myelography in spinal subdural empyema. *Neuroradiology*. 1987;29(1):99.
34. Patronas NJ, Marx WJ, Duda EE. Radiographic presentation of spinal abscess in the subdural space. *AJR Am J Roentgenol*. 1979;132(1):138-139.
35. Theodotou B, Woosley RE, Whaley RA. Spinal subdural empyema: diagnosis by spinal computed tomography. *Surg Neurol*. 1984;21(6):610-612.
36. Georgakopoulos A, et al. Positron emission tomography in spinal infections. *Clin Imaging*. 2015;39(4):553-558.
37. Hazer DB, Ayhan S, Palaoglu S. Neurosurgical approaches to spinal infections. *Neuroimaging Clin North Am*. 2015;25(2):295-308.
38. Al Barbarawi M, et al. Management of intramedullary spinal cord abscess: experience with four cases, pathophysiology and outcomes. *Eur Spine J*. 2009;18(5):710-717.
39. Chan CT, Gold WL. Intramedullary abscess of the spinal cord in the antibiotic era: clinical features, microbial etiologies, trends in pathogenesis, and outcomes. *Clin Infect Dis*. 1998;27(3):619-626.
40. DiTullio MV Jr. Intramedullary spinal abscess: a case report with a review of 53 previously described cases. *Surg Neurol*. 1977;7(6):351-354.
41. Menezes AH, Graf CJ, Perret GE. Spinal cord abscess: a review. *Surg Neurol*. 1977;8(6):461-467.
42. Weng TI, et al. Intramedullary abscess of the spinal cord. *Am J Emerg Med*. 2001;19(2):177-178.
43. Applebee A, et al. Intramedullary spinal cord abscess in a healthy woman. *Neurology*. 2007;68(15):1230.
44. Hood B, et al. Intramedullary abscess of the cervical spinal cord in an otherwise healthy man. *World Neurosurg*. 2011;76(3-4):361.e15-361.e19.
45. Benzil DL, Epstein MH, Knuckey NW. Intramedullary epidermoid associated with an intramedullary spinal abscess secondary to a dermal sinus. *Neurosurgery*. 1992;30(1):118-121.
46. Dho YS, et al. Catastrophic intramedullary abscess caused by a missed congenital dermal sinus. *J Korean Neurosurg Soc*. 2015;57(3):225-228.
47. Ersahin Y. Intramedullary abscess of the spinal cord. *Childs Nerv Syst*. 2003;19(10-11):777.
48. Mohindra S, Sodhi HS, Aggarwal A. Management problems of intramedullary holocord abscess: an illustration in a pediatric case. *Childs Nerv Syst*. 2012;28(4):637-640.
49. Nicola Z, Antonio C, De Tommasi A. Cervical dermal sinus complicated with intramedullary abscess in a child: case report and review of literature. *Eur Spine J*. 2014;23(suppl 2):192-196.
50. Tewari MK, et al. Intramedullary spinal cord abscess: a case report. *Childs Nerv Syst*. 1992;8(5):290-291.
51. da Silva PS, de Souza Loduca RD. Intramedullary spinal cord abscess as complication of lumbar puncture: a case-based update. *Childs Nerv Syst*. 2013;29(7):1061-1068.
52. Byrne RW, von Roenn KA, Whisler WW. Intramedullary abscess: a report of two cases and a review of the literature. *Neurosurgery*. 1994;35(2):321-326.
53. Koppel BS, Daras M, Duffy KR. Intramedullary spinal cord abscess. *Neurosurgery*. 1990;26(1):145-146.
54. Maurice-Williams RS, Pamphilon D, Coakham HB. Intramedullary abscess—a rare complication of spinal dysraphism. *J Neurol Neurosurg Psychiatry*. 1980;43(11):1045-1048.
55. Amacher AL. Intramedullary epidermoid associated with an intramedullary spinal abscess secondary to a dermal sinus. *Neurosurgery*. 1992;31(5):979.

56. Gerlach R, et al. Large intramedullary abscess of the spinal cord associated with an epidermoid cyst without dermal sinus. Case report. *J Neurosurg Spine*. 2007;7(3):357-361.
57. Hardwidge C, Palsingh J, Williams B. Pyomyelia: an intramedullary spinal abscess complicating lumbar lipoma with spina bifida. *Br J Neurosurg*. 1993;7(4):419-422.
58. Silva RT, et al. Penetrating cervical spine injury and spinal cord intramedullary abscess. *Arq Neuropsiquiatr*. 2012;70(4):308-309.
59. Takebe N, et al. Intramedullary spinal cord abscess and subsequent granuloma formation: a rare complication of vertebral osteomyelitis detected by diffusion-weighted magnetic resonance imaging. *Neurosurg Focus*. 2014;37(2):E12.
60. Mohindra S, et al. Intramedullary abscess in association with tumor at the conus medullaris. Report of two cases. *J Neurosurg Spine*. 2007;6(4):350-353.
61. Thakar S, et al. Metachronous occurrence of an intramedullary abscess following radical excision of a cervical intramedullary pilocytic astrocytoma. *Neurol India*. 2013;61(3):322-324.
62. Arnaiz-Garcia ME, et al. Intramedullary cervical abscess in the setting of aortic valve endocarditis. *Asian Cardiovasc Thorac Ann*. 2015;23(1):64-66.
63. Durmaz R, et al. Multiple nocardial abscesses of cerebrum, cerebellum and spinal cord, causing quadriplegia. *Clin Neurol Neurosurg*. 2001;103(1):59-62.
64. Sverzut JM, et al. Spinal cord abscess in a heroin addict: case report. *Neuroradiology*. 1998;40(7):455-458.
65. Hoche A. Experimentella Beitrage zur Pathologie des Ruckenmarkes. *Arch Psych Nervenkr*. 1899;209:975-1108.
66. Galkin M. Zur Methodik der Injektion des Lymphysystems beim Subarachnoidalraum aus. *Ztschr D Ges Exper Med*. 1930;74:482-489.
67. Bartels RH, et al. Intramedullary spinal cord abscess. A case report. *Spine*. 1995;20(10):1199-1204.
68. Kendall MJ, Clarke SW, Smith WT. Spinal abscess due to *Listeria monocytogenes* in a patient with hepatic cirrhosis. *J Pathol*. 1972;107(1):9-11.
69. Lascaux AS, et al. Painful neck stiffness secondary to an intramedullary abscess of the spinal cord in a HIV infected patient: a case report. *J Neurol*. 2002;249(2): 229-230.
70. Sinha P, Parekh T, Pal D. Intramedullary abscess of the upper cervical spinal cord. Unusual presentation and dilemmas of management: case report. *Clin Neurol Neurosurg*. 2013;115(9):1845-1850.
71. Elmac I, et al. Cervical spinal cord intramedullary abscess. Case report. *J Neurosurg Sci*. 2001;45(4):213-215.
72. Foley J. Intramedullary abscess of the spinal cord. *Lancet*. 1949;2:193-195.
73. Arbelaez A, Restrepo F, Castillo M. Spinal infections: clinical and imaging features. *Top Magn Reson Imaging*. 2014;23(5):303-314.
74. Dorflinger-Hejlek E, et al. Diffusion-weighted MR imaging of intramedullary spinal cord abscess. *AJNR Am J Neuroradiol*. 2010;31(9):1651-1652.
75. Moritani T, et al. Pyogenic and non-pyogenic spinal infections: emphasis on diffusion-weighted imaging for the detection of abscesses and pus collections. *Br J Radiol*. 2014;87(1041):20140011.
76. Roh JE, et al. Sequential magnetic resonance imaging finding of intramedullary spinal cord abscess including diffusion weighted image: a case report. *Korean J Radiol*. 2011;12(2):241-246.
77. Watts J, et al. Magnetic resonance imaging of intramedullary spinal cord lesions: a pictorial review. *J Med Imaging Radiat Oncol*. 2014;58(5):569-581.
78. Ebner FH, et al. Intramedullary lesions of the conus medullaris: differential diagnosis and surgical management. *Neurosurg Rev*. 2009;32(3):287-300.
79. Fortuna A, Contratti F, Di Lorenzo N. Cervical intramedullary abscess (extirpation by means of microsurgical techniques). *J Neurosurg Sci*. 1979;23(2):159-162.
80. Murray JF, Schraufnagel DE, Hopewell PC. Treatment of tuberculosis. A historical perspective. *Ann Am Thorac Soc*. 2015;12(12):1749-1759.
81. Boachie-Adjei O, Squillante RG. Tuberculosis of the spine. *Orthop Clin North Am*. 1996;27(1):95-103.
82. Dehoux E, Awada A, Palkar V. Urinary retention revealing a tuberculoma of the conus medullaris in a patient with intracranial tuberculosis: case report. *Spinal Cord*. 1996;34(10):630-632.
83. World Health Organization (WHO). *Global Tuberculosis Report*. Geneva: WHO; 2015:8-53.
84. Lee DY, Kim SP, Kim IS. Coexistence of spinal intramedullary tuberculoma and multiple intracranial tuberculomas. *Korean J Spine*. 2015;12(2):99-102.
85. Garg RK, Malhotra HS, Gupta R. Spinal cord involvement in tuberculous meningitis. *Spinal Cord*. 2015;53(9):649-657.
86. du Plessis J, et al. Unusual forms of spinal tuberculosis. *Childs Nerv Syst*. 2008;24(4):453-457.
87. Vadivelu S, et al. A review of the neurological and neurosurgical implications of tuberculosis in children. *Clin Pediatr (Phila)*. 2013;52(12):1135-1143.
88. Torii H, et al. Intramedullary spinal tuberculoma—case report. *Neurol Med Chir (Tokyo)*. 2004;44(5):266-268.
89. Nussbaum ES, et al. Spinal tuberculosis: a diagnostic and management challenge. *J Neurosurg*. 1995;83(2):243-247.
90. Rao GP. Spinal intramedullary tuberculous lesion: medical management. Report of four cases. *J Neurosurg*. 2000;93(suppl 1):137-141.
91. MacDonnell AH, Baird RW, Bronze MS. Intramedullary tuberculomas of the spinal cord: case report and review. *Rev Infect Dis*. 1990;12(3):432-439.
92. Rhoton EL, et al. Intramedullary spinal tuberculoma. *Neurosurgery*. 1988;22(4):733-736.
93. Konar SK, et al. Tuberculous lumbar arachnoiditis mimicking conus cauda tumor: a case report and review of literature. *J Neurosci Rural Pract*. 2011;2(1):93-96.
94. Bucy PC, Oberhill HR. Intradural spinal granulomas. *J Neurosurg*. 1950;7(1):1-12.
95. Vlcek B, Burchiel KJ, Gordon T. Tuberculous meningitis presenting as an obstructive myelopathy. Case report. *J Neurosurg*. 1984;60(1):196-199.
96. Garg RK, Malhotra HS, Kumar N. Paradoxical reaction in HIV negative tuberculous meningitis. *J Neurol Sci*. 2014;340(1-2):26-36.
97. Bansal D, et al. Cervical intramedullary tuberculoma: acute presentation and rapid response to medical therapy. *J Trop Pediatr*. 2002;48(1):55-57.
98. Kalita J, Mistra UK. Intramedullary cervical tuberculoma. *Spinal Cord*. 1999;37:297-298.
99. Chang KH, et al. Tuberculous arachnoiditis of the spine: findings on myelography, CT, and MR imaging. *AJNR Am J Neuroradiol*. 1989;10(6):1255-1262.

100. Lin TH. Intramedullary tuberculoma of the spinal cord. *J Neurosurg.* 1960;17:497-499.
101. Ratliff JK, Connolly ES. Intramedullary tuberculoma of the spinal cord. Case report and review of the literature. *J Neurosurg.* 1999;90(suppl 1):125-128.
102. Tacconi L, et al. Intramedullary spinal cord abscess: case report. *Neurosurgery.* 1995;37(4):817-819.
103. Brooks WD, Fletcher AP, Wilson RR. Spinal cord complications of tuberculous meningitis; a clinical and pathological study. *Q J Med.* 1954;23(91):275-290.
104. Varatharajah S, et al. Update on the surgical management of Pott's disease. *Orthop Traumatol Surg Res.* 2014;100(2):229-235.
105. Kobayashi K, et al. Tuberculous meningitis with dementia as the presenting symptom after intramedullary spinal cord tumor resection. *Nagoya J Med Sci.* 2015;77(4):653-657.
106. Chittem L, Bommanakanti K, Alugolu R. 'Precipitation sign': a new radiological sign for spinal intramedullary tubercular abscess. *Spinal Cord.* 2014;52(suppl 1):S1-S2.
107. Genzen JR, Kenney B. Central nervous system *Aspergillus* infection after epidural analgesia: diagnosis, therapeutic challenges, and literature review. *Diagn Microbiol Infect Dis.* 2009;65(3):312-318.
108. Malani AN, et al. Magnetic resonance imaging screening to identify spinal and paraspinal infections associated with injections of contaminated methylprednisolone acetate. *JAMA.* 2013;309(23):2465-2472.
109. Moudgal V, et al. Spinal and paraspinal fungal infections associated with contaminated methylprednisolone injections. *Open Forum Infect Dis.* 2014;1(1):22.
110. Smith RM, et al. Fungal infections associated with contaminated methylprednisolone injections. *N Engl J Med.* 2013;369(17):1598-1609.
111. Voelker JL, Muller J, Worth RM. Intramedullary spinal *Histoplasma* granuloma. Case report. *J Neurosurg.* 1989;70(6):959-961.
112. Merwick Á, et al. Intradural extramedullary spinal *Candida* infection. *Practical Neurology.* 2015;15(5):400-404.
113. Ingwer I, et al. *Aspergillus fumigatus* epidural abscess in a renal transplant recipient. *Arch Intern Med.* 1978;138(1):153-154.
114. Kingsley DP, et al. Intradural extramedullary aspergilloma complicating chronic lymphatic leukaemia. *Br J Radiol.* 1979;52(623):916-917.
115. Pfausler B, et al. Syndrome of the anterior spinal artery as the primary manifestation of aspergillosis. *Infection.* 1995;23(4):240-242.
116. Stein SC, et al. Chronic mycotic meningitis with spinal involvement (arachnoiditis): a report of five cases. *Ann Neurol.* 1982;11(5):519-524.
117. McCaslin AF, et al. Thoracic spinal cord intramedullary *Aspergillus* invasion and abscess. *J Clin Neurosci.* 2015;22(2):404-406.
118. Tan LA, et al. Rapidly progressive quadriparesis heralding disseminated coccidioidomycosis in an immunocompetent patient. *J Clin Neurosci.* 2014;21(6):1049-1051.
119. Cravens G, et al. Spinal cord compression due to intradural extramedullary aspergilloma and cyst: a case report. *Surg Neurol.* 1989;31(4):315-318.
120. Van de Wyngaert FA, et al. Spinal arachnoiditis due to *Aspergillus* meningitis in a previously healthy patient. *J Neurol.* 1986;233(1):41-43.
121. Young RF, Gade G, Grinnell V. Surgical treatment for fungal infections in the central nervous system. *J Neurosurg.* 1985;63(3):371-381.

SECTION XIII

CHAPTER 92 Vascular Malformations of the Spinal Cord

John E. O'Toole
Paul C. McCormick

Vascular lesions of the spinal cord are a rare cause of neurologic dysfunction, representing less than 5% of all intraspinal pathology.[1] This heterogeneous class of entities encompasses a wide range of etiologic, anatomic, pathophysiologic, and clinical features. They occur throughout the spine and may affect any age group, although the vast majority present between the third and fifth decades of life.[1] Symptoms and signs result from ischemia, venous congestion, hemorrhage, or mechanical compression of the spinal cord and roots. Most spinal vascular lesions are characterized by an abnormal arteriovenous shunt, which may be located within the dura, on the spinal cord surface, within the substance of the spinal cord or, rarely, extradurally.[2–5] The shunt may take the form of a simple direct arteriovenous fistula (AVF) or a more complex nidus of dysmorphic arteries and veins without an intervening capillary bed. Whereas the latter lesions are typically congenital, the more common fistulous lesions are often acquired.[6]

The evaluation and management of spinal vascular lesions have evolved considerably over recent decades as a result of accumulating clinical experience and the role of selective spinal angiography and embolization therapies. A fundamental understanding of the anatomy and pathophysiology of these lesions coupled with refinements in endovascular and operative techniques has permitted successful definitive therapy with minimal morbidity in most patients harboring vascular shunts of the spinal cord.

Classification

Various nomenclature and classification systems have been employed in the description of spinal vascular lesions.[4,7–9] As a first approximation, these lesions can be broadly divided by the presence or absence of an arteriovenous shunt. The vascular lesions without a shunt are cavernous malformations, a lesion of capillary structure.[10] Spinal cord arteriovenous shunts are separated into four types on the basis of the location and angioarchitecture of the abnormal arteriovenous connection (Box 92.1). Types I and IV represent direct AVFs that occur within the dural root sleeve (type I) or on the spinal cord surface (type IV). Type II arteriovenous malformations (AVMs) are true congenital malformations, similar to their intracranial pial counterparts. Type III AVMs are also congenital but demonstrate extensive contiguous involvement of intramedullary, intradural-extramedullary, and extradural-paraspinal tissues.

Spinal Arteriovenous Fistula/Malformation

Type I

Type I AVFs, the most commonly occurring type of spinal vascular malformation, have also been termed long dorsal AVMs; single-coiled vessel AVMs; angioma venosum racemosum; dural AVF; micro-AVF; and, more recently, intradural dorsal AVF.[4,7,8,11–17] A more sophisticated understanding of the anatomy and pathophysiology of these fistulas has developed since the seminal description by Wyburn-Mason,[17] who characterized these as purely venous lesions. The advent of selective spinal angiography in the 1960s reclassified them as slow-flow AVFs. Early surgical treatment was directed at stripping the long dorsal vein off the spinal cord surface. It was assumed that tiny feeding vessels, too small to be seen angiographically, supplied this dilated vein throughout its length. This treatment approach did stabilize or improve symptoms in some patients, but postoperative neurologic deterioration was seen in many others. Kendall and Logue,[13] in 1977, correctly recognized these lesions as simple AVFs between a radicular or radiculomedullary artery and a medullary vein, with the fistulous connection located in the dural root sleeve (Fig. 92.1). The entire intradural portion of the malformation, therefore, represents the enlarged spinal cord venous system that has been pathologically engorged from retrograde flow from the fistula into the spinal cord veins (Fig. 92.2). These malformations are likely often acquired and arise predominantly at thoracic and thoracolumbar levels. As mentioned earlier, these shunts and their venous drainage are almost universally dorsally located, with ventral communications being exceedingly rare.[18]

Type II

These malformations are known as glomus, nidus, or simply intramedullary type AVMs.[4,7] They are angiographically and

BOX 92.1 Classification of Spinal Vascular Malformations

Lesions With Arteriovenous Shunts

Type I (dural root sleeve AVF)
Type II (glomus AVM)
Type III (juvenile AVM)
Type IV (intradural AVF)

Lesions Without Arteriovenous Shunt

Cavernous malformations
Hemangioblastoma (?)

AVF, arteriovenous fistula; AVM, arteriovenous malformation.

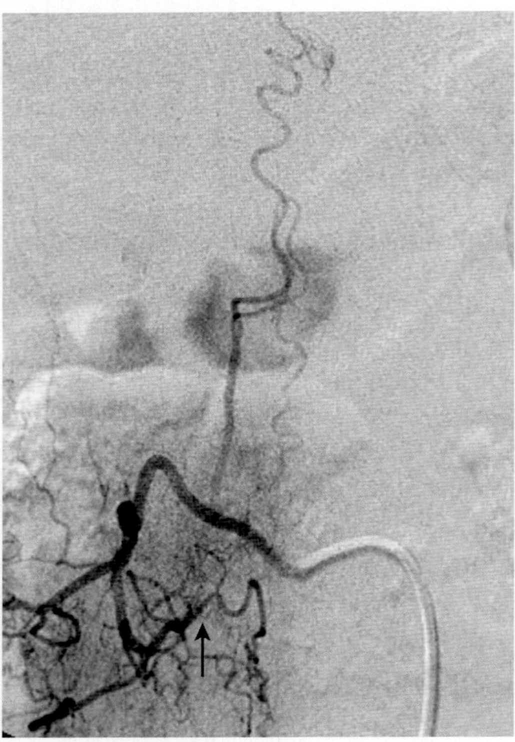

FIG. 92.1 Anteroposterior view of right L1 selective angiography demonstrates the typical fistula (*arrow*) of a type I AVF and the characteristic intradural medullary draining vein that extends on the dorsal surface of the spinal cord over many rostral segments.

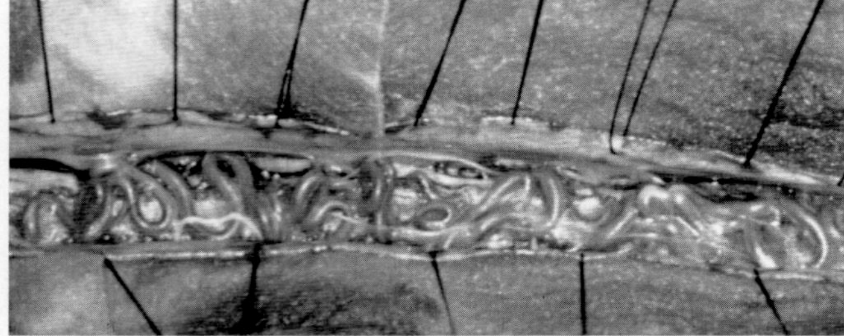

FIG. 92.2 Intraoperative image of a type I arteriovenous fistula shows an enlarged coiled vein on the dorsal spinal surface. (From Youmans JR. *Neurological Surgery*. 3rd ed. Philadelphia: WB Saunders; 1990.)

operatively well-defined lesions consisting of a distinct conglomeration of dysmorphic arteries and veins in direct communication without an intervening capillary bed (Figs. 92.3 and 92.4).[19,20] The location of the nidus may be completely or partially intramedullary and only rarely is confined to the epipial tissue of the cord. These latter lesions are sometimes referred to as perimedullary type II AVMs and most commonly occur dorsally at the cervicomedullary junction (Fig. 92.5).

Typical type II AVMs may arise anywhere within the spinal cord but predominantly are found at the cervical and lumbar enlargements or the conus medullaris. Type II AVMs of the cervical spinal cord frequently have multiple feeding vessels of anterior spinal, posterior spinal, and radiculomedullary arteries, whereas type II AVMs of the thoracic spinal cord or conus are often supplied via a single enlarged branch of the anterior spinal artery. Latent anastomotic channels invariably exist, however, which may emerge after proximal ligation or endovascular occlusion of the primary feeding vessel (Fig. 92.6).

Type III

Also known as juvenile or metameric AVMs, type III malformations are fortunately rare. These lesions do not possess a discrete nidus but rather consist of diffuse arteriovenous shunts with variable degrees of involvement of the spinal cord, vertebral, and paraspinal tissues (Fig. 92.7). Other metameric anomalies of associated organs and the skin are commonly associated with these lesions.

Type IV

Type IV malformations are completely intradural fistulas, variably referred to as perimedullary AVF, macro-AVF, or intradural ventral AVF.[4,7,8,12,21,22] Most occur in the thoracolumbar region as a fistula between the anterior spinal artery (ASA) and anterior spinal vein on the ventral spinal cord surface. Gueguen and colleagues[23] as well as Anson and Spetzler[12] subdivided these arteriovenous shunts according to the complexity and size of the lesion. A type IV-A malformation is a small, simple direct fistula with a single ASA feeder. Type IV-B lesions are medium-sized fistulas and have additional smaller feeding vessels arising from either the ASA or posterior spinal artery. Type IV-C fistulas are giant sized and demonstrate several enlarged ASA and posterior spinal artery feeding branches with dilated venous outflow. The subtypes may represent progressive changes resulting from venous congestion, thrombosis, collateral vessel recruitment, or ischemia. The sporadic nature of these malformations suggests an acquired rather than congenital nature, but their rarity makes their etiology difficult to determine.

Pathophysiology and Symptomatology

The pathophysiology of vascular malformations reflects localized derangements in spinal cord blood flow that are related

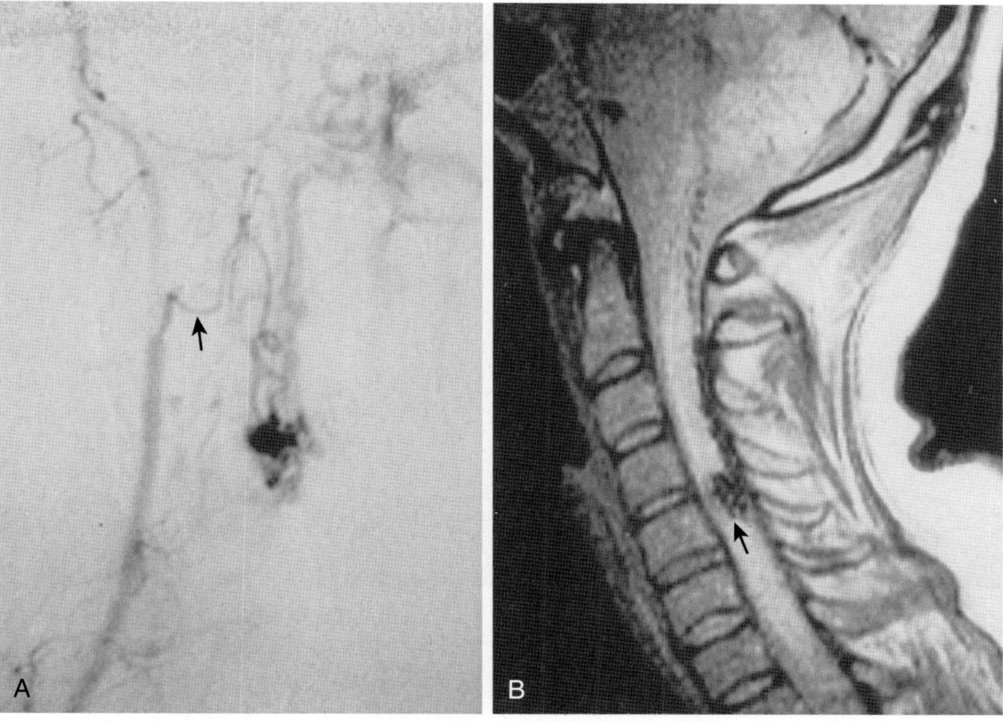

FIG. 92.3 (A) Selective spinal angiography reveals type II arteriovenous malformation of the cervical spinal cord supplied by a branch of the anterior spinal artery (*arrow*). (B) Sagittal magnetic resonance imaging demonstrates intramedullary location of the lesion (*arrow*). (From Youmans JR. *Neurological Surgery*. 3rd ed. Philadelphia: WB Saunders; 1990.)

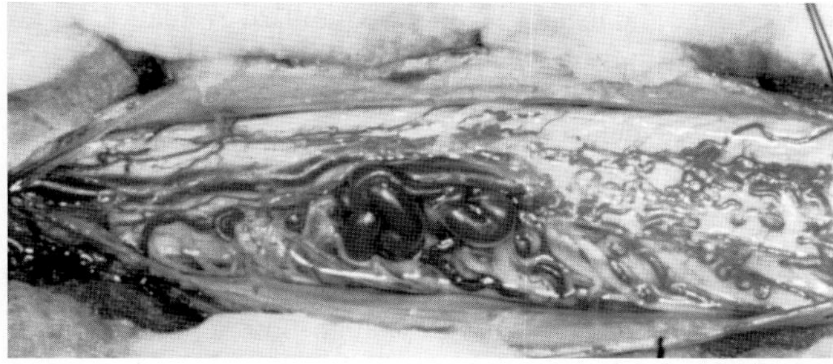

FIG. 92.4 Intraoperative image of a type II arteriovenous malformation shows a dorsally superficial arterialized vein overlying the intramedullary nidus that expands the circumference of the spinal cord. (From Youmans JR. *Neurological Surgery*. 3rd ed. Philadelphia: WB Saunders; 1990.)

primarily to the specific type of malformation. Similarly, the presenting symptoms and signs of spinal vascular malformations depend on whether the pertinent pathophysiologic process is venous congestion, hemorrhage, ischemia, or localized mass effect. Each type of lesion is discussed separately in this section, but, in general, relatively slow-flow lesions have typically chronic progressive courses indicative of high venous pressures, whereas high-flow lesions often have more abrupt presentations related to hemorrhage or ischemia.

Type I

Type I AVFs produce progressive spinal cord ischemia from venous hypertension.[7,11,15,16,24–28] Despite slow flow through the shunt, intradural venous pressures become markedly elevated and may approach systemic mean arterial pressure. Because spinal cord perfusion pressure is equal to mean systemic arterial pressure minus venous pressure, progressive spinal cord ischemia may ensue. The elevation of intraspinal venous pressures during activity or exercise accounts for the reversible ischemic symptoms often seen in these patients. Venous hypertension may be further exacerbated by structural changes, such as reductions in venous diameter and compliance secondary to intimal thickening and hyalinization seen with chronic exposure to high intravenous pressures (Fig. 92.8). Episodic acute neurologic deterioration in these patients may occur as a result of venous thrombosis. In rare cases, patients may present with subarachnoid hemorrhage mimicking that of intracranial aneurysm rupture.[29,30]

It follows, then, that type I AVFs produce symptoms usually in middle and advanced adult years with a mean age at symptom onset around 50 years. Men are four to five times more commonly affected than women. The majority occur in the thoracic or thoracolumbar region. Symptoms typically arise insidiously with back and leg pain and mild sensorimotor dysfunction. In early stages, symptoms may mimic those of neurogenic claudication secondary to spinal stenosis. Neurologic examination, however, often reveals mixed upper and lower motor neuron disease and patchy sensory loss, clearly differentiating the clinical picture from degenerative lumbar stenosis. The natural history of type I AVFs produces an inexorable progression of symptoms occasionally punctuated by episodes of acute worsening, as in the classic Foix-Alajouanine

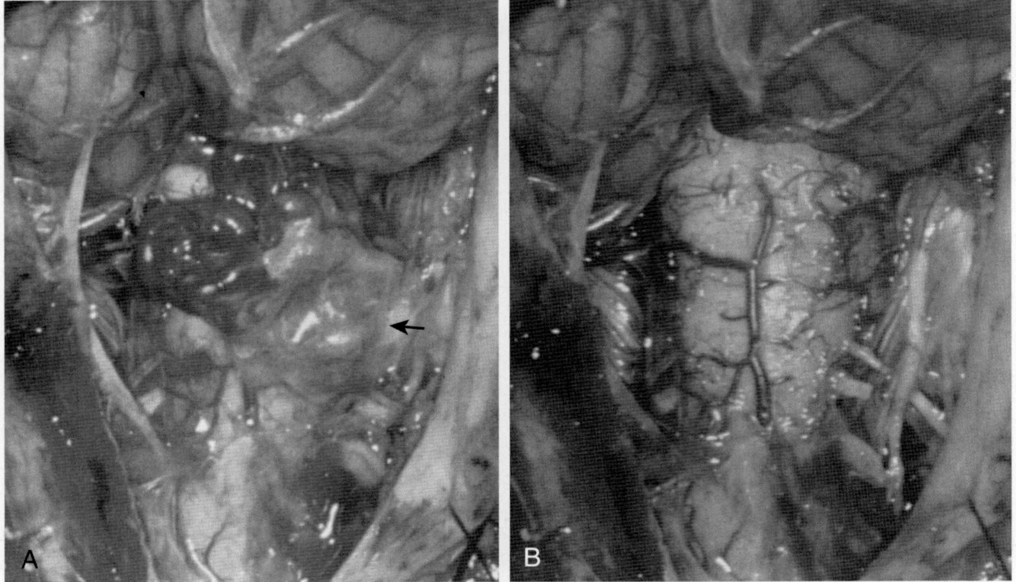

FIG. 92.5 Intraoperative photographs (A) before and (B) after surgical resection of a dorsal cervicomedullary junction type II AVM with associated venous aneurysm (*arrow*). (From Youmans JR. *Neurological Surgery*. 3rd ed. Philadelphia: WB Saunders; 1990.)

syndrome. If untreated, these lesions lead to significant disability and wheelchair dependence in most patients within 6 months to 3 years after symptom onset.[15]

Numerous investigators have demonstrated that preoperative neurologic status is the most important predictor of posttreatment outcomes.[28,31–33] Median time from symptom onset to diagnosis in modern series ranges from 15 to 23 months.[32–36] If type I AVFs are treated early in their course, symptoms are often reversible. However, in more chronic cases, progressive ischemia ultimately leads to irreversible neuronal loss and infarction. Therefore, definitive treatment should be administered as early in the disease as possible because function is unlikely to improve in the presence of severe incapacity.

Type II

As in types III and IV, type II AVMs are high-flow lesions in which the AVM nidus acts as a low-resistance sump siphoning blood away from the surrounding normal spinal cord producing ischemia. In addition to such "vascular steal" mechanisms, the high pressure and flow characteristics through these dysmorphic vessels render them susceptible to hemorrhage, in most cases on the venous side of the malformation, often from a venous aneurysm. Finally, enlarged tortuous feeding vessels or draining veins may cause localized mass effect with compression of the spinal cord or spinal roots, resulting in myelopathy or radiculopathy, respectively.

Type II AVMs present in childhood or adult years. An acute presentation from subarachnoid hemorrhage or intramedullary hemorrhage is most common.[16] As mentioned earlier, the presence of venous aneurysms seems to increase the risk of a hemorrhagic event. The acute onset of severe neck or back pain ("coup de poignard"[37]) approximates the level of the malformation and is typically the first symptom of AVM hemorrhage. The occurrence and progression of neurologic deficit are variable and dependent on the location and severity of the hemorrhage. For example, typical headache and nuchal rigidity may be the only symptoms of a spinal subarachnoid hemorrhage and usually lead to the standard evaluation for an intracranial ruptured aneurysm.[38] On the other hand, objective deficits are typically seen with intramedullary hemorrhage. These deficits evolve over minutes to hours; some degree of recovery is usually seen after incomplete lesions.

Types III and IV

Similar to type II AVMs, these high-flow lesions produce symptoms due to vascular steal/ischemia, hemorrhage, and mass effect. Type III AVMs have been associated with genetic syndromes such as Klippel-Trenaunay-Weber.[39] Type IV lesions have an equal incidence in males and females. Symptoms may arise at any age, although most patients present in childhood and early to middle adult years. Associations with hereditary hemorrhagic telangiectasia (Rendu-Osler-Weber disease) and Kartagener syndrome have been noted in younger patients.[7,8,40,41]

Radiology

Selective spinal angiography remains the gold standard for the definitive diagnosis and characterization of spinal vascular malformations. This imaging study identifies the locations and flow characteristics of vascular shunts as well as the sites of critical radiculomedullary arteries (e.g., artery of Adamkiewicz).[13,20-22,42-46] Its inherently invasive nature, however, has led to the development and use of alternative modalities as

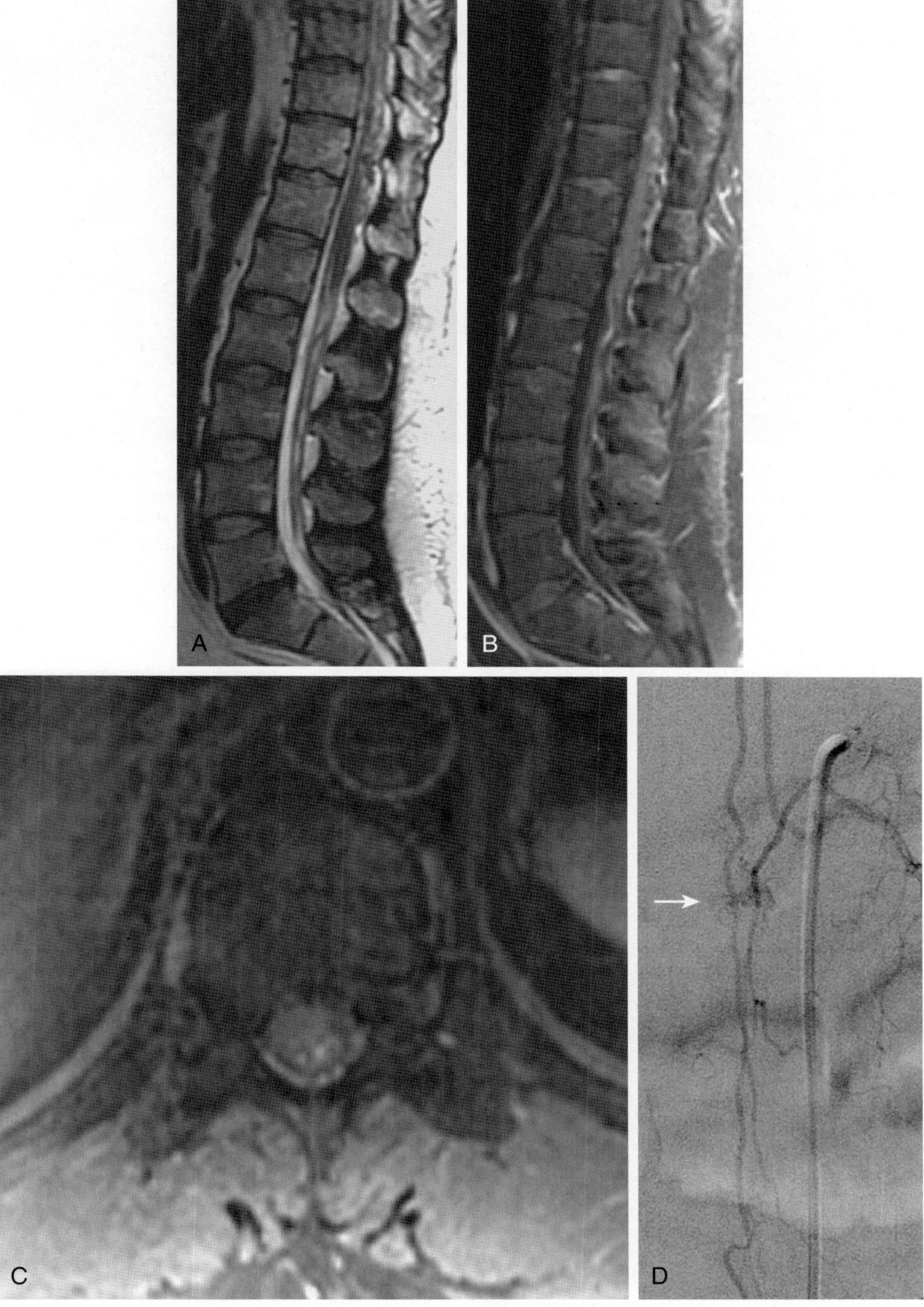

FIG. 92.6 (A) Sagittal T2-weighted magnetic resonance image (MRI) demonstrates numerous serpiginous flow voids over the dorsal surface of the lower thoracic spinal cord in a patient who had undergone prior embolization of a type II arteriovenous malformation (AVM) in this region. (B) Sagittal and (C) axial T1-weighted MRI with gadolinium show enhancing nidus of vessels in the substance of the cord at the level of the T10–T11 disc space. (D) Selective angiographic injection of the left T10 artery reveals the AVM nidus (*arrow*) and the associated shunting into the medullary venous system rostrad and caudad.

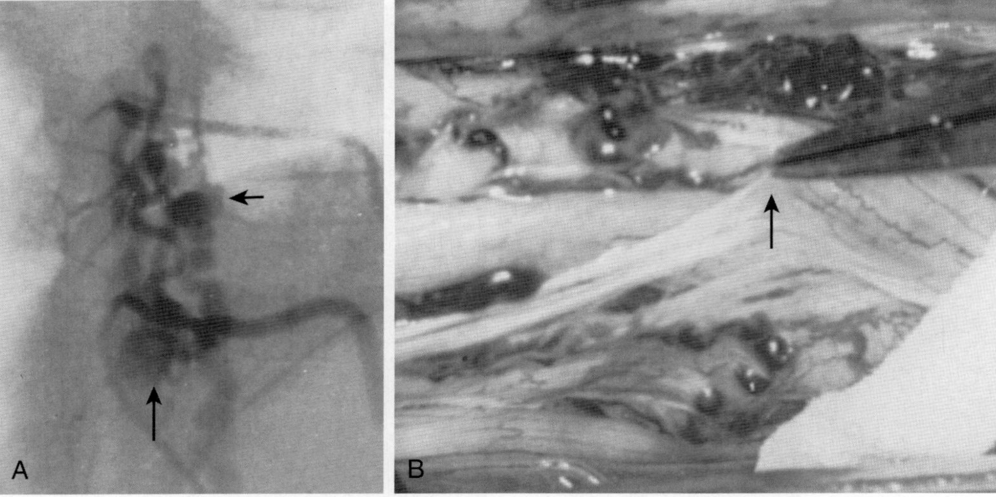

FIG. 92.7 (A) Spinal angiogram shows the intramedullary and extramedullary nature of a type III AVM (*arrows*). (B) Intraoperative image of another type III AVM demonstrates the dorsal, dorsolateral, and ventral location of the lesion permeating the intramedullary and extramedullary compartments and preventing safe resection. The cord is rotated by grasping the dentate ligament (*arrow*). (From Youmans JR. *Neurological Surgery*. 3rd ed. Philadelphia: WB Saunders; 1990.)

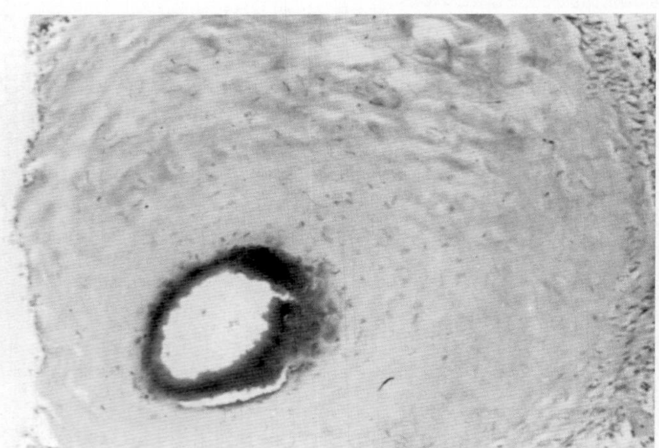

FIG. 92.8 Histologic cross-section of a vessel from a spinal cord vascular malformation demonstrates hyalinization and endarteritis obliterans with a minimal lumen. (From Youmans JR. *Neurological Surgery*. 3rd ed. Philadelphia: WB Saunders; 1990.)

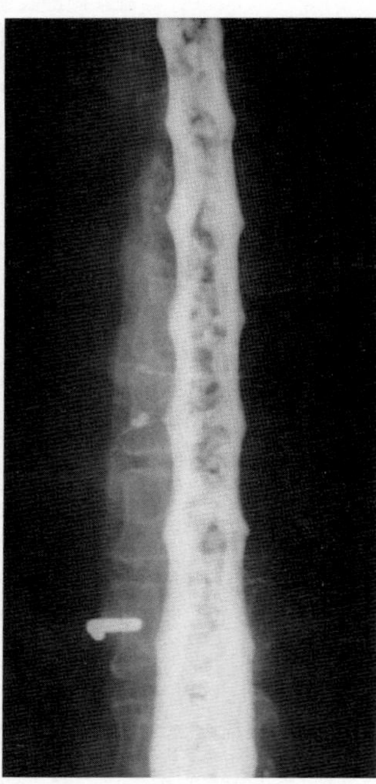

FIG. 92.9 Anteroposterior thoracic myelography reveals a typical long serpentine filling defect characteristic of type I arteriovenous fistula. (From Youmans JR. *Neurological Surgery*. 3rd ed. Philadelphia: WB Saunders; 1990.)

screening procedures. These currently include magnetic resonance imaging (MRI), magnetic resonance angiography (MRA), computed tomographic (CT) angiography (CTA), and CT myelography. Myelography has a long history in the diagnosis of spinal AVMs, particularly for type I AVFs, in which the characteristic serpentine filling defect on the dorsal spinal cord surface is often apparent (Fig. 92.9). These enlarged vessels are commonly identified on screening magnetic resonance scans (Fig. 92.10). If the filling defect extends toward a neural foramen, the level and side of the fistula may be suggested. The dilated venous filling defect should be differentiated from the venous dilatation seen rostral to high-grade extradural stenotic blocks.

MRI and MRA are useful for the initial screening of AVFs and are critical in the evaluation of intramedullary malformations, particularly with regard to operative planning and understanding the relationship of the malformation to the normal spinal cord. As with CT myelography, both MRA and CTA may permit more targeted selective angiography.[47,48]

Three-dimensional angiography is also emerging as a potential aid in angiographic delineation of the structural

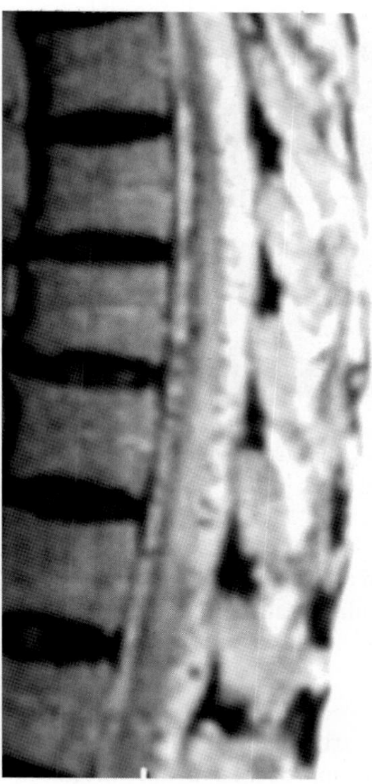

FIG. 92.10 T2-weighted sagittal magnetic resonance image of the spine demonstrates multiple signal voids on ventral and dorsal aspects of the spinal cord.

anatomy of spinal vascular malformations and their relationship to the surrounding spine and normal vessels.[49]

Treatment

Successful treatment of spinal vascular malformations requires the total obliteration or excision of the abnormal shunt. [11,12,14,15,21,26,38,44–46,50–52] Procedures that only partially reduce the shunt or address only proximal feeders may provide temporary benefit but all too often lead to delayed recurrences.

Surgical Therapy: General Considerations

The surgical approach to spinal cord vascular malformations depends on the level and anatomic position of the lesion. Nevertheless, the majority are dorsal or dorsolateral and therefore can be approached via a standard posterior laminectomy of appropriate number of levels. In general, routine perioperative antibiotics and corticosteroids are administered at the time of surgery. Neurophysiologic monitoring, including somatosensory evoked potential and motor evoked potential, are also routinely used. Whereas authors such as Malis[53] have described the use of the sitting or oblique positions for the posterior removal of malformations, we prefer the prone position for all such laminectomies. Although the sitting position decreases venous pressure and respiratory excursions, it also precludes the effective use of an assistant during the operation. With the patient in the prone position, the surgeon and assistant work together across the operating table.

The laminectomy is centered over the extent of the lesion, as identified on preoperative imaging. The bony exposure should be moderately wide and the dura opened with preservation of the arachnoid until the lesion can be visualized. The operating microscope is used from the time of dural opening. Malformations with an extramedullary component are immediately apparent, with the exception of small type IV fistulas on the ventral surface of the cord. Those lesions with a primarily intramedullary location (e.g., type II or cavernous malformations) are often identified by a bulging or discoloration of the spinal cord. The techniques for the removal of these latter lesions are similar to those used with intramedullary spinal cord tumors and are described in greater detail later.

For complex cases, intraoperative confirmation of shunt elimination may be obtained. The standard method employed is intraoperative angiography.[54,55] This, however, has its limitations with regard to both patient positioning and image resolution. For types I and IV fistulas, some authors have described the use of intraoperative micro-Doppler ultrasound or infrared imaging of spinal vascular blood flow to demonstrate successful obliteration of the shunt.[56–58]

After satisfactory occlusion or removal of the vascular shunt, hemostasis is meticulously achieved and a primary dural closure is performed. Should the latter not be possible, a dural substitute, either as onlay or sutured graft, may serve to reduce the risk of cerebrospinal fluid leak and postoperative scarring from the paraspinal musculature.

Endovascular Therapy: General Considerations

The role of endovascular techniques in the treatment of spinal vascular malformations continues to evolve. Advances in catheter technology, image resolution, and embolization materials have allowed increasing success and safety in the elimination of certain vascular lesions. The wide variety of embolic materials used in the endovascular treatment of spinal vascular malformations includes *N*-butyl cyanoacrylate, Onyx, polyvinyl alcohol, coils, cellulose acetate polymer, and trisacryl gelatin microspheres.[33,59–62]

The more widespread use of liquid adhesive embolic agents such as *N*-butyl cyanoacrylate and ethylene vinyl alcohol copolymer (Onyx Micro Therapeutics Inc) has generally been associated with more durable results and less recanalization as compared with particulate embolic materials (e.g., polyvinyl alcohol). Both neurophysiologic monitoring and pharmacologic provocative testing have emerged as important adjuncts in the endovascular treatment of spinal vascular malformations. Somatosensory evoked potentials and motor evoked potentials and testing with intraarterial injections of agents such as amobarbital (Amytal) and lidocaine have been shown to allow safer embolization of spinal AVMs.[62–64]

Whether endovascular techniques occupy a primary or adjunctive role depends not only on the type of vascular lesions but also on institutional experience. Whereas embolization may clearly be the procedure of choice for extradural fistulas and type III vascular malformations,[2] surgery remains the gold standard for type II lesions. For types I and IV lesions, some authors advocate initial treatment attempts with embolization,

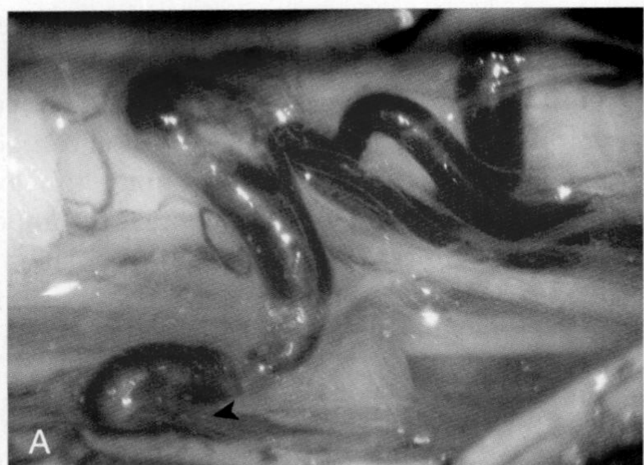

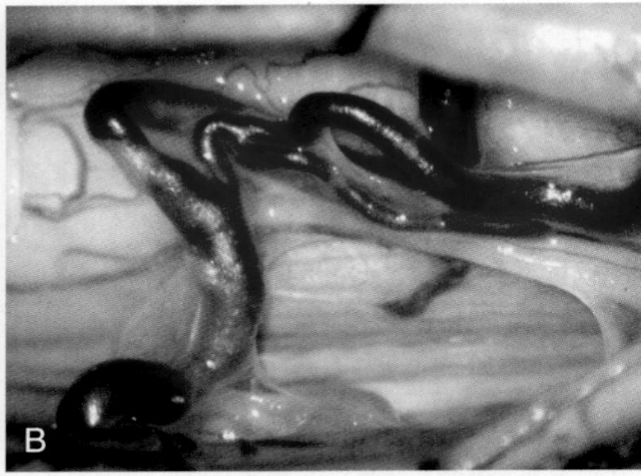

FIG. 92.11 (A) Intraoperative image of a type I arteriovenous fistula shows a T5 feeder arterializing dorsal spinal veins. Note the lateral dural entry point of the draining vein (*arrowhead*). (B) After coagulation of the vein at the dural entry point, the spinal venous system is noticeably less engorged.

reserving surgery for failures, but others prefer surgery as first-line treatment.

Type I

Treatment of type I dural AVFs has been simplified over the years. Operative stripping of the long dorsal vein off the spinal cord surface was recognized as a tedious and unnecessary procedure that was responsible for neurologic morbidity due to removal of normal spinal cord venous drainage. Currently, these lesions are treated by simpler and more refined surgical technique or by endovascular occlusion.

Operatively, type I shunts may be treated by excision of the dural fistula or interruption of the intradural draining vein (Fig. 92.11).[11,24,25] This can easily be accomplished via a two-level hemilaminectomy and partial medial facetectomy, exposing the dural root sleeve and foramen. A paramedian longitudinal dural incision allows exposure of the intradural nerve root and initial segment of the associated draining vein of the shunt. Simple interruption of the draining vein is the generally preferred technique, particularly in circumstances in which the radicular artery that supplies the fistula also supplies a spinal cord medullary artery. This, fortunately, occurs in less than 10% of cases. In cases of more complex or recurrent type I AVFs, fistula excision definitively prevents reestablishment of retrograde intradural venous drainage through collateral longitudinal extradural venous channels at adjacent radicular levels. Several millimeters of the feeding radicular artery and intradural draining vein may be cauterized, divided, and contiguously excised along with a small window of dura on the root sleeve. This dural defect can be primarily repaired with sutures. The wound is then closed in layers in a typical fashion.

Outcomes following the treatment of type I AVFs are generally good, with most reports demonstrating neurologic improvement or stabilization in 70% to 99% of patients.[31,32,36,65–68] Interestingly, motor and gait disturbances seem to improve to a greater degree than sensory or sacral deficits.[31,65] Surgery produces a 98% fistula obliteration rate, and endovascular embolization produces a 25% to 66% obliteration rate.[32,35,36,66,68–70] In general, then, for most type I lesions, we recommend surgery as a primary therapy to avoid the progressive myelopathy associated with a delay in definitive treatment that can be seen with endovascular treatment failures.

Type II

As mentioned earlier, type II lesions are classic AVMs and, as such, are often approached in an interdisciplinary manner using both endovascular and operative techniques. Endovascular occlusion of primary feeding vessels may reduce the overall shunt and assist removal at open surgery.

The type II malformations that form a simple nidus in a perimedullary location are the easiest to understand and treat. Circumferential interruption of their feeding arteries at the exact margin of the glomus is the surgical technique of choice. Interruption of the venous side of an AVM first can lead to hazardous elevations in pressure in the remaining venous drainage system, producing either excessive bleeding around the AVM or rupture of associated venous aneurysms.

Malformations that are largely intramedullary are similarly treated incorporating techniques used for intramedullary spinal cord tumors. The locus of the lesion is visualized, and a myelotomy is made over the dorsal surface of the malformation identifying both rostral and caudal poles of the malformation. Typically, irrigating bipolar cautery is used during the obliteration of the malformation. Only the largest vessels are clipped; from a practical point of view, this means clipping few or no arteries because the application of metallic clips to intramedullary lesions often proves difficult or dangerous. As expected, the AVM is approached from the arterial side first, serially coagulating and dividing arterial contributions to the AVM as it is gently peeled away from the cord substance on its venous pedicle, which is ligated just prior to final removal. As mentioned earlier, early interruption of the venous drainage should be avoided. Aneurysmal venous dilatations are prone to rupture even with minor surgical manipulation. Bipolar cautery can be used to shrink these venous aneurysms, but care must be taken not to violate the thin vessel wall. In some cases, the venous aneurysm may be gently teased out of the cord (Fig. 92.12).

In any case, the removal of the malformation and associated aneurysms leaves a surgical defect similar to that seen with

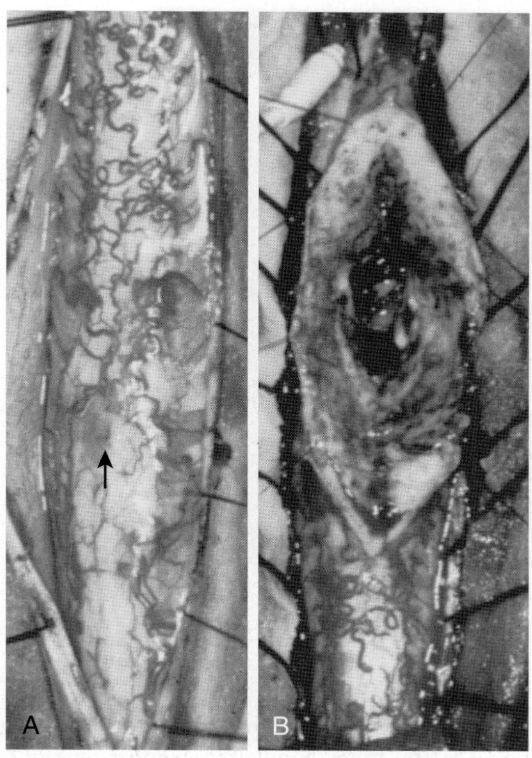

FIG. 92.12 (A) Intraoperative image demonstrates a large type II arteriovenous malformation (AVM). The *arrow* indicates a partially thrombosed venous aneurysm within the substance of the cord. (B) Total extirpation of the AVM and venous aneurysm was achieved via midline myelotomy. (From Youmans JR. *Neurological Surgery*. 3rd ed. Philadelphia: WB Saunders; 1990.)

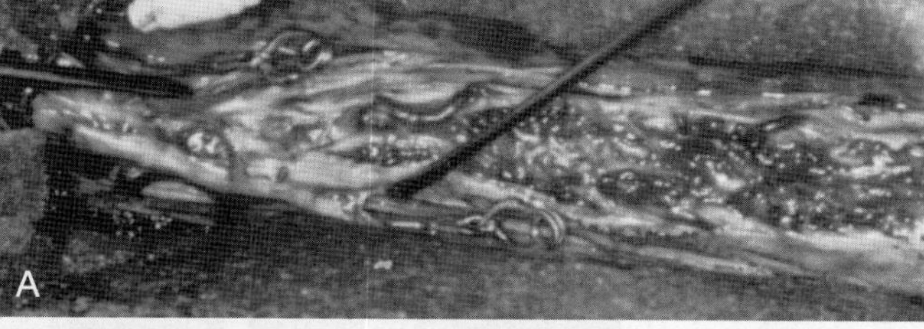

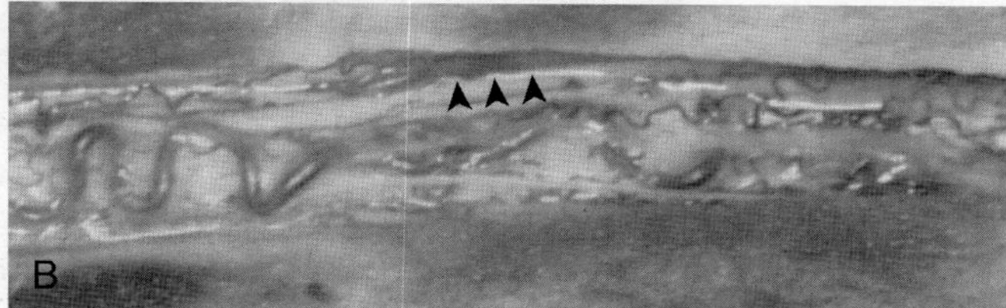

FIG. 92.13 Intraoperative images demonstrate interruption of (A) bilateral (*clips*) or (B) single (*arrowheads*) arterial feeders to type III arteriovenous malformations without radical excision of the extensive malformations. (From Youmans JR. *Neurological Surgery*. 3rd ed. Philadelphia: WB Saunders; 1990.)

excision of intramedullary tumors. It is indeed remarkable how thin the remaining spinal cord substance can appear and yet still produce functional neurologic outcomes postoperatively.

Type III

These lesions are the most difficult to treat. They penetrate the spinal cord, and histologic examination indicates violation of presumably functional cord tissue interspersed with vascular channels of the malformation. These AVMs do not have well-defined margins and comprehensively involve the intramedullary, intradural-extramedullary, and extradural compartments over many spinal segments. Although these are generally unresectable lesions, partial treatment through endovascular embolization, surgical decompression, and limited arterial ligation may produce some clinical benefit (Fig. 92.13).[4]

Such improvements are usually not durable, however, and the significant risk associated with aggressive treatment of type III AVMs must be carefully weighed before initiating any invasive therapies.

Type IV

Treatment of type IV AVFs depends particularly on the size and complexity of the lesion.[21,22] For small type IV-A shunts, surgical ligation of the fistula is definitive. Adequate exposure of these ventral intradural shunts often requires more aggressive posterior or posterolateral bone removal including facetectomy, as well as spinal cord rotation with suture retraction of the dentate ligament. Alternatively, anterior or anterolateral approaches to such ventral lesions may be used, with special attention paid to the need for spinal reconstruction and the attendant risk of cerebrospinal fluid fistulas.[71,72] Intraoperative intravenous administration of near-infrared indocyanine can be useful in assessing the completeness of the resection of difficult spinal cord vascular malformations.[73]

For more complex, higher-flow lesions (types IV-B and IV-C), endovascular obliteration of the shunt may be the preferred primary treatment or at least a preoperative adjunct.[22,40,74]

Cavernous Malformations

Cavernous malformations are benign congenital vascular lesions that occur in every organ system, including the brain and spinal cord. Pathologically, cavernous malformations consist of endothelial-lined capillary-like chambers and sinusoids without intervening neural tissue. They are slow-flow lesions without a direct arteriovenous fistula. Hemosiderin-stained neural tissue is often present at the peripheral margin of these malformations, indicative of prior hemorrhage or vascular leakage.

The etiology of cavernous malformations is unclear. Most are sporadic and solitary, but up to 10% to 15% of patients have more than one lesion, either in the spinal cord or brain.[75] A similar percentage of patients have a family history of cavernous malformations supporting a genetic risk factor.

Pathophysiology and Symptomatology

Based on the prevalence of cavernous malformation, it is likely that the vast majority of these lesions are incidental and asymptomatic throughout life. Therefore, the discovery of an incidental spinal cord cavernous malformation does

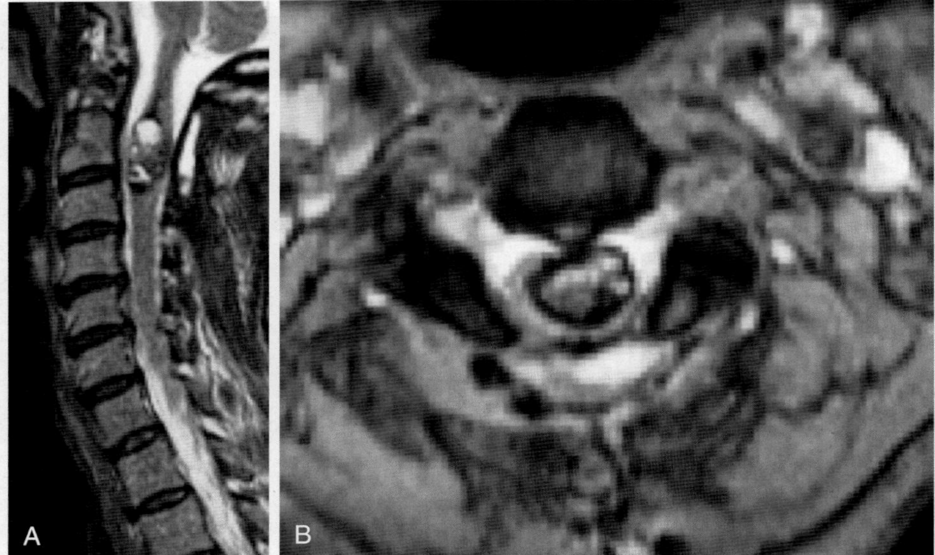

FIG. 92.14 T2-weighted (A) sagittal and (B) axial magnetic resonance imaging shows heterogeneous mass consisting of intralesional hemorrhagic/blood products surrounded by a well-defined low-signal hemosiderin margin.

not require consideration of treatment or periodic imaging surveillance. Symptomatic cavernous malformations generally present with acute hemorrhage and neurologic deficit. The deficits are generally mild to moderate in severity and often demonstrate significant improvement over the following weeks to months. The occurrence of an acute hemorrhage increases the risk of further hemorrhagic events.[76]

Radiology

Because cavernous malformations are slow-flow capillary lesions without arteriovenous shunting, angiography is usually unrevealing. Fortunately, due to the often enlarged blood-filled interstices of cavernous malformations, MRI is usually both characteristic and diagnostic for these lesions. T1- and T2-weighted MRI are particularly useful. On T1-weighted images, these lobulated masses tend to be isointense and hyperintense with an edge of hypointensity, which represents the reactive gliotic capsule. On T2-weighted images, the lesions are also heterogeneous, with a predominant hyperintensity surrounded by a hypointense rim after hemorrhage (Fig. 92.14). The heterogeneity is one of the characteristics of these lesions, which gives them the classic "popcorn" or "mulberry" appearance.[77]

Treatment

The treatment for symptomatic cavernous malformations is surgery. Neither radiosurgery nor embolization has been shown to be effective. As previously noted, surgery is usually not performed for asymptomatic lesions. The decision to recommend surgery for symptomatic lesions depends on an individualized patient evaluation that considers the severity of the symptoms as well as the risk of future hemorrhage and the risk of surgical intervention. For small, dorsally located lesions that reach the surface of the spinal cord, the risk of surgery is quite low. On the other hand, large and/or ventral lesions present a greater surgical risk.

The surgical technique for cavernous malformation resection depends on the relationship of the lesion to the spinal cord. For pial-based lesions, a circumscribing pial incision allows detachment and delivery of the cavernous malformation from the superficial substance of the spinal cord. Deeper intramedullary lesions are exposed by a midline myelotomy. Although unencapsulated, these malformations are generally well circumscribed and present a clear dissection plane.[10] Uncommonly, a more diffuse lesion permeates the spinal cord tissue and precludes surgical removal. Epidural cavernous malformations are exceedingly rare entities, but treatment follows that of other well-demarcated extradural pathologic processes.[78]

Summary

Vascular malformations of the spinal cord are rarely encountered, even in tertiary care centers with specialized microsurgical and endovascular staff. Nevertheless, these lesions produce a high rate of incapacity in a relatively young group of patients.

The primary aim in the treatment of spinal cord vascular malformations is obliteration or excision of the abnormal arteriovenous shunt. This is routinely achieved with the current techniques available in microsurgery and endovascular therapy for most malformations of types I, II, and IV. As with the excision of most cavernous malformations, successful treatment can be accomplished with preservation of neurologic function. Type III AVMs remain a clinical challenge awaiting novel approaches for treatment. The role of new therapeutic modalities, such as stereotactic radiosurgery (e.g.,

CyberKnife), in the management of these lesions has only begun to be explored.[79]

Outcomes in the care of patients with spinal vascular malformations have become quite satisfactory in most cases. Still, a poor preoperative neurologic condition predicts a poor outcome. Therefore, it is critical to recognize these lesions early in their clinical course and institute proper therapy by a surgical and endovascular team versed in the treatment of spinal, intramedullary, and vascular diseases.

PEARLS

1. Successful treatment of spinal vascular malformations requires total obliteration or excision of the abnormal shunt.
2. Type I AVFs may be treated by excision of the dural fistula or, more typically, by simple interruption of the intradural draining vein.
3. Surgical resection of type II AVMs should proceed in the same manner as removal of intramedullary spinal cord tumors, with identification of rostral and caudal poles of the glomus and circumferential interruption of the feeding arteries along the margin.
4. Alternative surgical approaches to standard posterior laminectomy, including anterior corpectomy and reconstruction, may be considered in the treatment of ventral lesions such as type IV-A fistulas.
5. More complex lesions often require interdisciplinary approaches using both endovascular and surgical techniques to achieve satisfactory radiographic and clinical results.

PITFALLS

1. In the embolization or surgical interruption of malformations, care must be taken not to sacrifice feeding radicular arteries that also supply spinal cord medullary arteries.
2. In the surgical resection of type II AVMs, arterial feeders should be eliminated first because early interruption of the venous drainage may produce excessive bleeding or venous aneurysm rupture.
3. With the exception of select cases, both surgical and endovascular treatments for type III AVMs infrequently provide long-lasting benefit and should therefore be cautiously applied, if at all, to these difficult entities.

KEY POINTS

1. Vascular malformations of the spinal cord are divided into four types. Types I and IV represent direct AVFs that occur within the dural root sleeve (type I) or on the spinal cord surface (type IV). Type II AVMs are intramedullary lesions similar to their intracranial counterparts. Type III AVMs have extensive involvement of intramedullary, intradural-extramedullary, and extradural-paraspinal tissues.
2. Preoperative neurologic status is the most important predictor of posttreatment outcomes, particularly for type I AVFs. Early diagnosis and treatment are critical to favorable outcomes in spinal vascular malformation patients.
3. Spinal vascular malformations should be entertained in the differential diagnosis of progressive myelopathy of uncertain etiology. Therefore, advanced diagnostic imaging, including spinal MRA or CTA to screen for such lesions, must be considered in the radiographic evaluation of such patients. Selective spinal angiography may then be used in a targeted manner to better assess suspicious regions of interest.
4. Endovascular embolization has a 33% to 75% failure rate in the obliteration of type I AVFs. Therefore, surgery should largely be considered as the primary treatment modality. In any practice setting in which embolization represents first-line treatment for these lesions, early and deliberate follow-up angiography is required to detect possible recurrence.

KEY REFERENCES

1. Cenzato M, Versari P, Righi C, et al. Spinal dural arteriovenous fistulae: analysis of outcome in relation to pretreatment indicators. *Neurosurgery*. 2004;55:815-822.
   This study describes the relevance of pretreatment conditions to neurologic outcome in the interdisciplinary treatment of a moderately large series of type I AVFs.
2. Spetzler RF, Detwiler PW, Riina HA, Porter RW. Modified classification of spinal cord vascular lesions. *J Neurosurg Spine*. 2002;96:145-156.
   This well-illustrated and comprehensive review provides a classification of all vascular disease seen within the spinal cord from authors with extensive experience treating these patients.
3. Steinmetz MP, Chow MM, Krishnaney AA, et al. Outcome after the treatment of spinal dural arteriovenous fistulae: a contemporary single-institution series and meta-analysis. *Neurosurgery*. 2004;55:77-87.
   These authors combine their own single-institution retrospective experience treating type I AVFs with a metaanalysis of the literature to demonstrate 98% and 46% success rates for surgery and embolization, respectively.
4. Wyburn-Mason R. *The Vascular Abnormalities and Tumours of the Spinal Cord and Its Membranes*. London: Henry Klimpton; 1943.
   This is Wyburn-Mason's original text, which is of historical interest in the progression of our understanding of spinal vascular malformations.

REFERENCES

1. Youmans JR, ed. *Neurological Surgery*. 2nd ed. Philadelphia: WB Saunders; 1982.
2. Rodesch G, Lasjaunias P. Spinal cord arteriovenous shunts: from imaging to management. *Eur J Radiol*. 2003;46:221-232.
3. Chuang NA, Shroff MM, Willinsky RA, et al. Slow-flow spinal epidural AVF with venous ectasias: two pediatric case reports. *AJNR Am J Neuroradiol*. 2003;24:1901-1905.
4. Spetzler RF, Detwiler PW, Riina HA, Porter RW. Modified classification of spinal cord vascular lesions. *J Neurosurg Spine*. 2002;96:145-156.
5. Kim LJ, Spetzler RF. Classification and surgical management of spinal arteriovenous lesions: arteriovenous fistula and arteriovenous malformations. *Neurosurgery*. 2006;59:S195-S201.
6. Vankan Y, Demaerel P, Heye S, et al. Dural arteriovenous fistula as a late complication of upper cervical spine fracture: case report. *J Neurosurg Spine*. 2004;100:382-384.
7. Rodesch G, Hurth M, Alvarez H, et al. Angio-architecture of spinal cord arteriovenous shunts at presentation: clinical correlations in adults and children. The Bicetre experience on 155 consecutive patients seen between 1981-1999. *Acta Neurochir (Wien)*. 2004;146:217-226.
8. Rodesch G, Hurth M, Alvarez H, et al. Classification of spinal cord arteriovenous shunts: proposal for a reappraisal—the Bicetre experience with 155 consecutive patients treated between 1981 and 1999. *Neurosurgery*. 2002;51:374-379.
9. Marsh WR. Vascular lesions of the spinal cord: history and classification. *Neurosurg Clin N Am*. 1999;10:1-8.
10. McCormick PC, Michelsen WJ, Post KD, et al. Cavernous malformations of the spinal cord. *Neurosurgery*. 1988;23:459-463.

11. Afshar JK, Doppman JL, Oldfield EH. Surgical interruption of intradural draining vein as curative treatment of spinal dural arteriovenous fistulas. *J Neurosurg*. 1995;82:196-200.
12. Anson JA, Spetzler RF. Classification of spinal arteriovenous malformations and implications for treatment. *Barrow Neurol Inst Q*. 1992;8:2-8.
13. Kendall BE, Logue V. Spinal epidural angiomatous malformations draining into intrathecal veins. *Neuroradiology*. 1977;13:181-189.
14. McCormick PC, Stein BM. Management of spinal vascular malformations. In: Barnett HJM, Mohr JP, Stein BM, Yatsu FM, eds. *Stroke: Pathophysiology, Diagnosis, and Management*. 2nd ed. New York: Churchill Livingstone; 1992:1135-1143.
15. Oldfield EH, Di Chiro G, Quindlen EA, et al. Successful treatment of a group of spinal cord arteriovenous malformations by interruption of dural fistula. *J Neurosurg*. 1983;59:1019-1030.
16. Rosenblum B, Oldfield EH, Doppman JL, Di Chiro G. Spinal arteriovenous malformations: a comparison of dural arteriovenous fistulas and intradural AVM's in 81 patients. *J Neurosurg*. 1987;67:795-802.
17. Wyburn-Mason R. *The Vascular Abnormalities and Tumours of the Spinal Cord and Its Membranes*. London: Henry Klimpton; 1943.
18. Niimi Y, Setton A, Berenstein A. Spinal dural arteriovenous fistulae draining to the anterior spinal vein: angiographic diagnosis. *Neurosurgery*. 1999;44:999-1003.
19. Doppman JL. The nidus concept of spinal cord arteriovenous malformations: a surgical recommendation based upon angiographic observations. *Br J Radiol*. 1971;44:758-763.
20. Houdart R, Djindjian R, Hurth M. Vascular malformations of the spinal cord: the anatomic and therapeutic significance of arteriography. *J Neurosurg*. 1966;24:583-594.
21. Barrow DL, Colohan AR, Dawson R. Intradural perimedullary arteriovenous fistulas (type IV spinal cord arteriovenous malformations). *J Neurosurg*. 1994;81:221-229.
22. Mourier KL, Gobin YP, George B, et al. Intradural perimedullary arteriovenous fistulae: results of surgical and endovascular treatment in a series of 35 cases. *Neurosurgery*. 1993;32:885-891.
23. Gueguen B, Merland JJ, Riche MC, Rey A. Vascular malformations of the spinal cord: intrathecal perimedullary arteriovenous fistulas fed by medullary arteries. *Neurology*. 1987;37:969-979.
24. Aminoff MJ, Logue V. Clinical features of spinal vascular malformations. *Brain*. 1974;97:197-210.
25. Aminoff MJ, Logue V. The prognosis of patients with spinal vascular malformations. *Brain*. 1974;97:211-218.
26. Logue V. Angiomas of the spinal cord: review of the pathogenesis, clinical features, and results of surgery. *J Neurol Neurosurg Psychiatry*. 1974;42:1-11.
27. Rodriguez FJ, Crum BA, Krauss WE, et al. Venous congestive myelopathy: a mimic of neoplasia. *Mod Pathol*. 2005;18(5):710-718.
28. Kataoka H, Miyamoto S, Nagata I, et al. Venous congestion is a major cause of neurological deterioration in spinal arteriovenous malformations. *Neurosurgery*. 2001;48:1224-1229; discussion 1229-1230.
29. Aviv RI, Shad A, Tomlinson G, et al. Cervical dural arteriovenous fistulae manifesting as subarachnoid hemorrhage: report of two cases and literature review. *AJNR Am J Neuroradiol*. 2004;25:854-858.
30. Koch C, Gottschalk S, Giese A. Dural arteriovenous fistula of the lumbar spine presenting with subarachnoid hemorrhage: case report and review of the literature. *J Neurosurg Spine*. 2004;100:385-391.
31. Cenzato M, Versari P, Righi C, et al. Spinal dural arteriovenous fistulae: analysis of outcome in relation to pretreatment indicators. *Neurosurgery*. 2004;55:815-822.
32. Atkinson JLD, Miller GM, Krauss WE, et al. Clinical and radiographic features of dural arteriovenous fistula, a treatable cause of myelopathy. *Mayo Clin Proc*. 2001;76:1120-1130.
33. Ushikoshi S, Hida K, Kikuchi Y, et al. Functional prognosis after treatment of spinal dural arteriovenous fistulas. *Neurol Med Chir (Tokyo)*. 1999;39:206-212.
34. Jellema K, Canta LR, Tijssen CC, et al. Spinal dural arteriovenous fistulas: clinical features in 80 patients. *J Neurol Neurosurg Psychiatry*. 2003;74:1438-1440.
35. Schick U, Hassler W. Treatment and outcome of spinal dural arteriovenous fistulas. *Eur Spine J*. 2003;12:350-355.
36. Westphal M, Koch C. Management of spinal dural arteriovenous fistulae using an interdisciplinary neuroradiological/neurosurgical approach: experience with 47 cases. *Neurosurgery*. 1999;45:451-457; discussion 457-458.
37. Kreppel D, Antoniadis G, Seeling W. Spinal hematoma: a literature survey with meta-analysis of 613 patients. *Neurosurg Rev*. 2003;26:1-49.
38. Kasdon DL, Wolpert SM, Stein BM. Surgical and angiographic localization of spinal arteriovenous malformations. *Surg Neurol*. 1976;5:279-283.
39. Alexander MJ, Grossi PM, Spetzler RF, McDougall CG. Extradural thoracic arteriovenous malformation in a patient with Klippel-Trenaunay-Weber syndrome: case report. *Neurosurgery*. 2002;51:1275-1278, discussion 1278-1279.
40. Mont'Alverne F, Musacchio M, Tolentino V, et al. Giant spinal perimedullary fistula in hereditary haemorrhagic telangiectasia: diagnosis, endovascular treatment and review of the literature. *Neuroradiology*. 2003;45:830-836.
41. Rosenow J, Rawanduzy A, Weitzner I Jr, Couldwell WT. Type IV spinal arteriovenous malformation in association with familial pulmonary vascular malformations: case report. *Neurosurgery*. 2000;46:1240-1244.
42. Cogen P, Stein BM. Spinal cord arteriovenous malformations with significant intramedullary components. *J Neurosurg*. 1983;59:471-478.
43. Djindjian R. Embolization of angiomas of the spinal cord. *Surg Neurol*. 1975;4:411-420.
44. Houdart R, Djindjian R, Hurth M, Rey A. Treatment of angiomas of the spinal cord. *Surg Neurol*. 1974;2:186-194.
45. Kunc Z, Bret J. Diagnosis and treatment of vascular malformations of the spinal cord. *J Neurosurg*. 1969;30:436-445.
46. Stein BM. Arteriovenous malformations of the brain and spinal cord. In: Hoff J, ed. *Practice of Surgery*. New York: Harper & Row; 1979.
47. Pui MH. Gadolinium-enhanced MR angiography of spinal arteriovenous malformation. *Clin Imaging*. 2004;28:28-32.
48. Terae S, Kudo K, Asano T, et al. CT angiography with multidetector-row helical CT in spinal arteriovenous malformation. *Clin Imaging*. 2004;28:23-27.
49. Prestigiacomo CJ, Niimi Y, Setton A, Berenstein A. Three-dimensional rotational spinal angiography in the evaluation and treatment of vascular malformations. *AJNR Am J Neuroradiol*. 2003;24:1429-1435.

50. Krayenbuhl H, Yasargil MG, McClintock HG. Treatment of spinal cord vascular malformations by surgical excision. *J Neurosurg*. 1969;30:427-435.
51. McCormick PC. Vascular tumors and vascular malformations of the spine. In: Vinken PJ, Bruyn GW, eds. *Handbook of Clinical Neurology*. Amsterdam: Elsevier; 1996.
52. Yasargil MG, DeLong WB, Guarnaschelli JJ. Complete microsurgical excision of cervical extramedullary and intramedullary vascular malformations. *Surg Neurol*. 1975;4:211-224.
53. Malis LI. Microsurgery for spinal cord arteriovenous malformations. *Clin Neurosurg*. 1979;26:543-555.
54. Benes L, Wakat JP, Sure U, et al. Intraoperative spinal digital subtraction angiography: technique and results. *Neurosurgery*. 2003;52:603-609.
55. Schievink WI, Vishteh AG, McDougall CG, Spetzler RF. Intraoperative spinal angiography. *J Neurosurg Spine*. 1999;90:48-51.
56. Nakagawa A, Hirano T, Uenohara H, et al. Use of intraoperative dynamic infrared imaging with detection wavelength of 7-14 microns in the surgical obliteration of spinal arteriovenous fistula: case report and technical considerations. *Minim Invasive Neurosurg*. 2004;47: 136-139.
57. Padovani R, Farneti M, Maida G, Ghadirpour R: Spinal dural arteriovenous fistulas: the use of intraoperative microvascular Doppler monitoring. *Br J Neurosurg*. 2003;17:519-524.
58. Iacopino DG, Conti A, Giusa M, et al. Assistance of intraoperative microvascular Doppler in the surgical obliteration of spinal dural arteriovenous fistula: cases description and technical considerations. *Acta Neurochir (Wien)*. 2003;145:133-137.
59. Warakaulle DR, Aviv RI, Niemann D, et al. Embolisation of spinal dural arteriovenous fistulae with Onyx. *Neuroradiology*. 2003;45:110-112.
60. Rodiek SO. Successful endovascular treatment of a spinal dural arteriovenous fistula with trisacryl gelatin microspheres. *Minim Invasive Neurosurg*. 2002;45:173-176.
61. Schaat TJ, Salzman KL, Stevens EA. Sacral origin of a spinal dural arteriovenous fistula: case report and review. *Spine*. 2002;27:893-897.
62. Sugiu K, Meguro T, Nakashiama H, Ohmoto T. Successful embolization of a spinal perimedullary arteriovenous fistula with cellulose acetate polymer solution: technical case report. *Neurosurgery*. 2001;49:1257-1260.
63. Niimi Y, Sala F, Deletis V, et al. Neurophysiologic monitoring and pharmacologic provocative testing for embolization of spinal cord arteriovenous malformations. *AJNR Am J Neuroradiol*. 2004;25:1131-1138.
64. Sala F, Niimi Y, Berenstein A, Deletis V. Neuroprotective role of neurophysiological monitoring during endovascular procedures in the spinal cord. *Ann N Y Acad Sci*. 2001;939:126-136.
65. Jellema K, Tijssen CC, van Rooij WJ, et al. Spinal dural arteriovenous fistulas: long-term follow-up of 44 treated patients. *Neurology*. 2004;62:1839-1841.
66. Steinmetz MP, Chow MM, Krishnaney AA, et al. Outcome after the treatment of spinal dural arteriovenous fistulae: a contemporary single-institution series and meta-analysis. *Neurosurgery*. 2004;55:77-87.
67. Song JK, Vinuela F, Gobin YP, et al. Surgical and endovascular treatment of spinal dural arteriovenous fistulas: long-term disability assessment and prognostic factors. *J Neurosurg Spine*. 2001;94:199-204.
68. Narvid J, Hetts SW, Larsen D, et al. Spinal dural arteriovenous fistulae: clinical features and long-term results. *Neurosurgery*. 2008;62:159-167.
69. Eskandar EN, Borges LF, Budzik RF Jr, et al. Spinal dural arteriovenous fistulas: experience with endovascular and surgical therapy. *J Neurosurg Spine*. 2002;96:162-167.
70. Van Dijk JM, TerBrugge KG, Willinsky RA, et al. Multidisciplinary management of spinal dural arteriovenous fistulas: clinical presentation and long-term follow-up in 49 patients. *Stroke*. 2002;33:1578-1583.
71. O'Toole JE, McCormick PC. Midline ventral intradural schwannoma of the cervical spinal cord resected via anterior corpectomy with reconstruction: technical case report and review of the literature. *Neurosurgery*. 2003;52:1482-1485.
72. Hida K, Iwasaki Y, Ushikoshi S, et al. Corpectomy: a direct approach to perimedullary arteriovenous fistulas of the anterior cervical spinal cord. *J Neurosurg Spine*. 2002;96:157-161.
73. Raabe A, Beck J, Gerlach R, et al. Near-infrared indocyanine green video angiography: a new method for intraoperative assessment of vascular flow. *Neurosurgery*. 2003;52:132-139.
74. Hida K, Iwasaki Y, Goto K, et al. Results of the surgical treatment of perimedullary arteriovenous fistulas with special reference to embolization. *J Neurosurg Spine*. 1999;90: 198-205.
75. Batra S, Lin D, Recinos PF, Zhang J, Rigamonti D. Cavernous malformations: natural history, diagnosis and treatment. *Nat Rev Neurol*. 2009;5:659-670.
76. Badhiwala JH, Farrokhyar F, Alhazzani W, et al. Surgical outcomes and natural history of intramedullary spinal cord cavernous malformations: a single-center series and meta-analysis of individual patient data. *J Neurosurg Spine*. 2014;21:662-676.
77. Hegde A, Mohan S, Tan KK, Lim CC. Spinal cavernous malformations: magnetic resonance imaging and associated findings. *Singapore Med J*. 2012;53:582-586.
78. Nagi S, Megdiche H, Bouzaidi K, et al. Imaging features of spinal epidural cavernous malformations. *J Neuroradiol*. 2004;31:208-213.
79. Ryu SI, Chang SD, Kim DH, et al. Image-guided hypo-fractionated stereotactic radiosurgery to spinal lesions. *Neurosurgery*. 2001;49:838-846.

CHAPTER 93 Vascular Anatomy of the Spine, Imaging, and Endovascular Treatment of Spinal Vascular Diseases

J. Diego Lozano
Ajit S. Puri
Ajay K. Wakhloo

Normal Vascular Anatomy of the Spine

An accurate and thorough understanding of the normal vascular anatomy of the spine and spinal cord is vital for the safe and appropriate performance of spinal angiography and endovascular intervention. Learning these skills is challenging because diagnostic spinal angiography is less commonly performed than cerebral angiography and is being gradually replaced by magnetic resonance angiography (MRA). In this section, we provide the reader with a concise overview of the vascular anatomy of the spinal cord and paraspinal structures as a basis for understanding spinal vascular diseases, their clinical classifications, and the approaches to treating them.

Arterial Supply

The arterial supply to the spine has a segmental distribution to the derivatives of each embryologic somite, including the paraspinal soft tissues, bone, and dura. In contrast, due to variability in the spinal cord arterial supply, the overall supply to each metamere is highly variable. The metameric arterial supply arises from a variety of parent vessels, including the vertebral arteries, aorta, iliac arteries, and others.

The spinal blood supply can be divided into a macrocirculation, which includes the vasculature of paraspinal structures up to the cord surface, and a microcirculation, which involves perforators to the cord beyond the anterior and posterior spinal arteries (ASA and PSA).[1,2]

Macrocirculation (Paraspinal Structures and Spinal Cord Surface)

Analogous to the cerebral blood supply, the pattern of blood supply to the spinal cord is based on the pattern of its embryologic development, which occurs from the outside in at each segmental level. The segmental levels are first manifest as primitive precursors termed *somites*. In the first few weeks after conception, the embryo is divided into 42 to 44 somites along the rostral-caudal direction. Of these, 31 somites persist through development, corresponding to the 31 pairs of spinal nerves (8 cervical, 12 thoracic, 5 lumbar, 5 sacral, 1 coccygeal). The derivatives of each somite and corresponding portions of the neural crest and neural tube are collectively referred to as a *metamere*.

The segmental arteries are numbered according to the nerve that they accompany in the neural foramen. Through their branches, they supply all the ipsilateral derivatives of their corresponding metamere: skin, muscle, bone, spinal nerve, dura, and spinal cord (Fig. 93.1). In the embryonic stage of development, each segmental artery has a branch supplying the cord. By the end of fetal development, most branches have regressed, and only a few contribute significantly to spinal cord perfusion. Of the initial 62 metameric arteries (31 pairs), 4 to 8 will end up supplying the ASA (diameter, 0.2 to 0.5 mm), and 10 to 20 will supply the PSA (diameter, 0.1 to 0.4 mm). Most of the segmental arteries end up supplying the related nerves, dura, vertebral body, and paraspinous muscles. The process of regression of the spinal cord blood supply is more pronounced caudad. The dominant artery supplying the spinal cord is named the artery of Adamkiewicz (AKA).

The simplified algorithm for the vascular supply at each segmental level is: major arterial trunk (vertebral artery, aorta) → spinal/segmental artery → radiculomedullary artery (ventral radicular artery) and radiculopial artery (ventral or dorsal artery) → pial network, paired posterior or single anterior spinal arteries.

Radicular arteries originate from the following major arterial trunks[1]:

Cervical: Vertebral arteries, ascending cervical branch of the thyrocervical trunk, deep cervical branch of the costocervical trunk, occipital and ascending pharyngeal branches of the external carotid artery

Thoracic: Branches of the costocervical trunk, internal thoracic artery of the subclavian artery, intercostal branches of the aorta

Lumbosacral-coccygeal: Lumbar branches of the aorta, median sacral artery of the aorta, lateral sacral branches of the internal iliac arteries, iliolumbar branches of the common iliac arteries

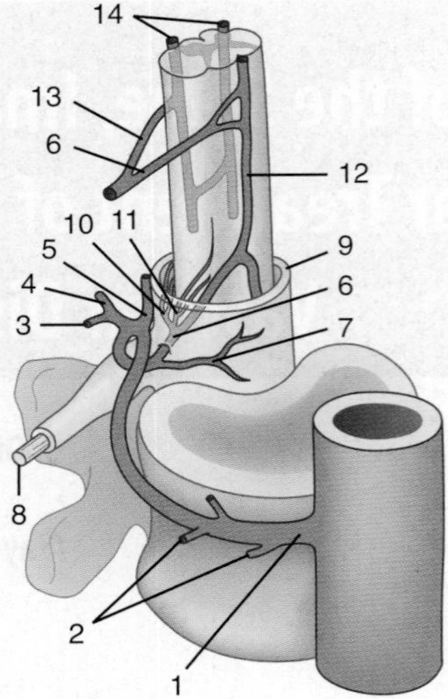

FIG. 93.1 A segmental artery and its branches, which supply all the ipsilateral derivatives of its corresponding metamere: muscle, skin, bone, spinal nerve, and spinal cord. *1,* Segmental artery; *2,* somatic branches for vertebral body supply; *3,* intercostal artery or muscular branch; *4,* dorsospinal trunk; *5,* paravertebral longitudinal anastomosis; *6,* radiculomedullary artery; *7,* dorsal somatic branch; *8,* spinal nerve; *9,* dural sheath; *10,* radicular branches to the dorsal nerve root; *11,* radicular branches to the ventral nerve root; *12,* anterior spinal artery; *13,* radiculopial artery; *14,* posterior spinal arteries. (From Mathis JM, Shaibani A, Wakhloo AK. Spine anatomy. In: Mathis JM, ed. *Image-Guided Spine Interventions*. New York: Springer-Verlag, 2004.)

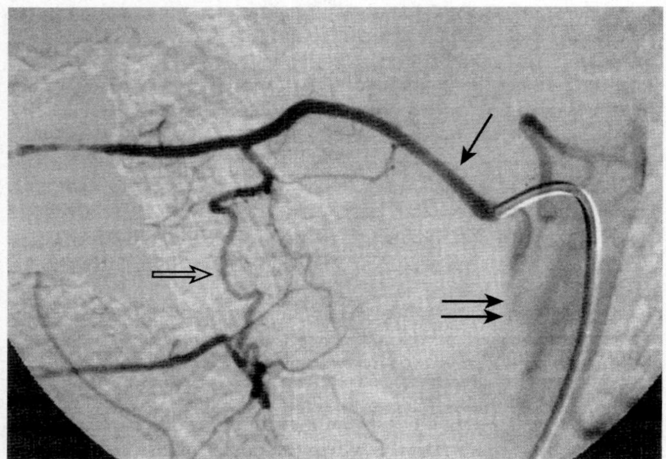

FIG. 93.2 Selective intercostal artery injection (*single arrow*) shows a longitudinal pretransverse anastomosis (*open arrow*) between the arteries of adjacent segments. Note reflux of contrast agent into the abdominal aorta (*double arrows*). (From Mathis JM, Shaibani A, Wakhloo AK. Spine anatomy. In: Mathis JM, ed. *Image-Guided Spine Interventions*. New York: Springer-Verlag, 2004.)

The segmental arteries form paraspinal and extradural anastomoses in the craniocaudal extension, which can be subdivided as follows[1]:

Ventrolateral: Ascending cervical artery of the thyrocervical trunk

Pretransverse: Anterior to transverse processes, such as the vertebral or lateral sacral arteries (Fig. 93.2). The latter supply the sympathetic nervous system in the thoracolumbar area.

Dorsal longitudinal: The branches to the midline insertion of the spinous process muscles, such as the deep cervical artery of the costocervical trunk

At each level, segmental arteries provide blood supply to the ventral and dorsal nerve roots through radicular arteries (see Fig. 93.1). Some of the radicular branches, however, supply not only the nerve root but also the spinal cord. These branches give rise to (1) the pial/coronal arterial network or the PSA and are called radiculopial arteries or (2) the anterior pial network and to the ASA and are named radiculomedullary arteries.

The dominant longitudinal blood supply to the spinal cord is provided ventrally by a single ASA and dorsally by paired PSAs. These two systems are connected via a superficial network of small pial arteries. The flow in spinal arteries can be bidirectional and depends on the size of the radiculomedullary and radiculopial arteries as well as the timing of the systolic pulse waves traveling within the aorta or vertebral arteries and being propagated into the segmental arteries at different levels.

As described earlier, radicular arteries originate from each segmental artery and supply the dorsal and ventral nerve roots after giving off branches to the paraspinous musculature, vertebral body, and dura. At the C1 level, radicular branches may be absent. Normally, radicular arteries are not seen on digital-subtracted angiograms because of the current limits of spatial resolution.

Radiculopial arteries supply the nerve roots by means of smaller branches and then run ventral to either the dorsal or the ventral nerve root to supply the pial network. Although they anastomose with pial branches of the ASA, they do not supply the ASA directly. There are more dorsal than ventral radiculopial arteries, and the dorsal radiculopial arteries are the dominant supply to the PSA. Their number varies from three to four in the cervical region, from six to nine in the thoracic region, and from zero to three in the lumbosacral region.

Radiculomedullary arteries are the dominant supply to the ASA. After giving off their radicular branches to the nerve roots, they run along the ventral surface of the nerve root, occasionally give off pial collateral branches, and continue to the ASA. On average, there are two to four radiculomedullary arteries in the cervical region, two to three in the thoracic region, and zero to four in the lumbosacral region. The largest radiculomedullary artery of the thoracolumbar segment is also known as the artery of Adamkiewicz (AKA; diameter, 0.55–1.2 mm). In 75% of patients, the AKA arises between T9 and T12, more commonly on the left. When its origin is above T8 or below L2, another major contributor to the ASA can be found either caudad or craniad. In 30% to 50% of cases, it also contributes significantly to the PSA. Generally, a pair of arteries arise in the cervical region from the intradural segment of each vertebral artery that fuse to one Y-shaped ASA. The typical hairpin anastomosis between the radiculomedullary arteries and the ASA is found angiographically at the lower

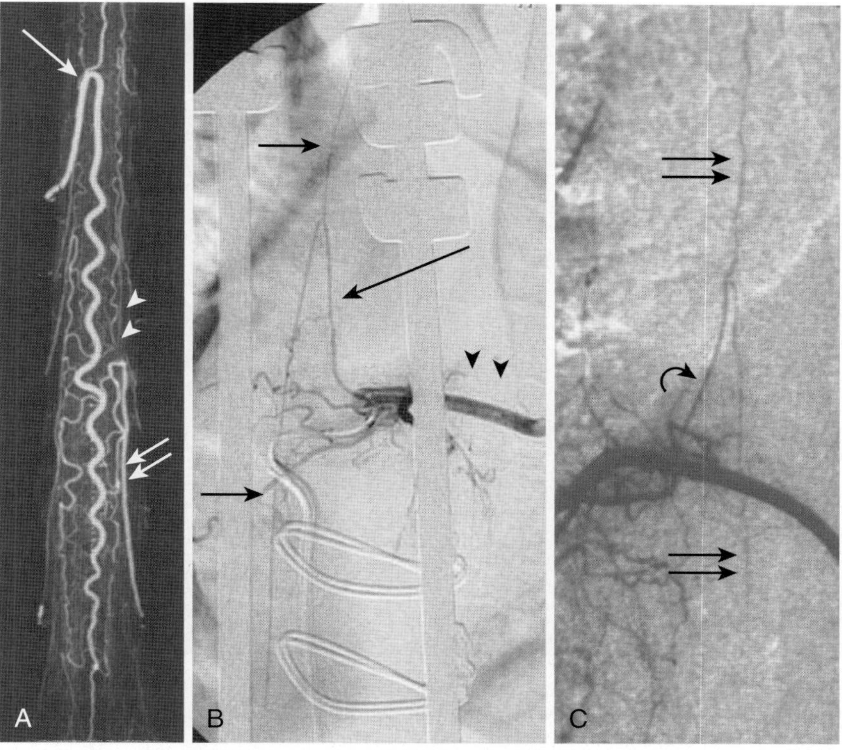

FIG. 93.3 (A) Microradiograph of the spinal cord vasculature shows the typical hairpin anastomosis between the radiculomedullary artery (artery of Adamkiewicz) and the anterior spinal artery (*single arrow*) found at the lower thoracic and the upper lumbar levels. A large radiculopial artery is seen (*double arrow*) with supply to the posterior spinal artery (*arrowheads*). (B) Left T10-intercostal arteriogram (*arrowheads*) shows the radiculomedullary artery (*long arrow*) and the anterior spinal artery (*short arrows*). (C) Injection of an intercostal artery shows a radiculopial artery (*curved arrow*) and the right posterior spinal artery (double arrows); note the smaller radius of the hairpin shape. (A, from Lasjaunias P, Berenstein A. *Surgical Neuroangiography, Vol. 3: Functional Vascular Anatomy of Brain, Spinal Cord and Spine*. Berlin: Springer-Verlag, 1990.)

thoracic and lumbar levels (Fig. 93.3). There is only one ASA, which continues from its Y-shaped origin to the artery of the terminal filum (diameter, 0.5–0.8 mm). The ASA is located in the subpial space in the ventral sulcus of the spinal cord, dorsal to the vein; it may be partly absent or not visible angiographically, especially at the thoracic level. Because of a lack of fusion during embryologic development, a short nonfused cervical segment may be present.

Identifying these small normal spinal arterial vessels has been a significant technical challenge in the development of noninvasive spinal imaging. Recent studies using newer techniques for contrast-enhanced MRA have shown success rates of 82.4% to 100% for detection of the ASA.[3,4] Identification of the ASA remains a challenge. Sheehy et al. reported detection rates of 96% (48 of 50 patients) for the cervical segment of the ASA.[5] Other studies of contrast-enhanced MRA at higher field strength have successfully depicted abnormally dilated ASAs in the setting of spinal vascular malformations, but reliable detection of the normal thoracolumbar ASA remains elusive.[6–8]

Microcirculation (Spinal Cord Perforators)

The circulation distal to the subpial ASA, the pial network, and the PSA can be divided into centrifugal (from the center of the cord out toward the surface) and centripetal (from the cord surface toward the center of the cord) systems.[1] The centrifugal system, also known as the sulcocommissural system, consists of 200 to 400 sulcocommissural arteries, which are located within the ventral sulcus of the spinal cord and originate from the ASA (Fig. 93.4). These arteries penetrate the sulcus similarly to brain perforators and enter the central gray matter, where they branch into radially oriented small arteries that run toward the white matter. Each sulcocommissural artery usually supplies one-half of the cord. The sulcocommissural system supplies most of the spinal cord gray matter and the ventral half of the white matter. Before entering the cord substance, each sulcocommissural artery anastomoses craniad and caudad with neighboring sulcocommissural arteries (see Fig. 93.4). Complex, longitudinally oriented anastomoses are also seen within the white and gray matter. Whereas the sulcocommissural arteries initially run horizontally, they take an ascending course with the growth and disproportionate elongation of the spinal column. The spinal cord territory supplied by the ASA versus the PSAs is comparatively as large as the proportion of a cerebral hemisphere supplied by the internal carotid arteries versus the vertebrobasilar system. An occlusion of the sulcocommissural artery at the lumbar segment in primates can cause severe damage to the ventrolateral two-thirds of the cord at the occluded and adjacent levels.[9]

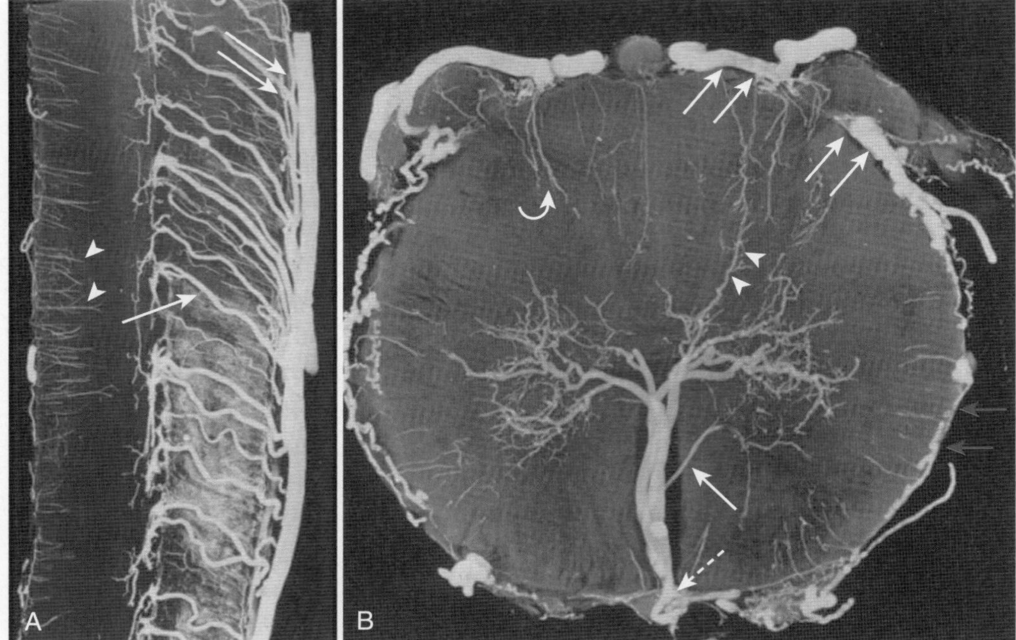

FIG. 93.4 Microradiographs of injected spinal cord vasculature. (A) Midsagittal plane shows ascending sulcocommissural arteries (*single arrow*) within the ventral sulcus of the spinal cord originating from the anterior spinal artery (*double arrows*) and dorsal perforators originating from posterior spinal arteries (*arrowheads*). (B) Axial plane shows the sulcocommissural artery and anterior perforators that supply the gray matter (*single arrow*). Intramedullary anastomoses between anterior and posterior perforators (*arrowheads*); posterior pial network and posterior spinal arteries (*double arrows*); superficial pial anastomoses between the anterior and posterior spinal arteries (*red arrows*); anterior spinal artery (*dashed arrow*); lateral perforators to white matter originating from pial network (*curved arrow*). (From Thron AK. *Vascular Anatomy of the Spinal Cord: Neuroradiological Investigations and Clinical Syndromes*. Berlin: Springer-Verlag, 1988.)

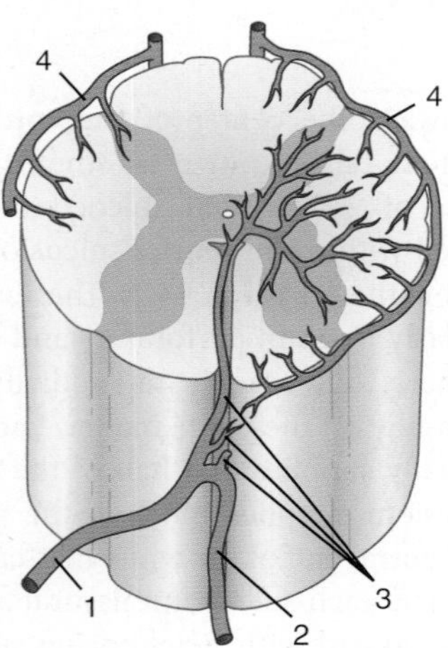

FIG. 93.5 Centrifugal and centripetal arterial network with intramedullary anastomoses. *1*, radiculomedullary artery; *2*, anterior spinal artery; *3*, sulcocommissural artery; *4*, coronal arterial system originating from the posterior spinal artery. (From Mathis JM, Shaibani A, Wakhloo AK. Spine anatomy. In: Mathis JM, ed. *Image-Guided Spine Interventions*. New York: Springer-Verlag, 2004.)

The centripetal system includes a pial network and the PSAs (Fig. 93.5). At the craniocervical junction, this system receives its blood supply directly from the intradural vertebral arteries or from the posterior inferior cerebellar arteries near their origins. At all other levels, radiculopial arteries provide the blood supply to the centripetal system. Radial branches of the pial network and the PSAs extend around the circumference of the cord and anastomose with the ASA. The radial arteries and the PSAs give off perforating branches to the cord all along their courses. These short perforating branches enter the white matter in a radial fashion and extend to a portion of the gray matter. Intramedullary anastomoses with branches of the sulcocommissural arteries exist. Pial anastomoses also exist in the longitudinal axis between the anterior and posterior vascular system. These anastomoses, however, are relatively small and cannot provide adequate craniocaudal supply to the anterior spinal cord in the case of ASA occlusion. Dependent on the location and size of a pial arteriovenous fistula (anterior or posterior) or a medullary (within the spinal cord) arteriovenous malformation (AVM), the blood supply can originate from the ventral and/or the dorsal vasculature and, therefore, from the centrifugal and/or centripetal system.

Somatic Arteries (Arterial Supply to the Vertebral Body)

The segmental artery is centered at the level of the intervertebral disc and the corresponding nerve (Fig. 93.6). It gives rise to an ascending somatic branch and a descending somatic branch. Each vertebral body is supplied by the descending somatic branches of the segmental arteries above and the ascending branches of the segmental arteries below. Because of extensive anastomoses, an injection in any one of these four

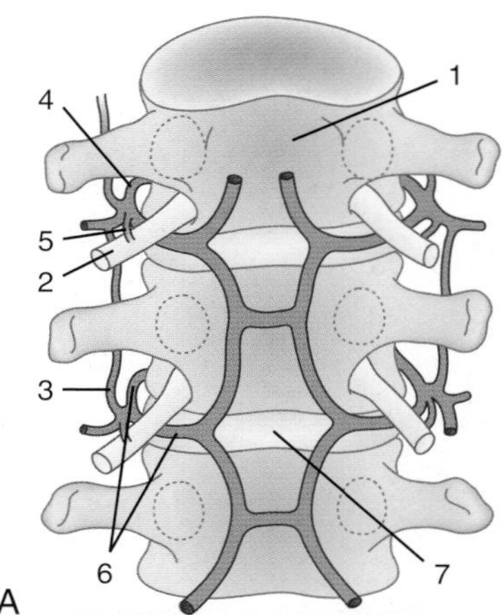

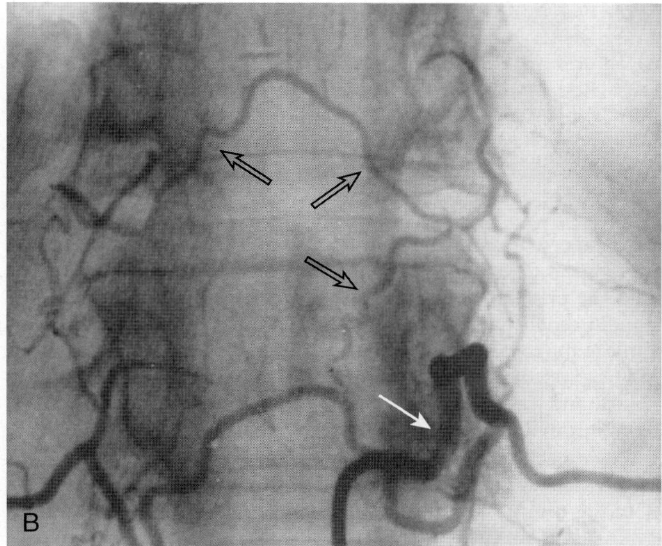

FIG. 93.6 Vertebral body blood supply. (A) Schematic illustration and (B) lumbar artery (*white arrow*) angiograph of the hexagonal anastomoses of dorsal somatic branches (*open arrows*). *1*, vertebral body; *2*, nerve root; *3*, pretransverse longitudinal anastomosis; *4*, segmental artery; *5*, radicular artery; *6*, segmental artery; and *7*, corresponding disc. (From Mathis JM, Shaibani A, Wakhloo AK. Spine anatomy. In: Mathis JM, ed. *Image-Guided Spine Interventions*. New York: Springer-Verlag, 2004.)

segmental arteries may enhance the entire vertebral body. On angiograms in frontal projection, the arterial network on the posterior surface of the vertebral body has a characteristic hexagonal shape. Tumor blush or vascular bone metastases should not be confused with the normal angiographic blush of the vertebral body.

Venous Drainage

After passing through the capillary network, blood is transported from the deepest parts of the spinal cord toward the surface (Fig. 93.7). Venous drainage of the cord can be divided into an intrinsic system, which runs in proximity to the centrifugal arterial system, and an extrinsic system, which runs in proximity to the centripetal arterial system. Unlike in the arterial blood supply, there is no dominance of the dorsal or ventral venous return. Dorsal and ventral sulcocommissural veins, which collect the venous outflow from the central gray matter, are a part of the intrinsic venous system. The venous perforators draining into the radial veins, which drain into the dorsal and ventral longitudinal collecting veins, belong to the extrinsic system. These longitudinal collecting veins finally drain into the radicular veins that run along the nerve roots and empty into the ventral epidural venous plexus. In addition to the main dorsal and ventral draining veins, there are short intersegmental lateral longitudinal veins linking adjacent radial veins. However, these lateral longitudinal venous channels are not large enough to form a functional dominant craniocaudal drainage, as do the dorsal and ventral systems.

The main ventral longitudinal venous channel is known as the anterior median vein. Flow in the thoracic longitudinal channels is bidirectional. The most cranial portion drains into the cervical region and, from there, partly via the anterior medullary vein into the median anterior pontine vein and the transverse pontine vein and, finally, into the superior petrosal sinus. The most caudal part drains into the lumbar region. There can be multiple longitudinal venous channels, especially in the thoracic region and ventrally.

The radicular (radiculomedullary) veins drain either into spinal nerve venous channels in the neural foramina or into a dural venous pool. Both venous systems eventually empty into the ventral epidural venous plexus (Fig. 93.8). The epidural venous system has a prominent ventral and a smaller dorsal component. The ventral epidural veins receive venous drainage from the vertebral bodies through anterior and posterior venules, the spinal cord via radiculomedullary veins, and the dura. They are also involved in some cerebrospinal fluid resorption via arachnoid granulations along the nerve root sleeves. The ventral epidural venous plexus forms a valveless, retrocorporeal hexagonal anastomotic plexus, which is continuous longitudinally. The direction of flow within this plexus is multidirectional and depends on the location of the contributing veins at each anatomic level.

The cervical portion of the plexus drains into the vertebral veins, which finally empty into the innominate veins. At the thoracic level, blood drains into the intercostal veins, which empty into the azygous and hemiazygous systems and subsequently the superior vena cava. In the lumbar segments, venous drainage involves the ascending lumbar vein on the left, the azygous and hemiazygous systems, and the left renal vein. At the sacral and coccygeal level, blood empties into sacral veins, the lateral sacral veins, and subsequently into both internal iliac veins.

Imaging and Endovascular Intervention of the Spine

Classification

Various classifications have been suggested over the past several decades for spinal vascular shunts (SVSs) based on angiographic features, pathophysiology, and neuroanatomy.[10–13] However, these classifications vary, may create confusion, and can be of little value for the endovascular approach to treating

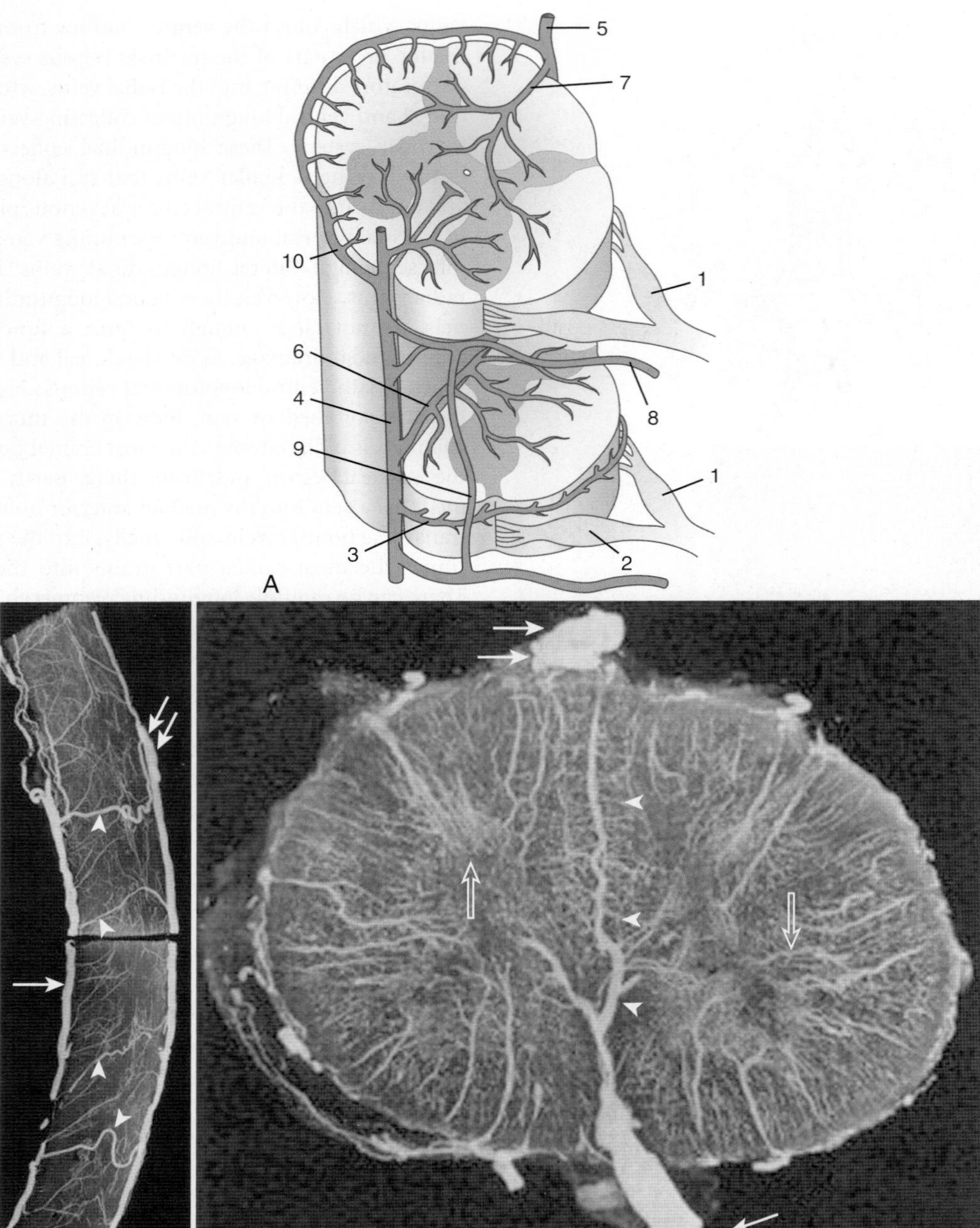

FIG. 93.7 Deep and superficial venous drainage of the spinal cord. (A) Schematic illustration: *1,* dorsal nerve root; *2,* ventral nerve root; *3* and *10,* radial/coronal veins; *4,* anterior median vein; *5,* posterior median vein; *6,* intramedullary anastomosis; *7,* dorsal sulcal vein; *8,* radiculomedullary vein; *9,* ventral longitudinal vein. (B) Midsagittal and (C) axial microradiographs of injected specimen. Multiple intramedullary anastomoses (*arrowheads*) between the ventral (*single arrow*) and dorsal (*double arrows*) median veins. Radially oriented deep venous system (*open arrows*) draining into the superficial pial venous network and intramedullary anastomoses. (A, From Mathis JM, Shaibani A, Wakhloo AK. Spine anatomy. In: Mathis JM, ed. *Image-Guided Spine Interventions*. New York: Springer-Verlag, 2004; B and C, From Thron AK. *Vascular Anatomy of the Spinal Cord: Neuroradiological Investigations and Clinical Syndromes*. Berlin: Springer-Verlag, 1988.)

most vascular abnormalities. To facilitate the understanding of spinal vascular shunts, we will address these lesions according to their location with respect to the spinal cord, including the paraspinal soft tissue (Table 93.1). Vascular lesions consisting of a single direct connection between the feeding artery and the draining vein are known as arteriovenous fistulas (AVFs) or arteriovenous shunts (AVSs). However, when multiple connections are present at the precapillary level, they are called arteriovenous malformations (AVMs). The core of an AVM that appears angiographically and anatomically as a conglomeration of vessels, because of the superimposition of connections between arteries and veins and lack of spatial resolution, is defined as the nidus. Most of the spinal vascular malformations are congenital, may grow over time, and

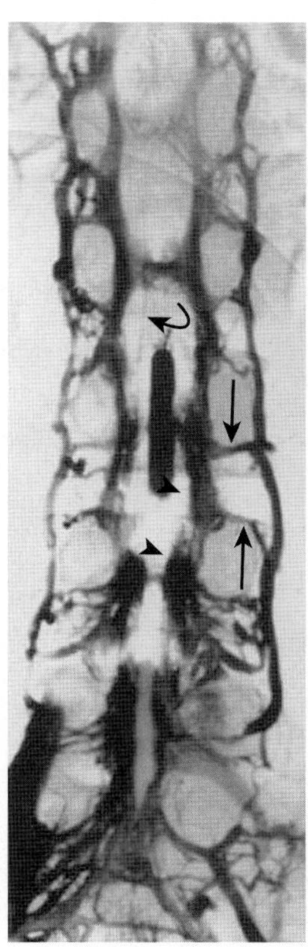

FIG. 93.8 Venography of lumbosacral epidural venous plexus. The emissary radicular veins (*arrows*) connect the epidural venous plexus (*arrowheads*) with the longitudinal paravertebral efferent system. Reflux is seen in the radiculomedullary vein (*curved arrow*). (From Lasjaunias P, Berenstein A. *Surgical Neuroangiography, Vol 3: Functional Vascular Anatomy of Brain, Spinal Cord and Spine*. Berlin: Springer-Verlag, 1990.)

become symptomatic only in adulthood. In this chapter, we focus on AVSs, AVMs, spinal artery aneurysms, neoplastic vascular lesions, aneurysmal bone cysts, vertebral hemangiomas, and vascular metastatic disease.

Imaging

Magnetic resonance imaging (MRI) is noninvasive, does not expose the patient to ionizing radiation, and should be the primary diagnostic tool in the evaluation of spinal vascular disease. MRI is able to delineate the spinal cord and paraspinal structures; the flow voids within vascular malformations; and the presence of edema, hemorrhage, venous congestion, and other associated processes. For patients without a known or presumptive diagnosis of spinal vascular disease, MRI remains the initial imaging modality of choice due to its ability to depict the broad range of vascular and nonvascular spinal diseases that may be the cause of a patient's neurologic symptoms. For instance, a recent study by Germans et al. found that MRI may be of utility in identifying spinal vascular malformations in patients with cerebral angiogram–negative subarachnoid hemorrhage.[14] While extremely sensitive in detecting signal abnormalities, particularly in the T2-weighted sequences, in the spinal cord and spinal canal, a differential diagnosis for spinal cord lesions seen on MRI must always be considered.[15]

Spinal AVSs can be strongly suggested on MRI; however, conventional digital subtraction angiography (DSA) remains the gold standard for evaluation of spinal vascular diseases and is necessary for visualizing the detailed anatomy and architecture of SVSs, including arterial feeders and venous return. Angioarchitectural changes characterized on angiography may suggest aging of the lesion.[16] Angiography will also give an estimate of the blood flow velocity within a malformation and help to guide an endovascular intervention. The addition of three-dimensional rotational angiography (3DRA) allows for better delineation of substructures of spinal AVSs, such as associated arterial or venous aneurysms, and their relationship to the shunt. It is particularly useful in delineating intramedullary from perimedullary shunts/malformations and in visualizing nidal and venous aneurysms.[17] 3DRA helps to assess feeding arteries for planned endovascular procedures, although reduced spatial resolution and limited temporal resolution limit its value for high-flow lesions. Superselective 3DRA may overcome some of these limitations (Fig. 93.9).

Noninvasive imaging of SVSs was initially attempted using phase contrast and time-of-flight MRI techniques.[18,19] Later studies with first-pass gadolinium-enhanced MRA and computed tomography angiography (CTA) show a better definition of the arterial and venous systems of the shunt.[7,8,20,21] In the most recent of these studies, Mull et al. were able to reliably distinguish between spinal dural AVF and spinal AVM in addition to identifying a large proportion of the clinically relevant vascular anatomy in each case. MRA not only allows for a proper pretherapeutic overview of the regional and lesional anatomy that will serve as a roadmap for treatment but also serves as posttherapeutic examination following endovascular treatment.[22] Development of time-resolved spinal MR angiographic techniques with a temporal resolution of 3 to 6 seconds and spatial resolution of about 1 to 3 mm seem to provide sufficient temporal and spatial resolution to identify, localize, and follow patients suspected of having an SVS.[23] Further improvement in spatial and temporal resolutions will allow MRA to become the premier diagnostic modality for spinal vascular disease.

With the advancement of multidetector technology, CTA has recently become a reasonable imaging modality for those patients for whom MRI is not an option, such as those with indwelling ferromagnetic material, unable to tolerate long imaging times, or for whom MRI is not available.[24,25] CTA may offer several important advantages over MRA. Higher spatial resolution allows for better visualization of submillimeter-sized vessels. Several studies have demonstrated feasibility of imaging the AKA using CTA, even in children.[25,26] Unlike MRI, which usually relies on suppressing surrounding tissues to optimize small vessel imaging, CTA can also be useful in the co-visualization of anatomic structures (spinal cord, bones) to improve localization of vascular lesions.

Ongoing investigations using 320-detector-row CT scanners and more recent techniques, such as four-dimensional CT (4D-CT), offer new diagnostic methods for assessing AVS in real time. In a recent study, 4D-CT was able to detect all AVM lesions previously detected by conventional DSA, including their size, location, feeding arteries, and draining

TABLE 93.1 Classification of Spinal Vascular Diseases

Anatomic Classification	Etiology	Pathophysiology	Clinical Presentation
Vascular Shunts			
Paraspinal AVS (M): e.g., traumatic vertebrovertebral AVF	Congenital/acquired	Cord compression (enlarged veins)	Progressive myelopathy
Epidural AVS (M)	Acquired	Cord compression (enlarged veins), vascular steal, venous congestion	Progressive myelopathy
Dural AVS (F): single (type IA), multiple (type IB)	Acquired	Venous hypertension/cord compression; hemorrhage is rare	Progressive myelopathy, pain
Pial AVS (F): low flow, moderate, high flow (type IVA, IVB, and IVC)	Congenital	Cord compression (enlarged veins), hemorrhage, vascular steal, venous hypertension, venous varix	Progressive myelopathy
Extradural-intradural (metameric, juvenile) AVM (type III)	Congenital	Cord compression, hemorrhage, vascular steal	Pain, progressive myelopathy
Intramedullary AVM (type II)	Congenital	Intramedullary hemorrhage, subarachnoid hemorrhage, cord compression, vascular steal	Acute and progressive myelopathy, pain
Neoplastic Vascular Lesions			
Cavernous angioma	Congenital	Cord compression (mass effect), repetitive bleeding	Acute and progressive myelopathy
Hemangioblastoma	Congenital/acquired	Asymptomatic, cord compression	Asymptomatic, myelopathy
Syndromes With Spinal AVM			
Osler-Weber-Rendu syndrome	Hereditary (autosomal dominant)	Venous hypertension, mass effect, vascular steal, subarachnoid hemorrhage	Myelopathy, radiculopathy
Cobb syndrome	Congenital	Cord compression, hemorrhage, vascular steal	Pain, progressive myelopathy
Klippel-Trenaunay (KT) and Parkes-Weber (PW) syndromes	Congenital	Cord compression (enlarged veins, hemorrhage, vascular steal)	Progressive myelopathy
Vertebral Vascular Lesions			
Aneurysmal bone cysts	Congenital/acquired	Hemodynamic imbalance, cord compression	Pain, progressive myelopathy
Vertebral hemangiomas	Incidence increases with age	Asymptomatic, cord compression	Pain, myelopathy, radiculopathy
Miscellaneous			
Spinal artery aneurysms	Congenital/acquired	Subarachnoid hemorrhage	Subarachnoid hemorrhage symptoms
Hypervascular metastatic lesions	Acquired	Pathologic fractures, cord compression	Acute and progressive myelopathy

AVF, arteriovenous fistula; AVM, arteriovenous malformation; AVS, arteriovenous shunt; F, fistula; M, malformation.

veins.[27] However, other studies suggest that for the localization of spinal dural AVFs, 3.0 Tesla dynamic contrast-enhanced MRA may be more reliable than multidetector CTA.[28]

In addition, exposure to ionizing radiation and the need for nephrotoxic iodinated contrast agents limit widespread application of CTA for the assessment of spinal vascular disease in the clinical setting.

In summary, advanced multidetector CT imaging and 3.0 Tesla contrast-enhanced MRA are considered, safe, rapid, and noninvasive modalities that have the potential to clearly show the extension of SVSs, feeding arteries, and fistulas.[29] Studies have also shown the sensitivity of MRA for depicting dural AVF; defining the level of the blood supply indirectly via enlarged draining veins will help to focus and reduce the time that catheter angiography takes.[18,20,30]

Catheter-Based Angiography and Intervention

Unlike what is conventionally believed, with modern catheter techniques and when performed by a trained physician, spinal diagnostic angiography should not bear a higher rate of complications than a diagnostic angiography of the peripheral system. Infrequently, minor asymptomatic iliac or aortic dissections may be encountered in elderly patients with significant atherosclerotic disease. Frequently, angiography is used prior to a planned surgery to locate the AKA (or radicularis magna) as the major supply to the anterior spinal cord. If a vascular lesion, especially a dural AVF, is suspected, a more thorough angiography may be required. This includes angiograms of the aortic arch, descending aorta, abdominal aorta, and pelvic system. In cases of brain AVS with drainage into the spine or cervical spinal cord AVM/AVS, the vertebral arteries, thyrocervical trunk, and deep ascending cervical arteries are also studied.

If an intervention is planned, a 5-Fr or a 6-Fr guide catheter is preferred for the coaxial microcatheter placement; if the region of interest is located higher, a long femoral sheath bypasses the often tortuous aortic/iliac system. Infrequently, the guide catheter may need to be changed over an exchange wire for a stable position within the intercostal or lumbar

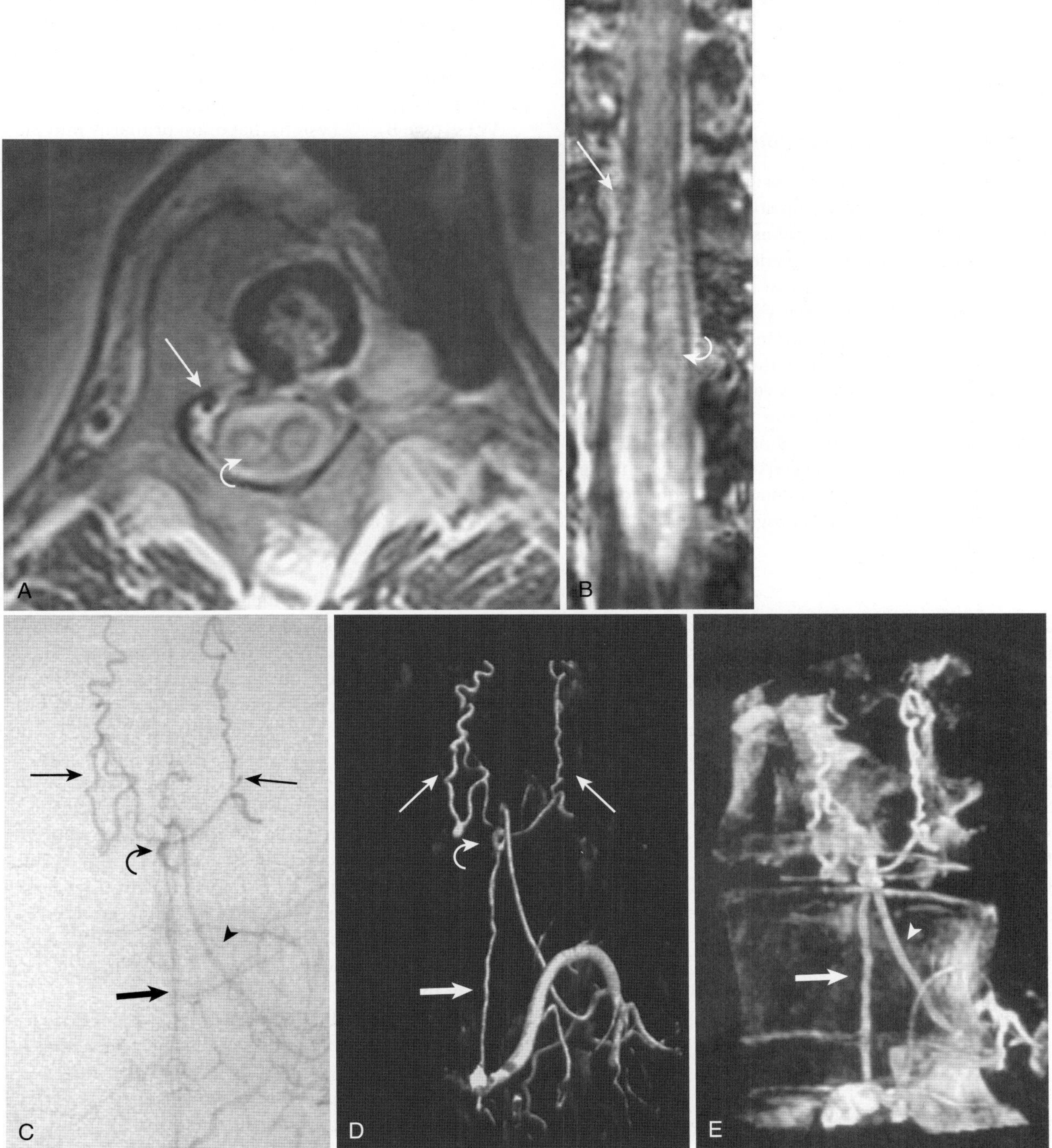

FIG. 93.9 A 50-year-old patient presented with paraparesis. Pial arteriovenous malformation (AVM) is associated with a split cord malformation type II (diastematomyelia). (A) Axial and (B) coronal magnetic resonance images show the split cord (*curved arrow*) and some enlarged vasculature (*arrows*). A significant cord swelling and edema is seen. (C) Superselective injection of the artery of Adamkiewicz (*arrowhead*) and three-dimensional rotational angiography (D and E) show the pial AVM, the typical hairpin turn of the anterior spinal artery (*large arrows*), and apically directed drainage into two main arterialized and congested dorsolaterally located longitudinal veins (*arrows*).

artery. Because it is easier and less traumatic to straighten the proximal part of the segmental arteries, we prefer hydrophilic-coated exchange glide wires. A range of microcatheters, including flow-guided catheters and microwires, are available for the interventional procedures. The selection has to be tailored to the size of the vessel and the embolic material used.

For diagnostic purposes, heparin is not given. For interventional procedures, heparin may be given, although rarely, to prevent inadvertent thrombosis, especially if catheters are navigated within the spinal cord vasculature. In select cases of high-flow AVSs with blood supplied from ASA or PSA, patients are administered aspirin and/or clopidogrel (Plavix) after the embolization to prevent a retrograde thrombosis of the ASA after reduction of the AVS.

Spinal Vascular Disorders

Paraspinal Arteriovenous Malformations and Shunts

Paraspinal AVSs/AVMs are rare lesions presenting with a female preponderance. They are mostly found at the thoracic or cervical level, present frequently as a fistula, and drain in enormous ectatic veins located outside the spine (Fig. 93.10). The patient can present with progressive neurologic symptoms and an audible bruit. The pulsatile venous ectasia can erode the bone, enlarge the neuroforamina, invaginate into the spinal canal, and directly compress the cord, thus mimicking an extradural tumor. If paraspinal veins communicate with intradural radicular veins and the perimedullary venous plexus, the pathologic venous drainage can create venous engorgement with congestive myelopathy.[31] Paraspinal vertebrojugular fistulas can be traumatic in origin, commonly seen after motor vehicle accidents, or iatrogenic, after placement of transjugular central lines.

Imaging

MRI shows a serpiginous flow void signal corresponding to feeding artery and/or large draining veins, located outside the spine. Spinal angiography shows the supplying artery, which is usually a branch of an intercostal artery at the thoracic level or a branch from the vertebral artery when the AVM is at the cervical level.[32,33] Paraspinal shunts may drain into paravertebral, epidural, or intradural venous systems. In the case of a high-flow AVM(F), distal flow within the parent artery (e.g., vertebral artery) may be absent owing to the presence of shunt and steal from the contralateral vertebral artery or cervical branches. In traumatic cases, the vertebral artery can be involved directly.

Treatment

The fistulas are occluded either by placement of a covered stent within the artery or by embolization of the AVF with detachable balloons or coils, acrylate injection, Onyx, or a combination of these materials (see Fig. 93.10).[34–36]

Epidural Arteriovenous Shunts

Also known as spinal extradural arteriovenous fistula (SEDAVF), these are rare vascular shunts anatomically distinct from the typical spinal dural arteriovenous fistula. SEDAVFs are typically supplied by radicular branches with a fistulous connection to the spinal ventral epidural (also termed extradural) venous plexus and are usually slow-flow lesions. They can be a source of neurologic morbidity as a result of venous engorgement and mass effect or venous hypertension due to recruitment of intradural perimedullary veins.[37] Cases of subarachnoid hemorrhage (SAH) as a presentation of these lesions have also been described.[38,39] Cervical SEDAVFs affect younger patients and are associated with neurofibromatosis (NF-1) and SAH.[37] Lumbosacral lesions affect an older patient population with a male sex predilection; these patients tend to present with generally worse neurologic deficits, likely due to their tendency to have intradural venous drainage.[37] SEDAVFs are described in two distinct subtypes: extradural AVFs with retrograde parenchymal drainage (type A) and pure extradural AVFs (type B).[40,41] Lesions that drain primarily into the ventral epidural venous plexus and secondarily into the intradural/medullary venous system have been reported. Most of the reported cases are sacral, with arterial supply from the lateral sacral arteries.[42]

Imaging

Using conventional MRI, it is difficult to distinguish dural from epidural shunts. The diagnosis is determined when MRA identifies the draining veins as serpentine, linear, or curved structures around the surface of the cord.[31] Intravenous injection of gadolinium–diethylenetriamine pentaacetic acid (Gd-DTPA) enhances the dilated veins and allows a better delineation.

Treatment

The ideal treatment of a type A SEDAVF is obliteration of shunts leading to the successive disappearance of the epidural venous lake as well as extradural and intradural drainers. Endovascular treatments include transvenous and transarterial embolization. Transvenous embolization may achieve a dramatic and definitive cure for this subtype of SEDAVF by means of occluding the fistula located on the venous site through epidural venous lake. One limitation, however, is the technical challenges associated with such access. The endovascular treatment of these shunts consists of a supraselective infusion of acrylate or Onyx with obliteration of the most proximal part of the draining vein and the feeding artery or a surgical obliteration of the arteriovenous connection.[37,41]

Although considered an alternative option, transarterial embolization is limited, as SEDAVFs usually have more feeders than a classical spinal dural AVF. Transarterial embolization risks incomplete obliteration of the draining veins, which could lead to further recruitment of feeders with recanalization of the lesion.

Microsurgical obliteration with sole drainer occlusion can lead to complete obliteration of the epidural venous lake and provide satisfactory outcomes in cases of a type A SEDAVF with a single draining vein. When facing a case with multiple intradural draining veins or recurrent SEDAVF, complete shunt occlusion by coagulating the epidural venous lake or a multimodal approach with endovascular procedures may be a feasible option.[43]

Dural Arteriovenous Shunts

Also known as dorsal intradural AVF or type I spinal AVM, this type represents the most common of spinal vascular lesions, accounting for about 70% of all arteriovenous shunts of the spine, and should be in the differential diagnosis in an adult presenting with gradually worsening myelopathy. Most authors have classified this lesion as type A if fed by a single arterial feeder and type B if fed by two or more feeders. The most common location for these malformations is between T4

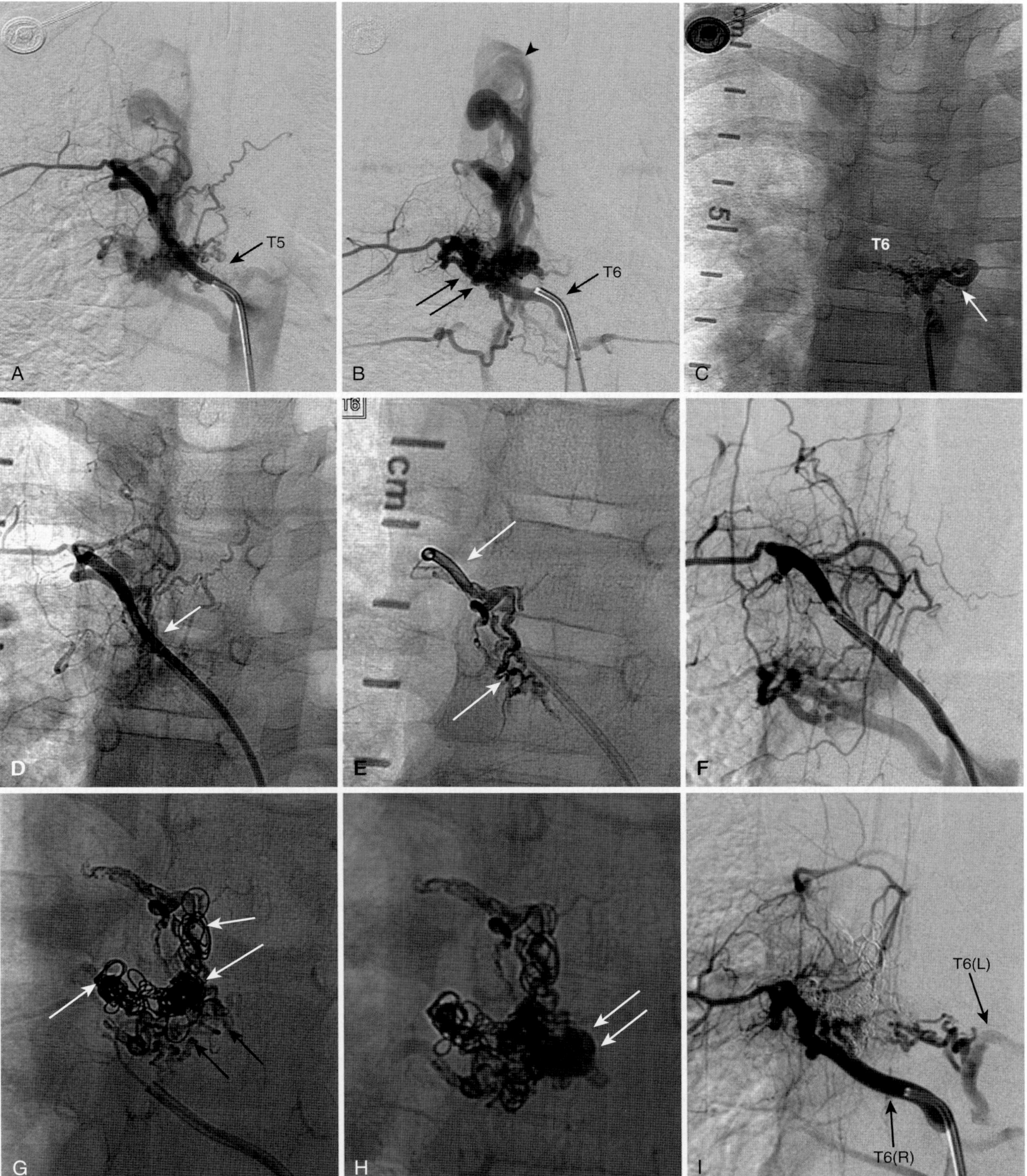

FIG. 93.10 An 8-year-old female was originally scheduled for surgery after presenting with progressive thoracic scoliosis, back pain, and growth disturbance. A vascular malformation was detected on preoperative magnetic resonance imaging/magnetic resonance angiography, which subsequent digital subtraction angiography found to be a congenital paraspinal arteriovenous malformation (AVM) at the T6 level. This was treated through an endovascular approach. (A–C) Selective angiograms show bilateral supply through several intercostal feeders (*arrows*) with drainage into the superior vena cava via the azygos vein (*arrowhead*). (D) Embolization begins at the T5 intercostal level with infusion of liquid embolics (E) to reduce AVM shunt (*arrows*). (F) Follow-up angiography shows flow reduction through the AVM. (G) Further embolization at the T6 level using transarterial placement of coils into the venous outflow (*arrows*) to reduce the shunt and capture the additional liquid embolics (*black arrows*). (H) Continued infusion of the embolic material into the AVM nidus with penetration of the venous pouch (*arrows*). I, Follow-up angiography of the right T6 intercostal artery (with reflux into the left T6 intercostal artery) shows a complete obliteration of the AVM.

and L3, with the peak incidence occurring between T7 and T12.[44,45] Although rare, possibly owing to the helpful effect of gravity on venous drainage above the level of the right atrium, dural shunts may occur above the level of the heart. When present, cervical spinal dural AVSs, particularly high cervical shunts, have unique angioarchitectural characteristics different from those seen in the other spinal regions.[46] Cervical spinal dural AVSs, similar to other locations, seem to be more prevalent in men (male/female ratio, ~ 2 : 1), with an average age in the mid-fifties, and with predominant arterial supply arising from the vertebral artery.[47] Hemorrhagic presentation of a thoracolumbar dural AVS is considered extremely rare.[48] However, previous reports have shown that cervical spinal dural AVSs may be more frequently associated with SAH.[49,50] It is also important to emphasize that spinal AVSs at any level can manifest with congestive myelopathy of the conus; thus, a complete spinal angiogram is necessary.[51] Spinal AVSs also may rarely be located in the sacral region and have a higher tendency of recurrence compared to their thoracolumbar counterparts.[52]

In general, spinal dural AVSs are composed of tiny arterial connections between the dural branch of a radicular artery (only rarely of a radiculomedullary artery) at the level of the proximal nerve root and a radiculomedullary vein (Fig. 93.11). Branches of adjacent radicular arteries may be involved in blood supply because of an extensive intradural collateral network. The arterialized radiculomedullary vein then transmits the increased flow and pressure to the valveless coronal venous plexus and longitudinal spinal veins. Subsequently, the radiculomedullary vein is enlarged and tortuous. The mean intraluminal venous pressure is increased to 74% of the systemic arterial pressure.[53,54] The normal venous pressure in the coronal venous plexus is 23 mm Hg and approximately twice that of the epidural venous plexus, which is necessary for venous drainage. In one series, the mean venous pressure in the coronal venous plexus was measured at 40 mm Hg.[10] Because the venous hypertension affects the normal venous return and extends into venules, it finally causes a venous infarction of the spinal cord. The progressive myelopathy often leads to paraplegia and bowel, bladder, and sexual dysfunction, with gradual worsening over months to a few years. Most of the patients become severely disabled within 3.5 years.[10,55–57] The majority of patients (79–85%) are men, and 86% of patients are 41 years of age or older at presentation.[44,45,58,59] The mean age at presentation is 55 years old; however, patients as young as 1 month of age have been reported as a result of hereditary hemorrhagic telangiectasia.[60] The most common presentation is progressive paraparesis, with sensory changes and complaints of back and leg pain.[61] The progression is usually continuous, but it can also present in a stepwise fashion or a waxing-waning course with gradual progression. In 10% to 20% of patients, the presentation is an acute exacerbation. The symptoms can be exacerbated by any physical activity that increases intraabdominal pressure and thus central venous pressure, as well as by an upright posture (impaired venous drainage due to hydrostatic pressure). A brain dural AVS of the posterior fossa (e.g., tentorial dural AVS) can mimic a spinal dural AVS if the venous drainage takes the pontomedullary path into the spinal cord venous system (Fig. 93.12). These dural brain AVSs have been classified as type V.[62] Thus, a diagnostic cerebral workup of the posterior circulation and both internal and external carotid arteries is a part of the spinal angiography. The most common misdiagnosis for these lesions is transverse myelitis, ischemic spinal cord infarction, disc disease, and spinal cord tumors.

Imaging

MRI identifies draining vessels as serpentine areas of flow void within the spinal canal on T2-weighted images. In axial T1- and T2-weighted MR images, dilated coronal veins with a low signal located around the spinal cord are visible. Enlarged radiculomedullary veins on dynamic contrast medium–enhanced MRA help to guide catheter angiography and help to reduce the contrast load for the patient.[18] The spinal cord can appear enlarged and hypointense on T1-weighted images; the flame-shaped spinal cord edema that spares the cord periphery can be well appreciated on T2-weighted images. Because it represents venous infarction, contrast medium enhancement within edematous changes is considered prognostically bad for recovery of neurologic function. Spinal

FIG. 93.11 Dural arteriovenous fistula (AVF; intradural AVF, type I spinal arteriovenous malformation [AVM]). (A and B) A single location and single arterial feeder (type IA) and multiple dural arterial supply (type IB): *1*, dural branches of radicular artery supplying AVM within the dura; *2*, arterialized radiculomedullary vein; *3*, dilated posterior median vein. (C) Intraoperative image of a dural AVF after opening of the dura shows an arterialized and congested posterior median vein (*arrow*) and a markedly swollen spinal cord. (D) Contrast medium–enhanced T1-weighted magnetic resonance (MR) image shows a nonspecific, diffuse, flame-shaped enhancement and swelling of the spinal cord (*curved arrow*) and dilated posterior median vein (*arrow*). (E) Three-dimensional time-of-flight MR angiogram in the coronal plane shows congested radiculomedullary vein (*single arrow*) and dorsal median vein (*double arrows*). (F) A microcatheter has been navigated through an intercostal artery (*arrowheads*), and superselective angiography of the radicular artery (*long arrow*) delineates the dural AVF (*curved arrow*), the retrograde draining and congested radiculomedullary vein (*double arrows*), and the congested dorsal median vein (*large arrow*). (G) After embolization, a plain spine radiograph shows *N*-butyl-cyanoacrylate cast within the radicular artery (*arrow*), the point of fistulization (*curved arrow*), and the radiculomedullary vein (*double arrows*). (H) Control angiography of the intercostal artery (*arrow*) shows a complete dural AVF obliteration.

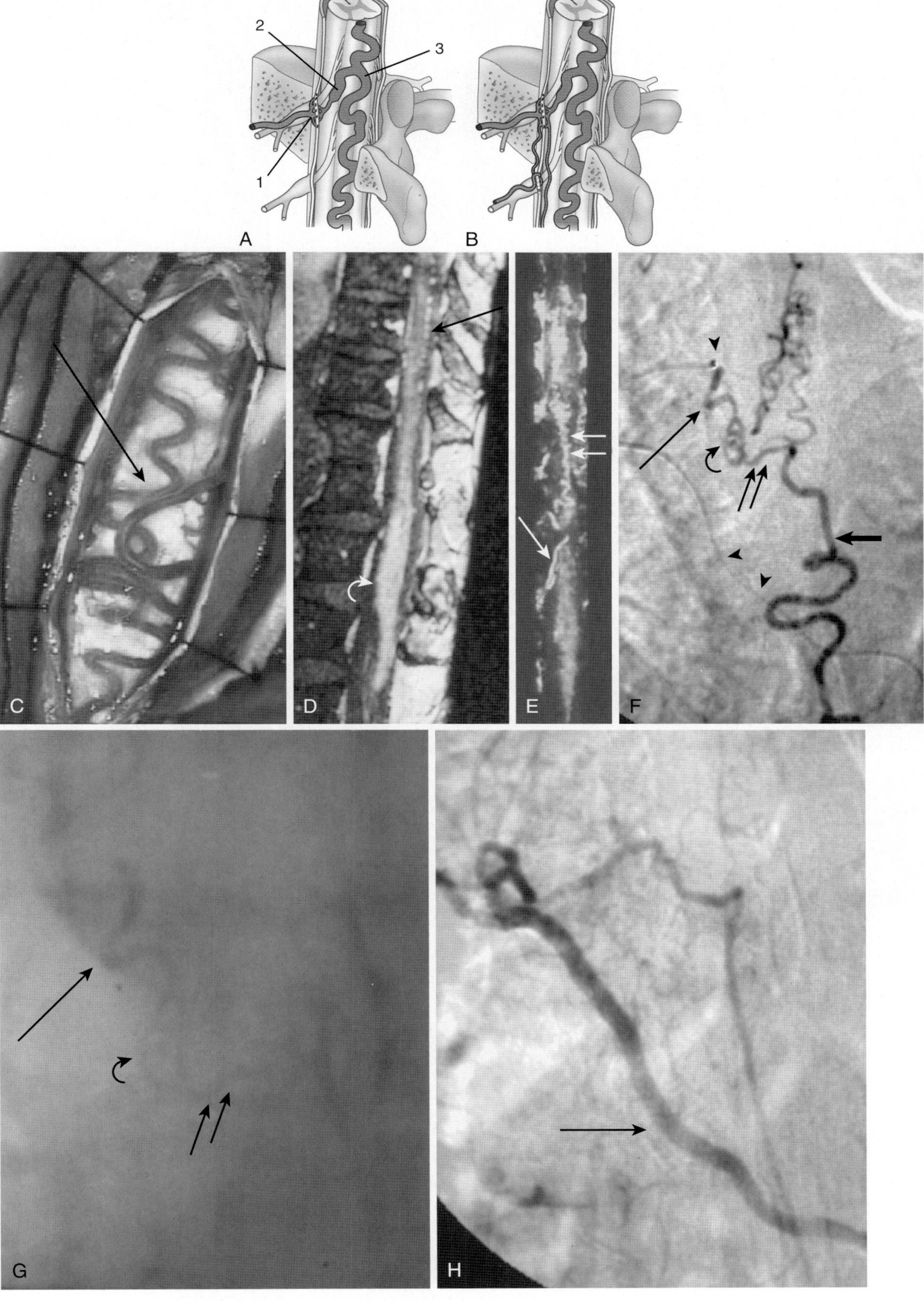
2
3
1
A
B
C
D
E
F
G
H

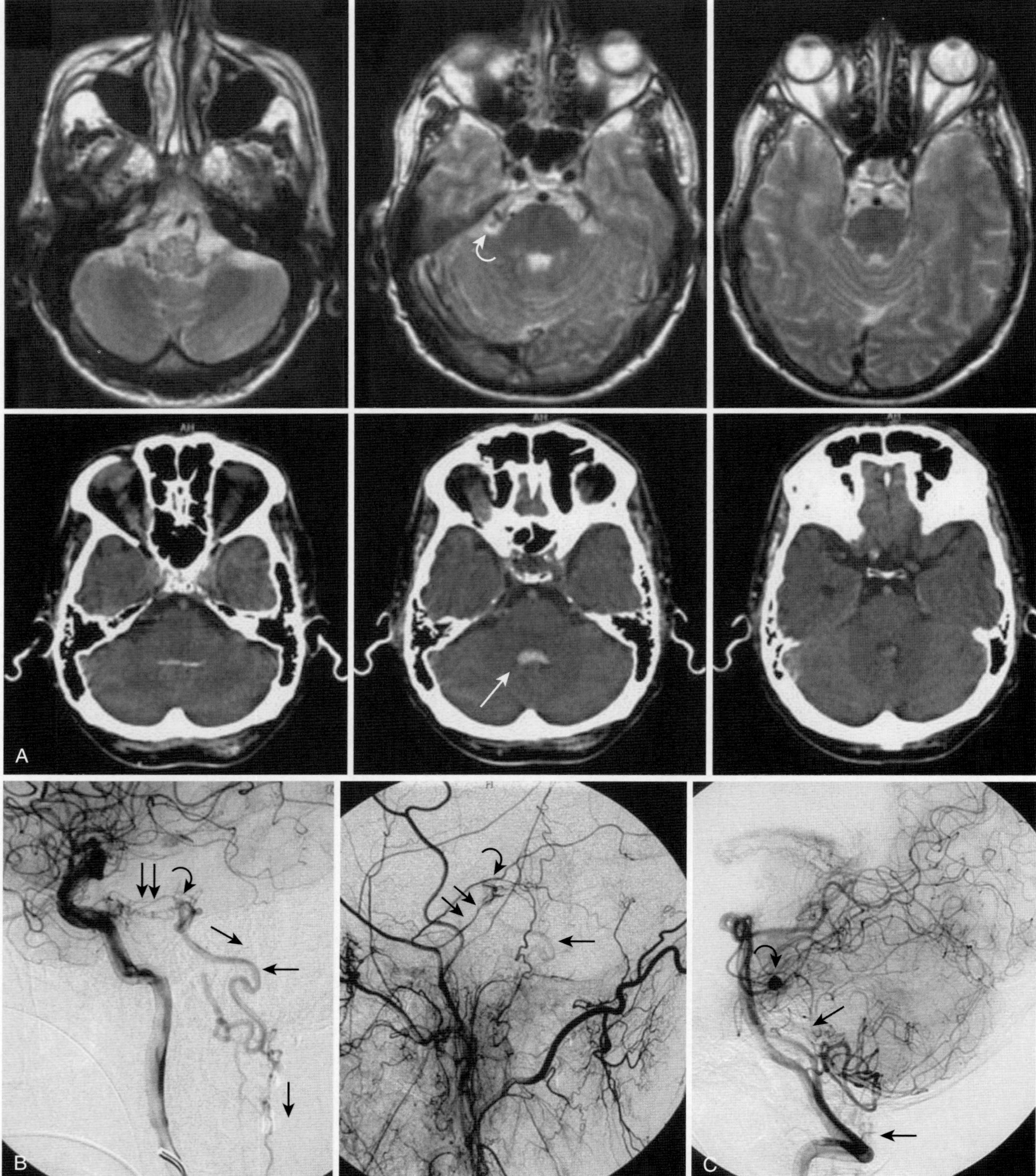

FIG. 93.12 A 55-year-old neurologically intact man presented with an intraventricular hemorrhage associated with a tentorial dural arteriovenous shunt (AVS) with drainage into the congested spinal venous system. (A) Axial T2-weighted magnetic resonance images and computed tomographic scans show hemorrhage into the fourth ventricle (*arrow*) and abnormal vascular structure anterior to the cerebellopontine angle (*curved arrow*). (B) Right internal and external carotid artery angiograms show dural branches originating from the meningohypophyseal trunk and the middle meningeal artery (*double arrows*) with filling of a tentorial dural AVS (*curved arrows*). Note early retrograde filling of congested median anterior pontine vein, transverse pontine vein, lateral pontine vein, and posterior and anterior median medullary veins (*single arrows*). (C) Left vertebral artery injection shows additional supply of the AVS via the tentorial branch (artery of Davidoff and Schechter) originating from the right superior cerebellar artery and early venous drainage into the spinal canal (*arrows*); an associated superior cerebellar artery aneurysm is seen (*curved arrow*).

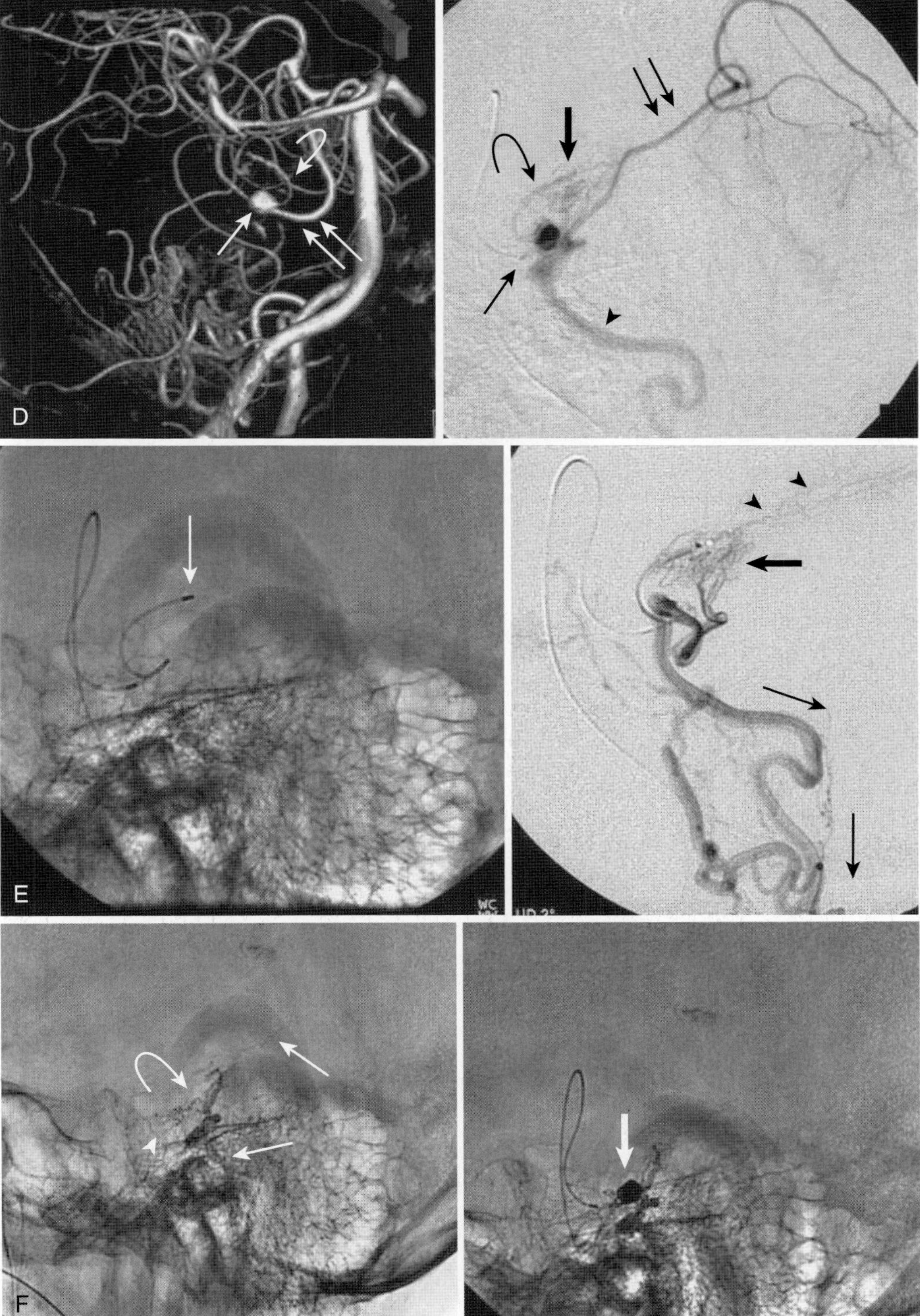

FIG. 93.12, cont'd (D) Three-dimensional angiography and superselective injection of the right superior cerebellar artery (*double arrows*) proximal to the aneurysm (*single arrows*) show the tentorial AVS (*large arrow*) fed by dural artery (*curved arrows*), the tentorial malformation, and the early filling of congested median anterior pontine vein (*arrowhead*). (E) Catheterization of dural artery through the aneurysm (*white arrow*) and filling of the AVS (*large arrow*) and tentorial dural veins (*arrowheads*). Note early venous drainage into the spinal canal (*single arrows*). (F) *N*-butyl cyanoacrylate infusion with filling of the AVS nidus (*curved arrow*), dural veins (*arrows*), and retrograde dural arteries originating from the internal carotid artery (*arrowhead*). Coiling of the superior cerebellar artery aneurysm (*large arrow*) in the same session.

Continued

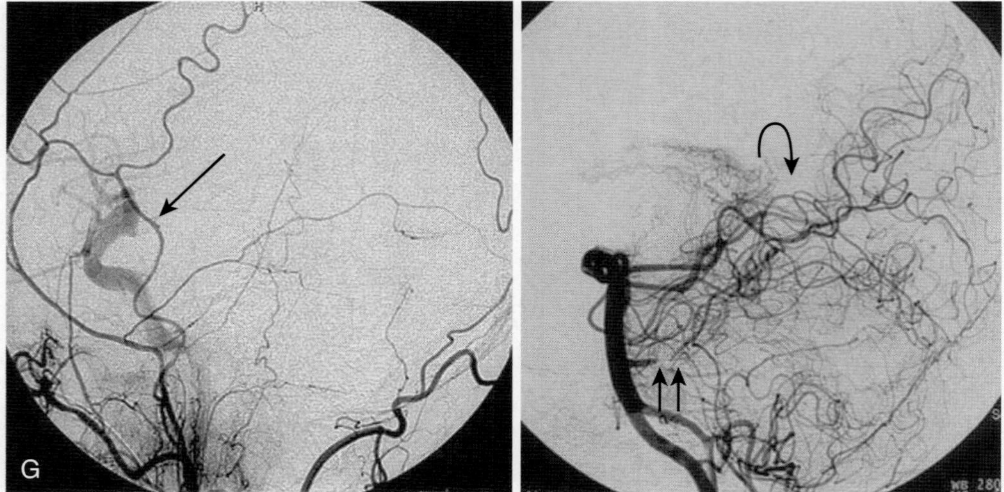

FIG. 93.12, cont'd (G) Control injection of the common carotid artery and the vertebral artery shows complete obliteration of the dural malformation and no filling of the meningohypophyseal dural branches (*single arrow*) and the aneurysms (*double arrows*, coil artifact superimposed on the superior cerebellar artery). Note the patency of the artery (*curved arrow*).

angiography shows a direct shunting of contrast agent from the radiculomeningeal artery supply into the extensive and tortuous draining radiculomedullary and perimedullary venous systems. The draining vessels are the coronal venous plexus situated along the dorsal surface of the spinal cord. Angiography also helps to delineate the ASA and guide the embolization. AVS feeding vessels can originate anywhere from vertebral artery to lateral sacral arteries (Fig. 93.13).

Last, normal cerebrospinal fluid pulsations typically dorsal to the cord on T2-weighted images may mimic a dural malformation.

Treatment

A cure can be achieved by opening the dura at the affected level and surgically disconnecting the radiculomedullary vein from the dural arterial supply.[61] Microsurgical treatment can be performed with exceedingly high obliteration rates and long-term postoperative improvement of preexisting deficits in the majority of cases.[63,64] Despite recent advances in endovascular techniques and materials, there is a subgroup of patients for which surgery remains the best treatment option.[65]

Alternatively, an endovascular intervention in experienced hands is very safe and effective. Endovascular therapy entails the infusion of *N*-butyl cyanoacrylate (NBCA) into the radiculomedullary vein after selective microcatheterization of the feeding artery.[66,67] Complete obliteration has been reported in up to 90% of patients, but with recurrence rates of up to 23%.[59] In pediatric patients, endovascular treatment (even partial but targeted) also appears to be a safe and stable therapeutic alternative in the management of spinal dural AVSs.[68] The availability of newer acrylate and liquid embolic agents and more experienced physicians has diminished the recurrence rate significantly. The consensus among interventional neuroradiologists at this time is that the successful treatment of these malformations consists of acrylate penetration of the fistula and the proximal radiculomedullary draining vein without entering the spinal cord draining system (see Fig. 93.11). The protocol used in some centers is an endovascular approach as the first line of treatment because of its noninvasive nature, low complication rate, and the ability to obtain immediate angiographic control and confirmation of obliteration. Factors determining the success of endovascular treatments among patients with spinal dural AVFs seem to include the presence of antegrade flow toward the draining vein and injection of NBCA glue less than 30%; these factors were associated with higher chance of draining vein penetration and, therefore, successful endovascular spinal dural AVF obliteration as reported in a recent single-center experience.[69] If the acrylate should not penetrate the radiculomedullary veins, the patient requires a surgical disconnection; the radiopaque acrylate mixture then can be used as a landmark for fluoroscopic-guided intraoperative localization. Alternatives for liquid embolic agents include Onyx; however, it has been associated with a higher recurrence rate, and possibly because of its deeper penetration into smaller vessels potentially connecting to the ASA or PSAs, considered less suitable for the endovascular embolization of spinal dural AVFs.[70]

Pial Arteriovenous Shunts

Also called ventral intradural AVF, perimedullary fistula, or type IV spinal AVM, a pial AVS is a direct fistula between the ASA and the coronal venous plexus (Fig. 93.14). Radiculopial supply may also be involved. Based on the size of the AVF and the blood flow, three different subtypes (A, B, and C) have been described.

Subtype A (Merland subtype I) is a small shunt with slow flow, with moderate venous hypertension.[71] There is no enlargement of the ASA and only minimal dilatation of the ascending draining vein.[10,72] The location of the fistula can be difficult to find, but it is characterized generally by the point at which a vessel caliber change between the smaller artery

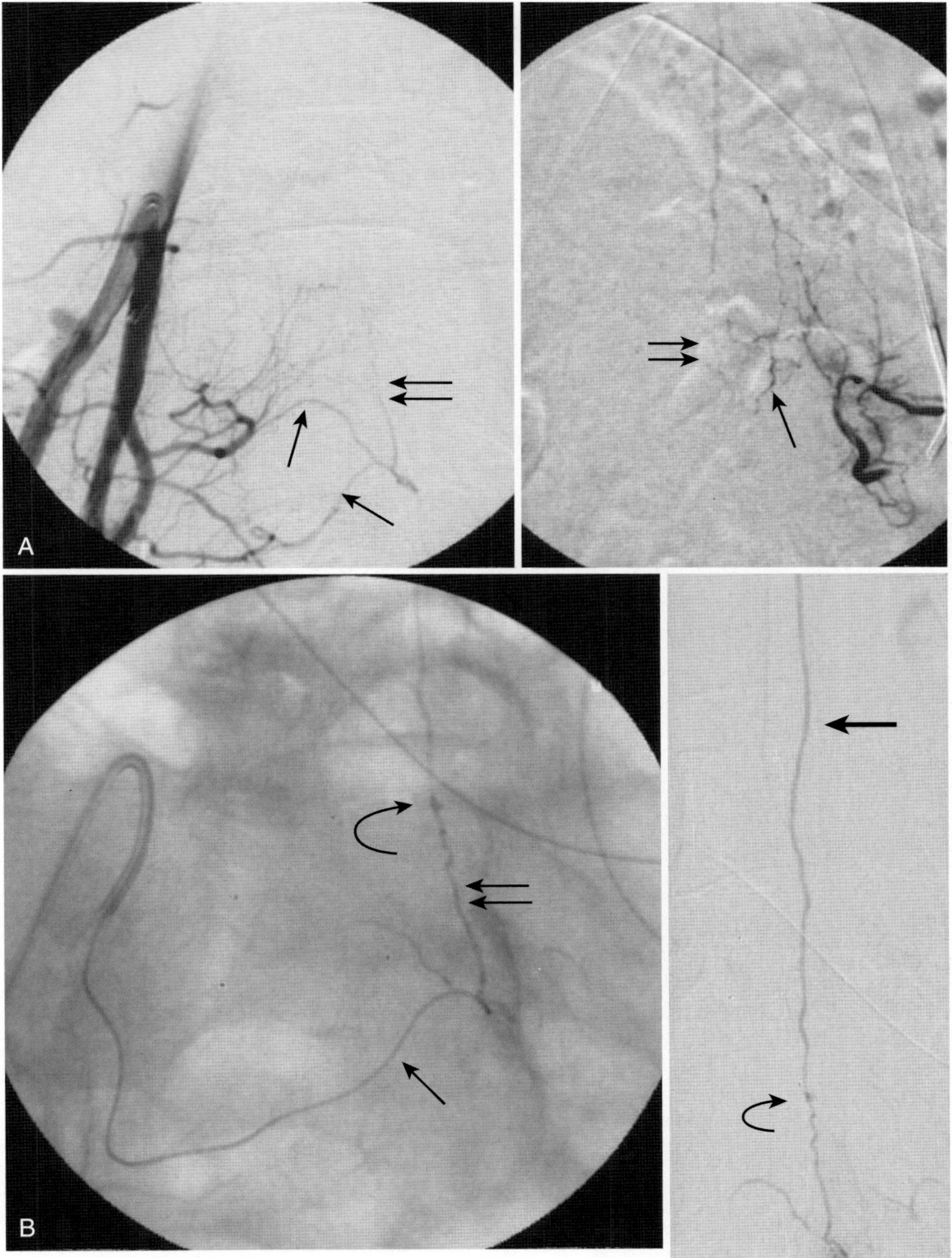

FIG. 93.13 Sacral dural arteriovenous shunt in a 60-year-old man who presented with paraparesis and bowel and bladder dysfunction. (A) Right internal iliac artery angiogram shows lateral sacral arteries (*arrows*) filling the dural artery of the filum (*double arrows*). (B) Superselective angiogram through the lateral sacral artery shows the spinal dural arteriovenous fistula within the end of the thecal sac (*curved arrow*) and the ascending vein along the cauda equina (*thick arrow*).

and the larger ectatic vein is seen.[73] Owing to the change from a higher arterial impedance to a lower venous one, a change in blood flow pattern and velocity can be observed on high-speed angiograms.[74,75] The ASA is the only feeder, and the AVF is typically located along the anterior aspect of the conus medullaris or proximal filum terminale.[71]

Subtype B (Merland subtype II) is a moderate-sized (intermediate) shunt with moderate enlargement of the feeding artery(ies) and the draining veins.[71] The location of the fistula is marked by venous ectasia.[73] This is a high flow rate shunt; associated flow-related arterial and venous aneurysms may be present. There are several abnormally dilated feeding arteries, composed of the ASA and one or two arteries from the dorsolateral pial network (PSA), all of which converge on the fistula. These are typically located at the level of the conus. Blood returns via tortuous and dilated ascending perimedullary veins.[71]

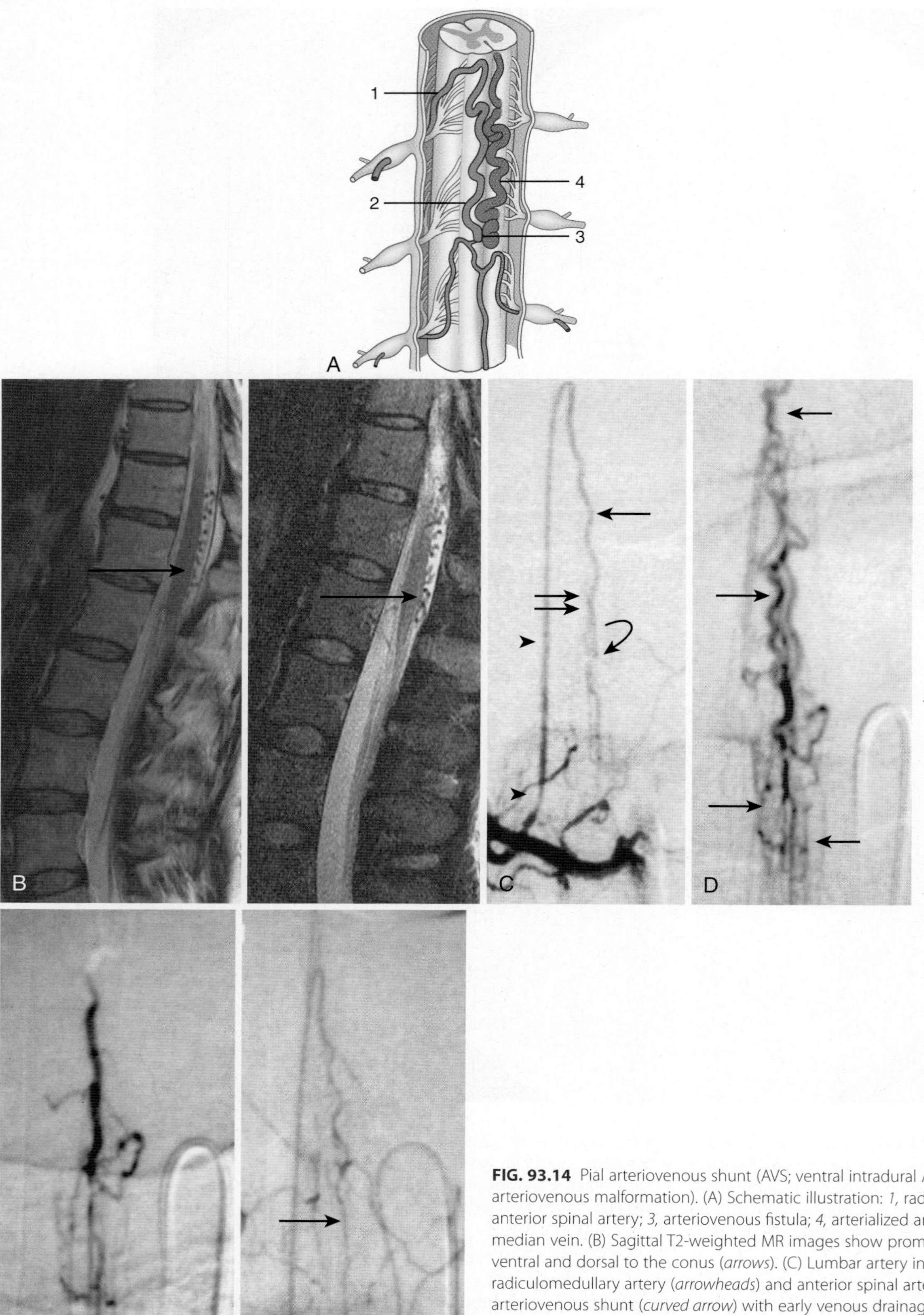

FIG. 93.14 Pial arteriovenous shunt (AVS; ventral intradural AVF or type IV spinal arteriovenous malformation). (A) Schematic illustration: *1,* radiculomedullary artery; *2,* anterior spinal artery; *3,* arteriovenous fistula; *4,* arterialized and congested anterior median vein. (B) Sagittal T2-weighted MR images show prominent intradural vessels ventral and dorsal to the conus (*arrows*). (C) Lumbar artery injection shows an enlarged radiculomedullary artery (*arrowheads*) and anterior spinal artery (*single arrow*) and an arteriovenous shunt (*curved arrow*) with early venous drainage (*double arrows*). (D) Congested ventral and dorsal veins as well as the venous plexus at the conus level (*arrows*). (E) Microcatheter angiography of the anterior spinal artery before embolization with *N*-butyl cyanoacrylate shows the congested venous system. (F) Two-year follow-up angiography after embolization shows a persistent AVS obliteration and patency of the anterior spinal artery (*arrow*). (A, Courtesy R.F. Spetzler; B–F, courtesy P.K. Nelson, New York University.)

Subtype C (Merland subtype III) is a giant fistula with very large arterial feeder(s) from the ASA and dorsolateral pial network (PSA) converging into the fistula and draining directly into a giant venous ectasia, often embedded within the substance of the cord.[71] These fistulas are rare, although, in at least one large series, they were the largest subtype of ventral intradural AVF.[71,73] The location of the fistula is more difficult to ascertain because of the giant, ectatic draining vein.[73] The giant, ectatic draining vein usually drains into the local metameric efferent veins, which are also dilated.[71] These lesions are typically located at the thoracic or cervical levels.

The clinical signs and symptoms may be due to vascular steal, especially with higher flow, venous hypertension, and mass effect with venous enlargement and aneurysm formation, as well as hemorrhage.[10] More than 90% of patients present with neurologic deficits. They almost always appear before age 40 years and often present during the first decade, with mean age at diagnosis being between 11.5 and 13.5 years. SAH is the presenting sign in approximately 40% of patients, but according to some authors only subtype C fistulas present as hemorrhage.[73,76] Occasionally, hematomyelia has also been reported.[77] Paraparesis or paraplegia is the most common sign, with progressive deterioration over time. Radiculomyelopathy or radiculopathy can also be present, presumably owing to mass effect from dilated venous structures. These lesions can be seen anywhere along the spine. When the fistula is located ventrolaterally or posterolaterally, a significant involvement of the dorsolateral pial network (PSA) is present.

Imaging

MRI reveals low-signal feeding and draining vessels within the spinal cord by identifying flow voids on T1 and T2 weighting (see Fig. 93.14). Additionally, sagittal and coronal T1-weighted images characterize the malformation by revealing the low signal nidus and enlarged ASA. On contrast medium–enhanced scans, pial vessels and epidural plexus can be appreciated. The spinal cord can appear enlarged and may show patchy enhancement on T1 weighting. It will appear hyperintense on T2 weighting, which corresponds to venous infarction, edema, or gliosis. Lumbar canal stenosis with engorged venous plexus or tortuous intradural roots may mimic a pial AVS. Other enhancing spinal cord masses—such as ependymoma, astrocytoma, or paraganglioma—must be considered in the differential diagnosis.

Treatment

Type A and B fistulas have traditionally been treated by microsurgery. In subtype A, the blood supply occurs through a minimally dilated ASA with slow flow; thus, endovascular treatment is difficult to achieve and microcatheterization might be hazardous. Endovascular reports, on the other hand, are limited. Oran et al. reported the treatment of five patients with type A fistulas using flow-directed catheters and NBCA; the authors were able to achieve complete fistula obliteration in four of the five cases, with the last patient requiring surgery.[78] There were no complications and all treated patients improved clinically. In select cases, a polyvinyl alcohol (PVA) particle embolization from a catheter positioned proximally may be considered if a coil- or acrylate-assisted occlusion of the fistula is not feasible.

In subtype B, a higher flow and a larger feeding artery facilitate the endovascular catheterization of the fistula and a curative acrylate infusion. In a report of 20 patients treated for AVSs, Lundqvist and colleagues reported treating two patients with subtype B fistulas using PVA embolization.[79] Both patients showed clinical improvement, but no long-term follow-up was documented.

Surgical treatment for type C lesions is generally considered high risk given the risk of intraoperative hemorrhage; thus, endovascular treatment is generally favored.[80] Both transarterial and transvenous treatment routes as well as direct venous puncture have been described.[76,81,82] Because of this high flow in subtype C, detachable balloons or fibered coils have been used in the past for a permanent obliteration of the fistula. NBCA may be used safely for a complete closure either alone or in conjunction with coils (see Fig. 93.14).[71,76,83,84]

Other embolic agents, such as Onyx, appear to have a similar safety profile as other, more commonly used materials when endovascularly treating spinal AVSs. A case report utilizing Onyx for endovascular embolization of pediatric spinal perimedullary fistula included two successfully treated patients with adequate clinical outcomes and without any permanent critical complications.[85]

Conus Medullaris Arteriovenous Shunts

A new category of spinal AVSs proposed recently is characterized by multiple feeding arteries, multiple niduses, and a complex venous drainage. These lesions are composed of multiple direct AVSs with feeders from the ASA and PSA as well as a glomus-type nidus that is usually extramedullary/pial. However, the conus medullaris AVS can occasionally be intramedullary.[10] They are always located in the conus medullaris and cauda equina and can extend along the entire extent of the filum terminale. Symptoms can be caused by venous hypertension, venous compression of the cord/cauda equina, or hemorrhage (subarachnoid or hematomyelia). Because of its location, this type of SVS is frequently associated with radiculopathy in addition to myelopathy.[86]

Treatment

Optimal treatment of conus medullaris AVSs involves aggressive embolization followed by microsurgical resection.[71,76,83,86,87]

Extradural/Intradural Arteriovenous Shunt

The rare form of an extradural and intradural AVS is also known as spinal arteriovenous metameric syndrome (SAMS) or juvenile AVM, or type III AVM (Fig. 93.15). SAMS is known for its formidable angioarchitecture and presumed poor natural history.[88–90] If all derivatives of the metamere (i.e., skin, muscle, bone, dura, and cord) are involved, it is known as Cobb syndrome.[90] While most patients with SAMS suffer from intradural spinal vascular pathology, there has been a recent report of SAMS affecting the epidural space and paraspinal space, leaving the intradural space unaffected.[91] It is

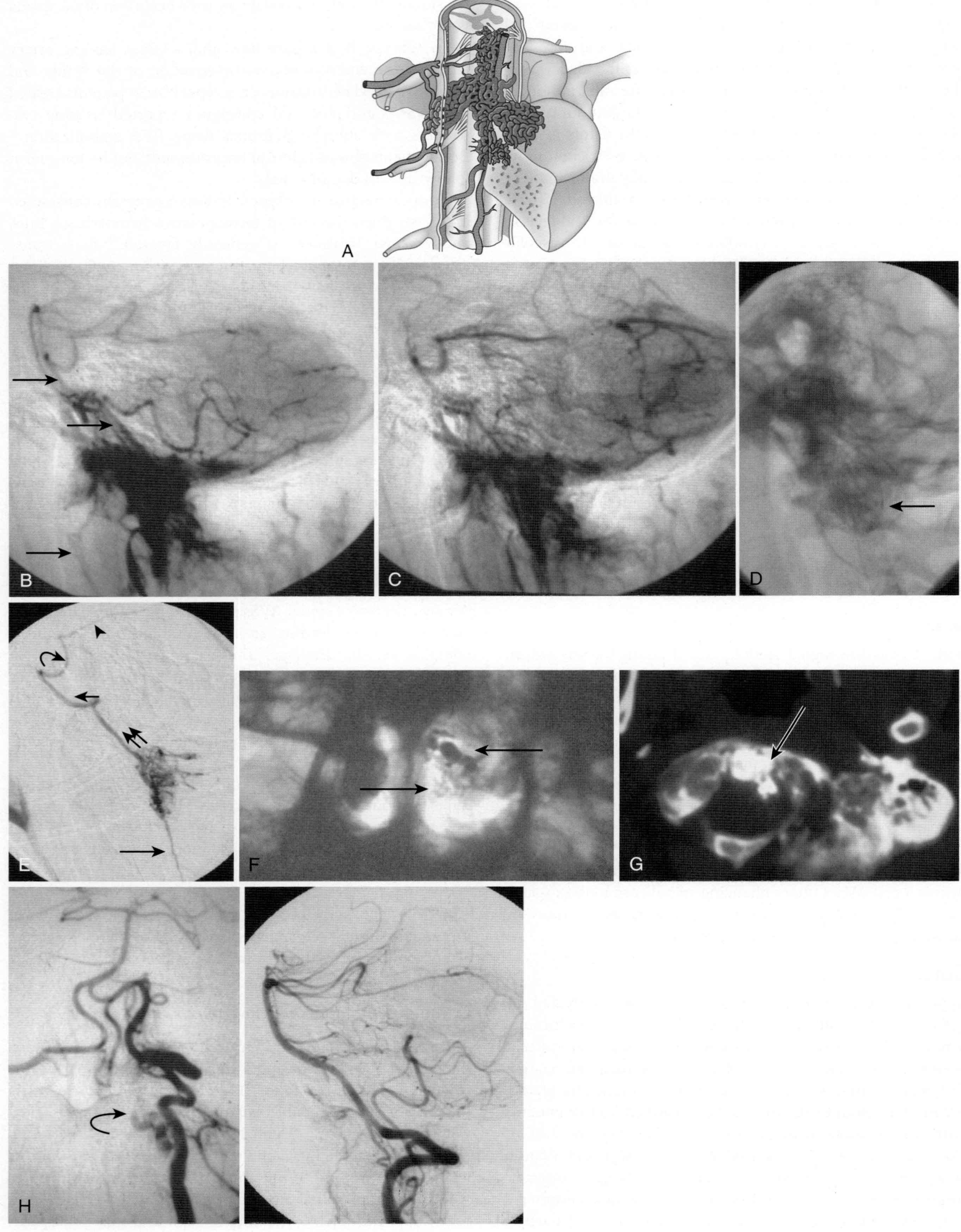
A
B
C
D
E
F
G
H

FIG. 93.15 Extradural/intradural arteriovenous malformation (AVM; metameric/juvenile AVM or type III spinal AVM). (A) Schematic illustration shows involvement of all derivatives of the metamere (i.e., skin, muscle, bone, dura, and cord). The blood supply involves branches of segmental arteries. (B–H) A 42-year-old man presented with neck pain, headaches, and recurrent cerebrospinal fluid rhinorrhea associated with a metameric AVM. Arterial (B) and venous (C) phase vertebral artery angiograms show extensive vascularity with early venous drainage (*arrows*) of the spinal cord, dura, soft tissue, and vertebral body at the craniocervical junction. (D) Superselective placement of a microcatheter into the anterior spinal artery (*arrow*). (E) Anterior spinal artery angiogram shows AVM of the spinal cord at the craniocervical junction with caudal drainage into the anterior median vein (*arrow*) and apical drainage through the anterior median medullary vein (*double arrows*) into the median anterior pontine vein (*short arrow*), and through the transverse pontine vein (*curved arrow*) into the superior petrosal vein (*arrowhead*). (F) Embolization of the spinal cord supply through the anterior spinal artery with *N*-butyl cyanoacrylate cast of the AVM nidus (*arrows*). (G) Control axial computed tomographic scan shows the acrylate cast adjacent to the dens (*arrow*) and delineates the dysplastic appearance of the left occipital condyle, the atlanto-occipital joint, and both lateral masses of the atlas associated with the AVM. (H) Left vertebral artery control angiograms in frontal and lateral projections after multiple staged embolizations through C1 muscular branch (*curved arrow*), the thyrocervical artery (not shown), and anterior spinal artery show an extensive devascularization of the malformation. (A, Courtesy R.F. Spetzler.)

estimated that SAMS accounts for approximately 6% to 19% of all spinal cord AVM cases.[11,92]

Imaging

MRI and MRA or three-dimensional CT enhanced with contrast medium reveals a large vascular mass involving the spinal cord. CT might show scalloping of posterior vertebral elements and widening of the interpedicular space. The AVM nidus will have an extradural and intradural extension. The spinal cord can be enlarged with heterogeneous signal on T1 weighting and hyperintense on T2 weighting corresponding to ischemia, edema, or gliosis. Old blood products can easily be depicted on T2-weighted, gradient-recalled echo sequences. Aortography and selective spinal angiography depict huge vertebral, paravertebral, spinal, and visceral angiomas. Differential diagnoses include intramedullary neoplasms, medullary AVMs, and some perimedullary AVMs.

Treatment

Because of the complex nature of the malformation, their management remains in the format of case reports even to date.[93] A combined endovascular and surgical approach is recommended.[10] In some patients, however, we have been successful with staged endovascular acrylate embolization, achieving curative results (see Fig. 93.15). The subgroup of SAMS with exclusively extradural AVMs can also achieve good treatment outcomes compared with SAMS with intra- and extradural extension.[91]

Intramedullary Arteriovenous Malformations

Also known as type II or classic spinal cord AVM, intramedullary AVMs are the second most common type of spinal vascular malformation, accounting for approximately 20% to 30% of all spinal vascular shunts. The angioarchitecture of these lesions is similar to that of the classic brain AVM, with multiple arterial feeders, a nidus located within the cord parenchyma, and draining veins. The nidus can be compact, known as glomus type, or diffuse, known as the plexiform or juvenile type, the latter of which should not be confused with the metameric type of AVM. The arterial feeders are usually multiple branches of the ventral spinal axis (ASA) and/or dorsolateral pial network (PSA). Medullary AVMs can be high flow, high pressure, and low resistance.[10] These lesions also tend to exhibit both nidal and feeding artery aneurysms.

In their most recently proposed classification, Spetzler and associates subdivided these lesions into those with a compact, glomus-type nidus and those with a diffuse nidus.[10] The natural history is difficult to ascertain, but the majority of patients present before the age of 40 years.[73] The most common presentation is an acute myelopathy due to intramedullary hemorrhage and/or SAH.[10,73] A proportion of patients present with intermittent or progressive myelopathy with deterioration of limb function or bowel and bladder function. The progressive myelopathy can be due to vascular steal, venous hypertension, or venous compression.[10] Pain can also be a common presenting symptom in these patients. If left untreated, patients can be expected to experience an episodic but progressive deterioration due to repetitive bleeding.[10] In one 8-year study of 60 patients, 36% of patients younger than 41 years and 48% of patients aged 41 to 61 years were wheelchair-bound within 3 years of diagnosis.[94] Based on Djindjian's original series of 150 patients, 13% of patients at the 5-year follow-up, 20% of patients at the 10-year follow-up, and 57% of patients at the 20-year follow-up had experienced clinical deterioration.[95]

A recent publication also aimed to describe the clinical features, outcome after treatment, and natural history of nidus-type II versus type IV spinal AV shunts (fistulous), suggesting that progression of clinical presentation from hemorrhage to congestive myelopathy during follow-up after treatment was noted predominantly in those patients who had AVMs of the nidus type. Complete obliteration could be achieved more often in the fistulous type than in the nidus type. Overall, these entities appear to demonstrate different clinical features and obliteration rates, which may affect their long-term prognosis.[96]

Imaging

Similar to brain AVM, spinal cord AVM appears on MRI as a conglomerate of dilated, perimedullary and intramedullary located vessels that are shown on T2-weighted sequences as flow voids and on T1-weighted images, depending on their flow velocity and direction, as mixed hyperintense/hypointense tubular structures. A venous congestive edema within the spinal cord with concomitant swelling of the cord may be present on T2-weighted images. Intraparenchymal hemorrhage and subarachnoid hemorrhage may appear as hyperintense spinal cord signal on T2 weighting, representing ischemia, edema, or gliosis.[97] Selective spinal angiography is necessary to define the exact type of AVM and to plan subsequent treatment (Fig. 93.16).

Treatment

Reports of embolization of intramedullary AVMs are rare.[98] Biondi et al. reported a total of 35 patients with thoracic AVMs who underwent a total of 158 PVA embolizations.[98] Although clinical improvement was reported in 63% of patients, recanalization was frequently observed due to the embolic agent used. Twenty percent of patients also were reported to demonstrate neurologic decline following embolization (seven of the 35 patients). Despite this, the endovascular approach is the treatment of choice, because a surgical resection is difficult to achieve and has a high intraprocedural risk, especially if the lesion lies on or within the ventral portion of the spinal cord.[98,99] Part of the difficulty of the surgical approach to treating these AVMs is the intramedullary location and the blood supply via tiny perforators arising from sulcocommissural branches or PSA. On the other hand, a staged endovascular occlusion of the proximal draining vein with NBCA as a more permanent embolic agent may be curative (see Fig. 93.16).[100] PVA has been described as safer for palliative embolization to obtain a temporary symptomatic effect, but it may not provide a permanent cure, as stated earlier.[98,101,102] Other embolic liquid agents, such as Onyx, have been utilized; reported preliminary evidence suggests that Onyx may be more effective than particles.[103] If a surgical resection is planned, embolization before surgery may be helpful.

Alternative treatments include radiosurgery and stereotactic radiosurgery. The latter appears to provide an effective and safe alternative treatment option to conventional radiation therapy, although the literature remains limited.[104,105]

Spinal Artery Aneurysms

Aneurysms of the spinal arteries are extremely rare. In more than 3000 spinal angiograms reviewed by Djindjian, only one isolated aneurysm was found.[106] No clear predilection site appears to exist for spinal aneurysms at any specific segment of the spinal artery.[107] Contrary to intracranial aneurysms, the location of spinal artery aneurysms is often unrelated to arterial branching sites. SAH of spinal origin is a rare event and accounts for less than 1% of all cases reported in the literature. Because of spontaneous obliteration of the aneurysm, the spinal angiography may remain negative.[107]

Imaging

Spinal artery aneurysms are rare, because significant experience with MRI exists. Single case reports have depicted SAH and associated aneurysm on contrast medium–enhanced T1 and T2 weighting as a focal lesion. A spontaneous thrombosis and aneurysm regression may be demonstrated on follow-up MR studies.[107]

Treatment

Because many of the reported spinal aneurysms have a fusiform rather than a saccular shape, standard surgical treatment using clips is often not possible. Endovascular treatment with fibrin glue may be achieved.[107] However, because of the limited experience with these aneurysms, and given that they may spontaneously occlude, a wait-and-see strategy appears justified and may be more adequate than emergency surgical or endovascular intervention.[107]

Neoplastic Vascular Lesions

Cavernous Malformations

Spinal cord cavernous malformations are uncommon vascular lesions that occur more frequently in females than in males, with a mean age of 36.4 years at diagnosis.[108] Cavernoma or cavernous angioma is a well-circumscribed, blue-reddish (mulberry-like) nodule. Microscopically, it is composed of dilated capillaries consisting of a simple endothelial layer with thin fibrous adventitia. Typically, there is no neural parenchyma centrally and the lesion is surrounded by a variable degree of gliosis and a pseudocapsule.[109] Within the lesion, there is often evidence for hyalinization, thrombosis in various stages of organization, calcification, cholesterol crystals, and

FIG. 93.16 Intramedullary arteriovenous malformation (AVM; type II spinal AVM). (A) Schematic illustration: *1*, radiculopial artery; *2*, AVM nidus; *3*, arterialized and ectatic posterior median vein. (B–F) A 21-year-old, otherwise healthy man presented with acute headaches and neck pain. (B) Computed tomography scan confirmed an extensive hemorrhage (*arrows*). Sagittal T1-weighted and axial T2-weighted magnetic resonance images show extensive intramedullary flow voids at the craniocervical junction. (C) Left vertebral artery angiogram in lateral and frontal projections shows an AVM nidus (*arrows*) and early drainage into the lateral pontine vein (*arrowheads*).

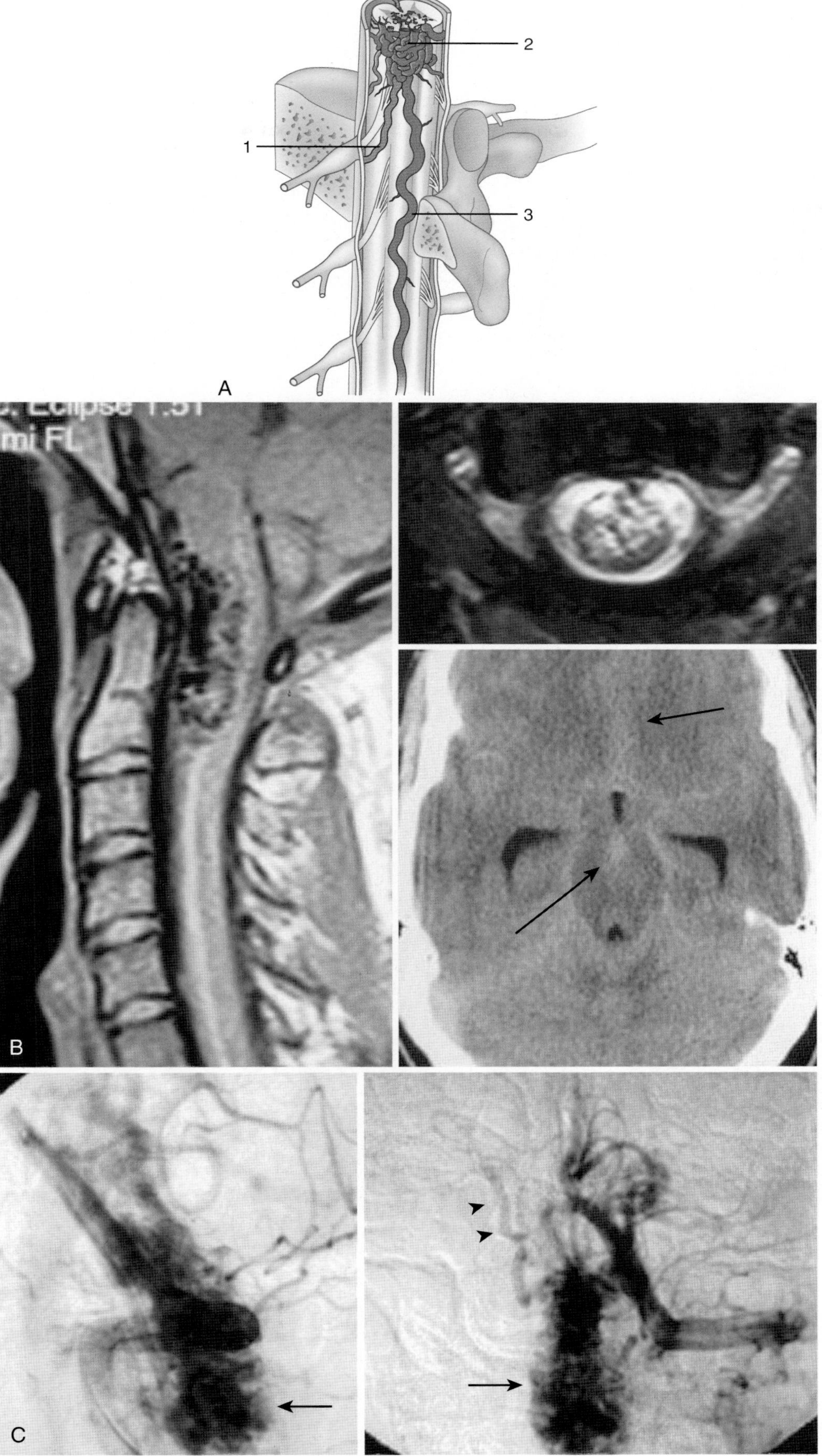

Continued

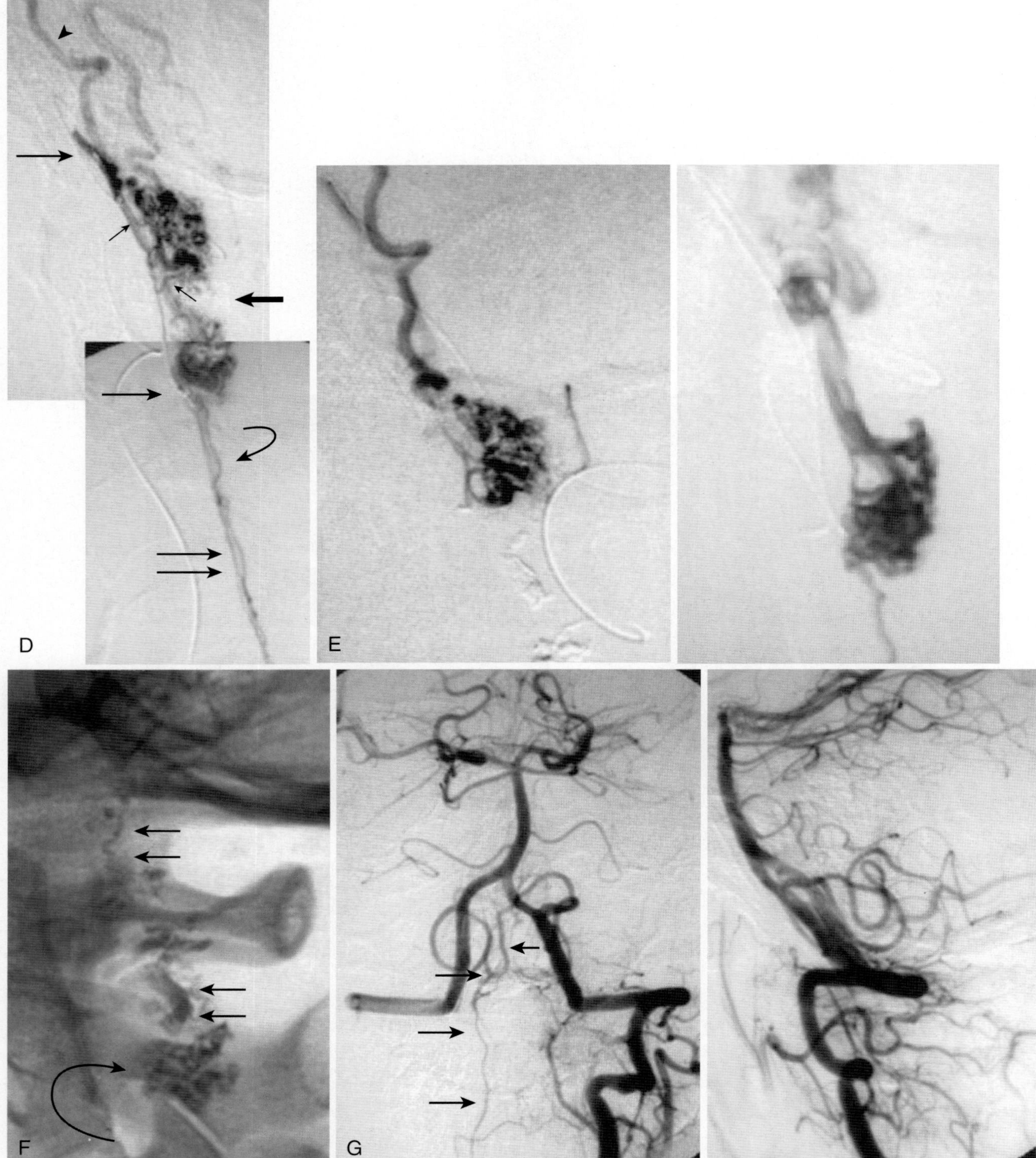

FIG. 93.16, cont'd (D) Microcatheterization of the anterior spinal artery and contrast medium injection at different levels (*arrows,* photomontage of two levels) after partial embolization (*large arrow*) delineate the detailed architecture of the glomus-shaped malformation supplied through sulcocommissural arteries (*small arrows*). Note the close relationship between the straight anterior spinal artery (*double arrows*) and the ectatic and elongated anterior median vein (*curved arrow*). (E–F) Superselective angiograms through sulcocommissural arteries of two different AVM compartments and staged *N*-butyl cyanoacrylate embolization with intranidal acrylate cast (*curved arrow*) and penetration of AVM draining veins (*double arrows*). (G) Left vertebral artery follow-up angiograms 6 months after complete obliteration show mild displacement of the patent anterior spinal artery (*arrows*) associated with the intramedullary AVM mass.

cysts.[110] The clinical course is variable, ranging from slowly progressive symptoms caused by a small hemorrhage or progressive symptoms due to repeated bleeding or mass effect due to capillary proliferation and vessel dilatation. Diagnosis is made by typical findings on MRI, whereas angiography is negative. Thus, cavernomas are often called angiographically occult vascular malformations.

Imaging

Cavernomas of the spine have a characteristic appearance on MRI, resembling those of the brain. They appear as well-defined lesions, with a hypointense rim on T2- or proton density–weighted images and often a hyperintense center on T2-weighted images. The hypointense rim is due to magnetic susceptibility artifacts from hemosiderin deposits.[97,111] The complex reticulated core with its typical mulberry-like appearance represents hemorrhage in different stages of evolution. T2-weighted gradient recalled echo images will show intense blooming due to susceptibility effects. Enhancement after instillation of a contrast agent may be present.

Treatment

Currently, there is no role for an endovascular approach. A conservative approach or surgical resection has been proposed. The noncapsulated lesions are well circumscribed and present a clear surface plane for dissection.

Hemangioblastoma

A hemangioblastoma is a true neoplasm of blood vessels, usually benign. It can arise either spontaneously or can be associated with von Hippel-Lindau syndrome.[112] In the spinal cord, hemangioblastomas constitute 3.3% of all intramedullary tumors and most commonly present in the fourth decade.[113] Up to 30% of patients with spinal cord hemangioblastomas have von Hippel-Lindau syndrome. The majority of spinal hemangioblastomas (79%) are singular. The thoracic cord is the most common site, followed by the cervical cord.[113]

Imaging

Because these tumors are typically quite vascular, serpentine areas of signal void may be seen that represent feeding arteries or draining veins associated with the tumor nidus. The administration of paramagnetic contrast agent dramatically improves visualization of the tumor nidus, often allowing its differentiation from the adjacent edematous spinal cord. Diagnostic angiography shows a hypervascular mass supplied by medullary arterial feeders. In the case of high blood flow velocity, they may resemble AVMs of the cord. However, unlike in spinal AVMs, there is no direct arteriovenous shunting and no individual vessels within the lesion that would be characteristic of a nidus (Fig. 93.17).

Treatment

A preoperative embolization significantly reduces the risk of a surgical resection (see Fig. 93.17).[114,115]

Systemic Syndromes Associated With Spinal Vascular Malformations

Osler-Weber-Rendu Syndrome (Hereditary Hemorrhagic Telangiectasia)

This autosomal-dominant syndrome consists of two genotypes (types 1 and 2). Type 1 is associated with mucocutaneous telangiectasia, pulmonary AVF, and AVSs of the central nervous system. The associated spinal AVSs are most often seen in the pediatric population and are always pial AVF (subtype C, ventral intradural AVF, or type IV). The endothelial cells in this syndrome lack the molecule endoglin and form abnormal vessels, especially after injury.[11]

Cobb Syndrome

This is the synonym for the complete manifestation of the metameric type of spinal vascular malformation (see also extradural/intradural AVM).[116]

Klippel-Trenaunay and Parkes-Weber Syndromes

These syndromes consist of vascular malformations involving primarily the lower limbs, with the following dominant features: cutaneous capillary malformation, varicose veins, and limb hypertrophy. Klippel-Trenaunay syndrome is composed mainly of venous anomalies; Parkes-Weber syndrome has more AVSs.[116] A spinal cord involvement with pial AVF or AVM can be present.

Treatment

Staged embolization and surgical resection, if feasible, is recommended.

Capillary Malformation–Arteriovenous Malformation Syndrome With Spinal Involvement

Capillary malformation–arteriovenous malformation (CM-AVM) is a recently identified autosomal-dominant disorder in which arteriovenous lesions have been reported in the brain, limbs, and face. Only half a dozen patients with CM-AVM and spinal AVSs have been described.[117] It has been suggested that some patients with AVSs of the neural axis, previously diagnosed as Cobb syndrome and hereditary hemorrhagic telangiectasia, might have CM-AVM syndrome.[118]

Treatment

Staged embolization and surgical resection, if feasible, is recommended.

Miscellaneous Vascular Lesions of the Vertebrae

Vertebral Hemangiomas

Vertebral hemangiomas are benign vascular malformations of the bone, with a well-known and well-described appearance on conventional radiography, CT, and MRI. The incidence

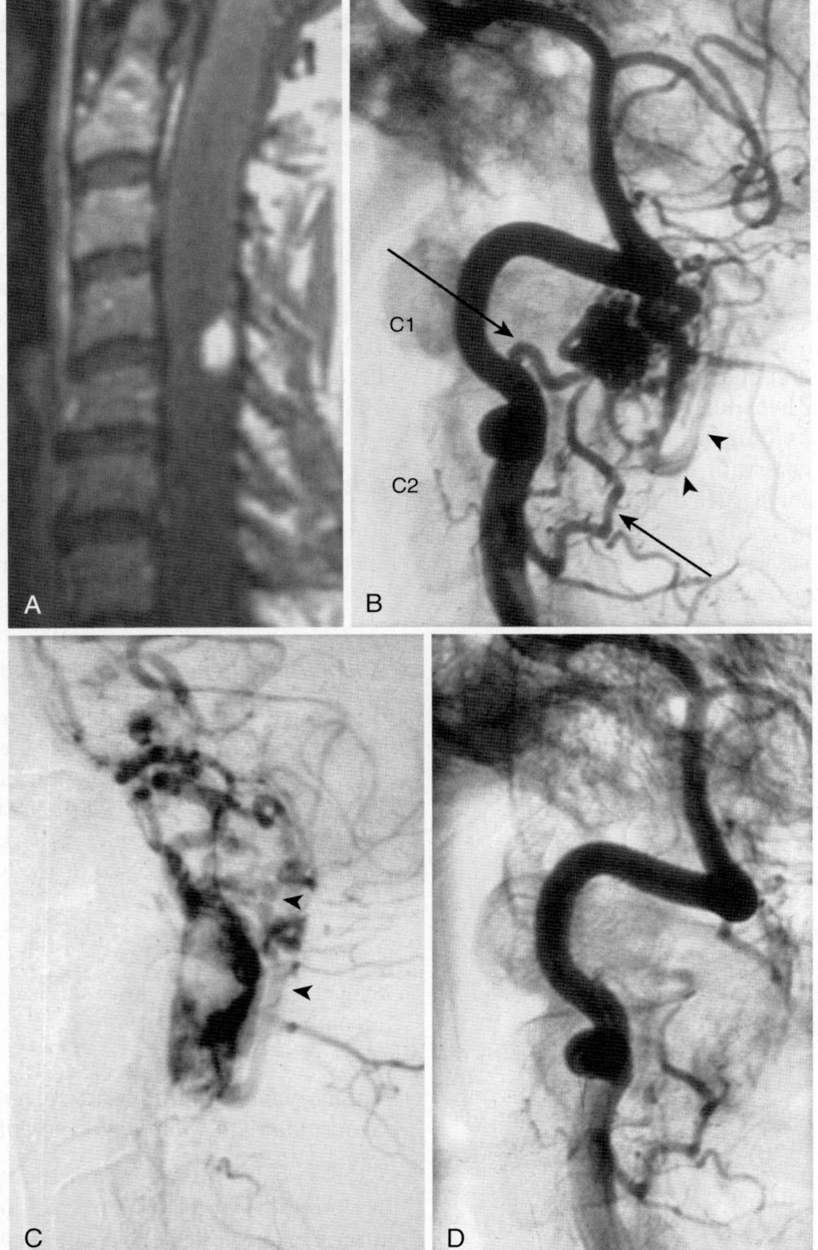

FIG. 93.17 (A) Sagittal T1-weighted magnetic resonance image after contrast medium instillation shows homogeneous enhancement of a dorsally located hemangioblastoma with spinal cord swelling. (B) Arterial and (C) capillary phases of vertebral angiography of a recurrent craniocervical hemangioblastoma show the extensive blood supply to the tumor (different patient than in A) through C1 and C2 muscular branches (*arrows*) and early drainage via dilated posterior median veins into the cranium (*arrowheads*). (D) Control angiography after extensive devascularization using microcatheter technique and polyvinyl alcohol particles.

of hemangiomas is variable, depending on age, but has been reported at around 11% with increasing age. Up to 30% of patients have multiple lesions. Pathologically, they are considered to be postcapillary vascular dysembryogenetic malformations. Microscopically, they are divided into capillary, cavernous, and mixed types.[119,120] Most of these lesions are asymptomatic and are incidental findings on MRI. Less than 1% of hemangiomas become symptomatic.[119] They may present as neurologic symptoms associated with cord compression or radiculopathy. A complete involvement of the vertebral body, including the body, pedicles, and laminae, is present in up to 65% of cases. A smaller number of patients show a partial body and pedicle/posterior element involvement (23.2%), and 11.8% have involvement of the body only. There is a female predominance (3 : 1), and young affected adults often present with cord compression and/or radiculopathy. Most of the lesions are in the thoracic spine (>70%).[119–121] Fox and coworkers noted that neck or back pain often preceded the neurologic symptoms, and thoracic myelopathy was the most common neurologic presentation.[120] An additional known risk factor for development of neurologic symptoms is pregnancy, with symptoms developing in the third trimester, possibly owing to the role of estrogen and/or increased venous pressure from abdominal distention and pressure of the growing uterus on the venous structures.[120] The mechanism for cord compression can be epidural extension of the lesion from the bone into the spinal canal, expansion of the bony vertebra by the hemangioma, a pathologic fracture of the vertebra, epidural hematoma from bleeding from the lesion, or compression by enlarged feeding arteries or draining veins.[120] Djindjian and coworkers characterized vertebral hemangiomas into three groups (types A, B, and C) based on clinical and imaging characteristics.[116]

Imaging

The lesions are commonly seen incidentally on imaging studies, particularly on MRI. On T1-weighted images, they present as increased signal intensity because of adipose tissue interspersed among the bone trabeculae.[122] An intense contrast medium enhancement is seen in the frequently mottled-appearing vertebral body. Extraosseous components, which contain only small amounts of adipose tissue, often display a lower signal on T1-weighted images. On T2-weighted images, both intraosseous and extraosseous components present increased signal intensity, which may be difficult to differentiate from metastasis. Pathologic fracture may be present.

Type A

These lesions present as signs and symptoms of cord compression. Imaging shows an extraosseous extension of the lesion, usually related to an insufficiency fracture associated with the lesion weakening the vertebral body (Fig. 93.18). Angiography shows dense opacification of the vertebral body via enlarged somatic branches of a normal-sized intercostal/segmental artery. The appearance of the lesion in the vertebral body is described as dense "pools" of contrast agent appearing in the midarterial phase and persisting into the venous phase.

Treatment

The usual treatment for these lesions consists of a preoperative embolization of the lesion with PVA particles and/or NBCA infusion directly into the hemangioma and operative decompression of the spinal cord/canal, possibly with a resection of the lesion and spinal reconstruction and stabilization. Doppman and colleagues made the important observation that even in these lesions with epidural extension, the lesion does not penetrate the dura but is confined by the periosteum, which results in the characteristic bilobed posterior margin of these lesions, indented centrally by the posterior longitudinal ligament.[119] Additional treatment options for these patients for whom timely treatment is a medical necessity is the technique of percutaneous transpedicular injection of ethanol.[120] With current CT or MRI technology, a percutaneous approach through the pedicle can be accomplished. The tip of the needle is usually positioned at the vertebropedicular junction. Contrast medium–enhanced CT or MRI may be helpful for the intervention. After needle placement, contrast agent is injected to show the opacification of the lesion. Subsequently, dehydrated ethanol opacified with metrizamide powder is forcefully injected. Anesthesia is recommended because of the pain associated with ethanol injection. For lower thoracic and upper lumbar lesions, the AKA has to be delineated on arterial angiograms before an intervention to prevent inadvertent cord ischemia. An improvement of symptoms can be seen within 1 to 2 days after the treatment. Follow-up MRI shows the shrinkage of lesions.

Type B

These lesions are associated with local pain and tenderness over the involved vertebral body and/or radicular signs. Imaging does not reveal any extraosseous extension. The angiographic appearance is similar to type A lesions, which are generally large. The first step in the evaluation of these lesions is to exclude the more common causes of back pain with the help of imaging and physical examination.[120] Imaging further helps to exclude involvement of the posterior element, cortical disruption, and epidural spread of the lesion. In the absence of these findings, percutaneous vertebroplasty with polymethyl methacrylate (PMMA) is the treatment of choice. Other treatment options include the endovascular transarterial embolization of the lesion using particles or NBCA or ethanol. Embolization can be effective in as high as 60% to 100% of patients treated.[120] Reizine and associates suggested that if a painful lesion is located in the cervical or lumbar spine without involvement of the posterior elements or cortical disruption, these lesions could be considered as nonevolutive (without potential for future growth causing cord compression).[123] On the other hand, if a painful lesion is located in the thoracic spine, especially in a young patient, and shows involvement of the posterior elements, cortical disruption, or soft tissue extension, it should be considered for potential growth and future cord compression.

Type C

These lesions represent the vast majority of hemangiomas, which are incidental findings and not associated with any symptoms. The angiogram shows only normal vertebral body enhancement.[73] Unless the patient develops symptoms (i.e., pain and/or neurologic deficits), follow-up imaging or additional studies are not necessary.[120] An exception can be made for very large lesions in a young patient, with the chance of further growth. A yearly follow-up may be considered, but no treatment is needed unless symptoms develop.

Aneurysmal Bone Cysts

Aneurysmal bone cysts are benign lesions of bones that primarily affect young people; 80% of patients present when younger than the age of 20 years. There is no sex predilection. Although aneurysmal bone cysts can occur at any location, 90% are seen in the spine. Within the spine, most lesions

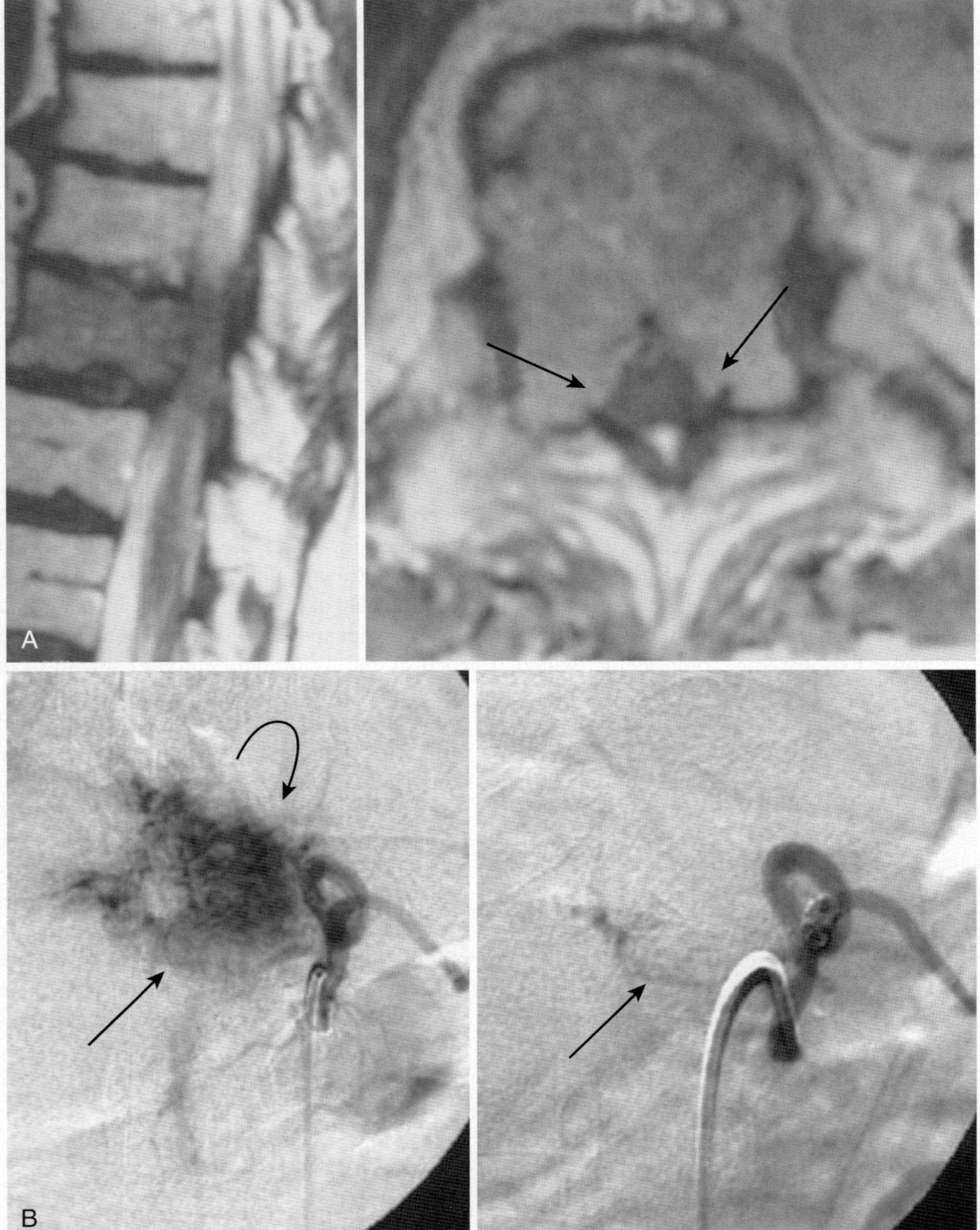

FIG. 93.18 (A) Fast spin-echo T2-weighted magnetic resonance image shows a thoracic vertebral body hemangioma with narrowing of the spinal canal. Axial contrast T1-weighted image shows enhancing extraosseous epidural extension of the hemangioma with cord compression (*arrows*). (B) Left intercostal artery angiogram shows hypervascularity of the vertebral body (*curved arrow*) with blood supply through multiple somatic branches (*arrows*). Control angiogram after particle embolization shows extensive devascularization of the hemangioma. (From Shaibani A, Wakhloo AK. Endovascular therapy of the spine. In: Mathis JM, ed. *Image-Guided Spine Interventions*. New York: Springer-Verlag; 2004.)

involve the posterior elements; however, the vertebral body can also be involved. Additionally, aneurysmal bone cysts can involve two contiguous vertebral bodies.[106] With regard to pathogenesis, most authors believe that a hemodynamic imbalance or abnormality within the bone is the etiologic factor, especially with regard to impaired venous drainage.[124,125] Some have suggested the presence of a congenital vascular abnormality in cases of de novo aneurysmal bone cysts and an impairment of venous drainage by a secondary factor (associated lesions or trauma) in other cases.[126]

Imaging

The radiographic appearance of aneurysmal bone cysts is characteristic (Fig. 93.19). Pathologically, the lesions consist of enlarged, septated, but communicating spaces within the bone, containing venous blood under higher than normal

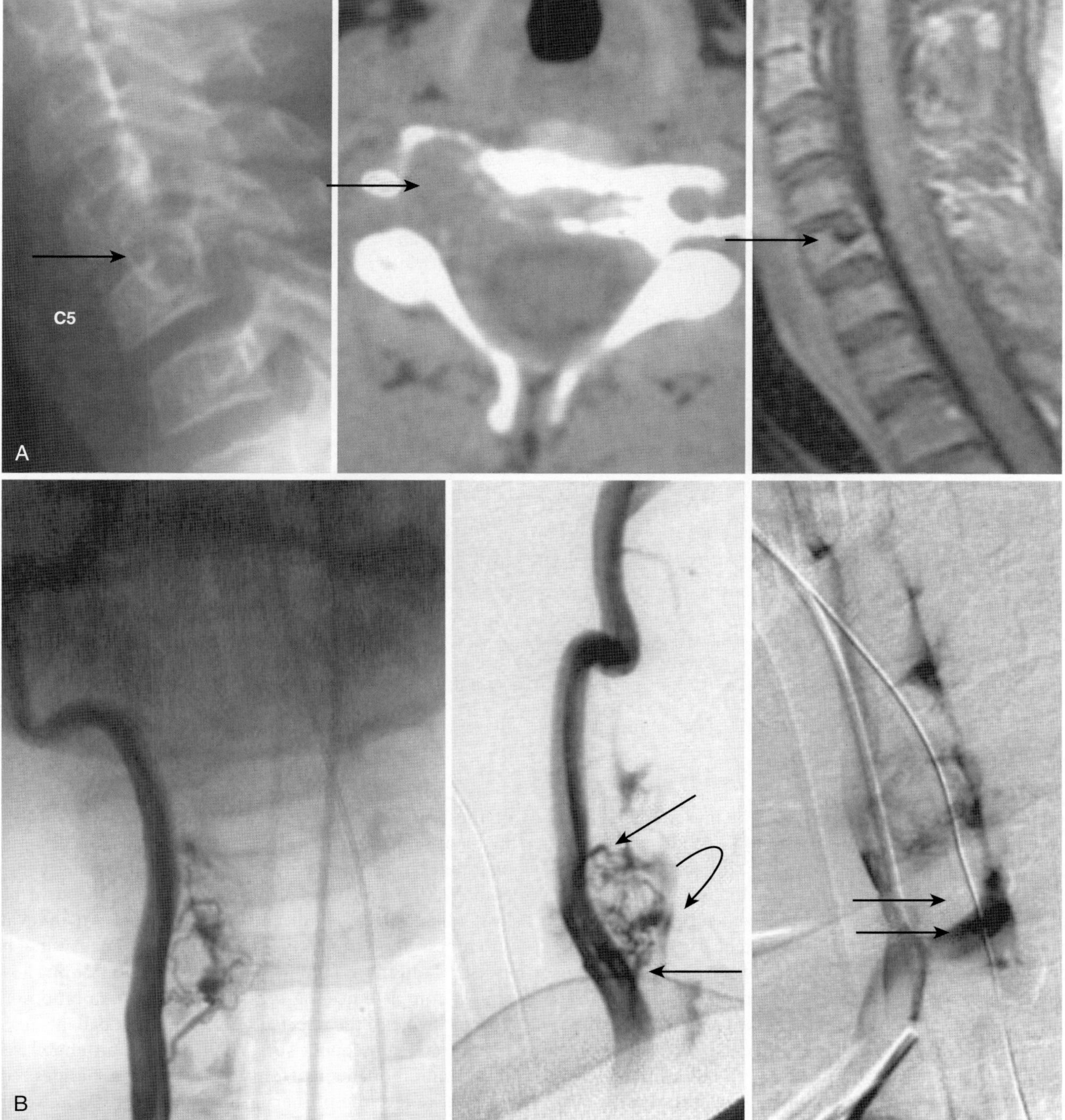

FIG. 93.19 An 11-year-old boy presented with intractable neck pain associated with an aneurysmal bone cyst. (A) Plain lateral spine radiograph, axial computed tomographic scan, and T1-weighted magnetic resonance image show the typically well-defined and calcified lesion within the C5 vertebral body (*arrows*). Note widening of the transverse foramen and a thinning of the spinal nerve sulcus and the anterior tuberculum. (B) Right vertebral artery angiograms in frontal and lateral projection (arterial and venous phase) show multiple enlarged somatic branches originating from two major radicular arteries (*arrows*). Note persistent filling of a hypervascular area with patchy collection of contrast material (*curved arrow*) and delayed washout into the epidural venous plexus (*double arrows*).

Continued

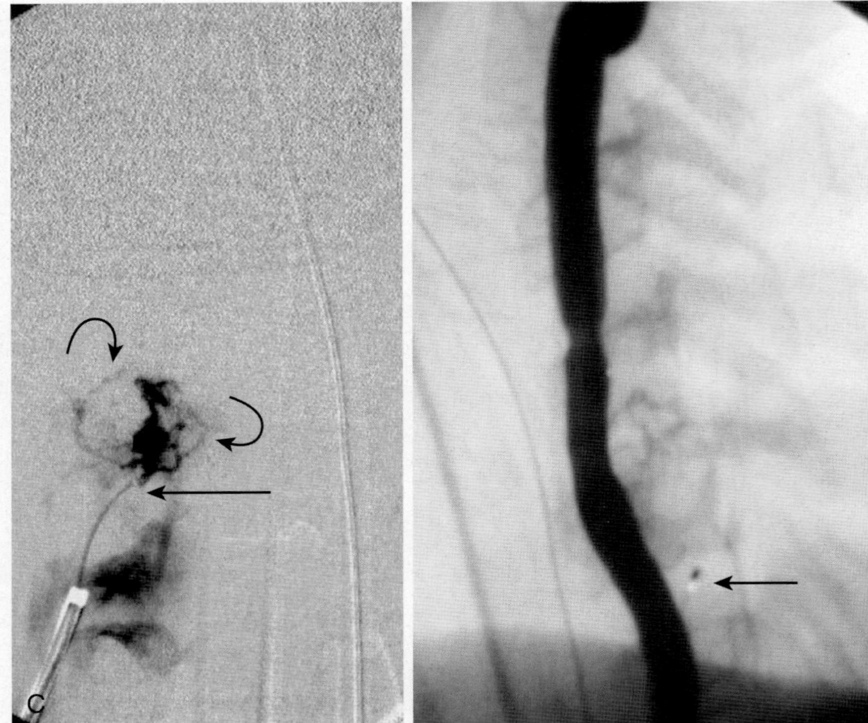

FIG. 93.19, cont'd (C) Superselective catheterization of the proximal radicular artery (*arrow*) and filling of multiple somatic branches (*curved arrows*). Polyvinyl alcohol particle embolization and subsequent control angiography of vertebral artery shows a near-complete devascularization; microcatheter is still in the radicular artery (*arrow at right*). Note mild vasospasm of vertebral artery related to a balloon test occlusion before embolization. (From Shaibani A, Wakhloo AK. Endovascular therapy of the spine. In: Mathis JM, ed. *Image-Guided Spine Interventions*. New York: Springer-Verlag; 2004.)

venous pressure. Fluid/fluid levels may be present on T1- and T2-weighted images resulting from blood products. Because of a rim of periosteum, a hypointense rim around the mass may be seen. The expansile remodeling of the vertebral body and the thinned cortex with absent tumor matrix can be appreciated very well. CT is excellent for finalizing the diagnosis. The lining of the spaces consists of a fibro-osseous patchwork and some giant cells.[106] Other differential diagnoses include osteoblastoma, metastases, and telangiectatic osteogenic sarcoma. Interestingly, up to one-third of aneurysmal bone cysts are found in conjunction with other lesions, such as fibrous dysplasia, osteoblastoma, or chondrosarcoma,[126] whereas others may be associated with previous trauma.[125] Angiographically, there is no pathognomonic pattern for aneurysmal bone cysts (see Fig. 93.19). Findings can vary from a faint or moderate vascularity to a dense vascularity with a rich network of dilated, tortuous feeding vessels and a dense stain of the lesion within the vertebral body.[106] Djindjian described arteriovenous shunting in some lesions, whereas others have described patchy collections of contrast agent within the cystic spaces, persisting into the late venous phase.[127]

Treatment

The most common approach to symptomatic aneurysmal bone cysts is surgery, whether with curettage or with resection of the lesion and reconstruction of the spine, if necessary. In many cases, owing to the vascularity of the lesion, the operating surgeon will request a preoperative angiography and embolization of the lesion to decrease intraoperative blood loss, which can be significant (see Fig. 93.19). An endovascular embolization can be the sole therapy for aneurysmal bone cysts.[128] Long-term follow-up data after embolization show an almost complete healing of the lesion and restoration of the normal shape of the affected bone. Thus, the patient may not require any subsequent surgery. If present, an endovascular embolization of an aneurysmal bone cyst can, besides reduce the size, relieve the primary pain symptom.[129] More recently, percutaneous injection of PMMA under fluoroscopic guidance has been advocated for cure. Resection of the lesion and resection of the spine is the treatment of choice when the lesion is symptomatic and if interventional treatment is not considered. In many cases, to decrease intraoperative blood loss, preoperative angiography and embolization may be necessary.

Spinal Metastasis

Neoplastic and metastatic lesions can involve the vertebral bodies as well as intramedullary and extramedullary structures. The goal of an endovascular treatment remains a devascularization before a planned surgery or biopsy (Fig. 93.20).

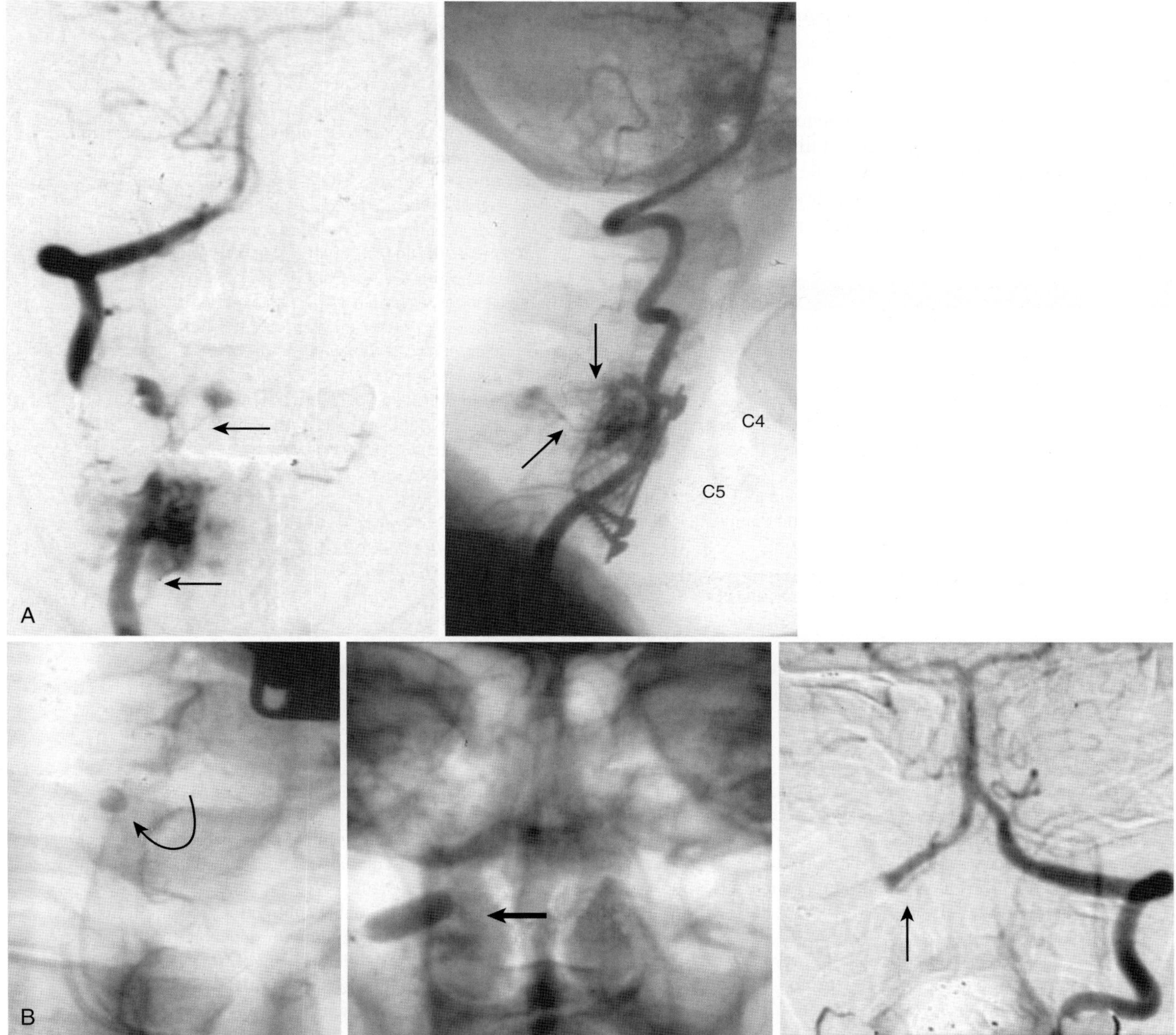

FIG. 93.20 Metastatic recurrence of a thyroid cancer after previous surgery and anterior stabilization. (A) Right vertebral artery angiograms in frontal and lateral projections show hypervascular lesion of C4 and C5 vertebral bodies supplied through multiple enlarged somatic branches (*arrows*). (B) Before planned preoperative embolization (not shown), a balloon test occlusion is carried out with a nondetachable balloon (*curved arrow*) followed by a permanent vertebral artery occlusion with a detachable balloon (*thick arrow*). Note excellent filling of the posterior circulation and the right intradural vertebral artery through the contralateral side. To minimize the dead space and prevent distal emboli, the balloon is placed just proximal to the origin of the right posterior inferior cerebellar artery (*thin arrow*).

This significantly reduces blood loss and improves the surgical resection.[130–133] Because the embolization is performed using Gelfoam, PVA, or occasionally dehydrated ethanol, attention has to be paid to a potential supply of radiculomedullary/pial arteries to the ASA or PSA. An embolization can, rarely, lead to tumor necrosis with subsequent swelling and spinal cord compression; a preprocedural high-dose corticosteroid medication has been suggested.[134] On rare occasions and in nonsurgical patients, embolization helps to reduce pain and to treat radicular compression.[135] Although a reduction of tumor growth may be seen, embolization for spinal metastasis and malignant spinal tumors is not curative.

Imaging

Metastases can present as a variety of different signal characteristics on MRI. Blastic metastases can appear hypointense on T1- and T2-weighted images if they are sclerotic. Lesions may uptake contrast agent depending on the amount of sclerosis. Lytic metastases may be hypointense on T1 and T2 weighting but enhance diffusely.

Treatment

An endovascular or direct percutaneous embolization of a vertebral body metastasis or malignant tumor can be achieved. The latter can be performed under CT or fluoroscopic guidance using NBCA,[136] PMMA, or dehydrated ethanol.[137,138] Use of PMMA can also provide biomechanical stability of the vertebral body.[139]

PEARLS

1. The hairpin-shaped junction between the radiculomedullary artery and the ASA has a larger radius than the one between the radiculopial artery and the PSA.
2. Owing to a generally singular large blood supply of the ASA through the AKA, the ventral spinal cord is more susceptible to ischemia than the dorsal part, which has an extensive collateral blood supply.
3. Because brain dural malformations may drain into the spinal canal, a cerebral angiography completes the diagnostic evaluation for a spinal vascular malformation.

PITFALLS

1. A spinal dural malformation can mimic a transverse myelitis.
2. Negative cerebral angiography in SAH may miss a spinal AVM or an aneurysm of the ASA.
3. Normal vertebral body vascularity can infrequently appear as a hypervascular metastatic lesion.

KEY POINTS

1. The hairpin-shaped junction between the radiculomedullary artery and the ASA has a larger radius than the one between the radiculopial artery and the PSA.
2. Owing to a generally singular large blood supply of the ASA through the AKA, the ventral spinal cord is more susceptible to ischemia than the dorsal part, which has an extensive collateral blood supply.
3. Because an intracranial dural fistula may drain into the spinal canal, a cerebral angiography completes the diagnostic evaluation for a spinal vascular malformation.
4. Ischemic changes of the spinal cord associated with a spinal dural fistula can mimic a transverse myelitis, a spinal cord tumor, or an ischemia related to a cord compression due to a disc herniation.
5. Negative cerebral angiography in SAH may miss a spinal AVM or an aneurysm of the ASA.
6. Normal vertebral body vascularity can infrequently appear as a hypervascular metastatic lesion.

KEY REFERENCES

1. Berenstein A, Lasjaunias P. *Surgical Neuro-angiography, Vol 5: Endovascular Treatment of Spine and Spinal Cord Lesions*. - New York: Springer-Verlag; 1992:125-127.
   The authors summarize the endovascular approach to spinal vascular disorders.
2. Biondi A, Merland JJ, Hodes JE, et al. Aneurysms of spinal arteries associated with intramedullary arteriovenous malformations: II. Results of AVM endovascular treatment and hemodynamic consideration. *AJNR Am J Neuroradiol*. 1992;13:923-931.
   This article is a summary of a vast experience in endovascular treatment of spinal AVMs.
3. Djindjian R. Clinical symptomatology and natural history of arteriovenous malformations of the spinal cord: a study of the clinical aspects and prognosis based on 150 cases. In: Pia H, Djindjian R, eds. *Spinal Angiomas: Advances in Diagnosis and Therapy*. Berlin: Springer-Verlag; 1978.
   This is an excellent summary of spinal AVMs from one of the pioneers in this field.
4. Lasjaunias P, Berenstein A, Ter Brugge KG. *Surgical Neuroangiography*. 2nd ed. Berlin: Springer-Verlag; 2001.
   This is an excellent reference book for spinal vascular anatomy.
5. Merland JJ, Reizine D, Laurent A, et al. Embolization of spinal cord vascular lesions. In: Viñuela F, Halbach VV, Dion JE, eds. *Interventional Neuroradiology: Endovascular Therapy of the Central Nervous System*. New York: Raven Press; 1992:153-165.
   This chapter reflects the experience from one of the leading schools in endovascular treatment of the spine.
6. Saraf-Lavi E, Bowen BC, Quencer RM, et al. Detection of spinal dural arteriovenous fistulae with MR imaging and contrast-enhanced MR angiography: sensitivity, specificity, and prediction of vertebral level. *AJNR Am J Neuroradiol*. 2002;23:858-867.
   This paper shows the value of MRI in detecting spinal dural malformation, which is the most common vascular disorder of the spine and often a diagnostic dilemma.
7. Spetzler RF, Detwiler PW, Riina HA, et al. Modified classification of spinal cord vascular lesions. *J Neurosurg Spine*. 2002;96(suppl):145-156.
   This is an excellent update on the most recent proposed classification on spinal cord vascular disorders.

REFERENCES

1. Lasjaunias P, Berenstein A, terBrugge KG. *Surgical Neuroangiography, Vol 1: Clinical Vascular Anatomy and Variations*. 2nd ed. Berlin: Springer-Verlag; 2001.
2. Krauss WE. Vascular anatomy of the spinal cord. *Neurosurg Clin N Am*. 1999;10(1):9-15.
3. Hyodoh H, et al. Double-subtraction maximum intensity projection MR angiography for detecting the artery of Adamkiewicz and differentiating it from the drainage vein. *J Magn Reson Imaging*. 2007;26(2):359-365.
4. Nijenhuis RJ, et al. Magnetic resonance angiography and neuromonitoring to assess spinal cord blood supply in thoracic and thoracoabdominal aortic aneurysm surgery. *J Vasc Surg*. 2007;45(1):71-77.
5. Sheehy NP, Boyle GE, Meaney JFM. Normal anterior spinal arteries within the cervical region: high-spatial-resolution contrast-enhanced three-dimensional MR angiography. *Radiology*. 2005;236(2):637-641.
6. Bowen BC. MR angiography of spinal vascular disease: what about normal vessels? *AJNR Am J Neuroradiol*. 1999;20(10):1773-1774.
7. Farb RI, et al. Spinal dural arteriovenous fistula localization with a technique of first-pass gadolinium-enhanced MR angiography: initial experience. *Radiology*. 2002;222(3):843-850.
8. Binkert CA, Kollias SS, Valavanis A. Spinal cord vascular disease: characterization with fast three-dimensional contrast-enhanced MR angiography. *AJNR Am J Neuroradiol*. 1999;20(10):1785-1793.
9. Yoss RE. Vascular supply of the spinal cord: the production of vascular syndromes. *Med Bull (Ann Arbor)*. 1950;16(11):333-345.

10. Spetzler RF, et al. Modified classification of spinal cord vascular lesions. *J Neurosurg*. 2002;96(suppl 2):145-156.
11. Rodesch G, et al. Classification of spinal cord arteriovenous shunts: proposal for a reappraisal—the Bicêtre experience with 155 consecutive patients treated between 1981 and 1999. *Neurosurgery*. 2002;51(2):374-379.
12. Geibprasert S, et al. Dural arteriovenous shunts: a new classification of craniospinal epidural venous anatomical bases and clinical correlations. *Stroke*. 2008;39(10):2783-2794.
13. da Costa L, Dehdashti AR, terBrugge KG. Spinal cord vascular shunts: spinal cord vascular malformations and dural arteriovenous fistulas. *Neurosurg Focus*. 2009;26(1):E6.
14. Germans MR, et al. Spinal vascular malformations in non-perimesencephalic subarachnoid hemorrhage. *J Neurol*. 2008;255(12):1910-1915.
15. Bou-Haidar P, Peduto AJ, Karunaratne N. Differential diagnosis of T2 hyperintense spinal cord lesions: part A. *J Med Imaging Radiat Oncol*. 2008;52(6):535-543.
16. Rodesch G, et al. Angio-architecture of spinal cord arteriovenous shunts at presentation. Clinical correlations in adults and children. The Bicetre experience on 155 consecutive patients seen between 1981-1999. *Acta Neurochir (Wien)*. 2004;146(3):217-226.
17. Prestigiacomo CJ, et al. Three-dimensional rotational spinal angiography in the evaluation and treatment of vascular malformations. *AJNR Am J Neuroradiol*. 2003;24(7):1429-1435.
18. Saraf-Lavi E, et al. Detection of spinal dural arteriovenous fistulae with MR imaging and contrast-enhanced MR angiography: sensitivity, specificity, and prediction of vertebral level. *AJNR Am J Neuroradiol*. 2002;23(5):858-867.
19. Mascalchi M, et al. Spinal vascular malformations: MR angiography after treatment. *Radiology*. 2001;219(2):346-353.
20. Luetmer PH, et al. Preangiographic evaluation of spinal dural arteriovenous fistulas with elliptic centric contrast-enhanced MR angiography and effect on radiation dose and volume of iodinated contrast material. *AJNR Am J Neuroradiol*. 2005;26(4):711-718.
21. Mull M, et al. Value and limitations of contrast-enhanced MR angiography in spinal arteriovenous malformations and dural arteriovenous fistulas. *AJNR Am J Neuroradiol*. 2007;28(7):1249-1258.
22. Condette-Auliac S, et al. MRI and MRA of spinal cord arteriovenous shunts. *J Magn Reson Imaging*. 2014;40(6):1253-1266.
23. Ali S, et al. Time-resolved spinal MR angiography: initial clinical experience in the evaluation of spinal arteriovenous shunts. *AJNR Am J Neuroradiol*. 2007;28(9):1806-1810.
24. Backes WH, Nijenhuis RJ. Advances in spinal cord MR angiography. *AJNR Am J Neuroradiol*. 2008;29(4):619-631.
25. Ou P, et al. CT angiography of the artery of Adamkiewicz with 64-section technology: first experience in children. *AJNR Am J Neuroradiol*. 2007;28(2):216-219.
26. Yamaguchi S, et al. Multi-detector-row CT angiography as a preoperative evaluation for spinal arteriovenous fistulae. *Neurosurg Rev*. 2007;30(4):321-326.
27. Wang H, et al. The diagnosis of arteriovenous malformations by 4D-CTA: a clinical study. *J Neuroradiol*. 2014;41(2):117-123.
28. Oda S, et al. Comparison of dynamic contrast-enhanced 3T MR and 64-row multidetector CT angiography for the localization of spinal dural arteriovenous fistulas. *AJNR Am J Neuroradiol*. 2014;35(2):407-412.
29. Cao JB, et al. Clinical application and diagnostic value of noninvasive spinal angiography in spinal vascular malformations. *J Comput Assist Tomogr*. 2014;38(3):474-479.
30. Pattany PM, Saraf-Lavi E, Bowen BC. MR angiography of the spine and spinal cord. *Top Magn Reson Imaging*. 2003;14(6):444-460.
31. Rodesch G, Lasjaunias P. Spinal cord arteriovenous shunts: from imaging to management. *Eur J Radiol*. 2003;46(3):221-232.
32. Chen CJ, et al. Small isolated paraspinal arteriovenous fistula. *AJNR Am J Neuroradiol*. 1997;18(2):359-361.
33. Cognard C, et al. Paraspinal arteriovenous fistula with perimedullary venous drainage. *AJNR Am J Neuroradiol*. 1995;16(10):2044-2048.
34. Goyal M, et al. Paravertebral arteriovenous malformations with epidural drainage: clinical spectrum, imaging features, and results of treatment. *AJNR Am J Neuroradiol*. 1999;20(5):749-755.
35. Han SS, Love MB, Simeone FA. Diagnosis and treatment of a lumbar extradural arteriovenous malformation. *AJNR Am J Neuroradiol*. 1987;8(6):1129-1130.
36. Martinez-Galdamez M, et al. Paraspinal arteriovenous malformation Onyx embolization via an Ascent balloon. *J Neurointerv Surg*. 2014;6(3):e19.
37. Huang W, Gross BA, Du R. Spinal extradural arteriovenous fistulas: clinical article. *J Neurosurg Spine*. 2013;19(5): 582-590.
38. Chuang NA, et al. Slow-flow spinal epidural AVF with venous ectasias: two pediatric case reports. *AJNR Am J Neuroradiol*. 2003;24(9):1901-1905.
39. Cosgrove GR, Theron J. Vertebral arteriovenous fistula following anterior cervical spine surgery. Report of two cases. *J Neurosurg*. 1987;66(2):297-299.
40. Clarke MJ, et al. Spinal extradural arteriovenous malformations with parenchymal drainage: venous drainage variability and implications in clinical manifestations. *Neurosurg Focus*. 2009;26(1):E5.
41. Rangel-Castilla L, et al. Spinal extradural arteriovenous fistulas: a clinical and radiological description of different types and their novel treatment with Onyx. *J Neurosurg Spine*. 2011;15(5):541-549.
42. Niimi Y, Berenstein A. Endovascular treatment of spinal vascular malformations. *Neurosurg Clin N Am*. 1999;10(1):47-71.
43. Niizuma K, et al. Surgical treatment of spinal extradural arteriovenous fistula with parenchymal drainage: report on 5 cases. *Neurosurgery*. 2013;73(suppl 2):E287-3.
44. Oldfield EH, et al. Successful management of spinal dural arteriovenous fistulas undetected by arteriography. Report of three cases. *J Neurosurg*. 2002;96(suppl 2):220-229.
45. Oldfield EH, et al. Successful treatment of a group of spinal cord arteriovenous malformations by interruption of dural fistula. *J Neurosurg*. 1983;59(6):1019-1030.
46. Onda K, et al. High cervical arteriovenous fistulas fed by dural and spinal arteries and draining into a single medullary vein: report of 3 cases. *J Neurosurg Spine*. 2014;20(3):256-264.
47. Kim DJ, et al. Angiographic characteristics and treatment of cervical spinal dural arteriovenous shunts. *AJNR Am J Neuroradiol*. 2010;31(8):1512-1515.
48. Koch C, Gottschalk S, Giese A. Dural arteriovenous fistula of the lumbar spine presenting with subarachnoid hemorrhage. Case report and review of the literature. *J Neurosurg*. 2004;100(suppl 4):385-391.

49. Hashimoto H, et al. Spinal dural arteriovenous fistula with perimesencephalic subarachnoid haemorrhage. *J Clin Neurosci*. 2000;7(1):64-66.
50. Fassett DR, et al. Intracranial subarachnoid hemorrhage resulting from cervical spine dural arteriovenous fistulas: literature review and case presentation. *Neurosurg Focus*. 2009;26(1):E4.
51. Geibprasert S, et al. Cervical spine dural arteriovenous fistula presenting with congestive myelopathy of the conus. *J Neurosurg Spine*. 2009;11(4):427-431.
52. Sasamori T, et al. [Sacral dural arteriovenous fistula: report of 4 cases]. *No Shinkei Geka*. 2011;39(5):505-511.
53. Eskandar EN, et al. Spinal dural arteriovenous fistulas: experience with endovascular and surgical therapy. *J Neurosurg*. 2002;96(suppl 2):162-167.
54. Hassler W, Thron A, Grote EH. Hemodynamics of spinal dural arteriovenous fistulas. An intraoperative study. *J Neurosurg*. 1989;70(3):360-370.
55. Merland JJ, Reizine D. Treatment of arteriovenous spinal-cord malformations. *Semin Intervent Radiol*. 1987;4(4): 281-290.
56. Merland JJ, et al. Embolization of spinal cord vascular lesions. In: Vinuela F, Halbach VV, Dion JF, eds. *Interventional Neuroradiology: Endovascular Therapy of the Central Nervous System*. New York: Raven Press; 1992:153-165.
57. Merland JJ, Riche MC, Chiras J. Intraspinal extramedullary arteriovenous fistulae draining into the medullary veins. *J Neuroradiol*. 1980;7(4):271-320.
58. Niimi Y, et al. Embolization of spinal dural arteriovenous fistulae: results and follow-up. *Neurosurgery*. 1997;40(4):675-682.
59. Van Dijk JMC, et al. Multidisciplinary management of spinal dural arteriovenous fistulas: clinical presentation and long-term follow-up in 49 patients. *Stroke*. 2002;33(6):1578-1583.
60. Cullen S, et al. Spinal arteriovenous shunts presenting before 2 years of age: analysis of 13 cases. *Childs Nerv Syst*. 2006;22(9):1103-1110.
61. Atkinson JL, et al. Clinical and radiographic features of dural arteriovenous fistula, a treatable cause of myelopathy. *Mayo Clin Proc*. 2001;76(11):1120-1130.
62. Cognard C, et al. Cerebral dural arteriovenous fistulas: clinical and angiographic correlation with a revised classification of venous drainage. *Radiology*. 1995;194(3):671-680.
63. Ropper AE, Gross BA, Du R. Surgical treatment of Type I spinal dural arteriovenous fistulas. *Neurosurg Focus*. 2012;32(5):E3.
64. Rangel-Castilla L, et al. Contemporary management of spinal AVFs and AVMs: lessons learned from 110 cases. *Neurosurg Focus*. 2014;37(3):E14.
65. Chibbaro S, et al. Surgical management of spinal dural arteriovenous fistulas. *J Clin Neurosci*. 2015;22(1):180-183.
66. Rodesch G, et al. Embolization of spinal cord arteriovenous shunts: morphological and clinical follow-up and results—review of 69 consecutive cases. *Neurosurgery*. 2003;53(1):40-49.
67. Rodesch G, et al. Spinal cord intradural arteriovenous fistulae: anatomic, clinical, and therapeutic considerations in a series of 32 consecutive patients seen between 1981 and 2000 with emphasis on endovascular therapy. *Neurosurgery*. 2005;57(5):973-983.
68. Rodesch G, et al. Spinal cord arteriovenous malformations in a pediatric population children below 15 years of age. The place of endovascular management. *Interv Neuroradiol*. 1995;1(1):29-42.
69. Su IC, et al. Factors determining the success of endovascular treatments among patients with spinal dural arteriovenous fistulas. *Neuroradiology*. 2013;55(11):1389-1395.
70. Clark S, et al. Spinal dural arteriovenous fistulas—presentation, management and outcome in a single neurosurgical institution. *Br J Neurosurg*. 2013;27(4): 465-470.
71. Mourier KL, et al. Intradural perimedullary arteriovenous fistulae: results of surgical and endovascular treatment in a series of 35 cases. *Neurosurgery*. 1993;32(6):885-891.
72. Bao YH, Ling F. Classification and therapeutic modalities of spinal vascular malformations in 80 patients. *Neurosurgery*. 1997;40(1):75-81.
73. Hodes JE, et al. Spinal vascular malformations: endovascular therapy. *Neurosurg Clin N Am*. 1999;10(1):139-152.
74. Wakhloo AK, et al. A novel approach to flow quantification in brain arteriovenous malformations prior to enbucrilate embolization: use of insoluble contrast (Ethiodol droplet) angiography. *J Neurosurg*. 1998;89(3):395-404.
75. Rudin S, et al. Microdroplet tracking using biplane digital subtraction angiography for cerebral arteriovenous malformation blood flow path and velocity determinations. *AJNR Am J Neuroradiol*. 1999;20(6):1110-1114.
76. Ricolfi F, et al. Giant perimedullary arteriovenous fistulas of the spine: clinical and radiologic features and endovascular treatment. *AJNR Am J Neuroradiol*. 1997;18(4): 677-687.
77. Saliou G, et al. Risk factors of hematomyelia recurrence and clinical outcome in children with intradural spinal cord arteriovenous malformations. *AJNR Am J Neuroradiol*. 2014;35(7):1440-1446.
78. Oran I, Parildar M, Derbent A. Treatment of slow-flow (type I) perimedullary spinal arteriovenous fistulas with special reference to embolization. *AJNR Am J Neuroradiol*. 2005;26(10):2582-2586.
79. Lundqvist C, et al. Spinal arteriovenous malformations: neurological aspects and results of embolization. *Acta Neurol Scand*. 1990;82(1):51-58.
80. Ducruet AF, et al. Endovascular management of spinal arteriovenous malformations. *J Neurointerv Surg*. 2013;5(6):605-611.
81. Casasco A, et al. Endovascular treatment of cervical giant perimedullary arteriovenous fistulas. *Neurosurgery*. 2012;70(1):141-149.
82. Gueguen B, et al. Vascular malformations of the spinal cord: intrathecal perimedullary arteriovenous fistulas fed by medullary arteries. *Neurology*. 1987;37(6):969-979.
83. Cho KT, et al. Treatment of spinal cord perimedullary arteriovenous fistula: embolization versus surgery. *Neurosurgery*. 2005;56(2):232-241.
84. Phadke RV, et al. Endovascular treatment in spinal perimedullary arteriovenous fistula. *Interv Neuroradiol*. 2014;20(3):357-367.
85. Honarmand AR, et al. Use of Onyx for endovascular embolization of pediatric spinal perimedullary (type IV) fistula: case report. *Clin Neurol Neurosurg*. 2013;115(10):2260-2263.
86. Wilson DA, et al. Multimodality treatment of conus medullaris arteriovenous malformations: 2 decades of experience with combined endovascular and microsurgical treatments. *Neurosurgery*. 2012;71(1):100-108.

87. Touho H, et al. Treatment of type II perimedullary arteriovenous fistulas by intraoperative transvenous embolization: case report. *Surg Neurol.* 1995;43(5):491-496.
88. Heros RC, et al. Direct spinal arteriovenous fistula: a new type of spinal AVM. *J Neurosurg.* 1986;64(1):134-139.
89. Kim LJ, Spetzler RF. Classification and surgical management of spinal arteriovenous lesions: arteriovenous fistulae and arteriovenous malformations. *Neurosurgery.* 2006;59(5 suppl 3):S195-S201.
90. Cobb S. Haemangioma of the spinal cord: associated with skin naevi of the same metamere. *Ann Surg.* 1915;62(6):641-649.
91. Elkordy A, et al. Exclusively epidural spinal metameric arteriovenous shunts: case report and literature review. *Spine J.* 2015;15(3):e15-e22.
92. Niimi Y, et al. Spinal arteriovenous metameric syndrome: clinical manifestations and endovascular management. *AJNR Am J Neuroradiol.* 2013;34(2):457-463.
93. Gross BA, Du R. Spinal juvenile (Type III) extradural-intradural arteriovenous malformations. *J Neurosurg Spine.* 2014;20(4):452-458.
94. Aminoff MJ, Logue V. Clinical features of spinal vascular malformations. *Brain.* 1974;97(1):197-210.
95. Djindjian R. Clinical symptomatology and natural history of arteriovenous malformations of the spinal cord: a study of the clinical aspects and prognosis based on 150 cases. In: Djindjian R, Pia H, eds. *Spinal Angiomas: Advances in Diagnosis and Therapy.* Berlin: Springer-Verlag; 1978.
96. Lee YJ, et al. Clinical features and outcomes of spinal cord arteriovenous malformations: comparison between nidus and fistulous types. *Stroke.* 2014;45(9):2606-2612.
97. Krings T, et al. Spinal vascular malformations. *Eur Radiol.* 2005;15(2):267-278.
98. Biondi A, et al. Embolization with particles in thoracic intramedullary arteriovenous malformations: long-term angiographic and clinical results. *Radiology.* 1990;177(3):651-658.
99. Medel R, Crowley RW, Dumont AS. Endovascular management of spinal vascular malformations: history and literature review. *Neurosurg Focus.* 2009;26(1):E7.
100. Acewicz A, et al. Endovascular treatment of cervical intramedullary arteriovenous malformation. *Neurol Neurochir Pol.* 2014;48(3):223-227.
101. Biondi A, et al. Aneurysms of spinal arteries associated with intramedullary arteriovenous malformations. II. Results of AVM endovascular treatment and hemodynamic considerations. *AJNR Am J Neuroradiol.* 1992;13(3):923-931.
102. Biondi A, et al. Aneurysms of spinal arteries associated with intramedullary arteriovenous malformations. I. Angiographic and clinical aspects. *AJNR Am J Neuroradiol.* 1992;13(3):913-922.
103. Corkill RA, Mitsos AP, Molyneux AJ. Embolization of spinal intramedullary arteriovenous malformations using the liquid embolic agent, Onyx: a single-center experience in a series of 17 patients. *J Neurosurg Spine.* 2007;7(5):478-485.
104. Sinclair J, et al. Multisession CyberKnife radiosurgery for intramedullary spinal cord arteriovenous malformations. *Neurosurgery.* 2006;58(6):1081-1089.
105. Park HK, Chang JC. Review of stereotactic radiosurgery for intramedullary spinal lesions. *Korean J Spine.* 2013;10(1):1-6.
106. Berenstein A, Lasjaunias P, terBrugge KG. *Surgical Neuroangiography: Endovascular Treatment of Spine and Spinal Cord Lesions.* Berlin.: Springer-Verlag; 1992:33.
107. Berlis A, et al. Solitary spinal artery aneurysms as a rare source of spinal subarachnoid hemorrhage: potential etiology and treatment strategy. *AJNR Am J Neuroradiol.* 2005;26(2):405-410.
108. Canavero S, et al. Spinal intramedullary cavernous angiomas: a literature meta-analysis. *Surg Neurol.* 1994;41(5): 381-388.
109. Rigamonti D, et al. Cavernous malformations and capillary telangiectasia: a spectrum within a single pathological entity. *Neurosurgery.* 1991;28(1):60-64.
110. Maraire JN, et al. Cavernous malformations: natural history and indications for treatment. In: Batjer HH, ed. *Cerebrovascular Disease.* Philadelphia: Lippincott-Raven; 1997:669-690.
111. Zevgaridis D, et al. Cavernous haemangiomas of the spinal cord. A review of 117 cases. *Acta Neurochir (Wien).* 1999;141(3):237-245.
112. Neumann HP, et al. Central nervous system lesions in von Hippel-Lindau syndrome. *J Neurol Neurosurg Psychiatry.* 1992;55(10):898-901.
113. Sze G. Neoplastic disease of the spine and spinal cord. In: Atlas SW, ed. *Magnetic Resonance Imaging of the Brain and Spine.* Philadelphia.: Lippincott-Raven; 1996:1377-1378.
114. Tampieri D, Leblanc R, TerBrugge K. Preoperative embolization of brain and spinal hemangioblastomas. *Neurosurgery.* 1993;33(3):502-505.
115. Eskridge JM, et al. Preoperative endovascular embolization of craniospinal hemangioblastomas. *AJNR Am J Neuroradiol.* 1996;17(3):525-531.
116. Djindjian R, et al. Vertebral hemangiomas and metameric angiomatosis (Cobb's syndrome). In: Nadjmi M, Piepgras U, Vogelsang H, eds. *Angiography of Spinal Column and Spinal Cord.* Stuttgart: Georg Thieme; 1981.
117. Yis U, et al. Capillary malformation-arteriovenous malformation syndrome with spinal involvement. *Pediatr Dermatol.* 2014;31(6):744-746.
118. Thiex R, et al. A novel association between RASA1 mutations and spinal arteriovenous anomalies. *AJNR Am J Neuroradiol.* 2010;31(4):775-779.
119. Doppman JL, Oldfield EH, Heiss JD. Symptomatic vertebral hemangiomas: treatment by means of direct intralesional injection of ethanol. *Radiology.* 2000;214(2):341-348.
120. Fox MW, Onofrio BM. The natural history and management of symptomatic and asymptomatic vertebral hemangiomas. *J Neurosurg.* 1993;78(1):36-45.
121. Jayakumar PN, Vasudev MK, Srikanth SG. Symptomatic vertebral haemangioma: endovascular treatment of 12 patients. *Spinal Cord.* 1997;35(9):624-628.
122. Ross JS, et al. Vertebral hemangiomas: MR imaging. *Radiology.* 1987;165(1):165-169.
123. Reizine D, et al. Vertebral arteriovenous fistulas. Clinical presentation, angiographical appearance and endovascular treatment. A review of twenty-five cases. *Ann Radiol (Paris).* 1985;28(6):425-438.
124. Lichtenstein L. Aneurysmal bone cyst. A pathological entity commonly mistaken for giant-cell tumor and occasionally for hemangioma and osteogenic sarcoma. *Cancer.* 1950;3(2):279-289.
125. Ameli NO, et al. Aneurysmal bone cysts of the spine. Report of 17 cases. *J Neurosurg.* 1985;63(5):685-690.
126. Bonakdarpour A, Levy WM, Aegerter E. Primary and secondary aneurysmal bone cyst: a radiological study of 75 cases. *Radiology.* 1978;126(1):75-83.

127. Lum C, terBrugge KG. Intervention in vascular lesions of the vertebrae. *Semin Intervent Radiol.* 2002;19:245-256.
128. Cigala F, Sadile F. Arterial embolization of aneurysmal bone cysts in children. *Bull Hosp Jt Dis.* 1996;54(4):261-264.
129. Radanović B, et al. Therapeutic embolization of aneurysmal bone cyst. *Cardiovasc Intervent Radiol.* 1989;12(6):313-316.
130. Broaddus WC, et al. Preoperative superselective arteriolar embolization: a new approach to enhance resectability of spinal tumors. *Neurosurgery.* 1990;27(5):755-759.
131. King GJ, et al. Surgical management of metastatic renal carcinoma of the spine. *Spine.* 1991;16(3):265-271.
132. Gellad FE, et al. Vascular metastatic lesions of the spine: preoperative embolization. *Radiology.* 1990;176(3):683-686.
133. Hilal SK, Michelsen JW. Therapeutic percutaneous embolization for extra-axial vascular lesions of the head, neck, and spine. *J Neurosurg.* 1975;43(3):275-287.
134. Jensen ME, et al. *Preoperative and palliative embolization of vertebral body metastases.* In: Proceedings of the 31st Annual Meeting of the American Society of Neuroradiology; 1993. Vancouver, British Columbia.
135. Evans AJ, et al. Vertebral compression fractures: pain reduction and improvement in functional mobility after percutaneous polymethylmethacrylate vertebroplasty: retrospective report of 245 cases. *Radiology.* 2003;226(2):366-372.
136. Gangi A, Kastler BA, Dietemann JL. Percutaneous vertebroplasty guided by a combination of CT and fluoroscopy. *AJNR Am J Neuroradiol.* 1994;15(1):83-86.
137. Chiras J, et al. Percutaneous injection of an alcoholic embolizing emulsion as an alternative preoperative embolization for spine tumor. *AJNR Am J Neuroradiol.* 1993;14(5):1113-1117.
138. Heiss JD, Doppman JL, Oldfield EH. Brief report: relief of spinal cord compression from vertebral hemangioma by intralesional injection of absolute ethanol. *N Engl J Med.* 1994;331(8):508-511.
139. Cotten A, et al. Preoperative percutaneous injection of methyl methacrylate and N-butyl cyanoacrylate in vertebral hemangiomas. *AJNR Am J Neuroradiol.* 1996;17(1):137-142.

CHAPTER 94 Syringomyelia

David M. Benglis Jr
Andrew Jea
Steve Vanni
Ashish H. Shah
Barth A. Green

Syringomyelia, or cavitation within the substance of the spinal cord without an ependymal lining, has been recognized for more than 300 years as a pathologic entity. Etienne is credited for the first pathologic description in 1564 in *La Dissection du Corps Humain*; he described a cystic lesion in the spinal cord that contained a "fluid, reddish, like the fluidity of that of the ventricles."[1]

Portal, in 1804, first appreciated and connected the clinical syndrome of an intramedullary cyst with the pathologic changes of the spinal cord.[2] Ollivier then coined the term "syringomyelia," combining the Greek words for "tube or pipe" and "marrow." He documented a connection between the fourth ventricle and this cystic structure, which he believed to be a congenital anomaly.[1,3]

The classic clinical description of syringomyelia is described as a dissociated, suspended segmental sensory loss, consisting of loss of sensation to pain and temperature and preservation of sensation to proprioception and light touch. Slowly progressive distal motor dysfunction may also occur. A syrinx may extend to the medulla and cause lower brain stem and cranial nerve dysfunction, termed *syringobulbia*.

Those ependymal-lined cavities that appeared to be pathologic dilatations of the central canal were termed *hydromyelia*. Some authors viewed hydromyelia, in which the central canal was dilated but preserved, and syringomyelia, with or without a connection to the central canal, as stages of a common process. Unification of the terms resulted in the concept of syringohydromyelia or hydrosyringomyelia.[1–4]

In 1973, Barnett published the first English-language monograph on syringomyelia.[5] He proposed a classification based on a variety of clinical and experimental observations and studies. The classification scheme consisted of two broad categories: (1) communicating syringomyelia (e.g., Chiari I malformation, Chiari II malformation, basilar arachnoiditis) and (2) noncommunicating syringomyelia (e.g., occurring with spinal dysraphism, spinal cord trauma, spinal cord tumor, spinal arachnoiditis; Box 94.1).

Over the last 20 years, experimental and clinical work, including that of Oldfield and Milhorat and their colleagues,[6–12] has helped to clarify the pathophysiology and treatment of this complex syndrome.[6–13] Nevertheless, a definite understanding of the etiology of syringomyelia has yet to be clarified.

Etiology, Pathology, Pathophysiology, Prominent Theories

Historical Perspective—Early Theories of Syringomyelia

Although the pathophysiology of syringomyelia has not yet been completely defined, the association between syringomyelia and congenital abnormalities was appreciated long ago. Baulmer was credited initially for establishing this relationship in 1887.[14] Schlesinger further substantiated this association in 1895 by noting congenital abnormality in one-third of the cases of syringomyelia that he had reviewed.[15]

Ollivier d'Angers formulated and Leyden further refined the developmental theory of syringomyelia formation.[15] These authors stated that syringomyelia must be considered a congenital disorder associated with embryonic maldevelopment, specifically, incomplete occlusion of the primitive fold. This improper fusion of the two folds of the primitive medullary groove allowed the abnormal lining of germinal cells to persist, resulting in simple hydromyelia.

Another theory implicates environmental fetal exposure in the pathophysiology of syringomyelia. Kahler and Pick in 1879 theorized that chronic intrauterine inflammation resulted in gliosis and aberrant development of the spinal cord that subsequently led to syrinx formation. On the other hand, in 1910, Haener proposed that events during the act of birth (e.g., trauma) may arouse neural activity in abnormally enclosed tissue, with resultant syrinx formation.[16] None of these claims were formally substantiated in case series.

W.J. Gardner: Hydrodynamic Theory—"Water Hammer"

In a series of landmark papers, W.J. Gardner expounded his hydrodynamic theory of the pathophysiology of

BOX 94.1 Types of Syringomyelia and Associated Abnormalities

Communicating

Chiari I malformation
Chiari II malformation
Basilar arachnoiditis

Noncommunicating

Occult spinal dysraphism
Spinal cord trauma
Spinal cord tumor
Spinal arachnoiditis

syringomyelia.[17–25] Gardner's theory was the first among three prominent current theories. He based his theory on three observations: (1) dye injected into the ventricular system was recovered from the syrinx at operation, (2) fluid withdrawn from the syrinx at operation strongly resembled cerebrospinal fluid (CSF) found in the ventricular system, and (3) experimental hydrocephalus produced by obstruction of the normal outflow of CSF from the fourth ventricle resulted in the formation of syringomyelia that was in communication with the ventricular system.[26]

Syringomyelia could be explained by failure of the embryonic rhombic roof to fenestrate during a critical period of development. The inability of CSF in the fourth ventricle to gain the usual access to the subarachnoid space during the 6th to 8th weeks of embryogenesis forced the hindbrain to herniate through the foramen magnum. A Chiari malformation was thereby created, and the failure of the CSF to expand the subarachnoid space resulted in communicating hydrocephalus. Gardner believed that the effect of the hindbrain malformation was to increase the obstruction to outflow at the foramen of Magendie and deflect the pulse wave of CSF into the opening of the central canal at the obex.

The pulse wave effect of the diverted CSF acted as a water hammer, gradually dilating the central canal or dissecting the substance of the spinal cord around the canal and creating a syrinx. From the perspective of Gardner, a congenital hindbrain defect that obstructed the CSF flow from the fourth ventricle to the subarachnoid space was the sine qua non of syringomyelia. Ball and Dayan[27] and West and Williams[28] questioned Gardner's theory and the necessity of a direct communication to the fourth ventricle for production of a syrinx. To support this statement, Milhorat and colleagues demonstrated in large autopsy studies that the majority of syrinxes did not communicate with the fourth ventricle and that the central canal was not patent in most normal adult patients.[10]

B. Williams: Craniospinal Pressure Dissociation Theory

Williams proposed an alternative theory to explain syrinx formation and speculated that a partial block of the spinal subarachnoid space produced a pressure differential between the ventricular system and the spinal subdural space during Valsalva-type maneuvers. He explained that venous distention associated with these maneuvers produced an increased intracranial pressure that was not evenly distributed to the lumbar subarachnoid space because of a more proximal subarachnoid block. This pressure difference was labeled *craniospinal pressure dissociation*, and the lower pressure in the lumbar theca caused fluid to be drawn into the syrinx. This phenomenon was termed *suck*.

Williams also believed that the cavity enlarged after its initial formation as the result of compression of the lower end of the cavity with the rapid filling of the epidural venous plexus during a cough or sneeze. The fluid in the syrinx was then propelled rostrally, dissecting the central canal or pericentral parenchyma of the spinal cord. Williams applied the term *slosh* to this part of his theory to explain syrinx extension.[29]

E. Oldfield: Abnormal Pulse Wave Theory

Oldfield and colleagues used magnetic resonance imaging (MRI) with and without cardiac gating, intraoperative ultrasonography, and direct intraoperative observation of the exposed hindbrain and documented the downward movement of the cerebellar tonsils during systole.[13] This group interpreted the data as obviating the necessity of a direct communication with the fourth ventricle, as advocated by Gardner. Moreover, they observed that the syringomyelic cord did not enlarge with Valsalva maneuver and that venous pressure had little to do with syrinx elongation, disputing the Williams suck and slosh theory. These authors proposed that the abnormal pulse wave in the spinal subarachnoid space, caused by the partial obstruction by the hindbrain, placed pressure on the spinal cord and dissected the central canal, causing the cyst to enlarge.

The ingress of CSF within the spinal cord parenchyma has recently been suggested to enter through dilated Virchow-Robin spaces. The blockage of flow creates eddylike currents analogous to a boulder in a rapidly flowing river. These forceful currents enter the cord parenchyma and first create microscopic changes (i.e., myelomalacia). They later develop into more confluent macrocystic cavities by dilation of the central canal and/or peripheral areas of the spinal cord.

Milhorat and colleagues proposed that normal CSF flow was from the spinal subarachnoid space through the parenchyma of the spinal cord into the central canal.[12] The CSF then flowed into the fourth ventricle outlet at the obex. Their theory was supported with a rodent model of syringomyelia. They injected kaolin into the central canal of rats, causing stenosis of the proximal central canal through an inflammatory reaction. A resultant syrinx was formed. These authors suggested that syrinx formation was due to disruption of normal CSF flow by the inflammatory stenosis (Fig. 94.1).

Communicating Syringomyelia

In 1896, Chiari published an addendum to an earlier work in which he described anomalies associated with hydrocephalus. In this latter publication, there were descriptions of patients with hydromyelia. Gardner and Goodall found that a majority of patients undergoing surgical decompression for symptomatic Chiari I malformation had a concurrent syringomyelia (Fig. 94.2).[23] Gardner and colleagues demonstrated,

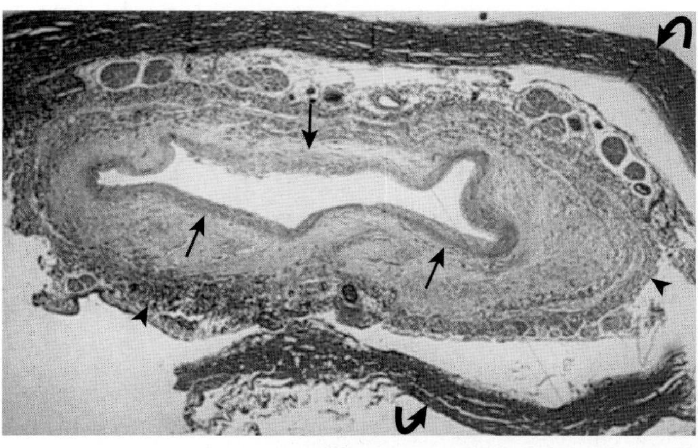

FIG. 94.1 Posttraumatic cord cyst. A low-power (×1.25) microscopic section image of a posttraumatic syringomyelia. There is a large, centrally located syrinx in the parenchyma of the spinal cord, which is surrounded by a thick wall of reactive astrocytes (*arrows*). The pia is thickened, and there are tissue changes that involve the spinal roots (*arrowheads*). The dura is also thickened (*curved arrow*). (From Madsen PW, Falcone S, Bowen B, Green BA. Post-traumatic syringomyelia. In: Levine A, Garfin S, Eismont F, Zigler J, eds. *Spine Trauma*. Philadelphia: WB Saunders; 1998.)

at operation, communication between the syrinx of the upper cervical cord and the ventricles in patients undergoing suboccipital craniectomy and cervical laminectomy for decompression.[21] Indigo-carmine was injected into the patient's lateral ventricle, and colored CSF was recovered by direct puncture of the cervical syrinx.

Appleby and colleagues established that a "communicating" type of syringomyelia could also be acquired from chronic arachnoiditis involving the basal cisterns and obstructing the outflow of CSF from the fourth ventricle.[30]

Noncommunicating Syringomyelia

Syringomyelia Associated With Spinal Arachnoiditis

The association between spinal arachnoiditis and syringomyelia was first reported by Vulpian in 1861 and by Charcot and Joffroy in 1869. Some authors believed that occlusion of blood vessels supplying the cord from profound arachnoid scarring was the underlying pathophysiologic process for intramedullary cavitation.[31–33]

As previously described, Williams implicated craniospinal pressure dissociation, secondary to obstruction of the subarachnoid space, as the factor responsible for cyst formation and extension in this disease entity.[34] In 2004, Chang and colleagues explained that the blockage of the spinal subarachnoid CSF pathway produces a relative pressure gradient inside the spinal cord distal to the blockage point that induces CSF leakage into the spinal parenchyma and the formation of syringomyelia.[35] Barnett and Milhorat considered this type of syringomyelia to be of the "noncommunicating" type because no connection between the cyst and fourth ventricle could be demonstrated.[13,36] Koyanagi and colleagues reviewed a series of 15 patients who underwent various shunting procedures for syrinx treatment caused by spinal arachnoiditis. Although neurologic improvement was found in a decent percentage of patients (60%), many required additional shunting procedures over time due to catheter blockage or failure.[37]

Additionally, there are some reports of dorsal septae/web that block CSF flow in the subarachnoid space, causing decreased pulsatile flow in the subarachnoid space. This pressure gradient may augment the CSF inflow into the syrinx. Lysis of these septae should improve CSF flow dynamics and reduce the size of the syrinx.[38,39]

Syringomyelia Associated With Spinal Cord Tumors

The association between syringomyelia and spinal cord tumors has been well established. In 1875, Simon was the first to report the simultaneous occurrence of syringomyelia and spinal cord tumors.[40] Proposed mechanisms for syrinx formation in this environment include (1) edema; (2) blockage of the perivascular spaces, with resultant tissue fluid stasis; (3) cavitation secondary to disturbance of blood supply to the spinal cord; and (4) spontaneous hemorrhage or autolysis of the mass.[32,41,42] Other authors contend that syringomyelia associated with a spinal cord tumor is due to a direct effect of the neoplasm.[15,40,43–45] Some authors believed that this disordered gliosis observed with tumor presence was also the underlying pathophysiologic cause even in cases not associated with an intramedullary neoplasm. This led some physicians to recommend radiation therapy as a rational but extreme form of primary therapy.[46] Today, the use of radiation therapy should be restricted only for primary therapy of a known neoplasm or as an adjunct to surgical resection of tumor (Fig. 94.3).

Spinal Cerebrospinal Fluid Dynamics in the Presence of a Neoplasm

Total or subtotal obstruction of CSF flow by an intramedullary or sometimes extramedullary/intradural tumor may be a significant factor for the development of syringomyelia. The subarachnoid and extracellular space of the central nervous system should be considered as a single-fluid compartment with no barrier to fluid movement between them. Interference with this normal CSF flow influences extracellular fluid flow out of the spinal cord. The high ratio of syrinx cavities associated with intramedullary tumors may be attributable to their simultaneous influence on the subarachnoid and extracellular spaces. Fluid transudation from tumor vessels, breakdown products of tumor cells, and in some cases active secretion also raise the protein content and thus the viscosity of the extracellular fluid, contributing to further aberrances on normal flow dynamics.[47] Less commonly, intramedullary cysts can present in association with an extramedullary neurofibroma or meningioma. The removal of the extramedullary mass lesion is usually followed by a spontaneous collapse of the associated syrinx.

Syringomyelia and Spinal Cord Tumors—Clinical Studies

In a surgical series of 100 intramedullary tumors, 45% of patients presented with an associated syrinx.[48] A syrinx was more likely to be found rostral to the tumor. Ependymomas

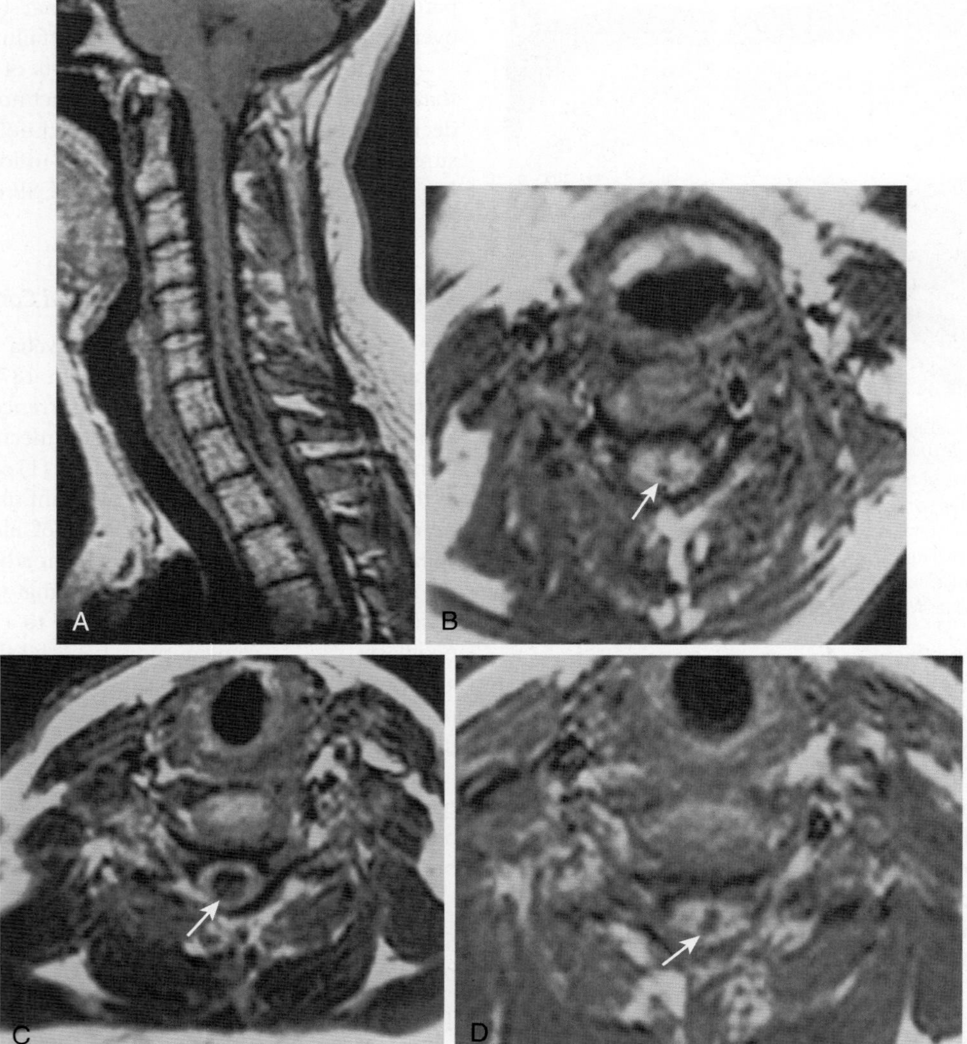

FIG. 94.2 Communicating syringomyelia (syringohydromyelia) with associated Chiari I malformation. (A) T1-weighted sagittal image shows ectopia of the cerebellar tonsils and an intramedullary cystic cavity extending from C2 to T2. (B–D) T1-weighted axial images demonstrate the central location of the cyst (*arrow*) at C5–C7.

and hemangioblastomas were the most common tumor types to be associated with a syrinx. Astrocytomas, on the other hand, tended to demonstrate syrinxes less often. The higher the spinal level, the more likely a syrinx was encountered.

Syringomyelia Associated With Spinal Cord Trauma

The pathophysiologic basis for the formation and extension of syrinxes of the injured spinal cord remains the subject of considerable debate. However, a constant factor in all cases is the alteration of normal CSF flow dynamics. The onset of signs and symptoms of progressive posttraumatic cystic myelopathy ranges from as early as 2 to 3 months following injury to as long as 30 years after injury.[49] Approximately 4% to 10% of patients suffering a traumatic spinal cord injury develop progressive spinal cord dysfunction associated with an expanding syrinx.[25,47,50] Nevertheless, some patients with posttraumatic radiologic syringomyelia may not exhibit any symptoms (intact motor and sensory function) in the chronic setting. Many patients with no symptoms have been identified who suffered injuries more than 20 years ago, suggesting potential spinal cord plasticity.[51]

Posttraumatic Syringomyelia—Human Studies

Milhorat's large autopsy study demonstrated that syrinxes associated with trauma had distinctly different histopathologic findings and were associated with different clinical symptoms when compared with those lesions that were in communication with the fourth ventricle or those cavities that appeared to be isolated dilatations of the central canal.[13] These syrinxes involved the parenchyma of the cord asymmetrically, were not associated with the central canal, and often extended to the pial surface. Examination of pathologic specimens revealed nonreversible damage to spinal nuclei and tracts,

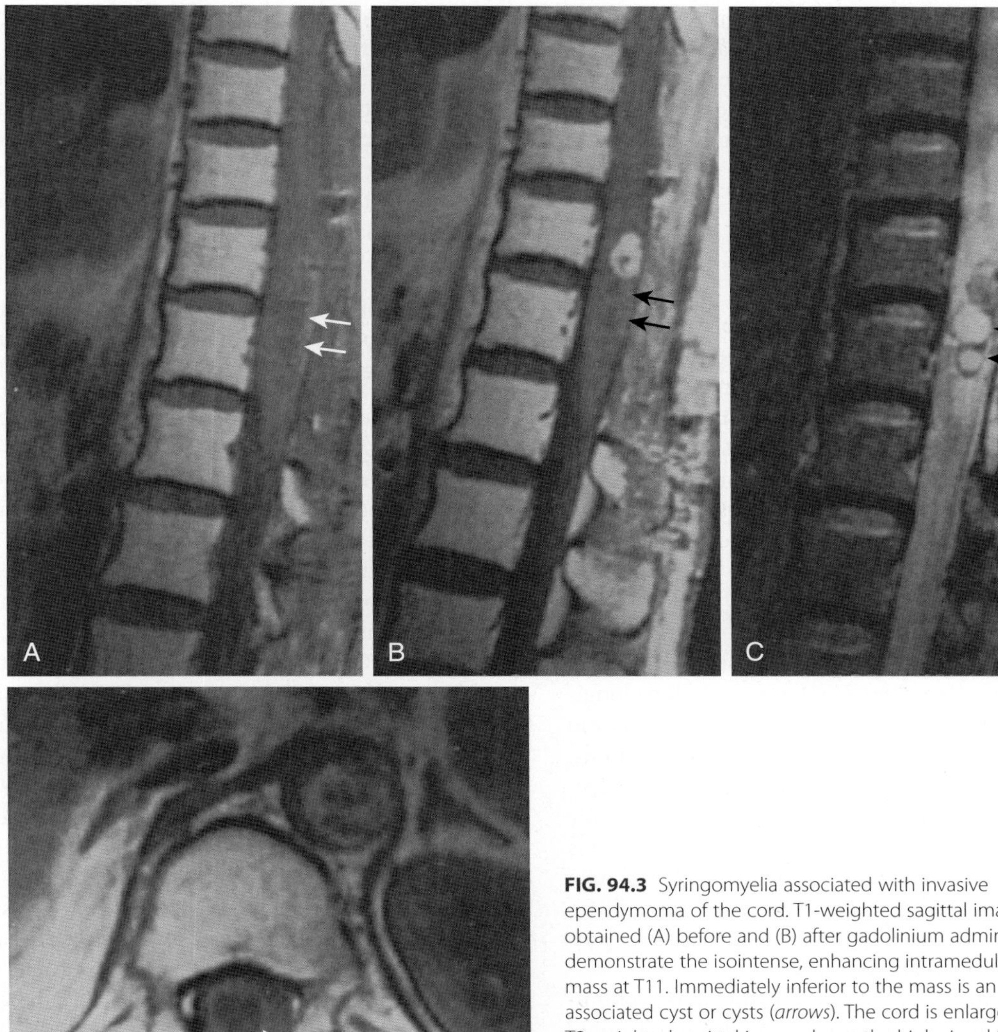

FIG. 94.3 Syringomyelia associated with invasive ependymoma of the cord. T1-weighted sagittal images obtained (A) before and (B) after gadolinium administration demonstrate the isointense, enhancing intramedullary mass at T11. Immediately inferior to the mass is an associated cyst or cysts (*arrows*). The cord is enlarged. (C) T2-weighted sagittal image shows the high signal intensity of fluid within the cysts (*arrows*) and relatively low signal intensity of the tumor. (D) T1-weighted axial image shows the eccentrically located cystic cavity (*arrows*), containing low-signal-intensity fluid, within the enlarged cord.

including focal necrosis, central chromatolysis, and wallerian degeneration.

Posttraumatic Syringomyelia—Mechanisms of Development

The possible factors implicated in the production of the initial cystic lesions in posttraumatic spinal cords included ischemia secondary to arterial and/or venous obstruction, tissue breakdown from lysosomes or other intracellular enzymes, liquefaction of a prior hematoma, mechanical damage from compression of the substance of the cord at the time of initial injury, or tethering by delayed formation of extensive subarachnoid adhesions and/or a bony gibbus.[13,52–60]

Similarly, the mechanism for the extension of the syringomyelia remains a matter of controversy leading to several mechanisms being proposed. Some view the rostral and caudal extension of the syrinx, which produces late neurologic symptoms, as a result of a one-way valvelike trapping effect of the subarachnoid space into the cavity.[10,61–63] Less frequently observed presentations of posttraumatic cysts include patients with a history of a herniated cervical or thoracic disc with resultant ventral compression from a bony or soft gibbus and disturbance of normal CSF flow. Spinal puncture with injection of an irritative dye (e.g., methylene blue) can cause an ascending arachnoiditis that may develop associated subarachnoid and/or intramedullary cysts. Patients who have subarachnoid hemorrhage may also develop spinal cord tethering with associated intramedullary or subarachnoid cysts.

Asano and colleagues[64] suggested that posttraumatic syringomyelia may be classified into two types. These authors contend that successful reestablishment of normal CSF flow dynamics by untethering the spinal cord stops the progression of clinical decline and, in some cases, may return valuable lost function. A preoperative distinction could be made on the basis of the presence (high-pressure type) or absence (low-pressure type) of the flow-void sign on T2-weighted MRI. With a midline myelotomy, fluid within a high-pressure syrinx would pour out, resulting in sustained neurologic improvement. In the low-pressure type, drainage of the syrinx would not collapse the expanded spinal cord and the surgical outcome would be modest at best.[64]

Clinical Features

The onset of syringomyelia is commonly between the ages of 25 and 40 years. Males are somewhat more affected than females. Syringomyelia most often affects the cervical or thoracic spinal cord yet sometimes extends rostrally into the medulla.

Hydrocephalus may be found in 10% to 33% of patients but is more likely related to an associated Chiari malformation.[28] This frequent association supports the concept of a hydrodynamic mechanism for the formation of syringomyelia.

Syringomyelia—Physical Examination

Clinical features are variable and dependent on the anatomic structures involved in a cross-sectional area as well as longitudinally. Anterior horn involvement results in weakness and wasting, especially in the upper extremities, and fasciculations. Posterior horn and decussating spinothalamic fiber involvement result in loss of pain and temperature sensation, usually in a suspended, segmental distribution, involving the arms and trunk, sparing the legs. Patients may occasionally feel pain that is characterized as boring or lancinating. The large fibers of the dorsal columns are usually unaffected; therefore, proprioception and light touch are preserved.

The autonomic pathways of the interomediolateral column may be affected, resulting in Horner syndrome, trophic changes of the skin, a neurogenic bladder, and dyshidrosis, although these manifestations are usually less frequent and rare. Corticospinal tract involvement may give spastic paraparesis. Patients experience a loss of deep tendon reflexes in the upper extremities. A skeletal survey may reveal congenital anomalies, including basilar impression and invagination, Klippel-Feil deformity, and spina bifida occurring primarily at C1.[65] Developmental scoliosis may occur as a result of cord cavitation and is probably not an unassociated congenital lesion.[66] Although discussed extensively in the literature, painless joint destruction (Charcot joints) occur in less than 5% of patients with syringomyelia.[67]

Cranial nerve involvement is seen with syringobulbia. Most often, signs and symptoms are unilateral. CN XII involvement results in tongue weakness and atrophy. CN XI dysfunction can result in weakness and wasting of the sternocleidomastoid and trapezius muscles, whereas CN IX and X involvement produces dysphagia and dysarthria. CN VII involvement results in a facial palsy, and involvement of the spinal tract of CN V produces sensory loss of pain and temperature of the face in an "onion skin" distribution, as well as reduced corneal sensation and reflex.

The clinical course of syringomyelia is usually insidious, worsening over several years to decades. Alternatively, the patient may worsen in an abrupt stepwise fashion, punctuated by intervals of clinical stability.[68] The prognosis of untreated syringomyelia is compatible with modified but productive survival for decades in 50% of surviving patients.[69] The remainder become incapacitated and die as a direct result of the pathologic process. Seki and Fehlings designed a rodent model to further elucidate the role of posttraumatic syringomyelia in spinal cord injury.[70]

Presentation of Progressive Posttraumatic Cystic Myelopathy (Severe Form of Posttraumatic Syringomyelia)

This syndrome is associated with single or multiple connected or separated spinal cord cysts or cystic cavities that may be located in the intramedullary, subarachnoid, or both compartments. A spinal cord fissure may also be associated with this distinct clinical entity. Cysts may result from a variety of causes, including high-velocity missile injuries that cause quadriplegia or paraplegia to relatively minor traumas associated with transient or minor neurologic deficits. Postsurgical patients or patients with a history of arachnoiditis, subarachnoid hemorrhage, meningitis, or multiple "spine blocks" form the second most common category of posttraumatic spinal cord cysts. Most patients in this group present with a history of a prior surgery (e.g., for an intraspinal mass). They have typically undergone an intradural spinal procedure, which results in local tethering of the spinal cord or more diffuse blockage of flow in the subarachnoid space.

The onset of signs and symptoms of progressive posttraumatic cystic myelopathy have ranged from as early as 2 to 3 months following the initial precipitating event to as long as many years later. The symptoms are listed here in order of decreasing frequency:

1. Motor loss
2. Sensory loss
3. Local or radicular pain (nondeafferentated, neurogenic, "burning" pain)
4. Increased spasticity and tone
5. Hyperhidrosis (above level of lesion)
6. Autonomic dysreflexia
7. Sphincter loss or sexual dysfunction
8. Horner syndrome (may be alternating)
9. Respiratory insufficiency (usually related to changes in position)
10. Change in motor "tone" (increased or decreased)

At presentation, the signs and symptoms may be unilateral or bilateral and may alternate from side to side with changes in position. They may also present as a solitary sign or symptom or in any combination. The increased utilization of noninvasive MRI has more frequently identified asymptomatic cases compared with previously employed imaging techniques.

Diagnosis

Diagnosis of syringomyelia was based on clinical presentation and course in the late 19th and early 20th centuries. This disorder was difficult for physicians to diagnose at that time because it had an insidious onset and a variable clinical course, and modern imaging techniques were unavailable. Intramedullary neoplasms, as well as demyelinating diseases (multiple sclerosis, amyotrophic lateral sclerosis), disorders of metabolism and nutrition (subacute combined degeneration in vitamin B_{12} deficiency), infectious causes of spinal cord dysfunction (tabes dorsalis from syphilis), and degenerative disease (cervical spondylosis leading to stenosis and cervical myelopathy), could all serve as confusing mimickers of a syringomyelic process.[1] In a majority of patients, the classic finding of segmental weakness and atrophy of the hands and arms, with loss of tendon reflexes and segmental dissociated sensory loss, could not be found.[71] Furthermore, in some chronic patients, no clinical correlates could be found despite severe radiologic evidence of syringomyelia.[51]

Imaging and Electrophysiologic Evaluation in Syringomyelia Diagnosis

Currently, the diagnostic test of choice for syringomyelia is MRI.[72] The initial MRI examination includes, as a minimum, sagittal and axial views of the lesion plus the adjacent spinal cord and/or brain stem in T1-weighted images. The addition of T2-weighted and/or mixed proton density images can complement the T1-weighted images (Fig. 94.4) and is almost necessary for evaluation of syringomyelia. Gadolinium-enhanced images are considered an essential part of the workup to detect tumors and differentiate between scar and disc material, especially in postoperative or posttraumatic cases.[73] Inclusion of the entire rostrocaudal extent of each cyst or cysts is important.

In addition to conventional MRI, a new generation of MRI software technology is currently available. Cine MRI is a real-time, motion picture–like analysis of spinal fluid flow dynamics in and around the spinal cord cyst.[74–76] Cine MRI works on the basis of imaging flow as it changes with the cardiac cycle, allowing radiologists to view CSF outflow obstructions or flow voids within the spinal canal. Magnetic resonance angiography is another technological advance that can be helpful in cases of syringomyelia associated with vascular lesions.

Spinal instrumentation, bullet fragments, or the inability of the patient to tolerate the enclosed space of the scanner degrades the ability of the MRI to provide adequate anatomic assessment. In these cases, a CT myelogram in combination with immediate and delayed high-resolution CT is performed. Difficulty in differentiating myelomalacia or an intramedullary tumor from a confluent syrinx is a limitation of this technique.[77]

Roser and colleagues have used electrophysiologic monitoring (e.g., the presence of silent periods with analysis of spinothalamic pathways) to assist in early diagnosis of syringomyelia that will likely become symptomatic and exclude patients with benign hydromyelia.[78] In a follow-up clinical study, the authors reviewed a group of patients with idiopathic syrinxes (e.g., not caused from Chiari I malformations, tumors, craniocervical junction abnormalities, scoliosis, trauma).[79] Conduction studies performed included somatosensory evoked potentials and motor evoked potentials, and detection of spinothalamic pain pathways with silent period studies were all negative in this idiopathic group. The major presenting symptom of these patients was pain (e.g., radicular, neuropathic, musculoskeletal), which prompted the original MRI examination. Over time, these patients tend to do better with conservative treatment than those in nonidiopathic groups.[80]

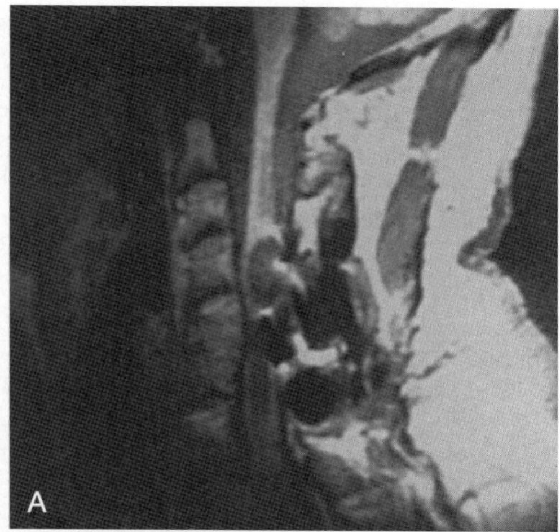

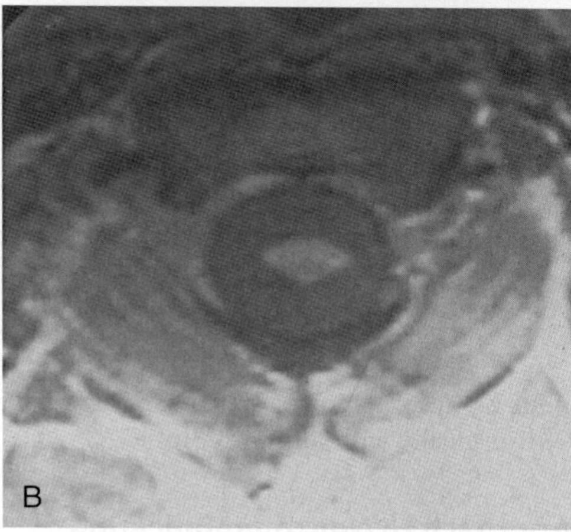

FIG. 94.4 Syringomyelia associated with trauma. (A) T1-weighted sagittal image shows an enlarged cord, with an intramedullary cyst, from C4–C7 in this patient with C5 and C6 fractures. Ferromagnetic artifacts from wires placed during a previous posterior fusion partially obscure the dorsal aspect of the canal from C4–C6. Superior to C3, the cord is narrowed and no cyst is present. (B) T1-weighted axial image at C2 confirms the narrowed anteroposterior diameter of the cord, secondary to dorsal tethering of the cord by scar tissue at C4.

Treatment

The treatment of syringomyelia continues to be controversial. There is no universally accepted method of intervention or consensus on the benefit of therapy. The first report of successful surgical therapy of syringomyelia was by Abbe and Coley in 1892.[81] They performed a three-level laminectomy and opened the dura to expose the cyst and aspirated clear fluid from the lesion, which then collapsed. This report was significant not because of clinical improvement with cyst

TABLE 94.1 Surgical Series Reporting Results of Syringomelia Shunting Procedures

Reference	No. Patients	Procedure	Follow-up	Clinical Results
Tator et al.[105] (1982)	20	Syringosubarachnoid shunting	5 y (average)	75% excellent; 25% deterioration
Barbaro et al.[61] (1984)	34	15 syringoperitoneal shunting 19 syringosubarachnoid shunting	1.5–12 y	Syringoperitoneal shunt: 53% good, 27% fair, 20% poor Syringosubarachnoid shunt: 32% good, 26% fair, 42% poor
Suzuki et al.[92] (1985)	29	Syringoperitoneal shunt	1 y (average)	76% improved; 17% unchanged; 7% deteriorated
Padovani et al.[91] (1989)	29	Syringosubarachnoid shunting	5 y (average)	31% improved; 59% stabilized; 10% deteriorated
Hida et al.[49] (1994)	10	Syringosubarachnoid shunting; syringoperitoneal shunting	NA	30% shunt malfunction
Sgouros et al.[84] (1995)	73	56 syringoperitoneal shunting 14 syringosubarachnoid shunting	NA	Only 53.5% syringoperitoneal and 50% syringosubarachnoid patients were stable at 10 y; 15.7% complication rate; 5% shunt obstruction
Asano et al.[64] (1996)	5	Syringosubarachnoid shunting	NA	40% obstruction; 20% deterioration
Schaller et al.[106] (1999)	10	Syringoperitoneal shunting	4 mo (average)	30% shunt obstruction or infection
Batzdorf et al.[94] (1998)	42	Syringosubarachnoid, syringoperitoneal, syringopleural shunting	NA	50% shunt failure
Isik et al.[107] (2013)	44	Syringopleural shunting	9.1 y	88% clinical improvement; 16% serious complications
Fan et al.[108] (2015)	26	Syringopleural shunting	27.4 mo	92% radiologic and clinical improvement

NA, not available.

drainage but because it showed that syringomyelia could be approached surgically without morbidity.

Direct Approach to Noncommunicating Syringomyelia

Methods

If surgery for syringomyelia-associated spinal arachnoiditis and deteriorating neurologic status is attempted, then the reconstruction of an alternative subarachnoid pathway around the area of adhesion is essential.[67] A wide laminectomy, intradural exploration with limited dissection of adhesions to establish free communication with the subarachnoid space above and below the area of adhesion and an expansile duraplasty are performed.

Preoperative drainage of an intramedullary cyst may be accompanied by rapid neurologic improvement, whereas surgical removal of an associated tumor routinely decompresses the syrinx.[58] One must also be attentive to delayed development of syringomyelia after spinal surgery because it may account for postoperative neurologic deterioration in some patients.[82]

Surgical intervention for a posttraumatic cyst was first undertaken with good results by Freeman in 1955.[83] An essential component of the surgery is untethering the spinal cord and nerve root adhesions, as well as reduction of any bony gibbus or soft tissue mass at the site of injury. This may first require a posterior approach for intradural exploration and untethering of the cord and root adhesions, followed by an anterior approach to remove any bony gibbus or soft tissue mass. Others include reconstruction of the subarachnoid space with a surgical meningocele and the addition of a syringosubarachnoid shunt in order to maintain the patency of the cyst in the subarachnoid space.[61,83–85] However, shunt failure rates as high as 5% to 50% have been reported (Table 94.1). The introduction of a foreign body in the form of a shunt tube, as well as surgical trauma, may also result in fixation of the cord to the dura by scar tissue and neurologic deterioration, therefore negating a lasting benefit from an untethering procedure.[77]

Poussepp and Elsberg have been given credit for development of the midline myelotomy (the "Elsberg-Poussepp operation") for treatment of spinal cord cysts.[86] Frazier, on the other hand, performed a paramedian myelotomy attempting to marsupialize the syrinx into the subarachnoid space.[87]

A 2-mm vertical myelotomy is usually performed in the midline at the dorsal median raphe. In the case of an eccentrically located cyst, the myelotomy is placed at the dorsal root entry zone rather than in the midline. In patients with "double-barreled" or multiloculated cysts, more than one myelotomy and shunt tube may be required. Whenever a syringosubarachnoid shunt is placed, several centimeters of shunt tubing should protrude from the myelotomy opening and into the distal subarachnoid space (at least 1–2 cm to prevent formation of granulation tissue over the lower end). If severe scarring with tethering of the spinal cord or obliteration of the subarachnoid space from a previous trauma or surgery is encountered, placement of a subarachnoid shunt tube in the conventional dorsal position is not adequate because of increased vulnerability to obstruction by scar tissue. In this situation, the distal shunt catheter may need to be placed in the ventral subarachnoid space by passing the shunt tubing laterally and caudally between the nerve roots.

TABLE 94.2 Surgical Series Reporting Results of Procedures on Noncommunicating Syrinxes

Reference	No. Patients	Procedure	Follow-up	Clinical Results
Adelstein[109] (1938)	86	Laminectomy; myelotomy	NA	76% improved; 12% worsened
Pitts et al.[110] (1964)	33 (46 procedures)	Laminectomy; laminectomy + myelotomy; laminectomy + drainage	2–31 y	16% good; 49% fair; 36% poor
Love et al.[111] (1966)	35	Laminectomy; laminectomy + syrinx aspiration; laminectomy + syringosubarachnoid shunt	1–10 y	29% excellent; 34% good or unchanged; 23% poor; 14% lost to follow-up
Anderson et al.[112] (1985)	11	7 laminectomy + syrinx aspiration; 4 laminectomy + syringotomy	11.8 y (range, 1.3–18.5 y)	18% improvement; 9% no progression; 73% deterioration
Lee et al.[113] (2001)	45	Laminectomy + untethering + duraplasty; laminectomy + syringosubarachnoid shunting + duraplasty	22.5 mo (range, 12–84 mo)	73% satisfactory; 20% unchanged; 7% deteriorated

NA, not available.

In cases of diffuse arachnoiditis, the shunt tubing should be placed in either the pleural or peritoneal space. In patients with previous abdominal surgery, use of laparoscopic approach to lyse abdominal adhesions helps facilitate distal shunt placement. The advances in laparoscopic techniques have reduced the incidence of syringopleural shunts. Syringosubarachnoid shunts work best when oriented so that fluid drains dependently in the upright position.

Meticulous hemostasis is important because blood at the surgical site may result in accelerated scarring and obstruction of the shunt tubing postoperatively. After untethering surgeries, careful technique must be utilized to maintain patency of the dorsal meningeal leaflet; the use of expansile duraplasty techniques (e.g., regenerative tissue matrices) and dural tenting may be helpful to prevent retethering of the spinal cord after these surgeries.[88] After the initial shunting procedure, intraoperative ultrasonography is important to ensure that the entire cystic cavity is collapsed and that the shunt tubing is in good position. Electromyographic monitoring complements motor and somatosensory evoked response monitoring to warn of compromise of the spinal cord or nerve roots.

Results

A recent review of surgery, through various approaches and techniques, for syringomyelia found that the reported effectiveness of surgical intervention had not changed in the past 100 years (except for a reduction in the observed mortality rate), with 67% to 76% of patients improving neurologically postoperatively.[89] Barnett,[36] in contrast, reported that management of patients with arachnoiditis was unrewarding, whether medical or surgical therapy was attempted. He considered both steroids and lysis of adhesions to be ineffective in the treatment of this disorder.

A recent article by Falci and colleagues reported on a large surgical series of posttraumatic spinal cord tethering patients (many with syrinxes) at a single center over the course of 10 years.[90] Surgeries were performed by a single surgeon using a consistent technique of spinal cord detethering, expansile duraplasty, and, when indicated, cyst shunting. No significant change was noted on preoperative versus postoperative American Spinal Injury Association sensory and motor index scores; however, outcome questionnaires resulted in significant benefits of self-assessment of arrest of functional loss and improvement of motor or sensory complaints.

Although effective in a number of small surgical series, the placement of a syringoperitoneal or syringosubarachnoid shunt is of questionable value.[37,84,85,89,91,92] The optimal treatment and determination of the indications for surgery await further research with relevant experimental models and a well-designed, multicenter clinical trial.

Tables 94.1 and 94.2 list some of the major surgical series in treating noncommunicating syringomyelia, represented most prominently by posttraumatic syringomyelia, with lysis of adhesions and/or shunting of the syrinx. Overall, they show surgical treatment of posttraumatic syringomyelia to be of modest reward. Many patients show short-term recovery of neurologic function, only to deteriorate again in long-term follow-up.

Indirect Approach to Communicating Syringomyelia

Methods

Gardner championed a new approach to the patient with a posterior fossa herniation (Chiari I malformation) on the basis of his hydrodynamic theory of syringomyelia formation.[22] The operation advocated for a suboccipital craniectomy for decompression of the cerebellar tonsillar herniation and closure of the communication between the syrinx and the fourth ventricle by plugging the obex with a piece of muscle.

Others have questioned the necessity and advisability of using an obex plug. Batzdorf argued that a plug in the obex was not necessary and potentially blocked a drainage path for the syrinx following bony decompression at the skull base and expansile duraplasty.[93,94] In addition, he advocated a limited suboccipital craniectomy to prevent downward herniation of the cerebellar tonsils postoperatively.

Tonsillar resection has been proposed as a useful adjunct to foramen magnum decompression to obtain simultaneous restoration of free CSF flow at the foramen of Magendie, hindbrain decompression, and relief of the "pistonlike" action of the tonsils. Several important issues aiming at prevention of postoperative arachnoiditis are as follows: (1) meticulous dissection of the pia mater covering the tonsils from the arachnoid layer, (2) subpial aspiration of the tonsils using the ultrasonic aspirator and creating a wide aperture in the lower fourth ventricle, and (3) suture of the arachnoid and duraplasty using a pericranial graft.[95,96] However, one study found that none of the patients who had coagulation of the tonsils showed clinical improvement versus 77% of patients without tonsillar manipulation.[27]

The majority of syrinxes associated with hindbrain malformations are not communicating but are isolated both rostrally and caudally by central canal stenosis. A posterior decompression alone may not effectively treat the syrinxes. An additional drainage-type procedure may be effective in these specific cases.[97–99] A long-term follow-up study (median, 88 months) by Aghakhani and colleagues followed 157 surgically treated patients with Chiari I malformation and syringomyelia.[100] More than 90% of the individuals showed improvement or stabilization in both clinical grade and syrinx size following surgery. Clinical worsening was more likely with greater age, increased syrinx size, severe motor deficits, or arachnoiditis at diagnosis.

The main objective in the surgical treatment of Chiari I malformation and related syringomyelia is to restore normal CSF dynamics at the craniovertebral junction by posterior fossa decompression. However, this decompression should be small enough to avoid downward migration of the hindbrain into the craniectomy defect. Current techniques to achieve these goals include not only posterior fossa decompression but also posterior fossa reconstruction.[101,102] Intraoperative monitoring of CSF flow dynamics through ultrasound or intraoperative MRI have been proposed to evaluate the degree of posterior fossa decompression and restoration of CSF flow. However, recently, it has been demonstrated that ultrasound and intraoperative MRI are limited in their ability to detect changes intraoperatively.[103]

One study questioned the need for early interventional surgery for incidentally identified syringomyelia associated with Chiari I malformations.[104] The long-term clinical courses of patients with asymptomatic, incidentally identified syringomyelia associated with Chiari I malformation were observed to be benign. The study concluded that unless changes in neurologic or MRI findings are detected, early interventional surgery is not necessary.

Results

Table 94.3 lists some of the large surgical series in treating communicating syringomyelia, represented by syringomyelia associated with Chiari I malformations. Overall, these studies show that posterior fossa decompression and/or reconstruction through a variety of techniques leads to effective neurologic improvement or halting of neurologic deterioration in 60% to 90% of cases.

Because substantial differences among the reported methods advocated by groups treating syringomyelia continue, a multicenter clinical trial must be organized before optimal treatment can be established.[89]

Conclusion

Although technological advances in noninvasive imaging methods have improved the ability to diagnose syringomyelia, effective therapy for these lesions has not similarly evolved. The accumulated experience of surgical therapy for these lesions has affirmed that the use of a foreign body (shunt tube) is not optimal and that reinsertion of the shunt or the lysis of adhesions frequently causes the production of additional scar tissue. On the other hand, surgical treatment of communicating syringomyelia associated with Chiari malformations, like its pathophysiology, is more established and better understood, leading to more rewarding surgical results and clinical outcomes. The research laboratory holds the key to the ultimate solution for the problem of syringomyelia.

PEARLS

1. MRI is the diagnostic test of choice for syringomyelia. Fast spin-echo techniques increase the amount of information culled from T2-weighted information in the presence of metallic artifact. Cine MRI sequences may provide valuable additional information regarding alterations in CSF flow dynamics.
2. Shunting and/or stenting of intramedullary cysts should always proceed from the caudal end, the tube directed rostral.
3. Expansile duraplasty with cadaveric dural allograft or an alternatively equivalent dural substitute is necessary to reconstruct the subarachnoid space and create an environment in which the spinal cord is less likely to tether dorsally.
4. Real-time intraoperative ultrasonography with sagittal and axial images is useful in ensuring that the entire cyst cavity is collapsed and the shunt tube is in good position.
5. For long cervicothoracic cysts or multilobulated complex cysts, the possibility exists that a single tube will not traverse the entire cyst. In these instances, more than one catheter may be necessary.
6. Postoperative positioning in a prone or semiprone posture while a patient is in bed for the first 30 days following an untethering surgery may lessen the possibility of retethering.
7. Preoperative placement of a lumbar or C12 subarachnoid drain for 3 to 5 days of postoperative CSF diversion may lessen the chance of a pseudomeningocele or postoperative CSF leak.
8. If during a spinal cord untethering procedure it is noted that the dura is densely adherent to a dorsal or dorsolateral area of spinal cord, it is preferable to cut around this area, leaving a free island of dura attached to the spinal cord rather than risking parenchymal damage.

PITFALLS

1. The optimum treatment for syrinxes is yet to be determined.
2. Lysis of adhesions and/or the placement of a syringoperitoneal or syringosubarachnoid shunt are of questionable value in cases of idiopathic or posttraumatic syrinxes; in contrast, posterior fossa decompression for Chiari I malformation has excellent success in treating communicating syrinxes.
3. Development of syringomyelia after surgery for a spinal tumor may account for delayed neurologic deterioration in some patients.
4. Dense arachnoiditis may preclude the use of a dorsal syringosubarachnoid shunt; in this case, the distal catheter may

TABLE 94.3 Surgical Series Reporting Results of Procedures on Chiari Malformations/Communicating Syringomyelia

Reference	No. Patients	Procedure	Follow-up	Clinical Results
Paul et al.[114] (1983)	71	Suboccipital craniectomy + C1–C3 laminectomy + duraplasty	4 y (range, 6 mo–9 y)	82% with early improvement, dropping to 61% at late follow-up
Pillay et al.[115] (1991)	35	31 posterior fossa decompression + plugging of obex; 2 posterior fossa decompression + syringosubarachnoid shunt; 2 syringosubarachnoid shunt only; 1 transoral resection of dens	3.4 y (average)	63% improvement; 31% unchanged; 6% deteriorated
Menezes et al.[116] (1991)	131	Posterior fossa decompression + fourth ventricle to subarachnoid shunt + plugging of obex	NA	85% improvement
Hida et al.[117] (1995)	70	33 foramen magnum decompression; 37 syringosubarachnoid shunting only	60 mo (range, 6 mo–12.5 y)	82% improvement in foramen magnum decompression group; 97% improvement in syringosubarachnoid shunt group
Guyotat et al.[96] (1998)	75	42 foramen magnum decompression; 16 foramen magnum decompression with third ventricle shunting; 9 foramen magnum decompression with syringosubarachnoid shunting; 8 foramen magnum decompression with tonsillar resection	52 mo (average)	47% improvement; 24.2% stabilization; 25.7% deterioration; 3% death
Hida et al.[118] (1999)	16 (pediatric)	7 foramen magnum decompression; 9 syringosubarachnoid shunting only	73 mo (range, 13–136 mo)	88–90% improved; 10–12% unchanged; 0% worsened
Blagodatsky et al.[119] (1999)	102	44 Gardner operation; 11 Gardner operation with tonsillar resection; 32 craniocervical reconstruction with syringotomy and ventriculosubarachnoid shunt; 15 Gardner operation with syringotomy	4.6 y (range, 2–8 y)	67.6% improvement; 20% stabilization; 9.8% deterioration
Sakamoto et al.[102] (1999)	43	20 expansile suboccipital cranioplasty + plugging of obex; 20 expansile suboccipital cranioplasty; 4[a] expansile suboccipital cranioplasty + intraarachnoid procedure	NA	91% improvement; 9% unchanged; 0% deteriorated
Depreitere et al.[120] (2000)	22	Suboccipital craniectomy + C1 laminectomy + C2–C3 laminectomy + tonsillar coagulation	Early: 56 days (average); late: 18 mo (range, 4–42 mo)	76% improvement in early follow-up, dropping to 68% improvement in late follow-up; 26% deterioration in late follow-up
Goel et al.[121] (2000)	145	31 posterior fossa decompression; 21 posterior fossa decompression + duraplasty; 83 posterior fossa decompression + syringosubarachnoid shunt/ thecoperitoneal shunt; 7 syringosubarachnoid/ thecoperitoneal shunt only; 3 transoral surgery	NA	76% improvement; 18% no change; 5% worsening
Sindou et al.[73] (2002)	44	Craniocervical decompression with extreme lateral resection of posterior rim of foramen magnum and expansile duraplasty with arachnoid preservation	4 y (range, 13 mo–10 yr)	82% resume normal life; 18% did not return to full work and/or a completely normal life
Asgari et al.[122] (2003)	31	Suboccipital craniectomy + duraplasty + tonsillar coagulation + C1 laminectomy + C2 laminectomy	35 mo (range, 6–60 mo)	42% improvement; 42% unchanged; 16% deteriorated
Dones et al.[123] (2003)	27	Suboccipital craniectomy + laminectomy + syringosubarachnoid shunt + duraplasty	52 mo (range, 3–138 mo)	0-75% improvement
Navarro et al.[124] (2004)	96 (110 procedures)	71 posterior fossa decompression; 38 posterior fossa decompression + duraplasty + tonsillectomy; 1 transoral odontoidectomy	2.3 y (range, 0.17–9.8 y)	68–72% success (dropping to 61% if tonsillectomy by thermal shrinkage was performed)
Arruda et al.[125] (2004)	60	Craniovertebral decompression + tonsillectomy + duraplasty	At least 6 mo	45–60% improvement

[a]One patient with recurrent syringomyelia after other procedure.
NA, not available.

need to be placed in the ventral subarachnoid space, pleural cavity, or peritoneum.

5. Demyelinating diseases (multiple sclerosis, amyotrophic lateral sclerosis), vitamin B_{12} deficiency, tabes dorsalis, apoptosis from a post-poliolike syndrome, and cervical myelopathy from spondylosis and stenosis are difficult to differentiate clinically from a syringomyelic process.

KEY POINTS

1. Two types of syringomyelia exist: communicating and noncommunicating.
2. Surgical treatment of communicating syringomyelia associated with Chiari malformations is more established and the pathophysiology better understood.

3. Ependymomas and hemangioblastomas are the most common tumor types to be associated with syrinxes.
4. Approximately 4% to 10% of patients suffering a traumatic spinal cord injury develop progressive spinal cord dysfunction associated with an expanding syrinx.
5. Cine MRI is a real-time, motion picture–like analysis of spinal fluid flow dynamics in and around the spinal cord cyst.

KEY REFERENCES

1. Gardner WJ. Anatomic anomalies common to myelomeningocele of infancy and syringomyelia of adulthood suggest a common origin. *Cleve Clin Q.* 1959;26:118-133.
   Gardner's publication was a classic paper and the first of the three prominent theories to survive to modern clinical practice.
2. Williams B. On the pathogenesis of syringomyelia: a review. *J R Soc Med.* 1980;73:798-806.
   Wlliams' theory on the pathogenesis of syringomyelia challenged the original concepts brought about by Gardner.
3. Oldfield EH, Muraszko K, Shawker TH, Patronas NJ. Pathophysiology of syringomyelia associated with Chiari I malformation of the cerebellar tonsils. Implications for diagnosis and treatment. *J Neurosurg.* 1994;80:3-15.
   Oldfield, using intraoperative ultrasound techniques, revealed that an abnormal pulse wave was created in the spinal subarachnoid space, potentially creating enlargement of a cystic syringomyelic cavity.
4. Falci S, Charlotte I, Lammertse D. Posttraumatic spinal cord tethering and syringomyelia: surgical treatment and long-term outcome. *J Neurosurg Spine.* 2009;11:445-460.
   This paper reported on a large surgical series of posttraumatic spinal cord tethering patients (many with syrinxes) at a single center over the course of 10 years.
5. Schurch B, Wichmann W, Rossier AB. Posttraumatic syringomyelia (cystic myelopathy): a prospective study of 449 patients with spinal cord injury. *J Neurol Neurosurg Psychiatry.* 1996;60:61.
   This is a large, prospective series on 449 patients with spinal cord injury, 20 of whom (4.45%) were diagnosed with posttraumatic syringomyelia. The authors followed the clinical course of this group (10 remained stable, while 10 clinically worsened).

REFERENCES

1. Finlayson A. Syringomyelia and related conditions. In: Joynt RJ, ed. *Clinical Neurology*. Vol. 3. Philidelphia: JB Lipincott; 1989.
2. Williams B. Progress in syringomyelia. *Neurol Res.* 1986;8(3):130-145.
3. Ballantine HT, Ojemann RG, Drew JH. Syringohydromyelia. In: Krayenbuhl H, Maspes PE, Sweet WH, eds. *Progress in Neurological Surgery*. S. Karger AG; 1971:227-245.
4. Hoffman HJ, Neill J, Crone KR, Hendrick BE, Humphreys RP. Hydrosyringomyelia and its management in childhood. *Neurosurgery*. 1987;21(3):347-351.
5. Barnett HJ. The epilogue. In: Barnett HJ, Foster JB, Hudson P, eds. *Syringomyelia. Major Problems in Neurology*. Philidelphia: WB Saunders; 1973:302-313.
6. Milhorat TH, Johnson RW, Milhorat RH, Capocelli AL, Pevsner PH. Clinicopathological correlations in syringomyelia using axial magnetic resonance imaging. *Neurosurgery*. 1995;37(2):206-213.
7. Milhorat TH, Johnson WD, Miller JI. Syrinx shunt to posterior fossa cisterns (syringocisternostomy) for bypassing obstructions of upper cervical theca. *J Neurosurg.* 1992;77(6):871-874.
8. Milhorat TH, Johnson WD, Miller JI, Bergland RM, Hollenberg-Sher J. Surgical treatment of syringomyelia based on magnetic resonance imaging criteria. *Neurosurgery*. 1992;31(2):231-245.
9. Milhorat TH, Kotzen RM, Anzil AP. Stenosis of central canal of spinal cord in man: incidence and pathological findings in 232 autopsy cases. *J Neurosurg.* 1994;80(4):716-722.
10. Milhorat TH, Miller JI, Johnson WD, Adler DE, Heger IM. Anatomical basis of syringomyelia occurring with hindbrain lesions. *Neurosurgery*. 1993;32(5):748-754.
11. Milhorat TH, Nobandegani F, Miller JI, Rao C. Noncommunicating syringomyelia following occlusion of central canal in rats. *J Neurosurg.* 1993;78(2):274-279.
12. Oldfield EH, Muraszko K, Shawker TH, Patronas NJ. Pathophysiology of syringomyelia associated with Chiari I malformation of the cerebellar tonsils. *J Neurosurg.* 1994;80(1):3-15.
13. Milhorat TH, Capocelli AL, Anzil AP, Kotzen RM, Milhorat RH. Pathological basis of spinal cord cavitation in syringomyelia: analysis of 105 autopsy cases. *J Neurosurg.* 1995;82(5):802-812.
14. Tamaki K. Pathogenesis of syringomyelia. *Arch Neurol Psychiatry*. 1938;40(4):748.
15. Poser C. *The Relationship Between Syringomyelia and Neoplasm*. Springfield, IL: Charles C. Thomas; 1956.
16. Mackay RP. Syringomyelia and intramedullary tumor of the spinal cord. *Arch Neurol Psychiatry*. 1935;33(6):1255.
17. Gardner WJ. Anatomic anomalies common to myelomeningocele of infancy and syringomyelia of adulthood suggest a common origin. *Cleve Clin J Med.* 1959;26(3):118-133.
18. Gardner WJ. Diastematomyelia and the Klippel-Feil syndrome: relationship to hydrocephalus, syringomyelia, meningocele, meningomyelocele, and iniencephalus. *Cleve Clin J Med.* 1964;31(1):19-44.
19. Gardner WJ. Hydrodynamic mechanism of syringomyelia: its relationship to myelocele. *J Neurol Neurosurg Psychiatry*. 1965;28(3):247-259.
20. Gardner WJ. Myelocele: rupture of the neural tube? *Clin Neurosurg.* 1968;15:57-79.
21. Gardner WJ, Abdullah AF, McCormack LJ. The varying expressions of embryonal atresia of the fourth ventricle in adults. *J Neurosurg.* 1957;14(6):591-607.
22. Gardner WJ, Angel J. The cause of syringomyelia and its surgical treatment. *Cleve Clin J Med.* 1958;25(1):4-8.
23. Gardner WJ, Goodall RJ. The surgical treatment of Arnold-Chiari malformation in adults. *J Neurosurg.* 1950;7(3):199-206.
24. Gardner WJ, McMurray FG. "Non-communicating" syringomyelia: a non-existent entity. *Surg Neurol.* 1976;6(4):251-256.
25. Griffiths ER, McCormick CC. Post-traumatic syringomyelia (cystic myelopathy). *Paraplegia*. 1981;19(2):81-88.
26. McLaurin RL, Bailey OT, Schurr PH, Ingraham FD. Myelomalacia and multiple cavitations of spinal cord secondary to adhesive arachnoiditis; an experimental study. *AMA Arch Pathol.* 1954;57(2):138-146.
27. Ball M, Dayan A. Pathogenesis of syringomyelia. *Lancet*. 1972;300(7781):799-801.
28. West RJ, Williams B. Radiographic studies of the ventricles in syringomyelia. *Neuroradiology*. 1980;20(1):5-16.
29. Williams B. On the pathogenesis of syringomyelia: a review. *J R Soc Med.* 1980;73(11):798-806.

30. Appleby A, Bradley WG, Foster JB, Hankinson J, Hudgson P. Syringomyelia due to chronic arachnoiditis at the foramen magnum. *J Neurol Sci*. 1969;8(3):451-464.
31. Caplan LR, Norohna AB, Amico LL. Syringomyelia and arachnoiditis. *J Neurol Neurosurg Psychiatry*. 1990;53(2):106-113.
32. Liber AF, Lisa JR. Rosenthal fibers in non-neoplastic syringomyelia. *J Nerv Ment Dis*. 1937;86(5):549-558.
33. Nelson J. Intramedullary cavitation resulting from adhesive spinal arachnoiditis. *Arch Neurol Psychiatry*. 1943;50(1):1.
34. Williams B. The distending force in the production of "communicating syringomyelia". *Lancet*. 1969;294(7613):189-193.
35. Chang HS. Theoretical analysis of the pathophysiology of syringomyelia associated with adhesive arachnoiditis. *J Neurol Neurosurg Psychiatry*. 2004;75(5):754-757.
36. Barnett HJ. Syringomyelia associated with spinal arachnoiditis. In: Barnett HJ, Foster JB, Hudgson P, eds. *Syringomyelia. Major Problems in Neurology*. Philadelphia: WB Saunders; 1973:220-244.
37. Koyanagi I, Iwasaki Y, Hida K, Houkin K. Clinical features and pathomechanisms of syringomyelia associated with spinal arachnoiditis. *Surg Neurol*. 2005;63(4):350-355.
38. Chang HS, Tsuchiya T, Fujisawa N, Oya S, Matsui T. Syringomyelia associated with arachnoid septum at the craniovertebral junction, contradicting the currently prevailing theory of syringomyelia formation. *Acta Neurochir (Wien)*. 2012;154(1):141-145.
39. McCormick PC. Dorsal arachnoid web. *Neurosurg Focus*. 2014;37(suppl 2):Video 8.
40. Barnett HJ, Rewcastle N. Syringomyelia and tumors of the nervous system. In: Barnett HJ, Foster JB, Hudgson P, eds. *Syringomyelia, Major Problems in Neurology*. Philadelphia: WB Saunders; 1973:261-301.
41. Feigin I, Ogata JUN, Budzilovich G. Syringomyelia. *J Neuropathol Exp Neurol*. 1971;30(2):216-232.
42. Russell DS. Capillary hæmangeioma of spinal cord associated with syringomyelia. *J Pathol*. 1932;35(1):103-112.
43. Ferry DJ, Hardman JM, Earle KM. Syringomyelia and intramedullary neoplasms. *Med Ann Dist Columbia*. 1969;38(7):363-365.
44. Peerless SJ, Durward QJ. Management of syringomyelia: a pathophysiological approach. *Clin Neurosurg*. 1983;30:531-576.
45. Sloof J, Kernohan J, MacCarty C. *Primary Intramedullary Tumors of the Spinal Cord and Filum Terminale*. Philadelphia: WB Saunders; 1964.
46. Conway LW. Hydrodynamic studies in syringomyelia. *J Neurosurg*. 1967;27(6):501-514.
47. Rossier AB, Foo D, Shillito J, Dyro FM. Posttraumatic cervical syringomyelia. *Brain*. 1985;108(2):439-461.
48. Samii M, Klekamp J. Surgical results of 100 intramedullary tumors in relation to accompanying syringomyelia. *Neurosurgery*. 1994;35(5):865-873.
49. Hida K, Iwasaki Y, Imamura H, Abe H. Posttraumatic syringomyelia. *Neurosurgery*. 1994;35(5):886-891.
50. Schurch B, Wichmann W, Rossier AB. Post-traumatic syringomyelia (cystic myelopathy): a prospective study of 449 patients with spinal cord injury. *J Neurol Neurosurg Psychiatry*. 1996;60(1):61-67.
51. Awai L, Curt A. Preserved sensory-motor function despite large-scale morphological alterations in a series of patients with holocord syringomyelia. *J Neurotrauma*. 2015;32(6):403-410.
52. Cushing HW. Hematomyelia from gunshot wounds of the spine. *Am J Med Sci*. 1898;115(6):654-682.
53. Fairholm DJ, Turnbull IM. Microangiographic study of experimental spinal cord injuries. *J Neurosurg*. 1971;35(3):277-286.
54. Holmes G. The Goulstonian Lectures on spinal injuries of warfare: delivered before the Royal College of Physicians of London. *BMJ*. 1915;2(2865):769-774.
55. Kao CC, Chang LW. The mechanism of spinal cord cavitation following spinal cord transection. *J Neurosurg*. 1977;46(2):197-209.
56. Kao CC, Chang LW, Bloodworth JMB. The mechanism of spinal cord cavitation following spinal cord transection. *J Neurosurg*. 1977;46(6):757-766.
57. Mair WGP, Druckman R. The pathology of spinal cord lesions and their relation to the clinical features in protrusion of cervical intervertebral discs (a report of four cases). *Brain*. 1953;76(1):70-91.
58. McVeigh JF. Experimental cord crushes. *Arch Surg*. 1923;7(3):573.
59. Wolman L. The disturbance of circulation in traumatic paraplegia in acute and late stages: a pathological study. *Paraplegia*. 1965;2(4):213-226.
60. Woodard JS, Freeman LW. Ischemia of the spinal cord. *J Neurosurg*. 1956;13(1):63-72.
61. Barbaro NM, Wilson CB, Gutin PH, Edwards MSB. Surgical treatment of syringomyelia. *J Neurosurg*. 1984;61(3):531-538.
62. Stoodley MA, Jones NR, Brown CJ. Evidence for rapid fluid flow from the subarachnoid space into the spinal cord central canal in the rat. *Brain Res*. 1996;707(2):155-164.
63. Williams B. Simultaneous cerebral and spinal fluid pressure recordings. *Acta Neurochir (Wien)*. 1981;59(1-2):123-142.
64. Asano M, Fujiwara K, Yonenobu K, Hiroshima K. Post-traumatic syringomyelia. *Spine*. 1996;21(12):1446-1453.
65. Dyste GN, Menezes AH, VanGilder JC. Symptomatic Chiari malformations. *J Neurosurg*. 1989;71(2):159-168.
66. Hall PV, Lindseth RE, Campbell RL, Kalsbeck JE. Myelodysplasia and developmental scoliosis. *Spine*. 1976;1(1):48-56.
67. Schlesinger EB, Antunes JL, Michelsen WJ, Louis KM. Hydromyelia. *Neurosurgery*. 1981;9(4):356-365.
68. Zager EL, Ojemann RG, Poletti CE. Acute presentations of syringomyelia. *J Neurosurg*. 1990;72(1):133-138.
69. Boman K, Iivanainen M. Prognosis of syringomyelia. *Acta Neurol Scand*. 1967;43(1):61-68.
70. Seki T, Fehlings MG. Mechanistic insights into posttraumatic syringomyelia based on a novel in vivo animal model. *J Neurosurg Spine*. 2008;8(4):365-375.
71. Honan WP, Williams B. Sensory loss in syringomyelia: not necessarily dissociated. *J R Soc Med*. 1993;86(9):519-520.
72. Pojunas K, Williams AL, Daniels DL, Haughton VM. Syringomyelia and hydromyelia: magnetic resonance evaluation. *Radiology*. 1984;153(3):679-683.
73. Sindou M, Chávez-Machuca J, Hashish H. Cranio-cervical decompression for Chiari type I-malformation, adding extreme lateral foramen magnum opening and expansile duroplasty with arachnoid preservation. Technique and long-term functional results in 44 consecutive adult cases—comparison with literature data. *Acta Neurochir (Wien)*. 2002;144(10):1005-1019.
74. Li AE, Wilkinson MD, McGrillen KM, Stoodley MA, Magnussen JS. Clinical applications of cine balanced

steady-state free precession MRI for the evaluation of the subarachnoid spaces. *Clin Neuroradiol.* 2015;25(4):349-360.

75. McGirt MJ, Nimjee SM, Fuchs HE, George TM. Relationship of cine phase-contrast magnetic resonance imaging with outcome after decompression for Chiari I malformations. *Neurosurgery.* 2006;59(1):140-146.
76. Wang CS, Wang X, Fu CH, et al. Analysis of cerebrospinal fluid flow dynamics and morphology in Chiari I malformation with cine phase-contrast magnetic resonance imaging. *Acta Neurochir (Wien).* 2014;156(4):707-713.
77. Steinmetz AP, Aschoff A, Kunze S. The iatrogenic tethering of the cord. *Acta Neurochir (Wien).* 1993;123(219).
78. Roser F, Ebner FH, Liebsch M, Dietz K, Tatagiba M. A new concept in the electrophysiological evaluation of syringomyelia. *J Neurosurg Spine.* 2008;8(6):517-523.
79. Roser F, Ebner FH, Sixt C, Hagen JM, Tatagiba MS. Defining the line between hydromyelia and syringomyelia. A differentiation is possible based on electrophysiological and magnetic resonance imaging studies. *Acta Neurochir (Wien).* 2009;152(2):213-219.
80. Nakamura M, Ishii K, Watanabe K, et al. Clinical significance and prognosis of idiopathic syringomyelia. *J Spinal Disord Tech.* 2009;22(5):372-375.
81. Abbe R, Coley WB. Syringo-myelia, operation-exploration of cord-withdraw of fluid-exhibition of patient. *J Nerv Ment Dis.* 1892;19(512).
82. Quencer RM, Morse BM, Green BA, Eismont FJ, Brost P. Intraoperative spinal sonography: adjunct to metrizamide CT in the assessment and surgical decompression of posttraumatic spinal cord cysts. *AJR Am J Roentgenol.* 1984;142(3):593-601.
83. Freeman LW. Ascending spinal paralysis. *J Neurosurg.* 1959;16(1):120-122.
84. Sgouros S, Williams B. A critical appraisal of drainage in syringomyelia. *J Neurosurg.* 1995;82(1):1-10.
85. Sgouros S, Williams B. Management and outcome of posttraumatic syringomyelia. *J Neurosurg.* 1996;85(2):197-205.
86. Edgar R, Quail P. Progressive post-traumatic cystic and non-cystic myelopathy. *Br J Neurosurg.* 1994;8(1):7-22.
87. Frazier CH. Shall syringomyelia be added to the lesions appropriate for surgical intervention? *JAMA.* 1930;95(25):1911.
88. Klekamp J. Treatment of syringomyelia related to nontraumatic arachnoid pathologies of the spinal canal. *Neurosurgery.* 2013;72(3):376-389.
89. Aschoff A, Donahuer E, Huwel N. Evaluation of syrinx-surgery: a critical comment in requirements for reliable follow up studies. *Acta Neurochir (Wien).* 1993;123(224).
90. Falci SP, Indeck C, Lammertse DP. Posttraumatic spinal cord tethering and syringomyelia: surgical treatment and long-term outcome. *J Neurosurg Spine.* 2009;11(4):445-460.
91. Padovani R, Cavallo M, Gaist G. Surgical treatment of syringomyelia: favorable results with syringosubarachnoid shunting. *Surg Neurol.* 1989;32(3):173-180.
92. Suzuki M, Davis C, Symon L, Gentili F. Syringoperitoneal shunt for treatment of cord cavitation. *J Neurol Neurosurg Psychiatry.* 1985;48(7):620-627.
93. Batzdorf U. Chiari I malformation with syringomyelia. *J Neurosurg.* 1988;68(5):726-730.
94. Batzdorf U, Klekamp J, Johnson JP. A critical appraisal of syrinx cavity shunting procedures. *J Neurosurg.* 1998;89(3):382-388.
95. da Silva JA, Holanda MM. Basilar impression, Chiari malformation and syringomyelia: a retrospective study of 53 surgically treated patients. *Arq Neuropsiquiatr.* 2003;61(2B):368-375.
96. Guyotat J, Bret P, Jouanneau E, Ricci AC, Lapras C. Syringomyelia associated with type I chiari malformation a 21-year retrospective study on 75 cases treated by foramen magnum decompression with a special emphasis on the value of tonsils resection. *Acta Neurochir (Wien).* 1998;140(8):745-754.
97. Bejjani GK, Cockerham KP, Rothfus WE, Maroon JC, Maddock M. Treatment of failed adult Chiari malformation decompression with CSF drainage: observations in six patients. *Acta Neurochir (Wien).* 2003;145(2):107-116.
98. Logue V, Edwards MR. Syringomyelia and its surgical treatment—an analysis of 75 patients. *J Neurol Neurosurg Psychiatry.* 1981;44(4):273-284.
99. Rascher K, Donauer E. Experimental models of syringomyelia—personal observations and a brief look at earlier reports. *Acta Neurochir (Wien).* 1993;123(3-4):166-169.
100. Aghakhani N, Parker F, David P, et al. Long-term follow-up of Chiari-related syringomyelia in adults. *Neurosurgery.* 2009;64(2):308-315.
101. Sahuquillo J, Rubio E, Poca M-A, et al. Posterior fossa reconstruction. *Neurosurgery.* 1994;35(5):874-885.
102. Sakamoto H, Nishikawa M, Hakuba A, et al. Expansive suboccipital cranioplasty for the treatment of syringomyelia associated with Chiari malformation. *Acta Neurochir (Wien).* 1999;141(9):949-961.
103. Bond AE, Jane JA Sr, Liu KC, Oldfield EH. Changes in cerebrospinal fluid flow assessed using intraoperative MRI during posterior fossa decompression for Chiari malformation. *J Neurosurg.* 2015;122(5):1068-1075.
104. Nishizawa S, Yokoyama T, Yokota N, Tokuyama T, Ohta S. Incidentally identified syringomyelia associated with Chiari I malformations: is early interventional surgery necessary? *Neurosurgery.* 2001;49(3):637-641.
105. Tator CH, Meguro K, Rowed DW. Favorable results with syringosubarachnoid shunts for treatment of syringomyelia. *J Neurosurg.* 1982;56(4):517-523.
106. Schaller B, Mindermann T, Gratzl O. Treatment of syringomyelia after posttraumatic paraparesis or tetraparesis. *J Spinal Disord.* 1999;12(6):485-488.
107. Isik N, Elmaci I, Isik N, et al. Long-term results and complications of the syringopleural shunting for treatment of syringomyelia: a clinical study. *Br J Neurosurg.* 2013;27(1):91-99.
108. Fan T, Zhao X, Zhao H, et al. Treatment of selected syringomyelias with syringo-pleural shunt: the experience with a consecutive 26 cases. *Clin Neurol Neurosurg.* 2015;137:50-56.
109. Adelstein LJ. The surgical treatment of syringomyelia. *Am J Surg.* 1938;40(2):384-395.
110. Pitts FW, Groff RA. Syringomyelia: current status of surgical therapy. *Surgery.* 1964;56:806-809.
111. Love JG, Olafson RA. Syringomyelia: a look at surgical therapy. *J Neurosurg.* 1966;24(4):714-718.
112. Anderson NE, Willoughby EW, Wrightson P. The natural history and the influence of surgical treatment in syringomyelia. *Acta Neurol Scand.* 1985;71(6):472-479.
113. Lee TT, Alameda GJ, Camilo E, Green BA. Surgical treatment of post-traumatic myelopathy associated with syringomyelia. *Spine.* 2001;26(suppl):S119-S127.

114. Paul KS, Lye RH, Strang FA, Dutton J. Arnold-Chiari malformation. *J Neurosurg*. 1983;58(2):183-187.
115. Pillay PK, Awad IA, Little JR, Hahn JF. Symptomatic Chiari malformation in adults: a new classification based on magnetic resonance imaging with clinical and prognostic significance. *Neurosurgery*. 1991;28(5):639-645.
116. Menezes AH. Chiari I malformations and hydromyelia complications. *Pediatr Neurosurg*. 1991;17(3):146-154.
117. Hida K, Iwasaki Y, Koyanagi I, Sawamura Y, Abe H. Surgical indication and results of foramen magnum decompression versus syringosubarachnoid shunting for syringomyelia associated with Chiari I malformation. *Neurosurgery*. 1995;37(4):673-679.
118. Hida K, Iwasaki Y, Koyanagi I, Abe H. Pediatric syringomyelia with Chiari malformation: its clinical characteristics and surgical outcomes. *Surg Neurol*. 1999;51(4):383-391.
119. Blagodatsky MD, Larionov SN, Alexandrov YA, Velm AI. Surgical treatment of Chiari I malformation with or without syringomyelia. *Acta Neurochir (Wien)*. 1999;141(9):963-968.
120. Depreitere B, Van Calenbergh F, van Loon J, Goffin J, Plets C. Posterior fossa decompression in syringomyelia associated with a Chiari malformation: a retrospective analysis of 22 patients. *Clin Neurol Neurosurg*. 2000;102(2):91-96.
121. Goel A, Desai K. Surgery for syringomyelia: an analysis based on 163 surgical cases. *Acta Neurochir (Wien)*. 2000;142(3):293-302.
122. Asgari S, Engelhorn T, Bschor M, Sandalcioglu IE, Stolke D. Surgical prognosis in hindbrain related syringomyelia. *Acta Neurol Scand*. 2003;107(1):12-21.
123. Dones J, De Jesús O, Colen CB, Toledo MM, Delgado M. Clinical outcomes in patients with Chiari I malformation: a review of 27 cases. *Surg Neurol*. 2003;60(2):142-147.
124. Navarro R, Olavarria G, Seshadri R, et al. Surgical results of posterior fossa decompression for patients with Chiari I malformation. *Childs Nerv Syst*. 2004;20(5):349-356.
125. Arruda JA, Costa C, Tella OI Jr. Results of the treatment of syringomyelia associated with Chiari malformation: analysis of 60 cases. *Arq Neuropsiquiatr*. 2004;62(2a):237-244.

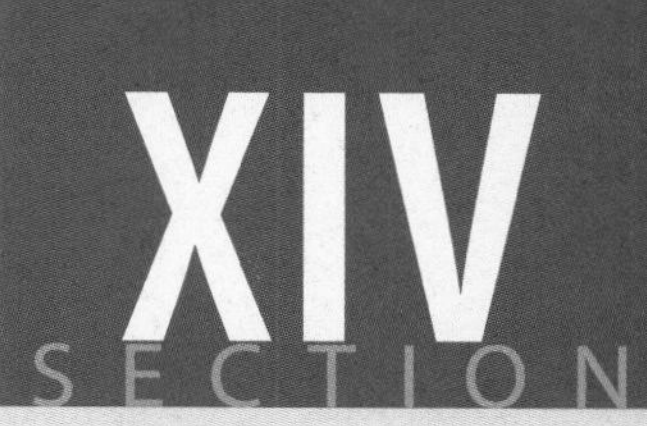

SECTION XIV

COMPLICATIONS OF SPINAL SURGERY

95 CHAPTER Intraoperative Spinal Cord and Nerve Root Injuries

Theodore D. Koreckij

Introduction

Neurologic injury is one of the most dreaded complications associated with spine surgery. Depending on the location, injury can be relatively minor (nerve root) to completely debilitating (spinal cord injury). Luckily, the frequency of devastating neurologic complication is rare. Nonetheless, increasing complexity of surgery is typically associated with increased risk of neurologic injury. Injury can occur at any stage in the operative procedure. Only with careful attention to detail can we hope to reduce risk.

In general, iatrogenic neurologic injury typically occurs either due to mechanical injury or secondary to ischemia. Mechanical injury can be caused by multiple mechanisms of compression. This compression can be the direct result of instrumentation either during decompression or by the malposition of a spinal implant (e.g., screw, cage). Additional compression could also be caused by an expanding postoperative hematoma or hemostatic agent. Another possible means of direct compression can occur as a result of deformity corrective measures resulting in neural element compression. Deformity correction can also result as a vascular occlusion via segmental artery thrombosis and subsequent spinal cord injury.

This chapter focuses on neurologic injuries associated with patient positioning, approach-related neurologic injuries, and those associated with common surgical techniques utilized within spine surgery. A separate section is devoted to discussion of iatrogenic neurologic injury in both pediatric and adult deformity correction surgery.

Preoperative Position

A chapter on discussion of intraoperative neurologic injury in spine surgery would not be complete without a discussion of injuries associated with patient positioning. As with any neurologic injury in surgery, incorrect patient positioning can result in a mechanical injury from direct pressure and/or ischemic insult due to prolonged hypothermia and controlled hypotension, as is frequently utilized in spine surgery.

The overall rate of neurologic injury from improper positioning from all surgery is estimated at 0.14%, with approximately 40% occurring in the brachial plexus.[1] Abduction of the upper limb in prone position to greater than 90 degrees can result in traction of the brachial plexus between the clavicle and first rib. The ulnar nerve can also be frequently affected if pressure is not offloaded at the elbow. Also at risk during prone positioning is the lateral femoral cutaneous nerve, with injury resulting in lateral thigh pain and paresthesias (meralgia paresthetica). In a prospective study of 105 patients undergoing elective spine procedures, injury to the lateral femoral cutaneous nerve was found in 20% of patients. In 89% of the patients, the nerve completely recovered within 3 months of surgery. Two patients still had pain and hypoesthesia of the anterolateral thigh 1 year after surgery.[2]

Visual field disturbance or loss is another feared neurologic injury that is attributed in part to patient positioning. The incidence of perioperative blindness has been reported at a rate between 0.05% and 1%.[3] Recovery is often limited, with a significant number of patients experiencing persistent significant visual loss. Perioperative blindness can be caused by cortical blindness, central retinal artery occlusion, and—from a neurologic standpoint—ischemic optic neuropathy, with the last being most commonly implicated. With ischemic optic neuropathy, several perioperative and intraoperative risk factors have been implicated, such as hemodilution, blood loss, facial edema, and surgical time. Preoperative medical comorbidities, such as diabetes and small vessel disease, also play a role.[4] Only very weak evidence is present in the literature to guide surgeons in prevention and treatment for it.

Cervical Spine Surgery

In the cervical spine, there exists a risk for both nerve root injury and spinal cord injury. The rates vary with the surgical approach utilized and whether instrumentation is performed.

Anterior Cervical Spine Surgery

Since Robinson and Smith first described the approach to the anterior cervical spine in 1955, anterior cervical surgery has become the preferred choice in the treatment of most cervical pathologies (Fig. 95.1). During the approach, the recurrent

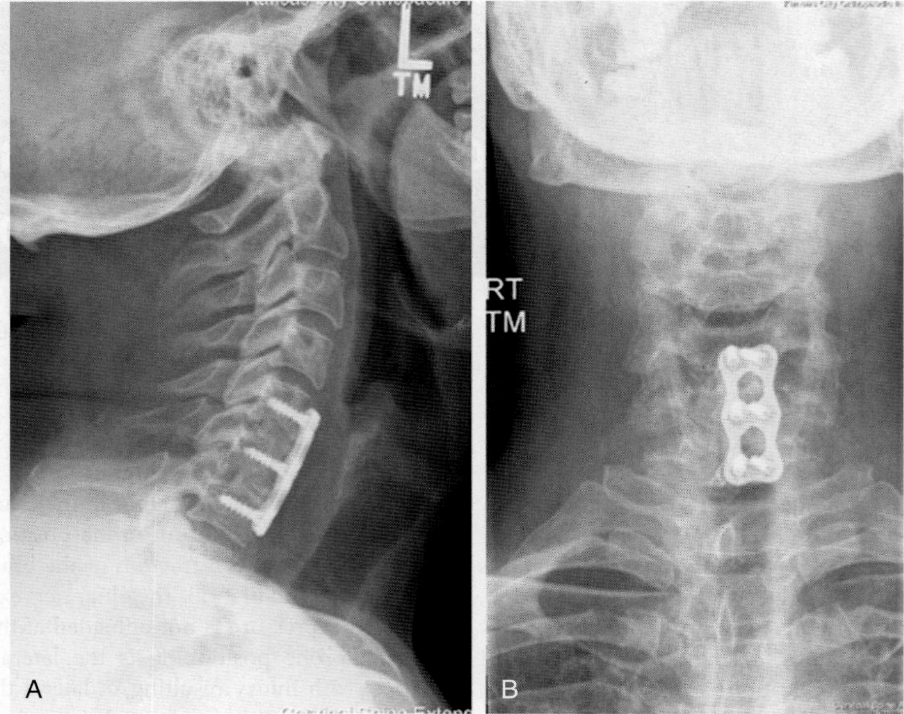

FIG. 95.1 Lateral (A) and anteroposterior (B) radiographs depicting two-level instrumented anterior cervical discectomy and fusion through the standard Smith-Robinson approach.

laryngeal nerve (RLN) is at risk in its path running between the esophagus and trachea, with injury resulting in unilateral vocal cord paralysis. The reported rates of RLN injury have ranged from 0.8% to as high as 11%.[5–7] It has been heavily debated regarding which is the appropriate side of neck to approach the cervical spine. Various reasons for a surgeon to choose one side over another include surgeon comfort and previous neck surgery, while some have cited anatomic considerations.[8] Classic anatomic teaching has shown that the left recurrent laryngeal nerve traverses in a more midline course and is less likely to be encountered in a left-sided approach compared to a right-sided approach, where it travels in a more lateral course on its path to the tracheoesophageal groove. Beutler et al. compared a consecutive series of 328 anterior cervical spine fusion procedures, 173 procedures completed from the right side and 155 completed from the left.[9] The overall incidence of RLN injury was 2.1%. The incidence of RLN injury with reoperative anterior cervical fusion surgery was 9.5%. They reported no difference in incidence of RLN injury with the side of surgical approach and surmised that the surgeon may safely approach the cervical spine from the side of personal preference and experience.

Another neurologic structure at risk during the anterior approach to the cervical spine is the sympathetic chain. It is found between the posterior lateral pharyngeal and carotid regions. The cervical sympathetic chain comprises three ganglia. The superior ganglion is at C2–C3; the middle ganglion is adjacent to C6; and the stellate ganglion lies in the costotransversopleural fossa.[10] Damage to the sympathetic chain, the stellate ganglion in particular, can result in Horner syndrome. Horner syndrome is characterized by the classic triad of miosis, partial ptosis, and loss of hemifacial sweating. It has a reported incidence between 0.2% and 4%.[11–13] Resolution typically occurs over several weeks to 1 month. Raising the medial edge of the longus colli muscle without excessive traction is the key to prevention.

The most dreaded complication in cervical spine surgery is injury to the spinal cord itself. Fortunately, the reported incidence is quite low, with a reported rate of less than 1%.[14–16] In a 1989 survey of members of the Scoliosis Research Society, rates of spinal cord injury following anterior cervical surgery were lower than those reported with posterior procedures.[17] Preoperative neurologic status and reason for surgery play a clear role in risk of injury. Myelopathic patients appear to be the most at risk, not surprisingly, as there is little room for error during canal decompression. In a study of over 1000 patients, Fountas et al. reported a worsening of myelopathy in 3 patients (0.2%).[18]

The most common reason to perform anterior cervical surgery is recalcitrant radicular pain. Unfortunately, worsening radiculopathy is a known complication following anterior cervical surgery. In a series of 450 consecutive cases of cervical discectomy without fusion, a worsening radiculopathy was noticed in 1.3% of patients.[13] In a single surgeon's experience of over 1500 cases of discectomy with fusion, a worsening radiculopathy at the index level of operation occurred in 14 patients (0.88%).[19]

The most common worsening radiculopathy following cervical surgery is a C5 palsy. More often associated with posterior cervical surgeries, there are reports of C5 palsy following anterior cervical surgery, most commonly following cervical corpectomy. Saunders et al. reported one case of C5 palsy in a retrospective review of 40 patients undergoing multilevel corpectomies.[12] Wada et al. found a slightly higher rate of 4% with an average of 2.5 levels of corpectomy.[20] In a retrospective series of 563 anterior cervical surgeries, Ikenaga and colleagues reported a 3.25% incidence of C5 palsy, all occurring in patients with opacification of posterior longitudinal ligament or suffering from cervical spondylotic myelopathy.[21]

Posterior Cervical Spine Surgery

There are several types of posterior cervical surgery. Some of the more commonly used posterior cervical procedures include posterior foraminotomy, laminoplasty, laminectomy, and laminectomy with fusion and instrumentation.

The rate of neurologic injury following posterior foraminotomy is very low. In a retrospective review of 95 operative levels, Skovrj et al. reported one case of radiculitis.[22] Jagannathan et al. report a 1.2% incidence of neurologic injury, all cases being a C5 palsy following a C4–C5 foraminotomy.[23] Grieve et al. reported a slightly higher incidence of worsening radiculopathy after surgery (7%) in 77 patients undergoing one-level posterior foraminotomies.[24] There were no cases of spinal cord injury reported in these studies. The complication profile of this procedure will be at the forefront of discussions due to renewed interest in the technique given the development of minimally invasive access and concern for adjacent-level disease with anterior cervical discectomy and fusion.

Laminoplasty and laminectomy are both widely used procedures to address multilevel spinal stenosis and myelopathy. The most commonly encountered neurologic complication is a C5 palsy. A large systematic review of over 103 studies and over more than 8500 patients looking specifically at the rate of C5 palsy during laminoplasty found that 16% of the studies reported a C5 palsy rate of greater than 10% (534 patients), 41% reported a rate of 5% to 10% (1006 patients), 23% reported a rate of 1% to 5% (857 patients), and 12.5% reported a rate of 0% (168 patients).[25] Another review specifically addressing the rate of C5 palsy with various techniques of posterior cervical surgery showed an overall incidence of 5.8%. The incidence after open-door laminoplasty, double-door laminoplasty, and laminectomy was 4.5%, 3.1%, and 11.3%, respectively.[26] In a systematic review comparing laminectomy versus laminoplasty for cervical spondylotic myelopathy, C5 paresis was found in 9 of 176 (5.11%) patients treated with laminoplasty and 12 of 157 (7.64%) patients treated with laminectomy with no significant difference found between the rates of injury.[27]

Despite the well-known risk of C5 palsy following cervical decompression, there is no definitive explanation for why it occurs. Its presentation after surgery can appear acutely or in a delayed fashion, occurring up to 2 months after the index procedure.[28] It will manifest clinically as deltoid weakness and potential biceps weakness with sensory loss. It typically presents unilaterally; on rare instances, however, bilateral paresis is apparent. Aside from actual iatrogenic mechanical injury to the nerve during surgery, several other causes have been reported in the literature. Tethering of the nerve results from shifting of the spinal cord,[29] spinal cord ischemia,[30] and reperfusion injury of the spinal cord.[31] Intraoperative spinal cord monitoring (discussed in further detail elsewhere in this text) has been shown to be a valuable tool for intraoperative detection of impending C5 palsy.[32] However, not all cases of C5 palsy are detected intraoperatively with monitoring, which supports the theory that some cases of C5 palsy occur after surgery is complete.[33]

The addition of instrumentation to spine surgery increases the rate of a number of complications. Theoretically, too long a screw placed through an anterior cervical plate could result in neurologic injury by direct spinal cord compression; no literature could be found describing this complication as yet.

However, the use of lateral mass fixation in posterior cervical surgery has been reported in multiple studies as a cause of iatrogenic neurologic injury (Fig. 95.2). Lateral mass screws are frequently used to augment posterior fusion techniques. Although not currently Food and Drug Administration (FDA)-approved for this application, lateral mass screws have been widely used over the last several decades. The original technique was first described by Roy-Camille in the late 1970s. Since that description, various authors have attempted to modify the technique in attempt to improve screw purchase and reduce complications related to screw malposition.[34–36] Al Barbarawi et al. reviewed a total of 2500 screws placed in 430 patients with a range of pathologies. They report a total of five screws requiring removal for worsening radiculopathy. They also reported 20 patients overall with a worsening C5 radiculopathy following surgery that resolved over time, although two patients did undergo screw revision at the C5 level.[37] In a 2013 systematic review of the complications associated with lateral mass screw fixation, Coe et al. reviewed 20 articles from the literature and found the overall rate of neurologic injury to be 3.9%.[38] The incidence was inclusive of C5 palsy and radiculopathy. The rate of injury attributed to screw malposition was 1.0%. These authors further reported the rate of nerve root injury per screw placement (N = 5771) to be 0.17%. Not surprisingly, given the trajectory of lateral mass screws, there were no reported cases of spinal cord injury.

A less commonly used technique of instrumentation within the cervical spine, at least in North America, is pedicle screw fixation. The concerns with this technique are the small pedicle diameters and risks associated with medial and lateral perforation. With medial or caudal perforation, there is risk to the spinal cord and nerve roots; with lateral perforation, there is risk of vertebral artery injury. In light of these risks, the interest in transpedicular screw fixation centers on improved biomechanical properties compared to lateral mass screws. Transpedicular screw fixation has been shown to have far superior pullout strength than lateral mass screws.[39] Despite its technical demands, this use of this technique has not been shown to have a significantly greater risk of neurologic injury compared to other posterior fixation techniques. Abumi et al. reported on 180 patients and 712 screws.[40] These authors attributed two cases of nerve root injury to screw malposition. One case of nerve root injury resolved with observation, whereas one case of muscle weakness required screw removal,

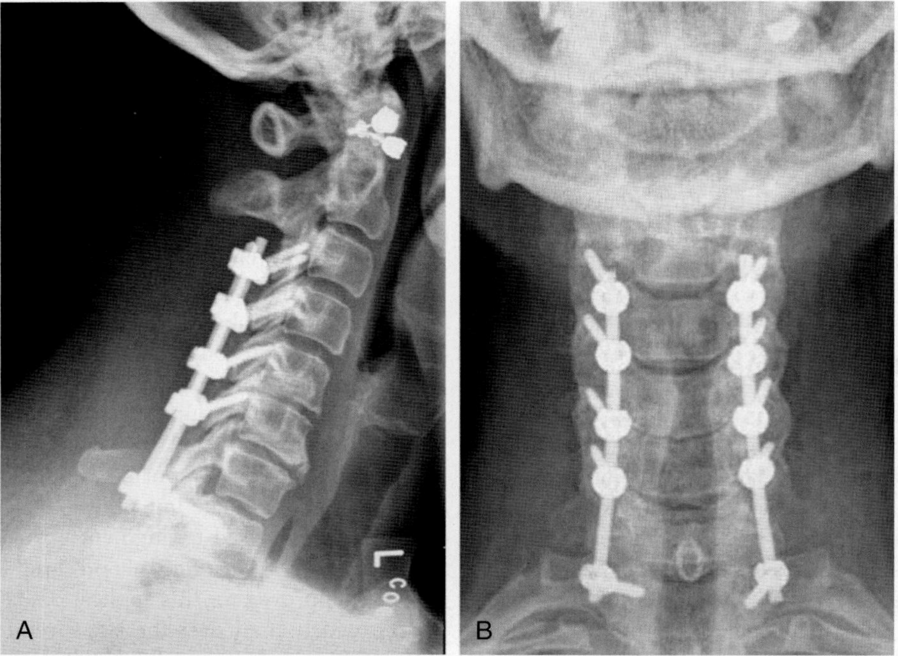

FIG. 95.2 Lateral (A) and anteroposterior (B) radiographs depicting C3–T1 instrumented laminectomy and fusion. C3–C6 received lateral mass screw fixation, C7 was skipped due to small lateral masses, and T1 received pedicle screw instrumentation.

with subsequent improvement in strength. In another study evaluating placement of cervical pedicle screws, 94 screws were implanted in 26 patients. Eight screws (9%) had a critical breach based on postoperative computed tomography (CT) evaluation. Three screws passed through the intervertebral foramen, causing temporary paresis in one case and a new sensory loss in another. In the latter patient, revision surgery was performed. Most screw malposition complications occurred in screws placed from C3 to C5.[41] This is not surprising, as anatomic studies have shown smaller pedicles at C3 and C4 compared to C5 and C6.[42] In a systematic review comparing 10 studies of lateral mass screw fixation and 12 studies of pedicle screw fixation, there was a 0.19% incidence of nerve injury per lateral mass screw placed and 0.31% per pedicle screw placed.[43] In the largest study to date, a review of 283 patients and more than 1000 pedicle screws revealed nerve root irritation attributed to pedicle screw insertion in three patients, all of whom required screw removal. There were no cases of spinal cord injury reported.[44]

Thoracolumbar Spine Surgery

Lumbar spinal stenosis is the most common reason for spine surgery today. The surgical treatment of stenosis without instability is usually a laminectomy or laminotomy. However, in the presence of instability (i.e., spondylolisthesis), most spine surgeons would agree that decompression (direct or indirect) coupled with fusion gives the best and most durable results. Again, the addition of instrumentation will present an additional risk for neurologic injury; there exists an exhaustive array of literature on iatrogenic neurologic complications following anterior and posterior lumbar spine surgery. Recently, transpsoas or lateral approaches to lumbar spine have become popular, with neurologic complications being mainly attributed to the approach. A discussion of the rates of neurologic injury in pediatric and adult scoliosis surgery are also discussed in this section.

Posterior Lumbar Surgery

Lumbar disc herniations are treated nonoperatively in the majority of cases. However, in those patients nonresponsive to conservative treatments, microdiscectomy is an option. In a systematic review of 42 studies investigating the rate of complications following microdiscectomy, the neurologic complications of a nerve root injury occur between 0.9% and 2.6% of cases depending on surgical technique utilized.[45] A Cochrane review revealed similar neurologic complication rates with no differences among the technique utilized.[46]

In the setting of lumbar stenosis without instability, a laminectomy can offer sustained symptomatic relief.[47] As with many procedures in spine surgery, there are a number of ways to achieve decompression. The standard open bilateral laminectomy has a proven track record, but the push to minimally invasive procedures has seen the development of techniques to perform the same procedure through smaller incisions and through the use of unilateral approaches. A Cochrane review comparing standard open laminectomy to bilateral laminotomy revealed no difference in neurologic complications. One recent study of 500 lumbar laminectomies by Bydon et al. found a 2.61% incidence of postoperative weakness.[48] However, in a recent publication, Nerland et al. reported no neurologic complications in 885 patients following standard and minimally invasive laminectomy techniques.[49]

Aside from iatrogenic mechanical injury, postoperative hematoma is a concern following any spinal surgery and, if missed, can lead to devastating consequences. A missed cauda equina syndrome can result in permanent sensory, motor, bowel, and bladder complications. Although there is typically some evidence of hematoma seen on postoperative CT/magnetic resonance imaging scans, the majority of these are asymptomatic.[50] Kou et al. found a 0.1% incidence of symptomatic hematoma in a retrospective review of approximately 12,000 cases, finding multilevel surgery and preoperative coagulopathy as risk factors.[51] Similarly, Awad et al. performed a retrospective review of over 14,000 spine procedures over an 18-year period.[52] They reported an overall incidence of symptomatic hematoma of 0.32%. In their study, intraoperative variables associated with symptomatic hematoma were more than five decompressed levels, hemoglobin less than 10 g/dL and blood loss greater than 1 L.

From the posterior approach, the anterior column can be accessed. This can be accomplished through a posterior lumbar interbody fusion (PLIF), in which the facets bilaterally are preserved, or through the more commonly utilized transforaminal lumbar interbody fusion (TLIF), which removes a facet unilaterally for placement (Fig. 95.3). The need for these additional procedures when performing a standard posterolateral fusion remains hotly debated and is beyond the scope of this chapter. The impetus for development of TLIF stemmed from the complications associated with the PLIF secondary to the need for significant dural retraction during placement. Increased radicular pain is the most commonly encountered neurologic complication with these procedures. In a review of these techniques, the overall rate of neurologic injury was reported to be between 0% and 7%, with the majority of injuries being transient in nature.[53] Humphreys et al. compared the two techniques in a retrospective study of 40 TLIF and 34 PLIF patients. They reported no neurologic complications in the TLIF group compared to four cases of radiculitis in the PLIF group.[54] In another retrospective comparison at a single institution, PLIF was associated with a 7.8% incidence of nerve root dysfunction versus 2% in the TLIF group. All cases were transient and resolved in 3 months.[55]

Lateral Lumbar Surgery

Lateral lumbar surgery (or the transpsoas approach) has seen increased utilization since Ozgur et al. described the technique in 2006.[56] This technique allows access to the anterior column and has been utilized in single-level degenerative and scoliotic deformities. The main neurologic complications of the technique involve the approach to the disc space through the psoas musculature and the traversing lumbar plexus. There are a number of articles detailing the anatomy of the lumbar plexus.[57–59] These anatomic studies highlight that neurologic injury is at highest risk during access to the L4–L5 interspace. At this level, the intrapsoas path of the nerve trunks passes closest to the midline portion of the disc space and most in line with the exposure. As exposure continues cephalad, the traversing nerve trunks are found posterior to the midline of

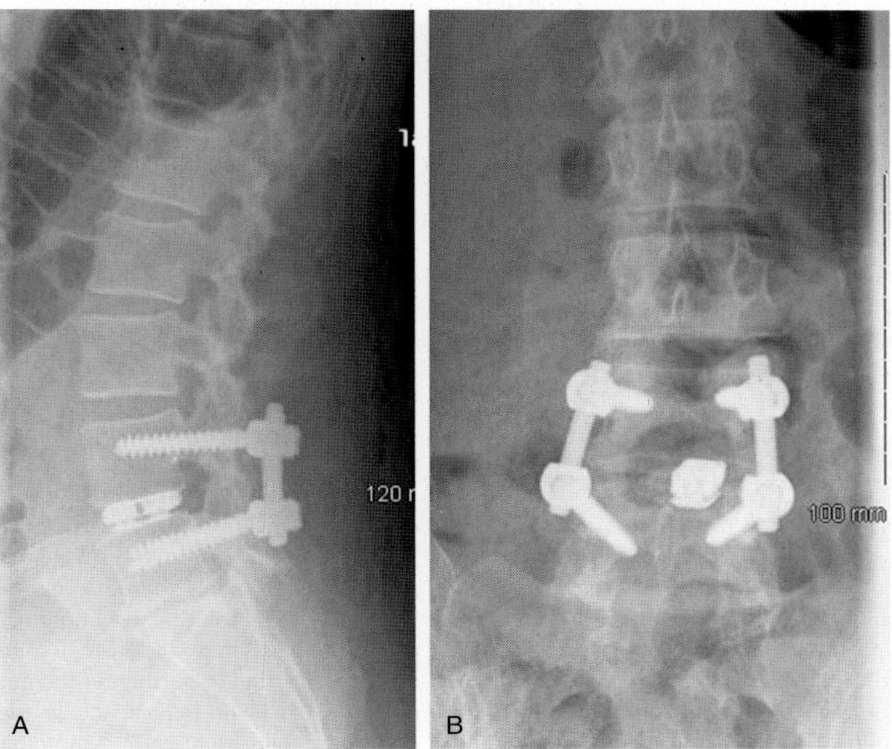

FIG. 95.3 Lateral (A) and anteroposterior (B) radiographs depicting an L4–L5 instrumented transforaminal lumbar interbody fusion.

the intervertebral disc and are not as frequently encountered during the approach.

The most commonly reported neurologic complication following the transpsoas approach is thigh dysesthesias. In one of the largest reported series utilizing the transpsoas approach, Rodgers et al. reported a 0.7% rate of neurologic injury secondary to the approach; all cases were transient in a study of over 600.[60] However, most other authors report higher rates. Anand et al. reported a 60% incidence of thigh paresthesia, all of which resolved within 6 weeks.[61] Cummock et al. report similar rates of dysesthesia, with 62.7% of patients (N = 59) complaining of thigh symptoms ranging from burning, aching, stabbing, or other pain (39.0%); to numbness (42.4%); to paresthesias (11.9%); and weakness (23.7%).[62]

In a review of the neurologic complications associated with this approach, Ahmadian et al. provided an excellent analysis of the literature. This was a review of 18 studies totaling over 2300 patients.[63] In their review, 304 patients (13.2%) were described as having possible lumbar plexus–related injuries. Motor weakness ranged from 0.7% to 33.6%, and sensory complications ranged from 0% to 75%. In addition to lumbar nerve root injury, the review also highlights possible injury to iliohypogastric, ilioinguinal, genitofemoral, subcostal nerves, and abdominal paresis with this approach.

Anterior Lumbar Surgery

The anterior lumbar fusion approach allows for better exposure of the disc space and thus a greater surface area for fusion. It also allows for improved ability to increase correction of sagittal deformity. Although the neural elements are not typically exposed, iatrogenic neurologic deficit has been described for anterior lumbar surgery, with reported prevalence ranging from 0.9% to 6.5%. In retrospective review of 471 anterior lumbar fusions, Sasso et al. reported intraoperative neurologic complications in two patients (0.9%).[64] Duggal et al. reported two cases of worsening radiculopathy (6%) in 33 patients under anterior lumbar interbody fusion for failed back syndrome.[65] In a review of iatrogenic neurologic injuries associated with lumbar fusion surgery, Ghobrial et al. report that the overall rate of neurologic deficit after anterior interbody fusions was 4.1%, although an overlap of lateral interbody fusion literature included in this review likely resulted in higher than expected rates of neurologic injury.[66]

Pediatric Deformity Correction

The development of the Harrington rod system for control of adolescent idiopathic scoliosis (AIS) was a major milestone in the treatment of scoliosis. Proximal and distal fixation of the curve is obtained and a distraction rod placed in between the fixation points. With the aid of a ratcheting mechanism, distraction was applied to the spine to correct the deformity. However, this technique was not without complications. In a 1975 report by the Scoliosis Research Society (SRS), the rate of spinal cord injury with the Harrington rod instrumentation was 0.72%. Half of these injuries resulted in complete paraplegia and the other half in partial paraplegia; one-third of the injured patients reported complete recovery, one-third reported partial recovery, and one-third reported no recovery.[67]

Advances in the field of spine surgery have spawned the development and increased utilization of segmental fixation with the use of a combination of hooks or pedicle screw instrumentation for the treatment of AIS. However, there remains risk of both spinal cord and nerve root injury. In a more recent review by the SRS, Coe and colleagues[68] examined cases reported from the years 2001 to 2003. Of the reported cases, 6716 cases were for AIS using either an anterior or posterior approach or combination. The reported rate of neurologic complications using an anterior approach was 0.26%, 0.32% for the posterior approach, and 1.75% when a combined approach was utilized. In total, there were 18 cases of incomplete spinal cord injuries, with nine (0.21%) occurring in the posterior group and nine (1.12%) in the combined group. No cases of spinal cord injury were reported in the anterior group. Complete neurologic recovery was reported in 11, incomplete recovery in six, and no recovery in one patient. However, there are inherent limitations associated with the SRS studies, as it is a volunteer database of retrospectively entered data by the members of the SRS. In a prospective study of more than 1300 patients, Diab et al.[69] reported two nerve root and four spinal cord injuries (overall complication rate of 0.38%). One nerve root injury was a position-related femoral neurapraxia, which resolved completely within 6 months. The other nerve root injury occurred below instrumentation and well after deformity correction. It too resolved completely with observation. All spinal cord injuries were incomplete, with complete resolution within 12 weeks.

As mentioned earlier, with the development of segmental fixation—namely, pedicle screw instrumentation—there has been an increased trend toward the use of posterior-only-based techniques.[70] There are a number of studies that highlight the rate of asymptomatic misplaced screws. Lehman et al. reported an 89.5% accuracy, based on CT assessment, in the placement of 1023 pedicle screws with no neurologic complications associated with misplacement.[71] In a systematic review of 21 studies with a total of 4570 pedicle screws in 1666 patients, 4.2% of screws were reported as malpositioned.[72] However, when CT scans were utilized to evaluate screw position, malposition rates were shown to be as high as 15.7%, which occurred in about 11% of patients in this review.

There are studies that highlight the additional risk of neurologic injury with the use of pedicle screws. In an earlier study, Lonstein et al. reported on complications using a combined total of 4790 screws.[73] They reported 11 screws used in nine procedures resulting in nerve root irritation (0.2%) manifesting as pain and/or weakness. Eight screws were removed, with resolution of symptoms in seven patients. One patient had residual weakness despite screw removal. In a more recent study reporting on the neurologic complications of more than 5900 pedicle screws placed using a freehand technique, there were eight symptomatic, misplaced pedicle screws (0.14%) in six of 481 patients (1.25%).[74] Three patients underwent revision surgery for radicular complaints, with

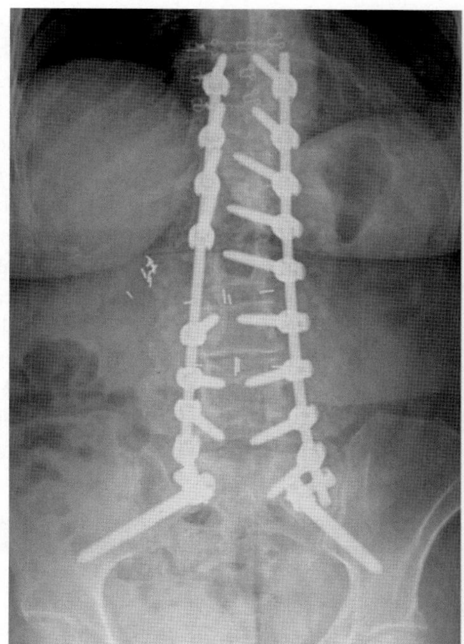
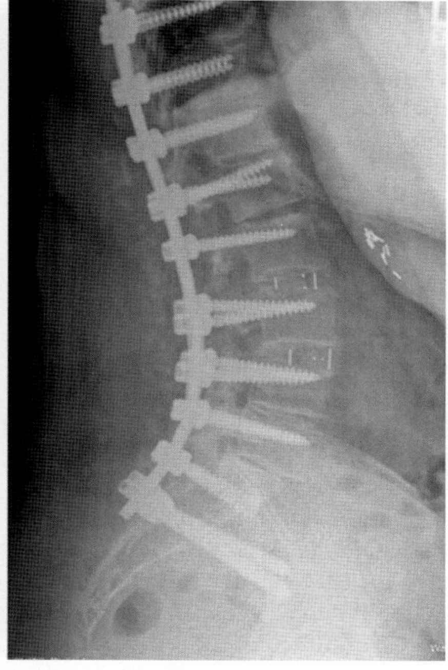

FIG. 95.4 Anteroposterior (A) and lateral (B) radiographs depicting surgical correction of adult degenerative scoliosis. T10–S1 pedicle screw instrumentation with alar-iliac pelvic screw fixation. Additional interbody fusions were placed at L2–L3 and L3–L4 at the apex of the curve to aid in curve correction.

complete resolution of their symptoms with screw removal. The remaining three patients had thoracic dermatomal pain not severe enough that they wished to undergo surgery. In this study, there was no reported case of spinal cord injury with screw instrumentation.

Adult Deformity Correction

With an ever increasing aging population and ever increasing life expectancy, the surgical treatment of adult degenerative scoliosis is becoming more frequent (Fig. 95.4). Adult degenerative scoliosis evolves from three main mechanisms: asymmetric disc and facet degeneration resulting in adult-onset scoliosis; the evolution of a curve present in adolescence; and scoliosis that is secondary to metabolic, arthritic, and posttraumatic disorders. In contrast to its adolescent counterpart, adult deformity is typically characterized by a rigid deformity and usually multiple levels of symptomatic stenosis requiring decompression. These patients may also have a sagittal imbalance; it is this sagittal imbalance, more so than the coronal deformity, that has been shown to be a major contributor to the poor quality of life in these patients.[75] The rigid deformity and sagittal imbalance often requires some form of osteotomy—Smith-Petersen osteotomy, pedicle subtraction osteotomy (PSO), or vertebral column resection (VCR)—depending on the plane and degree of deformity. The rate of complications associated with adult deformity is high. In the case of neurologic injury following adult deformity surgery, it typically presents immediately after surgery, but there are reports of delays in presentation of greater than 48 hours.[76]

There have been various articles published focusing on the incidence of complications and factors associated with increased risk. Carreon et al. found increasing age and the number of levels fused to be significant risk factors for the development of complications in patients greater than 65 years of age undergoing lumbar decompression and arthrodesis.[77] Daubs et al. reported on 51 consecutive patients older than 60 years of age undergoing an average of nine levels of fusion and instrumentation.[78] There was an overall perioperative complication rate of 37%. Four patients suffered a major neurologic deficit postoperatively with at least one suffering paraplegia secondary to a spinal cord infarct after surgery. Cho and colleagues reported seven patients with a postoperative neurologic deficit in a series of 166 patients undergoing surgery for degenerative scoliosis.[79] They did not report any significant spinal cord injuries. In a retrospective multicenter study, Charosky et al. reported on 306 patients undergoing adult deformity surgery.[80] They report a 7.5% incidence of postoperative neurologic complication. Eighteen peripheral nerve root deficits were reported in total. A significant motor deficit occurred in 11 cases, and a sensory deficit was seen in seven other patients. One patient presented with a cauda equina syndrome. Incomplete decompression and instrumentation malposition accounted for six cases of neurologic decline and an unknown cause in the remaining. In another study utilizing the SRS voluntary database on adult deformity cases between 2004 and 2007, 90 neurologic deficits (1.8%) were reported in the 4980 patients. Of these deficits, 71 were nerve root injuries, 11 were incomplete spinal cord injuries, one was a complete spinal cord injury, and five were cauda equina syndromes. For those neurologic complications with follow-up available, 23 nerve root injuries had complete recovery, 33 had partial recovery, and two had no recovery. For the incomplete spinal cord injuries, six had complete recovery and five had partial recovery. For the cauda equina injuries, one had a complete recovery, three had partial recovery, and one had no recovery.[81]

The addition of osteotomies to the index operation increases surgical time, bleeding, and rates of complications. In an early series of 33 patients undergoing PSOs, five patients (15%) developed transient neurologic deficits.[82] Buchowski et al. reported on the neurologic complications following 108 PSOs.[83] Deficits (defined as motor loss of two grades or more or loss of bowel/bladder control) were seen in 12 patients (11.1%) and were permanent in three patients (2.8%). With time, motor function improved by one grade in two patients and all three were able to ambulate. In addition to motor weakness, one patient developed a neurogenic bladder and weakness in the lower extremities 1 week following surgery, which gradually recovered over the course of several weeks following a wide decompression. In this study, the majority of these neurologic deficits were felt to be due to a combination of subluxation, residual dorsal impingement, and dural buckling. Auerbach et al. reported on 105 consecutive three-column osteotomies.[84] A total of 87 patients underwent a PSO and 18 had a VCR. They reported one optical deficit. Their rate of neurologic deficit with PSO procedures was 5.7% major permanent, 5.7% minor permanent, and 9.2% transient impairment. With VCR, one patient (5.6%) awoke with a transient sensory deficit. Suk et al.[85] reported on the outcomes of 70 patients who underwent VCR for severe spinal deformity. Postoperatively, there were six cases of cauda equina syndrome that resolved with emergent decompression. Two patients suffered complete permanent cord injury and four transient nerve root injuries that resolved without intervention.

Summary

Few complications are more dreaded after spine surgery than neurologic injury. There are ways to protect our patients against these injuries. First and foremost, it begins with a thorough patient examination and documentation of any preexisting neurologic deficits. Careful interpretation of preoperative imaging as it pertains to the patient's clinical picture will help to provide the best outcome with the least amount of risk. Once the decision for surgery is made, preoperative planning is of paramount importance. "We'll see when we get in there" is a recipe for disaster. In spine surgery, there are any number of ways to treat the same pathology and the types and rates of neurologic injury vary with procedure performed.

Intraoperative complications can occur from the moment anesthesia induction takes place. Constant dialogue between the surgeon and anesthesia team regarding blood pressure, perfusion, and body temperature are important in preventing spinal cord hypoperfusion. Intraoperative patient positioning, although commonly overlooked, is an extremely preventable source of neurologic complication. Once the surgery has started, the tenets of surgical technique must be adhered to at all times. Hands (both of them when possible) should be utilized and remain grounded to the patient when instrumenting the spine. Arm yourself with a command of anatomy; it can be a potent weapon against combating the changes associated with degenerative disease.

Luckily, the risk of neurologic injury is low for most spine surgeries. As expected, with an increase in case complexity, the degree and rate of neurologic injury increases. These risks must be tempered against the purported benefits of the surgery being entertained. The literature supports the notion that many deficits encountered after surgery are transient, although catastrophic neurologic complications can occur. A dialogue with the patient regarding these risks is also of paramount importance. Unfortunately, the risk of neurologic injury with spine surgery will never be eliminated. Knowledge of the risks and pitfalls of the surgery with careful attention to detail can help mitigate neurologic complications associated with spine surgery.

PEARLS

1. Careful inspection of preoperative imaging can help avoid neurologic injury.
2. Safe surgical technique cannot be emphasized enough (i.e., using two hands when instrumented the spine when possible, avoiding the passing instruments into already stenotic recesses).
3. Remain vigilant in postoperative assessment to identify neurologic injury.
4. Understanding that deformity surgery frequently involves both coronal and rotational deformity can help minimize pedicle screw malposition by obtaining appropriate intraoperative fluoroscopic images.

PITFALLS

1. Poor patient positioning can negate otherwise meticulous surgical technique and result in neurologic injury.
2. Lack of a preoperative plan, and adherence to it, is a recipe to create neurologic injury.
3. Neurologic injury happens. Avoidance will not make it go away. Order appropriate postoperative imaging and correct what can be corrected.

KEY POINTS

1. Neurologic injury in spine surgery can occur from improper patient positioning and becomes especially important as the duration of the surgical procedure increases.
2. The rate of spinal cord injury is very low across all type of spine surgery.
3. Some neurologic injuries are more likely to occur given the surgical approach; that knowledge is key to their avoidance.
4. C5 palsy is the most commonly encounter neurologic deficit after both anterior and posterior cervical surgery.
5. Revision surgery increases the risk of neurologic injury.
6. Neurologic injury can present in a delayed fashion (>48 hours after the procedure).
7. Not all neurologic injuries require action, but all should be acknowledged and documented.
8. CT analysis of pedicle screw placement highlights a high rate of misplacement. Luckily, the incidence of symptomatic pedicle screw, necessitating removal, is low.
9. The increasing complexity of surgery increases the risk of neurologic injury; d thus the need for increased instrumentation should be heavily weighed against it effect on patient outcomes.

KEY REFERENCES

1. Parks BJ. Postoperative peripheral neuropathies. *Surgery*. 1973;74(3):348-357.
2. Beutler WJ, Sweeney CA, Connolly PJ. Recurrent laryngeal nerve injury with anterior cervical spine surgery risk with laterality of surgical approach. *Spine*. 2001;26(12):1337-1342.
3. Rasouli MR, Rahimi-Movaghar V, Shokraneh F, Moradi-Lakeh M, Chou R. Minimally invasive discectomy versus microdiscectomy/open discectomy for symptomatic lumbar disc herniation. *Cochrane Database Syst Rev*. 2014;(9):CD010328.
4. Ahmadian A, Deukmedjian AR, Abel N, Dakwar E, Uribe JS. Analysis of lumbar plexopathies and nerve injury after lateral retroperitoneal transpsoas approach: diagnostic standardization. *J Neurosurg Spine*. 2013;18(3):289-297.
5. Hicks JM, Singla A, Shen FH, Arlet V. Complications of pedicle screw fixation in scoliosis surgery: a systematic review. *Spine*. 2010;35(11):E465-E470.
6. Buchowski JM, Bridwell KH, Lenke LG, et al. Neurologic complications of lumbar pedicle subtraction osteotomy: a 10-year assessment. *Spine*. 2007;32(20):2245-2252.

REFERENCES

1. Parks BJ. Postoperative peripheral neuropathies. *Surgery*. 1973;74(3):348-357.
2. Mirovsky Y, Neuwirth M. Injuries to the lateral femoral cutaneous nerve during spine surgery. *Spine*. 2000;25(10):1266-1269.
3. Stevens WR, Glazer PA, Kelley SD, Lietman TM, Bradford DS. Ophthalmic complications after spinal surgery. *Spine*. 1997;22(12):1319-1324.
4. Stambough JL, Dolan D, Werner R, Godfrey E. Ophthalmologic complications associated with prone positioning in spine surgery. *J Am Acad Orthop Surg*. 2007;15(3):156-165.
5. Grisoli F, Graziani N, Fabrizi AP, et al. Anterior discectomy without fusion for treatment of cervical lateral soft disc extrusion: a follow-up of 120 cases. *Neurosurgery*. 1989;24(6):853-859.
6. Yamamoto I, Ikeda A, Shibuya N, Tsugane R, Sato O. Clinical long-term results of anterior discectomy without interbody fusion for cervical disc disease. *Spine*. 1991;16(3):272-279.
7. Heeneman H. Vocal cord paralysis following approaches to the anterior cervical spine. *Laryngoscope*. 1973;83(1):17-21.
8. Ebraheim NA, Lu J, Skie M, Heck BE, Yeasting RA. Vulnerability of the recurrent laryngeal nerve in the anterior approach to the lower cervical spine. *Spine*. 1997;22(22):2664-2667.
9. Beutler WJ, Sweeney CA, Connolly PJ. Recurrent laryngeal nerve injury with anterior cervical spine surgery risk with laterality of surgical approach. *Spine*. 2001;26(12):1337-1342.
10. Ebraheim NA, Lu J, Yang H, Heck BE, Yeasting RA. Vulnerability of the sympathetic trunk during the anterior approach to the lower cervical spine. *Spine*. 2000;25(13):1603-1606.
11. Hankinson HL, Wilson CB. Use of the operating microscope in anterior cervical discectomy without fusion. *J Neurosurg*. 1975;43(4):452-456.
12. Saunders RL, Bernini PM, Shirreffs TG, Reeves AG. Central corpectomy for cervical spondylotic myelopathy: a consecutive series with long-term follow-up evaluation. *J Neurosurg*. 1991;74(2):163-170.
13. Bertalanffy H, Eggert HR. Complications of anterior cervical discectomy without fusion in 450 consecutive patients. *Acta Neurochir (Wien)*. 1989;99(1-2):41-50.
14. Tew JM, Mayfield FH. Complications of surgery of the anterior cervical spine. *Clin Neurosurg*. 1976;23:424-434.
15. Hilibrand AS, Schwartz DM, Sethuraman V, Vaccaro AR, Albert TJ. Comparison of transcranial electric motor and somatosensory evoked potential monitoring during cervical spine surgery. *J Bone Joint Surg Am*. 2004;86-A(6):1248-1253.
16. Emery SE, Bohlman HH, Bolesta MJ, Jones PK. Anterior cervical decompression and arthrodesis for the treatment of cervical spondylotic myelopathy. Two to seventeen-year follow-up. *J Bone Joint Surg Am*. 1998;80(7):941-951.
17. Graham JJ. Complications of cervical spine surgery. A five-year report on a survey of the membership of the Cervical Spine Research Society by the Morbidity and Mortality Committee. *Spine*. 1989;14(10):1046-1050.
18. Fountas KN, Kapsalaki EZ, Nikolakakos LG, et al. Anterior cervical discectomy and fusion associated complications. *Spine*. 2007;32(21):2310-2317.
19. Nanda A, Sharma M, Sonig A, Ambekar S, Bollam P. Surgical complications of anterior cervical diskectomy and fusion for cervical degenerative disk disease: a single surgeon's experience of 1576 patients. *World Neurosurg*. 2014;82(6):1380-1387.
20. Wada E, Suzuki S, Kanazawa A, et al. Subtotal corpectomy versus laminoplasty for multilevel cervical spondylotic myelopathy: a long-term follow-up study over 10 years. *Spine*. 2001;26(13):1443-1447.
21. Ikenaga M, Shikata J, Tanaka C. Radiculopathy of C-5 after anterior decompression for cervical myelopathy. *J Neurosurg Spine*. 2005;3(3):210-217.
22. Skovrlj B, Gologorsky Y, Haque R, Fessler RG, Qureshi SA. Complications, outcomes, and need for fusion after minimally invasive posterior cervical foraminotomy and microdiscectomy. *Spine J*. 2014;14(10):2405-2411.
23. Jagannathan J, Sherman JH, Szabo T, Shaffrey CI, Jane JA. The posterior cervical foraminotomy in the treatment of cervical disc/osteophyte disease: a single-surgeon experience with a minimum of 5 years' clinical and radiographic follow-up. *J Neurosurg Spine*. 2009;10(4):347-356.
24. Grieve JP, Kitchen ND, Moore AJ, Marsh HT. Results of posterior cervical foraminotomy for treatment of cervical spondylitic radiculopathy. *Br J Neurosurg*. 2000;14(1):40-43.
25. Duetzmann S, Cole T, Ratliff JK. Cervical laminoplasty developments and trends, 2003-2013: a systematic review. *J Neurosurg Spine*. 2015;23(1):24-34.
26. Gu Y, Cao P, Gao R, et al. Incidence and risk factors of C5 palsy following posterior cervical decompression: a systematic review. Shamji M, ed. *PLoS One*. 2014;9(8):e101933.
27. Lao L, Zhong G, Li X, Qian L, Liu Z. Laminoplasty versus laminectomy for multi-level cervical spondylotic myelopathy: a systematic review of the literature. *J Orthop Surg Res*. 2013;8:45.
28. Nassr A, Eck JC, Ponnappan RK, et al. The incidence of C5 palsy after multilevel cervical decompression procedures: a review of 750 consecutive cases. *Spine*. 2012;37(3):174-178.
29. Tsuzuki N, Abe R, Saiki K. Zhongshi L. Extradural tethering effect as one mechanism of radiculopathy complicating posterior decompression of the cervical spinal cord. *Spine*. 1996;21(2):203-211.
30. Rovira M, Torrent O, Ruscalleda J. Some aspects of the spinal cord circulation in cervical myelopathy. *Neuroradiology*. 1975;9(4):209-214.

31. Chiba K, Toyama Y, Matsumoto M, et al. Segmental motor paralysis after expansive open-door laminoplasty. *Spine*. 2002;27(19):2108-2115.
32. Fan D, Schwartz DM, Vaccaro AR, Hilibrand AS, Albert TJ. Intraoperative neurophysiologic detection of iatrogenic C5 nerve root injury during laminectomy for cervical compression myelopathy. *Spine*. 2002;27(22):2499-2502.
33. Tanaka N, Nakanishi K, Fujiwara Y, Kamei N, Ochi M. Postoperative segmental C5 palsy after cervical laminoplasty may occur without intraoperative nerve injury: a prospective study with transcranial electric motor-evoked potentials. *Spine*. 2006;31(26):3013-3017.
34. Cooper PR, Cohen A, Rosiello A, Koslow M. Posterior stabilization of cervical spine fractures and subluxations using plates and screws. *Neurosurgery*. 1988;23(3):300-306.
35. An HS, Gordin R, Renner K. Anatomic considerations for plate-screw fixation of the cervical spine. *Spine*. 1991;16(10 suppl):S548-S551.
36. Xu R, Haman SP, Ebraheim NA, Yeasting RA. The anatomic relation of lateral mass screws to the spinal nerves. A comparison of the Magerl, Anderson, and An techniques. *Spine*. 1999;24(19):2057-2061.
37. Al Barbarawi MM, Allouh MZ. Cervical lateral mass screw-rod fixation: surgical experience with 2500 consecutive screws, an analytical review, and long-term outcomes. *Br J Neurosurg*. 2015;1-6.
38. Coe JD, Vaccaro AR, Dailey AT, et al. Lateral mass screw fixation in the cervical spine: a systematic literature review. *J Bone Joint Surg Am*. 2013;95(23):2136-2143.
39. Jones EL, Heller JG, Silcox DH, Hutton WC. Cervical pedicle screws versus lateral mass screws. Anatomic feasibility and biomechanical comparison. *Spine*. 1997;22(9):977-982.
40. Abumi K, Shono Y, Ito M, et al. Complications of pedicle screw fixation in reconstructive surgery of the cervical spine. *Spine*. 2000;25(8):962-969.
41. Kast E, Mohr K, Richter H-P. Börm W. Complications of transpedicular screw fixation in the cervical spine. *Eur Spine J*. 2006;15(3):327-334.
42. Ebraheim NA, Xu R, Knight T, Yeasting RA. Morphometric evaluation of lower cervical pedicle and its projection. *Spine*. 1997;22(1):1-6.
43. Yoshihara H, Passias PG, Errico TJ. Screw-related complications in the subaxial cervical spine with the use of lateral mass versus cervical pedicle screws: a systematic review. *J Neurosurg Spine*. 2013;19(5):614-623.
44. Hojo Y, Ito M, Suda K, et al. A multicenter study on accuracy and complications of freehand placement of cervical pedicle screws under lateral fluoroscopy in different pathological conditions: CT-based evaluation of more than 1,000 screws. *Eur Spine J*. 2014;23(10):2166-2174.
45. Shriver MF, Xie JJ, Tye EY, et al. Lumbar microdiscectomy complication rates: a systematic review and meta-analysis. *Neurosurg Focus*. 2015;39(4):E6.
46. Rasouli MR, Rahimi-Movaghar V, Shokraneh F, Moradi-Lakeh M, Chou R. Minimally invasive discectomy versus microdiscectomy/open discectomy for symptomatic lumbar disc herniation. *Cochrane Database Syst Rev*. 2014;(9):CD010328.
47. Lurie JD, Tosteson TD, Tosteson A, et al. Long-term outcomes of lumbar spinal stenosis: eight-year results of the Spine Patient Outcomes Research Trial (SPORT). *Spine*. 2015;40(2):63-76.
48. Bydon M, Macki M, Abt NB, et al. Clinical and surgical outcomes after lumbar laminectomy: an analysis of 500 patients. *Surg Neurol Int*. 2015;6(suppl 4):S190-S193.
49. Nerland US, Jakola AS, Solheim O, et al. Minimally invasive decompression versus open laminectomy for central stenosis of the lumbar spine: pragmatic comparative effectiveness study. *BMJ*. 2015;350:h1603.
50. Teplick JG, Haskin ME. Review. Computed tomography of the postoperative lumbar spine. *AJR Am J Roentgenol*. 1983;141(5):865-884.
51. Kou J, Fischgrund J, Biddinger A, Herkowitz H. Risk factors for spinal epidural hematoma after spinal surgery. *Spine*. 2002;27(15):1670-1673.
52. Awad JN. Analysis of the risk factors for the development of post-operative spinal epidural haematoma. *J Bone Joint Surg Br*. 2005;87-B(9):1248-1252.
53. Chrastil J, Patel AA. Complications associated with posterior and transforaminal lumbar interbody fusion. *J Am Acad Orthop Surg*. 2012;20(5):283-291.
54. Humphreys SC, Hodges SD, Patwardhan AG, et al. Comparison of posterior and transforaminal approaches to lumbar interbody fusion. *Spine*. 2001;26(5):567-571.
55. Mehta VA, McGirt MJ, Garcés Ambrossi GL, et al. Trans-foraminal versus posterior lumbar interbody fusion: comparison of surgical morbidity. *Neurol Res*. 2011;33(1):38-42.
56. Ozgur BM, Aryan HE, Pimenta L, Taylor WR. Extreme Lateral Interbody Fusion (XLIF): a novel surgical technique for anterior lumbar interbody fusion. *Spine J*. 2006;6(4):435-443.
57. Davis TT, Bae HW, Mok JM, Rasouli A, Delamarter RB. Lumbar plexus anatomy within the psoas muscle: implications for the transpsoas lateral approach to the L4-L5 disc. *J Bone Joint Surg Am*. 2011;93(16):1482-1487.
58. Park DK, Lee MJ, Lin EL, et al. The relationship of intrapsoas nerves during a transpsoas approach to the lumbar spine: anatomic study. *J Spinal Disord Tech*. 2010;23(4):223-228.
59. Banagan K, Gelb D, Poelstra K, Ludwig S. Anatomic mapping of lumbar nerve roots during a direct lateral transpsoas approach to the spine: a cadaveric study. *Spine*. 2011;36(11):E687-E691.
60. Rodgers WB, Gerber EJ, Patterson J. Intraoperative and early postoperative complications in extreme lateral interbody fusion: an analysis of 600 cases. *Spine*. 2011;36(1):26-32.
61. Anand N, Baron EM. Khandehroo B, Kahwaty S. Long-term 2- to 5-year clinical and functional outcomes of minimally invasive surgery for adult scoliosis. *Spine*. 2013;38(18):1566-1575.
62. Cummock MD, Vanni S, Levi AD, Yu Y, Wang MY. An analysis of postoperative thigh symptoms after minimally invasive transpsoas lumbar interbody fusion. *J Neurosurg Spine*. 2011;15(1):11-18.
63. Ahmadian A, Deukmedjian AR, Abel N, Dakwar E, Uribe JS. Analysis of lumbar plexopathies and nerve injury after lateral retroperitoneal transpsoas approach: diagnostic standardization. *J Neurosurg Spine*. 2013;18(3):289-297.
64. Sasso RC, Best NM, Mummaneni P V, Reilly TM, Hussain SM. Analysis of operative complications in a series of 471 anterior lumbar interbody fusion procedures. *Spine*. 2005;30(6):670-674.
65. Duggal N, Mendiondo I, Pares HR, et al. Anterior lumbar interbody fusion for treatment of failed back surgery syndrome: an outcome analysis. *Neurosurgery*. 2004;54(3):636-643.
66. Ghobrial GM, Williams KA, Arnold P, Fehlings M, Harrop JS. Iatrogenic neurologic deficit after lumbar spine surgery: a review. *Clin Neurol Neurosurg*. 2015;139:76-80.
67. MacEwen GD, Bunnell WP, Sriram K. Acute neurological complications in the treatment of scoliosis. A report of

the Scoliosis Research Society. *J Bone Joint Surg Am.* 1975;57(3):404-408.
68. Coe JD, Arlet V, Donaldson W, et al. Complications in spinal fusion for adolescent idiopathic scoliosis in the new millennium. A report of the Scoliosis Research Society Morbidity and Mortality Committee. *Spine.* 2006;31(3):345-349.
69. Diab M, Smith AR, Kuklo TR. Neural complications in the surgical treatment of adolescent idiopathic scoliosis. *Spine.* 2007;32(24):2759-2763.
70. Vigneswaran HT, Grabel ZJ, Eberson CP, Palumbo MA, Daniels AH. Surgical treatment of adolescent idiopathic scoliosis in the United States from 1997 to 2012: an analysis of 20,346 patients. *J Neurosurg Pediatr.* 2015;16(3):322-328.
71. Lehman RA, Lenke LG, Keeler KA, Kim YJ, Cheh G. Computed tomography evaluation of pedicle screws placed in the pediatric deformed spine over an 8-year period. *Spine.* 2007;32(24):2679-2684.
72. Hicks JM, Singla A, Shen FH, Arlet V. Complications of pedicle screw fixation in scoliosis surgery: a systematic review. *Spine.* 2010;35(11):E465-E470.
73. Lonstein JE, Denis F, Perra JH, et al. Complications associated with pedicle screws. *J Bone Joint Surg Am.* 1999;81(11):1519-1528.
74. Dede O, Ward WT, Bosch P, Bowles AJ, Roach JW. Using the freehand pedicle screw placement technique in adolescent idiopathic scoliosis surgery: what is the incidence of neurological symptoms secondary to misplaced screws? *Spine.* 2014;39(4):286-290.
75. Savage JW, Patel AA. Fixed sagittal plane imbalance. *Glob Spine J.* 2014;4(4):287-296.
76. Auerbach JD, Kean K, Milby AH, et al. Delayed postoperative neurologic deficits in spinal deformity surgery. *Spine.* 2015;41(3):E131-E138.
77. Carreon LY, Puno RM, Dimar JR, Glassman SD, Johnson JR. Perioperative complications of posterior lumbar decompression and arthrodesis in older adults. *J Bone Joint Surg Am.* 2003;85-A(11):2089-2092.
78. Daubs MD, Lenke LG, Cheh G, Stobbs G, Bridwell KH. Adult spinal deformity surgery: complications and outcomes in patients over age 60. *Spine.* 2007;32(20):2238-2244.
79. Cho SK, Bridwell KH, Lenke LG, et al. Major complications in revision adult deformity surgery: risk factors and clinical outcomes with 2- to 7-year follow-up. *Spine.* 2012;37(6):489-500.
80. Charosky S, Guigui P, Blamoutier A, Roussouly P, Chopin D. Complications and risk factors of primary adult scoliosis surgery: a multicenter study of 306 patients. *Spine.* 2012;37(8):693-700.
81. Sansur CA, Smith JS, Coe JD, et al. Scoliosis Research Society morbidity and mortality of adult scoliosis surgery. *Spine.* 2011;36(9):E593-E597.
82. Bridwell KH, Lewis SJ, Edwards C, et al. Complications and outcomes of pedicle subtraction osteotomies for fixed sagittal imbalance. *Spine.* 2003;28(18):2093-2101.
83. Buchowski JM, Bridwell KH, Lenke LG, et al. Neurologic complications of lumbar pedicle subtraction osteotomy: a 10-year assessment. *Spine.* 2007;32(20):2245-2252.
84. Auerbach JD, Lenke LG, Bridwell KH, et al. Major complications and comparison between 3-column osteotomy techniques in 105 consecutive spinal deformity procedures. *Spine.* 2012;37(14):1198-1210.
85. Suk S-I, Kim J-H, Kim W-J, et al. Posterior vertebral column resection for severe spinal deformities. *Spine.* 2002;27(21):2374-2382.

96 CHAPTER Spinal Dural Injuries

Arya G. Varthi
Glenn Russo
Peter G. Whang

Anatomy and Pathophysiology

The meninges cover the brain and spinal cord. They consist of dura mater, arachnoid, and pia mater. The dura has three distinct layers: a fibroelastic outer layer, a fibrous middle layer, and a cellular inner layer.[1] Although there is controversy regarding the orientation of dural fibers, there is substantial evidence that they run longitudinally, as evidenced by their higher ultimate stress in this plane.[2] Cerebrospinal fluid (CSF) is produced by the choroid plexus in the lateral third and fourth ventricles of the brain. CSF formation occurs at a rate of 0.3 to 0.6 mL/min, which is the daily equivalent of 500 mL (Fig. 96.1).[3]

Incidence

High-energy thoracolumbar spinal trauma can lead to dural tears. Several authors have reported an incidence of dural tears between 10% and 19% in patients sustaining lumbar or thoracic burst fractures.[4,5] In a retrospective review of 45 patients with lumbar burst fractures, Ozturk et al.[4] reported a 19% rate of traumatic dural tears. Similarly, in an analysis of 60 patients with a surgically treated thoracic or lumbar burst fractures, Cammisa et al.[5] found an 18% rate of traumatic dural tears. Ozturk et al.[4] assessed their outcomes for L3–L5 burst fractures with associated greenstick lamina fractures and found a 25% rate of dural tears (Fig. 96.2). The authors recommended exploring the greenstick lamina fractures to avoid potential injury to neural elements. Other authors have also commented on the important association between traumatic dural tears and neurologic deficits due to nerve root avulsion or entrapment within the fracture.[5–8]

Dural tears can occur during elective spine surgery for degenerative spine disorders, with a higher rate reported during revision surgery. Incidental durotomies occur due to dural laceration during dissection of adherent, fibrotic, or calcified tissue. The dura in revision surgeries is more likely to tear because of adhesions in the epidural space, scarring, fibrosis, and loss of surgical landmarks. Dural tears are also more likely because of absence of dural lining due to prior injury or compression. Risk factors for durotomy in primary surgery include severe spinal stenosis (in these patients, the dura can be very thin or frankly eroded), adhesions, fibrosis, or redundancy.

The reported incidence of incidental durotomy varies. In a retrospective review of 2144 patients, Cammisa et al. reported a 3.1% rate of incidental durotomy,[9] with a higher incidence (8.1%) in revision surgeries. Stratifying by levels, authors have reported a 1% rate of dural tears with cervical surgeries[10] compared with a 7.6% rate for primary lumbar surgeries[11] and a 15.9% rate for revision lumbar surgeries.[11] Overall, revision spine procedures have a higher incidence of durotomy, with reported rates between 8.1% to 15.9%.[3,11,12]

The risk of incidental durotomy varies depending on the type of spine surgery; in the Spine Patient Outcomes Research Trial, Weinstein et al. found that the rate of durotomy increased from 4% for patients undergoing lumbar discectomy to 8% for patients undergoing decompression for lumbar stenosis to 11% for patients undergoing lumbar decompression and fusion for spondylolisthesis.[13–15]

Risk Factors

Surgeon experience and patient age have been implicated as risk factors for dural tears. In one prospective study, the authors found a higher dural tear rate in cases with residents and noted that Kerrison rongeurs were the tool most commonly used to create the accidental durotomy.[16] These authors also noted a higher dural tear rate in older patients and postulated that anatomic changes such as narrowing of spinal canal, thickening of the ligamentum flavum, increased osteophyte formation, and shortening of the spine with redundant dura[16] increased the risk of durotomy in these patients. Other studies have identified ossification of the yellow ligament, synovial cysts, postoperative scarring, excessive traction on severely herniated discs, and anatomically incorrect screw placement as significant risk factors for dural tears.[17,18]

Computed tomography (CT) myelograms can be useful diagnostic studies but have a risk of dural tear and CSF leak (Fig. 96.3). The incidence of dural tears following these

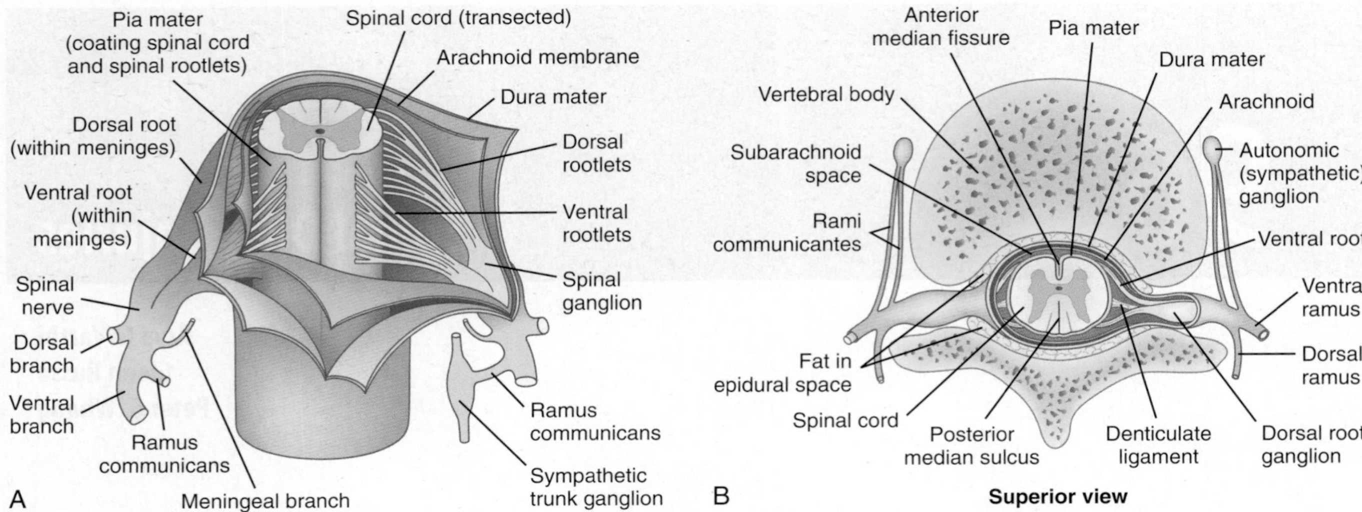

FIG. 96.1 Anatomy of the spinal cord and dura.

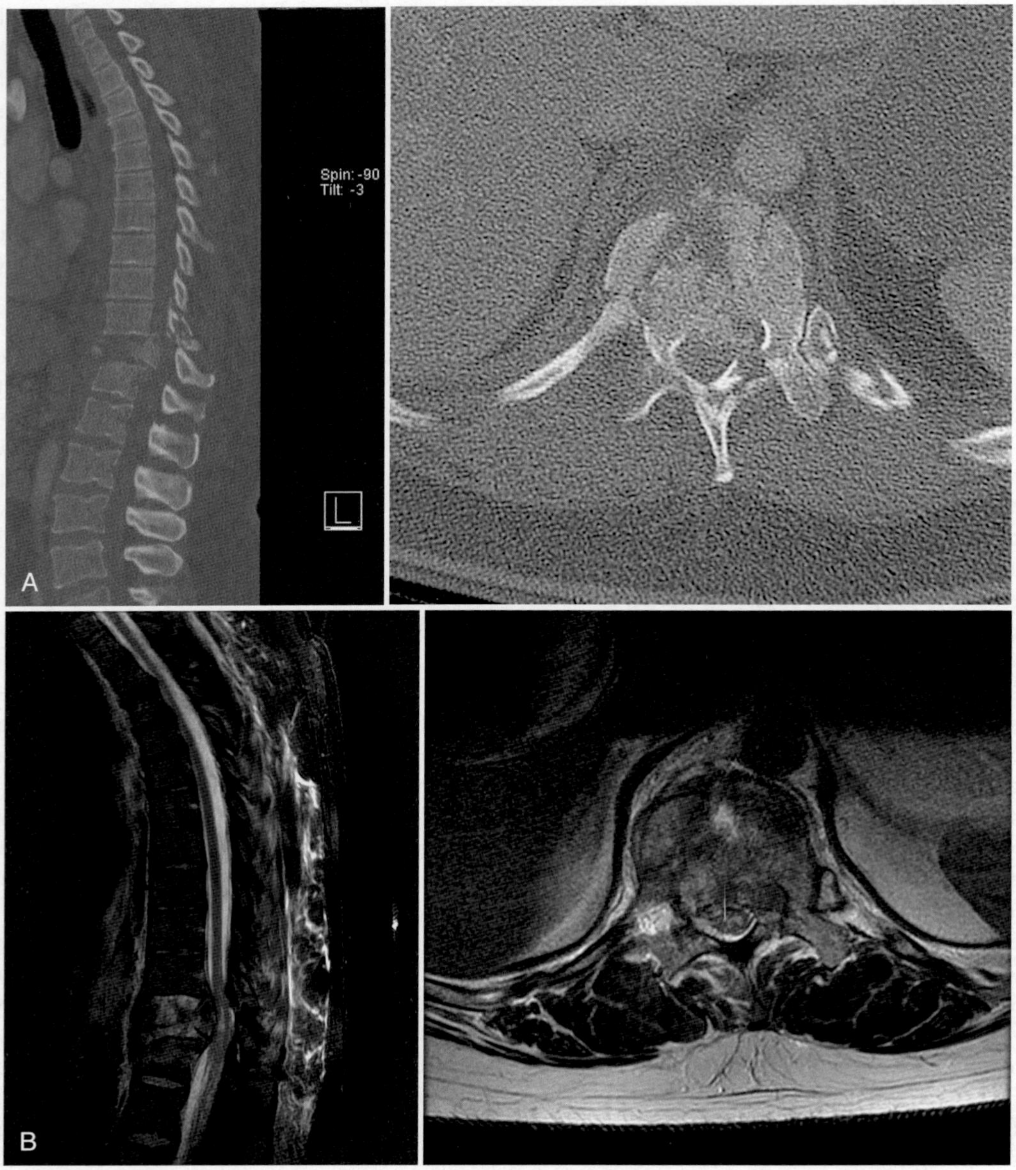

FIG. 96.2 (A) Computed tomography and (B) magnetic resonance images demonstrating a burst fracture with an associated dural injury.

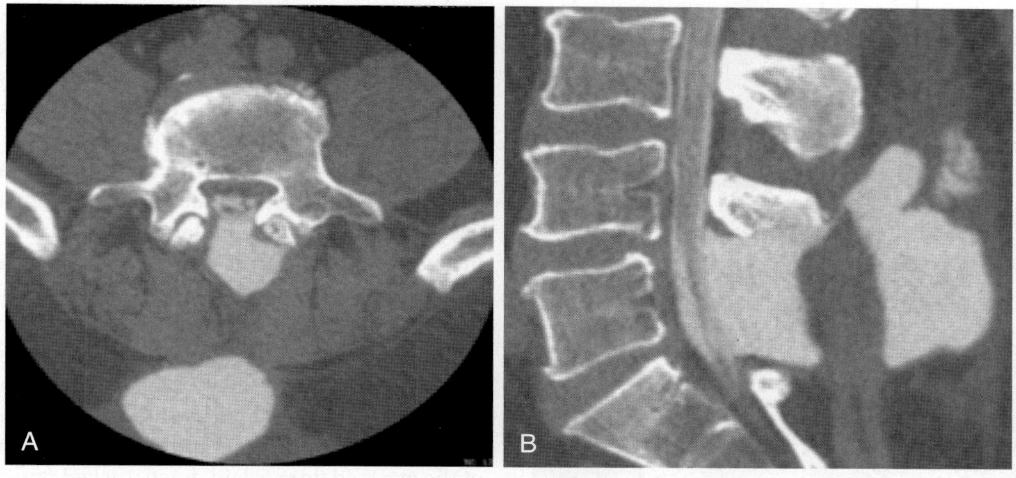

FIG. 96.3 (A) Anterior and (B) lateral myelograms demonstrating a dural injury and associated cerebrospinal fluid leak.

procedures varies widely and has been reported to be between 2% and 75%, as measured by postdural puncture headache.[19] The incidence of postdural puncture headache decreases with use of water-soluble contrast and smaller needles.[20] Durotomies associated with CT myelograms are different than those seen in surgical cases because in durotomies associated with CT myelograms, the puncture hole in the dura is surrounded by normal anatomy that contains the CSF leaking from the defect. This is in contrast to a traumatic or iatrogenic durotomy, as in these situations the anatomy is distorted with significant dead space and injured or decompressed tissue.

Ossification of the posterior longitudinal ligament is the biggest risk factor for durotomy during cervical spine surgery and usually occurs during resection of the posterior longitudinal ligament with a Kerrison rongeur or power burr. According to one study, patients with ossification of the posterior longitudinal ligament are 13.7 times more likely to sustain dural tears[10] than patients with other pathology who undergo a cervical spine procedure. The second most common risk factor for a cervical spine durotomy is revision cervical spine surgery.[10]

Diagnosis

Prompt diagnosis of dural tears is important for management.[18] Ideally, dural tears should be identified intraoperatively. Dural tears can range from a pinhole without leakage to a large defect. Sometimes dural tears are visible but often are not. If the tear is not visible, CSF leakage is likely indicative of a dural injury. CSF leakage manifests as a pulsatile light swirl of fluid within a bloodier field. Repeat bleeding from an area with prior hemostasis should increase suspicion for a dural tear because loss of dural turgor releases the tamponade effect on epidural veins.[18]

Dural tears are sometimes only identified postoperatively. These late-presenting tears are less common, with a frequency of 0.28%.[9] In some cases, the dural tear is not recognized intraoperatively due to incomplete breach of the arachnoid membrane. These tears can worsen postoperatively due to increased intradural pressure. In other cases, a dural tear is recognized intraoperatively but is inadequately repaired.

Patients with a dural tear present with a postdural puncture headache that increases in severity with standing. These headaches occur because the dural tear and associated CSF leak decrease the CSF pressure, causing caudal displacement of neural contents. This displacement stretches the meninges and results in a severe headache.[21] Patients with these headaches often have associated vertigo, blurred vision, nausea, vomiting, fevers, and infection. In addition, there is an association between postdural puncture headaches and intracranial hypotension, tonsillar herniation, subdural hematoma, and hygroma formation.[22–25]

The CSF that leaks from the torn dura can form a pseudomeningocele or a myelocutaneous fistula. Persistently clear or serosanguineous wound drainage following spinal surgery is indicative of a myelocutaneous fistula, which typically occurs on postoperative days 1 to 7. Myelocutaneous fistulas can lead to superficial infections, deep infections, and meningitis. One way to confirm a diagnosis of myelocutaneous fistula is to perform a β_2-transferrin assay on the fluid. Studies have demonstrated this test to have a high sensitivity and specificity.[18]

Magnetic resonance imaging (MRI) is the imaging study of choice in the diagnosis of a CSF leak (Fig. 96.4). In a retrospective review of 24 patients with a CSF leak, Johnson et al. found that MRI had a 100% sensitivity in identifying the location of the CSF leak.[26] MRI is sensitive to presence of CSF accumulation and pseudomeningoceles. Radionuclide cisternography is a new and promising test in the diagnosis of dural tears. One study reported an 84% sensitivity and 98% specificity in detecting difficult-to-find CSF leaks in patients with CSF rhinorrhea.[27]

Treatment

Proper technique is critical for the repair of dural tears. Prompt, watertight primary repair is the gold standard to prevent the complications from a persistent dural tear, which include CSF

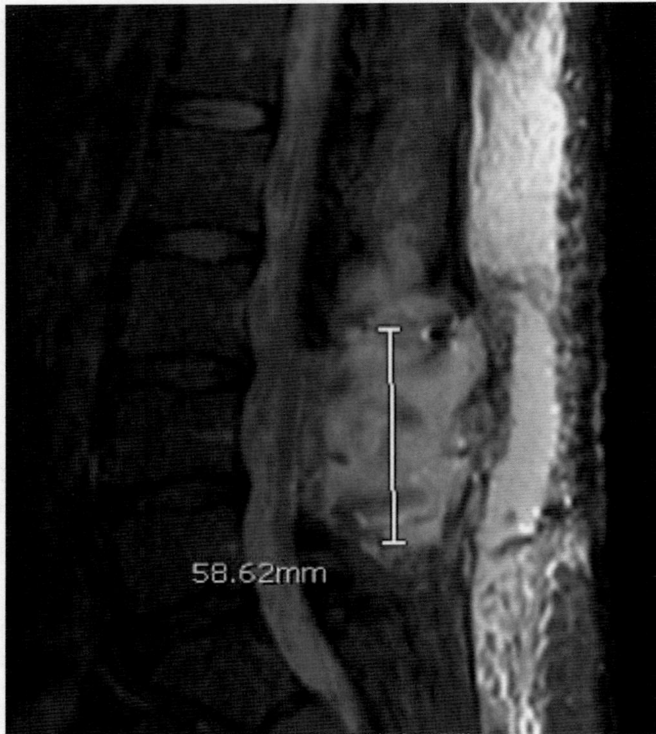

FIG. 96.4 Magnetic resonance image demonstrating extraaxial cerebrospinal fluid collection.

fistula, pseudocyst formation with associated risk of meningitis, nerve root entrapment and cranial nerve palsy, mass effect, and delayed wound healing.[18,28] The principles of dural repair have previously been described by Eismont.[28] The surgeon who cannot visualize the dural tear effectively may need to resect more bone to expose and repair the tear.[28] The entire extent of the tear must be identified and nerve roots should be gently pushed aside using a blunt instrument if necessary. Even if only the outermost layer of dura is torn, the surgeon should perform a primary repair; increased intraabdominal pressure postoperatively can cause the arachnoid to burst and result in delayed CSF leak.[18] Eismont recommended that surgeons use magnification for better visualization and argued that microscopes also allow for better illumination. Again, to improve visualization, surgeons should ensure that they have a dry surgical field through judicious use of bipolar electrocautery, oxidized regenerated cellulose, and absorbable gelatin sponges, and surgeons should suction through a Frazier tip or cottonoid pledget.[28] This maneuver avoids inadvertent suctioning of exposed nerve rootlets.

Primary repair of the dura has been described using multiple different sutures and techniques. Khan et al. repaired 338 lumbar durotomies using a 4-0 silk suture in a locking fashion, with a 98.2% success rate.[11] Other authors have described repairing durotomies with a 5-0 Gore-Tex suture with a similar success rate.[18] None of these techniques has documented superiority. The most important factor in dural repair is achieving a watertight closure. The strength of the dural repair should be tested with a Valsalva maneuver performed by the anesthesiologist prior to skin closure.[28] Surgeons should perform a tight fascial closure to prevent CSF from collecting at the skin. In fact, Eismont recommends against the use of subfascial drains to prevent this potential problem.[28] However, more recent data indicate that drains are safe even in the presence of a dural tear.[29]

In situations in which the surgeon is unable to close the dural tear primarily without undue tension, a graft should be used. Fat grafts are a popular option because they are impermeable to water, can be harvested via the same incision, do not adhere to neural elements, and help prevent scar formation. The two main methods for performing a fat graft are fat plugs and the onlay method. In a fat plug, the fat is placed in a dural defect, a separate incision is made to pass suture to the fat plug, and then the fat is sutured to the edge of the dural defect.[30] In the onlay method, a large piece of fat covering all of the exposed dura is laid down, tucked underneath the bone, and sutured to the dura.[31] Onlay grafts can be supplemented with muscle and fascia as needed.[31] For anterior tears, fat can also be used to fill disc space. Posterior application allows for circumferential coverage (Fig. 96.5).

Fibrin glue and collagen matrices can be used as adjuncts to augment dural repairs. Fibrin glues contain fibrinogen and factor XIII as well as thrombin and calcium. The glues have a hemostatic effect by simulating the final steps of the clotting cascade. Autogenous fibrin glues are commonly used but have a significant cost and the literature to date has not definitively shown improved outcomes in dural repairs with use of this product (although some data show a decrease in postoperative wound drainage).[32] Commercially available collagen matrices function as a graft. Multiple studies have shown these products to be an effective means of closing dura without increased risk of infection or adverse events.[33–35] These products do not need suture fixation and are replaced by natural collagen in 2 to 3 months.[33–35]

Various dural substitutes have also been investigated. The use of xenografts has been limited by the risk of disease transmission. Autologous grafts, such as the tensor fascia lata and lumbodorsal fascia, are safer from a disease transmission standpoint but obviously place a greater burden on operating room resources (e.g., longer operating room time, incision, blood loss). In children, the quantity of autologous grafting materials may be inadequate. Collagen sponges have a role as supplements to other materials as dural substitutes but are not watertight and cannot be used in isolation. Research is currently being conducted into the possible use of other collagen and synthetic materials as dural substitutes.[36–38]

Closed subarachnoid drainage is an option for primary treatment of a dural tear or can be used as an adjunct to other treatment methods. In closed subarachnoid drainage, patients have preferential drainage of CSF through the catheter instead of the dural tear. If this is used as adjunct, it protects a surgeon's dural repair.[39] Several studies report a good success rate with closed subarachnoid drainage. However, patients treated with this method have an increased risk of local infection or meningitis, both of which can develop despite the use of prophylactic antibiotics.[39,40]

There are less data regarding the optimal management of cervical dural tears than lumbar dural tears. However, cervical

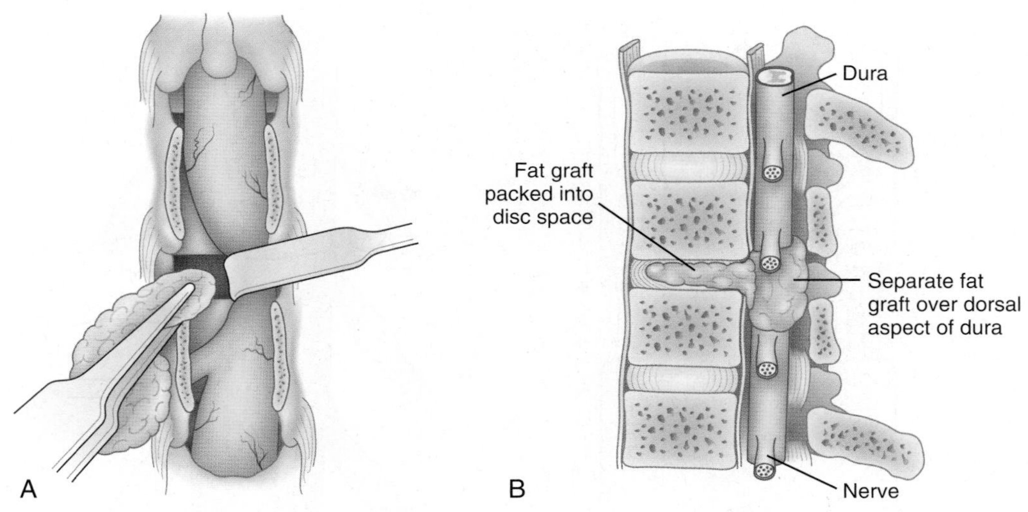

FIG. 96.5 Circumferential patch technique using a 360-degree fat enclosure to seal an anterior durotomy. (A) Fat is inserted and packed into the anterior disc space to seal the anterior leak. B. A separate sheet of fat is placed posteriorly, making contact with the anterior fat to create a ring of fat around the dura. The fat is then covered with fibrin glue and an absorbable hemostat. (Modified from Black P. Cerebrovascular fluid leaks following spinal surgery: use of fat grafts for prevention and repair. Technical note. *J Neurosurg*. 2002;96[2 suppl]:250–252.)

tears can be problematic—surgeons are often unable to repair them primarily due to the limited exposure afforded in an anterior cervical discectomy and fusion. One set of authors recommended utilizing Gelfoam for small tears and subarachnoid drains for larger tears.[10] Another set of authors reports a 98% success rate using an epidural blood patch for cervical dural tears when performed more than 24 hours after the index procedure.[20] The diagnosis of small cervical dural tears can be challenging due to the lack of classic symptoms, such as positional headache, nausea, or photophobia.

Postoperatively, patients who undergo dural repair may be placed on strict bed rest. The position of the patient on the bed is dictated by the goal of decreasing pressure to the affected area. Patients with cervical dural tears should rest in an upright position while patients with a lumbar dural tear should rest in a supine position. There is no clear protocol for how long to keep patients on strict bed rest. Canine studies demonstrate fibroblastic bridging of the dura on postoperative day 6 and dural healing at postoperative day 10.[41] In humans, several authors have reported excellent results with a shorter length of bed rest. In a review of 88 patients with lumbar dural tears, Wang et al.[29] kept patients on bed rest for an average of 2.9 days and reported good to excellent results in 76 of the 88 patients. Other authors have advocated for no mandatory bed rest after dural repair.[42] Hodges et al. retrospectively reviewed 20 patients with dural repairs who were not placed on mandatory bed rest.[42] The authors found that 15 patients had no symptoms and concluded that most patients who sustain an incidental durotomy that is able to be repaired may be treated successfully without mandatory bed rest. Many surgeons recommend individualizing postoperative bed rest according to the patient and the strength of the dural repair.

The treatment of late-presenting dural tears has traditionally involved surgical management with primary closure of the incidental durotomy[43] (Fig. 96.6). However, several authors advocate for nonsurgical measures to be used first in an attempt to avoid the risk associated with reoperation. These measures include bed rest, abdominal binders (focal compression for pseudomeningoceles),[44] and/or closed subarachnoid drains. In fact, some studies have shown that lumbar drainage of 120 to 360 mL/day for 3 to 5 days can lead to a 90% to 92% success rate.[39,40,45] In patients with a myelocutaneous fistula, bed rest, a watertight skin closure, and some form of ancillary CSF diversion have been reported to facilitate complete resolution of symptoms.[40,45] Epidural blood patching has also been reported for treatment of fistulas and pseudomeningoceles[46–48] (Fig. 96.7). Additional options include the use of a percutaneously injected fibrin sealant or a subfascial epidural drain.[43]

Outcomes

Primary dural repair has a failure rate of 5% to 10%.[35] The usual suspected mechanism is leakage from a suture hole. Some studies are investigating sutureless techniques, but there are currently no clear recommendations.[35] Sutureless techniques are a source of active study due to the increasing popularity of minimally invasive spine surgery. Shibayama et al. reported on seven patients treated with a microendoscopic dural repair technique.[36] The technique involves creating a patch graft from polyglactin mesh, which is then glued to the dura using a fibrin. The authors reported good results at 12-month follow-up.

Many studies show no long-term sequelae, no increased risk of postoperative infection, and no neural damage or arachnoiditis if a dural tear is repaired promptly.[9,29] Jones et al.[49] retrospectively reviewed the long-term outcomes for 17 patients who sustained an incidental durotomy during lumbar

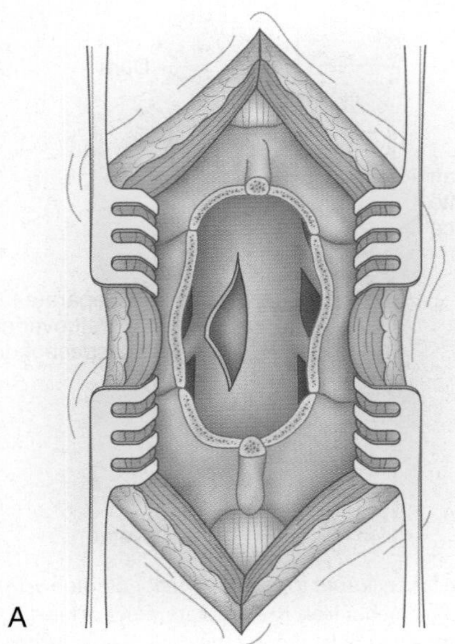

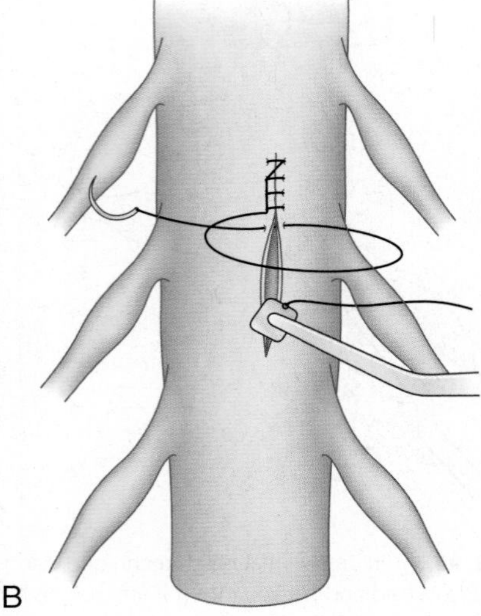

FIG. 96.6 Incidental durotomy and repair. (A) Multilevel laminectomy with longitudinal dural tear. (B) Repair of dural tear with running suture. Commonly used sutures include 4-0 silk and 5-0 Gore-Tex.

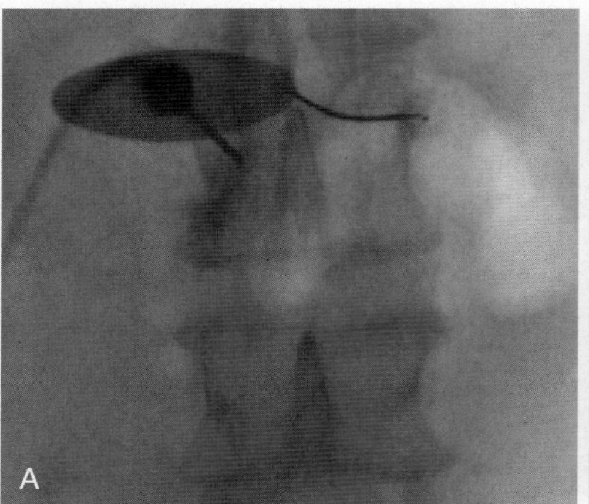

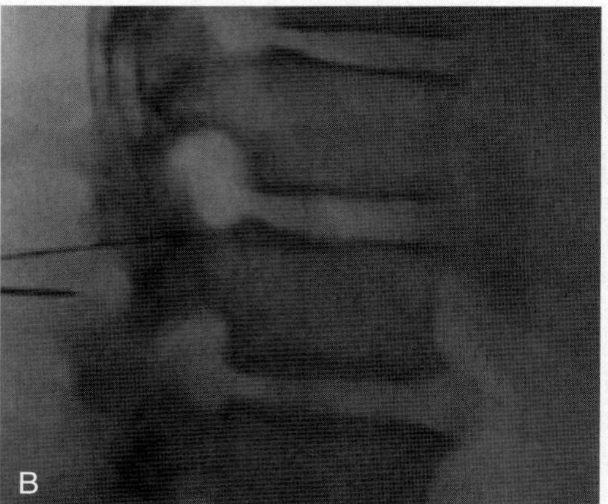

FIG. 96.7 Fluoroscopic images obtained during an attempted blood patch.

spine surgery and found no adverse change in patients' relief of back pain, leg pain, and success of surgery relative to 433 patients who did not sustain a dural tear. However, other studies have indicated that patients with dural tears have worse outcomes with a higher risk of postoperative back pain and headaches.[50] The morbidity of a durotomy has been reported to be lower for younger patients and patients receiving lumbar discectomy.[51]

Summary

Dural tears are one of the most common complications of spine surgery and are the second-most cited cause of malpractice lawsuits in spine surgery.[52] Therefore, it behooves the treating spine surgeon to counsel patients preoperatively regarding the possibility of this complication and to provide reassurance that when dural tears are properly treated there are no long-term sequelae.

KEY REFERENCES

1. Cammisa FP Jr, Eismont FJ, Green BA. Dural laceration occurring with burst fractures and associated laminar fractures. *J Bone Joint Surg Am*. 1989;71(7):1044-1052.

   These authors performed a retrospective analysis of 60 patients with thoracic or lumbar burst fractures. They found that patients with associated lamina fractures had a significantly higher risk of dural injury and neurologic deficit due to entrapment of neural elements.

2. Sin AH, et al. Predictive factors for dural tear and cerebrospinal fluid leakage in patients undergoing lumbar surgery. *J Neurosurg Spine*. 2006;5(3):224-227.

   This study prospectively compared the outcomes of patients who had a durotomy during lumbar spine surgery with patients who did not have this complication. Patients with durotomy had longer length of stay but did not have a higher rate of other complications.

3. Eismont FJ, Wiesel SW, Rothman RH. Treatment of dural tears associated with spinal surgery. *J Bone Joint Surg Am*. 1981;63(7):1132-1136.

This paper described the complications seen in patients with chronic cerebrospinal fluid leakage and was one of the first papers to describe different techniques for durotomy repair.

4. Kitchel SH, Eismont FJ, Green BA. Closed subarachnoid drainage for management of cerebrospinal fluid leakage after an operation on the spine. *J Bone Joint Surg Am.* 1989;71(7):984-987. *This retrospective review describes the use of a subarachnoid shunt in patients with persistent cerebrospinal fluid wound drainage postoperatively. Fourteen of 17 patients were treated successfully.*

5. Saxler G, et al. The long-term clinical sequelae of incidental durotomy in lumbar disc surgery. *Spine.* 2005;30(20):2298-2302. *This retrospective review of 450 patients who underwent lumbar spine surgery demonstrated no difference in long-term clinical outcomes in the 17 patients who had a durotomy compared with nondurotomy patients.*

REFERENCES

1. Vandenabeele F, Creemers J, Lambrichts I. Ultrastructure of the human spinal arachnoid mater and dura mater. *J Anat.* 1996;189(Pt 2):417-430.
2. Runza M, et al. Lumbar dura mater biomechanics: experimental characterization and scanning electron microscopy observations. *Anesth Analg.* 1999;88(6): 1317-1321.
3. Johanson CE, et al. Multiplicity of cerebrospinal fluid functions: new challenges in health and disease. *Cerebrospinal Fluid Res.* 2008;5:10.
4. Ozturk C, Ersozlu S, Aydinli U. Importance of greenstick lamina fractures in low lumbar burst fractures. *Int Orthop.* 2006;30(4):295-298.
5. Cammisa FP Jr, Eismont FJ, Green BA. Dural laceration occurring with burst fractures and associated laminar fractures. *J Bone Joint Surg Am.* 1989;71(7):1044-1052.
6. Andreychik DA, et al. Burst fractures of the second through fifth lumbar vertebrae. Clinical and radiographic results. *J Bone Joint Surg Am.* 1996;78(8):1156-1166.
7. Miller CA, Hunt WE. Variation of impaction fracture of lumbar spine. *J Neurosurg.* 1982;56(4):603.
8. Pickett J, Blumenkopf B. Dural lacerations and thoracolumbar fractures. *J Spinal Disord.* 1989;2(2):99-103.
9. Cammisa FP Jr, et al. Incidental durotomy in spine surgery. *Spine.* 2000;25(20):2663-2667.
10. Hannallah D, et al. Cerebrospinal fluid leaks following cervical spine surgery. *J Bone Joint Surg Am.* 2008;90(5):1101-1105.
11. Khan MH, et al. Postoperative management protocol for incidental dural tears during degenerative lumbar spine surgery: a review of 3,183 consecutive degenerative lumbar cases. *Spine.* 2006;31(22):2609-2613.
12. Stolke D, Sollmann WP, Seifert V. Intra- and postoperative complications in lumbar disc surgery. *Spine.* 1989;14(1):56-59.
13. Weinstein JN, et al. Surgical versus nonsurgical treatment for lumbar degenerative spondylolisthesis. *N Engl J Med.* 2007;356(22):2257-2270.
14. Weinstein JN, et al. Surgical versus nonoperative treatment for lumbar disc herniation: four-year results for the Spine Patient Outcomes Research Trial (SPORT). *Spine.* 2008;33(25):2789-2800.
15. Weinstein JN, et al. Surgical vs nonoperative treatment for lumbar disk herniation: the Spine Patient Outcomes Research Trial (SPORT) observational cohort. *JAMA.* 2006;296(20):2451-2459.
16. Sin AH, et al. Predictive factors for dural tear and cerebrospinal fluid leakage in patients undergoing lumbar surgery. *J Neurosurg Spine.* 2006;5(3):224-227.
17. Epstein NE. The frequency and etiology of intraoperative dural tears in 110 predominantly geriatric patients undergoing multilevel laminectomy with noninstrumented fusions. *J Spinal Disord Tech.* 2007;20(5):380-386.
18. Bosacco SJ, Gardner MJ, Guille JT. Evaluation and treatment of dural tears in lumbar spine surgery: a review. *Clin Orthop Relat Res.* 2001;389:238-247.
19. Peterman SB. Postmyelography headache rates with Whitacre versus Quincke 22-gauge spinal needles. *Radiology.* 1996;200(3):771-778.
20. Turnbull DK, Shepherd DB. Post-dural puncture headache: pathogenesis, prevention and treatment. *Br J Anaesth.* 2003;91(5):718-729.
21. Vakharia SB, et al. Magnetic resonance imaging of cerebrospinal fluid leak and tamponade effect of blood patch in postdural puncture headache. *Anesth Analg.* 1997;84(3):585-590.
22. Chadduck WM. Cerebellar hemorrhage complicating cervical laminectomy. *Neurosurgery.* 1981;9(2):185-189.
23. Friedman JA, et al. Cerebellar hemorrhage after spinal surgery: report of two cases and literature review. *Neurosurgery.* 2002;50(6):1361-1363.
24. Sciubba DM, Kretzer RM, Wang PP. Acute intracranial subdural hematoma following a lumbar CSF leak caused by spine surgery. *Spine.* 2005;30(24):E730-E732.
25. Zimmerman RM, Kebaish KM. Intracranial hemorrhage following incidental durotomy during spinal surgery. A report of four patients. *J Bone Joint Surg Am.* 2007;89(10):2275-2279.
26. Johnson DB, et al. Magnetic resonance imaging in the evaluation of cerebrospinal fluid fistulae. *Clin Radiol.* 1996; 51(12):837-841.
27. Aydin K, et al. Localization of cerebrospinal fluid leaks by gadolinium-enhanced magnetic resonance cisternography: a 5-year single-center experience. *Neurosurgery.* 2008;62(3): 584-589.
28. Eismont FJ, Wiesel SW, Rothman RH. Treatment of dural tears associated with spinal surgery. *J Bone Joint Surg Am.* 1981;63(7):1132-1136.
29. Wang JC, Bohlman HH, Riew KD. Dural tears secondary to operations on the lumbar spine. Management and results after a two-year-minimum follow-up of eighty-eight patients. *J Bone Joint Surg Am.* 1998;80(12):1728-1732.
30. Mayfield FH, Kurokawa K. Watertight closure of spinal dura mater. *J Neurosurg.* 1975;43(5):639-640.
31. Black P. Cerebrospinal fluid leaks following spinal surgery: use of fat grafts for prevention and repair. *J Neurosurg.* 2002;96(2 suppl):250-252.
32. Nakamura H, et al. The effect of autologous fibrin tissue adhesive on postoperative cerebrospinal fluid leak in spinal cord surgery: a randomized controlled trial. *Spine.* 2005;30(13):E347-E351.
33. Narotam PK, et al. Collagen matrix duraplasty for cranial and spinal surgery: a clinical and imaging study. *J Neurosurg.* 2007;106(1):45-51.
34. Biroli F, et al. Novel equine collagen-only dural substitute. *Neurosurgery.* 2008;62(3 suppl 1):273-274.
35. Narotam PK, et al. Collagen matrix (DuraGen) in dural repair: analysis of a new modified technique. *Spine.* 2004;29(24):2861-2867.
36. Shibayama M, et al. Patch technique for repair of a dural tear in microendoscopic spinal surgery. *J Bone Joint Surg Br.* 2008;90(8):1066-1067.

37. Messing-Junger AM, et al. Effectiveness and handling characteristics of a three-layer polymer dura substitute: a prospective multicenter clinical study. *J Neurosurg.* 2006;105(6):853-858.
38. Link MJ, Converse LD, Lanier WL. A new technique for single-person fascia lata harvest. *Neurosurgery.* 2008;63(4 suppl 2):359-361.
39. Kitchel SH, Eismont FJ, Green BA. Closed subarachnoid drainage for management of cerebrospinal fluid leakage after an operation on the spine. *J Bone Joint Surg Am.* 1989;71(7):984-987.
40. Shapiro SA, Scully T. Closed continuous drainage of cerebrospinal fluid via a lumbar subarachnoid catheter for treatment or prevention of cranial/spinal cerebrospinal fluid fistula. *Neurosurgery.* 1992;30(2):241-245.
41. Cain JE Jr, et al. The histomorphologic sequence of dural repair. Observations in the canine model. *Spine.* 1991; 16(8 suppl):S319-S323.
42. Hodges SD, et al. Management of incidental durotomy without mandatory bed rest. A retrospective review of 20 cases. *Spine.* 1999;24(19):2062-2064.
43. Hughes SA, et al. Prolonged Jackson-Pratt drainage in the management of lumbar cerebrospinal fluid leaks. *Surg Neurol.* 2006;65(4):410-414.
44. Leis AA, Leis JM, Leis JR. Pseudomeningoceles: a role for mechanical compression in the treatment of dural tears. *Neurology.* 2001;56(8):1116-1117.
45. McCallum JE, Tenicela R, Jannetta PJ. Closed external drainage of cerebrospinal fluid in treatment of postoperative CSF fistulae. *Surg Forum.* 1973;24:465-467.
46. Elbiaadi-Aziz N, et al. Cerebrospinal fluid leak treated by aspiration and epidural blood patch under computed tomography guidance. *Reg Anesth Pain Med.* 2001;26(4): 363-367.
47. Lauer KK, Haddox JD. Epidural blood patch as treatment for a surgical durocutaneous fistula. *J Clin Anesth.* 1992;4(1): 45-47.
48. Maycock NF, van Essen J, Pfitzner J. Post-laminectomy cerebrospinal fluid fistula treated with epidural blood patch. *Spine.* 1994;19(19):2223-2225.
49. Jones AA, et al. Long-term results of lumbar spine surgery complicated by unintended incidental durotomy. *Spine.* 1989;14(4):443-446.
50. Saxler G, et al. The long-term clinical sequelae of incidental durotomy in lumbar disc surgery. *Spine.* 2005;30(20):2298-2302.
51. Deyo RA, et al. Morbidity and mortality in association with operations on the lumbar spine. The influence of age, diagnosis, and procedure. *J Bone Joint Surg Am.* 1992;74(4):536-543.
52. Goodkin R, Laska LL. Unintended "incidental" durotomy during surgery of the lumbar spine: medicolegal implications. *Surg Neurol.* 1995;43(1):4-12.

CHAPTER 97 Vascular Complications in Spinal Surgery

Matthew L. Webb
Jonathan N. Grauer

Introduction

A vascular complication may be defined as an injury to a blood vessel and the sequelae of that injury, which may be the direct or indirect result of the procedure, surgical approach, or operative technique. For the purposes of this chapter, a vascular complication may arise directly from vascular injury or indirectly as a consequence of the injury. Mechanisms of blood vessel injury include laceration, traction, instrumentation malpositioning, and compression.[1] The spectrum of manifestations of vascular injuries include hemorrhage from laceration or traction of a vessel wall[2]; aneurysm or arteriovenous fistula resulting from vessel wall injury; blood flow interruption at the macroscopic end organ level or ischemia on a microscopic level[3]; embolization of air, plaque, or clot; and thrombosis or direct injury from instrumentation, including erosions from instrumentation in contact with pulsatile arteries and malpositioned screws (Fig. 97.1).[4] The most common vascular complication in spinal surgery, however, is direct laceration of a vessel resulting in acute bleeding.

Vascular complications associated with spinal surgery continue to increase in frequency, although the rate of increase is decelerating. From 1997 to 2003 the frequency of vascular complications reportedly quadrupled,[5] but from 2003 to 2010 the rates of vascular complications have increased by less than 50%.[6] This could be a result of an increasing frequency of anterior approaches to the thoracolumbar spine or an early trend toward increased documentation and reporting.[3,7-24] Between 2003 and 2010 the rates of venous thromboembolism, hemorrhagic anemia, and postoperative shock increased by about 150% in thoracic spine surgery, whereas the rates of these complications increased by less than 50% in cervical and lumbar spine surgery.[6]

It is also possible that vascular complications are underreported and the true incidences are impossible to know. For example, multiple reviews of cervical spine surgery have reported no vascular complications,[22,25] but in a questionnaire study that covered 5641 cases, vertebral artery injuries were noted in 0.14% of cases.[26] A hypothetical example of this underreporting would be a laceration of the left common iliac vein occurring during an anterior lumbar spinal exposure at L4–L5. The vascular and spinal surgeons recognize this injury and rapidly isolate and repair it. Although intraoperative blood loss is increased, there may be no other sequelae. Some surgeons do not consider this a complication, but rather a routine risk of exposure of the lumbosacral spine and therefore may not note or report it. A recent review of a prospective database of 1262 consecutive anterior approaches to the thoracolumbar spine found a 1.11% rate of injury to a major vessel.[27] It could also be that with increasing awareness and vigilance the real rate of these injuries has, in fact, decreased.

The consequences of vascular complications in spinal surgery can be severe. Three consequences include brisk bleeding leading to hemorrhagic shock,[28] interrupted vascular supply to vital organs such as the spinal cord or brainstem,[29,30] and secondary injury as a result of inadequate visualization caused by bleeding.[31] Poor visualization due to inadequate hemostasis can lead to spinal cord or nerve root injury. These consequences are not mutually exclusive and often occur in series or combination. The primary sequelae of bleeding often result from injury to, or disruption of, major blood vessels adjacent to the vertebral bodies. All these complications have consequences that may be irreversible, and for this reason prompt recognition and management are essential when these complications occur.

Prevention should be the primary focus in the discussion of vascular complications of spine surgery. Prevention of vascular complications is assisted by knowledge of the normal vascular anatomy and common variants,[32] including a knowledge of the relationships between particular blood vessels and bony landmarks,[33,34] by careful preoperative planning, and by the use of gentle intraoperative techniques with appropriate illumination and magnification. This chapter emphasizes the vascular anatomy of the spine and highlights the spectrum of spinal vascular injuries, how they may be recognized early and, most importantly, how they may be prevented.

Cervical Spine

Anterior Cervical Vascular Complications

Exposure of the anterior cervical spine commonly uses an approach medial to the sternocleidomastoid muscle and

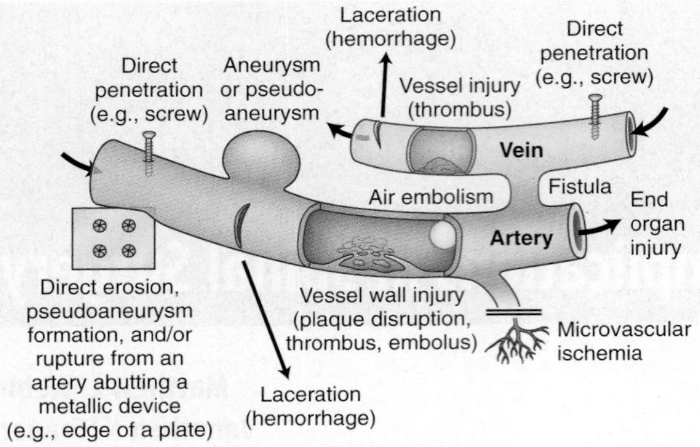

FIG. 97.1 Spectrum of vascular injuries, complications, or sequelae associated with modern cervical, thoracic, and lumbosacral spine surgery.

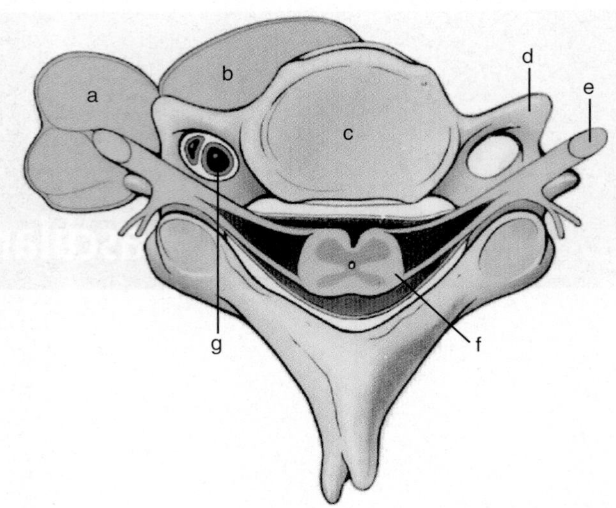

FIG. 97.2 Cross-sectional representation of the cervical spine at C5. The anterior scalenus muscle (*a*), the longus colli muscle (*b*), the vertebral body (*c*), and the transverse foramen (*d*) are noted. The cervical nerve root (*e*) and the spinal cord (*f*) are seen relative to the anterior vertebral body (*c*) and musculature (*a*, *b*). The vertebral artery (*g*) is noted within the transverse foramen. The vertebral artery enters the sixth cervical foramina and continues proximally to become the basilar artery. Injury to the vertebral artery may occur when releasing or dissecting the longus colli muscles. It may also be injured in discectomies that involve dissection in the lateral aspect of the disc near the uncovertebral joint (not shown).

carotid sheath (Smith-Robinson approach).[32] Vascular complications in the cervical spine are much less often the result of direct injury and much more often the result of improper and excessive retraction.[35-56] Although the absolute incidence of vascular injuries from anterior cervical spinal surgery is not known, they are rare events. For example, no vascular injuries were reported in reviews of 500[22] and 450 cases,[25] and a retrospective questionnaire study of 5641 cervical spine cases found an incidence of vertebral artery injury of only 0.14%.[26] Another review reported four cases of carotid artery injury during anterior cervical fusion. In those cases involving laceration of the carotid artery, all of these injuries were repaired primarily and no permanent neurologic sequelae occurred.[57] Although another case series cautioned that the vessels of the carotid sheath were at "some risk" from the self-retaining retractor, no cases of vascular injury were reported.[58] In order to prevent carotid artery injury, self-retaining blunt blades should be carefully placed deep to the longus colli muscles medially and laterally and not against the carotid sheath.

Vertebral artery injuries are also rare but are more common than carotid artery injuries. As a historical example, a single vertebral artery injury was reported in 175 cases of interbody fusion from 1976 to 1990 at a single institution.[59] The artery was sacrificed and there were no adverse consequences for the patient. Another case series reported four cases of vertebral artery injuries in 2015 anterior cervical spine cases for a case series incidence of 0.3%,[60] and another series reported 167 anterior cervical discectomy and fusions for degenerative disease technique without any major vascular injuries.[61] Despite these reports, the overall incidence of vertebral artery injury in cervical spine surgery is nearer to 1.4%,[62] with the lowest risks during anterior approaches to the subaxial cervical spine (0.3–0.5%)[51,60,63] and the greatest risks during posterior instrumented procedures of the upper cervical spine (4–8%).[53,64]

Treatment of the vascular injuries during anterior cervical spine exposure involves recognition, control of bleeding, repair, ligation, and endovascular stents when indicated. Although primary repair of the vertebral artery and common carotid artery is desirable, endovascular techniques are becoming the standard of care.

Vertebral Artery

The vertebral artery and vein are at risk from both anterior and posterior exposures of the cervical spine (Fig. 97.2). This is a unique feature of the cervical vascular anatomy. The vertebral artery is integrated with the spinal column passing through the vertebral foramen at levels superior to C7 and classically coursing anterior to posterior at C1–C2.[65] Detailed anatomic studies have presented the diversity of vertebral artery size, variations, and anomalies.[66] Vertebral artery injuries result in either hemorrhage, vertebral basilar insufficiency stroke, or both[51,65,67]; have classically been thought to occur in fewer than one in 200 anterior cervical surgeries[51]; and have been known to have devastating consequences. For example, vertebral artery injury during anterior cervical discectomy and fusion has been reported to have resulted in permanent neurologic deficits despite immediate identification of the laceration, control of bleeding, and primary repair.[68] As with other vascular complications of spine surgery, prevention is the best strategy for managing injuries of the vertebral artery.

During anterior exposure the vertebral arteries are at risk of injury by dissection lateral to the longus colli muscles, whereas during anterior discectomy any dissection beyond the lateral margins of the disc and lateral to the uncinate processes puts the vertebral artery at risk (Figs. 97.3 and 97.4).[51,69] Prevention of vertebral artery injuries laterally begins with careful dissection of the longus colli muscles. The anatomic relationship of the vertebral artery in the transverse foramina has been well described.[70-73] Beginning at C6 and proceeding to C2, the vertebral artery is tethered to the transverse foramina by a fibroligamentous mesh connected to the adventitia of the

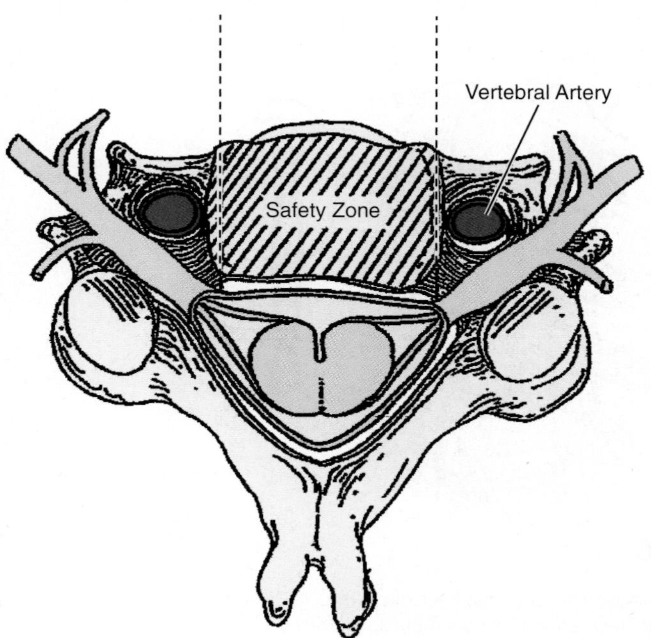

FIG. 97.3 Axial view of the cervical vertebrae showing the extent of anterior decompression that can safely be performed via a corpectomy. Decompression medial to the lateral aspect of the vertebral body border (i.e., medial to the uncinate process) avoids the transverse formina and the vertebral arteries.

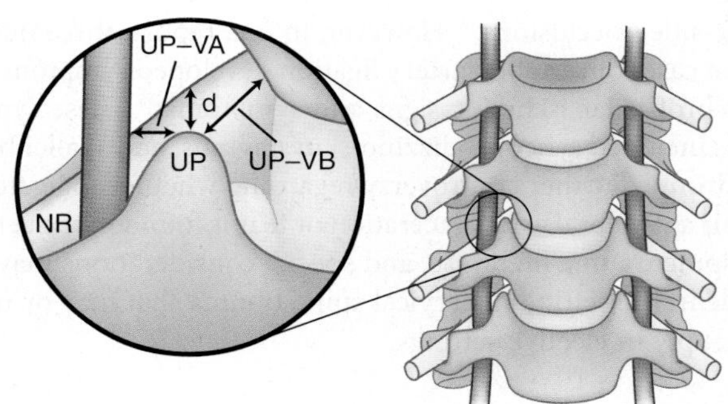

FIG. 97.4 Relationship of the vertebral artery to the uncinate process. The distance (*d*) from the tip of the uncinate process to the vertebral body (*UP–VB*), the distance from the tip of the uncinate process to the vertebral artery (*UP–VA*), and the distance from the tip of the uncinate process up to the nerve root (*UP–NR*) are presented to illustrate the risk of vertebral artery injury in the neural foramina near the uncovertebral joint.

vertebral artery, the vertebral body, and the superior margin of the transverse foraminal bony extension (Fig. 97.5). These relationships have implications if anterior vertebral artery laceration repair is attempted, especially for mobilizing and controlling the artery proximal and distal to the laceration.

It is recommended that the medial edge of the muscles be coagulated and a blunt periosteal elevator be used to mobilize the muscles laterally. To prevent injury to the vertebral artery, this periosteal elevator should never be directed posteriorly. The vertebral artery may also be injured by excess lateral dissection in the intervertebral space lateral to the uncinate processes (C3–C6); it is especially important to be aware of this risk in cases that require extensive dissection such as corpectomy (see Fig. 97.3). Care should be taken that dissection

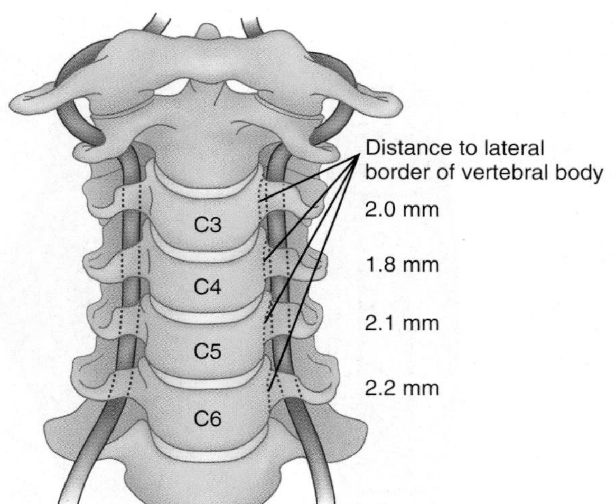

FIG. 97.5 Projection of the vertebral arteries traversing foramina on the anterior aspects of the lower cervical vertebrae. Note that the vertebral artery enters at C6 and becomes progressively more medial to the C3–C4 level. At that level it is 1.8 mm lateral to the uncinate process. This is important to understand during anterior cervical decompression surgery.

or bony resection remain medial to the uncinate process, sparing the medial border of the transverse foramen unless otherwise necessary (e.g., in tumor resection). To this end, it is important to note that the medial margin of the longus colli muscle is the most consistent landmark for the lateral extent of bony dissection. Furthermore, to avoid injury to the vertebral artery during corpectomy, most authors recommend a preoperative midline radiograph or computed tomography (CT) scan for any abnormalities of the vertebral artery in the transverse foramina. The availability of three-dimensional (3D) reconstructions of CT angiography (CTA) has greatly enhanced the value of imaging for preoperative planning,[74] especially in cases of variant or anomalous vertebral arteries that may deviate medially, either originating from the aorta[75,76] or otherwise ascending outside of the vertebral foramen.

It is also important to note that the association between cervical spine trauma and the vertebral artery has been increasingly recognized and studied. A recent review of three level I trauma centers found that 21% of patients with a cervical spine injury underwent screening for vertebral artery injury using CTA. Of those screened, a vertebral artery injury was found in 17%, and of those with a vertebral artery injury, neurologic events secondary to vertebral artery injury occurred in 14%.[77] These findings highlight the importance of preoperative CTA to investigate the course and patency of the vertebral arteries, especially in cases of cervical spine trauma.

If the vertebral artery is lacerated during the anterior dissection, the bleeding should be stopped by tamponade and the dissection carried laterally by mobilizing or dividing the longus colli muscles. This approach to the vertebral artery and cervical nerves, described by Verbiest, also exploits the interval medial to the sternocleidomastoid muscle and carotid sheath. However, unlike the Smith-Robinson approach, Verbiest's exposure proceeds lateral to the longus colli muscle.[78] The surgeon should be aware that this lateralization puts the cervical sympathetic trunk at greater risk of injury, especially at

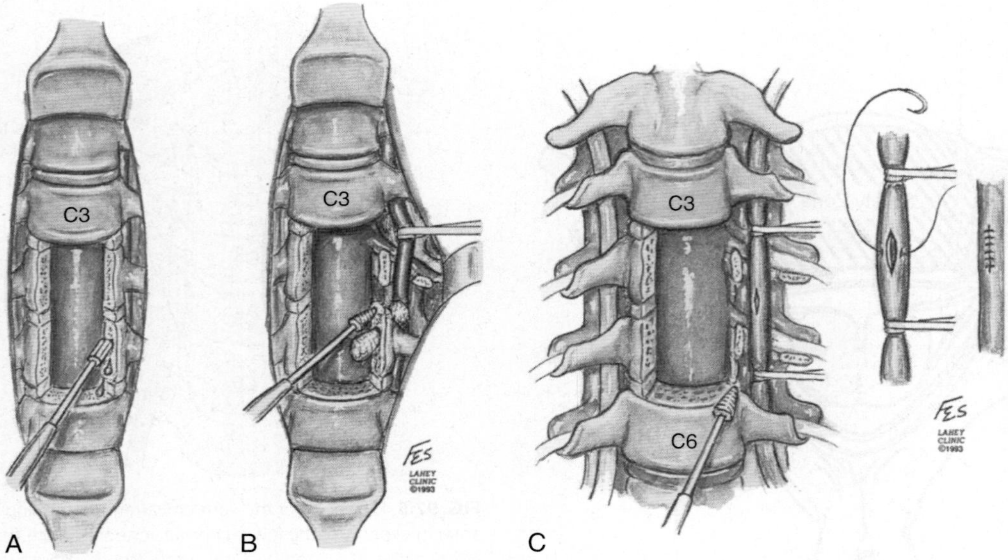

FIG. 97.6 (A) Surgical technique of repair of the vertebral artery. The trough has been cut in the C4–C5 bodies. The burr is angulated laterally to get slightly more exposure. The bleeding area is tamponaded. The bone anterior to the transverse foramen is drilled away to expose the vertebral artery. The C4, C5, and C6 nerve roots are exposed and protected. (B) Elastic loops have been placed around the vertebral artery proximal and distal to the laceration. (C) Laceration is repaired with interrupted sutures of 7-0 polypropylene. (From Pfeifer BA, Friedberg SR, Jewell ER: Repair of injured vertebral artery in anterior cervical procedures. *Spine.* 1994;19:1471–1474.)

lower cervical spinal levels, and Horner syndrome (ipsilateral ptosis, miosis, and anhidrosis) may result.[79] The costotransverse lamellae and fibroligamentous attachments can be removed to allow adequate exposure for primary vascular repair (Fig. 97.6A).[80] If primary repair is chosen, the artery should first be exposed proximal to the laceration, and vessel loops should be used for occlusion (Fig. 97.6B).[80] The nerve roots should be identified and protected. Once the artery is exposed and controlled, the laceration can be repaired, if possible (Fig. 97.6C).[80] The repair may require the assistance of an experienced vascular surgeon, and spinal stability should be ensured after this additional required exposure. Cross clamping of the injured vertebral artery may be required during the repair, and cross clamp duration should be minimized to decrease the likelihood of infarct resulting from vertebrobasilar ischemia.

Many authors support repair of the vertebral artery injury.[60,80,81] Others have ligated the lacerated vertebral artery.[25,65,82,83] The ability of the patient to tolerate unilateral occlusion of the vertebral artery without sequelae is supported by a study of nine patients with traumatic occlusion of the vertebral artery. Only two developed neurologic deficits, both of which were transient.[84] If the vertebral artery is to be sacrificed, it should first be studied by intraoperative angiography to ensure that the patient's anatomy will allow such a maneuver.[65,82,85] The presence or absence of neurologic deficit depends in part on the collateralization of the vertebral artery of the circle of Willis and the patency of the contralateral vertebral and basilar arteries.[25,37] A classic anatomic study reported that occlusion of the vertebral artery led to brainstem ischemia or infarct in 3.1% of left-sided occlusions compared with 1.8% of right-sided occlusions.[66] However, in one report, three out of seven cases of vertebral artery ligation developed symptomatic vertebrobasilar ischemic signs and symptoms.[51] These symptoms included syncope, dizziness, nystagmus, and Wallenberg syndrome. Further controversy regarding whether to ligate or repair a vertebral artery laceration or tear is found in the cervical spine trauma literature, and special considerations may be made in the setting of cervical spine trauma that may or may not apply in elective settings.

Carotid Artery

The common carotid artery is also at risk as the surgeon develops the dissection plane and during retraction for the deep anterior cervical spine exposure (Smith-Robinson approach). Identification of the carotid artery by palpation and gentle finger dissection helps minimize injury of this major vessel. Proper placement of self-retaining retractors requires medial-to-lateral mobilization of the longus colli muscles along the anterolateral aspect of the vertebral bodies. Blunt-tipped blades of these self-retaining retractors must be positioned deep to these muscles, and only enough tension should be applied to retract these muscles away from the vertebral body and disc margins to aid visualization of the vertebra and vertebral disc.

Compromise of carotid artery blood flow risks causing central nervous system ischemia (i.e., ischemic stroke),[86,87] and prolonged retraction of the artery could lead to thrombosis. Some authors have noted a progressive decrease in carotid blood flow secondary to the use of self-retaining retractors.[88] A study of 15 cases showed that ipsilateral carotid

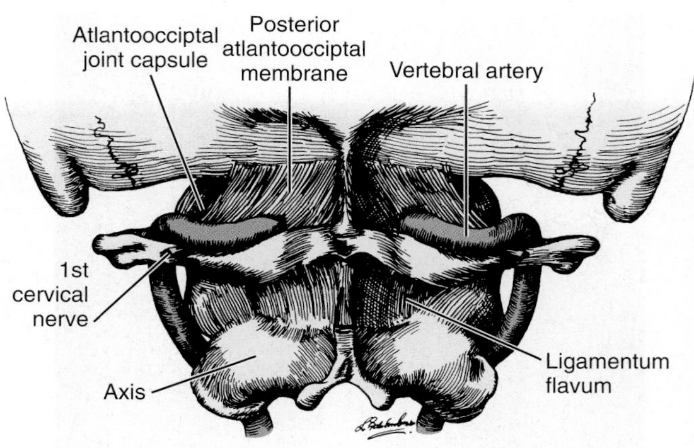

FIG. 97.7 Diagram showing the vertebral arteries coursing over the posterior arch of C1. The medial extent is usually 1.5 to 2 cm lateral to the midline.

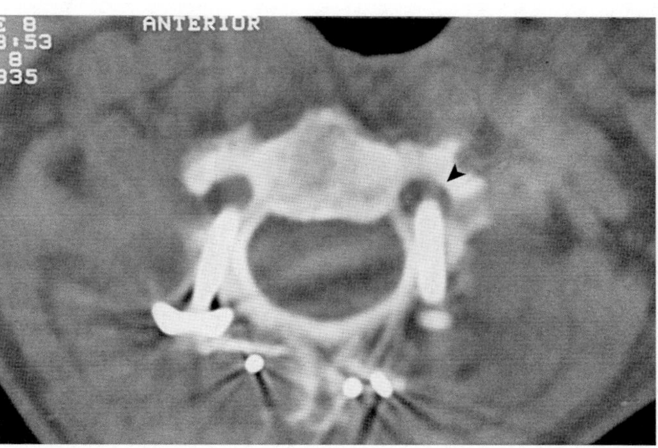

FIG. 97.8 Computed tomography shows a malpositioned C2 screw violating the transverse foramen (arrowhead), fortunately without ill effects or vascular sequelae.

artery blood flow decreased an average of 14% to 70% as measured by duplex ultrasonic flow as the anterior cervical discectomy and fusion procedure proceeded and the arterial cross-sectional area progressively decreased as the surgical duration increased. The diminished blood flow remained laminar at all times and rapidly returned to baseline postoperatively. Younger patients showed a greater drop in blood flow compared with older patients and those with atherosclerotic arteries.

A general strategy to prevent carotid artery ischemia is the intermittent release and repositioning of the retractors,[89] but this repositioning should be done carefully because manipulation of an atherosclerotic artery may dislodge plaques with the unintended consequence of embolic ischemic stroke.

Posterior Cervical Vascular Complications

The vertebral artery and venous plexus are the primary vascular structures at risk during posterior cervical approaches the spine (Fig. 97.7). Posterior vertebral artery injuries are rare,[30,65,90] but multiple cases of posterior vertebral artery injury during posterior cervical spinal surgery are reported in the literature.[57,90-92] Cranial base surgery continues to pose significant challenges and limitations owing to the variations of this region's cerebrovascular anatomy and physiology.[90,93]

Instrumentation of the upper posterior cervical spine from the occiput to C2 puts at risk the vertebral artery, carotid artery, and hypoglossal or spinal accessory nerves depending on the technique. Malpositioning of the lateral mass screws may injure the vertebral artery within the transverse foramen (Fig. 97.8).[23,73,97] C1–C2 transarticular screws risk the vertebral artery, carotid artery, and hypoglossal nerve anteriorly in the C2 transverse foramen. Preoperative CT may aid prevention of inadvertent injury as screw insertion progresses across the C1–C2 facet.[67,95] Anomalies and anatomic variations of the geometry of the foramen and the position of the vertebral artery are common. C1 lateral mass screws put the vertebral artery at risk posteriorly and laterally, and they require meticulous technique for mobilization and protection.[21,96] Preventive strategies include knowledge of the bony landmarks, choice of

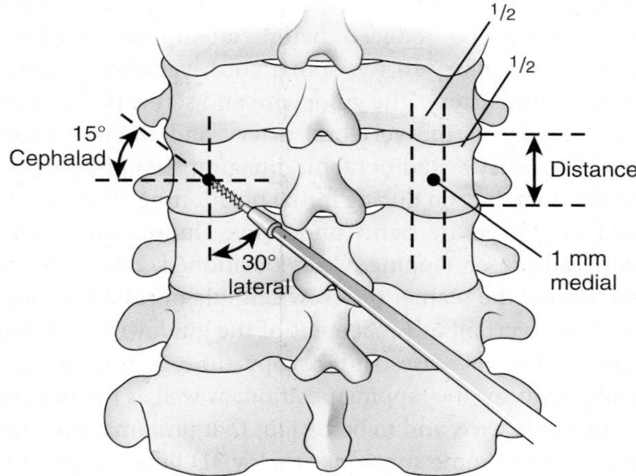

FIG. 97.9 Proposed angulation technique, approximately 15 degrees cephalad and 30 degrees lateral starting 1 mm medial to the midportion of the lateral mass. At C6 the vertebral artery is slightly more lateral to the starting point advocated by An and associates.[94] According to Lu and Ebrahaim,[65] the technique of An and associates describes safe angulation for the placement of lateral mass screws to avoid the anterior vertebral artery in the transverse foramina of C3-C6. (From An HS, Gordin R, Renner K: Anatomic consideration for plate-screw fixation of the cervical spine. *Spine.* 1991;16[Suppl]:S548–S551.)

appropriate screw lengths, and review of angles of insertion (Fig. 97.9).[94]

The vertebral artery and veins are directly anterior or slightly lateral (about 6 degrees lateral at C6) at the middle one-third of the lateral mass. Therefore, to avoid the vertebral artery the lateral mass screw should be started near the center of the mass and directed about 10 to 15 degrees lateral and 30 to 35 degrees cephalad. In contrast, the Magerl technique directs screws directly anterior from the central lateral mass and is more likely to injure a nerve or the vertebral artery. Studies have clearly identified the Magerl technique as most likely to injure the vertebral artery, with an incidence of 1.4% in a survey series of 5641 cases.[26] This technique should be avoided. A consecutive series of 43 patients reported no

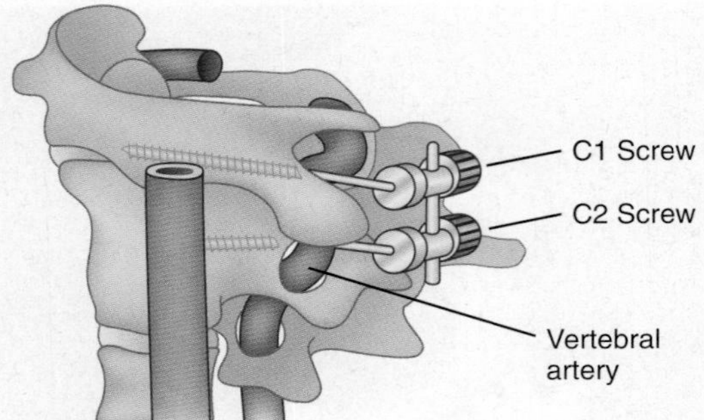

FIG. 97.10 Relationship of the vertebral artery to the C1–C2 posterior screw fixation, indicating how near to the internal carotid artery and the vertebral artery the C1 screw may be positioned.

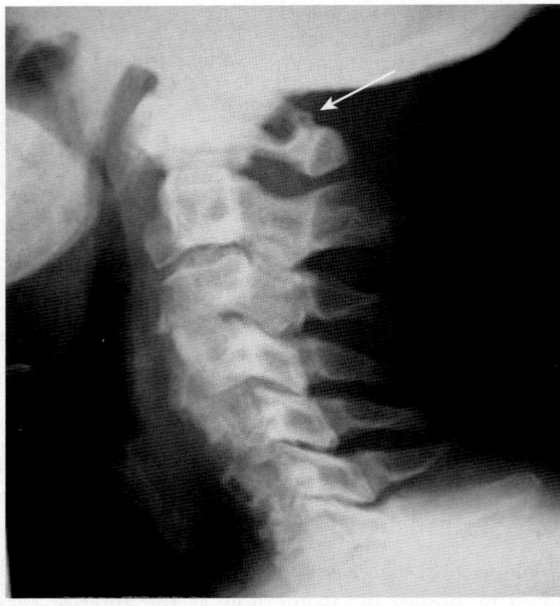

FIG. 97.11 Lateral cervical plain radiograph demonstrating the ponticulus ponticus (*arrow*). This has implications for C1–C2 surgery because the ponticulus ponticus is closely related to the certebral artery as it passes onto the posterior ring of C1. The incidence is common on plain films at about 15%.

vertebral artery injuries from lateral mass plating of the subaxial cervical spine.[97]

Placement of posterior C2 screws is routinely used to stabilize type II or high type III odontoid fractures. C1 and C2 injuries should be reduced before attempting fixation to reduce risk of injury to the spinal cord, vertebral artery, or interior carotid artery. The guidewire and screw tip both pose risks of injury to the vertebral artery and internal carotid artery (Fig. 97.10). Radiographic imaging should be used to minimize penetration during initial positioning. The C2 screw should be placed by hand under live fluoroscopy without power reaming or tapping. Once positioned, care should be taken to clear the reamer or screw cannula of residual bone to prevent inadvertent advancement of the guidewire. Although this procedure increases fluoroscopy time, it is essential to carefully monitor the tapping position, as well as the insertion over the guide wire, and to be certain that proximal migration does not occur. Some surgeons employ 3D fluoroscopy or CT image guidance in these cases.

Vertebral Artery

The vertebral artery is at greatest risk as it passes through the upper cervical spine. Most notably, the vertebral artery passes through the foramen of C2 as it extends cranially, then through the C1 foramen before coursing medially toward the midline on the superior aspect of C1.[65,82] In this area the vertebral artery occupies a groove on the posterior aspect of the posterior arch of C1; anatomic studies have shown that this groove is on average 18 mm lateral of midline, whereas the vertebral artery itself is on average 22 mm from midline.[98]

The vertebral artery is vulnerable because it passes between the C1 and C2 transverse foramina laterally. Lateral dissection along the caudal border of C1 should end on exposure of the dorsal ramus of C2. Due to this unique anatomy of the vertebral artery in the superior cervical spine, some authors have recommended that dissection should begin with identification of the posterior tubercle of the atlas, and that dissection of the posterior aspect of the posterior arch should remain within 12 mm of midline and the dissection should not extend beyond 8 mm of midline on the superior aspect of the arch.[99]

Cervical pedicle screws may be placed more safely at C6 or C7. The screws are started about 2 to 3 mm inferior to the superior articular facet and slightly lateral to the midline of the lateral mass. The screws should be angled medially 35 degrees at C6 or 30 degrees at C7. The C1–C2 technique, which is least likely to risk injury to the anterior vertebral artery, is the modified technique of C1 lateral mass screws and C2 intralaminar crossed screw fixation described in the literature.[100] In about 15.5% of patients, a false bony bridge called the *ponticulus ponticus* covers the vertebral artery as it passes onto the posterior C1 ring. This is easily noted on lateral cervical plain films (Fig. 97.11). It is important to recognize this common variant to avoid injury to the vertebral artery by dissection or C1 transosseous screw fixation.[101]

Vertebral artery injury posteriorly often occurs during lateral mass screw placement either from penetration or laceration by the drill, tap, screw, or probe. However, any technique that begins near or slightly inferior to the midline of the lateral mass and angles laterally and cephalad 15 to 30 degrees and uses screws that are 14 to 16 mm in length are unlikely to injure the vertebral artery or veins.[73,97] Of note, the average reported screw size for women was 14 × 3.5 mm compared with 16 × 3.5 mm for men. As with C2 screw placement, drilling should be done by hand and not under power. Also, caution should be used with the depth gauge. Care should be taken to not plunge and possibly pinch the vertebral artery with the curved end of the depth gauge.

C1 lateral mass fixation has proven to be safe, stable, and effective. The relationship of the vertebral artery at C1–C2 and its location to the triangular window of the pedicle of C1 have been emphasized in the literature (Figs. 97.12 and 97.13).[70-73] Primary clinical challenges are to identify the C2 root and the

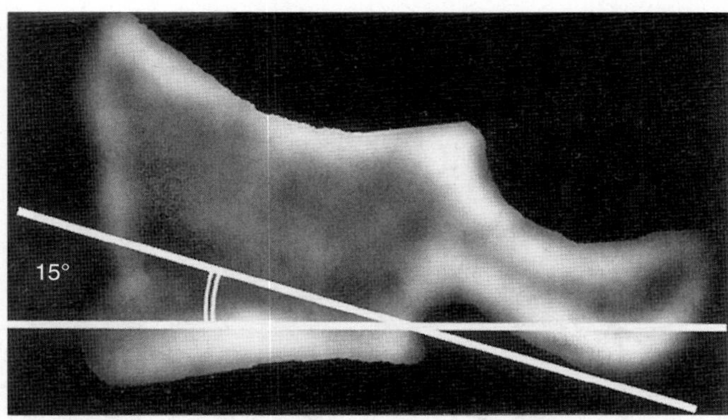

FIG. 97.12 Direction of C1 screw placement. Note that this is directed in approximately a 15-degree cephalad direction in relation to the transverse plane.

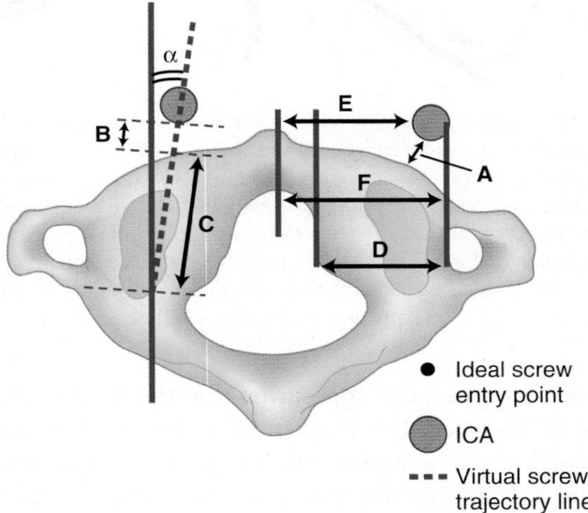

FIG. 97.13 Anatomic measurements and markings for the atlas and internal carotid artery. *A*, Shortest distance between C1 anterior cervical surface and the internal carotid artery. *B*, Shortest distance between C1 anterior cervical surface and the internal carotid artery on virtual screw (VS) trajectory line. *C*, VS line from the ideal screw entry point to the virtual exit point. *D*, Width of the C1 lateral mass. *C*, Distance from the C1 midsagittal line to the inner line of the transverse foramina; the angle made between the sagittal axis and the virtual axis line is labeled as alpha.

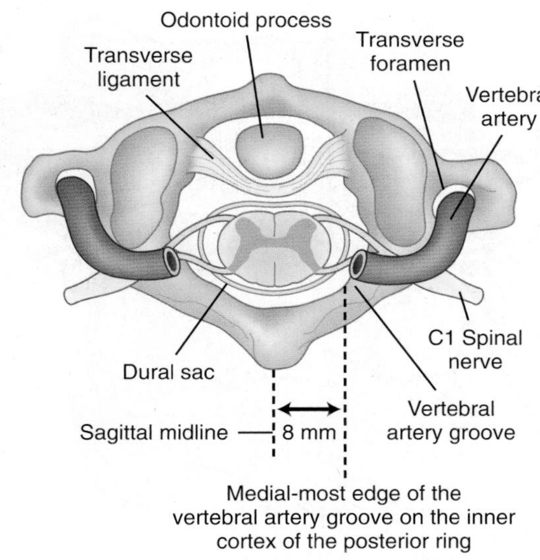

FIG. 97.14 Axial view through the superior aspect of the atlas (C1). Dissection of the superior aspect of the posterior rim of the C1 arch should remain within 8 mm of the midline.

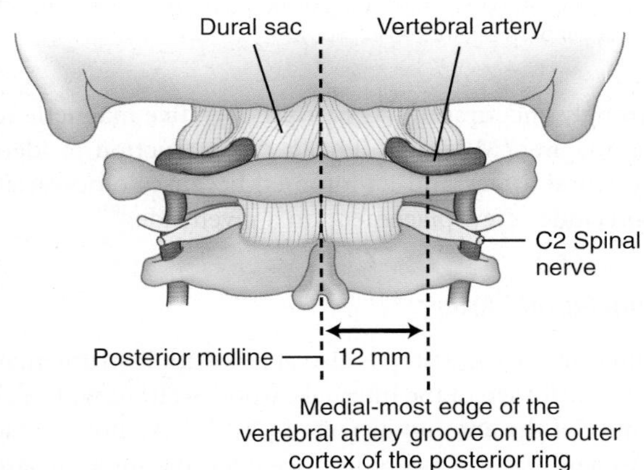

FIG. 97.15 Posterior view of the occipitocervical junction. Dissection on the posterior aspect of the posterior rim of C2 should remain within 12 mm lateral to the midline.

vertebral artery and to identify and control the venous plexus, which may project inferiorly between the vertebral artery and the posterior C2 dorsal ramus. Typically, the vertebral artery penetrates the ligamentum flavum 8 mm from the C1 tubercle and passes cephalad to the margin of the C1 posterior rim (Fig. 97.14). The level of the C1 lateral mass screw insertion at the inferior border of the C1 arch is typically 12 to 14 mm from the midline (Fig. 97.15). The ponticulus ponticus is a harbinger of injury to the vertebral artery along the cephalad margin, especially if the ponticulus ponticus is not appreciated during placement of C1 lateral mass screws (see Fig. 97.11).

C1 lateral mass screws should be started in the "window" of the lateral mass defined on the superior border by the C1 arch and the vertebral artery superior and on the inferior border by the C2 dorsal root ganglion (Fig. 97.16). This window is covered by a plexus of veins that should be coagulated and controlled. Removal of the inferior edge of the C1 arch often assists the placement of the C1 lateral mass or pedicle screw. The medial-most extension of the vertebral artery cephalad to the C1 ring is usually about 8 mm from the C1 tubercle but about 4 more mm lateral and caudal to the C1 ring; this is the optimal starting point for a C1 lateral mass screw.

Image guidance, including fluoroscopic or CT-based systems, increases patient safety during C1 lateral mass screw positioning given the high rate of vertebral artery anomalies in this area.[102] For example, one study found that 3.1% of patients lacked a vertebral artery on the right and 1.8% lacked a vertebral artery on the left, and 9.7% of patients had a significantly narrowed vertebral artery on the right and 5.7% had significant narrowing on the left.[66] This study also found two cases in which the vertebral artery branched directly into the posterior internal cerebellar artery.[66] Numerous minor and major variations are known to occur; for this reason surgeons

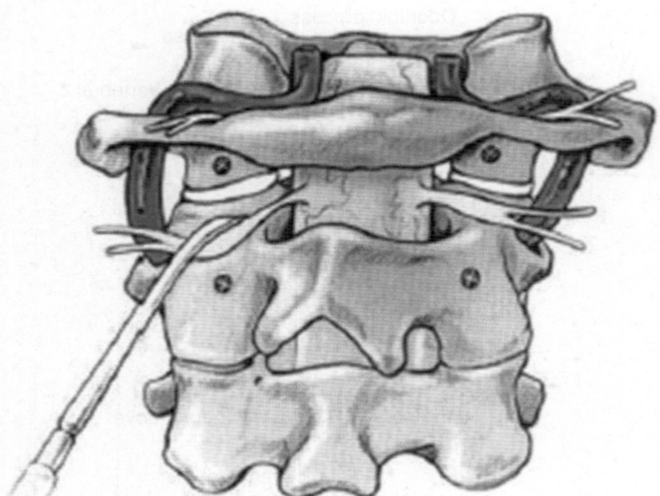

FIG. 97.16 Lateral mass fixation at C1 is safe, stable, and effective. Lateral mass screws at the C1 level should be started in the "window" of the lateral mass, the superior border of which is defined by the inferior aspect of the arch of C1 and the vertebral artery and the inferior border is defined by the C2 dorsal root ganglion. In this image, the starting point of the left C1 lateral mass screw is indicated by the top left circle with an "x" within it, the plexus of veins that covers the starting point has been removed, and the C2 dorsal root ganglion is retracted inferiorly.

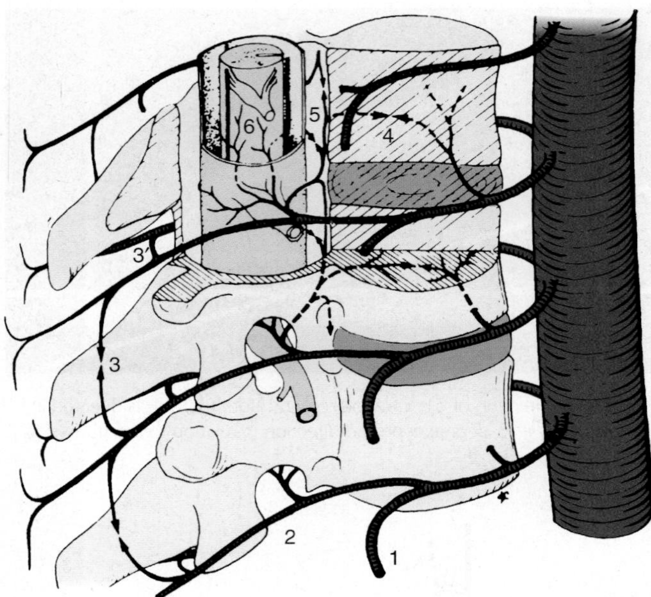

FIG. 97.17 Anastomoses of the dorsal branches of the spinal artery. *1,* Intercostal artery; *2,* dorsal branches of spinal artery; *3* and *3',* posterior anastomoses; *4,* vertebral anastomosis; *5,* retrovertebral anastomosis; and *6,* perimedullary anastomosis. Segmental vessels are shown exiting from the posterior aspect of the aorta. The vessels lie along the thoracic spine, across the midportion of the vertebral bodies. (From Lazorthes G, Gouaze A, Sadeh JO, et al. Arterial vascularization of the spinal cord: recent studies of the anastomotic substitution pathways. *J Neurosurg.* 1971;35:253–262.)

are strongly encouraged to order preoperative magnetic resonance imaging (MRI) or CT with reconstruction to identify the vertebral artery and its foramen because some variation may preclude screw placement on a given side.[103]

Internal Carotid Artery

The internal carotid artery is also at risk with instrumentation of C1 as the lumen of the internal carotid artery is within close proximity of the anterior aspect of C1.[104,105] Anatomic studies have shown that the mean distance from the internal carotid artery to C1 is on average 2.9 to 3.7 mm.[105,106] One study of 160 angiograms found that the internal carotid artery is never medial to of the lateral mass of C1, and with regard to the transverse foramen it was less often medial caudally than cranially.[106] For this reason some authors suggest that lateral mass screws that are angulated inferomedially are safer with respect to the internal carotid artery than screws placed in other trajectories. However, because of the risk of injury to this artery that is posed by a drill bit or the tip of a bicortical screw, some authors have recommended preoperative CTA before procedures in which C1 will be instrumented. If the internal carotid artery is found to be in close proximity to the anterior aspect of C1, it has been suggested that either a unicortical screw should be used or an alternative technique should be considered.[105]

Thoracic Spine

Anterior Thoracic Vascular Complications

Anterior exposure of the thoracic spine is well established and has many applications.[9,39,46,107-128] This can be done through open or thoracoscopic approaches for the treatment of a variety of disorders but is often used for scoliosis release, fusion, and instrumentation. The absolute incidence of vascular injuries from anterior thoracolumbar surgery may be as low as 1%. One retrospective review of 1262 consecutive patients from 1998 to 2010 found that injury to a major vessel occurred in 1.1% of cases.[27] Another review reported a 5.8% incidence of vascular complications in 207 open anterior thoracolumbar surgeries, with a mortality rate of 1%.[16] This report found a 3.4% incidence of direct vascular injuries of the segmental or intercostal vessels. Most had a delayed onset of sequelae, and one death occurred.

Among the potential vascular-related complications are injuries to the major vessels and their branches and the sequelae of interruption of the blood supply to the thoracic spinal cord (Fig. 97.17). Paraplegia secondary to unilateral vascular interruption of the thoracic segmental vessels is extremely uncommon. Bilateral disruption of the segmental blood supply, however, as in aortic surgery or dissection of aortic aneurysms, does confer a real risk of paraplegia.[24,129-134] There are many reports in the thoracic and vascular literature of the consequences of bilateral disruption of the blood flow to the thoracic cord during complex thoracic and thoracolumbar aneurysm reconstructive surgery. One study has shown that autoregulation of smooth muscle of the tunica media of the lower anterior spinal artery may further reduce blood flow to the cord after aortic cross clamping.[17]

Other procedures associated with spinal cord infarction include bilateral sympathectomies[20]; open thoracoscopy with pulmonary lobectomy[135]; open anterior surgery for tuberculosis in which bilateral vascular ligation or disruption occurs[133]; revision anterior scoliosis surgery, especially if approaching the previously undissected side of the anterolateral spine or if the curve has a significant kyphotic component[134,136]; and spinal angiography or magnetic resonance angiography (MRA) using the thoracic or abdominal aorta.[38,60,131] Video-assisted thoracoscopy (VAT) has been used for a variety of thoracic spine conditions.[111,112,117,137] One European meta-analysis found no vascular complications or paralyses associated with VAT.[138] A singular case of profound epidural bleeding occurred, but no incidence of segmental artery, aorta, or azygos vein injury was noted. Other studies of thoracoscopy have validated the utility and safety of VAT.[114,117,139-141]

Segmental Arteries

The relative importance of individual blood vessels that supply the spinal cord has been debated.[87] It was not until 1939 that it was determined that the segmental vessels that supply the spinal cord are indeed end arteries and that there are no anastomoses between the capillary beds.[37] The vessels that travel with the spinal nerve into the spinal canal do not seem to be important, as evidenced by a report in which three to 16 ipsilateral segmental arteries in a single patient were ligated without neurologic loss.[110]

Theoretically, the thoracolumbar spinal cord tolerates transient and permanent unilateral segmental blood flow disruption. However, bilateral segmental disruption, transient or permanent, is much more likely to cause spinal cord ischemia and consequent paraparesis or paraplegia. The precise incidence of spinal cord infarction and paraplegia due to vascular occlusion is not known, but the real incidence is very low. Morbidity and mortality statistics from the Scoliosis Research Society described an incidence of paraplegia of 1% due to indirect vascular compromise in more than 10,000 deformity cases.[65,142] Paraplegia rates are greater in adult patients and those treated with posterior instrumentation and fusion for severe scoliosis, kyphosis, kyphoscoliosis, or congenital scoliosis and kyphosis.[143] One case of vascular-induced paraplegia was reported in a series of more than 400 cases of anterior spinal surgery for tuberculosis,[133] and there is a cumulative series of more than 3000 extensive open anterior discectomies or partial corpectomies with unilateral ligation of thoracic segmental arteries without any cases of paraplegia.[110,116,119]

The transthoracic approach to the anterior thoracic spine usually requires mobilization of segmental arteries and veins over several vertebral levels.[69,110,116,119,144] A right-sided approach is recommended to avoid the pericardial structures because in 75% of people the artery of Adamkiewicz originates on the left side of the aorta between T8 and L1.[145] In cases of deformity, however, it is most advantageous to approach the convexity of the deformity, regardless of the side involved. The parietal pleura must be divided to gain access to the thoracic segmental and intercostal arteries.[146] This dissection should begin over the disc space because there are no vessels there. The individual vessels are identified and isolated with a right-angle hemostat and ligated, occluded with vascular clamps, or spared.[147] About 1 cm of segmental vessel should be maintained from the thoracic aorta or vena cava to avoid tearing injury to either of these large vessels. Although it has been shown that better collateralization and anastomotic substitution can occur as the segmental vessels are ligated or disrupted closer to the major vessels, the risk of catastrophic injury to the aorta or vena cava demands caution.[145] Inadvertent laceration or avulsion of the segmental vessels from the aorta or vena cava can result in rapid, voluminous bleeding. Bleeding should be immediately controlled by direct pressure proximal and distal to the defect, and repair of the aorta or vena cava should be assisted by a surgeon experienced in vascular surgery. It should also be noted that segmental vessels can also be injured by inadvertent avulsion or stretching,[16] and vascular injuries may present late (i.e., postoperative hemothorax).

It should be noted that unilateral ligation of thoracolumbar segmental arteries may be acceptable on the convexity of the deformity, but perhaps only in primary surgeries as certain complex revision surgeries may mimic bilateral ligation.[119] Cases in which there is significant kyphosis or kyphoscoliosis—especially in cases of multiple posterior procedures or prior surgeries—may increase the risk of paraplegia with unilateral ligation of particular segmental arteries. For this reason some authors have advocated spinal cord monitoring up to 20 minutes after ligation or clamping of a key segmental artery when the cord is at risk.[119] Winter and colleagues[119] describe a case of revision anterior scoliosis surgery in which the convexity was approached after prior anterior surgery from the concavity. The authors clamped a segmental artery and observed loss of somatosensory evoked potentials (SEPs). The spinal cord monitoring changes were reversible and the anterior discectomy was performed between the segmental vessels to spare spinal cord blood flow. This circumstance illustrates that bilateral thoracolumbar segmental vessel occlusion is associated with a small but definite risk of spinal cord infarction and permanent neurologic deficits. In any case, actual or indirect segmental vessel injuries should be avoided between T8 and L1 on the left. Spinal cord monitoring should be considered routine; motor evoked potentials (MEPs) are often used for this purpose. For monitoring on the anterior spinal cord MEPs are more precise than SEPs which primarily monitor the function of the dorsal columns of the spinal cord.

Artery of Adamkiewicz

Great attention has been given to the artery of Adamkiewicz, which is the largest of the segmental arteries supplying the thoracolumbar spinal cord (Fig. 97.18).[40,148-150] It originates on the left side in 80% of patients between T7 and L4 and is most often between T8 and L1 (92%).[150-153] Another study found that the artery of Adamkiewicz originates between T9 and T12 in 80% of patients and 100% of originations were between T8 and L2.[154] It is important to emphasize that in 10% to 12% of cases the artery of Adamkiewicz originates at L1–L2.[145,155] The artery of Adamkiewicz appeared between T5 and T8 in 15% of cases.[145] When the artery of Adamkiewicz appears in the midthoracic level, there is often a supplemental artery referred to as the arteria conus medullaris supplying the thoracolumbar cord. The thoracolumbar spinal cord has a rich anastomotic

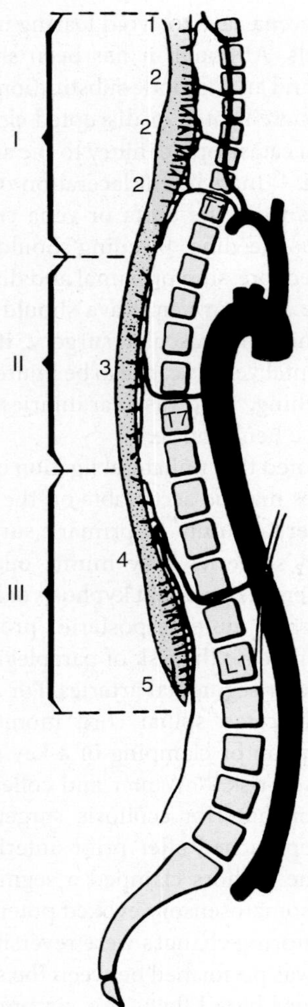

FIG. 97.18 Major arterial vessels supplying the spinal cord through the anterior spinal artery. The artery of Adamkiewicz is usually found in area *4*. *I*, Superior or cervicothoracic area; *II*, intermediate or midthoracic area; *III*, lower or thoracolumbar area. *1*, Anterior spinal artery; *2*, artery of the cervical enlargement; *3*, posterior spinal artery; *4*, artery of the lumbar enlargement; *5*, anastomotic loop of the conus medullaris. (From Lazorthes G, Gouaze A, Sadeh JO, et al. Arterial vascularization of the spinal cord: recent studies of the anastomotic substitution pathways. *J Neurosurg*. 1971;35:253–262.)

blood supply formed by both the anterior and posterior spinal arteries. The anterior spinal artery in the region of T4 to T9, however, is often small and can be incomplete.[145] The spinal canal was also the most narrow in the T4–T9 region, which could predispose to surgical complications, particularly in the face of a chronic low-reserve state of spinal fluid circulation.[30] Helical CT scans, MRA, and more contemporary spinal cord angiographic techniques have supported these prior anatomic studies.[134,150]

An elaborate study of the contributions of unilateral and bilateral vessel occlusion to paraplegia used a high-powered laser Doppler source with a Doppler flow meter placed in the vertebral body. Changes in the vertebral body blood flow were measured after ligation and occlusion of the segmental vessels.[156] Vertebral body flow may or may not correlate with the segmental vessel flow and is at best an indirect measurement, but this unique study is worth mention nonetheless. In 10 cases segmental vessels on one side were ligated as part of the index procedure and then the contralateral vessels were occluded or tamponaded from T7 to L3. A small decrease in blood flow of about 13% was recorded with ligation on one side, but there was a 75% loss of blood flow with bilateral blood flow disruption and all occlusions returned to baseline almost immediately after the patency of the vessels was restored. At T8, T10, T11, and L3 the authors noted there was no change in blood flow after bilateral occlusion; they attributed this to significant collateral circulation. The variability of spinal arterial vasculature underlies the importance of preserved blood flow with bilateral occlusion at any particular level in this study, but these findings highlight the relative safety of unilateral segmental artery occlusion relative to the risk of bilateral occlusion. A study of bilateral segmental vessel ligation in the watershed area of dogs found that paraplegia developed 100% of the time.[157] The human watershed area is T4 to T9. The artery of Adamkiewicz may be ligated in Rhesus monkeys without complications, but paraplegia follows when the anterior spinal artery (arterial median longitudinal artery) is simultaneously ligated.[148] These animal studies also emphasize the risk of paraplegia with bilateral segmental artery disruption.

Despite these reports, the artery of Adamkiewicz can be occluded under most circumstances. It is not uncommon in some scoliosis procedures that involve anterior instrumentation to perform an extensive ipsilateral sacrifice of these segmental arteries without significant sequelae.[110] No vascular or neurologic complications due to vascular injury were reported in 278 cases involving unilateral segmental ligation for anterior kyphotic deformity reconstructive surgeries with anterior Kostuik-Harrington instrumentation.[158] The authors of a report of more than 1200 consecutive anterior spinal cases with no cases of paraparesis or paraplegia related to the ligation of segmental vessels unilaterally recommend (1) vessel ligation unilaterally, (2) ligation on the convexity of the deformity, (3) ligation at the mid-body level, and (4) avoidance of hypotensive anesthesia.[119,159]

The risks of paraplegia and paraparesis in cardiothoracic surgery have been reduced by (1) limiting cross clamping times,[24,129] (2) avoiding hypotension,[24,129] (3) draining cerebrospinal fluid (CSF),[130,132] and (4) maintaining distal aortic perfusion by cardiopulmonary bypass.[24,130] CSF drainage or cooling has been proven to decompress the intradural space and improve blood flow to the cord via the artery of Adamkiewicz and other segmental vessels.[130,132] Other authors have noted that the keys to protecting neurologic function in regard to aortic surgery are to limit cross clamp time of the aorta to less than 30 minutes, reanastomose key intercostals, and cool the CSF.[154] Although there has been some debate about how to best prevent paraplegia, some general recommendations are to minimize cross clamping time and identify the artery of Adamkiewicz preoperatively. Spinal angiography or MRA may be used to identify this artery.

Most acute major vascular injuries during anterior thoracic or thoracolumbar surgery are direct injuries with immediate and profound blood loss that demands immediate attention. If the injury occurs during a minimally invasive approach the case should be converted to an open procedure. However, vascular complications may have a delayed presentation. For example, there has been a report of a delayed aortic rupture due to erosion of the aorta from a T12–L1 smooth rod anterior implant.[160] This occurred 20 months after a T11 burst fracture and repair in a middle-aged man presenting with nonspecific gastrointestinal symptoms. The tips of bicortical screws used in anterior instrumentation for thoracic scoliosis may also pose risks of major vessel injury because these vessels often closely approximate in the concavity of the curve of the spine.[118] These bleeding complications are due to excess length or depth gauging of the vertebral body screw hole. A calf model was used to study the placement of anterior thoracic vertebral body screws relative to the aorta at T6–T11 and to monitor at 3, 6, and 12 months. There were a number of penetrations into the aorta. Postmortem histology showed thinning of the aorta in 52%, and 60% had scarring with a trend of greater scarring with greater impregnation. In 96% of the cases with some screw contact, the aorta showed some cicatrix. The authors concluded that this histopathology was worrisome for late development of complications if the screw tip approached or entered the thoracic aorta.[161] Complications involving the aorta, however, are more characteristic of pedicle screw instrumentation after posterior approaches to the thoracic spine.

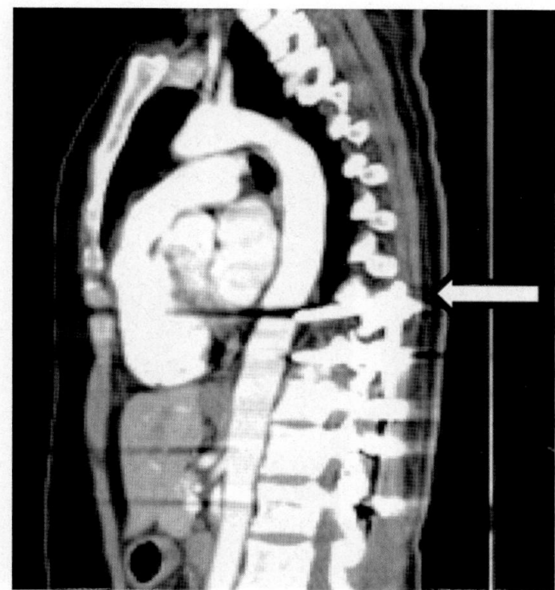

FIG. 97.19 Vascular complications during posterior thoracic spine surgery are rare. The most significant of these are iatrogenic injury to the structures of the posterior mediastinum by pedicle screws that breach the anterior cortex of the vertebral body. In this sagittal slice of a computed tomographic image with contrast, the tip of a thoracic pedicle screw (at the vertebral level indicated by the arrow) is seen in close proximity to the descending thoracic aorta.

Posterior Thoracic Vascular Complications

Typically, no major vessels are at risk during direct posterior midline thoracic exposure per se,[143,162] but the great vessels on the anterior aspect of the vertebrae may be placed at risk by instrumentation of the pedicles. If the anatomy is atypical, however, as in idiopathic right thoracic scoliosis, posterior exposure either during rib resection or aggressive posterolateral exposure may injure the intercostal arteries. Injury to an intercostal artery could lead to hemothorax with clinical dyspnea and hypoxia; in these cases thoracoscopy to ligate the vessel and drain the chest cavity could be considered. Although routine midline posterior cervical or thoracolumbar exposures may risk injury to segmental arteries anterior to the transverse processes, these complications are rare, and the characteristic vascular complication of this approach is iatrogenic injury to the great vessels by the tip of a pedicle screw.

Although studies have shown that the use of thoracic pedicle screws is safe,[163,164] their use is not universally accepted due to concerns about safety and complications,[165] and the reported rate of pedicle screw malpositioning is surprisingly high. Although one report of 4600 screws found a malpositioning rate of only 1.5%,[166] a more recent review of 4570 pedicle screws in 1666 patients who underwent corrective surgery for adolescent scoliosis found that 518 screws were malpositioned (5.2%). In studies that included systematic postoperative CT the rate of screw malposition was found to be as great as 15.7%[167] In this review 10 vascular complications were reported, but there were no irreversible sequelae. In fact, most reports of malpositioned pedicle screws describe no permanent consequences for the patient.[165-167]

Aorta

The range of complications related to pedicle screws include transient paresis, dural tear, infection, pneumothorax, pleural effusion, pedicle fracture, and screw loosening. Vascular complication during posterior thoracic spine surgery are rare. The most significant of these is iatrogenic injury to posterior mediastinal structures by screws that breach the anterior cortex of the vertebral body (Figs. 97.19 and 97.20).[168] Since instrumentation of the thoracic pedicles with pedicle screws has been recognized as the state of the art in the treatment of scoliosis,[169] multiple authors have reported injuries to the thoracic aorta; many of these are pseudoaneurysms, erosions, and otherwise delayed perforations of the thoracic aorta.[170-174] As pedicle fixation in the thoracic spine has become commonplace, the position of the screws relative to the canal and anterior vascular structures must be carefully considered.[175]

In the event of aortic disruption by a thoracic pedicle screw, endovascular repair of the aorta has been widely shown to be effective (Fig. 97.21).[176-180] Elective thoracotomy[181] and combined endovascular-thoracotomy procedures have also been described.[182,183] Even the use of biologic glue has also been reported to be successful in a few cases.[184] In any case of iatrogenic disruption of the vascular structures of the posterior mediastinum, consultation with an experienced vascular or cardiothoracic surgeon is advisable. The best strategy for these injures is to avoid them by selecting pedicle screws of appropriately short length that are placed using meticulous technique.[163]

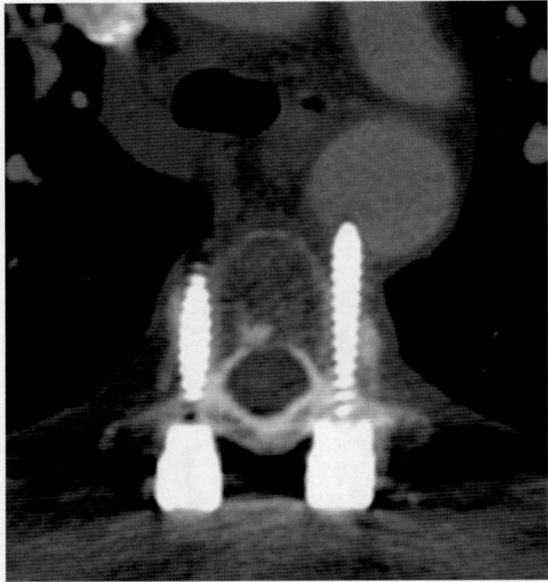

FIG. 97.20 The most significant of vascular injuries during posterior thoracic spine surgery are iatrogenic injuries to the structures of the posterior mediastinum by pedicle screws that breech the anterior cortex of the vertebral body. In this axial image of a computed tomographic scan, the tip of a left thoracic pedicle screw (on the right) is seen lateral to the cortex of the body of the vertebra; the screw tip is clearly impinging upon the descending aorta. If the position of this screw tip does not cause acute extravasation, then pseudoaneurysm, erosion, or otherwise delayed perforation of the thoracic aorta may occur.

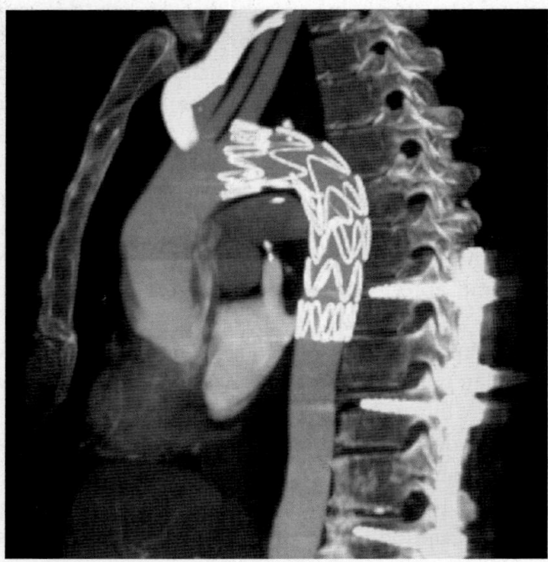

FIG. 97.21 In the event of aortic disruption by a thoracic pedicle screw, endovascular repair of the aorta has been shown to be effective. In this sagittal image an endovascular stent is visible in the arch of the aorta and the descending aorta at the level of the most superior thoracic pedicle screw.

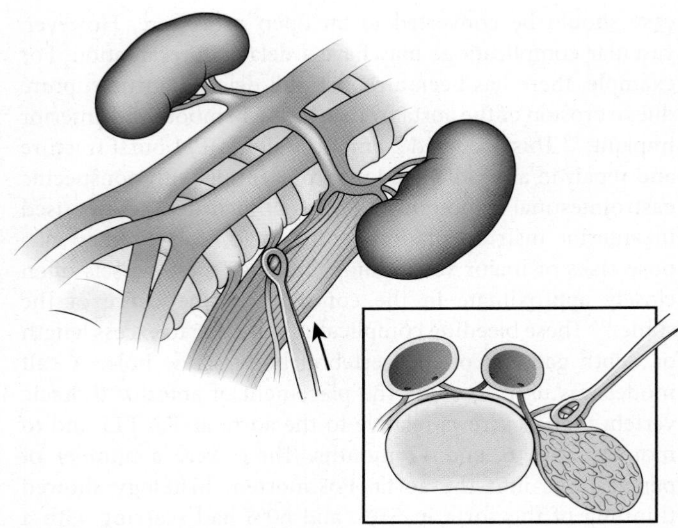

FIG. 97.22 Anatomic relationships among lumbar vessels, the aorta, and the inferior vena cava and the course in the retroperitoneum. In case of bleeding from lacerated lumbar vessel, the distal portion can be controlled by pressure exerted on the vessel between the overlying psoas muscle and spinal column (inset).

Lumbar Spine

Anterior Lumbar Vascular Complications

Anterior exposure of the lumbar and lumbosacral spine is often accomplished by a lateral retroperitoneal approach,[39,185] a transperitoneal approach,[186,187] or a paramedian hypogastric (mini-open, rectus-splitting, or minimally invasive anterior lumbar) retroperitoneal approach.[188] All these approaches directly address the vascular structures of the anterior lumbar spine and are best used for L1–L3 exposure[185,189-191]; for this reason some surgeons monitor left great toe pulse oximetry during these procedures to identify early and reversible left iliac artery occlusion. The rectus-splitting anterior or paramedian exposure, however, is limited to exposures from L3 to S1 due in large part to the branching of the renal arteries from the abdominal aorta (Fig. 97.22). Anatomic variants are common among these structures, especially the iliocaval bifurcation and the segmental vessels (Fig. 97.23). As with all anterior approaches to the spine, an appreciation for the prevalence and variety of vascular variations is the most important consideration for prevention of vascular injury. One review article emphasizes four key vascular components and considerations for anterior lumbar exposure that must be addressed: (1) the iliolumbar vein, (2) the left iliac vein, (3) the middle sacral vessels, and (4) the type of arterial retraction to optimize exposure but minimize the risk of blood flow alteration or displacement of plaque.[192]

The incidence of vascular injuries from anterior lumbar spinal surgery varies and is still believed to be underreported. Some case series have reported no complications, whereas one series of 102 consecutive cases performed by fellowship-trained vascular surgeons reported a 15.6% incidence.[35] Vascular injuries and complications during anterior lumbar

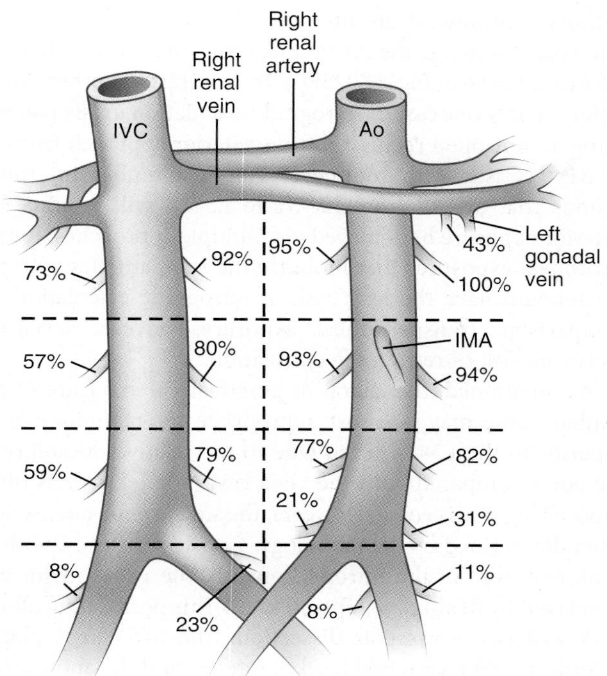

FIG. 97.23 Anatomic distribution of lumbar arteries and veins in the retroperitoneum. Numbers denote frequency (percent) of finding a certain branch among 102 consecutive retroperitoneal lymph node dissections. Ao, aorta; IVC, inferior vena cava.

exposures rarely result in serious sequelae unless the injury results in total disruption of the vascular supply to the lower extremity or viscera,[57] but depending on the spine surgeon's level of expertise and hospital credentialing, a collaborative effort with a surgeon experienced in vascular surgical techniques should be considered, especially in the ever more common anterior lumbar revision cases.[35,193,194] Prompt recognition and repair remain paramount and are the standard of care, and blood conservation techniques such as a Cell Saver with or without autologous blood donation have been recommended in anticipation of possible anterior thoracolumbar vascular complications.[195]

As anterior lumbar interbody fusion and arthroplasty techniques have gained wide acceptance, laparoscopic or rectus-splitting approaches have become less favored, especially for lateral exposure at levels L4–L5 and below.[1,39,133,186,188,192,194,196-200] This is partly because laparoscopic exposure of L3–L4 has been found to require significant aorta retraction, which has been demonstrated in more than nine out of 10 angiographically studied patients.[201] Multiple authors have found it possible, however, to access levels L3–L4 and above using a mini-open rectus-splitting exposure.[188,202] Although no difference in vascular complications was reported in a comparative study between a limited retroperitoneal approach and laparoscopic approach,[40] the rate of retrograde ejaculation was much greater in the laparoscopic cohort. Other studies confirm that the rates of postoperative ileus and retrograde ejaculation are reportedly greater with laparoscopic approaches than with open retroperitoneal techniques.[194] Bowel and bladder injuries have also been reported at a rate of 1.4%.[194] Due to these distinct disadvantages, laparoscopic and transperitoneal approaches have fallen out of favor.[197,203]

Although prevention is the primary objective, vessel injury during anterior lumbar surgery is not uncommon. In a review of 102 consecutive cases of anterior lumbar spinal surgery performed for a wide variety of lumbar spinal conditions and assisted by fellowship-trained vascular surgeons, the overall incidence of vascular injury was 15.6%.[35] All these injuries involved venous structures. There were 11 common iliac vein injuries, four inferior vena cava injuries, and one iliolumbar vein injury. All were identified and repaired primarily without any reported clinical significance. The incidence of venous injury differed by the extent of surgical approach. The hypogastric rectus-splitting approach was associated with a vascular complication rate of 18.4% versus a 7.7% injury rate with an anterolateral muscle-dividing retroperitoneal exposure. Multiple reviews of lumbar total disc replacement have found that the most common vascular complications are left common iliac vein laceration (5%), vena cava laceration (2%), and thrombosis of the left common iliac vein or left common iliac artery (<1%).[204] These studies emphasize that vascular problems may be relatively common with anterior lumbar spinal cases.

It is still somewhat controversial whether less-invasive approaches pose a greater or lesser risk of vascular injury. A series of 686 exposures reported a 1% incidence of arterial and venous injuries using a mini-open technique with minimal morbidity and mortality.[202] Many other authors have reported large series of anterior interbody fusions of the lumbar spine for degenerative disc disease and spondylolisthesis without major vascular injuries.[1,149,188,193,196,205–210] Regardless of the specific approach to the anterior lumbar spine, the rates of vascular injury are likely underreported and are best prevented with caution and a thorough understanding of the anatomy. If any of these approaches is chosen, it may be helpful to perform preoperative digital subtraction angiography or abdominal ultrasonography to confirm the level of the bifurcation of the aorta and vena cava, which may be particularly important for preoperative planning of total disc replacements.

Aorta and Vena Cava

Exposure of the L4–L5 level and above requires mobilization of the vena cava and aorta by sacrificing and ligating segmental vessels and the recurrent left iliolumbar vein. On the basis of MRI studies and clinical experience, some authors have suggested that there are three general anatomic patterns that are "best windows" to the L4–L5 interspace (Fig. 97.24A–C).[194] The aorta and vena cava, as well as the left common iliac vein and artery, may be mobilized together or independently to one side or the other in a caudal to cephalad manner, depending on the level of the iliocaval bifurcation (Fig. 97.25A–C).[194] For example, in cases with a low iliocaval bifurcation, the left common iliac vein is mobilized from left to right and the window to the L4–L5 disc is obtained by mobilizing the left common iliac artery to the left (see Fig. 97.25C). Given the relative frailty of the vena cava and the potential for tearing, laceration, or avulsion, there is no case in which the aorta,

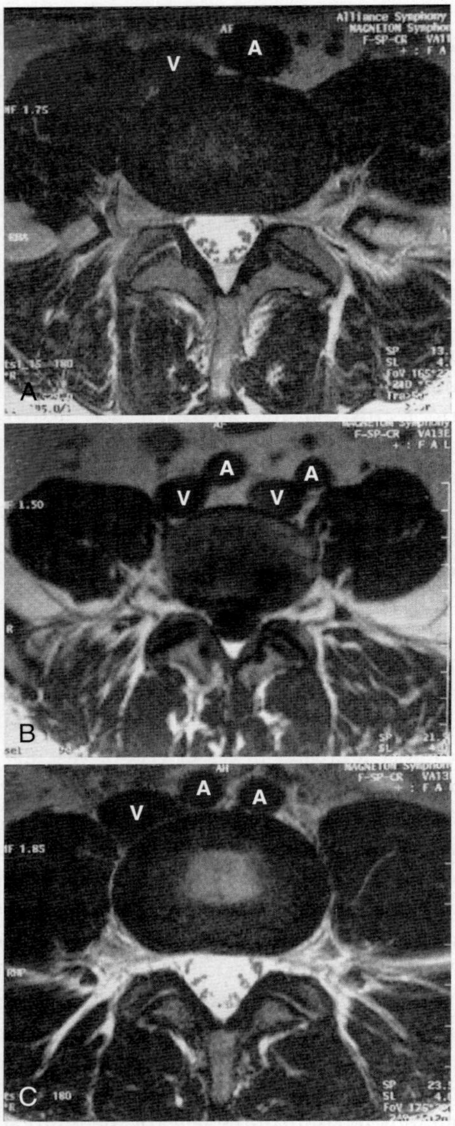

FIG. 97.24 (A) Axial magnetic resonance imaging (MRI) slice of the aorta (white A) and vena cava (white V). At this level, superior to the bifurcation of the aorta and the vena cava, surgical exposure of L4–L5 should be from the left side of the aorta. (B) Axial MRI slice of the arteries (white A's) and veins (white V's). At this level the aorta and vena cava have both bifurcated. In this case surgical exposure of L4–L5 is at the level inferior to the bifurcation of the aorta and vena cava. (C) At this level superior to the bifurcation of the vena cava and inferior to the bifurcation of the aorta, the vena cava (white V) and arteries (white A's) are indicated. Surgical exposure of L4–L5 in this case is between the left common iliac artery and the vein. (From Kleeman TJ, Michael Ahn U, Clutterback WB, et al. Laparoscopic anterior lumbar interbody fusion at L4-L5: an anatomic evaluation and approach classification. *Spine.* 2002;27:1390–1395.)

vena cava, or common iliac vessels are mobilized from right to left. As one extends the exposure to levels superior to L4–L5, the aorta and vena cava are almost always mobilized together from left to right.

There may be times in which a window needs to be created between the aorta and vena cava. A review of 139 cases warned that transperitoneal laparoscopic release and mobilization of the left segmentals of the aorta at L4–L5 were associated with a 16% rate of retrograde ejaculation.[194] For this reason the authors recommend an alternative exposure for the L4–L5 interspace between the aorta and vena cava in low iliocaval bifurcations (see Fig. 97.25D). In contrast, another series reported only one case of retrograde ejaculation in 684 patients using a mini-open rectus-splitting anterior approach from L2 to S1.[211] Cases with multilevel anterior lumbar interbody fusions that extend from L5–S1 to L3–L4 will require that anterior exposure be achieved via multiple approaches. Retroperitoneal exposures that mobilize the sympathetics with the peritoneum have the least risk of retrograde ejaculation. In comparison, transperitoneal exposures have a sevenfold increased risk of retrograde ejaculation.[212]

As mentioned, the lateral or anterolateral exposure of the lumbar spine may be most appropriate for pathology at or superior to the L3–L4 level. Due to the relative durability of the aorta compared with the vena cava, the left side is often chosen if all else is equal. However, the side of exposure is most often determined by the pathology. Considering the lateral or flank exposure of the retroperitoneum, the psoas major can be relaxed by flexing the hip and knee. This positioning allows safer and easier vascular dissection. The incision is placed according to the vertebral level of interest and the approach is carried to the retroperitoneal space. The psoas major is the key landmark guiding the deep dissection. Each segmental vessel is independently isolated over the vertebral body with a right-angle hemostat and is either clipped or ligated. Double ligation or clipping is preferred nearer the great vessels, leaving at least 1 cm of lumbar segmental vessel to minimize the risk of inadvertent injury to the aorta or vena cava. The use of clips versus suture ties is largely dependent on surgeon preference. Segmental vessels should be ligated over the center of the vertebral body because posterior ligation of the segmental vessels risks interference with foraminal or collateral blood flow. Furthermore, it is technically easier to control the vessels in this anatomic location. Regardless of the type of anterior exposure, access to the vertebral bodies and intervertebral discs requires identification, mobilization, control, and ligation or protection of the arteries and veins that cover the anterior lumbar spine.[1,22,39,94,133,186,188,192,194,196–201,213–231]

Retraction is always necessary after ligation and control of the left segmental vessels and the recurrent or ascending lumbar vein. Many surgeons use a retractor that affixes to the operating room table. It is important that this retractor be able to move with the patient and that the retractor adequately retract the peritoneal contents without undue stress on the great vessels.[232] Multiple factors aid in determining whether the great vessels may be safely incorporated into a fixed retractor setup, including patient age, weight, history of peripheral vascular occlusive disease, and vessel pliability. In most cases, the great vessels should not be incorporated into a fixed retractor because this may lead to complete occlusion of the aorta, vena cava, or common iliac arteries and veins.

Other possible events include laceration, embolization, vasospasm, and delayed deep vein thrombosis (DVT), which may also lead to significant complications. Although some authors have suggested Steinmann pin retraction (Fig. 97.26), some studies have found that this technique may increase the incidence of thrombosis.[233] With this technique, the incidence

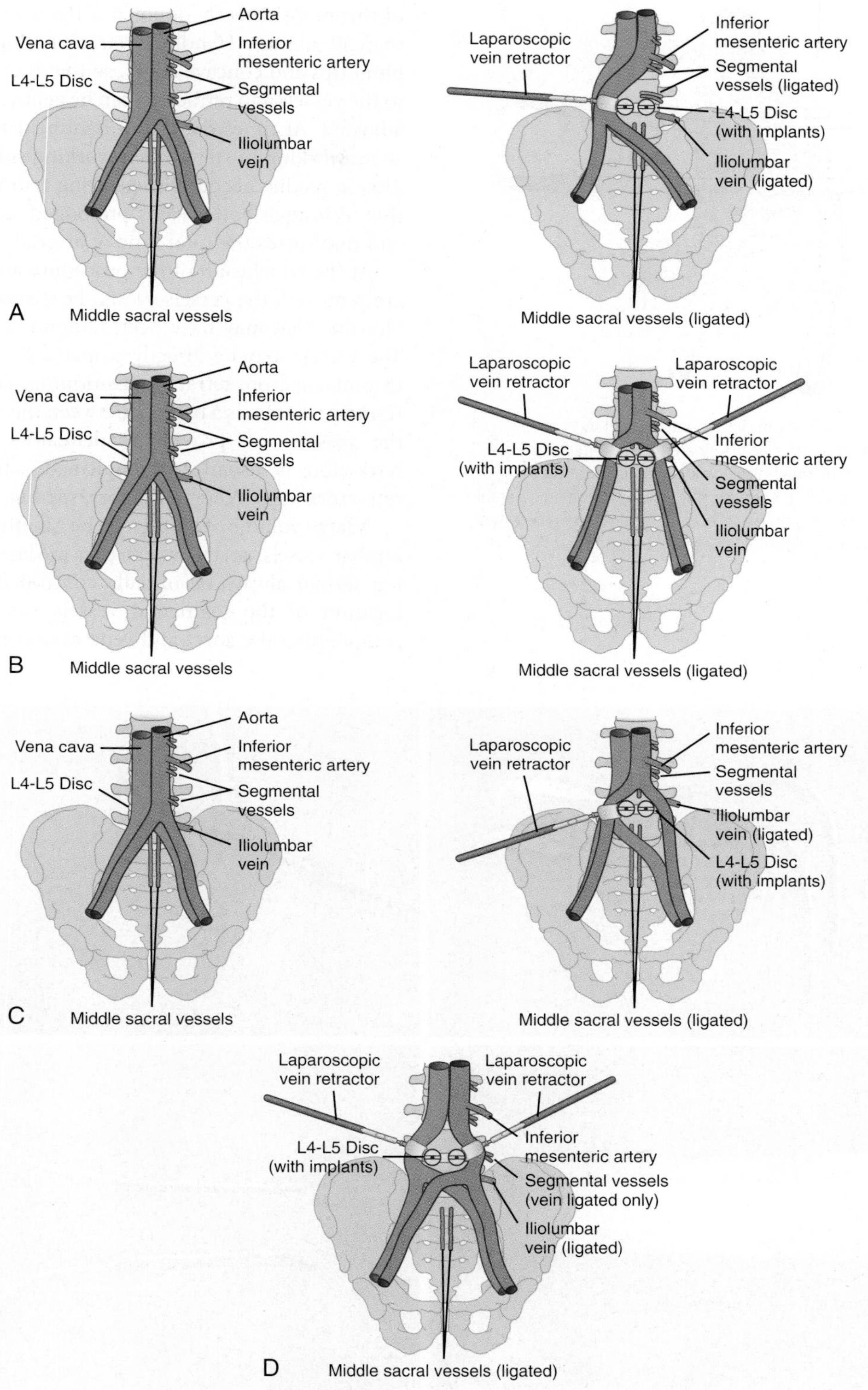

FIG. 97.25 (A) At this level, superior to the bifurcation of the aorta and the vena cava, surgical exposure of L4–L5 should be from the left side of the aorta. (B) At this level the aorta and vena cava have both bifurcated. In this case surgical exposure of L4–L5 is at the level inferior to the bifurcation of the aorta and vena cava. (C) At this level, superior to the bifurcation of the vena cava and inferior to the bifurcation of the aorta, surgical exposure of L4–L5 in this case is between the left iliac artery and the vein. (D) Proposed surgical exposure of L4–L5 at a level superior to the bifurcation of both the aorta and the vena cava with the aorta retracted to the left and the vena cava retracted to the right. (From Kleeman TJ, Michael Ahn U, Clutterback WB, et al. Laparoscopic anterior lumbar interbody fusion at L4-L5: an anatomic evaluation and approach classification. *Spine.* 2002;27:1390–1395.)

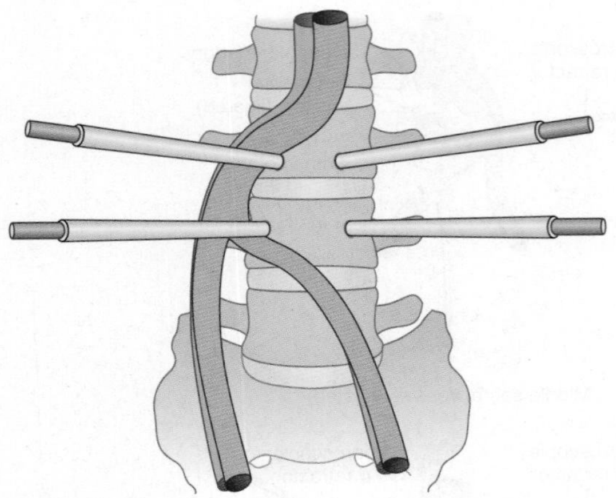

FIG. 97.26 Nonthreaded Steinmann pin retractors used to expose L3–L4. Note that the aorta and common iliac artery are under a great deal of tension and edge loading. This technique was originally described for exposure of the anterior vertebral body for discectomy maintaining stable fixation, but because of the tension placed on the arteries, this has been abandoned due to risk of thrombosis of the arterial blood flow.

of thrombosis nearly doubled if the pins were used for more than 30 minutes. Handheld retractors (Fig. 97.27) should have blunt tips and concave edges, so that they may be placed deep to the vessels and retraction can be gentle, variable, and readily adjusted. At times the use of handheld retractors will necessitate working in steps, often working side to side at the disc. This is readily accomplished using handheld retractors, and this technique both avoids prolonged, continuous retraction and minimizes the total time of arterial retraction.

At the conclusion of the procedure and once all retractors are removed, the vessels should be inspected for any obvious bleeding that may have been tamponaded by the retraction. The vessels may be directly palpated to exclude occlusion or thrombosis from retractor positioning. The choice of vascular retractor system is a balance between the risk of overstretching the vessels and providing adequate exposure.[234] Vascular retraction is usually accomplished safely using handheld retractors (e.g., Wiley retractors; see Fig. 97.27).

A large volume of blood may be rapidly lost if the segmental lumbar vessels, aorta, or vena cava are lacerated or torn. Bleeding should always be initially controlled by direct pressure. Ligation of the segmental vessels is assisted by carefully compressing the aorta and vena cava medially to identify the

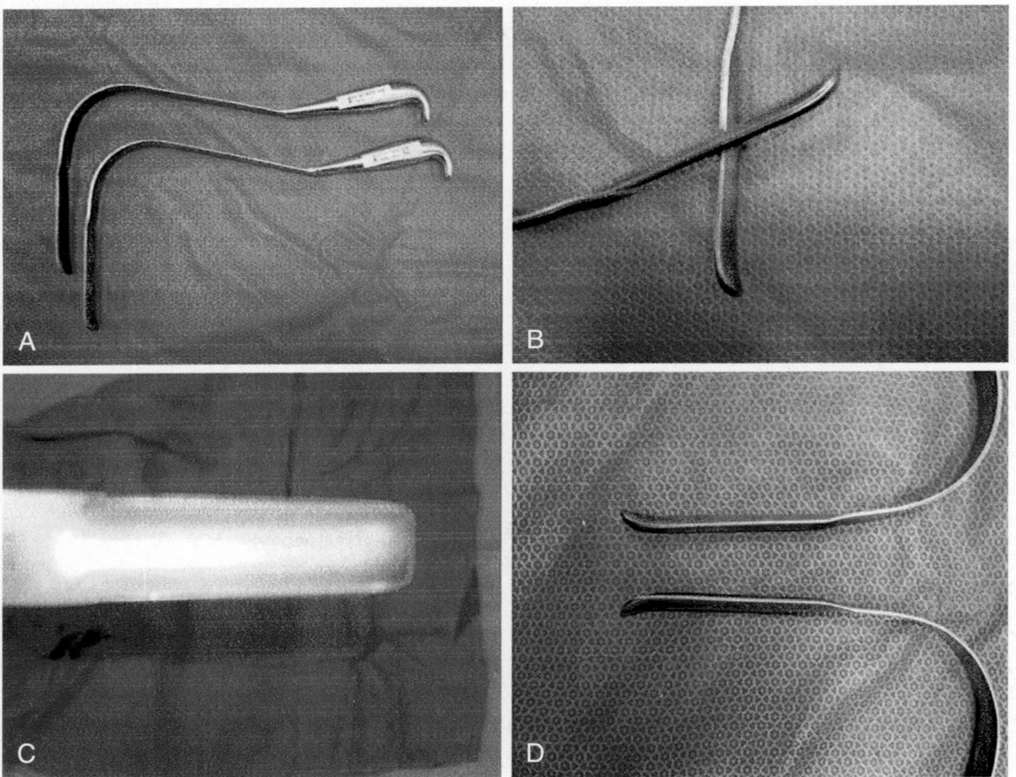

FIG. 97.27 (A) Two Wiley retractors with the handles to the right and the retracting components to the left. (B) Curved tips of the Wiley retractor allow for positioning under the artery while ensuring gentle retraction from side to side. (C) Retractor face showing that it is concave with smooth edges both at the tip and along the sides. (D) Wiley retractors are visualized with the retracting elements. The retracting ends are somewhat bulbous. They are concave toward each retractor and convex away from each retractor. There is a small, angled, blunt tip that allows it to be positioned under the vessel and mobilized safely off of the vertebral body or intervertebral disc. The major benefits of these retractors are that the amount of retractive force can be easily and immediately varied and they can be positioned without attachment to the table and without undue pressure on the arterial or vascular structures.

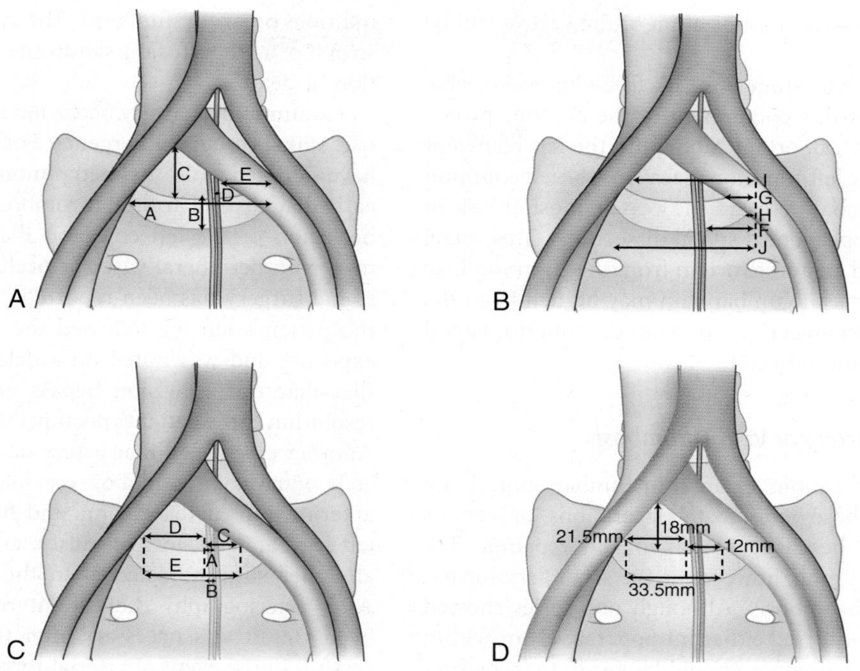

FIG. 97.28 (A–B) Direct measurements obtained from the cadaver. (A) *A*, Width of the L5–S1 disc; *B*, height of the L5–S1 disc at midline; *C*, distance from the bifurcation to the superior margin of the L5–S1 disc; *D*, the middle sacral artery at the L5–S1 disc; *E*, distance from the left side of the disc to the middle sacral artery at the superior margin of the L5–S1 disc. (B) *F*, Distance from the left side of the disc to the middle sacral artery at the inferior margin of the L5–S1 disc; *G*, distance from the left side of the disc to the left common iliac vein at the top of the L5–S1 disc; *H*, distance from the left side of the disc to the left common iliac vein at the bottom of the L5–S1 disc; *I*, distance from the left side of the disc to the right common iliac artery superior to the L5–S1 disc; *J*, distance from the left side of the disc to the right common iliac artery at the inferior margin of the L5–S1 disc. The *dotted line* represents the left side of the L5–S1 disc. (C) Calculated measurements. *A*, Middle sacral artery to midline at the superior margin of the L5–S1 disc; *B*, middle sacral artery to midline at the inferior margin of the L5–S1 disc; *C*, left common iliac vein to midline at the superior margin of the L5–S1 disc; *D*, right common iliac artery to midline at the superior margin of the L5–S1 disc; *E*, left common iliac vein to the right common iliac artery at the superior margin of the L5–S1 disc. (D) Accessibility to the L5–S1 disc space. The distance from the left common iliac vein to the right common iliac artery averaged 33.5 mm (range, 12 to 50 mm). The distance from the left common iliac vein to midline averaged 12 mm (range, −4 to 19.5 mm), whereas the distance from the bifurcation to the top of the L5–S1 disc space averaged 18 mm (range, 7 to 38 mm). (From Tribus CB, Belanger T. The vascular anatomy anterior to the L5-S1 disk space. *Spine.* 2001;26:1205–1208.)

bleeding source. Repair of the abdominal aorta and vena cava requires expertise in vascular surgery. While awaiting intraoperative vascular surgery consultation, bleeding should be controlled by direct pressure with a sponge or clamp. Primary repair is the standard of care except for segmental vessels, which can generally be sacrificed unilaterally. Successful repair often does not lead to any further complications, although the incidence of lower extremity DVT may be greater after vessel injury and repair.

Iliolumbar Vein

In anterior approaches to the lumbar spine the surgeon must work at the bifurcation of the abdominal aorta and at the formation of the common iliac veins from the vena cava (Figs. 97.28 and 97.29). The middle sacral vessels must be sacrificed for exposure of L5–S1. The left common iliac vein is vulnerable to laceration and tearing as it passes dorsal to the aortic bifurcation and becomes ventral and inferior to the left common iliac artery. If the bifurcation of the major vessels is more caudal at the L5–S1 disc level or if exposure above the

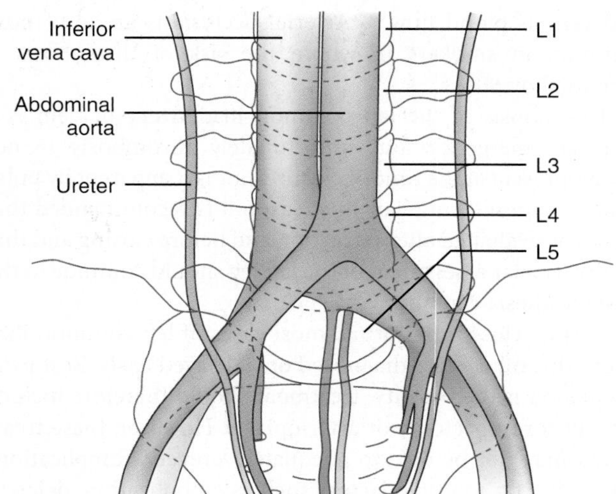

FIG. 97.29 Structures at risk during anterior approaches to the lumbar spine. (From Montorsi W, Ghiringhelli C. Genesis: diagnosis and treatment of vascular complications after intervertebral disc surgery. *Int Surg.* 1973;58:233–235.)

L4–L5 disc level is desired, mobilization of the vessels will be necessary.

It is important for the spine surgeon to be knowledgeable about the nuances of this component of the anterior procedure.[35] It is especially important to identify the left recurrent iliolumbar vein off the left common iliac vein. The left common iliac vein and iliolumbar vein are the vessels most at risk in lower left-sided retroperitoneal spinal dissections. This vessel is of variable size and anatomic origin from the common iliac vein. The left recurrent iliolumbar vein may branch from the left common iliac vein posteriorly or from the superior lateral margin of the left common vein.

Left Common Iliac Artery or Vein Thrombosis

Most vascular complications in anterior lumbar surgery are exposure related. These are mostly lacerations of venous structures that may be easily identified and repaired. The major risk to life and limb, however, is the secondary formation of an arterial thrombosis. Although one series showed that all thromboses occurred either intraoperatively or within 2 hours of surgery,[233] surgeons should be aware that the presentation of left common iliac artery thrombosis after anterior lumbar surgery has been reported to be delayed by hours to up to 13 days.[235] This type of occlusion may initially be mistaken for vasospasm.

Thrombosis of the left common iliac vein or artery is the most common vascular complication in single cases of total disc arthroplasty that involve two spinal levels.[236] This may be due to the relative immobility of the aorta and vena cava as they branch into the common iliac artery and vein at or near the L4–L5 disc space.[71] Thrombosis may occur secondary to any anterior lumbar procedure, but the risk may be greater in total disc arthroplasty because the entire anterior margin of the intervertebral disc must be visualized. At L5–S1, this may be accomplished relatively easily, but it is more difficult to achieve at L4–L5 and L3–L4 while preserving arterial and venous blood flow.[237] Arterial occlusions are also more common in smokers in whom the risk of thrombosis is increased by 80%.[233]

Thrombosis of the left common iliac artery or vein is a surgical emergency, but unfortunately thrombosis is not always present at the time of closure, nor is it apparent by pulse oximetry monitoring. For this reason it is recommended that pulses be evaluated after retraction and before closing and that neurovascular assessment of the left leg should continue in the postanesthesia care unit.[232,235]

Despite close monitoring, most cases of left common iliac artery thrombosis are diagnosed on a delayed basis. Restoring circulation is the priority; treatment should therefore include prompt thrombectomy or arterioplasty. However, these treatments may not be able to adequately prevent complications depending on multiple factors such as embolization, delay to diagnosis, and prolonged warm ischemia times of 6 to 8 hours or longer. In cases of prolonged warm ischemia, there are likely to be varying degrees of rhabdomyolysis and elevated compartment pressures for which prophylactic fasciotomy should be considered to prevent reperfusion syndrome and multiple organ dysfunction. The consequences may be catastrophic, as reperfusion syndrome could lead to leg amputation or death.

Common iliac artery occlusion or thrombosis is a rare but true spinal vascular emergency. For this reason some surgeons have adopted pulse oximetry monitoring of the left toe for early diagnosis of arterial thrombosis.[211] A case of thrombotic occlusion of the left common iliac artery in a 59-year-old man with peripheral vascular occlusive disease after anterior spinal surgery has been reported.[238] Vascular insufficiency of the patient's left leg followed the left lateral retroperitoneal exposure and was noted on a delayed basis postoperatively. Iliac-iliac open revision bypass grafting was required with resolution of the patient's postoperative neurologic complaints. Another case of left iliac artery occlusion presented immediately on awakening in a 67-year-old woman after a four-level anterior lumbar discectomy and fusion.[3] She presented with left leg paralysis, loss of pulses, and loss of sensation hours after her surgery, detected in the postanesthesia care unit. After arteriography the patient returned to surgery and a bypass graft was necessary after thrombectomy was unsuccessful. In the event of arterial thrombosis the goal should be prompt diagnosis, with a goal muscle ischemia time of less than 6 to 8 hours. If an iliac artery occlusion is suspected, emergent exploration or diagnostic angiography should be prioritized in the interest of minimizing warm ischemia time. Intraoperative angiography can be useful if the level or degree of occlusion is not apparent.

If an aortic or common iliac artery occlusion is surgically corrected, reperfusion syndrome may occur. Lower leg compartment syndromes are to be expected with reperfusion after warm ischemia durations of greater than 6 to 8 hours. Reperfusion syndrome is defined as an altered blood flow or ischemia that can further cause tissue and organ damage.[239] Exam findings may include early lower extremity sensory and motor deficits below the knee. In the initial phase, weakness in the L5 and S1 distributions is common. Ultimately there will be a pale, mottled, cool extremity, but pain to passive stretch of the compartments precedes these late findings and should greatly raise the suspicion for development of compartment syndrome.

Rhabdomyolysis with reperfusion is a potentially fatal late complication. In its most severe presentation, reperfusion syndrome can lead to multiple organ dysfunction with complicated interactions between antioxidants, complement, and serologic factors due to physiologic reactions to uncontrolled oxidative stress. Clinical effects of reperfusion syndrome include arrhythmias and myocardial stunning, strokes, gastrointestinal bleeds or infarction, and renal failure. The occurrence of many of these in combination is known as multiple organ dysfunction. Risk factors for multiple organ dysfunction include sepsis, major trauma, septic shock, aortic cross clamping, lower extremity ischemia, burns, circulatory shock and collapse, pancreatitis, and immunologic disorders. Multiple organ dysfunction has a high mortality rate. Optimal treatment may mitigate these effects. Ideally, reperfusion after arterial occlusion should occur in a controlled and closely monitored fashion and postoperative compartment pressure monitoring by serial examination of the extremities should be routine.

Posterior Lumbar Vascular Complications

Vascular complications in posterior lumbar spinal surgery are most often associated with lumbar discectomy.[229] However, there is a single case report of a vascular complication resulting in death after a lumbar laminectomy without discectomy for acquired spinal stenosis.[43] In that case a 62-year-old man developed high-output cardiac failure and hypovolemic shock with an expanding right retroperitoneal hematoma due to laceration of a segmental vessel caused by neuroforaminal probing. A blunt-tip gallbladder probe was used at L3–L4, tearing the right fourth segmental artery. Similarly, an 84-year-old patient undergoing kyphoplasty suffered an L4 segmental bleed requiring segmental angiographic embolization.[240] Notwithstanding these few cases, the majority of vascular complications in posterior lumbar spinal surgery occur during discectomy.

The incidence of lumbar vascular complications associated with lumbar discectomy is not known, but more than 300 cases of vascular complications associated with discectomy have been published, usually as case reports, or in small retrospective series.[2,12,15,28,29,36,41,57,129,150] These appear in periodicals of vascular and cardiovascular surgery, general surgery, orthopaedic surgery, neurosurgery, urology, and internal medicine; this variety emphasizes the complexity and spectrum of vascular and visceral injury that may complicate lumbar discectomy.

Aorta, Vena Cava, and Common Iliac Vessels

Vascular injury during lumbar discectomy occurs most commonly at the L4–L5 level, followed by the L5–S1 level. This reflects the frequency of symptomatic disc herniations at these levels, but the proximity of the anterior L4–L5 interspace to vascular structures also contributes to the incidence of vascular injury at this level. At the L4–L5 interspace the aorta, vena cava, common iliac vessels and branches are all at risk, but the left common iliac artery is the vessel most commonly injured (Fig. 97.30).[230] There are also reports of injury to the left recurrent iliolumbar vein and the superior rectal artery.[226,241] Vascular complications associated with lumbar discectomy occur in six categories: (1) laceration of the aorta or vena cava with immediate hypovolemic shock, (2) lacerations of the iliac vessels with or without immediate hypovolemic shock, (3) partial avulsion of a vessel wall with delayed hemorrhage or thrombosis, (4) injury incident to preexisting vascular disease such as an abdominal aortic aneurysm or atherosclerotic vessels, (5) false aneurysm and infected hematoma, and (6) arteriovenous fistula.[29] The instrument most commonly implicated in these injuries is the pituitary rongeur (Fig. 97.31).[9,119,242]

Risk factors for vascular injury during lumbar discectomy include (1) preexisting degenerative disc disease, (2) retroperitoneal inflammatory processes leading to adhesions between the vessels and the disc, (3) aggressive "total" discectomy, (4) increased intraabdominal pressure that may force vessel or viscera against or close to the disc (especially if anterior annular tears exist), and (5) revision discectomy when annular tears are common.[230] Annular tears are also a factor in primary discectomy and commonly occur anteriorly or laterally as part of degenerative disc disease.[243] Failure to appreciate disruption of the anterior anulus fibrosus may contribute to vascular injury during discectomy.[243-245] Adhesions may occur in anterior disc herniations and degenerative disc disease without prior anterior surgery, especially at L4–L5 and L3–L4 disc

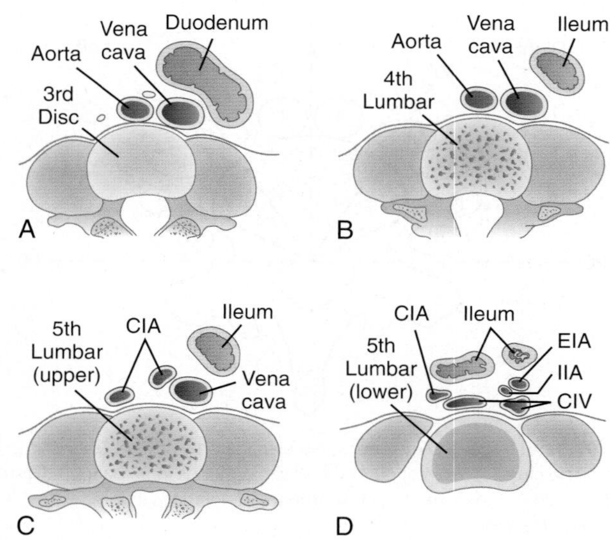

FIG. 97.30 Anatomic structures in the immediate vicinity, anteriorly, of the lower lumbar spine. (A) L3–L4 disc space. (B) L4 vertebral body. (C) L5 vertebral body. (D) Inferior end plate of L5. CIA, common iliac artery; EIA, external iliac artery; IIA, internal iliac artery; CIV, common iliac vein. (From Montorsi W, Ghiringhelli C. Genesis: diagnosis and treatment of vascular complications after intervertebral disc surgery. *Int Surg.* 1973;58:233–235.)

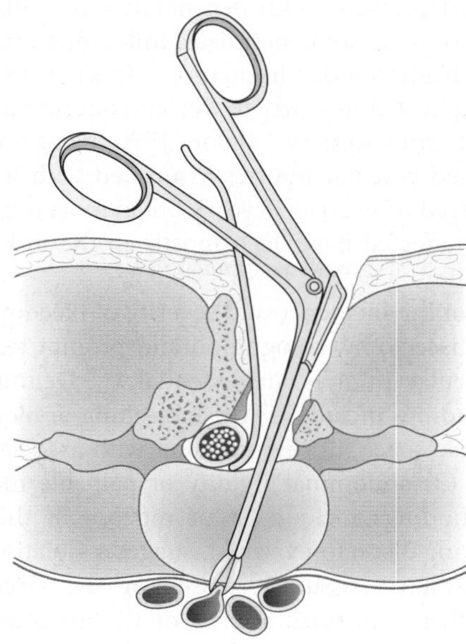

FIG. 97.31 Pituitary rongeur transgressing the anterior anulus and anterior longitudinal ligament, creating an injury to the anterior vascular structures. (From Montorsi W, Ghiringhelli C: Genesis: diagnosis and treatment of vascular complications after intervertebral disc surgery. *Int Surg.* 1973;58:233–235.)

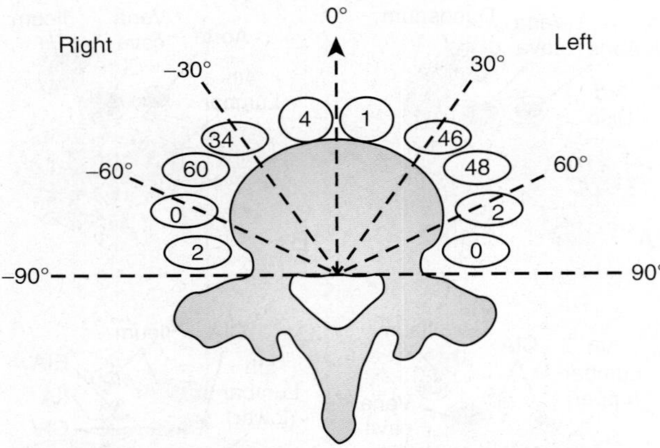

FIG. 97.32 Transverse prevertebral vascular anatomy at the L5–S1 disc level. Schematic representation of the vessel positions in 50 patients. (From Anda S, Aakhus S, Skaanes KO, et al. Anterior perforations in lumbar diskectomies. *Spine.* 1991;16:54–60.)

levels. Despite these multiple reports, injuries to the retroperitoneal vessels or viscera still occur (Fig. 97.32).

Prior surgery as a risk factor for vascular injury during discectomy is more important now than ever. As the rates of anterior lumbar surgeries have increased, it is not uncommon to find adhesion or inflammation changes around an unoperated intervertebral disc with degenerative disc disease. It is common to observe some peridiscal inflammation, especially at L4–L5 with anterior disc herniations. This peridiscal fibrosis has been implicated in injury to the left common iliac vein in patients with prior surgery.[36] Before 1990 the ages of patients who sustained vascular injuries associated with lumbar discectomy ranged from 20 to 58 years, but in more recent reports the patients affected have been mostly in the fifth and sixth decades of life.[2,12,15,28,29,36,57,129,137,160,242,246-255]

Because of the incidence and severity of bleeding sequelae in lumbar discectomy, recognition and prompt treatment of lumbar vascular injuries are essential.[2,247] Definitive intraoperative findings include (1) brisk bleeding or blood welling up in the disc space, (2) hypotension with associated tachycardia, and (3) abdominal rigidity or palpable mass. Other suspicious findings include fat or mucosa in the pituitary rongeur during discectomy, which suggests violation of retroperitoneal adipose tissue, a vessel, or the visceral wall.[2] However, other than brisk arterial or venous bleeding from the disc space, there are no pathognomonic signs of vascular injury.[247] Furthermore, less than 50% of reported cases noted bleeding from the disc space,[2] and fewer than 50% of vascular injuries during lumbar discectomy are recognized early.[256] Shevlin's test is an intraoperative test for a potential large anterior annular defect, especially in the face of unexplained hypotension during posterior lumbar discectomy. The test is performed by filling the wound with saline; if it escapes rapidly anteriorly, then an anterior disc defect is highly likely and may indicate a retroperitoneal vascular or visceral injury.[257] The test is not pathognomic but highly suggests an anterior annular defect allowing the flow of fluid into the retroperitoneal space.

Intraoperative hypotension unexplained by anesthetic effects is the most sensitive and early diagnostic finding. If bleeding from the disc space occurs intraoperatively in association with hypotension, pack the interspace, cover the wound with a sterile dressing, and start volume expanders or blood replacement immediately. A vascular or general surgeon should be called emergently, the patient should be turned to the supine position, and the abdomen should be prepped and draped for an extensive transperitoneal laparotomy. A generous longitudinal extensile abdominal incision has been suggested.[29] Options to surgically address the vascular injury include (1) direct suture repair, (2) resection of a damaged segment and graft or side-to-side repair, or (3) bypass graft or anastomosis when the injured segment of the vessel is ligated. If ligation of a major vein such as the internal or external iliac is required, thrombosis, lower extremity swelling, venous congestion, and thromboembolism are possible sequelae.[249]

It is not uncommon, however, for these injuries to go undetected during the procedure, only to be discovered in the recovery room. Therefore the surgeon should be vigilant for unexplained hypotension, tachycardia, and abdominal signs and symptoms during the perioperative period in order to promptly diagnose vascular injury.[247] The clinical presentation may mimic postoperative ileus, which is much more common; for this reason the surgeon must regard these symptoms with a high level of suspicion. The signs of shock, however, distinguish hemorrhage from paralytic ileus. Periodic education of recovery room staff has been recommended to help identify cases not apparent until after surgical lumbar discectomy, as well as other vascular complications such as iliac artery thrombosis and a pulseless or cold extremity. Unexplained hypotension, unusual abdominal symptoms, lower extremity pulse changes, leg swelling or engorgement, unexplained tachycardia, or a patient who appears in shock without a good explanation should represent warning signs of possible significant vascular injury. Using these principles, the incidence of vascular complications from routine and revision discectomy may be minimized.

To minimize the risk of a major vessel injury during lumbar discectomy, careful positioning and meticulous surgical technique are recommended.[8,229,258-260] Operations should be performed with adequate illumination and magnification. An operative microscope or loupes of ×2.5 to ×3.5 magnification are recommended. A limited or subtotal discectomy should be performed in most cases because the results of partial lumpectomy or discectomy are equivalent to a more aggressive and complete discectomy.[8] If not torn already, the posterolateral anulus is incised in a cruciate pattern with a scalpel blade inserted no more than 4 to 5 mm deep. The pituitary rongeur is inserted only under direct vision and limited to less than 2.5 cm in depth in most cases. More important than a depth measurement, however, is the feel of the instrument against the endplates before opening and closing the jaws of the pituitary rongeur.[2,28,250]

There is no clear consensus, however, as to the "safe" depth of penetration by a Kerrison or pituitary rongeur; recommendations range from 2.5 to 4.5 cm. Due to the oval geometry of the intervertebral disc, the angle and direction of insertion into the disc space also affect the safe depth of insertion (Fig. 97.32).[28,250] These depths also vary by the sex and build of the patient, the intradiscal pathology, and the interspace level

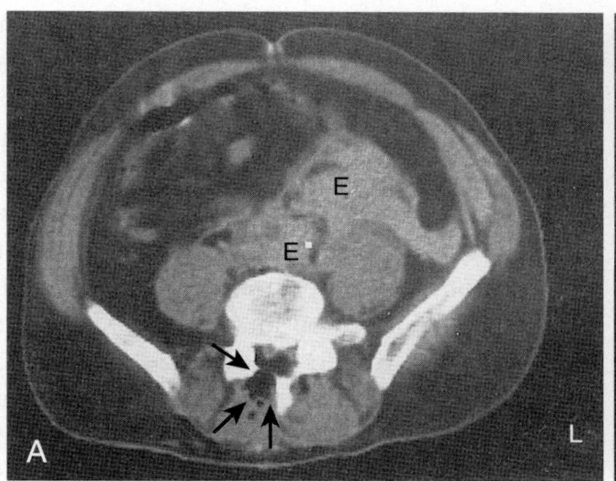

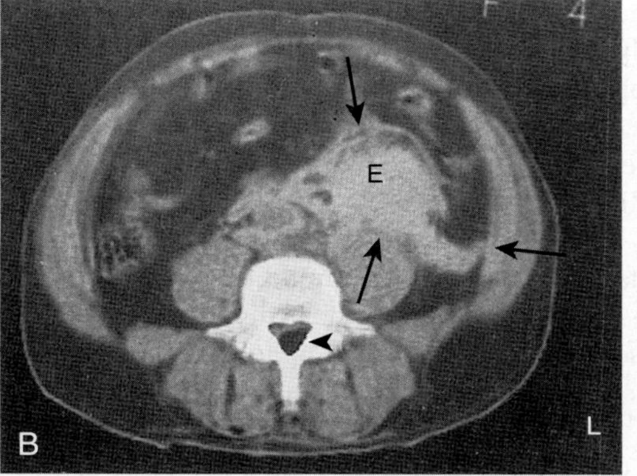

FIG. 97.33 Spontaneous hematic hyperdensity between cava and aorta (E). A hematoma is infiltrating the caudal aspect of the pararenal space. Arrows indicate air in the muscular tissue; arrowhead indicates air in the spinal canal at the hemilaminectomy site as a result of the recent surgical treatment (30 minutes).

because disc and endplate size vary by spinal level.[250] For example, instruments should not be inserted more than 2.5 to 3.75 cm below the posterior margin of the vertebral body at L2–L3 through L4–L5 and not more than 4 cm below the posterior vertebral margin at L5–S1. The marking scales on instruments by centimeters may improve the precision of this maneuver. Some authors have further suggested taking an intraoperative radiograph during the surgery for determination of depth as well as for documentation reasons.[2,250] Finally, and perhaps most importantly, the disc should be removed deliberately and patiently, and forceful or abrupt maneuvers should be avoided. Routinely, tactile perception should confirm that the pituitary rongeur is in contact with the vertebral endplates to ensure that the instrument is contained in the intervertebral disc space. Typically, the distance from the hinge jaw to the tip of the pituitary is about 1 cm. The surgeon should remember that the goal of discectomy is to relieve tension or compression of the nerve root, not to perform a total or subtotal discectomy per se; a 5% recurrence rate is preferable to even a single vascular injury during posterior limited discectomy. The potential for catastrophe resulting from direct vascular injury demands that the surgeon exercise careful and meticulous technique.

In summary, vascular injuries resulting from lumbar disc surgery are serious complications. Mortality rates vary and depend on the type of vascular injury[248,249,255] and the temporal relationships among injury, recognition, and treatment.[256] Early recognition and repair are not a guarantee of survival, especially in acute lumbar vascular injuries. These complications tend to manifest early and require emergent attention. Even if patients survive, long-term morbidity may occur from ischemic injury to cerebral or renal parenchyma, reperfusion injury, persistent pain with or without radiculopathy,[28,250] or even high-ouput cardiac failure in the case of arteriovenous fistula.[251]

Other Vascular Complications of Spine Surgery

Other vascular complications are less common or not necessarily characteristic of spine surgery, but are no less important; the relatively more common of these are discussed below.

Thrombosis and Thromboembolism

Thromboembolic disease in patients undergoing complex spinal surgery is being increasingly recognized.[16,35,65,127,158,159,194,261–269] Patients with thromboembolic disease or DVT may present asymptomatically or with lower extremity signs of calf pain, swelling, tenderness, positive Homans sign, or redness and induration along the course of the vein. Recent studies have attempted to quantify the incidence of thromboembolic disease in patients undergoing elective spinal surgery.[11,16,35,65,159,194,234,261–264] Using Doppler ultrasound imaging, one study found a 14% incidence of asymptomatic DVT 1 day after major adult spine surgery.[264] Pulmonary embolism (PE) can occur as well and may be present despite a negative venous Doppler ultrasound of the lower extremity. The diagnosis of DVT may be established definitively by invasive venography or secondarily by Doppler ultrasound. With high specificity and sensitivity, spiral CT of the chest has replaced the ventilation perfusion scan as the diagnostic test of choice for PE,[263,270] although the ventilation perfusion scan is still useful for patients with poor renal function who cannot tolerate intravenous contrast. Key factors in controlling postoperative thromboembolism include early mobilization, elastic stockings, and sequential compressive devices.

The risks of DVT and PE are associated with the type of surgery and operative time. Patients who undergo complex spinal reconstructive surgery—which often occurs in two stages—experience a greater incidence of lower extremity thromboembolism and PE. One study identified several factors that increase the risk of thromboembolism or PE in spine surgery.[242] These risk factors include inactivity, recumbency, increasing age, obesity, cigarette smoking, anterior spinal procedures, and iliac crest bone harvest. The authors of this study also reported that two-thirds of lower extremity DVTs occurred on the same side as the bone graft.[242] Another series found a 5.6% incidence of thromboembolic disease in 134 cases of cervical spine surgery compared with 26.5% of thoracolumbar cases.[263] A series of 686 anterior lumbosacral exposures found only a 1% incidence of thromboembolic disease,[202] which was similar to an incidence of 2% reported in another series of 60 anterior lumbar interbody fusion cases.[271]

The pharmacologic prevention of thromboembolic disease in patients undergoing spinal surgery must be balanced with the risk of bleeding complications. Traditional antithrombotic agents such as heparin, fractionated heparins, antiplatelet drugs, and warfarin are relatively contraindicated after spinal surgery due to the risks of epidural bleeding and epidural hematoma; these increased risks persist up to 4 weeks postoperatively. The use of aspirin (acetylsalicylic acid), however, is still debated.[11,262,270,272,273] A systematic review of the literature found that the overall risk of thromboembolism in patients not receiving chemical prophylaxis was 2.3% for degenerative conditions, 5.3% for deformity, and 6.0% for trauma.[274] This review also found that the risks of major bleeding with anticoagulation were low and varied from 0.0% to 4.3% depending on anticoagulant type.[274] The optimal timing of administration of anticoagulation is also unknown.

It is universally recommended, however, that intermittent pneumatic compression sleeves with elastic stockings be applied preoperatively and should be a primary mode of prophylaxis in patients undergoing all types of spinal surgery.[11,261,262,272,275] One study compared low-dose heparin with mechanical compression and alternating-day dextran and found both regimens reduced the incidence of thromboembolic disease by a factor of four.[261]

Patients with proven lower extremity thromboembolic disease or patients with symptomatic pulmonary emboli may best be managed with the placement of an inferior vena cava (IVC) filter.[264,275] Patients undergoing complex anterior spinal reconstruction who have two or more of the routine risk factors, such as obesity, sedentary lifestyle, and history of prior DVT or PE, may be considered candidates for prophylactic preoperative placement of a removable IVC filter.

It is ever more common that elderly patients presenting with surgical spinal disease will be taking oral anticoagulation agents such as warfarin for long-term anticoagulation after prosthetic heart valve, for chronic atrial fibrillation, or for other prophylactic reasons such as a history of transient ischemic attacks or other thromboembolic event. Novel oral anticoagulation agents such as the factor Xa inhibitors rivaroxaban and apixaban and the direct thrombin inhibitor dabigatran are also increasingly common and present unique challenges in perioperative reversal and monitoring.[276] Perioperative anticoagulation and the balance of risks of bleeding complications and thromboembolic events are complex issues and should be managed in consultation with the patient's medical and cardiac physicians. The biologic half-life of warfarin is 20 to 60 hours, and it is almost exclusively renally excreted. In general, warfarin should be stopped 5 to 7 days prior to surgery, allowing the prothrombin time and international normalized ratio to normalize, but this interval may vary dramatically in elderly patients with impaired renal function. Interim coverage with low-molecular-weight heparin is usually recommended to within 12 hours of surgery; heparin bridging may be appropriate in patients at high risk for thromboembolic events. When to restart warfarin is controversial, and opinions vary from a few days to a few weeks after surgery; epidural hematomas have been known to form long after spine surgery[277] in patients on warfarin[278] and low-molecular-weight heparin.[279]

The optimal timing of perioperative anticoagulation is unknown and the appropriateness of anticoagulation can be controversial.[274] For example, anticoagulation may be safer in shorter or limited surgical cases that do not involve laminectomy or corpectomy, but this intuition is not supported by evidence. A survey of 94 spine surgeons based on the perceived risk-to-benefit ratio of anticoagulation found that among surgeons who gave any prophylaxis, 12% did so within 24 hours, 15% after 24 hours, 22% after 48 hours, 13% after 72 hours, and 10% after 96 hours.[266] This study also identified a trend of placing IVC filters before surgery, and 77% of survey respondents would place an IVC filter in a high-risk patient in lieu of low-molecular-weight heparin.[266] This practice is supported by a study that implanted IVC filters in high-risk patients with (1) a history of DVT, (2) thrombocytophilia, or (3) malignancy; or those who had (4) been bedbound for more than 2 weeks, (5) were undergoing two- to three-stage multiple-day procedures, (6) anterior and posterior same-day surgery, (7) any procedures that would continue longer than 8 hours, or (8) who were experiencing significant intraoperative blood loss. In that study only one out of 74 patients in this high-risk group developed a PE.[280] A study of 100 circumferential cervical cases with only mechanical compression prophylaxis compared to historical controls anticoagulated with heparin found 1% PE and 1% DVT rates. Corpectomy cases had a slightly greater DVT rate of 2%, with a 7% PE rate. All thromboembolic events were nonfatal. The authors concluded that in high-risk cases IVC filters should be placed before surgery and intermittent stockings or sequential compression boots should be used during surgery.[281] Multiple studies support the use of IVC filters in high-risk patients.[282,283]

Epidural and Subdural Hematomas

Epidural hematomas can be catastrophic postoperative complications that may present with acute paraparesis or acute paraplegia.[9,90,277,285] Subdural hematomas may be similarly catastrophic and may occur without surgery. Subdural hematomas are generally the result of small arterial bleeding into the subarachnoid space, whereas epidural hematomas result from venous bleeding into the epidural space. For this reason subdural hematomas are more likely to be expansile. Risk factors for epidural and subdural hematomas include coagulopathy, thrombocytopenia, use of anticoagulation agents, poor intraoperative hemostasis, prolonged length of surgery, corpectomy, greater number of spinal levels treated, and ankylosing spondylitis.[65,67,284,286] Immediate evacuation of the hematoma and decompression of the neural elements are the gold standard of treatment. The prognosis of spinal epidural hematomas depends on the spinal level of the hematoma, the degree of deficit, and definitive surgical decompression occurring within 36 hours.[285-287] Hematomas with incomplete neurologic deficits may be delayed in treatment up to 48 hours.[288] Except in cases of vascular malformations, the degree of pressure and compression were the most important prognostic factors. In vascular cases, the extent of the arteriovenous malformations determined the volume of the bleed and subsequent amount of pressure induced.

Diagnosis is primarily made on clinical presentation. In a nonurgent clinical setting the diagnosis may be confirmed by ultrasound, CT, MRI, or myelography.[289] Spinal epidural hematomas typically present as severe back pain with or without radicular pain, and the thoracolumbar area is more involved than the cervical area. MRI is the diagnostic test of choice. The classic appearance of subdural and epidural hematomas on MRI is an isointense area on T1-weighted imaging that appears iso-high intensity on T2-weighted imaging. As the hematoma matures to become a clot, it loses water content and the T2-weighted images concomitantly decrease in intensity. A spontaneous epidural hematoma that is not associated with progressive or significant neurologic deficit can be managed nonoperatively. Any anticoagulation should be reversed and the hematoma should be monitored by serial imaging. Most symptomatic subarachnoid hematomas that are surgically decompressed within 12 hours will demonstrate neurologic improvements.

Coagulation studies should be ordered and corrected as needed with vitamin K and fresh-frozen plasma. Patients receiving warfarin, aspirin, heparin, factor Xa inhibitors, direct thrombin inhibitors, or any anticoagulation may experience subdural or epidural hematoma, especially if a laminectomy has been performed. Due to the risk of epidural hematoma, routine administration of warfarin, heparin, or low-molecular-weight heparin is not routine prophylaxis, but low-dose aspirin (81 mg) may be used with low risk of epidural hematoma.[284] Prevention of life-threatening consequences of PE is the most crucial issue in the management of thromboembolic disease. Mechanical compression devices are unlikely to cause bleeding problems, and along with early mobilization they are common prophylaxis for thromboembolic prevention in spinal surgery.[263] Removable IVC filters should be implanted preoperatively in high-risk cases or in patients who develop venous thrombosis above the popliteal fossa in the perioperative setting.[272,275]

Superior Mesenteric Artery Syndrome

The estimated incidence of superior mesenteric artery syndrome (SMAS) is 0.2% in deformity cases.[290] Wilkie syndrome and nutcracker syndrome are distinct varieties of SMAS. Wilkie syndrome occurs in patients with extreme malnutrition and weight loss that likely leads to external compression of the superior mesenteric artery.[291] Nutcracker syndrome is a rare condition characterized by the entrapment of the left renal vein between the superior mesenteric artery and the aorta. This discussion focuses on SMAS of the "cast syndrome" variety.

In cast syndrome the third part of the duodenum is compressed by the superior mesenteric artery, which causes intestinal obstruction.[292] Although cast syndrome is rare, it almost exclusively occurs in orthopedic patients who have had spinal surgery or who are in hip spica body casts.[293] The superior mesenteric artery classically branches anterior-inferiorly from the aorta at about the L1 spinal level at an acute angle such that the third part of the duodenum crosses between the aorta and the superior mesenteric artery. Corrective deformity surgery may further reduce the angle at which the superior mesenteric artery branches from the aorta, directly compressing the duodenum between the aorta and superior mesenteric artery (Fig. 97.34A).[294] These patients present with an upper gastrointestinal bowel obstruction (Fig. 97.34B).[294] This syndrome also has been described in adult paraplegics on a delayed basis or in adult hyperkyphotic corrections.[295]

A high index of suspicion is required to recognize this complication because most anterior spinal procedures are followed by some pain and at least some degree of ileus. SMAS may affect adults with kyphosis but is primarily seen in pediatric deformity cases. Low body mass index and a high degree of deformity correction are key risk factors for the development of SMAS.[295] Adult cases occur with significant corrections of kyphosis and have been reported as late as 24 days after the surgery.[296] Evaluation and diagnosis are usually established with abdominal films, CT, or MRI. Differential diagnoses include (1) postoperative ileus, (2) a large bowel obstruction, and (3) Ogilvie syndrome—a spastic pseudoobstruction.[297]

Initial treatment should include a nasogastric tube, restriction of oral intake, intravenous fluids, and electrolyte balance with or without hyperalimentation.[297,298] These patients may benefit from positioning left lateral decubitus with a slight Trendelenburg posture. Although the vast majority of cases resolve in 2 to 3 days with supportive measures, if the obstruction persists then intravenous hyperalimentation should be provided to prevent malnutrition with its attendant risk of wound problems. Most cases of SMAS resolve with this management, but direct surgical decompression may be necessary in cases that do not. If any external compressive device such as a cast or brace is present, a trial of compressive device removal should be attempted before surgical intervention is considered. Surgical decompression may include a duodenojejunostomy with or without release of the ligament of Treitz.[30] Gastrojejunostomy is an alternative.

Blindness via Indirect Vascular Injury

Indirect vascular complications may result from patient positioning during spinal surgery, but these are infrequent relative to the more common positioning-related injuries to peripheral nerves such as the ulnar nerve at the cubital tunnel or stretch injuries of the brachial plexus.[10,136,192] Sudden blindness may occur secondary to vascular complication in the retina and has been reported with prone positioning in posterior spinal surgery.[10,299,300] The etiologies of sudden blindness include thromboembolism to the retina, central retinal artery occlusion, and retinal vein thrombosis.[299] Embolism of clot, plaque, or air is rarely reported.[301]

Blindness secondary to these vascular complications of the retina are catastrophic and most often irreversible. Central retinal artery occlusion is directly related to pressure on the eye, whereas posterior ischemic optic neuropathy is associated with increased blood loss, prone position, and sustained

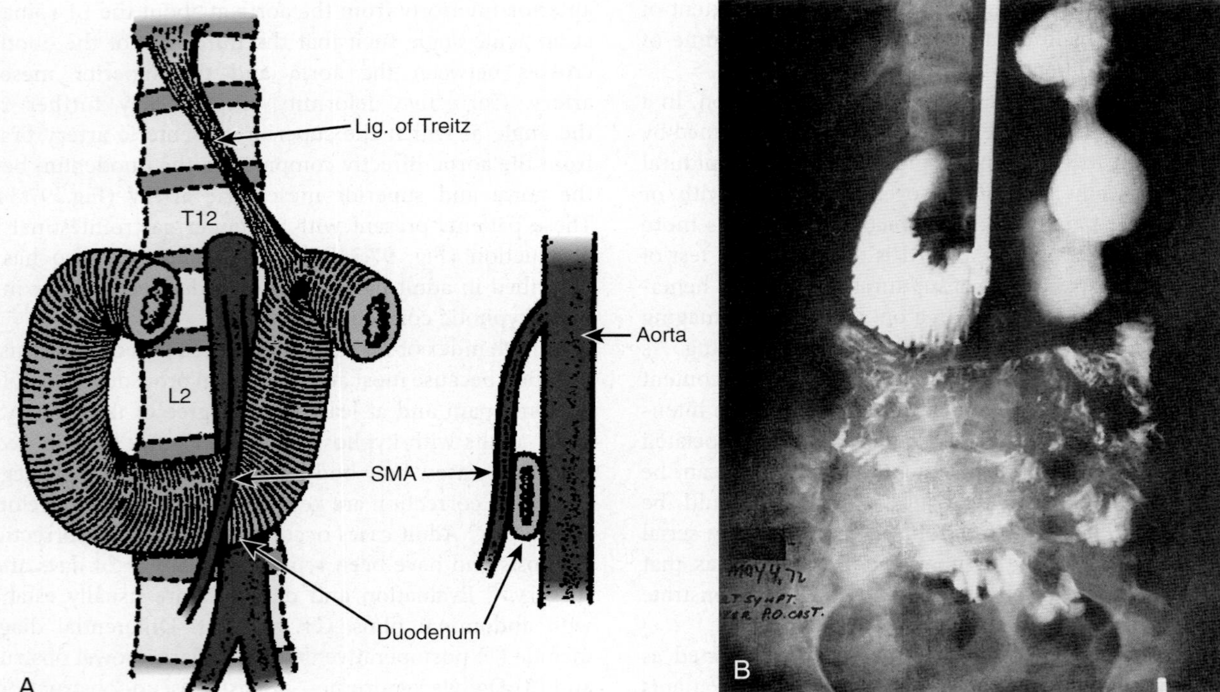

FIG. 97.34 Vascular compression of the duodenum. (A) Diagram of the third part of the duodenum showing the site of the duodenal compression. The third part of the duodenum passes between the superior mesenteric artery (SMA) anteriorly and the aorta and vertebral column posteriorly. Any reduction of the angle between the SMA and aorta will compress the duodenum. (B) Radiograph of a 16-year-old girl with idiopathic scoliosis and a 60-degree right thoracic curve. In a preoperative cast this was corrected to 19 degrees, and on the day of surgery the correction was 20 degrees. One week later a postoperative cast was applied and she ambulated. A day later she presented with nausea and vomiting. A Gastrografin swallow showed obstruction of the third part of the duodenum. The cast was removed, and the patient was kept supine with nasogastric suction to decompress the stomach. The obstruction resolved with this therapy, and a second postoperative cast was applied without recurrence of the obstruction. (A, From Skandalakis JE, Akin JT, Milsap JH, Gray SW. Vascular compression of the duodenum, part 2. Contemp Surg. 10:33, 1977.)

hypotension. Risk factors include (1) prolonged length of surgery, (2) increased intraoperative blood loss, (3) hypotension, and (4) direct ocular or periorbital pressure.[299,300] Preventive measures include eye protection, soft foam facial padding, managing intraoperative hypotension, and 20-degree reverse Trendelenburg positioning. If this complication does occur, ophthalmologic evaluation and treatment are recommended. The prognosis for restoration of sight, however, is very poor.

Iliac Crest Bone Graft

Autologous iliac crest bone graft is commonly used for arthrodesis of the cervical, thoracic, and lumbosacral spine.[80,143,158,186,193,200,202,206,207,209,302,303] Vascular injuries associated with concurrent iliac crest bone graft harvest most commonly involve the superior gluteal artery and vein in the sciatic notch[71] and less commonly the deep circumflex iliac artery.[304] Injury to the superior gluteal artery during harvest of a posterior iliac crest graft has been reviewed in the literature.[305] The incidence of this vascular injury is reportedly low but may be underreported.[303] Injury to these vessels is often the result of aggressive deep subperiosteal exposure of the gluteus maximus muscle from the posterior third of the iliac crest at the sciatic notch.

Injury to these vessels is usually direct, and bleeding can be profuse. Management options include packing, direct repair, ligation, or selective angiography and embolization. When possible, ligation is performed. This requires further exposure of the vessels by resection of the bone around the sciatic notch or rarely via exposure within the pelvis. An unrecognized or irreparable superior gluteal vessel injury may best be managed by selective endovascular embolization techniques postoperatively.[252,305] Partial injury of a vessel wall may result in an aneurysm.[304] In the case of aneurysm, selective endovascular embolization of the artery may be required if direct repair and hematoma evacuation are unsuccessful. Prevention of vessel injury is of course preferable to any post facto treatment option; therefore an understanding and appreciation of the vascular and anatomic relationships associated with the iliac crest bone graft harvest technique is the most effective strategy for managing the risk of these complications.

Conclusions

The risk of vascular complications during spinal surgery can be greatly reduced with thoughtful surgical planning and careful execution. Despite this, reports of vascular complications in cervical, thoracic, and lumbar surgery continue to increase in number. Knowledge of the vascular anatomy and common anatomic variants are the most important preventive measures.

In the cervical spine, the common carotid artery should be repaired if injured. Treatment of vertebral artery injuries is controversial; repair is preferred but is not always possible. As the availability of endovascular procedures expands, the standard of care is shifting toward endovascular repair with internal covered stents that plug the leak but maintain patency. In the thoracic spine, the segmental vessels should be preserved if possible or sacrificed only on one side as dictated by the pathology and approach. The artery of Adamkiewicz should be preserved if at all possible. The aorta is at particular risk for perforation by breach of the anterior cortex by a pedicle screw. In anterior lumbar surgery, the aorta, vena cava, common iliac vein, and iliolumbar vein are most at risk. Careful handling and meticulous technique will minimize the risk of venous injury. In the posterior lumbar spine, injury to the aorta, vena cava, and their branches should be avoided with careful surgical technique, especially in lumbar discectomy. If injuries occur to the abdominal aorta, vena cava, or the branches of the great vessels, early recognition and direct suture repair are the standard. This chapter emphasizes aspects of vascular anatomy, choice of approach, retractor placement, dissection planes, operative technique, and the importance of cooperation between the vascular surgeon and spine surgeon to aid in the prevention and treatment of these potentially serious and life-threatening vascular complications. Although the risks of these vascular complications or injuries can be minimized, they are still not uncommon even in the operating theaters of the most careful and prepared spine surgeons. For this reason adequate preparation should include preparation with the expectation that these vascular insults will occur. By preparing for these vascular complications, morbid or mortal sequelae may be prevented. Most spine surgeons understand these issues well and with the aid of vascular access surgeons they rarely encounter negative short- or long-term sequelae.

In summary, vascular complications of spinal surgery are, in fact, relatively common. In addition to the risks and injuries discussed above, harvesting bone graft from the iliac crest places the superior gluteal artery at risk. Thromboembolic complications after spine surgery are a particular area of concern, and much patient morbidity and mortality could be spared if these common complications could be effectively prevented. Epidural and subdural hematomas, superior mesenteric artery syndrome, and posterior ischemic optic neuropathy are unique vascular complications characteristic of spine surgery, and deserve special attention. The efforts of surgeons, clinicians, researchers, and health systems should approach these and all vascular complications with the primary goal of prevention.

Acknowledgment

We acknowledge the work of the authors of this chapter in the previous edition: Jeffrey L Stambough, MD, MBA, and Elisha K Clouse, RN, BSN, CCRP.

PEARLS

1. The vascular anatomy of the spine has numerous known anatomic variations and is prone to anatomic anomalies, especially in the upper cervical and at the lumbosacral junction. These vascular variations can significantly impact surgical planning in these areas; for this reason some surgeons have suggested careful review of preoperative axial imaging.
2. The vertebral artery is at greatest risk as it passes through the upper cervical spine. The vertebral artery passes through the foramen of C2 as it extends cranially, then through the C1 foramen before coursing medially toward the midline on the superior aspect of C1. The vertebral artery occupies a groove on the posterior aspect of the posterior arch of C1 that is on average 18 mm lateral of midline. Due to this unique anatomy of the vertebral artery in the superior cervical spine, some authors have recommended limited dissection in this area. Dissection of the posterior aspect of the posterior arch of C1 should begin with identification of the posterior tubercle of the atlas and should remain within 12 mm of midline and the dissection should not extend beyond 8 mm from midline on the superior aspect of the arch.
3. Anterior exposure of the lumbar and lumbosacral spine may be accomplished by a lateral retroperitoneal approach, a transperitoneal approach, or a paramedian hypogastric (mini-open, rectus-splitting, or minimally invasive anterior lumbar) retroperitoneal approach. All these approaches directly address the vascular structures of the anterior lumbar spine and are best used for exposure of L1–L3 levels. For this reason some surgeons monitor left great toe pulse oximetry during these procedures to identify early and reversible left iliac artery occlusion.
4. Some surgeons prefer hand-held retractors in the anterior approach lumbar spine. Hand-held retractors should have blunt tips and concave edges so that they may be safely placed deep to the vessels. Retraction should be gentle, variable, and readily adjusted. At times the use of hand-held retractors will necessitate working in steps, often working side to side at the level of the disc. This technique avoids both prolonged, continuous retraction and minimizes the total time of arterial retraction.
5. During an anterior approach to the lower lumbar spine, the middle sacral artery and vein must be ligated. The surgeon should not use these vessels as a central landmark because these vessels do not represent the midline of the L5–S1 intervertebral disc.
6. Vascular complications in posterior lumbar spinal surgery are most often associated with lumbar discectomy. The disc should be removed deliberately and patiently, and forceful or abrupt maneuvers should be avoided. Routinely, tactile perception should confirm that the Kerrison or pituitary rongeur is in contact with the vertebral end plates to ensure that the instrument is contained in the intervertebral disc space. The surgeon should remember that the goal of discectomy is to relieve tension or compression of the nerve root, not to perform a total or subtotal discectomy per se; a 5% recurrence rate is preferable to even a single vascular injury during posterior limited discectomy. The potential for catastrophe resulting from direct vascular injury demands that the surgeon exercise careful and meticulous technique.

PITFALLS

1. In about 15.5% of patients, a false bony bridge called the *ponticulus ponticus* covers the vertebral artery as it passes onto the posterior C1 ring. This is easily noted on lateral cervical plain

films. It is important to recognize this common variant to avoid injury to the vertebral artery by dissection or C1 transosseous screw fixation. The ponticulus ponticus is a harbinger of injury to the vertebral artery along the cephalad margin, especially if the ponticulus ponticus is not appreciated during placement of C1 lateral mass screws (see Fig. 97.11).

2. The vertebral artery is the main artery at risk in cervical spine surgery. As long as you stay medial to the uncinate process, it is highly unlikely that any injury will occur. Injury is likely to occur if the uncinate process is violated (usually by high-speed burring) or aggressively undercut during a foraminotomy.
3. Theoretically, the thoracolumbar spinal cord tolerates transient and permanent unilateral segmental blood flow disruption. However, bilateral segmental disruption, transient or permanent, is much more likely to cause spinal cord ischemia and consequent paraparesis or paraplegia. It should be noted that unilateral ligation of thoracolumbar segmental arteries may be acceptable on the convexity of the deformity, but perhaps only in primary surgeries, as certain complex revision surgeries may mimic bilateral ligation. Due to the well-known importance of the artery of Adamkiewicz, actual or indirect segmental vessel injuries should be avoided between T8 and L1 on the left.
4. Ligation of segmental vessels along the thoracolumbar spine is best accomplished by tying the artery in the middle of the vertebral body and along the convexity of a curve. If it is tied too close to the spine, the artery can retract and bleeding can be excessive, or it may in turn damage the blood supply to the neural elements. Conversely, if it is tied and cut too close to the vessel, an avulsion injury could occur. This would result in profuse bleeding and require expert vascular surgical repair.
5. Given the relative frailty of the vena cava and the potential for tearing, laceration, or avulsion, there is no case in which the aorta, vena cava, or common iliac vessels are mobilized from right to left. As one extends the exposure to levels superior to L4–L5, the aorta and vena cava are almost always mobilized together from left to right. In the anterior approaches to the lumbar spine, multiple factors aid in determining whether the great vessels may be safely incorporated into a fixed retractor setup. In most cases, the great vessels should not be incorporated into a fixed retractor; this may lead to complete occlusion of the aorta, vena cava, or common iliac arteries and veins. Many surgeons use a retractor that affixes to the operating room table. It is important that this retractor be able to move with the patient and that the retractor adequately retract the peritoneal contents without undue stress on the great vessels.
6. Although injury to the venous structures is more common during anterior lumbar surgery, the major risk to life and limb is the secondary formation arterial thrombosis. Although one series showed that all thromboses occurred either intraoperatively or within 2 hours of surgery, surgeons should be aware that the presentation of left common iliac artery thrombosis after anterior lumbar surgery has been reported to be delayed by hours to up to 13 days. This type of occlusion may initially be mistaken for vasospasm. Thrombosis of the left common iliac artery or vein is a surgical emergency. For this reason it is recommended that pulses be evaluated after retraction and before closing and the neurovascular assessment of the left leg should continue in the postanesthesia care unit. If the diagnosis is suspected, there is no need to proceed to arteriography. A pulseless left lower extremity can be assumed to be an occluded iliac artery, and urgent thrombectomy with or without further reconstruction should proceed.
7. Vascular complications in posterior lumbar spinal surgery are most often associated with lumbar discectomy. It is not uncommon, however, for these injuries to go undetected during the procedure, only to be discovered in the recovery room. Therefore the surgeon should be vigilant for unexplained hypotension, tachycardia, and abdominal signs and symptoms during the perioperative period in order to promptly diagnose vascular injury. The clinical presentation may mimic postoperative ileus, which is much more common; for this reason the surgeon must regard these symptoms with a high level of suspicion. The signs of shock, however, distinguish hemorrhage from paralytic ileus. Periodic education of recovery room staff has been recommended to help identify cases not apparent until after surgical lumbar discectomy.

KEY POINTS

1. In the discussion of vascular complications of spine surgery, prevention should be the primary focus. Prevention of vascular complications is assisted by knowledge of the normal vascular anatomy and common variants, including a knowledge of the relationships between particular blood vessels and bony landmarks. Through careful preoperative planning and the use of gentle intraoperative techniques with appropriate illumination and magnification, many of these complications can be avoided.
2. Vascular complications during posterior thoracic spine surgery are rare. The most significant of these is iatrogenic injury to posterior mediastinal structures by pedicle screws that breach that anterior cortex of the vertebral body. The best strategy for these injures is to avoid them by selecting pedicle screws of appropriately short length that are placed using meticulous technique.
3. Arterial and venous complications occurring in spinal surgery occur directly as a result of surgical dissection or indirectly as a result of manipulation or forces applied to soft tissues or spinal motion segments. Unrecognized vein injury tends to involve acute blood loss, whereas arterial injury tends to have subacute-chronic sequelae (thrombosis, embolization, fistulae, and/or aneurysm).
4. Most arterial and venous injuries in spinal surgery that occur from direct injury can be treated by ligation, primary repair, endovascular stenting, or selective embolization.
5. Arterial and venous injuries and vascular-related complications are increasingly reported in spinal surgery. This is due in large part to the increasing rates of anterior thoracolumbar spinal surgery. The most common vascular complication sequela is acute blood loss anemia.
6. Multiple reviews of lumbar total disc replacement have found that the most common vascular complications are left common iliac vein laceration (5%), vena cava laceration (2%), and thrombosis of the left common iliac vein or left common iliac artery (<1%). These studies emphasize that vascular problems may be relatively common with anterior lumbar spinal cases, but these rarely result in serious sequelae unless the injury results in total disruption of the vascular supply to the lower extremity or viscera. Depending on the spine surgeon's level of expertise and hospital credentialing, a collaborative effort with a surgeon experienced in vascular surgical techniques should be considered, especially in the ever more common anterior lumbar revision cases.
7. Prior surgery as a risk factor for vascular injury during lumbar discectomy is more important now than ever. As the rates of anterior lumbar surgeries have increased, it is not uncommon to

find adhesion or inflammation changes around an unoperated intervertebral disc with degenerative disc disease. It is common to observe some peridiscal inflammation, especially at L4–L5 with anterior disc herniations. This peridiscal fibrosis has been implicated in injury to the left common iliac vein in patients with prior surgery, and surgeons and patients should be aware of the increased risk of vascular injury during revisions surgery.

KEY REFERENCES

1. Peng CW, Chou BT, Bendo JA, Spivak JM. Vertebral artery injury in cervical spine surgery: anatomical considerations, management, and preventive measures. *Spine J.* 2009;9(1):70.
   Vertebral artery injury during cervical spine surgery is a rare but serious complication. This comprehensive literature review of vertebral artery injury during common anterior and posterior cervical spine procedures provides an overview of the surgical anatomy, management, and prevention of this injury. This review summarizes the findings of journal articles published on the topic after 2006. This review encourages review of preoperative MRI and/or CT scans and discusses endovascular repair as a treatment option when a vertebral artery injury is encountered.
2. Rampersaud YR, Moro ER, Neary MA, et al. Intraoperative adverse events and related postoperative complications in spine surgery: implications for enhancing patient safety founded on evidence-based protocols. *Spine.* 2006;31(13):1503.
   This prospective observational study assessed the incidence and clinical consequences of intraoperative adverse events from a wide variety of spinal surgical procedures with the hypothesis that most adverse events would not be identified through traditional practice audit approaches. Authors reviewed all nonmicrodiscectomy cases in a 1-year period and found that the overall incidence of intraoperative adverse events was 14%. A total of 23 adverse events led to postoperative clinical sequelae for an overall intraoperative complication incidence of 3.2%. In 10 cases blood loss exceeded 5000 mL (1.5%), and three cases involved suspected or actual vertebral artery injury (0.4%). The authors suggest that improved patient safety can only be maximized by independent practice audit and the development of prospective methods to record adverse event data so that enhanced, evidence-based, clinical protocols can be developed.
3. Kou J, Fischgrund J, Biddinger A, Herkowitz H. Risk factors for spinal epidural hematoma after spinal surgery. *Spine.* 2002;27(15):1670.
   To identify risk factors for the development of an epidural hematoma following spinal surgery, this case-control retrospective analysis compared patients with postoperative spinal epidural hematoma with patients who did not develop this complication. A single-institution review over a 10-year period identified twelve patients who demonstrated neurologic deterioration after surgery and required surgical decompression because of an epidural hematoma. All cases involved lumber laminectomies. Logistic regression identified multilevel procedures ($P = .037$) and the presence of a preoperative coagulopathy ($P < .001$) as significant risk factors. Age, body mass index, perioperative durotomies, and the presence of postoperative drains were not statistically significant risk factors.
4. Hicks JM, Singla A, Shen FH, Arlet V. Complications of pedicle screw fixation in scoliosis surgery: a systematic review. *Spine.* 2010;35(11):E465.
   This systematic review of the published literature on the use of pedicle screws in pediatric spinal deformity quantifies the risks and complications associated with pedicle screw instrumentation, particularly in the thoracic spine. The authors excluded articles dealing with neuromuscular scoliosis or bone dysplasia to focus mostly on adolescent thoracic idiopathic scoliosis. The review retrieved 21 studies with a total of 4570 pedicle screws in 1666 patients. Overall, 518 (4.2%) screws were reported as malpositioned. However, in studies in which postoperative computed tomography scans were done systematically, the rate of screw malposition was as high as 15.7%. Eleven patients underwent revision surgery for instrumentation malposition. There were no major vascular complications reported in these 21 studies. The authors identified nine case reports dealing with complications of pedicle screws. Such complications were mostly either vascular (10 cases) or neurologic (four cases) without any irreversible complications.
5. Glotzbecker MP, Bono CM, Harris MB, et al. Surgeon practices regarding postoperative thromboembolic prophylaxis after high-risk spinal surgery. *Spine.* 2008;33(26):2915.
   Although chemoprophylaxis for thromboembolic events is not routinely used after elective spinal surgery, it is more widely recommended in high-risk patients after spine surgery for trauma or tumors; however, there are no accepted treatment guidelines concerning this issue. This survey study gathered normative data across many practices regarding thromboembolic prophylaxis after high-risk surgery for tumors and trauma. This online survey has a 49% response rate. Regarding a safe time point to start chemoprophylaxis, the most common response was 48 hours after surgery (22%). However, individual responses varied widely. Some indicated they would start chemoprophylaxis before surgery, whereas others responded they would never use it. Sixty-three percent of surgeons based this decision on personal experience over evidence-based review of the literature. Respondents most commonly (47%) felt that the risk of clinically relevant postoperative epidural hematoma was between 1% and 5%. Those who felt the risk of epidural hematoma to be lower than 5% tended to initiate chemoprophylaxis earlier than those who estimated the risk to be higher than 5%. Thirty-seven percent felt the perceived risk for a DVT was 1% to 5%. Those who estimated the risk of DVT to be higher tended to initiate therapy earlier than groups that estimated the risk to be lower. These data were the first to demonstrate the wide variability of surgeons' practices regarding thromboembolic prophylaxis in high-risk spine surgery patients. This variability is likely a symptom of the glaring paucity of scientific evidence concerning the risk for symptomatic epidural hematoma, DVT, and PE and the efficacy and safety of specific chemoprophylactic protocols after spine surgery. This study highlights the need for more rigorous prospective evaluation of thromboembolic risk after spinal surgery and for the study of the efficacy and safety of currently available thromboembolic prophylaxis protocols.

REFERENCES

1. Flynn JC, Hoque MA. Anterior fusion of the lumbar spine. End-result study with long-term follow-up. *J Bone Joint Surg Am.* 1979;61(8):1143.
2. Goodkin R, Laska LL. Vascular and visceral injuries associated with lumbar disc surgery: medicolegal implications. *Surg Neurol.* 1998;49(4):358.
3. Raskas DS, Delamarter RB. Occlusion of the left iliac artery after retroperitoneal exposure of the spine. *Clin Orthop Relat Res.* 1997;(338):86.
4. Scroop R, Eskridge J, Britz GW. Paradoxical cerebral arterial embolization of cement during intraoperative vertebroplasty: case report. *AJNR Am J Neuroradiol.* 2002;23(5):868.
5. Ikard RW. Methods and complications of anterior exposure of the thoracic and lumbar spine. *Arch Surg.* 2006;141(10):1025.

6. Goz V, Weinreb JH, McCarthy I, et al. Perioperative complications and mortality after spinal fusions: analysis of trends and risk factors. *Spine*. 2013;38(22):1970.
7. Papadoulas S, Konstantinou D, Kourea HP, et al. Vascular injury complicating lumbar disc surgery. A systematic review. *Eur J Vasc Endovasc Surg*. 2002;24(3):189.
8. Balderston RA, Gilyard GG, Jones AA, et al. The treatment of lumbar disc herniation: simple fragment excision versus disc space curettage. *J Spinal Disord*. 1991;4(1):22.
9. Boukobza M, Guichard JP, Boissonet M, et al. Spinal epidural haematoma: report of 11 cases and review of the literature. *Neuroradiology*. 1994;36(6):456.
10. Eie N, Solgaard T, Kleppe H. The knee-elbow position in lumbar disc surgery: a review of complications. *Spine*. 1983;8(8):897.
11. Ferree BA, Stern PJ, Jolson RS, Roberts JM, Kahn A. Deep venous thrombosis after spinal surgery. *Spine*. 1993;18(3):315.
12. Freeman DG. Major vascular complications of lumbar disc surgery. *West J Surg Obstet Gynecol*. 1961;69:175.
13. Kraus DR, Stauffer ES. Spinal cord injury as a complication of elective anterior cervical fusion. *Clin Orthop Relat Res*. 1975;(112):130.
14. Laffont I, Bensmail D, Rech C, et al. Late superior mesenteric artery syndrome in paraplegia: case report and review. *Spinal Cord*. 2002;40(2):88.
15. Montorsi W, Ghiringhelli C. Genesis, diagnosis and treatment of vascular complications after intervertebral disk surgery. *Int Surg*. 1973;58(4):233.
16. Oskouian RJ, Johnson JP. Vascular complications in anterior thoracolumbar spinal reconstruction. *J Neurosurg*. 2002;96 (1 suppl):1.
17. Parke WW, Whalen JL, Bunger PC, Settles HE. Intimal musculature of the lower anterior spinal artery. *Spine*. 1995;20(19):2073.
18. Sen C, Eisenberg M, Casden AM, Sundaresan N, Catalano PJ. Management of the vertebral artery in excision of extradural tumors of the cervical spine. *Neurosurgery*. 1995;36(1):106.
19. Serrano Hernando FJ, Paredero VM, Solis JV, et al. Iliac arteriovenous fistula as a complication of lumbar disc surgery. Report of two cases and review of literature. *J Cardiovasc Surg (Torino)*. 1986;27(2):180.
20. Shallat RF, Klump TE. Paraplegia following thoracolumbar sympathectomy. Case report. *J Neurosurg*. 1971;34(4):569.
21. Song GS, Theodore N, Dickman CA, Sonntag VK. Unilateral posterior atlantoaxial transarticular screw fixation. *J Neurosurg*. 1997;87(6):851.
22. Tew JM, Mayfield FH. Complications of surgery of the anterior cervical spine. *Clin Neurosurg*. 1976;23:424.
23. Verbiest H. A lateral approach to the cervical spine: technique and indications. *J Neurosurg*. 1968;28(3):191.
24. Verdant A, Cossette R, Pagé A, et al. Aneurysms of the descending thoracic aorta: three hundred sixty-six consecutive cases resected without paraplegia. *J Vasc Surg*. 1995;21(3):385.
25. Bertalanffy H, Eggert HR. Complications of anterior cervical discectomy without fusion in 450 consecutive patients. *Acta Neurochir (Wien)*. 1989;99(1-2):41.
26. Neo M, Fujibayashi S, Miyata M, Takemoto M, Nakamura T. Vertebral artery injury during cervical spine surgery: a survey of more than 5600 operations. *Spine*. 2008;33(7):779.
27. Klezl Z, Swamy GN, Vyskocil T, Kryl J, Stulik J. Incidence of vascular complications arising from anterior spinal surgery in the thoraco-lumbar spine. *Asian Spine J*. 2014;8(1):59.
28. Anda S, Aakhus S, Skaanes KO, Sande E, Schrader H. Anterior perforations in lumbar discectomies. A report of four cases of vascular complications and a CT study of the prevertebral lumbar anatomy. *Spine*. 1991;16(1):54.
29. Bass J, Lach J, Fegelman RH. Vascular injuries during lumbar laminectomy. *Am Surg*. 1980;46(11):649.
30. Dommisse GF. The blood supply of the spinal cord. A critical vascular zone in spinal surgery. *J Bone Joint Surg Br*. 1974;56(2):225.
31. Freischlag JA, Sise M, Quinones-Baldrich WJ, Hye RJ, Sedwitz MM. Vascular complications associated with orthopedic procedures. *Surg Gynecol Obstet*. 1989;169(2):147.
32. Robinson RA, Southwick WO. Surgical approaches to the cervical spine. *Instr Course Lect*. 1960;17:299.
33. Moe JH, Purcell GA, Bradford DS. Zielke instrumentation (VDS) for the correction of spinal curvature. Analysis of results in 66 patients. *Clin Orthop Relat Res*. 1983;(180):133.
34. Riley LH. Surgical approaches to the anterior structures of the cervical spine. *Clin Orthop Relat Res*. 1973;(91):16.
35. Baker JK, Reardon PR, Reardon MJ, Heggeness MH. Vascular injury in anterior lumbar surgery. *Spine*. 1993;18(15):2227.
36. Bolesta MJ. Vascular injury during lumbar diskectomy associated with peridiskal fibrosis: case report and literature review. *J Spinal Disord*. 1995;8(3):224.
37. Bolton B. The blood supply of the human spinal cord. *J Neurol Psychiatry*. 1939;2(2):137.
38. Brillman J, Howieson J. Transient midbrain syndromes as a complication of vertebral angiography. Relationship to antecedent structural disease. *J Neurosurg*. 1974;41(1):71.
39. Burrington JD, Brown C, Wayne ER, Odom J. Anterior approach to the thoracolumbar spine: technical considerations. *Arch Surg*. 1976;111(4):456.
40. Kaiser MG, Haid RW, Subach BR, et al. Comparison of the mini-open versus laparoscopic approach for anterior lumbar interbody fusion: a retrospective review. *Neurosurgery*. 2002;51(1):97.
41. Lyness SS, Simeone FA. Vascular complications of upper cervical spine injuries. *Orthop Clin North Am*. 1978;9(4):1029.
42. Schellhas KP, Latchaw RE, Wendling LR, Gold LH. Vertebrobasilar injuries following cervical manipulation. *JAMA*. 1980;244(13):1450.
43. Smith DW, Lawrence BD. Vascular complications of lumbar decompression laminectomy and foraminotomy. A unique case and review of the literature. *Spine*. 1991;16(3):387.
44. Winter RB, Moe JH, Wang JF. Congenital kyphosis. Its natural history and treatment as observed in a study of one hundred and thirty patients. *J Bone Joint Surg Am*. 1973;55(2):223.
45. Murakami S, Mizutani J, Fukuoka M, et al. Relationship between screw trajectory of C1 lateral mass screw and internal carotid artery. *Spine*. 2008;33(24):2581.
46. Yamazaki M, Koda M, Aramomi MA, et al. Anomalous vertebral artery at the extraosseous and intraosseous regions of the craniovertebral junction: analysis by three-dimensional computed tomography angiography. *Spine*. 2005;30(21): 2452.
47. Takei H, Sagae M, Chiba K, Ogino T. The long-term follow-up of surgical treatment for cervical myelopathy with severe nape and upper arm pain caused by the anomalous vertebral artery: case report. *Spine*. 2008;33(17):E611.
48. Curylo LJ, Mason HC, Bohlman HH, Yoo JU. Tortuous course of the vertebral artery and anterior cervical decompression: a cadaveric and clinical case study. *Spine*. 2000;25(22):2860.
49. Peng CW, Chou BT, Bendo JA, Spivak JM. Vertebral artery injury in cervical spine surgery: anatomical considerations, management, and preventive measures. *Spine J*. 2009;9(1):70.

50. Hee HT, Majd ME, Holt RT, Whitecloud TS, Pienkowski D. Complications of multilevel cervical corpectomies and reconstruction with titanium cages and anterior plating. *J Spinal Disord Tech*. 2003;16(1):1.
51. Smith MD, Emery SE, Dudley A, Murray KJ, Leventhal M. Vertebral artery injury during anterior decompression of the cervical spine. A retrospective review of ten patients. *J Bone Joint Surg Br*. 1993;75(3):410.
52. Yonenobu K, Okada K, Fuji T, et al. Causes of neurologic deterioration following surgical treatment of cervical myelopathy. *Spine*. 1986;11(8):818.
53. Wright NM, Lauryssen C. Vertebral artery injury in C1-2 transarticular screw fixation: results of a survey of the AANS/CNS section on disorders of the spine and peripheral nerves. American Association of Neurological Surgeons/Congress of Neurological Surgeons. *J Neurosurg*. 1998;88(4):634.
54. Yonenobu K, Hosono N, Iwasaki M, Asano M, Ono K. Neurologic complications of surgery for cervical compression myelopathy. *Spine*. 1991;16(11):1277.
55. Pait TG, Killefer JA, Arnautovic KI. Surgical anatomy of the anterior cervical spine: the disc space, vertebral artery, and associated bony structures. *Neurosurgery*. 1996;39(4):769.
56. Cooney FD. Iatrogenic vertebral artery injury during anterior cervical spine surgery [author reply]. *Spine J*. 2003;3(1):89.
57. Hohf RP. Arterial injuries occurring during orthopaedic operations. *Clin Orthop Relat Res*. 1963;28:21.
58. Phillips DG. Surgical treatment of myelopathy with cervical spondylosis. *J Neurol Neurosurg Psychiatry*. 1973;36(5):879.
59. Schweighofer F, Passler JM, Wildburger R, Hofer HP. Interbody fusion of the lower cervical spine: a dangerous surgical method? *Langenbecks Arch Chir*. 1992;377(5):295.
60. Golfinos JG, Dickman CA, Zabramski JM, Sonntag VK, Spetzler RF. Repair of vertebral artery injury during anterior cervical decompression. *Spine*. 1994;19(22):2552.
61. Martín R, Carda JR, Pinto JI, et al. [Anterior cervical diskectomy and interbody arthrodesis using Cloward technique: retrospective study of complications and radiological results of 167 cases]. *Neurocirugia (Astur)*. 2002;13(4):265.
62. Rampersaud YR, Moro ER, Neary MA, et al. Intraoperative adverse events and related postoperative complications in spine surgery: implications for enhancing patient safety founded on evidence-based protocols. *Spine*. 2006;31(13):1503.
63. Burke JP, Gerszten PC, Welch WC. Iatrogenic vertebral artery injury during anterior cervical spine surgery. *Spine J*. 2005;5(5):508.
64. Madawi AA, Casey AT, Solanki GA, et al. Radiological and anatomical evaluation of the atlantoaxial transarticular screw fixation technique. *J Neurosurg*. 1997;86(6):961.
65. Lu J, Ebraheim NA. The vertebral artery: surgical anatomy. *Orthopedics*. 1999;22(11):1081.
66. Thomas GI, Anderson KN, Hain RF, Merendino KA. The significance of anomalous vertebral-basilar artery communications in operations on the heart and great vessels: an illustrative case with review of the literature. *Surgery*. 1959;46:747.
67. Lu J, Ebraheim NA, Yang H, Heck BE, Yeasting RA. Anatomic considerations of anterior transarticular screw fixation for atlantoaxial instability. *Spine*. 1998;23(11):1229.
68. Dickerman RD, Reynolds AS, Morgan BC, Zigler J. Vertebral artery injury. *J Neurosurg Spine*. 2007;7(1):112.
69. Harmon PH. Anterior excision and vertebral body fusion operation for intervertebral disk syndromes of the lower lumbar spine: three-to five-year results in 244 cases. *Clin Orthop Relat Res*. 1963;26:107.
70. Ebraheim NA, Lu J, Haman SP, Yeasting RA. Anatomic basis of the anterior surgery on the cervical spine: relationships between uncus-artery-root complex and vertebral artery injury. *Surg Radiol Anat*. 1998;20(6):389.
71. Ebraheim NA, Xu R, Farooq A, Yeasting RA. The quantitative anatomy of the iliac vessels and their relation to anterior lumbosacral approach. *J Spinal Disord*. 1996;9(5):414.
72. Ebraheim NA, Reader D, Xu R, Yeasting RA. Location of the vertebral artery foramen on the anterior aspect of the lower cervical spine by computed tomography. *J Spinal Disord*. 1997;10(4):304.
73. Ebraheim NA, Xu R, Yeasting RA. The location of the vertebral artery foramen and its relation to posterior lateral mass screw fixation. *Spine*. 1996;21(11):1291.
74. Sanchis-Gimeno JA, Blanco-Perez E, Larrazábal-Morón C, Mata-Escolano F. Anatomic variation of the vertebral artery. *Spine J*. 2016;16(11):e737.
75. Einstein EH, Song LH, Villela NL, et al. Anomalous origin of the left vertebral artery from the aortic arch. *Aorta (Stamford)*. 2016;4(2):64.
76. Wakita M, Takei R, Miyashita F, et al. Carotid ultrasound features of anomalous left vertebral artery originating from the aortic arch proximal to the left subclavian artery. *Neuroradiol J*. 2017;30(2):168-171.
77. Lebl DR, Bono CM, Velmahos G, et al. Vertebral artery injury associated with blunt cervical spine trauma: a multivariate regression analysis. *Spine*. 2013;38(16):1352.
78. Verbiest H. Anterolateral operations for fractures and dislocations in the middle and lower parts of the cervical spine. Report of a series of forty-seven cases. *J Bone Joint Surg Am*. 1969;51(8):1489.
79. Yin Z, Yin J, Cai J, Sui T, Cao X. Neuroanatomy and clinical analysis of the cervical sympathetic trunk and longus colli. *J Biomed Res*. 2015;29(6):501.
80. Pfeifer BA, Freidberg SR, Jewell ER. Repair of injured vertebral artery in anterior cervical procedures. *Spine*. 1994;19(13):1471.
81. Ernst E. Manipulation of the cervical spine: a systematic review of case reports of serious adverse events, 1995-2001. *Med J Aust*. 2002;176(8):376.
82. Lu J, Ebraheim NA, Georgiadis GM, Yang H, Yeasting RA. Anatomic considerations of the vertebral artery: implications for anterior decompression of the cervical spine. *J Spinal Disord*. 1998;11(3):233.
83. Landreneau RJ, Weigelt JA, Meier DE, et al. The anterior operative approach to the cervical vertebral artery. *J Am Coll Surg*. 1995;180(4):475.
84. Parbhoo AH, Govender S, Corr P. Vertebral artery injury in cervical spine trauma. *Injury*. 2001;32(7):565.
85. Ederli A, Sassaroli S, Spaccarelli G. Vertebral angiography as a cause of necrosis of the cervical spinal cord. *Br J Radiol*. 1962;35:261.
86. Chozick BS, Watson P, Greenblatt SH. Internal carotid artery thrombosis after cervical corpectomy. *Spine*. 1994;19(19):2230.
87. Gillilan LA. The arterial blood supply of the human spinal cord. *J Comp Neurol*. 1958;110(1):75.
88. Pollard ME, Little PW. Changes in carotid artery blood flow during anterior cervical spine surgery. *Spine*. 2002;27(2):152.
89. Cheung JP, Luk KD. Complications of anterior and posterior cervical spine surgery. *Asian Spine J*. 2016;10(2):385.

90. Molinari RW, Chimenti PC, Molinari R, Gruhn W. Vertebral artery injury during routine posterior cervical exposure: case reports and review of literature. *Global Spine J*. 2015;5(6):528.
91. Ye JY, Ayyash OM, Eskander MS, Kang JD. Control of the vertebral artery from a posterior approach: a technical report. *Spine J*. 2014;14(6):e37.
92. Oh CH, Ji GY, Yoon SH, et al. Delayed vertebral artery dissection after posterior cervical fusion with traumatic cervical instability: a case report. *Korean J Spine*. 2015; 12(2):79.
93. Origitano TC, al-Mefty O, Leonetti JP, DeMonte F, Reichman OH. Vascular considerations and complications in cranial base surgery. *Neurosurgery*. 1994;35(3):351.
94. An HS, Gordin R, Renner K. Anatomic considerations for plate-screw fixation of the cervical spine. *Spine*. 1991;16(10 suppl):S548.
95. Brockmeyer DL, York JE, Apfelbaum RI. Anatomical suitability of C1-2 transarticular screw placement in pediatric patients. *J Neurosurg*. 2000;92(1 suppl):7.
96. Stillerman CB, Wilson JA. Atlanto-axial stabilization with posterior transarticular screw fixation: technical description and report of 22 cases. *Neurosurgery*. 1993;32(6):948.
97. Wellman BJ, Follett KA, Traynelis VC. Complications of posterior articular mass plate fixation of the subaxial cervical spine in 43 consecutive patients. *Spine*. 1998;23(2):193.
98. Cacciola F, Phalke U, Goel A. Vertebral artery in relationship to C1-C2 vertebrae: an anatomical study. *Neurol India*. 2004;52(2):178.
99. Ebraheim NA, Xu R, Ahmad M, Heck B. The quantitative anatomy of the vertebral artery groove of the atlas and its relation to the posterior atlantoaxial approach. *Spine*. 1998;23(3):320.
100. Harms J, Melcher RP. Posterior C1-C2 fusion with polyaxial screw and rod fixation. *Spine*. 2001;26(22):2467.
101. Young JP, Young PH, Ackermann MJ, Anderson PA, Riew KD. The ponticulus posticus: implications for screw insertion into the first cervical lateral mass. *J Bone Joint Surg Am*. 2005;87(11):2495.
102. Bolger C, Wigfield C. Image-guided surgery: applications to the cervical and thoracic spine and a review of the first 120 procedures. *J Neurosurg*. 2000;92(2 suppl):175.
103. Schroeder GD, Hsu WK. Vertebral artery injuries in cervical spine surgery. *Surg Neurol Int*. 2013;4(suppl 5):S362.
104. Currier BL, Todd LT, Maus TP, Fisher DR, Yaszemski MJ. Anatomic relationship of the internal carotid artery to the C1 vertebra: a case report of cervical reconstruction for chordoma and pilot study to assess the risk of screw fixation of the atlas. *Spine*. 2003;28(22):E461.
105. Currier BL, Maus TP, Eck JC, Larson DR, Yaszemski MJ. Relationship of the internal carotid artery to the anterior aspect of the C1 vertebra: implications for C1-C2 transarticular and C1 lateral mass fixation. *Spine*. 2008;33(6):635.
106. Estillore RP, Buchowski JM, Minh do V, et al. Risk of internal carotid artery injury during C1 screw placement: analysis of 160 computed tomography angiograms. *Spine J*. 2011;11(4):316.
107. Zeidman SM, Ducker TB. Posterior cervical laminoforaminotomy for radiculopathy: review of 172 cases. *Neurosurgery*. 1993;33(3):356.
108. Bunnell WP. Anterior spinal fusion: experimental evaluation of technique. *J Pediatr Orthop*. 1982;2(5):469.
109. Crawford AH, Wall EJ, Wolf R. Video-assisted thoracoscopy. *Orthop Clin North Am*. 1999;30(3):367.
110. Dwyer AF, Schafer MF. Anterior approach to scoliosis. Results of treatment in fifty-one cases. *J Bone Joint Surg Br*. 1974;56(2):218.
111. Mack MJ, Regan JJ, Bobechko WP, Acuff TE. Application of thoracoscopy for diseases of the spine. *Ann Thorac Surg*. 1993;56(3):736.
112. Mack MJ, Regan JJ, McAfee PC, et al. Video-assisted thoracic surgery for the anterior approach to the thoracic spine. *Ann Thorac Surg*. 1995;59(5):1100.
113. Michele AA, Krueger FJ. Surgical approach to the vertebral body. *J Bone Joint Surg Am*. 1949;31A(4):873.
114. Newton PO, Shea KG, Granlund KF. Defining the pediatric spinal thoracoscopy learning curve: sixty-five consecutive cases. *Spine*. 2000;25(8):1028.
115. Picetti G, Blackman RG, O'Neal K, Luque E. Anterior endoscopic correction and fusion of scoliosis. *Orthopedics*. 1998;21(12):1285.
116. Riseborough EJ. The anterior approach to the spine for the correction of deformities of the axial skeleton. *Clin Orthop Relat Res*. 1973;(93):207.
117. Sucato DJ, Welch RD, Pierce B, et al. Thoracoscopic discectomy and fusion in an animal model: safe and effective when segmental blood vessels are spared. *Spine*. 2002;27(8):880.
118. Sweet FA, Lenke LG, Bridwell KH, Blanke KM, Whorton J. Prospective radiographic and clinical outcomes and complications of single solid rod instrumented anterior spinal fusion in adolescent idiopathic scoliosis. *Spine*. 2001;26(18):1956.
119. Winter RB, Lonstein JE, Denis F, Leonard AS, Garamella JJ. Paraplegia resulting from vessel ligation. *Spine*. 1996;21(10): 1232.
120. Hee HT, Khan MS, Goh JC, Wong HK. Insertion torque profile during pedicle screw insertion of the thoracic spine with and without violation of the pedicle wall: comparison between cylindrical and conical designs. *Spine*. 2006;31(22):E840.
121. Reddi V, Clarke DV, Arlet V. Anterior thoracoscopic instrumentation in adolescent idiopathic scoliosis: a systematic review. *Spine*. 2008;33(18):1986.
122. Higashino K, Katoh S, Sairyo K, et al. Pseudoaneurysm of the thoracoabdominal aorta caused by a severe migration of an anterior spinal device. *Spine J*. 2008;8(4):696.
123. Orchowski J, Bridwell KH, Lenke LG. Neurological deficit from a purely vascular etiology after unilateral vessel ligation during anterior thoracolumbar fusion of the spine. *Spine*. 2005;30(4):406.
124. Sucato DJ, Kassab F, Dempsey M. Analysis of screw placement relative to the aorta and spinal canal following anterior instrumentation for thoracic idiopathic scoliosis. *Spine*. 2004;29(5):554.
125. Maldonado TS, Rockman CB, Riles E, et al. Ischemic complications after endovascular abdominal aortic aneurysm repair. *J Vasc Surg*. 2004;40(4):703.
126. Sucato DJ, Duchene C. The position of the aorta relative to the spine: a comparison of patients with and without idiopathic scoliosis. *J Bone Joint Surg Am*. 2003;85-A(8): 1461.
127. Dickman CA, Rosenthal D, Karahalios DG, et al. Thoracic vertebrectomy and reconstruction using a microsurgical thoracoscopic approach. *Neurosurgery*. 1996;38(2):279.
128. Backes WH, Nijenhuis RJ. Advances in spinal cord MR angiography. *AJNR Am J Neuroradiol*. 2008;29(4):619.

129. Cambria RP, Clouse WD, Davison JK, et al. Thoracoabdominal aneurysm repair: results with 337 operations performed over a 15-year interval. *Ann Surg*. 2002;236(4):471.
130. Estrera AL, Rubenstein FS, Miller CC, et al. Descending thoracic aortic aneurysm: surgical approach and treatment using the adjuncts cerebrospinal fluid drainage and distal aortic perfusion. *Ann Thorac Surg*. 2001;72(2):481.
131. Feigelson HH, Ravin HA. Transverse myelitis following selective bronchial arteriography. *Radiology*. 1965;85(4):663.
132. Hill AB, Kalman PG, Johnston KW, Vosu HA. Reversal of delayed-onset paraplegia after thoracic aortic surgery with cerebrospinal fluid drainage. *J Vasc Surg*. 1994;20(2):315.
133. Hodgson AR, Stock FE, Fang HS, Ong GB. Anterior spinal fusion. The operative approach and pathological findings in 412 patients with Pott's disease of the spine. *Br J Surg*. 1960;48:172.
134. Takase K, Sawamura Y, Igarashi K, et al. Demonstration of the artery of Adamkiewicz at multi-detector row helical CT. *Radiology*. 2002;223(1):39.
135. Schepens MA, Defauw JJ, Hamerlijnck RP, De Geest R, Vermeulen FE. Surgical treatment of thoracoabdominal aortic aneurysms by simple crossclamping. Risk factors and late results. *J Thorac Cardiovasc Surg*. 1994;107(1):134.
136. Tarlov IM. The knee-chest position for lower spinal operations. *J Bone Joint Surg Am*. 1967;49(6):1193.
137. Mack JR. Major vascular injuries incident to intervertebral disk surgery. *Am Surg*. 1956;22(8):752.
138. Arlet V. Anterior thoracoscopic spine release in deformity surgery: a meta-analysis and review. *Eur Spine J*. 2000;9 (suppl 1):S17.
139. Huntington CF, Murrell WD, Betz RR, et al. Comparison of thoracoscopic and open thoracic discectomy in a live ovine model for anterior spinal fusion. *Spine*. 1998;23(15): 1699.
140. Caputy A, Starr J, Riedel C. Video-assisted endoscopic spinal surgery: thoracoscopic discectomy. *Acta Neurochir (Wien)*. 1995;134(3-4):196.
141. Connelly CS, Manges PA. Video-assisted thoracoscopic discectomy and fusion. *AORN J*. 1998;67(5):940.
142. MacEwen GD, Bunnell WP, Sriram K. Acute neurological complications in the treatment of scoliosis. A report of the Scoliosis Research Society. *J Bone Joint Surg Am*. 1975;57(3):404.
143. Bridwell KH, Lenke LG, Baldus C, Blanke K. Major intraoperative neurologic deficits in pediatric and adult spinal deformity patients. Incidence and etiology at one institution. *Spine*. 1998;23(3):324.
144. Majd ME, Castro FP, Holt RT. Anterior fusion for idiopathic scoliosis. *Spine*. 2000;25(6):696.
145. Lazorthes G, Gouaze A, Zadeh JO, et al. Arterial vascularization of the spinal cord. Recent studies of the anastomotic substitution pathways. *J Neurosurg*. 1971; 35(3):253.
146. Cook WA. Transthoracic vertebral surgery. *Ann Thorac Surg*. 1971;12(1):54.
147. Lowe TG, Betz R, Lenke L, et al. Anterior single-rod instrumentation of the thoracic and lumbar spine: saving levels. *Spine*. 2003;28(20):S208.
148. Di Chiro G, Fried LC, Doppman JL. Experimental spinal cord angiography. *Br J Radiol*. 1970;43(505):19.
149. Cloward RB. The treatment of ruptured lumbar intervertebral discs by vertebral body fusion. I. Indications, operative technique, after care. *J Neurosurg*. 1953;10(2):154.
150. Kawaharada N, Morishita K, Fukada J, et al. Thoracoabdominal or descending aortic aneurysm repair after preoperative demonstration of the Adamkiewicz artery by magnetic resonance angiography. *Eur J Cardiothorac Surg*. 2002;21(6):970.
151. Turnbull IM. Microvasculature of the human spinal cord. *J Neurosurg*. 1971;35(2):141.
152. Sandler AN, Tator CH. Review of the effect of spinal cord trama on the vessels and blood flow in the spinal cord. *J Neurosurg*. 1976;45(6):638.
153. Koshino T, Murakami G, Morishita K, Mawatari T, Abe T. Does the Adamkiewicz artery originate from the larger segmental arteries? *J Thorac Cardiovasc Surg*. 1999;117(5):898.
154. Cambria RP, Giglia JS. Prevention of spinal cord ischaemic complications after thoracoabdominal aortic surgery. *Eur J Vasc Endovasc Surg*. 1998;15(2):96.
155. Alpagut U, Dayioglu E. Anterior spinal artery syndrome after infrarenal abdominal aortic surgery. *J Cardiovasc Surg (Torino)*. 2002;43(6):865.
156. Hempfing A, Dreimann M, Krebs S, et al. Reduction of vertebral blood flow by segmental vessel occlusion: an intraoperative study using laser Doppler flowmetry. *Spine*. 2005;30(23):2701.
157. Kato S, Kawahara N, Tomita K, et al. Effects on spinal cord blood flow and neurologic function secondary to interruption of bilateral segmental arteries which supply the artery of Adamkiewicz: an experimental study using a dog model. *Spine*. 2008;33(14):1533.
158. Kostuik JP. Anterior Kostuik-Harrington distraction systems for the treatment of kyphotic deformities. *Spine*. 1990;15(3):169.
159. Faciszewski T, Winter RB, Lonstein JE, Denis F, Johnson L. The surgical and medical perioperative complications of anterior spinal fusion surgery in the thoracic and lumbar spine in adults. A review of 1223 procedures. *Spine*. 1995;20(14):1592.
160. Ohnishi T, Neo M, Matsushita M, et al. Delayed aortic rupture caused by an implanted anterior spinal device. Case report. *J Neurosurg*. 2001;95(2 suppl):253.
161. Faro FD, Farnsworth CL, Shapiro GS, et al. Thoracic vertebral screw impingement on the aorta in an in vivo bovine model. *Spine*. 2005;30(21):2406.
162. Chou SN, Seljeskog EL. Chapter 25. Alternative surgical approaches to the thoracic spine. *Clin Neurosurg*. 1973;20:306.
163. Kim YJ, Lenke LG, Bridwell KH, Cho YS, Riew KD. Free hand pedicle screw placement in the thoracic spine: is it safe? *Spine*. 2004;29(3):333.
164. Kim YW, Lenke LG, Kim YJ, et al. Free-hand pedicle screw placement during revision spinal surgery: analysis of 552 screws. *Spine*. 2008;33(10):1141.
165. Li G, Lv G, Passias P, et al. Complications associated with thoracic pedicle screws in spinal deformity. *Eur Spine J*. 2010;19(9):1576.
166. Suk SI, Kim WJ, Lee SM, Kim JH, Chung ER. Thoracic pedicle screw fixation in spinal deformities: are they really safe? *Spine*. 2001;26(18):2049.
167. Hicks JM, Singla A, Shen FH, Arlet V. Complications of pedicle screw fixation in scoliosis surgery: a systematic review. *Spine*. 2010;35(11):E465.
168. Vaccaro AR, Rizzolo SJ, Balderston RA, et al. Placement of pedicle screws in the thoracic spine. Part II: an anatomical and radiographic assessment. *J Bone Joint Surg Am*. 1995;77(8):1200.

169. Lenke LG, Kuklo TR, Ondra S, Polly DW. Rationale behind the current state-of-the-art treatment of scoliosis (in the pedicle screw era). *Spine*. 2008;33(10):1051.
170. Wegener B, Birkenmaier C, Fottner A, Jansson V, Dürr HR. Delayed perforation of the aorta by a thoracic pedicle screw. *Eur Spine J*. 2008;17(suppl 2):S351.
171. Sokolić J, Sosa T, Ugljen R, et al. Extrinsic erosion of the descending aorta by a vertebral fixator. *Tex Heart Inst J*. 1991;18(2):136.
172. Kakkos SK, Shepard AD. Delayed presentation of aortic injury by pedicle screws: report of two cases and review of the literature. *J Vasc Surg*. 2008;47(5):1074.
173. Choi JB, Han JO, Jeong JW. False aneurysm of the thoracic aorta associated with an aorto-chest wall fistula after spinal instrumentation. *J Trauma*. 2001;50(1):140.
174. Soultanis KC, Sakellariou VI, Starantzis KA, Papagelopoulos PJ. Late diagnosis of perforation of the aorta by a pedicle screw. *Acta Orthop Belg*. 2013;79(4):361.
175. Belmont PJ, Klemme WR, Dhawan A, Polly DW. In vivo accuracy of thoracic pedicle screws. *Spine*. 2001;26(21):2340.
176. Martín-Pedrosa JM, Gutiérrez V, González-Fajardo JA, Vaquero C. Endovascular treatment of thoracic aorta injury after spinal column surgery. *J Vasc Surg*. 2012;55(6):1782.
177. Minor ME, Morrissey NJ, Peress R, et al. Endovascular treatment of an iatrogenic thoracic aortic injury after spinal instrumentation: case report. *J Vasc Surg*. 2004;39(4):893.
178. Pesenti S, Bartoli MA, Blondel B, et al. Endovascular aortic injury repair after thoracic pedicle screw placement. *Orthop Traumatol Surg Res*. 2014;100(5):569.
179. Potter MQ, Lawrence BD, Kinikini DV, Brodke DS. Periaortic pedicle screw removal with endovascular control of the aorta and intraoperative aortography: a case report and review of the literature. *Evid Based Spine Care J*. 2013;4(2):149.
180. Tong X, Gu P, Yu D, Guo F, Lin X. An endovascular treatment of a thoracic aortic injury caused by a misplaced pedicle screw: Case report and review of the literature. *J Formos Med Assoc*. 2015;114(5):464.
181. Decker S, Omar M, Krettek C, Müller CW. Elective thoracotomy for pedicle screw removal to prevent severe aortic bleeding. *World J Clin Cases*. 2014;2(4):100.
182. Carmignani A, Lentini S, Acri E, et al. Combined thoracic endovascular aortic repair and neurosurgical intervention for injury due to posterior spine surgery. *J Card Surg*. 2013;28(2):163.
183. Colvard BD, Anaya-Ayala JE, Smolock CJ, et al. Hybrid approach for removal of an errant intra-vascular pedicle spinal fixation screw in the thoracic aorta. *J Vasc Surg*. 2012;56(1):201.
184. Deswysen Y, Labeau J, Kaminski L, Astarci P. Unusual management of thoracic aortic injury after spinal instrumentation: just glue it! *Aorta (Stamford)*. 2016;4(3):95.
185. Baniel J, Foster RS, Donohue JP. Surgical anatomy of the lumbar vessels: implications for retroperitoneal surgery. *J Urol*. 1995;153(5):1422.
186. Kozak JA, Heilman AE, O'Brien JP. Anterior lumbar fusion options. Technique and graft materials. *Clin Orthop Relat Res*. 1994;(300):45.
187. Lane JD, Moore ES. Transperitoneal approach to the intervertebral disc in the lumbar area. *Ann Surg*. 1948;127(3):537.
188. Dewald CJ, Millikan KW, Hammerberg KW, Doolas A, Dewald RL. An open, minimally invasive approach to the lumbar spine. *Am Surg*. 1999;65(1):61.
189. Capellades J, Pellisé F, Rovira A, et al. Magnetic resonance anatomic study of iliocava junction and left iliac vein positions related to L5-S1 disc. *Spine*. 2000;25(13):1695.
190. Parke WW, Whalen JL, Van Demark RE, Kambin P. The infra-aortic arteries of the spine: their variability and clinical significance. *Spine*. 1994;19(1):1.
191. Villano M, Cantatore G, Narciso N, et al. Vascular injury related to lumbar disk surgery. *Neurochirurgia (Stuttg)*. 1992; 35(2):57.
192. Watkins R. Anterior lumbar interbody fusion surgical complications. *Clin Orthop Relat Res*. 1992;(284):47.
193. Inoue S, Watanabe T, Hirose A, et al. Anterior discectomy and interbody fusion for lumbar disc herniation. A review of 350 cases. *Clin Orthop Relat Res*. 1984;(183):22.
194. Kleeman TJ, Michael Ahn U, Clutterbuck WB, Campbell CJ, Talbot-Kleeman A. Laparoscopic anterior lumbar interbody fusion at L4-L5: an anatomic evaluation and approach classification. *Spine*. 2002;27(13):1390.
195. Phillips WA, Hensinger RN. Control of blood loss during scoliosis surgery. *Clin Orthop Relat Res*. 1988;(229):88.
196. Crock HV. Anterior lumbar interbody fusion: indications for its use and notes on surgical technique. *Clin Orthop Relat Res*. 1982;(165):157.
197. Heim SE, Altimari A. Laparoscopic approaches to fusion of the lumbosacral spine: latest techniques. *Orthop Clin North Am*. 2002;33(2):413.
198. Heniford BT, Matthews BD, Lieberman IH. Laparoscopic lumbar interbody spinal fusion. *Surg Clin North Am*. 2000; 80(5):1487.
199. Regan JJ, Aronoff RJ, Ohnmeiss DD, Sengupta DK. Laparoscopic approach to L4-L5 for interbody fusion using BAK cages: experience in the first 58 cases. *Spine*. 1999;24(20):2171.
200. Sacks S. Anterior interbody fusion of the lumbar spine. Indications and results in 200 cases. *Clin Orthop Relat Res*. 1966;44:163.
201. Vraney RT, Phillips FM, Wetzel FT, Brustein M. Peridiscal vascular anatomy of the lower lumbar spine. An endoscopic perspective. *Spine*. 1999;24(21):2183.
202. Brau SA. Mini-open approach to the spine for anterior lumbar interbody fusion: description of the procedure, results and complications. *Spine J*. 2002;2(3):216.
203. Lieberman IH, Willsher PC, Litwin DE, Salo PT, Kraetschmer BG. Transperitoneal laparoscopic exposure for lumbar interbody fusion. *Spine*. 2000;25(4):509.
204. Freeman BJ, Davenport J. Total disc replacement in the lumbar spine: a systematic review of the literature. *Eur Spine J*. 2006;15(suppl 3):S439.
205. Reid JD, Weigelt JA. Forty-three cases of vertebral artery trauma. *J Trauma*. 1988;28(7):1007.
206. Cloward RB. Spondylolisthesis: treatment by laminectomy and posterior interbody fusion. *Clin Orthop Relat Res*. 1981;(154):74.
207. Collis JS. Total disc replacement: a modified posterior lumbar interbody fusion. Report of 750 cases. *Clin Orthop Relat Res*. 1985;(193):64.
208. Freebody D, Bendall R, Taylor RD. Anterior transperitoneal lumbar fusion. *J Bone Joint Surg Br*. 1971;53(4):617.
209. Sacks S. Anterior interbody fusion of the lumbar spine. *J Bone Joint Surg Br*. 1965;47:211.
210. Southerland SR, Remedios AM, McKerrell JG, Litwin D. Laparoscopic approaches to the lumbar vertebrae. An anatomic study using a porcine model. *Spine*. 1995;20(14):1620.

211. Brau SA, Delamarter RB, Kropf MA, et al. Access strategies for revision in anterior lumbar surgery. *Spine*. 2008;33(15):1662.
212. Smoljanovic T, Bojanic I, Rakovac M. Re: Sasso RC, Burkus JK, LeHuec JC. Retrograde ejaculation after anterior lumbar interbody fusion: transperitoneal versus retroperitoneal exposure. Spine (Phila Pa 1976) 2003;28:1023-6. *Spine*. 2010;35(14):E623.
213. Whitesides TE, Kelly RP. Lateral approach to the upper cervical spine for anterior fusion. *South Med J*. 1966;59(8):879.
214. Kratimenos GP, Crockard HA. The far lateral approach for ventrally placed foramen magnum and upper cervical spine tumours. *Br J Neurosurg*. 1993;7(2):129.
215. Di Fabio RP. Manipulation of the cervical spine: risks and benefits. *Phys Ther*. 1999;79(1):50.
216. Harmon PH. A simplified surgical technic for anterior lumbar diskectomy and fusion; avoidance of complications; anatomy of the retroperitoneal veins. *Clin Orthop Relat Res*. 1964;37:130.
217. Nguyen HV, Akbarnia BA, van Dam BE, et al. Anterior exposure of the spine for removal of lumbar interbody devices and implants. *Spine*. 2006;31(21):2449.
218. Maeng DH, Kim SY, Lee SH, Jang JS. Venovertebral vein: morphometric analysis and significance for the transabdominal spine surgeon. *J Spinal Disord Tech*. 2007;20(8):582.
219. Fantini GA, Pappou IP, Girardi FP, Sandhu HS, Cammisa FP. Major vascular injury during anterior lumbar spinal surgery: incidence, risk factors, and management. *Spine*. 2007;32(24):2751.
220. Jeon SH, Lee SH, Choi WC. Iliac artery perforation following lumbar discectomy with microsurgical carbon dioxide laser: a report of a rare case and discussion on the treatment. *Spine*. 2007;32(3):E124.
221. Barbaric ZL, Wegenius GA, Anderson GM. MR imaging: vascular anatomy of the abdomen. *Radiographics*. 1989;9(1):69.
222. Datta JC, Janssen ME, Beckham R, Ponce C. The use of computed tomography angiography to define the prevertebral vascular anatomy prior to anterior lumbar procedures. *Spine*. 2007;32(1):113.
223. Schwender JD, Casnellie MT, Perra JH, et al. Perioperative complications in revision anterior lumbar spine surgery: incidence and risk factors. *Spine*. 2009;34(1):87.
224. Bianchi C, Ballard JL, Abou-Zamzam AM, Teruya TH, Abu-Assal ML. Anterior retroperitoneal lumbosacral spine exposure: operative technique and results. *Ann Vasc Surg*. 2003;17(2):137.
225. Dula DJ, Fierro R, Gessner H, Snover WS. Vascular injury following disc surgery. *Am J Emerg Med*. 1986;4(5):406.
226. Bingol H, Cingoz F, Yilmaz AT, Yasar M, Tatar H. Vascular complications related to lumbar disc surgery. *J Neurosurg*. 2004;100(3 Suppl Spine):249.
227. Mayer HM. A new microsurgical technique for minimally invasive anterior lumbar interbody fusion. *Spine*. 1997;22(6):691.
228. Zdeblick TA, David SM. A prospective comparison of surgical approach for anterior L4-L5 fusion: laparoscopic versus mini anterior lumbar interbody fusion. *Spine*. 2000;25(20):2682.
229. Raptis S, Quigley F, Barker S. Vascular complications of elective lower lumbar disc surgery. *Aust N Z J Surg*. 1994;64(3):216.
230. Szolar DH, Preidler KW, Steiner H, et al. Vascular complications in lumbar disk surgery: report of four cases. *Neuroradiology*. 1996;38(6):521.
231. Sağdiç K, Ozer ZG, Senkaya I, Türe M. Vascular injury during lumbar disc surgery. Report of two cases; a review of the literature. *Vasa*. 1996;25(4):378.
232. Khazim R, Boos N, Webb JK. Progressive thrombotic occlusion of the left common iliac artery after anterior lumbar interbody fusion. *Eur Spine J*. 1998;7(3):239.
233. Kulkarni SS, Lowery GL, Ross RE, Ravi Sankar K, Lykomitros V. Arterial complications following anterior lumbar interbody fusion: report of eight cases. *Eur Spine J*. 2003;12(1):48.
234. Kossmann T, Jacobi D, Trentz O. The use of a retractor system (SynFrame) for open, minimal invasive reconstruction of the anterior column of the thoracic and lumbar spine. *Eur Spine J*. 2001;10(5):396.
235. Hackenberg L, Liljenqvist U, Halm H, Winkelmann W. Occlusion of the left common iliac artery and consecutive thromboembolism of the left popliteal artery following anterior lumbar interbody fusion. *J Spinal Disord*. 2001;14(4):365.
236. Hannibal M, Thomas DJ, Low J, Hsu KY, Zucherman J. ProDisc-L total disc replacement: a comparison of 1-level versus 2-level arthroplasty patients with a minimum 2-year follow-up. *Spine*. 2007;32(21):2322.
237. David T. Revision of a Charité artificial disc 9.5 years in vivo to a new Charité artificial disc: case report and explant analysis. *Eur Spine J*. 2005;14(5):507.
238. Marsicano J, Mirovsky Y, Remer S, Bloom N, Neuwirth M. Thrombotic occlusion of the left common iliac artery after an anterior retroperitoneal approach to the lumbar spine. *Spine*. 1994;19(3):357.
239. Eltzschig HK, Collard CD. Vascular ischaemia and reperfusion injury. *Br Med Bull*. 2004;70:71.
240. Biafora SJ, Mardjetko SM, Butler JP, McCarthy PL, Gleason TF. Arterial injury following percutaneous vertebral augmentation: a case report. *Spine*. 2006;31(3):E84.
241. Tsai YD, Yu PC, Lee TC, et al. Superior rectal artery injury following lumbar disc surgery. Case report. *J Neurosurg*. 2001;95(1 suppl):108.
242. Prothero SR, Parkes JC, Stinchfield FE. Complications after low-back fusion in 1000 patients. A comparison of two series one decade apart. 1966. *Clin Orthop Relat Res*. 1994;(306):5.
243. Lindblom K. Intervertebral-disc degeneration considered as a pressure atrophy. *J Bone Joint Surg Am*. 1957;39-A(4):933.
244. Birkeland IW, Taylor TK. Bowel injuries coincident to lumbar disk surgery: a report of four cases and a review of the literature. *J Trauma*. 1970;10(2):163.
245. Solonen KA. Perforation of the anterior annulus fibrosus during operation for prolapsed disc. *Ann Chir Gynaecol Fenn*. 1975;64(6):385.
246. Birkeland IW, Taylor TK. Major vascular injuries in lumbar disc surgery. *J Bone Joint Surg Br*. 1969;51(1):4.
247. Brewster DC, May AR, Darling RC, Abbott WM, Moncure AC. Variable manifestations of vascular injury during lumbar disk surgery. *Arch Surg*. 1979;114(9):1026.
248. Ezra E, Richenberg JL, Smellie WA. Major vascular injury during lumbar laminectomy. *J R Soc Med*. 1996;89(2):108P.
249. Franzini M, Altana P, Annessi V, Lodini V. Iatrogenic vascular injuries following lumbar disc surgery. Case report and review of the literature. *J Cardiovasc Surg (Torino)*. 1987;28(6):727.
250. Gower DJ, Culp P, Ball M. Lateral lumbar spine roentgenograms: potential role in complications of lumbar disc surgery. *Surg Neurol*. 1987;27(4):316.

251. Jarstfer BS, Rich NM. The challenge of arteriovenous fistula formation following disk surgery: a collective review. *J Trauma*. 1976;16(9):726.
252. Lee KH, Park JH, Chung JW, et al. Vascular complications in lumbar spinal surgery: percutaneous endovascular treatment. *Cardiovasc Intervent Radiol*. 2000;23(1):65.
253. Moore CA, Cohen A. Combined arterial, venous, and ureteral injury complicating lumbar disk surgery. *Am J Surg*. 1968;115(4):574.
254. Salander JM, Youkey JR, Rich NM, Olson DW, Clagett GP. Vascular injury related to lumbar disk surgery. *J Trauma*. 1984;24(7):628.
255. Seeley SF, Hughes CW, Jahnke EJ. Major vessel damage in lumbar disc operation. *Surgery*. 1954;35(3):421.
256. Desaussure RL. Vascular injury coincident to disc surgery. *J Neurosurg*. 1959;16(2):222.
257. Shevlin WA, Luessenhop AJ, Fox JL, McCullough DC. Perforation of the anterior annulus during lumbar discectomy. Case report. *J Neurosurg*. 1973;38(4):514.
258. An HS, Vaccaro A, Simeone FA, Balderston RA, O'Neill D. Herniated lumbar disc in patients over the age of fifty. *J Spinal Disord*. 1990;3(2):143.
259. Albert TJ, Balderston RA, Heller JG, et al. Upper lumbar disc herniations. *J Spinal Disord*. 1993;6(4):351.
260. Fraser RD. A wide muscle-splitting approach to the lumbosacral spine. *J Bone Joint Surg Br*. 1982;64(1):44.
261. Boström S, Holmgren E, Jonsson O, et al. Post-operative thromboembolism in neurosurgery. A study on the prophylactic effect of calf muscle stimulation plus dextran compared to low-dose heparin. *Acta Neurochir (Wien)*. 1986;80(3-4):83.
262. Ferree BA, Wright AM. Deep venous thrombosis following posterior lumbar spinal surgery. *Spine*. 1993;18(8):1079.
263. Oda T, Fuji T, Kato Y, Fujita S, Kanemitsu N. Deep venous thrombosis after posterior spinal surgery. *Spine*. 2000;25(22):2962.
264. West JL, Anderson LD. Incidence of deep vein thrombosis in major adult spinal surgery. *Spine*. 1992;17(8 suppl):S254.
265. Isley MR, Zhang XF, Smith RC, Cohen MJ. Intraoperative neuromonitoring detects thrombotic occlusion of the left common iliac arterial bifurcation after anterior lumbar interbody fusion: case report. *J Spinal Disord Tech*. 2007;20(1):104.
266. Glotzbecker MP, Bono CM, Harris MB, et al. Surgeon practices regarding postoperative thromboembolic prophylaxis after high-risk spinal surgery. *Spine*. 2008; 33(26):2915.
267. Lee HM, Suk KS, Moon SH, et al. Deep vein thrombosis after major spinal surgery: incidence in an East Asian population. *Spine*. 2000;25(14):1827.
268. Rokito SE, Schwartz MC, Neuwirth MG. Deep vein thrombosis after major reconstructive spinal surgery. *Spine*. 1996;21(7):853.
269. Brambilla S, Ruosi C, La Maida GA, Caserta S. Prevention of venous thromboembolism in spinal surgery. *Eur Spine J*. 2004;13(1):1.
270. Niemeyer T, Freeman BJ, Grevitt MP, Webb JK. Anterior thoracoscopic surgery followed by posterior instrumentation and fusion in spinal deformity. *Eur Spine J*. 2000;9(6):499.
271. Rajaraman V, Vingan R, Roth P, et al. Visceral and vascular complications resulting from anterior lumbar interbody fusion. *J Neurosurg*. 1999;91(1 suppl):60.
272. Cain JE, Major MR, Lauerman WC, et al. The morbidity of heparin therapy after development of pulmonary embolus in patients undergoing thoracolumbar or lumbar spinal fusion. *Spine*. 1995;20(14):1600.
273. Shaieb MD, Watson BN, Atkinson RE. Bleeding complications with enoxaparin for deep venous thrombosis prophylaxis. *J Arthroplasty*. 1999;14(4):432.
274. Cheng JS, Arnold PM, Anderson PA, Fischer D, Dettori JR. Anticoagulation risk in spine surgery. *Spine*. 2010;35(9 suppl):S117.
275. Armstrong RF, Addy V, Breivik H. Epidural and spinal anaesthesia and the use of anticoagulants. *Hosp Med*. 1999;60(7):491.
276. Levy JH, Faraoni D, Spring JL, Douketis JD, Samama CM. Managing new oral anticoagulants in the perioperative and intensive care unit setting. *Anesthesiology*. 2013;118(6): 1466.
277. Wong YW, Luk KD. Spinal epidural hematoma in a scoliotic patient with long fusion: a case report. *Spine J*. 2008;8(3):538.
278. Spanier DE, Stambough JL. Delayed postoperative epidural hematoma formation after heparinization in lumbar spinal surgery. *J Spinal Disord*. 2000;13(1):46.
279. Heppner PA, Monteith SJ, Law AJ. Spontaneous spinal hematomas and low-molecular-weight heparin. Report of four cases and review of the literature. *J Neurosurg Spine*. 2004;1(2):232.
280. Leon L, Rodriguez H, Tawk RG, et al. The prophylactic use of inferior vena cava filters in patients undergoing high-risk spinal surgery. *Ann Vasc Surg*. 2005;19(3):442.
281. Epstein NE. Intermittent pneumatic compression stocking prophylaxis against deep venous thrombosis in anterior cervical spinal surgery: a prospective efficacy study in 200 patients and literature review. *Spine*. 2005;30(22):2538.
282. Dearborn JT, Hu SS, Tribus CB, Bradford DS. Thromboembolic complications after major thoracolumbar spine surgery. *Spine*. 1999;24(14):1471.
283. Rosner MK, Kuklo TR, Tawk R, Moquin R, Ondra SL. Prophylactic placement of an inferior vena cava filter in high-risk patients undergoing spinal reconstruction. *Neurosurg Focus*. 2004;17(4):E6.
284. Kou J, Fischgrund J, Biddinger A, Herkowitz H. Risk factors for spinal epidural hematoma after spinal surgery. *Spine*. 2002;27(15):1670.
285. Morales Ciancio RA, Drain O, Rillardon L, Guigui P. Acute spontaneous spinal epidural hematoma: an important differential diagnosis in patients under clopidogrel therapy. *Spine J*. 2008;8(3):544.
286. Hauck EF, Nauta HJ. Spontaneous spinal epidural arteriovenous fistulae in neurofibromatosis type-1. *Surg Neurol*. 2006;66(2):215.
287. Matsumura A, Namikawa T, Hashimoto R, et al. Clinical management for spontaneous spinal epidural hematoma: diagnosis and treatment. *Spine J*. 2008;8(3):534.
288. Sasso RC, Smucker JD, Hacker RJ, Heller JG. Artificial disc versus fusion: a prospective, randomized study with 2-year follow-up on 99 patients. *Spine*. 2007;32(26):2933.
289. Dorsay TA, Helms CA. MR imaging of epidural hematoma in the lumbar spine. *Skeletal Radiol*. 2002;31(12):677.
290. Tsirikos AI, Jeans LA. Superior mesenteric artery syndrome in children and adolescents with spine deformities undergoing corrective surgery. *J Spinal Disord Tech*. 2005;18(3):263.
291. Bognár G, Ledniczky G, Palik E, et al. [Wilkie's syndrome]. *Magy Seb*. 2008;61(5):273.

292. Crowther MA, Webb PJ, Eyre-Brook IA. Superior mesenteric artery syndrome following surgery for scoliosis. *Spine*. 2002;27(24):E528.
293. Sprague J. Cast syndrome: the superior mesenteric artery syndrome. *Orthop Nurs*. 1998;17(4):12.
294. Altiok H, Lubicky JP, DeWald CJ, Herman JE. The superior mesenteric artery syndrome in patients with spinal deformity. *Spine*. 2005;30(19):2164.
295. Smith BG, Hakim-Zargar M, Thomson JD. Low body mass index: a risk factor for superior mesenteric artery syndrome in adolescents undergoing spinal fusion for scoliosis. *J Spinal Disord Tech*. 2009;22(2):144.
296. Derincek A, Wood KB, Muench CA. Superior mesenteric artery syndrome following correction of kyphosis in an adult. *J Spinal Disord Tech*. 2004;17(6):549.
297. Ahmed AR, Taylor I. Superior mesenteric artery syndrome. *Postgrad Med J*. 1997;73(866):776.
298. Munns SW, Morrissy RT, Golladay ES, McKenzie CN. Hyperalimentation for superior mesenteric-artery (cast) syndrome following correction of spinal deformity. *J Bone Joint Surg Am*. 1984;66(8):1175.
299. Stambough JL, Cheeks ML. Central retinal artery occlusion: a complication of the knee-chest position. *J Spinal Disord*. 1992;5(3):363.
300. Stevens WR, Glazer PA, Kelley SD, Lietman TM, Bradford DS. Ophthalmic complications after spinal surgery. *Spine*. 1997;22(12):1319.
301. Stauffer RN, Coventry MB. Anterior interbody lumbar spine fusion. Analysis of Mayo Clinic series. *J Bone Joint Surg Am*. 1972;54(4):756.
302. Graham JJ. Complications of cervical spine surgery. A five-year report on a survey of the membership of the Cervical Spine Research Society by the Morbidity and Mortality Committee. *Spine*. 1989;14(10):1046.
303. Moe JH. Complications of scoliosis treatment. *Clin Orthop Relat Res*. 1967;53:21.
304. Neo M, Matsushita M, Morita T, Nakamura T. Pseudoaneurysm of the deep circumflex iliac artery: a rare complication at an anterior iliac bone graft donor site. *Spine*. 2000;25(14):1848.
305. Lim EV, Lavadia WT, Roberts JM. Superior gluteal artery injury during iliac bone grafting for spinal fusion. A case report and literature review. *Spine*. 1996;21(20):2376.

98 CHAPTER Instrumentation Complications

Eeric Truumees

Introduction

The evolution of spinal instrumentation from simple wiring, to segmental, rigid fixation, to motion-preservation and dynamic implants has been powered by an improved understanding of spinal disease and its impact on the biomechanics of the spine. Coincident with that understanding have been improvements in metallurgy, perioperative spinal imaging, and a wealth of clinical outcomes data. Technical advances have also improved surgeons' ability to place implants in a safer and less morbid manner. These advances include imaging modalities from fluoroscopy to navigation to intraoperative axial imaging. Neurologic monitoring and tubular and minimally invasive retractor systems have also affected the incidence of soft tissue complications after spinal implant surgery. Overall, these advances affect the types of problems that can be addressed, procedural morbidity and the potential for medical complications, postoperative bracing or activity restrictions, and duration of muscle and overall surgical recovery.

These new implant categories offer a host of potential benefits to the patient. However, in some cases, our reach for more powerful spinal stabilization has exceeded our grasp and subjected our patients to a host of often unforeseen complications. More frequently, though, the plethora of treatment options has challenged surgeons' in-depth understanding of the specific goals for which the implant was designed. Simply put, even perfect placement of the wrong device will not afford the patient the optimal chance at recovery. Additionally, new tools have allowed us to treat conditions or patient populations previously considered unsuitable for surgery. The combination of higher-risk conditions, older and sicker patients, and a logarithmic increase in the number of implants placed ensures that implant-related complications remain an important topic for spine surgeons and learners.

This chapter highlights changing our evolving understanding of means to prevent and address these complications. For example, previous generations of spine surgeons were taught that "exposure is key." When difficulties in implant placement were encountered, increased dissection to improve access to and visualization of the surgical field was the most immediate means to reduce the risk of misplacement. While proper exposure and knowledge of spinal anatomy remain key features of a successful surgery, new tools have allowed safe implantation with a more limited exposure using image guidance. Additionally, the surgeon is assumed to have a general understanding of human spinal anatomy; however, optimal implant strategies increasingly require a detailed preoperative assessment of the specific patient's anatomy as gleaned from planar and axial imaging and often incorporating several modalities (e.g., radiographs and magnetic resonance imaging [MRI] or computed tomographic [CT] myelography and angiography). Another evolving critical concept in complication avoidance lies in suitable selection of the operative candidate, followed by preoperative optimization of that patient. Weight loss, smoking cessation, blood sugar control, and osteoporosis management are far more effective means of reducing global complication rates than any single change in intraoperative technique or modality.

Definitions and Classification

Complication can be a loaded term. It has different technical and emotional import for the patient, the surgeon, the medical board, the legal community, and other stakeholders.[1] While a number of definitions are readily available, most are inadequate, from a technical perspective, to demarcate issues along a spectrum from normal sequelae of the procedure to criminal negligence.

For example, some issues, while unfortunate, are a necessary correlate to the implant itself. These include soft tissue dissection and displacement. Even here, however, surgical morbidity may be affected by patient vulnerability, surgical technique, and implant bulk and placement. Most spinal implants span motion segments decreasing overall motion and increasing the loading on adjacent segments. However, proper surgical decision making may minimize the number of fusion levels. Intraoperative technical factors may affect the impact on adjacent segments (e.g., placement of the implant too near the adjacent disc space anteriorly or violation of the superior facet joint posteriorly by a pedicle screw). Interestingly, however, postoperative complaints of stiffness are not common in patients undergoing surgery for degenerative or deformity conditions.[2] In fact, in patients undergoing single-level fusion for degenerative disease, most reported less stiffness postoperatively.

In the pediatric population, spanning a motion segment may impact subsequent growth. In the context of congenital and early-onset deformity correction, arthrodesis and implant placement may impact later growth, including the crankshaft phenomenon, uneven growth of the trunk, and especially restrictive lung disease from inadequate thoracic growth.[3] Recently, increased attention has been focused on growing rods and VEPTR (Vertical Expandable Prosthetic Titanium Rib; DePuy Synthes). One recent study found that addition of a cross-link did not affect spinal canal area.[4] Another recent study found acceptable cervical alignment and growth within the fused areas in 40 children undergoing rigid atlantoaxial or occipitocervical fusion.[5]

Some issues are not ubiquitous but are extremely common and difficult to avoid, such as occipital numbness after placement of C1 lateral mass screws. Many are less frequent occurrences over which the treating physician may have limited control. A common example here is deep vein thrombosis after implant-related spine surgery in general, but also more specifically after placement of anterior lumbar cages or disc replacements. Careful exposure and handling of the iliac veins reduces, but does not eliminate, this risk. Wound infections and pseudarthrosis also fall into this category.

No spine surgeon likely has a 100% accuracy rate with transpedicular fixation in the lumbar spine. At some point, however, the "miss rate" exceeds an acceptable level. That level has changed as newer technologies, such as intraoperative navigation, have become available to assist the surgeon in difficult cases with limited landmarks. What is "acceptable" also varies by venue. In a medicolegal setting, a community standard is often used. But do we really have good data about these miss rates in a community setting?

Technical misadventures may also occur with inadvertent injury to the surrounding neurologic or vascular structures during implant placement. Some issues exceed even the term "complication." Major failures in surgical planning or technique, operating outside the scope of one's training, recommending surgeries for financial gain when little patient benefit can be expected, and an absence of informed consent may all reach the level of assault. Certainly, attorneys have been using pathways other than malpractice claims at an increasing rate.

To avoid this type of conflation, Sokol and Wilson describe a four part definition of "surgical complication"[1]:

1. A surgical complication is any undesirable and unexpected result of an operation. A scar need not be a complication. This will depend on whether it was expected. Our revised definition, however, does not specify the subject of the unpleasant result; hence a surgeon's needlestick injury would constitute a surgical complication. The solution is to specify the recipient of the surgical complication.
2. A surgical complication is any undesirable and unexpected result of an operation affecting the patient.
3. A surgical complication is any undesirable and unexpected result of an operation affecting the patient that occurs as a direct result of the operation.
4. A surgical complication is any undesirable, unintended, and direct result of an operation affecting the patient that would not have occurred had the operation gone as well as could reasonably be hoped.

Most spinal implant-related complications arise from failures in biology or biomechanics or from errors in surgical strategy or technique. Often, the most severe complications arise from a combination of these issues. Some complications require a failure in more than one area. In others, a deficit in one area can increase the risk of a complication in another.

Ultimately, implant failure rates are tied to the patient's underlying diagnosis. In one series of 289 patients treated for spinal metastatic disease, a 10.7% reoperation rate was reported. Of these, instrumentation failure accounted for 26%.[6] Another recent study found that durotomy was associated with a 2.2 times higher risk for pseudarthrosis.[7]

Implant-related complications vary with different patient demographics, including osteoporosis, spinal deformity, and previous surgery. Fujimori and others compared the safety and complication rates of pedicle screw placement between patients in three age-based cohorts: 0 to 5 years, 5 to 10 years, and 10 to 15 years of age.[8] In total, 5054 screws were placed, although far more were placed in the older age group (4219) than in the two younger cohorts. Although there were no neurologic complications associated with screw placement in this study, the overall complication rate ranged from 0.1% to 0.6% per screw, with the rates increasing as patient age decreased. Here, too, risk factors may span several of the groups in the failure taxonomy above. For example, osteoporosis or other bone quality issues, which are increasingly common in the aging population, confer risks across the spectrum from the biology of bone healing to the mechanics of spine fixation to technical issues encountered intraoperatively (poor bone quality limits tactile feedback and challenges intraoperative imaging, thereby increasing the risk of implant misplacement).

Biologic Failure

Biologic failure implies a disruption in the physiologic processes associated with healing from surgery. This disruption affects the ultimate success of the procedure and subjects the patient to possible revision surgeries or abject surgical failure. Common biologic issues complicating spinal implant surgeries include infection and other inflammatory issues, osteoporosis, and vascular issues. These issues may, singly or in combination, increase the risk of several adverse outcomes, including pseudarthrosis, implant loosening, bone failure and fracture, and adjacent-segment problems. These biologic risk factors are often driven by the individual patient's medical history. However, choices in spinal implants also have an effect on some of these phenomena (Fig. 98.1).

Infection and Inflammatory Conditions

In terms of direct impact, all surgeries expose the patient to the risk of infection. Surgeons typically are most concerned

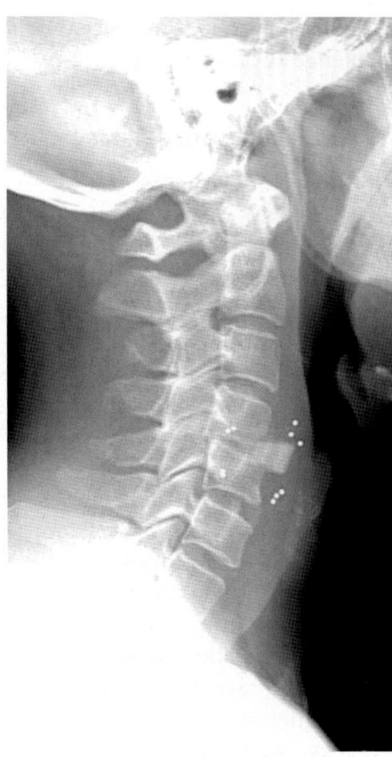

FIG. 98.1 Lateral cervical spine radiograph demonstrating anterior allograft bone displacement after fracture of resorbable anterior cervical plate with segmental collapse.

with wound infections and their sequelae, but urinary tract, pulmonary, and gastrointestinal (e.g., *Clostridium difficile* colitis) complications are also worrisome. The placement of foreign material into the patient's body has been shown to increase both the immediate postoperative infection rate and the risk of late, hematogenous implant seeding.[9]

Because spine surgeries incorporating implant placement are larger operations, it stands to reason that the incidence of infection and medical morbidity issues would be increased.[10,11] Certainly, the location of an infection has major consequences in terms of surgical accessibility and the risks of revision surgery. For example, abscess formation around anterior thoracolumbar implants may incorporate the major vessels.[12]

Infections may have an indirect impact on patient outcomes in that wound infections may lead to arachnoiditis, pseudarthrosis, correction loss, spondylodiscitis, adverse neurologic sequelae, and even death.[9]

Increasingly, the spine surgeon's implant selection may have an impact on the risk of infection. Bacterial adherence to spine implants (and even allograft bone) may generate biofilms that limit the ability of antibiotics or even open debridement procedures to eradicate the infection. The risk of bacterial adherence may vary depending on the implant material. Steel may carry higher risk than titanium for bacterial adhesion.[13] Titanium metal debris, in particular, excites an inflammatory reaction that either mimics or invites an infection.[14,15]

Loose or motion-preserving implants may exhibit fretting with wear debris or metal ion release. Metal-on-metal (MOM) bearing surfaces have recently received a great deal of attention. MOM total hip systems have been removed from the market due to metal debris–related osteolysis and implant loosening. MOM cervical and lumbar disc systems have been under investigation, but those systems have not progressed to market in the United States and are not marketed aggressively abroad.

Fusion systems may also lead to metal ion release, particularly when loose. One recent report found that in adolescent idiopathic scoliosis (AIS), increased serum metal ion levels were found immediately after surgery as part of the "putting in" rather than "wearing in" phase. The authors recommended thorough irrigation of the operative site prior to wound closure.[16] The same group reported that the surface area of the implants was directly related to postoperative serum levels of titanium and niobium in a series of 33 children.[17]

Serum ion levels may help identify radiographically subtle pseudarthrosis or other issues. For example, in long-term follow-up of AIS patients who underwent fusion with stainless steel implants, a serum chromium level above 0.6 ng/mL indicated a high risk of implant failure.[18] Use of positron emission tomography (PET)/CT has been reported to be effective in identifying postoperative infection in patients after instrumented spine procedures.[19,20] Newer generations of implants have sought to reduce this risk with changes in surface topography, eluting antibiotics, and even direct sintering of antibiotic molecules to the implant surface.

A common controversy relates to the retention or removal of spine implants in patients with wound infections. The presence of a biofilm on the implant may challenge the host's immune system and antibiotics to eradicate the infection while the implant remains in place. On the other hand, some authors suggest that mechanical stability is even more important as a predictor of ultimate healing.

In one recent study, a 51-patient cohort that had undergone posterolateral instrumented fusion complicated by wound infection was reported.[9] A total of 92.2% had at least one other medical problem. As with previous reports, the "most common infective culprit was *Staphylococcus* spp. found in 35 of 60 (58.3%) isolates, including 20 methicillin-resistant species. Gram-negative bacilli and polymicrobial infection were found significantly in patients presenting early-onset, deep-site infection and myonecrosis."[9] The infection was eradicated while preserving the implants in 41 of 51 cases (80.4%). The authors attributed this success to an early, aggressive approach.

The implants were removed in 10 cases (19.6%). This removal was attributed to delayed treatment and uncontrolled infection with implant loosening, correction loss, or late infection with spondylodesis. Delayed treatment, in this context, was typically more than 3 months. The authors did not correlate the number of debridement procedures with implant preservation. Poor outcomes were also reported in patients with significant comorbidities, malnutrition, severe trauma, neurologic deficits, and long-level instrumentation. Nearly one-third of the infected patients progressed to pseudarthrosis. Half of these patients were symptomatic and underwent successful revision surgery.

The authors concluded, in concert with most common recommendations, that retention of mechanically sound implants in early-onset infection permits fusion to occur, whereas delayed treatment, severe malnutrition, and multiple comorbidities will most likely result in a lack of effectiveness in eradicating the infecting pathogens.[9] Loose screws, on the other hand, can cause peridiscal erosion and incapacitating motion pain.

In another study of 817 consecutive patients undergoing instrumented lumbar fusion for degenerative disease, 37 (4.5%) developed postoperative infections at a median of 0.6 months.[21] Older age, diabetes, obesity, prior spine surgery, and length of hospital stay were each independently associated with an increased risk of developing infection. Only 3 (8%) required implant removal. Hikata and colleagues found that patients with high hemoglobin A1c levels had a 16.7% rate of postoperative infection compared to a 3.2% rate in patients without diabetes mellitus.[22] The authors recommended preoperative glucose control to reduce hemoglobin A1c to less than 7.0% before elective instrumented spine surgery. Proper nutritional support will also aid healing.[23]

The decision to place metallic implants during an initial debridement for osteomyelitis has also been controversial. A number of studies have suggested elevated but acceptable levels of postoperative surgical site infection or recurrent infection.[24-26] One recent study reported single-stage, single-level transforaminal interbody fusion for lumbar disciitis-osteomyelitis in 28 patients.[27] Good corrections of preoperative kyphosis and an 82.1% fusion rate were reported. Two recurrent infections were discovered, both in the first 2 months.

Bydon and colleagues compared the reoperation rate in 118 patients who underwent decompression alone versus decompression and instrumentation placement.[28] The reoperation rates (19.44% and 17.07%, respectively) were similar between the groups. The authors concluded that instrumentation of the infected spine is safe and should be considered when spinal integrity is compromised.

Arnold and others reported 94 patients with osteomyelitis who required implant placement during the initial treatment of the osteomyelitis. Of those, 23% failed at a median of 4 months postoperatively.[29] Addition of rifampin to the wound and chronic, suppressive antibiotics did not affect the failure rate. On the other hand, vancomycin powder is increasingly being placed in the wound as additional prophylaxis.[30]

Implant removal continues to be recommended for late (after 1 year) infection.[31,32] In one recent paper, implant retention was recommended in pediatric patients with both early and late infectons due to a lower pseudarthrosis and curve progression rate.[33]

One recent review recommended prophylactic flap coverage for high-risk implant cases.[34] Hyperbaric oxygen treatment has also been recommended.[35]

In patients with other spinal inflammatory diseases, typically spondyloarthropathies, the most important issues surround proper identification of the disease state, perioperative disease management, and a recognition that disease-modifying agents may adversely affect bone healing.[36] In addition, many spondyloarthropathies, such as ankylosing spondylitis, have a marked impact on spinal biomechanics. The bone is often demineralized due to aberrant loading patterns.[37] Autofusion leads to long lever arms that both increase the risk of unstable fracture and challenge successful operative restabilization.

Bone Quality and Osteoporosis

As with infection, poor bone quality can increase the risk of implant-related complications in several ways. Most importantly, poor bone quality requires careful consideration of operative strategy. Osteoporotic patients, for example, are often more fragile and not good candidates for larger, multisegmental spinal reconstructions. Unfortunately, from a mechanical point of view, these patients often require multipoint fixation and more aggressive correction of spinal alignment problems to avoid kyphotic collapse, adjacent-segment fracture, or implant failure.

With the aging of the population, type 2 osteoporosis is becoming more common. However, changes in hormone replacement practices have also increased the incidence of postmenopausal (type 1) osteoporosis. Often ignored are secondary causes of bone loss from other medications or medical problems (steroids, hyperparathyroidism). Such causes of type 3 osteoporosis are less responsive to medication management.[38]

Although newer medications offer patients better bone-building ability, these agents have among the highest noncompliance rates of any medication class. Even after the "bone decade," a sizable proportion of at-risk patients still make it to surgery without a preoperative assessment of bone mineralization.[39]

At a minimum, at-risk patients should have a dual-energy absorptiometry scan, although surgeons should carefully consider the trabecular architecture and cortical thickness on a preoperative CT scan as well. Surgeries can often be delayed to allow bone building. Perioperative administration of bisphosphonates, denosumab, and teriparatide have been studied in spinal fusion patients.[40,41] Teriparatide has been found to be most effective and can offer clinically relevant improvements in bone quality over 6 to 12 months of use.[42-44]

With a sense of the patient's bone quality in mind, potential changes in surgical strategy should be undertaken. In some elective conditions, the decision to move forward must be tempered by a realistic appraisal of the impact of fragility on the intended procedure's risk/benefit balance. In others, a delay to address bone quality is recommended. Such a delay is not likely to provide net gains for patients markedly incapacitated or nonambulatory due to their spinal pathology. In these patients, modifications to the surgical strategy must be considered. These considerations include types of bone anchors, number of anchors used, polymethylmethacrylate augmentation of screws, and avoidance of anterior/interbody procedures.[45-50]

Bone quality will limit the surgeon's ability to achieve distraction intraoperatively; in general, in the face of significant deformity, a spinal column–shortening approach is favored. Significant preload on bone anchors must be avoided (Fig. 98.2). Selection of motion-sparing approaches is compromised by early failure of the bone-implant junction.[51,52]

Intraoperatively, radiographic visualization may be compromised as well. The surgeon must be ready to abandon

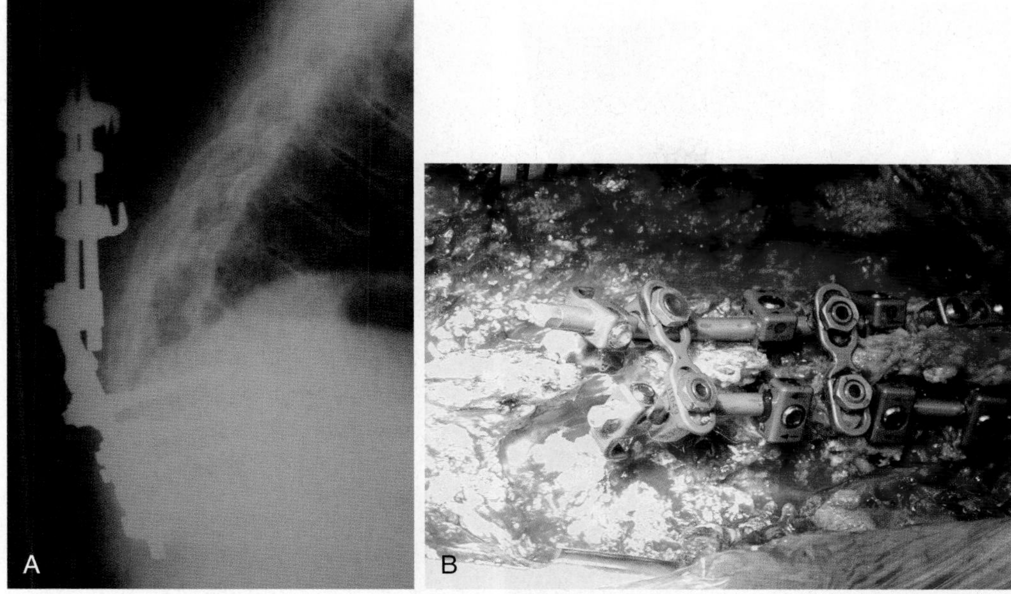

FIG. 98.2 (A) Lateral radiograph demonstrating a hook construct added to a previous transpedicular lumbar construct for an adjacent-segment osteoporotic burst fracture. (B) Intraoperative image of the displaced cranial hooks. In this case, greater anterior load sharing through corpectomy or polymethylmethacrylate augmentation could have been considered. Alternatively, a longer, more rigid cranial extension may have also prevented the failure.

percutaneous procedures if the proper landmarks cannot be visualized. Osteoporotic bone is vascular.[53] Late decortication, bone wax, blood product support, Cell Savers, and other techniques have been recommended to support these patients.

Postoperative concerns in osteoporotic patients include activity restriction and bracing to reduce implant stress. Osteoporotic bone likely progresses to union more slowly than healthy bone, but, even when fused, may be subject to higher bending forces. Implant removal is therefore discouraged, as late deformity progression and compression fractures have been described even within solid arthrodeses.[54,55]

Dysvascular Change

Vascular injury is a concern with implant misplacement, but subtler vascular embarrassment may lead to biologic failure of a spinal construct. Implant placement typically requires greater exposure and devascularization than decompression-only procedures. This devascularization may be particularly important in smokers and in surgeries in a previously irradiated bed (Fig. 98.3).[56-60]

Biomechanical Failure

As with biologic failure, biomechanical failure exists at the nexus between the patient's pathophysiology and the goals of the reconstructive procedure. Thus, this failure can arise from errors in surgical planning or from patient comorbidities. Biomechanical failure is typically expressed through one of several modes of failure, such as cage subsidence, rod fracture, or screw loosening or fracture.

Cage subsidence occurs when the loads through the cage exceed the carrying capacity of the bone on which it rests. Frequently, this failure is seen in patients with poor cancellous bone quality or when a hard cage subjected the host bone to a marked modulus of elasticity mismatch. Preoperatively, prevention may include selection of a wider cage supported by a larger portion of the vertebral endplate, especially the cortical ring. However, subsidence is seen even with wide lateral interbody fusions. In one recent study, 30% of patients had either grade I or II subsidence.[61]

Intraoperatively, careful endplate protection during preparation and placement will prevent the cage from sitting on softer subchondral bone. Postoperative loading should also be considered at each stage. Greater activity restrictions or bracing may be considered in larger patients. Cage failure is also more likely when there is ongoing instability in planes other than axial loading.[62] For example, posterior tension band failure leads to unloading of the posterior load-bearing columns and overloading of the endplate. This could be addressed with separate, posterior instrumentation.

Although late implant failure occurs because of failure of fusion or bone healing, early failure typically occurs for implant overloading. As such, early implant failure is typically related to failure to understand the direction or degree of spinal instability or errors in surgical strategy. For example, rod fractures are most common in stiff, adult spinal deformities at the level of spinal osteotomy (Fig. 98.4). In one recent series of 75 adults undergoing fusion for adult spinal deformity, 9.3% of those who had a pedicle subtraction osteotomy had a rod fracture compared with 2.6% of those who had a Smith-Petersen osteotomy.[63] The authors identified the following additional risk factors: pseudarthrosis at 1 year, sagittal

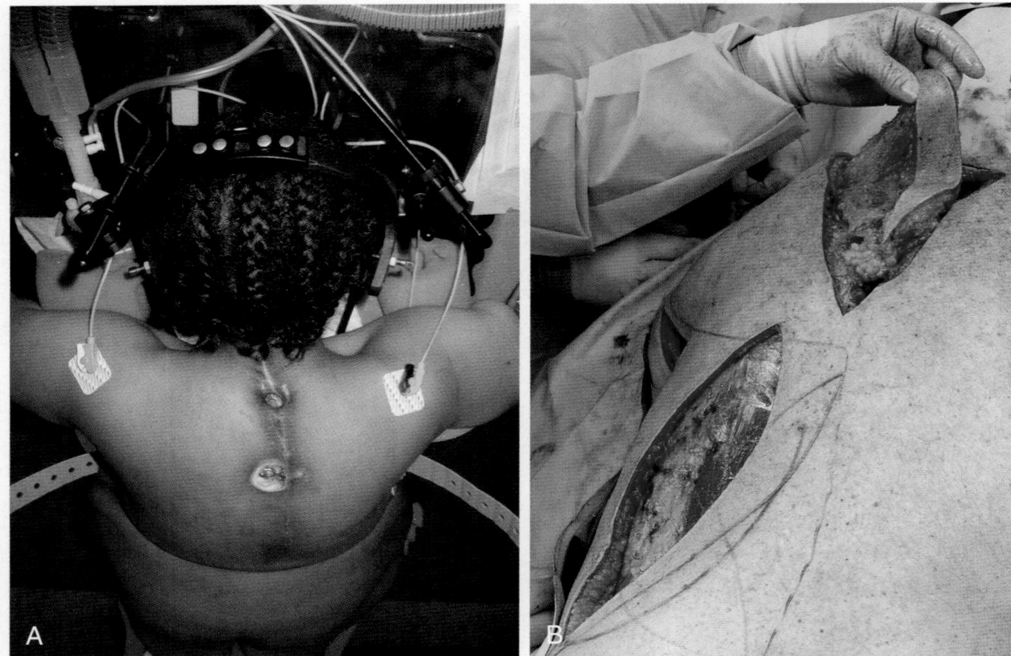

FIG. 98.3 Two patients with soft tissue coverage and healing problems. (A) Wound dehiscence and exposed implants. (B) Surgeon turning a flap to cover wound dehiscence after instrumented stabilization of a pathologic fracture in a previously irradiated wound bed.

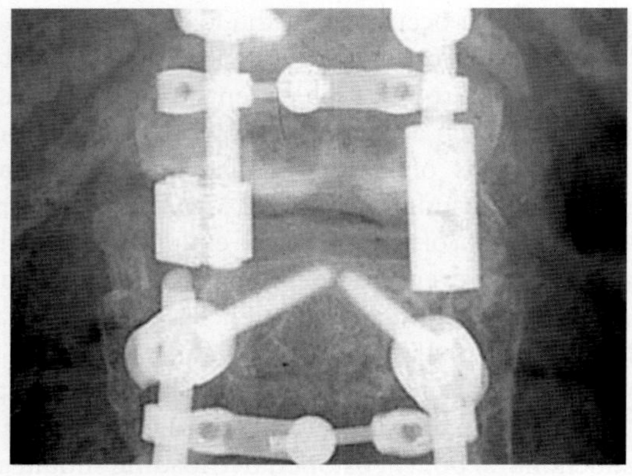

FIG. 98.4 Anteroposterior radiograph revealing rod fracture at the site of a previous fusion extension across the thoracolumbar junction. This high-stress area is more vulnerable to both slow fusion mass maturation and increased stress on the implants, especially where the rods meet the rod-to-rod connector. Potential solutions include attempts at anterior/interbody fusion and outrigger (or four-rod) constructs.

rod contour greater than 60 degrees, presence of dominoes and/or parallel connectors, and fusion construct crossing both thoracolumbar and lumbosacral junctions.

Unlike rods, bone anchors may fracture, loosen, or displace from the bone. In addition, polyaxial pedicle screws can exhibit disengagement between the screw and its tulip. Often motion or a 1-mm radiographic halo around the screw is used to define loosening. One recent study found that a change of 1.9 degrees of angulation between the pedicle screw axis and cranial endplate was 75% sensitive and 89% specific in detecting screw loosening on 6-month radiographs (Fig. 98.5).[64]

In late failure, bone healing and fixation failure are typically described in terms of a "race." Pseudarthrosis is often a multifactorial problem that involves the patient's biology and pathomechanics as well as the mechanical attributes of the fixation methodologies used. In some cases, the issue lies in the patient's biologic ability to heal in a reasonable time frame. The surgeon may choose to address this issue by adding autologous bone graft or bone morphogenetic protein (BMP).[65] BMP may be more effective in some areas compared with others. A higher than expected fusion failure rate of 10.8% was reported using recombinant human bone morphogenetic protein 2 (rhBMP-2) in a pediatric cohort undergoing occipitocervical and C1–C2 fusion surgery.[66] The same author group reported no increase in the risk of cancer at 4-year follow-up in 57 consecutive cases of rhBMP-2 use.[67]

In other patients, the problem lies in adequate stabilization of the motion segment. Depending on the patient population, pseudarthrosis leading to implant failure has become less common as fixation methods have evolved. In a series of 227 AIS patients undergoing posterior spinal fusion, a 2% rate of implant failure was noted.[31] Often, conversion to a more rigid form of fixation, such as transpedicular instrumentation or interbody cage placement, will successfully address the pseudarthrosis (Fig. 98.6).[68] Similarly, after anterior cervical discectomy, a posterior wiring or clamping procedure will often lead to union anteriorly.[69]

Even in challenging clinical scenarios, properly designed implant schemes exhibit low failure rates. In a cohort of 318 patients with spinal metastases undergoing separation surgery (which seeks to restore mechanical stability and remove only that part of the tumor in contact with the spinal cord). In this series, only 2.8% exhibited symptomatic implant failure that required revision.[70] Of those, failure was more common in women, in cases involving more than six contiguous

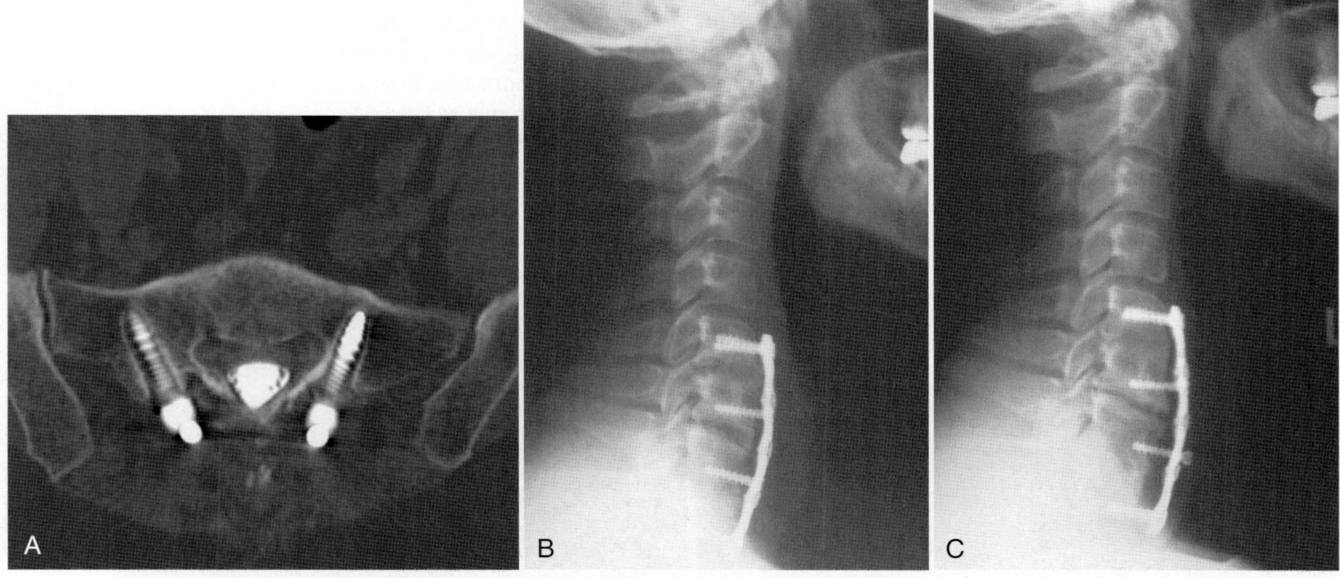

FIG. 98.5 (A) Loosening of cortical screws placed into the sacrum. The often-limited bone stock of the sacrum may challenge use of cortical trajectory screws. Transpedicular trajectories, particularly through the promontory anterior, might be considered. (B) Lateral radiograph performed shortly after surgery of an anterior cervical discectomy and fusion at C5–C6, C6–C7, and C7–T1. (C) This patient developed pseudarthrosis at the C6–C7 level with collapse and failure of the locking mechanism between the screw and plate, as evidenced by the screw backing out of the plate. The plate is also lifting off the spine. This patient developed recurrent neck pain and dysphagia. The complication includes biologic failure of the fusion and biomechanical failure of the plate-screw interface.

levels, and in patients who required concomitant chest wall resection.

Screw loosening is not necessarily diagnostic for fusion failure. Screws can loosen as part of a "dynamization" process. Additional issues complicate the biology of the bone-implant junction. For example, diabetics carry a higher risk of aseptic implant loosening.[71] These issues are more critical in dynamic stabilization approaches and likely decrease with solid segmental fusion.[72] Loose or fractured implants may migrate into other anatomic regions. Implant migration into the retroperitoneal space has been reported 6 years after instrumentation without fusion.[73] The authors cautioned against implant placement without concomitant spinal fusion.

These studies are complicated by the limitations of radiographic diagnosis of pseudarthrosis. Spinal implants often impede clear visualization of bone healing, especially stainless steel or trabecular metal. A recent review noted the limitations of radiographic studies in identifying pseudarthrosis due to the high rate of asymptomatic pseudarthroses and the number of conditions, such as adjacent-segment degeneration, that may mimic the symptoms of pseudarthrosis.[74] Dickson and colleagues, in a series of 171 consecutive pedicle subtraction osteotomy patients, identified 18 pseudarthroses, with two diagnosed more than 5 years after the index surgery.[75]

Errors in Surgical Strategy

Errors in surgical strategy are the easiest for the surgeon to remedy, but the remedy requires an in-depth understanding of spinal biomechanics and how various pathologies affect normal force transfer through the spine.

The surgeon must also estimate the degree to which intraoperative maneuvers will further affect the spine mechanically. From simple extensor muscle stripping to decompressive procedures (especially if the facets are resected), to more aggressive bone removal such as corpectomy or osteotomy, each step will further compromise "native" stability.

To properly select a reconstruction technique, the successful surgeon considers how various implant systems work to address those mechanical deficits. It has been noted that surgeons are often included in the "procedural" rather than "cognitive" group of physicians. This is unfair. While making a proper diagnosis in spine care is not always challenging, designing the correct treatment approach for the patient might be. All too often today, careful selection has given way to "more is better." But, "more" adds costs, time, and morbidity. Does every patient need a bone anchor at every level? Are lateral mass screws required, or will wiring suffice? Does every patient need an interbody cage?

Before surgery, the templating process for a surgeon anticipating an instrumented spinal reconstructive procedure must include the patient's goals and expectations, ability to participate in postoperative rehabilitation or bracing (if needed), and various pathologies as well as close assessment of the patient's regional anatomy. For example, the need for immediate loading and the advisability of bracing may be very different in spinal cord–injured or polytrauma patients. A two-level posterior cervical fusion at the occipitocervical junction for trauma requires a very different degree of operative immobilization and grafting than a similar procedure performed as a two-level subaxial procedure in a patient with marked spondylosis.

In other patients, especially in regard to the upper lumbar spine, the surgeon should ensure that the bone is large enough to safely contain a pedicle screw, for example. As with any surgery, a back-up plan must be ready in case the initial plan cannot be executed.

Aside from patient size and anticipated postoperative loading, regional mechanical considerations and overall spinal balance must also be considered. For example, stabilization across the thoracolumbar junction may require more levels of fixation than one at L4–L5.[76]

Independent of the surgical indication, the implant should seek to reverse the instability pattern presented by the pathophysiology. Typically, if a distraction force risks spinal column

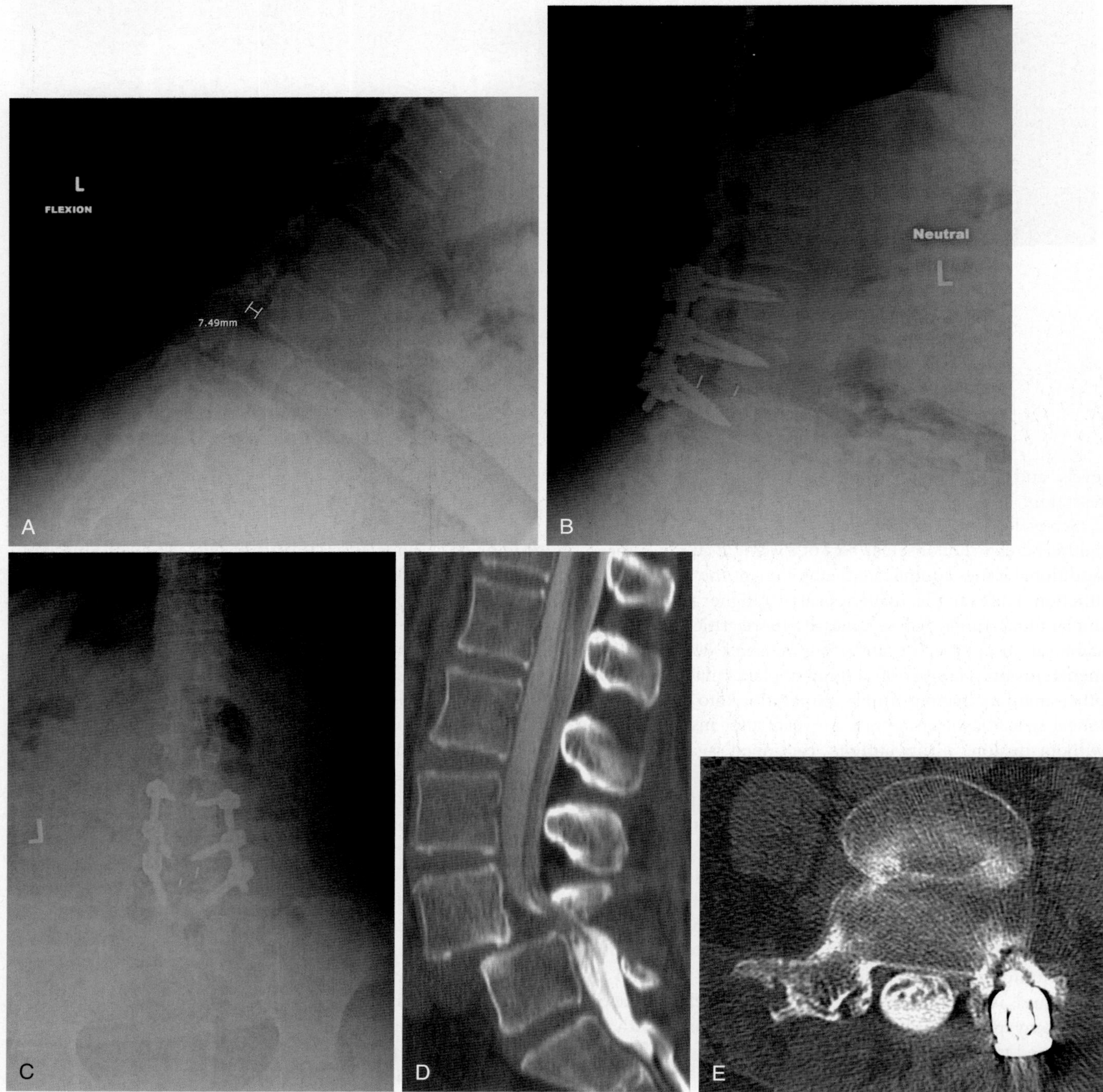

FIG. 98.6 (A) A 67-year-old osteopenic patient presented with back and leg pain associated with stenosis and a mobile anterolisthesis at L4–L5, as seen on lateral radiograph. Operative intervention included posterior decompression and fusion with interbody cage placement at L4–L5. (B–C) Follow-up radiographs revealed cage retropulsion into the canal. (D–E) Computed tomographic myelogram demonstrated the anterolisthesis with recurrent stenosis due to the slip and the cage.

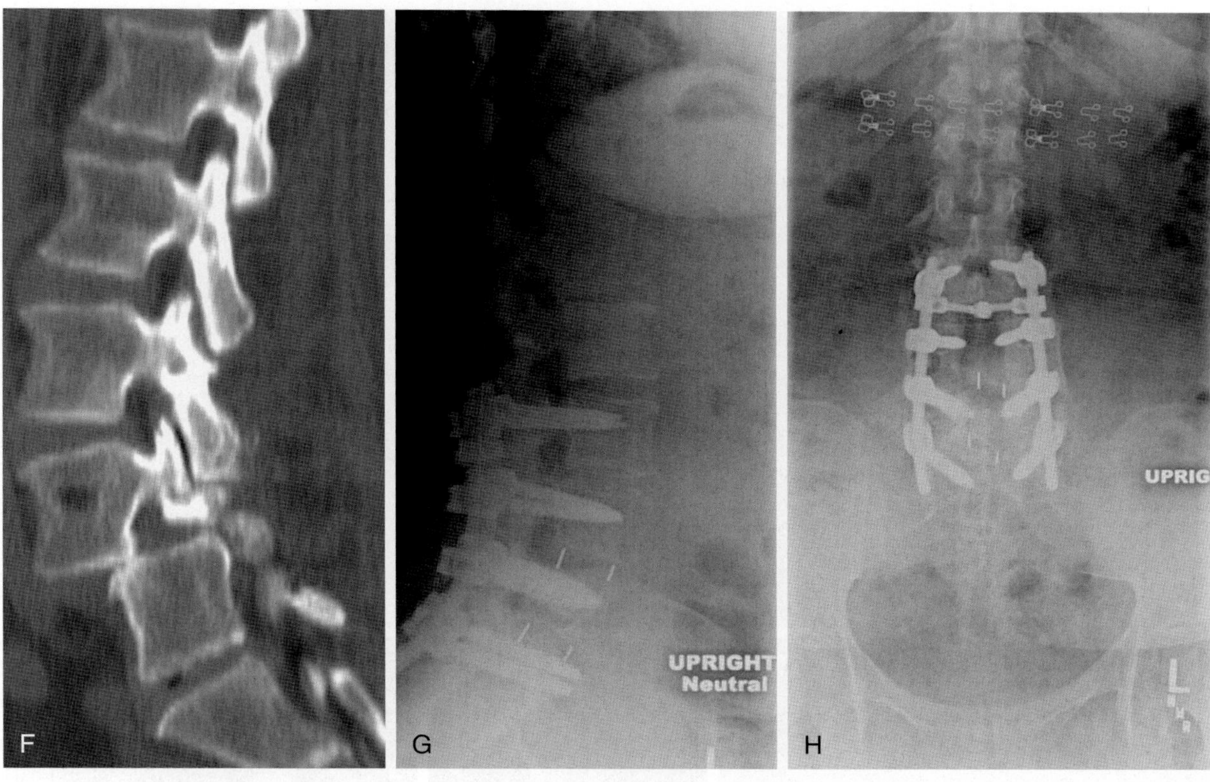

FIG. 98.6, cont'd (F) Parasagittal computed tomographic scan from another osteoporotic patient in whom unilateral fixation was used to treat a degenerative L4–L5 spondylolisthesis. A wide decompression with near-complete facetectomy was undertaken bilaterally and a pars fracture occurred postoperatively. (G–H) Revision surgery included bilateral instrumentation and extension cranially to L3 and caudally to the L5–S1 level. Given this patient's bone quality and significant, segmental instability, prevention might have included additional fixation at the time of the index surgery, protection of the midline elements or facets at L4–L5, or screw augmentation with polymethylmethacrylate.

stability, a tension band construct is used to convert those distraction forces into compression forces across the segment. These compression forces maintain alignment as well as promote bone healing.[77-79] The simplest of these constructs is posterior interspinous wiring. When the facets and anterior load-bearing column are intact, this method will be both least morbid and most cost effective.[78] However, facet injury or pars fracture subject the spine to additional shear loading, which a tension band wire cannot resist. In this setting, more rigid fixation, such as segmental screw-rod constructs, should be considered.

With increasing disruption of the vertebral body, load bearing is compromised. In this setting, even short-segment rigid screw-rod constructs may fail. Options include longer posterior constructs functioning in a bridging mode (e.g., an intramedullary nail when a bone defect is present) or direct restoration of anterior load-bearing capacity through corpectomy and cage or graft reconstruction.[80]

The degree of comminution requiring this type of extended construct continues to be debated; however, the involved region of the spine has a significant impact.[81,82] For example, in the cervical spine, depending on the level, nearly two-thirds of the load is borne through the articular pillars posteriorly.[83] Thus, if the lateral masses are intact, a corpectomy may only be required when additional canal decompression is desirable. Similarly, in the upper thoracic spine, an intact ribcage and sternum may act as a "fourth column" of the spine and transfer axial load bearing away from the compromised vertebral body.[84]

While bridging and tension band constructs may also be applied to the vertebral body anteriorly, the most common implant mode is a buttress. Here, axial forces are supported through partial conversion into a laterally directed force into the intact vertebral bodies into which the plate has been screwed. The buttress plate typically requires some ongoing anterior load-bearing capacity, either through fracture reduction or corpectomy and graft/cage placement. In this setting, the structural bone graft or cage acts as a strut to directly transfer load from the intact vertebral body above the injury to the intact vertebral body below (Fig. 98.7).

A final issue in complication avoidance through surgical strategy arises through the relationship between implant holding power and spinal alignment. It has been long established that implant failure rates increase when the spine is out of balance. The further from the patient's center of gravity, the greater the lever arm of body weight becomes on the construct.[85] Recently, considerable attention has been paid to concepts surrounding proper assessment and reconstruction of spinal alignment, especially sagittal balance.[86,87] Guler and others found a high rate of implant failure in S2 iliac screws

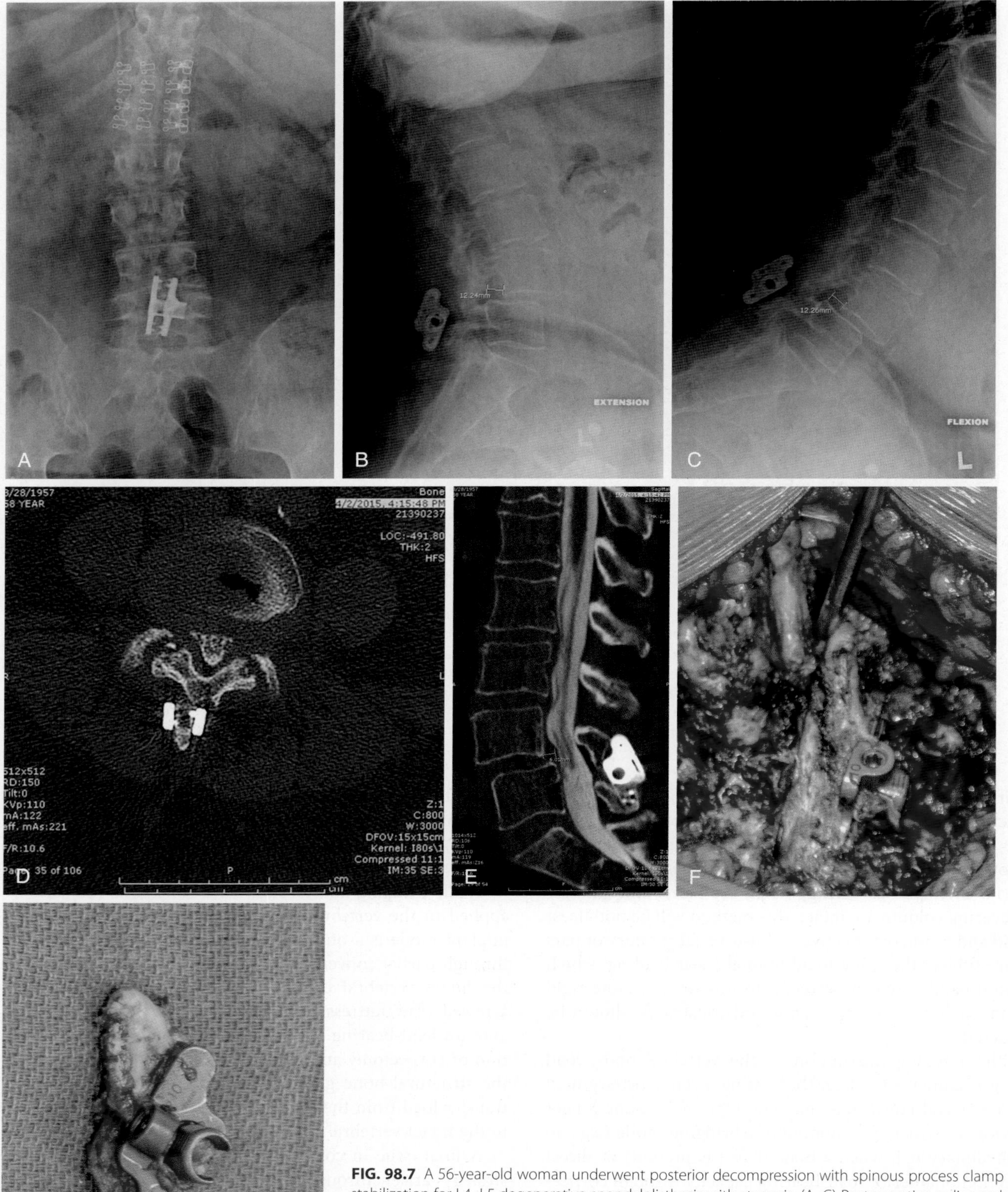

FIG. 98.7 A 56-year-old woman underwent posterior decompression with spinous process clamp stabilization for L4–L5 degenerative spondylolisthesis with stenosis. (A–C) Postoperative radiographs at 2 years, including flexion and extension views, reveal ongoing mobility. (D–E) Computed tomographic myelography revealed spinous process fracture of L4, ongoing stenosis, and no clear attempt at fusion. (F–G) The patient underwent surgery, which included removal of the fractured spinous process and loosened implant, revision decompression, and instrumented fusion with transpedicular instrumentation and an interbody cage. This complication could have been avoided by using the implant under its labeled indications.

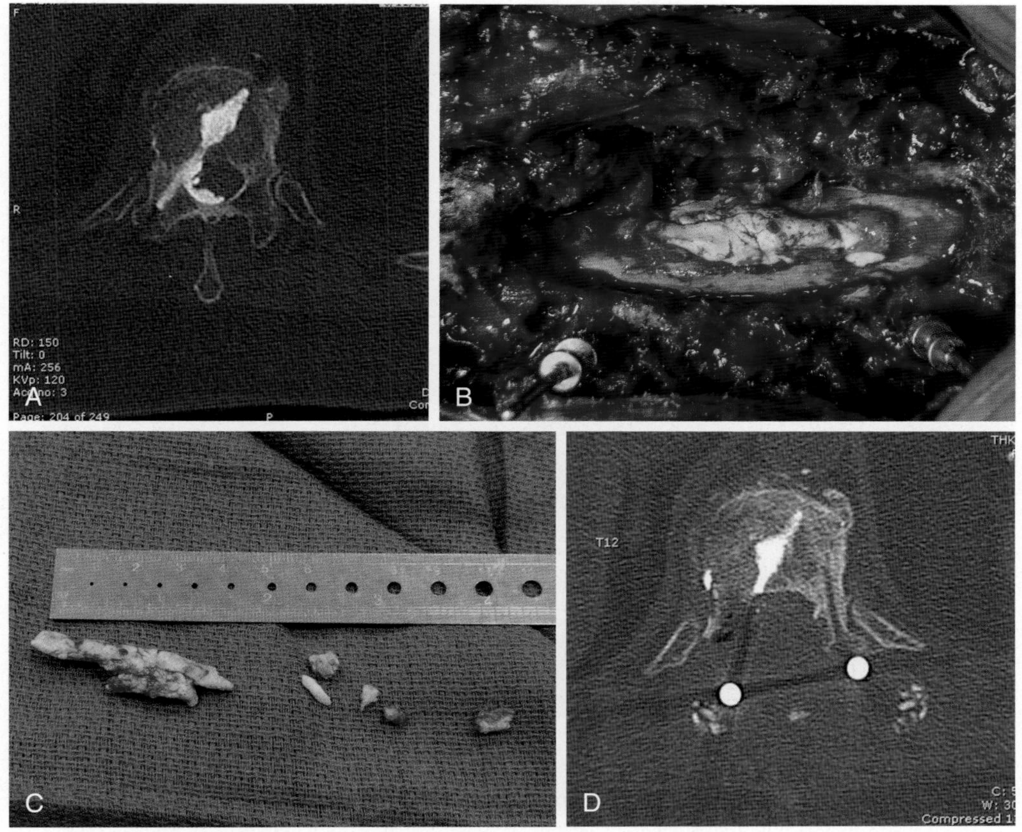

FIG. 98.8 A 72-year-old osteoporotic woman was referred from an outside hospital after reporting marked, lower extremity weakness (right greater than left) and thoracic radicular pain after a vertebroplasty procedure. (A) Computed tomography (CT) scan revealed polymethylmethacrylate (PMMA) incursion into the canal. (B) The patient was taken urgently to the operating room, where PMMA was found on the right side of the canal from anterior to posterior. (C) A wide decompression and pediculectomy were performed and the PMMA was removed. Due to the width of the decompression, a short-segment fusion was also performed. (D) Postoperative CT revealed a capacious canal. The risk of this complication is reduced by ensuring adequate intraoperative radiographic visualization of the posterior elements. When adequate radiographic images cannot be obtained, the procedure should be abandoned.

in long deformity cases, especially in older patients and those in whom lumbar lordosis restoration was inadequate.[88] In addition, the increased stresses to which the spine is subjected when out of balance may also affect rates of adjacent segment degeneration. A higher risk of subadjacent degeneration was reported below scoliosis fusions when the thoracic spine was fused in hypokyphosis (Figs. 98.8 and 98.9).[89]

Technical Error in Implementation of Surgical Strategy

The best conceived, optimal surgical strategy can be undone by imperfect execution. Several factors may influence this execution, including obscured landmarks, im proper lighting, lack of surgeon skill and experience, and inadequate exposure or fascial release. Although decompression procedures may suffer from technical complications from dural injury or inadequate decompression, instrumentation procedures are typically complicated by misplacement of the cage or screw.

Less-frequent technical errors include improper length or poor contouring of the rod, failure to properly torque the locking screws, material mismatch leading to a galvanic response, or failure to properly prepare or place the graft.

Screw and Wire Misplacement

Even in the hands of careful, experienced spine surgeons, implants may inadvertently be misplaced (Fig. 98.10). Such misplacement carries several direct and indirect risks for the patient. At worst, catastrophic cord or vascular injury may occur. At best, the screw simply offers less mechanical holding power than properly placed implants. Of course, most minor pedicle breaches are asymptomatic and may not affect healing or outcome.[90]

While less often performed as a stand-alone procedure today, wiring continues to be used as an adjunct to more rigid forms of fixation. Over time, younger surgeon familiarity with the technical nuances of wiring may be lost. Key issues include canal incursion when placing sublaminar wires and cut-through of the bone when overtensioning the wire.[91] Braided cables, while thicker, may reduce the risks of cut-through.

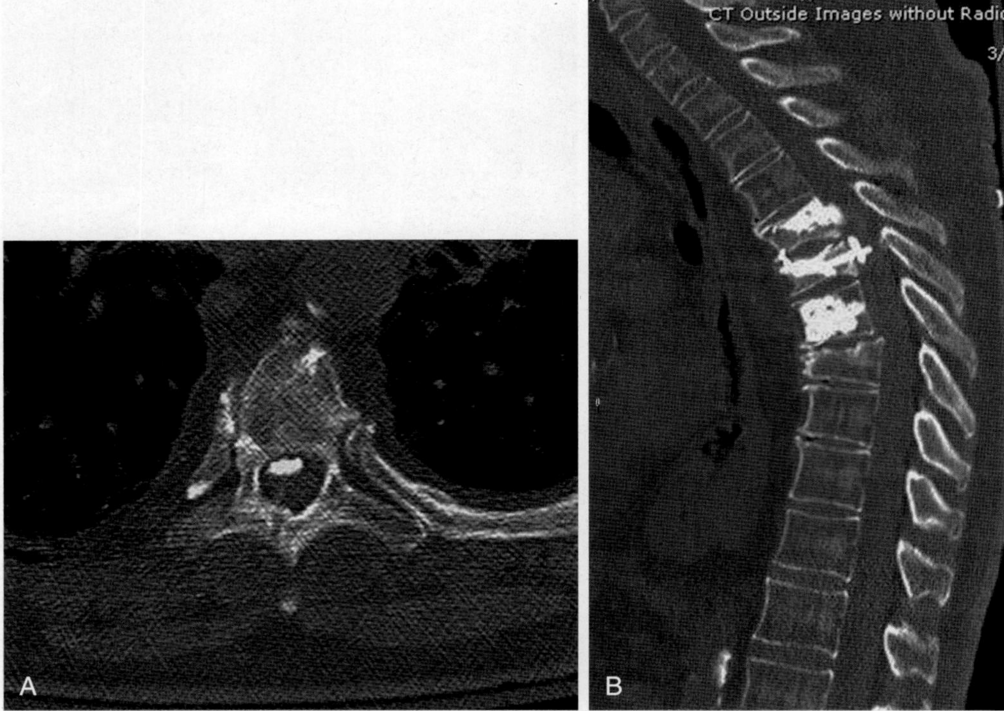

FIG. 98.9 A patient referred for new-onset lower extremity weakness after vertebroplasty. Although there was some polymethylmethacrylate in the canal, the apparent Jamshidi needle trajectory appeared to pass through the central canal. The patient was noted to be improving neurologically. Given the likelihood of direct cord trauma, the neurologic improvement and the patient's medical comorbidities, a nonoperative approach was selected. In patients with poor bone quality, adequate imaging must be available for percutaneous procedures to be safely performed. The surgeon must be ready to abort the procedure if adequate images are not available.

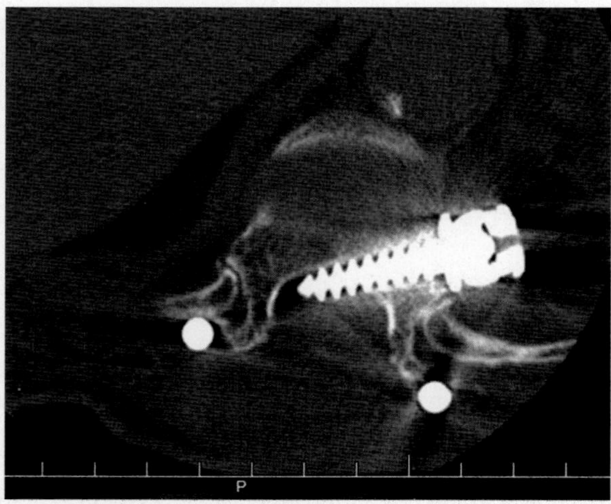

FIG. 98.10 This patient underwent anterior screw-rod reconstruction after a thoracic corpectomy. Clear incursion of the screw into the spinal canal was noted on postoperative computed tomographic scan. In these cases, careful attention to intraoperative position may decrease the risk of poor screw trajectory.

With screw placement, the risks vary widely by the type of screw and the level of the spine into which it is inserted. For example, although C2 and C7 pedicle screws have become commonplace, subaxial cervical pedicle screws between C3 and C6 continue, in most centers, to be reserved for revision or special cases only. Even a leading proponent of this technique, Kuniyoshi Abumi, recently wrote: "Even after surgeons became familiar with placement of cervical pedicle screws, screw malposition rate by freehand technique is high for patients with severe spondylotic conditions."[92] Reinhold and others[92a] noted that "several cadaver studies, even utilizing computerized image-guided systems, still showed high perforation rates from 18% up to 87.5%."

Cervical lateral mass screws, on the other hand, enjoy a relatively low rate of symptomatic misplacement. A recent large series of 430 patients with different cervical spine disorders who were treated with a total of 2500 lateral mass polyaxial screws were followed for up to 8 years.[93] No neurologic or vascular injury occurred, but five screws were repositioned.

Thoracic pedicle screws carry moderate risk, especially in patients with spinal deformity. One recent study of 218 thoracic pedicle screws placed for trauma in 28 patients found a 15.5% misplacement rate.[94] Pedicles less than 7 mm (and in particular those <5 mm) in diameter had higher misplacement rates, as did screws placed between T4 and T9.

As the most frequently placed spinal implants, lumbar pedicle screws are most familiar to spine surgeons. However, wound depth, spinal deformity, and level-to-level anatomic differences continue to challenge their accurate placement. A recent systematic review found that, despite intraoperative neurologic monitoring and intraoperating imaging, a 5.7% rate of new, postoperative neurologic deficits was reported.[95] When examining posterior decompression and fusion cases only, the rate was 1.9%, of which less than one-third was due to screw malposition.

Evolving Accuracy and Means of Detection

Regardless of the type of screw placed, a few tools are commonly used to improve accuracy. Historically, the intended screw track was sounded with a ball-tipped probe prior to screw insertion. Although this technique is still recommended, it is less frequently used alone. One study found that the accuracy of direct manual palpation of pedicle screw tracks with a ball-tipped probe was "disturbingly low."[96]

Radiographic confirmation of screw placement before wound closure also remains a commonly used measure. Plain radiographs are obtained after the implants have been placed. Acceptable accuracy rates continue to be reported for this technique.[97]

Direct placement under fluoroscopy or intermittent fluoroscopic assessment during the implantation process is more typically used today. In some centers, radiopaque markers are placed in the intended screw tracks before final implant placement.[98] Because these markers are much smaller than the screws, the pedicle itself is more readily appreciated on en face imaging (Fig. 98. 11). In addition, if a breach has occurred, it is typically much smaller than a screw diameter breach. These smaller fenestrations are less likely to cause nerve injury and allow more facile redirection.

The number of surgeons frequently using percutaneous screw placement techniques has increased over the past several years. One recent large series used postoperative CT imaging to assess placement of 724 open and 885 percutaneously placed screws.[4] The rate of breach was higher in the open group at 7.5% compared with 4.7% for the percutaneous group. The magnitude of breach was higher for the percutaneous group at 5.4 versus 3.7 mm. The authors concluded that percutaneous placement was adequately accurate when compared with open.

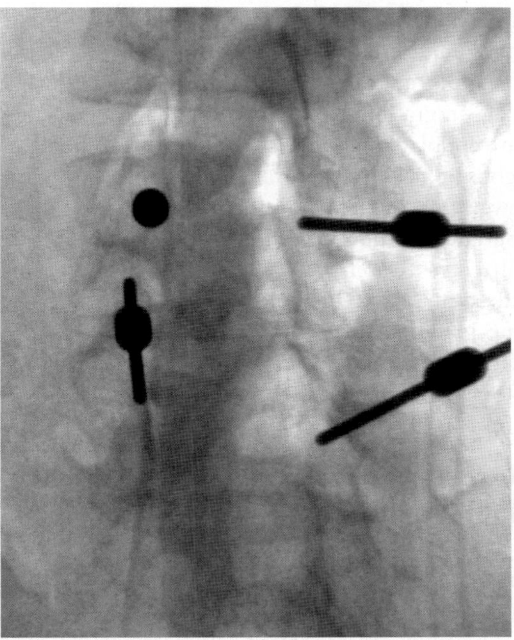

FIG. 98.11 When in doubt about the placement of spinal instrumentation, small markers can be placed into the proposed trajectory before large screws are inserted. This both reduces the risk of injury to the neural elements and decreases any violation of the pedicle that might compromise ultimate fixation. Particularly in scoliotic patients, a true en face view of the pedicle can ensure proper placement.

Similarly, the availability of intraoperative axial imaging and computerized navigation systems has increased. The relative benefit derived from these systems depends on the surgical indication. One recent series found no benefit in single-level instrumented fusions for degenerative spondylolisthesis.[99] On the other hand, a study of 260 patients found that navigation improved accuracy and pedicle filling, particularly in more complex reconstructions.[100] Another study of 145 patients found that the time required to use CT navigation systems and the accuracy of screw placement with those systems improved with time.[101]

Newer true-CT imaging has been reported. In one study of 170 screws placed in 23 consecutive patients, 18 to 34 minutes were added to the total operative time.[102] Seven screws were misplaced greater than 2 mm, resulting in an accuracy rate of 95.9%.

As with postoperative CT and MRI imaging, intraoperative imaging is distorted by metallic bloom artifacts. This bloom increases with screw size, but it is less with titanium than stainless steel and cobalt-chrome implants.[103] Certainly, intraoperative axial imaging, whether from cone-beam imaging or true CT, increases the radiation exposure to the patient compared with fluoroscopy.[104] By limiting live, intraoperative fluoroscopy, radiation exposure to the surgical team may be decreased.

Prevention

Several techniques can be used to decrease, but probably not eliminate, the risks of implant misplacement. First, prepare for the procedure with as complete an understanding of general spinal anatomy and the patient's individual anatomy as possible. Regional variations, autofusion, and congenital anomalies should be noted and understood before the skin incision. For example, any exposure of the posterior cervicocranium requires an understanding of the path of the vertebral artery. However, in some patients an aberrant course will increase the risk of certain types of screw placement. In addition, the disease state itself may impose additional risk to spinal instrumentation procedures. With severe, spondylotic collapse, the vertebral artery's course becomes tortuous and may medialize into the region in which a cervical corpectomy could be performed.[105] Metastatic disease may attract marked neovascularization that could risk intraoperative exsanguination if not recognized and addressed.

Proper implant sizing also requires a detailed knowledge of the host anatomy. Previously, various plastic templates could be used over hard copy radiographs and CT scans. Today, digital calipers can be used on picture archiving and communication systems to directly measure the optimal graft width or screw length. These measures can be verified intraoperatively.

Next, ensure proper intraoperative positioning. In the prone position, slight rotation of the body, especially in heavier patients, may result in improperly angled implants. In the lateral position, a patient drifting off true lateral may lead to excessively anterior implants that may direct screws into the canal or lead to late vessel erosions.

Intraoperatively, ensure adequate exposure and/or radiographic guidance. Running electromyography may signal implant misplacement, but directly stimulating the screws after placement may reduce the frequency with which patients with medial misplacements leave the operating room with implant impingement.[106,107]

New protocols combining navigation, intraoperative screw stimulation and, when stimulation suggests a breach, repeat CT scanning are being studied.[108]

Plate and Rod Issues

Technical errors may also affect plate or rod placement. In deformity cases, rod length estimates may inadequately account for contouring. Short rods risk screw-rod disengagement (Fig. 98.12).[109] Overlong rods, on the other hand, may cause impingement symptoms in the mobile regions of the spine above or below the fusion.

Overcontouring or undercontouring a plate or rod may also cause problems. Because most plates are placed in a buttress mode, undercontouring decreases the mechanical benefits of the plate. Undercontouring a posterior rod may lead to hypolordosis or other sagittal balance concerns.

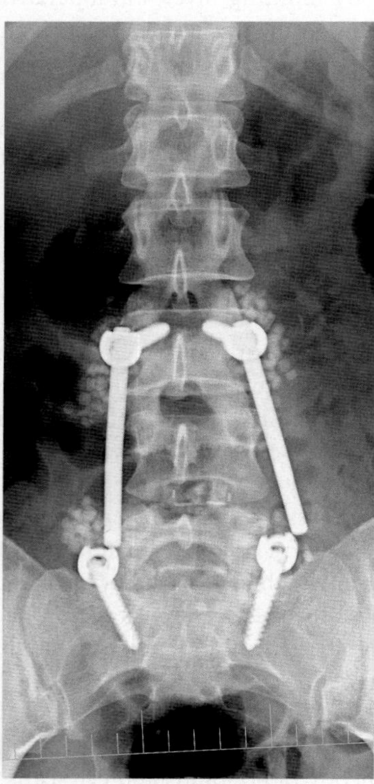

FIG. 98.12 Anteroposterior lumbar radiograph demonstrating implant failure from short rod placement. The locking screws did not adequately capture the rods, which subsequently disengaged as the patient moved. This complication can be avoided by ensuring at least a few millimeters of rod protrusion beyond the screw head. In this case, segmental fixation into L4 and L5 might also have decreased the stress on the screw-rod junction at S1.

Although a rod can be contoured to the idealized spinal alignment, the surgeon must ensure that adequate release (or osteotomy) has been performed. Otherwise, forcing the rod into the screw heads will excessively preload those screws and risk pullout. This is particularly true in patients with osteoporosis.

Especially in patients with complex deformities or staggered screw positions, the use of screw-rod connectors or multiple rods is preferred over acute rod bends. These rod bends, or repeated bending of the rod, lead to notch sensitivity and a greater chance of subsequent rod fracture.[110,111]

The surgeon must use caution when combining implants made from different metals.[112] Mixing stainless steel with titanium could lead to a galvanic response and early corrosion, although titanium has been used with cobalt-chromium alloy without significant corrosion or complications.

Graft and Cage Issues

Although grafting concerns are more pertinent to the larger discussion of spinal fusion, there are several issues directly relevant to complications of spinal instrumentation. First, as discussed above, the placement of spinal implants restricts the space available for bone grafting. If the graft bed is prepared after bulky polyaxial screws have been inserted, for example, optimal decortication may be difficult to achieve.

Second, in many settings structural allografts serve as spinal implants. These may be sophisticated, commercially machined corticocancellous spacers with specified degrees of lordosis, or they may be simple fibular segments or femoral rings. In this setting, the patient may be exposed to technical errors during insertion, such as those encountered with metallic and polyetheretherketone (PEEK) cages.

A tight interference fit for an interbody or corpectomy spacer is important to segmental stability and to prevent subsequent cage migration. However, oversized implants may injure the bony endplate or fracture on insertion. When harvesting autologous bone as a structural graft, use of a saw is associated with fewer graft failures than the use of osteotomes.[113]

Allograft handling depends on the form of the graft (lyophilized vs. fresh frozen). Adequate time for graft soaking is required to avoid brittle allograft splintering. Similarly, nonbone materials, especially PEEK and carbon fiber, may also shatter from impact during insertion or chronic overloading in the setting of pseudarthrosis.[114]

Important Structures Affected by Spinal Implant Impingement

Although this chapter cannot exhaustively cover the specific anatomic structures at risk with each spinal implant, a few general principles are important. Ultimately, spinal implants—through design, failure, or migration—may affect a number of perispinal tissues, including neurologic and vascular structures, the airway and esophagus, the bone and joints of the spine, and the spinal musculature (Fig. 98.13).

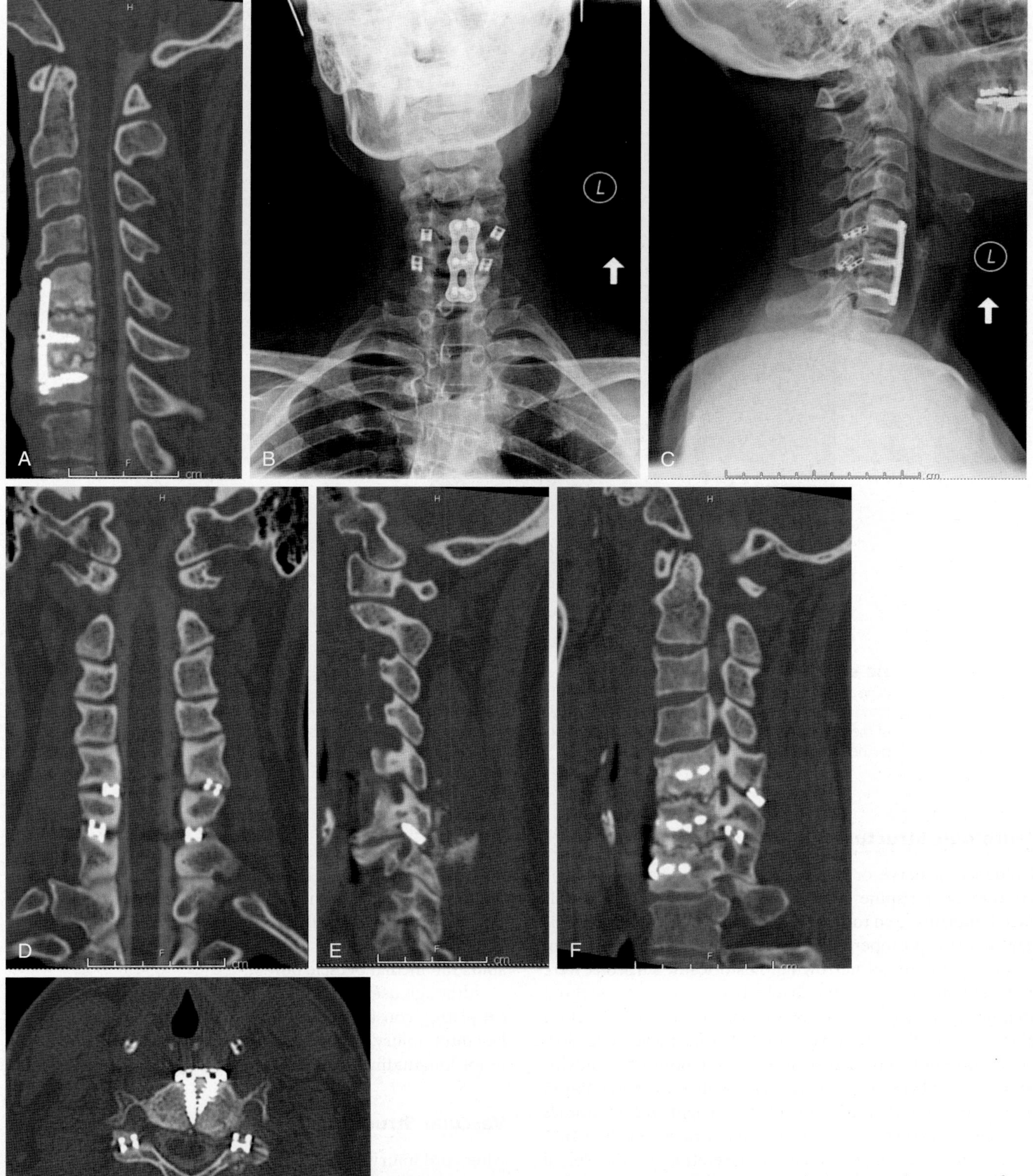

FIG. 98.13 This patient presented to the original surgeon with recurrent neck pain 1 year after two-level anterior cervical discectomy and fusion. (A) Computed tomography (CT) scan demonstrated pseudarthrosis. The patient was offered a minimally invasive posterior approach with facet joint spacers, as seen on the postoperative (B) anteroposterior and (C) lateral radiographs. Unfortunately, not only did the pain not improve, new left C7 radicular symptoms, including weakness, were reported. A later CT scan demonstrated anterior misplacement of the left C6–C7 facet implant. (D) Coronal, (E) parasagittal, (F) oblique, and (G) axial views are shown.

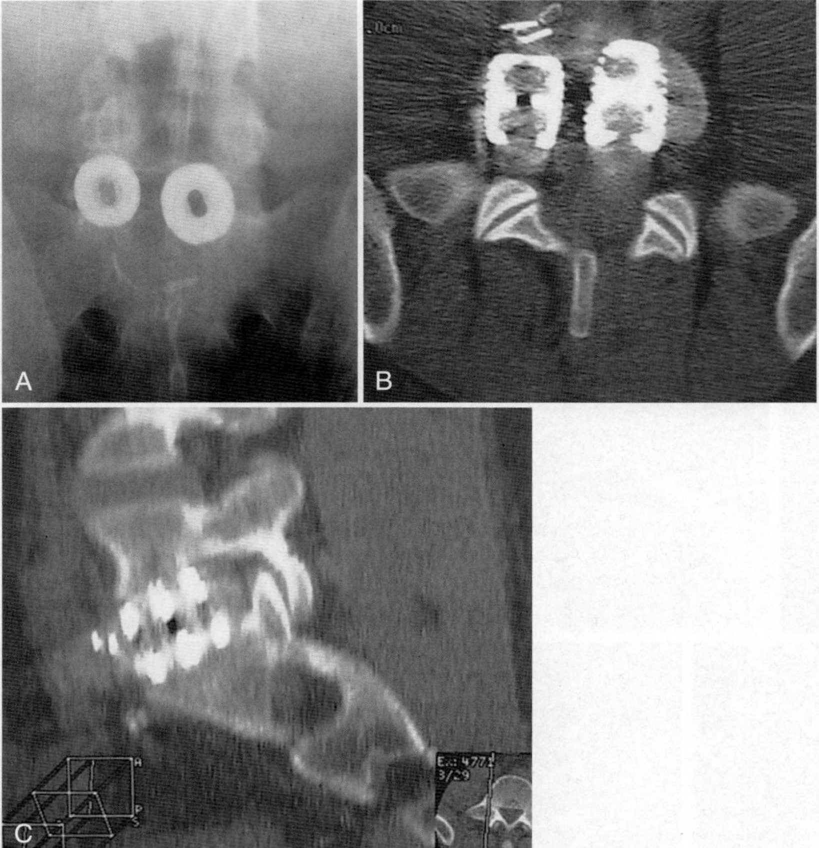

FIG. 98.14 (A) Anterior-posterior radiograph of an anterior interbody fusion with a pair of cages. Note that the cage on the left is laterally positioned and extends farther lateral than the pedicle. (B–C) Axial computed tomographic and sagittal reformatted images reveal that the laterally placed cage extends beyond the confines of the disc space and extends into the neuroforamina. It also appears that a disc fragment may have been pushed into the foramen.

Neurologic Structures

Avoidance of nerve or spinal cord injury is typically at the forefront of the spine surgeon's mind. However, even well-placed implants used to achieve reduction or improve lordosis may increase postoperative radiculopathy rates due to root traction or foraminal narrowing. Historically, surgeons were often taught to fuse spondylolisthetic segments without attempting reduction for fear of causing a nerve traction injury.[115] Over time, however, attempts to achieve better lordosis restoration and more anatomic reductions of spondylolistheses have been increaseing. With wide decompression of the foraminae and restoration of disc height, recent studies have reported acceptably low nerve injury rates (Fig. 98.14).[116]

Although any impingement or laceration of the spinal nerves or cord must be avoided, spinal implants may frequently contact the dura. It is unknown how often metallic or other material contact with the dura leads to adverse consequences. There are reports, for example, of late erosion of a cross-link into the dura.[117] In other cases, scar or implant encapsulation appears to protect the dura.

Medial screw misplacement frequently leads to a lateral durotomy. This area is difficult to access for direct repair and would typically require additional spinal destabilization and facet resection to reach. In one series of 695 patients, bone wax or simple screw placement was an adequate means of dural repair.[118] This is particularly important in the thoracic spine, where the pedicles are often narrow and the dura typically abuts the medial pedicle border.

Although use of bicortical screw fixation in anterior cervical plating constructs has decreased, there are no reports of late dural injury, perhaps due to the interposition of the posterior longitudinal ligament.

Vascular Structures

After cord injury, injury to one of the great vessels or vertebral arteries is the next most dreaded intraoperative complication of spine surgery. Potential injuries include laceration, impingement with late injury or fistula formation, impingement with vascular embarrassment of the vascular territory served by the vessel, and pseudoaneurysm formation (Fig. 98.15).

In many cases, screws have remained in contact with major vessels for long periods of time without sequelae. Foxx and colleagues monitored 33 screws in contact with major vessels

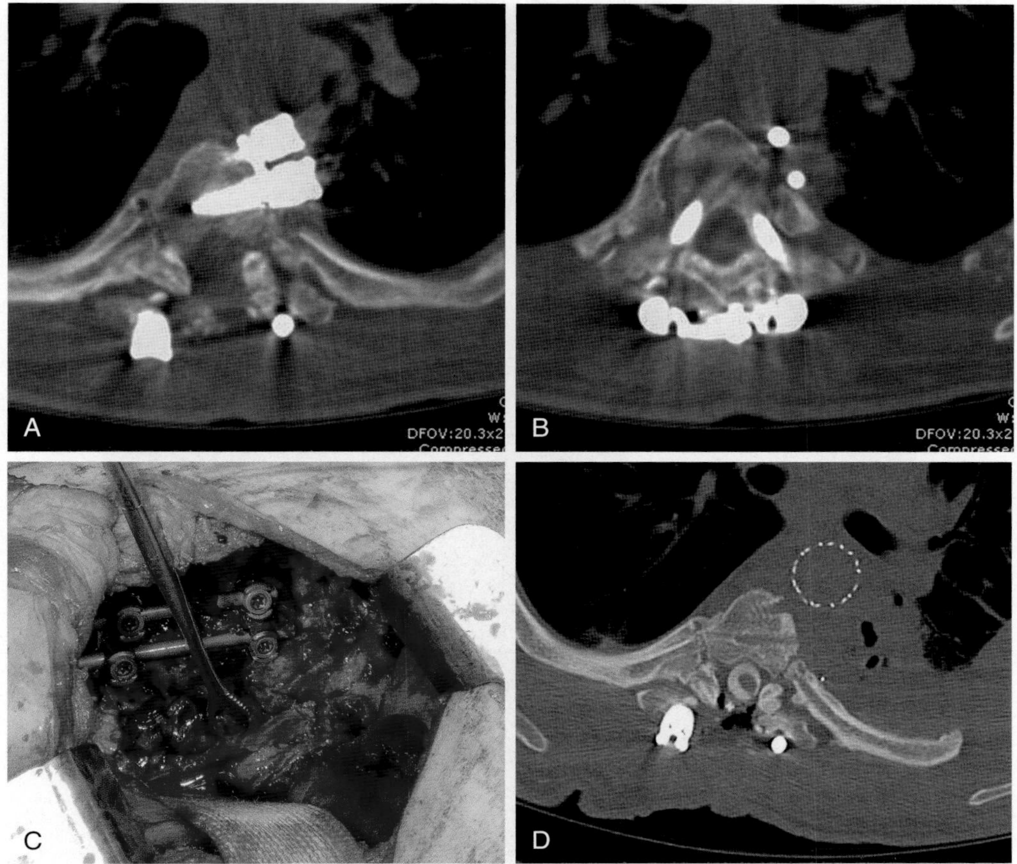

FIG. 98.15 This patient underwent anterior corpectomy with both anterior and posterior screw-rod reconstruction for a complex, neglected thoracic fracture-dislocation. Eight months after surgery, vascular symptoms consistent with an aortobronchial fistula were encountered. (A–B) Computed tomography (CT) demonstrated contact between the screw heads and the aorta. (C) The patient was taken to the operating room for vascular repair and anterior implant removal. (D) Follow-up CT scanning shows an aortic stenting and implant removal.

for a mean of 44 months without incident.[119] It should be noted that none of the screws penetrated or deformed the vessel in which it was in contact. The authors suggested that the "risk of repositioning a screw in contact with a major vessel but causing no symptoms must be weighed against the relative risk of leaving it in place."

However, the impact of implant contact on anterior vascular structures continues to be debated. Individual cases of acute hemorrhage, erosions, and pseudoaneurysm formation have been reported. Vertebral artery injury with screw placement is a well-known complication in cervical spine procedures. In one case, after resuscitation of massive intraoperative hemorrhage, a 7.0 cm postoperative pseudoaneurysm was reported.[120]

A case of lower extremity cyanosis beginning 15 days after transpedicular instrumentation placement for an L1 burst fracture was recently reported.[121] A 2.5 mm anterior perforation of the anterior cortex of L2 by the left pedicle screw was noted in association with complete obliteration of the infrarenal aorta.

Removal of anterior thoracolumbar implants is considered riskier due to the proximity of the major abdominal vessels. Recently, 617 consecutive anterior approaches were reported.[122] Implant removal cases, body mass index greater than 30, and multilevel exposures were found to be related to deep vein thrombosis, lymphedema, wound infection, and hospital readmission. These factors were not statistically related to major vessel injury. The authors concluded that reapproach of the thoracolumbar spine can be undertaken safely in patients with a body mass index less than 30 (Figs. 98.16 and 98.17).

Although posterior approaches in the thoracolumbar spine do not directly affect the vessels anteriorly, screw or cage placement may cause injuries. These injuries are very difficult to control in the absence of direct exposure. Posterior upper cervical approaches place the vertebral artery at risk, but screw placement anywhere above C7 increases that risk. As previously discussed, vertebral artery anatomy may preclude safe placement of some implant types in some patients or on some sides.

Anterior approaches to the spine risk direct injury during exposure or decompression. Although possible with any implant-related spine surgery, soft tissue injuries incurred during retraction, drilling, tapping, and placing screws or

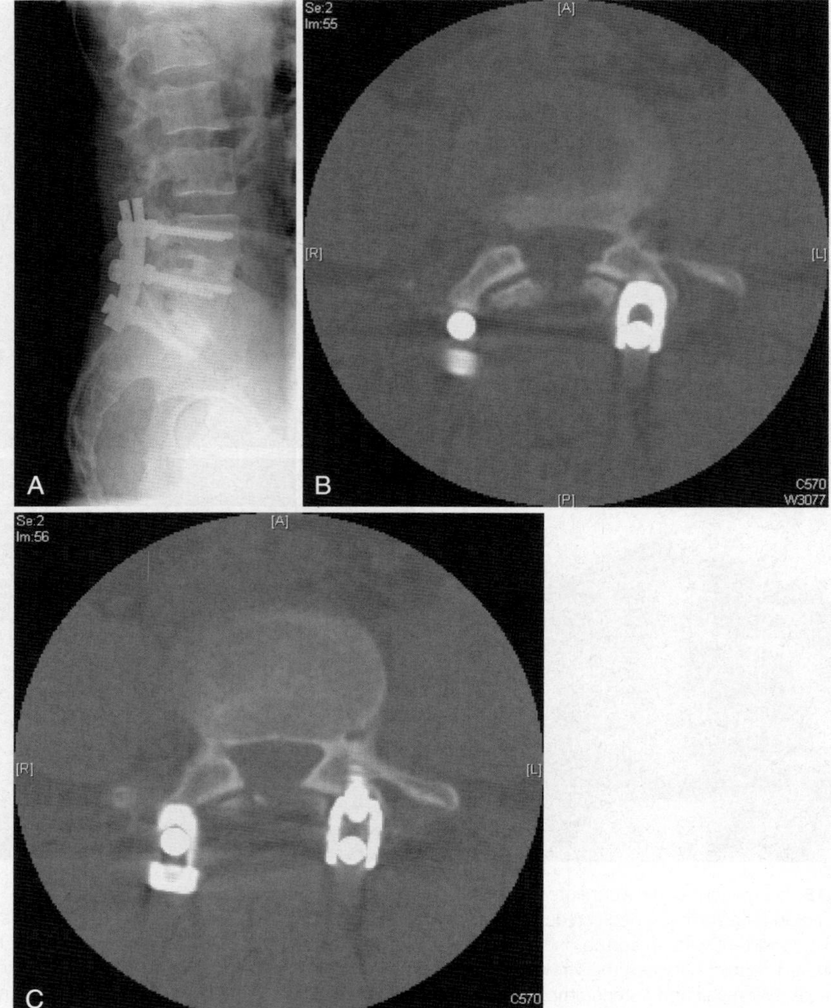

FIG. 98.16 (A) Lateral radiography of a patient who underwent a posterior fusion attempt at L4–S1 and then a later anterior fusion for a posterior pseudarthrosis. Note the position of the pedicle screws at L4; they appear to be set close to the mobile L3–L4 facet joint and traverse the pedicle parallel to its axis. (B–C) Axial computed tomography images at the L3–L4 facet/L4 pedicle level of the same patient. Note that the L4 pedicle screws violate the L3–L4 facet joints. Facet joint violation increases the patient's risk for adjacent-segment degeneration. The complication is an error in application and can be avoided by a more lateral entry point with a more medialized trajectory.

other hardware are more likely with anterior approaches, particularly anterior cervical approaches. Anterior thoracolumbar surgery often relies on lateral approaches. Typically, an approach from the left aortic side is favored due to the greater toughness of that vessel. Prevention is the key; full release of the soft tissues for proper exposure will decrease risk, as will use of drill and tap guides.

Bone and Joint

Implants may cause late disturbance to any bone or joint against which they abut. Four patients who underwent successful posterior C1–C2 fusion but reported pain on extension or crepitus were recently reported. Imaging revealed erosion of the occiput where the C1 fixation made contact with it.[123]

Another report recently described intradural migration of posterior cervical rods in a patient after open reduction and internal fixation of a C5–C6 fracture-dislocation in which no laminectomy had been performed.[124]

Screw placement may also affect adjacent-segment degeneration rates. In one recent study of 210 patents with a 9-year follow-up, patients with screws placed farther from the facet joint surface had lower rates of adjacent-segment degeneration (see Fig. 98.17).[125]

Other Soft Tissue Impingement

Spinal alignment can affect airway patency, especially with occipitocervical fusion procedures. One recent study suggested close attention to the occiput–C2 fixation angle to avoid

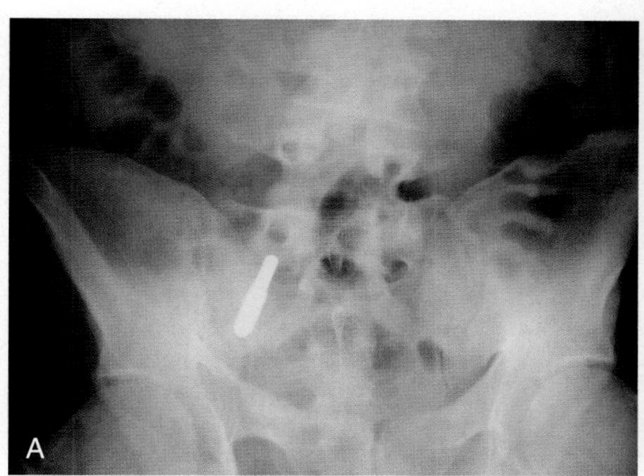

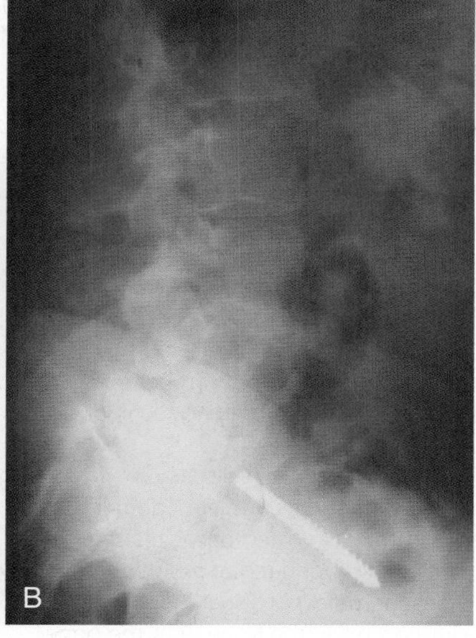

FIG. 98.17 During an attempt at removal of loose pedicle screws in the context of lumbar pseudarthrosis, one of the screws was inadvertently dislodged anteriorly. General surgery performed a combined retroperitoneal and transperitoneal removal of the screw.

airway obstruction, especially in patients with large tongues or micrognathia.[126] In this study, this angle tended toward flexion of 5 to 18 degrees in cases of airway obstruction.

In one series of 1789 patients undergoing anterior cervical discectomy and fusion, 74 underwent radiographic evaluation for dysphagia. Hardware or bone graft displacement was responsible for 18 of these cases and was more likely in the mid and upper cervical spine.[127]

The prominence of posterior screw-rod systems relative to the extensor compartment soft tissues of the spine has led some surgeons to recommend elective implant removal after soft tissue healing. The benefits of this additional surgery continue to be debated. In one recent series, implant removal was reported to reduce pain, especially in patients with higher pelvic incidence.[128] Fascial dehiscence and wound healing problems were reported in up to 9% of cases, however. One recent small study reported a decrease, but not elimination of, back pain in 80% of their heterogeneous patient cohort.[129]

Conclusions

Complications from spinal instrumentation are any undesirable and unexpected result stemming from placement of those implants. To be a significant complication, it must affect the patient and would not have occurred had implant placement "gone as well as could reasonably be hoped."[1]

Complication avoidance, and addressing complications once they occur, require a detailed understanding of the patient's underlying biology and the pathophysiology of his or her spinal condition. Expertise in spinal biomechanics and the ways in which various constructs affect the load bearing of the intact and diseased spine are required to select the most appropriate implants for the patient's condition. Once a primary (and back-up) strategy are in place, meticulous attention to detail during surgery will reduce the damage to surrounding healthy tissue and minimize the rate of implant malposition. A great surgeon will realize when aborting the current plan is required due to the patient's intraoperative hemodynamics, visualization difficulties, or unexpected findings.

Terrific tools, from intraoperative neurophysiologic monitoring to axial imaging and navigation, are now available. These will be helpful adjuncts, not mission-critical elements required for the surgery to proceed. These modalities have limitations, and the surgeon's instincts and deep understanding of spinal anatomy, mechanics, and physiology are key to reduce the complication rate.

KEY POINTS

1. Not all suboptimal outcomes of surgery are related to a complication.
2. Complication avoidance requires the following:
   - Preoperative attention to the patient's individual biology and anatomy. Bone quality assessment, smoking cessation, and perioperative glucose control, among other factors, can have a marked effect on complication rates.
   - Intraoperative attention to the patient's homeostasis. Support of appropriate hemoglobin levels and mean arterial pressure will reduce cardiopulmonary and, in some cases, neurologic complications.
   - Intraoperative attention to the patient's anatomy. Proper exposure and/or imaging guidance allow proper implant placement. The first step is proper intraoperative positioning.
   - Postoperative attention to the patient's recovery. Close attention to nutritional status, wound healing, spine loading and, when necessary, radiographic implant position and fusion progression allow early detection of minor problems before major complications ensue.

3. Avoiding late failure of spinal implants requires understanding forces to which the spine will be subjected, planes in which the spine is unstable, how the implants are meant to counteract these forces, and how instrumentation affects forces passing through structural grafts.
4. Most spine implants today are overengineered for their intended purpose. Thus fracturing of the implant itself is most likely a result of the following:
   - Iatrogenic weakness through notching or overbending. This can be reduced through consideration of bony anchor placement relative to the levels above and below and replacement of overbent rods.
   - Failure to achieve bony union. This can be reduced by careful attention to decortication and grafting technique and material.
   - Particularly high stress regions in a construct. This can be reduced by using thicker rods or plates, doubling the rods, or using hinged constructs at osteotomy sites, the occipitocervical junction, and regions with unreconstructed anterior load-bearing defects.
5. Most implant failure occurs in the bone or at the bone-implant junction. Methods to reduce this failure include the following:
   - Careful attention to fusion technique
   - Anterior interbody grafting at high-risk zones (e.g., lumbosacral junction)
   - Avoiding anterior interbody devices, when possible, in markedly osteoporotic patients
   - Augmenting the bone, when appropriate, with polymethylmethacrylate or other materials
   - Increasing the number of bone anchors (including hooks, tape, and cables)
   - Maximizing pedicle fill
   - Judicious use of bicortical fixation
   - Avoiding excessive preload on the implants
   - When necessary, perioperative antiosteoporotic medications and postoperative bracing

KEY REFERENCES

1. Sokol DK, Wilson J. What is a surgical complication? *World J Surg.* 2008;32(6):942-944.
   The term complication has always been loaded from a medicolegal standpoint. When used incorrectly to include any adverse surgical outcome or differently by different caregivers, it can lessen trust and weaken the therapeutic bond with the patient. In the era of surgeon report cards and value-based payments, a reasonable, uniform nomenclature has never been more important. This essay is a must-read for all surgeons.
2. Radcliff KE, Neusner AD, Millhouse PW, et al. What is new in the diagnosis and prevention of spine surgical site infections? *Spine J.* 2015;15(2):336-347.
   Postoperative wound healing and infection problems remain problematic. In this study, the authors discuss preoperative risk stratification and optimization, intraoperative prevention, and postoperative infection detection strategies.
3. Ohtori S, Inoue G, Orita S, et al. Comparison of teriparatide and bisphosphonate treatment to reduce pedicle screw loosening after lumbar spinal fusion surgery in postmenopausal women with osteoporosis from a bone quality perspective. *Spine.* 2013;38(8):E487-E492.
   With the aging of the population and increased survivorship among patients with metastatic disease and other conditions that compromise bone quality, achieving satisfactory fixation will be an increasing challenge. Ohtori and coworkers have published a number of studies examining postoperative antiosteoporotic management with bisphosphonates or teriparatide. In this study, 62 women undergoing one- and two-level decompression and fusion for degenerative spondylolisthesis were divided into three groups. These groups included teriparatide administration, bisphosphonate administration, and a control group. As expected, the slow mechanism of bisphosphonates did not yield appreciable improvements in screw-holding power over the control group. The teriparatide group, on the other hand, was found to have a much lower rate of screw loosening. Spine surgeons must increasingly be aware of bone density issues and address them preoperatively when possible. When more urgent surgery is required, postoperative antiosteoporotic management will likely reduce implant-related complications.
4. Kassis SZ, Abukwedar LK, Msaddi AK, Majer CN, Othman W. Combining pedicle screw stimulation with spinal navigation, a protocol to maximize the safety of neural elements and minimize radiation exposure in thoracolumbar spine instrumentation. *Eur Spine J.* 2016;25(6):1724-1728.
   Screw malposition remains a challenge in spine surgery. Aside from simply reducing the mechanical benefits of the screw, permanent nerve injury, durotomy, and unintended return to the operating room are among the sequelae of misplacement. A number of tools and techniques have been devised to improve screw placement rates. The authors of this study used a workflow that combines three-dimensional navigation and electromyographic screw stimulation to optimize screw placement before wound closure.
5. He B, Yan L, Guo H, et al. The difference in superior adjacent segment pathology after lumbar posterolateral fusion by using 2 different pedicle screw insertion techniques in 9-year minimum follow-up. *Spine.* 2014;39(14):1093-1098.
   Regardless of the initial indication for surgery, over the long term, adjacent-segment problems remain a serious concern. This study followed 210 patients with isthmic spondylolisthesis for a minimum of 9 years. They found that pedicle screw trajectories that position the implant farther from the joint surface significantly decrease the rate of adjacent-segment problems.

REFERENCES

1. Sokol DK, Wilson J. What is a surgical complication? *World J Surg.* 2008;32(6):942-944.
2. Hart RA, Marshall LM, Hiratzka SL, et al. Functional limitations due to stiffness as a collateral impact of instrumented arthrodesis of the lumbar spine. *Spine.* 2014;39(24):E1468-E1474.
3. Cunin V. Early-onset scoliosis: current treatment. *Orthop Traumatol Surg Res.* 2015;101(1 suppl):S109-S118.
4. Chapman TM, Blizzard DJ, Brown CR. CT accuracy of percutaneous versus open pedicle screw techniques: a series of 1609 screws. *Eur Spine J.* 2016;25(6):1781-1786. Erratum 2016;25(3):970.
5. Kennedy BC, D'Amico RS, Youngerman BE, et al. Long-term growth and alignment after occipitocervical and atlantoaxial fusion with rigid internal fixation in young children. *J Neurosurg Pediatr.* 2016;17(1):94-102.
6. Quraishi NA, Rajabian A, Spencer A, et al. Reoperation rates in the surgical treatment of spinal metastases. *Spine J.* 2015;15(3 suppl):S37-S43.
7. Bydon M, De la Garza-Ramos R, Abt NB, et al. Durotomy is associated with pseudoarthrosis following lumbar fusion. *J Clin Neurosci.* 2015;22(3):544-548.
8. Fujimori T, Yaszay B, Bartley CE, Bastrom TP, Newton PO. Safety of pedicle screws and spinal instrumentation

for pediatric patients: comparative analysis between 0- and 5-year-old, 5- and 10-year-old, and 10- and 15-year-old patients. *Spine*. 2014;39(7):541-549.
9. Chen SH, Lee CH, Huang KC, Hsieh PH, Tsai SY. Postoperative wound infection after posterior spinal instrumentation: analysis of long-term treatment outcomes. *Eur Spine J*. 2015;24(3):561-570.
10. Weinstein MA, McCabe JP, Cammisa FP Jr. Postoperative spinal wound infection: a review of 2,391 consecutive index procedures. *J Spinal Disord*. 2000;13(5):422-426.
11. Massie JB, Heller JG, Abitbol JJ, McPherson D, Garfin SR. Postoperative posterior spinal wound infections. *Clin Orthop Relat Res*. 1992;284:99-108.
12. Spivak JM, Petrizzo AM. Revision of a lumbar disc arthroplasty following late infection. *Eur Spine J*. 2010; 19(5):677-681.
13. Arens S, Schlegel U, Printzen G, et al. Influence of materials for fixation implants on local infection. An experimental study of steel versus titanium DCP in rabbits. *J Bone Joint Surg Br*. 1996;78(4):647-651.
14. Wang JC, Yu WD, Sandhu HS, et al. Metal debris from titanium spinal implants. *Spine*. 1999;24(9):899-903.
15. Cunningham BW, Orbegoso CM, Dmitriev AE, et al. The effect of titanium particulate on development and maintenance of a posterolateral spinal arthrodesis: an in vivo rabbit model. *Spine*. 2002;27(18):1971-1981.
16. Cundy WJ, Mascarenhas AR, Antoniou G, Freeman BJ, Cundy PJ. Local and systemic metal ion release occurs intraoperatively during correction and instrumented spinal fusion for scoliosis. *J Child Orthop*. 2015;9(1):39-43.
17. Cundy TP, Cundy WJ, Antoniou G, et al. Serum titanium, niobium and aluminium levels two years following instrumented spinal fusion in children: Does implant surface area predict serum metal ion levels? *Eur Spine J*. 2014;23(11):2393-2400.
18. Savarino L, Greggi T, Martikos K, et al. Long-term systemic metal distribution in patients with stainless steel spinal instrumentation: a case-control study. *J Spinal Disord Tech*. 2015;28(3):114-118.
19. Inanami H, Oshima Y, Iwahori T, et al. Role of 18F-fluoro-D-deoxyglucose PET/CT in diagnosing surgical site infection after spine surgery with instrumentation. *Spine*. 2015;40(2):109-113.
20. Wang Y, Cheung JP, Cheung KM. Use of PET/CT in the early diagnosis of implant-related wound infection and avoidance of wound debridement. *Eur Spine J*. 2016;25(suppl 1):38-43.
21. Chaichana KL, Bydon M, Santiago-Dieppa DR, et al. Risk of infection following posterior instrumented lumbar fusion for degenerative spine disease in 817 consecutive cases. *J Neurosurg Spine*. 2014;20(1):45-52.
22. Hikata T, Iwanami A, Hosogane N, et al. High preoperative hemoglobin A1c is a risk factor for surgical site infection after posterior thoracic and lumbar spinal instrumentation surgery. *J Orthop Sci*. 2014;19(2):223-228.
23. Klein JD, Hey LA, Yu CS, et al. Perioperative nutrition and postoperative complications in patients undergoing spinal surgery. *Spine*. 1996;21(22):2676-2682.
24. De la Garza-Ramos R, Bydon M, Macki M, et al. Instrumented fusion in the setting of primary spinal infection. *J Neurosurg Sci*. 2017;61(1):64-76.
25. Park KH, Cho OH, Lee YM, et al. Therapeutic outcomes of hematogenous vertebral osteomyelitis with instrumented surgery. *Clin Infect Dis*. 2015;60(9):1330-1338.
26. Talia AJ, Wong ML, Lau HC, Kaye AH. Safety of instrumentation and fusion at the time of surgical debridement for spinal infection. *J Clin Neurosci*. 2015;22(7):1111-1116.
27. Lu ML, Niu CC, Tsai TT, et al. Transforaminal lumbar interbody debridement and fusion for the treatment of infective spondylodiscitis in the lumbar spine. *Eur Spine J*. 2015;24(3):555-560.
28. Bydon M, De la Garza-Ramos R, Macki M, et al. Spinal instrumentation in patients with primary spinal infections does not lead to greater recurrent infection rates: an analysis of 118 cases. *World Neurosurg*. 2014;82(6):e807-e814.
29. Arnold R, Rock C, Croft L, Gilliam BL, Morgan DJ. Factors associated with treatment failure in vertebral osteomyelitis requiring spinal instrumentation. *Antimicrob Agents Chemother*. 2014;58(2):880-884.
30. Radcliff KE, Neusner AD, Millhouse PW, et al. What is new in the diagnosis and prevention of spine surgical site infections. *Spine J*. 2015;15(2):336-347.
31. Garg S, LaGreca J, Hotchkiss M, Erickson M. Management of late (>1 y) deep infection after spinal fusion: a retrospective cohort study. *J Pediatr Orthop*. 2015;35(3):266-270.
32. Lall RR, Wong AP, Lall RR, et al. Evidence-based management of deep wound infection after spinal instrumentation. *J Clin Neurosci*. 2015;22(2):238-242.
33. Khoshbin A, Lysenko M, Law P, Wright JG. Outcomes of infection following pediatric spinal fusion. *Can J Surg*. 2015;58(2):107-113.
34. Chieng LO, Hubbard Z, Salgado CJ, Levi AD, Chim H. Reconstruction of open wounds as a complication of spinal surgery with flaps: a systematic review. *Neurosurg Focus*. 2015;39(4):E17.
35. Onen MR, Yuvruk E, Karagoz G, Naderi S. Efficiency of hyperbaric oxygen therapy in iatrogenic spinal infections. *Spine*. 2015;40(22):1743-1748.
36. Sawin PD, Dickman CA, Crawford NR, et al. The effects of dexamethasone on bone fusion in an experimental model of posterolateral lumbar spinal arthrodesis. *J Neurosurg*. 2001;94(1 suppl):76-81.
37. Lu ML, Tsai TT, Lai PL, et al. A retrospective study of treating thoracolumbar spine fractures in ankylosing spondylitis. *Eur J Orthop Surg Traumatol*. 2014;24(suppl 1):S117-S123.
38. Niimi R, Kono T, Nishihara A, et al. A retrospective analysis of nonresponse to daily teriparatide treatment. *Osteoporos Int*. 2016;27(9):2845-2853.
39. Choma TJ, Rechtine G, McGuire RA, Brodke DS. Treating the aging spine. *Instr Course Lect*. 2016;65:269-279.
40. Tu CW, Huang KF, Hsu HT, et al. Zoledronic acid infusion for lumbar interbody fusion in osteoporosis. *J Surg Res*. 2014;192(1):112-116.
41. Ohtori S, Inoue G, Orita S, et al. Teriparatide accelerates lumbar posterolateral fusion in women with postmenopausal osteoporosis: prospective study. *Spine*. 2012;37(23):E1464-E1468.
42. Niimi R, Kono T, Nishihara A, et al. The relationship of BMD increases between the first 12 months and the latter 12 months by daily teriparatide treatment. *Calcif Tissue Int*. 2016.
43. Ohtori S, Orita S, Yamauchi K, et al. More than 6 months of teriparatide treatment was more effective for bone union than shorter treatment following lumbar posterolateral fusion surgery. *Asian Spine J*. 2015;9(4):573-580.
44. Ohtori S, Inoue G, Orita S, et al. Comparison of teriparatide and bisphosphonate treatment to reduce pedicle screw loosening after lumbar spinal fusion surgery

in postmenopausal women with osteoporosis from a bone quality perspective. *Spine*. 2013;38(8):E487-E492.
45. Truumees E, Demetropoulos CK, Yang KH, Herkowitz HN. Failure of human cervical endplates: a cadaveric experimental model. *Spine*. 2003;28(19):2204-2208.
46. Hasegawa K, Abe M, Washio T, Hara T. An experimental study on the interface strength between titanium mesh cage and vertebra in reference to vertebral bone mineral density. *Spine*. 2001;26(8):957-963.
47. Jost B, Cripton PA, Lund T, et al. Compressive strength of interbody cages in the lumbar spine: the effect of cage shape, posterior instrumentation and bone density. *Eur Spine J*. 1998;7(2):132-141.
48. Mattei TA, Rehman AA, Issawi A, Fassett DR. Surgical challenges in the management of cervical kyphotic deformity in patients with severe osteoporosis: an illustrative case of a patient with Hajdu-Cheney syndrome. *Eur Spine J*. 2015;24(12):2746-2753.
49. Goldstein CL, Brodke DS, Choma TJ. Surgical management of spinal conditions in the elderly osteoporotic spine. *Neurosurgery*. 2015;77(suppl 4):S98-S107.
50. Chang MC, Liu CL, Chen TH. Polymethylmethacrylate augmentation of pedicle screw for osteoporotic spinal surgery: a novel technique. *Spine*. 2008;33(10):E317-E324.
51. Glassman SD, Alegre GM. Adult spinal deformity in the osteoporotic spine: options and pitfalls. *Instr Course Lect*. 2003;52:579-588.
52. Huang RC, Lim MR, Girardi FP, Cammisa FP Jr. The prevalence of contraindications to total disc replacement in a cohort of lumbar surgical patients. *Spine*. 2004;29(22): 2538-2541.
53. Guzman JZ, Feldman ZM, McAnany S, et al. Osteoporosis in cervical spine surgery. *Spine*. 2016;41(8):662-668.
54. Dua K, Kepler CK, Huang RC, Marchenko A. Vertebral body fracture after anterolateral instrumentation and interbody fusion in two osteoporotic patients. *Spine J*. 2010;10(9):e11-e15.
55. Kim SK, Chung JY, Seo HY, Lee WG. Vertebral compression fracture within a solid fusion mass without trauma after removal of pedicle screws. *Spine J*. 2016;16(3):e219-e223.
56. Andersen T, Christensen FB, Laursen M, et al. Smoking as a predictor of negative outcome in lumbar spinal fusion. *Spine*. 2001;26(23):2623-2628.
57. Hilibrand AS, Fye MA, Emery SE, Palumbo MA, Bohlman HH. Impact of smoking on the outcome of anterior cervical arthrodesis with interbody or strut-grafting. *J Bone Joint Surg Am*. 2001;83-A(5):668-673.
58. Glassman SD, Anagnost SC, Parker A, et al. The effect of cigarette smoking and smoking cessation on spinal fusion. *Spine*. 2000;25(20):2608-2615.
59. McPhee IB, Williams RP, Swanson CE. Factors influencing wound healing after surgery for metastatic disease of the spine. *Spine*. 1998;23(6):726-732, discussion 732-723.
60. Wise JJ, Fischgrund JS, Herkowitz HN, Montgomery D, Kurz LT. Complication, survival rates, and risk factors of surgery for metastatic disease of the spine. *Spine*. 1999;24(18):1943-1951.
61. Ahmadian A, Bach K, Bolinger B, et al. Stand-alone minimally invasive lateral lumbar interbody fusion: multicenter clinical outcomes. *J Clin Neurosci*. 2015; 22(4):740-746.
62. Pitzen T, Matthis D, Steudel WI. The effect of posterior instrumentation following PLIF with BAK cages is most pronounced in weak bone. *Acta Neurochir (Wien)*. 2002;144(2):121-128, discussion 128.
63. Barton C, Noshchenko A, Patel V, et al. Risk factors for rod fracture after posterior correction of adult spinal deformity with osteotomy: a retrospective case-series. *Scoliosis*. 2015;10:30.
64. Aghayev E, Zullig N, Diel P, Dietrich D, Benneker LM. Development and validation of a quantitative method to assess pedicle screw loosening in posterior spine instrumentation on plain radiographs. *Eur Spine J*. 2014;23(3):689-694.
65. McAfee PC, Weiland DJ, Carlow JJ. Survivorship analysis of pedicle spinal instrumentation. *Spine*. 1991;16(8 suppl): S422-S427.
66. Sayama C, Willsey M, Chintagumpala M, et al. Routine use of recombinant human bone morphogenetic protein-2 in posterior fusions of the pediatric spine and incidence of cancer. *J Neurosurg Pediatr*. 2015;16(1):4-13.
67. Sayama C, Hadley C, Monaco GN, et al. The efficacy of routine use of recombinant human bone morphogenetic protein-2 in occipitocervical and atlantoaxial fusions of the pediatric spine: a minimum of 12 months' follow-up with computed tomography. *J Neurosurg Pediatr*. 2015;16(1):14-20.
68. Chun DS, Baker KC, Hsu WK. Lumbar pseudarthrosis: a review of current diagnosis and treatment. *Neurosurg Focus*. 2015;39(4):E10.
69. Toohey JS, Stromberg L, Neidre A, Ramsey M, Fogel GR. Treatment of cervical pseudarthrosis after Smith-Robinson procedure with Halifax clamp fixation. *J Surg Orthop Adv*. 2006;15(4):201-202.
70. Amankulor NM, Xu R, Iorgulescu JB, et al. The incidence and patterns of hardware failure after separation surgery in patients with spinal metastatic tumors. *Spine J*. 2014;14(9): 1850-1859.
71. Sanden B, Olerud C, Petren-Mallmin M, et al. The significance of radiolucent zones surrounding pedicle screws. Definition of screw loosening in spinal instrumentation. *J Bone Joint Surg Br*. 2004;457-461.
72. Wu JC, Huang WC, Tsai HW, et al. Pedicle screw loosening in dynamic stabilization: incidence, risk, and outcome in 126 patients. *Neurosurg Focus*. 2011;31(4):E9.
73. Bayri Y, Eksi MS, Dogrul R, Koc DY, Konya D. Migration of rod into retroperitoneal region: a case report and review of the literature. *Korean J Spine*. 2014;11(4):241-244.
74. Gruskay JA, Webb ML, Grauer JN. Methods of evaluating lumbar and cervical fusion. *Spine J*. 2014;14(3):531-539.
75. Dickson DD, Lenke LG, Bridwell KH, Koester LA. Risk factors for and assessment of symptomatic pseudarthrosis after lumbar pedicle subtraction osteotomy in adult spinal deformity. *Spine*. 2014;39(15):1190-1195.
76. Schreiber U, Bence T, Grupp T, et al. Is a single anterolateral screw-plate fixation sufficient for the treatment of spinal fractures in the thoracolumbar junction? A biomechanical in vitro investigation. *Eur Spine J*. 2005;14(2):197-204.
77. Segal D, Whitelaw GP, Gumbs V, Pick RY. Tension band fixation of acute cervical spine fractures. *Clin Orthop*. 1981; 159:211-222.
78. Lowry DW, Lovely TJ, Rastogi P. Comparison of tension band wiring and lateral mass plating for subaxial posterior cervical fusion. *Surg Neurol*. 1998;50(4):323-331, discussion 331-322.
79. al Baz MO, Mathur N. Modified technique of tension band wiring in flexion injuries of the middle and lower cervical spine. *Spine*. 1995;20(11):1241-1244.

80. Benzel E. *Biomechanics of Spine Stabilization: Principles and Clinical Practice*. New York: McGraw-Hill; 1995.
81. Benzel EC. Short-segment compression instrumentation for selected thoracic and lumbar spine fractures: the short-rod/two-claw technique. *J Neurosurg*. 1993;79(3):335-340.
82. Pellise F, Barastegui D, Hernandez-Fernandez A, et al. Viability and long-term survival of short-segment posterior fixation in thoracolumbar burst fractures. *Spine J*. 2015;15(8):1796-1803.
83. Yang K, King A. Mechanism of facet load transmission as a hypothesis for low back pain. *Spine*. 1984;9:557-565.
84. An HS, Vaccaro A, Cotler JM, Lin S. Spinal disorders at the cervicothoracic junction. *Spine*. 1994;19(22):2557-2564.
85. Wu SS, Hwa SY, Lin LC, et al. Management of rigid post-traumatic kyphosis. *Spine*. 1996;21(19):2260-2266, discussion 2267.
86. Luca A, Lovi A, Galbusera F, Brayda-Bruno M. Revision surgery after PSO failure with rod breakage: a comparison of different techniques. *Eur Spine J*. 2014;23(suppl 6):610-615.
87. Smith JS, Shaffrey E, Klineberg E, et al. Prospective multicenter assessment of risk factors for rod fracture following surgery for adult spinal deformity. *J Neurosurg Spine*. 2014;21(6):994-1003.
88. Guler UO, Cetin E, Yaman O, et al. Sacropelvic fixation in adult spinal deformity (ASD): a very high rate of mechanical failure. *Eur Spine J*. 2015;24(5):1085-1091.
89. Bernstein P, Hentschel S, Platzek I, et al. Thoracal flat back is a risk factor for lumbar disc degeneration after scoliosis surgery. *Spine J*. 2014;14(6):925-932.
90. Kast E, Mohr K, Richter HP, Borm W. Complications of transpedicular screw fixation in the cervical spine. *Eur Spine J*. 2006;15(3):327-334.
91. Sudo H, Abumi K, Ito M, Kotani Y, Minami A. Spinal cord compression by multistrand cables after solid posterior atlantoaxial fusion. Report of three cases. *J Neurosurg*. 2002;97(3 suppl):359-361.
92. Abumi K. Cervical spondylotic myelopathy: posterior decompression and pedicle screw fixation. *Eur Spine J*. 2015;24(suppl 2):186-196.
92a. Reinhold M, Magerl F, Rieger M, Blauth M. Cervical pedicle screw placement: feasibility and accuracy of two new insertion techniques based on morphometric data. *Eur Spine J*. 2007;16(1):47-56.
93. Al Barbarawi MM, Allouh MZ. Cervical lateral mass screw-rod fixation: surgical experience with 2500 consecutive screws, an analytical review, and long-term outcomes. *Br J Neurosurg*. 2015;29(5):699-704.
94. Gonzalvo A, Fitt G, Liew S, et al. Correlation between pedicle size and the rate of pedicle screw misplacement in the treatment of thoracic fractures: Can we predict how difficult the task will be? *Br J Neurosurg*. 2015;29(4):508-512.
95. Ghobrial GM, Williams KA Jr, Arnold P, Fehlings M, Harrop JS. Iatrogenic neurologic deficit after lumbar spine surgery: a review. *Clin Neurol Neurosurg*. 2015;139:76-80.
96. Donohue ML, Moquin RR, Singla A, Calancie B. Is in vivo manual palpation for thoracic pedicle screw instrumentation reliable? *J Neurosurg Spine*. 2014;20(5):492-496.
97. Parker SL, McGirt MJ, Farber SH, et al. Accuracy of free-hand pedicle screws in the thoracic and lumbar spine: analysis of 6816 consecutive screws. *Neurosurgery*. 2011;68(1):170-178, discussion 178.
98. Alhabib H, Nataraj A, Khashab M, et al. Pedicle screw insertion in the thoracolumbar spine: comparison of 4 guidance techniques in the intact cadaveric spine. *J Neurosurg Spine*. 2011;14(5):664-669.
99. Boon Tow BP, Yue WM, Srivastava A, et al. Does navigation improve accuracy of placement of pedicle screws in single-level lumbar degenerative spondylolisthesis? A comparison between free-hand and three-dimensional O-arm navigation techniques. *J Spinal Disord Tech*. 2015;28(8):E472-E477.
100. Luther N, Iorgulescu JB, Geannette C, et al. Comparison of navigated versus non-navigated pedicle screw placement in 260 patients and 1434 screws: screw accuracy, screw size, and the complexity of surgery. *J Spinal Disord Tech*. 2015;28(5):E298-E303.
101. Ryang YM, Villard J, Obermuller T, et al. Learning curve of 3D fluoroscopy image-guided pedicle screw placement in the thoracolumbar spine. *Spine J*. 2015;15(3):467-476.
102. Hecht N, Kamphuis M, Czabanka M, et al. Accuracy and workflow of navigated spinal instrumentation with the mobile AIRO CT scanner. *Eur Spine J*. 2016;25(3):716-723.
103. Elliott MJ, Slakey JB. CT provides precise size assessment of implanted titanium alloy pedicle screws. *Clin Orthop Relat Res*. 2014;472(5):1605-1609.
104. Dabaghi Richerand A, Christodoulou E, Li Y, et al. Comparison of effective dose of radiation during pedicle screw placement using intraoperative computed tomography navigation versus fluoroscopy in children with spinal deformities. *J Pediatr Orthop*. 2016;36(5):530-533.
105. Curylo LJ, Mason HC, Bohlman HH, Yoo JU. Tortuous course of the vertebral artery and anterior cervical decompression: a cadaveric and clinical case study. *Spine*. 2000;25(22):2860-2864.
106. Calancie B, Donohue ML, Harris CB, et al. Neuromonitoring with pulse-train stimulation for implantation of thoracic pedicle screws: a blinded and randomized clinical study. Part 1: methods and alarm criteria. *J Neurosurg Spine*. 2014;20(6):675-691.
107. Calancie B, Donohue ML, Moquin RR. Neuromonitoring with pulse-train stimulation for implantation of thoracic pedicle screws: a blinded and randomized clinical study. Part 2: the role of feedback. *J Neurosurg Spine*. 2014;20(6):692-704.
108. Kassis SZ, Abukwedar LK, Msaddi AK, Majer CN, Othman W. Combining pedicle screw stimulation with spinal navigation, a protocol to maximize the safety of neural elements and minimize radiation exposure in thoracolumbar spine instrumentation. *Eur Spine J*. 2016;25(6):1724-1728.
109. Gaines RW Jr. The use of pedicle-screw internal fixation for the operative treatment of spinal disorders. *J Bone Joint Surg Am*. 2000;82-A(10):1458-1476.
110. Abe Y, Ito M, Abumi K, et al. Scoliosis corrective force estimation from the implanted rod deformation using 3D-FEM analysis. *Scoliosis*. 2015;10(suppl 2):S2.
111. Yamanaka K, Mori M, Yamazaki K, et al. Analysis of the fracture mechanism of Ti-6Al-4V alloy rods that failed clinically after spinal instrumentation surgery. *Spine*. 2015;40(13):E767-E773.
112. Serhan H, Slivka M, Albert T, Kwak SD. Is galvanic corrosion between titanium alloy and stainless steel spinal implants a clinical concern? *Spine J*. 2004;4(4):379-387.
113. Jones AA, Dougherty PJ, Sharkey NA, Benson DR. Iliac crest bone graft. Osteotome versus saw. *Spine*. 1993;18(14):2048-2052.
114. Tullberg T. Failure of a carbon fiber implant. A case report. *Spine*. 1998;23(16):1804-1806.

115. Schwend RM, Waters PM, Hey LA, Hall JE, Emans JB. Treatment of severe spondylolisthesis in children by reduction and L4-S4 posterior segmental hyperextension fixation. *J Pediatr Orthop*. 1992;12(6):703-711.
116. Gandhoke GS, Kasliwal MK, Smith JS, et al. A multi-center evaluation of clinical and radiographic outcomes following high-grade spondylolisthesis reduction and fusion. *Clin Spine Surg*. 2016. Epub ahead of print.
117. Rahmathulla G, Deen HG. Spine fusion cross-link causing delayed dural erosion and CSF leak: case report. *J Neurosurg Spine*. 2015;22(4):439-443.
118. Feng B, Shen J, Zhang J, et al. How to deal with cerebrospinal fluid leak during pedicle screw fixation in spinal deformities surgery with intraoperative neuromonitoring change. *Spine*. 2014;39(1):E20-E25.
119. Foxx KC, Kwak RC, Latzman JM, Samadani U. A retrospective analysis of pedicle screws in contact with the great vessels. *J Neurosurg Spine*. 2010;13(3):403-406.
120. Guo S, Pan J, Li L, et al. Giant delayed pseudo-aneurysm following screw placement in C1 lateral mass. *Orthop Traumatol Surg Res*. 2014;100(6):691-694.
121. Blocher M, Mayer M, Resch H, Ortmaier R. Leriche-like syndrome as a delayed complication following posterior instrumentation of a traumatic L1 fracture: a case report and literature review. *Spine*. 2015;40(22):E1195-E1197.
122. Ballard JL, Carlson G, Chen J, White J. Anterior thoracolumbar spine exposure: critical review and analysis. *Ann Vasc Surg*. 2014;28(2):465-469.
123. Arizumi F, Moriyama T, Tachibana T, et al. Erosion in the occipital bone caused by the fixation instrument used for posterior atlantoaxial fusion—report of 4 cases. *Springerplus*. 2015;4:137.
124. Pulhorn H, Kareem H, Ulbricht C. Intradural migration of cervical posterior fixation rods. *Eur Spine J*. 2016;suppl 1: 6-10.
125. He B, Yan L, Guo H, et al. The difference in superior adjacent segment pathology after lumbar posterolateral fusion by using 2 different pedicle screw insertion techniques in 9-year minimum follow-up. *Spine*. 2014;39(14):1093-1098.
126. Huang M, Gonda DD, Briceno V, et al. Dyspnea and dysphagia from upper airway obstruction after occipitocervical fusion in the pediatric age group. *Neurosurg Focus*. 2015;38(4):E13.
127. Carucci LR, Turner MA, Yeatman CF. Dysphagia secondary to anterior cervical fusion: radiologic evaluation and findings in 74 patients. *AJR Am J Roentgenol*. 2015;204(4): 768-775.
128. Jentzsch T, Gomes de Lima V, Seifert B, Sprengel K, Werner CM. The benefits of elective spinal implant removal: a retrospective study of 137 patients. *Eur Spine J*. 2016;25(3):856-864.
129. Ak H, Gulsen I, Atalay T, Gencer M. Does the removal of spinal implants reduce back pain? *J Clin Med Res*. 2015;7(6):460-463.

CHAPTER 99 Postoperative Spinal Infections

Sohrab Pahlavan
Yu-Po Lee
Nitin N. Bhatia

Introduction

Postoperative spinal wound infections are relatively frequent problems that treating spine surgeons must know how to diagnose and address. Although strategies to reduce the occurrence of infection after spine surgery have seen some success, infection rates of up to 20% continue to be reported in the literature. These infections result in significant acute and chronic morbidity to the patient and cause significant financial drain to the patient and the health care system. Because of the relatively high incidence and difficulty in diagnosis, there must be a thorough understanding of the diagnostic and management principles in order to successfully treat these patients. Current treatment strategies need to be continually revisited in order to address commonly encountered microorganisms and potential resistance patterns that may develop.

Successful infection management begins preoperatively with aseptic technique and proper antibiotic prophylaxis administration. Additionally, a thorough preoperative workup with careful attention to potential patient risk factors is essential. The astute surgeon must have keen examination skills and the clinical sense to initiate the diagnostic workup for a postoperative infection when there is any significant suspicion, particularly with deep wound infections. The results from a diagnostic workup are often vague and difficult to interpret. The decision to treat an infection solely with medical therapy versus with aggressive surgical debridement continues to be a relatively controversial topic. Prompt and successful infection eradication has significant influence on the success of the original surgery and the ultimate patient outcome.

Incidence/Epidemiology

Postoperative wound infections are among the most common complications following spinal surgery. The incidence documented in the literature has historically been quite variable, with reported ranges from 0.5% to 20%.[1–7] This discrepancy is in part due to significant variation in case complexity, use of instrumentation, the definition of infection, and surgical approach. In general, increasing the complexity and invasiveness of the surgery correlates with a higher incidence of infection. More recently, however, a review of the Scoliosis Research Society Mortality and Morbidity database revealed superficial and deep infection rates to be 0.8% and 1.3%, respectively.[8] This contrast to older studies with higher infection rates underlines improvements in surgical technique and prophylaxis protocols.

Historically, lower-risk spinal surgeries include those that do not require instrumentation. Discectomy and laminectomy have reported incidences of infection of less than 3%. With the addition of instrumentation, however, the incidence of postoperative infection increases to greater than 12% in some studies.[9–19] A recent series demonstrated that infection rates in cases with implants were 28% higher than cases without implants (2.3% vs. 1.8%).[8] Specifically, lumbar discectomy has had a reported incidence of 0.7%, and using a microscope for the procedure increases the incidence to 1.4%. In the United States, the National Nosocomial Infections Surveillance System, a voluntary performance-measurement system orchestrated by the Centers for Disease Control and Prevention, has reported a 1.25% rate of surgical site infection following laminectomy and a 2.1% rate following laminectomy with noninstrumented fusion.[20] More recently, a large case series demonstrated an infection rate of 2.4% in decompression cases, whereas fusion cases had a significantly higher rate at 3.5%.[21]

Consistently throughout the literature, cases that require more extensive soft tissue dissection, longer operative time, greater blood loss, more significant soft tissue devitalization, or the creation of dead space have an increased infection rate.[22–25] In one study, an index of surgical invasiveness was found to be the strongest risk factor for infection, even when controlling for comorbidities and other known risk factors.[25] Another study comparing infection rates in patients undergoing discectomy alone and those undergoing discectomy and fusion showed infection rates of 1% versus 6%, respectively. In other reports, fusion without instrumentation has been associated with an infection rate ranging from 0.4% to 4.3%.[26] Historically, a general consensus has been that the use of devitalized bone graft material in fusions results in an infection rate from 1% to 5%. Olsen et al., however, found no increase in infection rates with the use of bone graft[27]; a systematic review of the literature supported their findings.[28]

As the use of instrumentation has become more commonplace, attention must be paid to a possible associated increased infection risk. Colonization of implanted devices occurs in upward of 50% of patients, although most do not display clinical symptoms of infection. Although implants rarely act as the initial source of infection, they may become a nidus for inoculation and subclinical growth of infectious organisms. The implant provides an avascular surface upon which bacteria can create a glycocalyx, which serves as a barrier to the host immune response and antibiotic treatment. In addition, micromotion can create metallosis and subsequent granulomas, which may become a potential site for bacterial colonization. Other theories postulate that local soft tissue inflammation and postoperative seromas may serve as a potential cause for the increased infection risk seen with instrumented fusions (Fig. 99.1). Historically, there has been wide variation in infection rates, but more recent literature reports elective instrumented surgical cases between 2.8% and 6%,[9,29,30] with a recent review of retrospective studies showing a rate between 2.1% and 8.5%.[31] Many authors feel that the actual infection risk with the use of spinal instrumentation is between 5% and 6%.[17–19,29,32]

Spinal trauma patients represent a unique population that have an increased risk for developing postoperative infections. The significant soft tissue devitalization and devascularization caused by the traumatic event result in local hypoxia, leading to tissue necrosis, edema, acidosis, and hematoma formation. This combination results in a medium optimal for bacterial proliferation isolated from the host defenses.[33] Systemically, the patient sustaining major trauma shows a hyperinflammatory state with alterations in the normally tightly controlled homeostasis of proinflammatory and antiinflammatory cytokine levels. The resultant imbalance leads to a state of immunosuppression that is thought to increase susceptibility to infection.[34] In addition, comorbid factors such as age,[35] medical conditions, poor nutritional status, and body habitus cannot be controlled for in the same manner that they are in elective surgery. The presence of complete neurologic injury significantly increases the risk of postoperative infection, while the presence of an infection decreases functional neurologic recovery.[36] In the largest clinical series investigating 256 surgically treated traumatic spinal injuries, the rate of postoperative wound infections was 9.4% compared with an infection rate of 3.7% seen in patients undergoing elective spinal surgery during the same time period at the same hospital.[37] Interestingly, one multicenter cohort study demonstrated an infection rate of 4.6%, concluding a similar rate to elective patients.[38] Other reviews have found postoperative infection rates in spinal trauma patients ranging from 9% to 15%,[9,39,40] which is greater than the previously discussed average infection rate seen in elective spinal surgeries. Furthermore, a systematic review demonstrated that the rate of nonsurgical infections also are higher in trauma patients compared to nonoperative controls.[41]

Anterior spinal procedures appear to be less susceptible to infection than posterior procedures. Infection rates following anterior cervical spinal surgery have been reported in the literature to be as low as 0% to 1%.[42–44] Anterior thoracic and lumbar surgery also display significantly less infection risk than their posterior counterparts, with rates 50% lower than those occurring after posterior surgery. The infection rates for anterior approaches are likely decreased by multiple factors, including better vascularity of the spinal column and decreased dead space creation. Combined anterior and posterior approaches are an independent risk factor for infection,[8] especially in cases of staged surgeries.[45]

With the rise in minimally invasive surgery (MIS) in spine surgery, several studies have examined its effect on surgical site infection (SSI) rates. Several studies have shown decreased rates of infections using MIS techniques. In one multicenter study reviewing 1388 cases, the infection rate was 0.74% for fusions, 0.10% for decompressions, and 0.22% overall.[46] MIS transforaminal lumbar interbody fusion procedures also have been reported to have lower infection rates compared to open procedures. Parker et al.[47] demonstrated an SSI rate of 0.6% in MIS compared to 4.0% with open techniques, while McGirt et al.[48] had a 4.6% SSI rate with MIS and 7% with open surgery. Some studies, however, have shown no differences in SSI rates between MIS and open techniques.[49,50] In a prospective series, there was no difference in infection rates for single-level transforaminal lumbar interbody fusion.[49] Interestingly, in the study by Parker et al.,[47] in the subgroup of single-level fusions, there also was no difference with MIS compared to open techniques. In light of these findings, specific conclusions regarding the effects of MIS on infection risks cannot be made; for multilevel fusions, however, there appears to be a benefit.[51]

Risk Factors

Patient risk factors play a pivotal role in influencing postoperative spinal infections. Many of these risk factors are modifiable if addressed prior to surgery. Others are nonmodifiable and have been shown to increase postoperative infection risk. Careful attention to these factors must be made in the preoperative workup because correcting them may have a significant impact on the ultimate outcome of the surgery.

Modifiable risk factors include smoking, obesity, surgery length, prolonged indwelling catheter use, length of hospital stay, and malnutrition. The patient and surgeon should work together to address these risk factors preoperatively. Poorly controlled diabetics are one of the highest-risk patient populations, with an estimated incidence of postoperative infections of 17%. A recent systematic review demonstrated that there was a statistically significant association between diabetes and SSI in five out of eight studies and in four out of five studies elevated blood glucose raised the risk of infection threefold.[28] A level II study also showed a 4.10 adjusted relative risk of SSI in diabetics.[52] It is thought that elevated blood glucose concentrations, particularly those above 200 mg/dL, can inhibit

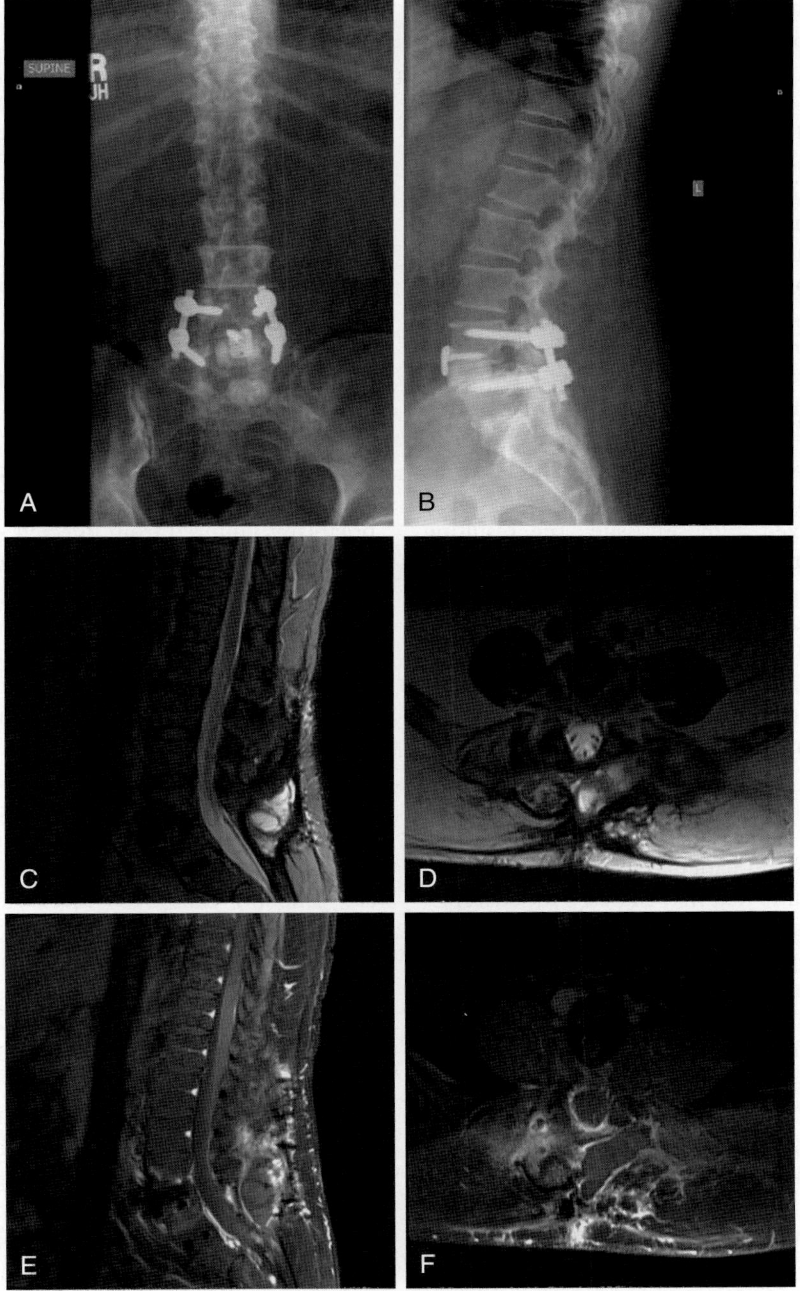

FIG. 99.1 (A) Anteroposterior and (B) lateral radiographs in a patient who had increasing low back pain and fevers following an anteroposterior lumbar decompression and fusion. (C) Sagittal T2 magnetic resonance image (MRI) shows postoperative fluid collection. (D) Axial T2-weighted MRI with loculated fluid collections posterior to the surgical site. (E) Sagittal T1-weighted MRI with contrast showing rim enhancement of the fluid collections, suggestive of infection. (F) Axial T1-weighted MRI with contrast with rim enhancement of the posterior fluid collection and diffuse contrast involvement of the soft tissue, suggestive of infection.

host immune response, including cellular chemotaxis and phagocytosis. In addition to creating a relatively immunocompromised state, poorly controlled diabetics are predisposed to chronic medical conditions, including hypertension, cardiovascular disease, and renal insufficiency. These medical issues predispose to poor tissue vascularity and can further increase postoperative infection and complication rates. Careful preoperative attention to tight blood glucose control and an assessment for other related factors may limit the risk of local infection and systemic morbidity in diabetics. In general, diabetics have increased complication rates, particularly with posterior lumbar surgery.

Malnutrition is an often underrecognized contributor to impaired healing potential of a patient. Approximately 25% of all elective lumbar fusion patients are malnourished.[53] In this same study, 11 of 13 complications in a group of 114 patients undergoing elective lumbar fusion were in malnourished patients, making them 15 times more likely to develop an infection. Serum albumin levels less than 3.5 g/dL, arm circumference less than 80% of normal, total lymphocyte count less than 1500/mm^3, recent weight loss greater than 10 pounds, transferrin levels less than 150 μg/dL, and abnormal skinfold measurements are all methods to evaluate nutritional status. Addressing the issue of malnourishment in the preoperative period is often underperformed and should be considered a major modifiable factor to limit poor healing.

Obese patients are also considered at high risk for developing postoperative infections.[54–56] Mehta et al. found that distribution of body mass actually is even more predictive of SSI than absolute BMI, with magnetic resonance imaging (MRI) measurements of skin-to-lamina distance and thickness of subcutaneous adipose layer being significant risk factors.[57] Overweight patients often require more extensive dissection through poorly vascularized adipose tissue. The resulting tissue devitalization and fat necrosis result in an environment favoring bacterial growth and proliferation. In addition, the increased operative time and blood loss necessary with obese patients increase their risk of infection. Obesity in itself is a risk factor for malnutrition, diabetes, and other medical comorbidities, further contributing to a poor healing environment with diminished immunogenic potential.

Smokers also have a significantly increased chance of developing postoperative infections.[22,23] Smoking cessation counseling should be a routine part of the preoperative meeting between surgeons and patients.

Nonmodifiable risk factors that may increase the susceptibility to infection must also be evaluated prior to surgery. Thorough assessment of a patient's medical history during the preoperative evaluation may reveal systemic comorbidities that should be identified and optimized prior to surgery. In all patients, preoperative infections, whether in the spine or elsewhere, should be addressed and treated prior to undergoing elective surgery.[11,29,42,58] Conditions such as rheumatoid arthritis, acquired immunodeficiency syndrome, adrenocortical insufficiency, long-term corticosteroid use, and malignancy may pose significant risk for developing postoperative infections.[59–61] A thorough discussion of potential complications associated with these confounding medical conditions is important during preoperative counseling. Medical optimization of these conditions may limit potential postoperative complications. Although age is not considered an independent risk factor, older patients are more likely to have comorbidities associated with an increased risk of postoperative infection.

Spinal surgeries for management of tumors are associated with a significantly higher rate of postoperative infections.[62,63] Patients treated with preoperative or postoperative local radiation are especially at risk.[64] Surgery performed through previously irradiated tissue increases the risk of infection and can make the surgery technically more challenging. It is generally recommended that elective spinal surgery occur 6 to 12 weeks following radiation of the surgical bed. In patients requiring postoperative radiation around the operative site, therapy should be delayed approximately 3 weeks to allow for adequate soft tissue healing.

Microbiology

Three potential sources are hypothesized to be responsible for postoperative infections: (1) direct inoculation during the operative procedure, (2) contamination during the early postoperative period, and (3) hematogenous seeding.[65–69] Of these, direct inoculation during the surgery is the most common, making aseptic technique and the appropriate use of prophylactic antibiotics of paramount importance.

Gram-positive cocci are the most common pathogens responsible for acute postoperative infections. The most commonly reported organism in the literature is *Staphylococcus aureus*, which causes greater than 50% of the infections in some reports.[29,43,55] Other common gram-positive species that cause postsurgical infections include *Staphylococcus epidermidis* and β-hemolytic streptococci. Common gram-negative organisms cultured from infected surgical sites include *Escherichia coli*, *Pseudomonas aeruginosa*, *Klebsiella pneumoniae*, *Enterobacter cloacae*, *Bacteroides*, and *Proteus* species. In cases of patients who are immunosuppressed, the surgeon must also be aware of the possibility of fungal infections, the management of which can greatly differ from bacterial infections.[70]

The microbiology of an infection can be influenced by the anatomic location of the surgery. Fecal contaminants are more likely to be involved in surgeries of the low lumbar or sacral regions. Bladder or fecal incontinence may predispose to gram-negative flora, especially with posterior lumbosacral incisions.

Infections that present greater than 1 year after surgery are generally caused by low-virulence organisms such as coagulase-negative staphylococcus, *Propionibacterium acnes*, and diphtheroids.[42,67] These organisms can be present as normal skin flora, and it is hypothesized that prolonged surgical wound drainage and inflammation may result in these infections. These low-virulent organisms are usually rapidly cleared by the host immune response with appropriate treatment and generally do not result in a clinical sepsis. In a retrospective review of postoperative infections presenting greater than 1 year after surgery, 10 of 11 patients with cultures incubated for greater than 1 week grew low-virulence skin organisms.[71] It is also critical to note that *Proprionibacterium acnes* cultures need to be kept for a minimum of 13 days.[72]

Hematogenous spread can also cause surgical site infections. These blood-borne infections are usually due to highly virulent organisms, including gram-negative bacteria. These infections are often associated with systemic illness and sometimes have grave consequences, such as multisystem organ failure. Due to repeated cannulization of the venous system, intravenous drug users have a higher incidence of gram-negative infections, as do patients who have prolonged hospital admissions.[55]

Diagnostic Modalities

Clinical Presentation

The most common presenting complaint for postoperative spinal infections is pain. Patients generally have an interval pain-free period immediately following the surgery for approximately 1 to 2 months and subsequently develop increasing pain over several weeks. The pain is classically out of proportion to what would be expected and may be associated with constitutional symptoms. Suspicion of a postoperative infection is frequently raised as the result of a change in the patient's clinical postoperative course from pain-free to painful.

Superficial wound infections generally present within 2 weeks of surgery, with local pain, erythema, drainage, and warmth. The examiner must always be cognizant of the possibility of an underlying deep infection. A presentation of superficial infection coinciding with constitutional symptoms may be an indication of a more serious deep infection that requires more aggressive treatment. Superficial wound infections in the early postoperative period that are not accompanied by increasing surgical site pain or systemic findings can frequently be treated with local wound care and oral antibiotics for approximately 2 weeks.

If a wound continues to drain after extensive local care or if the patient develops increasing operative site pain with the development of constitutional symptoms, it must be assumed that there is an underlying deep infection. Attention to physical examination findings at the local wound can be very informative to help define the extent of the infection and distinguish between superficial and deep infections. This difference is important when determining the course of treatment. Examination of the surgical site may reveal increased erythema, edema, tenderness to palpation, and drainage. The consistency and timing of the drainage also provides insight into the nature and depth of the infection. Clear, serosanguineous drainage might indicate an underlying seroma, while more copious purulent discharge indicates frank infection. Although characteristics have been defined in the literature, it can be very difficult to distinguish between deep and superficial wound infections. Furthermore, deep infections frequently have relatively unimpressive superficial findings, further confounding the diagnosis.

Systemic symptoms must also be taken into account when evaluating a wound infection. Fever is the most common constitutional symptom seen in these patients, although many patients with deep infections have no systemic symptoms. Early infection may be associated with high temperatures, chills, sweats, lethargy, or malaise. Sepsis can lead to multisystem organ failure and death if not addressed appropriately and rapidly, including possible urgent surgical debridement if the patient is medically stable to undergo surgery.

Late infections presenting more than 2 months after surgery can be difficult to diagnose because of the lack of obvious symptoms. Although the incision is healed, superficial skin changes such as erythema or tenderness may occur, although these findings are inconsistent. Increasing pain at the surgical site or the presence of constitutional symptoms should prompt suspicion of an underlying infection in either the early or late postoperative time periods.

In patients who have undergone anterior cervical surgery, the development of progressive difficulty with swallowing may indicate a retropharyngeal abscess. Patients can also present with minor drainage and skin changes, but fulminant infections leading to sepsis are not common in the anterior cervical subgroup.

Laboratory Testing

Laboratory studies are one of the first diagnostic tests used in suspected cases of postoperative infection. The initial blood workup should consist of a complete blood count including white blood cell count (WBC) with differential, erythrocyte sedimentation rate (ESR), and C-reactive protein (CRP). When used alone, many of these laboratory markers may be of little use. When taken together and repeated over time to display a trend, these markers quantify severity of infection and allow the clinician to monitor the response to treatment.

An elevated WBC is not an absolute indicator of infection. Pathogen virility and host response may cause variability in the WBC response to infection. In the early postoperative period, surgical stress can initiate intravascular leukocyte demargination that causes an increased WBC. Additionally, lack of significant elevation in WBC does not necessarily rule out an infection, especially in patients with immunosuppression.

The ESR elevates following spinal surgery and may not normalize until several weeks postoperatively. Variations in this time period to normalization have been reported. In one study, the ESR rarely elevated to levels greater than 25 mm/h and returned to baseline levels by the third postoperative week.[73] Another study showed that ESR elevation was prolonged and lasted up to 6 weeks postoperatively.[74] Peak ESR levels have been shown to correlate with the degree of invasiveness of the surgery, with more extensive surgeries causing higher ESR elevations than less invasive procedures.[75] The ESR level is a sensitive marker for infection, with up to 90% of cases of infections of the spine showing elevated values.[76] Furthermore, Carragee et al. found that a 25% drop in its value after 1 month of conservative treatment was an indicator for a good prognosis.[77]

As with the ESR, CRP values rise sharply during the initial postoperative period. Unlike the ESR, however, CRP decreases to baseline levels more rapidly. CRP levels generally peak on the third day postoperatively and return to baseline within 10 to 14 days. This rapid normalization makes CRP a more sensitive indicator of infection and a more useful diagnostic tool when determining the presence of infection, especially in the acute and subacute postoperative period.[74,75,78–80] An elevated ESR or CRP outside of this postoperative period can indicate a developing infection and can be used to monitor the efficacy of treatment.

When analyzed together, infectious laboratory markers provide a vital diagnostic tool to complement the initial clinical picture. Results may indicate a more severe infection than initially anticipated and dictate the need for a more aggressive diagnostic or therapeutic protocol. In addition, after the initiation of treatment, serial laboratory markers provide comparative interval data that indicate the response to treatment.

The precise and accurate identification of the culprit organism is a critical step in the treatment of a postoperative spinal infection. Cultures obtained from the superficial wound are

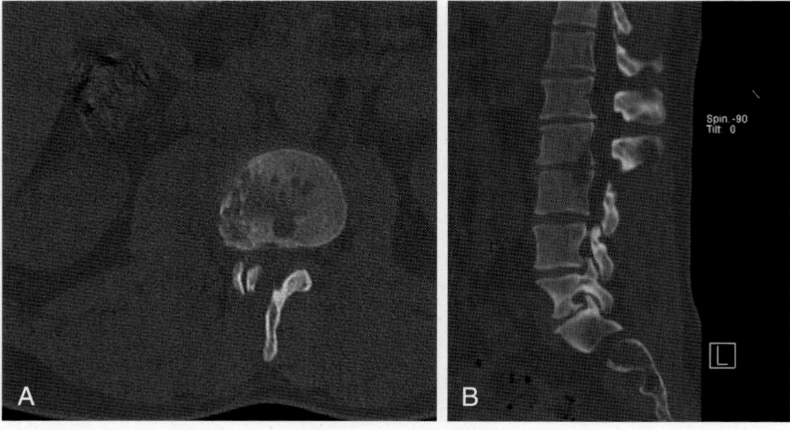

FIG. 99.2 (A) Axial and (B) sagittal computed tomography scan showing endplate lysis in a patient with postoperative discitis. Note the paravertebral soft tissue swelling in the right psoas muscle.

often contaminated with skin flora and can confuse the diagnostic workup. Some authors suggest early aspiration of a suspicious wound in order to attempt to isolate the infectious organism.[65] If there is no fluctuant mass to aspirate, as is often the case, computed tomography (CT) or fluoroscopic guidance can be used to accurately obtain a deep culture from the affected area. Frequently, fine-needle aspiration of the affected region does not provide ample tissue for an accurate diagnosis. We prefer to obtain a core-biopsy specimen in order to ensure that an adequate sample is provided to the laboratory. Blood cultures can reveal the responsible organism if taken in a septic individual prior to the initiation of antibiotics. While blood cultures are positive in 40% to 60% of cases of spontaneous spondylodiscitis,[76] the rate is considerably lower in postoperative infections.[81] If the blood cultures are positive and provide identification of an organism, it can be presumed that the same organism is the cause of the spinal infection and a biopsy of the spinal infection site may not be necessary. However, cases of polymicrobial infections that were missed using this method have been reported.[82] The most accurate cultures are those obtained during the surgical debridement prior to the administration of antibiotics. In many cases, however, such a surgical intervention is not necessary and these surgical cultures are not obtained.

Imaging

Plain radiographs are often the first imaging obtained during workup of a suspected infection. Findings on plain radiographs frequently can be quite subtle, and up to 4 weeks are often required to pass before radiographs show evidence of infection.[80] Inspection of the instrumentation for loosening or adjacent bony lysis may be clues of an infection. In cases of postoperative discitis, disc space narrowing is the first radiographic finding. This change generally occurs 4 to 6 weeks postoperatively. Early infectious disc space changes, however, may be difficult to distinguish from degenerative changes. Paravertebral soft tissue swelling may indicate the presence of an abscess, especially in the retropharyngeal space or paraspinal musculature. More significant radiographic findings—such as reactive bone formation, endplate destruction, osteolysis, and deformity—indicate a more significant infectious process and usually require at least 2 months to develop.

CT provides a more detailed view of spinal anatomy and may allow for earlier detection of postoperative infections than plain radiographs.[83] Endplate changes, bony lysis, and/or soft tissue fluid collections can indicate early infection (Fig. 99.2). As the infection progresses, more significant bony and intervertebral disc destruction may be seen. Implant-related artifacts may distort the detail and limit the usefulness of CT scans in patients with spinal instrumentation. CT-guided biopsies can also be utilized to provide an aspirate for culture or tissue biopsy from infected soft tissue or bone, as noted earlier.

Nuclear medicine studies are sometimes used to supplement other radiographic methods when working up a postoperative infection. Unlike MRI and CT, nuclear medicine studies are not limited by implant-associated artifacts. Bone scans are often nonspecific and may show generalized uptake around the surgical site in a postoperative spinal infection.[80] Although gallium-67 and technetium-99m scans provide early evidence of postoperative infections, their diagnostic value is somewhat compromised relative to studies evaluating the appendicular skeleton. Furthermore, when looking at postoperative infections specifically, gallium was not found to be helpful in differentiating infection from postoperative changes.[84] Indium 111–labeled WBC scans often have limited usefulness because of their poor specificity, particularly in the early postoperative period. Technetium-labeled ciprofloxacin, when combined with single-photon emission computed tomography, has been shown to have improved sensitivity and specificity over other nuclear medicine modalities, particularly if performed greater than 6 months after surgery.[85] ^{18}F-fluoro-D-deoxyglucose positron emission tomography has also been found to be a helpful adjunct for diagnosis in cases for which MRI is either not an option or inconclusive.[86] It is considered especially helpful in postoperative infections,[87,88] although availability and a relative lack of specificity remains an issue.

MRI with and without intravenous contrast is the most important imaging modality when evaluating postoperative spinal infections. Relative to other imaging modalities, MRI is

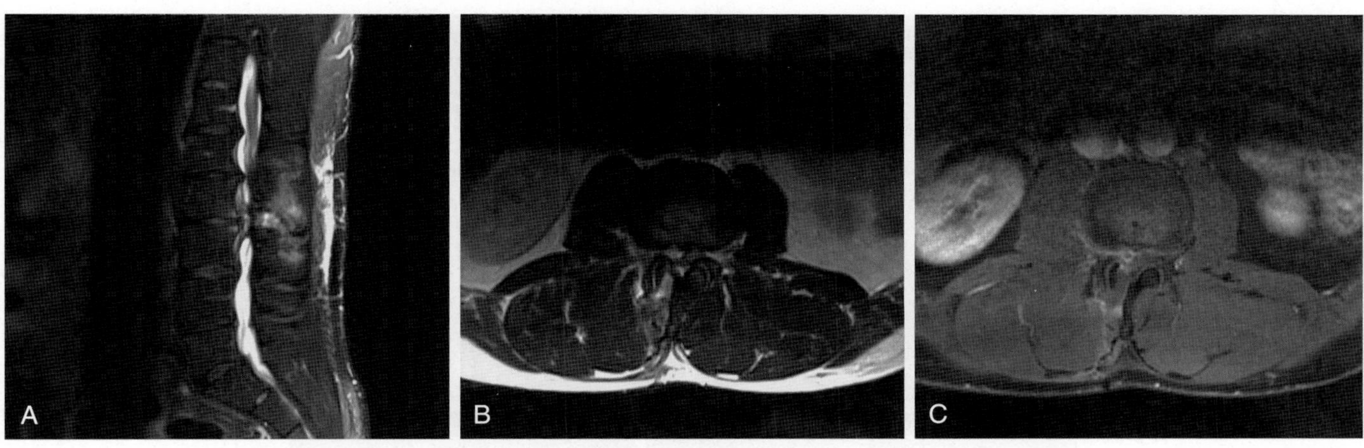

FIG. 99.3 Epidural abscess following a right L2–L3 microdiscectomy. (A–B) Note the compression of neural elements by the epidural abscess on the sagittal and axial T2-weighted magnetic resonance image (MRI). (C) On T1-weighted MRI with gadolinium contrast, the epidural abscess shows classic ring enhancement.

both highly sensitive (93%) and specific (96%) when evaluating spinal infections.[89–91] As with other imaging techniques, it may be difficult to distinguish nonpathologic postoperative changes from infections on MRI scans obtained in the early postoperative period. Thus, accuracy and reliability of the study is dependent on the elapsed time from the date of surgery, the level of clinical suspicion, and correlation with other diagnostic tools. Spinal instrumentation, particularly when composed of stainless steel, can cause significant MRI artifacts and severely limit the diagnostic utility of the study.

MRI can identify, with high sensitivity and specificity, postoperative osteomyelitis, discitis, and epidural abscesses. An epidural abscess displays a T1 isointense fluid collection with potential obliteration of the otherwise well-defined neural elements, and the T2-weighted images show significant increased intensity. Abscesses display ring enhancement on T1 images following the addition of intravenous (IV) gadolinium (Fig. 99.3). Osteomyelitis appears as areas of vertebral body and disc space hypointensity on T1-weighted images and hyperintensity on T2 images. In addition, there is a loss of definition between the vertebral bodies and the intervertebral disc space.[90–92]

Boden and associates compared the early postoperative MRI changes in noninfected individuals to those with confirmed discitis.[93] The most reliable difference seen in the discitis group was increased signal intensity of the adjacent vertebral body on T1-weighted images that was not present on preoperative studies. In addition, T2-weighted images showed increased signal intensity in the disc and adjacent marrow (Fig. 99.4). Only one of 17 control group patients displayed these signal intensity changes in the adjacent vertebral marrow. All cases of discitis displayed intervertebral disc signal enhancement with the addition of a contrast agent.

Classification

Classification systems for postoperative spinal infections are based on anatomic location, superficial versus deep infection, early versus late presentation, and comorbid medical conditions. These factors all play a significant role in the natural history of the infection and its response to treatment. With this stratification, management strategies may be tailored to the individual in an attempt to optimize treatment.

A classification scheme proposed by Thalgott and colleagues was adapted from the Cierny classification for the diagnosis and management of osteomyelitis.[94] Thalgott's classification scheme is based on the severity of infection and ability for host response. The severity of infection is divided into three groups: (1) superficial or deep infection with a single organism, (2) deep infection with multiple organisms, and (3) deep infection and myonecrosis with multiple or resistant organisms. Host response was divided into three physiologic classes: (A) normal systemic defenses, metabolic capabilities, and vascularity; (B) local or multiple systemic diseases, including cigarette smoking; and (C) immunocompromised or severely malnourished. Using this classification, Thalgott studied 32 patients with postoperative infections following fusion with instrumentation. Patients with group 1 infections were successfully treated with simple irrigation, debridement, and primary closure over a closed-suction drainage tube without an irrigant system. Patients with group 2 infections required an average of three irrigations and debridements and displayed greater success when treated with closed inflow–outflow suction irrigation systems when compared to simple suction drainage systems without constant inflow irrigation. Group 3 patients were difficult to manage and had poor overall outcomes. In addition, cigarette smoking was found to be a significant risk factor for developing postoperative infection.[94]

Prevention

The use of preoperative prophylactic antibiotics is routine for most spine surgeons. Although there is an increasing body of evidence-based medicine that supports the use of prophylactic antibiotics in spinal surgery, there is still no level I evidence

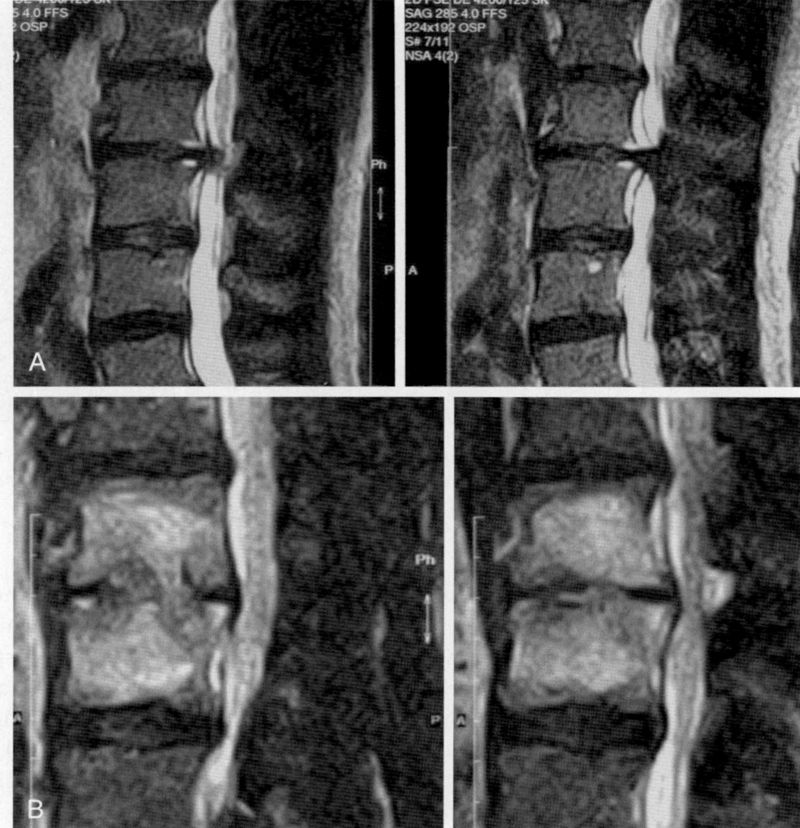

FIG. 99.4 (A) Preoperative sagittal T2-weighted magnetic resonance image (MRI) showing lumbar intervertebral disc herniation. Note the homogeneous bone marrow intensity throughout the lumbar spine. (B) Postoperative T2-weighted MRI showing diffusely increased signal within the disc and adjacent vertebral bodies.

clearly defining their efficacy. In a meta-analysis pooling data from six separate randomized controlled trials (RCTs), Barker and associates found an infection rate of 2.2% following the administration of antibiotics and 5.9% if antibiotics were not administered.[95] In a prospective RCT, Pavel et al.[96] compared infection rates following orthopaedic procedures with and without preoperative antibiotic prophylaxis with cephaloridine. In a subgroup analysis of spinal procedures, infection rates were 3% in patients treated with antibiotics and 9.2% in those without.[96] In another RCT comparing the efficacy of cefazolin relative to placebo in 141 patients, Rubinstein's group showed that the use of preoperative antibiotics decreased the incidence of postoperative infection from 12.7% in untreated controls to 4.3% in those receiving prophylactic antibiotics.[97] More recently, Shaffer et al. published an evidence-based clinical practice guideline based on the work of the Antibiotic Prophylaxis Work Group of the North American Spine Society.[98] They gave a relatively strong recommendation that patients undergoing spine surgery should receive antibiotic prophylaxis, although no specific recommendations regarding ideal agents or dosing schedules were given.

In order for antibiotics to be effective prophylactic agents, they must have antimicrobial action against the most common bacteria encountered and must be present in tissues adjacent to the surgical site in sufficient concentrations. Current recommendations suggested that antibiotic administration should begin 30 minutes to 1 hour preoperatively to ensure adequate antibiotic levels at the surgical site at the time of skin incision. With prolonged operative time, serum and tissue antibiotic levels decrease.[99,100] Some authors recommend repeating the dose of antibiotics after 4 hours of surgery; our group follows this protocol. The limited data regarding redosing patients intraoperatively and postoperatively do not show any significant differences in infection rates, however.[101–103] In a retrospective cohort, Dobzyniak and colleagues[101] compared infection rates in 433 patients who received preoperative and postoperative doses of antibiotics to 201 patients who received only a single dose of preoperative antibiotics. No significant differences in infection rates were detected in this study.

Because of their good coverage against the common bacterial agents encountered in spinal surgery, a limited side effect profile, and advantageous pharmacokinetics, cephalosporins are excellent candidates for prophylactic antibiotics. First-generation cephalosporins are good antibiotics for prophylactic administration as they have strong gram-positive coverage against the most common organisms that result in SSIs (*S. aureus* and *S. epidermidis*). In addition, they have action against common gram-negative organisms (*E. coli* and *Proteus*). Cefazolin continues to be the most commonly administered prophylactic antibiotic because it provides appropriate antimicrobial coverage, is relatively inexpensive, and reaches peak serum concentrations rapidly.

The human spine is a unique environment because of its combination of bony structures, intervertebral discs, and adjacent soft tissue musculature. Antibiotics used for the treatment of spinal infections need to be able to penetrate the involved structures to be maximally effective. Studies have documented the half-life and penetration of antibiotics into bone and intervertebral discs. Cefazolin displays a longer half-life in the serum and bone relative to other cephalosporins.[97,104,105] Human and animal studies evaluating the penetration of antibiotics into intervertebral discs have provided mixed results.[104–112] With increased age and decreased disc vascularity, systemic antibiotic penetration into the disc is impeded. In addition, the environment within a degenerating disc likely presents a barrier to obtaining consistent inhibitory levels of antibiotics. Penetration of antibiotics into the adult intervertebral disc depends on passive diffusion from adjacent bony structures and cartilaginous endplates as well as from the anulus fibrosus.[113] Studies have demonstrated the ability of cefazolin to penetrate the disc, although concentrations are higher in the anulus fibrosus relative to the nucleus pulposus.[104,106,107] There is evidence in the literature suggesting that the molecular charge of an antibiotic is an important determinant of its ability to diffuse into the disc. Studies have evaluated the penetration of negatively charged antibiotics into the positively charged disc when adequate serum concentrations are maintained.[104,106,114] Positively charged antibiotics, such as gentamicin and vancomycin, have been shown to freely penetrate the anulus fibrosus and nucleus pulposus, while negatively charged antibiotics such as penicillin are found in the anulus fibrosus but not the nucleus pulposus. The use of antibiotic delivery systems to circumvent this problem has been studied. In a prospective cohort study, Rohde evaluated the infection rate following discectomy in 1712 patients, 1134 of whom received prophylactic gentamicin-containing collagenous sponges at the cleared disc space.[115] Patients receiving the prophylactic antibiotic showed a 0% infection rate relative to a 3.7% infection rate in those who did not. Gentamicin-associated toxicity, however, makes it a suboptimal choice for routine surgical prophylaxis.

A recent prevention strategy that appears to have promising results is the use of antibiotic powder applied directly into the wound prior to closure at the conclusion of the case. Several studies have shown that local application of vancomycin powder significantly reduces rates of staphylococcal postoperative infections,[116–120] including cases in trauma patients[121] as well as posterior cervical spine cases.[122,123] In a rabbit model, Zebala et al.[124] showed that vancomycin powder was effective in eliminating staphylococcal contamination compared to controls. Furthermore, several studies have shown that the use of prophylactic antibiotic powder application not only helps lower postoperative infection rates but also is cost-effective overall.[125,126] The use of vancomycin powder is generally considered safe in both adults[116,117] and children.[127,128]

As a result of significant soft tissue disruption and the creation of a potential space, hematoma formation following spinal surgery is a frequent occurrence. Hematomas provide an excellent milieu for bacteria proliferation. In an attempt to address this potential complication, many surgeons utilize closed-suction devices during the postoperative course. The effectiveness of postoperative suction drains to prevent infection has not been clearly demonstrated in the literature. In a prospective randomized study examining 83 patients undergoing extensive lumbar spine surgery, no infections were reported in those who received and those who did not receive closed-suction drainage postoperatively.[129] Similar results are reported elsewhere in the literature.[130,131] In one study examining patients undergoing surgery for adolescent idiopathic scoliosis, patients without drains had no difference in infection rates compared to drained patients, while patients with drains had a significantly higher rate of blood transfusions.[132]

Antibiotic-resistant organisms have become an increasingly prevalent problem. Methicillin-resistant *S. aureus* (MRSA) is the most commonly isolated resistant organism. Many hospitals have initiated monitoring and regulatory strategies to identify emerging resistance patterns and have implemented specific prophylactic antibiotic protocols to control this growing problem. Infections caused by these resistant organisms are associated with significantly increased morbidity, mortality, and cost. Some of the risk factors associated with MRSA include prolonged use of antibiotics, previous exposure or infection with MRSA, indwelling catheter use, advanced age, and intensive care unit stay.

Irrigation solutions are often used intraoperatively in an effort to prevent or treat infections. Commonly used irrigants include solutions of bacitracin, iodine, chlorhexidine, neomycin, or a combination of triple antibiotics including neomycin, bacitracin, and polymyxin. There are no significant clinical data that clearly support the use of these antibiotic irrigants in spinal surgery. In vitro studies, however, have shown a significant reduction in bacterial counts with use of the additives.[133–135] Intraoperative anaphylactic reactions have been reported with the use of bacitracin irrigation,[136] especially when combined with cell-saver blood recycling devices, although these reactions are extremely rare. Irrigation can be delivered via pulsatile lavage, which may improve the removal of contaminants from bone and soft tissue. In vitro effects have shown significant reduction in bacterial colony counts, but the reported toxic effects on osteoblasts and osteoclasts by the pulsatile irrigation must be taken into account when using this technique. The merits of pulsatile lavage have recently come into question with in vivo studies showing better bacterial load reductions with low-pressure systems.[137] The literature studying the different types of irrigation focuses on the context of traumatic wounds and cannot necessarily be extrapolated to the prevention of SSIs.

Appropriate maintenance of the operating room environment is important to reduce the potential for contamination. Methods of decreasing airborne bacteria can be implemented in an attempt to decrease infection rates. Operating in a vertical laminar flow operating room has been suggested in the literature as a method of reducing infection rates and is utilized by some institutions. Gruenberg and colleagues described a significant reduction in infection rates in a retrospective study comparing conventional and vertical laminar flow operating rooms,[138] although more recent studies in the general surgical

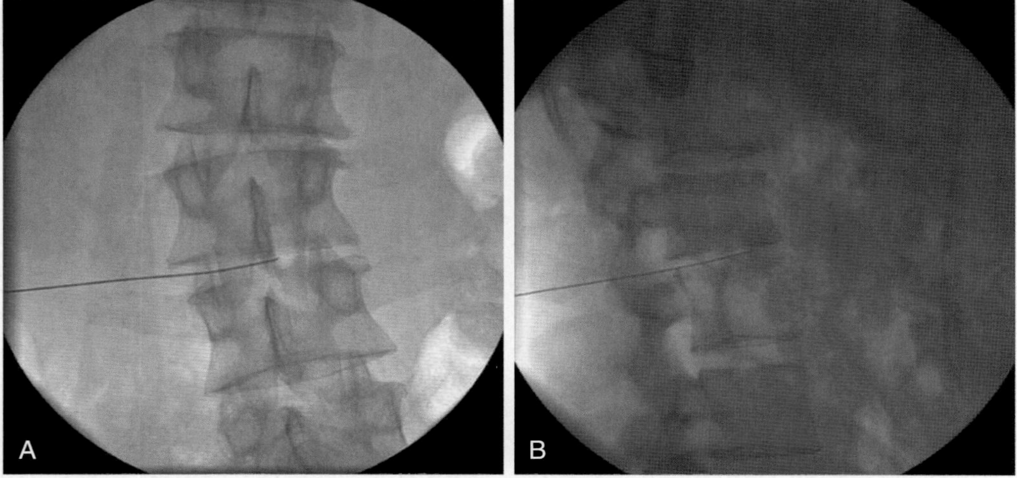

FIG. 99.5 Fluoroscopically guided biopsy of a postoperative disc space infection.

literature dispute this.[139,140] Basic principles of sterile technique should be adapted for every spinal procedure. Maintenance of a sterile field and double gloving with intermittent glove changes decrease the potential of surgeon contamination of the wound.[141] The use of an iodine-impregnated adherent plastic barrier over the operative field has been suggested by some authors as an additional method to decrease inoculation of the wound,[18] although a Cochrane review demonstrated no decrease in SSIs.[142] Limiting blood loss with meticulous attention to hemostasis, debridement of necrotic tissue, and periodic release of retractors help to minimize possible sites of infection.[143] In addition, flash sterilization of implantable devices is discouraged unless absolutely necessary.

Operating room behavior also plays a large role in preventing SSI. A large study of general-surgery SSIs found that a strict protocol of extensive antiseptic measures had no lower infection rates compared to a standard protocol.[144] It also found that increased SSI rates were attributable to minor violations in sterile technique rather than isolated gross violations. Other measures, such as covering the implants while not in use, have been found to decrease bacterial contamination, which could potentially lead to a lower rate of infection.[145]

Management

Successful treatment of postoperative spinal infections requires early diagnosis and appropriate medical and surgical management. Careful and early identification of a potentially catastrophic infection via clinical evaluation, laboratory testing, and imaging studies is helpful to enhance the chosen treatment regimen. The ultimate goal of any intervention is eradication of the infection, adequate wound closure, and maintenance of vertebral column stability. The approach to treatment often requires aggressive and sometimes repeated debridement in order to successfully prevent recurrence of infection. The treating surgeon must remain cautious when choosing conservative approaches, as these measures may not completely eradicate the infection.

The timing of infection in the postoperative spine is significantly influenced by the mode of inoculation and virulence of the organism. Early-presenting infections are generally a result of more virulent organisms such as MRSA and gram-negative bacteria[146] and are the result of intraoperative seeding. Delayed infections are typically caused by low-virulence organisms, such as skin flora, which may be introduced intraoperatively and subsequently adhere to instrumentation while encased in a glycocalyx biofilm.

The fundamental principles involved in the management of a postoperative infection include prompt diagnosis with isolation of a specific organism, if possible, and initiation of appropriate medical and surgical management. As previously discussed, image-guided biopsy can be used to provide specimens to accurately identify the offending organism. Our group generally performs a CT or fluoroscopically guided biopsy prior to proceeding with an open surgical biopsy (Fig. 99.5). Additionally, a minimum of two sets of blood cultures are sent on patients with a suspected spinal infection. If the blood cultures identify an organism, then that same organism can be presumed to be the cause of the spinal infection and invasive biopsies are not necessary. After an organism has been identified, appropriate antibiotic therapy should be initiated. Extremely superficial infections, such as a stitch abscess, can be treated with 2 weeks of oral antibiotics and close clinical follow-up. For any significant infection, however, a minimum of 6 weeks of IV antibiotics followed by 6 weeks of oral antibiotics are used. ESR and CRP measurements are used to monitor the response to treatment.

Most significant superficial and deep infections require surgical debridement in addition to IV antibiotic therapy. When surgical debridement is used, a meticulous approach must be taken to thoroughly eradicate the infection. The surgical treatment of a postoperative infection includes debridement of each layer of the wound. At each layer, assessment of tissue devitalization and possible communication with underlying planes must be assessed. In addition, appropriate specimens for staining and cultures should be taken from each layer prior to the initiation of intraoperative antibiotics. We routinely send all specimens for bacterial studies, including aerobic, anaerobic, fungal, and acid-fast studies. The surgical incision should excise all dermal margins that appear infected. In the underlying subcutaneous layers, infectious material may be encountered and must be appropriately removed along with all necrotic tissue. If the underlying deep fascial layers appear to be intact and the infection limited to the subcutaneous planes, some have advocated aspiration of the deep wound and exploration only if the Gram stain results are positive.[17] Other authors, however, recommend routine exploration and debridement of the deep layers to prevent missing a potentially disastrous deep infection. We follow this latter recommendation. In our experience, there is usually some communication between the superficial and deep surgical planes.

When involved with the infection, the deep fascial layers should be opened and all loose tissue and foreign material should be removed. After specimens for microbiologic studies have been obtained, broad-spectrum antibiotics can be initiated. Bone graft that appears to be significantly infected or is loosened by the debridement should also be removed.[18,19,94,143] If not obviously necrotic or infected, the bone graft should be left in place.

The need for repeat debridements depends on the extent of infection seen during the initial surgery. If Gram stain and culture results reveal multiple organisms, multiple debridements should be considered. Some advocate a "second look" irrigation and debridement 48 to 72 hours after the initial surgery in all cases. To better help surgeons stratify which patients could benefit from multiple irrigation and debridements, a predictive scoring model was developed using six factors, as described in Table 99.1. The final score groups patients into low, indeterminate, and high risk for needing multiple washouts.[147] Patients with higher risk are thought to potentially benefit from two-stage reconstructions.

Following sufficient debridement and irrigation of the wound, assessment of the wound and a plan for closure must be devised. There remains debate in the literature as to whether infected surgical wounds should be closed primarily after the initial surgical debridement versus a delayed staged closure with intermittent debridements.[18,71,148] We prefer a primary layered closure because wounds that remain open are susceptible to superinfection and wound contracture. In cases with significant myonecrosis that require multiple repeat debridements, primary closure may not be possible. Use of a closed-suction drain for a few days postoperatively is generally advocated. Closure over a suction irrigation system or packing the wound with a vacuum-assisted sponge system has been described.[42,149,150] In patients with significant infections or soft tissue involvement, the use of reconstructive soft tissue techniques—including flap coverage—may be necessary.

TABLE 99.1 Use of Postoperative Infection Treatment Score for the Spine (PITSS) to Predict Likelihood of Needing Two-Stage Reconstruction After Postoperative Infection

Predictors	PITSS Score
Spine Location	
Cervical	1
Thoracolumbar	2
Lumbosacral	4
Comorbidities	
None	0
Cardiovascular/pulmonary	1
Diabetes	4
Microbiology	
Gram positive	2
Gram negative or polymicrobial without MRSA	4
Polymicrobial with MRSA or MRSA alone	6
Distant Site Infection	
None	1
UTI/PNA	3
Bacteremia alone	5
Bacteremia with PNA/UTI	6
Instrumentation	
Yes	6
No	2
Bone Graft	
None	1
Autograft	3
Other (allograft, BMP and synthetic)	6

A higher PITSS score indicates a higher risk of the patient requiring repeat debridement. Scores between 7 and 14 correlate with low risk; scores between 15 and 20 correlate with intermediate risk; and scores between 21 and 33 correlate with high risk. BMP, bone morphogenic protein; MRSA, methicillin-resistant *Staphylococcus aureus*; PNA, pneumonia; UTI, urinary tract infection.

Spinal Instrumentation and Infections

The use of instrumentation in spinal procedures results in a greater risk of developing a postoperative infection. Reported infection rates following instrumented posterior lumbar fusion range from 2.8% to 20%, with most authors suggesting a true infection rate of approximately 5% to 6%.[11,16,17,43,146,151–159] In patients with extensive infections in the presence of instrumentation, even repeated surgical debridements along with intravenous antibiotics may fail to resolve the infection. The metallic implants provide a surface for the formation of a glycocalyx biofilm that is very difficult to penetrate with systemic antibiotics. During the debridement of infections with instrumentation, the implants should be routinely inspected. If the implants show obvious signs of loosening, they should be removed, and possibly replaced with new instrumentation if necessary. Removal of infected instrumentation that remains well fixed has long been debated in the literature. Some authors advocate complete removal of all instrumentation, independent of fixation and fusion status, because of the difficulty of eliminating the infection without removal,[18,66,71,160-162] especially in cases of adult deformity with delayed SSI.[163,164] Retention of spinal instrumentation, however, at the time of debridement has been recommended by many. Authors have described leaving well-fixed instrumentation in place following thorough debridement to prevent possibly catastrophic spinal instability.[11,16,17,43,146,151–159,165] Additionally, these authors have shown successful eradication of both anterior and posterior spinal infections with retained instrumentation. Vertebral

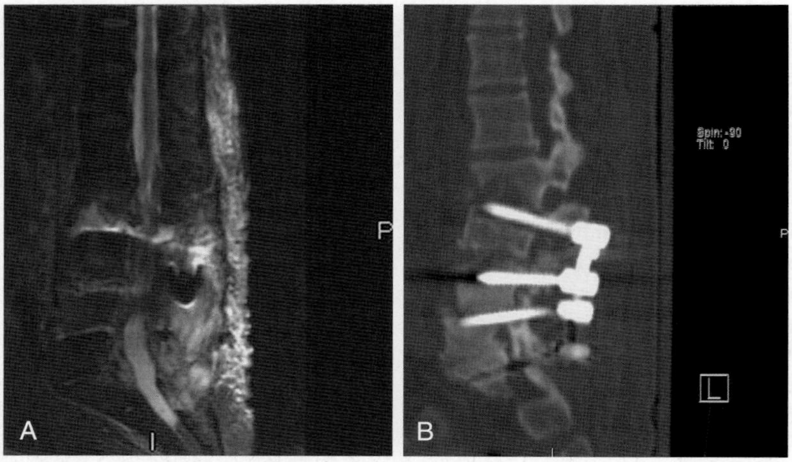

FIG. 99.6 Sagittal magnetic resonance image (MRI) and computed tomographic (CT) image in a patient with a lumbosacral instrumented fusion who developed a postoperative pyogenic infection. (A) Note increased signal within the L2–L3 disc space on MRI. (B) CT scan shows lack of solid arthrodesis and L2–L3 kyphosis. At the time of debridement, removal of the spinal instrumentation without reimplantation may lead to further spinal instability.

column malalignment, spinal cord compression, and paralysis are potential complications associated with instability if fusion is not complete at the time of instrumentation removal (Fig. 99.6). An approach taken by many is to administer long-term antibiotics to suppress the infection until a solid fusion is obtained. If the infection persists, the instrumentation can be removed after the arthrodesis has been achieved. One potential complication with this method is subsequent instability following instrumentation removal if the patient has an undetected pseudarthrosis. Titanium implants are less adherent to the bacterial glycocalyx, thus are favored over stainless steel implants if instrumentation needs to be reimplanted in an infected site.[166] If loose instrumentation is encountered during the debridement and there is a potential for spinal instability, the instrumentation should be replaced.

Discitis

Patients with postoperative disc space infections often develop symptoms after a relatively uneventful acute postoperative course. The most common presentation is increasing back pain that is out of proportion to physical examination and imaging findings. The pain can be associated with constitutional symptoms, including fevers, chills, and lethargy, or elevated laboratory markers. The presence of any new neurologic deficit should raise the suspicion for an epidural abscess or other space-occupying process. MRI with and without contrast is the diagnostic test of choice for patients with any postoperative infection, including suspected disc-space infection. The MRI scan, however, may not show positive findings until 5 days after the onset of infection. If clinical suspicion is high, repeat scanning may be necessary after several weeks. MRI findings typical of discitis include hypointensity on T1-weighted images and hyperintensity on T2-weighted images. Identification of the responsible organism either by percutaneous biopsy or blood culture may allow for more specific antibiotic coverage. If cultures are negative, treatment for the most commonly responsible organism, *S. aureus*, should be instituted. The majority of postoperative disc-space infections can be successfully treated with 6 weeks of intravenous antibiotics followed by 6 weeks of oral antibiotics. Surgical intervention may be indicated in the presence of systemic infection, increasing pain with a suboptimal response to antibiotic management, progressive destruction of the adjacent vertebral bodies, advancing neurologic deficit, or an epidural or paravertebral abscess. An anterior or posterior surgical approach can be utilized depending on the timing, original approach used for the primary surgery, and location of the most significant pathology.

Epidural Abscess

Epidural abscesses can have potentially devastating neurologic outcomes if not rapidly identified and treated. A major prognostic factor for a favorable outcome is early recognition and prompt intervention, particularly surgical debridement. Clinical and radiographic diagnosis may be difficult in the postoperative patient, and any neurologic deficit may not be apparent on initial presentation. With progression of the disease, the patient may show signs of increased back pain, systemic symptoms, and eventually neurologic deficit. The disease may progress rapidly, with paralysis potentially developing late in the course. Urgent surgical decompression is the treatment of choice for a progressive abscess. The surgical approach depends on the location of the abscess and the extent of involvement. Posterior canal epidural abscesses are usually best treated with a posterior decompression, such as a laminectomy. Anterior spinal canal epidural abscesses are frequently associated with granulation tissue from discitis or osteomyelitis, and anterior surgery may be necessary to eradicate the infection. More severe infections may require debridement from a combined anterior and posterior approach.

Complex Wound Closure

Severe postoperative spinal infections may result in significant soft tissue defects that require complex wound management. The goals of treating these complex wounds include obliteration of dead space, creation of adequate coverage for prominent bone or instrumentation, and enhancing vascularity for improved healing. Methods that may be utilized to treat these wounds include flap coverage and healing by secondary intention. Local, rotational, and free flaps are often utilized for coverage and have shown successful results. Even in complex wounds with deficient local tissue, muscle flaps can bring increased vascularity and adequate soft tissue coverage from distal sites to allow for healing while protecting instrumentation and bone graft.[24,167] The gold standard has been the trapezius muscle flap, although recent studies have also shown the paraspinous muscle flap to be efficacious for both thoracolumbar and cervical coverage.[168,169] Healing of complex wounds by secondary intention using vacuum-assisted closure devices has become popular. These devices create negative pressure in the wound, which results in increased vascularity and cellular proliferation. They help form granulation tissue over bone and instrumentation and have shown success in healing large open wounds.[170–172] Vacuum-assisted closure devices seem to be especially helpful adjuncts in closing spinal wounds infected with MRSA or multiple bacteria.[173] Prior to surgical intervention of patients who may require soft tissue reconstruction, it is critical that patients are optimized medically and nutritionally, and plastic and reconstructive surgeons should be involved prior to the surgical intervention.

Length of Antibiotic Treatment

Appropriate antibiotic treatment is critical to the successful eradication of any postoperative infection. Consultation with an infection specialist is usually obtained to assist in formulating a treatment plan. Once antibiotics have been initiated, close follow-up of the culture results is required to appropriately tailor the subsequent treatment regimen. During the treatment period, adjustment of the antibiotic might be necessary depending on the patient's response to treatment. Intravenous antibiotics are usually administered for approximately 6 weeks followed by approximately 6 weeks or longer of oral antibiotics. The specific time for treatment depends on the virulence of the infectious organism and its sensitivity to the antibiotics. Regular follow-up of infectious laboratory markers—including WBC, ESR, and CRP—assists in determining the response to treatment. In a prospective cohort study, patients with SSI after instrumented fusions were treated with operative debridement followed by 3 months of antibiotic therapy (2 weeks IV followed by 10 weeks oral). Using this standardized treatment protocol, there was a 94% success rate in eradicating infection.[174] Postsurgical spine infections with antibiotic-resistant organisms require special considerations, including patient isolation and treatment with appropriate antibiotics. Fortunately, new classes of antibiotics have been developed to supplement the previously limited options for treatment of infections such as MRSA and vancomycin-resistant enterococci.[172] Occasionally, prolonged antibiotic treatment may be necessary for suppression of infection in patients with retained instrumentation or recalcitrant infections.

Summary

Postoperative infections can occur following any type of spinal surgery. The consequences of these infections are devastating for the patient and the health care system. Preoperative medical optimization to prevent infections is a critical part of any surgical procedure. Routine preoperative antibiotic dosing and meticulous sterile surgical technique help to prevent iatrogenic seeding of the surgical site. Even with optimal preoperative and intraoperative care, postoperative infections can still occur. The treating surgeon must have a high index of suspicion in any patient who presents with increasing axial pain following a relatively pain-free postoperative period, especially when accompanied by systemic or incisional findings. MRI scan and laboratory testing help to confirm the diagnosis, and biopsy is useful to specifically identify the offending organism and appropriate antibiotics for treatment. In most patients, medical treatment with extended courses of antibiotics can treat the infection, although surgical debridement may be necessary if the infection does not respond to antibiotics or if there is neurologic deterioration, spinal instability, abscess formation, severe pain, or systemic signs/symptoms. Infections are associated with prolonged hospital stay, an increased rate of pseudarthrosis, and multiple subsequent operations; thus, the surgeon must take appropriate care to minimize infections and treat them rapidly if they do occur.

KEY POINTS

1. Spinal infection rates range from approximately 1% for microdiscectomies to 6% for instrumented decompression and fusions.
2. Surgeons can decrease postoperative infection rates by addressing comorbid conditions and preexisting conditions.
3. Postoperative spinal infections present most commonly with local pain, which can variably be accompanied by systemic symptoms.
4. ESR and CRP values can be followed to evaluate the severity of an infection and the response to treatment.
5. MRI scan with and without gadolinium contrast is the imaging test of choice for a suspected spinal infection.
6. Specific diagnosis of the offending organism via an image-guided biopsy or blood cultures should be obtained.
7. Treatment with IV antibiotics and possibly surgical debridement can eliminate the infection, even in the face of retained spinal instrumentation.

PEARLS

1. Appropriate preoperative medical optimization can decrease the rate of postoperative spinal infections.
2. Prophylactic surgical antibiotics should be used in addition to meticulous sterile technique.

3. Development of pain after a relatively pain-free postoperative period can signify the development of a postsurgical infection.
4. A multidisciplinary team, including infection specialists, spinal surgeons, and plastic surgeons, is needed to approach severe infections.

PITFALLS

1. Certain patient populations—including smokers, diabetics, and the malnourished—are at an increased risk for postoperative infections.
2. Infections can occur even in the late postoperative period, and vigilance must be maintained by the surgeon to avoid missing the often subtle development of these infections.
3. Certain common antibiotics have poor penetration into the nucleus pulposus; physicians must make antibiotic choices appropriate for these spinal infections.
4. Care must be taken when dealing with infections in patients with instrumented fusions. The instrumentation should be maintained as needed to prevent spinal instability and resultant neurologic deterioration. Bone graft should only be removed if infected.

KEY REFERENCES

1. Riley LH, Banovac K, Martinez OV, Eismont FJ. Tissue distribution of antibiotics in the intervertebral disc. *Spine*. 1994;19(23):2619-2625.
   This paper shows the effect that antibiotic charge can have on nucleus pulposus penetration, specifically with positively charged antibiotics, such as gentamicin, which show better penetration than negatively charged antibiotics, such as penicillin.
2. Brown MD, Brookfield KF. A randomized study of closed wound suction drainage for extensive lumbar spine surgery. *Spine*. 2004;29(10):1066-1068.
   This is a prospective randomized study that showed no benefit in reduction of infection by closed-suction drainage after lumbar spine surgery.
3. Boden SD, Davis DO, Dina TS, Sunner JL, Wiesel SW. Postoperative diskitis: distinguishing early MR imaging findings from normal postoperative disk space changes. *Radiology*. 1992;184(3):765-771.
   The authors evaluated the postoperative MRI findings in patients with documented postsurgical discitis versus another noninfected group to better characterize findings seen with postoperative disc space infections.
4. Thelander U, Larsson S. Quantitation of C-reactive protein levels and erythrocyte sedimentation rate after spinal surgery. *Spine*. 1992;17(4):400-404.
   This paper characterized the response of ESR and CRP to different kinds of spinal surgery and showed that CRP tended to normalize within 2 weeks after surgery and ESR normalized 3 to 6 weeks after surgery.
5. Weiss LE, Vaccaro AR, Scuderi G, et al. Pseudarthrosis after postoperative wound infection in the lumbar spine. *J Spinal Disord*. 1997;10:482-487.
   This paper demonstrated the dramatic negative effect a wound infection has on fusion rate, especially in fusion with allograft, fusion to the sacrum, and female gender.

REFERENCES

1. El-Gindi S, Aref S, Salama M, et al. Infection of intervertebral discs after operation. *J Bone Joint Surg Br*. 1976;58(1):114-116.
2. Ford LT, Key JA. Postoperative infection of intervertebral disc space. *South Med J*. 1955;48(12):1295-1303.
3. Lindholm TS, Pylkkanen P. Discitis following removal of intervertebral disc. *Spine*. 1982;7(6):618-622.
4. Stolke D, Sollmann WP, Seifert V. Intra- and postoperative complications in lumbar disc surgery. *Spine*. 1989;14(1):56-59.
5. Pilgaard S. Discitis (closed space infection) following removal of lumbar inervertebral disc. *J Bone Joint Surg Am*. 1969;51(4):713-716.
6. Wright TE, Orr RJ, Haberkern CM, Walbergh EJ. Complications during spinal anesthesia in infants: high spinal blockade. *Anesthesiology*. 1990;73(6):1290-1292.
7. Whitecloud TS 3rd, Butler JC, Cohen JL, Candelora PD. Complications with the variable spinal plating system. *Spine*. 1989;14(4):472-476.
8. Smith JS, Shaffrey CI, Sansur CA, et al. Rates of infection after spine surgery based on 108,419 procedures: a report from the Scoliosis Research Society Morbidity and Mortality Committee. *Spine*. 2011;36(7):556-563.
9. Rechtine GR, Bono PL, Cahill D, Bolesta MJ, Chrin AM. Postoperative wound infection after instrumentation of thoracic and lumbar fractures. *J Orthop Trauma*. 2001;15(8):566-569.
10. Brown EM, Pople IK, de Louvois J, et al. Spine update: prevention of postoperative infection in patients undergoing spinal surgery. *Spine*. 2004;29(8):938-945.
11. Glassman SD, Dimar JR, Puno RM, Johnson JR. Salvage of instrumental lumbar fusions complicated by surgical wound infection. *Spine*. 1996;21(18):2163-2169.
12. Graziano GP, Sidhu KS. Salvage reconstruction in acute and late sequelae from pyogenic thoracolumbar infection. *J Spinal Disord*. 1993;6(3):199-207.
13. Karlsson MK, Hasserius R, Olerud C, Ohlin A. Posterior transpedicular stabilisation of the infected spine. *Arch Orthop Trauma Surg*. 2002;122(9-10):522-525.
14. Jin D, Qu D, Chen J, Zhang H. One-stage anterior interbody autografting and instrumentation in primary surgical management of thoracolumbar spinal tuberculosis. *Eur Spine J*. 2004;13(2):114-121.
15. Labbe AC, Demers AM, Rodrigues R, et al. Surgical-site infection following spinal fusion: a case-control study in a children's hospital. *Infect Control Hosp Epidemiol*. 2003;24(8):591-595.
16. Li S, Zhang J, Li J, et al. Wound infection after scoliosis surgery: an analysis of 15 cases. *Chin Med Sci J*. 2002;17(3):193-198.
17. Perry JW, Montgomerie JZ, Swank S, Gilmore DS, Maeder K. Wound infections following spinal fusion with posterior segmental spinal instrumentation. *Clin Infect Dis*. 1997;24(4):558-561.
18. Richards BR, Emara KM. Delayed infections after posterior TSRH spinal instrumentation for idiopathic scoliosis: revisited. *Spine*. 2001;26(18):1990-1996.
19. Richards BS. Delayed infections following posterior spinal instrumentation for the treatment of idiopathic scoliosis. *J Bone Joint Surg Am*. 1995;77(4):524-529.
20. National Nosocomial Infections Surveillance (NNIS) System Report, data summary from January 1992 through June 2004, issued October 2004. *Am J Infect Control*. 2004;32(8):470-485.
21. Gruskay J, Kepler C, Smith J, Radcliff K, Vaccaro A. Is surgical case order associated with increased infection rate after spine surgery? *Spine*. 2012;37(13):1170-1174.
22. Veeravagu A, Patil CG, Lad SP, Boakye M. Risk factors for postoperative spinal wound infections after spinal decompression and fusion surgeries. *Spine*. 2009;34(17):1869-1872.

23. Pull ter Gunne AF, Cohen DB. Incidence, prevalence, and analysis of risk factors for surgical site infection following adult spinal surgery. *Spine*. 2009;34(13):1422-1428.
24. Mitra A, Harlin S. Treatment of massive thoracolumbar wounds and vertebral osteomyelitis following scoliosis surgery. *Plast Reconstr Surg*. 2004;113(1):206-213.
25. Cizik AM, Lee MJ, Martin BI, et al. Using the spine surgical invasiveness index to identify risk of surgical site infection: a multivariate analysis. *J Bone Joint Surg Am*. 2012;94(4):335-342.
26. Li YZ. [Wound infection after spinal surgery: analysis of 15 cases]. *Zhonghua Wai Ke Za Zhi*. 1991;29(8):484-486, 524-5.
27. Olsen MA, Nepple JJ, Riew KD, et al. Risk factors for surgical site infection following orthopaedic spinal operations. *J Bone Joint Surg Am*. 2008;90(1):62-69.
28. Schuster JM, Rechtine G, Norvell DC, Dettori JR. The influence of perioperative risk factors and therapeutic interventions on infection rates after spine surgery: a systematic review. *Spine*. 2010;35(9 suppl):S125-S137.
29. Massie JB, Heller JG, Abitbol JJ, McPherson D, Garfin SR. Postoperative posterior spinal wound infections. *Clin Orthop Relat Res*. 1992;284:99-108.
30. Hodges SD, Humphreys SC, Eck JC, Covington LA, Kurzynske NG. Low postoperative infection rates with instrumented lumbar fusion. *South Med J*. 1998;91(12):1132-1136.
31. Gerometta A, Rodriguez Olaverri JC, Bitan F. Infections in spinal instrumentation. *Int Orthop*. 2012;36(2):457-464.
32. Roberts FJ, Walsh A, Wing P, Dvorak M, Schweigel J. The influence of surveillance methods on surgical wound infection rates in a tertiary care spinal surgery service. *Spine*. 1998;23(3):366-370.
33. Kalicke T, Schlegel U, Printzen G, et al. Influence of a standardized closed soft tissue trauma on resistance to local infection. An experimental study in rats. *J Orthop Res*. 2003;21(2):373-378.
34. Gentile LF, Cuenca AG, Efron PA, et al. Persistent inflammation and immunosuppression: a common syndrome and new horizon for surgical intensive care. *J Trauma Acute Care Surg*. 2012;72(6):1491-1501.
35. Turnbull IR, Clark AT, Stromberg PE, et al. Effects of aging on the immunopathologic response to sepsis. *Crit Care Med*. 2009;37(3):1018-1023.
36. Failli V, Kopp MA, Gericke C, et al. Functional neurological recovery after spinal cord injury is impaired in patients with infections. *Brain*. 2012;135(Pt 11):3238-3250.
37. Blam OG, Vaccaro AR, Vanichkachorn JS, et al. Risk factors for surgical site infection in the patient with spinal injury. *Spine*. 2003;28(13):1475-1480.
38. Dubory A, Giorgi H, Walter A, et al. Surgical-site infection in spinal injury: incidence and risk factors in a prospective cohort of 518 patients. *Eur Spine J*. 2015;24(3):543-554.
39. Kornberg M, Rechtine GR, Herndon WA, Reinert CM, Dupuy TE. Surgical stabilization of thoracic and lumbar spine fractures: a retrospective study in a military population. *J Trauma*. 1984;24(2):140-146.
40. McAfee PC, Bohlman HH. Complications following Harrington instrumentation for fractures of the thoracolumbar spine. *J Bone Joint Surg Am*. 1985;67(5):672-686.
41. Ghobrial GM, Maulucci CM, Maltenfort M, et al. Operative and nonoperative adverse events in the management of traumatic fractures of the thoracolumbar spine: a systematic review. *Neurosurg Focus*. 2014;37(1):E8.
42. Weinstein MA, McCabe JP, Cammisa FP Jr. Postoperative spinal wound infection: a review of 2,391 consecutive index procedures. *J Spinal Disord*. 2000;13(5):422-426.
43. Levi AD, Dickman CA, Sonntag VK. Management of postoperative infections after spinal instrumentation. *J Neurosurg*. 1997;86(6):975-980.
44. Zeidman SM, Ducker TB, Raycroft J. Trends and complications in cervical spine surgery: 1989-1993. *J Spinal Disord*. 1997;10(6):523-526.
45. Pull ter Gunne AF, van Laarhoven CJHM, Cohen DB. Incidence of surgical site infection following adult spinal deformity surgery: an analysis of patient risk. *Eur Spine J*. 2010;19(6):982-988.
46. O'Toole JE, Eichholz KM, Fessler RG. Surgical site infection rates after minimally invasive spinal surgery. *J Neurosurg Spine*. 2009;11(4):471-476.
47. Parker SL, Adogwa O, Witham TF, et al. Post-operative infection after minimally invasive versus open transforaminal lumbar interbody fusion (TLIF): literature review and cost analysis. *Minim Invasive Neurosurg*. 2011;54(1):33-37.
48. McGirt MJ, Parker SL, Lerner J, et al. Comparative analysis of perioperative surgical site infection after minimally invasive versus open posterior/transforaminal lumbar interbody fusion: analysis of hospital billing and discharge data from 5170 patients. *J Neurosurg Spine*. 2011;14(6):771-778.
49. Park Y, Ha JW. Comparison of one-level posterior lumbar interbody fusion performed with a minimally invasive approach or a traditional open approach. *Spine*. 2007;32(5):537-543.
50. Kepler CK, Yu AL, Gruskay JA, et al. Comparison of open and minimally invasive techniques for posterior lumbar instrumentation and fusion after open anterior lumbar interbody fusion. *Spine J*. 2013;13(5):489-497.
51. Radcliff KE, Neusner AD, Millhouse PW, et al. What is new in the diagnosis and prevention of spine surgical site infections. *Spine J*. 2015;15(2):336-347.
52. Chen S, Anderson MV, Cheng WK, Wongworawat MD. Diabetes associated with increased surgical site infections in spinal arthrodesis. *Clin Orthop Relat Res*. 2009;467(7):1670-1673.
53. Klein JD, Hey LA, Yu CS, et al. Perioperative nutrition and postoperative complications in patients undergoing spinal surgery. *Spine*. 1996;21(22):2676-2682.
54. Cruse PJ, Foord R. A five-year prospective study of 23,649 surgical wounds. *Arch Surg*. 1973;107(2):206-210.
55. Wimmer C, Gluch H, Franzreb M, Ogon M. Predisposing factors for infection in spine surgery: a survey of 850 spinal procedures. *J Spinal Disord*. 1998;11(2):124-128.
56. Capen DA, Calderone RR, Green A. Perioperative risk factors for wound infections after lower back fusions. *Orthop Clin North Am*. 1996;27(1):83-86.
57. Mehta AI, Babu R, Karikari IO, et al. 2012 Young Investigator Award winner: The distribution of body mass as a significant risk factor for lumbar spinal fusion postoperative infections. *Spine*. 2012;37(19):1652-1656.
58. Stambough JL, Beringer D. Postoperative wound infections complicating adult spine surgery. *J Spinal Disord*. 1992;5(3):277-285.
59. Cruse PJ, Foord R. The epidemiology of wound infection. A 10-year prospective study of 62,939 wounds. *Surg Clin North Am*. 1980;60(1):27-40.

60. Calderone RR, Thomas JC Jr, Haye W, Abeles D. Outcome assessment in spinal infections. *Orthop Clin North Am.* 1996;27(1):201-205.
61. Mishriki SF, Law DJ, Jeffery PJ. Factors affecting the incidence of postoperative wound infection. *J Hosp Infect.* 1990;16(3):223-230.
62. Olsen MA, Mayfield J, Lauryssen C, et al. Risk factors for surgical site infection in spinal surgery. *J Neurosurg.* 2003;98(2 suppl):149-155.
63. McPhee IB, Williams RP, Swanson CE. Factors influencing wound healing after surgery for metastatic disease of the spine. *Spine.* 1998;23(6):726-732.
64. Omeis IA, Dhir M, Sciubba DM, et al. Postoperative surgical site infections in patients undergoing spinal tumor surgery: incidence and risk factors. *Spine.* 2011;36(17):1410-1419.
65. Sponseller PD, LaPorte DM, Hungerford MW, et al. Deep wound infections after neuromuscular scoliosis surgery: a multicenter study of risk factors and treatment outcomes. *Spine.* 2000;25(19):2461-2466.
66. de Jonge T, Slullitel H, Dubousset J, et al. Late-onset spinal deformities in children treated by laminectomy and radiation therapy for malignant tumours. *Eur Spine J.* 2005;14(8):765-771.
67. Richards BS, Herring JA, Johnston CE, Birch JG, Roach JW. Treatment of adolescent idiopathic scoliosis using Texas Scottish Rite Hospital instrumentation. *Spine.* 1994;19(14):1598-1605.
68. Viola RW, King HA, Adler SM, Wilson CB. Delayed infection after elective spinal instrumentation and fusion. A retrospective analysis of eight cases. *Spine.* 1997;22(20):2444-2450.
69. Heggeness MH, Esses SI, Errico T, Yuan HA. Late infection of spinal instrumentation by hematogenous seeding. *Spine.* 1993;18(4):492-496.
70. Pahlavan S, Bhatia NN. Fungal infections of the spine. *Semin Spine Surg.* 2016;28(3):163-172.
71. Clark CE, Shufflebarger HL. Late-developing infection in instrumented idiopathic scoliosis. *Spine.* 1999;24(18):1909-1912.
72. Butler-Wu SM, Burns EM, Pottinger PS, et al. Optimization of periprosthetic culture for diagnosis of *Propionibacterium acnes* prosthetic joint infection. *J Clin Microbiol.* 2011;49(7):2490-2495.
73. Kapp JP, Sybers WA. Erythrocyte sedimentation rate following uncomplicated lumbar disc operations. *Surg Neurol.* 1979;12(4):329-330.
74. Thelander U, Larsson S. Quantitation of C-reactive protein levels and erythrocyte sedimentation rate after spinal surgery. *Spine.* 1992;17(4):400-404.
75. Jonsson B, Soderholm R, Stromqvist B. Erythrocyte sedimentation rate after lumbar spine surgery. *Spine.* 1991;16(9):1049-1050.
76. Gouliouris T, Aliyu SH, Brown NM. Spondylodiscitis: update on diagnosis and management. *J Antimicrob Chemother.* 2010;65(suppl 3):iii11-iii24.
77. Carragee EJ, Kim D, van der Vlugt T, Vittum D. The clinical use of erythrocyte sedimentation rate in pyogenic vertebral osteomyelitis. *Spine.* 1997;22(18):2089-2093.
78. Fouquet B, Goupille P, Jattiot F, et al. Discitis after lumbar disc surgery. Features of "aseptic" and "septic" forms. *Spine.* 1992;17(3):356-358.
79. Meyer B, Schaller K, Rohde V, Hassler W. The C-reactive protein for detection of early infections after lumbar microdiscectomy. *Acta Neurochir (Wien).* 1995;136(3-4):145-150.
80. Silber JS, Anderson DG, Vaccaro AR, Anderson PA, McCormick P. Management of postprocedural discitis. *Spine J.* 2002;2(4):279-287.
81. Dufour V, Feydy A, Rillardon L, et al. Comparative study of postoperative and spontaneous pyogenic spondylodiscitis. *Semin Arthritis Rheum.* 2005;34(5):766-771.
82. Patzakis MJ, Rao S, Wilkins J, Moore TM, Harvey PJ. Analysis of 61 cases of vertebral osteomyelitis. *Clin Orthop Relat Res.* 1991;264:178-183.
83. Jevtic V. Vertebral infection. *Eur Radiol.* 2004;14(suppl 3):E43-E52.
84. Hadjipavlou AG, Cesani-Vazquez F, Villaneuva-Meyer J, et al. The effectiveness of gallium citrate Ga 67 radionuclide imaging in vertebral osteomyelitis revisited. *Am J Orthop.* 1998;27(3):179-183.
85. De Winter F, Gemmel F, Van Laere K, et al. 99mTc-ciprofloxacin planar and tomographic imaging for the diagnosis of infection in the postoperative spine: experience in 48 patients. *Eur J Nucl Med Mol Imaging.* 2004;31(2):233-239.
86. Gemmel F, Rijk PC, Collins JMP, et al. Expanding role of 18F-fluoro-d-deoxyglucose PET and PET/CT in spinal infections. *Eur Spine J.* 2010;19(4):540-551.
87. De Winter F, Gemmel F, Van De Wiele C, et al. 18-Fluorine fluorodeoxyglucose positron emission tomography for the diagnosis of infection in the postoperative spine. *Spine.* 2003;28(12):1314-1319.
88. Inanami H, Oshima Y, Iwahori T, et al. Role of 18F-fluoro-D-deoxyglucose PET/CT in diagnosing surgical site infection after spine surgery with instrumentation. *Spine.* 2015;40(2):109-113.
89. Vaccaro AR, Shah SH, Schweitzer ME, Rosenfeld JF, Cotler JM. MRI description of vertebral osteomyelitis, neoplasm, and compression fracture. *Orthopedics.* 1999;22(1):67-73.
90. Djukic S, Genant HK, Helms CA, Holt RG. Magnetic resonance imaging of the postoperative lumbar spine. *Radiol Clin North Am.* 1990;28(2):341-360.
91. Djukic S, Lang P, Morris J, Hoaglund F, Genant HK. The postoperative spine. Magnetic resonance imaging. *Orthop Clin North Am.* 1990;21(3):603-624.
92. Djukic S, Vahlensieck M, Resendes M, Genant HK. The lumbar spine: postoperative magnetic resonance imaging. *Bildgebung.* 1992;59(3):136-146.
93. Boden SD, Davis DO, Dina TS, Sunner JL, Wiesel SW. Postoperative diskitis: distinguishing early MR imaging findings from normal postoperative disk space changes. *Radiology.* 1992;184(3):765-771.
94. Thalgott JS, Cotler HB, Sasso RC, LaRocca H, Gardner V. Postoperative infections in spinal implants. Classification and analysis—a multicenter study. *Spine.* 1991;16(8):981-984.
95. Barker FG 2nd. Efficacy of prophylactic antibiotic therapy in spinal surgery: a meta-analysis. *Neurosurgery.* 2002;51(2):391-400.
96. Pavel A, Smith RL, Ballard A, Larson IJ. Prophylactic antibiotics in elective orthopedic surgery: a prospective study of 1,591 cases. *South Med J.* 1977;70(suppl 1):50-55.
97. Rubinstein E, Findler G, Amit P, Shaked I. Perioperative prophylactic cephazolin in spinal surgery. A double-blind placebo-controlled trial. *J Bone Joint Surg Br.* 1994;76(1):99-102.

98. Shaffer WO, Baisden JL, Fernand R, Matz PG. An evidence-based clinical guideline for antibiotic prophylaxis in spine surgery. *Spine J*. 2013;13(10):1387-1392.
99. Swoboda SM, Merz C, Kostuik J, Trentler B, Lipsett PA. Does intraoperative blood loss affect antibiotic serum and tissue concentrations? *Arch Surg*. 1996;131(11):1165-1171.
100. Polly DW Jr, Meter JJ, Brueckner R, Asplund L, van Dam BE. The effect of intraoperative blood loss on serum cefazolin level in patients undergoing instrumented spinal fusion. A prospective, controlled study. *Spine*. 1996;21(20):2363-2367.
101. Dobzyniak MA, Fischgrund JS, Hankins S, Herkowitz HN. Single versus multiple dose antibiotic prophylaxis in lumbar disc surgery. *Spine*. 2003;28(21):E453-E455.
102. Mastronardi L, Tatta C. Intraoperative antibiotic prophylaxis in clean spinal surgery: a retrospective analysis in a consecutive series of 973 cases. *Surg Neurol*. 2004;61(2):129-135.
103. Riley LH 3rd. Prophylactic antibiotics for spine surgery: description of a regimen and its rationale. *J South Orthop Assoc*. 1998;7(3):212-217.
104. Boscardin JB, Ringus JC, Feingold DJ, Ruda SC. Human intradiscal levels with cefazolin. *Spine*. 1992;17(6 suppl):S145-S148.
105. Guiboux JP, Cantor JB, Small SD, Zervos M, Herkowitz HN. The effect of prophylactic antibiotics on iatrogenic intervertebral disc infections: a rabbit model. *Spine*. 1995;20(6):685-688.
106. Fraser RD, Osti OL, Vernon-Roberts B. Iatrogenic discitis: the role of intravenous antibiotics in prevention and treatment. An experimental study. *Spine*. 1989;14(9):1025-1032.
107. Rhoten RL, Murphy MA, Kalfas IH, Hahn JF, Washington JA. Antibiotic penetration into cervical discs. *Neurosurgery*. 1995;37(3):418-421.
108. Scuderi GJ, Greenberg SS, Banovac K, Martinez OV, Eismont FJ. Penetration of glycopeptide antibiotics in nucleus pulposus. *Spine*. 1993;18(14):2039-2042.
109. Gibson MJ, Karpinski MR, Slack RC, Cowlishaw WA, Webb JK. The penetration of antibiotics into the normal intervertebral disc. *J Bone Joint Surg Br*. 1987;69(5):784-786.
110. Eismont FJ, Wiesel SW, Brighton CT, Rothman RH. Antibiotic penetration into rabbit nucleus pulposus. *Spine*. 1987;12(3):254-256.
111. Riley LH 3rd, Banovac K, Martinez OV, Eismont FJ. Tissue distribution of antibiotics in the intervertebral disc. *Spine*. 1994;19(23):2619-2625.
112. Currier BL, Banovac K, Eismont FJ. Gentamicin penetration into normal rabbit nucleus pulposus. *Spine*. 1994;19(23):2614-2618.
113. Urban JP, Holm S, Maroudas A, Nachemson A. Nutrition of the intervertebral disk. An in vivo study of solute transport. *Clin Orthop Relat Res*. 1977;129:101-114.
114. Walters R, Rahmat R, Fraser R, Moore R. Preventing and treating discitis: cephazolin penetration in ovine lumbar intervertebral disc. *Eur Spine J*. 2006;15(9):1397-1403.
115. Rohde V, Meyer B, Schaller C, Hassler WE. Spondylodiscitis after lumbar discectomy. Incidence and a proposal for prophylaxis. *Spine*. 1998;23(5):615-620.
116. Sweet FA, Roh M, Sliva C. Intrawound application of vancomycin for prophylaxis in instrumented thoracolumbar fusions: efficacy, drug levels, and patient outcomes. *Spine*. 2011;36(24):2084-2088.
117. Strom RG, Pacione D, Kalhorn SP, Frempong-Boadu AK. Lumbar laminectomy and fusion with routine local application of vancomycin powder: decreased infection rate in instrumented and non-instrumented cases. *Clin Neurol Neurosurg*. 2013;115(9):1766-1769.
118. Heller A, McIff TE, Lai S-M, Burton DC. Intrawound vancomycin powder decreases staphylococcal surgical site infections following posterior instrumented spinal arthrodesis. *J Spinal Disord Tech*. 2015;28(10):E584-E589.
119. Chiang H-Y, Herwaldt LA, Blevins AE, Cho E, Schweizer ML. Effectiveness of local vancomycin powder to decrease surgical site infections: a meta-analysis. *Spine J*. 2014;14(3):397-407.
120. Tubaki VR, Rajasekaran S, Shetty AP. Effects of using intravenous antibiotic only versus local intrawound vancomycin antibiotic powder application in addition to intravenous antibiotics on postoperative infection in spine surgery in 907 patients. *Spine*. 2013;38(25):2149-2155.
121. O'Neill KR, Smith JG, Abtahi AM, et al. Reduced surgical site infections in patients undergoing posterior spinal stabilization of traumatic injuries using vancomycin powder. *Spine J*. 2011;11(7):641-646.
122. Caroom C, Tullar JM, Benton EG, Jones JR, Chaput CD. Intrawound vancomycin powder reduces surgical site infections in posterior cervical fusion. *Spine*. 2013;38(14):1183-1187.
123. Strom RG, Pacione D, Kalhorn SP, Frempong-Boadu AK. Decreased risk of wound infection after posterior cervical fusion with routine local application of vancomycin powder. *Spine*. 2013;38(12):991-994.
124. Zebala LP, Chuntarapas T, Kelly MP, et al. Intrawound vancomycin powder eradicates surgical wound contamination: an in vivo rabbit study. *J Bone Joint Surg Am*. 2014;96(1):46-51.
125. Godil SS, Parker SL, O'Neill KR, Devin CJ, McGirt MJ. Comparative effectiveness and cost-benefit analysis of local application of vancomycin powder in posterior spinal fusion for spine trauma: clinical article. *J Neurosurg Spine*. 2013;19(3):331-335.
126. Emohare O, Ledonio CG, Hill BW, et al. Cost savings analysis of intrawound vancomycin powder in posterior spinal surgery. *Spine J*. 2014;14(11):2710-2715.
127. Gans I, Dormans JP, Spiegel DA, et al. Adjunctive vancomycin powder in pediatric spine surgery is safe. *Spine*. 2013;38(19):1703-1707.
128. Armaghani SJ, Menge TJ, Lovejoy SA, Mencio GA, Martus JE. Safety of topical vancomycin for pediatric spinal deformity: nontoxic serum levels with supratherapeutic drain levels. *Spine*. 2014;39(20):1683-1687.
129. Brown MD, Brookfield KF. A randomized study of closed wound suction drainage for extensive lumbar spine surgery. *Spine*. 2004;29(10):1066-1068.
130. Scuderi GJ, Brusovanik GV, Fitzhenry LN, Vaccaro AR. Is wound drainage necessary after lumbar spinal fusion surgery? *Med Sci Monit*. 2005;11(2):CR64-CR66.
131. Sasso RC, Williams JI, Dimasi N, Meyer PR Jr. Postoperative drains at the donor sites of iliac-crest bone grafts. A prospective, randomized study of morbidity at the donor site in patients who had a traumatic injury of the spine. *J Bone Joint Surg Am*. 1998;80(5):631-635.
132. Diab M, Smucny M, Dormans JP, et al. Use and outcomes of wound drain in spinal fusion for adolescent idiopathic scoliosis. *Spine*. 2012;37(11):966-973.

133. Dire DJ, Coppola M, Dwyer DA, Lorette JJ, Karr JL. Prospective evaluation of topical antibiotics for preventing infections in uncomplicated soft-tissue wounds repaired in the ED. *Acad Emerg Med.* 1995;2(1):4-10.
134. Rosenstein BD, Wilson FC, Funderburk CH. The use of bacitracin irrigation to prevent infection in postoperative skeletal wounds. An experimental study. *J Bone Joint Surg Am.* 1989;71(3):427-430.
135. Benjamin JB, Volz RG. Efficacy of a topical antibiotic irrigant in decreasing or eliminating bacterial contamination in surgical wounds. *Clin Orthop Relat Res.* 1984;(184):114-117.
136. Netland PA, Baumgartner JE, Andrews BT. Intraoperative anaphylaxis after irrigation with bacitracin: case report. *Neurosurgery.* 1987;21(6):927-928.
137. Owens BD, White DW, Wenke JC. Comparison of irrigation solutions and devices in a contaminated musculoskeletal wound survival model. *J Bone Joint Surg Am.* 2009;91(1):92-98.
138. Gruenberg MF, Campaner GL, Sola CA, Ortolan EG. Ultraclean air for prevention of postoperative infection after posterior spinal fusion with instrumentation: a comparison between surgeries performed with and without a vertical exponential filtered air-flow system. *Spine.* 2004;29(20):2330-2334.
139. Hooper GJ, Rothwell AG, Frampton C, Wyatt MC. Does the use of laminar flow and space suits reduce early deep infection after total hip and knee replacement?: the ten-year results of the New Zealand Joint Registry. *J Bone Joint Surg Br.* 2011;93(1):85-90.
140. Brandt C, Hott U, Sohr D, et al. Operating room ventilation with laminar airflow shows no protective effect on the surgical site infection rate in orthopedic and abdominal surgery. *Ann Surg.* 2008;248(5):695-700.
141. Short LJ, Bell DM. Risk of occupational infection with blood-borne pathogens in operating and delivery room settings. *Am J Infect Control.* 1993;21(6):343-350.
142. Webster J, Alghamdi AA. Use of plastic adhesive drapes during surgery for preventing surgical site infection. *Cochrane Database Syst Rev.* 2007;(4):CD006353.
143. Smilanich RP, Bonnet I, Kirkpatrick JR. Contaminated wounds: the effect of initial management on outcome. *Am Surg.* 1995;61(5):427-430.
144. Beldi G, Bisch-Knaden S, Banz V, Mühlemann K, Candinas D. Impact of intraoperative behavior on surgical site infections. *Am J Surg.* 2009;198(2):157-162.
145. Bible JE, O'Neill KR, Crosby CG, et al. Implant contamination during spine surgery. *Spine J.* 2013;13(6):637-640.
146. Bose B. Delayed infection after instrumented spine surgery: case reports and review of the literature. *Spine J.* 2003;3(5):394-399.
147. Dipaola CP, Saravanja DD, Boriani L, et al. Postoperative infection treatment score for the spine (PITSS): construction and validation of a predictive model to define need for single versus multiple irrigation and debridement for spinal surgical site infection. *Spine J.* 2012;12(3):218-230.
148. Hahn F, Zbinden R, Min K. Late implant infections caused by *Propionibacterium acnes* in scoliosis surgery. *Eur Spine J.* 2005;14(8):783-788.
149. Page CP, Bohnen JM, Fletcher JR, et al. Antimicrobial prophylaxis for surgical wounds. Guidelines for clinical care. *Arch Surg.* 1993;128(1):79-88.
150. Bhandari M, Adili A, Schemitsch EH. The efficacy of low-pressure lavage with different irrigating solutions to remove adherent bacteria from bone. *J Bone Joint Surg Am.* 2001;83-A(3):412-419.
151. Moe JH. Complications of scoliosis treatment. *Clin Orthop Relat Res.* 1967;53:21-30.
152. Lonstein J, Winter R, Moe J, Gaines D. Wound infection with Harrington instrumentation and spine fusion for scoliosis. *Clin Orthop Relat Res.* 1973;96:222-233.
153. Deckey JE, Court C, Bradford DS. Loss of sagittal plane correction after removal of spinal implants. *Spine.* 2000;25(19):2453-2460.
154. Wenger DR, Mubarak SJ, Leach J. Managing complications of posterior spinal instrumentation and fusion. *Clin Orthop Relat Res.* 1992;284:24-33.
155. Keller RB, Pappas AM. Infection after spinal fusion using internal fixation instrumentation. *Orthop Clin North Am.* 1972;3(1):99-111.
156. Benli IT, Acaroglu E, Akalin S, et al. Anterior radical debridement and anterior instrumentation in tuberculosis spondylitis. *Eur Spine J.* 2003;12(2):224-234.
157. Abbey DM, Turner DM, Warson JS, Wirt TC, Scalley RD. Treatment of postoperative wound infections following spinal fusion with instrumentation. *J Spinal Disord.* 1995;8(4):278-283.
158. Ha KY, Kim YH. Postoperative spondylitis after posterior lumbar interbody fusion using cages. *Eur Spine J.* 2004;13(5):419-424.
159. Picada R, Winter RB, Lonstein JE, et al. Postoperative deep wound infection in adults after posterior lumbosacral spine fusion with instrumentation: incidence and management. *J Spinal Disord.* 2000;13(1):42-45.
160. Rihn JA, Lee JY, Ward WT. Infection after the surgical treatment of adolescent idiopathic scoliosis: evaluation of the diagnosis, treatment, and impact on clinical outcomes. *Spine.* 2008;33(3):289-294.
161. McCarthy RE, Peek RD, Morrissy RT, Hough AJ Jr. Allograft bone in spinal fusion for paralytic scoliosis. *J Bone Joint Surg Am.* 1986;68(3):370-375.
162. Stevens DB, Beard C. Segmental spinal instrumentation for neuromuscular spinal deformity. *Clin Orthop Relat Res.* 1989;242:164-168.
163. Hedequist D, Haugen A, Hresko T, Emans J. Failure of attempted implant retention in spinal deformity delayed surgical site infections. *Spine.* 2009;34(1):60-64.
164. Núñez-Pereira S, Pellisé F, Rodríguez-Pardo D, et al. Implant survival after deep infection of an instrumented spinal fusion. *Bone Joint J.* 2013;95-B(8):1121-1126.
165. Ahmed R, Greenlee JDW, Traynelis VC. Preservation of spinal instrumentation after development of postoperative bacterial infections in patients undergoing spinal arthrodesis. *J Spinal Disord Tech.* 2012;25(6):299-302.
166. Sheehan E, McKenna J, Mulhall KJ, Marks P, McCormack D. Adhesion of *Staphylococcus* to orthopaedic metals, an in vivo study. *J Orthop Res.* 2004;22(1):39-43.
167. Dumanian GA, Ondra SL, Liu J, Schafer MF, Chao JD. Muscle flap salvage of spine wounds with soft tissue defects or infection. *Spine.* 2003;28(11):1203-1211.
168. Mericli AF, Mirzabeigi MN, Moore JH, et al. Reconstruction of complex posterior cervical spine wounds using the paraspinous muscle flap. *Plast Reconstr Surg.* 2011;128(1):148-153.
169. Mericli AF, Tarola NA, Moore JH, et al. Paraspinous muscle flap reconstruction of complex midline back wounds: risk factors and postreconstruction complications. *Ann Plast Surg.* 2010;65(2):219-224.

170. Yuan-Innes MJ, Temple CL, Lacey MS. Vacuum-assisted wound closure: a new approach to spinal wounds with exposed hardware. *Spine*. 2001;26(3):E30-E33.
171. Argenta LC, Morykwas MJ. Vacuum-assisted closure: a new method for wound control and treatment: clinical experience. *Ann Plast Surg*. 1997;38(6):563-576.
172. Clark NM, Hershberger E, Zervosc MJ, Lynch JP 3rd. Antimicrobial resistance among gram-positive organisms in the intensive care unit. *Curr Opin Crit Care*. 2003;9(5):403-412.
173. Ploumis A, Mehbod AA, Dressel TD, et al. Therapy of spinal wound infections using vacuum-assisted wound closure: risk factors leading to resistance to treatment. *J Spinal Disord Tech*. 2008;21(5):320-323.
174. Dubée V, Lenoir T, Leflon-Guibout V, et al. Three-month antibiotic therapy for early-onset postoperative spinal implant infections. *Clin Infect Dis*. 2012;55(11):1481-1487.

100

CHAPTER

Pseudarthrosis

SECTION XIV

Neil N. Patel
Martin H. Pham
Andre M. Jakoi
Jeffrey C. Wang

Introduction

Spinal fusions are one of the most common spine surgeries performed today. The number of spinal fusion surgeries performed has significantly increased over the past 2 decades. From 1998 to 2008, the rates of spinal fusion surgery have increased by 137%.[1] Although there have been significant improvements in spine surgery over the years, complications still exist. One prevalent complication is pseudarthrosis, which is the failure of an attempted fusion of the spine. Pseudarthrosis can be a significant problem that may be asymptomatic or lead to pain and disability and eventually the need for revision surgery. This chapter reviews prevention, evaluation, and management of pseudarthrosis of the cervical and lumbar spine.

Risk Factors

Fusion surgery is based on bony segments of the spine growing together. The biologic and biomechanical consideration of fusion surgery must be thoroughly understood to prevent pseudarthrosis. Three fundamental requirements are needed for bony fusion: a sufficient amount of osteogenic cells, an osteoconductive matrix that can act as a scaffold for new bone to form, and osteoinductive signals that promote bone formation. Along with that, it is imperative to have adequate blood supply to the fusion bed. Proper biomechanical stability also aids in limiting micromotion and strain to allow for bony fusion.

When there is a failure of fusion, or pseudarthrosis, it is due to an inadequacy of one or more of the requirements just listed. Patient-related factors and surgical technique play an important role as well. Thus, it is imperative to optimize all of those aspects to promote successful bony fusion.

Vitamin D deficiency has been linked to longer time to fusion with higher rates of nonunion.[2] Prevalence of vitamin D deficiency in patients undergoing spinal fusion is higher than the general population.[3,4] Preoperative analysis of vitamin D levels with appropriate treatment may aid in successful fusion.

Postoperative use of nonsteroidal anti-inflammatory drugs and steroids has been linked to increased pseudarthrosis rates.[5–9] Nonsteroidal antiinflammatory drugs inhibit osteogenic activity and, in turn, decrease fusion rates.[6] Cyclooxygenase-2 inhibitors, such as celecoxib, have not caused a statistically significant increase in pseudarthrosis rates.[7,8]

Smoking and use of nicotine products have been shown to significantly increase pseudarthrosis rates in both cervical and lumbar spinal fusions.[10–18] Brown et al. in 1986 reported fusion rates in smokers versus nonsmokers after undergoing a two-level lumbar laminectomy and posterolateral fusion.[11] All fusions were performed in situ without hardware or interbody devices. Nonsmokers had a pseudarthrosis rate of 8%, while smokers had a pseudarthrosis rate of 40%. Several other studies since then have validated the claim that smoking has a significant inhibitory effect on spinal fusions. A recent study by Bydon et al. analyzed the fusion rates of smokers versus nonsmokers in single-level and two-level instrumented posterolateral lumbar fusions and noted no difference in single-level fusion rates between smokers and nonsmokers.[12] However, two-level fusions showed a significantly higher pseudarthrosis rate in smokers versus nonsmokers (29.17% vs. 10.92%, respectively). Glassman et al. analyzed patients who had undergone single-level or two-level instrumented posterolateral lumbar fusion using iliac crest autograft to analyze the fusion rates of smokers versus nonsmokers versus previous smokers who quit.[13] The pseudarthrosis rate in smokers was almost double that of nonsmokers (26.5% vs. 14.2%, respectively). Previous smokers who quit postoperatively were noted to have a pseudarthrosis rate of 17.1%, trending toward the rate of the nonsmoking group. Hilibrand et al. evaluated smokers and nonsmokers who had undergone multilevel anterior cervical discectomy and fusion and noted solid bony fusions at all sites at a rate of 76% in nonsmokers and only 50% in smokers.[14] Beyond smoking, any use of nicotine products has been suggested to increase pseudarthrosis rates in rabbit models.[16,17]

Spinal Instrumentation and Its Effect on Fusion

Instrumentation of the spine has evolved significantly as we learn more about the biology and biomechanics of the spine. The main purpose of advances in technique and instrumentation is to improve results. Several studies have looked at the effects of spinal instrumentation on fusion rates and overall clinical outcomes.[19–44] The following is a brief overview of the effect of spinal instrumentation on the fusion rates. The advances in pedicle screws, interbody devices, cervical plates, and other spinal instrumentation are substantial and warrant an in-depth discussion, which is beyond the scope of this chapter.

Lumbar Spine

Several prospective randomized control studies have analyzed the effects of pedicle screw instrumentation on fusion rates.[19–24] Fischgrund et al. analyzed the fusion rates of single-level laminectomy and arthrodesis with and without pedicle screw instrumentation and noted a pseudarthrosis rate of 18% in the instrumented group compared to 55% in the uninstrumented group.[19] However, overall clinical outcomes were similar in both groups at 2 years. Kornblum et al. analyzed those same patients from the uninstrumented group to look at clinical outcomes at 5 to 14 years.[20] It was noted that clinical outcomes were significantly better in those patients with solid fusions compared to patients who had a pseudarthrosis (86% vs. 56%, respectively).

A prospective randomized study by Zdeblick et al. looked at the difference in fusion rates in uninstrumented, semirigid instrumented, and rigid instrumented posterolateral lumbar and lumbosacral fusions.[21] The uninstrumented group had a fusion rate of 65% compared to 77% in the semirigid instrumentation group and 95% in the rigid instrumentation groups. Rigid instrumentation had a statistically significant improved rate of fusion. Overall, pedicle screw instrumentation has been widely used to aid in rigidity in an attempt to increase fusion rates.

In contrast, Thomsen et al. performed a similar prospective randomized study and noted no difference in fusion rates with or without the use of pedicle screws.[22] Two other similar studies showed comparable results, with no difference in pain and functional outcomes and no difference in fusion rates.[23,24] These results contradict those of Fischgrund et al. and Zdeblick et al. Christensen et al. showed improved results with uninstrumented posterolateral fusions but noted that those individuals with diagnosed preoperative degenerative instability had better results with instrumented posterolateral fusions.[25]

Bono and Lee critically analyzed lumbar spinal fusion procedures and pseudarthrosis rates.[26] Their review noted a statistically higher fusion rate in instrumented posterolateral lumbar fusions. However, the overall clinical outcomes were similar. The Spine Patient Outcomes Research Trial also noted significantly improved fusion rates in pedicle screw instrumented posterolateral fusions versus uninstrumented fusions (85.29% vs. 67.24, respectively).[27]

Interbody fusion has become more common recently with the hypothesis that it aids in sagittal plane correction and provides another site for bony fusion to occur. Several randomized trials have analyzed the fusion rates and clinical outcomes of interbody fusion.[28,29] Christensen et al. showed that circumferential fusion with the use of an interbody cage resulted in significantly improved lumbar lordosis at 1-year follow-up and improved fusion rates with less reoperations.[28] Another study performed a similar randomized study with 2-year follow-up and noted that the overall clinical outcomes and fusion rates for posterolateral fusion versus interbody fusion were the same.[29] The Spine Patient Outcomes Research Trial noted no significant difference in fusion rates between instrumented posterolateral fusion and circumferential fusions with the use of an interbody device.[27] Several systematic reviews and meta-analysis studies suggest that circumferential fusions with interbody devices may increase fusion rates compared to posterolateral fusions alone.[30–33] Jalalpour et al. compared uninstrumented posterolateral fusion with transforaminal lumbar interbody fusion (TLIF) and concluded that, at 2-year follow-up, the TLIF group had better clinical outcomes.[34]

Controversy still remains regarding the use of pedicle screw instrumentation and interbody devices. There is data to suggest that fusion rates may be higher with the use of pedicle screws and interbody devices. However, good to excellent clinical outcomes can be achieved with or without instrumentation.[35,36]

Cervical Spine

Instrumentation in the cervical spine has also been analyzed to determine whether fusion rates and clinical outcomes are affected. Anterior cervical discectomy and fusion (ACDF) is the most common cervical spine surgery performed. Several studies have looked at the fusion rates with and without the use of plate fixation for ACDF.[37–44]

Wang et al. performed three studies analyzing the difference in fusion rates with and without use of plates in one-, two- and three-level ACDF.[37–39] The first study on single-level ACDF showed no statistical difference in fusion rates with the use of plate supplementation. However, graft collapse was significantly less in the patients with the use of plates. The second study noted significantly higher pseudarthrosis rates in the group without plates for two-level ACDF (0% in the plate group vs. 25% in the no-plate group). The third study analyzed three-level ACDF and showed a lower pseudarthrosis rate in the group with plates (18% in the plate group vs. 37% in the no-plate group). However, this difference was not statistically significant.

A meta-analysis performed by Fraser and Hartl analyzed the fusion rates of single-, two-, and three-level cervical procedures with and without use of a plate as well as ACDF versus corpectomy and fusion.[40] The data are summarized in Table 100.1.

Several studies have also shown no difference in fusion rates with the use of plate supplementation for single-level ACDF.[37,41,42] However, overall maintenance of cervical lordosis is better with the use of plates, with less graft collapse.[37,41,43]

TABLE 100.1 Cumulative Fusion Rates for Each Surgical Procedure

Type of Surgery	OUTCOME (NO. OF PROCEDURES) Fusion	Pseudarthrosis	Total (No. of Procedures)	Fusion Rate (%)
One-Level Procedures				
ACD	62	11	73	84.9
ACDF	1134	97	1231	92.1
ACDFP	329	10	339	97.1
Two-Level Procedures				
ACDF	337	85	422	79.9
ACDFP	174	10	184	94.6
One-level CORP	70	3	73	95.9
One-level CORPP	52	4	56	92.9
Three-Level Procedures				
ACDF	80	43	123	65.0
ACDFP	33	7	40	82.5
Two-level CORP	79	9	88	89.8
Two-level CORPP	51	2	53	96.2
Total	2401	281	2682	89.5

From Fraser JF, Hartl R. Anterior approaches to fusion of the cervical spine: a metaanalysis of fusion rates. *J Neurosurg Spine.* 2007;6:298–303.

The use of plates in ACDF procedures increases the fusion rates. This is especially true in multilevel ACDF procedures. When comparing multilevel ACDF to corpectomy, the fusion rates are similar.

ACD, anterior cervical discectomy; ACDF, anterior cervical discectomy and fusion; ACDFP, anterior cervical discectomy and fusion with plate placement; CORP, corpectomy; CORPP, CORP with plate placement.

Bone Grafting and Osteobiologics

Iliac crest autograft has long been considered the gold standard for bone grafting because of the osteogenic, osteoconductive, and osteoinductive nature of the graft. Yet, harvesting of iliac crest autograft can lead to a significant amount of donor site morbidity.[44]

The importance of graft material must be taken into consideration to effectively achieve the surgical goal of bony fusion. A recent systematic review of the literature on bone grafting materials found posterolateral lumbar fusion rates to be 79% with iliac crest bone graft, 52% with allograft alone, 89% with demineralized bone matrices, 87% with ceramics, 74% with autologous bone marrow, and 94% with bone morphogenetic protein.[45] A meta-analysis of anterior cervical pseudarthrosis showed a lower pseudarthrosis rate with the use of autograft (0.9%) compared to allograft (4.9%).[46] More recent advances in instrumentation, allografts, biologic substitutes, and cages have shown comparable overall fusion rates and results.[41,43] An in-depth discussion of the different types of graft options and osteobiologics, although important, is beyond the scope of this chapter.

Proper Surgical Technique

It is imperative that proper surgical technique is used when performing fusion surgery to allow for adequate bony fusion. This includes preparing the fusion bed surfaces meticulously by removing all soft tissue. When posterolateral fusion is attempted, after removal of all soft tissue at the fusion sites, proper decortication of the transverse processes and lateral facets with exposure of bleeding cancellous bone is paramount.[47]

Similar methodology needs to be implemented when performing an interbody fusion or ACDF. Removal of all disc material with subsequent scraping of the superior and inferior endplates to expose bleeding bone is ideal. One must be careful not to significantly violate the endplates, as that can lead to subsidence of the interbody device or graft, especially in osteoporotic bone.

Lumbar Pseudarthrosis

Evaluation

The reported rates in the literature of pseudarthrosis after lumbar fusion range from 5% to 35%, with significantly higher incidences in those patients being fused three or more spinal levels.[48–52] Considering that many patients with pseudarthrosis remain asymptomatic, the true incidence is likely underestimated in the literature.[53] A morphologic classification for posterolateral lumbar pseudarthrosis has been described, although it has not found significant clinical application yet (Fig. 100.1).[51,53,54]

Pseudarthrosis should be on the differential diagnosis for a postoperative lumbar fusion patient with back pain and/or neurologic symptoms. Accurately attributing low back pain to nonunion after lumbar spine surgery can be very difficult.[55–58] Worsening of symptoms with movement may also indicate a mechanical etiology, such as the instability associated with nonunion. Physical examination is usually nonspecific but may identify gross motion or find a spinal deformity present due to the loss of alignment from fusion failure.[51,53,59,60] Asymptomatic pseudarthrosis has been reported in as many as 50% of patients, making initial diagnosis difficult at times.[53]

Open surgical exploration is the gold standard for lumbar fusion evaluation because it allows for the direct visualization of bony fusion. However, it is highly invasive and recommended only in patients with a high suspicion of pseudarthrosis or hardware failure.[59–63] Noninvasive methods for establishing fusion status are preferable and much more practical than open surgery, but interpretation of fusion status can still be challenging.

The most common radiographic findings suggestive of pseudarthrosis are implant failure, loss of fixation, radiolucencies, and spinal deformity.[51,53,64,65] Successful fusion is often judged on plain films or computed tomography (CT) through continuous trabecular osseous bridging between vertebrae combined with absence of peri-implant radiolucency and the absence of motion on flexion-extension radiographs.[66–71] However, radiolucencies around pedicle screws may disappear over time and its presence does not always necessarily indicate a permanent pseudarthrosis.[72,73]

Some early pseudarthrosis patients may begin to successfully fuse 1 to 2 years after surgery and improvement can

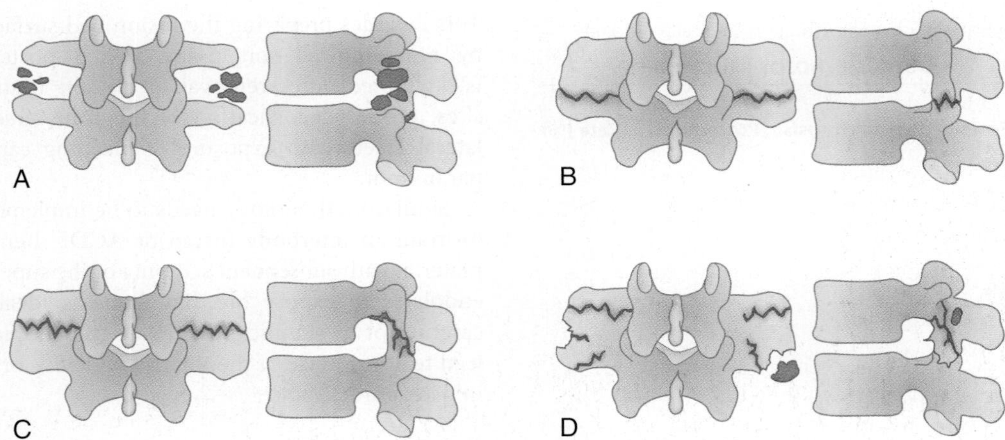

FIG. 100.1 Morphologic classification of posterolateral lumbar pseudarthrosis by Heggeness and Esses. (A) Atrophic: most severe case, involving gross atrophy and resorption of bone graft. (B) Transverse: most common, substantial mass of viable remodeled bone continuous with fusion mass of adjacent levels. (C) Shingle: substantial mass of mature bone graft is present, but defect is present and passes obliquely through the sagittal plane. (D) Complex: more than one adjacent defect in fusion mass. (From Chun DS, Baker KC, Hsu WK. Lumbar pseudarthrosis: a review of current diagnosis and treatment. *Neurosurg Focus.* 2015;39(4):E10; and Heggeness MH, Esses SI. Classification of pseudarthroses of the lumbar spine. *Spine (Phila Pa 1976).* 1991;16:S449–S454.)

continue for up to 4 or 5 years.[66] One study found that two-thirds of early pseudarthrosis cases had successful fusion 5 years after surgery. Pseudarthrosis has, in the past, been defined as the absence of solid bony fusion 1 year after the operation.[59,74] However, Tokuhashi et al. stated that, due to continued bone healing, it is not reasonable to diagnose a failure of osseous union within 1 year after posterior spinal surgery as pseudarthrosis and that instead it should be labeled as a "delayed union."[72] At 2 years postoperatively, if there is lack of successful bony fusion, it should be considered "indeterminate."[75] The final determination of a nonunion should be made 3 years after surgery.[66] Several studies show no difference in patient-reported outcomes in the first 1 to 3 years regardless of fusion status, and it is not until patients are followed long-term for greater than 5 years that radiographic pseudarthrosis impacts outcome, requiring intervention[19,20,53,76,77]

Plain radiography is commonly used as the first imaging evaluation of pseudarthrosis due to its rapid assessment and low cost. The US Food and Drug Administration guidelines for successful fusion include less than 3 mm of translational motion and less than 5 degrees of angular motion on flexion and extension radiographs.[53] For lumbar interbody fusion, Kuslich et al. suggested an angular change of greater than 7 degrees to indicate nonunion, 3 to 7 degrees as indeterminate, and less than 3 degrees to indicate fusion.[69] Other studies have proposed motion of 1 to 5 degrees to indicate fusion.[71] Bono et al. used a finite element analysis to show that less than 4.1 degrees of motion was most predictive of a solid fusion.[78]

The time to presentation of pseudarthrosis on plain films can vary. Kim et al. found an average time of 3.5 years to diagnosis of pseudarthrosis on plain radiographs.[65] Dickson et al. also found that only 73% of patients with confirmed pseudarthrosis was seen on plain films within the first 2 years postoperatively.[64] Studies have demonstrated a 62% to 68% correlation rate between preoperative evaluation of pseudarthrosis-negative plain films when compared with the gold standard of surgical exploration.[51,53,62,79–82]

CT has been shown to have the strongest correlation with intraoperative assessment of fusion status.[53,62,66,83,84] While there are currently no universal criteria or grading system to assess interbody bony fusion, many studies have defined pseudarthrosis through absence of bony trabeculation between adjacent vertebrae or periimplant radiolucency.[51,66,85,86] Although early literature on the use of CT for pseudarthrosis reported a correlation of 57% to 80% as compared to intraoperative findings,[62,87,88] there have since been considerable advances in CT technology with thin-slice sequence acquisition and 3-dimensional reconstruction techniques.[89] More recent published data have reported accuracy to be 74% to 96%.[63] Kanemura et al. used serial thin-cut CT examinations to show that a radiolucent zone of more than 1 mm around the interbody cages at 12 months was an early predictor of permanent pseudarthrosis.[66] Shah et al. also found that bridging trabeculation was found on 95% of CT scans versus only 4% of plain films.[85] Carreon et al. conducted two level 1 studies that showed the effective utility of CT imaging to assess fusion status.[63,90] Other studies have demonstrated that thin-section helical CT is more accurate in the detection of pseudarthrosis than plain film radiographs.[66,79,85,91-93]

Bone scan or bone scintigraphy is a nuclear scanning test that uses a small amount of a radioisotope (usually technetium-99m) with single-photon emission computed tomography to find tissue with high metabolic activity. In a series of 42 patients, Bohnsack et al. found bone scintigraphy to be only 88% accurate in diagnosing pseudarthrosis.[94] Similarly, McMaster and Merrick found in their series that there were a number of false positives due to the continued metabolic activity in both immature fusions and pseudarthrosis.[95]

Positron emission tomography (PET) scans also use a radioisotope tracer that emits positrons, such as fluorodeoxyglucose. Recently, its use for pseudarthrosis has been investigated. Foldager et al. showed in a porcine model that PET was a valid evaluation method to detect bone metabolic activity and fusion.[96] Recently, Peters et al. used ^{18}F-fluoride PET scans to discriminate between symptomatic and asymptomatic pseudarthrosis to serve as an indicator for revision surgery.[61] They found a significant difference between ^{18}F-fluoride activity in the lowest patient-reported clinical outcome group as compared to those in the highest group, concluding that ^{18}F-fluoride PET may be useful in diagnosing painful pseudarthrosis.

Because no noninvasive radiographic modality can yet approach the true gold standard of surgical exploration, it is recommended that multiple modalities be used to evaluate patients suspected of having pseudarthrosis.[79]

Management

Asymptomatic patients may benefit from a trial of conservative management with close clinical and radiographic follow-up. Those who require revision surgeries follow the primary principles of treatment that include replacement of any loose or ineffective instrumentation and regrafting.[51,59]

It remains controversial whether positive radiographic findings for pseudarthrosis in an asymptomatic patient make a clinical difference because these patients typically do not undergo revision surgery. Studies have shown that short-term (1–3 years) radiographic findings of nonunion have no impact on patient outcomes.[19,53,76]

DePalma and Rothman compared outcomes in patients with just radiographic evidence of pseudarthrosis.[49] There was no significant clinical differences between the two groups. It is still unclear why some patients with asymptomatic pseudarthroses maintain excellent clinical outcomes while others require significant management and treatment.[51,97,98] While nonunions can initially be asymptomatic on clinical follow-up, this complication may require revision surgeries up to 10 years after the index procedure.[19,20,99] Long-term follow-up in the initially asymptomatic failed lumbar fusion population is important.

Pseudarthrosis can be a cause of recurrent pain and disability and is one of the most common indications for revision lumbar surgery.[55,100,101] For those patients with pseudarthrosis who initially underwent just a posterolateral fusion (PLF), the placement of an interbody device or graft as a revision surgical treatment has been shown to be effective.

Circumferential fusion is the preferred method of treatment for pseudarthrosis and leads to higher fusion rates.[82,102–105] Noncircumferential revision surgery has been reported to have high rates of failure with persistence of the pseudarthrosis. Two studies analyzed the use of posterolateral fusion with instrumentation to treat their pseudarthrosis patients and found persistent pseudarthrosis in 51% and 45% of patients, respectively.[106,107] Studies utilizing circumferential fusion for treatment of pseudarthrosis have reported high fusion rates, ranging from 90% to 100% (Fig. 100.2).[82,103,105] Recently, Mobbs et al. conducted a prospective study to evaluate the utility of anterior lumbar interbody fusion (ALIF) as a salvage technique for lumbar pseudarthrosis. Twenty patients with failed TLIF or PLIF were treated with revision ALIF and demonstrated a 95% fusion rate at 1 year with improved clinical outcomes.[108]

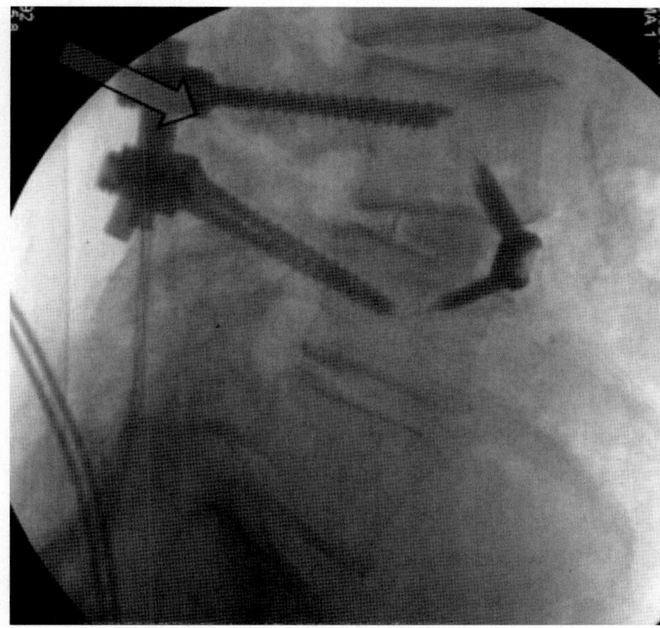

FIG. 100.2 Radiograph of patient with pseudarthrosis after failed prior posterior fusion treated with anterior lumbar interbody fusion (ALIF). Mobbs et al. noted 95% fusion rate after revision with ALIF in combination with improved clinical outcomes. (From Mobbs RJ, Phan K, Thayaparan GK, Rao PJ. Anterior lumbar interbody fusion as a salvage technique for pseudarthrosis following posterior lumbar fusion surgery. *Global Spine J.* 2016;6[1]:14-20.)

Surgical outcomes after revision surgery for pseudarthroses have been variable. Carpenter et al. reported 86 patients with lumbar pseudarthroses who underwent repair, of which a solid fusion was ultimately achieved in 81 patients (94%).[98] No association was noted between achievement of a solid fusion and clinical outcome score. Glassman et al. found that those patients who underwent PLF with instrumentation for nonunion improved the least in their Oswestry Disability Index scores compared to patients who underwent PLF for other indications.[109] Several other studies have shown that although revision surgery for pseudarthrosis may lead to high fusion rates, the overall clinical outcomes may not follow the same trend.[103,110]

Cervical Pseudarthrosis

Evaluation

Approximately one-third of patients with pseudarthrosis after anterior cervical fusion may be asymptomatic.[111] Symptomatic pseudarthrosis patients complain most consistently of neck pain with motion. Some may have neck pain since the time of surgery, while others develop new neck pain or symptoms up to 2 years after initial surgery. Nerve root compression with pain, sensory, and/or motor deficits in the upper extremities may also occur.

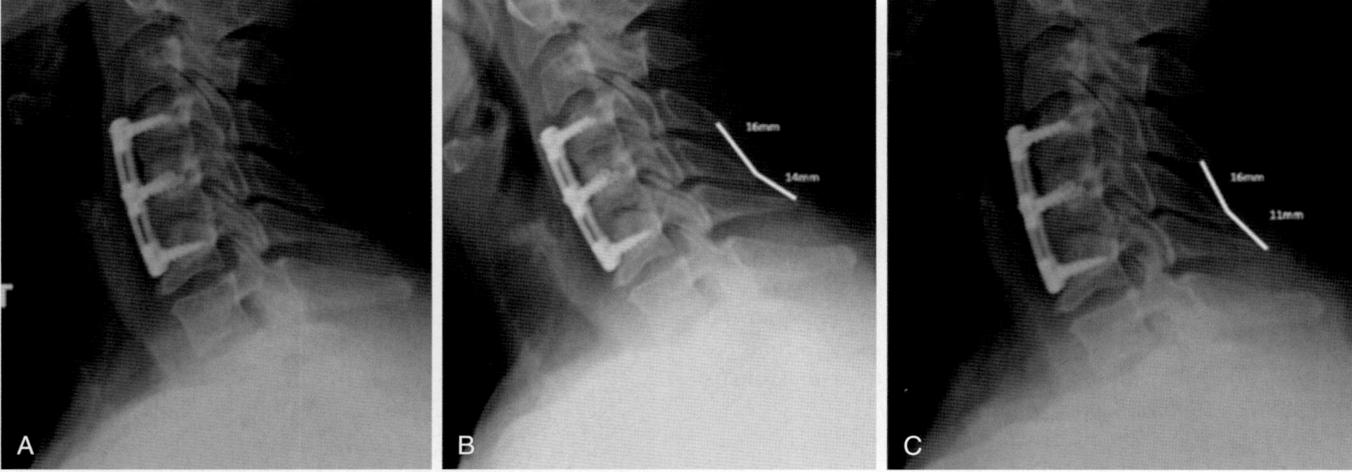

FIG. 100.3 (A) Neutral, (B) flexion, and (C) extension lateral films of a patient status post C4–C5, C5–C6 anterior cervical discectomy and fusion. C4–C5 appears consistent with union, C5–C6 appears consistent with pseudarthrosis. B and C demonstrate a greater than 2-mm increase in distance between spinous processes consistent with pseudarthrosis. (From Gruskay JA, Webb ML, Grauer JN. Methods of evaluating lumbar and cervical fusion. *Spine J.* 2014;14:531–539.)

As with the lumbar spine, the gold standard for diagnosing pseudarthrosis in the cervical spine is surgical exploration.[60] As surgical exploration is obviously invasive, other modalities have been used to aid in the diagnosis.

Plain radiographs are easily obtainable and are generally the first study used to evaluate a postoperative patient for pseudarthrosis. Utilization of flexion-extension lateral radiographs allows for the analysis of motion at the attempted fusion levels. Cannada et al. showed a change in interspinous process distance of more than 2 mm on flexion-extension radiographs correlated with pseudarthrosis, which was a better, more reproducible measure than Cobb angle (intervertebral angle; Fig. 100.3).[112] Song et al. analyzed fusion status on plain radiographs at differing magnification levels and noted that greater than or equal to 1 mm of spinous process motion at 150% magnification with adjacent-level motion of at least 4 mm provided pseudarthrosis diagnosis comparable to CT scan.[113] Screw loosening, implant failure, or periimplant radiolucency can also be analyzed with plain radiographs. A radiolucent line at the graft–vertebral body interface or lack of bridging osseous trabeculae may also suggest pseudarthrosis.[53,111,114,115]

Computerized motion analysis of plain radiographs can also be used in diagnosis.[83] A cutoff of greater than or equal to 1 degree of motion is noted to have a positive predictive value and negative predictive value similar to that found with CT scan. It was also noted that combining the two methods increased sensitivity and negative predictive value. Although the Food and Drug Administration guideline for diagnosis of pseudarthrosis of the cervical spine is 4 degrees of intervertebral motion, the use of 1 degree as the cutoff may be more reliable when using computerized motion analysis.[83,116]

As with the lumbar spine, CT scans allow for better analysis of bridging bony trabeculae to determine fusion. CT scan has been noted to determine pseudarthrosis at a higher, more accurate rate and have higher interobserver consistency (Fig. 100.4)[53,117–119] Thin-cut CT scan with reconstructions has been noted to be most accurate in evaluating for pseudarthrosis, yet it is still not 100%. It is best to combine all available imaging modalities and correlate that with the patient's symptoms to accurately diagnose pseudarthrosis. Surgical exploration still remains the gold standard.[119]

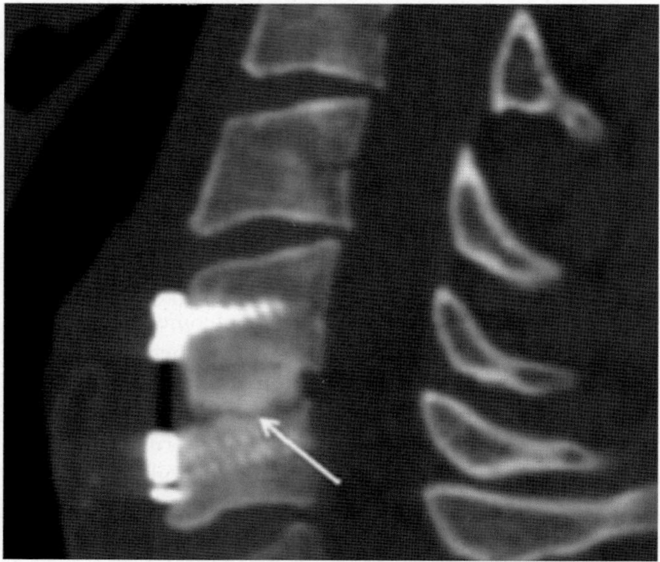

FIG. 100.4 Clearly notable lack of complete bony bridging between vertebral bodies after attempted anterior cervical discectomy and fusion. When evaluating for pseudarthrosis, thin-cut CT scan may be a useful diagnostic study. (From Gruskay JA, Webb ML, Grauer JN. Methods of evaluating lumbar and cervical fusion. *Spine J.* 2014;14:531–539.)

Management

Management of cervical pseudarthrosis is similar to that of the lumbar spine. Conservative management does have a role in asymptomatic patients, although close clinical and radiographic follow-up is needed in order to watch for progression or development of symptoms.[60,111,120,121]

Operative management of cervical pseudarthrosis can be done anteriorly or posteriorly. Phillips et al. analyzed 48 patients with cervical pseudarthrosis.[111] It was noted that 33% of patients with a radiographically diagnosed pseudarthrosis were asymptomatic and did not require surgical intervention. Of the 67% that were symptomatic, 28% of those had an asymptomatic period of at least 2 years before emergence of symptoms. The caudal-most level of a multilevel surgery was the most likely to have a pseudarthrosis (82%).

Brodsky et al.[122] performed a randomized study analyzing the fusion rates and clinical outcomes of the anterior versus posterior approach for treatment of patients with a diagnosis of symptomatic cervical pseudarthrosis. The anterior group achieved successful radiographic fusion in 76% with good to excellent clinical results in 59%; the posterior group achieved successful fusion in 94% with good to excellent clinical results in 88%.[122] Several other studies have shown similar results with higher rates of radiographic fusion after posterior repair of pseudarthrosis.[111,114,115,123,124]

In contrast, there is also data to suggest that anterior revision surgery is a viable option to manage cervical pseudarthrosis.[125–127] Tribus et al. showed 81% fusion rates with revision anterior cervical fusion,[126] while Coric et al. reported 100% fusion rates after anterior revision of pseudarthrosis.[127] There are special considerations that must be evaluated prior to revision anterior surgery. Scar tissue formation after the initial surgery may make the approach more challenging with obliteration of normal tissue planes if the revision approach is performed on the same side as the initial surgery. If the contralateral approach is considered to avoid scar tissue, vocal cord analysis must be performed to confirm adequate function of the recurrent laryngeal nerve on the side of the initial surgery.

Several systematic reviews and meta-analysis studies have analyzed the literature to evaluate the most effective management for cervical pseudarthrosis. They concluded that both anterior and posterior revision can lead to adequate fusion rates with good clinical outcomes, although posterior revision surgery has higher fusion rates.[121,128]

Cost of Pseudarthrosis

Economic value is increasingly becoming more important as a component of health care decision making. Limited data exist on the cost of pseudarthrosis and subsequently the cost of treatment and overall quality-of-life expenses. One study showed a total 2-year cost for revision surgery to be $41,631 with significant improvements in quality-adjusted life year (0.35) gained and concluded that revision surgery was modestly cost effective. Further research is required to fully explore the relationship between surgical intervention for pseudarthrosis of the spine and its potential financial implications.[129]

KEY REFERENCES

1. Glassman SD, Rose SM, Dimar JR, et al. The effect of postoperative nonsteroidal anti-inflammatory drug administration on spinal fusion. *Spine*. 1998;23:834-838.
   This study analyzed the effect of postoperative ketorolac administration on fusion rates and showed a statistically higher rate of nonunion with the use of ketorolac.
2. Brown CW, Orme TJ, Richardson HD. The rate of pseudarthrosis (surgical nonunion) in patients who are smokers and patients who are nonsmokers: a comparison study. *Spine*. 1986;11:942-943.
   This study analyzed the effect of smoking on lumbar laminectomy and fusion. This study showed pseudarthrosis rates of 40% in the smoking group and 8% in the nonsmoking group.
3. Fischgrund JS, Mackay M, Herkowitz HN, et al. Degenerative lumbar spondylolisthesis with spinal stenosis: a prospective, randomized study comparing decompressive laminectomy and arthrodesis with and without spinal instrumentation. *Spine*. 1997;22:2807-2812.
   This study showed the use of pedicle screw instrumentation for lumbar spondylolisthesis significantly improves fusion rates.
4. Bono CM, Lee CK. Critical analysis of trends in fusion for degenerative disc disease over the past 20 years: influence of technique on fusion rate and clinical outcome. *Spine*. 2004;29:455-463.
   This article critically analyzes the literature regarding lumbar fusions over a 20-year period to determine factors that may influence fusion rates and clinical outcomes.
5. Slappey G, Toribatake Y, Ganey TM, Ogden JA, Hutton WC. Guidelines to decortication in posterolateral spine fusion. *J Spinal Disord*. 1998;11(2):102-109.
   This cadaver study analyzed the intraosseous vascular structure of the lumbar spine to determine the most effective areas to decorticate in order to expose bleeding bone and marrow cells to the fusion bed.
6. Fraser JF, Hartl R. Anterior approaches to fusion of the cervical spine: a metaanalysis of fusion rates. *J Neurosurg Spine*. 2007;6:298-303.
   This metaanalysis compares the different types of anterior cervical surgeries to analyze fusion rates.
7. Chun DS, Baker KC, Hsu WK. Lumbar pseudarthrosis: a review of current diagnosis and treatment. *Neurosurg Focus*. 2015;39(4):E10.
   This article provides a comprehensive review of the methods of diagnosis and treatment for lumbar pseudarthrosis.
8. Gruskay JA, Webb ML, Grauer JN. Methods of evaluating lumbar and cervical fusion. *Spine J*. 2014;14:531-539.
   This article provides a comprehensive review of diagnosing lumbar and cervical pseudarthrosis with an overview of different imaging modalities that can be used.

REFERENCES

1. Rajaee SS, Bae HW, Kanim LE, Delamarter RB. Spinal fusions in the United States: analysis of trends from 1998 to 2008. *Spine*. 2012;37(1):67-76.
2. Ravidra VM, Godzik J, Dailey AT, et al. Vitamin D levels and 1-year fusion outcomes in elective spine surgery. *Spine*. 2015;40:1536-1541.
3. Ravindra VM, Godzik J, Guan J, et al. Prevalence of vitamin D deficiency in patients undergoing elective spine surgery: a cross-sectional analysis. *World Neurosurg*. 2015;83(6):1114-1119.
4. Stoker GE, Buchowski JM, Bridwell KH, et al. Preoperative vitamin D status of adults undergoing surgical spinal fusion. *Spine*. 2013;38(6):507-515.
5. Glassman SD, Rose SM, Dimar JR, et al. The effect of postoperative nonsteroidal anti-inflammatory drug administration on spinal fusion. *Spine*. 1998;23:834-838.

6. Dimar JR, Ante W, Zhang YP, Glassman SD. The effect of nonsteroidal anti-inflammatory drugs on posterior spinal fusion in the rat. *Spine*. 1996;21:1870-1876.
7. Long J, Lewis S, Kuklo T, Zhu Y, Riew KD. The effect of cyclooxygenase-2 inhibitors on spinal fusion. *J Bone Joint Surg Am*. 2002;84-A(10):1763-1768.
8. Reuben SS, Ekman FF. The effect of cyclooxygenase-2 inhibition on analgesia and spinal fusion. *J Bone Joint Surg Am*. 2005;87(3):536-542.
9. Sawin PD, Dickman CA, Crawford NR, et al. The effects of dexamethasone on bone fusion in an experimental model of posterolateral lumbar spinal arthrodesis. *J Neurosurg*. 2001;94:76-81.
10. Anderson MS, Christensen FB, Laursen M, et al. Smoking as a predictor of negative outcome in lumbar spinal fusion. *Spine*. 2001;26:2623-2628.
11. Brown CW, Orme TJ, Richardson HD. The rate of pseudarthrosis (surgical nonunion) in patients who are smokers and patients who are nonsmokers: a comparison study. *Spine*. 1986;11:942-943.
12. Bydon M, Garza-Ramos R, Abt NB, et al. Impact of smoking on complication and pseudarthrosis rates after single- and 2-level posterolateral fusion of the lumbar spine. *Spine*. 2014;39:1765-1770.
13. Glassman SD, Anagnost SC, Parker A, et al. The effect of cigarette smoking and smoking cessation on spinal fusion. *Spine*. 2000;25:2608-2615.
14. Hilibrand AS, Fye MA, Emery SE, Palumbo MA, Bohlman HH. Impact of smoking on the outcome of anterior cervical arthrodesis with interbody or strut-grafting. *J Bone Joint Surg*. 2001;83-A(5):668-673.
15. Lau D, Chou D, Ziewacz JE, Mummaneni PV. The effects of smoking on perioperative outcomes and pseudarthrosis following anterior cervical corpectomy. *J Neurosurg Spine*. 2014;21:547-558.
16. Silcox DH, Daftari T, Boden SD, et al. The effect of nicotine on spinal fusion. *Spine*. 1995;20:1549-1553.
17. Wing KJ, Fisher CG, O'Connell JX, Wing PC. Stopping nicotine exposure before surgery. *Spine*. 2000;25:30-34.
18. Hadley MN, Reddy SV. Smoking and the human vertebral column: a review of the impact of cigarette use on vertebral bone metabolism and spinal fusion. *Neurosurgery*. 1997;41(1):116-124.
19. Fischgrund JS, Mackay M, Herkowitz HN, et al. Degenerative lumbar spondylolisthesis with spinal stenosis: a prospective, randomized study comparing decompressive laminectomy and arthrodesis with and without spinal instrumentation. *Spine*. 1997;22:2807-2812.
20. Kornblum MB, Fischgrund JS, Herkowitz HN, et al. Degenerative lumbar spondylolisthesis with spinal stenosis: a prospective long-term study comparing fusion and pseudarthrosis. *Spine*. 2004;29:726-733.
21. Zdeblick TA. A prospective, randomized study of lumbar fusion: preliminary results. *Spine*. 1993;18: 983-991.
22. Thomsen K, Christensen FB, Eiskjaer SP, et al. 1997 Volvo Award winner in clinical studies: the effect of pedicle screw instrumentation on functional outcome and fusion rates in posterolateral lumbar spinal fusion: a prospective, randomized clinical study. *Spine*. 1997;22:2813-2822.
23. Moller H, Hedlund R. Instrumented and noninstrumented posterolateral fusion in adult spondylolisthesis, a prospective randomized study: part 2. *Spine*. 2000;25:1716-1721.
24. France JC, Yaszemski MJ, Lauerman WC, et al. A randomized prospective study of posterolateral lumbar fusion outcomes with and without pedicle screw instrumentation. *Spine*. 1999;24:553-560.
25. Christensen FB, Hansen EB, Laursen M, Thomsen K, Bunger C. Long-term functional outcome of pedicle screw instrumentation as a support for posterolateral spinal fusion: randomized clinical study with a 5-year follow-up. *Spine*. 2002;27:1269-1277.
26. Bono CM, Lee CK. Critical analysis of trends in fusion for degenerative disc disease over the past 20 years: influence of technique on fusion rate and clinical outcome. *Spine*. 2004;29:455-463.
27. Abdu WA, Lurie JD, Spratt KF, et al. Degenerative spondylolisthesis: does fusion method influence outcome? Four-year results of the Spine Patient Outcomes Research Trial. *Spine*. 2009;34:2351-2360.
28. Christensen FB, Hansen ES, Eiskjaer SP, et al. Circumferential lumbar spinal fusion with Brantigan cage versus posterolateral fusion with titanium Cotrel-Dubousset instrumentation: a prospective, randomized clinical study of 146 patients. *Spine*. 2002;27:2674-2683.
29. Hoy K, Bunger C, Niederman B, et al. Transforaminal lumbar interbody fusion (TLIF) versus posterolateral instrumented fusion (PLF) in degenerative lumbar disorders: a randomized clinical trial with 2-year follow-up. *Eur Spine J*. 2013;22:2022-2029.
30. Liu X, Wang Y, Qiu G, Weng X, Yu B. A systematic review with meta-analysis of posterior interbody fusion versus posterolateral fusion in lumbar spondylolisthesis. *Eur Spine J*. 2014;23:43-56.
31. Liu X, Wang Y, Qiu G, Weng X, Yu B. Meta-analysis of circumferential fusion versus posterolateral fusion in lumbar spondylolisthesis. *J Spinal Disord Tech*. 2014;27:E282-E293.
32. Liu X, Qui G, Weng X, Yu B, Wang Y. What is the optimum fusion technique for adult spondylolisthesis—PLIF or PLF or PLIF plus PLF? *Spine*. 2014;39:1887-1898.
33. Ye Y, Xu H, Chen D. Comparison between posterior lumbar interbody fusion and posterolateral fusion with transpedicular screw fixation for isthmic spondylolisthesis: a meta-analysis. *Arch Orthop Trauma Surg*. 2013;133:1649-1655.
34. Jalalpour K, Neumann P, Johansson C, Hedlund R. A randomized controlled trial comparing transforaminal lumbar interbody fusion and uninstrumented posterolateral fusion in the degenerative lumbar spine. *Global Spine J*. 2015;5:322-328.
35. Ekman P, Moller H, Tullberg T, Neumann P, Hedlund R. Posterior lumbar interbody fusion versus posterolateral fusion in adult isthmic spondylolisthesis. *Spine*. 2007;32:2178-2183.
36. Kim K, Lee S, Lee Y, Bae S, Suk K. Clinical outcomes of 3 fusion methods through the posterior approach in the lumbar spine. *Spine*. 2006;31:1351-1357.
37. Wang JC, McDonough PW, Endow KD, Kanim LEA, Delamarter RB. The effect of cervical plating on single-level anterior cervical discectomy and fusion. *J Spinal Disord*. 1999;6:467-471.
38. Wang JC, McDonough PW, Endow KD, Delamarter RB. Increased fusion rates with cervical plating for two-level anterior cervical discectomy and fusion. *Spine*. 2000; 25:41-45.
39. Wang JC, McDonough PW, Kanim LEA, Endow KK, Delamarter RB. Increased fusion rates with cervical plating for three-level anterior cervical discectomy and fusion. *Spine*. 2001;26:643-647.

40. Fraser JF, Hartl R. Anterior approaches to fusion of the cervical spine: a metaanalysis of fusion rates. *J Neurosurg Spine*. 2007;6:298-303.
41. Song K, Lee K. A preliminary study of the use of cage and plating for single-segment fusion in degenerative cervical spine disease. *J Clin Neurosc*. 2006;13:181-187.
42. Jacobs W, Willems PC, Kruyt M, et al. Systematic review of anterior interbody fusion techniques for single- and double-level cervical degenerative disc disease. *Spine*. 2011;36:E950-E960.
43. Vanek P, Bradac O, DeLacy P, et al. Comparison of 3 fusion techniques in the treatment of degenerative cervical spine disease. Is stand-alone autograft really the "gold standard"? *Spine*. 2012;37:1645-1651.
44. Silbar JS, Anderson DG, Daffner SD, et al. Donor site morbidity after anterior iliac crest bone harvest for single-level anterior cervical discectomy and fusion. *Spine*. 2003;28(2):134-139.
45. Hsu WK, Nickoli MS, Wang JC, et al. Improving the clinical evidence of bone graft substitute technology in lumbar spine surgery. *Global Spine J*. 2012;2:239-248.
46. Shriver MF, Lewis DJ, Kshettry VR, et al. Pseudarthrosis rates in anterior cervical discectomy and fusion: a meta-analysis. *Spine J*. 2015;15:2016-2027.
47. Slappey G, Toribatake Y, Ganey TM, Ogden JA, Hutton WC. Guidelines to decortication in posterolateral spine fusion. *J Spinal Disord*. 1998;11(2):102-109.
48. Berjano P, Langella F, Damilano M, et al. Fusion rate following extreme lateral lumbar interbody fusion. *Eur Spine J*. 2015;24(suppl 3):369-371.
49. DePalma AF, Rothman RH. The nature of pseudarthrosis. *Clin Orthop Relat Res*. 1968;59:113-118.
50. Grubb SA, Lipscomb HJ, Suh PB. Results of surgical treatment of painful adult scoliosis. *Spine*. 1994;19:1619-1627.
51. Chun DS, Baker KC, Hsu WK. Lumbar pseudarthrosis: a review of current diagnosis and treatment. *Neurosurg Focus*. 2015;39(4):E10.
52. Herkowitz HN, Sidhu KS. Lumbar spine fusion in the treatment of degenerative conditions: current indications and recommendations. *J Am Acad Orthop Surg*. 1995;3:123-135.
53. Gruskay JA, Webb ML, Grauer JN. Methods of evaluating lumbar and cervical fusion. *Spine J*. 2014;14:531-539.
54. Heggeness MH, Esses SI. Classification of pseudarthroses of the lumbar spine. *Spine*. 1991;16:S449-S454.
55. Dede O, Thuillier D, Pekmezci M, et al. Revision surgery for lumbar pseudarthrosis. *Spine J*. 2015;15:977-982.
56. Kim SS, Michelsen CB. Revision surgery for failed back surgery syndrome. *Spine*. 1992;17:957-960.
57. Ondra SL, Marzouk S. Revision strategies for lumbar pseudarthrosis. *Neurosurg Focus*. 2003;15:E9.
58. Steinmann JC, Herkowitz HN. Pseudarthrosis of the spine. *Clin Orthop Relat Res*. 1992;284:80-90.
59. Larsen JM, Capen DA. Pseudarthrosis of the lumbar spine. *J Am Acad Orthop Surg*. 1997;5:153-162.
60. Raizman NM, O'Brien JR, Poehling-Monaghan KL, Yu WD. Pseudarthrosis of the spine. *J Am Acad Orthop Surg*. 2009;17:494-503.
61. Peters M, Willems P, Weijers R, et al. Pseudarthrosis after lumbar spinal fusion: the role of (18)F-fluoride PET/CT. *Eur J Nucl Med Mol Imaging*. 2015;42:1891-1898.
62. Brodsky AE, Kovalsky ES, Khalil MA. Correlation of radiologic assessment of lumbar spine fusions with surgical exploration. *Spine*. 1991;16:S261-S265.
63. Carreon LY, Djurasovic M, Glassman SD, Sailer P. Diagnostic accuracy and reliability of fine-cut CT scans with reconstructions to determine the status of an instrumented posterolateral fusion with surgical exploration as reference standard. *Spine*. 2007;32:892-895.
64. Dickson DD, Lenke LG, Bridwell KH, Koester LA. Risk factors for and assessment of symptomatic pseudarthrosis after lumbar pedicle subtraction osteotomy in adult spinal deformity. *Spine*. 2014;39:1190-1195.
65. Kim YJ, Bridwell KH, Lenke LG, et al. Pseudarthrosis in adult spinal deformity following multisegmental instrumentation and arthrodesis. *J Bone Joint Surg Am*. 2006;88:721-728.
66. Kanemura T, Matsumoto A, Ishikawa Y, et al. Radiographic changes in patients with pseudarthrosis after posterior lumbar interbody arthrodesis using carbon interbody cages: a prospective five-year study. *J Bone Joint Surg Am*. 2014;96:e82.
67. Brantigan JW, Steffee AD, Lewis ML, Quinn LM, Persenaire JM. Lumbar interbody fusion using the Brantigan I/F cage for posterior lumbar interbody fusion and the variable pedicle screw placement system: two-year results from a Food and Drug Administration investigational device exemption clinical trial. *Spine*. 2000;25:1437-1446.
68. Blumenthal SL, Ohnmeiss DD. Intervertebral cages for degenerative spinal diseases. *Spine J*. 2003;3:301-309.
69. Kuslich SD, Ulstrom CL, Griffith SL, Ahern JW, Dowdle JD. The Bagby and Kuslich method of lumbar interbody fusion. History, techniques, and 2-year follow-up results of a United States prospective, multicenter trial. *Spine*. 1998;23:1267-1278.
70. Togawa D, Bauer TW, Brantigan JW, Lowery GL. Bone graft incorporation in radiographically successful human intervertebral body fusion cages. *Spine*. 2001;26:2744-2750.
71. McAfee PC, Boden SD, Brantigan JW, et al. Symposium: a critical discrepancy—a criteria of successful arthrodesis following interbody spinal fusions. *Spine*. 2001;26:320-334.
72. Tokuhashi Y, Ajiro Y, Umezawa N. Follow-up of patients with delayed union after posterior fusion with pedicle screw fixation. *Spine*. 2008;33:786-791.
73. Tokuhashi Y, Matsuzaki H, Oda H, Uei H. Clinical course and significance of the clear zone around the pedicle screws in the lumbar degenerative disease. *Spine*. 2008;33:903-908.
74. Turner JA, Ersek M, Herron L, et al. Patient outcomes after lumbar spinal fusions. *JAMA*. 1992;268:907-911.
75. McAfee PC. Interbody fusion cages in reconstructive operations on the spine. *J Bone Joint Surg Am*. 1999;81:859-880.
76. Herkowitz HN, Kurz LT. Degenerative lumbar spondylolisthesis with spinal stenosis. A prospective study comparing decompression with decompression and intertransverse process arthrodesis. *J Bone Joint Surg Am*. 1991;73:802-808.
77. Tsutsumimoto T, Shimogata M, Yoshimura Y, Misawa H. Union versus nonunion after posterolateral lumbar fusion: a comparison of long-term surgical outcomes in patients with degenerative lumbar spondylolisthesis. *Eur Spine J*. 2008;17:1107-1112.
78. Bono CM, Khandha A, Vadapalli S, et al. Residual sagittal motion after lumbar fusion: a finite element analysis with implications on radiographic flexion-extension criteria. *Spine*. 2007;32:417-422.
79. Choudhri TF, Mummaneni PV, Dhall SS, et al. Guideline update for the performance of fusion procedures for degenerative disease of the lumbar spine. Part 4: radiographic assessment of fusion status. *J Neurosurg Spine*. 2014;21:23-30.

80. Kant AP, Daum WJ, Dean SM, Uchida T. Evaluation of lumbar spine fusion. Plain radiographs versus direct surgical exploration and observation. *Spine*. 1995;20:2313-2317.
81. Sugiyama S, Wullschleger M, Wilson K, Williams R, Goss B. Reliability of clinical measurement for assessing spinal fusion: an experimental sheep study. *Spine*. 2012;37:763-768.
82. Albert TJ, Pinto M, Denis F. Management of symptomatic lumbar pseudarthrosis with anteroposterior fusion. A functional and radiographic outcome study. *Spine*. 2000;25:123-129.
83. Ghiselli G, Wharton N, Hipp JA, Wong DA, Jatana S. Prospective analysis of imaging prediction of pseudarthrosis after anterior cervical discectomy and fusion: computed tomography versus flexion-extension motion analysis with intraoperative correlation. *Spine*. 2011;36:463-468.
84. Cook SD, Patron LP, Christakis PM, et al. Comparison of methods for determining the presence and extent of anterior lumbar interbody fusion. *Spine*. 2004;29:1118-1123.
85. Shah RR, Mohammed S, Saifuddin A, Taylor BA. Comparison of plain radiographs with CT scan to evaluate interbody fusion following the use of titanium interbody cages and transpedicular instrumentation. *Eur Spine J*. 2003;12: 378-385.
86. Stauffer RN, Coventry MB. Anterior interbody lumbar spine fusion. Analysis of Mayo Clinic series. *J Bone Joint Surg Am*. 1972;54:756-768.
87. Laasonen EM, Soini J. Low-back pain after lumbar fusion. Surgical and computed tomographic analysis. *Spine*. 1989;14:210-213.
88. Rothem DE, Rothem L, Soudry M, Dahan A, Eliakim R. Nicotine modulates bone metabolism-associated gene expression in osteoblast cells. *J Bone Miner Metab*. 2009;27:555-561.
89. Lang P, Genant HK, Steiger P, Chafetz N, Morris J. [3-dimensional computed tomography and multiplanar CT-reformations in lumbar spondylodesis]. *Rofo*. 1988; 148:524-529.
90. Carreon LY, Glassman SD, Schwender JD, et al. Reliability and accuracy of fine-cut computed tomography scans to determine the status of anterior interbody fusions with metallic cages. *Spine J*. 2008;8:998-1002.
91. Santos ER, Goss DG, Morcom RK, Fraser RD. Radiologic assessment of interbody fusion using carbon fiber cages. *Spine*. 2003;28:997-1001.
92. Burkus JK, Sandhu HS, Gornet MF, Longley MC. Use of rhBMP-2 in combination with structural cortical allografts: clinical and radiographic outcomes in anterior lumbar spinal surgery. *J Bone Joint Surg Am*. 2005;87:1205-1212.
93. Lang P, Genant HK, Chafetz N, Steiger P, Morris JM. Three-dimensional computed tomography and multiplanar reformations in the assessment of pseudarthrosis in posterior lumbar fusion patients. *Spine*. 1988;13:69-75.
94. Bohnsack M, Gosse F, Ruhmann O, Wenger K. The value of scintigraphy in the diagnosis of pseudarthrosis after spinal fusion surgery. *J Spinal Disord*. 1999;12:482-484.
95. McMaster MJ, Merrick MV. The scintigraphic assessment of the scoliotic spine after fusion. *J Bone Joint Surg Br*. 1980;62-B:65-72.
96. Foldager C, Bendtsen M, Zou X, et al. ISSLS prize winner: positron emission tomography and magnetic resonance imaging for monitoring interbody fusion with equine bone protein extract, recombinant human bone morphogenetic protein-2, and autograft. *Spine*. 2008;33:2683-2690.
97. Adogwa O, Verla T, Thompson P, et al. Affective disorders influence clinical outcomes after revision lumbar surgery in elderly patients with symptomatic adjacent-segment disease, recurrent stenosis, or pseudarthrosis: clinical article. *J Neurosurg Spine*. 2014;21:153-159.
98. Carpenter CT, Dietz JW, Leung KY, Hanscom DA, Wagner TA. Repair of a pseudarthrosis of the lumbar spine. A functional outcome study. *J Bone Joint Surg Am*. 1996;78:712-720.
99. Mardjetko SM, Connolly PJ, Shott S. Degenerative lumbar spondylolisthesis. A meta-analysis of literature 1970-1993. *Spine*. 1994;19:2256S-2265S.
100. Hu RW, Jaglal S, Axcell T, Anderson G. A population-based study of reoperations after back surgery. *Spine*. 1997;22:2265-2270.
101. Martin BI, Mirza SK, Comstock BA, et al. Reoperation rates following lumbar spine surgery and the influence of spinal fusion procedures. *Spine*. 2007;32:382-387.
102. Buttermann GR, Garvey TA, Hunt AF, et al. Lumbar fusion results related to diagnosis. *Spine*. 1998;23:116-127.
103. Gertzbein SD, Hollopeter MR, Hall S. Pseudarthrosis of the lumbar spine. Outcome after circumferential fusion. *Spine*. 1998;23:2352-2356.
104. Hee HT, Castro FP Jr, Majd ME, Holt RT, Myers L. Anterior/posterior lumbar fusion versus transforaminal lumbar interbody fusion: analysis of complications and predictive factors. *J Spinal Disord*. 2001;14:533-540.
105. Slosar PJ, Reynolds JB, Schofferman J, et al. Patient satisfaction after circumferential lumbar fusion. *Spine*. 2000;25:722-726.
106. Lauerman WC, Bradford DS, Ogilvie JW, Transfeldt EE. Results of lumbar pseudarthrosis repair. *J Spinal Disord*. 1992;5:149-157.
107. West JL 3rd, Bradford DS, Ogilvie JW. Results of spinal arthrodesis with pedicle screw-plate fixation. *J Bone Joint Surg Am*. 1991;73:1179-1184.
108. Mobbs RJ, Phan K, Thayaparan GK, Rao PJ. Anterior lumbar interbody fusion as a salvage technique for pseudarthrosis following posterior lumbar fusion surgery. *Global Spine J*. 2016;6(1):14-20.
109. Glassman SD, Carreon LY, Djurasovic M, et al. Lumbar fusion outcomes stratified by specific diagnostic indication. *Spine J*. 2009;9:13-21.
110. Cassinelli EH, Wallach C, Hanscom B, Vogt M, Kang JD. Prospective clinical outcomes of revision fusion surgery in patients with pseudarthrosis after posterior lumbar interbody fusions using stand-alone metallic cages. *Spine J*. 2006;6:428-434.
111. Phillips FM, Carlson G, Emery SE, Bohlman HH. Anterior cervical pseudarthrosis natural history and treatment. *Spine*. 1997;22:1585-1589.
112. Cannada LK, Scherping SC, Yoo JU, Jones PK, Emery SE. Pseudoarthrosis of the cervical spine: a comparison of radiographic diagnostic measures. *Spine*. 2003;28: 46-51.
113. Song K, Piyaskulkaew C, Chuntarapas T, et al. Dynamic radiographic criteria for detecting pseudarthrosis following anterior cervical arthrodesis. *J Bone Joint Surg Am*. 2014;96:557-563.
114. Farey ID, McAfee PC, Davis RF, et al. Pseudarthrosis of the cervical spine after anterior arthrodesis: treatment by posterior nerve-root decompression, stabilization, and arthrodesis. *J Bone Joint Surg Am*. 1990;72:1171-1177.

115. Kuhns CA, Geck MJ, Wang JC, Delamarter RB. An outcome analysis of the treatment of cervical pseudarthrosis with posterior fusion. *Spine*. 2005;30:2424-2429.
116. Hipp JA, Reitman CA, Wharton N. Defining pseudarthrosis in the cervical spine with differing motion thresholds. *Spine*. 2005;30:209-210.
117. Ploumis A, Mehbod A, Garvey T, et al. Prospective assessment of cervical fusion status: plain radiograph versus CT-scan. *Acta Orthop Belg*. 2006;72:342-346.
118. Epstein N, Silvergleide RS. Documenting fusion following anterior cervical surgery: a comparison of roentgenogram versus two-dimensional computed tomographic findings. *J Spinal Disord*. 2003;16(3):243-247.
119. Buchowski JM, Liu G, Bunmaprasert T, Rose PS, Riew KD. Anterior cervical fusion assessments: surgical exploration versus radiographic evaluation. *Spine*. 2008;33:1185-1191.
120. DePalma AF, Cooke AJ. Results of anterior interbody fusion of the cervical spine. *Clin Orthop Relat Res*. 1968;60:169-186.
121. Kaiser MG, Mummaneni PV, Matz PG, et al. Management of anterior cervical pseudarthrosis. *J Neurosurg Spine*. 2009;11:228-237.
122. Brodsky AE, Khalil MA, Sassard WR, Newman BP. Repair of symptomatic pseudarthrosis of anterior cervical fusion: posterior versus anterior repair. *Spine*. 1992;17: 1137-1143.
123. Lowery GL, Swank ML, McDonough RF. Surgical revision for failed anterior cervical fusions: articular pillar plating or anterior revision? *Spine*. 1995;20(22):2336-2341.
124. Carreon L, Glassman SD, Campbell MJ. Treatment of anterior cervical pseudarthrosis: posterior fusion versus anterior revision. *Spine J*. 2006;6:154-156.
125. Newman M. The outcome of pseudoarthrosis after cervical anterior fusion. *Spine*. 1993;18(16):2380-2382.
126. Tribus CB, Corteen DP, Zdeblick TA. The efficacy of anterior cervical plating in the management of symptomatic pseudoarthrosis of the cervical spine. *Spine*. 1999;24(9):860-864.
127. Coric D, Branch CL Jr, Jenkins JD. Revision of anterior cervical pseudoarthrosis with anterior allograft fusion and plating. *J Neurosurg*. 1997;86(6):969-974.
128. McAnany SJ, Baird EO, Overley SC, et al. A meta-analysis of the clinical and fusion results following treatment of symptomatic cervical pseudarthrosis. *Global Spine J*. 2015;5:148-155.
129. Adogwa O, Parker SL, Shau D, et al. Cost per quality-adjusted life year gained of revision fusion for lumbar pseudoarthrosis: defining the value of surgery. *J Spinal Disord Tech*. 2015;28(3):101-105.

CHAPTER 101 Adjacent-Segment Disease

David M. Montgomery

Adjacent-segment pathology (ASP) is a common complication of spinal surgery. This chapter focuses on the causes, common clinical scenarios, and treatment options to avoid or treat ASP. Surgery changes the anatomy, physiology, kinematics, and biomechanics of the operated and contiguous elements of the spine. Nowhere are the influences of these factors more important than at the segments immediately above or below a surgical fusion. Short-term gratification from surgery can be tempered by long-term dissatisfaction when progressive degeneration causes symptoms to recur. Predicting the long-term outcome and assessing the risk/benefit ratio of surgery depends on accurate knowledge of the natural history of the patient and changes to the natural history from surgery. The dramatic increase in spinal fusion rates over the last 2 decades makes additional surgery for ASP much more common.[1] Expert treatment is guided by a thorough knowledge of the natural history, potential problems, complications, and treatment options for ASP.

Definition

ASP is an all-encompassing phrase describing abnormal changes to the spinal structures bordering an operative segment. ASP becomes important only when the pathology influences the clinical natural history. ASP can be thus be subdivided into radiographically detectable adjacent-segment degeneration (ASDeg) versus clinically relevant adjacent-segment disease (ASDis). The mere presence of radiographically detectable change to the spine does not equate to clinical relevance. Considerable research focuses on how surgery affects ASP with the ultimate goal of preventing, managing, or treating clinically relevant ASDis.

Natural History

Asymptomatic degenerative disc disease is common and parallels the normal spine aging process. The degenerative process is dynamic and progresses throughout life. Boden et al. evaluated lumbar spine MRI scans of asymptomatic volunteers. Degeneration or bulging discs were present in 35% of subjects 20 to 39 years old.[2] Degenerative changes, including disc herniations and spinal stenosis, increased to 57% of individuals over age 60 years. In a separate study, Boden et al. reported similar findings in the cervical spine.[3] Elfering et al. also showed that degenerative radiographic findings progress with age.[4] They prospectively reviewed MRI scans of asymptomatic volunteers over a 5-year timeline. A total of 41% of individuals showed advancement of degenerative changes without clinical symptoms. Clearly, progressive, asymptomatic degenerative changes to the spine are a normal part of the aging process.

The influence of surgery on the normal, expected degenerative process remains a subject of debate.[5] Surgical interventions are associated with ASDis, but whether these interventions significantly accelerate or cause the degeneration is debated.[6] Without randomized, controlled studies comparing surgical to nonsurgical patients, the significance of surgery on the degenerative process must be analyzed by less direct studies. Furthermore, the radiographic acceleration may not be clinically relevant. Radiographic adjacent-segment degeneration does not correlate well with symptomatic disease. In a study of postsurgical degenerative changes, Mannion et al. concluded that spinal fusion was associated with increased ASDeg but without influence on ASDis.[7]

Biomechanical and clinical outcome studies implicate surgery as an accelerating factor to ASDeg. Biomechanical studies demonstrate changes in adjacent-level intradiscal pressure and alterations of spine kinematics after a one-level fusion.[8] Other studies implicate excessive motion at adjacent spine segments. Torsional stresses due to spinopelvic imbalance alter disc stresses and physiology. All of these changes could theoretically alter the natural history of the adjacent disc.

Clinical outcome studies also implicate surgery as a contributing factor to ASP. The rate and severity of adjacent-level disc degeneration is not uniform after a fusion. Several independent studies show that the rate of ASDis varies depending on the type of surgery.[9] Laminectomy above the fusion, length of the fusion, type of fusion, instrumentation, and other factors change the rate of ASDis. The influence of surgical type on rate of ASDis links surgery to the degenerative process.

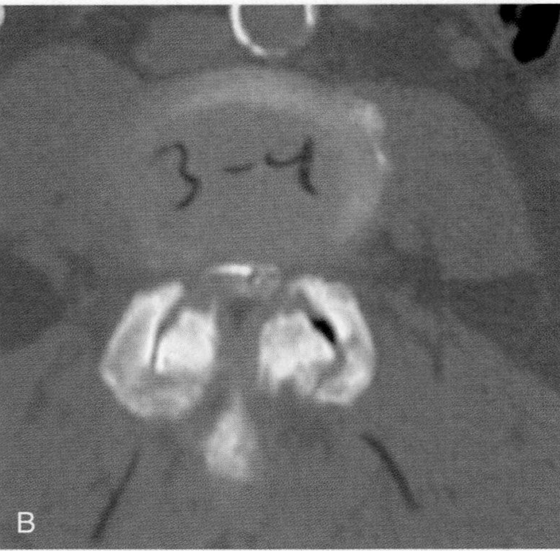

FIG. 101.1 Spinal stenosis at level above a fusion. (A) Lateral radiograph showing preexisting L4–L5 fusion. (B) Axial computed tomography/myelogram showing adjacent level stenosis at L3–L4.

BOX 101.1 Types of Adjacent-Level Degeneration

- Disc degeneration
- Disc herniation
- Spinal stenosis
- Spondylolisthesis
- Retrolisthesis
- Lateral listhesis
- Scoliosis
- Kyphosis
- Proximal junctional failure
- Proximal junctional fracture
- Sagittal imbalance
- Instability
- Facet degeneration
- Spondylolysis

Although the causes may be debatable, ASDeg and ASDis are realities of spinal practice. In a meta-analysis of the literature, Park et al. found that the incidence of symptomatic ASDis after spinal fusion ranged from 5.2% to 18.5% (Fig. 101.1).[9] The authors concluded that the biomechanical alteration of the levels adjacent to the fusion accelerated the natural history of ASDeg.

The normal spine starts to degenerate at an early adult age, then progresses throughout life. Most degenerative disease is asymptomatic, but for those who have symptoms, surgery may be necessary. Surgery alters the anatomy, physiology, biomechanics, and kinematics of the spine. Although debated, surgery likely accelerates ASDeg and ASDis, possibly leading to subsequent revision surgery.

Types of Adjacent-Level Degeneration

Box 101.1 lists the types of adjacent-level degenerative changes complicating patient management. The changes can occur alone or in combination. Management can range from observation to complex spinal reconstruction.

Etiology

The etiology of ASDeg is divided into several broad categories to help organize and stratify risk factors.

Biomechanical

Changes in motion, stress, strain, and stability influence the durability and strength of spinal structures. Surgical resection of posterior supporting elements—such as interspinous ligaments, facets, and paraspinous muscles—change the balance of forces aligning the spine. Malakoutian et al. reviewed published literature on kinematic changes at levels adjacent to a fusion.[10] They found that range of motion was affected more at the rostral end of the fusion than the caudal end. Range of motion increased 10% to 30% at the rostral end of a fusion. The findings are consistent with clinical prevalence of degenerative changes at the rostral segment in 70% to 100% of patients. They concluded that muscle damage from spine surgery may play a key role in ASDeg.

Fusions also alter the location of forces within the spine. The center of rotation of adjacent levels changes according to the type of fusion.[11] A posterior fusion displaces the center of rotation cephalad and posterior, increasing the stress on the facets. An anterior fusion displaces the center of rotation cephalad and anterior, increasing the shear and compressive stresses on the disc. A bilateral posterolateral fusion causes only slight increase in the facet joint stresses and had the least effect on the adjacent levels.

Other alterations in biomechanics include a change in disc pressure.[12] Fusions and spinal malalignment in the sagittal and frontal planes alter disc kinematics and accelerate degenerative changes.[8,13]

Genetic

The response of an intervertebral disc to similar mechanical factors is not uniform from patient to patient. Just as there is

BOX 101.2 Risk Factors for Adjacent-Level Degeneration

Age
Preexisting adjacent level disc degeneration
Adjacent-level facet degeneration
Ending fusion at L5
Length of fusion
Gender
Excessive distraction after posterior lumbar interbody fusion
Laminectomy adjacent to a fusion
Type of fusion
Sagittal imbalance
Body mass index
Instrumentation
Pelvic incidence/lumbar lordosis mismatch
Facet trophism and sagittal alignment
Osteoporosis
Iatrogenic muscle damage

a spectrum of radiographic degenerative changes in asymptomatic individuals, there is also a spectrum of adjacent-segment changes after the same type of fusion. Monozygotic twin studies comparing patients with dissimilar occupations attribute 26% to 72% of the difference in degenerative changes to genetic factors rather than environmental differences.[14] Gene expression response to mechanical loading is variable and can alter cellular metabolism of the disc.[15]

Physiology

Cell metabolism may be altered in adjacent discs as a response to immobilization. Cole et al. found in a canine study that disc metabolism was markedly altered adjacent to a fusion. Similar changes were not observed in a control group.[16]

Risk Factors

See Box 101.2 for a comprehensive list of risk factors implicated in the degenerative process.

Clinical Scenarios

Adjacent-Segment Disease After Laminectomy

By removing posterior stabilizing structures, a laminectomy alters spine kinematics.

Jansson et al. evaluated 9664 spinal stenosis patients over a 10-year period treated with a laminectomy and no fusion.[17] At 10-year follow-up, 11% of patients required a subsequent surgery. The study does not clarify the effect of laminectomy on ALDis acceleration, but does provide a baseline reoperation value for nonfusion surgical patients.

Adding a fusion to the laminectomy creates additional biomechanical stress to the adjacent level. Katz et al. studied surgically treated patients with spinal stenosis and 7- to 10-year follow-up.[18] The group was a mixture of laminectomy and laminectomy/fusion patients. Patients with spondylolisthesis 10 mm or greater had a fusion. Despite initial good results, 23% of patients required reoperation at 7- to 10-year follow-up. Adding a fusion to the laminectomy incrementally increased the reoperation rate at 10 years.

Lai et al. evaluated the magnitude of the laminectomy as a risk factor for ASDis after a spinal fusion.[19] A partial laminectomy with fusion was compared to a complete laminectomy with fusion. For both groups, the inferior facets at the fused level were partially resected and the adjacent-level facets were left intact. For the full laminectomy group, the entire spinous process and lamina of the upper vertebra and the supraspinous and interspinous ligaments connecting the upper vertebra to the adjacent segment were removed. For the partial laminectomy group, the structures were preserved except a portion of the upper lamina. After 6 years of follow-up, the authors concluded that the incidence of cranial segment instability was greater (24.3%) in the full laminectomy group than the partial laminectomy group (6.5%). The magnitude of the laminectomy influenced stability by removing the tension band stabilization effect of the supraspinous and interspinous ligaments.

Additional instability at adjacent segments has been documented when facetectomy is added to the laminectomy. In a cadaver study, segmental hypermobility was noted if more than 50% of the facet is removed.[20] Finite element analysis models confirm significant rotational instability if more than 75% of a facet is removed.[21] Aggressive facetectomy with the laminectomy creates concern for instability and subsequent ASDis.

Adjacent-Segment Disease After Lumbar Fusion

Lee, first noted clinically significant adjacent-level disease above various types of spinal fusions after an average symptom-free interval of 8.5 years.[22] The ASDis changes included degeneration of the facets, spinal stenosis, severe disc degeneration, spondylolisthesis, spondylolysis, and disc herniation. Schlegel et al. noted that pathology at segments not included in the fusion occurred at the adjacent segment 58% of the time.[23] These observations support biomechanical studies showing magnification of flexion, extension, and torsional strains at adjacent segments.[24]

Park et al. summarized the literature of adjacent-level disease after lumbosacral fusion.[9] Asymptomatic ASDeg ranged from 5.2% to 100%. Criteria for degeneration were based solely on radiographic criteria. Symptomatic ASDis ranged from 5.2% to 18.5%.

Radcliff et al. summarized available literature and concluded that the rate of ASDis is 2% to 3% per year.[6] Sears et al. further subdivided the rate based on the number of levels fused.[25] The mean annual incidence of ASDis after a single-level fusion is 1.7%. The rate increases to 3.6% after a two-level fusion and 5.0% after three- and four-level fusions. A laminectomy adjacent to a fusion increased the risk by 2.4 times. Stopping the fusion at L5 is associated with a 1.7 times risk of subsequent L5/S1 ASDis. Clearly, these numbers complicate the task of determining the number of levels to fuse in a patient with a single-level spondylolisthesis and multiple-level stenosis.

Treatment of adjacent-segment disease above a previous fusion can be complex and methods may vary. Treatment methods often center on a basic decision to extend the fused segments or merely decompress the adjacent level. Clinical decision making depends on factors such as presenting symptoms, neurologic status, relative complaint of back versus leg pain, stability, spinal balance, age, skill of the surgeon, and etiology of the ALDis.

Segmental instability above a fusion is reported in 45% of ASDis patients.[26] Thus, much of the literature on treating ALDis involves extending the length of the fusion.[27] The decompression can be very difficult in the presence of extensive scar due to a previous decompression. To avoid dural tears and excessive retraction of nerve roots, a destabilizing resection of the medial facets is advocated, thus necessitating a fusion. The role of an adjacent segment decompressive procedure alone is unclear but may be an option in a patient presenting with primarily neurologic complaints and a stable spine.[28] The lesser-magnitude surgery could delay an inevitable future complex spine reconstruction or avoid the fusion altogether. The difficulty of the decompression and the skill of the surgeon at revising previous decompressions and managing dural tears is a factor in the decision.[29] Clinical judgment, radiographs, and patient preference should guide operative treatment.[30]

Adjacent-Segment Disease After Scoliosis Surgery

Treating spinal deformities is a very challenging segment of spine surgery. Patients may present with pain, neurologic symptoms, and/or an abnormal appearance. Body self-image measurements point to an important psychological component related to patient satisfaction with outcome. The major goal of spinal deformity surgery is to create a stable spine and restore spinopelvic alignment.[31] Sagittal plane balance is the most important predictor of surgical outcome after deformity surgery.[32] The ability to stand upright rather than stooped forward or leaning to the side improves comfort as well as body image. Even in expert hands, only 23% of patients experience complete correction of their deformity at 1 year. Sagittal deformity is corrected completely in only 50% of cases. Dissatisfaction with a less than perfect spinal realignment can be further exacerbated by adjacent-segment disease.

Proximal junctional failure (PJF) is defined as a 10-degree or greater increase in the kyphosis angle of the upper instrumented vertebra (UIV) and the UIV +2. The incidence of proximal junctional kyphosis (PJK) is 32%.[33] (Fig. 101.2). Modes of failure include fracture of the UIV or UIV +1 in 56% of patients, ligament injury (35%), and implant pullout (9%).[34] The mode of failure depends on the level of the UIV. Soft tissue failure is more common for upper thoracic UIV. Fracture is more common for thoracolumbar UIV.[35] In a series of 1218 spinal deformity patients, PJF occurred in 5.6% of patients by 28 weeks postoperatively.[35] Another author reported PJF in 26% of patients by 5.3 years postoperatively.[36] PJF can worsen spinopelvic balance, cause chronic pain or neurologic deficit, and decrease patient satisfaction. As such, PJF is a major cause of outcome deterioration after adult deformity surgery. The decision to reoperate is surgeon dependent. In one study, revision surgery patients developing problems early in the postoperative period were younger and had a lower body mass index.[34] Risk factors for PJK include the length of fusion, patient age, osteoporosis, sagittal imbalance, and female gender.

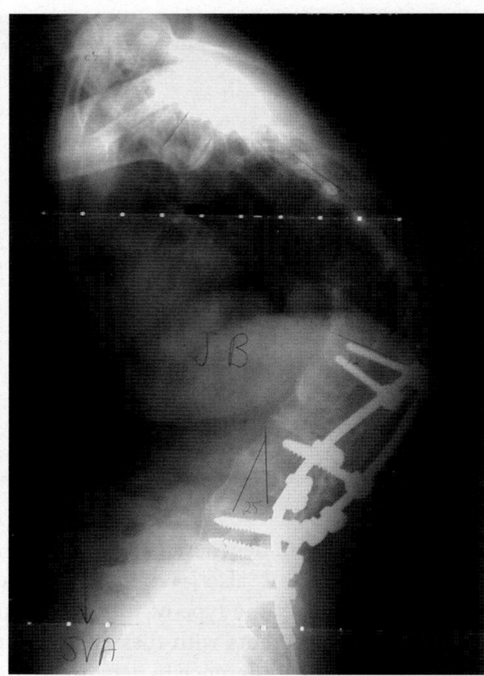

FIG. 101.2 Proximal junctional kyphosis causing a sagittal plane imbalance.

Adjacent-Segment Disease After Kyphoplasty

Vertebroplasty and kyphoplasty are minimally invasive procedures to augment vertebral compression fractures. Vertebroplasty involves injecting bone cement into the fractured vertebra. A kyphoplasty includes creation of a cavity within the fractured vertebral body and reestablishing vertical height before injecting the cement. Both procedures decrease the acute pain of fractures, thereby facilitating mobility and rehabilitation.[37–40] Short-term satisfaction can be compromised by long-term recurrent symptoms due to same-level disease and ASDis.

Bone cement injection into a fractured vertebra changes the strength and stiffness of the affected spinal element. The altered stiffness creates a stress riser at the adjacent segment.[41] The influence of vertebral augmentation on subsequent fractures and degeneration is a concern.

Fractures adjacent to a preexisting fracture occur with or without a vertebroplasty or kyphoplasty. Lindsay et al. studied the natural history of vertebral column fractures (VCF).[42] In patients with a previous VCF, the incidence of an additional fracture was 19.2% within the first year. This number does not differ significantly from patients treated with a kyphoplasty for the initial VCF.[43,44] The location of the subsequent fracture, however, may be altered.

The incidence of recurrent fracture after a kyphoplasty is 10% within the first 90 days after a kyphoplasty.[45] Trout et al. evaluated the location of subsequent fractures after a vertebroplasty.[46] Fractures adjacent to the treated level were 4.62 times that for nonadjacent-level fracture. In addition, adjacent-level fractures occurred sooner than nonadjacent-level fractures. Medium time for new adjacent fractures was 55 days compared to 127 days at nonadjacent levels.

The risk of subsequent-level fracture is related to osteoporosis, bone mineral density, severity and level of the fracture, and the presence of two preexisting fractures. One author found that the presence of vertebral body clefts within the fracture site is associated with a subsequent increased risk of fracture.[47] The development of a more compliant cement has been postulated as a method to reduce subsequent fractures.

Several studies have reported recompression at the site of the vertebroplasty/kyphoplasty.[48,49] Again, an association with intervertebral clefts has been postulated. Technical factors, such as poor contact of the cement with the endplate, may also be a factor.

In one study, new VCF occurred in 24% of patients by 1 year. Half of the fractures were at the adjacent level and only half were symptomatic. Most of the fractures occurred in the first 3 months.[50] The consensus of information indicates that subsequent fractures are not more common after a vertebroplasty/kyphoplasty but adjacent-level fractures are more numerous.

Adjacent-Segment Disease After Sagittal Imbalance Surgery

Patients with sagittal imbalance represent a unique subpopulation of patients with adult spinal deformity. Superior clinical outcomes have been linked to correction of spinopelvic balance. Glassman et al. noted that clinical outcome after spinal deformity surgery is highly correlated with sagittal vertebral axis (SVA) correction.[32] Patients with spinopelvic imbalance likewise present unique challenges and complications when compared to the general adult spinal deformity population. PJF is reported in 5.6% of the adult spinal deformity population.[35] The incidence of PJK is higher in patients with sagittal plane imbalance than in the general adult spinal deformity population. Smith et al. report an incidence of PJK in 35% of patients treated surgically for spinopelvic imbalance.[51] The most common mode of failure is fracture of the UIV. Only 37% of acute PJF patients required surgery. Surgery is less likely if the UIV is in the upper thoracic spine. PJK requiring surgical intervention was more common with an UIV at the thoracolumbar junction and least common when the UIV was in the upper thoracic spine.

Fixation to the pelvis is also a risk factor for developing postoperative PJK.[52,53] Eliminating motion at the caudal end of the construct may increase stress on the proximal junction. Interestingly, Smith et al. noted a higher rate of PJK with more complete correction of sagittal imbalance and a postoperative SVA less than 50 mm. The reason for increased PFK risk with more complete correction of spinopelvic balance is poorly understood. The large change in sagittal alignment from preoperative to postoperative status may cause significant anterior column stresses as the patient remains forward leaning in the postoperative period. The optimal correction of SVA in the deformity population remains to be determined.

Surgical Strategies to Treat/Avoid Adjacent-Segment Disease

Total Disc Replacement

Total disc replacement (TDR) has been proposed as a method to avoid or minimize ASDis. By preserving motion, biomechanical stresses at adjacent levels are closer to an unaltered spine than a fused spine. Noninferiority studies have shown that lumbar and cervical disc replacements provide equivalent results to traditional fusion methods for pain relief and improved function. These studies were important for gaining US Food and Drug Administration approval of the devices but did not answer the question about the influence on adjacent-level disease rates. More recent studies with long-term follow-up leave unanswered questions about the benefit of TDR. Zigler et al. evaluated 5-year follow-up data comparing TDR to circumferential fusion in the lumbar spine. Although radiographic degeneration (adjacent-level degeneration [ALDeg]) was lower in the TDR group (9.2%) compared to the fusion group (28.6%), the rate of surgery for adjacent-level disease (ALDis) was not statistically different between the groups.[54] Longer-term follow-up is needed to determine the effect of TDR on ALDis.[55]

Current support of TDR as a means to avoid ASDis is limited and awaiting additional level 1 and level 2 studies. Lower-level studies suggest TDR is an alternative to fusion.[56] The efficacy of disc replacement as a strategy to reduce ASDis requires further study.

Interspinous Devices

Interspinous stabilization devices have been developed as nonfusion alternatives to augment decompression surgery in the lumbar spine. These devices can be divided into static implants, such as blocks of bone, titanium or polyether ether ketone versus dynamic, flexible devices such as the Coflex (Paradigm Spine). The proported goals are to unload the facet joints, open the foramina, and protect the adjacent level. One device has been associated with a significantly higher reoperation rate (33%) compared to minimally invasive decompression and poor cost-effectiveness mainly due to the cost of the implant.[57,58] To date, there is no convincing evidence of improved outcome with the devices and no long-term data on the clinical effect on adjacent levels.[59–61]

Pedicle Screw–Based Dynamic Stabilization

Dynamic stabilization techniques provide partial rigidity to motion segments short of fully rigid fusions.[62] The theoretical concept is to allow enough rigidity to provide stability or prevent future instability but not enough rigidity to produce an acute stress riser at the junction of stabilized and nonstabilized segments.[63] Proponents of the techniques argue that a broad transition zone rather than an acute change in rigidity of the spine will reduce the rate of adjacent-level disease.[64] To date, the concept is unproven but has become popular due to dissatisfaction with traditional fusion techniques.

Dynamic stabilization devices work by providing a posterior tension band to the spinal element while allowing flexion and rotational motion.[65] An early device developed in Europe was the Graf ligament system. Pedicle screws are inserted above and below a motion segment, then linked by a nonelastic band.[66] Other systems have become available, including the Dynesys device (Zimmer Spine) but are marketed as fusion systems in the United States.[67,68]

Dynamic stabilization devices have become popular alternatives to traditional fusion surgery, especially outside of the United States.[69,70] The efficacy for prevention of ALDis remains uncertain, unproven, and requires further investigation.[71,72] Heo et al. studied ALDeg after a nitinol spring dynamic stabilization device insertion.[73] Using a modified Pfirrmann grading system of degeneration on follow-up MRI scans, 12% of cranial adjacent discs and 16% of caudal adjacent discs showed progressive degeneration at 2 years follow-up. The study was limited by an adequate control group, but was compared to symptomatic ASD in other studies of 2.5% per year or 16.5% in 5 years.[1,9,25] The authors concluded that dynamic stabilization may not prevent ALDeg. Other studies have noted a trend but no statistically significant evidence of reduction in symptomatic ALDis when comparing fusion to dynamic stabilization patients.[74] Dynamic stabilization device–related complications may actually increase the rate of reoperation rate. Long-term follow-up suggests that hyperextension and stabilization with the Graf device may narrow the spinal canal and exit foramina.[75] The benefit of dynamic stabilization on reduction of symptomatic ALDis reoperation rates remains theoretical and unproven for now.

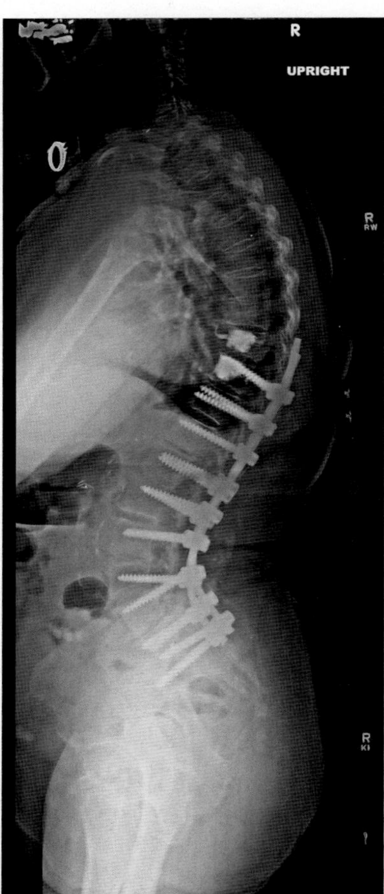

FIG. 101.3 Vertebroplasty augmentation of upper instrumented vertebra (UIV) and UIV+1 to help avoid proximal junctional kyphosis.

Bone Cement Augmentation of UIV and UIV+1

Vertebroplasty is a procedure to infiltrate a vertebral body with bone cement via a cannula inserted through the pedicle. When a cavity is created by inflating a balloon in the vertebral body and subsequently filled with bone cement, the procedure is called a kyphoplasty. Vertebral augmentation of the UIV and UIV +1 has been proposed as a strategy to lessen the rate of PJF or failure after spinal deformity surgery (Fig. 101.3).[76] Biomechanics data suggests that vertebroplasty or kyphoplasty reduces the rate of fracture in the osteoporotic spine, thus preventing or minimizing PJF.[77] In as separate study, vertebral augmentation in female patients over 60 years of age with fusions extending upward from L5 or S1 to the thoracolumbar junction (T9–L2) is cost-effective if a minimum of 9% of patients can avoid revision surgery.[78] The effectiveness of vertebral augmentation is still uncertain and requires better long-term study. Vertebral augmentation does not always prevent PJF (Fig. 101.4).[51]

Minimally Invasive Spine Surgery

The challenge of minimally invasive surgery (MIS) is to provide clinically significant improvement equivalent to open procedures. Advocates tout MIS as an alternative to open surgery that causes less tissue destruction.[79] Spinal fusion can alter the kinetics of the spine by destroying the facet, altering stabilizing muscle function, and altering the neurologic innervation to posterior stabilizing structures. MIS could theoretically lower rates of ASDis after fusion surgery by preserving normal anatomic structures and biomechanics.

Radcliff et al. evaluated ASDis in patients treated with an anterior lumbar interbody fusion followed by either open or percutaneous posterior pedicle screw instrumentation.[80] ASDis was diagnosed if a procedure such as an injection or reoperation was performed for new symptoms related to the adjacent level. At 3.8 years average follow-up, there was no difference between the two treatment groups. The overall rate of reoperation was 11.8%.

In a study comparing open versus MIS transforaminal lumbar interbody fusion patients, Yee et al. found no difference in the rate of ASDis between the two groups; however, there was a trend toward decreased risk of ASDis in the MIS group.[81] The numbers were small and follow-up of 33 months was short. Disruption of the facet joints is high even with percutaneous techniques. Patel et al. evaluated placement of percutaneous screws in a cadaver model.[82] Violation of the facet occurred in 58% of screws, with 17% being intraarticular. The minimizing effect of MIS on ASDis remains unproven.

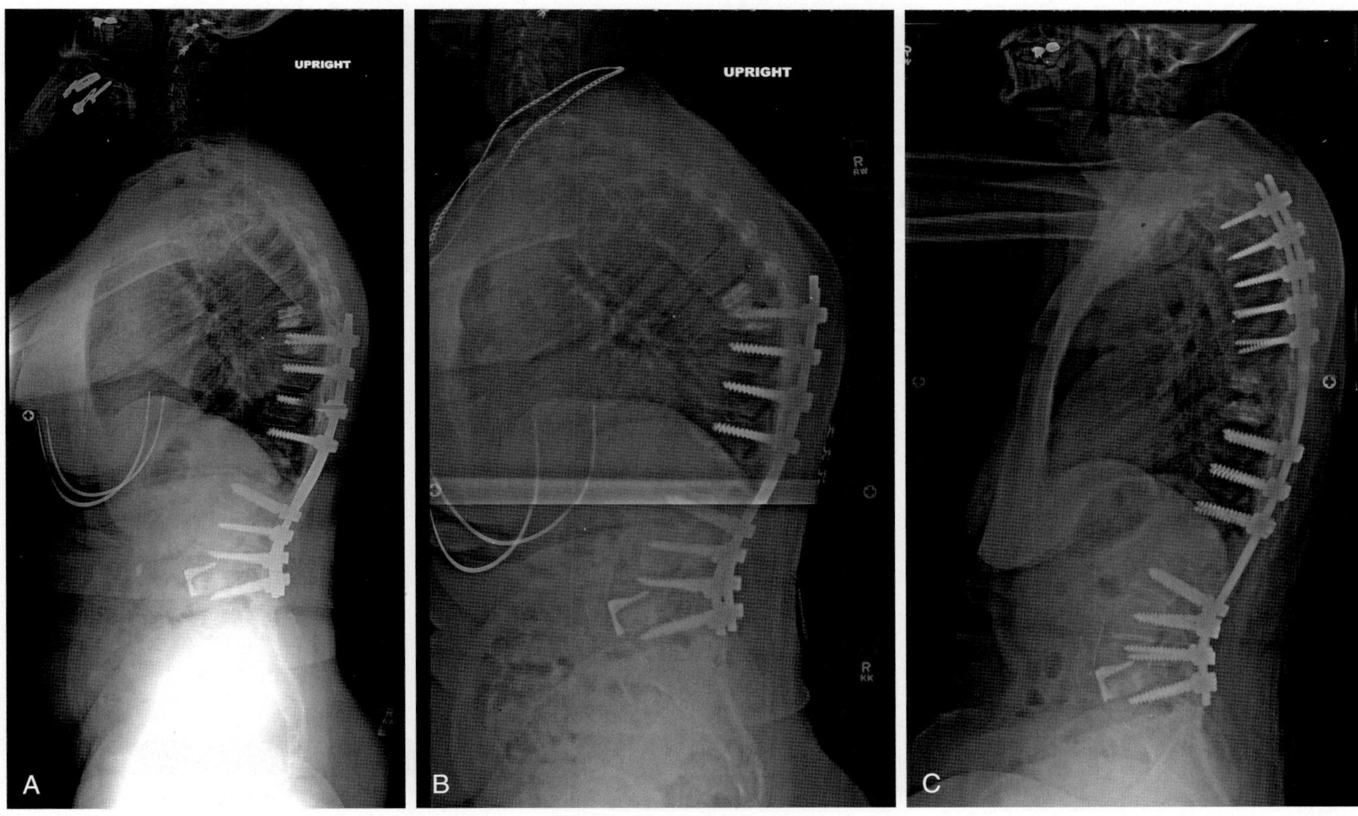

FIG. 101.4 Proximal junctional failure after fusion with cement augmentation of upper instrumented vertebra (UIV) and UIV+1. (A) Initial fusion with cement augmentation. (B) Three-month postoperative radiograph showing proximal junctional failure (PJF). (C) Reconstruction of PJF by proximal extension of fusion.

Lateral Interbody Fusion

Adjacent-level spinal stenosis is caused by facet and ligamentum flavum hypertrophy, buckling of the ligament, loss of disc height, foraminal stenosis, instability, and disc pathology. The traditional method of removing previous posterior implants; reinsertion of longer implants; and resecting bone, ligamentum, and disc is a major surgical procedure with considerable morbidity. The extreme lateral interbody fusion (XLIF) is a minimally invasive alternative for the patient with adjacent-level stenosis and minor deformity (Fig. 101.5). The XLIF procedure is performed through a small incision on the side of the torso. A channel is created with sequential dilators through the psoas muscle. A core of disc is removed and an implant is inserted across the disc space. The margins of the implant rest on the strong lateral pillars of the vertebral bodies, allowing stable distraction of the disc space. This strong distraction opens up the foramina and unbuckles the ligament flavum to indirectly decompress the central canal. The strong anterior longitudinal ligament is left intact to provide stability, unlike a traditional open anterior lumbar interbody fusion. Oliveira et al. showed that average foraminal area increased 24.7% and central canal area increased 33.1%.[83] The XLIF procedure provides a much less invasive decompression of the adjacent-level stenosis. In a study of 21 patients with stenosis at the rostral level to a fusion, back and leg pain scores were significantly reduced. Blood loss is minimal and open decompression of a scarred dural sac can be avoided.[84] Minimally invasive XLIF may be a surgical alternative to an open posterior revision decompression and stabilization.

Vertebroplasty for Proximal Junctional Fracture

Proximal junctional fractures at UIV+1 may require extensive spine reconstruction depending on the degree of deformity and neurologic status. For a select group of patients with a UIV+1 fracture and minimal deformity and no neurologic symptoms, vertebroplasty or kyphoplasty may be an option.

Yang et al. reported 87% patient satisfaction using the technique.[85] Average visual analog scale scores decreased from 80 preoperative to 26 one day postoperative after vertebroplasty for proximal junctional fracture above an instrumented fusion.

This technique is usually not possible at the UIV if the pedicle already contains a screw.

Cortical Bone Trajectory Screws to Add on to a Fusion

Adding on to a preexisting fusion may require a long exposure, extensive dissection through scar tissue, and reinstrumentation of the previous and new spinal segments. Connecting

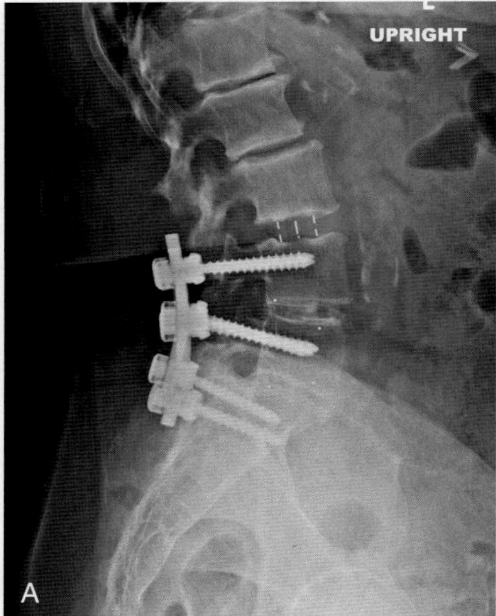

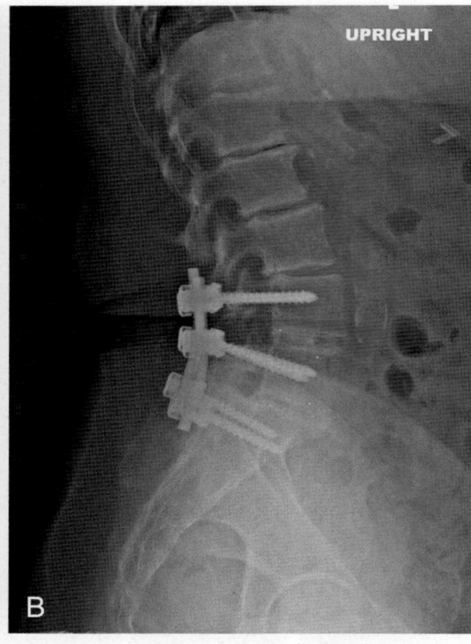

FIG. 101.5 Extreme lateral interbody fusion for adjacent segment stenosis. (A) Postoperative radiograph after extreme lateral interbody fusion. Notice the foramen distraction. (B) Preoperative radiograph showing collapse of L3–L4 disc space and foramen.

new implants on to old implants may require less exposure, but can be technically demanding. Connecting sleeves may loosen, causing the construct to fail. A novel approach using cortical bone trajectory screws has been described.[86] The technique involves adding a second screw to the old upper instrumented vertebrae. A cortical bone trajectory screw is added to the pedicle with a preexisting traditional pedicle screw. The technique requires image guidance and may be technically demanding. If successful, the technique requires only limited posterior exposure and allows a thorough decompression of the adjacent level stenosis.

Summary

Adjacent-level pathology is a reality of modern spine surgery. Proliferation of spinal fusions over the last decade has prompted much investigation into the causes, mitigating factors, and treatment of often very complex spinal problems. Minimizing unnecessary adjacent -evel destructive changes and providing a smooth transition of stresses at the margins of spine reconstructions are basic principles to mitigate future ASDis. Treating ALDis can challenge even a very skilled surgeon and requires an expert knowledge of revision techniques.

PEARLS

1. Revision surgery for adjacent-level disease occurs at an annual rate of about 2-3% per year.
2. Fusions accelerate adjacent-level degenerative disease.
3. The length of the fusion is a significant risk factor for future revision surgery.
4. Motion preservation strategies have not been proven to reduce the rate of revision surgery for adjacent-level disease.
5. MIS is not proven to lower the risk of ASDis.

PITFALLS

1. A laminectomy adjacent to a fusion increases the risk of ASDis by 2.4 times.
2. Proximal junctional failure (PJF) occurs in 26-32% of patients by five years follow up after adult spinal deformity surgery.
3. Fractures after kyphoplasty occur 4.6 times more often at an adjacent level than other levels.
4. PJK occurs more often in adult spinal deformity patients if they have a sagittal plane deformity.
5. PJK is more common with more complete correction of sagittal plane imbalance.

KEY POINTS

1. ALDis increases from 1.7% to 3.6% to 5.0% for one, two and three or four level fusions respectively.
2. Revision surgery above a fusion can consist of laminectomy alone or laminectomy plus extension of the fusion.
3. Segmental instability is reported in 45% of ASDis patients.

KEY REFERENCES

1. Park P, Garton HJ, Gala VC, et al. Adjacent segment disease after lumbar or lumbosacral fusion: review of the literature. *Spine.* 2004;29(17):1938-1944.
2. Sears WR, Sergides IG, Kazemi N, et al. Incidence and prevalence of surgery at segments adjacent to a previous posterior lumbar arthrodesis. *Spine J.* 2011;11(1):11-20.
3. Hostin R, McCarthy I, O'Brien M, et al. Incidence, mode and location of acute proximal junctional failures after surgical treatment of adult spinal deformity. *Spine.* 2013;38(12):1008-1015.
4. Sengupta DK. Dynamic stabilization devices in the treatment of low back pain. *Orthop Clin North Am.* 2004;35(1):43-56.
5. Lavelle WF, Cheney R. Recurrent fracture after vertebral kyphoplasty. *Spine J.* 2006;31(6):488-493.

6. Smith MW, Prokopis A, Lawrence BD, et al. Acute proximal junctional failure in patients with preoperative sagittal imbalance. *Spine J*. 2015;15(10):2142-2148.
7. Hart RA, Prendergast MA, Roberts WG, Nesbit GM, Barnwell SL. Proximal junctional acute collapse cranial to multi-level lumbar fusion: a cost analysis of prophylactic vertebral augmentation. *Spine J*. 2008;8(6):875-881.
8. Ghiselli G, Wang JC, Bhatia NN, Hsu WK, Dawson EG. Adjacent segment degeneration in the lumbar spine. *J Bone Joint Surg Am*. 2004;86(7):1497-1503.
9. Yee TJ, Terman SW, LaMarca F, Park P. Comparison of adjacent segment disease after minimally invasive or open transforaminal lumbar inter body fusion. *J Clin Neurosci*. 2014;21:1796-1801.
10. Wang MY, Vasudevan R, Mindea SA. Minimally invasive lateral interbody fusion for the treatment of rostral adjacent segment lumbar degenerative stenosis without supplemental pedicle screw fixation. *J Neurosurg Spine*. 2014;21:861-866.
11. Radcliff KE, Kepler CK, Maaieh M, et al. What is the rate of lumbar adjacent segment disease after percutaneous versus open fusion? *Orthop Surg*. 2014;6118-6120.
12. Hart R, McCarthy I, O'Brien M, et al. Identification of decision criteria for revision surgery among patients with proximal junctional failure after surgical treatment of spinal deformity. *Spine*. 2013;38(19):E1223-E1227.
13. Katz JN, Lipson SJ, Chang LC, et al. Seven to 10 year outcome of decompressive surgery for degenerative lumbar spinal stenosis. *Spine*. 1996;20(1):92-97.
14. Jansson KA, Nemeth G, Granath F, Blomqvist P. Spinal stenosis reoperation rate in Sweden is 11% at 10 years-a national analysis of 9664 operations. *Eur Spine J*. 2005;14:659-663.

REFERENCES

1. Ghiselli G, Wang JC, Bhatia NN, Hsu WK, Dawson EG. Adjacent segment degeneration in the lumbar spine. *J Bone Joint Surg Am*. 2004;86(7):1497-1503.
2. Boden SD, Davis DO, Dina TS, et al. Abnormal magnetic resonance scans of the lumbar spine in asymptomatic subjects. A prospective investigation. *J Bone Joint Surg Am*. 1990;72(3):403-408.
3. Boden SD, McCowin PR, et al. Abnormal magnetic-resonance scans of the cervical spine in asymptomatic subjects. A prospective investigation. *J Bone Joint Surg Am*. 1990;72(8):1178-1184.
4. Elfering A, Semmer N, Birkhofer D, et al. Risk factors for lumbar disc degeneration: a 5 year prospective MRI study in asymptomatic individuals. *Spine*. 2002;27:125-134.
5. Hilibrand AS, Robbins M. Adjacent segment degeneration and adjacent segment disease: the consequences of spinal fusion? *Spine J*. 2004;4(6Suppl):190S-194S.
6. Radcliff KE, Kepler KK, Jakoi A, et al. Adjacent segment disease in the lumbar spine following different treatment interventions. *Spine J*. 2013;13:1339-1349.
7. Mannion AF, Leivseth G, Brox JI, et al. ISSLLS Prize winner: long term follow up suggests spinal fusion is associated with increased adjacent segment disc degeneration but without influence on clinical outcome. *Spine*. 2014;39(17):1372-1383.
8. Dmitriev AE, Cunningham BW, Hu W, et al. Adjacent level intradiscal pressure and segmental kinematics following a cervicl total disc arthroplasty: an in vitro human cadaveric model. *Spine*. 2005;30(10):1165-1172.
9. Park P, Garton HJ, Gala VC, et al. Adjacent segment disease after lumbar or lumbosacral fusion: review of the literature. *Spine*. 2004;29(17):1938-1944.
10. Malakoutian M. *Degeneration and mechanics of the segment adjacent to a lumbar spine fusion: A biomechanical analysis (doctoral dissertation)*. Vancouver: University of British Columbia; 2014.
11. Yang SW, Langrana NA, Lee CK. Biomechanics of lumbosacral spinal fusion in combined compression-torsion loads. *Spine*. 1986;11:937.
12. Rao RD, David KS, Wang M. Biomechanical changes at adjacent segments following anterior lumbar inter body fusion using tapered cages. *Spine*. 2005;30(24):2772-2776.
13. Kumar M, Baklanow A, Chopin D. Correlation between sagittal plane changes and adjacent segment degeneration following lumbar spine fusion. *Eur Spine J*. 2001;10(4):314-319.
14. Battie MC, Videman T, Kaprio J, et al. The twin spine study: Contributions to a changing view of disc degeneration. *Spine J*. 2009;9:47-59.
15. Iatridis JC, MacLean JJ, Roughley PJ, Alini M. Effects of mechanical loading on intervertebral disc metabolism in vivo. *J Bone Joint Surg Am*. 2006;88(suppl 2):41-46.
16. Cole TC, Burkhardt D, Ghosh P, et al. Effects of spinal fusion on the proteoglycans of the canine intervertebral disc. *J Orthop Res*. 1985;3:277-291.
17. Jansson KA, Nemeth G, Granath F, Blomqvist P. Spinal stenosis reoperation rate in Sweden is 11% at 10 years-a national analysis of 9664 operations. *Eur Spine J*. 2005;14:659-663.
18. Katz JN, Lipson SJ, Chang LC, et al. Seven to 10 year outcome of decompressive surgery for degenerative lumbar spinal stenosis. *Spine*. 1996;20(1):92-97.
19. Lai PL, Chen LH, Niu CC, Fu TS, Chen WJ. Relation between laminectomy and development of adjacent segment instability after lumbar fusion with pedicle fixation. *Spine*. 2004;29(22):2527-2532.
20. Zdeblick TA, Zou D, Warden KE, McCabe R, Kunz D. Cervical stability after foraminotomy. A biomechanics in vitro analysis. *J Bone Joint Surg Am*. 1992;74(1):22-27.
21. Nataraja RN, Andersson GB, Patwardhan AG, Andriacchi TP. Study on effect of graded facetectomy on change in lumbar motion segment torsional flexibility using three-dimensional continuum contact representation for facet joints. *J Biomech Eng*. 1999;121(2):215-221.
22. Lee CK. Accelerated degeneration of the segment adjacent to a lumbar fusion. *Spine*. 1988;13(3):375-377.
23. Schlegel JD, Smith JA, Schleusener RL, et al. Lumbar motion segment pathology adjacent to thoracolumbar, lumbar and lumbosacral fusions. *Spine*. 1996;21(8):970-981.
24. Lee CK, Langrana NA. Lumbosacral spinal fusion: a biomechanical study. *Spine*. 1985;9:574.
25. Sears WR, Sergides IG, Kazemi N, et al. Incidence and prevalence of surgery at segments adjacent to a previous posterior lumbar arthrodesis. *Spine J*. 2011;11(1):11-20.
26. Lehmann TR, Spratt KF, Weinstein JN, et al. Long-term follow up of lower lumbar fusion patients. *Spine*. 1987;12:97-104.
27. Chen WJ, Lai PL, Niu CC, et al. Surgical treatment of adjacent instability after lumbar spine fusion. *Spine*. 2001;26(22):E519-E524.
28. Phillips FM, Carlson GD, Bohlman HH, Hughes SS. Results of surgery for spinal stenosis adjacent to previous lumbar fusion. *J Spinal Disord*. 2000;13(5):432-437.
29. Smorgick Y, Baker KC, Herkowitz H, et al. Predisposing factors for dural tear in patients undergoing lumbar spine surgery. *J Neurosurg Spine*. 2015;5:483-486.
30. Chou D, Dekutowski M, Hermsmeyer J, Norvell DC. The treatment of lumbar adjacent segment pathology after

SECTION XIV

a previous lumbar surgery: a systematic review. *Spine*. 2012;37(22S):S180-S188.

31. Moal B, Schwab F, Ames CP, et al. Radiographic outcomes of adult spinal deformity correction: a critical analysis of variability and failures across deformity patterns. *Spine Deform*. 2014;2(3):219-225.
32. Glassman SD, Berven S, Bridwell K, et al. Correlation of radiographic parameters and clinical symptoms in adult scoliosis. *Spine*. 2005;30:682-688.
33. DeWald CJ, Stanley T. Instrumentation-related complications of multilevel fusions for adult spinal deformity patients over age 65:surgical considerations and treatment options in patients with poor bone quality. *Spine*. 2006;31(19S):S144-S151.
34. Hart R, McCarthy I, O'Brien M, et al. Identification of decision criteria for revision surgery among patients with proximal junctional failure after surgical treatment of spinal deformity. *Spine*. 2013;38(19):E1223-E1227.
35. Hostin R, McCarthy I, O'Brien M, et al. Incidence, mode and location of acute proximal junctional failures after surgical treatment of adult spinal deformity. *Spine*. 2013;38(12):1008-1015.
36. Glattes RC, Bridwell KH, Linke LG, et al. Proximal junctional kyphosis in adult spinal deformity following long instrumented posterior spinal fusion: incidence, outcomes, and risk factor analysis. *Spine*. 2005;30(14):1643-1649.
37. Taylor RS, Taylor RJ, Fritzell P. Balloon kyphoplasty and vertebroplasty for Vertebral Compression fractures: a comparative systematic review of efficacy and safety. *Spine*. 2006;31(23):2747-2755.
38. Klazen CA, Lohle PN, de Vries J, et al. Vertebroplasty versus conservative treatment in acute osteoporotic vertebral compression fractures (Vertos II): and open-label randomized trial. *Lancet*. 2010;376(9746):1085-1092.
39. Eck JC, Nachtigall D, Humphreys SC, et al. Comparison of vertebroplasty and balloon kyphoplasty for treatment of vertebral compression fractures: a met-analysis of the literature. *Spine J*. 2008;8(3):488-497.
40. Garfin SR, Buckley RA, Ledlie J. Balloon kyphoplasty outcomes group balloon kyphoplasty for symptomatic vertebral body compression fractures results in rapid, significant, and sustained improvements in back pain, function, and quality of life for elderly patients. *Spine*. 2006;31:2213-2220.
41. Villarraga ML, Bellezza AJ, Harrigan TP. The biomechanical effects of kyphoplasty on treated and adjacent non treated vertebral bodies. *J Spinal Disord Tech*. 2005;18(1):84-91.
42. Lindsay R, Silverman SL, Cooper C, et al. Risk of new vertebral fracture in the year following a fracture. *JAMA*. 2001;285:319-323.
43. Harrop JS, Prpa B, Reinhardt MK, et al. Primary and secondary osteoporosis incidence of subsequent vertebral compression fractures after kyphoplasty. *Spine*. 2004;29(19):2120-2125.
44. Lee WS, Sung KH, Jeong HT, et al. Risk factors of developing new symptomatic vertebral compression fractures after percutaneous vertebroplasty in osteoporotic patients. *Eur Spine J*. 2006;15(12):1777-1783.
45. Lavelle WF, Cheney R. Recurrent fracture after vertebral kyphoplasty. *Spine J*. 2006;31(6):488-493.
46. Trout AT, Kallmes DF. New fractures after vertebroplasty: adjacent fractures occur significantly sooner. *AJNR Am J Neuroradiol*. 2006;27(1):217-223.
47. Trout AT, Kallmes DF, Lane JI. Subsequent vertebral fractures after vertebroplasty: association with intraosseous clefts. *AJNR Am Soc Neuroradiol*. 2006;27(7):1586-1591.
48. Heo DH, Chin DK, Yoon YS, et al. Recollapse of previous vertebral compression fracture after percutaneous vertebroplasty. *Osteoporos Int*. 2009;20:473-480.
49. Kim YY, Park CG, Rhyu KW. Recompression of vertebral bodies after balloon kyphoplasty for vertebral compression fractures—preliminary report. *J Korean Spine Surg*. 2009;16:89-94.
50. Voormolen MH, Lohle PN, Juttmann JR, et al. The risk of new osteoporotic vertebral compression fractures in the year after percutaneous vertebroplasty. *J Vasc Interv Radiol*. 2006;17(1):71-76.
51. Smith MW, Prokopis A, Lawrence BD, et al. Acute proximal junctional failure in patients with preoperative sagittal imbalance. *Spine J*. 2015;15(10):2142-2148.
52. Maruo D, Ha U, Inoue S, et al. Predictive factor for proximal junctional kyphosis in long fusions to the sacrum in adult spinal deformity. *Spine*. 2013;38:E1469-E1476.
53. Yagi M, King AB, Boachie-Adjei O. Incidence, risk factors, and natural course of proximal junctional kyphosis: surgical outcomes review of adult idiopathic scoliosis. Minimum 5 years of follow-up. *Spine*. 2012;37:1479-1489.
54. Zigler JE, Glenn J, Delemarter R. Five year adjacent level degeneration changes with single level disease treated using lumbar total disc replacement with ProDisc-L versus circumferential fusion. *J Neurosurg Spine*. 2012;17:504-511.
55. Tsung-Hsi Tu, Ziewacz JE, Mummaneni PV. Disc replacment versus fusion. *J Neurosurg Spine*. 2012;17:502-503.
56. Harrop JS, Youssef JA, Maltenfort M, et al. Lumbar adjacent segment degeneration and disease after arthrodesis and total disc arthroplasty. *Spine*. 2008;33(15):1701-1707.
57. Lonne G, Johnsen LG, Aas E, et al. Comparing cost-effectiveness of X-Stop with minimally invasive decompression in lumbar spinal stenosis: a randomized controlled trial. *Spine*. 2015;40(8):514-520.
58. Stromqvist BH, Berg S, Gerdhem P, et al. X-Stop versus decompressive surgery for lumbar neurogenic intermittent claudication: randomized controlled trial with 2-year follow-up. *Spine*. 2013;38:1436-1442.
59. Richter A, Schutz C, Hauck M, et al. Does a interspinous device (Coflex) improve the outcome of decompressive surgery in lumbar spinal stenosis? One year follow up of a prospective case control study of 60 patients. *Eur Spine J*. 2010;19(2):283-289.
60. Bono CM, Vacarro AR. Interspinous process devices in the lumbar spine. *J Spinal Disord Tech*. 2007;20(3):255-261.
61. Christie SD, Song JK, Fessler RG. Dynamic interspinous process technology. *Spine*. 2005;30(16S):S73-S78.
62. Sengupta DK. Dynamic stabilization devices in the treatment of low back pain. *Orthop Clin North Am*. 2004;35(1):43-56.
63. Schmoelz W, Huber JF, Nydegger T, et al. Dynamic stabilization of the lumbar spine and its effects on adjacent segments: an in vitro experiment. *J Spinal Disord Tech*. 2003;16(4):418-423.
64. Mulholland RC, Sengupta DK. Rational, principles and experimental evaluation of the concept of soft stabilization. *Eur Spine J*. 2002;11(suppl 2):198-205.
65. Nockels RP. Dynamic stabilization in the surgical management of painful lumbar spinal disorders. *Spine*. 2005;30(16S):S68 -S72.
66. Graf H. Lumbar instability; surgical treatment without fusion. *Rachis*. 1992;2:123-127.
67. Stoll TM, Dugois G, Schwarzenbach O. The dynamic neutralization system for the spine: a multi-center study of a novel non-fusion system. *Eur Spine J*. 2002;11(suppl 2):170-178.

68. Kim YS, Zhang HY, Moon BJ, et al. Nitinol spring rod dynamic stabilization system and Nitinol memory loops in surgical treatment for lumbar disc disorders: short-term follow-up. *Neurosurg Focus*. 2006;22(1):E10.
69. Grob D, Benini A, Junge A, et al. Clinical experience with the Dynesis semirigid fixation system for the lumbar spine: surgical and patient-oriented outcome in 50 cases after an average of 2-years. *Spine*. 2005;30:324-331.
70. Sengupta DK, Mullholland RC. Fulcrum assisted soft stabilization system: a new concept in the surgical treatment of degenerative low back pain. *Spine*. 2005;30:1019-1029.
71. Bono CM, Murali K, Vaccaro AR. Posterior pedicle fixation-based dynamic stabilization devices for the treatment of degenerative diseases of the lumbar spine. *J Spinal Disord Tech*. 2009;22(5):376-383.
72. Fu L, France A, Xie Y, et al. Functional and radiological outcomes of semi-rigid dynamic lumbar stabilization adjacent to single-level fusion after 2 years. *Arch Orthop Trauma Surg*. 2014;134(5):605-610.
73. Heo DH, Cho YJ, Cho SM, et al. Adjacent segment degeneration after lumbar dynamic stabilization using pedicle screws and a nitinol spring rod system with 2-year minimum follow-up. *J Spinal Disord Tech*. 2012;8:409-414.
74. Kanayama M, Togawa D, Hashimoto T, et al. Motion-preserving surgery can prevent early breakdown of adjacent segments: comparison of posterior dynamic stabilization with spinal fusion. *J Spinal Disord Tech*. 2009;22(7):463-467.
75. Kanayama M, Hashimoto T, Shigenobu K, et al. Adjacent segment morbidity after Graf ligamentoplasty compared with posterolateral lumbar fusion. *J Neurosurg*. 2002;96(suppl1):139-140.
76. Lattig F. Bone cement augmentation in the prevention of adjacent segment failure after multilevel adult deformity fusion. *J Spinal Discord Tech*. 2009;22(6):439-443.
77. Kayanja MM, Schlenk R, Togawa D, et al. The biomechanics of 1,2,and 3 levels of vertebral augmentation with polymethylmethacrylate in multilevel spinal segments. *Spine*. 2006;31:769-774.
78. Hart RA, Prendergast MA, Roberts WG, Nesbit GM, Barnwell SL. Proximal junctional acute collapse cranial to multi-level lumbar fusion: a cost analysis of prophylactic vertebral augmentation. *Spine J*. 2008;8(6):875-881.
79. Perez-Cruett MJ, Hussain NS, White GZ, et al. Quality of life outcomes with minimally invasive transforaminal lumbar inter body fusion based on long term analysis of 304 consecutive patients. *Spine*. 2014;39:E191-E198.
80. Radcliff KE, Kepler CK, Maaieh M, et al. What is the rate of lumbar adjacent segment disease after percutaneous versus open fusion? *Orthop Surg*. 2014;6118-6120.
81. Yee TJ, Terman SW, La Marca F, Park P. Comparison of adjacent segment disease after minimally invasive or open transforaminal lumbar inter body fusion. *J Clin Neurosci*. 2014;21:1796-1801.
82. Patel RD, Graziano GP, Vanderhave KL, Patel AA, Gerling MC. Facet violation with the placement of percutaneous pedicle screws. *Spine*. 2011;36(26):E1749-E1752.
83. Oliveira L, Marche L, Coutinho E, Pimenta L. A radiographic assessment of the ability of the extreme lateral inter body fusion procedure to indirectly decompress the neural elements. *Spine*. 2010;26S:S331-S337.
84. Wang MY, Vasudevan R, Mindea SA. Minimally invasive lateral interbody fusion for the treatment of rostral adjacent segment lumbar degenerative stenosis without supplemental pedicle screw fixation. *J Neurosurg Spine*. 2014;21:861-866.
85. Yang SC, Chen HS, Kao YH, et al. Vertebroplasty for symptomatic adjacent vertebral compression fracture. *J Spinal Disord Tech*. 2013;26(4):E130-E136.
86. Rodriquez A, Neal MT, Liu A, et al. Novel placement of cortical bone trajectory screws in previously instrumented pedicles for adjacent segment lumbar disease using CT image guided navigation. *Neurosurg Focus*. 2014;36(3):1-7.

CHAPTER 102 Failed Back Surgery Syndrome: Historical Perspective

Richard W. Easton

The Edwin Smith Papyrus (17th century BCE) described 48 cases of fractures, tumors, injuries, and wounds that occurred during the time period in which it was written.[1] The document also laid out a fairly complex method of examining and diagnosing the patients who were reported in the document. If that were not enough, the scrolls went on to further separate the injured patients who presented for treatment into three groups: treat, contend, and do not treat.

Historically, the patients were placed into the appropriate category only after careful evaluation by the treating person (physicians, priests, and others). The decision on whether to provide further care was made based on experiences with previous patients' outcomes and the presence or absence of an identifiable, treatable injury or lesion in the patient at hand. This system provided the most comprehensive health care identified for that time period and it serves as a model for our health care delivery today.

Nearly 1200 years later (460–370 BCE), Hippocrates was able to correlate the presence of low back pain with sciatica, the presence of pain down the leg.[2] In his description of the condition, Hippocrates noted that if a vertebra were injured or damaged, then patients would exhibit lower extremity pain and paralysis may follow. Nearly 2000 years later, in 1829, A.G. Smith performed one of the first decompressive laminectomies and exploration of the spine for sciatica. Joel E. Goldthwaite (1866–1961) described a patient with recurrent sciatica after surgery. He brought the patient back to surgery for an exploration and found nothing. This led him to conclude that the disc that was causing the pain went "back in place." This likely became one of the first explanations for the lack of pathology at the time of surgery.[3] Perhaps this is the time that failed back surgery syndrome (FBSS) was first described, albeit unknowingly.

What Is Failed Back Surgery Syndrome?

FBSS is the name given to a spectrum of patient complaints and symptoms that can occur in those who have undergone spinal surgery, decompressions, deformity surgery, and fusions.[4,5] FBSS is most often diagnosed when the outcome of the procedure does not meet or exceed the expectations of the surgeon and patient and the patient is left with residual back and/or leg pain or neck and/or arm symptoms.[6] This syndrome has been described by many names in the past, most recently "postlaminectomy syndrome." There has been confusion on the issue of what can be properly described as FBSS. In the strictest sense, only residual symptoms following a properly diagnosed and properly performed surgery are considered FBSS. Many authors have used the term "anatomically correct" to describe this proper execution of the correct treatment. When this fails to deliver relief, it is an FBSS. To the patient, however, surgical treatment that does not alleviate the problem is a failure. Therefore, the incidence of misdiagnosis and failed surgical treatment are included in the FBSS discussion. In fact, in recent years, there has been an increase in the number of cases of FBSS diagnosed as the number of surgeries on the spine have increased. The worldwide literature suggests that the incidence of FBSS is somewhere between 10% to 40% of surgical patients.[7] Those numbers are even more daunting since it has recently been estimated (from controlled randomized trials) that 5% to 50% of patients who have surgery will fail with regard to patient outcome and satisfaction following spine surgery.[8] Additionally, in 1997, there were over 317,000 lumbar surgeries performed in the United States[9]; by the year 2002, the number increased to over 1 million surgeries.[10] Fusion operations, as a subgroup, increased by over 220%. Multiple surgical procedures in the same area have been reported to have decreasing clinical success. The initial positive outcome was decreased to around 30% after the second surgery, 15% after the third, and to around 5% after the fourth surgery.[11] FBSS has a tremendous impact not only on the patients and families involved but also on the cost of health care delivery and society. There are many potential causes that land patients with the diagnosis of FBSS. These include, but are not limited to, poor patient selection, misdiagnosis and subsequent mistreatment, poor surgical technique or iatrogenic causes, permanent nerve damage, failure of fusion, failure or misplacement of instrumentation, and recurrence or progression of pathology.[12] The treatment of this diverse group of patients must be individually tailored depending on the underlying etiology. It is also important to identify those patients who potentially have a secondary agenda. These include worker's compensation patients or patients with litigation pending. The outcomes in these groups have been reported to be significantly worse when compared to controls.[13]

Economic Impact of Failed Back Surgery Syndrome

FBSS affects the ability of the patient to function and participate in family and societal settings. It prolongs the normal recovery phase by weeks to months to years. Its socioeconomic impact has been studied exhaustively relative to low back pain, but studies are lacking for determining the true cost of FBSS. It has been reported that the true impact of FBSS on an individual's quality of life and its economic cost to society are considerable. It is more disabling when compared to other chronic pain syndromes and chronic medical conditions such as heart failure and motor neuron diseases.[14] This inherently makes sense when one factors in the costs of multiple medical visits, the cost of the primary surgical procedure, and subsequent postoperative care. Added to those costs postoperatively are visits to the caregivers, physical therapy and inpatient rehabilitation, further postoperative diagnostic studies, continuing medications, pain management clinics, subsequent procedures, and the failure of the patient to return to the workplace.

Symptoms of Failed Back Surgery Syndrome

What then, are the primary complaints of patients in the postoperative period that would lead one to explore the possibility of FBSS? Patients who undergo surgery of the spine with or without fusions can have a variety of postoperative complaints; not all of them require further diagnostic workup. These patients sometimes require time after an operation to heal and for the symptoms that necessitated the initial procedure to subside. Attempts to resolve the symptoms during this period should be conservative and supportive without exposing the patient to invasive treatments. Guyer and colleagues[12] suggested a classification system based on the length of time between surgery and the onset of pain. Patients were placed into three groups: early (immediately after surgery to 3 weeks), intermediate (pain recurrence or new symptoms 1–6 months after surgery), and late (after 6 months of acceptable pain relief). The early group included wrong-level surgeries and failure to adequately address the pathology. The intermediate group was separated into gradual recurrence of pain versus after a specific, sometimes traumatic, event. The late group was more attributed to recurrent pathology at the level of surgery or the level above. It would be prudent to include the formation of scar tissue in this group as epidural fibrosis has usually reached its maximum around this time. This system seems as good as any proposed to date, as it allows for the clinician to focus the examination and diagnostic studies on the most likely issues causing the pain. It is, however, of the utmost importance to diagnose the cause of postoperative symptoms.

The diagnosis of FBSS crosses into many different specialties in medicine. First and foremost, it is the responsibility of the treating surgeon to confirm that he or she has, indeed, correctly performed the operation that was outlined to the patient in the period of conservative care and during the presurgical consultation. This involves not only reviewing the preoperative radiographic and diagnostic findings but also meeting with and listening to the patient and performing a complete and thorough physical examination. Sir William Osler's famous words "Listen to your patient, he is telling you the diagnosis," rings clearly here. The patient will frequently guide you to the appropriate area of concern if you take the time to get a complete history of the symptoms. This should be followed by a comprehensive examination of not only the affected area, to eliminate it as a possible source of the pain or symptoms, but a complete orthopaedic exam including the hips and knees. The presence or absence of associated medical conditions—such as heart disease, neuromuscular disease, and metabolic diseases—should also be ascertained. The use of other treatments for other diseases, such as chemotherapy or radiation therapy for cancer patients, is also critical information for the surgeon. A history of psychiatric disorders or depression and the patient's worker's compensation status should also be recorded. Diagnostic injections and electromyograms (EMGs) are sometimes also useful in determining the cause of postoperative pain.

Once the history and physical are complete, it is up to the surgeon to determine the appropriate diagnostic tests to be ordered. For example, when determining the cause of radicular symptoms after a decompressive procedure, diagnostic tests that allow visualization of the surgical site and the surrounding area should be ordered. Frequently, this will include magnetic resonance imaging (MRI) with or without gadolinium. Computed tomography (CT)/myelography can determine if there is any residual or recurrent compressive pathology centrally, laterally or extraforaminally or any additional pathology in the surrounding areas that was previously missed or not present. This can be very difficult to do, considering how hard it can sometimes be to identify an anatomic source of pain in patients without previous back surgery.[15,16]

If the history and physical examination are complete, the appropriate imaging studies and injections are performed, and the psychiatric evaluation is completed, it has been reported that a diagnosis can be reached in over 90% of the patients.[17] There is widespread agreement that the correct diagnosis is crucial to successful treatment of FBSS.[17–19]

The most common diagnosis in patients diagnosed with FBSS is foraminal stenosis, which is found in 25% to 29% of the patients. This was followed by a painful disc in 20% to 22%, and pseudarthrosis in 14%. Other causes include recurrent disc herniation in 7% to 12%, neuropathic pain in 10%, facet joint pain in 3%, and sacroiliac pain in 2%. Sagittal plane imbalance has also been implicated in recent studies of correctable causes of FBSS.[20] However, subsequent studies have shown an increase in the number of patients with residual pain due to sacroiliac joint dysfunction. The leading psychiatric factors identified were depression, substance abuse, and anxiety.[11]

When dealing with patients with FBSS, it is perhaps even more critical that the treating physician and patient have their plans and goals regarding outcomes of treatment aligned. A goal of improving the visual analog scale by 1.8 units (or approximately 50%) is an excellent starting point and has been shown to provide good results.[21]

Causes, Diagnosis, and Treatments of Components of Failed Back Surgery Syndrome

Foraminal or Lateral Recess Stenosis

There are many potential causes for residual back and leg pain in patients diagnosed with FBSS. Some are postsurgical complications and some are not. The primary cause of persistent radiculopathy after spine surgery is, for instance, inadequate decompression of the spine. This can occur centrally, in the lateral recess, or in the far lateral or foraminal areas of the spine. The incidence of this is reported to be between 25% and 29%.[22–24] When patients present with symptoms of persistent or new radiculopathy, the radiographic study of choice is MRI with and without gadolinium if there has not been a fusion with instrumentation (Fig. 102.1).[25] If the patient has had a fusion with instrumentation, then a myelogram and postmyelogram CT is indicated. Attention should be paid to not only the central canal but to the lateral recesses, especially the areas around the facet joints and the foraminal and extraforaminal areas. Lateral and far lateral stenosis can occur from hypertrophic facet joints, disc degeneration with loss of vertical height and subsequent foraminal collapse superior to inferior. Lateral and far lateral disc protrusions or herniations cause anterior to posterior narrowing. Far lateral discs can be easily missed if attention is not specifically paid to this area when reviewing diagnostic studies. EMGs are also useful to help delineate or define the involved levels. They are particularly useful when multiple levels are affected with degeneration or disc space collapse and when there may be residual stenosis at a single location on a single side or at multiple levels in multiple locations. The presence of ongoing denervation with radiographically proven stenosis is a strong indication for revision surgery.[26] Therapeutic and diagnostic injections can also aid in both treating and diagnosing the level of causative pathology. When the diagnosis of residual stenosis is made, the patient once again has treatment options. The first line of treatment can again be conservative care with physical therapy, nonsteroidal antiinflammatory drugs (NSAIDs), and antispasmodics and pain medication. This route is similar to the path they likely took when deciding on the initial procedure. If this does not relieve symptoms, then transforaminal, caudal, and epidural blocks can be used both therapeutically and diagnostically. Patients who respond to a single-level transforaminal block have an excellent chance of improvement or recovery with a revision decompression. If the injections fail, then the use of neurostimulation is an option. Finally, if the more conservative modalities fail to relieve symptoms, the surgical correction of the compressive pathology can be performed. Psychiatric evaluation prior to surgery is critical in this group, as chronic pain can lead to psychiatric pathology that can adversely affect the outcome. When performing revision decompression, particularly in the lateral recesses and transforaminal areas, care must be taken to not destabilize the area around the compressive pathology. Removal of greater than 50% of the facet joint has been shown to cause instability and could potentially necessitate future surgery, placing the patient right back into the FBSS group.

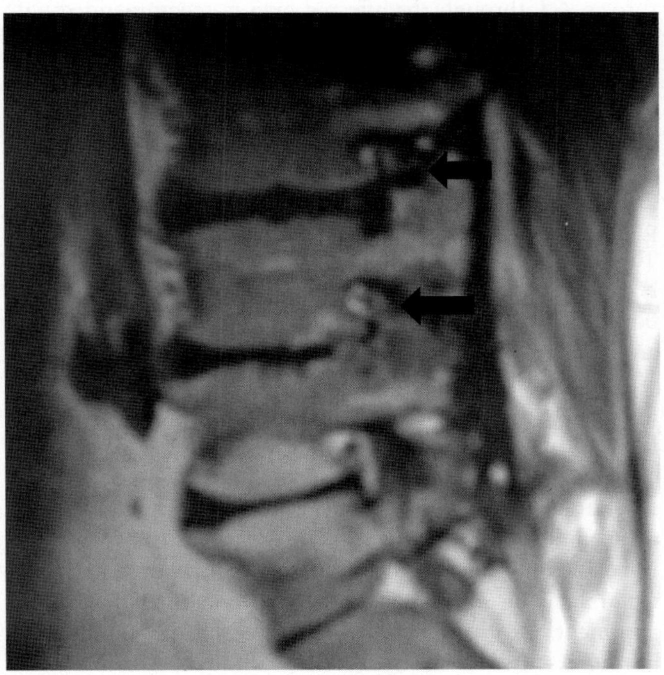

FIG. 102.1 Sagittal magnetic resonance image showing foraminal stenosis (*arrows*).

Painful Disc

The presence of a pathologically painful disc can cause a patient to report postoperative symptoms. The disc may be at the surgical level but can also be at an adjacent or nearby level. Generally, this should be ascertained prior to the initial surgical procedure and the issue should be addressed at the time of surgery. However, if the patient has persistent back pain postoperatively, the presence of a painful disc should be explored. MRI is once again the noninvasive study of choice for looking at disc morphology and the condition of the disc and endplates. Disc herniations and degenerative changes in and of themselves do not always cause back pain.[27] Recent evidence indicates that the presence of degenerative disc disease is not enough to correlate with low back pain. However, the presence of degenerative disc disease with endplate signal changes was highly associated with low back pain, particularly at the L3–L4, L4–L5, and L5–S1 levels.[28] These endplate signal changes, referred to as Modic changes, are more common in smokers and obese patients and are positive indicators of an increased risk of low back pain.[29] Additionally, the presence of narrowing of the disc space at two or more levels was more

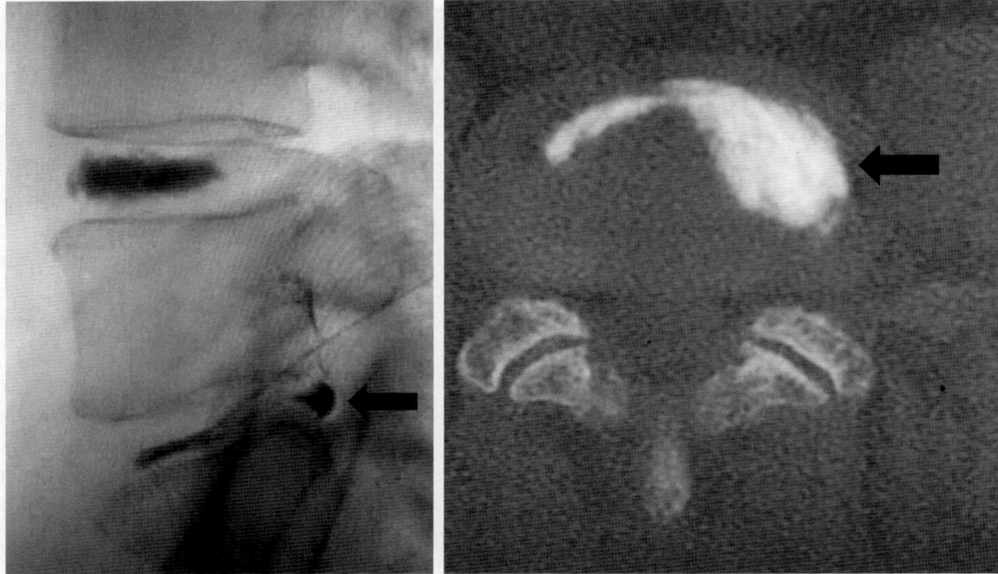

FIG. 102.2 Discogram (*left*) and postdiscogram computed tomography (CT) (*right*). Notice the posterior extravasation of dye at the L5–S1 level (*left, arrow*). This is consistent with a posterior annular tear. On the postdiscogram CT, the dye is contained at the level above the annular tear (*right, arrow*).

strongly associated with low back pain than other radiographic features (particularly when L5–S1 was excluded).[30]

Discography has been controversial in the past but may be useful in determining or confirming a painful disc (Fig. 102.2). Abnormal discs on MRI may or may not be pain generators. These discs should not provoke concordant pain when injected if normal but should if there is underlying pathology in the disc.[31] However, recent studies have shown that discography can lead to acceleration of the progression of degenerative changes in the disc.[32,33]

The presence of residual low back pain should also prompt the surgeon to investigate other nonspinal causes of low back pain. These include abdominal aortic aneurysms, renal stones or infections, sacral or vertebral insufficiency fractures in the elderly, tumors, and vascular problems.[34]

Once the diagnostic workup is completed and the patient has been informed that the disc is the pain generator, then a description of treatment options should be given to the patient. The patient may opt for conservative care with therapy and medications, blocks, or surgery. Surgical options include a standard fusion operation or artificial disc replacement, which recent studies have found to have similar results.[35] Artificial disc replacement surgery has slightly better results, however when used on single-level disease particularly on maintaining range of motion. Outcomes for both procedures are lower than fusions for the treatment of instability.[36]

Pseudarthrosis

The incidence of pseudarthrosis following lumbar spine surgery correlates with many variables.[37,38] Pseudarthrosis rates are predictably higher in smokers and nicotine users, diabetics, patients on NSAIDs, steroid users, and patients with systemic diseases and vascular insufficiency.[39–42] The number of levels fused and the type of fusion operation performed also affect the pseudarthrosis rate.[43–45] Interestingly, not all cases of pseudarthrosis are painful.[46]

The diagnosis of pseudarthrosis in FBSS begins with anteroposterior, lateral, and flexion-extension radiographs of the affected area. Lucency (bony absorption) around the hardware and motion within the fused levels on flexion-extension radiographs indicate bony absorption and pseudarthrosis. CT through the affected area is recommended with three-dimensional (3D) and coronal and sagittal reconstruction (Figs. 102.3 and 102.4). It is the study of choice to confirm or diagnose pseudarthrosis if the radiographs are equivocal. The use of bone scan with axial CT (single photon emission computed tomography [SPECT]) is extremely sensitive to pseudarthrosis but is not specific. This added sensitivity allows previously missed CT-tested pseudarthrosis to be diagnosed. This is particularly useful when there is not gross motion or bony absorption on plain radiograph and CT. Therefore, a bone scan with SPECT is the study of choice for patients who are otherwise difficult to diagnose for pseudarthrosis.

The surgical treatment for pseudarthrosis should be performed after optimizing the patient's chances for a successful fusion. This may involve removing as many of the correctable causes of pseudarthrosis as possible: in particular, cessation of smoking (which has a known negative impact on fusion)[47] and controlling blood sugar levels as tightly as possible to decrease infection and poor healing. The use of osteoinductive growth factors may be considered when treating pseudarthrosis. The treatment of this problem involves the physician and patient having discussions about risk factors and treatment options and their risks. The patient is largely responsible for increasing one's success rate by following the postoperative instructions.

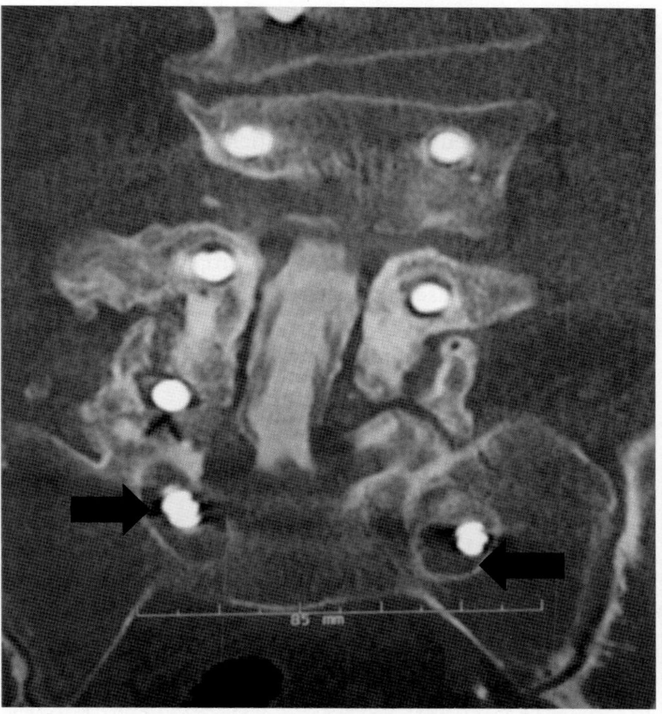

FIG. 102.3 Coronal computed tomographic (postmyelogram) images of an instrumented fusion with lucency around the pedicle screws (*arrows*), which indicates bony resorption and pseudarthrosis.

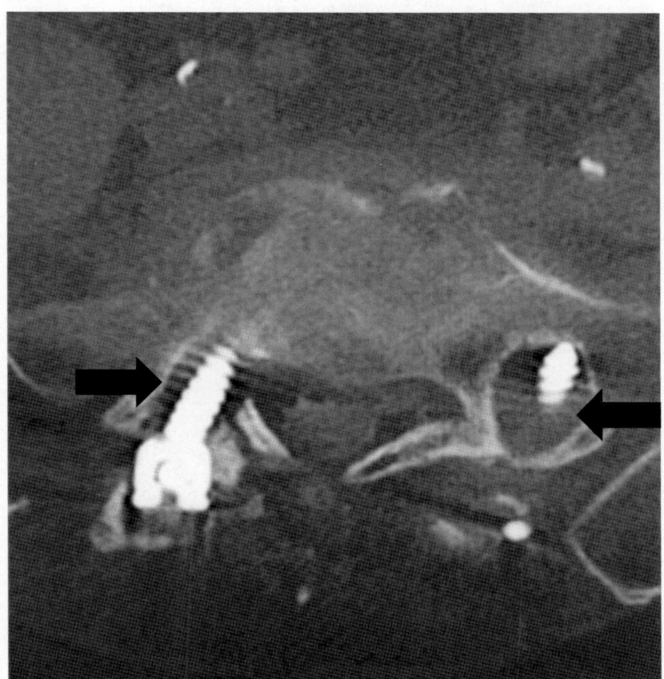

FIG. 102.4 Axial computed tomographic (postmyelogram) image showing lucency around the pedicle screws (*arrows*). This lucency indicates bony absorption and pseudarthrosis.

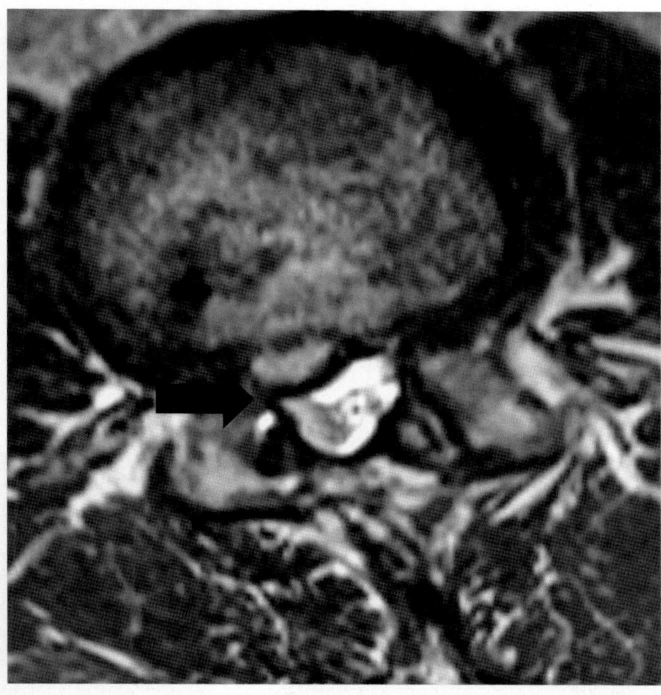

FIG. 102.5 Axial magnetic resonance image with recurrent disc herniation (*arrow*) causing nerve root and foraminal stenosis.

Recurrent Disc Herniation

Historically, the outcomes for the surgical treatment of herniated lumbar discs showed success rates from 70% to 95% (Fig. 102.5). Newer, larger studies now show that patients who have surgery for herniated lumbar discs have more improvement in physical function, higher satisfaction, better self-rated progress, and less pain than the nonoperative group.[48] Interestingly, there was no difference in work status between the surgical and nonoperative groups.

The recurrence of a disc herniation or the incomplete removal of the offending disc material during surgery can lead to postoperative back and leg pain that requires treatment and accounts for between 7% and 12% of the patients diagnosed with FBSS. In general, patients with recurrent disc herniation respond well to conservative care and should be treated as all herniated discs are—with conservative care prior to surgical intervention.[49] If conservative treatment fails to relieve symptoms, then selective injections (transforaminal or caudal blocks) can be tried. If all the conservative measures fail, then surgery is the best option. Once again, the surgeon should look closely for any associated pathology, especially instability that was either not identified preoperatively or iatrogenically created with an overexuberant decompression. Also, the surgeon should be very careful to critically inspect the foraminal and far lateral areas for residual or recurrent disc. If instability is present, a fusion operation is indicated. In the remaining patients requiring revision discectomy, the outcomes of revision discectomy and neurolysis in the lumbar spine are the same as a primary discectomy when assessed using the visual analog scales for back and limb pain and the Oswestry Disability Index.[50]

Neuropathic Pain, Epineural, Perineural, and Intradural Fibrosis (Arachnoiditis)

The diagnosis and treatment of postoperative fibrosis is complex, multimodal, and the subject of many papers, particularly in the pain medicine journals. These patients and their lengthy treatment can have a sustained negative economic impact and are very difficult to manage in a surgical practice. Neuropathic pain and intraspinal fibrosis are the cause of residual dermatomal pain postoperatively in approximately 7% to 10% of patients with FBSS. It is sometimes difficult to differentiate this pain from true radiculopathic pain due to compression of neural elements. Patients may actually have both pathologies to some degree or another. Neuropathic pain is characterized by a dysesthetic or burning pain in the back, buttock, and along one or two dermatomes. The pain may or may not be exacerbated by activity. Neuropathic pain may be due to systemic diseases (such as diabetes), medications (primarily chemotherapeutic agents), or postoperative epidural and perineural fibrosis and arachnoiditis (Fig. 102.6).

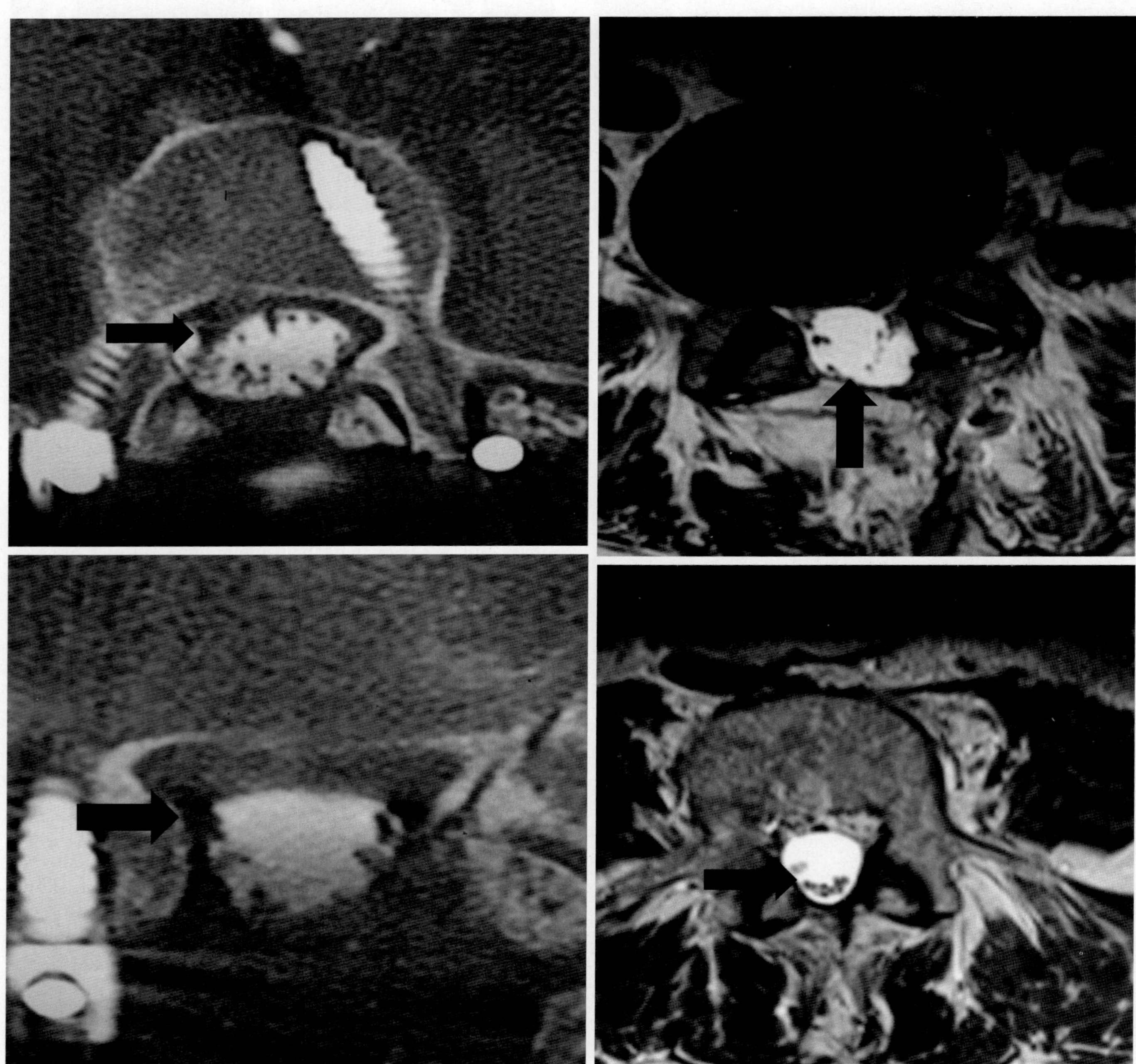

FIG. 102.6 Aggregation or clumping of the nerve roots, which indicates intradural fibrosis postoperatively (*arrows*). Also, the nerve roots are peripherally located, which gives the appearance of the "empty" sack.

The formation of scar tissue and adhesions following spine surgery is virtually universal. The role of this scar tissue as a pain generator is harder to determine; all patients develop some degree of scarring postoperatively but not all have persistent pain.[51] Generally, the diagnosis of fibrosis is made by myelogram with CT or with MRI with and without gadolinium.[52–54] These diagnostic studies may also be complemented with an EMG or diagnostic blocks or injections. However, these techniques are not very sensitive for detecting the severity and degree of adhesions.[55,56] Epiduroscopy has recently been used to evaluate and treat the spinal canal and to quantify the extent and severity of intraspinal scarring.[57] Epiduroscopy has also been reportedly used with some success in the treatment and prevention of these adhesions.[58] These studies have shown that the severity of intraspinal fibrosis is much higher than that reported on MRI.

This internal derangement and scarring of the nerves in the spinal canal and intrathecally is not generally thought to be surgically correctable and frequently requires treatment in a multidisciplinary pain clinic with a multidisciplinary approach. Even in the appropriate setting, neuropathic pain treatment may only provide partial relief in 40% to 60% of cases.[59] Pain clinics use many different modalities to treat this condition, including anticonvulsants (pregabalin and gabapentin), antidepressants (serotonin-norepinephrine reuptake inhibitors and tricyclic antidepressants), antiinflammatories, cannabis, dietary supplements, muscle relaxers, neuromodulators, spinal cord stimulation, intrathecal morphine pumps, oral opioids, and topical agents. The use of psychological evaluation and treatment should always be incorporated into these clinics. These patients can suffer from many different psychological illnesses due to their chronic pain.

Finally, there have been attempts to surgically treat this group of patients with open procedures, including neurolysis, free fat grafts, and hyaluronic acid. The results are generally poor.[60–62] Surgery should be performed in this group only if there is a documented associated surgically correctable lesion.

Facet Joint Pain

Pain originating from the facet joint after surgery accounts for less than 5% of the cases of FBSS. It is typically due to underlying arthritis as a pain generator, facet joint tropism, or fracture or instability that was previously not present or not recognized. There is a balancing act for adequate decompression of the central canal and lateral recesses, as overexcision of the facet joint can lead to thinning of the bone and the facet. This thin area can go on to fracture either in the facet or in the pars interarticularis. Similarly, complete excision of greater than 50% combined facets during a decompression at a single level can lead to instability.[63,64]

Facet joint tropism can also lead to postoperative pain if not correctly diagnosed prior to surgery (Fig. 102.7). Tropism is defined as a morphologic abnormality and/or a different coronal orientation between the right and left facet joints that can cause an asymmetrical stress on the joints.[65–68] This asymmetrical load can lead to the development of osteophytes, synovial facet cysts, and joint space narrowing with concomitant neuroforaminal narrowing.[69]

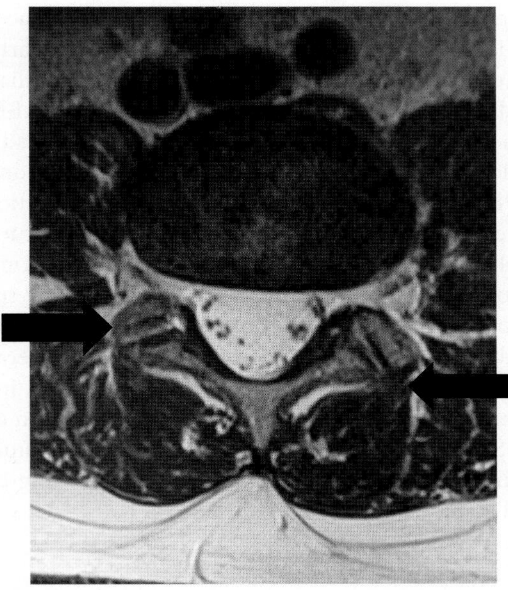

FIG. 102.7 Asymmetry between the angles of articulation of the facet joints at a single level *(arrows)*. This is referred to as facet joint tropism.

The diagnosis of conditions that affect the facet joints may be seen on plain radiographs with oblique and flexion-extension views but is best made using CT and myelography to assess the bony anatomy for arthritis, fractures, and morphology (tropism). This may be combined with MRI with gadolinium to assess the nerves and soft tissues and to delineate and define the extent of scarring. Bone scans with SPECT images are once again useful to localize the lesion if a fracture is suspected.[70]

Once diagnosed with a facet joint disorder, the initial treatment consists of physical therapy with an emphasis on core strengthening and avoidance of rotation and extension. Medications include NSAIDs, muscle relaxants, and preferably nonopioid pain medication. Interventional blocks can also be useful. Facet blocks can be used both therapeutically and diagnostically. If the facet joint can be localized with a block, then radiofrequency ablation can be attempted.[71,72] Surgical intervention is generally reserved for cases that have failed conservative care. The surgical treatment of choice is a fusion procedure for stabilization of the affected facet joint. Prior to surgical intervention, the patient and physician should discuss the diagnosis, options, and expected outcome to ensure that the expectations are aligned.

Sacroiliac Pain

The sacroiliac joint can be a cause of pain in the back, gluteal area, pelvis, thighs, and groin in the postoperative patient.[73,74] The incidence of pain referable to the sacroiliac joint after spine surgery is between 2% and 7%.[75] It is a diarthrodial joint with many ligaments and a complex innervation system of both the joint capsule and the ligaments. The sacroiliac joint is unique in that it has both hyaline cartilage and fibrocartilage.[76]

The diagnosis of pain emanating from the sacroiliac joint is based on physical examination (including the FABER test [flexion, abduction, and external fixation]) and radiologic evaluation with plain radiographs, CT scan, and bone scan with SPECT (Figs. 102.8 and 102.9). Diagnostic injections can help to confirm the disease. The presence of serologic markers may help in determining the presence of associated medical conditions such as ankylosing spondylitis and some spondyloarthropathies.[77] Treatment consists of conservative care with physical therapy, selective fluoroscopic sacroiliac therapeutic injections, the use of radiofrequency ablations, and, in some cases, surgical intervention for percutaneous or open arthrodesis.[78] Surgical intervention with percutaneous techniques is increasing in frequency and results are encouraging if strict surgical selection criteria are utilized.[79,80]

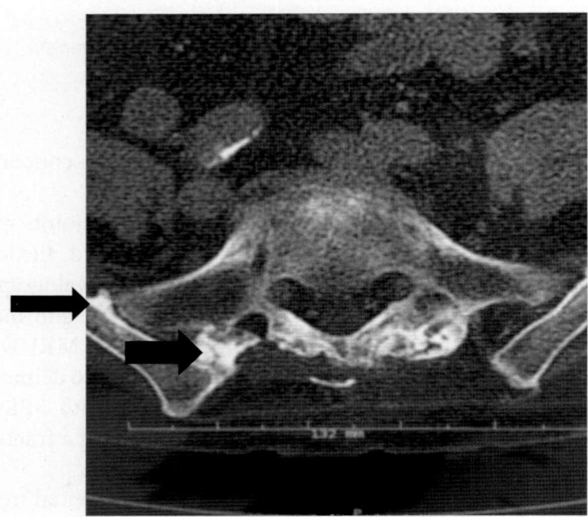

FIG. 102.8 Computed tomographic scan showing the presence of arthritis and a bone graft in the right sacroiliac joint (*arrows*).

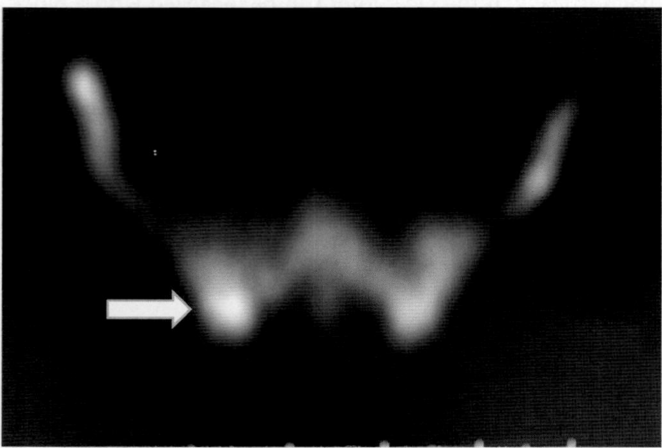

FIG. 102.9 Bone scan showing asymmetrical uptake between the right and left sides consistent with sacroiliitis (*arrow*).

Sagittal Plane Imbalance and Spinal Deformity

Collapse of the spine or sagittal plane deformity postoperatively can be a cause of surgical failure and postoperative pain. The instability and kyphosis can be a sequela of the surgery itself or iatrogenic in the case of long fusions without attention to balancing the sagittal plane. When performing a multilevel fusion, attention must be paid to the amount of lordosis in which the patient is fused. This condition can be further exacerbated by pseudarthrosis, junctional kyphosis, adjacent-level disease, and collapse and hip flexion contractures.[81,82] Likewise, when performing a multilevel decompression, care should be taken to not destabilize the spine. If the spine is fused, then adjacent levels should be evaluated for collapse and degeneration.[83,84] Diagnosis is made by physical examination and standing anteroposterior and lateral radiographs along with CT and MRI to look at adjacent levels for signs of disease. Sagittal plane deformity (Figs. 102.10 and 102.11) studies have demonstrated that the further the plumb line from C7 falls further anterior to the sacrum, results decline.[85]

Treatment for this condition can be conservative, but surgical intervention is frequently necessary to return the patient to optimal function. Osteotomies and derotational procedures are used to surgically correct the deformity.[86,87] Three major goals of surgery include (1) ensuring that the pelvic tilt is less than 20 degrees, (2) keeping the lumbar lordosis within 9 degrees of the pelvic incidence, and (3) correction of the

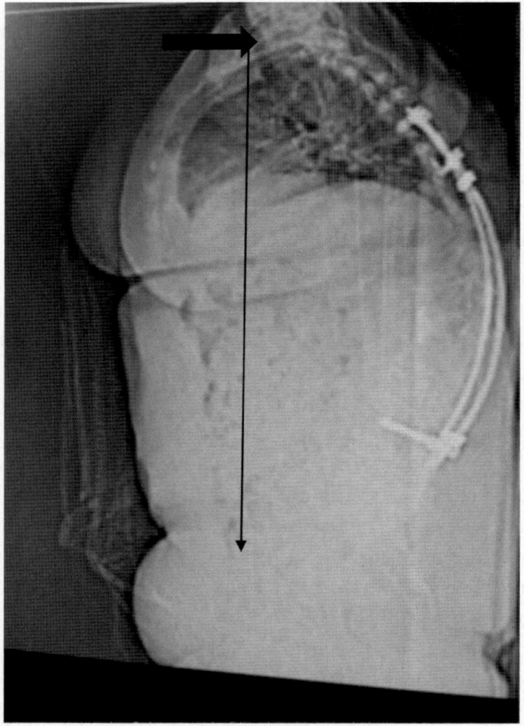

FIG. 102.10 A plumb line falling anterior to the sacral endplate, thus making the sagittal vertical axis >5 cm and indicating the presence of sagittal plane imbalance (*arrows*).

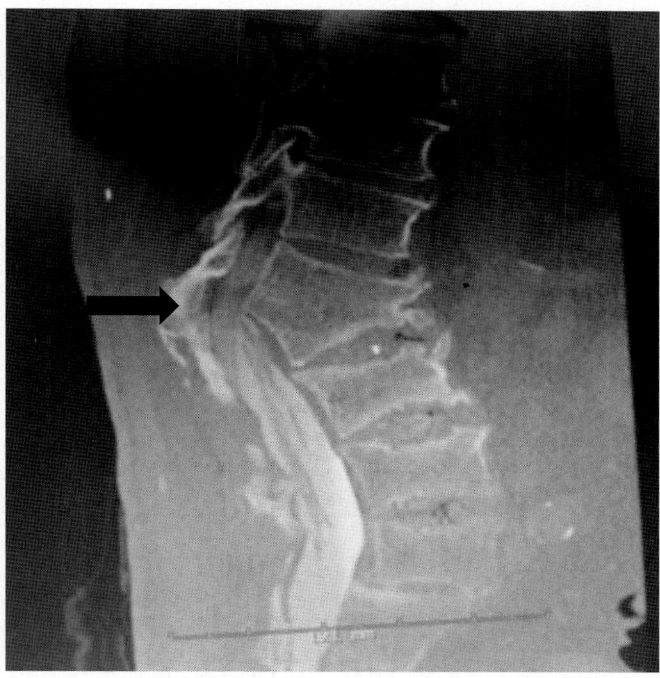

FIG. 102.11 Postosteomyelitis collapse of L1 onto L2. This creates an acute kyphosis and sagittal plane imbalance in the lumbar spine (*arrow*).

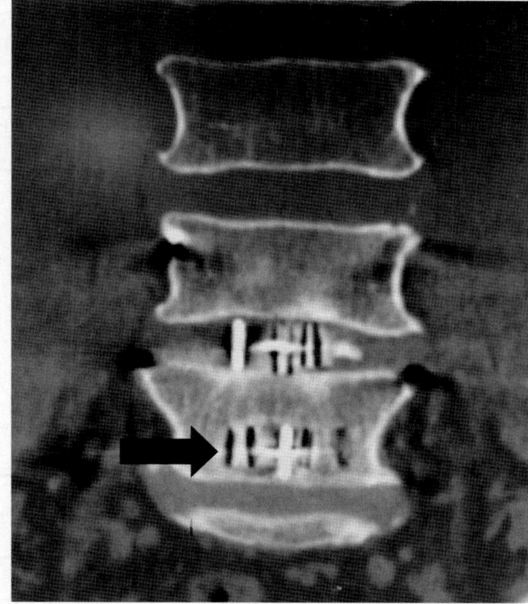

FIG. 102.12 Malpositioned interbody fusion device with failure to fuse the intended disc space. Note that the graft is in the vertebral body and not the disc space itself (*arrow*).

sagittal vertical axis to inside of 5 cm of neutral.[88] Attention must be paid to every detail of this corrective surgery. The patient should be informed of the problem, the options, and the proposed procedure with its risks and potential complications. Expectations should be discussed and psychological counseling offered if needed. The recovery is often lengthy, as with all revision surgeries.

Other Conditions

There are other reasons that patients have persistent pain and disability after back surgery. These include surgery on the incorrect level, malpositioned hardware, systemic diseases (such as lupus, rheumatoid arthritis, and ankylosing spondylitis), and infection. Generally, these situations are readily identifiable when the patient is seen in the postoperative period. Plain radiographs, CT scans, and MRI are useful in determining the levels and position of the hardware (Fig. 102.12). Bloodwork—such as a complete blood count, erythrocyte sedimentation rate, and C-reactive protein—and the presence or absence of immunologic markers are useful in identifying infections and in determining systemic diseases. A candid conversation with the patient is advised and correction of the condition should be offered if one is available. Referral to infectious disease or rheumatologic physicians may be helpful. In the case of malpositioned hardware or wrong-level surgery, a candid conversation about the issue is advised and correction of the problem as soon as possible is recommended. The best way to prevent wrong-level surgery is through direct and thorough conversations with the patient and family, surgical site marking and intraoperative radiography to verify levels.[89]

Summary

Revision surgery of the spine for the treatment of FBSS should only be considered in patients who have proven pathology with diagnostic studies and a failure to respond to conservative treatment or minimally invasive procedures (e.g., epidural blocks, facet blocks). Decision algorithms for the diagnosis and medical and surgical management of back pain and radiculopathy are shown in Figs. 102.13 and 102.14, respectively. Patients who have undergone surgical procedures of the spine can have tremendous improvement in their quality of life and return to normal activities if realistic expectations are discussed prior to the secondary procedure. However, there are those patients that fail to respond to correctly performed surgery. The cause of their pain may be anatomic or psychological.

The most common cause of true inoperable FBSS with radiculopathy is epineural and perineural fibrosis and arachnoiditis. Diagnosis of this problem is done using MRI with and without gadolinium and/or CT/myelogram. "Clumping of nerve roots" is a common radiographic description and is the term frequently used to describe fibrosis and adhesions within the nerve root. These findings, without the presence of any of the lesions described earlier, are in fact the true pathologic changes that should be used for giving patients the diagnosis of nonsurgical FBSS. Likewise, back pain persisting or increasing after surgery and without the presence of any of the correctable, diagnosable conditions described earlier should also be included in nonsurgical FBSS. Scar tissue and internal nerve damage are not correctable surgically, nor is back pain without a pathologic process.

It is also important to identify and refer for management those patients with psychiatric problems and secondary gain,

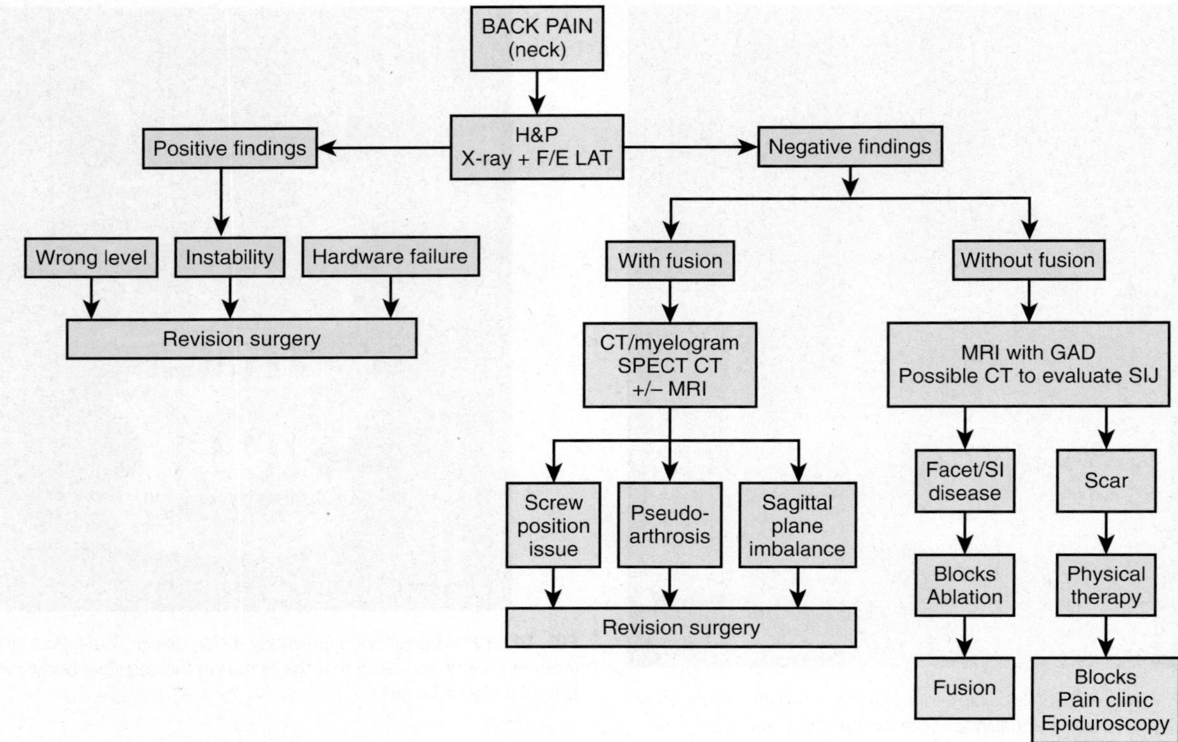

FIG. 102.13 Back pain algorithm. CT, computed tomography; F/E LAT, flexion/extension lateral; GAD, gadolinium; H&P, history and physical examination; MRI, magnetic resonance imaging; SIJ, sacroiliac joint; SPECT, single photon emission computed tomography.

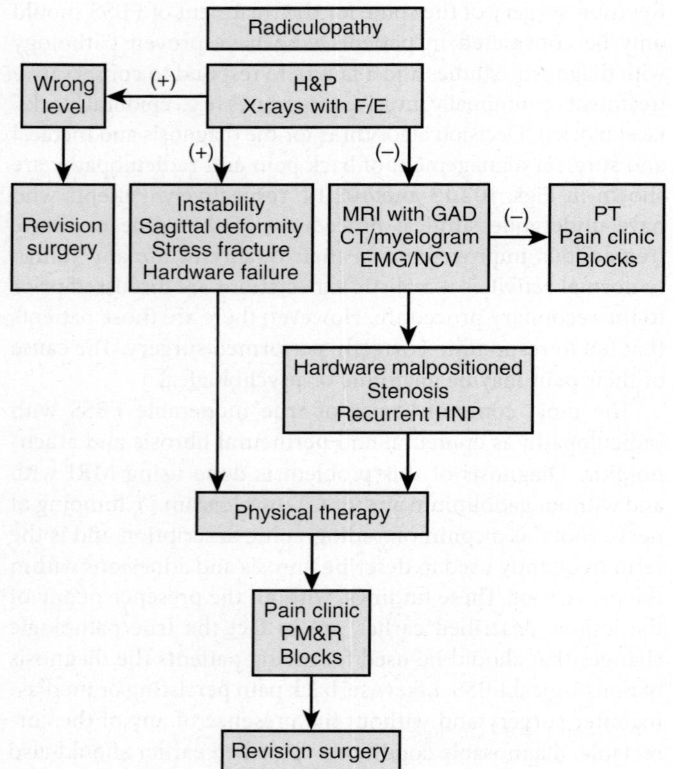

FIG. 102.14 Radiculopathy algorithm. CT, computed tomography; EMG, electromyogram; F/E, flexion/extension; GAD, gadolinium; H&P, history and physical examination; HNP, herniated nucleus pulposus; MRI, magnetic resonance imaging; NCV, nerve conduction velocity; PT, physical therapy; PM&R, physical medicine and rehabilitation.

as the presence of either of these conditions may also affect the overall outcome. In these groups of individuals, the surgeons are often left with dissatisfied patients who now live in the world of chronic pain and disability. It is the surgeons' obligation to exhaustively investigate the etiology of the residual symptoms.

If a surgically correctable lesion or problem is identified, then a treatment plan should be offered to the patient for the correction of the problem with its potential risks and complications in the hope of removing them from this stigmatized diagnosis. If no surgery is available for correction or improvement of the problem, then the patient should be referred to the appropriate setting for optimization of the condition.

KEY REFERENCES

1. Guyer RD, Patterson M, Ohnmeiss DD. Failed back surgery syndrome: diagnostic evaluation. *J Am Acad Orthop Surg.* 2006;14(9):534-543.
   This article provides a complete overview of steps to diagnose failed back surgery syndrome and a classification system.
2. Taylor RS, Taylor JT. The economic impact of failed back surgery syndrome. *Br J Pain.* 2012;6(4):174-181.
   This is an excellent cost analysis for failed back surgery syndrome.
3. Schofferman J, Reynolds J, Herzog R, et al. Failed back surgery: etiology and diagnostic evaluation. *Spine J.* 2003;5:400-403.
   This is a synopsis of the common causes of failed back surgery syndrome.
4. Bosscher H, Heavner J. Incidence and severity of epidural fibrosis after back surgery: an endoscopic study. *Pain Pract.* 2010;10(1):18-24.
   This article is about the prevalence of epidural scarring after back surgery.

REFERENCES

1. van Middendorp JJ, Sanchez GM, Burridge AL. The Edwin Smith papyrus: a clinical reappraisal of the oldest known document on spinal injuries. *Eur Spine J*. 2010;19(11):1815-1823.
2. Truumees E. A history of lumbar disc herniation from Hippocrates to the 1990s. *Clin Orthop Relat Res*. 2015;473(6):1885-1895.
3. Robinson JS. Sciatica and the lumbar disc syndrome: a historical perspective. *South Med J*. 1983;76:232-238.
4. Wilkinson HA. *The Failed Back Syndrome: Etiology and Therapy*. 2nd ed. Philadelphia: Harper & Row; 1991.
5. North RB, Campbell J, James CS, et al. Failed back surgery syndrome: 5-year follow-up in 102 patients undergoing repeated operation. *Neurosurgery*. 1991;28:685-691.
6. Waguespack A, Schofferman J, Slosar P, Reynold J. Etiology of long-term failures of lumbar spine surgery. *Pain Med*. 2002;3:18-22.
7. North RB, Ewend MG, Lawton MT, Kidd DH, Piantadosi S. Failed back surgery syndrome: 5-year follow-up after spinal cord stimulator implantation. *Neurosurgery*. 1991;28(5):692-699.
8. Taylor RS, Taylor RJ. The economic impact of failed back surgery syndrome. *Br J Pain*. 2012;6(4):174-181.
9. National Center for Health and Statistics. *National Hospital discharge survey. Series 13, No 144*. Washington, DC: Centers for Disease Control and Prevention; 1998.
10. Deyo RA, Mirza SK. Trends and variations in the use of spine surgery. *Clin Orthop Relat Res*. 2006;493:139-146.
11. Nachemson A. Evaluation of results in lumbar spine surgery. *Acta Orthop Scand Suppl*. 1993;251:130-133.
12. Guyer RD, Patterson M, Ohnmeiss DD. Failed back surgery syndrome: diagnostic evaluation. *J Am Acad Orthop Surg*. 2006;9:534-543.
13. Koerner JD, Glaser J, Radcliff K. Which variables are associated with patient-reported outcomes after discectomy? Review of SPORT Disc Herniation Studies. *Clin Orthop Relat Res*. 2015;473(6):2000-2006.
14. Taylor RS, Taylor JT. The economic impact of failed back surgery syndrome. *British Journal Pain*. 2012;6(4):174-181.
15. Saal J. General principles of diagnostic testing as related to painful lumbar spine disorders: a critical appraisal of current diagnostic techniques. *Spine*. 2002;27:2538-2545.
16. Deen HG Jr, Zimmerman RS, Lyons MK, et al. Analysis of early failures after lumbar decompressive laminectomy for spinal stenosis. *Mayo Clin Proc*. 1995;70:33-36.
17. Phillips FM, Cunningham B. Managing chronic pain of spinal origin after lumbar surgery: the role of decompressive surgery. *Spine*. 2002;28:2547-2553.
18. Cinotti G. Failures of surgery in lumbar spinal stensosis. Causes and management. *J Bone Joint Surg Br*. 1999;81B(suppl II):142.
19. Fritsch E, Heisel J, Rupp S. The failed back surgery syndrome: reasons, intraoperative findings, and long-term results: a report of 182 operative treatments. *Spine*. 2001;26:2521-2534.
20. Jang JS, Lee S, Min J, et al. Surgical treatment of failed back surgery syndrome due to sagittal imbalance. *Spine*. 2007;31(26):3081-3087.
21. Farrar JT, Young JP, LaMoreaux L, Werth JL, Poole RM. Clinical importance of changes in chronic pain intensity measured on an 11-point numerical pain rating scale. *Pain*. 2001;94:149-158.
22. Schofferman J, Reynolds J, Herzog R, et al. Failed back surgery: etiology and diagnostic evaluation. *Spine J*. 2003;5:400-403.
23. Waguespack A, Schofferman J, Slosar P, Reynolds J. Etiology of long-term failures of lumbar spine surgery. *Pain Med*. 2002;3:18-22.
24. Slipman CW, Shin CH, Patel RK, et al. Etiologies of failed back surgery syndrome. *Pain Med*. 2002;3:200-214.
25. Gopalakrishnan N, Nadhamuni K, Karthikeyan T. Categorization of pathology causing low back pain using magnetic resonance imaging (MRI). *J Clin Diagn Res*. 2015;9(1):17-20.
26. Coster S, de Bruijn SF, Tavy DL. Diagnostic value of history, physical examination and needle electromyography in diagnosing lumbosacral radiculopathy. *J Neurol*. 2010;257(3):332-337.
27. Simon J, McAuliffe M, Shamim F, Vuong N, Tahaei A. Discogenic low back pain. *Phys Med Rehabil Clin N Am*. 2014;2:305-317.
28. Teraguchi M, Yoshimura N, Hashizume H, et al. The association of combination of disc degeneration, end plate signal change, and Schmorl node with low back pain in a large population study: the Wakayama Spine Study. *Spine J*. 2015;15(4):622-628.
29. Mok FP, Samartzis D, Karppinen J, et al. Modic changes of the lumbar spine: prevalence, risk factors, and association with disc degeneration and low back pain in a large-scale population-based cohort. *Spine J*. 2016;16(1):32-41.
30. de Schepper EI, Damen J, van Meurs JB, et al. The association between lumbar disc degeneration and low back pain: the influence of age, gender, and individual radiographic features. *Spine*. 2010;35(5):531-536.
31. Walsh TR, Weinstein JN, Spratt KF, et al. Lumbar discography in normal subjects. *J Bone Joint Surg Am*. 1990;72A:1081-1088.
32. Carragee EJ, Don AS, Hurwitz EL, et al. 2009 ISSLS prize winner: does discography cause accelerated progression of degeneration changes in the lumbar disc: a ten-year matched cohort study. *Spine*. 2009;34(21):2338-2345.
33. Kim KS, Yoon ST, Li J, Park JS, Hutton WC. Disc degeneration in the rabbit: a biochemical and radiological comparison between four disc injury models. *Spine*. 2005;30(1):33-37.
34. Grangier C, Garcia J, Howarth NR, May M, Rossier P. Role of MRI in the diagnosis of insufficiency fractures of the sacrum and acetabular roof. *Skeletal Radiol*. 1997;26(9):517-524.
35. Wei J, Song Y, Sun L, Lv C. Comparison of artificial total disc replacement versus fusion for lumbar degenerative disc disease: a meta-analysis of randomized controlled trials. *Int Orthop*. 2013;37(7):1315-1325.
36. Carreon LY, Glassman SD, Howard J. Fusion and nonsurgical treatment for symptomatic lumbar degenerative disease: a systematic review of Oswestry Disability Index and MOS Short Form-36 outcomes. *Spine J*. 2008;8(5):747-755.
37. Gertzbein SD, Hallopeter MR, Hall S. Pseudoarthrosis of the lumbar spine. Outcomes after circumferential fusion. *Spine*. 1998;23:2352-2357.
38. Boden SD, Summer DR. Biological lesions affecting spinal fusion and bone regeneration. *Spine*. 1995;(suppl 24):12S-112S.
39. Bendo JA, Spival J, Moskovich R, et al. Instrumented posterior arthrodesis of the lumbar spine in patients with diabetes mellitus. *Am J Orthop*. 2000;29:617-620.
40. Carpenter CT, Dietz JW, Leung KY, et al. Repair of a pseudoarthrosis of the lumbar spine. A functional outcome study. *J Bone Joint Surg Am*. 1996;78:712-720.
41. Dimar JR Jr, Ante WA, Zhang YP, et al. The effects of nonsteroidal anti-inflammatory drugs on posterior spinal fusions in the rat. *Spine*. 1996;21:1870-1876.

42. Jenkins LT, Jones AL, Harms JJ. Prognostic factors in lumbar spinal fusion. *Contemp Orthop*. 1994;29:173-180.
43. Deguchi M, Rapoff AJ, Zdeblick TA. Posterolateral fusion for isthmic spondylolisthesis in adults: analysis of fusion rate and clinical results. *J Spinal Disord*. 1998;11:459-464.
44. Burkus JK, Dorchak JD, Sanders DL. Radiographic assessment of interbody fusion using recombinant human bone morphogenic protein type 2. *Spine*. 2003;28:372-377.
45. Buttermann GR, Glazer PA, Hu SS, et al. Revision of failed lumbar fusions. A comparison of anterior autograft and allograft. *Spine*. 1997;22:2748-2755.
46. Etminan M, Girardi FP, Khan SN, et al. Revision strategies for lumbar pseudoarthrosis. *Orthop Clin North Am*. 2002;33: 381-392.
47. Silcox DH 3rd, Daftari T, Boden SD, et al. The effect of nicotine on spinal fusion. *Spine*. 1995;20(14):1549-1553.
48. Weinstein JN, Lurie JD, Tosteson TD, et al. Surgical versus nonoperative treatment for lumbar disc herniation: four-year results for the Spine Patient Outcomes Research Trial (SPORT). *Spine*. 2008;33(25):2789-2800.
49. Stambough J. An algorithmic approach to recurrent lumbar disc herniation: evaluation and management. *Semin Spine Surg*. 2008;20:2-13.
50. Patel MS, Braybrooke J, Newey M, Sell P. A comparative study of the outcomes of primary and revision lumbar discectomy surgery. *Bone Joint J*. 2013;95-B(1):90-94.
51. Ozer AF, Oktenoglu Y, Sastani M. Preserving the ligamentum flavum in lumbar discectomy. *Neurosurgery*. 2006;59:126-133.
52. Miquel A, Court C, Pradel C, et al. Imaging of the postsurgical spine. *J Radiol*. 2010;91(9 Pt 2):1022-1034.
53. Hurme M, Katevuo K, Nykvist F, et al. CT five years after myelographic diagnosis of lumbar disc herniation. *Acta Radiol*. 1991;32:286-289.
54. Ross JS, Obuchowski N. MR evaluation of epidural fibrosis: proposed grading system with inter-observer variability. *Neurol Res*. 1999;21(suppl 1):S23-S26.
55. Richardson J, McGurgan P, Cheema S, et al. Spinal endoscopy in chronic low back pain with radiculopathy. *Anaest*. 2001;56:454-460.
56. Geurts JW, Kallewaard JW, Richardson J, Groen GJ. Targeted methylprednisolone acetate/hyaluronidase/clonidine injection after diagnostic epiduroscopy for chronic sciatica: a prospective, 1 year follow-up study. *Reg Anest Pain Med*. 2002;27:343-352.
57. Bosscher H, Heavner J. Incidence and severity of epidural fibrosis after back surgery: an endoscopic study. *Pain Pract*. 2010;10(issue1):18-24.
58. Richardson J, McGurgan P, Cheema S, et al. Spinal endoscopy in chronic low back pain with radiculopathy. *Anaesthesia*. 2001;56:454-460.
59. Dworkin RH, O'Connor AB, Backonja M, et al. Pharmacologic management of neuropathic pain: evidence-based recommendations. *Pain*. 2007;132(3):237-251.
60. Mayfield FH. Autologous fat grafts for the protection and repair of the spinal dura. *Clin Neurosurg*. 1980;27:349-356.
61. Abitbol J-J, Lincoln TL, Lind BI, et al. Preventing postlaminectomy adhesion: a new experimental model. *Spine*. 1994;19:1809-1844.
62. Songer MN, Ghosh L, Spencer DL. Effect of sodium hyaluronate on peridural fibrosis after lumbar laminectomy and discectomy. *Spine*. 1990;15:550-554.
63. Abumi K, Panjabi MM, Kramer KM, et al. Biomechanical evaluation of lumbar spinal stability after graded facetectomies. *Spine*. 1990;15(11):1142-1147.
64. Zander T, Rohlmann A, Klöckner C, Bergmann G. Influence of graded facetectomy and laminectomy on spinal biomechanics. *Eur Spine J*. 2003;12(4):427-434.
65. Jaumard N, Welch WC, Winkelstein BA. Spinal facet joint biomechanics and mechanotransduction in normal, injury and degenerative conditions. *J Biomech Eng*. 2011;133(7):71-110.
66. Sharma L, Kapoor D, Issa S. Epidemiology of osteoarthritis: an update. *Curr Opin Rheumatol*. 2006;18:147-156.
67. Berlemann U, Jeszenszky DJ, Buhler DW, Harms J. Facet joint remodeling in degenerative spondylolisthesis: an investigation of joint orientation and tropism. *Eur Spine J*. 1998;7:376-380.
68. Cyron BM, Hutton WC. Articular tropism and stability of the lumbar spine. *Spine*. 1980;5(2):168-172.
69. Gallucci M, Puglielli E, Splendiani A, Pistoia F, Spacca G. Degenerative disorders of the spine. *Eur Radiol*. 2005;15:591-598.
70. Mulconrey DS, Knight RQ, Bramble JD, Paknikar S, Harty PA. Interobserver reliability in the interpretation of diagnostic lumbar MRI and nuclear imaging. *Spine J*. 2006;6(2):177-184.
71. North R, Han M, Zahurak M, Kidd D. Radiofrequency lumbar facet denervation: analysis of prognostic factors. *Pain*. 1994;57:77-83.
72. Rashbaum R. Radiofrequency facet denervation: a treatment alternative in refractory low back pain with or without low back pain. *Orthop Clin North Am*. 1983;14:569.
73. Jung JH, Kim HI, Shin DA, et al. Usefulness of pain distribution pattern assessment in decision-making for the patients with lumbar zygapophyseal and sacroiliac joint arthropathy. *J Korean Med Sci*. 2007;22(6):1048-1054.
74. Daum WJ. The sacroiliac joint: an underappreciated pain generator. *Am J Orthop*. 1995;24:475-478.
75. Schwarzer AC, Aprill CN, Bogduk N. The sacroiliac joint in chronic low back pain. *Spine*. 1995;20(1):31-37.
76. Forst SL, Wheeler MT, Fortin JD, Vilensky JA. The sacroiliac joint: anatomy, physiology and clinical significance. *Pain Physician*. 2006;9(1):61-67.
77. Jee WH, McCauley TR, Lee SH, et al. Sacroiliitis in patients with ankylosing spondylitis: association of MR findings with disease activity. *Magn Reson Imaging*. 2004;22(2):245-250.
78. Ho KY, Hadi MA, Pasutharnchat K, Tan KH. Cooled radiofrequency denervation for treatment of sacroiliac joint pain: two-year results from 20 cases. *J Pain Res*. 2013;6:505-511.
79. Polly DW, Cher DJ, Wine KD, et al. INSITE Study Group. Randomized controlled trial of minimally invasive sacroiliac joint fusion using triangular titanium implants vs nonsurgical management for sacroiliac joint dysfunction: 12-month outcomes. *Neurosurgery*. 2015;77(5):674-691.
80. Waisbrod H, Krainick JU, Gerbershagen HU. Sacroilial joint arthrodesis for chronic lower back pain. *Arch Orthop Traumat Surg*. 1987;106:238-240.
81. Bridwell KH, Lenke LG, Lewis SJ. Treatment of spinal stenosis and fixed sagittal imbalance. *Clin Orthop*. 2001;384:35-44.
82. Sarwahi V, Boachie-Adjei O, Backus SI, et al. Characterization of gait function in patients with postsurgical sagittal (flatback) deformity: a prospective study of 21 patients. *Spine*. 2002;27:2328-2337.
83. Herkowitz HN, Abraham DJ, Albert TJ. Management of degenerative disc disease above an L5-S1 segment requiring arthrodesis. *Spine*. 1999;24:1268-1270.
84. Glassman SD, Pugh K, Johnson JR, et al. Surgical management of adjuvant level degeneration following lumbar spine fusion. *Orthopedics*. 2002;25:1051-1055.

85. Glassman SD, Bridwell K, Dimar JR, et al. The impact of positive sagittal balance in adult spinal deformity. *Spine*. 2005;30(18):2024-2029.
86. Smith-Peterson MN, Larson CB, Aufranc OE. Osteotomy of the spine for the correction of deformity in rheumatoid arthritis. *J Bone Joint Surg Am*. 1945;27:1-11.
87. Hehne HJ, Zielke K, Bohm H. Polysegmental lumbar osteotomies and transpedicled fixation for correction of long curved kyphotic deformities in ankylosing spondylitis. *Clin Orthop*. 1990;258:49-55.
88. Schwab F, Patel A, Ungar B, Farcy JP, Lafage V. Adult spinal deformity-postoperative standing imbalance: how much can you tolerate? An overview of key parameters in assessing alignment and planning corrective surgery. *Spine*. 2010;35(25):2224-2231.
89. Mody MG, Nourbakhsh A, Stahl DL, et al. The prevalence of wrong level surgery among spine surgeons. *Spine*. 2008;33(2):194-198.

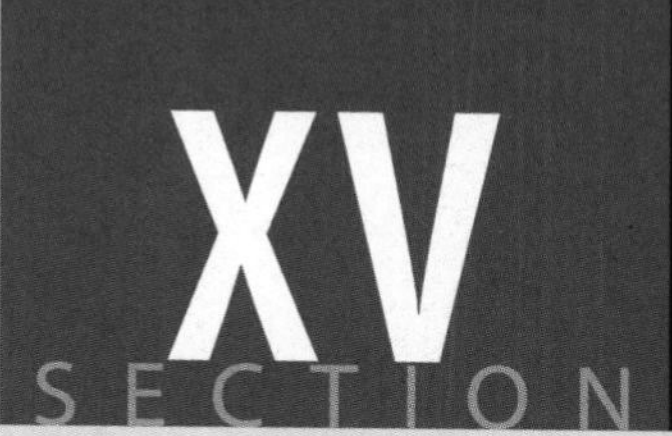
XV
SECTION

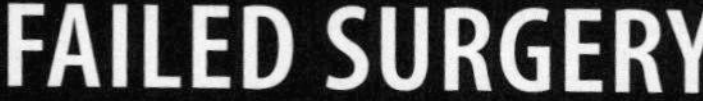
FAILED SURGERY

CHAPTER 103 Revision Spine Surgery

Michael J. Vives
Spencer Hauser
Saad B. Chaudhary

"A goal without a plan is just a wish"
– **Antoine de Saint-Exupéry**

The number of elective spinal surgeries performed yearly continues to increase at an accelerating pace.[1] Although advances in diagnostics, implant design, and biologic adjuncts have made these operations more predictable in outcome, a significant number of patients report persistent or recurrent symptoms. These patients represent a major challenge to spine care providers. In general, the odds for success continue to fall with each additional surgical undertaking. From a statistical standpoint, the second operation has a 50% chance of success, and after the second operation, patients are more likely to be made worse than better.[2] The risk of reoperation holds true independent of the index diagnosis, procedure performed, and comorbidities. As such, in the classic words of Waddell and colleagues, "caution and restraint are required when contemplating repeat back surgery."[3]

The term *failed back surgery syndrome* (FBSS) has been commonly used to describe patients who experience chronic disabling lower back pain and/or leg pain that persists or recurs following anatomically successful spinal surgery.[4] Similarly, patients who have undergone cervical procedures may report residual or recurrent neck and/or arm pain or myelopathic symptoms. FBSS has been shown to have considerable impact on an individual's health-related quality of life as well as a significant economic cost to society.[4] It is thus imperative to identify strategies to prevent these conditions as well as develop guidelines to manage established cases.[4] In order to improve the prospects for successful management, an algorithmic approach may be useful. Temporal factors relating to the symptoms may provide clues during the initial patient encounter. Beyond these considerations, general categorization of the symptom complex as being predominantly axial or radicular/claudicatory helps to focus the goals of treatment as the workup progresses. The patient's symptoms, physical findings, and diagnostics should be correlated to support a common diagnosis on which to base treatment recommendation and surgical strategy. Echoing Saint-Exupéry, the desire to address recurrent or persistent symptoms without a thoughtful plan is just wishful thinking. As such, each revision operation should include unique strategies to accomplish a specific goal beyond "redoing" the index procedure.

Patient Evaluation

A detailed history is mandatory to properly evaluate patients with persistent or recurrent pain after spinal surgery. Along with medical history, medications should be reviewed to rule out narcotic abuse. In addition, social history—including work history and motivation for return to work—should be elicited as well as involvement in litigation. This information can help predict functional outcome of revision surgery.[5] These histories may be quite complex, with lengthy and often emotional background stories. Despite these challenges, organization of the information and directed questions are essential to deriving specific points for further decision making.

The patient's main symptoms before the index surgery should be elicited as well as the index diagnosis and details of the patient's operative procedure. It is helpful to obtain the medical records and imaging studies that were performed before the previous surgical procedure to compare with the current situation. In some cases, after such careful analysis, an incorrect initial diagnosis may be identified.[6]

The time frame over which the new or recurrent symptoms develop may suggest their underlying etiology. Failure to achieve any pain-free interval after the primary surgery has been associated with incorrect preoperative diagnosis, wrong-level surgery, and inadequate decompression, particularly in the lateral recess or foraminal region.[7-9] Early onset of new radicular pain after surgery may suggest nerve root injury. If pedicle screws or interbody fusion devices have been placed, their position should be evaluated with computed tomography (CT).[6] In the intermediate postoperative period (1–6 months), mild new or recurrent pain may develop as patients progress through rehabilitation. Symptoms that develop suddenly after a specific inciting event may be from recurrent disc herniation or hardware failure. Recurrent symptoms of gradual onset in the intermediate time frame are often related to the development of scar tissue, such as epidural fibrosis or adhesive arachnoiditis.[2] Symptomatic pseudarthroses may also begin to manifest themselves toward the end of the 6-month postoperative period. Other causes of late postoperative pain include recurrent disc herniations or stenosis and the development of adjacent-level pathology. For the surgeon who may evaluate patients initially treated elsewhere, this timeline regarding the recurrence of symptoms is crucial to establishing the proper diagnosis.

A frequent cause of failed spine surgery is poor patient selection, which unfortunately is often more apparent in retrospect. Several authors have reported that psychological factors documented on the Minnesota Multiphasic Personality Inventory can be related to poor outcomes after spinal surgery.[10–12] Elevation of hypochondriasis, hysteria, and depression scales are most predictive. Poor results are also more likely in patients who exhibit abnormal pain behavior, receive worker's compensation, or are involved in litigation.[13,14] On the basis of a growing body of research demonstrating that these types of factors place patients at risk for poor outcomes, many insurance carriers, particularly within the worker's compensation system, are now requiring or strongly recommending presurgical psychological screening for potential spine surgery candidates.[15] The influence of these factors on outcome, however, is poorly understood. The combination of physical, psychosocial, and economic problems with which patients with FBSS present make individualized treatment plans necessary.

Another regrettably common cause of persistent symptoms is performance of the wrong surgical procedure. Wrong-level discectomy is the most common avoidable error in spine surgery. The North American Spine Society has advocated intraoperative radiographic localization in almost all cases to help prevent this misfortune.[9] However, wrong-level spine surgery can occur despite adhering to this protocol; up to 50% of spine surgeons may perform wrong-level spine surgery at some point in their career.[16] Another example of an improper procedure is to decompress only what appears to be the most stenotic level and leave other areas unaddressed, particularly in the lateral recess or foraminal region. Likewise, failure to identify the pain generator before performing an interbody fusion for discogenic pain can lead to disappointing results. Many patients will have one or two significantly abnormal discs on magnetic resonance evaluation but other areas with comparably mild changes, which may be surprisingly concordant at discography. In our own experience, such patients are advised against surgery.

Leg Pain Versus Back Pain

As with primary lumbar degenerative syndromes, differentiating the degree of axial back pain from radicular or neurogenic claudicatory symptoms is paramount to formulating an effective treatment plan. Although the diagnostic tests that follow will help identify the pathoanatomy, all of the findings should be kept in context with the patient's main complaint. An algorithm based on the patient's main complaint is presented in Fig. 103.1.

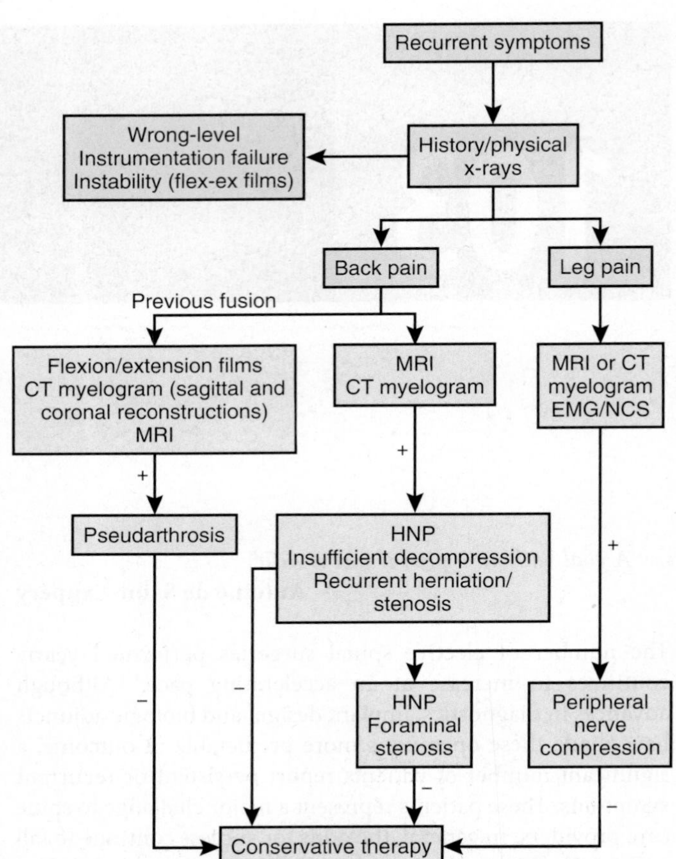

FIG. 103.1 Algorithm for approach to the patient with persistent or recurrent symptoms after lumbar spinal surgery. CT, computed tomography; EMG/NCS, electromyography/nerve conduction studies; flex-ex, flexion/extension; HNP, herniated nucleus pulposus; MRI, magnetic resonance imaging.

Physical Examination

The physical examination of patients with FBSS is similar to the initial examination for nonoperated patients. Posture, gait, and alignment—including sagittal balance while standing and sitting—should be observed.[5] Range of motion, tenderness, and nerve root tension signs should be elicited and a thorough neurologic examination should be performed. Although the physical examination findings of this condition may be nonspecific, a thorough examination may be helpful to exclude other conditions that may have similar presentations. In patients with leg pain, thorough examination of the hip and knee and assessment of distal pulses may reveal other potential causes of their symptoms. Nonorganic physical findings should be recorded, as described by Waddell.[17] More than two Waddell findings strongly predicts poor outcome, regardless of spinal pathology.[17]

Diagnostic Testing

Plain Radiography

Plain radiographs of the lumbar spine should include biplanar standing films. A coned-down lateral of the lumbosacral

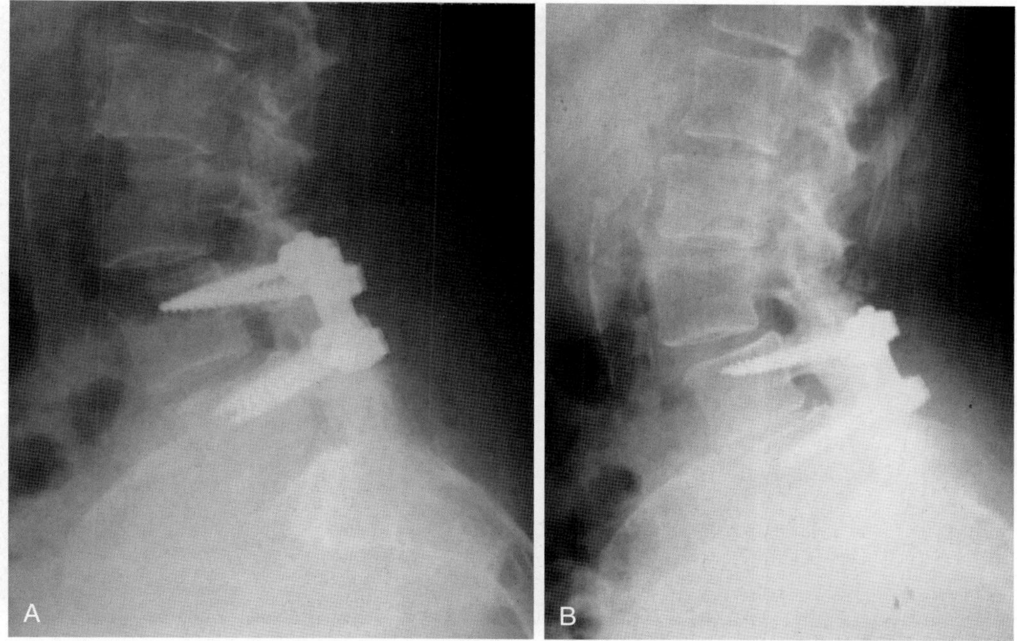

FIG. 103.2 Lateral plain radiographs after L4–L5 decompression and instrumented fusion for degenerative spondylolisthesis. Comparing the (A) early postoperative film with the (B) 7-year follow-up film shows that grade I spondylolisthesis has developed at the adjacent segment L3–L4.

junction and an anteroposterior Ferguson view may be particularly helpful in evaluating patients who have had previous surgery at the L5–S1 level. Patients with pain after a discectomy should be evaluated for iatrogenic pars fracture. Endplate rarefaction suggests a postoperative discitis. Previously placed spinal implants should be scrutinized for malposition, loosening, subsidence, or breakage. In addition to evaluation of disc height, endplate characteristics, and alignment, anterolisthesis or retrolisthesis at the adjacent levels should be noted (Fig. 103.2). Flexion-extension radiographs should be scrutinized for motion involving segments where fusion was attempted because gross motion detectable in this manner typically indicates pseudarthrosis. These films should also be evaluated for dynamic instability at levels adjacent to the previous surgery. The overall sagittal balance should be assessed on standing 36-inch radiographs with the hips and knees fully extended to eliminate any compensatory flexion that may mask deformity.[5] A flatback deformity from poorly contoured constructs or adjacent-segment degeneration (ASD) is best evaluated with this technique. A pelvis radiograph can assess for hip joint pathology that may be the source of groin or thigh pain.[5]

Advanced Imaging

CT with fine cuts and sagittal/coronal reconstructions can help delineate fusion status.[18] The adjacent levels should be carefully evaluated for hypertrophic facet arthropathy, spondylolysis, and pedicle stress fractures. Magnetic resonance imaging (MRI; Fig. 103.3) with and without gadolinium enhancement is the most sensitive test for evaluating neurologic compression at both the previously operated site and the adjacent levels.[19] Comparison of the enhanced and nonenhanced sequences can help differentiate epidural scar (enhancing) from recurrent disc herniations and hypertrophic ligamentum flavum (nonenhancing). In addition, gadolinium enhancement in the intervertebral disc and vertebral bodies may demonstrate the presence of postoperative infection.[5] With the advent of MRI, CT myelography is less commonly required but is still helpful in certain situations. Patients with contraindications to MRI, pronounced scoliosis, known stainless steel implants, or patients with substantial imaging artifact degrading magnetic resonance images can be better evaluated with CT myelography.

Diagnostic Injections

Selective nerve root injections have been shown to have both therapeutic and diagnostic efficacy in the management of patients with lumbar radicular pain.[20,21] However, following surgical manipulation of the spine and surrounding tissues, fibrosis and adhesions of the soft tissue can generate septations and eliminate the continuity that is required for spread of injected medications.[22] This may limit the therapeutic and diagnostic power of transforaminal injections in patients who have previously undergone surgery. Controlled studies documenting their predictive value in patients with FBSS are lacking. The authors have found them useful in situations in which MRI findings are equivocal and in situations in which multilevel pathology is present. The use of provocative discography is controversial and its role in the evaluation of previously operated discs is not universally accepted.[23] Some reports indicate that discography may predict surgical outcome for patients undergoing anterior lumbar interbody fusion (ALIF) for persistent pain after successful posterior fusion.[24,25] The role of discography in evaluating degenerated adjacent discs as pain generators is also unclear. Although this

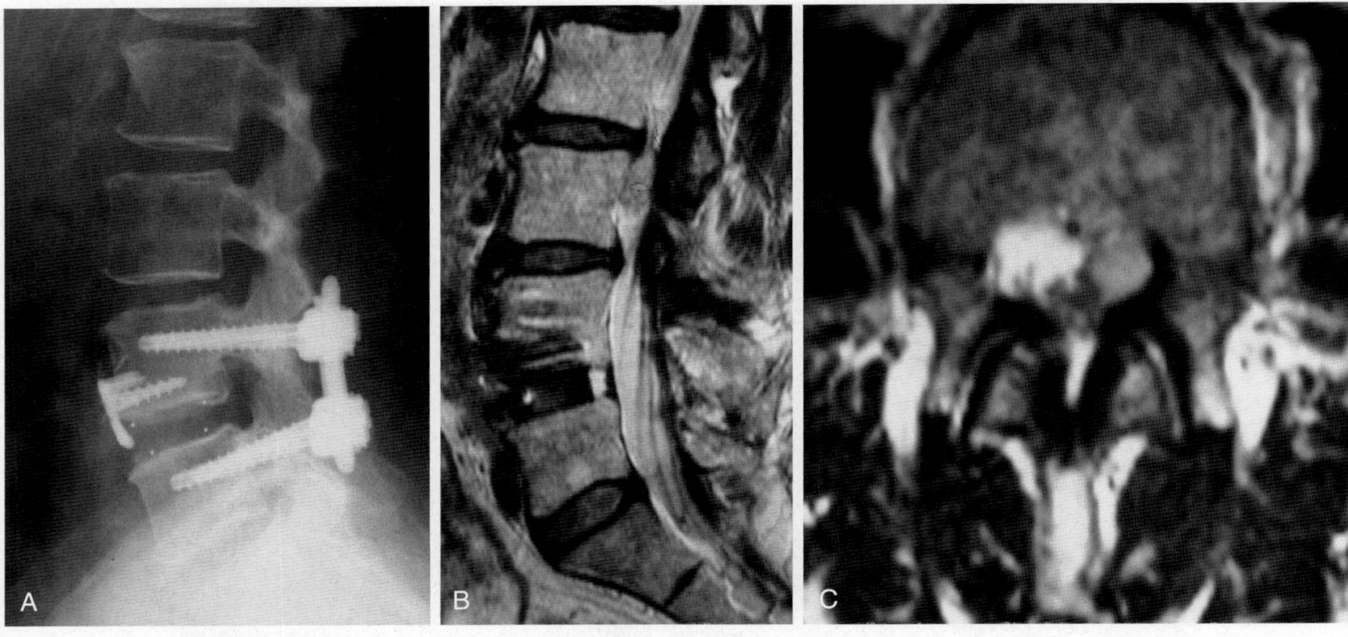

FIG. 103.3 (A) Lateral radiograph of a patient with newly recurrent symptoms of back and left thigh pain 18 months after an anterior L4–L5 fusion with percutaneous posterior fixation. (B) Sagittal magnetic resonance image (MRI) demonstrating an extruded disc herniation at L2–L3. (C) Axial T2 MRI demonstrating the extruded disc adjacent to the left L3 pedicle.

BOX 103.1 Conditions Amenable to Nonoperative Treatment

- Epidural scar/arachnoiditis
- Certain fractures (pedicle/pars/compression)
- Psychogenic factors
- Early discitis
- Extensive, multilevel degenerative disc disease
- Sacroiliac disease
- Peripheral nerve syndromes

has been suggested as a useful test in determining whether a degenerated segment below a long thoracolumbar fusion is a significant pain generator,[26] the role of provocative discography in the more common setting of adjacent-segment disease cranial to more limited lumbar procedures continues to be poorly defined.

Nonoperative Treatment

Nonoperative treatment will typically be involved to varying degrees in many patients with FBSS because measures such as physical therapy and pain medications are part of the usual postoperative regimen for most index lumbar procedures. When persistent complaints have triggered the workup outlined earlier, a diagnosis can be rendered in many cases. Several conditions may be amenable to nonoperative treatment (Box 103.1). The degree to which a patient's symptoms can be attributed to epidural scar formation is unclear. Epidural scar is an incidental finding in many patients who do not develop symptoms, and most surgeons feel that the scarring will inevitably return to some degree after revision, making the indication for repeat surgical intervention unclear. As new agents to help prevent proliferative epidural scarring are developed, the overall management of such patients may continue to evolve.

Nonoperative treatments may have a potential role in several other conditions. Fractures involving noninstrumented fusion masses, pedicles within the fused segments, or compression fractures cephalad to a fusion may be treated with bracing in the absence of frank instability. Postoperative discitis may be treated with biopsy, immobilization, and directed antibiotic therapy, but infection after instrumented fusions generally merits surgical intervention (see Chapter 100). Traditionally, sacroiliac symptoms were rarely treated with arthrodesis, and medical/physical therapy plus fluoroscopically guided injections were favored. Recently, minimally invasive techniques for sacroiliac fusion have been introduced, with studies reporting good outcomes at up to 5-year follow-up.[27,28] The success of this emerging technique is still dependent on making a proper diagnosis that the sacroiliac joint is the source of symptoms. Leg symptoms due to peripheral neuropathy should be managed medically; leg symptoms due to peripheral nerve compression may be amenable to bracing or specialized local care. Leg symptoms due to recurrent disc herniation or stenosis can be treated initially with physical therapy and nonsteroidals. Epidural injections may be offered as a treatment option; however, their effectiveness in the postoperative patient is less predictable. Transforaminal and caudal injections have some reported therapeutic success in uncontrolled studies.[29,30] Some have theorized that the presence of postoperative scar tissue interferes with dispersion of the injectate and leads to diminished effectiveness. Patients with diffuse degenerative disease and axial symptoms are typically advised to pursue intensive multidisciplinary rehabilitation combining physical training with cognitive behavioral interventions, vocational planning, and consultation with a specialist in chronic pain medical management.

Spinal cord stimulation has been used for more than 30 years to treat chronic pain, including FBSS. A thorough review is conducted in the chapter on interventional procedures for chronic pain. As one can imagine, it has been difficult to conduct well-designed trials to compare spinal cord stimulation to revision surgery. In a review of 583 studies of spinal cord stimulation published in 2004, the only class I randomized controlled trial did not include patients with FBSS.[31] A subsequent randomized controlled trial compared reoperation and spinal cord stimulation for patients with FBSS. Using at least 50% pain relief as a criterion for success, the authors reported that spinal cord stimulation was significantly more successful than reoperation.[32] A more recent randomized controlled trial by Coleman and colleagues[33] published in 2009 deemed spinal cord stimulation more successful than medical management for FBSS. They found that 48% of patients in the spinal cord stimulator group achieved the primary endpoint of 50% reduction of leg pain compared to 9% in the medical management group. The stimulator group also had less back and leg pain and greater treatment satisfaction at 6 months. The authors typically consider implantable spinal cord stimulators an option for patients with back and leg pain after spinal fusion when solid arthrodesis is apparent by imaging studies and all other potential causes of persistent pain have been excluded. A trial stimulator is typically done first and converted to a permanent device if the patient demonstrates a favorable response.

Surgical Treatment—Back Pain Predominant

Pseudarthroses and Failed Instrumentation

Although pseudarthroses are not always symptomatic, they do account for a considerable proportion of cases of FBSS. Likewise, instrumentation failure typically occurs in the setting of a pseudarthrosis; however, broken implants have been reported in cases of solid fusion. When either of these conditions is felt to be the cause of a patient's FBSS, any revision surgery should be carefully planned and executed. Patient selection is critical in determining who will benefit from a revision procedure. Factors such as smoking, diabetes, and worker's compensation result in diminished outcomes after both primary and revision surgeries.[34] There is no commonly accepted treatment algorithm for surgical management of pseudarthrosis. The surgical approach must be individualized on the basis of the location and etiology of the nonunion, the absence or presence of failing implants requiring revision (Fig. 103.4), the medical status of the patient (including any previous abdominal surgeries), and the surgeon's comfort level with specific techniques.

Nonunions after a posterior fusion that have adequate bone stock can often be managed by a revision posterior approach.[35] This should involve decortication of the pseudarthrosis and posterolateral fusion with instrumentation. At exploration of the fusion, the rods and screws are typically removed first. If the screw lengths and diameters are not known from the previous operative note, these should be determined from direct inspection and measurement. The posterolateral fusion masses are then exposed and any fibrous tissue associated with pseudarthrosis is debrided. If any question remains regarding the gross stability of the fused segments, we typically cannulate the previous pedicle screw holes with blunt probes or appropriately sized curettes and attempt to elicit segmental motion by cantilevering instruments. Use of a gouge to decorticate the previous fusion masses helps preserve any remaining bone stock. Because removing and replacing a pedicle screw results in a 34% decrease in pullout strength, some attempts must be made to improve purchase. If the anatomy permits, increasing the diameter of the screw by at least 1 mm or increasing the length by 5 to 10 mm can help improve fixation. Using a different pedicle screw system is beneficial because the screws will have a different thread pitch. In severely osteoporotic bone, polymethylmethacrylate can augment fixation strength. Achieving fusion can be challenging in such revision scenarios. As such, local bone is preferentially augmented by morsellized autograft harvested from the iliac crest. Allograft and demineralized bone matrix are used as extenders rather than graft substitutes. If both iliac crests have been previously used, other strategies for enhancing fusion should be considered. Options include electrical stimulation, bone marrow concentrates, or bone morphogenetic protein, although few studies have been performed to delineate their role in this circumstance.

When breakage of a pedicle screw is encountered, spanning that level with the addition of a crosslink is an option. If the affected level is at the end of the construct, extension of the fusion can be considered. If it is felt that reinstrumentation of the level with the broken screw is necessary, then screw removal is necessary. Commercially available screw removal sets are available, but most techniques involve removal of additional bone, thus, augmentation may be necessary. Careful patient selection is necessary to identify those patients who will benefit from a posterior or posterolateral strategy rather than a more involved procedure. West and colleagues[35] reported a 35% pseudarthrosis rate and a 47% clinical failure rate in patients with preexisting pseudarthrosis in whom posterior fusion and pedicle screw fixation were performed.

In cases of failed posterolateral fusion with inadequate bone stock (such as after a wide decompression), the interbody region may provide the best area of vascularized host surface for revision grafting. Excessive epidural scarring makes entry into the interbody space through virgin areas more desirable. ALIF permits placement of structural allografts or cages with large footprints. Using an anteroposterior approach in this situation has been associated with the best fusion rates; however, this comes at increased cost and increased risk of complications.[36] Also, not all of these patients improve clinically even after achieving a successful fusion.[34,37] Dede and colleagues[34] reported on clinical outcomes of revision surgery to fuse the pseudarthrosis site in patients who had previously undergone fusion on one or two lumbar motion segments for symptomatic degenerative disc disease or spondylolisthesis as the indication for the index surgery. Circumferential fusions made up the majority of revision surgeries and there was a fusion rate of 100%. However, only 50% of patients whose index procedure

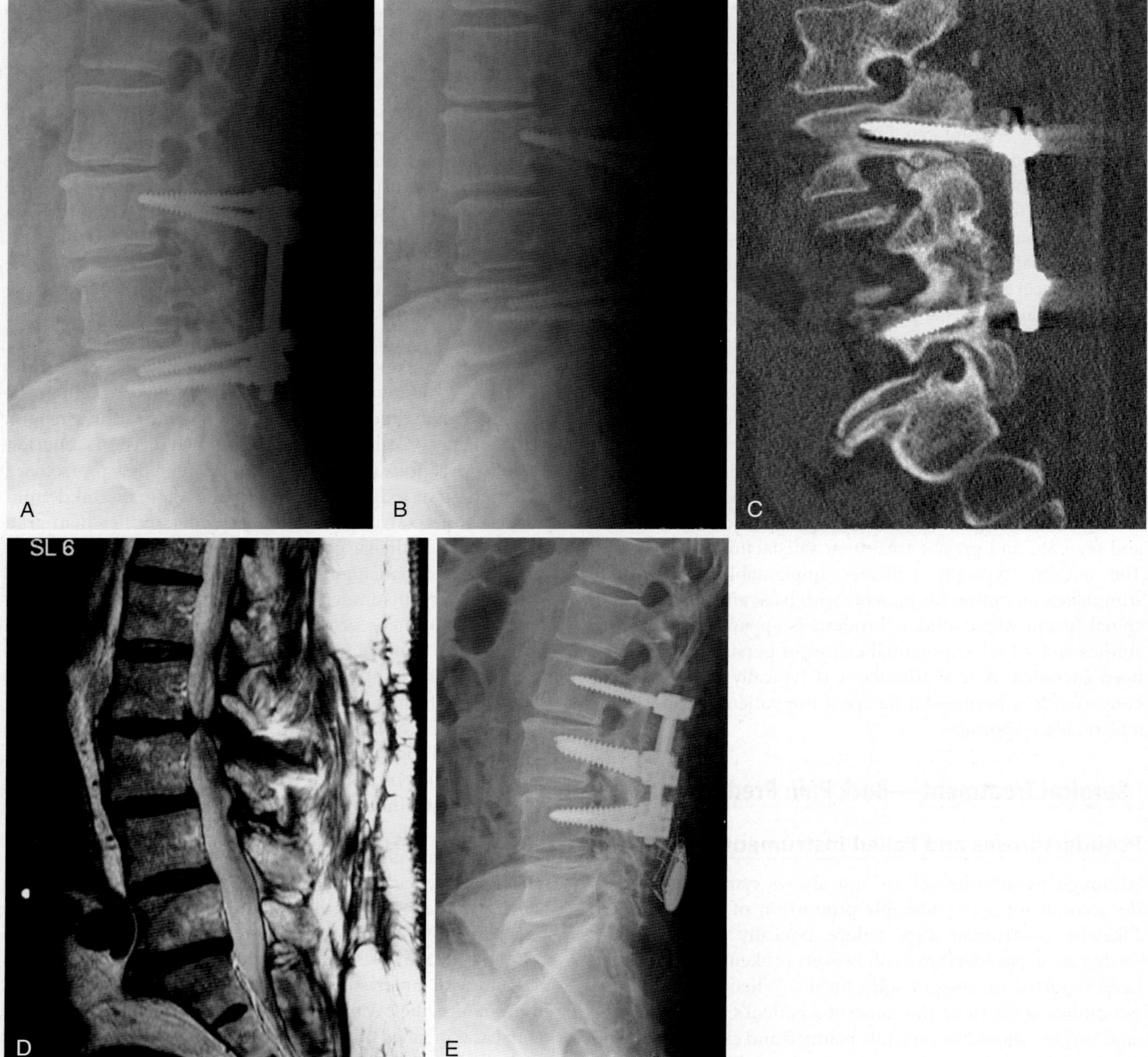

FIG. 103.4 (A) Neutral and (B) flexion lateral radiographs of a patient with a previous L3–L5 fusion and grossly loose screws at L3 evident. (C) Computed tomography showing solid fusion at L4–L5 but pseudarthrosis at L3–L4. (D) Magnetic resonance image showing adjacent-segment stenosis. (E) Postoperative radiograph showing revision L2–L4 decompression and fusion.

was for degenerative disc disease felt that their overall well-being had improved since revision surgery and 64% of those whose initial fusion was due to spondylolisthesis felt they had improved. For salvage of a single-level pseudarthrosis for which decompression is not necessary, ALIF followed by percutaneous pedicle screw fixation has been described, with radiographic fusion reported in 52 of 54 cases.[38]

In cases in which an anterior approach is problematic, a transforaminal lumbar interbody fusion (TLIF) is a good option[39,40] because the entry site to the interbody space may be less involved by postoperative scar. Studies examining this technique specifically for the management of pseudarthrosis, however, are lacking. Another increasingly popular technique, the lateral transpsoas interbody fusion, offers an additional approach to the interbody space without a formal anterior exposure (Fig. 103.5). This involves development of the plane between the posterolateral margin of the paraspinals and the peritoneal sac, followed by splitting the fibers of the psoas muscle. This technique requires high-quality intraoperative neurophysiologic monitoring of the nerve roots of the lumbar plexus[41] and intraoperative fluoroscopy. Although early reports of the technique have demonstrated

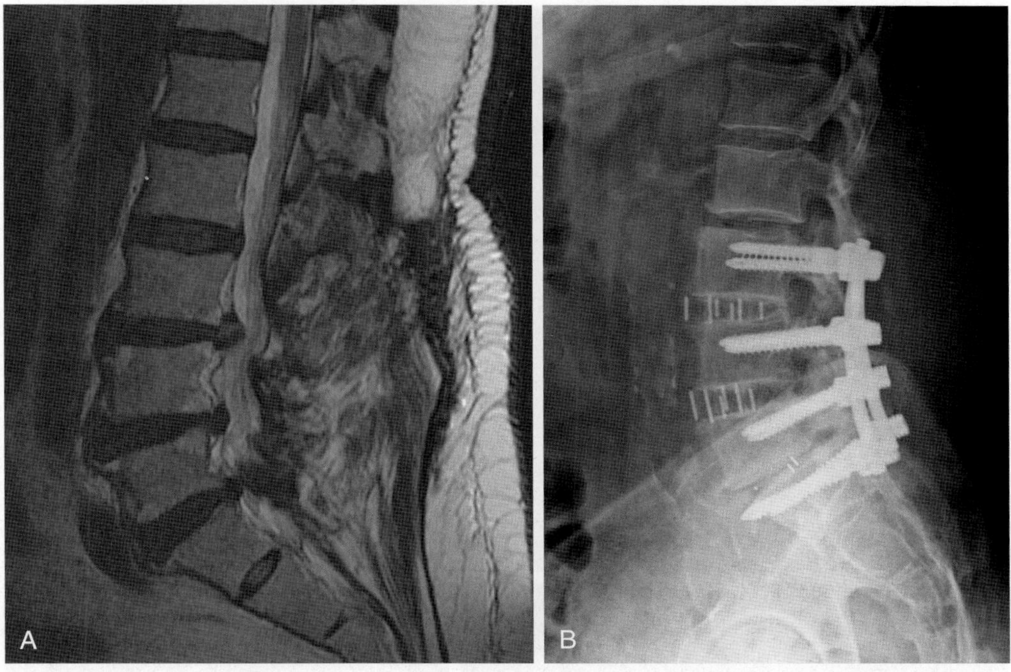

FIG. 103.5 (A) Sagittal magnetic resonance image of an obese patient previously decompressed from L3–S1 with recurrent back and leg pain. Recurrent stenosis with associated spondylosis is demonstrated. (B) Lateral radiograph after L3–L4 and L4–L5 lateral transpsoas interbody fusion, which was followed by a staged revision decompression, and L3–S1 fusion, including an L5–S1 transforaminal interbody fusion.

encouraging results with low complication rates,[42] data on this technique for revision arthrodeses are currently sparse. A study by Berjano and colleagues[43] looked at fusion rates in 53 patients who underwent lateral transpsoas interbody fusion. Patients with at least 1-year follow-up were evaluated clinically and by CT scan. They found a complete fusion rate of 87%, confirming that anterior interbody fusion by means of a transpsoas approach achieves high fusion rates with satisfactory clinical outcomes. Another study by Wang et al.[44] sought to determine if lateral interbody fusion without supplemental pedicle screws is effective in treating adjacent-segment disease in patients who had undergone previous lumbar fusion. They looked at postoperative numeric pain scale scores for leg and back pain and also obtained dynamic radiographs as well as CT scans in 21 patients who had undergone lateral interbody fusion for adjacent-segment disease. They found significant improvement of both leg and back pain scores. All patients had bridging bone on CT scan at last follow-up and there were no major complications noted. Technical aspects of these operations are covered elsewhere.

Revision of pseudarthroses after attempted posterior lumbar interbody fusion or TLIF can be challenging. We prefer to remove the cage from an anterior approach to the disc space (Fig. 103.6). Osteotomes are used to create planes adjacent to the cage and assist removal. The choice of implant to use for the ALIF is based on the defect left after removal of the cage. Whether a revision posterior fusion is required is then based on the integrity of the previously placed posterior implants and the overall segmental stability.

Anterior nonunions and failed lumbar disc arthroplasty present unique challenges. If the failed ALIF or arthroplasty device is not grossly unstable, a posterolateral fusion with instrumentation may suffice.[45,46] One study reported that removal of the prosthesis and circumferential fusion yielded slightly better results than posterior fusion at 1-year follow-up.[47] The authors, however, acknowledged that significant risks are inherent with removal of the arthroplasty device; thus, further studies are necessary to clarify management of this scenario. If the patient had a 360-degree fusion and the posterior fusion is solid, an isolated revision ALIF can be performed. The entire construct should be revised in cases of failed 360-degree fusions with both anterior and posterior pseudarthroses and unstable implants. Revision anterior lumbar procedures are technically demanding. Vascular injuries are common, for which an experienced surgeon or vascular surgeon should be considered.[48] Strategies to help navigate the hazards of the revision anterior approach have been recommended. A previous left retroperitoneal approach to L5–S1 may be best revised through a right retroperitoneal or transperitoneal approach. A previous left retroperitoneal approach to L4–L5 may be best revised through a transperitoneal or transpsoas approach.[49] Because retroperitoneal scarring may obscure the anatomy, other measures can be considered, such as preoperative ureteral stenting and intraoperative cannulation of the iliac veins with balloon catheters.

Painful Hardware

A small subgroup of patients may report recurrent pain despite intact implants, a solid fusion, and no other obvious pain generators. Implant removal in such cases remains controversial, particularly because the mechanism as to how the implants generate pain is not well understood. Some authors have

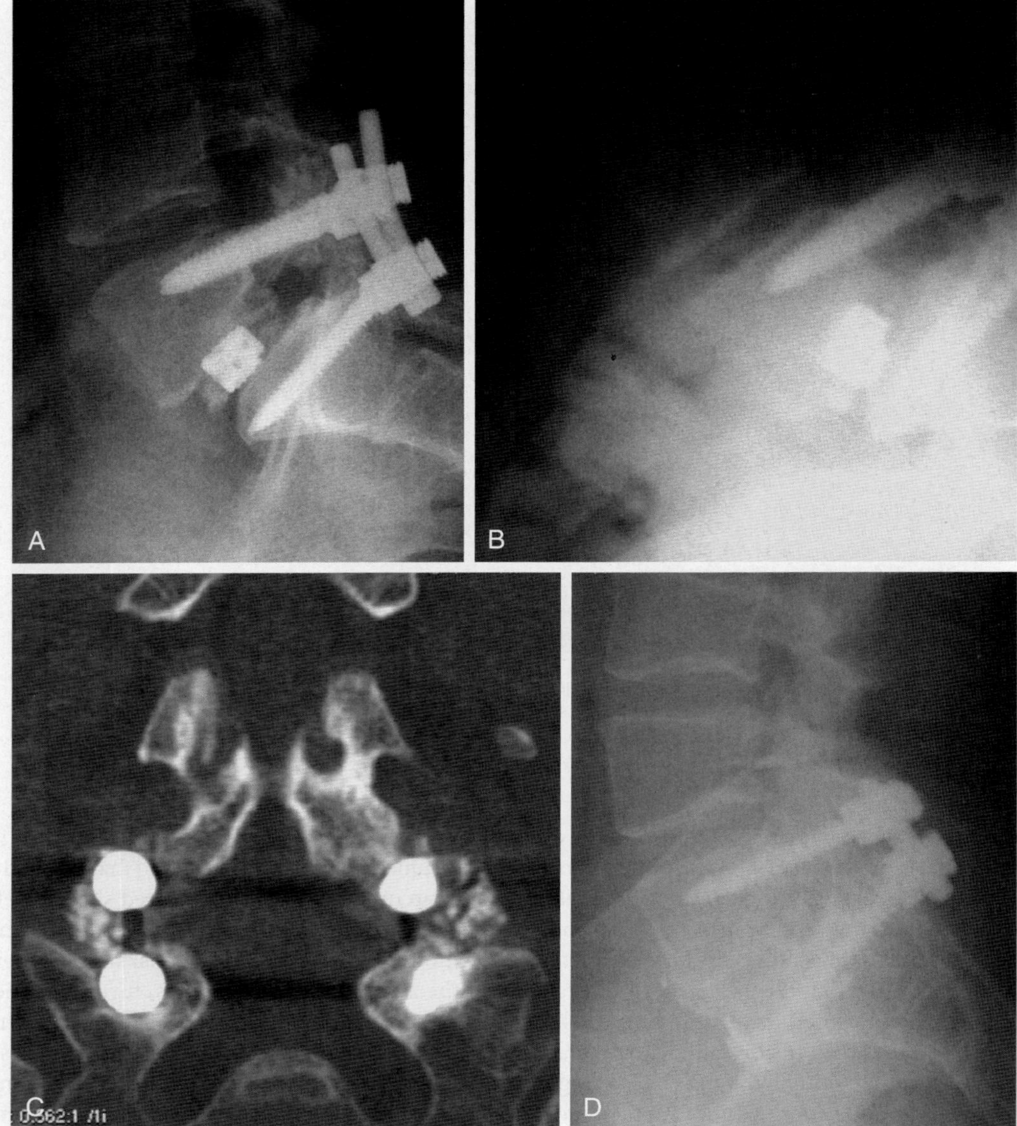

FIG. 103.6 (A) Lateral radiograph of a patient with a pseudarthrosis after L5–S1 transforaminal lumbar interbody fusion. (B) Flexion lateral view showing significant motion across the level of intended fusion. (C) Computed tomography scan showing incomplete posterolateral fusion masses. (D) Postoperative radiograph after anteroposterior revision fusion.

recommended injection of local anesthetic around the hardware as a diagnostic step.[50] For patients who report temporary relief of their pain with the injection, removal of the implants can be considered provided that the patient clearly understands that such an intervention may not have a predictable outcome. These authors reported an average 50% decrease in visual analog scale pain scores and functional improvement in 84% of 20 patients whose hardware was removed after a favorable response to diagnostic injection.[50]

Surgical Treatment—Leg Pain Predominant

The two most common situations in which revision surgery is required to treat recurrent leg pain are recurrent disc herniation and recurrent/residual stenosis. Because these surgeries have nuances quite distinct from their primary counterparts, some of their technical considerations are covered here.

Revision Discectomy

The first step in a revision discectomy is to carefully remove the pseudomembrane and scar tissue to identify the borders of the previous laminectomy.[51] The level of the dura in relation to the edge of the laminotomy should be determined from the preoperative imaging studies. If the spinous processes about the laminotomy site are preserved, these are convenient starting points to start elevating the pseudomembrane. Once the margins of the previous laminotomy have been cleared, a curved curette is used to carefully detach the scar from

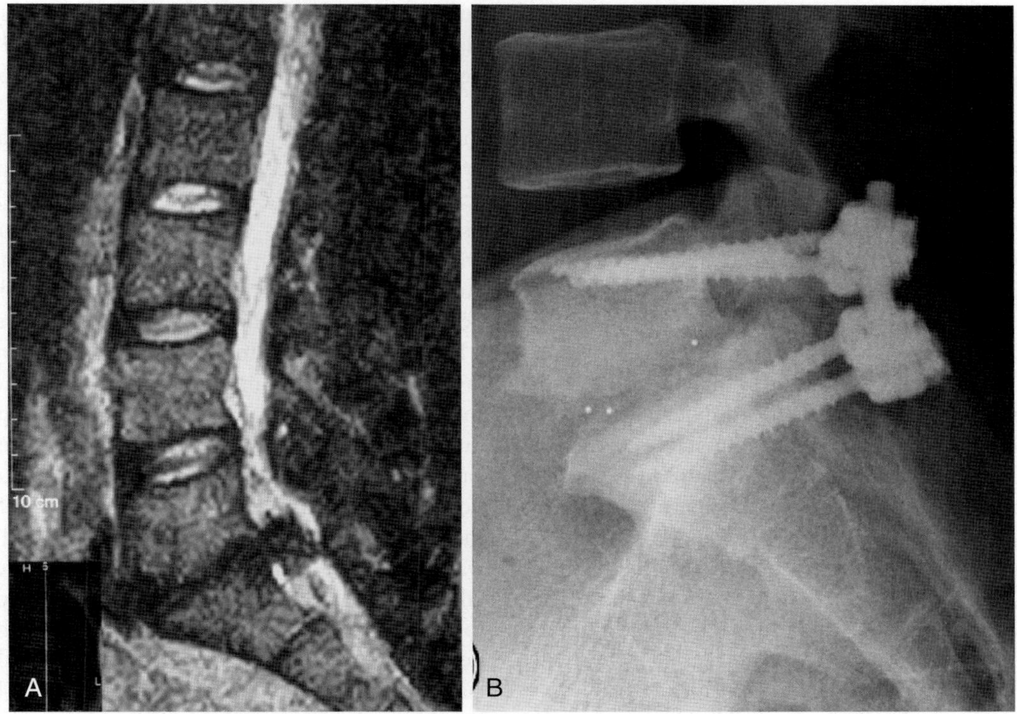

FIG. 103.7 (A) Sagittal magnetic resonance image of a patient with a third-time disc herniation at L5–S1. (B) Postoperative radiograph after revision discectomy and transforaminal lumbar interbody fusion.

the edges and then the undersurfaces of the lamina. Kerrison rongeurs are used to enlarge the laminotomy and identify normal dura. The pedicle can be palpated with a Penfield dissector or Woodson elevator and the traversing nerve root passing medial and exiting below can be identified. Mobilizing the nerve root from epidural scar should be done carefully. A reverse-angle curette firmly anchored on the surface of the disc just adjacent to the pedicle can be rotated toward the root to tease it free from adhesions and visualize the recurrent herniation. Once mobilization of the nerve root and visualization of the herniation is accomplished, the revision discectomy can be performed in a more standard manner.

Lubelski and colleagues[52] recently looked at quality-of-life outcomes after primary and revision discectomy. They found no preoperative quality-of-life differences between 116 patients who underwent primary discectomy and 80 patients who underwent revision discectomy. They found that both groups had significant improvements in quality of life, pain and disability, and psychosocial outcomes postoperatively; however, the improvement diminished after revision discectomy. Patel and colleagues[53] reported on a smaller cohort of 30 patients, comparing outcomes of revision discectomy with primary discectomy. All data were gathered from the same 30 patients who underwent both primary and revision surgery. Visual analog scales for lower limb and back pain were measured as well as Oswestry Disability Index scores. There was significant improvement in mean scores after both primary and revision discectomy, leading the authors to conclude that revision discectomy can give results as good as those seen after primary surgery.

Patients who develop a third-time herniation or those who report a significant component of back pain (in addition to leg pain) may require interbody fusion at the time of revision discectomy. A transforaminal interbody approach (Fig. 103.7) is favored by some because removing the facet and working more lateral to the traversing root requires less mobilization of the epidural scar.[54] A total of 73 patients who underwent a TLIF as revision for recurrent lumbar herniation after a previous discectomy were recently analyzed by Li and colleagues.[55] They studied clinical and radiologic outcomes as well as safety and effectiveness. They found significant improvement in clinical outcome measures postoperatively along with improved disc space height and stability at the fused level. Therefore, they recommend TLIF as safe and effective for treating recurrent lumbar herniations. Even with this strategy, dural tears are not infrequent and should be anticipated. An anteroposterior approach is favored by some in this situation, but we rarely advocate a stand-alone ALIF if leg pain is a significant part of the symptom complex. Although some have reported successful removal of extruded disc fragments at the time of ALIF, direct posterior neurolysis and decompression allow better intraoperative confirmation that the leg pain issue is effectively addressed.

Revision Laminectomy and Treatment of Adjacent-Level Stenosis

Preoperative Planning

A common and challenging cause of FBSS is recurrent spinal stenosis in the previously decompressed region or at the segment cranial to a previous decompression and fusion. Whether this adjacent-segment disease is the result of the normal progression of degenerative changes or biomechanical alteration caused by fusion remains controversial.[56] A subgroup analysis of the Spine Patient Outcomes Research Trial found that lumbar fusion and instrumentation were not associated with an increased rate of reoperation at the site of initial surgery or adjacent levels and that the only risk factor for reoperation after initial fusion for spinal stenosis was a duration of pretreatment symptoms of more than 12 months. Thus, reoperation may be related to the natural history of spinal degenerative disease.[57] As with primary lumbar spinal stenosis, nonoperative modalities should be the first-line treatment of recurrent disease. In those patients who are unresponsive to nonoperative modalities, revision surgery may be indicated. The primary goal is to ensure adequate neural decompression; the secondary goal is to stabilize and fuse unstable segments. As part of the overall surgical plan, an initial consideration is whether the previously operated area needs to be revised. Areas of residual or recurrent stenosis that could contribute to the patient's clinical complaints should be addressed at the time of reoperation. Likewise, a suspected pseudarthrosis should be formally explored. Because both of these require additional time and attention intraoperatively, advanced planning will promote efficient execution of the surgical plan.

The presence of a spondylolisthesis combined with stenosis at the adjacent segment should prompt strong consideration of extending the fusion. Retrolisthesis, rotatory listhesis, substantial hypermobility on flexion-extension films, or if iatrogenic destabilization is necessary for complete decompression are some situations that may also warrant extension of the fusion. We routinely extend the fusion at the time of decompression for junctional stenosis even in the absence of evidence of instability because motion can be considered one of the root causes of ASD.[58–60] Others, however, have reported that decompression alone in this setting can be effective.[61–63] Patients are typically advised of an increased incidence of durotomy and all other complications compared with the risk attendant with the index procedure.

Technical Aspects of Surgery

Imaging studies are reviewed to identify the borders of the previous decompression and the height and relation of the dura in relation to the bony margins. After the subcutaneous dissection is performed, the cranial edge of the previous decompression is exposed. In some cases, the landmark of the spinous process of this lamina may have been removed as part of the previous decompression; thus, great care is exercised until the bone is exposed. If there is any need to verify the anatomic level, an intraoperative lateral radiograph is taken. Exposure of the proximal "virgin" level is then performed in standard fashion. During exposure of the transverse processes of the adjacent level, the facet capsules are carefully preserved until those intended for fusion have been identified.

If it is necessary to explore a previous fusion or revise the decompression, these sites are carefully exposed. Dissection with electrocautery is directed obliquely toward the facets or instrumentation. Aggressive midline exposure may injure the vulnerable dura, but developing this initial plane too superficially can lead to a large dead space to close. If the fusion is to be explored, this can be done next, as described previously.

The cranial margin of the previous scar is generally where the stenosis is most severe. Even in cases in which an extensive revision of the previous decompression is unnecessary, the scar must be mobilized in this region. Working laterally, the pseudomembrane is carefully detached from the bony rim with a sharp, curved microcurette. After the initial release with curettes, the transition zone between scar and virgin dura can be progressively mobilized. In our practice, the cupped end of a Penfield No. 1 elevator is useful for this maneuver. The edge is placed directly along the bony rim; the wide surface helps to gradually develop the plane. Once the epidural scar and dura have been separated from the bone, the decompression can be performed. Kerrison rongeurs are usually effective; however, if the bone edge is broad and steep, efficient resection may be difficult. Using an osteotome or chisel to undercut the wall or create a thinner shelf of bone, a more controlled and effective use of the Kerrison rongeur is permitted. We have found a beveled-edge chisel to be helpful in that the bevel can help direct the initial pass laterally and can then redirect the cut downward by inverting the chisel edge. This can detach a long strip of bone as one piece, making it easier to remove.[64] Because many decompressions are performed, "pedicle-to-pedicle" palpation of the pedicle of the proximal segment from the previous decompression is helpful for orientation and to verify adequate decompression of the neural elements.

Because stenosis is often most severe centrally at the cranial margin of the previous decompression, it is sometimes helpful to defer detaching the scar in this region and first begin the laminectomy at the proximal end of the adjacent lamina. Because this differs from the conventional method of laminectomy (working caudal to cranial), great care should be exercised if this method is attempted. The lamina is thick and slopes ventrally at the cranial end; thus, it may be helpful to thin the bone with a rongeur or burr. A Penfield elevator can be used to release epidural adhesions beneath the lamina and gently displace the thecal sac ventrally while a Kerrison rongeur is used to remove the bone. As the previous laminectomy site is approached, it may be helpful to work laterally and use the chisel to undercut the medial portion of the inferior articular facet. Undercutting the superior facet of the previously decompressed segment often releases the neural elements across this stenotic zone laterally and indirectly decompresses the central region. The remaining central island of bone can then be steadied with a pituitary rongeur and released from the remaining scar with a curette. If an incidental durotomy is created, a primary repair is performed with a running nonabsorbable 6-0 Prolene suture.

Pedicle screws are then placed in the adjacent level using standard technique (Fig. 103.8). If the previous screws have been removed, they are replaced with larger-diameter screws or same-size screws with different thread pitch if this fits snugly in the pedicle. If the previous fusion involved multiple levels and appeared solid at exploration, the more distant levels may not require reinstrumentation. Achieving a solid fusion can be challenging in these cases. Whitecloud and

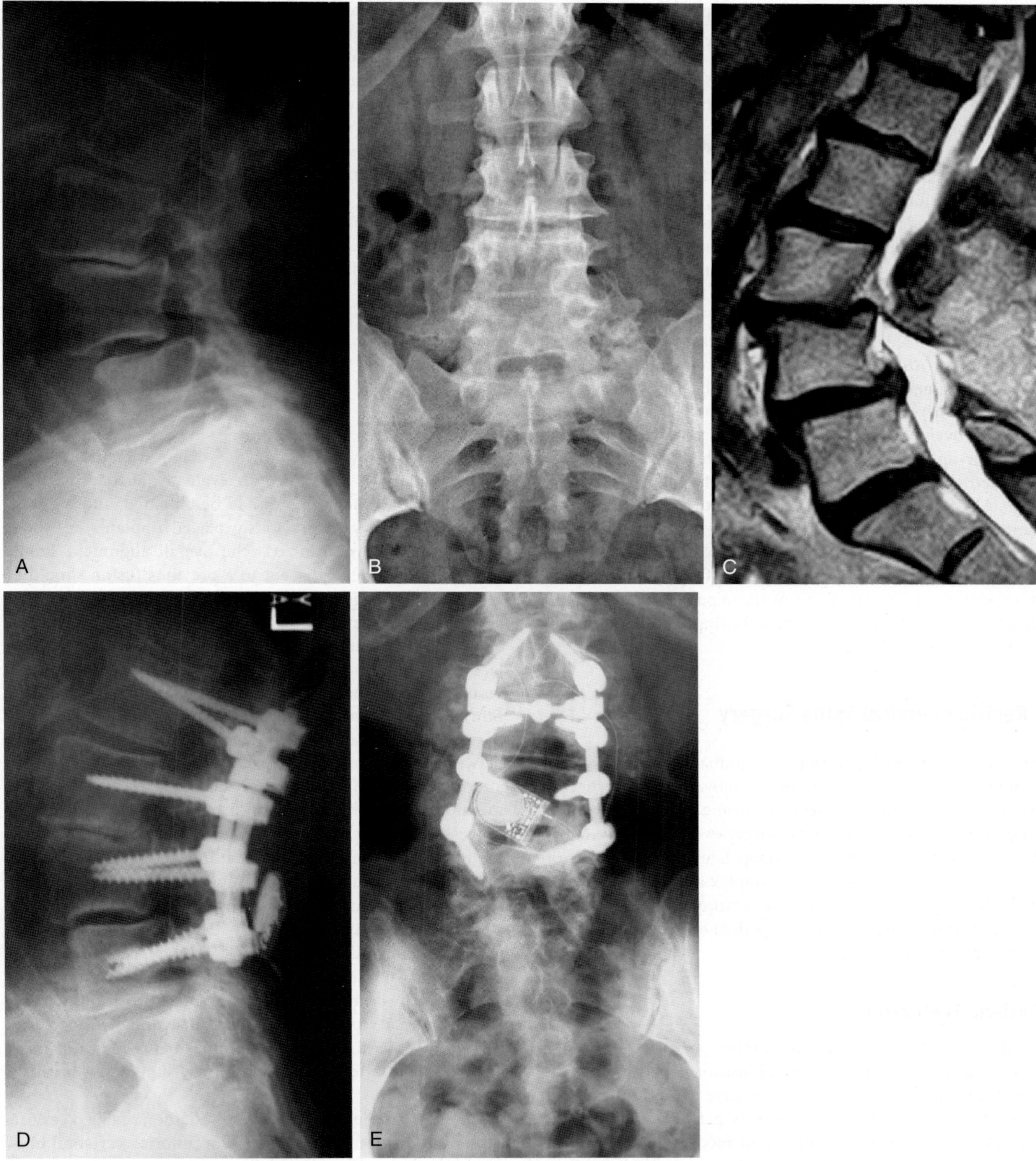

FIG. 103.8 (A) Lateral and (B) anteroposterior (AP) radiographs of a patient with a pseudarthrosis after previous L3–L5 decompression and noninstrumented fusion. (C) Magnetic resonance imaging showing junctional stenosis at L2–L3. (D–E), Lateral and AP radiographs after revision decompression and instrumented fusion with internal bone-growth stimulator.

colleagues[65] reported the results of patients undergoing decompression and fusion for ASD. Of cases in which noninstrumented fusion was attempted, 80% developed pseudarthroses compared with 17% of instrumented fusions. As such, we recommend segmental instrumentation and use of iliac crest autograft or other strategies for enhancing fusion, as discussed earlier.

The clinical outcomes for patients undergoing decompression and fusion for adjacent-segment stenosis are mixed. Phillips and colleagues reported the results of the 26 patients who underwent decompression or decompression and fusion for stenosis at the adjacent level.[63] Eleven of the 26 patients were either neutral or dissatisfied with their surgery. Other studies have reported more encouraging results. Schlegel and associates reported the results of 37 patients who were treated surgically for ASD.[62] Twenty-three patients were treated with decompression alone; 14 were treated with decompression and fusion. Twenty-six of the 37 patients reported good-to-excellent improvement of back and leg pain; however, the length of follow-up was limited to 2 years. Chen and colleagues[60] reported the results of 39 patients undergoing surgery for ASD. All of these patients were treated with a wide decompression and extension of their fusion, using instrumentation. At an average follow-up of approximately 5 years, 77% of patients had excellent or good results and their fusion rate was 95%. A sobering note was that five of these patients subsequently developed new disease at the neighboring segment, typically leading to a poor clinical result.

Revision Cervical Spine Surgery

In comparison with operations for lumbar degenerative conditions, cervical procedures have enjoyed relative success. Although "failed neck surgery syndrome" has not become a commonly used term, cervical surgeries occasionally fail to achieve their initial goal or develop late sequelae. Revision cervical spine surgery can be a complex and risky endeavor; thus, determining whether or not a patient is a candidate is essential. This section reviews the patient evaluation and treatment strategies for this condition.

Patient Evaluation

As discussed previously in the lumbar section, a thorough history must be obtained. Essential historical facts include the nature and duration of the preoperative symptoms and the type of operative procedure that was performed. Obtaining the patient's old imaging studies and medical records can be helpful in fully assessing the original problem leading to the index surgery. Recollection of the perioperative period after the initial surgery should then be pursued. Note should be made of any complications and the initial results of the surgery. Clarifying whether there was an initial period of improved pain or neurologic function versus unresolved or worsened symptoms can help establish if the appropriate procedure was performed. Questions regarding constitutional symptoms can assess for problems such as infection or tumor. Red flags, such as progressive weakness or unrelenting pain, may suggest an urgent or emergent situation. The patient should also be asked about hoarseness or swallowing difficulty that may be attributed to the initial procedure and may affect the surgical approach for the current problem. A full neurologic examination is required. Shoulder, elbow, and wrist pathology can mimic cervical spine pathology; thus, these conditions must be ruled out during patient evaluation to avoid unnecessary revision surgery.[66] This is especially true if the initial procedure did not provide any relief of the original symptoms. As with lumbar procedures, poor initial patient selection is one of the primary causes of failed surgery. Establishing the principal residual/recurrent problem as primarily axial neck pain, radiculopathy, or myelopathy is essential for formulating a treatment strategy. An algorithm for such patients is presented in Fig. 103.9.

Imaging

In addition to reviewing previous diagnostic studies, additional imaging is warranted to evaluate failed procedures. Upright plain radiographs should be obtained, and the position and integrity of previously placed implants and bone grafts should be scrutinized. The overall alignment should be noted. The levels adjacent to a previous fusion should be evaluated for degeneration. Flexion-extension lateral films should be performed to evaluate potential pseudarthrosis. Radiographic criteria suggesting a pseudarthrosis include lack of bridging bony trabeculae between graft and adjacent vertebral body and segmental motion on flexion-extension films.[67–69] Cannada and colleagues[70] conducted a study comparing measurement of Cobb angles and change in distance between the spinous processes for identifying pseudarthrosis after anterior cervical discectomy and fusion. They found that measurement of the change in distance between the spinous processes is more reproducible and accurate for diagnosing pseudarthrosis than the Cobb method. A change in distance of 2 mm or more was highly suggestive of pseudarthrosis. A more recent study published by Song and colleagues[71] in 2014 compared intraoperatively determined fusion status with dynamic radiographs and CT. They determined that interspinous motion greater than or equal to 1 mm should be used as the criterion to predict pseudarthrosis on dynamic lateral cervical spine radiographs. Instrumented posterior cervical fusions that develop pseudarthrosis may not move on flexion and extension but rather may show screw breakage or loosening.[66]

CT is an excellent modality for evaluation of failed cervical surgeries. Position of lateral mass or anterior vertebral body screws can be readily assessed. Bone status can also be assessed, especially if revision instrumentation is planned. Sagittal and coronal reconstructions are helpful for evaluating the position of interbody or strut grafts. Residual spondylotic bony compression or ossification of the posterior longitudinal ligament (PLL) can also be readily assessed. Findings on CT that are suggestive of a pseudarthrosis include absence of bridging trabeculae, bony lucency at the graft–vertebral body junction, or fracture and graft resorption. Buchowski and colleagues[72] conducted

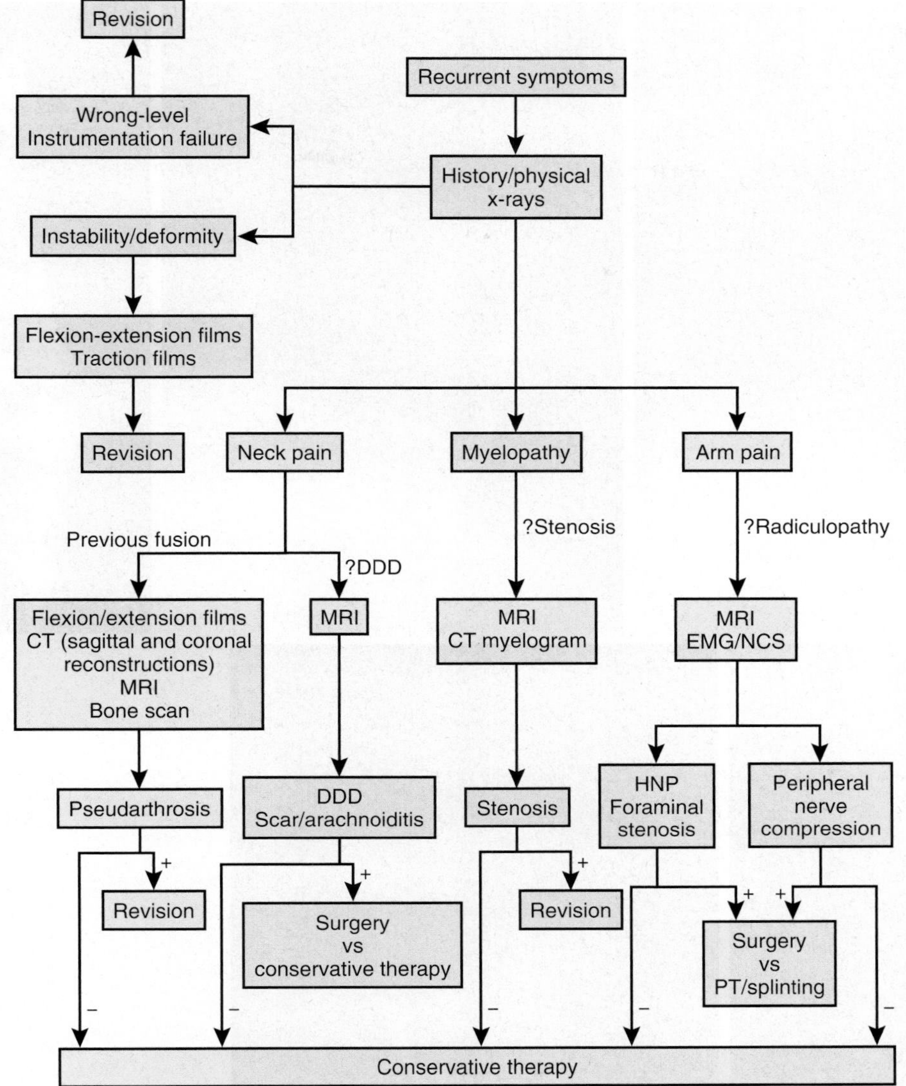

FIG. 103.9 Algorithm for approach to the patient with recurrent symptoms after cervical spine surgery. CT, computed tomography; DDD, degenerative disc disease; EMG/NCS, electromyography/nerve conduction studies; HNP, herniated nucleus pulposus; MRI, magnetic resonance imaging; PT, physical therapy.

a study assessing the reliability of plain radiographs, CT, and MRI to detect a pseudarthrosis after an anterior cervical fusion compared with intraoperative exploration. The study involved 14 patients, 8 of which were found to have pseudarthrosis at repeat surgery. Their results suggested that CT most closely agreed with intraoperative findings (Fig. 103.10).

MRI with and without gadolinium in patients who have had prior cervical surgery can differentiate recurrent disease and/or fluid collections from scar tissue, which is vascular and has high signal intensity on the T1-weighted image.[66] MRI can demonstrate missed soft disc herniations beneath the posterior longitudinal ligament. MRI can also delineate residual cord indentation at the vertebral body margins, cord atrophy, and gliosis. Levels adjacent to a previous fusion should be evaluated for soft disc herniation or internal disruption that may not be evident on plain radiographs. Findings on MRI should be closely correlated with previous images and with the patient's clinical presentation before any decision for revision surgery.

Nonspinal etiologies should be considered in cases in which the spinal imaging workup is equivocal. Reports of pain in the shoulder with overhead activities or impingement signs should prompt imaging of the shoulder.[73] Numbness in the hands, particularly at night, or positive findings on provocative tests of the carpal or cubital tunnel should raise suspicions of peripheral nerve compressive syndromes. These conditions, as well as peripheral neuropathies, may be further assessed by electromyography/nerve conduction studies.[74] Intrinsic conditions of the spinal cord can also mimic compressive myelopathies; consultation with a neurologist may be helpful in these cases.

Additional Testing

If there is concern for infection, a complete white blood cell count with differential as well as an erythrocyte sedimentation rate and C-reactive protein level should be obtained. These are

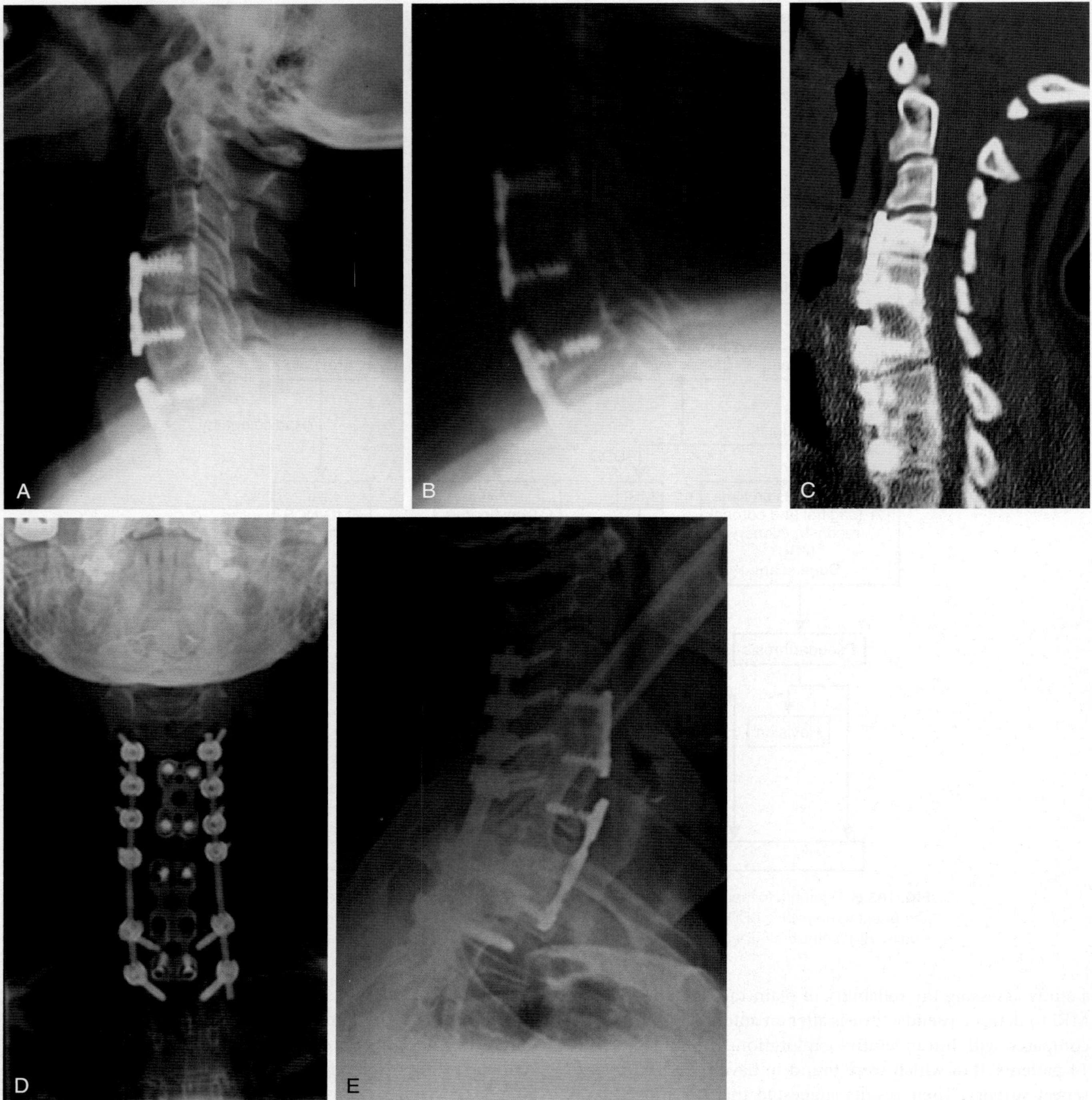

FIG. 103.10 (A) Lateral and (B) swimmer's view radiographs of a patient with pseudarthrosis at C6–C7 after multiple previous anterior cervical discectomies and fusions. Note broken screw at C6. (C) Sagittal reconstruction of computed tomography scan. (D–E), Anteroposterior and lateral radiographs after posterior C3–T2 fusion and C6–C7 foraminotomies.

discussed in greater detail in the chapter devoted to postoperative infections of the spine.

When planning revision anterior cervical spine surgery, it may be necessary to send the patient for vocal cord evaluation by an otolaryngologist to determine if there was injury to the recurrent laryngeal nerve during the initial procedure. It may also be necessary for patients to undergo preoperative evaluation of the esophagus if there is persistent dysphagia, prominent anterior instrumentation, or anterior instrumentation that is backing out.[66]

Early Postoperative Failure

Most of the conditions leading to early revision, including infection and hematoma, are discussed elsewhere as complications of anterior or posterior cervical procedures. An

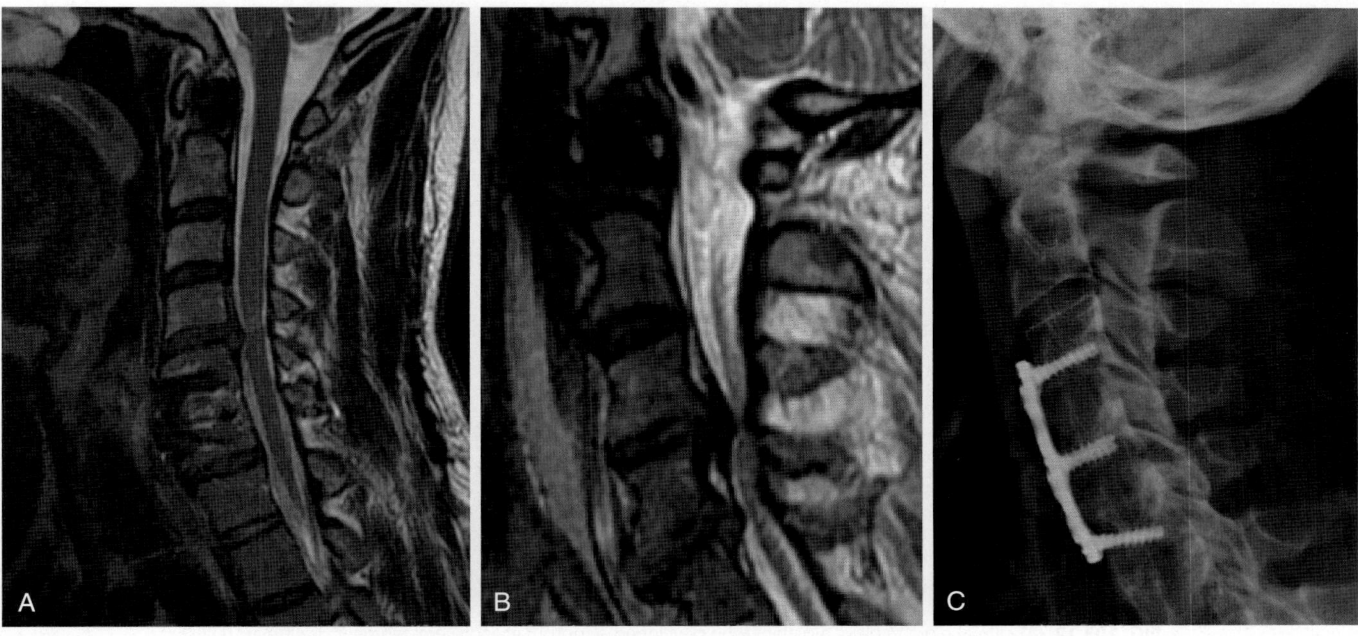

FIG. 103.11 (A) Sagittal magnetic resonance image (MRI) of a patient with recurrent pain and myelopathic complaints 4 years after previous C5–C6 fusion. Midline image shows a C4–C5 disc herniation above the fusion. (B) Paramedian sagittal MRI view also shows large C3–C4 herniated disc. (C) Postoperative lateral radiograph after removal of plate at C5–C6 and C3–C5 decompression and fusion.

occasional situation after anterior cervical discectomy and fusion can be a sequestered disc fragment that had penetrated the PLL. This may be demonstrated by MRI or CT myelography. To help avoid this occurrence, we recommend careful evaluation of the preoperative MRI and close scrutiny of the PLL in all cases. In most cases, we routinely open and resect the PLL even in the absence of an obvious defect or traversing disc material. If such a retained fragment is suspected of causing continued symptoms and is detected in the early postoperative period, the same approach can be used. Tissue planes can become obscured during the inflammatory phase of healing by as early as 3 weeks postoperatively. Once the spine is exposed, the previously placed plate and graft must be removed. In order to improve visualization in the depth of the disc space, partial or even complete corpectomy may be required. We find it helpful to distract across the segment with the use of Caspar pin distraction to tension the PLL. A straight microcurette can be used to create an opening between the vertically oriented fibers. After an opening has been created, a curved microcurette or blunt nerve hook can help develop the plane between the dura and PLL. The curette can be used to gently transect the fibers working serially toward each side, or a No. 1 Kerrison rongeur can be used if a plane was sufficiently developed. Even with loupes or an operating microscope, thin remaining layers of PLL can resemble the dura; thus, careful inspection is necessary to confirm the true extent of the decompression. After the offending fragment is removed, repeat grafting is necessary and plating (if desired) should be performed. If additional bone was removed, a new appropriately sized graft will be necessary; thus, a preoperative discussion of bone grafting options should be held.

Late Postoperative Failure

Historically, the most dramatic late postoperative failure after surgery for degenerative cervical conditions is postlaminectomy kyphosis. Other common conditions causing late failures include adjacent-segment disease, pseudarthrosis, and failed laminoplasty.

Adjacent-Segment Degeneration

Degeneration of segments adjacent to a prior fusion has been the subject of intense interest (Fig. 103.11). Concern about degeneration of neighboring motion segments has been one of the primary driving forces behind the development of nonfusion technologies. The classic study of this phenomenon was published by Hilibrand and colleagues in 1999.[75] In their series of 374 patients with extended follow-up, symptomatic adjacent-segment degenerative disease occurred at a rate of 2.9% per year over a 10-year period. In this series, more than two-thirds of all patients in whom the new disease developed failed nonoperative management. Wu and colleagues[76] published results from a retrospective study over 11 years to calculate the incidence of adjacent-segment disease after anterior cervical discectomy and fusion (ACDF) that required secondary fusion surgery. They found that repeat ACDF surgery for adjacent-segment disease occurred at a rate of 0.8% per year, much lower than previously reported. However, at the end of the 11-year cohort, a considerable portion of patients (5.6%) received a second operation. An even more recent study, published in 2014 by van Eck and colleagues,[77] included 672 patients who underwent ACDF over a 10-year period. Of these patients, 101 (15%) underwent revision surgery, 47

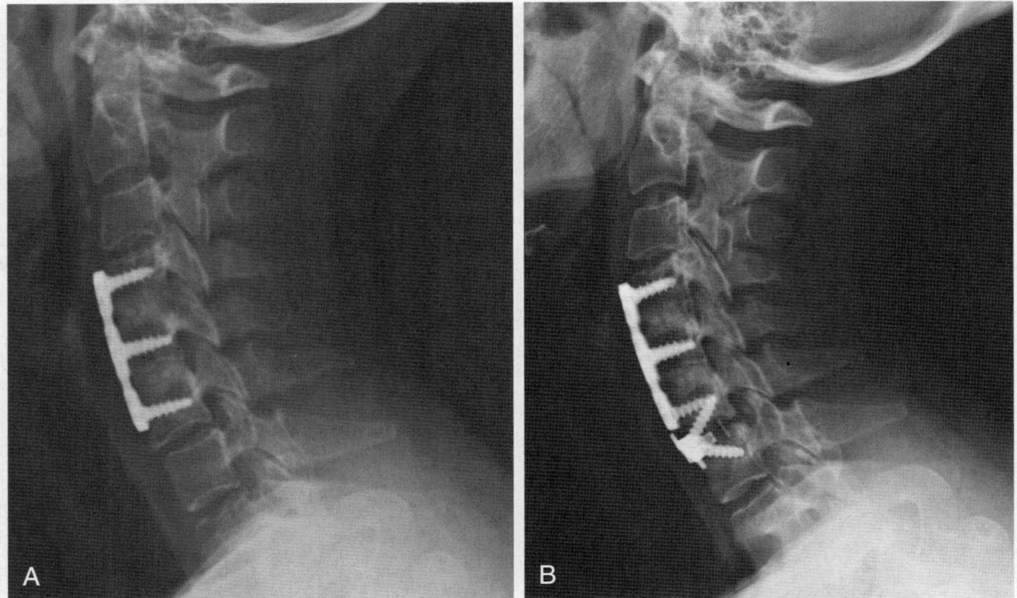

FIG. 103.12 (A) Lateral radiograph of a patient who developed symptomatic adjacent-segment disease at C6–C7 several years after a two-level anterior cervical decompression and fusion at C4–C5 and C5–C6. (B) Postoperative lateral radiograph after C6–C7 anterior cervical decompression and fusion using a stand-alone anchored cage to obviate the need for plate removal.

(47.5%) of which were due to adjacent-segment disease. Despite their modest odds for success, nonoperative measures are initially tried in the absence of a progressive neurologic condition. Nonoperative measures include physical therapy, nonsteroidal antiinflammatories, and injection therapy.[78,79]

Patients who fail nonoperative treatment should be considered for surgical intervention. Patients with radiculopathy due to a lateral disc herniation may be considered for a laminoforaminotomy provided that there is no substantial axial pain or instability. This procedure has demonstrated success as an index operation for patients with this pathology.[80] Its role for disease adjacent to an anteriorly fused segment is unknown, and theoretical concerns exist that abnormal stress transfer may lead to recurrent problems.

For patients with symptomatic adjacent-segment disease and substantial axial pain, bilateral radiculopathy, or myelopathy, anterior surgery should be considered. Although we preferentially use a left-sided approach for most primary cases, the decision to attempt reexposure through the same incision must be considered carefully. Obliteration of tissue planes leaves the trachea, esophagus, and vascular structures vulnerable. This issue may outweigh the risk of injury to the recurrent laryngeal nerve through a contralateral right-sided approach. Some have suggested otolaryngologic evaluation of vocal cord motility if a contralateral approach is entertained.[81] If a vocal cord is noted to be paretic from the previous approach, then the repeat approach should be same sided to avoid the possibility of injuring the contralateral intact recurrent laryngeal nerve. Hilibrand and colleagues[82] reported a fusion rate of 63% for nonplated interbody fusions for adjacent-segment disease using iliac crest autograft. The authors of that study suggested using a strut graft in hopes of increasing the likelihood of fusion. It is our strategy, however, to perform a plated interbody fusion for such adjacent-level procedures in hopes of improving the odds of fusion. If the previous fusion also used an anterior plate, removal may be required to allow proper position of the plate for the adjacent level. The specific design of the previously placed plate should be identified preoperatively so that appropriate instruments can be made available. Newer devices—such as threaded cages, staples, or cage-staple hybrids—have been introduced as alternatives that would obviate the need for plate removal/replating. (Fig. 103.12). Recent studies have attempted to compare their performance versus traditional methods,[83,84] but literature to document their suitability for revision situations is currently lacking. Cage dislocation and subsidence have been reported as complications associated with these devices. A study by Oh and colleagues[84] retrospectively compared the efficacy of two-level ACDF with cage alone and with cage and plate constructs with regard to clinical outcome and radiologic changes. Twenty-eight patients in the cage-alone group and 26 patients in the cage-and-plate group were assessed radiographically looking at fusion rate, kyphosis, disc height, and subsidence rate. Clinical assessment was also performed using Robinson's criteria. They found similar clinical outcomes in the two groups. Solid fusion was achieved in 96% of patients in each group, with shorter fusion durations in the cage-with-plate group. Segmental kyphosis was not statistically different between the groups. Subsidence occurred in 10 of 28 (35%) patients in the stand-alone group versus three of 26 patients (11%) in the cage-with-plate group. Overall, though cage-and-plate constructs result in shorter fusion duration and lower subsidence rate, both lead to similar clinical outcomes. Another study by Shi et al.[83] compared a cage-plate construct to a stand-alone anchored spacer in the treatment of three-level cervical spondylotic myelopathy. They too looked at clinical outcomes and radiographic parameters. They found similar results as the previously mentioned study with no differences observed in clinical outcomes and no significant differences in fusion rates. They did report significant differences between the groups with regard to cervical alignment, and they found subsidence at 9 of 54 (16%) levels fused using the stand-alone anchored spacer. They conclude that a plate-cage construct is superior to a stand-alone anchored spacer with regard to cervical alignment and subsidence; however, the stand-alone cage does have good clinical outcomes with high fusion rates.

Pseudarthrosis

The incidence of pseudarthrosis after anterior cervical interbody fusion ranges from 0% to 20% after single-level fusion.[85–89] The incidence has been reported to be as high as 50% after multilevel fusions.[90–92] The presence of a pseudarthrosis does not necessarily result in a failed operation,[93] but recent studies have suggested that successful bony fusion increases the likelihood of a favorable result.[94,95] In a retrospective study of 48 patients who developed pseudarthrosis after ACDF, 67% were symptomatic at latest follow-up or at the time of further surgery.[96] A younger age at the time of the ACDF increased the likelihood of the pseudarthrosis becoming symptomatic. In multiple-level ACDFs, the caudalmost operated level accounted for 82% of the pseudarthroses. Symptoms associated with pseudarthrosis include neck pain and a "radiculitis" or recurrent radiculopathy similar to the patient's preoperative symptoms.[94,95]

If patients are asymptomatic, treatment of pseudarthrosis may be nonoperative. Surgical management is indicated in those patients who have neck pain, neurologic symptoms, or instability.[97] Modifiable underlying factors that contribute to the risk of nonunion include metabolic abnormalities, smoking, and patient noncompliance with postoperative restrictions.[98,99] Once these issues have been addressed, the surgical approach must be selected. Both repeat anterior fusion and posterior laminoforaminotomy plus fusion have been described. The typical observation has been that the anterior pseudarthrosis eventually fuses as a posterior arthrodesis is achieved.[67] Published studies have reported success in 59% to 80% of patients treated with anterior repair of cervical nonunions.[95,99,100] As discussed in the previous section, a repeat anterior approach involves dissection through scar tissue with the associated risk of injuring the recurrent laryngeal nerve, carotid vessels, esophagus, and trachea.[101,102] Postoperative hoarseness and dysphagia are also not uncommon.[89,103,104]

Several studies have retrospectively compared posterior fusion versus anterior pseudarthrosis repair. Brodsky and colleagues[99] studied 34 patients being surgically treated for pseudarthrosis after anterior cervical fusion. Patients treated with a posterior fusion using wiring techniques had a 94% fusion rate, compared with 57% in patients who had revision anterior surgery. Lowery and colleagues[100] also reported a 94% fusion rate with posterior fusion in patients with anterior cervical nonunion compared with 57% fusion rate for revision anterior surgery. Carreon and colleagues[105] published a retrospective study of 120 patients undergoing repeat surgery for anterior cervical pseudarthrosis. Twenty-seven had repeat anterior procedures and 93 had posterior procedures. Patients in the anterior group had less blood loss and shorter average hospital stays. The anterior group had a 4% complication rate, while the posterior group had an 8% complication rate. All of the complications in both groups were wound or bone graft harvest site infections. Of the anterior revision group, 44% required an additional surgery for persistent nonunion, however, compared with only 2% in the posterior fusion group. The authors concluded that despite the higher blood loss, longer hospital stay, and higher complication rate, posterior fusion was preferable to anterior revision due to the higher fusion rate and much lower incidence of repeat revision surgery. More recently, McAnany and colleagues[106] performed a meta-analysis to assess the fusion rate and clinical outcomes of pseudarthroses treated with a posterior or a revision anterior approach. Sixteen studies reported fusion outcomes. The pooled fusion success was 86.4% in the anterior group and 97.1% in the posterior group; clinical outcomes did not differ between the groups. The authors concluded that symptomatic cervical pseudarthrosis can be effectively managed with either an anterior or a posterior approach.

Given these considerations, we typically use the posterior approach as our preferred method of treatment for anterior cervical pseudarthroses. This approach should have three components: decompression of the affected nerve root, initial stabilization with internal fixation, and achieving solid arthrodesis. Decompression can be achieved through a standard laminoforaminotomy. We typically focus on dorsally decompressing the nerve root rather than manipulating it and trying to remove ventral osteophytes or fibrous material. Lateral mass screws can be augmented by spinous process wiring if there is concern of the purchase after laminoforaminotomy. Posterior iliac crest autograft is usually preferred in order to maximize chances of a solid arthrodesis. In our practice, the main indication that warrants a repeat anterior approach is an anterior nonunion associated with unstable or prominently migrating anterior implants. There have been several reports of implants eroding through the esophagus in such cases left untreated.[107–110] At the time of such revisions, careful evaluation of the esophagus is necessary to detect perforation. Placement of dilute indigo carmine dye directly into the esophagus through a nasogastric or orogastric tube can aid in the detection of occult injuries. If dye is noted in the wound, then a defect is present and intraoperative consultation by a general or head and neck surgeon may be necessary.

Failed Multilevel Decompression for Cervical Myelopathy

The treatment goal in surgical management of patients with cervical myelopathy is to prevent further neurologic deterioration or promote recovery.[111] Barring the previously mentioned conditions, failure to improve after decompression may be due to advanced and irreversible neurologic changes, missed confounding diagnoses, or inadequate surgical decompression.[112] In these cases, further imaging studies should be performed to evaluate for any continued thecal sac compression. The study of choice is a gadolinium-enhanced MRI. In symptomatic patients, MRI may reveal continued anterior thecal sac compression in up to 40% of patients.[113] Myelography and postmyelography CT are also helpful when MRI findings are equivocal or for those patients who cannot undergo MRI.[114] Unfortunately, in the absence of focal dramatic findings, there are no good guidelines to select patients for repeat decompression.[113,115]

Two relatively common scenarios that can lead to disappointing results after multilevel surgery for myelopathy are progressive ossification of the PLL[116,117] and untreated or progressive kyphosis.[118–120] Both conditions are covered elsewhere in this text. In their absence, for selected cases for which further surgery is contemplated, we individualize the approach on the basis of the patient's previous operation. If the previous procedure was an anterior decompression, the posterior approach is safer and enables adequate visualization of each nerve root. A laminoplasty may be appropriate for residual myelopathy in the absence of neck pain or instability adjacent to the previously fused levels. Laminectomy and fusion may be more appropriate in patients who had previous multilevel corpectomies, instability above or below previous fusions, or those with significant axial pain. In patients who had previous posterior decompressions, an anterior approach may be indicated. Posterior cervical revision surgery is potentially dangerous because the anatomy is obscured by scar tissue and the potential for dural injury is high.[121] In some of these cases, limited decompression and anterior fusion of segments with large disc osteophyte complexes may be adequate to address residual symptoms.

PEARLS

1. Careful patient selection for primary surgery is the best way to limit the expansion of one's failed surgery population.
2. Nonoperative treatment should be attempted, where possible, before entertaining revision surgery because the overall outcome is less predictable.
3. Identify previously placed implants and have specific equipment available for their removal at the time of revision surgery.
4. Thoroughly discuss common complications and limitations of the revision procedure with patients preoperatively rather than after their occurrence.

PITFALLS

1. Failure to correlate imaging findings with the patient's clinical picture may lead to disappointing outcomes.
2. Modifiable risks for pseudarthrosis should be addressed before undertaking their repair.
3. Revision anterior lumbar surgery has a substantial risk of complications and requires expertise and careful planning. Transforaminal and lateral transpsoas approaches can be considered for adjacent-segment problems after previous anterior procedures.
4. Posterior approaches for anterior cervical pseudarthrosis may have higher complication rates but lower rates of future surgeries than anterior repairs.

KEY POINTS

1. Overall, revision surgery has a less favorable outcome than primary surgery regardless of the diagnosis.
2. Patient selection is the key to reducing the likelihood of revision surgery and for reducing the likelihood of repeat revision surgery.
3. Clarifying the patient's complaints as primarily axial or leg pain can be helpful for establishing a treatment approach for failed lumbar operations.
4. Both anterior and posterior cervical revision strategies have associated complications and limitations that should be thoroughly discussed with patients preoperatively.

KEY REFERENCES

1. Finnegan WJ, Tenlen JM, Marvel JP, et al. Results of surgical intervention in the symptomatic multiply-operated back patient. *J Bone Joint Surg Am*. 1979;61:1077-1082.
   This classic article details the declining chances for success with additional spinal procedures.
2. Albert TJ, Pinto M, Denis F. Management of symptomatic lumbar pseudarthrosis with anteroposterior fusion. *Spine*. 2000;25:123-130.
   This study demonstrates the favorable results of performing an interbody fusion for posterolateral lumbar nonunions.
3. Li Z, Tang J, Hou S, et al. Four-year follow-up results of transforaminal lumbar interbody fusion as revision surgery for recurrent lumbar disc herniation after conventional discectomy. *J Clin Neurosci*. 2015;22(2):331-337.
   This retrospective study demonstrates the safety and efficacy of TLIF for appropriately selected patients with recurrent lumbar disc herniation. They reported significant improvement of both back and leg pain VAS, ODI, and JOA scores at 4-year follow-up.
4. Hilibrand AS, Carlson GD, Palumbo MA, et al. Radiculopathy and myelopathy at segments adjacent to the site of a previous anterior cervical arthrodesis. *J Bone Joint Surg Am*. 1999;4:519-528.
   This study discusses the incidence and risk factors associated with adjacent-segment disease after anterior cervical fusion. It has been widely cited among proponents of motion-preserving technology.
5. McAnany S, Baird EO, Overley SC, et al. A meta-analysis of the clinical and fusion results following treatment of symptomatic cervical pseudarthrosis. *Global Spine J*. 2015;5(2):148-155.
   This metaanalysis compared outcomes of cervical pseudarthroses treated with either a posterior or revision anterior procedure. While clinical outcomes were similar, posterior fusion had a substantially higher pooled fusion rate.

REFERENCES

1. Weinstein JN, Lurie JD, Olson PR, et al. United States trends and regional variations in lumbar spinal surgery: 1992-2003. *Spine*. 2006;31:2707-2714.
2. Finnegan WJ, Tenlen JM, Marvel JP, et al. Results of surgical intervention in the symptomatic multiply-operated back patient. *J Bone Joint Surg Am*. 1979;61:1077-1082.
3. Waddell G, Kummel EG, Lotto WN, et al. Failed lumbar disk surgery and repeat surgery following industrial injuries. *J Bone Joint Surg Am*. 1979;61:201-207.
4. Taylor R, Taylor R. The economic impact of failed back surgery syndrome. *Br J Pain*. 2012;6(4):174-181.
5. Elgafy H, Vaccaro A. Rationale of revision lumbar spine surgery. *Global Spine J*. 2012;2:7-14.
6. Guyer RD, Patterson M, Ohnmeiss DD. Failed back surgery syndrome: diagnostic evaluation. *J Am Acad Orthop Surg*. 2006;14:534-543.
7. Crock HV. Observations on the management of failed spinal operations. *J Bone Joint Surg Br*. 1976;58:193-199.

8. Maistrelli GL, Vaughan PA, Evans DC, et al. Lumbar disc herniations in the elderly. *Spine*. 1987;12:63-66.
9. Wong DA. Present initiatives and future directions: how to best serve our patients and members. North American Spine Society Presidential Address, San Diego, CA. *Spine J*. 2004;4:8-14.
10. Block AR, Gatchel RJ, Deardorff WW, Guyer RD. *The Psychology of Spine Surgery*. Washington, DC: American Psychological Association; 2003.
11. Spengler DM, Freeman C, Westbrook R, Miller JW. Low-back pain following multiple lumbar spine procedures: failure of initial selection? *Spine*. 1980;5:356-360.
12. Wiltse LL, Rocchio PD. Preoperative psychological tests as predictors of success of chemonucleolysis in the treatment of the low-back syndrome. *J Bone Joint Surg Am*. 1975;57:478-483.
13. Klekamp J, McCarty E, Spengler DM. Results of elective lumbar discectomy for patients involved in the workers' compensation system. *J Spinal Disord*. 1998;11:277-282.
14. Taylor VM, Deyo RA, Ciol M, et al. Patient-oriented outcomes from low back surgery: a community-based study. *Spine*. 2000;25:2445-2452.
15. Block AR, Sarwer DB, eds. *Presurgical Psychological Screening: Understanding Patients, Improving Outcomes*. Washington, DC: APA Books; 2013.
16. Grimm B, Laxer E, et al. Wrong level spine surgery. *JBJS Rev*. 2014;2(3):e2.
17. Waddell G, McCulloch JA, Kummel E, Venner RM. Nonorganic physical signs in low-back pain. *Spine*. 1980;5:117-125.
18. Lang P, Genant HK, Chafetz N. Three dimensional computed tomography and multiplanar reformations in the assessment of pseudarthrosis in posterior lumbar fusion patients. *Spine*. 1988;13:69-75.
19. Ross JS, Masaryk TJ, Schrader M. MR imaging of the postoperative lumbar spine: assessment with gadopentate dimeglumine. *AJR Am J Roentgenol*. 1990;155:867-872.
20. Riew KD, Park JB, Cho YS, et al. Nerve root blocks in the treatment of lumbar radicular pain. A minimum five-year follow-up. *J Bone Joint Surg Am*. 2006;88:1722-1725.
21. Sasso RC, Macadaeg K, Nordmann D, et al. Selective nerve root injections can predict surgical outcome for lumbar and cervical radiculopathy. *J Spinal Disord Tech*. 2005;18:471-478.
22. Rahimzadeh P, Sharma V, Imani F, et al. Adjuvant hyaluronidase to epidural steroid improves the quality of analgesia in failed back surgery syndrome: a prospective randomized clinical trial. *Pain Physician*. 2014;17:E75-E82.
23. Carragee EJ, Chen Y, Tanner CM, et al. Provocative discography in patients after limited lumbar discectomy: a controlled, randomized study of pain response in symptomatic and asymptomatic subjects. *Spine*. 2000;25:3065-3071.
24. Weatherley CR, Prickett CF, O'Brien JP. Discogenic pain persisting despite solid posterior fusion. *J Bone Joint Surg Br*. 1986;68:142-143.
25. Barrick WT, Schofferman JA, Reynolds JB, et al. Anterior lumbar fusion improves discogenic pain at levels of prior posterolateral fusion. *Spine*. 2000;25:853-857.
26. Kostuik JP. Decision making in adult scoliosis. *Spine*. 1979;4:521-525.
27. Rudolf L, Capobianco R. Five-year clinical and radiographic outcomes after minimally invasive sacroiliac joint fusion using triangular implants. *Open Orthop J*. 2014;8:375-383.
28. Ledonio CG, Polly DW Jr, Swiontkowski MF, et al. Comparative effectiveness of open versus minimally invasive sacroiliac joint fusion. *Med Devices (Auckl)*. 2014;7:187-193.
29. Mavrocordatos P, Cahana A. Minimally invasive procedures for the treatment of failed back surgery syndrome. *Adv Tech Stand Neurosurg*. 2006;31:221-252.
30. Barre L, Lutz G, Southern D, et al. Fluoroscopically guided caudal epidural injections for lumbar spinal stenosis: a retrospective evaluation of long term efficacy. *Pain Physician*. 2004;7(2):187-193.
31. Turner J, Loeser J, Deyo R, et al. Spinal cord stimulation for patients with failed back surgery syndrome or complex regional pain syndrome: a systematic review of effectiveness and complications. *Pain*. 2004;108:137-147.
32. North RB, Kidd DH, Farrikhi F, et al. Spinal cord stimulation versus repeated lumbosacral spine surgery for chronic pain: a randomized, controlled trial. *Neurosurgery*. 2006;56:98-107.
33. Coleman S, Mackey S. Spinal cord stimulation compared with medical management for failed back surgery syndrome. *Curr Pain Headache Rep*. 2009;13(1):1-2.
34. Dede O. Revision surgery for lumbar pseudarthrosis. *Spine J*. 2015;15(5):977-982.
35. West JL 3rd, Bradford DS, Ogilvie JW. Results of spinal arthrodesis with pedicle screw-plate fixation. *J Bone Joint Surg Am*. 1991;73:1179-1184.
36. Albert TJ, Pinto M, Denis F. Management of symptomatic lumbar pseudarthrosis with anteroposterior fusion. *Spine*. 2000;25:123-130.
37. Lee Y, Sclafani J, Garfin S. Lumbar pseudarthrosis: diagnosis and treatment. *Semin Spine Surg*. 2011;23:275-281.
38. Lee SH, Kang BU, Jeon SH, et al. Revision surgery of the lumbar spine: anterior lumbar interbody fusion followed by percutaneous pedicle screw fixation. *J Neurosurg Spine*. 2006;5:228-233.
39. Potte BK, Freedman BA, Verwiebe EG, et al. Transforaminal lumbar interbody fusion: clinical and radiographic results and complications in 100 consecutive patients. *J Spinal Disord Tech*. 2005;18:337-346.
40. Lowe TG, Tahernia AD, O'Brien MG, et al. Unilateral transforaminal posterior lumbar interbody fusion (TLIF): indications, technique, and 2 year results. *J Spinal Disord Tech*. 2002;15:31-38.
41. Bengalis DM Jr, Vanni S, Levi AD. An anatomical study of the lumbosacral plexus as related to the minimally invasive transpsoas approach to the lumbar spine. *J Neurosurg Spine*. 2009;10:139-144.
42. Ozgur BM, Aryan HE, Pimenta L, et al. Extreme lateral interbody fusion (XLIF); a novel surgical technique for anterior lumbar interbody fusion. *Spine J*. 2006;6:435-443.
43. Berjano P, Langella F, Damitano M, et al. Fusion rate following extreme lateral lumbar interbody fusion. *Eur Spine J*. 2015;24(suppl 3):369-371.
44. Wang M, Vasudevan R, Mindea S. Minimally invasive lateral interbody fusion for the treatment of rostral adjacent-segment lumbar degenerative stenosis without supplemental pedicle screw fixation. *J Neurosurg Spine*. 2014;21:861-866.
45. Patel AA, Brodke DS, Pimenta L, et al. Revision strategies in lumbar total disc arthroplasty. *Spine*. 2008;33:1276-1283.
46. Bertagnoli R, Frank JF, Schneider SV. Complications and strategies for revision surgery in total disc replacement. *Orthop Clin North Am*. 2005;36:389-395.

47. Punt IM, Visser VM, Lodewijk WVJ, et al. Complications and reoperations of the SB CHARITE lumbar disc prosthesis: experience in 75 patients. *Eur Spine J*. 2008;17:36-43.
48. Nguyen HV, Akbarnia BA, van Dam BE, et al. Anterior exposure of the spine for removal of lumbar interbody devices and implants. *Spine*. 2006;31:2449-2453.
49. Leary SP, Regan JJ, Lanman TH. Revision and explantation strategies involving the CHARITE lumbar artificial disc replacement. *Spine*. 2007;32(9):1001-1011.
50. Alanay A, Vyas R, Shamie A, et al. Safety and efficacy of implant removal for patients with recurrent back pain after a failed degenerative lumbar spine surgery. *J Spinal Disord Tech*. 2007;20:271-277.
51. LaRocca H, Macnab I. The laminectomy membrane. *J Bone Joint Surg Br*. 1974;56:545-550.
52. Lubelski D, Senol N, Silverstein M, et al. Quality of life outcomes after revision lumbar discectomy. *J Neurosurg Spine*. 2015;22(2):173-178.
53. Patel M, Braybrooke J, Newey M, et al. A comparative study of the outcomes of primary and revision lumbar discectomy surgery. *Bone Joint J*. 2013;95-B:90-94.
54. Chen Z, Zhao J, AiGang L. Surgical treatment of recurrent lumbar disc herniation by transforaminal lumbar interbody fusion. *Int Orthop*. 2009;33:197-201.
55. Li Z, Tang J, Hou S, et al. Four-year follow-up results of transforaminal lumbar interbody fusion as revision surgery for recurrent lumbar disc herniation after conventional discectomy. *J Clin Neurosci*. 2015;22(2):331-337.
56. Miwa T, Sakawa H, Yamashita T, et al. Surgical outcomes of additional posterior lumbar interbody fusion for adjacent segment disease after single-level posterior lumbar interbody fusion. *Eur Spine J*. 2013;22:2864-2868.
57. Radcliff K, Curry P, Hilibrand A, et al. Risk for adjacent segment and same segment reoperation after surgery for lumbar stenosis: a subgroup analysis of the Spine Patient Outcomes Research Trial (SPORT). *Spine*. 2013;38(7): 531-539.
58. Dazley J, Dearing R, Bono C. Recurrent lumbar spinal stenosis: etiology and surgical management. *Semin Spine Surg*. 2013;25(4):283-294.
59. Hansraj K, O'Leary P, Cammisa F, et al. Decompression, fusion, and instrumentation surgery for complex lumbar spinal stenosis. *Clin Orthop Relat Res*. 2001;384:18-25.
60. Chen WJ, Lai PL, Chi-Chien N, et al. Surgical treatment of adjacent instability after lumbar spine fusion. *Spine*. 2001;26:E519-E524.
61. Ghiselli G, Wang JC, Bhatia NN, et al. Adjacent segment degeneration in the lumbar spine. *J Bone Joint Surg Am*. 2004;86:1497-1503.
62. Schlegel JD, Smith JA, Schleusener RL. Lumbar motion segment pathology adjacent to thoracolumbar, lumbar, and lumbosacral fusions. *Spine*. 1996;21:970-981.
63. Phillips FM, Carlson GD, Bohlman HH, et al. Results of surgery for spinal stenosis adjacent to previous lumbar fusion. *J Spinal Disord*. 2000;13:432-437.
64. Vives MJ, Bono CM, Garfin SR. Management of adjacent segment degeneration and spinal stenosis (scar). *Semin Spine Surg*. 2008;20:284-292.
65. Whitecloud TS, Davis JM, Olive PM. Operative treatment of the degenerated segment adjacent to a lumbar fusion. *Spine*. 1994;19:531-536.
66. Rihn J, Harrod C, Albert T. Revision cervical spine surgery. *Orthop Clin North Am*. 2012;43(1):123-136.
67. Farey ID, McAfee PC, Davis RF, et al. Pseudarthrosis of the cervical spine after anterior arthrodesis. *J Bone Joint Surg Am*. 1990;72:1171-1177.
68. Hilibrand AS, Dina TS. The use of diagnostic imaging to assess spinal arthrodesis. *Orthop Clin North Am*. 1998;29:591-601.
69. Martin GJ, Haid RW, MacMillan M, et al. Anterior cervical discectomy with freeze-dried fibula allograft: overview of 317 cases and literature review. *Spine*. 1999;24:852-859.
70. Cannada LK, Scherping SC, Yoo JU, et al. Pseudarthrosis of the cervical spine: a comparison of radiographic diagnostic measures. *Spine*. 2003;28:46-51.
71. Song K, Piyaskulkaew C, Chuntaropas T, et al. Dynamic radiographic criteria for detecting pseudarthrosis following anterior cervical arthrodesis. *J Bone Joint Surg Am*. 2014;96(7):557-563.
72. Buchowski JM, Liu G, Bunmaprasert T, et al. Anterior cervical fusion assessment: surgical exploration versus radiographic evaluation. *Spine*. 2008;33:1185-1191.
73. Manifold SG, McCann PD. Cervical radiculitis and shoulder disorders. *Clin Orthop Relat Res*. 1999;368:105-113.
74. Epstein NE, Epstein JA, Carras R. Coexisting cervical spondylotic myelopathy and bilateral carpal tunnel syndromes. *J Spinal Disord*. 1989;2:36-42.
75. Hilibrand AS, Carlson GD, Palumbo MA, et al. Radiculopathy and myelopathy at segments adjacent to the site of a previous anterior cervical arthrodesis. *J Bone Joint Surg Am*. 1999;4:519-528.
76. Wu C, Liu L. The incidence of adjacent segment disease requiring surgery after anterior cervical discectomy and fusion. *Neurosurgery*. 2012;70(3):594-601.
77. van Eck CF, Regan C, Donaldson WF, et al. The revision rate and occurrence of adjacent segment disease after anterior cervical discectomy and fusion: a study of 672 consecutive patients. *Spine*. 2014;39(26):2143-2147.
78. Weinstein SM, Herring SA, Derby R. Contemporary concepts in spine care. Epidural steroid injections. *Spine*. 1995;20:1842-1846.
79. Ellenger MR, Honet JC, Treanor WJ. Cervical radiculopathy. *Arch Phys Med Rehabil*. 1994;75:342-352.
80. Herkowitz HN, Kurz LT, Overholt DP. Surgical management of cervical soft disc herniation. A comparison between the anterior and posterior approach. *Spine*. 1990;15:1026-1030.
81. Winslow CP, Meyers AD. Otolaryngologic complications of the anterior approach to the cervical spine. *Am J Otolaryngol*. 1999;20:16-27.
82. Hilibrand AS, Yoo JU, Carlson GD, et al. The success of anterior cervical arthrodesis adjacent to a previous fusion. *Spine*. 1997;22:1574-1579.
83. Shi S, Liu Z, Li X, et al. Comparison of plate-cage construct and stand-alone anchored spacer in the surgical treatment of three-level cervical spondylotic myelopathy: a preliminary clinical study. *Spine J*. 2015;15(9):1973-1980.
84. Oh J, Kim TY, Lee HS, et al. Stand-alone cervical cages versus anterior cervical plate in 2-level cervical anterior interbody fusion patients: clinical outcomes and radiologic changes. *J Spinal Disord Tech*. 2013;26(8):415-420.
85. Aronson N, Filtzer DL, Bagan M. Anterior cervical fusion by the Smith-Robinson approach. *J Neurosurg*. 1968;29: 397-404.
86. Riley LH, Robinson RA, Johnson KA, et al. The results of anterior interbody fusion of the cervical spine. *J Neurosurg*. 1969;30:127-133.

87. Robinson RA, Walker AE, Ferlic DC, et al. The results of anterior interbody fusion of the cervical spine. *J Bone Joint Surg Am*. 1962;44:1569-1587.
88. Rogers WA. Fractures and dislocations of the cervical spine. An end-result study. *J Bone Joint Surg Am*. 1957;39:341-376.
89. Simmons EH, Bhalla SK. Anterior cervical discectomy and fusion. *J Bone Joint Surg Br*. 1969;51:225-237.
90. Conolly ES, Seymour RJ, Adams JE. Clinical evaluation of anterior cervical fusion for degenerative cervical disc disease. *J Neurosurg*. 1965;23:431-437.
91. Emery SE, Bolesta MJ, Banks MA, et al. Robinson anterior cervical fusion. Comparison of standard and modified techniques. *Spine*. 1994;19:660-663.
92. White AA, Southwick WO, Duponte R, et al. Relief of pain by anterior cervical spine fusion for spondylosis. *J Bone Joint Surg Am*. 1968;55:525-534.
93. Fernyhough JC, White JI, LaRocca H. Fusion rates in multi-level cervical spondylosis comparing allograft fibula and auto graft fibula in 126 patients. *Spine*. 1994;16:s561-s564.
94. Bohlman HH, Emery SE, Goodfellow DB, et al. Robinson anterior cervical diskectomy and arthrodesis for cervical radiculopathy. *J Bone Joint Surg Am*. 1993;75:1298-1307.
95. Newman M. The outcome of pseudarthrosis after cervical anterior fusion. *Spine*. 1993;18:2380-22383.
96. Phillips FM, Carlson G, Emery SE. Anterior cervical pseudarthrosis: natural history and treatment. *Spine*. 1997;22:1585-1589.
97. Koerner J, Kepler C, Albert T. Revision surgery for failed cervical spine reconstruction. *HSS J*. 2015;11:2-8.
98. Steinman JC, Herkowitz HN. Pseudarthrosis of the spine. *Clin Orthop Relat Res*. 1992;284:80-90.
99. Brodsky AE, Khalil MA, Sassard WR, et al. Repair of symptomatic pseudarthrosis of anterior cervical fusion: posterior versus anterior repair. *Spine*. 1992;17:1137-1143.
100. Lowery GL, Swank ML, McDonough RF. Surgical revision for failed anterior cervical fusion: articular pillar plating or anterior revision? *Spine*. 1995;20:2336-2341.
101. Beutler WJ, Sweeney CA, Connolly PT. Recurrent laryngeal nerve injury with anterior cervical spine surgery: risk with laterality of surgical approach. *Spine*. 2001;26:1337-1342.
102. Bertalanffy H, Eggert HR. Complications of anterior cervical discectomy without fusion in 450 consecutive patients. *Acta Neurochir (Wien)*. 1989;99:41-50.
103. Baron EM, Soliman AM, Gaughan JP, et al. Dysphagia, hoarseness, and unilateral true vocal fold motion impairment following anterior cervical discectomy and fusion. *Ann Otol Rhinol Laryngol*. 2003;112:921-926.
104. Winslow CP, Winslow TJ, Wax MK. Dysphonia and dysphagia following the anterior approach to the cervical spine. *Arch Otolaryngol Head Neck Surg*. 2001;127:51-55.
105. Carreon L, Glassman SD, Campbell MJ. Treatment of anterior cervical pseudarthrosis: posterior fusion versus anterior revision. *Spine J*. 2006;6:154-156.
106. McAnany S, Baird EO, Overley SC, et al. A meta-analysis of the clinical and fusion results following treatment of symptomatic cervical pseudarthrosis. *Global Spine J*. 2015;5(2):148-155.
107. Pompili A, Canitano S, Caroli F, et al. Asymptomatic esophageal perforation caused by late screw migration after anterior cervical plating: report of a case and review of relevant literature. *Spine*. 2002;27:E499-E502.
108. Fountas KN, Kapsalaki EZ, Machinis T, et al. Extrusion of a screw into the gastrointestinal tract after anterior cervical spine plating. *J Spinal Disord Tech*. 2006;19:199-203.
109. Gazzeri R, Tamorri M, Faiola A, et al. Delayed migration of a screw into the gastrointestinal tract after anterior cervical spine plating. *Spine*. 2008;33:E268-E271.
110. Lu DC, Theodore P, Korn WM, et al. Esophageal erosion 9 years after anterior cervical plate implantation. *Surg Neurol*. 2008;69:310-312.
111. Bernard TN Jr, Whitecloud TS III. Cervical spondylotic myelopathy and myeloradiculopathy. Anterior decompression and stabilization with autogenous fibula strut graft. *Clin Orthop*. 1987;221:149-160.
112. Emery SE, Bohlman HH, Bolesta MJ, et al. Anterior cervical decompression and arthrodesis for the treatment of cervical spondylotic myelopathy. Two to seventeen-year follow-up. *J Bone Joint Surg Am*. 1998;80:941-951.
113. Okamoto A, Shinomiya K, Furuya K, et al. Post-operative magnetic resonance imaging in patients with cervical myelopathy. *Spine*. 1991;16:s530-s533.
114. Fager CA. Evaluation of cervical spine surgery by postoperative myelography. *Neurosurgery*. 1983;12:416-421.
115. Martins AN. Anterior cervical discectomy with and without interbody graft. *J Neurosurg*. 1976;44:290-295.
116. Chiba K, Ogawa Y, Ishii K, et al. Long-term results of expansive open-door laminoplasty for cervical myelopathy-average 14-year follow-up study. *Spine*. 2006;31:2998-3005.
117. Masaki Y, Yamazaki M, Okawa A, et al. An analysis of factors causing poor surgical outcome in patients with cervical myelopathy due to ossification of the posterior longitudinal ligament: anterior decompression with spinal fusion versus laminoplasty. *J Spinal Disord Tech*. 2007;20:7-13.
118. Guigui P, Benoist M, Deburge A: Spinal deformity and instability after multilevel cervical laminectomy for spondylotic myelopathy. *Spine*. 1998;23:440-447.
119. Kaptain GJ, Simmons NE, Replogle RE, et al. Incidence and outcome of kyphotic deformity following laminectomy for cervical spondylotic myelopathy. *J Neurosurg*. 2000;93:199-204.
120. Albert TJ, Vaccaro AR. Postlaminectomy kyphosis. *Spine*. 1998;23:2738-2745.
121. Farcy JP, Weidenbaum M, Sola C. Surgical management of severe cervical kyphosis following extensive laminectomy. *Spine*. 1990;15:41-45.

CHAPTER 104 Failed Total Disc Arthroplasty

Andrew K. Simpson
Jack E. Zigler

Background

There have been multiple high-quality studies evaluating the safety and efficacy of both cervical and lumbar disc arthroplasty; the results of these studies have been favorable enough that surgeons are performing disc arthroplasty surgery with increased frequency. The aim of this chapter is not to delve into the vast amount of literature that addresses the safety, efficacy, and cost-effectiveness of arthroplasty versus fusion. Rather, the purpose of this discussion is to define the modalities of disc arthroplasty failure and help surgeons identify, prevent, and treat failed disc arthroplasty.

Spine fusions have been performed for decades prior to the development and implementation of disc arthroplasty procedures. Nonetheless, there continues to be a significant amount of controversy and practice variation with regard to the role of fusion for degenerative conditions. Thus, arthroplasty, as compared to fusion, is in its relative infancy. Two of the most common failure modalities unique to fusion surgery are pseudarthrosis and adjacent-segment disease. While we have long recognized the problem of pseudarthrosis, the role and relative importance of adjacent-segment disease has been less easily demonstrated. Disc arthroplasty was born out of the concept that eliminating motion from a mobile segment or joint is disadvantageous, which orthopaedic surgeons have long known and applied in the treatment of degenerative conditions of the appendicular skeleton—including the shoulders, hips, knees, and, more recently, in the ankles and wrists. In most of these cases, arthroscopy and arthroplasty are the first-line surgical treatment modalities, with fusion being reserved for salvage procedures.

Disc arthroplasty is a completely different procedure from fusion; as such, many of the complications and failure modalities are very different from those associated with fusion. Of the two most common failure modalities of fusion surgery, pseudarthrosis does not apply to disc arthroplasty and adjacent-segment disease has been shown to be significantly decreased following arthroplasty in both the cervical and lumbar spines. However, disc arthroplasty has its own set of unique failure modalities.

The increased utilization of disc arthroplasty over time dictates that there will be more patients undergoing these procedures with longer follow-up periods. Thus, the number of patients with disc arthroplasty failures will almost assuredly increase significantly over time. Currently, there is a relative paucity of literature from which to glean treatment recommendations for failed disc arthroplasty. Nonetheless, we recognize the future need for evidence-based treatment guidelines for the treatment of failed disc arthroplasty and have assembled what we consider to be the best practice recommendations for the prevention, diagnosis, and treatment of failed disc arthroplasty.

Prevention

The goal of this chapter is to identify and define the various modalities of disc arthroplasty failure as well as provide the clinician with strategies for therapeutic intervention and revision surgery. The technical aspects of primary disc arthroplasty will be reviewed and discussed elsewhere. The vast majority of disc arthroplasty failures can be prevented, as they are often derived from misjudgment in patient selection or technical shortcomings during the index procedure. Due to the fact that revision surgery in the anterior spinal column is fraught with much higher rates of approach-related complications, especially in the lumbar spine, attending to some of the most common missteps that lead to failures of disc arthroplasty is certainly merited. Specifically, we have found that the majority of failures can be traced back to improper indications, incomplete discectomy or endplate preparation, poor mobilization of the segment, or inappropriate implant sizing and placement.

Patient Selection

Proper patient selection for any spine intervention is at least as important, perhaps even more so, than perfect technical execution. Indicating patients for total disc arthroplasty is no exception. There are some conceptual differences in the treatment of cervical and lumbar disease; these differences play out when contrasting the literature for cervical and lumbar disc arthroplasty. Cervical disc arthroplasty is indicated for reconstruction following neurologic decompression. Lumbar arthroplasty is indicated for mechanical discogenic low back pain.

One inherent contrast is the fact that the majority of ventral neural compression is treated with anterior surgery in the cervical spine and posterior surgery in the lumbar spine. In the cervical spine, due to the fact that this is cord-level surgery, a great deal of radiculopathy is treated with anterior surgery, with the primary goal of surgery being neural decompression. Cervical fusion or disc arthroplasty is performed as a consequence of the subtotal discectomy necessary for adequate neural decompression. In the lumbar spine, however, neural compression in the absence of significant axial symptoms or instability is often treated with dorsal decompression alone. In the absence of instability or deformity, anterior surgery in the lumbar spine is typically reserved for treatment of axial symptoms, which, by nature, are much less predictable in terms of surgical outcome. These inherent differences between the treatment of cervical and lumbar disease are at least in part responsible for the much greater body of evidence supporting cervical disc arthroplasty outcomes. For the clinician, this means that indicating the proper patient for lumbar total disc replacement (TDR) is even more challenging.

Inclusion and exclusion criteria from US Food and Drug Administration (FDA) investigational device exemption studies identified the subsets of patients who would benefit from either fusion or TDR; 5- to 10-year follow-up of these patients has demonstrated durable and significant improvements in pain, impairment, and satisfaction scores.[1–5] There are multiple patient factors considered to be relative or absolute contraindications to disc arthroplasty, which have been demonstrated in the literature to be associated with higher rates of TDR failure. Patients with very poor bone quality—certainly those diagnosed with osteoporosis (T-score <2.5) but even those with osteopenia (T-score <1.0)—are more likely to have failures of the bone-implant interface. We routinely check densitometry on potential TDR patients and utilize more stringent criteria, avoiding lumbar TDR in most patients with a T-score less than −1.0 and avoiding cervical TDR when the T-score is less than −2.5. We often discover bone density abnormalities in otherwise healthy, relatively young patients. Patients with endocrine or metabolic bone diseases that might also affect bone formation are likely to have similar consequences. On the other hand, patients with an abundance of bone formation, such as diffuse idiopathic skeletal hyperostosis or ankylosing spondylitis, are also poor candidates for arthroplasty.

Ossification of the posterior longitudinal ligament is a contraindication to cervical TDR even if bridging autofusion has not occurred, as motion preservation is not only unnecessary but potentially deleterious, given the theoretical risk of continued osteophyte growth that may perpetuate further ventral neurologic compression. Hypermobility, either through inflammatory arthritides or systemic collagen disorders, is more likely to result in instability or supraphysiologic motion after disc arthroplasty. Obesity alters the biomechanical environment, especially for lumbar disc arthroplasty; it should be considered a relative contraindication, or even an absolute contraindication, at its extremes to motion preservation. Facet arthrosis or arthropathy, if symptomatic at the time of surgery, is likely to result in continued axial pain and should be thoroughly investigated with imaging as well as the clinical history and examination. Further, many surgeons in our practice will send patients for facet injections prior to considering lumbar disc arthroplasty, a negative response to which would certainly support the absence of symptomatic facet disease.

Instability is a contraindication to motion preservation. Pars fracture would be an extreme example of this and an obvious contraindication to disc arthroplasty. However, there were numerous failures in the early CHARITÉ trials for unrecognized pars defects.[6] More subtle instability is less easily defined and, as such, comes with a paucity of guidelines. Patients with more than a few millimeters of static spondylolisthesis, more than a few millimeters of intervertebral translation, or facet effusion on magnetic resonance imaging (MRI) scan ought to be evaluated carefully and may be considered relative contraindications to TDR. From the standpoint of global alignment, we consider lumbar sagittal imbalance and cervical kyphosis contraindications to disc arthroplasty, and decision making is based on the extent of kyphosis or sagittal imbalance, the patient's clinical symptoms, and the number of levels being addressed at surgery. Coronal deformity is more commonly encountered in the lumbar spine and we consider greater than 11 degrees of scoliosis an absolute contraindication to disc arthroplasty. In practice, however, we typically abide by more stringent criteria and avoid motion preservation in patients with greater than 5 degrees of coronal curvature (Fig. 104.1).

Discectomy and Endplate Preparation

Removal of the native disc is the initial procedural step for disc arthroplasty; performing a near-complete or radical discectomy is of paramount importance for a multitude of reasons, including neural decompression, exposure of stronger peripheral bone, and accurate implant sizing and placement. Shortcuts during discectomy will result in compounding technical challenges for the surgeon, while near-total discectomy will facilitate improved visualization, restoration of disc height and lordosis, better implant rim fit, sizing, and positioning. In the cervical spine, regional anatomic features make discectomy straightforward and near-complete removal of the disc and good visualization from uncus to uncus is rarely a technical challenge. In the cervical spine, it is our preference to remove the posterior anulus and posterior longitudinal ligament in order to confirm neural decompression, facilitate foraminotomy, and allow for parallel distraction of the endplates. This is perhaps a more technically demanding portion of the cervical discectomy and deserves careful attention as persistent foraminal compression, either static or dynamic, is the most common cause of neurologic failure after cervical disc arthroplasty. For patients with some uncovertebral spondylosis and bony foraminal narrowing, perhaps for whom a surgeon is pushing the indication for motion preservation,

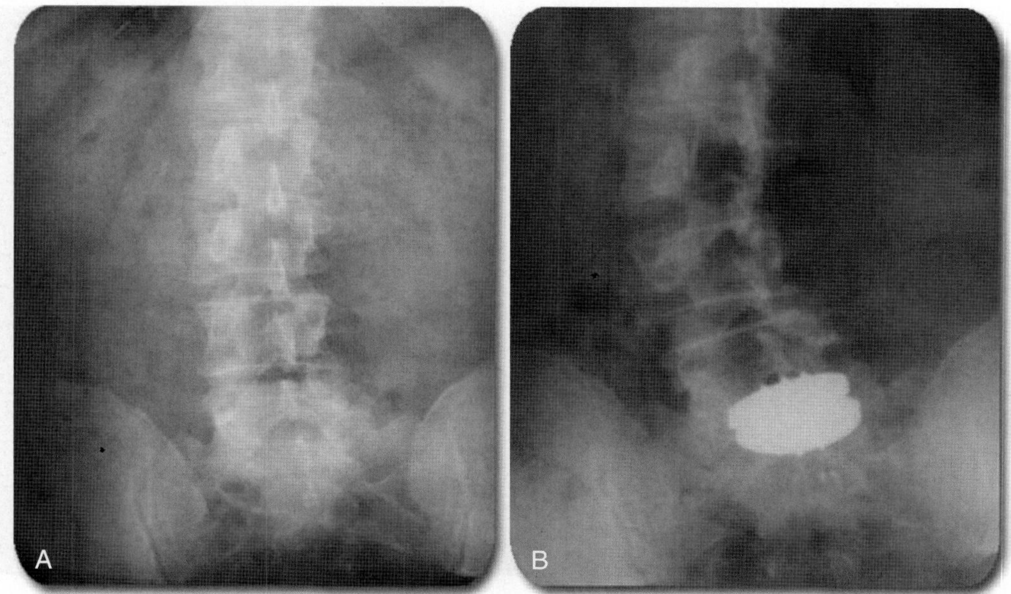

FIG. 104.1 (A) Preoperative radiograph of a patient with a mild coronal deformity. (B) Postoperative radiograph demonstrating significant coronal deformity progression after L5–S1 total disc replacement.

this portion of the procedure is even more important. Patients with significant disc space collapse and spondylosis requiring extensive bony resection are not indicated for arthroplasty. Following extensive decompression, they are at increased risk for implant subsidence and potential segmental ankylosis due to bone overgrowth with bridging osteophytes or heterotopic ossification.

Subtotal discectomy in the lumbar spine, on the other hand, is much more challenging, predominantly due to the regional vascular anatomy. Proper management of the great vessels is paramount for adequate visualization and exposure of the lateral aspects of the disc space. TDR requires even more thorough discectomy than anterior lumbar interbody fusion; thus, access surgeons and spine surgeons performing these procedures must be even more adept at the anterior approach to the lumbar spine and the mobilization of the great vessels. We prefer handheld retractors, which allow for intermittent and variable tension on the great vessels as needed during the procedure, though table-mounted retractor systems may be the only option for spine surgeons working without access assistance. In general, the most challenging portions of the disc to visualize and remove are the lateral and posterolateral portions, especially those ipsilateral to the operator. Adequate lateral discectomy is important for implant sizing and endplate coverage, while adequate posterolateral discectomy is important for preventing incomplete decompression and avoiding inadvertent displacement of disc material dorsally during prosthesis insertion. Visualization of the posterior portion of the disc space is often more challenging at L5–S1, especially in cases in which there are unfavorable pelvic parameters and greater sacral slope. Positioning the patient on an operative table with a break over the lumbosacral junction can help facilitate visualization and disc preparation. Flexing the operative table and utilizing Trendelenburg positioning can create segmental lordosis and bring the lumbosacral disc space into direct view. The posterior longitudinal ligament should be released on every case, and even resected if necessary to allow for parallel endplate distraction in patients in whom the posterior longitudinal ligament (PLL) is contracted and fibrotic.

Endplate preparation principles are similar in both the cervical and lumbar spine, with the goal being to remove the cartilaginous endplates down to the subchondral cortical bone. Violation of the cortical endplates and exposure of the cancellous bone weakens the bone-implant interface, increases the chance of subsidence, and may contribute to heterotopic ossification. There are subtle differences in technique that are implant-specific, more so than just keeled or nonkeeled; these subtleties are beyond the scope of this work. Nonetheless, the surgeon's familiarity with a particular implant and instrumentation is paramount.

Segmental Mobilization

The artificial disc implant does not confer motion. It allows and controls the segmental motion that the surgeon is able to gain at the time of discectomy and release both in the cervical and lumbar spine. In the cervical spine, a thorough discectomy and resection of the PLL along with decompression by minor symmetric uncovertebral joint resection generally mobilizes the segment adequately. Distraction pins and an intradiscal mechanical distractor also facilitate good segmental mobilization, with the TDR implant then functioning to control the motion. Failure to mobilize appropriately, "forcing" an implant into a tight disc space, or relying on bony endplate resection to accommodate an artificial disc replacement implant are all recipes for failure by lack of motion, subsidence, or bridging ossification.

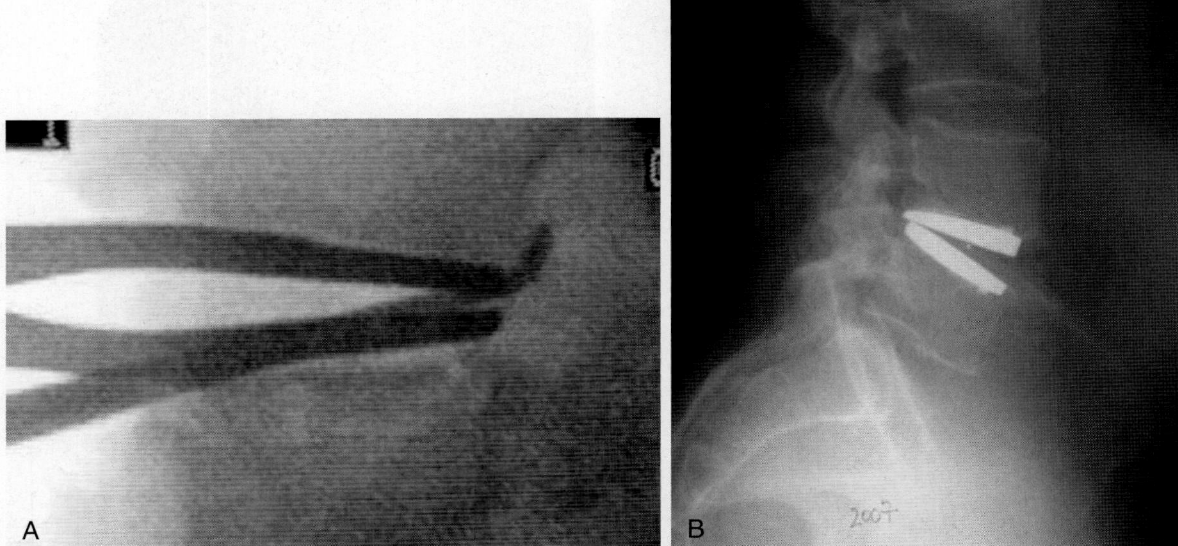

FIG. 104.2 (A) Intraoperative fluoroscopic image demonstrating posterior longitudinal ligament release with a curved curette. (B) Postoperative radiograph demonstrating poor implant positioning secondary to inadequate release of the posterior longitudinal ligament and posterior anulus.

The same principles apply to mobilization in the anterior lumbar spine, but the techniques are different. The spine surgeon must be comfortable working around the great vessels, there are no external distractor pins, and the visualization is more difficult due to the depths of the retroperitoneum compared to the anterior cervical spine. Mobilization is arguably the most critical step in lumbar arthroplasty technique, determining the effectiveness of motion preservation. Failure to adequately release the posterior longitudinal ligament and balance the lateral annular fibers without violating the endplates can result in early failure by implant subsidence, improper positioning, or even by anterior expulsion (Fig. 104.2).

Implant Sizing, Placement, and Alignment

The principles of implant sizing are similar for both cervical and lumbar disc arthroplasty, the most important of which is to use the largest-size footprint available that fits within the disc space and to slightly undersize the implant height to allow for improved motion range. The cortical bone in the periphery of the endplate is the strongest, meaning that smaller implant footprints result in higher contact stress on weaker bone.[7] In the cervical spine, there are instances in which a small portion of the medial aspect of the uncus must be reshaped in order to achieve appropriate fit. This occurs when one implant trial is undersized and the next-largest size impinges on the medial aspect of the uncus. In these instances, it is better to reshape the uncus than to undersize the implant. The identification of the midline is an important component of sizing and implant placement. It is important to identify the midline aspect of the disc space following appropriate-level verification. An anteroposterior fluoroscopic view is obtained early in the procedure and the midline is marked such that every part of the procedure, including the discectomy, is performed with reference to the midline. An implant that is not appropriately placed in the coronal plane can result in issues with direct nerve impingement on the ipsilateral side or perhaps under-distraction on the contralateral side and associated persistent stenosis. Sagittal plane implant placement is optimal when the posterior edge of the implant is in close continuity with the posterior aspect of the vertebral body, which typically results in proper placement of the center of rotation.[8] Sagittal plane sizing and placement is less commonly a source of technical shortcomings, as most surgeons utilize a predominance of lateral fluoroscopy during implant placement.

Implant lordosis is another parameter that can serve as a source of technical error leading to implant failure. The L5–S1 level presents a unique challenge, especially in patients with high sacral slope, in that the articulating surfaces of the implant may experience higher shear forces, resulting in higher rates of implant failure. Patients with higher, more vertical sacral inclination should be considered to have a relative contraindication to disc arthroplasty. Direct line-of-sight visualization of the posterior portion of the disc space may not be possible if a line drawn through the disc space on a lateral radiograph intersects below the pubic symphysis. In this situation, arthroplasty at the lumbosacral disc space may not be technically feasible and a fusion to better resist shear forces may be a more thoughtful surgical choice.

Failures of Total Disc Arthroplasty

Indications and Technique Issues

Poor patient selection, technical shortcomings, and device malpositioning are the most common causes of both cervical and lumbar disc arthroplasty failures.[9–12] Although there is sparse evidence for the management of TDR failures, the etiology of these failures has been thoroughly investigated in the literature through numerous investigational device exemption studies and longitudinal follow-up series. It is clear that the vast majority of TDR failures are the result of surgeon decision-making and technical missteps, which are preventable. The previous section presented in detail the most important strategies for avoiding these sources of TDR failure. Poor indications, failure to adequately mobilize the segment, and suboptimal implant positioning are the prime causes for poor postoperative results following arthroplasty.

Intrinsic Implant Failure

TDR implants by definition have moving parts, and are thus prone to intrinsic implant failures, ranging from issues with polyethylene wear to catastrophic material failures. Total implant failures, including dislocations and implant breakage or fracture, are extremely rare events that are limited essentially to case reports or very small series.[13–16] In these cases, there is often a significant technical shortcoming related to mismatch between implant and patient anatomy or implant/poly assembly, resulting in abnormal wear and early failure of the components.

While catastrophic implant failures are rare, perhaps a much more common but less elucidated issue is wear and wear particles. Polyethylene wear particles result in the activation of an inflammatory cascade that is associated with osteolysis and aseptic loosening of joint replacements. This has been well studied in the larger synovial joints of the appendicular skeleton as it applies to hip and knee replacement. In response to wear particles, macrophages release cytokines, including tumor necrosis factor-α and interleukin-1, which can activate osteoclasts and cause implant loosening.[17,18] The release of these cytokines may also result in the development of neuroinflammatory pain.[19]

The manufacturing processes and sterilization of polyethylene have been enhanced significantly over the last few decades, and wear issues have been greatly diminished with the use of partially cross-linked ultra-high-molecular-weight polyethylene. Polyethylene wear has been evaluated in a small number of retrieval studies for lumbar disc arthroplasty, and more recent-generation implants such as the Mobidisc (Zimmer Biomet) and Active-L (Aesculap) have demonstrated much lower rates of particulate debris compared with a previous study on an earlier-generation CHARITÉ III (DePuy Synthes) TDR (1–3 particles/mm^2 vs. 231 particles/mm^2).[20,21] The clinical role of particulate wear has not been described in the disc arthroplasty literature, although laboratory testing and measurement of particulate debris is part of every implant's FDA submission material. Polyethylene wear is a more significant problem in larger joints with greater surface area, biomechanical forces, synovial lining, and range of motion. This is perhaps why osteolysis and aseptic loosening is a less commonly recognized issue for lumbar and cervical disc arthroplasty. Nonetheless, one should consider that there may be some role of particulate matter and inflammatory cascade activation in TDR that, while too low to cause frank osteolysis, may be significant enough to result in neuroinflammatory pain and could be an underrecognized cause of persistent axial symptoms after total disc replacement.

Bone-Implant Interface Failure

Failures at the interface between the bone and TDR implant are the most common cause of mechanical failure seen in both the cervical and lumbar spine. Bone-implant issues range from a more subtle implant loosening, to subsidence, to outright vertebral fracture. Subsidence is a relatively common issue in both cervical and lumbar total disc arthroplasty from the standpoint of incidence and with regard to detection, as most patients undergo routine postoperative surveillance radiographs and many patients demonstrate some degree of implant subsidence, the majority of which are asymptomatic. TDR subsidence is contributed to by poor bone quality, implant undersizing, malpositioning, or endplate compromise during preparation or implant placement (Fig. 104.3). Subsidence of 1 to 3 mm is not uncommonly seen radiographically, but symptomatic and clinically relevant subsidence is much less common. However, it does account for a significant portion of early lumbar TDR failures. In evaluating complications from the early CHARITÉ disc, more than half of the failures were caused by device subsidence.[16] More modern implant designs with greater endplate coverage, in addition to surgeon education and improved techniques, have greatly reduced the incidence of clinically significant device subsidence.

Implant design plays a significant role in the bone–implant interface. Early biomechanical strength is dictated by the modality of implant fixation, whereas long-term stability of the bone–implant interface requires bony ongrowth. Specifically, prosthetic endplates may utilize teeth, keels, or screw fixation. Not surprisingly, biomechanical studies demonstrated that pullout strength was greatest for screws, followed by keels, followed by tooth ridges.[22] Thus, devices with smaller bone–implant anchors are more likely to mechanically loosen or migrate, especially in cases of malpositioning, in which the center of rotation of the device and the native spine are not concordant.

The use of keeled implants, though they provide increased early stability, introduces two well-described potential failure modalities. First, sagittal plane vertebral body fractures can occur secondary to deep keel cuts, which increases stress at the interface between the keel device and the bone. The risk of this complication is significantly heightened when multilevel TDR is performed with keeled devices. The intercalary vertebral body undergoes both cephalad and caudal keel cuts, and sagittal plane vertebral fractures have been described after multilevel keeled TDR in both the cervical and lumbar spine.[23,24] This is not a frequently encountered clinical issue. The second unique complication from keeled disc arthroplasty devices is a posterior vertebral body fracture that can occur when the keel cuts are too shallow in the anteroposterior dimension. Also, during implant insertion, the keel bottoms out dorsally and further attempts at positioning the implant more posteriorly result in a fracture of the posterior vertebral body, and possible displacement and neural compression.[25] This can occur with any implant, cervical or lumbar, if the

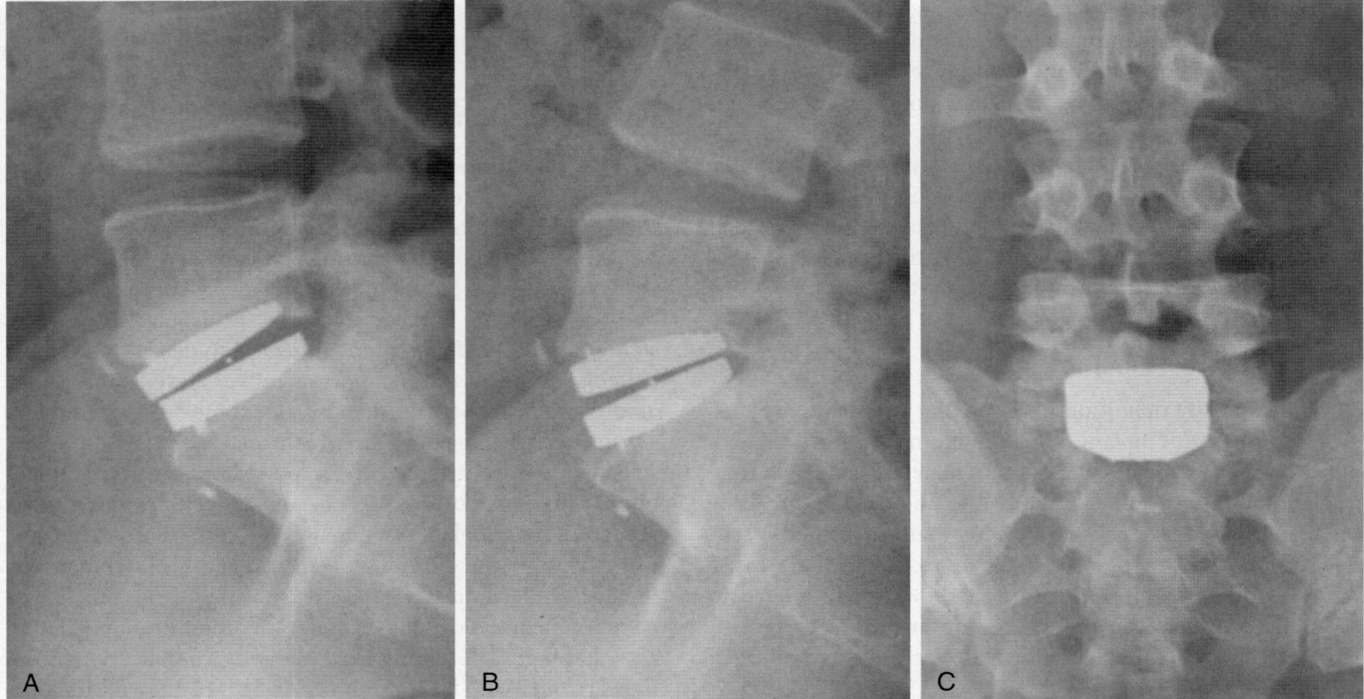

FIG. 104.3 (A) Flexion, (B) extension, and (C) anteroposterior radiographs of total disc replacement implant with endplate subsidence and loosening in a symptomatic patient.

surgeon does not carefully monitor the insertion trajectory fluoroscopically.

Host Response

There are several host responses to TDR that can result in failure modalities. The two most common types of host response include (1) osteolysis and its accompanying inflammatory reaction and (2) heterotopic ossification (HO). We discussed osteolysis in a previous section, as it is secondary to intrinsic implant wear characteristics. The remainder of this section addresses HO, as it has received a great deal of attention, particularly as it applies to cervical TDR.

HO is not an uncommon issue after cervical disc arthroplasty. As we obtain longer-term follow-up of patients after these procedures, we are likely to learn more about how they behave over time. On the spectrum of potential complications after TDR, even significant bridging HO resulting essentially in segmental fusion generally leads to a stable and clinically positive result. Outcomes of patients with bridging HO mirror those of patients with a successful anterior cervical discectomy and fusion (ACDF). We would argue that 10 years of motion preservation after disc arthroplasty and subsequent fusion would have still served the purpose of maintaining a more favorable biomechanical environment for the adjacent segments for a significant time. Nonetheless, significant HO and fusion defeat the technical purpose of a motion-preserving device.

The prevalence, temporal occurrence, and clinical significance of HO have been much more rigorously evaluated as it applies to cervical TDR. The most commonly utilized classification system for HO derives from McAfee and colleagues, which is a 4-point scale defining grade 4 HO as fusion.[26] Chen et al. performed a meta-analysis of HO after cervical disc arthroplasty and found that the pooled prevalence of any HO after 2 years was 58% and the prevalence of advanced HO (grades 3 and 4) after 2 years was 17%.[27] This meta-analysis also demonstrated that HO was not significantly related to clinical outcomes. Due to the fact that HO is quite common and there is significant interest in maintaining implant mobility, there has been a fair amount of investigational work in this arena. Heller et al. found evidence of early ossification on CT scans within the first several months of disc arthroplasty.[28] However, there are currently no clear evidence-based guidelines for the prevention of HO after cervical or lumbar disc arthroplasty procedures. Nonsteroidal antiinflammatory drugs (NSAIDs) have long been known to have inhibitory effects on bone healing. Tu et al. evaluated NSAID therapy in the postoperative period of cervical disc arthroplasty and found that the patients who are treated with NSAIDs—in particular, patients treated with cyclooxygenase-2 selective NSAIDs—had lower rates of HO at 2-year follow up, though the study was not powered enough to reach clear statistical significance.[29] We recommend thoughtful use of NSAIDs during the postoperative period, as the risks of therapy are minimal and outweighed by the potential benefit to motion preservation.

Deformity/Instability

Iatrogenic instability at the index level or iatrogenic deformity have been described as known complications after lumbar disc arthroplasty. Sagittal plane deformity and kyphosis are rarely encountered in the absence of catastrophic implant failure. Supraphysiologic motion and iatrogenic coronal deformity can occur, however, though with relative infrequency.

Supraphysiologic motion is an uncommon failure modality of total disc arthroplasty but occurs when postoperative motion exceeds the patient's preoperative motion arc and results in clinical instability and persistent axial pain from compensatory muscle spasm or facet capsular stretch. Patients will typically present with persistent dorsal pain originating from the paraspinal muscles and facet joints. Over time, many patients can develop compensatory facet hypertrophy, which can be diagnosed on advanced imaging with CT scan and MRI. This is a distinctly different entity than patients who had existing symptomatic facet disease that was merely missed during the preoperative evaluation. Nonetheless, the diagnostic evaluation of these patients is similar, and diagnostic facet injections are a useful objective tool. These patients may benefit from repeated therapeutic injections, radiofrequency rhizotomies, or ultimately from a posterior stabilization procedure.

Iatrogenic deformity is another form of instability that can occur after lumbar disc arthroplasty, particularly after multilevel procedures. As was mentioned earlier, significant coronal curvature (often described as more than 11 degrees) is an absolute contraindication to disc arthroplasty; however, even more subtle coronal plane deviations can be precipitated by disc arthroplasty, which fundamentally requires some removal of stabilizing structures, such as the anterior and posterior longitudinal ligaments and anulus. We tend to abide by more stringent coronal plane exclusion criteria and often avoid lumbar disc arthroplasty, especially multilevel procedures, in patients with even 5 degrees of coronal curvature. Some amount of asymmetrical disc collapse can generate coronal deformities that can be corrected through parallel endplate distraction; however, the condition of the lateral anulus and supporting structures is similarly compromised and even the most talented arthroplasty surgeons are at increased risk for precipitating deformity. Malpositioning of the implant in the coronal plane is capable of inducing deformity even in the context of normal preoperative alignment. During multilevel TDR, these errors are compounded, and surgeons are at increased risk of creating iatrogenic coronal deformities.

Neurologic Failure/Neural Impingement

Neurologic failure or persistent neural impingement is a failure modality more commonly encountered after cervical TDR by nature of the fact that cervical arthroplasty is typically performed for patients with primary radicular complaints. Incomplete neural decompression is one of the most common sources of failure following an arthroplasty procedure. Anterior cervical discectomy and fusion is a rather forgiving operation, and placement of a large interbody graft, even without direct foraminal decompression, is often enough to relieve the patient's preoperative radicular symptomatology. Disc arthroplasty, however, is a technically more challenging operation, as the surgeon is forced to limit bony resection, which reduces visibility. Further, due to the fact that arthroplasty preserves motion, there continues to be dynamic changes in the volume of the foramen with motion, which can exacerbate any residual foraminal stenosis. Additionally, coronal misplacement of an undersized implant can result in dynamic compression of the contralateral foramen and persistent or new radiculopathy.

In either the cervical or lumbar spine, failure to remove posterior disc material can result in displacement of that material into the neural canal or foramen and new postoperative radiculopathy. Patients who awake with new neurologic signs or symptoms after cervical or lumbar disc arthroplasty should be investigated in the acute setting with CT myelogram, as MRI is less helpful due to metal artifact (unless the implant is "MRI forgiving"). CT myelography will assess for disc or bone fragment in the neural canal or foramen, hematoma, or implant malposition. The immediate diagnosis of such complications is important, as it allows for an early revision of the anterior exposure and implant repositioning in the acute setting, which greatly diminishes the risk of revision anterior surgery.

Infection

Infection after total disc arthroplasty in the cervical or lumbar spine is a relatively uncommon complication; thus, there is very little literature with regard to evidence-based diagnosis and treatment modalities for these patients. Joint replacements in general, however, have been performed throughout the appendicular skeleton in large numbers and over many years; we can utilize the wisdom gained from joint arthroplasty to help guide us in the management of infection after disc replacement. In general, late infections of knee and hip replacements are most commonly treated in a staged fashion with implant removal, antibiotic therapy, and secondary exchange arthroplasty. However, multiple approaches to the anterior column of the cervical spine—and even more so lumbar spine—present a great deal of technical challenges and much higher risk of major complications. Additionally, there may be systematic differences between infections of the synovial joint space versus those in the anterior vertebral column.

The incidence of infection after total disc arthroplasty in either the cervical or lumbar spine is difficult to estimate, as the rarity of this complication precludes it from being well studied in most clinical series. At this point, the literature on infection after disc replacement is limited to case reports or as a single case in a cohort of TDR revision patients. As with any joint arthroplasty, there is a potential both for early and late infection. Patients will typically present with constitutional symptoms, axial pain, and perhaps some element of neurologic involvement. In most cases described in the literature, patients will also report gastrointestinal symptoms related to approximate anatomic structures, for instance, dysphagia in the cervical spine or a change in bowel habits in the case of lumbar anterior column infection. Laboratory values typically demonstrate an elevation in inflammatory markers, such as sedimentation rate and C-reactive protein, as well as elevation in white blood cell count. Depending on the acuity of the infection, imaging may demonstrate subtle findings or, if the duration of infection is longer, there may be periprosthetic involvement with subsidence or loss of fixation or perhaps a soft tissue fluid collection noted on advanced imaging.

The recommended treatment of periprosthetic total disc replacement infection requires implant removal, debridement, and conversion to a fusion procedure. Antibiotic therapies alone have limited if any role for the treatment of the prosthetic infections and risk further periprosthetic involvement and bony destruction, which may complicate the definitive therapeutic intervention. The potential morbidity of multiple anterior approaches to the cervical—and especially the lumbar—spine is much greater than that of multiple approaches to the knee or hip joint. This inherent difference dictates that the treatment algorithm for disc arthroplasty infection be different than for that of a peripheral joint replacement.

In cases of acute peripheral joint arthroplasty infection of limited duration, patients often do well with a more limited approach, with polyethylene exchange and debridement. Chronic infections of knee or hip arthroplasty prostheses are often treated with staged procedures, with initial debridement and delayed reimplantation. For disc arthroplasty infections, however, staged procedures would require multiple anterior approaches and limited polyethylene exchanges, even for acute infections, are at higher risk of failure. Based on these concepts, though with limited data, the best-practice recommendation for TDR infection is implant removal, debridement, and conversion to a fusion procedure, with or without supplemental dorsal fixation dependent on the status of the anterior column after debridement.

Diagnosis of Failed Disc Arthroplasty

History

The appropriate diagnosis and management of the patient with failed cervical and lumbar disc arthroplasty begins with a thorough discussion with the patient about the patient's history. It is often very helpful to understand the patient's symptoms prior to the disc arthroplasty procedure and whether the patient had a predominance of mechanical axial symptomatology or neurologic-mediated symptoms. Depending on the time from the initial surgery, the patient may or not be able to provide an accurate description of initial symptoms.

Next, it is important to understand the patient's response to the initial disc arthroplasty procedure in the immediate perioperative period, as well as how the patient progresses over time. For instance, the lack of any significant change after the procedure may indicate that the patient's initial surgical indications may have been misinterpreted or perhaps were not addressed during the procedure. A few examples of this may be a patient with significant mechanical axial symptoms that did not change after surgery, which could indicate that there is a component of facet or nondiscogenic-mediated pain that was not addressed or perhaps symptoms originating from a vertebral level that was not addressed. Another example may be a patient with significant radicular symptoms that did not change in the perioperative period, which could also indicate either an etiology from a different vertebral level or a technical shortcoming and incomplete foraminotomy or indirect foraminal decompression at the level of the surgery. On the other hand, the patient who does have a significant change in symptoms after the initial procedure and then experiences recurrence of prior symptoms or new symptoms is quite different. A significant change in symptoms after the index procedure would provide substantial evidence that the initial symptoms came from the operative level. In these cases, where there is a clear temporal period of symptomatic relief, the treating spine surgeon can be increasingly confident about both the etiology of symptoms and the potential reversibility with further surgical intervention.

Physical Examination

Physical examination of patients with failed disc arthroplasty, like that of all patients with spine pathology, is vital in understanding the potential etiology of the patient's symptoms. The neurologic examination in these patients is no different from that of any spine patient and is of utmost importance. Physical examination maneuvers evaluating axial symptoms are perhaps even more important, as differentiating the causal agent from the many potential pain generators can be challenging. For instance, a patient with more focal dorsal pain that is exacerbated with extension maneuvers and has tenderness over the facet joints is more likely to have facet-mediated pain and facet arthropathy. Contradistinctly, a patient with deep lumbodorsal pain exacerbated by flexion and sitting with no dorsal tenderness on examination may have pain from subsidence or implant loosening mediated by annular nociceptive fibers. While the specificity of the examination in and of itself may not be conclusive, in the context of a thorough history and concordant imaging findings, it is a fundamental part of the diagnostic algorithm for patients with pain after cervical or lumbar disc arthroplasty.

Imaging

Plain radiographs with dynamic views, MRI, and CT scan with or without myelogram are the most useful imaging studies for evaluating patients with failed disc arthroplasty. Plain radiography is useful for demonstrating implant size, positioning, and alignment. Many patients have these studies as part of routine postoperative surveillance. Dynamic views are important for assessment of functionality of the arthroplasty and to look for normal motion. These flexion and extension views may demonstrate limited motion from heterotopic ossification or autofusion or perhaps supraphysiologic motion, dynamic instability, or implant loosening. Lucencies at the bone–metal interface, endplate resorption, or subchondral cysts may be evident on plain radiographs. MRI is helpful for assessing the neural elements, though—depending on the type of implant used—the ventral spinal canal may be obscured by metal artifact. Nonetheless, MRI is still useful for evaluating the facet joints and looking for facet effusions or findings at the other vertebral levels that may be contributing to the patient's symptomatology. CT scan is useful for evaluating implant fixation and looking for more subtle loosening. Implant positioning and endplate coverage are better visualized on CT than compared to plain radiography. CT scan may also demonstrate bony abnormalities such as pars fractures and more carefully evaluate the bony elements of the facet joint. If the neural elements cannot be assessed clearly on the MRI scan, then the CT scan should be performed with myelography.

Interventional Procedures

Interventional diagnostic procedures are a valuable source of objective information in determining whether diagnostic imaging findings are clinically symptomatic. As it applies to failed disc arthroplasty, facet injections are often an integral part of the diagnostic workup. Patients with suspected pain from facet arthritis after disc arthroplasty are often sent at our institution for facet injections (intraarticular or medial branch blocks), which serve both a diagnostic and therapeutic purpose. A positive response to these injections is of great diagnostic value and confirms that the facet joints are the actual pain generator. Further, facet injections and rhizotomies may serve significant therapeutic value and can give some patients relief without requiring surgical intervention. Patients with very good transient relief after facet injections, but who fail to receive sustained resolution of their symptoms from repeated injections or rhizotomy, are likely to have good relief from further stabilization procedures. Surgeons should keep in mind, however, especially in the cervical spine, that the incidence of HO and auto-stabilization is not uncommon, meaning that dorsal-mediated symptoms at the level of disc arthroplasty may be self-limiting.

Revision Strategies

Revision strategy algorithms for failed disc arthroplasty are different for the cervical and lumbar spine due to the fact that revision anterior exposure in the cervical spine is associated with much less risk than that of the lumbar spine. For this reason, we will address revision strategies for cervical and lumbar TDR separately in this section.

Cervical Revision Strategies

The available approach options for revision of cervical TDR include anterior, posterior, or combined approaches. Due to the familiarity with the anterior cervical approach and the relative ease of anterior revision surgery, the vast majority of disc arthroplasty revisions in the cervical spine are performed with an anterior approach. The timing of revision surgery for the anterior cervical spine is not nearly as important as that for revision anterior lumbar surgery; however, for acute TDR failures, planning for revision surgery as soon as possible limits the amount of adhesions in the index surgical bed and makes reexposure less demanding. In the delayed setting, the principles of revision anterior exposure are the same as for any other procedure. One can choose to perform revision exposure through the ipsilateral side or may choose a contralateral approach if virgin territory is desired. Even in the absence of symptoms, consultation with an otolaryngologist is recommended to rule out subclinical vocal cord injury from the index procedure, especially if the surgeon is considering a contralateral approach.

Depending on the nature of the failure modality and the implant design, various revision strategies can be considered. For the most part, we recommend revision of cervical disc arthroplasty to fusion. There are rare instances when revision to another disc arthroplasty may be considered. One instance in which revision disc arthroplasty might be considered is in the acute setting when there is clearly an implant malposition or loosening that resulted in failure and when the index implant can be removed and replaced without significant damage to the endplates or vertebral bone loss. Even in these instances, patients should be informed and consent obtained for the potential need for ACDF as a bailout option. ACDF should be the default solution, as it allows the surgeon the technical freedom to remove significant portions of the vertebral body for safe explantation and can provide a more reliable result even in the context of endplate compromise, bone loss, and suboptimal interbody graft placement.

For the most part, choice of interbody graft and fusion implant can be left to surgeon preference, although one may want to consider supplemental anterior plate fixation rather than a stand-alone type device in the context of bone removal or bone loss. In cases requiring significant anterior bone removal, perhaps when severe subsidence results in kyphosis and corpectomy is necessitated, a combined approach with supplemental posterior fixation and fusion may be indicated.

Posterior approaches alone for cervical TDR failures have a relatively limited role and are rarely performed at our institution. Possible indications for posterior-only revision would certainly include patients who have an absolute contraindication to revision ventral approach or those with posterior column laxity with segmental kyphosis. One could also consider the posterior approach for isolated foraminotomy and decompression in patients with residual foraminal neural impingement.

Lumbar Revision Strategies

The treatment algorithm for the revision of failed lumbar disc arthroplasty is vastly more complex than its cervical counterpart owing mostly to the much higher technical difficulty and complication rates of revision access for anterior lumbar surgery. Healing in the retroperitoneum makes repeated access through the same tissue planes technically challenging after 2 to 3 weeks. Many access surgeons recommend waiting 3 to 6 months before considering access through the same approach once that early window has closed.

The incidence of vascular injury for primary anterior surgery is typically estimated at between 2% and 4%, while the incidence of vascular injury for revision approaches demonstrated in the CHARITÉ investigational device study was around 17%, with several other revision procedures aborted due to difficulty with vessel mobilization.[30–32] Very experienced access surgeons can now perform revision exposures with lower morbidity but still consider these as potentially high-risk surgeries. Full precautions should be taken, with large-bore intravenous access, ureteral stenting, groin access prepped and draped, and vascular trays in the operating room.

Retrograde ejaculation, which is a relatively rare event in primary anterior lumbar fusion performed through retroperitoneal approach (1.7%), has been reported in much higher rates, as high as 17.5%, if a transperitoneal approach is required for revision anterior surgery.[33,34] Ureteral injury is also an extremely rare event in primary lumbar access surgery, though it is much more susceptible in revision anterior retroperitoneal approaches, and we favor ureteral stent placement prior to any reexposure.

The most important factors that affect decision making with regard to lumbar TDR revision approaches include (1) time from the index procedure, (2) failure modality, (3) index surgical approach, (4) operative level, and (5) acceptability of arthroplasty implant positioning.

Timing, much more so than in cervical surgery, is paramount in determining the risk of revision anterior exposure. Within the first 1 to 2 weeks of the index procedure, there is minimal adhesion formation, and reexposure of the anterior lumbar spine incurs little incremental morbidity. For this reason, it is advisable to have the patient's follow-up in the early postoperative period with radiographic evaluation and to have a low threshold for revising implants with evidence of early migration or malpositioning. In this case, anterior revision is similar to cervical TDR revision in that lumbar TDR revision and reimplantation can be considered if this can be performed without significant damage to the endplates. However, revision to anterior lumbar interbody fusion ought to be considered the default, with few exceptions (Fig. 104.4).

The surgical level and the approach utilized for the index procedure also play a significant role in decision making and planning for possible revision anterior surgery. The typical vascular anatomy at L5–S1 makes it accessible from either the left or right retroperitoneal approach as well as a transperitoneal approach. Typically, a left-sided retroperitoneal approach is used for the index surgery; thus, revision strategy often employs a transperitoneal approach or right-sided retroperitoneal approach, the latter favored in cases of young males to avoid the elevated risk of retrograde ejaculation with a transperitoneal dissection. At L3–L4 or L4–L5, the revision left-sided retroperitoneal approach is typically employed, as the vascular anatomy makes other approaches less favorable. The situation is one of the most challenging for revision anterior exposure and is greatly benefited by the involvement of an experienced access surgeon. The far lateral, or transpsoas, approach does offer a potential alternative means to access failed disc arthroplasty through relatively virgin tissue planes likely not utilized during the index procedure. However, this approach is not viable at L5–S1 and may or may not be utilized at L4–L5, dependent on the patient's anatomy with regard to the psoas, vasculature, and iliac crest.

There are a few instances in failed lumbar TDR for which the revision anterior approach is a necessity. One of these instances is the case of prosthesis infection. As was mentioned earlier, the available evidence for this relatively rare complication demonstrates that device explantation and debridement are necessary for eradication of the infection. Another indication for revision through anterior approach is unacceptable implant position or migration, or component displacement, which may compress the anterior vascular structures. In the absence of these or other mitigating factors that necessitate implant removal or repositioning, a posterior approach is typically favored in order to avoid the relatively high morbidity of revision anterior surgery.

Posterior surgical options for failed lumbar TDR include decompression and/or instrumented posterior fusion. In cases in which there is failure due to neural impingement but the TDR implant is functioning well and in good position, a dorsal decompression is a suitable option. During this procedure, the surgeon must attend to maintenance of the stabilizing structures and avoid aggressive medial facetectomy or weakening of the pars. Posterior instrumentation and fusion is the most common salvage procedure for failed lumbar arthroplasty. For patients who present with persistent pain secondary to loosening, subsidence, instability, or facet arthrosis, who have failed exhaustive nonoperative modalities, and who do not have a clear indication for revision anterior surgery, posterior instrumented fusion is the recommended salvage procedure (Fig. 104.5). Biomechanical studies have suggested that pedicle screws combined with lumbar disc replacement are biomechanically similar to pedicle screws combined with interbody femoral ring allograft.[35] Conceptually, the disc arthroplasty prosthesis, if it is in an acceptable position, serves as a spacer implant that will maintain relative disc height during the fusion process. It will not serve as a biologic adjunct, however. For this reason, we tend to focus on optimizing the posterior biologic environment with thorough preparation of the posterolateral graft bed as well as decortication of the facet joints to serve as multiple potential fusion surfaces. In one of the largest series investigating outcomes after revision for failed lumbar TDR, Punt et al. compared posterolateral instrumented fusion alone versus an anteroposterior procedure with TDR explantation, interbody graft, and posterolateral fusion and found that both groups demonstrated similar clinical benefit, with no significant additional benefit afforded by TDR removal.[36]

Summary

Cervical and lumbar total disc arthroplasty has been demonstrated as a safe and effective alternative to fusion for treatment of cervical degenerative disc disease associated with myeloradiculopathy and for lumbar discogenic back pain in appropriately indicated individuals. Disc arthroplasty has thus become increasingly utilized. While surgeons are well acquainted with the diagnosis and management of failed fusion surgery, we are relatively unfamiliar with the treatment of failed disc arthroplasty. Nonetheless, we are likely to see more patients with failed disc arthroplasty in the future; this chapter attempts to provide spine surgeons with practical recommendations for the prevention, diagnosis, and treatment of disc arthroplasty failures.

The vast majority of failures are preventable and typically are the result of improper indications or technical shortcomings during the index procedure. They are largely avoidable by

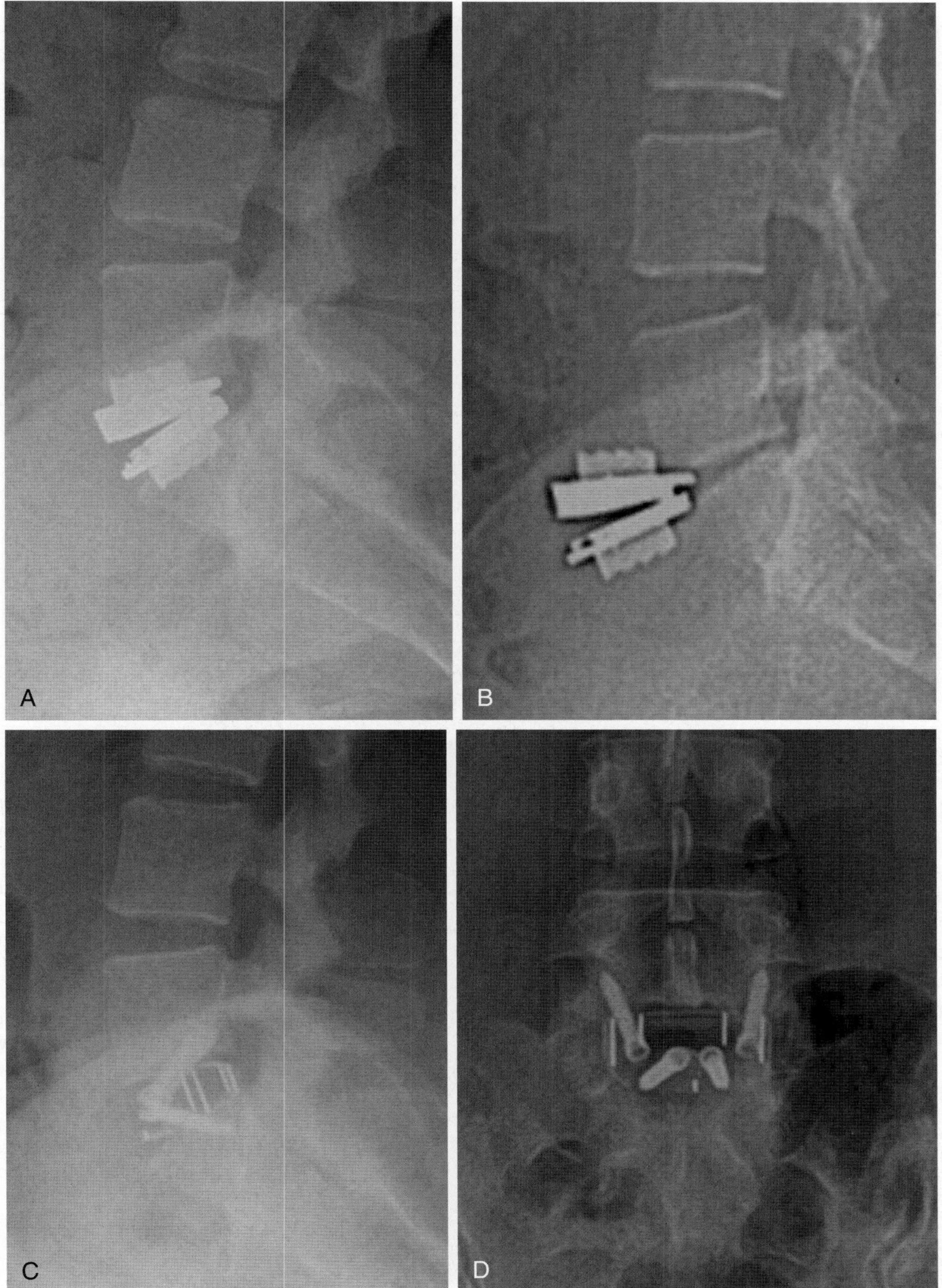

FIG. 104.4 (A) Immediate postoperative radiograph of total disc replacement in a suboptimal position. (B) Lateral scout image in the same patient, who presented with an acute increase in back pain in the immediate postoperative period with an anteriorly displaced device. (C) Lateral radiograph after device removal and revision to stand-alone anterior lumbar interbody fusion. (D) Anteroposterior radiograph after device removal and revision to stand-alone anterior lumbar interbody fusion.

surgical planning and technique. Careful attention to patient selection, especially for lumbar TDR, familiarity with the TDR implant and instrumentation, and thoughtful technical execution can greatly reduce the occurrence of TDR failures and the revision burden. When failures do occur, identifying the etiology through careful history, physical examination, imaging studies, and possibly with interventional modalities is paramount to effective treatment.

Surgical revision of cervical TDR failure is dominated by the revision anterior approach, whereas the much higher rate of morbidity with revision anterior lumbar approaches gives way to a much more complex surgical treatment algorithm.

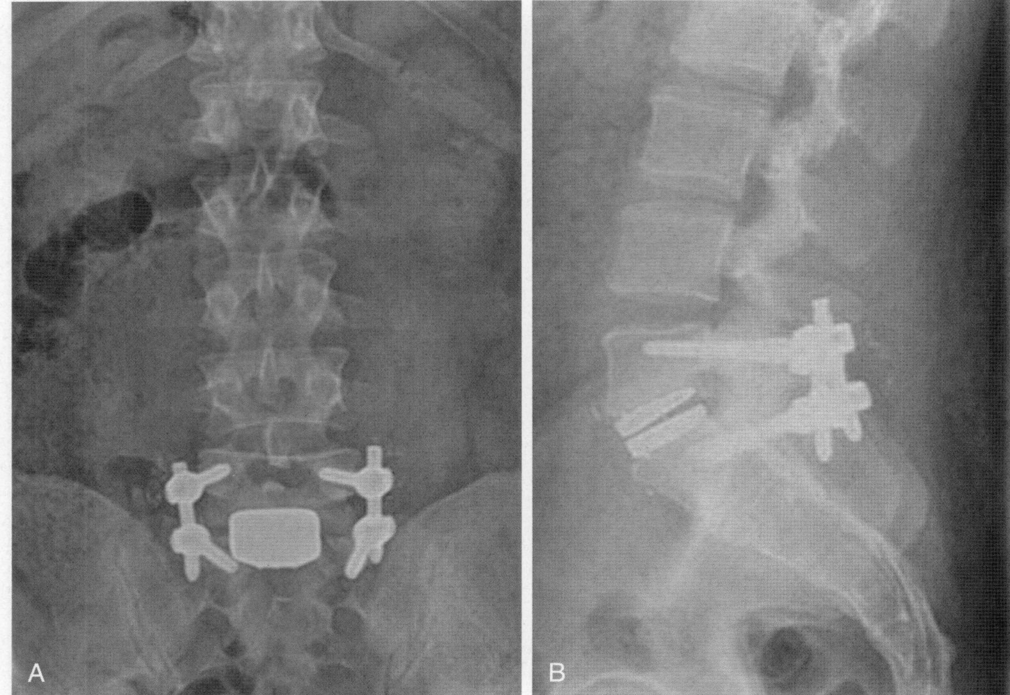

FIG. 104.5 Postoperative (A) anteroposterior and (B) lateral radiographs after posterior stabilization and fusion procedure for failed total disc replacement in acceptable alignment.

We recommend adherence to strict inclusion and exclusion criteria through the implementation of practice-based or institution-based protocols (including a preoperative dual-energy x-ray absorptiometry scan, CT scan, body mass index calculation, and so on) in order to reduce the incidence of failed disc arthroplasty. Using the FDA investigational device exemption criteria and the long-term follow-ups of patient cohorts selected within those criteria should reinforce the ability of arthroplasty to give a predicable result to our patients and help minimize arthroplasty failures.

KEY REFERENCES

1. Patel AP, Brodke DS, Pimenta L, et al. Revision strategies in lumbar total disc arthroplasty. *Spine*. 2008;33:1276-1283.
2. Park J, Chang H, Yeom JS, et al. Revision surgeries following artificial disc replacement of cervical spine. *Acta Orthop Traumatol Turc*. 2016;50:610-618.
3. Punt I, Willems P, Kurtz S, et al. Clinical outcomes of two revision strategies for failed total disc replacements. *Eur Spine J*. 2012;21:2558-2564.

REFERENCES

1. Blumenthal SL, McAfee PC, Guyer RD, et al. A prospective, randomized, multi-center FDA IDE study of lumbar total disc replacement with the CHARITÉ Artificial Disc vs. lumbar fusion: part I. Evaluation of clinical outcomes. *Spine*. 2005;30:1565-1575.
2. Gornet MF, Matthews HH, Burkus JK. *MAVERICK total disc replacement: a review of 12-month data from five investigational centers*. Proceedings of the NASS 20th Annual Meeting, Philadelphia, 2005.
3. McAfee PC, Cunningham BW, Holtsapple G, et al. A prospective, randomized, multi-center FDA IDE study of lumbar total disc replacement with the CHARITÉ Artificial Disc vs lumbar fusion: part II. Evaluation of radiographic outcomes and correlation of surgical technique accuracy with clinical outcomes. *Spine*. 2005;30:576-583.
4. Zigler JE. Clinical results with ProDisc: European experience and US investigational device exemption study. *Spine*. 2003;28:S163-S166.
5. Zigler JE, Burd T, Vialle EN, et al. Lumbar spine arthroplasty: early results using the ProDisc II: a prospective randomized trial of arthroplasty versus fusion. *J Spinal Disord Tech*. 2003;16:352-361.
6. McAfee PC, Geisler FH, Saiedy S, et al. Revisability of the CHARITÉ Artificial Disc Replacement: analysis of 347 patients enrolled in the US IDE Study of the CHARITÉ Artificial Disc. *Spine J*. 2005;5(4):1S.
7. Rauschning W. Pathoanatomy of lumbar disc degeneration and stenosis. *Acta Orthop Scand*. 1993;251:3-12.
8. Ishii T, Mukai Y, Hosono N, et al. Kinematics of the subaxial cervical spine in rotation: in vivo three-dimensional analysis. *Spine*. 2006;31:155-160.
9. Patel AP, Brodke DS, Pimenta L, et al. Revision strategies in lumbar total disc arthroplasty. *Spine*. 2008;33:1276-1283.
10. Bertagnoli R, Funk JF, Schneider SV. Complications and strategies for revision surgery in total disc replacement. *Orthop Clin North Am*. 2005;36:389-395.
11. Kostuik JP. Complications and surgical revision for failed disc arthroplasty. *Spine J*. 2004;4(6 Suppl):289S-291S.
12. Park J, Chang H, Yeom JS, et al. Revision surgeries following artificial disc replacement of cervical spine. *Acta Orthop Traumatol Turc*. 2016;50:610-618.

13. David T. Revision of a CHARITÉ artificial disc 9.5 years in vivo to a new CHARITÉ artificial disc: case report and explants analysis. *Eur Spine J*. 2005;14:507-511.
14. Mather P, Blackman M, Redla S, et al. Bilateral pedicle fractures following anterior dislocation for the polyethylene inlay of the Prodisc artificial disc replacement. *Spine*. 2005; 30:E311-E314.
15. Mayer HM, Wiechert K, Korge A, et al. Minimally invasive total disc replacement: surgical technique and preliminary clinical results. *Eur Spine J*. 2002;11:S124-S130.
16. Van Ooij A, Oner FC, Verbout AJ. Complications of artificial disc replacement: a report of 27 patients with the SB CHARITÉ disc. *J Spinal Disord Tech*. 2003;16:369-383.
17. Gallo J, Raska M, Mrazek F, et al. Bone remodeling, particle disease and individual susceptibility to periprosthetic osteolysis. *Physiol Res*. 2008;57:339-349.
18. Dumbleton JH, Manley MT, Edidin AA. A literature review of the association between wear rate and osteolysis in total hip arthroplasty. *J Arthroplast*. 2002;17:649-661.
19. Scholz J, Woolf CJ. The neuropathic pain triad: neurons, immune cells and glia. *Nat Neurosci*. 2007;10:1361-1368.
20. Austen S, Punt IM, Cleutjens JP, et al. Clinical, radiological, histological and retrieval findings of Activ-L and Mobidisc total disc replacements: a study of two patients. *Eur Spine J*. 2012;21(suppl 4):S513-S520.
21. Punt IM, Cleutjens JP, de Bruin T, et al. Periprosthetic tissue reactions observed at revision of total intervertebral disc arthroplasty. *Biomaterials*. 2009;30:2079-2084.
22. Cunningham BW, Hu N, Zorn CM, McAfee PC. Comparative fixation methods of cervical disc arthroplasty versus conventional methods of anterior cervical arthrodesis: serration, teeth, keels, or screws? *J Neurosurg Spine*. 2010; 12:214-220.
23. Datta JC, Janssen ME, Beckham R, Ponce C. Sagittal split fractures in multilevel cervical arthroplasty using keeled prosthesis. *J Spinal Disord Tech*. 2007;20:89-92.
24. Shim CS, Lee S, Maeng DH, et al. Vertical split fracture of the vertebral body following total disc replacement using ProDisc: report of two cases. *J Spinal Disord Tech*. 2005;18:465-469.
25. Shim CS, Shin HD, Lee SH. Posterior avulsion fracture at an adjacent vertebral body during cervical disc replacement with ProDisc-C: a case report. *J Spinal Disord Tech*. 2007;20: 568-572.
26. McAfee PC, Cunningham BW, Devine J. Classification of heterotopic ossification (HO) in artificial disc replacement. *J Spinal Disord Tech*. 2003;16:384-389.
27. Chen J, Wang X, Bai W, et al. Prevalence of heterotopic ossification after cervical total disc arthroplasty: a meta-analysis. *Eur Spine J*. 2012;21:674-680.
28. Tortolani PJ, Heller JG, Park AE, et al. Computed tomography (CT) scan assessment of paravertebral bone after total cervical disc replacement: prevalence, temporal relationships, and the effects of NSAIDs [abstract]. In: *Proceedings of the Cervical Spine Research Society*. 2003.
29. Tu TH, Wu JC, Huang WC, et al. Postoperative nonsteroidal anti-inflammatory drugs and the prevention of heterotopic ossification after cervical arthroplasty: analysis using CT and a minimum of 2-year follow-up. *J Neurosurg Spine*. 2015;22: 447-453.
30. Brau SA, Delamarter RB, Schiffman ML, et al. Vascular injury during anterior lumbar surgery. *Spine J*. 2004;4:409-412.
31. Escobar E, Transfeldt E, Garvey T, et al. Video-assisted versus open anterior lumbar spine fusion surgery: a comparison of four techniques and complications in 135 patients. *Spine*. 2003;28:729-732.
32. Sasso RC, Best NM, Mummaneni PV, et al. Analysis of operative complications in a series of 471 anterior lumbar interbody fusion procedures. *Spine*. 2005;30:670-674.
33. Sasso RC, Kenneth Burkus J, LeHuec JC. Retrograde ejaculation after anterior lumbar interbody fusion: transperitoneal versus retroperitoneal exposure. *Spine*. 2003;28:1023-1026.
34. Tiusanen H, Seitsalo S, Osterman K, Soini J. Retrograde ejaculation after anterior interbody lumbar fusion. *Eur Spine J*. 1995;4:339-342.
35. Cunningham BW, Hu N, Beatson HJ, et al. Revision strategies for single- and two-level total disc arthroplasty procedures: a biomechanical prospective. *Spine J*. 2009;9:735-743.
36. Punt I, Willems P, Kurtz S, et al. Clinical outcomes of two revision strategies for failed total disc replacements. *Eur Spine J*. 2012;21:2558-2564.

CHAPTER 105 Postoperative Deformity of the Cervical Spine

Andrew J. Pugely
Comron Saifi
K. Daniel Riew

Introduction

The evaluation and management of cervical spine deformity remains one of the most challenging issues within spinal surgery. Although multiple etiologies exist, iatrogenic malalignment represents a significant portion of cases. This chapter focuses on the evaluation of patients with postoperative cervical deformity, reviews preventive measures, and details our surgical approach. A series of case examples demonstrates our current techniques while emphasizing surgical principles.

The importance of global spinal alignment has been increasingly recognized. In deformity surgery, the cervical spine should not be viewed in isolation, but within the greater context of the cervicothoracic junction and overall spinal balance. More recent clinical and radiographic tools have been developed to aid in quantifying the nebulous complexities and building a surgical plan.

Assessment of Cervical Deformity

Clinical Evaluation

The clinical evaluation of a patient with postoperative cervical deformity should begin by understanding the nature of the disability. The impact of the deformity on the patient's activities of daily living is a critical component and should guide both nonsurgical and surgical management. A detailed surgical history is critical to preoperative planning. Previous surgical approach, instrumentation, and decompression areas should help guide surgical planning. Patients with previous anterior surgery should be considered for evaluation of vocal cord dysfunction to determine the innervation of the recurrent laryngeal nerve (RLN). Our preference is to approach the anterior spine opposite a previous surgery, unless RLN dysfunction is identified, as bilateral RLN palsies will result in loss of phonation.

The majority of patients have kyphotic deformities, but scoliosis is also common. The malalignment may be severe, and patients report inability to maintain horizontal gaze, difficulty eating, high fatigability, and pain. With loss of stability and normal alignment, pain can be severe and results from degeneration of the intervertebral discs and facet joints, increased stress on the posterior soft tissue complexes, and an often-dysfunctional posterior muscle complex. In addition to progressive pain and deformity, postoperative malalignment is often associated with neurologic dysfunction such as myelopathy and/or radiculopathy.

The physical exam should begin with a careful neurologic assessment. Progressive malalignment is commonly associated with myelopathy and radiculopathy. Bony and ligament overgrowth in response to instability hasten central and foraminal stenosis development. Furthermore, the draping and flattening of the spinal cord over the kyphotic vertebral bodies may also contribute to myelopathy and present as hand and gait disturbance. Evaluation of the patient's global and regional alignment allows for quantification of deformity severity. Measures such as the chin-brow vertical angle assess the lack of horizontal gaze.

Radiographic Evaluation

Standard evaluation in all spine patients should include static and dynamic radiographs of the cervical spine, including the cervicothoracic junction, as well as standing scoliosis films of the entire spine. We use the low-dose digital EOS Imaging system to obtain full-length standing films. Advanced imaging, including computed tomography (CT) and magnetic resonance imaging (MRI) of the operative region should also be obtained and allow for careful evaluation of the vertebral artery anatomy, areas of central and foraminal stenosis, the existing fusion mass, areas with previous laminectomies, and the presence of pseudarthrosis.

Radiographic measurements allow the surgeon to quantify the degree of deformity and set goals for operative correction. A variety of regional and global alignment parameters have been described and validated.[1,2] On the upright lateral radiograph, the C2–C7 sagittal vertical axis is the distance the center of C2 falls from the posterior-superior aspect of the C7 vertebral body. Cervical lordosis between C2 and C7 can be measured using a variety of techniques.[3] More recently other measurements to quantify deformity at the cervicothoracic junction and the global spine have been described[4] but are beyond the scope of this discussion. Overall, a thorough radiographic exam is critical to optimizing a safe and effective preoperative plan.

Deformity Prevention

The best treatment of postoperative cervical deformity is prevention. Iatrogenic malalignment can be produced during every step of a cervical spine operation. Errors in patient positioning, distractor placement, extent of decompression, instrumentation, selection or placement of bone graft, and even use of postoperative immobilization may all result in postoperative cervical deformity. Malalignment may occur after single-level or multiple-level operations, anterior or posterior operations, and decompression procedures with or without stabilization. The surgeon must pay meticulous attention to detail at every step of the procedure to prevent iatrogenic malalignment. This chapter reviews some of the common causes of iatrogenic malalignment of the cervical spine, outlines some techniques to avoid postoperative deformity, and discusses the treatment of postoperative cervical malalignment.

Preventing Iatrogenic Cervical Malalignment During Anterior Surgery

Positioning

The most common error of patient positioning for anterior surgery is to put the patient's neck into hyperlordosis. A rolled towel is often placed underneath the patient across the shoulders to extend the neck. Whereas moderate cervical lordosis is desirable, hyperlordosis such that the spinous processes are touching is, in general, excessive. If the patient is fused in this position he or she will often have severe interscapular and posterior cervical pain, especially if an extensive foraminotomy is not performed at the time of the procedure. Extension of the neck narrows the posterior neural foramen and may result in root compression. To avoid this complication, we routinely inspect the position with the patient supine to ensure that the neck is in a relatively neutral or slightly lordotic position. In addition, we examine the localizing radiograph to verify that the neck is in an acceptable amount of lordosis. If the patient's neck is hyperlordotic on this radiograph, we place Caspar distractor pins with the tips converging. When the distractor is placed over the pins, the amount of lordosis will be reduced (Fig. 105.1). At the end of the procedure, the goal is to have the neck in a normal lordotic configuration.

Coronal malalignment of the cervical spine may also occur. One potential cause of iatrogenic coronal deformity is taping one shoulder lower than the other during the initial patient positioning. Before prepping and draping, we routinely inspect the patient's head and shoulder positions to confirm that the cervical spine is aligned properly and that the shoulders are level. If a coronal deformity is introduced into the cervical spine at a single level, the adjacent levels will generally compensate for the malalignment with little effect on the overall balance. An instrumented fusion over multiple levels performed with the patient improperly aligned, however, may result in a postoperative deformity with clinical imbalance.

Finally, the surgeon must confirm that the patient is positioned in neutral axial rotation. Axial malalignment may occur as a result of slight rotation of the head. During the dissection and retraction, it is common for the surgeon

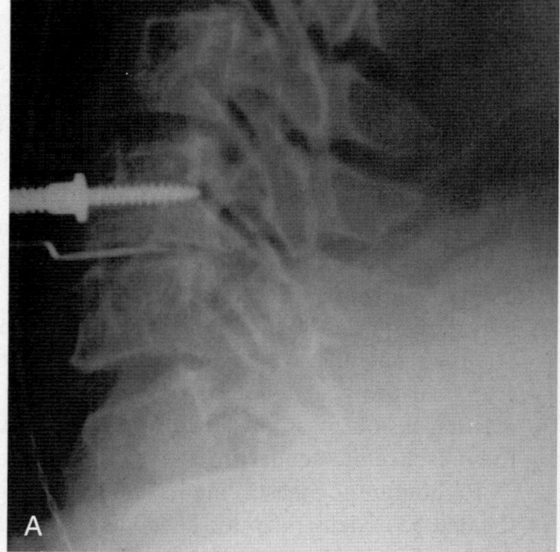

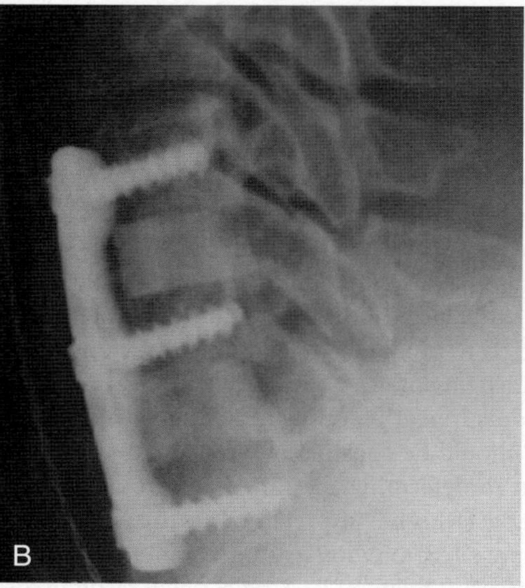

FIG. 105.1 (A) This intraoperative radiograph shows that the Caspar distraction pin has been placed into the body of C5 parallel to the caudal endplate. Note the hyperlordosis at C6–C7 with the touching spinous processes. A Caspar pin is then placed into C7 parallel to its rostral endplate. The tips of the pins converge. When the Caspar distractor is placed over the pins, it brings them into parallel alignment and reduces the lordosis. (B) Postoperative lateral radiograph shows correction of the hyperlordosis after graft placement and plating.

to inadvertently push the head away from the side of the approach. Some surgeons do this routinely to assist the exposure. If the surgeon is not aware that the head is rotated toward the contralateral side and puts a plate on, the segment will be fused in rotation. The rotational malalignment is obviously compounded when multiple segments are fused with instrumentation.

The surgeon can avoid creating a rotational deformity by using one of two techniques. The first is to ask the anesthesiologist to confirm that the nose is pointed straight up before placing any grafts and beginning the instrumentation. This, however, requires that the surgeon remember to ask the anesthesiologist. We prefer to use a more foolproof technique of routinely placing a tape across the forehead to prevent inadvertent rotation of the head during the operation. Another variation on this technique is to use commercially available head holders with an elastic chinstrap to stabilize the head. When performing high cervical approaches to C2–C3 or C3–C4, it is sometimes advantageous to rotate the neck to the contralateral side to gain better access to the spine. Under those circumstances, it is a good idea to write a reminder on the sterile drape to turn the head back into neutral alignment before grafting and plating are done.

Decompression

We routinely use Caspar distractor pins to open the disc space during anterior cervical surgery. Although the distractor is quite useful in exposing the disc space, the surgeon must be careful in placing the pins. If both pins are placed off center to one side, the disc space will open asymmetrically, causing segmental coronal angulation. If the pins are placed in an oblique position, the disc space will open asymmetrically and relative lateral translation of the vertebral bodies will occur. Finally, if the pins are placed in different planes, a rotational malalignment of the vertebra can occur (Fig. 105.2).

Failure to expose the entire disc space may increase the likelihood of performing an asymmetrical discectomy or corpectomy. Placing a graft asymmetrically on one side may result in a coronal plane deformity (Fig. 105.3). This can be avoided by exposing the intervertebral disc to the uncovertebral joints bilaterally before starting the decompression. These

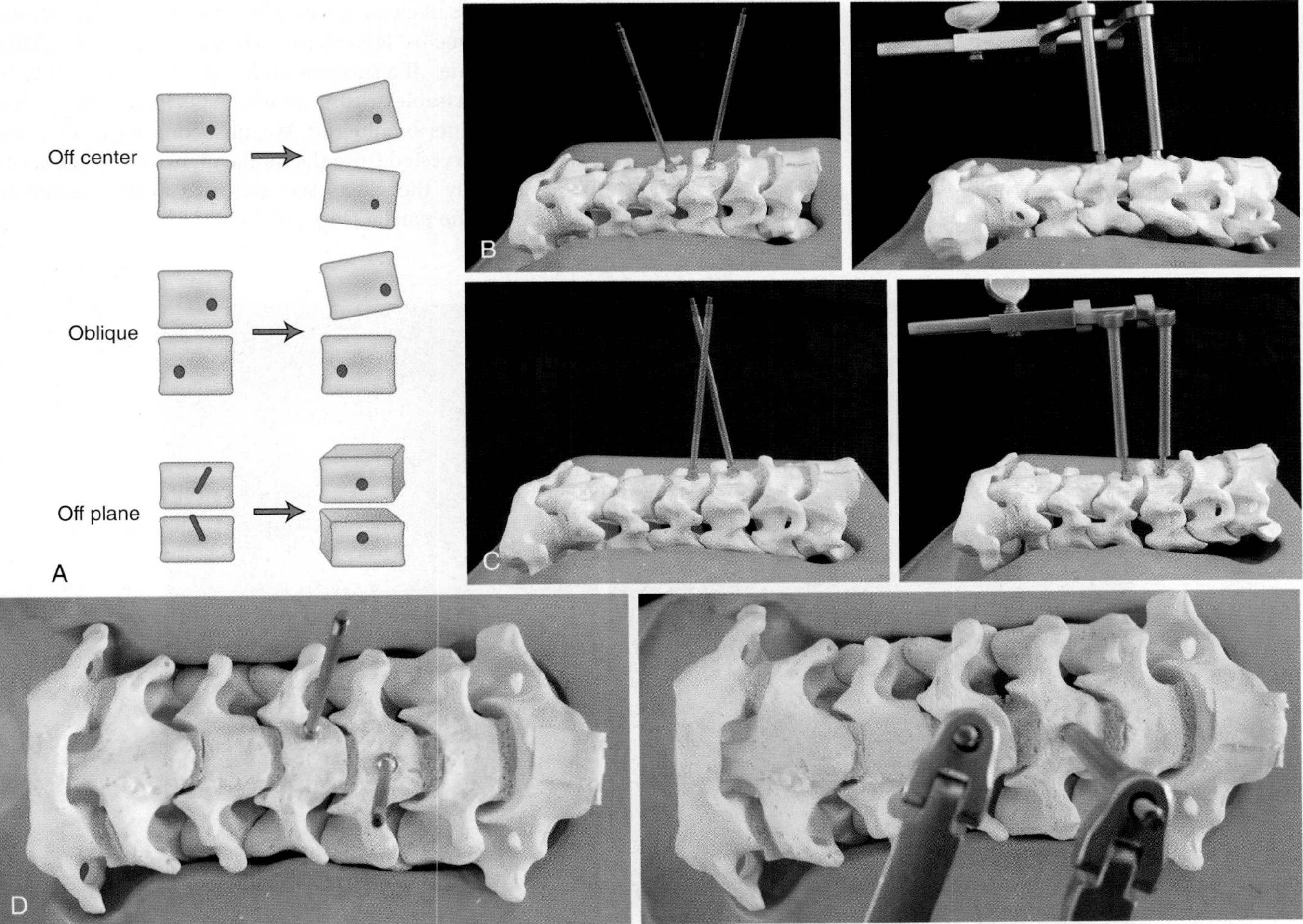

FIG. 105.2 (A) Misplacement of Caspar distraction pins may result in segmental deformity. Placing the pins off center may cause a coronal malalignment. (B) Converging pins will induce kyphosis when distraction is applied. (C) Conversely, diverging pins will induce lordosis. Pins placed obliquely off the midline will create a coronal deformity and a lateral listhesis when distraction is applied. (D) Distracting on pins that are off plane will create a rotational deformity.

lateral structures provide a fixed reference to the surgeon and assist in performing a symmetrical decompression and reconstruction.

The type of decompression performed also matters. Long corpectomies reconstructed with an allograft long bone can only be placed into a neutral or kyphotic position; because the graft is straight, it is impossible to produce lordosis. Kyphosis typically develops as the graft subsides into the endplates. To avoid this, we routinely use segmental decompression combining corpectomies at the levels that have retrovertebral compression with discectomies at levels that only have retrodiscal neural compromise (Fig. 105.4). For patients who have retrovertebral compression at more than one level, we perform a procedure that we call corpectomy-corpectomy: performing corpectomy at one level and skipping the next level, followed by a corpectomy at the third level (Fig. 105.5). This type of segmental decompression and fixation using several small grafts rather than one long strut graft allows for better preservation of cervical lordosis.

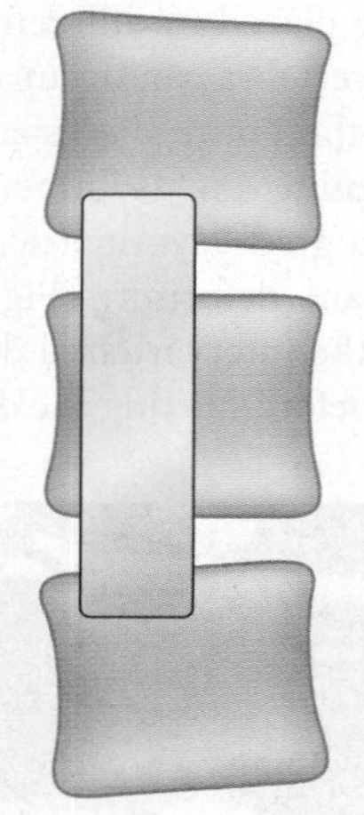

FIG. 105.3 Asymmetrical placement of graft may cause a coronal deformity.

Noninstrumented Fusion

A multilevel noninstrumented arthrodesis of the cervical spine can result in kyphosis as the grafts collapse or resorb (Fig. 105.6). Whereas the use of a plate does not absolutely guarantee the avoidance of kyphosis, most surgeons would agree that anterior cervical plates decrease the likelihood of postoperative kyphosis.[5,6]

Graft Selection

The type of graft material used can also influence the likelihood of postoperative kyphosis. In general, fresh-frozen allografts are less likely to collapse than freeze-dried bone, and freeze-dried bone is less likely to collapse than irradiated freeze-dried bone.[7] If a surgeon finds a piece of allograft to be fragile, it is advisable to use another specimen rather than implanting an inferior allograft. We most commonly use cortical allografts harvested from the fibula, ulna, radius, humerus, and occasionally the tibia. We also use dense cancellous allograft from the patella (Fig. 105.7).

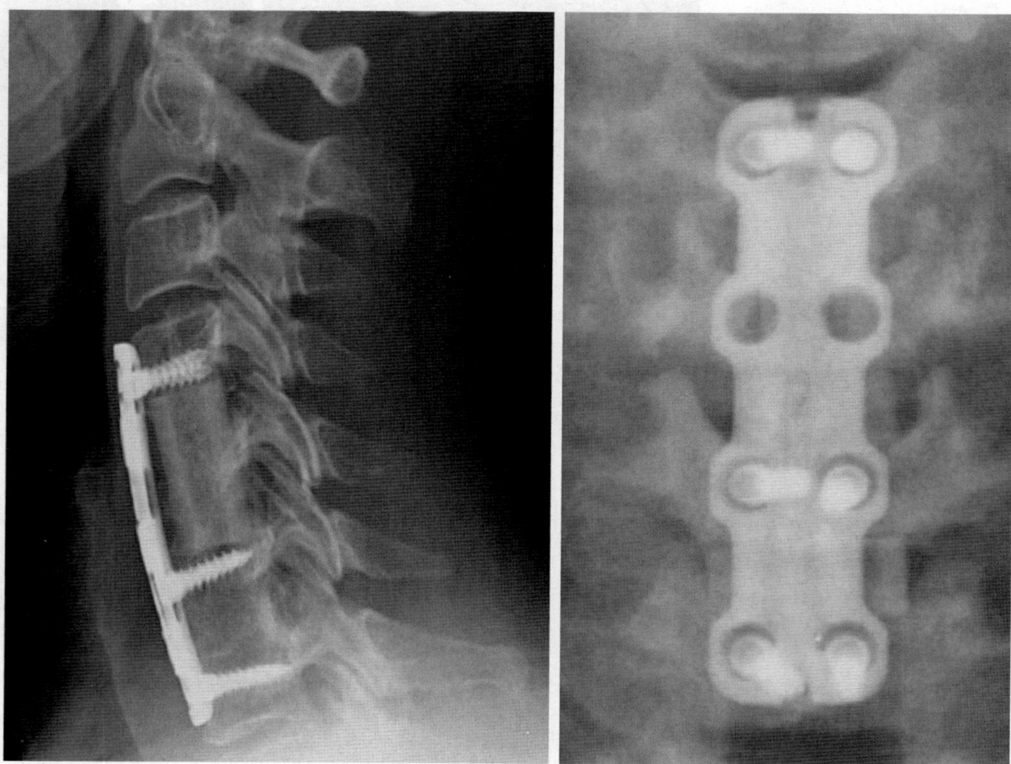

FIG. 105.4 Performing a corpectomy at one level and an adjacent discectomy (corpectomy-discectomy) provides more sites for fixation and allows the maintenance or establishment of lordosis.

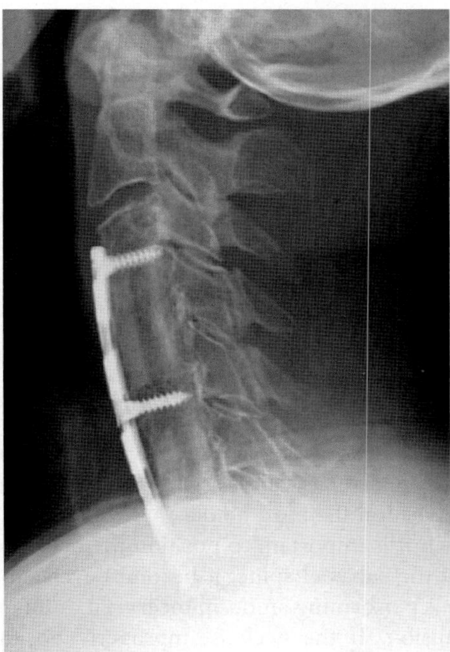

FIG. 105.5 Leaving a vertebral body intact between two corpectomies (corpectomy-corpectomy) provides an additional point of fixation in the middle of a long plate and allows for the maintenance or enhancement of lordosis.

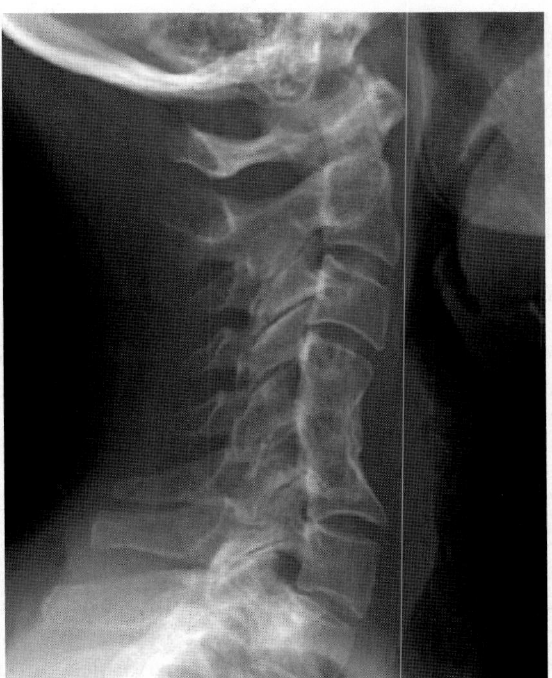

FIG. 105.6 This patient had been treated many years ago with an uninstrumented fusion from C4–C6. The graft appears to have resorbed or collapsed, resulting in segmental kyphosis. Notice the compensatory hyperlordosis at C6–C7.

The size of the graft also influences the propensity to develop postoperative kyphosis (Fig. 105.8). The grafts should be large enough to allow for 1 or 2 mm of subsidence without creating kyphosis. In addition, the more graft used per level, the less likely it is to collapse. For this reason, we routinely fill the disc space with as much graft as possible, which often means placing two allografts side by side (Fig. 105.9). More recently, we have moved to using iliac crest allograft. The width and depth of the disc spaces are measured preoperatively, and an allograft is hand selected and initially cut immediately before the skin incision. We prefer to fill the entire disc space, from uncinate to uncinate, with graft and we often insert a vertical "wedge" into a trough cut into the very lateral edge superior and inferior vertebral bodies. We have experienced higher union rates with this technique.

Anterior Instrumentation

Although judicious and careful use of anterior cervical plates can help avoid postoperative kyphosis, poor attention to detail can result in plate-induced malalignment. If a screw inadvertently perforates an adjacent disc space, it can result in rapid degeneration and collapse of that disc space. Even if the screw does not perforate the next disc space, placement of a plate within 5 mm of an adjacent level increases the likelihood of adjacent-level ossification development (Fig. 105.10).[8] The adjacent-level ossification can become quite profound, causing rapid deterioration of that adjacent disc space and resulting in kyphosis. The surgeon must be careful not to use a plate that is too long, especially when using dynamic or subsidence plates, because these will migrate toward the adjacent disc spaces as the grafts subside.

When performing anterior cervical fusions on a patient with preoperative cervical scoliosis, the surgeon must pay close attention to the overall alignment of the head, neck, and torso. Often, even in a patient with severe scoliosis, the spine rebalances itself such that the patient can hold the head in a neutral position. If the surgeon corrects the cervical scoliosis in a patient with severe thoracic curve, the head will be tilted to one side. This is analogous to correcting only the thoracic curve in a patient with a balanced and oppositely directed thoracolumbar curve, thereby causing shoulder asymmetry.

Patients who have long corpectomies are prone to graft extrusion. The reported incidence is as high as 9%.[9] Unfortunately, plates do not help prevent such complications (Fig. 105.11).[10] With static plates, extension of the neck loads the graft as the plate acts as an anterior tension band. In flexion the graft is unloaded because the anterior cervical plate acts as the center of rotation. In extension the inferior screws can pull out, and in flexion they can be driven into the next disc space, resulting in graft collapse or extrusion. To avoid these complications, we routinely perform circumferential stabilization in patients who undergo corpectomies at two or more levels. We also prefer a circumferential approach in patients with poor-quality bone who undergo single-level corpectomies.

Preventing Iatrogenic Cervical Malalignment During Posterior Surgery

Positioning

Positioning for posterior cervical procedures is just as critical as for anterior operations. We routinely use the Jackson frame (Mizuho OSI) to position our patients for posterior operations.

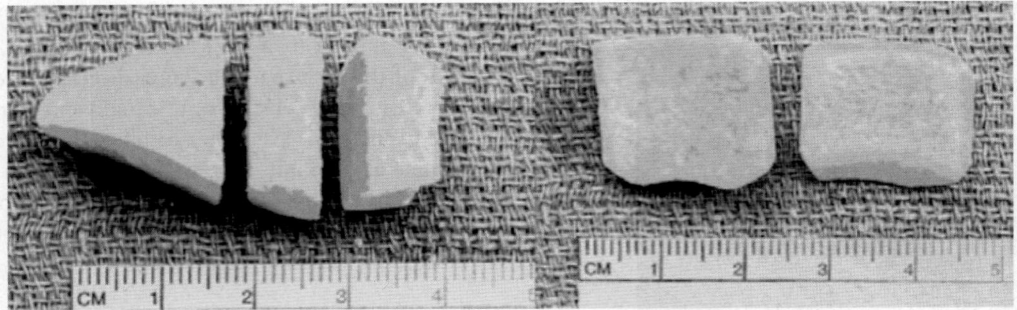

FIG. 105.7 Dense cancellous allograft may be obtained from the patella. This type of graft combines the structural integrity of cortical bone with the healing characteristics of cancellous bone.

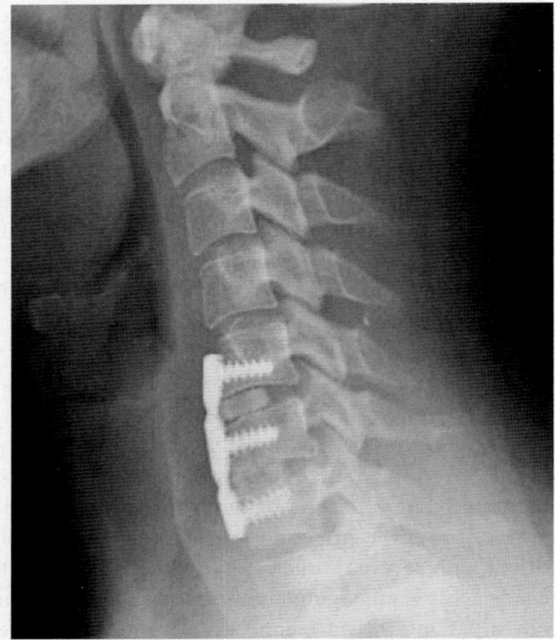

FIG. 105.8 This surgeon placed prefabricated grafts that are clearly undersized, resulting in segmental kyphosis.

We tape the shoulders down as for the anterior procedures. We also make sure that one shoulder is not pulled asymmetrically to prevent an iatrogenic coronal plane deformity. We place bolsters just underneath the clavicle and use Gardner-Wells (GW) tongs with bivector traction to allow us to position the neck in either flexion or extension. We check the position preoperatively to ensure that we can place the neck into an adequate amount of flexion and extension. Foraminotomies are best accomplished with the neck in maximal flexion, which unshingles the facets and exposes the underlying superior articular facet. If the neck is not adequately flexed during a foraminotomy, a large amount of the overhanging inferior articular facet must be resected to expose the underlying superior facet. This may weaken the structure and lead to a fracture. More commonly, it makes it difficult to place a lateral mass screw in patients who require fusion and decompression. Before fusion, we change the weight from the lower, or flexion, rope to the upper, or extension, rope. The advantage of using bivector tong traction is that the surgeon can easily alter the position of the neck intraoperatively. With fixed head holders such as Mayfield tongs, an assistant has to crawl under the table to reposition the head holder.

Although it is important to position the neck properly for fixation of the subaxial spine, it becomes even more critical when one is performing an occipitocervical or an occiput-to-thoracic fusion. If the neck is improperly positioned and instrumented, the resulting malalignment can be quite debilitating. Phillips and colleagues[11] measured the occipitocervical angle on 30 normal cervical spine radiographs of patients in flexion, extension, and neutral alignment. The occipitocervical angle was defined as the angle between the McRae line (the line connecting the basion and opisthion, which demarcates the foramen magnum on a lateral radiograph) and a line parallel to the rostral endplate of C3. The mean occipitocervical angle on the neutral radiographs was 44 degrees. Phillips and colleagues[11] recommend that when performing an occipitocervical fixation and fusion, the surgeon should try to fix the occiput and upper cervical spine in as close to this value as possible to provide the patient with a functional head position (Fig. 105.12). We concur with this for patients with occipitocervical fusions. However, when performing occiput-to-thoracic fusions, we prefer to fix the patient with 5 to 10 degrees of flexion compared with normal. This is because these patients are unable to bend their necks at all, and if they undergo fusion looking straight ahead they cannot look down to see their own bodies.

Decompression

Deformities can result from overly aggressive decompressions of the cervical spine. Even minimally invasive procedures such as posterior cervical foraminotomies can result in a postoperative deformity. If the procedure is performed through a small tubular retractor by a surgeon who is not intimately familiar with the microanatomy of the facet joint or who loses anatomic landmarks, too much of the facet may be resected. Zdeblick et al. demonstrated that resection of more than 50% of a facet can result in instability (Fig. 105.13).[12] To prevent this, the surgeon must always identify and visualize the lateral and medial aspects of the facet joint and take care to resect only the medial half of the joint.

A more common deformity-causing decompression is a laminectomy without a fusion. Laminectomies in children

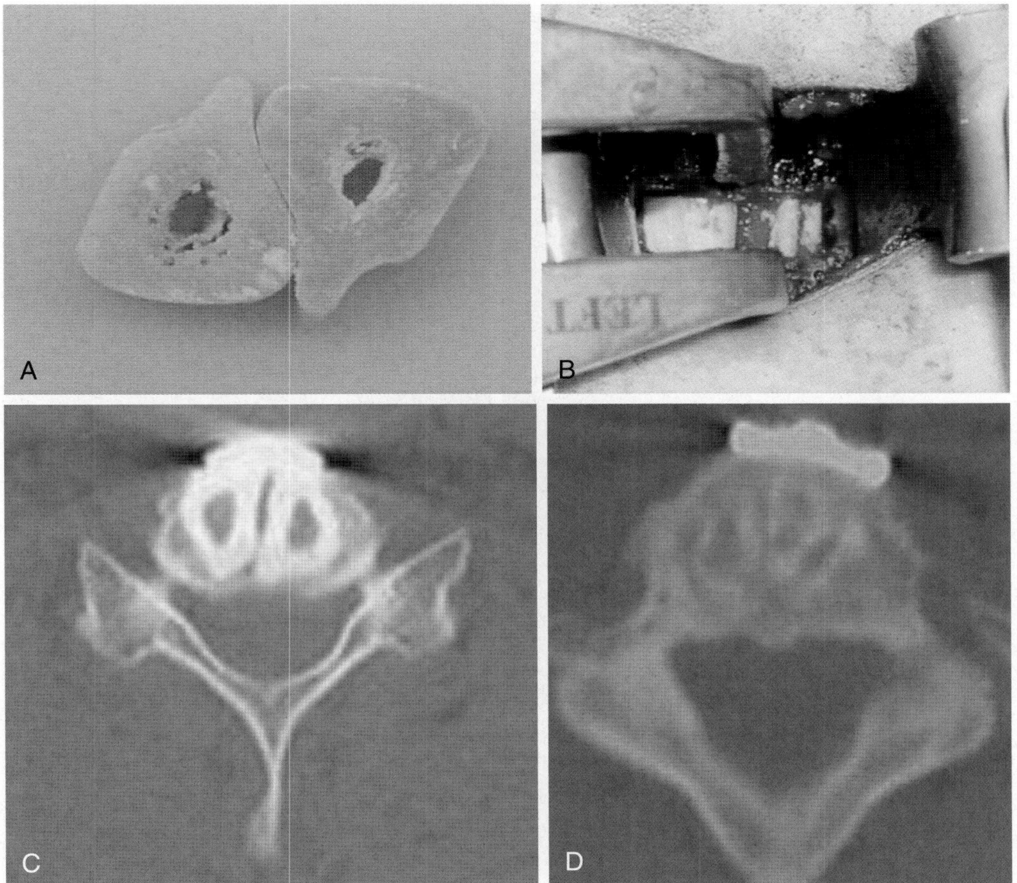

FIG. 105.9 When using cortical allografts, we prefer to use two or three grafts to maximally fill the disc space. (A) Double grafts before insertion. (B) Grafts in place. (C) Radiographic appearance of grafts. (D) At C6–C7 and below, three fibular grafts are occasionally necessary to fill the entire disc space.

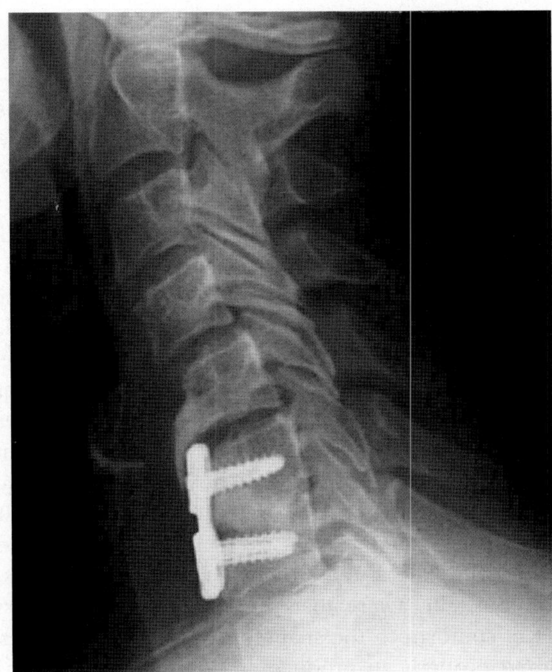

FIG. 105.10 If a plate is too close to the neighboring disc space, adjacent-level ossification disease may occur.

have been associated with a high incidence of postlaminectomy kyphosis (Fig. 105.14).[13] Even in adults it is difficult to predict when a patient might develop postoperative kyphosis. We therefore reserve complete laminectomies for patients who have significant anterior-stabilizing osteophytes with minimal range of motion of the cervical spine.

To avoid the complications associated with complete laminectomies, we prefer to perform laminoplasties. Laminoplasties are not without potential complications, however. It is possible to resect too much of the facet when performing foraminotomies along with laminoplasties that can result in instability and deformity. In addition, when performing a laminoplasty of C2, care must be taken to reattach the semispinalis cervicis muscle, which acts as the major extensor muscle of the neck. Failure to reattach this muscle can result in cervical kyphosis.

Noninstrumented Fusion

We believe that noninstrumented fusions of the posterior cervical spine are rarely, if ever, indicated. With safe and effective modern instrumentation, including lateral mass screws, spinous process wires/cables, and polyaxial screw-rod instrumentation, it is rare for us to find a situation in which we

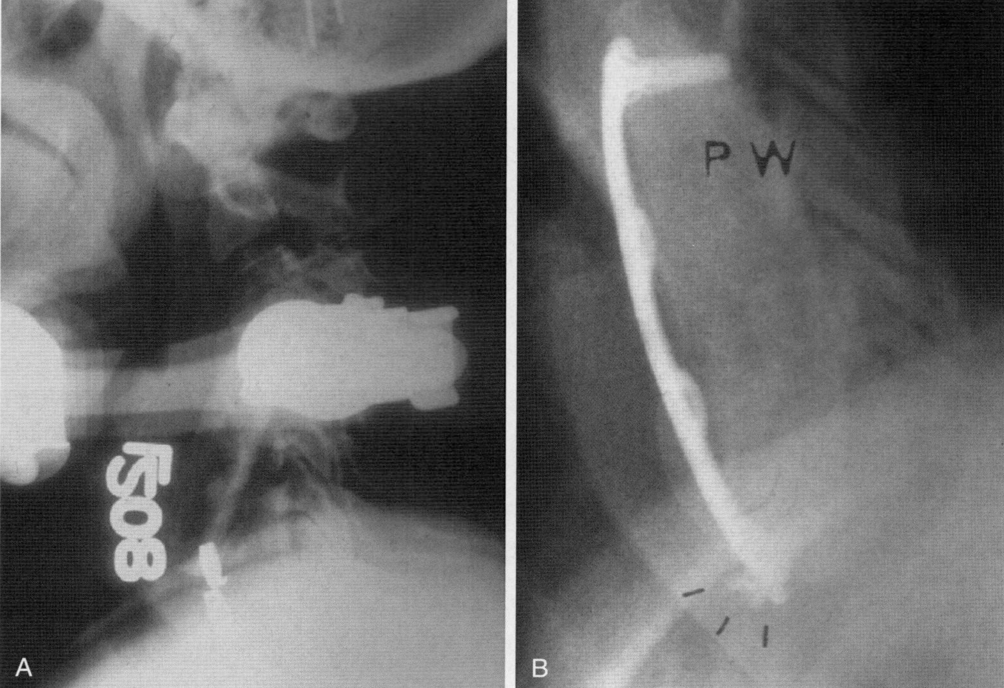

FIG. 105.11 (A) This patient had a two-level corpectomy. Graft extrusion occurred despite postoperative immobilization in a two-poster brace. (B) This lateral radiograph illustrates what can happen after a long corpectomy. The plate does not prevent subsidence and collapse of the graft and screw into the next disc space occurs.

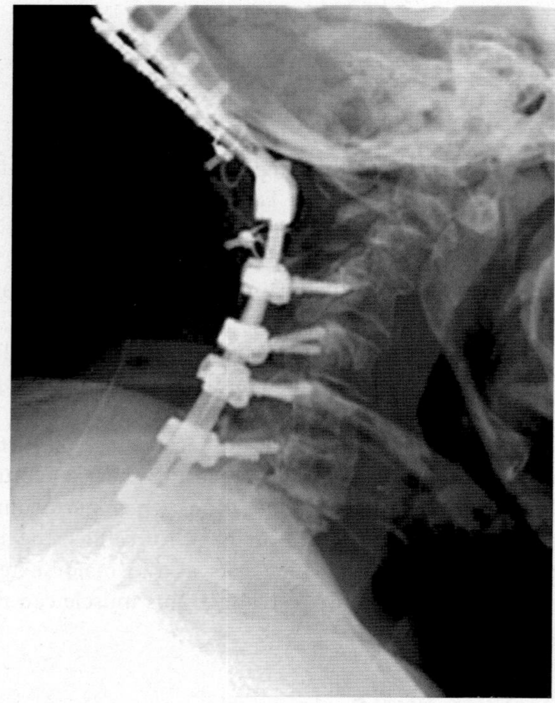

FIG. 105.12 It is important to position the patient properly before an occipitocervical or occipitocervicothoracic fusion to provide the patient with a functional position after fusion. We place the neck in slight flexion so that the patient can see his or her own body.

would consider a noninstrumented arthrodesis. A patient who undergoes a noninstrumented arthrodesis often has pain posteriorly, resulting in the loss of normal lordosis. As the spine fuses, it generally does so in a kyphotic or, at best, straight alignment (Fig. 105.15).

Inadequate Instrumentation

The use of inadequate instrumentation can result in postoperative malalignment. For example, in trauma cases in which patients have significant osteoligamentous disruption resulting in an unstable spine, the surgeon must achieve solid fixation with instrumentation to stabilize that segment. If the spinous processes and/or the lateral masses have been disrupted so that adequate bony purchase cannot be obtained, the fixation may have to be extended cranially and caudally until good purchase is located. Alternatively, circumferential stabilization can be performed. If the fixation is still inadequate, consideration should be given to immobilizing the patient in a halo vest. To the extent possible, all fixation points should be used. The greater the instability, the greater the necessity to obtain adequate bony purchase at multiple levels (Figs. 105.16 and 105.17).

When using lateral mass or pedicle screws and rods, the surgeon must be aware that the relatively flexible cervical spine will conform to the shape of the rod. If the rod is not contoured properly to produce an acceptable sagittal alignment, the cervical spine will conform to the rod and be fixed in a suboptimal alignment. Modern polyaxial screws allow for

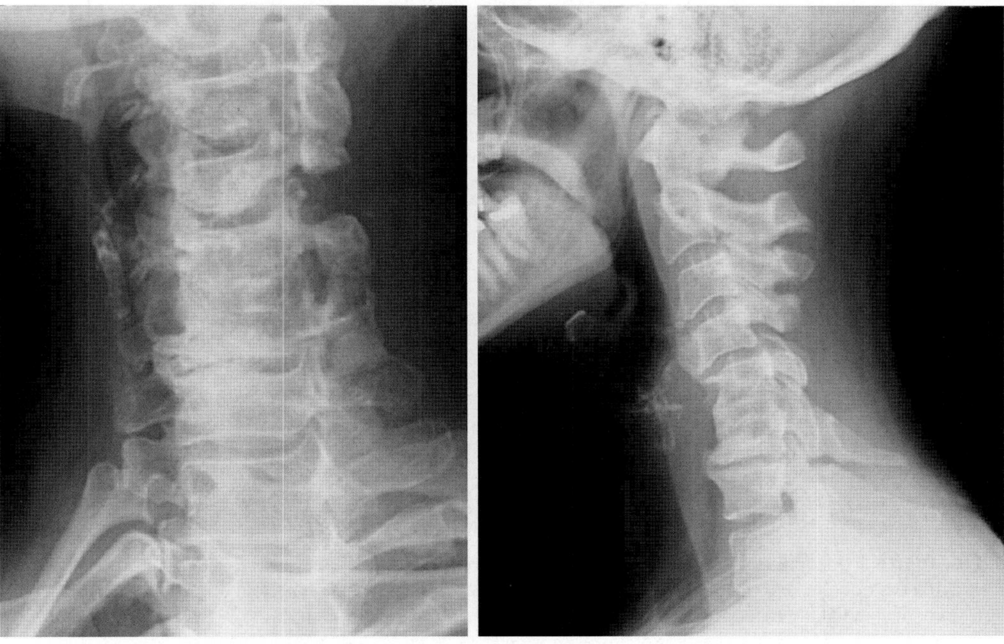

FIG. 105.13 Resection of more than 50% of the facet, particularly in the setting of a complete laminectomy, may lead to kyphosis.

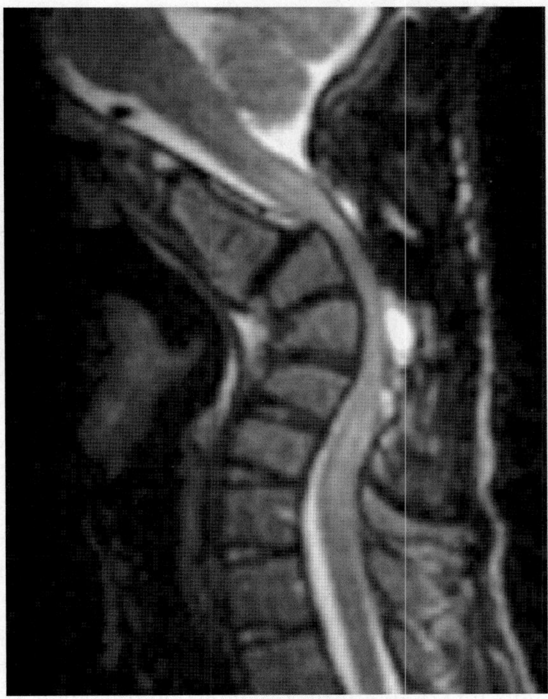

FIG. 105.14 Sagittal magnetic resonance image demonstrating cervical kyphosis in a patient who underwent multilevel laminectomies without fusion in childhood.

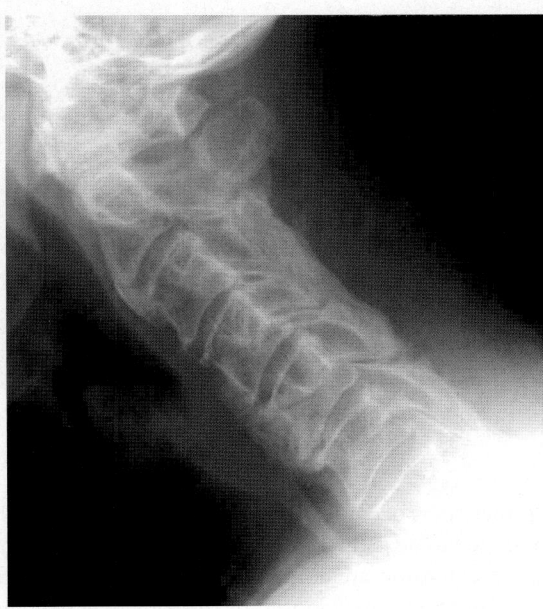

FIG. 105.15 A noninstrumented posterior cervical fusion with loss of cervical lordosis.

some mediolateral offset of the screw heads. However, if the screws are placed too far laterally or medially beyond the ability of the screw to accommodate the placement, lateral listhesis of one vertebral segment may occur. If the listhesis is extreme, it may even cause nerve root compression. This can be especially troublesome when attaching a C2 pedicle screw (directed from a lateral-to-medial direction) to a lateral mass screw at C3 (directed from a medial-to-lateral direction). The directional change of these screws is such that occasionally C3 must be bypassed and the rod placed from C2 down to a screw at C4. A similar situation arises when transitioning from a lateral mass screw at C6 or C7 to a pedicle screw at the adjacent caudal level.

Even when an arthrodesis is performed with the neck in lordotic alignment with adequate fixation, postoperative

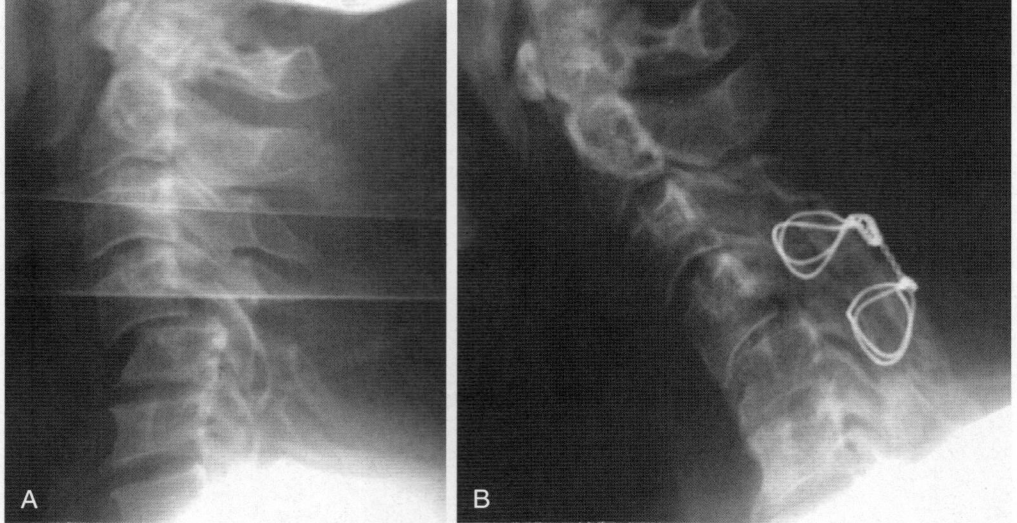

FIG. 105.16 Inadequate fixation after traumatic injury to the cervical spine may lead to iatrogenic deformity. This spine is not fully reduced, and these types of sublaminar wires are inadequate to maintain proper alignment. In addition, they are contraindicated in patients with neurologic deficits.

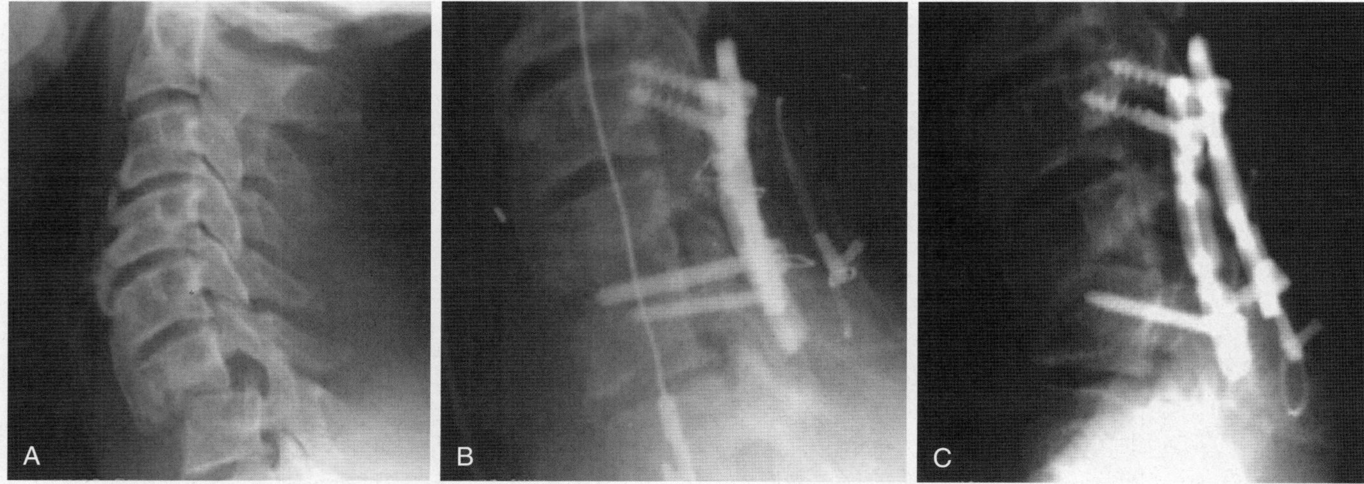

FIG. 105.17 All available fixation points should be used to reduce the likelihood of implant failure and deformity.

malalignment may occur. Patients with a preoperative kyphotic alignment due to degenerative disc disease who are fused with the neck in extension are at risk for developing postoperative kyphosis. The screws may loosen or the rods may bend as the spine settles back into its preoperative kyphotic alignment. Patients who have severe preoperative kyphosis or who have poor muscle control are often best treated with a circumferential procedure.

Surgical Treatment of Iatrogenic Deformity

Our surgical algorithm depends on multiple factors, including symptom pattern, deformity characteristics, previous surgeries, location of fusion mass, neurologic status, and clinical factors such as patient comorbidities. For patients deemed appropriate for maximal correction, the location of existing fusion mass drives our surgical planning. In addition to standard anterior/posterior decompression and instrumentation techniques, the deformity surgeon must often rely on spinal osteotomies or a combination thereof.

In general, we characterize cervical osteotomies as an anterior osteotomy (ATO), the posterior-based Smith-Petersen osteotomy (SPO), or a pedicle subtraction osteotomy (PSO). Additional classification systems, such as that proposed by Ames and the International Spine Study Group, have further subclassified cervical osteotomies for rigid deformity. In one of our recent publications, the results of 61 patients undergoing cervical osteotomy over a 10-year period were analyzed for corrective potential and blood loss.[14] On average isolated SPO, PSO, and ATO yielded 10, 35, and 17 degrees of angular correction, respectively, whereas an ATO with SPO provided at least equal correction of a PSO with less blood loss.

Cervical Osteotomy Description

Anterior Osteotomy

When approaching the anterior spine for rigid kyphosis, patient setup is critical for optimizing access. The patient is placed supine with a foam donut and sheets under the head. GW tongs are placed and traction initiated using 5 lb of weight. All patients with previous anterior surgery undergo the aforementioned evaluation. To approach the deformed spine a standard Smith-Robinson approach is used with a horizontal incision along Langerhans lines and extensive soft tissue dissection to allow access at least one to two levels above and below the desired area. Scoliotic spines are approached from the convex side where appropriate. Care must be taken to evaluate the preoperative MRI to determine the relationship of the vertebral artery to the costal processes and the foramen transversarium.

When performing an ATO, wide, symmetrical exposure of the anterior cervical spine is essential to a successful procedure. During exposure it is sometimes difficult to determine where the former disc space was. The best way to identify this is to elevate the longus colli muscles far laterally over the transverse processes. A Penfield No. 4 dissector can be used to palpate the lateral margin of the uncovertebral joint. This identifies where the old disc space used to be. To release the fusion mass and allow correction of the kyphosis, the entire width of the disc space must be exposed and drilled. The surgeon must be careful to maintain parallel surfaces of all osteotomies to prevent creating a new deformity. To achieve this, a total of four Caspar pins are placed perpendicular to the anterior plane above and below the levels of the resection to aid in generating lordosis. In the kyphotic spine, the pin tips will diverge while the insertion ends converge.

Once the area of interest is identified, a high-speed burr is then used to take down the fusion at the level of the original disc space. We routinely use a 3-mm carbide tip burr to perform this decompression. A diamond burr is not necessary and simply delays the case and increases the amount of heat production, which can injure the neural elements. Central bony resection is performed posteriorly to the level of the posterolateral ligament with the burr in constant motion. The lateral bony resection should be approached with extreme caution as the vertebral artery remains at risk for injury. The lateral border of the uncinate process is defined with a microcurette aimed medially to make room for placement of a Penfield No. 4 or 2 dissector or small cottonoid. With the lateral edge protected, the high-speed burr is used to resect the lateral bone from ventral to dorsal. Remaining bony shell can be removed with a microcurette. This can only be accomplished after burring all the way posteriorly through the fusion mass until the posterior longitudinal ligament is visualized. If the posterior longitudinal ligament has already been resected, there is usually still scar ventral to the thecal sac that protects it from inadvertent laceration by the burr. The bone should be resected uncinate to uncinate to allow closure without nerve root compression within the foramen. Asymmetric resection can also allow correction in the coronal plane. The degree of this osteotomy may range from partial uncovertebral joint resection to partial and complete corpectomy depending on corrective needs (Ames grade 1, 3, 4).

Once the ATO is complete, deformity correction is initiated by removing the sheets from underneath the patient's head while gently pressing on the forehead. We have found downward pressure on the head to be the safest technique and even capable of achieving correction through a posterior fusion mass. In addition, a vertebral body spreader (or Cobb) can be placed into the disc space itself. The disc space is then gradually distracted one click at a time, using all three devices. If the posterior fusion mass is not massive, it often has some plasticity such that placing enough extension moment on the anterior spine can bend it. Slow, steady distraction causes plastic deformation of the posterior fusion mass and achieves relative extension across the osteotomy. By slowly performing these maneuvers, one can often extend the disc space by 3 to 5 mm. An additional 10 to 20 lb are placed on the GW tongs if needed.

Once correction is achieved, a structural graft is placed in the anterior half of the disc space that has been created. A structural graft of maximal mediolateral width, shaped with the anterior height taller than the posterior, is sized to fit snugly into the expanded osteotomy site. The ideal graft has good contact with the anterior aspect of the vertebral bodies but has some room to settle into further lordosis following the subsequent posterior osteotomy. The graft should only occupy approximately the anterior two-thirds of the vertebral body so that there is no chance of retropulsion during the posterior operation. The surgeon should also ensure that the posterior aspect of the endplates behind the graft is not touching, because further extension can be obtained after the posterior osteotomy if needed.

An anterior plate with fixed-angle screws is used if the deformity has been completely corrected, but if further posterior correction is desired a trapezoid-shaped graft is placed in the anterior portion of the osteotomy site. A buttress plate at the lower level is placed to prevent graft extrusion during the posterior portion of the procedure. Alternatively, a dynamic cervical plate, which allows for translation, may be used to hold the graft(s) in place. By placing the graft on the anterior portion of the disc space during the anterior operation, the surgeon can hinge off of this graft and extend the spine after removing the dorsal fusion mass. For circumferential cases, this technique can sometimes prevent having to perform a three-part operation with an anterior, posterior, followed by a repeat anterior operation. Even if additional correction is not needed, we commonly augment the anterior procedure with a posterior arthrodesis and instrumentation.

Posterior Osteotomy

Posterior osteotomies range from partial to complete facet joint resection (SPO) to a closing-wedge pedicle subtraction osteotomy (PSO). Whether performed as the first procedure or as a second stage after an anterior surgery, the patient is placed in prone position using a GW bivector traction setup as previously described.

When performing an SPO, a midline posterior approach is performed with meticulous dissection to stay midline and minimize blood loss. In cases of previous posterior arthrodesis, all soft tissues are stripped from the spine. Any bone between the spinous processes is resected, and a thin Leksell rongeur can be used to take down the fusion mass over the facet joints. The remaining bone is then resected with a 3-mm high-speed burr. Lateral mass screws are then placed. The neck is then placed into a normal lordotic position using the extension rope of the bivector traction described earlier. If the spinous process or fusion mass is adequate, a cable connecting the cranial and caudal segments can be used to help extend the spine and hold it in the desired position until the rods are engaged into the lateral mass screws. Sufficient bone must be removed, both to allow correction of the deformity and to ensure that neural compression does not occur during this step. As in primary posterior procedures, the surgeon should use all available fixation sites to ensure a solid construct.

In performing a PSO, the same steps are taken with additional bone resection and closure required. We have been using PSOs less often given the corrective power of a combined ATO/SPO approach, for which blood loss and complications are significantly less. Nonetheless, a PSO can provide powerful angular correction and may be indicated in certain circumstances of severe cervical kyphosis, such as those where an anterior Smith-Robinson approach might not be safe. In general a cervical PSO is performed at C7 or below. Typically the vertebral artery will not be present in the foramen at C7, and the size of the canal and mobility of the C8 nerve root tend to result in a safer operation. Surgeons should appreciate that cervical PSO poses significant risk of cervical nerve palsies of the hand. For a detailed step-by-step description of the PSO technique, see the work by Wollowick and Riew et al.[15]

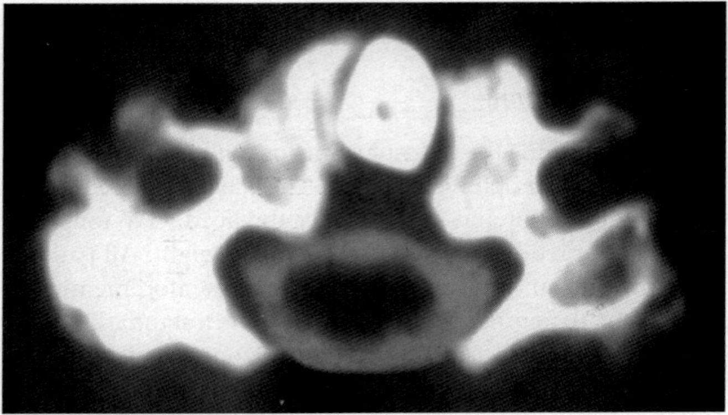

FIG. 105.18 This patient has had a laminectomy and subsequent corpectomy. Note that the two halves of the spine are connected only by soft tissue posteriorly and by the newly placed graft anteriorly.

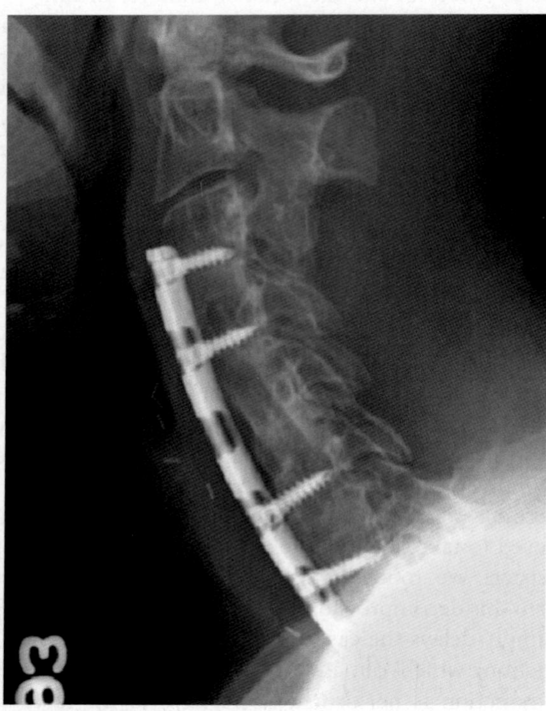

FIG. 105.19 This patient had a postlaminectomy kyphosis and myelopathy. There was cord compression behind C5, necessitating a corpectomy. At C3–C4, C6–C7, and C7–T1 there was only retrodiscal compression, which was decompressed with discectomies. With four fixation points above and six fixation points below the corpectomy, in a patient with good bone density, an anterior-only procedure was sufficiently rigid and stable to achieve a solid fusion with acceptable alignment.

Surgical Algorithm and Case Examples

Prior Laminectomies

A special situation arises when a patient who has previously undergone a laminectomy has persistent anterior compression and requires an anterior corpectomy with reconstruction. In these cases, we generally recommend a circumferential operation with anterior corpectomy followed by posterior stabilization with lateral mass instrumentation. Even with halo vest immobilization postoperatively, these patients are at a high risk for graft extrusion, collapse, and recurrent kyphosis.[16] Patients who have undergone a laminectomy and subsequently undergo an anterior corpectomy have two halves of the spine connected only by soft tissues (Fig. 105.18). These patients are extremely unstable to both rotation and flexion-extension forces. We strongly believe that in the majority of cases these patients are best treated with instrumentation circumferentially as well as adequate postoperative immobilization.

In patients who have excellent bone quality and who only require a single-level corpectomy, the surgeon can occasionally perform a single-level corpectomy at the level of retrovertebral compression and discectomies at the levels with only retrodiscal compression. If four screw points can be obtained above the level of the corpectomy and four to six points below, and if a rigid collar is used postoperatively, it may be possible to treat the patient with an anterior-only operation (Fig. 105.19). But for the majority of patients who have significant kyphosis and persistent stenosis requiring a cervical corpectomy, circumferential instrumentation is indicated. Because these patients have unstable cervical spines, the use of lateral mass instrumentation alone may result in failure, especially in patients with osteoporosis (Fig. 105.20).

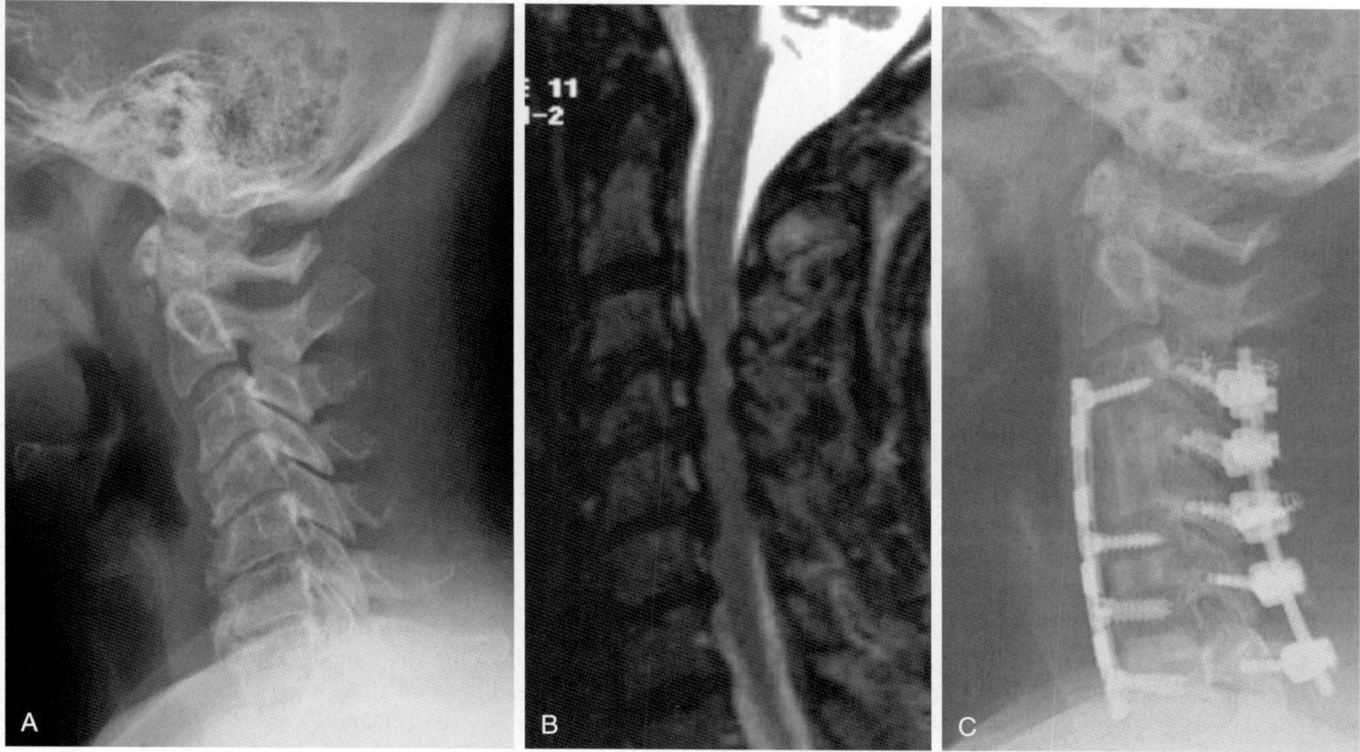

FIG. 105.20 This patient had congenital spinal stenosis, ossification of posterior longitudinal ligament, and kyphosis, the combination of which was causing myelopathy. After a laminectomy, she developed further kyphosis. We decompressed and instrumented her circumferentially. In someone with chronic kyphosis, there is a propensity for the kyphosis to recur, especially if the patient is osteoporotic. Adequate circumferential fixation is critical for preventing postoperative malalignment in such situations.

Prior Fusion

The fundamental principle of the treatment of iatrogenic cervical deformity is to approach the spine first from the side (anterior or posterior) with the previous fusion. Performing an osteotomy through the previous fusion provides the flexibility necessary to realign the spine. As discussed later, in cases of previous circumferential fusion, approaching the spine anteriorly first may allow the surgeon to perform a two-stage operation and avoid the need for a three-stage procedure. After the deformity is corrected, the surgeon must obtain solid fixation. Sometimes this can be accomplished with either anterior or posterior instrumentation, but often we prefer to use circumferential fixation for patients requiring osteotomies. Finally, the patient must be immobilized properly in the postoperative period.

Prior Anterior Fusion With No Posterior Fusion Mass

A patient with a previous anterior fusion and a kyphotic deformity is treated first with an anterior procedure. The nature of the prior operation, the nature of the deformity, and the location of neural compression, if any, all affect the surgeon's decision about whether to perform a discectomy, a corpectomy, or a combination procedure (e.g., corpectomy-corpectomy, corpectomy-discectomy).

Prior Posterior Fusion

In cases of previous posterior fusion, the posterior spine is approached first and osteotomies are performed through the fusion mass. Any bone between the spinous processes is resected, and a thin Leksell rongeur can be used to take down the fusion mass over the facet joints. The remaining bone is then resected with a 3-mm high-speed burr. Lateral mass screws are then placed. The neck is then placed into a normal lordotic position using the extension rope of the bivector traction described earlier. If there are adequate spinous processes or fusion mass, a cable connecting the cranial and caudal segments can be used to help extend the spine and hold it in the desired position until the rods are engaged into the lateral mass screws. Sufficient bone must be removed, both to allow correction of the deformity and to ensure that neural compression does not occur during this step. As in primary posterior procedures, the surgeon should use all available fixation sites to ensure a solid construct.

Case Study 1

This case (Fig. 105.21) illustrates what can be done if a patient has only a solid posterior fusion mass with no fusion anteriorly. This patient had undergone a posterior cervical fusion at an outside institution using wires. She presented to us several years later with severe neck pain, kyphosis, and persistent

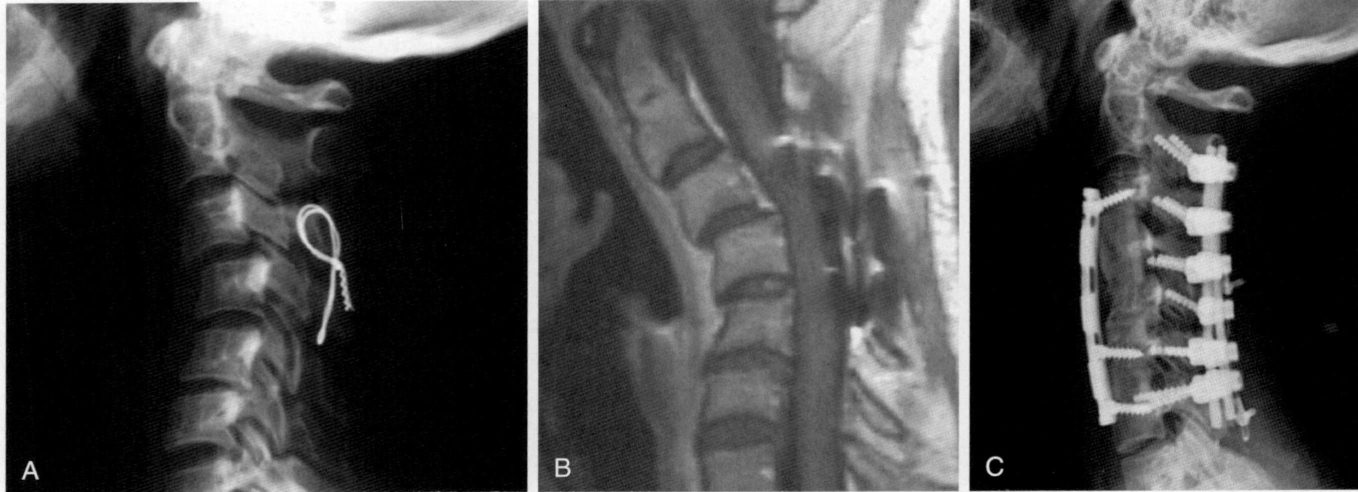

FIG. 105.21 Case study 1 in a patient with a solid posterior fusion mass with no fusion anteriorly. (A) Preoperative lateral radiograph. (B) Magnetic resonance image. (C) Postoperative lateral radiograph.

myeloradiculopathy. She was found to have disc protrusions at C5–C6 and C6–C7. She had retrovertebral compression behind C4 and retrodiscal compression at C5–C6 and C6–C7. We approached her posteriorly first and performed an osteotomy through the facet at C3–C4. We were then able to correct most of her kyphosis posteriorly using segmental instrumentation. We then turned her anteriorly and performed combinations of corpectomies and discectomies to restore her overall alignment and to decompress her C5–C6 and C6–C7 levels. She did quite well postoperatively with complete resolution of myeloradiculopathy and axial neck pain.

Case Study 2

This case (Fig. 105.22) illustrates the use of the fusion mass to achieve a solid fusion and obtain bony fixation points. This child was status post C1 and C2 laminectomy and occipitocervical fusion for congenital cervical anomalies. Unfortunately, the occipital fixation pulled out but the child went on to a solid fusion with the neck in kyphosis (see Fig. 105.22A). As the child continued to grow, C2 began to grow into the foramen magnum, causing compression of the pons. We performed an osteotomy of the fusion mass (see Fig. 105.22B). The bone between the foramen magnum and the fusion mass was resected, revealing the underlying thecal sac. Then the fusion mass was cut on the lateral margins down to about C3. At the caudal margin, a trough was created so that it could act as a hinge from which the fusion mass could be lifted dorsally to decompress the proximal spinal cord. We then extended the neck and dorsally lifted up the fusion mass (see Fig. 105.22C). The dorsal aspect of the skull at the level of the foramen magnum was in contact with the fusion mass. A small window was left centrally so that we could directly visualize the proximal cord to confirm that there was no compression. Occipitocervical instrumentation was then placed both laterally into the fusion masses and centrally into the fusion masses and the remaining spinous processes (see Fig. 105.22D). Normally such a small child would have poor fixation points. However, using any and all bony fixation points can allow for solid rigid fixation. The patient had a functional head position after surgery, and a solid fusion was obtained (see Fig. 105.22E and F).

Case Study 3

This case (Fig. 105.23) illustrates what can be done with a multiply operated patient with a problem with soft tissue coverage. In this case the patient had a C6 corpectomy and a posterior fusion from C4–C7 at another institution (see Fig. 105.23A). This was complicated by a postoperative infection, which necessitated that the wound be kept open and allowed to granulate in. At the time of her presentation to us, the spinous processes were still exposed (see Fig. 102.23B) and she reported intolerable neck pain. We treated her initially by placing her in a halo vest to extend the neck to decrease the tension on her wound. This allowed the wound to finish granulating in so that the spinous processes were covered. We operated on her once the erythrocyte sedimentation rate had normalized and we were sure that there was no further evidence of any infection. She was fused from C4–C7 and autofused from C7–T1. We approached her posteriorly first and took down the old fusion mass at C4–C5 and then reinstrumented her from C2–C6. We also fused and instrumented T1–T2 but did not attach the cervical and thoracic constructs because she had a solid fusion over this intervening area and because this was the area where she had the least amount of soft tissue coverage. We believed that dominoes at this level would have been too bulky in an area where she had little to no soft tissue coverage. We then turned her anteriorly and performed discectomies and fusions at C2–C3, C3–C4, and C4–C5. Because of the titanium cage that was placed anteriorly, we elected not to perform an osteotomy through the old fusion mass. Although we certainly could have achieved a better correction by taking down the old fusion mass at the C6 corpectomy site, this would have necessitated an anterior osteotomy followed by another posterior operation. We believed that this would have

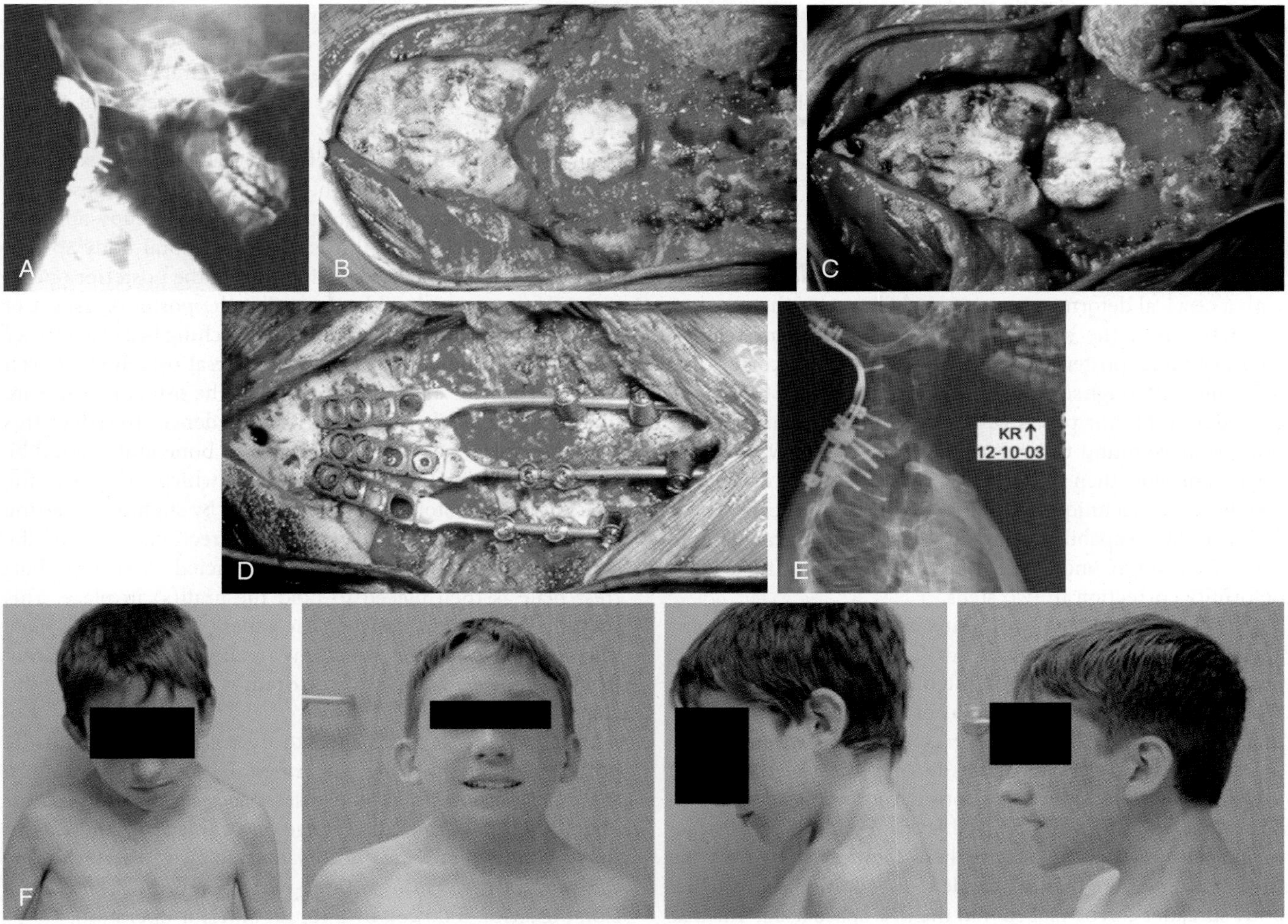

FIG. 105.22 Case study 2 illustrating use of a fusion mass to achieve a solid fusion and obtain bony fixation points. (A) Fusion in kyphosis after implants pulled out. (B) After osteotomy of fusion mass. (C) After closure of the osteotomy. (D) Multiple fixation points are obtained. (E) Postoperative radiograph. (F) Preoperative and postoperative images.

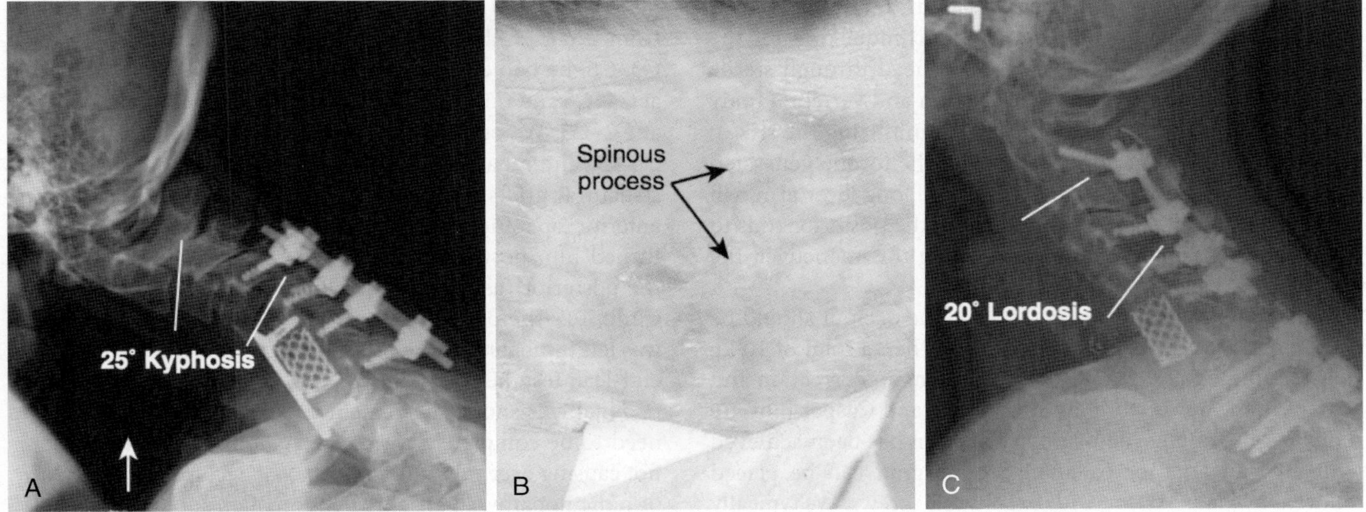

FIG. 105.23 (A) Preoperative lateral neutral radiograph. (B) Exposed spinous processes with friable skin that was stretched tight. (C) Postoperative lateral radiograph showing correction with kyphosis.

unnecessarily prolonged her case. The posterior operation was performed in 4 hours, and the anterior operation was performed in 1 hour and 45 minutes, allowing us to extubate the patient immediately postoperatively. We were able to correct her from 12 degrees of kyphosis to 4 degrees of lordosis over the C4–C5 segment (see Fig. 105.23C).

Prior Circumferential Fusion

A patient with solid arthrodeses anteriorly and posteriorly with a cervical deformity presents a challenge to the surgeon. In these cases, the surgeon often has to perform releases anteriorly and posteriorly before being able to correct the deformity. Although some surgeons recommend a "540-degree" procedure (anterior-posterior-anterior) for deformity correction, we have found that patients can be treated with a two-stage (anterior then posterior) procedure with acceptable results.[17] The technique uses the plasticity of the posterior fusion and the capability of modern anterior cervical plates to allow translation and angulation of the screws to achieve deformity correction in two steps.

The first part of the procedure is to approach the spine anteriorly and release the anterior fusion mass, as described previously. The osteotomy or osteotomies extend across the entire width of the fusion mass to ensure complete release and maximal flexibility. The posterior aspect of the vertebral body is resected slightly greater than the anterior aspect so that it can be closed down further. Thorough foraminotomies must be completed at all osteotomized levels. Four Caspar distractor pins are then placed across the osteotomy site(s): two on the right side and two on the left. In addition, a vertebral body spreader can be placed into the disc space itself. The disc space is then gradually distracted one click at a time, using all three devices. If the posterior fusion mass is not massive, it often has some plasticity such that placing enough extension moment on the anterior spine can bend it. Slow, steady distraction causes plastic deformation of the posterior fusion mass and achieves relative extension across the osteotomy. In patients with posterior instrumentation and fusion, a partial correction can still be obtainable during the anterior portion of the case. We use the same reduction technique of using the surgeon's hand against the patient's forehead through sterile sheets to assist the Caspar pin distraction and vertebral body elevator in deformity correction while minimizing the risk of vertebral body fracture or pin cut-out. The torque generated by the force of the surgeon's hand and the long lever arm will create a significant torque that can cause the posterior rods to bend into lordosis. By slowly performing this maneuver, the disc space can be extended by 3 to 5 mm.

After anterior deformity correction, the occiput should be resting on the table without any sheets. Then a total of 10 kg weight is placed on the GW tongs to maintain correction and stability, and the vertebral body spreader and Caspar pins are removed. If complete deformity correction has been achieved with only an anterior osteotomy, bone graft can be placed followed by plate fixation with fixed-angle screws. We typically augment anterior fixation with posterior screws placed in situ even if no further correction is needed.

If the deformity correction is not complete, a structural graft is placed in the anterior half of the disc space that has been created. A trapezoid-shaped structural graft, with the anterior height taller than the posterior, is sized to fit snugly into the expanded osteotomy site. The ideal graft has good contact with the anterior aspect of the vertebral bodies but has some room to settle into further lordosis after the subsequent posterior osteotomy. The graft should only occupy approximately the anterior two-thirds of the vertebral body so that there is no chance of retropulsion during the posterior operation. The surgeon should ensure that the posterior aspect of the endplates behind the graft is not touching because further extension can be obtained after the dorsal osteotomy. Given that the superior and inferior edges of the osteotomy site are often cancellous, there is a risk for subsidence. To reduce this risk, the largest possible surface area of bone graft should be used in the medial to lateral direction, which minimizes the stress at the osteotomy site. In addition, by slightly oversizing the graft in the cephalad-to-caudal direction, some of the anticipated subsidence can be counteracted. A cervical buttress plate is then placed to hold the graft(s) in place. This prevents graft extrusion when the patient is prone and is fixed only to one side of the osteotomy to allow further correction from the posterior approach. A drain is placed, and the anterior wound is closed.

The patient is then turned to a prone position, and the posterior osteotomies are performed. By placing the graft on the anterior portion of the disc space during the anterior operation, the surgeon can hinge off of this graft and extend the spine after removing the dorsal fusion mass. This technique can prevent performing a three-part operation with an anterior, posterior, followed by a repeat anterior operation.

Case Study 4

This case (Fig. 105.24) illustrates an anterior-posterior procedure to correct postoperative kyphosis in a patient with a circumferential fusion. This patient presented to us after having had six prior operations, including an anterior cervical discectomy and fusion from C3–T1 and a posterior fusion from C3–C7. Although he had achieved a solid fusion from C3–C6, he had a pseudarthrosis at C6–C7 and was kyphotic at C4–C5 and C5–C6. In addition, he had severe facet arthrosis at C2–C3. We performed anterior osteotomies at C4–C5 and C5–C6 and repaired the pseudarthrosis at C6–C7. We placed structural grafts at all levels and plated him anteriorly. The anterior operation took 3 hours and 20 minutes. We then turned him posteriorly and performed osteotomies through the posterior fusion mass. We fused and instrumented from C2 to T1. The posterior operation took 3 hours. The patient was left intubated overnight to protect his airway. Following a cuff-leak test, he was extubated.

Finally, it should be remembered that not all deformities need to be completely corrected. As long as the deformity is not causing excessive amounts of axial neck pain, myelopathy, or radiculopathy, a partial correction often suffices. Fig. 105.25 demonstrates a patient with rheumatoid arthritis and occipitocervical subluxation. This is best appreciated on the

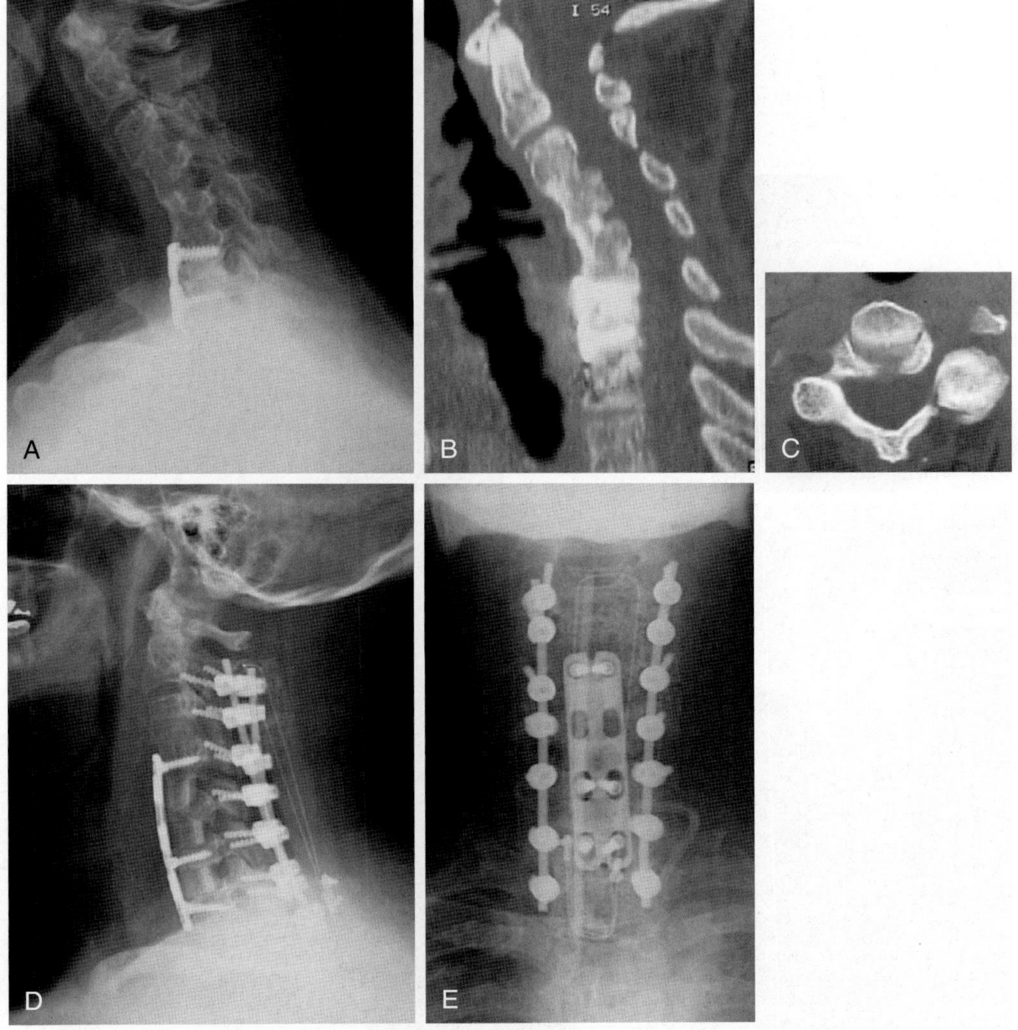

FIG. 105.24 (A) Lateral radiograph, (B) midsagittal computed tomography (CT) scan, and (C) axial CT scan through C2–C3 facet joint of a patient with six prior cervical spine operations. Postoperative (D) lateral and (E) posterior radiographs demonstrating circumferential fixation.

flexion-extension views of the upper cervical spine where the basion is anterior to the tip of the dens inflection and posterior to it in extension. The sagittal MRI shows an area of increased signal in the superior posterior aspect of the dens, just below the clivus. This represents the area of subluxation when the neck is in extension, as it was for this MRI. Because the patient had multilevel subluxations and an autofusion at C5–C6, which was in kyphosis, we elected to expedite the operation by performing decompressions and fusion circumferentially but not correcting the focal kyphosis at C5–C6. She also had numerous antibodies, which precluded the blood bank from being able to type and crossmatch her for any transfusions. We therefore performed a partial correction to achieve a modest improvement in the sagittal alignment. Because of the persistent kyphosis, it was not possible to contour a single plate, nor did we believe that it was absolutely necessary. Given that she had rheumatoid arthritis on corticosteroid therapy, we believed that circumferential stabilization would enhance the fusion rate. Indeed, the one area where she is not fused on the lateral radiograph is C7–T1, between the two plates. Although we did not get a perfect correction, we were able to achieve an excellent functional outcome without excessive blood loss or operative time.

Case Study 5

This patient (Fig. 105.26) underwent multiple failed anterior and posterior fusion procedures from C3–C7 at another institution. Her latest operation, an occipitocervical fusion to C7, resulted in pseudarthrosis, skull plate pullout, cervical kyphoscoliosis, and both chin-on-chest and ear-on-shoulder deformities with resultant pain and functional disability (see Fig. 105.26A–F). She underwent a posterior-only pedicle subtraction osteotomy and revision posterior spinal fusion from occiput to T4. To address both the coronal and sagittal plane deformities, a bigger wedge cut was made on the left side at C3–C4 and C7–T1. The pedicles of C4 and T1 were taken down bilaterally and correction achieved through these osteotomies. A large laminectomy was performed at C3, C4, C7, and T1, in addition to foraminotomies at C3–C4 and

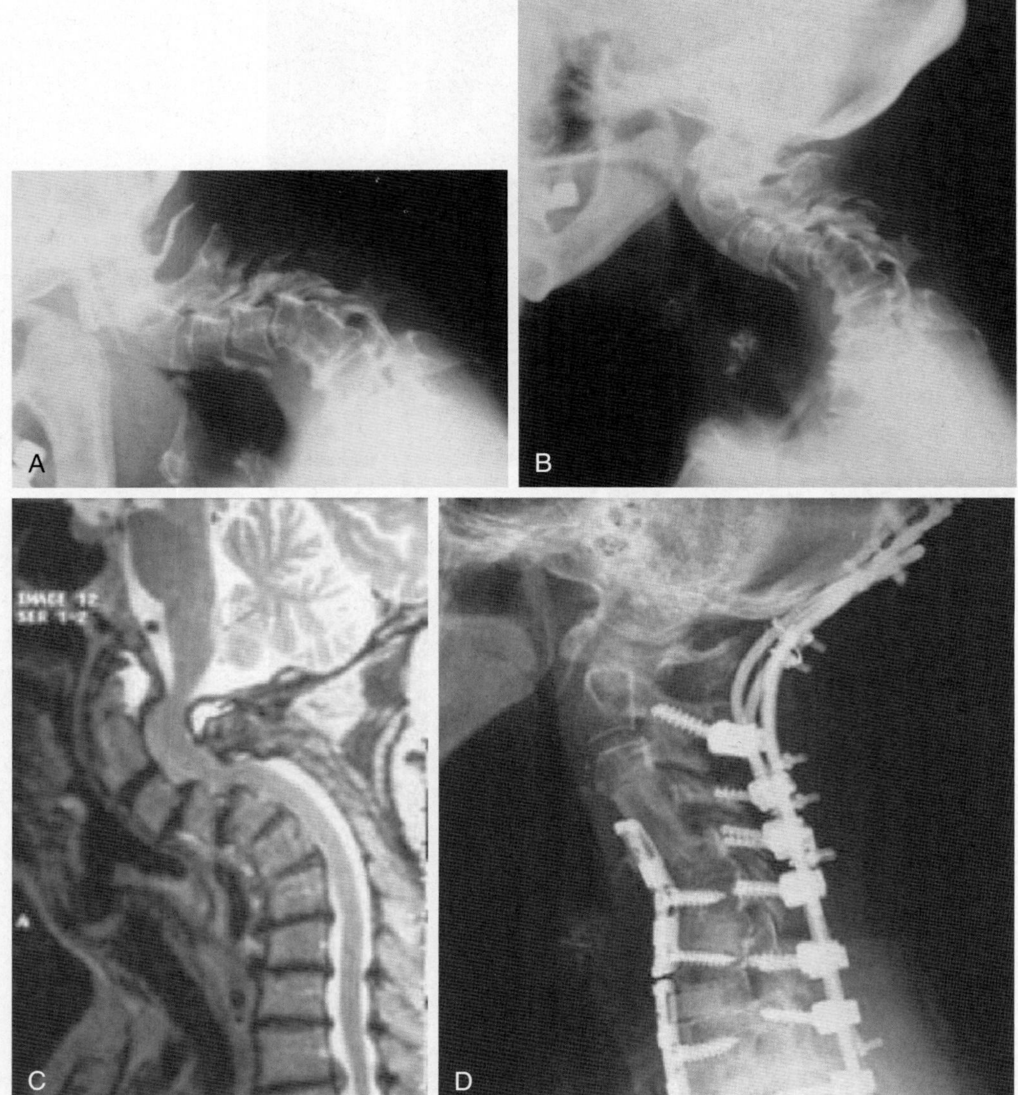

FIG. 105.25 (A) Flexion and (B) extension lateral radiographs of a patient with rheumatoid arthritis and occipitocervical subluxation. (C) Sagittal magnetic resonance image demonstrates severe cervical stenosis and occipitocervical subluxation. (D) Postoperative lateral radiograph. The focal kyphosis at C5–C6, where she had autofocused, was not corrected, but the overall cervical alignment and myelopathy were improved. Care was taken to make sure that the overall alignment was acceptable.

C7–T1. The deformity was then gently corrected by placing the neck in extension and shifting the traction weight to the extension rope from the flexion rope. At this point, permanent occipitocervical rods were placed. Visual inspection and intraoperative radiographs demonstrated excellent deformity correction in both planes (Fig. 105.26G–J).

Case Study 6

This patient had undergone five previous anterior and posterior surgeries, including posterior wound infection. She presented to us with postlaminectomy kyphosis and myeloradiculopathy, with obvious sagittal plane deformity adjacent to her previous distal cervical fusion (Fig. 105.27A–E). During the pedicle subtraction osteotomy at C7, after the pedicles of C7 had been completely taken down with C7 and C8 nerve roots free, an inadvertent vertebral artery injury was created and was immediately packed off (Fig. 105.27F). Bleeding was quickly controlled. Despite adequate bilateral decancellation, the neck was unable to be extended. Due to the injured vertebral artery, further left-sided decancellation would have been potentially unsafe. Therefore the decision was made to place temporary rods and close the posterior wound and perform an anterior osteotomy at C7 with C7 corpectomy. The patient was then placed in the prone position again for final correction and instrumentation as well as arthrodesis. She achieved excellent correction and experienced no untoward sequelae from the vertebral artery injury (Fig. 105.27G–K).

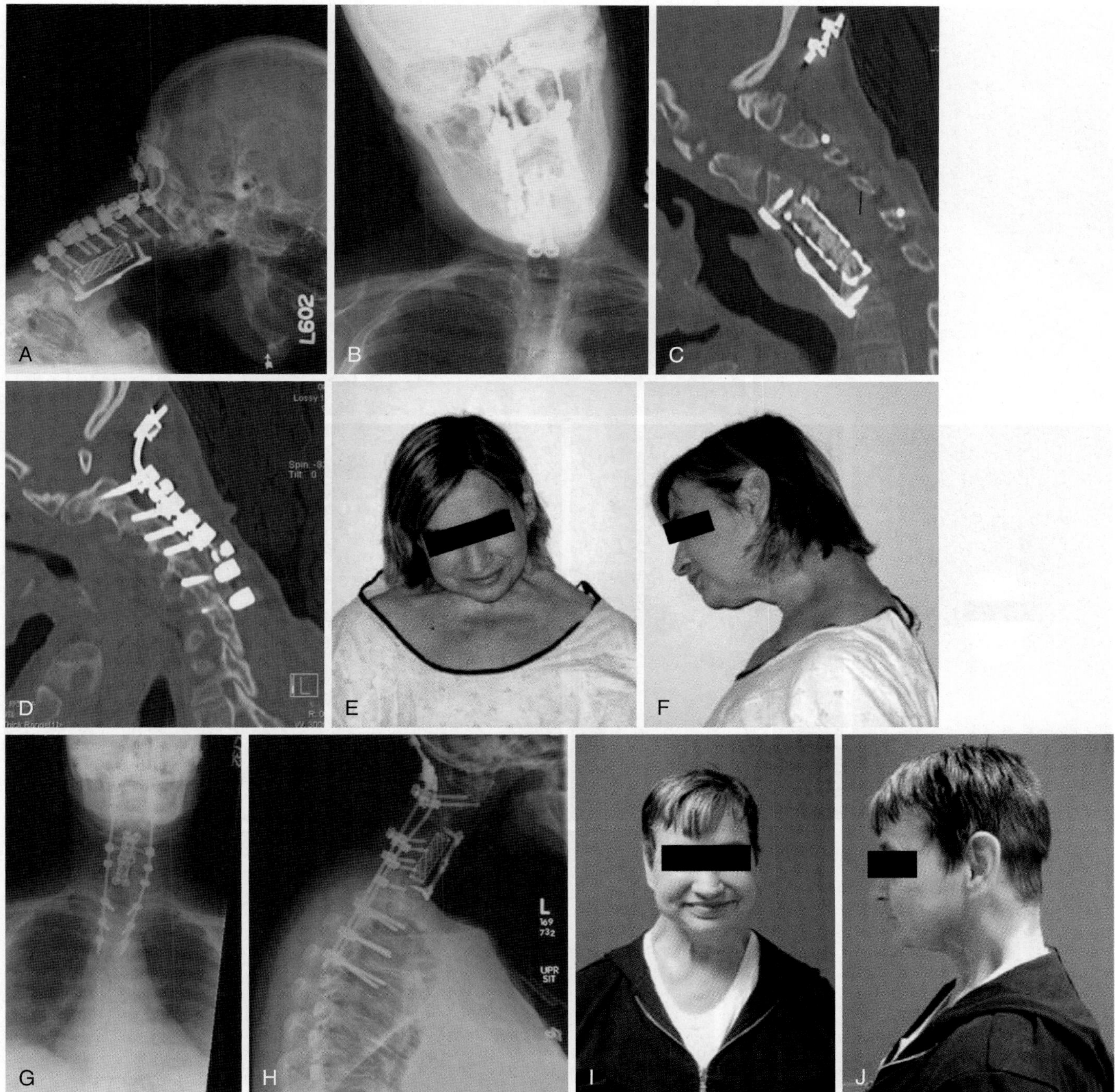

FIG. 105.26 Preoperative (A) lateral and (B) anteroposterior (AP) radiographs, (C–D) midsagittal computed tomography scan images, and (E–F) clinical images of a patient with chin-on-chest and ear-on-shoulder deformities. The patient underwent an asymmetric pedicle subtraction osteotomy at C4 and at T1 to correct her deformities in both the coronal and sagittal planes. Postoperative (G) AP and (H) lateral radiographs and (I–J) clinical images demonstrating excellent correction.

Case Study 7

This patient had been involved in a helicopter crash in the distant past and had sustained an unspecified cervical spine injury that was treated nonoperatively (Figs. 105.28A–E). He was then found to have developed a pseudomeningocele anteriorly but subsequent attempt at anterior surgical correction at another institution failed (the patient developed excessive bleeding and an arteriovenous fistula and the procedure was aborted), and the pseudomeningocele continued to enlarge. He then underwent laminectomies on the left side from C3–C7. On presentation to us, he had severe radicular symptoms, worsening pain, an enlarging pseudomeningocele, and rotational and coronal plane deformities. The patient underwent a corpectomy at C6, anterior cervical discectomy and fusion at C3–C4 and C7–T1, and repair of pseudomeningocele

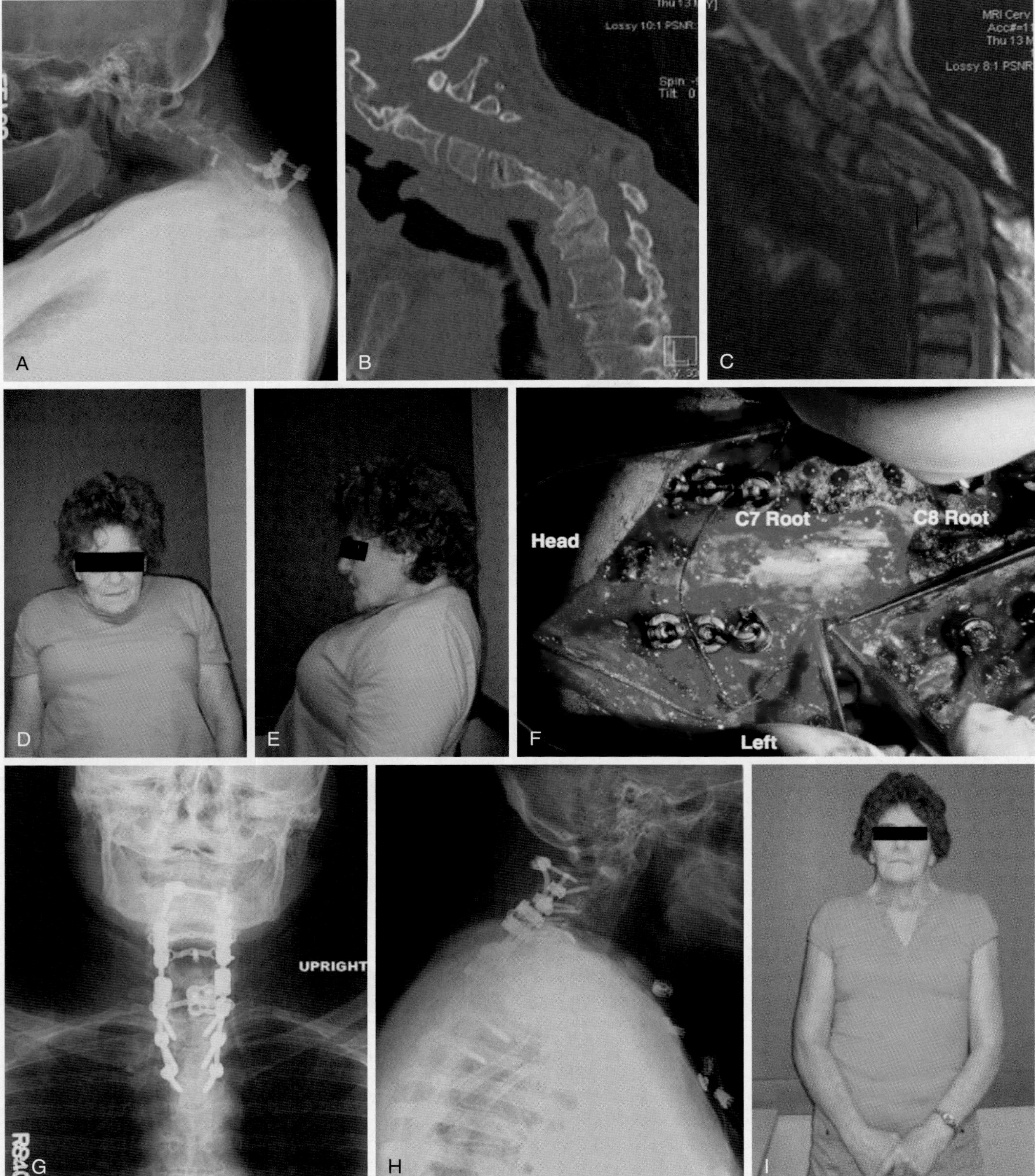

FIG. 105.27 (A) Preoperative lateral radiograph, (B) midsagittal computed tomography scan, (C) magnetic resonance image, and (D–E) clinical images of a patient with myeloradiculopathy resulting from postlaminectomy kyphosis. (F) Intraoperative image (of a different patient) showing the anatomic relationship between the exiting C7 and C8 nerve roots and the vertebral artery. (G) Anteroposterior and (H) lateral radiographs and (I–J) clinical images demonstrating excellent correction.

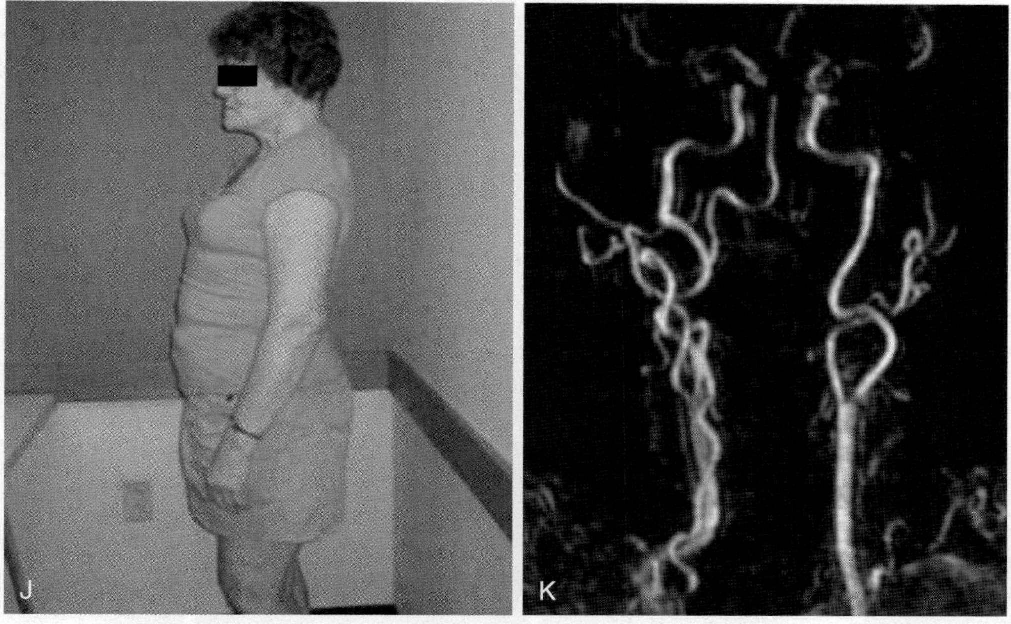

FIG. 105.27, cont'd (K) Postoperative angiogram revealing occluded vertebral artery.

(Fig. 105.28F–H). Following the anterior procedure, the patient was placed in the prone position for posterior cervical fusion from C2–T1. Copious amounts of bleeding were encountered despite the fact that the arteriovenous fistula had been embolized preoperatively. C2 laminar screws were used bilaterally, followed by placement of lateral mass screws from C3 bilaterally and from C4–C7 on the right side and pedicle screws at T1. The lateral masses on the left could not accept screws due to the bone deficiency from previous surgeries (Fig. 105.28I–J). The patient responded well and motor examination was normal until postoperative day 3, when he developed significant weakness of the left deltoid, biceps, and triceps, presumably from stretch injury related to correction of the coronal plane deformity. He was taken back to the operating room. Upon inspection of his construct, it was clear that the C2 screws had loosened and the left C3 screw had completely pulled out. The rods were removed and were contoured into a less-corrected (i.e., more scoliotic) position to reduce the stretch on the nerve roots. A third supplemental rod was placed to secure the tenuous posterior fixation using spinous process screws at C2, C7, and T1. We achieved further fixation of C2 using a short pedicle screw on one side and a pars screw on the other side (Fig. 105.28K–L). Allowing the cervical spine to relax back into a more scoliotic position enabled return of deltoid function on the basis of the intraoperative spinal cord monitoring data, so no further correction was attempted. The patient experienced dramatic improvement in his pain, made a complete neurologic and functional recovery, and was satisfied with his neck position.

Case Study 8

This patient with cerebral palsy had undergone numerous spinal operations before presenting to us, including multiple posterior and anterior procedures that were complicated by infections, wound dehiscence, instrumentation removal, myelopathy, and myelomalacia. He presented to us with significant ear-on-shoulder and chin-on-chest deformities in a wheelchair, with inability to achieve a horizontal gaze (Fig. 105.29A–B). He had collapse at C6–C7 following anterior C3–C6 fusion (Fig. 105.29C–F). We performed an osteotomy through C6 and C7 anteriorly, corpectomy of C7, with anterior cervical discectomy and fusion at T1–T2, T2–T3, and C2–C3. Using distraction on the Caspar pins, we were able to correct part of the kyphosis via plastic deformation of the posterior facets and lamina that had been fused. After placement of the trapezoidal grafts and buttress plates anteriorly to prevent graft extrusion, the patient was placed prone for posterior cervical fusion. C2 received a laminar screw on one side and a pedicle screw on the other. We performed a laminectomy at C6 and a Smith-Petersen osteotomy at C6–C7 after decompression. Next, the neck was corrected into a more neutral sagittal alignment, and the instrumentation was locked in place. An incomplete correction of his scoliosis was intentional in order to not put additional strain on the implants given the patient's extremely poor bone quality. His gaze, sagittal alignment, and to some extent his coronal alignment, although not perfect, were dramatically improved from baseline (Fig. 105.29G–J). When correcting coronal malalignment, root palsy on the concave side is common, increasing with greater correction. It may be advisable to correct the alignment in stages or accept some degree of undercorrection. Fortunately, in all of our cases, the root palsies have been transient.

Case Study 9

This patient presented with five previous cervical operations all done by different surgeons at an outside institution resulting in anterior cervical discectomy fusions from C3–C7, posterior cervical fusion from C3–T2, and kyphosis with

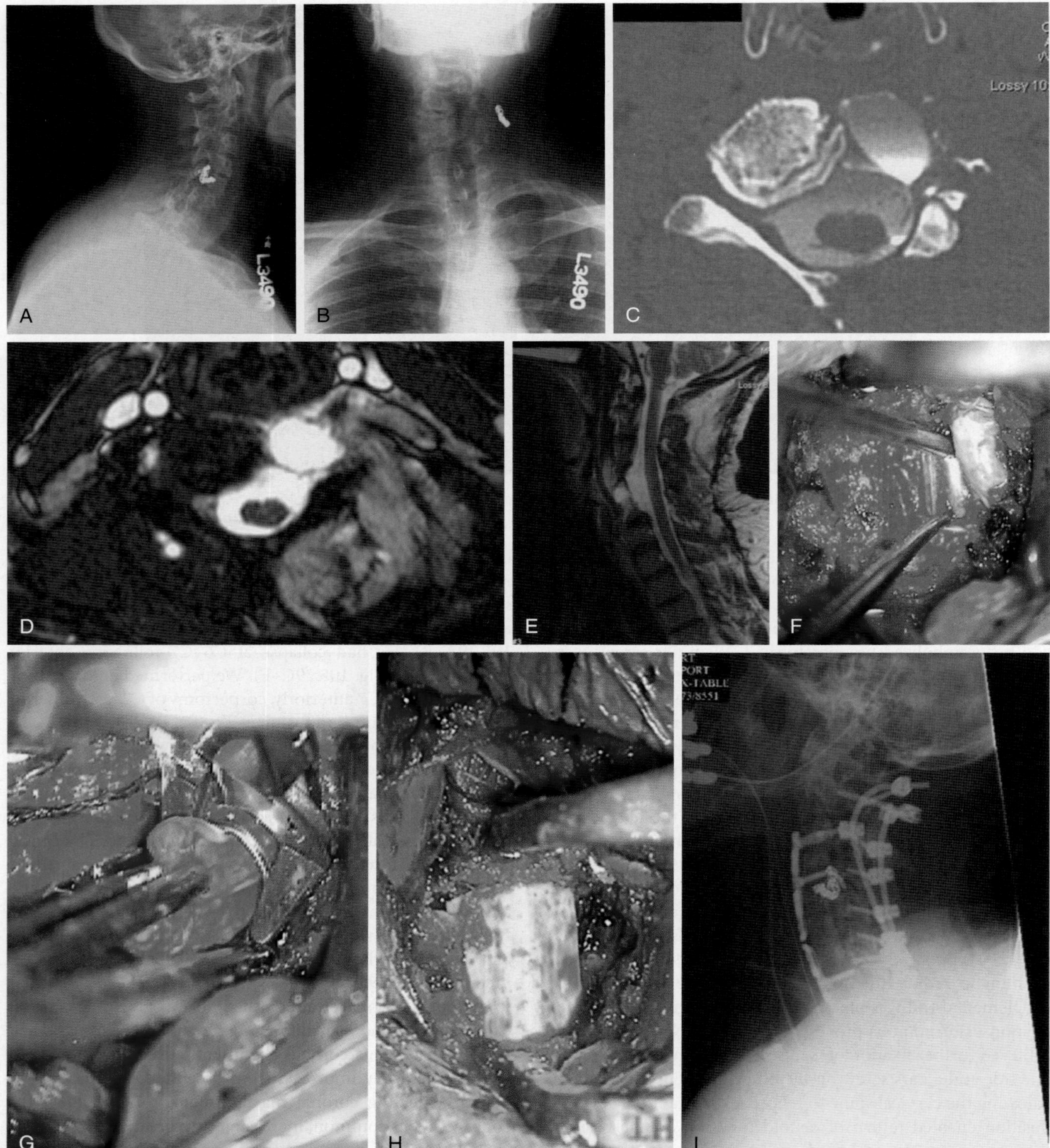

FIG. 105.28 Preoperative (A) lateral and (B) anteroposterior (AP) radiographs, (C) axial computed tomography myelogram, (D) magnetic resonance imaging (MRI), and (E) sagittal MRI of a patient with pseudomeningocele, radiculopathy, and disability after laminectomy and failed attempt at anterior repair. (F–H) Intraoperative images demonstrating pseudomeningocele repair. Initial postoperative (I) lateral and (J) AP radiographs.

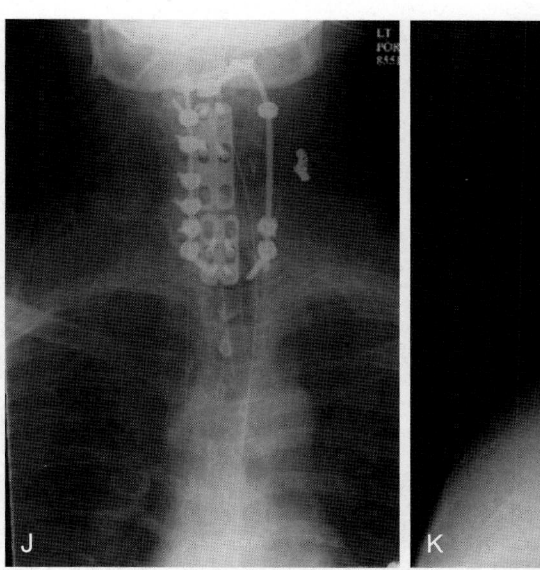

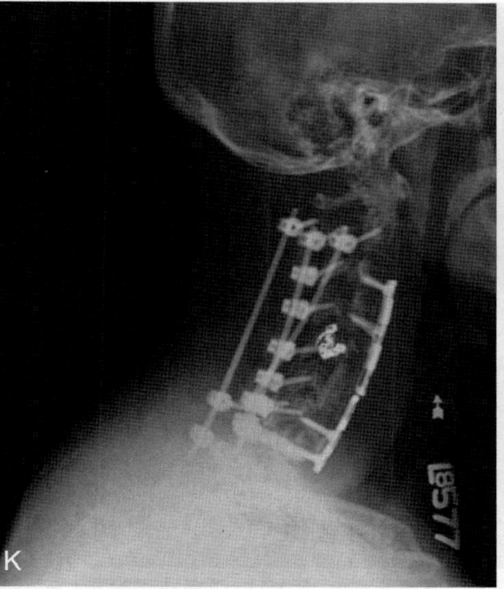

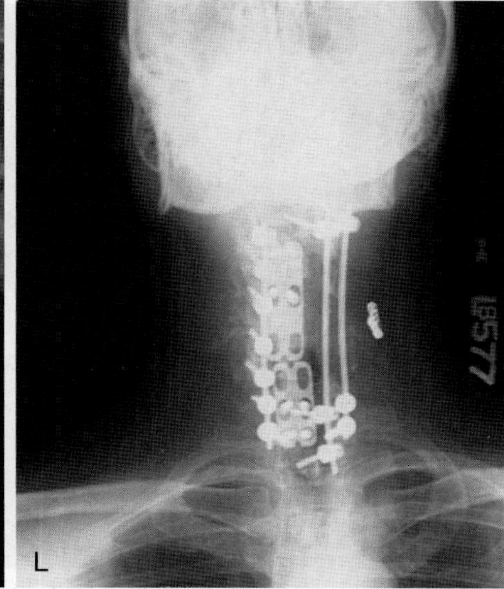

FIG. 105.28, cont'd Patient was taken back on postoperative day number 4 for progressive C5 palsy from overcorrection of coronal deformity. (K–L) Final postoperative radiographs, with supplemental C2, C7, and T1 spinous process screws and a third stabilizing rod.

laminectomies at T1 and T2. Unfortunately, the patient had become fused in kyphosis with a protracted neck. She complained of severe neck pain as well as her cervical deformity.

We approached the T2–T3 level first, took out the disc in its entirety, and then decorticated the end plate. We placed a low-profile stand-alone cervical interbody cage that was packed with fresh-frozen allograft bone, local autograft, and demineralized bone matrix. After tamping it in place, we fixed it with one 12 mm screw angled caudally. We then resected the T1–T2 disc in its entirety after visualizing the posterior longitudinal ligament. We reconstructed it with a 14 × 16 footprint 8 mm tall stand-alone cage packed with the same material as at T2–T3 level, fixed with one 14 mm screw. The C7–T1 level was solidly fused with some bony overgrowth. We did an anterior osteotomy through this as described above. We were able to open up the disc space in order to put in an 8 mm tall 14 × 16 stand-alone cage packed with the same material as the other levels.

We then turned the patient to a prone position. We removed the screws at C6, T1, T2 bilaterally, traded out the C6 screws, decided to go up to C5 and put in screws bilaterally into the lateral masses. She had a solid fusion at C7–T1, T1–T2, and even T2–T3 was fused. T3–T4 was not fused. We went ahead and took down the facet joint completely on the left side at C7–T1, removed the bottom 20% of the C7 pedicle, and decompressed the C8 nerve root because she had some decrement of her ulnar nerve on the left side. We then placed back the screws at C7 and T1 bilaterally. We performed SPOs at T2–T3 and T1–T2, taking down the facet joint until we were able to mobilize the two spaces. Thereafter, we put in bilateral pedicle screws at T1, T2, T3, and T4. We decided to take out the C5 screw on the left side so that we could take the cobalt-chrome rod and have everything fit. We extended the neck with GW tongs to reduce the kyphosis, and we put lateralizing connectors on the right at C6 and T1. Using a 3.5 mm diameter cobalt-chromium rod, we were able to obtain lordosis of the spine. Postoperatively the patient had good correction of her cervicothoracic alignment (Fig. 105.30).

Case Study 10

This patient presented with a history of a C5 cervical corpectomy done at an outside institution in the remote past with kyphotic collapse and autofusion at C6–C7 and C7–T1. He has a chin-on-chest deformity with kyphoscoliosis and spondylosis at C2–C3 and T1–T2. He reported severe neck pain and the inability to keep his head upright.

On anterior exploration, C6–C7 was solidly fused. We took down the fusion through an anterior osteotomy at C6–C7 and then put in a low-profile stand-alone cage packed with fresh-frozen allograft, local autograft, and demineralized bone matrix. The cage was secured with one 14 mm screw. Next, an osteotomy at C7–T1 was performed and the head was pushed down to correct the deformity at this level. Another low-profile stand-alone cage was used at this level with the same packing material and fixation as the C6–C7 cage. Next, a T1–T2 discectomy was done and reconstructed with the same cage, packing material, and screw as the prior levels.

The patient was then flipped prone. C2 pars screws were placed bilaterally followed by lateral mass screws on the left side at two levels and on the right side at three levels. Then pedicle screws were placed at T1, T2, and T3 bilaterally. We put a 3.5 mm diameter rod on the right side and a 3.2 mm diameter rod on the left. We also put translaminar screws at C7, T1, T2, and T3. We decorticated the facets and performed Ponte osteotomies at C6–C7 and C7–T1 using a ¼-inch osteotome, cutting into the facet joints bilaterally. We extended the neck and compressed the spinous process rods to get lordosis at C7 to T3. Lastly, we placed the other 3.2 mm titanium rod and, after compressing, put in facet screws at all levels (Fig. 105.31).

Text continued on p. 1930

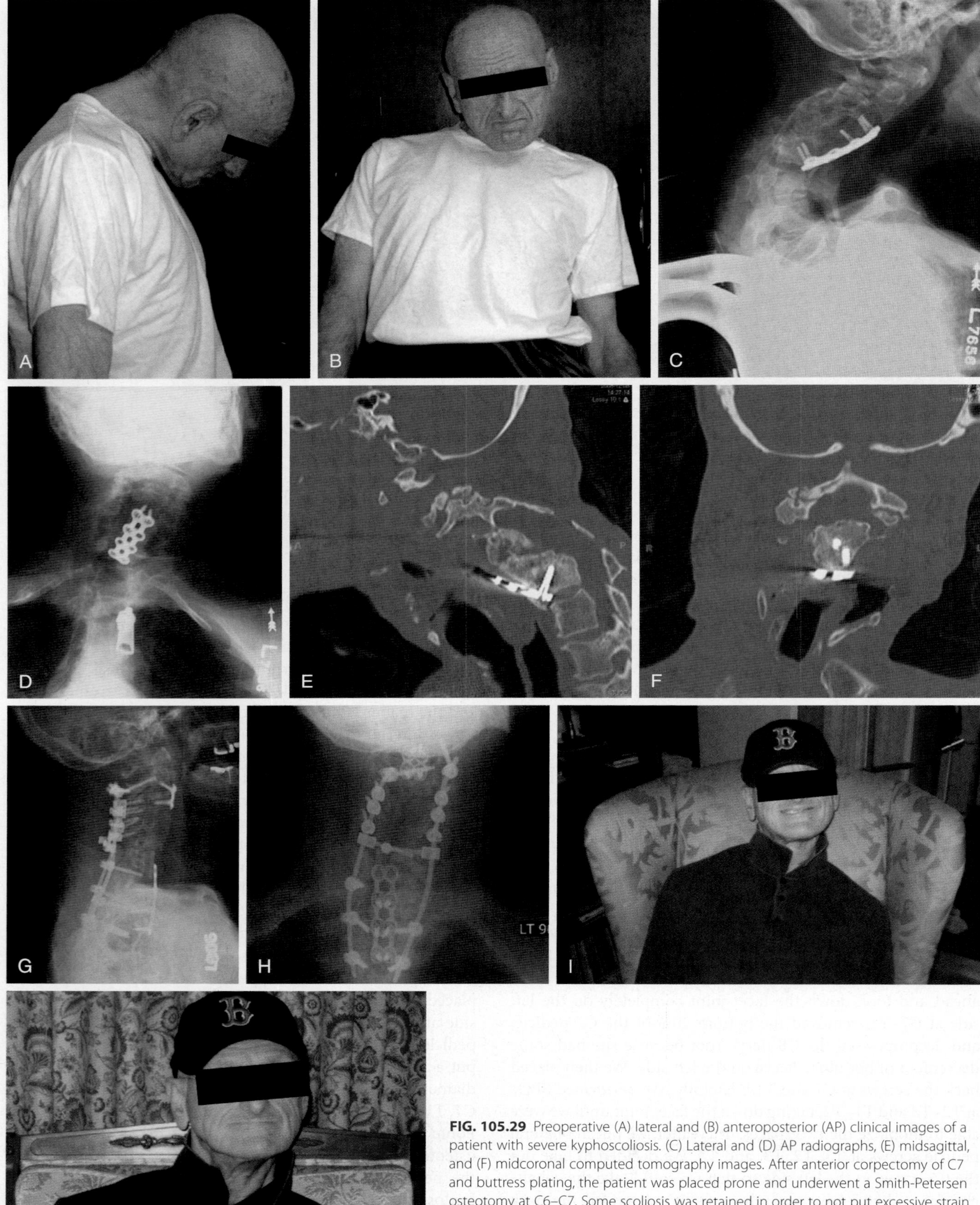

FIG. 105.29 Preoperative (A) lateral and (B) anteroposterior (AP) clinical images of a patient with severe kyphoscoliosis. (C) Lateral and (D) AP radiographs, (E) midsagittal, and (F) midcoronal computed tomography images. After anterior corpectomy of C7 and buttress plating, the patient was placed prone and underwent a Smith-Petersen osteotomy at C6–C7. Some scoliosis was retained in order to not put excessive strain on his implants given the patient's poor bone quality. Postoperative (G) lateral and (H) AP radiographs, and (I–J) clinical images revealing excellent correction of both planes with normalized horizontal gaze.

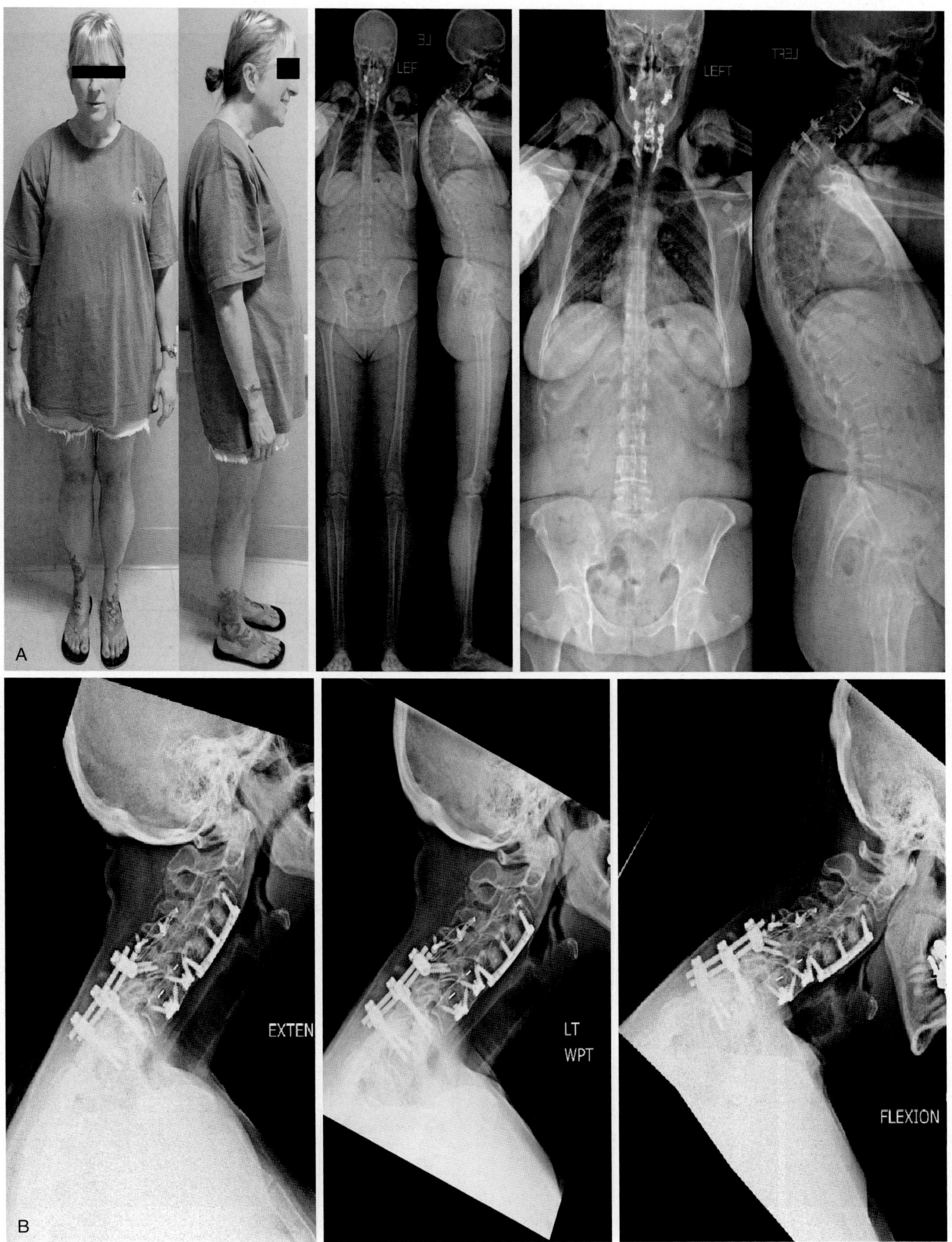

FIG. 105.30 (A) Preoperative EOS standing lateral, anteroposterior, clinical and radiographic images. (B) Preoperative flexion and extension laterals.

Continued

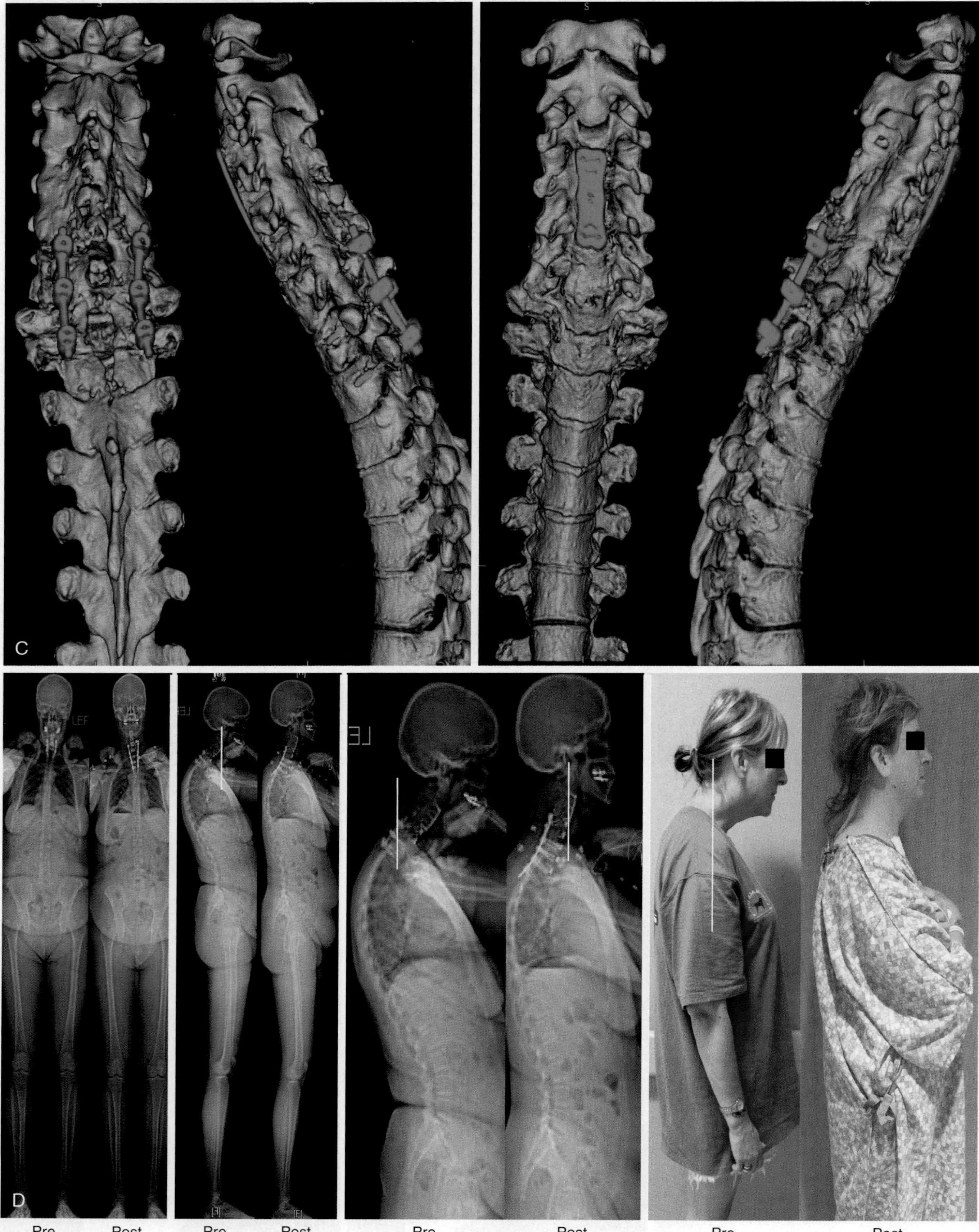

FIG. 105.30, cont'd (C) Preoperative three-dimensional computed tomographic reconstructions, and (D) postoperative radiographs (compared with preoperative) and clinical photographs revealing excellent correction of both planes with normalized horizontal gaze.

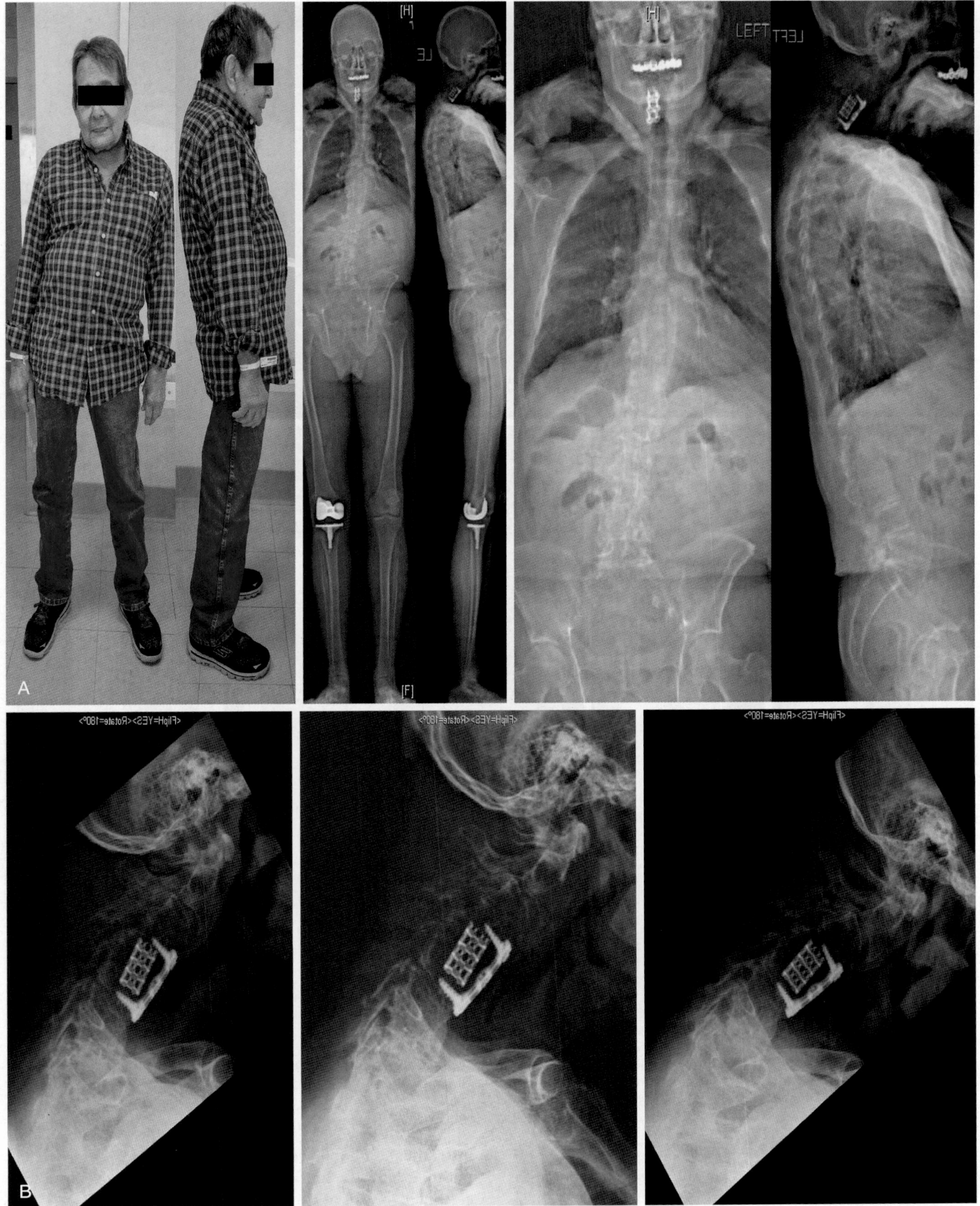

FIG. 105.31 (A) Preoperative EOS standing lateral and anteroposterior clinical images and radiographs. (B) Preoperative flexion and extension laterals.

Continued

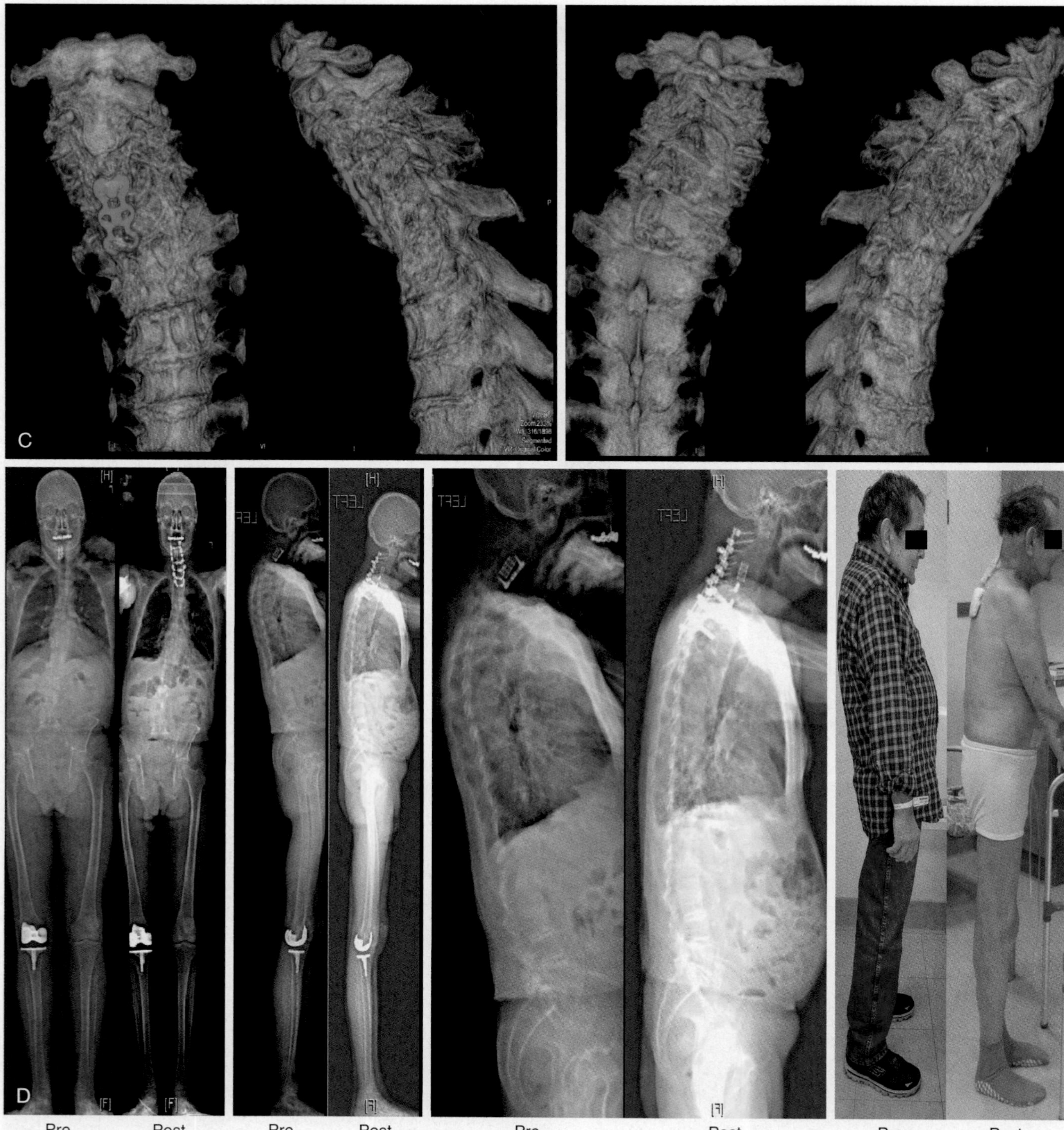

FIG. 105.31, cont'd (C) Preoperative three-dimensional computed tomographic reconstructions, and (D) postoperative radiographs (compared with preoperative) and clinical photographs revealing excellent correction of both planes with normalized horizontal gaze.

Case Study 11

This patient had multiple anterior and posterior operations done at several outside institutions. He developed kyphosis and intolerable pain. He had anterior cervical discectomy and fusion at C5–C7 with collapse at C6–C7 into kyphosis, posterior cervical laminectomy at C5, C6, and C7 with instrumentation followed by removal of instrumentation, and multiple anterior and posterior operative procedures with cervical kyphosis at C6–C7 and C7–T1.

An anterior osteotomy was performed at C6–C7, burring all the bone from uncinate to uncinate all the way back posteriorly until the posterolateral ligament was reached. After decompressing the C7 nerve root bilaterally, the C6–C7 space was expanded with Caspar distractors and by pushing down on the forehead after removing the sheets from under the back of his head. After doing this, there was good correction at C6–C7. We inserted fresh-frozen structural iliac crest allograft into the disc space, then fixed it in place with an anterior cervical plate with fixed-angle anterior screws. Two screws were placed into C6 and two screws into C7. Next, a C7–T1 discectomy was performed and low-profile cage was packed with fresh-frozen allograft, demineralized bone matrix, and local autograft and then placed in the prior disc space. We tamped it in place and fixed it with one 12 mm screw directed caudally. It should be noted that we did not perform an osteotomy at this level. Instead, we performed an anterior cervical thoracic discectomy and fusion at C7–T1.

Next, we flipped the patient prone and redecompressed C5, C6, and C7 because of scarring. Without this procedure, buckling of the scar on the posterior dura would have occurred with neck extension. We put in lateral mass screws at C4, C5, and C6 bilaterally and pedicle screws at T1, T2, and T3. We then burred down the C6–C7 facets, which had not broken but had plastically deformed. We then used an osteotome to complete the osteotomies bilaterally at C6–C7. At C7–T1, the facet joint was not fused on the right side. We performed an SPO by opening it up using a burr followed by an osteotome. On the left side, there was a small amount of fusion mass, which was taken down with a burr followed by a curved 0.25-inch osteotome to finish the osteotomy. We then placed 3.5 mm diameter titanium rods bilaterally with a side connector at T1 bilaterally. We used a spinous process cable at T1–T2 and T2–T3 to further extend the upper thoracic spine. We also used curved rods to help the cervical correction (Fig. 105.32).

PEARLS

1. Iatrogenic malalignment of the cervical spine may be prevented with careful intraoperative positioning using radiographic verification.
2. Bivector cervical traction using GW tongs allows the surgeon to place the cervical spine into a lordotic position for fusion after the exposure and decompression are completed.
3. The use of multiple small grafts (corpectomy-discectomy or corpectomy-corpectomy) allows for better preservation of cervical lordosis than does the use of a single longer graft.
4. Correction of iatrogenic cervical kyphosis in the presence of a circumferential fusion may be performed with an anteroposterior procedure with the use of an appropriately sized and shaped anterior graft and a plate that allows screw translation and angulation.

PITFALLS

1. Off-center placement of anterior cervical distraction pins, if not recognized, may create iatrogenic cervical malalignment in the coronal plane.
2. Aggressive decompressive laminectomies without fusion, particularly in children, may lead to iatrogenic cervical kyphosis.
3. A corpectomy at the same level as a previous laminectomy creates significant instability; circumferential fixation is usually necessary in this situation.

KEY POINTS

1. During anterior cervical procedures, if the patient is fused in hyperlordosis, he or she will often have severe interscapular and posterior cervical pain, especially if an extensive foraminotomy is not performed at the time of the procedure.
2. Caspar pin misplacement may lead to angular, rotational, or translational deformities.
3. Anterior cervical grafts should be large enough to allow for 1 or 2 mm of subsidence without creating kyphosis.
4. Correction of a cervical scoliosis, without appreciation for a severe thoracic curve, may lead to the head being tilted to one side. Therefore it is critical to pay close attention to the overall alignment of the head, neck, and torso.
5. The advantage of using bivector tong traction (i.e., flexion and extension) in posterior cervical fusion surgery is that the surgeon can easily alter the position of the neck intraoperatively. With fixed head holders such as Mayfield tongs, an assistant has to crawl under the table to reposition the head holder.
6. When performing a foraminotomy, it is critical to remove no more than 50% of the lateral mass to prevent iatrogenic instability.
7. Patients with a preoperative kyphotic alignment due to degenerative disc disease who are fused with the neck in extension are at risk for developing postoperative kyphosis; therefore circumferential fusion is often best in these situations.
8. Traumatic cervical spine injuries fixed with inadequate instrumentation or bony purchase may lead to postoperative malalignment.
9. Patients who have undergone a laminectomy and subsequently undergo an anterior corpectomy have two halves of the spine that are connected only by soft tissues. The significant instability that this introduces mandates circumferential fusion as well as adequate postoperative immobilization.
10. When circumferential treatment of iatrogenic cervical deformities is required, we generally prefer going in anteriorly, decompressing, and putting in undersized grafts and buttress plates to allow more correction posteriorly, then going in posteriorly to further correct and lock in the construct.
11. Correction of cervical scoliosis is associated with a high incidence of root palsies on the concave side. This is probably due to a stretch of the root or plexus and seems to recover over a period of weeks.

KEY REFERENCES

1. Hilibrand AS, Fye MA, Emery SE, et al. Increased rate of arthrodesis with strut grafting after multilevel anterior cervical decompression. *Spine*. 2002;27:146-151.
   This paper reports a higher rate of fusion among patients who underwent corpectomy with strut grafting compared with patients treated with multiple cervical discectomies and interbody grafts.
2. Kaiser MG, Haid RWJ, Subach BR, et al. Anterior cervical plating enhances arthrodesis after discectomy and fusion with cortical allograft. *Neurosurgery*. 2002;50:229-238.
   The authors report an increased rate of fusion after anterior cervical plating and discectomy with allogenic interbody graft with the use of a plate.
3. Riew KD, Hilibrand AS, Palumbo MA, et al. Anterior cervical corpectomy in patients previously managed with a laminectomy: short-term complications. *J Bone Joint Surg Am*. 1999;81:950-957.

SECTION XV

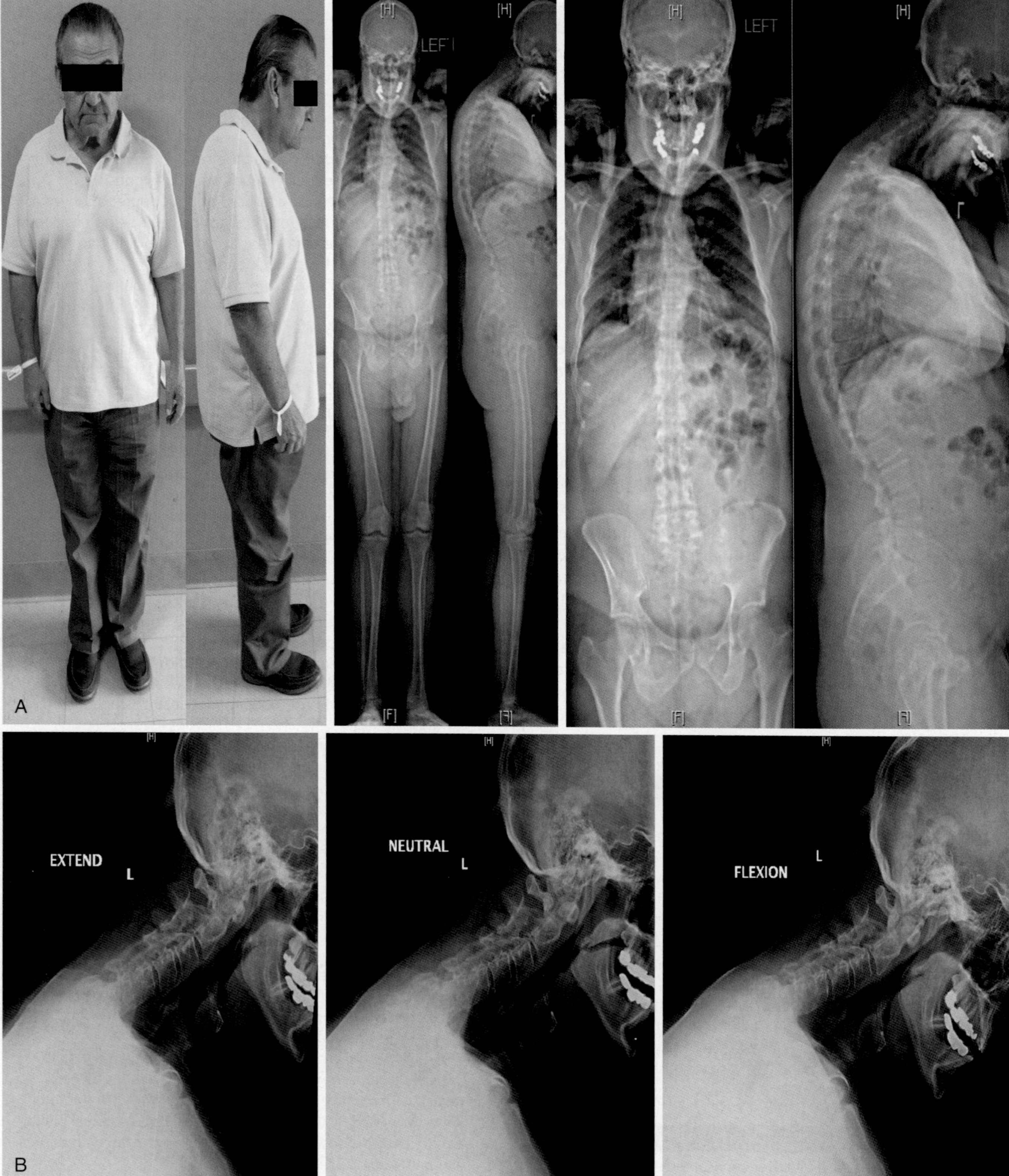

FIG. 105.32 (A) Preoperative EOS standing lateral and anteroposterior clinical images and radiographs. (B) Preoperative flexion and extension laterals.

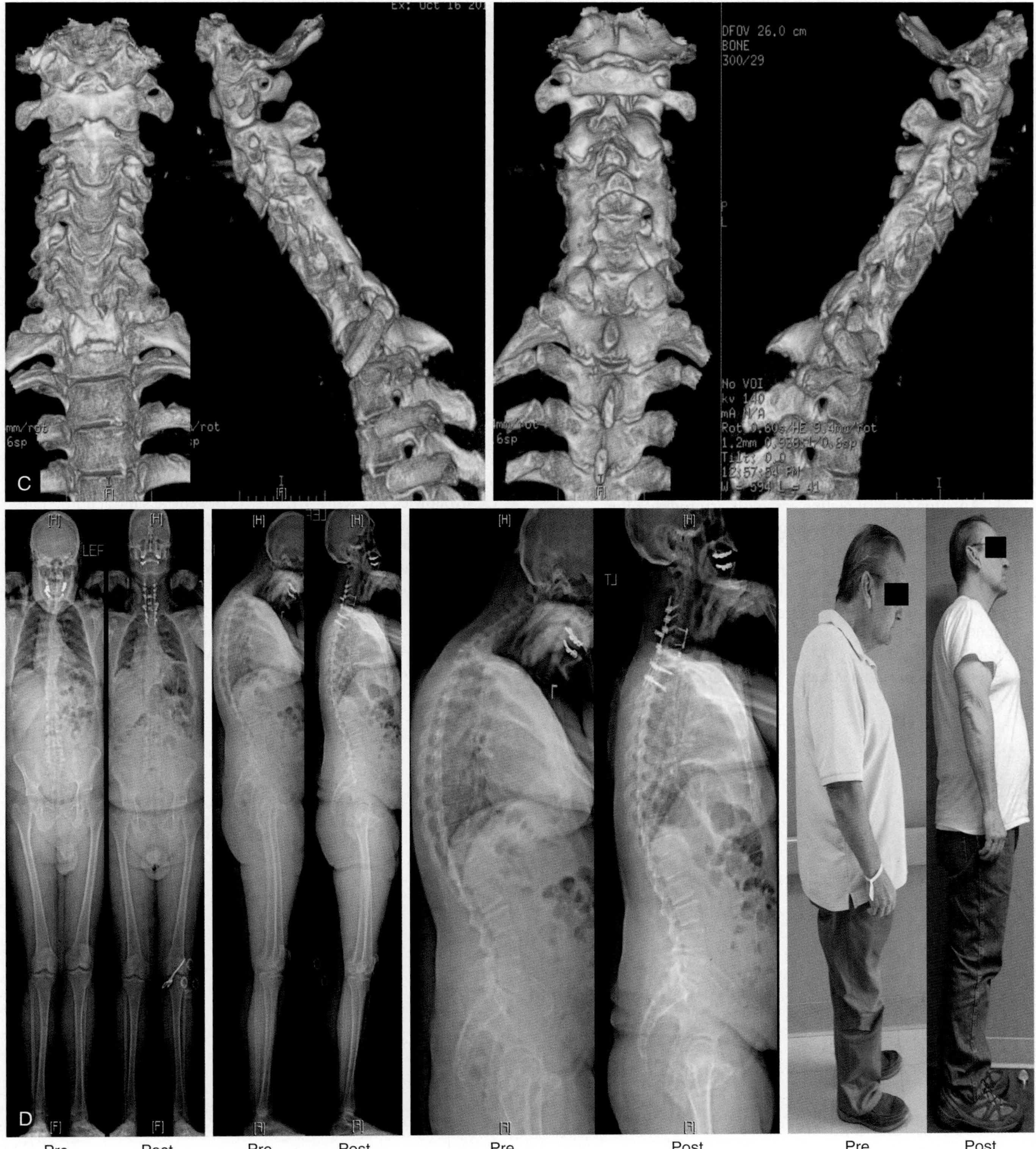

FIG. 105.32, cont'd (C) preoperative three-dimensional computed tomographic reconstructions, and (D) postoperative radiographs (compared with preoperative) and clinical photographs revealing excellent correction of both planes with normalized horizontal gaze.

The authors report a high rate of complications after corpectomy in patients who had a prior laminectomy and conclude that circumferential fixation may be necessary in these patients.

4. Zdeblick TA, Abitol JJ, Kunz DN, et al. Cervical stability after sequential capsule resection. *Spine.* 1993;18:2005-2008.
This paper describes the importance of limiting the extent of facetectomy to preserve segmental stability in the cervical spine.

REFERENCES

1. Ames CP, Smith JS, Scheer JK, et al. A standardized nomenclature for cervical spine soft-tissue release and osteotomy for deformity correction: clinical article. *J Neurosurg Spine.* 2013;19(3):269-278.
2. Ames CP, Smith JS, Eastlack R, et al. Reliability assessment of a novel cervical spine deformity classification system. *J Neurosurg Spine.* 2015;23(6):673-683.
3. Harrison DE, Harrison DD, Cailliet R, et al. Cobb method or Harrison posterior tangent method: which to choose for lateral cervical radiographic analysis. *Spine.* 2000;25(16):2072-2078.
4. Lee SH, Kim KT, Seo EM, et al. The influence of thoracic inlet alignment on the craniocervical sagittal balance in asymptomatic adults. *J Spinal Disord Tech.* 2012;25(2):E41-E47.
5. Kaiser MG, Haid RW Jr, Subach BR, Barnes B, Rodts GE Jr. Anterior cervical plating enhances arthrodesis after discectomy and fusion with cortical allograft. *Neurosurgery.* 2002;50(2):229-236.
6. Wang JC, McDonough PW, Endow KK, Delamarter RB. Increased fusion rates with cervical plating for two-level anterior cervical discectomy and fusion. *Spine.* 2000;25(1):41-45.
7. Vaccaro AR, Chiba K, Heller JG, et al. Bone grafting alternatives in spinal surgery. *Spine J.* 2002;2(3):206-215.
8. Park JB, Cho YS, Riew KD. Development of adjacent-level ossification in patients with an anterior cervical plate. *J Bone Joint Surg Am.* 2005;87(3):558-563.
9. Hilibrand AS, Fye MA, Emery SE, Palumbo MA, Bohlman HH. Increased rate of arthrodesis with strut grafting after multilevel anterior cervical decompression. *Spine.* 2002;27(2):146-151.
10. Vaccaro AR, Falatyn SP, Scuderi GJ, et al. Early failure of long segment anterior cervical plate fixation. *J Spinal Disord.* 1998;11(5):410-415.
11. Phillips FM, Phillips CS, Wetzel FT, Gelinas C. Occipitocervical neutral position. Possible surgical implications. *Spine.* 1999;24(8):775-778.
12. Zdeblick TA, Abitbol JJ, Kunz DN, McCabe RP, Garfin S. Cervical stability after sequential capsule resection. *Spine.* 1993;18(14):2005-2008.
13. Bell DF, Walker JL, O'Connor G, Tibshirani R. Spinal deformity after multiple-level cervical laminectomy in children. *Spine.* 1994;19(4):406-411.
14. Kim HJ, Piyaskulkaew C, Riew KD. Comparison of Smith-Petersen osteotomy versus pedicle subtraction osteotomy versus anterior-posterior osteotomy types for the correction of cervical spine deformities. *Spine.* 2015;40(3):143-146.
15. Wollowick AL, Kelly MP, Riew KD. Pedicle subtraction osteotomy in the cervical spine. *Spine.* 2012;37(5):E342-E348.
16. Riew KD, Hilibrand AS, Palumbo MA, Bohlman HH. Anterior cervical corpectomy in patients previously managed with a laminectomy: short-term complications. *J Bone Joint Surg Am.* 1999;81(7):950-957.
17. Sin AH, Acharya R, Smith DR, Nanda A. Adopting 540-degree fusion to correct cervical kyphosis. *Surg Neurol.* 2004;61(6):515-522, discussion 522.

CHAPTER 106 Arachnoiditis and Epidural Fibrosis

Robert F. Heary
Antonios Mammis

Spinal arachnoiditis is a nonspecific inflammatory process of the arachnoid layer of the spinal cord or cauda equina. Arachnoiditis was first described by Victor Horsley in 1909.[1] Since Horsley, numerous authors have described it with a variety of terms, including chronic spinal arachnoiditis, adhesive spinal arachnoiditis, meningitis serosa circumscripta spinalis, chronic spinal meningitis, spinal meningitides with radiculomyelopathy, lumbar adhesive arachnoiditis, spinal arachnoiditis, spinal fibrosis, and lumbosacral adhesive arachnoiditis. Furthermore, on the basis of specific radiographic or pathologic findings, arachnoiditis can be termed *arachnoiditis ossificans*, *calcific arachnoiditis*, or *pachymeningitis*.[1]

Anatomy

The arachnoid mater is an avascular membrane that lies between two vascularized membranes, the pia mater and dura mater. The arachnoid is attached to the underlying pia by numerous arachnoid trabeculae, creating a space between the arachnoid and the pia.[2] This space, or potential space in some instances, transmits arterioles and is referred to as the *subarachnoid space*. The arachnoid is composed of layers of squamous cells held together by a network of connective tissue. The arachnoid contains intercellular pores, which allow for the passage of molecules.[3]

Pathogenesis

A chronic infection or irritation can cause the arachnoid membrane to become thickened and adherent to both the overlying dura mater and the subjacent pia mater.[4] The pia-arachnoid carries the blood vessels to the spinal cord; this layer contains mesenchymal cells. In 1951, Smolik and Nash[5] recognized that when the outer arachnoid layer is injured, both the blood vessels and mesenchymal cells lend themselves to extensive proliferation. The ensuing reaction between the pia-arachnoid and the dura mater leads to obliterative arachnoiditis.

When the arachnoid membrane is exposed to an insult, an inflammatory response ensues, characterized by fibrinous exudates, neovascularization, and a relative paucity of inflammatory cellular exudates.[6,7] Vascular occlusive changes can lead to spinal cord ischemia.[4,8–11] The small perforating blood vessels that supply the portions of the white matter may be obliterated, with resultant necrosis and cavitation of the spinal cord parenchyma.[8,9,11] In addition to ischemia, blockage of venous return from the spinal cord or occlusion of cerebrospinal fluid (CSF) pathways may occur.[8]

The stages of progressive inflammation of the arachnoid that occur in lumbosacral arachnoiditis were described by Burton.[12] The initial stage, radiculitis, consists of an inflamed pia-arachnoid with associated hyperemia and swelling of the nerve roots. The second stage, arachnoiditis, is characterized by fibroblast proliferation and collagen deposition. During this stage, nerve root swelling decreases and the nerve roots adhere to each other and to the pia-arachnoid. The final stage, adhesive arachnoiditis, is the resolution of the inflammatory process and is characterized by dense collagen deposition. There is marked proliferation of the pia-arachnoid, as well as complete nerve root encapsulation, hypoxemia, and progressive atrophy. For reasons that are not fully understood, the adhesions occur preferentially on the dorsal segments.[1] The exact time course of these three phases has not been elucidated. Furthermore, it is not known how the specific causative insult for the development of arachnoiditis might affect the time course of each of the three phases.

Yamagami and colleagues[13] postulated that the pathologic changes in arachnoiditis may be secondary to diminished nutritional supply. They found that, in an experimental rat model, the development of arachnoiditis and neural degeneration directly corresponded to the magnitude of extradural inflammation and wound healing processes that occurred after laminectomy, with or without foreign bodies. Furthermore, adhesions of the arachnoid cause the nerve roots to lump together and, in doing so, these nerve roots are isolated from contact with the CSF, with resultant nutritional compromise.[13]

Etiology

In the first half of the 20th century, arachnoiditis was most often attributed to infectious causes.[8] Furthermore, arachnoiditis had been described mainly in the cervical and thoracic regions.[1] Since the 1950s, there has been a trend toward a higher incidence of arachnoiditis of noninfectious origin affecting the lumbar region.[1,8] The precise causes of spinal arachnoiditis are not clear and, likewise, the incidence and prevalence of spinal arachnoiditis in the general population is unknown.[8]

As stated previously, arachnoiditis was mainly of infectious origin in the first half of the 20th century. Syphilis, tuberculosis, and gonorrhea were the most prevalent causes.[1,14] Less common infectious causes include parasitic diseases and viral meningitis.[15,16] These infectious causes are important to differentiate from noninfectious causes of arachnoiditis because, in most cases, effective treatment is available for arachnoiditis of infectious origin. However, despite adequate treatment of the causative agent, scarring of the arachnoid membrane may lead to permanent damage.

There are a number of important noninfectious etiologies of arachnoiditis. In the 1940s, blood in the CSF following subarachnoid hemorrhage or surgery became the most prevalent cause of arachnoiditis.[1] Spinal arachnoiditis following subarachnoid hemorrhage continues to be common and is usually treated in a conservative fashion.[17] The breakdown products of hemoglobin form free radicals, and it has been postulated that these cause damage to nerves.[18,19] In experiments on dogs, it has been shown that injecting blood breakdown products into the subarachnoid space causes more meningeal inflammation than does the injection of fresh blood.[18] Cases of patients who have received epidural blood patches have given controversial results. Digiovanni and colleagues[20] described that the placement of an autologous blood patch into the epidural space produced no more inflammation than a standard lumbar puncture. Other authors, though, have described cases in which an epidural blood patch had allegedly been responsible for arachnoiditis.[21] Abouleish and colleagues[22] described 118 cases of epidural blood patches over a 2-year period. This group found 19 cases of axial back pain, two cases of radiculopathy, and no cases of arachnoiditis.[22]

Oil-based contrast media have been historically important causes of arachnoiditis. Iophendylate (Myodil, Pantopaque) is an oil-based contrast medium used in diagnostic myelograms. It was first used in the United States, in 1944, and its usage continued for 40 years. In Sweden, iophendylate was banned from clinical use in 1948 secondary to animal studies that identified it as a causative agent for arachnoiditis.[23] The incidence of arachnoiditis after the use of iophendylate is dose dependent and is quoted as 1%.[24] Iophendylate has a long half-life; thus, it is usually removed from the thecal space by aspiration at the conclusion of the myelogram.[8] Often, this removal process is not entirely successful and, in fact, incomplete removal of the contrast dye may produce further trauma and cause bleeding into the CSF.[4]

Guyer and colleagues[25] listed the following factors as influencing the development of arachnoiditis after myelography: the type of contrast agent used (the risk is greater with the oil-based medium than with the water-soluble medium and greater with the ionic medium than with the nonionic medium), the dosage of contrast medium, and the observation time after myelography (Fig. 106.1).

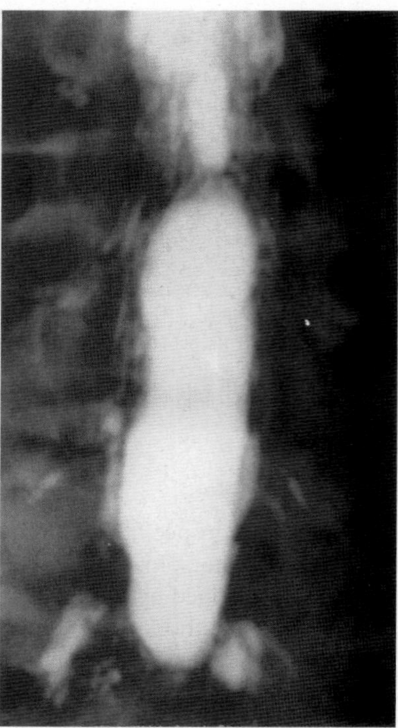

FIG. 106.1 Myelogram with oil-based medium demonstrating the marked lack of filling of nerve roots of adhesive arachnoiditis.

The use of intrathecal medications, either steroids or anesthetic agents, has been implicated as a cause of arachnoiditis. Intrathecal injection of corticosteroids was previously used for multiple sclerosis.[8] Epidural injection of corticosteroids for back pain is a common practice. One of the most commonly used agents is methylprednisolone acetate (MPA), which has been reported to cause arachnoiditis.[26–28] MPA is suspended in polyethylene glycol, which can cause arachnoiditis.[26–28] Furthermore, MPA is known to easily cross the intrathecal space, thus causing arachnoiditis.[28] Animal studies, though, have not shown MPA to cause significant meningeal inflammation after epidural injections.[29–31]

The use of intrathecal bupivacaine, with or without epinephrine, has also been reported to cause arachnoiditis. Boiardi and colleagues[32] described several cases of arachnoiditis after administration of bupivacaine with epinephrine. Gemma and colleagues[33] described a case of arachnoiditis after intrathecal administration of bupivacaine without epinephrine. It is unclear in these cases whether the arachnoiditis was triggered by the bupivacaine or other preservatives. Furthermore, it is unclear whether epinephrine plays a role in the pathogenesis of arachnoiditis.

A history of spinal surgery is a risk factor for arachnoiditis.[8] In particular, some investigators have specifically stated that surgery for a herniated intervertebral disc may lead to arachnoiditis.[5,7,25] Carroll and Wiesel[34] showed that a postoperative pain-free interval lasting between 1 and 6 months, followed by the gradual onset of leg pain, increases the likelihood that some scar tissue is responsible for the symptoms. Smolik and

Nash[5] showed that simple dural retraction for the visualization of a ruptured intervertebral disc may trigger arachnoiditis. Haughton and colleagues[35] showed that the nucleus pulposus of an intervertebral disc was able to cause focal arachnoiditis in monkeys.

Clinical Features

The diagnosis of arachnoiditis requires a detailed medical history and physical examination, as well as a review of confirmatory radiographic imaging studies. In obtaining a medical history from a patient with arachnoiditis, the clinician should seek three major characteristics of the pain. Pain of arachnoiditis is typically described as a burning pain that is constant and worsened by activity.[12] The pain of arachnoiditis may be located in the back or the lower limbs or both. The symptoms of arachnoiditis can vary from nonspecific back pain to radiculopathy and myelopathy.[36] Intractable pain that occurs secondary to arachnoiditis has a poorly localized pain pattern that is diffuse. In many patients, arachnoiditis is asymptomatic and is discovered as an incidental radiographic finding.[37] The pain symptoms of chronic arachnoiditis may be similar to those of other chronic pain syndromes, such as complex regional pain syndrome. The exact relationship of these pain syndromes has not been fully elucidated.

The physical examination findings in patients with arachnoiditis have been reviewed in two large clinical series. Burton followed 100 patients with arachnoiditis and found little motor weakness to be present.[12] These patients were commonly found to have a positive straight-leg raise sign, a tender sciatic notch, limited range of motion of the trunk, and paravertebral muscle spasms. Guyer and colleagues[25] followed 51 patients over more than 10 years and found that a decreased range of motion of the trunk was the most common finding on physical examination. In cases of chronic arachnoiditis with resultant syrinx formation, physical examination findings of syringomyelia are present. These include dissociative sensory loss and variable long tract signs.[8]

Radiographic Features

After a history and physical examination, radiographic imaging studies are used to confirm the clinical impression of arachnoiditis. Plain radiographs are not a useful diagnostic tool for detecting or confirming the presence of arachnoiditis.

On myelography, two distinct patterns of radiographic arachnoiditis can be differentiated. In type 1 arachnoiditis, there is pure adhesion of the nerve roots to the meninges with a homogeneous contrast pattern. No nerve root shadows are seen, and there is a rounded shortening of the nerve root pocket. In type 2 arachnoiditis, some proliferation is added inside the dural sac, which may be localized or diffuse.[38] The filling defects, narrowing, shortening, or occlusion of the spinal canal are also seen in this type of arachnoiditis. In early arachnoiditis, there is central nerve root clumping and thickening. As the arachnoiditis progresses, the nerve roots become adherent peripherally to the thecal sac and the terminal thecal sac appears "sleeveless" where the nerve roots do not fill it out in the normal pattern.[8] This finding can cause the thecal sac to appear empty.

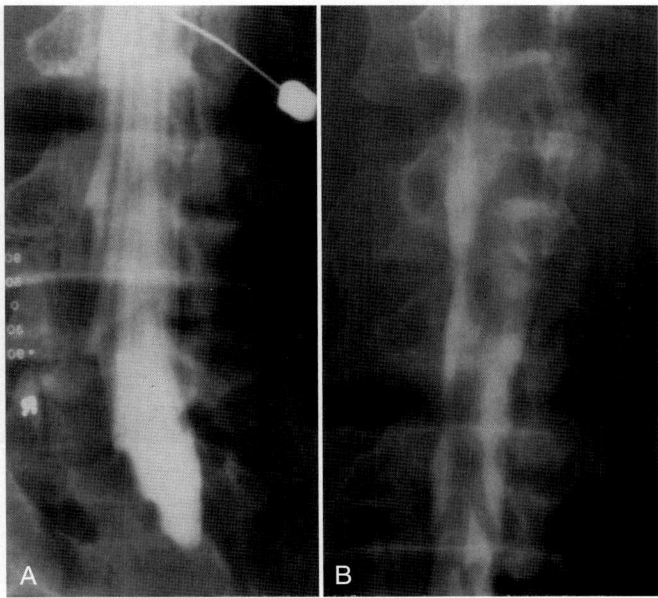

FIG. 106.2 (A) Myelogram demonstrating normal nerve root filling. (B) Myelogram of the same patient 7 years later. Clear evidence of arachnoiditis is shown by the thickened, "clumped" nerve roots that no longer show the normal filling of the nerve root sleeves.

On magnetic resonance imaging (MRI), one of three patterns is commonly found.[39] The first pattern is characterized by conglomerations of nerve roots, which are located centrally within the thecal sac. The second pattern is characterized by nerve roots that are clumped and attached peripherally to the meninges (Fig. 106.2). This appearance is similar to the empty sac appearance of myelography. The third pattern demonstrates increased soft tissue signal within the thecal sac with central obliteration of the subarachnoid space (Fig. 106.3).

At times, computed tomography or MRI reveals calcification or ossification of the spinal arachnoid in an entity called *arachnoiditis ossificans.* There are several subtypes of spinal arachnoiditis ossificans based on imaging characteristics. Type 1 has a semicircular arrangement, type 2 is circular, and type 3 demonstrates englobing of the caudal fibers.[40–42]

Spinal Epidural Fibrosis

Spinal epidural fibrosis is an entity observed after spine surgery that contributes to up to 14% of cases of failed back syndrome. Spinal epidural fibrosis is caused when fibroblasts from damaged paraspinal muscles enter the vertebral canal and proliferate, forming extensive epidural scarring.[43] This entity has been most typically described after cases of discectomy, whether open or percutaneous, as well as cases of implantation of spinal stimulating electrodes.[43,44]

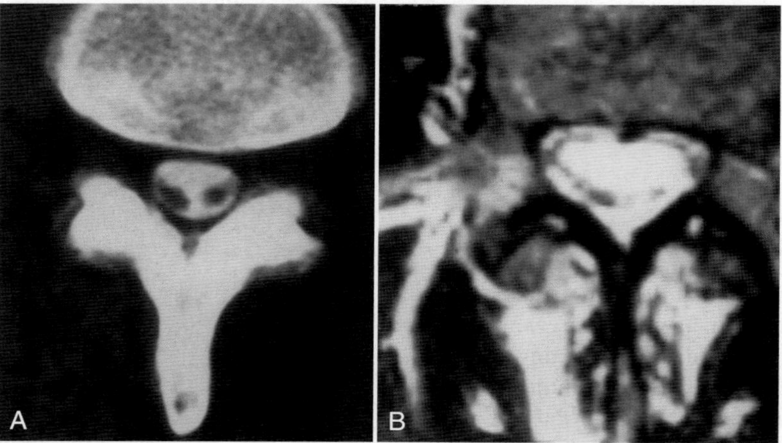

FIG. 106.3 (A) Computed tomographic myelogram demonstrating clumping of nerve roots in the thecal sac. (B) T2-weighted magnetic resonance imaging demonstrating the "empty sac" appearance of arachnoiditis. Note the peripheral location of the nerve roots within the thecal sac.

Treatment

A number of therapies are aimed at preventing or treating arachnoiditis or epidural fibrosis. Much of the research aimed at preventing failed back syndrome has dealt with strategies to prevent epidural fibrosis.

In a rat model of spinal epidural fibrosis, the administration of tissue plasminogen activator helped to prevent postlaminectomy epidural fibrosis. The presence of arachnoiditis was also less in the treatment group ($P < .01$).[45] Lee and colleagues[46] showed that the administration of 0.1 mg/mL of mitomycin C reduced epidural fibrosis after lumbar laminectomy in a rat model. This group made macroscopic, histologic, and MRI evaluations of the animals.[46] Epidural scarring was significantly reduced and dural adhesions were absent, while wound healing was not affected.

In a dog postlaminectomy model, it has been shown that a single fraction of 700 cGy external beam radiation helped to prevent epidural fibrosis and arachnoiditis. The authors demonstrated statistically significant reductions in the extent of fibrosis and density of fibroblasts. MRI confirmation of the efficaciousness of the therapy was also demonstrated.[47]

A recent study in humans aimed to evaluate the role of epidural steroids in preventing epidural fibrosis. Eighty-five of 178 patients received epidural steroids following discectomy. Patients were followed for 1 year and were assessed by questionnaires containing the pain scale. Application of epidural steroids resulted in less pain on the first and third days after surgery, resulted in shorter hospital stays, but did not prevent failed back syndrome or prevent epidural scar formation.[48]

The role of surgery in the treatment of arachnoiditis and epidural fibrosis is controversial. Surgical procedures that have been used to treat arachnoiditis include spinal fusion procedures, decompressive spinal procedures without fusion, neuroablative procedures, and implantation of spinal cord stimulators.[8]

A substantial body of literature exists that suggests open surgical procedures are not useful in the treatment of arachnoiditis. Carroll and Wiesel[34] found that no open surgical technique could eliminate the pathologic scar or significantly reduce the pain of arachnoiditis. Grahame and colleagues[37] also found that open surgical procedures had little or no effect on the long-term course of arachnoiditis.

Some groups argue for aggressive open surgical intervention for arachnoiditis and spinal epidural fibrosis. Shikata and colleagues[49] compared microlysis for arachnoiditis with and without spinal fusion. They found significant improvement in the clinical results when fusion was performed.

Spinal cord stimulation has been shown to have some benefit in patients with arachnoiditis. North and colleagues[50–54] have shown that spinal cord stimulation can be a successful therapy with proper patient selection. This group used temporary percutaneous electrodes as a screening technique before implantation of a permanent stimulator. A minimum of 50% pain relief with temporary electrodes over a 2- to 3-day course, as well as evidence of improved activity level and stable or decreased use of analgesics, was deemed satisfactory pain relief.[50–54]

Recent work has focused on minimally invasive techniques to treat arachnoiditis and spinal epidural fibrosis. A number of endoscopic techniques for adhesiolysis and promotion of CSF flow pathways have been developed with promising results.[55,56] Manchikanti and colleagues[57] demonstrated in a recent randomized controlled trial of spinal endoscopic adhesiolysis in chronic refractory low back pain and lower extremity pain that adhesiolysis with targeted delivery of local anesthesia and steroids is a successful technique in the treatment of arachnoiditis. This study demonstrated significant improvement in pain in 48% of subjects at 1-year follow-up.[57]

Summary

Arachnoiditis and epidural fibrosis are chronic conditions that result in significant morbidity. The long-term prognosis of these conditions is poor and there is no optimal management strategy that has been proven or widely accepted. Prevention of these conditions is ideal by avoiding agents that have been shown to lead to fibrosis and handling neural elements with care at surgery. In recent years, there has been a renewed interest in the management of arachnoiditis and spinal epidural fibrosis; as such, we have seen a number of promising experimental therapies. Pharmacologic therapy has shifted toward prevention and surgical therapy has shifted toward minimally invasive techniques. Although some surgeons advocate open surgical treatments to attempt to treat the *cause* of pain, we have found the best treatment results, as a whole, with the utilization of dorsal column stimulation to treat the *effects* of pain. Alternative treatments of the effects, including long-term use of narcotic medications, have been less effective in our hands. As these therapies and techniques are developed, there will be a need for more randomized, prospective, placebo-controlled, double-blind studies to determine the optimal methods for preventing and managing these devastating problems.

KEY POINTS

1. Spinal arachnoiditis is a nonspecific inflammatory process of the arachnoid layer of the spinal cord or cauda equina. When the outer arachnoid layer is injured, both the blood vessels and mesenchymal cells lend themselves to extensive proliferation. The ensuing reaction between the pia-arachnoid and the dura mater leads to obliterative arachnoiditis.
2. Spinal epidural fibrosis is caused when fibroblasts from damaged paraspinal muscles enter the vertebral canal and proliferate, forming extensive epidural scarring.
3. The progressive inflammation of arachnoiditis occurs in stages. The initial stage, radiculitis, consists of an inflamed pia-arachnoid with associated hyperemia and swelling of nerve roots. The second stage, arachnoiditis, is characterized by fibroblast proliferation and collagen deposition. The final stage, adhesive arachnoiditis, is the resolution of the inflammatory process and is characterized by dense collagen deposition.
4. Arachnoiditis can be caused by infectious etiologies, subarachnoid hemorrhage, epidural blood patches, myelography with oil-based medium, intrathecal injections of medications, and spinal surgery.
5. On myelography or MRI, arachnoiditis is characterized by clumping of the nerve roots. As the nerve roots become adherent peripherally, the thecal sac appears empty.
6. Treatment options for arachnoiditis or spinal epidural fibrosis include dorsal column stimulation, endoscopic adhesiolysis, external beam radiation, and open surgical adhesiolysis and spinal fusion.

KEY REFERENCES

1. Burton CV. Lumbosacral arachnoiditis. *Spine*. 1978;3:24-30.
   A description of the stages of progressive inflammation of the arachnoid that occur in lumbosacral arachnoiditis is provided.
2. Delamarter RB, Ross JS, Masaryk TJ, et al. Diagnosis of lumbar arachnoiditis by magnetic resonance imaging. *Spine*. 1990;15:304-310
   Morphologic changes of arachnoiditis are described in 24 patients undergoing MRI. Comparisons are made between MRI findings, CT myelography, and plain film myelography.
3. Guyer DW, Wiltse LL, Eskay ML, Guyer BH. The long range prognosis of arachnoiditis. *Spine*. 1989;12:1332-1341.
   The authors describe the factors influencing the development of arachnoiditis following myelography as the type of contrast agent used, the dosage of contrast medium, and the observation time after myelography.
4. North RB, Kidd DH, Zahurak M, et al. Spinal cord stimulation for chronic, intractable pain: experience over two decades. *Neurosurgery*. 2007;32:384-394.
   The authors describe that, with proper patient selection, spinal cord stimulation can be a successful therapy for arachnoiditis. Temporary percutaneous electrodes should be used as a screening technique before implantation of a permanent stimulator.
5. Smolik EA, Nash FP. Lumbar spinal arachnoiditis: a complication of the intervertebral disc operation. *Ann Surg*. 1951;133:490-495.
   A classic description of arachnoiditis as a complication of discectomy is provided.

REFERENCES

1. Rice I, Wee MYK, Thompson K. Obstetric epidurals and chronic adhesive arachnoiditis. *Br J Anaesth*. 2004;92:109-120.
2. April EW. *Clinical Anatomy*. 3rd ed. Philadelphia: Lippincott Williams & Wilkins; 1997:149-151.
3. Shantha TR, Evans JA. The relationship of epidural anesthesia to neural membranes and arachnoid villi. *Anesthesiology*. 1972;37:543-557.
4. Ransford AO, Harries BJ. Localised arachnoiditis complicating lumbar disc lesions. *J Bone Joint Surg*. 1972;54:656-665.
5. Smolik EA, Nash FP. Lumbar spinal arachnoiditis: a complication of the intervertebral disc operation. *Ann Surg*. 1951;133:490-495.
6. Delamarter RB, Ross JS, Masaryk TJ, et al. Diagnosis of lumbar arachnoiditis by magnetic resonance imaging. *Spine*. 1990;15:304-310.
7. Reigel DH, Bazmi G, Shih S-R, Marquardt MD. A pilot investigation of poloxamer 407 for the prevention of leptomeningeal adhesions in the rabbit. *Pediatr Neurosurg*. 1993;19:250-255.
8. Heary RF, Northrup BE, Barolat G. Arachnoiditis. In: Benzel EC, ed. *Spine Surgery*. 2nd ed. Philadelphia: Elsevier; 2005:2004-2012.
9. Mackay RP. Chronic adhesive spinal arachnoiditis. *JAMA*. 1939;112:802.
10. McLaurin RL, Bailey OT, Schurr PH, Ingraham FD. Myelomalacia and multiple cavitations of spinal cord secondary to adhesive arachnoiditis. *Arch Pathol*. 1954;57:138-146.
11. Sklar EML, Quencer RM, Green BA, Montalvo BM, Post MJ. Complications of epidural anesthesia: MR appearance of abnormalities. *Radiology*. 1991;181:549-554.
12. Burton CV. Lumbosacral arachnoiditis. *Spine*. 1978;3(1):24-30.
13. Yamagami T, Matsui H, Tsuji H, et al. Effects of laminectomy and retained extradural foreign body on cauda equina adhesions. *Spine*. 1993;18:1774-1781.
14. Poon TL, Ho WS, Pang KY, Wong CK. Tuberculous meningitis with spinal tuberculous arachnoiditis. *Hong Kong Med J*. 2003;9:59-61.
15. Hoffman GS. Spinal arachnoiditis. What is the clinical spectrum? *Spine*. 1983;8:538-540.
16. Jackson A, Isherwood I. Does degenerative disease of the lumbar spine cause arachnoiditis? A magnetic resonance study and review of the literature. *Br J Radiol*. 1994;67(801):840-847.
17. Kok AJ, Verhagen WI, Bartels RH, et al. Spinal arachnoiditis following subarachnoid haemorrhage: report of two cases and review of the literature. *Acta Neurochir*. 2000;142:795-799.

18. Jackson IJ. Aseptic hemogenic meningitis. *Arch Neurol Psych.* 1949;62:572-589.
19. Renk H. Neurological complications of central nerve blocks. *Acta Anaesthesiol Scand.* 1995;39:859-868.
20. Digiovanni AJ, Galbert MW, Wahle WM. Epidural injection of autologous blood for postlumbar-puncture headache II: additional clinical experiences and laboratory investigation. *Anesth Analg.* 1972;51:226-232.
21. Aldrete JA, Brown T. Intrathecal hematoma and arachnoiditis after prophylactic blood patch through a catheter. *Anesth Analg.* 1997;84:228-236.
22. Abouleish E, De la Vega S, Bledinger I, Tio T-O. Long-term follow-up of epidural blood patch. *Anesth Analg.* 1975;54:459-463.
23. Burton CV. Adhesive arachnoiditis. In: Youmans JR, ed. *Neurological Surgery*. 3rd ed. Philadelphia: WB Saunders; 1990:2856-2863.
24. Shaw M, Russell JA, Grossart KW. The changing pattern of spinal arachnoiditis. *J Neurol Neurosurg Psych.* 1978;41: 97-107.
25. Guyer DW, Wiltse LL, Eskay ML, Guyer BH. The long range prognosis of arachnoiditis. *Spine.* 1989;12:1332-1341.
26. Berg G, Hammar M, Moller-Nielsen J, et al. Low back pain during pregnancy. *Obstet Gynecol.* 1988;71:71-75.
27. Bernat JL. Intraspinal steroid therapy. *Neurology.* 1981;31:168-170.
28. Nelson DA. Dangers from methylprednisolone acetate therapy by intraspinal injection. *Arch Neurol.* 1988;45:804-806.
29. Abram S, Marasala M, Yaksh T. Analgesic and neurotoxic effects of intrathecal corticosteroids in rats. *Anesthesiology.* 1994;81:149-162.
30. Cicala RS, Turner R, Moran E, et al. Methylprednisolone acetate does not cause inflammatory changes in the epidural space. *Anesthesiology.* 1990;72:556-558.
31. Delany TJ, Rowlingson JC, Carron H, Butler A. Epidural steroid effects on nerves and meninges. *Anesth Analg.* 1980; 59:610-614.
32. Boiardi A, Sghirlanzoni A, La Mantia L, et al. Diffuse arachnoiditis following epidural analgesia. *J Neurol.* 1983;230:253-257.
33. Gemma M, Bricchi M, Grisoli M, et al. Neurologic symptoms after epidural anesthesia. Report of three cases. *Acta Anaesthesiol Scand.* 1994;38:742-743.
34. Carroll SE, Wiesel SW. Neurologic complications and lumbar laminectomy: a standardized approach to the multiply-operated lumbar spine. *Clin Orthop.* 1992;284:14-23.
35. Haughton VM, Nguyen CM, Ho K-C. The etiology of focal spinal arachnoiditis: an experimental study. *Spine.* 1993;18: 1193-1198.
36. Smith AS, Blaser SI. Infectious and inflammatory processes of the spine. *Radiol Clin North Am.* 1991;29:809-827.
37. Grahame R, Clark B, Watson M, Polkey C. Toward a rational therapeutic strategy for arachnoiditis. A possible role for d-penicillamine. *Spine.* 1991;16:172-175.
38. Jorgensen J, Hansen PH, Steenskov V, Oveson N. A clinical and radiological study of chronic lower spinal arachnoiditis. *Neuroradiology.* 1975;9:139-144.
39. Ross JS, Masaryk TJ, Modic MT, et al. MR imaging of lumbar arachnoiditis. *Am J Roentgenol.* 1987;149:1025-1032.
40. Chan CC, Lau PY, Sun LK, Lo SS. Arachnoiditis ossificans. *Hong Kong Med J.* 2009;15:146-148.
41. Domenicucci M, Ramieri A, Passacantilli E, et al. Spinal arachnoiditis ossificans: report of three cases. *Neurosurgery.* 2004;55:985.
42. Papavlasopoulos F, Stranjalis G, Kouyialis AT, et al. Arachnoiditis ossificans with progressive syringomyelia and spinal arachnoid cyst. *J Clin Neurosci.* 2007;14:572-576.
43. Smuck M, Benny B, Han A, Levin J. Epidural fibrosis following percutaneous disc decompression with coblation technology. *Pain Physician.* 2007;10:691-696.
44. Reynolds AF, Shetter AG. Scarring around cervical stimulating electrode. *Neurosurgery.* 1983;13:63-65.
45. Kemaloglu S, Ozkan U, Yilmaz F, et al. Prevention of spinal epidural fibrosis by recombinant tissue plasminogen activator in rats. *Spinal Cord.* 2003;41:427-431.
46. Lee JY, Stenzel W, Impekoven P, et al. The effect of mitomycin C in reducing epidural fibrosis after lumbar laminectomy in rats. *J Neurosurg Spine.* 2006;5:53-60.
47. Gerszten PC, Moossy JJ, Flickinger JC, et al. Inhibition of peridural fibrosis after laminectomy using low-dose external beam radiation in a dog model. *Neurosurgery.* 2000;46(6):1478-1485.
48. Hackel M, Masopust V, Bojar M, et al. The epidural steroids in the prevention of epidural fibrosis: MRI and clinical findings. *Neuro Endocrinol Lett.* 2009;30:51-55.
49. Shikata J, Yamamuro T, Iida H, Sugimoto M. Surgical treatment for symptomatic spinal adhesive arachnoiditis. *Spine.* 1989;14(8):870-875.
50. North RB, Campbell JN, James CS, et al. Failed back surgery syndrome: 5-year follow up in 102 patients undergoing repeated operation. *Neurosurgery.* 1991;28(5):685-690.
51. North RB, Ewend MG, Lawton MT, et al. Failed back surgery syndrome: 5 year follow-up after spinal cord stimulator implantation. *Neurosurgery.* 1991;28:692-699.
52. North RB, Kidd DH, Piantadosi S. Spinal cord stimulation versus reoperation for failed back surgery syndrome: a prospective, randomized study design. *Acta Neurochir Suppl.* 1995;64:106-108.
53. North RB, Kidd DH, Shipley J, Taylor RS. Spinal cord stimulation versus reoperation for failed back syndrome: a cost effectiveness and cost utility analysis based on a randomized controlled trial. *Neurosurgery.* 2007;61:361-368.
54. North RB, Kidd DH, Zahurak M, et al. Spinal cord stimulation for chronic, intractable pain: experience over two decades. *Neurosurgery.* 1993;32:384-394.
55. Warnke JP, Mourgela S. Adhesive lumbar arachnoiditis. Endoscopic subarachnoepidurostomy as a new treatment. *Nervenarzt.* 2007;78:1182-1187.
56. Warnke JP, Mourgela S. Endoscopic treatment of lumbar arachnoiditis. *Minim Invasive Neurosurg.* 2007;50:1-6.
57. Manchikanti L, Boswell MV, Rivera JJ, et al. A randomized, controlled trial of spinal endoscopic adhesiolysis in chronic refractory low back and lower extremity pain. *BMC Anesthesiol.* 2005;5:10.

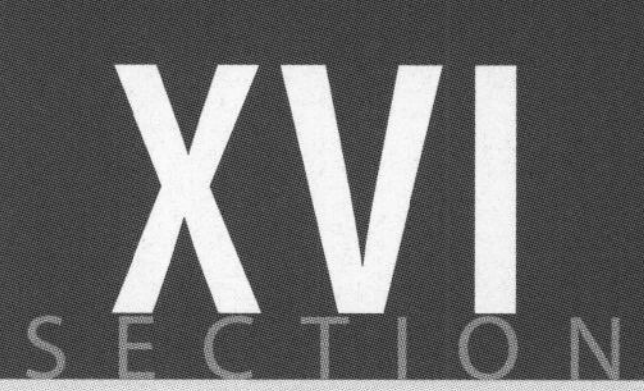

CHRONIC PAIN AND REHABILITATION

107 CHAPTER Chronic Pain: Basic Science

Aldric Hama
Shyam Gajavelli
Elizabeth A. Dugan
Jacqueline Sagen

Pain sensation is an important physiologic means by which an organism is informed about the immediate external environment and internal bodily function. The pain "experience" is the integration of a number of neurologic functions. In response to a brief painful stimulus, a rapid unconscious reflex and subsequent purposeful movement steer the organism away from the source of pain. The painful experience may be paired with a cue and remembered to generate avoidance behavior and evoke profound emotions. Pain from internal organs may signal either imminent or ongoing tissue damage, which can prompt a patient to seek medical attention. In a sense, acute pain assists survival.

However, chronic pain, pain that persists long after tissue healing due to injury or in tandem with disease, serves no useful biologic function.[1] Chronic pain leads to heightened anxiety and diminished social functioning.[2] The economic costs, in terms of both health care costs and lost productivity, are staggering and expected to rise even further as the population ages.[3-6] Thus there is a vital need to understand the mechanism of chronic pain and to develop mechanism-based analgesic therapies.

Chronic Spinal Cord Injury Pain

Chronic pain following spinal cord injury (SCI) is estimated to occur in 65% to 81% of SCI patients; approximately one third of those patients rate it as severe.[2,7] The addition of intractable pain to deficits in voluntary motor functions and autonomic dysfunction following SCI severely diminishes patient social and psychologic well-being.[8] To improve patient quality of life, pain relief is an important consideration along with other SCI-related complications in an overall treatment and rehabilitation strategy.

Despite increasing understanding of the cellular and molecular processes that mediate chronic pain in general, effective treatment for SCI pain in particular is lacking. At least two conditions thwart attempts to effectively ameliorate SCI pain. First, SCI pain is a heterogeneous condition with a number of possible interacting neurologic and inflammation-mediated mechanisms. Second, although chronic SCI pain shares striking similarities in terms of symptoms with other chronic pain states, such as peripheral nerve injury pain, distinct mechanisms distinguish chronic neuropathic SCI pain from that of other types of neuropathic pain. For example, there is a striking lack of parallelism between peripheral neuropathic pain and neuropathic SCI pain in terms of clinical pharmacology. The first steps toward effective analgesic treatment for SCI pain will involve not only careful clinical diagnosis but also consideration of SCI pain as a distinct chronic pain syndrome.

Spinal Cord Injury Pain Classification

The International Association for the Study of Pain has proposed a taxonomy that attempts to group SCI pain states to assist consistent clinical diagnosis and aid in designing effective pain management strategies (Table 107.1).[9] In addition, classification also aids researchers in designing appropriate experiments that will uncover mechanisms underlying SCI pain and hopefully uncover new analgesic targets.

As shown in Table 107.1, SCI pain can be divided into two general types, nociceptive and neuropathic. These pain types can be further divided by possible underlying pathologies. The classification of the various pain types (musculoskeletal, visceral, and neuropathic pain based on spinal lesion level) does not suggest definitive mechanisms, and the construct validity of the divisions has yet to be confirmed in clinical studies. However, such an uncomplicated taxonomy is a positive first step in systematically addressing the cause of SCI pain and developing useful therapies.

The first type of SCI pain, nociceptive pain, arises from stimulation of either somatic or visceral primary afferent nociceptors. Musculoskeletal pain has been characterized as dull, aching pain that worsens with movement and eases with rest.[7] In addition, this particular pain is localized to musculoskeletal structures. Examples of musculoskeletal pain sources

TABLE 107.1 Proposed International Association for the Study of Pain Classification of Pain After Spinal Cord Injury

Broad Type (Tier 1)	Broad System (Tier 2)	Specific Structures/Pathology (Tier 3)
Nociceptive	Musculoskeletal	Bone, joint, muscle trauma, or inflammation Mechanical instability Muscle spasm Secondary overuse syndromes
	Visceral	Renal calculus, bowel, sphincter dysfunction, etc. Dysreflexic headache
Neuropathic	Above level	Compressive mononeuropathies Complex regional pain syndromes
	At level	Nerve root compression (including cauda equina) Syringomyelia Spinal cord trauma/ischemia (central dysesthesia syndrome, etc.)
	Below level	Spinal cord trauma/ischemia (central dysesthesia syndrome, etc.)

From Siddall PJ. Management of neuropathic pain following spinal cord injury: now and in the future. *Spinal Cord.* 2009;47:352–359.

include injury to muscles or ligaments related to the initial injury, overuse of the shoulders and arms of a wheelchair-bound patient, and vertebral instability and osteoporosis due to SCI.[10] Given the initial challenges of novel self-propulsion and injury-associated pain, the onset of musculoskeletal pain is comparatively rapid (within weeks of the injury) and is the most commonly reported SCI-associated pain.[11] Chronic musculoskeletal pain has been noted long after the injury (at least 5 years) and could be associated with the long-term skeletal changes in posture due to injury.[7] Visceral pain has been described as spontaneous, dull, poorly localized, or cramping, apparently originating from deep visceral structures.[7] The occurrence of pain may or may not be coupled with visceral pathology and, unlike musculoskeletal pain, the onset of visceral pain may be months or years following SCI.[7,12] Although the incidence of chronic visceral SCI pain is low, the pain is described as either severe or excruciating.[7]

The second type of SCI pain is neuropathic pain, which results from trauma or disease to the nervous system. Neuropathic pain has been described as unevoked pain that is sharp, burning, shooting, stabbing, and electric, occurring continuously or as paroxysms. In addition to spontaneous pain, there may also be exaggerated painfulness evoked by nonnoxious stimulation (e.g., allodynia). Spontaneous and evoked neuropathic pain may occur at the level of injury due to a combination of damaged segmental spinal nerve roots or disinhibited spinal dorsal horn nociceptive neurons. About 40% of SCI patients experience at-level neuropathic pain.[7] In contrast to at-level pain, below-level pain appears to have a delayed onset after SCI, which could be due to dysfunction of brain regions postsynaptic to the spinothalamic tract.[7] Below-level pain is as severe and persistent as at-level neuropathic pain.[7] Despite a lack of cutaneous thermal detection (either cold or heat) below the lesion, below-level neuropathic pain occurs in about one-third of SCI patients. Interestingly, at-level and below-level cutaneous hypersensitivity correlates with the presence of below-level spontaneous pain, which suggests a common mechanism underlying these symptoms.[13,14] A positive correlation between spontaneous pain and cutaneous mechanical hypersensitivity of the painful area has been reported for other neuropathic pain states.[15] Such a correlation suggests that it may be possible to use defined stimuli to quantify spontaneous pain, beyond a subjective patient report, and objectively compare and contrast the efficacy of pain treatments.

General Mechanism

This chapter presents a general outline of the normal pain pathway. Detailed neuroanatomic and neurochemical schemes have been published elsewhere.[16] Noxious cutaneous stimuli (either thermal or mechanical) stimulate myelinated or unmyelinated small-diameter primary afferents, conducting the noxious signal to the spinal cord superficial dorsal horn (or, in the face, to the brainstem trigeminal sensory nucleus). Within the dorsal horn, excitatory neurotransmitters released from primary afferent central terminals stimulate postsynaptic dorsal horn neurons. A number of neuroactive substances (e.g., adenosine 5′-triphosphate [ATP]), excitatory amino acids, and neuropeptides activate their respective receptors on the postsynaptic neuron. By contrast, nonnociceptive, large-diameter, primary afferents terminate in the deep dorsal horn and also in the brainstem dorsal column nuclei.

Axons of dorsal horn nociceptive neurons ascend to the brain via a number of tracts. Axons of nociceptive neurons decussate in the spinal cord and ascend via the contralateral ventral funiculus (spinothalamic tract) and terminate in the ventroposterior lateral thalamus. The pain signal may be dispersed from the thalamic nucleus to various brain areas with diverse functions such as the sensory cortex, hypothalamus, limbic lobes, and motor nuclei. Although there are a number of indirect pathways between the spinal dorsal horn and brain, direct projections of dorsal horn neurons to a number of brain areas have also been reported.[17] By virtue of the numerous direct and indirect connections between nociceptive neurons to higher brain areas, pain evokes multiple physiologic and psychologic responses. Given human genetic diversity, it is apparent that the pain experience, as well as potential treatment strategies, differs among individuals and groups.[18,19]

In the normally functioning pain system, the excitatory component is counterbalanced by endogenous inhibitory components such that the initial pain sensation is not permanently propagated or does not evoke an exaggerated response. Primary afferents synapse with dorsal horn nociceptive neurons as well as inhibitory interneurons that, in turn, synapse with spinal nociceptive neurons, thus moderating pain transmission.[20] Also, axons of nociceptive spinal neurons that terminate in the brainstem activate serotonergic, catecholaminergic, and GABAergic (γ-aminobutyric acid) neurons, which in turn send axons down to the dorsal horn. Because terminals are found presynaptic to primary afferents and spinal nociceptive neurons, activation of these brainstem neurons leads to diminished pain perception. Direct application by intrathecal injection of inhibitory neurotransmitters and opioid neuropeptides reduces spinal nociceptive neuron responses to noxious peripheral stimulation and is antinociceptive in rats.[21] Analgesia is also observed in humans following intrathecal injection of similar substances (α-adrenergic, GABAergic, and opioid receptor agonists).[22] These findings show a considerable parallel between the human and rat spinal dorsal horn neurochemistry that further points out the utility of preclinical models in evaluating drugs for possible clinical use.

In contrast to the normal state, experimental evidence suggests that decreased inhibition, increased excitation, or a combination of both initiates and perpetuates a chronic pain state because of the pathology of the nervous system. For example, acute lumbar intrathecal injection of an antagonist to either the $GABA_A$ or $GABA_B$ receptor subtype or the glycine receptor leads to a transient yet robust hind paw hypersensitivity and vocalization in rats. This indicates that a tonic inhibition is present in the normal state, which dampens responses to peripheral stimulation. Similarly, intrathecal injection of an excitatory glutamate receptor agonist (e.g., *N*-methyl-D-aspartate [NMDA]) induces a long-lasting hind paw hypersensitivity.[23] The sustained excitation of nociceptive neurons may lead to increased intracellular cation levels, upregulation of second messenger systems, and gene expression.[16] These intracellular processes then lead to persistent hyperactivity and increased responsiveness to peripheral stimulation. Furthermore, such abnormal activity may be found throughout the pain neuraxis. Preclinical pain models have demonstrated considerable changes to normal neuroanatomy and neurochemistry following painful peripheral nerve injury or inflammation. For example, the central terminals of nonnociceptive primary afferents extend to spinal laminae normally receiving nociceptors, and these same afferents express neuropeptides typically found in nociceptors.[24,25] Changes in brain activity response to peripheral stimulation following an injury, including an SCI, have been observed.[26]

On the basis of findings in preclinical pain models, to attenuate clinical chronic pain states, it would be reasonable to increase inhibition (e.g., intrathecal $GABA_B$ receptor agonist baclofen) or decrease excitation (e.g., intrathecal NMDA receptor antagonist ketamine) at the level of the spinal cord, the first site of interaction between the peripheral nervous system and the central nervous system (CNS; see later).[22,27] Even though such acute measures may prove efficacious, they are temporary. It is likely that a number of regions within the nervous system may express abnormal excitation and that these changes have been made permanent via genetic and structural mechanisms. Cellular transplantation may be able to address some of these permanent changes and can be modified to target multiple aspects of CNS dysfunction. For example, transplantation of embryonic cells, such as neural progenitor cells or GABAergic neural progenitor cells, improves neuropathic pain symptoms, possibly through replacement of lost cells and promotion of increased inhibition.[28-38] Also, embryonic cells can be altered to continuously release endogenous analgesic substances, either through bioengineering or biomaterial platforms, which could be utilized to provide long-term pain relief.[39-48] This is particularly promising given the extensive preclinical and clinical research with cellular transplantation for functional recovery after SCI (for a review, see Yousefifard et al.[49]). Adjunct therapies, such as locomotor or cardiac training, may also improve long-term pain relief by targeting multiple aspects of SCI, including injury-evoked inflammatory processes, activation of endogenous analgesic systems, reduction of primary afferent sprouting, and normalization of neurotrophic factors within the spinal cord and affected musculature.[50-54]

Recombinant Analgesic Peptides

Naturally occurring peptides with analgesic properties are increasingly becoming the focus of preclinical pain research for several reasons, such as (1) their high specificity and affinity to pain-related target receptors, (2) their involvement as substrates of metabolism, and (3) their potential use in cellular and gene-based therapies. Vector-mediated delivery of possible analgesic molecules, such as opioid peptides, antiinflammatory cytokine interleukin-10, calcium channel binding peptide CBD3, brain-derived neurotrophic factor, and the GABA-synthetic enzyme GAD, have shown promising outcomes in rodent neuropathic pain models.[55-61] Herpes simplex virus–mediated opioid peptide gene delivery has recently undergone clinical trials for cancer pain.[48-62] A previous study described selection of promising therapeutic molecules.[63] Since then, exciting preclinical studies have demonstrated that naturally occurring peptides could be used to attenuate SCI-induced dorsal horn neuronal dysfunction underlying the SCI neuropathic pain state.

Intrathecal administration of histogranin, a peptide found in the medullary adrenal gland, ameliorated cutaneous hypersensitivity associated with neuropathic pain, possibly through reducing the activity of NMDA.[63-66] A recombinant synthetic version of histogranin, serine-histogranin (SHG), was expressed in vivo in rats by using a lentivirus expression system and reduced acute pain perception.[47] Naturally occurring μ-opioid receptor ligands, endomorphin-1 and -2 (EM-1 and EM-2) have also demonstrated efficacy in preclinical pain models. The preclinical findings of efficacy recently led to the initiation of a phase I clinical trial in which a viral vector delivered an opioid peptide gene to subjects with cancer pain.[48,62,67-69] Intraspinal injections of lentiviruses encoding SHG, EM-1 and EM-2, either singly or in combination, produced robust analgesic effects in SCI rats without decrement of efficacy over time (tolerance), as observed with some clinical analgesics.[70] Furthermore, the analgesic effects of the combination of SHG and EM appeared to be additive, which suggests a potential for greater analgesia with a combination compared with either peptides alone. The data suggest that delivery of therapeutic genes could be a useful approach in managing clinical neuropathic SCI pain.

The use of viruses to deliver therapeutic genes could be contraindicated in some patients. Thus, as an alternative, recombinant cell therapy offers the possibility of focal delivery of analgesic substances within the CNS. The recombinant cellular approach allows for the generation of genes encoding multiple copies of a peptide, which in turn allows for varying quantities of peptide to be produced. Genetically modified rat embryonic GABAergic cells expressing SHG significantly reduced thermal and mechanical hypersensitivity in rats with neuropathic SCI pain.[71] The GABAergic cells were capable of encoding from one to six copies of the SHG gene. Antinociception was observed, even when the cells were transplanted long after the injury.[71] Intrathecal injection of an antibody to SHG attenuated the antinociceptive effect of the transplants, demonstrating that significant amounts of SHG were released from the transplants. Levels of SHG released by the cells were confirmed by immunoblotting and immunocytochemistry.[71] These data highlight the potential use of gene and cellular therapies in providing long-lasting pain relief in patients with neuropathic SCI pain.

For obvious reasons, most experimental pain studies have focused on neural function. However, glial cells (e.g., microglia, astrocytes) vastly outnumber neurons in the CNS. Accumulating evidence indicates that glia have a key role in maintaining the neuropathic SCI pain state.[72] In the normal state, glia appear to maintain the homeostasis of the extracellular milieu. Because glia express receptors and ion channels, similar to neurons, they may respond to neuroactive substances. Following exposure to these substances, activated glia may release, in turn, a number of neuroactive substances and proinflammatory cytokines. The glial response following injury has been intensely characterized because modulating the response is believed to be crucial to promoting motor and sensory recovery.[73-75] Injury of the thoracic spinal cord leads to dramatic increases in microglia and astrocytes, not only at the site of injury, but also at the level of the lumbar enlargement several segments away.[76,77] Interestingly, similar increases in spinal glial activity in the lumbar spinal cord are observed in models of painful peripheral neuropathies.[78] Treatments designed to decrease glial function following SCI to improve motor function may also have a secondary effect of reducing SCI-induced pain. Such treatment studies should include sensory outcomes if the patient has SCI pain.

There is a compelling need for nonpharmaceutical treatment options for SCI patients through the identification of new and novel therapeutic strategies such as physical rehabilitation. Physical rehabilitation is a peripheral treatment that provides increased endogenous production of neurotrophic factors associated with spinal plasticity and functional recovery to the CNS, which can be difficult to deliver exogenously due to the impermeability of these neurotrophic factors across the blood-brain barrier.[79-82] Clinically, physical rehabilitation such as locomotor training (cycling and treadmill training) is prescribed to prevent muscle atrophy in the affected limbs and promote locomotor recovery in SCI patients.[83-88] However, aside from the known locomotor benefits, preclinical research has shown that moderate levels of locomotor training in rodent models of SCI provide partial reduction of neuropathic pain,[51,53] and increased levels of exertion under an intensive locomotor training protocol significantly reduced multiple symptoms of neuropathic pain not seen with moderate exertion.[54] These benefits are in part due to changes in endogenous opioid production, μ-opioid receptor expression, the bulbospinal serotonergic system, inflammatory markers, and aberrant sprouting of central terminals of nociceptive primary afferents.[53,89-99] Preclinical research findings suggest a dual role for physical rehabilitation to combat both neuropathic pain and locomotor dysfunction, thereby maximizing the potential for postinjury recovery, improving patient independence, and increasing productivity and participation in normal daily activities. Currently, physical rehabilitation is only prescribed to manage pain resulting from peripheral injury[100-103] and is rarely used for the management of central neuropathic pain.[104,105] Clinical trials in SCI patients are underway.[106,107]

Neuropathic Spinal Cord Injury Animal Models

The majority of preclinical SCI pain experiments have been done in rodents, not only because of the convenient availability of near-homogeneous subjects, but also because general clinical aspects of the histopathology following an SCI can be replicated in rats.[108] In addition, numerous analgesic treatments initially screened in peripheral injury chronic pain models have gone on to demonstrate clinical efficacy. Thus animal models of SCI pain may also be useful in both elucidating SCI pain mechanisms and developing novel clinical treatments.

Considerations

A degree of controversy exists surrounding the clinical relevance of rodent models of pain.[109] Such controversy plagues other fields of neurologic research as well.[110] The main clinical diagnosis of pain is based on the patient's verbal report, which would include pain severity, duration, and frequency. By contrast, in chronic pain models, a specific response to a given stimulus is interpreted as pain by experimenters. An exaggerated change in response to either nonnoxious or noxious (hyperalgesia) cutaneous stimuli is interpreted to mean a pathologic alteration in the underlying pain mechanism. However, such changes in sensory perception may not always be reported by patients, who primarily present with unevoked spontaneous pain.

An additional controversy that arises concerning animal models is deciding which would be best to use for preclinical research such that the information obtained could be readily translated into clinical practice. In terms of evaluating new therapeutics, predictive validity and reliability are crucial.[111] A model with predictive validity allows one to accurately foresee the effect of a treatment in humans.

If the animal displays behaviors that are analogous to clinical symptoms, the model is said to have face validity. In pain research, however, the outcome measures in preclinical and clinical situations may not be identical. Most preclinical analgesic drug studies measure changes in response to stimulation, whereas few clinical drug trials have solely used quantitative sensory testing. Despite the stark difference in outcome measures, the concordance between the animal and clinical results is between 61% and 88%.[112] In general, the high concordance suggests that the presence of cutaneous sensitivity (e.g., withdrawal threshold) is predictive of spontaneous pain (e.g., pain rating on a visual analog scale), but the wide range also indicates that some models may have better predictive value over others.

In an attempt to bridge the divide between clinical and preclinical outcome measures, basic scientists are working to quantify spontaneous pain-related behavior and changes in mood associated with chronic pain in animals.[7,109] As mentioned earlier, changes in affect may impair SCI rehabilitation, further degrading overall well-being. Some of the well-defined experimental methods used in other behavioral research fields such as psychiatry and drug addiction have been adopted to detect and quantify spontaneous pain-related behavior, with varying degrees of success.[113-115] For example, the University of Michigan developed a mechanical conflict-avoidance system (Coy MCS; Noldus Information Technology) that provides an operant method of pain testing that complements reflexive methods by addressing cognitive and motivational processing in rodents.[116] Given the current level of concordance between preclinical and clinical results and the difficulty of quantifying affect in animals, it is not entirely clear how much more translational or clinical value will be gained with the addition of nonspontaneous measures to current testing procedures.[110]

If a model has face validity, the assumption that follows is that it also has construct validity. Although it is desirable to mimic the clinical pathology in the rat, this may not always be possible. Demonstrating construct validity requires knowledge of the clinical mechanism, which is often lacking and incompletely understood. Also, as Geyer and Markou point out, the theoretical basis of neurologic disorders is constantly evolving.[110] Thus construct validity should not be the sole determinant to judge the usefulness of a model.

Finally, reliability refers to the "consistency and stability" of both the experimental procedure and the symptoms resulting from it.[110] On the one hand, this quality is highly desirable in basic science research because a highly predictable outcome following a manipulation reduces the chance of error and the need to use large numbers of subjects. On the other hand, clinical SCI is not homogeneous, and although many SCI patients have chronic pain, some do not.

Ultimately, the first consideration in choosing a model should be the scientific purpose of the model. Then, on the basis of the three main criteria (face, predictive, construct validity), the experimenter can determine whether the model is appropriate for the objectives.

Description of Spinal Cord Injury Models

Three general SCI injury models have been most frequently used: excitotoxin microinjection into the spinal cord parenchyma, acute trauma to spinal tissue, and photochemically induced ischemia of spinal vasculature. Each rat model displays distinct injury-induced, pain-related behaviors and histopathology—behaviors and pathologies that may not be observed in the other models. At the same time, a few general characteristics may be observed across models. The neurobiologic substrates that underlie SCI pain in one model could be specific to that model. On one hand, this may complicate efforts to develop analgesic treatments to cover a heterogeneous population. On the other hand, the heterogeneity of the clinical population and a diversity of mechanisms suggest that that there is no magic bullet and that numerous treatments for pain need to be developed.

Excitotoxin Injection

A series of microinjections of the nonsubtype selective glutamate receptor agonist quisqualate is placed into the deep dorsal horn of the thoracolumbar spinal cord.[117] The lesion leads to a dramatic necrosis of the deep dorsal horn but spares the superficial dorsal horn, thus preserving ipsilateral sensory input. Furthermore, syrinx formation is observed in these rats. Significant bilateral hind paw hypersensitivity to both thermal and mechanical stimuli is observed as early as 8 days following microinjection. Also, spontaneous grooming behavior, excessive hind paw scratching directed within the injected dermatome, begins about 2 days after microinjection and may progressively expand and worsen over time. The grooming behavior is suggestive of at-level unevoked pain. Both the grooming behavior and cutaneous hypersensitivity persist for weeks following injection.

The excitotoxic SCI model is unique in that the spinal cord lesion is generally restricted to the dorsal horn. Because of this selective destruction, there is little or no hind paw motor dysfunction. Several novel treatments have been tried in this rat model that attenuated pain-related symptoms, including grooming.[28,30,118] The predictive validity of this model is not known because extensive evaluation of clinically available analgesic drugs has yet to be done.

Acute Trauma to the Spinal Cord

Several methods of direct spinal injury lead to significant and long-lasting neuropathic pain–related symptoms. Following a laminectomy, the spinal cord at the thoracic level may be laterally hemisected, contused (e.g., New York University impactor), or compressed (e.g., vascular clip).

Following lateral hemisection of the spinal cord at level T13, rats develop bilateral hind paw hypersensitivity to heat (decreased withdrawal latency) and mechanical (decreased withdrawal threshold) stimuli beginning 10 days after injury.[119] Loss of ipsilateral hind limb function is also observed, but functional recovery begins about 7 days after injury. Despite mild-to-moderate hind paw dysfunction, as demonstrated by the Basso, Beattie, and Bresnahan (BBB) locomotor rating scores,[120] robust ipsilateral hind paw responses can be evoked in hemisected rats to observe the behavioral effects of therapeutics. In addition, a bilateral forepaw (above-level) hypersensitivity is observed beginning about 2 weeks after injury. A few clinically relevant analgesic drugs have been tested in these rats, along with novel treatments.[46,121] Systemic and intrathecal (catheter terminating at the spinal level T13) injection of morphine ameliorated hind paw mechanical hypersensitivity.[122] Intrathecal baclofen increased hind paw withdrawal thresholds in injured rats.[123] In contrast, intrathecal injection of the selective serotonin reuptake inhibitor (SSRI) fluvoxamine attenuated forepaw mechanical hypersensitivity to a greater degree than hind paw hypersensitivity.[124] The differing effect suggests a differential neuropharmacology between above- and below-level neuropathic pains. Hemisection of the spinal cord could be useful in comparing neurochemical and anatomic changes rostral or caudal to the lesion with the uninjured side. The lesion is relatively easy to generate and fairly consistent from rat to rat, which in part explains why this is the most commonly used SCI injury model.[125] However, the relevance of hemisection to clinical injury is not entirely clear because there are few human cases of spinal hemisection injuries.

Most spinal cord injuries are due to acute extradural impact and compressive forces.[108] These are traditionally modeled in animals using contusive impact devices in which the severity of the injury can be varied, resulting in locomotor dysfunction in a force-dependent manner.[126] In these animals, the effect of various intervention strategies can be examined.[125]

Even with standardized procedures and devices, it is still difficult to uncover a correlation between the degree of tissue damage and symptoms of neuropathic pain. Following a "moderate" contusion of the thoracic dorsal spinal cord, the forepaws develop hypersensitivity to heat and mechanical stimuli, but the sensitivity of the hind paws to these stimuli is variable.[127,128] A moderate contusion also yields long-lasting at-level hypersensitivity, whereas fewer rats with a severe injury displayed such hypersensitivity.[129] Hind limb functionality scores in moderately injured rats were considerably decreased but recovered such that scores were eventually the same as uninjured rats. Cutaneous hypersensitivity persisted, however, long after functional recovery.[129,130] Contusion injuries are the most commonly used SCI animal model for functional recovery research; however, this model may not be able to consistently produce below-level neuropathic pain.[72] Other studies have demonstrated significant at-level and below-level hypersensitivity with severe injury.[131,132] Clinical studies have yet to find a correlation among the extent of spinal cord injury, specific loss of certain tracts, or gray matter areas and pain.[133]

Similar to the excitotoxic SCI model, there has been little pharmacologic validation of either the hemisection or contusion model with clinical analgesic drugs, except for the anticonvulsant gabapentin.[134] The positive effect of an SSRI on above-level SCI pain in the hemisection suggests that this class of drug may be clinically useful. However, there is a lack of positive clinical evidence supporting the use of an SSRI in SCI pain.[27] In fact, the use of SSRI and tricyclic antidepressants such as amitriptyline may enhance SCI-induced spasticity, and tricyclic antidepressants may be contraindicated because of side effects such as urinary retention and constipation.[27,135] To increase confidence that novel analgesic interventions tested in these preclinical animal models will succeed in SCI patients, more pharmacologic validation studies are necessary.

Compression Injury

To mimic *circumferential compression,* a combination of impact and compression at multiple levels rather than a single point of the spinal cord, a modified aneurysm clip is used in which one jaw is slid under the anterior thoracic spinal cord, the other jaw is over the posterior cord, and the clip is closed for a given length of time (e.g., 1 minute).[136] Another important distinction of this model compared with others is the prolonged injury duration. A modified version of the circumferential compression model was used to evaluate several clinical analgesic drugs. As with other models, significant hind paw hypersensitivity to thermal and mechanical stimuli developed and hind limb locomotor function diminished; these effects were noted as early as 1 week after injury.[137,138] On the basis of a limited number of drugs, it appears that this model can distinguish analgesic from nonanalgesic drugs. For example, a sedating and anxiolytic dose of diazepam in SCI rats does not ameliorate hind paw hypersensitivity (Table 107.2). The antiarrhythmic sodium channel blocker mexiletine was not analgesic in clinical SCI pain and did not demonstrate efficacy in compression-injured rats (Table 107.3). In contrast, in an ischemic model of neuropathic SCI pain, mexiletine ameliorated mechanical hypersensitivity.[139]

TABLE 107.2 Drugs Evaluated in Rats With a Spinal Cord Compression Injury

		A_{50} Dose[a] (95% CL)		
Drugs (Route)	**Tested Dose (mg/kg)**	**Tactile**	**Heat**	**ED_{50} Rotarod[b]**
Amitriptyline (SC)	3, 10, 30	NS	NS	
Baclofen (SC)	1, 3, 10	3.8 (2.2–6.5)	4 (1.3–12.2)	2.1
Carbamazepine (SC)	2, 20, 60	NS	NS	
Diazepam (SC)	0.3, 1, 3	NS	NS	
Gabapentin (SC)	10, 30, 100	26 (16–42)	NS	128.6
Memantine (SC)	2, 6, 20	7.6 (3.4–16.7)	NS	2.4
Mexiletine (SC)	7.5, 25, 75	NS	NS	
Morphine (SC)	0.3, 1, 3	0.7 (0.5–1.2)	1.1 (0.4–2.7)	14.1
Rofecoxib (IP)	10	NS	NS	
Tramadol (SC)	10, 30, 100	20.6 (11.8–35.8)	ND	>20

From Hama A, Sagen J. Behavioral characterization and effect of clinical drugs model of pain following spinal cord compression. *Brain Res.* 2007;14:117–128.
[a]The A_{50} dose (mg/kg) is the 50% antinociceptive dose calculated at peak efficacy; N = 4-9 rats/dose.
[b]The 50% dose (mg/kg) that disrupted performance on the rotarod test.[230-233]
CL, Confidence limit; IP, intraperitoneal; ND, not determined; NS, no significant effect observed at any dose (P > .05) compared with vehicle treatment; SC, subcutaneous.

TABLE 107.3 Randomized Controlled Trials of Treatment of Spinal Cord Injury (SCI) Pain

Active Drug	Treatment Duration, Maximal Daily Dose, Study Design	Total No. SCI Patients	Outcome	NNT (95% CI)
Gabapentin	2–4 weeks, 1800 mg/day, crossover design	7	Equal to placebo	∞
Lamotrigine	2–9 weeks, 400 mg/day, crossover design	22	Equal to placebo	∞
Amitriptyline	6 weeks, 10–125 mg/day, parallel design	84	Equal to placebo	NA
Lidocaine (SA)	50–100 mg, crossover design	21	Better than placebo	3.5 (1.8–37)
Lidocaine (IV)	30 min, 5 mg/kg, crossover design	16/10	Better than placebo[a]	5 (1.6–∞)[b]
Mexiletine	2–4 weeks, 450 mg/day, crossover design	11	Equal to placebo	NA
Ketamine (IV)	60 + 120 μg/kg (20 min)	9	Better than placebo	NA
Alfentanil (IV)	7 + 12 μg/kg (29 min), crossover design	9	Better than placebo	NA
Morphine (IV)	20 min: 9–30 mg infusion, crossover design	15/9	Equal to placebo[a]	3 (1.6–40)[b]
Baclofen (IT)	50 μg, crossover design	7	Better than placebo	NA

IT, intrathecal; IV, intravenous; NA, not accessible from article; NNT, number of patients needed to treat to obtain one patient with 50% pain relief; SA, subarachnoid.
[a]Conclusion based on all patients in the study (SCI and stroke).
[b]Based on SCI patients. Individual references for each study in Finnerup and Jensen.[27]

A number of drugs were significantly antinociceptive, however, including systemic baclofen, morphine, and the anticonvulsants gabapentin and pregabalin.[140] Recent data from the rat spinal compression model suggest that memantine, tramadol (a cannabinoid receptor agonist), and the N-type voltage-gated calcium channel blocker ziconotide may be effective for neuropathic SCI pain (compare Tables 107.2 and 107.3).[138,141] While robust reduction of neuropathic SCI pain was obtained with exogenous cannabinoids, increasing synaptic levels of endogenous cannabinoids (e.g., anandamide) by blocking the degratory enzyme did not yield a comparable level of antinociception.[142] Clinical trials with appropriate controls are necessary to confirm the clinical utility of these drugs and establish predictive validity of the model.[143] Recent trials in patients with the anticonvulsant pregabalin (Lyrica) have reported some relief of pain symptoms in a number of chronic pain conditions, including SCI pain; however, adverse effects were also noted.[144-148] The pharmacologic data suggest a selective responsiveness to antinociceptive agents rather than generalized responses to ataxic or sedating drugs. The data also suggest differences between models (beyond the type of injury) in the mechanisms that maintain neuropathic SCI pain. Further drug efficacy comparisons between models are necessary to support this contention. In general, the diverse animal drug efficacy data imply that some drugs may be useful within specific populations of SCI patients.

Interestingly, drugs that have been shown to be efficacious for peripheral neuropathic pain, such as amitriptyline and the anticonvulsant carbamazepine, do not show efficacy in this model.[27,149] This suggests significant mechanistic differences between peripheral and central neuropathic pain and implies that distinct treatment approaches may be necessary depending on the injury, regardless of similarities in symptoms (e.g., allodynia).

Photochemical Ischemia

Ischemia in the CNS may lead to neuropathic pain.[2] Hao and colleagues[150] developed a neuropathic SCI pain model that did not involve mechanical destruction of CNS tissue. After intravenous injection of erythrosin B, laser irradiation of the thoracic vertebrae causes coagulation of the spinal blood vessels, which is limited to immediate spinal segments. A short-term (several days) mechanical hypersensitivity develops within the thoracic dermatome in which the ischemia occurred.[150] With greater ischemic damage, thoracic hypersensitivity reemerges several weeks after the initial hypersensitivity and persists for months. Furthermore, some of these animals (40%) mutilate their hind limbs ("autotomy"), suggesting the presence of below-level spontaneous pain or dysesthesia.[151]

Several clinical drugs have been evaluated in these rats.[139,151-154] The thoracic hypersensitivity was opioid sensitive and also suppressed with the antiarrhythmic drugs tocainide and mexiletine, the sedative pentobarbital, and gabapentin. However, clonidine and baclofen did not significantly affect hypersensitivity. In contrast, in clinical SCI pain, intrathecal clonidine and baclofen demonstrated efficacy, whereas (oral) mexiletine did not (see Table 107.3).[27,155,156] It is possible that at-level pain in these rats and the clinical neuropathic SCI pain are entirely different in terms of mechanism. The experimental approaches differ greatly as well; at-level pain was not specifically evaluated in the clinical trials, and there is a lack of below-level pain in this model. Other data using this model suggest that the NMDA receptor antagonist dextromethorphan could be useful in the treatment of SCI pain, as it appears to be for some types of peripheral neuropathic pain.[157] Ketamine, a drug with similar NMDA receptor channel blocking properties, has been shown to relieve neuropathic SCI pain.[158] The outcome of clinical studies using dextromethorphan will test the predictive value of the ischemia SCI model.

Dorsal Root Avulsion Model

The T13/L1 dorsal root avulsion model of spinal cord injury was developed specifically for the study of central pain and to minimize confounding complications, such as paralysis, urinary tract infections, and autotomy seen with SCI models that affect the ventral horn. This model results in tissue damage to Lissauer's tract, dorsal horn, and dorsal columns and induces robust and reliable hind paw mechanical allodynia associated with the L4–L6 spinal segments.[159,160] Two versions of the model have been developed for testing systemically or intrathecally administered pharmacologic agents. Pharmacologic administration of the phosphodiesterase inhibitor propentofylline, the macrophage migration inhibitory factor inhibitor ibudilast, and the Toll-like receptor 4 antagonist (+)-naltrexone each reversed below-level allodynia bilaterally in this model.[161] However, single administration was insufficient and administration of at least 1 to 2 weeks was required for reversal of pain symptoms. This may allow for interpretations of apparent drug failures after short-term dosing regimens.[161] Overall, this model provides an additional means to investigate below-level central neuropathic pain states associated with spinal cord injury.

Mechanism of Neuropathic Spinal Cord Injury Pain in Humans

Because of the ethical and technical limitations to human experimentation, there are few opportunities to directly observe the neural mechanism of chronic SCI pain in humans. The limited clinical data, however, reinforce the general preclinical finding in terms of increased spinal hyperexcitability following injury.

Using microelectrodes, spontaneous activity in dorsal horn neurons was recorded both rostrally and caudally to the injury in patients with SCI pain.[162,163] Similar activity in spinal neurons was also found in SCI rats.[164-166] In addition, dorsal horn neurons in rats displayed exaggerated excitation (central sensitization) to distal cutaneous stimulation, but analogous neurons have yet to be described in humans. Changes in CNS neural function have been observed beyond the spinal cord in both rats and humans.[167-169] The cause of the abnormal neural function is not known. One possibility is that, as observed in rats, lesions to dorsal gray matter lead to neuropathic SCI pain. On the basis of limited analyses of spinal lesions using magnetic resonance imaging, a significant distinction between patients with pain and pain-free patients and the extent of tract or gray matter damage was not observed.[133] Perhaps the temporal change in abnormal neural function parallels that of pain following SCI. A clinical time course study may not be technically feasible to address this issue, however.

At the cellular level, changes in excitatory or inhibitory neurotransmission may underlie abnormal activity of, for example, spinal neurons. Changes in neuropeptide content in the spinal dorsal horn following SCI in animals have been reported. An excitatory neuropeptide found in primary afferent nociceptors, calcitonin gene-related peptide (CGRP), was increased in the deep dorsal horn of the lumbar spinal cord, far removed from the thoracic injury site.[170,171] Both the spinal compression and hemisection models have significant below-level hypersensitivity to noxious and innocuous cutaneous stimuli, which are transiently ameliorated with a CGRP receptor antagonist.[121] The elevated CGRP content in the deep dorsal horn could partly underlie both increased neuronal activity and chronic pain. The CGRP content in the deep dorsal horn from SCI patients is also increased, although pain was not measured in these patients.[172] In the case of humans, then, the consequence of the change in neuropeptide content on sensation is not clear. The amelioration of neuropathic SCI pain with NMDA receptor antagonists such as ketamine and dextromethorphan indirectly suggests that glutamate receptor activity has a key role in maintaining pain. There is no direct evidence to demonstrate significant loss of GABAergic neurons, for example, in the spinal cord of neuropathic SCI pain patients. However, the indirect pharmacologic evidence such as analgesic effects with baclofen suggests that a loss of inhibition could be as important as the increase in excitation. Noninvasive magnetic resonance spectroscopy could be used to evaluate changes in inhibitory amino acids.[168,173]

Few clinical studies have evaluated the role of glia in clinical neuropathic SCI pain. Spinal cord tissue taken acutely following injury (15 to 60 days) exhibited marked microglia/macrophage infiltration proximal and distal to the injury.[174] A correlation between cellular activation and pain cannot be determined because the pain status of the patients was not determined. Although clinical data correlating possible dysfunction of brain nuclei with SCI pain are starting to emerge, postmortem tissue is currently the only way to evaluate in detail the neurochemical and anatomic processes following SCI.[167]

Currently, treatments for SCI pain are based more or less on trial and error rather than empirically. However, with increasing sophistication of medical imaging techniques combined with receptor-selective radioligands, it may be possible to observe and quantify the effect of SCI on neural areas that are pain related and assess the effect of treatment on these areas.[175] Drugs that are analgesic could be characterized by receptor-binding function as well as activity at defined pain-related areas.

Nonneural Molecular Targets for Spinal Cord Injury Pain

Although there are numerous interactions between glia and neurons following injury, research on chronic pain—SCI pain in particular—has been generally slanted toward neural events.[176,177] As a result, the development of novel analgesic drugs has focused on neural dysfunction. These include ziconotide and cannabinoids, both of which, coincidentally, are naturally based products.[143,178] Given that glia also express membrane proteins similar to those found on neurons, it is likely that drugs targeted to neurons may also affect glial function. This section summarizes a few of the cellular and molecular processes, with respect to glia, underlying the development of neuropathic SCI pain.

In addition to the sensitization of nociceptors and spinal dorsal horn neurons, an early and permanent "gliopathy" contributes to maintenance of neuropathic SCI pain. Gliopathy has been defined as the "dysfunctional and maladaptive" glia response to injury.[72] Like the response observed in neurons following injury, the glia response is persistent and elevated.

Gliopathy has also been reported in other neuropathic pain models.[179] Activated glia secrete proinflammatory cytokines, nociceptor sensitizers, and other substances that directly activate nociceptors and alter ion channel expression.[180,181] Glial nuclear factor–κB (NF-κB), a protein complex transcriptional factor with a key role in the cellular response to infection and stress, is presumed to be crucial in the intracellular process that underlies the long-term response to substances released from injured spinal cord. Activated NF-κB stimulates cytokine gene transcription. Knockout of glial NF-κB in mice reduced peripheral tissue injured–induced pain.[182] Nonsteroidal antiinflammatory drugs, glucocorticoids, and immunosuppressants inhibit the activation of NF-κB.[183] Early postinjury blocking of the NF-κB signaling cascade may attenuate the severity of later neuropathic SCI pain. It should be noted that NF-κB is also crucial in tissue healing. Thus an optimal, probably narrow, level of activation of NF-κB is necessary for recovery. In terms of SCI, the optimal level that will lead to both functional motor and sensory recovery remains to be defined.

Lipid Signaling

A number of proteins that have been identified by proteomic and genomic analyses in SCI can be functionally categorized in several groups, such as cell cycling, chemokines, cellular metabolism, lipid and protein degradation, neuronal survival, and regeneration.[184-187] In addition to cellular membrane formation, lipids also have important roles in extracellular and intracellular signaling. One such class of lipids is the lysophospholipids, lipids involved in cell proliferation and chemotaxis.

In addition to cytokines, NF-κB also induces transcriptional upregulation of ectonucleotide pyrophosphatase/phosphodiesterase 2 (ENPP2/autotoxin), the enzyme that produces lysophosphatidic acid (LPA).[188] Activation of the peripheral LPA1 receptor leads to demyelination and vascular remodeling, processes that in part mediate the initiation of nerve injury–induced pain.[189-191] In the spinal cord, LPA induces proliferation of astrocytes and also inhibits glutamate uptake by reactive astrocytes, thereby exacerbating glutamate neurotoxicity.[192] Because these pathologies are also observed following SCI and LPA activation appears to have a key role in initiating nerve injury–induced neuropathic pain, LPA may also contribute to the onset of neuropathic SCI pain. Antagonists to either the enzyme or the receptor may be useful in reducing the tissue pathology caused by LPA and perhaps ameliorating SCI pain. FTY720-phosphate (fingolimod), an immunosuppressant derived from the fungal product myriocin, has been demonstrated to have antitumor effects and is a potential treatment for multiple sclerosis.[193] It is an inhibitor of ENPP2 and a sphingosine-1-phosphate (S1P) receptor agonist. S1P activation leads to similar events observed with LPA, including the increased synthesis of prostaglandins, but FTY720-phosphate reduces pain following peripheral nerve injury.[193] A number of S1P receptor subtypes exist, so the effect of FTY720-phosphate could be mediated through one of these or via an entirely novel mechanism.

Glial Inhibitors

A number of intracellular or membrane targets modulate the glial response to injury. In spinal nociceptive neurons, glutamate excitotoxicity results in the upregulation of microglia-specific activator cysteine-cysteine chemokine ligand 21 (CCL21). This ligand is transported preferentially down axons and released.[194,195] The protein binds specifically to CXCR3 receptors expressed on microglia and not those found on neurons and astrocytes. The tetracycline derivative minocycline decreases microglia activation and expression of CCL21.[196] The presence of the microglia activator CCL21 is not restricted to the site of SCI but may be found rostrally in brain regions such as the thalamus.[196] Thus it is important to note here that an apparently discrete CNS lesion may lead to glia activation throughout the pain neuraxis, and systemic rather than localized treatment may be required to effectively treat neuropathic SCI pain.

On exposure to growth-inducing proinflammatory cytokines and nucleotides (e.g., ATP), glia begin to proliferate or reenter the cell cycle in a cyclin D1–dependent manner.[197,198] Cyclin-dependent kinases (CDKs) and cyclins assist the transition through various steps of the cell cycle. Postmitotic cells such as oligodendrocytes and neurons respond to these proliferation signals by undergoing apoptosis. CDK inhibitors that are under investigation as anticancer drugs (e.g., olomoucine, roscovitine, and flavopiridol) decrease spinal lesion volume following SCI.[199,200] These compounds also inhibited tumor necrosis factor (TNF)-α–mediated microglial proliferation. Antagonism of the Toll-like receptor, TLR4, by opioid inactive isomers (+)-naltrexone and (+)-naloxone, reverses neuropathic pain through blockade of downstream signaling leading to nitric oxide, TNF-α, and reactive oxygen species that may help explain the in vivo therapeutic effects of these antagonists.[201] Alvocidib, a flavopiridol derivative, reduced inflammation-induced peripheral tissue destruction.[202] The capsaicin-sensitive cation channel TRPV1 is found on peripheral nociceptors (as well as glia). CDK5 mediates TRPV1 phosphorylation, which leads to sensitized nociceptors. TNF-α, abundantly found in injured tissues, also sensitizes TRPV1 by a CDK5-mediated pathway.[203-206] Roscovitine, another nucleotide analogue, prevents activation of CDK2 and CDK5 and has been shown to be effective in attenuating inflammatory pain.[207,208] At higher concentrations, roscovitine could inhibit the activity of CDK5-inducible signal transduction pathway kinases such as extracellular signal-regulated kinase 1 (ERK1) and ERK2.[209] ERKs have been implicated in dorsal horn neural hyperexcitability and glial activation.[177] Cannabinoid receptor type 2 activation induces a microglial antiinflammatory phenotype and reduces migration through mitogen-activated protein kinase phosphatase induction and ERK dephosphorylation.[210,211] Thus prevention of injury-induced reinitiation of the glial cell cycle may be useful in limiting tissue damage as well as sensory dysfunction caused by overexpression of cytokines and other inflammatory mediators.

Propentofylline, a xanthine derivative with neuroprotective properties, has been shown to reduce neuropathic SCI pain via numerous possible mechanisms.[77,212] Propentofylline is both an adenosine reuptake inhibitor and phosphodiesterase (PDE) inhibitor.[213,214] Treatment of SCI rats with propentofylline leads to decreased glia activation and increased GABAergic function as indicated by increased protein expression of the enzyme that produces GABA in neurons, which coincided with decreased pain.[212] Similarly, ibudilast, another nonselective PDE inhibitor, suppressed glial cell activation and pain-related behavior following nerve injury.[215] Phosphodiesterase inhibitors, including sildenafil and minocycline, could be a novel class of analgesics for SCI pain; however, in recent clinical trials propentofylline failed to decrease postherpetic neuralgia.[211,216,217]

Finally, a membrane protein not involved in membrane electrical conduction may have potential as an analgesic target. The aquaporins (AQPs) are integral membrane proteins that are permeable to water and found in various mammalian cells.[218] AQP4 is highly expressed in brain and has been found exclusively in astrocytes.[219] Following SCI, these channels were found to be upregulated, which may partly explain the presence of numerous fluid-filled cavities (syrinx) within the injured spinal cord.[187,220] An SCI-induced increase in AQP1, found in neurons and ependymal cells, may also be involved in syrinx formation. The carbonic anhydrase inhibitor acetazolamide, a clinically used diuretic, may inhibit AQP4 function, reducing tissue damage and possibly SCI pain.[221,222]

It should be apparent that numerous short-term and long-term cellular processes are modulated following SCI and that addressing only one issue may not entirely control abnormal glial responses to injury. Drugs with multiple mechanisms may therefore be desirable over those with a specific mechanism.

The degree to which glial function can be attenuated to obtain pain relief is currently unknown. This problem also arises in blocking neurotransmission for pain relief—total block leads to anesthesia and adverse neurologic side effects. Likewise, complete block of glial function or completely destroying proteins associated with glial scarring following SCI leads to injury exacerbation.[223,224] Also, time to treatment would be an important consideration. Although immediate blockade of gliosis with cytokine-neutralizing antibodies or genetic manipulation significantly improved functional recovery after experimental SCI, few patients can be treated immediately following SCI.[225-227] In addition, neuropathic SCI pain emerges months or years following injury, making universal early treatment in all SCI cases questionable.[7] Further studies in terms of treatment timing and better understanding of the effects of novel glial inhibitors on eventual functional outcome are necessary.

Summary

The sheer amount of potential targets, time needed to evaluate these targets, and time required to create a safe drug may be discouraging for patients with SCI and their physicians. However, a number of clinically available drugs (and nontraditional substances) for other conditions may be useful in neuropathic SCI pain.

Despite the growing clarification of the mechanism underlying neuropathic SCI pain, the difficulty of providing effective pain relief persists. The experimental and clinical data point out that there are numerous neural and nonneural mechanisms that underlie the initiation and maintenance of neuropathic SCI pain. On one hand, preclinical research may eventually yield a multitude of treatments for treating neuropathic pain, whether they are orally consumed small molecules, cell-based therapies, or gene-based therapies. On the other hand, it is not entirely clear which of these enzymes or receptors can be effectively targeted by external intervention. Also, the most effective timing of the treatments, whether in parallel or in series, is not entirely clear.

A key test of the usefulness of a preclinical model is whether it can predict the clinical efficacy of a given treatment. Researchers believe that their models may be generalized to a given clinical situation, but this may lead to clinical failure on the basis of incorrect assumptions. Many of the neuropathic SCI pain mechanisms observed in rodents have yet to be demonstrated in humans. There should also be confidence that the animal end points and clinical end points are similar or the same. On the basis of a review of the preclinical and clinical literature, such confidence is lacking. If animal models are to shoulder the burden of producing novel treatments for neuropathic SCI pain, the validity of these models should be carefully ascertained. Failures and successes should be openly presented.[228,229]

Acknowledgment

The authors are supported by Buoniconti Fund, University of Miami Office of Research, Research Education, Innovative Medicine (RIM) Research Support Award and the State of Florida, Florida Department of Health.

KEY POINTS

1. *Gliopathy:* This concept stresses the contribution of nonneuronal cells to onset and maintenance of SCI-induced neuropathic pain. The dysfunctional and maladaptive glial response to injury sensitizes nociceptors and spinal dorsal horn neurons, thus contributing to the maintenance of neuropathic SCI pain. Pain treatments could have better outcomes if gliopathy is addressed. The beneficial effects of glial inhibition need to be timed and balanced to ameliorate pain—a complete ablation of glial response has similar outcomes as an unresolved glial response.
2. The molecular mechanism of chronic, neuropathic SCI pain is multifaceted, indicating that treatment aimed at several molecular targets rather than a single molecular target may be optimal.
3. Preclinical testing of a number of pharmacotherapeutics has uncovered similarities and differences in efficacy between neuropathic SCI pain and other chronic pain models. The data thus far suggest there are limited common mechanisms across pain states.

KEY REFERENCES

1. Falci S, Best L, Bayles R, et al. Dorsal root entry zone microcoagulation for spinal cord injury-related central pain: operative intramedullary electrophysiological guidance and clinical outcome. *J Neurosurg*. 2002;97(2 suppl):193-200.

Electrophysiologic identification of abnormal spinal dorsal horn neural activity below the level of lesion was investigated in neuropathic SCI pain patients. The presence of abnormal evoked or spontaneous neural activity was used to guide dorsal root entry zone lesioning.

2. Finnerup NB, Jensen TS. Spinal cord injury pain—mechanisms and treatment. *Eur J Neurol*. 2004;11:73-82.
A review of possible mechanisms of SCI pain and a listing of drugs that have been evaluated in randomized, placebo-controlled clinical trials for SCI pain.

3. Gwak YS, Crown ED, Unabia GC, et al. Propentofylline attenuates allodynia, glial activation and modulates GABAergic tone after spinal cord injury in the rat. *Pain*. 2008;138:410-422.
This study elucidates the potential of phosphodiesterase inhibitors as a novel class of analgesics for SCI pain.

4. Hulsebosch CE, Hains BC, Crown ED, et al. Mechanisms of chronic central neuropathic pain after spinal cord injury. *Brain Res Rev*. 2009;60:202-213.
This article introduces the concept of "gliopathy" and its contribution to maintenance of neuropathic SCI pain.

5. Lenz FA, Tasker RR, Dostrovsky JO, et al. Abnormal single-unit activity recorded in the somatosensory thalamus of a quadriplegic patient with central pain. *Pain*. 1987;31(2):225-236.
Early electrophysiologic identification of a supraspinal generator in below-level neuropathic SCI pain was investigated. Modern noninvasive equipment could be used to identify supraspinal activity in neuropathic SCI pain and possibly aid in the development of treatments.

6. Nesic O, Lee J, Unabia GC, et al. Aquaporin 1—a novel player in spinal cord injury. *J Neurochem*. 2008;105(3):628-640.
This study presents a molecule that has dual function. Use of inhibitors of such molecules should be carefully timed and balanced.

REFERENCES

1. Merskey H, Bogduk N. *Classification of Chronic Pain: Descriptions of Chronic Pain Syndromes and Definitions of Pain Terms*. 2nd ed. Seattle: IASP Press; 1994:240.
2. Bonica JJ. *Management of Pain*. 2nd ed. Philadelphia: Lippincott Williams & Wilkins; 1990:2120.
3. Straus BN. Chronic pain of spinal origin: the costs of intervention. *Spine*. 2002;27:2614-2619.
4. Mapel DW, Shainline M, Paez K, et al. Hospital, pharmacy, and outpatient costs for osteoarthritis and chronic back pain. *J Rheumatol*. 2004;31:573-583.
5. Allaire SH, Prashker MJ, Meenan RF. The costs of rheumatoid arthritis. *Pharmacoeconomics*. 1994;6:513-522.
6. Pentland W, McColl MA, Rosenthal C. The effect of aging and duration of disability on long term health outcomes following spinal cord injury. *Paraplegia*. 1995;33:367-373.
7. Siddall PJ, McClelland JM, Rutkowski SB, et al. A longitudinal study of the prevalence and characteristics of pain in the first 5 years following spinal cord injury. *Pain*. 2003;103:249-257.
8. Widerstrom-Noga EG, Felipe-Cuervo E, Yezierski RP. Chronic pain after spinal injury: interference with sleep and daily activities. *Arch Phys Med Rehabil*. 2001;82:1571-1577.
9. Siddall PJ, Yezierski RP, Loeser JD. Pain following spinal cord injury: clinical features, prevalence, and taxonomy. *Int Assoc Study Pain*. 2000;3:1-10.
10. Middleton JW, Leong G, Mann L. Management of spinal cord injury in general practice—part 2. *Aust Fam Physician*. 2008;37:331-332, 335-338.
11. Siddall PJ, Taylor DA, McClelland JM, et al. Pain report and the relationship of pain to physical factors in the first 6 months following spinal cord injury. *Pain*. 1999;81:187-197.
12. Kogos SC Jr, Richards JS, Banos JH, et al. Visceral pain and life quality in persons with spinal cord injury: a brief report. *J Spinal Cord Med*. 2005;28:333-337.
13. Finnerup NB, Johannesen IL, Fuglsang-Frederiksen A, et al. Sensory function in spinal cord injury patients with and without central pain. *Brain*. 2003;126(Pt 1):57-70.
14. Widerstrom-Noga E. Chronic pain and nonpainful sensations after spinal cord injury: is there a relation? *Clin J Pain*. 2003;19:39-47.
15. Attal N, Fermanian C, Fermanian J, et al. Neuropathic pain: are there distinct subtypes depending on the aetiology or anatomical lesion? *Pain*. 2008;138:343-353.
16. Millan MJ. The induction of pain: an integrative review. *Prog Neurobiol*. 1999;57:1-164.
17. Cliffer KD, Burstein R, Giesler GJ Jr. Distributions of spinothalamic, spinohypothalamic, and spinotelencephalic fibers revealed by anterograde transport of PHA-L in rats. *J Neurosci*. 1991;11:852-868.
18. Campbell CM, France CR, Robinson ME, et al. Ethnic differences in the nociceptive flexion reflex (NFR). *Pain*. 2008;134:91-96.
19. Tan EC, Lim Y, Teo YY, et al. Ethnic differences in pain perception and patient-controlled analgesia usage for postoperative pain. *J Pain*. 2008;9:849-855.
20. Millan MJ. Descending control of pain. *Prog Neurobiol*. 2002;66:355-474.
21. Yaksh TL, Hua XY, Kalcheva I, et al. The spinal biology in humans and animals of pain states generated by persistent small afferent input. *Proc Natl Acad Sci USA*. 1999;96:7680-7686.
22. Bennett G, Serafini M, Burchiel K, et al. Evidence-based review of the literature on intrathecal delivery of pain medication. *J Pain Symptom Manage*. 2000;20:S12-S36.
23. Yaksh TL. Behavioral and autonomic correlates of the tactile evoked allodynia produced by spinal glycine inhibition: effects of modulatory receptor systems and excitatory amino acid antagonists. *Pain*. 1989;37:111-123.
24. Neumann S, Doubell TP, Leslie T, et al. Inflammatory pain hypersensitivity mediated by phenotypic switch in myelinated primary sensory neurons. *Nature*. 1996;384:360-364.
25. Shortland P, Woolf CJ. Chronic peripheral nerve section results in a rearrangement of the central axonal arborizations of axotomized A beta primary afferent neurons in the rat spinal cord. *J Comp Neurol*. 1993;330:65-82.
26. Endo T, Spenger C, Hao J, et al. Functional MRI of the brain detects neuropathic pain in experimental spinal cord injury. *Pain*. 2008;138:292-300.
27. Finnerup NB, Jensen TS. Spinal cord injury pain—mechanisms and treatment. *Eur J Neurol*. 2004;11:73-82.
28. Brewer KL, Yezierski RP. Effects of adrenal medullary transplants on pain-related behaviors following excitotoxic spinal cord injury. *Brain Res*. 1998;798:83-92.
29. Eaton MJ, Wolfe SQ, Martinez M, et al. Subarachnoid transplant of a human neuronal cell line attenuates chronic allodynia and hyperalgesia after excitotoxic spinal cord injury in the rat. *J Pain*. 2007;8:33-50.
30. Hendricks WA, Pak ES, Owensby JP, et al. Predifferentiated embryonic stem cells prevent chronic pain behaviors and restore sensory function following spinal cord injury in mice. *Mol Med*. 2006;12(1-3):34-46.
31. Wolfe SQ, Garg M, Cumberbatch NM, et al. Optimizing the transplant dose of a human neuronal cell line graft to treat SCI pain in the rat. *Neurosci Lett*. 2007;414(2):121-125.

32. Eaton MJ, Wolfe SQ. Clinical feasibility for cell therapy using human neuronal cell line to treat neuropathic behavioral hypersensitivity following spinal cord injury in rats. *J Rehabil Res Dev*. 2009;46(1):145-165.
33. Braz JM, Sharif-Naeini R, Vogt D, et al. Forebrain GABAergic neuron precursors integrate into adult spinal cord and reduce injury-induced neuropathic pain. *Neuron*. 2012;74(4):663-675.
34. Jergova S, Hentall ID, Gajavelli S, Varghese MS, Sagen J. Intraspinal transplantation of GABAergic neural progenitors attenuates neuropathic pain in rats: a pharmacologic and neurophysiological evaluation. *Exp Neurol*. 2012;234(1):39-49.
35. Lee JW, Jergova S, Furmanski O, Gajavelli S, Sagen J. Predifferentiated GABAergic neural precursor transplants for alleviation of dysesthetic central pain following excitotoxic spinal cord injury. *Front Physiol*. 2012;3:167.
36. Braz JM, Wang X, Guan Z, Rubenstein JL, Basbaum AI. Transplant-mediated enhancement of spinal cord GABAergic inhibition reverses paclitaxel-induced mechanical and heat hypersensitivity. *Pain*. 2015;156(6):1084-1091.
37. Basbaum AI, Braz JM. Cell transplants to treat the "disease" of neuropathic pain and itch. *Pain*. 2016;157(suppl 1):S42-S47.
38. Shetty AK, Bates A. Potential of GABA-ergic cell therapy for schizophrenia, neuropathic pain, and Alzheimer's and Parkinson's diseases. *Brain Res*. 2016;1638(Pt A):74-87.
39. Krishna V, Konakondla S, Nicholas J, et al. Biomaterial-based interventions for neuronal regeneration and functional recovery in rodent model of spinal cord injury: a systematic review. *J Spinal Cord Med*. 2013;36(3):174-190.
40. Kanno H, Pressman Y, Moody A, et al. Combination of engineered Schwann cell grafts to secrete neurotrophin and chondroitinase promotes axonal regeneration and locomotion after spinal cord injury. *J Neurosci*. 2014;34(5):1838-1855.
41. Tian L, Prabhakaran MP, Ramakrishna S. Strategies for regeneration of components of nervous system: scaffolds, cells and biomolecules. *Regen Biomater*. 2015;2(1):31-45.
42. Jin Y, Bouyer J, Shumsky JS, Haas C, Fischer I. Transplantation of neural progenitor cells in chronic spinal cord injury. *Neuroscience*. 2016;320:69-82.
43. Lin XY, Lai BQ, Zeng X, et al. Cell transplantation and neuroengineering approach for spinal cord injury treatment: a summary of current laboratory findings and review of literature. *Cell Transplant*. 2016;25(8):1425-1438.
44. Brewer KL, Yezierski RP. Effects of adrenal medullary transplants on pain-related behaviors following excitotoxic spinal cord injury. *Brain Res*. 1998;798:83-92.
45. Eaton MJ, Wolfe SQ, Martinez M, et al. Subarachnoid transplant of a human neuronal cell line attenuates chronic allodynia and hyperalgesia after excitotoxic spinal cord injury in the rat. *J Pain*. 2007;8:33-50.
46. Hains BC, Johnson KM, Eaton MJ, et al. Serotonergic neural precursor cell grafts attenuate bilateral hyperexcitability of dorsal horn neurons after spinal hemisection in rat. *Neuroscience*. 2003;116:1097-1110.
47. Gajavelli S, Castellanos DA, Furmanski O, et al. Sustained analgesic peptide secretion and cell labeling using a novel genetic modification. *Cell Transplant*. 2008;17:445-455.
48. Wolfe D, Mata M, Fink DJ. A human trial of HSV-mediated gene transfer for the treatment of chronic pain. *Gene Ther*. 2009;16:455-460.
49. Yousefifard M, Rahimi-Movaghar V, Nasirinezhad F, et al. Neural stem/progenitor cell transplantation for spinal cord injury treatment. A systematic review and meta-analysis. *Neuroscience*. 2016;322:377-397.
50. Ditor DS, Latimer AE, Ginis KA, et al. Maintenance of exercise participation in individuals with spinal cord injury: effects on quality of life, stress and pain. *Spinal Cord*. 2003;41(8):446-450.
51. Hutchinson KJ, Gomez-Pinilla F, Crowe MJ, Ying Z, Basso DM. Three exercise paradigms differentially improve sensory recovery after spinal cord contusion in rats. *Brain*. 2004;127(Pt 6):1403-1414.
52. Nawoczenski DA, Ritter-Soronen JM, Wilson CM, Howe BA, Ludewig PM. Clinical trial of exercise for shoulder pain in chronic spinal injury. *Phys Ther*. 2006;86(12):1604-1618.
53. Detloff MR, Smith EJ, Quiros Molina D, Ganzer PD, Houle JD. Acute exercise prevents the development of neuropathic pain and the sprouting of non-peptidergic (GDNF- and artemin-responsive) c-fibers after spinal cord injury. *Exp Neurol*. 2014;255:38-48.
54. Dugan EA, Sagen J. An intensive locomotor training paradigm improves neuropathic pain following spinal cord compression injury in rats. *J Neurotrauma*. 2015;32(9):622-632.
55. Eaton MJ, Blits B, Ruitenberg MJ, Verhaagen J, Oudega M. Amelioration of chronic neuropathic pain after partial nerve injury by adeno-associated viral (AAV) vector-mediated over-expression of BDNF in the rat spinal cord. *Gene Ther*. 2002;9(20):1387-1395.
56. Milligan ED, Sloane EM, Langer SJ, et al. Controlling neuropathic pain by adeno-associated virus driven production of the anti-inflammatory cytokine, interleukin-10. *Mol Pain*. 2005;1:9.
57. Chen ML, Cheng C, Lv QS, et al. Altered gene expression of NIDD in dorsal root ganglia and spinal cord of rats with neuropathic or inflammatory pain. *J Mol Histol*. 2008;39(2):125-133.
58. Storek B, Reinhardt M, Wang C, et al. Sensory neuron targeting by self-complementary AAV8 via lumbar puncture for chronic pain. *Proc Natl Acad Sci USA*. 2008;105(3):1055-1060.
59. Beutler AS, Reinhardt M. AAV for pain: steps towards clinical translation. *Gene Ther*. 2009;16(4):461-469.
60. Kim J, Kim SJ, Lee H, Chang JW. Effective neuropathic pain relief through sciatic nerve administration of GAD65-expressing rAAV2. *Biochem Biophys Res Commun*. 2009;388(1):73-78.
61. Fischer G, Pan B, Vilceanu D, Hogan QH, Yu H. Sustained relief of neuropathic pain by AAV-targeted expression of CBD3 peptide in rat dorsal root ganglion. *Gene Ther*. 2014; 21(1):44-51.
62. Fink DJ, Wechuck J, Mata M, et al. Gene therapy for pain: results of a phase I clinical trial. *Ann Neurol*. 2011;70(2): 207-212.
63. NasiriNezhad F, Sagen J. NMDA antagonist peptide supplementation enhances pain alleviation by adrenal medullary transplants. *Cell Transplant*. 2005;14(4):203-211.
64. Lemaire S, Rogers C, Dumont M, et al. Histogranin, a modified histone H4 fragment endowed with N-methyl-D-aspartate antagonist and immunostimulatory activities. *Life Sci*. 1995;56(15):1233-1241.
65. Siegan JB, Hama AT, Sagen J. Suppression of neuropathic pain by a naturally-derived peptide with NMDA antagonist activity. *Brain Res*. 1997;755(2):331-334.
66. Hama AT, Siegan JB, Herzberg U, Sagen J. NMDA-induced spinal hypersensitivity is reduced by naturally derived

peptide analog [Ser1]histogranin. *Pharmacol Biochem Behav.* 1999;62(1):67-74.

67. Gross M, Liu B, Tan J, et al. Distinct effects of PIAS proteins on androgen-mediated gene activation in prostate cancer cells. *Oncogene.* 2001;20(29):3880-3887.
68. Hao S, Wolfe D, Glorioso JC, Mata M, Fink DJ. Effects of transgene-mediated endomorphin-2 in inflammatory pain. *Eur J Pain.* 2009;13(4):380-386.
69. Wolfe D, Wechuck J, Krisky D, Mata M, Fink DJ. A clinical trial of gene therapy for chronic pain. *Pain Med.* 2009;10(7):1325-1330.
70. NasiriNezhad F, Gajavelli S, Priddy B, et al. Viral vectors encoding endomorphins and serine histogranin attenuate neuropathic pain symptoms after spinal cord injury in rats. *Mol Pain.* 2015;11:2.
71. Jergova S, Gajavelli S, Pathak N, Sagen J. Recombinant neural progenitor transplants in the spinal dorsal horn alleviate chronic central neuropathic pain. *Pain.* 2016;157(4):977-989.
72. Hulsebosch CE, Hains BC, Crown ED, et al. Mechanisms of chronic central neuropathic pain after spinal cord injury. *Brain Res Rev.* 2009;60:202-213.
73. Bethea JR, Dietrich WD. Targeting the host inflammatory response in traumatic spinal cord injury. *Curr Opin Neurol.* 2002;15(3):355-360.
74. El Hokayem J, Cukier HN, Dykxhoorn DM. Blood derived induced pluripotent stem cells (iPSCs): benefits, challenges and the road ahead. *J Alzheimers Dis Parkinsonism.* 2016;6(5).
75. Deumens R, Koopmans GC, Joosten EA. Regeneration of descending axon tracts after spinal cord injury. *Prog Neurobiol.* 2005;77:57-89.
76. Detloff MR, Fisher LC, McGaughy V, et al. Remote activation of microglia and pro-inflammatory cytokines predict the onset and severity of below-level neuropathic pain after spinal cord injury in rats. *Exp Neurol.* 2008;212:337-347.
77. Gwak YS, Hulsebosch CE. Remote astrocytic and microglial activation modulate neuronal hyperexcitability and below-level neuropathic pain after spinal injury in rat. *Neuroscience.* 2009;161:895-903.
78. Hansson E. Could chronic pain and spread of pain sensation be induced and maintained by glial activation? *Acta Physiol (Oxf).* 2006;187:321-327.
79. Edgerton VR, de Leon RD, Tillakaratne N, et al. Use-dependent plasticity in spinal stepping and standing. *Adv Neurol.* 1997;72:233-247.
80. de Leon RD, Hodgson JA, Roy RR, Edgerton VR. Locomotor capacity attributable to step training versus spontaneous recovery after spinalization in adult cats. *J Neurophysiol.* 1998;79(3):1329-1340.
81. Edgerton VR, Tillakaratne NJ, Bigbee AJ, de Leon RD, Roy RR. Plasticity of the spinal neural circuitry after injury. *Annu Rev Neurosci.* 2004;27:145-167.
82. Gomez-Pinilla F, Ying Z, Roy RR, Hodgson J, Edgerton VR. Afferent input modulates neurotrophins and synaptic plasticity in the spinal cord. *J Neurophysiol.* 2004;92(6):3423-3432.
83. Jin Y, Tessler A, Fischer I, Houle JD. Fibroblasts genetically modified to produce BDNF support regrowth of chronically injured serotonergic axons. *Neurorehabil Neural Repair.* 2000;14(4):311-317.
84. Mehrholz J, Kugler J, Pohl M. Locomotor training for walking after spinal cord injury. *Spine.* 2008;33(21):E768-E777.
85. Marsh BC, Astill SL, Utley A, Ichiyama RM. Movement rehabilitation after spinal cord injuries: emerging concepts and future directions. *Brain Res Bull.* 2011;84(4-5):327-336.
86. Phillips AA, Cote AT, Warburton DE. A systematic review of exercise as a therapeutic intervention to improve arterial function in persons living with spinal cord injury. *Spinal Cord.* 2011;49(6):702-714.
87. Wang D, Ichiyama RM, Zhao R, Andrews MR, Fawcett JW. Chondroitinase combined with rehabilitation promotes recovery of forelimb function in rats with chronic spinal cord injury. *J Neurosci.* 2011;31(25):9332-9344.
88. Wirz M, Bastiaenen C, de Bie R, Dietz V. Effectiveness of automated locomotor training in patients with acute incomplete spinal cord injury: a randomized controlled multicenter trial. *BMC Neurol.* 2011;11:60.
89. Carr DB, Bullen BA, Skrinar GS, et al. Physical conditioning facilitates the exercise-induced secretion of beta-endorphin and beta-lipotropin in women. *N Engl J Med.* 1981;305(10):560-563.
90. Dey S. Physical exercise as a novel antidepressant agent: possible role of serotonin receptor subtypes. *Physiol Behav.* 1994;55(2):323-329.
91. Hicks AL, Martin KA, Ditor DS, et al. Long-term exercise training in persons with spinal cord injury: effects on strength, arm ergometry performance and psychological well-being. *Spinal Cord.* 2003;41(1):34-43.
92. Lo WC, Jackson E, Merriman A, Harris J, Clarke RW. 5-HT receptors involved in opioid-activated descending inhibition of spinal withdrawal reflexes in the decerebrated rabbit. *Pain.* 2004;109(1-2):162-171.
93. Kuphal KE, Fibuch EE, Taylor BK. Extended swimming exercise reduces inflammatory and peripheral neuropathic pain in rodents. *J Pain.* 2007;8(12):989-997.
94. Boecker H, Sprenger T, Spilker ME, et al. The runner's high: opioidergic mechanisms in the human brain. *Cereb Cortex.* 2008;18(11):2523-2531.
95. Valim V, Natour J, Xiao Y, et al. Effects of physical exercise on serum levels of serotonin and its metabolite in fibromyalgia: a randomized pilot study. *Rev Bras Reumatol.* 2013;53(6):538-541.
96. Bobinski F, Ferreira TA, Cordova MM, et al. Role of brainstem serotonin in analgesia produced by low-intensity exercise on neuropathic pain after sciatic nerve injury in mice. *Pain.* 2015;156(12):2595-2606.
97. Fuss J, Steinle J, Bindila L, et al. A runner's high depends on cannabinoid receptors in mice. *Proc Natl Acad Sci USA.* 2015;112(42):13105-13108.
98. Kim TW, Lim BV, Baek D, Ryu DS, Seo JH. Stress-induced depression is alleviated by aerobic exercise through up-regulation of 5-hydroxytryptamine 1A receptors in rats. *Int Neurourol J.* 2015;19(1):27-33.
99. Kim TW, Lim BV, Kim K, Seo JH, Kim CJ. Treadmill exercise alleviates stress-induced impairment of social interaction through 5-hydroxytryptamine 1A receptor activation in rats. *J Exerc Rehabil.* 2015;11(4):192-197.
100. Mannerkorpi K, Henriksson C. Non-pharmacological treatment of chronic widespread musculoskeletal pain. *Best Pract Res Clin Rheumatol.* 2007;21(3):513-534.
101. English AW, Wilhelm JC, Sabatier MJ. Enhancing recovery from peripheral nerve injury using treadmill training. *Ann Anat.* 2011;193(4):354-361.
102. Dobson JL, McMillan J, Li L. Benefits of exercise intervention in reducing neuropathic pain. *Front Cell Neurosci.* 2014;8:102.
103. Cooper MA, Kluding PM, Wright DE. Emerging relationships between exercise, sensory nerves, and neuropathic pain. *Front Neurosci.* 2016;10:372.

104. Henwood P, Ellis JA. Chronic neuropathic pain in spinal cord injury: the patient's perspective. *Pain Res Manag.* 2004;9(1):39-45.
105. Sadowsky CL, McDonald JW. Activity-based restorative therapies: concepts and applications in spinal cord injury-related neurorehabilitation. *Dev Disabil Res Rev.* 2009;15(2):112-116.
106. Norrbrink C, Lindberg T, Wahman K, Bjerkefors A. Effects of an exercise programme on musculoskeletal and neuropathic pain after spinal cord injury—results from a seated double-poling ergometer study. *Spinal Cord.* 2012;50(6): 457-461.
107. Galea MP, Dunlop SA, Davis GM, et al. Intensive exercise program after spinal cord injury ("full-on"): study protocol for a randomized controlled trial. *Trials.* 2013;14:291.
108. Bunge RP, Puckett WR, Becerra JL, et al. Observations on the pathology of human spinal cord injury. A review and classification of 22 new cases with details from a case of chronic cord compression with extensive focal demyelination. *Adv Neurol.* 1993;59:75-89.
109. Blackburn-Munro G. Pain-like behaviours in animals—how human are they? *Trends Pharmacol Sci.* 2004;25:299-305.
110. Geyer MA, Markou A. Animal models of psychiatric disorders. In: Bloom FE, Kupfer DJ, eds. *Psychopharamacology: The Fourth Generation of Progress.* New York: Raven Press; 1995:787-798.
111. Geyer MA, Markou A. The role of preclincal models in the development of psychotropic drugs. In: Davis KL, Charney D, Coyle JT, Nemeroff C, eds. *Neuropsychopharmacology: The Fifth Generation of Progress.* Philadelphia: Lippincott Williams & Wilkins; 2002:445-455.
112. Kontinen VK, Meert TF. Predictive validity of neuropathic pain models in pharmacological studies with a behavioral outcome in the rat: a systematic review. In: Dostrovsky JO, Carr DB, Koltzenburg M, eds. *Proceedings of the 10th World Congress on Pain.* Vol. 24. Seattle: IASP Press; 2003:489-498.
113. Hasnie FS, Breuer J, Parker S, et al. Further characterization of a rat model of varicella zoster virus-associated pain: relationship between mechanical hypersensitivity and anxiety-related behavior, and the influence of analgesic drugs. *Neuroscience.* 2007;144:1495-1508.
114. Kontinen VK, Kauppila T, Paananen S, et al. Behavioural measures of depression and anxiety in rats with spinal nerve ligation-induced neuropathy. *Pain.* 1999;80:341-346.
115. Mills CD, Grady JJ, Hulsebosch CE. Changes in exploratory behavior as a measure of chronic central pain following spinal cord injury. *J Neurotrauma.* 2001;18:1091-1105.
116. Lau D, Harte SE, Morrow TJ, et al. Herpes simplex virus vector-mediated expression of interleukin-10 reduces below-level central neuropathic pain after spinal cord injury. *Neurorehabil Neural Repair.* 2012;26(7):889-897.
117. Yezierski RP, Liu S, Ruenes GL, et al. Excitotoxic spinal cord injury: behavioral and morphological characteristics of a central pain model. *Pain.* 1998;75:141-155.
118. Yu CG, Fairbanks CA, Wilcox GL, et al. Effects of agmatine, interleukin-10, and cyclosporin on spontaneous pain behavior after excitotoxic spinal cord injury in rats. *J Pain.* 2003;4:129-140.
119. Christensen MD, Everhart AW, Pickelman JT, et al. Mechanical and thermal allodynia in chronic central pain following spinal cord injury. *Pain.* 1996;68:97-107.
120. Basso DM, Beattie MS, Bresnahan JC. A sensitive and reliable locomotor rating scale for open field testing in rats. *J Neurotrauma.* 1995;12:1-21.
121. Bennett AD, Chastain KM, Hulsebosch CE. Alleviation of mechanical and thermal allodynia by CGRP(8-37) in a rodent model of chronic central pain. *Pain.* 2000;86:163-175.
122. Kim J, Jung JI, Na HS, et al. Effects of morphine on mechanical allodynia in a rat model of central neuropathic pain. *Neuroreport.* 2003;14:1017-1020.
123. Gwak YS, Tan HY, Nam TS, et al. Activation of spinal GABA receptors attenuates chronic central neuropathic pain after spinal cord injury. *J Neurotrauma.* 2006;23:1111-1124.
124. Hains BC, Everhart AW, Fullwood SD, et al. Changes in serotonin, serotonin transporter expression and serotonin denervation supersensitivity: involvement in chronic central pain after spinal hemisection in the rat. *Exp Neurol.* 2002;175:347-362.
125. Rosenzweig ES, McDonald JW. Rodent models for treatment of spinal cord injury: research trends and progress toward useful repair. *Curr Opin Neurol.* 2004;17:121-131.
126. Stokes BT, Jakeman LB. Experimental modelling of human spinal cord injury: a model that crosses the species barrier and mimics the spectrum of human cytopathology. *Spinal Cord.* 2002;40:101-109.
127. Hains BC, Yucra JA, Hulsebosch CE. Reduction of pathological and behavioral deficits following spinal cord contusion injury with the selective cyclooxygenase-2 inhibitor NS-398. *J Neurotrauma.* 2001;18:409-423.
128. Mills CD, Hains BC, Johnson KM, et al. Strain and model differences in behavioral outcomes after spinal cord injury in rat. *J Neurotrauma.* 2001;18:743-756.
129. Siddall P, Xu CL, Cousins M. Allodynia following traumatic spinal cord injury in the rat. *Neuroreport.* 1995;6:1241-1244.
130. Vaysse L, Sol JC, Lazorthes Y, et al. GABAergic pathway in a rat model of chronic neuropathic pain: modulation after intrathecal transplantation of a human neuronal cell line. *Neurosci Res.* 2011;69(2):111-120.
131. Berrocal YA, Pearse DD, Andrade CM, et al. Increased spinal c-Fos expression with noxious and non-noxious peripheral stimulation after severe spinal contusion. *Neurosci Lett.* 2007;413:58-62.
132. Hubscher CH, Johnson RD. Chronic spinal cord injury induced changes in the responses of thalamic neurons. *Exp Neurol.* 2006;197:177-188.
133. Finnerup NB, Sorensen L, Biering-Sorensen F, et al. Segmental hypersensitivity and spinothalamic function in spinal cord injury pain. *Exp Neurol.* 2007;207:139-149.
134. Hulsebosch CE, Xu GY, Perez-Polo JR, et al. Rodent model of chronic central pain after spinal cord contusion injury and effects of gabapentin. *J Neurotrauma.* 2000;17: 1205-1217.
135. Stolp-Smith KA, Wainberg MC. Antidepressant exacerbation of spasticity. *Arch Phys Med Rehabil.* 1999;80:339-342.
136. Robins S, Fehlings M. Models of experimental spinal cord injury: translational relevance and impact. *Drug Discovery Today: Disease Models.* 2008;5:5-11.
137. Hama A, Sagen J. Behavioral characterization and effect of clinical drugs in a rat model of pain following spinal cord compression. *Brain Res.* 2007;1185:117-128.
138. Hama A, Sagen J. Antinociceptive effects of the marine snail peptides conantokin-G and conotoxin MVIIA alone and in combination in rat models of pain. *Neuropharmacology.* 2009;56:556-563.
139. Xu XJ, Hao JX, Seiger A, et al. Systemic mexiletine relieves chronic allodynialike symptoms in rats with ischemic spinal cord injury. *Anesth Analg.* 1992;74:649-652.

140. Yu J, Fu P, Zhang Y, Liu S, Cui D. Pregabalin alters nociceptive behavior and expression level of P2X3 receptor in the spinal dorsal horn in a rat model induced by chronic compression of the dorsal root ganglion. *Anat Rec (Hoboken)*. 2013;296(12):1907-1912.
141. Hama A, Sagen J. Antinociceptive effect of cannabinoid agonist WIN 55,212-2 in rats with a spinal cord injury. *Exp Neurol*. 2007;204:454-457.
142. Hama AT, Germano P, Varghese MS, et al. Fatty acid amide hydrolase (FAAH) inhibitors exert pharmacological effects, but lack antinociceptive efficacy in rats with neuropathic spinal cord injury pain. *PLoS ONE*. 2014;9(5):e96396.
143. Saulino M. Successful reduction of neuropathic pain associated with spinal cord injury via of a combination of intrathecal hydromorphone and ziconotide: a case report. *Spinal Cord*. 2007;45:749-752.
144. Guy S, Mehta S, Leff L, Teasell R, Loh E. Anticonvulsant medication use for the management of pain following spinal cord injury: systematic review and effectiveness analysis. *Spinal Cord*. 2014;52(2):89-96.
145. Mehta S, McIntyre A, Dijkers M, Loh E, Teasell RW. Gabapentinoids are effective in decreasing neuropathic pain and other secondary outcomes after spinal cord injury: a meta-analysis. *Arch Phys Med Rehabil*. 2014;95(11):2180-2186.
146. Onouchi K, Koga H, Yokoyama K, Yoshiyama T. An open-label, long-term study examining the safety and tolerability of pregabalin in Japanese patients with central neuropathic pain. *J Pain Res*. 2014;7:439-447.
147. Cardenas DD, Emir B, Parsons B. Examining the time to therapeutic effect of pregabalin in spinal cord injury patients with neuropathic pain. *Clin Ther*. 2015;37(5):1081-1090.
148. Parsons B, Emir B, Clair A. Temporal analysis of pain responders and common adverse events: when do these first appear following treatment with pregabalin. *J Pain Res*. 2015;8:303-309.
149. Finnerup NB, Otto M, McQuay HJ, et al. Algorithm for neuropathic pain treatment: an evidence based proposal. *Pain*. 2005;118:289-305.
150. Hao JX, Xu XJ, Aldskogius H, et al. Allodynia-like effects in rat after ischaemic spinal cord injury photochemically induced by laser irradiation. *Pain*. 1991;45:175-185.
151. Hao JX, Xu XJ. Treatment of a chronic allodynia-like response in spinally injured rats: effects of systemically administered excitatory amino acid receptor antagonists. *Pain*. 1996;66:279-285.
152. Hao JX, Xu XJ. Animal models of spinal cord injury pain and their implications for pharmacological treatments. *J Rehabil Med*. 2003;41(suppl):81-84.
153. Hao JX, Xu XJ, Urban L, et al. Repeated administration of systemic gabapentin alleviates allodynia-like behaviors in spinally injured rats. *Neurosci Lett*. 2000;280:211-214.
154. Kouya PF, Hao JX, Xu XJ. Buprenorphine alleviates neuropathic pain-like behaviors in rats after spinal cord and peripheral nerve injury. *Eur J Pharmacol*. 2002;450:49-53.
155. Glynn CJ, Jamous MA, Teddy PJ, et al. Role of spinal noradrenergic system in transmission of pain in patients with spinal cord injury. *Lancet*. 1986;2:1249-1250.
156. Taira T, Kawamura H, Tanikawa T, et al. A new approach to control central deafferentation pain: spinal intrathecal baclofen. *Stereotact Funct Neurosurg*. 1995;65:101-105.
157. Sang CN, Booher S, Gilron I, et al. Dextromethorphan and memantine in painful diabetic neuropathy and postherpetic neuralgia: efficacy and dose-response trials. *Anesthesiology*. 2002;96:1053-1061.
158. Eide PK, Stubhaug A, Stenehjem AE. Central dysesthesia pain after traumatic spinal cord injury is dependent on N-methyl-D-aspartate receptor activation. *Neurosurgery*. 1995;37:1080-1087.
159. Wieseler J, Ellis A, Maier SF, Watkins LR, Falci S. Unilateral T13 and L1 dorsal root avulsion: methods for a novel model of central neuropathic pain. *Methods Mol Biol*. 2012;851:171-183.
160. Wieseler J, Ellis AL, McFadden A, et al. Below level central pain induced by discrete dorsal spinal cord injury. *J Neurotrauma*. 2010;27(9):1697-1707.
161. Ellis A, Wieseler J, Favret J, et al. Systemic administration of propentofylline, ibudilast, and (+)-naltrexone each reverses mechanical allodynia in a novel rat model of central neuropathic pain. *J Pain*. 2014;15(4):407-421.
162. Falci S, Best L, Bayles R, et al. Dorsal root entry zone microcoagulation for spinal cord injury-related central pain: operative intramedullary electrophysiological guidance and clinical outcome. *J Neurosurg*. 2002;97(2 suppl):193-200.
163. Loeser JD, Ward AA Jr, White LE Jr. Chronic deafferentation of human spinal cord neurons. *J Neurosurg*. 1968;29:48-50.
164. Drew GM, Siddall PJ, Duggan AW. Mechanical allodynia following contusion injury of the rat spinal cord is associated with loss of GABAergic inhibition in the dorsal horn. *Pain*. 2004;109:379-388.
165. Wang J, Kawamata M, Namiki A. Changes in properties of spinal dorsal horn neurons and their sensitivity to morphine after spinal cord injury in the rat. *Anesthesiology*. 2005;102:152-164.
166. Yezierski RP, Park SH. The mechanosensitivity of spinal sensory neurons following intraspinal injections of quisqualic acid in the rat. *Neurosci Lett*. 1993;157:115-119.
167. Wrigley PJ, Press SR, Gustin SM, et al. Neuropathic pain and primary somatosensory cortex reorganization following spinal cord injury. *Pain*. 2009;141:52-59.
168. Pattany PM, Yezierski RP, Widerstrom-Noga EG, et al. Proton magnetic resonance spectroscopy of the thalamus in patients with chronic neuropathic pain after spinal cord injury. *AJNR Am J Neuroradiol*. 2002;23:901-905.
169. Lenz FA, Tasker RR, Dostrovsky JO, et al. Abnormal single-unit activity recorded in the somatosensory thalamus of a quadriplegic patient with central pain. *Pain*. 1987;31:225-236.
170. Christensen MD, Hulsebosch CE. Spinal cord injury and anti-NGF treatment results in changes in CGRP density and distribution in the dorsal horn in the rat. *Exp Neurol*. 1997;147:463-475.
171. Weaver LC, Verghese P, Bruce JC, et al. Autonomic dysreflexia and primary afferent sprouting after clip-compression injury of the rat spinal cord. *J Neurotrauma*. 2001;18:1107-1119.
172. Ackery AD, Norenberg MD, Krassioukov A. Calcitonin gene-related peptide immunoreactivity in chronic human spinal cord injury. *Spinal Cord*. 2007;45:678-686.
173. Grachev ID, Fredrickson BE, Apkarian AV. Brain chemistry reflects dual states of pain and anxiety in chronic low back pain. *J Neural Transm*. 2002;109:1309-1334.
174. Chang HT. Subacute human spinal cord contusion: few lymphocytes and many macrophages. *Spinal Cord*. 2007;45:174-182.
175. Borsook D, Becerra L. Phenotyping central nervous system circuitry in chronic pain using functional MRI: considerations

and potential implications in the clinic. *Curr Pain Headache Rep*. 2007;11:201-207.
176. Darian-Smith C. Synaptic plasticity, neurogenesis, and functional recovery after spinal cord injury. *Neuroscientist*. 2009;15:149-165.
177. Ji RR, Suter MR. p38 MAPK, microglial signaling, and neuropathic pain. *Mol Pain*. 2007;3(33).
178. Baastrup C, Finnerup NB. Pharmacological management of neuropathic pain following spinal cord injury. *CNS Drugs*. 2008;22:455-475.
179. Watkins LR, Hutchinson MR, Ledeboer A, et al. Glia as the "bad guys": implications for improving clinical pain control and the clinical utility of opioids. *Brain Behav Immun*. 2007; 21:131-146.
180. Binshtok AM, Wang H, Zimmermann K, et al. Nociceptors are interleukin-1beta sensors. *J Neurosci*. 2008;28:14062-14073.
181. Cramer SW, Baggott C, Cain J, et al. The role of cation-dependent chloride transporters in neuropathic pain following spinal cord injury. *Mol Pain*. 2008;4:36.
182. Fu ES, Zhang YP, Sagen J, et al. Transgenic glial nuclear factor-kappa B inhibition decreases formalin pain in mice. *Neuroreport*. 2007;18:713-717.
183. Yamamoto Y, Gaynor RB. Therapeutic potential of inhibition of the NF-kappaB pathway in the treatment of inflammation and cancer. *J Clin Invest*. 2001;107:135-142.
184. Kang SK, So HH, Moon YS, et al. Proteomic analysis of injured spinal cord tissue proteins using 2-DE and MALDI-TOF MS. *Proteomics*. 2006;6:2797-2812.
185. Ding Q, Wu Z, Guo Y, et al. Proteome analysis of up-regulated proteins in the rat spinal cord induced by transection injury. *Proteomics*. 2006;6:505-518.
186. Velardo MJ, Burger C, Williams PR, et al. Patterns of gene expression reveal a temporally orchestrated wound healing response in the injured spinal cord. *J Neurosci*. 2004;24:8562-8576.
187. Nesic O, Lee J, Johnson KM, et al. Transcriptional profiling of spinal cord injury-induced central neuropathic pain. *J Neurochem*. 2005;95:998-1014.
188. Li S, Zhang J. Lipopolysaccharide induces autotaxin expression in human monocytic THP-1 cells. *Biochem Biophys Res Commun*. 2009;378:264-268.
189. Inoue M, Ma L, Aoki J, et al. Autotaxin, a synthetic enzyme of lysophosphatidic acid (LPA), mediates the induction of nerve-injured neuropathic pain. *Mol Pain*. 2008;4:6.
190. Inoue M, Rashid MH, Fujita R, et al. Initiation of neuropathic pain requires lysophosphatidic acid receptor signaling. *Nat Med*. 2004;10:712-718.
191. Ueda H. Peripheral mechanisms of neuropathic pain—involvement of lysophosphatidic acid receptor-mediated demyelination. *Mol Pain*. 2008;4:11.
192. Shano S, Moriyama R, Chun J, et al. Lysophosphatidic acid stimulates astrocyte proliferation through LPA1. *Neurochem Int*. 2008;52:216-220.
193. Coste O, Pierre S, Marian C, et al. Antinociceptive activity of the S1P-receptor agonist FTY720. *J Cell Mol Med*. 2008;12:995-1004.
194. de Jong EK, Dijkstra IM, Hensens M, et al. Vesicle-mediated transport and release of CCL21 in endangered neurons: a possible explanation for microglia activation remote from a primary lesion. *J Neurosci*. 2005;25:7548-7557.
195. de Jong EK, Vinet J, Stanulovic VS, et al. Expression, transport, and axonal sorting of neuronal CCL21 in large dense-core vesicles. *FASEB J*. 2008;22:4136-4145.
196. Zhao P, Waxman SG, Hains BC. Modulation of thalamic nociceptive processing after spinal cord injury through remote activation of thalamic microglia by cysteine cysteine chemokine ligand 21. *J Neurosci*. 2007;27:8893-8902.
197. Neary JT, Kang Y, Shi YF. Cell cycle regulation of astrocytes by extracellular nucleotides and fibroblast growth factor-2. *Purinergic Signal*. 2005;1:329-336.
198. Sawynok J, Liu XJ. Adenosine in the spinal cord and periphery: release and regulation of pain. *Prog Neurobiol*. 2003;69:313-340.
199. Byrnes KR, Stoica BA, Fricke S, et al. Cell cycle activation contributes to post-mitotic cell death and secondary damage after spinal cord injury. *Brain*. 2007;130(Pt 11):2977-2992.
200. Diaz-Padilla I, Siu LL, Duran I. Cyclin-dependent kinase inhibitors as potential targeted anticancer agents. *Invest New Drugs*. 2009;27(6):586-594.
201. Wang X, Zhang Y, Peng Y, et al. Pharmacological characterization of the opioid inactive isomers (+)-naltrexone and (+)-naloxone as antagonists of toll-like receptor 4. *Br J Pharmacol*. 2016;173(5):856-869.
202. Sekine C, Sugihara T, Miyake S, et al. Successful treatment of animal models of rheumatoid arthritis with small-molecule cyclin-dependent kinase inhibitors. *J Immunol*. 2008;180: 1954-1961.
203. Utreras E, Futatsugi A, Rudrabhatla P, et al. Tumor necrosis factor-alpha regulates cyclin-dependent kinase 5 activity during pain signaling through transcriptional activation of p35. *J Biol Chem*. 2009;284:2275-2284.
204. Saikkonen B, Pareek TK, Agarwal N, et al. Conditional deletion of cyclin-dependent kinase 5 in primary sensory neurons leads to atypical skin lesions. *Cell Cycle*. 2008;7: 750-753.
205. Pareek TK, Kulkarni AB. Cdk5: a new player in pain signaling. *Cell Cycle*. 2006;5:585-588.
206. Pareek TK, Keller J, Kesavapany S, et al. Cyclin-dependent kinase 5 modulates nociceptive signaling through direct phosphorylation of transient receptor potential vanilloid 1. *Proc Natl Acad Sci USA*. 2007;104:660-665.
207. Yang YR, He Y, Zhang Y, et al. Activation of cyclin-dependent kinase 5 (Cdk5) in primary sensory and dorsal horn neurons by peripheral inflammation contributes to heat hyperalgesia. *Pain*. 2007;127:109-120.
208. Rossi AG, Sawatzky DA, Walker A, et al. Cyclin-dependent kinase inhibitors enhance the resolution of inflammation by promoting inflammatory cell apoptosis. *Nat Med*. 2006;12: 1056-1064.
209. Mizushima T, Obata K, Katsura H, et al. Intensity-dependent activation of extracellular signal-regulated protein kinase 5 in sensory neurons contributes to pain hypersensitivity. *J Pharmacol Exp Ther*. 2007;321:28-34.
210. Romero-Sandoval EA, Horvath R, Landry RP, DeLeo JA. Cannabinoid receptor type 2 activation induces a microglial anti-inflammatory phenotype and reduces migration via MKP induction and ERK dephosphorylation. *Mol Pain*. 2009;5:25.
211. Landry RP, Martinez E, DeLeo JA, Romero-Sandoval EA. Spinal cannabinoid receptor type 2 agonist reduces mechanical allodynia and induces mitogen-activated protein kinase phosphatases in a rat model of neuropathic pain. *J Pain*. 2012;13(9):836-848.
212. Gwak YS, Crown ED, Unabia GC, et al. Propentofylline attenuates allodynia, glial activation and modulates GABAergic tone after spinal cord injury in the rat. *Pain*. 2008;138:410-422.

213. Numagami Y, Marro PJ, Mishra OP, et al. Effect of propentofylline on free radical generation during cerebral hypoxia in the newborn piglet. *Neuroscience*. 1998;84: 1127-1133.
214. Kehlen A, Lauterbach R, Santos AN, et al. IL-1 beta- and IL-4-induced down-regulation of autotaxin mRNA and PC-1 in fibroblast-like synoviocytes of patients with rheumatoid arthritis (RA). *Clin Exp Immunol*. 2001;123:147-154.
215. Ledeboer A, Hutchinson MR, Watkins LR, et al. Ibudilast (AV-411). A new class therapeutic candidate for neuropathic pain and opioid withdrawal syndromes. *Expert Opin Investig Drugs*. 2007;16:935-950.
216. Syngle A, Verma I, Krishan P, Garg N, Syngle V. Minocycline improves peripheral and autonomic neuropathy in type 2 diabetes: MIND study. *Neurol Sci*. 2014;35(7):1067-1073.
217. Vanelderen P, Van Zundert J, Kozicz T, et al. Effect of minocycline on lumbar radicular neuropathic pain: a randomized, placebo-controlled, double-blind clinical trial with amitriptyline as a comparator. *Anesthesiology*. 2015; 122(2):399-406.
218. Agre P, Preston GM, Smith BL, et al. Aquaporin CHIP: the archetypal molecular water channel. *Am J Physiol*. 1993;265 (4 Pt 2):F463-F476.
219. Chen JM, Sepramaniam S, Armugam A, et al. Water and ion channels: crucial in the initiation and progression of apoptosis in central nervous system? *Curr Neuropharmacol*. 2008;6:102-116.
220. Nesic O, Lee J, Unabia GC, et al. Aquaporin 1—a novel player in spinal cord injury. *J Neurochem*. 2008;105:628-640.
221. Warner JS, Wamil AW, McLean MJ. Acetazolamide for the treatment of chronic paroxysmal hemicrania. *Headache*. 1994;34:597-599.
222. Woehlck HJ, Otterson M, Yun H, et al. Acetazolamide reduces referred postoperative pain after laparoscopic surgery with carbon dioxide insufflation. *Anesthesiology*. 2003;99:924-928.
223. Faulkner JR, Herrmann JE, Woo MJ, et al. Reactive astrocytes protect tissue and preserve function after spinal cord injury. *J Neurosci*. 2004;24:2143-2155.
224. Rolls A, Shechter R, Schwartz M. The bright side of the glial scar in CNS repair. *Nat Rev Neurosci*. 2009;10:235-241.
225. Okada S, Nakamura M, Mikami Y, et al. Blockade of interleukin-6 receptor suppresses reactive astrogliosis and ameliorates functional recovery in experimental spinal cord injury. *J Neurosci Res*. 2004;76:265-276.
226. Marchand F, Tsantoulas C, Singh D, et al. Effects of etanercept and minocycline in a rat model of spinal cord injury. *Eur J Pain*. 2009;13:673-681.
227. Peng XM, Zhou ZG, Glorioso JC, et al. Tumor necrosis factor-alpha contributes to below-level neuropathic pain after spinal cord injury. *Ann Neurol*. 2006;59:843-851.
228. Diguet E, Gross CE, Tison F, et al. Rise and fall of minocycline in neuroprotection: need to promote publication of negative results. *Exp Neurol*. 2004;189:1-4.
229. Gordon PH, Moore DH, Miller RG, et al. Efficacy of minocycline in patients with amyotrophic lateral sclerosis: a phase III randomised trial. *Lancet Neurol*. 2007;6:1045-1053.
230. Erichsen HK, Hao JX, Xu XJ, et al. Comparative actions of the opioid analgesics morphine, methadone and codeine in rat models of peripheral and central neuropathic pain. *Pain*. 2005;116:347-358.
231. Guneli E, Karabay Yavasoglu NU, Apaydin S, et al. Analysis of the antinociceptive effect of systemic administration of tramadol and dexmedetomidine combination on rat models of acute and neuropathic pain. *Pharmacol Biochem Behav*. 2007;88:9-17.
232. Medvedev IO, Malyshkin AA, Belozertseva IV, et al. Effects of low-affinity NMDA receptor channel blockers in two rat models of chronic pain. *Neuropharmacology*. 2004;47:175-183.
233. Patel S, Naeem S, Kesingland A, et al. The effects of GABA(B) agonists and gabapentin on mechanical hyperalgesia in models of neuropathic and inflammatory pain in the rat. *Pain*. 2001;90:217-226.

CHAPTER 108 Psychological Strategies for Chronic Pain

Sara Davin
Xavier F. Jimenez
Edward C. Covington
Judith Scheman

Pain is not what occurs at the periphery; it is what the brain perceives, and it is indisputably modifiable by emotions and beliefs. Actual damage is neither necessary nor sufficient for the perception of pain. Anger, depression, anxiety, fear, and other psychological variables can all increase the perception of both acute and chronic pain, as can believing it to be an indicator of a destructive process.

Back pain is an enormous problem for patients, health care providers, families, employers, and society.[1–3] Most patients seeking care from a spine specialist do so because of pain.[4] Because the natural history of most spine pain is self-limiting,[5,6] almost anything done will lead to the patient reporting a decrease in symptomatology in a matter of days or weeks (with the exception of bed rest, which has now been well shown to do more harm than good).[7] Most patients with back pain do not need to see a spine specialist; rather, they are seen by their primary care physicians. When it becomes persistent, it is commonly not attributable to any specific pathology or disease process.[8] Despite the fact that this has been well documented for over a decade, the idea that nonspecific low back pain must result from demonstrable pathology persists in the mind of patients and is often fostered by providers. This belief in and of itself may lead to the worsening of the pain. Patients who do go on to see a specialist often do so because the pain has persisted beyond the time of expected spontaneous resolution and they are worried. Of those patients whose pain does not resolve within a relatively short time, some will go on to develop chronic pain. The societal and individual costs of chronic debilitating pain are staggering. The economic burden of chronic low back pain has been estimated to range from $84.1 billion to $624.8 billion, with primary indirect costs attributable to lost work productivity.[9] It is likely that prompt recognition and intervention in cases with developing chronicity can lead to improved outcome with less need for extensive interventions.

With this context in consideration, this chapter will attempt to elucidate psychosocial factors that help contribute to the transformation of back pain into a disabling condition.

Pain Perception: Nervous System Attenuation and Amplification

Back pain is often ascribed to strains, sprains, annular tears, internal disc disruption, facet arthropathy, or bone pathology; however, it is often not explained by examination or imaging. Positive findings on an imaging test may be misleading, since patients with severe symptoms often have normal imaging, and patients with herniations, degenerated discs, bulges, osteophytes, and facet arthropathy are often without symptoms.[10,11]

To some extent, overreliance on imaging findings derives from the persistence of obsolete concepts concerning nociceptive pain. Essentially, these implied a more or less linear relationship between pain perception and peripheral stimulation; that is, a nociceptor is activated, the signal is transmitted to the dorsal horn (DH) of the spinal cord, and from there via the thalamus to the cortex, where pain is appreciated. Pain was seen as an analog representation of some event; for example, a child stepping on one's toe produces minimal pain, while an adult or an automobile would produce correspondingly greater pains. As a result, when a patient complained of severe pain and no appropriate pathology was found, the validity of the complaints was challenged.

More recent evidence shows that pain is a creation of the nervous system and not just a gauge of nociceptor activation. Nociceptive afferent signals are subject to marked attenuation and amplification by descending facilitatory and inhibitory tracts that have their action at the DH.[12] Further, the presence of prolonged nociceptive stimulation, inflammation, or nerve injury can lead to sensitization of the neurons that relay pain, death of inhibitory cells,[13,14] loss of tonic inhibition, and structural neuroplastic changes. Perhaps even more interesting, activation of immune cells, including glia[15] that were previously thought of as having only structural roles, produces exaggerated, widespread, and mirror-image pains.[16–18] DH molecular mechanisms of central sensitization include co-release of substance P and glutamate from afferent neurons, jointly activating *N*-methyl-D-aspartate receptors and thereby enabling temporal summation which can be reversed with *N*-methyl-D-aspartate receptor blockade.[19]

Patients with idiopathic chronic low back pain (CLBP) subjected to quantified thumb pressure report more pain and show more functional magnetic resonance imaging (MRI) activation in brain areas likely to reflect pain perception than do controls, suggesting that at least some portion of CLBP is related to central sensitization. Evidence also implicates central sensitization as a significant factor in whiplash-associated pain.[20] Thus, spine pain can result from local tissue pathology, central sensitization, or both. It is therefore unrealistic to expect that reports of chronic spine-related pain will necessarily correlate with the presence of severity of spine pathology. It should be further noted that in addition to such pain sensitization and facilitation, chronic pain syndromes are believed to develop as a result of faulty pain inhibition as well.[21] Pain inhibition involves processing via spinal-supraspinal-spinal loops[22]; implicated supraspinal structures include the prefrontal cortex, midbrain, and periaqueductal gray.[23] Evidence suggests the activation of healthy or adaptive pain inhibition with the use of exercise, for example, which has been demonstrated in back pain specifically.[24]

The interplay of cognitions and pain modulation is complex and of growing interest. It is known that guarding against the possibility of pain and anticipation of its occurrence activates cells in the rostroventral medulla that function to amplify incoming pain signals at the level of the DH. Animal models suggest that the simple facts of anticipating a pain sensation and expecting it to be important are sufficient to trigger these "on cells," in essence activating the "amplifiers" before the pain stimulus has even begun.[25]

Increasing evidence points to genetic variability in pain appreciation and in responses to endogenous and exogenous opioids.[26–28] Furthermore, there is compelling evidence that individual reporting of high/low pain in response to a standard stimulus demonstrates correspondingly high or low activation of the somatosensory cortex, anterior cingulate gyrus (a likely index of affective components of pain), and frontal cortex.[29]

To summarize, at least some forms of chronic back pain are likely secondary to this complex, multifactorial degree of central sensitization,[30] and instruments have been developed and validated for capturing and quantifying central sensitization (i.e., the Central Sensitization Inventory[31,32]). Further application of this inventory in both clinical and investigational contexts is warranted before systematic use, yet general consideration of central sensitization in back pain syndromes is certainly critical for any clinician managing this patient population.

Pain and the Psyche

Chronic pain syndrome is a term (not a diagnosis) that has fallen into disfavor with pain specialists but is still often used by others. It describes a condition of severe intractable pain with marked functional impairment and other behavioral changes that have no clear relationship to organic disorder. (Poor concordance between chronic pain and structural pathology does not, as noted earlier, challenge the authenticity of the pain.) Typically, these patients have inordinate use of medications and health care services, which are largely nonproductive. Thus, this is a nonspecific term for patients most typified by *abnormal illness behaviors,* primarily those of somatic preoccupation and regression into the sick role. The term is useful in that it properly directs therapy toward the reversal of regression and away from an exclusive focus on nociception. It does not, however, substitute for a careful diagnosis of the physiologic, psychological, and environmental factors that produce the syndrome.

Psychosocial vulnerabilities may precede or follow the development of low back pain, both proving to substantially contribute to overall outcomes. Carragee et al. followed 100 patients with mild CLBP and no prior spine-related disability for 5 years.[33] Moderate or severe Modic changes (degenerative changes noted on spine MRI) of the vertebral endplate were the only structural variable that weakly predicted adverse outcome. Provocative discography and baseline MRI predicted no outcome variables, but were weakly associated with pain episodes. Psychosocial variables strongly predicted long- and short-term disability and health care visits for low back pain. A model based on scores on the Modified Zung Depression Test, Modified Somatic Pain Questionnaire, Fear Avoidance Beliefs Questionnaire (physical activity subscale), and smoking status identified 100% of long-term disability subjects, 88% of all disability subjects, and 75% of subjects having a remission.

It is reasonable to posit a stress-diathesis model in which the degree of disability from a given degree of organic pathology will vary with the psychological reserves of the individual, the stresses of the workplace, and incentives/disincentives for recovery. Clearly, these variables overlap—the person with poor coping skills and limited education is unlikely to obtain the most desirable work situation.

Psychiatric Comorbidities

The most frequent psychiatric illnesses (excluding somatic symptom disorders) in pain center patients are anxiety disorders, depression, and substance abuse. In 200 CLBP patients entering a functional restoration program, Polatin et al. found that 77% of patients met lifetime diagnostic criteria and 59% demonstrated current symptoms for at least one psychiatric diagnosis.[34] The most common were those listed. A total of 51% met criteria for personality disorder. Substance abuse and anxiety disorders appeared to precede CLBP, while major depression could either precede or follow it. Studies vary as to the prevalence of psychiatric disorder; however, they tend to agree about those that are most common.

The prevalence of depression in chronic pain patients ranges from 10% to 83%. This extreme variance reflects variable settings, populations, and diagnostic criteria. In a Canadian general population survey of 118,533 people, CLBP was present in 9%. Major depression was present in 5.9% of those without pain and in 19.8% of those with CLBP. The rate of major depression increased in a linear fashion with pain severity.[35] It is likely that the arrow of causality can point in either direction, as there is evidence that pain predicts depression and depression predicts pain, and to similar degrees.[36]

In a probability sample of 5692 US adults, 35% of those with CLBP had comorbid mental disorders. Major depression was present in 12.6%, dysthymia in 5.6%, any anxiety disorder in 26.5%, and any substance use disorder in 4.8%. There was no increased prevalence of (nonalcohol) drug abuse.[37]

Major affective disorder can present with pain, in which case treatment of the mood disorder often provides relief. More commonly, however, depression appears as a consequence of pain, though not necessarily a direct result of it. Rudy et al. showed that the link between pain and depression could be mediated by perceived life interference (loss of gratifying activities) and loss of self-control.[36] Moreover, Strigo et al., in a study of the association of major depressive disorder and experimental pain, observed that anticipation of pain was associated with increased activity in the amygdala, anterior insula, and anterior cingulate cortex in patients with major depressive disorder when compared with normals.[39] This suggests that depressed patients experienced an affective response even before they experienced the painful stimulus. This was also associated with greater perceived helplessness. They posit that patients with major depressive disorder have an altered functional response within specific neural networks during the anticipation of pain that may lead to an impaired ability to modulate the painful experience as well as their emotional response to the pain.

There seems to be a vicious cycle in which pain behavior, loneliness, inactivity, helplessness, depression, withdrawal, loss of reinforcers and distractions, and pain are mutually reinforcing. Improving one element in this series often benefits the others. These issues, of course, are not resolved by pharmacotherapy, but do respond to successful rehabilitation.

Other Psychological Contributors to Chronic Pain

Anxiety adversely affects pain through a number of mechanisms, and it can be the major reason for failure of rehabilitation from CLBP. Phobic processes can promote a cycle of unnecessary self-protection and avoidance. Ultimately, this can lead to deconditioning in the individual with chronic pain. When people become afraid to move, disability and dysfunction can result as much from unwarranted fear as from the pain itself. Anxiety can also lead to muscle guarding and tension that lead to muscle shortening and other physiologic responses that worsen pain. Nociceptors that are normally unaffected by norepinephrine become sensitive to it following injury so that neuropathic pains are often exacerbated by anxiety as well as fear, anger, or excitement.

Pain catastrophizing is a cognitive–affective response to anticipated or actual pain, comprised of three domains (helplessness, magnification, and rumination).[40] It has been shown to markedly amplify pain and is associated with poorer outcome, heightened pain sensitivity, and impaired functioning.[41,42] This is the case for both acute and chronic pain.

Anger is associated with exacerbation of both acute and chronic pain. A number of authors have found associations between anger regulation, both expression and suppression, and severity of chronic pain.[43,44] In a study examining the effects of anger suppression in pain severity, Burns et al.[45] found that patients with CLBP who were told to suppress their anger toward a study confederate exhibited more pain behaviors and reported more pain than those who did not suppress their anger.

Recent research has looked at other psychological contributors to pain, such as guilt and various aspects of mood—including reactivity and positive affect—among those with CLBP. Serbic and colleagues explored the relations between pain-related guilt, lack of diagnostic certainty, and disability through structural equation modeling in CLBP patients. They found that pain-related guilt (especially social guilt) and diagnostic uncertainty contributed substantially to disability and mood.[46] While this study does not attribute causality to the associations, it does underscore the potential importance of addressing guilt through psychological strategies. Furthermore, low levels of positive affect combined with high negative affect among individuals with CLBP may increase the odds of comorbid fibromyalgia and worse functioning overall. Individuals with high levels of reactivity (high negative affect and high positive affect) have shown similar levels of pain, mood, and disability as those who are considered having a "healthy" balance of affect (high positive affect and low affect).[47]

Psychogenic Pain/Somatization: Diagnostic Considerations

Psychogenic pain is a concept whose existence is disputed and whose use has decreased with more modern understandings of the role of the nervous system in chronic pain. It was previously used when a medical explanation for pain was not identified. Similarly, the term *somatization* is used to refer to the presentation of physical symptoms with psychological underpinnings or influence. Clinically, patients may demonstrate behaviors that are incompatible with the degree of impairment that they describe. A plethora of complaints and marked functional impairment may coexist with well-preserved muscle definition. It may be that the term is used for several unrelated conditions, given that some diagnosed with psychogenic pain appear euthymic, animated, and sleep well, while others appear to suffer severely, cannot sleep, and even contemplate suicide. One clue to the presence of somatization is apparent reluctance to discuss nonsomatic issues. If asked about family, work, or politics, the response inevitably and rapidly diverges to talk about doctors, symptoms, and treatments. This is not typically seen even in severe physical illness. Another clue is the sense of immediacy in the recounting of the traumatic event—a minor remote event is described as though it occurred yesterday.

The American Psychiatric Association has historically grouped these disorders under the framework of "somatoform disorders," including diagnoses such as hypochondriasis, pain disorder, factitious disorder, and conversion disorder. The diagnostic terminology has changed multiple times, with the most recent revisions from the *Diagnostic and Statistical Manual of Mental Disorders, 5th edition* (*DSM-5*) being the "somatic symptom disorders."[48] This new classification system allows for a specifier, "with predominant pain," to account for those with pain symptoms. A diagnosis of somatic symptom disorder requires the presence of one or more somatic symptoms that cause distress or disruption in daily life, accompanied by an "excessive" psychological response (thoughts, feelings, behaviors), such as high levels of anxiety or preoccupation with symptoms for at least 6 months. Alternatively, if it is determined that psychological or behavioral factors contribute to adverse outcomes associated with the condition, a diagnosis of "psychological factors affecting pain condition" may be used.

There is evidence of a continuum between symptoms of posttraumatic stress disorder, dissociation, somatization, and affect dysregulation. These interrelated symptoms commonly follow major trauma, and there seems to be a hierarchy of traumas, such that natural disasters lead to fewer symptoms than do adult interpersonal traumas, with childhood trauma causing the most severe symptoms. Rome and Rome hypothesized that a process akin to kindling follows psychic trauma, leading to symptom amplification, spontaneous symptoms, anatomic spreading, and cross-sensitization.[49] These are processes that also characterize pain following neurologic trauma. They noted a melding of sensory and affective symptoms and a "polymodal allodynia" that rendered these people sensitized to both physical and emotional stressors. Most studies linking adult-onset chronic pain with childhood trauma have been retrospective. However, a study by Jones et al. looking prospectively at a 1958 British cohort of 7571 subjects found that, although adult onset of chronic pain was not associated with childhood surgery, it was associated with hospitalization for a motor vehicle accident, institutional care, maternal death, and familial financial hardship.[50] Strengthening directionality of their findings, they also found that the association was not explained by adult psychological distress or social class. Von Korff et al. also examined the effects of childhood psychosocial stressors and the onset of adult arthritis in a prospective study of 18,309 subjects from 10 countries participating in a World Mental Health Survey in the Americas, Europe, and Asia.[51] They found that, controlling for age, sex, and early onset of psychological disorders, subjects with significant childhood stressors had an increased risk of adult arthritis. Early-age onset of symptoms of depression and/or anxiety were associated with an increased risk of adult arthritis even after controlling for childhood stressors.

Other psychiatric conditions that may present with pain include hypochondriasis, dementia, psychosis, and factitious disorder. Experience suggests that new onset of conversion/somatization in the elderly is rare, and when present it may herald dementia. Malingering is by definition not a psychiatric illness. While thought to be uncommon in chronic pain (based on no data), it does occur.

Psychogenic Pain/Somatization: Pain Amplifiers

Multiple psychological factors affect both the perception of pain and ability to cope with it. Chronic stress increases both the perception of pain and disability. Distraction reduces pain awareness, while isolation and inactivity increases it and fosters self-preoccupation. Perhaps the major psychological factors that affect chronic pain are cognitions and incentives.

Cognitive theories of depression, anxiety, and pain hold that thoughts and beliefs are major determinants of affect, that is, how a person feels is less determined by events than by the person's interpretation of them. The individual who concludes from an unsuccessful job interview that the company has no openings reacts differently than the one who infers that he or she is undesirable and unlikely to find work. The terminal cancer patient who believes that "the surgeon got it all" will be more content than the healthy person who believes one's intractable pain is due to severe but undetected pathology. Maladaptive cognitions tend to be automatic and habitual; thus, they are rarely examined for validity. They are simply accepted.

Cognitive factors have an impact on pain in several ways. First, the adverse quality of pain is modified by its interpretation. Such "catastrophic" interpretations of pain as "the nerves are being crushed" or "the exercises feel like they're tearing something loose" impede coping. The situation can be worsened by health care providers who attribute the pain to incidental findings on imaging that may bear only a modest relationship to the pain. Chronic back pain, which is the leading cause of disability and absenteeism from the workplace, lacks a specific structural explanation in over 80% of cases. Additionally, it is often strongly driven by such psychosocial factors as fear of pain/reinjury, "catastrophizing," depression, and anxiety. Failure to address these issues in treatment of chronic back pain often leads to continued disability. Pain tolerance is reduced by thoughts emphasizing the averseness of the situation, the inadequacy of the person to bear it, or the physical harm that could occur. Such beliefs as "I will have a life again only after I am cured," "I can't go out to dinner if I am in pain," and "I shouldn't exercise if it hurts" have obvious impacts on adaptation.

Self-appraisal may be as important as appraisal of the pain itself. Those who feel unable to influence events eventually give up. Belief in personal helplessness fosters pain and disability; alternatively, a sense of self-efficacy promotes efforts to cope. Thus, perceptions of helplessness lead to depression, resignation, and passivity, which, in turn, increase disability and pain. Self-efficacy, the opposite of helplessness, has been repeatedly correlated with pain outcomes among a variety of chronic pain conditions, including CLBP.[52] "Locus of control" is a psychological construct that refers to one's sense of the determinants of future events. The perception that events are a consequence of the individual's own behavior (internal locus of control) is associated with better mood and function. Those with external locus of control tend to see future events as contingent on other people or "fate." People with chronic pain who have an external locus of control report depression and anxiety, feel helpless to deal with their pain, and often rely on maladaptive coping strategies such as excessive rest and eating. Decreased perception of self-control may explain much of the relationship between depression and pain.

Addiction

Of the problems that beset patients with chronic non-cancer pain (CNCP), perhaps none is more insidious and difficult to manage than addiction. It is more difficult to diagnose when it involves prescribed substances in the presence of CNCP than when it involves use of recreational substances. Certainly, when present, an addictive disorder magnifies complaints, impedes pain diagnosis, and confounds interventions, yet its treatment is essential, since addiction recovery seems to be the *sine qua non* for pain recovery. Nevertheless, such patients can be treated successfully, and they commonly demonstrate the same gratitude for their recovery as do addicted persons in whom pain is not a factor.

Diagnosing addiction in those with CNCP poses special challenges, in turn, also complicating empirical efforts to identify prevalence rates of addictive disorders in CNCP. Until recently, the *Diagnostic and Statistical Manual of Mental Disorders* (*DSM-IV-TR* version) utilized two diagnostic criteria, tolerance and physical dependence, which are virtually universal in chronic opioid and benzodiazepine therapy and do not distinguish the person with addictive disorder. Similarly, the International Classification of Disease (ICD) has been criticized for not accurately capturing addiction to prescribed medications and previous concordance rates between the *DSM* and ICD definitions were not favorable. While recent updates to the *DSM* (current version *DSM-5*) now specify that tolerance and withdrawal are not features of opioid use disorder in those taking opioids under medical supervision, there still lacks one common, unified definition for addiction. A third definition, proposed by the American Academy of Pain Medicine, American Pain Society, and American Society of Addiction Medicine, identifies addiction to be characterized by one or more of the following: loss of control over use, compulsive use, cravings, and continued use despite adverse consequences.[53] However, continued use despite adverse consequences is less obvious in addiction to prescribed drugs, since such consequences as irritability, drowsiness, poor concentration, regression, reduced libido, and economic losses can be attributed to pain.

Historically, the prevalence of addictive disorder in CNCP has been disputed due to poor quality of studies utilizing inconsistent assessment methods and diverse criteria to define addiction. Recent estimates (utilizing revised criteria from the *DSM-5*) suggest that up to 41% of individuals in an outpatient setting meet criteria for lifetime opioid use disorder.[53] In the first study to compare the three definitions/criteria for addiction (American Academy of Pain Medicine/American Pain Society/American Society of Addiction Medicine definition – "addiction," *DSM-5*, and ICD-10-11), 23.9% met criteria for addiction, 18.8% met ICD-11 criteria, and 17.8% met *DSM-5* criteria. Importantly, concordance rates were "substantial" between the three classifications ("addiction," ICD-11, and *DSM-5*).[54]

Diagnosis is also hindered by the lack of consensus as to what constitutes appropriate use. Opioid prescribing for CNCP, including back pain, has increased markedly over the past 15 years. One US survey reported a 660% increase in expenditures on opioids between 1997 and 2006; furthermore, rates of opioid prescribing for back and neck pain increased from 19% to 29% from 1999 to 2010.[55] It is a striking commonality across systematic reviews that the evidence for efficacy of opioids for chronic back pain is described as meager and unclear, with no evidence that they improve function. Furthermore, among random control trials for chronic back pain, there are no studies with long-term (beyond 4 months) follow-up and all have high dropout rates. When considering the risks of long-term opioid use and the lack of evidence regarding their benefit, the general recommendations have shifted markedly in the last 5 years.[56]

Clinical Observations and Clues to Addiction

For individuals with CNCP as well as those providers prescribing opioids, it can be unclear whether opioids are an asset or liability. An illusion of benefit results when the immediate effects of a drug obscure the deleterious effects of continuous use. Families who witness unwanted drug effects may believe them to be unavoidable and preferable to unrelieved suffering. Often, such patients, their families, and their physicians are surprised at the reduction in pain and suffering that often occurs after gradual elimination of the drug.

Clues to the presence of addiction in pain patients include frequent intoxication, mood changes, inattention to hygiene, inappropriate behaviors, and impaired coordination. Another indicator is provided when, despite generous analgesia, sick role behavior remains disproportionate to pathology. The patient who uses analgesics in a nonaddictive fashion, in contrast, is likely to have improved function. Combining other intoxicants with prescription drugs is an obvious clue. Urine toxicology facilitates the diagnosis of substance use disorder; however, it must be remembered that typical "dip stick" (immunoassay) technology may not identify synthetic or semisynthetic opioids and that gas chromatography/mass spectroscopy may be needed. Many states have enacted electronic prescription monitoring programs that can help identify aberrant use. Loss of control may be shown when patients who are incapable of rationing themselves use a month's supply in a few days, despite knowing they will have increased pain and withdrawal symptoms when their supply is depleted. Additional signs include multisourcing and family/physician concern about their medication consumption. Usually, a patient who has no history of alcohol or drug abuse who becomes physically dependent on benzodiazepines or analgesics in the course of pain treatment, who obtains the drugs legitimately, and who has not been drug impaired is not addicted. That is, the fact that chronic high-dose opioids are ineffective does not confirm the presence of an addictive disorder.

Conceptually, there are two issues: the treatment of addiction in pain patients and the treatment of pain in people with the disease of addiction. There seem to be no data as to which treatment should be first, but experience suggests that the pain patient who has an addiction to cocaine, marijuana, or alcohol often responds to traditional addiction care in a setting appropriate to the severity of the disease. In contrast, the person who has become iatrogenically addicted (and perhaps the person who has an "iatrogenic relapse" after a period of sobriety) seems to respond better if treatment is initiated in a pain treatment program. Acceptance of the diagnosis is facilitated when patients can interact with peers who have also developed addiction "through no fault of their own" and without engaging in illegal behaviors.

The treatment of pain in patients with comorbid addiction raises the question of whether to use opioids and, if so, how to protect the person's sobriety. Although it is considered unethical to withhold opioid analgesia from addicts,[57] patients should not be given useless or harmful treatments. Animal[58] and human[59] studies demonstrate that one of the most powerful stimuli to elicit resumption of dormant drug-seeking behavior is exposure to the drug of choice. This may explain the clinical impression that opioid therapy with recovering alcoholics is often more successful than is the case with recovering opioid addicts. Nevertheless, because of cross-addiction, a patient with any prior addiction is at heightened risk for new addiction, even to unrelated substances. This is supported by findings that most patients hospitalized for treatment of oxycodone addiction were found to have been treated previously for nonopioid substance use disorder.[60]

A distinction must be made between acute and chronic pain and between the patient who is actively engaging in substance abuse and the patient in recovery. There is no controversy regarding the treatment of *acute* pain in those with comorbid addiction. Opioids are appropriate, effective, and often essential. Acute injuries and surgery in addicts, even those in sustained recovery, may require more aggressive analgesia than in those with no addiction history, since tolerance is rapidly reestablished in the previously tolerant person or animal.

Patients in recovery may face surgery with trepidation, as they fear having to choose between unrelieved pain and addiction relapse. Some even refuse analgesia in an effort to preserve their sobriety. Experience suggests that this is unnecessary. Patients should be encouraged to inform the surgeon and anesthesiologist in advance of elective procedures that they are in recovery, may require higher than usual doses of analgesics, but wish to avoid their previous drug of choice, transition to long-acting oral agents as soon as possible, and arrange for safe use of opioids after discharge. The patients should increase their recovery work (e.g., 12-step meetings, meetings with addiction counselor) and should notify their addictionologist and sponsor of pending surgery so that support is in place. A spouse, friend, or sponsor can store opioids and bring a supply each day so that the patient is protected from the temptation of a supply of opioids within easy reach.

Appropriate treatment of comorbid pain and addiction remains controversial and there is little data on which to base therapy.[61] We must rely on "clinical wisdom" while remembering how often it has proved wrong when data became available.

Psychological Treatments

Many psychological treatments have been applied to chronic low back pain, as summarized in Table 108.1. Here we review these modalities and their relative efficacy.

Cognitive Behavioral Therapies

Cognitive behavioral therapy for pain (CBT-P) is predicated on the premise that pain-related beliefs and effectiveness of coping strategies impact the severity of emotional distress and physical disability. CBT-P has been shown to be effective in the treatment of chronic pain. Mirza and Deyo, in a review of randomized trials of fusion versus nonoperative care of CLBP, compared surgery, traditional nonoperative care, and CBT-P, and found that both surgery and CBT-P were better than unstructured, ill-defined nonsurgical care.[62] They concluded that CBT-P outcomes were comparable to surgical outcomes at 1 year and without the obvious risks associated with surgery. A consistent finding across systematic reviews of psychological approaches for chronic pain is that the effectiveness of CBT-P is best demonstrated for pain-related mood and function, with somewhat less of an effect on pain severity.[63] Techniques used in CBT-P include self-talk (both motivational and self-defeating), relaxation techniques, and distraction and positive coping strategies. Since stress can increase pain perception, learning to identify and manage stress can play an important role in the pain treatment. Often, patients come to the experience of pain with few coping mechanisms and major life stresses. Group, individual, and family therapy can help address stresses and teach new ways of managing pain and stress as an individual and as a larger family unit.

Mindfulness and Acceptance-Based Therapies

Mindfulness and acceptance-based therapies emphasize adaptation and lessened resistance to the pain experience. Rooted in a variety of philosophies, including Buddhism and theoretical models, such as the "Ironic Processes Model," these therapies teach individuals to adapt a nonjudgmental curious awareness to thoughts, feelings, and body sensations. These therapies are certainly supported by evidence that suppression of negative emotions increases self-reported pain and pain behaviors[45] as well as efforts to control or avoid unwanted experiences may actually increase suffering.[65] Techniques utilized in mindfulness and acceptance-based therapies, such as Acceptance and Commitment Therapy (ACT), include formal and informal meditation practice, experiential exercises modeling psychological "flexibility," and some of the central tenets of CBT.

Overall, the evidence for the efficacy of mindfulness-based treatments is still preliminary due to small to modest treatment effects and methodological limitations of studies (no control group, lack of control for nonspecific effects). However,

TABLE 108.1 Summary of Psychosocial Treatments and Clinical Recommendations for Chronic Low Back Pain

Psychological Treatment Modality	Summary of Empirical Findings	Clinical Recommendations
Cognitive behavioral therapy (CBT)	• Strongest impact on pain-related mood and function, with somewhat less of an effect on pain severity • Consistently superior to usual care • In chronic low back pain, CBT comparable to surgical outcomes at 1 year	• Low-risk, easy-to-understand treatment format • Suitable for a wide variety of ages and education levels • Can be generalized to also address dysfunctional thought patterns and behaviors related to comorbid depression, anxiety, and substance use • Acceptable "first-choice" treatment option in individuals who are treatment naïve
Psychodynamic therapy	• Evidence of improvements in psychiatric and somatic symptoms among patients with a variety of somatic medical conditions • Evidence of benefit in individuals with histories of trauma/abuse • No strong evidence exclusive to use in chronic pain	• May be useful in combination with other modalities in individuals who have history of extensive childhood trauma or attachment disorders
Mindfulness and acceptance-based therapies	• Historically, efficacy studies demonstrated small to moderate treatment effects with considerable methodological limitations. • Recent high-caliber study shows that benefits of mindfulness-based therapies equal those obtained in CBT in the chronic low back pain population.	• Offers patients an alternative way to understand and cope with chronic pain. • Consider use in those who are not receptive to other treatment modalities. • May be particularly suitable for individuals who struggle to achieve flexibility in thinking and emotional reactivity or those who struggle to accept that physical and emotional pain are components of the human experience.
Psychophysiologic and relaxation training	• Variable efficacy for psychophysiologic training/biofeedback in a variety of pain conditions but continues to be commonly used in the chronic pain population.	• Biofeedback offers a unique ability to objectify the stress response in a fairly simple, noninvasive manner and may be best suited to those individuals who demonstrate poor insight into the mind–body connection.
Family education and therapy	• Sufficient data support the education of family members of those with chronic pain. • Substantial research shows that solicitous partner responses worsen overall outcomes for individuals with chronic pain.	• Engage the family in treatment from the outset. • Provide education to the family on chronic pain as well as how their responses to pain may hinder or facilitate rehabilitation. • Encourage family members to reinforce positive, nonsick role behaviors and to ignore those behaviors that promote disability and illness. • Overprotection of the individual with chronic pain (including suggestions for rest or caution) impede overall improvements from chronic pain.
Interdisciplinary pain rehabilitation programs (IPRPs)	• IPRPs offer an intensive treatment intervention, combining pharmacotherapy, physical reconditioning, and psychological therapies. • Shown to be more effective than noninterdisciplinary rehabilitation for both chronic and subacute low back pain. • Substantial empirical evidence for the efficacy of IPRPs in chronic pain, with benefits lasting up to 10 years.	• IPRPs may be best suited to individuals with more severe levels of disability, deconditioning, and psychiatric comorbidities.

several recent studies offer promise. One systematic review and meta-analysis of meditation programs that included only randomized controlled trials and accounted for placebo effect found moderate evidence for its effects on mood and pain but no evidence that such benefits exceed those obtained from other psychological and medical treatments.[66] Another review of mindfulness-based therapies specifically for chronic pain reported small nonspecific improvements in pain and depression across 10 studies reviewed; however, significant and sustained improvements were demonstrated in pain acceptance, quality of life, and stress.[67] In a meta-analysis of 22 acceptance-based studies, including a combination of mindfulness and ACT, significant improvements were found for pain, depression, anxiety, physical well-being, and quality of life.[68] There have been few studies looking specifically at the use of mindfulness-based therapies for back pain. In a random controlled trial comparing mindfulness-based stress reduction to CBT and usual care among individuals with CLBP, Cherkin and colleagues found that mindfulness-based stress reduction and CBT showed equal benefits in terms of pain and function at 26 and 52 weeks, which exceeded usual care.[69] Thus, these relatively new therapeutic approaches appear to be a viable and complementary treatment option that offers patients an alternative way to conceptualize, understand, and cope with their pain experience. Their benefits may equal those found in CBT.

Psychodynamic and Interpersonal Therapies

Psychodynamic and interpersonal-oriented therapies emphasize relationships and attachment patterns. Psychodynamic therapy focuses heavily on early childhood experiences. While psychodynamic approaches produce improvements in psychiatric and somatic symptoms and reduce health care utilization among patients with a variety of somatic medical conditions, there is limited empirical support for their efficacy in chronic pain.[70] However, given the high rates of previous trauma and childhood stress in chronic pain, a psychodynamic approach may warrant consideration as a treatment approach in those with traumatic histories and attachment patterns.[71]

Education

Education may be one of the most critical of the "therapies" provided. It is often crucial because a patient's behavior and the family's reaction to the patient's disease may be based on faulty information or misconceptions. Education can clarify the problem and indicate the best response. It can be useful to interpret chronic pain as "real" but a "false alarm" that need not dictate activity.

Involving family in the education process is essential. Family members often feel confused and helpless in response to a loved one's pain. In turn, they may respond in ways that unintentionally reinforce the sick role, such as being overly protective or enabling. This dynamic reinforces dependency, overall reliance on others, and an external locus of control in the person with pain. Furthermore, criticism by family members for lack of positive health behaviors or for engaging in pain behaviors is related to greater physical dysfunction in the person with pain. Similarly, solicitous partner responses to pain behaviors are associated with overall poorer functioning. These findings are not isolated to clinical observations; they are also supported in the research.[72]

Psychophysiologic and Relaxation Training

Chronic uncontrolled stress amplifies pain and associated emotional distress. Thus, the direct target of these techniques is to teach individuals to self-regulate the stress response and the associated physiologic indicators. Relaxation techniques vary in nature but include deep breathing, progressive muscle relaxation, guided imagery, and visualization. All of these techniques can be used with or without psychophysiologic monitoring, such as in biofeedback. The benefits of relaxation training across a variety of health-related conditions are well established. In fact, the benefits of these techniques have been shown to go beyond a subjective sense of relaxation, such as by showing reductions in cortisol, adrenocorticotropic hormone, and norepinephrine in individuals who practice these techniques regularly.[73]

Relaxation techniques can have a direct effect on tense muscles and heightened arousal that is accompanied by the stress of pain. There is empirical evidence that relaxation training, self-hypnosis, and progressive muscle relaxation with or without biofeedback assistance offer favorable benefits in the treatment of pain.[74] However, systematic reviews evaluating the quality of the evidence for use of relaxation training and biofeedback therapy for pain generally exert caution in providing a "strong" recommendation for these therapies due to consistent methodologic flaws across studies.[75] In spite of the lack of gold standard studies, these therapies clearly offer a low-risk, simple, and drug-free method for slowing the cascade of stress hormones that often accompanies chronic pain.

The Role of Exercise

While exercise is not a specific psychological treatment, psychological status and physical fitness clearly have a reciprocal relationship, with each affecting the other. Fears of movement and exercise may present just as other "phobias" and when they persist lead to a vicious cycle of activity avoidance. A number of studies have addressed fear of movement in chronic pain, showing that those with so-called "kinesiophobia" report more pain, disability, and self-protective behaviors.[70] Conversely, even short bouts of exercise (10 minutes) have demonstrated immediate benefits on depression and anxiety in chronic pain patients.[71] Adding to this, graded exercise programs gradually reduce fears of harm from exercise and promote increased function.[72] In sum, exercise is an important component of psychological treatment of pain.

Interdisciplinary Pain Rehabilitation Programs

Interdisciplinary chronic pain rehabilitation programs are designed to help patients with disabling chronic pain restore function and quality of life. Interdisciplinary care is a team approach in which all the members of the team, including the patient, work together toward common goals. These programs have been shown to be more effective than noninterdisciplinary rehabilitation for both chronic and subacute low back pain.[73–75] Disciplines commonly involved in these programs include physical and occupational therapy, nursing, psychology, medicine, vocational rehabilitation, and chemical dependency counseling when needed. Some programs are intensive, 3 to 4 weeks long, and include active physical therapy and reconditioning, occupational therapy with an emphasis on body mechanics, group and individual psychotherapy, and medication management, while others are of variable duration and intensity. Some programs include weaning off of all habituating substances. When vocational and addiction needs are identified, these services can also be offered as part of the holistic approach to rehabilitation.

Summary

Psychosocial variables have been shown to have a significant impact on pain perception, and, in turn, disability due to pain. Pain intensity, the degree to which it interferes with activities, and the extent to which it disrupts mood all predict chronicity of back pain. Early identification of psychological vulnerabilities is essential to the overall outcome of patients with low back pain. Furthermore, psychological treatments offer a "low-risk" treatment option, with evidence of benefits that equal surgical interventions or exceed usual care. These therapies may be particularly important to utilize in the refractory patient or those with enhanced psychological vulnerabilities.

KEY POINTS

1. Pain is an unpleasant sensory, cognitive, and emotional experience associated with actual, potential, or perceived tissue damage.
2. The lifetime prevalence of back pain is essentially universal, yet the prevalence of disabling back pain is not. Psychological factors amplify pain, sometimes to disabling degrees.
3. Pain is not what occurs at the periphery; it is what the brain perceives. Actual damage is neither necessary nor sufficient for the perception of pain. Anger, depression, anxiety, fear, and other psychological variables can all increase the perception of both acute and chronic pain, as can believing pain to be an indicator of a destructive process.
4. Back pain is often ascribed to organic processes including strains, sprains, anulus tears, internal disc disruption, facet arthropathy, or bone pathology; however, it is often not explained by examination or imaging, and positive findings on imaging may be misleading.
5. The most frequent psychiatric illnesses (excluding somatic symptom disorders) in pain center patients are anxiety disorders, depression, and substance abuse. Addiction is prevalent and its treatment is essential, since addiction recovery seems to be the *sine qua non* for pain recovery.
6. Various psychotherapies—such as cognitive behavioral therapy, mindfulness and acceptance-based therapies, and relaxation training therapies—have shown efficacy in the treatment of chronic pain.
7. Interdisciplinary chronic pain rehabilitation programs have been shown to be more effective than noninterdisciplinary rehabilitation for both chronic and subacute low back pain.
8. *Pain is an unpleasant sensory and emotional experience associated with actual or potential tissue damage or described in terms of such damage.*—International Association for the Study of Pain 1973 consensus definition of pain

KEY REFERENCES

1. Mirza S, Deyo RA. Systematic review of randomized trials comparing lumbar fusion surgery to nonoperative care for treatment of chronic back pain. *Spine*. 2007;32(7):816-823.
This paper presents the results of five randomized trials that compared fusion to nonoperative treatment for chronic low back pain. They concluded that whereas surgery may be more efficacious than unstructured nonsurgical care, it may not be more effective than structured cognitive behavioral therapy.
2. Turk DC, Swanson KS, Tunks ER. Psychological approaches in the treatment of chronic pain patients. When pills, scalpels, and needles are not enough. *Can J Psychiatry*. 2008;53(4).
This article reviews the psychological models used to conceptualize the problem of chronic pain. It presents descriptions of treatments based on these models as well as evidence supporting their efficacy.
3. Chou R, Loser JD, Owens DK, et al. Interventional therapies, surgery, and interdisciplinary rehabilitation for low back pain: an evidence-based clinical practice guideline from the American Pain Society. *Spine*. 2009;34(10):1066-1077.
This paper presents the results of a systematic review of the literature by a multidisciplinary panel convened by the American Pain Society. It was designed to develop evidence-based guidelines on the use of interventional diagnostic tests and therapies, surgeries, and interdisciplinary rehabilitation for low back pain.
4. Carragee EJ, Alamin TF, Miller JL, et al. Discographic, MRI and psychosocial determinants of low back pain disability and remission: a prospective study in subjects with benign persistent back pain. *Spine J*. 2005;5:24-35.
These authors followed 100 patients with mild CLBP and no prior spine-related disability for 5 years. Moderate or severe Modic changes of the vertebral endplate were the only structural variable that weakly predicted adverse outcome. Provocative discography and baseline MR predicted no outcome variables but were weakly associated with pain episodes. Psychosocial variables strongly predicted long- and short-term disability and health care visits for LBP.
5. Hofbauer RK, Rainville P, Duncan GH, Bushnell MC. Cortical representation of the sensory dimension of pain. *J Neurophysiol*. 2001;86(1):402-411.
Numerous studies have presented evidence that multiple brain regions are activated during the experience of pain. This study used positron emission tomography to indirectly measure pain-evoked cerebral activity before and after hypnotic suggestions given to modulate the perception of perceived pain unpleasantness, thus separating the sensory and affective component of pain.

REFERENCES

1. Deyo RA. Descriptive epidemiology of low back pain and its related medical care in the United States. *Spine*. 1987;12:264.
2. Cassidy JD, Carroll LJ, Cote P. The Saskatchewan health and back pain survey. The prevalence of low back pain and related disability in Saskatchewan adults. *Spine*. 1998;23:1860.
3. Frymoyer JW, Cats-Baril WL. An overview of the incidences and costs of low back pain. *Orthop Clin North Am*. 1991; 22:263.
4. Deyo RA, Mirza SK, Martin BI. Back pain prevalence and visit rates: estimates from U.S. national surveys, 2002. *Spine*. 2006;31(23):2724-2727.
5. Croft PR, Macfarlane GJ, Papageorgiou AC, et al. Outcomes of low back pain in general practice: a prospective study. *BMJ*. 1998;316:1356.
6. Pengel LHM, Herbert RD, Maher CG, Refshauge KM. Acute low back pain; systematic review of its prognosis. *BMJ*. 2003;327:323.
7. Hagan KB, Jamtvedt G, Hilde G, Winnem MF. The updated Cochrane review of bed rest for low back pain and sciatica. *Spine*. 2005;30:542.
8. van Tulder MW, Assendelft WJ, Koes BW, Bouter LM. Spinal radiographic findings and non-specific low back pain. A systematic review of observational studies. *Spine*. 1997;22:427.
9. Gore M, Sadosky A, Stacey BR, Tai KS, Leslie D. The burden of chronic low back pain: clinical comorbidities, treatment patterns, and health care costs in usual care settings. *Spine*. 2012;37(11):E668-E677.
10. Boden SD, Davis DO, Dina TS, et al. Abnormal magnetic resonance scans of the lumbar spine in asymptomatic subjects. *J Bone Joint Surg Am*. 1990;72(3):403-408.
11. Jensen M, Brant-Zawadzld M, Obuchowski N, et al. MRI of lumbar spine in people without back pain. *N Engl J Med*. 1994;331:69-73.
12. Fields HL, Heinricher MM. Anatomy and physiology of a nociceptive modulatory system. *Philos Trans R Soc Lond B Biol Sci*. 1985;308:361-374.

SECTION XVI

13. Arvidsson J, Ygge J, Grant G. Cell loss in lumbar dorsal root ganglia and transganglionic degeneration after sciatic nerve resection in the rat. *Brain Res*. 1986;373:15-21.
14. Sugimoto T, Bennett GJ, Kajander KC. Transsynaptic degeneration in the superficial dorsal horn after sciatic nerve injury: effects of a chronic constriction injury, transection, and strychnine. *Pain*. 1990;42:205-213.
15. Watkins LR, Maier SF. Beyond neurons: evidence that immune and glial cells contribute to pathological pain states. *Physiol Rev*. 2002;82:981-1011.
16. Woolf CJ. Central mechanisms of acute pain. In: Bond MR, Charlton JE, Woolf CJ, eds. *Pain Research and Clinical Management*, Vol. 4, Procedures from the Fifth World Congress on Pain. Amsterdam: Elsevier; 1991:25-34.
17. Torebjörk HE, Lundberg L, LaMotte R. Neural mechanisms for capsaicin-induced hyperalgesia. *Pain*. 1990;41(suppl 1):S114.
18. Coderre TJ, Katz J, Vaccarino AL, et al. Contribution of central neuroplasticity to pathological pain: review of clinical and experimental evidence. *Pain*. 1993;52:259-285.
19. Staud R, Vierck CJ, Robinson ME, Price DD. Effects of the NMDA receptor antagonist dextromethorphan on temporal summation of pain are similar in fibromyalgia patients and normal controls. *J Pain*. 2005;6:323-332.
20. Curatolo M, Arendt-Nielsen L, Petersen-Felix S. Evidence, mechanisms, and clinical implications of central hypersensitivity in chronic pain after whiplash injury. *Clin J Pain*. 2004;20(6):469-476.
21. Staud R. Abnormal endogenous pain modulation is a shared characteristic of many chronic pain conditions. *Expert Rev Neurother*. 2012;12(5):577-585.
22. Swett JE, McMahon SB, Wall PD. Long ascending projections to the midbrain from cells of lamina I and nucleus of the dorsolateral funiculus of the rat spinal cord. *J Comp Neurol*. 1985;238:401-416.
23. Millan MJ. Descending control of pain. *Prog Neurobiol*. 2002;66:335-474.
24. Hoffman MD, Shepanski MA, Mackenzie SP, Clifford PS. Experimentally induced pain perception is acutely reduced by aerobic exercise in people with chronic low back pain. *J Rehabil Res Dev*. 2005;42(2):183-190.
25. Duncan GH, Bushnell MC, Bates R, et al. Task-related responses of monkey medullary dorsal horn neurons. *J Neurophysiol*. 1987;57(1):289-310.
26. Zubieta JK, Heitzeg MM, Smith YR, et al. COMT val 158 met genotype affects mu-opioid neurotransmitter responses to a pain stressor. *Science*. 2003;299(5610):1240-1243.
27. Uhl GR, Sora I, Wang Z. The mu opiate receptor as a candidate gene for pain: polymorphisms, variations in expression, nociception, and opiate responses. *Proc Natl Acad Sci USA*. 1999;96(14):7752-7755.
28. Devor M, Raber P. Heritability of symptoms in an experimental model of neuropathic pain. *Pain*. 1990;49: 51-67.
29. Coghill RC, McHaffie JG, Yen YF. Neural correlates of interindividual differences in the subjective experience of pain. *Proc Natl Acad Sci USA*. 2003;100(14):8538-8542.
30. Nijs J, Malfliet A, Ickmans K, Baert I, Meeus M. Treatment of central sensitization in patients with "unexplained" chronic pain: an update. *Expert Opin Pharmacother*. 2014;15(12):1671-1683.
31. Mayer TG, Neblett R, Cohen H, et al. The development and psychometric validation of the Central Sensitization Inventory. *Pain Pract*. 2011;12(4):276-285.
32. Neblett R, Hartzell MM, Mayer TG, Cohen H, Gatchel RJ. Establishing clinically relevant severity levels for the Central Sensitization Inventory. *Pain Pract*. 2017;17(2):166-175.
33. Carragee EJ, Alamin TF, Miller JL, et al. Discographic, MRI and psychosocial determinants of low back pain disability and remission: a prospective study in subjects with benign persistent back pain. *Spine J*. 2005;5:24-35.
34. Polatin PB, Kinney RK, Gatchel RJ, et al. Psychiatric illness and chronic low-back pain. The mind and the spine—which goes first? *Spine*. 1993;18:66-71.
35. Von Korff M, Crane P, Lane M, et al. Chronic spinal pain and physical–mental comorbidity in the United States: results from the national comorbidity survey replication. *Pain*. 2005;113:331-339.
36. Rudy TE, Kerns RD, Turk DC. Chronic pain and depression: toward a cognitive-behavioral mediation model. *Pain*. 1988;35(2):129-140.
37. DeGood DE, Kiernan B. Perception of fault in patients with chronic pain. *Pain*. 1996;64(1):153-159.
38. Deleted in review.
39. Strigo IA, Simmons AN, Matthews SC, Craig AD, Paulus MP. Association of major depressive disorder with altered functional brain response during anticipation and processing of heat pain. *Arch Gen Psychiatry*. 2008;65(11):1275-1284.
40. Osman A, Barrios FX, Kopper BA, et al. Factor structure, reliability, and validity of the Pain Catastrophizing Scale. *J Behav Med*. 1997;20(6):589-605.
41. Quartana PJ, Campbell CM, Edwards RR. Pain catastrophizing: a critical review. *Expert Rev Neurother*. 2009;9(5):745-758.
42. Weissman-Fogel I, Sprecher E, Pud D. Effects of catastrophizing on pain perception and pain modulation. *Exp Brain Res*. 2008;186(1):79-85.
43. Burns JW, Johnson BJ, Mahoney N, Devine J, Pawl R. Anger management style, hostility and spouse responses: gender differences in predictors of adjustment among chronic pain patients. *Pain*. 1996;64:445-453.
44. Bruehl S, Burns JW, Chung OY, Ward B, Johnson B. Anger and pain severity in chronic low back pain patients and pain free controls: the role of endogenous opioid blockade. *Pain*. 2002;99:923-933.
45. Burns JW, Quartana P, Gilliam W, et al. Effects of anger suppression on pain severity and pain behaviors among chronic pain patients: evaluation of an ironic process model. *Health Psychol*. 2008;5:645-652.
46. Serbic D, Pincus T, Fife-Schaw C, Dawson H. Diagnostic uncertainty, guilt, mood, and disability in back pain. *Health Psychol*. 2016;35(1):50-59.
47. Hassett AL, Goesling J, Mathur SN, et al. Affect and low back pain: more to consider than the influence of negative affect alone. *Clin J Pain*. 2016;32(10):907-914.
48. *Diagnostic and Statistical Manual of Mental Disorders*. 5th ed. Washington, DC: American Psychiatric Association; 2013.
49. Rome HP, Rome JD. Limbically augmented pain syndrome (LAPS): kindling, corticolimbic sensitization, and the convergence of affective and sensory symptoms in chronic pain disorders. *Pain Med*. 2000;1(1):7-23.
50. Jones GT, Power C, Macfarlane GJ. Adverse events in childhood and chronic widespread pain in adult life: results from the 1958 British Birth Cohort Study. *Pain*. 2009;143(1-2):92-96.
51. Von Korff M, Alonso J, Ormel J, et al. Childhood psychosocial factors and adult onset arthritis: broad spectrum risk factors and allostatic load. *Pain*. 2009;143:76-83.

52. Woby S, Watson P, Roach N, et al. Coping strategy use: does it predict adjustment to chronic back pain after controlling for catastrophic thinking and self-efficacy for pain control? *J Rehabil Med*. 2005;37:100-107.
53. Smith SM, Dart RC, Katz NP, et al. Analgesic, Anesthetic, and Addiction Clinical Trials, Translations, Innovations, Opportunities, and Networks (ACTTION) public-private partnership. Classification and definition of misuse, abuse, and related events in clinical trials: ACTTION systematic review and recommendations. *Pain*. 2013;154(11):2287-2296.
54. Boscarino JA, Hoffman SN, Han JJ. Opioid-use disorder among patients on long-term opioid therapy: impact of final DSM-5 diagnostic criteria on prevalence and correlates. *Subst Abuse Rehabil*. 2015;6:83-91.
55. Campbell G, Bruno R, Lintzeris N, et al. Defining problematic pharmaceutical opioid use among people prescribed opioids for chronic non-cancer pain: do different measures identify the same patients? *Pain*. 2016;157(7):1489-1498.
56. Martin BI, Turner JA, Mirza SK, et al. Trends in health care expenditures, utilization, and health status among US adults with spine problems, 1997-2006. *Spine*. 2009;34:2077-2084.
57. Deyo RA, Von Korff M, Duhrkoop D. Opioids for low back pain. *BMJ*. 2015;350:g6380.
58. Gardner EL. What we have learned about addiction from animal models of drug self-administration. *Am J Addict*. 2000;9:285-313.
59. Daley DC, Marlatt GA, Spotts CE. Relapse Prevention: Clinical Models and Intervention Strategies. In: Graham AW, Schultz TK, Mayo-Smith M, Ries RK, eds. *Principles of Addiction Medicine*. 3rd ed. Washington DC: American Society of Addiction Mdicine; 2003.
60. Potter JS, Hennessy G, Borrow JA, Greenfield SF, Weiss RD. Substance use histories in patients seeking treatment for controlled-release oxycodone dependence. *Drug Alcohol Depend*. 2004;76(2):213-215.
61. Nedeljkovic SS, Wasan A, Jamison RN. Assessment of efficacy of long-term opioid therapy in pain patients with substance abuse potential. *Clin J Pain*. 2002;18(suppl):S39-S51.
62. Mirza S, Deyo RA. Systematic review of randomized trials comparing lumbar fusion surgery to nonoperative care for treatment of chronic back pain. *Spine*. 2007;32(7):816-823.
63. Eccleston C, Morley SJ, Williams AC. Psychological approaches to chronic pain management: evidence and challenges. *Br J Anaesth*. 2013;111(1):59-63.
64. Deleted in review.
65. Wegner DM. Ironic processes of mental control. *Psychol Rev*. 1994;101(1):34-52.
66. Goyal M, Singh S, Sibinga EM, et al. Meditation programs for psychological stress and well-being: a systematic review and meta-analysis. *JAMA Intern Med*. 2014;174(3):357-368.
67. Chiesa A, Serretti A. Mindfulness-based interventions for chronic pain: a systematic review of the evidence. *J Altern Complement Med*. 2011;17(1):83-93.
68. Veehof MM, Oskam MJ, Schreurs KM, Bohlmeijer ET. Acceptance-based interventions for the treatment of chronic pain: a systematic review and meta-analysis. *Pain*. 2011;152:533-542.
69. Cherkin DC, Sherman KJ, Balderson BH, et al. Effect of mindfulness-based stress reduction vs cognitive behavioral therapy or usual care on back pain and functional limitations in adults with chronic low back pain: a randomized clinical trial. *JAMA*. 2016;315(12):1240-1249.
70. Shedler J. The efficacy of psychodynamic psychotherapy. *Am Psychol*. 2010;65(2):98-109.
71. Turk DC, Swanson KS, Tunks ER. Psychological approaches in the treatment of chronic pain patients—when pills, scalpels, and needles are not enough. *Can J Psychiatry*. 2008;53(4): 213-223.
72. Raichle KA, Romano JM, Jensen MP. Partner responses to patient pain and well behaviors and their relationship to patient pain behavior, functioning, and depression. *Pain*. 2011;152(1):82-88.
73. Chang BH, Dusek JA, Benson H. Psychobiological changes from relaxation response elicitation: long-term practitioners vs. novices. *Psychosomatics*. 2011;52(6):550-559.
74. Hofbauer RK, Rainville P, Duncan GH, Bushnell MC. Cortical representation of the sensory dimension of pain. *J Neurophysiol*. 2001;86(1):402-411.
75. Lee C, Crawford C, Hickey A. Active Self-Care Therapies for Pain (PACT) Working Group. Mind-body therapies for the self-management of chronic pain symptoms. *Pain Med*. 2014;15(suppl 1):S21-S39.

CHAPTER 109 Pharmacologic Strategies in Back Pain and Radiculopathy

Yashar Eshraghi
Nagy A. Mekhail

Back pain is a major health problem in the United States. About 70% to 85% of the population experiences back pain at some point in their lives, with the annual prevalence ranging from 15% to 45%. Usually, the clinical course is benign, with 95% recovering within a few weeks to months of onset. It is most common in middle-aged adults, with equal distribution in men and women. Back pain is the most frequent reason for activity limitation in people younger than 45 years and the second leading cause for doctor visits and absenteeism from work. The lower back is the primary site of pain in 85% of patients. It also has a major economic impact in the form of *direct costs* (costs incurred for physician services, surgery, medical devices, medications, hospital services, and diagnostic testing) and *indirect costs* (cost incurred from absenteeism and decreased productivity). The cost of treating low back pain has been increasing; total cost in the United States is estimated to exceed $100 to $200 billion per year. Two-thirds of the cost is indirect, due to lost wages and reduced productivity. The rate of back surgery in the United States has increased dramatically, especially for spinal fusion. From 1979–1981 to 1988–1990, the rate of hospitalizations with cervical spine surgery increased more than 45%, with the rates for cervical fusion surgery increasing more than 70%. The rate of hospitalizations with lumbar spine surgery increased more than 33%, with the rate for lumbar fusion surgery increasing more than 60%.[1–4]

Although often used in conjunction with other means of managing back pain, drug therapy remains a mainstay in the treatment of back pain. The ultimate endpoint of any therapeutic intervention is to overcome the pathophysiologic process responsible for pain generation. However, pharmacologic treatment of low back pain often aims to provide symptomatic relief.

It is important to recognize the nature and basic mechanisms of back pain before attempting to use pharmacologic agents. *Nociceptive* pain results from tissue injury and subsequent activation of peripheral nociceptors, whereas *neuropathic* pain arises from the nerve injury or dysfunction of central or peripheral nervous system elements. *Radicular pain*, or pain in the distribution of specific spinal nerve(s), is a form of neuropathic pain. It is frequently referred to as sciatica when it involves the lower extremities. *Radiculopathy* is the objective change of sensory or motor function due to conduction block in the axons of the spinal nerve or its roots as a result of irritation of the nerve by compression or inflammatory mediators. Neuropathic pain is notoriously difficult to treat. The paucity of well-designed, large, randomized, double-blind, and prospective placebo-controlled trials results in management decisions based on individual physician perspectives and experiences.[5–8] Most common drug therapies for back pain with or without radiculopathy include acetaminophen, nonsteroidal antiinflammatory drugs (NSAIDs), muscle relaxants, tramadol, antidepressants, opioids, and membrane-stabilizing medications. This chapter reviews the literature using an evidence-based approach whenever possible.

Acetaminophen

Acetaminophen, also known as *paracetamol,* is a *p*-aminophenol derivative with antipyretic and analgesic properties. It is frequently used as a first-line agent in acute low back pain and osteoarthritis due to its favorable gastrointestinal safety profile over aspirin and other antiinflammatory drugs.[9,10] No trial has evaluated acetaminophen versus placebo for chronic low back pain, and the only trial that compared paracetamol to no treatment did not show any favorable effects in acute low back pain.[11] In five trials, no significant difference was demonstrated between paracetamol at dosages up to 4 g/day and different NSAIDs for back pain of variable duration.[11–15] However, several systematic reviews of patients with osteoarthritis reliably showed acetaminophen to be slightly less effective in pain relief than NSAIDs.[16,17] The mechanism of action is not fully understood but is thought to have central and peripheral mechanisms. Acetaminophen is a weak inhibitor of cyclooxygenase enzymes (COX-l and COX-2) and may be a cloned COX-3 enzyme.[18] It has few side effects and is entirely metabolized in the liver. The maximum daily allowed dose of acetaminophen has been the subject of controversy. The pharmaceutical producer of the Tylenol brand of acetaminophen decreased the maximum daily dose of acetaminophen from 4000 mg/day to either 3000 mg/day or 3250 mg/day for consumers taking the 500-mg or 325-mg tablet preparations, respectively, which was not followed by many other manufacturers.[19] In order to diminish acetaminophen hepatotoxicity, the U.S. Food and Drug Administration (FDA) established regulations to limit prescription combination drug products to contain no more than 325 mg of acetaminophen per dosage unit.[20] Chronic administration f higher doses is associated with hepatotoxicity (especially in chronic ethanol users, malnourished, and fasting patients).[21]

Nonsteroidal Antiinflammatory Drugs

NSAIDs are the most frequently prescribed medications worldwide and are commonly used for treating back pain. They possess antipyretic, antiinflammatory, and analgesic effects, the latter two accounting for their use in arthritic and painful disorders. The mechanism of action of NSAIDs includes COX-l and COX-2 inhibition, resulting in decreased tissue levels of prostaglandins. NSAIDs that inhibit both COX-l and COX-2 include aspirin, ibuprofen, diclofenac, indomethacin, naproxen, and piroxicam. NSAIDs that selectively inhibit COX-2 include celecoxib, etodolac, meloxicam, and nimesulide.[22] In a systematic review of 65 randomized controlled trials of NSAIDs in low back pain, the authors concluded that NSAIDs were more effective compared with placebo but at the cost of significantly more side effects. There was moderate evidence that NSAIDs were more effective than acetaminophen for acute low back pain, but acetaminophen had fewer side effects. There was moderate evidence that NSAIDs were not more effective than other drugs for acute low back pain. There was strong evidence that various types of NSAIDs, including COX-2 NSAIDs, were equally effective for acute low back pain. The data suggested that NSAIDs were effective for short-term symptomatic relief in patients with acute and chronic low back pain without sciatica.[23] A systematic review of 13 trials found that NSAIDs are more beneficial than placebo in pain intensity. NSAIDs were slightly more effective than placebo as regards disability. However, the extent of the efficacy was minimal and the level of evidence was not significant.

NSAIDs can have serious side effects on various organ systems, including the gastrointestinal tract (gastroduodenal ulceration and bleeding), kidneys (renal insufficiency and hypertension), cardiovascular system (peripheral edema, hypertension, and congestive heart failure), and reproductive system (adverse pregnancy outcomes).[24–27] The risk of serious gastrointestinal complications, such as bleeding or perforation, is increased fourfold to fivefold with continued intake of nonselective NSAIDs, and the risk of developing renal failure is twofold. The risk of gastrointestinal complications is increased with age, history of peptic ulcer disease, concomitant corticosteroids, and anticoagulation therapy. Concomitant NSAIDs and anticoagulation therapy is not recommended, as it increases the risk of bleeding. The risk of acute renal failure increases with age, history of renal insufficiency, heart failure, hypertension, and use of diuretics or angiotensin-converting enzyme inhibitors.[28,29]

The toxicity associated with chronic NSAID administration limits its benefit-to-risk ratio. The discovery of isoenzymes of cyclooxygenase, COX-1 and COX-2 (predominant role in inflammation) led to the development of selective COX-2 inhibitors. COX-1 is responsible for generation of cytoprotective prostanoids and is constitutively expressed in platelets and gastroduodenal mucosa.[27,29] Thus, inhibition of COX-1 leads to the increased risk of gastroduodenal bleeding. Compared with nonselective COX inhibitors, the selective COX-2 inhibitors are associated with reduced gastrointestinal complications, provided that patients are not taking aspirin concomitantly.[26,29–31] Nonetheless, COX-2 inhibitors are just as effective analgesics as nonselective NSAIDs.[23] Misoprostol, a synthetic analog of prostaglandin E_1, exerts a gastrointestinal mucosal protective effect by increasing mucus, bicarbonate ion secretion, and increasing mucosal blood flow. Concomitant use of misoprostol or proton pump inhibitors with NSAIDs reduces the risk of gastrointestinal complications.[32] Misoprostol is available in tablet form in combination with diclofenac. Misoprostol should be used with caution in females of childbearing age because it can initiate uterine contractions and miscarriage.

The kidney constitutively expresses both COX-1and COX-2. This may explain why COX-2 inhibitors seem to exhibit a similar renal side effect profile to nonselective NSAIDs. It appears that renal side effects are consequent to the inhibition of COX-2 by NSAIDs.[25,30,31]

The cardiovascular effects of NSAIDs have caused a major stir since the introduction of selective COX-2 inhibitors (coxibs). There has been increased risk of cardiovascular events with patients using selective COX-2 inhibitors.[33–35] This resulted in withdrawal of rofecoxib and valdecoxib. Only celecoxib remains in the market. The possible mechanism of increase in cardiovascular risk seems to be due to the disruption of the normal balance between prothrombotic and antithrombotic prostaglandins. Thromboxane A_2 is a platelet activator and aggregator that is mediated by prostaglandin products of the COX-l isomer pathway. Prostaglandin I_2 vasodilates and inhibits platelet aggregation when the COX-2 isomer is activated.

Thrombotic cardiovascular events may follow when thromboxane A_2 predominates over prostaglandin I_2.[36] Coxibs use should be avoided in patients with increased cardiovascular risk, including patients with recent cardiovascular events, unstable angina, acute myocardial infarction, ischemic cerebrovascular events, and high blood pressure. If coxibs are indicated, the smallest effective dose for the shortest duration should be used. Naproxen may be a better alternative to coxibs.[37] Physicians should weigh the risk-to-benefit ratio when prescribing NSAIDs in all patients.

A diclofenac patch is available for topical use in acute musculoskeletal sprains. Use of topical patches for localized pain may reduce the risk of serious adverse events due to low systemic concentration.[38]

Muscle Relaxants

Skeletal muscle relaxants are commonly used for back pain. They are a heterogeneous group of agents that mainly act on the central nervous system (CNS). At therapeutic doses they seem to exert their effect through sedation and subsequent depression of the neuronal transmission.[39] Studies have shown that muscle relaxants are effective when used for short duration in treatment of acute low back pain. There is no evidence for long-term use of muscle relaxants in chronic low back pain.[36] In a systematic review of 30 trials, skeletal muscle relaxants were moderately superior to placebo for short-term pain relief. However, there was inadequate evidence to demonstrate the effectiveness of skeletal muscle relaxants for chronic low back pain and they were associated with more CNS adverse events compared to placebo.[40] Commonly used drugs include cyclobenzaprine, methocarbamol, metaxalone, carisoprodol, diazepam, tizanidine, baclofen, orphenadrine, and chlorzoxazone. The most common adverse effects are drowsiness and dizziness. Physicians should be aware of possible dependence and abuse of some of the muscle relaxants, such as diazepam and carisoprodol.[41]

Antidepressants

Antidepressants have been used widely for managing various painful conditions of neuropathic origin. Antidepressants differ in their effectiveness in pain control depending on whether they inhibit reuptake of serotonin (serotonergic antidepressants, such as paroxetine, fluoxetine, sertraline, and citalopram); norepinephrine (noradrenergic antidepressants, such as desipramine, and maprotiline); or both (serotonergic-noradrenergic antidepressants, such as amitriptyline, doxepin, imipramine, clomipramine, venlafaxine, and duloxetine). Serotonergic-noradrenergic antidepressants were found to be more effective than placebo in chronic low back pain.[42–44] The symptom reduction of these drugs in chronic low back pain seems to be independent of their effect on depression. There was conflicting evidence as to whether antidepressants improved the functional status of the patients with chronic low back pain.[5] In addition to chronic back pain, antidepressants exhibit an apparent antinociceptive effect in other musculoskeletal conditions, including osteoarthritis, rheumatoid arthritis, and fibromyalgia.[42,43] Antidepressants are associated with significant adverse events: drowsiness, dizziness, dry mouth, constipation, urinary retention, and weight gain.[45]

Duloxetine, a serotonin-norepinephrine reuptake inhibitor, has been approved for use in fibromyalgia and diabetic peripheral neuropathic pain.[46–51] A meta-analysis of four randomized, double-blind, placebo-controlled studies of duloxetine in the treatment of fibromyalgia showed it to be significantly superior to placebo in relieving pain. For chronic lower back pain, three trials showed lower pain intensity with duloxetine associated with lower pain intensity and better function versus placebo.[52–54] Adverse effects tend to be mild. The effectiveness of duloxetine compared to tricyclic antidepressants was not evaluated. The efficiency of antidepressants, particularly for radicular low back pain, has not been studied.

Opioids

Opioids remain the most potent analgesic and are a mainstay in the treatment of acute and chronic painful conditions of moderate to severe intensity. Although their analgesic efficacy is well established, their effect on functional improvement is controversial.[55–59] Nociceptive pain is more responsive to opioid therapy than is neuropathic pain. Opioids have been widely used for noncancer pain, including chronic low back pain and radiculopathy. However, some important issues need to be addressed with regard to opioid prescription for noncancer pain: the framework for opioid prescription, when to initiate opioid therapy, appropriate candidates for opioid therapy, and endpoint of treatment.[60] In general, there is low to moderate evidence to suggest that opioid analgesia is safe and effective for the treatment of patients with chronic low back pain, at least for the short duration. The evidence for functional improvement with opioids is limited, however. Opioids appear to be a reasonable treatment option for patients with moderate to severe chronic low back pain that is refractory to general rehabilitation, injections, and nonopioid analgesic medications; for patients with pain that is not directly treatable because of the structural disorder; or because of patient preference.[61,62] There are no long-term trials that have demonstrated the benefit of opioids for chronic lower back pain. However, cohort studies found a small decrease in pain with very minimal improvement or deterioration of disability following 6 to 12 months of opioid use.[63]

Opioids act by binding to the opioid receptors in the CNS and peripheral nervous system, referred to as μ, κ, and δ receptors. They are G-protein-coupled receptors that modulate ionic channels and intracellular pathways, leading to the various effects of the opioids. Most of the clinically used opioids exert their analgesic effects mainly through binding to μ receptors, although binding to κ and δ receptors may occur to varying degrees. Hydrocodone (class 3), morphine, oxycodone, and hydromorphone (class 2) are opioid agonists with relatively short duration of action that are useful for episodic or breakthrough pain. Some of the short-acting opioids are available in combination with acetaminophen, ibuprofen, or aspirin. Dosing may be limited by the toxicity of the companion drug. Meperidine use is not advisable because of low oral bioavailability and potential metabolite (normeperidine) accumulation and toxicity with prolonged administration. Agonist-antagonist opioids are not useful in chronic pain because they exhibit a ceiling effect, have reduced analgesic efficacy, can cause dysphoric reactions, and can reverse analgesia, precipitating withdrawal in patients treated with pure agonists. However, their addiction potential is much less compared with pure μ agonists.

Methadone is the potent opioid with a long half-life of more than 24 hours and is therefore used to block withdrawal and treat addiction and pain. For analgesia, it is best given every 6 to 8 hours on an as-needed basis rather than at fixed intervals. Because of its long half-life and large variability in its clearance, it tends to accumulate with repeated dosing. Caution should be exercised when increasing the dose and in the elderly.[64] The D-isomer of methadone exerts significant antinociception action in neuropathic pain models by blocking *N*-methyl-D-aspartate receptor.[65] Fentanyl is an intrinsically short-acting potent μ agonist that is available in a long-acting transdermal (reservoir) form. Onset is slow and stable blood levels are achieved 12 to 17 hours after application. An oral transmucosal form of fentanyl (oral transmucosal fentanyl citrate, fentanyl buccal tablet) has been used in managing breakthrough pain in opioid-tolerant cancer pain patients.[66] It has a rapid onset of action and should not be used in opioid-naïve patients. Longer-acting preparations of morphine and oxycodone are available in controlled-release formulations that provide a sustained effect over 12 to 24 hours.[67] The use of controlled-release preparations is recommended in chronic opioid therapy because it results in pain reduction comparable with the immediate-release form but with a significantly lower dosage and better quality of life. Some patients may need additional doses of opioids for breakthrough pain. These doses should not be greater than 10% to 20% of the total 24-hour dose of controlled-release medication. If the patient needs more than three doses for breakthrough pain in a 24-hour period, then the sustained-release dose may need to be increased.[68–72]

Side effects are common with opioids. They include constipation, urinary retention, nausea and vomiting, itching, sedation, decreased libido, cognitive blunting, and respiratory depression.[57,58] Constipation is the most common side effect. A high-fiber diet and a good bowel regimen is usually necessary when initiating opioid therapy.[71–73] Tolerance develops quickly to most of the opioid side effects, including sedation, nausea, and respiratory depression. Constipation, sweating, and urinary retention are resistant to tolerance. The cognitive effect of opioids is seen mostly in the beginning of opioid therapy initiation and does not persist beyond a few days. There is consistent evidence for lack of psychomotor abilities impairment in opioid-maintained patients.[61,74] The risk of cognitive dysfunction is highest with acute use and first prescription.

There are several concerns regarding opioid prescriptions, including side effects, physical dependency, tolerance, risk of addiction and abuse, diversion, and regulatory issues. *Physical dependence is* a state of physiologic adaptation resulting in withdrawal symptoms when a medication is abruptly stopped. Opioid withdrawal can result in flulike symptoms, nausea, diarrhea, sweating, mydriasis, tachycardia, hypertension, CNS arousal, and increased pain. Opioid withdrawal may be life threatening if the patient has significant coronary artery disease or metabolic disorder.[73] Tolerance is a phenomenon in which the patient develops resistance to the effects of medication with time. It occurs with opioid analgesia and also with its side effects. Patients need to be reassessed before increasing the dose if tolerance is suspected; increasing dosing requirement in cancer patients may relate to disease progression. If tolerance is significant, opioid rotation may be considered because of incomplete cross-tolerance among opioids.[60,75] Addiction is a neurobehavioral biologic disorder, with loss of control and continued use and craving of the drug despite harm. Important genetic, psychological, and sociocultural factors contribute to development of addiction. Patients with the highest risk of prescription opioid addiction are those with history (including family history) of substance or alcohol abuse.[76,77] Abuse refers to use of a drug outside the intended indication with potential for self-harm or harm to others. Pseudoaddiction refers to an addiction-like behavior by patients seeking higher doses of opioid to control undertreated pain. Pseudoaddiction resolves when a patient obtains adequate analgesia, whereas true addictive behavior does not improve (Table 109.1).[78]

TABLE 109.1 Pain Relief Versus Addiction[79]

Chronic Pain Patient	Addicted Patient
Not out of control with medications use	Out of control with medications use
Medications improve quality of life	Medications decrease quality of life
Concerned about medical problems	In denial about medical problems
Will follow the agreed-upon treatment plan	Does not follow the treatment plan
May have medications left over from the prior prescription	Short on medications, long on stories

From Savage SR. Addiction in the treatment of pain: significance, recognition, and management. *J Pain Symptom Manage.* 1993;8:265–278.

The guidelines for treatment of chronic pain with opioids include careful evaluation of the patient, a treatment plan that states the goal of therapy, informed consent, therapeutic trial, regular follow-up visits, consultation with specialists when necessary, and maintenance of good medical records.[61] Caution should be exercised while prescribing opioids to elderly patients; patients with a history of hepatic or renal impairment or marked respiratory depression; patients with a history of alcohol abuse or drug problems or diversion; and patients with secondary gain issues, such as pending disability or litigation. The goal of treatment should include partial analgesia, with the understanding that functional improvement may not occur. Adjuvant medications (NSAIDs, antidepressants, and anticonvulsants) may be used in conjunction with opioids to reduce the opioid requirement. Maintaining a high index of suspicion for abuse with patients who call frequently or lose prescriptions often and obtaining random urine toxicology screens are useful measures to avert abuse, addiction, or diversion problems with opioid therapy.

Tramadol

Tramadol is a nonscheduled opioid that is a synthetic analog of codeine. It is a weak μ receptor agonist with a receptor affinity of 6000-fold less than morphine. In spite of being a weak opioid receptor agonist, the relative potency of tramadol in acute pain ranges between 5% and 16% that of morphine. Tramadol inhibits uptake of norepinephrine and serotonin in the CNS, which may contribute to its additional analgesic effect. It does not inhibit cyclooxygenase, thus does not share the gastrointestinal or renal side effects of NSAIDs.[80–82] Tramadol has been shown to be effective in treatment of patients with chronic low back pain and provided greater pain relief compared to placebo.[62,83–89] It may be useful in neuropathic conditions, such as diabetic neuropathy and postherpetic neuralgia.[90]

The adverse effects of tramadol reflect its dual mechanism of action: opioid effects and monoaminergic effects (both of which cause dizziness, headache, sweating, and dry mouth). Clinically significant respiratory depression is almost never seen with clinically effective doses of tramadol and the risk of constipation is markedly low.[80,81] The effective oral dose is 200 to 400 mg/day in divided doses every 6 hours. Extended-release formulation and combination with acetaminophen are also available.[84,87,91]

Dosing must be reduced in elderly patients and in patients with significant renal and hepatic impairment.[82] Seizure is the most serious side effect of tramadol, which is predisposed by history of epilepsy, head trauma, metabolic disturbance, drug or alcohol withdrawal, and concurrent CNS infection. Seizures and serotonin syndrome may occur in patients taking tramadol and antidepressants, which inhibits serotonin uptake. Caution should therefore be used when tramadol and antidepressants are used concomitantly. Discontinuing antidepressants may be considered.[80,82,92]

Antiepileptics

Antiepileptics are most commonly used in the treatment of painful neuropathic conditions. FDA-approved anticonvulsants for specific conditions include carbamazepine (trigeminal neuralgia); gabapentin (postherpetic neuralgia); pregabalin (postherpetic neuralgia, diabetic neuropathic pain, and fibromyalgia); divalproex (migraine prophylaxis); and topiramate (migraine prophylaxis).[93] They exert their effect by blocking neuronal transmission through effects on various ion channels and receptors in the CNS and peripheral nervous system. Although anticonvulsants are commonly used to treat radicular pain, the data supporting the evidence of their use is inconsistent with some trials finding small or no effect and no antiepileptics are FDA approved for chronic low back pain.[5,45,94–100] Gabapentin is an alpha 2-delta ligand and acts on voltage-gated calcium channels. Dosing requires slow titration, starting at 100 to 300 mg per day up to a maximum of 3600 mg/day in divided doses.[5,101–103] Pregabalin is also an alpha 2-delta ligand that acts on voltage-gated calcium channels. It can be started with 50 to 75 mg twice daily and titrated up to 300 to 600 mg/day.[5,104–107] Topiramate blocks voltage-gated sodium channels, potentiates GABA transmission, and inhibits excitatory neurotransmission. Doses of 300 mg/day help reduce pain symptoms and improve mood and quality of life.[108,109] Topiramate is also associated with mild weight loss. The common side effects of gabapentin and pregabalin include somnolence, dizziness, confusion, ataxia, fatigue, peripheral edema, and weight gain. Side effects of topiramate include paresthesia, fatigue, weakness, sedation, dizziness, and diarrhea.[5] Dosage should be reduced and slower titration is necessary in elderly patients and in patients with significant hepatic and renal impairment.[110]

An algorithm for the management of acute and chronic low back pain with or without radiculopathy based on current available evidence is summarized in Fig. 109.1.

Other Treatments and Future Prospects

Oral and parenteral corticosteroids are frequently administered in acute back pain and radiculopathy, but their efficacy must be proven.[111–113] To counter the cardiovascular side

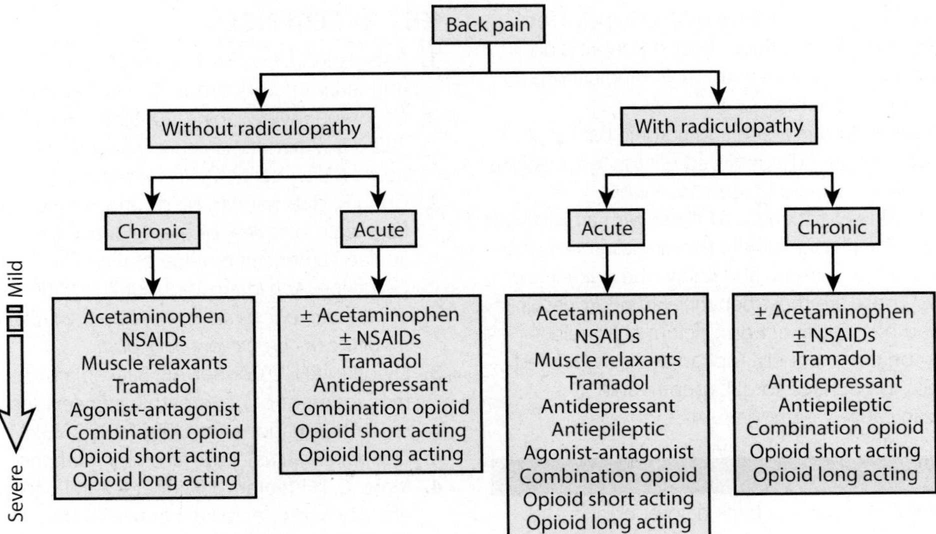

FIG. 109.1 Suggested algorithm for the pharmacologic management of back pain and radiculopathy. NSAIDs, nonsteroidal antiinflammatory drugs.

effects of NSAIDs, newer ones are being considered, including nitric oxide–NSAIDs, dual cyclooxygenase (COX) and lipoxygenase inhibitors, and anti-TNF-α therapy.[22] Newer tamper-resistant opioids are being developed to reduce abuse, misuse, and diversion. Multiple molecular entities have been developed, including glutamate antagonists, cytokine inhibitors, vanilloid-receptor agonist, catecholamine modulators, ion channel blockers, acetylcholine modulators, cannabinoids, opioids, adenosine receptor agonists, and others.[114,115] Systemic anti–nerve growth factor (anti-NGF) therapy demonstrated trivial benefit versus placebo for both pain relief and functional improvement of low back pain. With systemic administration of tanezumab (specific anti-NGF treatment), low evidence of a small to moderate but not clinically significant efficacy was found for pain relief of low back pain and functional improvement. In general, tanezumab and anti-NGF therapies showed moderate and low evidence of adverse effects and a greater risk of developing neurologic adverse effects versus placebo. Further research is required on the pathophysiology of anti-NGF therapies and adverse effects.[116] Molecular approaches to neuropathic pain include cell and gene therapies, antibodies, and ribonucleic acid interference–based treatments. Some of the novel targets for developing therapies for neuropathic pain include chemokine receptors, glial cells, and cytokines. Emergence of biologic approaches offers new therapeutic additions to address different painful conditions.[79,115,117] Despite the challenges in development of new medications for chronic lower back pain, new treatment options—such as gene and stem cell therapy—continue to surge.[118]

KEY POINTS

1. *Type of pain.* It is important to differentiate among nociceptive, neuropathic, and acute and chronic back pain.
2. *NSAIDs.* These are effective for short-term symptomatic relief in patients with acute and chronic back pain without sciatica. Avoid chronic use. Weigh the risk-to-benefit ratio, especially when using in elderly and high-risk patients.
3. *Muscle relaxants.* These are effective for acute low back pain but not chronic low back pain.
4. *Antidepressants.* These are beneficial in neuropathic pain. The analgesic effect is independent of their effect on depression. Consider potential drug interactions with other medications before prescribing antidepressants.
5. *Opioids.* These have been used in acute and chronic back pain. If chronic opioid therapy is planned, controlled-release formulations are recommended. Caution should be exercised while prescribing opioids to elderly patients and those with a history of alcohol or drug abuse. For chronic opioid therapy, establish goals of therapy, obtain informed consent, and follow the guidelines.
6. *Membrane stabilizers.* These are most beneficial in neuropathic pain. Gabapentin and pregabalin act on calcium channels. Topiramate acts on sodium channels. Topiramate is associated with mild weight loss as opposed to gabapentin and pregabalin, which can cause weight gain.

PEARLS

1. NSAIDs may be helpful in acute low back pain but not necessarily in radicular pain.
2. No evidence indicates that one NSAID is more effective than another.
3. NSAID effectiveness in chronic low back pain is questionable. COX-2 inhibitors may be as effective analgesics as nonselective NSAIDs.
4. Serotonergic-noradrenergic and noradrenergic antidepressants are effective in chronic low back and neuropathic pain relief.
5. The antinociceptive effect may be independent of the effect on depression.
6. Opioids are the most potent analgesics in nociceptive pain and are possibly useful in neuropathic pain.
7. Controlled-release preparations are recommended for chronic opioid therapy.
8. Opioids may be effective in treating pain, but functional improvement may not occur.
9. Most chronic pain patients are on stable doses of opioids for years.

PITFALLS

1. Chronic use of nonselective NSAIDs increases the risk of gastrointestinal bleeding and renal insufficiency.
2. COX-2 inhibitors decrease the risk of gastrointestinal bleeding but not the risk of renal failure.
3. COX-2 inhibitors might increase the risk of coronary events and should be used with caution in high-risk patients.
4. Muscle relaxants may not add to the analgesic effect of NSAIDs in acute low back pain.
5. Newer antidepressants have fewer side effects.
6. Caution should be taken when antidepressants are used concomitantly with tramadol.
7. Gradual, individualized titration is recommended when initiating treatment.
8. Avoid meperidine and agonist–antagonist opioids in patients with chronic pain.
9. Prior history of drug abuse is a strong indicator of prescription opioid abuse.
10. Differentiate between pseudoaddiction and addiction.
11. Follow guidelines for treatment of chronic pain with opioids, including obtaining informed consent and an opioid agreement.
12. Individualize a treatment plan, titrate medication slowly, and follow the patient closely at the initiation of treatment.

KEY REFERENCES

1. Roelofs PD, Deyo RA, Koes BW, et al. Non-steroidal anti-inflammatory drugs for low back pain: an updated Cochrane review. *Spine*. 2008;33:1766-1774.
   This is a systematic review of 65 randomized controlled trials to assess the effects of NSAIDs in the treatment of low back pain.
2. Chou R, Huffman LH. Medications for acute and chronic low back pain: a review of the evidence for an American Pain Society/American College of Physicians Clinical Practice Guideline. *Ann Intern Med*. 2007;147:505-514.
   Systematic reviews assess the benefit of different medications used for acute or chronic low back pain.
3. Dworkin RH, O'Connor AB, Backonja M, et al. Pharmacologic management of neuropathic pain: evidence based recommendations. *Pain*. 2007;132:237-251.
   This paper discusses the recommendations for neuropathic pain.
4. Maier C, Hildebrant J, Klinger R, et al. Morphine responsiveness, efficacy and tolerability controlled trial (MONTAS). *Pain*. 2002;97:223-233.
   This randomized, controlled trial concerns opioid use in noncancer pain.

5. Chang V, Gonzalez P, Akuthota V. Evidence-informed management of chronic low back pain with adjunctive analgesics. *Spine J.* 2008;8:21-27.
This paper reviews evidence for using adjuvant analgesics in management of back pain. This special issue of The Spine Journal (August 2008), titled "Evidence-informed management of chronic low back pain without surgery," contains other reviews on opioids, NSAIDs, muscle relaxants, and other analgesics.

6. Chou R, Deyo R, Friedly J, et al. *Noninvasive Treatments for Low Back Pain.* Rockville, MD: Agency for Healthcare Research and Quality; 2016 Available at: https://www.ncbi.nlm.nih.gov/books/NBK350276/.
This review examines the evidence on the comparative benefits and harms of noninvasive treatments for low back pain.

REFERENCES

1. Davis H. Increasing rates of cervical and lumbar spine surgery in the United States, 1979-1990. *Spine.* 1994;19(10):1117-1123.
2. Research on low back pain and common spinal disorders. *NIH Guide.* 1997;26(16). Available at: https://grants.nih.gov/grants/guide/pa-files/PA-97-058.html.
3. Katz JN. Lumbar disc disorders and low-back pain: socioeconomic factors and consequences. *J Bone Joint Surg Am.* 2006;88(suppl 2):21-24.
4. Luo X, Pietrobon R, Sun SX, Liu GG, Hey L. Estimates and patterns of direct health care expenditures among individuals with back pain in the United States. *Spine.* 2004;29(1):79-86.
5. Chang V, Gonzalez P, Akuthota V. Evidence-informed management of chronic low back pain with adjunctive analgesics. *Spine J.* 2008;8(1):21-27.
6. Wallace MS. Pharmacologic treatment of neuropathic pain. *Curr Pain Headache Rep.* 2001;5(2):138-150.
7. Dellemijn P. Are opioids effective in relieving neuropathic pain? *Pain.* 1999;80(3):453-462.
8. Bridges D, Thompson SW, Rice AS. Mechanisms of neuropathic pain. *Br J Anaesth.* 2001;87(1):12-26.
9. Koes BW, van Tulder MW, Ostelo R, Kim Burton A, Waddell G. Clinical guidelines for the management of low back pain in primary care: an international comparison. *Spine.* 2001;26(22):2504-2513.
10. Bijlsma JW. Analgesia and the patient with osteoarthritis. *Am J Ther.* 2002;9(3):189-197.
11. Milgrom C, Finestone A, Lev B, Wiener M. Floman Y. Overexertional lumbar and thoracic back pain among recruits: a prospective study of risk factors and treatment regimens. *J Spinal Disord.* 1993;6(3):187-193.
12. Evans DP, Burke MS, Newcombe RG. Medicines of choice in low back pain. *Curr Med Res Opin.* 1980;6(8):540-547.
13. Hickey RF. Chronic low back pain: a comparison of diflunisal with paracetamol. *N Z Med J.* 1982;95(707):312-314.
14. Nadler SF, Steiner DJ, Erasala GN, et al. Continuous low-level heat wrap therapy provides more efficacy than Ibuprofen and acetaminophen for acute low back pain. *Spine.* 2002;27(10):1012-1017.
15. Wiesel SW, Cuckler JM, Deluca F, et al. Acute low-back pain. An objective analysis of conservative therapy. *Spine.* 1980;5(4):324-330.
16. Towheed TE, Maxwell L, Judd MG, et al. Acetaminophen for osteoarthritis. *Cochrane Database Syst Rev.* 2006;(1):CD004257.
17. Zhang W, Jones A, Doherty M. Does paracetamol (acetaminophen) reduce the pain of osteoarthritis? A meta-analysis of randomised controlled trials. *Ann Rheum Dis.* 2004;63(8):901-907.
18. Botting RM. Mechanism of action of acetaminophen: is there a cyclooxygenase 3? *Clin Infect Dis.* 2000;31(suppl 5):S202-S210.
19. Krenzelok EP, Royal MA. Confusion: acetaminophen dosing changes based on NO evidence in adults. *Drugs R D.* 2012;12(2):45-48.
20. Food and Drug Administration (FDA) Center for Drug Evaluation and Research. *Organ-Specific Warnings: Internal Analgesic, Antipyretic, and Antirheumatic Drug Products for Over-the-Counter Human Use—Labeling For Products That Contain Acetaminophen. Guidance for Industry.* Silver Spring, MD: FDA; 2015 Available at: https://www.fda.gov/downloads/drugs/guidancecomplianceregulatoryinformation/guidances/ucm310477.pdf.
21. Bertin P, Keddad K, Jolivet-Landreau I. Acetaminophen as symptomatic treatment of pain from osteoarthritis. *Joint Bone Spine.* 2004;71(4):266-274.
22. Rao P, Knaus EE. Evolution of nonsteroidal anti-inflammatory drugs (NSAIDs): cyclooxygenase (COX) inhibition and beyond. *J Pharm Pharm Sci.* 2008;11(2):81s-110s.
23. Roelofs PD, Deyo RA, Koes BW, Scholten RJ, van Tulder MW. Non-steroidal anti-inflammatory drugs for low back pain. *Cochrane Database Syst Rev.* 2008;(1):CD000396.
24. Hernandez-Diaz S, Garcia-Rodriguez LA. Epidemiologic assessment of the safety of conventional nonsteroidal anti-inflammatory drugs. *Am J Med.* 2001;110(suppl 3A):20S-27S.
25. Appel GB. COX-2 inhibitors and the kidney. *Clin Exp Rheumatol.* 2001;19(6 suppl 25):S37-S40.
26. Hawkey CJ. NSAIDs and COX-2 inhibitors: what can we learn from large outcomes trials? The gastroenterologist's perspective. *Clin Exp Rheumatol.* 2001;19(6 suppl 25):S23-S30.
27. FitzGerald GA, Cheng Y, Austin S. COX-2 inhibitors and the cardiovascular system. *Clin Exp Rheumatol.* 2001;19(6 suppl 25):S31-S36.
28. Hernández-Díaz SRL. Association between nonsteroidal anti-inflammatory drugs and upper gastrointestinal tract bleeding/perforation: an overview of epidemiologic studies published in the 1990s. *Arch Intern Med.* 2000;160(14):2093-2099.
29. Hochberg MC. What have we learned from the large outcomes trials of COX-2 selective inhibitors? The rheumatologist's perspective. *Clin Exp Rheumatol.* 2001;19(6 suppl 25):S15-S22.
30. Bombardier C, Laine L, Reicin A, et al. Comparison of upper gastrointestinal toxicity of rofecoxib and naproxen in patients with rheumatoid arthritis. VIGOR Study Group. *N Engl J Med.* 2000;343(21):1520-1528.
31. Silverstein FE, Faich G, Goldstein JL, et al. Gastrointestinal toxicity with celecoxib vs nonsteroidal anti-inflammatory drugs for osteoarthritis and rheumatoid arthritis: the CLASS study: A randomized controlled trial. Celecoxib Long-Term Arthritis Safety Study. *JAMA.* 2000;284(10):1247-1255.
32. Targownik LE, Metge CJ, Leung S, Chateau DG. The relative efficacies of gastroprotective strategies in chronic users of nonsteroidal anti-inflammatory drugs. *Gastroenterology.* 2008;134(4):937-944.
33. Bresalier RS, Sandler RS, Quan H, et al. Cardiovascular events associated with rofecoxib in a colorectal adenoma chemoprevention trial. *N Engl J Med.* 2005;352(11):1092-1102.

34. Solomon SD, McMurray JJ, Pfeffer MA, et al. Cardiovascular risk associated with celecoxib in a clinical trial for colorectal adenoma prevention. *N Engl J Med*. 2005;352(11):1071-1080.
35. Nussmeier NA, Whelton AA, Brown MT, et al. Complications of the COX-2 inhibitors parecoxib and valdecoxib after cardiac surgery. *N Engl J Med*. 2005;352(11):1081-1091.
36. Malanga G, Wolff E. Evidence-informed management of chronic low back pain with trigger point injections. *Spine J*. 2008;8(1):243-252.
37. Vardeny O, Solomon SD. Cyclooxygenase-2 inhibitors, nonsteroidal anti-inflammatory drugs, and cardiovascular risk. *Cardiol Clin*. 2008;26(4):589-601.
38. Rainsford KD, Kean WF, Ehrlich GE. Review of the pharmaceutical properties and clinical effects of the topical NSAID formulation, diclofenac epolamine. *Curr Med Res Opin*. 2008;24(10):2967-2992.
39. Waldman HJ. Centrally acting skeletal muscle relaxants and associated drugs. *J Pain Symptom Manage*. 1994;9(7):434-441.
40. van Tulder MW, Touray T, Furlan AD, Solway S, Bouter LM. Muscle relaxants for non-specific low back pain. *Cochrane Database Syst Rev*. 2003;(2):CD004252.
41. Beebe FA, Barkin RL, Barkin S. A clinical and pharmacologic review of skeletal muscle relaxants for musculoskeletal conditions. *Am J Ther*. 2005;12(2):151-171.
42. Fishbain D. Evidence-based data on pain relief with antidepressants. *Ann Med*. 2000;32(5):305-316.
43. Teasell RW, Merskey H, Deshpande S. Antidepressants in rehabilitation. *Phys Med Rehabil Clin N Am*. 1999;10(2): 237-253.
44. Salerno SM, Browning R, Jackson JL. The effect of antidepressant treatment on chronic back pain: a meta-analysis. *Arch Intern Med*. 2002;162(1):19-24.
45. Chou R, Huffman LH, American Pain Society. American College of Physicians. Medications for acute and chronic low back pain: a review of the evidence for an American Pain Society/American College of Physicians clinical practice guideline. *Ann Intern Med*. 2007;147(7):505-514.
46. Acuna C. Duloxetine for the treatment of fibromyalgia. *Drugs Today (Barc)*. 2008;44(10):725-734.
47. Sumpton JE, Moulin DE. Fibromyalgia: presentation and management with a focus on pharmacological treatment. *Pain Res Manag*. 2008;13(6):477-483.
48. Wernicke JF, Pritchett YL, D'Souza DN, et al. A randomized controlled trial of duloxetine in diabetic peripheral neuropathic pain. *Neurology*. 2006;67(8):1411-1420.
49. Raskin J, Pritchett YL, Wang F, et al. A double-blind, randomized multicenter trial comparing duloxetine with placebo in the management of diabetic peripheral neuropathic pain. *Pain Med*. 2005;6(5):346-356.
50. Goldstein DJ, Lu Y, Detke MJ, Lee TC, Iyengar S. Duloxetine vs. placebo in patients with painful diabetic neuropathy. *Pain*. 2005;116(1-2):109-118.
51. Fishbain D, Berman K, Kajdasz DK. Duloxetine for neuropathic pain based on recent clinical trials. *Curr Pain Headache Rep*. 2006;10(3):199-204.
52. Skljarevski V, Ossanna M, Liu-Seifert H, et al. A double-blind, randomized trial of duloxetine versus placebo in the management of chronic low back pain. *Eur J Neurol*. 2009; 16(9):1041-1048.
53. Skljarevski V, Zhang S, Desaiah D, et al. Duloxetine versus placebo in patients with chronic low back pain: a 12-week, fixed-dose, randomized, double-blind trial. *J Pain*. 2010;11(12):1282-1290.
54. Skljarevski V, Desaiah D, Liu-Seifert H, et al. Efficacy and safety of duloxetine in patients with chronic low back pain. *Spine*. 2010;35(13):E578-E585.
55. Moulin DE, Iezzi A, Amireh R, et al. Randomised trial of oral morphine for chronic non-cancer pain. *Lancet*. 1996;347(8995):143-147.
56. Roth SH, Fleischmann RM, Burch FX, et al. Around-the-clock, controlled-release oxycodone therapy for osteoarthritis-related pain: placebo-controlled trial and long-term evaluation. *Arch Intern Med*. 2000;160(6):853-860.
57. Caldwell JR, Hale ME, Boyd RE, et al. Treatment of osteoarthritis pain with controlled release oxycodone or fixed combination oxycodone plus acetaminophen added to nonsteroidal antiinflammatory drugs: a double blind, randomized, multicenter, placebo controlled trial. *J Rheumatol*. 1999;26(4):862-869.
58. Schofferman J. Long-term opioid analgesic therapy for severe refractory lumbar spine pain. *Clin J Pain*. 1999;15(2):136-140.
59. Maier C, Hildebrandt J, Klinger R, et al. Morphine responsiveness, efficacy and tolerability in patients with chronic non-tumor associated pain—results of a double-blind placebo-controlled trial (MONTAS). *Pain*. 2002;97(3):223-233.
60. Savage SR. Opioid use in the management of chronic pain. *Med Clin North Am*. 1999;83(3):761-786.
61. Schofferman J, Mazanec D. Evidence-informed management of chronic low back pain with opioid analgesics. *Spine J*. 2008;8(1):185-194.
62. Chaparro LE, Furlan AD, Deshpande A, et al. Opioids compared to placebo or other treatments for chronic low-back pain. *Cochrane Database Syst Rev*. 2013;(8):CD004959.
63. Freund J, Kraus C, Hooper-Lane C. Clinical Inquiry: How effective are opioids for chronic low back pain? *J Fam Pract*. 2015;64(9):584-585.
64. Foley KM, Houde RW. Methadone in cancer pain management: individualize dose and titrate to effect. *J Clin Oncol*. 1998;16(10):3213-3215.
65. Shimoyama N, Shimoyama M, Elliott KJ, Inturrisi CE. d-Methadone is antinociceptive in the rat formalin test. *J Pharmacol Exp Ther*. 1997;283(2):648-652.
66. Messina J, Darwish M, Fine PG. Fentanyl buccal tablet. *Drugs of today*. 2008;44(1):41-54.
67. Reder RF. Opioid formulations: tailoring to the needs in chronic pain. *Eur J Pain*. 2001;5(suppl A):109-111.
68. Hale ME, Fleischmann R, Salzman R, et al. Efficacy and safety of controlled-release versus immediate-release oxycodone: randomized, double-blind evaluation in patients with chronic back pain. *Clin J Pain*. 1999;15(3):179-183.
69. Lazarus H, Fitzmartin RD, Goldenheim PD. A multi-investigator clinical evaluation of oral controlled-release morphine (MS Contin tablets) administered to cancer patients. *Hosp J*. 1990;6(4):1-15.
70. Cundiff D, McCarthy K, Savarese JJ, et al. Evaluation of a cancer pain model for the testing of long-acting analgesics. The effect of MS Contin in a double-blind, randomized crossover design. *Cancer*. 1989;63(11 suppl):2355-2359.
71. Hisgen WJ. Long-term opioid analgesia and chronic non-cancer pain. *WMJ*. 2001;100(5):17-21.
72. Portenoy RK. Opioid therapy for chronic nonmalignant pain: a review of the critical issues. *J Pain Symptom Manage*. 1996;11(4):203-217.
73. Brown RL, Fleming MF, Patterson JJ. Chronic opioid analgesic therapy for chronic low back pain. *J Am Board Fam Pract*. 1996;9(3):191-204.

74. Fishbain DA, Cutler RB, Rosomoff HL, Rosomoff RS. Are opioid-dependent/tolerant patients impaired in driving-related skills? A structured evidence-based review. *J Pain Symptom Manage*. 2003;25(6):559-577.
75. Nitschke R. The art of oncology: when the tumor is not the target—the power of silence. *J Clin Oncol*. 2002;20(7): 1952-1953.
76. Aronoff GM. Opioids in chronic pain management: is there a significant risk of addiction? *Curr Rev Pain*. 2000;4(2): 112-121.
77. Reid MC, Engles-Horton LL, Weber MB, et al. Use of opioid medications for chronic noncancer pain syndromes in primary care. *J Gen Intern Med*. 2002;17(3):173-179.
78. Weissman DE, Haddox JD. Opioid pseudoaddiction—an iatrogenic syndrome. *Pain*. 1989;36(3):363-366.
79. Savage SR. Addiction in the treatment of pain: significance, recognition, and management. *J Pain Symptom Manage*. 1993;8(5):265-278.
80. Bamigbade TA, Langford RM. Tramadol hydrochloride: an overview of current use. *Hosp Med*. 1998;59(5):373-376.
81. Shipton EA. Tramadol—present and future. *Anaesth Intensive Care*. 2000;28(4):363-374.
82. Gibson TP. Pharmacokinetics, efficacy, and safety of analgesia with a focus on tramadol HCl. *Am J Med*. 1996;101(1A): 47S-53S.
83. Schnitzer TJ, Gray WL, Paster RZ, Kamin M. Efficacy of tramadol in treatment of chronic low back pain. *J Rheumatol*. 2000;27(3):772-778.
84. Peloso PM, Fortin L, Beaulieu A, et al. Analgesic efficacy and safety of tramadol/acetaminophen combination tablets (Ultracet) in treatment of chronic low back pain: a multicenter, outpatient, randomized, double blind, placebo controlled trial. *J Rheumatol*. 2004;31(12):2454-2463.
85. Ruoff GE, Rosenthal N, Jordan D, et al. Tramadol/ acetaminophen combination tablets for the treatment of chronic lower back pain: a multicenter, randomized, double-blind, placebo-controlled outpatient study. *Clin Ther*. 2003;25(4):1123-1141.
86. Uberall MA, Mueller-Schwefe GH, Terhaag B. Efficacy and safety of flupirtine modified release for the management of moderate to severe chronic low back pain: results of SUPREME, a prospective randomized, double-blind, placebo- and active-controlled parallel-group phase IV study. *Curr Med Res Opin*. 2012;28(10):1617-1634.
87. Vorsanger GJ, Xiang J, Gana TJ, Pascual ML, Fleming RR. Extended-release tramadol (tramadol ER) in the treatment of chronic low back pain. *J Opioid Manag*. 2008;4(2): 87-97.
88. Lee JH, Lee CS, Ultracet ERSG. A randomized, double-blind, placebo-controlled, parallel-group study to evaluate the efficacy and safety of the extended-release tramadol hydrochloride/acetaminophen fixed-dose combination tablet for the treatment of chronic low back pain. *Clin Ther*. 2013;35(11):1830-1840.
89. Schiphorst Preuper HR, Geertzen JH, van Wijhe M, et al. Do analgesics improve functioning in patients with chronic low back pain? An explorative triple-blinded RCT. *Eur Spine J*. 2014;23(4):800-806.
90. Harati Y, Gooch C, Swenson M, et al. Double-blind randomized trial of tramadol for the treatment of the pain of diabetic neuropathy. *Neurology*. 1998;50(6):1842-1846.
91. Hair PI, Curran MP, Keam SJ. Tramadol extended-release tablets. *Drugs*. 2006;66(15):2017-2027.
92. Lewis KS, Han NH. Tramadol: a new centrally acting analgesic. *Am J Health Syst Pharm*. 1997;54(6):643-652.
93. Benzon HRJ, Wu C, eds. *Raj's Practical Management of Pain*. 4th ed. Philadelphia: Elsevier; 2008:660.
94. Baron R, Freynhagen R, Tolle TR, et al. The efficacy and safety of pregabalin in the treatment of neuropathic pain associated with chronic lumbosacral radiculopathy. *Pain*. 2010;150(3):420-427.
95. Baron R, Martin-Mola E, Muller M, et al. Effectiveness and safety of tapentadol prolonged release (PR) versus a combination of tapentadol PR and pregabalin for the management of severe, chronic low back pain with a neuropathic component: a randomized, double-blind, phase 3b study. *Pain Pract*. 2015;15(5):455-470.
96. Kalita J, Kohat AK, Misra UK, Bhoi SK. An open labeled randomized controlled trial of pregabalin versus amitriptyline in chronic low backache. *J Neurol Sci*. 2014;342(1-2):127-132.
97. Markman JD, Frazer ME, Rast SA, et al. Double-blind, randomized, controlled, crossover trial of pregabalin for neurogenic claudication. *Neurology*. 2015;84(3):265-272.
98. Romano CL, Romano D, Bonora C, Mineo G. Pregabalin, celecoxib, and their combination for treatment of chronic low-back pain. *Journal Orthop Traumatol*. 2009;10(4):185-191.
99. Yaksi A, Ozgonenel L, Ozgonenel B. The efficiency of gabapentin therapy in patients with lumbar spinal stenosis. *Spine*. 2007;32(9):939-942.
100. Atkinson JH, Slater MA, Capparelli EV, et al. A randomized controlled trial of gabapentin for chronic low back pain with and without a radiating component. *Pain*. 2016.
101. Yildirim KSM, Karatay S, et al. The effectiveness of gabapentin in patients with chronic radiculopathy. *Pain Clin*. 2003;15:213-218.
102. Backonja M, Beydoun A, Edwards KR, et al. Gabapentin for the symptomatic treatment of painful neuropathy in patients with diabetes mellitus: a randomized controlled trial. *JAMA*. 1998;280(21):1831-1836.
103. Rowbotham M, Harden N, Stacey B, Bernstein P, Magnus-Miller L. Gabapentin for the treatment of postherpetic neuralgia: a randomized controlled trial. *JAMA*. 1998;280(21):1837-1842.
104. Dworkin RH, O'Connor AB, Backonja M, et al. Pharmacologic management of neuropathic pain: evidence-based recommendations. *Pain*. 2007;132(3): 237-251.
105. Siddall PJ, Cousins MJ, Otte A, et al. Pregabalin in central neuropathic pain associated with spinal cord injury: a placebo-controlled trial. *Neurology*. 2006;67(10):1792-1800.
106. Dworkin RH, Corbin AE, Young JP Jr, et al. Pregabalin for the treatment of postherpetic neuralgia: a randomized, placebo-controlled trial. *Neurology*. 2003;60(8):1274-1283.
107. Tolle T, Freynhagen R, Versavel M, Trostmann U, Young JP Jr. Pregabalin for relief of neuropathic pain associated with diabetic neuropathy: a randomized, double-blind study. *Eur J Pain*. 2008;12(2):203-213.
108. Khoromi S, Patsalides A, Parada S, et al. Topiramate in chronic lumbar radicular pain. *J Pain*. 2005;6(12):829-836.
109. Muehlbacher M, Nickel MK, Kettler C, et al. Topiramate in treatment of patients with chronic low back pain: a randomized, double-blind, placebo-controlled study. *Clin J Pain*. 2006;22(6):526-531.
110. Tremont-Lukats IW, Megeff C, Backonja MM. Anticonvulsants for neuropathic pain syndromes: mechanisms of action and place in therapy. *Drugs*. 2000;60(5):1029-1052.

111. Friedman BW, Holden L, Esses D, et al. Parenteral corticosteroids for Emergency Department patients with non-radicular low back pain. *J Emerg Med.* 2006;31(4):365-370.
112. Deyo RA. Drug therapy for back pain. Which drugs help which patients? *Spine.* 1996;21(24):2840-2849.
113. Von Feldt JM, Ehrlich GE. Pharmacologic therapies. *Phys Med Rehabil Clin N Am.* 1998;9(2):473-487.
114. Gilron I, Coderre TJ. Emerging drugs in neuropathic pain. *Expert Opin Emerg Drugs.* 2007;12(1):113-126.
115. Jain KK. Current challenges and future prospects in management of neuropathic pain. *Expert Rev Neurother.* 2008;8(11):1743-1756.
116. Leite VF, Buehler AM, El Abd O, et al. Anti-nerve growth factor in the treatment of low back pain and radiculopathy: a systematic review and a meta-analysis. *Pain Physician.* 2014;17(1):E45-E60.
117. Dray A. Neuropathic pain: emerging treatments. *Br J Anaesth.* 2008;101(1):48-58.
118. Hsu E, Murphy S, Chang D, Cohen SP. Expert opinion on emerging drugs: chronic low back pain. *Expert Opin Emerg Drugs.* 2015;20(1):103-127.

CHAPTER 110 Physical Therapy: Art and Science of Practice

Eric A.K. Mayer
Ryan A. Tauzell

Introduction

Most spine specialists recognize that early mobilization (activation) of patients with neck or back pain is not harmful and is, in fact, necessary. Activity early in an acute course of neck/back pain shows 50% improvement of pain symptoms in greater than 90% of patients.[1] For this reason, physical therapy is the first-line treatment[2] and remains the backbone of spine care.[3] Most patients suffering an acute episode of back or neck pain recover in less than 1 week, and greater than 90% of patients are back to work before 90 days.[4] Yet, between 50% and 84%[5] of patients experience a recurrence of low back pain (LBP) within 1 year after recovering from a previous episode.[6] Therefore, in the face of recurrent pain, determining the most effective physical therapy intervention is beneficial for a surgeon's practice and the patient. This chapter provides insight into how this determination is made.

An unfortunate and too common analogy is that choosing a physical therapy (PT) clinic is like choosing a Starbucks; find the location closest to you and order. One franchise location makes the same coffee as any other location. The reliability of the Starbucks process produces a consistently similar quality product. This analogy would be correct if all physical therapists had high-reliability processes to create the similarly reproducible results as seen at Starbucks franchises.

The hypothetical clinical scenario required to mimic Starbucks outcomes would require all PT clinics to possess remarkable reliability in assessment procedures, formulation of diagnosis, and application of treatment. This putative process would then produce the same outcome from PT clinic to PT clinic. We all know these idyllic therapy outcomes are ridiculously untrue. Geography is usually destiny in the marked variability of outcomes for the same diagnosis.[7] Methods vary from clinic to clinic and even within a clinic. Clinician X utilizes significantly different methods than colleague Clinician Y, each defending one's approach with the same phrase: "…but it works for me." Meanwhile, neither is tracking outcomes to determine whether the same patient-centered results are being produced. The extensive variability within PT mirrors practice and cost variability throughout musculoskeletal medicine. PT as a mode of treatment and service delivery is a long way from the model employed by Starbucks. Nevertheless, some physical therapists strive to follow *evidence-based* assessment methods that lead to a valid reproducible diagnosis that, in turn, leads to reliable, predictably effective treatments that may be surgery sparing. Most important, these therapists can prove their effective and reliable methodology because they track patient outcomes and patient satisfaction scores in a problem-oriented record.

Readers of this chapter, as patient advocates, may ask themselves the following, taking this coffee-to-PT analog further. What if there *were* a "coffee shop" (PT clinic) that reliably produced a better cup of coffee? What if that cup of coffee cost less than others? And what if the overall experience of getting that coffee was superior to others? Would that be worth traveling somewhat farther to get? Would you refer a friend to that coffee shop? This analogy is the Institute for Healthcare Improvement triple aim: better care for individuals (quality and satisfaction), better health for populations, and lower per-capita costs.[8] Later in this chapter is a process describing exactly how to find the PTs who can reliably produce the best outcome at a lower cost with high patient satisfaction. It is, in fact, these professionals who will do the most to improve the spine surgeon's outcomes, patient satisfaction, and practice throughput.

Efficient spine surgeons' practices depend not on their skill in the operating room alone, but upon the skill of the physical therapist their patients see in the preoperative or perioperative period. A well-trained physical therapist utilizes a reliable assessment method that leads to a predictably effective treatment. The physical therapist then trains the patient in an independent functional program of self-assessment and self-treatment for long-term prevention of recurrence. This often empowers the patient to succeed and decreases the probability of multiple return visits for PT. The surgeon's office is also spared multiple unproductive patient visits. Due to the greater amount of time a physical therapist spends with a patient (compared to a surgeon), a therapist may have greater insight to hidden barriers preventing successful outcomes. A well-qualified physical therapist who determines that a patient is

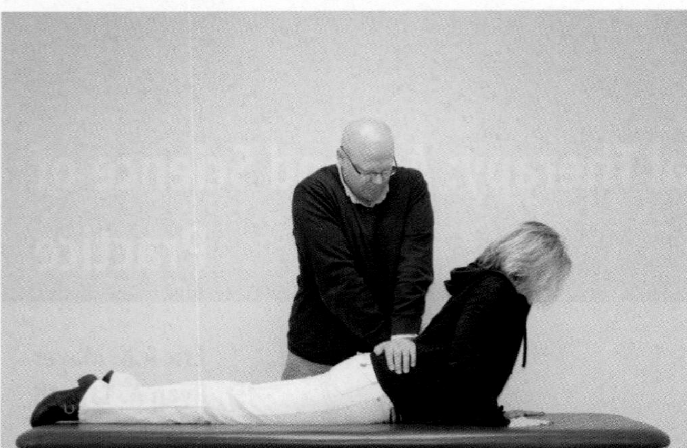

FIG. 110.1 Lumbar extension in lying with clinician overpressure is the specific exercise that produces the best response in symptom location, range of motion, neural tension signs, manual muscle testing, and reflex testing for this particular patient. All responses are capable of improving when the individual's specific corrective movement is performed. A thorough mechanical assessment determines the specific movement direction, load, and pressure required.

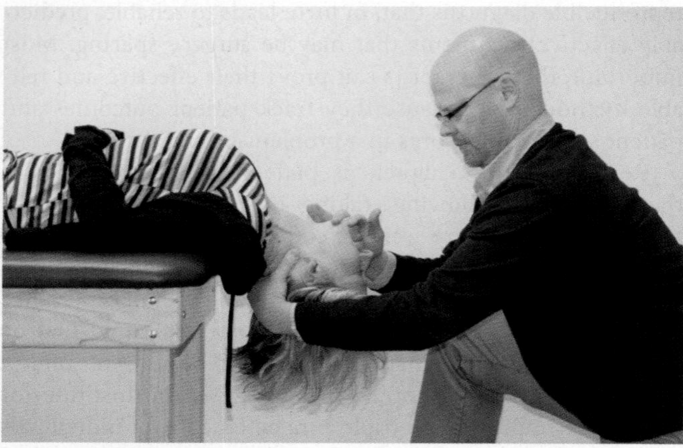

FIG. 110.2 Cervical traction with extension is initially required to allow this patient to return to specific loaded exercises. Again, a thorough mechanical assessment determines the specific direction, pressure, and load of the exercise based on the patient's history and response to movement.

not making satisfactory progress can also inform the surgeon about a patient's underlying biopsychosocial distress that may produce inferior surgical outcomes. Also, valuable mechanical information can be communicated to the surgeon by the physical therapist. For example, determining a reducible disc versus an irreducible disc is easily within the skill set of the mechanically trained physical therapist.[9] Effective and efficient spine practices thrive on collaboration and free communication between all team members. Patients are best served by a collaborative effort with the best trained therapists in the spine surgeon's geographic location (Figs. 110.1 and 110.2).

Guidelines for Selecting a Physical Therapist

The physical therapist with whom a surgeon chooses to collaborate must demonstrate skill in treating that surgeon's patient population. The therapist must possess a shared understanding of surgical indications and flags that may predispose patients to poor outcomes. In summary, the therapist must be a good fit for the surgeon's practice. The benefits of collaboration start early. Patients are seeking the spine surgeon's recommendations for all aspects of their care. Instructing patients to blindly find their own therapist can produce unreliable variability that can make surgical interventions less successful.[10] Hildebrandt et al. demonstrated that preoperative programs that do not change subjective feelings of disability in the patient produce inferior outcomes.[10] Simply referring patients to the in-house PT department at the spine surgeon's hospital/health system fails to guarantee quality treatment. Spine rehabilitation is not covered to the same extent in all PT programs and postgraduate training for PT also differs significantly.

Unless individual outcomes (not process measures) are measured by the therapist and used to inform practices, treatment efficacy provided will vary by clinic and even by clinician within the same clinic. Just like surgery, PT is not a standardized practice.

In order to judge the quality of a physical therapist, the spine surgeon is accountable for interviewing physical therapists to whom spine patients will be referred. By interviewing the physical therapist who will treat referred spine patients, the spine surgeon ensures that the patient is receiving the expected PT. Virtually all competent physical therapists want to collaborate with a spine surgeon. However, the physical therapists who are unwilling to accept an invitation for an interview with the surgeon often lack the skill set to treat the spine patient population. The physical therapists who do accept interviews should demonstrate spine-specific proficiency. Often, "bad actors" will be easily ruled out, utilizing an interview process. During this interview, the surgeon should identify several key data-driven factors. The more criteria the physical therapist meets, the better chance that therapist will provide highly effective and reproducible outcomes. Time spent screening therapists with the process described later will pay massive dividends by eliminating unproductive time in a busy surgeon's schedule. However, the spine surgeon may not have adequate preparation for such an efficient process. An alternative may be to choose the top one or two therapists in a practice and refer patients for a 6-month trial period, then request standard pre-post outcome data from each therapist (described later in this chapter). Occasionally, a surgeon's practice is in an area that has limited choice of PT clinics. This scenario is a golden opportunity for the spine surgeon to influence the type of continuing education for a PT clinic. The spine surgeon can request specific PT continuing education training on behalf of the patient population to ensure continuous quality improvement in nonoperative/postoperative patient care.

The interview process is comprised of 10 questions:

1. Does the physical therapist have experience treating spine patients? How many does the physical therapist treat per month? Spine patients are often the least sought out patients by physical therapists due to the perceived complexity and lack of outcomes associated with treatment. Experience with spine patients is an excellent start and simply indicates a lack

of avoidance of, if not interest in, this patient population. However, experience alone is not an indicator of treatment effectiveness. Continuation of questioning is required to determine effectiveness markers.

2. Does the physical therapist exclusively use active modes of treatment? Exercise and movement promotion are quintessential to the care of a spine patient. Passive modalities have little to no place in the care of the spine patient, with rare exceptions. Transcutaneous electrical neural stimulation (TENS) may possibly speed weaning from opioid pain medication use in the immediate postoperative period.[11] However, further use of low-value (high expense without any validated outcomes) modalities is generally inferior to active treatment. Ultrasound and various other modalities, including electrical stimulation, laser, massage, and traction, are inferior to the long-term outcome of active treatment and are discussed later in this chapter.
3. Is the physical therapist able to cite the reliability of the clinical protocol being used? Methods of PT practice are available that produce more reliable assessments and outcomes than others. Reliability is the most important first step toward validity. Any diagnosis produced by unreliable assessment methods is doomed to ineffective treatments and subsequent poor outcomes. A surgeon or physician may be unfamiliar with the phases of "usual care" physical therapy that lack reliability. Physical therapists who utilize methods with greatest reliability will be able to cite their evidence-based practice.
4. Does the physical therapist track the outcomes for quality assurance? The collection of meaningful data is imperative to determine if a process or intervention is producing an effect on the outcome. Here are some common standardized patient-reported functional outcome measures for the spine: the Oswestry Disability Index, Neck Disability Index, Pain Disability Questionnaire, Roland Morris Disability Questionnaire, and Pain Disability Index. A more recent measure, the Patient-Reported Outcomes Measurement Information System, utilizes computer-adaptive testing and scales that may allow greater breadth of outcome gathering without the burden of asking too many questions. Patient-centered perceptions of function are the most meaningful outcomes to track. In contrast to measuring pain scores, measuring functional perceptions more closely mirrors and predicts return to work and surgical outcomes than merely collecting visual analog scale pain scores measured at random intervals. In this patient population, a significant improvement in functional rating signals real gains for the patient and often meets the increasing regulatory burden with regard to *performance* measures.
5. Are the outcomes tracked for at least 1 year? High-value treatment interventions are durable. This means that a clinically significant improvement in outcome scoring should be durable for up to 1 year. Clinical effectiveness often requires education and patient buy-in for a gym-based or home-based exercise program. Patient adherence can be measured directly or through the proxy of the therapist's chosen outcome measures (see item 4) deployed to the patient at regular intervals for up to 1 year.[12] Long-term gains and surgical outcomes are tied to home program compliance.[13,14] The process of tracking outcomes requires other resources in addition to the usual clinical operation costs. Allocation of resources for outcome data tracking may be a strong indicator of that therapist's commitment to improving the patient's health.
6. Does the physical therapist take action to remediate deficiencies identified during outcomes tracking? Data are just numbers until utilized for a purpose. Whether therapists utilize the data for clinical decision making is what makes it meaningful. Clinical reasoning regarding a particular patient's care must occur based on trends in the collected data. Plans identifying and treating unexpected or deviant trends must be developed by the therapist to ensure safe and efficacious patient care. Addressing clinical nuances, including comorbidities confounding results, should heighten your confidence in your therapists' ability to handle a diverse patient population. Correct utilization of data enhances the patient's experience and improves therapist-to-surgeon communication.
7. Does the physical therapist participate in a regular quality control, continuous quality improvement, or a grand rounds process among clinicians (within or outside of the clinic) to identify patients not meeting expected outcomes so that changes can be implemented? Continuous quality improvement in some form is the most important learning tool as long as the format is a clinical case presentation or interactive workshop/small groups.[15] It is a mirror for the therapy practice to identify both best practices and deficiencies. Regular use of the process implies that the therapist is interested in communication and providing the surgeon and the patient with optimum outcome. This interdisciplinary approach improves the clinical experience for all clinicians involved as it centers care on each individual patient. The patient's treatment experience is enhanced when the knowledge base of senior/expert clinicians combines with innovative approaches and guidance of all stakeholders.
8. Does the physical therapist understand value? Can the physical therapist cite cost savings by reducing resource utilization (compared to community standard) while returning superior outcomes? This can be achieved through participation in a national registry (American Physical Therapy Association, Physical Therapy Outcomes Registry) or a national outcomes measurement tool such as Focus on Therapeutic Outcomes. Surgeons share responsibility with therapists to request access to deidentified claims data. This allows tracking of all regional entrances into the health care system. Comparisons of a practice's costs and outcomes against a regional benchmark is increasingly important. The cost of providing a service may not be readily accessible to all physical therapists. However, cost is directly related to the number of PT sessions that a patient receives per diagnostic ICD-10 code. Substitutes for the standard value formula (outcome/cost) exist. A simple formula is useful:

$$\text{Value} = \text{Outcomes}/\text{Visits}$$

Fewer visits and/or better outcomes increase value for patients and the value of that practice to the spine surgeons in their community. Newer time-driven activity-based costing tools are emerging as simple ways to make cost data actionable. Broadly speaking, the Value-Based Health Care Delivery initiative led by the Harvard Business School provides easy access to best-practice ideas while off-the shelf ideas may be accessed through a simple Internet search or through a national medical society.

9. Can the physical therapist present patient-level satisfaction scores? Collection of patient satisfaction questionnaires shows a dedication to patient-centered care. Improving the patient experience will reflect well on the surgeon who took time to identify a quality therapy practice. Conversely, poor patient experiences will be reflected in the surgeons' satisfaction scores as well. A willingness on the part of the therapist to identify areas of improvement is necessary in this increasingly data-driven marketplace. Patient satisfaction is a slippery slope and must be weighted in the face of other quality measures. Donabedian[16] concluded that access, administrative technical management, clinical technical management, interpersonal management, and continuity of care are domains that define patient satisfaction. Satisfaction ratings improve if the patient's expectations are met.[17] Dissatisfied patients are less likely to use professional advice, thus undermining both primary and secondary prevention.[18] Often, the most effective treatments bring a temporary increase in pain symptoms before gains are realized. Gentle guidance from the surgeon that effective therapy often hurts, but will not *harm*, the patient is a benefit for the patient, the therapist, and the surgeon's office staff. However, a skilled clinician who is cognizant of the patient experience can proactively educate and guide the patient through exercise regimens that ultimately produce the desired outcome. Through the use of collected data, patient satisfaction improves; this will, in effect, recruit more patients to whom the physical therapist can provide a high-quality service.
10. Finally, the surgeon should ask himself or herself the following: do I *trust* this person? If the interaction with the physical therapist does not feel right, patients will notice this as well. The late physician Leon Wiltse was famous for making difficult concepts understandable. After pioneering the use of quantitative testing (Minnesota Multiphasic Personality Inventory) to optimize surgical outcomes, he boiled down years of clinical acumen with a speech as President of the Association of Bone and Joint Surgeons on his famous "look 'em in the eye" test. If you do not trust what you see when you look the therapist in the eye, choose a different therapist.

Collaboration Between the Surgeon and the Therapist

After identifying a suitable physical therapist, the surgeon and the therapist can collaborate efficiently as members of the same patient care team. Each member has well-established roles—there are certain patient expectations from the spine surgeon and from the physical therapist.

Before the patient begins PT, the spine surgeon should prepare the patient for the PT experience. The patient–clinician relationship has a significant effect on health care outcomes.[19] However, the language used by the surgeon during this process has a *more* significant effect on the patient's outcome.[20] For example, visualize the following scenario as if you were the patient who has just been evaluated by the surgeon and compare the following statements: "You can try PT if you want; if it doesn't work, we might need to get an MRI." Or, "I have hand chosen the physical therapists I need you to see. They are experts in treating your particular problem. They will keep me up-to-date on your progress."

Words are very much a treatment by themselves. Words hold immense weight from a patient's perspective. Choose the words with which to treat patients wisely. In comparing the two statements, the first statement is spoken with pessimism, apathy, uncertainty, and a touch of callousness. The first statement creates a mindset for the patient implying failure in PT before even attempting it and that pathology will be proved with an MRI. This statement implies that improvement with PT means that the patient's condition was beneath the concern of a surgeon. Using language to inspire patients to work hard in PT is not just for the sake of the attempt, but instead has been shown to be good medicine.[21] The patients who attend PT without a bias or a chip on their shoulder experience greater progress, less lost work time, and fewer MRIs.[22] Physicians who employ the first statement are not merely uneducated regarding the importance of PT, their apathy contributes to low value and disreputable medical care.[23]

The tone in the second statement is spoken with confidence and empathy. It reflects very well on the surgeon, the therapist, and the patient. It relays the message that the surgeon is invested in the patient to the point that individualized care was selected with a specific hand-picked treatment. The trust engendered when a surgeon has already interviewed these particular clinicians is reinforced to the patient by the therapist. This simple and proper set-up offers hope to patients. Hopeful patients are more likely to take an active role in recovery, attend their first PT appointment, and return to activity more rapidly.[24] A positive attitude has a strong association with symptom resolution.[25] Better communication and interpersonal skills are able to detect problems earlier, can prevent medical crises and expensive intervention, and provide better support to patients. This may lead to higher-quality outcomes and better satisfaction, lower costs of care, greater patient understanding of health issues, and better adherence to the treatment process.[26]

In direct opposition is the uncertainty engendered when patients believe in the need to "fail" to get a definitive answer to the cause of their pain (receiving an MRI). Many patients falsely believe that an MRI, rather than clinical examination, is the best method to determine treatment.[27] A poorly educated patient fails to realize certain factors:

- The high sensitivity and low specificity of the MRI produces high false positives.[28–30]

- Asymptomatic or nonconcordant pathoanatomy is commonly found on the MRI.[31] The absence of pathology does not predispose the patient to a pain-free and fully functional existence.
- A thorough mechanical assessment by a well-qualified physical therapist can correlate pain complaints[32] with relevant imaging findings.[33]

In summary, a well-trained physical therapist, integrated by the surgeon into the care team, can educate the patient on fears, objectify pain responses to movement/positioning, return the locus of control to the patient, and identify and possibly decrease psychosocial factors associated with poor outcomes. A consistent message from all members of the patient care team instills confidence in the patient and improves both surgical and nonsurgical outcomes.

When the patient attends PT, the surgeon should have the following expectations. The physical therapist should treat this patient with an evidence-based, reliable method. This method should subgroup patients, then match the treatment to that patient's subgroup for a positive outcome.[34] A predictably positive outcome begins with a reliable, reproducible assessment process. The assessment method used by the physical therapist must exhibit both internal and external reliability. Without this reliability, every step thereafter fails due to unpredictable, nonspecific results.

The Quebec Task Force stated that the variability of methods producing an unreliable diagnosis is "the fundamental source of error" that ultimately results in poor outcomes.[35] Spratt reported that the process of establishing clinical validity required three imperatives: "The focus will be on a single diagnosis (D) that is unambiguously derived from a well-defined assessment (A), for which there is consensus for a single specific treatment (T), and where specific outcomes of treatment (O) are specified."[36] The result is the ADTO model, which requires hierarchical linkages between Assessment-Diagnosis, Diagnosis-Treatment and Treatment-Outcome. A predictably effective outcome is only possible with a reliable assessment method that produces classification subgroups.[37] While it may not be obvious to many physicians, classification subgrouping is the most important component in creating homogeneous groups of patients with similar treatment–response characteristics out of a population with heterogeneous symptoms of spine-related pain.[38–40]

Regardless of the classification system utilized for subgrouping, it must have the essentials described by the ADTO model. The subgrouping method must exhibit testable, reproducible reliability in all aspects of the clinical assessment, not just for certain self-limited assessed conditions. The therapist should be able to explain the assessment/classification system and should produce valid clinical diagnoses. The therapist must plan a predictably effective treatment for the diagnosis that produces superior outcomes compared to natural history and other common treatments for the same diagnosis.

When the therapist corresponds back to the surgeon following patient evaluation, the initial report should indicate to which subgroup the patient belongs and should include the clinical reasoning. Moreover, the therapist should indicate the *ability* to change symptoms, mechanics, concordant signs and/or neurologic signs via mechanical pressure and loading strategies. Equally important is communicating an *inability* to change these factors through varied mechanical pressure and loading strategies. Early determination of mechanical nonresponse facilitates rapid referral back to the surgeon for advanced imaging, injections, or surgery. Prolonged ineffectual care to maximize PT visits results in the patient losing confidence in the efficacy of therapy and exercise. A quality therapist decreases fear-avoidant behavior by ensuring rapid referral to the appropriate clinician.[41] Similarly, a quality therapist knows that time is a disability determinant. Therapists who determine in a short period of time whether a patient will respond or not respond are very valuable to a surgical practice.

Active Versus Passive Physical Therapy

Physical therapy for spine problems is an active process and very rarely requires bed rest beyond 24 hours.[42] Passive physical agents have shown no long-term effects on outcomes as stand-alone treatments.[43] Passive modalities have shown no place in the treatment of spine problems outside of the immediate postoperative time frame (when reducing opioid use may be advantageous).[44] Otherwise, there is no high-quality evidence to support the use of passive modalities such as TENS for the treatment of back pain.[45–47] The available evidence shows that in patients with chronic low back pain (CLBP), treatment with TENS is no more effective than treatment with a placebo and TENS adds no apparent benefit to that of exercise alone.[48] A Cochrane Collaboration systematic review concluded: "At this time, the evidence from the small number of placebo-controlled trials does not support the use of TENS in the routine management of chronic LBP."[46]

Therapeutic ultrasound is commonly used in the treatment of spine-related pain for thermal and nonthermal effects.[50] A Cochrane Library Review stated: "We did not find any convincing evidence that ultrasound is an effective treatment for low-back pain…." There is no existing high-quality evidence that ultrasound improves pain or quality of life: "Effects were so small they may not make any difference to patients' lives."[51] Therefore, the use of this common modality is highly discouraged.

Low-level laser and high-level laser are not recommended in place of or adjunct to conventional treatment.[52] Immediate pain improvements may be associated with low-level laser. However, evidence does not support the use of laser for improvement of function or reduction of disability for patients with chronic low back pain.[52]

Massage therapy for neck pain and LBP has shown no improvement in pain, dysfunction, or range of motion when compared to no treatment, inactive therapies, and active therapies.[54,55] However, massage therapy for LBP may be an effective treatment option compared to placebo or relaxation in the short term.[56] No evidence is available to support the long-term effectiveness of massage therapy for the treatment of acute, subacute, or CLBP.[57]

Lumbar traction in any form, alone or in combination with other treatments, has little or no impact on pain intensity, functional status, global improvement, and return to work. The use of traction as a treatment for nonspecific LBP, with or without sciatica, is not supported by the best available evidence.[58] Traction for neck pain shows no favorable results for pain or disability.[59,60]

Physicians should be aware that time spent performing passive physical modalities would be better spent performing effective movement-based treatment and cognitive behavior education. Though passive modalities are used regularly for the treatment of neck and low back pain, a spine surgeon should consider ordering active treatment with a specific note stating "no modalities" due to the lack of supportive evidence for passive modalities. The American Physical Therapy Association's top five Choose Wisely recommendations supports the use of active therapeutic approaches over passive treatment. They report the following: "There is limited evidence for use of passive physical agents to obtain clinically important outcomes for musculoskeletal conditions. A carefully designed active treatment plan has a greater impact on pain, mobility, function, and quality of life. Although there is some evidence of short-term pain relief for certain physical agents, the addition of passive physical agents should be supported by evidence and used to facilitate an active treatment program."[61]

Too often the phrase "but patients like it" is used to defend the overutilization of passive physical agents. This is when the collaborative surgeon–therapist relationship serves patient long-term interest. Even when patient expectations are taken into consideration, the surgeon can limit "passive" modalities while a collaborative therapist can explain the reasoning to the patient. The surgeon and physical therapist should not be driven by what the patient wants or feels is best. Analogous to physician satisfaction ratings being tied to prescriptions for narcotic pain medications, antibiotics, and MRIs, therapists who always meet patient expectations do not necessarily demonstrate best practices.[62] A false dilemma exists when health providers feel that fulfillment of patient expectations will improve satisfaction scores despite evidence that more effective treatment options exist. However, if the patient is able to experience positive rapid change with a movement-based treatment, there is a greater probability of compliance with an active plan of care and the perceived need for passive treatment diminishes.

Physical Therapy Levels of Care

As a final point, the spine surgeon should have a concept of *levels of care* when it comes to PT exercise interventions. The majority of this chapter has discussed the primary level of traditional PT care that is usually started in the mid-acute/subacute phase and is focused on range of motion, strengthening, and avoidance of deconditioning, with some emphasis on endurance and job-specific functional limitations. The patient population that responds to primary-level therapy is usually still at work, missing less than 6 weeks of usual activities, using limited or no opioid medication, experiencing minimal sleep interruption, and suffering relatively mild to moderate biopsychosocial distress with a variable component of fear avoidance. Much like limiting bed rest, there is very little evidence that formal conventional PT is necessary in the immediate acute period of 1 to 3 weeks.[63] Historically, advice for patients in the first 1 to 2 weeks of an acute spine-related pain process has been to remain active with gentle stretching, which may include performing yoga stretches or following a stretching booklet.[64] This antiquated advice remains common even as evidence-based practices encouraging PT evaluation are being incorporated into formal clinical guidelines.

LBP and neck pain have traditionally been considered to be self-limiting with a favorable prognosis. However, the treatment paradigm of self-guided nonspecific stretching, nonsteroidal antiinflammatory drugs, muscle relaxants, and reassurance of improvement is proving ineffective in a growing subpopulation that increasingly accounts for much of the indemnity costs. The recurrence rate of LBP within 12 months after initial episode has been reported to be as high as 84%.[65] Neck pain and LBP combined is now the number one cause of disability globally, moving up from the number two position.[66] The United States total cost (direct cost, indirect cost, intangible cost) associated with neck pain and LBP is estimated at over $600 billion and climbing.[67] The problem of neck pain and LBP is certainly not necessarily self-limited and has a mixed prognosis. Acute low back pain requires specificity of treatment as much as acute chest pain does. Disregarding acute low back pain as though it is not worthy of effort until there is a neurologic deficit may create later problems that can be more difficult to solve. Therefore, there is no better time than at the primary level to initiate specifically formulated, reproducible treatments. Paradigms of watchful waiting are proving ineffective and increasingly expensive. Specific, collaborative, and value-based treatment can save the patient from needless temporary disability in addition to modifying downstream costs associated with expensive advanced care.[68–70]

The spine surgeon should consider secondary-level therapy for patients who have been out of work for a prolonged period or who have inadequately recovered from a posttraumatic or postsurgical phase of healing. The overall goal of secondary-level care is reactivation. *Reactivation* is a term used for various active exercises to reverse deconditioning (termed "weak-link syndrome") while simultaneously addressing biopsychosocial factors, such as fear avoidance, which can result in aspects of "disability behavior."[71] Such patients have allowed enough time for tissue healing (casting, bracing, fracture healing, or surgery) and have a disproportionate amount of pain inhibition along with reduced range of motion and focal reduction in strength.[72] Patients exceeding more than 8 weeks of temporary total disability may have poor outcomes when referred to single-therapist, primary-level PT. Patient-reported outcome tools such as the STarT-Back tool, Pain Disability Index, and Pain Disability Questionnaire have each been shown to help triage patients to *primary-level* or *secondary-level* PT.[73] A commonly used instrument, the Oswestry Disability Index, showed relatively poor discrimination and responsiveness in head-to-head comparisons.[74]

Not all PT practices are capable of handling secondary-level PT. Capable practices have specialized training in assessment (commonly called physical capacity evaluations) and treatment often in the context of a work-hardening or work-conditioning program. Therapists who oversee these programs typically have specialized postgraduate training. These programs consist of increased treatment frequency and intensity with minimal to no passive modalities or manipulation. The focus of these programs starts with regaining full range of motion followed by rapidly introducing quota-based strengthening and endurance. Specific educational attention is placed on the injured area, with a particular focus on barriers to occupational/functional reintegration.

Finally, tertiary-level care usually combines interdisciplinary assessment and treatment for chronic disabling spinal disorders with specific focus on return to work/function and marked reduction of medical indemnity costs.[75] The preponderance of high-level medical literature supports a functional restoration approach.[76] Due to financial constraints of program administration, tertiary-level care may not be readily available in all surgeons' communities. Seeking consultation from a regional quaternary institution may be necessary. Of specific interest to the spine surgeon is evidence showing that patients with chronic disabling back pain who begin a functional restoration program before surgery have a high return-to-work rate when they complete the functional restoration program after surgery. This has been cited in several published disability guidelines outlining occupational injury.[77] Prior to placing a patient at maximal medical improvement, an evaluation at a tertiary-level therapy program often makes sense.

Summary

In summary, knowledge is power for the spine surgeon to effectively treat a broad sampling of patients with spinal disorders. Spine surgeons' ethical mandate is to advocate for their patients and to ensure that patients return to maximal vocational and avocational function from their injury. Historical benign neglect of recurrent disabling episodes will not be tolerated in an area of value-based, bundled-payment care. A shift to interdisciplinary collaboration is intended to embrace the triple aim—improving outcomes, improving patient experience, and reducing costs—in our increasingly value-driven health care environment. This chapter's intention is to provide high-level strategies to adequately assess the quality of therapy that the spine surgeon can recommend to patients in response to the need for high-value services that improve population health at a decreased cost.

KEY POINTS

1. Substantial variability exists in PT practice. A failed attempt at PT with one therapist does not necessarily mean that PT has, in fact, failed.
2. A formal interview of a physical therapist by the surgeon asking several key questions (contained in this chapter) will likely improve communication, therapy results, and surgical outcomes.
3. After acute injury, rest, particularly bed rest, for longer than 48 hours can be detrimental. Recommendation of prolonged rest after spine injury is associated with a higher rate of disability. Advising engaging in physical activity and acknowledging that the surgeon has specifically picked out a therapist or therapy actively engages patients in their own well-being and an activity-based PT program.
4. The use of *active* modes of therapeutic exercises is associated with a reduction in the duration of disability. Extremely limited evidence exists that use of passive therapies speeds patients' return to full function.
5. Pain is a poor guide for determining therapeutic duration and intensity. Exercise programs that promote/encourage/require patients' continuing with active therapy, even when their pain increased, had decreased work-related disability. Programs that encouraged pain to guide the dosage and intensity of therapy fared worse in primary and secondary outcome measures. Patients who stopped therapeutic activities due to pain seemed to experience an increase in behaviors such as taking painkillers, seeking health care, stopping work, limping, guarding, and talking about their pain. Pain intensity should not guide therapy and surgeons should reinforce patient questions regarding the difference between "hurt" and "harm."
6. Pain centralization and a patient's ability to obtain a directional preference with exercise are significant findings necessary to categorize patients for appropriate exercise. Categorizing patients and treating them appropriately results in a decrease in short-term (< 3 months) pain and disability for LBP compared with other standard treatments, such as nonsteroidal antiinflammatory drugs, educational booklet, and massage.
7. Monitoring of patients' functional and return-to-work outcomes by the therapist is important for quality assurance. Outcomes should be tracked for at least 1 year. The physical therapist should identify and remediate deficiencies in the PT program. The most effective strategies involve delivering exercise programs based on sound reproducible diagnostic methodology. Studies indicate favorable benefit from early use of aggressive PT (sports medicine model) and training that is quota based and not pain based in its progression.
8. The use of active treatment modalities instead of passive treatments is associated with substantially better clinical outcomes. Case series of patients with acute LBP treated by physical therapists who followed active therapy guidelines needed fewer treatment visits and had decreased cost, pain, and disability when compared to patients treated with a passive regimen of modalities and manipulation. A total of 64.7% of patients in the active-treatment protocol group deemed therapy a success compared to only 36.5% in the passive-treatment group.
9. Psychological support is important in overcoming fear beliefs about pain, injury, activity, and function. Moreover, active physical treatment, cognitive behavioral treatment, and a combination of each resulted in statistically equivalent and significant improvement. All demonstrated a statistically significant improvement over no treatment. (The cognitive treatment focused on behavioral reinforcement of increased physical activity.)
10. Patients who fail timely, single-therapist, active protocols should be considered for referral to a tertiary-level interdisciplinary functional restoration program. Delay in treatment is a leading cause of disability. Failure to improve with good, aggressive therapy does not necessarily imply a high surgical success rate for that patient.

KEY REFERENCES

1. Staal JB, Rainville J, Fritz J, et al. Physical exercise interventions to improve disability and return to work in low back pain: current insights and opportunities for improvement. *J Occ Rehabil.* 2005;15:491-505.
Physical exercise is not associated with an increased risk for injury recurrence. Despite numerous studies, more quantitative and qualitative investigations are needed to further clarify the requirements for a successful application and implementation of physical exercise interventions. The specific interventions and physical or behavioral effects may vary depending on content-related factors (e.g., type of exercises, dosage, frequency, skills of the health care providers) and contextual factors (e.g., treatment setting, compensation system). Patients' expectations and confidence in a specific treatment also influence physical exercise outcomes. Timing and goal setting are important in targeting work return with early application of quota-based therapy during the acute phase of work absenteeism.
2. Martin BI, Turner JA, Mirza SK, et al. Trends in health care expenditures, utilization, and health status among US adults with spine problems, 1997-2006. *Spine.* 2009;34:2077-2084.
Expenditures related to spine care have increased by 82%, and well health measures have decreased in the 10-year interval between 1997 and 2006. Overall, nearly 30% of the population state that they are somewhat limited in vocational activities by spine pain. This increased from 20% in 1995.
3. Videman T, Sarna S, Battie MC, et al. The long-term effects of physical loading and exercise lifestyles on back-related symptoms, disability, and spinal pathology among men. *Spine.* 1995;20:699-709.
Body shape and habitus have a greater effect on disc desiccation then serial physical loading, type of work, vocational activity, or lifestyle when analyzed with radiologic criteria for desiccation or degenerative changes.
4. Rainville J, Pransky G, Indahl A, Mayer EK. The physician as disability advisor for patients with musculoskeletal complaints. *Spine.* 2005;30:2579-2584.
Physicians play a key role in determining whether patients return to work in a timely fashion through their advice. Evidence exists that educating physicians changes the population prevalence of disabling spine injuries. Educational efforts to modify physician belief about back pain, injury, and the relation of hurt and harm seem to improve population outcomes. Physicians should be adequately educated to prevent advice that is detrimental to the patient's eventual functional recovery.
5. George SZ, Fritz JM, Bialosky JA, et al. The effect of a fear-avoidance based physical therapy intervention for patients with acute low back pain: results of a randomized clinical trial. *Spine.* 2003;28:2551-2560.
Patients with elevated fear-avoidance beliefs appeared to have less disability from fear-avoidance-based physical therapy when compared with those receiving standard care physical therapy.
6. Kool JP, Oesch PR, Bachmann S, et al. Increasing days at work using function-centered rehabilitation in nonacute nonspecific low back pain: a randomized controlled trial. *Arch Phys Med Rehabil.* 2005;86:857-864.
Pain is a poor predictor of therapeutic efficacy. Patients were split into two groups: (1) a function-based group that was encouraged to continue with therapeutic exercises despite the pain and (2) a pain-based group that was told to cease exercises when they had pain. Patients who were trained by a therapist to stop exercising because of pain fared worse in all measures than the function-based group. Additionally, the pain-based group exhibited additional behaviors such as stopping work, limping, guarding, talking about pain, taking pain killers, and seeking additional health care.
7. Fritz JM, Delitto A, Erhard RE. Comparison of a classification-based approach to physical therapy and therapy based on clinical practice guidelines for patients with acute low back pain: a randomized clinical trial. *Spine.* 2003;28:1363-1372.
For patients with acute, work-related low back pain, the use of a classification-based approach with four classification subgroups resulted in improved disability and return to work status after 4 weeks. The work return was statistically significant when compared with therapy based on other clinical practice guidelines. Patients with subjective and objective evidence of clinical instability were treated with a strengthening and stabilization exercise program. Classification systems with four different treatment approaches based on findings are used by physical therapists, yet indications for their application have not been adequately studied.
8. Ostelo RW, Costa LO, Maher CG, et al. Rehabilitation after lumbar disc surgery: an update Cochrane review. *Spine.* 2009;34:1839-1848.
Pain and function that failed to improve through back surgery should be treated with physical therapy or a functional restoration program. There is strong evidence for intensive exercise programs for functional status and faster return to work, and there is no evidence that they increase the reoperation rate.
9. Videman T, Gibbons LE, Kaprio J, Battié MC. Challenging the cumulative injury model: positive effects of greater body mass on disc degeneration. *Spine J.* 2010;10:26-31.
Contrary to popular belief, heavier body weight between twins and greater physical activity do not seem to increase disc desiccation or degenerative changes when followed over time with MRI. In fact, heavier twins who were more physically active in avocational activities seem to preserve MRI disc signal L1 and L4. This finding challenges the long-held belief in the cumulative injury model. The cumulative injury model seems to have no proof in favor of it, and there is fairly clear evidence with this article against this model.

REFERENCES

1. Coste J, Delecoeuillerie G, Cohen de Lara A, et al. Clinical course and prognostic factors in acute low back pain: an inception cohort study in primary care practice. *BMJ.* 1994; 308(6928):577-580.
2. Waddell G, Feder G, Lewis M. Systematic reviews of bed rest and advice to stay active for acute low back pain. *Br J Gen Pract.* 1997;47(423):647-652.
3. Deyo RA, Diehl AK, Rosenthal M. How many days of bed rest for acute low back pain? *N Engl J Med.* 1986;315(17): 1064-1070.
4. Pengel LH, Herbert RD, et al. Acute low back pain: systematic review of its prognosis. *Br Med J.* 2003;327(7410):323.
5. Pengel LH, Herbert RD, et al. Acute low back pain: systematic review of its prognosis. *Br Med J.* 2003;327(7410):323.
6. Stevens D, Maher CG, Pereira LSM, et al. Prevention of low back pain, a systematic review. *JAMA Int Med.* 2016;176(2): 199-208.
7. Weinstein JN, Lurie JD, et al. United States trends and regional variations in lumbar spine surgery: 1992–2003. *Spine.* 2006;31(23):2707-2716.
8. Berwick D, Nolan T, Whittington J. The triple aim: care, health, and cost. *Health Aff.* 2008;27(3):759-769.
9. Wetzel FT, Donelson R. The role of repeated end-range/pain response assessment in the management of symptomatic lumbar discs. *Spine J.* 2003;3:146-154.

10. Hildebrandt J, Pfingsten M, Saur P, Jansen J. Prediction of success from a multidisciplinary treatment program for chronic low back pain. *Spine*. 1997;22(9):990-1001.
11. Carroll D, Tramer H, McQuary B, Nye B, Moore A. Randomization is important in studies with pain outcomes: systemic review of transcutaneous electrical nerve stimulation in acute postoperative pain. *Br J Anesth*. 1996;77:798-803.
12. Zhang W, Moskowitz RW, Nuki G, et al. OARSI recommendations for the management of hip and knee osteoarthritis, Part II: OARSI evidence-based, expert consensus guidelines. *Osteoarthritis Cartilage*. 2008;16(2):137-162.
13. Vuori IM. Dose-response of physical activity and low back pain, osteoarthritis, and osteoporosis. *Med Sci Sports Exerc*. 2001;33(6 suppl):S551-S586.
14. McLean S, Burton M, et al. Interventions for enhancing adherence with physiotherapy: a systematic review. *Man Ther*. 2010;15(6):514-521.
15. Hebert R, Wright S. Re-examining the value of medical grand rounds. *Acad Med*. 2003;78:1248-1252.
16. Donabedian A. The quality of care: how can it be assessed? *JAMA*. 1988;260:1743-1748.
17. Hush J, Cameron K, Mackey M. Patient satisfaction with musculoskeletal physical therapy care: a systematic review. *Phys Ther*. 2010;91:25-36.
18. Goldstein M, Elliot S, Guccione A. The development of an instrument to measure satisfaction with physical therapy. *Phys Ther*. 2000;80(9):853-863.
19. Kelley J, Kraft-Todd L, et al. The influence of the patient-clinician relationship on healthcare outcomes: a systematic review and meta-analysis of randomized controlled trials. *PLoS One*. 2014;1-7.
20. Rainville J, Pransky G, Indahl A, Myer EK. The physician as disability advisor for patients with musculoskeletal complaints. *Spine*. 2005;30(22):2579-2584.
21. Rainville J, Ahern DK, Phalen L. Altering beliefs about pain and function in a functionally oriented treatment program for chronic low back pain. *Clin J Pain*. 1993;9:196-205.
22. Linton SJ, Vlaeyen J, Ostelo R. The back pain beliefs of health care providers: are we fear-avoidant? *J Occup Rehabil*. 2002;12:223-232.
23. Chou R, Qaseem A, Owens DK, Shekelle P. Diagnostic imaging for low back pain: advice for high-value health care from the American College of Physicians. *Ann Intern Med*. 2011;154(3):181-189.
24. Shaw WS, Pransky G, Fitzgerald TE. Early prognosis for low back disability: intervention strategies for health care providers. *Disabil Rehabil*. 2001;23:815-828.
25. Staal JB, Rainville J, Fritz J, et al. Physical exercise interventions to improve disability and return to work in low back pain: current insights and opportunities for improvement. *J Occup Rehabil*. 2005;15(4):491-505.
26. Ha J, Longnecker N. Doctor-patient communication: a review. *Oschsner J*. 2010;10(1):38-43.
27. Webster BS, Cifuentes M. Relationship of early magnetic resonance imaging for work-related acute low back pain with disability and medical utilization outcomes. *J Occup Environ Med*. 2010;52(9):900-907.
28. Brinjikji W, Luetmer P, Comstock B, et al. Systematic literature review of imaging features of spinal degeneration in asymptomatic populations. *Am J Neuroradiology*. 2015;36:811-816.
29. Okada E, Matsumoto M, Fujiwara H, Toyama Y. Disc degeneration of cervical spine on MRI in patients with lumbar disc herniation: comparison study with asymptomatic volunteers. *Eur Spine J*. 2011;20:585-591.
30. Jensen MC, Brant-Zawadzki MN, Obuchowski N, et al. Magnetic resonance imaging of the lumbar spine in people without back pain. *N Engl J Med*. 1994;331(2):69-73.
31. Jensen MC, Brant-Zawadzki MN, Obuchowski N, et al. Magnetic resonance imaging of the lumbar spine in people without back pain. *N Engl J Med*. 1994;331(2):69-73.
32. Long A, May S, Fung T. The comparative prognostic value of directional preference and centralization: a useful tool for front-line clinicians? *J Man Manip Ther*. 2008;16(4):248-254.
33. Albert H, Hauge E, Manniche C. Centralization in patients with sciatica: are pain responses to repeated movement and positioning associated with outcome or types of disc lesions? *Eur Spine J*. 2012;21(4):630-636.
34. Long A, Donelson R, Fung T. Does it matter which exercise? A randomized control trial of exercise for low back pain. *Spine*. 2004;29(23):2593-2602.
35. Quebec Task Force on Spinal Disorders, "Scientific approach to the assessment and management of activity-related spinal disorders,". *Spine*. 1987;12:S1-S59.
36. Spratt K. *Statistical Relevance. Orthopaedic Knowledge Update: Spine*. Vol. 2. Rosemont, IL: American Academy of Orthopaedic Surgeons; 2002:497-505.
37. Loisel P, Vachon B, Lemaire J, et al. Discriminative and predictive validity assessment of the Quebec task force classification. *Spine*. 2002;27(8):851-857.
38. Pransky G, Borkan J, Young A, Cherkin D. Are we making progress?: The tenth international forum for primary care research on low back pain. *Spine*. 2011;36(19):1608-1614.
39. Costa LC, Koes B, Pransky G, et al. Primary care research priorities in low back pain: an update. *Spine*. 2013;38(2):148-156.
40. van Tulder M, Furlan A, Bombardier C, et al. Updated method guidelines for systematic reviews in the Cochrane Collaboration back review group. *Spine*. 2003;28(12): 1290-1299.
41. Hartigan C, Rainville J, Sobel JB, et al. Long term exercise adherence following aggressive rehabilitation for chronic low back pain. *Med Sci Sports Exerc*. 2000;32:551-557.
42. Hagen K, Hilde G, Jamtvedt G, Winnem M. Bed rest for acute low-back pain and sciatica. *Cochrane Database Syst Rev*. 2004;(4):CD001254.
43. White N, Delitto A, Manal T, Miller S. The American Physical Therapy Association's top five Choosing Wisely recommendations. *Phys Ther*. 2015;95(1):9-24.
44. Unterrainer A. Postoperative and preincisional electrical nerve stimulation TENS reduce postoperative opioid requirements after major spinal surgery. *J Neurosurg Anesthesiol*. 2010;22:1-5.
45. Wellington J. Noninvasive and alternative management of chronic low back pain (efficacy and outcomes). *Neuromodulation*. 2014;17(S-2):24-30.
46. Khadilkar A, Odebiyi D, Brosseau L, et al. Transcutaneous electrical nerve stimulation (TENS) versus placebo for chronic low-back pain. *Cochrane Database Syst Rev*. 2008;(4):CD003008.
47. Johnson M, Paley C, Howe T, Sluka K. Transcutaneous electrical nerve stimulation for acute pain. *Cochrane Database Syst Rev*. 2015;(6):CD006142.
48. Deyo R, Walsh N, Martin D, Schoenfeld L, Ramamurthy S. A controlled trial of transcutaneous electrical nerve stimulation (TENS) and exercise for chronic low back pain. *N Engl J Med*. 1990;322:1627-1634.

49. Deleted in review.
50. Miller N, Smith N, Bailey M, et al. Overview of therapeutic ultrasound applications and safety. *J Ultrasound Med*. 2012; 31(4):623-634.
51. Ebadi S, Henschke N, et al. Therapeutic ultrasound for chronic low-back pain. *Cochrane Database Syst Rev*. 2014;(3):CD009169.
52. Poon TH, Carus C. The effectiveness of laser therapy on the management of chronic low back pain. *Int J Ther Rehabil*. 2016;23(9):432-443.
53. Deleted in review.
54. Cheng Y, Huang G. Efficacy of massage therapy on pain and dysfunction in patients with neck pain: a systematic review and meta-analysis. *Evid Based Complement Alternat Med*. 2014. Epub ahead of print.
55. Bervoets D, Luijsterburg P, et al. Massage therapy has short-term benefits for people with common musculoskeletal disorders compared to no treatment: a systematic review. *J Physiother*. 2015;61:106-116.
56. Kumar S, Beaton K, Hughes T. The effectiveness of massage therapy for the treatment of nonspecific low back pain: a systematic review of systematic reviews. *Int J Gen Med*. 2013; 6:733-741.
57. Furlan A, Giraldo M, Baskwill A, Irvin E, Imamura M. Massage for low-back pain. *Cochrane Database Syst Rev*. 2015;(9):CD001929.
58. Wegner I, Widyahening I, van Tulder M, et al. Traction for low-back pain with or without sciatica. *Cochrane Database Syst Rev*. 2013;(8):CD003010.
59. Yang J, Tam K, et al. Intermittent cervical traction for treating neck pain: a meta-analysis of randomized controlled trials. *Spine*. 2017;42(13):959-965.
60. Van der Heijden G, Beurskens A, Koes B, et al. The efficacy of traction for back and neck pain: a systematic, blinded review of randomized clinical trial methods. *Phys Ther*. 1995;75:93-104.
61. White N, Delitto A, Manal T, Miller S. The American Physical Therapy Association's top five Choosing Wisely recommendations. *Phys Ther*. 2015;95(1):9-24.
62. Frantsve L, Kerns R. Patient-provider interactions in the management of chronic pain: current findings within the context of shared medical decision making. *Pain Med*. 2007; 8(1):25-35.
63. Hayden J, Van Tulder MW, et al. Exercise therapy for treatment of non-specific low back pain. *Cochrane Database Syst Rev*. 2005;(3):CD000335.
64. Cramer H, Lauche R, Haller H, Dobos G. A systematic review and meta-analysis of yoga for low back pain. *Clin J Pain*. 2013;29(5):450-460.
65. Pengel L, Herbert R, Maher C, Refshauge K. Acute low back pain: systematic review of its prognosis. *Br Med J*. 2003;327:1-5.
66. GBD 2015 Disease and Injury Incidence and Prevalence Collaborators. Global, regional, and national incidence, prevalence, and years lived with disability for 310 diseases and injuries, 1990-2015: a systematic analysis for the Global Burden of Disease Study 2015. *Lancet*. 2016;388:1545-1602.
67. Dagenais S, Caro J, Haldeman S. A systematic review of low back pain cost of illness studies in the United States and internationally. *Spine J*. 2008;8:8-20.
68. Karlen E, McCathie B. Implementation of a quality improvement process aimed to deliver higher-value physical therapy for patients with low back pain: case report. *Phys Ther*. 2015;95(12):1712-1721.
69. Blackmore C, Mecklenburg R, Kaplan G. At Virginia Mason, collaboration among providers, employers, and health plans to transform care cut costs and improved quality. *Health Aff*. 2011;30(9):1680-1687.
70. Donelson R, Spratt K. The impact of a precise mechanical diagnosis for low back pain: a cost comparison with standard community care. *Spine J*. 2016;16(10):S301.
71. Smeets RJ, Vlaeyen JW, et al. Reduction of pain catastrophizing mediates the outcome of both physical and cognitive-behavioral treatment in chronic low back pain. *J Pain*. 2006;7(4):261-271.
72. Furlan AD, Pennick V, et al. 2009 updated method guidelines for systematic reviews in the Cochrane Back Review Group. *Spine*. 2009;34(18):1929-1941.
73. Hill JC, Whitehurst DG, Lewis M, et al. Comparison of stratified primary care management for low back pain with current best practice (STarT Back): a randomised controlled trial. *Lancet*. 2011;378(9802):1560-1571.
74. Garratt AM, Moffett JK, Farrin AJ. Responsiveness of generic and specific measures of health outcome in low back pain. *Spine*. 2001;26(1):71-77.
75. Garcy P, Mayer T, Gatchel RJ. Recurrent or new injury outcomes after return to work in chronic disabling spinal disorders: tertiary prevention efficacy of functional restoration treatment. *Spine*. 1996;21(8):952-959.
76. Mayer TG, Polatin P, Smith B, et al. Spine rehabilitation: secondary and tertiary nonoperative care. *Spine*. 1995;20(18): 2060-2066.
77. Mayer T, McMahon MJ, Gatchel RJ, et al. Socioeconomic outcomes of combined spine surgery and functional restoration in workers' compensation spinal disorders with matched controls. *Spine*. 1998;23(5):598-605.

CHAPTER 111 Functional Restoration in Chronic Spinal Pain

Tom G. Mayer
Randy Neblett
Peter B. Polatin

Functional Restoration Principles

Functional restoration is an intensive and goal-oriented form of interdisciplinary chronic pain management. It was originally developed at the Productive Rehabilitation Institute of Dallas for Ergonomics (PRIDE) to treat individuals with chronic spinal pain (CSP) who are disabled from performing important activities of daily living (ADLs), including work duties. It is now applicable to many forms of chronic pain in addition to CSP, which are injury related or involve the spine as a noninjury "target area" (see Chapter 108). The success of this treatment approach in restoring function to disabled individuals depends on several crucial principles common to all credible functional restoration programs, which include the following:

- Medical supervision: A functional restoration program has a medical director, or multidisciplinary medical team, providing medical supervision and consultation on related or comorbid medical issues.
- Quantitative assessment of physical and psychological function: Objective measurements of physical performance guide the measurement-driven physical training. Physical measurements are aimed at both the painful "weak link" body part(s) and whole-body functioning. A mental health assessment, including a clinical interview and validated self-report questionnaires (graded by severity levels to aid with clinical interpretation), help complete a whole-person functional assessment.
- Integrated interdisciplinary treatment team on site: A functional restoration program must have an integrated treatment team whose members are on site, full time, and dedicated entirely to the care of program patients.
- Outcome tracking: Because functional restoration is frequently a last option for CSP treatment, outcomes after the program represent the outcome of a full course of surgical and nonoperative therapies performed over an extended period of time. Objective, measurable outcomes (including socioeconomic variables and validated self-report questionnaires) are critical components of functional restoration programs and their quality assurance.

Irrespective of whether the CSP origin is injury related or not and surgically treated or not, virtually all such patients have, to a greater or lesser extent, several crucial pathologies in their multifactorial pain process. These include:

- A presumed musculoskeletal degenerative, postinjury or postoperative structural pain generator of a mechanical nature for which interventions and the passage of time have maximized healing beyond further correction or anticipated spontaneous recovery.
- A *deconditioning syndrome* of progressive inactivity resulting from pain (and associated psychological issues), with development of a spinal weak link relative to other uninvolved body parts. Deconditioning involves loss of motion, strength, endurance and coordination, and adversely affects function of adjacent body links.
- Development of psychosocial dysfunction (often including mood disorders, insomnia, fear-avoidance, posttraumatic stress, and central sensitization), which is sometimes accompanied by accentuation of premorbid psychiatric conditions.
- The frequent well-intentioned but often overdone tendency to overmedicate the pain, creating opioid-dependent "chemical copers," becoming progressively and comfortably accommodated to dysfunction and disability.
- Gradual decrease in commitment to social functions (e.g., work and family role) due to physical and motivational consequences of these factors, further reducing the patient's participation in family and community activities.

Functional restoration has *proven outcomes* that comprehensively deal with all of these CSP factors. Box 111.1 lists important components of a functional restoration program. Fig. 111.1 shows four treatment outcome variables, collected 1 year after completion of the PRIDE functional restoration program, over a 10-year span, from 1999 to 2008.

Introduction

It has been recognized for a long time that minimizing bed rest and maximizing an early return to activity are not harmful and

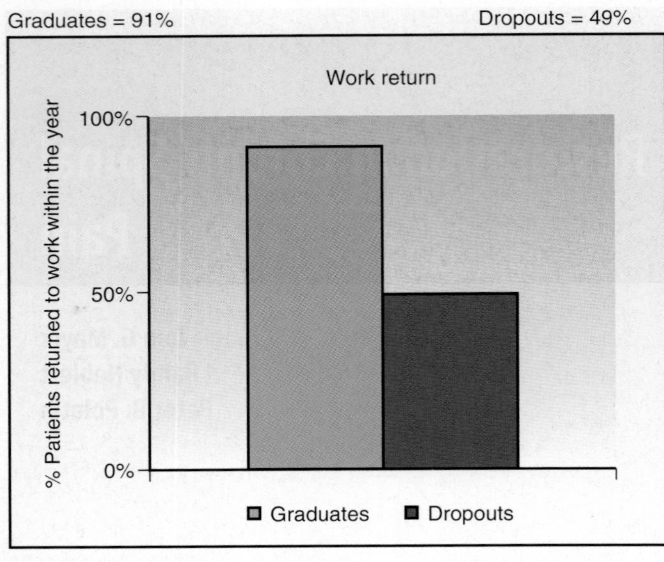

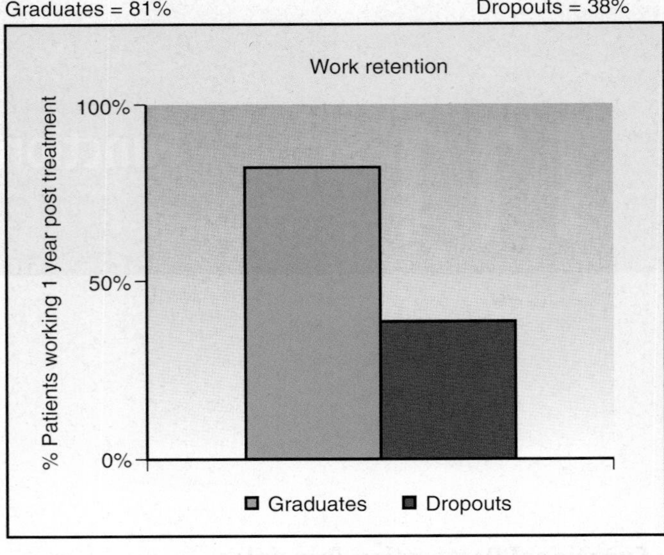

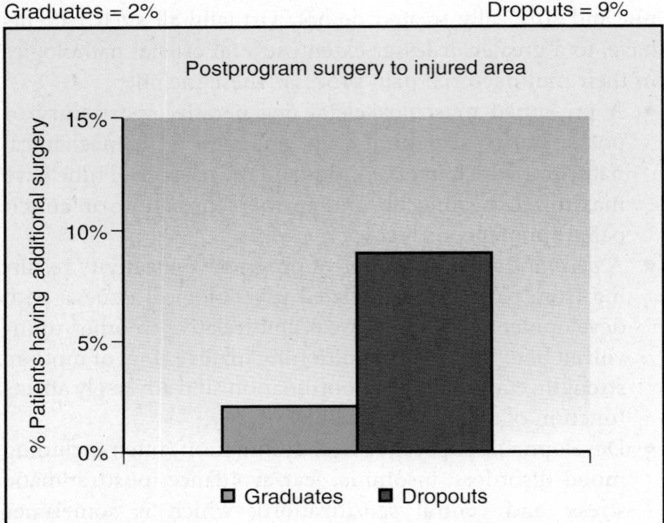

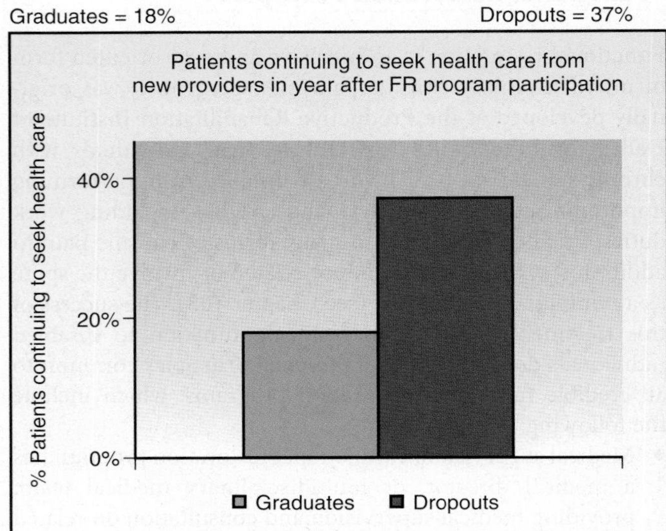

FIG. 111.1 Productive Rehabilitation Institute for Ergonomics (PRIDE) 10-year treatment outcomes (1999–2008). Data were collected from follow-up interviews and medical records 1 year after treatment discharge. FR, functional restoration.

BOX 111.1 Important Components of a Functional Restoration Program

- Quantification of physical capacity
- Quantification of psychosocial function
- Reactivation for restoration of fitness
- Measurement-driven reconditioning of the weak link functional unit
- Retraining in multiunit functional task performance
- Work simulation
- Multimodal disability management program
- Stress and pain management skills training
- Didactic classroom education
- Medication management with opioid taper
- Vocational/societal reintegration
- Formalized outcome tracking

show improved functional outcomes over "restful waiting" in 90% of patients who suffer an acute episode of low back and/or leg pain. Moreover, aggressive, quota-based rehabilitation appears to improve symptoms more rapidly than natural history in placebo-controlled trials.[1] Even without treatment, pain symptoms improve over 90 to 120 days in the majority of patients.[2] Despite medical advances, there is still a paucity of knowledge as to appropriate triage and disposition of the 10% of spinal pain patients who fail all single-provider interventions (including surgery) and absorb 80% to 90% of the money spent on spine care and associated medical issues.[3,4] Since the 1980s, integrated, interdisciplinary, advanced functional restoration rehabilitation has been recognized as the gold standard of care for treating patients who do not improve with other interventions. This chapter seeks to address the most challenging patients—those who fail to improve within 90 to 180 days with any single-provider modality—and who often receive increasingly aggressive and invasive interventions with unpredictable functional outcomes. Creating a best-practice model for this population is further complicated by the fact that CSP frequently does not correlate with radiologic findings nor do treatment outcomes correlate with radiologic criteria for success.[5,6]

A phasic nonoperative care model of primary, secondary, and tertiary modes of treatment of spinal disorders has become widely accepted. The concepts underlying this model have been identified in consensus panel documents provided by the North American Spine Society and national treatment guidelines.[7] Each mode brings with it greater expense but commensurately greater functional return in exchange for the increased cost. Briefly outlined, *primary care* refers to modalities applied during the acute injury phase, intended to modify symptoms during tissue healing. These include—but are not limited to—manual techniques, early single-specialty mobilization, and educational programs. So-called passive modalities may include immobilization after surgery, electrical stimulation, temperature modulation, and traction. Treatment is customarily provided by a single professional, with a limited number of treatments applied to a large number of acute-phase patients who appear clinically and radiologically appropriate.

Secondary care refers to therapy provided to a smaller number of patients not responding to initial symptom-modification treatment. Postacute or postoperative symptoms often require care plans focused on physical reactivation, combining quota-based exercise programs with education. Occasionally, additional passive modalities are employed for symptom modification. The main aim is to prevent late-phase deconditioning that is associated with prolonged inactivity in the transition from functional impairment to disability. In some cases, secondary care may have a degree of programmatic consolidation (e.g., work conditioning or work hardening), particularly toward the end of the postacute period. The lead role in secondary care is usually performed by physical and occupational therapists, with physicians, mental health professionals, social workers, disability managers, and/or chiropractors acting as consultants to ensure progress back to maximal function.

The small percentage of patients who fail to respond to secondary care, or those who fail to benefit from complex surgical procedures, become chronically impaired. These patients often respond positively to a *tertiary care* environment as the final option to regain lost function. When functional restoration, for one reason or another, is not made available, these patients are frequently consigned to opioids and repeated failed interventions, which are delivered with no strategy for functional recovery. Although tertiary rehabilitation is strongly advocated in national guidelines, physician awareness remains limited, as does the availability of tertiary care. Treatment management guidelines, such as the *Official Disability Guidelines*[8] (*ODG*) or from the American College of Occupational and Environmental Medicine,[9] identify evidence-based standards that are common to reputable tertiary-care programs. Increasingly, these guidelines, which define minimum standards of assessment and treatment, carry the weight of law in many large states and Canadian provinces. Although tertiary-level treatment is heterogeneous by nature, these guidelines help enforce minimum standards in configuration and outcomes for chronic pain management and functional restoration programs to meet the needs of a diverse population.

SECTION XVI

Which Patients Are Likely to Benefit From Functional Restoration?

As noted previously, the 10% of patients with injuries whose spinal pain becomes chronic accounts for 90% of the cost of health care utilization and disability benefits for this disease category.[10] The more chronic the spinal disorder becomes (the longer time passes after the injury without symptom resolution and return to normal functioning), the more likely that patients will become more severely disabled from normal ADLs. Chronic pain and disability are usually accompanied by psychosocial stress, social withdrawal, depression/anxiety, physical deconditioning, substantial losses (including loss of finances, sleep, and physical functioning), and declining coping skills. A biopsychosocial perspective views chronic pain and associated dysfunction as a complex interaction of biologic, psychological, and social variables, and is an essential concept in the treatment of this myriad of interacting symptoms.[11]

The inability to confront and overcome losses—combined with the downward spiral of pain, disability, and psychosocial distress—may lead CSP patients to overuse opioid medication, benzodiazepines, and other symptom-mediating medications, usually under the direction of a well-meaning physician who sees no other options. This single-modality approach can lead to further physical disuse and withdrawal from ADLs. Until very recently, it has become an increasing feature of the worker's compensation (WC) injury system that insurance carriers intentionally enable and encourage opioid dependence for chronically disabled CSP patients as an alternative to intensive rehabilitation and functional recovery. The carriers have been allowed to "cost shift" financial benefit responsibility to the federal government through Social Security Disability Income (SSDI) and health care to Medicare, while using various legal strategies to declare results of the injury "resolved," thus negating further responsibility for the state WC system. The more recent focus on the harmful effects of opioid addiction and the loss of worker productivity for a large segment of the working-age population receiving "permanent disability payments" under SSDI has begun a trend of the federal government pushing back, at least initially with Medicare set-asides.

Since Progressive Resistance Exercise programs were developed for the orthopedic rehabilitation of soldiers after World War II,[12,13] we have learned much about the secondary physical changes accompanying immobilization, disuse, and deconditioning in the spine and extremities. Spontaneous healing or surgical intervention may produce structural recovery of disrupted musculoskeletal tissues in a relatively short 6- to 12-week time period. In cases of severe injury, permanent tissue changes often remain after maximal tissue healing in the form of deformed bony structures or soft tissue instability and scarring. These structural pathologic changes may lead to permanent biomechanical derangements that can produce chronic pain. At its most severe, the structural changes may also include arthrofibrosis, perineural scarring, adhesive joint capsulitis, joint subluxations, and development of sympathetically mediated neuropathic pain syndromes.

One path for the development of CSP in many spinal injury patients is explained by the fear-avoidance model. Fear-avoidance is a nonadaptive style for coping with pain, involving avoidance of ADLs due to fear of increased pain and/or fear of injury/reinjury.[14,15] There is evidence that elevated fear-avoidance levels during the acute or subacute spinal pain phase can increase the risk that the pain will become chronic.[16,17] In contrast to spinal pain patients who engage in adaptive behaviors (attempt to "stay positive," maintain their mobility, and gradually increase their level of daily activities following their injuries), the fear-avoidant patient begins to catastrophize and anticipate increased pain and possible reinjury with increased activity. These dysfunctional thought patterns lead to overprotection of injured body parts, hypervigilance (overmonitoring of physical symptoms), decreased physical activity, decreased social interaction, and increased and exaggerated pain perceptions.[18] Chronically inhibited movement, physical disuse, and avoidance of normal ADLs will inevitably result in physical deconditioning, which is characterized by decreased elasticity of muscles and tendons, decreased range of motion (ROM) of joints, decreased muscle strength, weakness of the cardiovascular system, impairment of normal healing, and somewhat less common neuropathic or central pain phenomena (e.g., complex regional pain syndrome or central sensitization).[19,20] Fear-avoidance of increased movement and activity is self-reinforcing because attempts to increase activities very often result in pain flare-ups, muscle spasms, or muscle strains, due to the deconditioning syndrome.[10]

The deconditioning syndrome is usually reversible and correctable through training and education in contrast to many of the permanent structural changes referred to previously. Deconditioning involves loss of capsular elasticity, leading to progressive loss of joint motion (and sometimes even to complete rigidity or "frozen" joints).[21] Deconditioning also includes loss of neuromuscular function, leading to muscle fiber atrophy and attendant loses of strength, endurance, recruitment, and coordination. These localized musculoskeletal deficits in the injured, or target weak link, are often accompanied by more generalized aerobic capacity deficits. As the combination of structural and deconditioning pain and physical deficits take hold, inactivity and further deconditioning are accentuated in a vicious cycle of declining physical functioning.

In addition to physical deconditioning, central sensitization can become a contributing factor in chronic spinal pain. Central sensitization is a phenomenon in which neuronal dysregulation in the central nervous system results in hypersensitivity to both noxious and nonnoxious stimuli.[22] It has generally been associated with functional disorders, such as fibromyalgia, but it has become increasingly recognized that central sensitization is a factor for many CSP patients.[23,24] Evidence suggests that, after a painful spinal injury, a series of events (including hyperalgesia, allodynia, deficiency in descending and/or ascending central modulatory mechanisms, cognitive-emotional sensitization, and sensorimotor conflicts) occur in a subgroup of spinal pain patients, leading to central reorganization that maintains pain in the absence of ongoing peripheral nociception.[25] One longitudinal study found that spinal pain patients are more likely to develop widespread pain as regional spinal pain becomes more chronic.[23] Two separate studies conducted in functional restoration treatment populations found that 32% of CSP patients also met the American College of Rheumatology diagnostic criteria for chronic widespread pain,[26] and 23% of chronic musculoskeletal pain disorder patients met criteria for comorbid fibromyalgia.[27] Patients with central sensitization often develop central sensitivity syndromes (CSSs), with a long list of associated maladies that often result in disability and/or opioid dependence. These CSSs include fibromyalgia, chronic fatigue syndrome, irritable bowel syndrome, migraine headaches, myofascial pain, and others. The high likelihood of fear-avoidance and opioid dependence with these patients makes them excellent candidates for functional restoration.

Physical deconditioning, high pain sensitivity, psychosocial distress, and social withdrawal inevitably result in a high prevalence of psychopathology in many CSP patients.[28] Rates of both premorbid and postinjury psychiatric illness in the CSP population (e.g., major depression, substance abuse, anxiety disorders, personality disorders, childhood trauma) are much higher than for the US population in general.[29,30] An especially strong relationship has been found between chronic pain and major depressive disorder, in which comorbidity may reach over 50% as compared to US population estimates of 5% to 17%.[31] Furthermore, psychiatric symptoms (especially anxiety and substance disorders) have been found to precede the spinal injury for many CSP patients. In addition to psychiatric diagnoses, patient-reported symptoms of depression, anxiety, sleep disturbance, and perceived disability tend to be highly elevated for the average patient who enters functional restoration.[32–36]

With all of these factors leading to partial or total disability from work, recreation, or the family role, it is not at all surprising that many different groups of CSP patients are eligible for a functional restoration program. By its nature, it is especially suitable for work-related injuries, WC cases, or other types of *compensation injuries* (long-term disability, Social Security Disability, motor vehicle accidents). Patients who have become totally disabled from work by CSP are the most obvious candidates for functional restoration and are usually discovered and referred first. Delay in pursing surgical intervention or multiple surgeries sometimes leads to significant worsening of CSP by increasing the longevity of chronicity of disability, and these patients may present for treatment late. In today's competitive workplace and WC state systems, injured workers may be returned to duty prematurely and may have difficulty moving from part-time or light-duty work back to performing full-duty materials handling or positional requirements.

In addition to WC cases, functional restoration can be equally effective for treating patients with chronic pain and

BOX 111.2 Patients Likely to Benefit From Functional Restoration

- Worker's compensation injuries developing chronic partial/total disability
- Postoperative patients with long periods of disability and disuse due to prolonged surgical recovery
- Patients developing neuropathic or sympathetically mediated regional pain or radiculopathy disorders
- Central sensitization with a spinal target area
- Central sensitivity syndromes (e.g., fibromyalgia)
- Patients becoming deconditioned through fear-avoidance
- Patients developing disability primarily due to opioid dependence
- Patients enabled to disability by cost shifting to federal financial and health benefits

disability related to noncompensable injuries or pain of insidious onset.[37–39] In countries such as Sweden, where access to the best health care does not require an injury, the majority of CSP symptoms are reported by patients to begin insidiously rather than with a reported "incident or injury." In the United States, while a majority of patients report that their symptoms started from an "injury," a large subset of chronic pain patients begins insidiously and may be associated with various psychiatric or other comorbid conditions, often characterized by central sensitization and/or opioid dependence. Many patients with CSP from an insidious origin develop their disability slowly over years. Some patients develop spinal deconditioning through enforced disuse from other medical or nonmedical situations; these patients may develop disability due as much to the deconditioning as to the primary disease or other process that originally led to the inactivity. Once partial or total disability associated with a CSP disorder has developed, such patients are excellent candidates for functional restoration (Box 111.2).

The interaction of fear-avoidance of ADLs, social withdrawal, physical deconditioning, high pain sensitivity, opioid overuse, psychosocial distress, and psychopathology is complex. If all of these biopsychosocial factors are not addressed effectively, the treatment is likely to fail. When addressing these interacting factors, it is important to understand that many chronic spinal patients have lost hope and self-esteem. It is not simply a matter of prescribing an antidepressant and putting them into physical therapy (PT). Treatment success requires sustained encouragement and education from the treatment team to guide patients through the therapeutic process, which helps them "see the light at the end of the tunnel" and recognize that they have a chance for a more positive future and the ability to function successfully with normal ADLs, including sustained employment.

Interdisciplinary Functional Restoration Treatment Team

In a functional restoration program, a team of professionals works together with each patient toward a common goal of increasing physical and psychosocial functioning. Team members provide services within their individual disciplines to address the physical and psychosocial barriers that are preventing patients from reaching their full functional potential. In contrast to multidisciplinary treatment, in which all team members may or may not provide services in the same clinic and may or may not communicate regularly, all interdisciplinary team members in a functional restoration program provide treatment in the same facility. They communicate on a daily basis, both formally (in case conference meetings) and informally, and are always available to address patient needs as they arise. The functional restoration treatment team includes a supervising medical director, nursing staff, physical and occupational therapists, mental health professionals, and rehabilitation counselors (case managers).

The supervising medical director or multidisciplinary medical team helps to guide the rehabilitation program and treatment team. The physician must have a general background in sports medicine, musculoskeletal injury, psychoactive medications, disability management, and rehabilitation supervision. The medical director is usually assisted by a nurse "physician extender" or practitioner who must be able to educate patients on medical matters, triage musculoskeletal problems, provide medication control, and communicate with outside agencies about medical issues as they arise.

Both the physical and occupational therapists guide patients through mobility, strength, endurance, coordination, and core stability exercises while providing patient education on active pain management strategies. They supervise group stretch classes and gyms on a daily basis and work individually with patients as needed. The physical and occupational therapists may also have a team of exercise technicians who help monitor and guide patients through individual and group exercises. Physical therapists are responsible for ROM and strength assessments, and they supervise most of the progressive resistive exercises for individual joints or targeted weak link spine areas. Occupational therapists work more with whole-body functional activity simulation to help individuals overcome physical obstacles that are limiting productivity at work and home. They are also primarily responsible for functional capacity examinations at program admission and discharge. At the original PRIDE functional restoration program, the functional capacity evaluation (FCE), isokinetic testing, and other functional measurements are compared to a normative database (based on age, gender, and body mass index) to discover an initial tolerable training level in measurement-driven training. This is applied in the PT gym, where regional spinal or extremity weak links are trained, and in the occupational therapy (OT) gyms, where whole-person materials handling or positional requirements are trained. A computerized 75-step progressive resistance training program is also individualized to the patient population to ensure slow but steady recovery of function.

Mental health professionals are a vital component of functional restoration and can come from a variety of similar disciplines, including psychology, counseling, social work, and marriage and family therapy. They can provide a variety of services, including mental health assessments, supportive psychotherapy, psycho-education, and cognitive-behavioral therapy. They must address psychosocial factors, which can impede physical progress and return to optimal functioning.

Rehabilitation counselors/case managers oversee each patient's case. They must be knowledgeable about insurance coverage rules and federal and state WC guidelines. They communicate with payer sources and employers, provide vocational assessments and counseling, and facilitate referrals to state agencies for vocational assistance as needed. The case managers often function as team leaders within the program to identify the minority of patients who are progressing slowly (or not at all), highlighting the socioeconomic secondary gain issues that may be causing nonorganic illness behaviors, and setting up patient and family conferences to deal with crucial issues such as nonattendance, failures of cooperation and compliance, and patient frustration. They work closest with the supervising physician on behavioral issues during the program and provide documentation at the conclusion of the program on functional limitations, work return capabilities, and job plans. The case managers also supervise the outcome tracking process.

Functional Restoration Preliminaries

Initial Physician Evaluation

All team members must be involved from the outset in the initial assessment and quantification of barriers to the patient's recovery. This effort should be led by a medical director or physician member of the team, who, along with the nursing staff, performs an outpatient medical examination to review history, physical findings, and relevant radiologic or other diagnostic data. The intent of this visit is fourfold. First, the physician should look for medical barriers that were overlooked during previous evaluations and ensure that existing tissue damage is unlikely to improve with additional surgical intervention or activity limitation. Second, the physician should assess the degree to which psychosocial distress is causing other physiologic barriers such as insomnia, mood disorder, fear-avoidance, central sensitization, or inorganic signs that will undermine the success of the individual patient. Third, the physician should identify and document the patient's desired outcome from this intervention. Finally, a physician should make every attempt to establish a therapeutic relationship and provide education to overcome resistance to treatment. As the team leader, the physician should take care to avoid a confrontation at this meeting (this is occasionally the desired secondary gain outcome of some patients) by reassuring patients that they have a choice and that the shared outcome of this visit is that patients give the program a chance. Often, this is achieved by empowering patients to evaluate the program at the same time the program is evaluating them. Simultaneously, the physician should take note of specific declared goals of the patient and pass these along to the evaluating team to ensure early bonding through shared understanding that team members are aware of and supportive of the patient's functional goals. Additionally, this is the first opportunity for the physician and nursing staff to help clarify and guide the patient's treatment expectations, to make it plain that the primary outcome of the program is functional return, and to introduce the concept that disability is a choice.

A potentially useful component of the initial evaluation is the physician's proposal of the Surgical Option Process (SOP).[40,41] It comes into play if there is uncertainty or disagreement about whether a surgical option is likely to enhance recovery. In many cases, such uncertainty may bring the medical care sequence to a grinding halt related to this indecision. The SOP has recently been presented as an effective method of overcoming this recovery barrier. The patient who enters functional restoration with a surgical option agrees to participate in the first 50% of the program. At that point, an SOP determination meeting with the physician allows the patient to select the option to either *pursue or decline surgery.* If the patient decides to pursue surgery, the program is placed on medical hold while the patient pursues renewed surgical consultation and a pathway to a fresh determination of whether surgery is likely to be beneficial in the face of the patient's personal assessment that it is needed. Those who decline surgery simply complete the program. In a pilot and subsequent larger study, outcomes of the SOP have proven very promising.[40,41] In 70% of patients who elected to decline surgery, almost all (99%) continued to avoid surgical intervention over the postprogram year. Of the 30% who decided to pursue surgery, about half ended up receiving it, while the other half did not. Most of the patients failing to receive surgery after electing to pursue it were denied based on the determination by their surgeon or consultant (and rarely by a patient or an insurance carrier denial). Using the SOP model, delays in treatment that lead to further physical and psychosocial declines are avoided by the application of a decisive methodology.

If the patient is deemed appropriate for nonsurgical treatment, the physician should first initiate an interdisciplinary evaluation and then follow up with the patient in a second physician visit to go over the results. The results of this interdisciplinary evaluation determine whether a full or abbreviated functional restoration program will be requested. Lesser levels of care might still be feasible for patients who are working, have very limited disability, or have minimal psychosocial barriers and who have relatively high physical ability. Individual therapies, or work conditioning/hardening–equivalent treatments are available for those not requiring a full tertiary functional restoration program.

Interdisciplinary Evaluation

The functional restoration interdisciplinary team is in charge of the two-component evaluation. First, the Physical Department performs PT and OT individual assessments, followed by an FCE. The details of the FCE are discussed later in this chapter. Second, the Disability Management Team, consisting of mental health professionals and case managers, performs two critical interviews. The first is a formal mental health evaluation, while the second explores social and economic factors associated with the patient's disability, leading to identification of barriers to recovery and a plan to meet treatment goals. These components of preparing for a multimodal disability management process are also discussed later in the chapter. The results of this evaluation are shared with the patient at the second physician visit and are presented to referring physicians and payers during the treatment preauthorization process.

Second Physician Visit

The physician team leader takes the quantitative evaluations and initiates a frank discussion with the patient on the basis of firm data. It is hoped that the patient has bonded with one or more of the staff members in the course of the assessment process and has been impressed with the thorough assessment and milieu of function at the facility. If the patient agrees to proceed, the physician plans the length of the program on the basis of achieving maximum function. Instead of making patients "good as new," the team tries to focus patients on functional goals and manage their expectations toward reaching a functional plateau—possessing the physical strength and endurance to remain at a job and the psychological tools to control pain and cope with daily stressors. It is hoped that this important meeting will readjust patient expectations to internalize the concept of continued recovery after the program—keeping the patient focused on getting "good enough" rather than perfect. On the basis of objective data from the initial interdisciplinary assessment rather than simply relying on subjective pain reports, patients have set their own speedometer for the length and intensity of the treatment program. With the patient's agreement to participate in treatment, a comprehensive medication management strategy is also discussed with the patient. This strategy involves the use of medications specifically related to the findings of the initial evaluation to help control the identified problems (e.g., pain, inflammation, mood disorder, insomnia, neuropathic factors, cognitive issues, and/or central sensitization). It is important that patients understand that new medications and dosages may be prescribed at this point with the intention of reducing medication as pain recovery and functional improvement progress. Finally, the patient's agreement to enter the program is a tacit agreement to pursue functional posttreatment goals that are primarily vocational and societal but may also include familial and educational enrichment.

Insurance Preauthorization

It is a reality of current medical practice that almost every insurance system now requires preauthorization for complex treatments; functional restoration interdisciplinary programs are no exception. Over the past decade, this process has been streamlined to some degree by the acceptance of national guidelines that have been previously discussed.[8,9] Most state and federal worker's compensation carriers now have a preauthorization process, often delegated to a semi-independent vendor and guided by some type of state or federal rules. The peer review process involves submission of data for determination of authorization, usually overseen by a semi-independent physician evaluation, and often permitting a telephonic peer call between the requesting facility staff and peer reviewer. There is usually a single reconsideration appeal process inherent in the system. Whatever the methodology, the results of the physician assessment and interdisciplinary evaluation become integral to the approval or denial of the program within these systems. At this writing, such a formal preauthorization process is not generally part of group health coverage and the rules regarding interdisciplinary pain management are heterogeneous and arcane. There is also a large variation between what is permitted in hospital and outpatient settings. It is anticipated that the consolidation of national health care system reforms will ultimately create some standardization and clarity, but right now the ability of patients outside the WC system to participate in such programs may be limited in scope by financial barriers. In some states, state vocational rehabilitation agencies may provide some supplementation to medical insurance to assist patient rehabilitation for vocational recovery and preparation for retraining or work placement options.

Physical and Functional Capacity Assessment

For spine surgeons, the main principle to understand in tertiary level, interdisciplinary, functional restoration is that the usual way we assess activity tolerance (i.e., by endurance and pain) is, in this self-selected population, unreliable and counterproductive to functional return. As such, validated, reproducible quantitative measures of physical dysfunction must be employed to track functional gains. The FCE has become a popular term that denotes a variable set of methods and tests. Different methodologies for performing FCEs exist. They often lack specificity, physics-based principles of accuracy and precision, and comparisons to normative databases. Functional restoration requires true quantification of function because the absence of numeric data leaves physically inhibited patients and their care team enslaved by the cliché, "If it hurts too much, don't do it." An understanding of the principles of accuracy, precision, and sources of error is necessary when performing a quality FCE and interpreting the results.[42–44] In the PRIDE model of functional restoration, *physical capacity assessment* implies the assessment of the injured musculoskeletal spinal region, generally involving quantification through reproducibility of mobility, strength, and endurance of a given functional unit or around a given joint. On the other hand, the term *functional capacity assessment* implies measurement of whole-person performance—taking compensatory strategies into account in tasks that are specifically designed to stress the injured body parts (e.g., materials handling capability for lifting, carrying, or pulling, as well as tolerance of positions and activities such as sitting, standing, walking, and climbing). Research has focused on responsiveness of prerehabilitation functional measurements with retesting at the end of the program and comparison to specific normative databases.[43–48] Aided by a new generation of quantitative tools and an evidence-based consensus on techniques for FCEs, a reproducible prognostic FCE is now possible, even for difficult chronic pain patients.[49,50] This innovation permits an individual patient's comparison with both normative data and an absolute job requirement for materials handling and positional tolerances.

Range-of-Motion Assessment

Trunk motion is a compound movement combining intersegmental spine and hip motion components. A patient with a completely fused spine, but very loose hamstrings, can often bend forward to perform toe touches using hip motion alone. Although it is difficult to measure intersegmental motion nonradiologically, inclinometers may be used to separate the hip motion component from the lumbar spine motion component and derive valuable information.[51,52] The basic information on inclinometry originally came from British rheumatology, and the system has been used, in one form or another, in Europe for over 50 years.[53] As with all physical capacity measures, ROM information is only useful when compared with a normative database and contextualized by an identifiable effort factor. For lumbar ROM, the effort factor is the comparison between the hip motion component and the spine straight-leg raise test measurement.[52,54]

Contrary to the belief of many clinicians, a surprising amount of information can be obtained from visual observation of sagittal and coronal lumbopelvic motion. In subjects with normal spine and hips, forward bending occurs in a sequence (easier to recognize with the observer's hands on the top of the pelvis) in which the lumbar spine flexion occurs early and faster than the hip motion component. This represents an inborn physiologic strategy, recognizable by all familiar with "stoop labor," in which the spine "hangs on the ligaments" and then descends further through the action of the more powerful gluteal musculature around a hip access. When this pattern is interrupted in a patient population, it usually represents motion limited by pain or fear, but may also point to unrecognized segmental rigidity, spasm, or efforts to deceive the examiner. Segmental rigidity is an especially important finding. It is assessed through observation of coronal movement, which is often a source of pain, and is potentially correctable by exercise alone or the combination of exercise and facet injections at the rigid levels.[21,55]

Isolated Trunk Strength Assessment

Several devices are commercially available for assessing isometric, isotonic, or isokinetic trunk strength in various planes of motion. Most involve some type of pelvic stabilization, with application of force through a line projecting between the sternum and scapulae, thus representing trunk strength as torque (torsional force) around a pelvic fulcrum with a lever arm individualized to a subject's height. Cervical dynamic strength measurement devices have been seen in prototype form but are not currently available, leaving isometrics as the only cervical alternative. Isokinetic devices stabilize the variables of acceleration and velocity in order to provide torque as the primary independent variable. Isokinetic testing narrows the Gaussian distribution of values by limiting the number of independent variables, which, in our opinion, provides a more valid test. Isometric test models employing strain gauges have been used for more than 60 years. Though commercially available, dynamic isokinetic trunk strength testing has only been available since 1985. There is abundant literature demonstrating efficacy in identifying isolated motion-segment dysfunction (differentiating weakness and/or decreased endurance) and quantifying outcome improvements. Only a few commercially available isometric or isokinetic devices still exist. PRIDE currently uses a dynamometer connected to a sagittal semi-seated torso testing device[56] (Figs. 111.2 to 111.4).

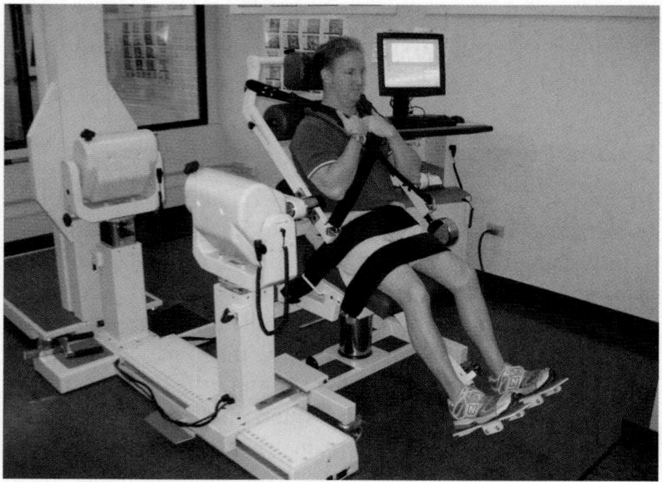

FIG. 111.2 A detachable sagittal trunk testing unit connected to a multidynametric system (Biodex 4; Biodex Inc.) that allows measurements of isolated trunk strength to be compared with normative databases related to age, gender, and body weight.

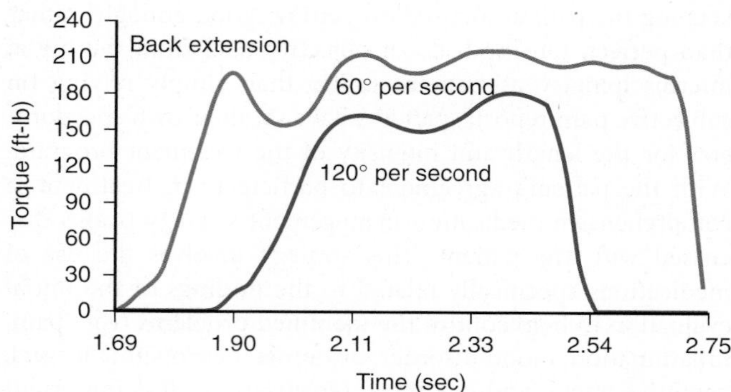

FIG. 111.3 Trunk extensor strength at two speeds (60 degrees and 120 degrees per second) for torque versus time for a normal subject on a Biodex 4 testing device.

Isolated trunk strength results from normal subjects have been compared with CSP patients with and without prior surgery.[38,45–47,57,58] Substantial differences have been shown between these groups, initially with incremental trunk strength improvement demonstrated during rehabilitation of chronically disabled spine pain patients[59,60] (see Figs. 111.3 and 111.4). The intent of all of the devices is to isolate and challenge the trunk strength component of the thoracolumbar functional unit by stabilizing above and below the area to be tested. The isolation of the vulnerable weak link portion of the vertebral biomechanical chain, linking the shoulder girdle to the pelvis, is intended to assess muscle strength and endurance just as measuring quadriceps and hamstrings is of prima facie importance to knee function. For any of the devices to be useful, the dynamometer must give accurate and reproducible

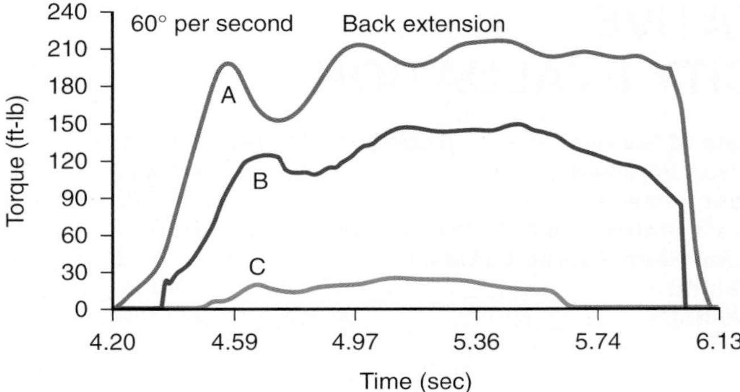

FIG. 111.4 Trunk extensor strength performance at 60 degrees/sec (Biodex 4; Biodex Inc.) demonstrating changes in strength curves anticipated during functional restoration (torque vs. time). *A*, Typical curve for a normal subject maintaining force throughout the contraction. *B*, Typical postrehabilitation patient curve demonstrating slower onset of torque (impulse) and lower torque, but with force well sustained through the contraction. *C*, Typical prerehabilitation patient demonstrating physical inhibition (also termed *fear-avoidance* or *kinesophobia*) with low impact, maximum torque, and ability to sustain torque through the predetermined test distance/time.

measurements and the testing protocol must conform exactly to the one that was employed when the normative database was created. The normative database can then be used to express the individual's results as a percent of normal.[43,45]

Cardiovascular Fitness Assessment

The inactivity that leads to deconditioning and a regional spinal motion/strength weak link in patients with CSP also reduces cardiovascular fitness, creating a feed-forward effect on decreasing weak-link endurance and overall functional tolerance. Treadmill, bicycle, and upper body ergometry have long been used to measure the cardiovascular response to a measured workload. Significant deficits in aerobic capacity are frequently present in chronic and postoperative CSP patients. These deficits are somewhat proportional to the duration of disability and the degree of inactivity.[61] Because inactivity may also produce deconditioning of arms and legs, the patient may quit the ergometry test due to limb fatigue rather than reduced cardiovascular fitness. However, these alternative scenarios can usually be distinguished either by interval monitoring of the heart rate delta achieved at the point of voluntary test termination or by comparing the upper and lower body ergometric results. In most deconditioned patients who are exerting full effort, an exaggerated heart rate response to relatively low workloads is customarily the limiting factor of the test. Such testing leads to a determination of the extent to which aerobic capacity training and/or lower and upper extremity strength training need to be added to the functional restoration program.

Whole-Body Task Performance (Functional Capacity) Assessment

The whole-body task performance assessment, usually the province of the occupational therapist, requires a skilled eye and a highly burnished insight. Whereas quantification of the isolated lumbar region has multiple internal checks, the whole-body materials handling performance component effort is subject to interference by a number of psycho-socioeconomic factors. A patient may demonstrate limited ability to lift, carry, push, or pull due to weakness, fear-avoidance, or chronic fatigue but may also avoid performing well on these tasks because of perceived financial secondary gain.[62] Physically, whole-body performance problems may be entirely due to the injured lumbar spine or may have to do with comorbid problems in the arms, upper back, or legs. Detecting the reason for suboptimal whole-body performance can sometimes be difficult. The whole-body performance assessment is divided into two major subsections that can be classified as *materials handling* and *positional tolerance*. These functional requirements can be compared to job descriptions, household tasks, or recreational demands to determine specific functional capabilities.

Lifting capacity has long been the gold standard for spine-related, materials-handling functional capacity. It is still the measurement of greatest concern to those medical and nonmedical personnel who judge the patient's work capacity or vocational suitability. The isometric lift task employed in the National Institute of Occupational Safety and Health guidelines is still in wide use and has a large comparative database, though it does not quite rectify the inherent lack of generalizability of isometric measurements. To give the full picture of any materials-handling task, several measures—including isometric, isokinetic, and isoinertial[63–66]—may be combined. All whole-person tests are standardized to provide interpretable, quantifiable information to assess the proximity to job-specific task performance, keeping the patient accountable to a specific outcome of choice. Within the domain of whole-body task performance, the subdomains of materials handling (e.g., floor-to-waist lifting, waist-to-shoulder lifting, carrying, pushing, pulling) and positional tolerance (e.g., sitting, standing, balance, stair/ladder climbing, reaching, squatting, walking, kneeling, or reaching) each have to be assessed and collated. Repeated longitudinal testing adds validity to programmatic compliance and credibility to the physician's attestation of task-specific suitability to the prospective employer. In addition, longitudinal studies, demonstrating sufficiently large differences in prerehabilitation and postrehabilitation performance measures, are an effective demonstration of the program's relevance and validity.[44,57,60]

A quantitative FCE has been developed for use in the PRIDE program. Examples of pre- and postrehabilitation FCE reports are provided in Figs. 111.5A and 111.5B, respectively. The patient entered the treatment program with 28 months of injury-related total disability and 12 months following L5–S1 fusion. His job of injury, in construction, required a very heavy physical demand level. He was terminated from his job of injury while in treatment and chose a target job goal of construction project manager. As can be seen in Fig. 111.5A, the patient tested at a below sedentary level in the initial FCE, in large part due to his inability to do any floor-to-waist lifting. Chronic pain patients are frequently so physically inhibited by their psychosocial comorbidities that "0" scores on one or more tests are not uncommon at the

QUANTITATIVE FUNCTIONAL CAPACITY EVALUATION

Name:		**Date of Service:**	01/04/2017 11:50am-3:50pm
SS#:		**Areas Involved:**	Lumbar
Age:	36	**Test:**	FCE PRE
Gender:	M	**Work Status:**	Initially full duty, off since approx. 8/14
DOI:	08/06/2014	**Total Hours Worked a Day:**	8-12
F-Class	WC	**Height:**	72 in.
Target Job Title:	Construction	**Weight:**	241 lbs.
Target DOT Category:	Very Heavy		

HISTORY

Purpose of FCE:

1. Quantification of safe functional abilities
2. Return to work and job placement decisions
3. Intervention and plan of care

Chief Complaint: Stiffness and soreness in low back, especially with cold or rainy weather

Surgery: 1/16 L5/S1 360 Fusion

Additional Health Problems: HTN (prior medication)

Mechanism of Injury: Shoveling asphalt and had a pop in low back

Patient reports difficulty or pain with:

- Balancing -"so much worse than prior"
- Climbing stairs
- Climbing ladder -unsure
- Crawling
- Kneeling -unsure, at least not prolonged
- Reaching overhead
- Sensation -numbness in left quadriceps
- Squatting -difficult with repetition
- Standing -very difficult
- Stooping -very difficult/painful
- Walking -after 1 hour, slight limp is noticed
- Twisting -difficult if with weight
- Carrying -unsure
- Lifting -unsure
- Pushing -unsure
- Pulling -unsure
- Reaching forward
- Reaching below waist

Job or Positional Demands:

Continuous:	Bending, Squatting, Stooping, Walking, Gripping, Twisting, Carrying, Lifting, Pushing, Pulling, Crouching, Kneeling, Reaching forward, Reaching below waist
Frequent:	Driving, Climbing ladder, Crawling
Occasional:	Pinching, Climbing stairs, Reaching overhead

PHYSICAL ASSESSMENT

	ROM	STRENGTH
Lumbar Spine:	Severely Deficient	Extremely Deficient
Biodex Lift (Lower Body):		Extremely Deficient
Biodex Lift (Upper Body):		Severely Deficient
Pile (Lower Body):		Extremely Deficient
Pile (Upper Body):		Severely Deficient
Gait:	Not functional relative to job demand	
Aerobic Fitness:	Low	

Patient able to complete some of the assessments.

Patient experienced moderate difficulty with the assessments.

Patient required frequent rest breaks throughout the assessments.

FIG. 111.5 (A) The quantified pain survey filled out by the patient.

PAIN LEVEL

Pre Test:	5 / 10	**Minimum level of pain reported during testing:**	5 / 10
Post Test:	6.5 / 10	**Maximum level of pain reported during testing:**	6.5 / 10

CONSISTENCY OF EFFORT

Variable based on:

- Heart rate monitoring
- Clinical observation
- Severe pain perception
- Inhibition

PHYSICAL DEMAND LEVEL (PDL)

Initial Job PDL Required:	**Very Heavy**
Lift: Floor to Waist	100+ lbs. Occasional / 50+ lbs. Frequent
Lift: Waist to Shoulder	100+ lbs. Occasional / 50+ lbs. Frequent
Carry	100+ lbs. Occasional / 50+ lbs. Frequent
Push (measured force)	100+ lbs. Occasional / 50+ lbs. Frequent
Pull (measured force)	100+ lbs. Occasional / 50+ lbs. Frequent
Tested PDL:	**Below Sedentary**
Lift: Floor to Waist	0 lbs. Occasional
Lift: Waist to Shoulder	8 lbs. Occasional / 0* lbs. Frequent
Carry	18 lbs. Occasional / 0* lbs. Frequent
Push (measured force)	36 lbs. Occasional / 0* lbs. Frequent
Pull (measured force)	36 lbs. Occasional / 0* lbs. Frequent

POSITIONAL TOLERANCE

Non-Material Handling Summary:

- Initial job demands met: None
- Initial job demands not met: Bending, Walking, Climbing stairs, Twisting, Climbing ladder

RECOMMENDATIONS/CONCLUSIONS

- FCE results are considered self-limited with some testing due to observed inhibition.
- *Patient required seated rest break between each test, so frequent tolerance was not demonstrated at this time.
- Patient did not meet lifting requirement for job.
- Patient did not meet carrying requirement for job.
- Isolated tests for ROM and/or strength identified deficits which will make it difficult or unsafe to perform bending, walking, twisting or climbing.
- Due to observed inhibition, fear avoidance, physical function limited by pain, and length of injury, this patient is a candidate for a pain management program.

A

FIG. 111.5, cont'd

Continued

initial FCE. The extreme deficits of trunk strength that he demonstrated in the Biodex lift test and the Progressive Isoinertial Lifting Evaluation indicated that he was unable to develop torque, which was likely due, at least in part, to pain inhibition. After completing the functional restoration program, however, his physical demand level had increased to heavy, which met the demands of his target job (see Fig. 111.5B). The principles underpinning an FCE in a chronic pain population are discussed in an American Medical Association book on FCEs by Galper and colleagues.[49]

In summary, quantification of physical function is a relatively new, important, but still underused tool in assessing patients with CSP. Quantification of physical functional capacity requires patient motivation, but because an effort factor can be identified by a skilled therapist with each physical capacity test, suboptimal effort can be recognized and used to evaluate and address patient fear-avoidance beliefs, hyperalgesia, or motivational barrier.

Mental Health Assessment

As stated previously, CSP is often accompanied by significant psychosocial distress, fear-avoidance of ADLs, social withdrawal, high pain sensitivity, opioid overuse, loss of self-esteem, anger, depression/anxiety, and a sense of helplessness and loss of control. These factors can inhibit functional recovery and a return to normal ADLs and can impede success in the

PRIDE

QUANTITATIVE FUNCTIONAL CAPACITY EVALUATION #4

Name:		**Date of Service:**	02/23/2017 9am-12pm
SS#:		**Areas Involved:**	Lumbar
Age:	36	**Test:**	FCE POST
Gender:	M	**Work Status:**	Terminated from job of injury.
DOI:	08/06/2014	**Total Hours Worked a Day:**	8+
F-Class	WC	**Height:**	72 in.
Target Job Title:	Construction Project Manager	**Weight:**	241 lbs.
Target DOT Category:	Heavy		

HISTORY

Purpose of FCE:

1. Quantification of safe functional abilities
2. Return to work and job placement decisions
3. Case management and case closure

Surgery: 1/16 L5/S1 360 Fusion; Prior non-related ORIF to L LE and L shoulder.

Additional Health Problems: ADHD controlled by medication. Labile hypertension not medicated.

PHYSICAL ASSESSMENT

	ROM	STRENGTH
Lumbar Spine:	Normal Range	Mildly Deficient
Biodex Lift (Lower Body):		Mildly Deficient
Biodex Lift (Upper Body):		Normal Range
Pile:		Mildly Deficient
Gait:	Within normal limits	
Aerobic Fitness:	Low	

Patient able to complete all of the assessments.

Patient experienced no difficulty with the assessments.

Patient required no breaks throughout the assessments.

CONSISTENCY OF EFFORT

Reliable based on:

- Heart rate monitoring
- Clinical observation
- Competitive behaviors
- Absence of pain behaviors
- Mild pain perception

FIG. 111.5, cont'd (B) When a "0" score occurs during physical testing, indicating that the patient is unable to demonstrate any force, it is rated as either "below sedentary" in the determination of the physical demand level (PDL), or "extremely deficient" under the isolated spinal region joint mobility or strength measures.

functional restoration program. The mental health assessment helps identify biopsychosocial barriers (depression, cognitive distortion, substance dependence, stress) so that they can be effectively addressed in treatment. The goal is not to "cure" psychosocial barriers but to provide therapeutic interventions to assist the patient in overcoming these barriers while in the functional restoration program, with the ultimate goal of maximizing successful rehabilitation and return to vocational, avocational, familial, and societal productivity. The most important mental health assessment tool is the clinical interview. Self-report tests can also be very helpful in the initial patient evaluation, in monitoring therapeutic progress during the course of treatment, and measuring final outcomes at the conclusion of the treatment program. Both of these assessment strategies are detailed in the next sections.

Clinical Interview

The clinical interview, performed by a trained and experienced mental health professional, has two primary goals. First, the interviewer seeks to identify the patient's goals and motivation for change, biopsychosocial factors that are contributing to the

PHYSICAL DEMAND LEVEL (PDL)

Initial Job PDL Required:	**Very Heavy**
Lift: Floor to Waist	100+ lbs. Occasional / 50+ lbs. Frequent
Lift: Waist to Shoulder	100+ lbs. Occasional / 50+ lbs. Frequent
Lift: Shoulder to Overhead	100+ lbs. Occasional / 50+ lbs. Frequent
Carry	100+ lbs. Occasional / 50+ lbs. Frequent
Push (measured force)	100+ lbs. Occasional / 50+ lbs. Frequent
Pull (measured force)	100+ lbs. Occasional / 50+ lbs. Frequent
Target Job PDL Required:	**Heavy**
Lift: Floor to Waist	80 lbs. Occasional / 40 lbs. Frequent
Lift: Waist to Shoulder	80 lbs. Occasional / 40 lbs. Frequent
Lift: Shoulder to Overhead	80 lbs. Occasional / 40 lbs. Frequent
Carry	80 lbs. Occasional / 40 lbs. Frequent
Push (measured force)	80 lbs. Occasional / 40 lbs. Frequent
Pull (measured force)	80 lbs. Occasional / 40 lbs. Frequent
Tested PDL:	**Heavy**
Lift: Floor to Waist	103 lbs. Occasional / 62 lbs. Frequent
Lift: Waist to Shoulder	82 lbs. Occasional / 49 lbs. Frequent
Lift: Shoulder to Overhead	82 lbs. Occasional / 49 lbs. Frequent
Carry	82 lbs. Occasional / 49 lbs. Frequent
Push (measured force)	100+ lbs. Occasional / 68 lbs. Frequent
Pull (measured force)	100+ lbs. Occasional / 86 lbs. Frequent

POSITIONAL TOLERANCE

Non-Material Handling Summary:

- Initial job demands met: Bending, Pinching, Reaching Overhead, Reaching Forward, Reaching Below Waist, Squatting, Stooping, Walking, Climbing stairs, Gripping, Twisting, Climbing ladder, Crawling, Crouching, Kneeling
- Target job demands met: Bending, Pinching, Reaching Overhead, Reaching Forward, Reaching Below Waist, Squatting, Stooping, Walking, Climbing stairs, Gripping, Twisting, Climbing ladder, Crawling, Crouching, Kneeling

RECOMMENDATIONS/CONCLUSIONS

- FCE results are considered valid.
- Lifting recommendations are based on testing and performance during program.
- Recommend that patient continue with an Independent Home Exercise Program to address flexibility and strength of lumbar musculature.
- Perform job duties in the Heavy physical demand category.
- The patient is seeking employment in construction project management. No restrictions for this alternate job plan.

B

FIG. 111.5, cont'd

patient's disability, and risk factors predicting treatment failure. The second objective is to begin building a therapeutic alliance to help the patient overcome obstacles and maximize treatment success. Specifically, the clinical interview assesses personal/family medical, psychiatric, and substance abuse history; the presence of depression/anxiety, sleep disturbance, and fear-avoidance beliefs; and history of cognitive disorders. Financial, interpersonal, and work-related stressors are evaluated (including job losses, job change, and job satisfaction). In addition, secondary gain issues, including pending litigation, are identified, which may affect the patient's trust, motivation, and treatment success.

Self-Report Questionnaires

Self-report questionnaires, which have more recently been termed patient-reported outcome (PRO) measures, are easy to use and can provide a helpful adjunct to the clinical interview. Periodic retesting can provide relevant information about the patient's self-perceived psychosocial response to treatment. A wide range of clinical PRO measures can assess specific psychosocial factors related to CSP. Though subjective and qualitative, they provide a method for quantifying and monitoring the levels of psychosocial distress that patients are experiencing. Test results can help screen for more serious psychopathology, including psychosis and suicidal ideation, which demand an immediate therapeutic response. Repeated self-report testing can also be a helpful measure of clinical progress. Lack of positive change as patients progress through treatment is a red flag for the treatment team, requiring a closer reevaluation of the patient's motivations, perceived response to treatment, trust in the treatment team, and alignment with therapeutic goals.

PRO scores have also been used with the concept of a minimum clinically important difference (MCID) in a number of recent studies.[67–69] The MCID concept can be used with both anchor-based and distribution-based approaches.[70,71] The fallacy of comparing one self-report measure with another and other pitfalls of the MCID concept are being raised as the MCID concept gains greater popularity.[72,73]

Symptoms that are commonly assessed by PRO measures in a functional restoration program are pain severity, depressive symptoms, anxiety symptoms, fear-avoidance beliefs, sleep disturbance, central sensitization symptoms, and perceived disability. Though the specific tests that are used in a functional restoration program are somewhat based on preferences of the psychology staff and medical director, it is important to choose measures with good psychometrics that are validated and published in peer-reviewed journals. Some popular PRO measures that have been found to be useful in the assessment of CSP patients are reviewed below. Note that it is beyond the scope of this chapter to review all available measures.

Pain Drawing

Pain drawings allow patients to provide a visual representation of their painful body areas. It is a basic and vital tool to help physicians understand a patient's presenting pain symptoms. Some versions of the pain drawing allow for quantification of the total percent of body area in which one is experiencing pain and the subjective characteristics of the pain.[74]

Function/Disability Questionnaires

Perhaps the most commonly used tool for low back pain is the Oswestry Disability Index (ODI).[75] With a score range between 0 (no disability) and 100 (completely bedridden), the ODI assesses one's level of pain and level of disability with functional tasks, including lifting, ability to care for oneself, ability to walk, ability to sit, sexual function, ability to stand, social life, sleep quality, and ability to travel. The Pain Disability Questionnaire[32,33] is a newer instrument useful not only for the lumbar spine, like the ODI, but for all other musculoskeletal conditions. It also includes a psychosocial component, vital in the assessment of CSP patients. Its responsiveness has been demonstrated and it is now being used in the most updated version of the American Medical Association Guides to the Evaluation of Permanent Impairment.[76]

The West Haven-Yale Multidimensional Pain Inventory (WHYMPI/MPI) is a 52-item, 12-scale questionnaire designed to assess important components of the chronic pain experience, including pain severity, perceived interference in daily functioning due to pain, perceived life control, affective distress, and self-perceptions about how significant others respond to one's pain and functional limitations.[77] MPI score profiles can indicate a patient's pain-coping style (adaptive coper, interpersonally distressed, or dysfunctional). A dysfunctional MPI coping style has been shown to be associated with decreased work productivity and excess health care utilization after completing a functional restoration treatment program.[78]

Mood Questionnaires

The Beck Depression Inventory (BDI) was developed by Aaron T. Beck, one of the founding fathers of cognitive-based psychotherapy.[79] It evaluates important components of depression, including cognitive factors, sleep disturbance, weight change, irritability, sexual dysfunction, and anhedonia. A cognitive/somatic BDI ratio can help guide psychoeducation and cognitive-behavioral therapy.[80] The BDI consists of 21 items, rated on a 0 to 3 Likert scale, with a total score from 0 to 63. Since its original publication, it has been revised several times.

The Inventory of Depressive Symptoms (IDS) is designed to assess all Major Depressive Disorder symptom domains specified in the Diagnostic and Statistical Manual of Mental Disorders.[81,82] The original version has 30 items (though only 28 items are summed for a total score) with a score range of 0 to 84. A shorter, 16-item self-report version (Quick Inventory of Depressive Symptoms), was later developed.[83] Both versions are also available in a clinician-administered format. An alternative (and older) clinician-administered depression measure is the Hamilton Rating Scale for Depression (HRSD).[84,85]

Some mood questionnaires are designed to assess anxiety symptoms. For instance, the Beck Anxiety Inventory (BAI) is a similar format to the BDI, with the same number of items and scoring system.[86] Unlike the BAI, the Pain Anxiety Symptom Scale (PASS) was designed to specifically measure pain-related anxiety.[87] Several versions are available, but the most commonly reported version has 20-items, rated on a 5-point scale from 0 (never) to 5 (always).

Sleep Disturbance Questionnaires

Insomnia is a very commonly reported problem with CSP patients. Though insomnia has traditionally been assumed to be simply a symptom of pain or depression, there is evidence that insomnia can occur independently of pain and depressive symptoms in CSP patients.[35] Several instruments are available to measure parameters of sleep disturbance and its effect on daily functioning. The Pittsburgh Sleep Quality Index is a comprehensive (and relatively long) scale that assesses seven sleep-related components, including sleep quality, latency, duration, habitual sleep efficiency, sleep disturbances, use of sleep medicine, and daytime dysfunction.[88] A much more concise measure is the Insomnia Severity Index.[89] This 7-item questionnaire assesses both nighttime and daytime components of insomnia with a 5-point Likert scale, from "not at all" to "extreme problems." Total scores indicate severity categories from *no clinical insomnia* to *severe clinical insomnia*. Studies have found that more severe patient-reported insomnia on the Insomnia Severity Index is associated with more severe patient-reported pain, depressive symptoms, disability, higher opioid use, and worse work outcomes 1 year after completing a functional restoration program.[34] The Epworth Sleepiness Scale, also a relatively short questionnaire, assesses the likelihood of a person dozing off or falling asleep in eight common life situations.[90]

Fear-Avoidance Questionnaires

As the association between CSP and fear-avoidance beliefs and behaviors is becoming more universally recognized, self-report measures of fear-avoidance have increased in popularity. Several scales are available that measure specific components of fear-avoidance. Perhaps the most studied is the Tampa Scale of Kinesiophobia (TSK).[91,92] Kinesiophobia refers to fear of movement and activity resulting from a feeling of vulnerability to pain and (re)injury. Several versions of the TSK are available, including the original 17-item version, and more recent 13- and 11-item versions. Severity ranges for the TSK-13, designed to help with clinical interpretation, have recently been developed.[93] They indicate four levels of severity of kinesiophobia symptoms, including subclinical, mild, moderate, and severe. The Fear-Avoidance Beliefs Questionnaire consists of 16 items with two subscales specific to fear-avoidance beliefs about work and general physical activity.[94] Because most of the items on the Fear-Avoidance Beliefs Questionnaire are specific to work activities, its use appears limited to individuals who are currently working or who have recently been off work due to pain. Because pain-related anxiety is a component of fear-avoidance, the PASS, which was mentioned in the previous section, is often viewed as a fear-avoidance measure.[87] More recently, the Fear-Avoidance Component Scale was developed to assess the important cognitive, emotional, and behavioral components of the evolving fear-avoidance model.[95,96] The Fear-Avoidance Component Scale consists of 20 separate items, covering common fear-avoidance beliefs and behaviors, scored from 0 ("completely disagree") to 5 ("completely agree"), resulting in a total possible score of 100.

Quality-of-Life Questionnaires

The Short Form-36[97] has achieved wide acceptance as an outcome measure in many areas of medicine and has been used in longitudinal studies of quality-adjusted life years for many diseases. It has 36 items that assess eight self-perceived health dimensions, with two global, comprehensive scores summarizing physical and mental health.

Personality Questionnaires

The Minnesota Multiphasic Personality Inventory (MMPI),[98–100] later revised into the MMPI II,[101] is the grandfather of self-report questionnaires for assessing personality and psychopathology. Because it has more than 500 self-report items and often has low patient acceptance, its use in chronic pain assessment appears to have declined over the years. By itself, it does not offer much help in choosing among treatment options. However, as part of a comprehensive evaluation, using several other assessment tools, the MMPI can add valuable information.[102]

Psychiatric Assessment

The Structured Clinical Interview for Diagnostic and Statistical Manual of Mental Disorders (SCID) uses a standardized interview format to assess for psychiatric disorders.[103] Because the rate of psychiatric illness is so high in chronically disabled patients, whether lifetime or secondary to the effects of disability, this instrument can be very useful for the assessment of psychopathology in CSP patients. It is considered the gold standard for psychiatric diagnoses in published research. However, because it is so comprehensive and is clinician administered, it is somewhat costly and time consuming to use. Therefore, many mental health professionals in functional restoration programs choose not to use it. Because of the cost and time commitment of the SCID, the Patient Health Questionnaire was developed.[104] This questionnaire is self-administered by the patient and easy to employ in a physician office. Though the results of this test can be a helpful guide in evaluating CSP patients for mental disorders, it cannot replace the expertise of a trained clinician in performing a clinical interview.[105]

Other Symptom Inventories

Broader symptom inventories are also available. For instance, the Symptom Checklist-90-Revised helps assess a broad range of self-reported psychological problems and symptoms of psychopathology.[106] The Brief Symptom Inventory is a related measure, with fewer items (53 vs. 90).[107] More recently, an 18-item version, the Brief Symptom Inventory-18 was introduced.[108] The Central Sensitization Inventory[109] is a relatively new measure, designed to assess psychophysiologic symptoms related to central sensitization and central sensitivity syndromes, which are known to be related to CSP.[23,24] It has 25 items, scored on a 4-point Likert scale, which rates the prevalence of symptoms from "never" to "always." Five severity levels, from "subclinical" to "extreme," can help with clinical interpretation.[110] Clinical research suggests that patients with CSSs can respond well to interdisciplinary biopsychosocial treatment interventions, but they tend to show poor treatment responsiveness to invasive medical procedures. High scores on the CSI can alert care providers to evaluate patients for central sensitization/central sensitivity syndromes before engaging in expensive and invasive diagnostic procedures.[111,112]

Treatment Components of Functional Restoration

Sports Medicine Concepts and Physical Training

The physical part of the interdisciplinary approach is centered around a quantitative, quota-based, measurement-driven, sports medicine approach to comprehensive rehabilitation. The principles of sports medicine have evolved from individualized rehabilitation of the competitive athlete to a conceptual and methodologic framework that connotes active treatment protocols for all individuals with physical deconditioning who want to return to higher levels of function. Much of the initial work and evidence was done with rehabilitation of injured limbs, but these concepts are clearly applicable to the spine as well.

Restoration of physical function has to begin with regaining the mobility of the weak link injured or target area(s). Loss of joint mobility may be associated with joint pain. Because muscles spanning the rigid joint cannot be stretched adequately, relieving muscle spasm pain can become difficult. Motion training is taught by physical therapists to be done frequently with low repetitions (every hour or 2 hours), both in and outside of treatment (as homework), to allow the patient to "ratchet up" the motion. Antiinflammatory medications and occasional joint injections to facilitate mobilization (not specifically for pain relief) can be beneficial in regaining motion.

Muscular strength and endurance can be restored through a variety of exercise modalities. As stated earlier in this chapter, dynamic muscle training has been shown to be the most efficient method of training. It involves distinct subcategories: isotonic, isokinetic, eccentric, and isoinertial, sometimes termed *psychophysical* (free weights).[113] *Isotonic* exercises are those in which the same force is applied throughout the dynamic range and is often inappropriately used for exercises in which a changing lever arm actually alters the applied torque. This type of exercise is most often associated with variable-resistance devices, using a cam to equalize muscular demands throughout the dynamic ROM. *Isokinetic* training devices require a sophisticated dynamometer that limits the speed to a preset value. In this mode, speed and acceleration are controlled, allowing almost unlimited torque around a central axis, which, in turn, eliminates the effect of acceleration on work. These devices accommodate a force application that provides injury protection, at least in the *concentric* (muscle shortening while contracting) type of contraction. Unlike variable resistance devices, however, high-speed training is possible for development of agility. Pure *eccentric* training is far to the right on the force–speed curve and can produce rapid strength gains with a correspondingly higher likelihood of injury at high forces or high speeds with little ability to provide external control for injury prevention. Finally, *isoinertial* (psychophysical) strength training, using free weights, is limited to those postures in which weight can be attached to the body or held in the hands, usually against gravity.

While professional athletes may often go "too far" and risk recurrent tissue injury, the vast majority of CSP patients are inhibited in physical performance due to their psychological profile and pain hypersensitivity (which is sometimes related to opioids and other medications), so that they will usually underperform. This is when a specific measurement-driven training program, individually based on age, gender, and height/weight perimeters, can be effective in progressing the patient in a stepwise fashion aimed at a predetermined goal. At PRIDE, a 75-step program allows safe but orderly individualized training that progresses patients despite pain, even if they have failed previous PT and OT reconditioning attempts from other providers. The patient's ability to progress in a strengthening program while overcoming pain symptoms helps develop patient confidence in one's future, and one's ultimate triumph over disability. Once the weak link target body part(s) have begun progressing in the PT gyms, the occupational therapists can more effectively coordinate each involved weak link with whole-person strengthening and coordination for functional capacity progression. Exercises that specifically simulate motion and loads of a sport or work activity have been shown in multiple studies to be an effective training tool that is robustly protective against reinjury.[114] Psychophysical and variable resistance lifting devices enable both concentric and eccentric contraction capability.

Secondary effects of a functional restoration program are also critically important. Physical training appears to have a specific beneficial effect on pain (possibly through increased synthesis of specialized neurotransmitters) and has been demonstrated to increase remodeling of scar and adhesions, while improving cartilage nutrition. Mobility that maximizes flexibility through the entire functional range appears to be the key to functional return. Combining improved ROM with normal strength and endurance provides a synergistic benefit of protecting functional motion with increased biomechanical efficiency. This development of protective muscular mechanisms is particularly important when a return to normal joint architecture can no longer be anticipated.

Thus, the specific physical conditioning programs that combine stretching, strengthening, cardiovascular fitness, endurance, and agility show the best and most consistent functional outcomes with less risk of future injury.[115] The application of these exercises is individualized on the basis of quantitative testing of function (noted earlier in this chapter), with the specificity and intensity of exercise changing to minimize the likelihood of injury and to maximize improvement in specific deficits to function. A variety of weight equipment is used in the program (Fig. 111.6). Finally, a posttreatment *fitness maintenance program* must be established and tailored to the physical and psychological makeup of the patient to ensure compliance when building on the initial gains made after graduating the intensive supervised program.

Psychosocial and Educational Interventions

In a functional restoration program, there is a strong relationship between gains in mental health and gains in physical health. For instance, meeting specific achievable physical goals in the gyms provides a shared sense of success between the patient and care team that allows the patient to overcome fear of further injury and to increase daily activity levels. The patient's perception of the meaning of pain may change over the course of treatment. Instead of the pain being perceived as frightening, distressing, and something to avoid at all costs, it can be perceived as merely an annoyance to be worked through and managed as one pursues ADLs. The relationship between mental and physical gains can create a feed-forward cycle of reconditioning in which gains in one area spur gains in the other. For example, as the collaboration of the patient and care team achieves functional returns of strength, flexibility, aerobic capacity, and simulation of actual work activities, increased feelings of self-confidence and self-efficacy, along with decreased feelings of distress and helplessness, naturally follow. The patient can learn that increased function, despite pain, can improve pain perception (though possibly not in a 1:1 fashion). Physical success is often accompanied by improvements in affect, mood, sleep, and thought processes, with a concomitant reduction in psychophysiologic symptoms of depression, anxiety, and pain perception. In the end, the team has provided an environment in which the rewards for being well far exceed perceived rewards for being sick.

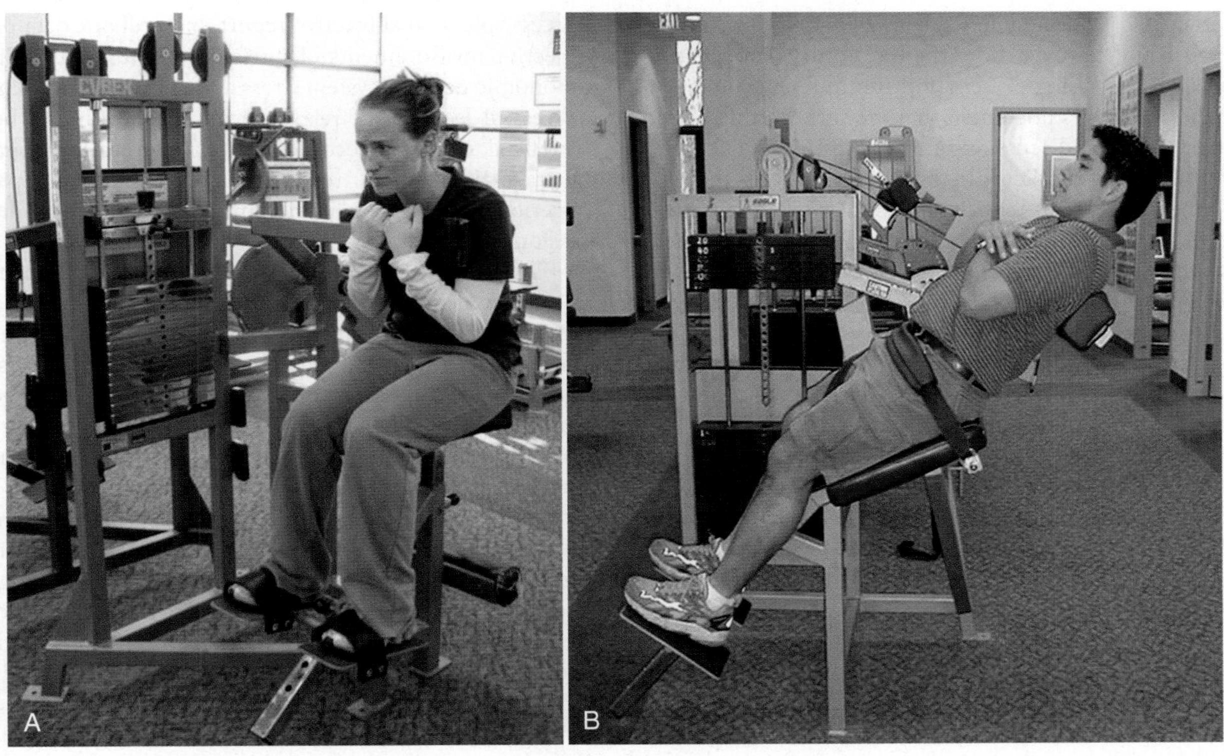

FIG. 111.6 (A) Abdominal and (B) back extension weight machines used for trunk strengthening.

Ultimately, as a result of functional restoration, CSP patients can shift their behavior away from an unrealistic dependency on a medical system in a vain attempt to "cure" the source of chronic pain, and to move toward independence in achieving the highest level of function possible. Some specific psychobehavioral therapeutic strategies are detailed next.

Psychotherapy

Two forms of psychotherapy are most often used in a functional restoration program: client-centered psychotherapy and cognitive-behavioral therapy (CBT).[116,117] A trusting therapeutic alliance is essential for both of these therapies to be effective. As with the physical component of functional restoration, the ultimate therapeutic goal of psychotherapy is to help patients achieve maximum psychological and physical functioning.

In client-centered psychotherapy, the therapist provides a supportive environment to allow patients to discuss their feelings and concerns without judgment. Many CSP patients feel isolated and report that they have no one to talk to about their pain-related experience. They often report that friends and family members are tired of hearing about it. They often get stuck in a cycle of ruminating about their injuries, struggling to get the medical help they need, and raging about the unfairness of their situation. The goal of client-centered psychotherapy is to allow CSP patients to tell their story and process their situation, while the therapist engages in active listening. CSP patients may have to repeat their stories and process their situation multiple times before they are ready to begin to let go of past injustices and begin to focus on improving their mental and physical functioning through the functional restoration treatment approach.

Unlike traditional psychotherapies, CBT is more structured and directive. Treatment focuses more on teaching and less on just talking. There is less focus on the past and more focus on making positive changes in the present and ultimately the future. The goal of CBT is to analyze and modify the interactions between thoughts, behaviors, emotions, and physiology. Negative and distorted thoughts, irrational belief systems, and dysfunctional behaviors can contribute to depression/anxiety, exacerbation of physical symptoms, and chronic pain-related disability. Negative and dysfunctional thoughts and behaviors can become habits, occurring outside of the patient's awareness. CBT follows an educational model. It is assumed that dysfunctional thoughts and behaviors have been learned; thus, they can be unlearned and replaced with more functional thoughts and behaviors. Through CBT interventions, CSP patients can become aware of their own dysfunctional thoughts/behaviors and how they are contributing to their current disability. CBT aims to teach specific cognitive and behavioral skills for managing stress and improving emotional and physical health. Stress management training, relaxation training, assertiveness training, and training to recognize and challenge negative/dysfunctional thoughts are commonly utilized in functional restoration. CBT usually involves homework to actively involve patients in their own treatment outside of therapy sessions.

Providers involved with the CBT approach must be aware of unique factors common in work-related injuries and the adversarial WC state and federal laws that have grown in developed countries over more than a century. Patients may perceive a risk of losing present and future financial benefits if their care providers document that they are "getting better" from their CSP. The discussion of reality testing in CBT for a "better future" may conflict with the perceived loss of the "bird in the hand" of current financial benefits or promises within the specific WC jurisdiction on a future "pot of gold" financial settlement. When the psychological and case management team recognizes treatment resistance, financial secondary gain is the most common cause. Other causes include secondary gain of relief from other family and social obligations or opioid and benzodiazepine dependence.[118] The managers of the interdisciplinary psychosocial interventions must be on the lookout for treatment resistance and utilize a number of counseling and educational strategies to combat the perception that improving function will have negative effects for the patient. The ability of the treatment team to reassure patients during counseling is vital to the achievement of functional restoration goals.

Stress Management and Self-Regulation Training

It is well known that stress can exacerbate pain and many CSP patients have poor coping strategies for managing stress (see Chapter 108). CSP patients often get into a perpetuating cycle of increased pain, increased emotional/cognitive reactivity, and increased tension. Stress management training can encompass a wide range of cognitive-behavioral strategies—from assertiveness, to time management, to mindfulness meditation, to paced diaphragmatic breathing. Self-regulation training, which is often a component of stress management, refers to a group of behavioral techniques for learning to gain some level of control over one's psychophysiology and ultimately over distressing psychological and physical symptoms. Common self-regulation techniques, which are offered in a functional restoration program, are relaxation training and biofeedback.[119]

Relaxation training involves learning and practicing specific techniques for focusing the mind and regulating the emotional, cognitive, and physiologic components of stress, which can disrupt the pain cycle and provide CSP patients with behavioral tools for self-managing stress and pain. A number of different relaxation techniques are available, including progressive muscle relaxation, body scanning, guided imagery, self-hypnosis, and meditation. Focus on slow diaphragmatic breathing can be incorporated in any of these techniques. The effectiveness of these techniques for stress and pain control is determined by the skill of the therapist in teaching them and the preferences and skill of the patient in learning them. Relaxation training often involves scripted inductions. Guided relaxation inductions can be performed live during treatment, either in a group or with individual patients. When done in an individual session, guided relaxation inductions can be modified to fit the individual needs and preferences of the patient. Biofeedback monitoring of physiologic responses can provide an excellent adjunct to relaxation training. Instead of judging a patient's relaxation success solely on subjective report, biofeedback data provide objective measurements of muscular tension and indices of autonomic nervous system stress and relaxation. To maximize successful learning of relaxation techniques, it can be very beneficial to provide recorded relaxation exercises for patients to practice outside of treatment and to monitor the patient's experience and success with home practice during individual sessions.

Biofeedback is a process in which biologic information is measured and fed back to a patient and a clinician. In chronic pain rehabilitation, the purpose of biofeedback training is to help patients learn increased awareness and control over biologic processes, with the ultimate goal of gaining independent control over pain and pain-related symptoms. A recent meta-analysis of 21 studies determined that biofeedback training for chronic low back pain, either alone or in conjunction with other therapeutic interventions, resulted in significant reductions in muscle tension and improvements in pain intensity, depression, and cognitive coping.[120] Effective biofeedback training must be performed by a trained clinician, preferably one who is certified through the Biofeedback Certification International Alliance (www.bcia.org). A variety of biofeedback modalities are used in chronic pain management and physical rehabilitation, including autonomic nervous system measures (breathing, heart rate, skin conductance, and hand temperature), central nervous system measures (electroencephalography), and biomechanical measures (force and pressure).[121] Surface electromyography (SEMG) is one of the oldest and most utilized biofeedback modalities in chronic pain rehabilitation.[122] SEMG measures the electrical activity generated by muscle action potentials, which are rapid electrical signals that travel along the surface of the motor endplate, resulting in a muscle contraction. SEMG allows the patient and clinician to have direct and immediate access to muscle functioning that is not possible with manual palpation or visual observation. SEMG can be used to help patients activate inhibited muscles, but it is most often used to teach patients how to better recognize and relax tense muscles, which may be contributing to pain.[121] CSP patients very often demonstrate a deficiency in their ability to discriminate between changes in muscle tension. They often develop muscle bracing habits and imbalanced postural adjustments in response to pain, which often occur outside of the patient's awareness. It has been suggested that these deficits may lead patients to believe that elevated muscle tension levels are in a normal range, which may preclude adjustments to lower tension levels.[123] SEMG biofeedback training can help patients to recognize and correct habitual muscle bracing habits and postural imbalances, to recalibrate their awareness of normal muscle relaxation, and to disrupt the pain/tension cycle. More recently, SEMG biofeedback has been used in functional restoration to help CSP patients stretch more effectively by helping them overcome pain and fear-related movement inhibition and increasing muscular relaxation skill when stretching.[124] As an adjunct to functional restoration, this SEMG-assisted stretching protocol has been shown to result in increased spinal ROM and associated self-report improvements in pain and disability.[125,126]

BOX 111.3 Some Educational Topics Taught in Function Restoration Classes

Anatomy and physiology related to pain and deconditioning
Nutrition for good health and weight loss
Pain-related medications, including opioids, antiinflammatories, muscle relaxants, hypnotics, and psychotropics
Specific exercise topics, including core strengthening, posture, use of a Swiss ball, use of therapeutic bands
How quantification is used in a functional restoration program to guide progression of physical treatment
Worker's compensation law
Concepts of stress, its relationship with pain, and strategies for managing stress
Common emotional correlates to chronic pain, including depression, anger, and worry
Common cognitive correlates to chronic pain, including negative and irrational thinking
Sleep education, including behavioral strategies for improving sleep success
Family dynamics and chronic pain
Assertiveness training

Didactic Classes

Education is a key component of functional restoration. Patients participate in didactic education each day of the program. Treatment team members from all departments participate in classes. See Box 111.3 for examples of class topics.

Case Management

Case management is an important and often underused component of the rehabilitative process. The case manager will meet with the patient regularly in order to assist in following the process and reaching treatment goals. The case manager's responsibilities include maintaining family contact; functioning as an administrative liaison with referring and consulting physicians' offices; updating rehabilitation nurses, insurance carriers, and lawyers; and maintaining relationships with state agencies. The most critical role for case managers involves movement from disability back to function, particularly when disability is associated with work-related injuries or when patients are receiving compensation (state/federal WC, long-/short-term disability, or SSDI benefits). Private and state vocational rehabilitation services can help patients reintegrate vocationally; the case manager's contacts with those resources are extremely valuable. It is important for communication to be open to all stakeholders in the patient's rehabilitation process as medicolegal, administrative, and financial concerns play an increasing role in modern society.

Case managers not only provide counseling regarding issues of treatment resistance (secondary gain financially or medication dependence) but must negotiate with patients as to how they can improve all aspects of their future once time-limited aspects of their case have resolved. This is sometimes difficult if major outside forces are actually encouraging disability and dysfunction. The most common secondary gain issues that need to be negotiated relate to compensation injuries such as WC or motor vehicle accidents, for which a patient may be paid financial benefits for being disabled (WC disability benefits or short-/long-term disability) until the treatment process has been deemed to be over, through a concept now generally known as maximum medical improvement. Until that declaration is generally accepted, patients may wish to live on the disability money rather than going back to work and reengaging in normal ADLs. Patients with secondary gain issues may demonstrate exaggerated pain behaviors and inconsistent physical performance with exercise and assessment. Case managers in a functional restoration program have a major tool unavailable to therapists in other treatment programs, because measurement-driven training and quantitative functional measurements show which patients are actually doing the physical training to improve themselves and which patients are dragging their feet. This recognition allows more focused "reality therapy" conversations to deal with secondary gain issues.

Over the past decade or more, many insurance carriers have encouraged patients to treat pain with high-dose opioids as a policy rather than focusing on rehabilitation designed to result in work return. A liberal federal policy of allowing "cost shifting" WC claims onto SSDI financial benefits and Medicare for medical benefits has been partially to blame. Greater federal attention and national concerns about the dangers of prolonged opioid dependence on society in general are contributing to some gradual reversal of these policies. Nonetheless, the concept of a lifetime of "free money" for disability under SSDI is appealing to some disaffected workers. Combine lack of work options and motivation with physician management consisting of high-dose opioids for addictive personalities, and the "secondary gain" of SSDI, even at a young age, can be appealing to some patients. The settlement of claims for permanent partial disability has undergone a change in many state venues, but a pot-of-gold mentality and encouragement from the plaintiff's attorneys can also be a cause of treatment resistance. Recognition of short- and long-term goals by the case manager and reality-based discussion with the patient can often overcome the treatment resistance and result in a long-term plan for tapering opioids, settling claims, and moving back to some type of work (even if it involves supplementing SSDI payments).

Medical Techniques Accompanying Functional Restoration

Interventional Procedures

Pain management for CSP often consists solely of repetitive injection procedures, prolonged opioid and benzodiazepine use to cover pain symptoms, and frequent use of spinal cord stimulators or drug pumps. These passive interventions used in isolation generally foster persistent dependence, disability, and dysfunction, thus are not considered best practices by current national treatment guidelines for CSP. However, occasional use of interventional procedures that facilitate functional improvement may be something for the multidisciplinary medical supervisory staff to consider. The first issue that interventions are likely to impact positively in a functional restoration program is the loss of mobility in the lumbar and cervical spine, termed *segmental rigidity*. This observable physical finding is similar to the pain associated with any fibrosed and contracted joint in the extremities and appears to arise in the spine from similar processes of joint contracture, primarily involving the facet joints. When a reasonable trial of exercise alone fails to restore intersegmental motion (usually in the lower lumbar spine or bracketing a lumbar or cervical fusion procedure), then the combination of facet injections at the rigid segments, with specific stretching exercises performed frequently, can result in measurable improvement in motion.[54,55] As in the example of the extremities, once intersegmental motion is restored and "ratcheted up" effectively, atrophic muscles can be more effectively strengthened, muscle spasm relieved, and multijoint coordination restored.

When perineural scarring from injury or surgery affects distal extremity function, or there is entrapment to neuropathy, perineural injections are commonly utilized. The CSP equivalent is the epidural steroid injection, often related to a specific nerve root and best treated with a transforaminal injection technique. When arm or leg radicular pain persists despite stretches to facilitate nerve mobilization, the epidural steroid injection is a useful technique to reduce pain and facilitate exercise participation. Sacroiliac joints may occasionally become inflamed through deconditioning and biomechanical imbalances. Certain provocative tests can help in the diagnosis of sacroiliac dysfunction and injections combined with specific exercises can allow faster progress in functional restoration. Finally, but only very occasionally, sympathetically mediated pain may be related to a spinal disorder, and a cervical or lumbar sympathetic block may help the rehabilitation process.

Functional restoration can take place in the presence of a spinal cord stimulator or a drug pump. However, they are rarely implanted in conjunction with a functional restoration program. More often, once the benefits of the functional restoration program are achieved, patients are more likely to request removal of these devices than to seek their implantation.

Medical Psychopharmacology

An awareness of common comorbid pain and neuropsychiatric disorders is necessary for more effective pharmacotherapeutic treatment of the CSP patient in the functional restoration setting. As discussed earlier, psychosocial factors (mood disorders, fear-avoidance, insomnia, posttraumatic stress, and the like) frequently accompany CSP and can exacerbate pain symptoms. Central sensitization is also a common cause of CSP through central mechanisms, often diagnosed as central sensitivity syndromes (such as fibromyalgia, myofascial pain, and chronic fatigue syndrome). Central sensitization and CSSs may respond to the same antidepressant medications as do mood disorders that accompany CSP. Chronic widespread pain or fibromyalgia may be premorbid or appear as a result of a traumatic injury.[26,27] Treatment agents include serotonin norepinephrine reuptake inhibitors (SNRIs) such as high-dose venlafaxine, desmethylvenlafaxine, duloxetine, and milnacipran, the latter two being approved by the US Food and Drug Administration (FDA) for this condition. Standard doses of these medications usually suffice and can serve a dual purpose. These agents generally offer a more benign side-effect profile than tricyclic antidepressants (TCAs), which have long been the mainstay for treatment for this condition.[127] Cyclobenzaprine has also been shown to be useful for some patients.[128] Pregabalin in higher doses than used for neuropathic pain (225–300 mg/day, usually divided into twice daily dosing) is effective, as is gabapentin in standard doses.

We favor the use of the secondary amine group TCAs (nortriptyline, desipramine, and protriptyline), which act primarily as norepinephrine reuptake inhibitors and have less sedative, anticholinergic, and orthostatic effects when compared with the tertiary amine group. The latter agents combine serotonergic and adrenergic effects and include amitriptyline, clomipramine, imipramine, and doxepin. All TCAs can be effective for chronic pain in low dosages. If the patient is suffering from comorbid depression, however, full clinically effective dosages should be used. There is less evidence to suggest that selective serotonin reuptake inhibitors (SSRIs)—such as fluoxetine, paroxetine, sertraline, citalopram, escitalopram, bupropion, and mirtazapine—are useful for chronic pain, but they may be effective in some patients who have developed mood disorders.

The SNRIs, TCAs, and SSRI antidepressants are all effective as well for frequently encountered comorbid anxiety disorders in this population. This includes panic disorder, generalized anxiety disorder, posttraumatic stress disorder, and the surprisingly common obsessive compulsive disorder. Effective use of these agents will reduce anxiety and therefore secondarily reduce muscular tension and pain perception. It may allow for easier tapering of sedatives/hypnotics, benzodiazepines (BZDs), and opioids.

Patients who are dependent on high-dose carisoprodol or short-acting BZDs can be converted to diazepam as per standard dosage converting tables and tapered using three-times-daily doses over 4 to 5 weeks. Patients taking BZDs in sizable doses over 6 months may be able to tolerate a 10% reduction every 1 to 2 weeks. For patients requiring muscle relaxants to tolerate functional restoration, we prefer antispasticity agents—such as baclofen and tizanidine—to centrally acting agents. The former agents may have analgesic properties as well.

Many CSP patients present with comorbid radiculopathy amenable to pharmacologic treatment. Again, the standard multipurpose pain agents—such as low-dose TCAs, SNRIs, pregabalin, and gabapentin—are useful for many patients. For second-line agents, we favor a neuromodulator such as low-dose oxcarbazepine, which may be given at bedtime, and topiramate, which has also been found to be effective. Some patients may require polypharmacy, using agents with different pharmacologic mechanisms of action for treatment of chronic neuropathic pain. Sodium channel blockers (such as mexiletine and lidocaine 5% patches) can be effective in some patients,[129] and a multitude of anticonvulsant medications (such as lamotrigine and levetiracetam) can occasionally be useful in patients who have failed first- and second-line therapies.[130]

Patients with more severe personality disorders, comorbid psychotic disorders, chemical dependency disorders, and treatment-resistant affective disorders may benefit from atypical neuroleptics, such as risperidone, ziprasidone, olanzapine, quetiapine, or asenapine. These agents, usually at low doses, may have a mitigating effect on anxiety, hyperarousability, emotional lability, and—particularly for quetiapine—refractory insomnia. They may occasionally have analgesic effects in some patients.[131] However, because most of them have the potential for metabolic syndrome as a side effect, it is important to monitor the body weight of patients for whom they are prescribed. Along with many other psychotropic agents, including antidepressants and antipsychotic agents, there can be a risk of QT interval prolongation in some patients, particularly females and those over the age of 65 years, so that an electrocardiogram is recommended at the beginning of such treatment.[132]

Opioid tapering presents possibly the greatest challenge in the pharmacologic treatment of the pain patient. Past experiences and second-hand knowledge of opiate withdrawal cause considerable distress in patients who fear that they will be forced to go "cold turkey." The chronic pain patient is inherently different than the habitual recreational heroin and pain pill user. It is incumbent on the practitioner that the patient be treated with compassion, dignity, and respect and be provided a comfortable tapering process, because patients initially experience increases in pain from exercise and reconditioning. For safety and hyperalgesia concerns, patients on high-dose opiates may need to be tapered significantly before being able to partake in a more aggressive measurement-directed reconditioning. Patients on low-dose opiates may be continued on their originally prescribed agent with dose reductions of 10% per day or 25% every 3 days, because this is usually tolerated well in terms of withdrawal. Chronic pain patients, however, generally need more time to become accustomed to the new sensation that they are experiencing and will be more comfortable with a 2- to 3-week tapering process. Adjunctive use of low-dose clonidine and/or BZDs may reduce symptom severity.

Sublingual buprenorphine is a good choice for substitution and tapering of opiate-dependent CSP patients. Buprenorphine is an opiate receptor, partial μ-agonist/κ antagonist. It is less potent than morphine but more tightly bound to the opiate receptor and dissociates more slowly from the receptor, thereby minimizing withdrawal symptoms in physically dependent patients. Buprenorphine is FDA approved in the United States in the sublingual form for the treatment of opiate dependence. It is combined with naloxone (Suboxone) to prevent intravenous abuse and is also available as buprenorphine alone as Subutex. It is FDA approved in intramuscular form as an analgesic agent (Buprenex). This agent is available in lower doses in sublingual tablet form and in a patch form as an analgesic agent.[133]

It is legal in all US states to taper pain patients' opioid medications to avoid withdrawal symptoms. Unless a special certification is obtained, it is not legal to detoxify a substance abuser with buprenorphine. In our experience, patients treated with buprenorphine experience significantly reduced cognitive, sedative, and euphoric effects and can experience mood enhancement and a smooth, uncomplicated withdrawal process. This can allow them to safely participate in functional restoration physical training in a timely manner. Buprenorphine is a moderate analgesic that can enhance the patient's ability to continue in treatment because it appears to be less associated with opioid-induced hyperalgesia than most other agents. When using buprenorphine, it cannot be given until the patient is in mild withdrawal because it preferentially displaces other opioids from the receptor site and precipitates a full and rapid withdrawal state.[134]

Recently, there have been several recommendations generated with regard to the use of opioids, of which the pain physician should be aware:

1. The short-acting opioid/Tylenol or nonsteroidal antiinflammatory drug combinations have been reclassified as Schedule II, requiring a triplicate or C2 prescription.
2. The US Department of Health and Human Services has published Guideline NCG9597 (2010) (http://www.guideline.gov/content.aspx?id=43745&search=narcotics#Section420), which has specific recommendations for use of opioids before and after surgery and during the acute, subacute, and chronic phases after an injury associated with pain. The recommended upper dose of narcotics should not exceed 120 morphine-equivalent dose (MED), unless prescribed by a pain specialist. The National Academy of Medicine (formerly the Institute of Medicine) has even more recent 2015 guidance that lowers the acceptable opioid dosage for chronic pain to 50 to 60 MED.
3. A national guideline, the *ODG*, has instituted a list of "N" second-line and "Y" first-line drugs that may be used within the WC system. Allowable narcotics include only the short-acting opioids (codeine, hydromorphone, hydrocodone, morphine, oxycodone), tramadol, buprenorphine, and naloxone. It also recommends a CSP maximum of 50 to 90 MED.

Functional Restoration Program Treatment Phases

Initial Treatment Phase

The program's initial phase often involves patient accommodation to scheduled attendance at a full day of program activities. This simple concept is often more difficult than it seems and requires time to rebuild activity tolerance. Atrophy is not just limited to the body but usually includes attention, mood, sleep success, and motivation to engage in ADLs. The early physical portion concentrates on rapidly advancing mobility and a home program of stretching, walking, and cardiovascular exercise to aid transition to the intensive phase. Detoxification or tapering down from medications such as opioids, muscle relaxants, and anxiolytics, as well as alcohol use, is facilitated by the gradual increase in patient confidence as early progress is achieved. The basic principle is to utilize whatever medications are needed to deal with the assessment findings early in the program and then taper medication later in the program as functional improvement occurs.

Depending on the duration of the chronic pain, the psychological comorbidities and the degree of conditioning, patients may fail to tolerate full days of back-to-back reconditioning in an intensive program. Moreover, various real barriers to attendance need to be considered, including problems with transportation, childcare or elder care, financial limitations, and dependence on the availability of care providers. Over the past decade, changes in WC systems have encouraged many employers to maintain patients at light-duty or part-time work rather than having them out of work on total disability. This means that there are more programs involving a stay-at-work treatment approach, in which the rehabilitation process needs to be organized around work responsibilities on the job.[135] All of these factors mean that functional restoration attendance may be part or full time, ranging from 1 to 5 days per week. Patients usually begin trying to do twice-weekly full days, increasing to three times a week quickly, and assessing their tolerance for further increases in attendance.

Intensive Phase

This phase is the most team intensive because the biopsychosocial multimodal disability management that is the hallmark of a program requires excellent interstaff communication. A crucial component of the intensive phase of functional restoration is the initiation of measurement-driven therapy (MDT). The measurements of the quantitative FCE (and repeated physical testing) set training levels in a progressive resistance strength-building and endurance-building computerized process, individualized to age, gender, and body mass. MDT is quota-based and a necessary component of a sports medicine reconditioning model. It is especially critical when an injury or pain target area has become a weak link relative to other body parts. In traditional PT and OT, dealing with a weak link is usually limited by the patient's pain tolerance, and therefore becomes pain-driven therapy. At some point, lacking other measurements to override the patient's pain perception, pain complaints for the CSP patient force the therapist to back down on attempts to recondition the weak link, limiting progress in the group of chronic pain patients unable to push through the chronic pain. This failure to respond to pain-driven therapy is usually the critical factor that selects out the candidate for functional restoration and is usually associated with a poor performance on initial FCE for those patients. The use of MDT provides a counterweight to pain perception and its psychological accompaniment (e.g., fear-avoidance, physical inhibition, and hyperalgesia).

The intensive phase is when most didactic classes and CBT interventions for stress management and pain control techniques are provided. This is also when most of the planning for vocational reintegration and a transition back to a more normal life takes place. The further decrease in use of habituating medication and stabilization of psychotropic medication is a crucial part of this phase, leaving patients with a stable and low-dose medication management plan at program discharge to cover the various aspects of their CSP. The usual maximum program length of 160 hours may be abbreviated for CSP patients with shorter periods of disability or those who are currently working part time or light duty and participating in a stay-at-work approach during their rehabilitation. For those with more chronic disability and very high opioid levels, programs of greater length may be justified. Short refresher programs may be appropriate for patients who have undergone postprogram surgeries. Every patient's functional restoration program ends with discharge testing, involving an FCE and repeat of the self-report questionnaires, to demonstrate the change that has occurred over the course of program participation and to help determine continued objective functional limitations.

Postprogram Long-Term Care Plan

Following program discharge, patients enter a long-term care plan (LTCP) phase. This open-ended process is handled by program physicians and nurse practitioners but supported by functional restoration program team members. Case managers usually assist patients in their work transition back to full-duty or modified-duty work, often with assistance from state or federal vocational rehabilitation agencies and other community resources. When appropriate, mental health professionals facilitate a connection to community resources for management of ongoing psychiatric or cognitive issues. The physical staff provides each patient with an individualized fitness maintenance program based on each patient's physical capacity at program discharge.

As part of the LTCP, patients may be offered the opportunity for quarterly visits to the supervising physician, who can provide medications to assist in meeting postprogram goals (work return, home exercise, and decreased health utilization). The opportunity to meet with specific members of the treatment team, as needed, for symptom exacerbations for focused interventions consistent with functional restoration philosophy is important for maintaining cost-effectiveness. The most positive therapeutic outcome, however, is for patients to develop a perception of independence and self-efficacy with their own ability to manage their chronic pain and related physical limitations so that ongoing medical management for pain is no longer required. In addition to routine LTCP quarterly visits, until the CSP condition has stabilized, patients may occasionally call in for flare-ups of pain. The shortest possible pharmacologic or interventional procedures are utilized to "keep molehills from becoming mountains."

Outcome Tracking Phase

This important program phase allows continued evaluation of long-term effectiveness of the program both from the patient's point of view and for the facility's continuous quality improvement initiative. Effort is made during the postdischarge phase to reinforce patient independence with fitness maintenance and pain management strategies so that return visits to the physician are minimized to maintenance evaluations only. It is important to educate patients about the willingness of team members to help with problems that arise after the program. Patient perception of an environment of care that extends beyond program discharge leads to a high rate of compliance in telephone tracking, which is performed at approximately 1 year after discharge. A high patient contact rate, in turn, allows performance of 1-year follow-up studies such as has been performed at PRIDE.[57,60] Fig. 111.1 contains some PRIDE treatment outcome variables, collected over a span of 10 years.

The PRIDE Research Foundation has published numerous studies in peer-reviewed publications that demonstrate the effectiveness of the functional restoration treatment approach. Through many years of data collection, a large clinical database of thousands of patients has allowed analyses of admission-to-discharge treatment responsiveness of clinical variables and the association of clinical variables with 1-year socioeconomic outcomes, measured at program discharge. Treatment responsiveness and outcome studies have been published on objective measures (such as functional capacity examination scores[136]), demographic factors (such as length of disability, age, or gender[137–139]), self-report variables (including pain severity, perceived disability, insomnia, depressive symptoms[32–35,140,141]), and external factors (such as state economic factors in work outcomes[142]). Published studies have investigated treatment responsiveness between patients with neck, lower extremity, and upper extremity problems with those with lumbar injuries[143–148] and between pretreatment lumbar discectomy and fusion.[20] Alternative treatment approaches, including the SOP, have been studied to accommodate patients who are uncertain about whether or not to have surgery.[40,41] Novel treatment approaches have been studied and published, such as the use of biofeedback training for surface electromyography-assisted stretching with CSP patients.[124,149–151] The cost of treatment for injured workers who receive treatment more quickly following the injury versus workers with a longer period of time between injury and treatment has been investigated.[152] Additional studies have investigated opioid use,[153,154] prerehabilitation psychological status, and comorbid psychiatric disorders at program admission and discharge.[28,102]

KEY POINTS

1. Spinal disorders are the second-leading cause for doctors' visits in the United States. The vast majority of spinal pain episodes are self-limited and improve without interventions or advanced imaging as long as the deleterious effects of immobilization, disuse, and disability are avoided. However, rehabilitation is sometimes necessary for returning to function after CSP develops.
2. A small minority of CSP patients account for the large majority of costs related to spinal disorders. Greater than 90% of spinal patients miss less than 2 days of work, leaving about 10% of patients who account for over 80% of lost work days. It has been shown that earliest possible intervention is most cost-effective, avoiding the secondary complications of progressive physical deconditioning and worsening psychosocial distress. For this reason, prolonged delay in performing appropriate imaging and diagnostic tests for surgical intervention is unwarranted, and an SOP may be helpful in decisively determining a surgical plan with shared decision making when surgical indications are not crystal clear. When surgery is not indicated, recommendations for engaging in the appropriate level of nonoperative care are identified in national treatment guidelines, such as the *ODG* or those developed by the American College of Occupational and Environmental Medicine and the North American Spine Society. When spine care physicians identify patients with CSP, especially when it is associated with significant disability from ADLs, referral to a functional restoration program should be strongly considered.
3. Patients with chronic spinal pain and disability must be assessed and treated from a biopsychosocial perspective. For this patient population, the interaction of fear-avoidance of ADLs, social withdrawal, physical deconditioning, high pain sensitivity, opioid overuse, psychosocial distress, and psychopathology is complex. If all of these biopsychosocial factors are not addressed effectively in treatment (as is done in a functional restoration program), the treatment is likely to fail.
4. Quantifying motion, strength, effort, psychological distress, employer disharmony, familial stress, secondary gain, and intrusive thoughts is the only way to prevent these variables becoming barriers to recovery. In addition to the well-known development of a deconditioning syndrome and chronic pain, psychosocial problems, discussed extensively in this chapter, and other medical comorbidities (e.g., neuropathic pain, postoperative scarring, postconcussive cognitive deficits, posttraumatic stress) can add even more challenges to the recovery process. Financial secondary gain and opioid dependence are both strongly associated with treatment failure, and the recognition of these additional barriers to recovery should motivate the spine care provider to consider an interdisciplinary program referral rather than continuing with lesser levels of care.
5. Functional restoration has demonstrated successful treatment outcomes replicated at multiple treatment sites for over 30 years through objective responsiveness measures of strength, ROM, and physical/psychological function, with total posttreatment return-to-work rates approaching 90% and 1-year work retention rates greater than 80%. Completion of a functional restoration program is also associated with low rates of future health utilization, additional surgeries, new claimed injuries, and medication use when compared with control or drop-out groups.
6. Interdisciplinary care is team driven and personnel intensive. A physician team leader must be a good diagnostician and an excellent integrator of disparate information. The team leader must assimilate quantified data from physical and occupational therapists, case managers, and mental health professionals to create an environment of function to help patients return to productive, contributing members of society.

KEY REFERENCES

1. Mayer T, Gatchel R, Mayer H, et al. A prospective two-year study of functional restoration in industrial low back injury: an objective assessment procedure. *JAMA*. 1987;258:1763-1767.
Follow-up to the 1985 Volvo award-winning study that demonstrates return-to-work and 1-year and 2-year work retention rates were far superior to nontreatment and a small treatment-decline group in a prospective matched cohort-control study. Rates of work return were 85% in the treatment group and 39% in the control group. Additionally, rates of new surgeries were 9% in the treatment group and 20% in the comparison group. Finally, the treatment group demonstrated 50% to 80% greater strength gains and range-of-motion gains with objective measurement tools compared with the control group. These objectively measured gains confirmed the statistically significant findings of greater work retention and decreased health care utilization seen in the treatment group compared with the

control group. Measurable functional gains that corresponded to work retention and the decreased health utilization served as a strong addition to the existing proof-of-concept study. Objective quantifiable measurements that corresponded to hard data outcomes served as an additional demonstration of the efficacy of the tertiary-level functional restoration.

2. Mayer T, Polatin P, Smith B, et al. Spine rehabilitation: secondary and tertiary nonoperative care. *Spine J*. 2003;3(3 suppl):28S-36S.
Discussion of rationale and formulation of a standard of care for spine rehabilitation. With the recognition of a bimodal distribution of cost and disability, ensuring prompt reactivation with minimal cost (first 90 days) is best suited for the vast majority of patients. A minority (20–40%) may need additional interventions (secondary care) aimed at reactivation and reeducation to prevent further disability. A small minority, which incidentally accounts for almost 90% of health costs associated with spine pain, will need interdisciplinary care (tertiary-level care), which is the only evidence- and outcome-proven way of decreasing disability and increasing return to work in this population.
3. DeLorme TL. Restoration of muscle power by heavy-resistance exercises. *J Bone Joint Surg*. 1945;27:645-667.
This groundbreaking article discusses in detail the implications of resistance exercise applied to an injured motion segment. The implications of this paper in the field of rehabilitation medicine cannot be overstated and are often referenced as the DeLorme principles. The primary finding of this far-reaching observational study shows resistance exercise can provide both endurance and power (strength). Next, resistance exercise is safe even when applied to an injured motion segment. Atrophy and muscle dysfunction from disuse can often lead to increased pain. Finally, following a quota-based resistance program can lead to improved function, strength, and endurance.
4. Kidner C, Mayer T, Gatchel R. Higher opioid doses predict poorer functional outcome in chronic disabling occupational musculoskeletal disorders. *J Bone Joint Surg Am*. 2009;91:919-927.
In a highly successful tertiary-level functional restoration program, very high levels of preprogram opioid narcotic use greater than 120 mg of morphine equivalents per day was associated with approximately 20% worse return-to-work rate (76% vs. 94%) within 1 year after treatment discharge compared with the nonopioid group. Work retention at 1-year follow-up was even lower (55% in the very high opioid group and 85% in the nonopioid group). Moreover, at 1 year after treatment, the group reporting the highest opioid use was 11.6 times as likely to be receiving Social Security disability income or Supplemental Security Income compared with the nonopioid group. These differences were true even though effective weaning and maintenance off opioids was voluntarily undertaken by all patients during the functional restoration program.
5. Seidel S, Aigner M, Ossege M, et al. Antipsychotics for acute and chronic pain in adults. *Cochrane Database Syst Rev*. 2008;(4):CD004844.
Meta-analysis of data from five of 11 randomized controlled trials showed that in selected patients with comorbid psychiatric conditions, use of atypical antipsychotics as an adjunct medicine shows significant reduction in mean pain intensity compared with placebo. Due to the risk of extrapyramidal side effects, care should be taken until further double-blind placebo control studies can be performed to better elucidate risk/benefit profile.
6. Mayer T, Gatchel R, Brede E, Theodore B. Lumbar surgery in work-related chronic low back pain: can a continuum of care enhance outcomes? *Spine J*. 2014;14(2):263-273.
Recent studies have found that worker's compensation (WC) patients with low back injuries who undergo lumbar fusion surgeries have relatively poor return-to-work rates of 26% to 36%, reoperation rates of 22% to 27%, and high rates of persistent opioid use 2 years after surgery. WC populations have also been found to have poorer lumbar spinal surgery outcomes than non-WC patients. This study compared groups of WC patients with different lumbar surgeries who then completed a functional restoration program: those with previous lumbar fusions (n = 331), those with previous nonfusion lumbar spine surgeries (n = 233), and a comparison group with no previous lumbar surgeries (n = 349). Postrehabilitation work-return rates (81–85%) and work retention rates 1 year later (81–75%), were statistically similar among the three groups, as were single-digit rates of reoperation or recurrent injury. These results suggest that early referrals to interdisciplinary rehabilitation of patients who do not respond to usual postoperative lumbar surgical care may accelerate recovery and achieve socioeconomic outcomes that are comparable to nonoperated patients.
7. Theodore B, Mayer T, Gatchel R. Cost effectiveness of early vs. delayed functional restoration for chronic disabling occupational musculoskeletal disorders. *J Occup Rehabil*. 2015;25(2):303-315.
Three groups of chronic pain disorder patients with worker's compensation claims and different lengths of disability (time between injury and treatment) were compared on functional restoration treatment outcomes. All three groups demonstrated comparable work outcomes 1 year after completing treatment. For patients who entered functional restoration treatment within 8 months of injury, there was an estimated 64% savings in medical costs and up to 80% savings in disability benefits and productivity losses compared with patients who entered treatment more than 18 months after injury. Overall, early rehabilitation resulted in estimated cost savings of up to 72% (or almost $170,000 per worker's compensation claim).
8. Brede E, Mayer T, Shea M, Garcia C, Gatchel R. Facilitating unequivocal and durable decisions in workers' compensation patients eligible for elective orthopedic surgery. *J Pain*. 2014;15(1):49-58.
This study introduced a surgical option process to improve functional restoration program (FRP) outcomes for patients with chronic musculoskeletal pain disorders who are undecided about elective orthopedic surgery. This surgical option process allows patients with unresolved surgical options to participate in an FRP for half of the normal treatment hours (approximately 80 hours) before deciding whether to pursue surgery. From a group of 245 patients with surgical options, the majority of patients declined surgery (n = 164) and were invited to complete the FRP. The remainder elected to pursue surgery and ultimately did undergo surgery (n = 43) or did not (n = 38). Within the year following treatment completion, less than 1% of patients who had declined surgery at program midpoint reversed their original decision and underwent surgery. The patients whose decision to have or not have surgery was accommodated demonstrated significant psychosocial improvement and excellent work return outcomes, which were similar to FRP patients without a surgical option. Patients who did not undergo surgery usually did so because they did not wish to accept the risk, or their surgeons thought better of performing new surgery at a surgical consultation after program midpoint. Those patients mostly completed the treatment program and had outcomes close to those for the other two groups. These results suggest that the addition of a formal surgical option process to an FRP can facilitate patients' decisive surgical decisions and help prevent delayed recovery.

9. Fore L, Perez Y, Neblett R, et al. Improved functional capacity evaluation performance predicts successful return to work one year after completing a functional restoration rehabilitation program. *PM R.* 2015;7(4):365-375.
A consecutive sample of 354 patients with chronic musculoskeletal pain disorders completed a functional restoration program. Each patient participated in a functional capacity evaluation (FCE) at admission and discharge from treatment. The results of each FCE yielded the physical demand level (PDL) at which patients were functioning. Overall, 96% of the patients demonstrated improvement in their PDLs from admission to discharge. A majority of patients (56%) were able to achieve a discharge PDL that was comparable to their estimated job-of-injury lifting requirement or higher. Discharge PDLs predicted both work return and work retention 1 year later, with higher discharge PDLs being associated with better work outcomes.

10. Asih S, Neblett R, Mayer T, Gatchel R. Does patient-reported insomnia improve in response to interdisciplinary functional restoration for chronic disabling occupational musculoskeletal disorders? *Spine.* 2014;39(17):1384-1392.
Insomnia was assessed with the Insomnia Severity Index (ISI), a validated patient-reported measure of insomnia symptoms, in a group of 262 patients with chronic pain disorders. They were assessed both at admission and at discharge from a functional restoration program. The degree of insomnia at admission significantly predicted program completion, so that patients reporting more severe insomnia were more likely to drop out of treatment. Insomnia improved for most of the patients who completed treatment, but a relatively high percent of patients (36.6%) continued to report clinically significant insomnia at program discharge. Patients who reported more severe insomnia at discharge also reported more severe pain, sadness, and disability, and were using more opioids, sleep sedatives, and antidepressants than patients who reported less severe insomnia at discharge. One year later, only 56% of the patients who reported the most severe level of insomnia at discharge were working, whereas 71% to 93% of those who reported less severe insomnia were working. Compared with patients who reported minimal insomnia at treatment discharge, those who reported severe insomnia were 10.4 times less likely to be working 1 year after completing treatment.

11. Jordan K, Mayer T, Gatchel R. Should extended disability be an exclusion criterion for tertiary rehabilitation? Socioeconomic outcomes of early versus late functional restoration compensation spinal disorders. *Spine.* 1998;23(19):2110-2117.
This was the first scientific article to look at the relationship between socially relevant outcomes and the length of disability before admission to a functional restoration program. Outcome variables, collected 1 year after treatment discharge, were compared between groups of patients with occupational injuries who entered and completed a functional restoration program with different lengths of work disability between time of injury and time of treatment admission. A short-term disabled group (between 4 and 8 months of disability) was compared with longer term disabled groups, extending beyond 5 years. No differences among the groups were found in the number of posttreatment new surgeries to the injured body part(s), visits to new providers, or new lost-time injuries. Though significant differences were found between the shorter and longer term disabled groups in the rates of work return within the year after discharge and work retention at 1 year after discharge, the longer term disabled groups still demonstrated very good work outcomes. Compared with work return (93%) and retention (80%) of the short-term disabled group, the longer term disabled groups demonstrated work return from 72% to 87% and work retention from 63% to 80%. Previous studies have found that treatment outcomes deteriorate as patients accommodate to prolonged disability following work-related injuries. However, the results of the present study, in large part, did not support this assumption. These results demonstrate that disabled workers who complete a quality functional restoration program have a very good chance of achieving positive psychosocial outcomes, including return and maintenance of employment, regardless of their length of disability before beginning treatment.

REFERENCES

1. Deyo R, Diehl A, Rosenthal M. How many days of bed rest for acute low back pain? A randomized clinical trial. *N Engl J Med.* 1986;315(17):1064-1070.
2. Coste J, Delecoeuillerie G, Cohen de Lara A. Clinical course and prognostic factors in acute low back pain: an inception cohort study in primary care practice. *Br Med J.* 1994;308(6928):577-580.
3. Webster B, Snook S. The cost of 1989 workers' compensation low back pain claims. *Spine.* 1994;19(10):1111-1116.
4. Hashemi L, Webster B, Clancy E. Trends of disability duration and cost for workers' compensation low back pain claims (1988-1996). *J Occup Environ Med.* 1998;40(12):1110-1119.
5. Modic M, Obuchowski N, Ross J. Acute low back pain and radiculopathy: MR imaging findings and their prognostic role and effect on outcome. *Radiology.* 2005;237(2):597-604.
6. Deyo RA, Ciol MA, Cherkin DC, Loeser JD, Bigos SJ. Lumbar spinal fusion: a cohort study of complications, reoperations, and resource use in the Medicare population. *Spine.* 1993; 18(11):1463-1470.
7. Mayer T, Polatin P, Smith B, et al. Spine rehabilitation: secondary and tertiary nonoperative care. *Spine J.* 2003;3(3 suppl):28S-36S.
8. Official Disability Guidelines. (2016). *ODG Treatment Guidelines.* Available at http://www.worklossdata.com/treatment-guidelines.html.
9. American College of Occupational and Environmental Medicine. (2016). *Occupational Medicine Practice Guidelines.* Available at http://www.acoem.org/practiceguidelines.aspx.
10. Mayer T, Polatin P. Tertiary nonoperative interdisciplinary programs: the functional restoration variant of the outpatient chronic pain management program. In: Gatchel R, Mayer T, eds. *Occupational Musculoskeletal Disorders.* Philadelphia: Lippincott Williams & Wilkins; 2000.
11. Gatchel RJ, Peng YB, Peters ML, Fuchs PN, Turk DC. The biopsychosocial approach to chronic pain: scientific advances and future directions. *Psychol Bull.* 2007;133(4):581-624.
12. DeLorme T. Restoration of muscle power by heavy-resistance exercises. *J Bone Joint Surg.* 1945;27:645-667.
13. DeLorme T, Watkins A. *Progressive Resistance Exercise: Technic Medical Application.* New York: Appleton-Century-Crofts, Inc.; 1951.
14. Vlaeyen J, Linton S. Fear-avoidance and its consequences in chronic musculoskeletal pain: a state of the art. *Pain.* 2000; 85(3):317-332.
15. Crombez G, Eccleston C, Van Damme S. Fear-avoidance model of chronic pain: the next generation. *Clin J Pain.* 2012;28(6):475-483.
16. Heymans M, van Buuren S, Knol D. The prognosis of chronic low back pain is determined by changes in pain and disability in the initial period. *Spine J.* 2010;10(10):847-856.

17. Asmundson GJ, Norton PJ, Norton GR. Beyond pain: the role of fear and avoidance in chronicity. *Clin Psychol Rev.* 1999;19(1):97-119.
18. Pincus T, Smeets R, Simmonds M. The fear avoidance model disentangled: improving the clinical utility of the fear avoidance model. *Clin J Pain.* 2010;26(9):739-746.
19. Bortz W. The disuse syndrome. *West J Med.* 1984;141(5):691-694.
20. Mayer T, McMahon M, Gatchel R. Socioeconomic outcomes of combined spine surgery and functional restoration in workers compensation spinal disorders with matched controls. *Spine.* 1998;23(5):598-606.
21. Mayer T, Gatchel R, Keeley J, et al. A randomized clinical trial of treament for lumbar segmental rigidity. *Spine.* 2004;29(20):2199-2205.
22. Yunus M. Central sensitivity syndromes: a new paradigm and group nosology for fibromyalgia and overlapping conditions, and the related issue of disease versus illness. *Semin Arthritis Rheum.* 2008;37(6):339-352.
23. Kindler L, Jones K, Perrin N. Risk factors predicting the development of widespread pain from chronic back or neck pain. *J Pain.* 2010;11(12):1320-1328.
24. Kindler L, Bennett R, Jones K. Central sensitivity syndromes: mounting pathophysiologic evidence to link fibromyalgia with other common chronic pain disorders. *Pain Manag Nurs.* 2011;12(1):15-24.
25. Roussel N, Nijs J, Meeus M. Central sensitization and altered central pain processing in chronic low back pain: fact or myth? *Clin J Pain.* 2013;29(7):625-638.
26. Mayer T, Towns B, Neblett R, Theodore B, Gatchel R. Chronic widespread pain in patients with occupational spinal disorders: prevalence, psychiatric comorbidity, and association with outcomes. *Spine.* 2008;33(17):1889-1897.
27. Howard K, Mayer T, Neblett R. Fibromyalgia syndrome in chronic disabling occupational musculoskeletal disorders: prevalence, risk factors, and posttreatment outcomes. *J Occup Environ Med.* 2010;52(12):1186-1191.
28. Dersh J, Mayer T, Theodore B. Do psychiatric problems first appear preinjury or postinjury in chronic disabling occupational spinal disorders? *Spine.* 2007;32(9):1045-1051.
29. Polatin P, Kinney R, Gatchel R. Psychiatric illness and chronic low back pain: the mind and the spine–which goes first? *Spine.* 1993;18(1):66-71.
30. Dersh J, Gatchel R, Mayer T, Polatin P, Temple O. Prevalence of psychiatric disorders in patients with chronic disabling occupational spinal disorders. *Spine.* 2006;31(10):1156-1162.
31. Blazer D, Kessler R, McGonagle K. The prevalence and distribution of major depression in a national community sample: the National Comorbidity Survey. *Am J Psychiatry.* 1994;151(7):979-986.
32. Anagnostis C, Gatchel R, Mayer T. The Pain Disability Questionnaire: a new psychometrically sound measure for chronic musculoskeletal disorders. *Spine.* 2004;29(20):2290-2302.
33. Gatchel R, Mayer T, Theodore R. The Pain Disability Questionnaire: relationship to one-year functional and psychosocial rehabilitation outcomes. *J Occup Rehabil.* 2006;16(1):75-94.
34. Asih S, Neblett R, Mayer T. Does patient-reported insomnia improve in response to interdisciplinary functional restoration for chronic disabling occupational musculoskeletal disorders? *Spine.* 2014;39(17):1384-1392.
35. Asih S, Neblett R, Mayer T, Brede E, Gatchel R. Insomnia in a chronic musculoskeletal pain with disability population is independent of pain and depression. *Spine.* 2014;14(9):2000-2007.
36. Choi Y, Mayer T, Williams M. What is the best screening test for depression in chronic spinal pain patients? *Spine J.* 2014;14(17):1175-1182.
37. Hazard R. Spine update: functional restoration. *Spine.* 1995;20(21):2345-2348.
38. Mayer T, Polatin P, Smith B. Contemporary concepts in spine care: spine rehabilitation: secondary and tertiary nonoperative care. *Spine.* 1995;18:2060-2066.
39. Cutler R, Fishbain D, Rosomoff H. Does nonsurgical pain center treatment of chronic pain return patients to work? A review and meta-analysis of the literature. *Spine.* 1994;19(6):643-652.
40. Brede E, Mayer T, Worzer W. Facilitating surgical decisions for patients who are uncertain: a pilot surgical option process within an interdisciplinary functional restoration program. *Spine J.* 2014;14(8):1686-1693.
41. Brede E, Mayer T, Shea M. Facilitating unequivocal and durable decision in workers' compensation patients eligible for elective orthopedic surgery: a surgical option process within an interdisciplinary functional restoration program. *J Pain.* 2014;15(1):49-55.
42. Mayer T, Kondrakse G, Beals S. Spinal range of motion: accuracy and sources of error with inclinometric measurement. *Spine.* 1997;22(17):1976-1984.
43. Brady S, Mayer T, Gatchel R. Physical progress and residual impairment quantification after functional restoration, part II: isokinetic trunk strength. *Spine.* 1994;19(4):395-400.
44. Curtis L, Mayer T, Gatchel R. Physical progress and residual impairment after functional restoration, part III: isokinetic and isoinertial lifting capacity. *Spine.* 1994;19(4):401-405.
45. Mayer T, Gatchel R, Keeley J. Optimal spinal strength normalization factors among male railroad workers. *Spine.* 1993;18(2):239-244.
46. Mayer T, Gatchel R, Keeley J, Mayer H, Richling D. A male incumbent worker industrial database, part I: lumbar spinal physical capacity. *Spine.* 1994;19(7):755-761.
47. Mayer T, Gatchel R, Keeley J. A male incumbent worker industrial database, part II: cervical spinal physical capacity. *Spine.* 1994;19(7):762-764.
48. Mayer T, Gatchel R, Keeley J, Mayer H, Richling D. A male incumbent worker industrial database, part III: lumbar/cervical functional testing. *Spine.* 1994;19(7):765-770.
49. Fore L, Keeley J, Mayer T. *Functional Capacity Evaluation for Patients with Chronic Pain: Guide to the Evaluation of Functional Ability.* Chicago: AMA Press; 2009: 291-312.
50. Galper J, Reese D, Shea R. *Use of Computerized Extremity and Trunk Tests in Functional Capacity Evaluation: Guide to the Evaluation of Functional Ability.* Chicago: AMA Press; 2009:117-129.
51. Keeley J, Mayer T, Cox R. Quantification of lumbar function part 5: reliability range of motion measures in the sagittal plane and in vivo torso rotation measurement technique. *Spine.* 1986;11(1):31-35.
52. Mayer T, Tencer A, Kristoferson S. Use of noninvasive techniques for quantification of spinal range of motion in normal subjects and chronic low-back dysfunctional patients. *Spine.* 1984;9(6):588-595.

53. Loebl W. Measurement of spinal posture and range in spinal movements. *Ann Phys Med*. 1967;9:103.
54. Mayer T, Gatchel R. *Functional Restoration for Spinal Disorders: The Sports Medicine Approach*. Philadelphia: Lea & Febiger; 1988.
55. Mayer T, Gatchel R, Keeley J. Lumbar segmental rigidity: can its identification with facet injections and stretching exercises be useful? *Arch Phys Med Rehabil*. 2000;81(9):1143-1150.
56. Biodex Medical Systems. *Dynamometers*. From http://www.biodex.com/physical-medicine/products/dynamometers.
57. Mayer T, Gatchel R, Kishino N. Objective assessment of spine function following industrial injury: a prospective study with comparison group and one-year follow-up. *Spine*. 1985;10(6):482-493.
58. Smith S, Mayer T, Gatchel R. Becker quantification of lumbar function part 1: isometric and multispeed isokinetic trunk strength measures in sagittal and axial planes in normal subject patients. *T Spine*. 1985;10(8):757-764.
59. Mayer T, Smith S, Keeley J. Quantification of Lumbar function part 2: sagittal plane trunk strength in chronic low back pain patients. *Spine*. 1985;10(8):765-772.
60. Mayer T, Gatchel R, Mayer H. A prospective two-year study of functional restoration in industrial low back injury: an objective assessment procedure. *JAMA*. 1987;258(13):1763-1767.
61. Protas E, Mayer T, Dersh J, et al. Relevance of aerobic capacity measurements in the treatment of chronic work-related spinal disorders. *Spine*. 2004;29(19):2158-2166.
62. Chaffin D. Human strength capability and low-back pain. *J Occup Med*. 1974;16:248-254.
63. Kishino N, Mayer T, Gatchel R. Quantification of lumbar function part 4: isometric and isokinetic lifting simulation in normal subjects and low back dysfunction patients. *Spine*. 1985;10(10):921-927.
64. Mayer T, Barnes D, Nichols G. Progressive isoinertial lifting evaluation, part 2: a comparison with isokinetic lifting in a disabled chronic low-back pain industrial population. *Spine*. 1988;13(9):998-1002.
65. Mayer T, Barnes D, Kishino N. Progressive isoinertial lifting evaluation, part 1: a standardized protocol and normative database. *Spine*. 1988;13(9):993-997.
66. Mayer T, Gatchel R, Barnes D. Progressive isoinertial lifting evaluation: erratum notice. *Spine*. 1990;15:5.
67. Jaeschke R, Singer J, Guyatt GH. Measurement of health status: ascertaining the minimal clinically important difference. *Control Clin Trials*. 1989;10(4):407-415.
68. Crosby R, Kolotkin R, Williams G. Defining clinically meaningful change in health-related quality of life. *J Clin Epidemiol*. 2003;56(5):395-407.
69. Copay A, Subach B, Glassman S. Understanding the minimum clinically important difference: a review of concepts and methods. *Spine J*. 2007;7(5):541-546.
70. Spratt K. Minimal clinically important difference based on clinical judgment and minimally detectable measurement difference: a rationale for the SF-36 Physical Function Scale in the SPOT Interventional Disc Herniation Cohort. *Spine*. 2009;34:1722-1731.
71. Gatchel R, Mayer T. Testing minimal clinically important difference: additional comments and scientific reality testing. *Spine J*. 2010;10(4):330-332.
72. Gatchel R, Mayer T. Testing minimal clinically important difference: consensus or conundrum? Clinical study. *Spine J*. 2010;10(4):321-327.
73. Theodore R. Commentary: methodological problems associated with the present conceptualization of the minimum clinically important difference and substantial clinical benefit. *Spine J*. 2010;10(16):507-509.
74. Mooney V, Cairns D, Robertson J. A system for evaluating and treating chronic back disability. *West J Med*. 1976;124:370-376.
75. Fairbank J, Cooper J, Davies J. The Oswestry low back pain disability questionnaire. *Physiotherapy*. 1980;66:271-273.
76. Rondinelli R. Rondinelli R, ed. *American Medical Association Guides to the Evaluation of Permanent Impairment*. 6th ed. Chicago: AMA Press; 2008.
77. Kerns R, Turk D, Rudy T. The West Haven-Yale Multidimensional Pain Inventory (WHYMPI). *Pain*. 1985;23(4):345-356.
78. Asih S, Mayer T, Williams M. Does classification of chronic musculoskeletal disorder patients into psychosocial subgroups predict differential treatment responsiveness and 1-year outcomes after a functional restoration program? *Clin J Pain*. 2015;31(12):1036-1045.
79. Beck A, Ward C, Mendelson M. An inventory for measuring depression. *Arch Gen Psychiatry*. 1961;4:561-565.
80. Wesley L, Gatchel R, Garofalo J, Polatin P. Toward more accurate use of the Beck depression inventory with chronic back pain patients. *Clin J Pain*. 1999;15:117-121.
81. Rush A, Giles D, Schlesser M. The Inventory of Depressive Symptomatology (IDS): preliminary findings. *Psychiatry Res*. 1986;18(1):65-87.
82. Rush A, Gullion C, Basco M. The Inventory of Depressive Symptomatology (IDS): psychometric properties. *Psychol Med*. 1996;26(3):477-486.
83. Rush AJ, Trivedi MH, Ibrahim HM, et al. The 16-Item Quick Inventory of Depressive Symptomatology (QIDS), clinician rating (QIDS-C), and self-report (QIDS-SR): a psychometric evaluation in patients with chronic major depression. *Biol Psychiatry*. 2003;54(5):573-583.
84. Hamilton M. A rating scale for depression. *J Neurol Neurosurg Psychiatr*. 1960;23:56-62.
85. Hamilton M. Development of a rating scale for primary depressive illness. *Br J Soc Clin Psychol*. 1967;6:278-296.
86. Beck A, Epstein N, Brown G. An inventory for measuring clinical anxiety: psychometric properties. *J Consult Clin Psychol*. 1988;56(6):893-897.
87. McCracken L, Zayfert C, Gross R. The Pain Anxiety Symptom Scale: development and validation of a scale to measure fear of pain. *Pain*. 1992;50(1):67-73.
88. Buysse D, Reynolds C, Monk T. The Pittsburgh Sleep Quality Index: a new instrument for psychiatric practice and research. *Psychiatry Res*. 1989;28(2):193-213.
89. Bastien C, Vallieres A, Morin C. Validation of the Insomnia Severity Index as an outcome measure for insomnia research. *Sleep Med*. 2001;2(4):297-307.
90. Johns M. A new method for measuring daytime sleepiness: the Epworth Sleepiness Scale. *Sleep*. 1991;14(6):540-545.
91. Miller R, Kori S, Todd D. The Tampa Scale: a measure of kinesiophobia. *Clin J Pain*. 1991;7(1):51-52.
92. Vlaeyen JW, Kole-Snijders A, Boeren RG, van Eek H. Fear of movement/(re)injury in chronic low back pain and its relation to behavioral performance. *Pain*. 1995;62(3):363-372.
93. Neblett R, Hartzel M, Mayer T. Establishing clinically meaningful severity levels for the Tampa Scale for Kinesiophobia (TSK-13). *Eur J Pain*. 2015;20(5):701-710.

94. Waddell G, Newton M, Henderson I. A fear-avoidance beliefs questionnaire (FABQ) and the role of fear-avoidance in chronic low back pain and disability. *Pain.* 1993;52(2):152-168.
95. Neblett R, Mayer T, Hartzell M, et al. The Fear-Avoidance Components Scale (FACS): development and psychometric evaluation of a new measure of pain-related fear avoidance. *Pain Pract.* 2016;16(4):435-450.
96. Neblett R, Mayer TG, Williams MJ, et al. The Fear-Avoidance Components Scale (FACS): responsiveness to functional restoration treatment in a chronic musculoskeletal pain disorder (CMPD) population. *Clin J Pain.* 2017;[Epub ahead of print].
97. Ware J, Sherbourne C. The MOS 36-Item Short-Form Health Survey (SF-36). I. Conceptual framework and item selection. *Med Care.* 1992;30(6):473-483.
98. Hathaway SR, McKinley JC. A multiphasic personality schedule (Minnesota): construction of the schedule. *J Consult Psychol.* 1940;10:249-254.
99. Hathaway SR, McKinley JC. *Manual for the Minnesota Multiphasic Personality Inventory.* Minneapolis: University of Minnesota Press; 1942.
100. Schiele B, Baker A, Hathaway S. The Minnesota Multiphasic Personality Inventory. *Lancet.* 1943;63:292-297.
101. Butcher JN, Graham JR, Ben-Porath YS, et al. *MMPI-2: Manual for Administration and Scoring, rev.* Minneapolis: University of Minnesota Press; 2001.
102. Gatchel R, Mayer T, Eddington A. MMPI Disability Profile: the least known, most useful screen for psychopathology in chronic occupational spinal disorders. *Spine.* 2006;31(25):2973-2978.
103. First M, Spitzer R, Gibbon M. *Structured Clinical Interview for DSM-IV Axis I Disorders.* New York: New York State Psychiatric Institute; 1995.
104. Spitzer R, Kroenke K, Williams J. Patient Health Questionnaire Primary Care Study Group, validation and utility of a self-report version of Prime-MD: the PHQ primary care study. *JAMA.* 1999;282(18):1737-1744.
105. Asih S, Mayer T, Bradford E, et al. The potential utility of the Patient Health Questionnaire as a screener for psychiatric comorbidity in a chronic disabling occupational musculoskeletal disorder population. *Pain Pract.* 2016;16(2):168-174.
106. Weiner IB, Craighead WE. *Symptom Checklist-90 revised. Corsini Encyclopedia of Psychology.* ed 4. Hoboken: NJL John Wiley & Sons; 2010;1743-1744.
107. Derogatis L, Melisaratos N. The Brief Symptom Inventory: an introductory report. *Psychol Med.* 1983;13(3):595-605.
108. Derogatis L, Unger R. *BSI 18: Brief Symptom Inventory 18: Administration, Scoring, and Procedure Manual.* Minneapolis: NCS Pearson; 2001.
109. Mayer T, Neblett R, Cohen H. The development and psychometric validation of the Central Sensitization Inventory. *Pain Pract.* 2012;12(4):276-285.
110. Neblett R, Hartzell MM, Mayer TG, Cohen H, Gatchel RJ. Establishing clinically relevant severity levels for the Central Sensitization Inventory. *Pain Pract.* 2017;17(2):166-175.
111. Neblett R, Cohen H, Choi Y. The Central Sensitization Inventory (CSI): establishing clinically significant values for identifying central sensitivity syndromes in an outpatient chronic pain sample. *J Pain.* 2013;14(5):438-445.
112. Neblett R, Hartzell M, Cohen H. Ability of the Central Sensitization Inventory to identify central sensitivity syndromes in an outpatient chronic pain sample. *Clin J Pain.* 2015;31(4):323-332.
113. Eriksson E. Sports injuries of knee ligaments: their diagnosis, treatment, rehabilitation and prevention. *Med Sci Sports.* 1976;8:133-144.
114. Hagglund M, Walden M, Ekstrand J. Lower reinjury rate with a coach-controlled rehabilitation program in amateur male soccer: a randomized controlled trial. *Am J Sports Med.* 2007;35(9):1433-1442.
115. Askling C, Karlsson J, Thorstensson A. Hamstring injury occurrence in elite soccer players after preseason strength training with eccentric overload. *Scand J Med Sci Sports.* 2003;13(4):244-250.
116. Molton I, Graham C, Stoelb B. Current psychological approaches to the management of chronic pain. *Curr Opin Anaesthesiol.* 2007;20(5):485-489.
117. Turk D, Swanson K, Tunks E. Psychological approaches in the treatment of chronic pain patients—when pills, scalpels, and needles are not enough. *Can J Psychiatry.* 2008;53(4):213-223.
118. Dersh J, Polatin P, Leeman G, Gatchel R. The management of secondary gain and loss in medicolegal settings: strengths and weaknesses. *J Occup Rehabil.* 2004;14(4):267-279.
119. Shaffer F, Moss D. Biofeedback. In: Chun-Su Bieber E, Bauer B, eds. *Textbook of Complementary and Alternative Medicine.* 2nd ed. Abingdon, UK: Informa Healthcare; 2006.
120. Sielski R, Rief W, Glombiewski JA. Efficacy of biofeedback in chronic back pain: a meta-analysis. *Int J Behav Med.* 2017;24(1):25-41.
121. Giggins O, Persson U, Caulfield B. Biofeedback in rehabilitation. *J Neuroeng Rehabil.* 2013;10:1-11.
122. Criswell E. *Cram's Introduction to Surface Electromyography.* 2nd ed. Sudbury, MA: Jones and Bartlett; 2011.
123. Flor H, Fürst M, Birbaumer N. Deficient discrimination of EMG levels and overestimation of perceived tension in chronic pain patients. *Appl Psychophysiol Biofeedback.* 1999;24(1):55-66.
124. Neblett R, Mayer T, Brede E. Correcting abnormal flexion-relaxation in chronic low back pain: responsiveness to a new biofeedback training protocol. *Clin J Pain.* 2010;26(5): 403-409.
125. Neblett R, Mayer T, Gatchel R. A clinical guide to surface EMG-assisted stretching as an adjunct to chronic musculoskeletal pain rehabilitation. *Appl Psychophysiol Biofeedback.* 2003;28(2):147-160.
126. Mayer T, Neblett R, Brede E. The quantified lumbar flexion-relaxation phenomenon (QLFRP) is a useful measure of improvement in a functional restoration program. *Spine.* 2009;34(22):2458-2465.
127. Ward N. Tricyclic antidepressant for chronic low back pain: mechanism of action and predictors of response. *Spine.* 1986;11(7):661-665.
128. Verdu B, Decoslerd I, Buclin T. Antidepressants for the treatment of chronic pain. *Drugs.* 2008;68(18):2611-2632.
129. Galer B, Jensen M, Mayer T. The lidocaine patch 5% effectively treats all neuropathic pain qualities: results of a randomized, double-blind, vehicle-controlled, 3-week efficacy study with use of the Neuropathic Pain Scale. *Clin J Pain.* 2002;18(5):297-301.
130. Jackson K. Pharmacotherapy for neuropathic pain. *Pain Pract.* 2006;6:27-33.
131. Seidel S, Aigner M, Ossege M, et al. Antipsychotics for acute and chronic pain in adults. *Cochrane Database Systematic Rev.* 2008;(4):CD004844.

132. Washington NB, Brahm NC, Kissack J. Which psychotropics carry the greatest risk of QTc prolongation? *Current Psychiatry*. 2012;11(10).
133. Johnson R, Strain E, Amass L. Buprenorphine: how to use it right. *Drug Alcohol Depend*. 2003;70:559-577.
134. Koppert W, Ihmsen H, Körber N. Different profiles of buprenorphine-induced analgesia and antihyperalgesia in a human pain model. *Pain*. 2005;118(1-2):15-22.
135. Howard K, Mayer T, Gatchel RJ. Effects of presenteeism in chronic occupational musculoskeletal disorders: stay at work (SAW) is validated. *J Occup Environ Med*. 2009;51(6): 724-731.
136. Fore L, Perez Y, Neblett R. Improved functional capacity evaluation performance predicts successful return to work one year after completing a functional restoration rehabilitation program. *PM R*. 2015;7(4):365-375.
137. Jordan K, Mayer T, Gatchel R. Should extended disability be an exclusion criterion for tertiary rehabilitation? Socioeconomic outcomes of early vs. late functional restoration in compensation spinal disorders. *Spine*. 1998;23:2110-2117.
138. Mayer T, Gatchel R, Evans T. Effect of age on outcomes of tertiary rehabilitation for chronic disabling spinal disorders. *Spine*. 2001;26(12):1378-1384.
139. Gatchel R, Mayer T, Kidner C. Are gender, marital status or parenthood risk factors for outcome of treatment for chronic disabling spinal disorders? *J Occup Rehabil*. 2005;15(2):191-201.
140. McGeary D, Mayer T, Gatchel R. High pain ratings predict treatment failure in chronic occupational musculoskeletal disorders. *J Bone Joint Surg Am*. 2006;88-A(2):317-325.
141. Anagnostis C, Mayer T, Gatchel R, Proctor T. The Million Visual Analog Scale: its utility for predicting tertiary rehabilitation outcomes. *Spine*. 2003;28(10):1051-1060.
142. Hartzell M, Mayer T, Neblett R. Does the economy affect functional restoration outcomes for patients for chronic disabling occupational musculoskeletal disorders? *J Occup Rehabil*. 2015;25(2):378-386.
143. Wright A, Mayer T, Gatchel R. Outcomes of disabling cervical spine disorders in compensation injuries: a prospective comparison to tertiary rehabilitation response for chronic lumbar spinal disorders. *Spine*. 1999;24(2):178-183.
144. Mayer T, Anagnostis C, Gatchel R. Impact of functional restoration after anterior cervical fusion on chronic disability in work-related neck pain. *Spine J*. 2002;2(4):267-273.
145. Mayer T, Gatchel R, Polatin P. Outcomes comparison of treatment for chronic disabling work-related upper extremity disorders and spinal disorders. *J Occup Environ Med*. 1999; 41(9):761-770.
146. Mayer T, Choi Y, Howard K, et al. Evaluation of functional restoration outcomes for chronic disabling occupational lower extremity disorders. *J Occup Environ Med*. 2013;55(12): 1489-1494.
147. Hartzell M, Mayer T, Asih S, et al. Evaluation of functional restoration outcomes for chronic disabling occupational cervical disorders. *J Occup Environ Med*. 2014;56(9):959-964.
148. Howard KJ, Mayer TG, Gatchel RJ. Comparison of chronic occupational upper extremity versus lumbar disorders for differential disability-related outcomes and predictor variables. *J Occup Environ Med*. 2012;54(8):1002-1009.
149. Neblett R, Mayer T, Gatchel R. Quantifying the lumbar flexion-relaxation phenomenon: theory, normative data, and clinical applications. *Spine*. 2003;28(13):1435-1446.
150. Neblett R, Mayer T, Gatchel R. Theory and rationale for surface EMG-assisted stretching as an adjunct to chronic musculoskeletal pain rehabilitation. *Appl Psychophysiol Biofeedback*. 2003;28(2):139-146.
151. Neblett R, Mayer T, Brede E, et al. The effect of prior lumbar surgeries on the flexion relaxation phenomenon and its responsiveness to rehabilitative treatment. *Spine J*. 2014;14(6):892-902.
152. Theodore B, Mayer T, Gatchel R. Cost effectiveness of early vs. delayed functional restoration for chronic disabling occupational musculoskeletal disorders. *J Occup Rehabil*. 2015;25(2):303-315.
153. Dersh J, Mayer T, Gatchel R. Prescription opioid dependence is associated with poorer outcomes in disabling spinal disorders. *Spine*. 2008;33(20):2219-2227.
154. Kidner C, Mayer T, Gatchel R. Higher opioid doses predict poorer functional outcome in chronic disabling occupational musculoskeletal disorders. *J Bone Joint Surg Am*. 2009;91(4):919-927.

SECTION XVI

CHAPTER 112 Surgical Procedures for the Control of Chronic Pain

F. Todd Wetzel
Charles N. Munyon
Michael Saulino

The results of conventional surgical therapy (e.g., deafferentation) for chronic benign pain syndromes are poor.[1,2] The results of so-called *neuromodulation therapy*, neurostimulation, and infusion techniques are continually improving, however, particularly in benign pain syndrome, which has typically been the most challenging to treat. Surgical experience with central deafferentation (e.g., cordotomy)[3–10] suggested that patients with neoplastic pain achieved satisfactory pain relief more frequently than those with benign pain. This is hardly surprising, as the effects of neural plasticity in patients with a longer lifespan should tend to confound the results of surgical interruption.[11] This was borne out in studies of cordotomy or dorsal rhizotomy.[12-18] A distinct characteristic of refractory benign pain is that it appears to follow lesions of the nervous system. This is in contrast to malignant pain, which is thought to be nociceptive.

Surgical intervention for chronic benign pain of lumbar origin is associated with high complication rates. The principles of such intervention, however, appear to be based on reasonable principles; these can be appreciated only with a basic understanding of neuropathologic mechanisms.

Mechanisms of Chronic Pain Production

The immediate effect of injury is to activate receptors in specific nerve fiber types. These include large myelinated Aβ fibers, small myelinated Aδ fibers, and small unmyelinated C fibers. The interaction of these afferents, primarily though not exclusively through the substantia gelatinosa, forms the basis for the gate control theory of pain. The cell bodies of primary nociceptive neurons are located in the dorsal root ganglion, with afferent synapses in layer I or V. Layer I cells are nociceptor specific and somewhat less discriminatory. Layer V cells respond to many inputs, mainly repetitive nociceptive stimuli and nociceptive input. The primary nociceptive neurons synapse on rostrally projecting second-order neurons in the dorsal horn, the theoretical target of the "gate."[19] After postinjury discharge, the next normal event would be for the fibers to return to rest. In the face of persisting injury, however, repeated firings are provoked; some receptors become more sensitive to subsequent stimulation and can, in fact, fire spontaneously. This sensitization can arise from direct change in the structure of the nociceptor[14,20,21] or as a response to substances released in its milieu.[22–25] As damaged tissue heals with scar formation, granulation tissue containing nerve sprouts and capillaries invades the area. This further changes the local environment and the sensitivity thresholds of the nerve endings. Such changes have relevance in the healing of surgical wounds such as those from laminectomy or spinal fusion; during healing, there may be significant pain problems generated by the wound itself. As would be expected from the nature of neuropathic pain, patients may note localized burning dysesthesias or even allodynia.

The compressed root is susceptible to such damage and all its ensuing consequences. Such roots are further subject to chemical irritation from the inflammatory process and to the resulting edema and ischemia. The end results of these pathologic processes are neural scar formation and demyelination.

The physiologic responses to nerve damage are complex and variable. Devor broadly classifies these into three groups.[26] The first, sensitization of the nociceptor endings, is characterized by a reduced threshold for activation. In such a state, nonnoxious stimuli may become capable of producing pain. Second, the nociceptive fibers themselves become a source of pain when they are activated at abnormal locations along their course; this is the phenomenon of ectopic electrogenesis. Third, pain could result from abnormal central processing of afferent impulses. In the setting of chronic spinal pain syndromes, the first two possibilities are most pertinent, with true central pain syndromes being uncommon.

Chemical[22,23,25] and mechanical[27–29] stimuli can invoke or modify repetitive discharge in the damaged nerve. Epinephrine and norepinephrine can both activate afferent fiber endings in neuromas; these responses are thought to be mediated by α-adrenergic receptors.[24,30,31] Sympathetic activity can produce abnormal sensation through neural transmitter release that stimulates afferent nerve sprouts possessing ectopic adrenergic chemosensitivity.[31] The abnormal sensations produced by these mechanisms may explain causalgia and other sympathetic dystrophies[32,33] along with the potential benefit of sympathectomy for such disorders.

The phenomenon of ectopic electrogenesis, which occurs in neuromas, can also develop in axons that have become demyelinated but remain in continuity. This issue relates directly to chronic low back and leg pain, in which a neuroma would not be expected to form, but in which demyelination of nerve roots is a known complication. Such demyelinated roots may exhibit either hyposensitivity or hypersensitivity. Spontaneous discharge has been shown to occur at sites of peripheral demyelination.[33] These discharge patterns are similar to those found in neuromas.[26] Consequently, nerves with regions of demyelination can demonstrate ectopic electrogenesis, which transfers nociceptor-like information into the central nervous system. Rhythmic firing, a characteristic of cell behavior not elicited until a certain threshold level of generation current is reached,[34] can be provoked in demyelinated regions by mechanical stimuli. This threshold characteristic is important because many injured nerves appear to be poised near the rhythmic firing threshold. As a consequence, brief or weakened stimuli can set off a prolonged discharge that may persist beyond removal of the stimulus.[26] In experimental preparations, tetanic stimulation produces this so-called *after-discharge,* which is followed by a period of prolonged electrical silence.[35] It is evident that this could have implications for pain relief from neuromodulation, such as spinal cord stimulation (SCS).

The dorsal root ganglion is mechanically quite sensitive in its normal state. Some discharge occurs spontaneously[36] even at baseline. Postdischarge, stimulation is common. This baseline excitability is heightened after peripheral nerve injury. In this instance, the dorsal root ganglion contributes ectopic barrages above and beyond those generated by the region of peripheral injury.[37,38] The state of excitability of the dorsal root ganglion is thus of clinical importance in root compromise.[33] In the chronically injured root, deafferentation in the form of ganglionectomy would, theoretically, remove this focus of irritability.

Damage to a peripheral nerve causes changes central to the lesion that may not be reversed by treating the original injury.[11] As noted earlier,[26,36] these central changes include heightened sensitivity of the dorsal root ganglion to mechanical distortion and to neurotransmitters. Axons central to a nerve lesion also diminish their conduction velocity. Cells in the dorsal root ganglion may degenerate, with consequent degeneration of central axons. This leads to substantial loss of afferent fibers, leading to deafferentation, which is another mechanism of pain. Additionally, the central terminals of C fibers change in response to peripheral nerve injury. The result is a failure of feedback mechanisms that produces prolonged depolarization and inhibition. Peripheral nerve section is thus followed by a reduction in inhibition of afferent fibers.[38] The cord "responds" to diminished input (deafferentation) by diminishing inhibitions to the remaining input.[39] The spinal cord itself thus becomes a location for continuing provocation of pain through mechanisms of chronic afferent barrage accompanied by reduced inhibition. Not surprisingly, many central ablative procedures, such as cordotomy, have been proposed as treatments for chronic pain syndromes. However, the role of these more central procedures in the treatment of chronic spinal pain syndromes is limited.

Variability in anatomy also creates additional levels of precision and uncertainty. Recently, Solmaz et al.[40] in a cadaveric study noted that there were an average of 4.8 ± 1.3 fibers consistent with intradural communication between dorsal rootlets of spinal nerves. The number of these intradural communications varied based on the level of the spine. All spanned one level, with the highest frequency in the cervical and thoracic areas. No cadaver had fewer than three, with some as high as seven. Clearly, such anatomic variation would compromise the results of any deafferentation procedure related to the dorsal rootlets.

Finally, the individual motion segment is richly innervated and thus capable of generating postinjury pain in the absence of frank neural compression.[41–46] Many of the procedures to be discussed are intended for the treatment of continued extremity pain caused by persistent neurogenic dysfunction; such procedures are usually unsuccessful in dealing with disorders of the motion segment per se. Thus, entities such as posttraumatic lumbar strain, postdecompressive segmental instability, and persistent discogenic pain are not well served by deafferentation procedures. Additionally, reversible sources of neural compression producing continued sciatica—such as disc herniation, lateral recess, or central or foraminal stenosis—must be meticulously excluded before the consideration of any of these procedures. Indeed, the most effective way to deal with the "failed back" (failed back surgery syndrome [FBSS]) is to avoid creating it by judicious treatment and surgery. Given the historical and current rates of spine surgery,[47] in the settings of favorable natural history of many degenerative syndromes,[48] it is unlikely that the incidence of FBSS will decrease.

The surgery for chronic pain in this setting has revolved around two concepts: deafferentation and enhancement of presynaptic inhibition. In the first case, the theoretical goal is diminution of the conduction of painful stimuli centrally by interrupting appropriate afferent pathways. Precise determination of these pathways can be difficult because of neuroplasticity, central mechanisms of continuing pain generation, and anatomic variation. In the second approach, enhancement of presynaptic inhibition, the goal is to achieve functional deafferentation by either chemical or physiologic means. Again, neuroplasticity complicates this approach.

Modulatory therapies that are germane to the concept of inhibition are nerve and cord stimulation and subarachnoid implants. Destructive therapies are essentially deafferentation procedures: rhizotomy and ganglionectomy. More central ablative procedures have no place in the current treatment of failed lumbar surgery syndromes. For example, the dorsal root entry zone lesion, produced by electrocoagulation, has been reported to yield a success rate of 54% to 82% in brachial plexus avulsion,[49–52] 50% in neurogenic pain from spinal cord injury, and nearly 60% in cases of postherpetic neuralgia, or complex regional pain syndrome.[53] However, in benign pain syndromes or arachnoiditis, dismal results have been reported.[54–57] Cordotomy[58] has been extensively studied in cases of neoplastic pain and can be of major benefit in this instance; some recent reports noted a 90% rate of pain relief in microendoscopically guided percutaneous procedures.[3,5,7,9,10] The procedure, in which the anterolateral pathways of the spinal cord are divided, thus interrupting pain and temperature transmission, has also been investigated for cases of lower cord or cauda equina injury. Porter and colleagues[8] reported a 62% rate of significant pain relief in follow-up ranging from 8 to 20 years. White and Sweet cited a 60% rate of pain relief in patients with cord injuries and in four of seven with cauda equina damage.[59] A recent review suggested that dorsal root entry zone, midline myelotomy, and anterolateral cordotomies, while continuing to be included in residency and fellowship training, should be "rarely used," particularly in benign pain syndromes, due to variability in results and the significant nature and frequency of complications (urinary incontinence, sexual dysfunction, and leg weakness). Additionally, genitourinary dysfunction rates of 8% to 92% have been reported.[5,6,8,9]

Deafferentation Procedures

Little attention in the recent literature has been focused on the use of rhizotomy as a treatment for chronic backache and sciatica. It has been widely investigated in other areas, however. As noted previously, results in tumor patients are generally superior to those achieved in chronic benign pain patients.[13,60–64] In a comprehensive review, Barrash and Leavens[65] analyzed dorsal rhizotomy for relief of tumor pain. Promising results of rhizotomy were noted in cases of central neoplasms as well as neoplasms involving the breast, colon, head and neck, lung, and rectal and urogenital systems. The problem of trigeminal neuralgia has been widely addressed as well. van Loveren and colleagues[66] reviewed their experience of 1000 patients with trigeminal neuralgia, comparing the techniques of percutaneous stereotactic rhizotomy and posterior fossa exploration. Of the 700 treated by percutaneous stereotactic rhizotomy, excellent or good results regarding pain relief were achieved in 125 patients treated with microsurgical vascular decompression or partial sensory rhizotomy. These favorable results were corroborated by the report of Bederson and Wilson[67] in 252 patients. Additionally, glycerol rhizotomy for trigeminal neuralgia has been investigated.[68–70] In general, good or excellent results are reported in 70% to 72% of the cases using this technique. Outcomes of intradural rhizotomy for neuropathic pain syndromes may be less favorable over time, however. A recent retrospective study of 55 patients treated by intradural cervical dorsal root rhizotomy for refractory occipital neuralgia reported a functional improvement of 57% at follow-up of 14 years. Interestingly, this is less than the rate reported for full pain relief (64%).[71]

Selective dorsal rhizotomy for spasticity in children with cerebral palsy, although controversial, has also been recommended. Cahan and colleagues[72] and Kundi and colleagues[73] emphasized the safety of the procedure, citing preservation of cortical somatosensory evoked responses. Good results have also been reported by others.[12,18,74–76] Intraspinal rhizotomy has been reported to diminish spasticity in patients with myelomeningocele.[77] Sacral rhizotomy in the treatment of hypertonic neurogenic bladder has also been investigated,[32,78–80] as has control of spasticity resulting from posttraumatic paraplegia.[81] Percutaneous radiofrequency rhizotomy resulted in improvement of spasticity in 24 of 25 patients in the series of Kasdon and Lathi.[82] In Turnbull's series, percutaneous rhizotomy improved lower extremity spasm in paraparetic patients who were not hospitalized.[83]

Taken in concert with the results presented for the disorders reviewed earlier, the outcome of rhizotomy for chronic lumbar pain syndromes is particularly grim. In the case of chronic pain patients, preservation of function is essential and the surgeon does not have the latitude to interrupt multiple roots, as is the case in many of the situations reviewed earlier. Additionally, the precise interpretation of pain reduction, which is necessarily subjective, complicates the evaluation of results of rhizotomy or ganglionectomy for chronic benign pain.

Rhizotomy and Ganglionectomy

Sectioning of the spinal nerves or excision of dorsal root ganglia can be accomplished at multiple levels. Rhizotomy may be performed by intradural section of the dorsal root, extradural section of the dorsal root, or extradural section of the mixed root (Fig. 112.1). Additionally, the median branch of the posterior primary ramus may be interrupted, although this is usually by a percutaneous technique, such as radiofrequency ablation (Fig. 112.2).

Sensory rhizotomy for the relief of chronic pain was first carried out by Abbe in 1888 but had been nearly abandoned by 1925 because of the relatively high failure rate and the subsequent interest in cordotomy.[12,84] Rhizotomy may be performed at this level to include selective sensory fibers or it may take the form of a complete rhizotomy. Characteristically, both ablative procedures are performed proximal to the ganglion.[15]

The goal of rhizotomy or ganglionectomy is denervation of the area in which pain is felt. It has frequently been assumed that root section should remove pain that is peripheral and circumscribed because the afferent territory of a few adjacent nerves presumably completely delineates the pain for that region.[15,85] Long-term results of rhizotomy fail to support this, however. In addition, results of selective sensory rhizotomy may be compromised because of the presence of denervation hypersensitivity, intersegmental cross-linking,[17,40] and overlapping dermatomes[86–89] and the presence of afferent unmyelinated axons in the ventral roots.[90,91] Intraoperative stimulation of these roots has been shown to provoke pain. If these ventral afferents comprise a significant portion of the ventral root, dorsal sensory rhizotomy may be providing insufficient deafferentation to interrupt pertinent sensory pathways.

One of the central problems in planning surgery for persistent limb pain is the precise delineation of the involved roots. Many authors have attempted to select patients on the basis of their response to individual nerve root sheath blockade as guided by electrophysiologic evidence of chronic radiculopathy and neurologic examination. Onofrio and Campa[17] reported their results in 286 cases of rhizotomy,

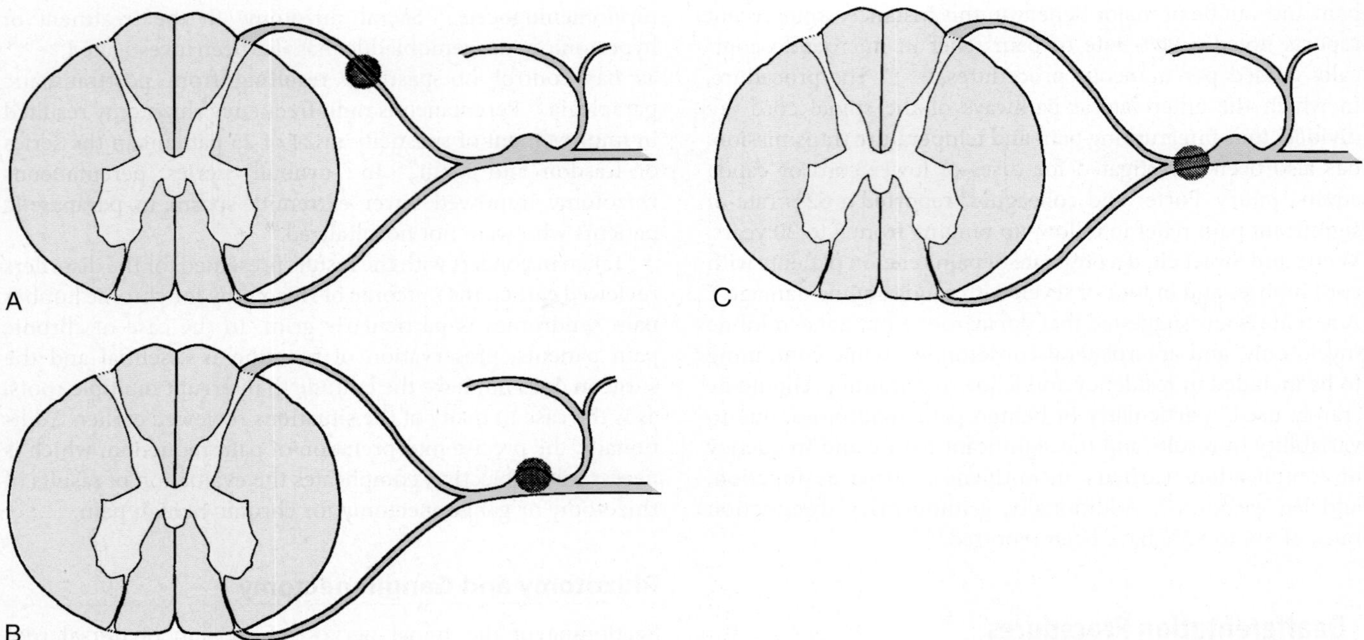

FIG. 112.1 Rhizotomy and ganglionectomy. The circular shaded areas the surgical lesions for (A) intradural rhizotomy, predominantly for use in cervical and thoracic areas; (B) extradural rhizotomy, predominantly used in the lumbosacral region; and (C) ganglionectomy. (From Wetzel FT. Chronic benign cervical pain syndromes: surgical considerations. *Spine*. 1992;17:S367–S374.)

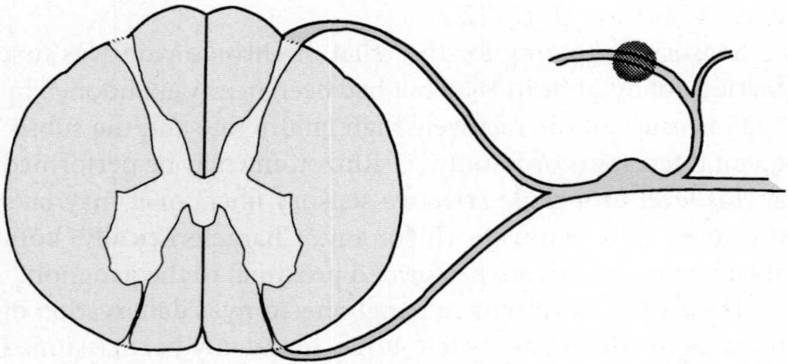

FIG. 112.2 Facet rhizotomy. The circular shaded area represents the surgical lesion created. (From Wetzel FT. Chronic benign cervical pain syndromes: surgical considerations. *Spine*. 1992;17:S367–S374.)

58 of which were lumbar. Only six of the 45 undergoing S1 rhizotomies reported long-term pain relief. Three of 13 patients who underwent lumbar rhizotomies had clinically successful results. These results were obtained despite consideration of dermatomal overlap and the use of selective nerve root blockade to plan the surgery. Loeser[16] reported similar results with a 14% success rate at 10 years. Arachnoiditis in the setting of failed disc surgery seemed to be correlated with poor results, and preoperative nerve root blocks provided little diagnostic or prognostic information. Loeser offered several reasons for these results, including incomplete root sectioning, inadequate numbers of roots divided, and a higher threshold of fibers in adjacent nerves, which may begin to produce chronic pain syndromes after the effects of local anesthetics from root blocks have worn off. He also speculated that central alterations may be important. Additionally, the utility of "diagnostic" nerve root blocks must be questioned. The selective root sheath injection appears to be nonspecific in not only a dermatomal sense but in a central and peripheral sense as well: several authors have reported on the ability of distal blocks to produce temporary relief.[92–94] Jain[95] believed that selective extradural sensory rhizotomy was not successful in the setting of arachnoiditis. Other authors have reported similarly discouraging results.[14,93,96]

In a compendium of results from multiple sources,[12] Dubuisson noted a 74% rate of immediate success following rhizotomy at L4, L5, and S1, which dropped to 33% 3 months after surgery.[15–17,63,95,96] These results are corroborated by the reports of others.[14,93,96] White, in reviewing a series of sensory rhizotomies for 10 patients with failed lumbar surgery, noted 80% good to excellent results. However, follow-up was variable, ranging from 4 months to 11 years, and no temporal specifics were reported. He did, however, agree that there was little pain relief when arachnoiditis was present.[61] Wetzel and colleagues[97] reported poor outcomes (14% success) in patients undergoing selective sensory rhizotomy at a mean follow-up of 2 years. All patients had undergone previously unsuccessful lumbar surgery.

Thus, it is difficult to recommend rhizotomy for the treatment of chronic benign lower extremity pain. Seemingly, the most reliable indication for rhizotomy is pain caused by deafferentation itself. Tasker and colleagues[32] reviewed 168 patients. The pain was divided into two groups: spontaneous and hyperpathic. In the latter, pain is induced by normally nonnoxious stimulation within adjacent areas of increased somatosensory thresholds. Overall, the pain in this group was nearly always causalgic or dysesthetic in quality and was associated with sensory loss. This was dramatically ameliorated by intravenous sodium thiopental, but not by morphine, and was usually relieved by proximal local anesthetic blockade. Various deafferentation procedures were reviewed, including rhizotomy, neurectomy, cordectomy, and cordotomy; each of these ablative procedures failed to relieve most patients of deafferentation pain. Hyperpathia, which occurred in incompletely deafferented areas, however, was partially relieved by surgical completion of the deafferentation, although the authors noted that pain may persist at the periphery of the sensory loss.

Sectioning of the dorsal root ganglion has been shown to provide the best results in terms of pain relief when performed for benign truncal neuralgias.[98] The results of ganglionectomy (see Fig. 112.1) at the caudal lumbar roots in cases of failed lumbar surgery are as disappointing as those reported for rhizotomy.[16,17,95,98,99] At this time, meaningful differentiation between rhizotomy and ganglionectomy as distinct therapeutic tools in this setting is impossible.

Technique

The patient is placed in a prone position under general anesthesia, and hemilaminectomy and partial facetectomy are used to expose the involved root. The root sheath is clearly identified and opened longitudinally for 8 to 10 mm proximal to the dorsal root ganglia. The dural septum, which separates dorsal and ventral roots, is identified, and a small nerve hook is passed between root filaments. Osgood and colleagues[98] noted that several distinct root fascicles are usually present. With electrocautery at a low setting, electrical stimulation is used to distinguish between motor and sensory fibers. As Bertrand has noted, however, caution must be used in relying on this test exclusively because chronically damaged roots may exhibit a higher threshold for motor excitation response than normal roots.[96] Thus, a wake-up test may be required. There are currently no reports in the literature on the use of somatosenory or motor evoked potentials to supplant this. When appropriate sensory fibers are identified, they can be sectioned with electrocautery or a microsurgical blade. Currently, there are no reliably described microsurgical or endosurgical techniques for rhizotomy or ganlionectomy in the particular instance of chronic benign lumbar pain syndromes, although endoscopic techniques have been described for facet rhizotomy.[100]

Facet Rhizotomy

Facet denervation is not nerve root surgery in the same sense that open rhizotomy is; rather, the theory behind this procedure involves destruction of the median branch of the posterior primary afferent nerve that supplies the facet joint (see Fig. 112.2). The median branch of the posterior primary ramus descends through a notch at the base of the transverse process and is covered by a ligament at the anteroinferior border of the facet joint at this level. This ligament is a continuation of the intertransverse membrane; it is here that several small twigs are given off to the facet joint. These twigs then enter the facet joint capsule.[46] Each posterior primary ramus supplies at least two facet joints, and each facet joint receives innervation from at least two spinal levels. Clinical features of facet joint syndrome have been described by several investigators. Mooney and Roberson are generally credited with one of the earliest descriptions.[44] Subsequent authors have attempted to improve the sensitivity and specificity of diagnosis and investigate diagnostic maneuvers, specifically response to facet blockade as selection criteria for facet rhizotomy[101] or even fusion.[102] Saal, in reviewing current diagnostic techniques, noted that the capacity of diagnostic facet blocks to correlate specifically with findings of the history and physical examination is limited.[103] Although a variety of signs and symptoms have been described as being associated with facet-mediated pain, these signs or symptoms are not specific enough to delineate a patient population suffering from facet-mediated pain per se.[104,105] Several studies have noted that the prevalence of facet pain among patients with chronic back pain is relatively low when measured by facet injection; however, the anesthetic response to a single uncontrolled block is as high as 50%, an unacceptably high false-positive rate.[106] It is generally felt that the gold standard by which facet joint blockade is judged is the appropriateness of the pain relief response based on duration of effect appropriate to the agent used for blockade and sustained relief by subsequent facet rhizotomy. This has been demonstrated in the cervical spine. In a study by Lord and colleagues,[107] patients experiencing neck pain from whiplash, who responded to facet blocks, were randomized into active and sham groups for radiofrequency lesioning. The median duration of pain relief in the active group was significantly greater than that in the sham group. No patients who failed to respond to blockade were included in the study.

Rees is generally credited with performing the first facet rhizotomies.[107] These were done percutaneously with a knife and reportedly resulted in immediate relief of symptoms in 998 of the 1000 patients who had facet pain in concert with the "intervertebral disc syndrome." Shealy[108] performed the procedure in North America but had an unusually high frequency of wound hematomas. This led to the adoption of a radiofrequency probe. Success rates as high as 90% were initially reported in previously nonoperated patients. That pain relief achieved by the interruption of afferent impulses of the facet joint has been suggested by the anecdotal reports of many authors who have noted immediate relief of pain in patients undergoing lumbar fusion.

Candidates for facet rhizotomy are those patients with back pain caused by facet dysfunction who have failed to respond to conservative therapy.[109] The key diagnostic maneuver is thought to be the facet block. This involves percutaneous insertion of a needle into the joint, under fluoroscopic guidance, followed by joint injection with lidocaine (Xylocaine) combined with steroids or contrast agents.[44,110,111] Patients in whom this procedure yields temporary relief may be candidates for facet rhizotomy.[109,110]

In the series of Shealy,[112] a satisfactory clinical result was noted in 79% of patients who had not had previous surgery. In patients who had undergone previous laminectomy, the success rate fell to 41%, and in those who had undergone previous fusion, success was only 27%. Of the 82 patients McCulloch followed from 6 to 20 months after facet rhizotomy, only 50% had satisfactory results.[113] Interestingly, three patients in this group required repeat surgery. Schaerer reported on 71 patients who underwent lumbar facet rhizotomy.[114] There were five distinct subgroups in his review: (1) lumbar facet disease without disc involvement (discography negative), (2) lumbar facet involvement with disc involvement (discography positive), (3) lumbar facet disease with discopathy and root signs, (4) facet signs with osteoarthritis, and (5) postlaminectomy pain. At a mean follow-up of 13.7 months, patients were evaluated using a pain profile. Thirty-five of 71 patients had satisfactory results. The highest percentage of success was in the author's first group—those who had a "pure" facet syndrome (seven of 15 patients). No attempt was made to determine statistically significant differences in outcome between these groups. Florez and colleagues[115] reported a series of 30 patients, achieving satisfactory results in 76%. Twenty-six of the patients were followed for 3 to 9 months. The best results were noted in patients without previous operations and those with shorter duration of symptoms. Oudenhoven[116] reported 377 patients with "pseudoradicular" pain in whom a lumbar facet syndrome was diagnosed by facet blocks. At a mean follow-up of 26 months, 83% were judged to be clinical successes. The author noted that a unilateral facet rhizotomy did not control pain and reported that 22% of patients who were judged to be clinical successes noted some return of symptoms at 18 to 24 months postoperatively. None of the authors reported any significant complications with the procedure. Lord and colleagues[117] reported on 19 patients who underwent cervical percutaneous neurotomy for neck pain of at least 3 months' duration following motor vehicle accidents. They found that results varied by level. Of the 10 patients who underwent C2–C3 rhizotomy, three obtained greater than 6 months of pain relief and one was pain free at the 4-month follow-up; the remaining six had return of symptoms over 3 weeks. Of the 10 who underwent more caudal neurotomies, seven obtained "clinically useful" pain relief. The authors noted that C2–C3 results may have been compromised by technical failure, including the relatively large diameter of the nerves and their variable course. In a recent level IV study, Duff et al.[118] reported that 63.64% of the patients in their series were pain free at 1 year. All patients had a mean of 1 year of pain relief.

With the recent interest in minimally invasive procedures, several studies have reported results of endoscopic rhizotomy of the lumbar spine. Jentzsch et al.[100] in a small series (four patients) reported that 75% had significant pain relief at 2 months. The sole study criterion was "chronic low back pain." Leon et al.[119] described a "360" technique of radiofrequency ablation of the medial branch of the posterior primary ramus and the internal joint capsule. In this level IV study of 73 patients, a mean decrease in 10 cm visual analog scale data from 7.3 to 1.7 with good to excellent outcomes was noted in 91.7 of the patients at 12 months.

One may be tempted to recommend this procedure after diagnosis of facet syndrome with facet arthrography and blockade. The current literature, however, does not substantiate the rates of clinical success (83%) reported earlier.[116] North and colleagues[101] retrospectively reviewed prognostic factors for facet rhizotomy and found that only 42% of those selected for rhizotomy by response to facet blockade had pain relief at 2 years postprocedure. Seventeen percent of those who experienced relief from blockade, but did not undergo rhizotomy, were improved. As noted previously, one randomized prospective study of rhizotomy for cervical pain noted a longer duration of relief in the active lesion group.[107] The reported complication rates are low,[120] and the apparent risk to the patient is minimal. There remain no convincing studies in the literature, however, suggesting that pain relief from the procedure is permanent.

Technique

The technique for this procedure is well described.[109,113] It is recommended that it be performed in the operating room or radiology department. Local anesthetic is adequate; the patient should be in the supine position for cervical rhizotomy or the prone position for thoracic and lumbar rhizotomy. Image intensification is required. Fourteen-gauge needles are placed unilaterally in the region of the appropriate facet(s) and nerves. A 5-mm, bare-tipped probe is then positioned in the area of the facet and the 14-gauge needle is partially withdrawn, leaving only the probe in the space between the superior facet and the transverse process immediately adjacent to the superior facet. The depth of the probe is controlled by lateral image intensification. A stimulation frequency of 100 Hz and from 0.1 to approximately 3 V is used to localize the tip away from the anterior ramus, as noted by the absence of paresthesia in the ipsilateral extremity. Once the depth is appropriate, stimulation adjacent to the posterior primary ramus reproduces a pain pattern familiar to the patient and the lesioning is then performed. A temperature-controlled lesion is produced by setting the controls at 25 V and 100 mA for approximately 60 seconds at 80°C. During the final 20 seconds, the amperage is slowly increased to the point where the milliamperage starts to diminish and voltage rises. This takes the temperature to approximately 90°C. After this, the probe is withdrawn, the wound dressed, and the patient mobilized. Alternatively, an endoscopic approach may be used as described earlier.[100] Whether or not the so-called "360" technique[100] is superior in the long run to the conventional deafferentation techniques is at this point unknown.

Sympathectomy

Sympathetic dystrophy represents a constellation of disorders of sympathetic nerve functions that accentuate or perpetuate chronic pain. Historically, Lankford[121] divided sympathetic dystrophy into two types, *causalgia* and *dystrophy,* based on the type of injury. More recently, Stanton-Hicks and colleagues[122] presented a revised taxonomic classification for reflex sympathetic dystrophy, regrouping the subtypes into a single entity, *complex regional pain syndrome (CRPS).* The diagnosis of CRPS requires regional pain and sensory changes following the index injury, coupled with skin color changes, temperature changes, abnormal sudomotor response, and edema. CRPS type I occurs without a specific nervous lesion and corresponds to sympathetic or traumatic dystrophy; type II refers to a discrete nervous lesion, equivalent to the former definition of causalgia. Obviously, many features of chronic spinal pain syndrome may fall into these various categories.

Given the multiplicity of complaints in patients with chronic extremity pain and the anatomic relationship of the sympathetic chain to the mixed lumbar root, the coexistence of autonomic dysfunction in the setting of chronic lumbar pain and radiculopathy is intuitively plausible. Patients with a pattern of persistent limb distress after spinal surgery may have signs and symptoms suggestive of sympathetic dysfunction. These include vasomotor changes, alterations in skin temperature, and joint stiffness.

The anatomic constancy of the sympathetic trunk with respect to the outer anulus has been well demonstrated by Bogduk and colleagues.[43] Pain fibers traveling lateral to the vertebral column in the sympathetic trunk may be prone to irritation owing to injury to the motion segment. Likewise, tears of the anulus fibrosus have been thought to be capable of producing a cold, painful limb on the ipsilateral side,[41] and Hodgson described a pattern of intractable lower extremity pain, associated with diminished temperature, in patients with failed lumbar surgery.[123]

Sympathectomy has been investigated in the treatment of limb distress of other causes, most notably vascular disease. Norman and House reported the results of lumbar sympathectomy for peripheral vascular disease in 153 patients.[124] Five years postoperatively, 67% of those who experienced claudication and 54% of those who experienced rest pain had avoided further surgery. Repelaer van Driel and colleagues[125] reported favorable results from sympathectomy in 66 patients who had suffered from lower limb ischemia. Jones also noted a beneficial effect of digital sympathectomy in treating ischemia of the hand in systemic disease.[126]

In the setting of persistent neurogenic dysfunction, however, the results of sympathectomy have been far less predictable. A central problem remains in establishing the diagnosis. The sine qua non for diagnosis remains response to sympathetic blockade.[42,92,127,128] Thermography has been suggested to be another diagnostic technique for detecting skin surface temperature changes associated with autonomic dysfunction.[93,129,130] Even with the use of both modalities, however, doubts have been raised regarding the validity of patient selection in chronic lumbar pain syndromes.[93]

Mockus and colleagues[131] reported on 34 patients who underwent lumbar sympathectomy. In 13, the precipitating incident was lumbar disc surgery. In this series, only one patient failed to obtain satisfactory relief. Wetzel and colleagues reported acceptable pain relief in only four of 17 patients at the 2-year follow-up. In this group, the patients' response to block was not as significant in predicting response to surgery as was their initial thermographic diagnosis.[93] Overall, including the results of even upper thoracic ganglionectomy, less than two-thirds of patients report satisfactory pain relief at 2 years with less than one-third reporting satisfactory pain relief at 5 years.[120] Thus, lumbar sympathectomy cannot be recommended with any conviction in the setting of chronic benign lumbar pain syndromes at this time.

Technique

The patient is positioned in the lateral decubitus position with the appropriate side up. A standard retroperitoneal approach is used, with a short transverse flank incision spreading each of the three layers of the anterior abdominal muscles, inferior to the level of the kidneys. This may be modified by a long, oblique incision from the twelfth rib to the lower abdomen, permitting access to the bodies of all the lumbar vertebrae. The lateral and inferior fibers of the latissimus dorsi and serratus posterior lie over the twelfth rib and may be partially transected. The distal half of the twelfth rib may be resected subperiosteally as well. The external oblique muscle is split in line with its fibers. The internal oblique and transverse abdominis are cut across their fiber in the same direction as the skin incision. Deep to the transversus is the peritoneum; posterior to this is the renal fascia. The renal fascia and the retroperitoneal fat must be dissected en bloc and taken anteriorly. The major dissection is posterior to the kidney, between Gerota's fascia and the quadratus lumborum and psoas.

The lumbar veins and arteries are anterior to the vertebral bodies, and mobilization is assisted with ligation of some of the segmental vessels. The sympathetic chain can then be plainly seen on the lateral aspect of the lumbar vertebra, with the most caudal ganglion usually at the L4 level. These ganglia should be dissected free from the underlying tissue, clipped, and removed. The wound is then closed in layers, with or without drainage as required.

Alternatively, sympathectomy can be performed endoscopically, even in the lumbar spine. Singh et al. reported reasonable results of endoscopic lumbar sympathectomy for plantar hyperhidrosis.[132] Fluoroscopically guided radiofrequency techniques have also been described in the thoracic spine.[133]

Stimulation Therapy

Epidural and Intraspinal Implants

Selective nerve root blockade (or epidural blockade) has been successfully used in many intraoperative and postoperative situations.[60,134–136] Likewise, implanted epidural narcotic reservoirs have been used in the treatment of intractable spinal and limb pain in a variety of neoplastic conditions.[137–142] Downing and colleagues[141] reported excellent relief of refractory pain in 23 cancer patients. In the series of Sjogren and colleagues,[143] 29 of 48 patients were able to be stabilized on epidural opioid treatment; of these patients, 21 were judged to be clinical successes. A tendency toward better relief of nonneurogenic pain was noted. In a large series reported by Liew and Hui,[144] good to excellent pain relief was obtained in 85% of patients. In patients who survived more than 3 months, the mean daily morphine requirement increased progressively from 3.5 to 19.5 mg per day, consistent with both drug tolerance and disease progression.

Overall, the results of intraspinal narcotics, usually morphine, are less consistent in benign pain than in pain from cancer. In an early report of 43 patients, 32 of whom had continuous delivery systems, Auld and colleagues[145] noted good to excellent pain relief in 65% of patients at greater than 2-year follow-up. Neither serious side effects nor evidence of addiction were observed. The same authors reported comparable results using a smaller system consisting of an epidural catheter and subcutaneous reservoir.[146] Prager recently summarized the current literature, noting comparable outcomes reported in most studies to date, with approximately 80% of cancer patients reporting greater than 50% pain relief and somewhat lower rates being reported for benign pain patients.[147]

The implantation of an indwelling narcotic reservoir is a promising technique for the management of benign refractory spinal pain syndromes; however, several notes of caution must be sounded. As previously noted, neuroplasticity in the setting of chronic benign pain tends to diminish the results of ablative therapies over time. In an earlier report, increasing narcotic requirements were seen in cancer patients.[144] Paice and colleagues[148] made a similar observation in chronic benign pain patients. In a multicenter study of 429 cases provided by 35 physicians, the temporal profile of drug use differed between cancer and noncancer patients: cancer patients had a higher initial dose, which increased quickly and then reached a plateau. Benign pain patients had a gradual, virtually linear increase in dose. Bearing this in mind, the following guidelines appear to be reasonable: an appropriate patient is one who is chronically disabled, not a surgical candidate, not appropriate for behavioral operant therapy, and psychologically sound. Whether a trial of electrical stimulation (discussed later) should precede consideration of an intraspinal implant is a matter of debate. Additionally, it appears to be the case that certain types of pain (e.g., nociceptive predominant) may be relatively stimulator resistant and are treated more effectively by intrathecal therapy.

For both intrathecal infusion and SCS, a psychologic assessment should be undertaken as a component of patient selection.[149] This analysis is best performed before initiating a trialing procedure. Certain mood and behavioral abnormalities are considered a contraindication for implantable device therapy (Box 112.1). It is important to recognize that the prevalence of depression, anxiety, and other mood disorders within a population of chronic pain patients is quite high and that these psychological abnormalities do not represent a contraindication for implantable pain technology.[150] The methodology for psychological clearance is not standardized. Some commonly used testing measures include the Minnesota Multiphasic Personality Inventory, Beck Depression Inventory, Sickness Impact Profile, and Oswestry Disability Index. Certain measures have failed to demonstrate significant prognostic value.[151] It is pertinent to note that psychological screening is not 100% effective in eliminating patients with significant psychopathology from trialing and implantation.[152,153] It may also be appropriate to maintain psychological interventions into the chronic phase of therapy because a synergistic effect on pain reduction has been reported with a combination of behavioral and interventional therapy.[154]

BOX 112.1 Psychological Contraindications for Implantable Pain Technology

1. Active psychosis
2. Major uncontrolled depression
3. Major uncontrolled anxiety
4. Abnormal illness behavior
5. Paranoid, schizoid, antisocial, or borderline personality disorder
6. Active suicidal behavior
7. Active homicidal behavior
8. Serious, unresolved alcohol or drug addiction problem
9. Serious cognitive deficits

Although several agents are commonly used for chronic intrathecal delivery, only three medications currently have US Food and Drug Administration (FDA) approval for long-term intrathecal use: baclofen, morphine, and ziconotide. Baclofen, a γ-aminobutyric acid (GABA)-B agonist,[155,156] has FDA approval for spasticity of both cerebral and spinal origin.[157,158] Although baclofen has shown some analgesic properties in animal studies, its utility in chronic pain is probably limited to musculoskeletal pain associated with spasticity and dystonias associated with CRPS.[159–162] Morphine, considered by many clinicians to be the first-line agent for intrathecal pain management, has been FDA approved for clinical use for more than 2 decades. Other opiates—such as hydromorphone, fentanyl, and sufentanil—have been used for chronic intrathecal delivery, but these agents lack formal FDA approval. Intraspinal opiates are thought to exert their therapeutic effect presynaptically by inhibiting calcium ion influx and postsynaptically by increasing potassium outflow.[163,164] The newest medication for intrathecal pain control is ziconotide, a synthetic form of ω-conotoxin MVIIa (Prialt; Élan Pharmaceuticals). This compound was originally isolated from the venom of the cone snail, *Conus magus*. This drug was formerly known as SNX-111 and is a 25-amino-acid peptide that blocks a neural-specific calcium channel on small myelinated and unmyelinated nociceptive afferents that are primarily localized in the superficial Rexed laminae (I and II).[165] The analgesic effect of ziconotide is produced when this channel blockade results in diminishing neurotransmitter release from these primary nociceptive afferents. Thus, the transmission of the pain signal never crosses the synaptic cleft from the primary afferents to the second-order neurons. Other commonly used agents for chronic intraspinal infusion include bupivacaine and clonidine. Intrathecal bupivacaine exerts its therapeutic action by directly inhibiting neuronal voltage-gated sodium channels and thus hindering nerve transmission. In general, the degree of blockade is related to the diameter, myelination, and conduction velocity of nerve fibers. Because the axons of pain-transmitting neurons tend to be thinner and poorly myelinated, bupivacaine can diffuse more readily into them than into thicker and more heavily myelinated nerve axons.[166] The mechanism of action for intrathecal clonidine, an α_2-adrenoceptor agonist, is not fully elucidated and may include interactions with *N*-methyl-D-aspartate receptors.[167]

Treatment algorithms for use of these agents, both in monotherapy and combination therapy, are far from standardized. It is important to recognize that although combination

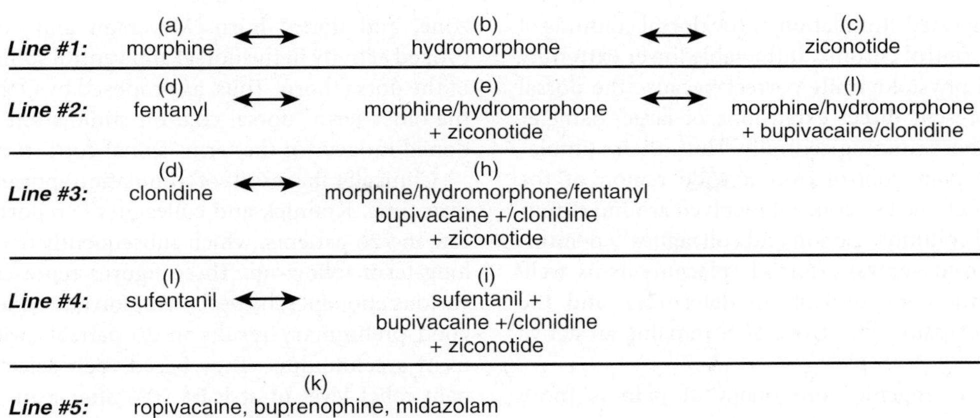

FIG. 112.3 2007 Polyanalgesic Consensus conference algorithm for intrathecal pain therapy. (Modified from Deer T, Krames ES, Hassenbusch SJ, et al. Polyanalgesic consensus conference 2007: recommendations for the management of pain by intrathecal (intraspinal) drug delivery: report of an interdisciplinary expert panel. *Neuromodulation*. 2007;10:300–328.)

therapy may have the therapeutic advantage of synergy between multiple agents, it also adds complexity with regard to stability, compatibility, and dosing adjustments. No combination therapy has FDA approval. One level of evidence-based decision making for intrathecal pain therapy is consensus statements of experienced clinicians. In January 2007, a consensus of experts convened to review the current medical literature and formulate updated guidelines for intrathecal pain therapy. The 2007 group recommended three first-line agents: morphine, hydromorphone, and ziconotide. Second-line agents include fentanyl monotherapy, as well as morphine or hydromorphone in combination with ziconotide; morphine or hydromorphone in combination with bupivacaine; and morphine or hydromorphone in combination with clonidine. The complete algorithm from this consensus panel is outlined in Fig. 112.3.[168]

Intrathecal delivery of medications can result in several potential adverse events, including sedation, cognitive impairment, nausea, vomiting, pruritus, urinary retention, constipation, hormonal dysfunction, and edema.[169] The majority of these problems can be managed with adjunctive care and/or adjustments of intrathecal delivery. However, the development of an inflammatory mass at the tip of the intraspinal catheter may require surgical intervention. These masses are called granulomas and were first described by North more than 2 decades ago.[170] The precise pathophysiology of these masses is not well understood. The relative contributions of drug dose, drug concentration, flow rate, continuous versus bolus dosing, catheter position, and cerebrospinal fluid dynamics remain somewhat unknown. Although several medications have been associated with granuloma development, morphine and increasingly hydromorphone are implicated in the majority of cases. There is consensus among experienced providers that high drug concentrations, especially for morphine, combined with low flow rate increase the risk of granuloma development. There is an increasing recognition of these masses with widespread use of magnetic resonance imaging, which makes prevalence reporting uncertain. The clinical presentation for granulomas ranges from asymptomatic to full-blown progressive myelopathy. Patients should be routinely queried for new-onset neurologic symptoms and undergo motor, sensory, and reflex examinations on a regular basis. This investigation is especially important in individuals who have demonstrated loss of pain control or new-onset pain complaints. Computed tomography myelography or magnetic resonance imaging with gadolinium contrast of the catheter tip region is necessary to confirm the diagnosis.[171] In asymptomatic and nonprogressive patients, weaning of intrathecal medications and initiation of saline infusion can produce spontaneous disintegration of the mass. In patients with progressive or severe neurologic compromise, urgent surgical decompression and excision are recommended.[172]

Technique

An epidural block of 0.5 to 1 mg of morphine mixed with saline is injected through a 22-gauge spinal needle. The degree and duration of pain relief are then noted in relation to side effects. Occasionally, an indwelling catheter of several days' duration may be required.

If a satisfactory response to the block is noted, an epidural or intrathecal catheter is placed subcutaneously through the T12–L1 or L1–L2 interlaminar space and brought through a subcutaneous tunnel to the flank. The tunnel is then taken anteriorly, where a pocket is created for the reservoir. The procedure can be done under local anesthesia.

Spinal Cord Stimulation

With the introduction of the gate control theory began a new era of thinking regarding chronic pain.[19] This theory held that low-threshold, primary, afferent fibers might be electrically activated peripherally, resulting in central suppression of nociceptive influences. Several authors[173,174] applied this idea to the treatment of pain in the distribution of a peripheral nerve, with encouraging results. Subsequently, Shealy and colleagues[175,176] suggested stimulation of the dorsal columns of the spinal cord to control chronic, intractable lower extremity pain. This seemed physiologically correct because the dorsal column fibers represent direct extensions of large-diameter primary afferent fibers running centrally. Thus, their stimulation should allow pain control over a wide region of the body.[86,177,178] Although the key concept revolved around stimulation of the dorsal columns, Larson and colleagues[179] demonstrated an effect from ventral electrode placements as well. Thus, active pathways are difficult to determine, and the physiologic basis of pain relief from SCS remains an active area of research.

Clinically, the neurogenic component of pain is more effectively treated than the nociceptive component; sympathetically mediated pain is more effectively treated than somatic pain. This suggests that the "gate" may be closed in the spinothalamic tract by activation of large-diameter afferents. Activation of supraspinal loops may provide ascending and descending inhibition. Additionally, direct stimulation or activation of descending pathways in the cord may block ascending impulses.[180] The mechanism by which SCS achieves the desired effect may not be limited to electrical depolarization of certain fiber populations. The work of Basbaum and Fields[181] has characterized a descending modulatory pathway; this lends credence to theories recommending the electrical and pharmacologic stimulation of *descending* pathways for the treatment of chronic pain. In this descending pathway, fibers from the midbrain and hypothalamus synapse in the dorsal pons and rostroventral medulla. Efferent, inhibitory impulses travel via the dorsolateral funiculus to synapses in the dorsal horn. These projections may functionally inhibit the target cells that give rise to the spinothalamic tract. The release of neuromediators in the dorsal horn has been documented in animal models. Linderoth and colleagues,[182,183] in a cat model, noted increased levels of substance P–like immunoreactivity in microdialysate from the dorsal horn after SCS. Release of serotonin was also noted, but no effects on extracellular levels of amino acids were detected. The authors speculate that serotonin release may be relevant for pain on the basis of the existence of descending neurons in the dorsolateral funiculus that store both substance P and serotonin and have a putative role in pain inhibition. Recent studies have also implicated GABA, demonstrating GABAergic activity following SCS.[182–184] Current thoughts on the neurochemistry of SCS have been elegantly summarized by Oakley and Prager.[180] SCS decreases dorsal horn excitability; releases dorsal horn GABA, substance P, serotonin, glycine, and adenosine; and reduces the release of glutamate, aspartate, and excitatory amino acids.

Initially, it was assumed that most of the effects of stimulation were attributed directly to stimulation of the dorsal columns. However, it has become clear that application of an electrical field to the dorsal epidural space may activate a larger number of neural structures. It is likely that paresthesias are elicited from intraspinal neural structures both inside and outside the cord. Barolat and colleagues[185] noted paresthesias ipsilateral to stimulating electrodes perceived as tingling sensations, reflecting stimulation of large myelinated fibers, involving the dorsal columns, dorsal roots, dorsal root entry zone, and dorsal horn. Meyerson and colleagues[186] noted evoked activity in the dorsal and ventral spinal cord at the level of the dorsal horn. Thus, as proposed by Oakley and Prager,[180] the older term "dorsal column stimulation" should be abandoned in favor of the term "spinal cord stimulation."

Clinically, the results of stimulation appear to have improved over time. Krainick and colleagues[187] reported a 38% success rate in 726 patients, which subsequently declined to 22.5% in long-term follow-up. These figures represent the results for various etiologies, however. Husson and colleagues[134] reported good preliminary results in 20 patients with radicular pain from arachnoiditis. They based their selection criteria on a pain relief level of at least 50% after a month of transcutaneous stimulation.[134] Wester,[135] in a series of 35 patients, 30 of whom were selected for implants, noted that 15 months postoperatively, 43.5% used the stimulator regularly. He found an increase in the amount of pain relief among patients with failed lumbar surgery syndromes and arachnoiditis. Young, in a series of 51 patients who underwent stimulator implantation, reported much less satisfactory results.[60] Twenty-five of the patients had undergone previous lumbar surgery; in all patients, pain had been present for at least 24 months. Thirty-seven patients underwent open laminectomy for implantation; 11 had electrodes placed percutaneously; and three, after an initial trial of percutaneous implantation, required open laminectomy. The author noted no major complications but stated that minor complications (e.g., paresthesia not in the desired location, infection, cerebrospinal fluid leak, lead migration, and breakage) required an additional 33 procedures. At a mean follow-up of 38 months, his results were disappointing. In the immediate postoperative period, 47% had significant relief, but no functional improvement (e.g., return to work) was noted in any patient. This raised the question of whether or not a spinal cord stimulator is an effective treatment for chronic benign pain.

Overall, with increased technical support, clinical experience, and the use of multichannel programmable devices, results have improved. Pain relief ranging from 0% to 85% has been reported.[55,112,140,185,187–213] All these studies, however, suffer from the same flaws: retrospective study design, variable definitions of criteria for success, and outcome comparisons independent of pain etiology. As the techniques and selection criteria have improved, an overall trend of increased maintenance of pain relief over time has been noted. Regarding efficacy in benign pain syndromes, the work of North and colleagues[206] appears to be illustrative. Successful outcomes, defined as 50% or greater pain relief, have been realized in 50% to 53% of patients with follow-up as long as 20 years.

Work by North and colleagues[188] bears special mention. In that prospective randomized study, SCS was compared with reoperation (laminectomy) for FBSS. Fifty-one patients were randomized into either stimulation or reoperation groups, with crossover permitted. Failure of stimulation was defined as crossover into the surgical group from the stimulator group, and failure of reoperation was defined as crossover into the stimulator group. Results for the first 27 patients reaching the 6-month crossover point showed a statistically significant ($P = .018$) advantage of SCS over reoperation. In a group of patients followed outside the study who opted for reoperation, 42% crossed over to SCS at 6-month follow-up. Kemler and colleagues[214] conducted a randomized prospective study to evaluate SCS in CRPS. Thirty-six patients were assigned to the SCS plus physical therapy group, while 18 received therapy alone. Of the 36, 24 had a successful trial and underwent implantation. At 6-month follow-up, patients in the SCS plus physical therapy group had significantly lower visual analog pain scale scores, although there were no functional differences between the groups.

Turner and colleagues[215] performed a meta-analysis of SCS for FBSS. In the 39 studies that met inclusion criteria, mean follow-up was 16 months, satisfactory pain relief (>50%) was reported by 59%, and complications occurred in 42%. All studies were case controlled. On the basis of these data, the authors concluded that no firm conclusions could be reached regarding efficacy or the effect of SCS on patient work status, disability, or medication use. It should be recalled that although this study did reflect the bulk of the available literature, it did not include either of the randomized prospective studies reviewed earlier.

The selection criteria for patients who may be candidates for SCS are of paramount importance. Krainick and colleagues[187] performed an initial trial with an electrode inserted into the arachnoid space using a small cannula. Stimulation was performed above the segmental level of pain for 30 minutes. In 73 patients, 28 obtained more than 50% pain relief. The value of a trial stimulation was also addressed by Nielson and colleagues.[178] In 96 of 221 patients who underwent a percutaneous trial, the stimulation was found to provide insufficient pain relief. Surprisingly, 28 of these 96 underwent permanent spinal cord stimulator implantation and, not surprisingly, failed to obtain *any* relief from the procedure.

Use of SCS to treat benign lumbar pain syndromes remains controversial. The most rigorous set of guidelines espoused for patient selection and technique are those of Krainick[177]: use of multiple electrodes, open epidural placement, localization of electrodes above the pain segments, absence of secondary gain, and localized rather than diffuse pain. These guidelines represent the ideal candidates for SCS. With the use of multiple electrodes to treat more complex pain syndromes, the open laminotomy or laminectomy approach is becoming more common, although percutaneous insertion may still be used as well (Fig. 112.4).[204,216]

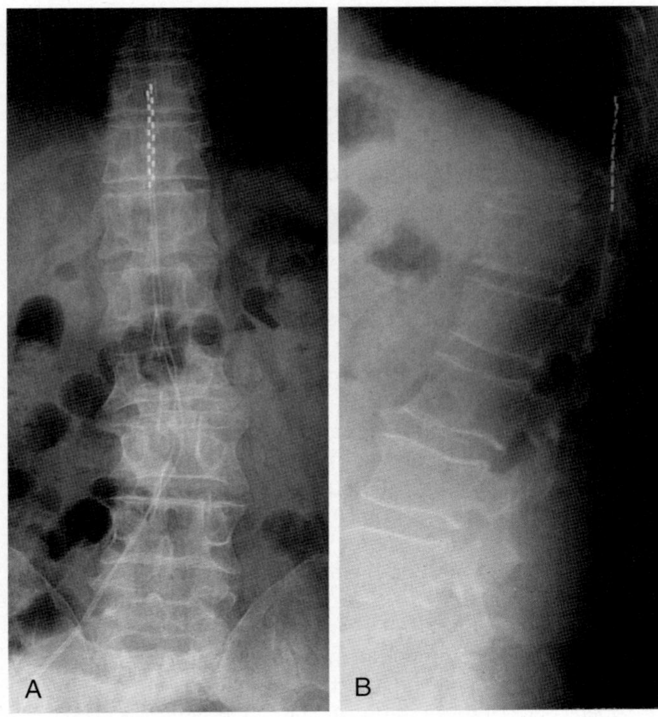

FIG. 112.4 (A) Note the symmetry around the midline and the thoracic placement. (B) Spinal cord stimulation, with multiple electrodes placed via a percutaneous epidural approach. These electrodes are in the optimal area for control of six to seven dermatomes involving the lower back and lower extremities.

Technique

Spinal cord stimulator implantation can be performed via several methods. These include percutaneous threading of the electrodes into the epidural space, epidural electrode insertion through an open laminotomy, and creation of an intradural pouch. The last is not clinically useful.

For most procedures, the patient is taken to the operating room and positioned prone. If the procedure is to be done percutaneously, local anesthesia with intravenous sedation is used. If an open laminotomy is preferred, the epidural space is directly visualized and the lead inserted. It is recommended that, for chronic lumbar pain syndromes, leads be inserted in the T12–L1 interlaminar space and traverse at least three levels cranially. This must be done under fluoroscopic control. The intradural pouch, well described by Burton, also requires an open laminotomy.[190]

Once the catheter is threaded, an unscrubbed assistant is given the lead to verify extension and efficacy of placement and to arrive at baseline parameters of stimulus intensity and frequency. After this, the lead is anchored in the fascia with a suture. A temporary lead extension is then tunneled and externalized for a trial. If a trial is done on the table and is successful, the lead and pulse generator are implanted permanently. A subcutaneous pouch and tunnel are created, and the lead is connected to the power source. The wounds are closed in a routine manner and compressive dressings are applied.

Summary

As can be appreciated in the previous discussion, the results of surgery for chronic lumbar pain syndromes are far from satisfactory. In ablative therapy, the results of rhizotomy and ganglionectomy are singly disappointing and can be recommended only when completion of the rhizotomy would result in alleviation of peripheral hyperpathia. Likewise, sympathectomy in the setting of chronic limb distress is unpredictable. The stimulatory therapies offer much more promise, with long-term outcome data available showing greater than 50%

pain relief in approximately 70%, with additional work required to determine the proper role of implantable narcotic reservoirs and of spinal cord stimulation. Overall, however, these results further underscore the need to emphasize careful preoperative planning before any lumbar surgery, with the objective of creating fewer chronic benign pain syndromes.

PEARLS

1. Most chronic pain syndromes are of mixed character, with nociceptive and neuropathic components. In general, nociceptive pain is aching, more difficult to localize, and narcotic responsive. In contrast, neuropathic pain tends to be burning or stabbing and generally refractory to narcotics except in high doses.
2. Perhaps the only reliable indication for a lumbar rhizotomy is a failed rhizotomy. In patients who underwent selective extradural sensory rhizotomy, they subsequently experienced significant peripheral hyperpathia. Completion of the rhizotomy resolved the pain in most cases.
3. For facet rhizotomy (medial branch of the posterior primary ramus) many authors advocate that not only the target facet but the rostral and caudal levels be lesioned as well due to intersegmental communication.
4. For patients with predominantly nociceptive pain, a subarachnoid implant (drug administration system or DAS) is usually more effective than spinal cord stimulation. The response of the patient to the epidural trial accurately predicts the response to the subarachnoid implant.
5. Patients with pure neuropathic pain syndromes often respond extremely well to spinal cord stimulation. Examples of this would be a unilateral "battered root" or complex regional pain syndrome. If a patient has a monoradiculopathy or unilateral pain, a trial can be performed with a permanent percutaneous electrode, which can remain in place with an extender following the trial so that the paresthesias do not have to be recaptured.

PITFALLS

1. In the rare instance of the central pain syndrome, no further peripheral surgery will be of benefit. The only way to diagnose a true central pain syndrome is persistence of pain despite a complete motor and sensory blockade distal to the level of spinal or epidural anesthesia.
2. All patients have large seromas following intrathecal pump implantation. This is particularly noticeable to the patient when he or she has difficulty feeling the reservoir itself or has a ballottable mass in the incision. This is normal. This should not be aspirated and the patient should be reassured.
3. For the first 6 to 12 weeks following implant, all SCS is positional. When the patient extends, the electrodes will move several millimeters closer to the cord as the dorsal cerebrospinal fluid space thins. Patients will experience paresthesias of increased intensity and perhaps different distribution. This positionality typically improves after 6 to 12 weeks; lead revision during this time should be avoided.

KEY POINTS

1. *The character of chronic pain:* Chronic pain differs from acute pain in many ways. In acute pain, after postinjury discharge, nociceptive fibers return to rest. In the case of persisting injury, repeated firings that can cause central changes are provoked as well. Thus, interruption of peripheral input (deafferentation) may not be effective treatment.
2. *Deafferentation procedures for chronic benign pain:* The results of surgical interruption of afferent circuits, regardless of the level, are generally poor and no longer in wide use. The exception to this may be facet rhizotomy (destruction of the medial branch of the posterior primary ramus by radiofrequency lesioning). The diagnosis of facet-mediated pain needs to be confirmed with appropriate facet blockade, with the duration of relief corresponding to the action of the anesthetic used. Recent studies show that when selected in this manner, results of cervical facet lesioning are superior to placebo.
3. *Neuromodulation:* Current medications approved by the FDA for long-term intrathecal (programmable pump) are baclofen, morphine, and ziconotide. Baclofen is useful in musculoskeletal pain associated with spasticity and dystonia, whereas morphine and ziconotide are useful for chronic pain. The latter is a nonnarcotic medication, a 25-amino-acid peptide that blocks a specific calcium channel.
4. *Neuromodulation:* Intrathecal delivery of medication via a programmable pump can result in several adverse events, the most problematic of which is the development of an inflammatory mass at the tip of the catheter. This may grow in size and require surgical intervention. Thus, the patient needs to be monitored for any neurologic changes. Habituation to medication may also occur, necessitating adjustment of the drug dosage, or even "drug holidays" in order to effectively manage the pain long term.
5. *Neuromodulation:* Spinal cord stimulation is effective predominantly in cases of neuropathic pain. Patients routinely undergo an epidural trial followed by permanent epidural implant via either percutaneous technique or laminotomy. By meta-analysis, satisfactory pain relief was reported by 59%. Randomized prospective studies comparing spinal cord stimulation to repeat laminectomy have shown a higher crossover rate from the surgical to the stimulation group than from stimulation to surgery.

KEY REFERENCES

1. Dubuisson D. Root surgery. In: Wall PD, Melzack R, eds. *Textbook of Pain.* 2nd ed. New York: Churchill Livingstone; 1989:784-789.
2. Loeser JD. Dorsal rhizotomy for the relief of chronic pain. *J Neurosurg.* 1972;36:745-750.
3. Howe JF, Loeser JD, Calvin WH. Mechanosensitivity of dorsal root ganglia and chronically injured axons: a physiological basis for the radicular pain of nerve root compression. *Pain.* 1977;3:25-41.
4. Wetzel FT, LaRocca SH, Adinolfi M. The treatment of chronic extremity pain in failed lumbar surgery. the role of lumbar sympathectomy. *Spine.* 1992;17:1462-1468.
5. Wetzel FT, Phillips FM, Aprill CN, et al. Extradural sensory rhizotomy in the management of chronic lumbar radiculopathy: a minimum 2-year follow-up study. *Spine.* 1997;22:2283.
6. North RB, Kidd DH, Campbell JN, Long DM. Dorsal root ganglionectomy for failed back surgery syndrome: a 5-year follow-up study. *J Neurosurg.* 1991;74:236-242.
7. North RB, Kidd DH, Zahurak M, Piantadosi S. Specificity of diagnostic nerve blocks: a prospective, randomized study of sciatica due to lumbosacral spine disease. *Pain.* 1996;65:77-85.
8. Schwarzer AC, Aprill CN, Derby R, et al. The false-positive rate of uncontrolled diagnostic blocks of the lumbar zygapophysial joints. *Pain.* 1994;58:195-200.
9. Lord SM, Barnsley L, Wallis BJ, et al. Percutaneous radio-frequency neurotomy for chronic cervical zygapophyseal-joint pain. *N Engl J Med.* 1996;335:1721-1726.

10. Prager JP. Neuraxial medication delivery: the development and maturity of a concept for treating chronic pain of spinal origin. *Spine*. 2002;27:2593.
11. Paice JA, Penn RD, Shott S. Intraspinal morphine for chronic pain: a retrospective, multicenter study. *J Pain Symptom Manage*. 1996;11:71-80.
12. North RB, Cutchis PN, Epstein JA, Long DM. Spinal cord compression complicating subarachnoid infusion of morphine: case report and laboratory experience. *Neurosurgery*. 1991;29:778-784.
13. Deer T, Krames ES, Hassenbusch S, et al. Management of intrathecal catheter-tip inflammatory masses: an updated 2007 consensus statement from an expert panel. *Neuromodulation*. 2008;11:77-91.
14. Oakley JC, Prager JP. Spinal cord stimulation: mechanisms of action. *Spine*. 2002;27:2574-2583.
15. North RB, Kidd DH, Lee MS, Piantodosi S. A prospective, randomized study of spinal cord stimulation versus reoperation for failed back surgery syndrome: initial results. *Stereotact Funct Neurosurg*. 1994;62:267-272.
16. Turner JA, Loeser JD, Bell KG. Spinal cord stimulation for chronic low back pain: a systematic literature synthesis. *Neurosurgery*. 1995;37:1088.

REFERENCES

1. Tasker RR, Dostrovsky JO. Deafferentation and central pain. In: Melzack R, Wall PD, eds. *Textbook of Pain*. 2nd ed. New York: Churchill Livingstone; 1989:154-186.
2. Tasker RR, DeCarvalho GT, Dolan EJ. Intractable pain of spinal cord origin: clinical features and implications for surgery. *J Neurosurg*. 1992;77:373-378.
3. Cowie RA, Hitchcock ER. The late results of antero-lateral cordotomy for pain relief. *Acta Neurochir (Wien)*. 1982;64: 39-50.
4. Tasker RR. Percutaneous cordotomy: the lateral high cervical technique. In: Schmidek HH, Sweet WH, eds. *Operative Neurosurgical Techniques: Indications, Methods and Results*. New York: Grune & Stratton; 1988:1191-1205.
5. Frankel SA, Prokop JD. Value of cordotomy for the relief of pain. *N Engl J Med*. 1961;264:971-974.
6. French LA. High cervical tractotomy: technique and results. *Clin Neurosurg*. 1974;21:239-245.
7. O'Connell JE. Anterolateral chordotomy for intractable pain in carcinoma of the rectum. *Proc R Soc Med*. 1969;62:1223-1225.
8. Porter RW, Hohmann GW, Bors E, French JD. Cordotomy for pain following cauda equina injury. *Arch Surg*. 1966;92:765-770.
9. Raskind R. Analytical review of open cordotomy. *Int Surg*. 1969;51:226-231.
10. Fonoff ET, Lopez WO, de Oliveria YS, Teixeria MJ. Microendoscopically-guided percutaneous cordotomy for intractable pain: case series of 24 patients. *J Neurosurg*. 2016;124:389-396.
11. Noordenbos W, Wall PD. Implications of the failure of nerve resection and graft to cure chronic pain produced by nerve lesions. *J Neurol Neurosurg Psychiatry*. 1981;44:1068-1073.
12. Abbe R. Intradural section of the spinal nerves for neuralgia. *Bost Med Surg J*. 1989;135:329-335.
13. Arens LJ, Peacock WJ, Peter J. Selective posterior rhizotomy: a long-term follow-up study. *Childs Nerv Syst*. 1989;5:148-152.
14. Bernard TN Jr, Broussard TS, Dwyer AP, LaRocca SH. Extradural sensory rhizotomy in the management of chronic lumbar spondylosis with radiculopathy. *Orthop Trans*. 1987;11:23.
15. Dubuisson D. Root surgery. In: Wall PD, Melzack R, eds. *Textbook of Pain*. 2nd ed. New York: Churchill Livingstone; 1989:784-789.
16. Loeser JD. Dorsal rhizotomy for the relief of chronic pain. *J Neurosurg*. 1972;36:745-750.
17. Onofrio BM, Campa HK. Evaluation of rhizotomy. review of 12 years' experience. *J Neurosurg*. 1972;36:751-755.
18. Oppenheim WL. Selective posterior rhizotomy for spastic cerebral palsy. A review. *Clin Orthop Relat Res*. 1990;253:20-29.
19. Melzack R, Wall PD. Pain mechanisms: a new theory. *Science*. 1965;150(699):971-979.
20. Beck PW, Handwerker HO, Zimmermann M. Nervous outflow from the cat's foot during noxious radiant heat stimulation. *Brain Res*. 1974;67:373-386.
21. Bessou P, Perl ER. Response of cutaneous sensory units with unmyelinated fibers to noxious stimuli. *J Neurophysiol*. 1969;32:1025-1043.
22. Fock S, Mense S. Excitatory effects of 5-hydroxytryptamine, histamine and potassium ions on muscular group IV afferent units: a comparison with bradykinin. *Brain Res*. 1976;105: 459-469.
23. Richardson BP, Engel G. The pharmacology and function of 5HT3 receptors. *Trends Neurosci*. 1986;9:424.
24. Korenman EM, Devor M. Ectopic adrenergic sensitivity in damaged peripheral nerve axons in the rat. *Exp Neurol*. 1981;72(1):63-81.
25. Levine JD, Gooding J, Donatoni P, et al. The role of the polymorphonuclear leukocyte in hyperalgesia. *J Neurosci*. 1985;5(11):3025-3029.
26. Devor M. Nerve pathophysiology and mechanisms of pain in causalgia. *J Auton Nerv Syst*. 1983;7:371-384.
27. Handwerker HO, Anton F, Reeh PW. Discharge patterns of afferent cutaneous nerve fibers from the rat's tail during prolonged noxious mechanical stimulation. *Exp Brain Res*. 1987;65:493-504.
28. Adriaensen H, Gybels J, Handwerker HO, Van Hees J. Nociceptor discharges and sensations due to prolonged noxious mechanical stimulation—a paradox. *Hum Neurobiol*. 1984;3:53-58.
29. Reeh PW, Bayer J, Kocher L, Handwerker HO. Sensitization of nociceptive cutaneous nerve fibers from the rat's tail by noxious mechanical stimulation. *Exp Brain Res*. 1987;65: 505-512.
30. Scadding JW. Development of ongoing activity, mechanosensitivity, and adrenaline sensitivity in severed peripheral nerve axons. *Exp Neurol*. 1981;73:345-364.
31. Wall PD, Gutnick M. Ongoing activity in peripheral nerves: the physiology and pharmacology of impulses originating from a neuroma. *Exp Neurol*. 1974;43:580-593.
32. Tasker RR, Organ LW, Hawrylyshyn P. Deafferentation and causalgia. In: Bonica JJ, ed. *Pain*. New York: Raven Press; 1980:305-329.
33. Howe JF, Loeser JD, Calvin WH. Mechanosensitivity of dorsal root ganglia and chronically injured axons: a physiological basis for the radicular pain of nerve root compression. *Pain*. 1977;3:25-41.
34. Calvin WH. Generation of spike trains in CNS neurons. *Brain Res*. 1975;84:1-22.
35. Lisney SJ, Devor M. Afterdischarge and interactions among fibers in damaged peripheral nerve in the rat. *Brain Res*. 1987;415:122-136.

36. Kirk EJ. Impulses in dorsal spinal nerve rootlets in cats and rabbits arising from dorsal root ganglia isolated from the periphery. *J Comp Neurol.* 1974;155:165-175.
37. Wall PD, Devor M. Sensory afferent impulses originate from dorsal root ganglia as well as from the periphery in normal and nerve injured rats. *Pain.* 1983;17:321-339.
38. Wall PD, Devor M. The effect of peripheral nerve injury on dorsal root potentials and on transmission of afferent signals into the spinal cord. *Brain Res.* 1981;209:95-111.
39. Wall PD. Introduction. In: Melzack R, Wall PD, eds. *Textbook of Pain.* 2nd ed. New York: Churchill Livingstone; 1989:13.
40. Solmaz B, Tatarli N, Ceylan D, Keles E, Cavdars S. Intradural communication between dorsal rootlets of the spinal nerves: their clinical significance. *Acta Neurochir (Wien).* 2015;157: 1069-1076.
41. O'Brien JP. Mechanisms of spinal pain. In: Melzack R, Wall PD, eds. *Textbook of Pain.* 2nd ed. New York: Churchill Livingston; 1989:244.
42. Walsh JA, Glynn CJ, Cousins MJ, Basedow RW. Blood flow, sympathetic activity and pain relief following lumbar sympathetic blockade or surgical sympathectomy. *Anaesth Intensive Care.* 1985;13:18-24.
43. Bogduk N, Tynan W, Wilson AS. The nerve supply to the human lumbar intervertebral discs. *J Anat.* 1981;132(Pt 1): 39-56.
44. Mooney V, Robertson J. The facet syndrome. *Clin Orthop Relat Res.* 1976;115:149-156.
45. Pallie W. The intersegmental anastomoses of posterior spinal rootlets and their significance. *J Neurosurg.* 1959;16:188-196.
46. Pedersen HE, Blunck CF, Gardner E. The anatomy of lumbosacral posterior rami and meningeal branches of spinal nerve (sinu-vertebral nerves); with an experimental study of their functions. *J Bone Joint Surg Am.* 1956;38-A:377-391.
47. Wynn Parry CB. The failed back. In: Melzack R, Wall PD, eds. *Textbook of Pain.* 2nd ed. New York: Churchill Livingstone; 1989:341-354.
48. Hakelius A. Prognosis in sciatica. A clinical follow-up of surgical and non-surgical treatment. *Acta Orthop Scand Suppl.* 1970;129:1-76.
49. Dieckmann G, Veras G. Plexus avulsion pain (neurogenic pain): high frequency coagulation of the dorsal root entry in patient with deafferentation pain. *Acta Neurosurg.* 1984;33(suppl):445-450.
50. Friedman AH, Bullitt E. Dorsal root entry zone lesions in the treatment of pain following brachial plexus avulsion, spinal cord injury and herpes zoster. *Appl Neurophysiol.* 1988;51:164-169.
51. Friedman AH, Nashold BS Jr, Bronec PR. Dorsal root entry zone lesions for the treatment of brachial plexus avulsion injuries: a follow-up study. *Neurosurgery.* 1988;22:369-373.
52. Thomas DG, Sheehy JP. Dorsal root entry zone lesions (Nashold's procedure) for pain relief following brachial plexus avulsion. *J Neurol Neurosurg Psychiatry.* 1983;46:924-928.
53. Chivukula S, Tempel ZJ, Chan CJ, et al. Spinal and nucleus caudalis dorsal root entry zone lesioning for chronic pain: efficacy and outcomes. *World Neurosurg.* 2015;84:494-504.
54. Wiegand H, Winkelmuller W. Treatment of deafferentation pain by high-frequency intervention on the dorsal root entry zone. *Dtsch Med Wochenschr.* 1985;110:216-220.
55. Nashold BS Jr, Ostdahl RH. Dorsal root entry zone lesions for pain relief. *J Neurosurg.* 1979;51:59-69.
56. Powers SK, Adams JE, Edwards MS, et al. Pain relief from dorsal root entry zone lesions made with argon and carbon dioxide microsurgical lasers. *J Neurosurg.* 1984;61:841-847.
57. Powers SK, Barbaro NM, Levy RM. Pain control with laser-produced dorsal root entry zone lesions. *Appl Neurophysiol.* 1988;51:243-254.
58. Spiller WG, Martin E. The treatment of persistent pain of organic origin in the lower part of the body by division of the anterolateral column of the spinal cord. *JAMA.* 1912;58:1489-1490.
59. White JC, Sweet WH, Hawkins R, Nilges RG. Anterolateral cordotomy: results, complications, and casues of failure. *Brain.* 1950;73:346-367.
60. Young RF. Evaluation of dorsal column stimulation in the treatment of chronic pain. *Neurosurgery.* 1978;3:373-379.
61. White JC. Posterior rhizotomy: a possible substitute for cordotomy in otherwise intractable neuralgias of the trunk and extremities of nonmalignant origin. *Clin Neurosurg.* 1965;13:20-41.
62. Scoville WB. Extradural spinal sensory rhizotomy. *J Neurosurg.* 1966;25:94-95.
63. Strait TA, Hunter SE. Intraspinal extradural sensory rhizotomy in patients with failure of lumbar disc surgery. *J Neurosurg.* 1981;54:193-196.
64. Toczek SK, McCullough DC, Gargour GW, et al. Selective sacral rootlet rhizotomy for hypertonic neurogenic bladder. *J Neurosurg.* 1975;42:567-574.
65. Barrash JM, Leavens ME. Dorsal rhizotomy for the relief of intractable pain of malignant tumor origin. *J Neurosurg.* 1973;38:755-757.
66. van Loveren H, Tew JM Jr, Keller JT, Nurre MA. A 10-year experience in the treatment of trigeminal neuralgia. Comparison of percutaneous stereotaxic rhizotomy and posterior fossa exploration. *J Neurosurg.* 1982;57:757-764.
67. Bederson JB, Wilson CB. Evaluation of microvascular decompression and partial sensory rhizotomy in 252 cases of trigeminal neuralgia. *J Neurosurg.* 1989;71:359-367.
68. Arias MJ. Percutaneous retrogasserian glycerol rhizotomy for trigeminal neuralgia. A prospective study of 100 cases. *J Neurosurg.* 1986;65:32-36.
69. Beck DW, Olson JJ, Urig EJ. Percutaneous retrogasserian glycerol rhizotomy for treatment of trigeminal neuralgia. *J Neurosurg.* 1986;65:28-31.
70. Bennett MH, Lunsford LD. Percutaneous retrogasserian glycerol rhizotomy for tic douloureux: part 2. Results and implications of trigeminal evoked potential studies. *Neurosurgery.* 1984;14:431-435.
71. Gande AV, Chivukula S, Moossy JJ, et al. Long-term outcome of intradural cervical dorsal root rhizotomy for refractory occipital neuralgia. *J Neurosurg.* 2015;18:1-9.
72. Cahan LD, Kundi MS, McPherson D, et al. Electrophysiologic studies in selective dorsal rhizotomy for spasticity in children with cerebral palsy. *Appl Neurophysiol.* 1987;50:459-462.
73. Kundi M, Cahan L, Starr A. Somatosensory evoked potentials in cerebral palsy after partial dorsal root rhizotomy. *Arch Neurol.* 1989;46:524-527.
74. Fasano VA, Broggi G, Zeme S. Intraoperative electrical stimulation for functional posterior rhizotomy. *Scand J Rehabil Med Suppl.* 1988;17:149-154.
75. Neville BG. Selective dorsal rhizotomy for spastic cerebral palsy. *Dev Med Child Neurol.* 1988;30:395-398.
76. Storrs BB, Nishida T. Use of the 'H' reflex recovery curve in selective posterior rhizotomy. *Pediatr Neurosci.* 1988;14:120-123.
77. McLaughlin TP, Banta JV, Gahm NH, Raycroft JF. Intraspinal rhizotomy and distal cordectomy in patients with myelomeningocele. *J Bone Joint Surg Am.* 1986;68:88-94.

78. Mulcahy JJ, Young AB. Percutaneous radiofrequency sacral rhizotomy in the treatment of the hyperreflexic bladder. *J Urol.* 1978;120:557-558.
79. Rockswold GL, Chou SN, Bradley WE. Re-evaluation of differential sacral rhizotomy for neurological bladder disease. *J Neurosurg.* 1978;48:773-778.
80. Rockswold GL, Bradley WE, Chou SN. Differential sacral rhizotomy in the treatment of neurogenic bladder dysfunction. preliminary report of six cases. *J Neurosurg.* 1973;38:748-754.
81. Laitinen LV, Nilsson S, Fugl-Meyer AR. Selective posterior rhizotomy for treatment of spasticity. *J Neurosurg.* 1983;58:895-899.
82. Kasdon DL, Lathi ES. A prospective study of radiofrequency rhizotomy in the treatment of posttraumatic spasticity. *Neurosurgery.* 1984;15:526-529.
83. Turnbull IM. Percutaneous lumbar rhizotomy for spasms in paraplegia. *Paraplegia.* 1983;21:131-136.
84. Wilkin RH: *Neurosurgical classics.* New York, Johnson Reprint Corp, 1968.
85. Davis L, Pollock LJ. The peripheral pathway for painful sensation. *Arch Neurol Psychiatry.* 1930;24:883-898.
86. Head H. On disturbances of sensation with especial reference to the pain of nerve disease. *Brain.* 1930;16:133.
87. Dykes RW, Terzis JK. Spinal nerve distributions in the upper limb: the organization of the dermatome and afferent myotome. *Philos Trans R Soc Lond B Biol Sci.* 1981;293: 509-554.
88. Foerster O. The dermatomes in man. *Brain.* 1933;56:1-39.
89. Sherrington CS. Experiments in the examination of the peripheral distribution of the fibers of the posterior roots of some spinal nerves. *Philos Trans R Soc Lond B Biol Sci.* 1898;190:45-186.
90. Coggeshall RE. Afferent fibers in the ventral root. *Neurosurgery.* 1979;4:443-448.
91. Sykes MT, Coggeshall RE. Unmyelinated fibers in the human L4 and L5 ventral roots. *Brain Res.* 1973;63:490-495.
92. Kilber RF, Nathan PW. Relief of pain and paraesthesiae by nerve block distal to a lesion. *J Neurol Neurosurg Psychiatry.* 1960;23:91-98.
93. Wetzel FT, LaRocca SH, Adinolfi M. The treatment of chronic extremity pain in failed lumbar surgery. the role of lumbar sympathectomy. *Spine.* 1992;17:1462-1468.
94. Xavier AV, McDanal J, Kissin I. Relief of sciatic radicular pain by sciatic nerve block. *Anesth Analg.* 1988;67:1177-1180.
95. Jain KK. Nerve root scarring and arachnoiditis as a complication of lumbar intervertebral disc surgery–surgical treatment. *Neurochirurgia (Stuttg).* 1974;17:185-192.
96. Bertrand G. The "battered" root problem. *Orthop Clin North Am.* 1975;6:305-310.
97. Wetzel FT, Phillips FM, Aprill CN, et al. Extradural sensory rhizotomy in the management of chronic lumbar radiculopathy: a minimum 2-year follow-up study. *Spine.* 1997;22:2283.
98. Osgood CP, Dujovny M, Faille R, Abassy M. Microsurgical ganglionectomy for chronic pain syndromes. technical note. *J Neurosurg.* 1976;45:113-115.
99. North RB, Kidd DH, Campbell JN, Long DM. Dorsal root ganglionectomy for failed back surgery syndrome: a 5-year follow-up study. *J Neurosurg.* 1991;74:236-242.
100. Jentzsch T, Sprengel K, Peterer L, Mica L, Werner CM. 3D navigation of endoscopic rhizotomy at the lumbar spine. *J Clin Neurosci.* 2016;23:101-105.
101. North RB, Kidd DH, Zahurak M, Piantadosi S. Specificity of diagnostic nerve blocks: a prospective, randomized study of sciatica due to lumbosacral spine disease. *Pain.* 1996;65:77-85.
102. Esses SI, Moro JK. The value of facet joint blocks in patient selection for lumbar fusion. *Spine.* 1993;18:185-190.
103. Saal JS. General principles of diagnostic testing as related to painful lumbar spine disorders: a critical appraisal of current diagnostic techniques. *Spine.* 2002;27(22):2538.
104. Revel M, Poiraudeau S, Auleley GR, et al. Capacity of the clinical picture to characterize low back pain relieved by facet joint anesthesia. proposed criteria to identify patients with painful facet joints. *Spine.* 1998;23:1972.
105. Revel ME, Listrat VM, Chevalier XJ, et al. Facet joint block for low back pain: identifying predictors of a good response. *Arch Phys Med Rehabil.* 1992;73:824-828.
106. Schwarzer AC, Aprill CN, Derby R, et al. The false-positive rate of uncontrolled diagnostic blocks of the lumbar zygapophysial joints. *Pain.* 1994;58:195-200.
107. Lord SM, Barnsley L, Wallis BJ, et al. Percutaneous radio-frequency neurotomy for chronic cervical zygapophyseal-joint pain. *N Engl J Med.* 1996;335:1721-1726.
108. Shealy CN. Percutaneous radiofrequency denervation of spinal facets. treatment for chronic back pain and sciatica. *J Neurosurg.* 1975;43:448-451.
109. Sluijter ME. Percutaneous facet denervation and partial posterior rhizotomy. *Acta Anaesthesiol Belg.* 1981;32:63-79.
110. Moran R, O'Connell D, Walsh MG. The diagnostic value of facet joint injections. *Spine.* 1988;13:1407-1410.
111. Destouet JM, Gilula LA, Murphy WA, Monsees B. Lumbar facet joint injection: indication, technique, clinical correlation, and preliminary results. *Radiology.* 1982;145:321-325.
112. Shealy CN. Dorsal column stimulation: optimization of application. *Surg Neurol.* 1975;4:142-145.
113. McCulloch JA. Percutaneous radiofrequency lumbar rhizolysis (rhizotomy). *Appl Neurophysiol.* 1976-1977;39:87-96.
114. Schaerer JP. Radiofrequency facet rhizotomy in the treatment of chronic neck and low back pain. *Int Surg.* 1978;63:53-59.
115. Florez G, Eiras J, Ucar S. Percutaneous rhizotomy of the articular nerve of Luschka for low back and sciatic pain. *Acta Neurochir (Wien).* 1977;(suppl 24):67-71.
116. Oudenhoven RC. The role of laminectomy, facet rhizotomy, and epidural steroids. *Spine.* 1979;4:145-147.
117. Lord SM, Barnsley L, Bogduk N. Percutaneous radiofrequency neurotomy in the treatment of cervical zygapophysial joint pain: a caution. *Neurosurgery.* 1995;36:732-739.
118. Duff P, Das B, McCrory C. Percutaneous radiofrequency rhizotomy for cervical zygapophyseal joint mediated neck pain: a retrospective review of outcomes in fifty-four cases. *J Back Musculoskeletal Rehabil.* 2016;29:1-5.
119. Leon JF, Ortiz JG, Foneseca EO, Martinez CR, Cuellar GO. Radiofrequency neurolysis for lumbar pain using a variation of the original technique. *Pain Physician.* 2016;19:155-161.
120. Whitworth LA, Feler CA. Application of spinal ablative techniques for the treatment of benign chronic painful conditions: history, methods, and outcomes. *Spine.* 2002;27:2607.
121. Lankford LL. Reflex sympathetic dystrophy. In: *Rehabilitation of the Hand.* 2nd ed. St. Louis: Mosby; 1989:509-532.
122. Stanton-Hicks M, Janig W, Hassenbusch S, et al. Reflex sympathetic dystrophy: changing concepts and taxonomy. *Pain.* 1995;63:127-133.
123. Hodgson AR. Mechanism of spinal pain. In: Melzack R, Wall PD, eds. *Textbook of Pain.* 2nd ed. New York: Churchill LivingstonE; 1989:245.

124. Norman PE, House AK. The early use of operative lumbar sympathectomy in peripheral vascular disease. *J Cardiovasc Surg (Torino)*. 1988;29:717-722.
125. Repelaer van Driel OJ, van Bockel JH, van Schilfgaarde R. Lumbar sympathectomy for severe lower limb ischaemia: results and analysis of factors influencing the outcome. *J Cardiovasc Surg (Torino)*. 1988;29:310-314.
126. Jones NF. Ischemia of the hand in systemic disease. the potential role of microsurgical revascularization and digital sympathectomy. *Clin Plast Surg*. 1989;16:547-556.
127. Wang JK, Johnson KA, Ilstrup DM. Sympathetic blocks for reflex sympathetic dystrophy. *Pain*. 1985;23:13-17.
128. Amadio PC. Pain dysfunction syndromes. *J Bone Joint Surg Am*. 1988;70:944-949.
129. Perelman RB, Adler D, Humphreys M. Reflex sympathetic dystrophy: electronic thermography as an aid in diagnosis. *Orthop Rev*. 1987;16:561-566.
130. Pochaczevsky R. Thermography in posttraumatic pain. *Am J Sports Med*. 1987;15:243-250.
131. Mockus MB, Rutherford RB, Rosales C, Pearce WH. Sympathectomy for causalgia. patient selection and long-term results. *Arch Surg*. 1987;122:668-672.
132. Singh S, Kaur S, Wilson P. Early experience with endoscopic lumbar sympathectomy for plantar hyperhidrosis. *Asian J Endosc Surg*. 2016;9:128-134.
133. Jain AK, Gupta K. Thoracic sympathectomy radiofrequency ablation. *Ann Card Anaesth*. 2015;18:612-616.
134. Husson JL, Meadeb J, Eudier F, et al. Treatment of chronic pain of the musculoskeletal system by epidural stimulation. *J Chir (Paris)*. 1988;125:522-524.
135. Wester K. Dorsal column stimulation in pain treatment. *Acta Neurol Scand*. 1987;75:151-155.
136. Meglio M, Cioni B, Prezioso A, Talamonti G. Spinal cord stimulation (SCS) in the treatment of postherpetic pain. *Acta Neurochir Suppl (Wien)*. 1989;46:65-66.
137. Coombs DW, Saunders RL, Gaylor M, Pageau MG. Epidural narcotic infusion reservoir: implantation technique and efficacy. *Anesthesiology*. 1982;56:469-473.
138. Onofrio BM, Yaksh TL, Arnold PG. Continuous low-dose intrathecal morphine administration in the treatment of chronic pain of malignant origin. *Mayo Clin Proc*. 1981;56:516-520.
139. St Marie B. Administration of intraspinal analgesia in the home care setting. *J Intraven Nurs*. 1989;12:164-168.
140. De La Porte C, Van de Kelft E. Spinal cord stimulation in failed back surgery syndrome. *Pain*. 1993;52:55-61.
141. Downing JE, Busch EH, Stedman PM. Epidural morphine delivered by a percutaneous epidural catheter for outpatient treatment of cancer pain. *Anesth Analg*. 1988;67:1159-1161.
142. Greenberg HS, Taren J, Ensminger WD, Doan K. Benefit from and tolerance to continuous intrathecal infusion of morphine for intractable cancer pain. *J Neurosurg*. 1982;57:360-364.
143. Sjogren P, Banning AM, Henriksen H. High-dose epidural opioid treatment of malignant pain. *Ugeskr Laeger*. 1989;151:25-28.
144. Liew E, Hui YL. A preliminary study of long-term epidural morphine for cancer pain via a subcutaneously implanted reservoir. *Ma Zui Xue Za Zhi*. 1989;27:5-12.
145. Auld AW, Murdoch DM, O'Laughlin KA. Intraspinal narcotic analgesia. pain management in the failed laminectomy syndrome. *Spine*. 1987;12:953-954.
146. Auld AW, Maki-Jokela A, Murdoch DM. Intraspinal narcotic analgesia in the treatment of chronic pain. *Spine*. 1985;10:777-781.
147. Prager JP. Neuraxial medication delivery: the development and maturity of a concept for treating chronic pain of spinal origin. *Spine*. 2002;27(22):2593.
148. Paice JA, Penn RD, Shott S. Intraspinal morphine for chronic pain: a retrospective, multicenter study. *J Pain Symptom Manage*. 1996;11:71-80.
149. Doleys DM. Psychological factors in spinal cord stimulation therapy: brief review and discussion. *Neurosurg Focus*. 2006;21:E1.
150. Carlsson AM. Personality characteristics of patients with chronic pain in comparison with normal controls and depressed patients. *Pain*. 1986;25:373-382.
151. North RB, Kidd DH, Wimberly RL, Edwin D. Prognostic value of psychological testing in patients undergoing spinal cord stimulation: a prospective study. *Neurosurgery*. 1996;39:301.
152. Ferrante FM, Rana MV, Ferrante MA. Conversion disorder mimicking Dejerine-Roussy syndrome (thalamic stroke) after spinal cord stimulation. *Reg Anesth Pain Med*. 2004;29:164-167.
153. Parisod E, Murray RF, Cousins MJ. Conversion disorder after implant of a spinal cord stimulator in a patient with a complex regional pain syndrome. *Anesth Analg*. 2003;96:201.
154. Molloy AR, Nicholas MK, Asghari A, et al. Does a combination of intensive cognitive-behavioral pain management and a spinal implantable device confer any advantage? A preliminary examination. *Pain Pract*. 2006;6:96-103.
155. Orsnes G, Crone C, Krarup C, et al. The effect of baclofen on the transmission in spinal pathways in spastic multiple sclerosis patients. *Clin Neurophysiol*. 2000;111:1372-1379.
156. Hill DR, Bowery NG. 3H-baclofen and 3H-GABA bind to bicuculline-insensitive GABA B sites in rat brain. *Nature*. 1981;290:149-152.
157. Ivanhoe CB, Tilton AH, Francisco GE. Intrathecal baclofen therapy for spastic hypertonia. *Phys Med Rehabil Clin N Am*. 2001;12:923.
158. Saulino M, Jacobs BW. The pharmacological management of spasticity. *J Neurosci Nurs*. 2006;38:456-459.
159. Slonimski M, Abram SE, Zuniga RE. Intrathecal baclofen in pain management. *Reg Anesth Pain Med*. 2004;29:269-276.
160. Dykstra DD, Mendez A, Chappuis D, et al. Treatment of cervical dystonia and focal hand dystonia by high cervical continuously infused intrathecal baclofen: a report of 2 cases. *Arch Phys Med Rehabil*. 2005;86:830-833.
161. Ward AB, Kadies M. The management of pain in spasticity. *Disabil Rehabil*. 2002;24:443-453.
162. van Rijn MA, Munts AG, Marinus J, et al. Intrathecal baclofen for dystonia of complex regional pain syndrome. *Pain*. 2009;143:41-47.
163. Pirec V, Laurito CE, Lu Y, Yeomans DC. The combined effects of N-type calcium channel blockers and morphine on A delta versus C fiber mediated nociception. *Anesth Analg*. 2001;92:239-243.
164. Yaksh TL, Rudy TA. Analgesia mediated by a direct spinal action of narcotics. *Science*. 1976;192:1357-1358.
165. Kristipati R, Nadasdi L, Tarczy-Hornoch K, et al. Characterization of the binding of omega-conopeptides to different classes of non-L-type neuronal calcium channels. *Mol Cell Neurosci*. 1994;5:219-228.
166. Tetzlaff JE. The pharmacology of local anesthetics. *Anesthesiol Clin North America*. 2000;18:217.

167. Roh DH, Kim HW, Yoon SY, et al. Intrathecal clonidine suppresses phosphorylation of the N-methyl-D-aspartate receptor NR1 subunit in spinal dorsal horn neurons of rats with neuropathic pain. *Anesth Analg.* 2008;107:693-700.
168. Deer T, Krames ES, Hassenbusch SJ, et al. Polyanalgesic consensus conference 2007: Recommendations for the management of pain by intrathecal (intraspinal) drug delivery: report of an interdisciplinary expert panel. *Neuromodulation.* 2007;10:300-328.
169. Ruan X. Drug-related side effects of long-term intrathecal morphine therapy. *Pain Physician.* 2007;10:357-366.
170. North RB, Cutchis PN, Epstein JA, Long DM. Spinal cord compression complicating subarachnoid infusion of morphine: case report and laboratory experience. *Neurosurgery.* 1991;29:778-784.
171. Deer T, Krames ES, Hassenbusch S, et al. Management of intrathecal catheter-tip inflammatory masses: an updated 2007 consensus statement from an expert panel. *Neuromodulation.* 2008;11:77-91.
172. McMillan MR. Intrathecal morphine and inflammatory masses. *Anesthesiology.* 2004;101:255.
173. Wall PD, Sweet WH. Temporary abolition of pain in man. *Science.* 1967;155:108-109.
174. Sweet WH, Wepsic JG. Treatment of chronic pain by stimulation of fibers of primary afferent neuron. *Trans Am Neurol Assoc.* 1968;93:103-107.
175. Shealy CN, Mortimer JT, Hagfors NR. Dorsal column electroanalgesia. *J Neurosurg.* 1970;32:560-564.
176. Shealy CN, Mortimer JT, Reswick JB. Electrical inhibition of pain by stimulation of the dorsal columns: preliminary clinical report. *Anesth Analg.* 1967;46:489-491.
177. Krainick JU. Spinal cord stimulation. In: Melzack R, Wall PD, eds. *Textbook of Pain.* 2nd ed. New York: Churchill Livingstone; 1989:924.
178. Nielson KD, Adams JE, Hosobuchi Y. Experience with dorsal column stimulation for relief of chronic intractable pain: 1968-1973. *Surg Neurol.* 1975;4(1):148-152.
179. Larson SJ, Sances A, Cusick JF, et al. A comparison between anterior and posterior spinal implant systems. *Surg Neurol.* 1975;4(1):180-186.
180. Oakley JC, Prager JP. Spinal cord stimulation: mechanisms of action. *Spine.* 2002;27(22):2574-2583.
181. Basbaum AI, Fields HL. Endogenous pain control mechanisms: review and hypothesis. *Ann Neurol.* 1978;4(5):451-462.
182. Linderoth B, Fedorcsak I, Meyerson BA. Peripheral vasodilatation after spinal cord stimulation: animal studies of putative effector mechanisms. *Neurosurgery.* 1991;28(2):187-195.
183. Linderoth B, Gazelius B, Franck J, Brodin E. Dorsal column stimulation induces release of serotonin and substance P in the cat dorsal horn. *Neurosurgery.* 1992;31(2):289-296.
184. Stiller CO, Cui JG, O'Connor WT, et al. Release of gamma-aminobutyric acid in the dorsal horn and suppression of tactile allodynia by spinal cord stimulation in mononeuropathic rats. *Neurosurgery.* 1996;39(2):367-374.
185. Barolat G, Massaro F, He J, et al. Mapping of sensory responses to epidural stimulation of the intraspinal neural structures in man. *J Neurosurg.* 1993;78:233-239.
186. Meyerson BA, Cui JG, Yakhnitsa V, et al. Modulation of spinal pain mechanisms by spinal cord stimulation and the potential role of adjuvant pharmacotherapy. *Stereotact Funct Neurosurg.* 1997;68(1-4 Pt 1):129-140.
187. Krainick JU, Thoden U, Riechert T. Spinal cord stimulation in post-amputation pain. *Surg Neurol.* 1975;4:167-170.
188. North RB, Kidd DH, Lee MS, Piantodosi S. A prospective, randomized study of spinal cord stimulation versus reoperation for failed back surgery syndrome: initial results. *Stereotact Funct Neurosurg.* 1994;62:267-272.
189. Blume H, Richardson R, Rojas C. Epidural nerve stimulation of the lower spinal cord and cauda equina for the relief of intractable pain in failed low back surgery. *Appl Neurophysiol.* 1982;45:456-460.
190. Burton C. Instrumentation for dorsal column stimulator implantation. *Surg Neurol.* 1974;2:39-40.
191. Clark K. Electrical stimulation of the nervous system for control of pain: University of Texas Southwestern Medical School experience. *Surg Neurol.* 1975;4:164-166.
192. de la Porte C, Siegfried J. Lumbosacral spinal fibrosis (spinal arachnoiditis). its diagnosis and treatment by spinal cord stimulation. *Spine.* 1983;8:593-603.
193. Devulder J, De Colvenaer L, Rolly G, et al. Spinal cord stimulation in chronic pain therapy. *Clin J Pain.* 1990;6:51-56.
194. Hoppenstein R. Electrical stimulation of the ventral and dorsal columns of the spinal cord for relief of chronic intractable pain: preliminary report. *Surg Neurol.* 1975;4:187-194.
195. Kumar K, Nath R, Wyant GM. Treatment of chronic pain by epidural spinal cord stimulation: a 10-year experience. *J Neurosurg.* 1991;75:402-407.
196. Deleted in review.
197. Law JD. Targeting a spinal stimulator to treat the "failed back surgery syndrome." *Appl Neurophysiol.* 1987;50:437-438.
198. Leclercq TA, Russo E. Epidural stimulation for pain control. *Neurochirurgie.* 1981;27:125-128.
199. LeDoux MS, Langford KH. Spinal cord stimulation for the failed back syndrome. *Spine.* 1993;18:191-194.
200. LeRoy PL. Stimulation of the spinal neuraxis by biocompatible electrical current in the human. *Appl Neurophysiol.* 1981;44(4):187-193.
201. Meglio M, Cioni B, Rossi GF. Spinal cord stimulation in management of chronic pain: a 9-year experience. *J Neurosurg.* 1989;70:519-524.
202. Meilman PW, Leibrock LG, Leong FT. Outcome of implanted spinal cord stimulation in the treatment of chronic pain: arachnoiditis versus single nerve root injury and mononeuropathy. *Clin J Pain.* 1989;5:189-193.
203. Mittal B, Thomas DG, Walton P, Calder I. Dorsal column stimulation (DCS) in chronic pain: report of 31 cases. *Ann R Coll Surg Engl.* 1987;69:104-109.
204. North RB, Ewend MG, Lawton MT, Piantadosi S. Spinal cord stimulation for chronic, intractable pain: superiority of "multi-channel" devices. *Pain.* 1991;44:119-130.
205. North RB, Ewend MG, Lawton MT, et al. Failed back surgery syndrome: 5-year follow-up after spinal cord stimulator implantation. *Neurosurgery.* 1991;28:692-699.
206. North RB, Kidd DH, Zahurak M, et al. Spinal cord stimulation for chronic, intractable pain: experience over two decades. *Neurosurgery.* 1993;32:384.
207. Pineda A. Dorsal column stimulation and its prospects. *Surg Neurol.* 1975;4:157-163.
208. Richardson RR, Siqueira EB, Cerullo LJ. Spinal epidural neurostimulation for treatment of acute and chronic intractable pain: initial and long term results. *Neurosurgery.* 1979;5:344-348.

209. Shelden CH, Paul F, Jacques DB, Pudenz RH. Electrical stimulation of the nervous system. *Surg Neurol.* 1975;4:127-132.
210. Siegfried J, Lazorthes Y. Long-term follow-up of dorsal cord stimulation for chronic pain syndrome after multiple lumbar operations. *Appl Neurophysiol.* 1982;45:201-204.
211. Simpson BA. Spinal cord stimulation in 60 cases of intractable pain. *J Neurol Neurosurg Psychiatry.* 1991;54:196-199.
212. Vogel HP, Heppner B, Humbs N, Schramm J, Wagner C. Long-term effects of spinal cord stimulation in chronic pain syndromes. *J Neurol.* 1986;233:16-18.
213. Waisbrod H, Gerbershagen HU. Spinal cord stimulation in patients with a battered root syndrome. *Arch Orthop Trauma Surg.* 1985;104:62-64.
214. Kemler MA, Barendse GA, van Kleef M, et al. Spinal cord stimulation in patients with chronic reflex sympathetic dystrophy. *N Engl J Med.* 2000;343:618-624.
215. Turner JA, Loeser JD, Bell KG. Spinal cord stimulation for chronic low back pain: a systematic literature synthesis. *Neurosurgery.* 1995;37:1088.
216. Law JD. A new method for targeting a spinal stimulator: quantitatively paired comparisons. *Appl Neurophysiol.* 1987;50:436.

Index

Page numbers followed by "*f*" indicate figures, "*t*" indicate tables, and "*b*" indicate boxes.

A

B

F

G

H

J

K

N

P

Q

R

S

U

V

W